Principles and Practice of Hospital Medicine

NOTICE

Principles and Practice of Hospital Medicine

Sylvia C. McKean, MD, SFHM, FACP
Associate Professor of Medicine
Harvard Medical School
Boston, Massachusetts

John J. Ross, MD, CM, FIDSA
Assistant Professor of Medicine
Harvard Medical School
Hospitalist Service, Brigham and Women's Hospital
Boston, Massachusetts

Daniel D. Dressler, MD, MSc, SFHM
Associate Professor and Director of Education
Section of Hospital Medicine
Associate Program Director
J. Willis Hurst Internal Medicine Residency Program
Emory University School of Medicine
Atlanta, Georgia

Daniel J. Brotman, MD, FHM, FACP
Associate Professor of Medicine
The Johns Hopkins School of Medicine
Director, Hospitalist Program
The Johns Hopkins Hospital
Baltimore, Maryland

Jeffrey S. Ginsberg, MD, FRCP(C)
Professor of Medicine
McMaster University
Saint Joseph's Hospital
Hamilton, Ontario

McGraw Hill Medical

New York Chicago San Francisco Lisbon London Madrid Mexico City
Milan New Delhi San Juan Seoul Singapore Sydney Toronto

Principles and Practice of Hospital Medicine

3 4 5 6 7 8 9 0 CTP/CTP 16 15 14

ISBN 978-0-07-160389-8
MHID 0-07-160389-1

This book was set in Myriad Pro by Thomson Digital.
The editors were James Shanahan and Cindy Yoo.
The production supervisor was Sherri Souffrance.
Project management was provided by Aakriti Kathuria, Thomson Digital.
The design coordinator was Armen Ovsepyan; the designer was Alan Barnett;
the cover designer was Mary McKeon.
Cover photo credit: Jetta Productions. Woman and doctor looking at electronic tablet.
China Translation & Printing, Ltd. was printer and binder.

Library of Congress Cataloging-in-Publication Data

Principles and practice of hospital medicine / by Sylvia C. McKean ... [et al.].
p. ; cm.
Includes bibliographical references.
ISBN-13: 978-0-07-160389-8 (hardback)
ISBN-10: 0-07-160389-1 (hardback)
I. McKean, Sylvia C.
[DNLM: 1. Clinical Medicine. 2. Hospitals. 3. Hospitalization. 4. Inpatients. WX 162]
362.11—dc23

2011038621

CONTENTS

SECTION 13 Pregnancy

SECTION 14 Psychiatry

SECTION 15 Addiction

SECTION 16 Pulmonary and Allergy Immunology

SECTION 17 Renal

SECTION 18 Rheumatology

EDITORS

Sylvia C. McKean, MD, SFHM, FACP
Part I
Part II
Part IV
Part V
Part VI, Sections 7, 12, 13, 14, 15, 20

John J. Ross, MD, CM, FIDSA
Part VI, Sections 4, 5, 10, 11, 17, 18

Daniel D. Dressler, MD, MSc, SFHM
Part VI, Sections 1, 2, 3, 6, 16

Daniel J. Brotman, MD, FHM, FACP
Part IV

Jeffrey S. Ginsberg, MD, FRCP(C)
Part III
Part VI, Sections 8, 9, 19

CONTRIBUTORS

Meredith C.B. Adams, MD [96]
Fellow, Department of Anesthesiology
Division of Pain Medicine
The Johns Hopkins University
Baltimore, Maryland

Kush Agrawal, MD [99]
Emory University School of Medicine
Department of Internal Medicine
Resident Physician
Atlanta, Georgia

G. Caleb Alexander, MD, MS [32]
Section of General Medicine and McClean
Center for Clinical Medical Ethics
Department of Medicine
University of Chicago
Chicago, Illinois

Anne E. Allan, MD [143]
Derm Dx
Boston, Massachusetts

Alpesh Amin, MD, MBA [23]
Professor and Chairman
Department of Medicine
Executive Director
Hospitalist Service
University of California
Irvine, California

Sonia Anand, MD, PhD, FRCP(c) [73, 263]
Professor of Medicine
Heart and Stroke Foundation of Ontario
Michael G. DeGroote Chair in Population Health Research
McMaster University
Hamilton, Ontario

Daniel A. Anaya, MD [50]
Staff Surgeon, Surgical Oncologist and Research Scientist
The Houston Center for Quality of Care and Utilization Studies
Michael E. DeBakey VA Medical Center
Assistant Professor
Division of Surgical Oncology
Michael E. DeBakey Department of Surgery
Houston, Texas

Douglas S. Ander, MD [122]
Associate Professor
Department of Emergency Medicine
Assistant Dean for Medical Education
Director Emory Center for Experiential Learning
Emory University School of Medicine
Atlanta, Georgia

Kristina Antonson, MD, PhD [94]
University of California Davis Department of Psychiatry
and Behavioral Sciences
Sacramento, California

Farnaz Arabshahi, RN, FNP [218]
Family Nurse Practitioner
Emory University Hospital
Atlanta, Georgia

Doris J. Armour, MD, MBA [66]
Assistant Professor
Department of Rehabilitation Medicine
Emory University
Atlanta, Georgia

Kelly Armstrong, PhD [34]
Senior Clinical Ethicist
Memorial Health System
Adjunct Assistant Professor
Department of Medical Humanities
SIU School of Medicine
Springfield, Illinois

Vineet M. Arora, MD, MAPP [9]
Assistant Professor
Department of Medicine
Associate Director
Internal Medicine Residency
Assistant Dean for Scholarship and Discovery
Pritzker School of Medicine
University of Chicago
Chicago, Illinois

Cameron Ashbaugh, MD [203]
Assistant Professor of Medicine
Harvard Medical School
Brigham and Women's Health
Boston, Massachusetts

Stanley Ashley, MD [44, 45, 46, 47]
Frank Sawyer Professor and Vice Chairman
Department of Surgery
Brigham and Women's Hospital
Boston, Massachusetts

Saima Aslam, MD, MS [196]
Assistant Professor
Section of Infectious Diseases
University of California
San Diego, California

Andrew Auerbach, MD, MPH [269]
Division of Hospital Medicine
University of California
San Francisco, California

Mark Ault, MD [114]
Director
Division of General Internal Medicine
Cedars Sinai Medical Center
Los Angeles, California

Vasilis C. Babaliaros, MD [131]
Gruentzig Cardiovascular Center
Emory Hospital
Atlanta, Georgia

Lindsey R. Baden, MD [198]
Assistant Professor of Medicine
Harvard Medical School
Division of Infectious Diseases
Brigham and Women's Hospital
Boston, Massachusetts

Meridale V. Baggett, MD [76]
Instructor in Medicine
Harvard Medical School
Inpatient Clinician Educator Service
Department of Medicine
Massachusetts General Hospital
Boston, Massachusetts

James L. Bailey, MD [250]
Professor
Emory University School of Medicine
Atlanta, Georgia

John Baillie, MB, ChB, FRCP(Glasg.), FACG, FASGE [157]
Professor of Medicine
Director
Hepatobiliary and Pancreatic Disorders Service
Wake Forest University Baptist Medical Center
Winston-Salem, North Carolina

Puneet Bains, MD, FRCPC [184]
Fellow, Medical Oncology
British Columbia Cancer Agency
Vancouver, British Columbia

Julio A. Barcena, MD [130]
Case Western Reserve University
Louis Stokes Cleveland VA Medical Center
Cleveland, Ohio

Robert B. Baron, MD, MS [37]
University of California
San Francisco, California

Thomas Barrett, MD [269]
Portland VA Medical Center and the
Oregon Health and Science University
Portland, Oregon

Thomas E. Baudendistel, MD [39]
Hospital-Based Services (HBS)\Assistant Program Director,
Internal Medicine Residency
Kaiser Permanente Oakland Medical Center
Oakland, California

Rabih Bechara, MD [117, 243]
Chief, Interventional Pulmonology
Emory University School of Medicine
Atlanta, Georgia

Nicole M. Bedi, RD, LDN, CNSC [54]
Team Leader Dietitian
Brigham and Women's Hospital
Boston, Massachusetts

Laurence Beer, MD, FHM [123]
Associate Site Director for Quality Improvement
Emory University Hospital
Section of Hospital Medicine
Atlanta, Georgia

Elie F. Berbari, MD [201]
Training Program Director
Division of Infectious Diseases
Associate Professor of Medicine
College of Medicine, Mayo Clinic
Rochester, Minnesota

Todd L. Berger, MD, FACEP [120]
Associate Professor
Program Director
Emergency Medicine Residency
University of Texas Southwestern
Austin, Texas

Colm Bergin, MD, FRCPI, FRCP [202]
Consultant, Physician in Infectious Diseases
St. John's Hospital, Dublin
Senior Lecturer in Clinical Medicine
Trinity College
Dublin, Ireland

David M. Berkowitz, MD [243]
Assistant Professor of Medicine
Director
Interventional Pulmonology
Emory University Hospital Midtown
Emory University School of Medicine
Atlanta, Georgia

Rachelle E. Bernacki, MD, MS [97, 215]
Director of Quality Initiatives
Pain and Palliative Care Program
Dana Farber Cancer Institute
Harvard Medical School
Boston, Massachusetts

Nicholas Beshara, JD, MPH [36]
Harvard University School of Public Health
Boston, Massachusetts

Robert A. Bessler, MD [21, 26]
Sound Physicians
Tacoma, Washington

Deepak L. Bhatt, MD, MPH, FACP [124]
Chief of Cardiology, VA Boston Health Care System
Director
Integrated Interventional Cardiovascular Program
Brigham and Women's Hospital and the VA Boston
Health Care System
Senior Investigator, TIMI Study Group
Harvard Medical School
Boston, Massachusetts

John P. Bilezikian, MD [247]
Professor of Medicine
Professor of Pharmacology
Columbia University
College of Physicians and Surgeons
New York, New York

Courtney Bilodeau, MD [224]
Attending Physician
Division of Obstetric and Consultative Medicine
Women's and Infants Hospital of Rhode Island
Providence, Rhode Island

Peter M. Black, MD, PhD [63, 64]
Franc D. Ingraham Professor of Neurosurgery
Harvard Medical School
Founding Chair
Department of Neurosurgery
Brigham and Women's Hospital
Children's Hospital Boston
Boston, Massachusetts

Morris A. Blajchman, MD, FRCP [177]
Chair, NHLBI TMH CTN Steering Committee
Professor Emeritus
Departments of Pathology and Medicine
McMaster University
Hamilton, Ontario

Ioannis A. Bliziotis, MD [185]
Internal Medicine Practitioner
Third University Department of Medicine
Sotiria Hospital and Senior Reseacher
Alfa Institute of Biomedical Sciences
Athens, Greece

Arline D. Bohannon, MD [165]
Assistant Professor of Internal Medicine
Virginia Commonwealth University
Richmond, Virginia

Peter A. Boling, MD [165]
Professor of Medicine
Virginia Commonwealth University
Richmond, Virginia

Marcy B. Bolster, MD [256, 257]
Professor, Department of Medicine
Director
Rheumatology Fellowship Training Program
Medical University of South Carolina
Charleston, South Carolina

Kenneth Boockvar, MD, MS [169]
Associate Professor
Brookdale Department of Geriatrics and Adult Development
Mount Sinai School of Medicine and Geriatrics Research
Education and Clinical Center
James J. Peters VA Medical Center
New York, New York

Ghada Bourjeily, MD [222]
Assistant Professor of Medicine
The Warren Alpert Medical School of Brown University Women and Infants Hospital
Department of Medicine
Pulmonary and Critical Care
Providence, Rhode Island

Christine Bradway, PhD, CRNP [172]
Assistant Professor of Gerontological Nursing
CE Program Director, Gerontology
Nurse Practitioner Program
University of Pennsylvania School of Nursing
Philadelphia, Pennsylvania

John M. Braver, MD [109, 110]
Assistant Professor, Harvard Medical School
Director
Gastrointestinal Radiology
Brigham and Women's Hospital
Boston, Massachusetts

Ursula C. Brewster, MD [248]
Assistant Professor of Medicine
Section of Nephrology
Yale University School of Medicine
New Haven, Connecticut

Jared R. Brosch, MD, MS [199]
Department of Neurology
Indiana University School in Medicine
Indianapolis, Indiana

Daniel J. Brotman, MD, FHM, FACP
Associate Professor of Medicine
The Johns Hopkins School of Medicine
Director, Hospitalist Program
The Johns Hopkins Hospital
Baltimore, Maryland

Katherine L. Brown, MD, MPH [146]
Boston University
Department of Dermatology
Boston, Massachusetts

Tina Budnitz, MPH [5]
Senior Advisor
Society of Hospital Medicine
Philadelphia, Pennsylvania

Robert Burakoff, MD, MPH [154]
Clinical Chief, Division of Gastroenterology
Director
Center for Digestive Health
Associate Professor of Medicine
Boston, Massachusetts

Amanda L. Caissie, MD, PhD [216]
Department of Radiation Oncology
University of Toronto
Toronto, Canada

Mitchell S. Cappell, MD, PhD [162]
Professor of Medicine
Oakland University William Beaumont School of Medicine
Chief of Gastroenterology
William Beaumont Hospital
Royal Oak, Michigan

Alexander R. Carbo, MD, SFHM [6, 38]
Assistant Professor of Medicine
Harvard Medical School
Hospital Medicine Program
Beth Israel Deaconess Medical Center
Boston, Massachusetts

Teresa L. Carman, MD [84]
Director
Vascular Medicine
University Hospitals Case Medical Center
Assistant Professor of Medicine
Case Western Reserve University School of Medicine
Cleveland, Ohio

Jeffrey Carter, MD [52]
Assistant Professor of Medicine
University of Colorado School of Medicine
Aurora, Colorado

Heather X. Cereste, MD [33]
Assistant Professor of Medicine and Public Health
Division of Medical Ethics
Weill Cornell Medical Center
Assistant Attending Hospitalist Medicine
New York Presbyterian Hospital Center
New York, New York

Matthew E. Certain, MD [132]
Fellow, Department of Cardiology
Emory University School of Medicine
Atlanta, Georgia

Marisa Cevasco, MD, MPH [44]
Resident, Department of Surgery
Brigham and Women's Hospital
Boston, Massachusetts

Walter W. Chan, MD, MPH [154]
Instructor in Medicine
Division of Gastroenterology
Hepatology and Endoscopy
Brigham and Women's Hospital
Harvard Medical School
Boston, Massachusetts

Arjun S. Chanmugam, MD, MBA [77]
Associate Professor
Department of Emergency Medicine
Director of Education
The Johns Hopkins University School of Medicine
Baltimore, Maryland

Kenneth K. Chen, MD, FRACP [223]
Fellow, Department of Obstetric Medicine
Women and Infants Hospital
Alpert Medical School
Brown University
Providence, Rhode Island

Hugo Quinny Cheng, MD [43]
Clinical Professor
Division of Hospital Medicine
Department of Medicine
University of California – San Francisco
San Francisco, California

Stephen K. Chia, MD, FRCPC [182]
Associate Professor of Medicine
Department of Medical Oncology
British Columbia Cancer Agency
University of British Columbia
Vancouver, British Columbia

Nishay Chitkara, MD [136]
NYU School of Medicine
Department of Medicine
Division of Pulmonary and Critical Care Medicine
New York, New York

Jennifer Christie, MD [153]
Emory University
Alexander, Georgia

Elbert B. Chun, MD [126]
Emory University School of Medicine
Associate Director, Hospital Medicine
Emory Orthopedic and Spine Hospital
Atlanta, Georgia

Cheryl R. Clark, MD, ScD [3]
Director of Health Equity Research and Intervention
Center for Community Health and Health Equity
Hospitalist, Brigham and Women's and Faulkner Hospitals
Division of General Medicine and Primary Care
Boston, Massachusetts

John O. Clarke, MD [95]
Assistant Professor of Medicine
Director of Esophageal Motility
Division of Gastroenterology
The Johns Hopkins University
Baltimore, Maryland

Stephen D. Clements Jr., MD [132]
Professor of Medicine, Cardiology
Emory University School of Medicine
Atlanta, Georgia

Steven L. Cohn, MD, FACP [42, 51]
Director – Medical Consultation Service
Kings County Hospital Center
Clinical Professor of Medicine
SUNY Downstate
Brooklyn, New York

Eric D. Collins, MD [233]
Assistant Professor of Clinical Psychiatry
Medical Director
Substance Abuse Services
Columbia University Medical Center
New York, New York

Darwin L. Conwell, MD, MS [156]
Associate Physician
Brigham and Women's Hospital
Associate Professor of Medicine
Harvard Medical School
Boston, Massachusetts

Zara Cooper, MD, MSc [44, 45, 46, 47, 139]
Instructor, Department of Surgery
Brigham and Women's Hospital
Division of Trauma
Burns and Critical Care
Harvard Medical School
Boston, Massachusetts

Darin J. Correll, MD [49]
Director
Postoperative Pain Management Service
Department of Anesthesiology
Perioperative and Pain Medicine
Brigham and Women's Hospital
Instructor of Anesthesia
Harvard Medical School
Boston, Massachusetts

Douglas B. Coursin, MD, FCCP [151]
Professor of Medicine and Anesthesiology
University of Wisconsin School of Medicine
Madison, Wisconsin

Lisa Criscione-Schreiber, MD [256, 257]
Assistant Professor of Medicine
Division of Rheumatology and Immunology
Duke University
Durham, North Carolina

Mark Crowther, MD, ChB, MRCP, FRCPath [72]
Consultant Haematologist
Department of Haematology
Worcester Royal Hospital
Worcester, United Kingdom

Mark A. Crowther, MD, MSc, FRCPC [70, 72]
Professor, Department of Medicine
McMaster University
Academic Division Director, Hematology
McMaster University
Head of Service (Hematology) and
Senior Clinical Research Advisor
St. Joseph's Health Care
Hamilton, Ontario

J. Randall Curtis, MD, MPH [140]
Professor, Department of Medicine
Division of Pulmonary and Critical Care
University of Washington
Seattle, Washington

Sonye K. Danoff, MD, PhD [241]
The Johns Hopkins University School of Medicine
Division of Pulmonary and Critical Care Medicine
Baltimore, Maryland

J. Ashley Davidson, MD [182]
Medical Oncologist
Fraser Valley Cancer Centre
British Columbia Cancer Agency
Surrey, British Columbia

David B. De Lurgio, MD, FACP [129]
Associate Professor of Medicine
Emory University School of medicine
Director of Clinical Electrophysiology
Emory University Hospital
Atlanta, Georgia

Steven B. Deitelzweig, MD, MMM, SFHM [265]
System Chairman
Department of Hospital Medicine
Vice President of Medical Affairs
Ochsner Health System
New Orleans, Louisiana

Paul F. Dellaripa, MD [254]
Assistant Professor
Harvard Medical School
Department of Rheumatology Brigham and Women's Hospital
Boston, Massachusetts

E. Patchen Dellinger, MD [50]
Professor of Surgery
University of Washington School of Medicine
Chief, Division of General Surgery
University of Washington Medical Center
Seattle, Washington

Gina DeSevo, PharmD [171]
Assistant Professor
Department of Pharmacy Practice
Jefferson School of Pharmacy
Thomas Jefferson University
Philadelphia, Pennsylvania

Lorenzo Di Francesco, MD, FACP, FHM [91]
Associate Professor of Medicine
Program Director, J. Willis Hurst Internal Medicine
Residency Program
Assistant Chief of Medicine
Grady Memorial Hospital
Emory University School of Medicine
Atlanta, Georgia

Marco P. Donadini, MD [61, 62]
Research Fellow
McMaster University Resident
Department of Clinical Medicine
University of Insurbia
Varese, Italy

Shira Doron, MD [187]
Attending Physician
Division of Geographic Medicine and Infectious Diseases
Tufts Medical Center
Assistant Professor of Medicine
Tufts University School of Medicine
Boston, Massachusetts

James D. Douketis, MD, FRCPC, FACP, FCCP [58, 59, 60, 61, 62]
McMaster University
St. Joseph's Health Care Hamilton
Hamilton, Ontario

Aeron Doyle, MDCM, FRCPC [48]
Clinical Assistant Professor
Department of Anesthesiology
Pharmacology, and Therapeutics
University of British Columbia
Vancouver, British Columbia

Daniel D. Dressler, MD, MSc, SFHM [99]
Associate Professor and Director of Education
Section of Hospital Medicine
Associate Program Director
J. Willis Hurst Internal Medicine Residency Program
Emory University School of Medicine
Atlanta, Georgia

Catherine E. DuBeau, MD [170]
Division of Geriatrics
University of Massachusetts Medical Center
Worchester, Massachusetts

Sydney Dy, MSc, MD [219]
Harry J. Duffey Family Pain and Palliative Care Program
Johns Hopkins Kimmel Cancer Center
Baltimore, Maryland

John Eikelboom, MBBS, MSc, FRACP, FRCPA, FRCPC [261]
Associate Professor
Department of Medicine
McMaster University
Hamilton, Ontario

Elwaleed A. Elhassen, MD [249]
Fellow, Division of Renal Diseases and Hypertension
School of Medicine
University of Colorado
Denver, Colorado

William J. Elliott, MD, PhD [253]
Professor of Preventive Medicine
Internal Medicine and Pharmacology
Head, Division of Pharmacology
Pacific Northwest University of Health Sciences
Yakima, Washington

John M. Embil, MD, FRCPC [145, 193]
Associate Professor
Departments of Medical Microbiology and Internal Medicine
Section of Infectious Diseases
University of Manitoba
Winnipeg, Manitoba

Scott Enderby, DO, SFHM [21]
Sound Physicians
Tacoma, Washington

Joseph C. English III, MD [141]
Associate Professor of Dermatology
Clinical Vice Chairman of Quality and Innovation
Department of Dermatology
University of Pittsburgh
Pittsburgh, Pennsylvania

Mary Eno, MD, MPH [232]
Kaiser Permanente Southern California
South Bay Department of Addiction Medicine
Los Angeles, California

Greg Erens, MD [65]
Assistant Professor
Department of Orthopedic Surgery
Emory University
Atlanta, Georgia

Manuel A. Eskildsen, MD, CMD [172]
Assistant Professor of Medicine
Division of Geriatric Medicine and Gerontology
Department of Medicine
Emory University School of Medicine
Atlanta, Georgia

Laura Evans, MD, MSc [136]
Assistant Professor of Clinical Medicine
Department of Medicine
Division of Pulmonary and Critical Care Medicine
New York University School of Medicine
New York, New York

Matthew E. Falagas, MD, MSc, DSc [185]
Director
Alfa Institute of Biomedical Sciences (AIBS)
Adjunct Associate Professor of Medicine
Tufts Medical School
Boston, Massachusetts
Director
Infectious Diseases Clinic Henry Dunant Hospital
Athens, Greece

James C. Fang, MD, FACC [130]
Professor of Medicine, Case Western Reserve University
Associate Chief, Division of Cardiovascular Medicine
University Hospitals Case Medical Center
Director
Heart Failure and Transplantation
University Hospitals Case Medical Center
Cleveland, Ohio

Harrison W. Farber, MD [244]
Professor of Medicine
Boston University School of Medicine
Director
Pulmonary Hypertension
Boston Medical Center
Boston, Massachusetts

Claire Farel, MD, MPH [195]
Clinical and Research Fellow
Division of Infectious Diseases
Brigham and Women's Hospital and
Massachusetts General Hospital
Boston, Massachusetts

Durathun Farha, MD [89]
Internal/Vascular Medicine Staff Physician
General Internal Medicine and Preoperative Center
Lahey Clinic
Burlington, Massachusetts

Jeanne M. Farnan, MD, MHPE [9]
Assistant Professor, Department of Medicine
Pritzker School of Medicine
Chicago, Illinois

Kevin Felner, MD [138]
Assistant Professor
Department of Medicine/Division of Pulmonary and Critical Care
NYU School of Medicine
VA Harbor Medical Center
New York, New York

Joseph J. Fins, MD, FACP [33, 208]
Chief, Division of Medical Ethics
Professor of Medicine
Professor of Public Health
Professor of Medicine in Psychiatry
Weill Cornell Medical College
Director of Medical Ethics and Attending Physician
New York Presbyterian Hospital-Weill Cornell Center
New York, New York

Leslie A. Flores, MHA [25]
Partner, Nelson Flores Hospital Medicine Consultants
Senior Advisor
Society of Hospital Medicine
La Quinta, California

John A. Flynn, MD, MBA, FACP, FACR [75]
D. William Schlott, MD
Professor of Medicine
Clinical Director
Division of General Internal Medicine
The Johns Hopkins University School of Medicine
Baltimore, Maryland

Ryan M. Ford, MD [158]
Transplant Hepatology Fellow, Emory Transplant Center
Emory University
Atlanta, Georgia

Vance G. Fowler Jr., MD, MHS [197]
Associate Professor
Division of Infectious Diseases
Department of Medicine
Duke University Medical Center
Durham, North Carolina

Graeme Fraser, MD, MSc (HRM), FRCPC [179, 180]
Hematologist
Juravinski Cancer Centre
Assistant Professor
Department of Oncology McMaster University
Hamilton, Ontario

Allison S. Friedenberg, MD [140]
Clinical Instructor
Division of Pulmonary and Critical Care
New York University School of Medicine
New York, New York

Joseph M. Furman, MD, PhD [82]
Professor
Departments of Otolaryngology
Neurology, Bioengineering and Physical Therapy
University of Pittsburgh School of Medicine
Director
Divisions of Balance Disorders
Pittsburgh, Pennsylvania

Michael Gardam, MSc, MD, CM, MSc, FRCPC [204]
Medical Director
Tuberculosis Clinic and Infection Prevention and Control
University Health Network
Assistant Professor
Alla Lana School of Public Health
University of Toronto
Toronto, Ontario

Steven Garlow, MD, PhD [225]
Associate Professor
Chief of Psychiatry
Emory University Hospital
Atlanta, Georgia

Neil Gesundheit, MD, MPH [41]
Associate Professor
Department of Medicine
Stanford University School of Medicine
Stanford, California

Sharlene Gill, MD, MPH [184]
Associate Professor of Medicine
BC Cancer Agency
University of British Columbia
Vancouver, British Columbia

Jeffrey S. Ginsberg, MD, FRCP(C) [69, 71, 261]
Professor of Medicine
McMaster University
Saint Joseph's Hospital
Hamilton, Ontario

Richard S. Gitomer, MD, FACP [16]
Chief Quality Officer
Emory University Hospital Midtown
Assistant Professor
Department of Internal Medicine
Emory University School of Medicine
Atlanta, Georgia

Jeffrey J. Glasheen, MD [52]
Associate Professor of Medicine
Director
Hospital Medicine Section
University of Colorado Denver
Denver, Colorado

Rachel Goodwin, MD, MSc, FRCPC [181]
Fellow, NCIC Clinical Trials Group
Queen's University
Kingston, Ontario

Steven M. Gorbatkin, MD, PhD [250]
Atlanta Veterans Affairs Medical Center
Atlanta, Georgia

Mark L. Graber, MD, FACP [8]
Professor and Associate Chair
Department of Medicine
SUNY Stony Brook
Chief, Medical Service, VA Medical Center Northport
Northport, New York

Norman D. Grace, MD [53]
Professor of Medicine
Tufts University School of Medicine
Lecturer on Medicine, Harvard Medical School
Director of Clinical Hepatology
Division of Gastroenterology and Hepatology, Brigham and Women's Hospital
Boston, Massachusetts

Yonatan H. Grad, MD, PhD [200]
Clinical and Resident Fellow
Division of Infectious Diseases
Massachusetts General Hospital and
Brigham and Women's Hospital
Boston, Massachusetts

Lisa M. Grandinetti, MD [141]
Assistant Professor
Department of Dermatology
University of Pittsburgh Medical Center
Pittsburgh, Pennsylvania

Stephen B. Greenberg, MD, MACP [206]
Senior Vice President and Dean of Medical Education
Baylor College of Medicine
Chief, Medicine Service
Ben Taub General Hospital
Professor, Baylor College of Medicine
Houston, Texas

Norton J. Greenberger, MD, MACP [74]
Clinical Professor of Medicine
Harvard Medical School
Senior Physician, Brigham and Women's Hospital
Boston, Massachusetts

Anne F. Gross, MD [231]
Massachusetts General Hospital/McLean
Boston, Massachusetts

Stephanie Grossman, MD, FHM, FAACP [218]
Assistant Professor
Department of Medicine
Emory University
Director of Palliative Care
Emory University Hospitals
Atlanta, Georgia

Angela S. Guarda, MD [228]
Associate Professor
Department of Psychiatry and Behavioral Sciences
Johns Hopkins School of Medicine
Director
Eating Disorders Program
The Johns Hopkins Hospital
Baltimore, Maryland

Debbie Gunter, RN, FNP, ACHPN [218]
Palliative Care Nurse Practitioner
Emory University Medical Center
Atlanta, Georgia

Richard D. Guthrie Jr., MD [265]
Regional Medical Director, Ochsner Clinic
New Orleans, Louisiana

Emily R. Hajjar, PharmD, BCPS, CGP [171]
Assistant Professor
Department of Pharmacy Practice
Jefferson School of Pharmacy
Thomas Jefferson University
Philadelphia, Pennsylvania

Lakshmi K. Halasyamani, MD, SFHM [7]
Vice President
Quality and Systems Improvement
Saint Joseph Mercy Health System
Member of Trinity Health
Ann Arbor, Michigan

Caleb P. Hale, MD [24]
Hospitalist and Instructor in Medicine
Harvard University School of Medicine and Beth Israel Deaconess Medical Center
Boston, Massachusetts

Sarah P. Hammond, MD [198]
Instructor of Medicine
Harvard Medical School
Division of Infectious Diseases
Brigham and Women's Hospital
Boston, Massachusetts

Joseph T. Hanlon, PharmD, MS [171]
Professor
Department of Medicine (Geriatrics)
Pharmacy and Therapeutics, and Epidemiology
University of Pittsburgh
Health Scientist, GRECC/CHERP
Pittsburgh Veterans Affairs Health System
Pittsburgh, Pennsylvania

Timothy P. Hanna, MD, MSc, FRCP(C) [181]
Clinical Fellow Radiation Oncology
Cancer Centre of Southeastern Ontario
Kingston, Ontario

Daniel J. Hanson, MD, FHM [20]
Virginia Mason Medical Center
Seattle, Washington

Caroline N. Harada, MD [166]
Assistant Professor of Medicine
Division of Gerontology, Geriatrics, and Palliative Care
University of Alabama at Birmingham
Birmingham, Alabama

Kimberly A. Hardin, MD, MS, FAASM [94]
Associate Professor of Clinical Medicine
Department of Internal Medicine
Division of Pulmonary
Critical Care, and Sleep Medicine
University of California, Davis
Sacramento, California

Gwendolynn Harrell, RN, CHPN [218]
Palliative Care
Emory University
Atlanta, Georgia

Carson R. Harris, MD [98]
Associate Professor
Department of Emergency Medicine
University of Minnesota Medical School
Minneapolis, Minnesota

Robert S. Harris, MD [135]
Assistant Professor
Department of Anesthesiology
Emory University School of Medicine
Atlanta, Georgia

Abel Po-Hao Huang, MD [63, 64]
Attending Neurosurgeon
National Taiwan University Hospital
Yun-Lin Branch
Clinical Lecturer
College of Medicine
National Taiwan University
Taipei, Taiwan

Meghan Hayes, MD [220, 222]
Assistant Professor of Medicine (Clinical)
Warren Alpert Medical School at Brown University
Division of Obstetric Medicine
Department of Medicine
Women and Infant's Hospital
Providence, Rhode Island

Margaret M. Hayes, MD [88]
Department of Internal Medicine
The Johns Hopkins University School of Medicine
Baltimore, Maryland

Catherine P.M. Hayward, MD, PhD [176]
Professor
Department of Pathology and Molecular Medicine
McMaster University
Head, Regional Specialized Coagulation
and Hemostasis Laboratory
Hamilton Regional Laboratory Medicine Program
Hamilton, Ontario

Katherine L. Heilpern, MD [120]
Professor and Chair
Department of Emergency Medicine
Emory University School of Medicine
Atlanta, Georgia

Michael Heisler, MD, MPH [133]

Galen V. Henderson, MD [210]
Assistant Professor of Neurology
Harvard Medical School
Brigham and Women's Hospital
Boston, Massachusetts

H. Franklin Herlong, MD [159]
Associate Professor of Medicine
Division of Gastroenterology
The Johns Hopkins University School of Medicine
Baltimore, Maryland

Heather L. Herrington, MD [166]
Assistant Professor of Medicine
Division of Geriatrics
Gerontology and Palliative Care
University of Alabama at Birmingham
Birmingham, Alabama

LeRoi S. Hicks, MD, MPH [3]
Assistant Professor in Medicine
Instructor in Health Care Policy
Brigham and Women's Hospital and
Department of Health Care Policy
Harvard Medical School
Boston, Massachusetts

Stacy Higgins, MD, FACP [4]
Assistant Professor
Division of General Medicine
Department of Medicine
Emory University School of Medicine
Atlanta, Georgia

Keiki Hinami, MD, MS [30]
Instructor, Department of Medicine
Northwestern University Feinberg School of Medicine
Chicago, Illinois

C. Edward Hoffler II, PhD, MD [65]
South Arkansas Orthopedic Center
Pine Bluff, Arkansas

Fernando Holguin, MD, MPH [238]
Assistant Professor of Medicine
Pediatrics and Environmental Occupational Health
University of Pittsburgh
Pittsburgh, Pennsylvania

Anthony N. Hollenberg, MD [150]
Chief, Thyroid Unit
Division of Endocrinology
Diabetes and Metabolism
Beth Israel Deaconess Medical Center
Associate Professor of Medicine
Harvard Medical School
Boston, Massachusetts

Elizabeth H. Holt, MD, PhD [247]
Assistant Professor
Section of Endocrinology
Department of Medicine
Yale University
New Haven, Connecticut

John A. Hopper, MD [234]
Vice Chair for Education
St. Joseph Mercy Hospital
Clinical Associate Professor
Internal Medicine, Pediatrics,
Psychiatry and Behavioral Neurosciences
Wayne State University School of Medicine
Detroit, Michigan

Michael H. Hoskins, MD [129]
Fellow, Cardiac Electrophysiology
Division of Cardiology
Emory University School of Medicine
Atlanta, Georgia

Susy Hota, MD, MSc, FRCPC [204]
Faculty of Medicine
Division of Infectious Diseases
University Health Network
University of Toronto
Toronto, Ontario

Liangge Hsu, MD [111]
Assistant Professor of Radiology
Harvard Medical School
Brigham and Women's Hospital
Boston, Massachusetts

Grace C. Huang, MD [113]
Assistant Professor of Medicine
Harvard Medical School
Staff Hospitalist, Beth Israel Deaconess Medical Center
Boston, Massachusetts

Amy Huberman, MD [79]
Resident Physician
Department of Psychiatry
The Johns Hopkins University School of Medicine
Baltimore, Maryland

Margo S. Hudson, MD [148]
Instructor in Medicine
Division of Endocrinology Diabetes and Hypertension
Brigham and Women's Hospital
Boston, Massachusetts

Jeff C. Huffman, MD [231]
Medical Director, Inpatient Medical Psychiatry Unit
Massachusetts General Hospital
Assistant Professor of Psychiatry
Harvard Medical School
Boston, Massachusetts

Daniel P. Hunt, MD [76]
Associate Professor of Medicine
Harvard Medical School
Director
Inpatient Clinician Educator Service
Department of Medicine
Massachusetts General Hospital
Boston, Massachusetts

Robert W. Hurley, MD, PhD [96]
Chief of Pain Medicine
Associate Professor
Department of Anesthesiology,
Psychiatry, Orthopedics, and Neurology
Medical Director
UF Pain and Spine Center
Gainesville, Florida

Brian G. Hynes, MB, BCh, BAO, MRCPI [124]
Fellow in Interventional Cardiology
Department of Medicine
Massachusetts General Hospital
Boston, Massachusetts

Brian H. Hyett, MD [155]
Clinical and Research Fellow in Gastroenterology
Brigham and Women's Hospital
Boston, Massachusetts

Aubrey Orion Ingraham, MD [39]
Professor of Neurosurgery
Harvard Medical School, Founding Chair
Department of Neurosurgery
Brigham and Women's Hospital
Children's Hospital Boston
Boston, Massachusetts

Bertrand L. Jaber, MD, MS [251]
Associate Professor of Medicine
Tufts University School of Medicine
Boston, Massachusetts

Francine L. Jacobson, MD, MPH [101, 105, 106, 107, 108, 109, 110, 111, 112]
Thoracic Radiologist at Brigham and Women's Hospital
Assistant Professor
Department of Radiology
Harvard Medical School
Boston, Massachusetts

Shilpa H. Jain, MD [152]
Clinical Instructor
Department of Endocrinology Gerontology, and Metabolism
Stanford University School of Medicine
Stanford, California

Claudius D. Jarrett, MD [65]
Orthopedic Resident
Department of Orthopedic Surgery
Emory University School of Medicine
Atlanta, Georgia

Danielle Jones, MD [91]
Assistant Professor of Medicine
Emory University School of Medicine
Atlanta, Georgia

J. Ryan Jordan, MD [125]
Cardiovascular Disease Fellow
Emory University School of Medicine
Division of Cardiology
Atlanta, Georgia

Scott Andy Josephson, MD [207]
Assistant Professor of Neurology
Director
Neuro Hospitalist Program
University of California – San Francisco
San Francisco, California

Zahid Junagadhwalla, MD [131]
Gruentzig Cardiovascular Center
Emory University Hospital
Atlanta, Georgia

Peter J. Kaboli, MD, MS [269]
Director
Midwest Rural Health Resource Center
Iowa City, VA Medical Center
Investigator
Center for Research in the Implementation of
Innovative Strategies in Practice
HSR&D Center of Excellence
Iowa City, VA Medical Center
Associate Professor
Internal Medicine Carver College of Medicine
University of Iowa
Iowa City, Iowa

Laurence Katznelson, MD [152]
Professor of Neurosurgery and Medicine
Stanford University School of Medicine
Stanford, California

Farshid Kazi, MD, MPH [23]
Department of Medicine
University of California
Irvine, California

Clive Kearon, MB, MRCPI, FRCPC, PhD [259, 260]
Professor, Department of Medicine
McMaster University
Hamilton, Ontario

Robert T. Keenan, MD, MPH [255]
Assistant Professor
Director of Rheumatology and Immunology
Department of Medicine
Duke University School of Medicine
Durham, North Carolina

Gabor D. Kelen, MD, FACEP, FAAEM, FRCP [268]
Professor and Chair, Department of Emergency Medicine
The Johns Hopkins University School of Medicine
Baltimore, Maryland

Corey D. Kershaw, MD [134]
Assistant Professor of Medicine
Interstitial Lung Disease Program
Division of Pulmonary, Allergy, and Critical Care Medicine
Emory University School of Medicine
Atlanta, Georgia

Anna Kho, MD [91]
Assistant Professor of Medicine
Emory University
Atlanta, Georgia

Claude Killu, MD [114]
Assistant Clinical Professor of Medicine
David Geffen School of Medicine, UCLA
Los Angeles, California

Emmanuel S. King, MD, FHM [14]
Assistant Professor of Clinical Medicine
Director of Clinical Operations, Section of Hospital Medicine
University of Pennsylvania, Philadelphia School of Pennsylvania
Pittsburgh, Pennsylvania

Joyce E. King, MD [230]
Director
Inpatient Medicine Training
Family Medicine Residency Program
Franklin Square Hospital Center
Baltimore, Maryland

Jan-Michael A. Klapproth, MD [163]
Assistant Professor of Medicine, Emory University
Fellowship Program Director for Digestive Diseases
Atlanta, Georgia

Michael Klompas, MD, MPH, FRCPC [194]
Associate Hospital Epidemiologist
Brigham and Women's Hospital
Assistant Professor
Department of Population Medicine
Harvard Medical School and Harvard Pilgrim Health Care Institute
Boston, Massachusetts

Serena Koenig, MD, MPH [190]
Brigham and Women's Hospital
Harvard Medical School
Boston, Massachusetts

Elizabeth F. Krakow, MD,CM, FRCPC [179, 180]
Clinical Scholar in Hematology
McMaster University Medical Center and Hamilton Health Sciences
Hamilton, Ontario

Svetlana Krasnokutksy, MD [255]
New York University
School of Medicine
New York, New York

Harold Kudler, MD [267]
Mental Illness Research
Education and Clinical Center
Mid-Atlantic Veterans Service Network/Department of Psychiatry and Behavioral Sciences
Duke University Medical Center
Durham, North Carolina

Ricky Kue, MD, MPH, FACEP [268]
Major, Medical Corps, United States Army Reserve
Associate Medical Director
Boston EMS, Police and Fire
Assistant Professor
Department of Emergency Medicine
Boston University School of Medicine
Boston, Massachusetts

Mark S. Lachs, MD, MPH [167]
Irene F. and I. Roy Psaty Distinguished Professor of Medicine
The Weill Medical College of Cornell University
Co-Chief, Division of Geriatrics and Gerontology
Director of Geriatrics
New York Presbyterian Health System
New York, New York

Albert Q. Lam, MD [57]
Clinical and Research Fellow, Renal Division
Department of Medicine
Brigham and Women's Hospital
Boston, Massachusetts

Vijay H. Lapsia, MBBS, MD [245]
Fellow, Division of Nephrology
Hypertension and Renal Hypertension
University of Florida
Gainesville, Florida

Lucia Larson, MD [220]
Associate Professor of Medicine and Obstetrics and Gynecology
Alpert Medical School of Brown University
Director of Obstetric Medicine, Women's Medicine Collaborative
Department of Medicine, Women and Infants Hospital
Providence, Rhode Island

Brian Leber, MD, FRCP(C) [174]
Professor of Medicine, McMaster University
Hamilton, Ontario

Noah Lechtzin, MD, MHS [93]
The Johns Hopkins University School of Medicine
Department of Medicine
Division of Pulmonary and Critical Care
Baltimore, Maryland

Linda Lee, MD [78]
Clinical Director
Division of Gastroenterology and Hepatology
The Johns Hopkins University School of Medicine
Director
Johns Hopkins Integrative Medicine and Digestive Center
Lutherville, Maryland

Linda S. Lee, MD [160]
Gastroenterology Division
Brigham and Women's Hospital
Harvard Medical School
Boston, Massachusetts

Angel Rodrigo Leon, MD [128]
Associate Professor of Medicine
Chief of Cardiology, Emory University School of Medicine
Chief of Cardiology, Emory University Hospital Midtown
Atlanta, Georgia

Blair J. N. Leonard, MD, PhD, FRCP [174]
Senior Hematology Fellow, McMaster University
Hamilton, Ontario

Marcos Lepe, MD [252]
Research Assistant
Dorrington Medical Associates
Universidad Autonoma de Baja California
Houston, Texas

William I. Levin, MD [56]
Associate Professor of Medicine
Division of General Internal Medicine
University of Pittsburgh School of Medicine
Pittsburgh, Pennsylvania

Mitchell M. Levy, MD, FCCM, FCCP [140]
Rhode Island Hospital/Brown University
Providence, Rhode Island

Joseph Ming Wah Li, MD, SFHM, FACP [31]
Assistant Professor of Medicine
Harvard Medical School
BIDMC Hospital Medicine Program
Director
Hospital Medicine Program
Associate Chief, Division of General Medicine and Primary Care
Beth Israel Deaconess Medical Center
Boston, Massachusetts

Orfeas Liangos, MD [251]
Assistant Professor of Medicine
Tufts University School of Medicine
Boston, Massachusetts

Solomon S. Liao, MD [40]
Associate Clinical Professor, Hospitalist Program
Department of Medicine
University of California, Irvine
Orange, California

Desiree Lie, MD, MSED [40]
Clinical Professor
Department of Family Medicine
University of California, Irvine
Orange, California

Cindy Lien, MD [217]
Palliative Care Physician and Medicine Hospitalist
Beth Israel Deaconess Medical Center
Instructor in Medicine
Harvard Medical School
Boston, Massachusetts

Elaine C. Lin Liew, MD, FRCA [151]
Assistant Clinical Professor of Anesthesiology
University of Wisconsin-Madison School of Medicine
and Public Health
Madison, Wisconsin

David J. Likosky, MD, SFHM [207]
Hospitalist Department
Evergreen Hospital Medical Center
Clinical Faculty, Department of Neurology
University of Washington
Seattle, Washington

John L. Lin, MD [66]
Assistant Professor
Emory University, School of Medicine, Physiatry,
Internal Medicine, Shepherd Center
Atlanta, Georgia

Elizabeth Lindenberger, MD [169]
Assistant Professor
Brookdale Department of Geriatrics and Adult Development
Mount Sinai School of Medicine and
Geriatrics Research, Education and Clinical Center
James J. Peters VA Medical Center
Bronx, New York

Lori-Ann Linkins, MSc, MD [259, 260]
Associate Professor
Department of Medicine
McMaster University
Hamilton, Ontario

Rafael H. Llinas, MD [87]
Associate Professor of Medicine
Clinical Vice Chair of Neurology
The Johns Hopkins Hospital
Baltimore, Maryland

Lenny Lopez, MD, MPH, MDiv [3]
Assistant in Health Policy
Mongan Institute for Health Policy
Massachusetts General Hospital
Associate Physician
Brigham and Women's Hospital
Boston, Massachusetts

Courtney H. Lyder, MD, GNP, FAAN [144]
Dean and Professor of Nursing and Health Services
UCLA School of Nursing and Assistant Director
UCLA Health System
Los Angeles, California

William L. Lyons, MD [164]
Associate Professor
Division of Geriatric Medicine
Department of Internal Medicine
University of Nebraska Medical Center
Omaha, Nebraska

Benjamin D. Mackie, MD [132]
Cardiology Fellow
Emory School of Medicine
Atlanta, Georgia

James H. Maguire, MD, MPH [190]
Professor of Medicine
Harvard Medical School
Senior Physician
Division of Infectious Diseases
Brigham and Women's Hospital
Boston, Massachusetts

Scott Manaker, MD, PhD [28]
Associate Professor of Medicine; Vice Chair for Regulatory Affairs
Department of Medicine
University of Pennsylvania Health System
Philadelphia, Pennsylvania

Kimberly D. Manning, MD, FACP, FAAP [237]
Assistant Professor, Division of General Medicine
Emory University School of Medicine
Atlanta, Georgia

Gary Margolias, MD [135]
Assistant Professor of Anesthesiology
Emory University School of Medicine
Atlanta, Georgia

Alayne D. Markland, DO, MSc [170]
Assistant Professor
Department of Medicine
Division of Geriatrics, Gerontology, and Palliative Care
School of Medicine
University of Alabama
Physician, Birmingham Veterans Affairs Medical Center
Birmingham, Alabama

Leisa L. Marshall, PharmD, FASCP [10]
Clinical Professor, Mercer University College of Pharmacy and Health Sciences
Department of Pharmacy Practice
Atlanta, Georgia

Greg S. Martin, MD, MSc [134]
Associate Professor of Medicine
Associate Director for Critical Care
Division of Pulmonary, Allergy and Critical Care
Emory University School of Medicine
Atlanta, Georgia

R. Kirk Mathews, MBA [29]
CEO, Inpatient Management Inc.
St Louis, Missouri

Melissa Mattison, MD, SFHM, FACP [168]
Harvard Medical School
Beth Israel Deaconess Medical Center
Boston, Massachusetts

Saverio M. Maviglia, MD, MSc [17]
Assistant Professor
Department of Medicine
Harvard Medical School
Associate Physician
Department of General Medicine
Brigham and Women's Hospital
Principal Informaticist
Partners Health Care System
Boston, Massachusetts

Anne B. McBride, MD [94]
USD Department of Psychiatry and Behavioral Sciences
University of California, Davis
Sacramento, California

Timothy B. McDonald, MD, JD [35]
Professor, Anesthesiology and Pediatrics
Chief Safety and Risk Officer for Health Affairs
University of Illinois
Chicago, Illinois

Andrew McFarlane, MLT, ART [173]
Technical Specialist Molecular Hematology and Red Cell Disorders
Lecturer McMaster University
Department of Medicine
McMaster University Medical Centre
Hamilton, Ontario

Gerard M. McGorisk, MD, FACC, MRCPI [126]
Assistant Professor of Medicine
Emory University School of Medicine and Atlanta VA Medical Center
Atlanta, Georgia

Catherine McGorrian, MB, BCh, LRCP&SI, MRCPI [263]
Cardiologist
The Heart House
Mater Misericordiae University Hospital
Dublin, Ireland

Sylvia C. McKean, MD, SFHM, FACP [5, 100, 101, 102, 105, 107, 108, 109, 112]
Associate Professor of Medicine
Harvard Medical School
Boston, Massachusetts

Graham T. McMahon, MD, MMSc [148]
Brigham and Women's Hospital
Endocrinology, Diabetes and Hypertension
Boston, Massachusetts

Thomas E. McNalley, MD [258]
Acting Assistant Professor
Department of Rehabilitation Medicine
University of Washington
Seattle Children's Hospital
Seattle, Washington

Khalid Medani, MD [64]

Ashish Mehta, MD [242]
Assistant Professor of Medicine
Emory University School of Medicine and Atlanta VA Medical Center
Atlanta, Georgia

Niharika D. Mehta, MD [223]
Assistant Professor of Medicine (Clinical)
Warren Alpert Medical School at Brown University
Division of Obstetric Medicine
Department of Medicine
Women and Infant's Hospital
Providence, Rhode Island

Diane E. Meier, MD [215]
Department of Geriatrics and Palliative Medicine
Mount Sinai School of Medicine
New York, New York

Karina Meijer, MD, PhD [178]
Division of Haemostasis and Thrombosis
Department of Haematology
University Medical Centre Groningen
Groningen, Netherlands

David Meltzer, MD, PhD [19]
Associate Professor of Medicine Economics
Chief, Section of Hospital Medicine Public Policy Studies
Director
Center for Health and The Social Science
University of Chicago Medical Center
Chicago, Illinois

Andrew Mente, PhD [73]
Assistant Professor
Department of Clinical Epidemiology and Biostatistics
Population Health Research Institute
McMaster University
Hamilton, Ontario

Peter A. Merkel, MD, MPH [264]
Professor of Medicine
Section of Rheumatology and the Clinical Epidemiology Unit
Director
Vasculitis Center
Boston University School of Medicine
Boston, Massachusetts

Christian A. Merlo, MD, MPH [88]
Assistant Professor of Medicine
The Johns Hopkins University School of Medicine
Division of Pulmonary and Critical Care Medicine
Baltimore, Maryland

Nicole L. Metzger, PharmD, BCPS [10]
Clinical Assistant Professor
Mercer University College of Pharmacy and Health Sciences
Atlanta, Georgia

Ralph M. Meyer, MD, FRCP(C) [181]
Edith and Carla Eisenhauer Chair in Clinical Cancer Research
Director, NCIC CTG
Professor, Departments of Oncology
Medicine and Community Health and Epidemiology
Cancer Clinical Trials Division, Cancer Research Institute
Queen's University
Kingston, Ontario

Joseph J. Miaskiewicz, MD, FHM [103]
Director
North Shore Medical Center
Hospitalist Service
Salem, Massachusetts

Marc Miller, MD [102]
Assistant Professor of Medicine
Cardiac Arrhythmia Service
Mount Sinai School of Medicine
New York, New York

Chad S. Miller, MD, FACP, FHM [90, 92]
Director
Student Programs
Associate Program Director
Residency
Tulane University Health Sciences Center
Department of Internal Medicine
New Orleans, Louisiana

Elinor Mody, MD [118]
Division of Rheumatology
Brigham and Women's Hospital
Boston, Massachusetts

Rita F. Moldovan, DNP, MS, RN [219]
Clinical Nurse Specialist
Department of Medicine Nursing
The Johns Hopkins Hospital
Baltimore, Maryland

Paul A. Monach, MD, PhD [264]
Assistant Professor, Department of Medicine
Section of Pneumatology, and Vasculitis Center
Boston University School of Medicine
Boston, Massachusetts

Carmen Monzon, MD [223]
Clinical Assistant Professor
Department of Psychiatry
Warren Alpert Medical School at Brown University
Providence, Rhode Island

Luis F. Mora, MD [128]
Chief Resident
Emory School of Medicine
Atlanta, Georgia

Ian Morrison, PhD [1]
Health Care Futurist
Menlo Park, California

Ala Moshiri, MD, PhD [81]
Wilmer Eye Institute
The Johns Hopkins University School of Medicine
Baltimore, Maryland

John E. Moss, MD [121]
Fellow Physician
Mayo Clinic Pulmonary Critical Care
Jacksonville, Florida

Luisa Silvia Munoz-Price, MD [186]
University of Miami
Jackson Memorial Hospital
Miami, Florida

Mandakolathur R. Murali, MD [237]
Department of Medicine
Massachusetts General Hospital
Boston, Massachusetts

Daniel M. Musher, MD [189]
Professor of Medicine
Professor of Molecular Virology and Microbiology
Distinguished Professor
Baylor College of Medicine
Chief of Infectious Diseases
Michael E. DeBakey VA Medical Center
Houston, Texas

Jennifer S. Myers, MD, FHM [14]
Assistant Professor of Clinical Medicine
Department of Medicine
University of Pennsylvania School of Medicine
Patient Safety Officer
Hospital of the University of Pennsylvania
Philadelphia, Pennsylvania

Dale M. Needham, MD, PhD [79]
Assistant Professor
Pulmonary Critical Care Medicine, and
Physical Medicine and Rehabilitation
School of Medicine
The Johns Hopkins University
Baltimore, Maryland

John Nelson, MD, MHM [27]
Medical Director
Hospitalists Practice
Overlake Hospital
Bellevue, Washington

Karin J. Neufeld, MD, MPH [79]
Director of General Hospital Psychiatry –
The Johns Hopkins Hospital
Assistant Professor
Department of Psychiatry and Behavioral Sciences
The Johns Hopkins University School of Medicine
Baltimore, Maryland

Andrew Nevins, MD, MS [41]
Clinical Assistant Professor
Department of Medicine
Stanford University School of Medicine
Stanford, California

Tareck Nossuli, MD, PhD [262]
Cardiology Fellow, Section of Cardiovascular Medicine
The Lahey Clinic
Burlington, Massachusetts

Lars Osterberg, MD [269]
Chief, General Internal Medicine
VA Palo Alto Health Care System
Clinical Associate Professor of Medicine
Stanford University School of Medicine
Palo Alto, California

Karin Ouchida, MD [167]
Assistant Professor of Medicine
Montefiore Medical Center Division of Geriatrics
Albert Einstein College of Medicine
Bronx, New York

Thomas A. Owens, MD [197]
Associate Professor, Departments of
Internal Medicine and Pediatrics
Duke University Medical Center
Durham, North Carolina

David A. Oxman, MD [191]
Instructor of Medicine
Harvard Medical School
Associate Physician
Division of Infectious Diseases and
Surgical Critical Care
Brigham and Women's Hospital
Boston, Massachusetts

Menaka Pai, MD, FRCPC [58, 59, 60]
Consultant, Laboratory Hematologist
Hamilton Regional Laboratory Medicine Program
Clinical Scholar – Thrombosis and Hemostasis
McMaster University
Hamilton, Ontario

Jeremy Paikin, MD [70]
Internal Medicine Resident
McMaster University
Hamilton, Ontario

Susan M. Palac, MD [212]
Assistant Professor
Department of Neurology
Emory University School of Medicine
Atlanta, Georgia

Robert M. Palmer, MD, MPH [85]
Department of Medicine
University of Pittsburgh
Pittsburgh, Pennsylvania

Anand K. Pandurangi, MBBS, MD [226]
Professor of Psychiatry and Adjunct Professor of Radiology
Medical Director and Chairman Division of Inpatient Psychiatry
Virginia Commonwealth University
Richmond, Virginia

Miguel A. Paniagua, MD, FACP [172]
Assistant Professor
Department of Internal Medicine
Division of Gerontology and Geriatric Medicine
St Louis, Missouri

Christopher Parks, MD [117, 243]
Assistant professor of medicine
Division of Pulmonary Allergy and Critical Care Medicine
Emory University School of Medicine
Atlanta, Georgia

Nainesh C. Patel, MD, FACC [127]
Co-Director MI Alert/Hypothermia Program
Lehigh Valley Health Network
Allentown, Pennsylvania

Shella Patel, ANP, BSN, MSN [218]
Palliative Care Nurse Practitioner Emory University Hospital and
Emory University Hospital Midtown
Atlanta, Georgia

Timothy J. Patton, DO [141]

Jill M. Paulson, MD [150]
Clinical Fellow
Division of Endocrinology
Diabetes, and Metabolism
Beth Israel Deaconess Medical Center
Instructor in Medicine
Harvard Medical School
Boston, Massachusetts

Mark Perazella, MD, FACP, FASN [248]
Associate Professor of Medicine
Director Nephrology Fellowship Program
Medical Director
Physician Associate Program
Department of Medicine
Yale University School of Medicine
Director
Acute Dialysis Program Yale-New Haven Hospital
New Haven, Connecticut

Jason Persoff, MD, FHM [121]
Assistant Professor of Internal Medicine
Division of Hospital Medicine
Mayo Clinic
Jacksonville, Florida

Richard A. Perugini, MD [68]
Surgical Director, Weight Center
UMass Memorial Medical Center
Assistant Professor of Surgery
University of Massachusetts Medical School
Boston, Massachusetts

Brent G. Petty, MD [11]
Associate Professor
Departments of Medicine and of Pharmacology and
Molecular Sciences
The Johns Hopkins University School of Medicine
Baltimore, Maryland

Kurt Pfeifer, MD [55]
Associate Professor of Medicine
General Internal Medicine
Medical College of Wisconsin
Milwaukee, Wisconsin

Tania Phillips, MD, FACPC [146]
Clinical Professor
Department of Dermatology
Boston University School of Medicine
Boston, Massachusetts

Michael H. Pillinger, MD [255]
Associate Professor of Medicine and Pharmacology
Director of Rheumatology Training
New York University School of Medicine
Section Chief, Rheumatology
New York Harbor Health Care System
Department of Veterans Affairs
New York, New York

Michael J. Pistoria, DO, FACP, FHM [127]
Associate Chief
Division of General Internal Medicine
Assistant Program Director
Internal Medicine Residency Program
Lehigh Valley Health Network
Allentown, Pennsylvania

Carol Pohlig, RN, BSN, CPC, ACS [28]
Senior Coding and Education Specialist
Office of Clinical Documentation
University of Pennsylvania Health System
Pittsburgh, Pennsylvania

Raymond O. Powrie, MD, FRCP, FACP [221]
Professor of Medicine and Obstetrics and Gynecology
Alpert Medical School of Brown University
Chief of Medicine
Department of Medicine
Women and Infants Hospital of Rhode Island
Providence, Rhode Island

Jennifer C. Price, MD [159]
Division of Gastroenterology and Hepatology
Department of Medicine
Johns Hopkins School of Medicine
Baltimore, Maryland

Amir A. Qamar, MD [53]
Division of Gastroenterology
Brigham and Women's Hospital
Boston, Massachusetts

Susan Y. Quan, MD [95]
Osler Medicine Resident
The Johns Hopkins University Department of Medicine
Baltimore, Maryland

Marzouq Awni Qubti, MD [75]
Post Doctoral Fellow
Department of Medicine
Division of Rheumatology
The Johns Hopkins University School of Medicine
Baltimore, Maryland

Tammie E. Quest, MD [218]
Associate Professor
Department of Emergency Medicine
Emory University School of Medicine
Atlanta, Georgia

Timothy R. Quinn, MD, CH [143]
Derm Dx
Boston, Massachusetts

Ruma Rajbhandari, MD, MPH [119]
Global Health Equity Resident
Department of Internal Medicine
Brigham and Women's Hospital
Boston, Massachusetts

Anupama Ravi, MD [153]
Division of Digestive Diseases
Emory University
Atlanta, Georgia

Clare Rock, MD [202]
Infectious diseases fellow
Department of Infectious Diseases
University of Maryland
Baltimore, Maryland

Graham Wester Redgrave, MD [228]
Assistant Professor
Psychiatry and Behavioral Sciences
The Johns Hopkins University School of Medicine
Assistant Director of the Eating Disorders Program at Johns Hopkins
Baltimore, Maryland

John J. Reilly Jr., MD [56]
Vice Chair for Clinical Affairs
University of Pittsburgh Medical Center
Professor of Medicine, University of Pittsburgh
Pittsburgh, Pennsylvania

Christina M. Delos Reyes, MD [235]
Assistant Professor
Department of Psychiatry
University Hospitals Case Medical Center
Cleveland, Ohio

Joseph Rhatigan, MD [2]
Assistant Professor of Medicine
Department of Medicine
Division of Global Health Equity
Brigham and Women's Hospital
Harvard Medical School
Boston, Massachusetts

Malcolm K. Robinson, MD, FACS [54]
Assistant Professor of Surgery
Harvard Medical School
Department of Surgery
Brigham and Women's Hospital
Boston, Massachusetts

Selwyn O. Rogers Jr., MD, MPH [139]
Associate Professor
Department of Surgery
Brigham and Women's Hospital
Boston, Massachusetts

Karen L. Roos, MD [199]
John and Nancy Nelson Professor of Neurology
Professor of Neurosurgery
Indiana University School of Medicine
Indianapolis, Indiana

Alexander E. Ropper, MD [209]
Resident, Department of Neurosurgery
Brigham and Women's Hospital and Children's Hospital
Clinical Instructor in Surgery, Harvard Medical School
Boston, Massachusetts

Allan H. Ropper, MD, FRCP [209, 213]
Professor of Neurology, Harvard Medical School
Executive Vice Chair of Neurology,
Brigham and Women's Hospital
Boston, Massachusetts

Bradley T. Rosen, MD, MBA, FHM [115]
Medical Director
ISP Hospitalist Service
Proceduralist
Assistant Clinical Professor
Cedars-Sinai Medical Center and UCLA School of Medicine
Los Angeles, California

Karen Rosene-Montella, MD [223, 224]
Senior Vice President
Women's Services and Clinical Integration, Lifespan
Vice Chair of Medicine for Quality/Outcomes
Division Chief Obstetric Medicine
Professor of Medicine and Obstetrics and Gynecology
The Warren Alpert Medical School at Brown University
Providence, Rhode Island

John J. Ross, MD, CM, FIDSA [192, 200, 205, 213]
Assistant Professor of Medicine
Harvard Medical School
Hospitalist Service, Brigham and Women's Hospital
Boston, Massachusetts

Michael A. Ross, MD, FACEP [123]
Associate Professor
Medical Director of Observation Medicine
Department of Emergency Medicine
Emory University School of Medicine
Atlanta, Georgia

Joseph N. Rudolph, MD [211]
Mt. Sinai School of Medicine
New York, New York

Arturo P. Saavedra, MD, PhD [142]
Instructor in Dermatology
Harvard Medical School
Department of Dermatology
Brigham and Women's Hospital
Boston, Massachusetts

Cheryl A. Sadow, MD [110]
Staff Radiologist
Division of Abdominal Imaging and Intervention,
Brigham and Women's Hospital
Harvard Medical School
Boston, Massachusetts

Elianna Saidenberg, MD, FRCP(C) [177]
Assistant Professor
Department of Pathology and Laboratory Medicine
University of Ottawa
Director Special Hematology Laboratory, the Ottawa Hospital
Ottawa, Ontario

Bisan A. Salhi, MD [122]
Emory University Department of Emergency Medicine
Atlanta, Georgia

John R. Saltzman, MD [155, 161]
Associate Professor of Medicine
Harvard Medical School
Director of Endoscopy
Brigham and Women's Hospital
Boston, Massachusetts

Michael Sanatani, MD, FRCPC [183]
Assistant Professor of Oncology
Department of Oncology
Division of Medical Oncology
University of Western Ontario
London, Ontario

Kenneth E. Sands, MD, MPH [22]
Senior Vice President for Health Care Quality
Beth Israel Deaconess Medical Center
Assistant Professor, Harvard Medical School
Boston, Massachusetts

Kaveh Saremi, MD [214]
Clinical Neurophysiology Fellow
UC Irvine ALS and Neuromuscular Center
Orange, California

Lewis Satterwhite, MD [239]
Fellow, Pulmonary and Critical Care Medicine
Emory University School of Medicine
Atlanta, Georgia

Milda R. Saunders, MD, MPH [32]
Clinical Associate
Section of Hospital Medicine and Fellow
MacLean Center of Clinical Medical Ethics
University of Chicago Medical Center
Chicago, Illinois

Paul E. Sax, MD [195]
Clinical Director
Division of Infectious Diseases
Brigham and Women's Hospital
Associate Professor of Medicine
Harvard Medical School
Boston, Massachusetts

Sandra Schaap, MDiv [218]

Adam C. Schaffer, MD [36, 104]
Instructor, Department of Medicine
Brigham and Women's Hospital
Harvard Medical School
Boston, Massachusetts

Danielle B. Scheurer, MD, MSc, FHM [80, 188]
Assistant Professor of Medicine
Harvard Medical School
Hospitalist, Brigham and Women's Hospital
Director
General Medicine Service
Boston, Massachusetts

Gordon D. Schiff, MD [8]
Associate Director
Center for Patient Safety Research and Practice
Division of General Internal Medicine
Brigham and Women's Hospital
Associate Professor of Medicine
Harvard Medical School
Boston, Massachusetts

Nicholas D. Schiff, MD [208]
Professor of Neurology and Neuroscience
Weill Cornell Medical College
New York, New York

Lynn Schlanger, MD [250]
Emory University VA Medical Center
Atlanta, Georgia

Robert K. Schneider, MD [229]
Associate Professor, Departments of
Psychiatry and Internal Medicine
Virginia Commonwealth University and
McGuire VA Medical Center
Richmond, Virginia

Jeffrey L. Schnipper, MD, MPH, FHM [13, 149]
Director of Clinical Research
BWH, Academic Hospitalist Service
Associate Physician
Division of General Medicine
Brigham and Women's Hospital
Assistant Professor of Medicine
Harvard Medical School
Boston, Massachusetts

Robert W. Schrier, MD [249]
Professor of Medicine
Division of Renal Diseases and Hypertension
School of Medicine, University of Colorado
Denver, Colorado

David A. Schulman, MD, MPH, FCCP [242]
Assistant Professor
Division of Pulmonary, Allergy and Critical Care Medicine
Emory University School of Medicine
Atlanta, Georgia

Sam Schulman, MD, PhD [178]
Professor of Medicine, McMaster University
Department of Medicine
Thrombosis Service, HHS-General Hospital
Hamilton, Ontario

Richard M. Schwartzstein, MD [83]
Vice President for Education
Associate Chief, Division of Pulmonary and Critical Care Medicine
Director
Carl J. Shapiro Institute for Education and Research
Beth Israel Deaconess Medical Center
Ellen and Melvin Gordon Professor of Medicine and
Medical Education
Faculty Associate Dean for Medical Education
Director
Harvard Medical School Academy
Harvard Medical School
Boston, Massachusetts

Victor F. Seabra, MD [251]
Research Instructor in Medicine
Tufts University School of Medicine
Boston, Massachusetts

Julian L. Seifter, MD [57]
Physician, Department of Medicine
Brigham and Women's Hospital
Boston, Massachusetts

Daniel S. Shapiro, MD [266]
Director
Clinical Microbiology Laboratory
Lahey Clinic
Adjunct Associate Professor of Medicine
Boston University School of Medicine
Boston, Massachusetts

Philip Shayne, MD, FACEP [120]
Associate Professor and Residency Director and
Vice Chair for Education
Department of Emergency Medicine
Emory University School of Medicine
Atlanta, Georgia

Ann S. Sheehy, MD, MS [151]
Assistant Professor
Department of Medicine
University of Wisconsin-Madison School of Medicine
and Public Health
Madison, Wisconsin

Eugenie Shieh, MD [78]
The Johns Hopkins University School of Medicine
Baltimore, Maryland

Eric M. Siegal, MD, SFHM [137]
Section of Allergy, Pulmonary and Critical Care Medicine
University of Wisconsin School of Medicine and Public Health
Madison, Wisconsin

Mark Siegler, MD [32]
Lindy Bergman Distinguished Service Professor
Professor, Departments of Medicine and Surgery
Director
MacLean Center for Clinical Medical Ethics
University of Chicago Medical Center
Chicago, Illinois

Ross D. Silverman, JD, MPH [34]
Professor and Chair, Department of Humanities
Professor, Department of Psychiatry
Southern Illinois University School of Medicine
Springfield
Professor of Medical Jurisprudence
Southern Illinois University School of Law
Carbondale, Illinois

Ajay K. Singh, MD, MBA, FRCP [246]
Associate Professor of Medicine
Harvard Medical School
Brigham and Women's Hospital
Boston, Massachusetts

Gerald W. Smetana, MD, FACP [55]
Division of General Medicine and Primary Care
Harvard Medical School
Beth Israel Deaconess Medical Center
Boston, Massachusetts

Robert L. Smith, MD [138]
Associate Professor of Medicine
New York University
Chief, Critical Care Medicine
New York Harbor Health Care System (VA)
New York, New York

Scot T. Smith, MD [21]
Sound Physician
Tacoma, Washington

David R. Snydman, MD, FACP [187]
Chief, Division of Geographic Medicine and Infectious Diseases
Professor of Medicine, Tufts University School of Medicine
Tufts-New England Medical Center
Boston, Massachusetts

Magda Sobieraj-Teague, MBBS [261]
Department of Hematology
Flinders Medical Centre
Adelaide, Australia

Aaron Sodickson, MD, PhD [106]
Assistant Professor of Radiology, Harvard Medical School
Section Chief, Emergency Radiology
Director
Brigham NightWatch Program
Brigham and Women's Hospital
Boston, Massachusetts

Nathan Spell, MD, FACP [12, 15]
Chief Quality Officer
Emory University Hospital
Emory Health Care, Inc.
Associate Clinical Chief
General Internal Medicine
The Emory Clinic, Inc.
Assistant Professor
Department of Medicine
Emory University School of Medicine
Atlanta, Georgia

James R. Spivey, MD [158]
Associate Professor of Medicine
Clinical Director of Hepatology
Director of Liver Transplant
Emory University Hospital
Atlanta, Georgia

Christopher J. Standaert, MD [258]
Clinical Associate Professor
Departments of Rehabilitation Medicine, Orthopedics, and Sports Medicine and Neurological Surgery
University of Washington
Seattle, Washington

Gerald W. Staton, MD [239]
Professor of Medicine, Division of Pulmonary and Critical Care Medicine
Department of Medicine
Emory University School of Medicine
Atlanta, Georgia

Arlene Stecenko, MD [240]
Associate Professor of Pediatrics and Medicine
Emory University School of Medicine
Atlanta, Georgia

Samuel J. Stellpflug, MD [98]
Regions Hospital Clinical Toxicology Service and Department of Emergency Medicine
St Paul, Minnesota and Hennepin Regional Poison Center
Hennepin County Medical Center
Minneapolis, Minnesota

Theodore A. Stern, MD [231]
Professor of Psychiatry, Harvard Medical School
Chief, Psychiatric Consultation Service
Massachusetts General Hospital
Boston, Massachusetts

Ram M. Subramanian, MD [158]
Assistant Professor of Medicine and Surgery
Emory University School of Medicine
Atlanta, Georgia

Kuyilan Karai Subramanian, MD [246]
Research Fellow in Medicine
Harvard Medical School
Postdoctoral Fellow
Brigham and Women's Hospital
Renal Division
Boston, Massachusetts

Prem S. Subramanian, MD, PhD [81]
Associate Professor of Ophthalmology
Neuro-Ophthalmology and Orbital Disease
Wilmer Eye Institute
The Johns Hopkins University School of Medicine
Associate Professor of Surgery
Division of Ophthalmology
Associate Professor of Surgery
Uniformed Services University of the Health Sciences
Baltimore, Maryland

Jeffrey A. Tabas, MD [37]
Director of Outcomes and Innovations – Office of Continuing Medical Education
Associate Professor
Department of Emergency Medicine
USCF School of Medicine
San Francisco, California

Jennifer K. Tan, MD [147]
Harvard Medical School
Department of Dermatology
Boston, Massachusetts

Peter Terry, MD [241]
Clinical Assistant Professor of Surgery
Department of Surgery, SUNY Downstate Medical Center
Brooklyn, New York

Anjala V. Tess, MD, SFHM [38]
Assistant Professor of Medicine Harvard Medical School
Hospital Medicine Program
Beth Israel Deaconess Medical Center
Harvard Medical School
Boston, Massachusetts

Patrick J. Tighe, MD [96]
Fellow, Department of Anesthesiology
Division of Regional Anesthesia
University of Florida
Gainesville, Florida

Derrick J. Todd, MD, PhD [254]
Staff Physician
Division of Rheumatology
Immunology, & Allergy
Instructor of Medicine
Harvard Medical School
Boston, Massachusetts

David Tong, MD, MPH [240]
Assistant Professor
Division of Hospital Medicine
Department of Medicine
Emory University School of Medicine
Atlanta, Georgia

Anne C. Travis, MD, MSc [161]
Instructor, Harvard Medical School
Associate Physician, Brigham and Women's Hospital
Boston, Massachusetts

Glenn J. Treisman, MD, PhD [230]
Professor of Psychiatry and Behavioral Sciences
Professor of Medicine
The Johns Hopkins University School of Medicine
Baltimore, Maryland

Elly Trepman, MD [145]

Nicholas Tsapatsaris, MD [89, 262]
Associate Section, Head Cardiovascular Medicine – Lahey Clinic
Associate Clinical Professor of Medicine
Tufts University School of Medicine
Burlington, Massachusetts

Geoffrey Tsaras, MD, ChB, MPH [201]
Clinical Fellow, Division of Infectious Diseases
Mayo Clinic College of Medicine
Rochester, Minnesota

Shachi Tyagi, MD [162]
Senior Resident (PGY-III) in Internal Medicine
William Beaumont Hospital
Royal Oak, Michigan

Prashant Vaishnava, MD [102]
The Zena and Michael A. Wiener Cardiovascular Institute
The Mount Sinai Medical Center
New York, New York

Joseph Varon, MD, FACP, FCCP, FCCM [252]
Clinical Professor of Medicine
The University of Texas Health Science Center
Clinical Professor of Medicine
The University of Texas Medical Branch at Galveston
Houston, Texas

Sondra S. Vazirani, MD, MPH [269]
Hospitalist, VHA Greater Los Angeles Health Care System
Associate Clinical Professor of Medicine
David Geffen School of Medicine at UCLA
Los Angeles, California

Nicole F. Velez, MD [142]
Resident
Harvard Combined Dermatology and Medicine Residency
Boston, Massachusetts

Madeleine Verhovsek, MD, BSc [173]
Clinical Scholar, Department of Medicine
McMaster University
Hamilton, Ontario

Donald C. Vinh, MD, FRCP, FACP [193]
Division of Infectious Diseases
Department of Medicine
Department of Medical Microbiology
McGill University Health Centre
Montreal, Quebec

Adrian Visoiu, MD [85]
Clinical Assistant Professor
Division of Geriatric Medicine
Department of Medicine
University of Pittsburgh
Pittsburgh, Pennsylvania

Ruth Ann Vleugels, MD [147]
Director
Connective Tissue Disease Clinic
Brigham and Women's Hospital
Department of Dermatology
Harvard Medical School
Boston, Massachusetts

Grant L. Walker, MA [265]
System Vice President Supply Chain
Ochsner Health System
New Orleans, Louisiana

Ruth H. Walker, MB, ChB, PhD [211]
Physician, Department of Neurology
James J. Peters Veterans Affairs Medical Center
Bronx, New York

Allan J. Walkey, MD, MSc [244]
Division, Pulmonary and Critical Care Medicine
Boston University School of Medicine
Boston, Massachusetts

David A. Walton, MD, MPH [2]
Instructor of Medicine
Harvard Medical School
Research Physician, Brigham and Women's Hospital
Boston, Massachusetts

Sally Wang, MD, FHM [116]
Instructor, Harvard Medical School
Hospitalist, Brigham and Women's Hospital
Boston, Massachusetts

Annabel Kim Wang, MD [214]
Associate Professor (Neurology) UC-Irvine Als
and Neuromuscular Center
Orange, California

Tracy J. Wanner, MD [83]
Pulmonary and Critical Care Fellow
Beth Israel Deaconess Medical Center
Massachusetts General Hospital
Brigham and Women's Hospital
Boston, Massachusetts

Martha C. Ward, MD [225]
Resident Physician, Combined Internal Medicine/Psychiatry Residency Program
Emory University School of Medicine
Atlanta, Georgia

Theodore E. Warkentin, MD [175]
Professor
Department of Pathology and Molecular Medicine
Department of Medicine
Michael G. DeGroote School of Medicine
McMaster University
Regional Director
Transfusion Medicine
Hamilton Regional Laboratory Medicine Program
Hematologist, Service of Clinical Hematology
Hamilton Health Sciences
Hamilton, Ontario

Michael Weaver, MD, FASAM [236]
Associate Professor of Internal Medicine and Psychiatry
Virginia Commonwealth University School of Medicine
Richmond, Virginia

Kathryn Webert, MD, MSc, FRCPC [176]
Assistant Professor
Department of Medicine and Department of Molecular Medicine and Pathology
McMaster University
Hamilton, Ontario

Mohammad Wehbi, MD [163]
Assistant Professor of Medicine
Section Chief Gastroenterology/Atlanta VA Medical Center
Emory University Hospital, Emory University School of Medicine
Atlanta, Georgia

Steven E. Weinberger, MD, FACP [18]
Senior Vice President for Medical Education and Publishing
American College of Physicians
Adjunct Professor of Medicine, University of Pennsylvania
Philadelphia, Pennsylvania

Saul N. Weingart, MD, PhD [6]
Vice President for Quality Improvement and Patient Safety
Dana-Farber Cancer Institute
Associate Professor of Medicine
Harvard Medical School
Boston, Massachusetts

Natalie E. West, MD, MHS [93]
Postdoctoral Fellow
Department of Medicine
Division of Pulmonary and Critical Care Medicine
The Johns Hopkins Hospital
Baltimore, Maryland

Mary C. Westergaard, MD [77]
Instructor, Department of Emergency Medicine
The Johns Hopkins University School of Medicine
Baltimore, Maryland

Tosha B. Wetterneck, MD, MS [30]
Associate Professor, Department of Medicine
School of Medicine and Public Health
University of Wisconsin and Research Faculty
Center for Quality and Productivity Improvement
University of Wisconsin-Madison
Madison, Wisconsin

William Whang, MD [65]
Sutter Gould Medical Foundation
Modesto, California

Chad T. Whelan, MD [15]
Associate Professor of Medicine
Director
Division of Hospital Medicine
Loyola University Chicago, Stritch School of Medicine
Maywood, Illinois

Christopher Whinney, MD, FACP, FHM [67]
Interim Chairman
Department of Hospital Medicine
Cleveland Clinic
Clinical Assistant Professor of Medicine
Cleveland Clinic Lerner College of Medicine
Cleveland, Ohio

David Wiener, MD [245]
Professor of Medicine and Physiology
University of Florida College of Medicine and NF/SGVHS
Gainesville, Florida

Jeffrey G. Wiese, MD, FACP, FSM, SFHM [90, 92]
Professor of Medicine, Associate Dean
Graduate Medical Education
Tulane University Health Sciences Center
New Orleans, Louisiana

B. Robinson Williams III, MD [125]
Assistant Professor of Medicine
Division of Cardiology
Emory Heart and Vascular Center
Atlanta, Georgia

Patrick Willis, MD [131]
Gruentzig Cardiovascular Center, Emory Hospital
Atlanta, Georgia

Neil H. Winawer, MD, SFHM [237]
Associate Professor of Medicine
Emory University School of Medicine
Atlanta, Georgia

Eric Winquist, MSc, MD, FRCPC, FACP [183]
Professor, Division of Medical Oncology
Department of Oncology,
Schulich School of Medicine and Dentistry
University of Western Ontario
London, Ontario

Kristin R. Wise, MD [133]
Assistant Professor of Medicine,
Emory University School of Medicine
Assistant Director of Critical Care Services
Section of Hospital Medicine
Emory University Hospital Midtown
Atlanta, Georgia

Karl Wittnebel, MD, MPH [115]
Department of General Internal Medicine
Cedars Sinai Medical Center
Los Angeles, California

Patricia Wong, MD, MSCE [159]
Assistant Professor of Medicine
The Johns Hopkins University School of Medicine
Division of Gastroenterology
Baltimore, Maryland

Kenneth E. Wood, DO, FCCP [151]
Professor of Medicine and Anesthesiology
Senior Director of Medical Affairs
Director Critical Care Medicine and Respiratory Care
University of Wisconsin-Madison Hospital and Clinics
Madison, Wisconsin

Rollin M. Wright, MD, MA, MPH [85]
Assistant Professor, Department of Medicine
Division of Geriatric Medicine
University of Pittsburgh
Pittsburgh, Pennsylvania

Stephen C. Wright, MD [119]
Chief of Medicine, Faulkner Hospital
Clinical Professor of Medicine
Tufts School of Medicine
Lecturer on Medicine, Harvard Medical School
Boston, Massachusetts

Jacqueline J. Wu, MD [68]
Instructor, Department of Surgery
Brigham and Women's Hospital
Boston, Massachusetts

Bechien U. Wu, MD, MPH [156]
Director of Pancreatic Disorders Gastroenterology
Kaiser Permanente Los Angeles Medical Center
Los Angeles, California

Julius Yang, MD, PhD [24]
Hospitalist, Department of Medicine
Instructor of Medicine, Harvard Medical School
Director of Inpatient Quality
Silverman Institute for Health Care Quality and Safety
Beth Israel Deaconess Medical Center
Boston, Massachusetts

Raymond Young, MD [227]
Assistant Professor of Psychiatry and Behavioral Sciences
Program Director
Psychosomatic Medicine Fellowship Program
Emory University School of Medicine
Department of Psychiatry
Atlanta, Georgia

Julie S. Young, MD, MS [94]
Department of Veterans Affairs,
Northern California Health Care System
Primary Care Behavioral Medicine Clinic
Mather, California

Robert Young, MD [99]
Clinical Instructor
Division of Hospital Medicine
Feinberg School of Medicine
Northwestern University
Chicago, Illinois

Shanta M. Zimmer, MD [86]
Assistant Professor
Director
Translational Research Track, MSCR Program
Institute for Clinical Research Education
University of Pittsburgh
Pittsburgh, Pennsylvania

Camilla Zimmermann, MD, PhD, FRCPC [216]
Head, Palliative Care Services, University Health Network
Associated Professor, Department of Medicine
University of Toronto
Toronto, Ontario

Jennifer E. Zora, BS [238]
Student, Emory School of Medicine
Rollins School of Public Health
Atlanta, Georgia

SECTION REVIEWERS

Robert Barbieri, MD
Chairman
Obstetrics and Gynecology and Reproductive Biology
Brigham and Women's Hospital
Kate Macy Ladd Professor of Obstetrics
Gynecology and Reproductive Biology
Harvard Medical School
Boston, Massachusetts
Part VI, Section 13

Preetha Basaviah, MD, FHM
Clinical Associate Professor of Medicine, Stanford University
Course Director, Practice of Medicine, Stanford University
Palo Alto, California
Part I, Section 7

Richard Baum, MD
Chief, Division of Angiography and Interventional Radiology
Brigham and Women's Hospital
Associate Professor of Radiology
Harvard Medical School
Boston, Massachusetts
Part V, Section 3

Rachelle E. Bernacki, MD, MS
Director of Quality Initiatives
Pain and Palliative Care Program
Dana Farber Cancer Institute
Harvard Medical School
Boston, Massachusetts
Part VI, Section 12

Francine L. Jacobson, MD, MPH
Thoracic Radiologist at Brigham and Women's Hospital
Assistant Professor, Department of Radiology
Harvard Medical School
Boston, Massachusetts
Part V, Section 2

Ralph M. Meyer, MD, FRCP(C)
Edith and Carla Eisenhauer Chair in Clinical Cancer Research
Director, NCIC CTG
Professor, Departments of Oncology
Medicine and Community Health and Epidemiology
Cancer Clinical Trials Division, Cancer Research Institute
Queen's University
Kingston, Ontario
Part VI, Section 9

Karen Rosene-Montella, MD
Senior Vice President
Women's Services and Clinical Integration, Lifespan
Vice Chair of Medicine for Quality/Outcomes
Division Chief Obstetric Medicine
Professor of Medicine and Obstetrics and Gynecology
The Warren Alpert Medical School at Brown University
Providence, Rhode Island
Part VI, Section 13

Nathan Spell, MD, FACP
Chief Quality Officer
Emory University Hospital
Emory Health Care, Inc.
Associate Clinical Chief
General Internal Medicine
The Emory Clinic, Inc.
Assistant Professor
Department of Medicine
Emory University School of Medicine
Atlanta, Georgia
Part I, Sections 2 and 3

Michael Weaver, MD, FASAM
Associate Professor of Internal Medicine and Psychiatry
Virginia Commonwealth University School of Medicine
Richmond, Virginia
Part VI, Section 15

CHAPTER REVIEWERS

William Branch, MD
Carter Smith Senior Professor of Medicine
Director
Division of General Internal Medicine
Department of Medicine
Emory University School of Medicine
Atlanta, Georgia
Chapter 4, The Interface Between Primary Care and Hospital Medicine

Roy Brower, MD
Department of Pulmonary and Critical Care Medicine
The Johns Hopkins Hospital
Baltimore, Maryland
Chapter 219, Care of the Imminently Dying Patient

Hugo Quinny Cheng, MD
Clinical Professor
Division of Hospital Medicine
Department of Medicine
University of California – San Francisco
San Francisco, California
Chapter 63, Common Neurosurgical Conditions
Chapter 64, Common Complications in Neurosurgery

Henry E. Fessler, MD
Department of Pulmonary and Critical Care Medicine
The Johns Hopkins Hospital
Baltimore, Maryland
Chapter 219, Care of the Imminently Dying Patient

Tom H. Lee, MD, MSc
Professor of Medicine, Harvard Medical School
Brigham Internal Medicine Associates
Network President, Partners Health Care System
CEO, Partners Community Health Care, Inc.
Boston, Massachusetts
Chapter 19, The Economics of Hospital Care

Michelle Mello, JD, PhD
Professor of Law and Public Health
Department of Health Policy and Management
Harvard School of Public Health
Boston, Massachusetts
Chapter 36, Medical Malpractice

Jeffrey L. Schnipper, MD, MPH, FHM
Director of Clinical Research
BWH, Academic Hospitalist Service
Associate Physician
Division of General Medicine
Brigham and Women's Hospital
Assistant Professor of Medicine
Harvard Medical School
Boston, Massachusetts
Chapter 99, Syncope

Nancy Sinclair, RN MBA
Director
Assessment and Learning
School of Medicine University of New Mexico
Albuquerque, New Mexico
Chapter 229, The Suicidal Patient

Martin Solomon, MD
Medical Director, Brigham and
Women's Primary Care Associates of Brookline
Division of General Internal Medicine
Department of Medicine
Brigham and Women's Hospital
Boston, Massachusetts
Chapter 4, The Interface Between Primary Care and Hospital Medicine

Peter Stone, MD
Associate Professor of Medicine
Harvard Medical School
Co-Director, Samuel A. Levine Cardiac Unit
Director
Clinical Trials CVD Division
Department of Medicine
Director
Clinical Trials Center
Brigham and Women's Hospital Cardiovascular Division
Boston, Massachusetts
Chapter 100, Tachyarrthymias

Jane de Lima Thomas, MD
Attending Physician
Adult Palliative Care
Dana Farber Cancer Institute/Brigham and Women's Hospital
Boston, Massachusetts
Chapter 217, Domains of Care: Physical Aspects of Care

Richard Zane, MD
Vice Chairman, Department of Emergency Medicine
Brigham and Women's Hospital Medicine
Associate Professor of Emergency Medicine,
Harvard Medical School
Boston, Massachusetts
Chapter 120, The Principles and Practice of Emergency Medicine
Chapter 123, Co-management of Patients in the Emergency Department

PREFACE

The Principles and Practice of Hospital Medicine reflects the evolution of the specialty of Hospital Medicine at a time of increasing pressures to address the ills of our health care system and to provide quality patient care that is safe, effective, patient-centered, timely, efficient, and equitable—the six dimensions defined by the Institute of Medicine. Regardless of practice setting, all clinicians will be increasingly called upon to improve the care they provide for populations of patients. This requires optimizing the function of the entire health care team, structuring their programs to better meet demand, and aligning their performance measures with those of their hospital networks.

The first major part of this book, Systems of Care, introduces key issues in Hospital Medicine, patient safety, quality improvement, leadership and practice management, professionalism and medical ethics, medical legal issues and risk management, teaching and development. In general, most physicians have little formal training relating to complex hospital systems or human error. These sections provide a background for improving the hospital setting for patients through system redesign, training, and teamwork.

The second major part of this book, Medical Consultation and Co-Management, reviews core tenets of medical consultation, pre-operative assessment, and management of post-operative medical problems. Although hospitalists have already changed the health care system by their presence and up to 85% of hospitalists report that they co-manage surgical patients, most do not have a surgical background. Surgeons present key concepts relating to General Surgery, Neurosurgery, and Orthopedic and Bariatric surgery, and anesthesiologists cover key concepts of Anesthesia. Experts in anticoagulation from McMaster University, Canada, review perioperative anti-thrombotic management and prevention. These sections present a framework for improving the co-management of surgical patients with significant medical illnesses that make them vulnerable to post-operative complications.

The third major part, Clinical Problem-Solving in Hospital Medicine, introduces principles of evidence-based medicine, quality of evidence, interpretation of diagnostic tests, systemic reviews and meta-analysis, and knowledge translations to clinical practice. Each field of medicine challenges clinicians to recommend a course of action for a specific patient at a particular time. To efficiently and safely obtain the right information through examination and testing, physicians need to ask the right questions. Increasingly, physicians must process an enormous amount of data in the care of a single patient and do not have time to critically review the medical literature at each encounter. The purpose of these chapters is to provide a context for evidence-based medicine so that clinicians optimize how they access information tools that facilitate clinical decision-making at the point of care.

The fourth major part, Approach to the Patient at the Bedside, covers the diagnosis, testing, and initial management of common complaints that may either precipitate admission or arise during hospitalization. Hospitalized patients differ from their outpatient counterparts in many respects, including severity of primary systemic illness precipitating admission, multiple co-morbidities that do not fit into one subspecialty, the number and route of administration of prescription drugs, and vulnerability to hospital-acquired complications. Condensed accounts of patient cases presented in these chapters and throughout the book provide examples of asking questions, thinking critically, and diagnosing and assessing problems so that the reader may apply key concepts directly to patient care. As much as possible this approach offers evidence-based strategies that can be employed when clinicians encounter an unfamiliar patient who has developed a new problem that requires urgent evaluation.

The fifth major part, Hospitalist Skills, covers the interpretation of common "low tech" tests that are routinely accessible on admission, how to optimize the use of radiology services, and the standardization of the execution of procedures routinely performed by some hospitalists. Diagnostic testing is rarely without risk or financial cost and almost never completely accurate. The pursuit of diagnostic tests may also delay much needed treatment; thus, physicians cannot pursue every diagnostic avenue, even if patients want all the information. These sections review the process of how to incorporate simple test results into clinical decision-making, how to select imaging tests, and how to safely perform procedures.

The sixth major part, Clinical Conditions, reflects the expanding scope of Hospital Medicine by including sections of Emergency Medicine, Critical Care, Geriatrics, Neurology, Palliative Care, Pregnancy, Psychiatry and Addiction, and Wartime Medicine. Although there have been tremendous strides in the technology relating to the management of many diseases and in proven therapies, performance gaps still remain. The objective of this part of the book is to present current best practices and highlight opportunities for improvement.

The overarching goal of this first edition is to make available a comprehensive resource for trainees, junior and senior clinicians, and other professionals so that they can effectively work together to create opportunities to ensure the delivery of high-quality health care and value.

Sylvia C. McKean, MD, SFHM, FACP

ACKNOWLEDGMENTS

The editors of *The Principles and Practice of Hospital Medicine* would like to acknowledge and thank our publisher McGraw-Hill, specifically, James Shanahan, Editor-in-Chief and Associate Publisher; Cindy Yoo, Project Development Editor; Laura Libretti, Administrative Assistant; and the numerous people assisting them to complete this effort. We also express our gratitude to the many contributors who worked diligently to create a comprehensive resource for our readers and all the people who supported us, including family and friends. Finally, we wish to recognize physicians who took the time out of their busy schedules to review chapters and/or sections of the book that clearly benefited from their valuable expertise.

Sylvia C. McKean, MD, SFHM, FACP

John J. Ross, MD, CM, FIDSA

Daniel D. Dressler, MD, MSc, SFHM

Daniel J. Brotman, MD, FHM, FACP

Jeffrey S. Ginsberg, MD, FRCP(C)

PART I

The Specialty of Hospital Medicine and Systems of Care

SECTION 1 Key Issues in Hospital Medicine

SECTION 2 Patient Safety

SECTION 3 Quality Improvement

SECTION 4 Leadership and Practice Management Skills

SECTION 5 Professionalism and Medical Ethics

SECTION 6 Medical Legal Issues and Risk Management

SECTION 7 Teaching and Development

SECTION 1

Key Issues in Hospital Medicine

CHAPTER 1

The Face of Health Care Emerging Issues for Hospitalists

Ian Morrison, PhD

INTRODUCTION

No medical specialty has come so far so fast as hospital-based medicine. In little more than a decade the number of general internists specializing in hospital-based medicine (ie, hospitalists) has grown to include more than 30,000. Hospitalists find themselves at the center of change in health care delivery and are key architects of the redesign of acute care to improve quality, safety, and cost-effectiveness. How will the environment of health care evolve over the next 10 years, and what will this mean for hospitalists and the patients and institutions they serve?

THINKING ABOUT THE FUTURE

Although one cannot predict the future, one can think systematically about it. Futurists try to combine analysis and imagination to think through how the future may unfold. A critical tool is to identify the key forces that are, singly and in combination, creating change and shaping the future environment. They are the major trends or directions that can be seen emerging, and their forward progress or lack of it can be analyzed. At the same time, the future can be shifted radically by particular events; for example, 9/11, the economic meltdown of late 2008, the passage of health reform legislation are all events that radically shifted the direction of history. Such event-driven discontinuities are notoriously difficult to predict and are often difficult even to speculate about. Futurists use scenario approaches to describe the range of uncertainty and create plausible stories of how the future unfolds. This chapter describes a series of driving forces that will have direct and indirect effects on the hospitalist field: the quest for value in health care, the economic dislocation of the recession, and broader health reform.

KEY DRIVING FORCES

There are several key driving forces that will shape the future of health care no matter what. Each of these driving forces create strategic issues for hospitalists and the organizations and patients they serve.

THE QUEST FOR VALUE

Health systems around the world are struggling with the same issues. Aging populations, savvy patients demanding cutting-edge technology, and the need for timely and easy access to services, all of this against a backdrop of payers (whether government, employers, or individual patients) struggling to afford ever rising costs. While cost containment is the permanent ongoing work of many health systems around the world, the focus is increasingly on creating value, not just reducing costs. Health systems around the world, each in their own way, are trying to create as much value as possible. It is a simple equation to write, but it is difficult to optimize:

$$\text{Value} = \frac{(\text{Access} + \text{Quality} + \text{Security of benefits})}{\text{Costs}}$$

Where

Access = access to services enabled through insurance coverage, as well as timely and geographically proximate availability of health care services.

Quality = superior health outcomes enabled by cutting-edge technology, evidence-based care, and responsive customer service.

Security of benefits = assurance that health insurance benefits (and thus health care services) will be available when needed and that benefits cannot be taken away or lost because of change in job status, change in health status, or age.

Every health system around the world is an ugly compromise around this equation. Some systems, like that of the United Kingdom, curtail access to cutting edge technology by slowing the adoption of expensive and marginally effective medical technologies, placing greater emphasis on universal access and encouraging active utilization of primary care and preventive services. The United States, in contrast, has placed much higher emphasis on quality of inputs: high technology, well-trained professionals, modern facilities, and entrepreneurial institutions competing on innovative interventionalist approaches to disease care, rather than emphasizing care coordination, universal access, or primary care approaches.

There is no perfect system. But it is becoming increasingly clear that the United States has struck a very expensive bargain; it has been well documented in a series of studies that the United States spends more than all other health systems, and by many measures gets less health status improvement, than many other systems. This is not the venue in which to explore the reasons for wide differences in comparative performance between countries or within countries; suffice it to say that all health systems will be under increasing pressure to deliver higher performance per dollar, euro, pound, or yen. This places an enormous responsibility on those who design care processes to make the care of patients as efficient, effective, and appropriate as possible.

PRACTICE POINT

- Hospitalists are key architects of the redesign of acute care to improve quality, safety, and cost-effective performance. While cost containment is the permanent ongoing work of many health systems around the world, the focus is increasingly on creating value, not just reducing costs alone.

ECONOMIC DISLOCATION AND THE IMPACT ON HOSPITALS

Recent economic dislocation has changed the economics of health care and dramatically affected the financial challenges facing American hospitals. Many believed that health care would be immune to the effects of a worldwide economic storm, but there have been major impacts, and they will continue to affect the landscape of hospitals for some time to come. There are a number of key impacts from the recent economic downturn of 2008–09:

- *Reduces the ability to pay by all actors.* Health care is paid for by contributions from business, government, and individual households. In the final analysis, it all comes from households either in the form of forgone wage income (which goes to health benefits instead), as taxes, or as direct premium contributions or out-of-pocket costs paid by patients and their families. We talk about health insurance as if it were some magic pot of money that comes from somewhere else, but it is simply the collective contributions that families make directly or through taxes or forgone wages. In a recession, all actors have a reduced ability to pay: household incomes are down, business profits are constrained, and government revenues fall dramatically as a result.
- *Increases health care as a share of all spending by business, government, and households.* When household income drops as it has in both 2008 and 2009, this raises the relative burden of health care costs on individuals, business, and government alike. Health care has become an even more salient cost for all actors, particularly federal and state governments. This is partly because of the sharp reduction in tax revenues, but also because of the increasing demand for public programs such as Medicaid. For example in the state of Michigan, where unemployment reached 15% in late 2009, the Medicaid rolls doubled as more people lost health insurance and descended into poverty.
- *Pits health care deductibles and co-pays against other budget items.* At the consumer level, real trade-offs are being made where consumers are asking for generic drugs; cutting their pills in half, and forgoing doctor visits, tests, and elective procedures because of the cost sharing involved. This helps explain the observation that elective surgery volume is down in many parts of the country. (Although perverse as it may seem, the threat of major health insurance reform has brought about a counter-trend of "use it or lose it" among those with good coverage. "I'll have the elective surgery now, because my insurance might not be so generous in the future.") As the economy recovers, the consumer is unlikely to return to the same level of confidence as in the early 2000s, when buoyant housing markets fueled a credit card and home-equity-led consumption boom. While the American consumer has a short memory, this recession has been so severe that attitudes may be permanently altered, and consumers may be at a new norm of saving more and being more parsimonious in their discretionary expenditures, including elective health care.
- *Raises costs of capital for provider investment in information technology (IT) and clinical capital.* Capital markets were decimated by the economic meltdown, creating tremendous tightness and expense of the credit facilities available to many hospitals. Many American hospitals have been forced to postpone major capital projects, whether it be new construction, big-ticket clinical capital expenditures such as advanced imaging, or even IT investment (although the latter would seem like a short-sighted saving given the future incentives embedded in the stimulus bill to deploy electronic health records).
- *Impacts the NASDAQ dependent and Kaiser too.* Many hospitals (a third is a crude estimate) are in the category of being the NASDAQ dependent; namely, they lose money on their clinical care operations but make up the difference and maintain a financial surplus on the basis of their investment income. Even integrated care behemoths such as Kaiser have felt the sting of the stock market on their investment portfolio and the resultant impact on operating finances.
- *Brings Medicare trust insolvency date in closer.* Medicare actuaries are constantly adjusting their estimate of when the hospital trust fund reaches insolvency (currently in 2017), based on the challenging economic outlook. In the long run, this means that pressure on Medicare reimbursement rates will be incredibly intense, particularly as the first true baby boomers (those born in 1947) reach Medicare eligibility in 2012.
- *Increases unfunded liability of Medicare, Governmental Accounting Standards Board, and other retiree health benefits.* There is somewhere between $1 and $2 trillion of unfunded retiree health benefit obligations that have been promised to public employees. Similarly, private employers with such retiree health benefits have experienced a need to increase funding for such schemes because of the drop in values in the investment accounts supporting these obligations to future retirees. Again the likelihood is that benefits will have to be scaled back in their generosity, cost-sharing will have to be increased, state and local taxes will have to be raised significantly, or promises will have to be broken. All of these alternatives are ugly and may result in pressure to reduce reimbursement levels to providers associated with these benefits.

- *Constrains federal and state budgets.* Tax revenues down, demand for government services up, is a recipe for deficits. The depth of the state budget crisis is being reached in late 2009. Some large states like California have astronomical budget deficits to close (in California's case, a $60 billion dollar deficit) with a combination of furloughs, service cuts, program reductions, eligibility reductions, and elaborate fiscal shell games. At the federal level the deficit is climbing toward $2 trillion. These are exceptionally challenging times, but the federal deficits and the long-term legacy of the economic crisis on the states' finances will inevitably constrain the ability to pay for health care in the future and cause greater pressure for innovation to make health care cheaper. If hospitals can't break even on Medicare payment rates today, good luck in 2020.
- *Sucks oxygen from big health care reform?* Against this dismal economic background, one might argue that health care reform and expansion of coverage could not be enacted, yet health reform has made its way through the legislative process and has become the law of the land. There are four key reasons why health reform has focused on coverage expansion. First, without reform the number of uninsured and underinsured will skyrocket as temporary stimulus measures expire (such as one-time Medicaid grants and COBRA extensions) and as employment and incomes recover slowly. Second, the base of the Democratic Party had very high expectations of President Obama and the Democratic Congress to deliver on health reform. While the fights were bitter and partisan, in the final stages, the president appealed to the core values of the Democratic Party that brought sufficient support to pass historic reform legislation. Third, stakeholders such as insurers, pharmaceutical companies, physicians, and others feared that by not supporting reform today they would face a much more Draconian and punitive reform in the future. And, fourth, absent some meaningful start on bending the cost curve of health care the challenge to pay for health care for all the country's citizens (never mind all its residents) may be insurmountable in the decade ahead. And so to health reform and its aftermath.

PRACTICE POINT

- Hospitalists will need to design care processes to make the care of patients as efficient, effective, and as appropriate as possible. Hospitalists will play a key leadership role in incorporating them in daily clinical practice across the continuum of care with particular attention being paid to best practices in handoffs to other care settings, integration with emerging medical home models, and in post-discharge care to prevent avoidable errors and readmissions. Hospitalists can and should be at the center of this all-important work of reengineering health care delivery for higher performance.

HEALTH REFORM

Major health reform has passed. On March 2010 President Obama signed the following into law:

- The Health care and Education Reconciliation Act
- The Patient Protection and Affordable Care Act

Although the effect that the legislation will have on the practice of Hospital Medicine is still unknown, payment incentives will attempt to reward quality of care to promote enhanced value for patients while reducing unnecessary costs. The laws extend health insurance coverage to 32 million people, an estimated 95% of legal U.S. residents by the end of the decade. Expansion of Medicaid, subsidized by the federal government, will cover half of this expansion, and private health insurance purchased through new insurance exchanges will cover the rest. U.S. citizens will be required to have health insurance or pay a penalty, and insurers cannot deny coverage in most instances. The laws also close a gap in prescription-drug coverage for seniors. The cost savings will depend on how the laws are implemented. Reducing readmission rates through improvement in the discharge process is one example of how hospitalists may play a pivotal role in reforming health care systems.

The new health reform will not be fully implemented until 2014, and it will face innumerable legal, political, and implementation challenges in the months and years ahead, but the passage of comprehensive health reform is a significant turning point for the American health care system. The final legislation is a form of what I have labeled the New American Compromise. (The Old American Compromise was managed competition, the elegant conception of Alain Enthoven of Stanford University that was the intellectual foundation of much of the health reform initiatives of the late 1980s and 1990s). Key elements of the New American Compromise are as follows:

- *Shared sacrifice.* Health care is both a right and an obligation: you have the right to expect access to health insurance but you have the obligation to participate in paying for it. A good example of this principle was embodied in the American Hospital Association's health policy platform, which used the tagline: "Health care for All, Paid by All." Shared sacrifice was also the rhetoric behind both the successful Massachusetts health reform efforts and the failed bid by California to adopt similar sweeping state legislation.
- *Strategic incrementalism.* Incrementalism is going from one bad idea to another bad idea, and this has been the hallmark of American health policy. But strategic incrementalism steps toward a broader vision, in this case universal coverage (or near universal coverage), by building on existing programs. The health care law involves both expansion of private insurance coverage as well as expansions of Medicaid and the State Child Health Insurance Program (SCHIP).
- *Compel participation.* There is no such thing as voluntary universal coverage, anywhere in the world. For universal coverage to be achieved individuals and employers need to be compelled to participate. (And even then we should expect a significant number of people to cheat. The Dutch do not cheat, they are a pretty civic-minded bunch, but we Americans would cheat. Even Liberals cheat: We all listen to National Public Radio (NPR) and nobody pledges.) The legislation provides tax credits and incentives for employers of a certain size to offer insurance. Most importantly, however, the legislation mandates that individuals have to be enrolled in health insurance (with some exemptions). A combination of penalties, fees, and reporting of coverage on tax returns is designed to enforce the mandate. The legislation includes tax credits and subsidies for lower-income households to purchase, and smaller employers to provide, health insurance benefits. And the legislation includes unique fees, taxes, and stakeholder concessions to raise revenues to cover the subsidies.
- *Restructure/regulate insurance market.* The legislation includes the creation of a health insurance exchange that will create new insurance marketplaces at the state level for the individual and small group insurance market. In addition, the legislation includes tough new regulations guaranteeing issuance and terms of offer of health insurance.
- *Public plan.* The most contentious aspect of reform has been the possible creation of a public plan to compete with private insurers. The public option proved politically unpalatable to the U.S. Senate and was dropped to gain final passage in the Congress.

- *Major seeds of change in reimbursement reform.* The legislation also contains some major seeds of change in reimbursement reform. Whether it be pilots and incentives to encourage the formation of accountable care organizations; or pay for performance schemes to discourage so-called never events or avoidable errors or hospital readmissions; or bundled payment pilots, these seeds of change could radically alter the incentives facing hospitals and, in turn, perhaps broaden and transform the role of hospitalists. In particular, hospitalists will be centrally involved in implementing the coordination of care required under these new incentives and may likely become designers of the clinical processes and protocols necessary for hospitals to flourish in the new reimbursement environment.

The bottom line of health reform may well be for hospitals and hospitalists to expect more patients at lower per unit levels of reimbursement, and with different incentives. All this underscores the need for innovation in practice to achieve higher-value care.

OTHER KEY ISSUES

While the quest for value, economic dislocation, and health reform are the three major driving forces for the future, it is important to introduce a few other forces that will have considerable effects on the future of hospitals and hospitalists:

- *Increased transparency.* More measurement and reporting of cost and quality information on providers will challenge all of health care to improve performance. It is likely in the future that quality and cost measurement and reporting will become more widespread, more comprehensive, and more focused on outcomes rather than just process measures, and they will incorporate measures across the continuum of care. Hospitalists will be at the center of designing and implementing such measures and will play a key leadership role in incorporating them in daily clinical practice.
- *Increased consumer expectations.* Patients and families continue to expect higher levels of quality, engagement, and responsiveness from health care institutions. Responsiveness to patients and families and engagement of patients and families in the management of chronic conditions will be increasingly important.
- *Coordination across the continuum of care.* Just as hospitalists have made great strides in the coordination of care within an institution on behalf of patients and families, they will be asked to play a greater role in coordinating care across the continuum of care, with particular attention being paid to best practices in handoffs to other care settings, integration with emerging medical home models, and postdischarge care to prevent avoidable errors and readmissions.
- *Growing physician stress.* Physicians are under pressure on their time because of reimbursement, regulation, and malpractice pressures, as well as overload of measurement and performance review. All of this leads to growing alienation and stress. As other physicians opt out of their nonclinical duties in the hospital due to increased stress and alienation, hospitalists will be asked to play ever greater roles in hospital staff leadership. A key challenge will lie in establishing appropriate compensation arrangements with hospital administration for these increased duties.
- *New emerging clinical technology.* Emerging clinical technology continues to offer new opportunities and challenges in the location and nature of care. As less invasive tools are developed and new technology allows more care to be moved to the ambulatory setting the role of hospitalists and intensivists will need to morph with the changing technological landscape.
- *New information technology.* Greater emphasis on the use of IT across the continuum of care has been turbocharged by the interest in health information technology (HIT) in the United States and elsewhere. The global deployment of HIT will present new opportunities for hospitalists to manage their patients, coordinate with other caregivers and monitor, evaluate, and continuously improve performance.
- *Evidence-based medicine and evidence-based policy.* More emphasis is being placed on the evaluative sciences, including issues such as comparative effectiveness research. Hospitalists may be asked to increasingly play the role of arbiter of comparative effectiveness information for the institutions they serve.
- *Care reengineering as the central work.* All of these forces mean that reengineering of clinical care processes to deliver high-quality, cost-effective care becomes central work in health care. Hospitalists have and will develop the combination of skills and training to be the leaders in redesign of acute care for the future. Hospitalists can and should be at the center of this all-important work of reengineering health care delivery for higher performance. We the patients wish you well.

SUGGESTED READING

Davis K, Schoen C, Schoenbaum SC, Doty MM, et al. Mirror, Mirror on the Wall: An International Update on the Comparative Performance of American Health care. New York, *The Commonwealth Fund*, May 2007.

CHAPTER 2

Global Health and Hospital Medicine

Joseph Rhatigan, MD
David A. Walton, MD, MPH

INTRODUCTION

> Disparities of outcome in and between countries are now the major challenges in medicine... What branch of medicine is not forced to confront the growing outcome gap that promises to shield the privileged while the world's bottom billion continue to die from readily preventable and treatable diseases?
>
> *Paul Farmer*

For many years, the global public health community viewed hospital-level health care delivery to be an inefficient drain on the health systems of low-income countries. The Primary Health Care Movement of the late 1970s sought to bolster community-level primary preventive health care services in low-income countries, oftentimes at the expense of hospital-level services. At that time, urban referral hospitals in many low and middle-income countries consumed large portions of national health budgets (often in the range of 40–60%) while providing little of the overall health care service delivery (often less than 5%). Furthermore these hospitals were not accessible to the large rural populations of these countries and were seen as preferentially benefiting the wealthier members of these societies.

In the mid-1990s, many global health leaders began to reexamine this view and to recognize that hospitals, especially district or primary-level hospitals that provide more accessible services at lower costs than referral hospitals, could be important drivers of improved health care delivery at all levels of the health system. Shortly after this, in the early 2000s, the creation of the Bill & Melinda Gates Foundation, the Global Fund to Fight AIDS, Tuberculosis and Malaria (GFATM) and the U.S. President's Emergency Plan for AIDS Relief (PEPFAR) led to massive increases in health sector funding in many low-income countries and a concomitant expansion of health care service delivery. As the global health community struggles to use this money effectively and equitably to improve the health of the poorest and sickest populations, the role of hospital-level services in global public health strategy is being closely examined.

This chapter provides an overview of the role of hospital-level health services in global public health programs and explores the link between Hospital Medicine and global health. It briefly describes global health and the global burden of disease, discusses the global disparities in health and in access to health care services, examines the role of district and referral hospitals in the health systems of low-income countries, describes how these hospitals function in the strategies to combat the leading public health problems facing these countries, and discusses the human resource crisis facing many countries. The chapter provides an example of how global public health programs can strengthen access to hospital-level services by examining a program in Haiti that one of the authors (DW) helps to lead. The conclusion reflects on common themes in global health and Hospital Medicine and how U.S.-based hospitalists can become involved in global health efforts.

GLOBAL HEALTH AND THE GLOBAL BURDEN OF DISEASE

The term *global health* refers to the study and practice that is concerned with improving health and achieving health equity for all people worldwide, with an emphasis on addressing those problems that are transnational. As the World Health Organization defines it, health is a state of complete physical, mental, and social well-being

TABLE 2-1 Leading Causes of Death by Income Group, 2004

	Disease or Injury	Deaths (Millions)	Percent of Total Deaths		Disease or Injury	Deaths (Millions)	Percent of Total Deaths
	World				*Low-income countries**		
1	Ischemic heart disease	7.2	12.2	1	Lower respiratory infections	2.9	11.2
2	Cerebrovascular disease	5.7	9.7	2	Ischemic heart diseases	2.5	9.4
3	Lower respiratory infections	4.2	7.1	3	Diarrheal diseases	1.8	6.9
4	COPD	3.0	5.1	4	HIV/AIDS	1.5	5.7
5	Diarrheal diseases	2.2	3.7	5	Cerebrovascular disease	1.5	5.6
6	HIV/AIDS	2.0	3.5	6	COPD	0.9	3.6
7	Tuberculosis	1.5	2.5	7	Tuberculosis	0.9	3.5
8	Trachea, bronchus, lung cancers	1.3	2.3	8	Neonatal infections†	0.9	3.4
9	Road traffic accidents	1.3	2.2	9	Malaria	0.9	3.3
10	Prematurity and low birth weight	1.2	2.0	10	Prematurity and low birth weight	0.8	3.2
	Middle-income countries				*High-income countries*		
1	Cerebrovascular disease	3.5	14.2	1	Ischemic heart disease	1.3	16.3
2	Ischemic heart diseases	3.4	13.9	2	Cerebrovascular disease	0.8	9.3
3	COPD	1.8	7.4	3	Trachea, bronchus, lung cancers	0.5	5.9
4	Lower respiratory infections	0.9	3.8	4	Lower respiratory infections	0.3	3.8
5	Trachea, bronchus, lung cancers	0.7	2.9	5	COPD	0.3	3.5
6	Road traffic accidents	0.7	2.8	6	Alzheimer and other dementias	0.3	3.4
7	Hypertensive heart disease	0.6	2.5	7	Colon and rectum cancer	0.3	3.3
8	Stomach cancer	0.5	2.2	8	Diabetes mellitus	0.2	2.8
9	Tuberculosis	0.5	2.2	9	Breast cancer	0.2	2.0
10	Diabetes mellitus	0.5	2.1	10	Stomach cancer	0.1	1.8

COPD, chronic obstructive pulmonary disease.
*Countries grouped by gross national income per capita - low-income ($825 or less), high income ($10 066 or more).
†This category also includes other non-infectious causes arising in the perinatal period, which are responsible for about 20% of deaths shown in this category.
Reproduced, with permission, from World Health Organization, *The Global Burden of Disease: 2004 Update*, WHO press: Geneva, 2008, page 12.

and not merely the absence of disease or infirmity. This chapter focuses on the health of populations that have limited resources, since it is these populations whose well-being is the most at risk.

There are many ways one can try to measure the health of a population. Some indicators attempt to assess the well-being of populations, whereas others assess impediments to health, such as the burden of disease. Because the vast majority of hospitals focus on providing health services to those suffering from disease, we will briefly review how disease burden is measured. (The World Health Organization regularly publishes reports on the global burden of disease. The following information comes from *The Global Burden of Disease: 2004 Update*, WHO, Geneva, 2008.)

Mortality is one method of assessing the burden of disease (see **Table 2-1** for a list of leading causes of death worldwide). Using this measure a few facts are worth highlighting:

- Of every 10 deaths, 6 are due to noncommunicable conditions; 3 to communicable, reproductive, or nutritional conditions; and 1 to injuries.
- Cardiovascular disease are the leading cause of death worldwide, accounting for 32% of all deaths in women and 27% of all deaths in men.
- 9.5 million children under the age of five die each year; 99% of these children die in low and middle-income countries. The vast majority of these are preventable deaths. Undernutrition is an underlying cause of about a third of these deaths.
- Almost one in five deaths worldwide are of children under 5 years of age.
- 500,000 women die of pregnancy-related complications each year, accounting for 15% of deaths of women of child-bearing age worldwide.
- There are great differences in life expectancy and cause of death between high and low-income countries. In high income countries more than two-thirds of all people live beyond the age of 70 and predominantly die of chronic diseases. In low-income countries less than a quarter of all people reach the age of 70, and people predominantly die of infectious diseases. Over a third of all deaths are among children.

PRACTICE POINT

- In high-income countries, more than two-thirds of all people live beyond the age of 70 and predominantly die of chronic diseases. In low-income countries, less than a quarter of all people reach the age of 70 and people predominantly die of infectious diseases. More than a third of all deaths are children.

By only accounting for death and not years of life lost, mortality data alone do not give a full picture of the global burden

TABLE 2-2 Leading Causes of Burden of Disease by Disability Adjusted Life-Year (DALYs), Countries Grouped by Income, 2004

	Disease or Injury	DALYs (Millions)	Percent of Total DALYs		Disease or Injury	DALYs (Millions)	Percent of Total DALYs
	World				*Low-income countries**		
1	Lower respiratory infections	94.5	6.2	1	Lower respiratory infections	76.9	9.3
2	Diarrheal diseases	72.8	4.8	2	Diarrheal diseases	59.2	7.2
3	Unipolar depressive disorders	65.5	4.3	3	HIV/AIDS	42.9	5.2
4	Ischemic heart disease	62.6	4.1	4	Malaria	32.8	4.0
5	HIV/AIDS	58.5	3.8	5	Prematurity and low birth weight	32.1	3.9
6	Cerebrovascular disease	46.6	3.1	6	Neonatal infections and other†	31.4	3.8
7	Prematurity and low birth weight	44.3	2.9	7	Birth asphyxia and birth trauma	29.8	3.6
8	Birth asphyxia and birth trauma	41.7	2.7	8	Unipolar depressive disorders	26.5	3.2
9	Road traffic accidents	41.2	2.7	9	Ischemic heart disease	26.0	3.1
10	Neonatal infections and other†	40.4	2.7	10	Tuberculosis	22.4	2.7
	Middle-income countries				*High-income countries*		
1	Unipolar depressive disorders	29.0	5.1	1	Unipolar depressive disorders	10.0	8.2
2	Ischemic heart disease	28.9	5.0	2	Ischemic heart disease	7.7	6.3
3	Cerebrovascular disease	27.5	4.8	3	Cerebrovascular disease	4.8	3.9
4	Road traffic accidents	21.4	3.7	4	Alzheimer and other dementias	4.4	3.6
5	Lower respiratory infections	16.3	2.8	5	Alcohol use disorders	4.2	3.4
6	COPD	16.1	2.8	6	Hearing loss, adult onset	4.2	3.4
7	HIV/AIDS	15.0	2.6	7	COPD	3.7	3.0
8	Alcohol use disorders	14.9	2.6	8	Diabetes mellitus	3.6	3.0
9	Refractive errors	13.7	2.4	9	Trachea, bronchus, lung cancers	3.6	3.0
10	Diarrheal diseases	13.1	2.3	10	Road traffic accidents	3.1	2.6

COPD, chronic obstructive pulmonary disease.

*Countries grouped by gross national income per capita.

†This category also includes other non-infectious causes arising in the perinatal period apart from prematurity, low birth weight, birth trauma and asphyxia. These non-infectious causes are responsible for about 20% of DALYs shown in this category.

Reproduced, with permission, from World Health Organization, *The Global Burden of Disease: 2004 Update*, WHO press: Geneva, 2008, page 44.

of disease. Over the past decade, the concept of the disability-adjusted life-year (DALY) has become the widely accepted measure of the global burden of disease. The DALY is based on years of life lost from premature death and years of life lived in less than full health. By accounting for years of healthy life lost to illness, it has replaced cruder estimates of disease burden such as total mortality and disease incidence and prevalence. DALYs for a disease or injury are calculated as the sum of the years of life lost due to premature mortality in the population and the years lost due to disability for incident cases of the disease or injury. Years of life lost are calculated from the number of deaths at each age multiplied by a global standard life expectancy for each age. (See **Table 2-2** for a ranking of global disease burden by DALY). Following are some important points to consider:

- In low and middle income countries infectious diseases account for over half of the burden of disease.
- DALYs are at least two times higher in Africa than in any other region and are mostly due to premature deaths.
- Children bear more than half the disease burden in low-income countries.
- Income levels are associated with major differences in the burden of disease, with poor populations suffering significantly higher DALYs than wealthier populations.
- Considerable variation exists between regions in the burden of disease.

GLOBAL DISPARITIES IN HEALTH AND ACCESS TO HEALTH SERVICES

Poverty remains one of the most important root causes of poor health worldwide, and the global burden of poverty continues to be high. Of the 6.8 billion people alive today, 43%, or about 2.7 billion, live on less than U.S. $2 a day, and 17%, or about 1.1 billion, live on less than U.S. $1 a day. Comparing national health indicators to gross domestic product (GDP) per capita among nations shows a clear relationship between higher GDP and better health, with only a few outliers. Numerous studies have also demonstrated the link between poverty and health within countries.

One such health indicator, the maternal mortality ratio (MMR), measures how many women die in childbirth for every live birth. The MMR varies widely worldwide and is often very high in low-income countries. Leading causes of maternal mortality are obstructed labor, hypertensive conditions, hemorrhage, and peripartum infections. All these conditions are treatable with access to hospital-level services such as operating rooms and blood banks. The maternal mortality rate therefore is a rough measure of how much access a population has to these hospital-level services. In high income countries the rate is often 5–10 maternal deaths for every 100,000 live births. Worldwide it averages 401 maternal deaths for every 100,000 live births, and throughout sub-Saharan Africa it averages 1000 maternal deaths per 100,000 live births.

HOSPITAL-LEVEL HEALTH CARE DELIVERY IN LOW-INCOME COUNTRIES

In many low-income countries, governments provide a majority of the medical services through a network of health care delivery units organized in a hierarchical order following the administrative division of the country. The district is often the smallest unit of health care organization (similar to a county in the United States), comprising between 100,000 and a million people, and is often administered by a single-level governmental division. Within each district, first contact with the medical system usually occurs at either a health post in very rural areas or a health center. Health centers are typically staffed by either nurses only or nurses and clinical officers (a clinical officer is similar to a physician assistant in the United States and has 2–3 years of medical training). Health centers provide a package of curative and preventive services, including family planning, vaccinations, prenatal care, outpatient primary health care, attended simple deliveries, minor surgical procedures (but usually not cesarean sections), HIV testing, and tuberculosis (TB) testing. Health centers may have 5–10 beds available for women in labor and for patients requiring straightforward medical admissions, one example being intravenous fluid replacement to replete volume losses from severe diarrhea. Patients requiring more complicated services are usually referred to a district hospital (sometimes called a primary-level hospital). Most districts will have at least one district hospital that generally has between 70 and 200 beds and is staffed by generalist physicians, clinical officers, and nurses. A district hospital usually provides more surgical services (such as appendectomy and C-sections, uncomplicated orthopedic care, and expanded obstetrical services), basic radiographic imaging, pediatric services, inpatient medical services, and basic rehabilitative services.

Higher-level care is provided at referral hospitals. In some countries there are both secondary-level hospitals at the regional or provincial level and tertiary-level hospitals at the national level, whereas in others, all care beyond the district hospital is provided by national-level tertiary care hospitals. (See **Figure 2-1** for a diagram representing a common form of health care facility organization.)

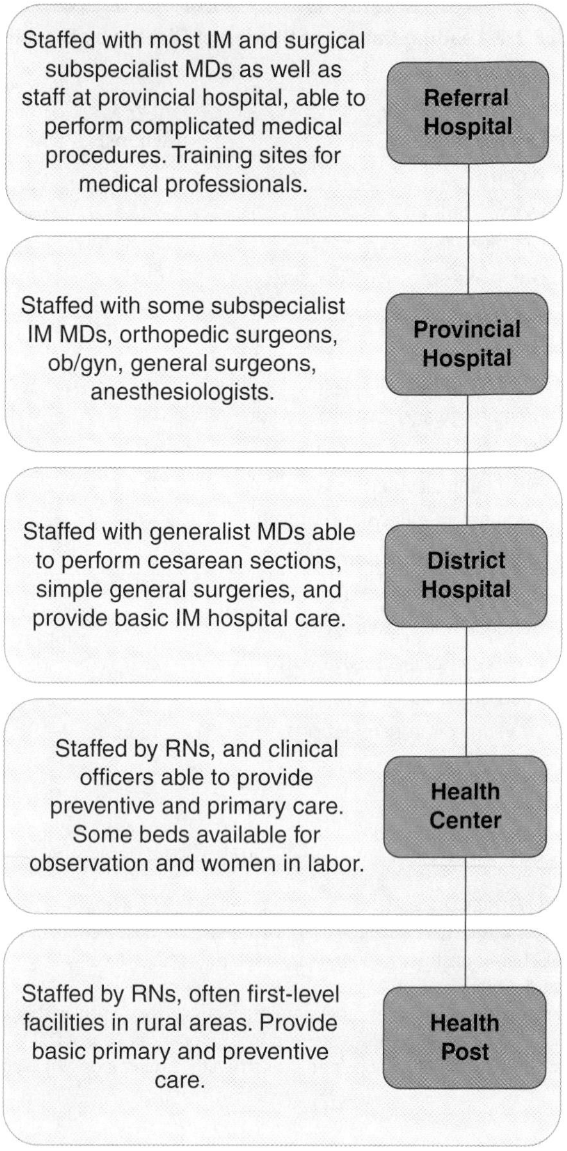

Figure 2-1 *A common form of health care facility organization.*

THE ROLE OF THE DISTRICT HOSPITAL IN HEALTH CARE DELIVERY

For much of the past 25 years, public health leaders have given a low priority to strengthening the provision of hospital-level services in low-income countries. The reasons for this are manifold, including a desire to use limited resources to improve primary health care and make it more accessible to large rural populations; the perceived overinvestment of limited public health budgets in hospitals that yielded little measurable benefits to the overall health of the populations; and the disparities in access to hospital-level care between wealthy and poor segments of the population. Detractors have been particularly critical of referral or tertiary-level hospitals as responsible for consuming a disproportionate share of national health budgets without contributing significantly to the health of large segments of the population. Other commentators have emphasized the critical role tertiary-level facilities play in professional education and provision of specialty care and have cited the inherent inefficiencies in providing care for complex, low-frequency medical conditions.

Over the past decade, the primary level or district hospital has increasingly been seen as a key component of the public health provision of basic health care. This has been especially true in the movement to improve maternal and child health. As discussed earlier, maternal and child deaths remain major public health problems in most low-income countries. Most public health efforts to lower maternal mortality advocate for skilled birth attendants to be present at the time of delivery. Skilled birth attendants are able to manage minor complications and identify more serious problems such as obstructed labor or peripartum sepsis. The treatment of these conditions and other leading causes of maternal mortality, such as peripartum hemorrhage and hypertensive disorders, requires hospital-level services such as access to operating rooms, blood banks, intravenous medications, and medical professionals skilled at performing cesarean sections and managing these obstetrical complications. Therefore, the district hospital that can provide these services is a necessary and valuable part of this strategy.

The district hospital has similarly been an important part of the strategy to lower child mortality. To accomplish this, the World Health Organization has implemented a program called Integrated Management of Childhood Illness (IMCI) in over 75 countries. The program uses standardized guidelines for the evaluation and treatment of sick children presenting to a primary health clinic. The guidelines help practitioners discern which children can be safely treated in the clinic and outpatient setting and which need to be referred to a district hospital. The success of the IMCI approach has been seen as reinforcing the role of the district hospital as a key component of robust primary health care systems.

THE HUMAN RESOURCE CHALLENGE

An increasingly worrisome barrier to improving medical service delivery in resource-poor settings is the lack of trained medical personnel. Even in countries that produce enough doctors, nurses, and technicians to care for the population, lack of medical staff can cripple programs. In what has been termed the "brain drain," doctors, nurses, pharmacists, and other medical professionals leave their home countries to pursue opportunities abroad, leaving behind health systems that are understaffed and underresourced. The World Health Organization recommends at least 20 physicians and 100 nurses per 100,000 people, which is widely regarded as a conservative suggestion. Despite these recommendations, many poor countries, beset by poverty, political instability, and the legacy of colonialism, fall short of those goals. Haiti only has 24 physicians per 100,000 people; over half of the countries in sub-Saharan Africa have fewer than 10 per 100,000. By comparison, the United States has approximately 267 physicians per 100,000 people, and Cuba boasts 630 per 100,000, the highest in the hemisphere.

Despite the sobering nature of these figures, these national aggregates fail to capture the stark disparities in health care professionals that exist within countries. Rural communities often fare much worse than urban centers in both accessibility of care and availability of trained medical staff. For example, in Malawi, although 90% of the population is rural, over 95% of clinical officers are based in urban facilities. Similar disparities are found in the majority of sub-Saharan African nations. These rural–urban disparities translate to critical shortages of medical staff in areas that often have the greatest need.

Biosocial analyses of the brain drain have demonstrated that the flight of qualified health care workers is not simply due to opportunities for higher remuneration. An internal review of the staff at a program one of the authors (DW) works at in rural Haiti identified several key reasons why Haitian physicians and nurses have chosen to work there: the ability to evaluate patients with modest but effective diagnostic tools; infrastructure to hospitalize patients who are in need of acute care; and a robust formulary of essential medications. One of the other most oft-cited reasons was the ability to treat patients regardless of their ability to pay, which is in stark contrast to many other heath care facilities in the country. Similar findings have been demonstrated elsewhere. These findings all suggest that the "brain drain" of trained health professionals from the developing world is due in large part to the lack of systems and tools that allow them to do the meaningful work they were trained to do.

SYNERGIES BETWEEN COMMUNITY- AND FACILITY-BASED CARE

Lessons learned in the public health response to TB and HIV offer insights regarding the synergy between community-based and facility-based care. A great deal of evidence suggests that the most successful TB and HIV treatment outcomes are seen when community-based care is offered to patients. The benefits of this type of care delivery model extend well beyond HIV and TB. Complex and chronic diseases (eg, congestive heart failure, insulin-dependent diabetes, chronic infectious diseases) are better managed with well-trained, paid, and supported community health workers (CHWs), as evidenced by decreased hospitalization, closer follow-up, and decreased morbidity and mortality.

Community health workers provide an essential bridge between facility-based medical services and the population these services target. By integrating CHWs into disease prevention and treatment programs, they can become important providers of primary care to populations that have difficulty accessing medical facilities due to physical, social, and economic barriers. However, community health workers can only function as part of a robust health care delivery system that provides adequate supervision, supplies, information management, and higher-level medical care.

PRACTICE POINT

- Community health workers provide an essential bridge between facility-based medical services and the population these services target. In areas where there are too few hospital-level health services, community-based care can extend the reach of diagnostic and therapeutic interventions. The most successful tuberculosis and HIV treatment outcomes are seen when community-based care is offered to patients.

The role of the hospitals and health centers cannot be underestimated, especially in resource poor settings. Coordination of CHWs, evaluation and management of acute and chronic disease, and hospitalization must be accomplished at health centers and hospitals. However, in our experience, community-based care, in coordination with hospital-level health services, has a synergistic effect on health outcomes in such settings. The effectiveness of the physical health care infrastructure is enhanced by taking advantage of the oft-ignored human infrastructure in these communities. In areas in which there are too few hospital-level health services, community-based care can extend the reach of diagnostic and therapeutic interventions.

STRENGTHENING HOSPITAL-LEVEL AND PRIMARY CARE IN HAITI

To illustrate the role hospital-level health services play within global health programs, we will use the example of one such project in Haiti that one of us (DW) has been extensively involved in while practicing Hospital Medicine part time in the United States.

Haiti is Latin America's oldest independent nation, born of a slave revolt that began in 1791. Over 95% of its population is descended from African slaves, and Haiti's history has been characterized by ongoing political strife. Haiti is the most impoverished nation in the Western Hemisphere, with an estimated 80% of the population living on less than U.S. $2 per day. There are profound inadequacies in health care, education, and housing. Haiti has the highest infant, maternal, and child mortality in the Western Hemisphere, and life expectancy hovers at 52 years of age.

Partners In Health (PIH), a small nongovernmental organization (NGO) based in Boston, and its partner organization, Zanmi Lasante (ZL), based in Haiti, have been working in the Central Plateau of Haiti for over two decades. This region is home to 550,000 people, most of them living in villages and in small towns, with poor access to potable water, paved roads, electricity, and health care.

In 2002 GFATM awarded Haiti a multiyear grant to expand HIV and TB services. PIH, a recipient of a portion of the grant, was given a mandate by the Haitian Ministry of Health (MOH) to carry out the expansion in the Central Plateau. The first "expansion" site was the small town of Lascahobas, an agricultural market center without industry or tourism that is located 2 hours from the border of the Dominican Republic. At that time, the only existing health infrastructure for the catchment area of 60,000 was a small ambulatory clinic run by the MOH. The staff included one doctor, one nurse, and five nurse's aides. There was no capability for hospitalization, care was fee-for-service, there were few medications available, and electricity and running water were unreliable. The clinic saw 12–20 patients per day. The nearest district-level hospital was an 8-hour trip on the back of a donkey, the primary mode of transportation.

Rather than implement a "vertical" system, solely providing care for the targeted diseases of HIV and TB, PIH and ZL sought to strengthen primary health care and hospital-based care by integrating TB and HIV services within a "basic minimum package" of services, which included the following:

- Training and capacity building for community-based care of chronic disease (HIV, TB, heart failure, diabetes, etc.)
- Community-based care delivered by village health workers
- Construction of an inpatient facility for medicine and pediatrics
- Electricity and running water available at all times
- A formulary of essential medications for inpatients and outpatients
- A laboratory
- Plain film X-ray capacity
- MOH staff along with PIH-trained staff
- Program capacity for diagnosis and care of TB, HIV, and sexually transmitted infections
- Program capacity for prenatal care and women's health
- Twenty-four-hour care
- A maternity ward
- Emergency services

A rapid referral system was established for cases that could not be dealt with at the clinic (eg, surgical emergencies, complications of labor). The referral hospital (a district-level hospital) and the clinic were connected via satellite Internet connection (at the time, there was no cellular telephone access in the Central Plateau). Messages sent were received in real time by on-call surgical teams, and the clinic provided transportation of patients.

In addition to the "basic minimum package," large-scale efforts were undertaken to increase vaccination among children and infants, as well as creating access to potable water for villages in the catchment area. Mobile clinics were conducted for communities that were located at the periphery of the catchment area (and often on mountainous terrain).

The results were as dramatic as they were rapid. Patient visits went from 20 to 150 per day in less than 3 months and plateaued at 250–350 after approximately 12 months. Rates of vaccination, diagnoses of HIV and TB, and prenatal visits increased dramatically. The 15-bed inpatient facility was at 100% capacity daily. It soon became apparent that, despite the rehabilitated infrastructure, the amount of patients seen was too large for the space available. After several years, additional funding was procured for the construction of a new hospital that would be owned by the Haitian MOH. Careful attention was paid to organization of patient flow, infection control in the wards and large waiting areas, inpatient capacity, and expanded laboratory capacity during the design phase. Once all medical and pediatric services were moved to the new hospital, the old clinic was renovated to create a hospital dedicated solely to women's health (see **Figures 2-2** and **2-3**).

Today the acute care hospital has a staff of 12 physicians and residents who see approximately 400 patients daily. Inpatient capacity, which now exceeds 60 beds, has an average census of 100%. At the women's health hospital, the number of deliveries has tripled, prenatal visits have doubled, and average daily patient encounters exceed 160 per day. A small operating room for emergency cesarean sections was built and is fully supplied. Cellular phone service has been installed in the Central Plateau, which has facilitated an already rapid referral system to the nearest district-level hospital.

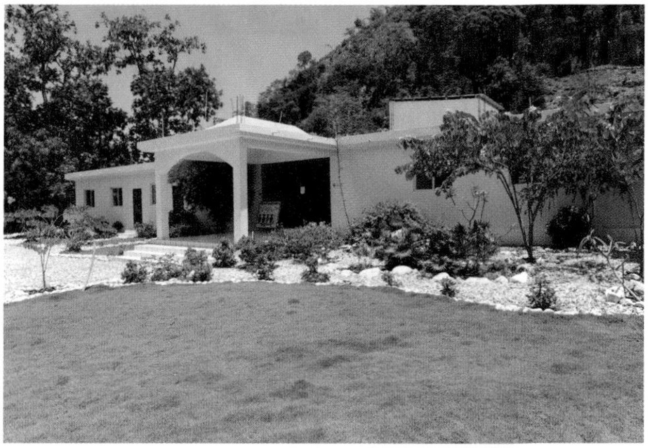

Figure 2-2 *The new hospital near Lascahobas (in Lacolline).*

PIH and ZL's experience in Haiti has demonstrated that "vertical" funding for HIV-related public health programs can strengthen primary health care and hospital-level services when used wisely. Although the primary funding for the clinic in Lascahobas was to expand AIDS care and prevention, by using this money strategically, PIH and ZL were able to strengthen the overall health system in Lascahobas, including primary health care and access to hospital-level care, in addition to delivering improved HIV care.

Such examples illustrate what we could achieve with many of the large investments being made today in global health. For instance, the reauthorization of the U.S. President's Emergency Plan for AIDS Relief (PEPFAR II) will invest U.S. $48 billion over the next 5 years to treat HIV/AIDS, TB, and malaria worldwide. This money will also be increasingly used to build sustainable, local capacity and, if used wisely, will improve overall health care service delivery in the nations in which PEPFAR operates.

CAREERS IN U.S. HOSPITAL MEDICINE AND GLOBAL HEALTH

We work in an academic hospitalist group with many colleagues who share a commitment to global health and Hospital Medicine and who have chosen careers that bridge these worlds. The practice of Hospital Medicine in the United States requires many of the same skills that are needed to deliver medical care in resource-limited settings. Both require expertise in team building and system thinking; comprehensive knowledge of general internal medicine and engagement with experts beyond one's area of practice; the facil-

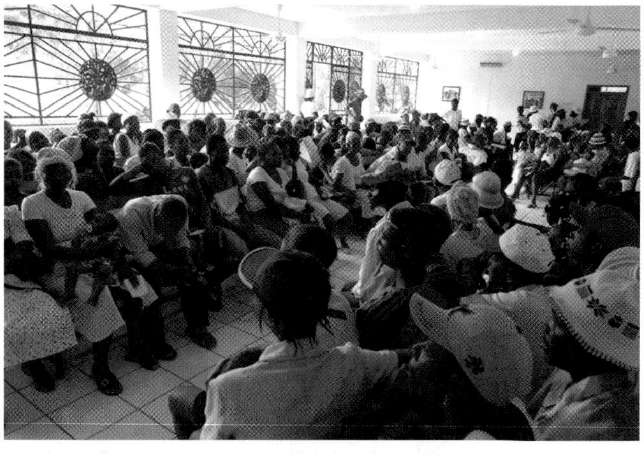

Figure 2-3 *The new hospital waiting room.*

ity to establish a therapeutic alliance rapidly with a diverse set of patients; and an understanding of the social, cultural, and economic factors that shape the prevention and treatment of disease in the patients we serve. In addition, because Hospital Medicine is usually practiced in blocks of time with no responsibility for patient care beyond the time one is "on-service," hospitalists can work overseas for extended periods of time between these blocks without compromising the care of their patients.

PRACTICE POINT

- The practice of Hospital Medicine in the United States requires many of the same skills that are needed to deliver medical care in resource-limited settings. Both require expertise in team building and system thinking; comprehensive knowledge of general internal medicine and engagement with experts beyond one's area of practice; the facility to rapidly establish a therapeutic alliance with a diverse set of patients; and an understanding of the social, cultural, and economic factors that shape the prevention and treatment of disease in the patients we serve.

For hospitalists wishing to explore opportunities in global health work, we suggest Edward O'Neil's book, *A Practical Guide to Global Health Service* (American Medical Association). We recognize that not all of our colleagues have the time or disposition to spend extended periods of time away from their home; however, we firmly believe that helping to address the issues discussed here and finding some solidarity with the populations most in need can be achieved in many ways: by studying and discussing these issues in the hospitals we work in, through financial support for organizations engaged in this work, by supporting advocacy efforts to advance the global health agenda, and through engagement in local projects that help the underserved living in nearby communities.

SUGGESTED READINGS

English M, Lanata CF, Ngugi I, Smith PC. The district hospital. In: Jamison DT, Breman JG Measham AR, et al, eds. *Disease Control Priorities in Developing Countries. 2nd ed.* New York: Oxford University Press; 2006:1211–1228.

Farmer P. *Pathologies of Power: Health, Human Rights and the New War on the Poor.* Berkeley: University of California Press; 2005.

Hensher M, Price M, Adomakoh S. Referral hospitals. In: Jamison DT, Breman JG Measham AR, et al, eds. *Disease Control Priorities in Developing Countries. 2nd ed.* New York: Oxford University Press; 2006:1229–1243.

O'Neil Jr E. *Awakening Hippocrates: A Primer on Health, Poverty and Global Service.* Chicago: American Medical Association; 2006.

O'Neil Jr E. *A Practical Guide to Global Health Service.* Chicago: American Medical Association; 2006

World Health Organization. *The Global Burden of Disease: 2004 Update.* Geneva: WHO Press; 2008.

CHAPTER 3

Racial/Ethnic Disparities in Hospital Care

Lenny Lopez, MD, MPH, MDiv
Cheryl R. Clark, MD, ScD
LeRoi S. Hicks, MD, MPH

INTRODUCTION

Racial and ethnic disparities in care have been consistently documented in the treatment and outcomes of many common clinical diseases. The 2003 Institute of Medicine (IOM) report, "Unequal Treatment: Confronting Racial and Ethnic Disparities in Health Care," defines disparities as differences in the treatment that are not directly attributable to access-related factors, clinical needs, patient preferences, or appropriateness of intervention (**Figure 3-1**). The elimination of health care disparities is a high priority for the federal government and several academic organizations.

Documented disparities of disease prevention and treatment include rates of vaccination, cancer screening, secondary prevention of myocardial infarction (MI), transplant surgery, curative surgery, and angioplasty. Disparities in health outcomes include cardiovascular disease, HIV/AIDS, diabetes, cancer, asthma, pregnancy outcomes, mental health, and hospitalization.

Specific examples include the following (**Table 3-1**):

- A higher risk of stroke, heart failure, and renal failure associated with hypertension (African Americans)
- A higher rate of complications from diabetes (African Americans and Native Americans)
- Later-stage colon, breast, and prostate cancer at presentation (African Americans)
- Less aggressive evaluation and treatment: curative lung cancer resection, cardiac catheterization, peripheral angioplasty, renal transplantation (African Americans)
- Diabetic more likely to receive amputations (African Americans)
- Higher death rates per 1000 hospital admissions in low mortality diagnosis related groups (African Americans, Hispanics, and the uninsured)

The observed racial/ethnic health care disparities have multifactorial etiologies. Patients face multiple barriers as they engage the health care system: (1) personal and family; (2) access to the health care system (structural, financial, types of services); and (3) the quality of the available providers (**Figure 3-2**). These barriers can occur individually or in combination to have an additive effect on health outcomes.

PRACTICE POINT

- Disparities in health outcomes include: cardiovascular disease, HIV/AIDS, diabetes, cancer, asthma, pregnancy outcomes, mental health, and hospitalization. Hospitalists can significantly influence the health status of African American and Latino patients if they comprehend their health care needs, communicate effectively, and advocate for additional local and institutional resources to ensure optimal discharge back to the community.

Historically, disparities in hospital care originated in the policy of hospital segregation during the first 66 years of the 20th century. Before the creation of Medicare, the Hospital Survey and Construction Act of 1946, commonly known as "Hill-Burton," was the largest federal grant program in health care. This law was intended to increase the number of hospital beds throughout the country. However, this was the only federal legislation in the 20th century that explicitly permitted use of federal funds to provide racially

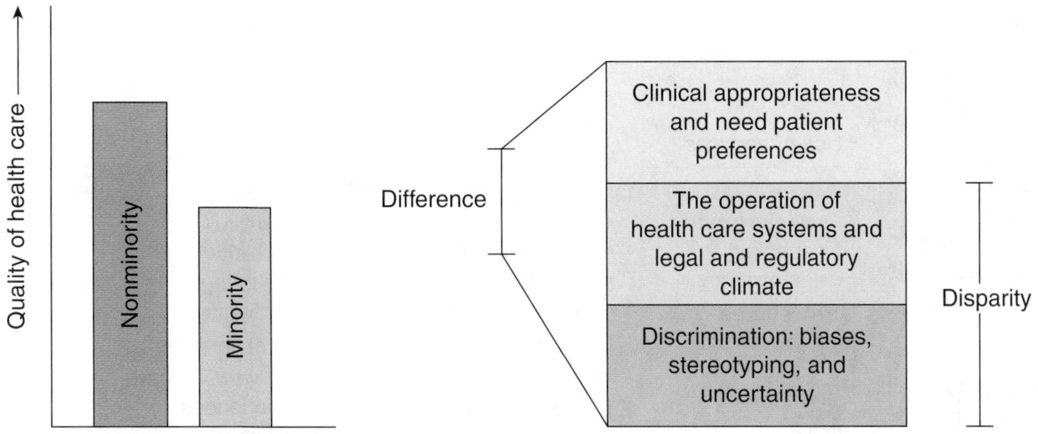

Figure 3-1 *Defining differences, disparities, and discrimination in populations with equal access to health care. (Reproduced, with permission, from Smedley BD, Stith AY, Nelson AR. Unequal treatment. Confronting racial and Ethnic Disparities in Health Care. Washington, DC: National Academies Press; 2002.)*

TABLE 3-1 Racial/Ethnic Disparities in Disease Prevention, Treatment, and Outcomes*

Conditions Where Minorities Documented with Greater Rates Compared to Whites
Cardiovascular disease: hypertension, stroke, congestive heart failure
Incidence and mortality from HIV
Type 2 diabetes: Prevalence Amputations Hospitalizations
Malignancy: Advanced stage breast cancer Advanced stage colon cancer Advanced stage prostate cancer
Pregnancy outcomes: Infant mortality Low birth weight Maternal mortality
End-stage renal disease
Preventable hospitalizations
Conditions Where Minorities Documented with Lower Rates Compared with Whites
Cardiovascular procedures: Cardiac catheterization Peripheral artery angioplasty Implantable cardiac defibrillators
Adult vaccinations
Solid organ transplantations
Secondary prevention for myocardial infarction
Curative surgery for lung cancer
Inadequate hemodialysis
Renal transplantation
Receipt of recommended care for acute myocardial infarction
Receipt of recommended care for pneumonia
Receipt of recommended care for congestive heart failure
Receipt of recommended care for type 2 diabetes
Satisfaction with hospital care
Age-adjusted life expectancy

*Adapted from *Unequal Treatment* and Agency for Health Care Research and Quality. National Health Care Disparities Report 2009. Agency for Health Care Research and Quality, U.S. Department of Health and Human Services.

exclusionary services ("separate but equal") thus augmenting the wide divide in poor-quality hospital services and facilities for African Americans. Hospital segregation ended with President Johnson signing into law the Medicare bill on July 9, 1965. The Medicare bill was tied to Title VI of the Civil Rights Act of 1964, which banned discrimination in any activities that used federal funds for training, employment, or construction. Because of this legal requirement, more than 95% of hospitals desegregated their facilities by the first day Medicare was implemented on July 1, 1966, in order to receive Medicare reimbursement.

The elimination of health care disparities is a high priority for the federal government, and many academic organizations are beginning to take steps to educate physicians about this problem. Hospitalists can significantly influence the health status of these patients if they comprehend their health care needs, communicate effectively, and advocate for additional local and institutional resources to ensure optimal discharge back to the community. To date, existing data suggest that the type of hospital facility and its location explain some of the observed racial and ethnic disparities in health care services; less is known, however, about disparities in hospital care. This chapter reviews the racial disparities in hospital care that can be impacted by hospitalists and proposes directions for future research.

MECHANISMS AND ETIOLOGY

INTERINSTITUTIONAL AND INTRAINSTITUTIONAL VARIATIONS IN CARE

Although where patients receive care likely explains some of the observed racial and ethnic disparities in health care service, prior studies suggest that hospital-level factors may play an important role in creating disparities in care. In addition, minorities live disproportionately in parts of the country that have lower-quality hospitals and fewer primary care physicians.

Safety-net hospitals predominantly serve poor and underserved patients and provide care for a disproportionate number of racial and ethnic minorities in the United States. Multiple studies have shown that these hospitals often provide a lower quality of care. This decreased quality is likely due to shortages of resources, nurse staff, technical support such as health information systems, and capital to make improvements. These hospitals have increased post-MI mortality rates and decreased performance measure scores for acute MI, lower performance on national quality process indicators for acute myocardial infarction (AMI), congestive heart failure (CHF), and pneumonia, and higher postoperative colon cancer mortality rates. In addition, they tend to have smaller gains over time on process measures

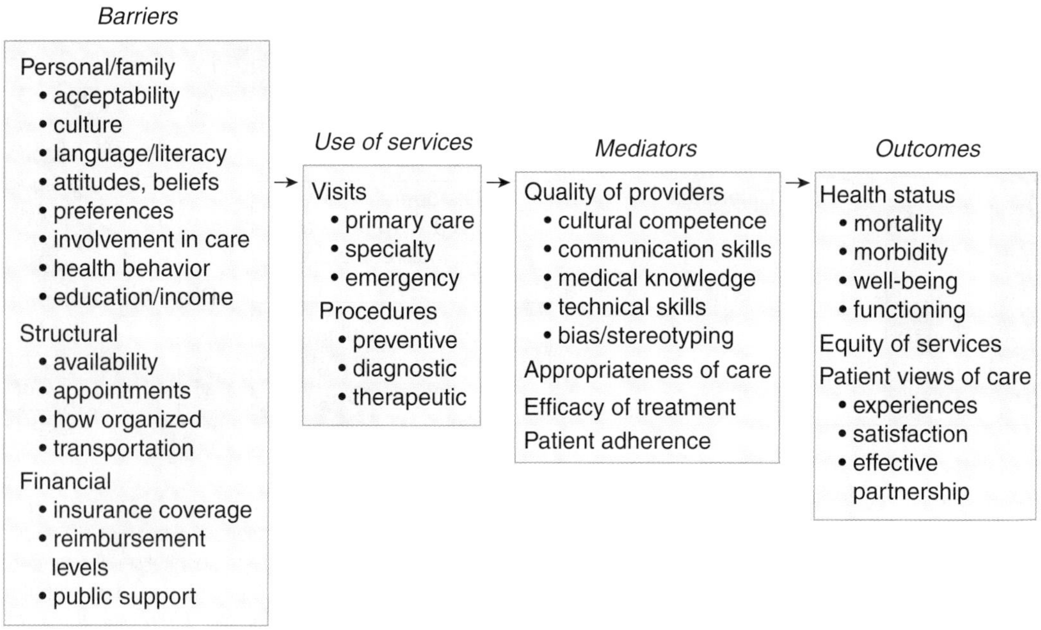

Figure 3-2 *Barriers and mediators of racial/ethnic health care disparities. (Adapted, with permission, from Cooper LA, Hill MN, Powe NR. Designing and evaluating interventions to eliminate racial and ethnic disparities in health care. J Gen Intern Med 2002;17:477–486. Copyright 2002 Society of General Internal Medicine.)*

for AMI, CHF, and pneumonia and are less likely to achieve high-performing status.

A large proportion of minority patients receive their care in a small number of hospitals and these facilities seem to provide a lower quality of care for common medical and surgical conditions. One study demonstrated that 90% of Hispanic and black Medicare beneficiaries receive their care at 25% of the 4500 acute care hospitals in the United States. Another study found significant racial/ethnic disparities in clinical processes for AMI, congestive heart failure, and pneumonia explained primarily by hospital factors and not individual patient characteristics. They also found that lower-performing hospitals tended to serve a larger proportion of minority patients. Similar findings have been demonstrated using national Hospital Quality Alliance (HQA) patient-level data. Other national studies demonstrate that African Americans go to hospitals that have lower rates of evidence-based medical treatments and worse risk-adjusted mortality after AMI, are less likely to receive optimal care for pneumonia as measured by national HQA measures, and have higher operative mortality risks for eight different procedures because the hospitals they attend have higher mortality rates for all patients.

In addition to differences in quality of care based on institution, data suggest that among patients hospitalized in the same institutions, racial and ethnic disparities in care often exist. Several studies have demonstrated significant racial and ethnic differences in utilization of cardiovascular procedures for patients hospitalized within the same institutions. For example, African Americans have a lower rate of coronary artery bypass procedures than whites, even with similar presentation and clinical features.

DIFFERENTIAL UTILIZATION OF MEDICAL PROCEDURES AND TECHNOLOGY AVAILABILITY

Racial differences in the utilization of medical procedures are well documented, especially for "referral-sensitive" procedures and invasive, costly procedures such as coronary revascularization. The reasons for these differences are complex and may reflect differences in clinical presentation, medical decision making, differential access to providers and institutions providing procedures, and differential care at hospitals.

Studies have demonstrated that Caucasian patients more often receive renal transplantation, cardiac surgical procedures, total joint replacement, and other procedures than do African Americans. African Americans are less likely to receive coronary revascularization compared to whites, even in hospitals with revascularization services. Additionally, African Americans are less likely to be transferred from hospitals without revascularization services to those with these cardiac services, and, even when they are transferred, they are still less likely to receive revascularization compared to Caucasians. These differences in procedure use have been associated with increased African American mortality rates. Finally, procedure volume has been shown to be a proxy for quality of care. African Americans and Hispanics tend to get care at low-procedure-volume hospitals with low-volume surgeons and cardiologists. A study of coronary artery bypass surgery (CABG) surgery outcomes in New York State found that African Americans and Asians were more likely to receive care from surgeons with higher risk-adjusted mortality. African Americans at low-volume hospitals have greater risk-adjusted mortality than Caucasian patients after elective aortic abdominal aneurysm (AAA) repair, CABG, and carotid endarterectomy (CEA).

Technology availability likely contributes to low performance. Hospitals with a high proportion of African American inpatients may have lower rates of adoption of new technologies. In general, safety-net providers are slower to adopt new technologies than non-safety-net providers. Providers and hospitals that invest in technology score higher on standard quality measures. However, national studies have demonstrated that providers who cared for uninsured and Medicaid African American and Hispanic patients are less likely to use electronic health records. These differences underscore the need to provide higher funding of public and other safety-net hospitals in order to reduce disparities in health care by ensuring the delivery of high-quality care for all patients.

PATIENT EXPERIENCES

Perceived provider attitude (both physicians and nonphysicians), including perceptions of provider prejudice, by minority patients has been shown to have a direct relationship to patient decision making and perceived quality and satisfaction. Reports of patient experiences with health care are therefore important correlates with quality. There are significant differences in hospitalized patients' self-reported experiences among different groups. African American and Latino patients are less satisfied with their hospital care, particularly in the dimension of having their preferences respected consistent with prior studies demonstrating racial/ethnic differences in satisfaction with provider communication and management. Both African American and Hispanic patients report that perceived attitudes of social workers and nursing staff have an important direct relationship on their perceived satisfaction and quality. Hispanic patients correlate high satisfaction with care when well-qualified medical interpreters are available.

These findings have several important implications for prioritizing quality improvement efforts in improving patient satisfaction with care. First, physicians and hospital staff should strive to better understand and address the expectations of African American and Latino patients. Second, hospital administrators should include allied health professionals and social workers in addition to nurses and physicians in training on patient-centered and culturally appropriate counseling techniques and communication. All clinicians should use medical interpreters when English is not the first language. Finally, hospitals should collect satisfaction data stratified by race and ethnicity in order to better tailor quality improvement (QI) efforts.

PRACTICE POINT

- Hospital administrators should include allied health professionals and social workers in addition to nurses and physicians in training on patient-centered and culturally appropriate counseling techniques and communication. All clinicians should use medical interpreters when English is not the patient's first language.

PRACTICE POINT

- Hospitals should collect satisfaction data stratified by race and ethnicity in order to better tailor quality improvement (QI) efforts.

FUTURE DIRECTIONS

Given the high number of minorities served at a small number of hospitals nationwide, improving hospital quality of care is one important approach to ameliorating health care disparities. The implementation of the hospitalist model of inpatient care and the adoption and implementation of health information technology (HIT) hold promise of being two important drivers of high quality.

ROLE OF HOSPITALISTS

Hospitalists are specialists in the general medical care of hospitalized patients. Their activities include patient care, teaching, research, and leadership related to inpatient care. The number of hospitalists continues to grow significantly across the nation; as a result, this specialty will care for increasing numbers of hospitalized underserved patients. Existing literature has demonstrated that hospitalists are associated with lower inpatient costs and shorter lengths of stay compared to general internists and family physicians, and such savings did not have a detrimental effect on rates of death or readmission. Importantly, hospitalists are associated with providing higher-quality inpatient care because of closer adherence to treatment guidelines and better postdischarge follow-up. A recent national study has demonstrated that hospitals with hospitalists were associated with better performance on quality indicators for AMI, pneumonia, and the composite domains of disease treatment, diagnosis, counseling, and prevention controlling for hospital characteristics such as size, location, ownership type, and staffing availability. These findings suggest that hospitalists, as specialists in inpatient hospital care, are important drivers of high-quality care. There are, however, no data reported on the performance of hospitalists compared to other providers relating to their care of different ethic groups.

Previous research using national quality measures has found substantial variability and room for improvement in the care of hospitalized patients across medical conditions. With the continued growth of the hospitalist inpatient care model, further research is needed to delineate the specific hospitalist model characteristics associated with improved quality and outcomes of care. The hospitalist model of inpatient care should be considered an essential component of quality improvement for hospitals seeking to improve inpatient care. This is especially true for public/municipal hospitals and smaller hospitals, which have been shown to be consistently associated with lower quality and which provide care for the disproportionate number of racial/ethnic minority patients.

HOSPITALISTS AND THE ROLE OF HEALTH INFORMATION TECHNOLOGIES AND QUALITY IMPROVEMENT

Hospitalists are often leaders of HIT and QI at their institutions. HIT refers to a conglomeration of technologies such as electronic health records (EHRs), computerized physician order entry, electronic clinical decision support tools, and clinical documentation, such as physician notes and discharge summaries. Many experts expect that HIT such as EHRs could significantly improve the efficiency and quality of health care. Recent national evidence shows very low levels of adoption of HIT in U.S. hospitals. In addition, it is likely that HIT adoption will impact institutions differentially, especially underresourced facilities such as those serving minority populations. A recent national survey indicates early evidence of an emerging digital divide, with minimal use of EHRs among hospitals that provide care to large numbers of poor patients. These same hospitals lagged behind others in quality performance as well, but those with EHR systems seemed to have eliminated the quality gap.

Despite a low level of implementation, research has demonstrated that HIT has the potential to increase the quality of care provided and augment patient safety. As hospitalists help establish and structure HIT systems, a focus on disparity reduction is important. HIT will facilitate the collection of race/ethnicity and language data in order to appropriately stratify collected data. However, HIT alone is not likely to improve quality significantly without additional interventions. Stratified data will address the long-standing problem of not having enough race/ethnicity data available for clinical and research purposes. Stratified data will also allow for targeted QI activities. HIT is an essential component of QI, and there is a strong evidence base that three types of HIT, decision support, alerts/reminders/prompts, and computerized provider order entry (CPOE), are associated generally with improved quality outcomes. In addition, HIT applications such as registries and quality reporting/auditing/feedback are associated with improved quality of care. These quality reports should be stratified by race/ethnicity. The design and implementation of HIT should include language service needs. Language barriers have been associated with decreased quality of care and an increased risk for adverse events. Language stratified data could also be linked to electronic medical record (EMR) alerts that assure the necessary ancillary services (ie, interpreters) are provided when needed.

CONCLUSION

Racial/ethnic disparities in hospital care and outcomes are based in a tradition of hospital segregation that has residual, significant, and persistent effects. A growing body of literature has demonstrated disparities in processes of care, utilization of procedures, clinical outcomes, and patients' experiences. These disparities are due in large part to differences in access to higher-quality hospitals; however, variation in intrainstitutional care has also been documented.

It is incumbent among policy makers, hospital administrators, and clinicians to develop strategies to achieve racial/ethnic equity in care. These strategies should include (1) examining within-institution differences in care, outcomes, and patient experience based on patients' race/ethnicity; (2) improving infrastructure and quality within largely minority-servicing institutions; and (3) developing QI initiatives focused on cultural competency and targeting high-risk racial/ethnic groups.

SUGGESTED READINGS

Agency for Healthcare Research and Quality. *National Healthcare Disparities Report 2009.* www.ahrq.gov/qual/nhdr09/nhdr09.pdf. Accessed July 19, 2010.

Groeneveld PW, Laufer SB, Garber AM. Technology diffusion, hospital variation, and racial disparities among elderly Medicare beneficiaries 1989–2000. *Med Care.* 2005;43:320–329.

Hasnain-Wynia R, Baker DW, Nerenz D, et al. Disparities in health care are driven by where minority patients seek care. Examination of the Hospital Quality Alliance Measures. *Arch Intern Med.* 2007;167:1233–1239.

Hicks LS, Ayanian JZ, Orav EJ, et al. Is hospital service associated with racial and ethnic disparities in experiences with hospital care? *Am J Med.* 2005;118(5):529–535.

Hicks LS, Tovar DA, Orav EJ, Johnson PA. Experiences with hospital care: perspectives of black and Hispanic patients [published online ahead of print April 15, 2008]. *J Gen Intern Med.* 2008;23(8):1234–1240.

Jha AK, DesRoches CM, Shields AE, et al. Evidence of an emerging digital divide among hospitals that care for the poor [published online ahead of print October 26, 2009]. *Health Aff (Millwood).* 2009;28(6):w1160–1170.

Jha AK, Orav EJ, Li Z, Epstein AM. Concentration and quality of hospitals that care for elderly black patients. *Arch Intern Med.* 2007;167:1177–1182.

Jha AK, Orav EJ, Li Z, Epstein AM. The characteristics and performance of hospitals that care for elderly Hispanic Americans. *Health Aff.* 2008;27:528–537.

López L, Hicks L, Cohen AP, McKean S, Weissman JS. Hospitalists and the quality of care in hospitals. *Arch Intern Med.* 2009;169:1–6.

Werner RM, Goldman LE, Dudley RA. Comparison of change in quality of care between safety-net and non-safety-net hospitals. *JAMA.* 2008;299:2180–2187.

CHAPTER 4

The Interface Between Primary Care and Hospital Medicine

Stacy Higgins, MD, FACP

INTRODUCTON

It is estimated that the United States currently has over 222,000 practicing active generalists that are either office or hospital based. This includes trained internists, family physicians, and pediatricians who provide primary care to the great majority of the U.S. population. Physicians in family medicine, general internal medicine, and general pediatrics are the foundation of U.S. health care, providing 52% of all ambulatory care visits, much of the inpatient care, 80% of visits for hypertension and 70% of visits for chronic obstructive pulmonary disease (COPD) and diabetes. Yet it is expected that there will be a significant shortage of primary care physicians over the next 20 years because the U.S. population is expected to increase by 18% between 2005 and 2025, and the population over age 65 (which utilizes the health care system twice as often as younger adults) will increase by 73%.

STATE OF PRIMARY CARE

At the same time, the number of medical school graduates who plan to enter general internal medicine has decreased annually since its peak in 1998, by nearly 40% overall in 2009. Increasing numbers of graduates who are entering general internal medicine are choosing to practice Hospital Medicine exclusively. More women are entering medical school and the physician workforce (at a nearly 50% expected even representation by 2025), and women are more likely than their male counterparts to work in part-time positions. Finally, the number of hours working and patients seen by older physicians who are approaching retirement is unlikely to be matched by the newly graduated physicians that are their replacements.

Between the growth of the population over age 65 and the decrease in physicians practicing outpatient primary care, there is expected to be an outpatient physician shortage by 2025. An expected 30% increase in ambulatory care visits for adults will significantly increase the workload for those who primarily practice outpatient medicine. Deficits of 35,000 to 44,000 adult generalists are expected by 2025, threatening the foundation of primary care for adults. Geographic differences in physician supply indicate that shortages will be more acute in rural areas. These numbers do not take into account health care reform, with the provision of universal coverage. This will add an additional 31 million people into a system that is already challenged, with expected increases in wait time for visits and further increasing workload on primary care providers.

Compare this to the physician workforce in Great Britain and Canada. The United States spends the most per capita on health care in the world, accounting for 15% of gross domestic product (GDP), yet, according to the World Health Organization, it ranks 37th in the world in several leading health indicators. In comparison, Canada spends about half as much per capita, and health care spending accounts for 10% of the GDP. One of the differences quoted between the two systems is access to primary care providers who act as "gatekeepers" to specialty care, helping to keep costs down. The number of physicians entering primary care in Canada is rising faster than those entering specialty fields, up from 96 per 100,000 in 2002 to 98 per 100,000 in 2006 (Canadian Institute for Health Information). In Great Britain, the National Health Service provides 90% of the health care to its population, and about 6% of GDP is spent on medical services. In Great Britain, nearly 50% of medical school graduates will enter the field of general practice.

In response to the aging population with its anticipated increase in health care utilization, the Association of American Medical Colleges called for a 30% increase in the number of medical students across the country. However, an increase in the number of medical students does not equal an increase in primary care providers 10 years from now. U.S. medical students have chosen primary care in declining numbers over the past 10 years for a variety of reasons, including less income as compared to procedural-based specialists, high debt burdens from medical school, the perception of primary care having less prestige with high work-related stresses (work harder for less money), and medical education favoring training in nonprimary care fields. Initial plans for a primary care career may be deterred by a chaotic resident clinic experience, and inadequate training in ambulatory topics.

GROWTH OF HOSPITAL MEDICINE

Contrast the growth of primary care with the growth of Hospital Medicine, which is the fastest-growing field in medicine. Since 1996, the number of physicians who identify themselves as hospitalists has grown to nearly 30,000, similar to the number of cardiologists, and second only to the number of primary care physicians in the United States. The precedent of this "site-based" specialty was set by Emergency Medicine and critical care medicine, where physicians manage a wide variety of diagnoses but limit their care to a specific location within the hospital. In the U.S. health care system several factors have contributed to the rapid expansion of Hospital Medicine, including economics, quality, and changes in residency training.

- In the early 1980s, Medicare changed its reimbursement of inpatient care from a daily rate to using diagnosis-related groups (DRGs) giving fixed payments for a given diagnosis. This created an incentive for hospitals to support strategies that would safely shorten length of stays, thereby decreasing hospital costs.
- The growth of managed care in the early 1990s often increased panel sizes for primary care physicians (PCPs), and therefore the number of patients seen daily. This drove inpatient care to the extremes of the day before or after their outpatient schedule. Care of patients in the hospital was seen by some as a barrier to the efficiency of inpatient care, often resulting in an increased average length of stay, a major driver of health care costs. At the same time, there was insufficient coordination of care provided by consulting subspecialists, further increasing costs and duration of stay. Hospitalists, who dedicated their time to patients in the hospital, fulfilled a growing need.
- In 1999, the Institute of Medicine (IOM) released "To Err Is Human" and in 2001 "Crossing the Quality Chasm," drawing national attention to the issue of quality. Hospitals are expected to be the leading force in improving quality and safety gaps nationwide. Often, hospital administrations turned to the new workforce of hospitalists who spent all of their work time in the hospital, monitoring care across several spectrums. This new workforce was often recently out of training and open to new ideas, practiced by evidence-based guidelines, and interested in team-based solutions to address quality issues. Quality improvement quickly falls into the domain of Hospital Medicine. Subsequent studies support that hospitalists lower cost (primarily by decreasing length of stay) while maintaining quality.
- In 2003, the Accreditation Council for Graduate Medical Education (ACGME) instituted the 80-hour resident work week, and in 2008 there was a shift toward increased emphasis on ambulatory medicine. Academic hospitals, which may have been resistant to the use of hospitalists prior to this time, now see hospitalists as a means to cover work that can no longer be performed by residents. Hospitalists are hired to cover "nonteaching" services in academic centers, and to supervise midlevel providers. With the sure advent of further limitation on resident work hours based on IOM recommendations, hospitalists will continue to fill in these gaps.

In the past few years, hospitalists have expanded their role of caring for inpatient internal medicine patients to include surgical patients. Surgeons are thus able to focus their time in the operating room (similar to PCPs focusing on care of patients in the office). Furthermore, reported hospital quality measures such as antibiotic use, venous thromboembolic prophylaxis, pain management, and preventive care are viewed as medical issues better managed by hospitalists. In addition, this allows surgical residents, under the same ACGME duty-hour restrictions as medical residents, to spend their time on becoming technically competent. Finally, with the aging of the population, many patients on the surgical service have increasingly complex medical issues that require comanagement by a trained internist.

The rapid growth of the field of Hospital Medicine occurred without clear guidelines as to the knowledge and skills necessary for successful practice. Early on, hospitalists functioned as internists in the hospital, focused on acute care in internal medicine, the same type of care as delivered during residency. Over time, the role of the hospitalist has changed from traditional medical consultant to comanager of patients admitted to other services (surgery, neurology, obstetrics); hospitalists are key players in the development of practice guidelines and implementation of information systems such as the electronic medical record and computerized physician order entry; and hospitalists are leaders in health care economics, including quality improvement and utilization review work.

In 2006, the Society of Hospital Medicine developed *The Core Competencies in Hospital Medicine: A Framework for Curriculum Development*, standardizing the expectations for training and professional development. The competencies have written learning outcomes and are divided into three sections: clinical competencies, procedures, and health care systems, with learning objectives categorized as knowledge, skills, and attitudes. The development of this curriculum can serve to address some of the deficiencies in residency-based education for those pursuing a career in Hospital Medicine.

In September 2009, the American Board of Internal Medicine (ABIM) recognized Hospital Medicine as a focused practice within internal medicine, with a separate maintenance of certification (MOC). This was done with the recognition that the practice of Hospital Medicine had reached a state of maturity within the field of internal medicine, demonstrated by the large number of physicians who self-identify as hospitalists, the growing number of general internists who no longer practice in the hospital setting, and acknowledgment of the value that hospitalists bring to improving patient care in the hospital setting. Recognizing the knowledge, skills, and attitudes needed beyond those developed in residency training, an internist pursuing an ABIM focused practice in Hospital Medicine program must complete training in internal medicine, be ABIM certified, and engage in a practice primarily focusing on Hospital Medicine for at least three years before sitting for the MOC.

Since 1996, the hospitalist model of inpatient care has experienced tremendous growth, and it is now seen as unusual for PCPs to admit and care for their patients in the hospital. Support for hospitalists delivering the majority of inpatient care comes from demonstrated reduction in resource use, including decreased hospital costs and length of stay, while preserving patient satisfaction. Initially, there was resistance on the use of hospitalists by PCPs with concerns over the loss of camaraderie that comes from being in a hospital and interacting with other specialists, as well as the feeling by PCPs that they would be abandoning ill patients to be cared for by strangers at a time when they need their regular physician the most. PCPs have now come to accept the hospitalist model as the standard of care and report that the use of hospitalists has decreased workload, while not affecting income. Hospitalists are the go-to caretakers for inpatients—they are able to provide round-the-clock care and facilitate and coordinate care of multiple consultants, and they are taking the lead in improving the overall system of care through quality improvement. In addition, for PCPs with busy practices, the need to cancel appointments or curtail the workday to attend to admitted patients is eliminated with the hospitalist model, resulting in increased availability of outpatient doctors to their patients.

Despite this, concern over the potential for discontinuity of care and disruption of the physician–patient relationship remains paramount. For outpatient doctors who have practiced medicine in both eras, "visiting patients (in the hospital) now feels like entering a foreign world." In an opinion piece (*Annals of Internal Medicine*), Dr. Howard Beckman describes, "when I agreed to the hospitalist system, I believed that I would be a member of my patients' hospital team.... However that fantasy has yet to be fulfilled. My belief that hospitalist care would result in abandoning my patients has largely been validated."[1] In the inaugural issue of the *Journal of Hospital Medicine*, Dr. Christine Cassel identified that continuity of care, continuing relationships, and efficient management of resources over the entire trajectory of a patient's illness, and not just during a hospitalization, has not been addressed by the field of Hospital Medicine. She urged for partnering of those who practice Hospital Medicine with others across the continuum of care, to ensure that patients, especially the most vulnerable, receive the service they need while in the hospital and after discharge.

PRACTICE POINT

- Hospitalists should partner with others across the continuum of care to ensure that patients, especially the most vulnerable, receive the service they need while in the hospital and after discharge.

The remainder of this chapter identifies some of the issues that remain as barriers in the interface between the primary care doctor and the hospitalist, with the goal to improve care of the patient, include both PCP and hospitalist input, and maintain quality utilization of the health care system.

COMMUNICATION BETWEEN THE OUTPATIENT PRIMARY AND ADMITTING HOSPITAL PHYSICIAN

When the hospitalist movement began, much of the concern, which continues today, was that input from the PCP is unavailable during crucial decision making for patients admitted to a hospital-based physician. Reasons for this are varied, including the hospitalist not contacting the PCP, the PCPs not making themselves available to discuss the patients, or, increasingly common, the patient being uninsured and not having a PCP. At times, PCPs may not want to be integrated as a member of the inpatient team because they are too busy with their outpatient practice, they feel comfortable working with hospitalists, and they want to defer all care to the hospitalist. In making decisions such as do not resuscitate (DNR) and withdrawal of care, the patient and family may be much more trusting and comfortable with their long-term physician who knows them not only in the setting of an acute illness but in the context of their routine life. It is critical that these issues are discussed prior to hospitalization, documented in the patient's chart, and communicated to the inpatient physician.

Much of it comes down to adequate, bidirectional communication between the hospitalist and the outpatient physician from the moment of admission. Initially the burden is on the outpatient physician to communicate with the admitting physician about the patient, providing a current list of outpatient medications and key past medical and social history that can influence the hospitalization course, particularly in situations where there is not an EMR link. Key to positive communication is the PCP acknowledging the legitimacy of the hospitalist and understanding that the hospitalist will direct care while the patient is hospitalized. The hospitalist must recognize the role of the PCP as long-term care provider who is familiar with the complete patient, outside of the acute, presenting illness. Essentially, this boils down to mutual respect. Where three are systems such as EMRs that can facilitate communication, PCPs should ensure medication lists are updated within them at each visit.

It is also important for patients and their family not to feel abandoned upon hospitalization. Physician groups that contract with a hospitalist group to provide inpatient care should educate their patients (perhaps via brochures available in the waiting room) on the role of hospitalists should they be admitted. A telephone call, or a visit if feasible, by the PCP to the patients and their family during this fragile time is an ideal way to reassure patients that the hospitalist and primary physician are in communication with each other and working in conjunction. A simple explanation from the hospitalist at admission on the respective roles of the PCP and hospitalist can also suffice and set the patient at ease. Admission is also a time for dialogue between the hospitalist and outpatient physician as to when and how often to be contacted regarding care of the patient. In enhancing communication between the PCP and the hospitalist, it is important not to make it onerous for either party, but to assess ideal timing and mechanisms of communication. Communication should occur on admission, prior to discharge, and with any changes in clinical status or major interventions, but this may vary from one physician to the next. Although e-mail may be the preferred method of communication for both personal and professional matters, when it comes to patient care, a phone call or face-to-face discussion allows a dialogue between physicians rather than a one-way report. Systems must be in place to facilitate communication by phone and prevent wait time on hold and the frustration of missed calls. Likewise, hospitalists need to be reassured that covering physicians will relay key information to the PCP. Covering physicians may not appreciate a phone call because they may not know the patient. The best system might be a combination of EMR and dedicated nurse hospitalist lines in the primary care practice. This way the hospitalist can be reassured that the voice message will make its way to the PCP while he or she awaits a return call.

Likewise the hospitalist service should inform the PCPs as to which hospitalist is taking care of their patient. Additionally, PCPs should be able to page one easily remembered number to ask the admitting hospitalist who the attending physician will be. Alternatively, a confidential group e-mail with the expectation that the responsible hospitalist will respond promptly might be used. With appropriate safeguards regarding patient confidentiality, e-mail communication may be preferred by some PCPs and hospitalists as well as patients' families who appreciate frequent updates and easy access to caregivers.

Hospitalist groups might wish to develop standards for communication and periodically assess their PCP groups to see if they are satisfied with the communication. Certainly, hospitalists should alert PCPs to new diagnoses such as cancer, test results that adversely impact prognosis, and all transitions, including imminent transfers to the intensive care unit. Ideally, PCPs should be informed of a pending discharge so they can raise certain issues and help determine best follow-up.

As Hospital Medicine services mature and more systems are in place, such as EMR, the relationship of the service with PCPs will likely evolve, and hospitalists may find that they are working more independently and that the communication is more likely to be initiated by them than by the PCP. However, it will always be important for hospitalists to be apprised of critical information not necessarily documented in the medical record, such as baseline functioning and personal beliefs.

PRACTICE POINT

- Bidirectional communication with primary care physicians should occur on admission, prior to discharge, and with any changes in clinical status or major interventions. It will always be important for hospitalists to be apprised of critical information not necessarily documented in the medical record such as baseline functioning and personal beliefs.

Patients should be promptly returned to the care of their PCPs postdischarge. Even though they may not need a follow-up visit within 10 to 14 days for the condition that led to hospital admission, in general, an early follow-up visit reestablishes the relationship, facilitates medication reconciliation, and provides opportunities to assess patient progress.

DISCHARGE SUMMARIES

Discharge summaries are used as a means to communicate the hospital course, discharge diagnoses, and medications, as well as to provide needed follow-up to the outpatient physician. However, discharge summaries should not be the only means of communication. The Joint Commission (TJC) requires that discharge summaries be completed within 30 days of hospital discharge, and that they include key elements such as reason for hospitalization, procedures performed, and condition at discharge. It has also been shown that when the physician receives the discharge summary prior to seeing the patient in follow-up, it is less likely that the patient will be readmitted to the hospital.

Since discharge summaries can only help direct patient care if they are received by the physician prior to follow-up, it is essential that this information be passed on in a timely manner. While the TJC requirement is 30 days, patients are usually seen in follow-up prior to this time. In a meta-analysis conducted by Kripalani, et al, direct communication between hospital physicians and PCPs during the discharge period occurred less than 20% of the time. Relying on the arrival of a discharge summary to communicate the hospital course also proved to be unreliable, with about 75% of patients contacting or being treated by their PCP before the physician had received a summary, and 25% of summaries never reaching the PCP. In contrast, hand delivery of a discharge letter by the patient to the PCP, or delivery of a letter via U.S. mail, increases the likelihood of arrival as well as shortens transit time, with the majority arriving prior to the patient contacting the physician, and an over 90% eventual arrival rate. Other modes of delivery that would increase timeliness include direct facsimile to the outpatient office, via EMR if the outpatient physician is within the same system, and e-mail.

Content of the discharge summaries is as important as timeliness. In the same meta-analysis conducted by Kripalani, et al, PCPs reported the following information as most important for providing adequate follow-up care: main diagnosis, pertinent physical findings, results of procedures and laboratory tests, discharge medications with reasons for any changes from prior medications, any adverse reactions to treatment, details of follow-up arrangements made, information given to the patient and family, test results pending at discharge, and specific follow-up needs. High-risk medications such as warfarin, insulin, or pain medication should have explicit, detailed information. Antibiotics and other time-limited medications should have a specific stop date. Inclusion of the hospitalist's contact information and that of key consulting specialists is also a crucial component of the discharge summary, so that direct communication between physicians continues as needed in this vulnerable time period.

Standardization of the summary, with structured subheadings to organize and highlight pertinent and relevant information, as well as pending results and discharge instructions, would greatly ensure that the discharge summary fulfills its role as a vital tool for transfer of information. The increasing use of EMRs across the country allows for prepopulation of many of these subheadings, such as diagnosis, admitting physician, and discharge medications, to ensure these important components are included in the discharge summary.

PRACTICE POINT

- Timely delivery of the discharge summary can direct post hospital care and help prevent re-admission. Consider hand delivery of the summary to the PCP by the patient, or via US mail or fax to the office. Content of the summary should include admission diagnosis, test results, pending and recommended tests, and a medication reconciliation, along with the discharge physicians contact information.

EVENTS AFTER DISCHARGE AND BEFORE FOLLOW-UP

Patients are being discharged from the hospital faster than ever before to complete their convalescence at home, often with workups to be completed as an outpatient. Patients are discharged with pending test results, with a significant risk for abnormal results that would warrant a change in management. Notably, in many cases, neither inpatient nor outpatient physician follows up on the results because they are ordered by one care provider (hospitalist or resident) but returned after discharge, when the care has been transferred to the PCP. Workup errors occur when an outpatient test or procedure recommended or scheduled by the inpatient physician is not followed up on by the outpatient provider for similar reasons. Both of these lapses in care lead to increased likelihood of the patient's being rehospitalized within 3 months of discharge, increasing overall health care costs. Any pending tests or incomplete workups must be included on the discharge summary for the PCP to follow up, and ideally, the hospitalist who ordered the tests should check on the pending test results as well.

The period immediately following discharge is a particularly vulnerable time for patients as they continue to recover from the inciting illness, try to coordinate postdischarge care, and manage any changes in medication prior to seeing their PCP. On discharge, patients should be told whom to contact with questions about medications, scheduled tests, or a change in clinical course. This contact should be the PCP, but it is contingent on the PCP having received the discharge summary and a contact number for the hospitalist. The hospitalist should also be available to the PCP in a timely manner as questions arise.

SCHEDULING THE FOLLOW-UP

With the high risk for readmission in the 30 days following discharge, patients should be followed more closely during this time for potential interventions that could prevent readmission or visits to the emergency department. The ideal interval before scheduled follow-up in the office depends on multiple factors, including condition on discharge, whether there are test results to be checked, and the patient's age, but there should be a firm follow-up appointment on discharge, which in most cases should not be more than 14 days hence. Conversely, the PCP has the obligation to contact patients who have missed postdischarge follow-up appointments.

INVOLVEMENT OF THE PATIENT AND CAREGIVERS

Especially during high census conditions, the discharge process is a hectic time; patients and families may receive cursory discharge instructions that have not adequately allowed for feedback of instructions or questions. In addition, the discharge process can be a confusing one for recovering patients who subsequently direct questions to the PCP about the hospitalization, procedures performed, and medication changes. If patients are discharged to extended care facilities, they may not receive any discharge instructions at the time of transfer.

In 2004, Coleman and colleagues designed a "Care Transitions Intervention" to improve care transitions by providing patients and their caregivers with the tools to more actively participate in the transition from hospital to home. Using four "pillars," a personal health record is created to facilitate communication between the patient and the PCP across all settings. Use of the care transitions intervention has been shown to significantly reduce the rates of rehospitalization at a significant cost savings to the health care system.

CONCLUSION

The Society of Hospital Medicine has included care transitions as a critical core competency for hospitalists: "Transitions of Care refers to specific interactions, communication, and planning required for patients to safely move from one service to another."[2] For optimal care of the patient, bidirectional communication needs to occur between the PCP and the hospitalist, with the patient and caregiver central to all discussions. This should decrease the marginalization of the PCP, increase the efficiency of the hospitalist, and ease the fears of patients and their family, with the ultimate goals of increasing patient satisfaction, decreasing rehospitalizations, and minimizing utilization of the health care system.

SUMMARY RECOMMENDATIONS

- Prior to admission or their becoming seriously ill, PCPs should actively engage in end-of-life planning with their patients and document these decisions in the medical record. For patients with chronic illnesses who are declining, the prognosis should be discussed. These communications should be incorporated into the initial discussion with the admitting hospitalist.
- Outpatient physician groups should educate their patients on the use of hospitalists for their admitted patients and reassure their patients that bidirectional communication occurs.
- Medication lists must be updated at every outpatient visit.
- On admission, the hospitalist should inform the PCP of the admission and the admitting diagnosis. If the PCP sent the patient to the hospital for admission or is made aware of the admission through the emergency department, the PCP should initiate communication with the admitting hospitalist. Primary care and Hospital Medicine practices should work together to develop communication systems to facilitate this process.
- A checklist of critical information that should be communicated at each care transition should be developed and should include home medications, chronic conditions, and social factors.
- Discussion on what would precipitate further communication (major tests, change in condition, etc); best method of communication (phone, fax, e-mail); and timing should be established on admission.
- The PCP should contact the family and/or caregivers during the admission, informing the family of the role of the hospitalist and that the hospitalist and PCP are a team and in contact with each other.
- Time and care should occur with discharge, recognizing that the postdischarge period is when the patient is most vulnerable for readmission. Hospitalists and members of the hospital multidisciplinary care team must ensure that patients and their family have been informed of any changes to medications and reasons for the change, tests pending on discharge, what to do in the event of a change in condition, and concrete plans for follow-up.
- The hospitalist should include the PCP in discharge planning, communicating discharge medications, any incomplete workups, tests pending, and when the patient is expected in follow-up. It should be clearly established in writing who is responsible for following up on pending tests and incomplete workups.
- PCPs are obligated to contact patients who did not keep their postdischarge appointment and should emphasize the importance of follow-up after hospitalization.

SUGGESTED READINGS

Cassel C. Hospital Medicine: an important player in comprehensive care. *J Hosp Med.* 2006;1:3–4.

Coleman EA, Williams M. Executing high-quality care transitions: a call to do it right. *J Hosp Med.* 2007;2:287–290.

Colwill J, Cultice J, Kruse R. Will generalist physician supply meet demands of an Increasing and aging population? *Health Aff.* 2008;27:W232–241.

Coleman EA, Parry C, Chalmers S, Min S. The care transitions intervention. *Arch Intern Med.* 2006;166:1822–1828.

Glasheen J, Goldenberg J, Nelson J. Achieving Hospital Medicine's promise through internal medicine residency redesign. *Mt. Sinai J Med.* 2008;75:436–441.

Goldman L, Pantilat S, Whitcomb W. Passing the clinical baton: 6 principles to guide the hospitalist. *Am J Med.* 2001;111:36S–39S.

Hauer K, Durning S, Kernan W. Factors associated with medical students' career choices regarding internal medicine. *JAMA.* 2008;300:1154–1164.

Kripalani S, Jackson A, Schnipper J, Coleman EA. Promoting effective transitions of care at hospital discharge: a review of key issues for hospitalists. *J Hosp Med.* 2007;2:314–323.

Kripalani S, LeFevre F, Phillips C, Williams M, Vasaviah P, Baker D. Deficits in communication between hospital-based and primary care physicians: implications for patient safety and continuity of care. *JAMA.* 2007;297:831–841.

REFERENCES

1. Beckman H. Three degrees of separation. *Ann Intern Med.* 2009; 151:890–891.
2. Dressler D. Transitions in care. The core competencies in Hospital Medicine: a framework for curriculum development by SHM, Editors Pistoria M, Amin A, Dressler D, et al. *J Hosp Med.* 2006;1(suppl 1):96.

CHAPTER 5

The Core Competencies in Hospital Medicine

Tina Budnitz, MPH
Sylvia C. McKean, MD, SFHM, FACP

INTRODUCTION

Initially, the hospitalist movement arose to reduce length of stay by having dedicated physicians in the hospital most of the time. Over time, the role evolved, and it became clear that hospitalists could improve the quality of inpatient care, promote patient safety, and educate the next generation of physicians. Although the term *hospitalist* was coined in 1996, over the subsequent decade there remained considerable variability in the definition of *hospitalist* and the scope of work attributed to that role from one practice setting to the next. At the same time that Hospital Medicine leaders embraced the importance of evidence-based care and systems improvement—especially around transitions of care and the well-publicized safety and quality issues facing hospitalized patients—they were recruiting physicians from traditional residency programs that had not adequately prepared them for their new roles. In fact, the Accreditation Council for Graduate Medical Education (ACGME) acknowledged training gaps in six main competency areas for evaluation of medical trainees: patient care, medical knowledge, practice-based learning improvement, interpersonal and communication skills, professionalism, and systems based learning.

The Society of Hospital Medicine (SHM) recognized the need to define specific competencies of a hospitalist to establish performance standards, differentiate Hospital Medicine as a unique subspecialty, and create a framework for training programs. SHM hoped that the creation of a document detailing core competencies would further serve to standardize training programs, highlight training gaps within internal medicine residency programs, and identify the professional development needs of practicing hospitalists. In 2006, SHM developed and published *The Core Competencies in Hospital Medicine: A Framework for Curriculum Development*. This document is a compendium of competencies for the practice of Hospital Medicine and was developed by SHM in conjunction with more than 100 hospitalists and physician leaders from university and community hospitals, teaching and nonteaching programs, and for- and not-for-profit programs throughout the United States (**Figure 5-1**).

Table 5-1 illustrates how the SHM core competencies align with ACGME outcome requirements.

Since the publication of TCCs in 2006, the evolution of the field of Hospital Medicine continues to present new opportunities not only for growth but for the development of expertise in areas not integrated into residency training. Hospitalists now specialize in the management of medical subspecialty patients, neurology patients, obstetrics, palliative care, critical care, and surgical comanagement. Tertiary care settings have increasingly become large intensive care units with step-down capacity for every patient whose preexisting comorbidities shape recovery. Hospitalists working in community settings may in fact become the teachers of the next generation of residents and medical students as they increasingly rotate through these settings. Although it may not be possible to predict the next stage of evolution, hospitalists are uniquely positioned to support accountable care and optimize integration and performance for the communities their hospitals serve. TCCs are the first step in the process of defining expectations for this young specialty and serve as a template for future educational initiatives.

TABLE 5-1 Two Chapters as Examples of How to Meet ACGME Outcome Requirements

Care of Vulnerable Populations Competencies	ACGME Core Competencies	Transitions of Care Competencies
Development of a formal curriculum around vulnerable populations reflects attitudes that care should be patient centered.	Patient care	Utilize the most efficient, effective, reliable, and expeditious communication modalities in patient transitions.
Teach that for vulnerable populations "business as usual" may be inadequate, and additional resources may be required to reach target goals.		Organize and effectively communicate medical information in a succinct format for receiving clinicians.
Expect students to proactively arrange for these services and provide feedback when this does not occur.		Recognize the impact of care transitions on patient outcomes and satisfaction.
Identify the key factors that lead to vulnerability, describe the needs of populations served and local resources available to ameliorate barriers to Health Care provision.	Knowledge	Describe information that should be retrieved and communicated during each care transition (eg, key elements involved in signing out a patient moving to the intensive care unit or going home).
Use the core competencies to develop activities, reading lists, bedside teaching, didactic sessions, and innovative educational forums.		Distinguish available levels of care for patient transition and select the most appropriate option (eg, Long Term Acute Care, rehab, Skilled Nursing Facility, psych facility, other facilities).
Formally evaluate social history-taking skills and construction of patient-centered care plans through direct observation and feedback sessions, attending rounds and bedside discussions	Practice-based learning and improvement	Inform receiving physician of pending tests and determine who is responsible for follow-up on results.
Solicit patient feedback on the trainee's performance.		Incorporate quality indicators for specific disease states into care plans.
Develop a social curriculum which reflects attitudes that trainees should be taught interpersonal and communication skills and professional role modeling.	Interpersonal and communication skills	Communicate with patients and families to explain their condition, ongoing medical regimen, follow-up care, and available support services
Use interpreters to effectively educate patients about their problems and engage them in their treatment.		Prepare patients and families early in the hospitalization for anticipated care transitions.
Make hidden goals and expectations explicit through role modeling and informal discussions.	Professionalism	Appreciate the value of real-time interactive dialogue between clinicians during care transitions.
Taking a resident on a home visit can be a particularly powerful way to promote professionalism.		Maintain availability to discharged patients for questions between discharge and follow-up outpatient visit.
Resident research projects might relate to the study of disparities of Health Care, especially among black and Latino populations at your institution.	System-based practice	Lead, coordinate, or participate in initiatives to develop and implement new protocols to improve or optimize care transitions (eg, medication reconciliation form development).
During ambulatory rotations, trainees would be expected to report on local resources, develop a social curriculum that could be used to teach trainees, standardize communication for vulnerable patients in their residency clinic.		Engage stakeholders (eg, inpatient clinicians, outpatient clinicians, nurses, administrators) in hospital initiatives to continuously assess the quality of care transitions.

Data from TCC, Chapter 3.2 and 3.24, Pistoria MJ, Amin AN, Dressler DD, McKean SM, Budnitz TB, eds. The core competencies in Hospital Medicine: a framework for curriculum development by The Society of Hospital Medicine. *The Journal of Hospital Medicine*. 2001;1(S1):1–55.

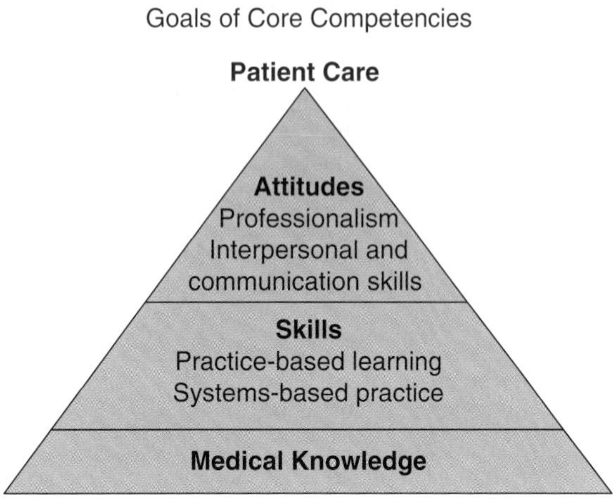

Figure 5-1 *The Goals of the Core Competencies.*

WHAT ARE THE CORE COMPETENCIES IN HOSPITAL MEDICINE?

TCCs standardize expected learning outcomes for teaching Hospital Medicine in medical school, postgraduate (ie, residency, fellowship), and continuing medical education programs, while allowing flexibility for curriculum developers to customize instructional strategies and context, as they integrate the most timely literature and evidence into medical content.

TCCs are divided into three sections: Clinical Conditions, Procedures, and Systems in Health Care. Within each section, chapter topics were selected based on relevance to Hospital Medicine; impact in terms of prevalence, economic costs, and effect on hospital systems. Each chapter demonstrates how the approach and orientation of hospitalists differ from those of traditional clinicians rotating through the hospital. The Procedures section acknowledges local and regional variations in who performs inpatient procedures, but it is limited to the core set of procedures most likely to be performed or supervised by a hospitalist. The goal is to provide some standardization of procedure performance for hospitalists.

PRACTICE POINT

TCC example of pain management

- "Explain the indications and limitations of nonpharmacologic methods of pain control available in the inpatient setting."
- The above competency standardizes the expectation that a physician be familiar with the nonpharmacologic pain control methods available, relate the evidence base for each approach, and local resources available; and apply those factors to determine the best option for a specific patient. At the same time, the competency allows an instructor to create curricula based on the most recent evidence-based literature on pain control options and tailor content around options available at that specific institution.

The Systems in Health Care section and the category Systems Organizations and Improvement in the other two sections describe mastery of multiple competencies across categories. The Systems in Health Care section includes clinical concepts that cross several disciplines such as care of the elderly patient, infection control, nutrition, and palliative care; and educational concepts such as hospitalist as teacher, patient education, and evidenced-based medicine; and organizational topics such team approach, transitions of care, patient safety, and quality improvement. Within each clinical, procedural, and systems chapter, TCCs highlight the expectation that hospitalists lead, coordinate, or participate in patient care and workflow efficiency improvement efforts. Recurring themes include an emphasis on the multidisciplinary approach, teamwork, inpatient quality and safety, and patient-centered communication to ensure safe and efficient care transitions and handoffs.

WHAT IS COMPETENCY-BASED EDUCATION AND HOW WAS IT APPLIED TO THE CORE COMPETENCIES?

Competency-based education focuses on articulating specific learning outcomes and measurable levels of proficiency rather than summarizing general outcomes or learning processes.

PRACTICE POINT

TCC palliative care example

- "Understand methods of palliation" and "Increase understanding of palliative care approaches" are not carefully conceived competency-based objectives. In these examples, it is unclear what exactly constitutes "understand," or how you would measure whether the learning objective had been achieved. Does generating a generic list of pharmacologic options for any category of patient qualify as understanding? Or, is the desired outcome something of a higher proficiency, such as the ability to develop a patient-specific palliation plan that takes into account functional status and patient- and family-established goals for pain management?

Using well-written competencies, educators can clearly articulate expected outcomes and design evaluation strategies to gauge not only "understanding" of a concept, but competency at a specific level. Competencies are often classified within three domains of outcomes: cognitive (knowledge), psychomotor (skills), and affective (attitudes).

PRACTICE POINT

Example of palliative care competencies in each category

- Knowledge: Describe the mechanisms that cause pain.
- Skill: Conduct a physical examination to determine the likely source of pain.
- Attitude: Promote the ethical imperative of accounting for patient-centered goals of care and frequent pain assessment and adequate control.
- System organization and improvement: Lead, coordinate, or participate in efforts to establish or support existing multidisciplinary pain control teams.

The authors of TCCs of Hospital Medicine added a fourth domain of competencies, "system organization and improvement," to emphasize the important role hospitalists play in shaping care processes at the system level.

PRACTICE POINT

Example of modification of palliative care competences

By the end of the training experience, physicians should be able to do the following:

- Explain the indications and limitations of opioid pharmacotherapy.
- Determine the appropriate route, dosing, and frequency for pharmacologic agents based on patient-specific factors.
- Promote the ethical imperative of accounting for patient-centered goals of care and frequent pain assessment and adequate control.

TABLE 5-2 The Cognitive Domain Levels of Proficiency

Knowledge: the lowest level of learning outcomes The ability to recall or repeat specific information based on memorization
Comprehension: the lowest level of understanding The ability to grasp the meaning of subject matter
Application: a higher level of proficiency The ability to apply rules, guidelines to new and concrete circumstances
Analysis: The ability to understand content and organizational structure and to criticize content
Synthesis: The ability to design or formulate something new based on available data
Evaluate: the highest level of proficiency requiring knowledge, comprehension, application, analysis, synthesis, and conscious value judgments The ability to judge the value of a project based on clearly defined criteria

When structured appropriately, a competency will indicate what a learner should be able to do as well as the level of proficiency that should be attained (**Tables 5-2** and **5-3**).

These examples clearly show the outcome and the level of proficiency that are expected. The first option, "explain the indications," requires less processing then the second. It can be taught by lecture, webinar, and reading assignments. It can be evaluated verbally or on written exam by simply restating the competency as a question. For example, please explain the indications and limitations of opioid pharmacotherapy.

The second competency, "Determine the appropriate route," indicates that learners are expected to obtain a higher level of proficiency. In this example, learners must apply what is known about the pharmacologic agents, the patient, and the specific disease and risk profile to develop a plan. Evaluation of this competency would require observing or assessing a treatment plan developed for a specific case study or patient. Similarly, instruction should provide opportunities to practice application of concepts to patient-specific examples.

The third competency, "Promote the ethical imperative," is an attitudinal competency. The verb, *promote* indicates that not only are learners expected to be knowledgeable about the value of determining patient-centered goals and closely monitoring pain control plans, but they are also expected to possess the motivation and ability to encourage others to adopt similar clinical care habits. Instruction for this competency would require exposing learners to scenarios that allow them to explore and discuss perspectives and values and develop empathy. Learners need to see instructors modeling behaviors and deconstruct how the behaviors led to or prevented specific outcomes. Evaluation of this competency would require a longer term observation.

TABLE 5-3 Levels of Proficiency: An Example Using the Topic Congestive Heart Failure

Knowledge: The second-year medical student is able to recite the causes of congestive heart failure (CHF) or list the different randomized controlled trials studying different drugs for the treatment of CHF.
Comprehension: The third-year student is able to predict the consequences of untreated CHF or explain which drugs are preferable in the treatment of CHF based on knowledge of the medical literature.
Application: The fourth-year student is able to use the American College of Cardiology practice guideline on CHF to consistently appropriately test and treat patients with CHF.
Analysis: The intern is able to detect hypothyroidism and CHF by history and physical examination of a patient and connect their relationship to the patient's presenting complaint of shortness of breath.
Synthesis: The senior resident is able to develop a research proposal involving patients with CHF to address unanswered questions and possibly create a new scheme for classifying CHF.
Evaluation: The senior attending cardiologist is able to judge the value of the research project and recommend revisions of the methodology.
Skills: The hospitalist is able to diagnose CHF on the basis of a chest X-ray and triage the patient appropriately based on triage criteria that incorporate a 2-minute bedside assessment of the hemodynamic profile looking for evidence of low perfusion and/or congestion at rest.
Attitudes: The hospitalist assumes responsibility for patient care, shows appreciation for and respect for cultural differences, adheres to practice-based guidelines, provides comprehensive patient and family education, demonstrates effective communication with the primary care physician, cardiologist, and other members of the care team so that the patient has a safe transition to home.
Systems-based approach: The hospitalist recognizes the importance of consulting with interdisciplinary teams (eg, social work to obtain a scale for daily weights, nutrition to advise on a low-salt diet, pharmacy to review and reconcile medications that might negatively impact CHF, and physical therapy to assess ability to climb stairs) to facilitate discharge planning and to reduce the chances of readmission. The hospitalist may also lead a hospital interdisciplinary initiative to improve the performance measures relating to prevention of deep venous thrombosis, readmission, and assessment of ejection fraction.

HOW ARE THE CORE COMPETENCIES USED IN HOSPITAL MEDICINE?

The core competencies are used to facilitate training of residents and medical students and form the backbone for initiatives to credential hospitalists. Since 2010, the American Board of Internal Medicine (ABIM) has conferred Internal Medicine Certification with a Focused Practice in Hospital Medicine. In order to be eligible for the Focused Practice in Hospital Medicine program, graduates of internal medicine residencies need to demonstrate the knowledge, skills, and attitudes defined by TCCs and acquired through practice dedicated to the hospital setting. SHM has created resources and educational programs based on TCCs, including resource rooms to guide improvement efforts, and mentored implementation programs to assist hospitalists in obtaining additional ABIM recognition.

Although TCCs provide a content framework for defining professional standards for Hospital Medicine, it is not a stand-alone document and cannot be a static document. The medical education community should continually develop and update competency-based curricula, training, and evaluation strategies to reflect evolutions in the science and practice of Hospital Medicine. Curricula should be accompanied by more robust evaluation strategies to assess the impact on individual learners and identify training gaps. This requires critically reviewing evaluation tools, providing hospital-specific data to physicians, identifying and lowering barriers to improvement, developing automatic reminder systems, and encouraging participation in quality improvement research. Educators should consider feedback from multiple sources, including receiving clinicians, nurses, care coordinators, and consultants. New and improved curriculum in health care systems and structured portfolios should promote competence as a physician and ultimately improve patient care.

To serve as an effective tool, future revisions of TCCs will take into account how the field and practice of Hospital Medicine has evolved and the skills required of hospitalists to provide exceptional patient care and clinical care leadership into the future. Over time, there will always be opportunities to refine competencies in areas such as information transfer, care transitions, and communication with physicians, other hospital staff, and most importantly our patients.

RESOURCES FOR HOSPITALISTS

Journal of Hospital Medicine

In 2006 the Society of Hospital Medicine published with Wiley the only peer-reviewed, indexed journal devoted to Hospital Medicine, the *Journal of Hospital Medicine* (*JHM*). *JHM*'s Impact Factor score, 3.163 is a tremendous achievement for a journal in its 5th year of publication and ranks JHM 21st in the field of medicine, general and internal subject categories. The following link covers aims/scope:

http://www3.interscience.wiley.com/journal/111081937/home/ProductInformation.html.

The following links discuss ethics and peer review:

http://www3.interscience.wiley.com/journal/111081937/home/ForAuthors.html

http://www.acgme.org/outcome/e-learn/

http://www.acgme.org/outcome/e-learn/module4_CurriculumTemplate.doc

SUGGESTED READINGS

Dressler DD, Pistoria MJ, Budnitz TB, McKean SC, Amin AN. The core competencies in Hospital Medicine: development and methodology. *The Journal of Hospital Medicine*. 2001;1(S1): 48–56.

McKean SC, Budnitz TB, Dressler DD, Amin AN, Pistoria MJ. How to use the core competencies in Hospital Medicine: a framework for curriculum development. *The Journal of Hospital Medicine*. 2001;1(S1):57–67.

Pistoria MJ, Amin AN, Dressler DD, McKean SM, Budnitz TB, eds. The core competencies in Hospital Medicine: a framework for curriculum development by The Society of Hospital Medicine. *The Journal of Hospital Medicine*. 2001;1(S1): 1–55.

SECTION 2

Patient Safety

CHAPTER 6

Principles of Patient Safety

Alexander R. Carbo, MD, SFHM
Saul N. Weingart, MD, PhD

INTRODUCTION

Patient safety is defined as freedom from accidental medical injury. Identifying such "adverse medical events" as a source of human suffering, the World Health Organization in 2002 recognized that the need to improve patient safety was a fundamental principle of all health systems. The concept of patient safety offers a positive spin on the more emotionally laden concept of medical error. Traditionally regarded as the result of incompetent or poorly prepared or motivated clinicians, medical error is now understood as a product of poorly designed systems of care that contribute to harm. The modern view of medical error is that patient safety can be produced only in organizations that take a systems-based approach to the problem, recognizing the inherent limits of human performance and the need to engineer the care delivery process in a way that is based on scientific principles. Nowhere is this issue more pressing than in the acute care hospital.

DEFINING THE PROBLEM

Patient safety emerged as a public health problem following the November 1999 release of *To Err Is Human* by the Institute of Medicine (IOM). This report described the epidemic of medical errors in the United States, accounting for as many as 98,000 unnecessary deaths per year. The IOM report described an approach to understanding this problem that relied on developments in human factors engineering and cognitive psychology. By focusing on methods to diagnose and improve systems of care, the report pointed to a novel approach for addressing this epidemic.

The IOM report provoked a broad response. The President of the United States directed the federal health care agencies to review and implement the recommendations outlined in the report. The agency responsible for research on quality of care issued $50 million in research grants. Accreditation agencies such as The Joint Commission developed standards and goals related to patient safety that would be required of hospitals. A group of Fortune 500 companies organized themselves into a consortium called the Leapfrog Group in order to encourage these organizations to purchase health care for their employees from organizations that met high standards for patient safety, including the use of intensivist physicians and electronic order entry systems. Advocacy groups such as the Institute for Health Care Improvement created campaigns and collaborative partnerships to spread patient safety–related improvements. And local, regional, and state organizations banded together to cooperate on initiatives to reduce medical errors. In short, the *To Err Is Human* report helped to crystallize a movement in the United States (and abroad) that brought a new intensity of purpose to enhancing patient safety and reducing medical errors.

HOSPITALIZED PATIENTS

Much of the early work on patient safety focused on hospitalized patients. This occurred for several reasons. Inpatients were judged to be particularly vulnerable by virtue of their acute illness, comorbidities, and the intensity of the interventions delivered. Hospitalized patients were more accessible to investigators for study. And improvements that affected the system of care were more readily developed and deployed in the hospital compared to settings such as ambulatory care, with fewer centralized resources to support measurement and improvement initiatives.

Given the central place of the acute care hospital in efforts to study and improve patient safety, hospitalist physicians are particularly well positioned to serve as patient safety champions in their organizations. Hospitalists are close to the delivery of care, so that they are knowledgeable about how errors and injuries occur. They understand how current systems may contribute to harm. And they are likely to have an informed perspective about the kinds of improvements that are likely to be both feasible and effective. Physician involvement is a critical component of successful improvement projects, and hospitalists are well equipped to participate in a meaningful way.

PRACTICE POINT

- Physician involvement is a critical component of successful safety improvement projects, and hospitalists are well equipped to participate in a meaningful way.

SCOPE OF THE PROBLEM

EPIDEMIOLOGY OF ERROR

Medical error was long regarded as a rare phenomenon. In the 1980s and 1990s, however, sentinel cases brought widespread attention to this problem. Among the most widely publicized cases was that of Libby Zion, a young woman who died at New York Hospital in 1984 after she was prescribed meperidine and a monoamine oxidase inhibitor—a fatal combination. Ten years later, Betsy Lehman, a young mother and *Boston Globe* reporter, died of an accidental chemotherapy overdose due to an ambiguous medication order.

A series of subsequent studies found that errors were common, especially among patients admitted to the hospital through the emergency department. The first large, epidemiologic study of medical errors was reported in the 1991 *New England Journal of Medicine*.[4] The Harvard Medical Practice study examined over 30,000 medical records of patients hospitalized in New York State in 1984. Investigators learned that 3.7% of patients had an "adverse event" defined as an injury due to medical care. These patients had serious adverse events, including those that extended the patient's hospitalization, or resulted in death or disability. These medical injuries resulted from surgical and medical care at similar rates, though the events that occurred on the medical service were more often judged to be preventable. Indeed, about one in four events was found to be the result of negligence: care that fell below community standards of medical care.

The Medical Practice Study was an affront to the concept that medical injuries are rare events. Although critics challenged the results, the findings have proven robust. Replications of the Medical Practice Study in Colorado and Utah (in the United States), Canada, United Kingdom, Australia, Spain, and France all show substantially similar results. Five to 10% of hospitalized patients experience an adverse event due to medical care during their hospitalizations, and many are preventable. Researchers extrapolated the Colorado and Utah study results to calculate the 44,000–98,000 excess deaths reported in the IOM's *To Err Is Human* report.

VULNERABLE PATIENTS

Although all hospitalized patients are at risk of medical errors, certain groups seem to be at particular increased risk. The youngest young and the oldest old are particularly vulnerable, perhaps due their reduced physiological reserve.[6] An error affecting a sick, elderly person may be more likely to result in injury than in a younger person with fewer comorbidities. The same is true for young children. The need to calculate weight-based medication doses confers on children an increased risk due to medication errors.

Other patients at high risk include those undergoing neuro-, thoracic, or vascular surgery. These are inherently risky procedures and often performed on individuals with multiple or serious underlying comorbidities. Patients admitted urgently are at higher risk than elective admissions. In addition, the number of interventions a patient experiences increases the opportunities for a mishap. In the Adverse Drug Event Prevention study, Bates and colleagues reported that the highest rates of adverse drug events were among patients in the medical intensive care unit. This was due to the greater number of medications and doses these patients received.

Medication-related errors and adverse drug events are an area of special interest to researchers and practitioners, since these events account for the greatest proportion of adverse events among admissions to the medical service. Studies that examined adverse drug events among hospitalized patients identified a consistent list of medications that account for a disproportionate share of serious incidents: anticoagulants, antibiotics, chemotherapy agents, narcotics and sedatives, and insulin.

EMERGING AREAS OF RISK

Adverse drug events have been a particularly fruitful area of work in patient safety, resulting in the dissemination of improvements in electronic order-entry systems, pharmacy safe practices, and guidelines for use of high-alert medications. Researchers are now beginning to tackle the problem of diagnostic error. This interest is driven in part by the prominence of missed and delayed cancer and myocardial infarction diagnoses among malpractice claims. Research has focused on the development of methods to understand lapses in critical processes of care, such as communicating and interpreting critical test results, and ensuring timely completion of referrals. Other thought leaders have focused attention on how doctors think. Can we train clinicians to avoid premature closure of diagnostic options by maintaining a broad differential diagnosis? How can we help them to avoid common mistakes, such as confirmation bias or premature conclusions?

Another emerging area of particular interest to Hospital Medicine physicians involves the risks associated with handoffs and transitions of care. Hospital Medicine practice is rife with opportunities to transition patient care to other hospitalists at the end of the shift or the week, to coordinate care with subspecialists and with colleagues in nursing and pharmacy, and to interact with the referring community practitioner. Research shows that hospital discharge is a particularly vulnerable time for patients, and a time when errors may occur for a variety of reasons. Failure to reconcile medications at discharge may lead to confusion on the part of patients. Handoffs to community physicians may fail to occur if the hospital discharge summary is delayed or incomplete. Recommended tests and procedures following discharge are often missed. Promising approaches to address these problems include standardization of handoffs through the use of templated sign-out forms, electronic communication with referring providers, and hospitalist-staffed postdischarge follow-up clinics.

Creating effective interventions relies on a solid understanding of the nature of error in health care, the methods to assess risk in health care organizations, and the tools that are used to develop patient safety improvements. These topics are the focus of the remainder of this chapter.

PRACTICE POINT

- Creating effective interventions relies on a solid understanding of the nature of error in health care, of methods to assess risk in health care organizations, and of the tools that are used to develop patient safety improvements.

NATURE OF ERROR IN HEALTH CARE

Human error is a complex phenomenon, but one that has recently come into better focus. Students of human error have argued that both human and systems factors contribute to error. By "human factors" we mean the environmental, work conditions, organizational, and individual characteristics that influence work performance. Experts conceive of human performance in several categories: skills, rule-based actions, and performance that relies on novel problem solving. When skills, knowledge, and rules break down or are misapplied, errors occur. These so-called active failures can further be subdivided into errors of execution and errors of planning.

Skills are stereotyped behaviors that require little conscious thought. When misapplied (errors in execution), they result in slips. For example, choosing an antibiotic to treat infection but inadvertently setting the wrong rate on the infusion pump would be an example of a slip. Knowledge and application of rules require conscious thought; when misapplied (errors in planning), they result in mistakes. For example, recognizing the infection but choosing to treat with a diuretic would be a mistake.

Everyone is prone to slips and mistakes. We can reduce the frequency of these errors through education and training. However, no one is infallible, and therefore, no one is immune from error. In fact, certain conditions can increase the risk of harm. Workers are more likely to make slips and mistakes when they are tired or overworked, bored, distracted, intoxicated, or ill.

Although all humans err, the impact of mistakes is more serious for individuals whose decisions and behaviors have a consequential effect on others. Military and commercial aviation, nuclear power, and health care are examples of industries where error can be catastrophic. In these settings, researchers and organizational leaders have begun to focus on the systems in which individuals work in order to design defenses that identify, intercept, and prevent errors before they result in harm.

A system is defined as a set of interdependent processes designed to accomplish a common aim. Certain characteristics of systems can allow or facilitate individuals' performance of unsafe acts. These characteristics are often called latent conditions or latent factors. Examples of latent factors include poor training, duty schedules that provide little time for sleep, lack of adequate supervision, lack of sufficient supplies, and a culture that discourages cooperation and teamwork. Analysts often focus on latent factors that represent design flaws for a particular process and that, in turn, allow unsafe acts to result in harm.

PRACTICE POINT

- A system is defined as a set of interdependent processes designed to accomplish a common aim. Certain characteristics of systems can allow or facilitate individuals' performance of unsafe acts. These characteristics are often called "latent conditions" or "latent factors."

Consider the case of a physician who failed to follow up on a radiology report showing a new lung nodule. The unsafe act must be understood in the context of the latent factors that contributed to the error. Was the physician overworked, covering for vacationing colleagues? Was there a consistent approach in place for the practice for follow-up of test results? Did a radiologist attempt to contact the ordering clinician unsuccessfully? Multiple latent factors typically contribute to an accident—and few are apparent until after an accident occurs. When a series of latent failures align, harm can result. This model of organizational failure has been described by British psychologist James Reason as the "Swiss cheese model."

Errors in medicine can be classified in other ways, into categories such as diagnostic errors, medication errors, and communication and transition errors. It is important to examine the underlying contributions of human and systems factors to each. of these categories. These issues will be addressed in subsequent chapters.

ORGANIZATIONAL ASSESSMENT

Health care organizations need ways to assess their performance with respect to patient safety. An organizational assessment has several components, including the measurement of errors, analysis of critical incidents, and implementation of safeguards to mitigate or prevent harm.

Hospitals use a variety of tools and techniques to measure patient safety. Most hospitals have voluntary reporting systems for reporting accidents or "close-call" errors that might have resulted in harm. This approach is in widespread use, in part due to government and accreditation agency requirements. Certain serious events must be reviewed internally and reported to the appropriate external oversight agency. Most hospital pharmacy departments use a similar approach, reporting "interventions" that pharmacists perform when they clarify or correct a clinician's order. Pharmacy interventions and safety incidents together represent an important source of data about errors and injuries, but these methods are subject to reporting bias. Busy clinicians often do not have time to complete these reports and may be less likely to report their own errors than those performed by colleagues upstream in the care process. In some organizations, an increasing number of incident reports is interpreted appropriately as a sign that safety is taken seriously by front-line clinicians.

Given the limitations of incident reporting and pharmacy interventions, hospital leaders and patient safety researchers have examined a variety of alternative approaches. Direct observation of clinicians at the point of care is a fruitful strategy but requires a tremendous amount of time and effort to maintain. Chart review methods are also well established but potentially resource intensive. Since not all errors result in harm, recent measurement tools have been developed to focus on harm events. The Institute for Health care Improvement Global Trigger Tool allows for the identification of adverse events, based on clues seen in the medical record.

Some organizations have access to sophisticated tools that can screen electronic medical records for possible errors or adverse events. These tools examine medication records for events—such as an order for antidote drugs like diphenhydramine, naloxone, and epinephrine—that may signal the presence of an adverse event. The U.S. Agency for Health Care Research and Quality has developed a set of Patient Safety Indicators (PSIs). The PSIs screen administrative records for adverse events based on diagnosis and procedure codes that are included in electronic discharge abstracts.

Once a critical incident or set of incidents has been identified, health care organizations need to cull the lessons that can be learned from these events. Traditionally, this has been the subject of the Morbidity and Mortality Conference, though the focus of M&M has often been on individual performance rather than systems factors that contributed to errors. In contrast, the root cause analysis is a systematic and structured approach to identify the latent conditions that contributed to an error. Root cause analyses, performed properly, create a nonpunitive environment for organizations to learn about the causes of errors and injuries and, in turn, to develop initiatives that prevent these errors from happening again.

These and other tools that help to identify problems and reduce errors will be further described in subsequent chapter 12.

EFFECTIVE ORGANIZATIONAL STRUCTURE SUPPORTING PATIENT SAFETY

No single model has emerged for an "ideal" patient safety program in hospitals. There are, however, several key components of an effective program. Effective programs must have methods to detect errors, analyze events, and implement improvements. In addition, effective programs build a culture in the organization that fosters an environment where reporting, analyses, and improvement initiatives can flourish. Buy-in from senior leadership and physician engagement are particularly important ingredients of the mix.

PRACTICE POINT

- No single model has emerged for an "ideal" patient safety program in hospitals. Effective programs must have methods to detect errors, analyze events, and implement improvements. In addition, effective programs build a culture in the organization that fosters an environment in which reporting, analyses, and improvement initiatives can flourish. Buy-in from senior leadership and physician engagement are particularly important ingredients of the mix.

Recent interest has also turned to the role that hospital governance plays in supporting safe patient care. The Institute for Health Care Improvement, in their 5 Million Lives campaign, recommended "Getting Boards on Board" in an effort to "fully engage the governance leadership in quality and safety." Hospital boards can drive safe care by using the following approaches:

- *Setting aims*: Set a specific aim to reduce harm. Make an explicit, public commitment to measurable quality improvements.
- *Getting data and hearing stories*: Select and review progress toward safer care... at every board meeting, grounded in transparency.
- *Establishing and monitoring system-level measures*: Identify a small group of organization-wide "roll-up" measures of patient safety that are continually updated and are made transparent to the entire organization and its customers.
- *Changing the environment, policies, and culture*: Commit to establish and maintain an environment that is respectful, fair, and just.
- *Learning, starting with the board*: Develop the board's capability and learn about how "best in the world" boards work with executive and medical staff leaders to reduce harm.
- *Establishing executive accountability*: Oversee the effective execution of a plan to achieve aims to reduce harm, including executive team accountability for clear quality improvement targets.[1]

In addition to the concepts previously discussed, patient safety can be improved by engaging senior leadership, and by making data-driven decisions regarding improvement efforts.

Hospitals also benefit from building robust services to support a comprehensive patient safety plan. These services include the appointment of patient safety officers, risk managers, and individuals to support data acquisition, data management, and process improvement efforts. These are usually housed under the rubric of Health Care Quality, though the specific details will differ from organization to organization.

QUALITY IMPROVEMENT

Although patient safety is a cornerstone of medical care, the notion of "quality" in health care includes several other important components. The IOM has defined six dimensions by which quality in health care can be evaluated:

- *Safe*: avoiding injuries to patients from the care that is intended to help them
- *Effective*: providing services based on scientific knowledge to all who could benefit, and refraining from providing services to those not likely to benefit
- *Patient-centered*: providing care that is respectful of and responsive to individual patient preferences, needs, and values, and ensuring that patient values guide all clinical decisions
- *Timely*: reducing waits and sometimes harmful delays for both those who receive and those who give care
- *Efficient*: avoiding waste, including waste of equipment, supplies, ideas, and energy
- *Equitable*: providing care that does not vary in quality because of personal characteristics such as gender, ethnicity, geographic location, and socioeconomic status.[2]

In this formulation, safety is one of several components of high-quality care.

How does a health system improve its performance in one or more of these domains? Many organizations rely on the Model for Improvement, which is an approach used to promote organizational change.[3] The basic steps in the Model for Improvement include the following:

- Setting aims
- Establishing measures
- Selecting changes
- Small tests of change, as in the plan-do-study-act (PDSA) model
- Implementing changes
- Spreading changes

After setting aims, measures must be established to determine whether improvement results from the changes that have been implemented. Unlike measurement in research, measurement in quality improvement is used to bring new knowledge into daily practice. It consists of small tests of change, with many sequential tests, and just enough data gathered in each round of testing to see if changes result in improvement. There are three fundamental types of measures:

- *Outcome measures*: evaluate the end result of a given system or process
- *Process measures*: evaluate the steps involved in a process
- *Balancing measures*: evaluate whether changes in one area result in (unintended) changes elsewhere

The process is then continued with the implementation and spread of change. These concepts of the Model for Improvement and Principles of Measurement will be discussed in greater detail in subsequent chapters 14 and 15.

QUALITY IMPROVEMENT AND SAFETY RESEARCH

Quality improvement and patient safety have intersected in recent years, as quality improvement methods have been applied to solve patient safety problems. For example, health leaders used the PDSA model to develop medication safety improvements for anticoagulants and other high-alert medications. Rapid-cycle improvements have led to innovation in communication of critical test results and handoff communication. As researchers understood the value of human factors principles and system-based design, patient safety leaders have embraced and promulgated "best practice" interventions that rely on these concepts. Key principles include the concepts of standardization and reliability, appropriate redundancy, use of communication, and teamwork tools. Best practice recommendations have been incorporated into recommendations and standards put forth by The Joint Commission and the National Quality Forum. Recognizing that there are limits to human performance, researchers have investigated the use of forcing functions as prompts. Attention has also been focused on the limits of human performance during times of fatigue, with efforts to reduce these effects. In addition, much has been made of the role of expanding information technology in promoting quality improvement and patient safety. Each of these concepts will be expanded upon in subsequent chapters.

CONCLUSION

Patient safety has emerged as a major public health problem. The epicenter of work in the area has focused on hospital care, given the multiple interventions delivered there and the vulnerability of the patient population. An enlightened view of patient safety frames medical errors as a problem of designing systems that identify errors and learn from them, and that build interventions that prevent errors and mitigate harm. A focus on errors as the product of incompetent clinicians is inaccurate and unproductive. Organizations that measure errors and injuries, that learn from them, and that apply quality improvement techniques to address them in turn produce safer care for their patients.

SUGGESTED READINGS

Agency for Healthcare Research and Quality. Patient safety indicators fact sheet. http://www.qualityindicators.ahrq.gov/downloads/psi/2006-Feb-PatientSafetyIndicators.pdf. Accessed December 12, 2009.

Bates DW, Cullen DJ, Laird N, et al. Incidence of adverse drug events and potential adverse drug events: implications for prevention. ADE Prevention Study Group. *JAMA.* 1995;274:29–34.

Brennan TA, Leape LL, Laird NM, et al. Incidence of adverse events and negligence in hospitalized patients. Results of the Harvard Medical Practice Study I. *N Engl J Med.* 1991;324:370–376.

Forster AJ, Murff HJ, Peterson JF, et al. The incidence and severity of adverse events affecting patients after discharge from the hospital. *Ann Intern Med.* 2003;138:161–167.

Gandhi TK, Kachalia A, Thomas EJ, et al. Missed and delayed diagnoses in the ambulatory setting: a study of closed malpractice claims. *Ann Intern Med.* 2006;145:488–496.

Groopman JE. *How Doctors Think.* New York: Houghton Mifflin; 2007.

Kohn LT, Corrigan J, Donaldson MS, eds. *To Err Is Human: Building a Safer Health System.* Report of the Committee on Quality of Health Care in America. Washington, DC: National Academy Press; 2000.

Reason J. Human error: models and management. *BMJ.* 2000;320:768–770.

Resar RK, Rozich JD, Classen D. Methodology and rationale for the measurement of harm with trigger tools. *Qual Saf Health Care.* 2003;12(suppl 2):ii39–ii45.

Sharpe VA, Faden A. *Medical Harm.* Cambridge: Cambridge University Press; 1998.

Thomas EJ, Petersen LA. Measuring errors and adverse events in health care. *J Gen Intern Med.* 2003;18:61–67.

Thomas EJ, Studdert DM, Burstin HR, et al. Incidence and risk factors for adverse events and negligent care in Utah and Colorado in 1992. *Med Care.* 2000;38:261–271.

Weingart SN, Wilson RM, Gibberd RW, et al. Epidemiology of medical error. *BMJ.* 2000;320:774–777.

World Health Assembly. Quality of care: patient safety. Resolution WHA55:18. 18 May 2002. http://apps.who.int/gb/archive/pdf_files/WHA55/ewha5518.pdf. Accessed December 12, 2009.

REFERENCES

1. Conway J. 5 Million Lives Campaign: getting boards on board: engaging governing boards in quality and safety. *Jt Comm J Qual Patient Saf.* 2008;34:214–220.
2. Institute of Medicine, Committee on Healthcare in America. *Crossing the Quality Chasm: A New Health System for the 21st Century.* Washington, DC: National Academy Press, 2001.
3. Langley GL, Nolan KM, Nolan TW, et al. *The Improvement Guide: A Practical Approach to Enhancing Organizational Performance.* San Francisco, CA: Jossey-Bass; 1996.

CHAPTER 7

The Role of Hospitalists in Creating a Culture of Safety

Lakshmi K. Halasyamani, MD, SFHM

INTRODUCTION

The publication in 1999 of the Institute of Medicine report, *To Err Is Human*, informed the public that almost 100,000 patients a year die as a result of medical errors. Since that time, there has been lively debate and dialogue about the accuracy of that measure, but more importantly there has been concerted national attention to develop strategies that will mitigate the rate of medical errors.

The growth of Hospital Medicine has coincided with the increased focus on quality and patient safety in health care. This has resulted in a unique opportunity for hospitalists to be both leaders and participants in identifying the facilitators for and barriers to creating and sustaining a culture of safety. As Hospital Medicine grows in size, scope, and accountability, the role of hospitalists in improving care and safety must also continue to expand.

KEY ELEMENTS OF SAFETY CULTURE

An organization that has a robust culture of safety encourages all of its members to view their role and work through a lens of personal accountability and systems improvement. The identification of patient care concerns is encouraged at all levels and in all dimensions of the organization, and is reviewed with the goal of redesign to optimize safety. In a safe culture responsible actions are taken to improve care instead of inaction manifested by complaining and refusal to be part of solutions.

An organization committed to patient safety has leaders who are visibly dedicated to change and reporting. When organizational leaders do not openly value safety as the paramount goal, staff members are often unwilling to report adverse events and unsafe conditions because they fear a punitive response or believe reporting will not result in any review or change. As an organization moves to begin to promote a culture of safety, a key first step is to address the overt and subtle ways that reporting issues has had punitive consequences. For example, staff who report patient care concerns may not be included in committees or councils, or their opinions may be downplayed because the focus is on maintaining the status quo rather than actively identifying care concerns in an ongoing manner. However, the shift from a punitive approach to one that emphasizes safe system design must balance the role of the system with individual accountability to adhere to established standards and processes.

Marx has identified four behavioral concepts that are important to understanding the interrelationship between discipline and patient safety: human error, negligence, intentional rule violations, and reckless conduct. A systems approach to improving care primarily addresses the errors that occur as a result of human error without any intention to harm or disregard an established standard. As one reviews negligent actions, intentional rule violations, and reckless conduct, the review of the systems within which these events occur must be balanced with individual accountability and intention. Ultimately, an organization that has a robust culture of safety has processes to review and fix systems and to address individual accountability.

Patient safety leadership walk rounds is a process by which organizational leadership makes regular visits to patient care units and clinical areas to collect information from the teams that are doing the bedside work. During walk rounds, leaders should ask questions such as the following: When was the last time you saw the possibility for an adverse event to occur? What safety issues keep you up at night? When an error is made on the unit, is it always reported? Why or why not? Including and engaging frontline staff in this way can create an environment of collaboration between senior leadership and bedside caregivers. However, conducting these rounds is just one aspect of a program committed to understanding and improving patient safety issues. The information collected during walk rounds must be connected to the other mechanisms within the organization to identify issues. Furthermore, the data must drive organizational priorities, the development of improvement plans, and the disciplined attention to the implementation and monitoring of those plans.

In addition to consistent patient safety leadership, another critical element to a culture that values safety is multidisciplinary team training. Team training is the backbone of aviation safety, and the formation of multidisciplinary work groups is central to quality improvement initiatives. However, the translation of multidisciplinary team training in the context of clinical care delivery at the bedside is in its early stages of development and widespread adoption. Much of the current literature focuses on closed environments such as emergency departments, intensive care units, labor and delivery suites, or operating rooms. Team training can take place with the assistance of sophisticated simulation software or in simulation centers. Although these tools are valuable and help to facilitate teamwork training, the value of team training must be realized at the bedside across a variety of settings and teams, most of which do not have access to technology or dedicated simulation centers.

A third essential element to a safe culture is the consistent involvement of patients/families/caregivers in the care design and delivery. Organizations measure and report patient satisfaction, but rarely is the focus to improve patient satisfaction linked with patient safety initiatives. However, when one examines patient care concerns and complaints, the issues identified often include communication among the care team, which includes the patient/family/caregivers. The inclusion of patients in the design of care delivery can help to align patient-centeredness with patient safety.

ASSESSING SAFETY CULTURE

The elements discussed related to the development of a culture of safety are measurable and assessed in survey tools that are administered to employees within the health care organization. Examples of such tools include the Agency for Health Care Research and Quality's (AHRQ's) culture of safety survey called the Hospital Survey on Patient Safety and the Safety Attitude Questionnaire (SAQ).

In 2004, The AHRQ released the Hospital Survey on Patient Safety Culture (HSOPS), which is a staff survey designed to help hospitals assess the culture of safety in their organizations (www.ahrq.gov/qual/patientsafetyculture/hformtxt.htm). Since then, this survey has been implemented in a variety of inpatient settings in the United States and internationally. As a way to compare scores across hospitals, the AHRQ funded the development of a comparative database in 2006. The database consists of data submitted by organizations that have administered the survey. Reporting data to the database is voluntary; however, it is a very important tool with which to understand how safety culture is changing over time, both within an organization and across myriad organizations (www.ahrq.gov/qual/hospsurvey09).

The SAQ survey was developed by Sexton and colleagues at the University of Texas at Austin. It has been used in over 500 hospitals in the United States, the United Kingdom, and New Zealand and has been psychometrically validated for use in critical care, operating rooms, pharmacy, ambulatory clinics, labor and delivery, and general inpatient settings. The SAQ elicits caregiver attitudes through analytically derived scales that include teamwork climate, job satisfaction, perceptions of management, safety climate, working conditions, and stress recognition.

These are two examples of surveys that assess patient safety culture. The link between survey results and clinical outcomes has only been demonstrated with the SAQ tool. Favorable scores on the SAQ were associated with lower ventilator-associated pneumonia rates, fewer medication errors, shorter lengths of stay, lower bloodstream infection rates, and lower risk-adjusted patient mortality rates. In addition to these patient outcomes, favorable scores on the SAQ have also been associated with lower nursing turnover rates. Recent studies show a strong correlation between walk rounds implementation and improvement in SAQ scores of the individuals directly involved in walk rounds.

HOSPITALISTS AND A CULTURE OF SAFETY

Hospitalist leaders and clinicians have a key role to play in supporting and contributing to an organization's culture of safety through involvement in identification of patient care issues, system redesign, and personal accountability in displaying behaviors that contribute to and sustain a safe culture.

PRACTICE POINT

- Hospitalist leaders and clinicians support and contribute to an organization's culture of safety through their involvement in identification of patient care issues, system redesign, and personal accountability.

Hospitalists, as frontline care providers, understand the obvious and more subtle issues that are in play during the complex set of processes involved in delivering reliable and safe patient care. By entering issues into error-reporting systems and bringing issues to relevant organizational teams and committees, the work that hospitalists perform every day can be evaluated through a lens of safety. In addition, as members of interdisciplinary teams, hospitalists can also begin to break down institutional silos so that true care team partnerships may develop.

Care problem identification is an important step in fostering a culture of patient safety, but it is only the first step. If problematic issues, once identified, are not addressed in a timely fashion, the end users who have taken the initiative to bring issues to light will quickly find that their efforts do not result in any responsive actions, and they will stop reporting. The link between identification and action is, therefore, crucial and must be developed and communicated.

The process of reviewing care issues involves multidisciplinary participants and the use of quality improvement tools such as root cause analysis (RCA) and failure modes and effects analysis (FMEA) (for more information on these tools see Chapter 12). Hospitalists can be key participants in review processes and ultimately in redesigning efforts and developing specific interventions and tools. As end users of tools developed, hospitalists' feedback into the tools themselves can be pivotal in the usefulness of the tool and ultimately the effectiveness of the interventions.

In many instances, intervention development and implementation are viewed as the final steps once a care issue is identified. However, the subsequent implementation is actually the key in transforming an unsafe practice into a safer one. The successful translation of a tool and process to the bedside is an outcome that hinges on the integration of a safety culture and redesign process. The safety culture values the identification of care issues and concerns with a thoughtful and participatory review. The redesign process engages the key stakeholders. One without the other results in incomplete translation and ongoing safety and care concerns.

Peter Drucker, the late father of modern management, has said that "culture eats strategy for breakfast"; this proverb also applies when one is referring to a safety culture. His perspective that "in a knowledge-based or service-based workforce, the system must serve the worker" is highly relevant as we review health care delivery systems and the roles of the team members who provide bedside care. The system within which teams work is a reflection of the culture that pervades the organization, and that culture can either be a tremendous enabler of progress or can serve as a limiting reagent that keeps an organization from achieving its potential and its desired outcomes.

An institutional focus on evidence-based practice interventions separate from a conversation about safety culture may lead to improvements in the utilization of specific medications or diagnostic studies, however it does not address the more complex but ubiquitous care concerns that cannot be so easily categorized. For example, a patient with an acute myocardial infarction may have received a percutaneous intervention promptly, but the subtle post-procedure changes in blood pressure might be ignored or missed unless the team is collectively aware and mindful of medication side effects, interactions, and dosing. Although tools such as checklists and alerts can assist bedside caregivers and standardize, specific processes and aspects of care, for complex care delivery they cannot replace the critical thinking and collaboration that both individuals and teams must possess.

Hospitalists as both frontline care providers and leaders within the organization have an opportunity to influence patient safety at multiple levels: the individual, team, and system. To this end, each hospitalist can implement a routine process which reviews key issues in the daily care of patients that can lead to hospital-acquired conditions and infections, such as falls, pressure ulcers, venous thromboembolic disease, and inappropriate Foley catheter use. In addition, if there are protocols or other standard work processes available, the hospitalist should utilize them routinely. If the tool is flawed or can be enhanced, the hospitalist has an obligation to inform the team that has developed the tool so it can be improved. At the individual level, the hospitalist has the opportunity to make a personal commitment to utilizing standard processes. Hospitalists can also help to facilitate smooth care transitions and handoffs at shift and service change by participating in established processes and valuing the important work of information transfer.

PRACTICE POINT

- At the individual level, the hospitalist has the opportunity to make a personal commitment to utilizing standard processes.
- At the team level, the hospitalist can help set a tone that promotes team dialogue and sharing of information. As members of interdisciplinary teams, hospitalists can also begin to break down institutional silos.
- At the systems level, hospitalists can enter issues into error-reporting systems and bring issues to relevant organizational teams and committees. Hospitalists can participate in or lead the development of information technology–based tools and the development, implementation, and adherence to practice standards that promote collaboration. Connecting the executive suite to the bedside is a unique perspective that hospitalist leaders can provide.

At the team level, the hospitalist can help to shape interdisciplinary communication by participating in team rounds, and by engaging the bedside nursing caregivers to the key clinical issues and concerns for the patient. The hospitalist is a member of the team and can help set a tone that promotes team dialogue and sharing of information. This communication fosters a greater sense of care integration and decreases non-value-added work. Many of the team-dynamic issues are uncovered in multidisciplinary team training. Hospitalists should participate in team training whenever they can and encourage the training as part of a successful patient safety program.

Finally, the hospitalist has an opportunity to participate in improving systems of care. At organizations that have electronic health records and computerized physician order entry, the hospitalist can participate in or lead the development of information technology–based tools. In addition, the hospitalist can participate in physician leadership groups that can address the development, implementation, and adherence to practice standards that promote collaboration and a culture that values team member participation. Individual hospitalists can impact the system by reporting errors and concerns within the organization's quality and patient safety structure. System-level change can only come about through interdisciplinary engagement and respect among team members. Although these ideals are discussed in interdisciplinary leadership forums, the proof of their existence is at the bedside. Frequently, when clinical care issues are reviewed, the lack of interdisciplinary communication and coordination is identified as one of the critical root causes. A summary of hospitalist strategies to improve patient safety is shown in **Table 7-1**.

TABLE 7-1 Summary of Key Hospitalist Strategies to Improve Patient Safety

Individual Strategies	Team Strategies	System Strategies
Adherence to established standards and protocols	Foster a collaborative environment by encouraging team communication	Participate in processes to standardize care delivery
Summarizing daily the care plan to the patient/family/caregiver	Adhere to standards of communication and practice established by the team	Identify patient safety issues and processes such as root cause analysis and failure modes and effects analysis
Participating in interdisciplinary team rounds	Support and participate in multidisciplinary team training	Serve as champions of evidence-based practice
Routine communication with nursing about the patient's care issues and concerns		Develop systems that foster and promote individual accountability
Routine communication at point-of-care transitions such as discharge and at shift and service change		Participate in the development of systems to improve care transitions
View oneself as a role model of collaborative practice		

THE ROLE OF THE PATIENTS AND CAREGIVERS IN PATIENT SAFETY

Recently, there has been increased attention on the role of patients and their caregivers in care delivery and patient safety. Thus far, patient/caregiver involvement has generally been as champions of initiatives and as advocates for culture change. The Joint Commission and other organizations have launched campaigns, such as Speak Up, encouraging patients/caregivers to ask questions and speak up about any care concerns.

However, it is not always clear to patients/caregivers what to speak up about. As physicians who care for acutely ill patients, hospitalists are fully aware of the importance of patient/caregiver communication about the care plan. However, often there is little coordination or integration of the patient/caregiver into care planning. As there is more attention paid to the specific behaviors and interventions that care teams should execute, is there not an opportunity to orient patients/caregivers to those priorities as well?

For example, in many hospitals there are initiatives launched to improve hand hygiene and reduce hospital-acquired infections and adverse events (such as falls and pressure ulcers). However, frequently patients/caregivers are unaware of these initiatives, the role they might play in keeping themselves safe, and whether or not the staff is adhering to recommended standards of practice. There is a tremendous opportunity for hospitalists to help shift the paradigm from patients/caregivers as passive recipients of care to active, engaged members of the team who understand the standards to which team members need to adhere (wash hands, round hourly, turn the patient) and help to support those standards.

HOSPITALIST LEADERSHIP AND PATIENT SAFETY

Leaders of Hospital Medicine programs can be a critical voice in advancing the goals of patient safety within an organization. Often, Hospital Medicine leaders interact with other clinical leaders in the organization and can both help to identify critical patient care issues and help to create a framework that shifts the focus from individual blame to system redesign. Interdisciplinary partnerships and leadership alignment at all levels of the organization are essential to understanding the factors contributing to a lack of a culture of safety and also in identifying the elements that can lead to its growth.

An organization's quality and safety infrastructure reflects the priority placed on both the identification of care concerns and their review and implementation. Hospitalist leaders have a tremendous opportunity to participate in the structure in place and work to refine it so that it supports safe care at the bedside. Connecting the executive suite to the bedside is a unique perspective that hospitalist leaders can provide. Furthermore, because of hospitalist engagement and collaboration with a wide range of clinical stakeholders, their contributions can be representative of the team of care providers.

In addition to working with organizational leaders, Hospital Medicine program leaders are in the position of evaluating the performance of individual hospitalists. Performance evaluations should include feedback from other physicians and nonphysicians on an individual's teamwork skills, responsiveness to care concerns, and participation in initiatives to improve care and safety.

SUGGESTED READINGS

Amin AN, Owen MM. Productive interdisciplinary team relationships: the hospitalist and the case manager. *Case Management.* 2006;11:160–164.

Barrett J, Gifford C, Morey J, Risser D, Salisbury M. Enhancing patient safety through teamwork training. *J Healthc Risk Manag.* 2001;21(4):57–65.

Colla JB, Bracken AC, Kinney LM, Weeks WB. Measuring patient safety climate: a review of surveys. *Qual Saf Health Care.* 2005;14(5): 364–366.

Frankel A, Grillo SP, Pittman M, et al. Revealing and resolving patient safety defects: the impact of leadership WalkRounds on frontline caregiver assessments of patient safety. *Health Services Res.* 2008;43(6):2050–2066.

Leonard M, Frankel A. Make safety a priority: create and maintain a culture of patient safety. *Healthcare Executive.* Mar/Apr 2006.

Nielson PE, Goldman MB, Mann S, et al. Effects of teamwork training on adverse outcomes and process of care in labor and delivery: a randomized controlled trial. *Obstet Gynecol.* 2007;109(1):48–55.

O'Leary KJ, Liebovitz DM, Baker DW. How hospitalists spend their time: insights on efficiency and safety. *J Hosp Med.* 2006;1:88–93.

Ranji SR, Shojania KG. Implementing patient safety interventions in your hospital: what to try and what to avoid. *Med Clin N Am.* 2008;92:275–293.

Sexton JB, Thomas EJ, Helmreich RL. Error, stress, and teamwork in medicine and aviation: cross sectional surveys. *BMJ.* 2000;320:745–749.

Thomas EJ, Sexton JB, Helmreich RL. Discrepant attitudes about teamwork among critical care nurses and physicians. *Crit Care Med.* 2003;31(3):956–959.

CHAPTER 8

Diagnostic Errors

Gordon D. Schiff, MD
Mark L. Graber, MD, FACP

INTRODUCTION

A diagnostic error is any mistake or failure in the diagnostic process leading to a misdiagnosis, a missed diagnosis, or a delayed diagnosis. This is an operational definition that includes any failures in the process of care, including timely access in eliciting or interpreting symptoms, signs, or laboratory results; formulating and weighing differential diagnosis; or lack of timely follow-up and specialty referral and evaluation. A diagnostic error is a construct that is usually based on reference to a subsequent test, clinical outcome, consultant's diagnosis, or autopsy—gold standards that are themselves often imperfect or unavailable. Errors in diagnosis-related processes are ubiquitous, ranging from a trivial failure to ask an "insignificant" historical question to overlooking minor lab abnormalities, to switching specimens between two patients, to more serious errors in interpretation of data, which may or may not have adverse clinical consequences in terms of labeling a patient with an erroneous diagnosis or impacting clinical actions or outcomes. Detecting diagnostic errors is critical to correction of the ongoing care for a current patient, as well as for learning how to avoid similar errors in the future.

Although there is a paucity of data on the prevalence of diagnostic errors in everyday practice, studies using a wide range of approaches suggest that the error rate is not small, conservatively 10–15% for many diagnoses. Selected examples and rates from these studies are summarized in **Table 8-1**. These studies, however, have serious limitations. To better quantify the frequency and types of diagnosis errors and their clinical outcomes we need research to supplement these indirect and retrospective data with more direct, more encompassing (ie, looking at more than just one diagnosis or patients who die), prospective studies, similar to those that have been done with medication errors. This is necessary not only to determine the magnitude of the problem in various settings but also to gauge the effectiveness of interventions. Unfortunately, we lack reliable, validated, and efficient methods for carrying out such studies. We believe one future role for hospitalists will be to contribute to ongoing surveillance to help characterize the incidence and types of such errors.

It can be difficult to reach consensus about what constitutes a diagnostic error, and additional problems arise in judging its significance. Clearly we are most interested in learning from errors where there is an evidence-based consensus about the error and opportunities for its prevention. However, in a given case it is often not clear, even in retrospect, what *is* the correct diagnosis, or whether it could or should have been established earlier in the patient's evaluation. More importantly, but often even more subject to conflicting reviewer judgment and limited evidence, are questions relating to outcomes. Would an earlier or different diagnosis in a given case have resulted in a more favorable outcome, and would different diagnostic decisions or strategies prevent similar errors and improve outcomes in the future?

DIAGNOSIS, DIAGNOSTIC ERRORS, AND HOSPITALISTS: THE CHALLENGES

Diagnosis and diagnostic error play a special role in Hospital Medicine. Hospitalist physicians are in a pivotal position to either correct or perpetuate erroneous diagnoses given to patients in the ambulatory setting or emergency department. In addition, hospitalists must coordinate effective and efficient workups of

TABLE 8-1 Estimated Incidence of Diagnostic Error

Type of Study	Study Example
Autopsy	Major unexpected discrepancies that would have changed the management are found in 10%.
Patient surveys	One-third of patients reported experience with a diagnostic error involving themselves, a family member, or close friends.
Second reviews—radiology	10–30% of breast cancers are missed on mammography.
Second reviews—pathology	6171 pathology specimens at Johns Hopkins were reread: major changes in prognosis or treatment were found in 1.4%.
Lab errors	9% overall error rate, including pre- and posttest errors.
Standardized patients	Internists misdiagnosed 13% of patients presenting with common conditions in clinic.
Error databases	Of voluntary reports by Australian physicians, 34% were diagnostic errors, and these were judged to be the serious and least preventable.
Malpractice data	Diagnostic errors are the leading category of cases in most large organizations.
"Look back" reviews in specific diseases	Subarachnoid hemorrhage—30% misdiagnosed initially.

undiagnosed problems or ones arising during the course of a hospital admission. Each day hospitalist clinicians must make numerous assessments on an array of diagnosis-related issues, including interpretation of changes in clinical status; deciding which tests to order and interpreting their results; deciding the likelihood that a new finding represents underlying diseases, as opposed to, say, a drug reaction; assessing the response to therapy (and recalibrating diagnostic likelihoods based on response or failure to respond); and skillfully sharing assessments and diagnostic uncertainties with patients and families. As the directors of the inpatient stay, the success of these endeavors falls squarely on the shoulders of the hospitalist.

Research from cognitive psychology has shown that clinicians use two differing modes of diagnostic thinking, as illustrated in **Figure 8-1**. The first, labeled "System 1" by cognitive scientists, commonly referred to as "intuition," is based primarily on rapid pattern recognition. At a subconscious and automatic level, many diagnoses are the result of quick recognition by experienced clinicians who have seen similar cases in the past. A simple example would be the visual recognition of a unilateral vesicular rash following a typical dermatome distribution, instantly diagnosed as herpes zoster. System 1 cognition is instantaneous, effortless, and very often correct. Unfortunately, it is also error prone, especially in relation to System 2 processing, the more conscious, deliberate, systematic, and analytical process that comes into play when we do not recognize an immediate solution. System 2 processing is also typically effective and correct, but invariably slower and can require more work. Using the framework of this dual process theory, we can understand how certain diagnostic errors simply reflect the acceptance of the first reasonable possibility that comes to mind (System 1), instead of pausing to consciously review other possibilities (System 2). Prematurely closing the thinking process in this way has been found to be a leading cause of diagnostic errors. On the other hand, given the efficiency of System 1 thinking, we would never make it through our rounds list if we worked exclusively in the mode of System 2.

Evidence shows that clinicians apply these approaches in remarkably varying and often idiosyncratic ways. Although most decisions are, in theory, based on clinical experience and an extensive understanding of the pathophysiology of disease, in reality decision making is a highly variable process, susceptible to a physician's personal bias, tolerance of risk, institutional culture, and available time. Over the past 30 years a body of literature has demonstrated that these and other generic cognitive biases play a strong role in medical decision making—biases that can distort weighing of information and diagnostic assessments. **Table 8-2** lists some of the common heuristics used to arrive at a diagnosis, and their potential pitfalls. These primarily affect System 1 cognition, but they can also influence System 2 processing.

While there is agreement that these sorts of errors exist, there is little evidence or consensus about what should be done to minimize their distorting influences. Some argue that humans are "hard wired" to use these mental shortcuts, so it would be more fruitful to concentrate improvement efforts on systems and environmental changes to block or minimize their likelihood or impact. An alternative approach is cognitive "de-biasing"—training that would increase self-awareness and develop skills to resist succumbing to these biasing influences. Regardless of how amenable these influences are to such training, it is likely that a physician who is at least consciously aware of their potential mischief is better off than one who lacks such self-awareness.

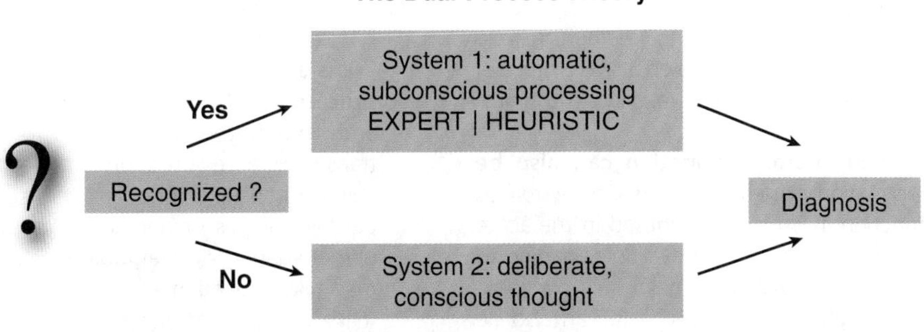

Figure 8-1 *The dual-process model of clinical reasoning.*

TABLE 8-2 Common Heuristics and Biases in Clinical Diagnosis

Heuristic	Description	Pitfall	Example
Availability	Estimating what is most likely by what is more common, recent, or more vividly recalled	Detracts from considering a broad and accurately calibrated differential	Overweighing brain tumor as cause of headache after recently missing a case
Representativeness	Pattern matching to the classic case	Overlooks accurate consideration of base rates of disease	Tendency to ascribe an unusual presentation to a rare disease rather than an atypical presentation of a common disease
Anchoring	Favoring initial information and impressions	Discounts subsequent information that may be critical	Failure to rethink a diagnosis suggested from the emergency department
Search satisficing (Premature closure)	Tendency to accept the first reasonable diagnosis that explains all the facts	Derails search for or consideration of alternate diagnoses	Delayed diagnosis of aortic dissection in a patient with chest pain thought to have angina
Confirmation bias	Seeking out and disproportionately weighing tests and facts that support prior beliefs and hypotheses	Selective and biased history gathering and testing strategies and interpretations	Dismissing symptoms as "nonorganic" in patient with known psychiatric diagnosis
Hindsight bias	Inclination to retrospectively view a diagnosis that was missed as obvious	Blame upstream clinicians for failing to diagnose what others "would never have missed"	In hindsight interpreting myriad celiac sprue symptoms as classic and unmistakable

DIAGNOSIS: CHALLENGES FOR HOSPITAL MEDICINE

Atop these "cognitive" factors, hospitalists face unique and increasing stresses that add to the challenges of reaching accurate and timely diagnoses. These stressors, which are at times painfully obvious and at other times more subtle and unrecognized, call for a constant sense of heightened awareness and vigilance to avoid their potential adverse impact. These special challenges facing inpatient clinician diagnosis include the following:

1. **Lack of prior knowledge of the patient**, particularly a patient's baseline mental status, functional ability, as well as the trust that derives from a longer-term relationship with a patient and family. This deficit goes beyond merely missing a particular piece of information from the history, but rather often means that important contextual information about patients and their daily activities, social situation, and health-related behaviors, beliefs, and barriers are often missing or deficient in Hospital Medicine doctor–patient relationships.
2. **Missing past medical data and illness course**, particularly when acutely ill patients are admitted with inadequate knowledge or capacity to give a good history and/or prior medical records are not readily accessible. Sorting out acute from chronic symptoms and illnesses is perhaps the most important diagnostic contribution an experienced hospital physician can make, yet this role is handicapped when key data are lacking. Complicating this problem is the ever-increasing reliance on shift coverage by both trainees and staff, increasing the likelihood that no one physician has a comprehensive picture of how the patient's illness has evolved or responded to initial management.
3. **In addition to missing data, information can also be misleading.** Interpretation of derangements of electrolytes or renal or liver function may be compromised in the acute setting if baseline comparisons are not available, leading to the pursuit of transient or trivial abnormalities or overlooking more subtle but significant changes. Data can also be compromised by therapy started earlier (eg, negative cultures when antibiotics were started in the emergency department, clean-catch urine culture specimens that are not properly collected, or urine electrolytes sent after intravenous fluids or diuretics are started).
4. **Prioritization and diagnostic focus**, vital for sorting out urgent problems and discerning causal relationships, is complicated in the setting of an acutely ill admitted patient. A major challenge is distinguishing which problems require rapid and definitive diagnosis and urgent intervention (eg, a seeding abscess or leaking aneurysm) versus which are secondary and can be put aside (eg, anemia, elevated blood pressure or blood glucose) while more urgent concerns are addressed. Triage and management decisions at times end up taking priority over diagnosis.
5. **Divergent, conflicting, and sometimes excessive information** from multiple sources, including data from the lab, imaging, and consultants. Given the plethora of data collected during the inpatient phase and because tests and advice are imperfect, this poses challenges and traps; for example, lesions that are seen on computed tomographic (CT) scans but not magnetic resonance imaging (MRI) or ultrasonography, or vice versa. Similarly, consultants will each assess a patient and make diagnostic recommendations from their own vantage point. Collating and reconciling such input when the patient's clinical situation is evolving can challenge the most experienced hospitalist diagnostician.
6. **Transfers can fragment and complicate the diagnostic process.** Handoffs in general are of concern (see Chapter 7), and we note the particular case of intensive care unit (ICU) transfers where attention to stabilization of critical organ failure often takes priority over keeping track of the entire patient and his or her problems. Monitoring or correcting hemodynamic or metabolic parameters in these settings may take precedence over connecting various findings to make explanatory diagnoses. Wading through thick charts

of critically ill patients with multisystem failure makes it easy to overlook (or even stop searching for) underlying or iatrogenic diagnoses.

7. **Trainees and diagnosis.** Relying on secondhand data or uncritically accepting trainees' assessments can pose serious risks. Independently assessing the patient with fresh data collection and thinking is the obvious antidote. However, this often is not possible because delegating and distributing some of this data collection and assessment, rather than completely duplicating efforts, is necessary for efficiency. Thus rounding each day entails skillful balancing of these trade-offs.
8. **Inexperience of hospitalists themselves.** Because the specialty is so young and workloads often grueling, we are less likely to find more senior physicians and experienced diagnosticians practicing Hospital Medicine. While often better versed on the latest medical advances, more junior physicians are less likely to have seen various disease presentations compared to more senior physicians, handicapping freshly minted hospitalists' diagnostic repertoire and judgment.
9. **Base rate distortions.** While some may argue that hospitalists are well calibrated for the "prior probability" of diseases in the inpatient setting, it is clear that rates of many diagnoses are, depending on the diagnosis, either much more or much less frequent than in the "outside" ambulatory world, from which hospitalists are more insulated. This could promote overdiagnosis of rarer conditions and neglect of more common diseases.
10. **Decline of the autopsy and other "feedback" mechanisms.** In earlier eras autopsies were performed on nearly every patient dying in the hospital. This opportunity to learn has nearly vanished as many hospitals have autopsy rates approaching zero with a concomitant atrophy of clinical-pathology correlation conferences. In the absence of this traditional feedback mechanism as well as severed longitudinal/continuity relationships, hospitalists have diminished opportunities to learn from patient outcomes and errors that become evident only over time. Readmitted patients whose diagnosis was missed at an earlier admission are seldom cared for by the same physician or team, again inhibiting feedback and learning from errors. Misplaced overconfidence, considered to be one of the contributors to diagnostic error, is an inevitable result.
11. **Higher thresholds required to justify hospital admission** means that patients with "easier" diagnoses are more often managed as outpatients. Inpatients typically present with more comorbidities and longer medication lists, contributing to the challenge of inpatient diagnosis. In addition, the increasing use of novel, powerful drugs, chemotherapy, and immunosuppressant drugs expands the range and likelihood of more exotic diagnoses.
12. **Lower threshold of patients remaining in the hospital**, the "sicker and quicker" phenomenon driven by pressures to minimize length of stay. Unlike earlier times when patients remained in hospital until a diagnosis was established, often for prolonged stays to "work up" their unexplained illnesses, patient stays are now truncated and diagnostic shortcuts are common. Gone is the opportunity for leisurely conferencing about academic diagnostic questions posed by challenging patients. Simply having time to reflect, rethink, and recognize that a diagnosis might be wrong or insufficient to explain the patient's findings or clinical course is a luxury squeezed out of our busy schedules. Thus venues for reaching better diagnoses have been lost in the more rapid throughput of compressed hospital stays.

PRACTICE POINT

Major factors contributing to diagnostic error in the inpatient setting:

1. Lack of prior knowledge of the patient
2. Missing past medical data and illness course
3. Misleading information
4. Complicated prioritization and diagnostic focus
5. Divergent, conflicting, and sometimes excessive information
6. Frequent handoffs and transfers of care from one team to another
7. Trade-offs requiring delegation and assessment necessary for efficiency
8. Inexperience of trainees and hospitalists
9. Base rate distortions due to differing experience from the ambulatory world where the rarer diseases are much less frequently seen
10. Decline of autopsy and other "feedback" mechanisms due to severed longitudinal continuity relationships
11. Multiple comorbidities, long medication lists, increasing use of novel powerful drugs, chemotherapy, and immunosuppressant drugs
12. Pressures to lower length of stay and discharge sicker patients to other settings

NEW PARADIGMS FOR PREVENTING AND MINIMIZING DIAGNOSTIC ERROR

Lessons from both outside and inside medicine have been applied to the challenge of making diagnosis more reliable. The following sections taken together represent an overlapping group of concepts that are relevant to hospitalists' approaches to the problem.

SITUATIONAL AWARENESS

To understand how high levels of quality and safety are achieved in danger-fraught situations, researchers and quality science engineers have studied so-called high-reliability organizations such as nuclear reactors or aircraft carriers. These organizations are highly adept at diagnosing problems at their earliest possible stage; a key enabling factor is situational awareness. The term refers to expert-level knowledge and heightened perception of all the environmental factors critical to making decisions in complex, dynamic situations, particularly those where information flow is critical. This error-prevention concept is equally applicable to clinicians seeking to recognize and prevent diagnosis errors.

Armed with an extensive knowledge base, familiarity with their patient's problems, and situational awareness of the 12 stressor factors listed earlier, hospitalists can take concrete steps to blunt these risks. For example, being aware of the inherent discontinuity problems of newly admitted patients, extra care can be taken at the transition points to counteract the dangers of inadequate communication and coordination. Recognition that a hospitalist's initial bedside encounter with a patient may be compromised by the lack of a longstanding trusting relationship, actionable knowledge of the patient's baseline level of functioning, or an appreciation of family dynamics, hospitalists can employ countermeasures to protect against these weak spots. These can take the form of triangulating the history (eg, with the patient, family, and primary care provider), or simply spending more time ensuring that the chronology and complaints are clear and consistent.

Hospitalists can also turn these weaknesses into strengths by using the opportunity to take a fresh look at the patient's problems, medications, and course of illness to identify factors that the busy outpatient provider may not have had a chance to uncover, weigh, or investigate. "Fresh eyes" are the key to detecting errors in many settings, and hospitalists are ideally poised to serve this function for the patients they inherit during their hospital stay. Requesting inpatient specialty consultations, or even asking another hospitalist colleague to review a case, offers another valuable way to engage "fresh eyes." Seeking out and weighing second opinions benefits the patient and promotes a culture of sharing and open discussion that strongly promotes a culture of safety. However, beware of the "curbside" consultation, that may introduce diagnostic error with its cursory nature.

INEVITABILITY AND MULTIFACTORIAL NATURE OF ERRORS

The historic Institute of Medicine report *To Err Is Human* recognized the futility of trying to prevent errors by striving for absolute perfection in our health care systems and clinical decision making and by punishing those who fall short. Instead, and seemingly paradoxically, the goal of dramatically reducing errors is best achieved by accepting that errors are inevitable, ubiquitous, and multifactorial and then by addressing the sources of error. Disease features (eg, atypical presentations, insidious course), patient-related characteristics (non–English speaking, competing diagnoses, failure to agree or adhere to recommended diagnostic tests), sometimes chaotic practice environments, and cognitive limitations all conspire to make diagnosis difficult. Diagnostic errors typically involve multiple breakdowns in both the cognitive- and system-related elements, and in one recent study averaged six distinguishable elements per case.

The major system-based factors relevant to successful, accurate, and timely diagnosis are listed in **Table 8-3**. System flaws can contribute to diagnostic errors directly (eg, lost test results, expertise not available) and indirectly, by creating an environment that detracts from optimal clinical consideration. Workload stress, fatigue, and the constant distractions that are commonplace on the ward are all examples of environmental conditions that degrade the quality of clinical decision making. Hospitalists are ideally positioned to identify system-related contributions to error and should play an active role in bringing these to the attention of quality improvement staff, helping whenever possible to ameliorate these problems. The Institute of Medicine identified repair of system-related flaws as the most effective approach to improving safety in health care.

These insights have multiple practical implications, including reorienting attention and redirecting energies toward these underlying causes and complexities of diagnosis failure. By identifying the leading factors contributing to such errors, specific prevention strategies can be better targeted, replacing more general exhortations to "have a high index of suspicion" for particular diseases.

TABLE 8-3 System-Related Factors That Contribute to Diagnostic Error

Domain	Example of Related Errors
Communication	Failure to communicate a pending test result to the next caregiver
Coordination of care	Lack of medical record availability
Availability of expertise	Discrepancies between preliminary and final radiological interpretations
Culture of safety	Repeated instances of the same error type aren't recognized or addressed
Supervision of trainees	Misdiagnosis by unsupervised trainees on overnight tours
Human factor elements	Work pressures, distractions, fatigue
Reliability of diagnostic services	Over reading incidental findings

FREEING ERRORS FROM BLAME BUT NOT LEARNING AND ACCOUNTABILITY

Establishing a "just culture" where people can feel comfortable reporting mistakes and errors without fear of reprisal or personal risk is a prerequisite for sharing and learning from errors. This does not mean individuals are not held accountable for their actions, but when difficult diagnoses, information deficits, and flawed systems play such important underlying roles, staff must be engaged in nonpunitive ways. Since many diagnosis errors are hidden, only a culture that seeks out, shares (including with patients), and learns from errors can be truly accountable. Controversy about the right balance of individual versus system responsibility and accountability represents a healthy tension, one that manifests itself at the bedside of every patient. The hospitalist is in a perfect position to be the doctor to sick patients as well as sick hospitals. This synergizing of clinicians going the extra mile to take responsibility for accurate diagnoses (including documentation and communication yet to be discussed) with behaviors that result in system problems and fixes being identified in real time, is at the core of a culture of diagnosis learning and improvement.

PRACTICE POINT

- The hospitalist is in a perfect position to be the doctor to sick patients as well as sick hospitals. This synergizing of clinicians who go the extra mile to take responsibility for accurate diagnoses (including documentation and communication) with behaviors that result in system problems and fixes being identified in real time is at the core of a culture of diagnosis learning and improvement.

Collective learning is essential and should be based on multilevel sharing of diagnostic error cases at "morbidity and mortality" conferences, safety rounds, and institutional quality improvement discussions. These discussions help identify organizational vulnerabilities and patterns of repeated errors and nurture academic inquiry. Many diagnoses are "straightforward" until uncertainties and test limitations are more introspectively and deeply probed. Learning from autopsies remains an invaluable tool to promote awareness of diagnostic error, and hospitalists should ardently strive for obtaining autopsies (and maintaining relationships that would enable such consent) wherever possible. When autopsies are obtained, safety lessons are enhanced by sharing the findings widely upstream to the physicians who cared for the patients or even radiologists whose interpretation can now be correlated with pathologic diagnoses.

DIAGNOSTIC UNCERTAINTY—EMBRACE RATHER THAN ESCHEW

As embodied in a number of the preceding precepts, uncertainty is a fundamental attribute of diagnosis. However, we lack the required infrastructure, temperament/reflexes, and patient expectations to optimally respond to diagnostic uncertainties. Indecisiveness is considered a sign of weakness, and patients who want answers will seek them elsewhere if we fail to provide them. We are insufficiently mindful of limitations of tests or the variability of symptom and disease presentation. Nuanced, qualified considerations slow us down in starting definitive treatment and prevent us from offering quick and short explanations to patients. Clinical notes are perhaps the greatest area of concern and frustration. Busy physicians lack time for extensive documentation of differential diagnosis and recording of complex diagnostic reasoning; and even if we did have time, our colleagues might balk at wading through lengthy notes. Yet thinking out loud (in notes) can be our opportunity, or what some would even term a "forcing function" to collect our thoughts, pause to think, and convey that thinking for others to error check.

PATIENT ENGAGEMENT IN DIAGNOSIS AND ERRORS

Unlike medication errors, where an undetected or unshared error and any minor consequences may quickly fade from patient awareness, many diagnosis errors have the potential to linger. Months later, when the cancer or the tuberculosis infection is finally diagnosed, it will be harder to ignore previous mistaken explanations for symptoms or findings. Although many ailments are self-limited or respond to nonspecific treatment despite an erroneous diagnosis, the loss of opportunity for specific, early treatment can be problematic, particularly if the problem is cancer, infection, or various other conditions where earlier intervention matters. This is now being increasingly recognized by the courts as a legitimate malpractice claim. More constructively, rather than view patients defensively, hospitalists should see and welcome patients as true partners in the diagnostic process. From contributing an accurate and thorough history to being alert and questioning when they fail to improve as expected or new problems arise, to hearing out and helping weigh our diagnostic uncertainties, patients are our best partners and the most important elements of a reliable diagnostic system.

ERRORS AT TRANSITIONS

Like other medical errors, diagnostic error fault lines are weakest at transitions of care. When patients are contacted postdischarge, in addition to medication errors, there is a significant rate of tests not being followed up or diagnostic information that is not optimally communicated to future caregivers. Rarely is there feedback to the inpatient-caring clinician, and in many hospital systems patients can be readmitted with no feedback or even awareness that the patient has returned to the original team. Particularly when the readmission diagnosis represents a missed complication or a prior diagnosis proven wrong, such feedback is essential for learning. Even when the patient is continuously in the hospital but the clinician team rotates off duty, downstream findings are rarely systematically fed back to upstream clinicians; missed diagnosis or autopsy results are usually heard about haphazardly.

On admission, critically reevaluating all major and active diagnoses a patient carries (from past admissions, the emergency department, or ambulatory MDs) is essential to ensure that these labels are still accurate and consistent with new clinical and laboratory data. The opportunity to nondefensively question or explore a previous diagnosis should be a routine element of handoffs.

At discharge, there must be complete and organized communication of diagnostic information tests and workups, clearly designating tests done but pending at discharge or scheduled to be performed postdischarge (see also Chapter 9). And hospital cultures and systems of care need to be "hard-wired" to ensure that feedback to prior caregivers in the case of diagnosis error is systematic rather serendipity.

THE CENTRAL ROLE OF SKILLFUL DOCUMENTATION

A wealth of diagnostic thinking risks being squandered unless this is thoughtfully summarized and recorded. Thoughtful documentation is essential to convey and synthesize the diagnostic thinking, consultative opinions, and, most importantly, unanswered questions at the conclusion of a hospitalization. A key element is an accurate and thorough problem list to ensure that problems are not lost, left hidden, or unexplained. At a minimum this entails adding all new significant clinical findings or test abnormalities, reorganizing/consolidating problem lists when unifying diagnosis or explanations are established, inactivating inactive problems, and ensuring that the recorded list is "interoperable" so that it can be shared by other caregivers. Capturing the richness of diagnostic consideration, while avoiding undesirable practices that overload notes with copious copied or outdated information, is another new challenge in the age of electronic records.

PRACTICE POINT

- Thoughtful documentation is essential to convey and synthesize the diagnostic thinking, consultative opinions, and most importantly, unanswered questions at the conclusion of a hospitalization. A key element is an accurate and thorough problem list to ensure that problems are not lost, left hidden, or unexplained.

DIAGNOSIS CHECKLIST AND BEHAVIORS TO AVOID ERROR

Checklists have proven benefit in reducing error in a wide range of high-complexity tasks; and given the uncertainties and challenges involved in medical decision making, using a checklist has substantial potential to minimize these errors as well. The checklist presented in **Figure 8-2** focuses on the key error-prone steps in the process of diagnosis and incorporates the concepts of error prevention reviewed earlier. Although the steps aren't necessarily followed in this order, medical decision making typically begins with directly interviewing and examining the patient, and if the diagnosis is not immediately evident, to begin differentiating the leading possibilities with diagnostic tests. An error in any one of these steps can lead to diagnostic error, and multiple breakdowns are common. A recent study of diagnostic errors found that three-quarters reflected breakdowns in just two steps: testing (44%) and synthesis (32%).

THE HISTORY AND PHYSICAL EXAMINATION

Obviously, hospitalists have substantial expertise in obtaining an accurate history and physical examination; but the importance of these steps bears reemphasis in an age of increasing reliance on sophisticated diagnostics. There is no substitute for obtaining a firsthand history from the patient. By various estimates, the correct diagnosis is made from the history alone in up to 90% of cases. Be especially wary of diagnostic errors in patients who cannot provide a coherent, detailed history (eg, infants and children, adults who have altered mental status, or non–English speaking or intubated patients).

Beware of group-think and "pass-through" diagnoses. Teams are susceptible to group-think when the impressions of the original clinician who interviews and examines the patient are accepted at face value by the group without independent verification, and this error propensity is magnified by the possibility that the first interviewer is a junior-level trainee. Pressures of group conformity also work against independent analysis.

Errors can also arise from framing and anchoring effects at transitions of care if you fail to retake the history and rethink the case. In an ideal world, the patient sequentially transitioned from an office visit to the emergency department to the inpatient setting would have three independent evaluations, a process that would tend

A Checklist for Diagnosis

Obtain YOUR OWN, COMPLETE medical history.

Perform a FOCUSED and PURPOSEFUL physical examination.

Generate some initial hypotheses and differentiate these with appropriate additional questions, physical examination, or diagnostic tests.

Pause to reflect—Take a diagnostic time-out:

- Was I comprehensive?
- Did I consider the inherent flaws of heuristic thinking?
- Was my judgment affected by any other biases?
- Do I need to make the diagnosis NOW, or can I wait?
- What's the worst-case scenario? What are the "don't miss" entities?

Embark on a plan, but acknowledge uncertainty and ENSURE A PATHWAY FOR FOLLOW-UP.

Figure 8-2 *A checklist for diagnosis.*

to minimize diagnostic error. In reality, downstream clinicians may simply accept the patient's history or physical findings passed on by an upstream colleague, a process that is inherently error-prone.

INITIAL HYPOTHESES AND DIFFERENTIATING THESE WITH APPROPRIATE DIAGNOSTIC TESTS

The skillful use of diagnostic testing is a key step in discounting alternative choices and arriving at the best diagnosis. With the many advances in the reliability of diagnostic testing per se, most errors in this stage involve shortcomings in communicating test results, choosing an appropriate test strategy, or failing to understand all the implications of test results. Every test has false-positive results that suggest diseases that are not really present, and worse, false-negative results that lead us to dismiss entities that are truly causal and potentially treatable. Avoiding these traps requires extensive familiarity with the characteristics of the tests themselves, and a partnership with the clinical directors of the clinical lab and imaging services. Staff in the clinical lab can provide invaluable help in choosing appropriate tests and making sure they are performed and interpreted correctly. Similarly, radiologists can typically provide a great deal more guidance in a conversation than would be included in their written report.

PAUSE TO REFLECT—TAKE A DIAGNOSTIC "TIME-OUT"

Short of getting a second opinion in every case, reflecting on the plausibility of the working diagnosis is the best tool you have to avoid diagnostic errors. Do I have enough facts, and are my facts reliable? Was my thinking flawed in any way? Are there unexplained findings that don't fully fit with the working diagnosis? Was I unduly influenced by my biases? Did I give the case enough time and consideration?

Recall that the top two cognitive errors are context errors and premature closure. Both of these problems reflect the same pathologic process: failing to think broadly enough about other possible diagnoses. Efforts to consider other options and to think broadly will therefore be successful in either case, and several different approaches have potential value:

- *Consider the opposite*: Carl Popper argued that refutation of alternatives was the strongest proof of a hypothesis. To use this approach in practice, just ask: "Why can't this be something else?" Tests that rule out alternative possibilities can be more valuable than tests directed at simply confirming your original suspicions.
- *Try "prospective hindsight"*: Derived from military planners, in this technique you look into the future and see that your working diagnosis is not correct. What did you miss, and what else should you have considered?
- *Keep an eye on decision support tools*: A growing number of Web-based differential diagnosis generators are now available, such as DXplain, Isabel, and DiagnosisPro. Many others types of computerized decision supports are becoming available in the form of alerts, instant access to reference materials (info buttons), or visual aids (dermatology tools such as Visual Dx). These stimulate consideration of diagnostic possibilities that might not otherwise have come to mind, and have the potential to address some of the inherent flaws in System 1 (intuitive) reasoning.

The habit of reflective practice can help avoid diagnostic errors from faulty intuitive cognition, but there is a price to be paid, starting with the extra time and effort. A more serious concern is that second guessing ourselves might lead us away from the correct diagnosis to one that is wrong. Reflective practice may also generate more diagnostic testing and the possibility of additional errors, including cascade effects, where an incidental finding or false-positive result leads to further investigations and the chance of harm if the tests are invasive. The challenge is to determine the point of equipoise, so that the net benefit of reflection outweighs the potential costs and problems. Hospitalists share in the collective professional responsibility to ensure that resources are not used wastefully, and the quest for diagnostic certainty needs to be counterbalanced and tempered by this obligation.

EMBARK ON A PLAN, BUT ACKNOWLEDGE UNCERTAINTY AND ENSURE A PATHWAY FOR FOLLOW-UP

Diagnosis needs to be recognized as a probabilistic exercise; absolute certainty is rarely realistic. Moreover, a diagnosis commonly matures over time, reflecting the progress of diagnostic tests and the evolution of the patient's symptoms or signs. This longitudinal dimension of diagnosis is quite real and underappreciated; it requires that a process should be established to refine or reconsider an initial diagnosis at later points in time. This dynamic aspect of diagnosis also mandates that patients need to be empowered to raise any "signals" they have concerns about. Perhaps the most important yet underdeveloped diagnosis safety net is active follow-up and feedback. Checking back to see how patients are doing needs to be more systematic, delegated, and automated. Patients and their families need to be educated in understandable and ongoing ways, sharing with them the diagnostic thinking, any remaining uncertainties, and their role in bringing to attention changes in their symptoms or in the response to treatment that would signal the need to rethink a diagnosis or management.

CONCLUSION

While diagnosis errors will never be eliminated, it is often possible to prevent, interrupt, or mitigate more serious patient harm. Through a combination of early recognition, avoiding commitment to irreversible courses of action whenever this is feasible, and keeping the door open to continuously rethink the diagnosis, the consequences of making an incorrect diagnosis can be minimized. Timely seeking of second options, sharing uncertainties with colleagues and patients, and the use of diagnosis checklists and decision-support tools can likewise serve to dampen or interrupt a cascade that might otherwise result in a wrong diagnosis and accompanying treatment errors.

SUGGESTED READINGS

Agency for Healthcare Research and Quality. Becoming a high reliability organization: operational advice for hospital leaders. Rockville, MD: 200808-0022. AHRQ Publication 08-0022, 2008. http://www.ahrq.gov/qual/hroadvice.

Berner ES, Graber ML. Overconfidence as a cause of diagnostic error in medicine. *Am J Med*. 2008;121(5A):S2–S23.

Croskerry P. A universal model of diagnostic reasoning. *Acad Med*. 2009;84:1022–1028.

Croskerry P. The importance of cognitive errors in diagnosis and strategies to minimize them. *Acad Med*. 2003;78:775–780.

Forster AJ, Murff HJ, Peterson JF, Gandhi TK, Bates DW. Adverse drug events occurring following hospital discharge. *J Gen Intern Med*. 2005;20(4):317–323.

Graber ML, Franklin N, Gordon RR. Diagnostic error in internal medicine. *Arch Int Med*. 2005;165:1493–1499.

Graber ML, Franklin N, Gordon R. Reducing diagnostic error in medicine: what's the goal? *Acad Med*. 2002;77:981–992.

Schiff GD. Minimizing diagnostic error: The importance of follow-up and feedback. Am J Med 2008;121 (5A):S38-S42.

Schiff GD, Bates DW. Can electronic clinical documentation help prevent diagnostic errors? *N Engl J Med*. 2010;362:1066–1068.

Schiff GD, Hasan O, Kim S, et al. Diagnostic error in medicine—analysis of 583 physician-reported errors. *Arch Int Med*. 2009;169(20):1881–1887.

CHAPTER 9

Communication and Transition Errors

Vineet M. Arora, MD, MAPP
Jeanne M. Farnan, MD, MHPE

INTRODUCTION

The increasing fragmentation of health care has resulted in more care transitions. This fragmentation includes by site (emergency rooms, ambulatory clinics, nursing facilities, rehabilitation) or physician specialty, which can be either organ-based (eg, cardiologists, nephrologists) or site-specific specialties (eg, Emergency Medicine physicians, critical care physicians). Hospitalists, of course, are the newest site-specific specialty to arrive on the health care scene. Increasingly, hospital care has become a field that focuses on the elderly, with over 50% of patients admitted to hospitals being older and often with several comorbidities.

This fragmentation has resulted in a greater need for care coordination and a focus on transitions, particularly for elderly patients. For example, the average primary care physician who sees 100 Medicare patients coordinates with 99 other doctors in 53 different practices. Moreover, 40% of hospitalized Medicare patients do not have a simple "hospital to home" transition, instead having brief stays at either a rehabilitation facility or a skilled nursing facility. Unfortunately, prior literature has illustrated that communication between hospital-based physicians and outpatient physicians is poor. While two-thirds of primary care physicians believe the use of hospitalists is a good idea, roughly half were satisfied with their experience communicating with hospitalists, and few received discharge summaries in a timely fashion to facilitate safe and effective management of their patient in the ambulatory setting.

In addition to care transitions in and out of the hospital, hospital care itself has become increasingly fragmented due to increased numbers of handoffs with the implementation of resident duty hour restrictions and the adoption of the familiar shift-work systems utilized by hospitalists. For example, for a typical patient, a member of the patient's primary team is present in the hospital only 50% of the time. Hospitalized patients are passed between doctors an average of 15 times during a single 5-day hospitalization.

Despite the ubiquitous nature of handoffs and care transitions, numerous studies suggest that care transitions and handoffs are plagued by communication errors, which ultimately can lead to patient harm. As a result of these concerns, prevention of handoff errors has been the subject of numerous policy and patient safety initiatives. Namely, The Joint Commission made implementing a "standardized approach to handoffs" a national patient safety goal for acute care hospitals in 2006. That same year, the World Health Organization labeled prevention of "handover errors" as one of the top five patient safety solutions, giving it equal footing with such high-priority solutions as hand hygiene. Physician groups have also taken notice. In 2009, six medical societies representing four different specialties (Emergency Medicine, geriatrics, general internal medicine, Hospital Medicine) came together for an unprecedented collaboration to acknowledge the importance of care transitions through creation and approval of a Transitions of Care Consensus Policy Statement for care transitions. The general tenets of effective handoffs include such principles as accountability, communication, timely interchange of information, and involvement of the patient and family members, among others.

Hospitalists have also played leading roles in advancing care transitions. The flagship organization for hospitalists, the Society of Hospital Medicine, has made handoffs part of its core competencies of Hospital Medicine. Going one step further, the Society of Hospital Medicine also convened a task force and released recommendations for hospitalist handoffs. The Society of Hospital Medicine, in partnership with the Hartford Foundation, has also created Project BOOST (Better Outcomes for Older Adults through Safe Transitions) to help delineate the components of effective discharge for hospitalized older patients.

Despite these initiatives, handoffs remain problematic and error prone. One of the biggest challenges to understanding handoffs is trying to delineate the many types of handoffs. To understand strategies for effective handoffs, it is first critical to understand the types of handoffs and the properties of handoffs that are associated with increased risk to patients.

PATHOPHYSIOLOGY: THE TAXONOMY OF TRANSITIONS

The handoff is

> a fluid, dynamic exchange that is subject to distraction, interruptions, fluctuates on aptitude of and confidence in off-going and on-coming clinician and is contingent on the on-coming clinician's confidence in the quality, completeness of the information.
>
> *Cook, et al. (2000)*

While the scope of Cook's definition refers primarily to shift change, the term *handoffs* has taken on a life of its own, with the term being used synonymously with a broader set of care transitions, such as admission, discharge, and even communication between outpatient physicians. Using this approach, we have divided handoffs into those that are either entirely intrahospital or those that are extrahospital—that is, they involve some component outside of the index hospital.

EXTRAHOSPITAL OR FACILITY HANDOFFS

ADMISSION

Hospital admission is a complex process that could include triaging a patient to the inpatient ward of a hospital from the admission source, such as (1) a home, (2) an emergency room, (3) a clinic, or (4) a skilled nursing facility. The admission process itself includes multiple handoffs, such as from Emergency Medicine Services (EMS) personnel to the Emergency Medicine physician, and from Emergency Medicine staff to hospital staff. *Because the emergency room is considered to be an ambulatory care site, the handoff from the emergency room to the hospital ward is considered extrahospital.*

DISCHARGE

Discharge is also a complex process by which a patient exits the hospital after the need for acute care is resolved or lessened. The patient could be discharged either to home for independent living, home with temporary or permanent home health services, or to another facility for ongoing care, which can either be temporary (eg, acute or subacute rehabilitation) or more permanent (eg, skilled nursing facility, hospice unit). Clinical responsibility and follow-up care for the patient can be transferred from a hospital-based clinician (eg, hospitalist, ward attending) to a primary care physician, or one physician could assume care of both the inpatient and the outpatient setting. This type of handoff also necessitates that caregivers and patients assume a higher level of ongoing responsibility for a patient, and therefore often involves active preparation of caregivers and patients to assume the care of the patient. Several social factors, such as family or caregiver support, home health services, and patient ability to live independently may influence how and where a patient is eventually discharged.

INTERHOSPITAL TRANSFER

Transfer from one hospital to another is typically due to either insurance reasons, patient preference; or the need for a higher level of care at a secondary or tertiary care hospital.

INTRAHOSPITAL HANDOFFS

Shift change

Shift change is the transfer of content and professional responsibility from one clinician to another at the end of the shift. One important distinction among shift changes is whether the outgoing clinician is assuming ongoing care of this patient or the handoff is just a temporary coverage for emergencies until the primary team returns. In the case of the latter, the covering physician is often accepting a handoff only to manage overnight emergencies, but planning and execution of care are largely on hold.

- *Signout*: A type of shift change that often preferentially refers to a primary team who is assuming care of the patient and transfers care temporarily to another clinician and that primary team member will return to assume care of patient. Can also refer to the written document used to transfer information.
- *Cross-coverage*: The care that a clinician provides when "covering" a patient whose daily responsibility is assumed by another clinician or team.

Service change

A service change is a permanent transfer of content and professional responsibility at the end of one's on-service time or rotation to a new physician or team of providers who will assume ongoing care of the patients. This service handoff is often more extensive and includes description of the initial reason for the patient's need for hospitalization, hospital course to date, current status, and anticipated plan of care, including discharge.

Service transfer

Service transfer is the change of service of a patient from care of one group of clinicians to an entirely different group of clinicians, usually from a different specialty or ward, to receive a different service that is unique to the receiver's specialty or ward. This could include an "escalation of care" due to worsening patient illness (transfer to the intensive care unit) or transfer to a subspecialty service for a specific management issue (transfer from medicine team to surgical team for procedure and postoperative care).

Lastly, it is important to acknowledge that outside of the United States, in Europe and Australia, the most frequently used term to describe handoffs is actually *handover*.

RISK STRATIFICATION OF HANDOFFS

In considering the various risks associated with these handoffs, a white paper from University HealthSystem Consortium suggests that the following three questions be used to triage risk to patients during handoffs: (1) Is the patient physically moving? (2) Is the handoff permanent (more than just a few hours or a night)? (3) Is the patient unstable? If the answer to any of these questions is a yes, then the risk is inherently higher. Therefore, the highest risk transitions may be admission—the patient is unstable, moving, and it is a "permanent handoff," meaning more than just a few hours. Another example would be the interhospital transfer of a patient from a lesser acuity hospital to a hospital to receive intensive unit care.

In addition to these questions to stratify risk during handoffs, another philosophy that has emerged is the concept of "common ground"—or rather how much knowledge do the incoming and outgoing clinicians already share about the patient? When a receiver may not know a patient at all, the handoff may be at greater risk due to the high degree of uncertainty that can cloud the initial evaluation of a patient. Uncertainty is a definite risk for patients and has been demonstrated to lead to patient harm or near misses and inefficient work in both resident signouts and hospitalist service

TABLE 9-1 Questions to Risk Stratify Handoffs—If Yes, to Any, Inherently Higher Risk

1. Is the patient physically moving?
2. Is the handoff permanent (more than just a few hours or a night)?
3. Is the patient unstable?
4. Is this the first time the receiver is hearing about a patient?

changes. Therefore, handoffs are inherently risky when the receiver does not have any a prior knowledge of the patient (**Table 9-1**).

CORE COMPONENTS OF HANDOFFS

Regardless of the transition involved, handoffs have the common goal of creating a shared mental model between the sender and the receiver. Certain core elements of handoffs include the following.

VERBAL COMMUNICATION

A handoff typically has some element of verbal communication, either face-to-face or over the phone. The goal of verbal communication is often to build a shared mental model for a patient, with a focus on anticipatory guidance and tasks to be done. During shift change in hospitals, this handoff is often called a *signout*. During admission, this could take the form of a report given over the phone between the emergency room physician and the hospital-based physician. When a patient is being discharged, this verbal communication is more often happening between hospital-based physicians and the patient and caregivers.

WRITTEN COMMUNICATION

There is usually some form of a written communication (or "transition record") that supplements the verbal handoff with additional information that could become important at a moment's notice, such as the patient's primary care physician or code status. During shift change in many academic teaching hospitals, this written communication is known as the signout. For discharge, this would be known as the discharge summary.

TRANSFER OF PROFESSIONAL RESPONSIBILITY

A handoff is more than just the transfer of information; it is also the transfer of professional responsibility. As such, some acknowledgment of the accountability for a patient's care is an important feature of successful handoffs.

CORE STEPS TO THE HANDOFF PROCESS

In addition to the core components of a handoff, it is important to consider the core steps to the process of handoffs. In thinking about handoffs as a process, one can conceptualize four basic phases to the process. Modified from a consensus paper for Emergency Medicine handoffs, these four phases would include the following (**Figure 9-1**):

1. *Pre-handoff*: Sender organizes and updates written information for handoff.
2. *Arrival*: Sender stops patient care tasks to conduct handoff. This step also includes the negotiation between sender and receiver for time and place of handoff.
3. *Dialogue*: A specific verbal exchange that takes place between sender(s) and receiver(s). This verbal exchange could either be face-to-face (often preferred) or over the phone in cases when an in-person handoff is not possible.
4. *Posthandoff*: Receiver integrates new information and assumes ongoing care of patient(s).

DIFFERENTIAL DIAGNOSIS OF FAILED HANDOFFS

Understanding the content and process of handoffs is essential to understanding how handoffs may fail. Each step in the process of handoffs is prone to failure as outlined here.

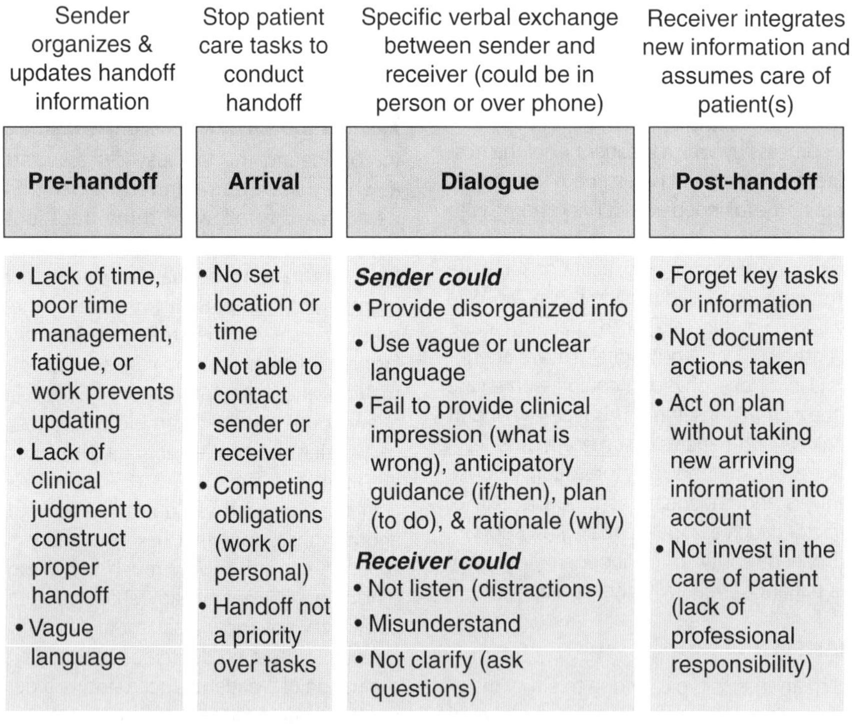

Figure 9-1 *Core steps in handoff process and possible failures.*

PREHANDOFF FAILURES

Since the focus of the prehandoff phase is to create and update the written communication for the handoff, failures in this phase lead to errors in the transition record. Often the inability to carry out the pre-handoff phase is due to lack of time, ineffective time management, workload, or forgetting to do so.

Failing to update the written communication can result in either omissions (information not present) or commissions (information provided is incorrect). For example, in one study of written signouts, 80% contained at least one medication omission and 40% one commission. Over half had the potential to cause significant harm to a patient. Although omissions were more common, commissions, such as including medications that were not actively being used in the patient's care, were more serious. Examples included anticoagulants, intravenous (IV) antibiotics, narcotics, and hypoglycemics (insulin, etc). In another study, the worst event associated with written signout was resuscitating a patient who was in fact not a full code, but whose code status in the written signout was not updated to "Do Not Resuscitate." The same phenomenon holds true for admission and discharge. In one study, 40% of admitted patients had a regularly used medication omitted on their home medication list. Of those discrepancies between inpatient and regularly used home medications, 38% were judged to be serious or to have the potential to cause moderate to severe patient harm. Similar problems also occur during discharge.

For these reasons, written communication that is linked to the electronic health record is often preferred. In addition to omissions and commissions in the written communication, the use of vague language such as "today," "tomorrow," or "yesterday" can result in confusion as can the use of nonstandard abbreviations that either are not understood or can be mistaken for something else (eg, HL for hyperlipidemia, which is often perceived as Hodgkin lymphoma).

ARRIVAL FAILURES

Arrival failures include not arranging a specific location or time to meet for a handoff. Even with a telephone handoff, if a time is not specified, the sender or receiver may fail to make contact at the handoff time. In addition, inability to contact the sender or receiver is a problem that has been reported. For example, hospital-based physicians report difficulty finding contact information for primary care physicians not readily available in their system, often resorting to Internet searches to locate contact information such as telephone numbers or clinic addresses. Work demands (busy clinical work, operating room, clinic, etc) or personal issues (late to work or having to leave work early due to family illness) can also compromise the arrival phase of a handoff. This is especially likely if the handoff does not take explicit priority over other clinical tasks. For example, the sender could be ready to arrive to the handoff but the receiver could be in the operating room.

DIALOGUE FAILURES

Similar to arrival, the dialogue phase of handoffs could result in failures from either the sender or the receiver. For example, the sender could provide disorganized information; use vague or unclear language; or fail to provide clinical impression (what is wrong with the patient), anticipatory guidance (if *x* occurs, then do *y*), plan (to do overnight), and rationale (why). On the other hand, receivers could fail to listen due to either inattention or external distractions. They could also misunderstand the information or fail to clarify any items they misunderstood through the use of questions.

Data from routine studies of human communication suggest that senders often overestimate how well receivers will understand them. Interestingly, this worsens the more familiar two people are with one another. This "egocentric heuristic" can lead to communication errors due to the use of vague language. For example, a husband may tell a wife, "Meet me there after work" but not clarify where "there" is or whether he means after her workday ends or after his workday ends. In his mind, he understood what he was trying to say, but he did not effectively communicate it. This same problem applies in handoffs. A recent study of pediatric handoffs demonstrates that 60% of the time, the most important piece of information about a patient was not communicated despite the sender believing it had been. In addition, the rationale for to-do actions was often not provided. A common example reported was that the covering intern was told to "check the CBC (complete blood count)" but not given any reason for doing so or what to do with abnormal results.

In addition to failures on the part of senders and receivers, information transmission can be hampered due to noisy, distracting settings that discourage conversation, the hierarchal nature of medicine (which can discourage open discussion between providers), language barriers, lack of face-to-face communication, and time pressures that lead to a hurried dialogue.

POSTHANDOFF FAILURES

In the most extreme form, attitudinal barriers, such as a receiver refusing to accept a handoff for a patient, can occur. This could be a refusal at either the individual, team, or hospital level. The key question is, Does the oncoming clinician have the same investment in the patient care as the outgoing clinician? Sometimes this is not the case. For example, night float or nocturnists may adopt an attitude that the patients they are caring for are "not their patients" and that their job is just to hold down the fort until the day team arrives. It is also possible that the physician who is leaving the service may no longer be invested in the ongoing care of the patient or patients, especially those who have been passed from physician to physician in multiple service changes.

STRATEGIES FOR IMPROVEMENT

Numerous and diverse strategies to improve handoffs in a variety of settings have been suggested. Due to the diverse nature of handoffs as described in the preceding taxonomy of handoffs, some strategies are applicable or more relevant to certain settings. Next we summarize some of the most common strategies employed to improve extra- and intrahospital handoffs.

EXTRAHOSPITAL HANDOFFS

One of the primary aims of an inpatient hospitalization is to deliver quality care to patients who are admitted for an acute complaint. However, the success of the hospital care plan implemented is dependent upon maintaining communication between the hospital-based physician and the patient's primary care physician (PCP). Ensuring that the patient's course and treatment, including addition of new medications and follow-up planning, are relayed to the PCP establishes continuity of care between both patient care arenas. Maintaining communication with the patient's PCP throughout the hospitalization is particularly important given that PCPs often regard the communication as ineffective and desire a role in their patients' hospital care. In addition to the PCP, it is critical to empower the patient and caregivers to assume responsibility for their care outside of the hospital.

Several strategies may be employed to improve extrahospital transitions. The three major strategies that have been employed to date include structured templates, medication reconciliation, and patient empowerment.

PRACTICE POINT

- Three major strategies that have been employed to date to improve transitions of care include structured templates, medication reconciliation, and patient empowerment.

Standardized or structured templates

Standardizing the nature of the information relayed across transitions, including medications, pending and completed test results, and major findings, ensures adequate follow-up and ease of resumption of patient care for the outpatient physician. Employing a standardized approach to communication of medications, pending test results, and hospital course can enable more coherent communication.

As patients are discharged, accurate, timely, and complete communication of the patient's hospital course is required for maintaining continuity of care. Successful strategies for easing this transition include establishing required content relayed to the PCP via discharge checklistsor via electronic health record tools that document the essentials of the patient's hospital stay. In fact, the Society of Hospital Medicine has developed a discharge checklist that can be used for this purpose.

Medication reconciliation

When a patient moves in and out of the hospital, medication reconciliation ensures that an up-to-date medication list is maintained. Ensuring the appropriate addition, continuation, and discontinuation of medications at the time of admission and discharge is an important strategy to prevent adverse medication errors and improve care transitions. In fact, the critical nature of medication reconciliation has been recognized as the 2005 national patient safety goal from The Joint Commission, and both the Institute of Health Care Improvement, as part of its' 100,000 Lives Campaign, and the Massachusetts Coalition for the Prevention of Medical Errors have developed tools to assist in the medication reconciliation process.

Patient coaching or empowerment

Empowering patients and their caregivers to take an active role in their own health care is also a helpful strategy to improve patient care during transitions. In fact, previous studies have demonstrated lower readmission rates and lower hospital costs for geriatric patients who received the Care Transitions Intervention, an educational intervention that encourages patients to take an active role in their care and provides tools and guidance from a "transition coach" to promote communication at discharge. In addition, Project RED or Reengineered Discharge provides hospitalized patients with a computer station to interface with "Louise," an e-avatar care transitions coach to assist them with understanding their discharge process.

■ INTRAHOSPITAL HANDOFFS

In the effort to improve in-hospital handoffs, The Joint Commission made standardized handoff communications the subject of a 2006 national patient safety goal requiring institutions to "implement a standardized approach to handoff communication, including an opportunity to ask and respond to questions." Critical elements to be included in this standardized model are that the process is interactive, timely, up-to-date, and contains minimal interruptions. Evidence for these goals emerges from the experience of other industries, trials of technological solutions, or communication practices in health care.

Standardized or structured templates

The importance of the implementation of a standardized strategy is critical for both the verbal and the written component of the intrahospital handoff. The use of standardized language during the verbal handoff helps to ensure transmission of consistent information and allows for interactivity in the handoff. One popular model is the Situation Briefing model (SBAR), which is a technique that originated in the U.S. Navy to ensure the relay of critical information. SBAR has been used successfully by allied health professionals, such as in nursing. Other mnemonics that have been used include SIGNOUT?, ANTICipate, HANDOFF, and IPASSTHEBATON. A recent systematic review of handoff mnemonics yielded 46 articles detailing 24 handoff mnemonics; few were evaluated or validated in research settings.

With respect to ensuring the transmission of accurate and updated information in the written component of the handoff, structured templates, such as computer-aided and electronic health record (EHR)-aided signouts, have been used at several institutions with success. In fact, Petersen and colleagues demonstrated a trend toward reduction of preventable adverse events after the implementation of a computerized signout system. With respect to ensuring the inclusion of critical content, Lee and colleagues demonstrated in a randomized, controlled trial that a standard signout guide resulted in improved written signout quality. However, using a standardized template for communication does not mean it is updated and has the correct or most pertinent information for the covering physician. Not only is it critical to ensure that the information included in the written signout is accurate, it is equally important to ensure adequate time to perform this update.

Face-to-face verbal update with interactive questioning

Studies of shift changes in other industries highlight that the use of face-to-face verbal update with interactive questioning is critical in conducting an effective handoff. Studies of health care professionals demonstrate general agreement with this principle. Moreover, face-to-face verbal update is often suggested as a recommendation for inpatient handoffs.

PRACTICE POINT

- Major strategies to improve intrahospital handoffs include standardized or structured templates, face-to-face verbal update with interactive questioning, an emphasis on anticipatory guidance and tasks to be done, and use of read-back.

Emphasize anticipatory guidance and tasks to be done

Receivers of intrahospital handoffs often state that they need only the pertinent information—what may happen and what to do about it. Unfortunately, the actual practice is often that the sender provides too much information or too little information. As a result, emphasis on these items can be especially helpful to hone receiver understanding of the patient. Indeed, one study shows that after the receipt of an intrahospital handoff, receivers are more likely to remember "if/then" items or "to-do" items more than general knowledge items about a patient. Moreover, the Society of Hospital Medicine Handoffs Task Force recommends that "insight on what to anticipate and what to do is the focus of the verbal exchange" and that "anticipated events are clearly labeled" and "tasks to be done are highlighted" for incoming hospitalists.

Use of read-back

Read-back allows the physician receiving the handoff to check the information received from the sender. Use of read-back is also a Joint Commission requirement for receipt of critical lab tests. Use of read-back has been shown to reduce the number of laboratory reporting errors during requested read-back of lab results. Although performing a read-back of the entire verbal handoff could be cumbersome and undesirable, the use of focused read-back can enhance memory for the high-priority items of a verbal handoff, namely tasks to do, and to clarify anticipatory guidance as already highlighted.

COMPLICATIONS

Numerous complications can arise from suboptimal handoffs. In general, these can be grouped into uncertainty in medical decision making that could lead to inefficient work processes, negative outcomes for patients, and frustration by patients and by clinicians.

UNCERTAINTY IN MEDICAL DECISION MAKING

Several studies suggest that poor handoffs often result in uncertainty during patient care decisions. Our work has documented this uncertainty in both extra- and intrahospital transitions, including among residents and hospitalist physicians. In both settings, this uncertainty often results in unnecessary or repeat work in an attempt to recover missing information that was not present in the handoff. For example, PCPs describe having to "piece together" the patient's hospital course from whatever limited data are available (eg, labs, prescriptions, home health, etc) when no discharge summary is available and when they were not notified regarding a patient's hospital stay. Likewise, hospitalists resort to obtaining information in the chart or from others, including the patient, after suboptimal service change. This uncertainty is often associated with negative patient outcomes outlined in the next section.

Negative patient outcomes

After a poor handoff, patients can suffer from a multitude of negative outcomes. For example, poor discharges could result in readmission or an emergency room visit, medication errors, or missed tests or follow-up appointments. For example, many patients are discharged from an inpatient stay with pending test results, and physicians are often unaware of test results requiring follow-up after discharge. Furthermore, hospitalized seniors whose PCPs were not aware of their hospitalization suffered twice as many postdischarge problems (eg, readmission, difficulty with follow-up appointments, problems with medications, etc) than those patients whose PCPs were aware of their hospitalization.

After poor intrahospital transitions, patients could also suffer from medication errors or delays in needed tests or therapies. Inadequate shift change has been associated with transfer to the intensive care unit and delays in tests or other care. Likewise, after inadequate service change, hospitalists perceived patient length of stay to be prolonged due to unclear information transmitted on plan of care, delay in indicated testing because of miscommunication, and unavailability of the physician leaving service to clarify confusion.

Frustration with care transitions

Although the most important negative consequences of poor handoff communication are patient related, relationships between clinicians and between clinicians and patients may also be impacted. For example, PCPs, inpatient physicians, and patients all express frustration when information is not readily available or identifiable during a patient admission or discharge. Moreover, patients expect that communication during handoffs, especially extrahospital transitions, is occurring. In fact, patients believe that physicians are obligated to communicate about their plan of care during handoffs. Unfortunately, because the reality may differ from the expectation, patients express frustration and even hostility with "having to repeat their story" or clarify issues due to suboptimal communication between their physicians. Patients also report frustration due to the negative outcomes of poor care transitions.

CONCLUSION

Ensuring safe and effective handoffs is critical to patient safety and the delivery of quality care. These handoffs occur during times of patient care transition and include both extra- and intrahospital transitions. To ensure the continued provision of safe care during these transitions, providers should be aware of the types of transitions and the ways in which these transitions represent vulnerability for patients and their safety. With this knowledge, employing strategies to ensure effective communication is critical to the delivery of safe patient care during transitions.

SUGGESTED READINGS

Arora VM, Farnan JM. Care transitions for hospitalized patients. *Med Clin North Am*. 2008;92(2):315–324.

Arora VM, Manjarrez E, Dressler DD, et al. Hospitalist handoffs: a systematic review and task force recommendations. *J Hosp Med*. 2009;4(7):433–440. Accessed May 11, 2011.

Cheung DS, Kelly JJ, Beach C, et al. Improving handoffs in the emergency department. *Ann Emerg Med*. 2010;55(2):171–180.

Coleman EA, Parry C, Chalmers S, et al. The care transitions intervention: results of a randomized controlled trial. *Arch Intern Med*. 2006;166(17):1822–1828.

Cook RI, Render M, Woods DD. Gaps in the continuity of care and progress on patient safety. *BMJ*. 2000;320(7237):791–794.

Halasyamani L, Kripalani S, Coleman E, et al. Transition of care for hospitalized elderly patients—development of a discharge checklist for hospitalists. *J Hosp Med*. 2006;1(6):354–360.

Hinami K, Farnan JM, Meltzer DO, et al. Understanding communication during hospitalist service changes: a mixed methods study. *J Hosp Med*. 2009;4(9):535–540.

Jack BW, Chetty VK, Anthony D, et al. A reengineered hospital discharge program to decrease rehospitalization: a randomized trial. *Ann Intern Med*. 2009;150(3):178–187.

Kripalani S, LeFevre F, Phillips CO, et al. Deficits in communication and information transfer between hospital-based and primary care physicians: implications for patient safety and continuity of care. *JAMA* 2007;297(8):831–841.

Philibert I, Leach DC. Re-framing continuity of care for this century. *Qual Saf Healthcare*. 2005;14(6):394–396. Accessed May 11, 2011.

Riesenberg LA, Leitzsch J, Little BW. Systematic review of handoff mnemonics literature. *Am J Med Qual*. 2009;24(3):196–204.

Snow V, Beck D, Budnitz T, et al. American College of Physicians; Society of General Internal Medicine; Society of Hospital Medicine; American Geriatrics Society; American College of Emergency Physicians; Society of Academic Emergency Medicine. Transitions of Care Consensus Policy Statement American College of Physicians–Society of General Internal Medicine–Society of Hospital Medicine–American Geriatrics Society–American College of Emergency Physicians–Society of Academic Emergency Medicine. *J Gen Intern Med*. 2009;24(8):971–976.

UHC Best Practice Recommendation: Patient Hand Off Communication White Paper May 2006. University HealthSystem Consortium.

CHAPTER 10

Medication Errors

Nicole L. Metzger, PharmD, BCPS
Leisa L. Marshall, PharmD, FASCP

INTRODUCTION

Medication therapy is becoming increasingly more complex as new drugs are developed and more therapeutic targets are elucidated. In addition, polypharmacy (≥ 5 scheduled medications) has become exceedingly common in geriatric patients and in patients with chronic disease states. As the complexity of drug therapy and the number of medications increase, patients are at a high risk for medication errors and adverse drug events (ADEs), or injuries resulting from medication. The National Coordinating Council for Medication Error Reporting and Prevention (NCC MERP) defines a medication error as "any preventable event that may cause or lead to inappropriate medication use or patient harm while the medication is in the control of the health care professional, patient, or consumer."[1] The Institute of Medicine (IOM) simplifies the definition by stating that a medication error is "any error occurring in the medication-use process."[2] Medication errors are particularly problematic when they lead to preventable ADEs, or injuries resulting from medication. The IOM estimated in 2006 that 25% of medication errors led to preventable ADEs. While the majority of ADEs are nonpreventable, it is still imperative that hospitalists recognize the seriousness of preventable ADEs and how these ADEs can be prevented.

INCIDENCE

Accounting for the true number of medication errors and ADEs is difficult since many go unrecognized or are not reported. Even though many databases are anonymous and nonpunitive, many professionals do not report medication errors and ADEs out of fear; institutions then cannot identify system failures and address the problems. In 2006, the IOM released *Preventing Medication Errors: Quality Chasm Series* and published staggering statistics about the number and cost of medication errors. The IOM estimated that each hospitalized patient experiences an average of one medication error daily. Though not all of these medication errors result in preventable ADEs, the IOM estimated that 1.5 million ADEs occur annually with 390,000–450,000 occurring within the hospital setting. Another study at a large academic medical center found that 2 of every 100 admitted patients experienced a preventable ADE resulting in $2.8 million in additional costs to the institution. Due to underreporting and underrecognition, these estimates likely underestimate the true number of medication errors and ADEs. Billions of additional dollars are spent each year as a result of medication errors and preventable ADEs. Identifying common error types and implementing strategies that reduce preventable errors and ADEs are the first steps to reducing the number and cost of errors.

COMMON ERROR TYPES

There are two ways to classify medication errors: commission errors that result from an action (ie, wrong dose or wrong route) and omission errors that result from no action (ie, missed doses or untreated indications). Both of these error types may occur during any step in the medication use process; however, most errors occur during prescribing and medication administration.

PRESCRIBING ERRORS

Background

Hospital prescribing errors occurred at a rate of 0.3 per patient per day as reported by the IOM in 2006. Another study reported that approximately 1% of prescribing errors resulted in harm to hospitalized patients.[3] Commission-related prescribing errors include selecting the wrong drug, wrong dose, wrong route of administration, wrong frequency, wrong dosage form, or entering an order on the wrong patient. Prescribing errors of omission include missing pertinent patient information (allergies, height, weight, previous ADEs, diagnoses, and home medications). Writing a safe medication order involves several steps, and physicians can reduce prescribing errors by clearly printing handwritten orders and including all necessary components: medication name, dose, route, frequency, and any special instructions, while avoiding ambiguous abbreviations and phrases. The physician can improve accuracy and completeness by taking additional time to review the order prior to signing it and sending it to the pharmacy.

Drug information

Prescribing errors and preventable ADEs may also arise from deficits in convenient drug information. The Internet program Epocrates provides a free drug information database that is downloadable to handheld devices, allowing convenient and efficient access to dosing guidelines and basic drug information. More comprehensive drug information databases, such as Lexi-Drugs by Lexi-Comp and Micromedex by Thomson Reuters, are available for purchase and download to handheld devices. Some health care institutions have subscriptions to these databases that allow providers to download handheld versions free of charge. In addition, physicians may consult with pharmacists for help with complex medication reconciliation, polypharmacy minimization, complicated medication selection and dosing, and drug information requests. The pharmacist can provide valuable information regarding medication therapy management, therapeutic drug monitoring, and drug interactions. Team-based or unit-based clinical pharmacists can provide point-of-care drug information, are experts on safe medication use, and can aid physicians in appropriate drug selection and dosing. The Institute for Safe Medication Practices (ISMP) publishes a list of high-alert medications that generate significant patient harm when used incorrectly (**Table 10-1**). Prescribers should exercise caution when prescribing these agents and ensure that the patient orders are clearly, accurately, and appropriately written. Prescribers should also comply with institution-specific cautions and guidelines for prescribing high alert medications.

Computerized physician order entry

Benefits: Computerized physician order entry (CPOE) has been shown to reduce inpatient prescribing errors; however, the evidence is limited. One study reported that CPOE could decrease serious medication prescribing errors by up to 55%.[4] A systematic review of multiple studies evaluating CPOE showed that 23 of 25 studies reported a significant relative risk reduction in medication errors, 6 of 9 studies reported a significant relative risk reduction in potential ADEs, and 4 of 6 studies reported a significant relative risk reduction in ADEs. Though the authors reported several study limitations and included studies with weak designs, the overall conclusion was that CPOE appears effective in reducing medication errors and ADEs.[5] Data regarding error severity are scant; however, some literature reports CPOE decreases both major and minor prescribing errors. Computerized physician order entry provides the prescriber with preset choices for commonly used medications and doses, which may aid in proper dose selection and reduce errors in order writing. Prescribers may also benefit from a CPOE-based clinical decision support system, such as allergy and drug interaction screening, dosing calculators, and drug information resources, which can result in safer medication and dosing selection. A subgroup analysis from a systematic review of CPOE studies showed that 14 studies with advanced clinical decision support systems reported greater relative risk reductions in medication errors compared to studies with limited to no decision support.

Risks: Though CPOE systems may reduce many types of medication errors, they may also be responsible for generating new error types. Overuse of low-importance and irrelevant clinical decision support alerts may lead to prescriber alert fatigue, which results in prescribers ignoring potentially serious alerts. High-sensitivity alerts should be implemented for critical warnings to minimize alert fatigue. Prescribers may accidentally select the wrong medication from the drop-down menu, especially when look-alike medications are listed in alphabetical order. Many institutions have included "Tall Man" letters into their CPOE systems to reduce the likelihood of a prescriber selecting the wrong drug (eg, levoFLOXACIN and leveTIRACETAM or hydrALAzine and hydrOXYzine). Duplicate orders have been a reported problem with CPOE systems since order entry screens may make it difficult to see what has already been entered for a patient. Computerized physician order entry alone will not alleviate all types of errors. A study in France showed that even after implementation of CPOE with a clinical decision support system, team-based pharmacists were still able to identify 33 drug-related problems per 100 admissions. Pharmacists sent identified drug-related problems through CPOE to a patient's medical record for physician review. Therefore, the authors of the study recommended the inclusion of pharmacists on medical rounds to identify drug-related problems.[6]

TRANSCRIBING ERRORS

Background

Transcribing errors occur when a written or verbal order is inappropriately translated and dispensed. Transcribing errors often result from illegible handwriting, look-alike/sound-alike medications, and inappropriate abbreviations. Computerized physician order entry can significantly reduce transcription errors by eliminating handwritten orders and prompting prescribers to enter all pertinent information to avoid ambiguous or incomplete orders.

Look-alike/sound-alike medications

The Joint Commission compiles lists for problematic look-alike/sound-alike medications based on specific practice settings. **Table 10-2** lists problem medications for the hospitalist. The look-alike/sound-alike medications pose significant risk for generating medication errors, especially when combined with illegible handwriting and unclear verbal communication. In addition, the U.S. Food and Drug Administration (FDA) utilizes people and computer software to review medication names submitted for new drugs prior to approval to reduce the number of look-alike/sound-alike medications. The FDA also monitors medication error reports resulting from drug name confusion on approved drugs. The FDA may require pharmaceutical companies to change a product's brand name after initial marketing when errors based upon the product name being too similar to another product already on the market are reported. For example, Altocor (lovastatin) was being confused with Advicor (lovastatin/niacin) and, subsequently, Altocor's name was changed to Altoprev. Galantamine, an acetylcholinesterase inhibitor for Alzheimer disease, was initially marketed as Reminyl but was subsequently changed to Razadyne when errors resulted from confusion with Amaryl (glimepiride), a sulfonylurea for diabetes.

Communication clarity

These safeguards help to reduce the risk of medication errors; however, clear written and verbal communication is also imperative. The Joint Commission publishes a "Do Not Use" list to reduce use of error-prone abbreviations and symbols in medical practice,

TABLE 10-1 ISMP High Alert Medication List

Classes/categories of medications
Adrenergic agonists, IV (eg, epinephrine, phenylephrine, norepinephrine)
Adrenergic antagonists, IV (eg, propranolol, metoprolol, labetalol)
Anesthetic agents, general, inhaled and IV (eg, propofol, ketamine)
Antiarrhythmics, IV (eg, lidocaine, amiodarone)
Antithrombotic agents (anticoagulants), including warfarin, low-molecular-weight heparin, IV unfractionated heparin, Factor Xa inhibitors (fondaparinux), direct thrombin inhibitors (eg, argatroban, lepirudin, bivalirudin), thrombolytics (eg, alteplase, reteplase, tenecteplase), and glycoprotein IIb/IIIa inhibitors (eg, eptifibatide)
Cardioplegic solutions
Chemotherapeutic agents, parenteral and oral
Dextrose, hypertonic, 20% or greater
Dialysis solutions, peritoneal and hemodialysis
Epidural or intrathecal medications
Hypoglycemics, oral
Inotropic medications, IV (eg, digoxin, milrinone)
Liposomal forms of drugs (eg, liposomal amphotericin B) and conventional counterparts (eg, amphotericin B deoxycholate)
Moderate sedation agents, IV (eg, midazolam)
Moderate sedation agents, oral, for children (eg, chloral hydrate)
Narcotics/opiates, IV, transdermal, and oral (including liquid concentrates, immediate and sustained-release formulations)
Neuromuscular blocking agents (eg, succinylcholine, rocuronium, vecuronium)
Radiocontrast agents, IV
Total parenteral nutrition solutions
Specific medications
Colchicine injection*
Epoprostenol (Flolan), IV
Insulin, subcutaneous and IV
Magnesium sulfate injection
Methotrexate, oral, nononcologic use
Opium tincture
Oxytocin, IV
Nitroprusside sodium for injection
Potassium chloride for injection concentrate
Potassium phosphates injection
Promethazine, IV
Sodium chloride for injection, hypertonic (greater than 0.9% concentration)
Sterile water for injection, inhalation, and irrigation (excluding pour bottles) in containers of 100 mL or more
Background
Based on error reports submitted to the USP-ISMP Medication Errors Reporting Program, reports of harmful errors in the literature, and input from practitioners and safety experts, ISMP created and periodically updates a list of potential high-alert medications. During February–April 2007, 770 practitioners responded to an ISMP survey designed to identify which medications were most frequently considered high-alert drugs by individuals and organizations. Further, to assure relevance and completeness, the clinical staff at ISMP, members of our advisory board, and safety experts throughout the U.S. were asked to review the potential list. This list of drugs and drug categories reflects the collective thinking of all who provided input.

*Although colchicine injection should no longer be used, it will remain on the list until shipments of unapproved colchicine injection cease in August 2008. For details, please visit www.fda.gov/bbs/topics/NEWS/2008/NEW01791.html.

Used with permission from the Institute of Safe Medication Practices.

as listed in **Table 10-3**. For example, the popular abbreviation *QD*, has been mistaken for *QOD* or *QID* during order transcription. Therefore, The Joint Commission recommends using "daily" in order to improve clarity. Abbreviations help to simplify and expedite the order-writing process, but taking a couple of extra moments to ensure order clarity by printing neatly and spelling out any potentially confusing instructions may minimize the risk for medication errors. For verbal orders and critical test results, The Joint Commission mandates the "read-back and verify" method, which requires the person receiving the verbal order to write down the order and then read the entire order back to the provider and ask for confirmation of accuracy. Providers may find it frustrating when they are in a hurry to have a nurse or pharmacist read back an entire order; however, this crucial step allows a double check prior to order entry and dispensing. For example, a verbal order was called in to an outpatient pharmacy for levofloxacin 500 mg

TABLE 10-2 Look-Alike/Sound-Alike Medications for Hospitals—The Joint Commission

Generic Name
Concentrated morphine liquid and conventional morphine liquid
Ephedrine and epinephrine
Hydromorphone and morphine injection
Hydroxyzine and hydralazine
Insulin preparations
Liposomal daunorubicin and doxorubicin and conventional daunorubicin and doxorubicin
Liposomal amphotericin B and conventional amphotericin B
Meformin and metronidazole
Oxycodone CR (OxyContin) and Oxycodone IR
Vinblastine and vincristine

National patient safety goal: identify and, at a minimum, annually review a list of look-alike, sound-alike drugs used in the organization, and take action to prevent errors involving the interchange of these drugs 2006–2008. The Joint Commission. (Accessed January 4, 2010 at http://www.jointcommission.org/NR/rdonlyres/C92AAB3F-A9BD-431C-8628-11DD2D1D53CC/0/LASA.pdf.)

po daily for 10 days. The outpatient pharmacist transcribed the order as levetiracetam 500 mg po daily. It wasn't until the pharmacist read back the order that the error was identified. The error likely occurred due to the sound-alike nature of the generic medication names and the similar dosing. Without utilizing the "read-back and verify" strategy, the patient would have experienced a serious medication error, likely resulting in an ADE.

DISPENSING ERRORS

Potential causes

Dispensing errors occur after transcription has taken place and may include the pharmacist sending the wrong medication or wrong dose to the floor or labeling a medication with the incorrect patient's name. Dispensing errors may occur during the compounding of specialized medication dosage forms or in the preparation of intravenous medications. Look-alike/sound-alike medications also increase the likelihood of medication errors. Many institutions have chosen to separate look-alike/sound-alike medications on the pharmacy shelves to avoid dispensing errors and have also included "Tall Man" lettering to differentiate between products whose names are similar.

Inappropriately labeled medications may also lead to medication errors. The Joint Commission, in National Patient Safety Goal (NPSG) 03.04.01, requires that all medications be labeled with the medication name, strength, amount, and expiration date and that unlabeled or inappropriately labeled medications be discarded. This should be enforced in all areas of the hospital, such as the intravenous admixture room or on the floor after a nurse draws up an intravenous medication into a syringe and does not administer it immediately. In addition, with the advent of floor-based, computerized dispensing cabinets, such as Pyxis, there have been serious medication errors where the wrong medication was stocked by pharmacy technicians. Six infants were injured in Indiana in 2006 and three were killed when adult-strength heparin (10,000 units/mL) was stocked by mistake in the neonatal intensive care unit instead of heparin flushes (10 units/mL). Dispensing errors occurred before the advent of computerized cabinets and occur with floor stock systems as well. Recently another heparin overdose occurred and was widely publicized in California when actor Dennis Quaid's infant twins were administered heparin flushes from an adult concentration vial. Though the vials were labeled differently, they looked alike. One product displayed a light blue label and the other displayed a dark blue label, thus increasing the potential for dispensing and administration-related errors.

Error prevention strategies

Dispensing errors can have devastating consequences for patients and, thus, it is imperative that pharmacists adopt a thorough and consistent approach to verifying medications prior to floor delivery. Thorough pharmacist review, if done correctly, can reduce dispensing errors. Institutions need reliable processes in place to avoid dispensing errors for high-risk medications. At the least, pharmacists should use two identifiers to compare an order with the dispensed product to ensure it is labeled for the correct patient. Pharmacists should review the drug name, dose, route, frequency, and expiration date on each order and dispensed product prior to sending the medication to the floor for patient administration. Allergy, laboratory review, drug interaction, and therapeutic duplication screening should be performed by the pharmacist prior to entering and/or verifying medication orders. Checklists and forcing functions built into the dispensing process for high-risk medications can reduce the chance for human error. Chemotherapeutic agent orders should require two pharmacists to independently review the order and double check any dosing calculations to avoid life-threatening errors. Distractions in the order entry/verification and dispensing areas should be minimized. There should be institutionwide quality assurance measures that ensure that once the pharmacist checks a prescription it is delivered to the right patient or stocked in the appropriate dispensing cabinet drawer.

TABLE 10-3 Unapproved Abbreviations by The Joint Commission

Unapproved Abbreviation	Substitution	Explanation
U (unit)	Use "unit"	May be confused with "0," "4," or "cc"
IU (International Unit)	Use "International Unit"	May be confused with "10" or "IV"
QD, q.d., qd (every day) Q.O.D, QOD, q.o.d, qod (every other day)	Use "daily" Use "every other day"	May be interchanged mistakenly. Periods may be confused with "I"
Trailing zero (X.0 mg)*	Use "X mg"	Decimal point is omitted
Lack of leading zero (.X mg)	Use "0.X mg"	Decimal point is omitted
MS (morphine sulfate)	Use "morphine sulfate"	Confused with magnesium sulfate
MSO_4 and $MgSO_4$	Use "morphine sulfate" or "magnesium sulfate"	Confused for one another

*Trailing zeros can be used in laboratory result reporting, imaging measurements, and catheter/tube sizing. They should not be used in medication orders or medication-related documentation.

Official do not use list.

ADMINISTRATION ERRORS

Background

Administration errors and prescribing errors are the two most common types of medication errors. In one study, prescribing or ordering errors accounted for 56% of preventable ADEs, and administration errors accounted for 34% of preventable ADEs.[7] The Institute of Medicine estimated in 2006 that each hospitalized patient experiences one administration-related error each day based on an administration error rate of 11% combined with the average patient receiving 10 or more medication doses per day.[2] Administration errors may include being administered the wrong medication, being administered the correct medication but the wrong dose, route, time, frequency, or rate of administration. Administration errors also include inappropriate mixing of medications upon administration, inappropriate crushing of medications, and giving the medication to the wrong patient. Administration errors are less likely to be "near misses" than other types of errors since administration is the final step in the medication use process.

Error prevention strategies

Patient identifiers and order instructions: To ensure that medications are administered to the correct patient, The Joint Commission's NPSG 01.01.01 requires that two patient identifiers be used to confirm a patient's identity before medication administration. In addition, prescribers should include specific instructions for administration to reduce order ambiguity and improve patient safety. For example, a prescriber may minimize rates of hypotension and bradycardia with intravenous antihypertensive medications by specifying hold parameters, such as hold for BP < 110/60 mm Hg or HR < 60 bpm. Another example is providing specific instructions to the nurse for administration of opioid pain relievers. Instead of prescribing range dosing, for example, oxycodone 5 mg: 1–2 tablets every 6 hours as needed for pain, the physician may elect to write the following: give oxycodone 5 mg po every 6 hours as needed for pain score of 4–7 and give oxycodone 10 mg po every 6 hours as needed for pain score of 8–10. These instructions provide the nurse with specific guidelines for safer medication administration.

Administration technology: Advances in technology have also improved medication administration safety. Automated dispensing cabinets, computerized intravenous infusion pumps, electronic medication administration records (eMAR), and bar coding have all been touted to improve the safety of medication administration.

Automated dispensing cabinets: Automated dispensing cabinets, such as Pyxis and Acu-DoseRx, have been adopted by the majority of U.S. hospitals, according to a 2008 survey conducted by the American Society of Health-System Pharmacists (ASHP).[8] The majority of hospitals with automated dispensing cabinets use patient-specific profiles, which only allow the nurse to remove ordered medications for a given patient. Some emergency medications are available via nurse override and can be removed before a physician order is entered and verified. Benefits to automated dispensing cabinets may include: minimizing the time between order verification by the pharmacist and medication administration, decreasing labor costs, decreasing dispensing errors, and improving the medication charge capture. Automated dispensing cabinets require identification and passwords for access providing a trail for controlled substances and other high-cost, high-risk medications. Lexi-Comp, a drug information database, is available for some automated dispensing cabinet models, allowing nurses to access information about administration, ADEs, and monitoring parameters prior to administering the medication to a patient. However, drug-information databases must be updated, and nurses must use their own clinical knowledge and judgment in addition to the information provided by drug information programs. Automated dispensing cabinets have streamlined medication dispensing and may prevent medication errors.

Smart pumps: Computerized intravenous infusion pumps, or "smart" pumps, are point-of-care devices that contain institution-specific, electronic drug libraries with set dosing ranges and alerts that provide safeguards against improper use of intravenous medications. Approximately 60% of hospitals reported implementing smart pump technology and 80% of hospitals with 600 or more beds had smart pumps in a 2008 survey by ASHP.[8] Traditional pumps can be programmed incorrectly by nurses, for example, if they mistakenly input milligrams instead of micrograms or insert a decimal point in the wrong place. These errors can have life-threatening consequences. In contrast, smart pump libraries alert the nurse when an entered medication is outside of the programmed range. There are varying levels of alerts. Some alerts, "soft alerts," require a nurse to confirm the programmed rate before proceeding, whereas others contain "hard" stops that require the nurse to reprogram the pump before any medication is infused. Many smart pumps require a nurse to verify the patient's weight, drug name, diluent volume, drug amount, dose, route, and infusion rate. One smart pump will allow programming for up to four intravenous medications simultaneously. Drug names scrolling across the pump along with the infusion rate have replaced older methods of identification, such as handwritten labels on colored tape to identify the infusing medications. Smart pumps also contain continuous quality improvement logs that record near misses and overrides that are downloadable for clinician review.

Electronic medication administration records and bar code–enabled point-of-care technology: Use of eMAR in combination with bar code–enabled point-of-care technology (BPOC) is a method of ensuring medication administration safety. This combination reduces the risk of order transcription errors on paper MARs, includes real-time updates, and requires a nurse to verify a patient's identity and electronically cross-reference the eMAR prior to medication administration. Color coding is used in eMARs to signal it is time to administer a medication, a medication is overdue, or a medication needs charting. The FDA requires all prescription medications and commonly used over-the-counter medications in hospitals to have bar codes to minimize medication errors, though a 2008 survey of hospitals reported only 25.1% have implemented BPOC.[8] A unique bar code is assigned to unit dose medications, nurses, and patient wristbands, and the data associated with each of those bar codes are electronically stored. With a BPOC system, a pharmacist enters an order that appears on an eMAR; and the nurse is then required to log on, scan the patient's wristband, and scan the medication to be administered. The scanned medication is compared in real time with the patient's eMAR, and if a mismatch occurs between the patient identification, medication name, dose, route, or administration time the nurse receives an alert. An eMAR and BPOC system, if used properly, should prevent the wrong patient from getting a medication; the wrong dose, drug, route, or frequency from being administered; or the patient receiving discontinued orders, thus significantly reducing the risk of administration-related errors. A study conducted at Brigham and Women's Hospital showed that implementation of BPOC decreased potential ADEs from 0.19% of dispensed doses to 0.07% of dispensed doses, leading to a total decrease of 7260 potential ADEs annually.[9] A follow-up cost-benefit analysis revealed that BPOC could prevent 517 ADEs annually, leading to a 5-year net benefit of 3.49 million dollars. A second study at Brigham and Women's Hospital further supported the use of BPOC to reduce medication errors and potential ADEs. The investigators compared the number of transcription errors and administration errors, both timing-related and nontiming-related, in units without BPOC to those with BPOC. There was a 41.4% relative reduction in nontiming administration errors (11.5% vs 6.8%, $P<0.001$) and a 50.8% relative reduction in potential ADEs due to nontiming administration errors (3.1% vs 1.6%, $P<0.001$) in units that implemented BPOC technology.[10] The authors also observed a significant reduction in timing-related administration errors and elimination of transcription errors in units with BPOC. Benefits to implementing BPOC technology also include improved inventory management, billing, and real-time documentation. Though data are limited, the eMAR and BPOC combination appears to be a cost-effective solution for preventing administration errors and ADEs.

PRACTICE POINT

Error prevention strategies for prescribing and administration include:

- Two patient identifiers to confirm a patient's identity before medication administration
- Specific instructions for administration to reduce order ambiguity and improve patient safety
- Administration technology
- Automated dispensing cabinets and smart pumps
- Electronic medication administration records (eMAR) in combination with bar code–enabled point-of-care technology (BPOC)

MONITORING ERRORS

Medication monitoring errors may result from inadequate or inappropriate drug monitoring. Medications with narrow therapeutic indices, such as lidocaine, digoxin, theophylline, valproic acid, carbamazepine, phenytoin, tacrolimus, cyclosporine, sirolimus, aminoglycosides, and vancomycin, require therapeutic drug monitoring to ensure efficacy and safety. Institutions provide these services in different capacities. Some institutions require physicians to order serum concentrations and interpret levels based on laboratory normal ranges. Other institutions require pharmacy consults for drug levels to be monitored, and some automatically have pharmacists monitoring drug concentrations through team- or unit-based clinical pharmacists or a pharmacy protocol. It is important for physicians to understand how drug concentrations are monitored at their institution and request a pharmacist's help in ordering or interpreting drug concentrations when necessary. A French study reported that 12.2% of pharmacist interventions involved medication monitoring, and 78.2% of these recommendations were accepted by physicians.[11] The timing of a level can determine whether a level is therapeutic. For example, if a vancomycin trough concentration is ordered without regard to when the dose is administered, it will not be reliable. Many times phenytoin concentrations are obtained and are not adjusted for a patient's renal function or serum albumin, leading to incorrect dosing. Refer to the patient case for information about reconciliation and monitoring medication errors that led to a preventable ADE. Monitoring errors can also be errors of omission, such as forgetting to obtain serum concentrations, failing to order an international normalized ratio (INR) when the patient is receiving warfarin, or failing to check a methadone patient's QT interval. Monitoring errors can lead to dire consequences if concentrations are subtherapeutic or supratherapeutic, resulting in therapy failure or toxicity.

RECONCILIATION ERRORS

Definition and risk

Medication reconciliation is a process of active decision by health care professionals at each patient transition to a different level of care (eg, nursing home stay to hospitalization), whether to continue, discontinue, or alter each patient medication order. Reconciliation errors may occur when a patient's home medications are incorrectly recorded or pertinent medications are omitted. A study evaluating medication discrepancies upon hospital admission found that over 50% of patients experienced at least one unintended discrepancy, of which, omitted home medications was the most common.[12] The Joint Commission mandates medication reconciliation (NPSG 8) in order to reduce the number of medication errors and adverse events. Medication reconciliation is required upon hospital admission, transfer to another level of care, and discharge. Many times patients are admitted overnight and cannot provide a reliable history for medication reconciliation. Considerable effort should be made by physicians, nurses, pharmacists, and patients to ensure that the admission medication reconciliation is complete and accurate.

Patient involvement

Another way that physicians can decrease reconciliation errors of commission and omission is by actively involving the patient. The Joint Commission recommends engaging patients in their care to improve safety (NSPG 13). Encourage patients to be proactive and involved in their medical care and to maintain an accurate and complete list of prescription and over-the-counter medications and nutritional and herbal products. Patients who take ownership of their medication therapy and can provide detailed and accurate lists to each physician are less likely to experience medication reconciliation–related errors. Having a complete and accurate medication list for each patient improves patient diagnosis, treatment, and monitoring. Missing an important medication, such as phenytoin, may lead to seizures, or improperly documenting a patient's warfarin dose may increase the patient's risk of bleeding.

Discharge counseling

Discharge medication counseling by a pharmacist may also decrease the number of preventable ADEs after discharge. In a study of 178 patients randomly assigned to receive discharge counseling and follow-up from a pharmacist compared with standard of care, the pharmacist identified 45 patients in the intervention arm (49%) who had medication-related errors resulting from inaccuracies in the admission medication reconciliation.[13] The same study illustrated that pharmacist-provided discharge counseling to reconcile medications and explain medication instructions and side effects, coupled with pharmacist follow-up after discharge, reduced the number of preventable adverse drug events. The Society of Hospital Medicine endorses a program called Better Outcomes for Older Adults through Safe Transitions (BOOST), which recommends risk stratifying patients upon admission. The program recommends discharge counseling for high-risk patients with polypharmacy (>5 scheduled medications) and/or problem medications (warfarin, insulin, digoxin, and aspirin/clopidogrel) to reduce the number of medication errors and preventable ADEs. By improving medication reconciliation, providing patient counseling, and involving patients, medication errors can be reduced.

CLASSIFICATION OF MEDICATION ERRORS

The National Coordinating Council for Medication Error Reporting and Prevention (NCC MERP) provides information about categorizing and defining medication errors (**Figures 10-1** and **10-2**).

QUALITY IMPROVEMENT

BACKGROUND

Reducing the number of medication errors and preventable ADEs involves an integrated multidisciplinary approach. Technology can be implemented to reduce the risk of medication errors and improve patient safety. The IOM recommends improving communication

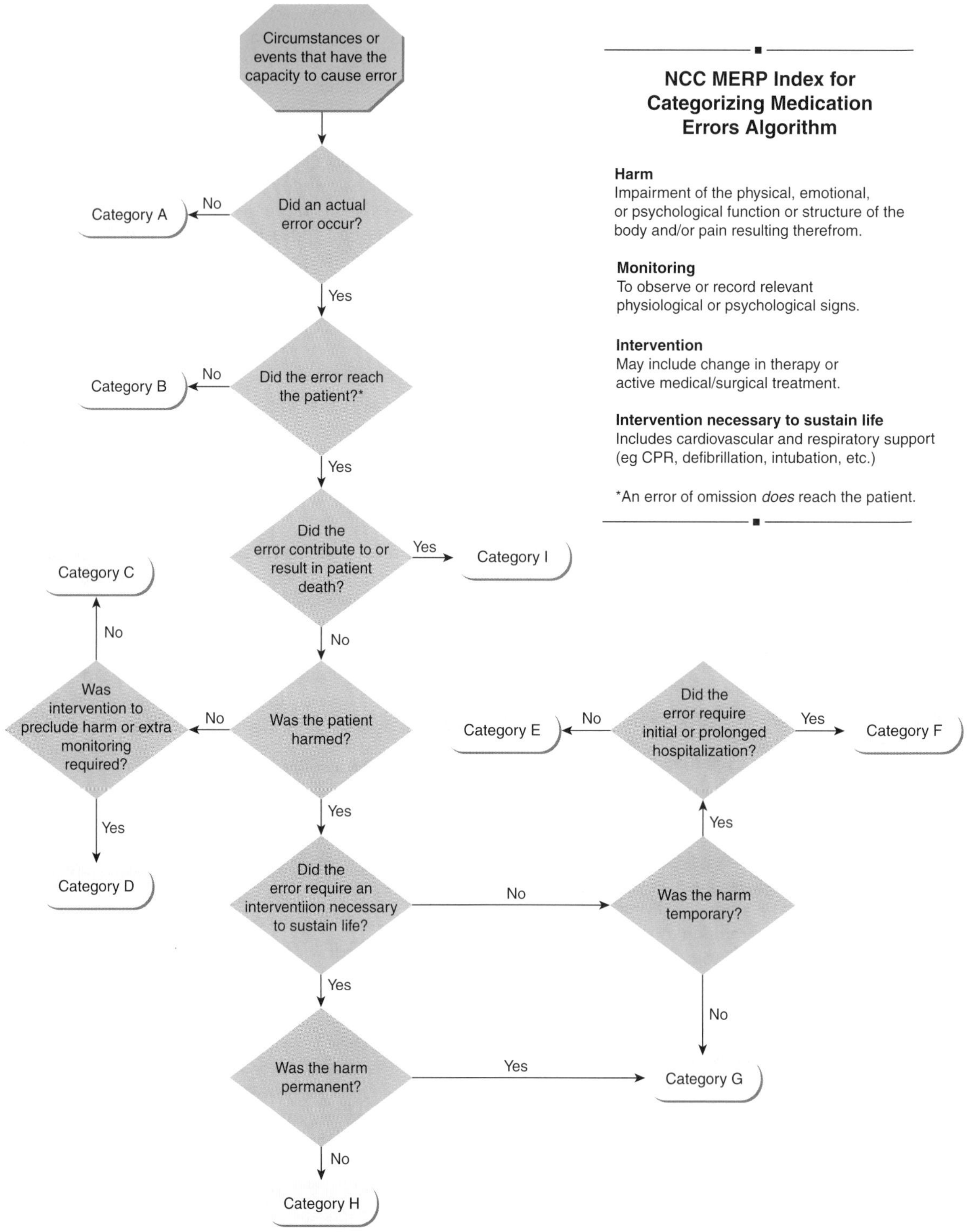

Figure 10-1 *NCC MERP Index for Categorizing Medication Errors Algorithm. (Reprinted, with permission, from the National Coordinating Council for Medication Error Reporting and Prevention, Copyright 2001.)*

between providers and between providers and patients to decrease the rate of preventable ADEs. Patients are encouraged to be empowered in regard to their care. Health care professionals should encourage all patients to ask questions about medications prescribed, dispensed, and administered. For example, inpatients are encouraged to ask nurses what medications are being administered and ask the physician the reasons why they were prescribed in order to give them a chance to identify potential errors.

Recognizing the barriers to safe medication use is important for error reduction. Patient barriers may include limited health care literacy, affordability, and/or cultural attitudes toward health care and communication. Medication counseling with an assessment of a patient's understanding through teach-back methods is a strategy to reduce errors. Government agencies are encouraged by the IOM to enhance the public's medication understanding and provide patient-friendly educational resources. The IOM states that

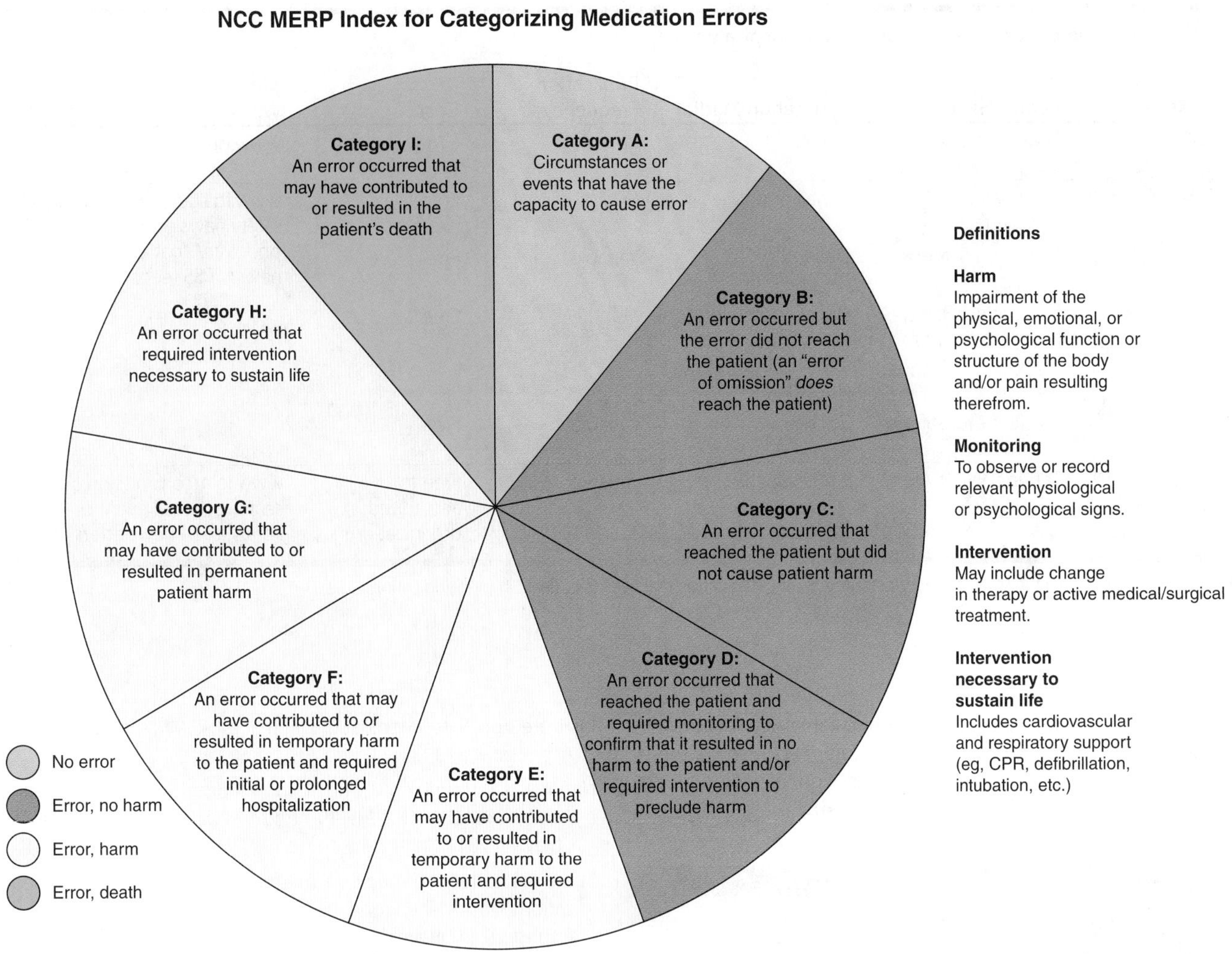

Figure 10-2 *NCC MERP Classification. (Reprinted, with permission, from the National Coordinating Council for Medication Error Reporting and Prevention, Copyright 2001.)*

patients have a right to expect providers to notify them of a clinically significant error and what ramifications to expect. Empowering the patient is an important proactive approach to detecting and preventing errors.

> **PRACTICE POINT**
>
> - Recognizing the barriers to safe medication use is important for error reduction. Patient barriers may include limited health care literacy, affordability, and/or cultural attitudes toward health care and communication. Medication counseling with an assessment of a patient's understanding through teach-back methods is a strategy to reduce errors.

ERROR REPORTING

Once an error or ADE occurs, reporting the error is an important quality improvement step. Many institutions have their own voluntary, nonpunitive, electronic reporting for medication errors and ADEs. These institutional reports are forwarded to a multidisciplinary quality assurance committee that investigates reports and identifies potential system failures. The goal for this process is to provide institutionwide change to prevent future errors and ADEs. In some institutions, mandatory reporting systems are implemented to increase reporting of medication errors; however, while mandatory reporting may produce more events to analyze, concerns over the punitive nature of this system and the decreased focus on system failures may limit its usefulness. In addition to voluntary error reporting databases, the IOM recommends implementing computerized ADE detection and direct observation of medication administration to improve error detection. National databases, such as the FDA's MedWatch and ISMP's Medication Errors Reporting Program, are also available to providers. Reporting errors promotes safety awareness and results in institutional or national practice changes that improve patient safety. The Joint Commission reviews institutions' responses to sentinel events during accreditation. Sentinel events may include but are not limited to ADEs and are defined as "unexpected occurrences involving death or serious physical or psychological injury, or the risk thereof."[14] The serious nature of sentinel events requires prompt investigation and action to prevent future events.

TABLE 10-4 Medication Safety Resources for Hospitalists

Publisher	Report Name	Publication Media	Publication Frequency	Cost	Website
ISMP	ISMP Medication Safety Alert!	E-mail	Biweekly	$160.00	www.ismp.org
FDA	Drug Safety Newsletter	E-mail or online	Quarterly	Free	www.fda.gov, search "drug safety newsletter," "safety podcasts," "patient safety news," "RSS feeds"
	FDA Drug Safety Podcasts	Online	Variable	Free	
	FDA Patient Safety News Broadcasts	Online, subscribe to mailing list to get a monthly e-mail with video links	Monthly	Free	
	RSS feeds for safety information	Online	Variable	Free	
The Joint Commission	Sentinel Event Alert	E-mail, online	Variable	Free to accredited organizations	www.jointcommission.org, search sentinel event or library, then newsletters

FDA, Food and Drug Administration; ISMP, Institute for Safe Medication Practices; RSS, Real Simple Syndication.

Several agencies publish reports that highlight safety issues with medications in an effort to keep providers informed. Many of these reports are available through e-mail subscription, providing timely and efficient access to information (**Table 10-4**).

PRACTICE POINT

- Once an error or ADE occurs, reporting the error is an important quality improvement step. The goal for this process is to provide institution wide change to prevent future errors and ADEs.

CONCLUSION

Errors in the medication use process increase morbidity and mortality for patients and increase costs to institutions. A better understanding of common error types and the error-prone steps in the medication use process may minimize error risk. Most errors occur during prescribing and medication administration. When patient care providers follow institutional policies and procedures fewer prescribing and administration errors should occur. In addition, providers who take an active role in medication safety or quality improvement committees in their institution and encourage medication and ADE reporting will raise awareness of the importance of this issue among coworkers and enhance safety through improvement of medication processes. Useful references include the medication safety resources from the Institute for Safe Medication Practices, the Food and Drug Administration, and The Joint Commission, which are updated regularly on medications involved in recent errors in the institutional setting.

SUGGESTED READINGS

Aspden P, Wolcott J, Bootman JL, et al. *Preventing Medication Errors: Committee on Identifying and Preventing Medication Errors*. Board on Health Care Services. Washington, DC: National Academies Press; 2007.

Institute for Safe Medication Practices (ISMP). www.ismp.org. Accessed May 11, 2011.

National Coordinating Council for Medication Error Reporting and Prevention (NCC MERP). http://www.nccmerp.org. Accessed May 11, 2011.

Strategies to reduce medication errors: working to improve medication safety. The Food and Drug Administration. (Accessed August 26, 2009 at http://www.fda.gov/Drugs/ResourcesForYou/Consumers/ucm143553.htm.)

The Joint Commission. http://www.jointcommission.org. Accessed May 11, 2011.

REFERENCES

1. National Coordinating Council for Medication Error Reporting and Prevention (NCC MERP). http://www.nccmerp.org. Accessed May 11, 2011.
2. Aspden P, Wolcott J, Bootman JL, et al. *Preventing Medication Errors: Committee on Identifying and Preventing Medication Errors*. Board on Health Care Services. Washington, DC: National Academies Press; 2007.
3. Reckmann MH, Wesbrook JI, Koh Y, et al. Does computerize provider order entry reduce prescribing errors in hospital inpatients? A systematic review. *J Am Medl Inform Assoc.* 2009;16:613–623.
4. Bates DW, Leape LL, Cullen DJ, et al. Effect of computerized physician order entry and a team intervention on prevention of serious medication errors. *JAMA*. 1998;280:1311–1316.
5. Ammenwerth E, Schnell-Inderst P, Machan C. The effect of electronic prescribing on medication errors and adverse drug events: a systematic review. *J AM Med Inform Assoc.* 2008;15:585–600. doi:10.1197/jamia.M2667.
6. Bedouch P, Allnet B, Grass A, et al. Drug related problems in medical wards with a computerized physician order entry system. *J Clin Pharm Thera.* 2008;34:187–195. doi:10.1111/j.1365-2710.2008.00990.x.

7. Bates DW, Cullen DJ, Laird N. Incidence of adverse drug events and potential adverse drug events. *JAMA*. 1995;274:29.

8. Pedersen CA, Schneider PJ, Scheckelhoff. ASHP national survey of pharmacy practice in hospital settings: dispensing and administration—2008. *Am J Health-Sys Pharm*. 2009;66: 926–946.

9. Poon EG, Cina JL, Churchill W, et al. Medication dispensing errors and potential adverse drug events before and after Implementing Bar Code Technology in the Pharmacy. *Ann Intern Med*. 2006;145:426–434.

10. Poon EG, Keohane CA, Yoon CS, et al. Effect of bar-code technology on the safety of medication administration. *New Engl J Med*. 2010;326:1698–1707.

11. Bedouch P, Charpiat B, Conort O, et al. Assessment of clinical pharmacists' interventions in French hospitals: results of a multicenter study. *Ann Pharmacother*. 2008;42:1095–1103.

12. Cornish PL, Knowles SR, Marchesano R, et al. Unintended medication discrepancies at the time of hospital admission. *Arch Intern Med*. 2005;165:424–429.

13. Schnipper JL, Kirwin JL, Cotungo MC, et al. Role of pharmacist counselling in preventing adverse drug events after hospitalization. *Arch Intern Med*. 2006;166:565–571.

14. Sentinel event policy and procedures. (Accessed August 7, 2009 at The Joint Commission. http://www.jointcommission.org/SentinelEvents/PolicyandProcedures/.)

CHAPTER 11

Principles of Evidence-Based Prescribing

Brent G. Petty, MD

INTRODUCTION

Medications are the principal tools doctors use to maintain health, reverse illness, and extend patients' survival, hopefully with good quality of life. Yet medications can also cause serious illness and fail to have the desired effect if they are used improperly. Additionally, medications can be extraordinarily expensive, and the cost to individual patients, to hospitals, and to our health system can become almost prohibitive. So the proper use of medications is critically important.

PRINCIPLES OF RATIONAL THERAPEUTICS

Before any medication is ordered in a hospital or prescribed for an outpatient, the prescriber needs to consider the (1) efficacy, (2) safety, and (3) cost of the medication, in that order of importance. Without efficacy for the condition being treated, no medication should be given. "It's not likely to be harmful" is no justification for trying something without demonstrated efficacy for the patient's problem, unless the intervention is in the setting of a clinical trial or the patient is informed of off-label use without evidence of benefit.

PRACTICE POINT

- Before any medication is ordered in a hospital or prescribed for an outpatient, the prescriber needs to consider the (1) efficacy, (2) safety, and (3) cost of the medication, in that order of importance. Without efficacy for the condition being treated, no medication should be given. There is a risk of toxicity with virtually all medications, so there must be a consideration of risk and benefit before starting or continuing medications.

EVIDENCE FOR EFFICACY

The quality of medical studies supporting the use of medications varies widely. In recent years, the quality of data has been graded by the groups reviewing the literature and making recommendations, such as the *Chest* guidelines for anticoagulation (**Table 11-1**). These grading systems consider the methodologies of the studies as well as the strength of the results.

Among the difficult issues with clinical trials is whether they can be extrapolated for all drugs in the same class. In general, extrapolation across a class is somewhat hazardous, as drug formulation, absorption, duration of effect, and sometimes drug interactions differ among drugs in the same class. Even with HMG CoA reductase inhibitors, whose effects on LDL cholesterol are mostly affected by drug potency and can often be equated through adjustment of dose, the efficacy related to clinical outcomes and adverse effects may vary. Thus what is true for one drug in a certain class may not be true for other drugs in the same class.

Another issue regarding the validity of clinical trials is the use of "surrogate markers" in place of "hard clinical end points." An example is a reduction of HIV RNA levels as a surrogate for medication efficacy instead of prolonged survival in patients with AIDS. Some surrogate markers have been demonstrated through rigorous clinical studies to be closely associated with hard clinical end points, providing assurance that they can be trusted as substitutes. Other surrogate markers have less data to justify their use as substitutes. A recent study points out the hazard of surrogate markers: a study of

TABLE 11-1 Grading System for Evaluating Evidence

	Strength of Recommendation	
	1 (Strong)	2 (Weak)
Quality of Literature		
A (High)	1A—Strong recommendation, high-quality evidence. Consistent evidence from RCTs without important limitations or exceptionally strong evidence from observational studies	2A—Weak recommendation, high quality evidence. Consistent evidence from RCTs without important limitations or exceptionally strong evidence from observational studies
B (Moderate)	1B—Strong recommendation, moderate-quality evidence. Evidence form RCTs with important limitations (inconsistent results, methodological flaws, indirect or imprecise), or very strong evidence from observational studies	2B—Weak recommendation, moderate-quality evidence. Evidence from RCTs with important limitations (inconsistent results, methodological flaws, indirect or imprecise), or very strong evidence from observational studies
C (Low)	1C—Strong recommendation, low or very low quality evidence. Evidence for at least one critical outcome from observational studies, case series, or from RCTs with serious flaws or indirect evidence	2C—Weak recommendation, low or very low quality evidence Evidence for at least one critical outcome from observational studies, case series, or from RCTs with serious flaws or indirect evidence

RCT, randomized controlled trial

interleukin-2 therapy in patients with HIV infection showed a substantial and sustained elevation of CD4+ cell count over a period of 7–8 years average follow-up, but no improvement in survival or the incidence of opportunistic infections.

Another common outcome strategy in clinical trials is "composite end points," combining as an "event" any one of several conditions, such as cardiac death, nonfatal myocardial infarction, and admission to a hospital for unstable angina. Obviously, all of these conditions are defensible as outcomes in patients with coronary artery disease, but they are decreasingly reliable as "hard clinical end points" for an intervention intended to influence the course of coronary artery disease. Especially when one of the three conditions contributing to the composite end point is the result of variable clinician judgment (eg, when to admit a patient for unstable angina), the reliability of the composite end point decreases.

SAFETY

Throughout all phases of drug development before drug approval (phases I, II, and III), safety is assessed, but at best these studies involve only a few thousand study subjects for the vast majority of drugs. With this number of patients, only side effects of moderate frequency (around 1–10 per thousand) will be identified. More rare (and often more serious) side effects may only become recognized with much more extensive use, involving tens of thousands of people. The experience with drugs such as troglitazone emphasizes the importance of postmarketing reporting of toxicities associated with newly approved medications to MedWatch and/or to the manufacturer.

There is a risk of toxicity with virtually all medications, so there must be a consideration of risk and benefit before starting or continuing medications. In many cases, the toxicity emerges without warning ("idiosyncratic"), such as rashes in response to sulfa drugs. These "adverse drug events" are usually unpredictable and are not considered "medication errors." In other cases, the possible toxicities of medications can be identified and treated before they become clinically dangerous (eg, hypokalemia with loop diuretics or hyperkalemia with ACE inhibitors). These adverse drug events are not medication errors either, unless the patient is not monitored appropriately with occasional serum potassium measures.

COST

The cost of medical care seems to steadily rise. The contribution of medication cost to overall health care expenses more than doubled from 4.7% in 1982 to 10.5% in 2002. Interestingly, while drug costs continue going up, the rate of increase in the cost of prescription drugs has decreased over the past 2 years, increasing only 4% from 2006 to 2007. Individuals sometimes find that they are unable to afford their medications, and as a result these patients often go without them. This "economic noncompliance" increases during difficult economic periods or when people have fixed incomes and must choose between paying for these medications or their food or mortgage. If hospitals and health systems could pay less for their medications, they would have more funds available for capital improvements or expanded personnel services.

Clinical trials have increasingly been including assessment of the quality of life saved, not just the survival rate. The measure of quality-adjusted life years (QALYs) is a standard and internationally recognized method to assess the relative benefit of medical interventions. It combines duration of survival and the quality of life during each year of life. Although one treatment might help someone live longer, it might also have serious side effects (eg, it might make them feel sick or put them at risk of other illnesses). Another treatment might not extend survival but it may improve quality of life (eg, by reducing pain). The quality of life rating can range from 0 (worst possible health) to 1 (best possible health). Having the QALY measurement allows one to consider cost effectiveness—that is, how much the drug or treatment costs per QALY. This is the cost of providing a year of the best quality of life available, which could be one person receiving one QALY, but is more likely to be a number of people receiving a portion of a QALY—for example, four people receiving 0.25 QALY. In this example, cost effectiveness is expressed as dollars per QALY.

Cost effectiveness analysis is another increasingly popular approach. This is another increasingly popular approach to assess the impact of intervention that may have financial benefit. For example, aspirin's cost is much lower than the cost of caring for the heart attacks it prevents. Sometimes the benefit is secondary or indirect. For example, acetylcholinesterase inhibitors are reported to cause a temporary delay in the cognitive decline of patients with dementia.

If this delay in cognitive decline can prevent a patient from requiring institutionalization or full-time care at home for a period of months or years, the costs of such care may be much more than the cost of the medication.

Policy makers including governmental bodies, payers, and influential foundations are interested in maximizing cost effectiveness. They are convinced, with some justification, that many practices and interventions might well be replaced with less costly approaches, without diminishing the quality of the care and the benefit our patients derive.

OTHER FACTORS THAT INFLUENCE MEDICATION SELECTION

PATIENT PREFERENCES AND VALUES

With rare exception, prescribers have a number of possible medications for managing diseases, and each may cause likely responses (good or bad) in addition to the intended response. In all cases, the patient's inclination to accept the proposed therapy should be considered.

The very choice of initiating medication treatment or not should be weighed. It is always an option in medicine to do nothing (offer no treatment), and sometimes no treatment is the best option. For example, in a patient with an acute inferior wall myocardial infarction who develops a Mobitz I block (Wenkebach), the occasional missed beat is of no clinical consequence, creates no risk for the patient, and almost always resolves without intervention. Treating such a problem with atropine or a pacemaker would be a mistake, introducing some risk of toxicity or complication for no clinical benefit, so no treatment is the best approach for such patients.

PRACTICE POINT

- The very choice of initiating medication treatment or not should be weighed. It is always an option in medicine to do nothing (offer no treatment), and sometimes no treatment is the best option.

The prescriber should also consider coexisting medical conditions that might likewise benefit from the same therapy, as this may magnify the benefit of the medication without adding additional risk of toxicity. For example, in a patient with hypertension who also suffers from frequent migraine headaches, a beta blocker or verapamil might be favored over other medications because they may reduce the frequency and/or severity of the migraine episodes at the same time the blood pressure is being reduced.

Patients with potentially life-threatening conditions (eg, metastatic cancer) are often treated with potent medications with the potential of side effects that are not only miserable but may also be life threatening. When treatments are similar in efficacy but differ in types of toxicities, the patients' preferences are important, since hair loss may be more adverse for some patients than risk of infection or incidence of diarrhea. Tailoring the medications used in such cases preserves the patient's autonomy and properly respects their right to choose among reasonable options.

PRACTICE POINT

- When treatments are similar in efficacy but differ in types of toxicities, the patients' preferences are important. Tailoring the medications used in such cases preserves the patient's autonomy and properly respects his or her right to choose among reasonable options.

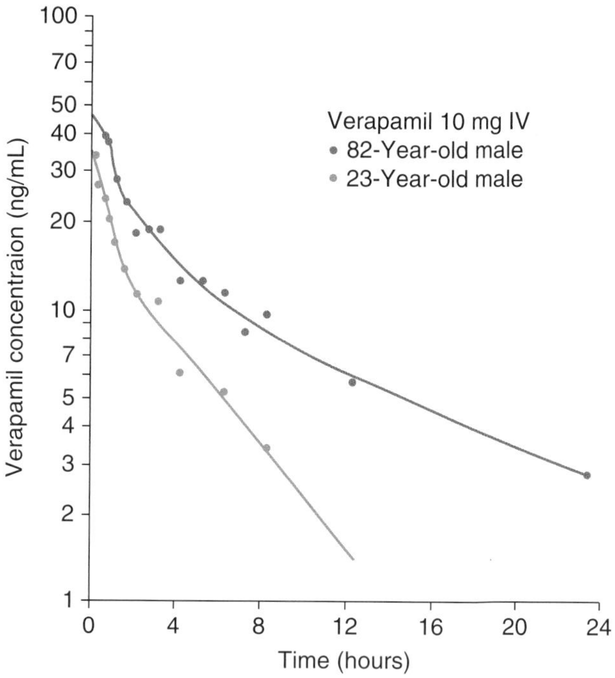

Figure 11-1 *Altered pharmacokinetics in the elderly. (Reproduced, with permission from Schwartz JB. Clinical pharmacology. In: Hazzard WR, et al., eds. Principles of Geriatric Medicine and Geronotology. 3rd ed. New York: McGraw-Hill; 1994.)*

INDIVIDUAL RISK

Sometimes patient characteristics create special susceptibility to adverse events. A good example relates to the toxicity seen with the nucleoside reverse-trancriptase inhibitor abacavir, which causes a hypersensitivity reaction in about 5–10% of patients. This reaction usually occurs in the first 2 months of treatment and is sufficiently severe that it requires discontinuation of the drug. The symptoms include fever, rash, and respiratory, gastrointestinal, and constitutional symptoms. The reaction was found to be associated with the HLA-B*5701 gene variant. Investigators in Australia have demonstrated that screening with genotyping before instituting abacavir therapy was effective in reducing the number of such reactions. In fact, there were no hypersensitivity reactions in the HLA-B*5701–negative patients. This is one of the best examples of the value of pharmacogenomics biomarkers to enhance our treatment of patients with medications.

The elderly make up an important group of patients. Patients age 65 or over constitute about 15% of the U.S. population, but they consume around 30% of the medications prescribed. The natural deterioration of both renal and hepatic function with age makes the elderly more susceptible to toxicity from regular use of medications. The altered pharmacokinetics with verapamil is but one example. **Figure 11-1** demonstrates the difference in elimination after an intravenous dose of verapamil in an 82-year-old man compared to a 23-year-old man. Not only is the elimination delayed, but the peak blood concentration is higher, perhaps related to a modest change in volume of distribution, which can occur with age. **Figure 11-2** shows the relationship of age and intravenous diazepam dose needed to achieve adequate sedation for a procedure. As predicted by pharmacokinetics, the dose needed for an elderly person is less than that needed for a younger patient. But **Figure 11-3** reveals additional information that is even more important. It shows the relationship of age and plasma concentration of diazepam needed to achieve adequate sedation for a procedure. Note that the

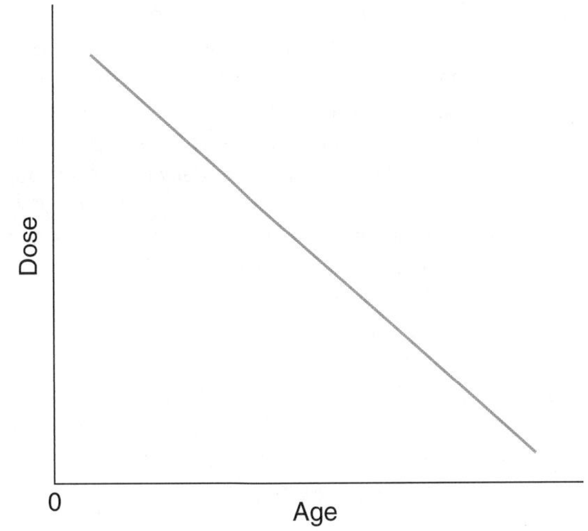

Figure 11-2 *Relationship of age and dose required to achieve a desired effect.*

concentration required diminishes steadily with advancing age, demonstrating that the elderly are more sensitive to diazepam than younger patients. So for both of these reasons (delayed elimination and increased sensitivity to the medication), dosing diazepam is best accomplished with additional caution in elderly patients. While this relationship between medication concentration and age is not seen with all benzodiazepines, starting at low doses and increasing slowly, according to individual patient response, is an especially good principle when prescribing medications for the elderly.

ASSESSING THE EVIDENCE

The strongest studies that direct medical practice are clinical trials that are well-designed, randomized, controlled, "blinded" or "masked," and prospective. Each of these elements is important to increase the likelihood that the results of the study can be accepted rather than be the result of chance. The study question is framed as a null hypothesis, which is often not what the investigators actually expect to find. In fact, most investigators begin with the expectation of showing a difference between the test compound and either standard treatment or inactive (placebo) treatment. So, for example, if one were comparing the effect of two HMG, CoA reductase inhibitors ("statins") on serum cholesterol, a null hypothesis could be, "There is no difference between atorvastatin and rosuvastatin in patients with hypercholesterolemia and symptomatic coronary artery disease." Then the study is conducted with a sufficient sample size to attempt to disprove the null hypothesis with a certainty of at least 95% that the degree of difference between the two drugs is a true difference and not just the result of chance (alpha or type I error = 0.05). More frequently now than in the past, it seems that the investigators expect that there will not be a significant difference between the two arms, or what is called a noninferiority study. Confirming that two medications are equivalent or noninferior requires a larger sample size than that for confirming that they are different. The beta, or type II, error is normally set at 0.2, but when investigators want more certainty that the observed similarity is more likely to be true than just the result of chance, the beta error may be reduced to 0.1.

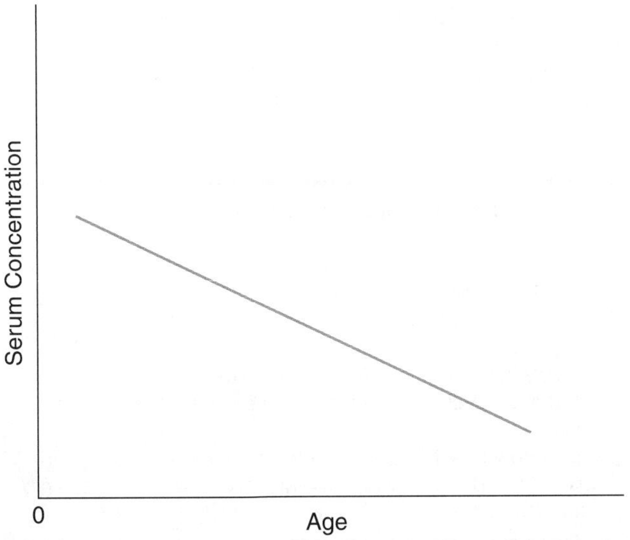

Figure 11-3 *Relationship of age and plasma concentration required to achieve a desired effect.*

Once the study is completed with the intended sample size, the results are analyzed. The most balanced approach is to assume that either of the two groups could be superior to the other, which leads to a two-tailed statistical test. It is especially interesting to see how each arm performed compared to the predicted response. The analysis can determine whether one group had a more favorable outcome than the other, and by how much they differed. The difference is statistically significant if it is less likely than 5% to have reached that difference through chance alone. The 5% threshold is, of course, arbitrary as a level to embrace an observation with absolute conviction versus 6% to discount as nothing very meaningful. In fact, when the difference reaches a 6% degree of certainty for being beyond a chance finding, it seems inappropriate to say that the performance of the groups was "not different." The truth is that the groups' performance *was* different, but that difference did not reach the level of statistical significance. In such cases, one often hears the term *trend* used to describe the difference, and the difference would likely have reached statistical significance if the sample size were larger *and* the proportional responses held the same levels with additional subjects.

Too often readers ignore the methods sections of published papers, giving their limited time instead to the abstract, a few figures or tables in the results, and the highlights of the discussion section. This approach may save time, but it ignores the critical information about characteristics of the study population recruited, what kinds of patients were excluded, how other medications were managed, and many other aspects that ultimately determine whether the results of the study are valid and whether they can be applied to any other population/patient group besides those enrolled in the study. The paper rises or falls on its methods, so results or conclusions are not valid if the procedures involved with conducting the study are seriously flawed.

The decisions about which specific drugs are included in a hospital's formulary are usually made by a multidisciplinary formulary committee, which includes physicians and other prescribers, nurses, pharmacists, and others. This group reviews the available data on efficacy, safety, and cost of products proposed to be added to or removed from the hospital formulary. To be an effective member of such a committee, an individual would need to understand the importance of efficacy, safety, and cost as they relate to the population of patients served by the hospital. Clear thinking is essential. It is especially important for the committee members to consider the hospital's welfare as opposed to advocacy for individual patients or a small group of patients. Workflow issues for all members of the care team are important. Likewise, the incremental cost of one product compared to another may influence whether sufficient money is available to hire or maintain staff members. It is the balance of these multiple issues that makes the work of the formulary committee interesting and important.

PRACTICE POINT

- To be an effective member of a multidisciplinary formulary committee, an individual would need to understand the importance of efficacy, safety, and cost as they relate to the population of patients served by the hospital. It is especially important for the committee members to consider the hospital's welfare as opposed to advocacy for individual patients or a small group of patients. Workflow issues for all members of the care team are important. Likewise, the incremental cost of one product compared to another may influence whether sufficient money is available to hire or maintain staff members. It is the balance of these multiple issues that make the work of the formulary committee interesting and important.

During the hospitalization, the patient may receive a different drug than what they were taking at home before admission. This may be the result of provider preference or formulary restriction. Hospital formularies are either open or closed, and may have additional restrictions. Open formularies allow prescribers to order any marketed product, and the patient will get whatever specific product was ordered. Closed formularies limit the selection of medications to a small number of products within either a chemical class or an indication class. For example, rather than having all H2-receptor blockers and proton pump inhibitors on the hospital's formulary, the hospital may restrict the choice to ranitidine or omeprazole. These determinations are generally made based on the assumptions of (1) equal, or at least adequate, efficacy; (2) no worse toxicity profile for the selected product; and (3) substantial cost savings.

When the history, physical examination, and relevant laboratory data have been obtained, treatment begins. The treatment may be either specific (based on the establishment of a specific diagnosis) or empiric (based on the best guess of diagnosis using the available evidence and considering the usual etiology responsible for the condition, such as the most likely bacterial pathogens for a community-acquired pneumonia). The initiation of new medication in the hospital or in the outpatient setting must be framed on the background of the medication that the patient previously had taken. The process of considering the immediate previous medications (the patient's "home medications") when ordering new treatment is called medication reconciliation. Home medications may not always have been taken at a patient's house, as the patient may have come to the hospital from a nursing home or may have been transferred from another hospital. Medication reconciliation is not simply copying the home medications onto the hospital's order sheet, but rather a thoughtful consideration of the value of each medication in light of the patient's new medical condition. There should be a conscious decision, for each and every medication, whether to stop, continue, or modify administration of the drug.

PRACTICE POINT

- Medication reconciliation is not simply copying the "home medications" onto the hospital's order sheet, but rather a thoughtful consideration of the value of each medication in light of the patient's new medical condition. There should be a conscious decision, for each and every medication, whether to stop, continue, or modify administration of the drug.

At the time of transfer to a new service or level of care, and at the end of the patient's hospitalization, another medication reconciliation should occur. This one differs from the one at admission because the consideration of medications to prescribe upon transfer or at discharge should take into account not only the medications the patient was taking in the hospital just before transfer or discharge, but the home medications. The purpose of this dual consideration is to avoid costly and potentially hazardous duplication of medications. As already explained, a patient may receive one proton pump inhibitor while in the hospital (eg, pantoprazole), which is different than the one taken at home (eg, omeprazole) or the one that might be prescribed at discharge (eg, lansoprazole). Patients have been known to be taking supplies of both warfarin and Coumadin following hospital discharge because one had been provided by prescription from the family doctor and the other was prescribed by the hospital doctors. Since generic and brand products may look different, it is not hard to understand how patients may not recognize the hazardous duplication.

PRACTICE POINT

- At the time of transfer to a new service or level of care, and at the end of the patient's hospitalization, a second medication reconciliation should occur. This one differs from the one at admission because the consideration of medications to prescribe upon transfer or at discharge should take into account not only the medications the patient was taking in the hospital just before transfer or discharge, but the "home medications." The purpose of this dual consideration is to avoid costly and potentially hazardous duplication of medications.

THERAPEUTIC DRUG MONITORING

Treatment of any patient should follow the "ideal therapeutic algorithm" (**Table 11-2**). First, the prescriber should have a therapeutic goal in mind, whether it is to lower the blood pressure to a certain point, reduce the hemoglobin A1c below a certain threshold, or drive the LDL cholesterol down under 100 mg/dL. With the goal in mind, an appropriate agent is selected, and then an appropriate dose of the agent is chosen. When relevant patient characteristics or concomitant medications are known, the dose may be individualized somewhat. After allowing a sufficient period of time for the intervention to reach a substantial or peak effect, which may be days or weeks, a repeat measurement is performed and is compared to the pretreatment reading and the therapeutic goal. Then, whatever the starting dose may have been, adjustments in the dose may well be needed to achieve the therapeutic goal. After the response to the new dose is observed, another adjustment in dose, or adding or substituting another medication, can be considered. All the while there is monitoring for evidence of adverse effects.

TABLE 11-2 Ideal Therapeutic Algorithm

1. Determine the therapeutic goal.
2. Choose an appropriate agent.
3. Choose the appropriate dose, individualizing for each patient when possible.
4. Know when/how to monitor for effectiveness and safety, including the essential criteria for appropriate therapeutic drug monitoring.
5. Know how to adjust the therapy (eg, increase the dose, add another medication, switch to another agents, etc) to attain the therapeutic goal and avoid toxicity.

From Petty BG. Rational Therapeutics course, The Johns Hopkins University School of Medicine.

TABLE 11-3 Criteria for Appropriate Therapeutic Drug Monitoring

1. Medication concentration or effects can be measured reliably and accurately.
   AND
2. The efficacy of medication treatment can be enhanced by achieving a certain concentration or effect range.
   AND/OR
3. The toxicity of medication treatment can be reduced by maintaining a certain concentration or effect range.

Therapeutic drug monitoring is a term that usually implies the measurement in some body fluid of a substance that is either the medication that is being monitored or a related substance. Therapeutic drug monitoring is best employed when certain criteria can be met (**Table 11-3**). If measuring a physiological result (eg, prothrombin time) or a drug concentration is part of the monitoring, one must be confident that the laboratory to be used can measure the item accurately and in a timely fashion. Then it must be known that the efficacy of the drug is enhanced or the toxicity of the drug is reduced by adjusting the dose of the medication. If the efficacy or toxicity of a medication cannot reliably be improved by adjusting the dose to achieve a result in the therapeutic range, then therapeutic drug monitoring is not of value. We should avoid the temptation to measure drug concentrations just because we can. Achieving and maintaining results in the therapeutic range should reduce the risk of toxicity or improve efficacy, or both.

It should be emphasized that measuring drug concentrations in plasma or serum establishes individual patient pharmacokinetics. One well-done drug concentration is more valuable than any algorithm that seeks to predict concentration or effect using patient characteristics, comorbidities, or other factors. Poorly done therapeutic monitoring may produce results that are misleading, and in this way are worse than having no testing at all. The duration of an infusion and the correct timing of the sample after the infusion are critical to having results that can be assessed in light of published data and guidelines. Especially hazardous is drawing blood samples for drug concentrations too soon after an intravenous dose of drug, which may put the sample in the period of the alpha half-life or distribution phase, rather than in the beta half-life or elimination phase, which is a more predictable and interpretable portion of the drug elimination curve. On the other hand, especially with oral medications, checking drug concentrations after too few doses are given to have the concentrations at or near steady state can lead to an underestimation of the adequacy of a dose, and a premature increase to a higher dose may lead to serious toxicity when the drug concentration does achieve steady state at a level too high for safety.

PRACTICE POINT

Measuring drug concentrations in plasma or serum establishes individual patient pharmacokinetics.

- One well-done drug concentration is more valuable than any algorithm that seeks to predict concentration or effect using patient characteristics, comorbidities, or other factors.
- Poorly-done therapeutic monitoring may produce results that are misleading, and in this way are worse than having no testing at all. The duration of an infusion and the correct timing of the sample after the infusion are critical to having results that can be assessed in light of published data and guidelines.

ROLE OF PHARMACISTS IN ASSISTING WITH MEDICATION ORDERING

More hospitals are employing pharmacists to assist prescribers in their management of patients. These trained professionals are especially knowledgeable about medication issues, including indications for medications, their doses (in both normal and physiologically impaired patients), drug–drug and drug–food interactions, and other important matters in medication use. They are familiar with resources that can help identify medications, including foreign and generic products. Some serve on hospital policy-making committees because of their perspectives related to drug dispensing and monitoring. In some hospitals, they see patients with conditions such as hypertension and evaluate the propriety of the patients' medications, the patients' knowledge of their medications and how to use them, and the most likely adverse events that the patients may encounter. Pharmacists round with care teams and provide information on medications during the discussions about the patients. Anticoagulation monitoring clinics can be staffed by pharmacists in some states. Pharmacists, like nurses, are the physicians' compatriots, and can help physicians avoid making serious errors. As important team members, they should be heeded, respected, and appreciated.

MANAGEMENT OF DRUG SAMPLES

The topic of drug samples is only a portion of the larger topic of the relationship of prescribers and hospitals to the pharmaceutical industry. Whether to allow samples in a practice or hospital at all can be very controversial. At balance is the advantage of "free" medication for those patients who can't afford it versus the clear marketing motivation of the suppliers of the samples. Samples may be allowed in the offices of individual practitioners or in the clinical space of a multidisciplinary group. Some hospitals have centralized samples into the pharmacy to be dispensed to the medically indigent with special prescriptions, while other hospitals have forbidden samples altogether. There are justifications on all sides of this issue, but if samples are allowed in an office, practice, or hospital, their use should be documented in each case they are dispensed, the patient should be supplied with product information (eg, from a pharmacy), and expiration and recalls should be monitored.

Samples are not the only strategy used by industry to influence prescribing and medication-ordering habits. Direct-to-consumer advertising, gifts, grants, support of clinical investigation, journal advertising, and even unrestricted donations to hospitals and medical schools have the potential to introduce a sense of obligation and indebtedness in those of us who influence the specific medications our patients receive. The issue is complicated, but we must concede that we all have biases, and that we should institute measures to minimize our biases or their effects. We must act as objectively as possible for the benefit of our patients.

"Academic detailing" is a concept that has been proposed to help reduce undue influence from industry. Academic detailing involves the distribution of knowledge from trusted medical personnel, often the leaders of academic departments or divisions, government advisers (eg, from the U.S. Food and Drug Administration, Centers for Disease Control and Prevention, or National Institutes of Health), or other external experts that can be invited into hospitals to educate the hospitals' medical staffs on the pros and cons of various medications. Leaders and other members of the hospital's formulary committee, as well as leaders and members of the hospitalist group at the hospital, may be considered for academic detailing if they have appropriate knowledge about the medications under discussion and are free from conflicts of interest that would potentially affect their opinions.

SUGGESTED READINGS

Guyatt GH, Cook DJ, Jaeschke R, et al. Grades of recommendation for antithrombotic agents. *Chest.* 2008;133(suppl):123S–131S.

Hoffman JM, Shah ND, Vermeulen LC, et al. Projecting future drug expenditures—2009. *Am J Health-Syst Pharm.* 2009;66:237–257.

INSIGHT-ESPRIT Study Group and SILCAAT Scientific Committee. Interleukin-2 therapy in patients with HIV infection. *N Engl J Med.* 2009;361:1548–1559.

Mallal S, Phillips E, Carcosi G, et al. HLA- B*5701 screening for hypersensitivity to abacavir. *N Engl J Med.* 2008;358:568–579.

Petty BG. Trends in medication use: implications for medication errors. *J Pharmacist Fin Econ Pol.* 2006;15:137–174.

Reidenberg MM, Levy M, Warner H, et al. Relationship between diazepam dose, plasma level, age, and central nervous system depression. *Clin Pharm Ther.* 1978;23:371–374.

www.nice.org.uk/newsroom/features/meaningeffectiveness andcosteffectivenesstheqaly.jsp. Accessed November 13, 2009.

CHAPTER 12

Tools to Identify Problems and Reduce Risks

Nathan Spell, MD, FACP

INTRODUCTION

Every organization needs a structure and a toolkit to support improving safety and quality. Since what cannot be seen cannot be fixed, robust identification of adverse events and sources of risk (risk to patients, to staff, and to the reputation of the organization) should be a priority of every hospital. This chapter begins with discussion of structures and tools to identify adverse events and risk-prone conditions. Once identified, the hospital and staff must then determine the priority items and which techniques will be applied to reducing adverse events and risks. Let us define a few terms for this chapter. Adverse events are instances of harm to patients resulting from medical care. Errors may be characterized as resulting from a flawed plan or from failure of a plan to be completed as intended. Not all adverse events result from error, and not all errors result in harm. A near miss is an error or system failure that is either intercepted before reaching the patient or causes no harm if it does reach the patient. Risk reduction efforts may focus on error prevention or on harm prevention. This chapter will not promote one approach over the other, as these principles and tools apply to both.

PRACTICE POINT

- Every organization needs a structure and a toolkit to support improving safety and quality. Since what cannot be seen cannot be fixed, robust identification of adverse events and sources of risk (risk to patients, to staff, and to the reputation of the organization) should be a priority of every hospital.

THE ROLE OF THE CULTURE OF SAFETY IN IDENTIFYING PROBLEMS

Where the culture of safety is healthy, it is easy to see that safety is a priority. People working in the area have a focus on safe practices and supporting one another in being safe and in delivering safe care. They may exhibit a "preoccupation with failure" as described by Weick and Sutcliffe, such that there is a general awareness of and attention to risks. Instead of ignoring small, nagging concerns, workers share those concerns with others, and team members rally to help resolve the concerns. When safety is a priority, physicians respond supportively to concerns about risks to patient safety and do not seek to blame when an error happens. When safety is a priority, staff supervisors and system leaders routinely inquire about safety concerns and take the time to listen, seek a deeper understanding of causes, and demonstrate their commitment to safety through action and by communication back to staff on the response to adverse events and concerns. Questions in **Table 12-1** can be useful to assess the effect of culture on identifying problems. See Chapter 7 for a more thorough treatment of culture of safety.

RISK IDENTIFICATION AS PART OF A SAFETY PLAN

Hospitals must be intentional about the identification of patient safety risks. The National Quality Forum identifies and promotes safe practices in health care (see http://qualityforum.org). Among these is the presence of leadership structures and systems to ensure awareness of safety failures in the organization and the performance gaps that need attention. Government and commercial health care purchasers, insurance providers, and hospital accreditation organizations provide strong incentives for hospitals to invest in

TABLE 12-1 The Effect of Culture on Identifying Problems

Questions to Assess the Culture of Safety
Are people comfortable reporting errors they witness?
Are people willing to report their own errors?
Do staff members freely discuss their concerns about patient safety?
Are supervisors receptive to these concerns?
Do people fear retribution for reporting or being blamed for adverse events?
Do staff members feel that leaders care about patient and staff safety?
Can people give examples of actions to improve safety that resulted from reports of adverse events or concerns?
Questions to Assess Leaders' Commitment to Safety
Are leaders visible in the hospital where patient care is delivered, asking staff about their concerns for safety?
Do leaders ensure that staff members do not suffer retribution for reporting?
Is there an identified patient safety officer who reports to system leaders or to the board?
Is safety regularly on the agenda at meetings of hospital departments, medical staff, and leaders?
Are adequate resources applied to identification and analysis of adverse events and risks?

infrastructure supporting the identification, analysis, and correction of risk-prone areas. Because information about errors and risks comes from many potential sources, hospitals face challenges to bringing this disparate information together in a meaningful way.

One of the chief challenges is that only a small fraction of true errors are detected by most methods, especially those based on human reporting. Computerized data mining methods tend to greatly increase the number of potential errors identified, but the specificity of these reports can be low. For example, a rule to identify nephrotoxicity from medications may look for a rise in the serum creatinine during hospitalization. Most of the cases identified will not result from an adverse drug event, and additional resources will be required to further investigate.

PRACTICE POINT

- Only a small fraction of true errors are detected by most methods, especially those based on human reporting. Bringing together the multiple sources of information allows for a broader view, and this effort benefits from having a central safety committee or a safety officer to whom the information funnels.

Knowing that the detected errors are but a sample of true errors and risk points, hospital safety leaders must decide whether there is value to applying additional resources to enhance detection. Bringing together the multiple sources of information allows for a broader view, and this effort benefits from having a central safety committee or a safety officer to whom the information funnels.

METHODS OF IDENTIFYING ADVERSE EVENTS AND ERRORS

Some methods are reactive and retrospective, being generated in response to specific events that come to attention. In contrast, systematic methods tend to identify latent or hidden errors or risk points and are more often proactive. Both types of approaches are necessary in the overall strategy to identify risks.

REACTIVE METHODS

Event-reporting systems

Event-reporting systems rely on workers bringing events to attention through their reports. In a healthy culture of safety, workers report freely and openly, with few barriers. Workers do not fail to report events that seem to represent small harms or risks of harm, because they are aware that these are important opportunities to learn. Indeed, a robust reporting system will collect a significant number of system failures or errors that were successfully intercepted or that did not result in harm, known as near misses. Near misses are golden opportunities to identify risk-prone conditions or processes and to intervene before harm results. An effective reporting system enhances the engagement of frontline staff in patient safety by providing an identified channel for their observations. To be effective, workers must be aware of the system and the value that leaders place on their reports. Timely acknowledgment and expressions of appreciation reinforce the desired reporting behaviors.

Ease of reporting is key to maintaining a low reporting threshold. Paper reports and verbal reports via telephone recording have advantages of speed, though the information has to be transcribed and aggregated separately. Electronic reporting systems may prompt for more precise and complete information from each report and may produce structured reports from which data are more easily analyzed. Electronic systems may also enable immediate notification of appropriate personnel. For instance, an event reported as causing significant patient harm may generate an automated communication to a risk manager, safety officer, or hospital leader, facilitating the response to the event.

How leaders and managers respond to aggregate data from event-reporting systems will send strong signals to the staff and to physicians. Because event reports are dependent on willingness to report and are unlikely to reflect true incident rates, leaders and managers should exercise caution in inferring that a high number of events reported represents worse safety in one area versus another. In fact, the number of reports may be more indicative of the culture of safety than of safety itself. However, it is human nature to conclude that higher numbers of reports indicates worse safety. Managers may worry that reports reflect poorly on their performance and discourage use of the reporting system. Leadership attention to the use of data for learning rather than for judging is critical to the reporting system effectiveness.

The options for reporter identity protection deserve intentional thought when designing an event reporting system. An open system makes no attempt to protect the reporter's identity, so colleagues and supervisors can know who reported. This kind of system can work where the culture of safety is strong enough that there is no retribution for reporting and, in fact, reporting is rewarded, whether by peer appreciation or formal recognition. Where the reporter is identified, an event report can be followed by further investigation, and an open and frank discussion of the event promotes learning. If reporters face criticism or retaliation in even a few instances, however, willingness to report can be severely affected.

A confidential reporting system allows identification of the reporter only to responsible system administrators who can follow up on the event with the reporter. Confidential reporting may overcome reluctance of some people to report and enhance detection of some kinds of sensitive issues. For example, a person reporting inappropriate sexual comments or behavior may be reluctant to have his or her identity known to the person whose behavior is being reported. Through attempts to protect the identity of the reporter, however, the investigation may have more limited scope that fails to obtain the whole picture.

Anonymous reporting serves to fully protect the reporter's identity and thus may expand reporting of sensitive events and reporting in work areas where a climate of fear exists. If inadequate information was submitted to identify the event, however, further investigation and learning are severely hampered. To the other extreme, if the reporter gave full information in a detailed report and few people are fully aware of the event, it may be impossible to maintain anonymity. Where necessary to provide for anonymous reporting, efforts to improve the culture of safety will ideally allow movement toward a more open reporting system.

Patient complaints and concerns

Patient complaints and concerns are another source of reports, whether submitted by patients or families or by staff members on behalf of them. The view from patients and families can be very valuable and complementary to the insights of staff members. These reports are more likely to reflect the level of service, compassion, communication, and partnering with patients and families. The reports are not likely to be anonymous and bring with them a duty to respond back to the patient or family. As with reports from staff members, treating the information as a learning opportunity can shape how frontline workers respond to complaints. While the volume and content of patient complaints and concerns may predict the likelihood of legal action, it may be difficult to draw actual conclusions about patient safety from rates of complaints.

Claims analysis

Analysis of medicolegal claims may be a tempting source of information, but it is less likely to generate useful ideas to improve patient safety than other methods. Since the vast majority of patients harmed through medical care do not bring claims, this subset is idiosyncratic. Deep understanding of any given event degrades rapidly with time, and investigation of an event should have occurred long before a claim was filed if the event was known earlier.

SYSTEMATIC METHODS

Patient safety walk rounds

Scheduled rounding in patient care areas by leaders can be an effective method to accomplish several goals, including promotion of a culture of safety. As described by Frankel and colleagues, structuring the content of rounds and recording the comments and concerns of staff members can yield valuable insights. Past events deserving of investigation and concerns about ongoing risks to patients may be heard by the leadership team. These reports stimulated by the visit of leaders may not have been collected through other means.

Morbidity and mortality conferences

Morbidity and mortality (M&M) conferences are a time-honored tradition in medicine. Discussion of patient death, complications, or harm resulting from care provides a learning opportunity for the attendees. Too often, perhaps due to the confidential nature of many conferences, the learning stops at the door, and feedback to the larger system does not happen. Additionally, the discussion of failures may be inhibited if the culture is not open, and the lack of a structured process of case review may lead to wide variation in the conclusions drawn from case review.

Structuring case reviews, identifying underlying causes of failures, and assigning responsibility for making system changes is an approach to making the M&M conference benefit the larger system.

Trigger tools

Adverse events and errors that surface through reporting systems and complaints poorly represent the rate at which such problems occur in a hospital. Structured reviews of medical records can identify problems that have not been reported and provide a rate estimate. One such method has been developed by the Institute for Health Care Improvement (IHI). Triggers are explicit criteria or clues to the presence of an adverse event, stimulating a deeper review of the record. Applying the tool to a random sample of hospital discharges can give an estimate of the rates of common sources of harm to patients. These rates can be tracked over time, and the information obtained may be used by the hospital to set improvement priorities.

Monitoring of high-risk processes

Some processes of care are inherently risky—provision of moderate sedation, performing invasive procedures, responding to cardiopulmonary arrests, and the like. Monitoring the processes of care and the outcomes can identify deviations from standard practice that may pose undue risks and point to steps that need to be strengthened. Using the example of cardiopulmonary resuscitation (CPR), the hospital may have a mechanism to review that the right complement of personnel responded to the emergency, that a team leader was identified, that the patient was correctly assessed, that the correct resuscitation algorithms were followed, and that the medications and other therapies were correctly administered. The results of CPR reviews and the outcomes of the resuscitation attempts are then reported to the appropriate hospital representative or committee.

In a hospital with a robust culture of safety, the insights from monitoring are shared and lead to actions to address deficiencies. Suppose, for example, resuscitation monitoring identifies that patients with difficult airways are not managed as well late at night as during the daytime hours when an anesthesiologist is available. This insight should be reviewed by hospital leaders who can determine the actions needed to provide better airway management at night. One solution may be to train and certify Hospital Medicine physicians to manage difficult airways.

Mining electronic data

Hospitals are rich in electronic data that can be mined for possible adverse events. Every hospital has administrative systems to support billing. Among the diagnosis codes are those that may indicate safety problems, such as codes for accidental puncture or laceration of an organ and for foreign body left in during a procedure. Since October 2008, hospitals routinely indicate whether conditions were present on admission. Reviewing diagnoses such as pressure ulcers and deep vein thromboses that were not indicated as present on admission may identify opportunities for improvement in these Patient Safety Indicators (see Chapter 15).

Electronic laboratory and pharmacy systems can be used to identify potential adverse events for further review. Instances of acute renal failure occurring after admission to the hospital may be identified by searching the laboratory data for patients in whom the serum creatinine has risen significantly. Errors in warfarin management may be identified among patients in whom vitamin K is administered. As electronic medical records become more widely used and record ever more of the details of the care of inpatients, much more robust and sophisticated data mining will be possible.

Failure modes and effects analysis

Failure modes and effects analysis (FMEA) is a prospective technique to anticipate the ways in which a process or equipment may fail and to prioritize the efforts to prevent failures. With roots in the military, FMEA is widely used in manufacturing and more recently is being applied to health care delivery. While there are a number of models, including Health Care Failure Modes and Effects Analysis used in the Veterans Health Administration, FMEA generally follows these steps.

1. **Choose the target for analysis.** Because conducting FMEA requires expertise and the commitment of significant time and resources, a hospital must select where to apply the technique. A frequent consideration is to focus where prior problems have occurred. One example is to identify and prevent errors in the placement and use of nasogastric tubes. FMEA can help a hospital safely implement a new technology such as bar coding the steps of medication preparation, distribution, and administration.
2. **Assemble the team.** To understand the process or equipment in fine detail, it is critical to identify team members with expertise from all disciplines that use, interact with, or maintain the process or equipment. A trained facilitator should be part of the team, as FMEA has a specific structure.
3. **Describe the process or use of equipment to be analyzed in detail.** This is best done graphically, beginning with a high-level flow diagram that serves as a framework for analysis. The flow diagram allows team members to share a mental model of the process steps. From the high-level diagram, the team can develop a detailed understanding of the different steps and supporting processes. When important gaps in the description cannot be filled in by team members, additional information is sought.
4. **Identify the ways that failure may occur (failure modes).** Drawing upon the expertise of team members and upon data where available, the team identifies vulnerabilities and underlying causes among the process steps or equipment functions.
5. **Prioritize the failure modes.** The team must decide where to focus attention for improvement or process redesign among the failure modes found in the previous step. To prioritize, most FMEA models apply a grading scale (eg, 1–10) to several aspects of each failure mode and its causes:

   Severity. The effect of each failure is described and assigned a grade. A low grade indicates a failure that would have minor consequences or is easily recoverable and the highest-grade failure effect is catastrophic (would cause grave harm and cannot be stopped once the failure occurs).

   Frequency. The probability of occurrence of the failure mode or its causes is also graded. Low-grade frequency suggests a very rare event and high grades more likely events.

   Risk of escaping detection. Failures that are immediately obvious allow for early detection and the opportunity to recover or to mitigate the effects. Easily detected failures receive a low score for risk of escaping detection. Other failures may be detected through routine inspection some time after occurrence. The highest score goes to failures that are not detected until the outcome (failure effect) has happened.

   Multiplying the grades of severity, frequency and risk of escaping detection for each failure mode produces a risk priority number. The failure modes can then be ranked, with the highest risk priority numbers indicating where the team should focus attention. Because this ranking process is imprecise, the results provide a guide rather than a prescription for the next steps.
6. **Determine the action steps.** If the FMEA leads the team to the conclusion that the process is far too unsafe to continue, a complete redesign may be necessary. Or, the team may conclude that bringing in a new piece of equipment is unjustified given the risks associated with it. More commonly, the team will identify ways to eliminate causes of failures, to provide earlier warning of failures, or to mitigate the effects of failures in service of improving overall safety.

RETROSPECTIVE INVESTIGATION OF EVENTS

Root cause analysis

Root cause analysis (RCA) is complementary to FMEA. It is a retrospective technique that provides a robust structure to review an adverse event or near miss. RCA is reactive; FMEA is proactive. But, the ultimate goal of each technique is to identify ways to prevent future adverse events. See **Table 12-2** for a comparison of these two techniques.

Effective RCA requires a detailed, intimate understanding of the event being studied and necessitates the participation or interview of people directly involved in the event. Because RCA is usually performed in response to a recent adverse event, emotions of people involved may be fragile. A poorly performed RCA that permits blaming of individuals can seriously undermine the culture of safety. RCA done well results in learning the underlying (root) causes of human failures, process failures, or equipment failures. Focus on correcting the root causes of failure fosters safer care of patients and a safer work environment for employees.

Conducting RCA requires a trained facilitator and an investment of time and resources. Hospitals will have to select where to focus this tool. Serious adverse events, such as the unexpected death of a patient related to an error, are obvious targets for RCA. However, near misses that reveal a potentially serious process failure should also be considered for RCA. A patient who recognizes that his chemotherapy has been mixed incorrectly because it is the wrong color may have prevented a serious medication error. RCA of this

TABLE 12-2 Comparison of FMEA and RCA

Failure Modes and Effects Analysis (FMEA)	Root Cause Analysis (RCA)
Prospective technique to predict the ways a process or equipment may fail and to plan prevention efforts	Retrospective technique to analyze an incident for the underlying causes of failure and to identify potential solutions
Steps:	Steps:
1. Choose target for analysis	1. Assemble the team
2. Assemble the team	2. Set the atmosphere
3. Describe the process in detail	3. Describe the events in detail
4. Identify the failure modes	4. Identify root causes
5. Prioritize the failure modes	5. Identify solutions to prevent recurrences
6. Determine the action steps	6. Report findings and recommendations to leaders

error may reveal weaknesses in the chemotherapy mixing process that need to be fixed. Root cause analysis will generally follow these steps:

1. **Assemble the team.** Some hospitals have an existing team for conducting RCAs. This team rarely has firsthand knowledge of the event being reviewed and will probably not have an intimate understanding of the focused work processes and environment of those involved in the event. The team will add members with such knowledge or will gain that knowledge through extensive interviews. More commonly, a team is brought together specifically for the RCA. In addition to the trained facilitator, the team should be interdisciplinary and involve people who work closely with the processes being evaluated. Some experts advise against including people directly involved with the event as team members because of their potential difficulty with being objective and open in such a forum. If those with direct involvement are invited to join the RCA team, the facilitator must be sensitive to this conflict and create an atmosphere conducive to openness. Hospital leaders, when possible, can strengthen team function by participating and supporting improvement opportunities that result from the RCA. If a leader does not participate directly, knowing that a leader will closely focus on the team recommendations can also lend weight to the RCA.
2. **Set the atmosphere.** In teams brought together for the RCA, the leader or facilitator may be the only person formally trained or experienced in the technique. Setting the atmosphere by providing an orientation to the process and laying out ground rules for the conduct of the RCA can be critical to success. Among the ground rules should be a prohibition against finger-pointing and personal attacks. While humans may have erred, directing blame at an individual stifles learning. Rather, for every failure point, ask, Why? or What conditions existed to permit this failure? Human error alone should not be an acceptable root cause. Another useful ground rule is to avoid speculation. Where gaps in understanding occur, the team should seek additional information.
3. **Describe the events.** Create a detailed flow diagram or a timeline of the sequence of events. The team seeks additional information to fill in gaps in understanding.
4. **Identify root causes.** Using structured questions as in the triggering and triage questions of the VA National Center for Patient Safety (see http://www4.va.gov/NCPS/rca.html) creates a more complete analysis by prompting consideration of categories of causes, including environmental conditions, equipment function, policies and procedures, training, communication, and fatigue. Again, digging deeper with each question and not accepting human error or procedural violation as a root cause are essential to identifying preventable causes.
5. **Identify solutions to prevent recurrences.** Using standardization and reliability science (see Chapter 16) will create more robust actions. Consider where similar vulnerabilities exist in the organization and generalize the learning where possible.
6. **Report findings and recommendations to leaders.** This step will help secure leadership support for actions needed.

Incident investigations

Most adverse events and near misses will not be investigated with an RCA, simply because the hospital is not capable of responding to all with this level of investigation. Still, the personnel performing the investigations should be seeking root causes of problems, identifying solutions, and generalizing to other areas. The results of incident investigations should feed back into the safety structure of the hospital through the safety committee or safety officer so that further action may be taken.

Peer review

Peer review processes are intended to judge the competence of health professionals. As such, peer review is fundamentally different from the investigations already described. This approach focuses not on problems in the health care system, but on individual performance. Peer review usually occurs as a physician or other provider is newly hired or granted specific hospital privileges to confirm competence or in response to some concern raised about performance. Concerns may arise in response to a particular incident or outcome or in response to data compiled over time. For instance, an unexpectedly high rate of procedural complications or resource utilization compared with peers may prompt closer review.

Peer review may generate insights about an error-prone process or other system problems that can be fed into the hospital safety or quality improvement structure. Judgments about the professional competence of individuals are managed through hospital medical staff governance structures.

As a strategy for reducing errors, peer review follows a "person approach" that is weak to the extent it assumes that human competence and behavior are responsible for most errors. Reliance on human perfection flies in the face of what is known about human performance in a variety of tasks (see Chapter 16), and the personal approach to error reduction undermines a culture of safety when individuals are blamed for errors and outcomes. The goal of peer review should be to ensure that health professionals are able to function to a level commensurate with the specific privileges granted. A "system approach" to error reduction assumes that most errors result from flaws in the system in which people work. The focus turns to creating a system that recognizes human fallibility and yet can prevent harm to patients.

Peer review also encompasses the behavioral norms expected of health professionals. Behavior that is disruptive to safe patient care or that threatens the safety of employees, such as verbal abuse of employees, lying about events in the care of patients, throwing public temper tantrums directed at others, or making unwanted sexual advances, must be dealt with by leaders. Failing to do so contributes to fear among employees and distrust of leaders, undermining the culture of safety.

RESPONDING TO IDENTIFIED ERRORS AND RISK POINTS

PRIORITIZATION

Health care delivery is an inherently complex and dangerous field. Patients enter hospitals with conditions that may be either known or mysterious. The methods we apply to diagnosis and therapy involve sharp objects, ionizing radiation, and toxins, delivered in a team setting where we must plan and communicate clearly across professional disciplines and across multiple handoffs. Danger, it seems, is everywhere. The challenge then lies in deciding which problems to tackle first and which problems to set aside.

Frontline employees bring their expertise about the risks they encounter. They should collaborate with the safety officer or committee that has a broader view of the problem areas in the hospital. The broader view comes from formal assessments of high-risk areas or processes, as with the FMEA technique, and from the accumulated experiences of risks and errors collected from the reporting system and other methods already discussed. When appropriate, local problems can be addressed with local solutions by the people who do the work. The hospital safety officer or committee will decide where and how to apply the more resource-intensive efforts to improve safety.

AVOIDING OVERREACTION AND UNINTENDED CONSEQUENCES

In the face of an adverse event, it can be tempting to apply intense focus and impose a quick solution. Indeed, when a serious continuing risk of harm is found, an immediate safeguard is appropriate. Reacting quickly to every danger, though, may cause loss of focus on higher-priority risks. Ill-considered solutions can overburden employees to the point of paralysis or can introduce additional harms. As an example, computerized order entry systems permit checking for drug–drug interactions as a safety feature. System administrators can select the level of interaction (severe, moderate, minor) at which an alert interrupts the prescribing process. If, in response to an adverse drug event, the level is set to include all potential interactions, the number of interruptions may overwhelm prescribers. As a result, cognitive errors may increase and prescribers may ignore more serious drug alerts. The net effect may well be to increase risks.

CONCLUSION

A robust safety plan helps to manage the complex and dangerous environment that is inpatient medical care delivery. It sets strategy and tactics for engendering a safe culture, identifying and investigating harms and risks, and prioritizing improvement efforts. The tools described in this chapter support the execution of a safety plan.

SUGGESTED READINGS

Berenholtz SM, Hartsell TL, Pronovost PJ. Learning from defects to enhance morbidity and mortality conferences. *Am J Med Qual.* 2009;24:192–195.

DeRosier J, Stalhandske E, Bagian JP, et al. Using health care failure mode and effect analysis: the VA National Center for Patient Safety's prospective analysis system. *Jt Comm J Qual Saf.* 2002;27(5):248–267.

Frankel A, Graydon-Baker E, Neppl C, et al. Patient safety leadership walkrounds. *Jt Comm J Qual Saf.* 2003;29(1):16–26.

Griffin FA, Resar RK. *IHI Global Trigger Tool for Measuring Adverse Events.* 2nd ed. IHI Innovation Series white paper. Cambridge, MA: Institute for Healthcare Improvement; 2009.

Hickson GB, Federspiel CF, Pichert JW, et al. Patient complaints and malpractice risk. *JAMA.* 2002;287(22):2951–2957.

Leonard M, Frankel A, Simmonds T. *Achieving Safe and Reliable Healthcare: Strategies and Solutions.* Chicago, IL: Health Administration Press; 2004.

Reason J. Human error: models and management. *BMJ.* 2000;320: 768–770.

Root Cause Analysis page. VA National Center for Patient Safety website. http://www4.va.gov/NCPS/rca.html. Accessed November 21, 2009.

Weick KE, Sutcliffe KM. *Managing the Unexpected: Assuring High Performance in an Age of Complexity.* San Francisco, CA: Jossey-Bass; 2001.

SECTION 3
Quality Improvement

CHAPTER 13

Quality Improvement and Safety Research

Jeffrey L. Schnipper, MD, MPH, FHM

INTRODUCTION

Hospitalists are often asked to participate in or lead quality improvement (QI) initiatives, locally and nationally. Because data collection and feedback are part of any QI effort (see Chapter 12), and because the results of these efforts are often published, the hospitalists who lead these efforts often ask (or are asked by others) the question: "Is this research?" The short answer is that QI research is different from standard QI efforts in many respects. In this chapter, we will address the differences between standard QI efforts and QI research, some reasons to do QI research, the appropriate time to do QI research (for you and for the scientific question at hand), how "rigorously" to conduct QI research, getting started with the process, the ingredients for a successful project, and issues related to study design and methods that are either unique to or are particularly relevant to QI research.

This chapter will address both "quality improvement" and "patient safety" research. The two terms are often used interchangeably, and often the line between them is gray (eg, is an effort to increase beta-blocker use to prevent a second myocardial infarction an issue of quality improvement or safety?). That said, "safety" is often used in the context of rare incidents where there is a strong link between an error and its associated outcome (eg, wrong-site surgery). The issues regarding both types of research are often the same, but we will make special mention of those additional issues unique to patient safety research that take account of the rarity of many safety events.

PRACTICE POINT

- Collecting, analyzing, and reporting data does not turn a QI project into research. The important characteristic of QI research, as opposed to standard QI efforts, is that the question to be answered is not "can we improve care here?" but "does this intervention work in general?" If the goal is to design and test a novel intervention to improve care (or to test an established intervention in a novel setting), to establish whether a particular intervention works in a wide variety of settings such that it might become a new standard of care, and/or to learn generalizable lessons about how to successfully implement such an intervention, then it is research.

OVERVIEW OF QI RESEARCH

QI VS QI RESEARCH

As noted above, QI research is not just writing up the results of a QI project. In fact, writing up the results should be part of almost all QI efforts so that other institutions can learn from your experience and you can earn "academic credit" for having done the work. The recently published SQUIRE Guidelines (http://www.squire-statement.org/) provide detailed advice on how to write up such results. Some of the content unique to these reports (as opposed to conventional research manuscripts) include the following:

- Introduction: description of the local problem and the intended improvement
- Methods: discussion of any ethical issues, planning the intervention, and planning the study of the intervention
- Results: description of the environmental context, a timeline of the intervention, degree of success in implementation,

how and why the plan evolved, and lessons learned from that evolution
- Discussion: issues of maintaining improvement over time, causal mechanisms regarding the specific components of the intervention, and how environmental context played a role in the success (or failure) of the intervention and its implementation

As noted above, collecting, analyzing, and reporting data does not turn a QI project into research. For example, in a standard QI project, results over time may be displayed using run charts with statistical process control limits, with results plotted over time, a central line at the mean, and limit lines at 3 standard deviations (SD) above and below the mean. In a chart with 25 data points, the chance of a point being outside the 3 SD lines, indicating "special cause variation," is 6.5%, similar to the 0.05 threshold for statistical significance in standard statistical tests. Such charts allow participants in a QI effort to see whether their interventions are working, whether the improvements seen are likely to be due to chance, and to help guide further improvements to the intervention.

The important characteristic of QI research, as opposed to standard QI efforts, is that the question to be answered is not "can we improve care here?" but "does this intervention work in general?" Human subject research is defined as "a systematic investigation, including research, development, testing, and evaluation designed to develop or contribute to generalizable knowledge." "Generalizable knowledge" can be further defined as "enduring knowledge about the nature and function of human beings." If the only goal of a QI effort is to improve local compliance with currently recognized best practices (or a safety effort designed to reduce medical errors) using recognized procedures, without adding to existing knowledge about the general nature and function of human beings, then it is not research. On the other hand, if the goal is to design and test a novel intervention to improve care (or to test an established intervention in a novel setting), to establish whether a particular intervention works in a wide variety of settings such that it might become a new standard of care, and/or to learn generalizable lessons about how to successfully implement such an intervention, then it is research.

WHY AND WHEN TO CONDUCT QI RESEARCH

There are many reasons to conduct QI research. These include general reasons, such as expanding the body of medical knowledge and helping your patients; local reasons, such as answering a burning question important for your institution or your practice; and personal reasons, such as professional satisfaction or to provide balance to your clinical duties. The important question to ask yourself is whether these reasons are enough to motivate you to do the work required. QI research requires a great deal of work and, especially at the beginning of a research career, may come as an addition to an already full clinical schedule. But if you are motivated, the rewards can be considerable.

The second issue is whether it is the right time scientifically to conduct QI research. An analogy to drug trials may be useful. In phase 1 of quality improvement, the question is usually, "Can this intervention work in at least one place?" This is analogous to early research and development work in a pharmaceutical company and phase I/II clinical trials that look for safety and efficacy in a limited number of carefully selected patients. In this phase, interventions are often not well defined. The best approach in this phase is to do standard QI work, iterative refinement of the intervention using Plan-Do-Study-Act cycles, and to monitor improvement using run charts (see Chapter 12). In other words, it is not time to do QI research yet. However, some of the groundwork for later research can be done at this time. For example, in addition to optimizing the intervention itself, measures of process and outcome can be developed, and measures of environmental context and intervention fidelity (see below) can also be developed.

In phase 2, the primary questions are the following:

- Does this intervention work outside of its original location?
- Does it require refinement?
- How likely is it to work?
- What is the magnitude of benefit?
- Is it cost-effective?
- Should this intervention be spread widely?

This is the perfect time to conduct a more rigorous evaluation, analogous to phase III drug trials (often randomized controlled trials) needed for FDA approval. This is the right time to do QI research and is the subject of the rest of this chapter.

PRACTICE POINT

- In "Phase I" of quality improvement, the question is usually "can this intervention work in at least one place?"
- In "Phase 2," a more rigorous evaluation is required to answer the question of whether an intervention that might work is ready for widespread use. This is time for QI research.
- In "Phase 3," QI interventions proven effective in Phase 2 are disseminated widely.

Once an intervention has been proven to work, the goal is to spread the intervention widely. This usually requires adaptation to each local environment, ideally using lessons learned from prior work (eg, what are the most effective components of the intervention?; and how can implementation be optimized?). This is "Phase 3." Again, this is a time for standard QI methods, now focused on local adaptation of the intervention and making the micro- and macro-environment more conducive to effective implementation. If the prior QI research was well done, then lessons about how, why, and where an intervention works have already been answered to help guide this process.

In summary, the time to do rigorous QI research is during phase 2 of an intervention: It might work, but is it ready for widespread use? The more novel, expensive, or risky the intervention, the greater the need to study it as rigorously as possible in order to know whether the benefits truly outweigh the risks and costs.

SHOULD QI RESEARCH BE CONDUCTED RIGOROUSLY?

The best ways to think about and conduct QI research are not without controversy. There are some, such as Pawson and Tilley and Dr. Donald Berwick of the Institute for Health Care Improvement, who would argue that all QI is local. QI efforts are inherently complex behavioral interventions and need different approaches than just testing a pill. Randomized controlled trials purposefully control for environmental context in the name of unbiased outcome assessment. And yet, it is precisely the context and the process that are most important to evaluate, because they reveal how, why, and where an intervention is successful. Proponents of this approach argue for more case studies and "formative evaluation" to better understand these issues.

However, ignoring stronger study designs can lead to gross overestimation of treatment effects. Observational before-after studies are inherently confounded by temporal trends (ie, general improvement over time), co-interventions (other interventions that may affect the outcome), and biased by the Hawthorne effect (improvement that comes when people know they are being watched). And studies that compare those who volunteer to implement an intervention early to those who do not may be completely confounded by inherent differences between implementation and control sites. QI research is not so different from all biomedical research in that the interventions need a degree of certainty before institutions invest time, money, and resources in their implementation. It is particularly important to know how likely an intervention is to be successful. For example, if an intervention is very successful at one hospital but not successful in the next 10 that are studied, that is very different from an intervention that is successful in 75% of the hospitals in which it is evaluated.

We therefore advocate for strong study designs when appropriate and possible, as discussed below. But we also advocate complementing this work with "mixed methods" (ie, quantitative and qualitative research) that look carefully at contextual factors, intervention fidelity (ie, how faithfully an intervention is implemented as designed), and barriers and facilitators to successful implementation (see Conceptual Model of QI Research, below). Lastly, not every study can (or should be) a randomized controlled trial.

CONCEPTUAL MODEL OF QI RESEARCH

Celia Brown and Richard Lilford wrote a series of articles in 2008 describing an approach for rigorously evaluating patient safety interventions based on the recommendations of a network sponsored by the Medical Research Council, United Kingdom that echoes this sentiment. Their conceptual framework is shown in **Figure 13-1**. It is based on the Donabedian "structure-process-outcome" model and provides additional detail for studies of patient safety interventions. They note that such interventions may be aimed at *management processes*, such as nurse to patient ratios and time allocated to professional development, and/or *clinical processes*, such as washing hands between patients. The effectiveness of an intervention should be observed at all points to the right of the intervention. *Patient outcomes* may be "hard" (such as hospital readmission or patient mortality), which are clearly relevant but may be relatively insensitive to change. Surrogate outcomes, process measures, and error rates are more sensitive to change and should complement hard outcome measurement.

Observations at the point of intervention should be used to assess the *fidelity* with which the intervention was implemented and how it has been adapted over time. If an intervention is not implemented with high fidelity, it is unlikely to cause improvements in outcomes, even if they are observed. And when improvement is not seen, low fidelity may explain those findings even if the intervention were theoretically efficacious.

Observations to the left of the intervention provide information about environmental *context* and may explain differences among sites. Organizational *structure* may influence management processes, which in turn affect *intervening variables* such as morale, safety culture, teamwork, and provider knowledge and beliefs. These variables then influence clinical processes. If an intervention, implemented with high fidelity, improves all downstream processes and outcomes (even if some are not statistically significant), then it increases the likelihood that the intervention itself was really the cause of the improvement.

GETTING STARTED

ASKING THE RIGHT QUESTION

Initial challenges to beginning a QI research project may include psychological (getting over the fact that you are not a "researcher"), scientific (developing a good research question), and logistical (choosing study designs that are feasible). The most important first step is choosing the right research question, ie, the uncertainty about something in the population that the investigator wants to resolve by making measurements on his or her study population. There is no shortage of these. Good research questions are indeed everywhere and may be provoked by your clinical experience, by the advent of new technologies, by acknowledging the need to improve, and/or by maintaining a healthy skepticism about prevailing beliefs. Developing questions is an iterative process, and we recommend consulting early and often with advisors and colleagues.

A good research question has the following attributes:

1. The study that can answer the question is feasible: adequate number of subjects, availability of adequate technical expertise, affordable in time and money.
2. The question is interesting: it confirms, extends, or refutes previous findings (this implies that you have done the background reading on the subject).
3. The question is relevant: it has implications for clinical knowledge, practice, or policy.
4. The question can be answered ethically.

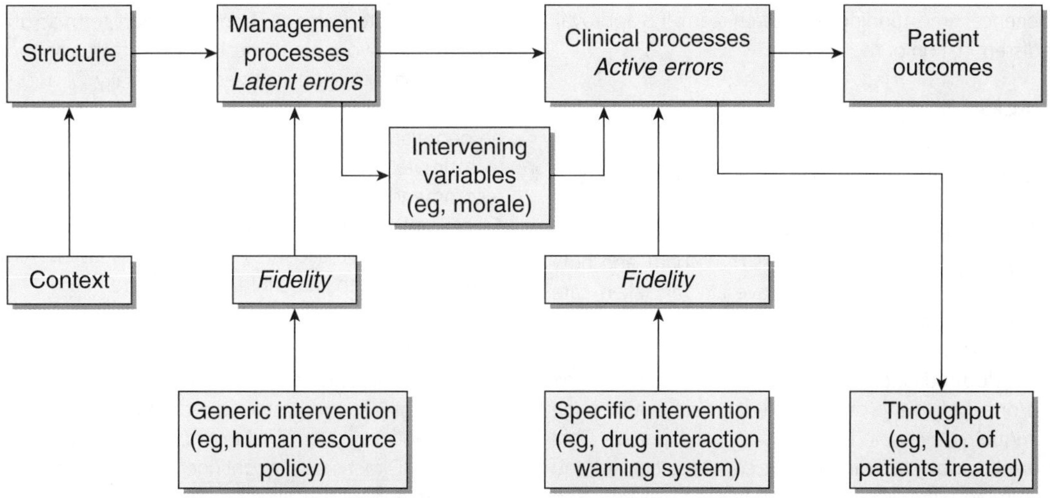

Figure 13-1 *Conceptual Framework for Evaluating Patient Safety Interventions. Observations can be made at all points in the chain to provide information on context, fidelity, and quality and safety outcomes. (Brown C and Lilford R, 337, a2764, 2008, with permission from BMJ Publishing Group Ltd.)*

Research questions often start out vague (eg, "Are fewer nurses bad for patients?"). To carry out a study, these questions need to be refined so that they become measurable. That is, your hypothesis needs to be testable. This means getting specific about three elements: the patient population, the intervention, and the outcome. Using the above example, a refined research question might be "for medical inpatients, is there an association between the patient-to-nurse ratio and in-hospital mortality?"

PRACTICE POINT

- A good research study must be feasible, relevant, confirm, extend, or refute previous findings, and be ethically answered. To carry out a study, the research questions need to be refined so that they become measurable. There are 2 attributes that make a research study useful to others: (1) internal validity, meaning that the results of the study reflect reality and can be believed, and (2) external validity, or generalizability, meaning that the results can be applied to other patients or settings.

PLANNING YOUR RESEARCH

Once a research question has been refined, the next steps are to develop a specific aim (or aims) and a hypothesis. The specific aim is what (exactly) you want to do. For example, "Determine the effects of an enoxaparin guideline on the appropriate use of enoxaparin." The hypothesis is the a priori, testable expectation for what you think is going to happen (or has happened). For example, "implementing an enoxaparin guideline will increase appropriate use of enoxaparin."

The next step is to develop a study proposal. Writing everything down in a standardized way serves several purposes: it forces you to address all the issues that may come up with a study's design and execution; it provides a convenient way for you to explain your study to others, get feedback, and refine your methods; and it is necessary for Institutional Review Board (IRB) approval and to obtain funding if needed (but we recommend developing a study proposal even if you do not intend to apply for funding). **Table 13-1** provides a list of the elements of a research proposal, both in "research speak" and their English translations.

TABLE 13-1 Outline of a Research Proposal

Research Speak	English Translation
Research question	What questions will the study address?
Background and significance	Why are these questions important? What do we already know about them?
Aims and hypothesis	What do you plan to do? What do you expect to happen?
Subjects: Inclusion/exclusion criteria Consent	Who will you study? How will they agree to participate?
Design	How will you actually do the study? What is your "protocol"?
Data sources	Where will you get your data? What do you plan to collect?
Outcome variables	Which data are key to your question (or hypothesis)?
Predictor variables (covariates)	Which will confuse (or confound) the issue?
Statistical issues	How large is the study and how will it be analyzed?
Human subjects	How will you maintain ethical standards? How will you protect patients' rights?

INGREDIENTS FOR A SUCCESSFUL RESEARCH PROJECT

Once you have a good research idea, what else do you need to turn it into a successful project? The basic components are data, research training or experience, time, funding, a research team, IRB approval, and a plan for dissemination of the results.

DATA SOURCES

Data can come from a wide variety of sources, including institutional data, publicly available data, data from collaborators, and data you collect yourself. Every institution collects data for billing, public reporting, and other purposes. The keys are to find out who leads this effort, whether and how you can access these data, and how clean they are (eg, whether the owners have already taken care of issues like missing or erroneous data, misspellings, and other features that make research quality analyses possible). Publicly available data have obvious advantages, but it can sometimes be time consuming and/or expensive to obtain, and data sets can be large and unwieldy, requiring a certain level of statistical expertise. Data you collect yourself is obviously under your complete control and can be designed to answer your exact question but takes time and resources to collect. Data from collaborators is sometimes the best of all worlds if such opportunities are available and you are interested in the questions the data can answer.

RESEARCH TRAINING AND EXPERIENCE

You *can* do research, but it helps to have some background. This background can take many forms, from mentors and collaborators, short-term programs, all the way to degree programs and fellowships. In our experience, a summer-long program in research methods (such as those at the Harvard School of Public Health and at the University of California, San Francisco School of Medicine), followed by a research project done in close collaboration with an experienced mentor, is often enough to pave the way for further collaborative research projects and/or small independent projects.

TIME

One of the most challenging ingredients to obtain is time. Unless you have protected time built into your schedule or you can negotiate for protected time up front, the short-term solution is often an investment of your own time. However, if you can prove your ability to successfully conduct projects, especially QI and safety projects of inherent value to the institution, then protected time can often be negotiated the second time around. An important early step is to estimate the time needed to complete a research project. We recommend designing a timeline as part of your initial proposal. An example is shown in **Figure 13-2**. You should consult early with someone else to make sure the timeline is feasible. Almost all studies take more time that you initially anticipate!

FUNDING

The degree of funding required, if any, will depend on the project. Be sure not just to consider direct costs but also the opportunity costs of you and your collaborators (ie, time taken away from other activities). Direct costs might include the paid effort of research assistants and statisticians, office supplies and incidentals, etc. As with a timeline, it is never too early to design a preliminary budget and share it with others for refinement. A sample budget is shown in **Table 13-2**. Line items include personnel costs (salary and fringe

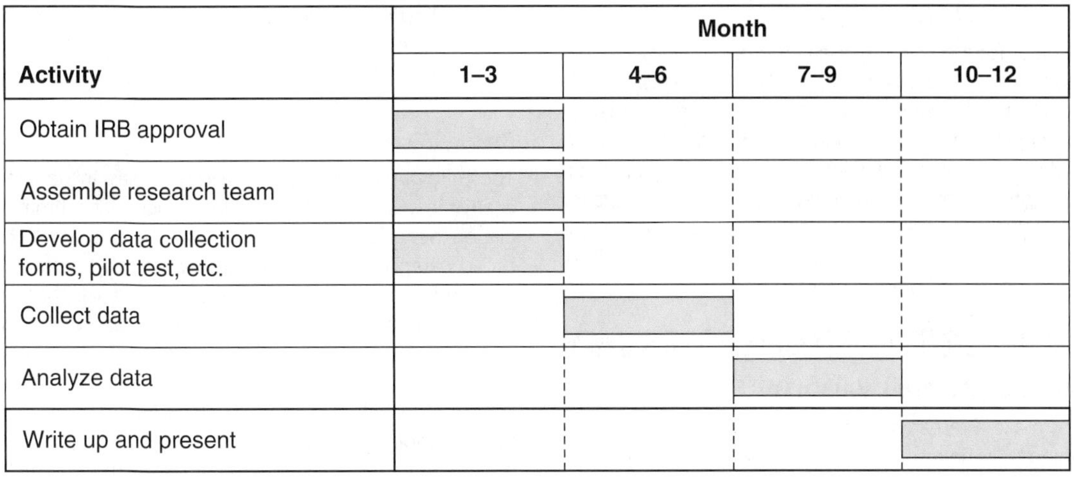

Figure 13-2 *Sample Timeline.*

for employee effort, hourly or daily fees for consultants), equipment, travel, and miscellaneous costs like office supplies, software, computer hardware, and photocopying.

Potential sources of funding depend on the scale of the project and the purpose of the study. For most QI and safety projects, the first place to start is usually your institution, especially if the costs are modest ($50,000–$100,000). If you can link your research question to financial and performance priorities of your hospital, internal funding becomes more likely. Internal sources include division or department funds, hospital-wide research grants, funding from the risk management organization at the hospital, and charitable giving. For questions less closely linked to hospital priorities or for larger projects, external funding is often required. Sources include foundations such as the National Patient Safety Foundation, the Commonwealth Found (US), and the Robert Wood Johnson Foundation; governmental sources such as Veterans Affairs, Agency for Health Care Research and Quality, and National Institutes of Health; statewide or national QI or safety initiatives; and industry, including pharmaceutical companies and device makers. Relationships between physicians and industry are definitely under more scrutiny than in the past, but some companies are still willing to fund investigator-initiated projects if priorities are closely aligned.

RESEARCH TEAM

The research team can, and should, be multidisciplinary, as is true of QI teams in general. One economical way to find collaborators is to work with medical students and housestaff, as long as the work can be done around their busy schedules (a good example of this kind of work is retrospective chart review). Paid research assistants are often required for daily, prospective data collection. Lastly, it is never too early to involve a statistician—they can help determine sample size (and therefore costs and feasibility of the study) and help resolve other methodologic issues before they become problems.

TABLE 13-2 Sample Budget

Item	Description	% Time	Amount
Principal investigator	Oversees project	20%	$30,000
Co-investigator	Research collaborator	10%	$15,000
Consultant	Specialized assistance	5%	$5000
Research assistant	Collects data	50%	$15,000
Statistician	Cleans, analyzes data	10%	$10,000
Travel to SHM	Presentation of findings		$1500
Office supplies	Copying, faxes, etc.		$500
Total			$77,000

SHM, Society of Hospital Medicine.

IRB APPROVAL

Institutional Review Board approval is often the source of much angst and controversy. To complicate matters, there is yet to be consensus on when IRB approval is needed. Some recent clarity was provided by Lynn, et al. in a 2007 article in *Annals of Internal Medicine*, "The ethics of using QI methods in health care." They note the characteristics of activities that are likely to be both QI and human subjects research, such as

1. Issues that go beyond current best practice
2. Allocation of patients to different treatments
3. Deliberately delayed feedback of data to avoid bias
4. Key involvement of researchers without commitment to ongoing QI at that site
5. Funding by parties outside the clinical setting

PRACTICE POINT

- QI research (as opposed to QI efforts alone) is human subjects research (HSR) and IRB approval is therefore required.

For our purposes, QI research (as opposed to QI efforts alone) is human subjects research, as noted in the introduction. IRB approval is therefore required. However, in many cases, it is possible to obtain expedited approval with waiver of patient consent on the grounds that the studies are of minimal risk, that patient confidentiality will be rigorously protected, that the study could not be practicably done if patient consent were required, and that the rights of patients will not be adversely affected by waiver of consent and authorization. As with your research proposal, begin the IRB application process early and have others with experience look through it (human research committees often have consultants who can help with this). Interview forms and consent forms will need to be created as part of this process. Do not worry if these are not finalized—amendments can always be submitted later. Lastly, as part of the IRB approval process, study staff must complete training in the ethical treatment of research subjects. Each institution has its own specific requirements.

DISSEMINATION PLAN

The last ingredient for a successful research project is a dissemination plan. Research in a vacuum is not useful. You have a responsibility to let others know the results of your study, positive or negative. Besides manuscripts, other study products might include detailed descriptions of your interventions, software specifications, data collection instruments (surveys and interview guides), etc. Outlets for dissemination include not only peer-reviewed journals but presentations at your own institution and professional society meetings, reports to your funders, and press releases.

STUDY DESIGN ISSUES IN QI AND SAFETY RESEARCH

INTERNAL AND EXTERNAL VALIDITY

Two attributes make a research study useful to others: (1) internal validity, meaning that the results of the study reflect reality and can be believed; and (2) external validity, or generalizability, meaning that the results can be applied to other patients or settings. Without internal validity, generalizability is a moot point, so in a sense internal validity is the more important of the two attributes.

THREATS TO INTERNAL VALIDITY

Chance

There are three main threats to the internal validity of a study: chance, confounding, and bias. Chance means that the results were simply due to the "luck of the draw." Type 1 error is when the null hypothesis is rejected due to chance when in fact it is true (for example, drug A is found to be better than drug B when in fact the two are equal). This can be thought of as a false-positive study. By convention, the threshold for type 1 error in most studies (known as alpha) is set at 0.05. When the *P* value from a statistical test is below this threshold, we call the difference statistically significant. Another way to think of this is to say that for every 20 studies that find a statistically significant difference, one of those studies is wrong simply due to chance.

Type 2 error results in accepting the null hypothesis when in fact it is false (eg, concluding that drug A and drug B are no different from each other when in fact drug A is better). The threshold, called beta, is typically set at 0.10 for definitive studies and 0.20 for preliminary studies—2 to 4 times higher than alpha. In other words, the medical scientific community has implicitly decided that it is more acceptable to have a false-negative study than a false-positive study. This makes sense for drug trials when the consequence of a positive study is FDA approval. It is less clear whether this argument holds for QI research. Statistical *power* is 1 minus beta. So, a study with 90% power means there is a 10% chance that it will not find a difference when in fact one exists, simply due to chance.

Confounding

Confounding is the second threat to internal validity. A confounder is a third factor ie, not the exposure or the outcome, associated with the exposure of interest (like the QI intervention you are studying) that independently causes the outcome of interest. For example, the earliest work in the epidemiology of lung cancer found a strong association with alcohol consumption. The confounder, of course, was cigarette smoking: something associated with alcohol use (people smoke in bars) that causes the outcome of interest (lung cancer). Confounding has to do with the science of what is being studied. Managing confounding requires knowledge of what factors could cause the outcome(s) you are studying. In QI research, major confounders include temporal trends (ie, general improvement with time, a problem with before-after studies), cointerventions (ie, other interventions that affect your outcome, implemented at the same time but apart from your intervention), and "indication" (ie, in nonrandomized studies, the reasons why sites choose to implement an intervention that may be strongly related to the outcomes being studied).

Bias

The third threat to internal validity is bias. In general terms, bias is error in a study that results in an incorrect estimate of the association between the exposure and the outcome. There are two broad categories: selection bias, which is an error in the process of identifying the study populations; and, much more common, observation or information bias, which is an error in measurement of the exposure and/or the outcome. There are many types of information bias, each with its own story: recall bias, interviewer bias, loss to follow-up, misclassification, etc. Unlike confounding, bias has more to do with human nature and how the study is conducted. In QI research, one major bias is the Hawthorne effect, or changes in measurement caused by participants' knowledge that they are being observed. Another potential bias arises when the intervention itself affects measurement. For example, in early studies of rapid response teams (RRTs), patients whose status was Do Not Resuscitate (DNR) were often excluded from the outcome of in-hospital mortality. When RRTs approached patients in extremis, one common activity was verifying code status. In several cases, patients and their caregivers decided to change code status to DNR. These patients were therefore excluded from the outcome. But before the advent the RRTs, these patients would have been included in outcome assessment because no one verified their code status at that time. A before-after study could find a difference in mortality simply because the intervention altered who was in the denominator for outcome assessment.

MANAGING THREATS TO INTERNAL VALIDITY

Table 13-3 provides ways to manage the threats to internal validity while the study is being designed (ie, before data are collected) and/or while the study is being analyzed (after data are collected). For example, during the study design phase, chance is managed using power and sample size calculations. If alpha and beta are chosen and the effect size can be estimated (ie, how beneficial the intervention will be), then the sample size can be calculated. Effect size may be estimated from preliminary studies, or more conservatively, may be chosen as the smallest effect that would be considered "clinically significant" by clinical experts. Conversely, if the sample size is fixed (eg, the ward has a known daily census and the study must be completed in 6 weeks), then statistical power to detect different effect sizes can be calculated. Once a study is completed, the effect of chance is derived using tests of statistical significance (ie, calculation of *P* values).

TABLE 13-3 Managing Threats to Internal Validity

Threat to Validity	Study Design (Before)	Analysis (After)
Chance	Power calculations	Statistics
Confounding	Randomization	Stratification
	Picking comparable groups	Multivariable regression
Bias	Blinding, prospective data collection, valid instruments, thorough follow-up	Unable to manage (although sometimes direction and magnitude can be estimated)

During the study design phase, confounding can be managed most effectively through randomization (confounding cannot exist if the confounder is evenly distributed among those who do and do not receive the intervention). Anything short of randomization is going to be less effective at managing confounding, but attempts can still be made to pick patient populations that are as comparable as possible (eg, medical wards from medium-sized, non-teaching community hospitals in the suburbs). During the data analysis phase, confounding can be managed with stratification (eg, looking at the effect of alcohol on lung cancer in smokers separately from the effect in nonsmokers). This is very effective if there are only one or two major confounders, but is impractical when the list of confounders is large (*N* confounders means 2^N subgroups to analyze, each with a very small sample size). The purpose of multivariable (sometimes called multivariate) analysis is to simultaneously "adjust" for multiple confounders at once. But keep in mind that confounding can still exist, either because of incomplete adjustment, inaccurate measurement of the confounder, or existence of other unmeasured confounders.

During the study design phase, bias can be minimized by employing principles of sound study design: blinding to intervention status (not just "double-blind," but as many people involved in the study as possible: patients, research assistants, outcome assessors, statisticians, etc), prospective data collection, valid data collection instruments such as surveys and questionnaires, and thorough follow-up for all endpoints. Once the study has been conducted, bias cannot be "adjusted for" during the data analysis phase, although sometimes its direction and magnitude can be estimated. For example, to estimate the impact of loss-to-follow-up, some experts recommend assuming that everyone who received the intervention and was lost to follow-up did poorly, while everyone who received usual care and was lost to follow-up did well. Even large effect sizes can crumble under the weight of such assumptions if the loss to follow-up rate is large. On the other hand, poor data collection instruments often create noise and bias "towards the null" (ie, finding no difference). Therefore, if a difference is found, it is probably not the result of such bias. Because bias cannot really be adjusted for after the fact, it is important to manage study design issues up front, before any data are collected.

IMPROVING GENERALIZABILITY

Improving the generalizability of a study is a less complex matter. Guidelines include the following: (1) describe your patient population well, so that others can determine whether their patient populations are comparable; (2) describe your interventions well, so that others can determine what they would need to do to replicate your experience; and (3) describe your environmental context well, so others can determine whether a comparable intervention could be implemented in their settings. A common question related to generalizability is whether interventions should be maximally customized to the particular site where it is being studied. Such an approach increases the chances of success, but it may come at the price of generalizability. The answer should depend on which aspects of the study site are unique. Ideally, during phase 1 work, exactly which features need to be customized (and how) has already been determined; and these customizations can then be specified in advance.

TYPES OF STUDIES USED IN QI RESEARCH

There are several study designs that are appropriate for quality improvement and safety research. These include randomized controlled trials (with randomization at either the individual patient level or "clustered" by physician, ward, service, or hospital), before-after studies, interrupted time series, "stepped wedge," and observational cohort studies (prospective and retrospective). Each has its advantages and disadvantages and each is more or less appropriate for different situations. Not all QI research needs to be a randomized controlled trial to provide valid information.

Randomized controlled trials

The main advantage of a randomized controlled trial (RCT) is that it minimizes confounding by ensuring that potential confounders are equally distributed in the different arms of the study. This is true regardless of whether the confounders are known or can be measured. To the extent that RCTs require prospective data collection and at least allow the possibility of some blinding, they minimize bias as well, although also required are valid data collection instruments and thorough follow-up. And these studies still require adequate sample size to deal with chance. Note that the outcome may be conducted at one point in time (after the intervention has been implemented in those sites randomized to receive it) or as relative improvement over time (preintervention to postintervention). The latter may be preferred if you suspect large variation in baseline performance and especially if the same patients are going to be followed for the entire study period. All RCTs should be analyzed on an "intention-to-treat" basis, meaning that outcomes are measured according to the original intent of the randomization, regardless of what treatment (if any) was actually received. This preserves the sanctity of the randomization and is particularly important in QI studies, where the factors that lead to successful implementation or compliance with an intervention may independently predict positive outcomes. However, RCTs may not always be feasible or ethical. You may have limited control over who receives a QI intervention or you may be required (eg, for regulatory reasons) to provide it to everyone. It is often not ethical to study potentially harmful interventions with an RCT. And for outcomes that are rare or take a long time to develop, RCTs may be prohibitively expensive to conduct. Rare outcomes are particularly an issue with safety (as opposed to QI) studies. The best times to use an RCT are when an intervention can be randomized; there is particularly big concern for temporal trends, cointerventions, and other confounders that may not be known or cannot be measured; when the costs or potential risks of the intervention is high (such that they need to be balanced against a precise estimate of benefits); the target outcome is of high value (such as mortality); many settings will be affected by the results (eg, possible incorporation into a regulatory requirement); and any other situation that requires a precise estimate of effects and costs.

PRACTICE POINT

The best times to use an RCT are when

- An intervention can be randomized
- There is a significant concern for temporal trends, co-interventions, and other confounders
- Multiple settings will be affected by the results
- The situation requires a precise estimate of effects and costs

Cluster randomization

Cluster randomized trials are a type of RCT in which the unit of randomization is larger than the individual patient. For example, in a recent trial of a medication reconciliation intervention, we randomized by both medical team and floor so that we had clean separation of both nurses and doctors in the two arms of the study. The advantages are that it avoids treatment group "contamination" (ie, clinicians who change their behavior even with control patients because they have been exposed to or know about the intervention), it facilitates implementation of the intervention (eg, service-wide educational efforts), and administrative convenience. The major disadvantage is loss of statistical power. When patients of one physician, for example, are treated similarly to each other but different from the patients of another physician, this results in "intra-class correlation." This reduces the effective sample size, depending on the degree of the correlation and the size of the clusters (eg, the number of patients per physician). This correlation therefore needs to be anticipated and estimated in advance and used when making estimates of required sample size. Nevertheless, this is the preferred study design in many cases, especially when there are big advantages to training and implementation, the threat of contamination is high, the intervention requires it, the cluster size is small, and/or when the advantages are otherwise worth the loss in power.

RCTs, whether clustered or not, may suffer from issues of generalizability in that not every patient or health care setting may be willing to participate in one. In general, this is a sacrifice worth making in the name of internal validity, if feasible and appropriate to do so. As noted above, describing your patients, intervention, and environment well goes a long way toward alleviating these concerns.

Stepped wedge

The stepped wedge is a study design in which an intervention is sequentially rolled out to different groups at different times, such as different floors of a hospital (**Figure 13-3**). The order of the rollout is randomized to avoid confounding by indication (ie, those most ready for the intervention get it first). Each group serves a different amount of time in the usual care and intervention arms. This approach allows adjustment for temporal trends and also minimizes confounding because each group serves as its own control. Thus, the stepped wedge provides the advantages of a control group but is more practical than an RCT, especially if the intervention requires a gradual rollout anyway. The disadvantages are practical constraints regarding implementation, logistical challenges, and the risk of contamination (eg, colleagues hearing about the intervention occurring on a different floor).

Time series

Before-after studies and interrupted time series may be more feasible than RCTs when you have limited control over who receives the intervention and when they receive it. In a simple before-after study, outcomes are measured at one point before the intervention and one point after the intervention (eg, use of measures to prevent venous thromboembolism before and after a mass email reminder is sent out). This is probably the most common QI research study design, but unfortunately is one of the worst. It is very sensitive to temporal trends and to cointerventions. Much preferred is an interrupted time series (ITS), in which repeated observations (at least 3) are made prior to and after the intervention is implemented. The effect of the intervention can then be measured over and above temporal trends (although it still does not adjust for cointerventions). ITS is useful if the intervention needs to be given to everyone, all at once. Because there is no control group, one disadvantage is lack of generalizability, especially if the study site is particularly enthusiastic and well equipped to conduct the intervention. Another disadvantage is that the analysis assumes that the intervention is implemented once and does not change over time. However, newer sophisticated analytical techniques, such as random effects models with nonlinear time-by-intervention effects, can take into account such phenomena as continuous improvement over time (eg, as the intervention is refined) and/or reaching a plateau due to a ceiling effect (inability to improve further because quality is already so high).

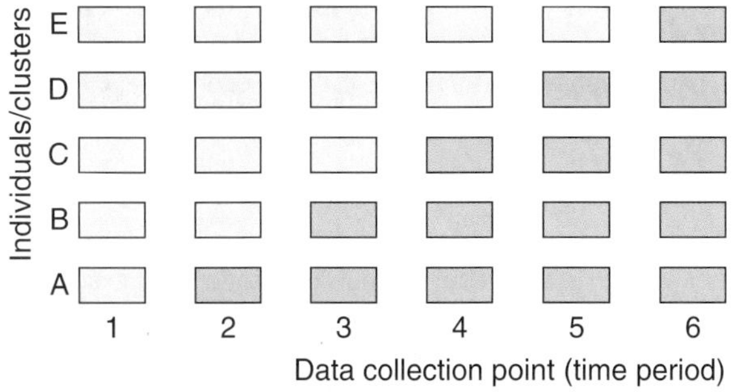

Figure 13-3 *Stepped Wedge Study Design. The intervention is rolled out to individuals or clusters sequentially over time, from blank cells (usual care) to shaded cells (intervention). (Brown C and Lilford R, 337, a2764, 2008, with permission from BMJ Publishing Group Ltd.)*

Cohort studies

A word of caution is in order about observational cohort studies, in which sites that choose to implement an intervention are compared with sites that choose not to. Because of potentially large differences in baseline rates of quality, the analysis should never be a simple comparison of outcomes at one point in time (eg, after implementation in the intervention arm). However, even if the analysis incorporates baseline rates by comparing improvement over time, these types of studies are potentially flawed. Those sites that are "early adopters" are often very different from those that are not in terms of culture of quality and safety, leadership, organizational structure, etc. These confounders may have large effects on the ability to implement and improve outcomes in response to an intervention. These confounders are also pervasive, potentially unknown, and difficult to measure. This confounding may be a fatal flaw to internal validity. A better approach is to deliver the intervention to as many groups as possible (to improve generalizability) and do an ITS.

Summary of study design issues

In conclusion, the optimal study design for a QI or safety study depends on answers to several questions.

1. Is it feasible and ethical to have a control group?
2. Do you have control over who gets the intervention and when?
3. Does the intervention need to be implemented all at once or gradually?
4. Can/should the intervention be delivered to individual patients, or does it make more sense to deliver it to a higher level (eg, physician, floor, service)?
5. Are the outcomes rare or do they take a long time to develop?
6. Are the costs and risks of the intervention low?
7. Will the results be used to promote widespread adoption of this intervention?

Table 13-4 illustrates how the answers to these questions may influence your choice of study design.

ADVANCED TOPICS AND CONTROVERSIES IN QI RESEARCH

One controversy in QI research is whether the interventions should be held fixed while they are being studied. On the one hand, such an approach allows for better description of the intervention, makes it clear "what" is being studied, and makes analyses easier to conduct. On the other hand, this approach does not allow for standard continuous quality improvement methods and may therefore limit the effectiveness of the intervention. The answer may depend on how much customization is considered necessary for a given intervention. In a phase 2 study, an intervention may already be optimized and it may be appropriate to hold it fixed. But even under

TABLE 13-4 Questions that Influence Choice of Study Design

Question	Preferred Study Designs: If Yes	Preferred Study Designs: If No
Is it feasible and ethical to have a control group?	RCT or clustered RCT	ITS Stepped wedge
Do you have control over who gets the intervention and when?	RCT or clustered RCT Stepped Wedge	ITS
Does the intervention need to be implemented all at once?	RCT or clustered RCT ITS	Stepped wedge
Can/should the intervention be delivered to individual patients?	RCT (randomization by patient)	Clustered RCT
Are the outcomes rare or do they take a long time to develop?	Multicenter ITS	RCT or clustered RCT
Are the costs and risks of the intervention low?	ITS Before-after studies	RCT or clustered RCT
Will the results be used to generate a requirement for adoption of this intervention?	RCT or clustered RCT	ITS Before-after studies

ITS, interrupted time series; RCT, randomized controlled trial.

these circumstances, we would still recommend a long pilot period that allows for continuous QI methods and/or a multiphase study in which improvements to an intervention are planned for at periodic intervals. For example, a study of a novel software application should likely be conducted as a multiphase study since changes to software often take a while and "version 1" of software is almost never ideal.

Another controversy is whether an intervention can be different at each site. Under some circumstances it may be desirable to standardize the goals and functions of the intervention rather than the exact form and structure. This allows for flexibility and maximizes the chances of success at each site. Such an approach may be preferred when the intervention is complex and when baseline achievement and environment are very different from site to site. Such an approach is recommended by Hawe and colleagues. For example, for a recently proposed multisite study of medication reconciliation, we chose to standardize the components of the intervention along functional lines (eg, "improve access to sources of preadmission medication information"). This was necessary because each site was different in terms of its current processes, its local strengths and weaknesses, and its environment. On the other hand, it makes the description of the intervention and the analysis more difficult.

One way to improve the analytic approach to both these issues (continuous improvement over time and different interventions at each site) is to break down an intervention into its component parts and quantify the degree to which the intervention achieves each goal at any point in time. Using random effects models, the outcomes for each patient are then a function of the site, the time period, and the "score" for each component of the intervention. In this way, the degree to which each component contributes to the success of the intervention can be quantified. Again using the above multicenter medication reconciliation study as an example, we developed a 0–4 score for each of the 15 components of medication reconciliation; and these will serve as predictors of the number of medication discrepancies per patient.

Not all ideas regarding QI and safety research are controversial. For example, it always makes sense to have adequate sample size to adequately answer your study question, to describe your interventions well, use unbiased measurement tools to collect data, look at both processes and outcomes, look at potential unintended consequences of your intervention, and examine environmental context and intervention fidelity. Studies are most successful when study design issues are anticipated and managed early, well before data are collected. Therefore, get the help of experts in study design and statistics as soon as your study question has been refined.

CONCLUSION

Regarding study design, chance, confounding, and bias are the major threats to the internal validity of a study. It is far better to minimize these when designing your study than to deal with them later at the analysis phase. Different study designs address these issues to different degrees. More formal study designs, such as cluster-randomized controlled trials, are preferred (if possible and ethical) when the benefits of the intervention are not self-evident or the intervention is costly and not without risk. But other study designs, such as stepped wedge and interrupted time series, are also excellent study designs depending on the situation.

Interesting research questions are everywhere. As a hospitalist, you are often in an ideal position to recognize these questions, so take advantage of that. Choose the right time to do research, both personally and for the research question. Plan your study in advance and get the help and training you need. Don't be afraid of the IRB: they can actually help you with your proposal, but allow enough time for the process to occur. You *can* do QI research, and by getting started, you may find that the rewards and the potential impact of your work on large patient populations are well worth the effort.

SUGGESTED READINGS

Benneyan JC, Lloyd RC, Plsek PE. Statistical process control as a tool for research and healthcare improvement. *Qual Saf Health Care.* Dec 2003;12(6):458–464.

Brown C, Hofer T, Johal A, et al. An epistemology of patient safety research: a framework for study design and interpretation. Parts 1–4. *Qual Saf Health Care.* Jun 2008;17(3):158–181.

Brown C, Lilford R. Evaluating service delivery interventions to enhance patient safety. *BMJ.* 2008;337:a2764.

Donabedian A. Explorations in quality assessment and monitoring. In: Griffith JR, ed. The definition of quality and approaches to it assessment. Washington, DC: Health Administration Press; 1980:4–163.

Dumas JE, Lynch AM, Laughlin JE, Phillips Smith E, Prinz RJ. Promoting intervention fidelity. Conceptual issues, methods, and preliminary results from the EARLY ALLIANCE prevention trial. *Am J Prev Med.* Jan 2001;20(1 Suppl):38–47.

Hawe P, Shiell A, Riley T. Complex interventions: how "out of control" can a randomised controlled trial be? *BMJ.* Jun 26 2004;328(7455):1561–1563.

Lynn J, Baily MA, Bottrell M, et al. The ethics of using quality improvement methods in health care. *Ann Intern Med.* May 1 2007;146(9):666–673.

Ogrinc G, Mooney SE, Estrada C, et al. The SQUIRE (Standards for QUality Improvement Reporting Excellence) guidelines for quality improvement reporting: explanation and elaboration. *Qual Saf Health Care.* Oct 2008;17(suppl 1):i13–i32.

Pawson R, Tilley N. Realistic Evaluation. London: Sage Publications, Ltd; 1997.

Stetler CB, Legro MW, Wallace CM, et al. The role of formative evaluation in implementation research and the QUERI experience. *J Gen Intern Med.* Feb 2006;21(suppl 2):S1–S8.

CHAPTER 14

Principles and Models of Quality Improvement: Plan-Do-Study-Act

Emmanuel S. King, MD, FHM
Jennifer S. Myers, MD, FHM

INTRODUCTION

Achieving quality in health care requires a focus on continuous performance improvement. Physicians pride themselves on being subject matter experts in their focused area of medical practice. Although such knowledge is critical for developing changes that result in improvement, alone it is not sufficient to produce fundamental changes in the delivery of health care. Physicians who practice in complex hospital and health care systems must acquire another kind of knowledge in order to develop and execute change.

W. Edwards Deming, an American statistician and professor who is widely credited with improvement in manufacturing in the United States and Japan, has described this knowledge as a "system of profound knowledge" (**Figure 14-1**). This knowledge is composed of the following items: appreciation for a system, understanding variation, building knowledge, and the human side of change. These concepts are not taught in many medical school, yet are essential for physicians and other health care providers who are passionate about improving the systems around them.

All hospitalists have witnessed changes that did not result in fundamental improvements within their hospital systems: the computerized order set that was successfully implemented but never revised based on prescribers' feedback, the paper checklist for medication reconciliation that never gets filled out, or the new rounding system that worked for the first few weeks but then failed to become a standard part of practice due to physician variation or lack of commitment. These are all examples of *first-order changes*—changes that only returned the system to the normal level of performance. In quality improvement work, individuals must strive for *second-order changes*, which are changes that truly alter the system and result in a higher level of system performance. Such changes impact how work is done, produce visible, positive differences in results relative to historical norms, and have a lasting impact. Although the model for improvement described below may seem simple, it is actually quite demanding when used properly; and the process is essential to both learning and ultimately changing complex systems.

PRACTICE POINT

- In quality improvement work, individuals must strive for second-order changes, which are changes that truly alter the system and result in a higher level of system performance. Such changes impact how work is done, produce visible, positive differences in results relative to historical norms, and have a lasting impact.

PLAN-DO-STUDY-ACT AS A TOOL FOR QUALITY IMPROVEMENT

The Plan-Do-Study-Act (PDSA) model is a commonly used tool in quality improvement (QI) science. Shewart and Deming described the model many years ago when they studied quality in other industries. This model first appeared in health care when Berwick described how the tools could be applied and emphasized an iterative approach to change. Using a "trial-and-learning approach" in which a hypothesis is tested, retested, and refined, the PDSA cycle allows for controlled change experiments on a small scale

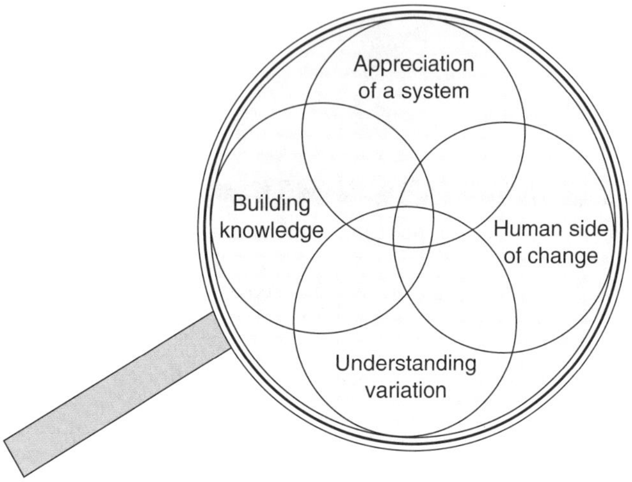

Figure 14-1 *Deming's System of Profound Knowledge. (Reproduced, with permission, from Langley GJ, et al. The Improvement Guide: A Practical Approach to Enhancing Organization Performance, 2nd ed. San Francisco, CA: Jossey-Bass; 2009.)*

before expansion to a larger system. The four repetitive steps of PDSA—plan, do, study, and act—are carried out until fundamental improvement, which can be exponentially larger than the original hypothesis, takes place (**Figure 14-2**).

PRACTICE POINT

- Using a "trial-and-learning approach" in which a hypothesis is tested, retested, and refined, the 4 steps of PDSA—plan, do, study, and act—are carried out repetitively until fundamental improvement, which can be exponentially larger than the original hypothesis, takes place.

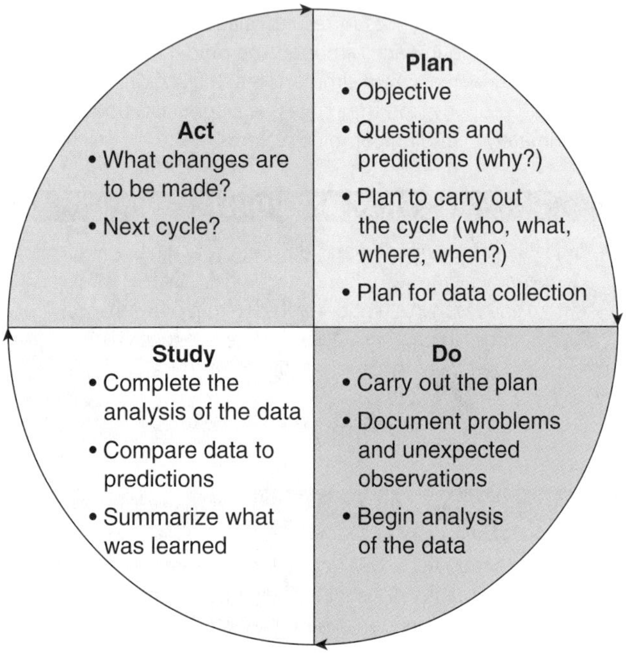

Figure 14-2 *The Plan-Do-Study-Act Cycle. (Reproduced, with permission, from Langley GJ, et al. The Improvement Guide: A Practical Approach to Enhancing Organization Performance, 2nd ed. San Francisco, CA: Jossey-Bass; 2009.)*

PLAN

During the Plan phase, the team generates broad questions, hypotheses, and a data collection plan. It is critically important during this period to define expectations and assign tasks and accountability to every team member. In the planning phase of the PDSA cycle, it is prudent to invest significant time and develop a well-framed question by reviewing related research and local projects and defining meaningful process and outcome measurements. Broad questions at the outset of a PDSA cycle can include "What are we trying to accomplish?" and "What changes can we make that will result in an improvement?" The ideal data collection tool answers the question: "How will we know that a change is an improvement?" It is also helpful for the team to generate predictions of the answers to questions early on. This aids in framing the plan more completely, to uncover underlying assumptions or biases before any testing, and to enhance learning in the Study phase by providing a baseline point of comparison.

Teams new to QI frequently will struggle with the question, "How do we measure improvement?" Defining discrete process measures is a good starting point when using PDSA. Process measures are used to assess whether the cycle is being carried out as planned. This is in contrast to outcome measures which are used to track success or failure and focus on the specific outcome that the team is trying to achieve (see Chapter 15).

DO

The Do phase in PDSA is a period of active implementation. It involves observation of the process, feedback on the process from end-users, and rigorous data collection. An overarching goal of this phase is to capture and document not only compliance with the new process, but also deviations, defects, or barriers in the process. There are always aspects of quality improvement projects that do not go as planned, and flexibility and open-mindedness are critical to maximize learning from improvement. The quality of the Do phase is intimately related to the quality of the Plan phase. A pitfall for many novice QI teams is to give in to the temptation to jump straight to implementing change without spending a significant amount of time planning. A poorly conceptualized improvement plan, an absence of a sound data collection model, or unclear accountabilities can have adverse effects on the implementation or "do" phase of a new initiative.

STUDY

Analysis of available process and outcome metrics and a qualitative appraisal of the process are the key activities in the Study phase. Time should be set aside to perform a critical review of the data collected and compare it to historical data (when available) and baseline predictions. Close attention should be paid to possible defects in any element of the process, including the data collection plan. If such issues are uncovered, the team may need to revise the initial data collection tools and overall plan. Thoughtful review of all trials, even those that were clearly unsuccessful based on metrics, is a critical and valuable process for the team. In fact, the "failures" in a PDSA cycle can yield unanticipated and improved directions. As the Study phase progresses, time should be spent considering if a follow-up PDSA cycle is planned and exactly what elements to include in that cycle.

ACT

The final component in a PDSA cycle is Act. The team should convene for a feedback and action planning session. Frontline workers in the system that is being changed should be included for honest input. A team approach rather than a "top-down" approach facilitates an open review of successes and failures. An action plan that encompasses lessons learned in the first three steps should then be put into motion. During this stage decisions are made about repeating certain test cycles after improvements are made or "spinning off" new test cycles based on the original one.

RAPID CYCLE, CONTINUOUS, AND SEQUENTIAL PDSA

In its most basic form, the PDSA model described above can be applied to change a single process. However, teams in health care often confront problems that require multiple changes, in parallel or succession, in order for improvement to happen. Caution is advised when initiating several PDSA cycles simultaneously, especially if there are significantly different data collection plans or if the team is inexperienced in QI methods. An alternative is a sequential PDSA model in which one PDSA cycle feeds into the next. This approach, in which teams continually change and refine their processes based on data evaluation and feedback, is called "continuous quality improvement." Experienced QI teams strive to utilize this approach. Rapid cycle PDSA is a continuous QI process that lends itself well to projects that are focused on relatively small scale changes. It is typically used by seasoned QI teams who are familiar with the PDSA model and who wish to implement rapid change.

CASE 14-1

AN EXAMPLE OF PDSA IN ACTION

To illustrate the PDSA model for improvement, a real QI project is presented here from start to finish. A hospitalist group sought to implement a new discharge planning toolkit aimed at improving transitions in care through risk assessment at the time of hospital admission. The assessment was accomplished through the use of a tool designed to predict a patient's individual risk for readmission to the hospital. One of the first team goals was to create a new process to coordinate and request risk-specific interventions from other teams (eg, nurse educators, pharmacists, a nurse for postdischarge follow-up phone calls) for patients deemed "high risk for hospital re-admission or transition in care problems" by the screening tool.

Cycle 1

Plan

In this phase, the QI team leaders decided that their priorities were (1) small-scale change, (2) gaining "buy-in" from frontline users of the toolkit, and (3) winning an early "victory" to establish the initiative. Given these priorities, the team decided to use sequential, rapid-cycle PDSA for the project. The initial goal was to pilot a screening tool drafted by an external group. A weekly meeting was convened that included representative users of the tool and assigned specific responsibilities and tasks with due dates to each team member. At baseline, the biggest barriers to overcome were the perception that the new tool was extra work, introducing a paper-based tool in a largely electronic health care environment, and lack of a tight infrastructure tying the requests to existing risk-specific interventions. Based on these concerns, the team reduced the number of interventions on the initial tool. A data collection plan was started and included both quantitative process metrics (eg, compliance rates with the tool, frequency of risk factors identified on the tool) and qualitative data from the users of the tool.

Do

The new tool was piloted for 2 weeks, during which time data was collected and feedback was solicited from the frontline team.

Study

After 2 weeks, the data showed that overall compliance with the tool was moderately high, but that two risk factors, health literacy and depression, had unexpectedly low percentages. On further inquiry, members of the team admitted that when they performed the risk screen, they paused on those two questions and frequently left them blank, concerned that it might take too much time during the admission process and frustrate new users of the tool.

Act

The team decided to make another edit to the tool before the second PDSA cycle. The health literacy and depression screening questions were removed based on feedback, with a plan to reintroduce them when the tool was more embedded in the hospital admission workflow.

Cycle 2

Plan

The second cycle focused on follow-up data collection with the health literacy and depression screening questions removed from the tool, to test the theory that this would improve compliance. The data collection plan was to track overall compliance with the tool for a 2-week period. In order to isolate any improvement as a result of this one small change, no other changes were made during this time.

Do

The new version of the tool was implemented.

Study

Compliance rates significantly increased from moderately high to very high, and the risk factor screening data remained unchanged. Qualitative feedback from frontline users was that the risk screening process was more streamlined and acceptable.

Act

A brief but successful cycle 2 ended with a plan to add an intervention checklist to the tool in the next phase.

Cycle 3

Plan

The goal of cycle 3 was to associate risk-specific interventions (education, follow-up phone calls, and social work interventions) with a patient's individual risk factor profile. To meet this goal, the team implemented a new version of the tool that included the risk-specific intervention requests and tracked request type and volume. A 2-week cycle was planned with continued weekly meetings during this time.

Do

Implemented a tool that allowed for interventions to be requested at the time of risk factor screening.

Study

After 2 weeks, the data showed stable high compliance with the form, stable risk factor data, but very low utilization of intervention requests. At feedback meetings, frontline users stated that at the time of admission, they were not ready to place a request for an intervention. They felt that intervention requests should be discussed in a multidisciplinary team on a follow-up hospital day when more information was available.

Act

Discharge planners on the team suggested that the intervention request process be integrated into daily discharge planning rounds, during which the entire patient care team (physician, nurse practitioner, registered nurse, discharge planners, patient service representative, and social worker) discussed each patient on the service. A nurse practitioner and patient service representative drafted paper forms that could be used to communicate requests for each of the interventions to the appropriate personel and to document completion of the task. The next phase would trial this new process.

Cycle 4

Plan

Cycle 4 was focused on implementing and studying the new discharge rounds process to request risk-specific interventions. The frequency of intervention requests in each category was added to the existing process metrics. Since this was a more substantial change than before and involved more than just one team of frontline users, a 4-week cycle duration was chosen.

Do

Clinicians continued to screen patients using the risk screening tool, intervention request forms were kept on hand during discharge rounds, and the patient service representative and discharge planners prompted the teams to request interventions based on patient risk factors. The requests were forwarded to the appropriate personnel (registered nurse, pharmacist, nurse educator), who then documented completion of the intervention on the form.

Study

Compliance rates and risk factor data remained steady, but there was a significant increase in intervention requests in all categories. However, documentation of completion of the intervention was low. It was determined that the documentation requirements were unfamiliar to the intervention teams, which was an oversight.

Act

For the next cycle further improvements in documentation of intervention completion and a reintroduction of the health literacy and depression screening questions was planned.

LESSONS LEARNED

The case study illustrates several important points for successful use of the PDSA model. First, the engagement and involvement of the end users of new QI tools and processes is critical to the success of any improvement project. These users are experts in the process who often know what should be tested next, and perfect champions when changes are disseminated on a larger scale. While it may be impossible to address or fix every problem that they identify, hearing their input, implementing changes based on their suggestions, and giving praise for their involvement and patience is an important skill for leaders of QI. Second, flexibility and creative thinking, skills that are used frequently in clinical care, are also essential in QI. In the case study, several barriers were identified such as: concerns about paper forms, perception that certain risk factors would halt the risk screening process, and lack of infrastructure around the systematic documentation of interventions. As these barriers became apparent, the team remained flexible and changed a part of the new process without compromising the integrity and team goals of the project.

PRACTICE POINT

Critical to the success of any quality improvement project:

- Engagement and involvement of the "end" users of new QI tools and processes
- Flexibility and creative thinking

ALTERNATIVE MODELS OF QUALITY IMPROVEMENT

In addition to the PDSA model described above, there are other frameworks that have been used to design and execute quality improvement projects. Adopting one specific framework (as opposed to adopting several) allows an organization to learn a common language and approach to improvement. Six Sigma and Lean are two common frameworks that will be briefly described.

Six Sigma was developed by Motorola in the mid 1980s and focused on reducing variations in process. Six Sigma has evolved into a number of conceptual frameworks. One of the more popular frameworks uses the acronym DMAIC. DMAIC stands for **d**efine QI goals, **m**easure the current process and develop a baseline, **a**nalyze cause and effect of factors, **i**mprove the process on the basis of the analysis and transition to standard processes, and **c**ontrol the process to ensure that variances are corrected before they result in defects.

Lean manufacturing (or just "Lean") was adapted from the Toyota Production Systems and is focused on continuously reducing waste in operations and enhancing the value proposition to customers. The Lean approach is based on a few key principles: defining from the customer perspective, identifying the activities required to provide the customer with a product or service, producing the products or services only when needed by customers, and pursuing perfection in the process. See Chapter 20.

CONCLUSION

Plan-Do-Study-Act has remained a fundamental tool for continuous quality improvement. Once comfortable applying this iterative approach, hospitalists can affect both small- and large-scale changes in their health care systems.

SUGGESTED READINGS

Berwick D. Developing and testing changes in delivery of care. *Ann Intern Med.* 1998;128:651–656.

Berwick D, Nolan T. Physicians as leaders in improving health care: a new series in Annals of Internal Medicine. *Ann Intern Med.* 1998;128:289–292.

Langley GJ, Moen RD, Nolan KM, Nolan TW, Norman CL, Provost LP. *The Improvement Guide: A Practical Approach to Enhancing Organizational Performance*. 2nd ed. San Francisco: Jossey-Bass; 2009.

Shewhart WA. Statistical Method from the Viewpoint of Quality Control. Washington, DC: Dover; 1986.

Tague N. *The Quality Toolbox*. 2nd ed. Milwaukee, WI: Quality Press; 2005.

Varkey P, Reller K, Resar R. Basics of Quality Improvement in Health Care. *Mayo Clin Proc.* 2007;82(6):735–739.

CHAPTER 15

Measurement and Measures in Hospital Medicine

Chad T. Whelan, MD
Nathan Spell, MD, FACP

INTRODUCTION

In this chapter we will discuss measuring quality of care—general principles of measurement, measures for judging quality, and measures used for the local management and improvement of care—with a focus on measures of particular interest to Hospital Medicine physicians.

THE INTEREST IN MEASURING QUALITY

MEASUREMENT FOR PERFORMANCE ASSESSMENT

The era of accountability has arrived in medicine. Consumers, purchasers, and providers of health care are increasingly interested in health care quality and safety. Health care value, in which value is a function of quality ÷ cost, is being closely scrutinized as the increasing cost of health care has outpaced inflation over several decades without a demonstrated concomitant increase in quality and safety.

PRACTICE POINT

- Without measurement, it is impossible to know if something is good or bad, the same or different. It is also impossible to know if efforts to improve care have been successful without measuring the impact of a change. The default position should always be to measure.

Consumers want a high-value product. Selection pressures allow consumers of health care to choose between providers. Historically, the primary decision maker in assessing quality has been the individual patient, with no access to data and little understanding of how to assess quality of care. Reputation and word of mouth have been used to assess quality, and patients tend to follow the advice of their doctors when being referred for additional medical care. As health care costs increase, purchasers of health care on a larger scale look for more objective ways to assess quality. Research reflected in the Dartmouth Atlas of Health Care has demonstrated tremendous geographic variation in costs and outcomes within the United States. Paradoxically, higher expenditures on health care in the United States have not been associated with improved outcomes.

These factors provide the foundation for the push from large-scale purchasers of health care to demand that providers be able to objectively demonstrate the quality of care they provide. The Leapfrog Group, a consortium of health insurance purchasers, encourages hospitals to voluntarily report a variety of measures and makes the resulting quality ratings available to the public (www.theleapfroggroup.org). The Centers for Medicare & Medicaid Services (CMS) and increasing numbers of commercial insurance companies provide incentives for hospitals and physicians to measure and report their health care quality. These purchasers apply selection pressures to improve quality by considering quality performance when choosing network providers or by paying differential rates for performance or participation in quality assessment. Beyond incentives, the mere fact of public reporting has influenced health care providers to turn attention and resources to improvement of quality and safety. *Performance measures* are markers of care used for public reporting or for incentive payment.

Organizations comparing performance commonly use one of two methods. The first is to compare one hospital's performance against that of peer organizations. This is the method used in

CMS's public reporting and is frequently reported as a ranking among peers (often by percentile). This method allows for a direct comparison of quality between hospitals. Two cautionary notes are important. First, when there is a small range between organizations in performance, ranking may overstate differences in quality. Second, without performance targets the highest ranked hospitals have little incentive to improve, and overall performance by hospitals may be mediocre.

Another approach is to compare a provider's performance with a benchmark; the provider either hits a target or does not. Targets are usually set arbitrarily (90% performance being a common target). When targets are set too high, care that is unnecessary may be provided to hit the targets. For example, consider the CMS Core Measure of percentage of patients with pneumonia receiving the first dose of antibiotics within six hours of arrival to the hospital. The level of scrutiny required to achieve 99% compliance with this measure may result in an unacceptable number of patients without pneumonia being treated with antibiotics in the effort not to miss a single patient with the diagnosis. In addition, this effort can divert attention away from other important aspects of clinical care.

PRACTICE POINT

The 3 fundamental types of measures evaluate:

- The end result of a given system or process (outcome measures)
- The steps involved in a process (process measures)
- If changes in one area result in (unintended) changes elsewhere (balancing measures)

MEASUREMENT FOR LOCAL QUALITY IMPROVEMENT

Internal audiences use measurement to improve care and to manage local performance. Pressures to improve quality may come from the external sources mentioned above or from internal sources such as risk assessments, clinical leaders, or the board. At the most basic level, constantly seeking to improve is at the core of our professional ethic in medicine. Comparison with prior performance, peers, or benchmarks can all be used for local improvement. Measurement within an organization may also serve to reduce variation. In general, reducing variation within a process leads to better outcomes, as described in Chapter 16.

Measurement forms the basis for scorecards, summaries of measures in multiple domains that are used by organizations to assess performance and to track progress. At the highest levels of the organization, a summary scorecard is commonly used to assess leadership performance toward achieving strategic goals. Components of the organization, such as sections of Hospital Medicine, can also be judged by such scorecards. See **Table 15-1** for examples of candidate measures.

TABLE 15-1 Example Measures for a Hospital Medicine Scorecard

Domain	Candidate Measures
Efficiency	Length of stay
	Rate of discharge before noon
	Timeliness of response to consultation requests
Quality	Performance on CMS Core Measures
	Risk-adjusted mortality rate
	Readmission rate
	Glycemic control
Safety	Percentage of use of medication reconciliation
	Rate of infections related to central venous catheters
	Rate of appropriate prophylaxis against venous thromboembolism
	Use of computerized provider order entry systems
Patient satisfaction	Performance on the Hospital Consumer Assessment and Health Care Systems survey questions about doctors
	Overall patient satisfaction scores
Financial	Contribution to hospital margin
	Controlling costs within budget
	Judicious use of expensive tests (MRI, etc)

MEASUREMENT IS THE FOUNDATION OF QUALITY

Without measurement, it is impossible to know if something is good or bad, the same or different. Individuals and organizations too often make decisions about health care without data. A patient who is about to undergo an elective hip replacement is likely to rely on suggestions from friends or a physician about which surgeon should do the procedure. Imagine instead if patients reviewed surgical outcomes and volumes to inform their decision. Large-scale consumers have started incorporating these types of objective quality measures into their decisions about health care purchasing and contracting. Instead of contracting with provider groups solely based on hospital affiliation and market share, they are considering things such as surgical volumes, readmission rates, complication rates, and patient satisfaction. While the science behind this measurement is still in its infancy, it is clearly moving to a more rational way of assessing care to make choices about which provider is the best for your needs.

It is also impossible to know if efforts to improve care have been successful without measuring the impact of a change. As discussed in Chapter 14, measurement is the answer to the question, "How do we know we are improving?" Too often we rush to "fix the problem" without a plan to measure the impact. It is only months or years later when the problem again surfaces that people go back and look to see why the solution was not as successful as hoped for. Without assessing an intervention, there is a real risk in wasting investment and efforts. There are some times when the luxury of measurement is not available or not needed because the results are so readily apparent. In organizations that make quality a high priority, these occasions should be rare. The default position should always be to measure.

KEY CONCEPTS IN MEASUREMENT

A basic understanding of core concepts in measurement is essential before trying to measure quality. These are outlined below.

MEASUREMENT RIGOR

In general, the higher the stakes of measurement, the greater the rigor required of the measures. Less rigor is generally required of measures chosen for local process improvement than for performance measures. Measures for local improvement must be "good enough" to show the direction and magnitude of change while being able to be obtained in a timely fashion, with sufficient frequency to be useful for tests of change, and with acceptable ease and expense. For example, assume that a team seeks to increase the proportion of discharge orders entered before noon on the day of discharge. Keeping a data collection form at the nurses' station for all discharging physicians to record the time of discharge order may be adequate to determine whether the process change this week has caused improvement over the results of last week. Excessive demands for measurement accuracy in this situation may slow the pace of improvement without yielding a better outcome. In contrast, measures used to evaluate the performance of individual physicians or of a section of Hospital Medicine for the purpose of incentive payment need a higher degree of accuracy. Still greater rigor is required of measurements submitted to CMS for Core Measure performance. Highly specific rules for chart abstraction are in place and subject to validation by external reviewers. This level of rigor has to do with the honesty of the data collection for public reporting, but it does not guarantee that the measures are internally valid predictors of health outcomes. Chapter 13 addresses specific measurement issues related to the rigor needed for research in quality improvement.

PRACTICE POINT

- In general, the higher the stakes of measurement, the greater the rigor required of the measures. Objective measures are those that someone external to the event can assess. A reliable measure will give the same result in the same situation. Validity is an assessment of how well what you are measuring accurately assesses quality. Balancing measures assess the unintended consequences of a change. Most quality improvement projects should have balancing measures as part of the assessment of the project.

OBJECTIVITY AND SUBJECTIVITY

Objective measures are those that someone external to the event can assess. Examples would include inpatient mortality rates, 30-day readmission rates, and length of stay. Subjective measures are qualitative measures reflecting personal experiences. Patient satisfaction with aspects of care, staff engagement scores, and self-reported understanding of informed consent are examples of subjective measures. Only those people involved in the process can provide this information. Both subjective and objective measures can be reliable and valid or unreliable and invalid. Both subjective and objective measures can be useful when measuring health care quality.

RELIABILITY

Reliability is related to reproducibility. A reliable measure will give the same result in the same situation. Reliability can be improved with better specification around the measurement, improving tools used to capture data, and training the individuals responsible for measurement. For example, do different observers of hand hygiene practices share the same understanding of how to score a provider on compliance with hygiene rules when unable to fully observe actions in a patient's room?

VALIDITY

Validity is an assessment of how well what you are measuring accurately assesses quality. For example, accurate medication instructions for patients being discharged from the hospital result in fewer adverse drug events at home. Medication reconciliation performed well should result in an accurate medication list for patient discharge (see Chapter 10 for further discussion). Measuring only the rate of use of medication reconciliation functions upon patient discharge without measurement of accuracy may not produce a valid proxy for medication safety.

STABILITY AND VARIABILITY

Any process has variability, and health care is no exception. While reducing variability is generally a good thing, there will always be some random variation. It is important to distinguish between random variation and systematic change. Traditional medical training emphasizes classic statistics as a way to distinguish random chance from statistically significant change with a major emphasis on *P* values. In quality improvement/measurement, tools such as control charts may be more useful. Based on statistical theory, these charts use locally generated data to identify what is normal variation and when a systematic change is seen. They are useful for assessing change over time. They are also useful for monitoring the sustainability of any improvement that has led to a new baseline. Use of statistical process control charts requires enough measurements for the application of valid statistical methods and the expertise to use the methods. A run chart, a simple line plot of measurements over time as they are generated, provides a quick and easy way to monitor a process. While lacking in statistical power, a run chart helps a team understand basic process performance in real time.

Statistical power to detect meaningful differences must be considered when applying measures of quality to smaller and smaller sectors of an organization. A critical decision in measurement is at what level performance will be measured—at the medical center level, between groups within the medical center (physician groups, nursing units, etc), or at the individual level. Currently, public reporting done by CMS is done at the medical center level. However, there is clearly a move toward individual physician-level reporting. While it is possible to measure performance at any level, this choice has implications that are important to understand. In general, the more refined (closer to the individual level) the measures are, the greater the variability in the measure, reflecting the smaller sample size. While some variability between individuals is certainly related to differences in practice patterns, some of it will also be related to factors that are unrelated to practice patterns. Consider trying to assess outcome and process measures for the diagnosis of pneumonia among individual physicians who may be admitting 10 to 20 patients with pneumonia per year compared with the performance of an entire Hospital Medicine group that admits 200 patients per year with the diagnosis. It is much more likely that random effects influence individual physician performance measures than those of the entire group.

RISK AND SEVERITY ADJUSTMENT

"My patients are sicker than theirs." This response is so common it can easily be seen as an excuse rather than an explanation. Yet, it is essential to take into account differences in patient populations when trying to compare two hospitals or even two individual physicians. Mortality rates of hospitals require adjustment, for instance. Compare a well-staffed hospital in an affluent community with a hospital of similar size in an underserved area on the mortality rate for patients admitted with community-acquired pneumonia. Patient factors such as poverty, nutrition, access to good primary care, and presentation with more advanced disease may create a higher risk of death at the hospital in the underserved area. Likewise, consider the mortality rate for pneumonia at a tertiary referral center. The most severely ill patients from a community hospital may be transferred to the tertiary center, and the average patient with pneumonia at the tertiary center is more likely to have severe comorbid illnesses. In order to address patient-specific and system-specific differences, risk and severity adjustment are needed. There are various validated methodologies for accounting for both patient-level and system-level differences. Typically, these methods will take into account patient characteristics such as age, gender, comorbid conditions (usually from billing data), severity of illness (diagnosis-related group weighting), and systems characteristics such as urban/rural, payer mix, academic/nonacademic, and bed size. These outcome measures may be presented as adjusted outcome rates or ratios of observed/expected outcomes. While these adjustments are necessary, it is important to recognize that we are in the very early stages of learning how to do risk and severity adjustment. For example, two organizations that provide quality assessment for academic medical centers are CMS and University HealthSystem Consortium. Their severity adjustment methods are different and, depending on the methods used, medical centers can vary widely in their performance in measures relative to their peer institutions. So, while not everybody's patients can be sicker, it is important to recognize and adjust for differences.

MEASUREMENT CATEGORIES

"We need to improve our process." "What do their outcomes look like?" Process and outcomes are categories of measurement that are helpful in assessing health care quality.

Most hospitals currently report on their quality of care for patients with pneumonia as part of the CMS value-based purchasing initiative, Core Measures. Patients with pneumonia benefit from receiving evidence-based care. What type of measures could be used to assess the quality of pneumonia care for the purposes of comparing hospitals and physicians or for improving the care delivered within a medical system?

OUTCOME MEASURES

Patients care about outcomes, the final result of what happens to them. Ultimately, all improvement efforts should be directed toward achieving results that patients care about better or obtaining the same results more efficiently. Patients who present with pneumonia care about whether they are likely to survive the hospital stay (in-hospital mortality) and beyond (30-day mortality), whether they will have to return to the hospital after discharge (30-day readmission rates), whether they can do everything they could at home before admission (quality of life or functional status), and whether they were treated with respect by caring staff (patient satisfaction). All of these patient-centric questions are outcomes. However, they can be challenging to measure. Most patients with pneumonia severe enough to be hospitalized do well. To show differences between providers to a meaningful degree requires that the adverse outcome happens frequently enough that you can find a difference. When event rates are infrequent, it is more difficult to demonstrate meaningful differences. Some of these outcome measures are relatively easy to capture, such as in-hospital mortality. Many are far more difficult. Thirty-day mortality and readmission rates (if other institutions are included) are not routinely available, with the exception of some aggregated data or for payer-specific populations. Measuring quality of life or functional status requires significant resources that most institutions find challenging to commit to, especially when it requires tracking patients after discharge. Despite all of these challenges with outcome measurements, they remain the most important to most observers.

PROCESS MEASURES

Process measures are more commonly used to assess health care quality. These are measures of the steps in the process of care that lead to better patient outcomes. In patients with pneumonia many medical interventions improve outcomes, including timely administration of the correct antibiotics, smoking cessation among cigarette users, and immunization against influenza. Assessments of each of these medical interventions performed in the hospital are process measures, as are all of the CMS Core Measures. Conceptually, if a process measure gets better, the outcome is likely to improve as well, though the strength of this association has not been well proven for all measures. Process measures are generally more responsive to change and easier to track than outcome measures. Process measures are helpful when trying to improve efficiency and reduce variability and as surrogate measures when there is a clear causal link between the process measure and the outcome measure of interest. However, using process measures when the causal association is not robust can lead to major efforts at improving processes that have little value. A recent example of this is in the area of inpatient hyperglycemia management. While the evidence for a causal effect of tight glycemic control on patient outcomes was still controversial, many hospitals across the country dedicated major efforts at improving glycemic control. With the release of additional studies raising questions about the benefits of tight glycemic control in most hospitalized patients, medical centers have stepped back from their quality improvement efforts in the area of tight glycemic control.

BALANCING MEASURES

Whenever a change is made, there are intended consequences and unintended consequences. *Balancing measures* assess the unintended consequences. These are used primarily in the improvement process and are less useful when measuring for selection pressure. Balancing process measures in the pneumonia example might include the number of patients who receive antibiotics unnecessarily or the number of patients with a delay in identifying an alternative diagnosis due to the intense focus on early identification of patients with pneumonia. Balancing outcome measures could include the costs of care (lower or higher) or adverse reactions to unnecessary antibiotics. Most quality improvement projects should include balancing measures as part of the assessment of the project.

COMPOSITE MEASURES

To this point we have discussed measurement of unique outcomes or processes. Measures may also be grouped to provide additional perspectives on health care delivery. *Composite measures* combine disparate measures into a single score, communicating overall performance simply and possibly providing a better understanding of the overall reliability of complex systems than consideration of individual measures alone. Component measures may rise or fall over time, but the overall composite measure can be used to set goals and to judge performance. As an example, the University HealthSystem Consortium Quality and Accountability scorecard ranks academic hospitals based on a composite measure derived from weighted scores for risk-adjusted mortality, Core Measure bundle performance, readmission rates, and other measures.

Inherent in creation of a composite measure is the arbitrary nature of weighting applied to the components of the measure and the scaling of the individual measures so that they can be combined into the single score. A Hospital Medicine group, for instance, may be assessed year to year in overall performance by the use of an index reflecting aspects of clinical quality, safety, efficiency, patient satisfaction and compliance with administrative expectations. While composite measures facilitate comparisons and simplify communication about health care quality, they come with several caveats. They are only as good as the weakest of their component measures in terms of validity, accuracy, and meaningfulness; and poorly derived composite measures mislead the audience when comparing performance between institutions. To address this concern, the National Quality Forum has developed a consensus framework for composite measure evaluation when applied to performance measures.

BUNDLED MEASURES

The components of a composite measure may reflect a variety of care processes and outcomes in quality, safety and efficiency; or the components may be selected to describe performance across a single diagnosis or care process. *Bundled measures* apply to this latter case. For example, the CMS Core Measures consist of diagnosis-specific bundles of measurements. The care of a patient with pneumonia may be assessed with a series of individual measures, such as time to initial antibiotics, whether blood cultures were obtained before first antibiotic administration, correct selection of antibiotics, whether counseling was offered to smokers, whether vaccines were administered (if appropriate), etc. On each of these individual measures, the hospital will be scored by how well it performs. However, for a given patient, the care was "perfect" only if the hospital achieved 100% of the applicable measures for that patient. In other words, the hospital "failed" the pneumonia core measure bundle for that patient if it failed to deliver on any of these measures. One can easily see that hospital performance on most of these individual measures must be well above 90% in order for the reported hospital pneumonia bundle to meet a 90% target. Thus, the bundle measurement reflects care provided from the individual patient perspective and can be a useful way to measure performance.

PRACTICE POINT

- All improvement efforts should be directed toward making the results that patients care about better, or achieving the same results more efficiently. Process measures are helpful when trying to improve efficiency and reduce variability, and as surrogate measures when there is a clear causal link between the process measure and the outcome measure of interest. However, using process measures when the causal association is not robust can lead to major efforts at improving processes that have little value.

CONCLUSION

As clinicians we have become very comfortable with measurement in the clinical arena. As hospitalists and leaders in quality, it is important that we become equally as comfortable with understanding measurement in this area. Many of the concepts are familiar; it is simply a reframing of the understanding of measurement that changes when trying to assess the quality of health care, and without measurement, understanding the value of health care is impossible.

SUGGESTED READINGS

Berwick DM, James B, Coye MJ. Connections between quality measurement and improvement. *Med Care.* 2003;41:I-30–I-38.

Donabedian A. *Evaluating the quality of medical care.* Milbank Q. 1966;44:166–206.

Institute of Medicine. *Crossing the quality chasm: a new health system for the 21st century.* Washington, DC: National Academy Press; 2001.

McGlynn E, Asch S. Developing a clinical performance measure. *Am J Prev Med.* 1998;14(supp3):14–21.

National Quality of Care Forum. *Bridging the gap between theory and practice: Exploring outcomes management.* Chicago: National Quality of Care Forum;1994.

Pronovost PJ, Nolan T, Zeger S, Miller M, Rubin H. How can clinicians measure safety and quality in acute care? *Lancet.* 2004;363: 1061–1067.

Sehgal AR. The role of reputation in US News and World Report's rankings of the top 50 American hospitals. *Ann Intern Med.* 2010;152:521–525.

CHAPTER 16

Standardization and Reliability

Richard S. Gitomer, MD, FACP

CASE 16-1

INADEQUATE STERILIZATION OF SURGICAL INSTRUMENTS

Midway through the wound debridement, the scrub nurse noted that the sterilization indicators had not changed colors—the surgeon was operating with instruments that had not been properly sterilized. The subsequent root cause analysis revealed that the sterile processing technician, at the end of his shift, forgot to push the button to start the autoclave. The arriving technician on the next shift assumed the autoclave had finished the cycle, and not noticing that the sterilization indicator on the cart had not changed color, removed the cart with the unsterilized trays and placed them on the shelf for use.

INTRODUCTION

In 1999, the Institute of Medicine (IOM) highlighted two studies from the 1980s that suggested between 44,000 and 98,000 patients die every year due to preventable medical errors.

The subsequent IOM report, *Crossing the Quality Chasm,* noted, "The current systems cannot do the job. Changing systems of care will." The report went on further to describe the six aims of safety, effectiveness, efficiency, patient-centeredness, timeliness, and equity. With these aims, the IOM has defined the ultimate vision for the U.S. health care system.

The limitations of the current health care system were further highlighted by Elizabeth McGlynn's study in 2003. In that study, her group found that patients only receive 55% of the care warranted by medical evidence. Furthermore, they found that the likelihood that an individual patient would receive all appropriate care was 2.5%.

HUMAN FACTORS

THE INDIVIDUAL

A main contributor to the performance shortfall is the limitation of human performance. **Table 16-1** shows expected human error rates in conditions under no undue time pressure or stress. Note that "under very high stress when dangerous activities are occurring rapidly," the error rate can be as high as one in four. Therefore, system designs that depend on perfect human performance are destined to fail. Furthermore, systems designed to function in conditions of high stress with frequent dangerous activities have a higher burden in order to ensure a favorable outcome.

As defined by the Federal Aviation Administration, "Within the FAA, human factors entail a multidisciplinary effort to generate and compile information about human capabilities and limitations and apply that information to equipment, systems, facilities, procedures, jobs, environments, training, staffing, and personnel management for safe, comfortable, and effective human performance."

When accounting for human factors it is helpful to consider the human and the system separately. Reliable systems must compensate for the limitations of human performance. In addition, organizational characteristics can negatively or positively impact human performance.

TABLE 16-1 Nominal Human Error Rates for Selected Activities

Activity (Assume no Undue Time Pressure or Stresses)	Rate
Error of commission, eg, misreading a label	.003
Error of omission without reminders	.01
Error of omission when item is embedded in a procedure	.003
Simple arithmetic errors with self-checking	.03
Monitor or inspector fails to recognize an error	.1
Personnel on different shifts fail to check the condition of hardware unless directed by a checklist	.1
Error rate under very high stress when dangerous activities are occurring rapidly	.25

PRACTICE POINT

- Organizational characteristics can negatively or positively impact human performance. When accounting for human factors, it is helpful to consider the human and the system separately.

When redesigning systems to improve performance and reduce adverse events, hospitalists should recognize the factors that may negatively impact human performance so that the design can account for the expected vulnerability.

There are limitations to human memory. On the average, a person is able to keep seven, plus or minus two, elements in short-term memory. A frequent system vulnerability is the reliance on human memory to retrieve key information at the time it is needed. In reliable systems, key information is made available at those key times, rather than relying on human memory.

Rushed people cut corners. Over time, the repeated short cuts result in a narrowing safety margin. The natural tendency to cut corners and the repeated experience of no negative outcome reassures the individual that they remain within an appropriate level of safety, or reliability. This is described as "normalization of deviance."

A glaring example of normalization of deviance was the1986 shuttle Challenger explosion 72 seconds after lift-off. The subsequent investigation found that the cause of the explosion was the failure of the O-rings that were part of the rocket engines. On previous launches there was evidence of damage to the O-rings. The following quote from the "Report of the Presidential Commission on the Space Shuttle Challenger Accident" illustrates how normalization of deviance led to the disaster. NASA and Morton Thiokol accepted escalating risk apparently because they "got away with it last time." As Commissioner Richard Feynman observed, the decision making was

> a kind of Russian roulette.... [The Shuttle] flies [with O-ring erosion] and nothing happens. Then it is suggested, therefore, that the risk is no longer so high for the next flights. We can lower our standards a little bit because we got away with it last time... You got away with it, but it shouldn't be done over and over again like that.

Normalization of deviance occurs because of the natural human tendency to slip into believing that despite short cuts, adequate safety or reliability margins remain. In health care, normalization of deviance is often a barrier when trying to implement a standard checklist for the insertion of a central line, an intentional pause with completion of a checklist before a procedure to ensure safety or other quality and safety interventions.

Stress impacts human performance by causing tunnel vision and filtering, selectively disregarding what is believed to be irrelevant information. This causes a loss of pattern recognition that humans use to rapidly discern complex situations. Fatigue negatively impacts human performance by impacting both short-term and long-term memory. The impact is similar to having a blood alcohol level of 0.1%. Other factors that commonly degrade health care worker performance include multitasking, interruptions, and environmental factors.

THE ORGANIZATION

James Reason described characteristics that impact an organization's capacity to support or impede an individual's ability to function reliably. Human error can be addressed from an organizational perspective using the "person approach" or the "system approach."

The person approach focuses on the actions of the frontline staff who commit errors. The errors, it is believed, are due to flawed mental processes that can be voluntarily corrected with enough motivation, attention, and vigilance. The institutional response is focused on correcting the variation in human behavior. Frequently, the responses engender fear of disciplinary measures, threat of litigation, retraining, naming, blaming, and shaming, so that the individual will focus more intently on the task at hand and not make a similar error. Often, new policies and procedures are written to ensure the correct behavior. In short, the person approach implicitly assumes that bad things happen to bad people.

The fundamental premise of the system approach is the anticipation of human fallibility. Human errors are to be expected. The errors are seen as consequences of an inadequate system design. It is believed that most errors occur because system barriers and defenses that are "upstream" lead to undesired outcomes.

PRACTICE POINT

- The fundamental premise of the "system approach" is the anticipation of human fallibility. Human errors are to be expected. The errors are seen as consequences of an inadequate system design. It is believed that most errors occur because system barriers and defenses that are "upstream" lead to undesired outcomes. Reliable systems must compensate for the limitations of human performance.

The person approach is somewhat appealing on several levels. It is emotionally satisfying to blame an individual for an adverse event. In addition, divorcing the unsafe act from the organization is clearly in the best interests of the managers, but these benefits come at a great cost—the willingness of staff to report errors. Contrast this with the experience that in 90% of aviation maintenance mishaps, the worker is found blameless. In order to improve, it is important to perform a detailed analysis of incidents and near misses. Without a reporting culture, this information never surfaces (see Chapter 7).

Conversely, the system approach recognizes human fallibility and system designs are successful despite human error. In reliable organizations, admission of errors and near misses is reinforced. Leadership in reliable organizations realizes that early detection of latent conditions that promote human error is essential in creating reliable systems.

Most organizations create barriers and defenses when designing systems of care; however, each barrier and defense is not perfect and has unique vulnerabilities. Reason describes this as a slice of Swiss cheese, yet these vulnerabilities are dynamic. Sometimes the holes are larger; other times they are located in a different place. For example, if one of the barriers is a second person checking the dose of insulin, this step may be less reliable on a specific day because the nurse was up late the night before with a sick child.

In many circumstances, when one barrier fails, a second is able to catch the defect, and the outcome is not compromised. In Reason's model, the defect may pass through one slice of Swiss cheese but is caught by the next slice. However, there are times when all the holes of multiple slices of Swiss cheese line up and the outcome is compromised: the patient is harmed.

Implicit in Reason's system approach to human error is the importance of culture. Reason notes that high-reliability organizations have a reporting culture. It is essential for the staff to feel safe surfacing errors and near misses. In high-reliability organizations leadership accepts the accountability to create safe environments that facilitate successful outcomes. The staff member is accountable to make safe choices by following the processes that they helped to create. The staff is also accountable for surfacing existing and potential opportunities for defects. If all live up to these accountabilities, the leadership response to error is supportive of the staff with a focus on identifying the source of the defect and developing a remedy to prevent its occurrence in the future.

RELIABILITY

As suggested in *Crossing the Quality Chasm*, new systems of care are required to achieve the level of reliability necessary to ensure that all patients receive the care they deserve. The new systems of care will need to account for human factors on the organizational level as well as at the individual process level.

THE ORGANIZATION

The health care industry has a level of complexity that matches, if not exceeds, other industries. The fact that humans execute most key processes challenges the reliability of the system. The complex systems, the dynamic environment, and the human involved with the process execution are major reasons for the reliability gap described at the beginning of this chapter. There are principles that can be gleaned from other complex organizations that can help overcome the reliability gap.

Karl Weick has described organizational characteristics he found in his study of complex organizations that function at a high level of reliability. The organizations include nuclear power plants, nuclear aircraft carriers, and the airline industry. He describes those industries as having mindfulness. He defines mindfulness as "a rich awareness of discriminatory detail." Individuals functioning in high-reliability organizations are aware of context, can discriminate details, and how the current situation differs from expectations. The five principles of mindfulness include preoccupation with failure, reluctance to simplify interpretations, sensitivity to operations, commitment to resilience, and deference to expertise.

Preoccupation with failure is a relentless focus on potential failure modes and how they can be prevented. An example in health care might be a detailed examination of an order set looking for ambiguities or potential error traps. A preoccupation with failure helps overcome the natural tendency to drift into unsafe or unreliable behaviors.

Mindful organizations resist the tendency to normalize unwanted occurrences into expected events. This reluctance to simplify interpretations helps to maintain safety and reliability margins. Repeated normalization of occurrences, or a lack of focus on these events, over time, can result in a major problem that could be avoided if the initial interpretation had been more focused. For example, resisting attributing a medication error to a nurse failing to use the "five rights" (right patient, right medication, right dose, right route, right time) because she did not focus. A mindful organization might ask if the process for executing the "five rights" is robust, and if there are adequate barriers to prevent error.

Sensitivity to operations reflects a deep understanding of the processes at a frontline level. This reflects knowing what really happens in the messy world of reality, not what policy is, or what is supposed to happen. In a mindful organization, there is enough familiarity with the process that when the pneumococcal vaccine rates are low, it is not surprising that the root cause relates to the complexity of the screening tool has induced many nurses to incorrectly determine that there are no indications for the vaccine to be administered.

Highly reliable organizations realize that all systems can fail. But, these organizations have a relentless focus on not allowing that failure to compromise the overall performance. A key element of the commitment to resilience is that the specific key failure modes may not be anticipated. A preoccupation with failure might result in the development of a medical rapid response team to attend to deteriorating patients before they arrest. But, simulation exercises to ensure a high-functioning team in an acute situation would be an intervention that demonstrated a commitment to resilience from an occurrence that might not be anticipated.

In highly reliable organizations decision-making authority seamlessly flows to the person with the best information to make the decision. The deference to expertise might be exhibited on an aircraft carrier where a seaman can stop the activities on the flight deck because he sees a condition that might be unsafe for the landing planes. In the ICU, a nurse might "stop the line" if she does not see all components of the central line insertion bundle.

Other organizations may not have all the complexities of health care organizations, but the five principles of mindfulness are directly applicable to health care. Organizations that exhibit these characteristics have a culture that promotes reliability.

THE RELIABILITY GAP

Weick paints a nice picture of what reliability looks like at the level of the organization. But, what does reliability look like at the level of the process? Reliability is intentional, and there are principles that guide the design of reliable processes.

Due to the complexity of health care delivery the causes of failure are frequently multifactorial. Understanding these causes helps shape the interventions. While not exhaustive, the following three explanations highlight key impediments to process reliability.

While readily acknowledging human fallibility, many health care providers expect perfection of themselves. In addition, there is often a feeling that the only way to ensure reliability is to rely on no one else. From this high standard comes an overreliance on vigilance and hard work. The reality of human factors, however, prevents the individual from performing reliably.

Individual providers tend to look at their personal delivery of health care one patient at a time. Ideally, the provider customizes a plan for the individual patient based on personal experience and the medical evidence. However, due to the limitations of human factors, and the paucity of high-level evidence for much of the care of the average practitioner, there is high variation in how patients are treated from one to the next.

While understandable, this lack of standardization comes at a cost—complexity. It is no longer possible for an individual to deliver the full spectrum of reliable care to an individual patient, as demonstrated by McGlynn and colleagues. Teams are essential for the delivery of reliable care. The more variation from patient to patient in a care plan, the greater the level of complexity for the rest of the

TABLE 16-2 Levels of Reliability

Level of Reliability	Typical Processes Infrastructure
<80% >2 defects in 10	Chaos
10^{-1} (80%) 2 defects in 10	No articulated common process Reliance on training and reminders
10^{-2} (95%) 1–5 defects in 100	Intentionally designed Utilizes principles of human factors engineering
10^{-3} (99.5%) 1–5 defects in 1000	Well-designed system with attention to process, structure, and outcomes

care team. The consequence of unwarranted variation is increased complexity and lower reliability.

This is not to say that standardization in a "cookie cutter" approach is required to reduce complexity. Rather, standardize what is "standardizable." Doing so relieves the care provider of the mundane and allows focus on those parts of the care plan that do require additional attention or expertise. For the rest of the care team, work is less complex because the reduced unwarranted variation allows them to plan and anticipate. Standardization allows the ICU nurse to plan for extubation in the postoperative patient who is progressing as expected. The standardization also frees the hospitalist to focus on other patients who are not progressing as expected that require an adjustment to the standardized protocol.

A third reason for the reliability gap is that many current processes fail to account for human factors. Process design based on human infallibility is inherently unreliable. The following section describes an approach to process design that facilitates accounting for human factors.

MEASUREMENT

Reliability is measured as the proportion of successes out of the opportunities. The definitions in **Table 16-2** reflect a standard way to describe levels of reliability and the infrastructure required to achieve those levels.

As suggested in Table 16-2, each level of reliability is associated with typical interventions. Interventions that result in 10^{-1} (1 to 2 defects in 10) reliability rely on vigilance and hard work. Examples of these interventions include:

1. Common equipment, standard order sheets, multiple choice protocols, and written policies/procedures
2. Personal check lists
3. Feedback of information on compliance
4. Suggestions of working harder next time
5. Awareness and training

Processes that result in 10^{-2} (1 to 5 defects in 100) reliability use principles based on human factors and reliability science. While more robust, these interventions tend to be more resource intensive. They include:

1. Building decision aids and reminders into the system
2. Facilitating desired action by defaults (scientific evidence)
3. Utilizing redundant processes
4. Incorporating scheduling in design development
5. Taking advantage of known habits and patterns in the design
6. Standardizing the process based on clear specification and articulation.

THE PROCESS

The reliability design strategy as described by a group at the Institute for Health Care Improvement consists of four steps:

1. Segmentation
2. Standardization
3. Detection and mitigation
4. Redesign the process based on the defects identified

PRACTICE POINT

- Reliable process design, regardless of the improvement methodology, is an effective approach to closing the reliability gap. When redesigning systems to improve performance and reduce adverse events, hospitalists should recognize the factors that may negatively impact human performance so that the design can account for the expected vulnerability. Closing that reliability gap requires focused multidisciplinary team involvement to develop and oversee the process redesign.

Segmentation

When embarking on an improvement project it is often helpful to divide the population into smaller groups in order to simplify the tests of change. Process improvement requires taking general knowledge or procedures and making them relevant in the local context. Unlike research, it is not possible to remove confounding variables. However, with segmentation the confounding variables can be controlled until the appropriate time.

To illustrate the power of segmentation consider implementation of congestive heart failure discharge instructions, which should include information about diet, when to call the primary provider, follow-up, daily weights, and discharge medications. The improvement team might consider segments based on familiarity of the medical and nursing staff with the care of patients with congestive heart failure. Clearly, there is a greater level of comfort on the cardiology floor than on the orthopedic floor. One might consider a continuum of comfort as follows: cardiology floor, general medicine floor, general surgery floor, and orthopedic floor.

Segmenting this way, and choosing to start the work on the cardiology floor, allows the team to focus on the process of delivering the discharge instructions without having to manage the barriers of knowledge deficit and comfort with the medications. Once the process for delivering the instructions is well defined and operational, the team can move on to the other floors and directly address the unique barriers, rather than trying to address the barriers while determining the correct process.

The segments should have the following qualities:

1. A design theme that helps simplify the improvement activity (knowledge, geography, willingness to participate, patient characteristics)
2. A reasonable volume so that there are enough opportunities to perform tests of change
3. Clear-cut defined boundaries so that there is no confusion about the population of patients being addressed.

Standardization

Standardization yields several key benefits. First, it improves reliability by reducing complexity, as described above. Second, it helps provide an infrastructure where roles and responsibilities are clearly defined. A standard infrastructure also allows for simplification of training, and competency testing. Standardizing key processes allows consistent implementation of evidence-based medicine.

Lastly, it simplifies identification of defects that can be analyzed for redesign, and facilitates performing tests of change.

The standardization step should be refined by serial tests of change. The reliability goal for the standardization step is 80%. If the step is less than 80% reliable the defects will overwhelm the detection and mitigation step, which tends to be more resource intensive.

In order to reliably deliver the congestive heart failure discharge instructions to the segments identified above, the team might explicitly assign roles and responsibilities and use checklists embedded in the discharge work flow. The check lists, how the process flows, and who has which responsibilities would be the subject of a series of tests of change until the process is 80% reliable.

Detection and mitigation

The value of the detection and mitigation step is that it helps reduce the complexity of the standardization step. Since the standardization step need only capture 80% of the opportunities, it is not necessary to develop contingencies for lower-frequency occurrences. If the standardization step had to include those contingencies, it would be too complex and therefore less reliable.

The detection and mitigation step includes two processes. The first process reliably captures the defects from the standardization step utilizing 10^{-2} level interventions. The second process mitigates the defect, using 10^{-1} level interventions.

The detection and mitigation step for the congestive heart failure example might be a hard stop prior to discharge, where the discharging nurse checks for all the key elements of the discharge. If any were missing, the provider responsible would be contacted to immediately remedy. You can see that if this happens too frequently, the nurse would be overwhelmed and the process would not be sustainable. Hence, it is necessary for the standardization process to have at least an 8 in 10 level of reliability.

Process redesign based on defects identified

In pursuit of continuous improvement the fourth step in the reliability design strategy is to examine the defects identified in the previous step and feed the learning back into the design of the standardization and detection and mitigation steps.

Once the processes in the first segment achieve an acceptable level of reliability, the team should move on to the next easiest segment. Now that the processes have been defined and tested, work in the next segment can focus on the barriers unique to the new segment. Attacking the segments from easiest to hardest allows the team to gain experience and further refine the process, which simplifies the work in even the most difficult segment.

Whenever, the nurse executing the detection and mitigation step identifies a defect (incomplete instructions) the cause is logged. These defects are tracked and the information is fed back to the design team to improve the previous two processes.

CONCLUSION

As highlighted by the IOM reports and McGlynn's work, patients are regularly experiencing preventable harm and are not receiving all of the care that is intended. Closing that reliability gap requires focused multidisciplinary team involvement to develop and oversee the process redesign. Understanding human factors and having a structured model for increased reliability is essential. Reliable process design, regardless of the improvement methodology, is an effective approach to closing the reliability gap.

SUGGESTED READINGS

Committee for Evaluating Medical Technologies in Clinical Use. *Assessing Medical Technologies*. Washington: National Academies Press; 1985:p. 5.

Committee on Quality of Health Care in America, Institute of Medicine. *Crossing the Quality Chasm: A New Health System for the 21st Century*. Washington, DC: National Academy Press; 2001.

Kohn LT, Corrigan J, Donaldson MS. *To Err Is Human: Building a Safer Health System*. Washington, DC: National Academy Press; 2000.

Marx D. *Patient Safety and the "Just Culture": A Primer for Health Care Executives*. New York: Trustees of Columbia University in the City of New York, Columbia University; 2001.

McGlynn EA, Asch SM, Adams J, et al. The quality of health care delivered to adults in the United States. *N Engl J Med*. 2003;348:2635.

Nolan T, Resar R, Haraden C, Griffin FA. *Improving the Reliability of Health Care. IHI Innovation Series white paper*. Boston: Institute for Health Care Improvement; 2004. (Available on http://www.IHI.org)

Reason J. Human error: models and management. *Brit Med J*. 2000;320:768.

Resar R. http://www.ihi.org/IHI/Topics/Reliability/ReliabilityGeneral/EmergingContent/SegmentPresentationandDesignTable.htm

Weick KE, Sutcliffe KM: *Managing the Unexpected: Resilient Performance in an Age of Uncertainty*. 2nd ed. San Francisco: John Wiley & Sons, Inc.; 2007.

Vaughan D. *The Challenger Launch Decision: Risky Technology, Culture, and Deviance at NASA*. Chicago: University of Chicago Press; 1996.

CHAPTER 17

The Role of Information Technology in Hospital Quality and Safety

Saverio M. Maviglia, MD, MSc

INTRODUCTION

The practice of medicine is at heart an exercise of collecting, filtering, summarizing, managing, analyzing, and acting upon information. This information comes directly from the patient's narrative history, but also from family and caretakers, and other providers. It also is derived from diagnostic interventions, including the physical examination, laboratory tests, radiologic exams, and procedures. Combined with reference knowledge about physiology, pathology, pharmacology, and other basic science disciplines, the physician makes an expert assessment of the patient's conditions and risks, and then recommends an action plan. Information about this plan must be communicated and coordinated with a larger team and with the patient and their family, executed, and then information about how the patient responds fed back in order to make adjustments over time. If this flow of information is compromised or hampered at any point in this cycle, then the potential for quality and safety problems emerges. Given this intense information-rich environment that the clinician must navigate, especially in the inpatient setting, it is clear that the judicious application of information technology (IT) can greatly empower the hospitalist in providing high quality and safe patient care; and conversely, that injudicious application of IT can promote errors and adverse outcomes.

Information technologies that impact patient safety and quality of care can be grouped into three major categories. First, there are the interventions that impact care as it is delivered in real time—this class is generally called *decision support* because it involves clinicians while they are making diagnostic and therapeutic decisions. The second class of information technologies, broadly known as *surveillance*, monitors the immediate downstream care processes to detect anomalies and unintended consequences so that effective corrective action may be taken quickly. The last general category of IT for safety and quality is *data mining*, or retrospective analysis of large repositories of data, such as patient registries, electronic health records, and administrative databases in order to detect meaningful patterns and signals that may help inform ways to improve the previous two types of information systems. Data mining overlaps with classical epidemiological health services outcomes research. This classification of information technologies is analogous to the distinctions between primary, secondary, and tertiary modes of disease management, which may be more familiar to clinicians.

DECISION SUPPORT

As defined above, decision support is any type of information system that intends to direct, guide, or alter medical decision making as it occurs in real time. This may occur via passive delivery of knowledge, such as quick access to online digital references, drug compendia, clinical calculators, or differential diagnosis tools. In this case, the user must voluntarily choose to activate the service. This type of decision support is usually well received by busy clinicians, because the clinician is motivated to get a question answered. However, passive decision support does not address latent information needs, or knowledge deficits unknown to the clinician.

Decision support may also occur via active knowledge delivery, such as alerts to avoid unsafe or undesired behavior, or reminders to promote desired behavior; the service is activated automatically. Usually, the intended behavior is evidence based, such as avoiding drug combinations that have been shown to result in adverse effects; but it can also be policy driven, such as to promote some medications over others based on formulary or insurance criteria. As active decision support is often interruptive, clinician acceptance of this information is variable, depending upon the perceived usefulness of the information provided and the manner in which it is displayed.

There are certain decision support systems which fall somewhere between active and passive, by facilitating workflow. Examples include messaging systems such as sign-out applications and secure email or text paging, electronic medication reconciliation applications, and results management programs. The ideal decision support interventions combine both approaches, by facilitating the desired workflow(s) and impeding the alternatives. These decision support interventions, which are often anticipatory, simultaneously make it "easy" to do the right thing, and hard to do the wrong thing. For example, compare two ways to implement decision support for optimal drug dosing. The first, more common approach is to analyze medication orders after they are entered; compare them to rules that assess patient factors such as age, gender, and comorbidities such as renal dysfunction; and then display a series of corrective alerts. The second approach does as much of the patient-specific calculations as possible up front, so that only the most reasonable medication alternatives for a given indication are offered in the first place, with default dose and frequency pre-calculated to match the patient's condition. Only the prescriber who chooses to override the defaults is interrupted to provide an override reason. Of course, the more sophisticated consultative approach to delivering decision support requires more data in computable form about a patient, as well as more complicated and nuanced rules, than the typical critical approach.

Evidence suggests that decision support can successfully influence provider behavior, improve process measures, increase quality of care, and reduce errors and adverse events. However, the way decision support is implemented can dramatically affect effectiveness. For example, when influenza vaccination reminders were first implemented at one inpatient site, the effect was minimal; but when the alert was changed to a complete prewritten order, and the default was set to "accept" instead of to "decline," the inpatient vaccination rate increased from 1% to 51% (Dexter PR, et al. *N Engl J Med.* 2001, 345(13):965–970).

PRACTICE POINT

- Evidence suggests that decision support can successfully influence provider behavior, improve process measures, increase quality of care, and reduce errors and adverse events. However, the way decision support is implemented can dramatically affect effectiveness. Poorly implemented systems can have unintended adverse consequences on health care providers or promote error.

More problematic is the growing recognition that poorly implemented systems can have unintended adverse consequences on health care providers, to the point of inciting clinician revolt, such as occurred at Cedars-Sinai Medical Center in Los Angeles in 2003 (Ornstein C. Los Angeles Times. January 22, 2003). Worse yet, computerized provider order entry, coupled with decision support, can potentially promote errors Koppel R, et al. *J Am Med Inform Assoc.* 2005;293(10):1197–1203. Therefore, the behavior of such systems must be continually scrutinized, and the information they provide must never be accepted blindly.

SURVEILLANCE

Surveillance IT is analogous to secondary prevention or care—it is meant to detect complications of care early so that the consequences can be prevented or ameliorated. The most prevalent example, which is still relatively rarely implemented in practice, is adverse event detection. This requires an electronic monitoring system that oversees all digital transactions in a health information system, such as new orders, new lab results, and new patient encounter records; a repository of rules that define potential events and the actions that should be taken; and a variety of effector systems to carryout the actions, such as texting or e-mail alerting. Collectively, these components form what is commonly known as an event engine. As an example, the monitoring system registers all new lab results, including an individual patient's falling platelet level. A rule in the repository defines a clinically significant rapid rate of decline (for example, an absolute drop of 50,000 or a relative drop of 30% over 2 days; or of 50,000 or 50% over 3 days) in the right clinical context (the patient has a current active order for a heparin-containing medication), to generate a response (alert the responsible clinician the next time she logs into the system, or text page a backup clinician if this does not occur within 24 hours). It is clear from this example that the effectiveness of this surveillance system is only as good as the breadth of events that can be monitored, the granularity with which rules can be authored to define clinically significant events, and the breadth of interventions available for actions.

Surveillance systems can collect and analyze quality-related data, as well as safety data. Such systems, sometimes called profiling or detailing systems, have been long utilized by pharmaceutical companies to direct and tailor marketing efforts, but they can also be used to track how often a hospitalist utilizes nonformulary medications, or how well a provider is achieving quality of care metric goals, such as percentage of their diabetic patients who get periodic eye and foot exams, or rates of resource utilization such as MRI imaging for headaches. This information can be shared with just the relevant provider, or with an entire practice, either de-identified or not. The most sophisticated profiling systems present the data in a quality dashboard that the provider can query dynamically in real time and link the data to relevant actions, such as emailing patients, flagging them for call back appointments, or automatically referring patients to a disease management program.

In addition to patient-specific and provider-specific event engines, surveillance systems have also been developed to work at the population level. For example, there are monitoring systems that track aggregated data about visits to regional emergency rooms, including chief complaints, to detect early signals of disease outbreaks such as from influenza or bioterrorism.

DATA MINING

The final class of IT that can be brought to bear on quality and safety is the retrospective analysis of large datasets to look for trends and patterns and their relationship or association with significant events, interventions, or behaviors. This traditionally has been called health services research, and can focus on either health care outcomes (mortality, morbidity, readmissions, adverse event rates) or their process-based proxies (frequency of deep vein thrombosis [DVT] prophylaxis measures, rate of compliance with recommended guidelines, or proportion of completed discharge summaries within 24 hours). Both are valid indicators of quality and safety effectiveness, though hard outcomes are often preferred, but usually more difficult to measure and influence. For example, measuring the effect of an intervention on incidence of DVT would be ideal, but in practice would require significant manual data collection by chart abstraction, and may be too infrequent an event in the time window allowed for study to make statistically sound conclusions. Instead, measuring how the intervention impacts the number of orders for subcutaneous heparin, especially where such orders are placed via CPOE, is much easier and a more common event.

The newest direction this type of research has taken is the combination of large datasets from different disciplines, to look for new and sometimes unanticipated or counterintuitive associations. Because of the increasing likelihood of chance alone being responsible for observing such relationships between data when multiple statistical tests are performed with the same data, this type of knowledge discovery requires large collections of data, runs the risk of uncovering statistically significant but clinically irrelevant patterns, and should always be considered hypothesis generating rather than confirming or refuting. A satirical but very true example is that if one were to measure how frequently lung cancer patients carry matches compared to patients without lung cancer, one might be tempted to conclude that carrying matches is a very dangerous activity. Another example is that if test results are defined to be in the normal range when they lie within the 95th percentile of results from a healthy population, then a battery panel of 20 tests will have at least one false positive result almost two-third of the time.

THE HOSPITALIST'S ROLE

There is great opportunity for clinicians such as hospitalists, who are often experts in workflow and systems thinking (whether by formal training or simply by experience), to help guide implementations of decision support interventions within their practice sites in order to increase the chance of success and minimize the chance of failure. Even after successful implementation of information technologies, there is ongoing need for clinicians to provide feedback about what works, what does not, and what could be done to improve the system. A higher level of involvement of hospitalists is to provide subject matter expertise to tweak rules and author new ones to make the decision support more specific, relevant, and effective. This never-ending work to keep the content of rules in line with ever changing knowledge has emerged as a new field of its own called knowledge management.

PRACTICE POINT

- Knowledge management requires keeping the content of rules in line with ever-changing knowledge and creating new ones to make decision support more specific, relevant, and effective. Even after successful implementation of information technologies, there is ongoing need for clinicians to provide feedback about what works, what does not, and what could be done to improve the system.

SUGGESTED READINGS

Ash JS, Berg M, Coiera E. Some unintended consequences of information technology in health care: the nature of patient care information system-related errors. *J Am Med Inform Assoc.* 2004;11(2):104–112.

Bates DW, Cohen M, Leape LL, Overhage JM, Shabot MM, Sheridan T. Reducing the frequency of errors in medicine using information technology. *J Am Med Inform Assoc.* 2001;8(4):299–308.

Fieschi M, Dufour JC, Staccini P, Gouvernet J, Bouhaddou O. Medical decision support systems: old dilemmas and new paradigms? *Methods Inf Med.* 2003;42(3):190–198.

Jung E, Li Q, Mangalampalli A, et al. Report central: quality reporting tool in an electronic health record. *AMIA Annu Symp Proc.* 2006:971.

Kaushal R, Shojania KG, Bates DW. Effects of computerized physician order entry and clinical decision support systems on medication safety: a systematic review. *Arch Intern Med.* 2003;163(12): 1409–1416.

Schedlbauer A, Prasad V, Mulvaney C, Phansalkar S, Stanton W, Bates DW, et al. What evidence supports the use of computerized alerts and prompts to improve clinicians' prescribing behavior? *J Am Med Inform Assoc.* 2009;16(4):531–538.

Sittig DF, Wright A, Simonaitis L, et al. The state of the art in clinical knowledge management: an inventory of tools and techniques. *Int J Med Inform.* 2010;79(1):44–57.

SECTION 4

Leadership and Practice Management Skills

CHAPTER 18

Principles of Leadership

Steven E. Weinberger, MD, FACP

INTRODUCTION

Physicians are frequently called upon to take on leadership roles. These roles can come in various forms, ranging from academic leadership roles (eg, division or department chief or chair) to educational leadership roles (eg, clerkship or residency program director) to leadership roles in a practice setting (eg, director of a practice group). Although some of the desired skills and competencies for the leader may be specific to particular roles and responsibilities, others are more generic and applicable to any of these leadership positions. In this chapter, I will concentrate initially on the generic aspects of leadership and conclude by discussing some of the challenges that are more specific to hospitalists and to the hospital environment. In addition, instead of trying to review the voluminous leadership literature, I will present a personal perspective, based upon my own experiences in a variety of leadership positions over many years. I will divide the discussion of leadership into four components: the personal attributes that a leader should demonstrate, the skills that should be acquired, a suggested approach for trying to reach a goal, and leadership challenges for hospitalists in the hospital environment.

LEADERS VS MANAGERS

Before considering the important attributes of a leader, it is worthwhile to understand the distinction between a *leader* and a *manager*. Much has been written about these differences, which can be readily summarized and understood by any of several descriptions or aphorisms:

- Leaders have followers; managers have subordinates. Individuals voluntarily follow a leader because of the qualities of the leader; subordinates work for managers because of the reporting relationship and the organizational authority vested in the manager.
- Leaders lead people; managers manage tasks.
- Leadership is doing the right thing; management is doing things right.
- Managers focus on tactics and tasks; leaders focus on strategy and direction.

In fact, however, these distinctions often blur in the setting of actual roles and responsibilities in the workplace. The individuals who are most successful in assuming roles with greater authority and responsibility are those who are both effective leaders and effective managers. A leader who does not have good management skills can generate visionary ideas but be unable to implement or operationalize them. A manager who does not have good leadership skills will be unable to mobilize and motivate a supportive team.

PRACTICE POINT

- The individuals who are most successful in assuming roles with greater authority and responsibility are those who are both effective leaders and effective managers. A leader who does not have good management skills can generate visionary ideas but is unable to implement or operationalize them. A manager who does not have good leadership skills will be unable to mobilize and motivate a supportive team.

Some activities and responsibilities of a physician leading a group of hospitalists can readily illustrate the differences between leadership and management. "Managing" the group means assuring that the patients are covered, that transitions of care are effectively handled, that chart and billing documentation is complete and accurate, and that teaching responsibilities are assigned and well integrated with patient care responsibilities. In contrast, "leading" the group means exploring and developing ideas for improving the system and its productivity, improving quality of care, developing the skills of the team, and facilitating the professional development of the team members.

For the purposes of this chapter, I will primarily use the terms "leadership" and "leadership skills," recognizing, however, that we are really considering both leadership and management skills. In the medical leadership positions that are likely to be assumed by readers of this chapter, success will hinge upon both leadership and managerial qualities and the importance of each in reinforcing the other. Therefore, my approach to discussing leadership and management qualities will be one of lumping rather than splitting.

DESIRABLE ATTRIBUTES OF THE LEADER

PRACTICE POINT

Qualities of successful leaders include:

- Professional integrity and honesty
- Openness and transparency in communicating to all constituencies, including receiving and providing feedback
- Willingness to recognize others' contributions and support their professional development
- Ability to create and maintain a positive work environment

It should go without saying that a leader must demonstrate professional integrity, including honesty. High standards of integrity and honesty are a prerequisite for obtaining the respect of colleagues, superiors, and subordinates. The leader sets the model of behavior for the rest of the team, and lack of professional integrity exhibited by the leader will soon be mirrored by cracks in professionalism among others.

The leader needs to be an effective communicator; openness and transparency in communicating to all constituencies assure that everyone is on the same page. A commonly held perception of a talented leader is often someone who can communicate both values and vision, including a set of goals and how those goals might be achieved. However, that is only part of the communication equation, which also involves establishing and transmitting expectations for others. It is critical that subordinates, trainees, and team members understand the expectations being placed on them, including how and on what basis they are being judged.

Communication must also occur on a two-way street, ie, the leader must be an excellent listener as well. If the leader is unable or unwilling to hear what others have to say, he or she will be doomed to failure. Without ideas and feedback from others, the leader will invariably make mistakes of both commission and omission that can be avoided by hearing the ideas and opinions of others and considering all perspectives when making important decisions.

Another important aspect of communication relates to feedback. The effective leader provides feedback in a constructive, professional manner. This feedback must be based on established expectations, not on the subordinate's or trainee's ability to read the leader's mind and guess what he wants. In addition, the feedback should be done in a way that is formative, ie, giving the receiver of the feedback an opportunity to, and advice on how to improve performance. Providing only summative feedback at the end of a responsibility or task allows no room for improvement and often proves frustrating to the person receiving the feedback.

An effective leader remembers that her success is determined by the contributions or development of the people she leads or trains. The leader must acknowledge the contributions of others and not always take credit for success. Nothing is so demoralizing to a team member as the feeling that his contributions are not being recognized and that someone else is taking credit for his work or accomplishments. At the same time, a successful leader is cognizant of, and aims to promote the professional development of the individuals for whom she is responsible. For example, true success for an academic leader is often determined as much by the ultimate careers of the individuals trained by the leader, as it is by the academic contributions of the leader himself. Supporting the professional development of one's trainees is one of the most important and enduring legacies that a leader can leave to the profession.

Finally, an intangible but critical quality of a successful leader is the ability to create and maintain a positive work environment. The leader needs to establish a workplace tone that is positive, in which people feel they are supported and a "can do" attitude prevails. Productivity of the individuals for whom a leader is responsible is dependent upon their interest in, and commitment to the team and to the shared goals and vision that have been defined by the leader. A setting in which individuals are competitive with each other, where back-biting is common, and people feel they do not respect and share the values of their colleagues and the leader, is not an enjoyable workplace. It is also one that will never reach its true potential.

LEADERSHIP SKILLS

PRACTICE POINT

Effective leaders should have the following skills:

- A high level of competence in the particular field related to the leadership role
- The ability to negotiate effectively
- A working familiarity with balance sheets and with revenue and expense statements
- The ability to run meetings that make good use of the participants' time and expertise

An important prerequisite for a successful leader is a high level of competence in the particular field related to the leadership role. For example, an educational leader must be accomplished as a teacher and educator in order to command the necessary respect of trainees and other educational colleagues. Similarly, a clinical leader must be highly regarded as an excellent clinician in order to have credibility with other clinicians.

Another important skill that leaders must acquire is the ability to negotiate effectively. This topic is covered extensively in a later chapter in this section, but it is important to stress that leaders must exercise their negotiation skills in many settings—when dealing with superiors, dealing with subordinates, or dealing with third parties with whom there is no reporting relationship. Physicians have typically not been trained in negotiation, but there are fortunately a number of excellent and readily accessible resources that can provide valuable guidance to the previously untrained leader.

Many leaders have responsibility for budgets, and a working familiarity with balance sheets and with revenue and expense statements is therefore useful. Although providing such financial training is beyond the scope of this chapter, a valuable resource that can provide basic training in the principles of accounting is a short, easy to read, programmed text used in many business schools.

Finally, the responsibility of running meetings often accompanies leadership roles. Everyone has participated in meetings that run effectively, where the participants feel they have not wasted their time, and they leave the meeting with a well-defined action plan. On the other hand, everyone has also participated in meetings that are poorly organized, do not make best use of participants' time, and do not have a well-defined purpose or outcome. Several important pointers:

- Meetings should ideally have an advance agenda sent to the participants, so that they can prepare appropriately.
- Meetings should start on time, and they should end on time (or early). Time is an incredibly valuable commodity, and meeting participants become distracted and resentful when time is wasted at the beginning of a meeting or when a meeting runs overtime and potentially affects their subsequent commitments.
- Meetings should be interactive and make good use of the participants' time and expertise. A successful meeting is not a monologue provided by the meeting coordinator. Rather, it involves active engagement and participation by all attendees, so that the participants feel they have contributed to the meeting and have not just been wasting their time.
- Successful meetings are wrapped up effectively, typically with a summary as well as a well-defined action plan. Everyone should understand the outcome of the meeting and the expected action plan, including the assignments that have been meted out to individuals and the timeline according to which they should be completed.

REACHING A GOAL

In trying to generate ideas and complete desired tasks necessary to reach a goal, the successful leader may find it helpful to remember a set of principles. At the outset, the leader needs to establish the goal and communicate it to others. In other words, the leader must define the destination before anyone can plot the route of how to get there. Once the goal is established, the leader must recognize that she does not need to generate all the ideas. Good work is typically done in teams in which everyone is encouraged to share ideas, no matter how crazy or far-fetched they may initially seem. In addition, not all good ideas need to come from within the team. One can adopt and build upon ideas and successful initiatives that have been developed by individuals outside the organization. The "not invented here" attitude often precludes an open mind to accepting ideas that have worked successfully in other settings.

The ideas necessary to reach a goal are often not grand and sweeping ones. A series of small steps, each of which can be judged and modified as necessary based upon the outcome achieved, is often more successful than a single, revolutionary idea that does not allow for opportunities to provide mid-course assessment and correction.

In making plans for a project or reaching a goal, the leader often needs to establish a team of individuals who will be working together. Assembling the right people is critical for a successful outcome. Team members need to be chosen based upon their skills, their interest in and enthusiasm for the project, their ability to work well with others on the team, and their openness in providing ideas and feedback about how things are going.

In making the best use of the team members, the leader must be willing to delegate responsibility appropriately. From the time of their training, physicians are often used to feeling that they need to take full responsibility for a patient, and this attitude of individual responsibility and accountability should often be modified when one assumes leadership responsibilities. Members of a team work best when they feel that responsibility has been bestowed upon them. Delegating responsibility is not a sign of weakness; rather, appropriate delegation demonstrates an understanding of how to share responsibility, engage others, make best use of available resources, and capitalize on each person's strengths.

As a project progresses, the leader must critically assess interim outcomes. Based on these outcomes, the leader must be willing to reassess the plan and adjust accordingly. The leader and the team members should also recognize that not all plans will be successful. A plan that does not succeed should not necessarily be viewed as a failure. Important lessons are often learned and new ideas generated based upon unanticipated problems or unexpected results.

LEADERSHIP CHALLENGES IN THE HOSPITAL ENVIRONMENT

Hospitalists who are in leadership positions or who are expected to effect change are often confronted with challenges that arise specifically from working in the hospital environment. Besides dealing with physicians, hospitalists are constantly working with nonphysician personnel and administrators whose management and reporting structure is quite independent of the physicians at the institution. A hospitalist leader who is trying to effect change but is not part of the hospital's administrative hierarchy may have difficulty shaping opinions and getting buy-in from a group of nursing leaders or from nonphysician hospital administrators. Even among physician leaders at the hospital, issues that arise are often centered around a competition for resources, so that the interpersonal relationships become adversarial rather than cooperative.

An additional challenge confronted by hospitalists stems from the fact that they are often young, and if they are female or from a minority group, may find it difficult to break into a hospital hierarchy that tends to be older, male, and Caucasian. A young woman who goes on staff as a hospitalist at the institution where she completed her residency may find it hard to shake the image of being a resident rather than a staff member and colleague. On the other hand, a young hospitalist who takes a position at an institution where he did not train may find it difficult to parachute in as a newcomer unfamiliar with a particular hospital's culture and personalities.

Although there is no tried and true way to overcome those challenges, a number of suggestions may be helpful. First, it is extremely valuable to obtain the trust and support of a more senior, well-respected person, ideally a current physician leader at the institution. Such an individual not only can serve as a mentor and advisor to guide the hospitalist in charting a path through treacherous waters, but he can also smooth the way for the young hospitalist to become accepted by the more established hospital hierarchy. For example, the support and trust from a well-respected division chief or department chair can be invaluable in easing the way for a hospitalist to deal with an older, potentially intimidating chief of surgery or hospital chief operating officer.

Second, as mentioned earlier in this chapter, it is critical for any clinician leader, particularly a hospitalist leader, to be viewed by both physician and nonphysician staff as an outstanding clinician. It is very difficult to have credibility in the hospital environment, particularly from physician colleagues and from nursing staff, if one is viewed as a "clinical lightweight." The hospitalist's conscientiousness, clinical skills, decision-making ability, communications skills, and professionalism all contribute to the individual's reputation and ability to command respect from others at the institution.

Third, it is important when trying to effect change and garner support from both physician and nonphysician staff to initially establish, promote, and focus on the principles underlying the proposed plan. Although it is easy for a hospital administrator to argue with a specific proposal, it is much more difficult to take a position against an ultimate goal of improving the quality and safety of patient care, improving hospital systems and efficiency, or improving the financial performance of the hospital.

Finally, it is important for the hospitalist to seek out defined leadership roles. Such roles can obviously be within the hospital community, eg, by serving on committees. However, establishing a presence and reputation outside the institution, eg, through involvement at regional and national levels, can only help the hospitalist's reputation and credibility within her own hospital setting.

FINAL WORDS

The concept of being a "born leader" has clearly given way to a philosophy that leadership skills can be learned. It is perhaps based on this premise that so many books and articles have been written about every possible aspect of leadership. Yet, it is fair to say that many personal qualities and aspects of personality do have an impact on potential success as a leader. When placed in a position with leadership responsibilities, it is valuable to take some time to self-reflect upon personality traits and how they will likely influence leadership style. In addition, one should try to assess what additional skills she needs to acquire to be an effective leader. Even though physicians are often placed in either clinical or academic leadership positions, they have not typically received leadership training. Recognizing the interplay between personal style and leadership skills, and acknowledging the importance of self-reflection on successes and failures as a leader will serve to make one an increasingly effective leader over time.

PRACTICE POINT

- To become an increasingly effective leader over time, it is important to recognize the interplay between personal style and leadership skills, and acknowledge the importance of self-reflection on successes and failures as a leader.

SUGGESTED READINGS

Breitner LK, Anthony RN. *Essentials of Accounting*. 10th ed. Upper Saddle River, NJ: Prentice Hall; 2009.

Fisher R, Ury W, Patton B. *Getting to Yes: Negotiating Agreement Without Giving In*. 2nd ed. New York: Penguin Books; 1991.

Shell GR. *Bargaining for Advantage: Negotiation Strategies for Reasonable People*. 2nd ed. New York: Penguin Books; 2006.

CHAPTER 19

The Economics of Hospital Care

David Meltzer, MD, PhD

INTRODUCTION

The economics of health care is an important concern in countries around the world, and is a particular area of concern in the United States. Hospital care constitutes about one-third of total health care expenditures, and patients who have been hospitalized often have very high costs after discharge, including for rehospitalization, skilled nursing facility, and home health use. Hospitals are increasingly being held responsible for managing these costs. As a result, hospitalists must have a good understanding of the economics of hospital care and the effects that hospitalists can have on health care costs. Many of the most important issues in the economics of hospital care, such as the critical role of health care technology, are relevant to many other aspects of health care economics. However, hospital care has certain fairly unique elements that deserve particular attention.

THE ECONOMICS OF HEALTH CARE

Health care now consumes about 1 in 6 dollars spent in the United States, up from 1 in 12 dollars in 1960. This increase in spending is not a problem in and of itself; growth in a sector of the economy can be highly desirable if it reflects the development of valuable new technologies (eg, computers). However, in the case of health care there are good reasons to question whether increases in spending have been consistently worthwhile. One reason for concern is that much of health care spending is covered by insurance. Insurance helps ensure that high cost, unpredictable health care is available to people when they need it. However, insurance also causes individuals to consume health care even when it might not be otherwise worthwhile for them. Moreover, because patients may not easily understand many of the complex decisions about their care, often spending may not align well with their underlying preferences. While many efforts are being made to better inform and empower patients to participate in their medical decisions, health care providers, hospitals, insurers, and policy makers must make decisions that patients cannot fully participate in and that influence patient care. Social institutions, such as licensure, accreditation, public reporting of outcomes, and market competition may also help ensure that these parts of the health care system act more effectively as agents of patients.

Indeed, while there is evidence that the value of increased health care spending on average has far exceeded the cost, there is also evidence that a sizable fraction of medical interventions provide little health benefit. The United States spends more per capita on health care than any other country, but many countries achieve comparable or better population health outcomes. These cross-national differences cannot be attributed completely to differences in the health care systems across countries. Nevertheless, the efficiency with which resources are used within these health care systems is a critical concern when seeking to maximize the health outcomes given available resources. Tools such as medical cost-effectiveness analysis are often used to assess how the cost of care compares to the health benefits produced. One metric for assessing cost effectiveness is the incremental cost-effectiveness ratio, which is calculated by dividing the change in costs resulting from an intervention by the change in life years lived, usually adjusted for quality of life. Whereas the decisions that people make about their own health suggest that people may value a one-year increase in life expectancy at about $50,000 to $200,000, some commonly used medical interventions cost more than $1 million per life year saved. Many interventions may not produce any health benefits, regardless of costs. The emerging field of comparative effectiveness research seeks to compare the effectiveness of health care interventions to determine when specific interventions should be utilized. While the appropriate role of costs and cost-effectiveness analysis in comparative effectiveness research is controversial, the concept that both costs and effectiveness of medical interventions are important policy concerns is widely accepted.

APPROACHES TO CONTROL HEALTH CARE EXPENDITURES

A wide range of approaches have been proposed to control health care expenditures. These include market-based approaches such as making patients and providers more sensitive to costs by limiting what services will be covered or how much of their costs will be paid. Consumer-side market incentives at the point of care, such as copayments, have been proven to reduce expenditures in numerous contexts, including the RAND Health Insurance Experiment. However, the ability to control the spending of high-cost consumers through copayments is limited by the high economic burdens these create for these individuals and their families. This limitation is especially important because health care costs are highly concentrated; more than 90% of all health care costs are borne by the top 50% of users. Within Medicare, the top 5% of users constitute 50% of spending. Since hospitalized patients are typically among these high-cost users, consumer-side cost sharing often has little effect on hospital spending because hospitalized patients often will have reached caps on out of cost payments.

Another approach to controlling health care spending is to reduce payments to providers. The extent to which this is possible is limited by the need for providers to maintain their financial solvency, but will generally reduce expenditures in the short run and place downward pressure on long run cost growth if it is maintained. Nevertheless, in a fee-for-service environment, reducing payments to providers may cause providers to engage in "demand inducement" in which they increase the quantity of services provided in order to make up for lost revenue. Indeed, this is one reason that many health economists believe that controlling health care costs will require paying for all of health care with fixed payments to cover all of a person's care over a defined period of time (capitation). Indeed, the single most important cost containment approach for hospitals has been the use of prospective payment for hospital care, in which hospitals are paid a fixed amount of money for a hospitalization for a given condition. We return to these ideas in the following section. Market-based approaches remain important under capitation because competition among providers may encourage providers to be more efficient in order to offer greater value to patients. Even in more regulated systems such as single-payer national health insurance systems, such competition between providers may increase quality and allow reductions in costs over time.

THE ORGANIZATIONAL STRUCTURE OF HOSPITALS

Most hospitals in the United States are not-for-profit institutions operated by staff employed by the hospital and acting under the supervision of a board that typically includes community leaders, physicians, patients, and others representing the diverse stakeholders that have interests in the operation of the hospital. To maintain their not-for-profit status and associated tax advantages, not-for-profit hospitals cannot make profits and must demonstrate evidence of the benefits they create for their community. Such community benefits can be hard to define, and even not-for-profit hospitals may be heavily influenced to make decisions that benefit hospital managers and staff more than patients. For-profit hospitals do not have the same community benefit obligations as not-for-profit hospitals and are less likely to provide types of care that are not profitable. However, the differences in services between for-profit and not-for-profit hospitals are often less than one might expect. Even government safety net hospitals, such as county hospitals, may face economic incentives to provide care for which insurance coverage is better. In general, payment rates in the United States are highest for private insurance, followed by Medicare, then Medicaid. Under the Emergency Medical Treatment and Active Labor Act (EMTALA), hospitals must ensure the provision of care for persons without insurance who face immediate life-threatening conditions. As an unfunded mandate, EMTALA has adverse effects on the financial well being of some hospitals that serve low income communities and the availability of emergency and hospital services in those communities.

The compensation of physicians varies across hospitals, with physicians in many for-profit and not-for-profit hospitals being paid through the professional fees that they bill, while physicians in government hospitals, academic medical centers, and hospitals owned by staff-model HMOs are more often paid a salary. Often, physicians working fee-for-service have unpaid institutional obligations, such as caring for uninsured patients or serving on committees, while physicians paid by salary will also have incentives for productivity. Thus, the differences in these means of paying physicians may not always be as large as they would seem.

Nevertheless, understanding the organizational structure of a hospital is essential to understanding how various policy changes may affect hospital care. For example, hospital managers will tend to want hospital resources to be very heavily used, while physicians may prefer that the hospital has excess capacity so that they and their patients can more easily access care. Decisions regarding the adoption of costly new technologies may have similar dynamics among physicians and hospitals. One exception is when hospitals can be paid more for care that is provided using an expensive new technology. In these cases, in areas with many hospitals, hospitals may compete with each other to attract doctors by buying costly new technologies in what has been termed a "medical arms race" (Zwanziger and Melnick 1988). This contrasts with the typical expectation that competition will drive down costs as more efficient organizations drive less efficient ones out of business. In recent years, as payment policies have been less generous, hospital competition has been associated with lower costs.

THE PAYMENT OF HOSPITALS

Before the 1980s, almost all hospitals were retrospectively paid fee for service for the care that they provided. This meant that when the patient received more care, for example by staying an extra day in the hospital, the hospital would receive more payment. Since rates typically covered the cost of hospital care plus some profit, hospitals had incentives to provide more care in order to increase profits or produce surplus revenue in excess of costs to help them achieve other parts of their mission. Not surprisingly, hospital costs grew rapidly.

In the 1980s, Medicare changed its reimbursement policy for hospital care to the Medicare Prospective Payment System (PPS), which paid hospitals a fixed amount for the hospital care of a specific group of conditions, which Medicare termed a Diagnosis Related Group (DRG). With hospital length of stay as a major driver of costs, hospitals could make more money if they reduced length of stay to allow them to care for more patients with a fixed amount of resources, and both hospital length of stay and costs fell dramatically. PPS raised several concerns, however, including the possibility that hospitals would admit healthy patients who did not have to be hospitalized but would have short lengths of stay and be very profitable, and the possibility that hospitals would discharge patients too quickly, resulting in bad outcomes.

To address these issues, Medicare established peer review organizations (PROs) to monitor for inappropriate utilization and low quality care. While there has been some evidence of inappropriate utilization and a tendency to discharge patients "sicker and quicker" (Kosecoff, Kahn et al 1990) under PPS, the PROs and subsequent utilization and quality initiatives suggest that the net cost advantages of PPS are large compared to these concerns. It should be noted that PPS has also been shown to occasionally reduce care and impair outcomes for the sicker people within any diagnostic grouping. This might be predicted because these sicker-than-average patients in a diagnostic group become less profitable under prospective payment. This may be one reason that prospective payment has never been fully prospective. For example, PPS does not provide the same reimbursement for the treatment of a heart attack regardless of whether bypass is or is not performed. To do so would be to produce financial penalties for performing bypass that likely would be harmful for patients. Similarly, PPS provides some extra "outlier" payments for patients with exceptionally long hospital length of stay relative to other patients with similar diagnoses.

PPS is also especially important to hospitalists because it increased the incentives for hospitals to reduce length of stay, making the potential benefits of hospitalist efforts to shorten the average length of stay more attractive to those hospitals. PPS also raised the average acuity of hospitalized patients, making the physical presence of hospitalists in the hospital more important. Thus, Medicare PPS probably contributed to the rapid growth of hospitalists. That said, there is also strong evidence that the number of hospitalists grew because they offered primary care physicians (PCPs) a way to avoid costly trips to the hospital to see an increasingly smaller number of hospitalized patients as primary care practice increasingly came to focus on preventive care. This suggests the potential for exciting new models of care in which a new type of hospitalist physician provides primary care and hospital care for a highly selected group of patients at high risk of hospitalization.

EFFECTS OF HOSPITALISTS ON HOSPITAL COSTS

Shortly after the term hospitalist was defined in the mid-1990s, reports began to be published describing reductions in hospital length of stay and costs due to hospitalists. Reviews of the subsequent literature have largely confirmed these early findings, though not all studies have found savings. Some factors have been suggested to affect the reductions in hospital costs from hospitalists, including hospitalist experience, which may be a particular concern because of the relative youth of the field and relatively high rates of burnout and turnover among hospitalists.

While several of these studies rely on natural experiments in which patients are assigned to hospitalist or nonhospitalist physicians based on a predetermined call schedule, a limitation of many of these studies is that patients may be assigned nonrandomly to physicians based on patient attributes that may be difficult to control for and may predict hospital resource utilization. This is especially a concern when attempting to understand the effects of hospitalists on costs for patients who would otherwise be cared for in the hospital by their own primary care physician. All of the studies with a design resembling random assignment are limited to academic medical centers, where the comparison is between having a hospitalist attending who is not the patient's PCP or a nonhospitalist attending who is also not the patient's PCP. To the extent one believes that receiving hospital care from a doctor who has an ongoing relationship to the patient (such as the patient's PCP) may be valuable, this limitation of the literature is a major one. There are also relatively few studies that characterize well how hospitalists may affect resource utilization after hospital discharge.

There is also a literature suggesting that hospitalists may produce resource savings when they serve as comanaging physicians with surgical or medical specialists. Such models are supported by the fact that both the hospitalist and the subspecialist can bill for their services in most settings. Whether such models would be economically attractive in settings in which both physicians could not bill for their time is not clear.

It is worth noting that many studies of the effects of hospitalists on resource utilization focus on length of stay. This is typically appropriate because length of stay is the largest determinant of hospital costs; most of the costs of hospital care are fixed costs and most hospitals operate close to capacity. However, in cases in which hospitals are not close to capacity and costs are fixed, or if staffing is easily varied, reductions in length of stay may not have the same implications for the cost per case as they more typically would. Correctly estimating the costs of care and savings or costs from specific programs in the context of hospitals is extremely difficult. Activity-based accounting systems, which attribute all the costs in the hospital to specific activities of patient care that can then be allocated across patients, are considered state-of-the-art in estimating hospital costs. However, these systems can be applied in many different ways across institutions that require that the resulting estimates of costs be considered with caution.

SYSTEM EFFECTS OF HOSPITALISTS

In addition to the direct effects of hospitalists on costs through the patient care they provide, hospitalists may also have effects on costs by helping to develop systems that address important clinical and economic needs of hospitals. These may include roles in designing and implementing utilization review and bed flow positions, health information system innovations such as computerized order entry, and efforts to reduce costly errors or improve adherence by developing quality indicators that are increasingly tied to economic incentives. Numerous studies suggest that medical errors are costly and that costly practices that might be reduced by improved information systems are common in hospital care. A growing literature also suggests that specific strategies to reduce errors and/or influence practice patterns through health information systems may produce cost savings. Such findings are neither universal nor completely compelling at this point, but it is likely that better implementation of these systems may produce more compelling results in the future, and hospitalists are very well situated to play such a role in that implementation. Economic incentives to reduce readmission are another major example of an area in which hospitalists are well situated to help a hospital respond to incentives to reduce resource use. In teaching hospitals, hospitalists may also improve the education of house staff in cost-effective approaches to patient care, which would reduce resource use by those residents even when they are no longer working with hospitalists. Even in settings in which PCPs continue to come to the hospital to direct patient care on a daily basis, hospitalists may decrease length of stay and costs by providing needed clinical expertise at times when the PCP cannot be present.

ACCOUNTABLE CARE ORGANIZATIONS AND THE FUTURE OF HOSPITALISTS

While retrospective reimbursement of health care provides attractive incentives for the provision of needed care, it can lead to excess provision of care. As a result, there is great interest in moving toward models in which payment is made prospectively for the care of an individual over a defined period of time. (Fisher, Staiger et al 2007) Medicare PPS was a step in that direction, but did not include costs incurred after discharge, potentially increasing the incentive for early discharge and increased rates of readmission. Similarly, the fact that PPS does not include physician fees in the payment for hospital care can increase incentives for consultation, the use of comanagement models, and even extended hospital length of stay from the physician perspective.

The Patient Protection and Affordable Care Act (PPACA) (United States. Congress. House. Committee on Ways and Means., United States. Congress. House. Committee on Energy and Commerce. et al, 2010) includes a spectrum of strategies to address these potentially perverse incentives, with penalties for rapid readmissions as a first step and payment of a fixed fee to care for a patient over a defined period of time at the other end of the spectrum. Under PPACA, Medicare is already charged to implement reductions in inpatient payment rates for hospitals that exceed targeted readmission rates. The maximum penalty will rise to 3% of payments by Federal Fiscal Year 2013. The Medicare Acute Care Episode (ACE) demonstration project will be a 5-year effort beginning in 2015 to test the effects on resource use and outcomes of providing a single payment to hospitals to cover all the hospital, physician, and other post-acute care costs for the 30 days before and 30 days after an acute episode of illness. In addition to requiring study of the effects of such "bundled payment" strategies, PPACA also mandates that Medicare establish infrastructure to begin to establish accountable care organizations that will assume full responsibility for the care of patients over a defined period of time in exchange for a fixed payment. The economic advantages of such a payment system in terms of cost reduction, integration of care, and avoidance of the perverse incentives for excess use created by retrospective fee-for-service systems are suggested by the successes of some staff model HMOs in these domains. However, it remains to be seen whether the successes of such models in cost containment can be easily replicated in other settings.

PRACTICE POINT

- To date, hospitalists have largely sought to establish their value case based on their ability to reduce inpatient costs, to generate inpatient revenue, and to improve hospital performance on established inpatient quality indicators that may be tied to increased patient demand or that rewards under pay for performance. However, the expected changes in reimbursement toward greater bundling and capitation will force hospitalists to build value cases based on new metrics, such as the total cost of care, reductions in readmissions, and improved long-term outcomes.

Payment reforms under PPACA may have important implications for hospitalists. Already, hospitals are increasingly looking to hospitalists and others to develop new systems to reduce readmissions. Bundled payment systems that combine hospital and professional fees could also change the incentives for comanagement models by eliminating the ability to obtain additional revenue by having multiple physicians treat a hospitalized patient on a given day. Bundled payments that include professional fees might also lead to complex negotiations between hospitalists and hospitals about payment for hospitalists. Full capitation models would reduce the extent to which Medicare physician fee schedules drive physician reimbursement, and might lead to further changes in the relative earnings of specialists and generalists. Although the effects of such changes are difficult to predict, it seems likely that specialty reimbursement would be particularly reduced. Primary care physicians might also find themselves facing increasing competition from nonphysician providers who might provide elements of primary care at lower cost. Together, these pressures might drive increasing numbers of young physicians into Hospital Medicine, which would probably put downward pressures on hospitalist earnings. Increases in health insurance coverage due to health care reform and the aging of the baby boomers might increase demand, somewhat offsetting these forces. In addition to these macro-level effects on hospitalist earnings, individual hospitalists may find their earnings strongly affected by the extent to which they can provide evidence of their ability to reduce costs and improve outcomes.

THE NEW VALUE CASE FOR HOSPITALISTS

To date, hospitalists have largely sought to establish their value case based on their ability to reduce inpatient costs, to generate inpatient revenue, and to improve hospital performance on established inpatient quality indicators that may be tied to increased patient demand or that rewards under pay for performance. However, the expected changes in reimbursement toward greater bundling and capitation will force hospitalists to build value cases based on new metrics, such as the total cost of care, reductions in readmissions, and improved long-term outcomes. Efforts to reduce cost of care are likely to take many forms, including programs to reduce readmission, skilled nursing facility use, and emergency department use after discharge, disease management programs, and palliative care programs that may reduce costs at the end of life. The history of similar efforts suggests that programs in these areas are likely to vary in their efficacy. For example, the Study to Understand Prognoses and Preferences for Outcomes and Risks of Treatments (SUPPORT), which was intended to improve care at the end of life for patients at high risk of death, did not improve care, outcomes, or resource use. More recently, the results of the Massachusetts General Hospital Care Management for High Cost Beneficiaries Project suggested savings of $3,600 per year for an aggressive case management system designed to support the care of high-cost Medicare beneficiaries. These studies will likely be followed by many more in the coming years that will aim to test new strategies to improve care. Many of these strategies are likely to include either public reporting of outcomes or financial incentives for hospitals to meet specified quality indicators or economic objectives. To date, public reporting and pay-for-performance programs have shown mixed results, again underscoring the importance of carefully evaluating these programs as they are implemented. However, such evaluations have encountered many challenges, including measurement issues, and the potential to more easily improve outcomes by changing patient mix rather than truly improving care. Under PPACA, a Patient Centered Outcomes Research Institute will be established with a mission to assess the comparative effectiveness of alternative health care strategies, including new models of care. In addition, the Center for Medicare and Medicaid Services (CMS) will receive support to establish a CMS Innovation Center that will expand its ability to develop and test new models of care. Hospitalists will likely play important roles in many of these models of care.

PRACTICE POINT

- Hospitalists who can help their institutions address the economics challenges ahead may be highly sought after and compensated if they can demonstrate the value of their expertise. Hospitalists can do this by practicing effective and cost-effective medicine and by helping their institutions to become more efficient in their clinical operations.

HEALTH DISPARITIES AND HEALTH REFORM

Disparities in health outcomes by race and ethnicity, socioeconomic status, and across geographic areas are well documented in the United States. Health disparities are mulitfactorial, including patient, provider, and system factors, many of which are noneconomic. Nevertheless, an important effect of health care reform that may affect health disparities is that health care reform is expected to expand health insurance coverage for many Americans who were previously uninsured. This should improve access to care for these individuals, but the overall increase in demand for health care may create additional challenges for insured persons who are seeking access in some areas, unless increases in the supply of care are sufficient to meet these needs. Decreases in reimbursement for services may encourage increased supply of care if providers seek to make up lost revenue with increased volume. However, if declines in reimbursement are sufficiently large, supply might constrict and access could be reduced. Because much of the cost of the uninsured has been covered by cross-subsidies from better insured patients, decreased payments for Medicare patients may make it more difficult for institutions to cover the cost of the uninsured. Plans to progressively cap the deductibility of employer contributions for health insurance may also decrease the extent to which cross-subsidies for care of the uninsured are feasible. Thus, cost-containment measures in health care reform may increase health care disparities unless the expansions in coverage created by health care reform can adequately maintain revenue for providers. This provides some insight into the importance of coverage expansions as an area of early emphasis within the overall implementation of health care reform; it is likely that later phases will place a greater emphasis on cost control and that the increases in access achieved in the initial stages of health care reform will help make such cost control measures possible while minimizing the instability of the health care system as payment reductions occur.

CONCLUSIONS AND IMPLICATIONS FOR PRACTICING HOSPITALISTS

The national need to reduce health care spending is likely to place major downward pressures on all payments in the health care system in the coming years, including physician reimbursement. Hospitalist roles, such as comanagement, that are supported by current physician payment mechanisms may become less attractive with increasing bundling of payments. On the other hand, hospitalists who can help their institutions address the economic challenges ahead may be highly sought after and compensated if they can demonstrate the value of their expertise. Hospitalists can do this by practicing effective and cost-effective medicine and by helping their institutions to become more efficient in their clinical operations.

SUGGESTED READINGS

Fisher ES, Staiger DO, Bynum JP, Gottlieb DJ. Creating accountable care organizations: the extended hospital medical staff. *Health Affairs*. 2007;26(1):W44–W57. Epub 2006 Dec 5.

Harris JE. Internal organization of hospitals–some economic implications. *Bell J Economics*. 1977;8(2):467–482.

Investigators SP, Connors AF, et al. A controlled trial to Improve care for seriously ill hospitalized patients. *JAMA*. 1995;274(20): 1591–1598.

Kosecoff J, Kahn KL, Rogers WH, et al. Prospective payment system and Impairment at discharge–the quicker-and-sicker story revisited. *JAMA*. 1990;264(15):1980–1983.

McClellan M, Engelberg Center for Health Care Reform at Brookings, et al. Implementing comparative effectiveness research priorities, methods, and impact. Washington, D.C.; Engelberg Center for Health Care Reform at Brookings: The Hamilton Project; 2009.

Meltzer D, Manning WG, Morrison J, et al. Effects of physician experience on costs and outcomes on an academic general medicine service: results of a trial of hospitalists. *Ann Intern Med*. 2002;137(11):866–874.

Meltzer DO, Chung JW. US trends in hospitalization and generalist physician workforce and the emergence of hospitalists. *J Gen Intern Med*. 2010;25(5):453–459.

Newhouse JP, Rand Corporation Insurance Experiment Group. *Free for All?: Lessons from the Rand Health Insurance Experiment*. Cambridge, Mass.; Harvard University Press; 1993.

United States Congress House Committee on Ways and Means, United States Congress House Committee on Energy and Commerce et al. *Compilation of Patient Protection and Affordable Care Act : as amended through November 1, 2010 including Patient Protection and Affordable Care Act health-related portions of the Health Care and Education Reconciliation Act of 2010*. Washington; U.S. Government Printing Office; 2010.

Zwanziger J, Melnick GA. The effects of hospital competition and the Medicare Pps Program on Hospital Cost Behavior in California. *J Health Econ*. 1988;7(4):301–320.

CHAPTER 20

Use of Lean Principles in Hospital Process Improvement

Daniel J. Hanson, MD, FHM

INTRODUCTION

Lean manufacturing, referred to commonly as "lean," comes from the Japanese manufacturing process management philosophy derived mostly from the Toyota Motor Company. Lean was popularized in the 1990s with the publication of the best seller *The Machine That Changed the World*, a book authored by Massachusetts Institute of Technology research scientists studying global manufacturing practices. This book by Womack, Jones, and Roos describes the manufacturing techniques behind Toyota's success and shows how, when implemented, these systems resulted in defect reduction, improved cost efficiency, higher productivity, and greater customer satisfaction. The results were remarkable: cars with one-third the defects, built in half the factory space, using half the man-hours. *The Machine That Changed the World* explained what lean production is, how it really works, and how it inevitably spread beyond the auto industry. It was not until 2001 that health care organizations began applying lean principles to processes outside of manufacturing.

In 1999, the Institute of Medicine Report, *To Err is Human*, challenged organizations to find better tools to effectively address cost and quality challenges. Those looking outside of health care for fresh approaches were impressed with the results seen in manufacturing companies using lean. The challenge would be to translate manufacturing tools into health care processes.

LEAN MANUFACTORING TRANSLATED INTO HEALTH CARE

Like manufacturing, health care delivery systems are often large, complex organizations with widespread waste and inefficiencies. For this reason the Toyota production system methods are attractive to health care leaders. Lean methods place the customer first, are obsessed with highest quality, safety, and staff satisfaction while succeeding economically. Beyond broad management ideals, the comparison to health care becomes less obvious. How can manufacturing cars be like caring for patients? It turns out that every manufacturing element is a production process. Health care is a combination of complex production processes: admitting a patient, performing surgery, or sending out a bill. Each involves thousands of processes, many of them very complex. All involve the concepts of quality, safety, customer satisfaction, staff satisfaction, and cost effectiveness. In health care, failing to deliver in any area not only causes dissatisfaction, but may even lead to patient harm.

INTRODUCTION TO LEAN PRINCIPLES

In a sequel book on lean, Womack and Jones provided 5 principles of lean production: defining value, value stream, flow, pull, and perfection. For simplification, this chapter will discuss value and value stream together. When improving any process using lean methods, it is important to study that process with respect to each of these five principles.

DEFINING VALUE

Defining value is the first step in "leaning" any process. Hence, one first identifies what is valuable within the process, as determined by the customer of the process. In identifying value, waste is automatically identified as that which is not valuable. Since the ultimate customer of any process in health care is the patient, it is important to ask "what would the patient be willing to pay for?" In auto manufacturing, car sales make this apparent. In health care, it has been

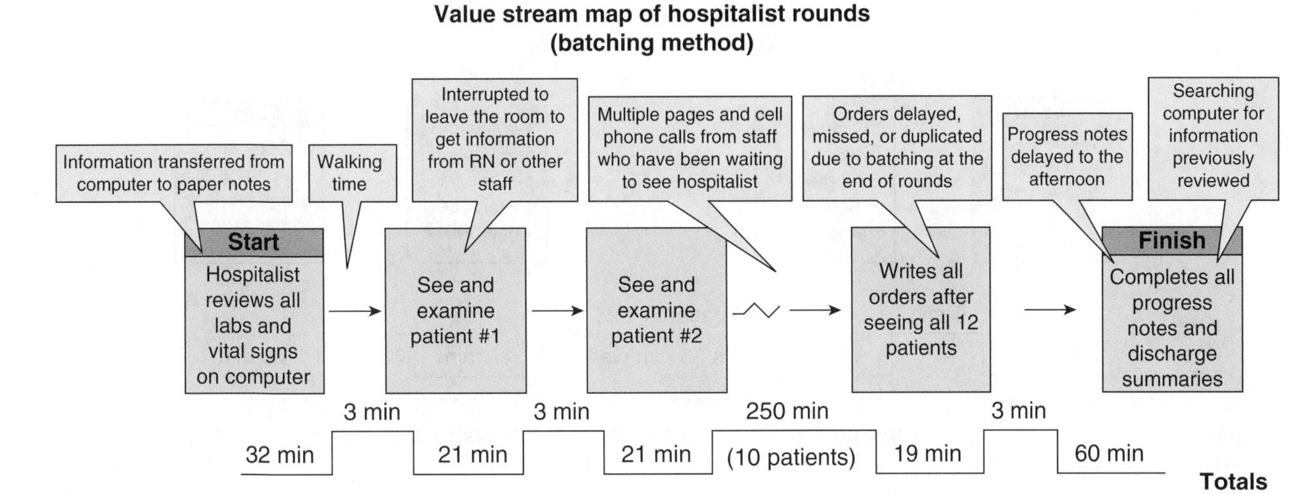

							Totals
Value added work	15 min	20 min	20 min	200 min	15 min	25 min	295 min (71%)
Nonvalue added work	20 min	4 min	4 min	50 min	7 min	35 min	120 min (29%)

Lead time (time from start of process to finish) = 415 min (36 min/patient/day)

Figure 20-1 *Represents a value stream map for hospitalist rounds performed with batching of previsit labs and vitals, order writing, and progress notes. The blue caption boxes signify examples of waste in the process. (Reproduced, with permission, from the Virginia Mason Medical Center, 2010.)*

historically less obvious. Does the process or task being improved change the form, fit, function, or satisfaction of the patient? If not, perhaps it does not add value. Using lean we can actually map out each step of an entire process in order to see the value and waste. This activity is called value stream mapping.

VALUE STREAM

A value stream is a series of specific actions necessary to complete a task or create a product from beginning to end. Value stream maps are created to visually communicate where value and waste occur in any process. Creating a value stream map involves making observations about a process, noting each step and its sequence, and measuring the time it takes for each step to occur (**Figure 20-1**). In Figure 20-1, note that the products measured are documentation and orders completed on a panel of hospitalized patients. Non-value-added activities are denoted and the time wasted performing these activities is measured. Non-value-added activities will need to be eliminated if the process is to be improved.

Waste

Waste can be categorized into 7 types in health care processes:

Overproduction: Any time a process causes a task to be performed more than necessary, production waste occurs. Examples of overproduction waste include ordering unnecessary labs, delivering 2 lunch trays to the same patient, or administering IV medications when oral medications would have been adequate.

Time-on-hand: This type of waste refers to waiting. Any time a patient is waiting for a medication, a procedure, or a provider it is considered waste. The hospital rounding example in Figure 20-1 illustrates time-on-hand waste as patients, families, and nurses waiting for the hospitalist to round and write orders. Also, the consultant may be waiting for the hospitalist's progress note.

Transportation: Unnecessary transport of people, equipment, or supplies is considered transportation waste. Examples include having to transport a patient to another facility to acquire an MRI or ordering a procedure kit but not using it.

Processing: This form of waste is associated with unnecessary handling, clerical work, cognitive effort, and time spent working on a process or task. An example of processing waste is seen in Figure 20-1 as the provider copies information from computer screen to paper and then back into a computer-generated progress note. Another example is searching for information that may have already been reviewed earlier in the day.

Stock on Hand: Excessive inventory is a form of waste. Examples include storing large quantities of expensive medications or other costly supplies for weeks or months before they are used.

Movement: Here, waste is as simple as a provider having to walk 20 feet to pick up a chart or walking to multiple wards to see patients.

Defective Products: Any time a process creates a product that is defective, whether it is harmful or not to the patient, it is waste. Providing the wrong dose of a medication, documentation errors, or wrong-site surgery are all examples of defective product waste.

PRACTICE POINT

- The 7 wastes in health care are overproduction, time-on-hand, transportation, processing, stock on hand, movement, and defective products.

FLOW

Once all types of waste have been identified and attempts have been made to eliminate such waste from a value stream, focus shifts to make the remaining steps flow in continuous movement toward the finished product. Natural tendencies are to see work in separate compartments of function and location. Again, hospital rounding is a good example. Before rounds, providers often review all lab results and vitals on all patients, followed by physical examinations, and

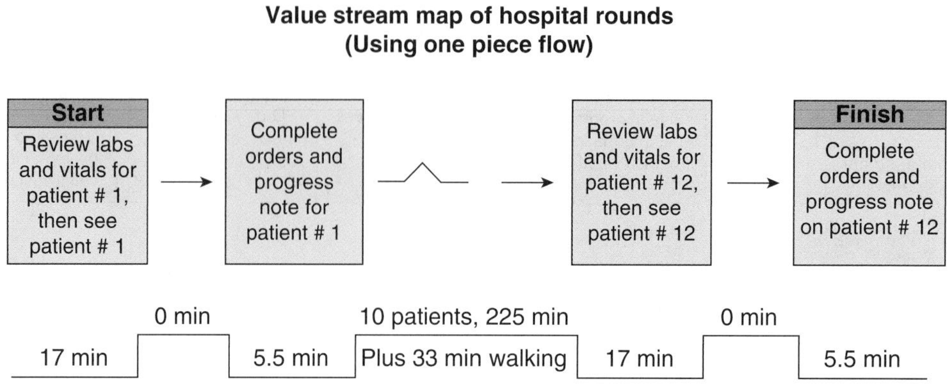

Rapid process improvement workshop progress report							
Team Name: Hospitalists							
Process summary: Reduce the nonvalue added time in the hospitalists' daily rounds through creation of one piece flow, standard work, and elimination of interruptions.							
Metrics	**Baseline**	**Target > 50%**	**Day 2**	**Day 3**	**Day 5**	**Final**	**Percent change**
Lead time – Time it takes to complete rounds on 12 patients	415 min	350 min	270 min	320 min	290 min	270 min	35%
Quality – Percent of patients w/ completed rounds by 12 PM	66%	100%	80%	90%	100%	100%	34%
Quality – Number of defects (interruptions, unnecessary pages, delayed progress notes, and orders).	14	7	8	9	5	5	64%
Walking distance – Hospital daily walking distance	2.09 miles	1 mile	1.9 miles	1.9 miles	1.9 miles	1.9 miles	9%

Figure 20-2 *Demonstrates the use of a 5-day rapid process improvement workshop (RPIW) to eliminate the waste identified in the value stream in Figure 20-1. (Reproduced, with permission, from the Virginia Mason Medical Center, 2010.)*

later, by completion of progress notes and orders. This is an example of performing work in batches. Batching seems efficient to the worker as long as he or she remains steadily busy. However, from the perspective of patients, this method is inefficient. Batching leads to delayed patient progress. Tasks are more efficiently and accurately completed when the product (patient wellness) is worked continuously rather than in batches. This is referred to as one-piece flow. Using this method, providers look up labs and vitals at the time they see each individual patient and complete all relevant orders and progress notes before moving on to the next patient.

With lean, the focus is always on the product. In health care, the product is simply the patient becoming more independent from our care. Patient needs, rather than those of the provider, come first. In contrast, when work is batched, mistakes, defects, and waste occur. When a process is initially forced into continuous flow it may be difficult to maintain. Barriers to flow will become obvious and, once exposed, are considered waste. Once this waste is eliminated, continuous flow may be achieved and maintained successfully. In essence, demanding flow exposes waste during the actual process of trying to maintain continuous flow (**Figure 20-2**). Figure 20-2 demonstrates how waste can be eliminated and how the rounding process can be improved by converting to one-piece flow.

■ PULL

Pull is a term used to describe the ideal operational sequence of a process in which downstream goods or services are not provided until the precise moment they are needed, not too soon nor too late. The pull of a product through a sequential process is best described by imagining that each step in that process is connected by a single thread that pulls the product, step by step, toward completion. Processes that "push" rather than "pull" create waste by producing too much product or the wrong product. Hospitals are managed as push production processes in which operating rooms, clinics, and emergency departments each push patients into the hospital. Often, patients are diverted elsewhere because hospitals frequently lack the ability to manage demand. In a pull system, each process in a chain of events is a customer of the preceding process. When pull is applied to health care, the underlying principle is that each process will receive the next patient exactly when it is ready. When patients are received too soon they often wait and providers feel pressured to perform work in nonstandard ways that may encourage mistakes or lapses in quality. Receiving a patient late requires providers to wait, which is also costly. True pull systems create continuous flow in which patients receive the exact care they need at the exact moment they need that care. At the same time, each provider's work pace is ideal, without being rushed or idle. It is conceptually possible to design a hospital with pull of admissions and discharges. Ideally, a hospital with pull processes throughout would allow continuous admission and discharge coordination such that admissions could be expected and planned in a way that eliminated waiting and diversion. This is no small task, as elective surgeries, clinic visits, and emergency care would require precise orchestration with discharges. This is why true pull processes are difficult to implement in health care systems today. Presently, pull systems are most prevalent in supply systems (**Figure 20-3**), where they can be easily implemented.

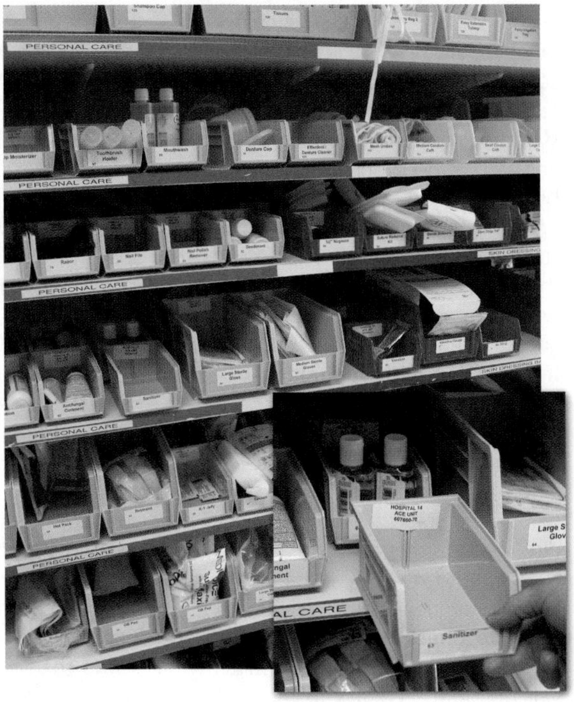

Figure 20-3 *Is an example of a hospital supply room using a pull system. Each supply bin, when empty, is removed and acts as a signal to: (1) pull the bin behind it forward and (2) a worker to resupply the empty bin and place it back behind the forward bin.*

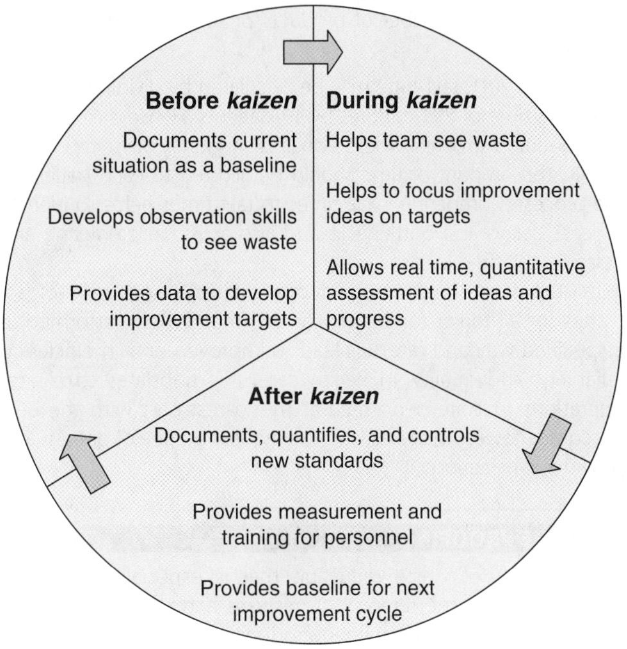

Figure 20-4 *Demonstrates the flow of change (kaizen) as managed using standard operations. (Reproduced, with permission, from the Virginia Mason Medical Center, 2010.)*

PERFECTION

The ultimate goal of lean is perfection by way of relentlessly ridding processes of all waste. When organizations successfully use lean methodology, a vision of perfection is developed that creates energy and urgency for change. This inertia must be checked by the perspective that powerful improvements unfold in many rapid, small cycles of change. Toyota refers to these small cycles of change as "kaizen," a Japanese term referring to continuous improvement. In an organization with robust lean efforts, kaizen is occurring in multiple ways throughout the organization, simultaneously. These improvement events, often called rapid process improvement workshops (RPIWs), must be well managed in an effort to maximize any benefits. One lean management method commonly utilized is called standard operations.

PRACTICE POINT

- The ultimate goal of lean is perfection by way of relentlessly ridding processes of all waste. When organizations successfully use lean methodology, a vision of perfection is developed that creates energy and urgency for change. Powerful improvements unfold in many rapid, small cycles of change. In health care, this translates to clinical operations that are performed at the lowest cost with the best outcomes, fewest mistakes, and the highest degree of patient and provider satisfaction.

Standard operations

Standard operations is a specified plan that often serves as the foundation for continuous process improvement. It is a plan of measuring and analyzing that documents the current state, allows development of waste visualization, and provides data useful in setting improvement goals. While making improvements, standard operations allows the team to assess and test ideas and measure progress. When the kaizen cycle is complete, standard operations documents new standards and provides new methods of measurement and training for the new baseline process (**Figure 20-4**). Managing change using standard operations ultimately leads to the most efficient process for any task. Standard operations demands that the work is performed with the best method and the highest quality each time, and with minimal variation and maximum reliability. Standard operations also ensures the highest output at the lowest possible cost. The components of standard operations are standard work, time, takt time.

Standard Work: When tasks are standardized to a repeatable cycle, abnormal conditions, mistakes, and waste become apparent. In addition, training becomes simplified and the work may be easily measured. Creating standard work occurs by documenting processes and procedures. Documentation and observations should occur at the actual work location, where the physical layout, sequence of work, and flow of providers, patients, and materials can be noted.

Time: Two time components that are measured are cycle time and lead time. Cycle time is the amount of time required for one worker or machine to complete one cycle of work. Lead time is the entire time required to provide a service or product, starting when that service or product is requested and ending upon delivery. Cycle time is depicted in Figure 20-1, using hospitalist rounding as an example, where cycle time begins with rounds on patient 1 and ends when rounding on patient 2 begins. Lead time, in the same example, begins with the start of rounds on patient 1 and ends with the conclusion of rounds on patient 12.

Takt Time: Takt is a German term meaning "rhythm" or "beat." Takt time is the amount of time necessary for a system to deliver a single product or service at the precise rhythm or rate demanded by customers. Market demand fluctuations influence takt time, which is calculated by dividing time available by the number of products or services needed during that time.

In Figure 20-1, takt time may be calculated by dividing the total rounding time of 295 minutes by 12 patients. Hence, takt time for this rounding process would equal 24 minutes, 30 seconds and ideally, this amount of time should be allotted to each patient in the process. Comparing cycle times to takt times helps to identify process delays and bottlenecks and also assists in predicting and balancing staffing levels.

In summary, standard operations creates a sequence of activities for a worker (or set of workers) that, when performed in a specified way and rate, will lead to improvements in efficiency, reliability, and quality. In health care, this translates to clinical operations that are performed at the lowest cost with the best outcomes, fewest mistakes, and the highest degree of patient and provider satisfaction.

MISTAKE PROOFING

One element of waste reduction that is especially applicable to health care is the removal of mistakes and defects. We know that health care is rife with opportunities to improve systems and processes. Between 2005 and 2007, lapses in patient safety resulted in 92,882 potentially preventable deaths and cost Medicare $6.9 billion. At the Toyota Motor Company in the 1960s, quality managers recognized that the statistical quality methods used by most manufacturers were important tools but did not go far enough to reduce defects to the ultimate goal of 0. Toyota realized long ago that organizations with aspirations for near perfect quality will only approach their goal if the expectation is perfection itself. Over time, Toyota has developed a systematic way of categorizing processes based on how mistakes are discovered and how quickly they are corrected. Toyota processes have further evolved to catch mistakes by inspection and, consequently, correct them early in the process. Some processes have been redesigned so that mistakes do not occur at all (**Figure 20-5**).

Categories of inspection are as follows:

No inspection: Here, no inspection occurs and mistakes are discovered by the customer. This is the least desirable system. This results in dissatisfaction, patient complaints, injuries, or lawsuits.

End of the Process Inspection: Inspections are performed at the end of the process and mistakes are caught by an inspector just before reaching the patient. Inspectors at this level are often unreliable and wasteful. These inspectors are farthest downstream in the process, which impacts their ability to provide the necessary feedback to remedy mistakes at the source. This type of inspection system relies on human diligence, training, and other human factors.

Self-Inspection with Judgment: Here, mistakes are found by the actual provider who made the mistake. That provider then self-corrects the error. An example would be the oncology nurse who finds her own mistake in chemotherapy dosing just before administration and corrects the dose. Mistakes discovered at this stage are more efficiently handled than mistakes discovered further downstream. However, these mistakes still contribute to wasteful delays. This type of inspection requires human attention and diligence.

Successive Check: With this type of inspection, mistakes are discovered by the next downstream worker who then provides prompt feedback to the upstream worker who made the mistake. A good example of successive check inspection is when an inappropriate medication is ordered for a patient and the nurse or pharmacist catches the mistake and notifies the ordering provider.

Self-inspection with Warning: In this case, the provider who makes a mistake receives an immediate warning, which may or may not be ignored. An example is a computer-generated alert that warns of an adverse drug reaction. With this method, inspections occur 100% of the time but mistakes are still possible if the provider ignores the warning.

Inspection with Control: Here, the ability to make a mistake is entirely prevented by design of the process or by a forcing function that halts the process until the mistake is corrected. This is the ultimate goal of all mistake proofing. Examples

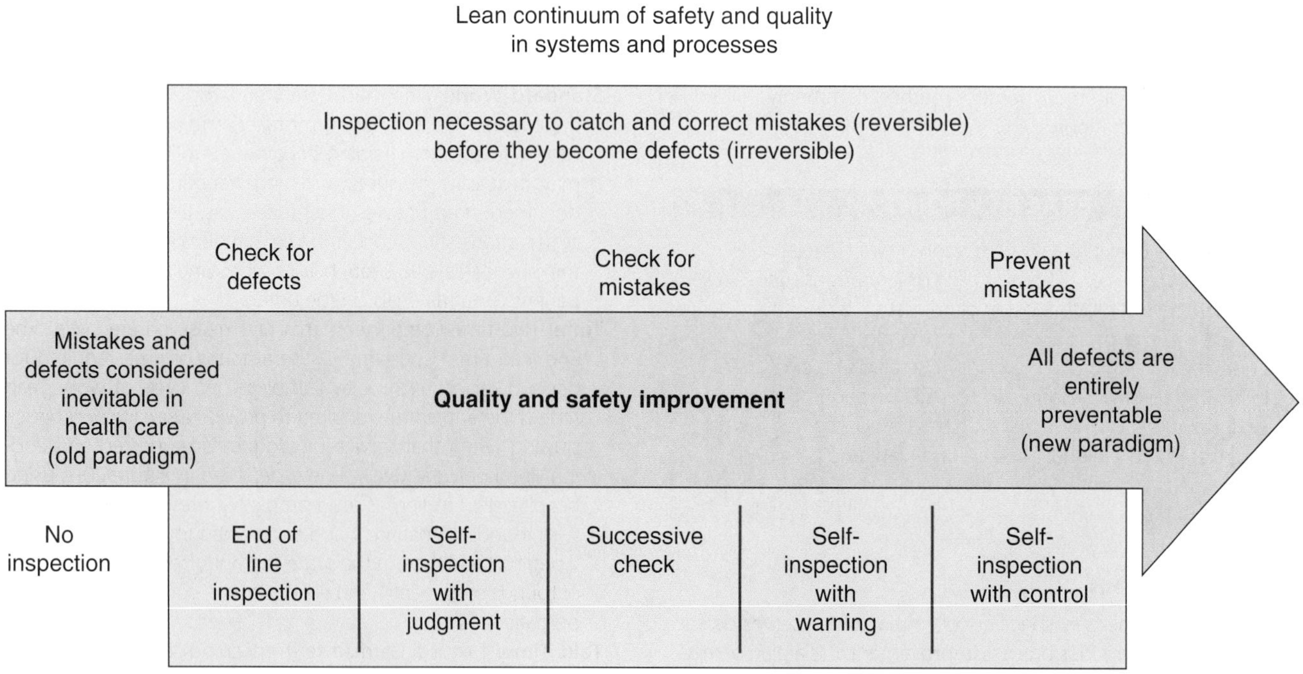

Figure 20-5 *Demonstrates the relationship of progressive inspection types to improved processes mistake proofing. (Reproduced, with permission, from the Virginia Mason Medical Center, 2010.)*

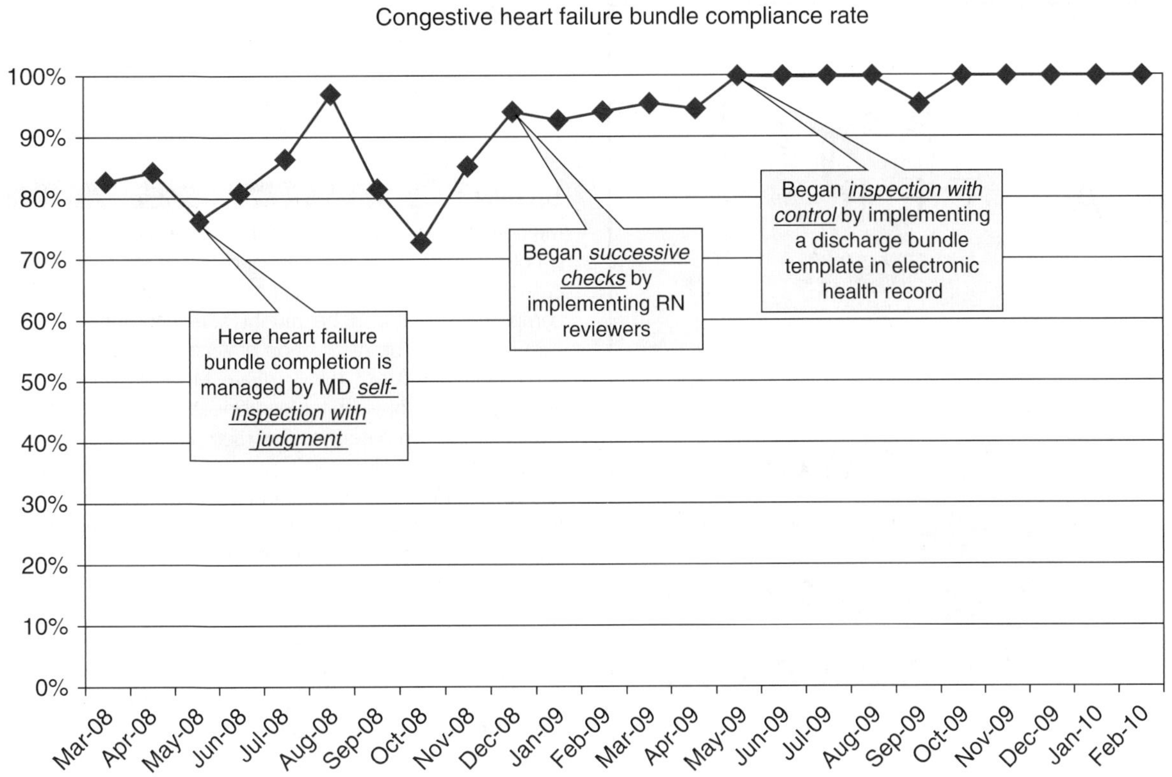

Figure 20-6 *Demonstrates an example of a process (completion of heart failure bundle) with improved outcomes (compliance rates climb to 100%) with the progression of the use of more reliable inspection types. (Reproduced, with permission, from the Virginia Mason Medical Center, 2010.)*

include anesthesia gas hoses that only connect with the correct supply nozzle or defibrillators that will not discharge until synchronized with the ECG, or "electrocardiogram" to prevent initiation of ventricular arrhythmias.

Mistake proofing is recognized as one of the most powerful lean tools because it provides a framework in which we no longer accept that medical mistakes and injuries are inevitable. Mistake proofing provides methods to not only improve systems, but to also perfect them. Once an organization can monitor and correct mistakes through continuous improvement methods, systems will improve and become defect free. The cost (rework, time, harm, poor morale, money) of managing mistakes and defects can be eliminated (**Figure 20-6**).

Organizations striving for 0 defects must cultivate a safe atmosphere in which all levels of staff are empowered to judge the quality of the work performed by both themselves and their coworkers and are encouraged to report concerns. It is necessary for each health care worker to have full license and accountability to be sure that all products of their work are defect free and that mistakes are not passed along downstream.

CONCLUSION

Recognizing that the U.S. health care expenditure per household is nearly double the cost of most other developed countries without comparable health outcomes, it is imperative that health care leaders vigorously pursue innovative management tools that have been shown to provide cost savings and quality improvement. Since 2001, lean principles have become widely used among many health care organizations throughout the United States and Europe, evidenced by the presence of numerous, relevant quality improvement publications, national medical meeting agendas, and lay press articles. While lean methodology has clearly transformed the manufacturing world, it appears that, perhaps health care may be its next major beneficiary.

PRACTICE POINT

- Recognizing that the U.S. health care expenditure per household is nearly double the cost of most other developed countries without comparable health outcomes, it is imperative that health care leaders vigorously pursue innovative management tools that have been shown to provide cost savings and quality improvement.

SUGGESTED READINGS

HealthGrades Sixth Annual Patient Safety in American Hospitals Survey, April, 2009. Pages 1–8.

Kim CS, Spahlinger DA, Kin JM, et al. Lean health care: what can hospitals learn from a world-class automaker? *J Hosp Med.* 2006;1(3):191–199.

Organization for Economic Co-operation and Development: Policy Brief: Economic Survey of the United States, 2008, December 2008, p. 10.

Shingo S. *Zero Quality Control: Source inspection and the Poka-Yoke System.* Tokyo: Japan Management Association; 1985.

Tatikonda L. *Commentary: Better Management Could Reduce Healthcare Costs.* The Oshkosh Northwestern. Oshkosh WI, Oct 27, 2009. http://www.thenorthwestern.com.

Virginia Mason Medical Center Archives. *RPIW The Hospitalists Role.* Seattle WA: Virginia Mason Medical Center; 2003.

Virginia Mason Medical Center Kaizen Promotion Office. *Lean Certification Modules.* Seattle WA: Virginia Mason Institute; 2009.

Womack J, Jones D, Roos D. *The Machine That Changed the World.* New York: Free Press; 1990.

Womack J, Jones D. *Lean Thinking: Banish Waste and Create Wealth in Your Corporation.* New York: Simon & Schuster; 1996.

CHAPTER 21

Teamwork in Leadership and Practice-Based Management

Scot T. Smith, MD
Scott Enderby, DO, SFHM
Robert A. Bessler, MD

INTRODUCTION

Multidisciplinary care refers to the active collaboration between various members in the health care system to deliver optimal care for every hospitalized patient. Successful teamwork is a core competency that can be taught and incorporated into patient care processes. The Association of American Colleges (AAMC), the Accreditation Council for Graduate Medical Education (ACGME), and the Society of Hospital Medicine (SHM) require specific teamwork-related competencies for medical students, residents, and hospitalists. Hospitalists can improve multidisciplinary care of hospitalized patients by demonstrating group dynamic skills, conducting effective multidisciplinary team rounds, evaluating performance, providing feedback, teaching about error and how teamwork and communication can reduce error, and by leading quality improvement initiatives.

The U.S. health care system is a highly organized and complex system. Over the last three decades of the public safety movement there have been landmark studies and published reports about individual and systemic failures that have not only cost lives but wasted billions of U.S. dollars while delivering unsafe care. Although different solutions may be debated, it is clear that the U.S. health care system will need to be redesigned to deliver the highest quality of care possible. Sweeping change requires effective teamwork on every level, hospital networks, hospital, hospitalist service, and direct multidisciplinary patient care.

In general, most physicians have little formal training relating to complex hospital systems or human error and lack insight into their own limitations during conditions of stress, lack of sleep, or conflicting demands. Strong hierarchy, power differentials, lack of clarity requiring specific tasks and roles, and lack of coordination are common teamwork and communication failures in health care. Lessons learned from the aviation industry can be applied to the delivery of hospital care, and hospitalists can take steps to reduce the likelihood of (1) individual error resulting from physiological and psychological limitations of human beings and (2) team errors resulting from failure to act or deviation from established standards. Although it is not possible to eliminate individual error, systems can be designed that reduce the likelihood of error and make hospitals a safer environment for patients. Working in teams and serving as the hub of communication network in the hospital, hospitalists are ideally poised to change the culture of "how we do things around here" by serving as clinical role models and as leaders of patient safety on the multidisciplinary care team. Without effective teamwork and medical leadership, however, these complex systems have been shown to be less effective in producing quality outcomes.

THE MULTIDISCIPLINARY HEALTH CARE TEAM

The hospitalist team is a unit of professionals that directly provides care and so most directly impacts the patient experience and the quality of care. Composition of the team varies, but a team typically may include a hospitalist, consulting physician(s), nurse, case managers or a social worker, and a pharmacist.

Individuals have particular tasks based on their particular specialties, but the hospitalist team depends on each other for situational awareness and goal success strategies. Situational awareness is a common, accurate understanding of the patient's condition, needs, clinical trajectory, and feelings based on the multiple perspectives of team members. The team only obtains situational awareness when these perspectives are communicated within the team. Without the perspectives of team members, no individual—including the hospitalist—truly has situational awareness. Decisions made, orders written, even conversations with patients without the perspectives of others on the team are less likely to promote coordinated, high quality care.

PRACTICE POINT

Limit your blind spots and those of your team

Unless you must, don't deliver care without situational awareness.

Create workflow scenarios that allow multiple team members' perspectives before making decisions, writing orders, and interacting with the patient.

At a minimum, round with the patient's nurse before you see the patient.

Communicate your perspective to the team. The team relies on the hospitalist for clinical perspective. At a minimum ask:

- What problems are being addressed and is each problem getting better or worse?
- What is being done for the patient (tests, evaluation by consultants, interventions, medication changes, etc) and why?
- What does the patient need to be safer?
- What does the patient need to feel better?
- What does the patient need for safe, timely discharge?

Goal success is an optimal patient experience. The team relies on each other to provide best practice care by limiting unnecessary variation in practice, enhancing patient satisfaction with the hospitalization experience, and discharging the patient as safely and as soon as possible. Variability in performance can be reduced by using appropriate protocols, order sets, checklists, and institutional processes to address a patient's problems.

PRACTICE POINT

Limit unnecessary variation in practice

Reliable systems make quality more likely by making the right thing more likely:

- If there isn't clear evidence supporting a particular choice, the team should consistently use institutional therapeutic choices (eg, for antibiotics, VTE prophylaxis, etc)
- Set reliable times for rounds.
- Use institutional order sets.

PRACTICE POINT

Provide care that satisfies the patient

- Improve the patient's perception of your team. Patients often feel that their care team is not coordinated or not talking to each other.
- Specifically, address your coordination with nurses, other physicians, pharmacists, therapists, etc.
- Let patients know that you are aware of and approve of what others on the team are doing.

Limiting the risks associated with prolonged unnecessary hospitalization should be a stated goal of the hospitalist team. In support of that goal, each team member—*as they round on their patients and decide whether to discharge now or not*—must determine whether the benefits of continued hospitalization outweigh the inherent risks of continued hospitalization. Each team member should be encouraged to articulate the rationale for their decision to the rest of the care team.

PRACTICE POINT

Discharge the patient safely and as soon as possible

Discharge the patient safely and as soon as possible. Hospitalization exposes patients to a host of physical and psychological risks; including:

- Blood stream infections
- Respiratory infections
- Urinary infections
- Adverse drug events
- Pressure ulcers
- Falls
- Functional decline
- Anxiety

A hospitalist typically leads the inpatient care team. As the leader, the hospitalist is responsible for goal clarity, role clarity, communication, and team cohesiveness. Effective teamwork requires the willingness of the team members to work toward a shared goal. Goal clarity requires explicitly stating what defines success for the team and a quality outcome for the patient.

- What medical conditions are or are not being treated as an inpatient?
- What is the goal of treatment?
- What is the endpoint of hospitalization?
- What is the reason for each test, intervention, change?

PRACTICE POINT

Be explicit about goals

Write the goal in the patient chart. For example:

- "Chest Pain: The patient has multivessel CAD and demand ischemia. He declines intervention other than medication changes. I am titrating nitrates and beta blockers. My goal for discharge: pain free at rest and while walking slowly in room, tolerating medication without orthostatic symptoms."

Role clarity requires explicitly identifying who will do what on the team.

- Who on the care team is responsible for which aspects of care?
- Who is discussing which issues with the patient?
- Which consultant is managing which problem?
- Who is writing orders for what?

Effective communication requires fostering the sharing of essential information across the hospitalist team. The team leader is responsible for demonstrating techniques that encourage specific teamwork behaviors that ensure that roles are clearly defined, timely and accurate information is shared, and plans are discussed and mutually agreed upon. Effective teamwork can reduce the number of medical errors through improved communication and better coordination of care.

- What method will the team use to communicate; for example: by reading each other's chart notes, by phone, face-to-face
- How often will members communicate; for example: during rounds, only as needed, every afternoon before going home?
- What tone and language will be used to decrease barriers and misunderstandings?

PRACTICE POINT

Structure your communication

Make team communication more reliable by:

- Using checklists
- Setting predictable rounding times
- Using agreed-upon care protocols
- Use structured communication such as SBAR

Situation: the specific problem:
"Mrs. Johnson has a headache and is hypotensive."

Background: the specific history that may relate to the current situation:
"She fell last night and did not have a CT of her head; she does take anticoagulants."

Assessment: the analysis of the problem:
"I believe she has a bleed in her head."

Recommendation/Request: the team member makes a recommendation and request of another:
"Dr. Smith, please see her immediately."

Cohesiveness requires recognition of a shared purpose, defined roles, and task interdependence. As the facilitator of optimal team function, the leader limits disruption and fragmentation of the team that can occur with any dynamic and complex process. This requires active listening and frequent communication with all members of the team, sharing decision-making responsibilities, and proactively providing opportunities for everyone to contribute according to their abilities, including patients and families.

- How do we help each other succeed?
- How do we eliminate what pulls us apart?

TEAM COMMUNICATION WITH PRIMARY CARE PROVIDERS, PATIENTS, AND FAMILIES IS A BIDIRECTIONAL PROCESS

Hospitalists generally define themselves as specialists of the medical care of hospitalized patients. Mistakenly, however, hospitalists may believe that they do not need either the input of the outpatient practitioner(s) or to partner with them. This is another silo mentality that neither fosters high quality care nor patient satisfaction. From a patient perspective, care does not begin with admission and end with discharge, and many patients wish that their practitioners have an ongoing role in their care during hospitalization. Ensuring that primary care providers are involved at various points in the continuum of care is a major quality issue.

Based on experience, we know that the quality of communication from the hospitalist to the community physician is paramount. The inpatient health care team must understand and synthesize outpatient goals into the initial hospital care plan and then proactively communicate with the outpatient team as the hospitalization proceeds. The hospitalist-leader should focus the inpatient team on processes in the transition of patients to other settings, ensure accuracy and thoroughness of documentation, and optimize communication before discharge actually takes place to increase the likelihood that discharge orders are carried out as intended.

The first step in understanding outpatient goals is identifying the leader of outpatient care. This simple act can be challenging. Some patients have established primary care providers; some have multiple specialists; many have no outpatient care providers. The hospitalist team must develop a discharge plan that supports outpatient goals to the greatest extent possible; then communicate that plan to patient's outpatient care team.

PRACTICE POINT

Outpatient goals

On admission ask, actively listen, and communicate key information:

- Talk to the patient. Who is the primary outpatient provider? What are the patient's own goals of care?
- Talk directly to the outpatient team and confirm outpatient goals.
- Talk to nonproviders (eg, family, friends, etc) identified by the patient. What are their goals?

Transitions in care are inherently risky events and effective discharge planning begins on the day of admission. Inadequate preparation can compromise care, contribute to medication errors, and create a sense of discontinuity for the patient and those who provide their longitudinal care. Hospitalists must focus on improving not only the substance of transitions, but also the experience of the transition for patients, their families, and primary care physicians. From day one of hospitalization, communicate with family, nurses, primary care providers, and others who will provide longitudinal care of the patient during and after hospitalization. The hospitalist should determine with the receiving community physician how communication should take place, telephone, e-mail, page, or fax; how often; by whom; what communication should occur; and determine the level of involvement of the outpatient practitioner in discharge decisions rather than simply relying only on discharge summaries to transfer information.

Importantly, the hospitalist-led team must also communicate to patients and their families in clear next steps with regard to their continued diagnosis, treatment, timing of anticipated discharge, and care beyond the hospital. To do this effectively, the team should have a shared understanding about all of the issues impacting the patient, diagnostic findings, and management plans. The patient's primary care nurse should not be overlooked as a key communicator of information to patients and families. The team leader should include the patient's nurse in rounds and update that nurse regularly. Likewise, patients and families are important members of the care team and should be informed and actually have an opportunity to ask questions and give consent to treatment. Patients should not receive conflicting information from doctors, nurses, consultants, and other members of the team. The information provided should be structured in straightforward simple language in accordance with the patient's literacy, utilizing interpreters when English is not the primary language.

Patient satisfaction surveys provide information that can be used to improve team performance. Sound Physicians, for example, surveys the patients of our primary care providers following discharge. In one survey conducted through the Sound Physicians' patient call center, we learned that nearly 9% of patients indicated inadequate communication from the hospitalist was a primary source of dissatisfaction. They conveyed that doctors did not always explain information in a way they could understand and others felt their physician did not listen to them. This type of direct feedback is the basis we use in educating hospitalists on the importance of providing patient-centered care. It also enables leaders to mentor team members and to set expectations for the desired performance, educating the service on how to effectively provide patient-centered care, and mentoring hospitalists who have lower scores.

PRACTICE POINT

Consistent, understandable patient education

On admission identify the appropriate family contact and make sure to update him or her daily as well as the patient, if appropriate, of:

- Provisional diagnosis
- Areas of uncertainty
- Planned diagnostic workup, consultation
- Management plan
- Anticipated date and time of discharge and to what setting
- What to do if something goes wrong and patient does not respond as anticipated

Answer any questions and confirm that the patient's family contact understands what you have said.

Daily make sure multidisciplinary team rounds include a review of:

- Provisional diagnosis
- Planned diagnostic work
- Management plan
- Anticipated date and time of discharge and to what setting
- What to do if something goes wrong

Answer any questions and confirm understanding and consensus.

Continuously update the primary nurse and other members of the team when:

- There is a change in plan
- There are results of a diagnostic workup
- There are new diagnoses
- There is a new complication

Listen to concerns and address them.

On the day of discharge summarize prior conversations:

- Medication changes and the reasons for changes
- New medications
- Diagnostic studies, the results and pending results
- Consultations performed during hospitalization and specific ongoing recommendations post discharge
- Who to contact if there is an unexpected problem

Provide written materials to complement verbal instructions that the patient should bring with him to the PCP's office.

THE ROLE OF THE DIRECTOR OF A HOSPITALIST SERVICE

Typically a hospitalist team is led by a chief hospitalist or medical director who provides daily clinical management of the team. In this role, the chief hospitalist is also the liaison to the hospital administration. The chief hospitalist has responsibility for the performance of the hospitalist service, provides administrative support for the service, develops schedules for hospitalists that reflect manageable workloads, and typically serves on hospital committees including pharmacy and therapy, critical care, safety, utilization review, The Joint Commission, Hospital Consumer Assessment of Health care Providers and Systems (HCAHPS) Survey, and compliance review boards.

The comprehensive hospitalist service is a team of physicians, midlevel professionals, and business managers. Depending on the institution, the hospitalist team may be employed by the hospital or part of an independent group of hospitalists, a member of a large multispecialty group practice, or affiliated with a larger regional or nationally-based hospitalist organization. A small percentage of hospitalists are *locum tenens* physicians who fill an important temporary role when teams require assistance.

Hospitalist leaders have the opportunity to set clinically appropriate and standardized care. As a result, teams of hospitalists have the ability to improve the quality of care of a larger group of hospitalized patients by delivering measurable and consistent quality care. To be effective, hospitalist leaders should

- ***Set clear expectations.*** Effective leaders provide teams with clear performance expectations. When the team understands how the leader measures excellence, they know what is expected of them.

  In addition to their clinical responsibilities, all hospitalists should understand the hospital's key initiatives and the areas in which the hospitalist team is going to be accountable to key hospital administrators including the chief executive officer (CEO), chief financial officer (CFO), chief medical officer (CMO), and chief nursing officer (CNO). Using metrics provides an objective method for communicating consistently on team performance measured against team goals. Hospitalist leaders should focus their hospitalist teams on delivering measurable quality improvements by reducing unnecessary practice variability.
- ***Delegate responsibility.*** The hospitalist leader delegates responsibilities to team members and establishes open lines of communication. When teams have a clear understanding of expectations, there is no room for ambiguity. Establishing open and honest communication encourages teamwork and collaboration. Frequently, hospitalist programs are carried on the back of the medical director. This model is destined to fail as it usually is the result of a lack of physician engagement with other physicians. Even with limited clinical responsibilities, the medical director must have superb delegation skills to reduce the potential for burnout.
- ***Empower team members.*** Excellent leaders empower hospitalist team members to get involved. When teams feel supported to make decisions they become more effective as a group. This also helps to develop future leaders by providing them the opportunity to learn decision-making skills within the framework of the team.
- ***Deal with conflicts swiftly.*** Effective leaders must be capable of dealing with conflicts immediately and removing roadblocks that can impair the effectiveness of the team.
- ***Ensure resources are available.*** Leaders ensure their teams have the necessary resources to do their work effectively. In Hospital Medicine the leader has to compete with the other hospital priorities and resources. The successful leader can navigate competing priorities without the emotion that often overtakes individual members of the team in the desire to help change a process.
- ***Recognize the impact of workload on quality.*** When the hospitalist workload is based on manageable encounters, hospitalists are more apt to deliver very consistent, high quality care. There is no national body of evidence that supports the ideal workload. The right workload depends on a myriad of factors including the following:
  - Does the physician already know the patients on his or her rounding list? How many new patients are there?
  - What kind of support staff is available to help the physicians?
  - What administrative duties does the physician have during the work day? Is there specialty backup coverage?
  - Does the physician have to do the procedures?
  - How efficiently does the hospital run?

We believe for the average hospitalist starting at 7:00 AM, with a 12–15 patient case load, and admitting or consulting on a few more during the day is the range in which a physician can give great care but can also be refreshed after a good night's rest to come to work again the next day. This workload enables the hospitalist to be an effective manager of the patients' care and communicate with the various stakeholders in a nonhurried and thorough fashion, improving the accuracy and satisfaction in the communication experience.

- ***Commit to develop team members.*** Hospitalist leaders provide professional development opportunities for their team members. Effective teams benefit from growth and advancement and from group incentives that drive performance excellence. Most physicians lack formal leadership training. Providing didactic skill development opportunities, access to professional coaches, and an ongoing support network are keys to successful professional growth for all team members, including the leader.
- ***Embrace diversity of teams.*** Today's hospitalist teams are diverse and require leaders who recognize and embrace different points of view. With a variety of cultural backgrounds, skill levels, training and team roles, it is important that the leader promote acceptance and openness when dealing with different situations.
- ***Measure and recognize performance.*** Measuring performance and providing objective feedback to team members drives continuous improvement. Effective leaders provide training and coaching to team members. They also find ways to recognize and reward performance excellence and improvement for both the team and individuals. Most physicians feel they have "arrived" after medical school and residency. Most are not used to a performance evaluation as part of being on a physician team. Tools, such as the 360 degree evaluation, provide feedback on specific areas that will make the individual and the team more effective. The hospitalist should be presented the metrics that matter to the patient and to the institution consistently.
- ***Recruit the right people to your hospitalist service.*** Recruiting the right team is another important factor in developing an effective hospitalist team. Taking time to evaluate candidates for both clinical and technical competency, as well as chemistry with the team, is critical for ensuring the success of effective teams. Evaluate the candidate's communication style and skills of the rest of the team. A well orchestrated interview agenda allows all team members to have time to interact with the candidate. It is important to have a cross-section of data points to assess compatibility of the candidate with the existing team. Finally, be sure to reach out to individuals who worked with the candidate previously to get a comprehensive picture of the candidate you are considering.
- ***Solicit feedback from members of the team to improve operations.*** A strong sense of team has been associated with higher retention.

  Physicians have many allegiances, including their outside interests and families, their hospital, their medical group, and their team. If a team is functioning well, members want to stay and make the team stronger.

With the average age of the hospitalist at 37 years of age and the average age of the hospitalist leader at 41 years of age, there is a significant need to develop leaders and not wait for leaders to evolve. A respected and effective hospitalist leader is a prerequisite to achieving a highly functioning hospitalist team. The field of Hospital Medicine has recognized this need and the Society of Hospital Medicine (SHM) recently established the Fellow in Hospital Medicine (FHM and SFHM) recognition. While specific traits are identified in the FHM and SFHM charters, they are typically skills acquired by hospitalists who have benefited from mentors or coaches and/or completed additional training. New in 2011 SHM will also provide certification in leadership in Hospital Medicine (leadership fundamentals and advanced leadership).

The effective hospitalist leader must inherently be a good manager. Managing a team includes allocating resources skillfully, meeting deadlines and obligations, and serving multiple stakeholders. It also requires effective communication, conflict management, and deft delegation ability. Masters-degree-level work, such as an Masters in Medical Management (MMM), Masters in Business Administration (MBA) or Masters in Health care Administration (MHA) can help hone these skills. Alternatively, SHM advanced leadership courses offer strategies and tools for personal leadership excellence and for developing a winning team and strengthening your organization.

ALIGNING HOSPITALISTS WITH HOSPITAL GOALS

The successful hospitalist service has teams assigned to drive performance that are aligned with hospitals goals and report on the results to hospital administration regularly. The most common hospital initiatives are in the areas of quality, operations, satisfaction, and financial performance. The hospitalist teams that will survive and thrive in the next decade will master the role of managing effective hospitalist teams that drive real value and measurable results for their hospital partner.

In order to improve outcomes, it is necessary for hospitalists to have clear and functional processes that incorporate utilization of best practices. They should be encouraged to identify ways to reduce variables in patient care, and importantly, they must be good stewards of their time and resources and focus on what matters most. Effective prioritization and time management are critical for driving improvements in all outcomes, whether clinical, satisfaction, or financial performance.

Each hospitalist service should determine benchmark performance expectations for their hospitalist team around admissions, discharge planning, processes for signing off care between shifts, and creating and managing care pathways. While there is a plethora of data sets that can be measured to drive performance, it is essential for hospitalist service teams to identify metrics that can be used to drive performance improvement and consistently measure them. Whether measuring continuous quality improvements, satisfaction, or efficiency, teams cannot improve unless their performance is measured. Once performance is measured, it can be managed. Performance measurements also can be used to provide reward systems to reinforce the behaviors.

The Hospital Consumer Assessment of Health care Providers and Systems (HCAHPS) survey developed by the Centers for Medicare and Medicaid Services (CMS) asks questions directed largely at the patient's experiences in the hospital. The survey probes efficacy of the health care team's communication with patients, instruction about medications, quality of nursing services, adequacy of planning for discharge, and pain management. Responses are reported in six composite domains, largely focused on the effectiveness of communication. The HCAHPS score is meant to reflect the patient's perception of the quality of the care they received in the hands of the doctors, nurses, and by the hospital. The following three broad goals shaped the HCAHPS instrument to produce data about patients' perspectives of care that allow:

1. objective and meaningful comparisons of hospitals on topics that are important to consumers,
2. the creation of new incentives for hospitals to improve quality of care, and

3. accountability in health care by increasing the transparency of the quality of hospital care provided in return for the public investment.

The average scores reflect the entire hospital experience, but the hospitalist team can significantly influence HCAHPS survey results and improve patient satisfaction scores. The 2008 *New England Journal of Medicine* article, "Patients' Perception of Hospital Care in the United States," by Ashish K. Jha, et al, concludes that the current level of communication and care leaves plenty of room for improvement. In this study, 63% of hospitals received a rating of 9 or 10 from patients and 89% scored their experience at 7 or better. The quality of hospital care continues to be highly variable, signaling an opportunity for the hospitalist team to take the leadership role in driving quality improvements and ratings that reach 90% or more consistently.

While the objectives of the CMS' HCAHPS instrument were carefully considered and the tool skillfully designed, the results pose challenges in interpretation. Many consider the HCAHPS data to be flawed due to the multivariate nature of the patient's course of care. Nevertheless, tracking and communicating data on clinical performance, however flawed, is a starting point and has previously prompted improvements in the quality of clinical care in hospitals.

When the hospitalist actively participates in the patient's transition of care from hospital to home or to a skilled nursing facility, data shows that satisfaction scores skyrocket. In addition, typically the family, case manager, nursing staff, and primary care physicians' satisfaction scores also increase. There also should be expectations set for hospitalist relations and assessments with critical partners including emergency physicians, primary care providers, and specialists. These relationships must be monitored on a regular basis to ensure cooperative integration is being achieved.

With bundling of payments and more scrutiny on readmissions, hospitals may prioritize resources to reduce readmission rates. Hospitalist leaders can develop communication standards to reduce practice variation, identify patients at increased risk for readmission, and work with other hospital leaders to redesign the systems in place that do not promote safe transitions. For example, the University of Pennsylvania attributed a drop in readmissions from a high of 15% to 5% in the short period from the fall of 2008 to February 2009 to implementation of tools from the SHM Project BOOST, including the "7P" checklist. The checklist tool simplifies the major modifiable risk factors to consider for readmission to the hospital. There are seven risk factors tied to suggested interventions for problem medications, principal diagnosis, depression, polypharmacy, poor health literacy, patient support, and prior hospitalization.

PROJECT BOOST

Project BOOST (Better Outcomes for Older adults through Safe Transitions) is one effort to improve the care of older patients as they transition from inpatient care to an outpatient facility or home. The SHM, working with Blue Cross and Blue Shield of Michigan and the University of Michigan, is launching a multisite implementation of the program seeking to:

- Avoid unplanned or preventable hospital readmissions and emergency department visits within 30 days of hospital discharge.
- Improve facility patient satisfaction scores.
- Improve patient satisfaction associated with discharge.
- Improve communication between inpatient and outpatient providers.
- Improve patient and family education about disease management and risk issues.
- Identify patients at high risk and mitigate that risk with multidisciplinary risk mitigation tools and strategies; including
    - *Discharge coordination/communication with follow-on providers*
    - *Patient and caretaker disease and disease management education including a "teach-back" strategy to ensure comprehension*
    - *Medication reconciliation including a review of interactions between discharge medications and previously prescribed medications interactions*
    - *Essential team members include nurses, case managers, patient educators, hospitalists*

To be effective, Project BOOST requires multidisciplinary teamwork, coordinating seamless transitions of care by utilizing the combined expertise of team members. This has significant economic and quality implications.

Hospitalist teams must be integrated into these processes. When the team is evaluated as part of the process, individual outliers are identified and receive the necessary training and mentoring to improve individual performance. Equally as important, the hospitalist can help improve institutional performance. High performance teams are indispensable to high performance hospitals. Examples include the following:

- ***A High-Functioning Team Becomes the Lifeblood of the Hospital.*** Hospitalist who improve the quality of the hospital, improve the quality of patient care. Physicians who work in such hospitals are involved in everything from the dietary needs of patients, to the workflow, to access to CT results 24 hours per day. Many hospital CEOs cannot imagine life without a hospitalist team helping to carry their hospital forward.
- ***An Effective Team Builds the Brand of the Hospital.*** An engaged and committed team is essential in building the hospital's brand. By reaching out to community providers, improving referrals, and making surgeons want to practice at their hospital the hospitalist contributes significantly to the overall brand value of the hospital in the community. It is often the hospitalist who the family and patient see more than specialists or other hospital staff. It is incumbent on the hospitalist to ensure that the hospital's success is largely dependent on the hospitalist and his or her interaction with others.
- ***Employing a Service-Focused Mindset.*** Hospitalists are one of the most visible groups in the hospital. The team that is service-oriented and prioritizes quality patient care and communication high on the list will be a sought-after change agent in the hospital. The hospitalist team that can demonstrate effective communications and satisfaction as well as a commitment to patient education is an invaluable resource to the hospital.

CONCLUSION

By virtue of their presence, hospitalist teams have changed the system of health care delivery in the United States. Hospital Medicine is now a major cost center in the U.S. health care system. Although the variety of impending solutions to remedy our nation's health care ills range from insurance reform to health care IT solutions, one common important resource has emerged, namely, the active leadership of hospitalists engaged to design and implement sweeping improvements in the quality, satisfaction, and efficiency of care delivered for hospitalized patients. Today, hospitalist teams play a more significant role in recognizing the needs of patients and their families and have developed ways to demonstrate accountability. Hospitalists impact the majority of clinical decisions made on behalf of hospitalized patients and therefore directly determine how medical resources are utilized and drive health outcomes and costs on medical care collectively.

SUGGESTED READINGS

Bohmer R. *Designing Care: Aligning the Nature and Management of Health Care*. Boston, MA: Harvard Business Review Press. 2009.

Goleman D. What Makes a Leader? *Harvard Business Review*. 2004: 43–52.

Jha A, Orav J, Zheng J, et al. Patients' Perception of Hospital Care in the United States. *N Engl J Med*. 2008;359:1921–1931.

Khatri N, Baveja A, Boren SA, Mammo A. Medical Errors and Quality of Care: From Control to Commitment. *California Management Review*. 2006:115–141.

Lee TH, Mongan JJ. *Chaos and Organization in Health Care*. Cambridge, MA. MIT Press; 2009.

Lee TH. Turning Doctors into Leaders. *Harvard Business Review*. 2010: 50–58.

Sehgal NL, Green A, Arpana R, Vidyarthi, Blegen M, Wachter R. Patient whiteboards as a communication tool in the hospital setting: A Survey of practices and recommendations. *Journal of Hospital Medicine*. 2010:(5).

CHAPTER 22

Patient Centered Care

Kenneth E. Sands, MD, MPH

INTRODUCTION

Patient centeredness is increasingly referenced as a core value in the provision of care and the concept of patient-centered care is moving from innovation to expectation and in some cases, even regulation. But what exactly does it mean to be providing patient-centered care, and how does one achieve this, at either the individual or institutional level? This chapter explores the term *patient centered*, and current thinking about how to strengthen the partnership between patients and providers in the delivery of care. Throughout, emphasis is given to those innovations most relevant to the hospitalized patient.

DEFINING PATIENT-CENTERED CARE

While the term *patient centeredness* now appears commonly in both medical literature and lay media, one may encounter a variety of definitions for this phrase. Perhaps the most "official" definition is the one proposed by the Institute of Medicine (IOM) in the landmark 2001 document *Crossing the Quality Chasm*, which describes patient centeredness as "providing care that is respectful of and responsive to individual patient preferences, needs, and values, and ensuring that patient values guide all clinical decisions."[1] The IOM goes on to describe patient centeredness as one of the six key "aims for improvement" for quality of care. As such it is presented as an intrinsic value, fundamental and irrefutable, as opposed to a system property with a known association with better outcomes. The concept has been advanced in the form of slogans such as "Nothing about me without me" or "Every patient is the only patient." Overlapping terms appear in both lay literature and medical literature, including *patient partnering* and *family-centered care*. In this chapter the term "patient centered" will be used to encompass the general concept of making care delivery more responsive to the needs and wishes of the individual patient and his or her family.

The construct presumes that care delivery under current models is not adequately patient centered. The IOM "Chasm" report conceptualizes the health care delivery system as in evolution from a clinician-centric, poorly coordinated and nonevidence-based model to a patient-centric, integrated system that consistently applies scientifically supported interventions. In early stage clinician-centric models, the patient plays a passive role as decisions regarding choice, timing, and settings of care delivery are the exclusive domain of the providers, and those same providers decide what information reaches the patient. Stories abound in lay and medical literature of patients feeling at the mercy of the medical system, unable to exert control over their own care. However, it is hard to find a quantitative assessment of the current state of patient centeredness (or lack thereof) in the U.S. health care system. Some insights can be gleaned from national results of the Hospital Consumer Assessment of Health Care Providers and Systems (HCAHPS) inpatient survey distributed by the Centers for Medicare and Medicaid Services (CMS), in which more than a quarter of patients report "never" receiving communication about new medications and their side effects, and more than 15% give the lowest possible score to questions about the responsiveness of hospital staff (composite scores, 2007 data).

The IOM describes the fully evolved stage of organizational development as the patient and family being part of the health care team with full access to information and the ability to exercise as much control over care as desired. What specific actions can an institution take to advance toward this model? These will be discussed below, divided into three key system properties: (1) free flow of information, (2) responsiveness to individual patient needs, and (3) patient participation in system design.

FREE FLOW OF INFORMATION

Patients are not truly partners in their own care if information, either about themselves or the care they are receiving, is only selectively available. The need for full transparency is represented as two "rules for redesign" as stated by the IOM:

- Knowledge is shared and information flows freely.
- Transparency is necessary.

The first rule recognizes that patients should have the ability to receive complete and understandable information about their condition, in real time. The second rule establishes that patients are entitled to information about the care itself, including the performance of the health care system and its providers, as well as the approach to care and its justification. While these concepts may seem self-evident, the health care system traditionally has not been configured in alignment with these rules. Prior to passage of The Health Insurance Privacy and Portability act (HIPPA), exchange of medical documentation required that a patient obtain a subpoena. Today, care still remains far from transparent: published reports suggest the majority of hospitalized patients cannot even identify the physician in charge of their care, let alone the details of the care plan.

PRACTICE POINT

- Patients should have the ability to receive complete and understandable information about their condition, in real time. Patients are entitled to information about the care itself, including the performance of the health care system and its providers, as well as the approach to care and its justification.

In the interest of better information exchange with patients, innovations are appearing. Some of these innovations change long-standing traditions of care delivery as currently practiced.

Open communication of the plan of care

For the typical hospital inpatient, the formal mechanisms for discussing, developing, and implementing the plan occur without patient involvement. Communication of the plan of care is a separate responsibility of the physician, occurring most often as an unstructured verbal communication. Thus there is no system that guarantees that the patient understands the plan, or has had the chance to ask questions. However, new approaches that provide structure to these exchanges, and thus more reliable sharing of information, are appearing in the interest of both patient centeredness and patient safety. For example, the Veterans Health Administration has introduced "The Daily Plan," a structured document containing information such as medications, scheduled procedures, and diet, reviewed with the patient each day of his or her hospitalization. The expectation is that The Daily Plan will improve provider-patient information exchange in both directions, provide an opportunity for patients to ask questions and share concerns, and identify problems that might cause risks to safety. Early reported experience shows that the large majority of patients receiving such a plan perceive a better understanding of their hospitalization, a better ability to ask questions, and a higher level of comfort with their hospital stay. Similar positive findings have been seen by introducing structured patient involvement with hospital discharge planning. A key element of these new models is some mechanism for "closed-loop communication," meaning there is verification that the communication has been received, understood, and any remaining questions have been answered.

PRACTICE POINT

- For the typical hospital inpatient, the formal mechanisms for discussing, developing, and implementing the plan occur without patient involvement. Verbal communication of the plan of care as a separate responsibility of the physician does not guarantee that the patient understands the plan, or has had the chance to ask questions. Approaches that provide structure to these exchanges, and thus more reliable sharing of information, are in the interest of both patient centeredness and patient safety.

Several hospitals have actually embedded patient communication into the work model by adapting bedside "rounds" to include the patient and/or family member. In a typical format, the patient and/or family member is oriented to the process of rounds and is given the option to participate. On rounds, the patient/family member is introduced to the members of the team, hears the presentation of the clinical situation, and is invited to participate in developing the plan. Teaching, including discussion of the condition and demonstration of physical findings, occurs with the patient's permission. For patients, such programs have been associated with higher satisfaction, better clinical outcomes, and shorter lengths of stay. Health care workers, in turn, have reported higher satisfaction with work and with the quality of teaching.

Disclosure and apology in setting of adverse events

Flow of information should not stop if care does not go as planned. Patients who experience an adverse event are ethically entitled to receive information about that event, and respond favorably to "I'm sorry" in those situations in which apology is indeed appropriate. For decades, conventional wisdom held that full disclosure and apology in association with adverse events would increase risk of litigation, and clinicians were thus typically coached to provide the patient as little information as possible in the wake of an adverse event. The reality seems to be quite the opposite: interviews with patients pursuing a lawsuit frequently cite a failure to receive open and honest communication as a factor in their decision to sue. Encouragingly, several institutions that have pursued aggressive programs in disclosure, apology (when there is culpability), and early settlement have witnessed a coincident decrease in malpractice expense.

Establishing a best practice for disclosure and apology requires that an institution establish an unambiguous position on the topic and communicate that position to the workforce. Mechanisms must be put in place to educate and support clinicians in the process of disclosure and apology. For any given clinician, personal involvement in disclosing error to a patient will be a rare event, so systems for "just-in-time" support and training must be available. Many institutions address this by creating a resource group with specific interest and training in best practices for disclosure and apology. Physicians, nurses, social workers, and patient safety professionals could all potentially serve in such a role. In the setting of an adverse event, the expert resource can support the clinicians involved and help determine the best timing, setting, and participants for communicating the event.

PRACTICE POINT

- Establishing the best practice for disclosure and apology when care does not go as planned requires that an institution establish an unambiguous position on the topic, and communicate that position to the workforce. Mechanisms must be put in place to educate and support clinicians in the process of disclosure and apology.

Access to medical documentation

Medical documentation has traditionally been the purview of the clinicians and not the patient. The passage of HIPPA in 1996 established that patients must be permitted to review and amend their medical records, but access to the record is still largely based on an exception process, the record being provided when there is an active request by the patient, which in practice occurs rarely. On the other hand, surveys show that when given the option to view the clinical record, the large majority of patients will accept. Many institutions are responding with systems that allow patients to directly access elements of clinical documentation electronically, but this is often limited to objective content such as problem lists, medication lists, and test results. Ready access to clinician documentation has been more controversial, although a formal, multi-institutional trial of active sharing of physician outpatient notes is underway as of this writing. The clinical impact of more open access to documentation has been hard to quantify. Increased patient confusion and anxiety, often cited in the past as reasons for not sharing information, appears to occur relatively rarely. At the same time, a clear benefit in terms of patient satisfaction or clinical outcomes has been hard to demonstrate in a controlled fashion. Patients identify factual errors in the record quite often, but whether these translate into actual changes in clinical care has not been determined. Such systems need to be designed to maintain appropriate levels of security, privacy, and restriction of access.

Access to information on clinical performance

There is a slow but undeniable trend toward greater sharing of information on clinical performance with the lay community. Health care institutions have been criticized for resisting this trend on the basis that clinical performance data is too difficult to correctly interpret, cannot be adequately risk adjusted, and/or will perversely impact clinician behavior. Thus, much of the initial effort to make performance data public has been involuntary, driven by regulators, creditors, or insurers, each of which may have its own unique requirements for public reporting of clinical performance. As a result, clinical information available in the public domain can vary dramatically from state to state. At a federal level, the patient can find a growing list of measures of hospital performance disseminated by the Centers for Medicare and Medicaid Services (CMS) via its Web site, www.hospitalcompare.hhs.gov.

Simultaneously, many institutions are now choosing to voluntarily share information on clinical performance (**Figure 22-1**). This trend is most readily apparent as a component of hospital Web sites, but some hospitals are also choosing to share information in the form of mailings or posted material within the facility (illustration). Reasons to pursue this strategy likely vary by institution, but might include (1) the ability to provide context and explanation to information already being shared elsewhere, (2) the ability to determine and expand the portfolio of information being shared, (3) the belief that sharing clinical performance information is a good business strategy, and (4) the belief that sharing clinical

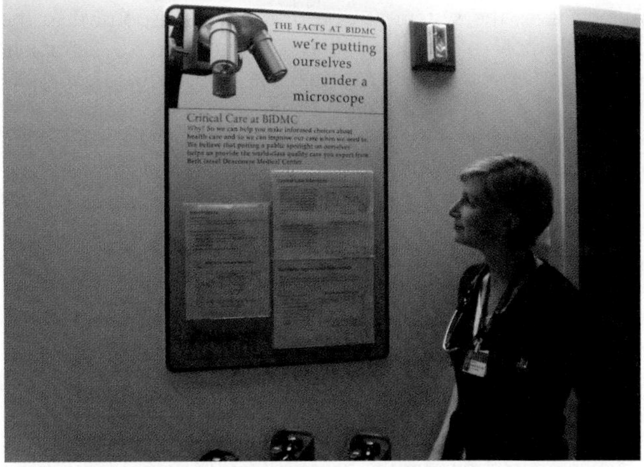

Figure 22-1 *Public display of performance on several clinical outcomes outside of an intensive care unit. The format allows for the information to be continuously updated. (Courtesy of Beth Israel Deaconess Medical Center, Boston, MA.)*

performance information is consistent with institutional values. The result is that a current survey of hospital Web sites will demonstrate a broad range of approaches to transparency; some provide a great breadth of information on performance, others almost none. Some hospitals provide metrics with a minimal amount of explanatory information, while others appear to go to great lengths to make the information accessible and available to a lay audience.

Little data is available regarding the degree to which patients use clinical performance data to make decisions regarding their own care. The data that does exist suggests that public opinion strongly favors the concept of public sharing of performance data, despite the fact that few consumers, at least currently, are directing their care on the basis of objective, publicly reported metrics.

RESPONSIVE TO INDIVIDUAL PATIENT NEEDS

Assuming the first ideal has been met and there is complete transparency and flow of information, how much control does the patient have over the plan of care or the ways in which that plan is carried out? Systems of care delivery have largely evolved in response to the needs of providers and the design of the payment system. The patient thus encounters a care delivery model that is confusing to navigate, inconvenient, lacking in capacity to respond to individual needs, and severely fractured between care delivery settings. A system that is truly responsive to the individual patient requires the capability to fully elicit individual patient preferences and then the capacity to customize care in response to those preferences.

PRACTICE POINT

- A system that is truly responsive to the individual patient requires the capability to fully elicit individual patient preferences, and then the capacity to customize care in response to those preferences. The concept of patient centeredness extends beyond the approach to the individual patient, and includes as a tenet that patients have a voice in the design of the care delivery system itself.

Appreciative of individual needs

At one level, the system can be made more responsive to the patient simply by ensuring that clinicians have a complete understanding of individual preferences. Unfortunately, despite the central role of interpersonal communication in almost every aspect of care delivery, evidence suggests that clinician-patient communication is often imperfect, and communication skills have only recently been recognized as a core competency by entities such as the Accreditation Council for Graduate Medical Education and The National Board of Medical Examiners. Training can in fact lead to improved communication skills, allowing the clinician to better identify the unique needs and values of the patient, while simultaneously improving patient understanding of his/her clinical situation.

Since needs and preferences may be linked to individual ethnic and religious traditions, patient centeredness requires that providers have an appreciation for this context. Cultural competence refers to the provider's ability to bridge cultural differences in the provider-patient relationship, through understanding and respect of the patient's beliefs and awareness of one's own biases. Cultural competency is most often discussed as a strategy for decreasing the persistent inferior clinical outcomes among minority populations (a topic beyond the scope of this chapter), but it is equally clear that cultural competency will also promote patient centeredness. Like communication, cultural competency is teachable; training programs in cultural competency are on the increase, and in fact are mandated for physicians in many states. In addition, institutions with significant numbers of patients from specific ethnic communities should look for ways to partner with that community to develop a shared appreciation of specific needs and preferences and developing appropriate institutional supports.

Capacity to respond to individual needs

Full appreciation of the unique needs of the individual is only meaningful if the system can customize care in response to those needs. This requires ceding some control to the patient. For example, many hospitals are eliminating restrictions on visiting hours in favor of open access for the patient's family. Family presence during invasive procedures and resuscitation events is now endorsed by several professional societies.

Programs that allow patients or family members to activate rapid response teams are now well described. Sometimes called "Condition H" or "Code Help," the concept was initially advanced for the pediatric setting, where serious adverse events have occurred in the presence of a concerned parent who was unable to bring immediate assistance to the bedside. The same principal has now been extended to the adult setting. A typical response team will include both a physician and nurse, and in some models may include critical care specialists and/or patient representatives. It is not unusual for clinicians to initially express resistance to the concept, citing concerns that patients and family members will overuse "code help" for inappropriate, nonurgent issues. However, the experience of institutions that have implemented response teams is that the option is used prudently and allows earlier interception of potential adverse events as well as other important issues such as inadequate pain control or communication problems. Successful implementation of a "code help" program requires patient and family education of the system and its purpose, a well structured activation mechanism, and a predefined set of individual responders. Protocols that define the mechanism for recording the incident and debriefing with the patient and family should also be established.

Incorporation of individual needs takes on a special significance when the patient has a "preference-sensitive" condition, meaning a condition with multiple potential approaches to management. Chronic back pain, prostate cancer, breast cancer, and depression are all examples of conditions in which patient preference might be the final determinant of the best care plan. Such situations call for informed, shared decision making, a term for the process of educating the patient about treatment options, associated outcomes and potential complications, and incorporating the expressed values of the patient into the final treatment plan. Informed shared decision making can be supported by decision aids, that is, structured materials such as a videotape or printed algorithm that help to illustrate treatment options and associated risks and benefits.

INVOLVING PATIENTS IN SYSTEM DESIGN

The concept of patient centeredness extends beyond the approach to the individual patient, and includes as a tenet that patients have a voice in the design of the care delivery system itself. In what might be described as a traditional model for hospital administration, the patient is seen as a consumer of services, without any formal role as part of hospital operations. The patient thus has little or no ability to advocate for system change, and the institution lacks the voice of the patient in the design of care processes. This is beginning to change as hospitals move to involve patients in operational activities, either by creating positions for patients or family members on existing hospital committees and/or creating a separate Patient/Family Advisory Council (PFAC) function. Indeed the presence of a PFAC is now mandated by regulation in some states. An institution may have a single PFAC or multiple PFACs based on a desire for specific patient involvement in discreet service lines.

A role for patient/family participation has been described for a myriad of institutional processes, including strategic planning, facility redesign, research oversight, ethics, care coordination, education, finance, credentialing, leadership search, information technology, process improvement, patient safety, service excellence, and personnel practices. Whether the plan is to involve patients on existing operational committees and/or to create one or more PFACs, a successful model for patient involvement in the design of care should begin with a vision and a plan that addresses a number of key issues:

- What are the goals for including a patient in this design process?
- What is the organizational model for patient involvement?
- What criteria will be used for selecting patient participants?
- What are the expectations of the patient participants?
- What is the selection process?
- How long is a term of service and are there term limits?
- What is the orientation process for patients to a hospital administrative role?
- What are the expectations for attendance?
- What criteria will be used to assess the performance of patient participants, and/or the PFAC committee itself?

An up-front strategy to define these issues is likely to be rewarded with a smooth-functioning program for patient involvement in hospital operations.

SUGGESTED READINGS

Berwick DM. What "patient-centered" should mean: confessions of an extremist. *Health Affairs.* 2009;28(4):w555–w565.

Gerteis M, Edgman-Levitan S, Daley J, et al. *Through the Patient's Eyes: Picker/Commonwealth Program for Patient Centered Care.* San Francisco, CA: Jossey-Bass; 1993.

Johnson B, Abraham M, Conway J, et al. *Partnering with Patients and Families to Design a Patient- and Family-Centered Health Care System: Recommendations and Promising Practices*. Bethesda, MD: Institute for Family-Centered Care and the Institute for Healthcare Improvement; 2008.

Lazare A. Apology in medical practice: an emerging clinical skill. *Journal of the American Medical Association*. 2006;296: 1401–1404.

Peto R, Tenerowicz LM, Benjamin EM, et al. One system's journey in creating a disclosure and apology program. *Joint Commission Journal on Quality and Patient Safety*. 2009;35(10): 487–492.

Teutsch C. Patient-doctor communication. *Med Clin N Am*. 2003;87: 1115–1145.

REFERENCE

1. Institute of Medicine. *Crossing the Quality Chasm: a New Health System for the Twenty-first Century*. Washington, D.C.: National Academy Press; 2001.

CHAPTER 23

Finance in the Health Care Sector

Farshid Kazi, MD, MPH
Alpesh Amin, MD, MBA

INTRODUCTION

Hospital spending accounts for a disproportionate portion of health care expenditures in the United States and hospitals will continue to be under constant pressure to improve efficiency with increasingly limited resources. Understanding the flow of money in health care has become an integral part of medicine. As health care reform reshapes a competitive environment, hospitals, hospitalist leaders, and practitioners need a common language and framework as they navigate hospital operations, set budgets for their employees, and achieve financial success. Hospitalists and hospitalist medical directors must be fiscally savvy in order to survive the challenging world of health care. Although a hospital administrator carries out much of the detailed analysis, the hospitalist medical director is responsible for the operation of the practice, which includes managing the Hospital Medicine's group budget. Beyond billing, the director should be informed of the status of all other revenue resources, including capitated payments, stipends, and other monies.

This chapter will introduce readers to commonly used hospital financial terminology and theory so that they may more effectively communicate with hospital administrators and develop a strategic plan for their practices. This chapter will present the topic of finance in health care in three sections: (1) health care payment schedules, (2) health insurance models, and (3) health care finance. Although the technical aspects of finance can be daunting, this chapter will provide a general overview for understanding reimbursement methods, insurance company models, and revenue maximization techniques.

HEALTH CARE PAYMENT SCHEDULES

How Medicare, Medicaid, and insurance companies reimburse hospitals influence cash flow, income statements, and budgeting. Below are some of the generally accepted payment methods in the health care industry.

CAPITATION

Under this type of payment system a health care provider is paid a fixed payment per member covered for a fixed period of time regardless of service utilization. For example, insurance company X will pay Dr. A $200 per member enrolled in insurance company X per month regardless of whether Dr. A sees the patient or not. In this payment method, the doctor must cover all costs associated with delivering health care in his office or health care setting including laboratory tests, imaging, and office visits. This payer schedule effectively shifts financial risk to the provider. The downside of this system is that risk is shifted to the provider. If the patient mix provided by the insurance company happens to require extensive medical resources during a specific period, all costs that supersede the lump-sum cash provided by the insurer must be paid out-of-pocket by the provider. The upside is the potential for profiting if a provider can make cost effective medical decisions to optimize medical care because all leftover cash from the lump sum payment is retained as profit.

FEE-FOR-SERVICE

Under this type of payment system, insurers reimburse a set fee for each service rendered. Typically, the reimbursement is a set percentage of the actual cost, which is a prenegotiated rate. Under this payment schedule, the provider is free to make medical decisions without having to consider costs. The financial risk is primarily assumed by the insurer. The downside of this system is there is no incentive to reduce health care costs by the provider. As a result, premiums for this type of insurance are typically much higher. The upside is the provider takes no financial risk in taking care of these patients.

PROSPECTIVE PAYMENT SYSTEM (PPS)

Originally developed by the government to help incentivize health care cost control and increase health care delivery efficiencies, this system of reimbursement gives a fixed, predetermined amount for various services. Unlike the capitation system, which provides a fixed amount per patient covered, the PPS reimburses a fixed sum for specific services. This fixed sum is derived from a classification system set forth by the government that varies depending on the health care setting. For example, Medicare will reimburse hospitals a fixed sum for each patient based on a diagnosis-related group (DRG). Therefore, if a patient is admitted for "community acquired pneumonia," Medicare will reimburse the hospital X dollars based on the DRG scale regardless of the length of stay (LOS). This method has since been adopted by some insurance companies as well.

HEALTH INSURANCE MODELS

In the United States today there are four main types of health insurers: Medicare, Medicaid, Health Maintenance Organizations (HMOs), and Preferred Provider Organizations (PPOs).

MEDICARE

President Lynden B. Johnson established Medicare in 1965 as part of the Social Security Act. It was originally designed as a government entitlement that provided health care for U.S. citizens age 65 and older who met defined criteria. Since then, Medicare has expanded to cover specific congenital or permanent disabilities. The details of eligibility, benefits, and premiums are beyond the scope of this chapter; however, it should be noted that there are four parts to Medicare. Each part has an optional enrollment and varies in copayments as follows:

Part A: Covers all inpatient hospital stays.

Part B: Covers services and products not covered by Part A. These typically include outpatient health care including imaging, laboratory tests, and durable medical equipment.

Part C: Allows beneficiaries to select a private health insurance to supplement their Medicare insurance. Through this program, Medicare pays a capitated fee to the private insurance companies, who then provide expanded medical coverage to the enrollee (ie skilled nursing facilities, prescription drugs, etc). In return however, the enrollee is usually limited to certain providers with whom the insurance company contracts. Furthermore, not all insurance companies provide the same supplemental benefits and therefore have different premiums.

Part D: Offers prescription drug coverage. Implemented in 2006, anyone enrolled in Parts A and B may sign up for Part D.

It is important to note that Medicare reimbursement schedules are different for the various parts. Part A is a PPS while Part B is based on a complex formula that includes relative value units (discussed in more detail later), geography, and inflation. Regardless of the reimbursement method, Medicare sets the standard within the health care industry annually. All insurance companies look to Medicare reimbursement schedules to negotiate their own reimbursement schedules with providers. This is why Medicare cuts in reimbursements over the past 10 years have had such a profound effect on finance within the health care industry. The delicate balance of controlling costs while adequately reimbursing for health care services is a constant struggle within the United States.

MEDICAID

Created in 1965 alongside Medicare, Medicaid is a means-tested, needs-based social welfare program. As opposed to Medicare, Medicaid is governed by individual states and funding is shared by both the state and federal governments. Most states have different rules and regulations governing the reimbursement schedules. Some states outsource the insurance to private companies under a capitation system.

HMO

HMOs are a type of managed care organization structured to emphasize primary care. The goal is to make every enrollee visit a primary care physician (PCP) on a regular basis in an effort to minimize the emergent issues that arise with undiagnosed, untreated, chronic medical problems. "Gatekeepers" have traditionally been associated with HMOs and refers to the PCP's role as the referral center for specialized care. Enrollees are not covered for any care given outside an emergent situation without preapproval or referral from their PCP. In theory this minimizes overutilization of highly expensive resources and maintains affordable premiums.

PPO

PPOs are also a type of managed care organization structured in a similar fashion to HMOs except that PCP referrals are not required in order to visit a specialist. PPOs have contracts with PCPs and specialists with whom an enrollee can schedule an appointment at any time at discounted rates. This allows greater flexibility in the enrollee's choice and ability to obtain second opinions. However, these insurance companies typically charge higher premiums and still require preapproval for any nonemergent hospitalization or procedures.

> **PRACTICE POINT**
>
> **Payer mix**
>
> - Many hospitalist practices care for a large number of unassigned patients without a primary care physician and/or medical insurance. This could mean a poor payer mix.
> - Traditionally, professional fee revenues for inpatient, nonprocedural care is low.
> - Ninety-seven percent of Hospital Medicine groups receive financial support from 1 or more outside groups in addition to collections from professional fees. Minimal subsidy funds might be expected if hospitalists only work weekday hours, are not responsible for emergency or unassigned patients, and have an excellent payer mix.

HEALTH CARE FINANCE

Health care finance can be broken up a number of ways, but the following is a description of the key aspects of financial reporting, utilization review, and productivity management. This section should lay the groundwork for understanding the financial goals of both hospitals and hospitalist groups.

FINANCIAL REPORTS

Financial reports can be difficult to decipher or seem unnecessary for smaller groups, but the reality is sustainability and growth cannot occur without utilization of financial reports. Expanding a hospital or hospitalist group requires knowledge of its revenue cycles, benchmarks, and opportunities for improvement. For the astute administrator, financial reports contain a plethora of information that is helpful in guiding strategic planning and financial decisions.

TABLE 23-1 Income Statement

	Current Quarter	Year-to-Date % Δ
Income		
Pre-op clinic visits		
Inpatient admissions		
Procedures		
Consults/Referrals		
Grants and Stipends		
Total Revenue		
Expenses		
Salaries		
Insurance		
Rent		
Office Supplies		
Malpractice insurance		
Employee benefits		
Depreciation		
Total Expenses		
Net Profit (Loss)		

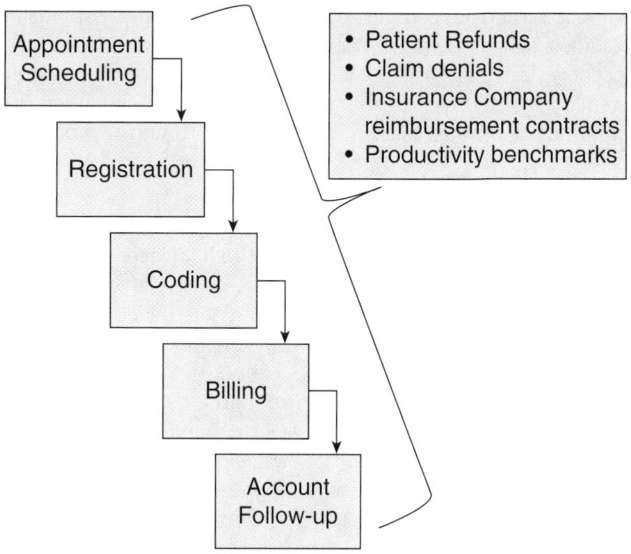

Figure 23-1 *The Revenue Cycle.*

For most businesses, financial information is organized into 4 main documents: (1) the balance sheet, (2) the income statement, (3) statement of retained earnings, and (4) statement of cash flows. For the purposes of this chapter we will use the income sheet and the statement of cash flows to highlight some fundamental aspects of medical finance.

Income statement

The income statement is also referred to as the profit loss statement and it typically contains information about a company's income, expenses, and profits. This report is used by investors, tax accountants, and managers alike to assess how a practice or hospital is transforming revenue into profits (or losses). Put simply, the income statement displays in table format a practice's net revenues (all sources of income) minus net expenses (including write-offs, depreciation, and taxes) to ultimately show a net profit. **Table 23-1** provides an abbreviated example of an income statement.

The income statement provides a road map for all sources of revenue in a practice over a given time period. The goal in evaluating an income statement is to compare it to your projected budget and then identify areas for expense reduction/revenue gains.

Increasing a hospitalist group's revenue does not necessarily equate to increasing the number of procedures or patient encounters. From a productivity and efficiency perspective, a medical practice's revenue is dependent on a number of interconnected processes that together are referred to as the revenue cycle. Take a hospitalist group's preop clinic for example. The process begins when a patient calls to schedule an appointment and ends with collection of the charges due. See **Figure 23-1** for details.

Each step in the revenue cycle is crucial to a hospital's or practice's bottom line (revenue) and must be evaluated on a regular basis. Below are some descriptions of each stage of the cycle and its importance:

- *Appointment scheduling* requires resources and missed appointments mean wasted resources. Support staff must be trained to deal with the constantly changing schedules of both physicians and patients to maximize the number of patients seen on any given day. Increasing the number of visits and procedures while minimizing the number of missed appointments is critical to increase overall revenue. While some practices may not require a high volume of patients to suit their business model, all practices require an efficient scheduling system to maximize revenue.
- *Registration* includes all the steps required to prepare a patient prior to the scheduled physician encounter such as recording basic information, updating medical records, measuring vitals, confirming medications, and placing patients in private rooms. All these steps must be done in a smooth and efficient manner in order to have the patient ready to be seen by the physician on time.
- *Coding* is a key part of the revenue cycle both for compliance and billing matters. All charting and subsequent coding must be compliant with Medicare and other guidelines in order to be reimbursed. Furthermore, the variability among physicians in coding for the similar office visits must be minimized through chart reviews and education. These chart reviews can be done both internally within a practice and by a third party source providing valuable insight to various physicians, their documentation techniques, and areas for efficiency improvement.
- *Billing* is the process of converting all documentation and coding to bills. There are a number of information systems, internal tracking methods, and electronic billing programs that must be evaluated and kept up to date to ensure proper revenue collection.
- *Account follow-up* ties up all the loose ends and concludes the revenue cycle. This last step is crucial for balance billing and monitoring overdue accounts. Improper payments or late payments can pose significant effects on cash flow and therefore, proper systems must be in place to maximize the conversion of billing to revenue.

The box in the upper right hand corner of Figure 23-1 includes examples of other factors that may not fit into any specific step of the revenue cycle. Claim denials or negotiating reimbursement contracts can have a sizable impact on a practice's revenue. Therefore, all factors contributing to the revenue cycle cannot be forgotten when evaluating an income statement discrepancy between an operating budget and revenue realized.

PRACTICE POINT

Professional fee collections

- Expect hospital administrators to conduct a formal financial analysis of their hospitalist programs, examining revenues, expenses, and return on investment.
- Hospital Medicine groups need to maximize their professional fee collections by
  - Creating production incentives for hospitalists.
    - Hospitalists who are compensated based on production generate approximately 18% or more RVUs annually than those who do not have a production component to their compensation.
  - Capturing and reporting all charges.
    - Build billing into the day-to-day operations of the practice.
  - Ensuring adequate documentation of a more intensive level of service and selection of the appropriate code.
    - Ongoing education is required to ensure compliance with current regulatory issues.

While this example focuses on the revenue cycle of a preoperative clinic, it is easily applicable for both hospitals and hospitalist groups. Hospitals must examine their revenue cycles for both elective admissions as well as admissions through the emergency room. Similarly, hospitalist groups constantly evaluate their revenue cycles for all inpatient admissions and consultations.

Overall, an income statement is simple in theory. It provides the reader with an understanding of a practice's income and expenses. Ideally, income should outweigh expenses and result in a net profit. While the numbers can give the reader a snap shot of the practice's profits or losses, these income statements are best utilized internally by a hospital or group practice to identify methods for streamlining processes, increasing production, and optimizing revenue. In the next section we will discuss the statement of cash flows to highlight key revenue indexes used by medical administrators to maximize the income statement.

Statement of cash flows

As the name indicates, this financial report lays out the movement of cash in and out of a practice over a given period of time. While the income statement takes into account all noncash transactions such as depreciation or claim denials, the statement of cash flows only accounts for cash or cash equivalents. The report typically breaks up cash flow into 3 categories: operations, investments, and financing (see **Table 23-2**'s simplified example). This report is used to assess a group's short-term liquidity and is often used by lenders, investors, payroll departments, and administrators.

Increasing liquidity means increasing flexibility in dealing with unforeseen financial situations such as periods with abnormally high claim denials. Cash flow is one of the most important financial reports to understand for small and large groups. The ability to pay bills, employees, and debts is mandatory in order to continue as a business.

DASHBOARD REPORTS

While the statement of cash flows and the income statement are only two examples of financial reports, they both highlight the important role financial statements play in the health care industry. The main goal in reviewing these documents internally is to identify areas for improvement or growth. Revenue, as discussed previously, is dependent on a number of interconnected processes that must be streamlined and efficient in order to maximize profits. Since financial statements are typically made every quarter, they lend themselves to a more action-reaction method of managing your practice. In contrast, dashboard reports are produced monthly (or as frequently as you want) and allow for continuous adjustments in a practice to avoid catastrophe.

TABLE 23-2 Statement of Cash Flows 2009–2010

Cash flows from operating activities etc
Accounts receivable
Grants receivable
Inventory
Reimbursements
Payroll
Benefits
Cash flows from investing activities:
Furniture
Equipment
Website purchase
EMR investment
Building purchase
Cash flows from financing:
(Uncommonly used for medical practices)

PRACTICE POINT

Overhead

- The hospitalist leader should assess overhead based on the resources actually consumed. The cost of billing and collection, malpractice insurance, and limited clerical support may be estimated as 20 % of revenue.
- Inappropriate overhead may occur in hospitals that charge hospitalist groups the same overhead that office physicians or others pay. Hospitalist collections should not ordinarily support office-based expenses of support staff and building or equipment costs.
- A high overhead rate (for example, more than 50%) may result in insufficient funds to pay hospitalists a competitive salary.

Dashboard reports are analogous to car dashboards and their ability to convey real-time information about performance and potential problems. Therefore, all well managed practices should have tools and resources to track performance and produce accurate, timely reports. As with scientific research, data should be methodically collected to guide informed decision-making. Regardless of whether you are a CEO of a large hospital or small independent hospitalist, you must equip yourself with the proper tools to make informed decisions. While most management information systems utilized by physicians are capable of producing dashboard reports, not all are, so it may be useful to inquire about these tools prior to making new upgrades or purchases.

Table 23-3 shows some commonly used metrics for dashboard reports by both hospital and physician groups. Some metrics have obvious utility, but some of the less intuitive measurements are described below.

- *Work Relative Value Units* (RVUs) are a tool used by Medicare to standardize reimbursements based on the organization's resource based relative value scale (RBRVS). It is beyond the scope of this chapter to explain the methodology of how RVU numbers are generated. Any procedure, encounter, or

TABLE 23-3 Commonly Used Metrics for Dashboard Reports

Physician Groups	Hospitals
Work RVUs	Work RVUs
Charge collections	Charge collections
Payer mix	Cost per case
Number of admissions	Contribution margin
Consults	Length of stay index
Office visits	Case mix index
Procedures	Readmission rates
Coding variances	Mortality index

TABLE 23-4 MGMA 2010 Report

Physicians at 100% Billable Activity	WRVUs
90th percentile	7176
75th percentile	5419
50th percentile	3860
25th percentile	2363
Median	3860

diagnosis is assigned a *relative value* with an RVU number based on physician work, practice expense, and malpractice expense. RVUs are a way to standardize productivity between all specialties. However, RVUs do not equal revenue and cannot be used as such. Caution must be used when evaluating a group's financial performances largely based on work RVUs. Instead, they are best used to compare productivity between physicians or groups. Furthermore, one should be cautious in utilizing work RVUs for hospitalists the same way they are utilized for areas in which opportunities exist to market and increase business like primary care or ENT. Hospitalists do not control the number of patients that come into the hospital and variations exist day by day. The Medical Group Management Association publishes industry metrics annually and **Table 23-4** contains some of the industry averages for work RVUs in 2009.

Hospital managers and group practices can utilize industry standards to evaluate their own productivity and make appropriate changes. Some groups use these standards to give feedback to physicians on how they compare to others while other groups use RVUs to encourage productivity by providing financial incentives for reaching specific percentiles.

- *Payer mix* evaluation is crucial to understanding gross revenue and developing long-term strategies. Evaluating trends can help augment contract negotiations and help guide areas of growth (see **Table 23-5**).
- *Length of stay (LOS) index* is the ratio of the actual LOS to the expected LOS. The expected LOS is a standard number based on industry expectations set forth primarily by Medicare but this can vary with specific insurance groups as well. The goal is to have this ratio less than one.
- *Case Mix Index (CMI)* is the average weight of all diagnosis related groups (DRGs) among a hospital's Medicare volume. To understand the importance of the CMI, you must first understand the DRG system. DRG is a system used by Medicare to assign patients with a specific diagnosis from approximately 500 groups. Each DRG is subsequently used in a prospective payment system to reimburse hospitals for specific admissions. DRGs are primarily concerned with utilization of resources, not with severity of illness or patient prognosis. Strictly speaking, it is an evaluation of cost to the hospital. To further standardize DRGs, the Centers for Medicare and Medicaid assign a relative weight (RW) to each DRG based on its resource utilization. Therefore, not all DRGs are treated equally.
- To calculate CMI for a specific time period, use the simple formula: [Total DRGs + Total RW] / Total DRGs. Ideally, the goal is to maximize CMI, which means your hospital deals with complex cases and difficult procedures. This in turn results in higher reimbursements from CMS. Even minor changes in a hospital's CMI can result in significant changes in revenue.
- *Coding Variances* can be used as one metric of productivity. Physicians often under code, and identifying this as an opportunity for education can provide a legitimate increase in revenue. **Table 23-6** shows physician "A" clearly under coding compared to his colleagues. Coding habits should also be compared to the standards published in your geographic area and specialty to further guide management. All coding should also have internal/external reviews to ensure compliance.

PRACTICE POINT

Society of Hospital Medicine (SHM) and medical group management association (MGMA) data

- In general, hospitalists who care for adult patients receive roughly 5% to15% more compensation than internists in traditional practice.
- Compensation and productivity metrics vary significantly across regions.
- National survey data should not solely guide compensation for a particular practice.
- Compensation of physicians in the local marketplace is a more useful benchmark.
- Higher-than-average productivity and/or a significant shortage of hospitalist staffing in a region will likely influence compensation.

TABLE 23-5 Payer Analysis

	June		July		August	
	Gross	% of Total	Gross	% of Total	Gross	% of Total
Aetna						
Blue Shield						
Cigna						
Uninsured						
Total						

TABLE 23-6 Coding Variances (Compared to Previous Month, %)

Physician	Level 1	Level 2	Level 3	Level 4	Level 5
A	4.12	3.14	−2.23	−2.20	−0.40
B	1.12	1.40	2	1.70	0.20
C	0.60	0.90	1.80	0.45	0.30
Total	5.84	5.44	1.37	−0.05	0.10

CONCLUSION

This chapter was designed to provide the introductory lexicon and basic principles guiding finance in health care. While there are many books published on each specific part of this chapter, true grasp of the information comes only with implementation of theoretical approaches. Much like taking care of patients, repetition and constant reading help elucidate the intricacies of health care finance.

SUGGESTED READINGS

Graban Mark. *Lean Hospitals: Improving Quality, Patient Safety, and Employee Satisfaction*. Boca Raton: CRC; 2009.

Huss WH, Coleman M. *Start Your Own Medical Practice: a Guide to All the Things They Don't Teach You in Medical School about Starting Your Own Practice*. Naperville, IL: Sphinx Pub; 2006.

Reiboldt Max. *Financial Management of the Medical Practice*. Second ed. Chicago, IL: American Medical Association; 2002.

CHAPTER 24

Strategic Planning: Demonstrating Value and Report Cards of Key Performance Measures

Caleb P. Hale, MD
Julius Yang, MD, PhD

INTRODUCTION

The field of Hospital Medicine has enjoyed tremendous growth over the past decade. Although partially driven by manpower needs derived from resident duty-hour restrictions and the declining availability of primary care physicians to oversee inpatient care, the widespread adoption of Hospital Medicine practice over the last ten years has also been fueled by the concomitant growth of the health care quality movement. The compelling need for improvement in the quality of care delivery in U.S. hospitals, heralded in two seminal Institute of Medicine reports, one in 2000 (*To Err is Human*) and the other in 2001 (*Crossing the Quality Chasm*), created an important platform upon which hospitalists could offer potential value to hospitals, patients, and referring primary care providers as a new field of inpatient specialists offering both the clinical and operational expertise needed to achieve optimal outcomes in hospital-based care.

The definition of "value" in Hospital Medicine has evolved over the last 10 years. The need to demonstrate some concept of "value" to key stakeholders (hospitals, patients, and referring primary care physicians) has been valid since the inception of the field, given that a significant proportion of hospitalist groups rely in some measure upon institutional fiscal support to exist. Hospitals, in particular, have been very much interested in understanding their "return on investment" for their financial commitments to hospitalist groups. Early studies demonstrated that hospitalist-driven care was associated with reduced lengths of stay and enhanced adherence with payor-defined "core measures" of performance. Fiscal value was a primary driver of early adoption of hospitalist medicine practices as lower lengths of stay of medical inpatients implied greater capacity for inpatient volume growth in high-margin specialties, and adherence to payor-defined performance measures meant hospitals could qualify for incentive payments (or avoid disincentive penalties) related to their quality of care delivery. As public reporting of hospital performance evolved, however, there has been increasing focus on clinical outcomes and patient satisfaction survey results as valid measures by which to compare hospitals; such attention has quickly translated into new domains by which the "value" of hospitalist-driven care can be assessed.

PERFORMANCE ASSESSMENT FOR HOSPITALISTS

Despite a number of studies designed to assess the quality of hospitalist-driven care, there remains a relative paucity of compelling evidence thus far that hospitalist care is necessarily more likely to result in improvements in meaningful outcomes such as mortality, readmission rates, or the quality of patients' hospital experience. In an increasingly financially constrained, and in some regions increasingly competitive, operating environment it may therefore be incumbent upon individual hospitalist groups to be able to demonstrate the value of their work in order to deliver an anticipated "return on investment" to sponsoring institutions through specific measures derived from their groups' own practice and measured at their own institutions.

A useful framework to assess value may be found in the Institute of Medicine's 2001 *Crossing the Quality Chasm* report, in which 6 "aims" for quality health care were defined: safe, efficient, effective, equitable, timely, and patient-centered. The various domains of hospitalist practice can be summarized to match this framework, and in many cases a variety of established metrics are readily available to most institutions in order to assess actual performance within each of these aims.

In considering the concept of performance assessment for hospitalists, hospital leaders should determine how process and outcome-based metrics might be applied: to individual hospitalists, a given hospitalist group, or to the hospital as a whole. The applicability of measurement at the level of the individual hospitalist depends on the nature of staffing and shared management of each patient over the course of the typical hospital admission. In many shift-based models, a number of consecutive hospitalists might be involved in the care of a single patient over the course of one hospitalization. If an ACE-inhibitor has not been prescribed during a hospitalization for a patient with chronic systolic heart failure and no contraindications, to whom might accountability lie (the admitting hospitalist, the daily rounding hospitalist who saw the patient early in the admission, or the discharging hospitalist)? In many instances, metrics applied at the group level might prove most useful by serving to identify opportunities for group directors to implement group-level interventions to enhance suboptimal outcomes. Metrics at the hospital level might apply for those groups whose members have achieved positions of departmental or hospital leadership, with the expectation that hospital-wide practice would improve once standards and innovations introduced and implemented by hospitalist staff are ultimately adopted by all services within a given hospital.

Another important consideration in determining the value of a Hospital Medicine group is clarifying whether there is an expectation for clinical processes and outcomes to improve only for patients admitted under hospitalists' care, or whether hospitalists are expected to contribute to system-wide transformation to improve outcomes across services for all admitted patients. In many academic medical centers, hospitalists play a central role in both undergraduate and graduate medical education, with the ability to provide individual instruction and mentorship as well as potentially contributing to curriculum and/or administrative leadership to improve educational programs overall at a given institution. In both clinical and educational impacts, therefore, hospitalists might be expected to be responsible for (and accountable to) outcomes at both the individual patient/learner level as well as system-wide performance.

PRACTICE POINT

- As public reporting of hospital performance evolved, there has been increasing focus on clinical outcomes and patient satisfaction survey results as valid measures by which to compare hospitals; such attention has quickly translated into new domains by which the "value" of hospitalist-driven care can be assessed. In an increasingly financially constrained, and in some regions increasingly competitive, operating environment, it may therefore be incumbent upon individual hospitalist groups to be able to demonstrate the value of their work in order to deliver an anticipated "return on investment" to sponsoring institutions through specific measures derived from their groups' own practice and measured at their own institutions.

There remains active investigation and debate as to which data actually represent meaningful metrics of hospital-based practice. Hospitalist groups are often largely reliant on existing hospital-level administrative databases, generally designed around payor-defined incentives and requirements for participation. Such data has traditionally emphasized process-based metrics (eg, whether pneumococcal vaccination was administered to appropriate at-risk populations) but have recently expanded to include well-defined clinical outcomes such as disease-specific mortality and readmission rates. Whether current process-based metrics alone sufficiently or accurately reflect the quality of care delivery has come under increasing scrutiny (especially given resources required to collect and report such metrics), and concurrent focus on associated clinical outcomes helps to ensure that such process-based performance predictably correlates with actual patient outcomes. Given the resources typically required to collect and report such metrics, most hospitalist groups will by necessity rely on data abstracted from existing hospital-based administrative measures for their own reporting and quality assurance purposes. The utility of such data, however, depends in part on the particular hospitalist group's clinical scope of practice, as standard disease-specific reporting may or may not coincide with those conditions primarily managed by that hospitalist group. For example, if the majority of heart attack patients are admitted to a cardiologist-led subspecialty service, hospital-level metrics of compliance with aspirin on arrival may not reasonably reflect hospitalist practice at that institution. Depending on the extent of quality assurance programs at a given institution, acquisition of more detailed information regarding practice performance typically requires design and application of dedicated reporting instruments focused on specific outcomes. Given the often prohibitive administrative resources needed for such data collection, this chapter primarily focuses on strategies to assess hospitalist performance derived largely from data that might reasonably be expected to be collected by hospitals for purposes of payor and/or regulatory compliance.

The issue of risk adjustment may also be important, especially if data is intended to offer valid comparison with either prior performance (eg, has length of stay declined because of better physician performance or because of declining acuity?) or with outside hospital/hospitalist groups (ie, "our patients tend to be sicker than theirs..."). Such risk adjustment may or may not be straightforward at an institutional level, but would typically be applied to publicly-reported data when comparing outcomes across institutions. Risk adjustment for comparison of outcomes within a given institution over time might be accomplished using case-mix index versus diagnostic-related groups (DRG)-specific measurements versus more formal assessment of acuity and comorbidity (using established tools such as the Charlson score).

SIX AIMS FOR HEALTH CARE AS DESCRIBED BY THE INSTITUTE OF MEDICINE

SAFETY

Patient safety may be defined as "the avoidance, prevention, and amelioration of adverse outcomes or injuries stemming from the processes of health care." The complexity and fast pace of the inpatient environment certainly presents major challenges to ensuring a "safe" episode of care (free of iatrogenic infection, injury, or error), and the hospitalist is in many ways ideally suited, due to his/her clinical area of focus, systems expertise, team leadership, and committed time within the operational environment of the hospital ward, to being a champion of patient safety for his/her patients as well as for the hospital in general.

As safety science continues to develop within health care, a number of adverse outcomes have been recognized as avoidable through reliable practice of evidence-based prevention measures. Such outcomes include infections acquired as a consequence of hospital-based procedures or exposures; falls related to debility, delirium, concurrent illness, or medication effects; thromboembolic events; as well as less frequently encountered but potentially devastating incidents such as wrong-site surgery, transfusion of mismatched blood type, or patient suicide. Such events are included on the National Quality Forum's Serious Reportable Events list, which may be used by hospitals as a basis for reporting outcomes to regulatory and oversight bodies. The safety performance of a given Hospital Medicine group can thus be assessed through the frequency of safety "failures" involving patients admitted to that group.

An important consideration when reviewing safety performance metrics, however, is the likelihood of a historical bias toward "under-reporting" of safety-related adverse events at most institutions. Should the result of hospitalist quality improvement efforts ultimately succeed in fostering greater transparency and better reporting of adverse events, this may initially paradoxically drive up the rate of reported serious adverse events, regardless of the actual frequency of such events before and after the introduction of the hospitalist group.

EFFECTIVE

The Institute of Medicine's second aim for health care quality improvement is effectiveness, described as the provision of services based on scientific knowledge. In the context of the practice of Hospital Medicine, this could be interpreted to mean the provision of evidence-based medicine as demonstrated by adherence to consensus-based clinical guidelines.

In 2003, the Centers for Medicare and Medicaid Services (CMS) began the Reporting Hospital Quality Data for Annual Payment Update (RHQDAPU) program, which based an annual incentive payment on the public reporting of a set of quality of care measures including process of care measures, outcome of care measures, and survey data on patients' perspectives of care; all designed by the Hospital Quality Alliance (HQA), a collaboration between the Center for Medicare Services (CMS), provider organizations, and participating acute care hospitals nationwide. These data are publically available through the Hospital Compare Web Site (www.hospitacompare.hhs.gov), and as of Fiscal Year 2009, 96% of hospitals participated in the reporting program and received the full incentive payment update for Fiscal Year 2010. The included process of care measures reported to the CMS are derived from evidence-based clinical guidelines for several of the most common diagnoses requiring inpatient care among Medicare and Medicaid recipients. Examples of "process of care measures" specifically relevant to a hospitalist's common clinical practice include: prescription of an angiotensin converting enzyme (ACE) inhibitor or angiotensin receptor blocker (ARB) for left ventricular systolic dysfunction, pneumococcal and influenza vaccination for pneumonia, and appropriate antibiotic selection for pneumonia. Relevant "outcome of care" measures include the 30-day risk-adjusted mortality rates following hospitalizations for pneumonia and heart failure. These indexes of quality may be appropriate surrogate measures of effective clinical care, and the HQA data are often referenced as the existing national standard of quality. As nearly all acute care hospitals already acquire and report these measures both publically and to the CMS, evaluation of the clinical effectiveness of hospitalists or a hospitalist group within an institution through these metrics would not place an undue additional burden on administrative resources available to the group performing a self-evaluation by this method.

Despite a strong association between these individual process of care measures and patient outcomes in specific subgroup analyses (as in the use of ACE inhibitors in left ventricular systolic dysfunction), the association between these discrete processes of care and risk adjusted mortality rates applied to hospitalist care may be confounded by the multiple and likely independent variables contributing to overall mortality rates. Indeed, a recent study by Lopez, et al 2009 found a positive correlation between the HQA process of care measures not only for the presence of hospitalists, but also in direct relation to nurse staffing ratios—a measure that has previously been demonstrated to impact patient mortality rates.

PATIENT CENTERED

The third aim of health care quality improvement as outlined by the IOM is patient-centered care, defined as providing care that is respectful of and responsive to individual patient preferences, needs, and values, and ensuring that patient values guide all clinical decisions.

The degree of patient centeredness of care is difficult to measure, but is perhaps best evaluated through surveys of patient satisfaction. The National Consumer Assessment of Health care Providers and Systems Hospital Survey (H-CAHPS) is a 27-question survey across 10 domains of patient perspectives on hospital care, administered by the CMS and publically reported on the Hospital Compare Web site. Questions address patient experiences of the care provided by doctors and nurses, with specific attention paid to perspectives on being treated with "courtesy and respect," being "listened carefully to," and "having things explained in a way you could understand." In-hospital medical care warrants special attention to this domain of quality as the nature and severity of illnesses requiring hospitalization frequently involve serious and difficult clinical decision making on the part of clinicians (frequently hospitalists) in collaboration with patients and their families. These survey data are widely reported by acute care hospitals in order to obtain the full incentive payment from the CMS as detailed above, and as such, may be a readily available measure of the degree of patient centered care as provided by hospitalists within an institution.

TIMELY

This aim for health care quality improvement includes efforts to reduce the sometimes harmful delays in the delivery of care. The hospitalist model of practice offers several advantages in the timely delivery of care. Hospitalist groups frequently provide in-house night time and weekend physician coverage, the absence of which remains a source of delays to patient care in the traditional model of on-call physician coverage during off hours. In addition to the extraordinary availability of hospitalists for inpatient care, hospitalists are frequently instrumental in the development and administration of efforts to improve hospital throughput and the efficiency of patient flow by methods such as the active triaging of patients in emergency departments, leading daily multidisciplinary rounds focused on resource and bed management, and discharge planning. Furthermore, the availability of hospitalist physicians often enhances timeliness of response in urgent or emergent clinical scenarios, through staffing and leadership of hospitals' rapid response teams or "code blue" resuscitation teams.

Several measures that are often recorded in acute care hospitals that may serve in part as surrogate measures of the timeliness of care provided by hospitalists include emergency department wait times for patients admitted to the hospitalist service; time that the emergency department spends "on diversion" due to overcrowding (if hospitalists are involved in emergency department throughput facilitation); nursing satisfaction survey data in regard to the responsiveness of hospitalist staff; and length of stay measures for hospitalist admissions. Patient satisfaction survey data may also include domains relating to the timeliness and availability of hospitalist staff. The H-CAHPS instrument administered by the CMS and described above does not have questions focused specifically on doctor timeliness; however, several of the global domain questions included such as those that pertain to the overall rating of the hospital, the likelihood to recommend the hospital, and the physician-specific metric of perception of being treated with courtesy and respect are likely heavily influenced by physician timeliness and availability.

■ EFFICIENT

Improvements in efficiency in health care as described by the IOM require the avoidance of waste, including waste of equipment, supplies, ideas, and energy. Multiple studies have demonstrated improvements in resource utilization during inpatient care following the implementation of hospitalist programs, predominantly through reductions in cost per admission and average length of stay (LOS) when hospitalists are compared against traditional, outpatient-based primary care provider models. These cost savings per admission and the potential increases in annual hospital patient volume facilitated by reductions in average LOS frequently substantiate a return on investment argument, financially justifying the implementation of hospitalist programs despite their near universal requirement for significant financial subsidy from their originating institutions. As the waste of equipment, supplies, and energy cautioned against by the IOM are likely to drive up costs and lengths of stay, the measures of cost per admission and admission duration appear to be reasonable measures of health care efficiency. Another measure of the efficiency of care provided by hospitalists can be found in hospital readmission rates. Thirty-day, risk adjusted, all cause readmission rates following hospitalizations for pneumonia and heart failure are two of the outcome of care measures included in the HQA quality metrics, and publically on the hospital compare Web site of the Centers for Medicare and Medicaid Services. Heart failure and pneumonia are among the most common admitting diagnoses managed by hospitalists, and as such, these publically available data on readmission rates may serve as useful evaluative tools when examining the efficiency of care as provided by a hospitalist group.

■ EQUITABLE

Equitable health care as described by the IOM involves care that does not vary in quality because of personal characteristics such as gender, ethnicity, geographic location, or socioeconomic status. Hospitalists are often the admitting physician for patients requiring hospitalization who do not have a primary care doctor (unassigned patients). Many of these patients have no usual care provider as a direct result of being uninsured or underinsured. Without a default physician to assume the care of these unassigned patients, harmful delays and barriers to the equitable delivery of quality care to this often indigent demographic can result. Hospitalists fulfilling this need can help to ameliorate discrepancies that may originate based on socioeconomic status.

Equitable health care requires a standard of quality among all demographics of health care consumers without variance based on gender, ethnicity, or socioeconomic background. As such, the measures of the quality of hospitalist care proposed and outlined in the sections above, including those pertaining to the other five aims health care quality improvement (safety, effectiveness, patient centeredness, timeliness, and efficiency) should be stratified by gender, ethnicity, and if possible, by socioeconomic status in the evaluation of the equity of care as provided by hospitalists.

MEASURING AND DEMONSTRATING REFERRING PROVIDER SATISFACTION

Evaluating and demonstrating the perceptions of and degree of satisfaction with hospitalist care and services among referring providers (predominantly community-based primary care physicians) is important to both Hospital Medicine groups and to their sponsoring institutions, Targeted interventions to optimize referring provider satisfaction are crucial to maintaining and improving market share in today's competitive health care environment. This is most commonly accomplished through locally and independently developed survey-based instruments periodically administered by the hospitalist group to referring providers. An appropriate survey typically includes rating or opinion scale-based questions assessing referring providers' perceptions of hospitalist care in the domains of communication (timeliness, clarity, collegiality, degree of collaboration); quality of care (clinical decision making, coordination of care, patient and family satisfaction); and perceived value and utility to the referring provider (quality of care provided to the provider's patients, ease and satisfaction with primary care practice). Open-ended questions soliciting specific comments are also generally included. Responses gathered through these instruments should be periodically evaluated and communicated to the hospitalist group as a whole in the development of targeted interventions to improve referring provider satisfaction.

PRACTICE POINT

- Hospital Medicine groups and their sponsoring institutions should evaluate and demonstrate the degree of satisfaction referring providers have with hospitalist care and services. Targeted interventions to optimize referring provider satisfaction are crucial to maintaining and improving market share in today's competitive health care environment.

CONTRIBUTIONS TO SYSTEMS IMPROVEMENT

In addition to providing high quality care to individual hospitalized patients through direct clinical oversight, hospitalists have increasingly assumed responsibility for the design and implementation of systems-based interventions to improve the quality of care delivery to all patients within a given hospital or health care system. Within a health care organization, hospitalists can provide instrumental leadership and insight into quality improvement efforts through participation in hospital committees, direct organizational leadership positions, or through project-based quality improvement efforts.

Hospitalists contribute to system-level quality improvement and hospital stewardship through direct membership and leadership on committees such as medical peer review committees, pharmacy and therapeutics committees, resuscitation committees, health information management committees, clinical informatics committees, and medical executive committees, among others. Additionally, in some health care organizations hospitalists have assumed direct leadership positions, serving not only as directors of Hospital Medicine programs, but also as medical directors of patient care units, palliative care services, rapid response team services, medical consult services, and others. Finally, project-based quality improvement activities may provide an important venue by which hospitalists can translate insights from their direct clinical work into the design and implementation of specific, focused system improvements targeting specific patient care processes or specific patient populations. Examples might include developing disease-specific inpatient care protocols, checklists to enhance reliability and standardization of care delivery, and communication interventions to improve the quality of care transitions at discharge. No matter the specific project or organizational involvement, documenting such participation at any level—direct leadership, committee membership, or project-based workgroups—in summary format allows for stakeholders throughout the organization to easily recognize the extent of a hospitalist group's contribution to the health system as a whole.

CONTRIBUTIONS TO MEDICAL EDUCATION AND SCHOLARSHIP

Analogous to their contributions to systems-based quality improvement, hospitalists at academic medical centers often play a central role in the inpatient educational experience of medical students,

TABLE 24-1 Hospital Medicine Performance Report Card (FY 2009)

Productivity	Average annual work RVUs: 3020 Average annual admissions and consultations: 575
Safety	Catheter-associated bloodstream infection: 0.6 per 1000 patient-days Catheter-associated urinary tract infection: 0.4 per 1000 patient-days Ventilator-associated pneumonia: 0.9 per 1000 patient-days Falls with injury: 0.6 per 1000 patient-days Pressure ulceration: 3.2 per 100 patients
Effectiveness (Medicare Core Measures)	**Heart failure:** Discharge instructions provided: 90% Evaluation of LV systolic function: 95% ACE-I or ARB prescribed for LV systolic dysfunction: 90% Smoking cessation counseling provided: 95% 30-day risk adjusted mortality rate: better than the U.S. national rate **Pneumonia:** Pneumococcal vaccination provided: 86% Initial antibiotics within 6 hours of arrival: 94% Appropriate antibiotics: 88% Influenza vaccination provided: 85% Smoking cessation counseling provided: 90% 30-day risk adjusted mortality rate: better than the U.S. national rate
Patient Centeredness (H-CAHPS)	Percent of time doctors "always treated patients with courtesy and respect": 82 Percent of time doctors "always listened carefully to patients": 78 Percent of time doctors "always explained things in a way patients could understand": 79
Timeliness	Average ED LOS for admitted patients: 5.3 hours Discharges before 2 PM: 36% Rapid response team/cardiopulmonary arrest events staffed: 552 In-hospital MD staff availability: 24 hours/day, 365 days/year
Efficiency	Average length of stay: 4.8 days Average cost per admission: $8120 Average Case-Mix Index: 1.20 30-day risk adjusted readmission rate for pneumonia: better than the U.S. national rate 30-day risk adjusted readmission rate for heart failure: better than the U.S. national rate
Equity	**Percentage of patients seen by payor status:** Uninsured: 6%; Medicaid: 14%; Medicare: 32%; other: 48% **Measures of safety, effectiveness, patient centeredness, timeliness, and efficiency as described above, stratified by self-reported race where available (white vs. nonwhite):** No significant differences
Referring provider satisfaction	**Average scores among surveyed referring providers on a 5-point scale (1 = strong disagreement, 3 = neither agree nor disagree, 5 = strong agreement):** Hospitalists communicate with me regarding my patients in a timely fashion: 4.2 Hospitalists demonstrate sound clinical decision making in the care of my patients: 4.4 Hospitalists involve me in a collaborative fashion in the care of my patients: 4.0 My patients verbalize satisfaction with hospitalist services: 4.0 Utilization of hospitalist services improves the care of my patients: 4.1
Systems Improvement and Administration	**Committee Leadership:** Medical Peer Review Committee, Medical Patient Care Committee, ED-Medicine Operations Committee, Resuscitation Committee, Medication Safety Committee, Health Information Management Committee **Committee Participation:** Nurse-Physician Partners Committee, Ethics Oversight Committee, Volume-Operations Committee, Network Development Committee, Medical Executive Committee, Patient-Family Advisory Committee, Falls Prevention Committee, Delirium Prevention Committee **Projects and Working Group Leadership:** Hand Hygiene Working Group, Catheter-Associated UTI Prevention Project **Projects and Working Group Participation:** Catheter-associated BSI Working Group, Heart Failure Working Group, Clinical Handoffs Project, Readmissions Working Group

(continued)

TABLE 24-1 Hospital Medicine Performance Report Card (FY 2009) (*continued*)

Education (AY 2008–2009)	**Administration/Leadership:** Graduate: Associate director of internal medicine residency Undergraduate: Third year clerkship coordinator **Instruction:** Clinical teaching assignments: 32 ward service months/year Classroom teaching assignments: GI physiology course section leader Medical Simulation: Team training course faculty, procedure training faculty **Evaluation:** Number of evaluations submitted regarding housestaff: 58 Number of evaluations submitted regarding medical students: 60 **Invited presentations:** Continuing Medical Education: courses in Geriatric Medicine and Patient Safety Graduate: 18 Undergraduate: 14 **Scholarship:** Grants awarded: 3 Publications in peer reviewed journals: 3 Publications in non-peer reviewed journals: 12 Scholarships awarded: 6 Academic advancement: 3 promotions

interns, and residents. Such contributions may originate from involvement in administrative oversight for a residency program or medical student clerkship program, or through individual hospitalist participation in the direct education, supervision, mentoring, guidance, and support of front-line learning teams. The quality of a hospitalist as an educator can be assessed through documented feedback and evaluation performed by a group of learners, such as residents or medical students, and the extent of participation in clinical education measured in terms of months "on-service" as teaching or ward attending, the number of invited lectures or presentations delivered, or the number of evaluations of students and housestaff that the hospitalist has submitted to the training program.

Research activity may be an important component of an individual hospitalist's and/or hospitalist group's academic contributions. Clinical research designed to inform or improve the care of hospitalized patients may form the basis for future innovation relevant to the care of patients within the hospitalist's health care system and beyond. Research activity can be reported in terms of grant funding, publication in peer-reviewed journals, and presentations at local or national meetings. Such activity not only extends the scope of medical knowledge in a broad sense, but may have important local benefits by enhancing the medical center's reputation and standing as an active site of research and innovation.

PRACTICE POINT

- A "performance report card" summarizing performance measures and contributions of the hospitalist service can serve as a valuable tool in the development of targeted goals for quality improvement and in demonstrating the value of a Hospital Medicine practice to key stakeholders.

CASE 24-1

The director of the hospitalist program at Bayside Medical Center has been asked to attend a meeting with the department chair and CFO of the medical center in one week. Aware of greater scrutiny on hospital operating costs due to dropping payor reimbursements, the director will have to justify the extent of nonprofessional salary support provided by the medical center to his hospitalist service. To further complicate matters, a hospitalist program currently providing care for inpatients at a nearby community hospital, well regarded in terms of efficiency, has explored the possibility of extending their practice to cover patients at Bayside. How can the director of Bayside's hospitalist program demonstrate the value of his service to key stakeholders within the medical center?

The director will need to demonstrate the tremendous value that his group provides to the medical center in terms of the care provided to medical inpatients, adherence to evidence-based and payor-defined guidelines, utilization of resources, patient and provider satisfaction, student and resident education, and systems-based improvements. He therefore seeks the assistance of the hospital's data specialists regarding existing measures of hospital performance that can be analyzed in terms of hospitalist-specific care. He then prepares a concise summary "Performance Report Card" to assist in his discussion with the chairman and CFO (**Table 24-1**).

With the performance report card in hand, the value of the hospitalist group to the department of medicine and Bayside Medical Center are readily apparent at a glance to the chairman and CFO. They congratulate the director for strong leadership of the group, and pledge continued support of the group's clinical and nonclinical efforts.

Evidence Based References

Institute of Medicine. *Crossing the Quality Chasm: A New Health System for the 21st Century*. Committee on Quality of Health Care in America. 2001; National Academy Press. Washington, D.C. http://books.nap.edu/openbook.php?record_id=10027&page=1. Accessed September 9, 2009.

Institute of Medicine. *To Err Is Human: Building a Safer Health System*. Kohn LT, Corrigan JM, Donaldson MS, Eds. 2000; National Academy Press. Washington, D.C. http://books.nap.edu/openbook.php?record_id=9728&page=R1. Accessed March 20th, 2010.

Rauch D. Provider Satisfaction. In: Flores L, ed. *Measuring Hospitalist Performance: Metrics, Reports, and Dashboards*. A White Paper Written and Produced by The Society of Hospital Medicine's Benchmarks Committee. The Society of Hospital Medicine (2006):46–49. http://www.hospitalmedicine.org. Accessed March 25, 2010.

The National Quality Forum. http://www.qualityforum.org/. Accessed March 20th, 2010.

U.S. Department of Health and Human Services. Hospital Compare Web Site. http://www.hospitalcompare.hhs.gov/. Accessed September 10, 2009.

U.S. Department of Health and Human Services. Centers for Medicare and Medicaid Services. Hospital Quality Initiatives. Reporting Hospital Quality Data for Annual Payment Update (RHQDAPU). http://www.cms.hhs.gov/HospitalQualityInits/08_HospitalRHQDAPU.asp#TopOfPage. Accessed September 12, 2009.

U.S. Department of Health and Human Services. Centers for Medicare and Medicaid Services. Hospital Care Quality Information from the Consumer Perspective (H-CAHPS). H-CAHPS survey instrument. http://www.hcahpsonline.org/surveyinstrument.aspx. Accessed September 9, 2009.

CONCLUSION

The value of hospitalists and Hospital Medicine has traditionally been demonstrated through financial benefits including reductions in average length of stay and cost per admission, substantiating a return on investment for sponsoring institutions that support internal Hospital Medicine programs. In the past decade, however, an increasing emphasis on the quality and safety of health care as championed in two formative reports of the Institute of Medicine: *To Err is Human* (2000) and *Crossing the Quality Chasm* (2001), has created a medium for the expanded demonstration of the value of Hospital Medicine through the domains of health care quality and safety. The six aims for health care in the twenty-first century as outlined in *Crossing the Quality Chasm*: safe, effective, patient centered, timely, efficient, and equitable, provide a framework for evaluating and demonstrating the value of hospitalist care. Hospitalists not only augment the quality of health care through efforts to target these quality indicators, but also through contributions to systems improvement, medical education, and research. In the measurement and evaluation of hospitalist performance through the above domains, it is helpful to rely on metrics that are commonly obtained through existing administrative databases, so as not to place an undue financial burden on the often limited administrative resources available to hospitalist groups in the evaluation of their own performance. A "performance report card" summarizing these measures and contributions can serve as a valuable tool in the development of targeted goals for quality improvement and in demonstrating the value of a Hospital Medicine practice to key stakeholders.

SUGGESTED READINGS

Aiken LH, Clarke SP, Sloane DM, et al. Hospital Nurse Staffing and Patient Mortality, Nurse Burnout, and Job Satisfaction. *JAMA*. 2002;288(16):1987–1993.

Howell E, Bessman E, Kravet S, et al. Active Bed Management by Hospitalists and Emergency Department Throughput. *Ann Intern Med*. 2008;149:804–810.

Jha AK, Zhonghe Li MA, Orav EJ, et al. Care in U.S. Hospitals – The Hospital Quality Alliance Program. *N Engl J Med*. 2005;353: 265–274.

Lindenauer PK, Remus D, Roman S, et al. Public Reporting and Pay for Performance in Hospital Quality Improvement. *N Engl J Med*. 2007;356:486–496.

Lindenauer PK, Rothberg MB, Pekow PS, et al. Outcomes of Care by Hospitalists, General Internists, and Family Physicians. *N Engl J Med*. 2007;357;25:2589–2600.

Lopez L, Hicks LS, Cohen AP, et al. Hospitalists and the Quality of Care in Hospitals. *Arch Intern Med*. 2009;169(15):1389–1394.

Meltzer D, Manning WG, Morrison J, et al. Effects of Physician Experience on Costs and Outcomes on an Academic General Medical Service: Results of a Trial of Hospitalists. *Ann Intern Med*. 2002;137:866–874.

Miller JA, Nelson J, Whitcomb WF. *Hospitalists: A Guide to Building and Sustaining a Successful Program*. Chicago, IL: Health Administration Press; 2008:19–60.

Needleman J, Buerhaus P, Mattke S, et al. Nurse-staffing levels and the quality of care in hospitals. *N Engl J Med*. 2002;346(22): 1715–1722.

CHAPTER 25

Negotiation and Conflict Resolution

Leslie A. Flores, MHA

INTRODUCTION

Hospitalists face the potential for conflict every day. They work in highly complex organizations in which in order to be successful they must interact effectively with a wide variety of individuals in what is often a challenging, emotionally charged environment. They must learn to navigate not only the formal organizational bureaucracy of rules, systems, and processes, but also the informal political hierarchy that influences power and decision making. Often, they must do so with little or no formal training in conflict management at an early stage in their medical careers. In addition, they may encounter conflicts between what referring physicians would like them to accomplish during hospitalization and the needs of the hospital to expedite care to the outpatient setting.

Hospital Medicine is also a young, evolving specialty that has enjoyed unprecedented exponential growth by serving the needs of multiple competing stakeholders. Few mentors or seasoned clinicians have specialized in Hospital Medicine, and as such they may not have a complete understanding of the specialty or even have career advancement of hospitalists on their radar screen. The potential exists for the service obligations of hospitalists to overwhelm opportunities for professional development, and this may promote career dissatisfaction, turnover, and symptoms of burnout. Leaders of hospitalist services may find themselves isolated as they advocate for the professional development of members of the service while meeting the service expectations of their employers or supervisors. The professional medical society for hospitalists, the Society of Hospital Medicine (SHM), is rapidly developing flexible support resources for hospitalists relating to business practice, career satisfaction, core competencies and role expectations. Until these standards become widely disseminated and health care services become better designed and hence less prone to error, hospitalists will continue to work in a hospital environment where they will increasingly be expected to perform as change agents at a time when change may not be welcome by others at their institutions.

For the purposes of this chapter, it will be important to distinguish between *disagreements* and *conflicts*. Disagreements happen regularly in human interactions, and occur whenever two or more individuals have differing opinions about something. A disagreement need not devolve into a conflict, and many do not. Conflicts arise when a party perceives that another party has negatively affected or will negatively affect agendas that the first party cares about. Conflicts are defined as processes that occur when tensions develop, that is, the emotions associated with a disagreement become so elevated that they impede the ability of the parties to interact with each other effectively.

Almost all conflict is a result of unmet expectations. For hospitalists, this commonly arises when there is a lack of understanding or a difference in expectations about the role of hospitalists. Hospitalists may assume that primary care physicians have explained to patients that someone else will be seeing them in the hospital. Patients and families, however, may not understand why their primary care physician is not present in the hospital and directing their care. Emergency Medicine physicians may expect the hospitalist to respond promptly to take a complicated social admission off their hands whereas hospitalists may feel that it is the role of the emergency room physicians to discharge patients who do not require admission. Emergency Medicine physicians and staff may expect for patients be triaged to hospital floors (to reduce their emergency department length of stay or avoid diversion) before critical information is available, or may expect hospitalists to care for patients in the emergency department when no beds are available. Meanwhile, floor nurses may expect hospitalists to be immediately available to address nonurgent requests. Primary care physicians may want patients to remain in the hospital until the workup is complete due to lack of resources in the outpatient setting and/or patient/family demands, whereas hospitalists are under pressure to discharge patients who do not require acute hospitalization. There may be differences of opinion among specialists and generalists regarding diagnosis, workup, and treatment or the role of the hospitalists in management. All physicians expect to be treated professionally, to have some autonomy over clinical decision making, and to have a reasonable work-life balance. Hospital administrators and employers, however, may require hospitalists to do nonphysician tasks or solve problems for other physician groups without taking into account the perspectives of the hospitalists or staffing needs for time-consuming tasks. When such expectations go unmet, people get frustrated or angry. They often respond in ways that then result in frustration or anger on the part of others. Emotions on both sides become elevated, and the stage is set for a conflict.

PRACTICE POINT

- Almost all conflict is a result of unmet expectations. For hospitalists this commonly arises when there is a lack of understanding or a difference in expectations about the role of hospitalists.

The most common reasons that expectations go unmet include

- **Lack of *clarity* about what is expected, or about how the expectation will be met**. It is easy to assume that because one's expectations are clearly understood by oneself, they are clear to others as well. Even when expectations are carefully explained, the other party may hear or interpret things differently than the speaker intends. The other party may also react more to the emotional aspect of the presentation or who is doing the talking rather than to the content.
- **Lack of *agreement* about what is expected or how to achieve it.** The high degree of complexity in error prone health care systems, stress and pressure, and the need for rapid change are important sources of potential conflict. Sometimes each party's expectations are clearly understood by the other party, but they simply disagree with each other about the desired outcome, the method, or both. This can occur if the parties have competing needs or interests that are perceived to be in opposition. For example, although resident work hour restrictions are clearly delineated in the academic setting, stress and pressure develop for hospitalists when the increased service obligations resulting from such restrictions conflict with the need for professional advancement. The emergence of rapid response teams involving hospitalists as first responders may also create conflict if hospitalists do not have the resources to handle their other tasks such as admissions, discharges, and essential communication due to interruptions in their workflow. Changing hospital processes to promote efficiency and recruitment of additional staff to meet challenges takes time and money.

In addition, age, gender, and cultural differences may play a role in the development and management of conflict. A generational gap may result in different work expectations, a paternalistic view of who is actually in charge, or resistance to changing to the new work requirements. Men and women may have different expectations of their work, and often have different ways of responding to stress, emotion, and conflict. In the United States, men often tend to use a competing or forcing style when faced with conflict, whereas women often tend to use compromising, accommodating, and avoiding.

A key aspect of cultural differences is the degree to which a person tends to identify most strongly with the group of which he or she is a part (a "collectivist culture") as opposed to identifying with the self (an "individualistic culture"). Individualistic cultures, which are the dominant cultures found in North America and Western Europe, value autonomy, creativity, and personal initiative. Most of the rest of the world is composed of collectivist cultures, which instead value conformity and harmony. A meta-analysis of studies on culture and conflict resolution styles found that people in individualistic cultures tend to choose forcing as a conflict style more often and people who come from collectivistic cultures tend to choose withdrawing, compromising, or problem-solving styles instead.

THE POTENTIAL BENEFITS OF CONFLICT

Conflicts are inevitable in human interactions. The increasingly complex and collaborative nature of the work that hospitalists do increases the likelihood that interpersonal conflicts will arise. These conflicts can be destructive if not effectively managed. But a healthy approach to conflict management acknowledges that not all conflict is entirely negative. There are potential benefits that may be derived from conflicts under certain circumstances. DeChurch and Marks (2001) reported that the ways in which groups handle conflict help to determine whether or not benefits were realized, noting that "the relationship between task conflict and group performance was positive when conflict was actively managed and negative when it was passively managed." This suggests that Hospital Medicine physicians will be well served to develop effective conflict management skills that can help them increase the likelihood that the conflicts they will inevitably face may yield positive results. In order to do so, it will be important for hospitalists to think strategically about how one may extract the maximum benefit from conflicts that do occur. Some of the potential benefits of appropriately-managed conflict include:

- **Catalyst for Change.** Conflicts can force needed change by surfacing problems that otherwise might not be recognized, and by elevating latent issues to a level that demands attention. This can be especially valuable in tradition-bound, change-resistant organizations.
- **Improved Outcomes.** Similarly, conflicts can ultimately yield improved outcomes, because they can facilitate learning in the search for better solutions and bring to the forefront useful information and emotions that lie below the surface. An individual may learn more about herself, about the other person, and about the situation.
- **Balance.** Healthy conflict helps to ensure that balance is maintained among competing needs and perspectives.
- **Increased Accountability.** Because conflicts involve strong emotions, a healthy conflict resolution usually involves careful articulation of what the parties have agreed to do to resolve it, and a significant degree of accountability to ensure that the agreements are followed through.
- **Improved Relationships.** When people skillfully manage a conflict between them in healthy, respectful ways, it can actually serve to strengthen their relationship going forward. They end up understanding each other better, and building greater trust because they have demonstrated that they can overcome differences.

KEY PRINCIPLES IN CONFLICT MANAGEMENT

This chapter offers five key principles that represent a good start for those who wish to build better conflict management skills (**Table 25-1**). However, more detailed treatments of all of these principles and others are contained in the references at the end of this chapter.

TABLE 25-1 Five Key Principles of Effective Conflict Management

1. Commit to *Confronting*
2. Attend to the *Conditions*.
3. Identify One's Personal *Contribution*
4. *Consider* what is Underlying Others' Behavior
5. *Clarify*

1. **Commit to *Confronting*.** Most people tend to shy away from conflict. It is tempting to believe that the problem will go away by itself if left alone; that others will soften their positions, forget about the issue, or change their minds, if given enough time. But when pressed, most people will acknowledge this is simply a convenient excuse for avoiding a confrontation that they fear could become uncomfortable or out-and-out unpleasant. Another important reason that people avoid conflict is their fear that openly confronting the situation will make things worse, rather than better. They may worry about handling the confrontation badly and unintentionally causing the situation to deteriorate, or they may fear that the conflict is intractable and that no matter how carefully and skillfully the situation is handled, the outcome will be negative.

In fact, conflicts cannot be resolved if they are not confronted. They may be glossed over or pushed into the background, but not truly resolved. And such conflicts are likely to surface again, often in unanticipated and damaging ways. Thus a willingness to acknowledge the existence of a conflict and to step up and confront it is a precondition to effectively managing the conflict.

PRACTICE POINT

- A willingness to acknowledge the existence of a conflict and to step up and confront it is a precondition to effectively managing the conflict. This requires an open and honest discussion of the issue, usually face-to-face, with the goal of understanding the root causes (the unmet expectations) that led to the conflict and addressing them.

In this context, the term "confrontation" is not intended to mean an angry, emotional exchange of verbal attacks. Instead, "confrontation" refers here to an open and honest discussion of the issue, usually face-to-face, with the goal of understanding the root causes (the unmet expectations) that led to the conflict and addressing them. The remaining principles in this section are intended to assist the confronter, once the decision to confront has been made, to carefully plan the confrontation (when time permits), and to handle it successfully.

2. **Attend to the *Conditions*.**[1] Patterson, et al (2002) note that there are two components to every successful crucial conversation: the actual ***content*** of the conversation, and the ***conditions*** under which the conversation occurs. Most people, when planning to confront or actually engage in a confrontation (a "crucial conversation"), think primarily about the content of the conversation: "What is this conflict about? What steps will resolve it? What points do I need to be sure to make? What will I say to get my points across? What will the other person say?"

People skilled in conflict management realize that the conditions matter just as much as—in fact, maybe more than—the content does. What types of conditions matter? The physical conditions matter a great deal. Is the conversation taking place in a private place instead of in public? Are the people involved in the conversation sitting or standing so they can engage each other at eye level, or is one person sitting with the other standing over him? Is there a desk or other impediment between the participants? Is the room too large or too small, too hot or too cold to be comfortable?

Psychological conditions matter even more. The hospitalist who wishes to be skilled at conflict management must learn to pay attention to what the other person or people involved in the conflict are experiencing emotionally. Are they feeling attacked or are they feeling safe? Do they feel that the hospitalist respects them and has their best interests at heart, or do they feel that their interests will be ignored or belittled? Do they sense that the hospitalist is going to push her agenda or opinion and ignore theirs, or do they believe the hospitalist is willing to listen and take their point of view into consideration? Do they feel that the hospitalist's opinion matters or that dialogue should occur at a "higher level" with senior physician leaders to the exclusion of hospitalists?

Before the actual content—what the conflict is about and how it should be resolved—can be effectively addressed, the skilled conflict manager must take steps to set up conditions that allow all parties to feel comfortable, safe, and heard. The necessary steps to creating these positive conditions involve ensuring mutual respect among the parties, and identifying or creating a mutual purpose. In other words, do others believe the hospitalist sees them as individuals worthy of the respect and consideration due to every human being, and do they believe that the hospitalist is mindful of their interests as well as his own in seeking an acceptable resolution?

PRACTICE POINT

- Before the actual content—what the conflict is about and how it should be resolved—can be effectively addressed, the skilled conflict manager must take steps to set up conditions that allow all parties to feel comfortable, safe, and heard. The necessary steps to creating these positive conditions involve ensuring mutual respect among the parties and identifying or creating a mutual purpose.

3. **Identify One's Personal *Contribution*.**[2] By definition, conflicts occur when emotions get in the way of resolving disagreements. This is true not only of others with whom a hospitalist may come in conflict, but of the hospitalist himself. Another important competency for skilled conflict managers is the ability to step back from their own emotions and assess their personal contribution to the situation; in other words, what impact are their own biases, assumptions, emotions, and actions having on the conflict itself, and on their approach to managing it? Do they truly intend to seek mutually acceptable solutions or do they just want to win?

For example, the person seeking to manage a conflict must pay attention not only to what others are experiencing emotionally but also to what he is experiencing emotionally himself. He needs to ask, "Am I feeling safe or am I under attack? Do I believe the others involved in this conflict will listen to me and take my interests into consideration, or not?" However, simply identifying one's own emotional state is not adequate. Effective conflict managers should also have the self-awareness to understand how their emotions will tend to influence their behavior in the confrontation. These tendencies are described as a person's "style under stress."

TABLE 25-2 Style Under Stress Test

1.	Rather than tell people exactly what I think, sometimes I rely on jokes, sarcasm, or snide remarks to let them know I'm frustrated.	T	F
2.	When I've got something tough to bring up, sometimes I offer weak or insincere compliments to soften the blow.	T	F
3.	Sometimes when people bring up a touchy or awkward issue I try to change the subject.	T	F
4.	When it comes to dealing with awkward or stressful subjects, sometimes I hold back rather than give my full and candid opinion.	T	F
5.	At times I avoid situations that might bring me into contact with people I'm having problems with.	T	F
6.	I have put off returning phone calls or e-mails because I simply didn't want to deal with the person who sent them.	T	F
7.	In order to get my point across, I sometimes exaggerate my side of the argument.	T	F
8.	If I seem to be losing control of a conversation, I might cut people off or change the subject in order to bring it back to where I think it should be.	T	F
9.	When others make points that seem stupid to me, I sometimes let them know it without holding back at all.	T	F
10.	When I'm stunned by a comment, sometimes I say things that others might take as forceful or attacking, comments such as "give me a break!" or "that's ridiculous!"	T	F
11.	Sometimes when things get heated I move from arguing against others' points to saying things that might hurt them personally.	T	F
12.	If I get into a heated discussion, I've been known to be tough on the other person. In fact, they might feel a bit insulted or hurt.	T	F

Excerpted with permission from Patterson K, Grenny J, McMillan R, et al. *Crucial Conversations: Tools for Talking When Stakes are High*. New York, NY: McGraw-Hill; 2002.

The Style Under Stress Inventory[3] in **Table 25-2** is based on the concept of *conversational safety,* and will assist individuals in assessing their own personal style under stress. In completing the questions, one should answer "T" for true or "F" for false, based on one's most frequent tendencies when in conflict situations. People feel safe in a crucial conversation if they believe that they will be listened to respectfully and if they do not feel attacked or ignored. They feel that the other people have their interests at heart, or at least that others' interests and their own are not diametrically opposed without room for finding common ground. The inventory is designed to help people understand how they tend to behave when they do not feel safe in a crucial conversation.

Individuals responding "true" for several of the first 6 questions are said to be *going to silence* when under the stress of a challenging conflict situation. This means they will tend to try to downplay or sugarcoat an issue, or even avoid it outright by changing the subject or disengaging when they do not feel safe. In such cases, they may believe that they have raised an issue and articulated their concerns, but others may be left confused or unaware of how strongly the person feels about the issue because of his *silence* tendencies. On the other hand, answering "true" to some or all of questions 7 through 12 means the person tends to *go to violence* when feeling unsafe in a conversation. These people will often try to force their opinion on others by controlling the conversation and either prevent others from speaking or belittle their contributions when they do.

Both silence and violence may be extremely damaging, when the goal of the conversation is to confront disagreements and work toward mutually acceptable solutions. When people understand their own silence or violence tendencies, they can begin to pay attention to how they are responding during conflict situations. They can look for evidence that they are not feeling safe and then step back to assess the impact their silence or violence is having on the conversation and adjust their interactions accordingly. As awareness of these tendencies grows over time, people can begin to anticipate situations in which safety may be at risk and to proactively develop plans to manage their own tendencies to go to silence or violence.

When thinking about one's personal contribution to a conflict situation, one should also be cognizant of one's own assumptions and biases about the others involved in the conflict, and especially one's beliefs about others' intentions. For example, it is usually helpful to consider the problem of *intent* versus *impact*. When analyzing a conflict, one should consider asking, "Is it the *impact* (ie, the outcome) of the other person's behavior that is bothering me so much, or is it what I believe about the person's *intentions*?"

This distinction is important because humans tend to overemphasize dispositional factors such as personality type or motives, and to discount situational factors such as external stressors, when interpreting the behavior of others; this phenomenon is known by psychologists as *the fundamental attribution error* or *correspondence bias*. Because of this bias, the emotions a person experiences about a disagreement, and thus the level of conflict that ensues, may be heightened as a result of presumed negative intentions on the part of others ("that surgeon is just lazy") and discounting the circumstantial factors that may be influencing others' behavior ("that surgeon is under real pressure to produce good outcomes, and doesn't have the training or experience to manage these complex medication regimens").

The fundamental attribution error may be exacerbated by a related tendency known as *the actor-observer bias* in which one tends to attribute others' behavior to their dispositions but to attribute one's own behavior to the circumstances ("that family member lost her temper because she's a demanding jerk, but I only lost my temper because she pushed me over the edge"). Self-awareness is critical for effective conflict management, especially awareness of one's own assumptions and biases.

PRACTICE POINT

- Self-awareness is critical for effective conflict management, especially awareness of one's own assumptions and biases.

4. ***Consider* What is Underlying Others' Behavior.** One of the keys to effective conflict management is the ability to understand why others respond the way they do in conflict situations (taking into account both dispositional factors and situational factors), and to modify one's interactions accordingly. The concept of conversational safety applies to the other parties involved in a conflict situation, as well as to oneself. Skilled conflict managers become adept at not only reading and adjusting their own behaviors, but also at looking for signs that others aren't feeling safe. Hospitalists may become more understanding of the anger expressed by patients' families, the controlling or snide comments from other medical staff members, or the sugar-coated change of subject by the hospital administrator when they understand that these behaviors often result from others' fear that they will be treated with disrespect, attacked, or ignored. If they can then work to address those underlying fears (part of paying attention to conditions) before launching into the content of the conversation, they will be more successful.

PRACTICE POINT

- One of the keys to effective conflict management is the ability to understand why others respond the way they do in conflict situations (taking into account both dispositional factors and situational factors), and to modify one's interactions accordingly. When someone acts in ways that contribute to a heightened level of conflict, it is worth considering whether that person has underlying human needs that are going unmet and that are contributing to his or her challenging behavior.

Another way of thinking about this issue is to anticipate that the more significant the conflict, the greater the chance that people will respond to it emotionally rather than logically. While it is not a clinically accurate model, it may be useful to think of peoples' brains as having a logical core, surrounded by a layer of emotion (see **Figure 25-1**). Every interaction a person has, no matter how logical it is, passes through this emotional filter on its way in or out.

For most people and under normal circumstances, the layer of emotion surrounding the logical core is relatively thin and the information from the interaction passes through it in both directions, informed by the emotion but not substantially altered by it. In a conflict situation, however, the emotional layer surrounding the logical core inflates like a balloon. In this situation, the expanded emotional layer takes over and prevents logical conversation and data from passing through. The person is responding from her emotion, rather than from logic. Hospitalists may be attempting to have a very logical conversation with a family member, assuming that they are addressing the family member's logical core. But the hospitalists' logical words can't get through the inflated emotional layer. The hospitalists are talking logic, and the family members are responding from emotion; no wonder they can't relate to each other. In such situations, it is necessary to let some air out of the balloon—to give the emotional layer a chance to deflate—before it will be possible to re-engage the logical core in problem solving or conflict resolution.

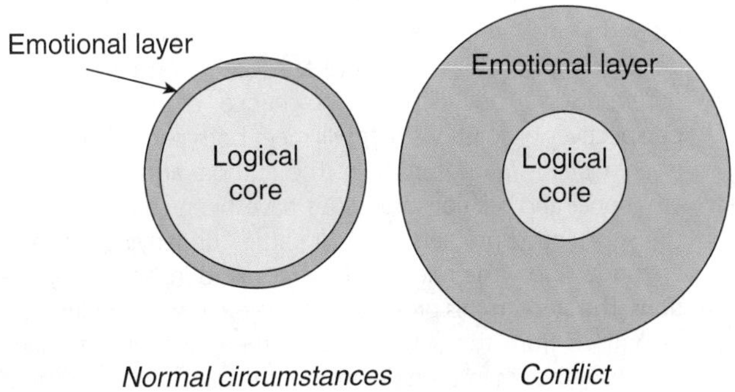

Figure 25-1 *Logic and Emotion Diagram.*

In addition to the overwhelming influence of emotion on how others respond to conflict situations, Heifetz and Linsky (2002) have argued that there are powerful and universal human needs that influence behavior, sometimes in dysfunctional or disruptive ways:

> Every human being needs some degree of power and control, affirmation and importance, as well as intimacy and delight.... We all have hungers, which are expressions of our normal human needs. But sometimes those hungers disrupt our capacity to act wisely or purposefully. Perhaps one of our needs is too great and renders us vulnerable. Perhaps the setting in which we operate exaggerates our normal level of need, amplifying our desires and overwhelming our usual self-controls. Or, our hungers might be unchecked simply because our human needs are not being met in our personal lives.[4]

When someone acts in ways that contribute to a heightened level of conflict, it is worth considering whether that person has underlying human needs that are going unmet, and that are contributing to his or her challenging behavior.

5. ***Clarify.*** When confronting another person about a conflict situation, effective communication skills are essential. It is important to focus on ensuring clarity, both in what one is attempting to convey, and in understanding the other person's point of view. Important communication skills include
   - *Setting the Stage.* Keeping in mind the principles of mutual respect and mutual purpose, it may be valuable to start out by communicating one's own positive intentions to the other person(s) in a way that builds toward these goals.
   - *Managing Expectations.* Hospitalists should clearly communicate what their own expectations were in the situation that gave rise to the conflict, and seek to understand what the other person's expectations were. This will create a foundation for further dialogue about the differences between what each party expected and what actually occurred.
   - *Active Listening.* Active listening skills involve not just hearing what the other person says, but also
     - actively engaging the other person with eye contact and body language;
     - working to enable the other person to feel comfortable sharing potentially difficult information;
     - listening "between the lines" for what *isn't* being said, as well as what *is* being said;
     - acknowledging the reality and legitimacy of the other person's emotions;
     - paraphrasing and reframing to ensure understanding of the other person's perspective;
     - asking questions and probing to understand root causes;
     - staying focused on the other person, rather than one's own planned response.
   - *Joint Problem-Solving.* Engaging all parties to the conflict in joint problem solving will help to clarify what needs to happen to resolve the conflict, and what the alternatives are for moving forward out of conflict. It will also help build mutual support of and commitment to the agreed-upon approach.

- *Articulating Next Steps.* Establishing a clear path of next steps and assigning responsibilities are vital components of a clear and effective communication process. It is worth talking both about the expected outcome, and about the method or process by which the outcome will be achieved: it is not uncommon for new conflicts to arise inadvertently when two parties believe they understand *what* will happen, only to clash over *how* it will be accomplished.

PRACTICE POINT

- When confronting another person about a conflict situation, effective communication skills are essential. It is important to focus on ensuring clarity, both in what one is attempting to convey, and in understanding the other person's point of view. Important communication skills include setting the stage, managing expectations, active listening, joint problem solving, and articulating next steps.

STRATEGIES FOR EFFECTIVE CONFLICT MANAGEMENT: CONFLICT RESOLUTION AND NEGOTIATION

1. **The Talking Stick.** Stephen Covey (1989) highlighted the importance of empathetic communication in describing the principle, "Seek first to understand, then to be understood." Covey (2004) further described the use among Native American cultures of the Talking Stick as a tool to help people resolve differences by creating greater mutual understanding and respect.[5] The Talking Stick is passed from one person to another, and only the person who is holding the Talking Stick is allowed to present her perspective. This ensures that only one person talks at a time, and increases the ability of others to listen because they are not permitted to argue or make their own points until the person holding the Talking Stick has finished.

The most powerful aspect of the Talking Stick, however, is that the person holding it does not relinquish it until she is satisfied that she has been fully understood by the others. It is the responsibility of the listeners to listen carefully and with empathy, and to ensure that the speaker feels understood—not necessarily agreed with—just understood. Once the speaker is satisfied that others understand him, she passes the Talking Stick on and assumes the responsibility to listen and make the next speaker feel understood. Covey describes the value of the Talking Stick as follows:

> This way, all of the parties involved take responsibility for one hundred percent of the communication, both speaking and listening. Once each of the parties feels understood, an amazing thing usually happens. Negative energy dissipates, contention evaporates, mutual respect grows, and people become creative. New ideas emerge. Third alternatives appear.

One does not need to use a physical Talking Stick to gain these benefits. It is possible to establish a framework for interacting in which the parties agree that they will alternate the responsibilities of talking and listening until both feel fully understood. This process can be very effective in facilitating the resolution of conflicts between hospitalists and other specialists regarding scope and service issues. Some parties may be able to do this independently, while others may benefit from facilitation by a third party mediator.

2. **Unhappy Patients and Families: Take the HEAT.** Some of the most challenging conflicts that hospitalists must manage are those that involve the unmet expectations of patients and families. Keeping in mind the role of emotion in conflict, Byham (1993) recommends the following approach for those who are responsible for addressing the needs of unhappy patients and families, as summarized by the acronym "Take the HEAT"[6]:
   - ***H**ear them out.* Active listening without interrupting, disagreeing, or defending is the crucial first step. Angry patients and family members need to be able to express their emotions in order to let some of the air out of the emotional balloon.
   - ***E**mpathize.* As with Covey's Talking Stick example, patients and families need to feel understood. It is not necessary to agree with them, but it is important to acknowledge their feelings and to attempt to understand the issue from their perspective.
   - ***A**pologize.* Byham points out that even if one does not wish to admit fault, it is important to apologize for the situation, and for the fact that the patient's expectations were not met.
   - ***T**ake responsibility for action.* Once the emotional balloon has been deflated, it is often possible to re-engage the patient or family member on a logical basis. A good way to make this transition is to take some concrete action, either to resolve the problem on the spot or to demonstrate a desire to improve the situation.
3. **Principles of Effective Negotiation.** Hospitalists frequently find themselves in potential conflict situations in which negotiation is an effective strategy for addressing the issue. These may include formal negotiations such as the development of professional service agreements, employment contracts, or incentive compensation metrics, or they may be less formal interactions such as working with specialists to define admitting responsibilities or comanagement services. Strong negotiation skills are also valuable for hospitalists working on medical staff committees or quality improvement projects when the diverse interests of many parties must be reconciled.

In traditional negotiations, each party stakes out a formal position and then proceeds to bargain from that position, using various tactics to "win" points that bring the final compromise outcome closer to this position. By contrast, the Principled Negotiation model developed by Fisher and Ury (1981) focuses on understanding all the parties' underlying interests and on identifying objective, fair options that can satisfy everyone.[7] The four tenets of Principled Negotiation are as follows:

- *Separate the People from the Problem.* This principle addresses the role of emotions and relationships in influencing one's perceptions about the negotiation. The authors suggest that negotiators seek to identify when relationships (either as friends or adversaries) may be getting in the way of seeking the best outcome, and that negotiators address these emotional aspects directly and openly with the goal of moving beyond them into objective and collaborative problem solving.
- *Focus on Interests, not Positions.* It is crucial to look beyond the formal stance a person has taken and attempt to understand his underlying interests, the "root causes" of his position. By understanding all parties' basic interests (both one's own and the other person's), one increases the chances of identifying new perspectives or solutions that will meet both parties' interests.
- *Invent Options for Mutual Gain.* The authors argue that once emotional and relationship issues have been separated from the substantive problem, and all parties' underlying interests are understood, the role of the parties is to invent better options. The steps in this process are: separating the identification of options from the act of judging them, looking for many options rather than a single answer, focusing on options that result in mutual gains, and then coming up with ways to make the decisions easy.

- *Insist on Using Objective Criteria.* Finally, Fisher and Ury acknowledge that despite one's best efforts, negotiators will sometimes face situations in which interests are truly in intractable conflict and mutually acceptable options may not be available. In these cases, effective negotiators will insist that decisions be made using objective, usually externally validated, criteria.

In addition to the tenets of Principled Negotiation outlined above, it is important to recognize that when the issues are complex, even the best and most carefully documented negotiation will probably fail to anticipate every nuance that may arise going forward. For example, when hospitalists negotiate and memorialize a "service agreement" with a group of specialists to define who will admit which types of patients, invariably a patient will present who does not fit neatly into any of the categories specified in the service agreement. If the potential for this to occur is not acknowledged and planned for up front, additional conflicts may arise despite the parties' careful efforts. The most valuable asset in such situations is a strong underlying relationship of mutual trust and respect that will enable the parties to resolve these issues on a case-by-case basis. The bottom line is that even the best negotiation skills and most clearly drafted documents cannot substitute for strong relationships.

CONCLUSION

Conflict is inevitable in human interactions, and the potential for serious conflict will grow as the complexity of interactions increases. The extremely challenging milieus in which hospitalists practice are rife with misunderstandings, disagreements, and unmet expectations, placing hospitalists at risk for conflict on a daily basis. Therefore the ability to understand and effectively manage conflict should be a core competency for all hospitalists. The first step in building effective conflict management skills is to understand the causes and potential benefits of conflict. Next, hospitalists should learn and apply key principles of conflict management; and finally, hospitalists need to develop competence and confidence in implementing useful strategies for managing different types of conflict.

SUGGESTED READINGS

Covey SR. *The 7 Habits of Highly Effective People.* New York, NY: Simon and Schuster; 1989:235–260.

DeChurch LA, and Marks MA. Maximizing the benefits of task conflict: The role of conflict management. *International Journal of Conflict Management.* 2001;(12):4–22.

Gilbert DT, and Malone PS. "The correspondence bias." *Psychological Bulletin.* 1995;(117): 21–38.

Holt JL, and DeVore CJ. Culture, gender, organizational role, and styles of conflict resolution: A meta-analysis. *International Journal of Intercultural Relations.* 2005;(29):165–196.

Jones EE, and Nisbett RE. *The Actor and the Observer: Divergent Perceptions of the Causes of Behavior.* New York, NY: General Learning Press; 1971.

Patterson K, Grenny J, McMillan, R, Switzler A, et al. *Crucial Conversations: Tools for Talking when Stakes are High.* New York, NY: McGraw Hill; 2002.

Ross L. "The intuitive psychologist and his shortcomings: Distortions in the attribution process." iIn Berkowitz L, (ed.) *Advances in Experimental Social Psychology.* (10:173–240), Orlando, FL: Academic Press; 1977.

Thomas KW, Thomas GF, Shaubhut N. Conflict styles of men and women at six organization levels. *International Journal of Conflict Management.* 2008;(19):148–166.

Triandis HC. *Individualism and Collectivism.* Boulder, CO: Westview Press; 1995.

REFERENCES

1. Patterson K, Grenny J, et al. *Crucial Conversations: Tools for Talking when Stakes are High.* New York, NY: McGraw Hill; 2002:45–51 and 68–74.
2. *Ibid.* 32–34 and 51–62.
3. The authors provide a free expanded version of the Style Under Stress Inventory online at https://www.vitalsmarts.com/styleunderstress.aspx, along with additional guidance on interpreting the results.
4. Heifetz RA, and Linsky M. *Leadership on the Line: Staying Alive through the Dangers of Leading.* Boston, MA: Harvard Business School Publishing; 2002: p.164.
5. Covey SR. *The 8th Habit.* New York, NY: Simon and Schuster; 2004:197–201.
6. Byham WC. *Zapp! Empowerment in Health Care.* New York, NY: Random House; 1993:145–146.
7. Fisher R, and Ury W. *Getting to Yes: Negotiating Agreement Without Giving In.* Boston, MA: Houghton Mifflin; 1981:16–98.

CHAPTER 26

Building, Growing, and Managing a Hospitalist Practice

Robert A. Bessler, MD

INTRODUCTION

According to the Society of Hospital Medicine (SHM), the number of hospitalists has increased from approximately 5,000 hospitalists in 2005 to more than 30,000 hospitalists in 2010. Despite this explosive growth and the fact that the majority of hospitals now have hospitalist programs, not all of them have been successful in establishing a thriving organization with staying power. The need for financial support of hospitalist programs and overextension of services coupled with recruitment issues, turnover, and leave of absences may lead to excessive workloads and possibly burnout. The overall annual turnover percentage of hospitalists is high, approximately 22% nationwide, despite opportunities to improve retention of physicians within a practice (SHM data). None of these issues are unique to Hospital Medicine and have been experienced by other geographically localized specialties including Emergency Medicine and critical care.

Patients and their families continue to express confusion about the role of hospitalists in their care and may misconstrue the term "hospitalists" for "hospice." Too often, hospitalists assume patients understand their presence at the bedside and neglect to take the time to explain their role as the *internal medicine physician* or family medicine physician responsible for patient care, assuming responsibility for everything from admission to discharge, including making patient rounds and ordering all needed tests and procedures. This failure in communication may leave patients and families feeling that their primary care provider has abandoned them, which may erode the patient hospitalist and patient-primary care provider relationship.

This chapter will explore the specific components essential to building, growing, and managing a thriving hospitalist practice with staying power.

STRATEGIC PLANNING

It is important to have a strategic plan for the practice around growth and the types of hospitals and programs best aligned with agreed upon goals and objectives. For example, strategic planning may require not aligning with all groups requesting support of the hospitalist team. If a group does not fit your strategic profile or geography, it may be best to decline the opportunity to manage a program. Depending on the goals of the practice, certain approaches may not promote patient satisfaction or continuity of care goals, as for example, when a hospital simply wants your team to cover admissions during the "off hours" that residents are not covering and then transfer patients to residents or surgeons during "peak hours." Obstacles of geographic distance requiring a day of travel of the core management team present an additional burden that make it best to pass up the opportunity without key management team members in place. Therefore, each hospitalist group should critically evaluate whether the growth into a new hospital makes sense based on the values and goals of the organization.

STRATEGIC PLANNING PROCESS

Before starting a practice it is critical to determine what factors predict the success or failure of strategic plans and those that the group defines as the business and financial motivators that impact on the decision to build, expand, and manage a hospitalist service.

In order to **build** a hospitalist practice, hospital leaders should:

- Define the clients, need for the program, the scope of services, and the type of employment model.

PRACTICE POINT

The hospitalist practice must start with a strategic planning process.

- *What are the goals of the practice?*
- *Where will the practice be located?*
- *Can we recruit to the location?*
- *What outcomes and metrics are we able to commit to as a group?*

- Articulate the mission, vision, values, and key value drivers of the practice.
- Determine the size of the program needed and the cost of the program.
- Set the compensation model.

After a program is up and running, successful practices may be faced with unprecedented **growth**. Hospital leaders will need to:

- Set expectations and priorities for growth.
- Define key stakeholders.
- Plan for growth.
- Assess the evolving needs of the service, such as using midlevel providers and the pros and cons of caps on services.
- Determine the skills in a hospitalist practice and the need for additional physician training.
- Reassess the compensation model as the needs of the service change.

From the building stage forward, there is a constant need for outstanding **management** to ensure a hospitalist practice thrives by using the steps provided in the following tables: (**Tables 26-1, 26-2,** and **26-3**)

- Define the right leadership and structure.
- Create an ownership mentality.
- Setting up the right processes.
- Tracking and reporting actionable data.
- Promoting outreach to the physician community and facilitating transitions of care.

TABLE 26-1 Building a Hospitalist Program: Key Factors to Consider

Characteristics	Examples
Recruiting	• Is the location conducive to recruiting hospitalists? Do they need to recruit a leader?
Compensation plan	• What is the market rate?
Patient encounters per physician	• What is the number of patients at 7 AM census? • What total number of patient encounters will physicians manage per day?
Schedule	• Is a tradition block schedule feasible? • Do you offer additional vacation days?
Management support	• What local support is required? • What regional support is required?
Tools to support communications, charge capture, scheduling, metrics	• How will hospitalists record charges? • Is there a convenient method to communicate to PCPs? • How will you demonstrate improvement in performance? • How will the group demonstrate quality?
Clinical processes development	• What best practices does the group adopt? • How do the processes impact care?

TABLE 26-2 Growing a Hospitalist Program: Core Values and Goals

Characteristics	Examples
Quality	• Measure length of stay • Measure readmissions rate • Measure CMS core measures • Measure time of discharge • Measure case mix index
Satisfaction	• Measure patient satisfaction • Measure nursing satisfaction • Measure PCP satisfaction • Measure specialist satisfaction • Measure administrative staff satisfaction
Efficiency	• Determine how to improve admission and discharge efficiency
Innovation	• What tools can be developed to support the team's core values?
Teamwork	• Determine how the team interacts with monthly and quarterly meetings. • How do you organize in teams? • What is the role of midlevel providers?
Leadership	• Is there a leadership development training path? • Is there a medical director or chief hospitalist on the site? • Are there regional leaders for clinical and business operations?
Financial	• Does the group charge a fee for services? • What are the overhead costs to manage the practice? • Is there a clear return on investment for the hospital to retain services of the group?
Integrity	• What guidance does the team provide to the physicians in the group? • How do we manage the impact of actions, values, methods, measures, principles, expectations, and outcomes of the team? • What criteria are used to assess integrity of candidates?
Research	• Is the group involved in research? • Is there support for data collection and analysis? • What funding is available to the group to support research?
PCP satisfaction	• How does the group measure PCP satisfaction? • Does the group reach out to the PCPs? • How does the group track referrals from PCPs?
Nursing satisfaction	• How does the group measure nursing satisfaction? • Does the group interface with nursing? • How does the group track nursing impact on outcomes?
Specialist satisfaction	• How does the group measure specialist satisfaction? • Does the group reach out to the specialist? • How does the group track referrals from specialists?

TABLE 26-3 Managing a Hospitalist Program: Key Strategies for Effective Management

Characteristics	Examples
Recruiting	• How does the group identify new hires? • Does the group use a recruiting agency?
Overhead	• What percentage of revenue is allocated to support programs (overhead)? • Do costs incorporate utilization of midlevels, nurses, support staff, and locums?
Training	• What allocation of resources does the group have for CME training? • How are new group members trained? • How are leaders mentored?
Growth	• Does the group want to expand? • Is the group capable of taking on additional patients at the primary site?
Service lines	• Does the group focus on acute care contracts with traditional hospitalists? • Does the group provide intensivists services? • Are there other service lines to consider: surgicalists, laborists, academic hospitalists?
Improvement strategies	• Where is the group's focus on quality? Efficiency? Satisfaction?

BUILDING A HOSPITALIST PRACTICE

Building a hospitalist practice starts with defining the clients and the need for a hospitalist program. In many community hospitals, a hospitalist program is created to care for the unassigned patient population. But even the definition of an unassigned patient is subject to much interpretation. For example, at many hospitals in the Puget Sound region of Washington State, an unassigned patient is any patient showing up in the emergency department (ED) and requiring admission who does not have a primary care doctor that admits patients at the hospital. In contrast, in Orlando, Florida, an unassigned patient is only defined as a patient who has no primary care doctor. In Orlando, if a patient has a primary care provider but that doctor does not have admitting privileges, it is standard practice to call the primary care provider to identify who will care for the patient in the hospital.

PRACTICE POINT

The *needs assessment*, from the perspective of the hospital might include:

- PCP and/or surgical dissatisfaction
- Admission and management of unassigned patients
- Admission and management of overflow patients due to American College of Graduate Medical Education (ACGME) work hour restrictions
- High inpatient census and long average length of stay (ALOS)
- Low reported performance measures
- External regulation (rapid response teams, code teams, etc)

In addition to covering the unassigned patient population, many hospitalist services cover those primary care providers (PCPs) who do not want the responsibility of admitting their own patients. There are two main forms of coverage relationships: coverage arrangements for 24 hours per day, 7 days per week; and coverage which is more like a house staff model in which the hospitalist admits the patients but then turns the care back over to the PCP the next day. These latter models continue to decline in numbers because of difficulty with recruitment of high quality doctors motivated to build a meaningful career with a resident-type model.

Hospitalist programs may also be created to manage medical specialty and surgical patients, usually after establishment of the initial hospitalist program.

It is essential to determine which patients the hospitalist group will manage, the scope of services, and whether additional training for some of the program members will be required. According to SHM, 78% of practicing hospitalists are trained in general internal medicine, and another 4% in an internal medicine subspecialty, most commonly pulmonary or critical care medicine. About 3% of hospitalists are trained in family practice; about 8% in pediatrics; and 2% in med-peds. The remaining 5% are nonphysician providers, usually nurse practitioners and physician assistants. If the medical patients are the first priority regardless of their demographic, leaders then need to consider severity of illness.

In most community hospitals today, hospitalists manage ICU patients in large part due to the shortage of critical care physicians (less than 5,000 in the U.S.). In general, the larger the hospital the less ICU medicine a hospitalist performs. Many hospitals have mandatory ICU consults after a set number of days or hours in the ICU or they provide specific guidelines on managing ventilated patients. The most popular model may be a hybrid arrangement in which access to a critical care physician occurs during the day and for emergencies but in-house at night. In such cases the hospitalist commonly does the work around admissions and daily visits with a consult and a follow-up visit by the pulmonary critical care physicians.

With the labor shortage being even more severe for critical care, hybrid models, along with the advent of telemedicine, are likely to take on even more ICU coverage responsibilities in the future. In general, leapfrog compliance guidelines drive a dedicated intensivist model, typically mandated in regional and tertiary hospitals.

"Code coverage" also defines the scope of the hospitalist practice. Many hospitals provide a separate code team, made up of the Emergency Medicine physician or in-house intensivist plus respiratory therapy, nurses, technicians, and pharmacists. Increasingly, hospitalists are being asked to partake in responding to the code process and arranging patient transfers to the ICU. In general, emergency physicians have more training and chances to keep their skills sharp around the procedures of a code, including intubation, starting central lines, and transvenous pacing. Typically, while an Emergency Medicine physician may respond first, a hospitalist with advanced cardiac life support (ACLS) training assumes leadership of the code.

Whether the hospitalist scheduled for the night shift is actually in the hospital or at home on call for emergencies also defines the scope of practice. Hospital-employed and hospital-contracted models tend to have in-house coverage while physicians who are part of a private fee-for-service group without a hospital contract tend to be available as an on-call physician available from home. Variables that impact the decision beyond economics include the volume of cross-coverage patients, the number of admissions per night, coexisting resident coverage, and the response time of the physician, if on call from home.

DEFINING THE TYPE OF EMPLOYMENT MODEL

There are several common employment models for hospitalist practices: employed by a private practice, by a hospital, by a multispecialty group, by a health plan/HMO, or a multisite or national practice. Among the multisite or national practice subgroups there are staffing solutions that specialize in Emergency Medicine, anesthesia, and a host of other physician specialists. Some of these multi-site specialty practices will hire hospitalists who work as independent contractors alongside the specialist. Among the national hospitalist groups there is a wide spectrum of employment arrangements ranging from those offering ownership and partnership to those that operate solely with independent contractors.

DEFINING THE MISSION, VISION, VALUES, AND KEY VALUE DRIVERS OF YOUR PRACTICE

It is critically important to define the mission, vision, and values of the practice from its inception. The leaders and hospitalists should take this task seriously. Schedule time to discuss and debate what is important to the group and leadership. The process of constructing your program's mission and vision statement should not be taken lightly. This process can take weeks to develop. Start by establishing dedicated time and secure an environment that is conducive to having uninterrupted, frank discussions. Enlist the input of all team members.

A **mission statement** explains the overall purpose of the hospitalist practice. The mission statement articulates what the organization does right now, in the most general sense. In this way, the mission also sets parameters for what the organization, through omission, does not do. Example of a mission statement: "The Hospitalist Group of Hilltop builds healthy relationships between St. John's Hospital and primary care providers in the community through public education and direct assistance services."

By comparison, the **vision statement** articulates the future of the organization and the community that it serves. The vision statement, when compared with the current reality of the organization or the community, implies the work still needs to be accomplished. In this way, it lends credibility and motivation to the mission statement. Example of a vision statement: "The Hospitalist Group envisions a group practice that drives improvements in patient outcomes including evidence that reflects our value to hospitals in our community."

On a yearly basis the practice should define key value drivers that articulate the focus of the organization and those areas that require organizational focus in order for the business to grow. Key value drivers (KVDs) should be set by the leaders with input from the entire team. KVDs must be easy to remember, measurable, and achievable. The behaviors that support the key values should also be clearly defined. In doing so, those in the practice will have a clear understanding of expectations even prior to joining the practice. These behaviors should be reinforced through the compensation and promotion practices of the group to make the practice values meaningful and alive on a daily basis. Typically teams evaluate progress on KVDs monthly or quarterly.

ESTABLISHING METRICS AND SETTING NEW GOALS FOR PERFORMANCE AND OUTCOMES

Standard performance metrics including average length of stay, core measures, case mix index, cost per case, and discharge efficiency are expected by hospital administration. It is essential to meet with the hospital and obtain agreement on which initiatives the hospitalist team will focus. Establish a data collection and reporting mechanism and the frequency of assessments. There are practice metrics that are becoming increasingly important to hospitals including (**Figure 26-1**)

- PCP referral volume and referral patterns
- Patient satisfaction and referral ratings
- Physician recruiting efficiency
- Physician retention rates
- 30-day same diagnosis readmission rates

MARKETING YOUR HOSPITALIST SERVICES

The best marketing generates word-of-mouth public relations based on how satisfied your patients are as well as the nursing and other hospital staff. An effective campaign requires all hospitalists on the team be fully engaged with the practice's mission.

In addition to the passive marketing that comes from word-of-mouth marketing, it is important to develop a marketing plan. A typical marketing plan for a practice includes initiatives that drive patient satisfaction to generating awareness in the community through PCP outreach. Create a budget that supports the plan.

PRACTICE POINT

Your marketing plan should include segments that target the following areas:

- **Identify Your Target Markets:** *Decide which target markets you want to canvas. You can either target referrals in specific geographic areas or by targeting outreach to specialists*
- **Develop a Public Relations Plan:** *Launch a new program with press releases, open house events, or broadcast the addition to new physicians through flyers or direct mail campaigns*
- **Create a Promotion/Awareness Plan:** *You can develop practice-branded written articles on a variety of topics that convey answers to patients' questions using topics such as What is a Hospitalist? or Improving Patient's Health Literacy. Use these in a mailing to your community or have the hospital place your articles in their newsletter.*
- **Develop Patient Satisfaction Tools:** *Create large, oversized business cards with photos of physicians, hospitalist brochures with photos of engaged, friendly physicians; consider Web-based information to share with patients.*
- **Create Recruiting Advertisements for Physicians:** *Provide your recruiter with materials about the job or special information about the location. Place them in hospitalist journals as print advertisements and classified ads.*
- **Conduct Market Research:** *Conduct market research in your local area to be sure you know what the local market is paying for hospitalists and places they practice and who might be interested in joining your practice in the area.*
- **Profile Your Team:** *Utilize a website and direct mail with photography of your team or host an open house or educational event.*

DESIGNING THE MODEL

It is essential to determine the size of the practice needed. The volume of patients who will be seen on a daily, nightly, and monthly basis determines the size of the practice. Next, assess the number of physicians required to meet the needs of the practice based on that estimated patient volume. The number of physicians depends on what is considered an acceptable workload of patients to manage per day, per night, and per month. To determine the number of patients, define the average number of admissions per day. If the emergency department uses a tracking tool, review the data to project the number of unassigned patients based on historical data. In many hospitals, this data is not accessible prior to initiating a program. Historically, the ward clerks simply entered the admitting physician's name in the hospital information system without mention of the fact that the patient did not have a primary care physician. It is essential to have a way to track the types of patients by referral type (eg, by PCP, unassigned, or consultations) when the hospitalist program begins operation.

In addition to determining the volume of unassigned patients, estimate the number of PCPs interested in turning over care. The only risk of double counting is if no hospitalist program existed prior to a new program starting up. Typically, in that scenario, the primary care provider was also likely cover unassigned patients.

After determining the number of admissions per year, divide the admissions by 365 days per year to obtain a rough estimate of the number of physicians required. Then take the average length of stay for the patients and add 1 extra for the day of discharge. Take this

Quarterly dashboard
Sample hospital report

Encounters/Month	
Month of data	May 2009
Value	1,505
Goal	1,200
Variance	306

GMLOS	
Month of data	May 2009
Value	3.79
Benchmark	3.49
Variance	0.5

GMLOS: CMS GMLOS	
Month of data	May 2009
Value	88.3%
Benchmark	80%
Variance	8.30%

Case mix index	
Month of data	May 2009
Value	1.32
Benchmark	1.3
Variance	0.02

Time of discharge order	
Month of data	May 2009
Value	66.2%
Benchmark/Goal	70%
Variance	–3.80%

Core measures	
Month of data	May 2009
Value	80%
Goal	82%
Variance	–2%

Total direct cost per dschg	
Month of data	May 2009
Value	$5,347
Goal	$5.250
Variance	147

Combined HCAHPS score	
Month of data	May 2009
Value	77.8%
Goal	79%
Variance	1.20%

Other PCP volume	
Month of data	May 2009
Value	220
Goal	150
Variance	70

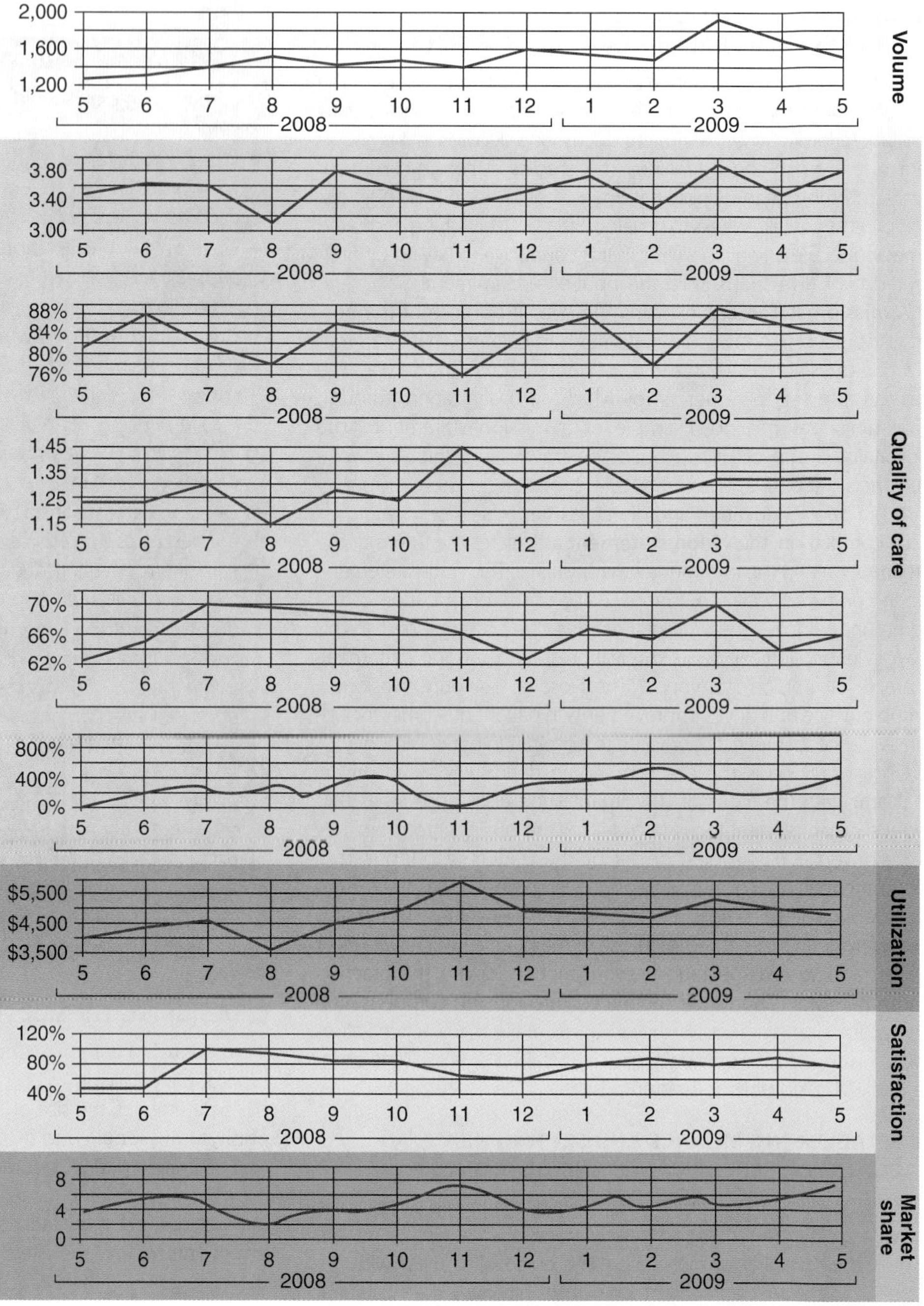

Figure 26-1 *A dashboard organized by volume of patients, quality, utilization, satisfaction performance, and market data indicators.*

number and multiply it by the number of admissions per day to determine the 7:00 AM census. For example, if there are 5 admissions per day with an average 4-day length of stay, the 7:00 AM census would be calculated as 5 × (4 ALOS + 1) = 25 patients at 7:00 AM. With the 7:00 AM census determined, calculate the number of the physicians per morning required for the hospitalist program.

There is much debate over the most appropriate census for the physician who begins rounding at 7:00 AM. In general, based on a typical mix of a few ICU patients and the balance of the load being medical patients, a hospitalist can manage 15 patients safely and efficiently. This number varies considerably due to the different agendas, acuity of patients, concomitant responsibilities such as rapid response teams, code teams, teaching, and goals of practices. In order to achieve a goal of early discharge and multiple visits a day with a considerable amount of committee involvement, hospitalists can maintain a census in the range of 12 to 15 patients. If the goal is productivity, and in some cases the use of nonphysician providers and physician extenders, the volume per hospitalist may be as high as 20 patients per day. Some practices define the census as the number of encounters per day, which include new admissions as well as discharges.

In a pure productivity-driven private practice model, the night shifts are often covered from home (eg, only coming back to the hospital for emergencies). This typically also means that the day shift doctors might share night call, even after working all day. In many practices today, the night shift is covered by a separate physician, nocturnists, due to the volume of admissions at night and the volume of cross-cover work needed.

In general, the billing revenues of a nocturnist will be lower than a day-shift hospitalist's.

A highly prevalent hospital-employed and national group practice model includes a schedule in which the hospitalist physician is on duty for 12 hours, 7 days a week and the following week the physicians is off for 7 days. There are also hybrid arrangements in which the physician works about the same total number of hours per month but with shorter periods of time on duty. In such a model, a 7:00 AM census of 25 to 30 patients would likely have 6 full-time physicians. In contrast, a private group model may take every fourth night of call from home, which could be managed with four full-time physicians on the team. The marketplace supply and demand for physicians and goals of various clients (eg, a hospital, HMO, or payor) often dictates the type of model required.

DETERMINING THE COST AND DIRECT COST OF THE HOSPITALIST PROGRAM

Calculating the cost of a hospitalist program includes direct labor costs: salaries of the physicians, benefits cost, malpractice coverage, and billing costs. The volume of patient visits, the payer mix, and the distribution of CPT codes reported determine the direct patient care revenues of the practice. The medical director who typically has responsibility for driving hospital outcomes will determine any additional revenues. According to a survey conducted by the Society of Hospital Medicine in 2008, 95% of hospitalist programs required some sort of subsidy or fee to help with the payer mix of the unassigned patients, night call coverage in-house, and for those organizations that focus on driving performance through service offerings. The ranges of fees hospitals pay range from $0 per year to $200,000 per physician annually. Fees are typically based on scope of work and payer mix.

SETTING THE COMPENSATION MODEL

In conjunction with determining the cost of the program, a compensation model must be established. In the past decade two significant challenges drove hospitalist compensation: an imbalance of supply and demand was coupled with a rapid rise of salaries, which started to escalate in 2001. This phenomenon has created a significant compression in salaries. Often the least experienced physician's compensation is closely aligned with the most experienced physicians in the practice. This compensation compression creates a dichotomy in the reward system with respect to physician skill and experience levels creating challenging team dynamics. There are two primary models: a pure productivity model and a pure salary model. Many salary models also include a component of compensation focused on productivity and quality metrics as well as outcomes, as described in chapter 27.

Recruiting a team of physicians and hiring a leader is a critical core competency for every hospitalist practice as discussed in chapter 29. Acquiring effective recruiting techniques is an area of investment that should not be minimized or overlooked in the development of a strong hospitalist practice.

GROWING A HOSPITALIST PRACTICE

SETTING PRIORITIES FOR GROWTH

Once the practice is launched, priorities must be established for the growth of the hospitalist program. If the unassigned patients are already covered in the practice, the next step could be a myriad of other opportunities, including contracting with PCP practices. It is essential to understand the scope of growth and prepare in advance of the patients' arrival. Many practices have failed or imploded by taking on more growth than they could handle. If there is a desire to handle 15 more patients per day with a 7 days on/7 days off model, it might be as simple as figuring out the need to hire 2 more physicians. But, if the program is already quite busy and adding 3 to 4 new admissions per day is in the growth plans, adding an admitting shift may be called for as well.

PRACTICE POINT

Use these common areas of practice management and determine whether you are prepared to grow.

Reflect about your hospitalist practice:

- *What are your priorities?*
- *What are your goals and core values?*
- *What effort can you invest to grow?*

What are the expectations of external interests?

- Performance measures
- Satisfaction of outside primary care physician groups
- The Joint Commission requirements
- ACGME
- Public performance reporting, obtaining ≥ 90% core measure scores

What is your work environment saying about the practice?

- Patient safety, quality, satisfaction
- Efficiency of care
- Career satisfaction which integrates core values:
  - Service excellence and patient safety
  - Continuous quality improvement and innovation
  - Professional growth, leadership, and scholarship

What are the expectations of hospital management?

- Caring for unassigned/uncompensated patients
- Reducing ALOS for top 10 DRGs by hospitalist discharge volume
- 24/7 service demands
- Reducing practice variation of hospitalists
- Hospitalist training on palliative care, end-of-life, and other medical specialties
- Development of a comanagement consultative service or a preoperative testing center
- Improvement of patient ED to floor times and/or care of admitted patients in the ED, management of a chest pain unit or rapid admission team
- Improvement of chart documentation for core measures (such as smoking cessation counseling)
- Improvement of billing for services provided
- Leadership of rapid response teams for ill inpatients

Does the practice have these evaluations and measurements in place?

- Report card for hospitalists
- Primary care physician survey
- Multiyear strategic planning, quarterly reports
- Hospitalist career satisfaction survey
- Hospitalist annual retreat with management to establish goals
  - Develop a 3-year plan for a hospitalist service that mirrors the hospital's multiyear plan
  - Create a meaningful, motivating, and achievable blueprint for clinical enterprise
  - Proactively support mission of patient care, quality improvement, and patient-centered care.

DEFINING KEY STAKEHOLDERS

The key stakeholders in the practice need to be clearly defined. Certainly the doctors in the practice are key stakeholders, but in many practices the hospital administration is also a key stakeholder. Identifying priorities is much like a game of chess. For example, if you choose to help solve another primary care group's needs before helping the orthopedic group with comanagement needs there may be repercussions. You should expect that the hospital administrator will want to weigh in on how this decision impacts the hospital and its development plans.

USING NONPHYSICIAN PROVIDERS

Another key decision for program growth is how to use nonphysician providers in the practice. While this topic is covered in the literature, there are plenty of mixed opinions on the use of midlevel providers in the inpatient setting. We have found two main areas of optimal benefit in our practices.

The first benefit for incorporating nurse practitioners (NPs) and physician assistants (PAs) is in very small programs of four full-time physicians with a daily census that can have dramatic swings around the average. The cost of an NP or PA provider is about one-half the labor cost of a physician and this can be a cost-effective way to leverage the existing physician coverage.

There is also a benefit from the use of nonphysician providers in very large programs, particularly in the management of surgical patients for their comorbid conditions. Many practices have incorporated nonphysician providers due to the physician shortage and a failure to recruit and retain high quality physicians. One unique challenge is that many nonphysician providers' value comes from their experience. A nonphysician provider practicing in the acute care setting for 10 years is much more likely to be able to function as a midlevel hospitalist than a new graduate nonphysician provider. For hospitalist physicians there is clearly value and competency in new a physician starting to work directly upon completing their training.

TYPES OF PHYSICIANS USED IN THE PRACTICE

Another area of importance in growing a hospitalist practice involves the types of physicians utilized. It is becoming more common to have family medicine-trained hospitalists practicing alongside internal medicine hospitalists in the same practice. Much has been debated on this topic and about 8% of hospitalists nationwide are family medicine trained. Factors that go into the determination to hire them include their comfort level with ICU patients and their experience managing the higher-level acuity patients. Another challenge is their ability to navigate the local politics associated with an internal medicine outpatient practice referring its inpatient practice to a family medicine physician. We have found that the experience of the provider trumps all board certification. There are plenty of internal medicine physicians not qualified to be hospitalists as well.

THE PROS AND CONS OF CAPS ON SERVICES

During the hospitalist practice growth phase, the group must be able to handle all of the new patients it agreed to accept or have a Plan B. Plan B might include a floodgate that closes in the form of a cap. This has been achieved at some hospitals to maintain safe and effective volumes. Two types of caps exist including those requiring a backup system. The backup system can be the existing hospitalists at a very high labor cost to a hospital or the new group of primary care physicians who have asked for coverage; this group may need to agree to occasionally provide coverage at the hospital. The latter group of physicians tends to be a short-term patch; they can quickly lose their skills and credentialing in the inpatient setting. Ideally, if the hospitalist group has agreed to accept a new group of patients, they need to have the capacity 24 hours per day, 7 days per week. A "sick call" rotation to cover anticipated maternity and paternity leaves as well as unexpected absences in a "young" specialty may have the benefit of allowing hospitalists to focus on career development, especially quality improvement initiatives, when they are not seeing patients, and not overwhelming them with service obligations.

MANAGING THE HOSPITALIST PRACTICE

SELECTING THE RIGHT LEADERSHIP AND STRUCTURE

There is a shortage of high quality physician leaders in the United States. To properly manage the practice, it is critical to appoint the most capable physician leader and establish an effective practice structure. The hospitalist leaders' roles are complex; they not only serve the hospitalists' team but also play significant roles within the hospital. In these roles, hospitalist directors are the most connected to how things actually work on a daily basis. Strong hospitalist physician leaders must lead by example. They must have effective organizational skills, be great communicators, and seek win-win situations for the hospitalist team, medical staff, and hospital. Hospitalist leaders also need to be aware of the professional goals of their members and delegate some responsibilities so that each member can also flourish and find a professional niche within the organization. Hospitalist directors may become isolated in their role, so it is important to ensure that they have advocates or mentors who can promote their agendas as well as provide counselling related to hospital politics. See Chapter 18 on Leadership.

Many hospitalist programs include a version of shift work. This type of schedule combined with the Generation Y culture in medical school today, *centered on work hours and patient volume restrictions,* have led to a unique challenge in Hospital Medicine. Many physicians seek outright employment models. They value time off at a very high level and it can be a challenge to engage them in what matters to make a practice successful. Ensuring the right job fit begins with the initial job interview during which performance expectations are clearly articulated.

CREATING AN OWNERSHIP MENTALITY

Like any small business, an ownership mentality is essential to the success of the hospitalist practice. How to instill the ownership mentality starts in the hiring process. Those applicants who take initiative and give solid examples of times in their career where they got involved, did things because they did not think anyone else could do it better, and were passionate about those experiences are telling. These are typically indicators that the physician is the type of hospitalist who will make the practice great. Defining the behaviors that support the values of the practice and then evaluating and rewarding those behaviors will go a long way to reinforcing what is important. For example, if participating in hospitalist committees is important, it can be rewarded as part of how the productivity dollars are allotted. Leading a hospital committee or playing a leadership role within the medical staff could be rewarded to an even greater extent.

SETTING UP THE RIGHT PROCESSES

Part of managing the practice is ensuring that the right processes are in place. Processes should be established for physician scheduling to daily case management meetings. Hospitalist processes should be highly sophisticated to drive improvements in utilization, documentation, discharge planning, and prospective quality metric monitoring. All of these processes require a tremendous amount of time, energy, and in many cases, technology and infrastructure to drive clinical and financial performance for the hospital and hospitalist practice. The scope of processes is beyond the scope of this chapter but this is a core competency that should not be overlooked in the management of an effective hospitalist program. Hospitalist leaders can promote simple solutions that make it easy for clinicians to communicate at transition points such as setting up dedicated phone lines in primary care practices so that the hospitalists do not waste valuable time trying to reach PCPs. Post discharge follow-up phone calls can be delegated to nonhospitalists such as case managers.

THE VALUE OF DATA TRACKING AND REPORTING

The well-known saying "you can't manage what you don't measure" is quite true in Hospital Medicine. It is essential to define what is important to the practice and measure those outcomes that matter most. Many require sophisticated technology solutions and partnerships with the hospital to obtain data. Benchmarking performance and then creating an action plan to improve upon areas is an effective approach that should be evaluated on a monthly and quarterly basis.

Metrics that matter on the revenue side of the equation include:

- Volume
- Work RVUs total
- Work RVU/CPT code
- Payer mix
- Collections per encounter (accrued)
- Charges
- Collections per month

On the labor cost side of the equation, there are a myriad of labor cost metrics. However, cost per shift is a commonly used metric that helps to effectively manage the performance of the practice, inclusive of benefits for the providers.

Outside of financial performance of the practice, there exist three main areas of performance monitoring: quality, utilization, and satisfaction.

For quality, most practices manage core measure performance. Readmission rate is also measured. In the coming years, it is likely that hospitals will be financially penalized for readmissions that occur within 7 to 14 days of the patient's prior admission. This will take added focus and processes, as the etiology surrounding readmissions is so multifactorial. Mortality and complication rates will take on added importance in the years ahead as well.

Utilization is a challenge for the average practice without a deep investment in infrastructure. Discharge order time by physician and utilization of the follow-up CPT codes to discharge codes are other great measures of throughput for the average hospitalist. The more follow-up visits a doctor has within a group compared to the same number of discharges of his or her peers could indicate the physician holds on to patients longer. Clearly, to be statistically valid, a large enough sample size will be needed to compare to peers, regardless. Other important metrics include cost per case by major DRG group.

The third pillar of a high quality hospitalist program is to measure satisfaction. Patient, PCP, nurse, and hospital administration satisfaction are key areas to track. Surveys and call centers are effective tools to track and analyze performance and test the effectiveness of improvement initiatives.

By identifying the parameters for measurement, any hospitalist service can develop a hospitalist scorecard to clarify the vision and strategy of the service by gaining consensus regarding what will be measured and reported. The scorecard requires setting targets, aligning strategic initiatives, allocating resources, and establishing milestones. Once these goals have been set, a process of communication and education of the members of the service must take place about the goals and linking rewards to performance measures. There are pitfalls relating compensation to quality of care if the candidate measure is not attainable or if the performance measure is linked to flawed data. Computer-generated data is much easier to obtain than chart review but is often based on the discharging physician, which may or may not reflect an individual's performance. Supplemented with primary care satisfaction data and chart review of key quality indicators such as transfers to intensive care units and/or readmissions, the hospitalist service can initiate rapid cycle improvements and educational initiatives, the impact of which can be tracked over time.

PHYSICIAN OUTREACH TO THE COMMUNITY OF PHYSICIANS

A successful practice ideally includes the community of physicians raving about the hospitalist group they partner with for their inpatient coverage. Many practices have imploded by not building relationships with the community of primary care providers and specialists. An outreach plan and daily communication on shared patients are essential to building the bridges necessary to the medical staff. Nothing is more important to this communication than a phone call at discharge linking the patient back to the community physician and, as a bonus, having the opportunity for the hospitalist to let the community doctor know what a great job he or she did for the patient during the hospitalization. Faxing, electronic messaging through an EMR, or e-mailing in an HIPAA-compliant way all of the necessary information on discharge is also an essential element to this process.

TRANSITIONS OF CARE BACK TO THE COMMUNITY

In the near future, it will also be essential to link the inpatient hospitalization to the continuum of care in the post-acute environment for those patients not discharged directly home. With the advent of bundled payments for hospitals and the penalties associated with readmissions for the same diagnosis within a specified time frame, there will be a clear need to improve the transition of care to the skilled nursing, long-term acute care, rehabilitation, and assisted living environments. Many successful practices are already on the forefront of this by placing partner physicians in these facilities on the same hospitalist platform as their acute care partners.

INTEGRATION TO THE POST-ACUTE PHYSICIAN

Finally, for those patients discharged from the hospital back to their home, it is essential that the hospitalist ensures a smooth transition. The window of time from when patients are discharged from acute care until they have a follow-up visit with their PCP is an especially risky timeframe for adverse outcomes and readmissions. Instituting a patient call-back program to check on patients post-discharge, having a way to track this data, and intervening in the care pathway when necessary is an essential process for a high quality hospitalist program.

CONCLUSION

The creation of new hospitalist practices is likely to continue in the coming decade with the changes forthcoming in our health care delivery system. Building, growing, and managing a successful and thriving hospitalist practice can be accomplished by focusing on certain essential elements.

SUGGESTED READINGS

Dye CF. *Leadership in Healthcare: Essential Values and Skills*. Chicago, IL: Health Administration Press; 2010.

Kaufman KP. *Best Practice Financial Management: Six Key Concepts for Healthcare Leaders*. Chicago, IL: Health Administration Press; 2006.

Levoy B. *222 Secrets of Hiring, Managing, and Retaining Great Employees in Healthcare Practices*. Sudbury, MA: Jones and Bartlett Publishers; 2006.

Lee BD, Herring JW. *Growing Leaders in Healthcare: Lessons from the Corporate World*. Health Administration Press. Chicago, IL: Health Administration Press; 2009.

Maccoby M. *Leaders We Need: And What Makes Us Follow*. Boston, MA: Harvard Business School Publishing; 2007.

Murphy S. *Building and Rewarding Your Team: A How-To Guide for Medical Practices*. Englewood, CO: MGMA; 2008.

Nemeth C. *Improving Healthcare Team Communication*. Burlington, VT: Ashgate Publishing; 2008.

Simone KG. *Hospitalist Recruitment and Retention: Building a Hospital Medicine Program*. Hoboken, NJ: Wiley-Blackwell; 2009.

Zahaluk DW. *The Ultimate Practice Building Book: How To Regain Control Of Your Practice, Achieve A Competitive Advantage In Your Local Market, And Reconnect With The Joy Of Medicine In The New Healthcare Economy*. Bloomington, IN: Trafford Publishing; 2007.

CHAPTER 27

Designing a Hospitalist Compensation and Bonus Plan

John Nelson, MD, MHM

INTRODUCTION

Hospitalist compensation can be thought of as consisting of two components: the amount of total compensation, including all elements such as base salary and bonus (sometimes referred to collectively as total W-2 wages); and the method by which it is earned. Both the amount and method of hospitalist compensation have evolved significantly over the last 10 to 15 years. However, the attributes of a desirable compensation plan have remained unchanged.

NECESSARY ATTRIBUTES OF A WELL-DESIGNED COMPENSATION PLAN

EASY TO UNDERSTAND

Any compensation plan should be simple enough that the hospitalist can explain it from memory. Complicated formulas used as the basis for paying a quality bonus or end-of-year "profit distribution" are problematic if the hospitalists do not fully understand them. A significant value of a salary bonus is to influence and reward behavior, but if the method of calculating the bonus is hard to understand then it is likely to be much less effective in bringing about this change. Disputes and resentment may arise when a doctor has misunderstood the formula and anticipated a larger bonus than the one that was paid.

PRACTICE POINT

Any compensation plan should:

- Be simple enough that the hospitalist can explain it from memory
- Be easy to defend in public
- Comply with all laws and regulations
- Have the ability to be modified over time
- Reward good work

EASY TO DEFEND IN PUBLIC

Despite efforts to keep the details of a compensation plan private, it will nearly always become public information either through a member of the practice talking about it to others at the "home" hospital or elsewhere. Or it could become public during a malpractice suit. In either case, the practice should think carefully in advance whether it could lead to significant embarrassment. For example, a financial reward for hospitalists' reducing length of stay could be seen as an incentive to send patients home so aggressively that some are sent home before they are ready. This could be very embarrassing and damaging information if it were made public.

COMPLIES WITH ALL LAWS AND REGULATIONS

The laws and regulations governing physician compensation and the financial relationships between doctors and hospitals or other entities are complex and always changing. It is important to ensure that any proposed compensation plan is reviewed by someone knowledgeable in these areas. Despite good intentions, it can be easy to inadvertently violate a legal requirement when designing a compensation plan.

CAN BE MODIFIED OVER TIME

Even if a compensation plan seems perfect today, it is very likely that the practice will evolve within just a few years so that the plan is no longer a good match with current reality, and it may even cause problems and inhibit the ability of the practice to make necessary adjustments in scheduling and other areas. For example, compensating hospitalists at a set dollar amount per shift worked may be reasonable today, but it might not be long before the schedule will need to change so that some shifts are longer or shorter and no longer match the single shift rate in the compensation plan. Because big changes to a compensation plan are difficult and time consuming, a practice might decide to simply keep the compensation plan as it is and forgo making the needed scheduling changes. In this case, the compensation plan is an impediment to effective practice operations. Compensating hospitalists based on hours of work or productivity, though having problems of their own, will in many practices come closer to automatically adjusting to other changes such as scheduling adjustments and changes in patient volume.

REWARDS GOOD WORK

Ideally, a compensation plan should encourage and reward the performance and behaviors that the practice desires. This might mean that a portion of total compensation is tied to the doctor's citizenship in the practice, or to performance on quality measures or other domains. The amount of money at stake, and the thresholds that trigger payment to the doctor must be planned carefully to ensure that they influence behavior and are not seen as too easy or too difficult to reach.

AMOUNT OF HOSPITALIST COMPENSATION

The amount of total hospitalist salary, including salary and bonus or incentive payments, has been rising steadily since the Society of Hospital Medicine[1] (SHM) first began collecting data in 1997. Some of this increase can be explained by increases in salary to keep up with inflation. A portion of the increase can be explained by increases in average hospitalist productivity; hospitalists are either working harder or more efficiently, which has likely had a role in increasing salaries. But probably the most significant factor leading to increases in salary is the excess demand for hospitalists that has outstripped the supply of doctors to fill the positions. This has led many organizations to increase salaries and provide incentives such as a sign-on bonus.

Table 27-1 provides the most recent national mean and median hospitalist compensation data available prior to the publication of this book. National measures of central tendency are only a starting point and a thorough understanding of the data requires a review of parameters like standard deviation, percentile rank, and so forth. It is also critical to understand the survey population, how terms were defined and the questions were asked, and to review subsets of the data based on region of the country, employer (eg, private practice or hospital employed), and other domains.

In locales where there are many open hospitalist positions, local market forces such as one's metropolitan area may be more influential than national surveys in determining competitive compensation levels for a particular practice. That is, knowledge of compensation and workload at the nearest hospitals may be just as important, or more important, than the results of national surveys. The compensation for nonhospitalist work can be influential also. For example, internists working as hospitalists typically earn more than the average for internists in office practice in the same area.

[1]Originally named the National Association of Inpatient Physicians.

TABLE 27-1 Compensation and Workloads for Hospitalists that Care for Adult Patients. From SHM and MGMA State of Hospital Medicine 2011 Report Based on 2010 Data

	Median	Mean
Salary	$220,619	$225,760
Retirement Benefits	$16,500	$19,990
Encounters	2,236	2,376
Work RVUs	4,166	4,257

MGMA, Medical Group Management Association; SHM, Society of Hospital Medicine. Note that salary includes all direct compensation (eg, W2 wages) including any salary bonus or incentive compensation.

PRACTICE POINT

- Knowledge of compensation and workload at the nearest hospitals may be just as important, or more important, than the results of national surveys.

SOURCES OF DATA ON HOSPITALIST COMPENSATION AND WORKLOAD

The figures provided in Table 27-1 are provided for illustration purposes, and will be of limited value soon after this book is published. However, an understanding of sources of data on hospitalist compensation and workload will ensure that one knows where to turn at any time for the most recent data.

The two largest surveys of hospitalist compensation, workload, and other metrics have been conducted biannually by SHM and annually by the Medical Group Management Association (MGMA). Beginning in 2010 and thereafter, these two organizations will conduct a joint annual survey that will benefit from SHM's in-depth understanding of the work of hospitalists and the relevant metrics, as well as MGMA's extensive expertise in conducting surveys and analyzing and reporting data. Survey results will be available through either organization.

Additionally, SHM will periodically conduct focused surveys to more fully understand various issues such as hospitalist turnover, the role of nonphysician providers in hospitalist practice, and scope of clinical practice.

There are many other sources of hospitalist survey data, including the American Medical Group Association (AMGA) and many consulting and recruiting firms that publish national or regional data. All of these are valuable data points, but it is important to understand survey methodology, sample size, and other parameters for each.

METHOD OF HOSPITALIST COMPENSATION

A reasonable way to think about the various methods or formulas used to compensate hospitalists is to think of them as consisting of up to three distinct elements:

- A fixed component, often called a base salary
- A productivity component based on patient care workload or production, for example as measured by work RVUs or billable encounters
- A performance-based component, which may be a function of performance on quality measures or citizenship, and so forth

These three components can be combined in nearly any proportion to create a reasonable compensation method. Most practices are best served by choosing one of the following combinations in **Figure 27-1**.

There are other potential salary elements, such as an end-of-year profit distribution, but these are applicable only in certain types of practices and will not be discussed here.

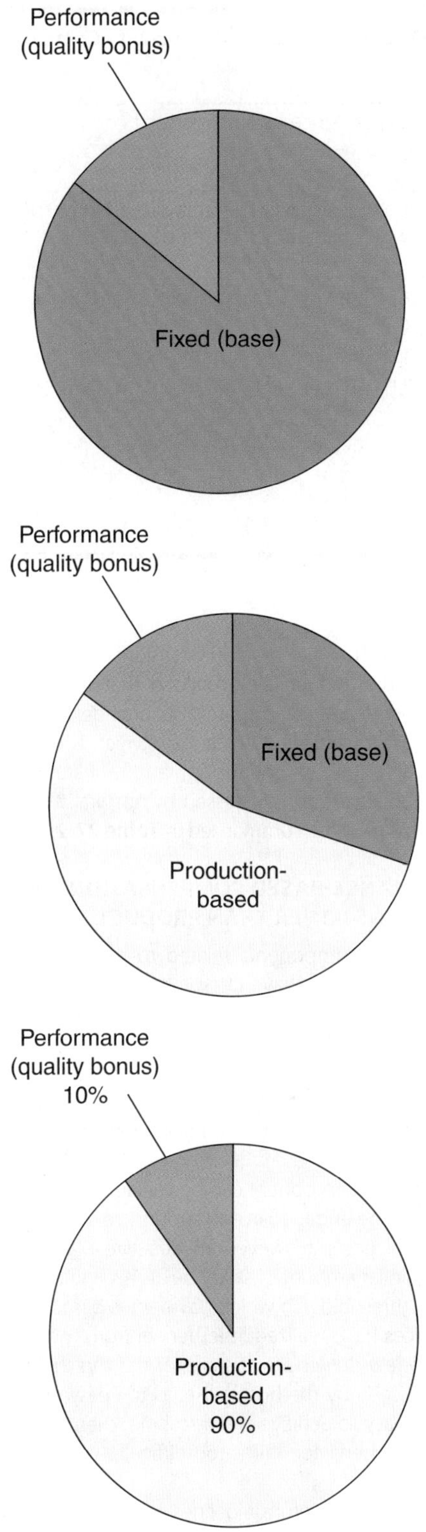

Figure 27-1 *Some sample methods to illustrate how the three common salary elements can be combined. The size of each pie slice is for illustration only, and not meant to represent ideal ratios.*

FIXED, OR "STRAIGHT" SALARY

A fixed salary has the advantages of being known to all parties in advance, eliminating uncertainty in budgeting, and providing certainty for the hospitalist. Anecdotal experience shows that a fixed salary is quite attractive to recent residency graduates, yet it is not a good choice for most practices because it doesn't reward or encourage good performance, and as workloads and other practice attributes (eg, number and length of shifts) change it often becomes badly mismatched to new situations.

PRACTICE POINT

- Fixed salary compensation is not a good choice for most practices because it doesn't reward or encourage good performance, and as workloads and other practice attributes (eg, number and length of shifts) change it often becomes badly mismatched to new situations.
- Production compensation has the advantage of allowing each doctor to work more or less than others in the group, and encourages all in the group to be attentive to optimal staffing and scheduling as well as be attentive to business practices such as proper current procedural terminology (CPT) coding. A significant weakness in compensating hospitalists, or any health care provider, solely on production is that it is a system of paying for doing more but not doing better.
- A performance component can be valuable in encouraging each doctor to become engaged in and supportive of hospitalist practice or institutional goals. However, an effective plan requires that a meaningful dollar amount of salary be at risk, and careful choices of metrics and thresholds on which payment is based must be made.

SHM surveys from 1997 to 2008 show a fixed salary was the most common method in use in 1997, but since then its popularity has steadily declined in favor of a combination of fixed and variable elements. The variable elements may be based on either production or quality performance, or both.

PRODUCTIVITY-BASED COMPENSATION

Most physicians in any specialty are compensated through fee-for-service payments—a form of productivity-based compensation. SHM surveys have shown that the portion of hospitalists with salaries based entirely on their individual production has remained stable at approximately 6% for several years.

A typical compensation plan based entirely on production might look like:

$$\text{compensation} = (\text{collected professional fees} + \text{other support (if any)}) - \text{overhead}$$

The "other support" in the formula is most commonly money paid by the hospital in which the hospitalists see patients.

Production compensation has the advantage of allowing each doctor to work more or less than others in the group, and encourages all in the group to be attentive to optimal staffing and scheduling, as well as being attentive to business practices such as proper current procedural terminology (CPT) coding.

A significant weakness in compensating hospitalists or any health care provider solely on production is that it is a system of paying for doing more but not doing better. That is, it incentivizes volume

TABLE 27-2 Concerns About Productivity Compensation Often Expressed by Hospitalists, and an Alternative View of Each Issue

Concerns	An Alternative View
Unreasonably risky since hospitalists can't control daily fluctuations in patient volume	Hospitalist groups have reasonably precise control of workload and compensation over long periods of time by managing staffing levels
Will disrupt cohesive group culture; will lead to hospitalists competing with one another for the next patient	Makes it much easier to trade work between group members (eg, one may want to work less, and another may want to work more to increase income)—*promotes* group cohesion
It is just a way to get hospitalists to work unreasonably hard, leading to poor patient care and burnout	It provides each doctor some flexibility to make individual choices about how hard he/she wants to work
Will lead to increased patient length of stay since hospitalists can increase income by keeping patients in the hospital longer	Increased length of stay is a risk, but anecdotal experience shows this is very uncommon unless a practice is overstaffed (ie, too many providers for the patient volume)
Will adversely affect recruiting	Candidates are unlikely to be attracted to productivity compensation unless the hospitalist currently in the group sees it as a good thing; a practice can provide a minimum salary guarantee for the first one to two years a doctor is in the practice

and not quality. This may lead an occasional hospitalist to take on an unreasonable and unsafe workload that must be dealt with by the practice leadership. It can also provide a financial reward to a hospitalist for high length of stay, which is out of alignment with hospitals' goal of optimizing length-of-stay management. Additional concerns often expressed by hospitalists about productivity compensation are summarized in **Table 27-2**.

PERFORMANCE-BASED COMPENSATION (RELATED TO DOMAINS OTHER THAN PRODUCTIVITY)

Hospitalist salary components related to performance on quality or citizenship measures have been increasing in popularity. These components are often referred to by a term like *quality bonus* or something similar. They may be based on quality targets such as performance on Centers for Medicare and Medicaid Services (CMS) Core Measures, with patients, and/or referring physician satisfaction, proper CPT coding, committee participation, meeting attendance, and so forth.

A performance component can be valuable in encouraging each doctor to become engaged in and supportive of hospitalist practice or institutional goals. However, an effective plan requires that a meaningful dollar amount of salary be at risk, and careful choices of metrics and thresholds on which payment is based must be made. Many practices have realized little benefit from their quality bonus because too few dollars are at stake, or the thresholds that trigger payment are seen by the hospitalists as too easy or too difficult to reach. If it is easy to achieve the threshold, then there will be little or no effect on behavior. If it is too difficult, then the doctors may ignore it.

There are several useful guidelines for creating a performance-based compensation component.

Choice of metric on which to base compensation

Performance metrics used as a basis for compensation should usually be those that have already been routinely measured and discussed, and all parties are familiar with how the data is collected and analyzed, including any weakness in it. It may be very appealing to use a new metric that has not routinely been measured in the past, but all too often flaws in the data collection and analysis process become evident leading to a lack of trust and potential conflict over whether the goals have been met. The available data may show that no payment is due, but the hospitalists may be critical of flaws in the data and argue that payment is due despite the data or that the analysis should be repeated. It is usually best to avoid such contentious and stressful metrics.

Good metrics include those that hospitals are already required to measure and report, such as performance on core measures and patient satisfaction.

Setting the payment threshold(s)

Setting a single performance threshold that triggers payment of all available dollars is usually problematic. If performance falls just under this threshold the hospitalists may insist that the analysis be repeated, or that every patient chart is reviewed to see if it should be removed from the data set if a nonhospitalist was responsible for the performance outcome.

Instead, payment for most metrics will usually work best if paid on a predetermined scale from no payment to the maximum amount available. For example, if patient satisfaction for hospitalist patients is currently at 70%, and the goal is 75%, then the portion of dollars paid could be determined by subtracting the baseline or lower limit (70% in this example) from actual performance (assume it is 73.8%) as a measure of percentage of improvement toward the goal. In this example, the patient satisfaction improved 76% ($[3.8 \div 5] \times 100$), so 76% of the available dollars will be paid.

Group- vs. individual-based metrics

Most performance metrics are difficult to attribute to individual hospitalists and lend themselves to payment to all members of the group, often prorated based on the portion of full-time work done by the individual. For example, it might be desirable to create a quality bonus for appropriate use of β-blockers in acute myocardial infarction. But many or most patients will have been cared for by more than a single hospitalist, and there is usually no good way to attribute credit or blame to a single individual.

Payment intervals

It may take a year to accumulate a valid sample size for many metrics, meaning an annual calculation of payment is most appropriate. But some measures allow more rapid accumulation of a valid sample and could be paid as often as quarterly. More frequent payment based on a quality metric is usually very complicated and time consuming, making it impractical.

Number of metrics

The number of metrics should be kept small enough that the dollar amount of payment available for each remains significant. This will usually mean no more than three or four metrics should be part of a performance compensation component at a time. The practice might value excellent performance on 25 metrics or more, but including all of them in a bonus plan will usually prove unwieldy and ineffective. However, it is very reasonable to change the metrics used in the plan every year or so.

CONCLUSION

All hospitalist practices should seriously consider including a performance-based compensation element that might range from 5% to 20% of total annual salary. They will need to think carefully about how to apportion the remaining (largest) portion between a fixed and production-based component. These can be thought of as opposite ends of a continuum and it is reasonable to be entirely fixed or entirely production-based, or anywhere in between. The practice history, goals, and culture will have a significant influence in determining the best choice.

CHAPTER 28

Clinical Documentation for Hospitalists

Scott Manaker, MD, PhD
Carol Pohlig, RN, BSN, CPC, ACS

INTRODUCTION

The medical record of an individual patient serves numerous functions. Ideally, the record should provide a comprehensive historical vehicle promoting excellence in care delivery to a patient, transcending communication barriers, and facilitating care coordination among multiple disparate providers and facilities (such as hospitals). The medical record also serves as the basis for a variety of financial, legal, and administrative functions including the documentation for both professional and facility fee reimbursement, quality and safety assessments (including pay for performance), malpractice litigation and disability determinations, and community-based care and public health initiatives.

Currently, the medical record of an individual patient is fragmented, with various pieces shared only sometimes among numerous providers. Hospitalists typically care for a patient during a single episode of facility-based care. Fortunately, the proliferation, adoption, and increasing interoperability of electronic medical records (EMRs), and their evolution into personalized health records, holds promise for consolidation and availability of all relevant clinical information to each provider participating in the care of a single patient.

SOME GENERAL PRINCIPLES

This chapter focuses upon the documentation requirements incumbent upon hospitalists for professional fee billing of their clinical services. Some general principles of physician documentation warrant discussion despite this focus, and apply to both paper and electronic medical records.

The documentation of physician services should always comprise the essential components of a patient's chief complaint, history, physical examination, and medical decision making. The concerns of both patient and provider should be clearly recorded, including expectations (realistic or not) and satisfaction (and dissatisfaction). All diagnostic test orders and results should reside in the chart, as well as documentation of various specific services (eg, physical, occupational, speech, or rehabilitation therapy; home health services, durable medical equipment needs, and social work evaluations).

PRACTICE POINT

- The documentation of physician services should always comprise the essential components of a patient's chief complaint, history, physical examination, and medical decision making. The concerns of both the patient and provider should be clearly recorded, including expectations (realistic or not) and satisfaction (dissatisfaction).

Corrections

At some point in time, every medical record requires a correction. In a paper document, draw a single line through the inaccurate portion and write a correction nearby, dating and signing the revision. The original entry thereby remains legible for future reference. For example, consider misidentification of a right swollen knee joint, when actually it is on the left: when the physician recognizes the mistaken documentation, the *right* side should have a single line drawn through it (ie, overstrike text) and a note written nearby indicating that the *left* side is the accurate side. Sign and date these changes on the day of correction. Methods and appearances of corrections and amendments in electronic medical records continue to evolve, but all incorporate password-protected signatures with electronic date- and time-stamped entries.

Late-entry documentation

Like corrections, addenda or late entries can be made at any time and labeled as such, with a dated and timed signature. Also, explain why the entry was made late and not contemporaneously. For example, following a hospital visit, a hospitalist responds to a rapid response call and neglects to document the visit in the hospital medical record. When recognized the next day, document the hospital visit as a late entry and specify that the care was delivered the previous day.

AN OVERVIEW OF HOSPITAL PAYMENT SYSTEMS

As the most prominent payer in the United States, Medicare payment systems are of paramount importance to understand. Fortunately, Medicare policies are established by the Centers for Medicare and Medicaid Services (CMS) and available online through the CMS On-Line Manual System, so that everyone can in principle understand how claims are processed and payments are made. Medicare policies are largely consistent across the United States, and many private payers follow CMS's lead to a greater or lesser extent. However, remember that regional Medicare contractors develop local coverage determinations from CMS payment policy, and can create idiosyncratic interpretations of the documentation guidelines for evaluation and management (E/M) services. One such example would be the nuanced medical decision making (see below) evaluations implemented by Trailblazer Medicare. Similarly, various third party payers have the right, as allowable under their contract with physician groups, to create unique documentation mandates and payment policies. Facilities also generate requirements, such as a history and physical are required before a procedure, which do not comprise medically necessary, billable physician services.

Medicare pays hospitals for inpatient services using an inpatient prospective payment system (IPPS), which relies primarily on the diagnosis in order to group the services delivered to an inpatient into a Medicare severity-diagnosis related group (MS-DRG). Many diagnostic categories have two or three severity levels, differentiated by the presence or absence of a specified set of complications and comorbidities (CCs) or major complications and comorbidities (MCCs). Hospitals and other facilities frequently request hospitalists to clarify, expand, or specify their clinical documentation to ensure the assignment of a hospitalization to the proper MS-DRG. This single MS-DRG payment covers all facility services during the inpatient stay. Many payers have adopted a similar mechanism of providing a single, fixed payment for an entire hospitalization, often referred to as a case rate.

Some non-Medicare payers still reimburse hospitals and facilities with a fixed payment for each day, commonly described as a per diem rate. The daily payment potentially varies depending upon the types of services provided to the patient (eg, intensive care versus skilled nursing care). Other payment models are likely to emerge as a result of health care reform, including the evolution of accountable care organizations and the emergence of patient-centered medical homes.

AN OVERVIEW OF PHYSICIAN PAYMENT SYSTEMS

Physician services are typically reported using the American Medical Association (AMA) *Current Procedural Terminology* (CPT), fourth edition, which lists descriptive terms and identifying codes to report medical services and procedures. CPT provides a uniform language to accurately describe all medical, surgical, and diagnostic services and procedures. Even physicians receiving capitated payments still typically report CPT codes for their services.

Hospitalists predominantly report E/M codes (CPT 99201-99499), which for Medicare exceed $32 billion annually and account for more than 40% of the Medicare physician fee schedule allowed charges. Other bedside procedures and diagnostic testing, sometimes performed by hospitalists, are found in CPT. In selecting the proper E/M code, the site and nature of service determine the *visit category*; and the key components of history, physical examination, and medical decision making determine the specific level of CPT code within a visit category.

Many payers are now adopting Medicare's recognition and regulation of nurse practitioners and physician assistants as nonphysician providers, independently able to provide, document, and bill for E/M services. The number of nonphysician providers performing hospitalist services is rapidly increasing. Therefore, when we refer to *providers* throughout this chapter, we include both physicians and these qualified nonphysician providers functioning in an independent billing role.

DIAGNOSIS CODING

The International Classification of Diseases, Ninth Revision Clinical Modification (ICD-9) codifies every disease, disorder, condition, symptom, and health care encounter. Payers initially determine the *medical necessity* of services and procedures based upon the ICD-9-CM code(s) that accompany every provider and hospital claim. Each entry into the medical record should clearly state the diagnoses considered and addressed in the service. The successor International Classification of Diseases, Tenth Revision (ICD-10), which has been available for more than 10 years, is slated for implementation in 2013.

THE KEY COMPONENTS OF PHYSICIAN E/M DOCUMENTATION

Selecting an E/M level focuses upon the content of the three key components: history, physical examination (PE), and medical decision making (MDM). Time is considered a fourth key component, but only affects the E/M level when counseling and/or coordination of care dominate more than 50% of the physician's total visit time (see below). When counseling and/or coordination of care involves less than 50% of the physician's total visit time, both time and the nature of the presenting problem are only considered as contributory factors and do not determine the E/M level.

PRACTICE POINT

- Selecting an evaluation and management (E/M) level focuses upon the content of the three key components: history, physical examination, and medical decision making. Time only affects the E/M level when counseling and/or coordination of care dominate more than 50% of the physician's total time.

Two sets of documentation guidelines have been elaborated by Medicare and largely adopted by other payers. The earlier 1995 guidelines are the most widespread, and generally applicable to hospitalists along with most medical and surgical specialists. The later 1997 guidelines elaborate specialty-specific physical examinations, as well as clearly articulate detailed physical examination requirements lacking in the 1995 guidelines. Several nuanced differences also exist between the two guidelines in aspects of history. The 1995 guidelines will be described in detail throughout this section, and the 1997 guidelines are highlighted below in a separate section for completeness.

HISTORY

The elements of history include the chief complaint (CC), history of present illness (HPI), review of systems (ROS), and the past, family, and social histories (PFSH). A chart note may not segregate these elements into unique subtitled areas, but rather the information may be interspersed amid the written, typed, or even dictated narrative.

Chief Complaint (CC)

Typically, the reason for the visit is often quoted from the patient's own words as a sign or symptom, such as, "my belly hurts." Always document a CC in the progress note, even absent an acute complaint, such as, "pneumonia follow-up." Avoid statements lacking a specific clinical reference (eg, "post-op visit Day #3").

History of Present Illness (HPI)

The HPI conveys information about the CC, from either the origin (at an initial encounter) or the interval between sequential patient encounters. This information is arbitrarily allocated into eight elements: location, quality, severity, duration, timing, context, modifying factors, and associated signs/symptoms. The HPI is then quantified as *brief* (one to three elements) or *extended* (four or more elements). For example, consider this extended HPI: "Patient complains of increased (severity) pedal (location) edema that began two days ago (duration). Less able to walk. No chest pain (associated signs/symptoms)."

Review of Systems (ROS)

The ROS refers to signs or symptoms experienced in conjunction with the CC. Fourteen systems are recognized: constitutional, eyes, ears/nose/mouth/throat, cardiovascular, respiratory, gastrointestinal, genitourinary, musculoskeletal, integumentary (which includes the breast), neurologic, psychiatric, endocrine, hematologic/lymphatic, and allergic/immunologic. Medical necessity, as deemed by the treating provider in light of the patient's current or previous conditions, determines the number of systems required for review.

An ROS may be problem pertinent, extended, or complete. A *problem-pertinent* ROS documents one system directly related to the CC. An *extended* ROS requires documentation of two to nine systems, that is, the system that is directly related to the CC, along with one or more additional systems. A complete ROS documents 10 or more individual systems. When obtaining a complete ROS, to decrease the amount of time spent listing each system individually, both the 1995 and 1997 (see below) E/M documentation guidelines allow the physician to comment on the positive and pertinent negative systems, with an additional comment that the "remainder is negative." However, insurers may not accept alternative phrases, and even some Medicare contractors (eg, Trailblazers Medicare) require individual documentation of each system.

Past, Family, and Social Histories (PFSH)

The past history includes documentation of previous illnesses, hospitalizations, surgeries, medications, allergies, and immunizations. The family history provides information regarding potential hereditary illnesses. The social history may list details of the patient's substance use (tobacco/alcohol/illicit drugs), sexual history, employment status, level of education, marital status, or living arrangements.

A *pertinent* PFSH includes a comment in any one of the three histories (ie, past, family, or social). Full credit for a *complete* PFSH requires a comment in each history (ie, past, family, and social). When reporting initial hospital, observation, or nursing facility care, consultations, and new office, home, and domiciliary visits, a complete PFSH comprises one comment documented in each of the three histories. In contradistinction, emergency department (ED) services or established patient visits in the home, domiciliary, office, or other outpatient area require one comment in two of the three histories for credit as a complete PFSH.

TABLE 28-1 Levels of History

History Level	HPI	ROS	PFSH
Problem-focused	Brief (≤ 3)	None	None
Expanded problem-focused	Brief (≤ 3)	Problem pertinent (1)	None
Detailed	Extended (≥ 4)	Extended (2–9)	Pertinent (1)
Comprehensive	Extended (≥ 4)	Complete (≥ 10)	Complete (2 or 3)*

*All three for new patient encounters; 2 of 3 for subsequent or ED encounters.

Providers may review and comment that the "family history is noncontributory" and still receive credit for the family history from most insurers. Certain Medicare contractors, such as Trailblazers Medicare and Wisconsin Physicians Service Insurance Corporation, prohibit this terminology and require specific documentation regardless of clinical relevance (eg, "family history negative for liver disease"). Also note that with subsequent services, both for hospital care and nursing facility visits, indicating an "interval history" does not require redocumentation of the PFSH unless it is clinically relevant.

Determination of history level

The number of historical elements present in the chart note determines the level of history (**Table 28-1**). If all of the requirements are not met for a given level of history, select the level associated with the *deficient* element. For example, a comprehensive history requires documentation of the CC, ≥ 4 HPI elements, ≥ 10 ROS, and a complete PFSH. If the ROS only includes documentation for 9 systems, a comprehensive history cannot be selected; report a service that requires only a detailed history: CC, ≥ 4 HPI elements, 2-9 ROS, and a pertinent PFSH.

Other circumstances

A PFSH obtained during an earlier encounter does not need to be rerecorded if the provider demonstrates review and updating of the previous information. Update the history by describing any new information or noting the absence of change, along with the date and location of the earlier PFSH; this earlier PFSH must be contained in the body of the medical record. CPT requires only an *interval* history for subsequent hospital or subsequent nursing facility visits, and it is usually unnecessary to record information about the PFSH, which is unlikely to change in these settings. For established outpatient encounters, documentation regarding the PFSH is unnecessary when PE and MDM are used as the basis for the level of the encounter, unless the patient provides the physician with updated information.

Most auditors disallow a single statement as both an HPI element and ROS element. The ROS and/or PFSH may be recorded by ancillary staff, or on a form completed by the patient. The provider must annotate, supplement, or confirm this information recorded by others, either by a reference to the history form in the progress note or by initialing and dating the form.

If unable to obtain history from the patient, the record should describe the patient's condition or the circumstance that precludes obtaining a history. For example, "... patient sedated and paralyzed, unable to obtain additional history." However, reviewers expect providers to incorporate historic information to the extent possible, from all reasonably available sources (eg, old records, emergency medical services documents, other provider documentation, or conversations).

Finally, although the physician may collect all of the information required for a complete ROS, the most common underdocumentation error is failure to document at least 10 systems. The second most common mistake is a missing family history or social history.

PRACTICE POINT

- Although the physician may collect all of the information required for a complete review of systems, the most common underdocumentation error is failure to document at least 10 systems. The second most common mistake is a missing family or social history.

PHYSICAL EXAMINATION (PE)

Individual PE elements will be assigned to body areas (head and face, neck, chest, abdomen, genitalia/groin/buttocks, back/spine, and each extremity) or organ systems (constitutional, eyes, ears/nose/mouth/throat, cardiovascular, respiratory, gastrointestinal, genitourinary, musculoskeletal, integumentary, neurologic, psychiatric, and hematologic/lymphatic/immunologic). Providers may document specific findings (eg, "abdomen soft") or make a generalized comment (eg, "HEENT normal"). Abnormal findings must be specifically documented, such as "S_3"; however, a comment indicating "abnormal" without elaboration is insufficient.

The PE documented in the medical record is categorized as problem-focused, expanded problem focused, detailed, or comprehensive. One comment in an area constitutes a *problem-focused exam*. The distinction between the expanded problem-focused and detailed examination under the 1995 Guidelines is the greatest ambiguity in physical examination documentation. Both the *expanded problem-focused* and *detailed* exams require documentation of two to seven systems. However, "detailed" is defined as an extended examination of the affected body area or organ system, in addition to other symptomatic or related organ systems. The number of required comments regarding the affected body area or organ system to consider the examination detailed has never been defined by either CPT or Medicare. Attempting to decrease ambiguity and variability among auditors, Highmark Medicare Services scores a detailed exam using the "4 × 4" rule: 4 elements examined in 4 body areas or 4 organ systems (totaling 16 documentation elements). In contrast, Trailblazers Medicare and some other contractors suggest using the 1997 guidelines (discussed later) for detailed exam requirements.

The *comprehensive* examination is a general multisystem examination or a complete examination of a single organ system. Medicare requires the minimum documentation for the general multisystem examination to include one comment in each of eight systems; of course, additional comments in each system and more than eight systems may be described, as clinically indicated. For example, a comprehensive examination may be documented as follows: "P=76, BP=120/80, RR=12 (constitutional); HEENT normal (eyes and ENMT); neck supple (musculoskeletal); regular rate and rhythm (cardiovascular); lungs clear (respiratory); soft abdomen (gastrointestinal); no icterus (integumentary), normal gait (neurological)." The requirements for a comprehensive single organ system still remain undefined for use with these 1995 guidelines.

MEDICAL DECISION MAKING (MDM)

The complexity of MDM drives selection of a level of service. MDM is categorized as *straightforward, low, moderate,* or *high*. Three categories must be considered to determine the level of MDM complexity: the number of diagnoses, the amount and complexity of data, and the risk to the patient.

TABLE 28-2 Valuation of Diagnostic and Treatment Options

Number of Diagnoses/ Treatment Options	Points per Problem
Self-limited/minor problem (stable, improved, or worsening)	1 (max = 2 problems)
Established problem (stable or improving)	1
Established problem (worsening)	2
New problem, without additional workup	3 (max = 1 problem)
New problem, with additional workup planned	4

Number of diagnoses considered

This first category identifies the number of diagnoses and/or management options considered in the encounter, based upon the documentation. Up to four points are assigned to each problem, with more points assigned for new problems than for established problems, and a new problem requiring additional workup (ie, diagnostic testing) given the maximum four points. Established problems identified as worsening receive a higher value than stable or improving problems. A self-limited or minor problem (eg, sunburn) receives minimal credit as these issues typically do not warrant a defined plan of care (**Table 28-2**).

New problems require initiation of a care plan, while established problems may require modification or continuation of a care plan. An *established* problem has been previously considered by the physician or provider group (to allow for cross coverage and handoffs between same specialty providers in the same group). Note that credit is given for a problem considered, although not primarily under treatment by the physician. For example, in a patient receiving steroids for an inflammatory disease, the hospitalist receives credit for noting the potential adverse consequence upon serum lipids, even if a cardiologist is primarily treating the dyslipidemia. Similarly, a chronic condition such as diabetes, cared for by an endocrinologist, is categorized as a *new* problem to the hospitalist newly treating the patient during an admission for ketoacidosis.

Established patients may also have *new* problems. For example, an asthmatic with a resolving flare may experience heartburn. This additional new complaint of heartburn may be considered *new* if commented upon in the progress note and no prior care plan for gastroesophageal reflux exists.

Physicians receive credit only for issues considered in the care plan. Diagnoses merely listed in the assessment and plan without elaboration of the care, or simply ascribing the care to others (eg, "diabetes – per endocrinologist") are considered part of the patient's *problem list* in the PFSH. Additionally, new hospitalizations warrant new care plan development, and physicians can receive *new problem* credit even if the patient has been previously hospitalized by the same group. This is a nuance of inpatient and observation care only.

Data considered

The second category of determining the MDM complexity is the amount and/or complexity of data reviewed or ordered by the provider during the patient encounter. Both the type and source of information considered are valued (**Table 28-3**).

Ordering and/or reviewing of pathology/laboratory, radiology, and medicine data each provide separate but equal credit. Irrespective of the test volume in each category, only one point is allocated per category (ie, pathology/laboratory, radiology, or medicine) for the

TABLE 28-3 Valuation of Data Considered

Amount and/or Complexity of Data Ordered/Reviewed	Points
Review and/or order of clinical test(s)	1
Review and/or order of test(s) in the pathology/laboratory section of CPT	1
Review and/or order of test(s) in the radiology section of CPT	1
Review and/or order of test(s) in the medicine section of CPT	1
Decision to obtain old records and/or obtain history from someone (nonhealth care provider) other than the patient	1
Review and summarize old records, obtain additional history, or discuss the case with another health care provider	2
Independent visualization of actual image, tracing, or specimen	2

encounter. For example, the provider ordering a dozen serologic collagen vascular studies in the morning may also review the three results received in the afternoon; nonetheless, only one point is granted for this care. A single, separate point may be assigned each to pathology/laboratory, radiology, and medicine data, respectively, are cumulative in nature, and the chart note should refer to all the data reviewed or ordered to capture all of the provider work. In other words, if the chart note comments upon a radiology result (one point) and an echocardiogram order (one point), two points may be awarded for the amount of data in that encounter. Independently visualizing images, tracings, or specimens is considered separately, and additional to reviewing the formal interpretation, as long as the chart note clearly documents this occurrence (ie, "...films and report reveal..."). Without such specific reference distinguishing personal review of the images and of the formal interpretation, an auditor only provides minimal credit for merely reviewing the report.

Providers also receive credit for the additional effort of obtaining information from sources other than the patient or old records, such as conversations with other health care professionals. The chart note should specifically mention the source, along with the information reviewed (eg, "...spouse confirms loud snoring").

TABLE 28-4 Table of Risk

Level of Risk	Presenting Problem(s)	Diagnostic Procedure(s) Ordered	Management Options Selected
Minimal	• One self-limited or minor problem (eg, cold, insect bite, tinea corporis)	• Laboratory tests requiring venipuncture • Chest X rays • ECG/EEG • Urinalysis • Ultrasound (eg, echocardiography) • KOH prep	• Rest • Gargles • Elastic bandages • Superficial dressings
Low	• Two or more self-limited or minor problems • One stable chronic illness (eg, well-controlled hypertension, noninsulin dependent diabetes, cataract, BPH) • Acute uncomplicated illness or injury, (eg, cystitis, allergic rhinitis, simple sprain)	• Physiologic tests not under stress (eg, pulmonary function tests) • Noncardiovascular imaging studies with contrast (eg, barium enema) • Superficial needle biopsies • Clinical laboratory tests requiring arterial puncture • Skin biopsies	• Over-the-counter drugs • Minor surgery with no identified risk factors • Physical therapy • Occupational therapy • IV fluids without additives
Moderate	• One or more chronic illnesses with mild exacerbation, progression, or side effects of treatment • Two or more stable chronic illnesses • Undiagnosed new problem with uncertain prognosis (eg, lump in breast) • Acute illness with systemic symptoms (eg, pyelonephritis, pneumonitis, colitis) • Acute complicated injury (eg, head injury with brief loss of consciousness)	• Physiologic tests under stress (eg, cardiac stress test, fetal contraction stress test) • Diagnostic endoscopies with no identified risk factors • Deep needle or incisional biopsy • Cardiovascular imaging studies with contrast and no identified risk factors (eg, arteriogram, cardiac catheterization) • Obtain fluid from body cavity (eg, lumbar puncture, thoracentesis, culdocentesis)	• Minor surgery with identified risk factors • Elective major surgery (open, percutaneous, or endoscopic) with no identified risk factors • Prescription drug management • Therapeutic nuclear medicine • IV fluids with additives • Closed treatment of fracture or dislocation without manipulation
High	• One or more chronic illnesses with severe exacerbation, progression, or side effects of treatment • Acute or chronic illnesses or injuries that pose a threat to life or bodily function (eg, multiple trauma, acute MI, pulmonary embolus, severe respiratory distress, progressive severe rheumatoid arthritis, psychiatric illness with potential threat to self or others, peritonitis, acute renal failure) • An abrupt change in neurologic status (eg, seizure, TIA, weakness, sensory loss)	• Cardiovascular imaging studies with contrast with identified risk factors • Cardiac electrophysiological tests • Diagnostic endoscopies with identified risk factors • Discography	• Elective major surgery (open, percutaneous, or endoscopic) with identified risk factors • Emergency major surgery (open, percutaneous, or endoscopic) • Parenteral controlled substances • Drug therapy requiring intensive monitoring for toxicity • Decision not to resuscitate or to de-escalate care because of poor prognosis

Risk to the patient

The third MDM category assesses the *patient's* risk of complications, morbidity, or mortality, with respect to the presenting problem, diagnostic procedures ordered, or management options chosen. Four levels of patient risk exist (minimal, low, moderate, and high), with examples of each risk type included in Medicare's "Table of Risk" (**Table 28-4**). The limited number of examples serves as illustrative references for common clinical scenarios, but not as a comprehensive list.

When determining the level of risk, consider comorbidities as well as the plan of care in assessing a patient's risk, thereby potentially increasing the complexity of MDM. Similarly, diagnostic studies or alternatively, procedures under consideration or excluded based upon excessive risk, impact the complexity of MDM (eg, "...will defer MRI, as potential morbidity of transport to magnet exceeds risks of empiric treatment"). Although many bulleted items on the table may pertain to a particular chart note, the single bulleted item in any risk category associated with the highest risk determines the patient's risk level. For example, a note documenting the monitoring of liver function tests to assess for statin toxicity comprises high risk (drug therapy requiring frequent monitoring for toxicity). However, remember risk does not equal complexity: risk is but one category (among three) of MDM and not the sole contributor to complexity.

Assigning MDM complexity

Based upon the chart note, points are assigned for diagnoses managed and data considered, and patient risk is assessed. The final result of MDM complexity hinges on the two highest-valued categories. In other words, *two of the three categories must meet or exceed the requirements assigned to a specific level of complexity* to select that level, as illustrated in **Table 28-5**.

To illustrate the assignment of MDM complexity, consider the following example. The chart note considers three stable established diagnoses (three points), several blood tests (one point), and high patient risk. The lowest of the three categories (data considered) is eliminated, and the lower of the two remaining categories (number of diagnoses) determines the moderate MDM complexity for the note. While most contractors utilize the same standardization when assigning points, beware of contractors (eg, Trailblazers Medicare) who impose different standards.

1997 GUIDELINES

Medicare issued a second set of revised documentation guidelines for E/M services in 1997. MDM and the level categories remained unchanged from the prior 1995 documentation guidelines, as detailed above. While ambiguity plagues many aspects of the 1995 guidelines, excessive proscription limits the 1997 guidelines. The 1997 guidelines made a single minor revision to the history, while the physical examination content received extensive modification.

TABLE 28-5 Levels of Medical Decision Making

Complexity	Diagnosis or Treatment Option Points	Data Points	Risk Level
Problem-focused	≤ 1 (minimal)	≤ 1 (minimal)	Minimal
Low	2 (limited)	2 (limited)	Low
Moderate	3 (multiple)	3 (multiple)	Moderate
High	4 (extensive)	4 (extensive)	High

The requirements for each level of physical examination were heavily revised, and specialty-specific single organ system examinations defined. In response to widespread complaints from the physician community, CMS allowed physicians to document using either the 1995 or 1997 guidelines, according to their individual preference, and directed auditors to review the physician documentation based on the set of guidelines most favorable to the physician for the E/M code reported for the encounter. Most physicians, including hospitalists, find the 1995 guidelines most applicable.

History

The 1997 guidelines do not limit the provider to identifying individual factors associated with the CC (eg, duration, timing, context). Rather, a provider may document the status of one or more chronic conditions; this option is most useful to subsequent hospital visits. A brief HPI documents one or two conditions, while an extended HPI documents a minimum of three conditions. Some reviewers allow this option only if applying the 1997 guidelines to the entire note.

Physical examination

The 1997 guidelines allow a provider to select either a general multisystem examination or any one of the single organ system examinations. Hospitalists typically utilize the general examination, which specifies examination elements to perform and document. *Negative* or *normal* comments remain acceptable for the 1997 guidelines, along with the mandate to specify comments on any abnormal findings. Documentation in the medical record of 1 to 5 specified (referred to as *bulleted*) physical examination elements comprises a *problem-focused* examination; 6 to 11 bulleted elements defines the *expanded problem-focused* examination; and a *detailed* examination requires 12 or more bulleted items.

Two important, major differences distinguish the 1997 *comprehensive* examination (**Tables 28-6** and **28-7**) requirement from the 1995 guideline. First, for the 1997 general multisystem exam, the provider must perform all the elements specified in at least nine organ systems or body areas. Second, the provider needs to document only a minimum of two elements from each of those nine systems or areas.

DETERMINING LEVEL OF SERVICE

For both the 1995 and 1997 guidelines, assign a specific level to each of the three key components. Rate history and examination each as either problem-focused, expanded problem-focused, detailed, or comprehensive. Rate the complexity of MDM as either straightforward, low, moderate, or high. CPT correlates specific levels of the key components with certain levels of most E/M services.

Initial patient encounters (initial hospital care, CPT 99221-99223; initial observation care, CPT 99218-99220; consultations, 99241-99245 and 99251-99255) require consideration of all three key components. Consider only two of the key components for subsequent hospital (CPT 99231-99233) or observation visits (CPT 99224-99226). The lowest component of the two or three key components required determines the visit level. For example, a level three initial hospital service (CPT 99223) includes a comprehensive history, comprehensive exam, and high-complexity decision making (**Table 28-8**). If the documentation merely supports a detailed level of history, yet meets the requirements for a comprehensive examination and high-complexity decision making, report only a level one initial hospital service (CPT 99221). In contrast, if a subsequent hospital visit note contains a complete examination and high-complexity MDM, then report CPT 99233 and history need not even be considered. When selecting visit levels for services that only consider two key components, MDM should be one of those two key components. While not stated in the documentation

TABLE 28-6 1997 General Multisystem Physical Examination

System/Body Area	Elements of Examination
Constitutional	• Measurement of *any three of the following seven* vital signs: (1) sitting or standing blood pressure, (2) supine blood pressure, (3) pulse rate and regularity, (4) respiration, (5) temperature, (6) height, (7) weight (may be measured and recorded by ancillary staff) • General appearance of patient (eg, development, nutrition, body habitus, deformities, attention to grooming)
Eyes	• Inspection of conjunctivae and lids • Examination of pupils and irises (eg, reaction to light and accommodation, size, and symmetry) • Ophthalmoscopic examination of optic discs (eg, size, C/D ratio, appearance) and posterior segments (eg, vessel changes, exudates, hemorrhages)
Ears, Nose, Mouth, and Throat	• External inspection of ears and nose (eg, overall appearance, scars, lesions, masses) • Otoscopic examination of external auditory canals and tympanic membranes • Assessment of hearing (eg, whispered voice, finger rub, tuning fork) • Inspection of nasal mucosa, septum, and turbinates • Inspection of lips, teeth, and gums • Examination of oropharynx: oral mucosa, salivary glands, hard and soft palates, tongue, tonsils, and posterior pharynx
Neck	• Examination of neck (eg, masses, overall appearance, symmetry, tracheal position, crepitus) • Examination of thyroid (eg, enlargement, tenderness, mass)
Respiratory	• Assessment of respiratory effort (eg, intercostal retractions, use of accessory muscles, diaphragmatic movement) • Percussion of chest (eg, dullness, flatness, hyperresonance) • Palpation of chest (eg, tactile fremitus) • Auscultation of lungs (eg, breath sounds, adventitious sounds, rubs)
Cardiovascular	• Palpation of heart (eg, location, size, thrills) • Auscultation of heart with notation of abnormal sounds and murmurs Examination of: • carotid arteries (eg, pulse amplitude, bruits) • abdominal aorta (eg, size, bruits) • femoral arteries (eg, pulse amplitude, bruits) • pedal pulses (eg, pulse amplitude) • extremities for edema and/or varicosities
Chest (Breasts)	• Inspection of breasts (eg, symmetry, nipple discharge) • Palpation of breasts and axillae (eg, masses or lumps, tenderness)
Gastrointestinal (Abdomen)	• Examination of abdomen with notation of presence of masses or tenderness • Examination of liver and spleen • Examination for presence or absence of hernia • Examination of anus, perineum, and rectum, including sphincter tone, presence of hemorrhoids, rectal masses • Obtain stool sample for occult blood test when indicated
Genitourinary	**Male:** • Examination of the scrotal contents (eg, hydrocele, spermatocele, tenderness of cord, testicular mass) • Examination of the penis • Digital rectal examination of prostate gland (eg, size, symmetry, nodularity, tenderness) **Female:** Pelvic examination (with or without specimen collection for smears and cultures), including • Examination of external genitalia (eg, general appearance, hair distribution, lesions) and vagina (eg, general appearance, estrogen effect, discharge, lesions, pelvic support, cystocele, rectocele) • Examination of urethra (eg, masses, tenderness, scarring) • Uterus (eg, size, contour, position, mobility, tenderness, consistency, descent or support) • Adnexa/parametria (eg, masses, tenderness, organomegaly, nodularity) • Examination of bladder (eg, fullness, masses, tenderness) • Cervix (eg, general appearance, lesions, discharge) • Uterus (eg, size, contour, position, mobility, tenderness, consistency, descent or support) • Adnexa/parametria (eg, masses, tenderness, organomegaly, nodularity)
Lymphatic	Palpation of lymph nodes in two or more areas: • Neck • Axillae • Groin • Other

(continued)

TABLE 28-6 1997 General Multisystem Physical Examination (*continued*)

System/Body Area	Elements of Examination
Musculoskeletal	• Examination of gait and station • Inspection and/or palpation of digits and nails (eg, clubbing, cyanosis, inflammatory conditions, petechiae, ischemia, infections, nodes) Examination of joints, bones, and muscles of one or more of the following six areas: (1) head and neck; (2) spine, ribs, and pelvis; (3) right upper extremity; (4) left upper extremity; (5) right lower extremity; and (6) left lower extremity. The examination of a given area includes: • Inspection and/or palpation with notation of presence of any misalignment, asymmetry, crepitation, defects, tenderness, masses, or effusions • Assessment of range of motion with notation of any pain, crepitation or contracture • Assessment of stability with notation of any dislocation (luxation), subluxation, or laxity • Assessment of muscle strength and tone (eg, flaccid, cog wheel, spastic) with notation of any atrophy or abnormal movements
Skin	• Inspection of skin and subcutaneous tissue (eg, rashes, lesions, ulcers) • Palpation of skin and subcutaneous tissue (eg, induration, subcutaneous nodules, tightening)
Neurologic	• Test cranial nerves with notation of any deficits • Examination of deep tendon reflexes with notation of pathological reflexes (eg, Babinski) • Examination of sensation (eg, by touch, pin, vibration, proprioception)
Psychiatric	• Description of patient's judgment and insight Brief assessment of mental status including: • Orientation to time, place, and person • Recent and remote memory • Mood and affect (eg, depression, anxiety, agitation)

guidelines, medical necessity underlies every physician service and is most appropriately demonstrated through MDM. Reporting subsequent services with MDM as a key component thereby precludes the allegation of an unwarranted high-level subsequent encounter based upon merely a comprehensive history and examination (eg, common cold).

TIME COUNSELING/COORDINATING CARE

CPT assigns most E/M codes a *typical* time to render a service, but importantly, the service duration need not last that length. For inpatient services, time accrues as unit or floor time in addition to face-to-face time. When more than 50% of the total service time involves counseling and/or coordination of care, the provider may select a code reflecting the total time spent with the patient, rather than the three key components. Time and the corresponding counseling details must be documented in the medical record when selecting the E/M code on the basis of time (eg, "25 of 40 minutes spent urging the patient to undergo a diagnostic biopsy"). Of course, record patient responses to counseling and all relevant history, examination, and MDM as necessary for good patient care.

TABLE 28-7 Levels of 1997 Physical Examination

Level of Exam	Performance and Documentation
Problem-Focused	*1 to 5* elements identified by a bullet.
Expanded Problem-Focused	*At least 6* elements identified by a bullet.
Detailed	*At least 2* elements identified by a bullet from *each of 6 areas/systems* OR *at least 12* elements identified by a bullet in *2 or more areas/systems.*
Comprehensive	Perform *all elements* identified by a bullet in *at least 9* organ systems or body areas and document *at least 2* elements identified by a bullet from *each of 9 areas/systems.*

INPATIENT CARE CODES

INITIAL HOSPITAL CARE

Only patients admitted to an inpatient hospital may receive initial hospital care (CPT 99221-99223) (Table 28-8); other CPT codes describe services provided to patients in other facility settings (eg, skilled nursing facility). The attending physician admitting the patient reports this service. Many payers now mandate consulting physicians to report this service for their initial encounter during a hospitalization (see Consultations below). Documentation requirements of all three key components (history, physical examination, and MDM) must be met.

CONSULTATIONS

A provider requesting an opinion or advice from another provider defines an inpatient consultation. The request for consultation need not originate from a physician but may also come from another qualified health care provider (eg, nurse practitioner, physician assistant, resident, etc) involved in the patient's care, as appropriate. Inpatient consultations (CPT 99251-99255) (**Table 28-9**) occur in the hospital or nursing facility, once per admission per specialty for both new and established patients. Similarly, outpatient consultations (CPT 99241-99245) (**Table 28-10**) occur in the emergency room or outpatient hospital settings, such as observation units. All three key components (history, physical examination, and MDM) must be met.

Effective January 1, 2010, CMS ceased recognizing consultation codes (CPT 99241-99255), and mandated the report of initial hospital care codes (CPT 99221-99233) in lieu of inpatient consultations and of new or established outpatient visits (CPT 99201-99215) in lieu of

TABLE 28-8 Levels of Initial Hospital Care

Initial Hospital Care	History	Examination	MDM	Time
99221	Detailed or comprehensive	Detailed or comprehensive	Straightforward or low	30 min
99222	Comprehensive	Comprehensive	Moderate	50 min
99223	Comprehensive	Comprehensive	High	70 min

outpatient consultations. New patients are defined as individuals who have not been seen within the last three years by a provider with the same specialty designation within the same provider group. Most managed Medicare programs and several other payers have implemented a similar consultation policy.

SUBSEQUENT HOSPITAL CARE

All admitting providers (and consultants) report subsequent hospital care (CPT 99231-99233) (**Table 28-11**) each day after an initial hospital care (or consultation) is reported. However, only one subsequent hospital care code per patient per day per specialty group will be reimbursed. Subsequent visits include surgical comanagement pre- and postoperative visits. Documentation of two of the three key components (history, physical examination, and MDM) must be met, unless reporting the visit based upon time.

Intrafacility transfers

For patients transferred from one attending physician or provider group to another during the same inpatient stay, the receiving provider cannot report a consultation. However, some payers may allow the reporting of an initial inpatient service (CPT 99221-99223) as an associated consequence of their abolition of consultations, but only when transferred from a different provider group or specialty.

Patients discharged from an acute inpatient stay and admitted to another location (eg, long-term acute care hospital, psychiatric care, hospice, or rehabilitative care outside or within the same physical plant) pose equally difficult coding dilemmas. Provider groups who provided care during the initial acute stay, and then participate in medically necessary postacute care, report their services as subsequent hospital care (CPT 99231-99233). They make also report an initial hospital care (CPT 99221-99223) service if they are the attending physician of record for the postacute care.

Hospice

Providers caring for patients reassigned to inpatient hospice must distinguish their services from those of the hospice-employed providers. Report these medically necessary E/M services (CPT 99231-99233) with the modifier GW (service unrelated to the terminal condition; eg, 99233–GW).

DISCHARGE DAY MANAGEMENT

Hospital discharge day management services (CPT 99238-99239) describe discharge care, and may only be reported by the attending of record at discharge. The discharge service must include face-to-face service and it may also include a final examination, a discussion of the treatment course and follow-up plans, and preparation of the discharge records, prescriptions, and referral forms. When payers allow the hospital-required discharge summary to serve as supporting documentation for discharge day management codes, include the date and details of the final face-to-face service. Providers from other groups report subsequent hospital care services (CPT 99231-99233) on the day of discharge.

The cumulative time for discharge day services represents only a single provider's time. If the discharge service requires 30 or more minutes on the patient's floor/unit by a single provider, report 99239 and specifically document the time (start/stop or total cumulative time); otherwise, report 99238.

OBSERVATION CARE

Report observation care services (CPT 99217-99236) for patients admitted to hospital outpatient units, often referred to as observation, 23-hour, or short stay units.

ADMISSION AND DISCHARGE FROM OBSERVATION CARE ON THE SAME DAY

Use CPT 99234-99236 (**Table 28-12**) to report observation care, if discharged on the same calendar day. Proper use of these codes depends upon individual payer regulations. For example, Medicare requires the patient to be in observation for at least eight hours on one calendar day. The provider must personally document the total amount of observation time.

Documentation of all three key components (history, physical examination, and MDM) must be met, and the physician must write two separate admission and discharge notes. If the patient is in observation for less than eight hours, only the initial observation care code (99218-99220) can be reported to Medicare with no discharge service reportable. Some insurers may not recognize CPT 99234-99236, and only allow a provider to report an initial observation code (99218-99220) under any circumstance.

TABLE 28-9 Levels of Inpatient Consultations

Inpatient Consultation	History	Examination	MDM	Time
99251	Problem-focused	Problem-focused	Straightforward	20 min
99252	Expanded problem-focused	Expanded problem-focused	Straightforward	40 min
99253	Detailed	Detailed	Low	55 min
99254	Comprehensive	Comprehensive	Moderate	80 min
99255	Comprehensive	Comprehensive	High	110 min

TABLE 28-10 Levels of Outpatient Consultations

Outpatient Consultation	History	Examination	MDM	Time (Face-to-Face)
99241	Problem-focused	Problem-focused	Straightforward	20 min
99242	Expanded problem-focused	Expanded problem-focused	Straightforward	40 min
99243	Detailed	Detailed	Low	55 min
99244	Comprehensive	Comprehensive	Moderate	80 min
99245	Comprehensive	Comprehensive	High	110 min

INITIAL OBSERVATION CARE

CPT 99218-99220 (**Table 28-13**) describe the initial day of observation care. All three key components (history, physical examination, and MDM) must be met for each of the observation admission codes. After admitting a patient to observation status, if the same provider group subsequently converts the patient to a hospital inpatient (ie, admits the patient) on the same calendar day, report *only* the appropriate admission service (99221-99223) for the calendar day. Similarly, if admitting a patient to observation following an office evaluation on the same day, report only the appropriate observation code.

Observation discharge care

Report discharge from observation with CPT 99217, typically on the calendar day following admission to observation. The provider must perform a final examination (albeit a minimal examination suffices) of the patient, discuss the course of treatment and ongoing care, and prepare the discharge records.

Subsequent observation care

In rare circumstances, a patient remains in observation for more than two calendar days. Report the second calendar day with the appropriate subsequent observation day service (CPT 99224-99226) (**Table 28-14**) and the observation discharge day code (99217) on the final (third calendar) day.

CRITICAL CARE SERVICES

Critical care services represent the care of the critically ill or injured patient, utilizing different sets of codes, depending upon the patient's age and/or condition. Adult critical care codes (CPT 99291-99292) are selected according to the time spent by the physician in directing the care of the patient, while the neonatal (CPT 99468-99469) and pediatric (CPT 99471-99476) critical care codes are chosen based upon the age of the patient and apply to the entire calendar day.

A critical illness or injury acutely impairs one or more vital organ systems, such that there is a high probability of imminent or life-threatening deterioration in the patient's condition. Critical care treats single- or multiorgan system failure to prevent clinically significant or life-threatening deteriorations, and requires the provider to devote his or her full attention to the patient; therefore, the provider cannot provide services to any other patient during that same time.

Adult critical care is a time-based service of minimum 30 minutes duration. Report CPT 99291 for the first 30 to 74 minutes of critical care; report CPT 99292 for each additional 30 minutes beginning with 75 minutes of critical care. Critical care occurs on the floor/unit, and need not occur solely at the bedside. Critical care time includes reviewing databases, chart notes, telemetry, laboratory studies and radiographic images, and conversations with other providers such as consultants and ancillary care providers. However, all time associated with separately reportable procedures (such as placement of central venous and arterial catheters, cardiopulmonary resuscitation, and thoracentesis, paracentesis, and lumbar puncture) must be excluded from critical care time.

PROLONGED CARE

The prolonged care codes (CPT 99354-99359) may be reported when the provider's visit extends more than 30 minutes beyond the typical time allotted by CPT for the service provided. These codes must be reported in addition to the primary E/M service. Medicare only reimburses the codes representing the physician's direct (face-to-face) contact during inpatient (CPT 99356-99357) and outpatient (CPT 99354-99355) visits. Other payers recognize these codes on an individual, contracted basis. No payer recognizes the non-face-to-face prolonged service codes (CPT 99358-99359).

TEACHING PHYSICIAN REGULATIONS

The teaching physician regulations define the circumstances under which a *physician* provider may bill for professional services rendered to a patient in a teaching setting. Generally, the teaching physician may report E/M services and procedures they either personally perform, or personally supervise a resident performing. However, under no circumstance can time spent teaching ever be used as a basis for reporting a service.

TABLE 28-11 Levels of Subsequent Hospital Care

Subsequent Hospital Care	History	Examination	MDM	Time
99231	Problem-focused	Problem-focused	Straightforward or low	15 min
99232	Expanded	Expanded	Moderate	25 min
99233	Detailed	Detailed	High	35 min

TABLE 28-12 Levels of Same Day Observation Admission and Discharge

Initial Observation Care and Discharge on Same Day	History	Examination	MDM
99234	Detailed or comprehensive	Detailed or comprehensive	Straightforward or low
99235	Comprehensive	Comprehensive	Moderate
99236	Comprehensive	Comprehensive	High

DEFINITIONS

Resident

The regulation defines a resident as any physician enrolled in an accredited graduate medical education program, at any year of postgraduate training. Students (medical, nursing, physician's assistant, or nurse practitioner) are never considered physicians-in-training, and the teaching physician regulations cannot apply to students. Similarly, nonphysician providers are not subject to the regulation, and may neither supervise residents nor be supervised under application of the regulation (see Nonphysician Providers later in this chapter).

Teaching physician

Any independently practicing physician may supervise residents. Neither an academic faculty appointment nor compensation for teaching is required; therefore, these regulations clearly apply to private practice physicians with resident participation in hospitalized inpatient services.

GC modifier

The GC modifier should be appended to every reported service with any participation by a resident, even if the entire service was provided and documented by the teaching physician, with the resident as a silent passive observer.

E/M SERVICES

Physical presence

The teaching physician must personally provide the critical or key portion of an E/M service and then participate in the management plan for that patient. Typically, the teaching physician will perform portions of the E/M service, partially overlapping the resident, or at a completely different time than the resident with no overlapping services. The teaching attending need not obtain or verify every element of the service provided by the resident.

Documentation

The teaching physician need not document the entire service, but rather a short linking (tethering) statement. However, this tethering statement must specifically reference the resident's note and demonstrate the teaching physician's physical presence, evaluation of the patient, and active involvement in the care plan (**Table 28-15**). Simply cosigning a resident note with a minimal statement of agreement is insufficient. Similarly, a scribed note authored by a student or resident cannot adequately identify the teaching physician as the provider of a clinical service.

Report the E/M service based upon the pooled documentation by the teaching physician and the resident, as well as any patient-completed history forms and the elements of past, family, and social history and any review of systems obtained from students. The teaching physician should specifically add any clinically relevant elements of history, physical examination, or medical decision making left out of the resident documentation and specify to which (among many possible) resident note(s) his or her statement links. In addition, although not required, teaching attendings should also directly sign the resident note with a comment referring the reader to the tethering statement in the medical record.

Electronic Medical Records (EMRs)

The 2006 update to the regulation specified additional documentation guidelines in EMRs. The teaching physician must personally add the tethering statement in a secured (ie, password-protected) manner. In addition, the composite EMR note, comprising the resident documentation tethered by the teaching physician, must contain some unique aspect of the patient encounter and not comprise entirely predetermined, unedited text (ie, a "macro").

PROCEDURES

Major procedures

The regulation defines a *major procedure* as typically requiring more than five minutes to perform. Therefore, most inpatient procedures performed by hospitalists (such as arthrocentesis, thoracentesis, paracentesis, and lumbar puncture) comprise a major procedure. The teaching physician must define and be physically present for the critical or key portion of the procedure, document their presence for the critical or key portion of the procedure, and be immediately available (eg, on the unit/floor) for the entire procedure. The critical or key portion(s) of the procedure may vary among different patients undergoing the same procedure, and the teaching physician may supervise the critical or key portion of only one procedure at a time. It is useful, albeit not mandatory, to specify the critical

TABLE 28-13 Levels of Initial Observation Care

Initial Observation Care	History	Examination	MDM
99218	Detailed or comprehensive	Detailed or comprehensive	Straightforward or low
99219	Comprehensive	Comprehensive	Moderate
99220	Comprehensive	Comprehensive	High

TABLE 28-14 Levels of Subsequent Observation Care

Subsequent Observation Care	History	Examination	MDM	Time
99224	Problem-focused	Problem-focused	Straightforward or low	15 min
99225	Expanded	Expanded	Moderate	25 min
99226	Detailed	Detailed	High	35 min

or key portion of the service. A resident statement of the teaching physician's physical presence is inadequate.

Minor procedures

The regulation defines a *minor procedure* as typically requiring less than five minutes to perform, and mandates the teaching physician be physically present for the entire procedure, with no overlap of another service.

TIME-BASED CODING

Many E/M services may be reported based upon counseling/coordinating or critical care time as discussed earlier. The regulation specifies that only time spent by the teaching attending in direct patient care accrues toward time-based coding; no instructional or didactic time may be included. The teaching physician must document his or her time (start/stop or total cumulative) and describe his or her service (counseling/coordinating inpatient care, providing critical care, discharge management). For example: "I spent more than 45 minutes personally urging Ms. Smith to undergo a biopsy to diagnose her breast mass as the cause of her hypercalcemia." A linking statement, while commonly made in the medical record, is inadequate for reporting time-based services, nor may a resident statement document the time spent by the teaching physician.

TABLE 28-15 Linking/Tethering Statements

Unacceptable examples of linking/tethering statements:
Agree with above. (*Legible signature*)
Rounded, review, agree. (*Legible signature*)
D/w resident. (*Legible signature*)
Seen and agree. (*Legible signature*)
Patient seen and evaluated. (*Legible signature*)
Legible signature alone.
Acceptable examples of linking/tethering statements:
I saw and evaluated the patient. D/w resident and agree with resident's findings and plan as documented in the resident's note.
See resident's note for details. I saw and evaluated the patient and agree with the resident's findings and plan, as written.
I performed a history and physical examination and management discussed with resident. Reviewed resident's note and agree with findings and plan of care.
See resident's note for details. Saw and evaluated patient and agree with the resident's findings and plan, as written.
I saw and examined the patient. Agree w/resident's note except murmur louder, so obtain an echocardiogram to evaluate.
I saw and evaluated pt. Agree w/resident's note except picture more consistent with pericarditis than myocardial ischemia. Will begin nonsteroidal treatment.

Data from *Medicare Claims Processing Manual*, Chapter 12, Section 100.

NONPHYSICIAN PROVIDERS

Physicians increasingly utilize nurse practitioners (NPs) and physician's assistants (PAs) as nonphysician providers (NPPs). Some NPP services may be incorporated into the clinical activities provided by the physician, while other clinical services can be performed and reimbursed independently. Several options for these services exist for Medicare, which we will describe in depth. Other insurers may mimic Medicare, or define completely separate, specific contractual mechanisms for addressing these services.

INDEPENDENT BILLING

The 1997 Balanced Budget Act (BBA) allowed for NPPs to independently bill for their services. NPPs must enroll and obtain a Medicare National Provider Identifier (NPI) and provider number to submit claims. Many payers enroll NPPs for independent billing in primary care practices; some may also recognize NPPs linked to hospitalist groups. Currently, only Aetna plans to consistently recognize all specialty NPPs for independent billing purposes and issue a provider number to any qualified NPP.

Services

NPPs may perform all services typically considered physician's services, within the limitations of their state-regulated scope of practice. Such services include E/M visits, many procedures, and performance of diagnostic testing; for each of these services, the NPP would generally perform and document the service exactly as a physician would. However, many states articulate different scopes of practice, supervisory requirements, documentation standards, and cosignature requirements for NPs distinct from PAs, and may require additional documentation beyond that of a physician. Facilities may further impose internal guidelines involving documentation standards or cosignature requirements.

Billing

NPs may directly bill Medicare and receive payment. In contrast, only the qualified employer of a PA may receive payment. Medicare limits reimbursement for NPPs to 85% of the Physician Fee Schedule; Aetna plans to similarly discount their services.

"INCIDENT TO" BILLING

Medicare allows NPPs to provide services "incident to" those of the physician, in the physician office setting. Qualifying "incident to" services include follow-up services typically performed by office staff, such as vital signs, injections, and simple dressing changes, as well as more advanced services within their state-regulated scope of practice. Medicare mandates the physician's physical presence in the office suite (direct supervision), during performance of all "incident to" services. "Incident to" services are not applicable to the majority of hospitalist services, characteristically provided in facility settings.

SHARED/SPLIT BILLING

In October 2002, CMS created a shared/split billing policy for NPP services provided in a facility setting and third party payers increasingly recognize variations of this policy. Under split/shared billing, both the physician and the NPP render *portions* of a service. The designated NPPs must have a Medicare provider number (see *Independent Billing* earlier in this chapter) linked to the same group practice as the sharing physician.

Services

Shared/split billing applies only to specified E/M services, and never procedures or diagnostic testing. Critical care and consultations performed by an NPP must be reported using independent billing. Services must occur in either the inpatient (place of service [POS] 21), hospital outpatient (POS 22), or emergency department (POS 23) sites of service. Services may be rendered concurrently or at separate times during the same calendar day, but both the NPP and the physician must each have a face-to-face encounter with the patient (or else the NPP must report the service as an independent provider).

Documentation

Shared/split service documentation must clearly identify the providers involved and evidence the physician's portion of the service. The NPP and the physician should each note their involvement in the patient's care. If the NPP and physician each write separate notes, the two notes should refer to each other such that the supporting documentation for the service rendered comprises the composite of both notes. Legible signatures and dates must accompany each provider's note.

Billing

Shared/split services may be reported under either the physician or the NPP provider number, but Medicare reimburses NPP services at 85% of the Physician Fee Schedule. The usual Medicare payment at 100% of the Physician Fee Schedule occurs if the physician provider number appears on the claim.

Non-Medicare payers

Insurers not recognizing the various Medicare billing options for NPP services typically do not issue NPP provider numbers. In order to obtain reimbursement for NPP services in this situation, delineate the details of these circumstances in the contract terms with each payer.

TEAM SERVICES

CARDIOPULMONARY ARREST

Hospitalists typically supervise, and at times partially perform, cardiopulmonary resuscitation (CPT 92950). A dedicated clinical resuscitation or code call team usually renders this complex, time-intensive effort. Most hospitals have a designated cardiopulmonary resuscitation form to achieve complete, optimal documentation of these expected but uncommon events. Simply signing a suitable form authenticates the supervision or performance of the cardiopulmonary resuscitation (CPR) service.

E/M service

Any E/M service provided on the same calendar day as CPR should be separately documented in the medical record. Correct billing of the E/M service requires appendage of a 25 modifier (eg, 99291-25) to demonstrate the service as separately identifiable from the procedure.

Other procedures

Certain procedures frequently accompany cardiopulmonary resuscitation, including endotracheal intubation (CPT 31500), chest tube insertion (CPT 32551), pericardiocentesis (CPT 33010), central venous catheter insertion (CPT 36556), and arterial puncture (CPT 36600). Remember each of these separately billable procedures also requires a separate procedure note for documentation, and that all time associated with these procedures must be excluded from any reported critical care time.

RAPID RESPONSES

Rapid responses assemble a multidisciplinary, critical care team to evaluate deteriorating patients outside of an intensive care unit. Also, at times, a patient, visitor, or employee in any location within the hospital may require a rapid response and transport to the hospital emergency room.

Inpatients

For rapid response services provided to inpatients, document the service provided in the medical record. Report an appropriate inpatient E/M service (including potentially critical care and use the hospital inpatient place of service (POS 21) on claim submissions.

Outpatients

For employees or visitors, as well as patients in observation status, use the outpatient hospital site of service (POS 22). Document an appropriate outpatient E/M service in the medical record. If the visitor or employee is admitted that same calendar day, both the site of service and the E/M code for the service may change.

MODIFIERS

As noted throughout the text above, at times certain modifiers must be appended to a CPT code to allow proper claims processing. Several modifiers are occasionally utilized by hospitalists.

25, SEPARATELY IDENTIFIABLE E/M SERVICE

Append this modifier to indicate performance of a significant, separately identifiable E/M service on the same day as a procedure, when performed by the same provider group. The E/M service must be medically necessary, beyond the usual preoperative and postoperative care associated with the procedure. The two chart notes (for the procedure and the E/M service) should clearly elaborate the rationale for the two services. For example, the procedure indication might be ascites while the E/M service provided evaluation and management of hepatic encephalopathy.

59, SEPARATELY IDENTIFIABLE PROCEDURE

Modifier 59 is most frequently employed with code pairs identified in the National Correct Coding Initiative (NCCI) edits, representing procedures typically bundled together. Do not use modifier 59 to bypass an NCCI edit without establishing the proper criterion for its appropriate clinical use with two procedures or services (other than an E/M service) as distinct or independent from each other, when performed on the same day. For example, following a large volume, therapeutic thoracentesis (CPT 32422) later that same day the patient develops an iatrogenic pneumothorax requiring chest tube insertion (CPT 32551); report both 32422-59 and 32551, after documenting two independent procedure notes.

■ GC, SEPARATELY IDENTIFIABLE E/M SERVICE

Append modifier GC to any E/M service or procedure in which a resident participated, under the direction of a teaching physician.

■ GV, PHYSICIAN NOT EMPLOYED BY HOSPICE

Use this modifier when the hospitalist serves as the attending physician, rather than the hospice physician.

TEMPLATED NOTES

Templated chart notes, whether formatted as preprinted paper progress notes with check boxes or electronically constructed as combinations of macros and click-boxes, are common, appropriate documentation tools. Such tools enhance legibility and facilitate efficient documentation in accord with the E/M guidelines. Unfortunately electronic notes often become the source for increasingly prevalent "cut-and-paste" errors, highlighting the need to balance efficiency with accuracy in providing safe, efficient care to complex patients.

■ AUDIT TOOLS

Audit tools are useful adjuncts to ensuring adherence to E/M billing guidelines, patient safety and quality initiatives, and other process assessments. Such tools are often custom designed in the context of chart reviews and institutional initiatives, or implementing coding and billing audits associated with practice compliance plans. CMS has not developed or endorsed any formal audit tool for E/M services, although several Medicare contractors (eg, Trailblazers and Highmark) make their E/M score sheets available to assist providers in adhering to documentation guidelines.

SUGGESTED READINGS

American Medical Association. Current Procedural Terminology (CPT) 2011. Chicago, IL: American Medical Association; 2009.

Association of American Medical Colleges. Medicare's teaching physician documentation instructions. Washington, DC: American Association of Medical Colleges; 2002. Available online at www.aamc.org/advocacy/library/teachphys/mtpdi.pdf.

Centers for Medicare and Medicaid Services. *Medicare Claims Processing Manual*. Bethesda, MA: Department of Health and Human Services; 2011. Available online at www.cms.hhs.gov/manuals/downloads/clm104c12.pdf.

Highmark Medicare Services: Specialty Exam Scoresheets. Camp Hill, PA: Highmark Medicare Services; 2011. Available online at www.highmarkmedicareservices.com/partb/reference/scoresheets.html.

Hoffman SA, Manaker S. Inpatient and outpatient consultations after elimination of payments for evaluation and management consultation codes. *Chest*. 2011;139:933–938.

Manaker S, Pohlig CA, Krier-Morrow D. *Coding for Chest Medicine 2011: Pulmonary, Critical Care and Sleep*. Northbrook, IL: American College of Chest Physicians; 2011.

Siegler EL, Adelman R. Copy and paste: a remediable hazard of electronic health records. *Amer J Med*. 2009;122:495.

Trailblazer Health Enterprises. *Evaluation and Management Coding and Documentation Reference Guide*. Dallas, TX: Trailblazer Health Enterprises; 2009. Available online at www.trailblazerhealth.com/Publications/Job%20Aid/coding%20pocket%20reference.pdf.

CHAPTER 29

Best Practices in Physician Recruitment and Retention

R. Kirk Mathews, MBA

INTRODUCTION

Much has been made of the fact that the practice of Hospital Medicine has become the fastest growing specialty in the history of American medicine. Most experts agree that there are approximately 30,000 physicians practicing as hospitalists as of 2010. The Society of Hospital Medicine reports a membership of approximately 10,000. Yet even with the rapid increase in hospitalist supply, the demand remains even greater. Many believe the demand will reach 40,000 hospitalists in the next several years.

As a result, recruiting competition for hospitalists is fierce. Therefore, it is imperative that hospitalist practices maintain a high performance recruiting function as a core competency. Recruiting physicians requires a good understanding of human nature, a proven process and the discipline to apply that process to a large number of candidates. It is hardly an exact science, yet there are several important principles that must be applied. This chapter will attempt to provide employers with a basic understanding of these principles as well as some tips and suggestions to enhance their recruiting performance.

SOURCING CANDIDATES

Many employers make the mistake of believing they are actively recruiting if they run a recruiting advertisement in medical journals or perhaps even if they have engaged a recruitment agency. In most cases, these are merely passive recruiting efforts. Actively trying to locate candidates through existing relationships and Internet recruiting will yield much better results. In the current competitive recruiting environment, it is critical that the employer have an aggressive candidate sourcing strategy.

Every good candidate sourcing strategy begins with the establishment of candidate parameters, including training requirements (MD, DO, internal medicine, family practice, etc). It is important for the employer to have a good understanding of their customer, the referring physicians, when establishing the candidate parameters. For example, the decision to hire family practice physicians as hospitalists should only be made with the approval of the referring medical staff.

The candidate sourcing plan should be thorough yet budget friendly. The following are all potential sources of candidates that should be considered by the employer.

EXISTING MEDICAL STAFF

Often, the best hospitalist that a hospital could hope to hire might already be on staff. Confidentially asking formal and informal medical staff leadership about who might be a good candidate could yield great low-cost results. Medical staff leadership will probably know which physicians are the best clinicians as well as who might be thinking about exploring a change in their practice situation.

MEDICAL STAFF REFERRALS

Hospitals must be intentional about asking existing medical staff members for referrals. Most physicians are so busy they will not take time to really think about colleagues who would be good hospitalists without frequent prompting. Of particular value are recent additions to the medical staff. Newly trained physicians will be aware of physicians coming behind them in the next graduating class and recently relocated experienced physicians will be aware of former colleagues that might be good candidates. Employers should approach these new members of the medical staff and intentionally "jog" their memory to uncover these referrals. Some employers offer a financial incentive for candidates hired as a result of a medical staff referral.

OTHER LOCAL/REGIONAL HOSPITALS

Recruiting physicians from other local hospitals can be very effective since these physicians have already made the decision to live in the area. If the hospital is a "friendly" competitor or a patient referral source, some political and/or business caution should be exercised. It is also advisable for the employer to be attentive to signs that the local competitors might also be recruiting their physicians.

JOURNAL ADVERTISING

This popular sourcing tool can produce candidates when used properly. Journal ads should be eye-catching and brief. No ad can provide enough information for a candidate to decide they want the job, but it can provide enough information for them to decide they do *not* want the job. The goal of any ad is to prompt the candidate to take action—either place a phone call or visit a Website to learn more. Some of the more popular journals for sourcing hospitalists include *The Hospitalist* (a publication of the Society of Hospital Medicine), *Annals of Internal Medicine*, and *The Journal of the American Medical Association*. The employer should also look for ways to leverage their journal ad investment. Many medical journals also offer online job boards. Often, job postings on these boards are discounted or free for employers who run print ads. In some cases, these boards are only accessible to employers who run print ads. Employers should evaluate the relative value of print ad vs Internet job postings and minimize their print investment (small black and white ad vs full page color) if they believe the online posting is more valuable.

ONLINE HOSPITALIST JOB BOARDS

Internet recruiting has dramatically changed the business of physician recruiting as many candidates now do most of their investigations online. These sites charge employers to post their ads. Some provide employers with CVs; others provide a more detailed candidate profile of those candidates visiting their site. The Society of Hospital Medicine has developed an excellent candidate sourcing tool with their Career Center at www.hospitalmedicine.org/careercenter. Other popular sites include Hospitalistjobs.com and Practicelink.com.

DIRECT MAIL

Direct mail has long been used to source physician candidates with varying degrees of effectiveness. Employers choosing to use direct mail should purchase a very targeted mailing list and design a mailer to prompt the candidate to action. Since direct mail campaigns usually generate a very low return, an inexpensive and colorful postcard is usually the most cost-effective direct mail tool.

CAREER FAIRS

Career fairs can be excellent sources of candidates for hospitals within a reasonable distance of the event. These sponsored events are designed to assist second and third year residents to get exposure to various employers. These fairs allow employers to begin the recruiting relationship with any given candidate "face to face." To enhance the return on the investment in such a fair, employers can contact (via e-mail, phone, or postal mail) residents in the area and arrange to meet them at the fair.

RESIDENCY PROGRAM RELATIONSHIPS

Employers should establish relationships with all the residency programs in their region. Getting to know the program directors of all the programs within 200 miles can yield outstanding low-cost results. Offering to provide a noon lecture or some other resource to the program director can be an excellent way to begin to develop the relationship. Such events also provide excellent exposure to the residents. This exposure is valuable for future recruiting—even exposure to first and second year residents.

> **PRACTICE POINT**
>
> - Employers should establish relationships with all the residency programs in their region. Getting to know the program directors of all the programs within 200 miles can yield outstanding low cost results.

RECRUITMENT FIRMS

Recruitment firms are only as good as the individual recruiter assigned to complete the assignment. Many employers choose to use recruitment firms to extend their reach on difficult-to-fill searches such as hospitalist positions. Contingency-based companies only charge a fee if they are successful. This is a risk-free approach but this financial relationship creates a candidate-focused recruiting effort. A contingency recruiter will locate a good marketable candidate and then "shop" him to a variety of potential employers. With no real obligation to the employer, recruiters are most likely to shop their candidates to their most attractive client locations, increasing their chances for a placement. Retained recruiting firms typically charge a monthly fee in return for monthly effort to fill the assignment. Retained firms rarely offer a guarantee of success, so the employer is taking the risk of making a significant investment without successfully hiring a candidate. Both types of firms can produce results, so it is important for employers to be very comfortable with the recruiter assigned to their search before they engage any recruiting firm.

In summary, a candidate sourcing plan is similar to an investment portfolio—diversity is good. Placing all the eggs in one basket is a high-risk approach to sourcing good candidates.

THE PRE-INTERVIEW CANDIDATE ASSESSMENT

This section is focused on completely assessing the candidate prior to extending an invitation for an onsite interview. Onsite interviews are time consuming and expensive, so the employer should be reasonably certain that they will want to extend an offer to the candidate *prior* to inviting a candidate to the interview. This should minimize the possibility of learning something about the candidate *during* the onsite visit (once the time and money have already been invested) that eliminates them from consideration.

However, prior to assessing any candidates, it is highly advisable for the employer to assess their own practice. Only in knowing their own practice well can they determine what candidate characteristics will create the best opportunity for a good long term fit. What skills/training are required in this practice? How do the physicians communicate? What is the governance structure, a democracy or a dictatorship? Are there strict policies in place or do physicians work things out informally or "on the fly"? How much social time do the physicians spend together? Understanding these things about their own practice should enable the employer to recruit and retain a better candidate.

> **PRACTICE POINT**
>
> - Prior to assessing any candidates, it is highly advisable for the employer to assess their own practice. Only in knowing their own practice well can they determine what candidate characteristics will create the best opportunity for a good long-term fit.

Accordingly every effort should be made to thoroughly assess the following aspects of each candidate prior to an onsite visit:

Training and clinical skills: Be aware of any gaps in the candidate's training. Gaps can be unavoidable in many cases, but they can also indicate a problem. Most candidates will be able to provide a thorough explanation for any gaps in their coverage without difficulty. Employers should verify the candidate's explanation whenever possible. They should also verify that the candidate has the skills (such as procedural skills) required for the practice.

Prior work experience: Discuss all prior work experiences with the candidate. Asking the candidate about the reasons for terminating each employment relationship can uncover a pattern of discontent or employer dissatisfaction. If the candidate has numerous previous jobs, constructing a timeline can be helpful to reveal any gaps or overlaps in their work experience, either of which will require further explanation/investigation.

Communication skills: Good verbal communication skills are critical for a hospitalist. Many employers make the mistake of talking too much when assessing a candidate (as well as during an onsite visit). It is important for the employer to set the stage with a question, and then to get off the stage and allow the candidate to speak as long as they wish. The employer should make note of both the content of the answers, as well as the ease and comfort with which the answers are provided.

Work ethic and workplace attitude: These are two of the more difficult candidate characteristics to evaluate, yet are among the most important to understand. Practices in which the physicians are mismatched in work ethic and workplace attitude are at the greatest risk of turmoil and turnover. The following are some questions that an employer can ask to help determine a candidate's work ethic and workplace attitude:

- How many patients do you feel you can comfortably see in one day?
- Describe a situation where you felt overworked.
- How hard to you like to work?
- When do you typically begin your workday?
- Describe a time when you were asked to work overtime without compensation.
- Describe any volunteer work that you have performed.
- What personal gratification do you get from your work?

Checking references: Unfortunately, the process of checking references has become less and less valuable. Most employers are afraid to say anything negative about the candidate for fear of legal recourse. As a result many have resorted to simply providing the dates of employment for the candidate and nothing more. Many residency program directors are hesitant to give a poor reference on a candidate because of the same legal concerns or perhaps because it would be a poor reflection on their program. As a result, they often prefer to only send a "To whom it may concern" form letter. When pressed, they will sometimes "rate" the candidate on a variety of topics. However, it is extremely rare for a program director to rate a candidate as "poor" in any category. The common practice seems to be rating the lesser candidates as "average." However, unfortunately, checking references remains a required element of any recruiting process, so how can an employer benefit from such a potentially flawed process? Here are a few tips to enhance the referencing process:

1. **Ask for specific references.** The employer should not simply rely on whomever the candidate decides to provide. The employer should always ask to speak with the candidate's supervisor or residency program director. Other potentially valuable references might come from the hospital administrator, a referring physician who has had patients cared for by the candidate, unit nurses who have worked with the candidate, and ED physicians who have worked with the candidate.
2. **Speak directly with the reference whenever possible.** There is much to be gained from listening carefully when the reference is questioned. "Pregnant pauses" and voice inflections are absent from reference letters and forms, but can speak volumes about what that person believes about the candidate.
3. **Describe the practice.** When speaking with a reference, the employer should describe their own practice and then ask how the candidate will perform in such a practice. The employer should not simply ask "yes or no" questions or only ask the reference to "rate" the candidate on a scale of 1 to 10. The employer should attempt to engage the reference in a meaningful dialogue about the candidate's strengths and weaknesses.

The employer should keep in mind that the goal of the referencing process is not to simply avoid a bad hire; the goal should be to determine whether the candidate can succeed in their practice and become a good long-term, productive member of the practice. The referencing process can be a valuable tool not only in the hiring process, but information uncovered in the referencing process can be valuable in managing the candidate once they are hired.

THE ONSITE VISIT/INTERVIEW

For most employers, the onsite visit/interview is when the practice leaders evaluate the candidate in order to determine if they will extend an offer of employment. However, in a high-performance recruiting process, the onsite visit will provide *confirmation* of an evaluation that has already been conducted. Only the final element of the candidate evaluation should be performed during the onsite visit, that is, a face-to-face confirmation of facts already reviewed. This approach allows the employer to focus on (what should be) the real goal of the onsite visit—convincing the candidate that they want this job!

This approach to recruiting is foreign to most employers but is best illustrated by considering how major universities recruit their star athletes. College coaches never invite anyone to visit their campus for official recruiting visits before they thoroughly examine them. A college coach will watch hours of game films of the prospective recruit. They will interview the candidate by phone. They will interview the recruit's high school coach, guidance counselor, and sometimes even their girlfriend! Only after they are convinced the athlete is someone they want to recruit do they invite them to campus for the official visit. During the visit, the recruit will briefly visit face-to-face with the head coach, and the rest of the visit is organized in such a way to convince the athlete that their athletic and academic goals can be achieved at that university.

When a physician candidate has "passed" the pre-interview assessment and there is a high likelihood that the candidate will receive an offer during the onsite, then (and only then) should the candidate be invited to an onsite visit. That visit should include the following elements:

Ice-breaker event: Often a meal, coffee, or an open-house type of event is best for an ice breaker. The event should be casual and informal with plenty of opportunity for discussion.

Business discussion: This is the time to review the financial elements of the position, including a review of the employment agreement. The employer should make sure the candidate has the opportunity to ask any questions about the financial arrangements including income, benefits, vacation, etc.

Community introduction: This should be more than a simple community tour and should include introductions to key people in the community that might play a role in the candidate's life upon their relocation. For example, if the candidate has children of junior high school age, a drive by the junior high school would be nice. However, making an appointment for the candidate to meet the junior high school principal is much better!

Time with future colleagues: Every onsite visit should provide time when the physicians can communicate with some of the other physicians in the practice about how the practice functions on a daily basis. The candidate should feel free to ask any questions they might have about practice operations.

Hospital tour: A hospital tour should include some time with key hospital leaders, both physician and nonphysician leaders. For example, even a brief hello and handshake with the hospital CEO can convey a valuable message to the candidate that the hospitalist program is important to the hospital.

Wrap-up discussion: The wrap-up discussion is perhaps the most important element of the onsite visit. This is the time to get the candidate's initial feedback from their visit and (most importantly) correct any false impressions that may have received. This is also time to directly ask the candidate if they want the job.

PRACTICE POINT

- When a physician candidate has "passed" the preinterview assessment and there is a high likelihood that the candidate will receive an offer during the onsite visit, then (and only then) should the candidate be invited to an onsite visit. It is critically important for employers to respond to candidate's questions and concerns in a very timely manner following the onsite visit. Every candidate should receive a follow-up phone call within a day or two of the visit.

Here are some tips to keep in mind when planning a candidate visit.

1. **Honesty is the best policy.** Since no practice is perfect and no community is utopia, the employer should never try to hide any deficiencies from the candidate. However, employers should take care not to unduly overemphasize a potential concern. This can happen inadvertently when every person who speaks with the candidate mentions a negative aspect of the community. They are doing so with the best of intentions and the candidate's best interest at heart, but in so doing might give more weight to the concern than is warranted. One way to avoid this is to assign one person to mention this concern and make sure the entire interview team understands who will be doing so.
2. **Control the agenda.** The employer should control the agenda with every member of the interview team well prepared for their role. The interview team should be composed of the very best the practice has to offer. The employer should hand select this team and avoid placing chronic complainers on the team.
3. **Always bring the candidate spouse.** The employer must understand they are recruiting the entire family, not just the physician. Often the spouse represents more than 50% of the decision to accept or decline an offer. If the candidate cannot bring their spouse on the visit, every effort should be made to set a different date when they will be able to attend.
4. **Avoid bringing the candidate's children.** Encourage the candidate to leave their children at home if at all possible. One (or both) of the parents will be distracted at some point during the interview if the children attend. If the candidate insists in bringing the children, arrange for child care during the visit so the parents can focus on the visit.
5. **Strive for a one visit process.** If the preinterview assessment and the on-site visit is *well structured and thorough*, the employer should be prepared to complete the process with only one visit from the candidate. Many employers make the mistake of thinking if they like the candidate on the first interview, they can bring them back for a second visit. In the current recruiting environment, they may not get a chance at a second trip. They should prepare the candidate to make a decision after the first visit because...
6. **Time kills all deals.** The candidate will rarely be more excited about the job than immediately following the visit. Because the competition is tremendous and the candidate's opportunities are many, the employer must act with a sense of urgency. This means responding to candidate questions immediately and providing a sample agreement during the interview and an executable agreement immediately following the visit.
7. **Expect the unexpected.** The employer should be flexible enough to allow for unexpected and unavoidable changes to the interview agenda.

FOLLOW-UP AND NEGOTIATIONS

Finally, it cannot be overemphasized that time kills all deals. It is critically important for employers to respond to candidate's questions and concerns in a very timely manner following the onsite visit. Every candidate should receive a follow-up phone call within a day or two of the visit.

When a candidate wants to negotiate one or more elements of the contract, the employer should implement "Big Picture Negotiations." Both parties are best served when each can consider specific contract requests in light of all requested contract concessions. The employer should inform the candidate of this policy and instruct them to thoroughly review the employment agreement, and present all concerns/requests at one time. This approach will help the employer from making a significant concession without knowing if another significant request will follow. If the candidate presents a long, unreasonable list of contract requests, the employer should be honest with the candidate and ask them which, if any, of the requests are "deal breakers." The employer should address these first, as it is very frustrating to work through a long list of relatively minor concerns only to see the deal fall apart at the end. These negotiations should always be conducted in an unemotional, businesslike manner. This will give the candidate confidence that the practice leaders handle difficult issues with professionalism.

A FEW WORDS ABOUT RETENTION, OR... WHY GOOD RECRUITING IS SO IMPORTANT!

One only needs to attempt to add up the total cost of physician turnover to understand the importance of good recruiting. "Getting it right the first time" is critically important in recruiting hospitalists. Consider the following scenario:

One of your hospitalists has just given notice that they will be leaving your practice in 120 days. What is the potential financial impact on your practice? The answer is found by adding up some (or all) of the sample expenses in **Table 29-1**.

PRACTICE POINT

- One only needs to attempt to add up the total cost of physician turnover to understand the importance of good recruiting. "Getting it right the first time" is critically important in recruiting hospitalists.

TABLE 29-1 Potential Financial Impact of Turnover

1. Malpractice tail: Is the practice responsible for all or part of the departing physician's tail? If so, this might be 2–3 times the most recent annual premium.	Up to $25,000
2. Will you engage a professional recruitment firm?	Up to $25,000
3. Candidate sourcing budget (journal ads, Internet job boards, etc)	$6,000
4. Candidate interview expenses (assuming four interviews to fill the position at $1500 per interview)	$6,000
5. Signing bonus	$15,000
6. Relocation expense allowance	$10,000
7. Time required of everyone in the practice to source, screen, and interview all potential candidates.	???
Subtotal	$87,000

The subtotal in Table 29-1 assumes the candidate is sourced, interviewed, signed, licensed, credentialed, and relocated all within 120 days in order to avoid any gap in physician coverage for your program. Depending on the desirability of your location and the availability of candidates interested in your location, this 120 days may be achievable. However, for many practices, 120 days is sadly only a dream. Some hospitals cannot even get hospital privileges granted in 120 days! If your remaining physicians cannot absorb the patient volume once their departing colleague is gone, the practice will be faced with locum tenens coverage that could cost up to $2,000 per day! For every month the position is unfilled, the practice must pay $60,000 in locums fees. It is easy to see how the $87,000 can quickly become $147,000 or $207,000. The cost of turnover is high! And this table does not even begin to try and calculate the cost of decreased collections (when locums docs are used or while the new doc is getting up to speed on the billing software, etc). Furthermore, losing an experienced hospitalist who has positive working relationships with your primary care physicians and a working knowledge of the hospital may further compound the financial impact and adversely affect the smooth functioning of the service.

The best protection against turnover is to recruit well the first time. Every practice should work really hard to make sure the candidate is a good fit for the practice during the recruitment phase of their relationship. However, every practice will experience turnover. Some more than others, but it will happen to everyone eventually. Here are a few tips to consider regarding retention:

1. Never stop recruiting your physicians! Hospitalists are too hard to come by, so never stop paying attention to the factors affecting their job satisfaction.
2. Create a work/life/compensation balance that makes sense and do everything possible to keep it in balance. If any one element of this three-sided scale is significantly out of balance with the other two for an extended period of time, turnover is inevitable.
3. Assign each new physician a mentor, a sort of big brother or big sister within the practice. This person should not only help the new physician navigate their new professional surroundings, but be available to advise the new physician on community issues such as neighborhoods, schools, and community resources.
4. Provide a physician feedback forum of some kind. Frustration will build when physicians feel like their issues are not being heard. They may not always get the answers they wanted, but fair-minded physicians will understand if they are at least allowed such a forum.
5. Use team-building exercises or events to avoid any one physician from feeling isolated within the group. Sometimes these can be social events and sometimes they might be professional retreats.

CONCLUSION

An understaffed hospitalist program will quickly become an unstable program with far-reaching consequences that are both clinical and financial. It is imperative that hospitalist programs become very proficient in recruiting the physicians they need to provide the outstanding care their patients deserve. Hopefully, this brief chapter will provide employers with an added nugget of advice that will help them improve the performance of their recruiting process.

SUGGESTED READING

Singer A, Swenson D, Wilcox G, et al. Confronting the Hospitalist Workforce Shortage. The Phoenix Group. 2008. www.phoenix-groupwhitepaper.com/docs/confronting_hospitalist_workforce_shortage.PDF

CHAPTER 30

For the Individual: Career Sustainability and Avoiding Burnout

Keiki Hinami, MD, MS
Tosha B. Wetterneck, MD, MS

INTRODUCTION

Hospital Medicine's successful growth in the United States concurrently poses challenges to its sustainability. Its growth has occurred in response to the demand of managed care for dedicated inpatient generalists to serve in various roles, including boundary spanners, communicators, quality enhancers, and care givers. The combination of roles and the often shifting work requirements demand flexibility from hospitalists who are also collectively working harder each year according to the biannual productivity surveys administered by the Society of Hospital Medicine. Moreover, many of the ranks are being filled by young physicians at the beginning of their medical careers. The characteristic stressors related to the work environment and demographics of the hospitalist workforce create conditions under which job burnout has emerged as a valid concern.

The scope of burnout among hospitalists was exposed in 1999 when a nationwide survey of the National Association of Inpatient Physicians (NAIP) identified 12.9% of respondents feeling "burned out" and an additional 24.9% "at risk of burnout." In 2005, a survey of hospitalist leaders ranking the top challenges to their groups identified 7 areas directly related to burnout situated at the top of the list (**Table 30-1**). Other site-based medical specialties like critical care and Emergency Medicine have seen burnout rates as high as 40% to 60% and have taken proactive steps in trying to reduce burnout rates through job design and focus on the individuals. Not in spite of, but because of its rapid growth leaders in the field have deliberated over the sustainability of hospitalist practice models. To retain the best physicians capable of delivering the highest quality of care, understanding burnout and ways to address it remains an essential task for the discipline.

WHAT IS BURNOUT?

DEFINITION

Burnout is a psychological syndrome leading to a worker's erosion of engagement with their job due to long-term exposure to emotionally demanding work. It is a condition observed predominantly, though not exclusively, among those in the helping professions, like health and social services, where direct, frequent, and intense interactions with people are common and where the outcomes of work are not totally dependent on the actions of the worker. The most frequently cited conceptualization of burnout comes from Christina Maslach and colleagues who describe three constitutive dimensions. The first, *emotional exhaustion,* is a literal depletion of the worker's energy due to the work demands. It may manifest in hospitalists as "compassion fatigue" or the tendency to distance themselves, cognitively and emotionally, from their work as they realize they cannot continue to give of themselves to patients and coworkers. In essence, it is a coping response to work overload. The second is *depersonalization*, marked by a detached emotional callousness or cynicism and manifests as indifference or dysfunctional attitudes and behaviors toward patients. It is often a protective response to emotional exhaustion. The final component of burnout, *diminished personal accomplishment*, is the erosion of a worker's sense of personal effectiveness, which brings on a feeling of powerlessness and the tendency to negatively evaluate oneself. This may manifest as a hospitalist not completing assigned tasks or worsening professional self-esteem. Emotional exhaustion is usually considered necessary for burnout to be diagnosed, the other components may occur in parallel, sequentially, or not at all.

TABLE 30-1 Top Challenges Facing Hospital Medicine Groups

Challenge to Hospitalist Groups	% Leaders Indicating Among Top 3 Challenges
Total hours/Work-life balance*	42%
Recruitment	35%
Daily workload*	29%
Expectation of hospital	23%
Reimbursement*	17%
Professional respect/ Job satisfaction*	17%
Career sustainability*	15%
Retention*	15%
Quality of care*	13%
Specialist availability	11%
Bed capacity	11%
Scheduling	11%

*Areas related to burnout.
Data from the biannual Society of Hospital Medicine Productivity Survey 2007–08.

Burnout is distinct from related concepts like stress, depression, and dissatisfaction. The definitions of each have been established empirically, and while they overlap significantly, burnout is specific to the context of the workplace as an ongoing emotional response to chronic demands and interpersonal stressors. Job dissatisfaction is a predictor of burnout; workers who are dissatisfied are more likely to be burned out. However, it is not fully clear whether dissatisfaction always precedes burnout or is a result of burnout (or other workplace conditions that also produce burnout). Individuals who are depression-prone have higher rates of burnout and even though burnout is specific to the workplace, it can also affect homelife. Job stress can be conceptualized by two models: the demand-control-support model and the effort-reward imbalance model. In the first model, job stress is more likely when there are high job demands (usually workload and time pressure), low control over job (autonomy in decision making, patient outcomes) and low support (from colleagues, supervisor, organization; inadequate resources). Given the high job demands inherent in the medical profession, control and support are important mediators. With effort-reward imbalance, there is a discrepancy between the demands and obligations of the job (effort) and the rewards offered like salary, career opportunities, esteem, and job security. For workers who are very committed to their jobs, this imbalance leads to job stress. Again, given the high demands associated with hospitalist jobs and the professional commitment displayed by most physicians, rewards are very important to mediate stress.

WHY IS BURNOUT IMPORTANT TO HOSPITALISTS?

Across a wide variety of professions, burnout has been associated with negative work outcomes including decreasing work hours or job turnover, decreased work effectiveness and productivity, reduced job and organizational commitment, and stress-related health outcomes such as alcohol and drug use or depression. In addition, the negative attitudes and actions of burned out workers can negatively impact others in and out of the workplace. These outcomes and the impact on Hospital Medicine are considered in depth in the proceeding section.

PRACTICE POINT

- Across a wide variety of professions, burnout has been associated with negative work outcomes including decreasing work hours or job turnover, decreased work effectiveness and productivity, reduced job and organizational commitment, and stress-related health outcomes such as alcohol and drug use or depression. In addition, the negative attitudes and actions of burned out workers can negatively impact others in and out of the workplace.

PHYSICIAN BURNOUT AND JOB PERFORMANCE

Burnout predicts poor physician job performance. For example, providers who are happy with their work are known to increase patients' satisfaction and adherence to physician advice. On the other hand, patients of depersonalized physicians have been shown to take longer to recover from their illness. Physicians in Great Britain report providing lower standards of care, being more angry and sometimes abusive with patients as a result of chronic stress. Similarly, burned out general internists and medicine residents have reported engaging in suboptimal patient care such as making errors not due to a lack of knowledge or inexperience. Additionally, a strong negative correlation has been found between emotional exhaustion and quality of care among hospital-based medical subspecialists in Israel.

Although the mechanisms connecting burnout to poor-quality patient care have not been empirically proven, one proposed causal pathway involves the providers' emotional state. One measure of emotions—positive affect—is associated with enhanced decision making and problem solving as well as higher levels of patient centeredness in health care providers. Therefore, burned out hospitalists may be less cognitively vigilant and less likely to put forth the extra effort necessary to deliver the highest quality, patient-centered care.

REDUCED ORGANIZATIONAL COMMITMENT AND JOB TURNOVER

Hospitals and practice groups recognize the need for physicians' commitment to their organization. Organizational commitment refers to employee identification with, and involvement in, a particular community, for example, a hospitalist group or the hospital in which they work. Higher levels of commitment are reflected in lower rates of turnover and are also believed to promote better job performance. Burnout is associated with decreased worker organizational commitment in health care professionals. In addition, being around burned out workers and having negative interactions with them may impact other workers organizational commitment. There is a definite association with burnout and job turnover in medicine. Other site-based specialties like critical care and Emergency Medicine physicians with high levels of burnout are feeling the impact of job turnover on the sustainability of their professions. Specifically, 39% of Emergency Medicine physicians in 2005 expressed their intention to leave practice within five years—a rate that exceeded the recruitment of new physicians through residency training in the same year. Given that turnover and recruitment are major challenges to hospitalist programs and the continued rapid growth of hospitalist programs in the United States, it is essential that burnout be minimized to ensure that experienced hospitalists remain clinically active in the profession to train the future workforce.

STRESS-RELATED HEALTH PROBLEMS AMONG PHYSICIANS

Like all health care providers, physicians experience high levels of job stress. A correspondingly high proportion of physicians, about 20%, are believed to suffer from depression. Burnout was the term originally coined by Herbert Freudenberger to describe patients afflicted by alcoholism and drug abuse in the 1970s, and it remains a feature of the 8% to 12% of health professionals who develop a substance-related disorder at some point in their lives. Suicide is another disturbing problem for health care providers. According to the Psychiatric Clinics of North America, male physicians are two times more likely to commit suicide than the average American, and female physicians are three times more likely. Although only a few studies have tied job burnout to the profound psychological and spiritual dislocation that predispose physicians to self-destructive behavior, the traditional lack of self-care among physicians, scarcity of resources for physician support, and burnout are understood to be related aspects of the same stress-related problem.

WHAT LEADS TO BURNOUT IN HOSPITALISTS?

The key features of hospitalist work and individual characteristics that are associated with burnout are summarized in **Table 30-2** and discussed in detail below.

WORKLOAD

Excessive workload is consistently confirmed as a source of burnout. In 2008, the average hospitalist documented 13.4 encounters per 12-hour shift with a mean of 2180 shift-hours annually, an increase in production compared with 2005. Cost and time pressures pose additional job demands on the typical hospitalist. Irregular night shifts, extended work weeks, and other nontraditional work patterns can predispose hospitalists to physical exhaustion. Some hospitalists engaged in nonclinical responsibilities spend additional time on administrative work, education, and research.

Both qualitative and quantitative work overload contribute to exhaustion by depleting the capacity of physicians to meet job demands. Numerous studies, including the Physician Worklife Study (PWS) of U.S. generalists and specialists, demonstrate the unfavorable effects of overload, time pressure, and resource scarcity on physician stress, burnout, and dissatisfaction. Workload is perceived variably by individuals and cannot be measured simply by the number of hours worked. A study by Shirom and colleagues found that work hours only indirectly predicted quality of care through perceived overload, suggesting other considerations mitigate the effects of physician work hours. One consideration is the protective effect of recovery time. Acute fatigue resulting from an especially demanding event at work does not necessarily lead to burnout, given recovery during restful periods at work or at home. When work overload is persistent, as opposed to sporadic, there is little opportunity to rest and restore balance. A sustainable workload or work-life balance, in contrast, provides opportunities to refine coping skills to draw energy from other restorative aspects of daily life.

TABLE 30-2 Characteristics Associated with Job Burnout

Job Characteristics	Individual Characteristics
Job demands: workload, time pressure, complex patients	Early career
Role conflict and role ambiguity	Male gender
Lack of job control/ autonomy	Not married
Lack of support or good relationships with colleagues and supervisors	Lack of social support outside of work
Lack of reciprocity from patients	Personality factors: external locus of control, low hardiness, low self-esteem
Lack of resources to do the job	
Lack of organizational commitment to hospitalist groups or individuals	

WORK ROLE AND AUTONOMY

The demand-control model of occupational stress offers a framework in which control of the work environment mitigates stress created by ongoing work demands. According to the 1999 NAIP survey, 97% of hospitalists reported being "highly autonomous" or "autonomous" in their clinical role. Since that time, the role of some hospitalists may have evolved in ways that diminish control over their work. Physician autonomy is reduced when their role is uncertain or unpredictable. This is often the case in hospitalist work where the work demands rise and fall erratically. A potential for role conflict exists, in theory, when hospitalists are required to reconcile their responsibilities as advocates both for the hospital and for the patient. Novel practice patterns, such as primary or comanagement of patients typically cared for by surgeons or specialists, also introduce the potential for role ambiguity and decreased autonomy.

Evidence linking burnout to autonomy in health care providers is taken from studies of nurses for whom role conflict and ambiguity are associated with emotional exhaustion. On the positive side, active participation in organizational decision making has consistently been found to be linked to higher levels of efficacy and lower levels of exhaustion. Control over workplace hazards increases employee's energy and health at work.

INTERPERSONAL CONTACTS

The typical hospitalist routinely interacts with many individuals at work. Whether patients, colleagues, or any number of coworkers on an interdisciplinary team, hospitalists are expected to communicate well and seamlessly coordinate care with other stakeholders. A central proposition of social exchange theory is that individuals pursue reciprocity in interpersonal relationships, and those who find themselves participating in an unreciprocated relationship will become distressed. Physicians who do not receive the intrinsically sought-after positive feedback from patients and coworkers are more likely to manifest signs of burnout.

A study by Bakker and colleagues examined the relationships between general practitioners and patients over a period of 5 years, and found that emotional exhaustion evoked negative attitudes toward patients. In turn, physicians who attempted to gain emotional distance from their patients as a way of coping with exhaustion were found to produce the demanding behaviors that they sought to avoid. Additional research establishes burnout's association with a greater exposure to patients with poor prognosis. Unlike traditional practitioners with whom patients have longitudinal relationships, clinical encounters with hospitalists are relatively brief. The difficulty of rapidly establishing rewarding relationships with patients may pose a unique risk for burnout among hospitalists. Hoff and colleagues found that favorable patient-related interactions, more than peer relations, predicted hospitalists' intent to stay in the career.

Coworker support augments the personal accomplishment dimension of burnout, reflecting the value physicians place on expert evaluation by peers. The PWS shows that support from colleagues has a significant protective effect against stress. To highlight the importance of coworker support, solo practitioners were found to be particularly susceptible to stress. Furthermore, Hoff and colleagues show that burnout in hospitalists is more closely associated with less favorable social relations involving colleagues and coworkers than negative experiences related to the economically induced pressures of the job, such as reduced autonomy and the use of financial incentives. In a study of nurses, burnout was found to be more prevalent among those with negative interpersonal contacts, especially negative contacts with supervisors. These studies suggest that working with adversarial or emotionally distant coworkers or having ineffective leadership may predispose hospitalists to burnout.

ORGANIZATIONAL CHARACTERISTICS

Hospitalist practice models are as diverse as the number of practices that exist in the Unite States. Although, hospitalist groups are unified in the goals of containing cost while improving quality of care, the organizational culture, incentive structures, hierarchies, and operating rules that govern job demands vary widely. All of these factors can influence individual hospitalists' fit with their organization. Additional negative impact on burnout can surface when organizations violate basic expectations of fairness and equity.

Various studies demonstrate how economic pressures adversely affect attitudes related to physician career quality and longevity. For instance, job satisfaction is negatively impacted by more restrictive forms of reimbursement such as capitation, less time available to spend with patients, and the use of financial incentives related to productivity.

The lack of fit between a hospitalist and his or her job is another determinant of burnout. A study by Shanafelt and colleagues found that physicians in an academic department of internal medicine were less likely to show burnout when they spent more time engaged in the activities—patient care, research, education, or administration—they found most meaningful. The practice of Hospital Medicine offers ample opportunities for physicians to pursue customized careers in unconventional areas of medicine like management and advocacy. While some hospitalists find the variety of activities to be satisfying, others risk mismatch when they commit to jobs to which they are not well suited.

Fairness refers to the extent to which work decisions are perceived to be just. When organizational policies are fair, emotional exhaustion correlates with job performance but when they are consistently unfair, poor job performance is prevalent even where employees show no signs of burnout. Hospitalists may perceive injustice through differential treatment of physician groups by hospitals. Disproportionate distribution of responsibilities or rewards among members of a hospitalist group can breed resentment that can affect quality of care and burnout status.

PERSONAL CHARACTERISTICS

Hospitalist jobs usually do not require special training beyond the typical hospital-based residency experience. As a result, it is an attractive career opportunity for young physicians who can feel proficient immediately out of residency training. However, studies consistently show that younger individuals are more susceptible to burnout compared with more experienced counterparts. The reason for this has not been studied thoroughly but one possible explanation is that younger people are more idealistic compared with veterans on the job. Young workers with high expectations of a job and organization and a desire to express their skills and abilities can become burned out when expectations are unmet.

Unmarried workers, especially men, seem to be more prone to burnout; and single workers seem to experience higher burnout levels than those who are divorced. Spouses can be protective of stress and burnout, presumably because social support can buffer the pathologic influences of stressful events. Social support, especially from informal contacts, is positively related to good health and efficacy, irrespective of the presence or absence of work stressors.

Individuals with certain psychological dispositions are more prone to burnout. Those with an internal locus of control attribute daily events to personal effort while those with an external locus of control attribute them to outside forces or chance. Not surprisingly, burnout is higher among those with an external locus of control. Persons with low self-esteem and low levels of resilience or hardiness are associated with higher burnout due to not being open to change and feelings of not being in control.

HOW CAN BURNOUT IN HOSPITALISTS BE ADDRESSED?

PREVENTION AND INTERVENTION

Considerable evidence supports the fact that organizational and job factors play a greater role in burnout than individual worker characteristics and may be more remediable. It can be said that the organization acts upon the physician, whose personality, coping style, early experiences, skills, and competencies filter or exacerbate its effects. Solutions to the burnout problem, therefore, should be addressed primarily at the level of the job or organization. The goal should be to balance the demands of the job with the control, reward, and support needs of the worker. This may not be an easy task; most burnout interventions in the past have focused on individuals rather than jobs or organizations because it is perceived to be easier and less expensive to change people. Nevertheless, given the newness and evolving nature of hospitalist programs and their relationships with organizations, job design should be a primary focus.

PRACTICE POINT

- Considerable evidence supports the fact that organizational and job factors play a greater role in burnout than individual worker characteristics and they may be more remediable. Solutions to the burnout problem, therefore, should be addressed primarily at the level of the job or organization.

The strongest evidence supports controlling job demands: workload and time pressure. But as stated above, simply reducing work hours or patient encounters does not alleviate the consequence of burnout and high demands are inherent to the medical profession. Addressing hospitalists' fit with their job in the other mismatched areas may be more effective. For example, some hospitalists may be able to tolerate greater workload if they have control over the work they do, value the work they are doing and feel they are doing something important, or if they feel well rewarded for their efforts. Creative scheduling may decrease perceived workload by introducing necessary time for recovery. Providing hospitalists with skills to care for nonmedical patients and to form better relationships with consultants may relieve the demands of comanagement.

Hospitalists are also social creatures, thus focusing on relationships are important. Fostering a mutually supportive organizational culture focused on common goals, and implementing systems to facilitate rewarding interpersonal interactions are likely to minimize burnout. Hospitalists who feel they are working as part of a cohesive team, supported and appreciated by those around them (other hospitalists, nurses, consultants, primary care providers, etc.), and who feel positively recognized by patients and families will have less burn out. These interventions may be particularly important in supporting younger hospitalists who are more vulnerable to emotional exhaustion.

At the individual level, hospitalists can learn coping skills for stress. Evidence suggests that skills to improve relaxation, time management, assertiveness, and social skills can be learned. Unfortunately, individual-oriented approaches do not consistently protect against burnout. Recruiting resilient individuals with interpersonal skills and favorable personality profiles may be a strategy for organizations. Although medical schools and training programs routinely select based on characteristics like personality, an exclusionary approach to burnout prevention may sacrifice diversity in the hospitalist workforce without addressing the underlying systems problem. The most durable and feasible interventions may involve tailoring practice models to individual needs, but evidence to guide such interventions is lacking. The fit of the job and the worker is key to job satisfaction and avoiding burnout.

CONCLUSION

The work of typical hospitalists is characterized by high work demands, decreased autonomy, and potentially difficult interpersonal interactions that puts them at risk for burnout. The consequences of burned-out hospitalists include poor job performance, dissatisfaction, turnover, and various health-related problems like depression and substance abuse. There is not adequate evidence to guide efforts to prevent or minimize the impact of burnout at this time. Organizational efforts to protect work-life balance and support vulnerable individuals from destructive behavior are worthwhile.

SUGGESTED READINGS

Bakker AB, Schaufeli WB, Sixma HJ, Bosveld W, Van Dierendonck D. Patient demands, lack of reciprocity, and burnout: a five-year longitudinal study among general practitioners. *J Organ Behav.* 2000;21:425–441.

Hoff T, Whitcomb WF, Nelson JR. Thriving and surviving in a new medical career: the case of hospitalist physicians. *J Health Soc Behav.* 2002;43:72–91.

Lindenauer PK, Pantilat SZ, Katz PP, Wachter RM. Hospitalists and the practice of inpatient medicine: results of a survey of the National Association of Inpatient Physicians. *Ann Intern Med.* 1999;30:343–349.

Linzer M, Manwell LB, Mundt M, Williams E, Maguire A, McMurray J, et al. Organizational climate, stress, and error in primary care: the MEMO study. In: Advances in patient safety: from research to implementation. AHRQ Publication No. 050021 (1). Rockville, MD: Agency for Healthcare Research and Quality; 2005, vol. 1: 65–77.

Maslach C, Leiter MP. Early predictors of job burnout and engagement. *J Appl Psychol.* 2008;93:498–512.

Shanafelt TD, West CP, Sloan JA, Novotny PJ, Poland GA, et al. Career fit and burnout among academic faculty. *Arch Intern Med.* 2009;169:990–995.

Shirom A, Nirel N, Vinokur AD. Overload, autonomy, and burnout as predictors of physicians' quality of care. *J Occup Health Psychol.* 2006;11:328–342.

Wetterneck TB, Linzer M, McMurray JE, Douglas J, Schwartz MD, Bigby JA, et al. Worklife and satisfaction of general internists. *Arch Intern Med.* 2002;162:649–655.

CHAPTER 31

Strategies for Cost-Effective Care

Joseph Ming Wah Li, MD, SFHM, FACP

INTRODUCTION

The increasing scrutiny on both the quality and the cost of health care in the United States promotes value-driven health care or the highest quality of care at the lowest cost. The perception that hospitalists provide high-value health care impels the continued growth in the field of Hospital Medicine. As the U.S health care system proceeds to reshape itself, hospitalists will continually be challenged to justify this perception by providing high-quality care in a cost-effective manner. The term *cost-effective* does not mean never spending any money or resources to diagnose, treat, and manage diseases. It does require being smart with decisions on how, when, and where to invest resources. The shotgun approach—ordering an entire battery of tests to rule out a multitude of diagnoses—does not generate cost-effective or even high-quality care. Ordering the right tests at the right time to safely diagnose conditions without needless waste entails not only critical thinking to ask the right questions to get the right information but also easily accessible decision-making support and multidisciplinary teamwork. Delivering cost-effective care in a complex hospital system with lots of moving parts starts with recognizing the relationship between the moving parts and identifying opportunities for improvement. This chapter will use examples to demonstrate how communication, multidisciplinary teamwork, and measurement can be incorporated into a hospitalist practice to deliver cost-effective care (**Table 31-1**).

PRACTICE POINT

- The term *cost effective* does not mean never spending any money or resources to diagnose, treat, and manage diseases. It does require being smart with decisions on how, when, and where to invest resources.

COMMUNICATION

> *"The single biggest problem in communication is the illusion that it has taken place."* (George Bernard Shaw, 20th-century Irish playwright)

THE PAGER

Most clinicians rely on the pager as an essential communication tool. A telephone line open for the recipient to return the page and an assumed response time for answering the page before leaving the area if an *unreasonable* amount of time has passed rest on both spoken and unspoken rules. What is considered a *reasonable* amount of time is subject to interpretation and to the urgency of the situation. Despite the foibles of numeric paging, it remains a vital system of communication in the American health care system because of its reasonable cost and lack of acceptable alternatives. Unlike numeric paging, text paging allows providers to send text messages via the computer keyboard and telephone operators. The recipient can receive information not only about the call back number but also identification of the caller, the urgency of the call, the specific problem, and whether a response is required. This allows recipients to prioritize their calls and decide when to respond. Text paging can not only improve the communication experience but vastly improve the efficiency of communication. No system is perfect, however, unless the participants follow explicit rules or communication standards

TABLE 31-1 Principles of Cost-effective Hospitalist Care

- Standardize whenever possible.
- Do it right, the first time—patient safety is imperative.
- Do what is necessary—do not waste your time on the other stuff.
- Timing is critical.
- Make it count more than once—why waste your time doing something more than once?
- Assess and improve—you cannot improve something that you cannot or do not measure.

TABLE 31-2 Keys to Effective Multidisciplinary Rounds

- Always start on time!
- Be prepared to participate.
- Remember that rounds are an investment of everyone's time.
- Keep to the topic at hand; do not stray.
- Follow a template.
- Write orders during rounds.
- Treat complicated cases as outliers and speak about those cases last.

agreed upon by the service. Choosing to send numeric messages without indicating the nature or urgency of the call also does not offer advantages over numeric paging.

MULTIDISCIPLINARY ROUNDS

Essential health care delivery calls for effective communication. How hospitalists communicate with patients and families and other providers not only impacts their relationships with others, but also their ability to provide cost-effective care. One process, multidisciplinary rounds, facilitates communication with the primary goal to expedite care. Health care teams, composed of hospitalists, nurses, and case managers, at a minimum, should conduct rounds at least once daily each morning as early as possible after the nursing shift change and the hospitalist-to-hospitalist handoff. Some hospitals have found it useful to include nurses' aides, pharmacists, physical and occupational therapists, social workers, and dieticians as well. During rounds, a hospitalist leads a brief discussion about the plan of care for each patient and solicits feedback from all participants. Discussions about each patient should last no longer than two to three minutes and are often shorter. For the occasional patient whose issues demand a longer discussion, that patient should be treated as an outlier and discussed at the end of rounds. Nonphysician providers should solicit physician orders *during* rounds. The team considers barriers to patient discharge with each discussion, identifies opportunities to improve care, and takes steps to overcome those barriers. Rounds conclude with the expectation that each participant has a clear understanding of each patient's care plan for that day and for the hospital stay. At the completion of rounds hospitalists should be able to prioritize their work by seeing the sickest patients first, followed by potential early discharges, then the remainder of old patients, followed by new admissions.

Consumers and payers now view both patient satisfaction and 30-day hospital readmission rates as surrogate markers of quality. Multidisciplinary rounds may help health care teams score well on these quality measures because effective interdisciplinary communication promotes a shared understanding of the patient's needs, expectations, and care plan that anticipates postdischarge needs. With sufficient forethought and discussion, providers are able to address these needs before the discharge day. This approach also minimizes sending mixed messages to the patient and family. The end result of effective interdisciplinary communication is not only more cost-effective care but also a more satisfied patient who is less likely to be readmitted to the hospital unnecessarily.

Multidisciplinary rounds beneficially provide everyone a forum for communication. A standardized process for focused interdisciplinary communication early in the day encourages participants to exchange essential information that will facilitate early patient discharges. The placement of multiple key stakeholders in the same room at the same time allows the team leader to communicate once rather than holding the same conversation with multiple providers, and minimizing interruptions throughout the day allows providers to provide more efficient care. All providers should make an effort to funnel communication toward rounds rather than stopping the doctor or nurse throughout day with questions and comments unless there is a critical update such as a cancelled discharge due to a new problem or unexpected test result. To optimize efficiency and to ensure that significant new information is incorporated into patient care plans, some hospitalist programs have found it useful to hold an additional brief huddle in the afternoon to review and possibly revise the plans which were discussed at morning rounds.

The act of holding rounds every morning is no panacea. In fact, if done incorrectly, multidisciplinary rounds can potentially lead to a paradoxical increase in costs. Such rounds require an investment of all providers' time and energy. Any wise investment derives greater savings than the cost put into the investment. Longer rounds lower the return on investment and divert members from other competing responsibilities. Ineffective rounds fail to reduce the number of pages being sent between providers in the immediate period of time subsequent to rounds. It is important to set expectations early, be vigilant for any signs of trouble, and address issues before the rounds spiral out of control. Examples include (see also **Table 31-2**):

1. **Late arrivals.** It is vitally important to set the expectation of prompt arrival. Otherwise, the start time for rounds will drift from day to day and waste time for those who do show up on time.
2. **Lack of preparation.** Participation at rounds requires that the current primary nurse and hospitalist have both received sufficient critical information from the overnight staff to effectively participate in rounds. Otherwise, participants will find themselves with nothing to say at rounds or worse, provide erroneous or useless information about each patient's clinical status.
3. **Exchange of extraneous information.** It is incumbent for the leader of rounds to keep the discussion pertinent and limit extraneous conversation. A standardized template to guide discussion about each patient may help focus the discussion such as using the mnemonic CARET:

   C – **C***ritical lab values?*
   A – *Did this patient receive special* **A***ttention overnight and, if so, why?*
   R – **R***enewals: what orders need to renewed or written?*
   E – **E***nd of hospital care: what is the barrier to discharge?*
   T – **T***elemetry: does this patient need it?*
4. **Excessive duration of rounds.** Lengthy rounds that postpone the day's work may be a symptom of inability to present patient information succinctly, lack of preparation or focus, or fatigue resulting in extraneous information. Using an egg

timer during each patient discussion will provide immediate feedback and create a sense of urgency for the group to finish the discussion about each patient within the allotted time. The absence of food or coffee and everyone standing will promote the expectation of work and the need to finish the dialogue.

SHARED KNOWLEDGE AND TEAMWORK

"Knowledge is power." (Francis Bacon, 16th-century English philosopher)

Organizing information saves time for retrieval of information at a later date, and saving time usually means saving money—certainly a cost-effective strategy. While most people can file things by alphabetical order, filing contents by themes or topics requires additional skills and education. Put another way, information can tell us "what", but application of knowledge is rich with "who, where, when, and why?"

PRACTICE POINT

Efficient communication requires:
- Text paging
- Multidisciplinary rounds
- Shared knowledge and teamwork
- Documentation templates

According to Wikipedia, a wiki is, "a website that allows the easy creation and editing of any number of interlinked web pages via a web browser." Think of a wiki as a Web site that anyone with access can not only review but also easily post information for others to see from home or at work (**Table 31-3**). Computers or smart phones can access this venue for shared knowledge. Wikis can provide providers with timely access to information necessary to do their job not only correctly but also efficiently. For example, a group's wiki can facilitate communication by providing not only a primary care provider's *information* that is available in the telephone book or on the Web but also information about the backline, including what time to use the backline and for what reasons. Shared, easily accessible knowledge and its application are invaluable to efficiency and standardization of care.

For many hospitals with high census conditions where efficiency is especially critical, patients' bed assignments in the hospital may in fact impact on length of stay. The process for allocation of hospital beds utilizes limited information which may include the need for telemetry monitoring and isolation as well as the intended service (general medicine hospitalist or nonhospitalist, surgery, and specialty services such as critical care, neurology, and oncology). Some hospitals try to geographically cohort all of a given hospitalist provider's patients on one or no more than two adjacent clinical care units. Not only does this process facilitates the development of multidisciplinary rounds—improbable if a service has 15 patients located on 10 different floors—this process promotes the sharing of patient-specific knowledge on the floor between the multiple clinical providers, facilitates communication to family members, and encourages the provision of cost-effective care. Although geographic localization promotes efficiency of care and teamwork, it may not be feasible when other patients, waiting in the busy emergency room for a bed, cannot be admitted to a floor. From a flow or throughput perspective, it would seem to make most sense to transfer patients into their rooms as quickly as possible wherever beds are available in the hospital to avoid emergency department diversion even if they do not require a private or negative airflow room. However, this process may not be the most efficient or cost effective if these patients subsequently have to be moved to different rooms to accommodate other patients who require admission to a limited resource, namely, private rooms. Shared information about anticipated discharges and specific information concerning patients waiting in the emergency department to be admitted may improve patient flow. This information should be continuously accessed and updated by multiple users such as emergency department, admitting, and floor nursing staff.

TABLE 31-3 Advantages and Disadvantages of a Wiki

Advantages
- Simple: you do not have to be a techie to contribute
- Easily accessible anywhere you have access to the World Wide Web
- Regulate access: anyone with access can contribute or edit (tracks every edit; easy to revert back)
- Instantaneous: no lag to update information

Disadvantages
- Requires connectivity to the Web
- Easily disorganized due to flexibility of structure
- Vulnerable to spam and vandalism if not properly maintained
- Provides readily accessible forum for potential bad apples and unfavorable ideas

TIMING AND ANTICIPATION

"A good hockey player plays where the puck is. A great hockey player plays where the puck is going to be." (Wayne Gretzky, legendary hockey player)

The experiences of U.S. companies in post–World War II Japan highlighted the importance of manufacturing efficiency and its impact on the bottom line. The Japanese manufacturing principle of "just in time" (JIT) is a strategy to improve a business's return on investment by reducing inventory and the costs associated with carrying inventory. Although many American companies have applied the Toyota Production System to their own processes, the U.S. health care system has been slow to adopt the Lean approach. In academic medical centers, residents commonly allocate a significant part of their days to performing tasks that could be provided by others, eg, putting in intravenous lines, transporting patients to the MRI scanner, and making postdischarge appointments for patients. From a cost perspective, the lower hourly wages of residents compared with nurses and other hospital staff may have promoted adoption of these inefficiencies. However, from a patient safety perspective and training perspective, it is no longer feasible, especially with new work hour restrictions; nor does it make sense for hospitalists to assume these "resident" tasks, which would only further contribute to the prohibitive waste already present in the medical system. Paying an unnecessary premium for work that can be done by nonphysicians should be replaced by a more cost-effective approach that requires matching responsibilities and roles with appropriately trained staff. Administrative assistants should make follow-up appointments; transport staff should transport patients, nurses should provide nursing care, and hospitalists should perform tasks appropriate for the specialty of Hospital Medicine (**Table 31-4**).

SURGE IN CLINICAL DEMAND

Proponents of the hospitalist model of care argue that hospitalists provide more timely care for hospitalized patients than outpatient providers. It is difficult to imagine primary care providers, typically working in their clinics removed from the hospital during the day,

TABLE 31-4 Just in Time Key Elements: Examples in Hospital Medicine

- Create an uniform workload: perform discharge paperwork the night before anticipated discharge
- Reduce lot sizes: minimize number of individual hospitalist providers necessary to meet clinical demand
- Work with vendors to reduce lead times: geographically cohort hospitalist patients
- Preventative maintenance: hold staff meetings and training sessions during the time of day when clinical demand is low
- Flexible workforce: all hospitalists capable of working all shifts
- Total quality control: peer review of work and processes

being able to meet expectations of immediate availability. However, hospitalists may not always provide more timely care than primary care providers, especially when they do not know the patients and have not yet communicated with primary care physicians. Twenty years ago, the majority of primary care providers visited their handful of hospitalized patients at 7 AM before quickly returning to their offices often located near the hospital. Nurses would likely have all of their marching orders for each patient typically by 8 AM It is difficult, however, to imagine hospitalists consistently having all the orders in the chart by 8 AM In fact, demands of critically ill patients on the attention of hospitalists may delay the evaluation and management of other patients for a number of hours. Meanwhile, nurses may be waiting for discharge orders for some patients ready for safe discharge that morning. Hospitalists typically face this surge in demand for their attention not only each morning but also in the late afternoon and early evening when the number of admissions from the emergency department peaks. Left unaddressed, these surges in clinical demand create problems for hospitalists that can potentially eliminate any possibility of cost savings to the hospital. At one time of the day, demand outstrips the supply; at another time of the day, hospitalists may seemingly have nothing to do depending on the census, which may be influenced at least in part by the admissions process of residents. How to solve this problem is a matter of controversy. Some have argued that hospitalists should simply provide additional staffing during the peak periods of clinical demand by creating job descriptions for hospitalist admitters and dischargers. Others have argued that during the lull periods of clinical demand, decrease staffing by having some doctors take hospital calls from home. While each plan has merits, neither plan, in and of itself, is a panacea for solving this problem of peaks and valleys in clinical demand. Asking providers, who have no real knowledge of their patients' hospital stay, to discharge patients they have never met creates new discontinuities of care, fraught with new risks. Simply controlling the volume of staffing does not address the issue of increased demand. To effectively address demand, clearly defining and understanding the nature of the demand being asked of hospitalists may lead to a reassessment of the role and responsibilities of hospitalists. The amount of time hospitalists spend in patients' rooms actually pales in comparison to the amount of time spent reviewing the patients' chart and studies, documentation of service, and communication with other providers, especially at the time of discharge. For some patients who will be transferred to rehabilitation facilities the next day, hospitalists may prepare the discharge paperwork the afternoon or night before, thereby eliminating a task peak clinical demand. Documentation templates may help streamline the admission and discharge processes, which ordinarily require immense paperwork and documentation. Rather than writing out the complete physical examination, utilization of a documentation template to provide the same information not only improves physician legibility but also improves efficiency and billing revenue for the hospital. Documentation templates have the added benefit of standardizing the expectations for each hospitalist note, thereby improving the quality of documentation without increasing the time to write the note.

ASSESSMENT

"Learning is like rowing upstream; not to advance is to drop back." (Chinese proverb)

The old management adage is that you cannot improve or manage what you cannot measure. As health care moves increasingly toward value-based purchasing, hospitalists must understand these concepts in order to not only thrive but to survive. Within the past 5 years, the Centers for Medicare and Medicaid Services has developed Core Measures to measure performance of acute care hospitals regarding a number of diagnoses. Patients and families can go on to the Web and see how their local hospital did on a number of performance metrics at www.hospitalcompare.hhs.gov. A similar Medicare Web site posts performance data regarding nursing homes called Nursing Home Compare. The Medicare program, Physician Quality Reporting Initiative, evaluates individual physician performance. The message is clear: you choose to perform self-assessment or external forces will publicly report data regarding your performance.

There is no agreement on how to measure the performance of hospitalist programs and individual members, but it is critical that everyone understands how they are being evaluated and that the process of measurement produces valid data. Because hospitalists often overlap each other in the care of their patients, it is easier to measure performance of the group than to measure individual performance. Some measures are simple but important to evaluate, such as the percentage of patients who received appropriate prophylaxis against venous thromboembolic disease, the percentage of patients who had a documented pain assessment, and the percentage of patients who had a documented code status. Performance on these measures with feedback can promote patient safety and satisfaction, and often improve the cost-effectiveness of care being delivered. It is much more expensive to treat hospital-acquired complications, such as a deep venous thrombosis or a pulmonary embolism, than to prevent them.

PRACTICE POINT

- There is no agreement on how to measure the performance of hospitalist programs and individual members, but it is critical that everyone understands how they are being evaluated and that the process of measurement produces valid data. Because hospitalists often overlap each other in the care of their patients, it is easier to measure the performance of the group than it is to measure individual performance.

Hospital readmission rates may also indicate quality as well as cost, but measurement is fraught with challenges. The rate of hospital readmission within 30 days will never be zero, but physicians should strive to eliminate all unnecessary or preventable 30-day hospital readmissions (**Table 31-5**). Review of a given provider or a group's 30-day hospital readmission rate should track readmissions over time and look at other factors such as patients' length of stay, case mix index (a measure of severity of illness), and social issues known to be associated with a higher risk of readmission such as homelessness or lack of insurance. Hospitals and payors, both of whom likely have a low operating margin, are already obtaining data that can be used to assess the value of the hospitalist service

TABLE 31-5 Risk Factors for Early Hospital Readmission

- Insurance status
- Social support: marital status
- Health condition: Charlson comorbidity index and SF-12 physical component score
- Hospital care utilization: more than one hospital admission within past year, current hospital length of stay of greater than two days

Data from Hasan O, Meltzer DO, Shaykevich SA, et al. Hospital readmission in general medicine patients: a prediction model. *J Gen Intern Med.* 2009;25(3):211–219.

to the institution. Hospitalists should be aware of the data collected and try to ensure that the data is not only valid but reflects measures that they can impact.

CONCLUSION

Value-driven health care is in its early stages but is here to stay. In order for hospitalists to succeed in this increasingly competitive environment, hospitalists will need to demonstrate not only the ability to improve the quality of care but also to practice in a cost-effective manner. Improvement in communication and teamwork processes will facilitate the delivery of cost-effective care. A commitment to measurement and continuous improvement is essential to helping hospitalist succeed in this environment.

SUGGESTED READINGS

Courtney M, Edwards H, Chang A, et al. Fewer emergency readmissions and better quality of life for older adults at risk of hospital readmission: a randomized controlled trial to determine the effectiveness of a 24-week exercise and telephone follow-up program. *J Am Geriatr Soc.* 2009;57(3):395–402.

Garasen H, Windspoll R, Johnsen R, et al. Intermediate care at a community hospital as an alternative to prolonged general hospital care for elderly patients: a randomised controlled trial. *BMC Public Health.* 2007;7:68.

Gillespie U, Alassaad A, Henrohn D, et al. A comprehensive pharmacist intervention to reduce morbidity in patients 80 years or older: a randomized controlled trial. *Arch Intern Med.* 2009, May 11; 169(9):894–900.

Graumlich JF, Novotny NL, Nace GS, Aldag JC. Patient readmissions, emergency visits, and adverse events after software-assisted discharge from hospital: cluster randomized trial. *J Hosp Med.* 2009;4(7):E11–E119.

Hasan O, Meltzer DO, Shaykevich SA, et al. Hospital readmission in general medicine patients: a prediction model. *J Gen Intern Med.* 2009;25(3):211–219.

Moher D, Weinberg A, Hanlon R, et al. Medical team coordinator and length of hospital stay. *Can Med Assoc J.* 1992;146:511–515.

Selker HP, Beshansky JR, Pauker SG, et al. The epidemiology of delays in a teaching hospital. *Med Care.* 1989;27(2):112–130

SECTION 5

Professionalism and Medical Ethics

CHAPTER 32

Principles of Medical Ethics

Milda R. Saunders, MD, MPH
G. Caleb Alexander, MD, MS
Mark Siegler, MD

WHY IS ETHICS IMPORTANT TO HOSPITAL MEDICINE?

Hospitalists, like all physicians, must master not only the clinical, but also the interpersonal and ethical dimensions of medical practice. Four features of Hospital Medicine generate particular ethical challenges for the practicing clinician. First, hospitalized patients often face urgent medical issues in the midst of uncertainty. Second, the patient and the hospitalist are usually strangers to one another, having met for the first time when the patient is admitted to the hospitalists' service. Decisions about code status, end-of-life care, or aggressiveness of care, difficult under the best circumstances, become even more difficult because hospitalists do not have the continuity of care many outpatient physicians have with their patients. Third, despite laudable efforts by many hospitalists to communicate with primary care providers, the absence of long-standing relationships with patients increases the challenge of knowing and representing their wishes and best interests during the course of clinical care. Finally, hospitalists' shift work also poses challenges to the communication and trust required for sound clinical decision making. Patients and family members may begin a conversation about the goals and plan of care with one hospitalist only to have to continue such a conversation with another covering physician.

Nevertheless, the ethical challenges that hospitalists face may also create opportunities to help navigate some of the most difficult clinical ethical issues in medicine. For example, the greater familiarity of hospitalists regarding decision making with the acutely ill may allow them to develop greater comfort and expertise with frequently encountered ethical dilemmas. The hospital setting also provides additional human resources to navigate the moral complexities of clinical care. These include interdisciplinary teams of nurses, social workers, chaplains, ethics consultants, and medical consultants that may be much harder to assemble in an outpatient setting.

This chapter will describe the purpose and principles of clinical ethics, explore frequently encountered inpatient clinical challenges that raise important ethical issues, and finally, highlight a number of ethical and professional issues that hospitalists face.

CLINICAL ETHICS AND ITS APPLICATION

Many fields of ethical inquiry focus on values, standards of conduct, and moral judgment. Clinical ethics provides a structured approach for identifying, analyzing, and resolving ethical issues in clinical medicine. In addition, it allows clinicians to speak in a common language about justifications for clinical decisions that have ethical implications.

PRACTICE POINT

- Clinical ethics provide a structured approach for identifying, analyzing, and resolving ethical issues in clinical medicine. In addition, clinical ethics allow clinicians to speak in a common language about justifications for clinical decisions that have ethical implications.

Traditionally, bioethics has been guided by four principles: respect for autonomy, beneficence, nonmaleficence, and justice. Autonomy, personal rule of the self, is the notion that individuals acting with understanding and intentionality, free from coercion or external control, can control what happens to their bodies. Beneficence is a positive duty to act for the benefit of others, while weighing the benefits and harms to the individual nonmaleficence requires the clinician to not intentionally cause harm. Justice is defined as fair, equitable, and appropriate treatment based on what is due to a person. While it is important to know and understand each of these principles, they do not provide a concrete way to solve the ethical dilemmas often faced by clinicians.

Clinicians are encouraged to use a deliberative process of clinical ethical analysis such as the four-quadrant model described by Jonsen and colleagues in *Clinical Ethics*. Similar to a SOAP note (Subjective, Objective, Assessment, and Plan) that provides a consistent, practical approach for organizing and discussing clinical problems, the four-quadrant model offers a structured heuristic for ethical analysis. By considering the four quadrants—medical indications, patient preferences, quality of life, and contextual features—clinicians can delineate the ethically relevant facts of the case, show where further information is needed, and begin to weigh and balance these four considerations to help reach a clinical-ethical decision that is right for the patient. While clinicians may still arrive at a decision that some might disagree with, the four-box model encourages clinicians to be deliberative and explicit in their reasoning. Each of the following cases illustrates some frequently encountered ethical issues as well as relevant concepts from clinical medical ethics.

CASE 32-1

BRAIN TUMOR BUT NO INTEREST IN TREATMENT

Ms. Taylor is a 39-year-old woman admitted with recent onset of blindness and a CT scan that indicates a large brain tumor. She is lucid, says she feels fine, and indicates that she would like to go home. Her husband asks you to treat his wife in whatever way you think would maximize her chances of survival and recovery.

Ms. Taylor is assessed by the admitting hospitalist. She is oriented to time, place, and person and is able to state why she was admitted, what the scan showed, and why both the physicians and her husband think she should be treated. She continues to demand that she be discharged from the hospital. She states that she does not believe in disease: it is all a plot of the medical-industrial complex to enslave the populace and conduct experiments. A psychiatry consult is requested for further evaluation, and she repeats her views to the psychiatry team. Further discussion with her husband indicates that she has had these beliefs for the past 10 years and has refused to see a physician since then. Ms. Taylor also explains that she dislikes hospitals and wants to spend her final days at home with her family. The psychiatrist indicates that she has decision-making capacity and thus has the right to refuse treatment.

Comments on Case 1. **Hospitalists must frequently obtain consent from patients for tests and therapies under challenging circumstances, eg, an ill, frightened patient whom one has just met. In order for patients to make informed decisions, to consent or refuse, they must have decision-making capacity as well as information about the risks, benefits, and alternatives. An important first step for clinicians is to assess whether the person has decision-making capacity for the decision at hand. In many cases, such as severe metabolic encephalopathy, the patients' decision-making capacity, or lack thereof, is apparent without any formal assessment. Other cases require a more in-depth discussion with patients, often with the assistance of psychiatry and ethics consultants.**

> **PRACTICE POINT**
>
> - By considering (1) medical indications, (2) patient preferences, (3) quality of life, and (4) contextual features, clinicians can delineate the ethically relevant facts of the case, show where further information is needed, and begin to weigh and balance these four considerations to help reach a clinical ethical decision that is right for the patient. While clinicians may still arrive at a decision that some might disagree with, this approach encourages clinicians to be deliberative and explicit in their reasoning.

This case, based on an actual clinical consultation, raises several questions. Why is the patient refusing treatment? Why does she not believe she is sick, especially given her recent blindness? What accounts for the discordant preferences of the patient and her husband? Most essentially for the clinician struggling to determine the best course of action, the case raises the question of whether the patient has the decision-making capacity to make the specific decisions at hand of refusing treatment for the brain tumor.

COMPETENCY AND DECISION-MAKING CAPACITY

Competency is a legal concept, a "yes/no" question decided by a judge on whether a person has the legal authority to make personal decisions, like financial or health care decisions. By contrast, decision-making capacity is a clinical concept that determines whether the person has the capacity to make his or her own health care decisions in a specific clinical circumstance. Decisional capacity is dynamic; it can change over time for an individual patient. It is also decision specific. For example, a patient may have had decisional capacity with regard to a decision to be admitted for acute chest pain, but in later lose decisional capacity to accept or refuse coronary bypass surgery.

Despite the centrality that decisional capacity plays in allowing patients to make autonomous choices, such as accepting or refusing treatment, there are no uniform and objective criteria to assess it. Generally, a person is thought to have decision-making capacity if he or she can communicate a choice, understand relevant information, appreciate the situation and its consequences, and manipulate information rationally. The stringency of the criteria is often based both on the probable risks and benefits of the proposed treatment, and the reasonableness of the choice. That is, a relatively low threshold for decisional capacity is required for a person to consent to antibiotics for an uncomplicated pneumonia since it is a high benefit, low risk decision and a reasonable choice. A more stringent assessment of decisional capacity is required for a person to refuse antibiotics for a neutropenic fever; it is a high-risk decision that most people would deem unreasonable. In emergent, life-threatening situations when patient's refuse a potentially life-saving intervention without giving a reason for refusal, physicians often may treat such patients and try to clarify decision-making capacity when the patient stabilizes. If uncertainty remains, clinicians should seek consultation and guidance from psychiatrists, ethics committees or consultants, and hospital attorneys.

INFORMED CONSENT

Informed consent, the willing acceptance of a medical intervention by a patient after adequate disclosure by the physician of the nature of the intervention, and its risks, benefits, and alternatives, is how respect for patient autonomy is operationalized. Many clinicians think consent consists of signing the consent form in order to receive a therapy (eg, blood or chemotherapy) or procedure; however, signing the consent form simply serves to document a consent process of discussion and negotiation that is ongoing. While most of the interventions performed on patients do not require consent documentation, they do require ongoing dialogue in order to give patients information and to obtain feedback.

INFORMED REFUSAL

Informed refusal is the rejection of a medical intervention by a patient after disclosure by the physicians about its risks, benefits, and alternatives. In situations where the intervention is elective or the potential benefit is low, refusal is usually not a major concern to clinicians. When the intervention is medically indicated, and expected to give the patient a large benefit, perhaps even saving the patient's life, the patient's autonomy (to consent or refuse) appears to be in opposition to the physician's beneficence. Refusal of consent in a situation that would potentially cause the patient harm requires further discussion. In many cases, the patient may simply need more information or reassurance about potential pain or harm. If the patient is able to articulate the reasons for the intervention, the potential risks of forgoing the intervention, and a coherent reason why he or she does not accept the intervention, then physicians must accept the patient's decision. Ideally the patient's refusal is consistent with a rational, coherent worldview, eg, as when a Jehovah's Witness refuses to accept blood products, or when a patient states "I do not want surgery for my brain tumor because at the end of my life I would prefer to be home with my family." Clinicians need not agree with the patient's reasons in order to acknowledge that they are logical and valid within the patient's belief system. Ultimately, competent adults have the right to make (what the treating clinician or others may deem to be) a bad decision.

CASE 32-2

A HUSBAND AS SURROGATE DECISION MAKER FACES TOUGH CALLS

Ms. Jenkins is a 45-year-old former dancer who is severely ill with necrotizing fasciitis that has required bilateral lower extremity amputation. When she presented earlier, she was unconscious and her husband consented to the surgery. She is being co-managed by a hospitalist and a critical care physician in the intensive care unit. She is intubated and requiring mechanical ventilation. Her husband indicates that she would not wish to live with amputations and requests discontinuation of her ventilator, which would likely result in her death. Her parents object.

Discussions with the husband reveal that his wife had seen news stories about people in a persistent vegetative state and indicated that she would not want to live like that. He also reports that she loved dancing more than anything, and would feel that after an amputation, life was not worth living. Her parents agree that she had stated similar things to them. The hospitalists, surgeons, and intensivists involved in the case feel that she has a good chance for a meaningful recovery in which she would regain the ability to interact with her environment and make her own decisions.

Mr. Jenkins explains that in requesting withdrawal of life support he was simply trying to honor what he believed to be his wife's wishes. He admits he is uncertain what to do. After talking with her parents, the physicians, and the social worker, he allows the patient to remain on a time-limited trial of life support for several weeks. She is extubated in 10 days. She has a prolonged course of physical therapy. Over time, she comes to accept life after amputation and never expresses a desire to die. She is currently the choreographer of a wheelchair dance troupe.

Comments on Case 2. **In the hospital setting, hospitalists will care for many patients who lack decision-making capacity, either temporarily or for prolonged periods of time. To help determine patients' wishes and preferences, hospitalists should be familiar with their state's rule for surrogacy and, if it is possible, ask patients on admission who can speak for them if they are unable to speak for themselves. Occasionally, surrogates may make irreversible decisions that run counter to medical recommendations or patient interests. It is important to try to resolve these disagreements "close to the bedside" by using family members, ethics consultants, chaplains, social workers, and only rarely, legal action.**

In this case the patient is currently unable to speak for herself as a result of her illness. She currently lacks decisional capacity, and physicians must rely on someone to speak on her behalf. She has no prior advance directives, either appointing someone to speak for her or making her wishes explicit for end-of-life care. According to her state's law, her husband is her presumed surrogate.

ADVANCE DIRECTIVES

There are two types of advance directives, living wills and a durable power of attorney for health care. A living will is a document that specifies what treatments a patient would like to receive or forgo in cases of terminal illness and decisional incapacity. Living wills often serve only as a general guide to the patient's wishes because they are formulaic and open to interpretation. A durable power of health care attorney (health care proxy) is a document that allows patients to name who can make their health care decisions in situations of decisional incapacity. The number of people with health care proxies is small, even among those with serious medical illness. Even for patients who have appointed a proxy, they may not have told the proxy of the appointment or discussed their wishes with them.

SURROGATES

Some patients may have permanent loss of decision-making capacity from conditions such as advanced dementia or permanently impaired consciousness. Other patients may lose decision-making capacity temporarily during a hospitalization due to delirium, encephalopathy, or medication. When a patient lacks medical decision-making capacity, medical decisions must be made by a surrogate, an authorized person acting on the patient's behalf. Unless the patient has specifically appointed a surrogate through a durable power of health care attorney, family members are considered the patient's surrogate. Many states have rules to designate the order of family surrogates (eg, first the spouse, then parents, children, siblings, etc). Despite these rules, there may still be conflicts about who should be the legitimate decision maker. For example, if a couple has been separated for more than 10 years, but never divorced, or if the patient has a common law wife or domestic partner (who is not legally acknowledged by that particular state). If a patient has several children, who by law are equal surrogates, but they disagree on what should be done, who should decide? In these cases, meetings between the clinical team and involved family are helpful to negotiate the difficult and often emotional disagreements. These situations often require frank communications among the involved parties, and may sometimes require the guidance of the hospital legal department or ethics consultants. All states have a provision to appoint guardians for patients who lack decisional capacity and have no apparent surrogates.

COMMUNICATION

After the clinician has obtained and assessed the clinical data, and developed a clinical strategy, these conclusions must also be discussed with the patient or surrogate. A central ethical obligation of clinicians is not simply to arrive at the answer but to communicate the recommendations to the patient or the patient's surrogate. This obligation is simple to accept on its face, but has important implications in clinicians' daily work. It means that clinicians must present information to patients that they are able to understand, in the language in which they are fluent, in terms that are understandable to them, and in a sufficient level of detail. While most clinicians endorse this principle, many physicians fall short in its implementation. The English-speaking physician who attempts to muddle through an explanation of an illness to a primarily Spanish-speaking patient has unwittingly erred. So too has the physician who explains a new diagnosis in overly technical terms that are not clear to the lay listener.

SUBSTITUTED DECISION-MAKING

Surrogates are asked to act on behalf of patients who have lost decision-making capacity. When a patient's preferences regarding the specific clinical decision at hand (eg, whether to initiate hemodialysis) are known to the surrogate, these should guide clinical decision making. More commonly, such specific wishes are not known, and the surrogate must act on the patient's behalf through a process of *substituted judgment*. When the patient has not specifically stated what he or she would want, a surrogate should use knowledge of the patient's values or beliefs to guide medical decision making. In cases where patient's wishes are unknown or unclear, then the surrogate must act in the patient's best interests.

As the legal surrogate acting in good faith, Mr. Jenkins is within his right to request that no further treatment be given. However, the clinical context is important because some of the patient's physicians believe the patient has a reasonable chance of meaningful recovery. In addition, they recognize that if she did not improve as expected, treatment discontinuation could still be considered.

WITHDRAWING AND WITHHOLDING

Many clinicians and surrogates believe that it is ethically different to withdraw care compared to initially deciding to withhold care. Often, once a trial intervention like mechanical ventilation or nasogastric tube feeding has been started, clinicians may feel that discontinuing it, even if the patient is not improving, is ethically impermissible. While recognizing that clinicians may feel there are psychological differences, ethical theory and many religious traditions draw no distinction between withdrawing and withholding. Both the law and clinical ethics allow clinicians to try an intervention for a limited amount of time and then withdraw it if the patient does not improve.

CASE 32-3

FUTILITY AND END-OF-LIFE CARE

Ms. Smith, a 74-year-old woman with metastatic non–small cell lung cancer, is admitted from home with worsening shortness of breath, fever, and chills. She has obstructive pneumonia from progressive disease despite four rounds of palliative chemotherapy. She is mostly bed bound and dependent on her homemaker and her daughter for most of her needs. The patient demands her regularly scheduled chemotherapy.

The hospitalist discusses the patient with the consulting oncologist. The oncologist states that although there are additional palliative regimens available, in trials, patients similar to Ms. Smith have not received a survival benefit and often have worse quality of life. Ms. Smith has several discussions with the oncologist, hospitalist, and palliative care team, and decides to forgo further chemotherapy and return home with hospice and palliative care services.

Comments on Case 3. **Hospitalists frequently care for patients with terminal medical conditions. Each new treatment or procedure should be considered in terms of the expected risks and benefits given the patient's prognosis, preferences, and goals of care. Hospitalists can play an important role in aggressive symptom management for terminally and chronically ill patients.**

This is a case of an elderly patient, who has poor performance status and disease progression despite multiple rounds of palliative chemotherapy; each of these diminishes the likelihood she will receive benefit from further chemotherapy.

FUTILITY

Physicians are under no ethical obligation to continue futile treatments regardless of patient or surrogate requests. Because of this important shift of the ethical demands in situations of futility, it is important to discuss its definition. Physiologically futile treatments offer no possibility of achieving their intended goals. Ambiguity may occur when physicians define something as futile when they simply mean it is unlikely to bring about the intended outcome; what constitutes probabilistic futility may range from < 1% to < 15%. Ambiguity in defining futility may also be due to disagreement on intended goals. In these situations, the therapy itself is effective, but will not achieve improvement of quality of life or restoration of health. For example, physicians may not want to offer dialysis to a septic neutropenic patient with metastatic cancer and multisystem organ failure. In this case, while dialysis is still an effective renal replacement therapy, it is unlikely to meaningfully change this patient's outcome. Some interventions in medicine truly are physiologically futile, implausible given the current state of medicine. However, most treatments that are considered futile should still be approached by weighing the benefits and harms in light of the goals of care.

END-OF-LIFE AND PALLIATIVE CARE

While most people would prefer to die at home, more than 50% of people in the United States die in the hospital. There are numerous ethical challenges in end-of-life care, including poor communication with patients or family about the imminence of their death due to physicians' poor prognostic ability, physicians' discomfort discussing death and dying, and not wanting to give up on the patient or cause them to give up hope. One way around these issues is to discuss end-of-life issues—specifically code status, treatment limitations, and health care proxy—with all patients who enter the hospital with an intact mental status and a serious medical condition. Although time consuming and often unnecessary, such regular discussions normalize the conversation for both physicians and patients, and increase the clinicians' likelihood of learning important information from patients while they are able to convey it.

Whether patients choose curative treatment or palliative care at the end of life, they need attention to symptom management. Clinicians caring for terminal patients may fear hastening their demise through aggressive pain control or sedation. The doctrine of double effect ethically justifies the aggressive use of medications even if they hasten death, if the intended purpose is to relieve pain and other symptoms and not to cause death.

CASE 32-4

MEDICAL MISTAKE?

Mr. Ramirez, a 78-year-old man with a history of diabetes and hypertension, is admitted with a transient ischemic attack with left-sided weakness and dysarthria. Per hospital protocol, he is monitored and given aspirin, dipyramidole, and a statin. His symptoms resolve. The following day, he awakens with new left-sided weakness and dysarthria. An MRI shows an acute ischemic neuro checks. In reviewing with the team what could have been done to prevent this poor outcome, it is revealed that nursing neuro checks were not ordered, therefore early treatment with tissue plasminogen activator could not be offered. On rounds, Mr. Ramirez asks the hospitalist attending to explain what this new weakness means and whether he could have prevented it. Prior to rounding on Mr. Ramirez, the hospitalist discussed his case with neurology and risk management. She explains to Mr. Ramirez he likely had a stroke during the night. While he was on optimal medical management, his stroke was not caught in time because he was not checked during the night.

Mr. Ramirez was living independently prior to his hospitalization. Due to Medicare insurance rules, he is no longer a candidate for acute rehab because he is unlikely to be discharged home after rehab. According to the social worker, unless he can get a family member to agree to care for him after discharge from rehab, he will have to go to a skilled nursing facility with less intense rehab, which will decrease his chances for a full recovery. Mr. Ramirez is clear that there are limits to what the medical team may discuss with his family members. Even though involving his family may result in a better outcome during both his rehab and eventual discharge, the medical team must respect his rights to autonomy and confidentiality.

On Friday Mr. Ramirez is medically ready for discharge. The social worker has arranged transfer to the nearby skilled nursing facility with which the hospital has an informal relationship. Discussions with the rehab physician lead the hospitalist to believe that Mr. Ramirez would receive better, more intensive and comprehensive, rehab at another facility that would not be able to accept him until Monday. The hospitalist discusses her concerns with the patient, and explains the potential hospital costs he may incur. He opts to wait until Monday for discharge. The director of utilization review, also the head of the hospitalist group, wants to know why Mr. Ramirez is not being discharged when he has already been accepted at a facility.

Comment on Case 4. Hospitalists, like other physicians, may face external challenges to the doctor-patient relationship. Hospitalists may encounter medical errors more frequently than their outpatient counterparts due both to the high complexity and acuity of hospitalized patients and the ability to see the immediate consequences of their decisions. Hospitalists have an opportunity to advocate for their individual patients interests, as well as working to change systems in the hospital to prevent medical errors, protect patient confidentiality, and avoid conflicts in interest.

ADDITIONAL ETHICAL AND PROFESSIONAL CHALLENGES

TRUTH-TELLING

Another ethical obligation of physicians is not to lie to or mislead patients. Clinicians' communication must not only be clear, it must also be complete. While very few clinicians would actually lie to a patient, at times providers may be tempted to withhold information or mislead a patient, either for the providers or the patient's best interest. One may not disclose a medical error for fear of losing the patient's trust and esteem. One may withhold a potentially devastating diagnosis or fail to discuss a grim prognosis to spare the patient emotional distress. One could also fail to disclose all reasonable treatment alternatives in order to steer the patient to the "appropriate" course. These actions, which may have a benevolent intent, are unethical.

DISCLOSURE OF ERROR

Hospitalists deal with medical complexity and uncertainty; like all physicians, they may also make mistakes. When medical errors occur, physicians are encouraged to inform the patient and to rectify the situation. When a serious medical error occurs, physicians are ethically obligated to disclose, often after discussing the situation with the medical-legal department within the hospital. When errors occur in a hospital setting, they often are the fault not only of an individual clinician's actions, but of a system failure. In addition to disclosing to patients, physicians should also file an incident report with the quality or oversight committee to help prevent future occurrences. Physicians may also notice mistakes made by others (eg, primary care physicians, treating physicians at another hospital). In these instances, the rules of disclosure are less certain. One may not want to speak ill of a colleague, especially if not all of the facts are known. In cases where serious harm has resulted, one should err on the side of disclosure.

CONFIDENTIALITY

Physicians are ethically and legally bound by confidentiality to not divulge information disclosed by a patient during a clinical encounter. This principle is often challenging to enforce in a hospital setting for many practical and ethical reasons. Computerized records and paper charts may be left unsecured and accessible by many people. On walk rounds patient information is often presented right outside the patient's door within hearing range of family or friends who may be visiting. Many of the workspaces and telephones are in semipublic areas where things can be overheard. Providers may also discuss patients in public places such as elevators and cafeterias. Protecting patient confidentiality may also be in conflict with other social needs such as the use of data for public health or research purposes, the ability to inform family members about patient conditions that may directly impact them, and the transition of care among providers.

CONFLICT OF INTEREST

A conflict of interest occurs when a person has an external motivation to perform actions that are at variance with the acknowledged duties of his or her professional role. Many conflicts of interest are financial, eg, physicians' incentives to refer within a group or physicians receiving gifts from a pharmaceutical representative. The presence of a conflict does not necessarily mean that physicians will act contrary to duty. Physicians are asked to explicitly report their conflicts. As hospitalists become more involved with utilization review, either as part of an oversight committee or through salary bonus tied to lower utilization and short stays, they may face additional conflicts of interest. While everyone benefits from the practice of efficient, cost-effective medicine, an overemphasis on getting patients in and out may compromise the doctor-patient relationship and patient care.

CONCLUSION

Although Hospital Medicine is a new and growing field, hospitalists do not need to invent new ethical principles. These principles and their application have been well established. Each field of medicine challenges clinicians to obtain the clinical facts, assess patient preferences, weigh risks and benefits, and recommend a course of action for a particular patient at a particular time. Hospitalists face important challenges and opportunities, some of them unique to the practice of Hospital Medicine, for providing efficient, effective, and ethically sound care to hospitalized patients.

SUGGESTED READINGS

Appelbaum PS, Grisso T. Assessing patients' capabilities to consent to treatment. *N Engl J Med.* 1988;319(25):1635–1638.

Beauchamp T, Childress J. *Principles of Biomedical Ethics* 6th ed. New York: Oxford University Press; 2008.

Ditto PH, Danks JH, Smucker WD, et al. Advance directives as acts of communication: a randomized controlled trial. *Arch Intern Med.* 2001;161(3):421–430.

Jonsen AR, Siegler M, Winslade W. *Clinical Ethics: A Practical Approach to Ethical Decisions in Clinical Medicine.* 7th ed. New York: McGraw-Hill; 2010.

Miles SH, Koepp R, Weber EP. Advance end-of-life treatment planning. A research review. *Arch Intern Med.* 1996;156(10):1062–1068.

CHAPTER 33

Common Indications for Ethics Consultation

Heather X. Cereste, MD
Joseph J. Fins, MD, FACP

"Hospital admission frequently occasions sensitive and highly charged decisions about issues such as code status, aggressiveness of interventions, and end-of-life care, to name a few, at a time when patients are sickest, most vulnerable, and least able to look after their own interests."[1]

INTRODUCTION

Nearly 2500 years ago, the Hippocratic writers decreed in the Epidemics, Bk. I, Sect. XI., "Declare the past, diagnose the present, foretell the future; practice these acts. As to diseases, make a habit of two things—to help, or at least to do no harm." The basic tenets of ethics apply to all medical specialties. Hospital Medicine does not constitute a novel relationship but one founded upon a long-standing tradition of practices and manifestations of professionalism in which the physician places the interests of the patient above his or her own, and practices with competence, integrity, and beneficence. How ethical principles are applied depends on the context of care. The ethical disputes that may be encountered are not unique to Hospital Medicine, but have a rich history in bioethics, social movements, and landmark court cases.

The nature of the doctor-patient relationship and the new dichotomy of the inpatient and outpatient settings continue to evolve as specialized care becomes more localized to geographic areas such as the emergency room, intensive care unit, most recently, general medical units, and in the future, the medical home. This fragmentation of the clinical encounter into a unit of hospitalization represents a departure from the time-honored, and almost mythic, longitudinal doctor-patient relationship of general practice and primary care.

Unlike the classic doctor-patient relationship, decision making in the hospital is generally more harried and of a more critical nature. Dedication to ethical practice preserves stability in a "crisis" and promotes a culture of trust necessary for advocacy and a sound doctor-patient relationship. Especially if patients do not understand the role of hospitalists, perceive that their primary care physicians have abandoned them, or have questions of trust due to cultural differences or other factors, the doctor-patient relationship may be in jeopardy. The ethics, expertise, and availability of the hospitalist balance patient-centered obligations with the need to maximize efficiencies within temporal constraints. The old adage "the secret of caring for the patient is caring for the patient" is aided when hospitalists do not make assumptions about their patients' priorities at the outset and evaluate each patient with a fresh perspective. Communication with the patient's outpatient doctor, familiarization with the medical record and meetings with patients and their intimates who may have essential information to share during the patient's illness is not only good clinical care but congruent with ethical practice.

PRACTICE POINT

- Having a longitudinal perspective from an outpatient colleague can help mitigate against diagnostic and prognostic errors that may occur when the object of one's practice is hospitalized patients. Consultation with an outpatient physician is also critical to build a trusting hospitalist-patient relationship. Patients may suspect potential conflicts of interest or dual agency between hospitalists as salaried hospital employees and patient needs.

There is an ethical mandate to optimize cooperation, or co-management, between doctors and other members of the health care team, an essential element of the hospitalist model. Hospitals have traditionally been places where different professional specialties have their own way of functioning, often in "splendid isolation." Hampered care coordination—and the splitting of the clinical team—has the potential to hinder the cultivation and maintenance of the therapeutic relationship. In all settings, trust is sustained by the appropriate use of consultants, an awareness of one's sphere of practice, and an appreciation for continuity of care. Being transparent and sharing the results of consultations with patients and their families will help promote a trusting and effective doctor-patient relationship.

This chapter will review key ethical concepts and standards in the context of Hospital Medicine and explain the role of ethics consultation to facilitate patient care.

HOSPITAL ETHICS COMMITTEES AND ETHICS CASE CONSULTATION

The Joint Commission requires that hospitals develop and implement a process to handle ethical issues in patient care but does not specify how this should be done. It may be done by an ethics consultant, an ethics committee, or on an ad hoc basis. Ethics committees consist of physicians, social workers, attorneys, theologians, and others representative of the immediate community that the hospital serves. Ideally, the committee should be intellectually rich with devoted members capable of ethics mediation. Importantly, the authority of ethics committees is limited to an advisory body that seeks to achieve a consensus through mediation. Recent surveys have demonstrated that ethics committees consult on a range of issues across the life cycle helping patients, families, and staff grapples with challenging questions that require expert assistance.

THE ETHICS COMMITTEE AT NEW YORK PRESBYTERIAN

Weill Cornell Medical Center typically conducts 150 to 200 consults a year. In a recent year, 62% pertained to end-of-life care issues, 40% related to family conflict, and the remainder was evenly distributed across treatment refusals, comorbid medical and psychiatric issues, pediatrics, geriatrics, and team conflict requiring mediation. Since the initiation of the service in 1994, case volume, acuity, and complexity has risen with a clear ICU predominance of 57% in 2008.

INFORMED CONSENT AND REFUSAL

Informed consent is the ethical lynchpin of modern medical ethics in which the dialogue between the patient and physician preserves the patient's voice in directing care. This doctrine is rooted in respect for persons and the promotion of autonomy and patient self-determination through an interpersonal process whereby physicians and patients interact with each other in order to select an appropriate course of medical care, with the patient critically assessing his or her own values and preferences (**Table 33-1**).

Once a patient has made a choice, consent must be maintained over time to remain the moral warrant for permission to infringe upon the patient's zone of privacy. Patients who provide consent retain the ability to revise that decision and withdraw it.

TABLE 33-1 Decision-making Capacity and Competence

- Ability to communicate a choice
- Understand the nature and consequences of the choice
- Manipulate rationally the information necessary to make the choice
- Reason consistently with previously expressed values and goals

PRACTICE POINT

Indications for ethics consultation

Ethical Issues
- Advance directive
- Brain death
- Capacity/informed consent
- Confidentiality
- Discharge/placement
- DNR
- Futility
- Isolated incapacitated patient
- Maternal/fetal conflict
- Medical error
- Pain management
- Refusal of recommended treatment
- Research ethics
- Resource allocation
- Surrogate decision making
- Transplant issues
- Truth telling
- Withdrawal of ventilator
- Withdrawal of other life sustaining therapy
- Withdrawal or withholding artificial nutrition and hydration
- Withholding of other life-sustaining therapy

Contextual Issues
- Cultural/ethnic/religious
- Communication
- Dispute/conflict
  - Intra-family
  - Intra-staff
  - Staff-family
  - Staff-patient
  - Patient or family in denial
  - Physician attitude toward treatment
- Quality of life

Data from Nilson EG, Acres CA, Tamerin NG and Fins JJ. Clinical Ethics and the Quality Initiative: A pilot study for the empirical evaluation of ethics case consultation. *Am J Med Qual.* 2008;23(5):356–364.

PRACTICE POINT

- Decision-making capacity is not a global assessment of cognitive ability or intelligence, or knowledge of serial sevens, but rather a discrete capability of understanding the consequences of specific choices offered and made. Determining decision-making capacity is a clinical judgment that is distinct from the juridical judgment of competence. Moreover, for a patient to be competent legally as dictated by law, he or she must possess both decision-making capacity and be of age or an emancipated minor.

While informed consent imposes responsibilities on both the patient and the hospitalist, it creates an opportunity to build a trusting doctor-patient relationship. A properly executed informed consent is founded upon mutual respect, good communication, and results in a shared agreement about the course of medical care. A relationship forged through the informed consent process can facilitate

TABLE 33-2 Informed Consent and Refusal

- Informed consent is a patient right.
- Not all patients retain this right, predicated on the ability to be self-determining, which requires capacity.
- Patients must have decision-making capacity to participate in informed consent.

realistic patient expectations and help prevent disputes. Barriers to the informed consent process include:

1. **Poor care coordination.** Mixed communication, or even contradictory information to the patient and/or family, may cause confusion undermining care decisions.
2. **Fragmentation of care.** Lack of clarity about one's overall condition may also encumber the patient's ability to make informed choices.
3. **Adaptation to the new set of potentially limited choices** imposed on the patient by hospitalization and progressive illness. This displacement of the locus of control, outside of the patient's prior sphere of autonomous decision making, requires both the patience and compassion of the hospitalist in order to help the patient understand how his experience of hospitalization might influence his response to illness.

The all too common refrain, "I consented the patient," mistakenly prizes outcome (agreement to a proposed procedure) over process (a clear and informed decision whether that choice resulted in the acceptance or refusal of a treatment). The importance of the informed consent process is the act of deliberation in making a sound medical choice (**Table 33-2**).

PRACTICE POINT

- Informed consent is neither the recitation of facts by the physician nor the placement of a signature on a document. Instead, informed consent is the provision of information to a capacitated patient or surrogate decision maker necessary to make a medical choice either to accept or refuse a medical intervention. For this process to have integrity there must be adequate disclosure in clear language of the nature and purpose of the contemplated procedure and associated risks and benefits. The decision need be noncoerced and voluntary and the patient or surrogate must be apprised of any alternatives to the proposed intervention, if there is one available.

Concern about patient decision-making capacity typically occurs with refusal rather than with agreement of a proposed therapy. The treatment refusal may be equated with a loss of decision-making capacity because the decision challenges the doctor's expert recommendation. Under the rubric of self-determination, patients retain the right to refuse treatments and physicians have a orollary obligation to be sure that the patient understands the consequences of that choice. Mere refusal by itself does not mean a patient lacks capacity for decision making.

The philosopher James Drane developed a capacity assessment tool to assist in the assessment of patient choices. Invoking a "sliding scale of competence," Drane sought to link the increasing gravity of a patient's decision with a progressive degree of explication. If a patient were to refuse life-sustaining therapy, he would have to more fully demonstrate his reasons, rationale, and appreciation of the consequences than if he were refusing an elective procedure. The level of decision-making capacity should be in accordance with the risks and benefits of the decision to be made. These reasons can be founded on personal, religious, or cultural beliefs. The stringency of the standard of capacity at each level is correlated with the dangerousness of the treatment decision. Refusal of care by a capacitated patient who is well informed needs to be respected, even if that refusal would lead to serious harm. This is ethically supported by the principle of autonomy and legally by the patient's right to privacy and dominion over one's self.

Every effort should be made to discern the patient's rationale for refusal of recommended treatment and counter any misinformation with appropriate facts. Ethics consultation may help resolve ethical issues when treatment refusals are made by a surrogate on behalf of an incapacitated patient.

TRUTH TELLING AND SHARING BAD NEWS

In our pluralistic society, some patients may prefer nondisclosure of medical information. In traditional Japanese culture, withholding of medical information is the norm founded upon *ishin denshin*, the Japanese term for the nonverbal communication of the truth. Many Islamic societies operate with less doctor-patient dialogue and a greater reliance on cultural and contextual clues in order to implicitly, versus explicitly, communicate information to the patient. In such contexts of overt nondisclosure, patients eventually deduce their status because they observe the nature of their treatments and the reactions of those around them (**Table 33-3**).

Part of the art in doctor-patient communication is titrating generic advice to the particular patient's willingness to know and use information. The burdens and benefits of "truth telling" and breaking bad news are weighed against the information necessary to make an informed treatment choice.

Approach the patient by stating that in this country standard practice requires sharing all medical information with the patient, unless he decides to delegate the dialogue and the implicit authority to make choices using that information to a surrogate as the health care agent.

THERAPEUTIC EXCEPTION OR PRIVILEGE

On that rare occasion when the risks associated with disclosure outweigh the benefits, practitioners can deliberately withhold information in contravention of the patient's self-determination and right to know. Typically, such a deviation from standard practice, referred to as "therapeutic exception" or "privilege," would involve a severely depressed patient who might become suicidal with grievous news. We recommend that a psychiatrist assess such cases and that the local ethics committee be involved in the deliberative process.

ADVANCE DIRECTIVES

Seventy percent of seriously ill patients are unable to decide treatment options at the end of life. The majority of these patients do not have advance directives at the time of hospitalization. By taking on

TABLE 33-3 Truth Telling

Truth telling and sharing bad news

- The physician is under an obligation to communicate specific information to the patient necessary for making informed and deliberate choices.
- While there is no precise metric to determine what patients need to know to make choices, most physicians adhere to a "reasonable person" standard with the provision of that amount of information that an "average" person would need to have to make a choice.
- Full medical disclosure is the norm for most Western people.

TABLE 33-4 Standards for Surrogate Decision Making

- First and foremost, adhere to the explicit wishes of the patient.
- If unknown, determine what decision the patient probably would have made based on the patient's values, beliefs, and past decisions as interpreted by the surrogate.
- When neither knowledge of expressed wishes nor inference of substituted wishes exists, make a best-interests judgment based on what a generic patient would want in a given circumstance.

discussions at the onset of care, practitioners can establish a doctor-patient/family relationship and mitigate many ethical dilemmas that could ensue should the patient deteriorate.

Advance directives allow the patient the opportunity to specify preferences in advance of incapacity through a living will and/or designate a surrogate to speak on his behalf through the identification of a "durable power of attorney" or "health care agent" or "proxy." With an advance directive, an incapacitated patient can be treated in accordance with his prior wishes. Such advance care planning can decrease speculation about what the patient would have wanted and decrease the moral angst associated with the proxy role, a burden that is often understated (**Table 33-4**).

When there is no surrogate (a health care agent) appointed by the patient or a guardian appointed by a court, ethical norms and the law assign standing to these surrogates:

1. The patient's spouse (and in many jurisdictions to domestic partners)
2. Thereafter, a relative such as an adult child, parent, sibling
3. Finally, a close friend

Each state may have its own hierarchy for this prioritization. We recommend the use of a health care agent over a living will, when there is a surrogate who the patient trusts. In the living will, an adult with capacity sets forth directions regarding medical interventions and other actions that should or should not be taken in specific circumstances if he becomes incapacitated in the future. Often ambiguous and difficult to interpret, this document may contain inherent contradictions and fail to anticipate possible scenarios. In contrast, embodying surrogacy in a designated surrogate—versus a document as in the case of living will—allows for more dynamic decision making and provides an individual who can interpret the patient's prior wishes in light of evolving circumstances and the patient-proxy covenant.

All 50 states recognize an advance directive as an extension of the patient's voice under the Patient Self-Determination Act (PSDA) of 1990, which requires health care institutions that participate in Medicare and Medicaid programs to ask patients whether they have an advance directive, inform patients of their right to complete an advance directive, and incorporate advance directives into the medical record.

Surrogates make decisions for incapacitated patients according to three distinct decision-making standards: patients' expressed wishes, substituted judgments, and best interests. When invoking substituted judgment, the surrogate places herself in the shoes of the patient and tries to make a decision as the patient would. When neither knowledge of expressed wishes nor inference of substituted wishes exist, the surrogate makes a decision based on what a reasonable person would make balancing benefits and burdens.

Even when surrogates consider the patient's values, the stress of the surrogate role coupled with family dynamics and imprecise prior patient wishes can lead to morally ambiguous situations. Conflicts can also arise between surrogates of equal standing, such as two sisters who cannot agree on their mother's care. A rigid hierarchical approach to surrogate decision making oversimplifies a process that is complex, dynamic, and personal. When two surrogates disagree, ask them to set aside their own preferences and articulate what each believes is in the patient's best interest. This minimizes potential conflicts of interest and may lead to a concordance of views. When this approach fails, hospitalists may give ethical—if not legal—precedence to that surrogate who has been assuming more of the care responsibilities.

Sometimes the conflict about goals of care arises from an incongruity between a written directive and an oral one. Given the objective reality of documentation, deference will more likely be given to a previous written rather than verbal directive, even if more contemporaneous verbal preferences emerge—which ethically would take precedence. Hence, all practitioners should clearly document, *in the medical record*, any and all articulations of preference on the part of the patient. The discharge summary should include documentation of advance care planning as a guide to future care.

ETHICS CONSULTATION AT THE END OF LIFE

Establishing clear goals of care and having a working awareness of the inherent conflicts and biases that may arise at life's end can help prevent conflict and enhance patient care at a time when comfort and tranquility are at a premium. Decisions to accept or refuse life-sustaining therapy are all predicated upon the aforementioned principle of self-determination as exercised through a process of informed consent or refusal. Clinicians need to distinguish responsibility and culpability when considering their role in helping patients die comfortably.

WITHHOLDING LIFE-SUSTAINING THERAPY: DO NOT RESUSCITATE ORDERS

Causality is least complex in cases where a decision is made to withhold life-sustaining therapy (LST). By withholding LST, we mean a decision to not institute an intervention that could prevent death or prolong a dying process. The prototypic example of withholding LST is a do-not-resuscitate (DNR) order, which, in the hospital setting, means the forgoing of cardiopulmonary resuscitation (CPR) or basic cardiac life support (BCLS) as well as advanced cardiac life support (ACLS) to patients who have sustained a cardiopulmonary arrest. When a patient, health care agent, or other surrogate consents to a DNR order, an intervention will not interrupt the natural course of events. In such cases, the cause of death is clearly the underlying disease process.

Unlike other treatments to *withhold* CPR requires consent, based on the *emergency presumption* of providing care if consent cannot be obtained. Traditionally, physicians are obligated to perform CPR unless there is a contrarian request for a DNR order, which constitutes an informed refusal.

Essentially, all patients who undergo cardiopulmonary arrest will receive CPR unless the patient or their surrogate consents to a DNR order. When a patient or surrogate provides consent, the order should be clearly placed into the medical record and the medical and nursing teams informed in a standard manner. The patient's DNR status should travel with the patient when he or she goes off the floor and be readily available for consultation should an event occur. A DNR order should be reviewed periodically and may be reversed by the patient at any time and by the surrogate decision maker if the decision does not undermine a patient's decision while capacitated.

Seventy percent to 80% of deaths occur with DNR orders in place for hospitalized dying patients. In the modern hospital, DNR orders take many forms, ensconcing the patient's *negative right to be left alone*. Despite the prevalence and resonance of a dying patient with DNR orders on a general medical ward, it is important to appreciate that DNR orders do not preclude other treatments or interventions. It solely applies to decisions about cardiopulmonary arrest. Ethically, patients with DNR orders may receive care in the intensive care unit (ICU) or in the operating room. DNR status should be honored across specialties and not impede access to appropriate palliative care if it can only be offered through an intensive care or operative intervention. Indeed, some assert that it is patently unethical to condition appropriate care upon the presence or absence of a DNR order.

In practice, institutions vary in their triage of patients with a DNR order regarding ICU or surgical care or other interventions requiring intubation such as endoscopy. The Task Force of the American College of Critical Care Medicine and the Society of Critical Care Medicine argues against ICU admissions, for example, noting that: "ICU admissions should be reserved for patients with reversible medical conditions who have a reasonable prospect of substantial recovery."

Significant variation may relate to how to precisely identify patients who have a "reasonable prospect of substantial recovery." Moreover, if allocation or scarce resources (eg, ICU beds) or cost containment motivates triage decisions, adherence for individual clinicians creates ethical conflicts because of their primary fiduciary obligation to the patient. Existing data suggests that the presence of a DNR order at the time of MICU consultation was significantly associated with the decision to refuse a patient to the MICU.

Because any arrest during surgery could be considered reversible, secondary to the procedure, physicians, patients, and/or surrogates should discuss DNR status prior to surgery. We echo the recommendation of the American College of Surgeons for a process of "required reconsideration" of the preexisting DNR order as part of the informed consent process for surgery. If the patient or surrogate rescinds the DNR order perioperatively, a decision is made to reinstitute it upon arrival in the recovery room or at a specified time interval after surgery.

If the patient, or surrogate, wants to maintain a DNR status during the procedure, this must be documented in the preoperative consent. If the patient dies in the OR, it is considered an "expected death" under the rubric that DNR situations result in the patient's demise. In some institutions the physicians may find honoring an intraoperative DNR order to be against their conscience. In these cases there should be a provision of conscientious objection and removal from the case, so long as the primary physician responsibility of nonabandonment is not breached.

Both decisions to treat patients with a DNR order in the ICU or in the surgical suite ultimately hinges on achieving clarity about the goals of care. In each care decision, there is a conflict between a negative right to be left alone (the DNR order *not* to resuscitate) and the positive right to needed care. This balance of negative and positive engagement makes sense when the goals cohere, such as in the example of a palliative colostomy for an obstructing colon cancer. In that case, the surgical diversion is meant to provide comfort to a dying patient who had a DNR order, an ethically balanced plan of care.

In summary, the choice to forgo cardiopulmonary resuscitation supports the patients' right to refuse medical care even if this refusal leads to death. Notably, surrogate decision makers make up close to 80% of DNR requests. Hospitalists and primary care physicians are encouraged to initiate DNR discussion with the patient or proxy as soon as possible, preferably not when patients are immediately faced with cardiopulmonary cessation and imminent death.

THE DO-NOT-INTUBATE (DNI) CONUNDRUM

Do-Not-Intubate (DNI) or partial DNR orders compromise the integrity of practitioners because they imply resuscitation without intubation as a medically efficacious intervention despite the marginal effectiveness of comprehensive cardiopulmonary resuscitation itself. Most patients who have asystole or a ventricular tachyarrhythmia requiring cardioversion and/or chest compressions will also need intubation. Restoration of a viable cardiac rhythm places clinicians in the untenable position of being unable to fully complete resuscitation efforts.

In our experience, a DNI decision suggests ambivalence about goals of care, ie, a desire to survive without remaining on a ventilator for a protracted period of time. We recommend that these patients be fully resuscitated and also complete an advance directive that would allow a withdrawal of the ventilator if they were to linger beyond an aforementioned time limit.

Some patients or their surrogates would choose to be DNR but desire intubation in nonarrest situations in order to "pull through an illness." This might occur in the management of a COPD exacerbation, acute congestive heart failure, or pneumonia. Analogous to patients who are DNR in the OR, such patients want to be palliated (as per the aforementioned, diverting colostomy for obstructive colon cancer) or treated for potentially reversible conditions (sepsis) while setting limits on resuscitation should they deteriorate and sustain a cardiac arrest or complete respiratory failure. Intubation of patients with DNR orders might be regarded as a time trial.

WITHDRAWING LIFE-SUSTAINING THERAPY

Accepted as a norm, dating from the blue-ribbon President's Commission for the Study of Ethical Problems in Medicine and Biomedical and Behavioral Research, there is no ethical distinction between withholding and withdrawing treatment. The statement that the removal of LST device *causes* a patient to die, especially if the death is closely related temporally, is a *misconstrual* of causality. Withdrawal of LST simply removes an impediment to death. The intent is freedom from interventions that are perceived as burdensome. Death after refusal or withdrawal of an intervention results from the underlying disease. A decision to withdraw life-sustaining therapies may be challenging due to:

- Transference and counter transference often embedded in end-of-life decisions
- Physicians reluctance due to a misconstrued view that there is an ethical, and certainly psychological, difference between withholding and withdrawal of LST
- A sense of failure or sense of culpability
- Uncertainty about prognostication
- Inadequate communication with patients and/or surrogates about goals of care
- Differences between how physicians and lay people view these decisions

State and federal law regulate who is entitled to authorize the plan when the patient cannot speak for himself regarding a decision to withdraw LST. In the wake of the U.S. Supreme Court decision in the *Cruzan* case and the federalism of the aforementioned Patient Self-Determination Act, each state can set an evidentiary standard about the amount of evidence from the patient's prior wishes or values, if known, would be necessary to grant authority to a surrogate or physician to withdraw the intervention. Although the Supreme Court in *Cruzan* observed that there is no difference between the withdrawal of artificial nutrition and hydration and the withdrawal of a ventilator, some religious traditions view the provision of food and water as normative obligations that require a higher degree of foreknowledge of the patient's wishes.

MEDICAL DEVICES AT LIFE'S END

When automated implanted cardioverter defibrillators (AICDs) and permanent pacemakers (PPMs) only provide stand-by interventions, we view deactivation of their resuscitative role as withholding of care. In contrast, when a patient is paced continuously with a permanent pacemaker, either in a PPM or as a function of the AICD, deactivation is defined as a withdrawal of LST. Deactivation decisions should adhere to evidentiary decision-making standards as consistent with applicable state law, and ethics consultation may provide expert guidance. In our view, consider disabling the AICD and/or the episodic functions of the PPM when a patient or surrogate consents to a DNR, given the similarity between internal and external defibrillation.

RELIEF OF SUFFERING AND PALLIATIVE SEDATION

Suffering is defined as an existential threat to the self and distinct from pain. Palliative sedation is defined as the use of specific sedative medications to relieve intolerable pain and suffering from refractory symptoms, even at the risk of death. Palliative sedation aims to control symptoms rather than to end life; archaic, misleading terminology such as "terminal sedation" should be avoided. Palliative sedation provides different levels:

1. Ordinary sedation (for relief of heightened anxiety or stress without reduction of consciousness)
2. Proportionate sedation (for reduction of patient's awareness of distressing symptoms with the minimum dose necessary to promote the patient's ability to engage with his family and his immediate environment)
3. Palliative sedation to unconsciousness (when less extreme measures have not relieved suffering)

The initiation of palliative sedation to unconsciousness often invokes ethical dilemmas due to confusion about physician-assisted suicide or euthanasia. The doctrine of double effect, originating from Catholic theology, refers to the doctrine where a physician uses a treatment, or gives a medication, for an intended effect where the potential outcome is good (eg, relief of a symptom), knowing that there could be an undesired secondary effect (such as death). Double effect distinguishes between the ethically mandated goal of treating intolerable patient suffering from hastening death by engaging in physician-assisted suicide or euthanasia. In all circumstances, the degree of sedation must be proportional to the severity of suffering and is given only after the process of informed consent has ensued with the patient and or surrogate.

MEDICAL FUTILITY

Broadly defined, medical futility can be broken down into several domains:

- Physiologic futility (when it is absolutely—or to a reasonable degree of medical certainty—impossible to achieve a physiologic effect such as CPR in the setting of persistent acidosis)
- Qualitative futility (when the patient's physiology may improve, but there is no patient-centered benefit)
- Quantitative futility (when the intervention has not worked in similar patients within an accepted confidence interval)

Disagreement about the effectiveness of ongoing care may evoke strong emotions on the part of patients, families, and physicians entrusted to provide care. Multiple prior admissions when the patient "pulled through" despite negative odds, many clinicians with disparate views about aggressiveness of care at the end of life, communication failures, and cultural differences all contribute to a family's view of the patient's overall condition, prognosis, and how they would want him to spend the end of his life. It is important to try and prevent these disputes through ongoing communication during the course of the illness, to be reflective about the implicit force of one's countertransference and avoid mixed messages from different physicians by ensuring coherent comanagement.

PRACTICE POINT

- Comanagement of patients by a hospitalist and a specialist, whether medical or surgical, requires both parties to see the patient in the hospital. If the primary specialist is out of the hospital, care must be transferred to the inpatient doctor just as a primary care physician transfers care to the inpatient doctor. The primary specialist should not be dictating management from afar.

The best way to overcome fragmentation is to have a meeting including all key clinicians involved (physicians, social work, nursing, etc), significant others designated by the patient, and family members. The aim of the discussion is to create a comprehensive factual understanding of patient's condition and prognosis. Then, after achieving a broad understanding of the medical facts, a fruitful discussion regarding both family and clinician expectations can ensue over the course of multiple meetings.

Ultimately, the imperative for members of the health care team rests on exploring the intricacy of their patient's history and values and appreciate that many surrogates may be reluctant to immediately accept a physician's prediction of medical futility. In these circumstances it is helpful to ask the surrogate to make judgments believed to be in the patient's best interest and to articulate goals of care. On many occasions a surrogate may desire something that is unachievable through the provision of care. Having the surrogate articulate these goals provides an opportunity for reality testing and an occasion to redirect a beneficent impulse, so long as practitioners appreciate why they are so potentially distressed by family demands for futile care.

CONCLUSION

At the epicenter of inpatient care, hospitalists should maintain clarity, mediate misunderstandings about the diagnosis, prognosis, or goals of care, and minimize the opportunity for conflict to arise by organizing the medical team through sound comanagement, without dominating it—all in the service of patient-centered care. Hospital ethics consultants and committees stand ready to provide assistance and remind us of the centrality of patient beneficence in all its many forms.

SUGGESTED READINGS

Berger JT, DeRenzo EG, Schwartz J. Surrogate decision making: reconciling ethical theory and clinical practice. *Ann Intern Med.* 2008;149(1):48–53.

Drane JF. Competency to give an informed consent. A model for making clinical assessments. *JAMA.* 1984;252(7):925–927.

Fins JJ. *A Palliative Ethic of Care: Clinical Wisdom at Life's End.* Sudbury, MA: Jones & Bartlett; 2006.

Guidelines for intensive care unit admission, discharge, and triage. Task Force of the American College of Critical Care Medicine, Society of Critical Care Medicine. *Crit Care Med.* 1999;27(3):633–638.

Hinami K, Farnan JM, Meltzer DO, Arora VM. Understanding communication during hospitalist service changes: a mixed methods study. *J Hosp Med.* 2009;4(9):535–540.

Kelley AS, Reid MC, Miller DH, Fins JJ, Lachs MS. Implantable cardioverter-defibrillator deactivation at the end of life: a physician survey. *Am Heart J.* 2009;157(4):702–708.

Kripalani S, Jackson AT, Schnipper JL, Coleman EA. Promoting effective transitions of care at hospital discharge: a review of key issues for hospitalists. *J Hosp Med.* 2007;2(5):314–323.

Kripalani S, LeFevre F, Phillips CO, Williams MV, Basaviah P, Baker DW. Deficits in communication and information transfer between hospital-based and primary care physicians: implications for patient safety and continuity of care. *JAMA*. 2007;297(8): 831–841.

Meltzer D. Hospitalists and the doctor-patient relationship. *J Legal Stud*. 2001;30(2):589–606.

Meuller PS, Hook C, Hayes DL. Ethical analysis of withdrawal of pacemaker or implantable cardioverter-defibrillator support at the end of life. *Mayo Clin Proc*. 2003;78:959–963.

REFERENCE

1. Pantilat SZ, Alpers A, Wachter RM. A new doctor in the house: ethical issues in hospitalist systems. *JAMA*. 1999;282(2):171–174.

SECTION 6

Medical Legal Issues and Risk Management

CHAPTER 34

Medical-Legal Concepts: Advance Directives and Surrogate Decision Making

Kelly Armstrong, PhD
Ross D. Silverman, JD, MPH

INTRODUCTION

Advance directives, such as living wills, health care powers of attorney, do-not-resuscitate orders, and mental health care directives, are written legal documents that offer patients the opportunity to reflect upon and provide direction for their future medical care. They are important and useful tools to facilitate discussions between patients, family members, and physicians about end-of-life care choices, and they provide guidance and legal protection in those situations when a patient is no longer capable of declaring her care preferences and critical and difficult treatment decisions need to be made. Following an advance directive facilitates making end-of-life care decisions at the patient's bedside rather than through contentious court proceedings. More importantly, advance directives are legal mechanisms that reinforce the fundamental professional and moral responsibility of health care providers and institutions to promote and protect patient autonomy, welfare, and dignity.

PRACTICE POINT

- Advance directives are legal mechanisms that reinforce fundamental professional and moral responsibilities of health care providers and institutions to promote and protect patient autonomy, welfare, and dignity. Advance directives are best thought of as the result and documentation of a patient-centered process aimed at extending the rights of patients to guide their medical care, even through periods when they are no longer able to directly participate in decisions about their own care.

This chapter offers an introduction to advance directives, examining the general structure of the various types of advance directives, when they may be triggered, what clinical circumstances and decisions they may cover, as well as the relative strengths and weaknesses of the different advance directive instruments. Every state has laws describing the types of advance directives available in its jurisdiction, the processes by which such documents may be created and triggered, how and where they can be employed, and the legal protections afforded to care providers and health care facilities that carry out care decisions when guided by such documents. These laws may be supplemented by policies and procedures adopted by your local hospital or health care facility to direct the use of advance directives in your particular setting. Given the unique idiosyncrasies found from state law to state law and facility policy to facility policy, the reader should note that not all varieties of advance directive instruments may be available in your particular locale, and the processes used to carry out a particular advance directive may diverge from what is described in this chapter.

PRACTICE POINT

- Every state has laws describing the types of advance directives available in its jurisdiction, the processes by which such documents may be created and triggered, how and where they can be employed, and the legal protections afforded to care providers and health care facilities that carry out care decisions when guided by such documents. These laws may be supplemented by policies and procedures adopted by your local hospital or health care facility to direct the use of advance directives in your particular setting.

CONCEPTUAL FOUNDATIONS

The 1960s and 1970s saw a movement toward greater patient participation in health care that resulted in new ways to ensure shared decision making between patients and their physicians. During this time, dramatic medical and technological advances underscored the importance of recognizing and incorporating the goals and values of all patients, while ethicists, the courts, and others came to a consensus that a decisionally capable patient has the right to accept or refuse any type of medical care. However, many persons feared a loss of control may occur if they became incapacitated and unable to make their own medical decisions. As a result, patients and potential patients became increasingly aware of the need to make provisions for their own future medical treatment.

PATIENT SELF-DETERMINATION ACT

In 1990, the U.S. Supreme Court heard the case of Nancy Cruzan, a 33-year-old woman diagnosed in a persistent vegetative state after a car accident in 1983. In the case of *Cruzan v. Commissioner, Missouri Department of Health*, 497 U.S. 261 (1990), Nancy's parents sought to have the feeding tube removed and allow Nancy to die. The Court found that decisionally capable patients have the right to refuse life-sustaining therapies, including nutrition and hydration. However, the Court also indicated that states could require third parties acting on behalf of patients who are no longer decisionally capable to submit evidence of the patient's wishes before granting a request to withdraw life-sustaining treatment.

Partly in response to the Cruzan decision, Congress passed the Patient Self-Determination Act in 1990. This law attempts to make it clear patients have the right to make decisions regarding their medical care. This includes the right to accept or refuse treatment and the right to complete an advance directive as evidence of their wishes. The law requires any health care provider participating in Medicare or Medicaid to provide all persons over the age of 18 with written information regarding the patient's right to accept or refuse treatment and right to complete an advance directive. Providers include hospitals, nursing homes, home health care providers, hospices, and health maintenance organizations, but not outpatient-service providers or emergency medical personnel. The Patient Self-Determination Act also requires health care providers to document whether patients have advance directives, establish policies to implement advance directives, and educate their staff and the community about advance directives. Patients should also be informed that having an advance directive is not required to receive medical care.

UNIFORM HEALTH CARE DECISIONS ACT

After the Cruzan decision, significant changes occurred in state laws across the United States regarding health care decision making. While every state passed legislation authorizing the use of at least one form of advance directive, there was very little uniformity between the laws. By 1993, state laws regarding health care decision making were often fragmented, incomplete, and sometimes inconsistent. Statutes in one state frequently conflicted both with other statutes from the same state, and with statutes from other states. With this confusion in mind, the Uniform Health care Decisions Act (UHCDA) was drafted in 1993. Under the UHCDA, any adult or emancipated minor may execute or provide an "advance health-care directive," which refers to either a "power of attorney for health care" or other "individual instruction." If an individual fails to execute a power of attorney for health care or if the agent is not available, the UHCDA authorizes health care decisions to be made by a "surrogate" to be selected from a priority list. The Act also recognizes an individual's authority to define the scope of any instruction or agency as broadly or as narrowly as the individual chooses.

ADVANCE DIRECTIVES

Advance directives empower individuals to make their goals, values, and treatment preferences known before a loss of decisional capacity may occur. The term *advance directives* refers to oral or written instructions about a person's medical care that provide guidance regarding medical treatment to health care professionals if and when the patient becomes unconscious or otherwise unable to make his or her own decisions. All 50 states, either through statute or case law, have provisions for honoring advance directives. Despite this, different jurisdictions utilize different standards, terminology, and limitations of authority. Physicians should become familiar with the local requirements for completing and honoring a legal advance directive.

The legal requirements for a valid advance directive vary from state to state, but in general any adult or emancipated minor with decisional capacity can execute an advance directive. In some rare instances an advance directive may have an expiration date, however in general an advance directive remains in effect until such time as the patient revokes it. Different states have different requirements for validly revoking an advance directive, but most recognize a decisionally capable person may revoke an advance directive at any time simply by making the intention to revoke clear to a lawyer or health care provider, either verbally or in writing.

Because of the additional effort required to complete a written directive, the written directive is generally held to have more power than oral statements; however, this should be evaluated on a case-by-case basis. Because not every medical situation can be anticipated, in some situations oral statements provoked by the situation of others or even a television program may be more directly relevant to the situation at hand.

> **PRACTICE POINT**
>
> - The written directive is generally held to have more power than oral statements, however this should be evaluated on a case-by-case basis. Because not every medical situation can be anticipated, in some situations oral statements provoked by the situation of others or even a television program may be more directly relevant to the situation at hand.

NONCONFORMING DOCUMENTS

While many state statutes contain standard or recommended language for advance directives, people are introduced to advance directives from a variety of sources, including financial planners, senior organizations, national agencies, and religious organizations, not to mention the Internet. Most state statutes explicitly acknowledge that versions of advance directives that do not contain the recommended statutory language, as well as some oral statements, may also be valid. Such nonconforming directives cannot be dismissed just because they do not contain the language recommended by statute. Evaluating directives that do not conform to the recommended language found in state statutes requires physicians to determine, with the assistance of the ethics committee or legal counsel if necessary, whether a nonconforming directive meets the state's standard of reliability. In other words, is it clear that the patient intended to document his or her wishes with the intention that such documentation would be relied upon and followed by the health care team? Such seriousness of purpose can be demonstrated by a variety of means

TABLE 34-1 Types of Advance Directives

Advance Directive	Type	Covered Activity
Living will	Instructional	End-of-life document for patients with a terminal illness who wish to forgo death-delaying procedures
Physician's orders for life-sustaining treatment/ medical orders for life-sustaining treatment	Instructional	Portable physician orders for life-sustaining treatment that apply across all emergency and care settings
Power of attorney for health care	Proxy	Appoints a person over the age of 18 to make decisions on behalf of the patient
Psychiatric advance directive	Combination	Allows patient to preauthorize certain types of mental health treatment in the event of acute psychiatric illness; also allows the patient to appoint someone to make mental health treatment decisions
"Five wishes"	Combination	Combines a living will, power of attorney for health care, and instructions for comfort care and personal matters

including if the document contains the patient's signature, if the document is witnessed, if the document was presented to the physician by the patient as an advance directive, or if the patient discussed the document with family members as evidence of the patient's wishes.

ADVANCE CARE PLANNING

When advance directives first came into existence, they were viewed as legal documents offering legal protection from unwanted treatment at the end of life. As the practice of medicine has become more patient centered, a greater focus has emerged on ensuring all medical decisions are not only clinically sound, but also based on the patient's personal goals for care. Advance directives are best thought of as the result and documentation of a patient-centered process aimed at extending the rights of patients to guide their medical care, even through periods when they are no longer able to directly participate in decisions about their own care.

Optimally, before completing an advance directive, individuals will have the opportunity to have a structured discussion with their physician or other clinician about their health care wishes and goals. Ideally, these conversations are held before the patient becomes ill, even though physicians cannot discuss with specificity every scenario that may occur. Advance directives may simply contain general preferences, or they may contain specific instructions about particular treatments. Those that contain only general preferences can be less helpful in guiding care than those with specific instructions because general preferences can require more interpretation in light of the current medical evidence. For example, a patient's statement "I don't want to live hooked up to machines," may mean the patient's does not want CPR, or it may mean the patient wants all aggressive therapies until such time as those therapies fail to restore the patient to an acceptable quality of life. A comprehensive process of advance care planning includes a discussion of possible or likely scenarios based on the patient's unique medical situation, a discussion of the patient's values and goals, documentation of the patient's values and goals, and a way to ensure that this information is available to present and future care providers. The advance directive as a document provides a legally recognized way to record this discussion.

TYPES OF ADVANCE DIRECTIVES

Although state statutes vary, there are three basic types of advance directives: instructional, such as living wills; proxy, such as a power of attorney for health care; and combination directives, which provide both instructions for care and name a proxy to make decisions.

INSTRUCTIONAL ADVANCE DIRECTIVES

Instructional directives provide consent or refusal for specific treatments that may need to be utilized when the patient is unable to make the decision, traditionally at the end of life (**Table 34-1**).

Living wills

Living wills are the most common instructional directive. A living will directs physicians to withhold or withdraw life-sustaining measures and to provide only comfort care if the patient has a terminal illness and life-sustaining measures are prolonging the dying process without a chance for recovery. The living will thus addresses only a small subset of medical situations and critics cite the typically vague language and difficulty physicians have predicting with certainty when a patient is at the end of life as primary reasons that the document has fallen out of favor in terms of utility. Nevertheless, the document can be helpful as a starting point for further discussion, and it serves as evidence of a patient's values, specifically that there are certain outcomes the patient would not wish to pursue. The living will is also a useful document for persons who do not have a designated agent or proxy since it speaks directly to the physician and does not require the consent of a designated agent or proxy in order for the physician to take action.

Some jurisdictions have placed restrictions on how the living will may be invoked. For example, Illinois and Missouri do not permit the withdrawal of artificial nutrition and hydration if the withdrawal would be the proximate cause of death (rather than the patient's terminal condition). Most states also have provisions invalidating the document if the patient is pregnant, and some states dictate that the power granted to a designated agent such as a power of attorney for health care takes precedence over the power provided in the living will. Physicians should refer to the specific statutes in their state for guidance.

As the first widely known advance directive, the living will is the most well known and physicians should be aware that many patients refer to all advance directives by the name "living will," and others may confuse the living will with a last will and testament. Care should be taken to verify the exact type of directive(s) the patient may have.

Do-not-resuscitate orders

Do-not-resuscitate (DNR) orders have become increasingly common in the care of the dying patient. The decision whether to resuscitate a patient who suffers a cardiac or respiratory arrest involves consideration not only of the potential clinical outcomes, but also the patient's preferences regarding the intervention and if the likely outcome is one that would be desired by the patient. In order to streamline care from the inpatient to outpatient setting, a majority of states now have legislation permitting the use of out-of-hospital DNR orders. These DNR orders are physician orders that direct health care professionals across all emergency, living, or health care settings to withhold or withdraw (if treatment has already begun in absence of the form) specific types of life-sustaining treatment, such as CPR or defibrillation, in the event of a respiratory or cardiac arrest.

Physician's orders for life-sustaining treatment (POLST)

POLST stands for physician's orders for life-sustaining treatment, and the POLST form has been adopted by several states. (Some states such as New York use the acronym MOLST for medical orders for life-sustaining treatment.) POLST addresses the desire some persons may have, particularly those persons who are experiencing a chronic or life-limiting illness, to avoid unwanted emergency medical care like CPR or a transfer to the hospital. POLST takes advance directives a step further by not only documenting a patient's treatment preferences, but also providing emergency and other medical personnel with clear physician orders to follow in the case of an emergency. Depending on the state, the POLST form has three or four sections outlining the patient's desire to have or refuse CPR, whether the patient would like to be taken to a hospital, and the types of medical interventions desired by the patient, including the provision of comfort care, antibiotics, or artificially administered nutrition. In those states that have adopted the POLST paradigm, the orders are valid in all emergency, living, and health care settings. If a patient presents the POLST document in a state that has not adopted the POLST paradigm, the document should be interpreted as strong and reliable evidence of the patient's known wishes regarding treatment.

Other types of instructional directives

Other types of instructional directives allow individuals to refuse specific therapies, such as blood transfusion or dialysis, for persons who have specific desires to refuse those types of therapy. For example, many Jehovah's Witnesses do want blood or blood products administered under any circumstances, even though death may be an outcome of the refusal. The instructional directive provides evidence of the patient's wishes, and many will specifically release the physician from any liability for following the directive.

PROXY ADVANCE DIRECTIVES

Proxy advance directives such as the power of attorney for health care allow a patient to appoint another person over the age of 18 to make health care decisions in circumstances when the patient is unable to make those decisions for himself or herself. The proxy advance directive is not limited to end-of-life decisions and is therefore a more useful document for the vast number of decisions that can be encountered throughout the lifespan. The only requirement before the instrument takes effect is the patient must lack decisional capacity regarding the decision at hand. Physicians should note that because decisional capacity is decision specific, a patient may have the capacity to make some decisions, but require assistance to make other types of decisions.

The person appointed by a power of attorney for health care is called a power of attorney or an "agent." Because a power of attorney has been directly appointed by the patient, a power of attorney typically has broad authority to make the same kinds of decisions as the patient unless that authority has been limited by the patient or by statute. Thus, in most states, a power of attorney can accept or refuse any type of treatment. Because the power of attorney can execute a broad range of powers, health care professionals and others should ensure the appointment of a power of attorney is executed without coercion or duress. Some states require the power of attorney to accept the agency in writing, while others restrict agency to a single individual in order to minimize the chances that disagreement or differences of opinion between two or more agents stall medical decisions. Physicians should refer to the specific statutes in their state for guidance.

COMBINATION ADVANCE DIRECTIVES

There is a growing trend in advance directives toward allowing persons to combine instructions regarding treatment preferences with appointing a decision maker to make proxy decisions. Many state forms now allow persons completing an instructional form to also specify or appoint a power of attorney at the same time. It is important to note that while many combination forms grant the proxy decision maker broad powers of decision making, the document may also contain a limitations or exclusions section that limits the types of decisions that the proxy decision maker can make on behalf of the patient.

Psychiatric advance directives

Psychiatric advance directives allow persons with mental illnesses to engage in advance planning with their physicians regarding potential future care. Persons with mental illnesses retain the right to refuse treatment, as long as they do not pose a serious risk of harm to themselves or others. However, during an acute episode of psychiatric illness an individual may become unable to make or communicate decisions about treatment. A psychiatric advance directive allows currently competent patients who may experience an acute episode of psychiatric illness in the future, to agree in advance to treatment they may refuse later when ill. Unlike many other types of advance directives that focus on empowering the patient to refuse unwanted interventions, psychiatric advance directives are generally "opt-in" documents where the patient may preconsent to inpatient hospitalization, medication, or other helpful treatment modalities. In addition to offering a clear written statement of an individual's treatment preferences, the psychiatric advance directive can also be used to assign decision-making authority to another person while the individual is incapacitated. Correctly executed and implemented directives not only promote individual autonomy and empowerment, they can eliminate the need for court involvement and assist in recovery by communicating to the physician and others the types of treatments that have or have not worked for the person in the past.

"Five wishes"

"Five wishes" is a combination advance directive introduced in 1996 that has become popular because of its easy-to-read language. It introduces the subjects of a living will, power of attorney, comfort care, spirituality, and other personal matters such as forgiveness and memorial plans in the form of five distinct but overlapping "wishes." The first two wishes—"the person I want to make care decisions for me when I can't" and "the kind of medical treatment I want or don't want"—are intended to serve as legal documentation fulfilling the requirements of many states' living will and power of attorney statutes.

HONORING ADVANCE DIRECTIVES

Today's health care providers, and physicians in particular, have the simultaneous responsibility of respecting patients' autonomous choices while protecting from harm those patients who are incapable of making an authentic or informed decision. For patients with variable or fluctuating capacity, circumstances may arise where the patient is capable of being involved in some, but not all, decisions. The minimum standard for decisional capacity is directly related to the risk involved in the decision. Thus, a patient may legitimately consent to a low-risk procedure such as a blood draw or CT scan, but need assistance with more complex decisions such as whether to have surgery. The presumption is that a coherent care plan should be established around the patient's known wishes whenever possible.

PRACTICE POINT

- For patients with variable or fluctuating capacity, circumstances may arise in which the patient is capable of being involved in some, but not all, decisions. The minimum standard for decisional capacity is directly related to the risk involved in the decision. The presumption is that a coherent care plan should be established based on the patient's known wishes whenever possible.

INFORMED CONSENT

Informed consent is, with rare exceptions, required before treatment can be provided to a patient. In order for consent to be valid, it must be given voluntarily in light of accurate and relevant information—in a language intelligible to the recipient—regarding the risks, benefits, and alternatives of the proposed interventions. In addition to providing information that the average reasonable person might desire, it is important that patients receive sufficient information within the priorities that have the most meaning for them. For instance, some religious belief systems require or preclude certain forms of medical treatment. Other patients may want to know how incapacitated they may be after a surgery, or how long they must wait before driving. Valid consent also requires the person giving consent to have sufficient decisional capacity to make the decision at hand.

PRACTICE POINT

- Most advance directives are not applicable when the patient has decisional capacity and is capable of exercising his or her right to accept or refuse medical treatment. Thus, a patient's oral statements made while the patient is decisionally capable should be followed even if those statements conflict with a written directive.

DECISIONAL CAPACITY

There are relatively few guidelines informing physicians and others when to conduct and document an explicit assessment of an individual's decisional capacity. However, assessments of decisional capacity should be ongoing and not restricted to instances where the patient disagrees with a physician's recommendation for treatment. Assessment and documentation may be warranted whenever the individual consents to complex or high-risk interventions, when the patient makes choices that do not appear prudent or when the decision is outside the patient's norms, or when the patient has marked cognitive deficits or other risk factors for impaired decisional capacity. Although some complex situations may call for a specialized assessment by a psychiatrist or ethicist, most capacity assessments can be completed by any physician responsible for obtaining consent to treat the patient.

PRACTICE POINT

The presumption is that patients can make their own decisions until they demonstrate otherwise. Although some complex situations may for call for a specialized assessment by a psychiatrist or ethicist, most capacity assessments can be completed by the physician obtaining consent to treat.

Decisional capacity assessments are not justified merely because the patient disagrees with a recommendation. However, assessments may be warranted when:

a. the individual consents to a high risk procedure
b. when the patient's choices do not appear prudent or are outside of the patient's norms
c. when the patient has marked cognitive deficits or other risk factors for impaired decisional capacity

It is important to note that because capacity may fluctuate over time, physicians may be dealing with a proxy decision maker for some aspects of treatment, and directly with the patient for other aspects. When reasonable, important decisions should wait until the patient regains decisional capacity (if expected), and decisions made by others should be reviewed with the patient if and when he or she regains capacity. The presumption is that patients can make their own decisions until they demonstrate otherwise. Therefore, each decision should be put before the patient and if the patient concretely demonstrates that he or she is unable to make the particular decision at hand, this should be carefully documented in the patient's medical record. Many jurisdictions also require documentation of the reason for the patient's incapacity and its expected duration.

Decisional capacity is functionally defined in light of a specific decision. As the risk of a proposed intervention increases, so too does the threshold standard for decisional capacity. For instance, the capacity needed to consent to routine labs would be lower than the capacity required for consent to open heart surgery. Grisso and Appelbaum have put forward the most frequently used model for assessing decisional capacity standards 1-4 in **Table 34-2**.

Some commentators have also indicated that under certain circumstances it may be prudent to add the fifth criterion, particularly if the decision being made by the patient represents a radical or abrupt change in treatment goals, or does not conform to what is known about the patient values or other decisions.

COMPETENCE AND DECISIONAL CAPACITY

Decisional capacity and competence are not synonymous. Competence is a legal designation that must be made by a court,

TABLE 34-2 Standards for Assessing Decisional Capacity

Assessing Decisional Capacity
1. The patient can make and communicate a choice.
2. The patient demonstrates understanding of his or her medical condition, prognosis, and the risks and benefits of the available treatment options.
3. The patient has the capacity for reasoned decision making.
4. The patient is able to apply his or her own values to the decision at hand.
5. *The patient's decision remains stable over time (if the situation allows), or the patient can make a reasoned explanation why the decision is not consistent with the patient's previously known wishes.*

whereas decisional capacity is determined by a physician or other clinician. Not all patients with a developmental, cognitive, or mental illness have impaired decisional capacity, even if they have been declared incompetent or have been appointed a guardian. On the contrary, there is significant variability in the decisional capacity among these patients. The examining clinician should evaluate each patient's capacity in light of the particular decision at hand.

PRACTICE POINT

- Competence is a legal designation that must be made by a court, whereas decisional capacity is determined by a physician or other clinician. Not all patients with a developmental, cognitive, or mental illness have impaired decisional capacity, even if they have been declared incompetent or have an appointed guardian. The examining clinician should evaluate each patient's capacity in light of the particular decision at hand.

PROXY DECISION MAKING

Physicians respect a patient's autonomy by recognizing that the patient's right to accept or refuse treatment remains even after he or she loses decision-making capacity. Patients who have lost decisional capacity may continue to communicate through their advance directives, or through a power of attorney or surrogate who interprets what the patient would choose in a given situation.

When medical decisions need to be made for a patient who lacks decisional capacity, physicians should first inquire whether the patient has documented any wishes in a written advance directive such as a POLST form or a durable power of attorney for health care. Optimally, the patient will have documented preferences that directly relate to the proposed treatment. However, this rarely happens. More commonly, a third party is necessary to represent the patient's interests and interpret the patient's known wishes and values in light of the current medical situation. If the patient has designated a decision maker in an advance directive such as a power of attorney for health care, the designated agent should be relied upon to make decisions. If the patient does not have a power of attorney or some other document that directs care, such as a POLST form or living will (or those documents exist but do not apply to the situation at hand), a surrogate should be appointed.

SURROGATE DECISION MAKING IN THE ABSENCE OF ADVANCE DIRECTIVES

Many states have established protocols for identifying a legal third-party decision maker in the absence of a documented advance directive. This third-party decision maker may be called a proxy or a surrogate, depending on the state. Most patients have not completed an advance directive and there should be no presumption inferred from the fact that an advance directive has not been executed. The guiding principle in appointing any surrogate is to find the person, or group of persons, who best know the patient's values and health care goals. This person or persons should be able to effectively communicate with the health care team, and be willing to make choices the patient would most likely make if he or she could speak for himself or herself.

Where they exist, state statutes generally indicate the family of the patient should be responsible for making medical decisions. The order of priority for appointing a surrogate is usually listed by degree of legal or blood relationship, with a court-appointed legal guardian of the patient first, then a spouse or domestic partner (in jurisdictions that recognize this status), adult children of the patient, a parent of the patient, an adult sibling, other family members, and finally a close friend of the patient (**Table 34-3**). While "family" is generally recognized as a biological or legal relationship, most states have not specifically addressed more complicated relational ties such as when the patient has full siblings, half siblings, and step siblings who all consider themselves to be close relatives of the patient on the same level of the surrogate hierarchy. If more than one person has the same level of priority (such as several adult children), consensus is preferred, but many states allow for a majority decision when consensus cannot be reached. The disagreeing party then has the option of turning to the court to assist in resolving the dispute. In states that do not appoint surrogates by statute, case law may offer guidance, or the physician or ethics committee can nominate the decision maker according to the standards of the institution.

TABLE 34-3 Priority Hierarchy for Appointing a Surrogate

Typical Order of Priority for Appointing a Surrogate in Absence of Applicable Advance Directive (Check Local Jurisdiction)
1. Court-appointed guardian
2. Spouse or domestic partner (where legally recognized)
3. Adult children
4. Either parent
5. Adult siblings
6. Other family members
7. A close friend of the patient

Guiding standards

Two basic principles should guide treatment decisions for decisionally incapable patients: respecting and promoting the patient's autonomy, and fostering the patient's well-being. All surrogates and care providers have an obligation to follow the informed verbal or written wishes of the patient and to act in the person's best interests. They should also take into account the person's values and goals if those are known. Three legal and ethical standards have been established to guide such decisions: (1) The highest standard is a directly relevant autonomous directive where the patient's wishes in regard to the decision at hand are known, either through documentation or discussion. (2) The most common standard used is substituted judgment where the proxy decision maker is tasked with making the decision he or she believes the patient would have made in this situation based on what is known about the patient's wishes, personal values and preference, and goals. (3) In the best interest standard, the patient's wishes are unknown or have never been known (such as cases involving infants), and the proxy decision maker must weigh the risks and benefits of all of the alternatives and make a decision that achieves the greatest net benefit from the perspective of the patient.

PRACTICE POINT

- There are two basic principles that should guide treatment decisions for decisionally incapable patients: respecting and promoting the patient's autonomy, and fostering the patient's well-being.

Confidentiality and HIPAA

Although medical care has always included the need to keep patients' medical information confidential, the Health Insurance Portability and Accountability Act (HIPAA) has further specified and codified the responsibility of health care providers. In order to make effective decisions, proxy decision makers need information about the patient's medical history and care. HIPAA regulations recognize this and entitle duly documented proxy decision makers to the same medical information as the patient in regard to the decision at hand. However, physicians should disclose only that information needed by the proxy to make an informed choice regarding the decision at hand. If possible and/or when directed by the patient, physicians should avoid discussing highly personal information such as sexually transmitted diseases, HIV status, chemical dependency, mental illness, or any history of sexual or physical abuse, unless such information is absolutely necessary in order for the proxy to make appropriate and informed decisions.

Scope of authority

The exact scope of a surrogate's decision-making authority varies by state. Patients may also document certain limits on the kinds of decisions that may be made by their surrogate. For example, some living wills state the surrogate decision maker cannot override specific instructions such as a request not to receive CPR. Some state laws also suggest the patient must assent to, or minimally not refuse, decisions made by the surrogate. This offers a layer of protection to those patients who may not reach the threshold for decisional capacity with respect to the decision at hand, but who are still aware of and engaged with what is happening to them. When there is disagreement between the patient and surrogate, and a clinically appropriate compromise that is acceptable to both parties cannot be found, it is advisable to contact the hospital's ethics committee.

Because the surrogate is often an individual whom the patient has not explicitly appointed to the role of decision maker, many states place restrictions on the types of end-of-life decisions that can be made by the surrogate. Broadly speaking, these restrictions may require the attending physician and one additional physician to document that the patient has a "qualifying condition," such as a terminal illness or permanent unconsciousness, before honoring a request by the surrogate to withhold or withdraw life-sustaining treatment.

Generally, a proxy decision maker for a decisionally incapable patient may conduct routine medical affairs for the patient including consulting with the patient's health care providers, providing verbal or written consent for medical procedures, applying for public benefits such as Medicare or Medicaid, authorizing the release of information and clinical records needed for continued care, and authorizing the transfer of the patient to or from health care facilities. Care should be taken that such activities are warranted by the patient's clinical condition, do not conflict with the patient's known wishes, and that they are undertaken by the proxy only when it is not expected that the patient will be returned to a decisionally capable state in the time necessary to assure continuity of care.

Conflicts

Occasionally, situations arise in which a surrogate makes a decision or requests an intervention that conflicts with either the patient's advance directive or other instructions the patient provided to the care team while the patient was still decisionally capable. For instance, it is not uncommon for a patient's child to request CPR be provided even when the patient has specifically requested a DNR order. Plans and treatment goals previously established between the patient and the physician should not be changed without concrete evidence that those decisions were made due to factual, conceptual, or clinical error. The primary responsibility of the physician is to the patient, and decisions made after the patient loses decisional capacity should further the continued interests of the patient. Additionally, surrogates are morally and legally required to make decisions that conform as closely as possible to those the patient would choose for himself or herself. Physicians thus are not obligated to follow requests by surrogates that do not comply with the patient's known wishes. If the physician is unable to resolve the conflict, it may be helpful to involve a third party to help mediate the situation such as an ethics consultant or committee, or hospital legal counsel. If an ethically, legally, and clinically sound agreement cannot be reached, court review may be necessary.

PRACTICE POINT

- Occasionally, a surrogate may request an intervention that conflicts with the patient's previous instructions (such as rescinding a DNR put in place by the patient). Physicians are not obligated to follow requests by surrogates that do not comply with the patient's known wishes. Assistance from the ethics committee or legal counsel may be necessary in order to resolve the conflict.

SPECIAL CASES

Implied consent

In health care, the principle of implied consent is sometimes colloquially referred to as "emergency consent" since it is most commonly invoked when the following conditions are met: (1) there is an emergency circumstance where the patient is unable to participate in the informed consent process (usually because the patient is unconscious), and there is no available evidence of the patient's wishes not to receive the therapy; (2) no other proxy decision maker is available to make decisions for the patient; and (3) the physician is compelled to immediately provide necessary treatment without which serious or irreversible harm to the patient's life or health may result. Thus, implied consent is presumed when a person needs help and cannot explicitly provide consent. Implied consent also refers to situations where the patient does not expressly state, either verbally or in writing that a procedure may be done, but his or her actions imply consent. A common example is when the patient extends an arm after being told that the physician wants to draw blood for laboratory analysis. Implied consent is legally accepted and provides a defense against claims of battery, but not against claims of negligence. Physicians should follow their institutions' documentation standards when relying on implied consent in the context of a medical emergency, and clearly identify why emergency treatment was necessary as well as the nature and immediacy of the threat.

Minors

The rights of minors to make decisions about their medical care have expanded over the past decade. While in general, a parent or legal guardian of a minor has to provide consent for treatment, some jurisdictions are granting older minors, especially those over the age of 16, broad leeway to make decisions about their medical treatment. Nearly all jurisdictions allow legally emancipated minors and minors who are pregnant or parents themselves to make medical decisions for their care and their own minor children. However, some states now have statutes or case law that allow mature minors to provide consent to procedures if they can demonstrate that they are mature enough to understand and appreciate the nature and consequences of a proposed medical procedure or treatment. Rather than reliance on an "all-or-none" phenomenon, the mature minor doctrine allows for individual assessment of the stability of the minor patient's value system along with their emotional and intellectual development. This approach recognizes that decisional capacity in a minor is a gradual process affected by personal characteristics and environment. The laws concerning the extent minors are allowed to make medical decisions for themselves vary from jurisdiction to jurisdiction, and most jurisdictions are reluctant to allow minors to refuse potentially life-sustaining treatment without involvement of the court. It is therefore advisable that each physician be familiar with the local statutes.

Artificial nutrition and hydration

Medical and legal issues abound when it comes to the use of artificial nutrition and hydration (ANH), particularly in the dying or permanently unconscious patient. The U.S. Supreme Court made it clear in its 1990 Cruzan decision that ANH is a medical treatment and a decisionally capable patient may refuse any and all types of medical treatment, including ANH and other types of life-sustaining treatment. Patients may also execute a specific instructional directive that references ANH and clearly communicates the patient's refusal of ANH. However, state laws are highly variable in regard to proxy decision-maker requests to withhold or withdraw ANH, and many living will laws expressly forbid the withholding or withdrawal of ANH as a means to shorten the dying process. Some states require "clear and convincing" evidence of the patient's wishes to forgo administration of ANH before a proxy request may be honored. Clear and convincing evidence would require either a written directive or evidence of a serious, reflective discussion with the patient on the subject. Other states have lesser evidentiary standards, and some include ANH within the parameters of life-sustaining treatment that may be terminated upon request of a proxy decision maker whenever the standards are met for withdrawal of life-sustaining treatment. Physicians should refer to the specific statutes in their state for guidance.

Physician-assisted suicide

The U.S. Supreme Court ruled in 1997 that states may maintain laws that prohibit or allow euthanasia and assisted suicide. A few states now allow terminally ill adult patients, who are decisionally capable and able to communicate their wishes, to end their lives through the voluntary self-administration of a lethal dose of medication prescribed by a licensed physician expressly for that purpose. In Oregon and Washington, the statutes are called the Death with Dignity Act. Patients must fulfill several requirements before receiving the medication, including initiating verbal and written requests, undergoing a second opinion consultation, receiving psychiatric intervention if the patient is perceived to be depressed, and undergoing a 15-day waiting period. This process is sometimes called "physician-assisted suicide" because patients self-administer the medication at a time of their choosing with the intention of ending their life. Because the patient actively takes steps to end his or her life, this is different than withholding or withdrawing medical treatment where barriers to the dying process are removed. This is also different than voluntary active euthanasia where the physician acts upon the voluntary request of a decisionally capable patient and the physician intentionally administers medications or other interventions to cause the patients death. In states that allow it, patients must request and self-administer the lethal medication. No state allows the medications to be administered or requested by a proxy decision maker, even where there is clear evidence of the patient's wishes.

SUGGESTED READINGS

Appelbaum PS. Assessment of patient' competence to consent to treatment. *N Engl J Med.* 2007;357:1834–1840.

Burns JP, Edwards J, Johnson J, Cassem NH, Truog RD. Do-not-resuscitate order after 25 years. *Crit Care Med.* 2003;31(5): 1543–1550.

Johnstone MJ, Kanitsaki O. Ethics and advance care planning in a culturally diverse society. *J Transcult Nurs.* 2009;20(4):405–416.

Jonsen AR, Siegler M, Winslade WJ. Clinical Ethics: *A Practical Approach to Ethical Decisions in Clinical Medicine.* 7th ed. New York: McGraw-Hill; 2010.

Scheyett AM, Kim MM, Swanson JW, Swartz MS. Psychiatric advance directives: A tool for consumer empowerment and recovery. *Psychiatr Rehabil J.* 2007;31(1):70–75.

Siegel MD. End-of-life decision-making in the ICU. *Clin Chest Med.* 2009;30:181–194.

Valvano TJ. Legal issues in sexual and reproductive health care for adolescents. *Clin Pediatr Emerg Med.* 2009;10:60–65.

Von Gunten CF, Ferris FD, Emanuel LL. The patient-physician relationship. Ensuring competency in end-of-life care: communication and relational skills. *JAMA.* 2000;284(23):3051–3057.

CHAPTER 35

Preventing and Managing Adverse Patient Events: Patient Safety and the Hospitalist

Timothy B. McDonald, MD, JD

INTRODUCTION

In November 1999 the Institute of Medicine (IOM) issued the report *To Err is Human*, detailing a problem of preventable medical errors that were killing as many as 98,000 inpatients per year. Specific types of medical errors highlighted in the IOM report include error in the administration of treatment, failure to order and follow-up on indicated diagnostic exams, and avoidable delays in care and treatment. Many years later problems still exist: nearly 2 million patients a year develop infections during their hospitalizations, and 90,000 to 100,000 of those infected die while hand-hygiene rates range from 30–70% at most acute care facilities. The IOM report also estimated that medical errors cost the U.S. $17 billion to $29 billion a year, and called for sweeping changes to the health care system to improve patient safety.

Improvements in patient safety have focused on addressing the root causes of these preventable patient harm events, specifically events related to poor communication, lack of teamwork, fragmentation of care, and a lack of leadership from the medical community. In addition, patient safety experts have also implored physicians and hospitals to approach patient harm events with transparent, open, and honest communication between caregivers and patients and families in order to learn from mistakes and poorly designed systems.

This chapter focuses on the important ways in which hospital-based physicians can actively participate in the prevention of patient harm and provide appropriate management and assistance when patient harm does occur.

PREVENTING ADVERSE PATIENT EVENTS

While there are many important ways that hospital-based physicians can proactively maximize the safety of their patients, most patient safety experts would agree that the areas of highest priority can fit into three broad domains: communication, teamwork, and leadership (see **Table 35-1**). Within each of these domains lies critical concepts and issues about which the highly reliable and safe-practicing physician must remain mindful.

PRACTICE POINT

- While there are many important ways that hospital-based physicians can proactively maximize the safety of their patients, most patient safety experts would agree that the areas of highest priority can fit into 3 broad domains: communication, teamwork, and leadership. Within each of these domains lie critical concepts and issues about which the highly reliable and safe-practicing physician must remain mindful.

COMMUNICATION

No chapter on patient safety and the prevention of patient harm is complete without a major focus on the role communication—or lack thereof—plays in serious patient safety events. The most common types of communication of high priority in patient safety are listed in Table 35-1.

Handoffs

Year after year The Joint Commission (TJC) publishes data showing 65–70% of all sentinel events are rooted in communication breakdowns. It appears that since the implementation of the

TABLE 35-1 Preventing Patient Safety Events

Communication	
	Handoffs within and between services
	Documentation in the electronic health record
	Managing critical test results
Teamwork	
	Multidisciplinary rounds
	Infection prevention
	Patient Triage
	Rapid Response Teams
Leadership	
	Hospital/Medical Center Committees
	Safety Culture

Accreditation Council for Graduate Medical Education (ACGME) resident physician work hour limitations the communication problems have increased, especially in the area of **handoffs,** when the responsibility of care is passed from one provider to the next. With this limitation of resident physician work hours the need and demand for hospital-based physicians to "fill the gaps" in patient care has increased substantially. Associated with that increase in demand, hospitalists in particular have recognized the imperative of a standardized, user-friendly, and reliable method of handing off care from one provider to the next.

The content and process for handing off in the inpatient setting has evolved as practitioners try to meet regulatory requirements while maintaining simplicity, efficiency, and usability of the various handoff tools that are available. Various pneumonic tools, such as **S**ituation, **B**ackground, **A**ssessment, **R**ecommendation (SBAR) have been devised to assist in the handoff process but have come and gone from institutional policies and guidelines as providers struggle with a reliable way to meet this important imperative. Hospitalists must play a role in designing and implementing a best practice handoff process appropriate for the context in which they work.

Vendors of electronic health records (EHRs) have also entered the arena with HER-based tools to facilitate the often onerous process of handing off care of large numbers of patients. Regardless of the chosen method, all hospital-based physicians must employ a reliable process to transmit necessary patient information from physician to physician. Defective or unreliable handoffs substantially increase risk of patient harm and the associated liability.

Documentation in the Electronic Health Record (EHR)

With the passage of the 2010 Health Care Reform Act, it has become increasingly clear that the use of electronic health records will become much more ubiquitous in the coming years. While patient safety benefits of EHRs are well documented, only recently have informatics experts been publishing the unintended, unsafe consequences related to their use.

One of the most glaring examples of an unintended, unsafe consequence to EHR implementation is the abuse of "cut and paste" or "copy and paste" functionality, the process by which entire sections of nursing or physician documentation are copied and pasted from past to present notes. Numerous published reports demonstrate cases in which erroneous information has propagated, almost "virally," throughout a patient's EHR through the use of copy and paste. This process creates unsafe conditions for the patient such as in the example of the erroneous propagation of a "faux" allergy to an important medication. Serious medical-legal consequences can result for those who continue to misrepresent medical information through subsequent "copies" of the erroneous information or for those who act upon this unreliable information. The credibility of physicians comes into question when they are forced to defend misinformation they have propagated throughout the medical record, such as a temperature of 1101.5°F or a blood pressure of 1180/60.

While the "copy and paste" functionality provides useful efficiencies for documentation of long lists of medications or past surgical procedures, hospital-based physicians must be aware of the deleterious consequences of the inappropriate use of this functionality and they should serve as positive role models and mentors throughout the organization for others who document in the EHR. From a patient safety and legal perspective, it is also incumbent upon the hospitalist to facilitate the correction of erroneous information encountered in the EHR.

Management of Critical Test Results

Critical-test results management cuts to the heart of the health care business. U.S. hospitals complete approximately 12 billion diagnostic tests every year. Most test results are within normal range and do not require follow up by the clinician. However, a small but important number of test results, approximately1% to 5% of a hospital's test volume, are abnormal or critical. Hospitals and hospital-based physicians have a professional, legal, and ethical obligation to ensure that these results are communicated to the responsible physician and appropriate action is taken.

Traditional systems to communicate and manage critical results are full of potential points of failure. In many hospitals, especially for hospital-based physicians, contact information changes on a regular basis. Radiology departments and the pathology lab may not have the correct contact information for the responsible physician. Faxes can be equally problematic as the receiving machine might be off or out of paper. And once communicated, the right person might not receive the information. Unfortunately, radiologists and laboratory technicians may spend hours or days trying to track down the appropriate physician for results communication. Not surprising, miscommunication of critical findings have been identified as the causative factor in 85% of radiology lawsuits. Appropriately, The Joint Commission (TJC) has deemed the management of critical test results as a national patient safety priority and requires hospitals and health care professionals to improve processes involved in such results. To improve the safety and quality of care their patients receive, hospitalists must play an integral role in the design and implementation of systems and processes to manage critical test results. At a minimum, in the hospital setting they must actively participate in a process to ensure the proper identification of responsible physicians and an efficient means for involving those responsible physicians in the communication and action based upon these results.

TEAMWORK

Multidisciplinary rounds

Data abounds on the value teamwork brings to the safe and effective delivery of health care. The days of a single physician effectively micromanaging a patient's entire hospital stay are long gone. Research has shown that physicians can mitigate the negative effects of the necessary fragmentation of health care delivery by participating in multidisciplinary rounds during which physicians, nurses, pharmacists, and other allied health professionals discuss the daily plan for the patient and coordinate the transition of care to the outpatient setting. Inclusion of the patient and family in these rounds also provides benefit.

Especially for complicated patients, multidisciplinary rounds have been demonstrated to reduce length of stay, decrease the incidence of medication errors, prevent hospital readmissions, and improve overall patient and family satisfaction related to the hospital stay. As health care reimbursement models transition to a "pay for performance" or "pay for quality" metric, hospitals and hospitalists will find multidisciplinary rounds fundamental to the business model of health care.

Infection prevention

All patient safety and quality organizations as well as health care regulators have identified heath care associated infections (HAIs) as a top priority. The human and financial toll of HAIs accounts for a large portion of preventable harm in the United States. Therefore, the elimination of any significant proportion of HAIs is paramount to control health care costs and preventing patient harm. The role of the hospitalist as an essential, active member of the health care team is central to the efforts to reduce HAIs.

Three easily identifiable areas of quality improvement related to prevention of HAIs include (1) hand hygiene, (2) prevention of catheter-associated urinary tract infections (CAUTIs), and (3) intravenous line-associated blood stream infections, especially those related to central lines (CLABSIs). With observed hand-hygiene rates in most hospitals hovering around an abysmal 40–50%, administrators struggle to find solutions. Many leaders have found the solution to the hand-hygiene dilemma in the active engagement of hospitalists in their institution-wide efforts. Numerous success stories show that hospitalist engagement, by actively promoting hand-hygiene within their team, has taken 40–50% compliance rates to a sustainable 90% or higher. From the patient perspective, these increases in hand-hygiene rates translate into substantial reductions in methicillin-resistant staph (MRSA) infections and other HAIs.

The involvement of hospitalists on daily rounds in which they are able to order the removal of nonessential foley catheters substantially reduces the incidence of CAUTIs. The same holds true for CLABSIs, in which the reduction in the days of use for invasive intravenous lines is also associated with a heath care-associated infection. With all these efforts, hospitalists are ideally situated to affect safety outcomes for their patients and others on their teams and in the institutions where they practice.

Patient triage and Rapid Response Teams (RRT)

As the frontline physicians accepting or coordinating inpatient hospital admissions, the hospitalist has an affirmative obligation to make certain newly admitted patients are placed on units and into beds that are appropriate for the level of care they need. Nonetheless, patients on appropriate wards or units will still deteriorate faster than the care professionals anticipate. When that happens, in the interest of patient safety, hospitals must have a process for rapidly summoning a team of professionals to assess the patient's current state of deterioration and to assist in a "re-triaging" process.

Whether activated by other physicians, nurses, patients, or family members, hospital-based physicians play an important role in the response to the deteriorating patient in many institutions. Effective and valuable physician members of a rapid response team, or any team assigned to respond to the clinically deteriorating patient, possess certain necessary attitudes and skills. As a leader of the team, the hospitalist must approach each "call for help" with a high degree of "mindfulness" in order to avoid premature closure based upon selective information provided to them by the care professionals previously caring for the patient. Regardless of whether the "call for help" or activation of the RRT seems appropriate after the initial response and investigation, it remains critical that the physician leader of the response team supports those who trigger the activation and helps prevent ridicule or criticism of those who asked for help.

The hospitalist must remain open minded while gathering all potentially important information that might be useful for arriving at solutions or treatments to reverse the deteriorating trend in condition. While carefully listening to other team members and caregivers, the leader of the team must be able to synthesize an approach that considers all the relevant factors, especially unexpected findings, and avoid the temptation to disregard information that might be inconsistent with their preliminary diagnosis—the concept of premature closure. They must remain cognizant of their own confirmation biases and strive to keep them in check. Not all chest pain is a myocardial infarction and not all wheezing is asthma!

From the skills perspective, a successful hospitalist RRT team leader must demonstrate competence in basic airway skills, use of emergency medications, and the ability to interpret electrocardiograms. The most important skill, however, rests in the ability of the hospitalist to function as an effective team leader with an ability to communicate clearly, concisely, and calmly and demonstrate a capacity to coordinate the activities of other care professionals they might be meeting for the first time.

The hospitalist also adds value by actively participating in hospital-wide committees that review the outcomes of rapid response team actions and other emergency cardiac care activities. Only then can they facilitate change in the processes the hospital puts in place for recognizing and responding to the patient with unexpected changes in clinical condition.

■ LEADERSHIP

Medical staff or hospital-wide committees

In recent years, The Joint Commission (TJC), the National Quality Forum (NQF), and the Centers for Medicare and Medicaid (CMS) have built standards and endorsed safe practices around medical staff and medical center leadership's responsibility and accountability for the safety and quality within their organizations. This focus provides the hospitalist with important opportunities to take leadership roles on medical staff and hospital committees, working groups, and task forces that focus on safety and quality. As physicians who concentrate wholly on hospital-based care, no group is better positioned to influence outcomes than hospitalists. They should work as solution seekers for the best ways to standardize handoffs, design the electronic health record, improve infection control practices, create accountabilities for the CMS Core Measures, and oversee team building and rapid response teams throughout the entire organization. Failure to engage in these efforts represents significant lost opportunities.

Safety culture

As hospitalists are clearly some of the most visible physicians in any organization, they bear a unique role and responsibility for promoting a robust "safety culture" within the organization and specifically in the units where they focus their practice. The Agency for Healthcare Research and Quality (AHRQ) identifies key features of a "safety culture" that includes the willingness of hospital staff to openly communicate concerns about patient care on their units. Units where staff express comfort when questioning physicians or other authority figures when they disagree or have concerns are considered units with a "safer" culture. Other positive attributes of "safe" units are those in which mistakes are openly discussed and those discussions focus on "systems" issues instead of blaming specific individuals.

The difference between the culture of one unit to that of another in the same hospital often correlates with the difference between the middle management communication styles of the associated units. Units with nursing managers and physician leaders who focus on open, honest, effective, and nonpunitive communication related to adverse patient events score higher on safety culture surveys than others. In addition, there is data to suggest that those units with positive safety culture survey results have a lower incidence of adverse patient events when compared to units with less positive surveys. To that end, the hospital-based physician is uniquely situated to foster a culture of curiosity, inquiry, and appropriate challenging of authority through role modeling and mentoring. By setting positive examples for other physicians and staff, the hospital can lead in the efforts to ensure all of the units in which they work strive toward a safe, patient-centered approach to medical care.

MANAGING PATIENT SAFETY EVENTS

THE PRINCIPLED APPROACH

Even when hospital-based physicians do their best to proactively maximize the safety of their patients, unintentional harm still occurs. Importantly, the integrity of the individual physician or institution rests on the response to patient harm as much as it does to prevention. When harm occurs there is a choice to deny, minimize, rationalize, and blame others, including the patient, or to approach each harm event with a commitment to an open inquiry and honest communication following harm—the "principled approach." The hospital-based physician is constantly presented with this choice.

It is well recognized that there are a multitude of barriers to honest communication following harm that include fear of litigation, humiliation, lost income, reputational damage, risk to privileges and license, and the uncertainty of outcome. Nonetheless, the "deny and defend" approach to patient harm and the delegation of managing harm to the legal community has arguably not prevented any of those feared outcomes and instead has damaged the reputation of the medical profession and prevented any learning following patient harm events. The "principled approach" to patient harm is arguably the smarter approach because it effectively addresses many of the reasons that patients sue (lack of communication, need for explanation, sense of dishonesty or "hiding something") and provides a forum for learning and improving patient safety.

The principled approach to patient harm relies heavily on the hospital-based physician in at least 6 specific areas: (1) the immediate response, (2) reporting of harm, (3) communication, initially and in follow-up, (4) investigation, (5) identification of process and performance improvement opportunities, and (6) the necessary follow-up. See **Table 35-2**.

Responding and reporting

Responding to and the reporting of patient safety events are the first step in any principled process to patient harm. See **Table 35-3**.

TABLE 35-2 Principled Response to Patient Harm Events

Respond immediately
Reporting
Investigation
Communication
Performance improvement
Follow-up

TABLE 35-3 Immediate Response

Address current needs of patient and family
Contact Risk Management or Patient Safety Hotline
Identify care professionals for ongoing care
Identify key persons for patient/family communication
Preserve data, equipment, and so forth
Document "just the facts" in medical record or risk management report

Reporting triggers the institutional response process while the health care team responds to the immediate medical needs of the patient. Most hospitals encourage care professionals, especially physicians, to report any patient safety incident to its Safety and/or Risk Management Department. Reports are often made by telephone, hand-written, online, and in person. Hospitals are mandated by the Centers for Medicare and Medicaid (CMS) and The Joint Commission (TJC) to provide for a reporting process for patient harm events.

It is incumbent upon the hospital-based physician to understand and appreciate the reporting process used in any hospital where they work. Importantly, the hospitalist needs to recognize the importance of their role in taking care of the patient when harm occurs and ensuring that neither the patient nor the family is abandoned during this critical time.

Benefits of reporting

The benefits of rapid institutional reporting of patient safety events within the organization provide substantial incentive for all hospital-based physicians to report and encourage reporting harm events. These benefits include (1) the activation of the internal patient safety and risk management processes including a crisis management plan, if indicated, (2) the preservation of data and information, (3) the opportunity to trigger immediate support for patient, family, and care professional, (4) the initiation of a "quality committee" investigation and the "legal privilege" most states afford such investigations, and (5) the establishment of a communication link with the harmed patient and his or her family.

As with documentation in the medical record, when reporting a patient safety event, hospitalists should take care to provide only the necessary factual information to commence an investigation. They should avoid documenting speculation, hasty conclusions with incomplete facts, or "finger-pointing" in the report.

Investigation

As advocates for quality medical care and patient safety, hospitalists possess special skills for participating in the investigation of serious adverse outcomes (see **Table 35-4**). Patients and families want and deserve the "facts" after a harm event. An appropriate investigatory

TABLE 35-4 Investigation

Perform within context of authorized quality improvement process
Involve interprofessional personnel as indicated
Utilize a validated root cause analysis (RCA) process or tool
Incorporate organizational quality and patient safety personnel
Consider involving patients and families in RCA process

process is needed to provide them with the necessary information. The hospital-based physician should commit to participating in any institutional root cause analysis or other investigatory process following a serious harm event. Such investigations should try to avoid the traditional "shame and blame" approach to adverse events and instead focus on systems-based issues and identification of possible areas of improvement.

Nonetheless, prior to knowing all the facts, patients and families are still entitled to effective communication in the early aftermath of a harm event.

Communication

Once harm occurs, honest and effective communication helps maintain trust between the patient and family and care professionals. With their easy availability, often 24 hours a day, the hospitalist is uniquely positioned to facilitate such communication. After all, for the patient who has experienced an unexpected outcome, every hour that goes by without effective communication constitutes more harm.

Honest and effective communication after a harmful adverse event is not just the right thing to do, but the smart thing to do as well. Patients and families sue, in large part, because they perceive a lack of transparency, abandonment, or "cover-up." A transparent process with open lines of communication and disclosure of all pertinent information can mitigate those patient and family perceptions.

Disclosure of any actual error associated with the harm is a multifaceted process that requires careful planning, preparation, and coordination by physicians and hospital administrators. Given its complexity, physicians understandably fear that an inadequate or poorly executed disclosure of medical errors will only serve to frustrate frontline practitioners, ruin the reputation of the organization and individual practitioners involved in the incident, and encourage lawsuits.

Successful adverse event response programs that include "full disclosure" rely heavily upon integration between the clinical departments and hospital risk management. This integration ensures that the various stakeholders are "on board" or at least aware of the plan for communication after adverse events. The stakeholder list must include the medical malpractice insurance carriers for the various parties who might be affected. In order to provide a consistent approach to adverse events for providers, patients, and families, all of the steps involved in the response to harm should be preapproved by all appropriate stakeholders before implementation.

The process of communication after harm occurs generally falls in 3 phases: immediate, intermediate, and final or follow-up phase. See **Table 35-5**. The extent of hospitalist involvement in this type of communication will depend upon the relationship of the hospitalist with the patient and his or her family. Long-term close physician-patient relationships are conducive to multiple meetings and discussions wherein the hospitalist will quickly discover that "disclosure" is a process and not an event.

It is important that a liaison for the family is identified and appropriate empathy and assurance of nonabandonment is expressed at each visit. It is critical for the hospitalist to understand the difference between "empathy" and "apology." Empathy is the understanding or sharing of another person's emotions and feelings whereas an "apology" is admitting a mistake that caused harm. In medicine, there is an ethical imperative to express empathy when patients suffer harm but apologies should only be reserved for situations when it is clear mistakes or errors have caused the harm. Therefore, apologies carry real legal implications and should only be offered when the facts are clear and agreed upon by the stakeholders with knowledge of the event.

TABLE 35-5 Communication

Immediate	
	Express empathy
	Don't make promises you can't keep
	Disclose "known" facts
	Assure nonabandonment
	Identify persons (liaison) for follow-up
Intermediate	
	Ensure liaison presence
	Continue to express empathy
	Disclose facts discovered during investigation
	Ask and answer clarifying questions
	Apologize if consensus exists about error or substandard care causing harm
	Explain plan for prevention of future harm
	Offer ongoing contact and communication
Final or follow-up phase	
	Ensure liaison presence
	Answer additional questions
	Express empathy, apology, if indicated
	Discuss performance improvement measures
	Offer ongoing contact and support

Example of expression of empathy: "I am sorry your pneumonia has progressed to the point where despite our best efforts we now need to put a breathing tube in your windpipe to help you breathe."

Example of apology: "I am sorry I did not check your abnormally low blood sugar result this morning. If I had seen the result I could have given you some extra sugar to prevent your seizure this morning."

Process improvements

The value in a principled, transparent approach to adverse patient events lies in the ability to learn from mistakes within a rigorous, reflective environment that promotes performance improvement efforts designed to significantly improve the delivery of care. To be effective, hospital-based physicians must play a role in these performance improvement efforts that follow suboptimal care. Patients and families involved in adverse events caused by inappropriate care are intensely interested in learning the ways in which similar events are less likely to occur. Discussing these quality improvement measures with them also helps to maintain the trust and bond between patient and provider.

CONCLUSION

The evidence for abundant opportunities to improve patient care and prevent patient harm has become indisputable. Earlier estimates on the annual number of preventable deaths in hospitals far underestimated the actual number of deaths that could be prevented, especially from health care-associated infections. Moving forward it has become clear the mantra "no outcome, no income" or "no pay for low quality performance" is going to apply to a significant number of episodes of care. To that end, hospital-based physicians are ideally situated to positively influence issues in patient and quality of care outcomes through their active engagement on performance improvement efforts, their communication skills, and their ability to lead multidisciplinary efforts.

In addition, hospitalists can take a lead in providing honest, open, and effective communication to patients and families after unexpected adverse event outcomes. This transparent approach can be the catalyst, for the transformation of an organization's culture for effectively responding to the needs of patients, providers, and the health care system. Adopting a policy and practice of transparency related to harm events represents a major shift in organizational focus and will need the full support of hospitalists to fully implement. This approach will require strong and persistent endorsement by the kind of leadership that hospitalists can provide their organizations. The added value of transparency is found in the opportunity to rapidly learn from, respond to, and modify practices based on harm investigation with these now transparent events.

SUGGESTED READINGS

Boothman RC, Blackwell AC, Campbell DA Jr., Commiskey E, Anderson S. A better approach to malpractice claims? The University of Michigan Experience. *Journal of Health and Life Sciences Law*. 2009; 2(2):15–159.

Hickson GB, Federspeil CF, Pichert JW, Miller CS, Gauld-Jaeger J, Bost P. Patient complaints and malpractice risk. *JAMA*. 2002;287(22):2951–2957.

Institute of Medicine. *To Err Is Human: Building a Safer Health System*. Kohn LT, Corrigan JM, Donaldson MS, Eds. Washington, D.C.: National Academy Press; 2000.

Leape LL, Berwick DM. Five years after To Err Is Human: what have we learned? *JAMA*. 2005;293(19):2384–23890.

McDonald TB, Helmchen LA, Smith KM, Centomani NM, Gunderson A, Mayer DB, Chamberlin W. Responding to patient safety incidents: the seven pillars. *Qual Saf Health Care*. doi:10.1136/qshc2008.031633.

McDonald T. Error disclosure within a principled approach to adverse events. ASA Newsletter. 73(5):20–22, 2009.

National Quality Forum. *Safe Practices for Better Healthcare–2010 Update: A Consensus Report*. Washington DC.: NQF; 2010.

CHAPTER 36

Medical Malpractice

Adam C. Schaffer, MD
Nicholas Beshara, JD, MPH

INTRODUCTION

Medical malpractice is a serious concern for many physicians and a topic that often prompts intense debate. In this chapter, we review the elements of medical malpractice, as well as data about the frequency of both negligent medical care and actual claims of medical malpractice. Data that exist about how well the malpractice system does in achieving its purpose of deterring negligent medical care and compensating patients who are harmed by such negligence are reviewed. We also discuss malpractice issues that are of particular concern to hospitalists, and, most crucially, what can be done to try to reduce the risk of being the subject of a medical malpractice claim.

THE ELEMENTS OF MEDICAL MALPRACTICE

Medical malpractice is a form of negligence that applies to health care providers including doctors, nurses, and institutional medical care providers like hospitals. At the core of negligence-based liability is the notion that individuals committing unintentional but reasonably avoidable acts that cause injury should be required to compensate the victims of those acts. To determine whether negligence is present in a given situation, courts require plaintiffs to prove four elements through a preponderance of the evidence: duty, breach, causation, and harm.

PRACTICE POINT

To determine whether negligence is present in a given situation, courts require plaintiffs to prove four elements through a preponderance of the evidence: duty, breach, causation, and harm.

- In the hospital setting, physicians have a duty to provide care with the same skill and diligence as a reasonably competent physician in the same specialty or field of practice would under similar circumstances.
- The question of whether a physician breached the duty of care, then, often hinges on competing testimony provided by expert witnesses as to the applicable standard of care and whether the conduct in question failed to meet that standard.
- To establish legal causation, the plaintiff must show that the breach was both the "cause in fact" and the "proximate cause" of the injury.

The duty of care in negligence claims is a hypothetical standard by which the court judges the conduct of the defendant to determine whether he or she had an obligation to act differently. In the hospital setting, physicians have a duty to provide care with the same skill and diligence as a reasonably competent physician in the same specialty or field of practice would under similar circumstances. Failure to meet this standard constitutes a breach of the physician's duty of care. In most cases, for this duty to exist, a physician-patient relationship must have been established.

In order to determine whether a physician has breached the duty of care, an expert witness must testify as to the applicable standard

The authors would like to thank Prof. Michelle M. Mello for her review of the manuscript and her thoughtful comments. The authors would also like to thank the National Practitioner Data Bank for assistance with data acquisition.

in court. In the majority of states, physicians are judged by a national standard of care that all physicians in the same specialty would be expected to follow. However, in a significant number of states, physicians are judged by what other physicians in the same specialty and in the same geographic area would have done in a particular situation. In either case, the relevant testimony must come from expert witnesses who have the education, training, or other credentials that would make them familiar with the applicable standard of care. The question of whether a physician breached the duty of care then, often hinges on competing testimony provided by expert witnesses as to the applicable standard of care and whether the conduct in question failed to meet that standard.

Even if a physician breaches this duty by failing to adhere to the standard of care, the plaintiff in a case cannot establish liability unless that breach is the actual cause of the injury. To establish legal causation, the plaintiff must show that the breach was both the "cause in fact" and the "proximate cause" of the injury. As articulated by Louisell, et al, a breach of the duty of care is the "cause in fact" of damages if the plaintiff can establish that the presence of the breach was the "deciding factor" in determining whether the damage would have occurred. Put differently, a breach of the duty of care would not be the "cause in fact" of harm if the harm would have occurred despite the negligent care of a physician. In addition to being the cause in fact of harm, a breach of the duty of care must also be the proximate cause in order to satisfy the causation element of negligence. To be the proximate cause of harm, the harm must be, by its nature, a foreseeable or direct consequence of a breach of the duty of care. Some courts require an additional or alternative finding that the breach was a "substantial factor" in causing the injury, especially when two or more parties may be responsible.

If the court or jury finds that a physician has breached a duty by failing to adhere to the applicable standard of care and that the breach is the cause in fact and proximate cause of a patient's injury, then the physician will be liable for damages. The measure of such damages is often highly dependent on the facts and circumstances surrounding the particular incident. Generally, a claimant can recover compensatory damages for both economic and noneconomic harm. Economic damages include current and future loss of earnings and the specific costs associated with treating the injury such as medical bills and drug expenses. Economic damages also include the costs of living with the injury such as modifications to the home to accommodate a wheelchair. Noneconomic damages most often include pain and suffering (physical and emotional) from the injury. In addition, courts may order punitive damages for injuries that are the result of malicious conduct or a willful disregard of patient safety. However, such instances are relatively rare.

Medical malpractice claims usually involve numerous medical personnel involved in every stage of the patient's care. Malpractice plaintiffs cast a wide net when filing suit for a number of reasons. First, it is often cost prohibitive to file an individual suit against each defendant because of the increased costs of legal discovery. Second, because most states employ a comparative negligence standard (meaning that total damages are calculated and then allocated to defendants based on their percentage of contribution of fault), it is difficult to allocate damages among separate claims. It is also more likely that naming multiple defendants will help the plaintiff narrow down which of the defendants was actually at fault (if any). Third, joining multiple defendants in the same suit allows plaintiffs to use the defendants' own knowledge and testimony to establish standards of care, cutting down on the costs of hiring independent expert witnesses. Finally, there may be jurisdictional rules that prohibit separate claims and require naming all the responsible parties in a single claim if a failure to do so would result in an unfair outcome or an increased burden on the judicial system.

THE EPIDEMIOLOGY OF MEDICAL MALPRACTICE

Information concerning the extent of medical malpractice is limited because of the inherent difficulties in identifying adverse events and determining which cases were the result of negligence. More reliable data may be obtained on the number of paid malpractice claims, since insurance companies are required to report them to a national database. However, malpractice claims are a crude measure of malpractice patterns because there is a poor correlation between negligence and claiming.

Overall, therefore, an analysis of malpractice trends is limited by the quality of the underlying data. Despite such limitations, there are some sources of data that can provide insight into trends regarding the payments made for malpractice. One useful source of information on medical malpractice is the National Practitioner Data Bank (NPDB), which was established by the Health care Quality Improvement Act of 1986. The Act was intended to improve the quality of medical care, in part by requiring the submission of malpractice claims to the NPDB, which can then be referenced by health care institutions when making hiring decisions. Based on NPDB data, **Figure 36-1** shows trends regarding the number of payments, the median payments, and the mean payments for medical malpractice for the period 1997–2008.

Some studies have analyzed the epidemiology of medical injury in specific states. Examining more than 30,000 records of patients hospitalized in New York State in 1984, the Harvard Medical Practice Study is the largest study to assess the rate of medical malpractice injuries and claims. In this study, Brennan, et al, showed that adverse events occurred in 3.7% of hospitalizations and of these adverse events, 27.6% were determined to be due to negligence. In a further analysis of the Harvard Medical Practice Study by Localio, et al, the overall rate of malpractice claims per discharge was 0.13%. In this study, the vast majority of adverse events did not result in a malpractice claim. Of the adverse events due to negligence that were identified, remarkably, only about 2% resulted in malpractice claims. The estimated ratio of negligence to claims was 7.6 to 1.

Testing the generalizability of the results of the Harvard Medical Practice Study, a subsequent, methodologically similar study by Thomas, et al, examined 15,000 hospital records from Utah and Colorado. In this study, which yielded comparable results to the

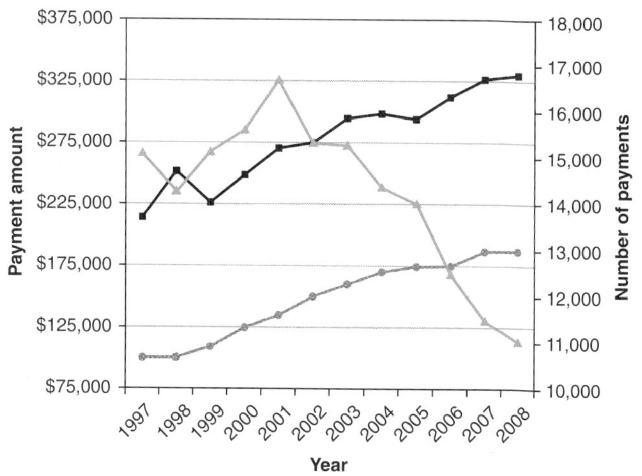

Figure 36-1 *The number of payments and the mean and median payment amounts for medical malpractice, by year, 1997 to 2008, based on the NPDB data (Data from the NPDB Annual Reports, and directly from the NPDB. Data from 2007 and 2008 are preliminary).*

Harvard Medical Practice Study, 2.9% of hospitalizations in each state involved adverse events. Of these adverse events, 32.6% were a result of negligence in Utah, and 27.4% were a result of negligence in Colorado. Additional analysis of these data by Studdert, et al, in 2000 showed that only about 3% of those patients who suffered a negligent injury filed a malpractice claim. Characteristics more common among patients who suffered negligence but did not file a malpractice claim include low income, uninsured, insured by Medicare or Medicaid, and age ≥75 years. Of those malpractice claims identified during the study period, 78% were made despite the absence of negligence and 56% were made despite the absence of an adverse event. The ratio of negligent adverse events to claims was 5.1 to 1 in Utah and 6.7 to 1 in Colorado.

The two main purposes of the medical malpractice system are to compensate patients who suffered injuries resulting from negligence, and to deter negligent behavior by imposing costs on physicians who practice negligently. These data call into question whether the medical malpractice system is achieving these objectives. Given the large number of adverse events due to negligence not leading to a malpractice claim, the medical malpractice system is not efficient at holding negligent physicians accountable, and many patients who have been injured as a result of malpractice are not receiving compensation. One implication of these data is that the rate of claims is a problematic metric to use in assessing quality of care, since most episodes of negligence do not lead to malpractice claims, and a significant number of malpractice claims are filed in the absence of negligence or injury.

A somewhat different picture emerges when the outcomes of claims are analyzed, rather than simply the filing of claims. Studdert, et al, in 2006 evaluated 1452 closed malpractice claims in which objective assessments were made by reviewers as to whether there were medical errors resulting in injury. Of those claims filed involving injuries, 63% were determined to be a result of error. In cases in which there was injury due to error, compensation was paid 73% of the time. In cases in which there were no errors, no compensation was paid 72% of the time. The authors of the study concluded that although the malpractice system does a reasonable job of providing compensation only when there is injury as a result of a medical error, the process has significant shortcomings. Namely, cases take a long time to come to resolution (five years, on average, from injury to disposition) and the monetary costs of litigating the claims are steep (54% of the compensation paid).

Thus the data show a very limited correlation between malpractice claims made and acts of actual malpractice. Based on the 2006 data from Studdert, et al, looking at the outcomes of claims, it appears that the majority of claims with merit result in compensation and the majority of meritless claims are denied compensation, which has also been observed in other analyses of outcomes of claims, as summarized by Baker. However, the system of determining which claims have merit is protracted and expensive.

AREAS OF MEDICAL MALPRACTICE OF SPECIAL CONCERN TO HOSPITALISTS

INTRODUCTION

Many of the potential areas of malpractice that concern hospitalists relate to the inherent discontinuity between inpatient and outpatient care. These areas include failure to follow up on incidental findings and appropriately addressing test results that may be pending at the time of discharge or may be altered upon final review (eg, by the attending radiologist or pathologist). This situation is exacerbated by the multiple handoffs of patient care that can occur when hospitalists work shifts. Moreover, in academic medical centers, tests may be ordered by resident physicians and the attending hospitalist may not even be aware that the test was ordered. Given that Hospital Medicine is a relatively young field with limited case law involving hospitalists specifically, cases applicable to hospitalists may be drawn from other fields of medicine in which physicians have temporary relationships with their patients, such as Emergency Medicine.

CASE 36-1

FAILURE TO FOLLOW UP ON AN INCIDENTAL FINDING

A 62-year-old male with a significant smoking history presented to the emergency department (ED) in November 1999 after a fall resulting in a left shoulder injury. The ED physician took X-rays of the chest and left shoulder, read them as showing no fracture, and discharged the patient home. Four days later, the attending radiologist read the X-ray as showing a left lung nodule, and a report of the X-ray was sent to the ED physician and primary care physician (PCP). The radiologist did not call either the ED physician or the PCP. The patient saw his PCP twice in December 2000 for back and shoulder pain and was sent for physical therapy. The patient presented to the ED in August 2001 with chest and shoulder pain. A chest X-ray was obtained, which the ED attending read as normal, but the radiologist noted a large mass in the left lung. This information was not conveyed to the patient's PCP. After another visit to his PCP in September 2001, the patient presented to the ED again in October 2001 with back and chest pain, and a chest X-ray showed a mass occupying the majority of his left lung. The patient died of metastatic disease soon thereafter. The patient's children filed suit against the PCP, ED physician, and radiologist, and the suit was settled for more than $500,000.

Adapted from Wright J, McCormack P. Failure to act on incidental finding. CRICO Forum 2007;25:6–7.

The preceding case illustrates the liability pitfalls that can result from inadequate communication among the physician ordering a radiologic study (the ED physician), the physician interpreting the study (the radiologist), and the physician who is best suited to follow up on the abnormal results (the primary care physician). This case had features that are common in ED cases leading to malpractice claims, as elucidated by Kachalia, et al, including the misreading of plain radiographs, the involvement of multiple individual failures, and process breakdowns.

Pending tests and incidental findings

Hospitalists frequently find themselves in the same position as the ED physician in the above case, ordering a study the final results of which may not come back until after the patient has been discharged. The same problem applies to laboratory tests. One study by Roy, et al, encompassing the hospitalist services at two academic medical centers found that 41% of patients had laboratory or radiology results pending at the time of discharge and in 9.4% of cases the results of these studies were considered potentially actionable. Seventy percent of the inpatient physicians and 45.8% of the outpatient physicians were unaware of these potentially actionable results.

The problem of pending test results at the time of discharge is best addressed at a systems level—for example, through a mechanism that automatically notifies the ordering provider of the final results of such tests. However, such systems are not widely in place and even when they are, physicians still often fail to follow up on clinically significant results. Consequently, physicians need to take responsibility for following up on the final results of the tests that they order.

Physicians may also be held responsible for responding to test results ordered by another physician when these results come back while that physician is on duty, as was held in *Siggers v. Barlow* (906 F.2d 241). Responding to these test results often means communicating with the patient's primary care physician (PCP) about what additional follow-up needs to occur, such as the need for serial imaging for an incidentally discovered pulmonary nodule. Discharge summaries, while important, are generally not adequate as the only means of communicating important findings that need to be followed up by the PCP. Kripalani, et al, and Pantilat, et al, identified a number of potential deficiencies in the discharge summary as the sole means of communicating with the PCP. These deficiencies include the possibility that the discharge summary does not reach the correct PCP (occurring 25% of the time), failure to include tests pending at discharge (occurring 65% of the time), and the PCP not receiving the discharge summary prior to follow-up (occurring 67% of the time). Therefore, hospitalists should contact PCPs directly regarding important test results or other matters that need to be followed up, by phone and/or letter, and this communication should be documented in the patient's chart.

Coordination of consultant care

The number of malpractice cases involving hospitalists specifically is not well documented, given that Hospital Medicine has not been recognized as a distinct specialty and so tallies of malpractice cases are usually not broken down by involvement of a hospitalist. Moreover, as with all malpractice cases, many cases involving hospitalists may be settled prior to trial, and so no public record of the matter may be generated. Reports to the National Practitioner Data Bank contain only limited details about cases. Despite these limitations, the few reported cases involving hospitalists are instructive in illustrating potential areas of malpractice liability distinct to hospitalists. These areas may not be captured by analyses relying on fields thought to have analogous malpractice liability concerns, such as Emergency Medicine.

One such potential area of malpractice liability concerns the use and coordination of consultants. Hospitalists list active coordination of consulting specialists as one of the benefits they bring to patient care. However, with this responsibility for coordination of specialists, and in their role of the attending physician of record for the patient, hospitalists are at risk of incurring malpractice liability based on the actions of the consulting specialists.

CASE 36-2

DOMBY v. MORITZ (2008 CAL. APP. UNPUB. LEXIS 1856)

A 67-year-old female with a history of hypertension checked her own blood pressure, found that it was elevated, and contacted her PCP. As instructed by her PCP, the patient took an extra dose of atenolol, after which she had an episode of syncope. She presented to the hospital, where she was bradycardic and so the ED physician gave the patient atropine and glucagon to reverse the effects of the atenolol. A partner of the patient's cardiologist was contacted and advised to put an external pacemaker on the patient, but the cardiologist did not see the patient. The patient was admitted to the ICU by a hospitalist. In anticipation that an internal pacemaker might be needed, the hospitalist reversed the patient's coumadin with fresh frozen plasma. The ICU nurses called the cardiologist to report that the patient was bradycardic and feeling unwell. The cardiologist never placed an internal pacemaker. The hospitalist was next contacted by the ICU nurses once the patient was in cardiac arrest. The patient's family filed suit against both the cardiologist and the hospitalist. The court ultimately found in favor of the hospitalist.

The preceding case, *Domby v. Moritz* (2008 Cal. App. Unpub. LEXIS 1856), illustrates this risk. In filing suit against both the cardiologist and the hospitalist, the family of the patient asserted that the hospitalist should have ensured that the cardiologist physically came in to evaluate the patient. Although the court ultimately found in favor of the hospitalist, this case illustrates that hospitalists have to take an active role in discussing the treatment plan with consultants and in clearly delineating who has responsibility for which aspects of the patient's care. It can be legally hazardous to consider a clinical decision "not my call" and exclusively within the purview of a specialist, because the hospitalist, as the attending physician of record, can face litigation based on the decisions made by the consulting specialists.

RISK FACTORS FOR MEDICAL MALPRACTICE CLAIMS AND STRATEGIES TO REDUCE THIS RISK

THE IMPORTANCE OF THE PHYSICIAN-PATIENT RELATIONSHIP AND COMMUNICATION

In considering ways to reduce the risk of facing a medical malpractice claim, a key question to ask is why patients decide to file claims, given that the vast majority of patients who are injured due to medical errors do not initiate a malpractice action. One study, by Beckman, et al, which examined 45 plaintiff depositions in medical malpractice cases, found that in 71.1% of cases there were significant relationship issues between the plaintiff and the defendant physician. The most common issue was the feeling by the patient of having been deserted by the physician. Examples include abandonment, and the physician being unavailable and sending associates such as residents in the place of the attending physician. Other relationship issues that were present in the examined depositions included: devaluing the patient (such as by discounting the patients' illness or pain); delivering information poorly (including failure to explain what was occurring); and failing to understand the patient's or family's perspective (such as by not asking for the patients' opinion).

The behavior of consulting specialists who are brought in after an adverse event has occurred may also influence whether a malpractice claim is filed. In 54.8% of cases, health care professionals raised questions about the care the patient had received, and in 70.6% of these cases, the health care professional who cast doubt on the quality of the care that had been provided by the defendant physician was a consultant who saw the patient after the adverse event. In a couple of cases, it was an acquaintance—who happened to be a health care professional but was not directly involved in the case—who suggested that the care received was substandard. Therefore, consultants seeing a patient after an adverse event need to be mindful that even an offhand remark on the care the patient has received may affect whether the patient pursues a malpractice claim.

These data suggest specific measures that can be taken to reduce the risk of a malpractice claim being filed. It is important to avoid those physician behaviors—such as creating conditions in which the patient may feel abandoned and not fully acknowledging the patient's concerns or discomfort—that were commonly seen in plaintiff malpractice depositions. Given the possibility that having associates such as residents or physician assistants see the patient runs the risk of the patient feeling abandoned, the attending physician should explain the expected involvement of associates up front. It may also be helpful to frame the care to the patient as being provided by a team, so the patient does not feel connected only to the attending physician. It is also important to ensure that patient expectations about the outcome of a procedure or treatment are realistic. The informed consent process is an opportune occasion to address the patient's expectations.

Strong communication skills are also important. Supporting the benefit of good communication skills in reducing litigation, another study by Lester, et al, found that physicians who exhibited "positive communication behaviors" such as making eye contact, acknowledging what the patient says, and spending more time with the patient, elicited reduced litigious feelings in observers. Hickson, et al, in 1994 showed that the patients of obstetricians with a high frequency of malpractice claims complained about these physicians' communication skills, including these physicians not listening and not providing information. The rate of these complaints about poor communication was significantly higher for physicians with a history of a high frequency of medical malpractice claims than for physicians with a better claims record.

On a systems level, it may be possible to identify physicians within an organization who are at increased risk of a malpractice claim. Physicians with an increased number of patient complaints have more risk management episodes, defined as both malpractice claims that are filed and incidents reported by staff members to the risk management department. One study by Hickson, et al, from 2002 retrospectively examined a cohort of 645 physicians, looking for an association between the number of unsolicited patient complaints and the number of risk management episodes. A small number of physicians generated a markedly disproportionate number of patient complaints, with 9% of the physicians garnering more than 50% of the complaints. There was a significant positive correlation between the number of complaints received and both the total number of risk management episodes and the number of lawsuits.

Similarly, another study by Stelfox, et al, found that scores from a commonly used survey of hospital satisfaction produced by Press Ganey Inc. were significantly associated with risk management episodes, which included both malpractice lawsuits and incidents identified by risk management as having the potential to result in a malpractice claim. The survey instrument included five questions asking patients to rank their inpatient attending physician in different areas, using a scale of 1 to 5 for each question, with a score of 5 denoting the highest rating. Each 1-point decrement on the survey correlated with a 5% increase in the rate of risk management episodes. The specific questions on the survey that had the strongest correlation with risk management episodes were those regarding the time the physician spent with the patient and the concern the physician showed for the patient's qualms. No significant correlation was found between the responses to questions on how satisfied the patient was with the physician's skill and the rate of risk management episodes. There was also a positive correlation between the rate of patient complaints and the rate of risk management episodes. Notably, a breakdown of complaints against physicians again suggested the crucial importance of good communication with the patient. Of the 483 complaints analyzed in the study, 75% of them concerned communication issues and 25% of them related to patient care matters. These two studies by Hickson, et al, and Stelfox, et al, show that by using data that are commonly collected by hospitals—number of complaints and the results of patient satisfaction surveys—it may be possible to identify physicians who are at elevated risk of being named in a malpractice action.

CASE 36-3

COMPLAINTS AGAINST DR. A

Dr. A is a physician who joined the hospitalist service four years ago. During his time as a member of the hospitalist group, his scores on the Press Ganey surveys have been in the lowest decile of physicians at the hospital. As the director of the hospitalist service, you receive a call from a manager in the patient relations department saying that Dr. A has been the subject of two complaints within the past six months. The patient relations manager says both complaints are very similar, and the complaints describe Dr. A as being unwilling to fully discuss his patients' medical conditions. The complaints further state that it seems like Dr. A is always trying to get out of the patients' rooms as quickly as possible and that he appears annoyed when the patients ask questions. One of the patients who complained wrote: "Dr. A just did not seem like he really cared about me or my many medical problems. I would not want him to take care of me again or any members of my family."

When you, as the director of the hospitalist service, meet with Dr. A about these issues, he seems irritated and explains that every physician has at least a few disgruntled patients and that is part of practicing medicine. Dr. A says he wants to make sure he sees all his patients and completes his billing forms promptly, and so he can't be expected to linger in patients' rooms. Dr. A further explains that if a patient asks a question that he deems important, then he makes sure to answer that question fully.

If it is possible to recognize physicians at increased risk of malpractice suits, such as Dr. A in the preceding case, then potentially actions can be taken to mitigate this risk. For example, physicians who receive a high number of complaints or with particularly low satisfaction ratings could undergo educational programs aimed at enhancing their patient-communication skills. One approach, advocated by Moore, et al, consists of a tiered intervention system. Initially, a physician who has been identified as being at high risk for being sued for malpractice is approached by a peer to discuss the issue. If that is not effective in improving the physician's complaint rate, then a plan for improvement is developed in conjunction with someone in authority, such as the department chair. If these efforts are still unsuccessful, meetings can be held with senior officials in hospital management, with the possibility of discipline or dismissal. Components of the plan to reduce the complaint rate (and so potentially also the risk of facing a malpractice action) can include enhancements to the management of the physician's practice, continuing medical education on the physician-patient relationship, and/or mental health evaluation.

DISCLOSING ERRORS TO PATIENTS

Physicians understandably are often conflicted about whether to disclose medical errors (also see Chapter 34). Historically, physicians have been hesitant to disclose mistakes for fear of inviting litigation over an error that may otherwise have gone unnoticed by the patient, and in order to avoid possible censure over having made a mistake. An opposing view holds that disclosing errors will help avoid the strain in the patient-physician relationship and the breakdown in communication that may occur after a mistake, and so may decrease the risk of litigation, or at least lead to smaller awards.

The empirical evidence is inadequate to clearly answer what effect disclosure of medical errors will have on the likelihood of malpractice litigation. Policy changes regarding notification of patients about medical errors implemented by some medical centers do provide examples of the possible consequences of disclosure policies. In 1987, the Lexington, Kentucky, Veterans Affairs Medical Center (VAMC), in reaction to two large malpractice payouts, decided to put into place a policy of proactively identifying and investigating cases of possible medical negligence. If medical negligence was found, the representatives from the Lexington

VAMC would have a face-to-face meeting with the patient or next of kin. At this meeting, hospital representatives would explain the situation, answer any questions, and offer restitution—the amount of which was based on a determination of actual loss. Claims assistance was also offered. Reviewing 15 years of experience with this full disclosure policy at the Lexington VAMC, Kraman, et al, concluded that this approach appeared to reduce the amount of overall malpractice payouts. Although the Lexington VAMC had an increased number of payouts, the average amount of these payouts was relatively small, at $14,500. This compares to a mean pretrial settlement amount of $98,000 for all medical centers in the VA system. Despite the Lexington VAMC being in the top quarter of all VAMCs in the number of tort claims filed, it was in the bottom quarter of all VAMCs in terms of total malpractice payouts. This VAMC experience has major limitations regarding its generalizability, because physicians in VAMCs do not pay individual malpractice premiums and as federal government entities VAMCs are not subject to punitive damages.

Several hospital systems and liability insurers have instituted programs that couple disclosure of unanticipated care outcomes with rapid offers of compensation in appropriate cases. The most widely discussed program is the one implemented by the University of Michigan Health System (UMHS) in 2002, described by Boothman, et al, In this program, unanticipated outcomes are promptly disclosed and investigated. The three principles the UMHS cites as defining their risk management approach are: (1) rapid offers of compensation when "unreasonable" care was the cause of the injury; (2) forceful defense of claims in which the care provided was reasonable; and (3) using knowledge gained from the incidents that are identified to try to prevent future injuries and claims. With this policy in effect, the UMHS saw a decrease in annual litigation costs, in the number of claims and lawsuits, and in the time to resolution of claims and lawsuits. Program administrators report that compared with August 2001 (prior to the error disclosure program going into effect), in August 2005 (after the error disclosure program had been in effect), annual litigation costs decreased from $3 million to $1 million; the number of claims and lawsuits decreased from 262 to 114; and the average time to resolution of claims and lawsuits dropped from 20.7 months to 9.5 months. These results were heralded in a 2006 article coauthored by then-Senators Hillary Rodham Clinton and Barack Obama. Of 419 UMHS medical school faculty who were surveyed, 98% of them approved of the change in approach to risk management.

Despite the encouraging reports from organizations implementing disclosure-and-offer programs, some uncertainty remains about disclosure as a risk management strategy, particularly when disclosures are not made in the context of compensation programs. A major legal concern about disclosure in the absence of some mechanism for awarding rapid and modest compensation is that, because most medical errors do not result in malpractice claims, aggressive disclosure of medical errors may prompt claims that would otherwise not have been filed. A theoretical modeling of this issue by Studdert, et al, in 2007 concluded that routine disclosure would have a 94% likelihood of increasing malpractice compensation costs. Regulatory protections that exist, such as state "apology laws" designed to allow physicians to apologize without having it used against them, may provide only very limited protection. These laws may prevent expressions of regret from being used against the physician, but not ancillary information surrounding that expression of regret, such as information about causation or fault.

Ultimately, one can expect to see progressively wider implementation of policies encouraging or even requiring error disclosure. The basis for this expectation is independent of the effect of error disclosure policies on malpractice costs, but is instead based on regulatory, public policy, and ethical considerations. Some states and accreditation organizations, such as The Joint Commission, are increasingly implementing standards requiring error disclosure. Error disclosure, with the accompanying ability to gather data on what types of mistakes are recurring, also supports the public policy goal of improving systems so as to reduce future errors. In 2005, then-Senators Hillary Rodham Clinton and Barack Obama introduced the National Medical Error Disclosure and Compensation (MEDiC) bill. The MEDiC bill would have provided grant and technical support to encourage disclosure of medical errors and offers of compensation in cases in which errors were made. Information from increased disclosure of medical errors would have been collected and used to inform safety initiatives. The bill was never enacted.

Disclosure of medical errors is generally considered the ethically appropriate course. Honesty is necessary to maintain a strong physician-patient relationship, and informed consent requires that patients be fully aware of the circumstances surrounding their treatment so they can decide about further care. Demonstrating this trend toward increasing disclosure of medical errors, a consensus statement from the Harvard-affiliated hospitals in 2006 expressed a commitment to full disclosure of medical errors in order "to change our systems to prevent future error" and because "it is the right thing to do."

PRACTICE POINT

- Disclosure of medical errors is generally considered the ethically appropriate course. Honesty is necessary to maintain a strong physician-patient relationship, and informed consent requires that patients be fully aware of the circumstances surrounding their treatment so they can decide about further care.

DEFENSIVE MEDICINE

Defensive medicine, as defined by a 1994 Office of Technology Assessment report, is "when doctors order tests, procedures, or visits, or avoid high-risk patients or procedures, primarily (but not necessarily solely) to reduce their exposure to malpractice liability." Defensive medicine can be categorized by whether it is positive, such as ordering of extra tests to try to forestall a malpractice claim, or negative, such as avoiding patients perceived as representing an increased malpractice risk. Some authors prefer the term "assurance behavior" in place of positive defensive medicine, and "avoidance behavior" in place of negative defensive medicine, so as to avoid the suggestion of approval or disapproval about defensive medicine.

Particularly in environments of high-liability stress, defensive medicine appears to be very common. A 2005 study by Studdert, et al, surveyed physicians in litigation-prone specialties (Emergency Medicine, general surgery, orthopedic surgery, neurosurgery, obstetrics/gynecology, and radiology) in Pennsylvania, which had experienced rapidly increasing malpractice premiums. Of the physicians who responded to the survey, 93% had engaged in defensive medicine and 42% were limiting the scope of their practice because of fear of liability. The most common type of defensive medicine in the survey was ordering extra tests, which 59% of physicians reported doing. This was especially common among emergency physicians, 70% of whom reported ordering extra tests. Physicians concerned about whether their malpractice insurance coverage was adequate and those who felt their insurance premiums were particularly onerous were especially likely to engage in defensive medicine. Common negative defensive medicine practices included avoiding high-risk patients, reported by 39% of physicians, and avoiding high-risk procedures, reported by 32% of physicians. Positive and negative defensive medicine practices have differing implications for the health care system. Positive defensive medicine has the potential to increase costs while offering modest, if any, benefits to patients. In contrast, negative defensive medicine may limit patients' access to certain medical services viewed as high risk, such as obstetrics.

Not only is defensive medicine common, but it is also expensive. Estimates of the costs of defensive medicine vary and are fraught with methodological limitations. One estimate by Anderson is that approximately 5–9% of health care spending can be labeled as defensive. A concern is that if defensive medical practice becomes common enough, it may become the standard of care, which could force all physicians to practice in a defensive manner.

Overall, there is no clear empirical evidence that defensive medicine affects patient outcomes. There are some theoretical arguments against the practice of defensive medicine. Patients who perceive that their physician is ordering a test or procedure for a defensive reason may react negatively to this and be more likely to file a claim in the event of an adverse outcome. Some forms of defensive medicine involve physical risk to the patient—for example, ordering unnecessary biopsies and other invasive procedures. Particularly for these cases, services ordered primarily to serve the desire of the physician for minimizing risk and not the medical needs of the patient are ethically suspect. However, if fear of malpractice causes physicians to lower their tolerance for the possibility that a significant finding, such as a cancer, could be missed, then this effect is not necessarily deleterious. Indeed, some tests ordered primarily or solely to benefit the physician (by reducing medicolegal risk) end up having clear benefit to the patient. In the aggregate, though, defensive medical practices are likely cost ineffective.

ADDITIONAL STRATEGIES TO REDUCE THE RISK OF A MALPRACTICE CLAIM

A number of different strategies can be employed to potentially reduce the risk of a malpractice action. As discussed above, good communication practices with patients and their families are crucially important. Feelings on the part of patients that the physician is unavailable or dismissive of the patients' concerns may increase the risk of a malpractice claim. Delegating important communication tasks should be avoided. Residents and other trainees may not provide complete information to patients, may not convey information in a sensitive manner, and may not carefully document the communications they do have with patients.

A 2007 case decided by the Massachusetts Supreme Judicial Court, described by Annas, highlighted the importance of informing patients about the potential side effects of their medications. The case, *Coombes v. Florio* (450 Mass. 182), concerned a 72-year-old patient on multiple medications including oxycodone, tamsulosin, and oxazepam, who was driving and fatally struck a 10-year-old boy. The boy's mother sued both the driver of the car and the driver's physician, Dr. Roland J. Florio. The Massachusetts court ruled that this was not a medical malpractice case, because the boy who was killed and his mother had no physician-patient relationship with Dr. Florio. Nonetheless, the court held that Dr. Florio could still be subject to a negligence claim, because he did have a duty to make the patient aware of the side effects of the medications the patient was taking so that the patient could make an informed decision about whether it was safe to drive. The court reasoned that if it was not safe for the patient to drive, then an accident, which might result in harm to parties other than the patient, was a foreseeable consequence. The court drew an analogy with a bar owner being found negligent when someone becomes inebriated at the bar and then drives and becomes involved in a fatal collision.

Inadequate communication among physicians, both between hospitalists, and between hospitalists and PCPs, is a significant liability concern for hospitalists. These communications should be standardized whenever possible. Handoffs of patient care between hospitalists should use a standardized form so that crucial information, such as diagnostic uncertainties and the status of communication with the PCP, is not overlooked. Although the discharge summary is not in and of itself adequate as the only means to communicate important information to a patient's PCP, it can be designed to help make sure the PCP receives important information arising from the hospitalization. For instance, the discharge summary can have standardized sections dedicated to tests pending at the time of discharge and issues requiring outpatient follow-up. Having these sections in all discharge summaries ensures that the person preparing the discharge summary addresses these areas and also gets PCPs accustomed to looking for this information in the discharge summaries. Even with standardized discharge forms, important issues requiring outpatient follow-up should still be directly communicated to the PCP, so as to minimize the chance that these matters get overlooked.

Checklists have been found to reduce complications and mortality in the surgical setting, and the benefits of checklists also extend to the medical setting. Checklists in Hospital Medicine have the potential to reduce errors that could give rise to a malpractice claim, such as the failure to use appropriate deep vein thrombosis (DVT) prophylaxis in a patient who subsequently develops a pulmonary embolus while in the hospital, or leaving a central venous catheter in a patient who then develops a catheter-related bloodstream infection. Checklists could also improve efficiency, such as by making sure a patient who needs a physical therapy evaluation receives one promptly. To enhance the effectiveness of a checklist in Hospital Medicine, other members of the care team, such as the nurses, should be involved in ensuring the components of the checklist have been met, and are empowered to raise the issue when the components of the checklist have not been met.

A practice that can be legally perilous is that of obtaining informal "curbside" consultations. Questions to consultants about a specific patient should generally be made as a formal request for consultation, not an informal "curbside" consultation. When consultants provide "curbside" consultations, they are usually not seeing the patient and evaluating all the data, so their assessment may be based on incomplete information. Moreover, a "curbside" consultation does not result in a note from the consultant in the chart, so the basis for the consultant's recommendations will not be part of the medical record. A consultant who formally sees the patient will also usually be able to continue to follow the patient as an outpatient, which can help with the transition of care to the outpatient setting and provide a resource to whom the patient's PCP can turn for assistance. If the name of a consultant who provides a "curbside" consultation is placed in the chart, then if a malpractice claim arises, it is likely that the consultant will be named in the claim.

Table 36-1 summarizes strategies designed to reduce the risk of a malpractice claim.

COPING WITH A MALPRACTICE CLAIM

Being the subject of a malpractice claim can be intensely stressful. Common reactions to being sued include anger, depressed mood, frustration, irritability, and insomnia. Samkoff and Gable have even compared physicians' reaction to a lawsuit with the five Kübler-Ross stages of grief: denial, anger, bargaining, depression, and then acceptance. Physicians are at risk of personalizing the claim and considering it an attack on their competence and character. Adding to the stress of a malpractice claim is that the process of adjudicating it is commonly protracted, often taking four to five years from the time of the adverse event to resolution of the case.

Approaches that can help physicians cope with the stress of a malpractice claim include discussing the stress with trusted friends,

TABLE 36-1 Strategies to Reduce the Risk of a Medical Malpractice Claim

Strategy	Explanation
Maintain open and empathetic communication with patients and their families	Inadequate or insensitive communication from the physician is commonly cited as a reason that patients file a malpractice claim. Good communication with the patient may reduce the likelihood that a malpractice claim is filed, especially in the event of an unexpected outcome.
Be careful about delegating communication	Delegating important communication tasks to trainees runs the risk of the information being conveyed in an insensitive manner, the communication not being well documented in the chart, and the patient taking offense that the attending physician did not care enough to come in person.
Standardize handoffs	Standardizing handoffs, such as by having predesigned handoff forms, helps ensure that important information, such as pending tests requiring follow-up, are communicated to the incoming physician.
Standardize discharge summaries	One way to make sure that the discharge summary contains crucial items, such as tests pending at the time of discharge and issues that require outpatient follow-up, is to have a standardized discharge template with sections prompting the inclusion of this information.
Directly communicate with PCPs	Important items requiring outpatient follow-up, such as an incidentally discovered lung nodule, should be communicated directly to the PCP by letter or telephone call, and this communication should be documented in the chart. A discharge summary alone is not adequate to communicate important follow-up matters.
Use checklists	Checklists can ensure that routine measures required for most patients, such as DVT prophylaxis, are not overlooked. Implementation of checklists should involve the entire care team.
Avoid "curbside" consultations	Consultants who provide "curbside" consultations make recommendations based on what may be incomplete information and there is no record of the consultation in the chart.
Recognize that hospitalists can be held responsible for consultants' decisions	When a consultant is negligent, the hospitalist, as the attending of record, is likely to be named in the claim. When a hospitalist has concerns about the decisions of a consultant, this should be discussed with the consultant. The responsibilities of the consultant should be clearly defined.
Collect and provide feedback to physicians	Negative feedback from patients about a physician, particularly about the physician's communication skills, can signal that this physician is at elevated risk of a malpractice claim. This feedback should be conveyed to the physician, and a plan to remedy the identified deficiencies should be made.

family, and colleagues. Discussions of specific details of the case should occur only in settings where privilege applies, such as with one's lawyer or with a therapist with whom one has a formal patient-clinician relationship. Open discussion with family about the accompanying stress can be especially helpful, since the stress of the malpractice claim is likely to affect family members. Colleagues should express support when they know an associate is facing a malpractice action. Some professional societies also offer specific counseling resources or referrals for physicians trying to deal with the stress of a malpractice action.

One of the reasons malpractice claims can be so stressful for physicians is that so much of their own identity revolves around their profession. Realizing this, the physician should attempt to depersonalize the claim. Most claimants have as their primary objective obtaining compensation, not vilifying the physician. Physicians dealing with a malpractice suit should use it as an occasion to assess whether they have appropriate balance between their professional lives and their leisure time. Spending time engaged in avocational pursuits, such as hobbies and time with friends, is important. Physicians should also have the lawyer representing them explain what the process of adjudicating the claim will entail, so that the process is demystified and surprises are minimized. The facts surrounding the case should be examined to see if there is a systems-level issue that can be addressed to help prevent future claims—for example, designing a system for reviewing incoming radiology studies if a radiographic finding was missed.

There are some specific pitfalls that must be avoided during the stress of malpractice litigation. Physicians facing a malpractice claim who do not have a formal PCP should obtain one, as a PCP can be helpful with medication for symptoms and referrals for counseling. Self-medication should be avoided. Insomnia is a common symptom arising from the stress of a malpractice claim, and physicians who feel medication is needed to treat insomnia should discuss this with their own physician, and should not self-prescribe or obtain medication from a colleague informally. One action that should never be taken is going back and altering any documents in an effort to assist one's defense. Not only is this unethical and potentially criminal, but also by the time a physician is aware that a malpractice claim may be filed, the filing party almost certainly has copies of the medical records and related documents.

CONCLUSION

Popular perceptions notwithstanding, the medical malpractice system appears to do a reasonable job of awarding compensation primarily in cases that actually involve an injury due to negligence. Nevertheless, the system is inefficient and expensive. In addition, most adverse events resulting from negligence never lead to claims or compensation, and meritless malpractice claims also remain a problem.

In seeking to avoid malpractice claims, physicians need to be conscientious about communicating with the patient so that the patient does not feel abandoned or devalued. Such breakdowns in communication between the physician and patient set the stage for a malpractice claim should an adverse event occur. Although case law involving hospitalists specifically is limited, issues hospitalists need to be careful about include coordinating the actions of consulting specialists, following up on pending tests, and communicating with PCPs about issues that require outpatient follow-up.

PRACTICE POINT

- In seeking to avoid malpractice claims, physicians need to be conscientious about communicating with the patient, so that the patient does not feel abandoned or devalued. Although case law involving hospitalists specifically is limited, issues hospitalists need to be careful about include coordinating the actions of consulting specialists, following up on pending tests, and communicating with PCPs about issues that require outpatient follow-up.

The future evolution of the medical malpractice system may be influenced by the effort at federal health care reform. The debate over health care reform is one in which reform of the medical malpractice system is frequently implicated. Many of the parties shaping the debate over health care reform are the same ones who have an important interest in the functioning of the medical malpractice system, so debates over reforming the health care system and reforming the medical malpractice system may well be intertwined.

Legal Citations:

Domby v. *Moritz*, 2008 Cal. App. Unpub. LEXIS 1856
Coombes v. *Florio*, 450 *Mass.* 182 (2007)
Siggers v. *Barlow*, 906 F.2d 241 (1990)
Beilke v. *Coryell*, 524 N.W.2d 607, 610 (N.D. 1994)
Hill v. *Medlantic Health Care Group*, 933 A.2d 314, 325 (D.C. App. 2007)
Kent v. *Pioneer Valley Hospital*, 930 P.2d 904, 906 (Ut. App. 1997)
Palandjian v. *Foster*, 842 N.E.2d 916, 921–22 (Mass. 2006)
Polozie v. *United States*, 835 F. Supp. 68, 72–74 (D. Conn. 1993)
Health Care Quality Improvement Act of 1986, Pub. L. No. 99–660, 100 Stat. 3743
(codified as amended in scattered sections of 42 U.S.C.).

Medical Malpractice and Hospital Medicine: Evidence Base and Literature

Background and Epidemiology

Baker T. Reconsidering the Harvard Medical Practice Study: conclusions about the validity of medical malpractice claims. *J Law Med Ethics.* 2005;33:501–514.

Brennan TA, Leape LL, Laird NM, et al. Incidence of adverse events and negligence in hospitalized patients. Results of the Harvard Medical Practice Study I. *N Engl J Med.* 1991;324: 370–376.

Brennan TA, Sox CM, Burstin HR. Relation between negligent adverse events and the outcomes of medical-malpractice litigation. *N Engl J Med.* 1996;335:1963–1967.

Danzon PM. *Medical malpractice: theory, evidence, and public policy*. Cambridge, Mass.: Harvard University Press; 1985.

Keeton P, Prosser WL. *Prosser and Keeton on the law of torts*. St. Paul, Minn.: West Pueblo Co.; 1984.

Localio AR, Lawthers AG, Brennan TA, et al. Relation between malpractice claims and adverse events due to negligence. Results of the Harvard Medical Practice Study III. *N Engl J Med.* 1991;325:245–251.

Louisell DW, Williams H. Medical malpractice litigation guide. Newark, NJ: Matthew Bender.

Mello MM, Brennan TA. The role of medical liability reform in federal health care reform. *N Engl J Med.* 2009;361:1–3.

Mello MM, Studdert DM. The Medical Malpractice System: Structure and Performance. In: Sage WM, Kersh R, eds. *Medical malpractice and the U.S. health care system*. New York: Cambridge University Press; 2006.

Studdert DM, Mello MM, Gawande AA, et al. Claims, errors, and compensation payments in medical malpractice litigation. *N Engl J Med.* 2006;354:2024–2033.

Studdert DM, Thomas EJ, Burstin HR, Zbar BI, Orav EJ, Brennan TA. Negligent care and malpractice claiming behavior in Utah and Colorado. *Med Care.* 2000;38:250–260.

Thomas EJ, Studdert DM, Burstin HR, et al. Incidence and types of adverse events and negligent care in Utah and Colorado. *Med Care.* 2000;38:261–271.

Areas of Medical Malpractice of Special Concern to Hospitalists

Alpers A. Key legal principles for hospitalists. *Am J Med.* 2001;111: 5S–9S.

Kachalia A, Gandhi TK, Puopolo AL, et al. Missed and delayed diagnoses in the emergency department: a study of closed malpractice claims from 4 liability insurers. *Ann Emerg Med.* 2007;49:196–205.

Kripalani S, LeFevre F, Phillips CO, Williams MV, Basaviah P, Baker DW. Deficits in communication and information transfer between hospital-based and primary care physicians: implications for patient safety and continuity of care. *JAMA.* 2007;297:831–841.

Pantilat SZ, Lindenauer PK, Katz PP, Wachter RM. Primary care physician attitudes regarding communication with hospitalists. *Am J Med.* 2001;111:15S–20S.

Roy CL, Poon EG, Karson AS, et al. Patient safety concerns arising from test results that return after hospital discharge. *Ann Intern Med.* 2005;143:121–128.

Wright J, McCormack P. Failure to Act on Incidental Finding. CRICO Forum 2007;25:6–7.

Risk Factors for Medical Malpractice Claims and Strategies to Reduce this Risk

Annas GJ. Doctors, drugs, and driving—tort liability for patient caused accidents. *N Engl J Med.* 2008;359:521–525.

Beckman HB, Markakis KM, Suchman AL, Frankel RM. The doctor patient relationship and malpractice. Lessons from plaintiff depositions. *Arch Intern Med.* 1994;154:1365–1370.

Fox BC, Siegel ML, Weinstein RA. "Curbside" consultation and informal communication in medical practice: a medicolegal perspective. *Clin Infect Dis.* 1996;23:616–622.

(continued)

Medical Malpractice and Hospital Medicine: Evidence Base and Literature (*continued*)

Risk Factors for Medical Malpractice Claims and Strategies to Reduce this Risk
Hales BM, Pronovost PJ. The checklist—a tool for error management and performance improvement. *J Crit Care*. 2006;21:231–235.
Hickson GB, Clayton EW, Entman SS, et al. Obstetricians' prior malpractice experience and patients' satisfaction with care. *JAMA*. 1994;272:1583–1587.
Lester GW, Smith SG. Listening and talking to patients. A remedy for malpractice suits? *West J Med*. 1993;158:268–272.
Moore IN, Pichert JW, Hickson GB, Federspiel C, Blackford JU. Rethinking peer review: detecting and addressing medical malpractice claims risk. *Vanderbilt Law Review*. 2006;59:1175–1206.
Stelfox HT, Gandhi TK, Orav EJ, Gustafson ML. The relation of patient satisfaction with complaints against physicians and malpractice lawsuits. *Am J Med*. 2005;118:1126–1133.
Disclosing Errors to Patients
Boothman RC, Blackwell AC, Campbell DA, Jr., Commiskey E, Anderson S. A better approach to medical malpractice claims? The University of Michigan experience. *Journal of Health & Life Sciences Law*. 2009;2:125–159.
Clinton HR, Obama B. Making patient safety the centerpiece of medical liability reform. *N Engl J Med*. 2006;354:2205–2208.
Gallagher TH, Studdert D, Levinson W. Disclosing harmful medical errors to patients. *N Engl J Med*. 2007;356:2713–2719.
Hebert PC, Levin AV, Robertson G. Bioethics for clinicians: 23. Disclosure of medical error. Canadian Medical Association Journal. 2001;164:509–513.
Joint Commission on Accreditation of Health Care Organizations. Health Care at the Crossroads: Strategies for Improving the Medical Liability System and Preventing Patient Injury; 2005.
Kachalia A, Shojania KG, Hofer TP, Piotrowski M, Saint S. Does full disclosure of medical errors affect malpractice liability? The jury is still out. *Jt Comm J Qual Saf*. 2003;29:503–511.
Kraman SS, Cranfill L, Hamm G, Woodard T. John M. Eisenberg Patient Safety Awards. Advocacy: the Lexington Veterans Affairs Medical Center. *Jt Comm J Qual Improv*. 2002;28:646–650.
Kraman SS, Hamm G. Risk management: extreme honesty may be the best policy. *Ann Intern Med*. 1999;131:963–967.
Massachusetts Coalition for the Prevention of Medical Errors. When things go wrong: responding to adverse events. A consensus statement of the Harvard hospitals. Boston, Massachusetts; 2006 March.
Studdert DM, Mello MM, Gawande AA, Brennan TA, Wang YC. Disclosure of medical injury to patients: an improbable risk management strategy. *Health Aff* (Millwood). 2007;26:215–226.
Defensive Medicine
Anderson RE. Billions for defense: the pervasive nature of defensive medicine. *Arch Intern Med*. 1999;159:2399–2402.
Kessler D, McClellan M. Do Doctors Practice Defensive Medicine? *The Quarterly Journal of Economics*. 1996;111:353–390.
Office of the Assistant Secretary for Planning and Evaluation, U.S. Department of Health and Human Services. Addressing the new health care crisis: reforming the medical litigation system to improve the quality of health care; 2003.
Sloan FA, Shadle JH. Is there empirical evidence for "Defensive Medicine"? A reassessment. Journal of Health Economics. 2009;28:481–491.
Studdert DM, Mello MM, Sage WM, et al. Defensive medicine among high-risk specialist physicians in a volatile malpractice environment. *JAMA*. 2005;293:2609–2617.
U.S. Office of Technology Assessment. Defensive medicine and medical malpractice. Washington, D.C.: United States Congress, Office of Technology Assessment; 1994.
Coping with a Malpractice Claim
Charles SC. Coping with a medical malpractice suit. *West J Med*. 2001;174:55–58.

SUGGESTED READINGS

Beckman HB, Markakis KM, Suchman AL, Frankel RM. The doctor-patient relationship and malpractice. Lessons from plaintiff depositions. *Arch Intern Med*. 1994;154:1365–1370.

Brennan TA, Leape LL, Laird NM, et al. Incidence of adverse events and negligence in hospitalized patients. Results of the Harvard Medical Practice Study I. *N Engl J Med*. 1991;324:370–376.

Kripalani S, LeFevre F, Phillips CO, Williams MV, Basaviah P, Baker DW. Deficits in communication and information transfer between hospital-based and primary care physicians: implications for patient safety and continuity of care. *JAMA*. 2007;297:831–841.

Localio AR, Lawthers AG, Brennan TA, et al. Relation between malpractice claims and adverse events due to negligence. Results of the Harvard Medical Practice Study III. *N Engl J Med*. 1991;325:245–251.

Moore IN, Pichert JW, Hickson GB, Federspiel C, Blackford JU. Rethinking peer review: detecting and addressing medical malpractice claims risk. *Vanderbilt Law Review*. 2006;59:1175–1206.

Stelfox HT, Gandhi TK, Orav EJ, Gustafson ML. The relation of patient satisfaction with complaints against physicians and malpractice lawsuits. *Am J Med*. 2005;118:1126–1133.

Studdert DM, Mello MM, Brennan TA. Medical malpractice. *N Engl J Med*. Jan 15 2004;350(3):283–292.

Studdert DM, Mello MM, Gawande AA, et al. Claims, errors, and compensation payments in medical malpractice litigation. *N Engl J Med*. 2006;354:2024–2033.

SECTION 7

Teaching and Development

CHAPTER 37

Principles of Adult Learning and Continuing Medical Education

Jeffrey A. Tabas, MD
Robert B. Baron, MD, MS

INTRODUCTION

Most physicians learn through informal approaches, including reading, point-of-care learning, and consulting colleagues. More formal adult learning occurs mainly through continuing medical education (CME). The approach to physician learning through CME is changing and hospitalists are poised to play a crucial role in its development. Hospitalists are increasingly the primary teachers in the hospital setting and play a major role in performance improvement. Modern CME integrates these two processes. In this chapter, we discuss principles of adult learning, the changing landscape of CME, and the resultant responsibilities and opportunities for hospitalists.

ADULT LEARNING

Adult learning is complex. Understanding the framework of adult learning theory can help inform curricular design, teaching, and evaluation. Of the many theories of adult learning, three are most influential: the behaviorist, cognitivist, and constructivist theories. No single theory fits the learning style of all adult learners, and most educators use elements from each.

Behaviorism, popularized by B. F. Skinner, focuses on using consequences to shape behavior. A desired behavior is rewarded with positive reinforcement, while undesired behavior is discouraged with negative reinforcement. This theory emphasizes that feedback is critical to learning.

Cognitivism tries to explain learning through information-processing models and minimizes the focus on the behavioral response. It highlights the importance of information that is appropriately organized by the educator and the development of problem-solving skills by the learner.

Constructivism, popularized by Jean Piaget, teaches that learners construct new knowledge from experiences they integrate into their own existing framework of understanding when the experience is consistent with that framework. When the experience is inconsistent with that framework, they either change their perceptions of the experience or reframe their internal model of understanding. This theory emphasizes the educator's role as facilitator instead of didactic teacher and the learner's need for a social and active learning process.

PRACTICE POINT

- Adults learn most effectively when they (1) perceive the relevance of educational material, (2) are actively engaged, (3) have input into choosing educational experiences and directing their own learning, and (4) have the chance to step back and reflect on their learning.

Together, these theories suggest that adults learn most effectively when they (1) perceive the relevance of educational material, (2) are actively engaged, (3) have input into choosing educational experiences and directing their own learning, and (4) have the chance to step back and reflect on their learning.

Moore has proposed that adult learning involves a five-stage process.[1] These are: "(1) recognizing an opportunity for learning; (2) searching for resources for learning; (3) engaging in learning to address an opportunity for improvement; (4) trying out what was learned; and (5) incorporating what was learned." Learning occurs not as a linear progression through these stages, but as a dynamic process with complex interactions that include revisiting and concurrence of various stages. CME may stimulate the first stage by providing the recognition that the opportunity for learning exists ("I did not know that continuous positive airway pressure [CPAP] decreases intubation in patients with congestive heart failure [CHF]") or the third stage by providing the learning needed to address the opportunity for improvement ("I developed the competence to appropriately select candidates for CPAP and the steps to implement it"). As described above, learners most readily progress through stages when they see relevance ("ICU beds are limited and I can save hospital resources by avoiding intubation"), are actively engaged ("The CME presentation used dynamic learning approaches such as case presentations, question and answer, or audience response systems"), have chosen the subject ("I want to learn how to implement CPAP"), and reflect on their learning experience ("Is this something that would work in my institution and do I need more learning to effectively implement this?").

CME EFFECTIVENESS

Recently, an expert panel described the effectiveness of CME based on a systematic review by the Johns Hopkins Evidence-Based Practice Center. The best available evidence suggests that CME is effective in achieving and maintaining knowledge, competence, and procedural skills, as well as improving practice behavior and clinical practice outcomes, if the activity is planned and implemented according to recommended approaches. Assessments show that interventions using live educational strategies are more effective than print, multimedia are more effective than single media, and multiple exposures are more effective than a single exposure. Simulation methods in medical education seem effective in disseminating psychomotor and procedural skills.

While current evidence supports the effectiveness of CME, a systematic review of the reliability and validity of the tools used to assess that effectiveness found that more evidence is needed to confirm their value. Some have pointed out that a rigorous approach to assessment would be best coordinated by a national entity dedicated to providing a concerted approach to examining CME effectiveness.

THE ROLE OF THE HOSPITALIST IN CONTINUING EDUCATION

Research reveals significant gaps between the medical care patients actually receive and the care they should be getting. Hospitals that have hospitalists provide care closer to the ideal—their care is associated with better performance measures, such as improved diagnosis, treatment, counseling, and prevention, as well as decreased length of stays and hospital costs. The hospitalist plays an essential role in closing the quality gaps through implementing guidelines and reporting and implementing quality measures. Much of that role involves changing physician behaviors, which is the essence of CME. Given that many nationally reported quality measures—heart failure, acute myocardial infarction, pneumonia, asthma, venous thromboembolism, and stroke care, among others—fall within the purview of the hospitalist, the hospitalist must be versed in the theory of CME and be prepared to deliver such activities.

PRACTICE POINT

- The hospitalist plays an essential role in closing the quality gaps through implementing guidelines and reporting and implementing quality measures. As teachers, hospitalists are expected to define practice gaps, provide process and outcomes data as a basis for self-assessment, teach performance improvement principles as a template for educational interventions, and incorporate point-of-care learning and teaching into their practice. Much of that role involves changing physician behaviors, which is the essence of CME.

THE CHANGING LANDSCAPE OF CME

Continuing medical education has traditionally used didactic lectures and reading followed by testing to confirm knowledge, with little heed paid to the importance of physician practice behaviors. The focus of modern CME has evolved from increasing knowledge to improving physician competence, physician performance, and patient outcomes. This is reflected in the drive to incorporate practice-based learning and improvement into all aspects of continuing education and accreditation. Driven by the link to quality in patient safety, the American Board of Medical Specialties has mandated that all specialty boards adopt practice performance assessment as the fourth component in maintaining certification. The American Board of Internal Medicine was one of the first specialty boards to adopt this requirement. The Federation of State Medical Boards has also discussed the value of performance improvement in maintaining licensure. As a result of this changing focus, the Accreditation Council for Continuing Medical Education (ACCME) has incorporated self-directed physician improvement and change as a desired outcome of CME activities. ACCME has developed the following systematic approach to ensure appropriate planning, implementation, and assessment of each CME activity:

1. Identify the professional practice gap—the difference between current practice and optimal performance—appropriate to learners of this activity. Current practice can be identified through auditing individual physicians or practice groups, or from reported hospital, regional, or national data involving registries or national quality measures. Performance can reflect patient outcomes, such as mortality or readmission rates, or process measures, such as counseling for smoking cessation in patients with pneumonia. Optimal performance can be determined through assessing practice guidelines, medical literature, national benchmarks, and the like. The difference between the two is the practice gap. Professional practice gaps are not limited to patient care but can also involve other areas, such as research or administrative practice.
2. Identify the educational needs—improved knowledge, competence, or performance—that should be addressed to close the practice gap. These can be determined by surveying learners, interviewing thought leaders in the content area, or reviewing literature, for example.
3. Identify which outcomes the activity is designed to improve—competence (strategies to apply knowledge), performance (what is done in practice), or patient outcomes—and how they will be measured (for example by looking at changes in hospital quality measures). Improved knowledge alone, which may be an educational need, is not an adequate outcome. For example, the educational need may be a lack of knowledge of the indications for CPAP in patients with CHF, but the outcome should be the ability

to apply that knowledge when presented with several case scenarios and appropriately select the patient that might benefit from the therapy.

4. Select an appropriate educational format to encourage this change (for example, a case-based lecture with spaced learning using follow-up e-mail reminders).
5. Identify the potential barriers to change, and describe how to address them.
6. Identify ways to cooperate and collaborate outside of the CME activity to help facilitate change, such as interaction with the quality department or other organizations.

PRACTICE POINT

- The focus of modern CME has evolved from increasing knowledge to improving physician competence, physician performance, and patient outcomes.

Educators who thoroughly understand and apply this approach will be better able to provide the quality learning needed to effect the desired improvements.

NOVEL FORMS OF CME: POINT-OF-CARE CME AND PERFORMANCE IMPROVEMENT CME

In 2005, the American Medical Association (AMA) implemented two new formats for CME: Internet Point-of-Care CME (PoCCME) and Performance Improvement CME (PICME). PoCCME is CME developed by an accredited provider that includes self-directed online learning. A physician answers a clinical patient question in real time using an evidence-based source and then documents the question, the sources consulted, and the resultant application to practice. For example, a physician needs to know the parameters used to determine when a patient with CHF can be weaned off CPAP. Working with an accredited provider, she goes online to determine the criteria for weaning, and then documents her question, sources, and how she will use the information. That physician can then receive PoCCME credits.

With PICME, a physician or group of physicians performs a three-step process in which they (1) learn how to measure performance and then assess their practice, (2) develop an intervention based on best practice, and (3) remeasure performance and then reflect on the impact of the intervention. PICME typically involves longer-term interventions and activities that require chart review or data collection. These activities may address the structure, process, or outcome of a physician's practice with direct implications for patient care. The goal is for CME to be an active process that occurs within the clinical care setting, as opposed to a more passive process in a nonclinical setting. It acknowledges that some process changes require systems-level change. Objectives include learning the performance improvement process, taking an active role in learning and change, and attempting to directly improve patient care processes and outcomes through an educational activity. For example, a hospitalist group identifies a gap between the observed catheter-related bloodstream infection (CRBSI) rate and the desired rate based on national guidelines. They develop a tool to self-report compliance with the central catheter insertion "bundle" and measure the rate of compliance. The group then implements a training activity and monitors the self-reported rate of compliance or subsequent CRBSI infection rates. If rates have not improved, they analyze their approach again, looking for other needs that can be addressed to improve these outcomes. While drawbacks to this approach are the prolonged effort and time required, these may not be any greater than the effort, time, and cost of traveling to a several-day live meeting, and may yield significantly greater improvements in care. With their established track record in patient safety and quality and the advent of PICME, hospitalists are a natural resource for implementing this new form of CME.

PRACTICAL IMPACT OF THE HOSPITALIST ON CME

The role of hospitalists in CME continues to expand. Programs have been developed for hospitalists as agents of change in venues ranging from university CME programs, to the Society of Hospital Medicine, to the Agency for Health care Research and Quality (AHRQ). Hospitalists should incorporate the principles described above into the CME planning and education process. This would include close collaboration and communication between educators and the institutional staff responsible for quality and safety initiatives. Approaches to planning internal CME such as grand rounds might include comparing hospital-quality data to national guidelines to identify gaps and then surveying physicians to identify needs related to those gaps. An example of a planned activity after identification of a practice gap and learning needs, such as for catheter-related bloodstream infection rates, might include hands-on skills workshops with trainers to improve techniques (performance) in central line insertion practices. CME activity assessment could include before-and-after surveys to determine whether the activity's content relates to their practice and how it has changed that practice. More robust assessment would include measuring changes in process or patient outcomes in conjunction with the hospital quality department.

In an example of such a hospitalist-based learning intervention, Kisuule and colleagues reported direct improvements in hospitalist antibiotic prescribing practices.[2] In this study, antibiotic prescribing patterns of 17 hospitalist practitioners were reviewed and classified as appropriate or inappropriate. The practitioners then reviewed inappropriate prescribing practices as well as current practice guidelines. Prescribing patterns before and after the intervention showed significant improvements.

Hospitalists are poised to play a major role in the future of CME. This will include use of interactive case-based learning, simulation, and other learning formats, in the same way we teach students and residents. It will also include defining practice gaps, providing process and outcomes data as a basis for self-assessment, teaching performance improvement principles as a template for educational interventions, and incorporating point-of-care learning and teaching into their practice.

SUGGESTED READINGS

Basow D. Internet Continuing Education. In *Continuing Education in the Health Professions: Improving Healthcare Through Lifelong Learning*. Presented Josiah Macy, Jr. Foundation Conference November 28, 2007. Accessible at http://www.josiahmacyfoundation.org.

Bordage G, Carlin B, Mazmanian PE. Continuing medical education effect on physician knowledge: effectiveness of continuing medical education: American College of Chest Physicians Evidence-Based Educational Guidelines. *Chest*. 2009;135(suppl 3): 29S–36S.

Davis D, Galbraith R. Continuing medical education effect on practice performance: effectiveness of continuing medical education: American College of Chest Physicians Evidence-Based Educational Guidelines. *Chest*. 2009;135(suppl 3):42S–48S.

Federation of State Medical Boards Special Committee on Maintenance of Licensure Draft Report on Maintenance of Licensure February 2008. http://www.fsmb.org/pdf/Special_Committee_MOL_Draft_Report_February2008.pdf. Accessed February 15, 2010.

Institute of Medicine. Redesigning Continuing Education in the Health Professions. http://iom.edu/Reports/2009/Redesigning-Continuing-Education-in-the-Health-Professions.aspx. Accessed December 18, 2009.

Mazmanian PE, Davis DA, Galbraith R. Continuing medical education effect on clinical outcomes: effectiveness of continuing medical education: American College of Chest Physicians Evidence-Based Educational Guidelines. *Chest*. 2009;135(suppl 3):49S–55S.

Measuring Improvement Using Clinical Measures, ACCME. http://education.accme.org/video/accme-interviews/measuring-improvement-using-clinical-measures. Accessed February 15, 2010.

Ratanawongsa N, Thomas PA, Marinopoulos SS, et al. The reported validity and reliability of methods for evaluating continuing medical education: a systematic review. *Acad Med*. 2008;83(3):274–283.

Regnier K, Kopelow M, Lane D, Alden E. Accreditation for learning and change: quality and improvement as the outcome. *J Contin Educ Health Prof*. 2005;25(3):174–182.

The Joint Commission Performance Measures Initiative. http://www.jointcommission.org/PerformanceMeasurement/PerformanceMeasurement. Accessed February 15, 2010.

REFERENCES

1. Moore D. How physicians learn and how to design learning experiences for them. In *Continuing Education in the Health Professions: Improving Healthcare Through Lifelong Learning*. Presented Josiah Macy, Jr. Foundation Conference November 28, 2007. Accessible at http://www.josiahmacyfoundation.org.
2. Kisuule F, Wright S, Barreto J, Zenilman J. Improving antibiotic utilization among hospitalists: a pilot academic detailing project with a public health approach. *J Hosp Med*. 2008;3(1):64–70.

CHAPTER 38

Setting a Learning Environment in the Hospital

Anjala V. Tess, MD, SFHM
Alexander R. Carbo, MD, SFHM

INTRODUCTION

Hospitalists serve as teachers and role models for students, trainees, and other hospital staff. Expertise in Hospital Medicine includes not only the clinical knowledge and skills pertinent to acute inpatient medicine but also the skills and attitudes of institutional safety practices. These practices may include delivery of safe handoffs, prevention of health care–associated infections with hand washing and antimicrobial resistance by evidence-based antibiotic prescribing, and actively engaging in institutional patient safety and quality improvement initiatives. Hospitalists' availability and physical proximity to learners clearly positions them to become effective educators. But hospitalists' success as teachers cannot rely on physical proximity alone. The structure of Hospital Medicine practice poses challenges: lack of time, competing demands between clinical work and education, and the pressure of duty hour restrictions. In addition, hospitalists face common hurdles of how to teach at multiple levels simultaneously, how to assess competence, and how to provide feedback. To succeed in the critical role of educator, hospitalists must establish a productive learning environment in which to work. This chapter will focus on applying some of these key principles and skills in medical education that the hospitalist will find useful in daily work.

GOALS AND EXPECTATIONS OF THE HOSPITALIST AS TEACHER

In order to meet the goal of effective teaching, hospitalists should first have a clear understanding of what expectations exist. The *Core Competences in Hospital Medicine: A Framework for Curriculum Development* by the Society of Hospital Medicine (SHM) sets expectations about the role of the hospitalist as teacher. These include the knowledge (eg, teachable moments and microskills), skills (eg, setting expectations and role modeling), and attitudes (eg, recognizing the needs of the learner) required for hospitalist educators. Hospitalists should reflect on how to apply these expectations as they manage patients with students, residents, physician assistants, nurse practitioners, and other members of the multidisciplinary team. Beyond serving as supervisor, explicit goals should include serving as a clinical role model: competent with clinical knowledge, demonstrating analytic ability and professionalism, and incorporating new knowledge into practice. Hospitalists should strive to support their teams by mentoring, showing interest and providing advice about careers, anticipating mistakes, and when they occur minimizing them in a nonblaming manner, and providing feedback. Teaching should be dynamic and engaging, flexible enough to meet the needs of different learners, balanced with variable clinical demands, and incorporate self-reflection.

A MODEL OF CLINICAL TEACHING

David Irby's observational study of "master teachers" is a useful reference for hospitalists who plan to teach. Irby proposes a model in which educators divide their teaching time into three phases: planning, teaching, and self-reflection. The objectives outlined in the *Core Competencies* should be kept in mind in each of these three phases. This framework adapts easily to one-on-one teaching, bedside teaching on rounds, and small group learning in team or attending rounds.

In the planning phase the teacher prepares the session by talking with learners ahead of time, gets to know them well enough to understand what they need, and sets priorities based on time and needs assessment. This focus on the trainee helps shift the emphasis away from what the teacher wants to teach to what the learners need.

In the teaching phase the teacher diagnoses both the learner and the patient. The teacher asks questions of the learner about the patient in order to make a clinical decision, and also questions the learner on what he or she understands so the teacher can tailor his or her teaching. The one-minute preceptor and varying questions are two potential strategies that hospitalists can easily incorporate into their clinical teaching (see Bedside Teaching below).

The last phase is self-reflection. The hospitalist should spend time at the end of a session or rotation to reflect on what went well in his teaching and what he can improve. It may include asking for feedback from learners, team members, and peers. This is an essential component of effective teaching as the individual hospitalist can continue to develop his or her teaching scripts and skills.

PRACTICE POINT

- Educators divide their time into three phases: planning, teaching, and self-reflection. Planning focuses on the trainee, thereby shifting the emphasis away from what the teacher wants or feels comfortable to teach to what the learners need. In the teaching phase the teacher diagnoses both the learner and the patient. Finally, self-reflection incorporates feedback from learners, team members, and peers to develop an effective strategy for improving teaching skills.

SETTING EXPECTATIONS WITH THE LEARNER

Adult learning theory espouses that learners need to clearly understand the expectations of them. For single teaching sessions, this can be accomplished with a brief introduction at the beginning of the session. The longer the teacher-learner relationship, the more formal the expectations sessions can be. Setting aside time to discuss specifics reinforces the importance of education, especially in times of busy service.

PRACTICE POINT

- Beyond serving as supervisor, explicit goals should include serving as clinical role model: competent with clinical knowledge, demonstrating analytic ability and professionalism, and incorporating new knowledge into practice. Setting clear and appropriately focused goals at the beginning of the rotation provides more effective assessment.

Expectations should cover not only the hospitalist's goals but also the learners' goals. The focus becomes learner-centric instead of teacher-centric alone. Partnering with the team around these goals helps members to become active participants in their own education. Expectations should include explicit details regarding roles and responsibilities of the team. Patient safety is clearly tied to effective teamwork and being explicit about this helps learners understand this concept as well. Topics to discuss could include the following:

- **Communication:** Contact numbers and expectations of when communication should take place within team.
- **Logistics on rounds:** Details such as start time, presenters of cases, and location of rounds should lead to a negotiated plan that provides autonomy to the learner and allows the hospitalist to sufficiently supervise care.
- **Teaching role for the residents or other senior members of the team:** With the close proximity of attending hospitalists on the medical units, the autonomy of more advanced learners or team members is at risk, as more junior team members will naturally come directly to the attending. Explicit attention to the residents and their role can help preserve autonomy.
- **Collective educational goals for the month:** A discussion should include a list of didactic topics and skills such as presenting or synthesizing assessments and plans at the bedside. This will help hospitalists plan their teaching in a learner-centric way.
- **Clinical expectations for how to function as a team:** Details such as who is responsible for the parts of clinical care including communication with patients, families, primary care physicians, and consultants should be discussed. Other patient safety issues such as follow-up of pending test results at discharge and attention to the group's behavior around hand hygiene or DVT prophylaxis should be agreed upon as well.
- **Expectations regarding documentation:** Expectations for admission, daily documentation, and discharge documentation are a key component of the teaching hospitalist's role. Few other teachers will be able to directly observe a student or house officer's daily work. Setting expectations early in the month will allow you to teach this critical skill and provide meaningful feedback.

One of the realities of practicing as a teaching hospitalist is that learners' schedules are not always synchronized with the teacher's schedule. As a result, hospitalists may have limited opportunities to assess and provide feedback. Setting clear and appropriately focused goals at the beginning of the rotation provides more effective assessment.

CASE 38-1

SETTING EXPECTATIONS

The hospitalist arrives at 8 AM to start rounds on the first day of the month. The team sees him arrive but does not gather for 15 minutes. Eventually the resident starts rounds and says, "Let's start at room 3." The intern pulls out his papers and says "This patient is a 78-year-old with congestive heart failure..." Rounds continue and the team sees all of the patients. Very little teaching is done on rounds and the students look bored. At the end the resident says, "Thanks. I guess we will see you tomorrow." Everyone walks away.

This case raises several questions:

- What is the structure of rounds?
- What are the roles of the team members?
- Does the team have a common understanding of the educational goals for the month?

The core issues include communication about the learner-teacher contract, logistics, and teaching role identification. The hospitalist has not set expectations or defined roles, and this lack of explicit goal setting makes it harder for the students to participate and learn. The resident may also not be able to fulfill his role as teacher on the team. Learners are often focused on completing the work of the day and may need to be prompted to think about team structure. The hospitalist may need to be explicit about roles and responsibilities.

Case follow-up

The hospitalist could have taken a different approach to address the role of defining and setting expectations. Though this may require an extra step at the beginning of the rotation, it saves time and contributes to safer care later.

As the intern launched into his presentation, the hospitalist could have said, "John, may I interrupt for a second before we get into this case? I just wanted to take five minutes to quickly orient us as a group. We will be working together for the next three weeks so I thought we should chat about how things can work most effectively for us as a team. Who should run rounds? What has worked for you in the past? I generally like presentations at the bedside every morning and have the resident run rounds. I will stand in the back, listen, observe and interject occasionally. But I am hoping Rita can lead and teach for most of the rounds…"

After agreement is reached, the team can also address logistics about communication: "I can be reached at this number. You don't need to call me for everything. I would like the resident to be the team leader here. But you should feel comfortable calling me anytime. I do want to hear if someone is deteriorating or undergoing a major procedure. I think we need to develop a clear plan of how we are going to communicate with our patients too."

The hospitalist can conclude goal setting with a summary of initial teaching roles and topics: "It sounds like John is interested in brushing up on the cardiac exam and Shirley wants to make sure we discuss antibiotics at some point. Please remind us to incorporate the cardiac examination and antibiotic therapy on every relevant patient during rounds. Let's start back with the patient. John, you were saying…"

TEACHING AT THE BEDSIDE

"Medicine is learned by the bedside and not in the classroom."[1]
(Sir William Osler)

Bedside teaching is a key component of education in the hospital setting. By going to the bedside with other members of the team, clinical teachers have the opportunity to assess the clinical status of the patient, evaluate the performance of the learners, and reinforce the value of the bedside exam and history. Hospitalists can role model critical thinking, professionalism, and communication while making clinical decisions with the team. In addition, by working closely with learners at the bedside hospitalists can better evaluate learners' knowledge and skills.

Studies have shown that hospitalists do not teach at the bedside as much as students would like. Many faculty, particularly younger faculty, may be intimidated by the prospect of bedside rounds. Clinicians may fear that they will overwhelm or confuse patients with bedside presentations. In contrast, studies have actually shown that patients have a favorable response to bedside teaching. Junior faculty may also feel the need to appear omniscient, and fear not having answers in front of trainees. However, humility reminds the rest of the team that no individual has all of the answers all of the time and this authenticity can actually help to involve learners in the discussion. "When no one is always right, no one needs to fear being wrong."[2]

While on rounds, both faculty and learners may feel the pressure of time constraints. This is especially true in the era of work-hours regulations and high patient turnover resulting in shorter length of stay. When the census is high, the team runs the risk of sacrificing teaching in the name of efficiency, when "card flipping" substitutes for bedside visits. This problem is exacerbated in systems in which the teaching hospitalist is also managing patients without learners and is pulled in multiple directions.

Hospitalists are expected to simultaneously teach students, interns, and senior medical residents, each with obviously varying levels of knowledge and skills. This "one room schoolhouse" can be challenging for a young hospitalist who may have only one or two years of experience. Similarly, as the academic year progresses, learners change; their needs are very different in July than in May.

Careful attention to the structure of rounding at the bedside can help address these challenges and facilitate learning for team members in an efficient manner:

- **Set expectations as a group:** Clear expectations of roles and responsibilities of team members and standards for team communication should be defined ahead of time. The team can then spend less time organizing the work and more time on the clinical care and teaching. Teaching that meets preidentified goals is learner centered and more effective. The hospitalist might ask the team what they are interested in learning this month and then look for teachable moments as they arise at the bedside.
- **Prepare the teaching session:** Preparing teaching points on both clinical concepts and process of care helps the hospitalist overcome the anxiety of teaching at the bedside. Briefly discussing cases with the resident on the night before rounds can generate a list of clinical topics to be used as teaching points on rounds. The hospitalist can use textbooks and online references to supplement her knowledge base prior to rounds. Review of online resources on how to perform parts of the physical exam can also help relieve anxiety around this area of clinical teaching.
- **Develop teaching scripts:** Teaching scripts are concise teaching points on given topics. The goal for bedside teaching is not to develop a long didactic piece. In Hospital Medicine, scripts include both clinical knowledge and insights into systems and processes of care. As a hospitalist gains more experience he can start to quickly incorporate it into his work and teaching, and as a result will feel more prepared to teach. Scripts also provide a method to manage different learners by targeting pieces of the script to different levels. While basic concepts in diagnosis may be aimed at students or early interns, more seasoned interns or residents may benefit from a sophisticated discussion about management. Irby suggests making three to five teaching points when teaching so as not to overwhelm the learners.
- **Diagnose the learner while teaching on rounds:** In order to teach most effectively and choose the right teaching point, the teacher needs to assess where the learner is in his understanding of a case or condition. The one-minute preceptor is a useful method of diagnosing the learner (see **Table 38-1**). Aagaard[3] showed that faculty who used the one-minute preceptor arrived at the patient's diagnosis sooner and established a better sense of the resident's competence. The use of increasing sophistication of questions can also reveal opportunities to teach at the bedside. Questions that focus on recall of medical knowledge tend to be closed and focused on facts (eg, "What are the risk factors for coronary artery disease?") Higher-order questions that ask for a diagnosis or plan emphasize synthesis and analysis and are more open (eg, "What do you think is causing her chest pain and why?") Since most teaching at the bedside occurs in a group setting, the hospitalist must be careful to be nonjudgmental in asking questions and correcting mistakes. By rotating the questions to each member of the team, hospitalists can also lead short discussions and create a supportive learning environment for everyone.
- **Think about the location of team members on rounds:** Once the expectations of each team member have been set, make sure that the presenter is situated in a position so that others can hear him. Make sure that the person charged with decision making is centrally located, so that he can hear input from each of the team members. In addition, make sure that those not directly involved in the case are situated such that they can still participate; this is particularly helpful when working with medical students.

TABLE 38-1 Diagnosing the Learner Using the One-Minute Preceptor

Step	Rationale	Example
Get a commitment.	This step transforms passive learners into active learners by engaging them in a two-way conversation, and allows the teacher to make an assessment of what the learner is thinking.	A student presents a case of a patient with chronic obstructive pulmonary disease (COPD) and CHF who is short of breath and wheezing on exam. At the end he mentions that they stopped the patient's ACE inhibitor. *Hospitalist: "What do you think is going on?"* *Student: "I think he has a CHF exacerbation."*
Probe for supporting evidence.	This step enables the teacher to diagnose the learner and understand his rationale. Sometimes a learner arrives at the correct answer but does not really understand why. By probing, the hospitalist is able to glean what concepts the learner already knows and whether the learner is correctly synthesizing data to arrive at a diagnosis or plan.	*Hospitalist: "Why do you think the patient has a CHF exacerbation?"* *Student: "Because the patient is wheezing, has an* S_3 *and edema. He seems overloaded to me. He also responded to furosemide with diuresis."*
Reinforce what was done well.	This step provides reassurance and validates the information that the learner has synthesized. It also serves to teach the others in the group.	*Hospitalist: "I agree that the diagnosis is most likely CHF because he exhibits several signs of volume overload."*
Give guidance about errors and omissions.	This step prevents the learner and others in the group from leaving with incorrect information. If mistakes are not corrected, the learner will likely commit the same mistake again. It is important when correcting a mistake that teachers not pass judgment. Instead, teachers should focus on facts as well as evidence from the literature and provide a rationale.	*Hospitalist: "I probably would not have held his ACE inhibitor though, because that is a key component of effective treatment for CHF."*
Teach a general principle.	Teaching should close with a teaching point at the appropriate level for this learner. If there are several questions and insufficient time to answer them, questions should be documented as "learning issues" for the team. This acknowledges the importance of these questions while permitting members of the team to direct their learning.	*Hospitalist: "ACE inhibitors have been shown to decrease mortality in CHF and so we should aim to put all patients with systolic heart failure on an ACE inhibitor. I generally like to start at the lowest dose and titrate up quickly to the highest dose the patient can tolerate without developing hypotension. This is a core measure of quality in heart failure patients. I will e-mail you a key paper on this if you are interested."*

Adapted, with permission, from Neher JO, Stevens NG. The one-minute preceptor: shaping the teaching conversation. *Fam Med.* 2003;35(6):391–393.

- **Role model lifelong learning:** Often questions arise on rounds to which the hospitalist will not know the answer. This provides opportunities to explicitly role model how to find new answers either through the literature or through consultation.

CASE 38-2

THE ACTIVE LEARNING ENVIRONMENT

During hospital rounds with your resident, the intern presents a patient's admission for increasing shortness of breath. The patient is complicated with multiple medical comorbidities including CHF and COPD. The vital signs are normal and the intern's findings on exam this morning include wheezes. During the entire presentation he is looking from his notes to you. He concludes with "We don't have time today, so we don't need to see her. As far as her shortness of breath, what would you like to do?" The entire team turns and looks at you.

This case raises several questions:

- Does the hospitalist have enough information to make a decision?
- How might the hospitalist gain a sense of the learner's understanding of the case?
- How can the learner be encouraged to become more active, and not defer decision making to the attending?
- How might the hospitalist involve the resident in the teaching and learning from this case?

To make the appropriate decision on this patient's case, the hospitalist clearly needs to examine and question the patient to distinguish between an exacerbation of COPD and CHF. By performing a focused cardiopulmonary exam on the patient, he can demonstrate key physical examination skills and "think out loud" to highlight what he is doing and why. The team can then make a clinical decision about this patient's heart failure and COPD regimen, keeping the goals of the hospitalist in line with the goals of the team. Lastly, by going to the bedside as a team, the hospitalist also has the opportunity to assess the learner's bedside manner, communication skills, professionalism, and clinical skills.

The hospitalist may not initially know what the intern is thinking about the case and by using the one-minute preceptor or specific questions the hospitalist can determine where the learner is as well. Without understanding what the learner knows, teachers run the risk of teaching too little or at too basic a level. Passive learners, such as the one described in this case, are a particular challenge for the hospitalist. When learners defer decision making to the hospitalist, it is challenging to evaluate them, particularly if time is limited. The role of the resident is also not well defined in this case, making the resident marginalized and passive. After expectations are set, it would be important to situate the student and the resident centrally, allowing the resident the opportunity to teach and to make decisions after the case presentation. The hospitalist could first query the student to determine the level of understanding and then turn to the resident to let him teach. This would turn a passive learning experience into an active one for both the student and the resident.

Case follow-up

The hospitalist should try to turn the passive atmosphere into an active one, and encourage the group to go and examine the patient.

"Well, John, I think we should go in and see her. I know we have a lot of patients but we can do a focused exam and this will give your resident a chance to review the cardiac exam in CHF, which you were interested in. Before we go in though, I want to hear what you think is going on."

GIVING FEEDBACK

Feedback and evaluation are critical components of the educational contract between learners and educators. Once expectations have been clearly delineated, feedback allows the teacher and learner to evaluate performance and to set goals for continued learning. Hospitalists have the critical responsibility of providing feedback to learners. Studies have shown that learners value and rate hospitalists favorably because of their ability to give feedback.

Faculty may be reluctant to deliver constructive feedback, however there are several key components that can help facilitate the process:

- **Timeliness:** Feedback should be timely at a mutually convenient time. In addition to real-time feedback, "formal" feedback can be provided midway though a rotation and again at the end of the rotation. By waiting until the end of the rotation, learners will not have the opportunity to act on observations and to make improvements.
- **Specificity:** Feedback should be specific and based on observations, not assumptions. Gross generalizations are rarely helpful, and will not change or reinforce behaviors. Instead, hospitalists should provide specific examples of how to achieve proficiency. This holds true for constructive feedback, in which specific details should focus on the behavior in question, without passing judgment on the individual.
- **Remediable:** Feedback should only focus on remediable issues. It should be within the learner's locus of control. For example, it is not fair to criticize learners for being absent from the wards when it is their course director who sets the schedule.
- **Process:** Though no two feedback sessions are the same, there are some basic elements that can be used to structure the process. Hospitalists may begin by asking for open-ended feedback from the learner. Learners often identify areas that teachers may not know how to broach, and understanding the learner's perspective may help the teacher to bring up these issues. In addition, reviewing the expectations and learner's self-assessment can help structure the feedback.

  Be sure to specifically address things that were done well, and make concrete suggestions about what to improve, setting new specific goals for the learner. The learner should be given time to clarify or ask a question about the observations; the purpose of feedback is for the learner to improve. The learner may have an initial negative reaction to feedback and may need a few moments to digest the details of the communication. Using facts rather than commentary about the individual helps learners to accept feedback. Hospitalists should then close with an opportunity to elicit feedback on their own performance, and about the learner's experience as a whole. This communication highlights that feedback is a life-long process that provides important opportunities for self-improvement.
- **Setting:** Feedback should be done in a quiet and private space, which can prevent distraction or interruption. This avoids situations in which constructive feedback is given in front of peers and respects the learner's need for privacy.

CASE 38-3

FEEDBACK

It is the last afternoon of a month's rotation with the resident team. Post call, the intern is trying to discharge her patients before the weekend. You enjoyed your month and felt that the intern had a solid fund of knowledge and connected well with her patients. Occasionally, however, she overlooked details and you caught several mistakes before discharge. Overall patient care did not suffer, but the process could have been more efficient. The hospitalist decides to give the intern this feedback.

The intern sits down at the nursing station with her attending. He says "You have been doing a great job, but I am concerned that you are forgetful. Three weeks ago you made a few mistakes on discharges." The intern looks around at the other interns in the area, becomes tearful and then quiet. She sits with arms folded, and after many long silences or one-word responses to further questions on her self-assessment, she stands and says "OK I have to go now. Is there anything else?"

This case raises several questions:

- Was this the best time and/or setting to give feedback?
- Did the hospitalist learn anything about the learner's self-assessment?
- How could the hospitalist have received feedback on his own teaching?

In this example, the process of providing feedback was not perceived as constructive. The intern received negative feedback in a public place, at the end of a post-call day, when she was tired and under stress to finish her work before the weekend. Once she felt humiliated before her peers the intern likely heard nothing more and could not absorb or reflect on what transpired. The hospitalist lost an opportunity of identifying extenuating circumstances that might have affected this intern's performance. The intern probably would not have informed him of any psychosocial stressors, illness, or personality conflicts in front of others. If identified, the hospitalist had a responsibility to communicate true concerns to the program director.

Perhaps the hospitalist could have provided feedback to the intern earlier in the rotation, so that it did not come as a surprise on the final day. "Forgetful" also seems like a judgment on this intern as an individual. Instead, specific examples of what was overlooked immediately after the initial events would probably have been more actionable. The hospitalist also did not take the opportunity to elicit specific feedback about his own performance, or about the learner's experience as a whole.

Case follow-up

This case demonstrates how important it is to provide feedback in a nonjudgmental manner with careful attention to the timing and location, so that the learner can have the space and time to absorb and reflect. The feedback is also not timely or specific.

In this particular example, the hospitalist probably should have checked to see if this was an appropriate time to give feedback. *"I know you are post-call and have a lot to do before leaving. Do you have time to meet today? I would like to exchange feedback."* If not, rescheduling to a later date is likely appropriate but do not leave the rotation without a scheduled time and place in hand or at least a plan to check back on a certain date. This is akin to the patient being discharged without a follow-up appointment: it is much more challenging to arrange later!

During the session, he could have begun with: *"How do you think this month went for you? Do you feel you met your own learning goals?"*

Once the learner has shared her self-assessment, the hospitalist could then have shared his observations: "I observed the way that you explained Mrs. Smith's heart failure regimen changes to her and to her family. You gave a clear explanation about why we discontinued hydrochlorothiazide and added furosemide and lisinopril to her regimen, and you patiently answered her questions regarding her other heart failure medications. I was concerned that some details were overlooked during the discharge process. On two occasions patients were discharged without ACE inhibitors."

After a pause to allow her to digest the information, "May I ask how you typically reconcile medications on discharge? How can we come up with a method to help remember key medications?"

After core suggestions are discussed, "May I ask for some feedback? How did my communication style work for you? Was I available enough? What could I have done differently?"

PRACTICE POINT

- By embracing their responsibility as teachers, hospitalists will become as central to the education of trainees as they are to the operation of medical centers as a whole.

CONCLUSION

In summary, hospitalists should embrace their role as inpatient teachers. Though not without challenges, it is a vital part of learners' development and central to hospitalists' identity as educators. Fortunately, the necessary skills become easier with practice and time. While actively prioritizing setting expectations and providing feedback, hospitalists can teach more efficiently and effectively. The role of the hospitalist at the bedside has become even more important as faculty presence on the wards has otherwise become limited. As discussed in a recent editorial, "The single best thing that can be done to augment patient safety and quality is to maximize the time the patient spends with his health care team; and the hospitalist, who is not in a rush to complete morning rounds in an effort to get to a clinic or an endoscopy suite, may be the person who has the time to prioritize bedside rounds as a part of the educational environment."[4] By embracing their responsibility as teachers, hospitalists will become as central to the education of trainees as they are to the operation of medical centers as a whole.

SUGGESTED READINGS

Ende J. Feedback in clinical medical education. *JAMA.* 1983;250(6):777–781.

Goldenberg J, Glasheen JJ. Hospitalist Educators: Future of inpatient internal medicine training. *Mount Sinai Journal of Medicine.* 2008;750:430–435.

Gonzalo JD, Masters PA, Simons RJ. Attending rounds and bedside case presentations: medical student and medicine resident experiences and attitudes. *Teach Learn Med.* 2009;21(2):105–110.

Hauer KE, Wachter RM, McCulloch CE, et al. Effects of hospitalist attending physicians on trainee satisfaction with teaching and with internal medicine rotations. *Arch Intern Med.* 2004;164:1866–1871.

Irby DM. How attending physicians make instructional decisions when conducting teaching rounds. *Acad Med.* 1992;67(10):630–638.

Lake FR, Vickery AW, Ryan G. Teaching on the run tips 7: effective use of questions. *MJA.* 2005;182(3):126–127, 205.

Lehmann LS, Brancati FL, Chen M, et al. The effect of bedside case presentations on patients' perceptions of their medical care. *N Engl J Med.* 1997;336(16):1150–1155.

Neher JO, Stevens NG. The one-minute preceptor: shaping the teaching conversation. *Fam Med.* 2003;35(6):391–393.

Pistoria MJ, Amin AN, Dressler DD, et al. The core competencies in Hospital Medicine: hospitalist as teacher. *JHM.* 2006;1(S1):72–73.

REFERENCES

1. Thayer WS. Osler the teacher. *Bull Johns Hopkins Hosp.* 1919;30:198–200.
2. Ende J. What if Osler were one of us? Inpatient teaching today. *J Gen Intern Med.* 1997;12(S2):S41–S41.
3. Aagaard E, Teherani A, Irby D. Effectiveness of the one-minute preceptor model for diagnosing the patient and the learner: proof of concept. *Acad Med.* 2004;79:42–49.
4. Wiese J. Productivity vs. production capacity: hospitalists as medical educators. *J Hosp Med.* 2009;4(8):460–462.

CHAPTER 39

Mentorship of Peers and Trainees

Aubrey Orion Ingraham, MD
Thomas E. Baudendistel, MD

INTRODUCTION

The word "mentor" comes from Homer's *Odyssey*, in which Troy-bound Odysseus entrusts his young son to the care of his close friend, Mentor. Mentor, a transitional figure in the youth's growth, acts as the son's guardian and wise advisor, and through their mutual relationship, the son develops his own identity. Ancient history is filled with examples of the importance of mentoring. Tradesmen in the Middle Ages were principally trained by dedicated mentors within their guilds. Chinese kings employed *Shang Jang*—literally, "the enlightened stepping aside to create room in the center for the next deserving person to step in and take charge"—to pass the crown to a successor.

Mentoring has been vital to the art and practice of medicine since Hippocrates. Good mentors have played key roles in the history of medicine and discovery, in the development of young doctors, and in the institutions that train physicians. Today's health care leaders point to the importance of mentoring in choice of career as well as career advancement and productivity. Yet, the available evidence shows that fewer than 50% of third- and fourth-year medical students and in some fields fewer than 20% of faculty members had a mentor.[1] Academic hospitalists in particular, but also hospitalists in the community, not only serve as mentors to trainees but also to other members of the multidisciplinary team. Because Hospital Medicine is a young specialty, peer mentorship is crucial to the success of the specialty (**Figure 39-1**).

PRACTICE POINT

- Because Hospital Medicine is a young specialty, peer mentorship is crucial to the success of the specialty. Recent surveys at several U.S. and Canadian medical schools highlight that lack of mentoring is a powerful predictor of delays in academic advancement. Faculty members derive personal and professional satisfaction from mentoring residents.

This chapter will summarize the existing literature on the benefits of mentoring in clinical medicine, highlight successful mentoring models and behaviors, and present a potential framework for mentoring clinician-educators and trainees in Hospital Medicine.

THE VALUE OF MENTORING IN MEDICINE

Just as Mentor in the *Odyssey* helped the son recognize a disguised Odysseus returning from Troy, a modern day mentor can recognize previously unseen qualities in the mentee or help open doors to unnoticed opportunities. Surveys of faculty and health care leaders and one recent systematic review identified several potential benefits of mentoring in medicine. Mentoring influences career choice, including medical students' specialty selections; promotes career advancement; increases academic productivity; develops physicians' leadership skills; shapes professional ethics; fosters development of academic departments, institutions, and professional societies; and increases career satisfaction. Clinician-educators who receive mentoring may be more likely to stay in an academic position and view the mentoring relationship as important to academic development and

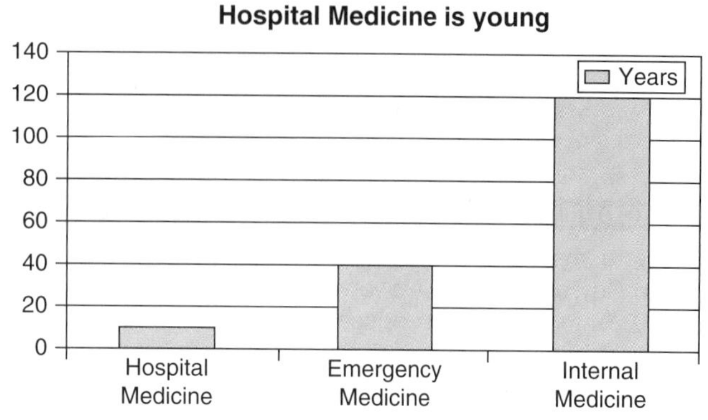

Figure 39-1 *Number of years various specialties have been accredited.*

promotion. The strongest evidence in support of mentoring has been demonstrated for clinician-scientists, who positively associated mentorship with scholarly productivity.

For house officers, mentoring has been promoted as one way to enhance resident satisfaction, improve career planning and readiness for future careers, and reduce stress and burnout. Medical residents clearly value mentoring. In one survey of 329 Internal Medicine house staff, 93% felt that mentoring helped in professional development, career advice, clinical assistance, research, and finding a job after residency (**Table 39-1**).

While most studies have focused on half of the mentorship pair, the mentee, available literature identifies potential benefits to the mentor.

Faculty members derive personal and professional satisfaction from mentoring residents. Mentoring residents may count toward promotion, result in special awards, and possibly advance scholarly productivity.

BARRIERS TO MENTORING FOR JUNIOR FACULTY AND RESIDENTS

Despite consistent reports of potential benefits of mentorships, data show that fewer than 50% of third- and fourth-year medical students and in some fields fewer than 20% of faculty members have a mentor. Clinician-educators are much less likely to identify a mentor than clinician-scientists and also less likely to serve as mentors. Despite their numbers among medical school faculty, clinician-educators account for only 28% of general internal medicine mentors. Most clinician-educator mentors volunteer for this activity and they say they already have as many mentees as they can handle. Unlike the situation for faculty researchers, objective criteria for academic advancement as a clinician-educator are wanting, and the contributions of clinician-educators have been lacking at many universities. Faculty cite competing time pressures, inadequate faculty development around mentoring, and lack of recognition of mentoring by promotions committees as factors dampening their willingness to mentor residents.

TABLE 39-1 Benefits of Mentoring

Benefits to the Mentee

- Increased advocacy for career development
- High-level career advice from experienced senior person
- Enhanced access to opportunities beyond the current level of the mentee, including:
  - research (grants, editing, publications, collaborations)
  - promotions
  - new job openings (within or outside the institution)
  - committee membership
  - roles in professional organizations
  - networking with key thought leaders
- Valuable, nonthreatening, feedback from "third party" who is separate from the employer-employee relationship
- Access to a role model of professionalism, ethics, and values
- More directed and formal timeline and framework for career success

Benefits to the Mentor

- Renewed sense of excitement for career brought about by revisiting own history of professional growth; participating in the professional and personal development of a colleague; and continuing professional legacy of shaping "the next generation" of physicians
- Enhanced recognition among peers and junior staff
- Cultivation of specific interpersonal skills (active listening, effective communication, modeling)
- Exposure to new ideas and opportunities, often leading to increased creativity and productivity (including publications and projects)
- Pride in a mentee's successes
- Enhanced personal growth
- Broadened network via mentee's collaboration and connection to other personnel, including cross-discipline and cross-department interactions
- Discussion and exploration of mentor's values with others
- An accurate perspective on barriers experienced by current junior staff
- Credit toward career advancement as a result of mentoring

Benefits to the Department

- Bolstered staff morale, motivation, institutional dedication, and career satisfaction
- Enhancement of productivity and creativity
- Discovery and development of personnel talent
- Ensurance of department's future survival through development of leadership
- Communication and demonstration of the department's values, goals, and expected personal and professional standards
- Reinvigoration of senior faculty
- Development of cross-departmental, national, and international networks

TABLE 39-2 A Good Mentor

- Maintains confidentiality
- Is knowledgeable and respected in his or her field
- Is approachable, nonthreatening, accessible, facilitative, empowering
- Challenges and debates mentee in a constructive way
- Employs a careful and dynamic balance between compassion and empathy, and impartiality and honesty
- Shows genuine interest and investment in a mentee's concerns, well-being, and future
- Asks questions that provoke critical thinking, reasoning, analysis, and contemplation
- Recognizes and admits limitations, then guides mentee to appropriate resource
- Recognizes importance of work-life balance in professional success
- Demonstrates confidence in a mentee
- Possesses strong interpersonal and negotiation skills
- Can listen actively and communicate clearly
- Avoids abuse of his or her influence or position
- Provides frequent and detailed feedback
- Encourages independent behavior, yet is available when needed
- Seeks opportunities for a mentee to assist with his or her own projects (if appropriate and relevant to mentee's goals)
- Expects and tolerates expressions of emotion from mentees at times of significant anxiety or frustration

Junior hospitalist clinician-educators often worry about identifying a niche of expertise and securing time and financial support for nonclinical activities. Hospitalists have championed many aspects of the inpatient arena, including patient safety, quality improvement, resource utilization, transitions of care, surgical comanagement, and ward teaching. This jack-of-all-trades approach, while valuable to the field, can be viewed on the individual faculty level by promotions committees as "master of none." A second tension exacerbates this problem. Hospitalist clinician-educators often cannot generate enough revenue from clinical duties to support unfunded nonclinical work, making it hard to secure protected time and financial compensation to develop expertise in education, scholarly activity, or administration.

To become more promotable, clinician-educators must ramp up their productivity during nonclinical time. The traditional clinician-educator paradigm—periods of active clinical work along with more relaxing nonclinical time—must be rethought. To paraphrase one department chair, just as diastole is now recognized as an active time of the cardiac cycle, so too must one view the nonclinical duties of clinician-educators. In some instances, clinical and nonclinical duties may overlap and provide a "two-for-one" opportunity; examples include teaching and clinical work as a ward attending, or committee work interspersed with clinical duties. For academic promotion, however, clinician-educators may need dedicated protected time and funding to support these interests. Grant funding for education research and medical school remuneration for course leadership or administrative roles provide limited support. When these resources fall short, hospitalists often turn to their division leaders for support, who in turn need to convince hospital leadership to support non-clinical activities of hospitalists.

Recent surveys at several U.S. and Canadian medical schools highlight that lack of mentoring is a powerful predictor of delays in academic advancement. Special academies in academic medicine and transparent advancement criteria for clinician-educators have recently been established to promote academic medicine as a desirable career path. Despite the benefits to faculty and trainees, less than half of internal medicine residents in 1 large survey established a mentoring relationship with a faculty member, and minority residents established mentorships much less often. House officers feared approaching senior faculty, failed to identify a mentor with similar personal or professional interests, and lacked awareness that residents could seek out mentors; only a minority felt they did not need a mentor.

THE MENTOR–MENTEE RELATIONSHIP

Meaningful definitions of mentoring identify core elements and specific behaviors of a successful mentoring relationship while honoring the intimate and unique aspects of a given mentoring pair. A useful definition states that mentoring is a protected relationship occurring between a more advanced career incumbent (mentor) and a younger novice (mentee). Jacobi defined key elements in such a relationship.[2] A mentoring relationship (1) focuses on achievement or acquisition of knowledge; (2) consists of 3 components: emotional and psychological support, direct assistance with career and professional development, and role modeling; (3) is personal in nature, involving direct interaction; (4) emphasizes the mentor's greater experience, influence, and achievement within an organization; and (5) is reciprocal, designed to enrich the professional and personal lives of both mentor and mentee. Importantly, mentorship is not just for the most junior in the medical profession; advancing career levels present different learning needs that can be addressed through ongoing mentorship.

While most interactions occur within the workplace, many find that meals, social events, shared hobbies, and professional meetings provide additional opportunities for career guidance. The effective mentoring relationship assumes an always professional and nonsexual, rather than personal, focus; mutual trust and respect allow for disagreement. **Table 39-2** illustrates the key qualities of a good mentor.

The best way to pair mentors with mentees is unknown. Mandatory mentor assignments engage all mentees in some form of advising, thus addressing vexing gaps in mentoring among physicians. There may be other advantages of formal mentoring programs over informal mentoring. More effective and enduring mentor–mentee relationships may result from independent partnerships.

MENTORING MODELS

Mentoring models include: (1) the traditional model of mentorship as a one-to-one relationship spanning an entire professional career at one academic institution, (2) collaborative group mentoring, (3) mentorship between one mentee and multiple mentors, (4) integrated peer mentoring, (5) networking at annual society meetings, (6) mentoring from a distance (telementoring), and combinations thereof. **Table 39-3** reviews mentoring models and the strengths and weaknesses of each.

A "closed model" of mentoring follows the rigid construct of a protégé who receives teaching and counsel from an older master

TABLE 39-3 Mentoring Models

	Description	Advantages	Disadvantages	Best Uses
Closed models: mentee seeks out mentoring from a senior person				
Assignment model	A new resident or junior faculty is immediately assigned a senior faculty member as his or her mentor by senior leadership in the department. The assignment is either chosen randomly, or may be based on information gleaned from prior interviews, application forms, or essays. Gender or race may factor into the dyad assignment.	Guarantees mentee engagement with a senior person. Mentor–mentee pairs can be matched for mutual personal or professional interests or gender.	Risks pairing participants who have little natural or mutual affinity. Mentee receives only one mentor's perspective.	Mentee preferring or requiring a mentor within the first several months of beginning an internship or career. Mentee starting at a large and multifaceted institution where informal selection of a mentor may take significant time to form.
Choice model	A new resident or junior faculty is required to choose a more senior faculty to serve as a mentor within several months of beginning employment.	Allows some self-selection between participants, which may be especially important for women and minority mentees.	Risks leaving a mentee without a mentor during an often stressful transition. Mentee receives only one mentor's perspective.	Mentee with issues of a sensitive or confidential nature seeking a confidante. Mentee with specific racial/ethnic preferences.
Open models: mentee seeks mentoring from multiple sources				
Multiple mentor model	A new resident or junior faculty actively seeks multiple mentors from different places, career levels, or career paths.	Provides flexibility and broad expertise for the mentee.	May create many "diluted" relationships. Less continuity with a given mentor. No central senior overseer, thus relies heavily on the mentee's level of self-motivation and management.	Mentee not certain of career trajectory and wants advice from senior faculty in multiple domains (teaching, administration, research, clinical) Mentee undertaking a project spanning several disciplines or departments.
Layered model	A new resident or junior faculty is immediately assigned to a group of similar-experienced peers, all of whom share one mentor. This mentor holds periodic meetings (attended by all mentees) to discuss topics. The mentor then further guides mentees to individual faculty for specific advising.	Allows some guided peer-to-peer mentoring and provides a flexible and broad network of potential senior advisors. Safe environment for idea sharing.	Provides less individually tailored and private counsel. Multiple mentee format may diminish mentor advocacy for individual mentee; output relies heavily on the mentee's level of self-motivation and management.	Mentee with undifferentiated career focus. Mentee desiring both a general mentor, and involvement in peer groups and projects spanning many disciplines. Junior mentee wishing to enhance networking.
Facilitated group/ Collaborative mentoring model	Residents or junior faculty attend structured group forums facilitated by senior faculty. Sessions include skill development, career planning, scholarly writing, role play, videotaping, group discussion, peer and facilitator feedback, narrative writing, and self-reflection.	Allows education across broad content areas relevant to junior mentees, and provides a broad network of potential senior advisors.	Provides less individually tailored and private counsel, and lacks content and scheduling flexibility. No central senior overseer, thus relies heavily on the mentee's level of self-motivation and management.	Junior faculty seeking to strengthen fundamental junior faculty skills in teaching, research, and publication. Junior faculty wishing to gain a broad understanding of the expertise and opportunities available at their institution.

due to assignment on initiation (assigned model), or due to more natural formation of a mentoring relationship within an expected time frame (choice model). "Open models" of mentoring occur when a proactive protégé seeks out mentoring from different sources.

Peer mentoring can serve important advising and networking functions. Peer mentoring can sometimes be at least as effective as the traditional master-protégé construct. The nonhierarchical nature of peer mentoring addresses problematic issues in senior-junior mentoring relationships such as power, dominance, dependency, and transference. Peer mentors also may be more readily available and provide a way to gain different perspectives and current information on diverse opportunities, especially in a young specialty such as Hospital Medicine, which has relatively few practicing senior hospitalists.

TIPS FOR SUCCESSFULLY MENTORING HOSPITALIST CLINICIAN-EDUCATORS

Successful mentoring behaviors for clinician-educators differ at each step in the mentoring relationship: preparing for mentoring, approaching a mentor for the first time, ongoing mentoring, and ending the mentorship. Overarching goals in mentoring clinician-educators include personal and career satisfaction and professional advancement. Novice mentors and junior faculty should receive structured faculty development to learn a core set of mentoring skills. **Table 39-4** elaborates further on key elements for success at each phase of mentorship.

One important element of successful mentoring is self-reflection, a key means by which both participants initiate personal, relationship, and practice improvements. By the mentor role modeling self-reflection and actively promoting self-reflection within the mentee, the mentee may internalize an important skill of a self-directed lifelong learner. The goal of self-reflection is to identify specific short- and long-term goals to aid future career development. To achieve this, the mentor needs to guide the mentee so the mentee can articulate personal strengths and weaknesses, and then transform the self-assessments into concrete goals for future career development.

PRACTICE POINT

- One important element of successful mentoring is self-reflection, a key means by which both participants initiate personal, relationship, and practice improvements. By the mentor role modeling self-reflection and actively promoting self-reflection within the mentee, the mentee may internalize an important skill of a self-directed lifelong learner. The goal of self-reflection is to identify specific short- and long-term goals to aid future career development. To achieve this, the mentor needs to guide the mentee so the mentee can articulate personal strengths and weaknesses and then transform the self-assessments into concrete goals for future career development.

For example, a junior faculty hospitalist might be an outstanding clinician and a great bedside role model, but may not receive strong evaluations of his or her didactic teaching. A mentor would first lead the mentee to recognize these areas of relative strength and weakness. Then, the mentor might suggest specific ways for the mentee to improve didactic teaching skill, or may encourage the mentee to seek experiences that maximize the mentee's strengths and

TABLE 39-4 Best-Practice Behaviors for Successful Mentoring

	Mentee	Mentor
Preparing for mentoring	• Assess your competencies in the roles you currently hold (preparation of clinician-educator portfolio may facilitate this). • As specifically as possible, define career goals (eg to be a successful clerkship director, to obtain funding for educational research, to achieve national recognition). • List specific activities and experiences you seek.* • Identify specific questions pertaining to the kinds of help you think you need. • Determine the key personal and professional qualities you desire or value in a mentor (see Table 39-2). • Consider seeking a mentor 1 level above you, and another 2 levels above your current career level.	• Be honest in assessing your availability to commit to a new mentee. • Consider requesting and reviewing an updated CV from your prospective mentee prior to meeting. • Enumerate the particular areas in which you might be of value to a mentee.*
First meeting	• Explain why you have chosen to approach the potential mentor. • Explain how the potential mentor has already helped you. • Explain your level-specific career goals and the similarities you see between your goals and the potential mentor's work. • Explain your current academic role and what you think you might need in terms of advice and guidance. • Verbally recognize and appreciate a potential mentor's time and energy. • Ensure you have the mentor's updated contact information and ask which method of communication he or she prefers. • Consider sending a thank you note after your first meeting.	• Befriend the mentee to diffuse the power dynamic. • Start with open-ended questions (eg, "What do you hope to gain from our work together?") • Be honest regarding your commitment and ability to effectively mentor that individual. • Recognize your limitations and provide alternative resources to those whom you cannot effectively mentor. • Summarize and confirm (eg "It sounds like I could best help you now by…Is this true?") • Ensure you have the mentee's updated contact information and ask which method of communication he or she prefers.

(continued)

TABLE 39-4 Best-Practice Behaviors for Successful Mentoring ***(continued)***

	Mentee	Mentor
Ongoing mentoring	• Determine the structure of meetings (eg, e-mail, in person, telephone). • When in doubt, always take the initiative. • Prepare and set the agenda for mentoring meetings. • Ensure meetings with your mentor are scheduled at regular intervals. • Keep your mentor aware of changes in goals, barriers encountered, and progress achieved in reaching your goals. • Seek and accept challenges and feedback. • Have realistic expectations of the mentee–mentor relationship. • Consider creating and following a written checklist or timeline to track progress.	• Assist mentee in establishing goals. • Listen to your mentee actively and patiently. • Refine mentee's specific goals, and push mentee for his or her "dreams" (what may seem unobtainable to mentee may seem achievable to you). • Hold mentee to high but obtainable standards. • Advocate for mentee. • Inform the mentee about new opportunities and suggest alternate resources for information about academic opportunities, political culture, and networking. • Protect the mentee from possible threats. • Use your experience, clout, and influence to serve as a champion for the mentee. • When you are unable to meet mentee's needs, refer mentee to another mentor. • Foster mentee development. • Commit your time and energy on a regular, ongoing, and flexible basis. • Recognize different mentee learning styles and tailor your approach: some mentees may need direct, task-oriented assistance, while others need help with problem solving or articulating ideas. • Assist in the mentee's identity development; consider how you will "wean" the mentee. • Collaborate with mentee if this helps promote mentee's agenda, not yours. • Credit the mentee for his or her diligence and creative output (includes authorship or grants). • Provide honest feedback in a constructive and caring manner. • Serve as role model and confidante. • Exhibit high professional and moral character. • Be responsive and available. • Follow through on promises. • Maintain confidentiality (except in rare circumstances as required by law, such as harassment, danger to self/others, professional misconduct).
Ongoing mentoring		• Seek out feedback from mentee. • Be nonjudgmental, accepting, and sensitive to personal differences (ie, gender, culture, or age-related differences). • Be comfortable sharing personal knowledge (medical and nonmedical), including failures.
Ending the mentoring relationship	• Talk about when the relationship should end (eg, a certain time point, or once certain goals are achieved). • Ask for advice on future advisors or mentors. • Thank your mentor.	• Talk about when the relationship should end (eg a certain time point, or once certain goals are achieved). • Offer suggestions for future mentors or directions of interest. • Thank your mentee.

*Common mentoring goals include: assistance with grant-writing or manuscript preparation, advice for promotion and advancement (including advice unique to women and minorities), building a network, research collaboration, teaching skills, negotiation, enhancing educator portfolio, improving understanding of organization politics, oral presentation skills, and work–life balance.

minimize exposure to areas of weakness. Importantly, the mentor should periodically request the mentee to evaluate the quality and effectiveness of the mentoring relationship.

Key questions to ask oneself include: What do I perceive as my strengths and weaknesses? How do these strengths and weaknesses compare with how others have evaluated me? What activities provide me the greatest source of career satisfaction? What activities would I like to do more or less of? Which senior faculty member's career path do I want to emulate? What specific roles do I see myself in within the next 3–5 years? 5–10 years? What obstacles stand in the way of my career goals? What skills or knowledge do I need to acquire to address my weaknesses or to be able to realize my career goals? What are the goals and vision of my supervisor (eg, chairperson) and do my interests and strengths align with these goals? If not, how can I demonstrate my value to the division or group?

DOCUMENTING CLINICIAN-EDUCATOR ACCOMPLISHMENTS: THE CLINICIAN-EDUCATOR PORTFOLIO

The clinician-educator "portfolio" enumerates and organizes a faculty member's educational activities and achievements for the purposes of academic promotion and self-reflection. Traditionally, decisions regarding academic promotion were based on information summarized in a *curriculum vitae (CV)* and letters of recommendation. The educator portfolio adds several elements: a novel structure to capture all clinician-educator activities, including those elements not traditionally captured in a CV; demonstration of the impact of the educator's activities on trainees, peers, the organization, and the field as a whole; and a vehicle for self-reflection.

The concept of the clinician-educator "portfolio" is analogous to an architect's or artist's portfolio. The educator portfolio includes faculty member's educational achievements, which have expanded from classic "teaching" duties to include a broader array of hospitalist activities: clinical duties, teaching and curriculum development, mentoring, scholarly productivity, leadership, and administration including quality improvement and patient safety (**Table 39-5**). Importantly, the portfolio often serves as the basis for professional review, academic promotion, as a "body of work" when meeting prospective employers, and as the basis for self-reflection. Ideally, the portfolio's format aligns directly with institutional promotion criteria, thus allowing chairpersons and promotion committees (members of which may not be clinicians) to appreciate the value of distinct activities.

Importantly, the portfolio is intended to complement, and not replace, the curriculum vitae. Whereas the curriculum vitae serves as a detailed outline, the portfolio goes further to exhibit the quality and breadth of accomplishments. For example, an effective portfolio often contains the actual curricula that a clinician-educator developed, manuscripts and miniaturized poster presentations that a faculty coauthored with mentees, a summary of numerical evaluations of the faculty by trainees, and detailed information on mentee outcomes resulting from the faculty member's mentorship. Commonly, a narrative on the faculty's medical education philosophy and career goals is included. Continuous maintenance of a portfolio ensures that important activities are captured as they occur. To emphasize the most significant accomplishments, we suggest a limit of 10 pages without attachments.

TABLE 39-5 Elements of a Clinician-Educator Portfolio

Category	Examples to Support this
Clinical activities	List of clinical duties and average time per week spent on each
Direct teaching	List of teaching activities (ward or ICU teaching, lectures, small group facilitation, resident report, clinic precepting, visiting professorships)
	Summary of evaluations from ward rotation, ideally with comparison to peer averages
	Teaching awards
Curricular design • Instructional development	Revision or implementation of new course, rotation, or program (eg, procedural simulation training, journal club curriculum, homeless clinic rotation) and how participation in course was evaluated
	Outcome assessments (eg, evaluations from course participants; end-of-course test scores or observed procedural competence)
Mentoring • Interns and residents • Medical students • Junior faculty • Peers	List of mentee names by academic year, with hours spent mentoring each and outcomes of mentoring (eg, implemented global health rotation in residency; nominated mentee for regional award; helped determine career choice, etc.)
	Collaborations with mentees: manuscripts, curricular change, research
	Participation in formal mentoring program locally, regionally, or nationally
	Formal evaluations by mentees, of the clinician-educator's mentoring abilities.
Educational administration and leadership	Admissions committees (for residency or medical school), including interviewing activity
	Course or clerkship director
	Education or curriculum design and oversight committees
	Dean's office or student affairs position
	Evaluation committee
	Program directing
	Elected positions and committee involvement in professional societies for medical education activity (eg, Association of Program Directors or Clerkship Directors in Internal Medicine; education committee work within professional society, such as Society of Hospital Medicine)
	Faculty development leader (eg, taught small group of faculty on ultrasound-guided central venous catheter insertion)
Educational scholarly activity	Grants for education research or education activity (eg, funding to design new curriculum)
	Publications (peer-reviewed publications, book chapters, editorials, opinion pieces, letters)
	Editing and peer reviewing of grants or manuscripts related to education research
	Test question writer (eg, for American Board of Internal Medicine or In Training Exam)
	Posters or oral presentations involving educational topics at society meetings
	Workshop moderator or presenter at society meeting (eg, promoting quality improvement activity in residency)
Hospital administration	Committee work: role on committee (eg, member, chairperson) and specific activities for that committee
	Quality improvement activities
	Patient safety activities (eg, peer review committee, root cause analyses)

TIPS FOR SUCCESSFULLY MENTORING RESIDENTS

Existing literature on mentoring in residency describes the value residents place on mentoring and the successful aspects of the resident-faculty mentorship relationship. Residents rated the following mentoring needs in decreasing order of importance: career advice, research options, confidential source of support, networking, role modeling of work-life balance, and faculty interaction. A case-control study of internal medicine attending physicians identified a few desirable attributes of faculty role models. Compared with a group of teaching attendings who were not given special recognition by house staff, internal medicine attending role models spent more time teaching and in actively fostering relationships with house officers, placed greater emphasis on the doctor–patient relationship and psychosocial aspects of care, and had received more formal training in teaching. Encouragingly, several of these behaviors may be modifiable with focused faculty development.

Other ideal mentor attributes include maintaining confidentiality; being approachable, accessible, and nonjudgmental; getting to know the mentee on a personal level; promoting the mentee's goals over the mentor's; providing opportunities for the mentee ("opening doors"); and encouraging self-reflection. Given the importance residents place on confidentiality in mentoring, program directors or other direct supervisors may not be ideal mentors, though they will subsume many of the advice and role-model functions of mentors.

Formally assigning mentors makes it easier for residents to identify mentors. Faculty development around mentoring and rewarding faculty may improve willingness of faculty to mentor residents. According to Ramanan, et al, meeting with mentors just twice a year satisfies residents, lessening concerns about time commitments.

Taken together, existing literature supports the following as ingredients for successful resident mentoring, as outlined in **Table 39-6**: formal assignment of faculty mentors that considers the needs of women and minorities; dedicated time for house staff and mentors to meet, at least twice annually; faculty development to augment mentoring skills; and buy-in from department heads that may include protected time, recognizing mentoring when considering promotions, and mentoring awards.

TABLE 39-6 Strategies to Promote Successful Mentoring of Trainees

- Formal assignments of faculty mentors that takes into consideration the needs of women and minorities
- Dedicated time for housestaff and mentors to meet: formal meetings at least twice annually with readily available access to mentor at other times
- Buy-in from department chairperson:
  - Ensure protected faculty time for mentoring
  - Establish bonuses or awards for successful mentoring
  - Explicitly recognize mentoring as criteria for faculty promotion
- Faculty development to augment mentoring skills around the following common topics for house staff mentees:
  - Helping residents apply for jobs after residency:
    - Preparing a curriculum vitae
    - Focusing the job search
    - Interviewing skills
    - Communication with potential employers
    - Negotiating strategies
    - Timeline
  - Assisting residents with the fellowship application process:
    - Advantages to applying during second- versus third-year of residency
    - Fellowship match through ERAS (how the process works, key deadlines)
    - Selecting faculty to write letters of recommendation
    - Preparing personal statements and curriculum vitae
    - Selecting programs to apply to (reputation, location, unique program aspects, when to consider programs outside the match)
    - Elements sought by fellowship directors
    - Interviewing skills
    - Lifestyle considerations in the specialty
  - Mentoring resident scholarly activity:
    - Preparing a clinical vignette abstract, poster, or case report
    - Giving oral presentations and speaking publicly
    - Establishing a quality improvement project
    - Writing effective review articles
    - Providing potential networking opportunities locally, regionally, nationally
    - Involving residents in professional societies
    - Submitting to the institutional review board
    - Providing resources for statistical support
  - Optimizing clinical and professional development:
    - Selection of elective rotations
    - Ethics, integrity, and professionalism
    - Interpersonal skills with physicians, nurses, and staff
    - Time management, organization, and efficiency
  - Providing resources for handling difficult situations (burnout, psychiatric illness, substance abuse, interpersonal conflicts, family/social stressors, career angst, financial stress, and medical errors)

SPECIAL MENTORING RELATIONSHIPS IN ACADEMIC MEDICINE: WOMEN AND MINORITIES

Women and minorities face hurdles in academic advancement, and the lack of mentors who mirror their personal and professional experiences may contribute to this problem. In a survey of full-time female internal medicine faculty, women with mentors published more and reported greater overall career satisfaction. Many studies detail the lower incidence of mentorship among women in academic medicine compared to men. Women are much less likely than men to describe a relationship with a mentor as a positive experience that influenced their careers. Additionally, compared to male mentees, female mentees were more likely to select women mentors, an important point considering there are fewer women than men among senior medical faculty and therefore a smaller pool of available women mentors. Mentoring, including using less traditional models, has been suggested as a way to address women's lack of advancement in academic medicine. Other reports have not found gender discrepancies in mentoring nor same-gender mentors to be essential.

How race and ethnicity contribute to forming mentor relationships has not been as well studied as gender, but researchers have found that members of traditionally underrepresented groups tend to be drawn to those who are racially similar. Blacks more than whites are willing to search beyond their immediate environment to seek same-race mentoring if it is not available locally, and like female mentors, minority mentors are in high demand. Increasing gender and minority diversity in medical schools make it even more likely that women and minority faculty will be called upon to be mentors. Successful mentoring of these groups holds promise for increasing their representation in medical school faculties.

CONCLUSION

Mentoring is as old as the field of medicine. Although quantifiable evidence of the value of mentoring is only beginning to emerge, research shows many benefits for the mentee and mentor, and even for the institution and profession. Mentoring may influence the career choice of trainees and junior faculty (including the decision to enter internal medicine or pursue an academic career), advance the career of clinician-educators (including women and minorities), improve retention of junior faculty in academic positions, and enrich the professional lives of both mentor and mentee.

Formally assigning mentors to junior clinician-educators and residents ensures that all mentees get some mentoring. No single mentoring model is superior, so the mentoring pair should use one that best meets the mentee's specific goals. Clinician-educator mentees should be encouraged to assemble their activities and achievements into an educator portfolio, a tool designed to enhance their chances of promotion at academic medical centers. Mentoring residents should ensure confidentiality (except in extraordinary circumstances) and therefore someone other than a program director or direct supervisor may best serve this function. Resident mentoring should focus on career planning and preparedness, networking, identifying opportunities for scholarly activity, role modeling of work-life balance, and supporting the resident.

SUGGESTED READINGS

Coates WC, Hobgood CD, Birnbaum A, Farell SE. Faculty development: academic opportunities for Emergency Medicine faculty on education career tracks. *Acad Emerg Med.* 2003;10:1113–1117.

Emans SJ. Community of Mentors, Guidelines for Mentors. Children's Hospital Boston, Office of Faculty Development, 2009. http://www.childrenshospital.org/cfapps/research/data_admin/Site2209/mainpageS2209P1.html. Accessed October 5, 2009.

Farrell SE, Digioia NM, Broderick KB, Coates WC. Mentoring for Clinical-Educators. *Acad Emerg Med.* 2004;11:1346–1350.

Garmel GM. Mentoring medical students in academic Emergency Medicine. *Acad Emerg Med.* 2004;11:1351–1357.

Ramanan R, Phillips R, Davis RB, Silen W, Reede J. Mentoring in medicine: keys to satisfaction. *Am J Med.* 2002;112:336–341.

Ramani S, Gruppen L, Kachur EK. Twelve tips for developing effective mentors. *Medical Teacher.* 2006;28:404–408.

The Educator's Portfolio, Academy of Medical Educators. University of California at San Francisco. February 2010. http://medschool.ucsf.edu/academy/Educators_Portfolio. Accessed October 7, 2009.

Zerzan JT, Hess R, Schur E, et al. Making the most of mentors: a guide for mentees. *Acad Med.* 2009;84:140–144.

REFERENCES

1. Sambunjak D, Straus SE, Marusic A. Mentoring in Academic Medicine: A Systematic Review. *JAMA.* 2006;296:1103–1115.
2. Jacobi M. Mentoring and undergraduate academic success: a literature review. *Rev Educ Res.* 1991;61:505–532.

CHAPTER 40

Cultural Sensitivity Training

Desiree Lie, MD, MSED
Solomon S. Liao, MD

INTRODUCTION

Cultural competence has been defined as "the ability to understand and respond effectively to the cultural and linguistic needs of patients in the health care encounter" or "a set of attitudes, skills, behaviors, and policies that enable organizations and staff to work effectively in cross-cultural situations. It reflects the ability to acquire and use knowledge of the health-related beliefs, attitudes, practices, and communication patterns of clients and their families to improve services, strengthen programs, increase community participation, and close the gaps in health status among diverse population groups." Cultural competency training recognizes both the individual patient-doctor relationship and population-based perspectives.

Despite published reports of disparities in health care for the uninsured, African American, and Hispanic population relative to Caucasians and those with private insurance, most graduates of U.S. internal residency programs have not received adequate training in culture competency at the start of their careers. Two specific accreditation standards (ED-21 and ED-22) now require the teaching of cross-cultural issues in medical schools, and states have begun to legislate inclusion of this teaching in continuing medical education (CME) for physicians to better address health care needs of the diverse U.S. population. An integrated, rather than stand alone, curricular strategy is considered the most effective way to deliver this training across the continuum of medical education. The Association of American Medical Colleges (AAMC) has provided a framework to isolate key domains and learning objectives that recognize under addressed issues within cultural competency teaching and to guide faculty. The AAMC recently revised six domains identified as: health disparities, bias and stereotyping, community strategies, cross-cultural communication skills, working with interpreters, and the culture of medicine, with the first three being least addressed by most schools. Attending faculty, fellows, or residents should integrate teaching in the 6 domains, take steps to assess teaching impact and improve future self-directed learning.

Most educational research supports the case-based, precepting approach as more effective than the formal lecture-based didactic method during clinical training. Despite limited time to provide didactic teaching, frequent direct contact with learners presents informal or hidden opportunities for "teachable moments" that inevitably occur throughout the workday. This chapter will focus on ways to integrate teaching into direct patient care activities and identify "teachable moments" that build on learners' existing knowledge and skills. Case studies will be used to (1) provide a framework to address cultural competency teaching, (2) identify potential missed opportunities for teaching, (3) demonstrate learner- and patient-centered strategies to integrate the teaching of cultural competence into the hospitalist rotation, (4) review methods for assessing and giving feedback to learners, and (5) provide resources to help faculty to improve the teaching of cross-cultural medicine.

CASE 1: ADDRESSING HEALTH DISPARITIES

Health disparities are differences in the prevalence, etiology, presentation of disease, and access to care that result in unequal outcomes for different groups of people. They can be attributed to the patient (attitudes, adherence, education, beliefs, and health literacy), the physician (lack of knowledge, bias, poor cultural skills) and the health system (insurance, hospitals, neighborhoods, access

CASE 40-1

TWO PATIENTS, SAME MEDICAL PROBLEM

Student SS presents a 45-year-old African American single mother with left ventricular dysfunction secondary to severe hypertension unresponsive to multiple drug regimens. Increasing shortness of breath and recurrent left chest pain brought her to the emergency department, where she was noted to have a blood pressure on admission of 210/98 mm Hg.

Student WM presents a 60-year-old white male smoker on a prepaid health plan. With history of multiple cardiovascular risk factors, he developed congestive heart failure 2 years ago. He is now functionally limited, lives alone, and receives disability income. His primary care physician's office directly admits him to the hospital for worsening dyspnea on exertion, progressive orthopnea, and bilateral leg edema.

Both patients had physical exam findings, chest x-rays, and B-type natriuretic peptide (BNP) levels consistent with acute heart failure. Acute myocardial infarction was successfully ruled out for both patients and both patients received loop diuretics. The attending recommends medication changes to optimize their heart failure management. The attending then moves on to the third admission of the night.

Five Minute precepting model

What are the missed teaching opportunities for culturally competent patient care here?

How else could the attending have responded to the students?

What teaching strategies can be used to facilitate learning about health disparities?

Evidence-based assignment

Before the next morning's rounds both students present a summary of one systematic review and one randomized trial addressing the black-white disparity in heart failure but report that they could not find a clinical practice guideline that addressed race.

---

to care, bias). Disparities resulting in adverse outcomes affect many patient groups including ethnic minorities, rural populations, the elderly, the young and those with disabilities, different sexual orientation, or religious beliefs. Recent research has uncovered a myriad of ethnic and gender disparities in the process and outcomes of care by physicians and hospitals. Physicians can reduce disparities in their own practices and communities by recognizing vulnerable populations and seeking opportunities to improve screening and diagnosis, patient education, and access to care for the underserved. See Chapter 3, Health Care Disparities.

QUESTIONS

- What are the missed teaching opportunities for culturally competent patient care?
- How else could the attending have responded to the students?
- What teaching strategies can be used to facilitate learning about health disparities?

This attending failed to use the example of two patients with a similar problem as an opportunity to teach about potential sources of disparity in heart failure outcomes. Using Socratic questioning to engage the students' interest in the topic, the attending might have framed specific questions as follows:

- (*Asking for information*): "Do you know if there are differences in risk for heart failure between African American and white patients? Are you aware of differences between Latinos, Native Americans, and Asians?"
- (*Open-ended questions*): "What are your thoughts about the long-term prognosis for these 2 patients?" "Are there differences in patient satisfaction between hospitalized African American and white patients? What factors might influence patient satisfaction?"
- (*Combination questions*): "What are some management strategies to ensure the best outcome for these two patients? Are they different because of the patient's race or insurance status?"
- (*Prediction questions*): "What is the impact of health insurance or the lack of insurance on their health?" "What is the data relating to neighborhood dimensions that may affect health? What if one of these patients was homeless?"
- (*Extension questions*): "What else can you do to improve care for these 2 patients?" "If you were given a grant to conduct cardiovascular research in health disparities, what would be your hypothesis for a new study? If you were a health policy maker how would you distribute funding to reduce this disparity?"
- (*Action question*): "What would you do if you were their primary care doctor?"
- (*Summarizing questions*): "What inferences can we make about health disparities and their causes from these two cases? How would you summarize what we have learned from this discussion?"

Knowledge gaps or inability to answer questions could generate learning using an evidence-based assignment. The attending might ask a search question, such as "Does race affect long-term outcomes of myocardial infarction, hospitalization, or mortality for patients hospitalized with their first episode of heart failure?" In preparation for the next morning's rounds the students would perform a focused literature search for the best and most recent practice guidelines or studies to present as practice pearls for reducing racial disparities in heart failure care. The students may be asked to define neighborhoods and report back on specific data about neighborhoods and homelessness in their city and how different boundaries carry different risks related to hepatitis, diabetes, and other diseases. The attending might explore the ethics of distributive justice, a discussion of how insurance coverage impacts health, and how physicians can address social determinants of health. This attending has now planted the seed of scientific inquiry into health disparities as a legitimate health outcomes research topic and an important health policy issue.

CASE 2: RECOGNIZING AND ADDRESSING BIAS AND STEREOTYPING

First noted in a study comparing the likelihood of referral of African American versus white, and male versus female patients, for angiography and more recently observed for thrombolysis decision-making, unconscious physician bias can potentially negatively impact clinical decision making despite evidence for best practice. Implicit bias against "fat people" among health care providers has been well documented and recognizing unconscious bias is one way to prevent the bias from adversely affecting outcomes of care.

ASSIGNMENT, FOLLOWED BY 1:1 OBSERVATION AND FEEDBACK

After assigning a few obese patients to the student, the attending observes a 10-minute counseling session by the student at the bedside of a patient before discharge. At the end he turned and asked the patient "So, how do you feel about losing weight? What will you do differently now?" The patient replies, "No doctor here has asked me about what I am willing to give up and what I cannot give up and shown such understanding about my emotional struggles with food. Maxwell has visited me every day and knows every detail about my diet and lifestyle now. Can I follow up with him?" The student smiles and says "Of course. I am in ambulatory medicine the next 6 weeks. Let me help you make an appointment." Thus, by being nonjudgmental and giving the student permission to recognize his own bias, the attending has also improved the student's skills in motivational counseling and given him new confidence in caring for obese patients. The likelihood of future self-directed learning in the student may also have increased.

CASE 40-2

NEGATIVE ATTITUDES ABOUT OBESITY

A third-year clerkship student, MT, presents a case of a 45-year-old obese, hypertensive man admitted 2 days ago with chest pain to rule out acute coronary syndrome. He now has no symptoms or signs of cardiac disease and his cardiac workup, including a stress echocardiogram, are negative. When asked about a management plan, the student responds "I really think this patient's problem is his obesity and he should not have been admitted just because he was so anxious. It's a waste of our scarce resources to manage these patients so aggressively when they refuse to lose weight." The attending ignores this comment and asks the student when he would discharge the patient.

Socratic questioning

What is the missed teaching opportunity for cultural competence here?

How else could the attending have responded to the student?

What teaching strategies can be used to help the student recognize that provider attitudes and bias and stereotyping impact patient outcomes?

QUESTIONS

In this second case, the attending missed the opportunity to identify bias and stereotyping and to teach about the impact of provider attitudes on patient outcomes. While demonstrating competence at presenting a history and physical examination, the student expressed a personal opinion revealing his feelings about obese patients. The attending could have explored the basis of the student's remark (professionalism), uncovered misconceptions about the management of acute chest pain (knowledge deficit), and lack of awareness about approaches to obesity management and the social determinants of illness (attitude). The 5-minute precepting model uses the following steps to address the student's learning needs:

- *Positive reinforcement*: "That was a well organized, focused, and pertinent presentation."
- *Probing question*: "Why do you think he has not lost weight?"
- *A commitment*: "If you were his primary doctor, what would you do to address his obesity?"
- *Correction of a mistake*: "The reasons we admitted him were the following. . . ."
- *Constructive feedback and teaching general principles*: "When we next see an obese patient, let's use the method you suggest (or that you do more research to find out about), to elicit his reasons for not losing weight and see if we can address motivation."

The educator might explore the student's negative bias toward obesity and how negative perceptions of the student as a professional who dislikes him may affect the patient's compliance. The attending might self-reflect by sharing "all of us have biases, some unconscious. I keep a private journal to reflect on these feelings and it helps me maintain my positive outlook and focus on the patient's best interests."

Follow-up strategies include assigning the student to

- perform a literature search on behavioral, pharmacologic, and surgical approaches to weight management, the impact of provider bias on patient behaviors and attitudes, or the impact of neighborhood on obesity;
- present "best practice" pearls to the team;
- use this information to obtain a detailed social history that may uncover risk factors for obesity; and
- care for more obese patients with the explicit goal of practicing ways to improve patient adherence to lifestyle advice and other interventions.

Evaluation would require direct observation of his counseling skills and ability to conduct motivational interviewing. While his internal attitude toward obese patients may not change, the student should be encouraged to demonstrate professional behaviors that enable patients to recognize obesity as a health risk and provide them with additional resources to enhance weight reduction.

CASE 3: CROSS-CULTURAL COMMUNICATION SKILLS/USING AN INTERPRETER

In the United States, one in five patients are reported to have difficulty communicating with their physicians, which leads to lower adherence and poor health-seeking behaviors resulting in poorer health outcomes. The problem is even greater among those who are not English-proficient. Federal law prohibits discrimination by language proficiency and some states such as California now mandate interpreter services in the health care setting under a language assistance bill. Improving language access has been shown to lead to improved care transitions and health outcomes in different settings.

CASE 40-3

BIAS AND STEREOTYPING

The attending hears a conversation between the clerkship student and intern. Student ML asks in a challenging tone "Why is this patient not receiving a narcotic medication for his renal pain like our other patients? He told me in Spanish his pain is 9 out of 10 and not relieved by the ibuprofen, and even I with my 'Spanglish' could understand that." Intern SM says "Delgado looks like a gang-banger demanding narcotics. I suspect he is drug-seeking. The interpreter was not available when I talked with him so I could not get much of what he was saying." Since she has not seen the patient yet, the attending leaves to see another patient.

Health care team dynamics

What is the potential teaching opportunity for cultural and linguistic competence here?

How else should the fellow respond to what she heard?

What teaching strategies can facilitate learning about cross-cultural communication and the need for working with interpreters?

Conflict management and role modeling

The intern conducts an interview working with an interpreter, incorporating the Kleinman questions and the LEARN model. The team initiated pain management with a morphine patient-controlled analgesic (PCA) pump. At the briefing, the interpreter shares information that this patient just lost his job, will soon lose his health insurance, and has concerns about how to care for his family. A Spanish-speaking social worker subsequently sees him. Both trainees volunteer to explore reasons behind variable use of interpreter services at their hospital and solutions to this problem. They also offer to jointly present the topic of language access and health outcomes at the next medical grand rounds with the hospital interpreters in this presentation. Thus, they disseminate what they have learned to the hospitalist group that includes residents, fellows, and faculty, with the potential to both benefit in-hospital patients and satisfy continuing medical education requirements.

PRACTICE POINT

- Role modeling reinforces those behaviors that are effective cross-cultural communication skills in an explicit way before, during, or after encounters. The ultimate goal will be that learners will adopt those behaviors in future.

Feedback

1. **Self-reflection.** During a private feedback session with the intern about his teaching skills, start with self-rating to assess the intern's insight into his own teaching skills."How effective do you think you were at teaching the student? Why do you think so?"
2. **Positive reinforcement.** Follow with an appropriate feedback sandwich. "It's really great that you took time out to explain what you were doing for this patient."
3. **Identification of specific behaviors and specific suggestions for improvement.** "However, not working with an interpreter and making an assumption based on his appearance may convey that you are making important clinical decisions without adequate information. Next time I suggest that you qualify the decision not to prescribe narcotics by letting the student know that you will consult with an attending and also request for a certified interpreter during the patient's hospitalization before making a final decision about narcotics."

■ QUESTIONS

Bi-directional-feedback. Close with "Would you like to summarize what we discussed today? How can I do better in giving you feedback?"

- What is the potential teaching opportunity for cultural and linguistic competence here?
- How else should the fellow respond to what she heard?
- What teaching strategies can facilitate learning about cross-cultural communication and the need for working with interpreters?

Case 3 presents a missed opportunity to teach cross-cultural and linguistic skills to both the intern and student and to improve pain management. Waiting until rounds and soliciting feedback on how each team member would manage the patient's pain may reveal differing opinions. However, reflecting "the culture of medicine," more junior students are likely to defer to their senior colleagues and choose not to disagree, and the teachable moment will have passed.

An alternative approach, taking on the role of the physician in charge of the team and the patient, might use **conflict management** tools to elicit common care goals for pain relief, treatment, and early discharge in a nonconfrontational, compassionate manner. Guiding questions about this patient's pain assessment explore ways to achieve the best patient outcomes. "How shall we resolve our lack of agreement concerning his pain?" An interviewing tool, such as the *Kleinman questions*, solicits the patient's perspective of his illness. Examples include "What do you think is the cause of your pain? What kind of treatment do you think you should receive? What results do you hope to achieve?" Another communication tool, the **LEARN** (listen, explain, acknowledge, recommend, negotiate) model, can help providers negotiate treatment plans with their patients. **Role modeling** includes reminding the team of the importance of taking the extra time to request the help of a certified medical interpreter by demonstrating how the use of effective interviewing skills of interpreters at the bedside with the team provides new information that is instrumental in pain management. At the end of the interview, a briefing outside the patient's room, including the interpreter's feedback, will reinforce those behaviors that are effective cross-cultural communication skills in an explicit way before, during, or after encounters.The ultimate goal will be that learners will adopt those behaviors in the future.

Feedback to learners should be ongoing and incorporate both positive and constructive components. Teaching combined with proximate and one-on-one feedback to learners given respectfully and in private, often reinforces learning and reflection and is more likely to promote behavior change than teaching alone.

ASSESSING YOUR LEARNERS AND YOUR OWN TEACHING SKILLS

These teaching cases represent teaching opportunities that do not require much additional time or resources. Key outcomes include increased knowledge about health disparities (Case 1), recognizing and reflecting on personal bias (Case 2), and the importance of using interpreters to assist in the delivery of patient-centered care, self-reflection, and providing feedback (Case 3).

Assessing the impact of education on cultural competence remains a challenge in the immediacy of one-on-one precepting and ward round teaching. Clinician-educators can employ several techniques to assess their learners' knowledge, attitudes, and skills that also reflect their own teaching effectiveness. Self-report is the most commonly used technique but may not be entirely objective. For example, an attending can ask after rounds or case presentations "What do you now know about health disparities that you did not know before rounds?" or "Please share one thing that you will do differently when you next interview a patient who does not speak English." Direct observation of skills using behavior checklists is more objective but can be time-consuming. Asking for evaluations from other team members including peers, nurses, and other health professionals can provide a more balanced perspective of the learner but is subject to bias toward social skills assessment rather than medical knowledge or skill assessment. In general, these sources should be used for formative rather than summative evaluation.

TABLE 40-1 Teaching Resources

U.S. Department of Health and Human Services, Office of Minority Health. National standards for culturally and linguistically appropriate services in health care. Washington, DC: 2000. Available at: http://www.omhrc.gov/assets/pdf/checked/finalreport.pdf The Commonwealth Fund, at www.commonwealthfund.org
The Centers for Disease Control and Prevention at www.cdc.gov
National Association of Public Hospitals and Health Systems. "Serving Diverse Communities in Safety Net Hospitals and Health Systems," The Safety Net 2003; 17(3): Fall. http://www.naph.org/Template.cfm?Section=The_Safety_Net_Archive&template=/ContentManagement/ContentDisplay.cfm&ContentID=3407
National Center for Cultural Competence, Georgetown University. "Self-Assessment Checklist for Personnel Providing Primary Health Care Services," http://gucchd.georgetown.edu/nccc/documents/Checklist%20PHC.pdf
Communicating Effectively Through an Interpreter (1998) (Available from the Cross Cultural Health Care Program, 270 South Hanford Street, Suite 100, Seattle, Washington 98134; Phone (206)-860-0329; Website www.xculture.org) Quality Interactions: A Patient-Based Approach to Cross-Cultural Care, Manhattan Cross Cultural Group and Critical Measures, http://www.criticalmeasures.net/cross_cultural/elearning.htm
Delivering Culturally Effective Care for Patients with Diabetes Medical Directions—The Virtual Lecture Hall and Department of Family Medicine, University of Arizona College of Medicine at the Arizona Health Sciences Center, http://www.i-3d.org/Educational_Resources/Other_Resources/Other_resources_3.aspx
Quality Care for Diverse Populations, Video/CD-ROM/Facilitator's Guide, Contributors: five video vignettes depicting simulated physician-patient visits in an office setting as a means to explore ethnic and sociocultural issues found in today's diverse health care environment. Produced by the American Academy of Family Physicians (AAFP), Bureau of Primary Health Care, Health Resources and Services Administration, June 2002. (AAFP Order Dept., 11400 Tomahawk Creek Parkway, Leawood, KS 66211; Phone (800)-944-0000; Fax (913)-906-6075)
Worlds Apart. A Four-Part Series on Cross-Cultural Health care. By Maren Grainger-Monsen, MD, and Julia Haslett, Stanford University, Center for Biomedical Ethics (available from Fanlight Productions, www.fanlight.com)
Unnatural Causes, video vignettes for teaching about health disparities, available at www.unnaturalcauses.org
Working Together to End Racial and Ethnic Disparities: One Physician at a Time, by the American Medical Association; 22-minute DVD featuring interviews with physicians, nurses, and patients who have experienced disparities in health care firsthand. It includes a **CD-ROM** with fact sheets covering components of health care disparities covering: quality of care, trust and stereotyping, cultural competence, language barriers and health literacy. A **Facilitation guide** is also included to stimulate audience discussion about health care disparities. Vignettes are useful for grand rounds, small group discussions, and/or large lectures. Available at http://www.ama-assn.org/ama1/pub/upload/mm/433/health_disp_kit.pdf or call the AMA at (800) 621-8335. Item #OP325305.
Educating Physicians on Controversies in Health (EpoCH) by the American Medical Association is a series of 5-minute informational Web streaming programs (free)—developed by the AMA and targeting primary care physicians. The objective of these programs is to inform physicians about the challenges and controversies at the interface of clinical medicine and public health and to offer possible strategies to address these in their practices. Topics include Racially tailored medicines, Language Barrier in Your Practice Health Care Disparities, Uninformed consent: What can happen when a patient does not understand the information you have provided? http://www.ama-assn.org/ama/pub/category/15369.html

TIPS FOR FACULTY DEVELOPMENT

Busy clinician-educators may keep updated in the area of health disparities and cultural competence by a combination of meeting attendance, self-directed learning, and peer discussion with feedback targeting his or her own areas of learning need. For example, a newly published article in one's professional journal describing racial or socioeconomic disparities could trigger an evidence-based medicine grand round discussion or debate. Statistics from one's own hospital (for example, race or gender-related morbidity data on readmission rates for congestive heart failure) or case reports (involving, for example, adverse outcomes in underserved or vulnerable populations) could trigger a literature review on documented diagnosis related disparities and effective strategies to address condition. Medical librarians may demonstrate techniques for conducting literature searches for health disparities data. Consulting regularly updated Web sites quickly provides useful information about health disparities. Soliciting input from colleagues and evaluations from students of one's own teaching skills in this area can be challenging but often rewarding (**Table 40-1**).

Continuing medical education is available on some Web resources and can be used to update and maintain knowledge and skills. Clinician-educators interested in designing and incorporating specific curricula into their own programs can consult with a diverse set of resources from Web modules, to videos, to CD-ROMs for use in their own classrooms. Lastly, "to teach is to learn twice," and being a speaker for issues of health disparities is another effective method for keeping current in the field.

Hospitalists should be role models by teaching cultural competency to their students and all members of their health care team. Hospitalists can educate trainees and other members of the team that steps to provide additional resources to reduce health care disparities actually improve clinical outcomes, including indicators of quality such as mortality and readmission rate. Hospitalists should take steps to improve the system of care for diverse populations and provide opportunities for trainees to become involved in quality improvement and research relating to disparities in health care. Measurement of performance gaps may become integral to physician education.

PRACTICE POINT

- Hospitalists should be role models by teaching cultural competency to their students and all members of their health care team.

SUGGESTED READINGS

Burgess D, van Ryn M, Dovidio J, Saha S. Reducing racial bias among health care providers: lessons from social-cognitive psychology. *J Gen Intern Med*. 2007;22(6):882–887.

Carter-Pokras, Baquet, What is a health disparity? Public Health Reports, Sept/Oct, 2002.

Flores, G. The impact of medical interpreter services on the quality of health care: A systematic review. *Med Care Res Rev*. 2005;62, 255–299.

Kleinman A, Eisenberg L, Good B. Culture, illness, and care: clinical lessons from anthropologic and cross-cultural research. *Ann of Int Med*. 1978;88:251–258.

Neher JO, Gordon KC, Meyer B, Stevens N. A five-step "microskills" model of clinical teaching. *J Am Board Fam Pract*. 1992;5:419–424.

Ngo-Metzger Q, Sorkin DH, Phillips RS, et al. Providing high-quality care for limited English proficient patients: The importance of language concordance and interpreter use. *J Gen Intern Med*. 2007;22(Suppl 2):324–330.

Ogden J, Flanagan Z. Beliefs about the causes and solutions to obesity: a comparison of GPs and lay people. *Patient Educ Couns* (2008) 71:72–78.

Problems include understanding doctor, feeling doctor listened, had questions but did not ask. Source: The Commonwealth Fund 2001 Health Care Quality Survey, available at www.commonwealthfund.org.

Teachman BA, Brownell KD. Implicit anti-fat bias among health professionals: is anyone immune? *Int J Obes Relat Metab Disord*. 2001;25(10):1525–1531.

Youdelman MK. The medical tongue: U.S. laws and policies on language access. *Health Aff* (Millwood). 2008;27:424–433.

WEB-BASED RESOURCES

Association of American Medical Colleges, available at http://www.aamc.org/meded/tacct/start.htm.

Federal Register: August 8, 2003 68(153):47311–47323; From the Federal Register Online via GPO Accesshttp://wais.access.gpo.gov; DOCID:fr08au03-California Language Assistance Bill, Senate Bill 853 available at: http://www.leginfo.ca.gov/pub/03-04/bill/sen/sb_0851-0900/sb_853_bill_20031009_chaptered.html.

Institute of Medicine. *Crossing the Quality Chasm*. Available at http://www.iom.edu/Reports/2001/Crossing-the-Quality-Chasm-A-New-Health-System-for-the-21st-Century.aspx.

Liaison Committee for Medical Education available at www.lcme.org.

Lie D, Boker J, Crandall S, et al. Faculty and medical student perceptions of cultural competence instruction: a study in seven schools using the Tool for Assessing Cultural Competence Training (TACCT). *Medical Education Online*. 2008:13.

Management Sciences for Health. The Providers' Guide to Quality and Culture. Available at http://erc.msh.org/mainpage.cfm?file=2.1.htm&module=provider&language=English.

U.S. Dept. of Health and Human Services, Think Cultural Health. Available at https://www.thinkculturalhealth.org/cc_legislation.asp.

CHAPTER 41

The Use of Patient Simulation in Medical Training: From Medical School to Clinical Practice

Andrew Nevins, MD, MS
Neil Gesundheit, MD, MPH

INTRODUCTION

During the past 20 years, teaching methods in medical education and clinical practice have shifted from a focus on factual knowledge to an emphasis on problem solving and a deeper understanding of principles. At the same time, there has been a sea change in how medical professionals develop their clinical skills, away from learning by direct patient contact toward simulated learning in which actors portray patients (standardized patients or SPs) or patient cases are reenacted electronically (virtual patients or VPs). Using SPs and virtual environments for clinical encounters reinforces principles that are best learned through tactile/experiential contact, boosts the confidence of the learner, and can enhance patient safety.

Apart from their value in teaching clinical skills, exercises using SPs and VPs can also help assess student proficiency. Most medical educators agree that assessments should cover all essential content and goals of a curriculum, often including mastering facts, practical skills, and problem solving. SP exercises have been used for more than 30 years in the U.S. to assess the ability of a student to conduct an appropriate history and physical examination. More recently, simulated environments have been used to assess a learner's "clinical reasoning"—the ability to integrate data, create a differential diagnosis of possible explanations for a patient's illness, and apply logic to make the best clinical decision. SP and virtual patient exercises can provide an ideal medium to test these skills. Indeed, multipronged assessments that test what a learner knows, through the use of pencil-and-paper exercises and what a learner can do by using SPs, VPs, or objective structured clinical examinations (OSCEs), provide a more comprehensive inventory of student skills than any single-assessment approach.

SP exercises and virtual patients can also be made more or less complex and so are suitable for teaching and assessing health care providers from novice to expert.

In this chapter we review the modern use of simulated environments, for both teaching and assessment purposes, at various levels of medical education. Simulation is increasingly used to teach principles and assess performance at all levels of medicine, from the beginning medical student attempting to master the medical interview, to multidisciplinary teams coordinating crisis care.

USING STANDARDIZED PATIENT SIMULATION TO TEACH AND ASSESS CORE CLINICAL SKILLS

Given that the best way to replicate a human being is with a human being, many aspects of the clinical world can be evoked using specially trained actors to portray patients with particular health conditions or concerns. Because of the special training they receive to consistently reenact patient presentations, these actors have been called "standardized patients" (SPs). They are able to give a predefined account of their condition and to answer a full range of questions about themselves in a consistent way.

In a typical SP exercise, a faculty member first develops a clinical script with specific objectives in mind. For example, one may wish to test a student's ability to obtain a focused history and perform a physical exam for a patient with abdominal pain. After the case is developed, a faculty panel reviews the script for medical accuracy. An actor is then trained to portray the medical facts of the case, including his or her character's specific condition and relevant past history. At the conclusion of the exercise, the SP completes a checklist describing which questions were asked and which physical exam maneuvers were performed (and whether they were performed correctly). The SP also provides a more subjective assessment of the student's communication skills. For a strictly formative exercise, training may involve memorizing a basic script over a few hours and providing direct feedback to the student. However, for "high-stakes" clinical examinations, actor training is often quite elaborate and detailed, involving multiple sessions over weeks to months, to ensure that the actors' portrayals are standardized—that they show a certain level of internal consistency—and can appropriately determine whether a specific question was asked or a specific physical exam maneuver was performed correctly.

Standardized patients may be used for both teaching and assessment purposes in multiple, interdependent domains of clinical skills (see **Figure 41-1**). These areas include history and physical examination skills, data interpretation and clinical reasoning, patient management, and working within multidisciplinary teams. These skill domains are progressively complex, and a learner must become proficient within one area in order to develop the next. Communication skills are key skills throughout these domains. If appropriately developed and supported, SPs and VPs can add to clinical skills instruction and assessment at all of these steps of medical education.

BASIC CLINICAL SKILLS: HISTORY AND PHYSICAL EXAMINATION

Most medical schools now use standardized patients to help acquire and assess basic clinical skills. Although used primarily at the medical school level, SPs can also reinforce these skills throughout the duration of medical training.

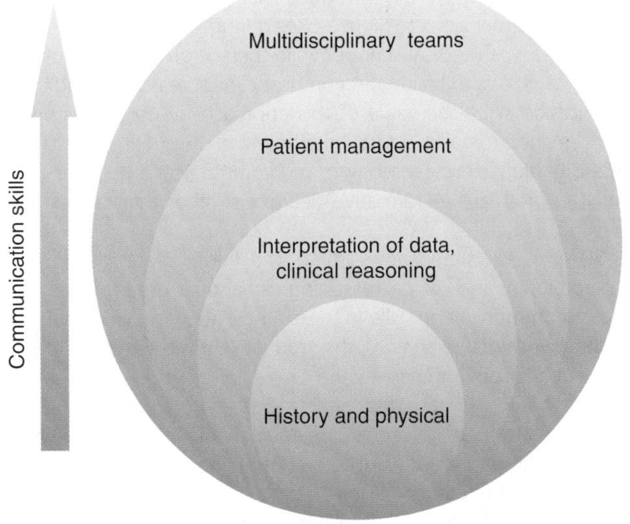

Figure 41-1 *The hierarchy of interdependent clinical skills that can be taught and assessed using standardized and virtual patients. The innermost circle shows the early skills of history taking and physical examination introduced in the first two years of medical school, which comprise foundational skills used by all physicians. The next circle includes skills in interpreting data and clinical reasoning that are emphasized later in medical school and become the cornerstone of clinical diagnostics. Beyond those are yet more advanced skills of patient management, required of all practicing physicians. The last circle emphasizes the growing interdisciplinary nature of clinical practice. Standardized and electronic patients and other simulated environments are being used increasingly at all levels of clinical training. The left arrow ("Communication skills") signifies that clinical mastery must be accompanied at each level by the simultaneous development of enhanced communication skills, which can also be taught, practiced, and tested using simulation.*

The SP approach has frequently been used when first teaching basic history and physical examination skills to entry level medical students. This allows novices to practice and hone their skills before direct patient contact. At this initial level, students need not specifically know how to interpret their results. Rather, the goals may simply be to become comfortable with the parts of a medical history and the mechanics of performing a focused or comprehensive physical examination; even something as basic as laying hands on the body can be daunting for some students. As students progress in their preclinical years and learn the physiology and pathophysiology of human disease, they begin to understand not just the mechanics but also the clinical implications of their questions and findings. Practicing symptom- or diagnosis-specific exercises with direct faculty and SP feedback can be truly valuable.

At Stanford, SP exercises during the first year of medical school mainly allow students to learn and practice parts of the medical history and physical examination and are formative, including feedback directly from the SP. Therefore, by the end of the first-year curriculum, students are comfortable obtaining a medical history and performing a basic physical examination. As students progress during their medical training, they have targeted practice for specific clinical scenarios and can further refine these skills and practice more advanced topics in a safe, constructive setting. For example, we rely on SP exercises to introduce topics such as obtaining a sexual history, discussing substance abuse, and motivational interviewing (eg, advocating for smoking cessation), allowing students to become more comfortable with unfamiliar or difficult themes. Similarly, more sensitive parts of a physical exam, such as genital or pelvic examinations, are often best first learned with a trained, standardized educator; pelvic educators (or "gynecological teaching associates") are common in medical schools and can also help clinical medical students and residents reinforce their skills.

As students master the mechanics of the history and physical examination, SP exercises developed primarily to instruct students may also be used for assessment. At Stanford we employ a series of SP-based "high-stakes" clinical examinations at various milestones in medical training. A more formative assessment at the end of the first year ensures that students have mastered basic history, physical examination, and communication skills before entering the second year. A similar, more complex examination toward the end of the second preclinical year serves as a benchmark. Having acquired additional scientific and clinical knowledge, students have learned to think in real time and ask the most salient questions and, understanding the implications of the history, then perform the most relevant maneuvers in a focused physical examination. This exam ensures that students enter their clinical clerkship training having mastered a set of essential history, physical examination, and communication skills. Finally, along with other medical schools in California, Stanford participates in a half-day clinical performance examination (CPX) after the first year of clinical training that evaluates students' performance in clinical and interpersonal skills. Successful completion of the CPX is a Stanford University School of Medicine graduation requirement.

The value of SPs in assessing history and physical examination skills has been increasingly recognized on a national level. The United States Medical Licensing Examination (USMLE) now includes a day-long clinical skills component for the Step 2 exam ("Step 2-CS") in which examinees interview and assess 12 standardized patients. As the role and importance of this examination evolves, medical schools may place more emphasis on exercises of this nature.

PART I

The Specialty of Hospital Medicine and Systems of Care

> **PRACTICE POINT**
>
> - Simulation is increasingly used to teach principles and assess performance at all levels of medicine, from the beginning medical student attempting to master the medical interview, to multidisciplinary teams coordinating crisis care. This real-time approach to potentially complicated scenarios can involve multiple learners at, varying levels and with instructor and self-directed feedback, may improve both medical skills and communication during multidisciplinary team encounters.

Although teaching and assessing basic clinical skills is largely completed in medical school, learners must retain these skills as they progress in their training. Recognizing that there may be gaps in knowledge gained at medical school, a decline in these basic clinical skills over time, or both, residency education is now reinforcing basic history and physical exam skills. In addition, as one moves forward in training, these exercises may become more complex, not only regarding reinforcing basic skills but also teaching more advanced topics in the history and physical examination. For example, the department of medicine at Stanford has instituted a program called the "Stanford 25," a new initiative designed to showcase and teach 25 basic physical exam skills and their diagnostic benefits to residents. While real patients are often used as illustrative examples, SPs have also been employed and provide an excellent opportunity to help teach and reinforce these essential skills at this level. In addition, since SPs are specifically trained to provide feedback, residents may receive additional training from the SP that they may not otherwise get from an actual patient.

At the most basic level, assessing communication skills focuses largely on subjective patient satisfaction scores and important feedback about how the patient "felt" about the student. So-called patient–physician interaction (PPI) scores reflect themes such as the ability to open and close an interview effectively, gather information in a straightforward way, listen actively, establish personal rapport, explore the patient's perspective, and consider the patient's comfort during the physical exam. As students progress in their training, SP exercises can also focus on more advanced communication skills, such as learning how to conduct a medical interview using an interpreter. Students may not even be aware of some of their own behaviors, or may feel uncomfortable in drawing out information from patients; using SPs is a safe environment in which to develop, practice, and get feedback about their communication style.

At Stanford, we conduct an SP baseline interview for all entering medical students, primarily used for self-reflection and feedback. During our SP exercises throughout the first year (and subsequent portions of the curriculum), patient communication skills are assessed using a standardized checklist that we train SPs to complete. We continue to assess these same PPI skills over time, permitting longitudinal assessment; this gives students the ability to reflect on their own performance as their skills develop and mature. As students and residents continue to develop their own styles during training, using SPs can be an effective way to practice and receive feedback on essential communication skills.

INTERPRETING DATA AND DEMONSTRATING CLINICAL REASONING SKILLS

SP exercises are widely used in the U.S. to help teach and assess history and physical examination skills, as described above. More recently, these exercises have been extended to teach more advanced skills—interpreting data and engaging in stage-appropriate clinical reasoning. Although clinical reasoning can also be assessed by pencil-and-paper exercises, SP exercises also challenge students by asking them to engage spontaneously in several levels of the reporter–interpreter–manager–educator (RIME) paradigm that describes how a trainee matures from being able to obtain information to knowing how to apply it.

At Stanford we have developed exercises ("interstation exercises") that students complete immediately after an SP encounter to teach and assess these more advanced skills. As an example, if an SP is portraying a patient with chest pain, the interstation exercise might test "next steps" in patient management. Students' responses depend on how accurately they performed the history and physical exam in the room as well as on their practical knowledge of how a patient with chest pain might best be managed. Clinical tests, such as electrocardiograms, chest X-rays, and cardiac enzymes, can be provided to give the student the typical information that a practicing physician might confront in real life. These simulations can therefore be extremely valuable. If a student misses the diagnosis (eg, does not recognize the injury current of a myocardial infarction on the ECG), formative feedback can be provided. This type of exercise would be expected to improve patient safety by making it less likely that the same mistake would be repeated.

Student knowledge of patient management can also be assessed using the SP format. In the example above, a student might be asked about next steps in managing a patient with a myocardial infarction. Should the patient be admitted to the hospital? If so, should the patient go to a monitored bed? Which medications might be started? Should the patient undergo cardiac catheterization? What would the student do if the patient developed a serious cardiac arrhythmia (ventricular tachycardia)? These are just some of the questions that can be asked, and a common case like this might be adapted to test learners from novice to expert.

At Stanford we typically introduce data interpretation and clinical reasoning dimensions to SP exercises during the second, third, and fourth years of medical school. While there is growing enthusiasm about using SPs to teach and reinforce clinical reasoning and communication skills, the value of this approach in assessing student performance remains unproven. Therefore using SPs to test data interpretation, clinical reasoning, and communication skills appears most appropriate in formative (learning) rather than assessment (testing) exercises.

SP exercises aimed at teaching and informally assessing data interpretation and clinical reasoning can also be used to teach and assess communication skills. In the example above (a patient with an acute myocardial infarction), the student might be expected to return to the room and convey the clinical information to the patient and describe next steps. More complex communication challenges can be created, such as in this case, the patient with a myocardial infarction who might not want to be hospitalized, or the patient who might agree to be hospitalized but asks that the student-physician disguise the reason when speaking with family.

MANAGING PATIENTS

SP- and virtual-patient exercises can also be developed to help medical students, residents, and physicians practice their patient management skills. At the medical student level, cases can be developed to fill gaps in the clinical curriculum caused by the unpredictability of patient presentations at hospital inpatient services or outpatient clinics. This ensures equal exposure to all clinical trainees and can round out what otherwise is sometimes a hit-or-miss exposure to important clinical cases. Cases can also be developed to represent patients with uncommon diseases so that all students meet a full spectrum of clinical challenges. In SP exercises, the management question often is, "What would your next step be?" In virtual patients (electronic exercises), the next step as well as subsequent steps of management can be tested as information is doled out in a stepwise (and potentially conditional) manner.

At Stanford we have used SP and virtual patient exercises to reinforce skills that benefit from practice and immediate feedback, such as resuscitation and communication. Resuscitation skills, both for adult and pediatric patients, are improved through having a learner practice "what if?" emergency scenarios. Mannequins are commercially available (for example, the Harvey cardiac simulator) that have been adapted to reenact various emergency settings, and cases have been developed by faculty to teach principles of resuscitation and assess learner competency. Likewise, certain topics involving physician–patient communication benefit greatly from a dress rehearsal, which can enhance the physician's effectiveness in comforting and reassuring the patient. Communication topics we have rehearsed in a standardized-patient format include breaking bad news (a case we have used at Stanford, for example, is informing a patient that he or she has a malignancy), using a medical interpreter to reinforce best practices for using an interpreter while effectively communicating with the patient, and discussing sensitive topics such as risk and preventing spread of sexually-transmitted diseases. One can envision many settings in which SP and virtual reenactments would be effective in practicing and improving other communication skills and allowing learners to share in decision making.

FUNCTIONING WITHIN A MULTIDISCIPLINARY TEAM

In addition to focusing on the individual learner or an individual patient encounter, SP exercises may also simulate encounters in which the participant is a member of a health care team. This real-time approach to potentially complicated scenarios can involve multiple learners at varying levels and, with instructor and self-directed feedback, may improve both medical skills and communication during multidisciplinary team encounters. For example, mock codes to help train rapid response teams demonstrate the interplay between internal medicine, anesthesia, nursing, and respiratory therapy and, combining this with the SP approach, can be expanded to involve the patient and family. Another scenario may involve a complicated hospital encounter in which general medicine, the patient's primary care physician, subspecialty consults, nursing, and social work might play a role; we have simulated such situations in the preclinical years successfully using a standardized family.

Other service industries, such as airlines and air traffic control, already routinely use this form of training to simulate complicated or high-risk scenarios. With continued technological advances, this kind of training in medical fields will continue to expand.

ACCEPTANCE OF STANDARDIZED AND VIRTUAL PATIENTS IN MEDICAL EDUCATION

For SP and virtual patients to be useful in medical education, the end users (students) must accept this teaching and assessment approach. We recently showed at Stanford that both SP and virtual patients were well accepted by second- and fourth-year medical students. Students particularly liked the ability of virtual patients to integrate abnormal physical findings, such as embedded heart murmurs (via audio files) and neurological abnormalities (via video clips). The VP format was better able to test seamlessly the more advanced skill of clinical reasoning, the ability of a student to create an appropriate initial differential diagnosis, based on the history and physical exam findings, and to refine that diagnosis based on results from laboratory and imaging studies.

Even though the VP case received relatively high scores, students rated the SP case higher as a "valuable learning experience." This may be because the SP exam allowed students to have spontaneous interactions, offered practice with a real physical exam, and gave students a chance to exercise their interpersonal skills. What was clear from our experience at Stanford was that SP and VP complemented each other as simulated learning exercises. Students found both types of exercises, when properly designed, challenging and rewarding.

MEASURING THE EFFECTIVENESS OF SIMULATION-BASED INSTRUCTION AND LEARNING

Despite the many uses of simulation-based instruction, as described herein, the effectiveness of simulation will require further study to define optimal settings for the use of this new technology. Simulation has been shown to be effective in teaching practitioners "quick thinking" required in resuscitations and in practicing acute decision-making that occurs in critical care units, both pediatric and adult. Simulation learning has been shown to improve the acquisition of manual skills needed during adult advanced cardiac life support, such as emergency intubation, and of cognitive skills during these emergencies, such as which medications to administer and when to defibrillate. A recent study showed that simulation training was superior in providing the knowledge and practical skills to manage a cardiac arrest when compared with training gained by reading and the use of other multimedia instruction.

There are few studies examining the value of simulation-based instruction to teach clinical reasoning at the medical student level. Testing and validating the appropriate uses of simulation-based learning will be necessary for this modality to be fully accepted and embraced in medical education.

FUTURE DIRECTIONS

Both standardized and virtual (electronic) patient simulations can be used for instruction and assessment in a variety of contexts. New technologies and continued acceptance of this approach will continue this growth trend.

The continuing development of digital technologies may further integrate the SP and electronic alternatives. For example, at Stanford we have used computer-based interstation exercises between patient encounters in SP-based exams. For example, a student may first conduct a history and physical exam for a patient complaining of shortness of breath, and immediately afterward complete a computer-based exercise on subject content related to that patient encounter, such as interpreting a chest radiograph or results of the patient's pulmonary function tests. Even closer integration of SP and computerized technologies may be in the offing; for example, one may see an SP in a clinical encounter, and then see a computerized version of the same "patient" after completing a set of online clinical reasoning exercises or a literature search.

In addition to computerized patients who provide a desktop-simulated encounter for an individual learner, an even more advanced variant of this approach lets multiple participants interact simultaneously with the same patient in a so-called "virtual world." In such a setting, each learner develops an online character representing his or her role in the simulated clinical environment. Each participant can then interact with other participants, and each may take on different roles in the clinical scenario created. In a virtual world, as with desktop simulations, information can be gathered and actions taken, and the patient's condition may improve or worsen. The virtual world can reenact interpersonal interactions between various clinicians and with the patient.

Part-task physical trainers are another burgeoning technology that focuses on a specific portion of a patient simulation or task to be performed. For example, urinary catheter trainers replicate genital anatomy, and students can physically learn the process of inserting a Foley catheter in either male or female patients; plastic models that replicate the pelvic structures of female patients allow for the practice of key components of the pelvic exam without causing discomfort to real patients. The most advanced of these part-task pelvic trainers contain electronic force sensors to let the student know exactly what parts of the anatomy they feel, and how hard they or their instruments pressed on various areas. Along these lines, a new trend may involve the combination of a part-task physical trainer with an SP. For example, there are part-task trainers for suturing deep cuts or lacerations. These consist of a pad of special soft plastic material with a cut in the surface. The pad can be strapped on the arm of an SP and then covered with appropriate clinical draping material. The student not only has to suture the wound but, as in real life, must do so while attending to the patient's needs and conversing with the patient. Our use of this type of part-task trainer at Stanford in a high-stakes clinical exam met with success and student acceptance.

Finally, although established at the medical school level, these approaches may become more commonly used at the resident or postdoctoral level as training and licensing programs continue to redefine competencies for accreditation. Simulated exercises can be mapped to Accreditation Council for Graduate Medical Education (ACGME) core competencies to assist in maintaining certification for residency and fellowship training programs. Simulated patient-based applications may also be used in continuing medical education (CME) programs for practicing clinicians and to assure continued skills for board certification and recertification. Indeed, simulated patient programs can be an important addition to the spectrum of clinical skills instruction throughout medical education.

CONCLUSION

Simulation is increasingly used to teach principles and assess performance at all levels of medicine, from the beginning medical student attempting to master the medical interview, to multidisciplinary teams coordinating crisis care. Both standardized and virtual (electronic) patient simulations can be used for instruction and assessment in a variety of contexts. Testing and validating the appropriate uses of simulation-based learning will be necessary for this modality to be fully accepted and embraced in medical education.

SUGGESTED READINGS

Barrows HS. An overview of the uses of standardized patients for teaching and evaluating clinical skills. *Acad Med.* 1993;68:443–451; discussion 51–53.

Gesundheit N, Brutlag P, Youngblood P, Gunning WT, Zary N, Fors U. The use of virtual patients to assess the clinical skills and reasoning of medical students: initial insights on student acceptance. *Med Teach.* 2009;31:739–742.

Hartmann CW, Meterko M, Rosen AK, et al. Relationship of hospital organizational culture to patient safety climate in the Veterans Health Administration. *Med Care Res Rev.* 2009;66:320–338.

Jones JS, Hunt SJ, Carlson SA, Seamon JP. Assessing bedside cardiologic examination skills using "Harvey," a cardiology patient simulator. *Acad Emerg Med.* 1997;4:980–985.

Pugnaire MP, Domino FJ, Alper EJ. Expanding the "standardized family" across three clerkships: a model for creating an interdisciplinary core curriculum in primary care. *Acad Med.* 2000;75:530–531.

Weinstock P, Halamek LP. Teamwork during resuscitation. *Pediatr Clin North Am.* 2008;55:1011–1024, xi–xii.

Windish DM, Price EG, Clever SL, Magaziner JL, Thomas PA. Teaching medical students the important connection between communication and clinical reasoning. *J Gen Intern Med.* 2005;20:1108–1113.

Youngblood P, Heinrichs L, Cornelius C, Dev P. Designing case-based learning for virtual worlds. *Simul Healthc.* 2007;2:246–247.

Zary N, Johnson G, Boberg J, Fors UG. Development, implementation and pilot evaluation of a Web-based Virtual Patient Case Simulation environment-Web-SP. *Med Educ.* 2006;6:10.

PART II

Medical Consultation and Co-Management

SECTION 1

Core Tenets of Medical Consultation

CHAPTER 42

Role of the Medical Consultant

Steven L. Cohn, MD, FACP

INTRODUCTION

Medical consultation has become an important component of Hospital Medicine. These consultations include preoperative evaluation, perioperative management, and medical care of patients on various nonmedical services. Previous surveys found that many primary care physicians and hospitalists felt inadequately trained in perioperative medicine, and as a result, this area received additional emphasis as part of the core competencies for Hospital Medicine. With the growth of the hospitalist movement, the role of the consultant has evolved from providing evaluation and advice to include comanagement of the patient in certain settings. The goal of this chapter is to review the role and responsibilities of the medical consultant, focusing on the principles of consultation and techniques to improve effectiveness.

GENERAL PRINCIPLES OF CONSULTATION

More than 25 years ago, Goldman and colleagues described the concepts for performing medical consultations. His "Ten Commandments" for effective consultation included the following:

1. Determine the question.
2. Establish urgency.
3. Look for yourself.
4. Be as brief as appropriate.
5. Be specific and concise.
6. Provide contingency plans.
7. Honor thy turf.
8. Teach with tact.
9. Talk is cheap and effective.
10. Followup.

These concepts, which incorporated many of the ethical principles described by the American Medical Association (AMA), are important and remain valid for the traditional consultation. However, some modifications are necessary to cover the new role of hospitalists as comanagers.

TYPES OF CONSULTATION

The traditional or standard medical consultation consisted of a formal request from the requesting physician to evaluate a patient and answer a specific question (**Table 42-1**). The consultant was expected to address the question and to provide advice and recommendations, but not to write orders or bring in other consultants; the requesting physician remained in control and responsible for the patient's overall care and treatment. The consultant also focused on the specific problem rather than looking for and addressing other issues. Consultations were requested only when necessary and not for routine management. The follow-up period was usually brief and did not involve daily visits for the duration of hospitalization.

This traditional role of the consultant has been changing over the past 5–10 years. A survey by Salerno and colleagues revealed that many surgeons wanted the medical consultant to assume more of a comanagement role. Specifically, they wanted the consultant to address all medical issues as necessary as well as to write orders and continue to follow the patient. Comanagement arrangements have most often been with orthopedic surgeons and more recently with neurosurgeons. Comanagement has potential advantages of decreasing length of stay and reducing complications. Surgeons and nurses often prefer comanagement; however, one possible

TABLE 42-1 Roles and Responsibilities of Different Types of Consultations

	Traditional	Comanagement	Curbside
MD in charge overall	Requesting physician	Shared responsibility	Requesting physician
Primary care of medical problems	Requesting physician	Medical—consultant Surgical—requesting physician	Requesting physician
Question addressed	Specific	Broader issues—other medical problems	Should not address either but offer to do formal consult or give only general advice
Order writing	No	Yes	No
Follow-up	Limited, as needed	Daily until discharge	No, no formal relationship

disadvantage is that the comanaging consultant may feel subservient to the surgeon and may be asked to assume responsibilities outside his area of training. This new role of comanagement will be discussed in detail in the next chapter.

Yet another type of consultation is the so-called "curbside" or informal consult in which the consultant is asked to provide an opinion or advice without personally seeing the patient. Although these should be avoided from a medicolegal standpoint, they occur frequently. Ideally the consultant should offer to perform a formal consult but if any advice is given, it should be generic and simple. The requesting physician should not refer to the consultant in the medical record if he has not seen the patient, and if he has had any contact with the patient, the consultant should write a note in the chart.

PRACTICE POINT

If the consultant is asked to provide an opinion or advice without personally seeing the patient (the "curbside consult"), the consultant should:

- Offer to perform a formal consult.
- Provide only generic and simple advice.
- Document any patient encounter in the chart.

The requesting physician should not refer to the consultant in the medical record if the consultant has not seen the patient.

DETERMINING THE QUESTION

In view of the multiple types of consultations, it is imperative that the requesting physician specify exactly what is being requested, and if there is any uncertainty, the consultant should clarify this question by communicating directly with the requesting physician. In addition to specifying the role of the consultant, the requesting physician should be specific as to the question being asked of the consultant. For example, a request for preoperative consultation may be for surgical risk assessment, a "green light" to proceed with anesthesia and surgery, a diagnostic or management issue, reassurance, or documentation for medicolegal purposes. As obvious as this may be, disagreement regarding the primary purpose for the consult still occurs between the requesting physician and the consultant. Several studies noted that the consult requests were vague and nonspecific (eg, clearance or evaluation), or did not even ask a question. Without clarifying the reason for the consult, the consultant may respond in a manner that fails to answer the question being asked by the requesting physician.

PRACTICE POINT

In view of the multiple types of consultations, it is imperative that the requesting physician specify:

- The expected role of the consultant
- The question to be answered by the consultant

If there is any uncertainty, the consultant should clarify this question by communicating directly with the requesting physician. The consultant should avoid making recommendations about the type of anesthesia and other areas outside his or her area of expertise.

ANSWERING THE QUESTION

Traditionally, the consultant restricted his or her advice to the specific problem or question. However, more frequently the consultant is addressing other issues noted during the evaluations. Assuming these other findings and recommendations are relevant and important, most surgeons are in favor of this approach. What the requesting physician does not want is a laundry list of things to do for minor problems or issues that do not need to be addressed during the current hospitalization.

If the consultation is for preoperative evaluation, the consultant needs to:

1. Assess the severity and degree of control of the patient's medical problems.
2. Estimate surgical risk.
3. Determine if the patient is in his or her optimal medical condition for surgery.
4. Decide whether further tests or interventions are indicated.
5. Make recommendations regarding the patient's medications and any necessary prophylaxis.

The consultant should avoid making recommendations about the type of anesthesia and other areas outside his or her area of expertise. Also, the consultant should refrain from using the term "cleared for surgery," even if consulted for that reason, as this implies a guarantee that the patient will not have a complication.

OPTIMIZING EFFECTIVENESS

Factors influencing or improving compliance

Various studies found a number of factors that have been associated with improved compliance with the consultant's recommendations (**Table 42-2**). In general, following Goldman's Ten Commandments or Salerno's modification (see **Table 42-3**) will result in effective consultation.

TABLE 42-2 Factors that Influence or Improve Compliance with Consultant Recommendations

Prompt response (within 24 hours)
Limit number of recommendations (≤ 5)
Identify crucial or critical recommendations (versus routine)
Focus on central issues
Make specific relevant recommendations
Use definitive language
Specify drug dosage, route, frequency, duration
Frequent follow-up including progress notes
Direct verbal contact
Therapeutic (versus diagnostic) recommendations
Severity of illness

Reproduced, with permission, from Cohn SL, Macpherson DS. Overview of the principles of medical consultation. In: Basow D, ed. *UpToDate*. Waltham, MA, 2009.

Determine and clarify the question: As noted, the reason for the consultation needs to be clearly defined by the requesting physician and understood and addressed by the consultant.

Punctual response: The consultant should be available to respond in a timely fashion, depending on the urgency of the consultation. Truly "stat" consults should be answered in less than 30 minutes, and in general, elective consults should be answered within 24 hours, preferably the same day they were requested.

Recommendations:

1. **Prioritize and limit:** The consultant should make specific, precise recommendations that should be listed in order of importance. Crucial or critical recommendations are more likely to be followed, as are those at the top of the list. For this reason, it was previously felt that the number of recommendations should be limited to no more than five, but more recently the feeling is to leave as many recommendations as needed to answer the consult and offer to help with writing and implementing them (comanagement). Therapeutic recommendations are more likely to be followed than diagnostic ones.
2. **Language:** The consultant should use definitive language, be specific with his recommendations, and provide contingency plans. For example, recommendations for medications should specify the drug name, dose, frequency, route of administration, and duration of therapy. The requesting physician should be told what response to expect, how long it will take, as well as how and when to adjust the medication dose if necessary.
3. **Communication:** Direct verbal communication with the requesting physician is crucial and preferable to just leaving a note in the chart. A quick call to the requesting physician will let him know that the consult has been answered, what the recommendations are, and what needs to be done so the orders can be written and the process expedited. It is also important to communicate with other members of the health care team to coordinate care.
4. **Follow-up:** Appropriate follow-up visits will reassess the patient's condition and ensure that recommendations were followed. The consultant should clearly document his findings

TABLE 42-3 Original and Modified Ten Commandments for Effective Consultations

1983 Commandments		2006 Modifications	
Commandment	Meaning	Commandment	Meaning
1. Determine the question.	The consultant should call the primary physician if the specific question is not obvious.	1. Determine your customer.	Ask the requesting physician how you can best help him or her if a specific question is not obvious; he or she may want comanagement.
2. Establish urgency.	The consultant must determine whether the consultation is emergent, urgent, or elective.	2. Establish urgency.	The consultant must determine whether the consultation is emergent, urgent, or elective.
3. Look for yourself.	Consultants are most effective when they are willing to gather data on their own.	3. Look for yourself.	Consultants are most effective when they are willing to gather data on their own.
4. Be brief as appropriate.	The consultant need not repeat in full detail the data that were already recorded.	4. Be brief as appropriate.	The consultant need not repeat in full detail the data that were already recorded.
5. Be specific.	Leaving a long list of suggestions may decrease the likelihood that any of them will be followed, including the critical ones.	5. Be specific, thorough, and descend from thy ivory tower to help when requested.	Leave as many specific recommendations as needed to answer the consult but ask the requesting physician if he or she needs help with order writing.
6. Provide contingency plans.	Consultants should anticipate potential problems; a brief description of therapeutic options may save time later.	6. Provide contingency plans and discuss their execution.	Consultants should anticipate potential problems, document contingency plans, and provide a 24-hour point of contact to help execute the plans if requested.
7. Thou shalt not covet thy neighbor's turf.	In most cases, consultants should play a subsidiary role.	7. Thou may negotiate joint title to thy neighbor's turf.	Consultants can and should comanage any facet of patient care that the requesting physician desires; a frank discussion defining which specialty is responsible for what aspects of patient care is needed.

(*continued*)

TABLE 42-3 Original and Modified ten Commandments for Effective Consultations *(continued)*

1983 Commandments		2006 Modifications	
Commandment	Meaning	Commandment	Meaning
8. Teach with tact.	Requesting physicians appreciate consultants who make an active effort to share their expertise.	8. Teach with tact and pragmatism.	Judgments on leaving references should be tailored to the requesting physician's specialty, level of training, and urgency of the consult.
9. Talk is cheap and effective	There is no substitute for direct personal contact with the primary physician.	9. Talk is essential.	There is no substitute for direct personal contact with the primary physician.
10. Provide appropriate followup.	Consultants should recognize the appropriate time to fade into a background role, but that time is almost never the same day the consultation note is signed.	10. Followup daily.	Daily written follow-up is desirable; when the patient's problems are not active, the consultant should discuss signing off with the requesting physician beforehand.

Modified, with permission, from Salerno, et al. *Arch Intern Med.* 2007;167:271–275 and data from Goldman L, Lee T, Rudd P. Ten commandments for effective consultations. *Arch Intern Med.* 1983;143(9):1753–1755.

and update recommendations in the medical record. There is no standard regarding how often the consultant needs to see the patient, but this should be determined by the patient's medical condition, type of surgery, and whether the requesting physician wants comanagement or not. When the patient is medically stable and there is no longer a need for the medical consultant, he should sign off and document this in the chart. Recommendations and arrangements for long-term follow-up can also be noted at this time.

PRACTICE POINT

The consultant should document:

- Specific and precise recommendations listed in order of importance
- Name, initial dose, frequency, route of administration, titration, and duration of recommended therapy

The consultant should provide:

- Prompt service.
- Direct verbal communication with the requesting physician upon completion of the initial consult
- Updates and follow-up as appropriate depending on requested role

CONCLUSION

The ideal medical consultant will "render a report that informs without patronizing, educates without lecturing, directs without ordering, and solves the problem without making the referring physician appear to be stupid." It is hoped that by following these principles, the medical consultant will be effective in providing useful information and recommendations to the requesting physician who will then implement them in an attempt to improve patient outcome.

SUGGESTED READINGS

Choi JJ. An anesthesiologist's philosophy on 'medical clearance' for surgical patients. *Arch Intern Med.* 1987;147(12):2090–2092.

Cohn SL. Overview of the principles of medical consultation. In: Basow D, ed. *UpToDate*. Waltham, MA: UpToDate; 2009.

Devor M, Renvall M, Ramsdell J. Practice patterns and the adequacy of residency training in consultation medicine. *J Gen Intern Med.* 1993;8(10):554–560.

Goldman L, Lee T, Rudd P. Ten commandments for effective consultations. *Arch Intern Med.* 1983;143(9):1753–1755.

Kleinman B, Czinn E, Shah K, Sobotka PA, Rao TK. The value to the anesthesia-surgical care team of the preoperative cardiac consultation. *J Cardiothorac Anesth.* 1989;3(6):682–687.

Kuo D, Gifford DR, Stein MD. Curbside consultation practices and attitudes among primary care physicians and medical subspecialists. *JAMA.* 1998;280(10):905–909.

Lee T, Pappius EM, Goldman L. Impact of inter-physician communication on the effectiveness of medical consultations. *Am J Med.* 1983;74(1):106–112.

Plauth WH, Pantilat SZ, Wachter RM, Fenton CL. Hospitalists' perceptions of their residency training needs: results of a national survey. *Am J Med.* 2001;111(3):247–254.

Rudd P, Siegler M, Byyny RL. Perioperative diabetic consultation: a plead for improved training. *J Med Educ.* 1978;53(7):590–596.

Salerno SM, Hurst FP, Halvorson S, Mercado DL. Principles of effective consultation: an update for the 21st-century consultant. *Arch Intern Med.* 2007;167(3):271–275.

CHAPTER 43

Definition, Principles, and Goals of Comanagement

Hugo Quinny Cheng, MD

INTRODUCTION

EMERGENCE OF HOSPITALIST COMANAGEMENT

Limitations of traditional medical consultation

While the traditional model for medical consultation still exists in many hospitals, particularly at academic medical centers, many surgeons and hospitalists have expressed concerns about its limitations. Traditional consultation requires the referring physician to recognize when a patient requires a consultant's input. However, a surgeon may not recognize when a patient is at high risk for medical complications, and thus fails to seek a consultation in a timely manner. Similarly, a hospitalist may identify important medical problems beyond the initial reason for consultation. The traditional consultation model, which limits the consultant to leaving recommendations, may also be inefficient if their implementation by the referring physician is delayed. To overcome these limitations, many hospitalists have taken on a more active role in caring for patients admitted for surgical or other specialty care. This new model has been termed *comanagement*.

GROWTH OF COMANAGEMENT

A 2005 survey by the Society of Hospital Medicine (SHM) found that 85% of Hospital Medicine groups performed comanagement. Several factors are driving the growth of comanagement. Demographic changes in the surgical population have been a major impetus for surgeons' demand for comanagement. As surgical volumes increase, surgeons must spend greater amounts of time in the operating room and have become less available to care for their patients on the floor. The availability of surgical house staff at teaching hospitals has also become increasingly limited due to tighter restrictions on resident duty hours. Simultaneously, surgical patients are older and sicker, and thus at greater risk for medical complications. Not surprisingly, many surgeons now feel that the traditional consultation model is too limiting. A study in 2007 found that only 41% of surgeons felt that consultants should limit their input to the initial consultation question, and only 37% believed that consultants should avoid writing orders without prior approval from the primary team. The majority of surgeons in this study desired a comanagement relationship with their consultant.

Medical centers have also pushed Hospital Medicine groups to adopt a comanagement role. Much of this impetus may arise from the desire to recruit and retain surgeons who demand medical comanagement. However, in some cases, hospital administrators have advocated for comanagement as a way to improve quality, safety, and cost efficiency in surgical patients, the same way that hospitalists have demonstrated these benefits in their own patients. Hospitals may also desire comanagement in response to nursing staff concerns about the limited availability of surgeons and specialists to respond to questions or address problems in their patients.

While not all hospitalists have been eager to pursue comanagement, many Hospital Medicine groups view it as a way to expand their role and demonstrate their value. Comanagement has also been seen as a potential source of revenue to hospitalist groups, both through increased professional fee collection as well as strategic support from the medical center.

TABLE 43-1 Differences Between Consultation and Comanagement

	Traditional Medical Consultation	Comanagement
Determination of hospitalist's responsibilities and scope of practice	Determined at time of referral or based on informal understanding	Previously negotiated formal agreement between hospitalist and specialist
Identification of patients	Hospitalist only sees patients referred by specialist	Hospitalist may see patients selected by predetermined clinical criteria without specialist referral
Identification of problems	Hospitalist only addresses problems identified by specialist	Hospitalist may choose which problems to address
Communication of assessment and recommendations	Hospitalist only communicates assessment and recommendations to specialist	Hospitalist communicates directly with patient when appropriate
Communication with nurses and other providers	Hospitalist does not address questions or concerns from nurses	Hospitalist directly responds to questions and concerns from nurses
Permission to write orders and request additional consultation	Hospitalist must obtain permission from specialist first	Prior discussion with specialist rarely needed
Role in discharge planning	Hospitalist has limited or no role	Hospitalist addresses medical problems at time of discharge
Role of hospitalist beyond direct patient care	None	Hospitalist may work with specialist in quality improvement, education, and research projects

DEFINITION OF COMANAGEMENT

There is no universally accepted definition of comanagement, and this moniker has been applied to a wide range of practice patterns. One definition, which encompasses most hospitalists' practice, is that comanagement is *a negotiated, collaborative relationship, which provides hospitalists with a broad scope of practice and also requires their increased responsibility for management of medical care in patients who are primarily being treated by a surgeon or other specialist*. This definition does not assume that the surgeon or specialist will serve as the admitting physician. The term has also been applied to situations in which the hospitalist acts as the admitting physician for surgical patients, a practice that is especially common in nonteaching hospitals. While some have argued that it is the specialist who is comanaging the patient in that scenario, rather than the hospitalist, much of this discussion will still be relevant. The specific protocols and attributes of comanagement services vary. However, many comanagement services have common features that distinguish them from traditional medical consultation (**Table 43-1**).

PRINCIPLES AND BEST PRACTICES IN COMANAGEMENT

FORMAL AGREEMENT

Even when a comanagement relationship evolves organically over time, a formal agreement between the hospitalist and specialist is a key feature for success. This agreement should be negotiated between the Hospital Medicine group and a champion for comanagement among the specialists. A written policy or protocol provides shared expectations for the hospitalist's roles and responsibilities. This is crucial for preventing disagreements and dissatisfaction that can arise from misunderstanding between hospitalist and specialist. If specialists become busier or if hospitalists demonstrate their value, the natural tendency is for both the number of comanaged patients and the depth of hospitalists involvement to grow. The formal agreement can provide the hospitalists with a degree of protection and predictability in terms of their workload by setting limits to the comanagement service's census or require provision of additional resources as the service grows.

PRACTICE POINT

- A formal agreement between the hospitalist and specialist is a key feature for success. A written policy or protocol provides shared expectations for the hospitalist's roles and responsibilities. This agreement should be negotiated between the Hospital Medicine group and a champion for comanagement among the specialists.

Ensuring good patient care, however, is the most important reason to develop a formal comanagement agreement. By its nature, comanagement entails fragmentation of care. The primary physician's responsibility to provide comprehensive care under a traditional care model is now being shared with another physician under comanagement. A formal, negotiated agreement helps to ensure that care is not omitted, duplicated, or in conflict. In some cases, these agreements must include multiple parties, such as when several subspecialists provide potentially overlapping care. For example, a neurosurgeon, a neurologist, and an intensivist, in addition to the comanaging hospitalist, will often jointly manage patients admitted with subarachnoid hemorrhage. The comanagement agreement should carefully define each specialist's roles and responsibilities.

PRACTICE POINT

- Ensuring good patient care is the most important reason to develop a formal comanagement agreement. By its nature, comanagement entails fragmentation of care. A formal, negotiated agreement helps to ensure that care is not omitted, duplicated, or in conflict.

TABLE 43-2 Examples of Patient Selection Criteria for Comanagement

	Surgical Population	Selection Criteria for Comanagement
Huddleston (2004)	Elective arthroplasty	Age > 75 years *plus* history of either: Any 1: diabetes, CHF, history of MI or coronary bypass grafting, CVA, dementia, severe COPD, immune suppression, severe renal insufficiency, sleep apnea, or severe peripheral arterial disease; *or* Any 2: HTN, arrhythmia, venous thromboembolism, coagulation disorder, mild COPD, mild renal insufficiency
Phy (2005)	Orthopedic surgery	All hip fracture patients
Simon (2007)	Pediatric orthopedic surgery	Pediatric spinal fusion patients with significant medical problems, including history of multiple medications, seizure disorder, nutritional concern, or significant social concerns
Pinzur (2009)	Orthopedic surgery (lower extremity reconstruction)	Stable medical comorbidities, including CAD, CHF, diabetes, or HTN; *or* Critical social issue
Auerbach (2010)	Neurosurgery	History of CAD, CHF, significant arrhythmia, ischemic stroke, chronic kidney disease, COPD, dementia, insulin-dependent diabetes, chronic anticoagulation

SELECTING PATIENTS AND PROBLEMS

Surgeons and other specialists may not recognize when a patient would benefit from medical consultation. Many comanagement protocols try to circumvent this problem by having the hospitalist follow patients who meet predetermined clinical criteria, even in the absence of a referral from the primary physician. Optimal patient selection criteria have not been elucidated, but they should be based on known risk factors for medical complications (**Table 43-2**). These risk factors may include specific admitting diagnoses or procedures (eg, hip fracture repair), demographic features (eg, over age 70), or the presence of specific medical comorbidities (eg, one or more revised cardiac risk index predictors). Determining appropriate selection criteria can be challenging. Comanagement probably has little benefit for healthy, low-risk patients, and overly inclusive criteria dilute the impact of hospitalists while overburdening them with work. Thus, attention should also be given to the projected number of patients that would be comanaged under the selection rules.

Most comanagement agreements also permit the hospitalist to identify which medical issues to address. The traditional consultation paradigm, which restricts the consultant's purview to a single question or problem, fails to take advantage of the hospitalist's particular skill at delivering comprehensive inpatient medical care. Thus, in developing a formal comanagement policy, it may be more important to delineate the issues that the hospitalists will *not* address. These might be problems that are beyond the hospitalist's training or experience. They may also include tasks that can be competently performed by other providers, and would represent an inappropriate use of the hospitalist's time.

SCOPE OF PRACTICE

Studies have found that 25–50% of recommendations by consultants at academic medical centers are ignored. By allowing the hospitalist to provide direct patient care including order writing, comanagement potentially improves efficiency of care. Thus, comanagement arrangements almost always allow the hospitalist to write orders and consult other physicians without prior permission from the specialist. However, the comanagement protocol should also specify any limitations on the hospitalist's scope of practice, such as requiring prior approval before ordering anticoagulants or invasive procedures. Protocols should also account for many hospitalists' reluctance to care for problems beyond their training including most surgical care, by formally limiting their scope of practice in these areas.

PRACTICE POINT

- It may be more important for a formal comanagement policy to delineate the issues that the hospitalists will not address. These might be problems that are beyond the hospitalist's training or experience. They may also include tasks that can be competently performed by other providers, and would represent an inappropriate use of the hospitalist's time.

COMMUNICATION

In the traditional consultation model, excellent communication skills are crucial because consultants must clearly convey their recommendations to referring physicians. Although comanaging hospitalists will more typically write orders than leave recommendations, proper communication under comanagement remains essential for good patient care. The comanagement agreement should set expectations for when verbal communication between the hospitalist and specialist is required, frequency of communication, and how the specialist (who may be in the operating room) can be reached. Hospitalists should also expect to receive inquiries from nurses, rehabilitation specialists, and other hospital staff when caring for comanaged patients. While this aspect of comanagement can increase efficiency of care, it can also lead to confusion among staff members about whom to call. Furthermore, being readily available to hospital staff can also burden the hospitalist with too many inquiries, many of which could be more appropriately addressed by other providers. Thus, the comanagement agreement should specify when the hospitalist should be called as opposed to the specialist. Regular meetings between the comanagement service director and nursing leadership can also help ensure that calls are appropriately directed.

TABLE 43-3 Examples of Outcome Measurements for Comanagement

Satisfaction Outcomes	Specialist and nursing perceptions of • Promptness of care • Availability of hospitalist • Quality of communication • Quality of discharge planning • Quality of overall care • Impact on provider's ability to deliver care
	Patient satisfaction (Press-Ganey survey results)
	Primary care provider satisfaction
	Hospitalist satisfaction
Efficiency Outcomes	Overall length of stay
	Time from admission to surgery
	Time from surgery to discharge
	Direct cost of care
	Appropriateness of bed utilization
	Cancellation of surgery
	Specialist's productivity
Clinical Outcomes	Mortality
	Medical complications
	Readmission
	Unplanned ICU admission
	Processes outcomes (eg, Joint Commission Core Measures)

GOALS OF COMANAGEMENT

Before embarking on the creation of a comanagement service, it is important to determine the service's goals as well as the likelihood of success in achieving them. The service agreement should describe these goals. Ideally, these goals should be measurable and their progress should be tracked. Typical goals for a comanagement service include those related to provider and patient satisfaction, efficiency of care, and improvements in clinical outcomes (**Table 43-3**).

> **PRACTICE POINT**
>
> • Before embarking on the creation of a comanagement service, it is important to determine the service's goals as well as the likelihood of success in achieving them. The service agreement should describe these goals. Ideally, these goals should be measurable and their progress tracked.

PROVIDER SATISFACTION

Since comanagement arrangements are often initiated at the behest of the specialist or the medical center, it is important to ensure that the providers served by the hospitalists are satisfied. Measurement of this outcome is easily achieved through the use of surveys. It may be useful to obtain baseline data on satisfaction prior to starting comanagement. Studies have found strong provider preference for a comanagement model. In a randomized trial of comanagement for elective arthroplasty patients at a tertiary care hospital, surgeons preferred the comanagement service to a traditional consultation service. The vast majority of surgeons felt that the comanagement model was either somewhat better or much better in terms of quality of communication between providers, ease of asking for advice from medical physicians, ease of providing high quality medical care, recognition of patients' postoperative medical needs, and promptness with which these needs are addressed. Interestingly, the nurses caring for arthroplasty patients were even more enthusiastic in their preference for comanagement than the surgeons. This may reflect the greater availability of the hospitalist under the comanagement model. There is less evidence for improvement in patient satisfaction under comanagement models. Medically complicated orthopedic surgery patients comanaged by a hospitalist were no more likely to recommend that hospital than those in a historical control. Other parties to consider surveying for satisfaction data include primary care providers and the hospitalists themselves.

EFFICIENCY OF CARE

Numerous studies have demonstrated that hospitalists improve efficiency of care, typically measured by cost of care and length of stay (LOS) compared to nonhospitalists. Some evidence exists that hospitalists also improve efficiency when co-managing surgical patients. Among patients admitted for hip fracture repair at a tertiary care hospital, those comanaged by a hospitalist underwent surgery an average of a half-day sooner and had an overall length of stay that was 2 days shorter compared to a historical control. There was no increase in 30-day readmission rates among comanaged patients. The benefits of comanagement on efficiency of care may be greater in more complicated patients. In the previous study, non-comanaged patients with more severe systemic illnesses were more likely to suffer a delay in time to surgery. This association was not seen in comanaged patients. At the same institution, comanaged elective arthroplasty patients did not have a reduction in observed LOS compared to non-comanaged patients, but their adjusted length of stay was a half day shorter. Overall direct medical costs did not differ among these arthroplasty patients. In contrast, a comanagement service for neurosurgery patients did not shorten LOS but was associated with a significant reduction in adjusted hospital costs. In pediatric patients undergoing spinal fusion, the introduction of selective hospitalist comanagement was associated with decreases in LOS and variability in LOS.

CLINICAL OUTCOMES

A retrospective analysis of nearly 85,000 patients found that perioperative complication rates did not differ much between hospitals with high and low adjusted mortality rates. This suggests that it is the timely recognition and appropriate management of these complications that has the greatest impact on mortality rates. In theory, a readily available hospitalist, experienced in recognizing and treating perioperative medical complications, can improve clinical outcomes in surgical patients. The evidence for whether this goal can be achieved through comanagement is mixed. Among elective arthroplasty patients randomized to comanagement, the risk of minor complications (urinary tract infection, electrolyte abnormalities, and fever) was reduced, but there was no effect on more serious complications or mortality. Among hip fracture patients at the same institution, hospitalist comanagement was not associated with changes in either perioperative or long-term mortality rates or the risk of complications, with the exception of delirium, which was actually more commonly reported in comanaged patients. This unexpected finding illustrates a pitfall of measuring complication rates, which is the potential for increased detection and documentation of complications by hospitalists, who may be more likely to order diagnostic tests and report complications. This detection and reporting bias makes it difficult to assess the impact of comanagement on less serious complications rates. Clinical outcomes measurements less likely to be affected by this bias include more severe complications, mortality, unplanned ICU admission, and readmission rates. In addition, it may be useful to track process outcomes such as compliance with core measures from the Joint Commission of Accreditation of Health care Organizations or other evidence-based strategies to improved patient safety. While less tangible than clinical endpoints, process measurements are less subject to confounding and they measure quality more directly.

PITFALLS OF COMANAGEMENT

PROBLEMS WITH SHARED RESPONSIBILITY

Despite its limitations the traditional consultation model offers the advantage of clarity with regard to responsibilities. The admitting physician is directly responsible for all aspects of a patient's care, and the consultant is primarily responsible to the referring physician. A comanagement arrangement, which includes shared (and sometimes overlapping) responsibility, can lead to uncertainty about who is in charge. A carefully considered comanagement protocol or policy can reduce this uncertainty, but not eliminate it entirely. Common pitfalls with shared responsibility include ethical conflicts, medicolegal risks, and disengagement of the specialist.

Ethical conflicts

Division of clinical responsibility between providers creates potential ethical conflicts. In a 1999 report, the Council on Ethical and Judicial Affairs of the American Medical Association recommended steps to avoid or resolve ethical conflicts that may occur under surgical comanagement:

1. Comanagement should only be undertaken for the benefit of the patient.
2. Physicians' responsibilities should be delineated according to their expertise and abilities.
3. One physician should ultimately be responsible for coordinating care, and other providers should communicate with this physician.
4. Patients should consent to comanagement and be informed about the credentials and responsibilities of each provider and the billing arrangement.
5. Physicians should avoid actual or perceived financial conflicts of interest that can arise from self-referral.
6. Referrals for comanagement should not be based on expected financial reciprocation or other self-serving bases. In particular, fee-splitting must be avoided.
7. Patient confidentiality must be safeguarded.

While not explicitly stated in the report, it is clear that one physician must ultimately have decision-making authority when there are irreconcilable differences of opinion about treatment.

Medicolegal risks

Comanagement potentially increases the medicolegal exposure of the hospitalist compared to traditional consultation. A traditional consultant has performed due diligence by adequately evaluating the patient and recommending appropriate management for the consultation question. Under comanagement, the hospitalist also assumes responsibility for ensuring that the management is appropriately carried out. In some cases, the hospitalist may be held partially liable for errors or negligence on the part of the surgeon, or vice versa, especially in gray areas in which medical and surgical care overlap. For example, who is at fault if a patient develops a pulmonary embolism in the absence of prophylaxis? The surgeon might assume that provision of prophylaxis is a medical issue, while the hospitalist believes that it is the surgeon's duty to document adequate hemostasis before anticoagulants are ordered. Another concern is being held responsible for following up on test results ordered by another provider. Is the hospitalist at fault for failing to review an abnormal ECG ordered by the surgeon? While routine communication between hospitalist and specialist and explicit delineation of roles in a comanagement agreement can reduce medicolegal risk, it is not possible to anticipate all contingencies. Acceptance of this risk may be an inevitable aspect of comanagement.

Disengagement of the specialist

Another concern of hospitalists is that comanagement agreements will foster clinical disengagement by the surgeon or other specialist. The diffusion of responsibility for a patient's progress or outcome to another physician may decrease the pressure to maintain the highest professional standards for availability and responsiveness. This problem may be particularly acute in comanagement arrangements in which the hospitalist is the admitting physician. In that situation, disengagement by the specialist leaves hospitalists to deal with surgical or other problems beyond their training.

HOSPITALIST DISSATISFACTION

In addition to the usual concerns about workload, sustainability, and compensation, comanagement can introduce specific problems that adversely impact career satisfaction. Unless care is taken, engagement in comanagement can lead to an unequal relationship, usually with the hospitalist as the lesser partner. This inequality is exacerbated if either physician perceives the hospitalist to be an employee of the specialist. Dissatisfaction can also occur when hospitalists' believe that comanagement is being undertaken for the surgeons' convenience rather than to fulfill a medical need that they are uniquely capable of addressing. Arrangements in which the hospitalist admits medically stable surgical patients can make comanagement feel like little more than a night and weekend admitting service for the specialist, unless the agreement clearly establishes more appropriate criteria for engagement. Similarly, comanagement services that ask the hospitalist to serve primarily as a replacement for residents or midlevel practitioners will also be demoralizing and impair a Hospital Medicine group's ability to recruit and retain high quality physicians.

FINANCIAL RISK

Very few hospitalist groups in the United States are entirely self-supported through professional fee revenue. The vast majority of groups require financial support, usually from the hospital. Little has been published about the revenue that can be generated by a comanagement service, but hiring additional providers for comanagement will likely incur further deficits. Thus, in developing a comanagement program, particular attention must be directed toward ensuring financial feasibility. This often requires a guarantee of financial support from parties that are encouraging the creation of a comanagement service, such as the hospital or the specialists.

PRACTICE POINT

- Particular attention must also be directed toward ensuring financial feasibility. This often requires a guarantee of financial support from parties that are encouraging the creation of a comanagement service, such as the hospital or the specialists.

In the United States, the billing codes for consultation have been eliminated along with their associated documentation requirements, such as the need for a written request for consultation. Initial encounters for the purpose of consultation (and possibly comanagement) will henceforth be billed under the same codes used for admission history and physical examination. The impact of this change on comanagement services is still uncertain. Elimination of the more lucrative consultation codes may decrease compensation for some services. However, elimination of the rigorous documentation requirements for consultation may also allow hospitalists to receive greater payment for their initial comanagement encounters, which often occur without a formal request for consultation. Understanding the regulations governing professional fee billing is crucial when estimating the revenue that is generated by a comanagement service, as well as when establishing the communication and documentation expectations required of both the hospitalist and specialist.

CONCLUSION

Comanagement is a negotiated, collaborative relationship, which broadens hospitalists' scope of practice but also requires their increased responsibility when managing medical care in patients admitted primarily for problems treated by surgeons or other specialists. The comanagement service agreement should specify the role of the hospitalists and may include patient and problem selection criteria, limits to order writing, communication protocols, as well as division of responsibilities. The agreement should also describe the goals of the comanagement service such as improvements in provider and patient satisfaction, efficiency of care, and clinical outcomes, and the process by which success at achieving these goals will be measured. While comanagement has the potential to improve care, it carries a unique set of pitfalls that arise from division of responsibility. Again, the comanagement service agreement should include provisions to minimize these risks and ensure the career satisfaction of participating hospitalists.

SUGGESTED READINGS

American Medical Association Council on Ethical and Judicial Affairs. Ethical implications of surgical comanagement. CEJA Report. 1999;5-I-99. Available at http://www.ama-assn.org/ama1/pub/upload/mm/369/ceja_5i99.pdf.

Auerbach AD, Wachter RM, CHeng HQ, et al. The impact of a hospitalist-neurosurgeon comanagement service on provider experience, patient outcomes, and resource use. *Arch Intern Med.* 2010;170:2004–2010.

Gaferi AA, Birkmeyer JD, Dimick JB. Variation in hospital mortality associated with inpatient surgery. *New England J Med.* 2009; 361:1368–1375.

Huddleston JM, Long KH, Naessens JM, et al. Medical and surgical comanagement after elective hip and knee arthroplasty. A randomized, controlled trial. *Ann Intern Med.* 2004;141:28–38.

Phy MP, Vanness DJ, Melton LJ, et al. Effects of a hospitalist model on elderly patients with hip fracture. *Arch Intern Med.* 2005;165: 796–801.

Salerno SM, Hurst FP, Halvorson S, et al. Principles of effective consultation: an update for the 21st-century consultant. *Arch Intern Med.* 2007;167:271–275.

Sharma G, Kuo Y, Freeman J, et al. Comanagement of hospitalized surgical patients by medicine physicians in the United States. *Arch Intern Med.* 2010;170:363–368.

Siegal EM. Just because you can, doesn't mean that you should: a call for rational application of hospitalist comanagement. *J Hosp Med.* 2008;3:398–402.

Simon TD, Eilert R, Dickinson LM, et al. Pediatric hospitalist comanagement of spinal fusion surgery patients. *J Hosp Med.* 2007;2:23–30.

Whinney C, Michota A. Surgical comanagement: a natural evolution of hospital practice. *J Hosp Med.* 2008;3:394–397.

SECTION 2
Key Issues Relating to Surgery

CHAPTER 44

Physiologic Response to Surgery

Marisa Cevasco, MD, MPH
Stanley Ashley, MD
Zara Cooper, MD, MSc

INTRODUCTION

Since 1932, when Cuthbertson first described the systemic response to lower-limb injury, our understanding of surgical physiology has grown significantly, resulting in improved perioperative management, decreased complications, more efficacious analgesia, and faster recovery times. Better control of the sympathoadrenal pathway, endocrine response, and fluid management results in less patient fatigue, shorter functional recovery, and decreased hospital stays. In this chapter we will review the surgical stress response, fluid and electrolyte balance, and organ-specific responses to surgery.

SURGICAL STRESS RESPONSE

Surgical stress response is the physiologic response to surgery and the name given to the hormonal and metabolic changes that follow surgery. This stress response has three key components: (1) sympathetic nervous system activation, (2) endocrine response with pituitary hormone secretion and insulin resistance, and (3) immunologic and hematologic changes including cytokine production, acute phase reaction, neutrophil leuokocytosis, and lymphocyte proliferation.

PRACTICE POINT

The surgical stress response has three key components:

1. Sympathetic nervous system activation
2. Endocrine response with pituitary hormone secretion and insulin resistance
3. Immunologic and hematologic changes including cytokine production, acute phase reaction, neutrophil leukocytosis, and lymphocyte proliferation

SYMPATHETIC NERVOUS SYSTEM

The sympathoadrenal response results from an increased secretion of catecholamines from the adrenal medulla. Circulating norepinephrine and epinephrine result in tachycardia and hypertension, and directly modify the function of numerous organs, including the liver, pancreas, and kidney. Gluconeogenesis is increased, glucagon production is stimulated, and water is retained to maintain fluid volume and cardiovascular homeostasis.

ENDOCRINE RESPONSE

The endocrine response includes changes in pituitary secretion with secondary effects on hormone secretion from target organs. The overall metabolic effect is increased catabolism, which mobilizes substrate to provide energy, and retention of salt and water to maintain fluid volume and cardiovascular homeostasis. Specifically, corticotrophin stimulates cortisol secretion from the adrenal cortex resulting in increased blood glucose levels, arginine vasopressin stimulates the kidney to retain water, and insulin secretion by the pancreas is often diminished (**Table 44-1**).

Cortisol secretion increases rapidly following the start of surgery. It results in protein breakdown, gluconeogenesis in the liver, and increased lipolysis. Blood glucose concentrations increase and are related to the intensity of the surgical injury. Consequently, longer and more drastic elevations in blood glucose are seen in cardiac surgery than in minor surgical procedures such as herniorrhaphy. The usual mechanisms that maintain glucose homeostasis are ineffective in

TABLE 44-1 Principal Hormonal Responses to Surgery

Endocrine Gland	Hormone	Change in Secretion
Anterior pituitary	ACTH	Increases
	Growth hormone	Increases
	TSH	May increase or decrease
	FSH and LH	May increase or decrease
Posterior pituitary	AVP	Increases
Adrenal cortex	Cortisol	Increases
	Aldosterone	Increases
Pancreas	Insulin	Often decreases
	Glucagon	Usually small increases
Thyroid	Thyroxine	Decrease

the postoperative period; cortisol promotes glucose production, there is a relative lack of insulin, and increased peripheral insulin resistance. Glycemic control is very important in surgical patients as the risks of perioperative hyperglycemia are well documented and include wound infection and impaired wound healing.

Protein catabolism is an important effect of increased perioperative cortisol concentrations. Both skeletal and visceral muscle are broken down to release amino acids for energy or to be used by the liver to form new protein including the acute phase reactants. This process results in weight loss, muscle wasting, and impaired healing. Studies have shown that surgical patients provided with nutritional supplements including glutamine and arginine, two essential amino acids, benefited from a faster recovery, fewer infections, and a shorter hospital stay.

■ IMMUNOLOGY

In addition to the endocrine response to surgery, other changes occur, most notably an increase in cytokine production and acute phase reactants. Cytokines are a group of low-molecular-weight proteins that include the interleukins and interferons, and they have a major role in the body's response to surgery and trauma. They are responsible for local effects of mediating and maintaining the inflammatory response to tissue injury. The main cytokines released after surgery are interleukin-1 (IL-1), tumor necrosis factor-α (TNF-α), and IL-6. The initial reaction of the body to surgery is to generate TNF-α and IL-1 from activated macrophages and monocytes in damaged tissues. This in turn stimulates the production of IL-6, the main cytokine responsible for the systemic changes known as the acute phase response. Cytokine production reflects the degree of tissue trauma; levels are lowest in laparoscopic and minimally-invasive procedures, and highest in major vascular procedures, joint replacements, and colorectal surgery. Cytokine levels peak 24-hours postoperatively and remain elevated for two to three days.

■ ACUTE PHASE RESPONSE

The acute phase response is characterized by systemic changes including fever, granulocytosis, and the production of acute phase proteins in the liver. Acute phase proteins, including C-reactive protein (CRP), fibrinogen, and α-2 macroglobulin, are inflammatory mediators, antiproteinases, and scavengers in tissue repair. D-dimer protein, a fibrin degradation product, will also be elevated in the postoperative period and may remain elevated for several weeks. Hematologic changes also occur along with the acute phase reaction, resulting in neutrophil leukocytosis and lymphocyte proliferation. Fever and leukocytosis can be expected in the first 48 hours after surgery, and should not prompt an infectious workup or antibiotic treatment in most cases.

FLUIDS AND ELECTROLYTES

■ FLUIDS

Patients often present for surgery after an overnight fast or inability to tolerate oral feeding, and will have a preexisting fluid deficit proportionate to the duration of the fast. This fluid deficit will be exacerbated by surgical wound losses and blood loss, although it may be partially replaced by careful intraoperative management by the anesthesia team. Obligatory fluid losses are proportional to the size of the surgical wound, and are due mainly to evaporative losses and internal redistribution of body fluids. This redistribution of fluids, also called "third-spacing," can result in massive fluid shifts and intravascular depletion, and manifests as postoperative hypotension, tachycardia, and decreased urine output. Burn injuries, peritonitis, and extensive surgical dissections or bowel resection cases may result in extracellular fluid translocating across serosal surfaces as ascites or into the bowel lumen; this translocated fluid does not readily equilibrate with the intracellular compartment, further exacerbating postoperative hypovolemia. Postoperative intravenous fluid replacement may be guided targeting urine output to 0.5 mL/kg/hr.

In a healthy adult on a normal diet, water input may be 1600 mL/day. A minimum intake of 500 mL/day is based on concentrating urine to a maximum of 1200 mOsm/kg when 600 mOsm of solute is excreted. In addition, oxidation provides 300 mL and fruits and vegetables 800 mL. To maintain balance with water output of 1600 mL/day, daily water losses may be approximated as follows: 500 mL from urine, 500 mL from skin, 400 mL from the respiratory tract, and 200 mL from stool. The typical Western diet provides 100–250 mEq Na+ per day. Maintenance fluids replace physiologic ongoing losses of water and electrolytes from urine, sweat, respiration, and stool. Replacement fluids correct water and electrolyte deficits from GI, urinary, skin, bleeding, third spacing, and losses during surgery.

Crystalloids are fluids that pass through the intravascular to extravascular interstitial fluid compartment. The predominant effect of volume from crystalloids is the interstitial space that accounts for 70–80% of the extracellular space. Normal saline (0.95 NaCl) in the amount of 1.1 liter will result in 275 cc into plasma and 825 cc into the interstitium. Normal saline is somewhat hypertonic to cells so that there will be some shift of fluid out of cells. Colloids are high-molecular-weight solutions that include plasma, hetastarch, albumin, and dextran. Hetastarch, albumin, and dextran are rarely used in the postoperative period. There has been no evidence to demonstrate that colloids are more effective in volume resuscitation than crystalloids; they are nearly 100 times more expensive on a per-volume basis and have been associated with adverse effects including allergic reactions in certain patients.

Maintenance fluids replace physiologic ongoing losses of water and electrolytes from urine, sweat, respiration, and stool. Replacement fluids correct water and electrolyte deficits from GI, urinary, skin, bleeding, third spacing, and losses during surgery. Crystalloids are the fluid of choice in both settings. Lactated Ringer's (LR) solution is typically the intravenous crystalloid of choice for fluid resuscitation in the first 48 hours. Intraoperative fluid losses are isotonic, thus a replacement-type solution such as LR with approximately 100 mL of free water per liter, 28 mEq/L of lactate, and 130 mEq/L of sodium is often used as it is the most physiologic solution when large-volume resuscitation is necessary. Potential disadvantages of LR include the interaction of calcium with various IV medications (such as aminocaproic acid and certain antibiotics) and concern for spurious lactate increase (although lactic acid levels should not be routinely drawn in postoperative patients unless there is a specific concern for tissue ischemia). By postoperative day three, ongoing fluid loss is primarily due to water loss and should be replaced by hypotonic solutions. Patients are then transitioned to maintenance-type solutions, such as D51/2NS + 20 mEq/L of potassium. Dextrose is provided to maintain tonicity and also to prevent ketosis and hypoglycemia during postoperative fasting or bowel rest. Dextrose in the amount of 1 gm provides 3.4 kcal, thus, 5% dextrose solution, (50 grams of dextrose/L) will provide 170 kcal. Three liters of 5% dextrose will provide nearly 900 kcal, which is enough to limit breakdown of endogenous proteins. Caution is advised regarding the administration of the hypertonic solution D5NS, which provides 560 Osm/L and will result in cell dehydration. In addition, in critically ill patients, glucose is metabolized to lactate and may result in metabolic acid production rather than metabolic energy production. Because of these significant adverse effects to dextrose administration, enteral and parenteral nutrition are better options in appropriate candidates (see Chapter 54).

PRACTICE POINT

Postoperative fluid replacement:

- Intraoperative fluid losses are isotonic.
  - Lactated Ringer's (LR) solution is typically the intravenous crystalloid of choice for fluid resuscitation in the first 48 hours.
- Ongoing fluid loss is primarily due to water loss by postoperative day three.
  - Patients are then transitioned to maintenance-type solutions, such as D51/2NS + 20 mEq/L of potassium.

Normal saline is often administered to patients who are hypotensive. Compared with plasma, the sodium, chloride, and osmolality is higher and the pH lower. The main disadvantage is that large volumes often cause a hyperchloremic metabolic acidosis. Three percent NS is occasionally used in patients with intracranial swelling; 3% NS should not be routinely used without receiving guidance from the neurosurgical or neurology team (**Table 44-2**).

ELECTROLYTES AND ACID BASE

Postsurgical patients often have electrolyte or acid-base imbalances, especially during prolonged periods of fasting as seen in patients recovering from bowel surgery. High-output nasogastric tubes, emesis, or enteric fistulas may result in hyponatremic, hypochloremic metabolic alkalosis. The leakage of exudates and transudates from large wounds, such as an open abdomen used to decompress an abdominal compartment syndrome, can also rapidly deplete both extracellular water and sodium. Nonosmotic ADH secretion from surgical stress and resuscitation with large volumes of LR will also contribute to postoperative hyponatremia. In these cases, hyponatremia should be treated by expanding the intravascular volume with an isotonic solution such as normal saline, which will correct the diluted serum sodium. Hypernatremia is less likely to develop in the immediate postoperative period, but may develop later in the hospital course, and is often associated with a relative lack of free water. Five percent dextrose (D5W) is the solution of choice for replacement of pure water deficits. Interventions to correct hypernatremia should decrease osmolality at a rate of 10–15 mEq per liter over 24 hours. Rapid rehydration can lead to brain swelling and permanent neurologic damage.

Potassium, the principal intracellular cation, plays a major role in cellular electrophysiology, and is integral to protein and carbohydrate synthesis. Serum potassium concentration should be closely monitored in the surgical patient. Surgical patients receiving blood transfusions may develop hyperkalemia from hemolysis of transfused products if they are administered at a rate greater than 100 mL/hr. Hypokalemia is more typically encountered in the postoperative setting, and is often associated with a metabolic alkalosis. Excessive renal losses of K^+ or uncompensated losses of gastrointestinal (GI) fluid are usually the causes of hypokalemia. Circulating β-2 agonists from the surgical stress response are also known to directly affect Na^+–K^+–ATPase activity and decrease serum [K^+]. Most patients are asymptomatic until plasma K^+ falls below 3.5 mEq/L; cardiovascular effects are most prominent and typically manifest as an abnormal electrocardiogram or arrhythmias. Patients undergoing cardiothoracic surgery and those with underlying cardiac disease should have their plasma potassium levels closely monitored and repleted to a level between 3.5–5.0 mEq/L for cardiac arrhythmia prophylaxis. Potassium replacement therapy is safest when administered orally; intravenous replacement should be reserved for patients unable to tolerate the oral formulation and should be administered gradually; the rate of intravenous infusion of K^+ should not exceed 20 mEq per hour.

Magnesium, another intracellular cation, is an important cofactor in many enzymatic processes. Only 1–2% of total body magnesium stores are in plasma, but surgical patients may develop weakness, muscle fasciculations, ataxia, or seizures with inadequate circulating volumes. Atrial fibrillation and ventricular dysrhythmias are also associated with hypomagnesemia, and administration of 2 grams of magnesium chloride following cardiothoracic surgery

TABLE 44-2 Intravenous Crystalloid Fluids Used in the Postoperative Period

Type of Fluid	Indications	Composition
LR	Typically used for the first 48 hours postoperatively; replacement fluids	130 mEq/L Na^+, 109 mEq/L Cl^-, 4 mEq/L K^+, 3 mEq/L Ca^{++}, 28 mEq/L Lactate, pH 6.4, 273 mOsm/L
D51/2NS+20K	Hypotonic maintenance fluids used after initial fluid resuscitation completed	50 gm dextrose; 77 mEq/L Na^+, 77 mEq/L Cl^-, 20 mEq K^+; pH 5.7; 452 mOsm/L
NS	Alternative to LR; watch for hyperchloremic metabolic acidosis	154 mEq/L Na^+, 154 mEq/L Cl^-, pH 5.7, 308 mOsm/L
½ NS	Hypotonic maintenance solution	77 mEq/L Na^+, 77 mEq/L Cl^-, pH 5.7
3% NS	Used in conjunction with neurosurgical or neurology teams to treat cerebral swelling	513 mEq/L Na^+, 513 mEq/L Cl^-, pH 5.7, 1027 mOsm/L
D5W	Free water; no role in resuscitation	50 gm dextrose, 278 mOsm/L
Human plasma	140 mEq/L Na^+, 103 mEq/L Cl^-, 4 mEq/L K^+, 5 mQ/L Ca^{++}, 2 mEq/L Mg^{++}, 25 mEq/L $HCO3^-$, pH 7.4, Osmolality 290 mOsm/L	

has been demonstrated to decrease postoperative cardiac events and mechanical ventilation time. Similar to potassium, serum magnesium concentration is decreased by catecholamines from the surgical stress response. Intravenous replacement is preferable, as enteral administration may result in a laxative effect.

Calcium, an important extracellular cation, should be monitored postoperatively, particularly in surgical oncology patients (who may have bony destruction due to metastasis or paraneoplastic syndromes), those with renal disease, or undergoing thyroid or parathyroid surgery. Although 98% of total body calcium is maintained in the bone, imbalance of extracellular calcium concentration may result in significant physiologic disturbances. Hypocalcemia may present with tetany, carpopedal spasm (Trousseaus sign), masseter spasm (Chvosteks sign), laryngospasm (stridor), paresthesias, or confusion. The diagnosis of hypocalcemia should be based on the laboratory value of plasma-ionized calcium, as the ionized portion is free and physiologically important. Hypercalcemia, on the other hand, will manifest as anorexia, vomiting, weakness, and polyuria, and may progress to lethargy, ataxia, or coma. It should be treated as a medical urgency, often with hydration and subsequent diuresis and occasionally with the addition of a bisphophonate or calcitonin.

SELECT ORGAN-SPECIFIC RESPONSES TO SURGERY

NEUROLOGY

Surgical patients are often elderly, naïve to narcotics, and with baseline comorbidities including impaired renal or hepatic clearance or cardiac disease. These factors, coupled with disrupted sleep, relative immobility, exposure to polypharmacy, and loss of the familiar home environment place patients at risk for developing postoperative delirium.

Postoperative delirium is characterized by impaired cognition, fluctuating levels of consciousness, altered psychomotor activity, and a disturbed sleep-wake cycle. It usually becomes apparent on the first or second postoperative day and symptoms become worse at night. Patients with preexisting cognitive impairment or those that are dependent on alcohol or sedatives are at an even greater risk for developing postoperative delirium. An increase of serum cortisol from the stress of surgery and anesthesia is also thought to contribute to postoperative confusion.

The rate of postoperative delirium may be as high as 60% in certain populations. It is more likely to occur in those patients undergoing cardiac surgery (particularly in cases with long cardiopulmonary bypass time and relative intraoperative cerebral hypoperfusion); orthopedic procedures (secondary to fat embolism); or ophthalmologic cases employing the use of anticholinergic drugs.

PRACTICE POINT

- The rate of postoperative delirium may be as high as 60% in certain populations. It is more likely to occur in those patients undergoing cardiac surgery, orthopedic procedures, or ophthalmologic cases employing the use of anticholinergic drugs. It may also result from acute alcohol withdrawal, which would require a different management approach.

Haloperidol is the drug of choice for treatment of acute delirium. Benzodiazepines may exacerbate delirium especially in elderly patients and in patients with liver disease. However, short-acting benzodiazepines should be prescribed to prevent alcohol withdrawal in patients who drink daily. Neither muscle relaxants nor physical restraints are particularly effective. Central nervous depressants, H2-antagonists, anticholinergics, digitalis, phenytoin, lidocaine, and aminophylline should be used with discretion. In general, drugs with short elimination half-lives are preferable to long-acting drugs (see Chapter 80).

CARDIOVASCULAR

Circulating catecholamines from the surgical stress response often result in tachycardia and hypertension. Perioperative beta-blockade should be employed in patients with a history of cardiac disease, targeting a heart rate between 60–70 beats per minute. For these patients, preoperative cardiac optimization often includes a statin and an aspirin. Hospitalists should be able to provide cardiac risk stratification and assist the surgical team in achieving optimal heart rate and blood pressure control through beta-blockade and antihypertensives. Hospitalists should also be able to identify which patients may benefit from intervention for unstable cardiac disease, including severe or critical aortic stenosis, atherosclerosis, and conduction system disease. As consultants, hospitalists would be expected to communicate with the patient's outside cardiologist if available (see Chapter 51).

For patients with aortic stenosis undergoing noncardiac operations, peripheral hypotension should be avoided. Hypotension decreases the coronary artery filling pressures, decreases oxygen supply, and may result in cardiac ischemia. Vasodilators such as nitroglycerin should particularly be avoided. For patients with valvular lesions or prosthetic cardiac valves, surgical procedures convey an increased risk for the development of bacterial endocarditis. Prophylactic antibiotics must be administered in the perioperative period according to American Heart Association (AHA) guidelines.

PULMONARY

Surgical patients are susceptible to postoperative pulmonary complications. Incentive spirometry, early mobility, and deep breathing exercises to expand lung volumes will help prevent postoperative complications such as atelectasis, tracheobronchitis, and pneumonia. Adequate pain control, especially epidural analgesia for thoracic or complex abdominal surgeries, will allay splinting. Limiting surgical time, performing a laparoscopic procedure instead of an open case, and the use of regional anesthesia instead of general anesthesia with an endotracheal reduces pulmonary complications. Patients with chronic obstructive disease or restrictive lung disease are at an increased risk of developing postoperative pulmonary complications and should receive aggressive medical therapy, including the use of inhaled short-acting beta-agonist and anticholinergic bronchodilator medications in appropriate patient populations. Systemic corticosteroid treatment, in short courses, also improves spirometry in patients with obstructive lung disease. Surgical outcomes are not adversely affected by perioperative inhaled corticosteroid administration when prescribed for obstructive lung disease. Inadequate treatment of active lung disease is a greater contributor to perioperative morbidity than systemic corticosteroid administration (see Chapter 54).

GASTROINTESTINAL

Ileus, or nonmechanical obstruction of the gastrointestinal tract persisting for greater than three days, is common in surgical patients. Hypomotility of the gastrointestinal tract secondary to uncoordinated propulsive action results in impaired transport of intestinal contents. Both gas and fluids accumulate within the bowel, leading to abdominal distension and discomfort, hiccupping (irritation of the phrenic nerve), nausea, and vomiting. Ileus most commonly occurs after intraabdominal surgeries, although it is also seen in patients undergoing retroperitoneal or extraabdominal surgery; those with sepsis; pneumonia; biliary or renal colic; or after a myocardial infarction.

Patients with metabolic abnormalities such as hypokalemia or hypomagnesemia are also predisposed to develop ileus.

In surgical patients, the stress response is thought to play a key role in promoting the development of postoperative ileus. Circulating catecholamines, third-spacing of fluids, and bowel wall edema all contribute to intestinal hypomotility. Surgical manipulation of the bowel also leads to activation of adrenoreceptors on inhibitory spinal reflex arcs, further delaying the return of bowel function; the use of thoracic epidurals blocking this reflex has been shown to prevent ileus.

Treatment of postoperative ileus is supportive in nature and includes hydration, correction of electrolyte imbalances, and discontinuation of medications that hinder bowel motility. Routine postoperative placement of nasogastric tubes in asymptomatic patients is unnecessary but is warranted in those with recurrent episodes of emesis. Studies have investigated the role of gum-chewing or early ambulation on the resolution of ileus but neither of these proposed therapies have demonstrated efficacy. Some advocate for early postoperative feeding to help diminish the occurrence of ileus, but this too has provided equivocal results. Ultimately, all nonmechanical obstructive ileus will resolve over time; the small bowel typically regains function first, followed by the stomach, and lastly by the large intestine (see Chapter 46).

PRACTICE POINT

- Treatment of postoperative ileus includes hydration, correction of electrolyte imbalances, and discontinuation of medications that hinder bowel motility. Routine postoperative placement of nasogastric tubes in asymptomatic patients is unnecessary but is warranted in those with recurrent episodes of emesis.

In terms of preventing ileus, the use of local or epidural anesthesia or a combination of local and opioid analgesia rather than systemic or epidural opioids, is effective. The elimination of ileus allows for the early use of enteral nutrition, which is an important factor in reducing the risk of infectious complications. Moreover, patients with ileus may have discomfort and pain, causing them to be less mobile and increasing their risk for pulmonary complications. Ileus also enhances catabolism because of poor nutrition, leading to impaired wound healing, prolonged hospital stays, and overall postoperative morbidity.

RENAL

Acute renal failure (ARF) has been defined as a precipitous decline in renal function associated with the accumulation of nitrogenous waste (azotemia). It is commonly associated with decreased urine production leading to oliguria or anuria, although nonoliguric forms also exist.

In the postsurgical patient, ARF is often initiated by perioperative hemodilution and hypovolemia. It is a common complication following cardiac surgery using cardiopulmonary bypass (CPB) but may also occur following general surgery procedures. Hemodilution from aggressive fluid resuscitation and hypovolemia from hemorrhage or inadequate volume replacement reduce the viscosity of capillary blood flow and redistribute blood from the renal medulla to the renal cortex, subjecting the medulla to ischemia. Constriction of the afferent and efferent arterioles by circulating catecholamines from the surgical stress response also contributes to ischemic injury. This renal tubular injury, otherwise known as acute tubular necrosis, is a histologic diagnosis characterizing most forms of perioperative intrinsic renal failure. Initiation of tubular injury may also be due to circulating nephrotoxins such as aminoglycosides, inhaled anesthetics, or radiocontrast agents administered in the perioperative period.

TABLE 44-3 Surgical and Medical Conditions Predisposing to ARF

Trauma	Vascular disease
Cardiopulmonary bypass	Hypotension
Underlying renal disease	Hypovolemia
Renal transplantation	Liver failure
Urologic surgery	Sepsis
Pigment nephropathy	Contrast agents
Drugs (eg, aminoglycosides)	

Once tubular damage is sustained, a number of factors contribute to maintenance of tubular damage. Intraluminal obstruction from cell swelling and sloughing, persistent vasoconstriction, back-leakage of luminal fluid across damaged tubular epithelium, and decreased glomerular capillary membrane permeability all add to nephron dysfunction and delayed renal recovery. The trauma or illness that led directly to the surgical procedure and preexisting medical conditions are also important risk factors in developing ARF (**Table 43-3**) (see Chapter 57).

CONCLUSION

In closing, patients undergoing surgery are subject to a series of metabolic and hormonal changes that alter normal physiology. This surgical stress response affects nearly every organ system and is dependent on the type and duration of surgery. Awareness of the physiologic changes expected in the postoperative period, and knowledge on how to manage them, will enable patients to recover quickly and potentially avoid complications. Close collaboration with the surgical team in the postoperative period is an important aspect of patient management.

SUGGESTED READINGS

Jamieson RA, Ledigham I, Kay AW, MacKay C. *Jamieson and Kay's Textbook of Surgical Physiology*. 4th Edition. Philadelphia, PA: Churchill Livingstone; 1988.

Kanani M, Elliott M. *Applied Surgical Physiology Vivas*. 1st Edition. London, England: Greenwich-Medical; 2004.

Morgan GE, Mikhail MS, Murray MJ. *Clinical Anesthesiology* (Lange Series). 4th Edition. New York, NY: McGraw-Hill; 2002.

Townsend CM, Beauchamp D, Evers MB, Mattox KJ, eds. *Sabiston Textbook of Surgery: The Biologic Basis of Modern Surgical Practice*. 18th Edition. Philadelphia, PA: Saunders; 2007.

CHAPTER 45

Perioperative Hemostasis

Zara Cooper, MD, MSc
Stanley Ashley, MD

INTRODUCTION

Postoperative bleeding is a dreaded surgical complication. More often than not you will hear, "It was dry when we closed…" as your surgical colleagues struggle to identify the source. Risk factors include trauma, coagulopathy, or factor deficiency, which may be congenital or acquired from malnutrition, antibiotic use, or liver disease. Hospitalized patients are commonly anticoagulated prior to surgery. Patients at risk should have a preoperative evaluation including a complete blood count, liver function tests, prothrombin time, activated partial prothrombin time, and international normalized ratio (**Figure 45-1**). Patients with platelet dysfunction from aspirin, antiplatelet agents, or uremia are also at increased risk of postoperative hemorrhage.

WORKUP

Surgical bleeding is usually from a blood vessel that was improperly occluded or was in spasm during surgery but is no longer in spasm and is bleeding into the surgical space. Nonsurgical bleeding is associated with coagulopathy and should be addressed medically with normalization of clotting factors that may require transfusion or other agents that are discussed in detail below.

Ideally, hemostasis is achieved before the patient leaves the operating room (OR). However, patients who have received anticoagulation during surgery or experienced large blood loss during surgery are at risk for ongoing bleeding or rebleeding. Significant blood loss is expected with cardiopulmonary bypass and vascular procedures in which intravenous anticoagulation is routinely administered intraoperatively, as well as hepatic, obstetric, and large orthopedic procedures. Emergent and urgent procedures are also associated with higher blood loss. These patients are placed at high risk due to coagulopathy and a bloody surgical field that can obscure the surgeon's ability to identify all bleeding points.

Postoperative bleeding should be suspected in any postoperative patient with hypotension, low urine output, or tachycardia. Even if these can be explained by other events, a complete blood count (CBC) is in order to rule out bleeding as a consideration. If bleeding is present, transfusion with blood and crystalloid to maintain blood volume are in order. Resuscitation should commence as you are looking for a source.

PRACTICE POINT

Postoperative bleeding should be suspected in any postoperative patient with hypotension, low urine output, or tachycardia.

- Surgical bleeding is usually from a blood vessel that was improperly occluded or was in spasm during surgery but is no longer in spasm and is bleeding into the surgical space.
- Nonsurgical bleeding is associated with coagulopathy.

Physical exam may reveal signs of shock as well as a tense or tender abdomen in the case of intra-abdominal bleeding, or a tense compartment after extremity surgery. Bleeding in the retroperitoneum may not be immediately obvious and should be suspected in aortic or prostate surgery. Bleeding may also not be obvious in obese patients. Drains left in the surgical bed may have bloody output. Cardiac and thoracic patients should have their chest tube output followed closely. If there is no chest tube in place, a chest X-ray

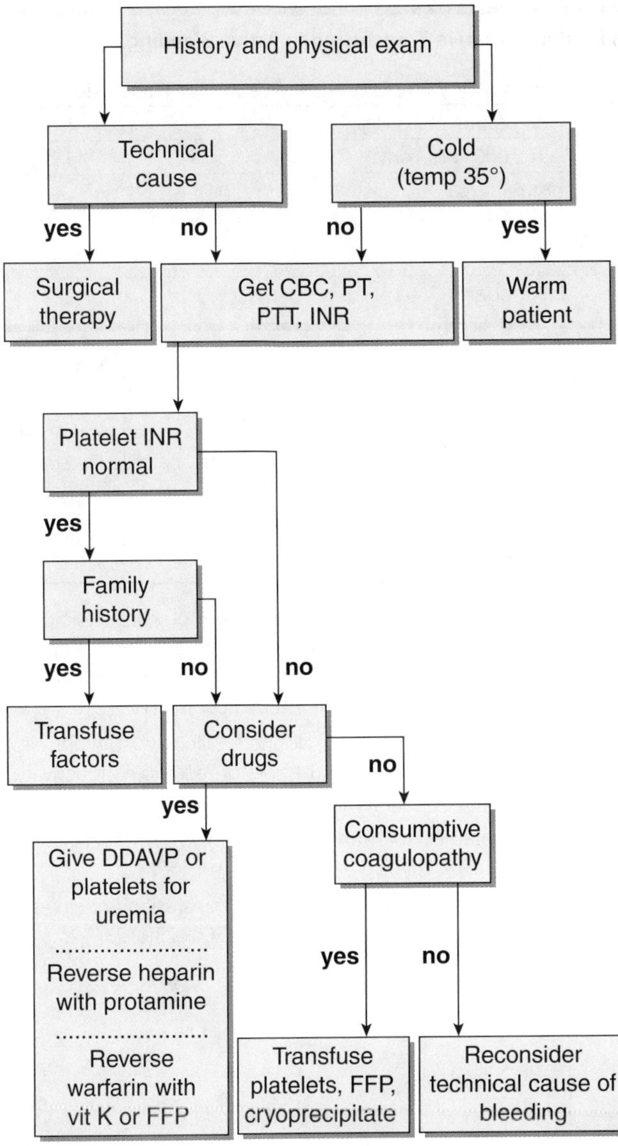

Figure 45-1 *Management of Post Operative Bleeding.*

will demonstrate a hemothorax. No matter the potential source, the operating surgeon should be notified immediately about any change in the patient's condition.

TREATMENT

If surgical bleeding is the source, then surgical correction is the only solution. However, patients with significant bleeding may also be coagulopathic and this should be addressed before the patient returns to the operating room if possible. A coagulation panel including prothrombin time (PT), partial thromboplastin time (PTT), and international normalized ratio (INR) should be ordered. If the patient had significant blood loss and transfusion in the OR, it is useful to check a fibrinogen level as these patients may require cryoprecipitate to improve clotting. Although spontaneous bleeding is rarely seen with a platelet count above 20,000, patients who are actively bleeding should have their platelets corrected to 100,000. It is important to keep in mind that patients who have been taking aspirin, antiplatelet agents, or have uremia may have a normal platelet count with a functional deficiency and could benefit from transfusion. Desmopressin can be used to partially reverse platelet dysfunction in patients with end-stage renal disease.

PRACTICE POINT

- If surgical bleeding is the source, then surgical correction is the only solution. However, patients with significant bleeding may also be coagulopathic and this should be addressed before the patient returns to the operating room if possible.

Patients who have an elevated PTT from intraoperative heparin administration may be reversed with protamine. The activated clotting time can be used to guide the appropriate dosage. Protamine is associated with allergic reactions and hypercoaguability, and caution should be used in its administration. This is especially the case in vascular and cardiac surgical patients who receive large boluses of heparin during surgery, and who are also at risk of graft thrombosis. Unfortunately, there is no reversal agent for low-molecular-weight heparin, which increases the risk of using it in the immediate postoperative period. Coagulopathy from Coumadin is usually reversed preoperatively with fresh frozen plasma and vitamin K. In the setting of profound hemorrhage with coagulopathy, recombinant factor VII may be used. This is very expensive and is associated with thrombus formation, and should not be prescribed to a surgical patient without surgical input.

Hypothermia exacerbates coagulopathy and so patients should be covered with warm blankets or convection blankets, and given warmed fluids until normothermia returns.

Bleeding from the wound itself often causes a great deal of excitement at the bedside but is often of little consequence. Usually a "skin bleeder" can be managed with a stitch or two, by holding pressure, or with bedside cautery. If the wound is bleeding at a good clip, a gauze dressing and tape will rarely do the trick and the person who placed it will often be alarmed to find a blood-soaked dressing when he or she returns. If the bleeding can't be stopped after 10–15 minutes of manual pressure, the surgeon should be notified.

PRACTICE POINT

- If the bleeding from a surgical wound cannot be stopped after 10–15 minutes of manual pressure, the surgeon should be notified.

Data does not support absolute transfusion triggers. The current American Society for Anesthesiologists guidelines for perioperative blood transfusions recommend following physiologic endpoints and clinical assessment. However, general transfusion guidelines (see **Table 45-1**) advise giving packed red blood cells when hemoglobin levels are less than 6 gm/dl, platelets when platelet levels are less than 50 × 109/L and, fresh frozen plasma (FFP) when the PT is greater than 1.5 × normal, the PTT is higher than 2 × normal and the INR is greater than 2.0. FFP should not be used for volume expansion alone. Cryoprecipitate is indicated for patients with congenital factor deficiencies, in massive transfusion, and if the fibrinogen level is less than 80–100 mg/dl with massive coagulopathy. There is insufficient data to guide transfusion above these thresholds. Resuscitation in the bleeding patient depends on the pace of the bleeding. Therapy should be guided by the potential for ongoing bleeding and physiologic endpoints such as heart rate, blood pressure, urine output, oxygen saturation, and electrocardiography. More advanced monitoring including echocardiography and invasive hemodynamic measurements can be used when appropriate. Ongoing shock and ischemia require transfusion regardless of the laboratory results. Volume replacement requires crystalloid and blood products; replacement with crystalloid alone can exacerbate coagulopathy. Rapid bleeding is usually associated with a more profound coagulopathy and more recent transfusion guidelines for trauma patients

TABLE 45-1 American Society of Anesthesiologists (ASA) Guidelines for Perioperative Transfusion in Active Bleeding

Therapy	Laboratory Value Indicates Transfusion	Laboratory Value Exceeds Indication for Transfusion
Packed red blood cells	Hemoglobin 6 g/dl	Hemoglobin 10 g/dl
Platelets	≤ 50,000 cells/mm³	≥ 100,000 cells/mm³
Fresh frozen plasma	PT ≥ 1.5 × normal PTT ≥ 2 × normal INR ≥ 2.0	normal
Cryoprecipitate	80–100 mg/dl and coagulopathy	Fibrinogen ≥ 150 mg/dl

recommend the replacement of packed cells, platelets, and fresh frozen plasma at a ratio of 1:1:1. Bleeding with a less profound coagulopathy should be treated as the laboratory values indicate.

Once hemorrhagic shock has been adequately addressed, there is no need for ongoing resuscitation. Volume replacement to supraphysiologic levels is associated with adverse outcomes such as volume overload, abdominal compartment syndrome, bowel edema and ileus, and respiratory failure with adult respiratory distress syndrome.

CONCLUSION

Postoperative bleeding is a feared surgical complication because reoperation, blood transfusion, and shock are all associated with poor outcome. Bleeding should be considered in any postoperative patients with tachycardia, hypotension, oliguria, or evidence of shock. Postoperative bleeding may be due to technical error, coagulopathy, or both. Physical exam and laboratory tests can guide management, and resuscitation should occur even as a source is sought. The surgical team should be involved in the workup and decision making as early as possible and should be called as soon as bleeding is suspected.

SUGGESTED READINGS

An updated report by the American Society of Anesthesiologists Task Force on Perioperative Blood Transfusion and Adjuvant Therapies. Practice guidelines for perioperative blood transfusion and adjuvant therapies. *Anesthesiology*. 2006;105:198–208.

Phillips LE, Zatta AJ, Schembri NL, Noone AK, Isbister J. Uncontrolled bleeding in surgical patients: the role of recombinant activated factor VIIa. *Curr Drug Targets*. 2009;10(8):744–770.

Spahn DR. Strategies for transfusion therapy. *Best Pract Res Clin Anaesthesiol*. 2004;18(4):661–673.

Spinella PC, Holcomb JB. Resuscitation and transfusion principles for traumatic hemorrhagic shock. *Blood Rev*. 2009;23(6):231–240.

CHAPTER 46

Postoperative Complications

Zara Cooper, MD, MSc
Stanley Ashley, MD

INTRODUCTION

There are many postoperative complications related to particular procedures that are beyond the scope of this text. Hospitalists caring for surgical patients should have an understanding of what surgical procedure was performed, the indication for that operation, and what perioperative concerns the operating surgeon has based on the circumstances of that particular patient or procedure. This should be part of the communication between the surgical and hospitalist staff. Here we will consider complications that are commonly associated with all surgical procedures.

PRACTICE POINT

- Hospitalists caring for surgical patients should have an understanding of what surgical procedure was performed, the indication for that operation, and what perioperative concerns the operating surgeon has based on the circumstances of that particular patient or procedure. This should be part of the communication between the surgical and hospitalist staff.

The prevention of postoperative complications should begin in the preoperative period. A thorough history and physical examination should identify conditions that increase the risk for bleeding, infection, and cardiopulmonary compromise. Elective surgery provides an opportunity to uncover and modify risk factors. Aspirin, antiplatelet agents, NSAIDS, and anticoagulant therapy are routinely held preoperatively to decrease bleeding risk.

PRACTICE POINT

- The prevention of postoperative complications should begin in the preoperative period.

POSTOPERATIVE FEVER

Low-grade postoperative fever occurs in as many as one-third of postoperative patients and is usually caused by postoperative inflammation, atelectasis, or hematoma absorption rather than infection. Fever from inflammation occurs earlier than fever from infection; 1.6 vs. 2.7 days in 1 series. Evaluation should include physical exam and a white blood cell count, and should otherwise be targeted toward specific signs and symptoms in the first 48 hours. After 48 hours, temperatures greater than 38.5°C without a clear source should prompt a complete fever workup including chest X-ray, blood, sputum, and urine cultures, and a white blood cell count. Pay particular attention to the surgical wound and sites of venous access as potential sources.

PRACTICE POINT

Postoperative fever

- Low grade postoperative fever occurs in as many as one-third of postoperative patients and is usually caused by postoperative inflammation, atelectasis, or hematoma absorption rather than infection.
- After 48 hours, temperatures greater than 38.5°C without a clear source should prompt a complete fever workup.

THE POST ANESTHESIA CARE UNIT (PACU)

After surgery, the patient will stay in the Post Anesthesia Care Unit (PACU) for close monitoring, to regain consciousness, and for physiologic recovery. Typical problems managed in the PACU include postoperative pain, hypertension, respiratory insufficiency, and postoperative nausea and vomiting (PONV). Patients with altered consciousness after general anesthesia may be unable to verbalize their pain, leaving caregivers to rely on physical signs such as hypertension, tachycardia, agitation, and tachypnea for diagnosis.

Pain, hypoxia, and elevated catecholamines contribute to hypertension and tachycardia. Give beta-blockers to patients at risk for postoperative myocardial ischemia and to avoid withdrawal in patients who used them preoperatively.

There a number of factors contributing to postoperative pulmonary insufficiency: type of anesthesia, type and duration of procedure, endotracheal intubation, and respiratory depression from narcotics. Immediately after surgery most patients will require some supplemental oxygen. However, dyspnea, tachypnea, wheezing, and signs of respiratory distress need to be addressed in the PACU. Upper abdominal procedures and thoracic procedures are commonly associated with pain, impairing respiratory effort and causing hypoxia and dyspnea. Patients with a low ejection fraction or diastolic dysfunction may have difficulty managing volumes of fluid received intraoperatively, and are at risk for postoperative pulmonary edema. Evaluate with physical exam and chest X-ray. Cardiac or thoracic surgical patients will usually have a chest tube postoperatively and it is important to keep in mind that a poorly functioning chest tube or residual pneumothorax can also cause respiratory distress. This can also be detected by physical exam and confirmed with a chest X-ray. All patients who have central lines placed intraoperatively require a postoperative chest X-ray to rule out pneumothorax.

Hypotension in the PACU may be related to hypovolemia, narcotic and benzodiazepine administration, and epidural anesthesia but is most worrisome for postoperative bleeding. Markers for hypovolemia include low urine output, signs of shock, and altered mental status, which can be masked by the residual effects of anesthesia. Invasive monitoring with a urinary drainage catheter, central line, or arterial line should be utilized if a patient remains hypotensive and he or she does not improve with volume. In the case of low urine output it is usually unwise to administer diuretics in the immediate postoperative setting; pulmonary edema due to capillary leak associated with perioperative inflammation can be seen in the setting of intravascular volume depletion. The premature administration of diuretics exacerbates intravascular depletion, hypotension, and inadequate end organ perfusion, and is rarely the correct first step in volume management.

PRACTICE POINT

Low urine output in the immediate postoperative setting

- Intravascular volume depletion may occur concurrently with pulmonary edema due to a capillary leak associated with perioperative inflammation.
- The premature administration of diuretics exacerbates intravascular depletion, hypotension, and inadequate end organ perfusion, and is rarely the correct first step in volume management.
- Postoperative oliguria (less than the equivalent of 0.5 cc/kg/hr) requires urgent evaluation for the possibility of urinary retention.

Medications and epidural anesthesia should not cause hypotension in the absence of hypovolemia. Although the instinct is to reduce the analgesia, hypotension in this case should also prompt administration of a fluid bolus to address underlying hypovolemia. Patients with hypotension require a thorough physical exam to look for sources of bleeding, and a hematocrit and coagulation panel to rule out hemorrhage and coagulopathy (see Chapter 45 Perioperative Hemostasis, Chapter 61 Perioperative Management of Patients who are Receiving Oral Anticoagulant Therapy, and Chapter 62 Perioperative Management of Patients who are Receiving Antiplatelet Therapy).

The causes for nausea and vomiting are multifactorial. Prior history of PONV increases the risk of recurrence, as do long procedures, volatile anesthetics, and procedures involving the inner ear, eye, and abdominal viscera. Patients at high to moderate risk benefit from prophylactic antiemetics, motility agents, or a scopolamine patch before emersion from anesthesia.

WOUND COMPLICATIONS

In a healthy patient wounds will take 6 weeks to heal completely and reach 80% of their previous tensile strength. Wounds closed primarily should be kept clean, dry, and covered for a minimum of 48 hours after surgery. Typically, operative dressings are removed on postoperative day 2 and thereafter patients can shower. Surgeons restrict postoperative activities to avoid stress on the wound for 4–6 weeks. Wet to dry dressing changes are used in contaminated wounds healing secondarily. The wet dressing provides a moist environment that encourages granulation. Removal of the dressing after it has dried provides mechanical debridement and keeps the wound clean. At the time of discharge, instructions include specifics relating to activity level, who and when to call should late wound complications become manifest, and instructions for follow-up.

SURGICAL SITE INFECTIONS

Surgical site infections (SSI) account for approximately 15% of nosocomial infections and are the most common infections after surgery. They are associated with a 7-day increased length of stay and more than $3000 in additional hospital costs. In 2006, a consortium of hospital and professional groups introduced the Surgical Care Improvement Project Guidelines (see **Table 46-1**) with the goal of decreasing postoperative complications 25% by 2010. These include measures for reducing SSIs.

SSIs are classified as superficial, deep, or organ space infections. Superficial infections are wound infections involving the skin and

TABLE 46-1 Surgical Care Improvement Project Module

1. Prophylactic antibiotic received within 1 hour prior to surgery
2. Prophylactic anantibiotic selection for surgical patients
3. Prophylactic antibiotics discontinued within 24 hours after surgery end time (48 hours for cardiac patients)
4. Cardiac surgery patients with controlled 6 AM postoperative serum glucose
5. Surgery patients with appropriate hair removal
6. Surgery patients on beta-blocker therapy prior to arrival who received a beta-blocker during the perioperative period
7. Surgery patients with recommended venous thromboembolism prophylaxis ordered
8. Surgery patients who received appropriate venous thromboembolism prophylaxis within 24 hours prior to surgery to 24 hours after surgery
9. Colorectal surgical patients who are normothermic (96.8–100.4) upon arrival (first 15 minutes) to post anesthesia care unit

subcutaneous tissues. Deep infections involve the fasica or muscle below. Deep space infections involve organs below the cutaneous and muscular layers. Despite the most rigorous aseptic technique, all wounds are contaminated to some degree and have some risk of infection. Even "clean" wounds without any evidence of gross contamination have a 1.5% risk of infection.

PRACTICE POINT

Wound infections

- Despite the most rigorous aseptic technique, all wounds are contaminated to some degree and have some risk of infection.
- Wound infections commonly occur between 5 and 10 postoperative days
  - Antibiotics are not necessary for simple wounds that have been drained.
  - Antibiotics alone will not cure a deep space infection.
  - A very high fever in a patient immediately postoperatively raises concern for a clostridial necrotizing wound infection and mandates an immediate surgical evaluation at the bedside.

Risk factors for wound infection include host- or patient-related factors and operative factors. Host factors include body habitus and prior comorbidities such as diabetes, prolonged disability, immune suppression, malnutrition, severity of underlying disease, and smoking history. Operative factors include operating room conditions, administration of antibiotic prophylaxis, and hypoxia or hypotension during the procedure. Prevention includes aseptic and meticulous surgical technique, including gentle handling of tissue, hemostasis, and avoiding excessive suturing. Infection rates are lower with clippers than razors, and hair should be removed just before incision. Prophylactic antibiotics, dosed by weight, and administered within 1 hour of incision, are used in contaminated and infected cases. In the event of significant contamination in the OR, wounds should be left open and managed with delayed primary closure or wet to dry dressings (see Chapter 50 Antimicrobial Prophylaxis in Surgery).

The hallmark signs of wound infection are fever, pain, heat, tenderness, and purulent drainage from the wound. Wound infection commonly occurs between 5 and 10 postoperative days; however, infections may occur before then. In fact, a very high fever in a patient immediately postoperatively raises concern for a clostridial necrotizing wound infection and mandates an immediate surgical evaluation at the bedside. Standard treatment of a wound infection is to open the wound and allow adequate drainage. Antibiotics are not necessary for simple wounds that have been drained.

Deep space infections require drainage percutaneously under CT guidance or during a return trip to the operating room. Antibiotics alone will not cure a deep space infection due to inadequate penetration of relatively remote, closed spaces. Anastomotic leaks typically occur between postoperative days 5 and 7 and are accompanied by abdominal pain, fever, and elevated white count. This constellation of symptoms after an enteric anastomosis should prompt a CT scan. Most often these leaks can be managed with percutaneous drainage. Inability to control the infection and sepsis requires operative drainage (**Table 46-2**).

DEHISCENCE, HEMATOMAS, SEROMAS

Wound dehiscence is disruption of any layer of the surgical wound. This rare complication results from increased pressure on the wound, insufficient wound closure, or poor healing. Patient factors associated with poor wound healing include: malnutrition, liver disease, diabetes, immunosuppression, and chronic steroid use. Serosainguinous fluid from the wound is considered a sentinel sign of dehiscence but is not always present. Management depends on the size and location of the wound as well as the patient's condition. Wound dehiscence in the abdomen is usually managed by urgent closure. A surgical emergency, evisceration, occurs when wound dehiscence leads to extrusion of abdominal contents.

Hematomas are usually caused by inadequate hemostasis during surgery and may cause wound elevation, pressure, pain, disruption, and infection. Risk factors for the development of hematomas include bleeding disorders and anticoagulant use. Patients may become alarmed by the benign skin discoloration that may be associated with hematomas. Hematomas following neck exploration may rapidly compromise the airway with tracheal deviation in the postoperative period. Precipitating factors include abrupt increases in intrathoracic pressure from coughing, emesis, or Valsalva maneuvers. Treatment involves rapid evacuation under sterile conditions.

Seromas are collections of serous fluid that form after procedures involving disrupted lymphatic flow and raised skin flaps. Examples include such procedures as inguinal hernia repair, groin exploration, and mastectomy. Suction drains may be left in place at the end of the procedure to increase tissue apposition and remove fluid. Compression dressings can also reduce the risk of seroma formation. Seromas increase the risk for wound disruption and infection but are not usually infected themselves and rarely present more than a nuisance. Management may be expectant, include serial aspirations, or rarely, a return to the operating room to ligate contributing lymphatics.

PULMONARY COMPLICATIONS

(See Chapter 55 Preoperative Pulmonary Risk Assessment). Limited chest excursion due to pain and small airway collapse due to

TABLE 46-2 Surgical Wound Classification

Wound Classification	Infection Risk	Procedure Type
Clean: No infection or inflammation Respiratory, gastrointestinal, biliary, and urinary tracts not entered	1.5%	Vascular surgery
Clean contaminated: Entry into respiratory, biliary, gastrointestinal, urinary tracts with minimal spillage No evidence of infection or major break in aseptic technique	10%	Appendectomy
Contaminated: Inflammation, gross spillage from GI tract, break in technique Fresh traumatic wound	20%	Foreign body in a wound
Dirty or infected: Purulent drainage, fecal contamination, perforated viscus, delayed or contaminated traumatic wound, presence of devitalized tissue	40%	Abscess, perforated viscus

airway secretions, blood clots, or poorly positioned endotracheal tubes cause atelectasis, which is an important risk factor for pneumonia. Incisional pain and somnolence from narcotics also impair pulmonary clearance. This is especially true for thoracic and upper abdominal procedures in which pain interferes with normal respiratory excursion causing splinting. Clinical findings include hypoxia and fever. Collapsed airways predispose patients to infection and pneumonia. Prevention includes adequate pain control, respiratory therapy, and early mobilization. When possible, encourage patients to get out of bed on the evening of surgery. Treatment of atelectasis includes encouraging coughing, deep breathing, and pulmonary toilet. Incentive spirometers (IS) are useful to engage patients in their own postoperative recovery; however, they are not more effective in preventing pneumonia or controlling costs than routine pulmonary toilet. IS are superior to no pulmonary therapy at all.

PRACTICE POINT

Atelectasis

- Prevention includes adequate pain control, respiratory therapy, and early mobilization.
- Treatment of atelectasis includes encouraging coughing, deep breathing, and pulmonary toilet.
  - Antibiotics are not necessary for simple wounds that have been drained.
  - Incentive spirometers (IS) are useful to engage patients in their own postoperative recovery; however, they are not more effective in preventing pneumonia, or controlling costs, than routine pulmonary toilet.
  - IS are superior to no pulmonary therapy at all.

Postoperative pneumonia occurs in 1.5% of patients after major noncardiac surgery, and increases the risk of postoperative mortality tenfold. Risk factors include emergent surgery, thoracic and upper abdominal procedures, abdominal aortic aneurysm repair, age, poor functional status, steroid use, recent weight loss, and recent alcohol use. Postoperative pneumonia is a clinical diagnosis revealed by fever, elevated white count, rales, or dullness on physical exam, positive sputum or tracheal aspirate, and infiltrate on chest X-ray. Aspiration commonly causes hospital-acquired pneumonia and the microbiology reflects tracheal rather than oral secretions. Patients with aspiration pneumonitis, without aspiration pneumonia, should not receive antibiotics. Patients with swallowing dysfunction, neuromuscular disorders, and altered sensoirum are at risk for aspiration. Nasogastric tubes are thought to increase the risk of aspiration because they interfere with oropharyngeal clearance and closure of the GE junction. However, a study comparing incidence of aspiration in patients fed via gastrostomy tube and nasogastric tubes did not show gastrostomy tubes to be superior in preventing aspiration pneumonia. As with other hospital infections, broad antibiotic coverage is recommended initially, tailoring therapy when sputum cultures are available (see Chapter 194 Healthcare and Hospital-Acquired Pneumonia). Prevention includes adequate pain control, respiratory therapy, and early mobilization. When possible, patients should be encouraged to get out of bed on the evening of surgery.

CARDIAC COMPLICATIONS

Postoperative myocardial infarction (POMI) is usually caused by rupture of an existing thrombus, and it is associated with very high mortality in high-risk groups. These lesions do not usually cause ischemia during preoperative testing, but create demand ischemia with surgical stress. Intraoperative risk factors for perioperative complications include operative site, large volume shifts, high blood loss, hypotension, and catecholamine surges. Poor functional status, prior ischemic heart disease, heart failure, diabetes, renal insufficiency, and high risk surgery all increase the risk of perioperative cardiac complications. Preoperative optimization is critical in patients with known risk factors (see Chapter 51 Preoperative Cardiac Risk Assessment and Perioperative Management). Increased risk is associated with emergency surgery, long operative times, high volume replacement, and the type of procedure. Vascular surgical patients are at highest risk because of the prevalence of coexisting coronary disease. Thoracic, orthopedic, head and neck, and intra-abdominal procedures are moderate risk, associated with 1–5% risk of a perioperative cardiac event. Intraoperative hypotension and large fluctuations in blood pressure, use of vasopressors, and catecholamine surges all increase the risk of demand ischemia. Trendelenberg positioning and intra-abdominal insufflation from laparoscopy decrease venous return contributing to demand ischemia.

Classic symptoms of chest pain and diaphoresis may be masked in the postoperative period due to the prolonged effects of anesthesia and narcotics. Physicians caring for patients at risk should have a low threshold for investigating a POMI when there is postoperative hypotension or hypoxia. Workup includes ECG and cardiac enzymes. If cardiac ischemia is present, the mechanism is usually not an acute coronary syndrome and the use of anticoagulants should be discussed with the operating surgeon. Recent surgery is a contraindication to the large doses of heparin used in the cardiac catheterization laboratory, but treatment decisions should be made on an individual basis.

Volume resuscitation can cause postoperative congestive heart failure and pulmonary edema in any patient. Resting tachycardia due to pain, anxiety, withdrawal states as well as hypovolemia may precipitate alveolar edema, especially in patients with diastolic dysfunction. In severe cases of flash pulmonary edema, patients will also have severe hypertension, which may be related to underlying renal artery stenosis. Postoperative heart failure should be treated with fluid restriction, diuretics, rate and blood pressure control, and afterload reducing agents as indicated.

Thoracic and cardiac surgery patients are at especially high risk for developing postoperative dysrhythmias. Atrial fibrillation and atrial flutter are most common and are associated with age, elevated catecholamines, beta blockade withdrawal, hypokalemia, hypomagnesemia, and volume shifts, which cause atrial stretch. Postoperative atrial fibrillation occurs in as many as 40%, 50%, and 60% of patients after CABG, valve replacement, or combined CABG/valve replacement, respectively. The highest incidence is on postoperative days 2 and 3. Arrythmias may also be associated with electrolyte abnormalities and large fluid shifts seen in lengthy abdominal procedures with significant third-spacing, such as abdominoperineal resection or hepatobilliary procedures, and in procedures with significant blood loss such as vascular or long orthopedic surgeries, (see Chapter 52 Cardiac Complications After Noncardiac Surgery).

GASTROINTESTINAL COMPLICATIONS

Postoperative ileus is expected after gastrointestinal surgery but it is also seen after other procedures associated with narcotic use and immobility. Ileus is associated with abdominal distention, nausea, belching, and inability to pass flatus. Resolution of the symptoms usually occurs within 5 days of surgery but can be longer, particularly in debilitated patients or those with significant narcotic use. It is wise to routinely prescribe stool softeners with narcotics. Classically, radiographs in ileus will demonstrate uniform distribution of air throughout the bowel, but this not always the case and differentiating ileus from obstruction on plain films can be difficult. Abdominal CT scan with enteric contrast has 100% sensitivity and specificity in distinguishing postoperative obstruction from ileus and is the test of choice.

PRACTICE POINT

Postoperative ileus

- Postoperative ileus is expected after gastrointestinal surgery but it is also seen after other procedures associated with narcotic use and immobility.
  - Resolution of the symptoms usually occurs within 5 days of surgery but can be longer, particularly in debilitated patients or those with significant narcotic use.
- Although vomiting may be seen with ileus, it can also herald a postoperative small bowel obstruction, a worrisome event after abdominal surgery.
  - Differentiating ileus from obstruction on plain films can be difficult.
- Involve general surgeons early in the management of postoperative colonic pseudoobstruction.

Although vomiting may be seen with ileus, it can also herald a postoperative small bowel obstruction which is a worrisome event after abdominal surgery. Intraperitoneal adhesion formation from postoperative inflammation is one of the most common causes of obstruction. Internal hernia is caused by small bowel trapped in an abdominal gutter, or a mesenteric defect created during surgery; it can be diagnosed with a CT scan, and should be managed with hydration, bowel rest, and nasogastric tube decompression as is typical for other episodes of small bowel obstruction. Postoperative obstructions occur in 1% to 10% of patients after abdominal surgery. They may be self-limited and do not always require reexploration.

Colonic pseudo-obstruction is associated with prolonged immobility and institutionalization. Old age, previous functional limitation, and orthopedic surgery are known risk factors. Patients present with signs of ileus, and radiographs demonstrate decompressed small bowel and uniformly dilated colon. As with small bowel obstruction, treatment involves hydration, bowel rest, and decompression. In refractory cases, neostigmine is an option but should only be administered with careful monitoring because it is associated with bradycardia. Severe cecal dilatation with perforation is a life-threatening complication of colonic pseudo-obstruction. In patients with acute dilatation, a cecum measuring more than 11 cm warrants decompression. This can be achieved surgically, with a cecostomy tube or cecal resection, or percutaneously, with a cecostomy tube placed by interventional radiology. Treatment depends on patient condition and local expertise. General surgeons should be engaged early in the management of postoperative colonic pseudo-obstruction.

DELIRIUM

Postoperative delirium is a common finding in older patients who demonstrate sensitivity to narcotics and anesthetics or who have a history of frequent alcohol use, dementia, or sundowning. Patients undergoing cardiovascular and thoracic surgery are at particular risk but delirium is seen after all major surgical procedures. The causes are multifactorial, including medications, disability, and loss of environmental cues, insomnia, and recovery from cardiopulmonary bypass after cardiac surgery.

Delirium presents with confusion, agitation, hallucination, and confabulation. Patients may present a risk to themselves and others by trying to get out of bed without assistance or trying to remove tubes and drains. Prevention entails maintaining a regular sleep-wake cycle, restoration of environmental clues such as daylight and clocks, and minimizing bright lights and loud noises. Some patients will respond well to reassurance and emotional support for their anxiety. When managing patients with postoperative psychiatric disturbances it is important to rule out organic causes of disease such as sepsis or stroke. Some patients will require benzodiazepines for alcohol withdrawal or antipsychotics to address hallucinations, agitation, or paranoia. It is best to start at low doses and titrate up as necessary because these medications can be heavily sedating, interfering with pulmonary function and physical therapy, both essential to postoperative recovery.

DEEP VENOUS THROMBOSIS AND PULMONARY EMBOLUS

Surgical patients are at high risk for venous thromboembolism (VTE) due to the surgical procedure itself, which results in prolonged immobility, hypercoagulability, and endothelial damage. Patients with known hypercoaguable states, prior VTE, and malignancy are at especially high risk. High-risk surgical procedures include orthopedic surgery, trauma, and neurosurgical treatment of head injury and brain tumors. Prophylaxis starts before surgery with the application of pneumatic compression devices and subcutaneous heparin prior to anesthetic induction. Unless there are clear contraindications, such as increased bleeding risk, patients should receive pharmacologic prophylaxis and compression stockings with pneumatic boots. Patients with severe peripheral vascular disease may develop digital ischemia from sequential compression devices, which should be avoided in these patients (see Chapter 58 and Chapter 59 VTE Prophylaxis of Surgical Patients).

Pulmonary embolus (PE) still causes considerable mortality in hospitalized patients. PE should be suspected in all surgical patients presenting with symptoms of dyspnea, tachycardia, and hypoxemia. The decision to start anticoagulation should be made with the operating surgeon (see Chapter 259 and Chapter 260 Diagnosis and Treatment of VTE).

URINARY TRACT INFECTIONS (UTI)

Urinary tract infections (UTI) are especially common after vaginal or urologic surgery and with the use of indwelling catheters. The most common pathogens are *Escherichia coli*, *Staphylococcus saprophyticus,* and *Proteus mirabilis*. However, hospitalized and immunosupressed patients are also susceptible to *Klebsiella, Proteus vulgaris, Candida albicans,* and *Pseudomonas*. Women and obese patients are at highest risk for postoperative UTI. The standard for prevention is the removal of indwelling catheters within 48 hours of insertion.

Common clinical findings include fever, leukocytosis, dysuria, hematuria, incontinence and/or urinary retention. Occasionally cloudy urine or pyuria will be present as well. Debilitated and elderly patients can present with altered mental status, which is a sign of urosepsis or systemic infection from a urinary tract source. A urinalysis and urine culture should be obtained before starting empiric antibiotic coverage. Asymptomatic bacteriuria should not be treated. Criteria for diagnosis are the same as for UTIs in the nonpostoperative period, nitrites and leukocyte esterase in the urinalysis and 10^5 CFU/ml of a single organism in the urine culture. Nosicomial UTIs are typically treated with antibiotics for longer than community-acquired UTI (see Chapter 205 UTI).

POST OPERATIVE URINARY RETENTION

Common risk factors for postoperative urinary retention include: male sex; prostatic enlargement; epidural, spinal, or prolonged anesthesia; antihistamine and narcotic use; and pelvic and perineal procedures. An overdistended bladder (>500 ml) and disruption of the neural pathways that control voiding impairs urinary contraction and micturition. Prophylactic catheterization in the operating room is recommended for any procedure lasting more than 3 hours and when interruption of the sacral plexus is anticipated (eg, abdominoperineal resection). If a catheter is not present, patients should be encouraged to void soon after the procedure. If the patient has not voided for more than 6 hours, it is appropriate to evaluate bladder size with an ultrasound or a catheter should be placed empirically. The treatment for bladder distention is catheterization and efforts to mitigate any contributing factors. Postoperative oliguria (less than the equivalent of 0.5 cc/kg/hr) requires urgent evaluation and treatment. Some patients may have repeated episodes of urinary retention in the postoperative period. In this case initiate appropriate pharmacologic treatment and plan for potential discharge with a urinary catheter and outpatient urologic follow-up.

CONCLUSION

In conclusion, postoperative complications are associated with significant morbidity, prolonged length of stay, and hospital costs. Careful assessment preoperatively, attention to surgical technique and anesthetic management intraoperatively, and a multidisciplinary approach to medication management, infection control, and patient mobility postoperatively all can reduce the risk of surgical complications. Hospitalists caring for surgical patients should be aware of the common complications discussed here, and the complications unique to procedures done for patients under their care. A postoperative course that is not marked by daily improvement should raise suspicion for postoperative complications and prompt communication with the operating surgeon.

SUGGESTED READINGS

Arozullah AM, Khuri SF, Henderson WG, et al. Development and validation of a Multifactorial risk index for predicting postoperative pneumonia after major noncardiac surgery. *Ann Intern Med.* 2001;135:847–857.

Barie PS, Eachempati SR. Surgical site infections. *Surg Clin North Am.* 2005;85(6):1115–1135.

Lawrence VA, Cornell JE, Smetana GW. Strategies to reduce postoperative pulmonary complications after noncardiothoracic surgery: systematic review for the American College of Physicians. *Ann Intern Med.* 200618;144(8):596–608.

Mattei P, Rombeau JL. Review of the pathophysiology and management of postoperative ileus. *World J Surg.* 2006;30(8):1382–1391.

CHAPTER 47

Surgical Tubes and Drains

Zara Cooper, MD, MSc
Stanley Ashley, MD

INTRODUCTION

Surgical drains are used to monitor for a postoperative leak or abscess, collect normal physiologic fluid or to minimize dead space. **Table 47-1** lists various types of drains, as well as their locations and indications. Although caregivers should know the location and purpose of drains, they should not manipulate surgical drains without input from the surgeon who placed them.

PRACTICE POINT

- Although caregivers should know the location and purpose of drains, they should not manipulate surgical drains without input from the surgeon who placed them.

TYPES AND USES OF SURGICAL DRAINS

CHEST TUBES

Chest tubes are placed in the pleural space to evacuate air or fluid. They can be as thin as 20 French or as thick as 38 French and are typically placed between the fourth and fifth intercostal space in the anterior axillary line. However, location may vary according to the type of surgery. The tubes can be straight or angled. Angled tubes are used primarily to collect fluid and are usually placed near the diaphragm.

The tubes are connected to a collecting system with a three-way chamber (**Figure 47-1**). The water chamber holds a tall column of water which prevents air from being sucked into the pleural space with inhalation. The suction chamber can be attached to continuous wall suction to remove air or fluid, or it can be left without suction on water seal. The third chamber is the collection chamber which should be marked at regular intervals to monitor fluid drainage.

Clinical indications for a chest tube include pneumothorax, hemothorax, or a persistent or large pleural effusion. Pneumothorax and hemothorax are emergent indications, but, in the operating room, chest tubes are usually placed after thoracic surgery or when the diaphragm has been violated and air has entered the pleural space. For large, loculated empyemas video-assisted thoracoscopic surgery (VATS) is preferable to chest tube drainage. A chest X-ray should be obtained after any chest tube insertion. Although chest tubes should be well secured, they can migrate, and it is wise to get a daily chest X-ray to document the location of the tube. Chest tubes are equipped with a radiopaque line, which should be visible on chest X-ray. There is a gap in the line on the tube that should be visible in the pleural space on the film. Respiratory variation in the fluid in the collecting tube will be seen if the tube is well placed. If the patient experiences ongoing pain, fever, or inadequate drainage, a chest computed tomographic (CT) scan can identify malpositioning of the tube. There is no indication for prophylactic antibiotics for chest tubes. If a chest tube needs adjustment, it can be pulled out, but it should never be advanced into the cavity. The tube that has been outside the chest is contaminated and poses an increased risk of infection once advanced into the pleural space.

Criteria for removal are often subjective and depend on the indication for placement. If the patient has a pneumothorax, air bubbles will be visible in the water chamber when the patient

TABLE 47-1 Surgical Tubes and Drains

Type	Location	Clinical Indication	Clinical Scenario
Chest tube	Pleural space Mediastinal space	Pneumothorax Hemothorax Pleural effusion	Trauma, cardiac surgery, malignant effusion
Nasogastric tube	Stomach	Intestinal decompression, gastric feeding	Small bowel obstruction, temporary dysphagia
Gastric tube (gastrostomy)	Stomach	Prolonged enteral access, or gastric decompression	Prolonged mechanical ventilation, malignant gastric outlet obstruction
Jejunal tube (jejunostomy)	Jejunum	Prolonged postgastric feeding in the setting of gastroparesis, gastric outlet obstruction, or high aspiration risk	Prolonged mechanical ventilation, malignant gastric outlet obstruction, recurrent aspiration pneumonia
Duodenal	Duodenum	Post gastric feeding in the setting of gastroparesis, gastric outlet obstruction or high aspiration risk	Mechanical ventilation, dysphagia, acute aspiration risk
Penrose drains	Peritoneal space, small surgical space	Used to maintain surgical tract for adequate drainage	
Closed suction drains Jackson Pratt Hemovac	Surgical space	Evacuate serous fluid or blood Prevent seroma formation Tissue apposition to improve wound healing Drain gastrointestinal secretions	Mastectomy, ventral hernia repair, plastic surgery flaps, gastrointestinal anastomoses
Vacuum-assisted closure device	Open wound	Accelerated wound closure	Open trunk or extremity wound

coughs. In this case the tube should be left on continuous suction to evacuate the air. Once the "air leak" has resolved, the chest tube may be placed on water seal to confirm that the pneumothorax is resolved and that suction is no longer required. Water seal mimics normal physiology. A chest X-ray should be obtained when the tube is changed from suction to water seal or vice versa. If the pneumothorax is not resolved the normal course is to put the tube back onto continuous suction. It is not advisable to clamp a tube when pneumothorax is suspected because it can precipitate a tension pneumothorax.

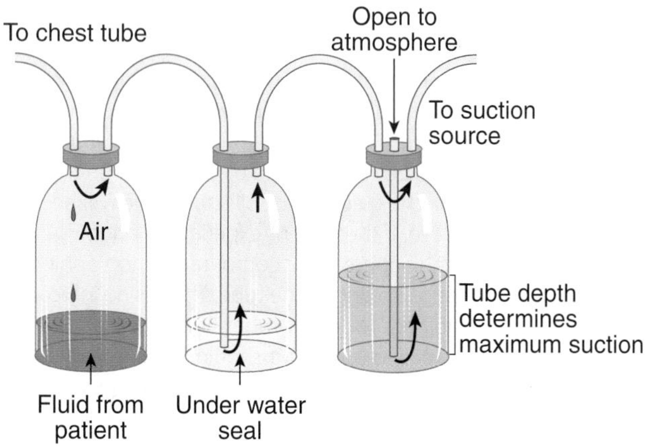

Figure 47-1 Chest drainage collection systems. *(Reproduced, with permission, from Hall JB, Schmidt GA, Wood LDH. Principles of Critical Care. 3rd ed. New York: McGraw-Hill; 2005: Fig. 95-4.)*

PRACTICE POINT

Chest tubes

- If a chest tube needs adjustment, it can be pulled out but it should never be advanced into the cavity. The tube that has been outside the chest is contaminated and poses an increased risk of infection once advanced into the pleural space.
- It is not advisable to clamp a tube when pneumothorax is suspected because it can precipitate a tension pneumothorax.
- Criteria for removal are often subjective and depend on the indication for placement.

In the event of a pleural effusion or hemothorax, the tube can usually be removed when the output is less than 100–200 mL per day, and the lung is expanded. This is subject to surgeon preference. Again, the tube should usually be taken off suction and placed on water seal to rule out pneumothorax prior to tube removal. Blood may clog chest tubes, rendering them ineffective. In this case the clot may be evacuated with suction tubing under sterile conditions by an experienced hand. In some cases an additional tube may be required.

PENROSE DRAINS

Penrose drains are often used to drain fluid or to keep a space open for drainage. Examples are drains to prevent seroma formation after ventral hernia repair or abdominal drains after debridement in infected pancreatitis. Because of their pliability they can easily be inched out, allowing drainage of the cavity and controlled closure.

In contrast with closed drains, they permit ingress as well as egress and may more easily permit colonization.

CLOSED SUCTION DRAINS

These are moderately stiff but pliable plastic drains that are used to collect fluid in a postoperative cavity (ie, Jackson Pratt and Hemovac). They are commonly used in postmastectomy patients to drain gastrointestinal anastomoses, after plastic surgery to prevent seroma formation and to promote tissue apposition, or after orthopedic procedures to collect blood. The hospitalist should notify the surgeon if a patient has bloody drainage and a falling hematocrit. If you are unsure if the drainage is blood or serous fluid, send a hematocrit count from the drain fluid to confirm composition. Typically drains used to collect blood will be left in place until the drainage is less than 20 mL. They are at high risk for clotting off and should be stripped frequently. Drains may be left in the operative space to monitor postoperative leakage; for example, they are sometimes left in place after a difficult rectal anastomosis, pancreatic resection, or cholecystectomy if a bile leak is anticipated. The value of anastomotic drainage is controversial in the surgical literature, and some suggest that they actually increase the risk of leak. If an infected collection is a concern, some surgeons prefer to wait and proceed with percutaneous drainage should the need arise. Drains are usually removed when output is minimal and can be left for weeks if necessary. This is left to surgeon discretion. Rare complications include erosion into surrounding tissues and inadvertent suturing of the drain in place such that reexploration is required to remove it.

NASOGASTRIC AND DUODENAL TUBES

Nasogastric tubes (NGTs) may be used for decompression or feeding and are most often used in the nonoperative management of small bowel obstruction or ileus. As obstruction or ileus resolves, the tube output should decrease, and symptoms of nausea, vomiting, and abdominal distention should improve. If resolution of bowel function is obvious, the NGT can be removed. If there is doubt, a trial of placing the NGT to gravity and checking the aspirate after 4 hours can be helpful. NGT output less than 100 mL indicates that gastric contents are progressing through the gastrointestinal tract and the obstruction has resolved.

PRACTICE POINT

Nasogastric tubes

- If resolution of bowel function is obvious, the NGT can be removed.
- If there is doubt, a trial of placing the NGT to gravity and checking the aspirate after 4 hours can be helpful. NGT output less than 100 cc indicates that gastric contents are progressing through the GI tract and the obstruction has resolved.

Persistently high output in a patient with some resolution of bowel function may suggest postpyloric placement, which can be confirmed on an abdominal X-ray. NGTs should be placed in the most dependent portion of the gastric lumen, and placement can be confirmed by chest or abdominal X-ray.

NGTs are sump pumps and have a double lumen, which includes an air port to assure flow. The air port should be patent for optimal functioning. The tube may be connected to continuous wall suction or intermittent suction. The former is thought to increase the risk for mucosal injury. Regardless of the suction type, the suction should be low to avoid mucosal avulsion. NGTs may also be helpful in gastric lavage and in diagnosing gastrointestinal bleeding. Bloody output indicates an upper bleed, proximal to the ligament of Treitz, whereas bilious output suggests a lower gastrointestinal bleed.

Duodenal tubes are small-bore tubes used when postpyloric feeding is preferable. Although type I evidence is lacking, convention suggests that postpyloric feeding reduces the risk of aspiration. Duodenal tubes are used exclusively for feeding and are placed through the nares. They are very narrow caliber and require a long wire for insertion. The wire should be removed as soon as placement is confirmed. They are very soft and flexible, but the wire used for placement makes them very stiff, increasing the risk of inadvertent insertion into the airway. Therefore, placement by an experienced operator is particularly important. In obtunded patients who cannot protect their airway, nasoenteric feeding tubes should be placed under laryngoscopic or bronchoscopic guidance to reduce the risk of airway intubation (see Chapter 119).

GASTROSTOMY AND JEJUNOSTOMY TUBES

Gastrostomy tubes are most commonly used for feeding but may also be used for decompression in the event of functional or anatomic gastric outlet obstruction. They are indicated when patients need prolonged enteral access in the case of prolonged mechanical ventilation or head and neck pathology that prohibits oral feeding. They are also rarely used for gastropexy, to tack an atonic or patulous stomach to the abdominal wall or to prevent recurrence of paraesophageal hernias. Initiation and advancement of tube feeds depend on the clinical picture. In severely injured or critically ill patients, tube feedings should be held until the patient is hemodynamically stable and resuscitation is complete. Patients with increasing vasopressor requirements are at risk of intestinal ischemia. Otherwise feedings should be initiated within 24 hours of injury and advanced to the goal rate within 48 hours. In patients who have had gastrointestinal surgery, initiating feedings is left to surgeon discretion, dependent on the procedure performed, the intraoperative events, and surgeon experience.

Patients with outlet obstruction or delayed gastric emptying can be hypersecretory, losing liters of fluid a day in gastric secretions. This may cause electrolyte abnormalities that need to be addressed with fluid replacement. The patient's intake and output should be monitored closely. Because of the stomach's generous lumen, gastric tubes rarely clog and are often easier to manage than other enteral feeding tubes. Tubes are placed percutaneously by interventional radiologists, endoscopically by surgeons and gastroenterologists, and via laparoscopy or laparotomy by surgeons. The latter is often reserved for patients with difficult anatomy or who are having laparotomy for another reason.

Surgical tubes and drains are used exclusively for feedings and are usually placed 10–20 cm distal to the ligament of Treitz. These tubes can be more difficult to manage because the lumen of the small bowel is smaller than the stomach, and the tubes are more apt to clog. Some prefer not to put pills down the tube to mitigate this risk. Routine flushes with water or saline are also helpful. In the event that they do get clogged, carbonated liquids, meat tenderizer, or enzymes can help dissolve the obstruction. If the tube has been in place for more than 2 weeks, it can easily be replaced at the bedside with a tube of comparable caliber. If the tube has not been in place that long, it requires replacement with radiographic guidance as the risk of creating a false lumen is high. Replaced tubes should always be confirmed radiographically. Over time, tubes can become loose and fall out. If they need replacement, the preceding guidelines apply. We caution against replacing with a bigger-lumen tube as this will just increase the defect in the abdominal wall and the risk for persistent leak of bowel contents onto the surrounding skin.

VACUUM-ASSISTED WOUND CLOSURE

Intermittent negative pressure therapy accelerates wound healing and minimizes infection by removing interstitial fluid, increasing blood flow, and reducing edema. The negative pressure is also thought to deform matrix cells, which increases proliferation, protein synthesis, and matrix formation.

The device includes a sponge, a suction device, and a drain, which are placed in the wound bed and secured with transparent adhesive. The adhesive must be well sealed to maintain vacuum suction. The drain is attached to a vacuum device that is set to a cyclical negative pressure, which keeps the sponge to suction and drains fluid from the wound. The pressure depends on the type and location of the wound. The sponge, which should be applied to a clean wound bed, is typically changed every 2–4 days and may be applied for acute and chronic wounds. The vacuum device is contraindicated in necrotic or malignant wounds and wounds with exposed vessels, nerves, anastomosis, or organs. Bleeding risk should be reconsidered before the vacuum device is used. A visiting nurse or nursing facility that will manage the wound after hospital discharge must know what the wound looked like at discharge, how frequently the vacuum should be changed, and the desired pressure level. Again, infection is a contraindication to using the vacuum and warrants removal and reevaluation of the wound.

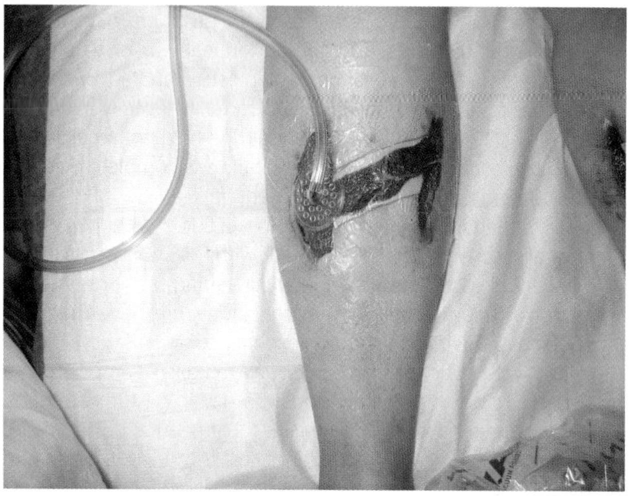

CONCLUSION

Postoperative bleeding is a feared surgical complication because reoperation, blood transfusion and shock are all associated with poor outcome. Bleeding should be considered in any postoperative patients with tachycardia, hypotension, oliguria or evidence of shock. Postoperative bleeding may be due to technical error, coagulopathy, or both. Physical exam and laboratory tests can guide management and resuscitation should occur even as a source is sought. The surgical team should be involved in the workup and decision making as early as possible and should be called as soon as bleeding is suspected.

PRACTICE POINT

Vacuum assisted wound closure

- Contraindications include necrotic or malignant wounds, and wounds with exposed vessels, nerves, anastomosis or organs. Infection warrants removal and reevaluation of the wound.
- Bleeding risk should be reconsidered before using the vacuum device.
- If a visiting nurse of nursing facility will manage the wound after hospital discharge he or she must know what the wound looked like at discharge, how frequently the vacuum should be changed, and the desired pressure level.

SUGGESTED READINGS

Bovill E, Banwell PE, Teot L, et al. International Advisory Panel on Topical Negative Pressure. Topical negative pressure wound therapy: a review of its role and guidelines for its use in the management of acute wounds. *Int Wound J.* 2008;5(4):511–529.

Symbas, PN Chest Drainage Tubes. *Surgical Clinics of North America* 1989;69(1):41–46.

Wiley W, Souba MP, Fink GJ, et al. *ACS Surgery: Principles and Practice.* WebMD; 2006.

SECTION 3

Anesthesia

CHAPTER 48

Anesthesia: Choices and Complications

Aeron Doyle, MDCM, FRCPC

INTRODUCTION

Hospitalists are often involved in perioperative patient care and should be familiar with techniques and complications of anesthesia, as well as preoperative and postoperative considerations. Current modalities include general anesthetics, neuraxial techniques (spinal and epidural), regional anesthetics (nerve blocks), and monitored anesthetic care (MAC), or so-called conscious sedation. Each mode of anesthesia has benefits and risks that must be weighed in view of the operative procedure and the condition and comorbidities of each patient. The administration of regional or local anesthetics does not preclude the necessity for general anesthesia in the event of unforeseen events or complications. Therefore, patients undergoing all but the most minor procedures should be assessed as potential candidates for general anesthesia.

PRACTICE POINT

Cardiovascular and psychiatric medications in the perioperative period

- Beta-blockers, calcium channel blockers, and amiodarone should be continued in the perioperative period. Patients who receive perioperative angiotensin-converting enzyme inhibitors and angiotensin receptor blockers may be at greater risk of intraoperative hypotension. Some authorities recommend holding these drugs on the day of surgery, particularly for operations with significant fluid shifts or using techniques associated with systemic inflammatory responses, such as cardiopulmonary bypass. It is traditionally recommended to stop monoamine oxidase inhibitors (MAOIs) two weeks prior to surgery. Patients who take MAOIs perioperatively are at risk of serotonergic toxicity and hypertension, especially with vasopressor use, as well as excessive sedation from inhibition of opioid metabolism by MAOIs. Some anesthesiologists continue MAOIs perioperatively, avoiding indirect-acting sympathomimetics such as ephedrine, and using narcotics such as morphine with lesser degrees of interaction with MAOIs, instead of meperidine. Tricyclic antidepressants (TCAs) and selective serotonin reuptake inhibitors (SSRIs) may be continued perioperatively. TCAs have rarely been associated with intraoperative hypotension, requiring norepinephrine for reversal. SSRIs are occasionally implicated in perioperative serotonin syndrome, particularly when given with serotonin 5-HT_3 receptor antagonists such as ondansetron, and phenylpiperidine opioids such as fentanyl.

GENERAL ANESTHESIA

General anesthesia is usually induced with a short-acting intravenous agent such as propofol and maintained with inhaled halogenated ethers or intravenous propofol. The mechanism of action of inhalational anesthetics remains unclear and may be a membrane effect, a receptor effect, or both. These agents may be used in conjunction with narcotics and muscle relaxants to achieve balanced anesthesia and may also be supplemented with inhaled nitrous oxide. Airway protection may be obtained by endotracheal intubation; airway patency, but not protection, may be ensured with a laryngeal mask airway, or oropharyngeal airway with mask.

Complications of general anesthesia include postoperative nausea and vomiting (PONV); aspiration; complications of intubation, such as dental, mucosal, or laryngeal trauma; atelectasis and complications of positive pressure ventilation, such as barotrauma; complications of positioning during surgery; and allergic or idiosyncratic reactions to anesthetic agents. Additionally, ischemic or thromboembolic events may occur perioperatively because of physiologic stresses from surgery or anesthesia.

PRACTICE POINT

Side effects of anesthesia induction

- Propofol is the most commonly used agent for anesthesia induction. A common side effect is hypotension from vasodilation and decreased cardiac output, which occurs in up to 16% of patients. Barbiturates such as methohexital and thiopental sodium are occasionally used for anesthesia induction but also have cardiovascular depressant effects. Etomidate and ketamine are sometimes used for anesthesia induction in patients at higher risk of hypotension from propofol, such as the elderly. Etomidate rarely has significant cardiovascular side effects, but it does inhibit 11-beta-hydroxylase, an enzyme involved in steroid synthesis, thus attenuating the adrenal stress response and potentially leading to postoperative hypotension. This effect may persist for up to 24 hours in elderly patients after a single dose for anesthesia induction. Ketamine does not depress respiratory drive, unlike most anesthetic agents, and it actually has bronchodilator effects that make its use attractive in patients with reactive airway disease. However, ketamine has side effects that make its use in elderly patients problematic, including increases in heart rate and blood pressure, myocardial depression that is masked by its sympathomimetic effects, postoperative delirium and hallucinations, and neurodegenerative apoptosis in animal models.

POSTOPERATIVE NAUSEA AND VOMITING

PONV occurs after approximately 10% of surgeries. Risk factors include younger age; female gender; intraabdominal, ophthalmic, or ear, nose, and throat (ENT) surgery; past history of PONV or motion sickness; and being a nonsmoker. Strategies to lower the risk of PONV include avoidance of general anesthesia in favor of regional anesthesia, use of propofol, avoidance of nitrous oxide and volatile anesthetics, minimization of opioids, and adequate hydration. Intraoperative prophylaxis and postoperative treatment may include central dopaminergic antagonists such as prochlorperazine, peripheral dopaminergic antagonists such as metoclopramide, serotonin 5-HT_3 receptor antagonists such as ondansetron, and corticosteroids such as dexamethasone. These agents may also be used as rescue agents after emesis to prevent further symptoms. PONV usually abates in 24–48 hours. The examination of a patient with presumed PONV should assess for bowel sounds and the presence or absence of abdominal distention to avoid missing a diagnosis of postoperative ileus.

ASPIRATION

Aspiration is the entry of gastric contents into the trachea and lower airways. It may occur prior to or during induction of anesthesia, intraoperatively if the airway is unprotected, or during emergence from anesthesia and postoperatively. A chemical pneumonitis usually results with severity increasing with lower pH or particulates. Risk factors include a full stomach, preexisting gastroesophageal reflux disease (GERD), obesity, intraabdominal obstruction or other pathology, pregnancy, and trauma. American Society of Anesthesiologists guidelines for nil per os (NPO) status preoperatively recommend two hours for clear fluids, six hours for a light meal (essentially toast and clear fluids), and eight hours for full meals. These guidelines are for healthy elective patients with no GERD or other risks. Routine antireflux prophylaxis is not recommended, but in patients with GERD, histamine H_2-receptor antagonists, proton pump inhibitors, physical antacids, or promotility agents such as metoclopramide may be indicated. Patients on these medications should have them ordered preoperatively.

COMPLICATIONS OF INTUBATION AND AIRWAY MAINTENANCE

In closed claim studies, the most common awards for anesthetic complications are those for dental trauma (approximately 1 in 5000). Laryngeal injury may have an incidence as high as 6% in general anesthesia but is usually minor and self-limiting, such as sore throat or vocal cord hematoma. Hoarseness lasting longer than 7 days should be evaluated by an otolaryngologist. Mucosal lacerations have an incidence of 1 in 1000, but again are usually self-limiting.

ATELECTASIS

Atelectasis, alveolar collapse generally in dependent areas of the lung, is common with general anesthesia, particularly in surgery involving the upper abdomen. Postoperative fever and hypoxia due to physiologic intrapulmonary shunt are typical manifestations. Mobilization is the most effective treatment, with chest physiotherapy and incentive spirometry generally having disappointing results. Continuous or bilevel positive airway pressure (CPAP or BiPAP) devices may be beneficial if tolerated by the patient.

POSITIONING COMPLICATIONS

Nerve injuries may occur as a complication of various positions under anesthesia. Ulnar neuropathies are the most common, with an incidence varying from 4–50/10,000 patients. Risk factors include male gender, extremes of body weight, and prolonged hospitalization. The common peroneal nerve may be injured by pressure at the fibular head in the lithotomy position (feet in stirrups). Brachial plexus injuries may occur from sternotomy and retraction of the chest wall during coronary bypass surgery. Compartment syndrome in the extremities may occur if tissue swelling causes obstruction of venous and lymphatic drainage, with failure of capillary perfusion and cell death. This may result from improper positioning, or more often from extensive and prolonged surgery. It presents as intractable pain, with examination revealing an absence of pulses. Surgical fasciotomies are required to decrease tissue pressure.

EYE INJURY

Eye injury is reported in up to 0.05% of patients postoperatively. The majority of cases are corneal abrasions. These resolve within days with topical antibiotics and rarely cause permanent visual impairment. Rarely, patients develop ischemic optic neuropathy or central retinal artery occlusion. Risk factors include prone or lateral position, prolonged surgery, hypotension, spine surgery, and anemia. Unfortunately, the prognosis for recovery is poor in these instances.

ALLERGIC AND OTHER REACTIONS

Anaphylactic reactions under anesthesia are rare but potentially life threatening. As many medications are given in the perioperative period, it may be difficult to determine the causal agent, which may include antibiotics, muscle relaxants, or latex. Opioids cause histamine release, resulting in redness and itching, but rarely anaphylaxis.

Malignant hyperthermia (MH) is a rare reaction triggered by inhalational anesthetics (except nitrous oxide) or succinylcholine (a depolarizing muscle relaxant). It generally presents with increased metabolic rate, acidosis, and finally rhabdomyolysis. Treatment consists of discontinuing triggering agents, the administration of dantrolene, and supportive care in an intensive care setting. MH is an autosomal dominant disorder, so patients with relatives with suspected or confirmed MH should receive nontriggering anesthetics.

Abnormalities of the enzyme pseudocholinesterase may result in the prolongation of action of the muscle relaxant succinylcholine, leading to postoperative weakness or paralysis. Heterozygous individuals may have mild prolongation, lasting 20 to 30 minutes, whereas homozygous individuals may require sedation and ventilation support for hours, depending on the dosage initially given. Succinylcholine should be avoided in these patients if possible.

ACUTE RENAL FAILURE

Acute renal failure, defined as a fall in creatinine clearance to 50 mL/min or less, occurs within the first week after major noncardiac surgery in approximately 0.8% of patients with previously normal renal function, with 0.1% of patients requiring renal replacement therapy. The development of postoperative acute kidney injury (AKI) is an independent predictor for hospital mortality. Preoperative predictors of AKI in various studies have included age, emergent surgery, liver disease, diabetes mellitus, an elevated body mass index, high-risk surgery, congestive heart failure, ischemic heart disease, peripheral vascular occlusive disease, and chronic obstructive pulmonary disease necessitating chronic bronchodilator therapy. Intraoperative strategies to minimize the risk of AKI include maintenance of euvolemia, avoidance of nephrotoxins, and maintenance of optimal blood pressures.

PERIOPERATIVE MYOCARDIAL INFARCTION

Myocardial infarction occurs in two distinct clinical settings in the perioperative period. Patients may develop an acute coronary syndrome related to plaque rupture. Major contributing factors are physiologic stress and high levels of catecholamines leading to tachycardia, hypertension, and coronary thrombosis, coupled with increased coagulability because of tissue trauma and cessation of antiplatelet agents. The other scenario is the patient with severe but stable coronary disease who develops subendocardial ischemia because of an imbalance between myocardial oxygen supply and demand. Causative factors may include tachycardia, hypotension or hypertension, anemia, and hypoxemia. In this latter setting, anesthesia may be a contributing factor, leading to hypotension and decreased cardiac output.

STROKE

Perioperative stroke has many contributing factors, including hypercoagulability from tissue trauma, emboli from vascular manipulation, temporary cessation of antiplatelet and anticoagulant drugs, and hypotension from bleeding or anesthetic agents. The risk of stroke is highest in vascular surgery: 1.4–3.8% in patients undergoing coronary artery bypass grafting (CABG), 7.4% in combined CABG and valve replacement, and 9.7% in multiple valve replacement. The risk of stroke in patients undergoing general surgery ranges from 0.08 to 0.7%. Atrial fibrillation, valvular disease, renal disease, and prior stroke are the most robust predictors of perioperative stroke in general surgery patients. Most perioperative strokes are embolic in origin, with only 9% being related to hypoperfusion. The risk of perioperative stroke may be increased when high doses of beta-blockers are begun just prior to surgery in patients who have not taken beta-blockers previously. Chronic beta-blocker use does not appear to increase the risk of perioperative stroke.

NEURAXIAL ANESTHESIA

Neuraxial anesthesia techniques include the introduction of medications, usually local anesthetics or opioids, into the subarachnoid space (spinal fluid) or epidural space. In the epidural space, a catheter may be inserted for injections or infusions. Local anesthetics then act on the spinal cord and nerve roots to inhibit sodium channel conduction and block nerve impulses. Opioids act directly on spinal cord receptors, as well as having varying degrees of rostral and systemic spread. The benefits of neuraxial anesthesia may include preemptive analgesia (the prevention of establishment of pain pathways), decreased sympathetic activation, hypercoagulability and inflammation caused by the stress of surgery, and potential avoidance of airway manipulation. Although there are short-term benefits of postoperative analgesia through an indwelling epidural catheter inserted just before surgery, there are conflicting mortality and morbidity benefits. Contraindications to neuraxial anesthesia include untreated sepsis, bacteremia, infection at the injection site, bleeding diatheses, increased intracranial pressure, and patient refusal.

Relative contraindications include preexisting neurological deficit, hypovolemia, left ventricular outflow obstruction such as aortic stenosis, and lack of cooperation or communication. Complications of neuraxial anesthesia include pain at insertion site, dural puncture headache, hypotension, high level of block, epidural or spinal hematoma or abscess, and pruritis from opioids.

DURAL PUNCTURE HEADACHE

Dural puncture headache results from persistent leakage of cerebrospinal fluid (CSF) following spinal anesthesia or inadvertent dural puncture during epidural anesthesia. It is typically positional and severe. Rates following spinal anesthesia are about 1 in 400. The risk is reduced by use of a smaller-gauge needle with a pencil-point tip, rather than a cutting tip. The risk also decreases with patient age. Dural puncture after epidural is operator dependent; a rate of 1 in 200 is usually quoted. Treatment includes bed rest, hydration, caffeine, and epidural blood patch if headache persists despite conservative therapy. Epidural blood patch involves injecting the patient's own blood into the epidural space to occlude and clot the CSF leak, with about 70% lasting success the first time performed. The procedure may be repeated if initial results are not satisfactory.

HYPOTENSION AND HIGH BLOCK

Hypotension occurs secondary to loss of vascular tone. It may be mitigated by preprocedural fluid loading and treated with vasopressors and fluid after it develops. In epidural anesthesia, incremental dosing may also limit hypotension, particularly in patients with a fixed cardiac output. High block occurs when nerve conduction is lost at a higher level than intended. It may result in perceived respiratory distress due to loss of chest wall proprioception, loss of diaphragm function at midcervical levels, and unconsciousness if the brain stem level is reached. Shock may ensue from profound vasodilation accompanied by block of cardioaccelerator sympathetic fibers. Treatment includes physiologic support and sedation until the block recedes.

HEMATOMA OR ABSCESS

Spinal hematoma or abscess may cause nerve root or spinal cord compression and constitutes a medical emergency, as decompression must occur within eight hours for reasonable chance of recovery. The overall rate of hematoma is 1:220,000 for spinals and 1:150,000 for epidurals but is higher in certain groups of patients

TABLE 48-1 Perioperative Management of Antiplatelet Drugs and Thromboprophylaxis in Patients Receiving Spinal or Epidural Anesthesia

Drug	Perioperative Management
Nonsteroidal anti-inflammatory drugs	No contraindication unless the patient is taking concurrent medications affecting clotting in the early postoperative period, such as oral anticoagulants, unfractionated heparin, and low-molecular-weight heparin
Clopidogrel	Stop 7 days before neuraxial block
Ticlopidine	Stop 14 days before neuraxial block
Glycoprotein (GP) IIb/IIIa inhibitors	Stop 8 hours (eptifibatide, tirofiban) to 48 hours (abciximab) before neuraxial block
Warfarin	Stop 4–5 days before procedure; document normal INR before initiation of neuraxial block; INR should be < 1.5 at the time of neuraxial catheter removal; neurologic assessment should be continued for 24 hours after catheter removal
Subcutaneous heparin	No contraindication with twice daily dosing and total daily dose ≤ 10,000 U; consider delaying dosage until after neuraxial block, especially if technical difficulty expected
Intravenous heparin	Heparinize 1 hour after neuraxial technique; remove catheter 2–4 hours after last heparin dose
Low-molecular-weight heparin (LMWH)	For patients on low (prophylaxis) dose LWMH, needle placement should occur at least 12 hours after last dose; for patients on high (treatment) dose LMWH, needle placement should be delayed at least 24 hours after last dose; postoperatively, administer LMWH no sooner than 24 hours after surgery, and remove catheter 2 hours before first LMWH dose
Fondaparinux	Avoid; if essential, use techniques employed in clinical trials (single injection, atraumatic needle placement, no indwelling neuraxial catheter)
Direct thrombin inhibitors	Insufficient information, avoid
Thrombolytics	Absolute contraindication

Data from Horlocker TT, Wedel DJ, Rowlingson JC, et al. *Reg Anesth Pain Med.* 2010;35:64–101.

and procedures. Half of all cases of epidural hematoma result in devastating, preventable, and permanent neurologic injury, even after prompt surgical intervention. As mentioned, bleeding diatheses are a contraindication to neuraxial anesthetics, but if time permits, a bleeding tendency may be corrected preoperatively with plasma or specific coagulation factors. The use of anticoagulant drugs significantly increases the risk of spinal hematoma. Unfractionated heparin may be reversed with protamine, but low-molecular-weight heparin must be held for 24 hours preprocedure. Platelet inhibitors should be held preoperatively, though low-dose aspirin is not contraindicated if no other anticoagulant is present. Specific perioperative anticoagulant therapy guidelines are published by the American Society of Regional Anesthesia and Pain Medicine (**Table 48-1**).

REGIONAL ANESTHESIA

In regional anesthesia, specific nerves or a nerve plexus is blocked to create a discrete area of anesthesia. These techniques may be utilized alone or in combination with sedation or general anesthesia and may involve a single injection of local anesthetic or the placement of a catheter to provide for multiple injections or infusions for postoperative analgesia. Traditionally, injections were guided by anatomical landmarks with or without electrical nerve stimulation to confirm proximity to the nerve. With the advent of ultrasound-guided techniques, the success rate of regional nerve blocks can be improved, and the risk of nerve injury lessened. Contraindications include infection at the injection site or patient refusal or inability to cooperate. Preexisting nerve injury or progressive neuropathies may also be contraindications. Certain block techniques may have specific contraindications, such as interscalene block and respiratory failure, as hemidiaphragm paralysis results. Complications of regional blocks include direct injury to nerve fibers by injection needles or local anesthetics, systemic anesthetic toxicity, and hematoma or abscess at the injection site. Anticoagulant guidelines are similar to those for neuraxial techniques.

MONITORED ANESTHETIC CARE

MAC, also referred to as conscious sedation or local-combined anesthesia, refers to the use of periprocedural sedation, with or without local, regional, or neuraxial anesthesia. Medications are the same as those used for induction of general anesthesia, including narcotics, benzodiazepines, and propofol. In some cases, only the dosage of sedative agents or the absence of airway maintenance distinguishes this from general anesthesia. Therefore, full monitoring, airway equipment, and resuscitative medications should be available. MAC does not preclude the need to sometimes progress to general anesthesia, and preoperatively should be treated similarly with regard to NPO status, medications, or resuscitation.

SUGGESTED READINGS

Bateman BT, Schumacher HC, Wang S, Shaefi S, Berman MF. Perioperative acute ischemic stroke in noncardiac and nonvascular surgery: incidence, risk factors, and outcomes. *Anesthesiology.* 2009;110:231–238.

Green L, Machin SJ. Managing anticoagulated patients during neuraxial anaesthesia. *Br J Anaesth.* 2010;149:195–208.

Horlocker TT, Wedel DJ, Rowlingson JC, et al. Regional anesthesia in the patient receiving antithrombotic or thrombolytic therapy: American Society of Regional Anesthesia and Pain Medicine evidence-based guidelines (third edition). *Reg Anesth Pain Med.* 2010;35:64–101.

Kheterpal S, Tremper KK, Englesbe MJ, et al. Predictors of postoperative acute renal failure after noncardiac surgery in patients with previously normal renal function. *Anesthesiology.* 2007;107:892–902.

Landesberg G, Beattie WS, Mosseri M, et al. Perioperative myocardial infarction. *Circulation.* 2009;119:2936–2944.

Poldermans D, Schouten O, van Lier F, et al. Perioperative strokes and beta-blockade. *Anesthesiology.* 2009;111:940–945.

Selim M. Perioperative stroke. *N Engl J Med.* 2007;356:706–713.

CHAPTER 49

Perioperative Pain Management

Darin J. Correll, MD

INTRODUCTION

Pain is the most common symptom of disease. It is defined as an unpleasant sensory and emotional experience, associated with actual or potential tissue damage. There are sound medical and legal reasons to treat pain aggressively in hospitalized patients. The Joint Commission, which certifies all health care institutions in the United States, mandates that all patients have the right to adequate pain assessment and management (**Table 49-1**).

In the inpatient setting, patients may be more concerned about pain relief than the outcome of their underlying illness. Poor pain control has adverse physiologic consequences that lead to worse outcomes (**Table 49-2**).

PRACTICE POINT

- Poor pain control has adverse physiologic consequences that lead to worse outcomes. In postoperative patients, better analgesia improves cardiovascular, respiratory, endocrine, immunologic, gastrointestinal, and hematologic status. Acute pain that is not satisfactorily treated may become persistent.

In postoperative patients, better analgesia improves cardiovascular, respiratory, endocrine, immunologic, gastrointestinal, and hematologic status. Acute pain that is not satisfactorily treated may become persistent.

PATHOPHYSIOLOGY: NOCICEPTIVE AND ANTI-NOCICEPTIVE PATHWAYS

Nociception, the perception of noxious stimuli, is a preconscious neural activity that is normally necessary, but not sufficient, for pain. It is more accurate to refer to nociceptive pathways, rather than pain pathways. The peripheral nerve fibers acting as nociceptors are lightly myelinated A-delta and unmyelinated C fibers, which are triggered or sensitized (peripheral sensitization) by several substances, including adenosine triphosphate (ATP), prostanoids, bradykinin, serotonin, histamine, and hydrogen ions. Heat, pressure, or nerve damage also results in activation.

The primary nociceptors synapse in the dorsal horn of the spinal cord (**Figure 49-1**), where the excitatory amino acids glutamate and aspartate and peptides such as substance P serve as neurotransmitters. Noxious impulses ascend in the lateral spinothalamic tract to the medial and lateral thalamus and spread to sensory regions of the cerebral cortex. Parts of the limbic system are also activated; presumably, this is where nociception is associated with emotion and arousal and becomes pain.

The nociceptive system has built-in positive and negative feedback loops. Prolonged firing of nociceptors enhances synaptic transmission to dorsal horn neurons. This process of *central* sensitization involves glutamine and a host of other mediators. Central sensitization is an adaptive response that prevents further injury during a vulnerable period of tissue healing. This heightened sensitivity generally returns to baseline over time. However, if central sensitization is prolonged beyond the healing phase, chronic pain may result.

Substance P–mediated nociception is antagonized by local production of endogenous opiates, such as enkephalins and endorphins, in the dorsal horn and the brain stem. Binding of narcotics to opiate receptors in these locations may account for the analgesic effects of these drugs. As well, powerful top-down, endogenous

TABLE 49-1 Joint Commission Pain Assessment and Management Standards for Hospitals

1. The hospital respects the patient's right to pain management.
2. The hospital educates all licensed independent practitioners on assessing and managing pain.
3. The hospital assesses and manages the patient's pain. The hospital conducts a comprehensive pain assessment that is consistent with its scope of care, treatment, and services and the patient's condition.
4. The hospital uses methods to assess pain that are consistent with the patient's age, condition, and ability to understand.
5. The hospital assesses and reassesses its patients. The hospital defines, in writing, criteria that identify when additional, specialized, or more in-depth assessments are performed for pain.
6. Based on the patient's condition and assessed needs, the education and training provided to the patient by the hospital include any of the following: discussion of pain, the risk for pain, the importance of effective pain management, the pain assessment process, and methods for pain management.

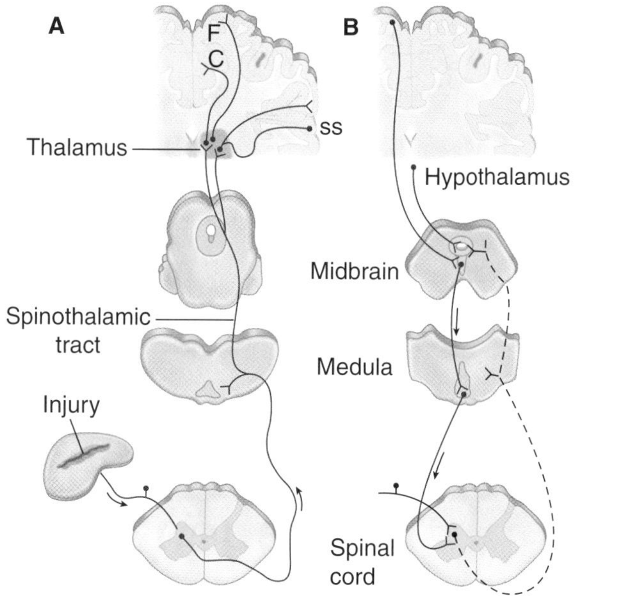

Figure 49-1 *Nociception transmission and pain modulatory pathways. A, Transmission system for nociceptive messages. Noxious stimuli activate the sensitive peripheral ending of the primary afferent nociceptor by the process of transduction. The message is then transmitted over the peripheral nerve to the spinal cord, where it synapses with cells of origin of the major ascending pain pathway, the spinothalamic tract. The message is relayed in the thalamus to the anterior cingulate (C), frontal insular (F), and somatosensory cortex (SS). B, Pain-modulation network. Inputs from frontal cortex and hypothalamus activate cells in the midbrain that control spinal pain-transmission cells via cells in the medulla. (Reproduced with permission from Fauci AS, Braunwald E, Kasper DL, et al. Harrison's Principles of Internal Medicine. 17th ed. New York: McGraw-Hill; 2008, Fig. 12-4.)*

mechanisms of pain modulation originate in the cortex and travel through brain stem and midbrain structures en route to the spinal cord. These descending pain control pathways are mediated by noradrenergic and serotonergic transmission, as well as endogenous opiates.

CHARACTERIZING PAIN INTENSITY

The most commonly used measures of pain intensity in the acute setting are single-dimension scales (**Table 49-3**). A numerical rating scale has the numbers 0 to 10 spaced evenly across a page, where 0 is "no pain at all" and 10 is "the worst pain imaginable." Patients are instructed to circle the number that represents the amount of pain they are currently experiencing. A common variation is the verbal numeric scale, where patients are asked to verbally state a number between 0 and 10 to correspond to their present pain intensity. Some people prefer to use words to describe the intensity of their pain; these are termed verbal descriptor scales. Another variant that may be useful in the elderly or cognitively impaired are scales with drawings of faces, ranging from a contented smiling face to a distressed-looking face.

TABLE 49-2 Physiologic Consequences of Uncontrolled Pain

Cardiovascular	Tachycardia, hypertension, increased cardiac workload
Pulmonary	Hypoxia, hypercarbia, atelectasis, decreased cough
Gastrointestinal	Decreased gastric emptying, nausea/vomiting, ileus
Renal	Urinary retention
Endocrine	Increased adrenergic activity, catabolic state, sodium/water retention
Immunologic	Impairment, slowed wound healing
Musculoskeletal	Splinting, contractures, decreased mobility (deep vein thrombosis)
Hematological	Increased coagulability
Neurological	Anxiety, fear, anger, fatigue, delirium

Single-dimensional scales are quick and simple to use, an important benefit in the acute setting when repeated measures are needed over a brief period of time. One disadvantage is that they attempt to assign a single value to a complex, multidimensional experience. Another is that patients can never know if the present experience is the "worst." If a value of "10" is chosen and the pain worsens, the patient has no means to express this.

Several multidimensional scales exist that attempt to assess various aspects of the patient's pain experience (eg, McGill Pain Questionnaire, Brief Pain Inventory). These multidimensional scales take into account the complex nature of pain. However, in the inpatient setting, they are too time consuming for rapid or repeated use. One compromise is to address a limited number of the dimensions of pain, using a few single-dimensional scales to address issues that are important to hospitalized patients—pain, anxiety, depression, anger, fear, and interference with physical activity.

DIAGNOSIS

HISTORY

The history of the patient in pain includes the pain's *location* and the presence of *radiation* from the primary site. *Intensity* should be determined using appropriate scales, as already described. The patient should describe the pain's *character* (eg, aching, burning, dull, electric-like, sharp, shooting, stabbing, tender, throbbing). This may provide clues to diagnosis (**Table 49-4**). Does the pain have a *pattern* (constant, intermittent, or better or worse at certain times of day) and *aggravating and alleviating factors*? Does the pain have an *impact on functional status*? Are the patient's activities of daily living affected

TABLE 49-3 Single-Dimension Pain Scales

Numerical rating scale:

0	1	2	3	4	5	6	7	8	9	10

Verbal descriptor scales:

No pain	None	Mild	Moderate	Severe	Worst pain imaginable

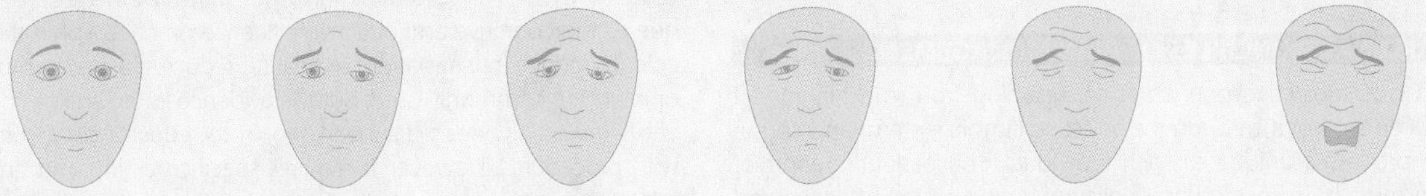

0	2	4	6	8	10

The Faces Pain Scale—Revised. From Pain 2001;93:173–183. Used with permission from IASP.

as an outpatient, or is it hampering their ability to cough, get out of bed, and ambulate while in the hospital? The patient's *prior analgesic history*, in particular, what therapies have either worked or not worked in the past, helps to decide what agents may be effective now. Exact doses of *ongoing analgesics* should also be determined.

Past medical history

The patient's medical history should be obtained. Medical conditions that cause pain include cancer, diabetes, osteoarthritis, rheumatoid arthritis, herpes zoster (shingles), and spinal cord injury. Psychological conditions may adversely impact a patient's pain experience and need appropriate diagnosis and therapy. These include anxiety (especially in acute pain states), depression (most prevalent in persistent pain states), fear, catastrophizing (assuming the worst-case scenario), and personality disorders. A family history that is positive for substance abuse in the patient's relatives is a risk factor for addiction in the patient. A social history positive for alcohol, tobacco, or other drugs may indicate a need to prescribe agents to prevent withdrawal (ie, benzodiazepines or nicotine patches). Even patients with a history of addiction still need to be appropriately treated for pain in the acute setting. In this setting, it may be useful to enlist the help of a psychiatrist or psychologist trained in addiction management.

PHYSICAL EXAMINATION

A directed *physical examination* of the painful site, and a generalized physical exam of the patient as appropriate, should be performed. Pain (especially acute) may be associated with tachycardia, hypertension, diaphoresis, and tachypnea. However, since sympathetic activation is a common and nonspecific finding in hospitalized patients, it offers little help in the diagnosis and treatment of pain in an awake, competent patient. These measures may be used as surrogates in patients who cannot express their pain experience. However, it is important to remember that patients may not exhibit any alterations in vital signs despite significant levels of pain, especially patients who have persistent pain.

PRACTICE POINT

- Patients may not exhibit any alterations in vital signs despite significant levels of pain, especially patients who have persistent pain. Since sympathetic activation is a common and nonspecific finding in hospitalized patients, it offers little help in the diagnosis and treatment of pain in an awake, competent patient.

TABLE 49-4 Determining the Mechanism and Treatment of Pain

Pain Mechanism	Character	Examples	Treatment Options
Somatic	Usually well localized and constant Aching, sharp, stabbing	• Laceration • Fracture • Burn • Abrasion • Localized infection or inflammation	• Heat/cold • Acetaminophen • NSAIDs • Opioids • Local anesthetics (topical or infiltration)
Visceral	Not well localized—constant or intermittent Generalized ache, pressure or cramping, can be sharp	• Muscles/spasm • Colic or obstruction (gastrointestinal or renal) • Sickle cell • Internal organ infection or inflammation	• NSAIDs • Opioids • Muscle relaxants • Local anesthetics (nerve blocks)
Neuropathic	Can be localized (ie, dermatomal) or radiating, can also be generalized and not well localized Burning, tingling, electric shock, lancinating.	• Trigeminal • Postherpetic • Postamputation • Peripheral neuropathy • Nerve infiltration	• Anticonvulsants • Tricyclic antidepressants • Muscle relaxants • NMDA antagonists • Neural/neuraxial blockade

NMDA, N-methyl-D-aspartate; NSAIDs, nonsteroidal anti-inflammatory drugs.

DIAGNOSTIC TESTING

Diagnostic tests to determine the etiology of pain may be useful in some situations (eg, radiographs to assess for fracture, magnetic resonance imaging (MRI) to diagnose nerve impingement in the spinal cord, or electromyography (EMG) to diagnose a neuropathy). However, normal test results should not be used to discount a patient's report of pain.

CARDINAL PRINCIPLES OF PAIN MANAGEMENT

Pain is a subjective phenomenon, resulting from the filtering of nociceptive input through the affective (limbic system) and cognitive processes unique to each individual. The patient's report of pain must be respected and believed. As pain is an affective and cognitive experience, the placebo response to analgesics is real and may be helpful. However, using the placebo response does not mean misleading patients, or administering an inactive substance to determine whether they are lying or to punish them. Rather, the placebo effect in contemporary medicine is that patient belief in a particular therapy makes it more likely to work. Physician attempts to truthfully "talk up" genuine attempts at analgesia are thus likely to enhance the effects. The reverse is also true. If a patient states that a particular therapy "never works for them," it is less likely to be effective.

The patient's pain level and degree of pain relief should be assessed appropriately and regularly. Pain should be treated quickly. Therapy should not be withheld while the diagnosis is unclear; pain treatment does not impede the ability to diagnose disease. A comprehensive plan should be used that addresses the multidimensional aspects of pain. This may require an interdisciplinary team approach (eg, hospitalist, pain specialist, anesthesiologist, surgeon, psychiatrist or psychologist, and physical therapist), especially for patients with persistent pain.

The analgesic plan should be discussed with the patient and, when appropriate, the patient's family. The patient's expectations for pain management should be understood, and patients should be offered reasonable goals for therapy. A multimodal approach for managing pain, employing both pharmacologic and nonpharmacologic measures, is better than using just one modality. This approach allows for optimal analgesia with the lowest incidence of side effects. Clinicians should be familiar with several agents within each class of analgesics, including possible side effects, because individual responses vary greatly.

PRACTICE POINT

- A multimodal approach for managing pain, employing both pharmacologic and nonpharmacologic measures, is better than using just one modality. This approach allows for optimal analgesia with the lowest incidence of side effects. In the absence of a contraindication, all patients in pain should be prescribed a nonopioid analgesic.

If pain is present most of the time or expected to last for an extended period of time (ie, more than a few weeks), long-acting agents or round-the-clock dosing of short-acting agents should be used. When long-acting drugs are used, immediate-release agents will also be needed for breakthrough pain. When pain is intermittent or expected to be of brief duration (ie, less than 2 weeks), then as-needed dosing of immediate release agents can be used alone.

TREATMENT

Pharmacologic and nonpharmacologic treatment measures are often used together. Pain medication falls into three categories: nonopioid analgesics, opioids, and adjuvant analgesics. Therapy should be individualized in a multimodal, stepwise approach, adding or changing agents when pain control is inadequate, and withdrawing agents as pain resolves (**Table 49-5**).

NONPHARMACOLOGIC MEASURES

Although scientific data on nonpharmacologic measures are limited, most have little risk. At a minimum, they may have placebo benefit, due to the cognitive and affective influence on pain. Application of cold (to reduce inflammation) or heat (to reduce spasms) to muscles or joints are commonly used, but the evidence for an analgesic benefit is mixed. Hypnosis has been shown to reduce pain associated with procedures. However, it requires specific training and time to administer. In the acute setting, the results with transcutaneous electrical nerve stimulation (TENS) are conflicting, with somewhat better evidence of effectiveness in the setting of chronic pain, particularly painful diabetic neuropathy. Relaxation and guided imagery have shown little evidence for any benefit in the acute setting. Attention techniques can be complicated in that one needs to determine which approach is better for a particular patient. Some patients do better when instructed to shift attention away from the pain, whereas others do better if instructed to attend to a particular portion of the pain (eg, the sensory component, as opposed to the emotional component). Acupuncture and electroacupuncture have been shown to be beneficial in the acute setting, reducing both pain and common side effects from opioid analgesics. However, these are labor intensive, and specific training is required.

NONOPIOID ANALGESICS

In the absence of a contraindication, all patients in pain should be prescribed a nonopioid analgesic. These agents have analgesic effects and are opioid sparing, leading to decreased side effects. They are the primary analgesics for low-intensity pain associated with headache or musculoskeletal disorders and are useful adjuncts in moderate to severe pain. These agents have a plateau effect, such that doses beyond the recommended range increase the incidence of side effects but do not improve analgesia.

Acetaminophen inhibits cyclooxygenase in the brain, which may account for its antipyretic actions. However, it does not inhibit peripheral prostaglandin synthesis. This explains its lack of side effects on gastric mucosa and platelets, but it also means that it is not active at peripheral sites of inflammation. In diseases where inflammation plays a major role in generating pain (eg, rheumatoid arthritis), acetaminophen is of little benefit. (The analgesic mechanism of acetaminophen is not well characterized but may involve facilitation of central downregulation of pain by serotonin, increasing levels of endogenous cannabinoids, or inhibition of nitric oxide synthesis in the spinal cord, which may interfere with substance P–related nociception.)

The nonacetylated salicylates (eg, choline magnesium trisalicylate) have a relatively low incidence of gastrointestinal bleeding, perhaps related to their lack of inhibition of platelet aggregation. The nonselective nonsteroidal anti-inflammatory drugs (NSAIDs) are potent anti-inflammatory analgesics with significant risk for gastrointestinal bleeding and renal insufficiency. No single NSAID appears to be more effective as an analgesic than any other, but as there is great interpatient variability in response, changing agents may be of benefit if one does not seem to be effective. The COX-2 selective NSAIDs have a reduced risk of peptic ulceration compared to nonselective NSAIDs, but an equivalent chance of renal toxicity. Celecoxib is currently the only COX-2 selective NSAID available in the United States. It should not be considered a first-line agent given its cost, and should not be used long term at high doses, as it may increase the risk of major cardiovascular events. **Table 49-6** lists the dosing regimens and adverse effects of selected nonopioid analgesics.

TABLE 49-5 Suggested Pain Management Schemes

The World Health Organization devised the analgesic ladder for the treatment of cancer pain. The concepts behind its use are helpful in the management of all types of pain, both persistent and acute.

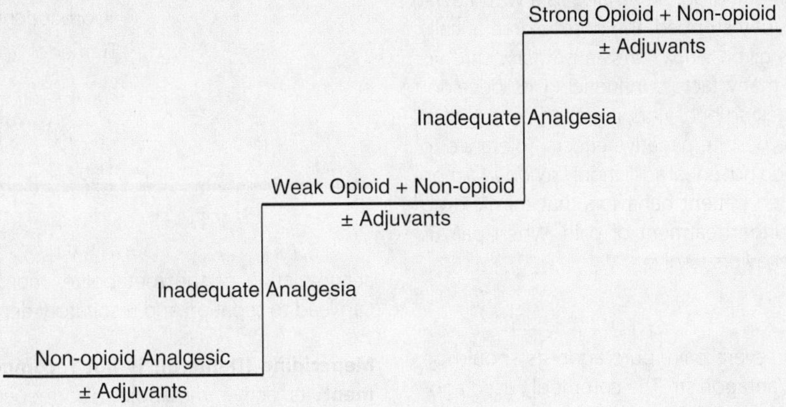

The World Federation of Societies of Anaesthesiologists devised another analgesic ladder to use for the treatment of acute/postoperative pain.

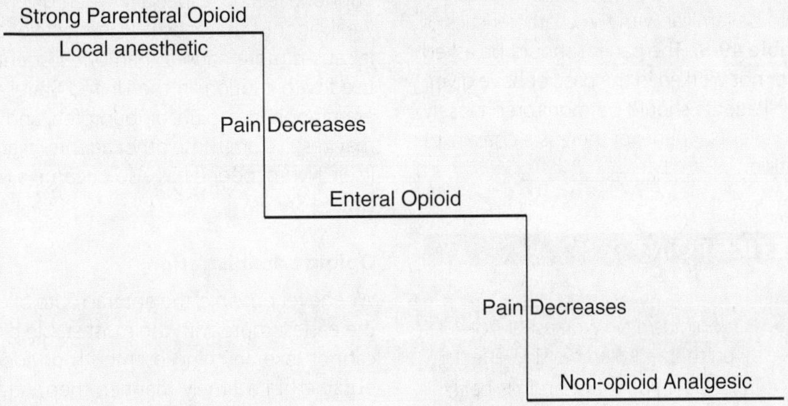

Data from World Health Organization. *Cancer Pain Relief*. Geneva, Switzerland: World Health Organization; 1986 and Data from *Charlton JE. WFSA Update in Anesthesia*. 1997;7:2–17.

TABLE 49-6 Select Nonopioid Analgesics

Agent	Adult Dosing	Maximum Daily Dose	Comments
Acetaminophen	650–1000 mg every 6 hours	4000 mg	Single doses above 1000 mg do not improve analgesia
Choline magnesium trisalicylate	1000–1500 mg twice a day	3000 mg	Caution in liver disease, avoid in severe liver disease
Diclofenac	50 mg twice a day-four times a days	200 mg	Low GI effect incidence, but possible increased renal effects, recent data suggest increased negative CV effects
Etodalac	200–400 mg every 6–8 hours	1000 mg	Low GI and renal effect incidence, safest NSAID in liver disease
Ibuprofen	400–600 mg every 4–6 hours	3000 mg	< 1500 mg daily has low risk of GI effects, possible increased renal effects, inhibits CV benefits of aspirin when given concomitantly
Ketorolac	30 mg every 6 hours	120 mg	High risk of renal and GI complications; use for no more than 5 days; 15 mg every 6 hours in renal impairment, age >65, weight < 50 kg
Nabumetone	750–1,500 mg daily or twice a day	1500 mg	Low GI effect incidence
Naproxen	250–500 mg every 6–12 hours	1500 mg	Possible increased liver and renal effects, probably least negative CV effects
Celecoxib	100–200 mg daily	200 mg	Use 100 mg dose if possible; long-term use has increased negative CV effects

CV, cardiovascular; GI, gastrointestinal.

OPIOIDS: TERMINOLOGY

Tolerance is the diminished response to a drug over time, such that, in order to maintain the same effect, the drug dose needs to be increased. *Dependence* is a state of physiologic adaptation that develops with continued use of a drug, presenting as a withdrawal syndrome if the drug is abruptly stopped, the dose is dramatically reduced, or an antagonist is given. *Addiction* is a primary, chronic, neurobiologic disease with many factors influencing its development. It manifests as drug-seeking behaviors, impaired control over the drug, and continued use despite negative effects. Tolerance to and dependence on opioids do not equal addiction! *Pseudoaddiction* denotes iatrogenically induced patient behaviors that mimic drug seeking, due solely to the undertreatment of pain. When pain is adequately managed, the behaviors resolve.

Opioid therapy basics

When treating moderate to severe pain, pure agonists should be used, as opposed to agonist/antagonists. The commonly used agonists are shown in **Table 49-7**.

Optimal analgesic dose varies widely among patients, even the opioid naïve. Side effects from opioids also vary widely between patients. It is therefore helpful to be familiar with the characteristics of several different agonists (**Table 49-8**). The patient should be asked which opioids have worked or not worked in the past, or have given them intolerable side effects. Patients should be monitored closely for effectiveness and adverse events whenever there is a change of agent or route of administration.

PRACTICE POINT

Opioids

- Patients should be asked which opioids have worked or not worked in the past, or have given them intolerable side effects.
- Whenever possible, the enteral route of administration is best, as it is the easiest route with the most stable pharmacokinetics. If a patient cannot take anything by mouth or adequate analgesia cannot be obtained in a timely manner, then intravenous (IV) administration should be used. Intramuscular administration should be avoided.
- If pain is present most of the time or expected to last for an extended period of time (ie, more than a few weeks), long-acting agents or round-the-clock dosing of short-acting agents should be used. When long-acting drugs are used, immediate-release agents will also be needed for breakthrough pain.
- Patients should be monitored closely for effectiveness and adverse events whenever there is a change of agent or route of administration.
- When pain is intermittent or expected to be of brief duration (ie, less than 2 weeks), then as-needed dosing of immediate release agents can be used alone.
- When a patient is competent, the use of an IV patient-controlled analgesia (PCA) offers the best overall pain management option for postoperative hospitalized patients.

Selecting an opioid

Codeine is not a good first choice due to the fact that 10–20% of the population lacks an active form of the enzyme (cytochrome P450 2D6) necessary to convert codeine into an active drug in the body (ie, morphine). All opioids should be used with caution in patients with renal or hepatic insufficiency; lower doses or longer dosing intervals are wise in this setting. Morphine is relatively contraindicated in patients with severe renal insufficiency due to the accumulation of the metabolite, morphine-6-glucuronide, which can lead to sedation and respiratory depression.

TABLE 49-7 Opioid Classification

Not Recommended	Weak	Strong
Meperidine	Codeine	Fentanyl
	Hydrocodone	Hydromorphone
	Tramadol	Methadone
		Morphine
		Oxycodone
		Oxymorphone

Meperidine (Demerol) is not recommended for pain management Its active metabolite, normeperidine, can accumulate in 24–48 hours to levels that produce nervous system excitation (tremors, muscle twitching, convulsions). Meperidine causes a strong euphoric feeling, especially when given by intravenous push. It is a weak agonist that is usually ineffective for more than mild pain, and it causes more nausea than other agents. Hydrocodone should be used with caution. In the United States, it is coformulated with acetaminophen, aspirin, or ibuprofen, and adverse events and toxicity may result from these other agents, in addition to the hydrocodone itself. Hydrocodone has also become a favored drug of abuse in the United States.

Opioid administration

Whenever possible, the enteral route of administration is best, as it is the easiest route with the most stable pharmacokinetics. If a patient cannot take anything by mouth or adequate analgesia cannot be obtained in a timely manner, then intravenous (IV) administration should be used. Intramuscular administration should be avoided. It is painful; there are wide fluctuations in absorption; it takes a long time to reach peak effect; there is a rapid fall-off of action thereafter. When a patient is competent, the use of an IV patient-controlled analgesia (PCA) offers the best overall pain management option (see later discussion).

Opioid dosing

Recommended starting doses for moderate to severe pain in the opioid-naïve are listed in **Table 49-9**. If a patient is not receiving enough pain relief at a given dose, subsequent doses should be increased by 25–50%. If a patient is having pain before the next dose is due, the dosing interval should be reduced, or the dose increased.

A switch to another opioid may be necessary in several circumstances. First, patients on therapeutic opioid doses who are not receiving any pain relief may not have a receptor population at which that particular opioid is effective. A different opioid may provide better analgesia. Second, if a patient is having intolerable side effects, rotation to a different opioid may provide relief. In this case, the patient's receptor population may bind a particular opioid in regions that cause side effects. Third, if a particular opioid cannot be given by the route of administration required, then changing to another opioid will be necessary. Finally, if a patient has been on an opioid for a long time and has developed tolerance, rotation to a different opioid may provide better analgesia, usually at less than the expected equianalgesic dose. A similar effect may also be seen in patients on long-term opioid therapy for chronic pain who have an episode of acute pain; better analgesia may also be experienced in this setting with a switch to a different opioid.

TABLE 49-8 Opioid Characteristics

Agonist	Route	Equianalgesic Dose (mg)	Onset (min)	Peak Effect (min)	Duration of Effect (h)
Morphine	IV	10	5–10	10–30	3–5
	Oral	30	15–60	60–120	4–6
	Oral CR	–	30–120	180–240	8–12
	Oral SR	–	30–120	480–600	8–24
Codeine	IM	120	10–30	90–120	4–6
	Oral	200	30–45	60	3–4
Hydromorphone	IV	1.5	5–20	15–30	3–4
	Oral	7.5	15–30	90–120	4–6
Oxycodone	Oral	20	15–30	30–60	4–6
	Oral CR	–	30–60	90–180	8–12
Methadone	IV	10*	10–20	60–120	4–6
	Oral	20*	30–60	90–120	4–12
Fentanyl	IV	0.1	< 1	5–7	0.75–2+
	TD	(See Table 49-11)	720–1,080	1,440–4,320	48–72
Oxymorphone	IV	1	5–10	30–60	3–6
	Oral	10	"meaningful relief" = 60		4–6

CR, controlled-release; IM, intramuscular; IV, intravenous; SR, sustained-release; TD, transdermal.

*These doses are based on single administrations and should only be used to convert between oral and IV methadone. If converting a patient who has been on a different opioid, use the following table that takes into account the dose-dependent potency changes seen with methadone:

Equianalgesic Conversion to Methadone§

Oral Morphine Equivalent That Patient is Taking	Oral Methadone (mg)	Oral Morphine (mg)
< 100 mg/day	1	4
101–300 mg/day	1	8
301–600 mg/day	1	10
601–800 mg/day	1	12
801–1000 mg/day	1	15
> 1000 mg/day	1	20

To determine the starting dose of oral methadone:

- Convert the patient's daily opioid dose into oral morphine equivalents.
- Convert the daily oral morphine equivalents to a daily oral methadone dose using the table.
- Reduce the calculated daily oral methadone dose by 33–50%.
- Divide the resulting reduced daily dose by 3.
- Prescribe this dose of oral methadone (in mg) every 8 hours.

§This table is not meant to be used to convert from methadone to other opioids. There is limited data on the conversion from methadone to other agents, and inadequate analgesia often results. Thus, if it is necessary to convert from methadone to another opioid agonist, it is best performed in stages, with close monitoring of the patient for effectiveness (eg, introduce the new agent over a 3-day period as the methadone dose is tapered by one-third each day).

Equianalgesic-dosing charts (see Table 49-8) are based on the relative potency of opioid agonists, as determined by single-dose clinical studies and experience. These calculations are estimates only, and clinical judgment is always required for use. Incomplete cross-tolerance exists between the various opioids. Patients may not be as tolerant to a new opioid agonist as they are to the one they were on previously. Thus, when converting between opioids, the calculated equianalgesic dose of the new agent must be reduced by 25–75% to prevent oversedation and respiratory depression. **Table 49-10** shows an example of opioid conversion.

Sustained-release or long-acting opioids

Episodic pain or pain expected to be of a brief duration should be treated with immediate-release agents alone. Sustained-release formulations should be initiated in the acute setting if pain is present most of the time, and pain is expected to last for an extended period of time (2–3 weeks or more). When using a sustained-release opioid, an immediate-release opioid equivalent to 10–15% of the 24-hour total every few hours on an as-needed basis should also be prescribed. If more than four to five rescue doses of immediate-release opioid are needed in 24 hours, the dose of sustained-release agent should be increased by 50–100% of the total 24-hour breakthrough dose used.

Transdermal fentanyl is not appropriate to treat acute pain, especially in the opioid-naïve. Its use in the acute setting may lead to severe respiratory depression from the delayed peak effect of the drug. It should only be used in patients already tolerant to opioids of comparable potency. **Table 49-11** gives recommendations for conversion from other opioids to transdermal fentanyl.

Methadone is also not appropriate as a first-line agent in the acute setting, especially in the opioid-naïve. Its use requires an understanding of the unique pharmacology of the drug, especially its extended duration of action and its dose-dependent potency. Also, as it takes several days to reach a stable plasma concentration, patients need to be monitored closely for efficacy and side effects. As methadone is a racemic mixture of a mu agonist and

TABLE 49-9 Recommended Starting Doses of Opioids for Adults Over 50 kg

Agonist	Oral	IV
Codeine	15–60 mg every 3–4 hours	n/a
Hydrocodone	5–10 mg every 3–6 hours*	n/a
Tramadol	50–100 mg every 4–6 hours†	n/a
Oxycodone	5–10 mg every 3–4 hours	n/a
Morphine	10–30 mg every 3–4 hours	5–10 mg every 2–4 hours
Hydromorphone	2–6 mg every 3–4 hours	1–1.5 mg every 3–4 hours
Oxymorphone	10–20 mg every 4–6 hours	1 mg every 3–4 hours

*Daily dose limited by acetaminophen component in available preparations.
†Maximum recommended 24-hour dose: 400 mg in adults < 75 years old; 300 mg in adults > 75 years old.

an N-methyl-D-aspartate (NMDA) antagonist (see later discussion), patients develop less analgesic tolerance. Patients must be made aware of the long duration of action of methadone, be warned not to take extra doses or mix it with other medications, and be familiar with signs of overdose.

PATIENT-CONTROLLED ANALGESIA BASICS

PCA is primarily intended as maintenance therapy. If the patient is in moderate to severe pain when it is begun, IV loading doses must be given to achieve comfort, because the incremental dosing of the PCA will not be effective in a reasonable period of time. The use of a PCA helps overcome the wide interpatient variation in opioid requirements by allowing the patient to control the dosing regimen. Morphine is the most common first-line agent. It is not the best choice in patients with renal insufficiency, due to accumulation of the active metabolite. Fentanyl has a quicker onset and shorter duration of action than morphine. This decreases the likelihood of oversedation, but the patient must activate the PCA more often, making it difficult for some patients to sleep at night. Hydromorphone is generally more effective in opioid-tolerant patients. Recommended starting doses in the opioid-naïve patient are listed in **Table 49-12**, along with suggestions for dose titration.

The lockout interval, or minimum time between doses, is typically set at 5–10 minutes. Even though the time to peak effect may be longer than this, in practice no major differences are seen with longer lockouts. There have also been no good studies to suggest that a particular lockout interval is better than any other.

A basal rate on the PCA may be needed in opioid-tolerant patients or in patients receiving fentanyl, given its short half-life. Basal rates are not recommended in the opioid-naïve, elderly, or patients with obstructive sleep apnea or morbid obesity. Basal rates should be decreased or discontinued if a patient is not activating the PCA, or if the patient is becoming excessively sedated.

COMPLICATIONS/OPIOID-INDUCED SIDE EFFECTS

Nausea, vomiting, pruritus, constipation, sedation, and respiratory depression are common opioid-related side effects. They occur more often in opioid-naïve patients, as tolerance eventually develops to all these effects, except constipation. Adverse effects can be ameliorated by changing the drug dose or schedule, switching to a different agent (side effects of different opioid agonists vary among patients), specific therapy to counteract the side effect, or adding another analgesic or adjuvant to allow a lower opioid dose.

Constipation should always be expected with opioids. Prophylactic use of stool softeners, such as docusate, and stimulant laxatives, such as senna preparations, is recommended. Nausea and vomiting can be treated with any of the available agents (eg, prochlorperazine, ondansetron, metoclopramide, promethazine), as none has been shown to be more or less effective. Metoclopramide is a promotility agent with limited antinausea effects and is most effective if there is vomiting. Promethazine or

TABLE 49-10 Example of Opioid Conversion

1. Patient used 15 mg of IV hydromorphone in the past 24 hours.
2. According to the equianalgesic table:

   1.5 mg of IV hydromorphone = 20 mg of oral oxycodone

   $$\frac{1.5 \text{ mg of IV hydromorphone}}{20 \text{ mg of oral oxycodone}} = \frac{15 \text{ mg of IV hydromorphone}}{X}$$

   X = 200 mg of oral oxycodone/day
3. Taking into account incomplete cross-tolerance, decrease the total daily opioid dose by 25–75%:

   200 − (0.25 × 200) = 150 mg of oral oxycodone/day

   200 − (0.75 × 200) = 50 mg of oral oxycodone/day
4. Dose initially every 4 hours:

   150/6 ≅ 25 mg oxycodone every 4 hours

   50/6 ≅ 8 mg oxycodone every 4 hours

   Therefore, order: oxycodone 10–25 mg every 4 hours as needed for pain.

TABLE 49-11 **Dose Conversion Guidelines from Another Opioid to Transdermal Fentanyl**

24-Hour Oral Morphine Equivalent Dose (mg/day)*	Transdermal Fentanyl Initial Dose (mcg/h)
60–134	25
135–224	50
225–314	75
315–404	100
405–494	125
495–584	150
585–674	175
675–764	200
765–854	225
855–944	250
945–1034	275
1035–1124	300

*Convert other opioid to oral morphine equivalents using an equianalgesic dose table.

This table should not be used to convert from transdermal fentanyl to another opioid because the conversion to transdermal fentanyl in this table is conservative. Therefore use of this table to convert from transdermal fentanyl to another opioid can overestimate the amount of the new agent, resulting in overdosage and respiratory depression.

TABLE 49-12 **Suggested Starting Patient-Controlled Analgesia Dose and Dose Changes**

	Morphine	Hydromorphone	Fentanyl
Staring PCA dose	1.0–1.5 mg	0.2 mg	20–25 mcg
PCA dose change	0.5 mg	0.1 mg	5–10 mcg

possibly a scopolamine patch may be effective if the patient has a history of motion sickness, or if nausea is provoked by movement, as opioids sensitize the inner ear labyrinthine system. Extreme caution must be used with promethazine because of its possibility to cause severe tissue damage if extravasation occurs. Pruritus is generally thought to be a central mu opioid receptor-related phenomenon. Diphenhydramine is only effective if the etiology is definitely due to histamine release, which is usually only the case for large doses of morphine given quickly, or a true allergic reaction. Nalbuphine 5 mg IV every 4 hours as needed is more effective in that it treats the cause, by antagonism of the central mu receptors. Sedation may be a troublesome side effect, particularly when using opiates to alleviate persistent pain in terminal illness. The proper treatment of respiratory depression from opioid agonists is described in **Table 49-13**.

ADJUVANT ANALGESICS

Adjunctive agents are useful for additional analgesia in opioid-tolerant patients, and have a particular role in the treatment of neuropathic symptoms and chronic pain. Examples of adjuvant analgesics with dosing guidelines and common side effects are listed in **Table 49-14**.

The most commonly used antiepileptics are gabapentin and pregabalin. They are effective for neuropathic pain and may have benefits in the acute setting as well. Antidepressants are also effective in neuropathic pain. Analgesic doses are lower than those for depression treatment, and the onset of analgesia is faster (days) than the antidepressant effects (weeks). Skeletal muscle relaxants are useful for muscle injury or spasms. The antispasmodic baclofen is useful for the treatment of pain with a spastic component or in certain neuropathic pain states. Antagonism of the NMDA receptor

TABLE 49-13 **Treatment of Suspected Opioid-Induced Respiratory Depression**

Suggested definition of respiratory depression:

- Oxygen saturation below 90% or decrease of more than 5% from baseline in patients with baseline oxygen saturation of < 90%.

  AND
- Respiratory rate less than 8 breaths per minute.

Primary, nonpharmacologic treatments of respiratory depression:

- If patient is taking effective breaths but at a rate of < 8 per minute:
  - Tactile and verbal stimulation, naloxone administration may not be essential.
- If patient is taking ineffective breaths and/or with a respiratory rate < 4 per minute:
  - May require ventilatory assist with bag-valve mask and supplemental oxygen. This should be instituted while diluting and administering naloxone.

Naloxone should only be considered in the following situations:

- Patient is unarousable or minimally arousable to tactile/verbal stimulation.
- Patient is requiring ventilatory assistance.

Proper naloxone dilution and dosing:

- 1 ampule (0.4 mg) of naloxone must be diluted with 9 mL saline to yield 0.04 mg per mL.
- Administer to patient in 1–2 mL increments (0.04–0.08 mg) at 2–3 minute intervals until response.
- If no change in respiratory depression after 0.4 mg naloxone has been titrated, consider another etiology other than opioid induced.
- If there is some, but not enough, improvement after 0.4 mg of naloxone has been titrated, continue titration.
- Naloxone's half-life is less than most of the opioid agonists, so be aware that rebound respiratory depression may recur. Therefore, be prepared for the need to readminister naloxone boluses or consider use of a naloxone infusion.

TABLE 49-14 Select Adjuvant Analgesics

Class	Agent	Adult Dosing	Side Effects/Comments
Antiepileptics	Gabapentin	Start with 300 mg orally every 8 hours, increase by 300 mg daily after a few days to a max of 3600 mg/day in divided doses	Dizziness and somnolence; do not stop abruptly
	Pregabalin	Start with 50 mg orally every 8 hours or 75 mg orally every 12 hours; in 1 week increase to max of 300 mg/day in divided doses	
Tricyclic antidepressants	Amitriptyline Nortriptyline	25 mg orally every night at bed time; increase to max of 150 mg/day in a single or divided doses	Anticholinergic symptoms (eg, dry mouth, confusion, sedation, and hypotension)
Local anesthetics	Lidocaine 2.5% and prilocaine 2.5% cream	2–2.5 gm per 10–25 cm^2 skin for 1–2 hrs before procedure	Localized skin reactions; rare cardiovascular and/or CNS toxicity; prilocaine may contribute to methemoglobinemia in patients treated with other agents known to cause this
	Lidocaine patch 5%	Up to 3 patches for up to 12 h within a 24 h period	Localized skin reactions; rare cardiovascular and/or CNS toxicity; only FDA indication is for treatment of postherpetic neuralgia
Glucocorticoids	Dexamethasone	4–8 mg orally every 8–12 hours	Typical steroid-induced side effects from long-term use (> 2–3 months) usually outweigh benefits; concomitant use with NSAIDs not recommended
Skeletal muscle relaxants	Cyclobenzaprine	5–10 mg orally every 8 hours	Long-term use can lead to the development of dependence
	Tizanidine	4–8 mg orally every 6–24 hours	
	Orphenadrine	100 mg orally every 12 hours 60 mg IV every 12 hours	
Antispasmodic	Baclofen	10 mg orally every 8 hours, titrate slowly to max of 80 mg/day in divided doses	Drowsiness; may impair renal function; abrupt discontinuation may cause seizures
NMDA antagonists	Ketamine	0.1–0.2 mg/kg/h IV	Sedation, dreams and hallucinations possible but infrequent at analgesic (low) dose, treat with the addition of benzodiazepine or dose-reduction
	Dextromethorphan	Start with 30–90 mg orally every 8 hours, increase to max of 360 mg/day in divided doses	Best dose and regimen not well defined
Alpha-2 Agonist	Clonidine	0.2 mg/day via a transdermal patch, left on for 1 week	Hypotension and sedation; monitor for rebound hypertension on discontinuation if used for > 1 week

CNS, central nervous system; FDA, U.S. Food and Drug Administration; NSAID, nonsteroidal anti-inflammatory drug.

has no primary analgesic effect, but it has opioid-sparing, opioid tolerance-reversing, and antihyperalgesic effects. Ketamine, in addition to being an NMDA antagonist, interacts with opioid and other receptors, and thus it has true analgesic properties in addition to the NMDA class effects. Ketamine use improves pain scores and has an opioid-sparing effect of up to 50%, although there are equivocal benefits in reduction of opioid side effects. The alpha-2 agonist, clonidine, has analgesic and opioid-sparing effects. Dexmedetomidine has documented opioid-sparing effects when given by IV infusion. It may have analgesic effects as well, although this effect may only occur at sedating doses, restricting its use to sedated intensive care patients. Glucocorticoids are used in cancer pain management to reduce inflammation from tumor invasion of nerves.

Benzodiazepines may reduce the insomnia and anxiety that often accompany acute pain. However, these agents do *not* have analgesic properties. They must be used with extreme caution in acute pain, especially when high doses of opioids are required, as significant sedation and respiratory depression can occur in the benzodiazepine-naïve patient. In the anxious patient with pain, adequate titration with analgesics should occur before the addition of a benzodiazepine.

ACUTE PAIN IN THE OPIOID TOLERANT

When opioid-tolerant patients experience an event resulting in pain escalation, opioid use is expected to be higher than mere replacement of what the patient was receiving before. The additional doses of opioids required may be much higher than in opioid-naïve patients. More complaints of pain and high pain scores should be expected. Discussion of reasonable goals and expectations of analgesic therapy with the patient is crucial. Multimodal therapy in this patient population is helpful to achieve the best pain control, and have the least escalation of home opioid dose as possible.

CONSULTATION

Involvement of a pain specialist may be appropriate in the patient with severe pain that remains uncontrolled after several escalations of drug doses and use of multiple classes of agents. Concomitant psychiatric illness may warrant input from a psychiatrist or psychologist. Certain diagnostic tests, such as diagnostic epidural injections, require an interventional pain physician. Physical therapy, surgery, complementary therapies, or invasive treatment modalities, such as epidural injections, intrathecal pumps, and spinal cord stimulators, will require referral to the appropriate provider.

DISCHARGE CONSIDERATIONS

Communication with the patient's primary care provider about the discharge analgesic plan is essential, especially if the prior analgesic regimen has been changed. Follow-up should be arranged to ensure effectiveness of the analgesic regimen, monitor for side effects after discharge, and taper the patient off analgesics, or reduce doses to baseline if the patient was on chronic analgesics before.

WEANING OPIOIDS

If the cause of pain is gone, patients need discontinuation of opioids in a manner that prevents the occurrence of withdrawal symptoms, such as abdominal pain, diarrhea, tachycardia, vomiting, diaphoresis, runny nose, muscle cramps, piloerection, anxiety, and irritability. When weaning a patient from long-acting agents, the dose of the long-acting agent should be decreased by 25–50% every 2 days. Once the patient is off the sustained-release form, the immediate-release agent can also be weaned. In weaning a patient from immediate-release agents, the opioid dose should be reduced by 50% for 2 days, and then reduced by 25% every 2 days thereafter until the total dose in oral morphine equivalents is 30 mg/day. The drug may be discontinued after 2 days on the 30 mg/day dose.

QUALITY IMPROVEMENT

Data on pain management quality should be collected periodically to assess the quality of care, to establish baseline data, and to identify areas in which care can be improved. The American Pain Society has proposed the following six quality indicators for hospital-based pain management: (1) pain intensity is documented with a numeric or descriptive rating scale; (2) pain intensity is documented frequently; (3) pain is treated by a route other than intramuscular; (4) pain is treated with regularly administered analgesics, and whenever possible, a multimodal approach is used; (5) pain is prevented and controlled to a degree that facilitates function and quality of life; and (6) patients are involved in the treatment plan and are informed and knowledgeable about pain management.

SUGGESTED READINGS

American Pain Society. *Principles of Analgesic Use in the Treatment of Acute Pain and Cancer Pain.* 6th ed. Glenview, IL: American Pain Society; 2008.

Gordon DB, Dahl JL, Miaskowski C, et al. American Pain Society recommendations for improving the quality of acute and cancer pain management. *Arch Intern Med.* 2005;165:1574–1580.

Gruener D, Lande SD, eds. *Pain Control in the Primary Care Setting.* Glenview, IL: American Pain Society; 2006.

Morrison RS, Meier DE, Fischberg D, et al. Improving the management of pain in hospitalized adults. *Arch Intern Med.* 2006;166: 1033–1039.

United States Food and Drug Administration/Center for Drug Evaluation and Research website. http://www.accessdata.fda.gov/scripts/cder/drugsatfda/index.cfm. Accessed April 3, 2010.

Whelan CT, Jin L, Meltzer D. Pain and satisfaction with pain control in hospitalized medical patients. *Arch Intern Med.* 2004;164: 175–180.

SECTION 4

Perioperative Assessment and Management

CHAPTER 50

Antimicrobial Prophylaxis in Surgery

Daniel A. Anaya, MD
E. Patchen Dellinger, MD

INTRODUCTION

Surgical site infection (SSI) is the most common complication in surgical patients. Significant advances have occurred over the last few decades resulting in better understanding of the relevant risk factors for SSI, and high-level evidence has identified specific preventive strategies that help reduce the incidence of SSI. With the introduction of asepsis and antisepsis, prophylactic antibiotics have had the most significant impact reducing the incidence of SSI. However, in order to achieve the benefits derived from their use and minimize potential undesired effects, practice of this strategy needs to follow specific basic principles.

This chapter reviews the epidemiology and clinical impact of SSI, describes the role of prophylactic antibiotics as a preventive strategy, and expands on the specific principles that guide their appropriate use. We will also summarize specific recommendations for different procedures while highlighting important aspects of different antibiotic regimens. Lastly, we will identify specific barriers to this practice and identify some health service interventions proven to improve past and current practice patterns when using antibiotic prophylaxis.

RATIONALE FOR USE OF ANTIMICROBIAL PROPHYLAXIS

SURGICAL SITE INFECTION EPIDEMIOLOGY AND RISK FACTORS

It is estimated that over 40 million surgical procedures are performed every year in the United States. SSIs complicate approximately 2–5% of these procedures, representing 38% of nosocomial infections occurring in surgical patients. Risk factors for SSI can be classified as patient-related factors and local/surgical factors, and can be stratified into modifiable or potentially modifiable, and nonmodifiable risk factors. Modifiable risk factors include elective operations in the presence of associated infections, prolonged preoperative hospital stays, seromas, dead space, foreign bodies, routine drain use, among others, and can be modified with the use of good surgical practice and specific preventive strategies. Nonmodifiable risk factors are most commonly patient related and have an important effect on the incidence of SSI for each individual patient. The wound class (Appendix 1) is a relatively good predictor of SSI and has traditionally been used to estimate the risk of SSI and as a benchmark for interinstitutional comparisons. However, with the more recent understanding of SSI and its multifactorial risk factors, different predictive scores, such as the National Nosocomial Infection Surveillance (NNIS) score, have been developed to better estimate the risk of SSI for each individual patient after considering the interaction between different risk factors (**Table 50-1**). Specific preventive measures have been identified and are used to decrease the risk of SSI. These include minimizing the presence of microorganisms (eg, prophylactic antibiotics), and optimizing the patient's ability to fight those still present at the surgical site, during the perioperative period.

IMPACT OF SURGICAL SITE INFECTION

The effect of SSI on patients and the health care system is significant. Patients with SSI are more prone to develop additional complications, including wound dehiscence, hernia, and complicated infections such as necrotizing soft tissue infections. Multiple

TABLE 50-1 National Nosocomial Infection Surveillance (NNIS) System Classification for Determining the Risk of Surgical Site Infection

Risk Factors	Points
Procedure duration ≥ 75th percentile of duration for that specific operation	1
Contaminated or dirty wound	1
American Society of Anesthesiology score III–V	1
Final Score	**Risk of Surgical Site Infection**
0	1.5%
1	2.9%
2	6.8%
3	13.0%

large, single-center, multicenter, and population-level analyses have revealed at least a twofold increased risk of postoperative mortality in patients with SSI. Additionally, SSI is associated with longer hospital stays (10–12 excess days), a higher risk of intensive care unit (ICU) admission, and a fivefold higher risk of hospital readmission. Similarly, the treatment of patients with SSI results in an excess cost of over $5000 per patient, representing a U.S. national cost between $130 and $845 million per year. As such, and given the availability of multiple preventive measures, SSI is not only considered a significant surgical complication but is also used as a health care quality indicator.

GOALS OF ANTIMICROBIAL PROPHYLAXIS

Based on the preceding considerations and high-level evidence-based data, antimicrobial prophylaxis is a preventive strategy used with the primary goal of reducing the risk of SSI. As such, antimicrobial prophylaxis is used as a preventive strategy when infection *is not present* but the risk of postoperative SSI *is present*. The efficacy and effectiveness of this practice are measured by its impact on the incidence of SSI, and its principles as well as developed guidelines are tailored toward achieving an improvement in this specific outcome. Additionally, the practice of antimicrobial prophylaxis should follow strict guidelines to maximize its benefits while minimizing undesired effects such as emergence of resistant bacteria or potential—although rare—side effects in individual patients at low risk of developing SSI.

PRACTICE POINT

Antimicrobial prophylaxis is used as a preventive strategy when infection is not present but the risk of postoperative SSI is present.

- The relative benefit of antibiotic prophylaxis holds for all cases, but the absolute benefit and the number needed to treat or prevent an SSI are less for procedures with a low baseline risk of infection.
- The decision to use prophylaxis should be based on a complex assessment of the risk of infection and the cost and morbidity of the infections that might occur for that procedure, all balanced against the cost of the prophylaxis including its price and the potential for adverse effects including allergies, superinfections, and the generation of bacterial resistance by overuse.

COMMON PRINCIPLES

INDICATIONS FOR ANTIBIOTIC PROPHYLAXIS

John Burke first described the value of prophylactic antimicrobials in the 1950s with animal studies that clearly demonstrated the principles of prophylaxis that are still followed today. Since then, many retrospective studies, prospective randomized trials, systematic reviews, and meta-analyses have confirmed the efficacy of prophylactic antimicrobials in decreasing the risk of SSI and established the basic principles. The magnitude of this effect directly relates to the magnitude of the risk of SSI. The majority of studies have focused on evaluating the efficacy of prophylactic antibiotics when used for specific operations. This has resulted in high-level data supporting their use for clean-contaminated and contaminated operations, and more controversial data for their use in operations classified as clean. However, the risk of SSI can vary significantly between patients undergoing similar surgical procedures. Various studies have shown that using a more comprehensive predictive tool (such as the NNIS score), the risk of SSI can in fact be higher for some patients with less contaminated wounds, depending on the presence of other risk factors. This has been supported by randomized trials and meta-analyses demonstrating a clinical benefit of using prophylactic antibiotics for breast, cardiac, orthopedic, and vascular surgery, as well as other clean operations.

More recently, Bowater and colleagues published a paper assessing the overall general benefit of prophylactic antibiotics independent of the specific operative procedure.[1] They performed a meta-analysis of available meta-analyses on the topic and collated the data from studies assessing their efficacy in different types of procedures. This paper concluded that the use of prophylactic antibiotics is an effective practice that reduces the risk of SSI, regardless of the operation, and the decision to use prophylaxis should take this into consideration.

The relative benefit of antibiotic prophylaxis holds for all cases, but the absolute benefit and the number needed to treat to prevent an SSI are less for procedures with a low baseline risk of infection. The decision to use prophylaxis should be based on a complex assessment of the risk of infection, the cost, and the morbidity of the infections that might occur for the procedure, all balanced against the cost of the prophylaxis, including its price and the potential for adverse effects such as allergies, superinfections, and the generation of bacterial resistance by overuse. Based on this type of reasoning, patients in whom a prosthesis (implantation of any foreign body) is to be used or for those having cardiac operations, for example, have long been considered appropriate cases to receive prophylaxis even though the procedures are "clean" and the relative risk of SSI is fairly low. Clearly, an SSI in a patient with a recent hip replacement or after a coronary artery bypass grafting (CABG) procedure has more morbidity than that presenting after removal of a subcutaneous lipoma of the trunk. With these considerations, the use of antimicrobial prophylaxis should be based on a preoperative risk assessment that takes into consideration other variables in addition to wound classification, as well as the potential consequences of this complication.

Based on existing data and the foregoing considerations, prophylactic antibiotics are indicated for the following:

- Clean-contaminated and contaminated operations
- Clean operations with a high risk of SSI
  - NNIS score ≥ 1 +/− other associated important risk factors
  - Immune-compromised host
  - Other clean operations with known increased risk of SSI, such as groin incisions and mastectomy

- Clean operations for which SSI has significant clinical consequences
  - Examples: operations involving placement of prosthesis (eg, joint replacements, mesh hernia repairs, etc), craniotomy, and cardiac and vascular operations

SELECTION OF ANTIMICROBIAL AGENT

The characteristics of the ideal agent for effective antibiotic prophylaxis include (1) appropriate bactericidal effect on the bacteria expected to be present at the surgical site, (2) adequate biodistribution in the surgical site, (3) low risk of potential side effects (allergic reactions, *Clostridium difficile* colitis, change in resistance patterns, etc), and (4) low cost. The majority of guidelines helping to choose the appropriate agent are based on randomized trials in which a specific antibiotic regimen has been tested for a specific procedure. We support the use of this evidence-based decision making. However, the vast majority of procedures are prone to SSI with similar species of bacteria, and similar types of antibiotics have been tested. If clinical trial data are not available for a specific procedure, it is reasonable to generalize from trial data on procedures with comparable bacterial flora and risk.

PRACTICE POINT

The characteristics of the ideal agent for effective antibiotic prophylaxis include:

1. Appropriate bactericidal effect on the bacteria expected to be present at the surgical site.
2. Adequate biodistribution in the surgical site.
3. Low risk of potential side effects (allergic reactions, *C difficile* colitis, change in resistance patterns, etc)
4. Low cost.

In general, the first consideration is to determine the class of wound and the most common bacteria causing SSI in each case. For clean wounds, skin flora with gram-positive bacteria are the most common pathogens causing SSI. For these operations, cefazolin is the most commonly used antibiotic, and it follows the four main principles already outlined. Alternatives to this agent include other first- or second-generation cephalosporins, oxacillin, and clindamycin, among others. For patients with documented and clinically relevant beta-lactam allergies, clindamycin or vancomycin is an adequate alternative. For procedures with expected gram (–) +/– anaerobic bacteria, such as most clean-contaminated and contaminated operations, coverage for these pathogens must guide antibiotic selection. Specific regimens include single agents such as ertapenem, cefotetan, and cefoxitin or multiple-agent regimens such as an aminoglycoside or a quinolone plus clindamycin or metronidazole (**Table 50-2**).

PRACTICE POINT

Selection of antimicrobial agent

1. Determine the class of wound and the most common bacteria causing SSI in each case.
2. Consider local resistance data from your hospital's surveillance systems.
   - A specific agent may be recommended for an operation based on national guidelines. However, if microbiologic data derived from local surveillance programs reveal that the expected flora have a high resistance rate to that agent, another antibiotic must be used.
   - Trending patterns of resistance to the different agents used can help identify emergence of resistance early, and can guide local protocols.

Local data derived from a hospital's surveillance systems are important and must be considered when choosing a prophylactic antibiotic. Although a specific agent may be recommended for an operation, based on national guidelines, if microbiologic data derived from local surveillance programs reveal that the expected flora have a high resistance rate to that agent, another antibiotic must be used. Similarly, trending patterns of resistance to the different agents used can help identify emergence of resistance early and can guide local protocols.

Recent concern in the lay press regarding methicillin-resistant *Staphylococcus aureus* (MRSA) infections has led to calls to use vancomycin routinely as a prophylactic agent for clean operations. Data for this are conflicting, however. One recent study randomized cardiac patients to vancomycin versus cefazolin in a hospital with a high rate of MRSA and found more MRSA infections in the cefazolin arm but more methicillin-sensitive *Staphylococcus aureus* (MSSA) infections in the vancomycin arm and no difference in overall rates between the two groups. A more reasonable approach has been described as screening patients for MRSA colonization preoperatively and choosing to use vancomycin for those in whom these bacteria are present. However, the logistics of information management in a program of this sort are problematic. Further studies are needed to better define the role for routine or selective use of vancomycin as a prophylactic agent in these procedures.

ANTIBIOTIC TIMING

PRACTICE POINT

Timing, dosage, and duration of prophylactic antibiotics

1. Administer antibiotics within one hour prior to incision time.
2. The chosen dose should accomplish adequate tissue levels throughout the whole operation.
   - Higher than standard doses are recommended for obese patients.
   - Current guidelines recommend redosing of antibiotics for procedures lasting two or more half-lives of the specific agent used.
3. There are no studies demonstrating superior efficacy of longer courses of prophylactic antibiotics in the postoperative period.
   - Specifically, for patients undergoing colorectal, other abdominal and gastrointestinal procedures, vascular, cardiac, gynecologic, urologic, orthopedic and head and neck operations, there is enough evidence supporting the use of short (<12–24 hours) regimens over longer ones, and in the majority of cases, significant evidence to recommend a single-dose strategy.

The importance of antibiotic administration before incision was the first key fact determined about prophylaxis. John Burke first described the direct relation between timing of prophylaxis—in relation to incision time—and effectiveness, and identified the decisive period to be as close to the incision time as possible.[2] More recently, other investigators have corroborated these findings, showing a linear increase in the rate of SSI as the time of prophylaxis administration gets further from the incision time. All studies show a dramatic rise in SSI when antibiotics are first given after incision. This probably results from the effect of both the serum and the tissue antibiotic levels at the time of operation, with the best and most persistent levels achieved when the antibiotic is given close to the incision time. Based on these principles, current guidelines recommend administering prophylactic antibiotics within one hour prior to incision time. The exceptions to this are vancomycin

TABLE 50-2 Recommended Antibiotic Prophylaxis Regimens for Different Types of Surgical Procedures Based on Published Guidelines and Most Current Available Data

Type of Surgical Procedure	Recommended Antibiotic Regimen	Alternative Regimens for ß-lactam Allergies
Cardiothoracic operations	Cefazolin Cefuroxime Cefamandole	Clindamycin Vancomycin
Vascular operations	Cefazolin Cefuroxime	Clindamycin Vancomycin
Gastrointestinal clean procedures and those involving entry into theupper gastrointestinal tract	Cefazolin	Ciprofloxacin Clindamycin Vancomycin
Biliary tract operations	Cefazolin Ampicillin/sulbactam Cefotetan	Ciprofloxacin
Appendectomy	Cefoxitin Cefotetan Ampicillin/sulbactam Cefmetazole Piperacilline/tazobactam Ertapenem Ciprofloxacin or an aminoglycoside + metronidazole or clindamycin	Ciprofloxacin or an aminoglycoside + metronidazole or clindamycin
Colorectal	Ertapenem Cefoxitin Cefotetan Cefazolin plus metronidazole Ciprofloxacin or an aminoglycoside + metronidazole or clindamycin	Ciprofloxacin or an aminoglycoside + metronidazole or clindamycin
Hip or knee arthroplasty	Cefazolin Cefuroxime	Clindamycin Vancomycin
Hysterectomy	Cefazolin Cefotetan Cefoxitin Cefuroxime Ciprofloxacin or an aminoglycoside + metronidazole or clindamycin	Ciprofloxacin or an aminoglycoside + metronidazole or clindamycin
Head and neck operations	Cefazolin ± metronidazole Clindamycin ± aminoglycoside	Clindamycin ± aminoglycoside
Urologic operations	Cefazolin	Ciprofloxacin
Craniotomy	Cefazolin Oxacillin Nafcillin	Vancomycin

Indications may vary based on the specific operation and standard principles of prophylaxis.

or fluoroquinolones, both of which require slow infusion and can begin two hours prior to the incision time to avoid undesired antibiotic-related side effects. In addition, when the operation involves placement of a proximal tourniquet, the antibiotic infusion must be completed before the tourniquet is inflated, to allow for adequate tissue levels at the surgical site.

ANTIBIOTIC DOSING

Antibiotic dose is another important factor related to the efficacy of this prophylaxis strategy. The chosen dose should accomplish adequate tissue levels throughout the whole operation. The most accurate way to assure this is to use doses based on body weight. Most weight-based recommendations are derived from the pediatric literature, making this approach somewhat cumbersome, and hence standard doses that fit within recommended parameters are commonly used for the majority of adult patients. However, weight-based recommendations can be helpful when using prophylactic antibiotics in patients with extreme body weights. Specifically, the standard dose may need to be decreased to avoid antibiotic toxicity in extremely thin or pediatric patients, particularly when

TABLE 50-3 Characteristics of Selected Antibiotics More Commonly Used for Surgical Site Infection Prophylaxis

Antibiotic	Recommended Weight-Based Dose	Standard Recommended Dose	Half-Life* (in Hours)	Recommended Redose Interval (in Hours)
Cefazolin	20–30 mg/kg	1–2 grams	1.2–2.5	2–5
Cefuroxime	50 mg/kg	1.5 grams	1–2	3–4
Clindamycin	3–6 mg/kg	600–900 mg	2–5.1	3–6
Vancomycin	10–15 mg/kg	1 gram	4–6	6–12
Cefoxitin	20–40 mg/kg	1–2 grams	0.5–1.1	2–3
Cefotetan	20–40 mg	1–2 grams	2.8–4.6	3–6
Cefepime	–	1–2 grams	2.2	4
Ciprofloxacin	400 mg	400 mg	3.5–5	4–10
Gentamicin	3–5 mg/kg	300 mg	2–3	6
Metronidazole	15 mg/kg	500–1000 mg	6–14	12
Piperacillin/tazobactam	–	3.375 grams	0.7–1.2	2–4
Ertapenem	–	1 gram	4	8

Reported values applicable to adults.
*Half-life calculated for normal renal function.

using antibiotics with a narrow therapeutic window. More frequently, however, appropriate doses must be selected to achieve adequate tissue levels in obese patients. A study by Forse and colleagues demonstrated that in obese patients undergoing bariatric surgery, a dose of cefazolin twice the standard dose (2 g vs 1 g) was necessary to achieve adequate serum and tissue levels, and this practice was associated with a lower rate of surgical site infection (5.6% vs 16.5%, $P < .03$). Based on this and other similar studies, higher than standard doses are recommended for obese patients. Additionally, studies have demonstrated the association between antibiotic serum and tissue levels and incidence of SSI in patient populations including cardiac and gastrointestinal operations.

Given the need for adequate antibiotic tissue levels throughout the whole operation, repeat dosing is a relevant issue. Randomized trials, large single- and multiple-institution analysis, and the NNIS score have repeatedly identified duration of operation as an important independent risk factor for SSI. The specific mechanisms behind this have not been completely clarified. However, subtherapeutic antibiotic tissue levels found at the end of long operations can at least partially explain this association. Although different cutoff times have been used to define "long operations," studies evaluating redosing of antibiotics for cardiac and gastrointestinal procedures lasting longer than three to four hours have shown a lower incidence of SSI when following this practice. Given variation in specific pharmacokinetic properties of different antibiotics, current guidelines recommend redosing of antibiotics for procedures lasting two or more half-lives of the specific agent used. Adjustments to this rule need to be considered for patients with renal insufficiency in which the half-life of most antibiotics is prolonged (**Table 50-3**).

DURATION OF ANTIBIOTIC PROPHYLAXIS

Although adequate intraoperative antibiotic tissue levels are necessary to decrease the risk of SSI, the same is not true for the postoperative period. By definition, the use of antibiotic prophylaxis is to prevent a surgical site infection; hence, when compared with antibiotics used for the treatment of an infection, different principles apply regarding duration of antibiotics. Despite an extensive body of evidence supporting the use of a single preoperative dose (and intraoperative redosing when indicated) over a multiple-dose strategy (ie, one preoperative dose with subsequent postoperative doses), this is perhaps one of the most difficult principles to translate into real-life practice. A recent analysis demonstrated that in current practice, antibiotics are continued for over 24 hours after the operation in over 50% of patients. Multiple studies in different populations of patients have evaluated the role of single- versus multiple-dose prophylaxis. Specifically, for patients undergoing colorectal, other abdominal and gastrointestinal, vascular, cardiac, gynecologic, urologic, orthopedic, and head and neck operations, there is enough evidence supporting the use of short (<12–24 hours) regimens over longer ones, and in the majority of cases, significant evidence to recommend a single-dose strategy. There are no studies demonstrating superior efficacy of longer courses of prophylactic antibiotics. McDonald and colleagues reported results of a systematic review based on 28 randomized trials totaling over 9000 patients and reported no difference in the overall rate of SSI with either approach. Based on these findings, the authors recommended the use of a single-dose practice and emphasized the equivalent benefit and decreased cost of this strategy, with the additional benefit of decreasing the emergence of infections caused by resistant pathogens.

SPECIFIC PROCEDURES

Different single- and multiple-antibiotic regimens have been evaluated for various procedures. Based on these data, the expected microorganisms at the surgical site of each specific procedure, and the similar pharmacologic characteristics of these regimens, different alternatives are recommended. Table 50-2 lists some of these alternatives by surgical type, and although this is a helpful guideline for choosing antibiotics, the decision of which antibiotic to use is dynamic and should incorporate published high-level data, the aforementioned principles, and other local and system-related aspects such as cost and antibiotic resistance data.

IMPLEMENTATION PRACTICES/QUALITY IMPROVEMENT

Given the relative high incidence of SSI, its clinical impact, and the significant burden to the health care system, preventive strategies have been receiving more attention by physicians, health care institutions, and policy makers. One strategy to focus efforts on the effective delivery of known preventive strategies is to classify all SSIs as *potentially preventable* (not all prevention measures used or used incorrectly) or *not apparently preventable* (all known preventive measures used appropriately). While it will probably never be possible to reduce the number of SSIs to zero, diligent effort should be able to achieve a zero rate of potentially preventable infections. A number of local and national guidelines, specific implementation strategies, and collaborative group approaches have been recently developed with the objective of improving current practice targeted to minimize the number of potentially preventable SSIs. In 2002, the Centers for Medicare and Medicaid Services (CMS) and the Centers for Disease Control and Prevention (CDC) implemented the National Surgical Infection Prevention (SIP) project, with the aim of decreasing undesired outcomes and costs derived from potentially preventable SSIs. The appropriate use of prophylactic antibiotics was identified as a crucial measure in preventing SSI, and three practice performance measures were developed: (1) antibiotic dose given within 60 minutes of incision time, (2) appropriate selection of antibiotic, based on national guidelines, and (3) discontinuation of antibiotics within 24 hours of the end of the procedure.

An examination of over 11,000 operations performed on Medicare patients around the United States revealed that only 56% had antibiotic prophylaxis given within one hour of incision time, and only 40% had the antibiotic discontinued within 24 hours after the operation ended. Multiple efforts have focused on improving practice patterns for the use of prophylactic antibiotics. Overall, practice patterns have improved over time, with more recent assessments revealing better—although still inadequate—compliance with the three SIP performance measures. Various interventions have been used to help improve substandard practice and generally focus on education/feedback interventions and detailed changes in the process of care. A recent study led by the CMS and the SIP collaborative group, involving 56 different hospitals, demonstrated that an intervention based on educational/feedback sessions, models of improvement, and methods of implementing and measuring changes resulted in significant improvement in the timing and duration of antibiotics as well as improved performance with other nonpharmacologic preventive measures, and led to a 27% drop in the rate of SSI when comparing the before and after study periods. Other studies implementing similar educational and process-of-care interventions have demonstrated similar findings, emphasizing the importance of information dissemination and culture change. Some investigators have focused on more specific interventions such as shifting the responsibility of providing the antibiotic from the preoperative nurse to the anesthesiologist, developing checklists and standardized printed preoperative prophylaxis orders, and using automated systems to improve practice of this strategy. All such interventions have resulted in equivalent success.

Gagliardi and colleagues recently published a systematic review assessing the factors likely to influence appropriate antibiotic prophylaxis. Their results support the implementation of interventions such as development of multidisciplinary pathways focused on improving individual physicians' knowledge, attitudes, and beliefs and promoting team communication, as well as the use of written and computerized order sets. However, they also emphasize the need for further research to better characterize the benefit of these strategies. These future efforts should ideally be carried on within a framework of regional and/or national collaborative groups, which have the advantage of overcoming some of the difficulties in translating knowledge to practice at a single-institution level.

Evidence and Literature

1. Antimicrobial Prophylaxis in Surgery: Clinical Guidelines from the American Society of Health-System Pharmacists, the Infectious Diseases Society of America, the Society of Health Care Epidemiology of America, and the Surgical Infection Society. *Am J Health System Pharm*. 2011. In press.
2. Anaya DA, Dellinger EP. Surgical infections and choice of antibiotics. In: Townsend CM, Beauchamp RD, Evers BM, Mattox KL, eds. *Sabiston Textbook of Surgery: The Biological Basis of Modern Surgical Practice*. 18th ed. Philadelphia, PA: Elsevier, Saunders; 2007. Antibiotic prophylaxis in surgery: a national clinical guideline.
3. Scottish Intercollegiate Guidelines Network 104, 2008. http://www.sign.ac.uk/pdf/sign104.pdf, Accessed March 2010.
4. Bratzler DW, Houck PM. For the Surgical Infection Prevention Guideline Writers Group. Antimicrobial prophylaxis for surgery: an advisory statement from the National Surgical Infection Prevention Project. *Am J Surg*. 2005;189:395–404.
5. Dellinger EP, Gross PA, Barrett TL, et al. Quality standard for antimicrobial prophylaxis in surgical procedures: Infectious Diseases Society of America. *Clin Infect Dis*. 1994;18:422–427.
6. Mangram AJ, Horan TC, Pearson ML, et al. The Hospital Infection Control Practices Advisory Committee. Guidelines for prevention of surgical site infection. *Am J Infect Control*. 1999;26:97–134.
7. Kirkland KB, Briggs JP, Trivette SL, Wilkinson WE, Sexton DJ. The impact of surgical-site infections in the 1990s. attributable mortality, excess length of hospitalization, and extra costs. *Infect Control Hosp Epidemiol*. 1999;20:725–730.
8. Finkelstein R, Rabino G, Mashiah T, et al. Vancomycin versus cefazolin prophylaxis for cardiac surgery in the setting of a high prevalence of methicillin-resistant staphylococcal infections. *J Thorac Cardiovasc Surg*. 2002;123(2):326–332.
9. Dellinger EP. Prophylactic antibiotics: administration and timing before operation are more important than administration after operation. *Clin Infect Dis*. 2007;44: 928–930.
10. Dellinger EP. What is the ideal time for administration of antimicrobial prophylaxis for a surgical procedure. *Ann Surg*. 2008;247:927–928.
11. Steinberg JP, Braun BI, Hellinger WC, et al. Timing of antimicrobial prophylaxis and the risk of surgical site infections: results from the Trial to Reduce Antimicrobial Prophylaxis Errors. *Ann Surg*. 2009;250(1):10–16.
12. van Kasteren ME, Mannien J, Ott A, Kullberg BJ, de Boer AS, Gyssens IC. Antibiotic prophylaxis and the risk of surgical site infections following total hip arthroplasty: timely administration is the most important factor. *Clin Infect Dis*. 2007;44(7):921–927.
13. Weber WP, Marti WR, Zwahlen M, et al. The timing of surgical antimicrobial prophylaxis. *Ann Surg*. 2008;247:918–926.
14. Zanetti G, Flanagan HL, Cohn LH, Giardina R, Platt R. Improvement of intraoperative antibiotic prophylaxis in prolonged cardiac surgery by automated alerts in the operating room. *Infect Control Hosp Epidemiol*. 2003;24: 13–16.
15. Bratzler DW, Houck PM, Richards C, et al. Use of antimicrobial prophylaxis for major surgery: baseline results from the National Surgical Infection Prevention Project. *Arch Surg*. 2005;140:174–182.
16. Dellinger EP, Hausmann SM, Bratzler DW, et al. Hospitals collaborate to decrease surgical site infections. *Am J Surg*. 2005;190:9–15.

CONCLUSION

Surgical site infection is the most common complication following surgical procedures. It is associated with significant impact on patient outcomes and health care resource utilization. The use of prophylactic antibiotics is recognized as a proven strategy to reduce the risk of this complication. Current guidelines for the appropriate use of antibiotic prophylaxis are well supported by level I data. Although different antibiotics are recommended for different operations, general principles for the use of prophylaxis can help guide the use of this preventive measure. Prophylactic antibiotics are indicated when there is a significant risk of SSI such as in clean-contaminated and contaminated operations, as well as for selected clean operations, based on the presence of other risk factors and the impact of SSI for each specific patient population. With few exceptions, antibiotics must be given within one hour prior to incision, using generous (but safe) doses, redosed for longer operations (usually at two to three half-lives), and should be discontinued within 24 hours of the end of the operation, if not at the end of the operation. When compliance with these principles improves, the incidence of SSI decreases. However, as in many fields in medicine, translation of knowledge into practice is not easy. Specific health service interventions focused at disseminating knowledge, promoting multidisciplinary participation, and standardizing orders for antibiotic prophylaxis have proven successful in this task. Further efforts should continue to assess specific interventions to continue to optimize current practice and should ideally be done within regional/national collaborative groups that help overcome intrinsic institutional barriers to appropriate practice.

SUGGESTED READINGS

Anaya DA, Dellinger EP. Challenges in prevention of surgical site infections. *Infect Med.* 2005;23(3):120–126.

Gagliardi A, Fenech D, Eskicioglu C, Nathens AB, McLeod R. Factors influencing antibiotic prophylaxis for surgical site infection prevention in general surgery: a review of the literature. *Can J Surg.* 2009;52(6):481–489.

Kilo CM. A framework for collaborative improvement: lessons from the institute for healthcare improvement's breakthrough series. *Qual Manag Health Care.* 1998;6(4):1–13.

McDonald M, Grabsch E, Marshall C, Forbes A. Single- versus multiple-dose antimicrobial prophylaxis for major surgery: a systematic review. *Aust N Z J Surg.* 1998;68(6):388–396.

REFERENCES

1. Bowater RJ, Stirling SA, Lilford R. Is antibiotic prophylaxis in surgery a generally effective intervention? Testing a generic hypothesis over a set of meta-analyses. *Ann Surg.* 2009;249: 551–556.
2. Burke JF. The effective period of preventive antibiotic action in experimental incisions and dermal incisions. *Surgery.* 1961;50: 161–168.

APPENDIX 1

Surgical wound classification based on degree of potential contamination, according to the Centers for Disease Control and Prevention (CDC) guidelines

CLEAN

An uninfected operative wound in which no inflammation is encountered and the respiratory, alimentary, genital, or uninfected urinary tract is not entered. In addition, clean wounds are primarily closed and, if necessary, drained with closed drainage. Operative incisional wounds that follow nonpenetrating (blunt) trauma should be included in this category if they meet criteria.

CLEAN-CONTAMINATED

An operative wound in which the respiratory, alimentary, genital, or urinary tracts are entered under controlled conditions and without unusual contamination. Specifically, operations involving the biliary tract, appendix, vagina, and oropharynx are included in this category, provided no evidence of infection or major break in technique is encountered.

CONTAMINATED

Open, fresh, accidental wounds. In addition, operations with major breaks in sterile technique (eg, open cardiac massage) or gross spillage from the gastrointestinal tract, and incisions in which acute, nonpurulent inflammation is encountered are included in this category.

DIRTY

Old traumatic wounds with retained devitalized tissue and those that involve existing clinical infection or perforated viscera. This definition suggests that the organisms causing postoperative infection were present in the operative field before the operation.

CHAPTER 51

Preoperative Cardiac Risk Assessment and Perioperative Management

Steven L. Cohn, MD, FACP

INTRODUCTION

Hospitalists and internists are frequently called upon to perform preoperative medical consultations, and cardiac risk assessment is what is most often requested. Preoperative evaluation is now part of the core curriculum for Hospital Medicine, but when surveyed a number of years ago, many hospitalists felt inadequately trained to do this.

Preoperative cardiac risk assessment has evolved over the past 40 years from a simple global assessment of a patient's physical status (the ASA classification) to multivariate risk analyses (Goldman, Detsky) to a simplified scoring system (Lee RCRI) to guidelines from the American College of Cardiology/American Heart Association, American College of Physicians (ACC/AHA, ACP). The most current of these is the ACC/AHA guidelines for perioperative cardiac evaluation and management, originally published in 1996 and updated in 2007 to incorporate the RCRI factors. Using these guidelines and selective cardiac testing (pharmacologic stress tests), physicians are now better able to provide a more accurate assessment of perioperative risk, and the focus has turned to risk reduction strategies. These include revascularization by coronary artery bypass grafting (CABG) or percutaneous coronary intervention (PCI), medical therapy (beta-blockers, alpha-agonists, statins), and other intraoperative measures (normothermia, anesthetic technique). Although surgical and anesthetic techniques have improved and perioperative cardiac events have decreased, operative mortality and cardiac morbidity remain significant, especially among high-risk patients or high-risk procedures.

This chapter reviews the current state of the art for perioperative risk assessment and risk reduction in patients with cardiac disease.

PREOPERATIVE RISK INDICES

Goldman and colleagues published the first large prospective multivariate analysis of preoperative cardiac risk. They identified nine independent predictors of death or major postoperative cardiac complications. These risk factors were assigned points based on their relative importance, and the event rates were correlated with the point total in this risk index. Detsky and colleagues modified this risk index by expanding the list of risk factors and combining this with the pretest probability of complications based on the risk of the surgery itself. Eagle and colleagues identified five factors—age, diabetes mellitus (DM), angina, myocardial infarction (MI), and heart failure—associated with perioperative cardiac events and used these to stratify risk and decide when to do further cardiac testing. Most recently Lee and colleagues identified and validated six factors associated with increased risk of perioperative complications. These factors were high-risk surgery, coronary artery disease (CAD), heart failure, cerebrovascular disease (stroke or transient ischemic attack), DM requiring insulin, and renal insufficiency (creatinine > 2.0 mg/dL). These studies, using simple clinical evaluation (history, physical examination, and basic laboratory studies) found many similar factors predicting increased risk of perioperative cardiac complications and helped refine preoperative risk stratification.

CLINICAL RISK FACTORS

PRACTICE POINT

- Active clinical conditions are unstable coronary syndromes (MI < 30 days, unstable or severe angina), decompensated heart failure, hemodynamically significant arrhythmias, or severe (symptomatic) valvular heart disease.

A detailed history and focused physical examination are key in clinical risk assessment, and a few basic diagnostic tests may also be helpful. Current risk assessment is usually based on the Lee RCRI and the ACC/AHA guidelines, which now include the RCRI factors. What the ACC previously defined as major clinical predictors are now called active cardiac conditions. These are unstable coronary syndromes (MI < 30 days, unstable or severe angina), decompensated heart failure, hemodynamically significant arrhythmias, or severe (symptomatic) valvular heart disease. The group previously called intermediate clinical predictors is now called clinical risk factors and includes five of the six Lee RCRI factors (MI > 30 days, stable mild angina, compensated or history of heart failure, DM, renal insufficiency, and stroke)—the type of surgery is considered separately. The so-called minor risk predictors in the 2002 guidelines were dropped with the exception of cerebrovascular disease, which was moved up to the clinical predictor group. These minor predictors included some factors typically associated with risk of developing CAD (hypertension, dyslipidemia, cigarette smoking), but most studies found that these factors were not significant predictors of postoperative cardiac complications.

PRACTICE POINT

- MI > 30 days, stable mild angina, compensated or history of HF, DM, renal insufficiency, and stroke significantly predict higher risk of postoperative cardiac complications as well as the surgical procedure. Although traditional risk factors for the development of coronary artery disease (hypertension, dyslipidemia, smoking) should be addressed at the time of discharge, they should not be incorporated into the risk assessment for postoperative cardiac complications.

PROCEDURAL RISK

Independent of the patient's clinical risk factors, the type of surgery has its own inherent risk that needs to be taken into account. This concept was used in Detsky's modified cardiac risk index and is also a factor in the ACC algorithm. For example, a patient undergoing cataract surgery, a low-risk operation, is unlikely to have a complication even if the patient's clinical risk is high. Conversely a patient with no clinical risk factors undergoing high-risk surgery, such as a Whipple procedure, is more likely to have a postoperative complication than would have been predicted based on clinical pretest probability alone. Therefore, the risk of the surgery itself may alter management and influence the decision to do further testing. The ACC defines three groups for surgical risk—vascular, intermediate, and low. The previous designation of high risk has been changed to vascular surgery to reflect that the preponderance of evidence for cardiac testing was done for patients undergoing aortic and major vascular surgery, and the approach to these patients may be somewhat different than that for nonvascular surgery. The intermediate risk category includes most intrathoracic, intraabdominal, head and neck, orthopedic, and urologic procedures as well as some lower-risk vascular procedures such as carotid endarterectomy and endovascular abdominal aortic aneurysm repair. Low-risk surgery includes procedures not invading the chest or abdomen such as endoscopic or superficial procedures, eye surgery, and breast surgery.

PRACTICE POINT

- The ACC defines three groups for surgical risk: vascular, intermediate, and low. Low-risk surgery includes procedures not invading the chest or abdomen.

FUNCTIONAL CAPACITY

Goldman and colleagues noted that patients with good exercise capacity, even with mild, stable angina, tend to do well. This follows the concept of the ischemic threshold in which a patient developing ischemia on a stress test at a lower exercise level and with a lower rate-pressure product is at higher risk than someone who can perform 8–10 metabolic equivalents (METS) before developing symptoms. Reilly and colleagues found that a patient's self-reported exercise capacity correlated with the risk of postoperative complications, and the ACC guidelines use this in their risk assessment algorithm.

PRACTICE POINT

- Because a patient's self-reported exercise capacity correlates with the risk of postoperative cardiac complications, clinicians should factor functional capacity into their risk assessement.

LABORATORY TESTS

Many preoperative screening blood tests are performed unnecessarily, but a few may be helpful in assessing cardiac risk. These include measures of renal function, blood urea nitrogen (BUN) and creatinine, and glucose (as a screen for diabetes). Unless serum potassium is significantly abnormal (3.0 or >5.5 mEq), it is unlikely to increase risk or alter management. Anemia has been noted as a risk factor in some studies, but there is no evidence that treating it with transfusions alters risk. An electrocardiogram (ECG) looking for evidence of CAD or conduction defects may be of value in at-risk patients. Other findings can either be identified by clinical exam (arrhythmias) or don't change management (left ventricular hypertrophy (LVH), nonspecific ST-T changes).

ACC/AHA ALGORITHM

The ACC developed a stepwise approach to preoperative cardiac risk evaluation using the information obtained from the history, physical examination, and laboratory tests (**Figure 51-1**). The underlying theme is to minimize testing and not to order a test if the result will not change management. The approach is as follows:

1. Is the surgery *emergent* (and I tend to include *urgent*, meaning within 24 hours)?

   If it is, time does not permit diagnostic testing or revascularization and the patient will proceed to surgery. In the short time period available, the physician can try to medically optimize the patient's problems.

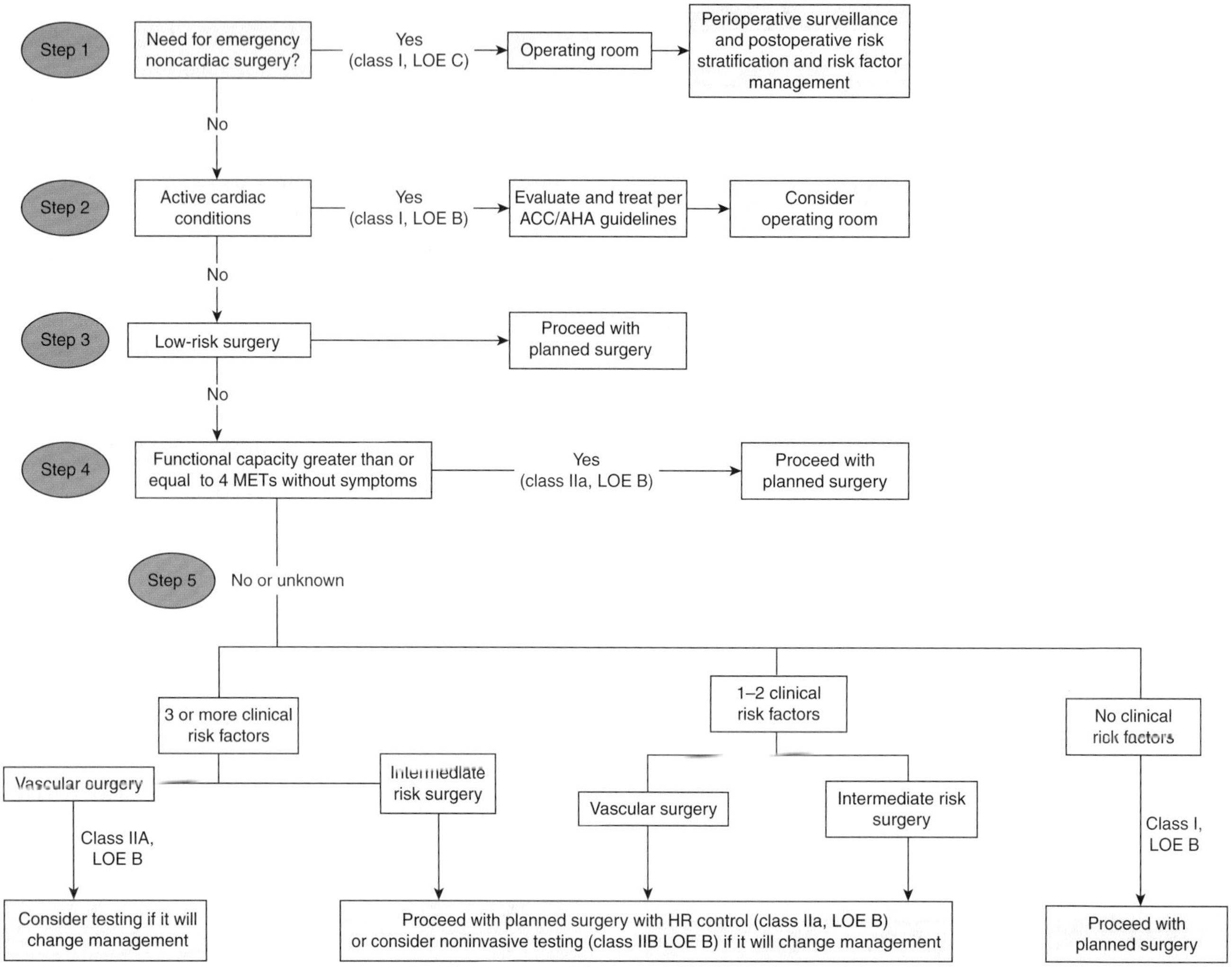

Figure 51-1 *ACC/AHA Cardiac Evaluation and Care Algorithm for Noncardiac Surgery. (Reproduced, with permission, from Fleischer LA, Beckman JA, Brown KA, et al. ACC/AHA 2007 guidelines on perioperative cardiovascular evaluation and care for noncardiac surgery: a report of the American College of Cardiology/American Heart Association Task Force on Practice Guidelines. J Am Coll Cardiol. 2007;54:e169.)*

2. Assuming surgery is not emergent, does the patient have any of the *active cardiac conditions*?

   If so, elective surgery should be delayed for further diagnostic workup and therapy. Most patients do not have these conditions.
3. Is the surgery low risk?

   If it is, the patient should proceed to surgery without any further testing or intervention because we cannot further reduce risk that is already low (<1%).
4. If not scheduled for low-risk surgery, does the patient have adequate exercise capacity (≥4 METS)?

   If so, for the most part, these patients will do well and do not need to undergo further cardiac testing.
5. Assuming the answers to all of the previous questions were no, the next step is to determine the patient's clinical risk factors.

   If there are no clinical risk factors, the patient should proceed to surgery with no further testing.

   If the patient has one or two risk factors, the guidelines recommend proceeding to surgery with heart rate control; however, they do say you can consider noninvasive testing (NIT) if the results will change management.

   The recommendations are the same for three risk factors and nonvascular surgery; however, for three or more risk factors and vascular surgery, the recommendation is to consider NIT.

This last step allows for individualizing management, but it is also somewhat vague and may lead to significant differences in opinion and approach.

DIAGNOSTIC TESTS

PRACTICE POINT

- The underlying theme of preoperative testing is to minimize testing and not to order a test if the result will not change management. A preoperative stress test may be considered for patients with a low functional capacity (< 4 METs) and with ≥ three clinical risk factors undergoing vascular surgery, but only if it will change management.

Stress tests were designed to diagnose CAD and myocardial ischemia and not to predict short-term events. Because the pathophysiology of perioperative MIs includes unstable plaque rupture or coronary thrombosis as well as myocardial ischemia related to coronary stenosis and an imbalance of oxygen supply and demand, stress tests are poor at predicting which patients are at increased risk for surgery. Although they are good at identifying a patient with CAD, they have a low positive predictive value (PPV), usually between 15 and 20% for perioperative MI, and most patients, even with an abnormal test, will not have a postoperative cardiac complication. On the other hand, a normal or negative stress test is usually associated with a high negative predictive value (NPV), ranging from 95 to 99%, indicating that there is a low likelihood that these patients will have a perioperative event.

Because many patients with cardiac disease undergoing surgery have suboptimal exercise capacity and would be unable to achieve 85% of their target heart rate on an exercise test, pharmacologic stress testing is usually used. Furthermore, if these patients had adequate exercise capacity, they probably would not be candidates for stress testing in the first place. The tests most commonly used are dobutamine stress echocardiography (DSE) and dipyridamole or adenosine nuclear imaging (usually thallium). These tests are effective in identifying CAD, but as noted earlier, are poor at identifying patients who will develop postoperative cardiac events and should be used selectively in conjunction with the patient's pretest probability for the results to be meaningful. The test characteristics are influenced by patient selection and pretest probability. In general, results are similar with DSE and dipyridamole thallium (DPT), and test selection should be based on the local expertise available; however, DSE tends to have fewer false-positives except in the case of left bundle branch block (LBBB) where DPT is preferred. On the other hand, DSE is preferred for patients with asthma or chronic obstructive pulmonary disease (COPD) because DPT can cause bronchospasm. Resting two-dimensional (2D) echocardiography is not recommended to predict perioperative ischemic complications and should only be used to evaluate valvular heart disease or heart failure.

WHO NEEDS STRESS TESTING BEFORE SURGERY?

The goal of NIT is to further refine clinical judgment and identify patients at significantly increased risk. Bayes theorem can be applied to preoperative evaluation to decide which patients might benefit from stress testing. A patient with a low pretest probability will usually remain at low risk for perioperative complications even if the NIT is positive. Similarly, a patient with high pretest probability will remain a relatively high-risk patient even if the stress test is negative (may represent a false-negative). Therefore, NIT should probably be restricted to intermediate-risk patients where a positive test can move a patient into a higher-risk category and a negative test can reclassify a patient as being at lower risk. The utility of this theoretical approach was supported by L'Italien and colleagues who showed that clinical assessment correlated with outcomes for low- and high-risk patients, and stress test results only changed the probability of complications (confirmed by outcomes) for intermediate-risk patients. Boersma and colleagues also demonstrated that the clinical risk score correlated with outcomes and was rarely changed by stress testing. However, a study by Poldermans and colleagues randomized intermediate risk patients, all of whom were treated with bisoprolol (titrated to a target heart rate of 60 to 65 beats per minute), to preoperative stress testing or no testing. They found no difference in perioperative MI or cardiac death regardless of whether they had a preoperative stress test assuming they were adequately beta-blocked. The results of this study beg the question of whether anyone needs NIT if they can be optimally treated medically.

WHEN IS PREOPERATIVE CORONARY ANGIOGRAPHY INDICATED?

The ultimate goal of the preoperative evaluation process is to identify the high-risk patient and intervene in some manner to reduce risk of postoperative complications. Assuming stress testing identifies a patient at high risk for postoperative complications, the next step should be to further define risk using cardiac catheterization with a goal of possible revascularization. Otherwise, if the patient is to be treated medically, the stress test was probably unnecessary as it did not change management. Potential candidates for coronary angiography are those high-risk patients with demonstrated ischemia on stress testing or those with unstable coronary syndromes (recent MI, severe angina, unstable angina) whose clinical risk is high enough to bypass stress testing and who have independent criteria for coronary angiography independent of their need for noncardiac surgery. If coronary angiography demonstrates significant anatomic lesions, a decision must be made regarding revascularization options—PCI or CABG.

RISK REDUCTION STRATEGIES

Once a patient has been identified as being at high risk, either by clinical evaluation or after stress testing or coronary angiography, the next step is to take measures to reduce that risk. The two main options include revascularization or medical therapy or both. The question is whether these therapies are effective.

CORONARY REVASCULARIZATION

Results from the Coronary Artery Surgery Study (CASS) showed that patients who underwent CABG, were symptom free, and then went on to have noncardiac surgery had a lower risk of postoperative mortality and nonfatal MI than similar study patients treated medically. This benefit was only for high-risk surgery, and the protective effect of CABG appeared to last for four to six years. However, the morbidity and mortality after CABG were not taken into account, and these patients did not have prophylactic CABG in preparation for noncardiac surgery. These results differ from those of the Coronary Artery Revascularization Prophylaxis (CARP) trial in which patients with stable cardiac symptoms scheduled to undergo elective major vascular surgery were evaluated by NIT, and those with abnormal tests went on to coronary angiography. Patients with suitable anatomy for revascularization were then randomized to medical therapy with or without revascularization (CABG or PCI). Exclusion criteria included >50% stenosis of the left main coronary artery, significant aortic stenosis, or left ventricular ejection fraction (LVEF) < 20%. Prophylactic revascularization was associated with a mortality of 1.7%, perioperative MI of 5.8%, and reoperation rate of 2.5%. In this particular study there were no perioperative strokes, but typically this occurs in up to 2%. A subgroup analysis of this study, as well as a recent meta-analysis showed that CABG appeared to be more protective than PCI, possibly because of a more complete revascularization. Because of the associated morbidity and mortality, prophylactic revascularization would only be expected to benefit patients at high risk undergoing high-risk surgery. However, DECREASE V, a small study of these very high-risk patients (three or more risk factors and extensive stress-induced ischemia on DSE undergoing major vascular surgery) in whom a previous study showed no benefit from perioperative beta-blockers, failed to demonstrate improved short- or long-term outcomes with revascularization in addition to optimal medical therapy. Criticisms of these studies raised concerns that the CARP trial patients did not have severe enough CAD, whereas the DECREASE V patients were too sick. Another recent trial found a benefit to routine versus selective cardiac catheterization for screening patients before elective aortic surgery. Intention-to-treat analysis showed decreased cardiac mortality and a similar trend in major adverse cardiac events

(MACE) in the routine cardiac catheterization group at 30 days and at follow-up four years later.

It was felt that prophylactic PCI, with its lower risk for adverse events than CABG, might be better, but there are no studies to confirm this. On the other hand, numerous studies and a meta-analysis reported an increased risk associated with noncardiac surgery soon after PCI. This is related to stent thrombosis in patients who have prematurely discontinued the recommended course of dual antiplatelet therapy and, to a lesser degree, bleeding in patients who were taking aspirin and clopidogrel. The ACC/AHA guidelines recommend delaying elective surgery for at least 2 weeks after balloon angioplasty, 4–6 weeks after placement of a bare metal stent (BMS), and 12 months after a drug-eluting stent (DES) in order to complete the course of aspirin and clopidogrel. Should surgery be required before these time intervals in a patient who had PCI, the recommended options, in priority order, are to try to perform the surgery on dual antiplatelet therapy if possible, to discontinue clopidogrel 5–7 days before surgery and continue aspirin, or to discontinue both aspirin and clopidogrel 5–7 days before surgery. The antiplatelet therapy should be resumed as soon as possible after surgery, assuming adequate hemostasis has been assured. The largest observational case series from Mayo Clinic supports these recommendations for BMS and DES.

PRACTICE POINT

The ACC/AHA guidelines recommend delaying elective surgery for patients with recent stent placement at least:

- Two weeks after balloon angioplasty
- Four to six weeks after placement of a bare metal stent (BMS)
- Twelve months after a drug-eluting stent (DES) in order to complete the course of dual antiplatelet therapy.

A more potent antiplatelet agent, prasugrel, was recently approved by the U.S. Food and Drug Administration (FDA), but there are as yet no clinical data regarding the outcomes of noncardiac surgery in patients treated with this drug. Other new antiplatelet agents are in clinical trials and are expected to be submitted for FDA approval shortly. One of these drugs, ticagrelor, is a potent yet reversible antiplatelet inhibitor, which may be promising for "bridging therapy" to minimize a patient's time off antiplatelet therapy before noncardiac surgery.

MEDICAL THERAPY

Beta-blockers

Early studies with prophylactic beta-blockers demonstrated beneficial effects. Mangano and colleagues used atenolol, started immediately preoperatively, titrated to a heart rate of 55–65 beats per minute and continued for < 7 days postoperatively, in 200 patients undergoing various operations. There was less ischemia in the atenolol-treated group but no reduction in short-term outcomes of death or nonfatal MI. However, surviving patients in the beta-blocker group went on to have fewer cardiovascular events by 2 years. Poldermans and colleagues used bisoprolol, started at least 7 days preoperatively, titrated to a heart rate between 55–65 beats per minute, and continued for at least 30 days postoperatively, in 112 patients with abnormal DSEs undergoing major vascular surgery. The trial was stopped early because the bisoprolol-treated group had a significant reduction in postoperative MI and cardiac death (3% vs 34%). Despite the small numbers of patients in these trials and methodologic criticisms, various agencies and society guidelines began recommending prophylactic beta-blockers.

Subsequent studies involving approximately 1500 patients (POBBLE, DIPOM, MaVS) using metoprolol, started at most 1 day before surgery and not titrated to a specific heart rate, showed no benefit in various cardiovascular outcomes. Lindenauer and colleagues using an administrative database of over 600,000 patients, reported that being on a beta-blocker within 2 days of surgery was associated with decreased in-hospital mortality in high- but not low-risk patients (stratified by RCRI score).

The POISE trial was expected to resolve this controversy but instead raised more questions. In this study over 8000 patients with athersclerotic heart disease (ASHD) or risk factors for it who were scheduled for various surgical procedures were randomized to metoprolol controlled release (CR) or placebo. Patients received the first dose (metoprolol CR 100 mg or placebo) 2–6 hours before surgery followed by a second dose (100 mg) within 6 hours after the end of surgery, and then a maintenance dose of 200 mg daily started 12 hours after the postoperative dose. The drug was withheld for heart rate < 45 beats per minute or systolic blood pressure (BP) < 100 mm Hg and then restarted at half the dose 12 hours later if BP and pulse improved. Primary outcome, a composite of cardiac death, nonfatal MI, and cardiac arrest, was significantly better in the metoprolol-treated group (see Figure 51-1) but was primarily due to a reduction in nonfatal MIs. However, this benefit came at the expense of a significant increase in stroke and total mortality (two of the secondary outcomes) in the treatment group, in part due to more episodes of hypotension and bradycardia. Mortality was increased in patients with sepsis, and stroke risk appeared to be increased in patients with prior strokes and intraoperative hypotension. This study generated significant commentary and criticism, mainly related to the high dose of metoprolol that was started shortly before surgery in beta-blocker-naïve patients, many of whom underwent emergency surgery or had sepsis. This tempered the enthusiasm for prophylactic beta-blockers.

The most recent beta-blocker study (DECREASE IV) using bisoprolol, started well in advance (median 34 days) of surgery and titrated to a heart rate between 50 and 70 beats per minute reduced cardiac death and nonfatal MI in intermediate risk patients. If beta-blockers are to be beneficial, it appears that they need to be started at least 7 days before surgery and titrated to a heart rate somewhere in the range of 55–70 beats per minute to minimize the risk of significant hypotension or bradycardia. Higher-risk patients or those undergoing vascular or higher-risk surgical procedures would be most likely to benefit.

Although the final answer isn't in, the ACC recently published a focused update on perioperative beta-blockers reflecting results from POISE and the new DECREASE.trials. The only remaining class I recommendation is to continue beta-blockers in patients already on them. Class IIa recommendations say that for patients undergoing vascular surgery, beta-blockers are probably recommended for patients at high cardiac risk (known CAD or ischemia on preoperative testing) and are reasonable for patients with two or more risk factors (besides surgery) undergoing vascular or intermediate. risk surgery. Class IIb recommendations state that usefulness of beta-blockers is uncertain in patients undergoing intermediate-risk or vascular surgery who have only one clinical risk factor (not CAD) and in patients undergoing vascular surgery with no clinical risk factors. Class III recommendations state that beta-blockers should not be given to patients with contraindications and also noted that high-dose beta-blockers started shortly before surgery without time for dose titration are not useful and may be harmful (Class III).

PRACTICE POINT

The 2007 ACC/AHA recommendations for administration of beta-blockers

Class I recommendations:

- Continue beta-blockers for patients already on them.

Class IIa recommendations:

- Probably recommended for patients at high cardiac risk (known CAD or ischemia on preoperative testing) undergoing vascular surgery.
- Reasonable for patients with two or more risk factors (besides surgery) undergoing vascular or intermediate risk surgery.

Class IIb recommendations:

- Usefulness uncertain for patients with only one clinical risk factor (not CAD) undergoing vascular or intermediate-risk surgery.
- Usefulness uncertain for patients undergoing vascular surgery with no clinical risk factors.

Class III recommendations:

- Do not prescribe for patients with contraindications.
- High-dose beta-blockers started shortly before surgery without time for dose titration are not useful and may be harmful.

Statins

In addition to lowering cholesterol, statins have a number of so-called pleotropic effects. These include reduced platelet aggregation, improved endothelial function, and reduced inflammation. It is thought that this latter effect in particular may help stabilize plaques and prevent plaque rupture, which might lead to an MI. Most observational studies report that perioperative statin use is beneficial in reducing postoperative cardiac complications and death in both cardiac and noncardiac surgery. A meta-analysis by Kapoor and colleagues confirmed this benefit; however, there are few randomized controlled trials. The first of these, a small study of 100 patients using atorvastatin 20 mg started 30 days before surgery, demonstrated a beneficial effect on a composite outcome including some weaker end points; however, the most recent study (DECREASE III) with almost 500 patients using fluvastatin 80 mg extended release before vascular surgery showed that the statin-treated group had less ischemia and a statistically significant reduction in the composite end point of cardiac death and nonfatal MI. This latter study also demonstrated that statins reduced LDL and total cholesterol, multiple inflammatory markers including C-reactive protein (CRP) and interleukin (IL)-6, but also were safe in that there were no cases of rhabdomyolysis or significant hepatic injury. Although no safety issues were found in a review of statin use in vascular surgery patients, the drug manufacturers still recommend discontinuing statins before surgery due to these potential safety concerns. However, the ACC recommends continuing them perioperatively as the potential benefit outweighs the theoretical risk. Based on the DECREASE III trial it appears that patients who are not on a statin but are scheduled for vascular surgery would benefit from starting a statin preoperatively. It is also likely that patients with independent indications for statins (CAD, DM, peripheral arterial disease (PAD), hyperlipidemia) undergoing high-risk surgery might benefit as well. Unanswered questions regarding perioperative statin use are whether this is a class effect, what dose should be used, how long in advance to start it prophylactically for it to be effective, and which patients are most likely to benefit from them.

OTHER CARDIOVASCULAR CONDITIONS

HYPERTENSION

Hypertension is at best a minor risk factor. Although various recommendations mention blood pressures (diastolic BP >110 mm Hg or systolic BP >180 mm Hg) when cancellation of elective surgery should be considered or which might be associated with increased risk, there is no hard evidence to support them. Hypertensive patients are more likely to have more labile blood pressure perioperatively and intraoperative hypotension. The etiology of the hypertension, and presence of end organ damage are more likely to be associated with any cardiac morbidity than the preoperative blood pressure itself. Most antihypertensive medications should be continued, including on the morning of surgery, with the possible exceptions of diuretics and angiotensin-converting enzyme (ACE) inhibitors or angiotensin receptor blockers (ARBs).

ARRHYTHMIAS

Hemodynamically significant arrhythmias are included in the active cardiac condition group in the ACC guidelines. These include tachyarrhythmias (rapid atrial fibrillation (AF), supraventricular tachycardia (SVT), ventricular tachycardia (VT)) as well as bradyarrhythmias (symptomatic sinus bradycardia, high-degree atrioventricular (AV) block) and should be evaluated and treated before elective surgery.

HEART FAILURE

Decompensated heart failure is an active cardiac condition requiring postponement of elective surgery in order to optimize medical therapy. Beta-blockers should not be started preoperatively in these patients, and in a subgroup analysis of the CIBIS II study, patients with heart failure had little benefit from beta-blockers.

VALVULAR HEART DISEASE

The lesion most likely to be associated with perioperative cardiac complications is symptomatic, severe aortic stenosis (AS). Patients with a systolic murmur suggestive of AS, particularly if they have chest pain, dyspnea, or syncope, should have a 2D echocardiogram performed. If they have symptomatic severe AS and the planned noncardiac surgery is elective, the recommendation is for valve replacement. Should the patient refuse or if the surgery is more urgent, it has been possible to get most of these patients through surgery successfully using medical therapy and intraoperative monitoring. Mitral stenosis, when associated with atrial fibrillation and heart failure, may also increase risk, but most of the other valvular lesions do not require surgical intervention before noncardiac surgery. Pulmonary hypertension is now being recognized as a risk factor as well, but studies are limited.

Endocarditis prophylaxis is only indicated for patients undergoing dental and upper respiratory procedures who have a prosthetic valve, previous endocarditis, complex congenital heart disease that has not been repaired (or was repaired in the past six months), or valvular disease in a transplanted heart.

CONCLUSION

Using the ACC guidelines, the patient can be classified as low-intermediate- or high-risk clinically. Combining this with the risk of the planned surgery, the physician can decide not only whether further testing is indicated but also whether it is likely to change management. Prophylactic revascularization is rarely necessary just to get a patient through surgery, and the majority of the patients will be managed medically. It is important for future studies to determine optimal use of beta-blockers, statins, and other therapies in order to have patients in their optimal medical condition prior to elective noncardiac surgery to reduce postoperative complications.

PART II Medical Consultation and Co-Management

Evidence

Preoperative Risk Indices and Clinical Risk Factors

Boersma E, Poldermans D, Bax JJ, et al. Predictors of cardiac events after major vascular surgery: role of clinical characteristics, dobutamine echocardiography, and beta-blocker therapy. *JAMA*. 2001;285(14):1865–1873.

Detsky AS, Abrams HB, Forbath N, Scott JG, Hilliard JR. Cardiac assessment for patients undergoing noncardiac surgery: a multifactorial clinical risk index. *Arch Intern Med*. 1986;146(11):2131–2134.

Eagle KA, Coley CM, Newell JB, et al. Combining clinical and thallium data optimizes preoperative assessment of cardiac risk before major vascular surgery. *Ann Intern Med*. 1989;110(11):859–866.

Foster ED, Davis KB, Carpenter JA, Abele S, Fray D. Risk of noncardiac operation in patients with defined coronary disease: The Coronary Artery Surgery Study (CASS) registry experience. *Ann Thorac Surg*. Jan 1986;41(1):42–50.

Goldman L, Caldera DL, Nussbaum SR, et al. Multifactorial index of cardiac risk in noncardiac surgical procedures. *N Engl J Med*. 1977;297(16):845–850.

L'Italien GJ, Paul SD, Hendel RC, et al. Development and validation of a Bayesian model for perioperative cardiac risk assessment in a cohort of 1,081 vascular surgical candidates. *J Am Coll Cardiol*. 1996;27(4):779–786.

Lee TH, Marcantonio ER, Mangione CM, et al. Derivation and prospective validation of a simple index for prediction of cardiac risk of major noncardiac surgery. *Circulation*. 1999;100(10):1043–1049.

Procedural Risk

Dripps RD, Lamont A, Eckenhoff JE. The role of anesthesia in surgical mortality. *JAMA*. 1961;178:261–266.

Eagle KA, Rihal CS, Mickel MC, Holmes DR, Foster ED, Gersh BJ. Cardiac risk of noncardiac surgery: influence of coronary disease and type of surgery in 3368 operations. CASS Investigators and University of Michigan Heart Care Program. Coronary Artery Surgery Study. *Circulation*. Sep. 16 1997;96(6):1882–1887.

Functional Capacity

Reilly DF, McNeely MJ, Doerner D, et al. Self-reported exercise tolerance and the risk of serious perioperative complications. *Arch Intern Med*. 1999;159(18):2185–2192.

Revascularization: CABG/PCI

Biccard BM, Rodseth RN. A meta-analysis of the prospective randomised trials of coronary revascularisation before noncardiac vascular surgery with attention to the type of coronary revascularisation performed. *Anaesthesia*. 2009;64(10):1105–1113.

McFalls EO, Ward HB, Moritz TE, et al. Coronary-artery revascularization before elective major vascular surgery. *N Engl J Med*. 2004;351(27):2795–2804.

Monaco M, Stassano P, Di Tommaso L, et al. Systematic strategy of prophylactic coronary angiography improves long-term outcome after major vascular surgery in medium- to high-risk patients: a prospective, randomized study. *J Am Coll Cardiol*. 2009;54(11):989–996.

Rabbitts JA, Nuttall GA, Brown MJ, et al. Cardiac risk of noncardiac surgery after percutaneous coronary intervention with drug-eluting stents. *Anesthesiology*. 2008;109(4):596–604.

Schouten O, van Kuijk JP, Flu WJ, et al. Long-term outcome of prophylactic coronary revascularization in cardiac high-risk patients undergoing major vascular surgery (from the randomized DECREASE-V Pilot Study). *Am J Cardiol*. 2009;103(7):897–901.

Ward HB, Kelly RF, Thottapurathu L, et al. Coronary artery bypass grafting is superior to percutaneous coronary intervention in prevention of perioperative myocardial infarctions during subsequent vascular surgery. *Ann Thorac Surg*. 2006;82(3):795–800; discussion 800–791.

Stent

Grines CL, Bonow RO, Casey DE, Jr, et al. Prevention of premature discontinuation of dual antiplatelet therapy in patients with coronary artery stents: a science advisory from the American Heart Association, American College of Cardiology, Society for Cardiovascular Angiography and Interventions, American College of Surgeons, and American Dental Association, with representation from the American College of Physicians. *J Am Coll Cardiol*. 2007;49(6):734–739.

Nuttall GA, Brown MJ, Stombaugh JW, et al. Time and cardiac risk of surgery after bare-metal stent percutaneous coronary intervention. *Anesthesiology*. 2008;109(4):588–595.

Risk Reduction Medical Strategies

Beta blockade

Bohm M, Maack C, Wehrlen-Grandjean M, Erdmann E. Effect of bisoprolol on perioperative complications in chronic heart failure after surgery (Cardiac Insuffi ciency Bisoprolol Study II (CIBIS II)). *Z Kardiol*. 2003;92(8):668–676.

Brady AR, Gibbs JS, Greenhalgh RM, Powell JT, Sydes MR. Perioperative beta-blockade (POBBLE) for patients undergoing infrarenal vascular surgery: results of a randomized double-blind controlled trial. *J Vasc Surg*. 2005;41(4):602–609.

Devereaux PJ, Yang H, Yusuf S, et al. Effects of extended-release metoprolol succinate in patients undergoing non-cardiac surgery (POISE trial): a randomised controlled trial. *Lancet*. 2008;371(9627):1839–1847.

Fleischmann KE, Beckman JA, Buller CE, et al. 2009 ACCF/AHA focused update on perioperative beta blockade. *J Am Coll Cardiol*. 2009;54(22):2102–2128.

Juul AB, Wetterslev J, Gluud C, et al. Effect of perioperative beta blockade in patients with diabetes undergoing major non-cardiac surgery: randomised placebo controlled, blinded multicentre trial. *BMJ*. 2006;332(7556):1482.

Lindenauer PK, Pekow P, Wang K, Mamidi DK, Gutierrez B, Benjamin EM. Perioperative beta-blocker therapy and mortality after major noncardiac surgery. *N Engl J Med*. 2005;353(4):349–361.

(*continued*)

Evidence (*continued*)

Risk Reduction Medical Strategies

Beta blockade

Mangano DT, Layug EL, Wallace A, Tateo I. Effect of atenolol on mortality and cardiovascular morbidity after noncardiac surgery. Multicenter Study of Perioperative Ischemia Research Group. *N Engl J Med*. 1996;335(23):1713–1720.

Poldermans D, Bax JJ, Schouten O, et al. Should major vascular surgery be delayed because of preoperative cardiac testing in intermediate-risk patients receiving beta-blocker therapy with tight heart rate control? *J Am Coll Cardiol*. 2006;48(5):964–969.

Poldermans D, Boersma E, Bax JJ, et al. The effect of bisoprolol on perioperative mortality and myocardial infarction in high-risk patients undergoing vascular surgery. Dutch Echocardiographic Cardiac Risk Evaluation Applying Stress Echocardiography Study Group. *N Engl J Med*. 1999;341(24):1789–1794.

Yang H, Raymer K, Butler R, Parlow J, Roberts R. The effects of perioperative beta-blockade: results of the Metoprolol after Vascular Surgery (MaVS) study, a randomized controlled trial. *Am Heart J*. 2006;152(5):983–990.

Beta blockade and Statin

Dunkelgrun M, Boersma E, Schouten O, et al. Bisoprolol and fluvastatin for the reduction of perioperative cardiac mortality and myocardial infarction in intermediate-risk patients undergoing noncardiovascular surgery: a randomized controlled trial (DECREASE-IV). *Ann Surg*. 2009;249(6):921–926.

Statin

Durazzo AE, Machado FS, Ikeoka DT, et al. Reduction in cardiovascular events after vascular surgery with atorvastatin: a randomized trial. *J Vasc Surg*. 2004;39(5):967–976; discussion 967–976.

Kapoor AS, Kanji H, Buckingham J, Devereaux PJ, McAlister FA. Strength of evidence for perioperative use of statins to reduce cardiovascular risk: systematic review of controlled studies. *BMJ*. 2006;333(7579):1149–1115.

Schouten O, Boersma E, Hoeks SE, et al. Fluvastatin and perioperative events in patients undergoing vascular surgery. *N Engl J Med*. 2009;361(10):980–989.

Schouten O, Kertai MD, Bax JJ, et al. Safety of perioperative statin use in high-risk patients undergoing major vascular surgery. *Am J Cardiol*. 2005;95(5):658–660.

Hypertension

Fleisher LA. Preoperative evaluation of the patient with hypertension. *JAMA*. 2002;287(16):2043–2046.

Valvular Heart Disease

Wilson W, Taubert KA, Gewitz M, et al. Prevention of infective endocarditis: guidelines from the American Heart Association: a guideline from the American Heart Association Rheumatic Fever, Endocarditis, and Kawasaki Disease Committee, Council on Cardiovascular Disease in the Young, and the Council on Clinical Cardiology, Council on Cardiovascular Surgery and Anesthesia, and the Quality of Care and Outcomes Research Interdisciplinary Working Group. *Circulation*. 2007;116(15):1736–1754.

SUGGESTED READING

Fleisher LA, Beckman JA, Brown KA, et al. ACC/AHA 2007 guidelines on perioperative cardiovascular evaluation and care for noncardiac surgery: a report of the American College of Cardiology/American Heart Association Task Force on Practice Guidelines (Writing Committee to Revise the 2002 Guidelines on Perioperative Cardiovascular Evaluation for Noncardiac Surgery) developed in collaboration with the American Society of Echocardiography, American Society of Nuclear Cardiology, Heart Rhythm Society, Society of Cardiovascular Anesthesiologists, Society for Cardiovascular Angiography and Interventions, Society for Vascular Medicine and Biology, and Society for Vascular Surgery. *J Am Coll Cardiol*. Oct 23 2007;50(17): e159–e241.

CHAPTER 52

Cardiac Complications After Noncardiac Surgery

Jeffrey Carter, MD
Jeffrey J. Glasheen, MD

INTRODUCTION

In the last 10 years, there has been a growing body of literature regarding the prevention of perioperative cardiac complications with important strides toward minimizing postoperative cardiac events. That said, cardiac complications do occur, and this chapter addresses their demographics, risk factors, and management. It is divided into sections of postoperative myocardial infarction, congestive heart failure, atrial fibrillation, and ventricular arrhythmias.

POSTOPERATIVE MYOCARDIAL INFARCTION

BACKGROUND

The combination of an aging, comorbid population with the rapid increase in surgical procedures has resulted in perioperative myocardial infarction (PMI) becoming a common and unfortunate reality. The incidence of PMI is dependent upon patient risk factors, the type of surgery, and the definition of MI. An early review of PMI in an unselected group of patients over the age of 40 years uncovered PMI rate of 1.4% compared to a 6.9% rate in patients selected for preoperative cardiac testing, presumably a higher-risk cohort. The largest study to date of operative cardiac outcomes, the PeriOperative Ischemic Evaluation (POISE) trial, found a 30-day MI rate of 5.7% in the control group undergoing noncardiac surgery. Meanwhile, the Coronary Artery Revascularization Prophylaxis (CARP) trial included a cohort of high-risk patients with known coronary artery disease undergoing vascular surgery and noted that 27% of patients experienced a postoperative troponin elevation. The overall risk and consequences of PMI are dependent upon patient- and procedure-related risk factors and it is thus imperative to risk assess (covered in Chapter 51), recognize, and appropriately manage PMI.

DIAGNOSIS AND PROGNOSIS

Perioperative MI was traditionally difficult to diagnose because the key biomarker, creatinine kinase-MB is routinely elevated in postoperative patients due to skeletal muscle trauma. Additionally, the key symptom of chest pain is often masked at least partially by anesthesia, analgesia, and sedation. Furthermore, electrocardiograms (ECGs) are infrequently obtained, missing subtle or transient changes. As a result, PMI was routinely overlooked or not recognized until complications occurred, often as late as postoperative day 5. This played a significant role in the traditionally high rates of morbidity and mortality of PMI. Short-term mortality with PMI is directly correlated to the level of troponin elevation and ranges from 3.5 to 25%. Moreover, even postoperative troponin leak negatively impacts long-term survival.

The advent of troponin testing, sensitive and specific for myocardial injury, greatly enhances the ability to diagnose PMI. Coupling a rise of cardiac biomarkers with signs of myocardial ischemia—such as consistent symptoms, ECG changes, or findings on coronary imaging—allows PMI to be reliably diagnosed. Most PMIs occur within 24 hours of surgery, but about 10% occur more than 1 day postoperatively. The reasons for this dichotomy can be explained by the two different mechanisms of PMI.

PRACTICE POINT

Postoperative MI usually occur within 24 hours of surgery but about 10% occur more than 1 day postoperatively.

- Short-term mortality is directly correlated to the level of troponin elevation and ranges from 3.5% to 25%. Moreover, even postoperative troponin leak negatively impacts long-term survival.
- The underlying pathology determines optimal management.
  - Type 1 postoperative MI with true ST-elevation MI is uncommon and generally treated as a traditional ACS. Risks of management (increased surgical site bleeding) and benefits (of restoring coronary blood flow) need to be carefully weighed with the surgical team prior to initiation of therapy.
  - Type 2 postoperative MI is best treated by restoring the oxygen supply-demand imbalance. Analgesics and beta-blockers are titrated to reduce the heart rate below 60 beats per minute.
- Recognition and treatment includes management of arrhythmias, volume resuscitation and transfusion.

PATHOPHYSIOLOGY

Type 1 PMI

Traditional MIs result from an acute coronary syndrome (ACS). More to the point, a vulnerable plaque experiences a spontaneous rupture. This is often associated with plaque inflammation in the face of high emotional or physiologic stress situations. These stressors are common in the perioperative setting where sympathetic tone is high due to release of catecholamines. Additionally, hemodynamic instability is common, and coronary vasoconstriction may occur. The end result is that intracoronary plaques may rupture, initiating the coagulation cascade and the resultant type 1 PMI.

Type 2 PMI

Type 2 PMI is associated with myocardial oxygen supply and demand imbalances and is more common in operative than in nonoperative settings. The main driver for type 2 PMI is tachycardia. Patients with significant coronary artery disease (typically >70% stenosis) and left ventricular hypertrophy (which increases myocardial demand) quickly overwhelm oxygenation delivery at elevated heart rates. The tachycardia is driven by myriad forces such as increased adrenergic tone, postoperative pain, systemic vasodilation, hypovolemia, and anemia. Electrocardiographically this presents as ST-depression rather than overt ST-elevation MI in the bulk of cases.

Type 2 PMI accounts for more than half of all PMIs. One study evaluating patients who died from PMI found that only 46% of patients had evidence of plaque rupture and thrombosis. The rest presumably died from complications of type 2 PMI. The pathophysiology of PMI explains why type 2 tends to occur within 3 days of surgery when the oxygen supply–demand balance is most impaired, whereas type 1 PMI from plaque rupture occurs with an even distribution over the 3 weeks following surgery.

MANAGEMENT

The management of PMI mirrors its pathophysiology. Type 1 PMI with true ST-elevation MI is uncommon and generally treated as a traditional ACS with the goal of revascularizing an acutely thrombosed artery. This management is complicated by increased risks of surgical site bleeding but generally involves anticoagulation and antiplatelet therapy along with coronary revascularization. These risks and benefits need to be carefully weighed with the surgical team prior to initiation of therapy. Beta-blockers and statin medications are also indicated.

Type 2 PMI is best treated by relieving the oxygen supply–demand imbalance. This includes reducing the adrenergic drive through pain control, beta-blockade, and maintenance of euvolemia. These former are best managed through the considered use of analgesics and beta-blockers to reduce the heart rate below 60 beats per minute, whereas the latter is accomplished by recognizing and treating the cause of hypovolemia.

Postoperative hypotension is commonly due to a combination of volume depletion and anesthetic agents and can be treated with IV fluids. However, other causes such as sepsis, arrhythmia, hemorrhage, cardiac failure, and pulmonary embolism should be considered and treated appropriately. Hypertension-induced type 2 PMI should be treated with beta-blockers and other antihypertensives as needed. Tachyarrhythmias such as atrial fibrillation with rapid ventricular response should be rate controlled or cardioverted as the situation dictates.

Postoperative anemia management to prevent and treat PMI is controversial as both postoperative anemia and liberal transfusion have been shown to "worsen outcomes." For example, a retrospective study found preoperative hematocrit levels <39% (hemoglobin ~13 g/dL) were associated with increased cardiac complications and mortality. Conversely, the medical literature generally shows no benefit and potential harm in transfusing critically ill patients with hemoglobin levels above 7 g/dL. However, a subgroup analysis of these data revealed that patients with ischemic heart disease appeared to do better with more liberal transfusion policies (ie, transfusion to >10 g/dL). Although not in the operative setting, another study found worse outcomes in patients who received a transfusion for hematocrit levels >25% (hemoglobin ~8 g/dL) in the setting of ACS. Furthermore, the protective effect of perioperative beta-blockers appears to be attenuated in the setting of surgical anemia where data support that beta-blocker use in the face of significant anemia worsens outcomes. While the data are murky, it appears a reasonable policy to transfuse patients with PMI or ACS and a hematocrit of <25% (hemoglobin 8 g/dL). Of course, patients who are hemodynamically unstable due to hemorrhage require volume resuscitation and transfusion with close monitoring in a critical care setting.

MONITORING

There is little data to guide the use of postoperative monitoring for PMI. However, PMI is a strong predictor of short- and long-term mortality, and early intervention appears to improve outcomes. Further, the typical symptoms of MI are often masked by the surgical state. Thus it is reasonable to monitor high-risk patients for PMI. The ACC/AHA 2007 perioperative cardiac guideline recommends an electrocardiogram (ECG) at baseline, immediately postoperatively, as well as daily for the first 2 postoperative days in those at high risk (see Chapter 51 for determining cardiac risk) for PMI. They further recommend limiting postoperative cardiac enzyme testing to those with symptoms or ECG findings consistent with ACS. Positive findings should result in increased vigilance and initiation of appropriate therapy and secondary prevention.

CONCLUSION

Postoperative MI is an unfortunate reality that is driven by the increasing frequency of surgical procedures in our aging, comorbid population. Despite prudent preoperative assessment, PMI still occurs and is often masked by the operative state. PMI more often occurs from oxygen supply–demand imbalances than ACS and as such is most often treated with a return to homeostasis. High-risk patients should undergo at least limited postoperative monitoring for PMI.

POSTOPERATIVE CONGESTIVE HEART FAILURE

BACKGROUND

CHF following noncardiac surgery is a common postoperative cardiac complication. The incidence depends on the patient population because it occurs after less than 5% of major surgeries but as frequently as 25% in patients with known cardiac disease. In a single-center series, the incidence of postoperative pulmonary edema was 7.6% with a mortality rate of almost 12%. By these numbers it is more common and perhaps more deadly than postoperative ischemic events. Many of the landmark perioperative cardiac outcomes trials such as POISE and the Dutch Echocardiographic Cardiac Risk Evaluation Applying Stress Echo (DECREASE) series do not include postoperative CHF in their combined cardiac end point. Nonetheless, it is an important postoperative complication that leads to increased morbidity, mortality, length of stay, and cost.

DEFINITION AND DIAGNOSIS

There is no formal definition of postoperative CHF. However, in trials that have included CHF as a major adverse cardiac event, it is defined as pulmonary edema. This is a reasonable definition because pulmonary edema, with its resulting dyspnea and hypoxemia, is the most common presenting syndrome. That said, all postoperative pulmonary edema is not CHF; there is a long list of noncardiac causes of airspace disease, including aspiration, acute respiratory distress syndrome (ARDS), and pneumonia to be considered. Once airspace disease has been identified, the evaluation should focus on volume status, including the amount of fluid infused in the perioperative period, examination of the neck veins for distension, and edema, particularly in the sacrum for patients who have been bedridden. A patient with pulmonary edema and such signs of volume overload should be considered to have postoperative CHF.

Risk factors for postoperative CHF include preexisting cardiac disease, particularly recent MI or unstable angina, diabetes, significant intraoperative hemodynamic changes (mean arterial pressure increase *or* decrease >40 mm Hg from preoperative baseline), and abdominal aortic aneurysm repair. A case series of fatal postoperative pulmonary edema in largely healthy patients found that the average positive fluid balance was 67 mL/kg/day positive, or about 7 liters. Interestingly, another prospective evaluation of the risk of development of postoperative CHF found that lower volumes of administered fluid and negative net fluid balance were associated with higher rates of postoperative CHF. These findings may be explained by the lower use of intravenous fluids in patients with a history of cardiac disease. Certainly the amount of fluids given in the perioperative period is an important historical fact, and despite these counterintuitive findings, it is reasonable to consider *more* intraoperative IV fluids to be a risk factor for postoperative pulmonary edema.

EVALUATION AND MANAGEMENT

Once it has been determined that a patient has CHF, initial evaluation should focus on early identification of myocardial ischemia. While all postoperative CHF is not ischemic in nature, postoperative MIs often have atypical presentations requiring a high degree of suspicion. Therefore, electrocardiography, cardiac monitoring, and serial cardiac enzymes are mandatory in the workup of postoperative CHF. Interestingly, patients with ischemia-induced postoperative CHF have increased risk of subsequent cardiac events, whereas those with nonischemic postoperative CHF do not. Patients with ischemia-induced postoperative CHF should be managed according to ACC/AHA guidelines. The benefits of antiplatelet medications or systemic anticoagulation must be weighed against the risks and consequences of surgical bleeding; these decisions are best made in concert with surgical colleagues.

Postoperative CHF typically occurs within the first 36 hours after surgery. Pulmonary edema occurring immediately after extubation, particularly in the post anesthesia care unit, could be a result of "negative pressure pulmonary edema." This is a poorly characterized clinical syndrome associated with postextubation laryngospasm. This leads to increased use of accessory muscles and greater negative intrathoracic pressures, which in turn causes pulmonary edema. The classic patient is a young healthy male undergoing surgery of the aerodigestive tract. Treatment is supportive, with diuretics, oxygen, continuous positive airway pressure (CPAP) and, occasionally, reintubation. Although one series revealed that nearly half of the patients with this entity required reintubation, the prognosis for a complete recovery is excellent.

> **PRACTICE POINT**
>
> Postoperative CHF typically occurs within the first 36 hours after surgery.
>
> - Once it has been determined that a patient has CHF, initial evaluation should focus on early identification of myocardial ischemia.
> - Patients with ischemia-induced postoperative CHF should be managed according to ACC/AHA guidelines, weighing the benefits of antiplatelet medications or systemic anticoagulation against the risk and consequences of surgical bleeding with surgical colleagues.

Nonischemic postoperative CHF still warrants further evaluation. ACC/AHA guidelines recommend, at a minimum, a complete history and physical as well as laboratory, ECG, chest radiography, and transthoracic echocardiography (TTE). Consideration for noninvasive or invasive coronary angiography should be reserved for patients presenting with ischemic CHF. While these guidelines are not specific to the postoperative setting, it is reasonable to apply them to this scenario.

Historical information should include preoperative symptoms of heart failure or angina, use of stimulant drugs and alcohol, as well as chemotherapeutic agents that increase the risk of development of CHF. Laboratory evaluation should include assessment of hepatic, thyroid, and renal function as well as complete blood counts, glycohemoglobin, and lipid testing. An exhaustive search for less common causes of CHF such as amyloidosis should be reserved for those in which the clinical scenario is suggestive of such an etiology.

Initial management of postoperative pulmonary edema consists of diuresis and discontinuation of IV fluids coupled with fluid and sodium restriction. Supplemental oxygen can be used as needed. If left ventricular systolic dysfunction is discovered during the workup, patients should be managed similarly to those in a nonoperative setting. This includes the addition of an ACE inhibitor and heart failure beta-blocker medications. Lipid lowering with statin medications is indicated should a patient's lipid profile warrant it. Aspirin as prevention of subsequent ischemic events is indicated, although surgical hemostasis needs to be considered in the timing of antiplatelet initiation.

In summary, CHF is a relatively common and serious postoperative cardiac complication that is best defined as cardiogenic pulmonary edema. Risk factors are preexisting cardiac disease, diabetes, and intraoperative hemodynamic changes. Large amounts of perioperative IV fluids most likely present an additional risk factor, although data are discordant on this issue, and "threshold" levels for the development of pulmonary edema are not well established. Ischemic and nonischemic CHF should be distinguished because this differentiation has the largest impact on subsequent prognosis. Ischemic CHF should be managed per current societal guidelines, weighing the benefits of anticoagulation and antiplatelet agents against the risks of surgical site bleeding. The evaluation and management of nonischemic postoperative CHF is similar to those encountered in other clinical settings and should follow current guidelines.

POSTOPERATIVE ATRIAL FIBRILLATION

INCIDENCE, RISK FACTORS, AND PREVENTION

Atrial fibrillation (AF) is the most common atrial arrhythmia following surgery. While it is a well known complication of cardiac surgery, affecting as many as 40% of coronary artery bypass procedures, it is also common following noncardiac surgery with an aggregate incidence of about 4.5%. Peak incidence of postoperative AF occurs on postoperative day 2, and it typically lasts 1 to 4 days. In 20–30% of cases it resolves without specific intervention, and less than 20% of patients will remain in AF at the time of discharge.

> **PRACTICE POINT**
>
> Peak incidence of postoperative atrial fibrillation occurs on postoperative day 2 and it typically lasts 1 to 4 days.
>
> - In 20–30% of cases it resolves without specific intervention and less than 20% of patients will remain in AF at the time of discharge.
> - For patients with a history of troublesome postoperative AF, only statin medications have been studied in a noncardiac surgical population and are therefore the recommended agent for prophylaxis.
>
> While the need for cardioversion is rare, most patients will require rate control. Initial rate control is best achieved via parenteral medications that slow conduction through the atrioventricular (AV) node. Published goals for rate control of ventricular response are a resting heart rate of 60–80 beats per minute (bpm) rising to 90–115 bpm with moderate exercise.
>
> - First-line agents include nondihydropyridine calcium channel blockers or beta-blockers.
> - For patients with a known or suspected accessory pathway, amiodarone is the first-line agent.
> - For patients with concomitant heart failure, IV digoxin or amiodarone are the preferred agents.
>
> For those patients who do not have resolution of their arrhythmia, they will need basic cardiac evaluation according to the American College of Cardiology/American Heart Association (ACC/AHA) guidelines for atrial fibrillation.
>
> - Stroke prophylaxis with anticoagulation hinges on balancing the risk of stroke and risk reduction from anticoagulation against the risk and consequences of surgical bleeding and whether the atrial fibrillation is persistent.

The risk factors for postoperative AF are similar to those following cardiac surgery. Patient-specific risk factors include advanced age, male sex, premature atrial contractions on preoperative ECG, valvular heart disease, American Society of Anesthesiologists class III or IV, CHF, hypertension, and preoperative hypokalemia. Abdominal aortic aneurysm repair, thoracic surgery, and abdominal surgery all carry increased risk of postoperative AF in comparison to orthopedic and other surgeries. In general, the "sicker" the patient or the "bigger" the surgery, the higher is the risk of postoperative AF.

Preoperative statin use prior to noncardiac thoracic surgery has been shown to reduce the risk of postoperative AF, an effect that has been attributed to the "pleiotrophic" or anti-inflammatory effect of statins. In the cardiac surgery population, concomitant use of beta-blockers, amiodarone, statins, and steroids is associated with decreased incidence of postoperative AF. Perioperative beta-blocker use is associated with an increased risk of death in low-risk patients and an increased risk of death and stroke when started immediately preoperatively in moderate- to high-risk patients and is therefore not recommended solely for prophylaxis of postoperative AF (see Chapter 51). For patients with a history of troublesome postoperative AF, only statin medications have been studied in a noncardiac surgical population and are therefore the recommended agent for prophylaxis.

EVALUATION AND MANAGEMENT

The initial step in management of atrial arrhythmias is to verify the specific diagnosis by ECG. AF is characterized by the absence of p waves and an irregularly irregular R–R interval. Initial management depends on the clinical status of the patient. Hemodynamically unstable patients, characterized by hypotension or signs of poor perfusion such as loss of consciousness, need immediate direct current electrical cardioversion. This is an uncommon clinical scenario, and this management should be reserved for life-threatening hemodynamic collapse.

While the need for cardioversion is rare, most patients will require rate control. Initial rate control is best achieved via parenteral medications that slow conduction through the atrioventricular (AV) node. First-line agents include nondihydropyridine calcium channel blockers or beta-blockers. For patients with a known or suspected accessory pathway, AV blocking agents can lead to faster ventricular response and are thus contraindicated. In these cases amiodarone is the first-line agent. For patients with concomitant heart failure, IV digoxin or amiodarone is the preferred agent. While postoperative AF may convert spontaneously or following initial rate control, patients with AF that persists beyond a few minutes will likely need long-acting oral medications. It is reasonable to use the oral equivalent of the agent that was successful with the initial rate control. Published goals for rate control of ventricular response are a resting heart rate of 60–80 beats per minute (bpm) rising to 90–115 bpm with moderate exercise. It is important to remember that AF is often a manifestation of an underlying perturbation such as infection or venous thromboembolism (VTE), and these diagnoses should be considered before escalating AV nodal blockade.

Anticoagulation is challenging in postsurgical patients with new AF where the risk of stroke and risk reduction from anticoagulation must be balanced against the risk and consequences of surgical bleeding. There are two decision points for the commencement of anticoagulation for postoperative AF. Some patients have a high enough stroke risk that it is appropriate to anticoagulate them upon diagnosis of AF. A helpful tool for risk stratification of stroke in AF is the 6-point CHADS2 score, which uses established stroke risk factors of *C*HF, *h*ypertension, *a*ge > 75, *d*iabetes and *s*troke (2 points). Current guidelines recommend perioperative bridging therapy for high-risk patients (CHADS2 score of 5 or 6), and it is therefore reasonable to consider acute anticoagulation of these patients suffering new postoperative AF. Of course, the risks and consequences of surgical bleeding must be weighed against the risk of stroke in the acute setting. For example, it may be reasonable to acutely anticoagulate a patient with new AF at high risk for stroke after a total hip replacement but not after intracranial surgery.

The second decision point occurs in patients with persistent postoperative AF, which often warrants long-term stroke prophylaxis. Formal definitions of "persistent" postoperative AF are lacking. Certainly AF present at discharge should be considered persistent.

Many patients, though, will fall into a gray area between the need for acute anticoagulation and those with AF at discharge. Examples include patients with extended (ie, longer than 24 hours) postoperative AF that resolves prior to discharge, or those whose subsequent evaluation reveals a high risk of intermittent AF. For these patients, reasonable strategies include ambulatory monitoring to detect continued AF, with or without a period of warfarin therapy, depending on risk. In general, a CHADS2 score of 2 or higher is an indication for chronic warfarin therapy. Patients with a CHADS2 score of less than 2 should have aspirin for stroke prophylaxis.

More than 80% of new postoperative AF will resolve by discharge. Patients who do not have resolution of their arrhythmia will need basic cardiac evaluation. The American College of Cardiology/American Heart Association (ACC/AHA) guidelines for AF list the minimum initial evaluation to include history and physical, ECG, Transthoracic Echocardiogram (TTE), and laboratory tests of thyroid, renal, and hepatic function. The goal of this evaluation is to best delineate whether this is paroxysmal AF that has been present in the past or is likely to recur in the future. The TTE is helpful for determining left ventricular function, atrial size, and valvular function—factors that will help guide decisions regarding stroke prophylaxis.

If a patient's symptoms resolve with rate control, the employed strategy should be continued. In this approach, no attempt is made at restoration of sinus rhythm, and the patient's ventricular rate is controlled with AV nodal blockade alone. Rhythm control strategy is aimed at restoration of sinus rhythm and can be accomplished via chemical or electrical cardioversion and subsequent antiarrhythmic medications. The rhythm control strategy mandates anticoagulation such that patients whose surgery precludes therapeutic anticoagulation are not candidates for cardioversion. Despite the theoretical benefit of rhythm control, it is not associated with lower rates of stroke and death, and there are inconsistent reports of improved quality of life.

ASSOCIATED CONDITIONS

Postoperative AF may occur in isolation or be associated with underlying systemic conditions. More than half of patients with AF after noncardiac surgery have a major underlying condition, with infection having the strongest association. For example, patients with postoperative AF have a relative risk of 7.4 for bacterial pneumonia and 6.2 for sepsis compared to those without arrhythmia. For patients in the surgical intensive care unit (ICU), the leading cause of death in patients with new-onset AF is sepsis. In general, the incidence of sepsis in patients with new postoperative arrhythmias is 20–30%, although this figure is primarily from surgical ICU data.

Primary cardiac events are less commonly antecedent to new AF. The relative risk of MI in patients with a new arrhythmia is 4.2. In colorectal surgery patients, both pulmonary edema and overall complications are more common in patients with new arrhythmias. Other postoperative complications associated with new-onset AF include pulmonary embolism, gastrointestinal bleed, cerebrovascular accident, hypokalemia, and anastomotic leakage.

Given the frequency of serious underlying etiologies, new AF following noncardiac surgery should be regarded as a possible harbinger of life-threatening postoperative complications. Thus appropriate evaluation of new postoperative arrhythmia warrants a complete evaluation of the patient with consideration of infectious, cardiac, and thrombotic complications.

SUMMARY

AF is the most common arrhythmia following noncardiac surgery, with patient-specific risk factors similar to those for AF in the general population. It typically occurs early in the postoperative course. Preoperative statin therapy is associated with a lower risk of developing AF in some surgical populations, but there are insufficient data to recommend this practice routinely, particularly in lower-risk patients. Beta-blockers are not recommended solely for prophylaxis of postoperative AF. Initial management of postoperative AF commences with verification of the diagnosis with an ECG. Hemodynamically unstable patients need emergent cardioversion. Patients with rapid ventricular responses require IV administration of nodal blocking agents followed by an oral equivalent. The decision to anticoagulate must balance stroke risk in the acute setting with the risk of operative bleeding. Telemetry surveillance for AF is indicated in patients requiring an ICU stay but is not otherwise routinely recommended. Patients with persistent AF will need adequate rate control and, should they remain symptomatic, consideration of cardioversion and subsequent rhythm control. A CHADS2 score of 2 or greater is an indication for chronic anticoagulation in most patients with persistent AF at the time of discharge.

POSTOPERATIVE VENTRICULAR ARRHYTHMIAS

Ventricular arrhythmias are uncommon following noncardiac surgery. Because of this, data are sparse regarding risk factors and outcomes. In the thoracic surgery population, one study found the incidence of nonsustained ventricular tachycardia (NSVT) to be 15%, but there were no episodes of sustained ventricular arrhythmias, nor did any of these episodes lead to hemodynamic instability. Importantly, nonischemic ventricular tachycardia (VT) following noncardiac surgery is not associated with worse long-term outcomes.

The most common scenario described in the literature for serious ventricular arrhythmias is following postoperative MI in patients with underlying heart disease. Fatal ventricular arrhythmias are included in the outcomes of major trials such as CARP and DECREASE-V, but the contribution of ventricular arrhythmias to the endpoint is not reported.

When confronted with a ventricular arrhythmia, the first decision point is to ascertain the patient's hemodynamic status. Unstable patients, defined as having hypotension or loss of consciousness, need emergent treatment as described in Advanced Cardiac Life Support (ACLS) protocols. Hemodynamically stable patients with ventricular arrhythmias need urgent evaluation for acute ischemia including 12-lead ECG and serial cardiac enzymes. Should this workup reveal myocardial ischemia, treatment according to published guidelines should be commenced. Significant electrolyte abnormalities, notably hypokalemia and hypomagnesemia, are reversible causes of ventricular arrhythmias and thus warrant prompt evaluation and repletion. In the setting of torsades de pointes, or polymorphic ventricular tachycardia with prolonged QT interval, empiric magnesium should be given. As QT prolongation is often a result of medication use, the patient's medication list should be reviewed and potentially offending medications discontinued. Hemodynamically stable but sustained VT requires antiarrhythmic drugs. A review of antiarrhythmic medications is beyond the scope of this chapter.

In summary, postoperative ventricular arrhythmias are an uncommon cardiac complication, but with potentially serious consequences. Hemodynamically unstable patients will need emergent defibrillation. Patients with ventricular arrhythmias need urgent evaluation for cardiac ischemia. Fortunately, nonischemic VT does not appear to negatively impact long-term prognosis.

SUGGESTED READINGS

Amar D, Zhang H, Heerdt PM, et al. Statin use is associated with a reduction in atrial fibrillation after non-cardiac thoracic surgery independent of C-reactive protein. *Chest.* 2005;128:3421–3427.

Amar D. Prevention and management of perioperative arrhythmias in the thoracic surgical population. *Anesthesiology Clinics.* 2008;26:325–335.

Arieff AI. Fatal postoperative pulmonary edema. *Chest*. 1999;115(5): 1371–1378.

Charlson ME. Risk for postoperative congestive heart failure. *Surg Gynecol Obstet*. 1991;171:95–105.

Dennis T. Mangano DT, Browner WS, Hollenberg M, et al. Long term cardiac prognosis following non-cardiac surgery. *JAMA*. 1992;268:233–239.

Devereaux PJ, Yang H, Yusuf S, et al. Effects of extended-release metoprolol succinate in patients undergoing non-cardiac surgery (POISE trial): a randomized controlled trial. *Lancet*. 2008;371: 1839–1847.

Fleisher LA, Beckman JA, Brown KA, et al. ACC/AHA 2007 guidelines on perioperative cardiovascular evaluation and care for non-cardiac surgery: a report of the American College of Cardiology/American Heart Association task force on practice guidelines. *Circulation*. 2007;116:e418–e500.

Fuster V, Rydén LE, Cannom DS, et al. ACC/AHA/ESC 2006 guidelines for the management of patients with atrial fibrillation. *Circulation*. 2006;114:700–752.

Go AS, Hylek EM, Chang Y, et al. Anticoagulation therapy for stroke prevention in atrial fibrillation. *JAMA*. 2003;290:2685–2692.

Landesberg G, Beattie WS, Mosseri M, Jaffe AS, Alpert JS. Perioperative myocardial infarction. *Circulation*. 2009:119:2936–2944.

CHAPTER 53

Preoperative Evaluation of Liver Disease

Amir A. Qamar, MD
Norman D. Grace, MD

INTRODUCTON

Evaluation of patients with liver disease prior to surgery is crucial to estimating perioperative morbidity and mortality and to improving outcomes. The operative risk of liver disease can be related to the rapid changes in liver function that can occur in acute hepatitis or can be related to chronic complications of portal hypertension and parenchymal liver disease in patients with cirrhosis. Therefore, establishment of a risk profile should be based on the etiology of the underlying liver disease and the degree of hepatic decompensation associated with the presence of cirrhosis and portal hypertension. This chapter explains how to assess and prepare patients with liver disease for surgery and provides a framework for predicting operative morbidity and mortality.

FACTORS ASSOCIATED WITH PERIOPERATIVE LIVER DISEASE

CHANGES IN HEPATIC BLOOD FLOW

The liver receives a dual blood supply from the portal vein and the hepatic artery. Unlike most other organs, the majority of hepatic oxygen supply in normal individuals is venous via the portal vein. Administration of anesthesia and surgery influences portal and hepatic blood flow. However, when flow through the portal vein is reduced, the hepatic artery vasodilates to increase oxygen supply to the liver. This compensatory vasodilatation appears to be reduced in response to a decrease in portal vein flow caused by changes in hepatic architecture as a result of fibrosis and nodular formation associated with cirrhosis. Due to intraoperative decreases in blood pressure and cardiac output, blood flow in patients with cirrhosis is further decreased in the portal vein and splanchnic vessels. Anesthetics in high doses reduce the hepatic artery's ability to vasodilate in response to these changes in portal blood flow.

These changes in hepatic blood flow may lead to hepatic ischemia and necrosis induced by hypotension when patients with cirrhosis undergo surgery or receive anesthetic agents. This phenomenon leads to the release of inflammatory mediators resulting in multiorgan system failure. In a study of 733 cirrhosis patients undergoing surgery, Ziser and colleagues found an 11.6% mortality rate. Intraoperative hypotension was among factors found to predict perioperative complications and decreased survival.

TYPE OF SURGERY

Postoperative morbidity and mortality in patients with cirrhosis are also influenced by the type of surgery.

> **PRACTICE POINT**
>
> Postoperative morbidity and mortality in patients with liver disease are related to the etiology and severity of liver disease.
>
> - Generally, patients with mild liver enzyme abnormalities without cirrhosis and most compensated Child-Pugh Class A patients can safely undergo surgery.
> - For all other patients, a careful assessment of the benefits of surgical intervention must be weighed against the risk of hepatic decompensation and mortality. These risks should be enumerated as part of the informed consent process.

> **PRACTICE POINT**
>
> Postoperative morbidity and mortality in patients with cirrhosis are related to:
> - Intraoperative hypotension
> - The type of surgery
> - The type of anesthesia
> - Severity of the liver disease

Abdominal surgery

During abdominal surgery, direct trauma due to surgical retraction can lead to hepatic injury. Manipulation of the splanchnic and portal vasculature may also reduce portal or hepatic flow leading to ischemic injury. In particular, patients with Child-Pugh class C cirrhosis who undergo abdominal surgery have been reported to have 75% perioperative mortality.

Cardiovascular surgery

Cardiovascular surgery, due to effects on portal and hepatic artery blood flow, is also associated with increased perioperative morbidity and mortality. The required perioperative pressor support and prolonged cardiopulmonary bypass are important contributors to hepatic injury.

Emergency surgery

Many patients who require emergency surgery may be hemodynamically unstable from systemic vasodilation (eg, sepsis) or hypotensive due to hemorrhage (eg, trauma, abdominal surgery), and their outcome is often poor. In a study by Demetriades and colleagues of 46 patients with cirrhosis who underwent emergency laparotomy, the postoperative mortality rate was 45%, which was significantly greater than that for noncirrhotic control patients.

Orthopedic surgery

There is little information in the literature regarding specific operative risks for patients with cirrhosis who may require surgery for orthopedic problems. Hsieh and colleagues reviewed 38 patients over a 20-year period who underwent hip arthroplasty. The 30-day complication rate was 26.7%. Advanced cirrhosis, age, elevated serum creatinine, low serum albumin, platelet count, ascites, hepatic encephalopathy, and increased operative blood loss were contributory factors to the high complication rate.

TYPE OF ANESTHETIC

Anesthetic agents may reduce hepatic blood flow by reducing cardiac output. Even spinal and epidural anesthesia may affect hepatic blood flow by reducing the mean arterial pressure. In patients with liver disease, effects on hepatic metabolism may lead to prolonged action of anesthetic agents or production of toxic radicals resulting in increased morbidity and mortality.

CAUSE AND SEVERITY OF LIVER DISEASE

Perioperative morbidity and mortality are influenced by the etiology and severity of the patient's liver disease. The presence of cirrhosis or acute hepatitis at the time of surgery adversely influences the outcome after surgery. Generally, patients with chronic hepatitis from any etiology without features of hepatic decompensation do very well with surgery, and specific precautions are not necessary. However, in patients with acute liver disease and compensated or decompensated cirrhosis, it is critical to assess the perioperative risk as part of informed consent. Acute hepatitis, especially alcoholic hepatitis, and decompensated cirrhosis are absolute contraindications to elective surgery. A number of scoring and staging systems have been suggested as useful in assessing the perioperative risk. However, the Child-Pugh score and the Model for End-Stage Liver Disease (MELD) score are most commonly used in clinical practice. Measurement of the hepatic venous pressure gradient (HVPG) has excellent prognostic value, but its use is confined to a limited number of academic medical centers. A recent study showed that patients with compensated cirrhosis with clinically significant portal hypertension, defined by an HVPG ≥ 10 mm Hg, were at significant risk of developing clinical decompensation defined as the occurrence of ascites, variceal bleeding, or hepatic encephalopathy.

> **PRACTICE POINT**
>
> - Acute hepatitis, especially alcoholic hepatitis, or decompensated cirrhosis are absolute contraindications to elective surgery. Patients with alcoholic liver disease should be abstinent for at least three months prior to surgery. They should be assessed for signs of alcohol dependence prior to surgery.

CHILD-PUGH SCORE

The Child-Pugh score combines the subjective and objective assessment of liver function (**Table 53-1**). In a recent study of 33 patients with cirrhosis compared with 31 age- and sex-matched control patients, the Child-Pugh score accurately predicted morbidity after cholecystectomy. In another study of 44 patients with cirrhosis who underwent cardiac surgery, a preoperative Child-Pugh score ≥ 8 was predictive of postoperative mortality. Ziser and colleagues using a large database, found that a high Child-Pugh score was associated with increased perioperative morbidity

TABLE 53-1 Child-Pugh Scoring System

	1	2	3
Bilirubin	< 2.0 mg/dL	2.0–3.0 mg/dL	> 3.0 mg/dL
Albumin	> 3.5 g/dL	3.5–2.8 g/dL	< 2.8 g/dL
Prothrombin time	< 4 seconds greater than control	4–6 seconds greater than control	> 6 seconds greater than control
Ascites	Absent	Mild–moderate	Moderate–severe
Encephalopathy	Absent	Mild (grade I–II)	Severe (grade III–IV)

Score 5–6: Child class A
7–9: Child class B
> 10: Child class C.

TABLE 53-2 Operative Mortality Rates in Patients Undergoing Abdominal Surgery Based on Child-Pugh Class

Child-Pugh Class	Risk of Operative Mortality
A	10%
B	30%
C	80%

Data from Garrison RN, Cryer HM, Howard DA, et al. Clarification of risk factors for abdominal operations in patients with hepatic cirrhosis. *Ann Surg.* 1984;199(6):648–655.
Data from Mansour A, Watson W, Shayani V, et al. Abdominal operations in patients with cirrhosis: still a major surgical challenge. *Surgery.* 1997;122(4):730–735.

and mortality. **Table 53-2** summarizes the operative mortality risk of patients with different Child-Pugh classes of cirrhosis who undergo abdominal surgery based on two important studies by Garrison and colleagues and Mansour and colleagues.

MELD SCORE

The Model for End-Stage Liver Disease (MELD) score is able to accurately assess short-term mortality in patients with cirrhosis. The scoring system uses the serum bilirubin, creatinine, and prothrombin time (international normalized ratio) to assess hepatic function. Recent data also suggest that the presence of hyponatremia is associated with an even further risk of mortality.

Teh and colleagues assessed 772 patients with cirrhosis who underwent major digestive, cardiac, or orthopedic surgery. They found that the 30-day mortality ranged from 5.7% for a MELD score <8 to 50% for a MELD score >20. **Table 53-3** summarizes the mortality risk for surgery in patients with different MELD scores preoperatively. Similar findings were reported by Perkins and colleagues where a preoperative MELD score ≥ 8 suggested a high risk of perioperative morbidity and mortality. However, Surman and colleagues were unable to find a MELD cutoff that would predict increased risk after cardiac surgery.

PATIENT ASSESSMENT

HISTORY AND PHYSICAL EXAMINATION

Hospitalists should perform an assessment of symptoms suggestive of hepatitis, including nausea, vomiting, jaundice, pruritis, night sweats, fevers, or weight loss. In patients with cirrhosis, recent gastrointestinal bleeding, an increase in abdominal girth, weight gain, changes in the sleep-wake cycle, or memory changes suggest a poorer prognosis. Any use of alcohol or illicit substances needs to be assessed.

TABLE 53-3 Preoperative MELD Scores and Seven-Day and Thirty-Day Mortality Rates

MELD Score	7 Days	30 Days
0–7 (*n* = 351)	1.9 (314)	5.7 (301)
8–11 (*n* = 257)	3.3 (236)	10.3 (219)
12–15 (*n* = 106)	7.7 (94)	25.4 (78)
16–20 (*n* = 35)	14.6 (29)	44.0 (19)
21–25 (*n* = 13)	23.0 (7)	53.8 (4)
≥26 (*n* = 10)	30.0 (6)	90.0 (1)

Reproduced, with permission, from Teh SH, Nagorney DM, Stevens SR, et al. Risk factors for mortality after surgery in patients with cirrhosis. *Gastroenterol.* 2007;132(4):1261–1269.

TABLE 53-4 Laboratory and Radiologic Testing

- Liver function tests and albumin
- Complete blood counts
- Prothrombin time and international normalized ratio
- Chemistry profile
- Abdominal ultrasound and Doppler study of hepatic vasculature
- Computed tomographic scan or magnetic resonance imaging
- Hepatic venography for hepatic venous pressure gradient

STUDIES

Table 53-4 lists laboratory and radiology studies that should be considered in the preoperative assessment of patients with liver disease to ascertain their perioperative risk.

PREOPERATIVE MANAGEMENT

The preoperative management of patients with cirrhosis involves aggressive treatment of portal hypertension and hepatic insufficiency to reduce operative morbidity and mortality. Depending on specific etiology of the liver disease, certain preoperative changes in management may be considered. Important general and etiology-specific management points are reviewed following here.

GENERAL MANAGEMENT

Coagulopathy

Hepatic insufficiency leads to inadequate production of factors II, V, VII, and IX, resulting in development of coagulopathy with an increased risk of perioperative bleeding. Thrombocytopenia in liver disease is multifactorial. Portal hypertension–induced sequestration of platelets further increases the risk of bleeding. Administration of platelets, fresh frozen precipitate, and cryoprecipitate should be administered prior to surgery to reduce the risk of bleeding during and after surgery. Recent data suggest recombinant factor VIIa may be used in situations of emergent uncontrollable bleeding in cirrhotic patients. However, this agent should be used with caution. In 2005, the U.S. Food and Drug Administration (FDA) issued a warning to health care practitioners that recombinant factor VIIa was associated with an increased risk of arteriothromboembolic events, including myocardial ischemia, myocardial infarction, cerebral ischemia, and cerebral infarction.

Varices

The risk of bleeding in patients with cirrhosis who have esophageal varices is approximately 8% per year. Once variceal bleeding occurs there is a 20% mortality associated with the bleeding event. Preventive therapies include the use of nonselective beta-blockers and endoscopic variceal ligation. There are no specific treatments to reduce the risk of perioperative variceal bleeding. A target hematocrit of 25 is recommended to prevent overtransfusion. In patients who do experience postoperative gastrointestinal bleeding, the use of antibiotics is recommended to reduce the risk of mortality from spontaneous bacterial peritonitis (SBP), in turn related to bacterial translocation, infection, and sepsis.

TABLE 53-5 Risk Factors for Morbidity and Mortality in Patients with Biliary Obstruction

- Hematocrit < 30
- Bilirubin > 11 mg/dL
- Blood urea nitrogen > 90
- Creatinine > 1.4 mg/dL
- Albumin < 3.0 g/dL
- Age > 65 years
- Aspartate aminotransferase (AST) > 90
- Malignancy

Ascites and spontaneous bacterial peritonitis

Ascites is the most frequent and generally the first event to occur in patients with cirrhosis and hepatic decompensation. Treatment includes salt restriction, the use of diuretics (including furosemide and spironolactone), and paracentesis. Transjugular intrahepatic portosystemic shunting (TIPS) in the management of ascites prior to surgery is not recommended except for patients who may be undergoing liver transplantation. For patients with hypoalbuminemia, ascites, or edema, perioperative fluid management should include the use of colloids such as albumin. In patients without the development of third-space accumulation of fluid, crystalloids (ie, saline) are appropriate.

Biliary obstruction

Biliary obstruction preoperatively is associated with increased morbidity and mortality and should be treated with decompression prior to surgery. Specific factors that increase operative risk are noted in **Table 53-5**.

Hepatic encephalopathy

Hepatic encephalopathy is provoked by a number of factors listed in **Table 53-6**. Care should be taken to reduce the risk of hepatic encephalopathy after surgery by avoiding specific precipitants (Table 53-6).

ETIOLOGY-SPECIFIC MANAGEMENT

Alcoholic liver disease

Patients with alcoholic liver disease should be abstinent for at least three months prior to surgery. They should be assessed for signs of alcohol dependence prior to surgery. If there is evidence of alcoholic hepatitis, surgery should be delayed until the hepatitis improves. Treatment with prednisone or pentoxyfylline should be considered in patients with evidence of significant hepatic dysfunction as assessed by a well-defined scoring system.

TABLE 53-6 Precipitants of Hepatic Encephalopathy

- Gastrointestinal bleeding
- Hypovolemia
- Renal failure
- Use of sedating agents
- Hypokalemia
- Alkalosis
- Trauma
- Infection
- Constipation
- Colon surgery

Hepatitis B and hepatitis C

Patients on treatment with nucleoside and nucleotide analogues for hepatitis B should continue treatment in the perioperative setting. Patients receiving interferon for either hepatitis B or C should hold or discontinue treatment due to its adverse effect on the immune system and platelet production.

Autoimmune hepatitis

Many patients with autoimmune hepatitis receive treatment with either prednisone or the purine analogue azathioprine. Treatment should be continued in the perioperative setting. Patients who are on or have recently been tapered off of steroids should be treated with stress dose steroids.

Alpha-1 antitrypsin deficiency and hemochromatosis

There are no specific treatments for alpha-1 antitrypsin deficiency. However, patients with this condition may have underlying lung disease and should be assessed for this prior to surgery.

Similarly, patients with hemochromatosis are at increased risk of a cardiomyopathy and should be assessed for cardiac dysfunction prior to surgery.

Wilson disease

Patients with Wilson disease are on long-term treatment including penicillamine, trientene, or zinc. Patients receiving penicillamine should continue treatment but the dose should be reduced.

RISK TO SURGEON

HEPATITIS B

Due to the increasing prevalence of viral hepatitis B and C, there is a risk to the surgeon in the event of inadvertent skin puncture injury or exposure to body fluids. Before the era of vaccination, 30% of surgeons reported an episode of acute hepatitis and 5% developed chronic hepatitis. All health care providers are now required to be immunized for hepatitis B. A small proportion of people do not respond to the vaccine and require a second round. In surgeons who mount a hepatitis B surface antibody response, no intervention is needed if a body fluid exposure or injury occurs. In individuals exposed to hepatitis B who lack immunity to the virus as determined by a negative HBsAb, hepatitis B virus (HBV) immunoglobulin and HBV vaccination should be done immediately. Health care providers should have their hepatitis B antibody status checked every 10 years to confirm continued immunity and should be retreated if immunity is lacking.

HEPATITIS C

No vaccine for hepatitis C is available. The presence of a hepatitis C antibody is not associated with immunity. Universal health precautions should be practiced by all health care providers to reduce transmission. Hepatitis C antibody status and viral RNA should be checked at the time of exposure to assess baseline status and then repeated in three to six months to rule out chronic infection. Antiviral therapy for individuals developing acute hepatitis C is associated with an excellent response.

CONCLUSION

It is important to stratify the operative risk of patients with liver disease based on the acuity, etiology, and severity of disease and the urgency and type of surgery to be undertaken. Generally, patients with mild liver enzyme abnormalities without cirrhosis and most compensated Child-Pugh class A patients can safely undergo surgery. For all other patients, a careful assessment of the benefits of surgical intervention must be weighed against the risk of hepatic decompensation and mortality. These risks should be enumerated as part of the informed consent process.

SUGGESTED READINGS

Centers for Disease Control and Prevention. Updated U.S. public health service guidelines for the management of occupational exposure to HBV, HCV, and HIV and recommendations for postexposure prophylaxis. *MMWR Morb Mortal Wkly Rep.* 2001;50:1–42.

Demetriades D, Constantinou C, Salim A, et al. Liver cirrhosis in patients undergoing laparotomy for trauma: effect on outcomes. *J Am Coll Surg.* 2004;199(4):538–542.

Garcia-Tsao G, Sanyal AJ, Grace ND, et al. Prevention and management of gastroesophageal varices and variceal hemorrhage in cirrhosis. *Hepatology.* 2007;46(3):922–938.

Garrison RN, Cryer HM, Howard DA, et al. Clarification of risk factors for abdominal operations in patients with hepatic cirrhosis. *Ann Surg.* 1984;199:648–655.

Hayashida N, Shoujima T, Teshima H, et al. Clinical outcome after cardiac operations in patients with cirrhosis. *Ann Thorac Surg.* 2004;77:500–505.

Hsieh PH, Chen LH, Lee MS, et al. Hip arthroplasty in patients with cirrhosis of the liver. *J Bone Joint Surg.* 2003;85-B:818–821.

Perkins L, Jeffries M, Patel T. Utility of preoperative scores for predicting morbidity after cholecystectomy in patients with cirrhosis. *Clin Gastroenterol Hepatol.* 2004;2(12):1123–1128.

Surman A, Barnes DS, Zein NN, et al. Predicting out after cardiac surgery in patients with cirrhosis: a comparison of Child-Pugh and MELD score. *Clin Gastroenterol Hepatol.* 2004;2(8):719–723.

Teh SH, Nagorney DM, Stevens SR, et al. Risk factors for mortality after surgery in patients with cirrhosis. *Gastroenterol.* 2007;132(4):1261–1269.

Ziser A, Plevak D, Wiesner RH, et al. Morbidity and mortality in cirrhotic patients undergoing anesthesia and surgery. *Anesthesiology.* 1999;90(1):42–53.

CHAPTER 54

Nutrition and Metabolic Support

Nicole M. Bedi, RD, LDN, CNSC
Malcolm K. Robinson, MD, FACS

INTRODUCTION

The importance of providing adequate nutrition as an adjunct to medical care was identified as early as the era of Hippocrates. Today, it is known that malnutrition is associated with increased infection rates, longer hospital length of stay, and increased hospital costs. Not surprisingly, malnutrition is also associated with increased mortality. For example, Correia and Waitzberg demonstrated that malnutrition is an independent predictor of mortality, morbidity and hospital expense after controlling for patient age and disease severity. Hence, it is imperative that the nutritional statuses of all patients be assessed throughout their hospitalizations in order to develop appropriate nutritional plans. This could potentially improve outcomes.

Unfortunately, the prevalence of malnutrition in the hospitalized patient was largely ignored until 1974 when Butterworth published his landmark paper entitled "The Skeleton in the Hospital Closet." Shockingly 30 to 50% of inpatients are malnourished upon admission, and they tend not to improve nutritionally, and frequently worsen, while hospitalized.

This chapter is designed to assist the hospital physician in identifying those patients at increased risk of malnutrition, as well as determining the most appropriate nutritional prescription.

NUTRITION EVALUATION AND SCREENING

Every patient should have a nutrition assessment when admitted to the hospital. This is usually done by a dietitian or a nurse making use of a nutrition screening questionnaire. The assessment process includes a combination of anthropometric measurements, history and physical examination, and laboratory analyses. Utilization of any one parameter is unlikely to yield a reliably accurate determination of nutritional status all of the time. However, when all of these parameters are considered in conjunction, one can generally get a good idea of a patient's nutritional status.

PRACTICE POINT

Every patient should have a nutrition assessment when admitted to the hospital.

- IBW for a woman may be estimated as 100 pounds for the first 5 feet plus an additional 5 pounds for every inch over 5 feet. The IBW for a man is 106 pounds for the 5 five feet plus an additional 6 pounds for every inch over 5 feet.
- Underweight is a BMI less than 18 kg/m^2, and overweight is a BMI greater than 25 kg/m^2.

Pitfalls to relying on body weight as an indicator of nutritional status include

- fluid overload states, which falsely elevate weight in a malnourished patient;
- obesity, which may mask significant weight loss.

ANTHROPOMETRIC MEASUREMENTS AND PHYSICAL ASSESSMENT

Classically, nutritional status is assessed with anthropometric measurements. These are a set of noninvasive, quantitative techniques for determining an individual's body fat composition by measuring specific dimensions of the body. This includes such parameters as height and weight, triceps skin-fold thickness, mid–upper arm circumference, and bodily circumference at the waist, hip, and chest. If such measurements fall below standard norms then one is considered malnourished. For example, health care professionals can compare a patient's weight to the "ideal" body weight (IBW) found in tables from various sources, such as the 1952 Metropolitan Life tables of IBW. Alternatively, one can use the Hamwi "rule of thumb," which was developed from the Metropolitan table. This rule states that the IBW for a woman is 100 pounds for the first 5 feet plus an additional 5 pounds for every inch over 5 feet. The IBW for a man is 106 pounds for the first 5 feet plus an additional 6 pounds for every inch over 5 feet.

Body mass index (BMI, weight in kilograms divided by height in meters squared) can also be used as a metric of IBW. A BMI less than 18 kg/m^2 is considered underweight, and overweight is a BMI greater than 25 kg/m^2. BMI is beginning to replace the other traditional indices of determining IBW because it is independent of gender and body frame size.

Patients who are deemed underweight by any of the foregoing assessments are at risk for developing nutritionally related complications, especially in the presence of acute illness or weight loss. However, one cannot assume that those patients who have a normal weight or who are overweight are well nourished. Acutely ill patients, who have received aggressive resuscitation, can accumulate several kilograms of fluid, which masks their true dry weight and therefore nutritional status. Thus the underweight weight patient may have a "normal" weight under such conditions. Similarly, patients with liver dysfunction and ascites, or renal dysfunction may have their true dry weight masked by excessive fluid retention. Therefore, the physical exam should include assessment for edema and ascites, and comparisons of weight over time should be based on best estimates of dry weight. Finally, even patients whose dry weight is in the obese range can be malnourished. Overweight and obese individuals may have unintentionally lost significant weight over a short period of time due to illness, during which time protein degradation and loss of lean body mass have occurred.

To avoid these pitfalls of determining nutritional status based on admission weight alone, the practitioner should first determine the presence or absence of unintentional weight loss in all patients. Unintentional weight loss has consistently been shown to be a reliable measure of malnutrition, especially in older adults. A loss of greater than 5% of one's usual body weight (UBW) in 1 month or 10% of UBW over 3 months is considered clinically significant even if one is initially obese. The practitioner should be wary of self-reported height and weight as they are notoriously inaccurate. Hence it is crucial to actually measure height and weight in all patients on admission if possible. Additional physical assessment should include evaluation of skin, hair, mouth, and nails for signs of nutrient deficiencies. Temporal or interosseous muscle wasting and clavicular prominence are classic signs of loss of lean body mass. Dry skin or rash, dry hair or hair loss, poor skin turgor, night blindness, glossitis, and muscle weakness may also point to micro or macronutrient deficiencies. The physician should also determine whether there has been a change in functional status, change in oral intake, or alteration of gastrointestinal (GI) function. These physical and history assessments combined with anthropometric measures assist the health care professional with identifying malnourishment.

PRACTICE POINT

- Unintentional weight loss has consistently been shown to be a reliable measure of malnutrition, especially in older adults. A loss of greater than 5% of one's usual body weight (UBW) in 1 month or 10% of UBW over 3 months is considered clinically significant even if one is initially obese.

LABORATORY DATA

Measurement of serum proteins is also frequently used in the nutrition screening process. Most commonly used are albumin and prealbumin (or transthyretin), but transferrin and retinol-binding protein (RBP) may also be monitored.

Albumin is a well-known marker of nutrition status. It is most useful as an indicator of chronic malnourishment, particularly in the outpatient setting. It is also negatively correlated with morbidity and mortality for inpatients. These positive features make albumin a favorite for nutritional screening. However, albumin is a poor marker of the return of nutritional status to normal in malnourished patients because of its 21-day half-life. One would not expect normalization of serum albumin for at least 14–21 days of adequate protein intake in the hospitalized, malnourished patient, and this is only after the primary pathological process has resolved.

PRACTICE POINT

Albumin is a poor marker of the return of nutrition status to normal in malnourished patients because of its 21-day half-life.

- One would not expect normalization of serum albumin for at least 14–21 days of adequate protein intake in the hospitalized, malnourished patient after the primary pathological process has resolved.

Prealbumin is a better marker of nutrition progress in the hospitalized patient due to its 3-day half-life.

- Determining the nutritional significance of a single low prealbumin level in the setting of a high CRP is unreliable.
- If the prealbumin remains depressed despite a return of CRP to normal, it suggests that the patient has inadequate nutrient intake.

In contrast to albumin, prealbumin has a 3-day half-life and is a better marker of nutrition progress in the hospitalized patient. Prealbumin has also been shown to be a useful nutrition screening tool, which correlates well with dietitian assessments of nutritional status. Thus, when available, many institutions prefer prealbumin as the laboratory parameter of choice for nutritional screening and monitoring. Transferrin and RBP have been shown to have similar responses to adequate protein intake as prealbumin, and may be substituted in facilities that do not have laboratory assays for prealbumin readily available.

Of note, all of the "nutrition" proteins are negative acute phase reactants. The liver decreases their production during acute illness or following surgery. Hence, a low prealbumin during such periods may be more reflective of an inflammatory condition alone rather than poor nutritional status. In order to optimize interpretation of prealbumin, one should analyze this lab value in concert with C-reactive protein (CRP). CRP, in contrast to prealbumin, is a positive acute phase reactant, which increases during inflammatory states. When CRP is high, prealbumin is usually low. Determining the nutritional significance of a single low prealbumin level in the setting of a high CRP level is unreliable. However, following the trend of several prealbumin and CRP measurements over time can provide useful information. In a patient who is recovering from illness and receiving adequate protein, one should see a reciprocal rise in prealbumin over time and a drop in CRP. If the prealbumin remains depressed despite a return of CRP to normal, it suggests that the patient has inadequate nutrient intake.

Hyper- or hypovolemia, steroid administration, alcoholism, liver and renal failure can also alter circulating nutrition protein levels independent of nutritional status. Measurement of these protein levels on the day of admission and prior to any medical interventions may provide the most relevant information regarding nutritional standing, while measurements several days into a hospital admission are less reliable.

In short, there are many nonnutritional factors that may alter the level of circulating nutritional proteins used to monitor nutritional status. Hence, although it is important to monitor such levels, physicians must use caution when interpreting these markers.

THE NUTRITION PRESCRIPTION

Following nutrition assessment, a nutrition prescription is made. No formal nutrition plan is necessary for patients who are well nourished and are not at risk for malnourishment on admission. However, these patients should be reassessed every 3 to 5 days for the development of such risks. All patients who are malnourished on admission, or who are at risk of developing malnutrition, should have a formal nutrition plan developed. This begins with determination of nutrient requirements.

DETERMINATION OF NUTRIENT REQUIREMENTS

While it is obvious that underfeeding the hospitalized patient is undesirable, it is less well appreciated that overfeeding calories is detrimental as well. Excess carbohydrate administration can result in hyperglycemia and excess carbon dioxide production, which is of particular concern in patients with lung disease who may retain CO_2 and have difficulty weaning from the ventilator. Long-term overfeeding may eventually lead to the development of hepatic steatosis. Overfeeding protein can increase ureagenesis and cause renal distress. Overfeeding fat can be immunosuppressive. Hence the goal is to determine nutrient needs precisely, avoid both under- and overfeeding of the hospitalized patient, and deliver macronutrients in the appropriate proportions.

The "gold standard" for determination of caloric requirements is indirect calorimetry, or a "metabolic cart" study. The metabolic cart measures oxygen consumption and carbon dioxide production and then calculates resting energy expenditure (REE) through utilization of the Weir equation. Indirect calorimetry provides a result, which already includes the additional caloric expenditure related to disease stress, but not the caloric expenditure related to activity. Hence the results of the metabolic cart study are increased by an activity factor to calculate the final daily caloric expenditure. Typically, activity factors range from 0 to 5% in intubated patients to as high as 30% in ambulatory patients.

Metabolic cart testing remains the only reliable way to determine caloric requirements for patients with a very low or high BMI, for those with amputations, and for those who have severe illness or injury such as multiple traumas or burns. Use of predictive equations to estimate caloric requirements in such patients can lead to highly inaccurate results. Unfortunately, metabolic cart studies require trained personnel and expensive equipment, so these studies are not available in all facilities.

The use of predictive equations is the most common method for determining caloric requirements. There have been many equations developed over the past century. The Harris-Benedict equation (HBE), developed in 1919, is based on studies of healthy volunteers and is the oldest and most widely used equation for determining basal metabolic rate (BMR), the basis for calculating daily caloric requirements. A recent meta-analysis, however, suggests that the Mifflin–St. Jeor equation may be more accurate than the HBE for determining caloric needs when the two equations are compared to indirect calorimetry. The HBE and Mifflin–St. Jeor equations do not factor in the increased caloric expenditure related to disease. This is in contrast to a metabolic cart study. Hence, once the BMR is determined via these predictive equations, an estimate of the additional caloric expenditure from activity *and* metabolic stress is factored in to determine the overall daily caloric requirement. Stress

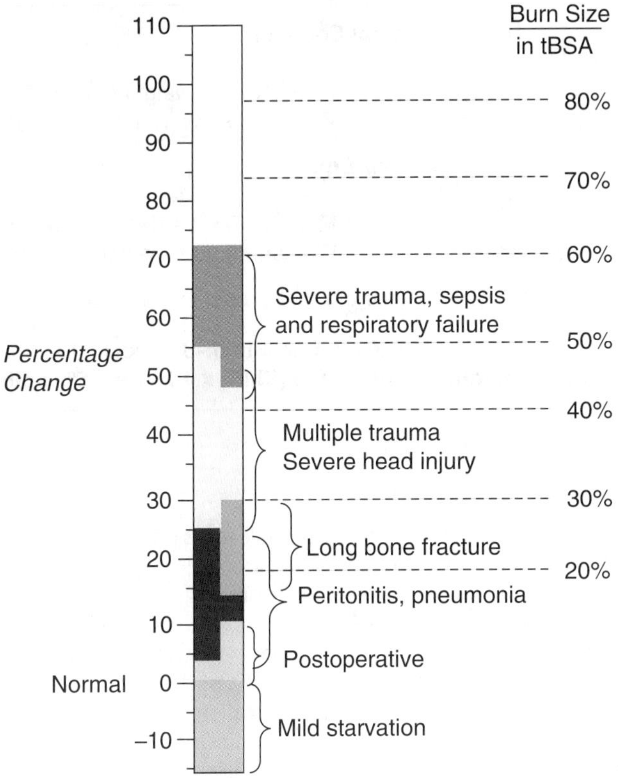

Figure 54-1 *Percent change in metabolic rate due to injury.*

factors can range from 10% in routine patients to 100% in severe burn patients (**Figure 54-1**).

Generally speaking, the actual body weight is used for caloric assessment. However, in patients who are greater than 120% of their ideal weight, the use of ideal weight is recommended. Some nutrition professionals will use an "adjusted weight" for obesity, although no routine standardized adjustment has been published (**Figure 54-2**). In addition to caloric prescription, providers should determine their patients' protein goals. Generally, hospital patients require between 1.2 and 1.5 g/kg of protein per day, with burn patients requiring up to 2.0 g/kg. Provision of protein over 2.0 g/kg/day of actual body weight is not beneficial and may place undue stress of the kidneys.

While the preceding methods for determining caloric and protein needs are recommended and more precise, a quick rule of thumb is to prescribe 25–30 calories/kg/day and 1.2 g protein/kg/day of ideal body weight. This yields reasonable results for most patients. The physician can follow weight trends, circulating proteins, and changes in medical or functional status, and tailor calorie goals up or down accordingly.

ROUTE OF FEEDING

The next component of the nutrition prescription is determining the route of feeding (**Figure 54-3**). Oral nutrition is the easiest, most physiologic, and therefore preferred route of nutrient delivery for hospitalized patients. But when patients cannot safely or adequately meet their nutrient requirements through oral diet alone, specialized nutritional support must be considered.

ENTERAL NUTRITION

Enteral nutrition (EN) is the term used to describe nutrient provision via the GI tract from the mouth to the jejunum and includes oral diets. However, for the purpose of this discussion, *enteral nutrition*

Harris Benedict Equation

Men: [13.75 x weight (kg)] + [5.00 x height (cm)] – [6.78 x age (y)] + 66.5
Women: [9.56 x weight (kg)] + [1.85 x height (cm)] – [4.68 x age (y)] + 655.1

Mifflin-St. Jeor Equation

Men: (9.99 x weight) + (6.25 x height) – (4.92 x age) + 5
Women: (9.99 x weight) + (6.25 x height) – (4.92 x age) – 161

EXAMPLE: A 45-year-old man presents a diverticular abscess with ileus. He is 6 feet tall (182.9 cm) and 176 lbs (80 kg).

BMR (using Mifflin-St. Jeor) = [9.99 x 80] + [6.25 x 182.9] – [4.92 x 45] + 5 = 1726
Calorie Requirement = 1726 (BMR) x 1.25 (ie, 25% activity factor) x 1.10 (ie,10% stress factor) = 2473 calories/day

Figure 54-2 *Equations for determining basal metabolic rate.*

will refer to feeding of patients via enteric tubes placed in the stomach or jejunum.

When evaluating patients for initiation of specialized nutritional support, one can follow the old adage "if the gut works, use it." Provision of nutrients into the GI tract preserves structural and functional integrity and maintains gut-associated lymphoid tissue. Relative and absolute contraindications to enteral feeding include major GI hemorrhage, peritonitis, severe ileus, bowel obstruction or fistulae distal to enteral access site, intestinal ischemia, and malabsorptive disorders with high-volume diarrhea (eg, short bowel syndrome, radiation enteritis, graft versus host disease of the GI tract).

ENTERAL ACCESS

After the decision is made to pursue EN support, the physician must determine the most appropriate access route. This decision is based on two major factors: (1) whether the patient requires short- or long-term feeding, and (2) whether gastric function is normal.

Nasoenteric tubes (NGTs) are the most commonly used access for patients who require short-term feeding because they can usually be placed noninvasively at the bedside. Occasionally, endoscopic or fluoroscopic guidance is required. If gastric function is normal, an NGT is placed. If gastric emptying is impaired or there is concern for aspiration of gastric contents, then a postpyloric nasoduodenal or nasojejunal tube should be considered. Lightweight, small-bore flexible tubes are available that offer the most comfort to the patient. However, their flexibility often does not allow for withdrawing fluid, thereby limiting one's ability to check gastric residuals. Smaller-bore tubes are also prone to clogging and therefore require frequent flushes with water.

When placing a nasal feeding tube at the bedside, it is essential to verify that the final position is within the GI tract and not in the lungs, particularly with small-bore tubes. Auscultation over the left upper quadrant and insufflating air into the NGT is a time-honored but notoriously unreliable practice for confirming gastric placement of a tube. Radiography remains the "gold standard" for confirmation

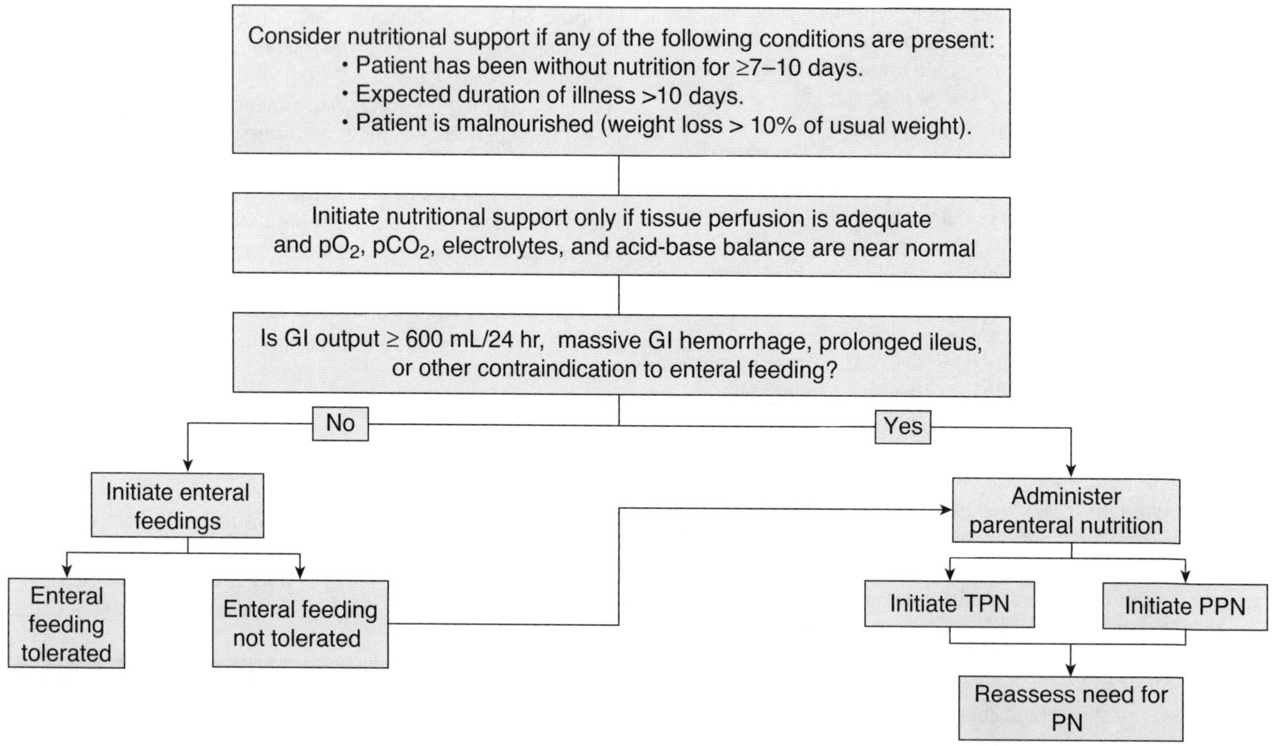

Figure 54-3 *Determining route of nutritional support.*

of enteral tube placement and can prevent the potentially lethal complication of infusing tube feeds into the lungs.

Patients who require long-term enteral access (eg, greater than 6 weeks) should be considered for gastrostomy or jejunostomy tube placement. Unless contraindicated, gastric feeding is preferred over jejunal feeding as the former allows for bolus feedings if desired. Feeds are allowed to flow by gravity into the gastrostomy tube in divided feeding doses, four to six times daily. In contrast, patients receiving jejunal feeding must receive continuous feedings via an infusion pump over a minimum of 10 to 12 hours. This is usually less desirable for the patient and caregivers. Gravity or bolus feeds directly into the jejunum provide too much solution at once and can precipitate diarrhea, dumping syndrome, bloating, and nausea and vomiting.

The most common method for placement of the gastrostomy tube (g-tube) is via fluoroscopy or percutaneous endoscopic gastrostomy (PEG) tube placement. Less commonly, g-tubes can be placed via open or laparoscopic surgical techniques. Relative contraindications for g-tube placement include significant ascites, history of gastric surgery that limits gastric size (eg, total gastrectomy) or prohibits access to the main stomach (eg, following weight loss surgery procedures such as gastric bypass), or intestinal obstruction distal to the stomach.

In patients who require more permanent jejunal feeding, percutaneous endoscopic gastrostomy tube placement with jejunal tube extension (PEG-J) is an option. This is perhaps the best option for patients who have poor gastric emptying or chronic reflux with aspiration, who would benefit from simultaneous gastric decompression and small bowel feeding. The disadvantage of the PEG-J is that the jejunal extension tube has a tendency to migrate back into the stomach and may need to be replaced. In patients who do not need both gastric and jejunal access, a standard jejunostomy may be preferred. Jejunostomy tubes are most often placed in the operating room via open or laparoscopic technique, although some surgeons and gastroenterologists are also performing percutaneous endoscopic jejunostomy (PEJ). Jejunal access is recommended for patients who have proximal intestinal obstructions, history of some gastric surgeries as already described, or poor gastric emptying, or who are at risk for aspirating stomach contents.

ENTERAL FORMULAS

There are standard and specialized enteral formulas that can be used to provide nutrition. Since all of these formulas have fixed macronutrient content, it may not be possible to deliver sufficient protein without overfeeding calories. Hence, one usually delivers the feedings at a rate to provide appropriate calories and then supplements protein with a protein modular (eg, Beneprotein).

Standard (ie, polymeric) enteral formulas are made up of intact protein, fats, and carbohydrates. Generally somewhere between 1 and 1.5 liters of solution will meet the dietary reference intakes for vitamins and minerals as well. Formulas are characterized by number of calories per milliliter and can be found in 1.0, 1.2, 1.5, and 2.0 cal/mL varieties. The more concentrated the formula (1.5 and 2.0 cal/mL), the higher the fat content and osmolarity. Concentrated formulas are designed for patients who require fluid restriction or who can only tolerate lower volumes of tube feeding infusion. However, concentrated formulas may be poorly tolerated due to their hyperosmolarity in patients with chronic diarrhea or malabsorptive disorders. In addition, concentrated formulas tend to provide inadequate free water at an average goal rate, which can lead to dehydration if additional fluid is not administered via feeding tube, or intravenously.

Elemental, "semi-elemental," or peptide based (eg, Peptimen, Vivonex, Optimental) formulas may help maximize absorption in patients with malabsorptive disorders. The formulas provide protein in the form of amino acids or di- or tripeptides, with simple sugars as well.

A recent area of interest in EN has been the tailoring of EN therapy to potentially improve outcomes. "Immune-enhancing diets" (IEDs) are formulas that are fortified with some combination of arginine, glutamine, omega-3 fatty acids, and/or antioxidant vitamins and are believed to enhance immunity, although this is controversial. It appears that IEDs may prevent infectious complications in postsurgical or head and neck cancer patients, and have been recommended for use in surgical intensive care unit (ICU) patients. Formulas with emphasis on omega-3 fatty acids may possibly improve outcome in those with acute respiratory distress syndrome and systemic inflammatory response syndrome of sepsis. These formulas, if deemed appropriate, are generally limited to use in ICU patients and not the general hospital patient population.

There are also specialty formulas for a variety of disease states such as pulmonary, renal, and liver dysfunction and diabetes. They all have their pros and cons, which are beyond the scope of this chapter except as described in the following sections. These formulas should be selected with caution because they are generally quite expensive, may not have a justifiable benefit for patients, and in some cases may even cause harm.

MONITORING ENTERAL FEEDING TOLERANCE

Feedings are typically started at a low rate, and gradually advanced to the infusion goal over a period of 24 to 48 hours. As this goal is approached, the patient is monitored for tolerance as assessed by the development of "high" gastric residuals and diarrhea. Patients are also evaluated for other symptoms such as nausea, vomiting, diarrhea, abdominal pain, and bloating. If signs and symptoms of intolerance develop, the feedings are held until the issue resolves. Persistent intolerance is an indication to consider an alternative plan. Patients receiving gastric feedings should be considered for post-pyloric feeding as this may improve most symptoms of intolerance with the exception of diarrhea.

Checking gastric residuals has traditionally been the hallmark for monitoring tube feeding tolerance and avoiding tube-feed-associated aspiration. However, several well-designed studies have failed to demonstrate a significant link to gastric residual volume (GRV) and aspiration risk. This has led to high variability in the use of GRV for monitoring tube feed advancement. Currently, the American Society for Parenteral and Enteral Nutrition (ASPEN) recommends monitoring of GRV for the first 48 hours of EN initiation. If the GRV is greater than 250 mL on two residual checks, the physician should consider a motility agent such as metoclopromide or erythromycin. If the gastric residual is greater than 500 mL the feedings should be held and the patient evaluated by a physician for abdominal distention, glycemic control, adequacy of motility agents if not already ordered, or consideration of small bowel feeding access.

PRACTICE POINT

The American Society for Parenteral and Enteral Nutrition (ASPEN) recommends monitoring of gastric residual volume (GRV) for the first 48 hours of enteral nutrition initiation.

- If the GRV is greater than 250 mL on 2 residual checks, the physician should consider a motility agent such as metoclopromide or erythromycin.
- If the gastric residual is greater than 500 mL, the feedings should be held and the patient evaluated by a physician for abdominal distention, glycemic control, adequacy of motility agents if not already ordered, or consideration of small bowel feeding access.

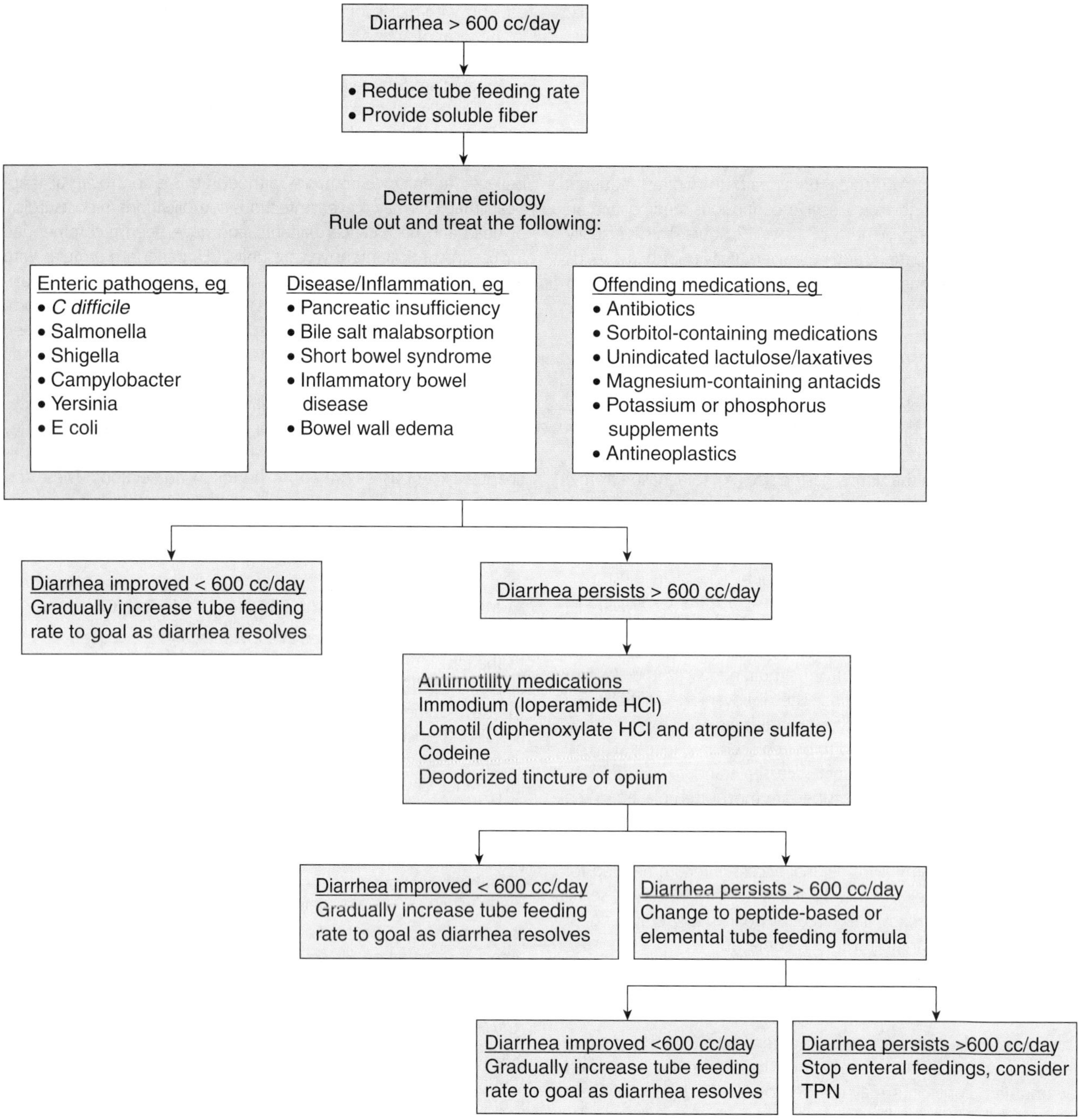

Figure 54-4 *Management of diarrhea in tube-fed patients.*

Patients at aspiration risk should also have the head of the bed elevated between 30 and 45 degrees at all times. It is important to note that even in patients who are tolerating tube feeds, aspiration of oropharyngeal secretions may occur. Hence, it is important not to assume that aspiration is related to tube feeds. In addition, the outdated practice of mixing blue food coloring with tube feeds as a way to monitor for "microaspiration" should be abandoned. Several reports indicate that this practice fails to improve aspiration detection and can increase morbidity and mortality.

Diarrhea is also a common problem with tube feed administration. It can be attributed to gastrointestinal pathogens, bowel edema or inflammation, malabsorptive disorders, and most commonly, medications such as antibiotics. When a patient develops diarrhea, the physician should send stool samples to rule out infectious causes such as *Clostridium difficile*. If infection is present, it should be treated. If the diarrhea is noninfectious, the patient's medication panel should be reviewed. Medications are the primary cause of diarrhea in up to 60% of cases. Sorbitol-containing medications, especially when administered via feeding tube, are known to cause diarrhea. If noninfectious diarrhea persists, soluble fiber (eg, Benefiber, banana flakes) may be added to the medication regimen, or the tube feeding formula can be changed to a fiber-containing formula. Antimotility agents (eg, loperamide) may also be prescribed (**Figure 54-4**).

PARENTERAL NUTRITION

Patients who cannot tolerate EN should be considered for initiation of parenteral nutrition (PN). However, it should be noted that PN is associated with higher rates of infectious and metabolic complications such as volume overload, hyperglycemia, and electrolyte abnormalities compared to EN. Because of these risks, PN appears to become beneficial only after the initial 10–14 days of hospitalization without adequate enteral feeding in patients who are well nourished at admission. As the duration of inadequate nutrition exceeds 14 days, the risk of nutritionally related complication rates increases, and the benefits of PN begin to outweigh the risks compared to those who continue to receive inadequate EN alone. At this point, PN should be considered. The threshold for initiation of PN may be less than 10–14 days depending on the degree of malnutrition at hospitalization and anticipated duration without adequate enteral intake.

Indications for PN include, but are not limited to, severe malabsorptive disorders (short bowel syndrome, graft versus host disease of the GI tract, radiation enteritis, inflammatory bowel disease), high output enterocutaneous fistulae if distal feeding access is not feasible, pancreatitis with enteral feeding intolerance, bowel obstruction, uncontrolled anastomotic leak following GI surgery, and prolonged postoperative ileus. The main contraindication to PN is the ability to safely and effectively feed via the enteral route.

PARENTERAL NUTRITION PRESCRIPTION AND MONITORING

PN solutions contain carbohydrate in the form of dextrose, protein as crystalline amino acids, and lipids from polyunsaturated long-chain triglycerides such as soybean oil or a safflower/soybean oil mixture. Vitamins, electrolytes, and trace elements are added to the formulation as needed. Electrolytes must be added at the appropriate concentrations to avoid "cracking" of lipid-containing PN. If cracking occurs, precipitates form in the solution, and the lipid emulsion separates into layers, making it unsafe for administration.

Physicians must carefully monitor patients for metabolic changes such as hyperglycemia or refeeding syndrome upon initiation of PN. Hyperglycemia may increase infectious complications, hospital length of stay, and cost. Refeeding syndrome is characterized by electrolyte abnormalities that occur during the reinstitution of carbohydrate calories to a starved patient. Serum phosphate, magnesium, and potassium depletion may develop and precipitate potentially life-threatening cardiac arrhythmias or neuromuscular complications. PN prescriptions typically provide from 1 to 3 liters of fluid per day depending on the physician's assessment of maintenance fluid requirements. A general rule of thumb is 30 mL per kilogram. Carbohydrates generally make up about 50–60% of the caloric prescription, at 3.4 calories per gram of dextrose. Protein generally provides about 15–25% of the calories at 4.0 calories per gram of amino acid. The current U.S. Food and Drug Administration (FDA)-approved lipid emulsions are primarily made up of omega-6-rich oils, which have been shown to be proinflammatory and potentially immunosuppressive. Hence, lipid provision should be limited to 20–25% of calories at 10 calories per gram of intravenous (IV) lipid.

It is advisable to start with a lower volume and concentration of dextrose when initiating PN to avoid metabolic complications. One liter of a 10% dextrose solution is a good starting point. Subsequently the volume, and dextrose, lipid, and protein concentrations are increased as needed in the metabolically stable patient to the eventual goal caloric and fluid provision (**Figure 54-5**). Blood sugar levels should be closely monitored and maintained below 180 mg/deciliter (dL), and abnormal electrolyte levels should be corrected, especially potassium, phosphate, and magnesium, before starting or advancing to the goal solution. Additionally, any patient who is at high risk for refeeding syndrome should receive IV thiamine replacement prior to initiation of total parenteral nutrition (TPN) to prevent development of Wernicke encephalopathy. The solutions should be administered using a volumetric pump set at a constant rate. In general, PN lipid infusion should not exceed 1 g/kg/day, and dextrose infusion should be less than 5 mg/kg/minute. Eventually the PN solution can be cycled nocturnally (generally between 10 and 16 hours) in long-term PN patients, once glycemic control is achieved. Once stable, patients can have lab monitoring decreased to once or twice weekly.

Patients receiving *long-term* PN may develop PN-associated liver dysfunction (PNALD). However, alterations that occur within the first 2 weeks of PN therapy generally resolve despite continuation of TPN. Alternate causes of liver function test (LFT) elevation should always be ruled out, such as hepatotoxic medications, biliary obstruction, and sepsis. PNALD should be a diagnosis of exclusion rather than the first thought in the acutely ill patient that has just been started on PN. Excess provision of IV dextrose or lipid, and deficiencies of carnitine and choline may increase the likelihood of PNALD. Provision of the appropriate amount of dextrose and carbohydrate, repleting carnitine and choline, and administering even small amounts of enteral nourishment may decrease the risk of developing PNALD. Finally, decreasing PN cycle time to less than 24 hours each day may allow for hepatic "rest" and decrease continuous insulin secretion, which may decrease fatty deposits in the liver.

PARENTERAL ACCESS

Central venous access is required for the administration of TPN because TPN solutions are hyperosmolar. Peripheral PN (PPN) solutions, which are available in some hospitals, have limited dextrose and amino acid concentrations in order to keep osmolarity lower. This improves tolerance of PN delivery via a peripheral vein. It also, of course, lowers caloric density, and therefore patients may require higher volume solutions to get close to their calorie requirement, which increases peripheral edema and cardiac stress. PPN is generally not a good long-term (greater than 3–5 days) solution for most patients.

The physician must also determine the most appropriate access device for PN. Percutaneous catheters that are placed in jugular, subclavian, or femoral veins may be used for PN administration. The femoral approach is generally undesirable because of increased infection risk, increased risk of deep venous thrombosis, and limitations on patient ambulation. This approach is only advised for patients who cannot receive alternate central access. Peripherally inserted central catheters (PICCs) are placed in the upper arm in the basilic or cephalic vein and threaded to the superior vena cava. A PICC line is the ideal catheter for a patient who requires TPN for 6 weeks or less, assuming the PICC is not required for another indication as well. PICC lines can be left in place for longer than 6 weeks if the patient does not develop infection or thrombosis. To reduce the risk of developing these complications, some suggest that tunneled (eg, Hickman or Broviac) catheters or completely subcutaneous catheters (eg, Port-a-cath or power ports) are indicated if it is known that central venous access will be necessary for longer than 6 weeks.

The most common complication associated with PN is the development of catheter-related bloodstream infections (CRBSIs). The use of single-lumen catheters, or dedicating one port of a multiport line to TPN alone, may reduce risk of CRBSI. Appropriate hygiene such as complete sterile barrier precautions at time of insertion, using appropriate dressing and chlorhexidine at insertion site, and regular changing of administration sets is recommended. No significant benefit has been demonstrated from the use of prophylactic antibiotics, use of heparin, or routine replacement of central lines.

Diagnosis of CRBSI is best achieved by culture of the catheter tip, or paired blood cultures from a peripheral vein and from the catheter. In the event of CRBSI, short-term lines should be removed and appropriate antibiotic therapy prescribed. Long-term lines may

Patient is a 45 year old man with diverticular abscess, as in Figure 54-2. Advancement to an oral diet has been unsuccessful for 10 days, and TPN is required.

A. Estimate nutrient requirements:

Calorie requirement: 2373 calories/day (see Figure 54-2)
Protein requirement: 1.5 g/kg/day = 80 x 1.5 = 120 grams/day
Fluid requirement: 30 mL/kg body weight = 80 x 30 = 2400 mL

B. Determine the solution

1. Protein content

120 g protein ÷ 2.4 Liters fluid = 50 g/L
50 g = 5% amino acids per liter
4 calories/g of amino acids x 120 g = 480 kcals of protein

2. Lipid content (*approximately 20–25% of non-protein kcals*)

2373 total calories – 480 protein calories from protein = 1893 non-protein kcals
20% of 1893 calories = 380 fat calories
Round to nearest 100 = 400 kcals lipid/day
2 kcals/mL of 20% lipid solution = 200 mL of 20% lipid

3. Carbohydrate (CHO) content (*approximately 50–60% of non-protein calories*)

2373 total calories – 480 protein calories – 400 fat calories = 1493 CHO kcals
1493 CHO kcals ÷ 3.4 kcals/g of dextrose = 439 g dextrose
439 g dextrose ÷ 2.4 L = 183 g dextrose/L
183 g dextrose = 18% dextrose per liter

4. Final solution*

2.4 liters of 18% dextrose, 5% amino acids, with 400 calories (40 grams) lipid/day.
* This assumes a triple mix (ie, mix of carbohydrate, lipid, and amino acids in one bag). Some institutions will hang lipid separately. Other institutions do not allow for customized solutions and have a limited selection of solutions from which the clinician chooses to get close to the calorie and protein needs of the patient.

Figure 54-5 *Parenteral nutrition calculation.*

be salvaged with the use of an antibiotic lock technique in which a concentrated antibiotic solution is instilled into the line or lumen and left for prolonged periods. However, lines should be removed in the event of septic shock, resistant bacteria or fungal infection, or other complicated infection.

SPECIAL CONSIDERATIONS

While a comprehensive discussion of all the complex nutrition issues that the hospitalist may face is beyond the scope of this chapter, a few of the more common situations that may be encountered are discussed briefly.

PANCREATITIS

Pancreatitis patients require no nutritional intervention in 80–90% of cases as most will resume an oral diet within 7 days of admission. EN remains the preferred route of nutritional support for the remaining patients because it is associated with a significant reduction in infectious morbidity, length of stay, and mortality compared to PN. EN can be appropriately achieved by feeding into the stomach or jejunum depending on gastric emptying. Of note, patients who are fed within the first 24–48 hours of admission may tolerate enteral feeding better than those who start feeding later, and such early feeding is associated with substantial outcome benefits. These benefits diminish in patients who start feeding as late as day 4.

PN should be considered in severe pancreatitis patients who cannot receive enteral feeding for prolonged periods. It is important to note, however, that PN may exacerbate the inflammatory response to pancreatitis if initiated too early and thus worsen outcome. Hence, ASPEN guidelines suggest not starting PN for 5 days in those with severe pancreatitis, even if enteral feeding is not possible.

PRACTICE POINT

- The main contraindication to parenteral nutrition is the ability to safely and effectively feed via the enteral route. ASPEN guidelines suggest not starting PN for 5 days in those with severe pancreatitis, even if enteral feeding is not possible.

RENAL DISEASE

Dialysis patients often have poor oral intake, increased nutrient losses in their dialysates, and increased catabolic stress. Thus malnutrition is common in this patient population. The Kidney

Disease Outcomes Quality Initiative (K/DOQI) guidelines recommend protein restriction for *outpatient* dialysis patients, but notably recommend that dialysis patients receive 1.2–1.3 g/kg of protein when hospitalized for acute illnesses. Provision of protein similar to that which is prescribed for patients with normal renal function is necessary for recovery. Many nutrition experts also believe that acutely ill patients who are predialysis should still receive 1.2–1.5 g/kg/day of protein to aid in the recovery process as well, even if this precipitates the need for dialysis. However, further study is needed to definitely decide how best to manage the predialysis patient population.

HEPATIC DISEASE

Malnutrition is also highly prevalent among patients with liver disease. Unfortunately, most traditional markers of nutrition status may be more reflective of diminished hepatic synthetic capacity rather than nutrition. In addition, anthropometric measurements can all be altered by fluid status. Previous thoughts regarding the benefits of protein restriction in those with hepatic encephalopathy have not been supported by more recent studies. For example, Cordoba and colleagues found no differences in outcomes of encephalopathy between those on normal and protein restricted diets, and that low protein diets in fact caused breakdown of lean body mass. Although much research has been devoted to the evaluation of diets supplemented with branch chain amino acids (BCAAs), the routine use of BCAA-enhanced formulas is only recommended for those with encephalopathy refractory to luminal-acting antibiotics and lactulose therapy, as these formulas may provide some benefit in coma grade.

PREOPERATIVE NUTRITION SUPPORT

Several papers indicate that malnourished patients suffer more postoperative complications than those who are adequately nourished. Weight loss of greater than 10% of body weight most consistently predicts adverse outcomes. Buzby and colleagues performed one of the most validated studies in this area. From their analyses, they developed a measure of perioperative complication risk, which they termed "Nutrition Risk Index" (NRI) and is calcated as follows:

$$\text{NRI: } 1.519 \times \text{the serum albumin level (in grams per liter)} + 0.417 \times (\text{current weight/usual weight} \times 100)$$

Patients were classified as borderline, mildly, or severely malnourished. The patients who met criteria for severe risk with an NRI of less than 83.5 benefited from preoperative feeding with TPN because they had fewer noninfectious surgical complications (wound dehiscence, pressure ulcers, GI bleeding, cardiac arrest, renal failure) compared to controls. Mildly malnourished patients did not experience the same benefit; rather they suffered additional infectious complications related to TPN. Hence, one can conclude that the malnourished patient may benefit from pre-oeprative feeding, while the well nourished individual may be adversely affected by this type of nutritional intervention.

Less is known about forced enteral feeding (eg, tube feeds) in a preoperative patient. However, as discussed earlier, there are many benefits to EN support over PN support. Therefore, in patients who do have some degree of malnutrition but do not meet NRI criteria for preoperative feeding, EN may be considered if possible. In those for whom enteral nourishment is not possible or is marginally tolerated PN should be considered. Additionally, nutrition support should be administered for a minimum of 10–14 days prior to surgery to provide optimal benefit. Feeding for less than that time frame would not be expected to allow enough time for nutrient stores to be replenished appreciably, and therefore would not be expected to provide significant improvement in outcome. Close consultation with the surgeon is required to determine both the optimal route of feeding and the timing of the operation.

NUTRITIONAL SUPPORT AT THE END OF LIFE

The use of artificial nutrition and hydration in the terminally ill patient is the topic of much debate. Small studies suggest that home PN can be associated with some survival benefit in select patients with slow-growing tumors (eg, carcinoid, certain sarcomas, or ovarian cancer) despite the onset of GI malabsorption or obstruction. Unfortunately, there is little solid data upon which to base strong recommendations for most other terminal illnesses. ASPEN clinical guidelines recommend PN be limited to patients who (1) are physically and emotionally able to participate in their own care; (2) have a life expectancy of >40–60 days; (3) have strong social and financial support; and (4) have failed trials of less invasive medical therapy such as appetite stimulants and EN. In patients with a limited prognosis (<2 months) artificial nutrition is not advised. Patients may be palliated with intravenous fluids and vitamins, but the experience of hospice health care providers suggests that symptoms related to dehydration and starvation in the terminally ill are generally well tolerated and produce few symptoms. Family members should be advised of this as they often falsely believe that withholding fluid and nutrition uniformly results in suffering.

Recommendations regarding forced tube feeding in the terminally ill who cannot tolerate oral feeding but have a functional GI tract are even less clear. Generally, one must weigh the risks of tube feeding complications versus the benefits. Such feeding may be appropriate with good functional status and life expectancy greater than 2 months. When adverse events and risks outweigh the benefits, one should consider ceasing nutritional intervention.

CONCLUSION

Malnutrition is prevalent in a significant number of hospitalized patients, but all too often nutrition is an afterthought. Because of the adverse effects of malnutrition on the host, it is now believed that appropriate nutrition intervention may improve outcome, decrease cost, and speed recovery. All patients should be screened for malnutrition, have nutrition plans put in place to prevent deterioration of nutritional status, and be aggressively treated for malnutrition when identified in those without a terminal illness. EN is the feeding route of choice, but parenteral nutrition can be life saving in those who cannot receive adequate nutrition by the enteral route for prolonged periods. Effective treatment of the hospitalized patients includes an effective, thoughtful nutrition plan.

SUGGESTED READINGS

Bankhead R, Boullata J, Brantley S, et al. Enteral nutrition practice recommendations. *JPEN J Parenter Enteral Nutr*. 2009;33:122–167.

Butterworth CE. The skeleton in the hospital closet. 1974. *Nutrition*. 1994;10:435–441.

Clinical practice guidelines for nutrition in chronic renal failure. K/DOQI, National Kidney Foundation. *Am J Kidney Dis*. 2000;35:S1–140.

Cordoba J, Lopez-Hellin J, Planas M, et al. Normal protein diet for episodic hepatic encephalopathy: results of a randomized study. *J Hepatol*. 2004;41:38–43.

Correia MI, Waitzberg DL. The impact of malnutrition on morbidity, mortality, length of hospital stay and costs evaluated through a multivariate model analysis. *Clin Nutr*. 2003;22:235–239.

Gramlich L, Kichian K, Pinilla J, Rodych NJ, Dhaliwal R, Heyland DK. Does enteral nutrition compared to parenteral nutrition result in better outcomes in critically ill adult patients? A systematic review of the literature. *Nutrition*. 2004;20:843–848.

McClave SA, Chang WK, Dhaliwal R, Heyland DK. Nutrition support in acute pancreatitis: a systematic review of the literature. *JPEN J Parenter Enteral Nutr*. 2006;30:143–156.

McClave SA, Martindale RG, Vanek VW, et al. Guidelines for the provision and assessment of nutrition support therapy in the adult critically ill patient: Society of Critical Care Medicine (SCCM) and American Society for Parenteral and Enteral Nutrition (A.S.P.E.N.). *JPEN J Parenter Enteral Nutr*. 2009;33:277–316.

Perioperative total parenteral nutrition in surgical patients. The Veterans Affairs Total Parenteral Nutrition Cooperative Study Group. *N Engl J Med*. 1991;325:525–532.

Pittiruti M, Hamilton H, Biffi R, MacFie J, Pertkiewicz M. A.S.P.E.N. Guidelines on parenteral nutrition: central venous catheters (access, care, diagnosis and therapy of complications). *Clin Nutr*. 2009;28:365–377.

Robinson MK, Trujillo EB, Mogensen KM, Rounds J, McManus K, Jacobs DO. Improving nutritional screening of hospitalized patients: the role of prealbumin. *JPEN J Parenter Enteral Nutr*. 2003;27:389–395.

CHAPTER 55

Preoperative Pulmonary Risk Assessment

Kurt Pfeifer, MD
Gerald W. Smetana, MD, FACP

INTRODUCTION

A comprehensive preoperative evaluation must include assessment of the risk of postoperative pulmonary complications. While few would argue this point, pulmonary risk is often underappreciated as clinicians typically focus the majority of their energy on the preoperative cardiac evaluation. Highlighting the risk of this approach, postoperative pulmonary complications occur with similar frequency and greater morbidity than cardiovascular complications.

Clinicians intuitively recognize several risk factors for pulmonary complications, but some predictors of postoperative respiratory problems are not obvious. Additionally, clinicians may struggle with the appropriate utilization of preoperative pulmonary diagnostic testing. Recently published risk indices and practice guidelines provide valuable assistance in the identification of risk factors and the performance of evidence-based preoperative evaluation.

POSTOPERATIVE PULMONARY COMPLICATIONS

Pulmonary complications following anesthesia and surgery result from central nervous system suppression and altered respiratory dynamics. Administration of sedating agents and neuromuscular blockade exposes the patient to the risk of aspiration. Furthermore, regardless of the type of anesthetic technique utilized, patients will experience a reduction in lung volumes perioperatively. Reduction in lung volumes is the primary mechanism that may lead to atelectasis and predispose a patient to the additional complications of pneumonia and respiratory failure. This reduction in lung volumes is greatest for patients undergoing thoracic and upper abdominal surgery. **Table 55-1** lists specific postoperative pulmonary complications and diagnostic considerations for each.

PATIENT-SPECIFIC RISK FACTORS

Several different patient characteristics increase postoperative pulmonary risk (**Table 55-2**). While most of these patient-specific factors are nonmodifiable, their identification is important for providing patients, surgeons, and anesthesiologists with an accurate assessment of perioperative risk and to identify patients for whom one should employ risk reduction strategies.

CHRONIC LUNG DISEASE

Multiple studies have identified chronic obstructive pulmonary disease (COPD) as a major risk factor for postoperative respiratory problems. In a recent systematic review, authors reported COPD to be a significant predictor of postoperative pulmonary complications; the pooled odds ratio was 1.79. Surprisingly, the risk attributable to COPD was lower than other patient-related risk factors. Other forms of chronic lung disease, including interstitial lung diseases and obesity hypoventilation syndrome, have not been sufficiently studied to definitively determine their impact on perioperative pulmonary risk. However, pulmonary hypertension has recently been shown to increase the risk for both postoperative pulmonary complications and perioperative mortality.

ADVANCED AGE

Advanced age is a more important predictor of pulmonary complications than COPD. Contrary to previous belief, this risk is not a result of the cumulative morbidities associated with aging. After

TABLE 55-1 Postoperative Pulmonary Complications

Atelectasis	• Potential cause of *mild* hypoxia. • Generally not a cause of postoperative fever or moderate to severe hypoxia.
Pneumonia	• Diagnostic criteria vary—utilize same as nosocomial pneumonia. • Often polymicrobial—common pathogens include *Pseudomonas, Staphylococcus aureus, Streptococcus pneumoniae*, and enteric gram-negative bacilli. • Though aspiration of secretions is a likely contributor to development, anaerobic bacteria rarely cause postoperative pneumonia.
Respiratory failure	• The inability to wean off ventilator support within 48 hours of surgery or unplanned reintubation. • Typically a combination of hypoxic and hypercapnic respiratory failure.
Chronic obstructive pulmonary disease (COPD) exacerbation	• Diagnostic criteria and assessment are the same as in the nonoperative population.

TABLE 55-2 Patient-Specific Risk Factors for Postoperative Pulmonary Complications

Major
Chronic lung disease
Advanced age (age > 50)
Functional dependence
Comorbid disease (ASA class ≥ 2)
Congestive heart failure
Pulmonary hypertension
Minor or Indeterminate
Obstructive sleep apnea
Acute alteration of mental status
Smoking
Abnormal chest examination
Abnormal chest radiography
Alcohol use > 2 drinks/day
Weight loss > 10% of body weight
Chronic corticosteroid use
Stroke (past history)
Preoperative blood transfusion

adjustment for these additional risk factors, age greater than 59 has an odds ratio of 2.09, whereas age greater than 69 carries an odds ratio of 3.04. Recognition of age, even in the absence of other comorbidities, as an important source of pulmonary risk is critical as the population ages and more elderly patients undergo surgical procedures. The consequence of these observations is that even healthy older patients are at risk for postoperative pulmonary complications. This stands in contrast to postsurgical cardiac complications, which are not more common among older patients after adjusting for comorbidities.

SMOKING

Cigarette smoking increases the risk of postoperative pulmonary complications, but the degree of risk elevation is actually less than that from COPD and age. Clinicians should consider a recent history of cigarette smoking to be at least a moderate predictor of pulmonary risk.

MEDICAL COMORBIDITIES

As the number of comorbid illnesses increases, so does the risk of perioperative complications. The American Society of Anesthesiologists (ASA) classification system is easy to use and predicts the risk of postoperative respiratory problems as well as overall morbidity and mortality. Compared with ASA class I patients (no comorbidities), patients with an ASA class of II or greater have a nearly fivefold increase in the rate of postoperative pulmonary complications. The risk increases with each higher ASA class.

FUNCTIONAL STATUS

Large multivariate studies have also identified dependence on others for assistance with activities of daily living as a significant risk factor for postoperative pulmonary complications. The contribution of functional dependence to perioperative pulmonary risk is similar to that of cigarette smoking and chronic lung disease.

CONGESTIVE HEART FAILURE

Congestive heart failure (CHF) is not only an obvious risk factor for perioperative cardiac complications but also a predictor of postoperative respiratory failure. Although the cause of respiratory failure may be CHF-related pulmonary edema, a history of CHF is nonetheless an independent risk factor for pulmonary complications with a relative risk estimated at 5.7 in the geriatric population.

OTHER RISK FACTORS

In addition to the previously described risk factors, several other patient characteristics have been less clearly linked to postoperative pulmonary complications. For instance, abnormal findings on chest examination and abnormal chest radiography have been associated with increased pulmonary risk in smaller, older studies but not in more recent large-scale multivariate analyses. Consumption of more than two alcoholic drinks per day within 2 weeks of surgery, recent weight loss exceeding 10% of total body weight, chronic corticosteroid use, preoperative transfusion of more than 4 units of blood, acute alteration of mental status, and a history of stroke were modest risk factors for postoperative pneumonia in the largest prospective study to date.

The role of obstructive sleep apnea (OSA) in postoperative complications has long been intuited but not confirmed in objective studies. In at least one study, OSA patients showed an upward trend in reintubation, hypercapnia, and hypoxemia as well as a statistically significant increase in unplanned intensive care unit (ICU) admissions. Other recent studies also suggest that patients identified as being at risk for but not formally diagnosed with OSA have an increased risk of postoperative pulmonary complications. For example, patients with at least two clinical features of OSA (snoring, crowded oropharynx, daytime somnolence, or witnessed apneas) who have abnormal overnight oximetry are more likely to develop postoperative hypoxemia or airway management problems than patients without these features. Until more data are available, it is reasonable to consider OSA at least a moderate risk factor for perioperative respiratory problems.

FACTORS NOT ASSOCIATED WITH INCREASED PULMONARY RISK

Notably absent from the described risk factors are four conditions often mistaken as predictors of postoperative pulmonary complications: well-controlled asthma, obesity, diabetes mellitus, and immunosuppression. Although a potential relationship between perioperative pulmonary risk and morbid obesity or asthma has been assumed by some clinicians, multivariate investigations have consistently found no such correlation. The current literature provides little data on the contributions of immunosuppression and diabetes mellitus to pulmonary surgical complications.

PROCEDURE-SPECIFIC RISK FACTORS

Patient characteristics impact perioperative pulmonary risk significantly, but procedure-specific factors are even greater predictors of postoperative pneumonia and respiratory failure (**Table 55-3**). Unlike the majority of patient-specific risk factors, some of these surgery-related factors may be modifiable.

SURGICAL SITE

The site of operation is the most important determinant of postoperative pulmonary risk. As expected, surgeries involving the respiratory system and adjacent areas carry the highest risk of postoperative pulmonary complications (**Table 55-4**). Head and neck operations are high-risk procedures due in part to impairment of the upper airway. Restriction of diaphragmatic motion by pain from abdominal procedures leads to reduced lung volumes, the precursor of pulmonary complications.

ANESTHETIC TECHNIQUE

Several studies have identified general endotracheal anesthesia (GETA) as an independent predictor of postoperative pulmonary complications. In comparable analyses, neuraxial blockade (spinal and epidural anesthesia) was associated with lower rates of postoperative morbidity and mortality compared with GETA. However, these data have been challenged recently and have important methodologic flaws. Recent randomized controlled trials have not consistently identified GETA as a risk factor. While these data suggest a potential risk reduction strategy, selection of anesthetic technique is the primary responsibility of the anesthesiologist. Medical consultants should collaborate with anesthesiologists to share their risk assessment and suggestions for risk reduction strategies.

POSTOPERATIVE CARE REQUIREMENTS

For some surgical procedures, postoperative care strategies may confer increased risk for respiratory problems. The risks of ventilator-associated pneumonia with mechanical ventilation and atelectasis and aspiration with prolonged bed rest are well documented in the nonoperative population and apply to postsurgical patients as well. Less recognized is the link between nasogastric (NG) intubation and postoperative pneumonia. Meta-analyses have demonstrated that the selective use of NG intubation only to control vomiting and abdominal distention, rather than routine use after abdominal surgery, is associated with a lower rate of pneumonia and atelectasis.

TABLE 55-3 Procedure-Specific Risk Factors for Postoperative Pulmonary Complications

Surgical site
- Head and neck
- Thoracic
- Abdominal
- Abdominal aortic aneurysm repair
- Neurosurgical
- Vascular

General anesthesia

Nasogastric intubation

Emergency surgery

Prolonged surgery (>3 hours)

TABLE 55-4 Pulmonary Complication Rate for Surgeries with Increased Pulmonary Risk

Surgery	Pulmonary Complication Rate
Abdominal aortic aneurysm repair	25.5%
Abdominal	14.2%
Head and neck	10.4%

Reproduced, with permission, from Smetana GW, Lawrence VA, Cornell JE. Preoperative pulmonary risk stratification for noncardiothoracic surgery: systematic review for the American College of Physicians. *Ann Intern Med.* 2006;144:581–595.

OTHER RISK FACTORS

Regardless of the surgical site or anesthetic technique, procedures performed on an emergent basis carry a higher risk of respiratory complications. Surgeries with duration greater than three hours are also associated with an increased risk for postoperative pneumonia and respiratory failure. Literature on the pulmonary risks with laparoscopic versus open surgeries is sparse, and decisions regarding such surgical approaches should be made based on other factors.

PRACTICE POINT

The strongest predictors of postoperative pulmonary complications are as follows:
- **Advanced age:** Beginning at age 50, perioperative pulmonary risk begins to increase and becomes particularly high in patients over the age of 70 years.
- **Surgical site:** A location anywhere from the mouth to upper abdomen disrupts the airway and/or normal respiratory dynamics.

DIAGNOSTIC STUDIES

A thorough history and physical examination are the cornerstones of the preoperative evaluation. In most instances, diagnostic testing adds little to the risk assessment as established by clinical evaluation. Testing has a role when the risk is uncertain after history and physical examination.

CHEST RADIOGRAPHY

Chest radiography is part of many clinicians' routine preoperative evaluation despite evidence that chest X-ray results rarely change perioperative management. Abnormalities on preoperative chest radiography are common, occurring on 10–20% of films. However, a minority of these findings are unexpected based on the clinician's physical assessment and history, and an even smaller number influence perioperative care. Use of chest imaging should be reserved for the same indications as in the nonoperative setting—evaluation of new or changed cardiopulmonary symptoms. The American College of Physicians perioperative pulmonary guidelines also suggest obtaining chest radiography in asymptomatic patients who are over the age of 50 and undergoing thoracic, upper abdominal, or abdominal aortic aneurysm repair.

ARTERIAL BLOOD GAS ANALYSIS

Early studies of preoperative arterial blood gas (ABG) analysis suggested that hypercarbia and hypoxemia predicted postoperative pulmonary complications. Subsequent reviews concluded that clinical assessment was equally accurate in predicting postsurgical respiratory problems. Taking into account that no arterial CO_2 or O_2 value is an absolute contraindication to surgery, clinicians should perform ABG analysis only if the results will significantly influence perioperative management (ie, excluding hypercarbia and respiratory acidosis in a patient with COPD and increased shortness of breath).

PULMONARY FUNCTION TESTING

Formal pulmonary function testing has a well-established role in the preoperative evaluation of patients before lung resection and surgical coronary revascularization. Its role in noncardiothoracic surgery is questionable. Analogous to ABG analysis, initial studies of preoperative spirometry suggested it was useful for predicting postoperative morbidity, but later data comparing spirometry to history and physical examination showed no clear incremental benefit from pulmonary function testing. Further, no spirometric values can be used as cutoffs to prohibit noncardiothoracic surgery. Indications for pulmonary function testing are the same as in the general setting: evaluation of unexplained respiratory symptoms and characterization of lung disease when it is unclear whether a patient's airflow obstruction is optimally reduced.

OTHER STUDIES

Analyses of large pools of noncardiothoracic surgery patients identified abnormal blood urea nitrogen (BUN) and albumin levels as strong predictors of postoperative pulmonary complications. Both elevated BUN (>21 mg/dL) and hypoalbuminemia (albumin level <35 g/dL) predict postoperative respiratory failure to a similar or greater degree than COPD and advanced age. The American College of Physicians recommends checking albumin levels in patients at increased perioperative pulmonary risk.

PRACTICE POINT

- Diagnostic testing rarely adds value to perioperative pulmonary risk assessment in noncardiothoracic surgery. A thorough history and physical examination is sufficient in almost all cases.

PREOPERATIVE PULMONARY RISK ASSESSMENT TOOLS

In recent years, the scientific community has paid more attention to the importance of postoperative pulmonary complications; the result has been the generation of practical risk assessment tools.

In 2000 and 2001, using a large administrative database and multivariate analysis, Arozullah and colleagues published risk indices for the quantification of postoperative respiratory failure and pneumonia risk. These indices allow a clinician to estimate a patient's perioperative pulmonary risk (**Table 55-5**). A similar risk index was later updated and revalidated for respiratory failure in general and vascular surgery patients. However, this index included some elements less familiar to the average hospitalist (ie, surgical work relative value units and wound classification) and was too complicated for use in daily clinical practice.

The American College of Physicians has also developed clinical guidelines for perioperative pulmonary risk assessment and reduction for patients undergoing noncardiothoracic surgery. Based on a systematic review of the available literature up to 2006, these guidelines corroborated previous risk indices and provide a valuable resource for performing an evidence-based preoperative evaluation.

PERIOPERATIVE PULMONARY RISK REDUCTION STRATEGIES

PREOPERATIVE SMOKING CESSATION

While smoking cessation is always a worthy agenda, its benefit before noncardiothoracic surgery is unclear. Studies investigating the impact of preoperative smoking cessation have shown variable results. Unexpectedly, most have shown no benefit of preoperative smoking cessation, and some have even suggested an increased risk of postoperative pneumonia and respiratory failure when smoking cessation occurred within eight weeks of surgery. The basis for this observation is not certain but may be the result of an increase in sputum production often seen in the first one to two months after successful cigarette cessation. While this remains a subject of inquiry, for now, smoking cessation should be considered primarily for long-term risk reduction rather than perioperative risk reduction.

ANESTHETIC AND ANALGESIC TECHNIQUES

Anesthesia considerations remain the purview of anesthesiology, but it is important for Hospital Medicine practitioners to understand potential risk reduction strategies related to anesthetic and analgesic techniques. Previous studies have shown that avoidance of long-acting neuromuscular blockade medications (pancuronium) can reduce the risk of postoperative pulmonary complications. Additionally, recent studies have strengthened the evidence that use of postoperative epidural anesthesia reduces the risk of postoperative respiratory failure, especially in abdominal aortic and coronary revascularization surgery. Data supporting the use of neuraxial (epidural or spinal) anesthesia as a risk reduction modality remain less convincing.

LAPAROSCOPIC SURGICAL APPROACH

Similar to anesthetic choices, the selection of laparoscopic versus open surgery is typically outside the scope of practice of Hospital Medicine practitioners. However, the hospitalist should advise the surgical team of a patient's pulmonary risk so that it can be part of the decision-making process. The available evidence is mixed, but some studies suggest lower rates of postoperative pulmonary complications for laparoscopic, rather than open, abdominal surgery. This may be particularly true after colorectal and bariatric surgery. When possible, a laparoscopic approach is one potential strategy to reduce the risk of postoperative pulmonary complications.

LUNG EXPANSION TECHNIQUES

The largest body of evidence for a perioperative pulmonary risk reduction strategy is for lung expansion techniques. Incentive spirometry, intermittent positive pressure breathing, deep breathing exercises, and continuous positive airway pressure reduce the risk of postoperative pulmonary complications. None of these strategies has been shown to be superior to another. Given the minimal risk associated with these techniques, the American College of Physicians recommends that incentive spirometry or deep breathing exercises be used for all patients with increased pulmonary risk. In a

TABLE 55-5 Risk Indices for Predicting Postoperative Pneumonia and Respiratory Failure

Risk Factor	Pneumonia Risk Score	Respiratory Failure Risk Score
Type of Surgery		
AAA repair	15	27
Thoracic	14	21
Upper abdominal	10	14
Neck	8	11
Neurosurgery	8	14
Vascular surgery	3	14
Age		
≥80 years	17	6
70–79 years	13	
60–69 years	9	4
50–59 years	4	–
Functional Status		
Totally dependent	10	7
Partially dependent	6	
BUN		
<8 mg/dL	4	–
22–30 mg/dL	2	–
>30 mg/dL	3	8
Albumin <3 g/dL	–	9
Weight loss >10% within 6 months	7	–
Chronic steroid use	3	–
Emergency surgery	3	11
General anesthesia	4	–
Alcohol use (>2 drinks/day within 2 weeks)	2	–
COPD history	5	6
Smoker within 1 year	3	–
Impaired sensorium	4	–
CVA history	4	–
Preoperative transfusion (>4 units)	3	–

Risk Class	Pneumonia Risk Score	Probability of Pneumonia	Respiratory Failure Risk Score	Probability of Respiratory Failure
1	0–15	0.2%	0–10	0.5%
2	16–25	1.2%	11–19	2.2%
3	26–40	4.0%	20–27	5.0%
4	41–55	9.4%	28–40	11.6%
5	>55	15.3%	>40	30.5%

BUN, blood urea nitrogen; COPD, chronic obstructive pulmonary disease; CVA, cerebral vascular accident.

Reprinted, with permission, from Arozullah AM, Conde MV, Lawrence VA. Preoperative evaluation for postoperative pulmonary complications. *Medical Clinics of North America.* 2003;87(1):158–159.

subsequent report, an intensive program of preoperative inspiratory muscle training significantly reduced pulmonary complication rates after coronary bypass surgery.

SELECTIVE NASOGASTRIC DECOMPRESSION

The American College of Physicians also recommends the use of NG tubes only as needed for postoperative nausea or vomiting, oral intake intolerance, or symptomatic abdominal distention. This recommendation results from observations that routine, rather than selective, NG decompression following abdominal surgery led to increased rates of pneumonia and atelectasis.

CONCLUSION

Postoperative pulmonary complications are an underrecognized source of significant surgical morbidity and mortality. Estimation of pulmonary risk is an essential part of the preoperative evaluation and includes assessment of both patient- and procedure-related risk factors. Most risk factors are not modifiable, but the preoperative pulmonary evaluation provides an accurate estimation of risk for patients and physicians that improves informed decision making. Moreover, identification of high-risk patients can heighten postoperative vigilance for respiratory failure and pneumonia and lead to the use of those strategies proven to reduce risk.

PRACTICE POINT

Why preoperative pulmonary evaluation matters

Most of the risk factors for postoperative pulmonary complications are nonmodifiable, and many of the available risk reduction strategies are either beyond the responsibility of the primary care physician/hospitalist (choice of anesthesia and surgical approach) or routinely utilized (incentive spirometry and deep breathing exercises). Thus preoperative pulmonary evaluation can be undervalued. However, identification of patients at increased pulmonary risk remains critical for the following reasons:

- Communication of increased pulmonary risk to the anesthesiologist and surgical team prompts consideration of risk reduction strategies under their control.
- Modification of the postoperative care unit team's triage decisions. For example, after a surgery that would usually be done as an outpatient, a high-risk patient may be admitted for extended observation.
- Heightened postoperative vigilance for respiratory problems. Specific examples of effects on management include the following:
  - Lower threshold for initiating workup for pneumonia in setting of postoperative fever (which would otherwise be attributed to benign, expected postoperative fever).
  - Admission to unit specializing in respiratory care or mobilization of respiratory therapy resources beyond the traditional scope.
  - Lower threshold for treatment of postoperative pneumonia when chest radiographs are equivocal.

SUGGESTED READINGS

Arozullah AM, Daley J, Henderson WG, Khuri SF. Multifactorial risk index for predicting postoperative respiratory failure in med after major noncardiac surgery. The National Veterans Administration Surgical Quality Improvement Program. *Ann Surg.* 2000;232: 242–253.

Arozullah AM, Khuri SF, Henderson WG, Daley J. Development and validation of a multifactorial risk index for predicting postoperative pneumonia after major noncardiac surgery. *Ann Intern Med.* 2001;135:847–857.

Chung F, Yegneswaran B, Liao P, et al. Validation of the Berlin questionnaire and American Society of Anesthesiologists checklist as screening tools for obstructive sleep apnea in surgical patients. *Anesthesiology.* 2008;108(5):822–830.

Hulzebos EHJ, Helders PJM, Favié NJ, De Bie RA, de la Riviere AB, Van Meeteren NLU. Preoperative intensive inspiratory muscle training to prevent postoperative pulmonary complications in high-risk patients undergoing CABG surgery. *JAMA.* 2006;296: 1851–1857.

Johnson RG, Arozullah AM, Neumayer L, Henderson WG, Hosokawa P, Khuri SF. Multivariable predictors of postoperative respiratory failure after general and vascular surgery: results from the Patient Safety in Surgery Study. *J Am Coll Surg.* 2007;204:1188–1198.

Lawrence VA, Cornell JE, Smetana GW. Strategies to reduce postoperative pulmonary complications after noncardiothoracic surgery: systematic review for the American College of Physicians. *Ann Intern Med.* 2006;144:595–608.

Leung JM, Dzankic S. Relative importance of preoperative health status versus intraoperative factors in predicting postoperative adverse outcomes in geriatric surgical patients. *J Am Geriatr Soc.* 2001;49:1080–1085.

Liu SS, Wu CL. Effect of postoperative analgesia on major postoperative complications: a systematic update of the evidence. *Anesth Analg.* 2007;104(3):689–702.

Qaseem A, Snow V, Fitterman N, et al. Risk assessment for and strategies to reduce perioperative pulmonary complications for patients undergoing noncardiothoracic surgery: a guideline from the American College of Physicians. *Ann Intern Med.* 2006;144(8):575–580.

Smetana GW, Lawrence VA, Cornell JE. Preoperative pulmonary risk stratification for noncardiothoracic surgery: systematic review for the American College of Physicians. *Ann Intern Med.* 2006;144: 581–595.

CHAPTER 56

Management of Postoperative Pulmonary Complications

William I. Levin, MD
John J. Reilly Jr., MD

INTRODUCTION

General internists practicing in the inpatient setting are frequently called upon to provide perioperative care to a broad spectrum of surgical patients, in either a consultative or a comanagement role. Although historically much emphasis has been placed on postoperative cardiac complications, postoperative pulmonary complications are known to occur with equal frequency. The Confederate general, Thomas "Stonewall" Jackson, wounded in the Battle of Chancellorsville in 1863, was perhaps the earliest recorded victim of a postoperative pulmonary complication, dying of pneumonia eight days after the successful amputation of his left arm. Postoperative pulmonary complications contribute significantly to morbidity, mortality, and health care costs. It is estimated that over 1 million patients undergoing nonthoracic surgery in the United States annually experience postoperative pulmonary complications. Pulmonary complications produce the highest attributable costs among common categories of postoperative complications and can result in a fivefold increase in the median cost of an operation. The presence of pulmonary complications after major surgery increased 30-day mortality from 2% to 22%, and 1-year mortality from 8.7% to 45.9% based on data from the National Surgical Quality Improvement Program (NSQIP). The most important postoperative pulmonary complications are atelectasis, pneumonia, respiratory failure, and exacerbation of underlying chronic lung disease, although earlier studies have also included transient and self-limited clinical findings. A general principle is that the closer the operative site is to the diaphragm, the higher the likelihood of postoperative pulmonary complications. Interventions to reduce the incidence of these complications depend on the aggressive application of preventive measures to high-risk patients. A recent systematic review characterized patient-related and procedure-related risk factors and provided evidence-based guidelines on preventive strategies.[1] This chapter focuses on the pathogenesis, early recognition, and evidence-based treatment of common postoperative pulmonary complications.

PRACTICE POINT

- A general principle is that the closer the operative site is to the diaphragm, the higher the likelihood of postoperative pulmonary complications.

ATELECTASIS

Atelectasis, or reversible alveolar collapse, is a common perioperative phenomenon and occurs in 90% of patients receiving general anesthesia. Computed tomographic (CT) studies have demonstrated collapse of 15–20% of the lung volume near the diaphragm. Dr. William Pasteur, a Swiss physician practicing in England in the early part of the last century, wrote extensively on the postoperative lung and noted, "when the true history of postoperative lung complications comes to be written, active collapse of the lung from deficiency of inspiratory power will be found to occupy an important position among determining causes." Most atelectasis appearing during general anesthesia resolves within 24 hours after surgery in normal subjects and is of little clinical significance. Atelectasis can persist for two days or longer after major surgery, including abdominal and thoracic surgery, and is thought to represent the starting point in a cascade of events that leads to the more serious complications of pneumonia and acute respiratory failure.

PATHOPHYSIOLOGY

The formation of perioperative atelectasis can be understood by considering the effect of surgery on normal respiratory mechanics as well as the mechanisms involved in alveolar collapse. The induction of anesthesia alters the distribution and timing of neural drive to the respiratory muscles, interfering with coordination of activity. The supine position and use of positive pressure ventilation alter the distribution of ventilation and lead to hypoventilation of dependent areas. Surgical trauma can produce reflex inhibition of the phrenic nerve from stimulation of the viscera, mechanical disruption of the intercostal or abdominal respiratory muscles, and voluntary limitation of respiratory motion from postoperative pain. The characteristic postoperative mechanical abnormality is a restrictive pattern with severely reduced inspiratory capacity, vital capacity (VC), and functional residual capacity (FRC), clinically demonstrated by rapid shallow respirations.

Pulmonary atelectasis occurs by three mechanisms: compression atelectasis, absorption (resorption) atelectasis, and loss of surfactant. Compression atelectasis results when the transmural pressure distending the alveolus is reduced, allowing the alveolus to collapse. During anesthesia, change in diaphragmatic function and chest geometry causes pressure from the abdomen to be transmitted into the thorax, resulting in compression of lung tissue. Resorption atelectasis describes collapse of alveoli related to absorption of gas from occluded or hypoventilated areas of the lung. Since oxygen is absorbed more rapidly than nitrogen, air with high inspired FiO_2 will be absorbed more rapidly, resulting in collapse. Surfactant function, important in stabilizing the alveoli, may be disrupted by anesthesia and mechanical ventilation. The physiologic consequence is ventilation-perfusion (V/Q) mismatch resulting in hypoxemia.

DIAGNOSIS—DOES THIS PATIENT HAVE ATELECTASIS?

Atelectasis is recognized by the finding of hypoxemia in an appropriate clinical scenario in the absence of other plausible diagnoses. The patient demonstrates dyspnea or tachypnea, and physical findings can include basilar rales and decreased breath sounds in the affected area. Atelectasis is often cited as a cause of postoperative fevers, but studies have demonstrated no association between atelectasis and fever and suggest that early postoperative fevers are more likely due to the inflammatory response to surgery.[2] Atelectasis is detected radiographically by opacification of a lobe or lobar segment and evidence of volume loss. The most reliable sign is displacement of the interlobar fissure, but other signs include elevation of the hemidiaphragm, mediastinal shift, and compensatory overinflation of adjacent aerated segments. There may be linear opacities ("plate-like") in the parenchyma in dependent portions of the lungs. Silhouette sign can be positive, with obliteration of adjacent boundaries. Posteroanterior (PA) and lateral images of the chest are preferred, and the ability of plain radiographs to detect atelectasis in recumbent critically ill patients is less certain. CT is sensitive in detecting areas of collapse, and may also reveal other pathology.

TREATMENT

Treatment of postoperative atelectasis centers on lung expansion techniques, shifting from supine position when possible, and adequate postoperative analgesia. The FRC has been identified as the single most important postoperative lung volume parameter, and efforts to restore normal pulmonary mechanics are beneficial. A simple posture change from supine to seated will increase FRC by 0.5 to 1.0 liters. Standing and early ambulation are also helpful when tolerated.

The goal of lung expansion maneuvers is to produce a large and sustained increase in transpulmonary pressure that distends the lung and reexpands the collapsed lung units. Techniques include incentive spirometry, deep breathing exercises, chest physical therapy, intermittent positive-pressure breathing (IPPB), and continuous positive airway pressure (CPAP). A recent systematic review found that for patients undergoing abdominal surgery, any type of lung expansion intervention improved outcome, with no one modality being superior. Incentive spirometry was the least labor intensive. IPPB is the most costly and was associated with unacceptable abdominal distension in a significant number of cases. CPAP is beneficial for patients unable to participate in incentive spirometry or deep breathing exercises. Another systematic review also found evidence that use of CPAP in patients undergoing abdominal surgery led to lower rates of postoperative atelectasis and pneumonia.

The effect of different types of analgesia in decreasing postoperative atelectasis has been examined. Studies have been heterogeneous and small, but a recent meta-analysis found a trend toward decreased postoperative atelectasis and pneumonia with the use of postoperative epidural analgesia in patients undergoing abdominal surgery. Postoperative epidural and patient-controlled intravenous analgesia both seem superior to on-demand delivery of opioids in preventing postoperative pulmonary complications. The potential benefit of epidural anesthesia must be weighed against bleeding risk from deep vein thrombosis (DVT) prophylaxis.

PRACTICE POINT

- Postoperative epidural and patient-controlled intravenous analgesia both seem superior to on-demand delivery of opioids in preventing postoperative pulmonary complications. The potential benefit of epidural anesthesia must be weighed against bleeding risk from DVT prophylaxis.

COMPLICATIONS

Mild hypoxemia from atelectasis is usually well tolerated, but more severe hypoxemia can affect end organs. Atelectasis itself may cause mild acute lung injury. Left untreated, atelectasis likely predisposes to the development of pneumonia and potentially respiratory failure.

POSTOPERATIVE PNEUMONIA

Pneumonia ranks as the third most common postoperative infection behind urinary tract infection (UTI) and wound infection. The incidence of pneumonia following major abdominal surgery ranges between 2% and 19% and is a principal factor in increased mortality. Development of hospital-acquired pneumonia is associated with a 30–50% increased risk of developing acute respiratory failure requiring mechanical ventilation and increases hospital stays by an average of 7–9 days at an excess cost of $40,000 per patient.

Postoperative pneumonia is a subset of hospital-acquired pneumonia (HAP), which is pneumonia occurring 48 hours or more after admission and not incubating at the time of admission. The major early management goal for postoperative pneumonia is to provide appropriate antibiotics in adequate doses based on the best prediction of suspected pathogens and resistance pattern.

The timing of onset of HAP is an important epidemiologic variable. Early-onset HAP, less than five days into admission, is more likely to be caused by antibiotic-sensitive bacteria unless other risk factors for multidrug-resistant (MDR) pathogens are present. Late-onset HAP, five or more days after admission, is more likely to be associated with MDR pathogens. Additional risk factors for MDR pathogens include acute care hospitalization for two or more days or antimicrobial

TABLE 56-1 Risk Factors for Multidrug-Resistant Pathogens

Antimicrobial therapy in the preceding 90 days
Current hospitalization of 5 days or more
High frequency of antibiotic resistance in the community
Presence of risk factors for health care-associated pneumonia (HCAP)
Hospitalization for 2 days or more in the preceding 90 days
Residence in a nursing home or extended care facility
Home infusion therapy
Chronic dialysis within 30 days
Home wound care
Family member with multidrug-resistant pathogen
Immunosuppressive disease and/or therapy

therapy within the preceding 90 days, nursing home or long-term care facility residence, home infusion therapy, chronic dialysis, wound care, family member with an MDR pathogen, and immunosuppression (**Table 56-1**). Hospital- and unit-specific microbiologic data are also very important in selecting appropriate treatment.

PRACTICE POINT

The timing of onset of HAP is an important epidemiologic variable.

- Early onset HAP, less than five days into admission, is more likely to be caused by antibiotic-sensitive bacteria unless other risk factors for multidrug-resistant pathogens (MDR) are present.
- Late onset HAP, five or more days after admission, is more likely to be associated with multidrug-resistant (MDR) pathogens.

The recent American Thoracic Society/Infectious Diseases Society of America (ATS/IDSA) guideline emphasizes ventilator-associated pneumonia (VAP) because it is more readily studied, but suggests it is reasonable to extrapolate the conclusions regarding risk factors for infection with specific pathogens to nonintubated, nonventilated HAP patients.

PATHOPHYSIOLOGY

The sequence of events in HAP begins with colonization of the oropharynx with pathogens, which can occur within 48 hours of admission. Sources of pathogens include contaminated health care devices, the environment, and transfer from other patients or staff. These pathogens must be aspirated from the oropharynx into the lower respiratory tract, and then overwhelm the natural host defense mechanisms. Microaspiration is known to occur in up to 45% of healthy subjects during sleep and can be worsened in postsurgical patients by decreased gag reflex, ineffective coughing, sedation, supine posture, especially during enteral feeds, and routine (rather than selective) use of nasogastric (NG) tubes. The host defenses are also affected in multiple ways by general anesthesia, including mechanical impairment of normal mucociliary transport and interference with function of alveolar inflammatory cells, including polymorphonuclear leukocytes, macrophages, lymphocytes, cytokines, antibodies, and complement.

The microbiology of early-onset HAP without MDR risk factors tends to mirror community-acquired pneumonia and includes *Streptococcus pneumoniae*, *Haemophilus influenzae*, methicillin-sensitive *Staphylococcus aureus*, and antibiotic-sensitive Enterobacteriaceae (**Table 56-2**). Pathogens in late-onset HAP or the presence of MDR risk factors also include methicillin-resistant *S aureus* (MRSA), *Pseudomonas aeruginosa*, extended-spectrum beta-lactamase (ESBL) -producing *Klebsiella*, and *Acinetobacter baumannii* (**Table 56-3**).

TABLE 56-2 Early-Onset Hospital-Acquired Pneumonia Without MDR Risk Factors

Potential Pathogen	Recommended Antibiotic
Streptococcus pneumoniae	Ceftriaxone
Haemophilus influenzae	or
Methicillin-sensitive *Staphylococcus aureus*	Levofloxacin, moxifloxacin, or ciprofloxacin
Antibiotic-sensitive enteric gram-negative bacilli	or
	Ampicillin/sulbactam
Escherichia coli	or
Klebsiella pneumoniae	Ertapenem
Enterobacter species	
Proteus species	
Serratia marcescens	

DIAGNOSIS—DOES THIS PATIENT HAVE POSTOPERATIVE PNEUMONIA?

The goal of diagnosis is to identify which patients have a pulmonary infection so that antibiotics are not delayed but that patients with noninfectious etiologies are not exposed unnecessarily to the antibiotics. All patients should undergo a comprehensive history and physical exam, chest X-ray (preferably PA and lateral), measurement of arterial O_2 saturation, complete blood count (CBC), electrolytes, liver function tests, and blood cultures. All ventilated patients should

TABLE 56-3 Late-Onset Hospital-Acquired Pneumonia or HAP with MDR Risk Factors

Potential Pathogens	Recommended Antibiotic Combination
Streptococcus pneumoniae	Antipseudomonal cephalosporin (cefepime, ceftazidime)
Haemophilus influenzae	or
Methicillin-sensitive *Staphylococcus aureus*	Antipseudomonal carbapenem (imipenem or meropenem)
Antibiotic-sensitive enteric gram-negative bacilli	or
Escherichia coli	Beta-lactam/beta-lactamase inhibitor (piperacillin-tazobactam)
Klebsiella pneumoniae	
Enterobacter species	
Proteus species	
Serratia marcescens	plus
Plus	Antipseudomonal fluoroquinolone (ciprofloxacin or levofloxacin)
Pseudomonas aeruginosa	
Klebsiella pneumoniae (ESBL)	
Acinetobacter species	or
Methicillin-resistant *Staphylococcus aureus*	Aminoglycoside (Amikacin, gentamicin, or tobramycin)
	plus
	Linezolid or vancomycin

TABLE 56-4 Centers for Disease Control and Prevention Criteria for Diagnosis of Nosocomial Pneumonia

Radiology	Signs/Symptoms/Laboratory
Two or more serial chest X-rays with at least one of the following:	At least one of the following:
New or progressive infiltrate	Fever (> 38°C) with no other source
Consolidation	Leukopenia (< 4000 WBC/µL) or leukocytosis (> 12,000 WBC/µL)
Cavitation	Mental status changes with no other cause in adult > 70 years old
	And at least two of the following:
	New onset of purulent sputum
	New-onset cough, dyspnea, tachycardia
	Rales or bronchial breath sounds (BS)
	Worsening gas exchange

have lower respiratory cultures obtained, ideally prior to starting antibiotics, to guide deescalation of therapy. Other processes that produce similar symptoms including congestive heart failure, atelectasis, pulmonary thromboembolism, drug reactions, pulmonary hemorrhage, and acute respiratory distress syndrome (ARDS) need to be considered.

The Centers for Disease Control and Prevention (CDC) criteria for diagnosis of nosocomial pneumonia in adults require radiologic as well as clinical and laboratory findings (**Table 56-4**). The recent ATS/IDSA guideline describes two diagnostic approaches to HAP: clinical and bacteriologic. The clinical approach bases the diagnosis on a new infiltrate on chest X-ray plus clinical evidence of infection. The bacteriologic strategy is based on lower respiratory tract samples and is more suited to ventilated patients where there is ready access to the lower respiratory tract. The presence of a new or progressive radiographic infiltrate plus two of three clinical features (fever, leukopenia or leukocytosis, and purulent secretions) yields a sensitivity of 69% with specificity of 75% and represents the most accurate clinical criteria for starting antibiotics.

PRACTICE POINT

- The presence of a new or progressive radiographic infiltrate plus two of three clinical features (fever as > 38°C, leukopenia or leukocytosis, and purulent secretions) yields a sensitivity of 69% with specificity of 75%, and represents the most accurate clinical criteria for starting antibiotics for HAP.

TREATMENT

Treatment strategies seek to balance the need to provide early, appropriate empiric antibiotic therapy with avoidance of excessive antibiotic exposure in both spectrum and duration. Delay in initiating appropriate antibiotics in VAP patients with severe sepsis has been shown to increase mortality, and initial inadequate drug selection, even when later adjusted, is also associated with worse outcome. Aggressive early therapy combined with deescalation of initial antibiotics based on clinical or microbiologic data is encouraged. Empiric drug selection takes into account the epidemiologic timing and presence of MDR risk factors, previous antibiotic exposure, and the institution-/unit-specific antibiogram.

For early-onset HAP without MDR risk factors, single-agent therapy is reasonable. Recommended agents include ampicillin/sulbactam, ceftriaxone, a fluoroquinolone, or ertepenem (see Table 56-2). For early-onset HAP with MDR risk factors or late-onset HAP, a three-drug regimen is recommended (see Table 56-3). This should include (1) an antipseudomonal cephalosporin (cefepime, ceftazidime) or antipseudomonal carbapenem (imipenem or meropenem) or piperacillin-tazobactam plus (2) an antipseudomonal fluoroquinolone or aminoglycoside plus (3) linezolid or vancomycin. Considerations in antibiotic selection might also include pharmacodynamic properties and mechanism of action. Fluoroquinolones and linezolid achieve high concentration in bronchial secretions. Aminoglycosides and fluoroquinolones are bactericidal in a concentration-dependent fashion, whereas vancomycin and beta-lactams are bactericidal in a time-dependent fashion. Aminoglycosides and the quinolones also have a postantibiotic effect and suppress antibiotic growth even after concentrations fall.

The patient should be reevaluated in 48–72 hours, and antibiotics narrowed or discontinued based on culture results and clinical response. Therapy lasting seven to eight days has been shown to be equally effective to longer courses in patients receiving an appropriate initial antibiotic regimen with a good clinical response. *Pseudomonas* and MRSA are the exception due to significant rates of recurrence and should still be treated with a longer course of antibiotics.

COMPLICATIONS

Patients who fail to respond or worsen should be reevaluated at 48–72 hours. Possible reasons for lack of response include the presence of a complication (empyema, lung abscess, drug fever), an alternate site of infection (*Clostridium difficile* colitis, line-related infection), wrong diagnosis (atelectasis, pulmonary embolism (PE), ARDS, pulmonary hemorrhage, neoplasm), or wrong organism (clinically unrecognized immunosuppression).

RESPIRATORY FAILURE

Acute respiratory failure is defined as the requirement for mechanical ventilation longer than 48 hours postoperatively or unplanned reintubation for cardiac or respiratory failure. It can be considered the most severe of the clinically significant postoperative pulmonary complications based on its impact on morbidity, mortality, and cost. Mortality data from the Department of Veterans Affairs National Surgical Quality Improvement Program showed an increase in 30-day mortality from 2.3% to 29.1% in patients with respiratory failure, and an increase in 1-year mortality from 9.3% to 55.9%. Another study found the rate of postoperative respiratory failure in patients undergoing general and vascular surgery to be 3%, with 30-day mortality of 26.5%. Pulmonary complications raised median hospital costs to $62,704 compared to $5,015 when the complications were absent, more expensive than thromboembolic, cardiovascular, or infectious complications.

PATHOPHYSIOLOGY

Postoperative acute respiratory failure results from the onset over minutes to hours of impaired pulmonary gas exchange severe enough to cause organ dysfunction or to threaten life. Respiratory failure can be broadly categorized as hypoxemic respiratory failure (respiratory insufficiency) or hypercapnic respiratory failure (ventilatory failure), and the two forms may coexist. Mechanisms underlying hypoxemic respiratory failure, defined as an arterial pO_2 of less than 60 mm Hg, include decreased FiO_2, hypoventilation, impaired diffusion, V/Q mismatch, and right-to-left shunt. Most hypoxemic hospitalized patients have some combination of V/Q mismatch and right-to-left shunt. A structural-anatomic classification that localizes the primary pathology to the alveoli, interstitium, cardiopulmonary vasculature, airways, or pleura may be helpful when trying to make a specific diagnosis. In the postoperative patient, the alveoli and interstitium can be affected by pulmonary edema, acute lung injury/ARDS, atelectasis, and pneumonia. The vasculature can be affected by pulmonary embolism or develop pulmonary hypertension due to hypoxic vasoconstriction and/or elevated left atrial pressures. The airways can be affected by exacerbations of COPD, asthma, and mucous plugging, and the pleura may be affected by pneumothorax or pleural effusion.

Hypercapnic respiratory failure, characterized by a pCO_2 greater than 45 mm Hg and respiratory acidosis, can be classified as drive failure or pump failure. Drive failure results when the patient's ventilatory effort is insufficient and can be caused by drug overdoses, general anesthesia, central nervous system (CNS) disease, and obesity hypoventilation syndrome. The most common contributors in the perioperative setting are residual sedation from general anesthesia or the effects of opioid analgesics on respiratory drive and level of consciousness. Pump failure results when ventilatory demand exceeds the patient's capability and can be caused by prolonged effect of neuromuscular blocking agents, underlying neuromuscular disorders, electrolyte abnormalities and metabolic disturbances, pleural disorders, chest wall abnormalities, and respiratory muscle fatigue. It can be aggravated by increased CO_2 production in the setting of a hypermetabolic postoperative state; this is especially true in patients with underlying loss of parenchyma (emphysema) who have a decreased alveolar surface area available for gas exchange.

DIAGNOSIS—WHAT IS CAUSING THIS PATIENT'S RESPIRATORY FAILURE?

Diagnostic workup should begin with the ABCs—airway, breathing, and circulation—and treatment initiated concurrently. Supplemental oxygen should be provided and intravenous (IV) access obtained, as well as cardiac monitoring and pulse oximetry. A focused history and physical exam will yield clues to the presence or absence of underlying cardiac and pulmonary disease. The hypoxemic respiratory failure patient will appear tachypneic and tachycardic, perhaps with central cyanosis. The hypercapnic respiratory failure with decreased ventilatory drive will appear hypopnic or apneic, in no respiratory distress. The ventilatory pump failure patient will appear in respiratory distress with rapid shallow ineffective respirations. All patients should receive a chest X-ray, electrocardiogram (ECG), and routine bloodwork including CBC and serum chemistries. An arterial blood gas should be obtained in order to calculate an A–a gradient, establish whether ventilatory failure is present, and determine acid–base status. Further diagnostic workup will be guided by the results of these initial studies. If the etiology is not apparent on initial evaluation, further testing might include CT angiography of the chest and echocardiography.

TREATMENT

The goal for management of acute postoperative respiratory failure is to quickly and correctly identify the underlying pathophysiologic process and provide targeted treatment that will avoid the need for intubation and mechanical ventilation. Hypoxemic respiratory failure has a broad differential diagnosis, and initial supportive care should be followed by treatment of the specific disease process identified. Pneumonia or other infection should be treated with prompt initiation of appropriate antibiotics after obtaining cultures. Volume overload and pulmonary edema can be treated with diuretics and additional cardiac evaluation. Bronchospasm should be aggressively treated with inhaled beta-agonists and anticholinergics with systemic corticosteroids as indicated. Suspected pulmonary embolism should be expeditiously evaluated and treated as the postoperative conditions allow.

TABLE 56-5 Noninvasive Ventilation—Indications and Contraindications

Indications	Contraindications
Clinical observations • Moderate to severe dyspnea • Tachypnea (> 24 for hypercapnic, > 30 for hypoxemic) • Accessory muscle use or abdominal paradox	Absolute • Respiratory arrest • Unable to fit mask
Gas exchange • Acute ventilatory failure: $PaCO_2$ > 45 mm Hg, pH < 7.35 • Hypoxemia: PaO_2/FiO_2 < 200	Relative • Medically unstable • Unable to protect airway • Excessive secretions • Agitated, uncooperative • Recent upper gastrointestinal or airway surgery • Multiple-organ failure

With hypercapnic respiratory failure, the most common cause of insufficient ventilatory drive is medication effect. Opioids are the most potent suppressor of both hypoxic and hypercapnic ventilatory drive, but other sedatives and hypnotics also cause respiratory depression. Respiratory arrest, inability to protect the airway, and severe respiratory acidosis mandate intubation. COPD exacerbation can also lead to respiratory muscle fatigue and can be treated with noninvasive positive pressure ventilation (NPPV).

The use of noninvasive mechanical ventilation to treat acute respiratory failure has recently been reviewed. When effective, it has been shown to decrease the need for intubation, the rate of complications, and the intensive care unit (ICU) length of stay. NPPV is indicated when there is a demonstrated need for ventilatory support and no contraindications (**Table 56-5**). There is level 1 evidence to support the use of NPPV in COPD exacerbations, cardiogenic pulmonary edema, weaning from ventilator in COPD, and immunosuppressed patients. There is level 2 evidence to support its use in postoperative respiratory failure, community-acquired pneumonia with COPD, asthma, extubation failure, and in do-not-intubate-status patients (**Table 56-6**). Indications include moderate to severe dyspnea, tachypnea > 24 breaths per minute, use of accessory muscles with abdominal paradox, pCO_2 > 45 with pH < 7.35, and hypoxemia. Contraindications include respiratory arrest, inability to tolerate/fit mask, medically unstable, uncooperative, unable to protect airway, excessive secretions, multiple organ failures, and recent upper airway or upper gastrointestinal (GI) surgery. Noninvasive ventilation (NIV) should be initiated early when indicated to take advantage of a therapeutic window of opportunity. Improvement is expected over the first one to two hours. If hypoxemia persists, then there may be a concomitant complication such as aspiration or pneumonia. After initial stabilization, a decision should be made regarding appropriate level of care. Determinants of this will include ability to manage the airway, method of oxygen delivery to maintain adequate O_2 status, and the intensity of nursing care required. Intubation should not be delayed in patients who fail an NIV trial.

COMPLICATIONS

Complications of postoperative respiratory failure include increased risks related to intubation, ventilator-induced acute lung injury progressing to ARDS, VAP, GI bleeding, and DVT.

TABLE 56-6 Evidence-based Medicine: Key References for Postoperative Pulmonary Complications

Study	Methodology	Results	Limitations	Bottom Line
Squadrone V, et al. Continuous positive airway pressure for treatment of postoperative hypoxemia. *JAMA.* 2005;293:589–595.	Multicenter, prospective, randomized clinical trial to compare the efficacy of CPAP with standard oxygen therapy in the treatment of postoperative hypoxemia	1332 patients enrolled; 209 underwent randomization; 10 patients in the control group and one patient in the CPAP group required intubation ($P = .005$)	Study included only patients suspected of atelectasis	Compared to standard treatment, early use of CPAP decreased the incidence of endotracheal intubation and other complications in patients with postoperative hypoxemia after major abdominal surgery.
Chastre J, et al. Comparison of eight versus 15 days of antibiotic therapy for ventilator-associated pneumonia in adults. *JAMA.* 2003;290: 2588–2598.	Randomized, double-blind trial to compare the outcomes of therapy with an 8-day or 15-day antibiotic regimen for a group of ICU patients with VAP	402 patients enrolled; no statistically significant benefit in outcome measures from prolonging antibiotics to 15 days	Trial was only double blinded through the first week of the study; a large subset of ICU patients were excluded from the study	For ICU patients who developed microbiologically proven VAP, no clinical advantage of prolonging antimicrobial therapy from 8 to 15 days. Exceptions include immunocompromised patients, those with inappropriate initial antibiotics, and those with a nonfermenting gram-negative bacillus
Ibrahim EH, et al. Experience with a clinical guideline for the treatment of ventilator-associated pneumonia. *Crit Care Med.* 2001;29: 1109–1115.	Prospective before and after study to determine if the implementation of a clinical guideline could increase adequacy of initial antimicrobial treatment in patients with VAP	102 consecutive patients with VAP prospectively evaluated; after the intervention there was an increase in adequate antibiotic prescribing, decrease in duration of treatment	Performed in a single MICU; small sample size	A simple guideline can increase the administration of adequate antibiotic therapy for VAP and decrease the duration of treatment without affecting mortality or length of stay
Taylor S, et al. Postoperative day one: a high risk period for respiratory events. *Am J Surg.* 2005;190:752–756.	Retrospective case-control analysis of inpatients having a narcotic-related respiratory event compared with controls	62 patients with narcotic-related respiratory events were compared with 62 controls; 77.4% occurred in the first 24 hours after surgery	Small sample size; more women were enrolled in the study	The first 24 hours after surgery represent a high-risk period for respiratory events caused by narcotics

CPAP, continuous positive airway pressure; ICU, intensive care unit; MICU, medical intensive care unit; VAP, ventilator-associated pneumonia.

COPD EXACERBATION

Patients with COPD have an elevated risk of developing postoperative pulmonary complications, including an exacerbation of obstructive lung disease. Ideally these patients will have had good preoperative risk assessment, with optimization of medical management and initiation of preventive measures such as lung expansion maneuvers and smoking cessation four or more weeks prior to the procedure (when applicable). Postoperative management consists of continuing the preventive measures as well as maintenance of home medications. Patients with COPD have a higher prevalence of comorbid conditions such as congestive heart failure and coronary artery disease (CAD), so they must be carefully evaluated should they become short of breath. There is also a high rate of concomitant PE with COPD, up to 20%, so this also needs to be ruled out.

PATHOPHYSIOLOGY

A COPD exacerbation is defined as an event in the natural course of the disease characterized by a change in the patient's baseline dyspnea, cough, and/or sputum that is beyond normal day to day variations, is acute in onset, and may warrant a change in regular medication in a patient with underlying COPD. Exacerbations are thought to be an inflammatory event, and the airway manifestations include edema, bronchospasm, and increased sputum production. Exacerbations are heterogeneous events caused by complex interactions between the host, respiratory viruses, airway bacteria, and environmental pollution, but in approximately one-third no cause is identified. Hyperinflation and bronchospasm lead to increased work of breathing. Progressive hypoxemia develops, producing a downward spiral that can progress to acute ventilatory failure when the respiratory muscles fatigue. COPD is associated with other comorbid conditions, including ischemic heart disease (HD), pneumonia, and diabetes mellitus (DM), as well as venous thromboembolism (VTE), and one of these can contribute.

DIAGNOSIS—DOES THIS PATIENT HAVE A POSTOPERATIVE EXACERBATION OF COPD?

Typical symptoms include increased breathlessness accompanied by wheezing and chest tightness, increased cough and sputum production, change in color and tenacity of sputum, and fever. Routine evaluation should include chest X-ray, routine labs, arterial blood gas, and ECG to differentiate COPD from other causes given the frequent comorbidities.

TREATMENT

Treatment of postoperative COPD exacerbation does not differ from typical treatment, except that other medical complications prevalent in the postoperative period, including PE and congestive heart failure, need to be carefully considered. Lung function can be optimized with inhaled short-acting beta-adrenergic and anticholinergic agents along with systemic glucocorticoids. A short course of antibiotics may decrease duration of exacerbation. There is currently no role for methylxanthines or chest physical therapy (PT). NPPV is the preferred method of ventilatory support and has been shown to improve outcomes in COPD exacerbations. Invasive mechanical ventilation is reserved for patients who have not responded to NPPV.

PRACTICE POINT

- Treatment of postoperative COPD exacerbation does not differ from typical treatment, except that other medical complications prevalent in the postoperative period, including PE and CHF, need to be carefully considered.

COMPLICATIONS

Complications of COPD exacerbation include pneumonia, progression to acute respiratory failure, and pneumothorax.

QUALITY IMPROVEMENT

Hospitalists can have a significant impact on processes of care related to postoperative medical management. Internists, surgeons, and anesthesiologists should work collaboratively to see that high-risk patients are identified and consistently receive appropriate preventive interventions for pulmonary complications, including smoking cessation and incentive spirometry training prior to surgery. Hospitalists can also play a role in training unit personnel in the rationale and technique for these treatments, as well as early mobilization out of bed. Institution- and unit-specific protocols for empiric antibiotic selection can be developed taking into account microbiology, sensitivity patterns, and formulary to ensure high rates of initial appropriate antibiotic regimens. Hospitalists can also participate in review of quality indicators such as rate of nosocomial pneumonia and postoperative respiratory failure, and provide guidance on institutional initiatives to reduce numbers.

SUGGESTED READINGS

American Thoracic Society. Guidelines for the management of adults with hospital-acquired, ventilator-associated, and healthcare-associated pneumonia. *Am J Respir Crit Care Med.* 2005;171:388–416.

Duggan M, Kavanagh BP. Pulmonary atelectasis: a pathogenic perioperative entity. *Anesthesiology.* 2005;102:838–854.

Ferreyra G, Long Y, Ranieri VM. Respiratory complications after major surgery. *Curr Opin Crit Care.* 2009;15:342–348.

Global strategy for the diagnosis, management, and prevention of chronic obstructive pulmonary disease. GOLD Executive Summary. *Am J Respir Crit Care Med.* 2007;176:532–555.

Johnson RG, Arozullah AM, Neumayer L, Henderson WG, Hosokawa P, Khuri SF. Multi-variable predictors of postoperative respiratory failure after general and vascular surgery: results from the patient's safety in surgery study. *J Am Coll Surg.* 2007;204:1188–1198.

Kieninger AN, Lipsett PA. Hospital-acquired pneumonia: pathophysiology, diagnosis, and treatment. *Surg Clin N Am.* 2009;89:439–461.

Lawrence VA, Cornell JE, Smetana GW; American College of Physicians. Strategies to reduce postoperative pulmonary complications after non-cardiothoracic surgery: systematic review for the American College of Physicians. *Ann Intern Med.* 2006;144:596–608.

Magnusson L, Spahn DR. New concepts of atelectasis during general anaesthesia. *Br J Anaesth.* 2003;91:61–72.

Nava S, Hill N. Non-invasive ventilation in acute respiratory failure. *Lancet.* 2009;374:250–259.

Qaseem A, Snow V, Fitterman N, et al. Clinical Efficacy Assessment Subcommittee of the American College of Physicians. Risk assessment for and strategies to reduce perioperative pulmonary complications for patients undergoing noncardiothoracic surgery: a guideline from the American College of Physicians. *Ann Intern Med.* 2006;144:575–580.

REFERENCES

1. Smetana GW. Lawrence VA, Cornell JE. Preoperative Pulmonary Risk Stratification for Noncardiothoracic Surgery: Systematic Review for the American College of Physicians. *Ann Intern Med.* 2006;144:581–595.
2. Barone JE. Fever: Fact and fiction. *J Trauma.* 2009;67:406–409.

CHAPTER 57

Assessment and Management of the Renal Patient

Albert Q. Lam, MD
Julian L. Seifter, MD

INTRODUCTION

The kidneys are responsible for a number of vital homeostatic processes, including the excretion of nitrogenous waste products, the regulation of fluid volume and electrolytes, acid–base balance, and the production of hormones important for blood pressure regulation, erythropoiesis, and bone metabolism. They are frequently affected by disease, both acute (occurring over days to weeks) and chronic (occurring over months to years), and the prevalence and incidence of these disease processes in the United States and globally are rising. Acute kidney injury (AKI), formerly known as acute renal failure, has become an increasingly common cause of hospitalization with an incidence of 5–7% among hospitalized patients. Chronic kidney disease (CKD) reportedly affects 13% of adults in the United States[1] and is associated with significant morbidity, mortality, and high costs of hospitalization. Furthermore, the recent advent of automatic reporting of estimated glomerular filtration rate (eGFR) with serum creatinine by hospital laboratories has resulted in more patients being identified as having impaired renal function. In order to provide the highest level of care for patients presenting with acute or CKD, the clinician should have a strong understanding of the fundamental issues relevant to their evaluation and management.

EVALUATION OF THE RENAL PATIENT

HISTORY AND PHYSICAL EXAMINATION

The evaluation of the patient with kidney disease begins with a thorough history and physical examination. The clinician should identify early on whether the renal disease is an acute or chronic condition. If previous medical records are available for the patient, this can be determined by quickly reviewing prior laboratory testing, with particular attention given to serum creatinine, blood urea nitrogen, and urinalyses. Patients who present on admission with AKI should be questioned about recent symptoms (eg, vomiting, diarrhea, edema, difficulty voiding, decreased appetite, weight changes) and events (eg, changes in oral intake, new medications, history of nonsteroidal anti-inflammatory drug [NSAID] use, administration of intravenous contrast, recent colonoscopy) that may help narrow the differential diagnosis of AKI. The presence of symptoms such as fever, rashes, arthralgias, epistaxis, and hemoptysis may be suggestive of an underlying systemic disease process such as vasculitis or other inflammatory conditions. For patients who develop AKI during their hospitalization, a thorough review of the most recent hospital events—including episodes of hypotension, recent diagnostic and therapeutic procedures, and initiation of new medications—should be performed. All patients presenting with acute or CKD should be questioned about symptoms associated with uremia, including fatigue, nausea, vomiting, pruritus, metallic taste, lethargy, and confusion, since the presence of these symptoms may indicate the need for dialysis.

A past medical history should be elicited to identify a prior history of kidney disease or other systemic diseases that could be relevant to the current presentation. In patients with CKD, who may or may not be presenting with an acute kidney-related problem, the clinician should establish the underlying cause, chronicity, and severity of the kidney disease. If the patient has end-stage renal disease (ESRD), information about the patient's nephrologist, outpatient dialysis unit, and regular dialysis schedule (including the timing of the last dialysis session) should be obtained and conveyed to the clinicians and other health care providers who will be facilitating the patient's dialysis during the hospitalization. The clinician should also obtain a complete and current list of the patient's medications, which should include prescription medications as well as all over-the-counter medications, herbal remedies, and supplements. A family history of kidney disease or other systemic illnesses should also be documented.

The physical examination starts with a careful assessment of the patient's vital signs. The presence of a fever should always raise suspicion for an infection, particularly in dialysis patients or immunosuppressed patients, but can also be observed in the setting of acute kidney diseases such as acute glomerulonephritis, vasculitis, and allergic interstitial nephritis. Blood pressure may be elevated (eg, in acute nephritic syndrome, malignant hypertension, scleroderma, long-standing kidney disease), normal, or low (eg, in volume depletion, sepsis, cirrhosis, heart failure). The clinician should closely review the patient's intake and output records to (1) ensure that the proper oral and intravenous fluids, if needed, are being administered to the patient at an appropriate frequency and rate depending on the patient's clinical context, and (2) to evaluate the patient for evidence of positive or negative fluid balances that could contribute to volume overload or depletion, respectively.

Key aspects of the physical examination include (1) determination of the patient's volume status, (2) identification of physical manifestations that can be associated with specific renal disease conditions, and (3) assessment for signs of uremia. Assessment of volume status is important for both the accurate diagnosis and management of most renal diseases. In the setting of prerenal acute kidney injury, for instance, the presence of hypervolemia (eg, elevated jugular venous pressure, pulmonary congestion, peripheral edema) could be suggestive of decreased renal perfusion from congestive heart failure or cirrhosis, whereas the presence of hypovolemia (postural pulse increase >30 beats/min, severe postural dizziness, dry axilla and/or mucous membranes) would be more consistent with a diagnosis of volume depletion from bleeding or gastrointestinal losses. To best assess the jugular venous pulsation, the patient should be reclined with the head elevated at 30–45 degrees, and the elevation of the right internal jugular vein above the sternal angle should be measured. Certain physical findings (eg, edema, abdominal bruits, palpable purpura, warm and swollen joints) can be associated with specific renal diseases. Palpable purpura may be observed in vasculitic processes such as Wegener granulomatosis, microscopic polyangiitis, or Churg-Strauss syndrome. Abdominal bruits in the patient with refractory hypertension and progressive renal failure may be suggestive of renovascular disease. A funduscopic examination can reveal arteriolar narrowing, hemorrhages, exudates, or papilledema—findings consistent with chronic hypertension. Only a comprehensive physical examination will enable the clinician to identify these and other particular findings (see **Table 57-1**).

PRACTICE POINT

Key aspects of the physical examination include

1. determination of the patient's volume status,
2. identification of physical manifestations that can be associated with specific renal disease conditions, and
3. assessment for signs of uremia.

Patients with uremia can have a number of different physical examination findings. Evidence of uremic pericarditis or pleuritis may be present, as manifested by a pericardial or pleural friction rub, respectively. The pericardial friction rub classically has three components, one systolic and two diastolic, and a scratchy or grating quality. Skin and nail changes may include uremic frost (fine residue of excreted urea remaining on the surface of the skin), skin hyperpigmentation, or "half-and-half" nails (sharp demarcation between proximal and distal nail halves). Patients who have fluid retention may have pulmonary congestion or peripheral edema. Neurological findings can include confusion, coma, asterixis, and sensory deficits. As with the clinical symptoms of uremia, the presence of these physical findings, especially the pericardial friction rub and neurological abnormalities, may indicate the need for dialysis.

LABORATORY TESTS

Serum electrolytes

Serum electrolytes are essential to the evaluation of the patient with both acute and chronic renal disease. Serum sodium concentration provides insight into the water balance of a patient and can identify patients with hyponatremia and hypernatremia, both of which can be seen in patients with kidney disease. Monitoring serum potassium levels is vital, since impaired renal function decreases renal potassium excretion and can lead to potentially life-threatening hyperkalemia in oliguric or anuric patients. The clinician should be aware that the serum potassium concentration might not be an accurate indicator of total body potassium stores, since the majority of total body potassium is confined to the intracellular fluid compartment. This is evident, for example, in patients with diabetic ketoacidosis whose labs reveal elevated serum potassium levels in spite of diminished total body potassium stores. Serum chloride and bicarbonate levels are useful to the assessment of volume and acid–base status. The serum anion gap can be calculated from serum sodium, chloride, and bicarbonate concentrations ($AG = Na^+ - [Cl^- + HCO_3^-]$) and used to narrow the differential diagnosis of metabolic acidosis. Serum calcium, phosphorus, and magnesium levels should also be monitored in patients with renal disease, as these electrolytes yield important information about renal tubular function and bone mineral metabolism. Hyperphosphatemia and hypocalcemia are commonly seen in patients with acute and chronic renal disease and contribute to the development of secondary hyperparathyroidism.

Blood urea nitrogen and creatinine

Serum blood urea nitrogen (BUN) and creatinine are both nitrogenous end products of metabolism that generally rise in the setting of renal disease. Urea is formed from ammonia derived from the breakdown of dietary and tissue proteins, whereas creatinine is a by-product of muscle creatine metabolism. Urea and creatinine are both freely filtered by the kidneys but handled differently in the tubular system; whereas urea is partly reabsorbed by the proximal tubule and inner medullary collecting duct, creatinine is secreted to a small extent by the tubules. Despite these tubular alterations, BUN and creatinine are still the most commonly used biomarkers of renal function. Neither of these tests, however, is ideal for the early detection of renal disease. Elevations in serum BUN can be seen in other nonrenal factors, such as high protein intake, upper gastrointestinal tract bleeding, and states of high catabolism (fever, corticosteroids, and burns). Serum creatinine can also be affected by a variety of factors, including muscle mass and medications that impair tubular creatinine secretion (eg, trimethoprim, cimetidine, older cephalosporins). Though BUN and creatinine have traditionally been used as the primary biomarkers of renal injury, their use may decrease in the future in favor of more sensitive and specific biomarkers, including neutrophil gelatinase-associated lipocalin (NGAL), kidney injury molecule-1 (KIM-1), and cystatin C.

TABLE 57-1 History and Physical Examination Findings in Renal Disease

Renal Disease	History	Physical Exam Findings
Prerenal acute kidney injury	• Volume depletion (hemorrhage, vomiting, diarrhea, diuretics, burns) • Heart failure • Cirrhosis • Medications (NSAIDs, ACE inhibitors/ARBs, cyclosporine, tacrolimus) • Radiocontrast exposure	• Orthostatic hypotension, dry mucous membranes and axillae • Elevated JVP, +S3, lung rales, edema (heart failure) • Jaundice, ascites, edema (cirrhosis)
Intrarenal acute kidney injury		
Glomerular	• Gross hematuria or cola-colored urine • Cough and hemoptysis (Goodpasture syndrome) • Epistaxis, sinusitis, hemoptysis, arthralgias, (Wegener, Churg-Strauss) • Rash, arthralgias (systemic lupus erythematosus) • Recent respiratory infection (postinfectious glomerulonephritis, IgA nephropathy)	• Fever, palpable purpura, arthritis (vasculitis) • Saddle-nose deformity (Wegener) • Oral ulcers, rash, arthritis, pericardial rub (SLE)
Interstitial	• Fever, arthralgias, rash • Medications (NSAIDs, antibiotics)	• Fever, skin rash
ATN	• Episode of hypotension • Medications (aminoglycosides, amphotericin B, cisplatin)	• Hypotension • Warm (early sepsis) or cold extremities (late sepsis)
Vascular	• Trauma, muscle necrosis (rhabdomyolysis) • History of multiple myeloma • History of atherosclerosis • Recent vascular intervention • Anticoagulation • Flank pain (renal vein thrombosis)	• Elevated BP • Livedo reticularis, ischemic extremities
Postrenal acute kidney injury	• Urinary urgency, hesitancy, oliguria or anuria • Gross hematuria • Flank pain, renal colic • History of nephrolithiasis • Medications (acyclovir, indinavir, anticholinergics)	• Distended bladder • Enlarged prostate • Palpable abdominal or pelvic masses
Nephrotic syndrome	• Weight gain • Foamy urine • Medications (NSAIDs, gold, penicillamine)	• Anasarca, ascites, edema
Uremia	• Fatigue, lethargy, confusion, seizures • Anorexia, nausea, vomiting • Pruritus, metallic taste, bleeding	• Asterixis • Pericardial or pleural friction rub • Half-and-half nails • Dry and atrophic skin, pallor, hyperpigmentation, ecchymoses, uremic frost

ACE, angiotensin-converting enzyme; ARB, angiotensin receptor blocker; BP, blood pressure; JVP, jugular venous pressure; NSAID, nonsteroidal anti-inflammatory drug; SLE, systemic lupus erythematosus.

Estimated glomerular filtration rate

All patients with kidney disease, both acute and chronic, should have their kidney function assessed by estimation of the glomerular filtration rate (GFR). GFR can be estimated by a few common methods, including (1) measurement of serum creatinine, (2) calculation of creatinine clearance, and (3) use of estimation equations such as the Cockcroft-Gault formula (creatinine clearance) or the Modification of Diet in Renal Disease (MDRD) equation (GFR). The normal GFR in a healthy adult is >90 mL/min. There is an expected decrease in GFR with age, of approximately 1 mL/min/year after age 35. Elderly patients may also have lower creatinine levels due to decreased muscle mass. Measurement of serum creatinine is the simplest to perform and has been the most frequently used surrogate for GFR. However, given that serum creatinine concentration can be affected by several factors, including an individual's muscle mass, dietary protein intake, and certain medications, it is not the most accurate method of estimating GFR. Both the Cockcroft-Gault and MDRD equations are relatively complex formulas that take into account serum creatinine as well as other defined factors such as age, race, gender, and weight. They were designed to estimate GFR in patients with established CKD and are most useful for this purpose. As these equations have yet to be well validated in specific populations, including individuals with normal or near-normal renal function, children and elderly individuals, and certain ethnic groups, they should be interpreted with caution in these patients. Furthermore, it is important to understand that serum creatinine and the estimation equations should only be used to approximate GFR in patients with *stable* kidney function (unchanging serum creatinine). If the clinician is uncertain about the accuracy of GFR estimation, a 24-hour urine collection can be performed to calculate creatinine clearance.

PRACTICE POINT

Laboratory testing

- Serum creatinine and the estimation equations should only be used to approximate GFR in patients with stable kidney function (unchanging serum creatinine).
- The examination of the urinary sediment by microscopy is one of the most valuable tests in the evaluation of the renal patient and can provide useful diagnostic information about both acute and chronic kidney disease.
  - Urine particles lyse easily after collection, and therefore urine samples should be examined within 2 to 4 hours of acquisition.
  - The pathognomonic finding of ATN on urinary sediment is the presence of coarse "muddy brown" granular casts, which represent extensive renal tubular epithelial cell injury.
- In the setting of acute kidney injury, a fractional excretion of sodium (FENa) in combination with clinical history and other lab tests may help differentiate between prerenal etiologies and acute tubular necrosis (ATN).
  - A FENa of < 1% can also be seen in a number of other diseases, such as contrast-induced nephropathy, pigment nephropathy due to rhabdomyolysis, acute glomerulonephritis, hepatorenal syndrome, early urinary obstruction, acute interstitial nephritis, and even ATN.
  - A FENa may be difficult to interpret in the setting of diuretic therapy.
- If the patient has a nonanion gap metabolic acidosis, one can calculate a urine anion gap (UAG) to help differentiate between gastrointestinal losses of bicarbonate (eg diarrhea) and renal tubular acidosis using the following formula: (urine Na^+ + urine K^+) – urine Cl^-.

Proteinuria

Proteinuria, one of the hallmarks of kidney damage, is most frequently detected qualitatively by urine dipstick, which grades proteinuria on a scale of concentration: trace, 1+ (30 mg/dL), 2+ (100 mg/dL), 3+ (300 mg/dL). Normal urine may test slightly positive if very concentrated. The urine dipstick is only capable of detecting albumin in the urine, which is the most abundant protein seen with glomerular proteinuria; thus the presence of other proteins such as immunoglobulin light chains will not be detected by dipstick alone. The finding of proteinuria by dipstick should prompt a more accurate quantification, either by a single random measurement of urine protein and urine creatinine concentration to determine the urine protein-to-creatinine ratio or by a 24-hour urine collection for protein and creatinine excretion rate. Small amounts of urinary albumin (30–300 mg/L) that cannot be detected by dipstick can be quantified by measuring a urine microalbumin concentration and normalized to a creatinine measurement in the same sample.

Hematuria

Hematuria is defined as the presence of red blood cells in the urine. In the absence of gross bleeding, hematuria is most commonly discovered on a urine dipstick (which detects the pseudoperoxidase activity of hemoglobin) or urinalysis. False-positive dipstick results are seen in the setting of hemoglobinuria, myoglobinuria, menstrual blood in the urine, vigorous exercise, and concentrated urine. If significant proteinuria or renal dysfunction is also present, the kidney should be considered the source of hematuria until proven otherwise, and a renal biopsy should be considered to establish a diagnosis. In the absence of these findings, microscopic hematuria is considered to be isolated hematuria. The differential diagnosis of isolated microscopic hematuria can be divided into renal (glomerular) or extrarenal (nonglomerular) processes. Immunoglobulin A (IgA) nephropathy, thin basement membrane disease, and Alport syndrome are three of the most common causes of glomerular hematuria, though any form of acute or chronic glomerulonephritis can be a potential source. Common etiologies of nonglomerular hematuria include urinary tract infections, kidney stones, urinary tract tumors, trauma, bladder polyps, cystic kidney diseases (eg, polycystic kidney disease, medullary cystic disease), and metabolic abnormalities such as hypercalciuria and hyperuricosuria. Hematuria associated with exercise, especially running, is usually a benign condition in which the bleeding source is likely renal pelvis. Hematuria associated with glomerular bleeding may or may not be associated with flank pain, and ureteral causes that obstruct the urinary tract can be a source of severe pain and renal colic. Hematuria in other cases is usually painless. In extrarenal hematuria, the red blood cells typically appear normal on urinary sediment, round and uniform, whereas in glomerular hematuria, the red blood cells may appear dysmorphic due to distortion from the passage through the glomerular filtration barrier. Imaging studies are indicated to search for a structural cause of hematuria. Detection of persistent extrarenal hematuria should prompt further workup and consultation with a urologist to identify the source of bleeding. In older individuals particularly, bladder cancer should be considered. In cases of isolated glomerular hematuria, a renal biopsy is not typically indicated, since the pathologic diagnosis rarely has any effect on the management or outcome.

Abnormal urinalysis

The examination of the urinary sediment by microscopy is one of the most valuable tests in the evaluation of the renal patient and can provide useful diagnostic information about both acute and CKD. Urine particles lyse easily after collection, and therefore urine samples should be examined within 2 to 4 hours of acquisition. Certain characteristic findings on urinalysis may point the clinician toward a specific diagnosis. The presence of red blood cells, when greater than 1–2 per high-power field, generally indicates hematuria (see Hematuria). White blood cells (pyuria), when greater than 2 per high-power field, can be observed with upper or lower urinary tract infections, contamination from genital secretions, or inflammation in the kidney, as in interstitial nephritis or acute glomerulonephritis. Urinary casts are cylindrical aggregates of protein and/or cells that form in the lumen of the distal convoluted tubule or collecting duct and are excreted into the urine. Hyaline casts, the most common type of cast, are acellular and consist primarily of Tamm-Horsfall mucoprotein produced by tubular epithelial cells. They can be seen in the setting of dehydration or vigorous exercise in normal patients who produce concentrated urine but can be seen in patients with proteinuria. Granular casts, the second most common type of cast, are usually formed from degenerating cellular casts or protein-containing lysosomes and can appear fine or coarse in texture. "Muddy brown" granular casts contain degenerating tubular epithelial cells and are commonly seen in acute tubular injury. Fatty casts are hyaline casts that contain lipid droplets and can be observed in patients with diseases causing lipiduria, such as the nephrotic syndrome. When red blood cells leak through the glomerular filtration barrier, they can form red blood cell casts in the tubular lumen, a finding that is consistent with acute glomerulonephritis. White blood cell casts are indicative of inflammation or infection in the kidney and can be seen in acute glomerulonephritis, interstitial nephritis, and acute pyelonephritis. Red blood cell casts and white blood cell casts are always pathologic findings and should prompt further evaluation of the patient for the clinical entities already mentioned.

Urine chemistries

Urine chemistries, consisting primarily of the urinary sodium, potassium, chloride, and creatinine, can be useful in the evaluation of a number of renal conditions. In the setting of acute kidney injury, a fractional excretion of sodium (FENa) in combination with clinical history and other lab tests may help differentiate between prerenal etiologies and acute tubular necrosis (ATN). The FENa can be calculated by the following formula: (urine $Na^+ \times$ plasma creatinine)/(plasma $Na^+ \times$ urine creatinine) $\times$ 100. A FENa of < 1% is commonly seen in prerenal causes of oliguria, and a FENa > 2% is usually indicative of ATN. There are limitations to the use of the FENa, however, since a FENa of < 1% can also be seen in a number of other diseases, such as contrast-induced nephropathy, pigment nephropathy due to rhabdomyolysis, acute glomerulonephritis, hepatorenal syndrome, early urinary obstruction, acute interstitial nephritis, and even ATN. Furthermore, a FENa may be difficult to interpret in the setting of a patient taking diuretics. In such cases, calculating a fractional excretion of urea (FEurea) may be a more sensitive test to differentiate prerenal AKI (FEurea < 35%) from ATN (FEurea 50–65%).

In the setting of a nonanion gap metabolic acidosis, one can calculate a urine anion gap (UAG) to help differentiate between gastrointestinal losses of bicarbonate (eg, diarrhea) and renal tubular acidosis using the following formula: (urine Na^+ + urine K^+) – urine Cl^-. A negative UAG is consistent with gastrointestinal losses, whereas a positive UAG is frequently seen with renal tubular acidosis.

Serum enzymes

Serum enzyme levels should be interpreted cautiously in patients with impaired renal function, especially those with ESRD undergoing hemodialysis or peritoneal dialysis. These patients frequently have elevations in various serum enzyme levels due to decreased renal clearance, though abnormally low levels can occasionally be encountered. Such lab abnormalities can confound the diagnosis of certain diseases, which are often detected by increases in the levels of these serum enzymes. Cardiac enzymes, including cardiac troponin T (cTnT), cardiac troponin I (cTnI), and the Muscle/Brain (MB) isoenzyme of creatine kinase (CK-MB), are commonly used to detect acute coronary syndromes and to appropriately triage patients to coronary care units. This is particularly relevant to patients with CKD and ESRD, in which cardiovascular disease is highly prevalent. However, patients with impaired renal function often have elevated levels of cardiac troponins and CK-MB even in the absence of acute myocardial injury. A large percentage of false-positive elevations in cTnT and CK-MB are seen in patients with ESRD when these markers are used to diagnose acute myocardial infarction (MI). The use of cTnI is less likely to be associated with false-positive elevations, and serial measurements of cTnI are currently the most specific marker of myocardial damage in patients with renal failure and suspected acute MI.

The serum levels of liver and pancreatic enzymes can also be affected in patients with renal failure. Serum aminotransferase levels are frequently found to be in the lower range of normal values in patients with CKD and ESRD. In the absence of liver disease, gammaglutamyl transpeptidase (GGT) levels are most often normal but may be elevated in a small percentage of patients. Serum alkaline phosphatase levels are often elevated in dialysis patients, usually as a result of coexisting bone disease. An isolated elevation in serum alkaline phosphatase may not correlate well with hepatobiliary disease in ESRD patients; however, if a chronically elevated alkaline phosphatase level is accompanied by an elevation in serum GGT or 5′-nucleotidase, one should be more suspicious of an obstructive or infiltrative hepatobiliary process. Elevations in both serum amylase and lipase levels can be observed in patients with CKD and ESRD, even when acute pancreatitis is not present. The levels of these pancreatic enzymes in these patients are commonly threefold to fivefold higher (but typically less than three times the upper limit of normal) and may make the accurate diagnosis of acute pancreatitis more difficult. The elevations are due primarily to decreased renal clearance of these enzymes, though in the case of serum lipase, the use of heparin during hemodialysis has also been found to contribute to elevated levels.

IMAGING STUDIES

Ultrasonography

Ultrasonography is a safe, noninvasive, rapid, and inexpensive diagnostic imaging modality used to study the kidneys. One distinct advantage of ultrasonography is that it requires neither ionizing radiation nor a potentially toxic intravenous contrast agent, which makes it a safe initial imaging study, especially for patients with known renal insufficiency. Renal ultrasonography can provide valuable information about kidney size, shape, and gross appearance. Normal adult kidneys are approximately 9–13 cm (4–5 inches) in length and 5–7.5 cm (2–3 inches) in width and should not differ by much more than 1 cm. With chronic injury, the renal parenchyma becomes replaced with fibrotic tissue and the renal cortex becomes thinner, causing diseased kidneys to shrink in size. In patients in which the chronicity of kidney disease is uncertain, the finding of smaller-sized kidneys on ultrasonography is suggestive of longstanding kidney disease. A number of conditions are associated with large kidneys, such as autosomal dominant polycystic kidney disease, urinary tract obstruction, HIV nephropathy, the early stages of diabetic nephropathy, and infiltrative diseases such as amyloidosis or kappa light chain nephropathy associated with multiple myeloma. Asymmetry in kidney size may indicate unilateral kidney disease, and the clinician must determine whether the smaller or larger kidney is abnormal. Increased echogenicity in the kidneys is a commonly reported and nonspecific finding, usually denoting medical renal disease. Renal ultrasonography can also identify the presence of cysts, stones, or masses in the kidney. In the patient presenting with acute kidney injury, renal ultrasonography can be useful in identifying obstructive uropathy, which usually manifests as hydronephrosis, although false-negative results can be seen in patients with early obstruction (less than 3–4 days), coexisting volume depletion, or obstruction caused by retroperitoneal fibrosis or compression by retroperitoneal or intraparenchymal tumor or blood.

Doppler ultrasonography

Doppler ultrasonography can provide information about the presence and flow of blood through the vessels of the kidney. High-velocity or disorganized flow patterns can be seen in patients with hemodynamically significant renal artery stenosis. In addition, information about the vascular resistive indices can be obtained; elevated resistive indices (> 0.80) in a stenotic kidney are suggestive of severe parenchymal disease and a low likelihood of response to revascularization. Given the potential toxicities of using iodinated contrast agents or gadolinium, particularly in patients with impaired renal function, Doppler ultrasonography has recently become more widely used as the initial imaging study to evaluate renal artery stenosis. It is important to note that the sensitivity of Doppler ultrasonography is highly operator dependent and can be affected by factors such as patient anatomy.

Computed tomography

Computed tomography (CT) can be instrumental to the evaluation of renal disease. In the evaluation of the patient with suspected renal colic, noncontrast helical CT scanning is currently the gold standard for diagnosing nephrolithiasis and can detect essentially all kidney stones with the exception of indinavir stones. Noncontrast can also be useful to detect ureteric obstruction in a patient with acute kidney injury, particularly when intravenous (IV) contrast is to be avoided due to nephrotoxicity. The administration of IV iodinated contrast permits the visualization of other disease processes. Imaging of the renal parenchyma is enhanced by IV contrast and facilitates the evaluation and detection of renal mass lesions such as renal cell carcinoma. CT angiography is one of the modalities of choice in evaluating the renal vasculature and can be used to diagnose suspected renal artery stenosis or aneurysms. CT urography allows imaging of the collecting system and can identify filling defects such as stones, blood clots, and tumors. The drawback to the use of iodinated contrast agents is the potential nephrotoxicity, especially in patients with preexisting renal impairment, diabetes, heart failure, or hypovolemia (see Contrast-Induced Nephropathy). In patients with ESRD who have residual renal function, administration of contrast dye can induce further tubular damage and lead to loss of the remaining renal function. As preservation of residual renal function in patients with ESRD has been shown to correlate with improved survival even after the initiation of dialysis, the use of contrast in these patients should be avoided if possible.

Magnetic resonance imaging

The primary role of magnetic resonance imaging (MRI) in renal imaging is in the evaluation of renal masses. MRI can effectively differentiate benign versus malignant lesions in the kidney, especially when CT scanning with intravenous iodinated contrast is contraindicated or if ultrasonographic and CT scans have been nondiagnostic. MR angiography (MRA), which involves the administration of intravenous gadolinium, has become the modality of choice in the evaluation of renovascular disease. According to one meta-analysis, gadolinium-enhanced MRA had a reported sensitivity of 97% and specificity of 85% for the detection of renal artery stenosis.[2] However, the use of gadolinium-based contrast agents in patients with moderate to severe CKD, especially those on dialysis, has been associated with the development of nephrogenic systemic fibrosis (NSF), a debilitating condition characterized by fibrosis of the skin, joints, eyes, and other internal organs. Given the risk of NSF, patients with an estimated GFR < 30 mL/min or requiring dialysis should not be administered gadolinium-based contrast agents. In these patients, Doppler ultrasonography may be a safer alternative study.

Radionuclide scans

Radionuclide studies are capable of providing functional information about the kidneys that is not detected by ultrasonography, CT, or MRI. Static radionuclide scans employ a radiolabeled tracer (eg, technetium 99m-DMSA) that binds to renal parenchymal cells but is not excreted into the tubules. These studies are most useful in quantifying the functional cortical tissue of each kidney and determining the percentage contribution of each kidney to total renal function. Dynamic radionuclide scans use tracers (eg, technetium 99m-DTPA, technetium 99m-MAG3) that are taken up by nephrons and then excreted into the collecting system. A diuretic such as furosemide is often administered just prior to injection of the tracer in order to ensure high levels of diuresis during the study. Dynamic scans can be used to evaluate potential renal tract obstructions as well as the response to treatment of the obstruction. Formerly used in the diagnosis of renovascular hypertension by providing a functional assessment, captopril renal scans have been more recently replaced by duplex Doppler ultrasonography, CT, and MRA, which have a higher sensitivity and specificity.

ACUTE KIDNEY INJURY

Acute kidney injury (AKI), formerly termed acute renal failure, is a sudden and sustained decline in renal function that results in the failure to excrete metabolic waste products, maintain fluid and electrolyte balance, and regulate acid–base homeostasis. AKI is an increasingly common cause of hospitalization, with 1% of all patients reported to have AKI upon admission to the hospital and 2–5% of inpatients subsequently developing AKI during their hospitalization. In spite of advances in intensive care and dialysis support over the last 50 years, the overall mortality rate of AKI continues to remain high, ranging from 20 to 90% depending on the severity of patient illness and the medical setting. The role of the hospitalist is to be able to acknowledge and diagnose common causes of AKI, to initiate management by identifying and treating reversible factors, to recognize when patients with AKI require dialysis as an intervention, and to know when to appropriately consult a nephrologist.

Numerous definitions covering the entire spectrum of severity of AKI have been previously proposed, but only recently have efforts been made to devise a more uniform definition for AKI. Two classification systems, the RIFLE and AKIN criteria, have defined and stratified AKI by stages of severity based on graded increases in serum creatinine and periods of decreased urine output (**Table 57-2**). The more recent AKIN criteria have proposed a definition for AKI that incorporates the prognostic significance associated with small changes in serum creatinine. The diagnosis of AKI can be established by (1) an abrupt (within 48 hours) absolute

TABLE 57-2 Definitions and Classification Systems for Acute Kidney Injury

RIFLE Stages	AKIN Stages	RIFLE Increase in Serum Creatinine	AKIN Increase in Serum Creatinine	RIFLE and AKIN Urine Output
Risk (R)	1	≥ 150 to 200%	≥ 0.3 mg/dL or ≥ 150 to 200%	< 0.5 mL/kg/h × > 6 hours
Injury (I)	2	> 200 to 300%	> 200 to 300%	< 0.5 mL/kg/h × > 12 hours
Failure (F)	3	> 300%	> 300% or acute renal replacement therapy	< 0.3 mL/kg/h × ≥ 24 hours
Loss (L)	Complete loss of kidney function for > 4 weeks			
End-stage kidney disease (E)	Need for renal replacement therapy for > 3 months			

AKIN, Acute Kidney Injury Network; RIFLE, Risk. Injury. Failure. Loss. ESRD.

TABLE 57-3 Etiologies of Acute Kidney Injury

Prerenal

Volume depletion
- True volume depletion
  - GI losses (vomiting, diarrhea)
  - Renal losses (diuretics, osmotic diuresis)
  - Skin losses (burns, sweating)
- Effective volume depletion
  - Congestive heart failure
  - Cirrhosis
  - Nephrotic syndrome

Vasoconstriction
- NSAIDs
- ACE inhibitors/ARBs
- Iodinated contrast agents
- Cyclosporine and tacrolimus

Hepatorenal syndrome

Hypotension

Postrenal

Prostatic hypertrophy

Obstruction
- Bladder outlet obstruction
- Stones
- Crystals (acyclovir, indinavir)
- Tumors
- Clots
- Retroperitoneal fibrosis

Intrarenal

Glomerular
- Acute glomerulonephritis
  - ANCA-associated vasculitis (Wegener granulomatosis, microscopic polyangiitis, Churg-Strauss syndrome)
  - Anti-GBM disease (Goodpasture syndrome)
  - Immune complex disease (lupus nephritis, poststreptococcal glomerulonephritis, cryoglobulinemia, IgA nephropathy)

Interstitial
- Drug-induced (NSAIDs, penicillin analogues and cephalosporins, rifampin, sulfa drugs)
- Autoimmune (SLE, Sjögren syndrome)
- Infections (legionella, leptospirosis, cytomegalovirus, streptococci)

Tubular
- Ischemic acute tubular necrosis
  - Hypotension
  - Sepsis
- Nephrotoxic acute tubular necrosis
  - Aminoglycoside antibiotics
  - Amphotericin B
  - Cast nephropathy (myeloma kidney)
  - Cisplatin
  - Iodinated contrast agents
  - Pigment nephropathy (hemoglobin, myoglobin)

Vascular
- Large vessel
  - Bilateral renal artery stenosis
  - Renal vein thrombosis
  - Renal thromboembolism
- Small vessel
  - Thrombotic microangiopathies (HUS, TTP)
  - Cholesterol atheroembolism
  - Malignant hypertension
  - Scleroderma renal crisis

ACE, angiotensin-converting enzyme; RB, angiotensin receptor blocker; GI, gastrointestinal; HUS, hemolytic uremic syndrome; NSAID, nonsteroidal anti-inflammatory drug; SLE, systemic lupus erythematosus; TTP, thrombotic thrombocytopenic purpura.

increase in serum creatinine of ≥0.3 mg/dL from baseline, (2) a percentage increase in serum creatinine of ≥50%, or (3) oliguria of ≤0.5 mL/kg/hour for >6 hours. Although both the RIFLE and AKIN classification systems have been validated in a variety of clinical settings, their utility at this time appears to be greater for research use than for the bedside.

AKI can be divided into three diagnostic categories based on the anatomic location of the cause of injury: prerenal, intrarenal, and postrenal (**Table 57-3**). It can be further subdivided into oliguric (urine output <400 mL/day) and nonoliguric (urine output >400 mL/day) AKI, with patients producing less than 100 mL urine/day considered to be anuric. These distinctions are important, given that epidemiological studies have found that oliguria in the setting of AKI is an independent predictor of mortality. Oliguric AKI is more characteristic of prerenal etiologies and urinary obstruction, while nonoliguric AKI is commonly seen in intrarenal causes of AKI. Anuria is uncommon and is usually associated with complete urinary tract obstruction, bilateral renal infarction, renal vein thrombosis, cortical necrosis, or high-grade ischemic acute tubular necrosis.

PRERENAL

Prerenal AKI is defined as a reduction in GFR that is caused by hypoperfusion of the kidney. In most cases of prerenal AKI, the kidneys are morphologically normal. The etiologies of prerenal AKI can be divided into conditions that cause volume depletion and conditions that induce renal vasoconstriction. True volume depletion may result from hemorrhage or gastrointestinal, urinary, or cutaneous fluid losses. "Effective" volume depletion refers to decreased effective circulating volume in the setting of normovolemia or hypervolemia and can result from marked vasodilatation as seen in the setting of sepsis, heart failure, cirrhosis, and third-spacing. Renal vasoconstriction is most often caused by medications, including angiotensin-converting enzyme (ACE) inhibitors, angiotensin receptor blockers (ARBs), NSAIDs, intravenous iodinated contrast agents, and the immunosuppressant drugs cyclosporine and tacrolimus.

Patients with prerenal AKI usually present with an elevated BUN and creatinine, and the ratio of BUN to creatinine is classically greater than 20:1. Urinalysis often reveals an elevated specific gravity and the absence of significant hematuria or proteinuria. The urinary sediment is typically bland but may show hyaline casts. The kidneys, able to respond appropriately to the reduction in renal perfusion, compensate by maximizing sodium and water reabsorption. Urine sodium is typically low, and the FENa and urea are < 1% and < 35%, respectively. Patients with prerenal AKI often respond favorably to volume resuscitation and discontinuation of any offending therapeutic agents.

Intrarenal

In all cases of intrarenal AKI, the primary abnormality is within the kidney. The causes of intrarenal AKI can be subdivided into four anatomic categories: glomerular disease, interstitial disease, tubular disease, and vascular disease. The clinician must integrate the elements of history, physical examination, and laboratory testing to distinguish between these categories, since appropriate treatment is dependent upon an accurate diagnosis. As in prerenal AKI, patients generally present with an elevated BUN and creatinine, though the ratio is usually normal (< 20:1). The FENa may be variable and cannot reliably distinguish between the different causes of intrarenal AKI. The urinalysis is frequently abnormal, and findings on the urinary sediment can provide clues to the location of the kidney injury. In some patients, the clinical presentation and laboratory evaluation are insufficient to establish a diagnosis, and a percutaneous renal biopsy may be indicated to better guide management.

The most common cause of intrarenal AKI is ATN, which is responsible for the majority of cases of AKI in hospitalized patients. ATN may be caused by either ischemic or nephrotoxic injury. Ischemic ATN is often associated with periods of prolonged hypotension and markedly reduced renal perfusion, which can be seen in the setting of heart failure, sepsis, or cardiac surgery. Nephrotoxic ATN can be caused by either endogenous (eg, heme pigments) or exogenous (eg, aminoglycoside antibiotics, amphotericin B, cisplatin, and iodinated contrast agents) toxins. The clinical course of ATN can be variable: while many patients typically experience an oliguric phase (onset within 24 hours of the renal insult and duration of 1–3 weeks) followed by a diuretic phase (increase in urine output that is indicative of renal recovery), some patients remain nonoliguric throughout. The pathognomonic finding on urinary sediment is the presence of coarse "muddy brown" granular casts, which represent extensive renal tubular epithelial cell injury. Due to impaired tubular sodium reabsorption, the urine sodium is > 40 mEq/L and the FENa is usually > 2%. Both ischemic and nephrotoxic ATN resolve in most cases, but dialysis is sometimes required when renal injury is severe. A recently noted cause of renal injury after colonoscopy follows use of preparations containing phosphate salts that precipitate in the kidney in volume-depleted patients or those with CKD. Alternative preparations are recommended.

The glomerular type of AKI involves acute inflammation of the glomeruli or glomerular vessels. Acute glomerulonephritis can be either renal-limited or associated with systemic illnesses such as infections (eg, poststreptococcal/postinfectious glomerulonephritis), autoimmune disorders (eg, systemic lupus erythematosus), or vasculitis (eg, cryoglobulinemia, Wegener granulomatosis). The urinalysis is always abnormal and classically reveals evidence of damage to the glomerular filtration barrier, with features such as proteinuria and the presence of dysmorphic red blood cells and red blood cell casts. Urine sodium and FENa may be low. The workup of acute glomerulonephritis should include serologic tests such as complement levels, antistreptococcal antibodies, antibodies against hepatitis B and C, antinuclear antibodies, antineutrophil cytoplasmic antibodies, antiglomerular basement membrane antibodies, and cryoglobulins. Definitive diagnosis, however, usually requires a renal biopsy.

Acute interstitial nephritis (AIN) is defined as inflammation of the renal interstitium that results in AKI. AIN is most often caused by medications (see Drug Toxicity) but can also be associated with infections (eg, legionella, leptospirosis, cytomegalovirus, streptococci) and autoimmune diseases (eg, systemic lupus erythematosus, Sjögren syndrome, sarcoidosis). Classic symptoms include fever, rash, and arthralgias, and the classic triad of fever, maculopapular erythematous rash, and eosinophilia is observed in only 10% of cases of AIN. Laboratory testing may reveal a FENa > 1%, but this is not always reliable. Urinalysis may show mild proteinuria (< 1 g/day), and the urinary sediment may reveal red blood cells, white blood cells, and white blood cell casts. Occasionally, urine eosinophils are observed with a Wright or Hansen stain, but this finding is neither highly sensitive nor specific for the diagnosis of AIN and can be seen in other inflammatory conditions. Definitive diagnosis can be established with a renal biopsy. Treatment of AIN is primarily the identification and cessation of the offending agent.

AKI can also be caused by acute vascular disease affecting either the large or the small renal blood vessels. Large-vessel diseases involve the renal arteries and veins and include bilateral renal artery stenosis, renal thromboembolism, renal artery dissection, and renal vein thrombosis. As a general rule, large-vessel disease must be bilateral in order to cause AKI, with the exception of unilateral disease in the patient with a solitary kidney. Patients may present with symptoms of renal infarction, complaining of acute flank pain and hematuria. Small-vessel diseases that can cause AKI include malignant hypertension, scleroderma renal crisis, and cholesterol atheroembolic disease. Patients with cholesterol atheroembolic disease often have a history of recent aortic instrumentation or surgical intervention or anticoagulation, and physical exam may reveal findings such as livedo reticularis on the skin overlying the lower extremities, characteristic toe or foot discoloration, or Hollenhorst plaques in the retina. The urinalysis in vascular AKI typically shows microscopic hematuria with or without proteinuria. Eosinophilia, eosinophiluria, and hypocomplementemia can also be seen in cholesterol atheroembolic disease. Imaging (eg, CT, MRI, or radionuclide studies) is often required to confirm the diagnosis of large-vessel disease.

Postrenal

In all patients presenting with AKI, urinary tract obstruction must be ruled out early, since timely intervention often improves or fully restores renal function. Obstruction to the flow of urine commonly occurs at the level of the prostate, particularly in adult men, but can occur at any location along the urinary tract. Upper urinary tract obstruction (ie, at the level of the ureters or renal pelvis) must be bilateral in order to cause AKI; the sole exception is unilateral obstruction in the patient with a solitary kidney. Common causes of postrenal AKI include prostatic hypertrophy or prostate cancer, obstructing kidney stones, urothelial tumors, and retroperitoneal fibrosis or malignancies. Patients with bilateral obstruction often present with oliguria (partial obstruction), polyuria (a sign of associated nephrogenic diabetes insipidus), or anuria (complete obstruction) and may report symptoms of flank pain, abdominal pain, renal colic, or hematuria. Ultrasonographic imaging usually reveals hydronephrosis, though this may be absent in cases of retroperitoneal or infiltrative diseases that encase the ureters or kidneys. CT and dynamic radionuclide studies can also be used to diagnose urinary obstruction. Treatment of postrenal AKI focuses on relief of the obstruction.

■ MANAGEMENT STRATEGIES

General principles

Management of AKI should be focused on treating and reversing the specific cause of injury. Patients with prerenal AKI, for example, should be given volume resuscitation to restore euvolemia. In patients with postrenal AKI due to urinary obstruction, treating the source of obstruction can improve and in many cases fully restore renal function. Currently, there are no effective pharmacologic therapies for the treatment of AKI, and treatment focuses more on supportive management. There are a number of basic principles of management that can guide the clinician managing AKI:

1. **Optimization of volume status and hemodynamic parameters.** Daily weights and intake and output should be monitored closely. Medications that can compromise renal perfusion, including ACE inhibitors, ARBs, NSAIDs, and calcineurin inhibitors, should be discontinued. Patients who are hypovolemic should be given volume accordingly, with either crystalloids, colloids, or blood products. With the exception of a few settings (eg, cirrhosis), the use of colloids has not been proven to have greater benefit than crystalloids in AKI. Vasopressors or inotropes should be considered in patients who remain hypotensive despite of volume resuscitation. In patients who are hypervolemic, the role of diuretics in the treatment of AKI is controversial. Although loop diuretics may be useful to treat volume overload in an oliguric patient, conversion of oliguric to nonoliguric AKI with diuretics has not been shown to improve survival or shorten the time to renal recovery. At high doses, loop diuretics may also lead to ototoxicity. Therefore, these medications should be used judiciously in patients with AKI.
2. **Close monitoring and management of renal function, acid–base status, and serum electrolytes.** Serum BUN, creatinine, and electrolytes should be monitored daily. If hyperkalemia is present, medical treatment with, for example, intravenous calcium gluconate, insulin, inhaled albuterol, and sodium polystyrene sulfonate (kayexalate) should be initiated. Specific treatment depends on the severity, the presence of oliguranuria and ECG abnormalities; dialysis may be necessary if electrocardiographic abnormalities are present. Potassium intake via diet, medications, and intravenous fluids should also be eliminated. Hyperphosphatemia can be treated with oral phosphorus binders such as calcium acetate, calcium carbonate, sevelamer hydrochloride, and sevelamer carbonate. Aluminum hydroxide is also highly effective at lowering phosphorus levels in severe cases, but its use should be limited to no more than 1–2 weeks due to the potential for aluminum toxicity. If acidemia is present, patients can be treated with intravenous fluids containing sodium bicarbonate.
3. **Appropriate adjustment of medication dosing.** All medications should be dosed to reflect the level of renal impairment, based on estimated GFR, or the need for dialysis (**Table 57-4**). Since eGFR can only be calculated when the serum creatinine is stable, a GFR of < 10 should be assumed for patients whose serum creatinine is acutely increasing. Importantly, narcotics can frequently accumulate in patients with renal impairment and, if necessary, should be used with caution.
4. **Avoidance of nephrotoxins.** Medications that are known to be nephrotoxic, such as NSAIDs, and aminoglycoside antibiotics, should not be administered to patients with AKI. Patients who take ACE inhibitors or ARBs on a chronic basis for hypertension or cardiovascular disease should stop these medications, at least temporarily until renal function has recovered. Intravenous iodinated contrast agents and gadolinium-containing agents should be avoided.
5. **Management of uremic bleeding.** Patients with severe AKI and uremia may develop bleeding diatheses due to uremic platelet dysfunction and can be treated with synthetic arginine vasopressin analogues (eg, intravenous DDAVP 0.3 mcg/kg × 1–2 doses). Hemodialysis is the definitive treatment and should be performed in cases of severe bleeding.
6. **Nutritional support.** Nutritional status is a major prognostic factor in patients with acute kidney injury. Malnutrition is highly prevalent in these patients and increases the likelihood of in-hospital mortality and complications, prolongs hospital stays, and increases the use of health care resources. Appropriate nutritional therapy is thus essential to the management of AKI, and consultation with an experienced dietitian may be of benefit. Hyperkalemia and hyperphosphatemia are common in patients with AKI, and a diet that is low in potassium and phosphorus should be instituted. Critically ill patients with AKI are in a highly catabolic state and at high risk for severe protein energy wasting. Nutritional support, parenteral or enteral, is frequently required in order to ensure adequate delivery of protein and energy, prevent further metabolic derangements and complications, improve wound healing, bolster the immune system, and decrease mortality.

It should be noted that, in spite of the available treatment modalities and advances in dialysis technology, mortality in patients with AKI remains high with a rate of approximately 50–80% in critically ill patients.

When to consult a nephrologist

There are a number of common clinical scenarios that are considered nephrologic emergencies, and evaluation by a nephrologist should be requested immediately. Delaying treatment may be life threatening. These scenarios include (1) volume overload in an oliguric or anuric patient; (2) hyperkalemia with serum potassium > 5.5 – 6 mEq/L and/or associated with changes on the electrocardiogram and other electrolyte abnormalities, especially in an oligoanuric patient; (3) toxic overdoses that can be treated with hemodialysis, including ethylene glycol, methanol, and lithium; (4) symptomatic or severe hyponatremia; (5) hypertensive crises; (6) rapidly progressive glomerulonephritis, as suggested by renal failure with the presence of red blood cells and/or red or white blood cell casts in the urinary sediment; and (7) microangiopathic hemolytic anemias including thrombotic thrombocytopenic purpura and hemolytic uremic syndrome.

PRACTICE POINT

Indications for emergent nephrology consultation include

- volume overload in an oliguric or anuric patient;
- hyperkalemia with serum potassium > 5.5–6 mEq/L and/or associated with changes on the electrocardiogram and other electrolyte abnormalities, especially in an oligoanuric patient;
- toxic overdoses that can be treated with hemodialysis, including ethylene glycol, methanol, and lithium;
- symptomatic or severe hyponatremia;
- hypertensive crises;
- rapidly progressive glomerulonephritis, as suggested by renal failure with the presence of red blood cells and/or red or white blood cell casts in the urinary sediment;
- microangiopathic hemolytic anemias including thrombotic thrombocytopenic purpura and hemolytic uremic syndrome.

Indications for renal biopsy

A percutaneous renal biopsy can be instrumental to the diagnosis of AKI as well as other kidney diseases. This procedure is typically

TABLE 57-4 Dosing Adjustments for Commonly Prescribed Medications in Patients with Impaired Renal Function

Drug	Usual Dose	GFR > 50 mL/min/1.73 m²	GFR 10–50 mL/min/1.73 m²	GFR < 10 mL/min/1.73 m²
Acyclovir (oral)	200–800 mg every 4–12 hours	100%	100%	200 mg every 12 hours
Allopurinol	300 mg daily	75%	50%	25%
Ampicillin/ sulbactam (Unasyn)	1.5–3 g IV every 6–8 hours	100%	1.5–3 g IV every 12 hours (GFR 15–29)	1.5–3g IV every 24 hours (GFR 5–14)
Cefazolin (Ancef)	500 mg–1.5 g every 8 hours	100%	Every 12 hours	50% every 24–48 hours
Ceftazidime (Fortaz)	1–2 g every 8–12 hours	100%	Every 12–24 hours	Every 24–48 hours
Ceftriaxone (Rocephin)	1–2 g every 24 hours	No adjustment needed		
Ciprofloxacin	400 mg IV or 500–750 mg orally every 12 hours	100%	50–75%	50%
Enoxaparin (Lovenox)	Prophylaxis: 30 mg SC every 12 hours	Usual dosage	30 mg SC daily (GFR < 30)	
	DVT treatment: 1 mg/kg SC every 12 hours or 1.5 mg/kg SC once daily		1 mg/kg SC every 24 hours (GFR < 30)	
Fluconazole (Diflucan)	200–400 mg every 24 hours	100%	50%	50%
Gabapentin (Neurontin)	300–600 mg three times daily	Usual dosage	400–1400 mg/day (divided twice daily) (GFR 30–59)	100–300 mg daily
			200–700 mg/day (GFR 15–29)	Not recommended
Levetiracetam (Keppra)	500–1500 mg every 12 hours	Usual dosage	250–750 mg every 12 hours (GFR 30–50)	
			250–500 mg every 12 hours (GFR < 30)	
			Hemodialysis: 500–1000 mg every 24 hours, supplemental dose of 250–500 mg recommended after dialysis	
Levofloxacin (Levaquin)	250–750 mg orally/IV daily	Usage dosage	500 mg initial dose, then 250 mg every 24 hours	500 mg initial dose, then 250 mg every 48 hours
Metformin (Glucophage)	500–1000 mg twice daily	Contraindicated in men with serum creatinine > 1.5 mg/dL and women with serum creatinine > 1.4 mg/dL or patients with GFR < 60		
		Should be temporarily discontinued 24–48 hours prior to administration of any radiocontrast agents and not restarted for 48 hours afterward due to the risk of developing lactic acidosis		
Metoclopramide (Reglan)	10–15 mg three to four times daily	Usual dosage	50%	25%
Piperacillin/ Tazobactam (Zosyn)	3.375 g IV every 6–8 hours	100%	2.25 g IV every 6 hours (GFR 20–40)	2.25 g IV every 8 hours
			2.25 g IV every 8 hours (GFR < 20)	
Simvastatin (Zocor)	10–80 mg daily	Usual dosage	Usual dosage	Start at 5 mg daily
Vancomycin	1 g IV every 12 hours	1 g IV every 12 hours	Start with 1 g IV every 12 hours (GFR 40–60)	
			Start with 1g IV every 24 hours (GFR < 40)	
			Determine dose by serum level monitoring	

DVT, deep vein thrombosis; GFR, glomerular filtration rate; IV, intravenous; SC, subcutaneous.

performed under ultrasonographic guidance with local anesthesia, though in morbidly obese patients a CT-guided biopsy can alternatively be performed. In the setting of AKI, a renal biopsy may be most helpful either when the diagnosis of acute glomerulonephritis is suspected or when the cause of renal failure is unknown. Other common indications for performing a renal biopsy include unexplained glomerular hematuria, significant proteinuria, and nephrotic syndrome. Absolute contraindications to percutaneous renal biopsy include uncontrolled moderate to severe hypertension, uncontrolled bleeding diathesis or severe anemia, an uncooperative patient, and a solitary functional kidney. Relative contraindications include anatomic abnormalities of the kidney that may increase the risk of the procedure, a skin infection overlying the biopsy site, active renal or perirenal infection, hydronephrosis, and the presence of multiple renal cysts or a renal tumor. The most common complication following percutaneous renal biopsy is bleeding, which if clinically significant is usually recognized within 12 to 24 hours postbiopsy. Other complications include pain, gross hematuria, and infection.

Chronic anticoagulation with warfarin is not a contraindication to renal biopsy; however, for each individual patient, the need and urgency for biopsy must be weighed against the risk of thrombosis if anticoagulation is stopped. In patients chronically taking aspirin or other antithrombotic agents, these medications should be held as soon as it is known that a biopsy will be performed (ideally 1–2 weeks prior to the procedure) and should not be resumed until 1–2 weeks after the procedure. Heparin should be stopped at least 6 hours prior to the biopsy and held for at least 12 to 24 hours postbiopsy.

Indications for dialysis

Dialysis is initiated to prevent and treat the life-threatening complications and uremic symptoms associated with the development of severe AKI. Generally accepted indications for the initiation of dialysis in the setting of AKI include (1) severe metabolic acidosis; (2) hyperkalemia, especially if electrocardiographic abnormalities are present; (3) volume overload refractory to the use of diuretics; and (4) uremic signs and symptoms, such as pericarditis, altered mental status, or seizures. The optimal timing of dialysis initiation has not been well established. Although a few retrospective and nonrandomized trials have found that earlier initiation of dialysis may improve survival, these results have yet to be tested in a large prospective randomized clinical trial.

SPECIFIC SYNDROMES

Postoperative renal failure

Postoperative AKI resulting in oliguria and/or an elevated serum creatinine level is one of the most common and serious complications of surgery, representing 18–47% of all cases of hospital-acquired AKI. It is associated with an increased risk for serious infections and sepsis, higher costs of hospitalization, and significantly increased mortality following both cardiac and noncardiac surgery. An estimated 0.1 to 30% of patients undergoing cardiovascular and thoracic surgeries develop postoperative AKI, and between 1 and 7% of these patients need renal replacement therapy. Furthermore, postoperative AKI that requires dialysis carries an in-hospital mortality rate of 60–80%.

The most common cause of postoperative AKI is ischemic ATN resulting from decreased renal perfusion during surgery. ATN can occur in a variety of surgical scenarios ranging from supra- or infrarenal aortic cross-clamping in vascular surgery to cardiopulmonary bypass during cardiac surgery. Common risk factors for the development of postoperative AKI include preexisting renal dysfunction, diabetes mellitus, advanced age (>65), major vascular surgery, cardiopulmonary bypass times greater than 3 hours, and recent exposure to nephrotoxic agents including contrast dyes, NSAIDs, and aminoglycosides. Patients may present postoperatively with either an acute elevation in serum creatinine or a reduction in urine output.

A number of principles can guide the evaluation and management of postoperative AKI:

1. **Identification of inciting factors.** Perioperative records and flowsheets should be thoroughly reviewed for evidence of hypotension, significant intraoperative or postoperative fluid losses (eg, blood and intravascular fluid losses, insensible losses, drainage losses, and third-spaced fluid losses), and the administration of potentially nephrotoxic agents (eg, NSAIDs for pain control or hydroxyethyl starches used for volume resuscitation).
2. **Hemodynamic monitoring.** Patients should have close perioperative hemodynamic monitoring, and if necessary, invasive monitoring with intra-arterial, central venous, or pulmonary arterial catheters should be used.
3. **Maintenance of adequate renal perfusion.** Though no optimal mean arterial pressure (MAP) has been established to ensure adequate renal perfusion, maintaining a MAP of at least >65 mm Hg and preferably >75–80 mm Hg is recommended.
4. **Optimization of volume status.** Intravenous fluid hydration should be administered to optimize renal perfusion in patients with volume depletion or hemodynamic instability. Patients who develop oliguria are often hypovolemic and should be given a fluid challenge. If they respond favorably with an improvement in urine output or hemodynamic parameters, more fluid challenges can be attempted.
5. **Avoidance of nephrotoxic agents.** Concomitant use of nephrotoxic medications is a risk factor for the development of postoperative AKI. If iodinated contrast agents must be used for diagnostic or therapeutic purposes, the smallest amount of nonionic iso-osmolar volume of contrast should be used. Other drugs such as NSAIDs, aminoglycosides, and amphotericin B should be avoided if possible. Patients who take ACE inhibitors or ARBs on a chronic basis should discontinue these medications prior to surgery, since chronic ACE inhibition reportedly increases the risk of postoperative AKI.
6. **Pharmacologic agents.** A variety of pharmacologic agents, including dopamine, fenoldapam, atrial natriuretic peptide, mannitol, calcium-channel blockers, and loop diuretics, have been tested for their ability to prevent postoperative AKI. The results of these studies are inconclusive, and there is insufficient evidence to recommend their use at this time.

Hepatorenal syndrome

Hepatorenal syndrome (HRS) is a functional form of AKI that occurs primarily in patients with cirrhosis and ascites. The pathophysiology of HRS is thought to be due to nitric oxide–induced vasodilation of the splanchnic circulation leading to marked intrarenal arterial vasoconstriction and a reduction in GFR. There are two types of HRS: type 1 HRS is the rapidly progressive form of the disease characterized by a doubling of the initial serum creatinine level to greater than 2.5 mg/dL over a period of less than 2 weeks. The prognosis of patients with type 1 HRS without liver transplantation is generally very poor. Type 2 HRS is a more moderate form of renal failure characterized by serum creatinine levels between 1.5 and 2.5 mg/dL and associated with a more indolent course and improved survival compared to type 1 HRS. Both type 1 and type 2 HRS can occur spontaneously or develop after a precipitating event, most commonly a bacterial infection such as spontaneous bacterial peritonitis (SBP). Diagnostic criteria for HRS were recently revised by the International Ascites Club in 2007 and now include the following: (1) cirrhosis with ascites; (2) serum creatinine >1.5 mg/dL; (3) no improvement in serum creatinine (decrease to ≤1.5 mg/dL) after at least 2 days with diuretic withdrawal and volume expansion with albumin; (4) absence of shock; (5) no current or recent treatment with nephrotoxic drugs; and (6) absence of renal parenchymal disease (proteinuria >500 mg/day, microhematuria with >50 red blood cells per high-power field, and/or abnormal renal ultrasonography). With proper medical treatment, HRS is potentially reversible. Type 1 HRS can be treated with vasoconstrictors (eg, terlipressin, midodrine in combination with octreotide, norepinephrine) combined with albumin. Transjugular intrahepatic portal shunt (TIPS) may be considered in patients with type 1 HRS with either partial response (decrease in serum creatinine to ≥50% of pretreatment value but not reaching the goal of ≤1.5 mg/dL) or no response (no decrease in serum creatinine or decrease to < 50% of pretreatment value) to medication. There is currently no definitive evidence demonstrating a benefit to using vasoconstrictors in patients with type 2 HRS. In patients being treated for SBP, prophylaxis with albumin is indicated, as this has been shown in one randomized clinical trial to reduce the incidence of HRS by 66% and significantly decrease in-hospital and 30-day mortality rates. The suggested dose of albumin is 1.5 mg/kg body weight on the first day, followed by 1 mg/kg body weight on the third day. Liver transplantation remains the treatment of choice for both type 1 and type 2 HRS.

Contrast-induced nephropathy

Contrast-induced AKI is a common complication seen in patients who have undergone diagnostic and/or therapeutic procedures involving the intravenous administration of an iodinated contrast medium. It is one of the most common causes of AKI acquired in the hospital setting, with reported incidence rates ranging from < 5 to > 30%. Contrast-induced AKI is commonly defined as an increase in serum creatinine (either an absolute increase of 0.5 mg/dL or a 25% increase from baseline) occurring within the first 24 hours after contrast exposure. The mechanism of injury involves renal vasoconstriction, impaired vasodilation, medullary hypoxia, and direct tubular cell damage. Preexisting renal impairment (eGFR < 60 mL/min) and diabetes mellitus are the two most important risk factors for developing contrast-induced AKI, though heart failure, hypovolemia, nephrotoxic drugs, and hemodynamic instability are other common risk factors.

A number of preventive strategies have been studied in patients at risk for contrast-induced AKI:

1. **Type of contrast agent.** The choice of contrast agent is important, since higher osmolar agents are associated with greater nephrotoxicity. In high-risk patients, nonionic iso-osmolar (eg, iodixanol) and low-osmolar (eg, iohexol, ioversol, iopamidol) contrast agents have been shown to have the least nephrotoxicity.
2. **Volume expansion.** Intravenous hydration is clearly beneficial in the prevention of contrast-induced AKI, though the optimal hydration fluid has yet to be determined. The current evidence indicates that isotonic fluids (either normal saline or sodium bicarbonate) are more protective than half-normal saline. Although initial clinical trials showed a benefit to using sodium bicarbonate over normal saline, more recent evidence has not confirmed these findings. The rate and timing of hydration are also unclear. If using normal saline, one possible regimen is 1 mL/kg for 6–12 hours before the procedure, followed by 1 mL/kg for 6–12 hours after the procedure. Alternatively, if using isotonic sodium bicarbonate (three 50 mL ampules each containing 50 mEq of sodium bicarbonate in 850 mL of 5% dextrose in water), one possible regimen is a bolus of 3 mL/kg for 1 hour prior to the procedure, followed by an infusion of 1 mL/kg for 6 hours after the procedure.
3. **N-acetylcysteine.** Though frequently used in the prevention of contrast-induced AKI, *N*-acetylcysteine has had inconsistent results in most clinical studies and meta-analyses. While some trials have reported significant protection, others have shown less substantial or even insignificant benefits. Given its relatively benign drug profile and its low cost, however, *N*-acetylcysteine is still often recommended as an adjunctive agent to IV hydration. In at-risk patients, it can be administered as 600 mg or 1200 mg orally twice daily on the day before and the day of the procedure.
4. **Diuretics.** The use of diuretics, particularly mannitol and furosemide, has not shown any benefit and may actually be harmful to patients.
5. **Hemodialysis/hemofiltration.** Although iodinated contrast agents are removable by dialysis, there is currently no definitive evidence to suggest that prophylactic hemodialysis or hemofiltration reduces the incidence of contrast-induced AKI.

Drug toxicity

Therapeutic agents frequently cause AKI in the hospital setting. The clinician should suspect drug toxicity when there is an acute rise in serum creatinine associated with the recent administration of a drug. As with the approach to AKI, the pathophysiology of drug nephrotoxicity can be divided into prerenal, intrarenal, and postrenal mechanisms. The most common mechanisms involve direct renal tubular injury resulting in ATN or renal interstitial inflammation leading to AIN. Other forms of injury include tubular obstruction due to precipitation of a drug, alterations in intrarenal blood flow, and, less commonly, glomerular disease. Drugs that are commonly associated with nephrotoxicity and their primary mechanisms of toxicity are listed in **Table 57-5**.

Drug-induced ATN is seen with the administration of medications that are excreted primarily by the kidneys, including aminoglycoside antibiotics, amphotericin B, and cisplatin (see Chemotherapy-Induced Nephrotoxicity). Aminoglycosides, commonly prescribed for the treatment of gram-negative bacterial infections, cause dose-dependent ATN with a frequency ranging from 10 to 20%. Neomycin causes the greatest nephrotoxicity; gentamicin, tobramycin, and

TABLE 57-5 Nephrotoxic Drugs in Acute Kidney Injury

Nephrotoxicity	Drugs
Prerenal	ACE inhibitors
	Angiotensin receptor blockers
	Cyclosporine
	IL-2
	Iodinated contrast agents
	NSAIDs
	Tacrolimus
Intrarenal	
• Acute interstitial nephritis	NSAIDs
	Penicillin analogues (nafcillin, oxacillin)
	Cephalosporins
	Sulfa drugs (sulfamethoxazole, thiazide diuretics)
	Rifampin
	Ciprofloxacin
	Proton-pump inhibitors
	Aminoglycoside antibiotics
• Acute tubular necrosis	Amphotericin B
	Cisplatin
	Iodinated contrast agents
	HIV medications (adefovir, ritonavir, tenofovir)
Postrenal	Acyclovir
	Analgesics
	Indinavir
	Methotrexate

ACE, angiotensin-converting enzyme; IV, human immunodeficiency virus; IL, interleukin; NSAID, nonsteroidal anti-inflammatory drug.

amikacin cause intermediate nephrotoxicity; and streptomycin causes the least nephrotoxicity. It should be recognized that aminoglycoside toxicity may follow oral administration of neomycin in cirrhotics, joint lavage after orthopedic procedures, and skin applications in burn patients. ATN typically develops 5–10 days after initiation of aminoglycoside treatment and is generally nonoliguric. The kidney injury is usually reversible with withdrawal of the drug, but renal replacement therapy may be necessary in some cases.

AIN is another frequently seen form of drug-induced nephrotoxicity that accounts for 3–15% of all drug-induced AKI. The most common offending agents include NSAIDs, penicillin analogues, cephalosporins, sulfonamides, rifampin, ciprofloxacin, and proton-pump inhibitors. While the onset of drug-induced AIN has been reported as early as a few days after a secondary exposure to a medication, it usually occurs 7–14 days and as late as weeks to months after a primary exposure. AIN is typically reversible with withdrawal of the drug, though renal recovery may take as long as weeks to months. Treatment of AIN with steroids has an unclear benefit, though some case series suggest that a short course of prednisone (1 mg/kg/day for up to 4 weeks) may increase the rate of recovery.

Drug-induced urinary obstruction generally results from the precipitation of drugs within the renal tubules or the ureters. Crystal-induced AKI and nephrolithiasis have been seen with medications such as acyclovir and indinavir. Certain analgesics containing aspirin, phenacetin, and caffeine may cause renal papillary necrosis, and sloughing of the necrotic tissue can lead to acute ureteral obstruction. Patients with drug-induced urinary obstruction may present with symptoms of renal colic and acute urinary tract obstruction. Management involves hydration, pain control, and discontinuation of the medication, although invasive removal of the stones may be required in severe cases.

A number of medications are known to modulate renal hemodynamics and cause a prerenal type of AKI. It is important to understand that intraglomerular capillary pressure and hence GFR are highly dependent on the vasomotor tone of both the afferent and the efferent arterioles. When renal perfusion is decreased, regulation of GFR involves vasodilation of the afferent arteriole and vasoconstriction of the efferent arteriole. Drugs that inhibit these compensatory mechanisms can further impair renal perfusion and lead to AKI. These agents include NSAIDs, ACE inhibitors, ARBs, cyclosporine, tacrolimus, and iodinated contrast agents (see Contrast-Induced Nephropathy). NSAIDs inhibit the production of prostaglandins, which are important mediators of afferent arteriolar vasodilation. In patients with normal renal function, this effect is largely inconsequential, but in those whose baseline renal perfusion is already impaired (eg, patients with heart failure or volume depletion), it can significantly reduce intrarenal blood flow and renal function. In contrast, ACE inhibitors and ARBs selectively block angiotensin II-mediated vasoconstriction of the efferent arteriole. A consequential increase in serum creatinine of up to 30% is acceptable with ACE inhibitors and ARBs, given the proven long-term renal protective effects of these medications, but more significant loss of renal function may be observed in patients with decreased renal perfusion or renovascular disease. Cyclosporine and tacrolimus, both calcineurin inhibitors widely used as immunosuppressants, cause intense afferent and efferent arteriolar vasoconstriction. Most patients taking these medications experience a reduction in GFR within weeks to months of starting therapy. As this effect is generally reversible and thought to be dose related, cyclosporine- or tacrolimus-induced AKI can usually be managed with a reduction in dose.

Chemotherapy-induced nephrotoxicity

Several therapeutic agents used to treat cancer are known to be toxic to the kidneys and may cause AKI. Factors such as intravascular volume depletion, simultaneous administration of other nephrotoxic drugs and/or iodinated contrast agents, urinary tract obstruction, and underlying renal disease may increase the potential of chemotherapy-induced nephrotoxicity. Cisplatin is one of the most well-established nephrotoxic chemotherapeutic agents. Commonly used in the treatment of a wide variety of malignancies, cisplatin can cause dose-related acute tubular necrosis and significant hypomagnesemia due to renal magnesium wasting. AKI may be reversible, though the repeated administration of cisplatin may lead to more chronic and irreversible kidney damage. Aggressive hydration with intravenous fluids, particularly isotonic normal saline, can increase urine volume and flow and function as prophylaxis against cisplatin toxicity. Newer-generation platinum compounds such as carboplatin and oxaliplatin have also been shown to cause acute tubular injury.

Methotrexate, an antimetabolite commonly used in the treatment of different malignancies, is not nephrotoxic at low doses (<0.5 to 1.0 g/m^2) but may have significant nephrotoxicity at higher doses (1 to 15 g/m^2). The mechanism of injury involves precipitation of the methotrexate in the tubules, causing direct tubular injury and leading to urinary obstruction. Prophylaxis with intravenous fluid administration and urinary alkalinization reduces the potential for toxicity. Dosing must be adjusted in patients with preexisting renal impairment.

Alkylating agents such as cyclophosphamide and ifosfamide are known to cause hemorrhagic cystitis and hyponatremia. Ifosfamide is more nephrotoxic than cyclophosphamide and can cause significant proximal tubular dysfunction, leading to a Fanconi-like syndrome including renal tubular acidosis and hypophosphatemia, and distal nephron toxicity resulting in nephrogenic diabetes insipidus. Interleukin-2, often used to treat renal cell carcinoma and metastatic melanoma, can cause reversible AKI by inducing a capillary leak syndrome that leads to interstitial edema and volume depletion. Treatment is focused on restoring intravascular volume and stabilizing hemodynamic parameters. **Table 57-6** lists several chemotherapeutic agents that commonly cause nephrotoxicity.

Cardiorenal syndrome

Cardiorenal syndrome (CRS) describes a set of acute or chronic conditions involving the heart and the kidney in which dysfunction of one organ leads to dysfunction of the other. Though it was previously thought that primary cardiac disease gave rise to renal dysfunction, evidence now suggests that renal impairment can also lead to cardiac dysfunction. A recently proposed classification system divides CRS into five subtypes: (1) type 1 CRS (acute worsening of cardiac function leads to acute kidney injury),

TABLE 57-6 Chemotherapeutic Agents and Mechanisms of Toxicity

Chemotherapeutic Agent	Mechanism of Toxicity
Alkylating agents	
• Cisplatin, carboplatin, oxaloplatin	Tubular injury, renal magnesium wasting
• Cyclophosphamide	Hemorrhagic cystitis, hyponatremia
• Ifosfamide	Proximal tubular dysfunction
Antimetabolites	
• Methotrexate	• Crystal-induced tubular injury with high-dose treatment
Biological response modifiers	
• Interleukin-2	• Capillary leak syndrome and volume depletion

(2) type 2 CRS (chronic abnormalities in cardiac function lead to CKD), (3) type 3 CRS (acute worsening of renal function causes acute cardiac dysfunction), (4) type 4 CRS (CKD contributes to decreased cardiac function, ventricular hypertrophy, diastolic dysfunction, and/or increased risk of adverse cardiovascular events), and (5) type 5 CRS (a systemic condition causes both cardiac and renal dysfunction). Type 1 CRS, which is a common occurrence, is most relevant to the discussion of AKI. Patients with type 1 CRS present with acute heart failure that leads to the development of AKI due to a reduction in renal perfusion. AKI tends to be more severe in patients with acute heart failure with systolic dysfunction compared to those with diastolic dysfunction. The early diagnosis of type 1 CRS is difficult, since at the time when an elevation in serum creatinine is detected, kidney injury has already occurred and little can be done therapeutically. Often, patients with type 1 CRS develop a decreased responsiveness to diuretic therapy, and the use of higher doses or combinations of diuretics can worsen the AKI. Patients with volume overload who are refractory to diuretics may need the removal of fluid through ultrafiltration. Other renal considerations in the heart patient include the possibility that potent vasodilating medications, such as hydralazine and calcium channel blockers, may manifest as edema, decreased urinary salt and water excretion, azotemia, and diuretic resistance. This syndrome occurs primarily in the patient with CKD or renovascular disease and can be thought of as a renal "steal" syndrome. Many drugs used in a cardiac setting are excreted by the kidney and may reach toxic systemic levels in renal disease. These include digoxin, procainamide, and morphine. The level of blood pressure reduction may have paradoxical effects on cardiac and renal function. For many reasons, management of patients with CRS is challenging, and involvement of a multidisciplinary team consisting of nephrologists, cardiologists, critical care physicians, and cardiac surgeons is recommended.

Rapidly progressive glomerulonephritis

Rapidly progressive glomerulonephritis (RPGN) is characterized by the acute onset of glomerular inflammation and progressive loss of renal function over a short period of time (days to weeks to months). Crescent formation within injured glomeruli is one of the pathologic hallmarks of this disease process. Patients may present with hypertension, azotemia, oliguria, proteinuria, and edema and typically have an active urinary sediment with dysmorphic red blood cells and red blood cell casts. RPGN is generally classified into three categories based on the cellular mechanism of disease and immunofluorescence pattern: type 1 (anti-GBM disease, linear pattern of IgG staining), type 2 (immune complex disease, granular pattern of IgG staining), and type 3 (pauci-immune disease, little or no immunofluorescent staining). Serological tests [eg, anti-GBM antibody, antineutrophil cytoplasmic antibodies (ANCAs), antinuclear antibody (ANA), complement levels] should be ordered, though definitive diagnosis frequently requires a renal biopsy. The diagnosis of RPGN should be considered a nephrologic emergency, and a nephrology consultation should be requested immediately to assist with renal biopsy and initiate appropriate treatment.

CHRONIC KIDNEY DISEASE

CKD affects approximately 13% of all adults in the United States. The Kidney Disease Outcomes Quality Initiative (K/DOQI) program defines CKD in adults as either (1) evidence of structural or functional kidney abnormalities, such as albuminuria, abnormal urinalyses, abnormal renal imaging, with or without decreased glomerular filtration rate (GFR); or (2) decreased GFR, with or without evidence of kidney damage, persisting for more than 3 months. GFR is most often determined by using estimating equations such as the Cockcroft-Gault or the MDRD formulas. Many hospitals now use these equations to routinely report eGFR whenever serum creatinine is measured. The National Kidney Foundation has stratified CKD into five stages of severity (**Table 57-7**). CKD and ESRD are associated with significant complications, including anemia, hypertension, bone disease, and acid–base and electrolyte disturbances, all of which are frequently encountered in the hospital setting.

TABLE 57-7 Staging of Chronic Kidney Disease

Stage	Description	GFR (mL/min/1.73 m²)
1	Kidney damage with normal or ↑ GFR	≥90
2	Kidney damage with mild ↓ GFR	60–89
3	Moderate ↓ GFR	30–59
4	Severe ↓ GFR	15–30
5	Kidney failure	< 15 or dialysis

GFR, glomerular filtration rate.

GENERAL INPATIENT MANAGEMENT

The management of a hospitalized patient with CKD or ESRD should be guided by a number of important general principles. First, the patient's nephrologist and dialysis unit, if applicable, should be contacted upon admission and discharge. This promotes communication between the outpatient and inpatient health care providers and facilitates continuity of care, often providing the hospitalist with the most current patient information, including patient history, medication regimen, vascular access history, and baseline parameters such as blood pressure and estimated dry weight. Second, admission orders should take into account the special needs of patients with CKD and ESRD. Vital signs should include regular blood pressure measurements, daily weights, and accurate measurements of intake and output. Unnecessary phlebotomy should be avoided, particularly in patients with anemia, and routine blood tests in dialysis patients can often be drawn at their dialysis sessions just prior to initiation. Third, all measures should be taken to protect the vascular access of ESRD patients who are receiving hemodialysis. Blood pressures and blood draws should be performed in the arm contralateral to the one with the vascular access. If blood must be drawn from the ipsilateral arm, it should be taken from the most distal vein possible, preferably from the dorsum of the hand. Given their increased risk of infection, hemodialysis catheters should be reserved for dialysis use only, and under no circumstances with the exception of life-threatening emergencies should a dialysis catheter be accessed for other purposes.

Patients with CKD frequently have altered drug metabolism due to changes in glomerular flow and filtration, tubular reabsorption and secretion, and renal bioactivation and metabolism. In addition, other factors such as drug absorption, bioavailability, distribution volume, and protein binding may also be altered and can influence the handling of medications in these patients. Inappropriate medication dosing can result in either drug toxicity or drug ineffectiveness. Upon admission to the hospital, the complete list of medications of a patient with CKD should be carefully reviewed, and particular attention should be given to medications that produce metabolites that can lead to prolonged pharmacologic effects in the setting of reduced renal clearance. All medications, especially those that are initiated during the hospitalization, should be appropriately dosed according to a patient's reduction in GFR.

As with all inpatients, nutrition is a vital part of the care of the hospitalized CKD patient and should be tailored appropriately to the patient's comorbidities. If available in the hospital, a registered renal dietitian can be of tremendous value in providing dietary recommendations during the hospitalization as well as in counseling patients on healthy eating habits following discharge. According to the K/DOQI guidelines, patients with CKD stages 1–4 should be on a low-sodium (< 2000 mg/day) diet in general, and potassium and phosphorus intake should be adjusted according to lab values. Provided that urine output is normal, there is no restriction on the amount of fluids in these patients' diets. Patients with ESRD should be placed on a diet that is low in potassium (2000–3000 mg/day), low in phosphorus (800–1000 mg/day), and low in sodium (< 2000 mg/day). Fluid intake should be limited to 1.5 to 2 liters daily to prevent large increases in interdialytic weight gain. Certain water-soluble vitamins are lost during hemodialysis and can be replaced with a daily multivitamin such as Diatx ZN (Pamlab, LLC), Dialyvite 3000 (Hillestad Pharmaceuticals), Nephplex Rx (Nephro-Tech, Inc.), Nephrocaps (Fleming Company), and Nephro-Vite Rx (Watson).

Hypertension

An estimated 50–75% of patients with a GFR < 60 mL/min/1.73 m^2 (CKD stages 3–5) have hypertension, and as renal function declines, hypertension becomes increasingly prevalent. Given the higher risk of cardiovascular morbidity and mortality associated with hypertension and CKD, the National Kidney Foundation Clinical Practice Guidelines for Hypertension recommend that in all patients with hypertension and CKD, blood pressure should be targeted to a systolic value of < 130 mm Hg and a diastolic value of < 80 mm Hg. The purpose of these goals is to decrease the risk for cardiovascular events and to delay the progression of CKD. ACE inhibitors and ARBs should be considered as first-line therapy for hypertension in CKD, given their antiproteinuric effects and long-term renoprotective effects. Diuretics, particularly loop diuretics, can be particularly useful in optimizing blood pressure. Loop diuretic doses should be titrated upward as tolerated until normalization of blood pressure is achieved or the patient develops symptoms or signs of overly aggressive diuresis (eg, lightheadedness, hypotension, rising BUN and creatinine). The effectiveness of thiazide diuretics decreases in patients with a GFR < 30 mL/min; however, these medications can be used synergistically with loop diuretics to improve diuresis in patients with refractory edema. Patients with ESRD on hemodialysis should have their morning doses of blood pressure medications held on dialysis days to prevent episodes of intradialytic hypotension and to facilitate volume removal during dialysis.

Anemia

Normocytic, normochromic anemia is a common complication of CKD and ESRD and impairs the quality of life of patients with CKD. It is primarily due to a deficiency in erythropoietin production by the kidneys, though other contributing factors to anemia in patients with CKD include iron deficiency, shortened red blood cell survival, uremic inhibitors of erythropoiesis, hemolysis, bleeding, loss of blood in hemodialysis circuits, and repeated blood draws. Anemia becomes more common as GFR decreases to < 60 mL/min/1.73 m^2. Treatment of anemia in CKD patients improves quality of life and decreases mortality. The National Kidney Foundation Disease Outcomes Quality Initiative (K/DOQI) Clinical Practice Guidelines and Clinical Practice Recommendations for Anemia in CKD, most recently updated in 2007, recommend that the hemoglobin target in dialysis and nondialysis patients with CKD generally be in the range of 11.0 to 12.0 g/dL. Treatment with an erythropoiesis-stimulating agent such as erythropoietin or darbepoietin alfa reduces the need for frequent blood transfusions and is recommended to achieve this target in anemic CKD patients. In nondialysis patients, levels above this target should be avoided, due to recent evidence demonstrating that these levels are associated with adverse cardiovascular outcomes. Therefore, the hemoglobin target in dialysis and nondialysis patients with CKD should not be > 39213.0 g/dL.

To ensure that anemic patients will respond to treatment with erythropoietin or darbepoietin, iron stores should be monitored regularly. Standard indices include a serum ferritin concentration, serum iron concentration, and total iron binding capacity. Iron deficiency in patients with CKD is defined as (1) transferrin saturation (TSAT) < 20%, or (2) serum ferritin < 100 ng/mL. Patients who meet either of these criteria should be given iron supplementation, either orally (eg, ferrous sulfate 325 mg three times daily) or intravenously (eg, iron sucrose, iron gluconate) to maintain a TSAT > 20–25% and serum ferritin between 200 and 500 ng/mL.

Bone metabolism

Renal phosphorus excretion is decreased in patients with CKD and can result in elevated serum phosphorus levels and lower serum calcium levels due to increased binding of phosphorus. Serum calcium and phosphorus levels should be followed regularly in the inpatient setting. Patients with CKD and/or ESRD with hyperphosphatemia should be placed on low phosphorus diets (< 800–1000 mg/day) during their hospitalization and should be counseled to limit their intake of foods that are high in phosphorus, such as dairy products, meats, dried beans and peas, and cola drinks. Hyperphosphatemia that cannot be adequately controlled by dietary modification alone should be treated with oral phosphorus-binding agents. Oral aluminum hydroxide, historically the first agent made available to treat hyperphosphatemia, is rarely used these days because of its long-term risk of aluminum toxicity and osteomalacia. It has been largely replaced by the calcium-containing (calcium acetate, calcium carbonate, and calcium citrate) and the non-calcium-containing phosphorus binders (sevelamer hydrochloride, sevelamer carbonate, and lanthanum carbonate). When administered with meals, these medications function to inhibit the gastrointestinal absorption of phosphorus; thus they are not effective at lowering serum phosphorus levels in patients who are not receiving any dietary intake. Calcium acetate has been demonstrated in a number of studies to be more cost-effective than sevelamer. However, in patients who develop extraskeletal calcifications or recurrent hypercalcemia from calcium-containing phosphorus binders, sevelamer and lanthanum are suitable, though more expensive, alternatives. Calcium-containing phosphorus binders and sevelamer or lanthanum can also be used in combination to treat hyperphosphatemia that is difficult to control with a single agent. Of note, sevelamer hydrochloride has been associated with metabolic acidosis; in these patients, substituting with sevelamer carbonate may be of benefit as this formulation does not decrease serum bicarbonate levels.

Acid–base and electrolytes

Patients with CKD may have a metabolic acidosis due to impaired acid secretion. Sodium bicarbonate should be administered to patients with serum bicarbonate concentrations < 22 mEq/L to prevent the complications of chronic metabolic acidosis, specifically bone disease and loss of lean body mass due to increased breakdown of skeletal muscle. Sodium bicarbonate can be given as oral tablets [650 mg (7 mEq) twice daily with meals] or alternatively in the form of baking soda (1/2 to 1 teaspoon dissolved in water or juice twice daily with meals). Patients may experience some abdominal bloating with bicarbonate treatment. Citrate salts should not be used as alkalinizing agents in CKD as they may increase aluminum absorption.

Electrolyte disorders are also common in patients with CKD and ESRD. When GFR decreases to < 15–20 mL/min, renal potassium excretion is impaired and hyperkalemia may occur. In patients who still produce adequate urine output, acute hyperkalemia can usually be managed medically with calcium gluconate (if electrocardiographic changes are present), insulin, inhaled albuterol, potassium-binding resins (eg, sodium polystyrene sulfonate), and loop diuretics. Patients with ESRD and oliguria or anuria will often require dialysis therapy to treat the hyperkalemia. Chronic management of hyperkalemia involves dietary potassium restriction; supplementation with loop diuretics and potassium-binding resins is usually not necessary but can be useful for long-term control. If resins are used, it should be noted that they can result in hypocalcemia, sodium overload, and malabsorption of other medications. If given as a retention enema they can cause colonic ulceration. These resins should not be given with aluminum hydroxide gels. Hypokalemia is less common in patients with CKD but can be caused by low potassium intake, diuretic use, or gastrointestinal losses.

The ability of the kidney to properly concentrate or dilute urine is reduced as renal function is progressively lost, and both hyponatremia and hypernatremia are common in patients with CKD. Hyponatremia may be due to impaired free water clearance or volume depletion through renal or extrarenal sodium losses. A careful assessment of volume status can guide appropriate treatment: patients who are euvolemic or hypervolemic will usually benefit from free water restriction and occasionally diuretics, whereas patients who are hypovolemic may require administration of intravenous normal saline. Hypernatremia can be seen in the setting of impaired water intake (eg, poor thirst mechanisms or decreased access to water) or excessive renal or extrarenal water losses. Hypernatremia may also accompany recovery from AKI as the high level of urea falls with the osmotic diuresis. Patients should be given free water, either orally or intravenously, to correct the water deficit.

Fluids

The management of a hospitalized patient with CKD or ESRD should be guided by a number of important general principles.

1. The patient's nephrologist and dialysis unit, if applicable, should be contacted upon admission and discharge.
2. The admission orders should take into account the special needs of patients with CKD and ESRD.
3. All measures should be taken to protect the vascular access of ESRD patients who are receiving hemodialysis.
4. All medications, especially those that are initiated during the hospitalization, should be appropriately dosed according to a patient's reduction in GFR.

PRACTICE POINT

- In ESRD patients with little or no urine production, oral fluid intake should be closely monitored and restricted to 1–1.5 L/day. Large interdialytic weight gains (> 4–5 kg) due to liberal fluid consumption or administration of intravenous fluids and medications can make volume removal during dialysis more difficult.

CONCLUSION

Acute and chronic kidney disease is common in hospitalized patients. Although consultation by an experienced nephrologist is often required in the care of these patients, a strong understanding of the issues presented in this chapter will facilitate the hospital clinician's ability to anticipate and independently manage issues that frequently arise during the hospitalization of the renal patient.

SUGGESTED READINGS

Bellomo R, Ronco C, Kellum JA, Mehta RL, Palevsky P. Acute renal failure—definition, outcome measures, animal models, fluid therapy and information technology needs: the Second International Consensus Conference of the Acute Dialysis Quality Initiative (ADQI) Group. *Crit Care*. 2004;8:R204–212.

Cohen RA, Brown RS. Clinical practice: Microscopic hematuria. *N Engl J Med*. 2003;348:2330–2338.

Coresh J, Selvin E, Stevens LA, Manzi J, Kusek JW, Eggers P, Van Lente F, and Levey AS. Prevalence of chronic kidney disease in the United States. *JAMA*. 2007;298:2038–2047.

Munar MY, Singh H. Drug dosing adjustments in patients with chronic kidney disease. *Am Fam Physician*. 2007;75:1487–1496.

Pannu N, Nadim MK. An overview of drug-induced acute kidney injury. *Crit Care Med*. 2008;36:S216–223.

Ronco C, Haapio M, House AA, Anavekar N, Bellomo R. Cardiorenal syndrome. *J Am Coll Cardiol*. 2008;52:1527–1539.

Salerno F, Gerbes A, Gines P, Wong F, Arroyo V. Diagnosis, prevention and treatment of hepatorenal syndrome in cirrhosis. *Gut*. 2007;56:1310–1318.

Sear JW. Kidney dysfunction in the postoperative period. *Br J Anaesth*. 2005;95:20–32, 2005.

Thadhani R, Pascual M, Bonventre JV. Acute renal failure. *N Engl J Med*. 1996;334:1448–1460.

Venkataraman R, Kellum JA. Prevention of acute renal failure. *Chest*. 2007;131:300–308.

REFERENCES

1. Coresh J, Selvin E, Stevens LA, et al. Prevalence of chronic kidney disease in the United States. *JAMA*. 2007;298:2038–2047.
2. Tan KT, van Beek EJ, Brown PW, van Delden OM, Tijssen J, Ramsay LE. Magnetic resonance angiography for the diagnosis of renal artery stenosis: a meta-analysis. *Clin Radiol*. 2002;57:617–624.

SECTION 5

Perioperative Antithrombotic Management and Prevention

CHAPTER 58

Venous Thromboembolism (VTE) Prophylaxis for Patients Requiring Nonorthopedic Surgery

Menaka Pai, MD, FRCPC
James D. Douketis, MD, FRCPC, FACP, FCCP

WHAT IS THE RISK FOR VENOUS THROMBOEMBOLISM IN PATIENTS REQUIRING NONORTHOPEDIC SURGERY?

EPIDEMIOLOGY

Each year, surgeons in the United States perform more than 46 million inpatient surgeries, the majority of which are nonorthopedic surgeries. Patients undergoing nonorthopedic surgeries are a heterogeneous group in terms of surgery type, comorbidities, and associated risk for venous thromboembolism (VTE), which comprises deep vein thrombosis (DVT) and pulmonary embolism (PE). Patients at low risk for VTE typically undergo surgical procedures lasting less than 30 minutes, are immediately mobile following surgery, or are already receiving therapeutic-dose anticoagulant therapy. All other surgical patients are considered to be at moderate or higher risk for VTE and merit some form of prophylaxis. VTE in the patient undergoing nonorthopedic surgery can cause significant morbidity and mortality and is a common cause of readmission to the hospital.

PATHOPHYSIOLOGY

Many factors contribute to VTE after nonorthopedic surgery (**Table 58-1**).

Trauma and surgery both contribute to venous injury and activation of the coagulation system. Postoperatively, patients may have persistently reduced mobility, which causes stasis of blood flow in the deep venous system. Patients undergoing certain types of surgery may also have independent risk factors for VTE, such as obesity in the bariatric surgical patient.

As in the orthopedic surgery setting, most episodes of postoperative DVT in nonorthopedic surgery are clinically silent. These unnoticed clots usually resolve spontaneously without administration of antithrombotic therapy. However, 25% to 50% grow and cause symptomatic DVT or PE.

WHICH PATIENTS UNDERGOING NONORTHOPEDIC SURGERY NEED VTE PROPHYLAXIS?

DOES THIS PATIENT UNDERGOING GENERAL SURGERY NEED VTE PROPHYLAXIS?

CASE 58-1

A 32-year-old mother of two comes to the emergency room with abdominal pain and nausea. An ultrasound confirms acute appendicitis, and the general surgeon at your center feels this patient should have an appendectomy within the next six hours. He feels she is at low operative risk, since she has no past medical history and is taking no medications, apart from an oral contraceptive pill. The general surgery resident phones you to ask if the patient needs VTE prophylaxis.

Data from studies done more than 20 years ago involving patients who did not routinely receive thromboprophylaxis found that rates of asymptomatic DVT in patients having general surgical procedures were between 15% and 30%, while rates of fatal PE occurred in 0.2% to 0.9% of patients. Current surgical practices, including improved perioperative care, rapid postoperative mobilization, and greater use of regional anesthesia have likely reduced these figures. However, general surgery patients are still considered to be at moderately high risk of VTE. Numerous randomized clinical trials and

TABLE 58-1 Factors that Increase Risk for Venous Thromboembolism in Surgical Patients

Surgical Factors
Antecedent trauma (as reason for surgery)
General anesthesia (compared with regional/local anesthesia)
Abdominal surgical approach (ie, compared with vaginal approach)
Open surgical approach (ie, compared with laparoscopic approach)
Use of the lithotomy position intraoperatively
Extrinsic venous compression intraoperatively
Extended duration of surgery (ie, > 1 hour)
Postoperative infection
Central venous catheterization
Immobility (confined to bed, needing assistance to ambulate)
Nonsurgical Factors
Increasing age
Pregnancy and the puerperium
Acute medical illness (eg, congestive heart failure, obstructive lung disease)
Acute ischemic stroke
Acute neurologic disease
Inflammatory bowel disease
Cancer (active or occult)
Sepsis
Previous VTE
Prior pelvic radiation
Inherited or acquired thrombophilia
Myeloproliferative disorders
Obesity
Drugs (eg, chemotherapy, hormonal therapy, erythropoeisis stimulating agents)

meta-analyses have shown that thromboprophylaxis with low-dose unfractionated heparin (LDUH) and low-molecular-weight heparin (LMWH) reduce the risk of asymptomatic DVT and symptomatic VTE by more than 60% in these patients.

PRACTICE POINT

The risk of thrombosis

- According to the ACCP 2008 guidelines, the type of surgery is the primary determinant of the risk of DVT, and the type and duration of anesthesia is generally determined by the surgical procedure.
  - The approximate DVT risk without prophylaxis is based on objectively confirmed rates of DVT in asymptomatic patients who did not receive prophylaxis.
  - There is a range of approximately 10–40% in general surgical patients, depending on the specific procedure, complications, and traditional risk factors.
- General anesthesia poses a greater risk of VTE than spinal or epidural anesthesia and the duration of anesthesia irrespective of the type of anesthesia influences VTE risk, with > 3.5 hours associated with the highest risk.
- Postoperative complications may further increase the risk.

Patients with no additional risk factors, who have short (< 30 minute) procedures, and who can mobilize postoperatively, do not require any specific thromboprophylaxis. All other patients should be evaluated for VTE prophylaxis. Patients at a low risk for bleeding should receive pharmacologic prophylaxis with low dose unfractionated heparin (LDUH), low molecular weight heparin (LMWH), or fondaparinux. There have been no trials that directly compare the two most popular dosing regimens of subcutaneous LDUH, 5000 units every 8 hours and 5000 units every 12 hours. There have been several trials comparing LMWH and LDUH, and both are considered equally efficacious. There is conflicting evidence regarding the safety of LMWH versus LDUH, but a recent meta-analysis showed that lower doses of LMWH were associated with less bleeding than LDUH. Our practice is to use the lowest recommended dose of heparin for prophylaxis, to minimize bleeding complications, and reduce the number of injections that a patient must receive. The selective factor Xa inhibitor fondaparinux has also been evaluated for major abdominal surgery. There does not appear to be any significant difference in VTE, major bleeding, or death when fondaparinux is compared with LMWH.

Mechanical thromboprophylaxis is an option in patients with a high risk of bleeding. However, graduated compression stockings (GCS) and intermittent pneumatic compression devices (IPC) are not as effective as pharmacologic prophylaxis, and do not appear to reduce the risk of proximal DVT or symptomatic PE. Though many use them as an "add-on intervention" in general surgery patients who are at particularly high risk of VTE, such as those with cancer, there is little evidence that they add to the protective effect of pharmacologic prophylaxis.

The evidence for extended thromboprophylaxis in general surgery is not as robust as in orthopedic surgery. One trial showed that the incidence of asymptomatic DVT in cancer surgery patients was lower in patients who had their LMWH continued for two to three weeks after hospital discharge; however, this trial only included patients undergoing cancer surgery. At this time, it is not recommended that all general surgery patients receive extended thromboprophylaxis. However, cancer patients who are at particularly high risk of VTE should be considered for postdischarge prophylaxis for two to three weeks.

PRACTICE POINT

A risk assessment does not have to be complicated.

- It is the number of risk factors that determines whether a patient is low, moderate, or high risk, not just the surgical procedure itself.
- Once you exceed three risk factors, the patient is high risk.

DOES THIS PATIENT UNDERGOING GYNECOLOGIC OR UROLOGIC SURGERY NEED VTE PROPHYLAXIS?

CASE 58-2

A 78-year-old man is undergoing a radical prostatectomy for prostate cancer. His past medical history is significant for type 2 diabetes mellitus, peripheral neuropathy, and a below-knee amputation performed 10 years ago. He has no history of bleeding. The urologist asks you if you are aware of any intraoperative or postoperative strategies to reduce this patient's VTE risk.

There are fewer randomized clinical trials of thromboprophylaxis in gynecologic surgery, with no data on combined mechanical and pharmacologic prophylaxis or extended duration thromboprophylaxis. However, the rates of DVT, PE, and fatal PE in major gynecologic surgery are similar to those in general surgery. For this reason, thromboprophylaxis recommendations are similar. There is data that otherwise low-risk patients undergoing benign gynecologic surgery benefit equally from continuously-used IPC versus LDUH twice daily. There is also data that cancer remains a significant thrombosis risk factor in gynecologic surgery, and that twice-daily dosing of LDUH may be less effective than thrice-daily LDUH or LMWH.

VTE is an important problem in major urologic surgery, with rates of postoperative symptomatic VTE between 1% and 5%. However, there has been only one methodologically rigorous randomized clinical trial in the last 20 years in this area. Again, thromboprophylaxis recommendations are similar to those in general surgery. It is known that open procedures (versus transurethral procedures) and the use of the lithotomy position are associated with increased VTE risk. Communication with the surgeon and the anaesthetist can modify these intraoperative factors and help reduce the patient's VTE risk.

DOES THIS PATIENT UNDERGOING CARDIAC OR VASCULAR SURGERY NEED VTE PROPHYLAXIS?

CASE 58-3

An 82-year-old woman is undergoing femorodistal bypass for longstanding peripheral arterial disease. She is an ex-smoker, and has a history of hypertension and hyperlipidemia. The patient is currently on aspirin and has been told that she will receive additional blood thinners at the time of her operation to keep her arteries from getting blocked. She has read about deep vein thrombosis, and wonders if she should receive any extra care to prevent this complication of surgery.

There is limited evidence for VTE prophylaxis in vascular surgery patients, with only four randomized clinical trials in this area (**Figure 58-1**). Three trials compared LDUH with no thromboprophylaxis. LDUH was not associated with a lower rate of proximal DVT, and bleeding rates were higher in those who received LDUH. The fourth trial compared LDUH 7,500 U every 12 hours with enoxaparin 40 mg once daily. There was no significant difference in rates of DVT detected by routine ultrasound screening or rates of major bleeding. Why does VTE prophylaxis not appear to have a benefit in vascular surgery patients? The most likely reason is that vascular surgery patients frequently receive antithrombotic agents such as intravenous heparin, and antiplatelet agents such as aspirin and clopidogrel, to prevent arterial occlusion after vascular reconstruction. These agents lower the risk of VTE, making routine use of additional anticoagulants redundant (and possibly harmful). At this time, routine thromboprophylaxis is not recommended in vascular surgery patients. Patients with additional VTE risk factors may receive prophylaxis with LMWH, LDUH, or fondaparinux.

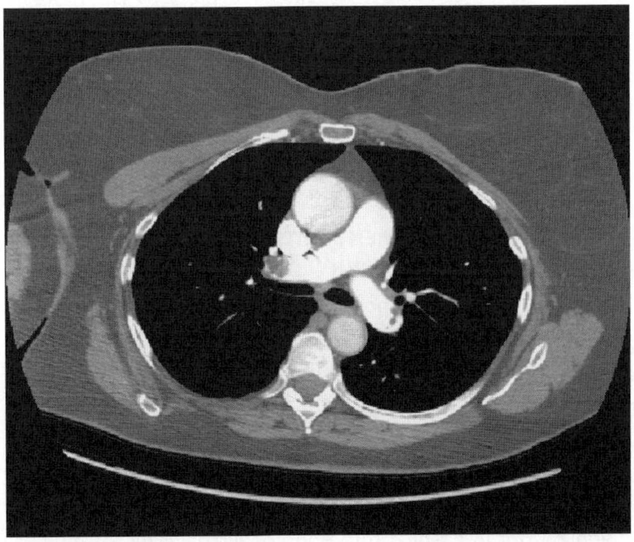

Figure 58-1 *Computed tomography pulmonary angiography showing emboli in both pulmonary arteries.*

There is also limited evidence for VTE prophylaxis in cardiac surgery patients. Like vascular surgery patients, these individuals receive antithrombotic agents such as intravenous heparin, and antiplatelet agents such as aspirin and clopidogrel. Patients who undergo cardiac valve replacement generally receive full-dose anticoagulation postoperatively, making pharmacologic VTE prophylaxis redundant. The incidence of symptomatic VTE after cardiac surgery is thought to range from 0.5% to 3.9%. Patients at highest risk are those on prolonged bed rest, those with prolonged hospitalization before surgery, and those with congestive heart failure. The risk of heparin-induced thrombocytopenia (HIT) also influences decision making regarding thromboprophylaxis. Approximately 20% of patients undergoing coronary artery bypass grafting (CABG) who develop a PE are diagnosed with HIT. HIT has been shown to be more common when LDUH is used, versus LMWH. It is uncertain if thromboprophylaxis should be administered to all cardiac surgery patients; however, in CABG patients who do not receive full-dose therapeutic anticoagulation postoperatively most physicians elect to use prophylactic-dose heparin or bilateral mechanical thromboprophylaxis (if the patient has not had saphenous vein grafting). Because the risk of HIT is high in cardiac surgery, LMWH is preferred over LDUH.

DOES THIS PATIENT UNDERGOING NEUROSURGERY NEED VTE PROPHYLAXIS?

Patients undergoing major neurosurgery are at a moderate risk for VTE, with rates of proximal DVT as high as 5% postoperatively. Those with malignant brain tumors are at particularly high risk. One prospective study of more than 250 patients with gliomas showed that 31% had symptomatic, venographically confirmed DVT within five weeks of their surgery. However, a major barrier to optimal VTE prophylaxis in neurosurgery patients is their risk of bleeding. Intracranial bleeding can have devastating clinical consequences, and for this reason, preoperative and early postoperative pharmacologic prophylaxis should be used with caution in craniotomy patients. Rates of intracranial hemorrhage appear to double when postoperative LMWH is compared to mechanical or no thromboprophylaxis (approximately 2% to 6% versus 1% to 3%). Most of these bleeds occur within the first two days after surgery. A reasonable approach that balances the risks of bleeding and thrombosis is to start mechanical thromboprophylaxis with IPC at the time of neurosurgery. Perioperative use of IPC is highly effective, reducing the risk of VTE by more than two-thirds. If a careful clinical assessment is stable and postoperative CT scan does not show bleeding at 24 to 48 hours, LMWH or LDUH can be added to further protect the patient from VTE. There is no evidence for extended prophylaxis in neurosurgery patients.

DOES THIS PATIENT UNDERGOING LAPAROSCOPIC OR BARIATRIC SURGERY NEED VTE PROPHYLAXIS?

Laparoscopic surgery is becoming an increasingly popular alternative to conventional open surgical procedures, due to decreased tissue trauma and faster recovery times. However, there are some unique features of laparoscopic surgery that increase thrombosis risk, including longer intraoperative time and pneumoperitoneum (which creates venous stasis in the lower extremities). Nevertheless, rates of symptomatic VTE following laparoscopic surgery are lower than in general surgery, less than 0.5% in most series. Rates of asymptomatic VTE are thought to be lower than 1%. For this reason, routine VTE prophylaxis is not recommended in laparoscopic surgery.

Bariatric surgery, which includes Roux-en-Y gastric bypass, gastric banding, vertical-banded gastroplasty, and biliopancreatic diversion, is also a growing field. More than 100,000 bariatric surgeries for morbid obesity are performed in the United States every year. Obesity is a known risk factor for VTE and puts bariatric surgery patients in a unique risk group. Rates of symptomatic VTE vary depending on the study quoted, anywhere from 0.8% to 2.4%. However, there is still insufficient high-quality evidence to make clear recommendations regarding VTE prophylaxis in bariatric surgery. Early ambulation and mechanical prophylaxis (either IPC or GCS) are widely accepted components of postoperative care in bariatric surgery patients. The American College of Chest Physicians' most recent guidelines also recommend LMWH, LDUH (three times daily), or fondaparinux be routinely used. Doses of LMWH and LDUH should be increased in obese patients.

WHAT PHARMACOLOGIC AND NONPHARMACOLOGIC STRATEGIES SHOULD BE USED FOR VTE PROPHYLAXIS?

Physicians have a number of options available when choosing the type of VTE prophylaxis in nonorthopedic surgery. Mechanical methods of prophylaxis, which include graduated compression stockings and intermittent pneumatic compression devices, are a safe option in patients with an increased bleeding risk (**Table 58-2**). However, they are inferior to pharmacologic prophylaxis and are insufficient protection against VTE in patients at high risk of thrombosis. All patients with an increased risk for bleeding should be reassessed regularly so pharmacologic prophylaxis can be started when the bleeding risk decreases to an acceptable level.

Pharmacologic prophylaxis should be the thomboprophylaxis strategy of choice in nonorthopedic surgery. Refer to **Table 58-3** for the recommended dose regimens. However, these doses may be inadequate in the bariatric surgery population. LMWH dosing in obese patients remains controversial.

PRACTICE POINT

Pharmacologic prophylaxis should be the thomboprophylaxis strategy of choice in nonorthopedic surgery.

- Mechanical methods of prophylaxis, which include graduated compression stockings and intermittent pneumatic compression devices, are a safe option in patients with an increased bleeding risk.
- However, they are inferior to pharmacologic prophylaxis, and are insufficient protection against VTE in patients at high risk of thrombosis.

TABLE 58-2 Contraindications to Thromboprophylaxis with Anticoagulants

Excessive active bleeding (beyond that expected after surgery)
At high risk for bleeding that precludes anticoagulants (eg, brain lesion)
Recent serious bleeding (eg, within 1 month)
Coagulopathy (eg, INR > 1.5, aPTT > 40)
Thrombocytopenia (eg, platelets < 75 x 10^9/L)

TABLE 58-3 Pharmacologic Prophylaxis Options in Nonorthopedic Surgery, with Accepted Doses

Fondaparinux (Arixtra) 2.5 mg SC once daily
Dalteparin (Fragmin) 2500 units or 5000 units SC once daily
Enoxaparin (Lovenox) 40 mg SC once daily or 30 mg SC every 12 hours
Nadroparin (Fraxiparine) 1900–3800 anti-Xa units SC once daily
Tinzaparin (Innohep) 3500 or 4500 anti-Xa units SC once daily
Heparin 5000 units SC every 12 hours or every 8 hours

Previous studies that have tried to address this issue have used anti-Xa levels as a primary outcome instead of clinical events. None of the currently available LMWH products have a "maximum dose," apart from dalteparin. Prospective nonrandomized studies have questioned the validity of dose limitation by showing that increasing the total daily dose of LMWH by 50% for patients with a BMI > 50 kg/m^2 can effectively increase patients' anti-Xa levels to the target prophylactic range (0.2–0.4 IU/mL). However, these studies used anti-Xa levels as a primary outcome instead of clinical events, and were not all sufficiently powered to detect bleeding. Higher doses of anticoagulant may be necessary to achieve an appropriate level of prophylaxis for obese patients (**Table 58-4**). Physicians must be cautious of bleeding complications as they increase LMWH dosing. Anti-Xa levels, though not a surrogate marker for bleeding risk, can provide a useful adjunct to close clinical monitoring.

WHAT ARE SOME PRACTICAL MANAGEMENT ISSUES FOR THE HOSPITALIST IN VTE PROPHYLAXIS?

CONSIDERATIONS UPON DISCHARGE FROM HOSPITAL

There is no evidence that patients undergoing nonorthopedic surgery benefit from routine DVT screening using Doppler ultrasound or venography. This strategy may pick up asymptomatic venous thrombosis in a small number of patients, but does not appear to reduce the rates of clinically significant events. There is also no robust evidence that VTE prophylaxis should be extended after hospital discharge. Patients at particularly high risk of thrombosis (eg, cancer surgery, prolonged immobility, and multiple other risk factors), may be candidates for extended prophylaxis for two to three weeks with injectable anticoagulants. The hospitalist can facilitate this transition by arranging nursing care at home, instructing the patient (or a caregiver) on injection technique and safe disposal of used needles, and clarifying who to call if bleeding develops. All patients should be educated about the signs and symptoms of VTE during their hospital stay and at the time of discharge.

QUALITY IMPROVEMENT INITIATIVES TO OPTIMIZE VTE PROPHYLAXIS

VTE prophylaxis in nonorthopedic surgery patients is a critical public health issue. In 2009, the U.S. Surgeon General cited VTE as one of the most preventable hospital-acquired illnesses, and issued a call to action to optimize its prevention. Though VTE prophylaxis in nonorthopedic surgery is based on scientific evidence, the quality and number of trials is limited compared to the orthopedic surgery population. There is also significant room for improvement in compliance rates with the American College of Chest Physicians' guidelines for in-hospital thromboprophylaxis. A recent multinational cross-sectional study demonstrated that compliance rates were approximately 85% in orthopedic surgery, but dropped to

TABLE 58-4 Summary of Recommendations for VTE Prophylaxis in Nonorthopedic Surgery

Setting	Average Bleeding Risk	High Bleeding Risk
General surgery	Low thrombosis risk: early and frequent ambulation Moderate thrombosis risk: fondaparinux, LMWH, LDUH High thrombosis risk: fondaparinux, LMWH, LDUH (3 times daily), plus mechanical prophylaxis. Consider post-discharge prophylaxis.	Moderate to high thrombosis risk: GCS, IPC
Gynecologic surgery	Low thrombosis risk: early and frequent ambulation Moderate thrombosis risk: LMWH, LDUH High thrombosis risk: LMWH, LDUH (3 times daily), plus mechanical prophylaxis. Consider post-discharge prophylaxis.	Moderate to high thrombosis risk: IPC
Urologic surgery	Low thrombosis risk: early and frequent ambulation Moderate to high thrombosis risk: Fondaparinux, LMWH, LDUH (2 to 3 times daily). Consider adding mechanical prophylaxis.	Moderate to high thrombosis risk: GCP, IPC
Vascular surgery	Low thrombosis risk: Early and frequent ambulation Moderate thrombosis risk: Fondaparinux, LMWH, LDUH	Moderate thrombosis risk: GCS, IPC
Coronary artery bypass surgery	LMWH LDUH	GCS IPC
Neurosurgery	IPC. Consider cautious addition of LMWH or LDUH.	IPC
Laparoscopic surgery	Low thrombosis risk: early and frequent ambulation Moderate to high thrombosis risk: Fondaparinux, LMWH, LDUH	GCS IPC
Bariatric surgery	LMWH, LDUH (3 times daily), fondaparinux. Consider adding mechanical prophylaxis.	GCS IPC

66% in gastric surgery, 59% in colon surgery, and 47% in urologic surgery. Concerted system-wide and local efforts must be made to increase the appropriate use of thromboprophylaxis in nonorthopedic surgery.

SUGGESTED READINGS

Agnelli G, Bergqvist D, Cohen AT, et al. Randomized clinical trial of postoperative fondaparinux versus perioperative dalteparin for prevention of venous thromboembolism in high-risk abdominal surgery. *Br J Surg.* 2005;92:1212–1220.

Bergqvist D, Agnelli G, Cohen AT, et al. Duration of prophylaxis against venous thromboembolism with enoxaparin after surgery for cancer. *N Engl J Med.* 2002;346:975–980.

Clagett GP, Reisch JS. Prevention of venous thromboembolism in general surgical patient: results of meta-analysis. *Ann Surg.* 1988;208:227–240.

Cohen AT, Tapson VF, Bergmann JF, et al. Venous thromboembolism risk and prophylaxis in the acute hospital care setting (ENDORSE study): a multinational cross-sectional study. *Lancet.* 2008;371(9610):387–394.

Collins R, Scrimgeour A, Yusuf S. Reduction in fatal pulmonary embolism and venous thrombosis by perioperative administration of subcutaneous heparin: overview of results of randomized trials in general, orthopedic, and urologic surgery. *N Engl J Med.* 1988;318:1162–1173.

Geerts WH, Bergqvist D, Pineo GF, et al. Prevention of venous thromboembolism: American College of Chest Physicians Evidence-Based Clinical Practice Guidelines (8th Edition). *Chest.* 2008;133(6 suppl):381S–453S.

Goldhaber SZ, Schoepf UJ. Pulmonary embolism after coronary artery bypass grafting. *Circulation.* 2004;109:2712–2715.

Mismetti P, Laporte S, Darmon JY, Buchmüller A, Decousus H. Meta-analysis of low molecular weight heparin in the prevention of venous thromboembolism in general surgery. *Br J Surg.* 2001;88(7):913–930.

Simone EP, Madan AK, Tichansky DS, et al. Comparison of two low-molecular-weight heparin dosing regimens for patients undergoing laparoscopic bariatric surgery. *Surg Endosc.* 2008;22(11):2392–2395.

Yu HT, Dylan ML, Lin J, Dubois RW. Hospitals' compliance with prophylaxis guidelines for venous thromboembolism. *Am J Health Syst Pharm.* 2007;64:69–76.

CHAPTER 59

Venous Thromboembolism (VTE) Prophylaxis for Patients Requiring Orthopedic Surgery

Menaka Pai, MD, FRCPC
James D. Douketis, MD, FRCPC, FACP, FCCP

WHAT IS THE RISK FOR VENOUS THROMBOEMBOLISM IN PATIENTS REQUIRING MAJOR ORTHOPEDIC SURGERY?

EPIDEMIOLOGY

In the United States, more than 540,000 total knee replacements and more than 230,000 total hip replacements are performed annually. In addition to patients undergoing hip fracture repair surgery, patients undergoing these major orthopedic surgeries are one of the highest risk groups for developing postoperative VTE, which comprises deep vein thrombosis (DVT) and pulmonary embolism (PE). Large randomized clinical trials have shown that patients' risk for developing proximal DVT, the thrombi that are most likely to cause PE, is 10% to 30%. Symptomatic VTE occurs in 1.3% to 10% of patients within 3 months of surgery, and after total hip replacement, 1 patient in 300 will die from PE if VTE prophylaxis is not used. Patients undergoing other types of orthopedic surgery are also at increased risk for VTE, and proximal DVT in these patients can also lead to life-threatening PE. VTE is also a common cause of readmission to the hospital. Moreover, hospital costs and hospital stay are doubled for patients who develop VTE after surgery. VTE is also associated with potentially serious long-term complications, including post-thrombotic syndrome, cardiorespiratory insufficiency, recurrent VTE, and bleeding associated with the use of treatment doses of anticoagulants.

PATHOPHYSIOLOGY

Many factors contribute to the development of VTE after major orthopedic surgery (**Table 59-1**). Trauma and surgery both contribute to venous injury and activation of the coagulation system. Postoperatively, patients may have impaired mobility, which causes stasis of blood flow in the deep venous system. Patients undergoing certain types of orthopedic surgery, such as joint replacement and hip fracture repair surgery, also tend to be older and typically have medical comorbid conditions. Increased age is recognized as an independent risk factor for VTE as well.

Most episodes of postoperative DVT are clinically silent, since they develop when patients are recumbent or have limited mobility. (Typically, clinical features of vein obstruction in ambulatory patients cause lower limb swelling and pain.) Although a considerable proportion of such thrombi will resolve spontaneously without administration of antithrombotic therapy, 25% to 50% of clots grow and cause symptomatic DVT or PE.

WHICH PATIENTS UNDERGOING ORTHOPEDIC SURGERY NEED VTE PROPHYLAXIS?

DOES THIS PATIENT UNDERGOING HIP FRACTURE REPAIR, HIP REPLACEMENT, OR KNEE REPLACEMENT NEED VTE PROPHYLAXIS?

CASE 59-1

A 76-year-old woman from a retirement home comes to the emergency room with a hip fracture, sustained after a fall out of bed. The orthopedic surgeon at your center feels she is at low operative risk, since she has no past medical history apart from breast cancer 2 years ago, which was treated with mastectomy, radiation, and chemotherapy. The patient is currently taking raloxifene, a selective estrogen receptor modulator, and vitamin B_{12}.

TABLE 59-1 Factors that Increase Risk for Venous Thromboembolism in Surgical Patients

Surgical factors
Antecedent trauma (as reason for surgery)
General anesthesia (compared with regional/local anesthesia)
Abdominal surgical approach (ie, compared with vaginal approach)
Open surgical approach (ie, compared with laparoscopic approach)
Use of the lithotomy position intraoperatively
Extrinsic venous compression intraoperatively
Extended duration of surgery (ie, > 1 hour)
Postoperative infection
Central venous catheterization
Immobility (confined to bed, needing assistance to ambulate)
Nonsurgical factors
Increasing age
Pregnancy and the puerperium
Acute medical illness (eg, congestive heart failure, obstructive lung disease)
Acute ischemic stroke
Acute neurologic disease
Inflammatory bowel disease
Cancer (active or occult)
Sepsis
Previous VTE
Prior pelvic radiation
Inherited or acquired thrombophilia
Myeloproliferative disorders
Obesity
Drugs (eg, chemotherapy, hormonal therapy, erythropoeisis stimulating agents)

Patients undergoing hip fracture repair, hip replacement, or knee replacement are considered to be at the highest risk for VTE among all orthopedic surgery patients. Prophylaxis is safe and effective in these patients. For this reason, VTE prophylaxis is routinely recommended.

DOES THIS PATIENT UNDERGOING ELECTIVE SPINE SURGERY NEED VTE PROPHYLAXIS?

CASE 59-2

A 68-year-old man is undergoing an elective laminectomy for lumbar decompression after years of back and leg pain. His past medical history is significant for type 2 diabetes mellitus, hypertension, and obesity. Last month, he also had a large upper GI bleed from a perforated gastric ulcer. The orthopedic surgeon asks you if he needs VTE prophylaxis, and if so, what kind.

Though patients undergoing elective spine surgery are at lower risk of VTE than those undergoing hip fracture surgery or lower-extremity joint replacement, they should be considered for VTE prophylaxis. Patients undergoing these surgeries tend to be less mobile in the postoperative period, and the surgeries themselves tend to be longer. They may have additional risk factors, such as advanced age, malignancy, presence of a neurologic deficit, previous VTE, or an anterior surgical approach. If a patient has none of these risk factors and can ambulate early and frequently, no additional thromboprophylaxis needs to be considered. However, if there are additional risk factors present, thromboprophylaxis should be used. There are no large randomized trials in this area, but the data suggest that postoperative low-dose unfractionated heparin (LDUH) and postoperative low molecular weight heparin (LMWH) are beneficial. If intermittent pneumatic compression devices (IPC) are used (for example, in patients at increased bleeding risk), they should be put on in the operating room, and continued postoperatively.

DOES THIS PATIENT UNDERGOING A MINOR ORTHOPEDIC PROCEDURE NEED VTE PROPHYLAXIS?

CASE 59-3

A 21-year-old college football quarterback is undergoing knee arthroscopy to investigate chronic knee pain after an injury on the field. He has no other medical history, and is not taking any medications. You are working with the orthopedic surgeon to determine if the patient needs VTE prophylaxis.

Knee arthroscopy, either to examine the knee or to perform minimally invasive surgery, is a very common orthopedic procedure. More than 5 million arthroscopies are performed in the United States every year. However, the risk of symptomatic VTE appears to be very low, at less than 1%. A systematic review concluded that the benefit of using LMWH compared with no prophylaxis in knee arthroscopy patients was similar to the harm. (Number need to treat = 20, number needed to harm = 17.) A recent randomized controlled trial that compared full-length graduated compression stockings to prophylactic LMWH showed that prophylactic LMWH for 1 week reduced a composite end point of asymptomatic proximal deep venous thrombosis, symptomatic venous thromboembolism, and all-cause mortality. However, nearly half of the events making up the composite outcome measure were distal vein thrombi, which have questionable clinical significance. At this time, routine thromboprophylaxis is not recommended after knee arthroscopy, unless the patient has other risk factors for clotting or has a complicated procedure that results in prolonged immobility.

Isolated distal leg injuries (occurring below the knee) that require orthopedic stabilization with a cast or splint but no surgical intervention are also very common problems in the orthopedic surgery setting. There have been a number of randomized clinical trials of prophylaxis in patients with these injuries. LMWH was not clearly shown to reduce the frequency of DVT compared with no prophylaxis. Practice patterns vary, but the most recent American College of Chest Physicians (ACCP) guidelines recommend that patients with isolated distal leg injuries do not receive routine thromboprophylaxis.

WHAT PHARMACOLOGIC AND NONPHARMACOLOGIC STRATEGIES SHOULD BE USED FOR VTE PROPHYLAXIS?

Physicians have a number of options available when choosing the type of VTE prophylaxis. In patients with an increased risk for bleeding (**Table 59-2**), pharmacologic prophylaxis may not be safe. Mechanical methods of prophylaxis, which include graduated compression stockings, intermittent pneumatic compression devices, and the venous foot pump, are a safer option. All of these methods work by increasing venous flow and reducing stasis. They are, in

TABLE 59-2 Contraindications to Thromboprophylaxis with Anticoagulants

Excessive active bleeding (beyond that expected after surgery)
At high risk for bleeding that precludes anticoagulants (eg, brain lesion)
Recent serious bleeding (eg, within 1 month)
Coagulopathy (eg, INR > 1.5, aPTT > 40)
Thrombocytopenia (eg, platelets < 75 x 10^9/L)

general, less effective than pharmacologic prophylaxis in high risk groups though; if they are not properly used, they are ineffective and if not properly fitted, lead to noncompliance by patients due to discomfort. Patients undergoing major orthopedic surgery should receive mechanical prophylaxis alone if they are at a high risk for bleeding. There is evidence for the efficacy of the venous foot pump and the intermittent pneumatic compression device in joint replacement surgery. There is no comparable evidence in hip fracture surgery. All patients with an increased risk for bleeding should be followed closely. If the bleeding risk decreases to an acceptable level, pharmacologic prophylaxis should be started as soon as possible.

Pharmacologic prophylaxis, though it carries a higher bleeding risk, is more effective than mechanical prophylaxis. It should be the thromboprophylaxis strategy of choice in major orthopedic surgery. There is evidence that LMWH, fondaparinux, and adjusted-dose warfarin administered to achieve a target INR of 2.5 (range of 2.0 to 3.0) are effective to prevent VTE after hip fracture surgery, as well as total hip and knee replacement. Refer to **Table 59-3** for the recommended dose regimens.

PRACTICE POINT

Choice of pharmacologic agent

- There is evidence that low-molecular-weight heparin (LMWH), fondaparinux, and adjusted-dose warfarin administered to achieve a target INR of 2.5 (range of 2.0 to 3.0) are effective to prevent VTE after hip fracture surgery, as well as total hip and knee replacement.
  - LMWH has been found to be superior to Vitamin K antagonists for major orthopedic surgery to prevent proximal, total DVT with no difference in bleeding or clinical PE.
  - Fondaparinux has been found to be superior in hip fracture but may be associated with more bleeding.
- Aspirin has no clear benefit in either hip or knee arthroplasty.
- Recommended duration depends on the duration of surgery.

TABLE 59-3 Pharmacologic Prophylaxis Options in Orthopedic Surgery, with Accepted Doses

Fondaparinux (Arixtra®) 2.5 mg SC once daily
Dalteparin (Fragmin®) 2,500 units or 5,000 units SC once daily
Enoxaparin (Lovenox®) 40 mg SC once daily or 30 mg SC every 12 hours
Nadroparin (Fraxiparine®) 1,900–3,800 anti-Xa units SC once daily
Tinzaparin (Innohep®) 3,500 or 4,500 anti-Xa units SC once daily
Heparin 5,000 units SC every 12 hours or every 8 hours
Warfarin (target INR 2.5, range 2.0–3.0)

TABLE 59-4 Summary of Recommendations for VTE Prophylaxis in Major Orthopedic Surgery

Setting	Average Bleeding Risk	High Bleeding Risk
Hip fracture surgery *Continue prophylaxis for 10 to 35 days*	Fondaparinux LMWH Adjusted-dose warfarin LDUH *Mechanical prophylaxis may be used in addition to one of the above anticoagulants*	GCS IPC VFP
Total hip replacement *Continue prophylaxis for 10 to 35 days*	Fondaparinux LMWH Adjusted-dose warfarin	IPC VFP
Total knee replacement *Continue prophylaxis for 10 to 35 days*	Fondaparinux LMWH Adjusted-dose warfarin IPC	IPC VFP

Many centers still use aspirin and low-dose unfractionated heparin (LDUH) in the setting of total hip and knee replacement. Aspirin does reduce the risk of DVT and PE when compared to placebo, but it provides much less protection against VTE than anticoagulants and, like anticoagulants, confers an increased bleeding risk when administered during the perioperative period. For these reasons, aspirin should not be the agent of choice for thromboprophylaxis after major orthopedic surgery. LDUH, 5000 units twice daily, is less effective than LMWH as thromboprophylaxis after joint replacement, and should not be considered the agent of choice in this setting either. There is a lack of high quality data on the efficacy of LDUH compared with LMWH after hip fracture surgery. A systematic review could not draw any conclusions regarding the superiority of one agent over the other, due to insufficient power. LDUH can be considered in the setting of hip fracture surgery, but most of these patients can safely receive LMWH, fondaparinux, or a vitamin K antagonist. A summary of the thromboprophylaxis recommendations for major orthopedic surgery is presented in **Table 59-4**.

A common problem in caring for patients with hip fracture is surgical delay. Logistical and patient factors can cause a delay between hip fracture and its surgical repair. This delay can significantly increase the risk for VTE, with more than 50% of patients having venographic evidence of DVT with a 48-hour delay, and more than 10% of such patients having venographic evidence of proximal DVT. Although there is no evidence that initiating thromboprophylaxis while patients are waiting for their surgery is effective to prevent VTE, it is reasonable to do so based on the aforementioned studies directly assessing risk and the biological premise that immobile patients who have sustained a hip injury and, therefore, possible adjoining venous injury, are at risk for VTE. Ongoing communication with the orthopedic surgeon and the use of a short-acting anticoagulant (LMWH, LDUH) in the interim period before hip fracture repair will ensure that the anticoagulant can be safely stopped once the patient is taken to surgery.

Time is an important issue when considering VTE prophylaxis in major orthopedic surgery, both the time that the prophylaxis is started, and the time that it is stopped. Patterns of practice regarding when prophylaxis is started vary around the world. European centers tend to start pharmacologic prophylaxis the night before surgery, while the North American practice typically is to start prophylaxis the day after surgery. A preoperative LMWH initiation strategy is thought to reduce DVT whereas postoperative initiation is thought to minimize bleeding. However, a review of studies in which initiation of LMWH for VTE prophylaxis was pre- or postoperative showed no apparent difference in rates of DVT (10.2% vs. 14.4%) or bleeding (1.4% vs. 2.5%) with either approach, though bleeding appeared higher (6.3%) for patients in whom LMWH was initiated within 6 hours of surgery. Hospitalists should discuss the timing of starting prophylaxis with orthopedic surgeons and anaesthetists at their site. In general, it is reasonable to initiate LMWH prophylaxis within 24 hours of surgery in most patients. The start of LMWH can be delayed for 1 to 2 days if there is greater than expected postoperative bleeding, typically manifested by excessive wound drainage. A distinction should be made between a decrease in hemoglobin before and after surgery, which is expected and due to surgical trauma, and a decrease in hemoglobin that occurs entirely in the postoperative period, which may indicate ongoing surgical site bleeding or an emerging intramuscular hematoma.

The duration of prophylaxis in major orthopedic surgery has been the subject of much recent study. There is now strong evidence from large randomized trials and systematic reviews that patients undergoing hip fracture surgery, total hip replacement, and total knee replacement should continue pharmacologic VTE prophylaxis for at least 10 days and up to 35 days after surgery. There is no evidence for extended prophylaxis in other orthopedic surgeries. Strategies to facilitate extended out-of-hospital prophylaxis are discussed in the penultimate section of this chapter.

WHAT ARE THE RISKS OF VTE PROPHYLAXIS IN PATIENTS UNDERGOING ORTHOPEDIC SURGERY?

The ACCP's Guidelines on Antithrombotic and Thrombolytic Therapy is a well-accepted resource that guides many clinicians' decisions about VTE prophylaxis. This document, which is based on high quality evidence (when available) and expert consensus, is now in its eighth edition. However, in December 2008, the American Association of Orthopedic Surgeons (AAOS) published a competing set of guidelines concerning the use of VTE prophylaxis in orthopedic surgery. The AAOS guidelines differ from the ACCP guidelines in several ways. In particular, they argue for less aggressive prophylaxis than the ACCP guidelines, and do not explicitly recommend *routine* VTE prophylaxis for total hip and knee replacement. A greater value is placed on bleeding risks than clotting risks. Recommendations for low dose warfarin, routine use of aspirin, and consideration of no VTE prophylaxis are made. Placement of a vena cava filter is also suggested as an option for patients with bleeding risks.

PRACTICE POINT

VTE prophylaxis in orthopedic surgery patients is a major patient safety issue.

- Acute PE is the second most common cause of death after THR (40 PEs/10,000 THRs).
- Symptomatic VTE often is diagnosed post-hospital discharge in 76% of THR patients who developed VTE and 47% of those who had TKR.

The publication of the AAOS guidelines generated a great deal of controversy. Several publications addressed its recommendations, and concluded that many of them were not based on evidence, and in some cases, actually went against high quality published data. However, before simply discarding the AAOS guidelines, one must consider the ideas behind it. Orthopedic surgeons have long expressed concerns about the bleeding risks surrounding anticoagulant therapy. Bleeding can be disastrous in the postoperative period, resulting in increased morbidity and mortality, increased rates of rehospitalization and reoperation, increased length of stay, and increased health care costs. However, analysis of numerous randomized trials has shown that the rates of major bleeding in anticoagulant versus placebo arm are similar. LMWH, when started immediately after elective knee replacement, may be associated with an increase in wound hematomas, but this relationship is not clear. It has also been suggested that anticoagulants increase the risk of wound infection. Two large cohort studies have shown that this is not the case, but the relationship remains controversial.

High-quality evidence has shown that VTE prophylaxis is both effective *and* safe in patients undergoing major orthopedic surgery. What should one do when faced with conflicting guidelines? Ongoing communication between physicians and surgeons, reliance on the most rigorous and evidence-based trial data, and an understanding of the true risks and benefits of venous thromboembolism prophylaxis is essential.

PRACTICE POINT

- High-quality evidence has shown that pharmacologic VTE prophylaxis is both effective and safe in patients undergoing major orthopedic surgery.
- When appropriately dosed, the risk of bleeding from heparin agents, fondaparinux, and adjusted-dose warfarin to achieve a target INR of 2.5 is very low.

WHAT ARE SOME PRACTICAL MANAGEMENT ISSUES FOR THE HOSPITALIST IN VTE PROPHYLAXIS?

CONSIDERATIONS UPON DISCHARGE FROM HOSPITAL

There is no evidence that patients undergoing orthopedic surgery benefit from routine DVT screening using Doppler ultrasound or venography. This strategy may pick up asymptomatic venous thrombosis in a small number (< 2.5%) of patients. However, a randomized clinical trial showed that it does not reduce the rates of symptomatic VTE.

At the time of discharge, it is more important to consider whether a patient would benefit from extended out-of-hospital prophylaxis. Patients undergoing hip fracture surgery, total hip replacement, and total knee replacement should continue pharmacologic VTE prophylaxis for at least 10 days and up to 35 days after surgery, even after discharge home. If a patient is discharged on an injectable anticoagulant and does not have nursing care at home, he or she (or a caregiver) should be educated on injection technique and safe disposal of used needles. Patients discharged on vitamin K antagonists should also be educated about their medication and a plan should be put into place regarding laboratory monitoring of the INR and dose adjustment of the vitamin K antagonist. All patients should be educated about the signs and symptoms of VTE.

QUALITY IMPROVEMENT INITIATIVES TO OPTIMIZE VTE PROPHYLAXIS

VTE prophylaxis in orthopedic surgery patients is based on scientific evidence and accepted clinical practice guidelines. It is also a major patient safety issue. When compared to other patient groups, orthopedic surgery patients do have higher rates of appropriate VTE prophylaxis; however there is tremendous room for improvement. Compliance rates with American College of Chest Physicians' guidelines for in-hospital thromboprophylaxis range from 50% to 70% in orthopedic surgery. A recent Canadian study showed that compliance rates with guidelines for out-of-hospital prophylaxis are even poorer, with less than 20% of eligible patients receiving thromboprophylaxis after discharge. A large number of system-wide and local strategies have been developed to increase the appropriate use of thromboprophylaxis. VTE prophylaxis has been highlighted in national standards of care in both the United States and the United Kingdom, and has become an important feature of hospital accreditation commissions and quality improvement campaigns worldwide. Many hospitals have successfully developed formal, active strategies and written policies for prophylaxis in high risk patients, such as those undergoing orthopedic surgery. Ideally, each hospital should have a formal policy and standardized protocols for thromboprophylaxis in at-risk hospitalized patients. Strategies such as computer decision support systems, preprinted order sets, and periodic audit and feedback have been shown to work. However, each patient's individual risk factors for clotting and bleeding must be considered when making decisions about prophylaxis. It is important for hospitalists to work closely with orthopedic surgeons to achieve the best patient outcomes.

SUGGESTED READINGS

American Academy of Orthopaedic Surgeons Clinical Guideline on Prevention of Symptomatic Pulmonary Embolism in Patients Undergoing Total Hip or Knee Arthroplasty. Adopted by the American Academy of Orthopedic Surgeons Board of Directors May 2007. Available at: www.aaos.org/research/guidelines/PE_guideline.pdf. Accessed May 24, 2009.

Camporese G, Bernardi E, Prandoni P, et al. Low-Molecular-Weight Heparin versus Compression Stockings for Thromboprophylaxis after Knee Arthroscopy: A Randomized Trial. *Ann Intern Med.* 2008;149(2):73–82.

Eikelboom JW, Karthikeyan G, Fagel N, Hirsh J. American Association of Orthopedic Surgeons and American College of Chest Physicians Guidelines for Venous Thromboembolism Prevention in Hip and Knee Arthroplasty Differ. What Are the Implications for Clinicians and Patients? *Chest.* 2009;135:513–520.

Geerts WH, Bergqvist D, Pineo GF, et al. Prevention of venous thromboembolism: American College of Chest Physicians Evidence-Based Clinical Practice Guidelines. 8th ed. *Chest.* 2008;133(suppl 6):381S–453S.

Khan NA, Quan H, Bugar JM, et al. Association of postoperative complications with hospital costs and length of stay in a tertiary care center. *J Gen Intern Med.* 2006;21:177–180.

MacDougall DA, Feliu AU, Boccuzzi SJ, Lin J. Economic burden of deep-vein thrombosis, pulmonary embolism, and post-thrombotic syndrome. *Am J Health Syst Pharm.* 2006;63(Suppl 6):S5–S15.

Otero R, Uresandi F, Cayuela A, et al. Use of venous thromboembolism prophylaxis for surgical patients: a multicentre analysis of practice in Spain. *Eur J Surg.* 2001;167:163–167.

Rahme E, Dasgupta K, Burman M, et al. Postdischarge thromboprophylaxis and mortality risk after hip-or knee-replacement surgery. *CMAJ.* 2008;178:1545–1554.

Strebel N, Prins M, Agnelli G, Büller HR. Preoperative or postoperative start of prophylaxis for venous thromboembolism with low-molecular-weight heparin in elective hip surgery? *Arch Intern Med.* 2002;162(13):1451–1456.

Yu HT, Dylan ML, Lin J, Dubois RW. Hospitals' compliance with prophylaxis guidelines for venous thromboembolism. *Am J Health Syst Pharm.* 2007;64:69–76.

CHAPTER 60

Venous Thromboembolism (VTE) Prophylaxis for Hospitalized Medical Patients

Menaka Pai, MD, FRCPC
James D. Douketis, MD, FRCPC, FACP, FCCP

WHAT IS THE RISK FOR VENOUS THROMBOEMBOLISM (VTE) IN HOSPITALIZED MEDICAL PATIENTS?

EPIDEMIOLOGY

VTE, which comprises deep vein thrombosis (DVT) and pulmonary embolism (PE), is a common cause of morbidity and mortality in hospitalized medical patients. The baseline incidence of asymptomatic VTE in hospitalized medical patients without anticoagulant prophylaxis is 7% to 15%. Linked administrative database studies indicate that 1.7% of hospitalized medical patients develop symptomatic VTE within 3 months of hospitalization. This is lower than in surgical patients, who have a risk of 2% to 3%. However, because of the sheer number of hospitalized medical patients when compared to surgical patients, the burden of illness is high. Approximately 50% to 70% of symptomatic VTE and 70% to 80% of fatal PE occur in medical patients, and recent hospitalization for medical illness accounts for 25% of all VTE diagnosed in the community. The quoted risk of 1.7% is also based on the risk in all medical patients, some of whom have a lesser illness severity. In prospective studies assessing medical patients who have at least one major risk factor for VTE such as severe cardiac or respiratory disease and do not receive VTE prophylaxis, the incidence of DVT as detected by venography is approximately 10% to 15%. In the absence of anticoagulant prophylaxis, the incidence of proximal DVT, which is the type of DVT most likely to embolize, is approximately 5% and the incidence of PE is 0.5%. VTE is associated with potentially serious long-term complications, including post-thrombotic syndrome, cardiorespiratory insufficiency, recurrent VTE, and bleeding associated with anticoagulant therapy. VTE is also a common cause of readmission to the hospital, and is associated with increased hospital costs and length of stay.

PRACTICE POINT

Risk of thrombosis

- Approximately 50% to 70% of symptomatic VTE and 70% to 80% of fatal PE occur in medical patients.
- Recent hospitalization for medical illness accounts for 25% of all VTE diagnosed in the community.
- In prospective studies assessing medical patients who have at least 1 major risk factor for VTE such as severe cardiac or respiratory disease and do not receive VTE prophylaxis, the incidence of DVT as detected by venography is approximately 10% to 15%.

PATHOPHYSIOLOGY

Hospitalization for an acute medical illness is independently associated with about an 8-fold increased risk for VTE. Chart audits have shown that nearly all hospitalized medical patients have at least one VTE risk factor, be it immobility, increased age, cancer (active or occult), or acute medical illness (eg, congestive heart failure, obstructive lung disease). Certain populations of hospitalized medical patients, such as those in the intensive care unit, have additional risk factors including central venous catheterization. (**Table 60-1**)

TABLE 60-1 Factors that Increase Risk for Venous Thromboembolism in Hospitalized Medical Patients

Increasing age
Immobility (confined to bed, needing assistance to ambulate)
Pregnancy and the puerperium
Acute medical illness (eg, congestive heart failure, obstructive lung disease)
Acute ischemic stroke
Acute neurologic disease
Inflammatory bowel disease
Cancer (active or occult)
Sepsis
Previous VTE
Prior pelvic radiation
Inherited or acquired thrombophilia
Myeloproliferative disorders
Obesity
Medications (eg, chemotherapy, hormonal therapy, selective estrogen receptor modulators, erythropoeisis stimulating agents)
Central venous catheterization (eg, PICC line, internal jugular line)

WHICH HOSPITALIZED MEDICAL PATIENTS NEED VTE PROPHYLAXIS?

DOES THIS GENERAL MEDICAL PATIENT NEED VTE PROPHYLAXIS?

CASE 60-1

A 76-year-old man from a retirement home comes to the emergency room with an acute exacerbation of congestive heart failure. He has a past medical history of hypertension, type 2 diabetes mellitus, and gout. He has no bleeding history and a baseline CBC, INR, aPTT, and creatinine are normal. The intern on the general medicine ward asks if this patient requires VTE prophylaxis, and if so, how effective it will be at preventing symptomatic events.

There is no standardized or validated risk stratification algorithm to guide VTE prophylaxis in medical patients. As a general guide, medical patients presenting with ischemic stroke, chronic heart failure, chronic obstructive pulmonary disease, cancer, history of prior VTE, sepsis, acute neurologic disease, or severe inflammatory disease should be given VTE prophylaxis. Immobility is considered a weaker risk factor, and is difficult to clearly define. However, patients who cannot ambulate without assistance still merit consideration for prophylaxis.

A recent meta-analysis has shown that pharmacologic prophylaxis is effective in reducing fatal PE, symptomatic PE, and symptomatic DVT by more than 50% with no increase in major bleeding compared with placebo in general medical patients. There is no effect on all-cause mortality, and the number needed to treat to prevent one symptomatic PE is high (more than 300). However, due to the large number of at-risk hospitalized medical patients, thromboprophylaxis still provides an opportunity to reduce morbidity in a significant number of patients. There does not appear to be a difference in bleeding rates of VTE rates between with low dose unfractionated heparin (LDUH), low molecular weight heparin (LMWH), and fondaparinux. Of note, fondaparinux and tinzaparin, though frequently used for VTE prophylaxis in medical patients, have not yet been approved for use in this population.

TABLE 60-2 Contraindications to Thromboprophylaxis with Anticoagulants

Excessive active bleeding
At high risk for bleeding that precludes anticoagulants (eg, brain lesion)
Recent serious bleeding (eg, within 1 month)
Coagulopathy (eg, INR > 1.5, aPTT > 40)
Thrombocytopenia (eg, platelets < 75 x 10^9/L)

PRACTICE POINT

Risk of bleeding associated with anticoagulant prophylaxis

- The risk for fatal bleeding is 0.02% to 0.5%, or 32% higher than in patients who do not receive prophylaxis. Prospective trials have shown that this difference is not statistically significant, but this finding may be because the studies were underpowered to show a difference in bleeding risk.
- There does not appear to be a difference in bleeding rates of VTE rates between LDUH, LMWH, and fondaparinux.

In patients with an increased risk for bleeding (**Table 60-2**), physicians commonly choose mechanical methods of thromboprophylaxis to increase venous flow and reduce stasis: graduated compression stockings (GCS), intermittent pneumatic compression devices (IPC), and the venous foot pump.

However, there are no randomized clinical trials evaluating mechanical thromboprophylaxis in general medical patients. In a placebo-controlled trial assessing GCS for DVT prophylaxis in patients with acute ischemic stroke, GCS did not provide additional therapeutic benefit for DVT prevention (10.0% vs. 10.5%) but conferred a 4-fold increased risk for skin breaks, ulceration, and blisters. Mechanical thromboprophylaxis should be considered inferior to pharmacologic prophylaxis in preventing VTE, and should only be used as an adjunct to pharmacologic prophylaxis, or as an option in patients with an unacceptably high bleeding risk. All patients with an increased risk for bleeding should be followed closely. If the bleeding risk decreases to an acceptable level, pharmacologic prophylaxis should be started as soon as possible.

PRACTICE POINT

Mechanical thromboprophylaxis

- Mechanical thromboprophylaxis is inferior to pharmacologic prophylaxis in preventing VTE.
- There are no randomized clinical trials evaluating mechanical thromboprophylaxis in general medical patients.
- It should only be used as an adjunct to pharmacologic prophylaxis, or as an option in patients with an unacceptably high bleeding risk.
- All patients with an increased risk for bleeding should be followed closely. If the bleeding risk decreases to an acceptable level, pharmacologic prophylaxis should be started as soon as possible.

DOES THIS CANCER PATIENT NEED VTE PROPHYLAXIS?

CASE 60-2

A 68-year-old woman is admitted to hospital with febrile neutropenia. She is currently receiving epirubicin and docetaxel for treatment of metastatic breast cancer. Her past medical history is significant for type 2 diabetes mellitus and obesity. On review of her laboratory investigations, you notice that her platelet count is reduced at 10 x 10^9/L. The oncologist asks you if she needs VTE prophylaxis, and if so, what kind.

Cancer confers a 6-fold increased risk of VTE, and active cancer accounts for 20% of all new VTE events in the community. Conventional chemotherapies, erythropoietin stimulating agents, angiogenesis inhibitors, and hormonal therapies (including selective estrogen receptor modulators and aromatase inhibitors) also increase the risk of VTE. Once patients with cancer develop VTE, it can be difficult to treat due to intercurrent illnesses, the need for invasive procedures, thrombocytopenia, and high VTE recurrence rates. It is, therefore, essential to carefully risk stratify patients and consider thromboprophylaxis when patients with cancer are admitted to hospital. It is unclear whether anticoagulant prophylaxis is effective to prevent VTE in cancer patients who are ambulatory. However, cancer patients with an acute medical illness, either cancer-related or otherwise, or who are bedridden should receive thromboprophylaxis in accordance with the recommendations for general medical patients.

PRACTICE POINT

- Cancer confers a 6-fold increased risk of VTE, and active cancer accounts for 20% of all new VTE events in the community. Once patients with cancer develop VTE, it can be difficult to treat, due to intercurrent illnesses, the need for invasive procedures, thrombocytopenia, and high VTE recurrence rates.

DOES THIS CRITICALLY ILL PATIENT NEED VTE PROPHYLAXIS?

CASE 60-3

A 32-year-old woman with meningococcal meningitis has been in the intensive care unit for 3 days. She is intubated and ventilated, and continues to require vasopressors. You are working with the intensivist to determine if the patient needs VTE prophylaxis.

Patients in the intensive care unit are particularly heterogeneous, both in terms of thrombosis risk and in terms of bleeding risk. Reflecting this heterogeneity, the rates of asymptomatic DVT (detected by ultrasound or venography) range from < 10% to nearly 100%. There are only 2 randomized trials of thromboprophylaxis in patients in the intensive care setting, 1 comparing LDUH to placebo, and the other comparing LMWH to placebo. Both significantly reduced the rate of DVT detected on routine screening, yielding a relative risk reduction of approximately 50%.

All patients admitted to the intensive care unit should have a routine assessment of risk for thrombosis and bleeding. Patients who have an acceptable bleeding risk should receive LMWH or LDUH, while those considered at high risk for bleeding should receive GCS and/or IPC. This latter group should be reassessed daily, and if the bleeding risk decreases to an acceptable level, pharmacologic prophylaxis should commence as soon as possible.

TABLE 60-3 Pharmacologic Prophylaxis Options in Hospitalized Medical Patients, with Accepted Doses

Dalteparin (Fragmin®) 5,000 units SC once daily
Enoxaparin (Lovenox®) 40 mg SC once daily or 30 mg SC every 12 hours
Nadroparin (Fraxiparine®) 1,900–3,800 anti-Xa units SC once daily
Heparin 5,000 units SC every 12 hours or every 8 hours

WHAT ARE THE RISKS ASSOCIATED WITH VENOUS THROMBOEMBOLISM PROPHYLAXIS?

The major risk of pharmacologic VTE prophylaxis is bleeding. In medical patients, bleeding may occur at the anticoagulant injection site (eg, rectus sheath hematoma) or at a remote site (eg, from an occult peptic ulcer that is predisposed to bleeding). The risk for fatal bleeding associated with anticoagulant prophylaxis is 0.02% to 0.5%, or 32% higher than in patients who do not receive prophylaxis. Prospective trials have shown that this difference is not statistically significant, but this finding may be because the studies were underpowered to show a difference in bleeding risk. Bleeding complications can be minimized by carefully assessing patients' individual bleeding risks *before* starting anticoagulants (**Table 60-3**). Patients should also be assessed regularly for signs and symptoms of bleeding while they are on anticoagulants.

The other important risk associated with pharmacologic VTE prophylaxis is heparin-induced thrombocytopenia (HIT). This rare but serious complication of heparin-derived anticoagulants is caused by antibody formation to the heparin-derived anticoagulant and an antigen on the patient's platelets. It is strongly associated with venous and to a lesser extent, arterial thrombosis, and can have devastating consequences. HIT is more common with LDUH compared to LMWH, and more common in surgical versus medical patients. In medical patients who received anticoagulant prophylaxis with LDUH, the risk for HIT was 1.4%. Data are lacking as to the risk for HIT in medical patients who are receiving LMWH but it is probably one-tenth the risk observed with LDUH. Irrespective of the anticoagulant administered, platelet counts should be monitored serially for all patients on anticoagulants and physicians should be watchful for signs and symptoms of arterial or venous thromboembolism that can herald the development of HIT.

PRACTICE POINT

Heparin-induced thrombocytopenia (HIT)

- HIT is more common with LDUH compared to LMWH, and more common in surgical versus medical patients.
- In medical patients who received anticoagulant prophylaxis with LDUH, the risk for HIT was 1.4%.
- Data are lacking as to the risk for HIT in medical patients who are receiving LMWH but it is probably one-tenth the risk observed with LDUH.

Overall, the risks of major bleeding and HIT are small in hospitalized medical patients, and are far outweighed by the benefits of pharmacologic VTE prophylaxis.

WHAT ARE SOME PRACTICAL MANAGEMENT ISSUES FOR THE HOSPITALIST IN VTE PROPHYLAXIS?

PHARMACOLOGIC PROPHYLAXIS IN THE SETTING OF RENAL INSUFFICIENCY

Renal impairment is a significant challenge in the administration of venous thromboprophylaxis. Drugs like LMWH and fondaparinux are primarily cleared by the kidney, and in the setting of reduced renal function, these drugs can accumulate and increase bleeding risk. Ongoing studies are evaluating the bioaccumulation of these anticoagulants and the clinical consequences. At this time, only prophylactic dose dalteparin has been shown not to bioaccumulate when the creatinine clearance is less than 30 mL/min. Before prescribing any renally cleared anticoagulant, physicians should measure a patient's serum creatinine and formally calculate the creatinine clearance (which depends on age and weight). If renal function is found to be impaired, an anticoagulant that does not bioaccumulate should be chosen. If this is not possible, the dose should be lowered and/or the anti-Xa level should be monitored.

PRACTICE POINT

Renal insufficiency

- Before prescribing any renally cleared anticoagulant, physicians should measure a patient's serum creatinine and formally calculate the creatinine clearance (which depends on age and weight).
- If renal function is found to be impaired, an anticoagulant that does not bioaccumulate should be chosen. If this is not possible, the dose should be lowered and/or the anti-Xa level should be monitored.

CONSIDERATIONS UPON DISCHARGE FROM HOSPITAL

There is no evidence that hospitalized medical patients benefit from routine DVT screening using venous ultrasound or venography and therefore, routine DVT screening at the time of hospital discharge cannot be recommended. The risk to benefit ratio of extended out-of-hospital prophylaxis is also unclear. Medical patients with chronic illness or who are to be transferred to a long-term care facility may have an ongoing increased thrombosis risk, making extended-duration prophylaxis an appealing option. A recent randomized trial compared extended-duration (5 weeks) and short-duration (10 days) VTE prophylaxis with enoxaparin, 40 mg once-daily, in 4,726 medical patients. Though extended-duration prophylaxis significantly decreased the risk for any VTE and symptomatic VTE, it increased the risk for major bleeding 4-fold. At this time, extended-duration prophylaxis is not recommended in medical patients. However, all patients should be educated about the signs and symptoms of VTE at the time of discharge and be instructed to seek urgent medical care if thrombosis is suspected.

QUALITY IMPROVEMENT INITIATIVES TO OPTIMIZE VTE PROPHYLAXIS

There is a significant gap between evidence for VTE prophylaxis and clinical practice in hospitalized medical patients. A recent international registry demonstrated that in a population of 15,156 hospitalize medical patients only 50% received any form of prophylaxis. A multicenter Canadian chart audit determined that 90% of acutely ill medical patients were eligible for some form of prophylaxis, while only 23% received it. What is rather astonishing is that only 16% of patients received appropriate prophylaxis.

Medical patients have repeatedly been shown to have the poorest rates of VTE prophylaxis among all hospitalized patients. Yet since 1998, the American College of Chest Physicians has given anticoagulant prophylaxis in at-risk hospitalized medical patients a Grade 1A recommendation, their highest level. Why is VTE prophylaxis underused in hospitalized medical patients? It is likely because medical patients are more heterogeneous than their counterparts on surgical wards. Their need for prophylaxis is not driven by a standardized type of surgery, but by their underlying diseases, their mobility status, and their reason for hospitalization. Health care providers may be unclear about the indications and contraindications for anticoagulant prophylaxis in a given patient.

Many organizations have also identified VTE as a major patient safety concern, including the U.S. Department of Health and Human Services, the World Health Organization, the World Alliance for Patient Safety, and the International Alliance of Patients' Organizations. VTE prophylaxis has also been highlighted as an important feature of hospital accreditation commissions and quality improvement campaigns worldwide. Evidence supports a multicomponent strategy to optimize VTE prophylaxis in hospitalized medical patients, including formal hospital policy, standardized preprinted order sets, computer decision support systems, electronic and human alerts, and periodic audit and feedback. Hospitalists are in an ideal position to champion appropriate VTE prophylaxis in hospitalized medical patients, at a local, national, and international level.

SUGGESTED READINGS

Alikhan R, Cohen AT. A safety analysis of thromboprophylaxis in acute medical illness. *Thromb Haemost.* 2003;89:590–591.

CLOTS Trials Collaboration, Dennis M, Sandercock PA, Reid J, et al. Effectiveness of thigh-length graduated compression stockings to reduce the risk of deep vein thrombosis after stroke (CLOTS trial 1): a multicentre, randomised controlled trial. *Lancet.* 2009; 373:1958–1965.

Cohen AT, Tapson VF, Bergmann JF, et al. Venous thromboembolism risk and prophylaxis in the acute hospital care setting (ENDORSE study): a multinational cross-sectional study. *Lancet.* 2008;371:387–394.

Cook D, Crowther M, Meade M, et al. Deep venous thrombosis in medical–surgical critically ill patients: prevalence, incidence, and risk factors. *Crit Care Med.* 2005;33:1565–1571.

Douketis J, Cook D, Meade M, et al. Prophylaxis against deep vein thrombosis in critically ill patients with severe renal insufficiency with the low-molecular-weight heparin dalteparin: an assessment of safety and pharmacodynamics: the DIRECT Study. *Arch Intern Med.* 2008;168:1805–1812.

Geerts WH, Bergqvist D, Pineo GF, et al. Prevention of venous thromboembolism: American College of Chest Physicians Evidence-Based Clinical Practice Guidelines (8th Edition). *Chest.* 2008; 133(suppl 6):381S–453S.

Kakkar AK, Levine MN, Kadziola Z, et al. Low molecular weight heparin, therapy with dalteparin, and survival in advanced cancer: the Fragmin Advanced Malignancy Outcome Study (FAMOUS). *J Clin Oncol.* 2004;22:1944–1948.

MacDougall DA, Feliu AU, Boccuzzi SJ, Lin J. Economic burden of deep-vein thrombosis, pulmonary embolism, and post-thrombotic syndrome. *Am J Health Syst Pharm.* 2006;63(20 Suppl 6):S5–S15.

Samama MM, Cohen AT, Darmon JY, et al. A comparison of enoxaparin with placebo for the prevention of venous thromboembolism in acutely ill medical patients. *N Engl J Med.* 1999; 341:793–800.

Turpie AG. Extended duration of thromboprophylaxis in acutely ill medical patients: optimizing therapy? *J Thromb Haemost.* 2007; 5:5–11.

CHAPTER 61

Perioperative Management of Patients who are Receiving Oral Anticoagulant Therapy

Marco P. Donadini, MD
James D. Douketis, MD, FRCPC, FACP, FCCP

INTRODUCTION

The perioperative management of patients who require interruption of a vitamin K antagonist (VKA) because of surgery or another non-invasive procedure is a common and sometimes challenging clinical problem. Bridging anticoagulation refers to the use of a short-acting anticoagulant, which is usually therapeutic-dose subcutaneous low-molecular-weight heparin (LMWH) such as enoxaparin 1 mg/kg twice-daily, administered during the time when a VKA is interrupted and there is no therapeutic anticoagulation. However, there is no standardized definition of 'bridging anticoagulation' and other treatment regimens, including low-dose (enoxaparin 40 mg once-daily) or intermediate-dose (eg, enoxaparin 40 mg twice-daily) LMWH regimens, have been used, particularly in selected patients at high risk for bleeding complications.

Although perioperative anticoagulant management may be straightforward in many cases, requiring simple interruption and postoperative resumption of VKA therapy, there are also many instances where management decisions may affect clinical outcomes, whether thromboembolic or bleeding. In all cases management decisions are anchored on weighing perioperative risks for thromboembolism and bleeding.

The objectives of this chapter are: 1) to stratify patients according to their risk for arterial or venous thromboembolism if VKA therapy is stopped and the risk for bleeding associated with surgery or procedure; 2) to provide a practical approach to the perioperative interruption and resumption of VKA therapy; 3) to provide a practical protocol for the administration of bridging anticoagulation when required.

CASE 61-1

A 54-year-old woman with rheumatic valvular heart disease requires hysterectomy (uterine fibroids). She has a St. Jude mechanical prosthetic valve in the mitral position and she Is on warfarin. The perioperative management of anticoagulant therapy should start with the assessment of her thromboembolic risk, which should be considered high in the presence of any mitral valve prosthesis.

The second step is represented by the assessment of bleeding risk, which can be considered not high because the type and location of surgery do not involve critical sites or major tissue injury or highly vascularized organ.

A preoperative bridging regimen is suggested here:

- Day -5: stop warfarin (may stop on day -6 if INR range is 2.5–3.5)
- Day -3: start therapeutic-dose heparin (SC LMWH or IV UFH)
- Day -1:
  - check INR if possible (if INR > 1.5, vitamin K 1–2 mg orally can be administered)
  - if SC LMWH was chosen, give the last dose in the morning (this dose must be reduced by 50% in case of once-daily dosing regimen)
  - if IV UFH was chosen, stop infusion 4 hours before surgery

A post-operative bridging regimen is suggested here:

- Day 0: after assessing surgical site hemostasis, warfarin can be resumed on the evening after surgery, if feasible
- Day +1 to +3: resume therapeutic-dose LMWH or UFH when hemostasis is secure, and in no case before 12 hours after surgery (typically on the morning afterwards)
- Day +5 to +6: stop LMWH or UFH when INR is therapeutic

TABLE 61-1 Stoke Risk in Atrial Fibrillation: CHADS$_2$ Score

Risk Criteria	Score
Congestive heart failure	1
Hypertension	1
Age ≥ 75 years	1
Diabetes	1
Prior Stroke or transient ischemic attack	2

TABLE 61-2 Stroke Risk According to CHADS$_2$ Score in Patients with Nonvalvular AF not Treated with Warfarin

CHADS$_2$ Score	Annual Stroke Rate (95% Confidence Interval)
0	1.9 (1.2–3.0)
1	2.8 (2.0–3.8)
2	4.0 (3.1–5.1)
3	5.9 (4.6–7.3)
4	8.5 (6.3–11.1)
5	12.5 (8.2–17.5)
6	18.2 (10.5–27.4)

A cautionary note: there are no randomized controlled trials that definitively guide the clinician regarding which patients must receive bridging therapy to avoid devastating thromboembolic complications and which patients should not due to increased risk of perioperative bleeding associated with bridging. Although most practitioners use the CHADS scoring system, clinical judgment is still required for each patient at the bedside. For patients with additional comorbidity that increases the risk of bleeding such as new renal failure, thrombocytopenia, or an elevated INR prior to warfarin administration, it is important to define the additional risk of increased bleeding and weigh that against the known risk of thromboembolic complications. Significant renal failure, thrombocytopenia, or elevated INR requires further investigation and treatment, usually prior to any initiation of anticoagulation.

PERIOPERATIVE THROMBOEMBOLIC AND BLEEDING RISK STRATIFICATION

THROMBOEMBOLIC RISK STRATIFICATION

Patients who are receiving oral anticoagulant therapy, usually with warfarin, represent a spectrum of thromboembolic risk that is determined primarily by the clinical indication for warfarin therapy and, secondarily, individual patient characteristics. The most frequent clinical indications for warfarin therapy are chronic atrial fibrillation (AF), mechanical heart valves (MHV), and venous thromboembolism (VTE). The principal thromboembolic risk is arterial in patients with atrial fibrillation or a mechanical heart valve, and venous in patients with prior VTE. When considering this risk, both the risk of such events and their clinical consequences should be considered.

Although there are no validated risk stratification schemes to quantify thromboembolic risk, a suggested risk classification scheme separating patients into high, moderate, or low risk categories for thromboembolism is outlined below and in **Tables 61-1** to **61-3**.

High risk for thromboembolism (> 10% per year):

- AF: CHADS$_2$ score of 5 or 6; recent (within 3 months) stroke or transient ischemic attack (TIA); rheumatic valvular heart disease
- MHV: mitral valve prosthesis; older generation (caged-ball or tilting disk) aortic valve prosthesis; recent (within 3 months) stroke or TIA
- VTE: prior VTE within past 3 months; severe thrombophilia (protein C, protein S, or antithrombin deficiency, antiphospholipid syndrome, combined thrombophilic abnormalities)

Moderate risk for thromboembolism (5–10% per year):

- AF: CHADS$_2$ score of 3 or 4
- MHV: aortic bileaflet valve prosthesis and 1 of the following: atrial fibrillation, prior stroke or TIA, other stroke risk factors (heart failure, hypertension, age ≥ 75 years, diabetes)
- VTE: prior VTE within past 3 and 12 months; nonsevere thrombophilia (heterozygous factor V Leiden or prothrombin mutation); recurrent VTE; active cancer (treated within 6 months or palliative)

TABLE 61-3 Suggested Risk Stratification Scheme for Perioperative Arterial and Venous Thrombembolism

	Indication for WARFARIN therapy		
Thrombotic Risk	Atrial fibrillation	Mechanical Heart Valves	VTE
High	• CHADS$_2$ score: 5 or 6 • Recent (< 3 months) stroke or TIA • Rheumatic valvular heart disease	• Any mechanical mitral valve prosthesis • Older aortic mechanical valve prosthesis (caged-ball, tilting disk) • Recent (< 6 months) stroke or TIA	• Recent (< 3 months) VTE • Severe thrombophilia†
Moderate	CHADS$_2$ score: 3 or 4	• Bileaflet aortic valve prosthesis with at least 1 risk factor*	• VTE within 3–12 months • Nonsevere thrombophilia§ • Recurrent VTE • Active cancer
Low	CHADS$_2$ score: 0–2 (without prior stroke or TIA)	• Bileaflet aortic bileaftlet without any risk factors*	VTE > 12 months

CHADS, Cardiac failure-Hypertension-Age-Diabetes-Stroke; TIA, transient ischemic attack; VTE, venous thromboembolism; WARFARIN, vitamin K antagonist.
*Risk factors: atrial fibrillation, cardiac failure, hypertension, age > 75 years, diabetes, stroke, or TIA.
†Severe thrombophilia: deficiency of protein C, protein S, or antithrombin, antiphospholipid syndrome, multiple abnormalities.
§Nonsevere thrombophilia: heterozygous factor V Leiden or factor II mutation.

Low risk for thromboembolism (< 5% per year):

- AF: $CHADS_2$ score of 0 to 2, without previous stroke or transient ischemic attack
- MHV: aortic bileaflet valve prosthesis without atrial fibrillation or any other stroke risk factors
- VTE: prior VTE more than 12 months before and no other risk factors (among above-mentioned)

In addition to this classification, which aims to quantify thromboembolic risk, the qualitative or clinical impact of an event should be considered. Thus, the impact of the arterial thromboembolic event, especially stroke, is likely to be greater than that of a recurrent venous event.

PRACTICE POINT

Thromboembolic risk stratification should take into account:

1. The risk of thromboembolism:
   - High > 10% per year
   - Moderate 5–10% per year
   - Low < 5% per year
2. The clinical impact of an event (with arterial embolism likely greater than recurrent venous thrombosis):
   - Embolic stroke can result in death or major disability in about 70% of patients.
   - Thrombosis of a mechanical heart valve is fatal in about 15% of patients.
   - Recurrent VTE is fatal in 4% to 9% of patients.

BLEEDING RISK STRATIFICATION

The risk for perioperative bleeding is determined primarily by the type of surgery that is planned and secondarily on patient-specific characteristics. In terms of surgical factors that determine risk for bleeding, these include the extent of surgery and associated tissue injury, the anatomical region involved, and whether hemostasis is actively attained, through suturing and cautery, or left to occur by secondary intent. The risk for bleeding should not only consider the anticipated amount of blood loss but also the clinical consequences of bleeding.

PRACTICE POINT

- Bleeding risk stratification should take into account not only the anticipated amount of blood loss from a surgical procedure but also the clinical consequences of bleeding.

Although there is no validated method to quantify perioperative bleeding risk, special attention is warranted for certain surgical or other invasive procedures associated with a high risk of bleeding. Such high-risk surgery can be summarized as follows:

- "Closed-space" surgery, which includes intracranial, spinal, retroperitoneal, and eye posterior chamber surgery
- Coronary artery bypass or heart valve replacement surgery in which bleeding into the pericardium can have life-threatening consequences
- Major vascular surgery such as aortic aneurysm repair and peripheral artery bypass in which there may be vascular tissue damage that is prone to bleeding
- Surgery associated with major tissue injury, such as major orthopedic surgery, reconstructive plastic surgery, and major cancer surgery, in which the extent of the surgery may predispose to postoperative bleeding

TABLE 61-4 Patient Stratification Scheme for Perioperative Bleeding

Very high risk
• Neurosurgery (intracranial or spinal surgery)
• Cardiac surgery (coronary artery bypass or heart valve replacement)
High risk
• Major vascular surgery (abdominal aortic aneurysm repair, aortofemoral bypass)
• Major urologic surgery (prostatectomy, bladder tumor resection)
• Major lower limb orthopedic surgery (hip/knee joint replacement surgery)
• Lung resection surgery
• Intestinal anastomosis surgery
• Permanent pacemaker insertion or internal defibrillator placement
• Selected invasive procedures (kidney biopsy, prostate biopsy, cervical cone biopsy, pericardiocentesis, colonic polypectomy)
Intermediate risk
• Other intra-abdominal surgery
• Other intrathoracic surgery
• Other orthopedic surgery
• Other vascular surgery
Low risk
• Laparoscopic cholecystectomy
• Laparoscopic inguinal hernia repair
• Dental procedures
• Dermatologic procedures
• Ophthalmologic procedures
• Coronary angiography
• Gastroscopy or colonoscopy
• Selected invasive procedures (bone marrow aspirate and biopsy, lymph node biopsy, thoracentesis, paracentesis, arthrocentesis)
Very Low Risk (warfarin interruption not needed)
• Single tooth extraction or teeth cleaning
• Selected skin biopsy or skin cancer removal
• Selected cataract removal

- Urologic surgery such as prostate and bladder surgery (including endoscopic surgery), in which high concentrations of urokinase in the urine can promote surgical site bleeding.

A suggested classification of bleeding risk can be considered in **Table 61-4**. In addition, some seemingly minor procedures should be considered with caution, since the risk of bleeding may be unexpectedly high. Such procedures include:

- Resection of colonic polyps especially large polyps (> 1 cm), in which the polyp stalk may be a source for ongoing bleeding;
- Biopsy of the prostate or kidney, in which endogenous urokinase production may promote bleeding, possibly for several days after the procedure; and
- Cardiac pacemaker or defibrillator implantation in which the unopposed layers of the subclavian pacemaker pocket are left to heal by secondary intent.

RISK FOR PERIOPERATIVE BLEEDING AND ITS CONSEQUENCES

The choice to stop warfarin therapy should take into consideration the risk and the clinical impact of perioperative bleeding. Some studies show an increased risk for bleeding when surgery is performed in patients who continue to receive warfarin therapy; in particular, this is likely to confer increased bleeding after major surgery associated with increased blood loss. Moreover, closed-space surgery (intracranial, intraspinal, retroperitoneal, posterior eye chamber) may result in bleeds associated with considerable morbidity and mortality.

THROMBOEMBOLIC RISK AFTER INTERRUPTION OF WARFARIN THERAPY

Based on prospective cohort studies using low-molecular-weight heparin (LMWH) as bridging therapy, patients who require temporary interruption of a warfarin during surgery have the following overall estimated crude risk for perioperative arterial thromboembolism: 0.83% associated with mechanical valves and 0.57% associated with atrial fibrillation. This risk is approximately 1% in studies that did not use any bridging anticoagulation. Finally, in patients with a prior VTE, the overall crude risk for perioperative venous thromboembolic events was 0.60%, again based on prospective cohort studies that used LMWH as bridging therapy. What is lacking in all of these assessments are prospective data on the risk for thromboembolism in patients who do not receive bridging therapy during warfarin interruption.

Another related aspect is the clinical impact of thromboembolic events: embolic stroke can result in death or major disability in about 70% of patients; thrombosis of a mechanical heart valve is fatal in about 15% of patients; recurrent VTE is fatal in 4% to 9% of patients.

Recent clinical practice guidelines recommend that when anticoagulant therapy needs to be interrupted, the use of bridging anticoagulation may be used according to the following broad scheme:

- *High risk patients*: therapeutic-dose heparin bridging therapy is recommended.
- *Intermediate risk patients*: therapeutic-dose *or* low-dose heparin bridging therapy is suggested.
- *Low risk patients*: low-dose heparin bridging therapy *or* no bridging is suggested.

PRACTICE POINT

Recent clinical practice guidelines recommend that when anticoagulant therapy needs to be interrupted, the use of bridging anticoagulation may be used according to the following broad scheme:

- High risk patients: therapeutic-dose heparin bridging therapy is recommended.
- Intermediate risk patients: therapeutic-dose or low-dose heparin bridging therapy is suggested.
- Low risk patients: low-dose heparin bridging therapy or no bridging is suggested.

Although low-dose LWMH regimens are appropriate for the prevention of postoperative venous thrombosis, it is possible but improbable that such dose regimens have comparable efficacy as therapeutic-dose regimens to prevent arterial thromboembolism such as stroke.

STOPPING AND RESUMING WARFARIN THERAPY PERIOPERATIVELY

An overview of the management of patients who require temporary interruption of a warfarin before surgery is provided in **Figure 61-1** and individual components of management are discussed below.

STOPPING WARFARIN THERAPY: WHEN AND HOW

Among oral anticoagulants, warfarin is the most commonly used preparation but other vitamin K antagonists such as acenocoumarol and phenprocoumon are also used, especially in European countries. Warfarin, which has a half-life of about 36–42 hours, should be stopped 5 days before surgery is planned (which corresponds approximately to 5 half-lives of warfarin) to allow elimination of any residual anticoagulant effect prior to surgery. This time duration may be longer when the targeted therapeutic range of INR is higher than 2.0–3.0, as for example for mechanical heart valves (target INR 2.5–3.5), or in elderly patients in whom a slower decay of the anticoagulant effect may occur.

This chapter focuses on the most commonly used oral anticoagulant drug, which is warfarin. It should be noted, though, that acenocoumarol has a half-life of about 6–8 hours and phenprocoumon of about 96–140 hours. Consequently, acenocoumarol should be stopped 2 days before surgery and phenprocoumon 10 days before surgery, which corresponds approximately to 5 half-lives of these drugs.

RESUMING WARFARIN: WHEN AND HOW

Warfarin takes about 48 hours to prolong the INR after surgery and about 5 days to attain a therapeutic INR (2.0–3.0) when it is reinitiated at usual dose after surgery. For this reason, it is suggested to resume warfarin 12 to 24 hours after surgery, assuming adequate postoperative hemostasis, since it is anticipated that full wound healing will have occurred by 48 hours later when an appreciable anticoagulant effect is expected.

BRIDGING THERAPY

TREATMENT REGIMENS

There is no standardized definition of bridging anticoagulation and more than 1 type of heparin dose regimen has been studied in prospective studies of perioperative anticoagulation. In terms of drug types, subcutaneous LMWH is the most commonly used drug for bridging and when adopted, therapeutic-dose LMWH is typically used more than low-dose regimens. Unfractionated heparin (UFH) is another drug regimen used for bridging therapy, although its use is less frequent because it is not easily manageable when the intravenous route is chosen. UFH can, however, be administered subcutaneously as a weight-based, twice-daily, fixed-dose (250 IU/kg) regimen although this approach has not been assessed in the perioperative setting.

In terms of drug dosage, both therapeutic-dose regimens (eg, enoxaparin, 1 mg/kg SC twice-daily) and low-dose (venous thrombosis prophylaxis) regimens (eg, enoxaparin, 40 mg once-daily) have been considered as bridging therapy, with therapeutic-dosing being the most commonly used regimen. The evidence that therapeutic-dose LMWH is efficacious to prevent arterial thromboembolism is indirect, since prospective studies assessing therapeutic-dose LMWH for the prevention of arterial thromboembolism did not have a no-bridging comparison group. However, a large trial assessing stroke prevention in patients with AF found that therapeutic-dose idraparinux, an antifactor Xa inhibitor with a similar mode of action as LMWHs was as effective as warfarin in preventing arterial thromboembolism. Although low-dose LWMH regimens are appropriate for the prevention of postoperative venous thrombosis, it is possible but improbable that such dose regimens have comparable efficacy as therapeutic-dose regiment to prevent arterial thromboembolism such as stroke.

Other LMWH bridging regimens include dalteparin 100 IU/kg twice-daily or 200 UI/kg once-daily or 5000 IU once-daily, and tinzaparin 175 IU/kg once-daily. UFH can be administered intravenously at a dose to maintain the activated partial

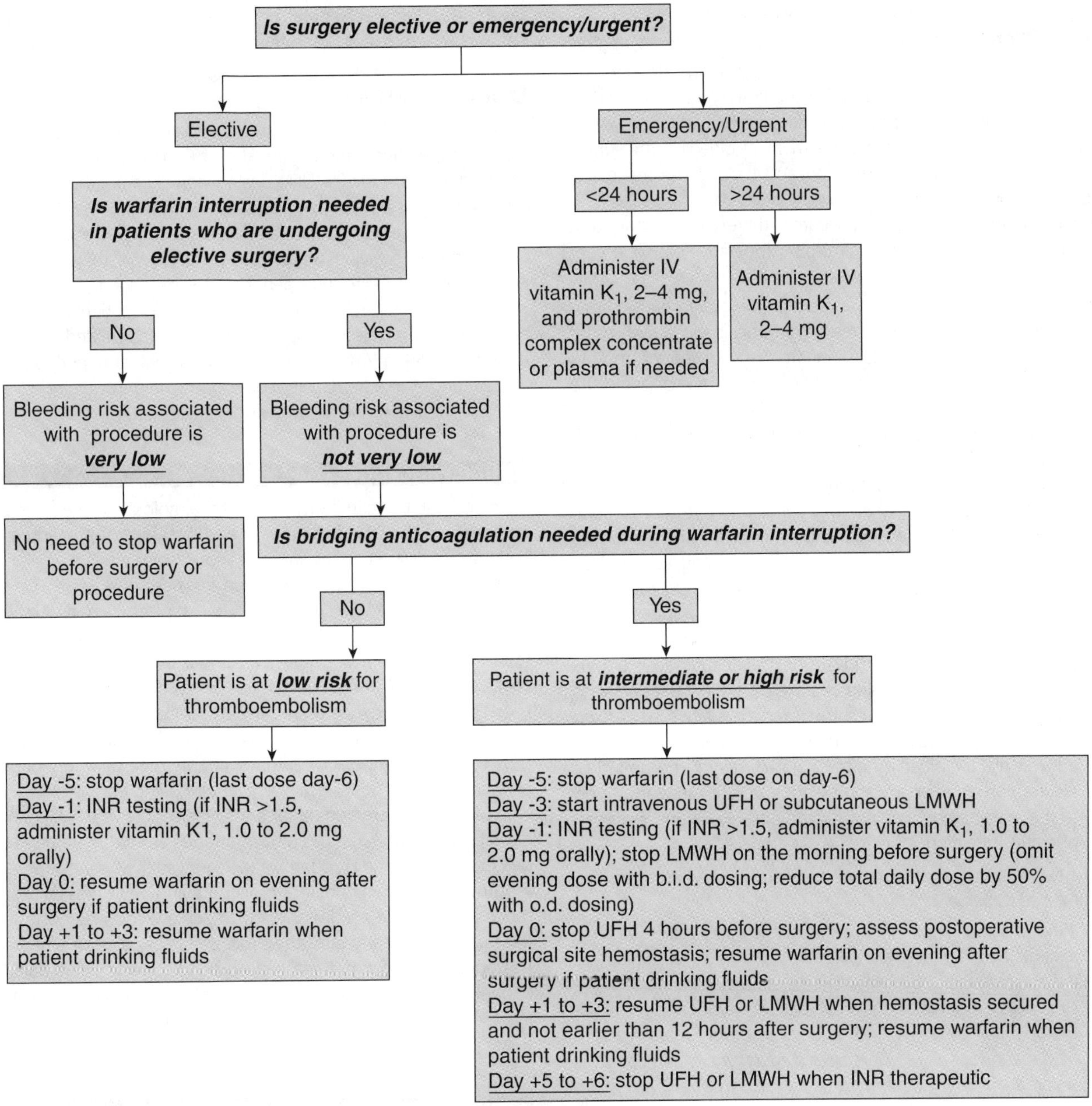

Figure 61-1 *Overview of perioperative management of warfarin therapy before and after surgery or other invasive procedures.*

thromboplastin time (aPTT) at 1.5–2.0 times the normal value or as a low-dose regimen, 5000 IU twice-daily.

STARTING AND STOPPING HEPARIN: PREOPERATIVE PERIOD

Since warfarin has a half-life of 36–42 hours, heparin could be started on the morning 2 days after warfarin interruption (or the third day before surgery). Once heparin administration has begun, it should be continued until an appropriate time before surgery, depending on the type of heparin (UFH or LMWH) and its dosage, as follows:

- *Intravenous UFH*: since its half-life is about 45 minutes, it should be stopped about 4 hours before surgery (corresponding approximately to 5 half-lives).
- *Subcutaneous LMWH*: since the elimination half-lives of LMWHs are about 4–5 hours, the last dose should be administered 20 to 25 hours before surgery or on the morning of the day before surgery (corresponding approximately to 5 half-lives).

Two studies have shown that preoperative, therapeutic-dose LMWH is frequently associated with a detectable anticoagulant effect during surgery. In 1 prospective cohort study, 30% of patients receiving therapeutic-dose LMWH (once-daily or twice-daily regimens, with the last dose given not less than 12 hours before surgery) resulted in a residual anticoagulant effect at the time of surgery. Moreover, a second study showed that 34% of patients who received a twice-daily regimen of therapeutic-dose LMWH (ie, enoxaparin, 1 mg/kg twice-daily), with the last dose given on the evening before surgery, had a substantial anticoagulant effect that was within the therapeutic range at the time of surgery. For these reasons, on the day before surgery, patients receiving therapeutic-dose LMWH as bridging anticoagulation should receive only the morning dose if a twice-daily regimen is used or they should reduce by 50% the total dose of LMWH if a once-daily regimen is used.

RESUMING AND STOPPING HEPARIN: POSTOPERATIVE PERIOD

An assessment of the risk for postoperative bleeding depends on 2 factors: (1) the anticipated surgical-related risk, which is defined by the type of surgery; and (2) the postoperative evaluation of wound hemostasis. Consequently, the assessment of bleeding risk, which largely drives the decision about when (and if) to resume anticoagulants in the postoperative period, is individualized.

Assuming that hemostasis is secured, there are 3 factors that clinicians should consider to minimize postoperative bleeding after anticoagulants are resumed:

- *How long has it been since the operation/procedure*: early (within 6 hours), low-dose LMWH resumption has been shown to be associated with higher bleeding rate than delayed resumption (12 to 24 hours); other studies have shown that delaying the resumption of therapeutic-dose LMWH until hemostasis is secured or avoiding it altogether in high risk patients is associated with a low risk for bleeding (1.0–2.9%), and also with a < 1% risk of arterial thromboembolism
- *Dose of anticoagulant when anticoagulation is resumed*: therapeutic-dose LMWH or UFH has been shown to be associated with a higher risk of major bleeding compared to low-dose LMWH or UFH regimen or no bridging (OR 4.4) in a prospective multicenter registry (data submitted for publication).
- *Flexibility in postoperative resumption of anticoagulant therapy*: a prospective bridging study using therapeutic-dose LMWH showed that major bleeding occurred in 20% of patients who had major surgery and resumed anticoagulation at a fixed time, within 24 hours after surgery; other studies demonstrate a lower risk for bleeding after major surgery if the timing of resumption of anticoagulation is not fixed but varies according to the anticipated bleeding risk and observed intra- and postoperative bleeding.

In general terms, postoperative bridging therapy strategies are summarized as follows:

- Minor surgery in patients receiving therapeutic-dose LMWH: resume this regimen approximately 24 hours after surgery (eg, the following day), when there is adequate hemostasis.
- High bleeding risk surgery in patients who are receiving therapeutic-dose LMWH: either delay resumption of therapeutic heparin for 48–72 hours after surgery, when hemostasis is secured; or administer only low-dose heparin when hemostasis is secured; or avoid the use of LMWH altogether.

In the postoperative period, after both warfarin and heparin have been resumed, the last step is considering the timing for stopping heparin. As previously pointed out, when warfarin is resumed at the patient's usual dose, therapeutic range is expected to be reached in 5–6 days and at this point heparin bridging can be stopped.

LABORATORY MONITORING

INR MONITORING

In the preoperative period, it is reasonable to have INR testing done 1 or 2 days before surgery, whenever feasible, to confirm a normal or near-normal INR. If INR is still elevated (eg, ≥ 1.5), low-dose oral vitamin K, 1 to 2 mg orally, can be administered. In this way, instances in which there is an elevated INR on the day of surgery can be avoided as this may lead to cancellation of the surgery or the need to administer a coagulation factor blood product replacement, typically fresh frozen plasma or prothrombin complex concentrates. In the postoperative period, it is reasonable to measure the INR once or twice during the initial 7–10 days after warfarin resumption, in order to determine whether therapeutic anticoagulation has been reached and heparin bridging can be stopped.

aPTT MONITORING

Intravenous UFH can be monitored both in the preoperative and postoperative periods with the aPTT. However, it should be noted that the use of a UFH dosing nomogram, which was not designed for use in the perioperative setting, may be misleading, and should be avoided, especially in the postoperative setting.

In patients receiving therapeutic-dose LMWH, there is not an established role for routine perioperative monitoring of antifactor Xa activity. However, for selected categories of patients, as for example moderate-to-severe renal insufficiency (calculated creatinine clearance <50 ml/min) or extreme body weight, perioperative assessment of anti-Xa activity could be of help in guiding LMWH management, as in the nonoperative clinical setting.

MINOR PROCEDURES

Minor dental, dermatologic, and ophthalmologic procedures can comprise up to 20% of all surgical and nonsurgical procedures in patients who are receiving antithrombotic drugs.

Two aspects are worth considering for these procedures. On the one hand, these minor procedures are typically associated with little blood loss (ie, bleeding might not be clinically relevant). On the other hand, they are often performed in a clinic or other out-of-hospital setting. If bleeding occurs when the patient is at home, it could generate concern and anxiety for her/him. Consequently, patients should be given instructions about bleeding, in particular how to recognize a bleeding that warrants medical attention and how to manage a nonclinically relevant bleeding episode.

In patients undergoing minor dental procedures, such as a single dental extraction, warfarin can be continued around the time of the procedure and an oral prohemostatic agent such as tranexamic acid mouthwash (1–2 hours before procedure and 2–3 times daily after procedure) can be coadministered to achieve local hemostasis in the immediate period after the procedure. For patients scheduled to undergo a minor dermatologic procedure, warfarin should be continued periprocedurally. The same holds for inpatients undergoing cataract removal, as this is an avascular procedure with minimal tissue injury and blood loss.

CONCLUSION

The management of patients who require interruption of a warfarin before an elective surgical or other invasive procedure requires an assessment of patients' risk for thromboembolism during warfarin interruption and their risk for bleeding associated with surgery. These considerations will determine whether patients receive bridging anticoagulation. In patients in whom bridging anticoagulation may be warranted, the risk for bleeding associated with the surgery or invasive procedure will determine when bridging is resumed after surgery. In recent years, considerable progress has been made in our understanding of the therapeutic benefits and risks of bridging anticoagulation through cohort studies and patient registries. However, several questions remain that are best addressed by randomized trials. Most important, perhaps, is the need to address whether bridging anticoagulation is needed in patients who require temporary interruption of warfarin, especially in patients at low to moderate risk for thromboembolism who constitute the majority of patients assessed and in whom best practice is uncertain. Additional unanswered questions relate to the timing of bridging anticoagulation before and after surgery and identifying types of surgery and procedures in which the risk for bleeding precludes bridging anticoagulation.

SUGGESTED READINGS

Amadeus Investigators, Bousser MG, Bouthier J, Büller HR, et al. Comparison of idraparinux with vitamin K antagonists for prevention of thromboembolism in patients with atrial fibrillation: a randomised, open-label, non-inferiority trial. *Lancet*. 2008;371:315–321.

Douketis JD, Berger PB, Dunn AS, et al. The perioperative management of antithrombotic therapy. American College of Chest Physicians evidence-based clinical practice guidelines (8th edition). *CHEST*. 2008;133:299S–339S.

Douketis JD, Johnson JA, Turpie AG. Low-molecular-weight heparin as bridging anticoagulation during interruption of warfarin: assessment of a stardardized periprocedural anticoagulation regimen. *Arch Intern Med*. 2004;164:1319–1326.

Douketis JD, Woods K, Foster GA, at al. Bridging anticoagulation with low-molecular-weight heparin after interruption of warfarin therapy is associated with a residual anticoagulant effect prior to surgery. *Thromb Haemost*. 2005;94:528–531.

Dunn AS, Spyropoulos A, Turpie AG. Bridging therapy in patients on long-term oral anticoagulants who require surgery: the Prospective Peri-operative Enoxaparin Cohort Trial (PROSPECT). *J Thromb Haemost*. 2007;5:2211–2218.

Kearon C, Ginsberg JS, Julian JA, et al. Comparison of fixed-dose weight-adjusted unfractionated heparin and low-molecular-weight heparin for acute treatment of venous thromboembolism. *JAMA*. 2006;296:935–942.

Kovacs MJ, Kearon C, Rodger M, et al. Single-arm study of bridging therapy with low-molecular weight heparin for patients at risk of arterial embolism who require temporary interruption of warfarin. *Circulation*. 2004;110:1685–1663.

O'Donnell MJ, Kearon C, Johnson J, et al. Preoperative anticoagulant activity after bridging low-molecular-weight heparin for temporary interruption of warfarin. *Ann Inter Med*. 2007; 146:184–187.

Torn M, Rosendaal FR. Oral anticoagulation in surgical procedures: risks and recommendation. *BR J Haematol*. 2003;123:676–682.

White RH, McKittrick T, Hutchinson R, et al. Temporary discontinuation of warfarin therapy: changes in the international normalized ratio. *Ann Inter Med*. 1995;1220:40–42.

Woods K, Douketis JD, Kathirgamanathan K, et al. Low-dose oral vitamin K to normalize the international normalized ratio prior to surgery in patients who require temporary interruption of warfarin. *J Thromb Thrombolysis*. 2007;24:93–97.

CHAPTER 62

Perioperative Management of Patients who are Receiving Antiplatelet Therapy

Marco P. Donadini, MD
James D. Douketis, MD, FRCPC, FACP, FCCP

INTRODUCTION

The perioperative management of patients who are receiving antiplatelet therapy is a common clinical problem given the large number of patients who are receiving these agents for treatment of coronary artery disease, cerebrovascular disease or peripheral arterial disease. Such patients may be receiving: acetylsalicylic acid (ASA) alone; clopidogrel alone; ASA and clopidogrel. Patients who are receiving antiplatelet drugs encompass a broad risk spectrum for cardiovascular events that depends on the clinical indication for antiplatelet therapy and whether patients are receiving treatment for the primary or secondary prevention of cardiovascular disease. There are no perioperative risk classification schemes that consider the benefits and risks of continuing or interrupting antiplatelet therapy.

The objectives of this chapter are: 1) to stratify patients according to their risk for acute coronary events if antiplatelet therapy is stopped and the risk for bleeding associated with surgery or procedure; and 2) to provide a practical approach to the perioperative interruption and resumption of antiplatelet therapy.

CASE 62-1

A 68-year-old man with a drug-eluting stent (DES) inserted 4 months ago (following myocardial infarction) requires surgery for removal of a parotid cancer. He is on aspirin and clopidogrel. The perioperative assessment of perioperative antiplatelet therapy should start from the assessment of his thromboembolic risk: given the recent DES implantation, the risk of stent-thrombosis if aspirin and/or clopidogrel are interrupted is very high (and associated also with high morbidity and mortality).

The second step is represented by the assessment of bleeding risk: this surgery involves a moderately vascular, nonclosed-space organ (parotid gland) with an expected small to moderate tissue injury and the potential for intraoperative cautery/suturing.

In this case, after balancing the high thrombotic risk (possibly associated with high morbidity and mortality) and the moderate bleeding risk, the suggested strategy is to continue aspirin and clopidogrel perioperatively.

Cautionary note: There are no randomized trials comparing continuation with interruption of antiplatelet drugs around the time of surgery and patient management should be based also as individual circumstances.

ASSESSING PERIOPERATIVE ATHEROTHROMBOTIC AND BLEEDING RISKS

PERIOPERATIVE ATHEROTHROMBOTIC RISK ASSESSMENT

Patients who are receiving antiplatelet drugs have a variable risk for atherothrombotic cardiovascular events, which depends to a large extent on the indication for the antiplatelet therapy. Although an overall risk classification scheme for atherothrombotic events does not exist, it is reasonable to consider patients who are receiving antiplatelet therapy as primary prevention against stroke or myocardial infarction as being at lowest risk for atherothrombotic events. On the other hand, patients considered at high risk for such events include those with a recent acute coronary syndrome, in particular within the past 3 months, and

TABLE 62-1 Risk for Thrombotic Cardiovascular Events in Patients not Adhering or Discontinuing ASA in Secondary Prevention or not taking ASA for Primary Prevention

Clinical Condition	Risk: Odds Ratio
Primary prevention*	1.1–1.2†
Secondary prevention in coronary heart disease	~2
Secondary prevention after coronary drug-eluting stent implantation	~90

*Population: healthy individuals or presence of cardiovascular risk factors.
†Risk for cardiovascular events in patients nonassuming vs. assuming aspirin.

those with a recent placement of a coronary stent, in particular within the past 6 weeks to 6 months (**Table 62-1**).

PRACTICE POINT

- Although an overall risk classification scheme for atherothrombotic events does not exist, it is reasonable to consider patients who are receiving antiplatelet therapy as primary prevention against stroke or myocardial infarction as being at lowest risk for atherothrombotic events. On the other hand, patients considered at high risk for such events include those with a recent acute coronary syndrome, in particular within the past 3 months, and those with a recent placement of a coronary stent, in particular within the past 6 weeks to 6 months.

BLEEDING RISK ASSESSMENT

Along with patient-specific characteristics, such as concomitant liver or kidney disease, an assessment of the perioperative bleeding risk depends largely on the type of surgery or procedure being performed. In assessing surgery/procedure-specific bleeding risk, 2 factors should be considered: the expected amount of blood loss; and the location of the surgery/procedure. Thus, the amount of bleeding is important as it can lead to local complications such as a wound hematoma or systemic complications such as cardiovascular collapse. The site of bleeding is also important if a procedure may involve the brain, spinal cord, or heart, as even a small amount of intracranial, spinal, or pericardial bleeding can have devastating clinical consequences.

Although there is no validated method to quantify perioperative bleeding risk, special attention is warranted for certain surgical or other invasive procedures associated with a high risk of bleeding. These can be categorized into 4 groups: (I) extensive surgery associated with substantial tissue damage such as major orthopedic surgery, reconstructive plastic surgery, and major cancer surgery; (II) urologic surgery such as prostate and bladder surgery (including endoscopic surgery); (III) "closed-space" surgery such as that which is intracranial, spinal, posterior chamber of the eye, and cardiac (coronary artery bypass or heart valve replacement) surgery; and (IV) major vascular surgery, such as aortic aneurysm repair.

CASE 62-2

A 62-year-old man with a history of non-ST-elevation myocardial infarction (NSTEMI) 5 years ago (treated only with medical therapy) requires neurosurgery for removal of a meningioma. Among other cardiovascular risk factors, he has hypertension and type 2 diabetes. During the last 3 years, he has not had any acute coronary syndrome-related symptoms.

The atherothrombotic risk should consider both the history of NSTEMI (5 years ago) and the absence of anginal or other cardiac symptoms in the last 3 years. In this case of stable coronary artery disease the thrombotic risk could be considered moderate. The bleeding risk associated with intracranial surgery is very high, because it is performed in a closed space.

After balancing the thrombotic and bleeding risk, the suggested antiplatelet management could be as follows:

- Day −7 to −10: stop aspirin to achieve < 10% residual antiplatelet effect at time of surgery (30–40% of residual antiplatelet effect at surgery would be present if aspirin is stopped at day −4 to −5)
- Day −1: no indication for platelet function assessment using platelet function assays
- Day +1: assess surgical site hemostasis and, if feasible, resume aspirin at the usual dose

Cautionary note: clinical judgment is still required for individual patient management.

A suggested classification of bleeding risk can be considered in **Table 62-2**. In addition, there are some minor surgeries or procedures that, on the surface, may not appear to confer an increased risk for bleeding but warrant caution when perioperative anticoagulation is used. Resection of colonic polyps, especially those with large sessile stalks, may confer significant bleeding since after

TABLE 62-2 Risk for Bleeding According to Type of Surgery

Very high risk • Neurosurgery (intracranial or spinal surgery) • Cardiac surgery (coronary artery bypass or heart valve replacement)
High risk • Major vascular surgery (abdominal aortic aneurysm repair, aortofemoral bypass) • Major urologic surgery (prostatectomy, bladder tumor resection) • Major lower limb orthopedic surgery (hip/knee joint replacement surgery) • Lung resection surgery • Intestinal anastomosis surgery • Permanent pacemaker insertion or internal defibrillator placement • Selected invasive procedures (kidney biopsy, prostate biopsy, cervical cone biopsy, pericardiocentesis, colonic polypectomy)
Intermediate risk • Other intra-abdominal surgery • Oher intrathoracic surgery • Other orthopedic surgery • Other vascular surgery
Low risk • Laparoscopic cholecystectomy • Laparoscopic inguinal hernia repair • Dental procedures • Dermatologic procedures • Ophthalmologic procedures • Coronary angiography • Gastroscopy or colonoscopy • Selected invasive procedures (bone marrow aspirate and biopsy, lymph node biopsy, thoracentesis, paracentesis, arthrocentesis)
Very low risk (antiplatelet drug interruption not needed) • Single tooth extraction or teeth cleaning • Selected skin biopsy or skin cancer removal • Selected cataract removal

the stalk is transected. In patients having a biopsy of the prostate or kidney, endogenous production of urokinase within the urinary tract may promote bleeding for up to 1 week after the procedure while healing takes place at the biopsy site. In patients having a cardiac pacemaker or defibrillator implantation, the subclavian pocket that is dissected between the fascial layers is left unopposed to heal by secondary intention making patients susceptible to pacemaker pocket hematoma.

CLINICAL CONSEQUENCES OF ANTIPLATELET THERAPY INTERRUPTION

In the perioperative management of patients on antiplatelet therapy, the risk for atherothrombotic cardiovascular events related to the interruption of such therapy is a first step in weighing the risks and benefits of interrupting or continuing antiplatelet therapy. In a nonoperative clinical setting, patients with coronary artery disease who stop or do not adhere to aspirin therapy have a 3-fold increased risk for major adverse cardiovascular events compared to those who continue aspirin. In patients with peripheral arterial disease, interruption of aspirin therapy also confers an increased risk for acute lower limb ischemia and stroke. Even though there are a few data regarding the mean time between aspirin interruption and subsequent cardiovascular events, some studies found this time window is approximately 1 week for acute coronary syndrome, 2 weeks for a cerebrovascular event, and 4 weeks for peripheral arterial ischemia.

PRACTICE POINT

Even though there are a few data regarding the mean time between aspirin interruption and subsequent cardiovascular events, some studies found this time-window is approximately

- 1 week for acute coronary syndrome
- 2 weeks for a cerebrovascular event
- 4 weeks for peripheral arterial ischemia.

PRACTICE POINT

Coronary artery disease

- In a nonoperative clinical setting, patients with coronary artery disease who stop or do not adhere to aspirin therapy have a 3-fold increased risk for major adverse cardiovascular events compared to those who continue aspirin.
- Interruption of antiplatelet therapy in patients with a recently implanted drug-eluting stent confers a 90-fold increase risk of adverse cardiovascular events related to stent thrombosis, including death and myocardial infarction.
- Both for bare-metal and drug-eluting stents, withdrawal of antiplatelet therapy while coronary reendothelialization is not complete, represents a major independent predictor of late-stent thrombosis, an event associated with high morbidity and mortality.
- In order to mitigate the risk for perioperative stent thrombosis, elective noncardiac surgery should be avoided during the period when stent endothelialization is still ongoing.

Peripheral arterial disease

- Interruption of aspirin therapy confers an increased risk for acute lower limb ischemia and stroke.

Patients who have undergone a coronary percutaneous intervention with the placement of a bare metal or drug-eluting coronary artery stent deserve special consideration. Interruption of antiplatelet therapy in patients with a recently implanted drug-eluting stent confers a 90-fold increase risk of adverse cardiovascular events related to stent thrombosis, including death and myocardial infarction. Both for bare metal and drug-eluting stents, withdrawal of antiplatelet therapy while coronary reendothelialization is not complete represents a major independent predictor of late stent thrombosis, an event associated with high morbidity and mortality.

BLEEDING RISK WITH CONTINUED PERIOPERATIVE ANTIPLATELET THERAPY

NONCARDIAC SURGERY

There are few randomized controlled trials or prospective cohort studies comparing benefits and risks of continuing and interrupting antiplatet therapy around the time of elective noncardiac surgery. In one placebo-controlled trial involving predominantly patients who had hip fracture repair surgery, aspirin use in the perioperative period conferred an increase for major bleeding with no apparent benefit in the prevention of cardiovascular events, including stroke and myocardial infarction. In abdominal or pelvic surgery, some retrospective studies found an increased risk for bleeding with perioperative continuation of aspirin, whereas one study did not find a difference in blood loss in patients who took aspirin before surgery compared to those who did not. In otolaryngologic surgery, patients given aspirin after tonsillectomy were found to have a 7-fold higher reoperation rate. Finally, in intracranial neurosurgery, perioperative aspirin use conferred an increased risk for postoperative intracerebral hematoma.

Considering clopidogrel, retrospective cohort studies have shown increased rates of bleeding with its perioperative continuation. In addition, one cohort study in patients undergoing bronchoscopy found increased rates of bleeding after biopsy in patients receiving clopidogrel or clopidogrel plus aspirin compared to no antiplatelet drugs.

CORONARY ARTERY BYPASS GRAFTING

Elective or urgent coronary artery bypass grafting (CABG) surgery is frequently required in patients on antiplatelet therapy (aspirin and/or clopidogrel). Minimizing the risk for perioperative bleeding in patients undergoing CABG surgery is important because of an increased risk for death and other adverse outcomes in patients who require blood transfusion in the perioperative period. If aspirin therapy is continued perioperatively, some observational studies found an increased risk for mediastinal bleeding, blood transfusion, and reoperation, although these findings were not found in other studies. Indeed, a large cohort study found perioperative continuation of aspirin to be associated with lower postoperative mortality without an increased risk of reoperation or blood transfusion. In the case of clopidogrel, there is good evidence from large clinical trials, mainly in patients with prior acute coronary syndromes, of an increased risk for blood transfusions and major bleeding when clopidogrel was continued around the time of CABG, although this risk diminished if it was interrupted approximately 5 days before surgery.

Ultimately, the surgeon will be in the best position to define the risk of bleeding. The medical consultant should try to define the risk for cardiovascular events related to interruption of antiplatelet therapy, and in many cases, this requires consultation with the patient's primary cardiologist.

INTERRUPTION AND PERIOPERATIVE RESUMPTION OF ANTIPLATELET THERAPY

The timing of interruption of antiplatelet drugs depends to a large extent on drug pharmacodynamics. Since both aspirin and clopidogrel irreversibly inhibit platelet function, the platelet lifespan may be considered as a measure for deciding when to interrupt antiplatelet therapy before surgery if the aim is to have hemostasis fully restored. Aspirin and clopidogrel irreversibly inhibit platelet cyclooxygenase-1 (COX-1) and adenosine diphosphate (ADP) receptors, respectively, so their effect persists for the lifespan of platelets, which is 7 to 10 days. Thus, for patients who require temporary interruption of aspirin or clopidogrel before surgery or an invasive procedure and require normalized hemostasis, it is suggested that these drugs are interrupted 7 to 10 days before surgery. After surgery, these agents should, in general, be resumed when there is adequate postoperative hemostasis. In some studies, dealing with patients with mechanical heart valves, aspirin has been resumed on the same day of surgery at the usual maintenance dose.

In the case of clopidogrel, data are lacking about its resumption after its interruption, also with regard to the starting dose. Resumption with a maintenance dose achieves maximal platelet function inhibition after 5 to 10 days, whereas a loading dose achieves this effect within 2 to 15 hours after administration. Therefore, the resumption dose of clopidogrel will depend largely on the presence or absence of a coronary stent, its type and time from its placement. In recent consensus group guidelines, resumption of aspirin or clopidogrel is suggested to be done at approximately 24 hours (or the next morning) after surgery, if there is adequate hemostasis.

A scheme for perioperative antiplatelet management in patients without a coronary stent may follow the suggested recommendations of consensus group guidelines (**Table 62-3**). Thus, in patients not at high risk for cardiovascular events, interruption of antiplatelet drugs is reasonable since the potential risks of continuing therapy are likely to outweigh any putative benefits. For patients at moderate to high risk for cardiovascular events, management can be determined based on the type of surgery or procedure they are to undergo. For noncardiac surgery, it is suggested to continue aspirin perioperatively, interrupting clopidogrel at least 5 days and, preferably, within 10 days before surgery. For CABG, it is suggested to continue aspirin perioperatively and if interrupted, to reinitiate aspirin between 6 hours and 48 hours after CABG. In clopidogrel-treated patients, this should be interrupted at least 5 days and preferably, within 10 days before CABG. Finally, for PCI, it is suggested to continue aspirin perioperatively and if clopidogrel is interrupted prior to PCI, resume it after PCI with a loading dose of 300 mg to 600 mg in accordance with usual post-PCI management recommendations.

ALTERNATIVE BRIDGING THERAPY STRATEGIES

Some antithrombotic drugs that provide some temporary inhibition of platelet function may be theoretically used as bridging therapy in the perioperative management of patients who are receiving antiplatelet therapy. However, evidence is lacking as to their efficacy and safety in this clinical setting.

In patients who require interruption of aspirin and/or clopidogrel during the perioperative period, administering unfractionated or low molecular weight heparin, in a similar way as is done in patients who require temporary interruption of vitamin K antagonists, may seem reasonable since these anticoagulants have some antiplatelet properties. However, there is no evidence of any cardioprotective effect when anticoagulants are used, temporarily, in lieu of antiplatelet drugs and therefore, this strategy is not recommended in current guidelines.

Alternative strategies that may be considered as putative bridging therapy during interruption of ASA and/or clopidogrel may include the use of short-acting glycoprotein IIb-IIIa inhibitors, new reversible ADP receptor antiplatelet inhibitors, or reversible COX-1 inhibitors. Studies are needed to assess the efficacy and safety of bridging therapy in patients who are taking antiplatelet drugs and until relevant data are available caution is required in the use of short-acting antithrombotic drugs in this clinical setting.

PATIENTS WITH CORONARY STENTS

In patients with recent placement of a coronary stent, the risk of stent thrombosis is high if antiplatelet therapy is discontinued prematurely. In such patients, coronary stent thrombosis is associated with high morbidity and mortality, typically with a large myocardial infarction or death in more than 50% of affected patients. In order to mitigate the risk for perioperative stent thrombosis, elective noncardiac surgery should be avoided during the period when stent endothelialization is still ongoing.

For bare metal stents, 6 weeks is considered to be the time period for stent endothelialization and consequently, elective noncardiac surgery should be postponed for a minimum of 6 weeks after stent placement. A longer time is required for reendothelialization of sirolimus- or paclitaxel-eluting stents compared to bare metal stents,

TABLE 62-3 Suggested Perioperative Management for Patients Receiving Antiplatelet Drugs

Clinical Scenario	Suggested Perioperative Management
Low risk for CV events and elective surgery	• Interruption of antiplatelet drugs should be considered
High risk for CV events and elective surgery	• Consider use of aspirin perioperatively • If patients are receiving clopidogrel, clopidogrel should be interrupted at least 5 and preferably 7–10 days before surgery
Coronary stent in place and elective surgery	• In patients with a bare metal coronary stent who require surgery within 6 weeks of stent placement, aspirin and clopidogrel should be continued in the perioperative period • In patients with a drug-eluting coronary stent who require surgery within 6–12 months of stent placement, aspirin and clopidogrel should be continued in the perioperative period where feasible
Undergoing CABG	• Aspirin should be continued up to and beyond the time of CABG • If aspirin is interrupted, it should be resumed 6–48 hours after surgery • Clopidogrel should be interrupted at least 5 days and, preferably, 10 days before surgery
Undergoing minor procedures	• In patients who are who are undergoing minor procedures (dental, dermatologic, ophthalmologic) and are receiving aspirin, consider continuing aspirin around the time of the procedure • If such patients are receiving combined aspirin-clopidogrel therapy, consider interruption of clopidogrel unless patients are at high risk for coronary stent thrombosis

but less is known about the timing of noncardiac surgery in these patients. After the placement of a drug-eluting stent, aspirin is recommended indefinitely and clopidogrel is recommended for at least 12 months. Thus, for patients who are receiving combined aspirin-clopidogrel therapy for at least 12 months after the placement of a drug-eluting stent. Elective surgery should be postponed for at least 6 months and, preferably, for 12 months after stent placement.

In recent consensus group guidelines, perioperative continuation of both clopidogrel and aspirin is recommended in patients who require urgent surgery within 6 weeks after placement of a bare metal stent and within 6–12 months after placement of a drug-eluting stent.

PATIENTS UNDERGOING MINOR PROCEDURES

Minor dental, dermatologic, and ophthalmologic procedures can comprise up to 20% of all surgical and nonsurgical procedures in patients who are receiving antithrombotic drugs.

Two aspects are worth considering for these procedures: on the one hand, these minor procedures are typically associated with little blood loss (ie, bleeding may be not clinically relevant), whereas, on the other hand, they are often performed in a clinic or other out-of-hospital setting. If bleeding occurs when the patients are at home, it could generate concern and anxiety for them and their families. Consequently, patients should be given instructions about bleeding, in particular how to manage it when it is not clinically relevant and how to recognize a bleeding that warrants medical attention.

Considering the available evidence, current consensus guidelines recommend continuing aspirin in case of minor dental procedures, minor dermatologic procedures, and cataract removal. In the case of clopidogrel, data are lacking for the perioperative management in the case of minor procedures.

In patients with coronary stents, the recommendations given for noncardiac surgery still apply for minor procedures: dual antiplatelet therapy should not be interrupted within 6 weeks from placement of a bare metal stent and within 12 months from placement of a drug-eluting stent.

In case of a minor procedure, for patients at lower risk, without a coronary stent, it is reasonable to interrupt clopidogrel 5 to 10 days before and to continue aspirin, given that combined antiplatelet treatment will increase bleeding risk above that of the risk with either drug alone.

CONCLUSION

The perioperative management of patients who are receiving antiplatelet drug therapy requires, as with patients who are receiving warfarin, an assessment of patients' risk for thromboembolism during drug interruption and their risk for bleeding associated with surgery. These considerations will determine whether patients continue or interrupt antiplatelet therapy. Modest progress has been made in our understanding of the therapeutic benefits and risks of perioperative antiplatelet therapy through observational studies. However, several questions remain that are best addressed by randomized trials. Most important, perhaps, is the need to address the safety of continuing antiplatelet therapy in patients with coronary stents who are undergoing surgery. Additional unanswered questions relate to the timing of interruption and resumption of antiplatelet drugs before and after surgery.

SUGGESTED READINGS

Berger JS, Roncaglioni MC, Avanzini F, et al. Aspirin for the primary prevention of cardiovascular events in women and men: a sex-specific meta-analysis of randomized controlled trials. *JAMA.* 2006;295:306–313.

Biondi-Zoccai GGL, Lotrionte M, Agostoni P, et al. A systematic review and meta-analysis on the hazards of discontinuing or not adhering to aspirin among 50279 patients at risk for coronary artery disease. *Eur Heart J.* 2006;27:2667–2674.

Burger W, Chemnitius J-M, Kneissl, et al. Low-dose aspirin for secondary cardiovascular prevention—cardiovascular risks after its perioperative withdrawal versus bleeding risks with its continuation—review and meta-analysis. *J Intern Med.* 2005;257:399–414.

Douketis JD, Berger PB, Dunn AS, et al. The perioperative management of antithrombotic therapy. American College of Chest Physicians evidence-based clinical practice guidelines (8th edition). *CHEST.* 2008;133:299S–339S.

Iakovou I, Schmidt T, Bonizzoni E, et al. Incidence, predictors, and outcome of thrombosis after successful implantation of drug-eluting stents. *JAMA.* 2005;293:2126–2130.

King SB 3rd, Smith SC Jr., Hirshfeld JW Jr., et al. 2007 focused update of the ACC/AHA/SCAI 2005 guideline update for percutaneous coronary intervention: a report of the American College of Cardiology/American Heart Association Task Force on Practice guidelines. *Circulation.* 2008;117:261–295.

Mangano DT. Multicenter study of perioperative ischemia research: aspirin and mortality from coronary bypass surgery. *N Engl J Med. 2002*;347:1309–1317.

Merrit JC, Bhatt D. The efficacy and safety of perioperative antiplatelet therapy. *J Thromb Thrombolysis.* 2002;13:97–103.

Pfisterer M, Brunner-La Rocca HP, Buser PT, et al. Late clinical events after clopidogrel discontinuation may limit the benefit of drug-eluting stents. *J Am Coll Cardiol.* 2006;48:2584–2591.

SECTION 6

Medical Management of Neurosurgical Patients

CHAPTER 63

Common Neurosurgical Conditions

Abel Po-Hao Huang, MD
Peter M. Black, MD, PhD

INTRODUCTION

Hospitalists increasingly comanage neurosurgical conditions as part of a multidisciplinary care team. This chapter will present the management of common neurosurgical conditions, including brain tumors, hydrocephalus, stroke and other vascular diseases, traumatic brain injury, spinal cord injury, and degenerative spine disease.

BRAIN TUMORS

Both primary and metastatic brain tumors can cause significant morbidity and mortality due to their location within the central nervous system. Recognition of the common symptoms including headache, seizures, and altered mental status is important for general physicians. MRI helps to define the location and extent of the tumor and provides a diagnosis. Surgery is often required to confirm the definite pathology and guide further treatment (**Table 63-1**).

Benign tumors (meningiomas, pituitary adenomas, acoustic neuromas) often have a favorable outcome with surgical resection or radiation therapy including stereotactic radiation. Skull base tumors are more difficult to handle with surgery alone and might require multimodality treatment. Primary malignant brain tumors (gliomas, medulloblastomas) benefit from radiation and chemotherapy. Brain metastases remain a frequent complication of systemic tumors but are temporarily controlled with surgery or radiation therapy. Unfortunately, the mortality rate from malignant brain tumors remains high.

CLINICAL PRESENTATION

Brain tumors can cause either focal or generalized neurological symptoms. Generalized symptoms include headache, nausea, and vomiting, which are suggestive of increased intracranial pressure. **Headache** occurs in about half of the patients. When focal headache occurs, it may indicate the precise location of the tumor. The headache may be more severe on awakening in the morning (the so-called "morning headache"). It can be difficult to differentiate from tension headache, cluster headache, and migraine. Seizures occur at presentation in 15–95% of patients with brain tumors, depending on the type of tumor. The seizures are mostly focal but may become generalized and cause loss of consciousness. **Focal neurologic deficits**, such as hemiparesis, aphasia, and visual loss, are usually subacute onset and progressive and may reflect the location of the tumor. Some tumors may also present with a **stroke syndrome**.

DIAGNOSIS

Brain CT typically demonstrates a mass lesion with variable contrast enhancement. MRI is the imaging study of choice in evaluating a brain tumor due to its high sensitivity and resolution. On T1-weighted images, most tumors are low signal intensity and may or may not enhance with contrast medium. Generally speaking, more contrast enhancement is observed with high-grade or malignant tumors. The sensitivity and specificity of these imaging study techniques are not high enough to make the diagnosis, and definitive diagnosis still requires a surgical biopsy or resection to examine the pathology. Because most primary brain tumors remain localized to the brain, systemic staging is not necessary. However, medulloblastoma, ependymoma, and germ cell tumors may spread via the cerebrospinal fluid pathway. Therefore, MRI of the spine should be performed for these patients to rule out cerebrospinal fluid seeding.

TABLE 63-1 Imaging Characteristics and Survival of Patients with (1) Glioblastoma Multiforme, (2) Low Grade Glioma, (3) Meningioma, and (4) Metastasis

	Imaging Characteristics	Survival
Glioblastoma multiforme	These tumors typically have irregular ring-like contrast enhancement; significant brain edema and the mass effect, which can be severe enough to cause herniation. They typically involve white matter and can spread across the corpus callosum and involve both hemispheres.	12–15 months
Low grade glioma	On MRI, these tumors are usually hypointense on T1-weighted imaging and hyperintense on FLAIR and T2-weighted imaging. These lesions rarely enhance. Cystic changes are not uncommon.	7.3–12.0 years
Meningioma	Adjacent to bone and usually have a "dural tail." This finding indicates that the tumor is anchored to the dura and growing along it. They have a characteristic diffuse pattern of enhancement.	5-year survival 69% 10-year survival 63%
Metastasis	These lesions are usually located in the white-grey matter junction and will avidly enhance contrast.	2.3–7.1 months

PRACTICE POINT

- The sensitivity and specificity of brain imaging studies techniques are not high enough to make the diagnosis, and definitive diagnosis still requires a surgical biopsy or resection to examine the pathology. Generally speaking, more contrast enhancement is observed with-high grade or malignant tumors.

PRACTICE POINT

- Because most primary brain tumors remain localized to the brain, systemic staging is not necessary. However, medulloblastoma, ependymoma, and germ cell tumors may spread via the cerebrospinal fluid pathway. Therefore, MRI of the spine should be performed for these patients to rule out cerebrospinal fluid seeding.

TREATMENT

Surgery

For meningiomas, pituitary adenomas, and vestibular schwannomas surgery is all that is needed. In gliomas, an aggressive resection of the tumor with preservation of the functional area appears to improve prognosis. Biopsy is generally reserved for patients with tumors in the eloquent region of the brain where resection might result in unacceptable neurologic deficit. The goal of surgery in patients with primary CNS lymphoma or germ cell tumors is biopsy only because these tumors are highly responsive to chemotherapy or radiotherapy. Recent advances in surgical technology have facilitated tumor removal with low perioperative morbidity. For example, infiltrative gliomas in the vicinity of functional brain regions can be aggressively removed if the surgery is performed with the patient awake during the operation to map critical regions such as the speech area. Another useful tool is navigation, using preoperative imaging to guide surgery within critical regions and allowing the surgeon to access the tumor safely and accurately. "Brain shift" due to cerebrospinal fluid egress after dural opening may occur and the images are not real-time. Intraoperative MRI provides the surgeon with real-time updated data on tumor volume and location so that he can achieve maximal resection of the brain tumor.

Radiation therapy

Radiotherapy, an important adjunct treatment for many patients with brain tumors, prolongs survival for most. Whereas whole-brain radiation may be administered for certain tumors, such as primary CNS lymphomas and multiple metastases, conformal radiation using multiple field techniques has become the standard of treatment for most patients with glioma. This type of radiation has been as effective and reduces the dose of radiation to normal brain tissue, therefore reducing radiation-related injury.

An important form of focal radiotherapy used to treat many benign and metastatic brain tumors, stereotactic radiosurgery (SRS) delivers a high radiation dose in a single fraction to an image-defined target while minimizing the radiation to the surrounding critical structures. SRS treatment spares normal structures by using conformal dose plans that deposit large radiation doses into the target with a rapid fall off of radiation at the edges of the dose plan. However, SRS seems to be less effective for infiltrative brain tumors. Fractionated stereotactic radiotherapy (SRT) combines the advantages of SRS with the biological benefit of fractionation. These advantages are helpful when treating lesions that are of greater volume (greater than three centimeters) or near vulnerable structures such as the optic nerves.

Chemotherapy

Chemotherapy provides only modest benefit for most patients with brain tumors, but exerts a crucial synergistic effect in combination with surgery and radiation therapy for patients with high-grade glioma. The most commonly used agent is temozolomide, which is an alkylating agent that penetrates the blood-brain barrier. Temozolamide exerts a modest increase in survival for patients with high-grade glioma. It may cause bone marrow suppression. Carmustine-impregnated degradable polymers (Gliadel wafer) placed within the resection cavity have been safe with a modest increase of survival for newly diagnosed high-grade gliomas and recurrent glioblastoma. Nitrosoureas also have modest antitumor activity in patients with oligodendroglioma. Platinum-based regimens have antitumor efficacy for medulloblastomas and germ cell tumors. High-dose methotrexate regimens are the current primary treatment for patients with primary CNS lymphomas. Currently, multiple agents that target different signaling pathways, such as epidermal growth factor receptor inhibitors and angiogenesis inhibitors, are under investigation and show promise in early clinical trials.

IMPORTANCE FOR GENERAL DOCTORS

Corticosteroids, anticonvulsants, and anticoagulants are important medications for the management of patients with brain tumors. Steroids should be started as soon as the diagnosis is made if there is mass effect or edema around the tumor. Corticosteroids are useful for decreasing vasogenic edema, thus controlling increased intracranial pressure. Their long-term use can result in substantial adverse effects. Patients who present with seizures should be treated with anticonvulsants. Anticonvulsants, such as phenytoin and carbamazepine, that induce hepatic cytochrome P-450 enzymes, increase the metabolism of many chemotherapeutic agents. For this reason anticonvulsants that do not induce these enzymes, such as levetiracetam, are generally preferred. It is not necessary to give prophylactic antiepileptic drugs in patients who have never had a seizure

Clinically apparent deep vein thrombosis or pulmonary emboli that require anticoagulation drugs may occur in 20–30% of patients with brain tumors. Conventional therapy with heparin and warfarin is usually effective and well tolerated. Patients receiving anticoagulants that are maintained within the therapeutic range do not appear to have a higher risk of intracranial hemorrhage than those without anticoagulants.

PRACTICE POINT

Management considerations for the internist caring for patients with primary brain tumors

- Steroids should be started as soon as the diagnosis is made if there is mass effect or edema around the tumor.
- It is not necessary to give prophylactic antiepileptic drugs to patients who have never had a seizure.
- Patients receiving anticoagulants that are maintained within the therapeutic range do not appear to have a higher risk of intracranial hemorrhage than those without anticoagulants.

NORMAL PRESSURE HYDROCEPHALUS

Normal pressure hydrocephalus (NPH) is an important cause of gait disturbance and memory loss in the elderly, perhaps involving as many as 5% of patients thought to have Alzheimer disease. It has been classically defined by dementia, gait disturbance, urinary incontinence, and ventricular enlargement.

PRACTICE POINT

Normal pressure hydrocephalus (NPH)

- It is an important cause of gait disturbance and memory loss in the elderly, perhaps involving as many as 5% of patients thought to have Alzheimer disease.
- The gait disturbance has been described as magnetic gait, gait apraxia, or a frontal ataxia.
  - The most characteristic appearance is the patient's feet being "stuck to the floor."
  - Other characteristic findings include short steps, broad-base and decreased stride length and height.
  - Postural instability is also frequently seen and patient may present with frequent falls.
- Improvement in gait usually occurs within 3 months and dementia within 6 months in 60–80% of patients following CSF shunt placement.

NPH is most prevalent in the sixth and seventh decade, although it can be seen at any age. When it occurs secondarily to other conditions such as subarachnoid hemorrhage, traumatic brain injury, and meningitis, this syndrome is referred to as secondary NPH. Otherwise, the term *idiopathic normal pressure hydrocephalus* (INPH) is used to describe the syndrome. Since the clinical presentation and progression of this disorder has great variation, its diagnosis often represents a challenge for clinicians. There is little consensus regarding the selection of patients for shunt implantation although various supplemental tests, including the CSF tap test, external CSF drainage, and measurement of CSF outflow resistance, have been applied to predict surgical response. In general, CSF shunting provides significant symptom improvement in 60–80% of patients with NPH.

CLINICAL PRESENTATION

Normal pressure hydrocephalus is classically described as having three characteristic features: gait disturbance, cognitive dysfunction, and urinary incontinence. There must also be ventricular dilation. Dysfunction of periventricular white matter tracts, particularly those related to frontal lobe connections, has been proposed as the mechanism for these clinical features.

Gait disturbance is the most prominent feature in early stage NPH and the most responsive deficit to a CSF shunting procedure. The gait disturbance has been described as magnetic gait, gait apraxia, or a fontal ataxia. The most characteristic appearance is the patient's feet being "stuck to the floor." Other characteristic findings include short steps, broad-based and decreased stride length, and height. Postural instability is also frequently seen and the patient may present with frequent falls.

The cognitive dysfunction of NPH includes decreased attention, recent memory difficulty and concentration, psychomotor slowing, and apathy. Features such as aphasia, agnosia, and apraxia are less seen in NPH patients.

TREATMENT

The treatment of choice for NPH is CSF shunting, usually from ventricle to peritoneum. Significant clinical improvement can be seen in 60–80% of patients.

The shunt system consists of a proximal catheter (ventricular catheter), a valve, and a distal catheter (can be peritoneal, pleural, or atrial). Many types of valves are available, including differential pressure valves and flow-limiting valves. In the former, the CSF shunting occurs only when the pressure difference across the valve is greater than a certain value. Fixed pressure valves are classified as low (2–5 cm H_2O), medium (5–10 cm H_2O), or high pressure (10–15 cm H_2O). With differential pressure valves there is the possibility of CSF overdrainage when the patient changes position from supine to upright. Therefore, the antisiphon device (ASD) was devised to solve the problem of gravity-dependent drainage. Flow-limiting valves provide a constant CSF flow rate over a range of pressure gradients. There is currently no evidence suggesting one shunt system works better or results in better outcomes than the others.

Recently programmable or adjustable valves have been developed. They have different pressure settings and allow adjustment of the pressure setting transcutaneously. Some of these shunt systems are susceptible to external magnetic fields including MRI and even small magnets. Therefore, patients with programmable shunts should have their shunt reprogrammed as soon as possible after MRI.

IMPORTANCE FOR GENERAL DOCTORS

NPH's triad of dementia, gait disturbance, and urinary incontinence, is an important cause of reversible gait disturbance and dementia in the elderly. The shunt procedure is simple with modest intraoperative and perioperative complications. Improvement in gait usually occurs within three months and dementia within six months. If gait worsening or general drowsiness occurs postoperatively, a head CT scan should be performed. A shunt series of plain X-ray films that visualize the entire shunt system is also helpful to exclude disconnection.

STROKE RELEVANT TO NEUROSURGERY

Cerebrovascular diseases or strokes are common and devastating disorders, causing approximately 200,000 deaths each year in the United States. Most cerebrovascular diseases are characterized by the sudden onset of a focal neurologic deficit. In this overview, we will cover stroke relevant to neurosurgery, including aneurysmal subarachnoid hemorrhage (SAH), intracerebral hemorrhage (ICH), and ischemic stroke. Other neurosurgical vascular topics such as carotid stenosis, cerebrovascular malformation, and moyamoya disease are not covered.

CLINICAL PRESENTATION

Aneurysmal subarachnoid hemorrhage

Many patients with aneurysmal SAH present with an acute onset of severe headache, often described by patients as the "worst headache of my life." Other patients might present with neck stiffness, seizure, and mental status changes. More severe patients may present in a coma or with severe neurologic deficit. The Hunt and Hess Scale is used as a clinical grading scale to describe the severity of SAH and the scale correlates well with long-term outcomes in these patients (**Table 63-2**). The diagnosis is by CT and angiography.

Intracerebral hemorrhage

ICH accounts for 10% of all strokes and the mortality rate is approximately 50%. Symptoms typically begin with sudden headache during activity. Nausea, vomiting, delirium, loss of consciousness, and seizures are also common. CT is diagnostic. Neurologic deficits are usually sudden and progressive. Most ICHs are hypertension-related with the common location in the putamen, thalamus, cerebellum, and brain stem. Large hemorrhages located in the putamen or thalamus may cause hemiparesis due to damage of the adjacent internal capsule. Patients with cerebellar ICH usually develop symptoms over several hours and are characterized by suboccipital headache, nausea, vomiting, and ataxia; they may also have hydrocephalus. Patients with brainstem hemorrhage usually present with coma or severe deficit. Patients with small ICH may present with focal neurologic deficits without a disturbance of consciousness or other features suggestive of increased intracranial pressure.

TREATMENT

Ischemic stroke

Malignant cerebral infarct occurs in a significant number of stroke patients with a high mortality rate due to progressive cerebral edema with herniation and brainstem compression. Decompressive craniectomy may be a life-saving procedure in selected patients when performed early (within 48 hours); especially in young patients (younger than 45), it may lead to satisfactory functional recovery.

TABLE 63-2 Hunt and Hess Scale

Asymptomatic, mild headache, slight nuchal rigidity	1
Moderate to severe headache, nuchal rigidity, no neurologic deficit other than cranial nerve palsy	2
Drowsiness/confusion, mild focal neurologic deficit	3
Stupor, moderate-severe hemiparesis	4
Coma, decerebrate posturing	5

The indication for craniectomy is individualized and should involve extensive discussion with the patient's family.

Subarachnoid hemorrhage (SAH)

Treatment of aneurysmal SAH patients consists of securing the aneurysm, management of vasospasm, hydrocephalus, and other potential medical complications. Microsurgical clipping and endovascular coiling are the two options to secure a ruptured aneurysm in order to prevent rebleeding. Endovascular coiling has been developed as an alternative to surgery and is performed through angiography to pack multiple coils into the aneurysmal dome to exclude it from the cerebral circulation. The International Subarachnoid Aneurysm Trial (ISAT) found that coiling had a more favorable outcome, but with a higher risk of rebleeding. Wide-neck aneurysms (in which the ratio of the neck diameter to that of the largest dome is more than 0.5), middle cerebral artery aneurysms, aneurysms that have normal branches arising from the dome, and giant aneurysms are better treated with surgical clipping as complications from coiling is higher in this group of patients.

Patients with large ICH and severe brain swelling should be surgically treated by hematoma evacuation and/or decompressive craniectomy. Currently, treatment decisions should be individualized.

Intracranial hemorrhage (ICH)

The International Surgical Trial in Intracerebral Hemorrhage (STICH) study included 1033 patients with supratentorial ICH and randomized these patients to either early hematoma evacuation or initial medical management. The result of the study showed that early hematoma evacuation does not improve outcome. However, about 26% of patients in the study failed medical treatment and required surgical evacuation of the hematoma. Recently, minimally invasive endoscopic hematoma evacuation has been performed increasingly and may prove beneficial in future trials.

Cerebellar hemorrhage with a diameter greater than three centimeters will require surgical evacuation as these hematomas usually cause brain stem compression. Without surgical treatment these patients usually deteriorate rapidly and die. Close clinical follow-up in the neurointensive care unit is suggested for alert patients without focal neurologic signs provided that the hematoma is less than three centimeters.

IMPORTANCE FOR GENERAL DOCTORS

Early diagnosis, intervention, and comprehensive neurointensive care can significantly improve outcomes in patients with cerebrovascular diseases. Recognition and proper management of potential medical complications after disease onset is crucial. These include vasospasm, hydrocephalus, seizure, electrolyte imbalance, neurogenic pulmonary edema, cardiac arrhythmia, and hypopituitarism.

TRAUMATIC BRAIN INJURY

Traumatic brain injury (TBI) occurs when an outside force traumatically injures the brain. It is a major cause of death and disability as a result of motor vehicle accidents, falls, or violence. TBI can be classified based on severity (Glasgow Coma Scale), mechanism (penetrating or closed), and other features (focal or diffuse). Diagnosis is suspected clinically and confirmed by imaging studies.

CLINICAL PRESENTATION

Head injuries can be classified as mild, moderate, or severe according to the Glasgow Coma Scale (GCS); GCS 14 or 15 is mild TBI, 9 to 13 is moderate TBI, and 3 to 8 is severe TBI. Patients with mild TBI may have headache, nausea, vomiting, confusion, or amnesia. Most patients with moderate or severe TBI lose consciousness.

DIAGNOSIS

Diagnosis is suspected clinically and confirmed by head CT scan in most cases. The common types of TBI are: concussion, diffuse axonal injury, brain contusions, and intracranial hematomas.

Concussion

Concussion is defined as a transient and reversible alteration in mental status lasting from seconds to less than six hours. Head CT is negative in these patients, although many might suffer from the so-called "postconcussion syndrome" that consists of symptoms such as nausea, headache, dizziness, and memory disturbance.

Diffuse axonal injury

Diffuse axonal injury (DAI) is often defined clinically as a loss of consciousness lasting longer than six hours in the absence of a specific focal lesion. It occurs when deceleration causes shear-type forces that result in diffuse disruption of subcortical axonal fibers. Head CT scan may be negative or may have small petechial hemorrhages in the white matter region. It is also the underlying injury in shaken baby syndrome.

Brain contusions

Contusions can impair a wide range of brain functions depending on their size and location. Their diagnosis is best made with CT. Larger contusions may cause brain edema and increased ICP. Contusions may enlarge, especially within the first days following the initial trauma, and cause neurologic deterioration.

Intracranial hematomas

Intracranial hematomas can occur in patients with TBI and may be epidural, subdural, subarachnoid hemorrhage, or intracerebral. These are usually apparent on head CT scans. Epidural hematomas (EDH) are collections of blood between the skull and dura mater. EDHs that are rapidly expanding are usually caused by arterial bleeding, most commonly due to damage to the middle meningeal artery by a temporal bone fracture. These patients usually require emergent surgical intervention.

Subdural hematomas (SDH) are hemorrhages between the dura mater and the pia-arachnoid mater. Acute subdural hematomas arise from tearing of the cortical vein or the bridging veins between the cortex and dural sinuses. These hematomas usually cause significant brain compression and elevated ICP. When these processes occur, mortality and morbidity are high even with aggressive surgical measures. As mentioned previously, chronic subdural hematomas produce symptoms gradually over several weeks or months after trauma and occur more often in elderly patients. In contrast to its acute counterpart, edema and increased ICP are unusual.

Intracerebral hematomas are hemorrhages within the brain parenchyma. They often result from contusion hemorrhage. Increased ICP, herniation, and brain stem compression can develop, particularly with temporal contusions.

Head CT is usually the initial imaging of choice in patients with TBI and should always be done in patients with more than transiently impaired consciousness, GCS score less than 15, focal neurologic deficit, persistent vomiting, seizures, a history of loss of consciousness, or clinically suspected fractures. On CT scan, contusions and acute bleeding appear hyper-dense compared with normal brain parenchyma. EDH classically appears as lenticular-shaped opacities often in the territory of the middle meningeal artery while SDH classically appear as crescent-shaped opacities overlying brain tissue. A chronic subdural hematoma appears hypodense compared with brain tissue, whereas a subacute subdural hematoma may be isodense in character. It is important to recognize the signs of mass effect and herniation on head CT scans because these patients usually require emergent surgical intervention. These signs include sulcal effacement, ventricular and cisternal compression, and significant midline shift (greater than five millimeters).

MRI may be useful later in the clinical course to detect more subtle contusions and DAI. It is usually more sensitive than CT for the diagnosis of very small acute or isodense subacute and isodense chronic subdural hematomas.

TREATMENT

Medical management

About 80% of TBIs are mild. Patients who have had loss of consciousness or have any abnormalities in mental or neurologic function and cannot be observed closely after discharge are generally observed in the emergency department or overnight in the hospital and follow-up CT is done in six hours. Patients who have no neurologic deficit but minor abnormalities on the head CT may need only a follow-up CT within 24 hours. With a stable CT and normal neurologic examination results, these patients may be discharged home.

Injury is severe in 10% of patients who have TBI and often require emergent intubation and mechanical ventilation, measures to control elevated ICP, and many require emergent neurosurgical intervention. For intractable increased ICP, consider CSF drainage, temporary hyperventilation (target $PaCO_2$ of 30 to 35 mm Hg), pentobarbital coma, or decompressive craniotomy. Subsequent management consists of adequate ventilation, oxygenation, and brain perfusion to avoid secondary brain injury. Current treatment protocols suggest that the cerebral perfusion pressure (CPP) value to target lies within the range of 50–70 mm Hg. Hypotonic fluids (for example 5% D/W) are detrimental because they contain excess free water that can worsen brain edema and elevated ICP. Other potential medical complications to be aware of include hyponatremia, hyperglycemia, seizure, and infection. Close neurologic monitoring using the GCS and pupillary response or ICP monitor should continue, and CT scan is repeated, particularly if there is an unexplained ICP rise.

Surgery

Intracranial hematomas may require urgent surgical evacuation to prevent or treat brain shift, compression, and herniation. However, patients with parenchymal mass lesions who do not show evidence for neurologic compromise, have controlled ICP, and no significant signs of mass effect on CT scan may be managed nonoperatively with intensive monitoring and serial imaging. Patients with small SDH can often be treated without surgery. Factors that suggest a need for surgery include a midline brain shift greater than five millimeters, compression of the basal cisterns, and worsening neurologic examination. Chronic subdural hematomas may require surgical drainage but much less urgently than acute SDH. Large or arterial EDHs are treated surgically, but small EDHs that are thought to be venous in origin can be followed with serial CT scans.

IMPORTANCE FOR GENERAL DOCTORS

Initial management of TBI patients consists of maintenance of adequate ventilation, oxygenation, circulation, and brain perfusion to avoid secondary brain injury. Early neurosurgical consultation is mandatory since many moderate or severe TBI patients may benefit from emergent surgical intervention.

Patients should be kept in euvolemic and normosmolar conditions since many measures to control ICP will disturb fluid balance. Osmotic agents, such as mannitol or glycerol, may be given to lower ICP and maintain serum osmolality. Finally, decompressive craniotomy can be considered for patients with refractory-increased ICP. This procedure is done by removing bone flap with duraplasty to allow the swollen brain to expand outward (rather than inward and compressing the brain). In patients with significant contusion, SDH, depressed skull fracture, or a GCS score < 10, prophylactic anticonvulsant should be administered. Serum levels should be measured to adjust the dose. If no seizures develop within one week, anticonvulsants should be stopped since their value in preventing late-onset seizures is not well established.

TRAUMATIC SPINAL CORD INJURY

Traumatic spinal cord injury (TSCI) is a serious problem that mostly affects young adults as a result of motor vehicle accidents, falls, or violence. Most TSCI occurs with mechanical injury to the vertebral column causing fracture, dislocation, ligament injury, disruption or herniation of the intervertebral disc, which in turn cause compression of the spinal cord with secondary injuries resulting from ischemic, inflammatory, and other mechanisms. Despite recent advances in the understanding of the pathophysiology, it remains a devastating condition with high morbidity.

CLINICAL PRESENTATION

Most patients present with pain at the site of the spinal injury. However, a majority of these patients have associated traumatic brain and systemic injuries that might obscure the patient's symptoms. Therefore, it is important for physicians to exclude TSCI in these patients since early diagnosis of the potentially reversible condition affects prognosis. About half of TSCIs involve the cervical cord and as a result present with motor deficit. The severity of cord syndromes are classified using the American Spinal Injury Association (ASIA) scale or the Frankel scale. In **complete TSCI** (ASIA grade A), sensation above the injured level is intact (ie, the C5 and higher dermatomes are spared in a C5–6 dislocation) and there will be no sensation in levels below. Similarly, there will be reduced muscle power in the level immediately below the injury. In the acute stage, reflexes are absent, there is no response to plantar stimulation, and muscle tone is flaccid. Urinary retention and/or priapism might be present and the bulbo-cavernosus reflex is usually absent.

In contrast, various degrees of sensory or motor function are preserved below the level of injury in **incomplete TSCI** (ASIA grades B through D). Sensation is preserved to a greater extent than motor function in most cases since the sensory tracts are located in more peripheral, less vulnerable areas of the cord. The anal sensation and bulbo-cavernosus reflex are preserved in most cases.

Common and clinically relevant syndromes of TSCI include central cord syndrome, anterior cord syndrome, and spinal shock.

Central cord syndrome is the most common type of TSCI with a fairly optimistic prognosis. This syndrome most often occurs in elderly patient with preexisting cervical stenosis or spondylosis after mild hyperextension injury. It is characterized by greater motor impairment in upper extremities compared with lower extremities, bladder dysfunction, and a variable degree of sensory loss below the level of injury.

Anterior cord syndrome is a condition in which the blood supply to the anterior or ventral two-thirds portion of the cord is interrupted. This more often represents a direct injury to the anterior spinal cord by prolapsed disc or bony fragments rather than direct vascular injury of the anterior spinal artery.

Spinal shock is defined as motor paralysis, loss of sensation, and absent bowel and bladder control, with initial loss but gradual recovery of spinal reflexes. This condition is often seen in patients with complete TSCI. Cervical TSCI can cause total loss of sympathetic innervations and patient might present with bradycardia and hypotension. Spinal shock may last several hours to several weeks.

Autonomic dysreflexia is caused by uninhibited sympathetic inhibition in patients with TSCI above T6. Patients might have extreme high blood pressure, headaches, profuse sweating, facial erythema, and urinary retention.

DIAGNOSIS

When the previously mentioned clinical manifestations are present and TSCI is suspected, imaging studies will help us to assess the severity and extent of the injury. Plain X-rays provide a rapid assessment of alignment and fractures. In the cervical spine, all cervical vertebrae and the top of T1 must be visualized. In muscular males with a cervical injury, pulling the shoulders down by pulling down on the wrists in a straight line and downward toward the feet may better allow visualization of the lower cervical vertebrae. A swimmer's view should be performed if the lower cervical levels and the top of T1 are not adequately visualized. Neurologic signs and symptoms of cervical spine injury in the setting of normal plain X-rays warrant further imaging studies such as CT or MRI.

CT with sagittal and coronal reconstructions may replace a plain X-ray for assessment when it is readily available since it has higher sensitivity for detecting spinal fracture when compared with plain X-rays. It also has advantages over X-rays in assessment of spinal canal patency. This is often the exam of choice (a cervical CT) when a head CT scan is required to rule out traumatic brain injury.

MRI provides a detailed study of the spinal cord as well as spinal ligaments, intervertebral discs, and paraspinal soft tissues. Its ability to assess bony injury is not superior to CT, however. MRI can provide valuable information regarding the extent and mechanism of TSCI, which can influence treatment and prognosis. It is also recommended in TSCI patients with a negative CT scan in order to detect occult ligamentous or disc injury or epidural hematoma.

TREATMENT

Methylprednisolone is the only treatment that has been suggested in clinical trials to improve outcomes in patients with acute, nonpenetrating TSCI. However, the evidence is limited, and its use is debated. The American Association of Neurological Surgeons and Congress of Neurological Surgeons concluded that the use of steroids in acute TSCI is recommended as a treatment option. The standard dose is 30 mg/kg IV bolus, followed by an infusion of 5.4 mg/kg per hour for 23 hours. Management of hyperglycemia and prophylactic treatment of peptic ulcer are important management considerations in patients receiving steroid treatment.

Patients with TSCI require urgent neurosurgical consultation to assess the necessity of decompression and stabilization. Currently there is no standard guideline regarding the role, timing, and method of decompression and stabilization in acute TSCIs. For cervical fracture with subluxation or dislocation, closed reduction methods are a treatment option. Since there are no evidence-based guidelines regarding the indications for or timing of surgery, surgery depends on a surgeon's experience and practice norms of the institute. Surgery may be considered for neural decompression, spinal stabilization, and reduction of dislocations. Neurologically intact patients with cervical SCI are not treated operatively unless there is significant spinal instability. Surgical indications for closed thoracolumbar fractures are more equivocal due to the difficulties defining spinal instability in these cases. The Thoracolumbar Injury Severity Score has been applied as a scoring system composed of three variables: the morphology of the injury, the integrity of the posterior ligamentous complex, and the neurological status of the patient (**Table 63-3**). A total score of less than four indicates a non-operative injury; more than, an operative injury. Patients with a score

TABLE 63-3 Thoracolumbar Injury Severity Score

Parameter	Points
Morphology	
Compression fracture	1
Burst fracture	2
Translational/rotational	3
Distraction	4
Neurologic involvement	
Intact	0
Nerve root	2
Cord, conus medullaris	
Incomplete	3
Complete	2
Cauda equina	3
Posterior ligamentous complex	
Intact	0
Injury suspected/indeterminate	2
Injured	3

of four have an injury that is operative at the surgeon's discretion. However, the efficacy of this algorithm remains to be prospectively evaluated.

The timing of surgical intervention is also controversial. In contrast to early concepts in which patients are usually managed by delayed surgery (more than five days) due to the assumed higher medical complication rate in patients with early surgery (within 72 hours), more contemporary studies suggest that medical complication rates are actually lower in patients who undergo early surgery, which allows for earlier mobilization and reduced intensive care unit and length of hospital stay. A systematic review analyzed published data regarding the timing of surgical decompression and concluded that early decompression, within 72 hours, can be performed safely without increasing systemic complications. However, an impact on neurologic recovery of early surgery could not be determined from the currently available literature. At this time, most surgeons consider neurologic deterioration after incomplete TSCI to be an indication for early surgery if there is no contraindication. The role of early surgery with a complete TSC is debatable given the overall ominous prognosis of these patients. While some operate for spinal stabilization in the early stage, most defer the surgery to a later stage.

IMPORTANCE FOR GENERAL DOCTORS

When TSCI is suspected thorough evaluation should be done as soon as possible. These include assessment of TSCI per se and associated injury, the necessity of traction reduction or surgical intervention, and the risk-benefit evaluation for the use of megadose methylprednisolone. When intubation is attempted in patients with cervical spinal cord injury, consider consultation of the anesthesiologist for a fiberoptic intubation, done with the patient awake to reduce any further cord injury that potentially could be caused by a regular intubation with neck movement and extension.

Patients with acute TSCI require admission to an intensive care unit for monitoring and treatment of potential life-threatening complications, including cardiovascular instability and respiratory failure. Patients should receive prophylaxis to protect against deep venous thrombosis and pulmonary embolism. Other long-term complications include pressure sore and respiratory or urinary tract infection.

Recognition of autonomic dysreflexia is important since this is a potential life-threatening condition that might occur in hospitalized patients. Treatment consists of antihypertensive treatment and immediate determination and removal of the triggering stimuli, for example, bladder catheterization in case of urinary retention. The condition can become chronic and recurrent. Long-term medical therapy may include alpha- or calcium channel blockers in these cases.

DISC HERNIATION

Spinal disc herniation occurs when there is a tear in the outer ring (annulus fibrosis) of an intervertebral disc with bulging out of the central content called nucleus pulposus. The bulging disc is usually posterolateral in position. Spinal disc herniations mostly occur in patients in their 30s or 40s when the nucleus pulposus is still a gelatin-like substance. Dehydration of the nucleus pulposus occurs with aging and greatly reduces the risk of herniation.

Spinal disc herniation is a common disease entity and can occur in any disc in the spine. Since lumbar and cervical disc herniations are the two most common types, we will be focusing on the clinical presentation and treatment of these two entities.

CLINICAL PRESENTATION

Clinical presentation of a herniated disc can vary depending on the location of the herniation and can range from little or no pain to severe and unrelenting neck or low back pain that will radiate into the regions served by compressed nerve roots. The most common cervical disc herniations occur between the C5/6 and the C6/7. The herniated disc may cause compression of the cord (causing myelopathy) or the nerve root (causing radiculopathy). Symptoms can affect the neck, shoulder girdle, scapula, shoulder, arm, and hand.

The most common levels for a lumbar herniated disc are L4–5 and L5-S1. The onset of symptoms is characterized by a sharp, burning, stabbing pain radiating down the posterior or lateral aspect of the leg to below the knee. Pain is generally superficial and localized, and is often associated with numbness or tingling. In more advanced cases, motor deficit, diminished reflexes, or weakness may occur. Generally, only the relatively uncommon central disc herniation provokes low back pain and saddle pain in the S1 and S2 distributions. A central herniated disc may also compress nerve roots of the cauda equina, resulting in difficult urination, incontinence, or impotence. This is the so-called "cauda equina syndrome" and emergency surgery to prevent permanent loss of function is indicated.

DIAGNOSIS

Diagnosis is made based on the history, symptoms, and physical examination. Motor, sensory, and reflex function should be assessed to determine the affected nerve root level. Examination of the cervical or lumbar spine by neurologic levels is helpful in locating the source of the patient's symptoms.

Nerve root tension signs are often used in the evaluation of patients suspected of having a herniated disc. In patients with cervical disc herniation, pain is exacerbated by neck extension and rotation or by the Spurling maneuver (patient's neck is extended, laterally bent, and held down) designed to elicit radicular symptoms. In the lumbar disc herniation, the straight-leg raising test is performed with the patient in the supine position. The physician raises the patient's leg. Normally, this position results in only minor tightness in the hamstrings. If nerve root compression is present, this test causes severe pain in the back of the affected leg and can reveal a disorder of the L5 or S1 nerve root. In some cases, when clinical diagnosis and localization is obscure, electromyogram and nerve conduction velocity (EMG/NCV) studies might provide more information. These studies measure the electrical impulse along nerve roots, peripheral nerves, and muscle tissue and may differentiate radiculopathy from myopathy and neuropathy.

Imaging studies provide valuable information that supports the diagnosis of disc herniation. Plain X-rays and CT have limited value. The gold standard imaging study for herniated disc is MR. It has the ability to demonstrate the severity of intervertebral disc damage, including annular tears and end plates destruction. As with all imaging studies, MRI can reveal degenerative and bulging discs in asymptomatic persons. Therefore, treatment decisions should be based on the clinical assessment with diagnostic test correlation.

TREATMENT

The majority of patients with herniated discs will improve in six weeks and do not require surgery. One study found that "after 12 weeks, 73% of patients showed reasonable to major improvement without surgery."[1]

Analgesics are often prescribed to alleviate the acute pain and allow the patient to begin exercising and stretching. Nonsteroidal anti-inflammatory medication is usually the first-line agent, but their long-term usage for patients with persistent pain is complicated by their possible adverse effects. Oral steroids may be useful in some cases. An alternative measure is epidural steroid injection. This technique, however, is now considered limited to short-term pain relief in selected patients only and in certain settings may result in serious complications. Rehabilitation, physical therapy, antidepressants, and exercise programs may all be useful adjuncts.

SURGERY

While most patients with a herniated disc may be effectively treated conservatively, some do not respond to conservative treatment or have symptoms that necessitate referral to a specialist. Any surgical decision should be firmly based on the clinical symptoms and corroborating results of diagnostic testing. Indications for referral include the following: (1) cauda equina syndrome, (2) progressive neurologic deficit, (3) profound neurologic deficit, and (4) severe and disabling pain refractory after four to six weeks of conservative treatment.

PRACTICE POINT

Indications for referral to a neurosurgeon for a herniated disc

- Cauda equina syndrome
- Progressive neurologic deficit
- Profound neurologic deficit
- Severe and disabling pain refractory to four to six weeks of conservative treatment.

Surgical results are satisfactory in approximately 75% to 95% of patients. The goals of surgery include relief of nerve compression allowing the neurologic recovery and relief of pain. For lumbar disc herniation, these goals could be achieved through microsurgical discectomy, open discectomy, and various minimally invasive techniques. Minimally invasive techniques include percutaneous manual nucleotomy, automated percutaneous lumbar discectomy, laser discectomy, endoscopic discectomy, microendoscopic discectomy, and nucleoplasty. These techniques involve smaller incisions and surgery with the aid of indirect visualization; they have the theoretical advantage of faster recovery and less pain compared to standard discectomy. Although all the minimally invasive techniques have been reported to yield high success rates, to date no studies have demonstrated any of these to be superior to microsurgical discectomy. Therefore microsurgical discectomy continues to be regarded as the standard. The primary surgical procedure may be combined with lumbar fusion surgery in selected cases. Anterior cervical discectomy and fusion is a common procedure performed in patients with cervical disc herniation. The disc removed in the lumbar or cervical region is frequently replaced by an artificial disc.

IMPORTANCE FOR GENERAL DOCTORS

Degeneration of the intervertebral disc from a combination of factors can result in herniation, especially in the lumbar and cervical regions. The presence of pain, myelopathy, radiculopathy, and other symptoms depends on the site and degree of herniation. A detailed history and neurologic examination, supplemented by MRI, can differentiate a herniated disc from another disease entity. Most patients recover within four weeks of symptom onset. Many treatment modalities have been suggested for disc herniation, but studies often provide conflicting results. Initial screening for serious pathology and close follow-up for complications, including neurologic defects or refractory pain are essential in the management of disc herniation.

SUGGESTED READINGS

Bratton SL, Chestnut RM, Ghajar J, et al. Guidelines for the management of severe traumatic brain injury. IX. Cerebral perfusion thresholds. *J Neurotrauma.* 2007;24 (Suppl 1):S59–64.

Gerber DE, Grossman SA, Streiff MB. Management of venous thromboembolism in patients with primary and metastatic brain tumors. *J Clin Oncol.* 2006;24:1310–1318.

Glantz MJ, Cole BF, Forsyth PA, et al. Practice parameter: anticonvulsant prophylaxis in patients with newly diagnosed brain tumors. Report of the Quality Standards Subcommittee of the American Academy of Neurology. *Neurology.* 2000;54:1886–1893.

Johnston SC, Higashida RT, Barrow DL, et al. Recommendations for the endovascular treatment of intracranial aneurysms: a statement for health care professionals from the Committee on Cerebrovascular Imaging of the American Heart Association Council on Cardiovascular Radiology. *Stroke.* 2002;33:2536–2544.

Saatman KE, Duhaime AC, Bullock R, Maas AI, Valadka A, Manley GT. Classification of traumatic brain injury for targeted therapies. *J Neurotrauma.* 2008;25:719–738.

Suarez JI, Tarr RW, Selman WR. Aneurysmal subarachnoid hemorrhage. *N Engl J Med.* 2006;354:387–396.

Teasdale G, Jennett B. Assessment of coma and impaired consciousness. A practical scale. *Lancet.* 1074;2:81–84.

Wijdicks EF, Kallmes DF, Manno EM, Fulgham JR, Piepgras DG. Subarachnoid hemorrhage: neurointensive care and aneurysm repair. *Mayo Clin Proc.* 2005;80:550–559.

Zink BJ. Traumatic brain injury outcome: concepts for emergency care. *Ann Emerg Med.* 2001;37:318–332.

REFERENCE

1. Vroomen PC, de Krom MC, Knottnerus JA. Predicting the outcome of sciatica at short-term follow-up. *Br J Gen Pract.* 2002;52: 119–123.

CHAPTER 64

Common Complications in Neurosurgery

Khalid Medani, MD
Abel Po-Hao Huang, MD
Peter M. Black, MD, PhD

INTRODUCTION

Regional complications, such as hemorrhage, infection, and hydrocephalus, or systemic complications, including deep vein thrombosis and septicemia, may follow neurosurgical procedures. Significant morbidity and mortality can result from delaying the diagnosis of these complications or deferring their management. Hospitalists need to be familiar with the most frequently encountered postoperative complications so that they can take immediate and appropriate actions to improve outcomes.

POSTOPERATIVE HEMORRHAGE

The incidence of postoperative hemorrhage in a survey of 4992 intracranial procedures done in 1988 was estimated to be 0.8%. Of these, intracerebral hemorrhage accounted for 60%, epidural hemorrhage 28%, subdural hemorrhage 7.5%, and intrasellar hemorrhage 5%. In a series of 1771 craniotomies, the incidence of postoperative hematomas requiring surgery was estimated to be 1.4%. Among these 0.7% were epidural, 0.2% subdural, and 0.5% were hemorrhages in the tumor bed. The later type of hemorrhage was fatal in two cases.

Early postoperative hemorrhage from whatever cause usually presents with drowsiness, focal neurologic deficit, or seizure. It can be diagnosed by an urgent CT and often necessitates immediate return to the operating room (OR). Late hemorrhage may be intraparenchymal or subdural at the procedure site or at a remote location. In traumatic brain injury (TBI), coalescence of multiple contusions and small hematomas may form a large hematoma that causes additional mass effect requiring immediate intervention.

PRACTICE POINT

Early postoperative hemorrhage from whatever cause usually presents with drowsiness, focal neurologic deficit, or seizure.

Late hemorrhage may be intraparenchymal or subdural at the procedure site or at a remote location.

- An intracerebral hemorrhage typically occurs in the bed of a resected tumor. The patient usually presents with symptoms and signs of increased ICP including headache, nausea, vomiting, and alteration in consciousness level. The clinical picture also may be variable according to the site of the hematoma.
- The suspicion of postoperative SDH should be raised when a patient develops neurologic deterioration while in the recovery room or in the intensive care unit.
- Ventricular hemorrhage due to continued ooze of blood into the ventricles may cause headache, vomiting, confusion, and alteration of the consciousness level depending on the severity of the hemorrhage. External ventricular drainage should be considered.

In traumatic brain injury (TBI), coalescence of multiple contusions and small hematomas may form a large hematoma that causes additional mass effect requiring immediate intervention.

Low platelet count, platelet dysfunction, and deficiency of clotting factors as in liver diseases may contribute to postoperative hemorrhage. Severe TBI patients should be screened for coagulopathy because of risk of disseminated intravascular coagulation (DIC) from tissue destruction and release of cerebral thromboplastin. Massive blood transfusion also can cause significant hemolysis, which impedes hemostasis. Hemorrhages are discussed below according to their sites.

SUBGALEAL HEMATOMA

Uncontrolled oozing from the main scalp arteries and deep muscles may cause subgaleal hematoma. Presenting as a soft fluctuant mass beneath the scalp, it usually does not require anything more than observation and resolves spontaneously. Rarely, if the hematoma is massive, neurosurgeons perform aseptic aspiration to avoid wound dehiscence.

EPIDURAL HEMATOMA

The evolution of epidural hematoma (EDH) is most commonly from bleeding, usually arterial, originating from epidural arteries or veins. Indications for surgery include increasing size or symptoms. Alteration of mental status is the most important symptom and an alarm signal to suspect postoperative EDH. The patient may become obtunded, develop contralateral hemiparesis, and contralateral pupillary dilation. An immediate CT scan without contrast confirms the diagnosis. In this setting, the patient should be taken immediately to the operating room for surgical evacuation of the hematoma and control of the bleeding.

SUBDURAL HEMATOMA

The incidence of postoperative subdural hematoma (SDH) may be reduced with the use of subdural drains. SDH following craniotomy is usually detected incidentally with a CT scan early in the postoperative period. If sufficient mass effect develops from the hematoma, clinical signs may follow within the next few hours. However, the suspicion of postoperative SDH should be raised when a patient develops neurologic deterioration while in the recovery room or in the intensive care unit. Immediate CT scan imaging should guide reoperation.

Asymptomatic patients with postoperative SDH without significant mass effect can be followed clinically and radiologically with the expectation that it will disappear. Rarely, it evolves into chronic SDH.

Patients with a ventricular shunt may develop a subdural hematoma with low pressure. The overall incidence of this type of SDH in adults is 4–23%. The subdural collection can be either ipsilateral to the shunt (32%), on the opposite site (21%), or bilateral (46%). If a nonprogrammable valve was used, it can be replaced with a higher-pressure unit. In nonshunt-dependent cases, the valve can be adjusted, replaced, removed, or temporarily tied. Insertion of an antisiphon device can be also considered.

PARENCHYMAL HEMATOMA

An intracerebral hemorrhage typically occurs in the bed of a resected tumor. The patient usually presents with symptoms and signs of increased intracranial pressure (ICP) including headache, nausea, vomiting, and alteration in consciousness level. The clinical picture also may be variable according to the site of the hematoma. CT scan is required for the diagnosis. The hematoma size on CT scan and presence of mass effect in addition to the clinical signs determine whether the hematoma is significant. If significant, reexploration with effort to secure hemostasis is required. The hematoma will increase its mass effect over hours to days after it is initially detected.

VENTRICULAR HEMORRHAGE

Ventricular hemorrhage due to continued ooze of blood into the ventricles may cause headache, vomiting, confusion, and alteration of the consciousness level depending on the severity of the hemorrhage. External ventricular drainage should be considered.

POSTOPERATIVE INFECTION

Infection is a potentially problematic postoperative complication. The incidence of postoperative infection is 0.8–7.0% with the use of antibacterial prophylaxis. Without prophylaxis, the incidence is higher. Cephalosporins are currently the preferred antibiotics used for prophylaxis when skin flora (*staphylococci*) are the likeliest pathogens. Vancomycin is an alternative. In 0.5% of postoperative infection cases, craniotomy is necessary to treat the infection. Presenting symptoms and their frequency in postoperative infection are summarized in **Table 64-1**.

Postoperative infections can include an infected intracranial device, meningitis, cranial osteomyelitis, brain abscess, subdural empyema, or local wound infection. The causative agents, clinical features, and appropriate management are discussed below for each type.

INFECTION OF INTRACRANIAL DEVICE (SHUNT INFECTION)

Shunt infection can be early or late onset. Early shunt infection occurs no later than six months following the device placement. The incidence of early and late infection per procedure is 7% and 6% respectively. *Staphylococci* are the most common pathogens involved in device infection. The most common route for an early infection is seeding of the device during the operative period. *S epidermidis* has been estimated to be the culprit in 60–75% of cases. This is followed by *S aureus* and gram-negative Bacilli. The latter contribute to 6–20% of causes. Late infection occurs almost always due to *S epidermidis or propionobacter*. It usually occurs due to indolent infection. Rarely, it results from seeding of a vascular shunt during a septicemic episode or colonization during an episode of meningitis.

Clinical features of shunt infection include nonspecific symptoms such as headache, lethargy, and intermittent fever. Meningeal symptoms are often not seen. Shunt dysfunction can also occur, and approximately 29% of patients presenting with shunt dysfunction are found to have positive cultures.

Diagnosis of shunt infection cannot be made on clinical features alone, and definitive diagnosis is made by culture of Cerebrospinal fluid (CSF) either through lumbar puncture or shunt tap. Blood workup will reveal total WBCs above 20,000/mm^3 in 30% of patients and increased Erythrosedimentation rate (ESR). Blood culture is positive in less than 33% of patients. CSF analyses reveal a WBC count usually less than 100 cells/mm^3. Gram stain is positive in only 50% of CSF samples, and CSF culture is positive in 60% of

TABLE 64-1 Presenting Symptoms and Their Frequency in Postoperative Infection

Symptom	Percentage
Fever	22%
Purulent discharge	17%
Changing mental status	18%
Headache	10%
Swelling	7%
Seizure	2%

cases. Head CT scan usually is not helpful, although ependymal enhancement may indicate ventriculitis. Abdominal ultrasound or CT may show a pseudocyst. Treatment of device infection with an antibacterial alone usually has a low success rate, and should be continued for 45 days. Shunt removal in addition to EVD is the preferred management. The removed device should also be cultured.

Intravenous vancomycin that covers both *S aureus* and *S epidermidis* is initially prescribed. CSF penetration of vancomycin results in a concentration of 18% that of the serum. Oral rifampin may be added to increase the coverage. Intraventricular antibiotic injection can be used adjuvant to intravenous therapy. Treatment for specific organisms includes intravenous nafcillin or cefazolin for methicillin-sensitive *Staphylococci*. Intravenous vancomycin plus oral rifampin and trimethoprim is preferred for *Multiple Resistant Staph Aureus* (MRSA). For *Enterococci*, *Corynebacterium*, and *Propionibacterium* species, intravenous ampicillin is preferred. Aerobic gram-negative rods are treated based on susceptibilities. If CSF cultures remain negative for three days, antibiotics should be continued for an additional 10–14 days, and then a new shunt can be replaced.

PRACTICE POINT

Shunt infection

- Clinical features of shunt infection include nonspecific symptoms such as headache, lethargy, and intermittent fever. Meningeal symptoms are often not seen. Shunt dysfunction can also occur, and approximately 29% of patients presenting with shunt dysfunction are found to have positive cultures.
- Diagnosis of shunt infection cannot be made on clinical features alone, and definitive diagnosis is made by culture of CSF either through lumbar puncture or shunt tap.

Postoperative meningitis

- Symptoms usually begin several days postoperatively and are indistinguishable from chemical meningitis. They include fever, meningismus, nausea, vomiting, and altered mental status.

Cerebral abscess

- Clinical symptoms are nonspecific for abscess and most are due to increased intracranial pressure from edema surrounding the lesion.
- Because of risk of transtentorial herniation, LP should be avoided.

Subdural empyema

- A collection of pus under the dura is a neurosurgical emergency. Rapidly spreading infection can lead to herniation and death.

Wound infections

- Readily observable and diagnosable, wound infections usually do not manifest before the second postoperative day, and they might not be detected for days or weeks following surgery.

POSTSURGICAL MENINGITIS

The incidence of meningitis following neurosurgical operations is 0.5–0.7% in clean procedures and 0.4–2% in contaminated procedures (eg, cerebral abscess, subdural empyema). Prophylactic antibiotics decrease the rate of postsurgical meningitis.

This complication can result from contamination during procedure (most common), skin breakdown, or hematogenous seeding. *S aureus* is the most common organism. Respiratory tract *flora* can occur in the sinus entry. Other pathogens include: *Enterobacteriaceae*, *Pseudomonas*, and *pneumococci*. Symptoms usually begin several days postoperatively. They include fever, meningismus, nausea, vomiting, and altered mental status. However, the same clinical feature can be found in chemical meningitis, which is more common. Posterior fossa surgery may lead to chemical meningitis due to irritation from blood breakdown when introduced into the subarachnoid space and also from the use of dural substitutes. It is characterized by CSF pleocytosis without positive cultures.

Because of the difficulty in confirming the diagnosis of postoperative bacterial meningitis and risk of serious morbidity and mortality from delay in therapy, the recommended approach is to start broad-spectrum antibiotic therapy for all patients who have symptoms suggesting bacterial meningitis. CSF should be obtained for culture before antibiotics are initiated. Intravenous vancomycin and ceftazidime should be started empirically. Gentamicin is added for pseudomonas. If the CSF culture remains negative and CSF WBC counts and chemistries do not suggest infection, then antibiotics can be stopped and steroids should be begun for presumed chemical meningitis.

CRANIAL OSTEOMYELITIS

Rarely, cranial osteomyelitis may follow cranial surgery because the skull is usually very resistant to osteomyelitis. It can also occur due to contagious spread from otitis media or sinusitis. Common pathogens include *S aureus* (the most common) and *S epidermidis*. Gram-negative organisms can also be involved in cases following sinusitis or otitis.

Patients may complain of pain, swelling, and local tenderness. If patients are febrile, underlying pus or subdural empyema may be present. Total white cell count and ESR are frequently normal.

The earliest manifestation of the infection on the skull x-ray is soft tissue swelling, which usually occurs 3–5 days after infection. Bony changes may become apparent after 7–10 days as spotty areas of demineralization interspersed with areas of normal bone. A CT scan is more useful in determining the extent of the disease and may show bony changes earlier than the plain film. MRI has limited use in diagnosing skull osteomyelitis but can demonstrate soft tissue changes adjacent to osteomyelitic foci. Radionucleotide bone scan with gallium-67 is a very sensitive test and considered the initial imaging modality of choice. A negative gallium-67 scan indicates cure of cranial osteomyelitis.

Treatment is surgical debridement of infected skull, excision of the involved bone or the alloplastic plate, and closure of the scalp without cranioplasty. This should be followed by aggressive antibacterial therapy intravenously for 1–2 weeks and then orally for 6–12 weeks. Most treatment failures are due to treatment less than four weeks. Until *MRSA* is ruled out, vancomycin and a third generation cephalosporin are the most preferred antibiotics. Cranioplasty can be done if there are no signs of infection for more than six months after the surgical debridement.

BRAIN ABSCESS

Postoperative cerebral abscess can result from different mechanisms: contagious spread from a suppurative focus, spread following cranial surgery or trauma through a dural break, hematogenous spread, or cryptogenic abscess with no primary source found. The most common mechanism is the contagious spread from otitis media or frontal sinusitis via a direct extension from osteomyelitis or emissary veins. Pathogens usually correlate with the primary source. In otitis media and mastoiditis, organisms are usually: *Streptococci*, *Bacteroides*, and *Enterobacteriaceae*. The later usually occur in mixed cultures. Following head injury, *Staphylococci* are the most common organisms, followed by *Streptococci*, mixed *Enterobacteriaceae*, and *Clostridia*. *S epidermidis* and *S aureus* are by far the most common pathogens following neurosurgical procedures.

Clinical symptoms are nonspecific for abscess and most are due to increased intracranial pressure from edema surrounding the lesion. These include headache, nausea, vomiting, and alteration of mental status. Fever only occurs in 50% of patients. Hemiparesis and seizure develop in 30–50% of cases. Nuchal rigidity and other focal symptoms can be present according to the location of the abscess. Blood work is usually not helpful in the diagnosis of brain abscess. The total white cell count is usually normal or mildly elevated in 60–70% of cases. ESR may be also normal and blood cultures are usually negative. CT scan is very sensitive for the diagnosis, but usually nonspecific. Diffusion-weighted MRI is the best diagnostic tool and is very helpful in differentiating cerebral abscess from necrotic tumor. MRI spectroscopy is also diagnostic for abscess when it shows elevated amino acids and acetate or lactate peaks. CSF sampling demonstrates an infectious pattern in only 50% of cases, and because of risk of transtentorial herniation LP should be avoided.

Treatment of cerebral abscesses is usually a combination of both medical and surgical approaches. Antibiotics alone are given for asymptomatic patients or apparent cerebritis. Surgical management consists of aspiration under CT guidance, or craniotomy for complete excision of the abscess. Initial antibiotic regimen consists of vancomycin in addition to a third-generation cephalosporin (eg, ceftriaxone or cefotaxime) and metronidazole (to cover *Bacteroides*). If *MRSA* has been ruled out in culture, vancomycin can be substituted with nafcillin. Parenteral therapy should continue for 4–6 weeks, often followed by prolonged oral therapy.

SUBDURAL EMPYEMA

This is the collection of pus under the dura and is a neurosurgical emergency. Rapidly spreading infection can lead to herniation and death. In most cases the source is an infection in the paranasal sinuses, middle ear, or mastoid air cells. Other sources include extension from cranial osteomyelitis, cranial trauma, surgical procedures, or infection of a subdural hematoma. Polymicrobial pathogens (usually with anaerobes) are commonly associated with sinusitis or otitis. Other organisms like aerobic *Streptococci*, *S pneumoniae*, *H influenzae*, *Staphylococci*, and Gram-negative bacilli can also be recovered. *S aureus* and facultative Gram-negative bacilli dominate in postoperative patients.

Clinical features include fever, which is the predominant symptom and occurs in 95% of cases. Focal headache and signs of meningeal irritation occur in more than 80% of cases, although associated meningitis occurs only in 14% of cases. Focal neurologic signs and seizures occur in 80% and 45% of patients respectively, and they are usually associated with rapid spread of infection. Postsurgical subdural empyema occurs insidiously in contrast to other types of subdural empyemas, which usually have an acute onset.

Diagnosis should be considered in all patients with meningeal signs and focal deficit. The diagnosis may be masked in patients with head injury or those previously having similar symptoms. CT scan with intravenous contrast is usually helpful, but MRI is the best diagnostic tool. CSF analysis is usually not helpful as meningitis is rare and lumbar puncture is potentially hazardous because of risk of herniation.

Treatment consists of emergency craniotomy and drainage of the pus to avoid herniation. The drained fluid (as well as blood sample) should be sent for aerobic and anaerobic culture. Antibiotics should be started immediately, which include a combination of vancomycin with a third generation cephalosporin (eg, cefotaxime). These are then modified according to the culture results. Antibiotic therapy should continue for at least three weeks.

TABLE 64-2 Treatment of Specific Postoperative Infections

Bacteria	Antibiotic
Staph aureus	Oxacillin or vancomycin
Meth-Resistant *Staph aureus* (MRSA)	Vancomycin
Staph epidermidis	Vancomycin
Gram-negative organisms	Ampicillin or ceftazidime
proprionobacter	Ceftazidime
E Coli	Gentamicin

WOUND INFECTION

Wound infections usually do not manifest before the second postoperative day and they might not be detected for days or weeks following surgery. They are generally caused by *S aureus* or skin flora such as *S epidermidis*. Occasionally, gram-negative aerobes such as *E coli* and *Pseudomonas aeruginosa* are involved, especially in patients who had open head trauma. Wound infections are readily observable and diagnosable. They ordinarily manifest with tenderness, erythema, and swelling. Systemic illness and toxicity can occur in infection with toxigenic strain of *S aureus*. Diagnosis is confirmed with wound aspiration or swabbing for culture and gram stain. Early and late skull X-ray or CT scan can be ordered to exclude osteomyelitis.

Systemic antibiotics should be initiated immediately and before culture and gram stain results. As most infections are due to gram-positive cocci, first-generation cephalosporin such as cephazolin is used as initial therapy. Occasionally, when there is pus accumulation, the wound needs to be opened, drained, irrigated, and then loosely closed over a drain (**Table 64-2**).

POSTOPERATIVE HYDROCEPHALUS

The incidence of postoperative hydrocephalus in cranial base surgery was estimated to be 8% in cranial base surgery for tumor resection. It usually results due to spillage of blood into subarachnoid space or ventricles because of inadequate hemostasis or extension of surgery into ventricles. Sometimes, it occurs due to swelling in the operative site and secondary sealing of the outlets of CSF (especially when surgery is done around the aqueduct or foramen of Monro). It can also result from CSF infection postoperatively, (ie, ventriculitis or meningitis). Focal hydrocephalus (trapped ventricle) develops when surgery is undertaken near the foramen of Monro. It can be due to a blood clot or residual tumor. Hydrocephalus also may occur two to four weeks postoperatively from progressive arachnoiditis caused by aseptic/bacterial meningitis or even subarachnoid hemorrhage from aneurysm.

Clinically, the patient presents with symptoms of increased ICP such as headache, nausea, and vomiting. Diagnosis is made on the basis of these symptoms in addition to findings on CT scan or MRI, which are very sensitive tests. Assessment of ventricular size prior to operation should establish a baseline for comparison with the postoperative image. A ventricular catheter may be used for treatment; it allows both ventricular drainage and ICP monitoring. Generally, if ventricular drainage requires more than a week in situ, it should be converted into a shunt, or a new ventriculostomy should be placed on the opposite side. The sooner the decision of shunt placement is made, the less likely systemic complication or shunt infection will occur. In the presence of meningitis or ventriculitis, ventricular drainage is important in controlling the pressure and draining the site of infection effectively.

TABLE 64-3 DVT Prophylaxis

Group	Estimated DVT Risk	Typical Patients	Recommended Prophylaxis
Low risk	< 10%	Age < 40 yrs, minimal risk factors. General anesthesia: < 30 min.	No prophylaxis, or PCB/TEDS.
Moderate risk	10–40%	Age ≥ 40 yrs, malignancy, prolonged bed rest, extensive surgery, varicose veins, obesity. General anesthesia: > 30 min, SAH, head injury.	PCB/TEDS, or Low-dose heparin if no ICH/SAH.
High risk	40–80%	History of DVT/PE, paralysis, brain tumor (especially meningioma or malignant glioma).	PCB/TEDS + low-dose heparin (if no SAH/ICH).

PCB, pneumatic compression boots; PE, pulmonary embolism; TEDS, TED, stocking.

PRACTICE POINT

Postoperative hydronephrosis

- Clinically, the patient presents with symptoms of increased ICP such as headache, nausea, and vomiting.
- Diagnosis is made on the basis of these symptoms in addition to findings on CT scan or MRI, which are very sensitive tests.

DEEP VEIN THROMBOSIS

The risk of deep vein thrombosis (DVT) in neurosurgical patients is estimated to be 19–50%. It is particularly high in neurosurgical patients because of the long operating time of some procedures, the prolonged bed rest, and the possible presence of a paralyzed limb. Coagulopathy also occurs in brain tumors and head injury due to release of brain thromboplastin; Without prophylaxis 28% of meningioma or glioma patients develop DVT and 8% pulmonary embolism. Specific neurologic risk factors for DVT include spinal cord injury, brain tumors, head trauma, and stroke. DVT and pulmonary embolism are covered elsewhere in this text. For neurosurgical purposes, the major issue is when anticoagulants may safely be administered. Although there are no class 1 data on this, we believe 72 hours is a reasonable time to consider anticoagulation after surgery; this number may vary depending on the vascularity and hemostatsis in a specific case (**Table 64-3**).

CSF LEAK (CSF FISTULA)

Trauma and surgery represent more than 70% of causes of CSF leak. In the majority of postoperative cases, CSF leak occurs immediately with an incidence of 8% in cranial base operations and may manifest months after the surgery.

A CSF fistula is clinically manifested as otorrhea or rhinorrhea in most of the cases. Otorrhea usually results from CSF leak through the mastoid air cells (especially after posterior fossa surgery and translabyrinthine approach for acoustic neuroma). Rhinorrhea can occur from the CSF leak through the sphenoid sinus (especially in posttranssphenoidal surgery), cribriform plate or ethmoidal roof (frontal fossa floor), frontal air cells, herniation into empty sella, and then into sphenoid air sinus. It can also result after temporal bone fracture or acoustic neuroma surgery through a leak into the middle ear, eustachian tube, and then nasopharynx. CSF can also leak through the skin following a surgical or traumatic wound. A spinal CSF leak can occur with a dural defect and presents as a fluid collection around the dura.

CSF appears as clear as water; it has a salty taste in rhinorrhea, a glucose level above 30 mg/dl, and is positive for β_2 transferrin (this protein can be detected by electrophoresis and it presents only in CSF and vitreous fluid, but not in tears, saliva, nasal exudates, or serum). Skull X-ray or CT scan may demonstrate signs of pneumocephalus.

Localizing the site of CSF fistula is a major step in the evaluation of this complication. In 90% of the time, a CT scan with intravenous contrast is sufficient to locate the site of the fistula. Water-soluble contrast CT cisternography (WS-CTC) is the procedure of choice to locate the site of the fistula. This is performed by intrathecal injection of radio-opaque contrast followed by CT scan. The test is indicated when there is no site identified on plain CT, when multiple bony defects are identified and it is essential to determine which site is leaking, or if a bony defect is seen on CT and no abnormal enhancement is seen in the adjacent brain parenchyma. Radionucleotide cisternography may be useful in leaks too slow or small to show up on WS-CTC. This is performed by a radionucleotide tracer followed by scintigram. MRI has a limited value in localization of CSF fistulae.

Sometimes a CSF leak can be followed expectantly. Prophylactic antibiotic use is controversial. Medical therapy is usually indicated, however. These measures include bed rest, avoiding straining (stool softening/avoid blowing the nose), acetazolamide, and modest fluid restriction. If the leak persists despite these measures, obstructive hydrocephalus and mass effect must be ruled out first with a CT scan or MRI, then lumbar puncture can be done once or twice daily, or continuous lumbar drainage (CLD) via catheter should be performed for 96 hours.

Surgical management is indicated for a persistent traumatic CSF leak of more than two weeks in duration in spite of nonsurgical measures, spontaneous or delayed onset leaks because of their high incidence of recurrence, and leaks complicated by meningitis. Surgical techniques aimed at sealing the leaks include different procedures: occlusion of the mastoid air cells with bone wax or muscle, reclosure of the dura, and the use of dural graft or fascia. Transnasal sellar injection of fibrin glue under local anesthesia may also be considered for leaks following transsphenoidal surgery.

CONCLUSION

Care of neurosurgical patients requires effective collaboration and communication in order to optimize quality of life following a neurosurgical injury. Although hospitalists will no doubt encounter a wide variety of neurosurgical issues and pathology, this chapter reviews complications typically encountered in the hospital setting. Hospitalists can play a critical role in the care of these patients who often have significant co-morbidities that increase their vulnerability to medical and surgical complications. If hospitalists engage in co-management services, the impact of their work should be measured to ensure agreed upon goals are achieved.

SUGGESTED READINGS

Kalfas IH, Little JR. Postoperative hemorrhage: A survey of 4992 intracranial procedures. *Neurosurgery*. 1988;23(55):343–347.

LeBeau J, Criessard P, Harispe L, et al. Surgical treatment of brain abscess and subdural empyema. *J Neurosurg*. 1973;38:198.

Post EM, Modesti LM. "Subacute" postoperative subdural empyema. *J Neurosurg*. 1981;55(5):761–765.

Sen C, Sekhar L. Complications of cranial base surgery. In: Post K, Friedman E, McCormick P, eds. *Postoperative Complications in Intracranial Neurosurgery*. New York, NY: Thieme; 1993.

SECTION 7

Medical Management of Orthopedic Surgery Patients

CHAPTER 65

Common Orthopedic Surgical Procedures

William Whang, MD
Greg Erens, MD
Claudius D. Jarrett, MD
C. Edward Hoffler II, PhD, MD

INTRODUCTION

The majority of inpatient orthopedics focus on the hip, knee, and spine. Improvements in orthopedic implants, techniques, and overall medical care have expanded indications for reconstructive efforts to restore function, reduce pain, and improve quality of life. This chapter reviews the most common major operations typically encountered in the hospital setting.

THE HIP

ANATOMY

The hip, a ball and socket joint with articular cartilage, provides for load bearing and low-friction motion. The bony architecture supported by a fibrocartilaginous labrum, joint capsule, and traversing muscle groups provides stability. These muscle groups load the hip joint at 2 to 3 times the body weight and are highly sensitive to any changes in hip center of rotation or length of the lever arms. Synovial fluid provides nutrition to the avascular cartilage. The femoral head receives blood from the ascending branches off the medial circumflex femoral artery. Disruption of this retrograde blood supply may lead to avascular necrosis.

Any surgical approaches require significant soft tissue dissection to reach the hip joint. The most commonly used and most extensile posterior approach provides excellent visualization of the femur and acetabulum. The sciatic nerve is the main structure at risk. With meticulous repair following dissection of the posterior capsule, dislocation rates have been dramatically reduced. The lateral and anterior approaches both leave the posterior joint capsule intact resulting in low instability rates. Lateral approaches require hip abductor dissection and may lead to abductor insufficiency and a Trendelenburg gait. Anterior approaches provide limited exposure to any posterior structures. Trochanteric osteotomy provides extensile exposure but risks nonunion. The specific approach is chosen based on pathology, patient factors, and surgeon preference.

TOTAL HIP ARTHROPLASTY

Total hip arthroplasty (THA) can dramatically relieve pain and improve function (**Table 65-1**). Surgical candidates have generally tried and failed a conservative course of weight loss, analgesics, assistive devices, therapy, and activity modifications. Preoperative radiographs should confirm destruction of the hip joint and allow for surgical planning. Other causes of "hip pain" should be ruled out. Arthritis often coexists in the hip and spine, with true hip pain perceived in the groin and anterior thigh.

THA involves removal of the diseased hip joint and implantation of a prosthetic hip. Autologous blood transfusion may be discussed preoperatively. Perioperative blood salvage is an option in complex cases. Regional anesthesia may be associated with better initial outcomes than general anesthesia. This decision should be made in accord with the patient and anesthesiologist. The most significant factor associated with risk of postoperative transfusion is preoperative hemoglobin.

The prosthetic hip consists of a femoral component, an acetabular component, and a bearing/coupling surface. Fixation of the prosthesis is either cemented or cementless. Cemented THA are more commonly used for lower demand patients, due to concerns regarding loosening in higher demand patients. Cemented fixation provides an immediate mechanical bond to the host bone and

TABLE 65-1 Hip Surgery

Hip Arthroplasty Procedures	Indication for the Procedure	Contraindications	Procedure	Comments
Primary total hip replacement	Degenerative joint disease, inflammatory arthritis, avascular necrosis, developmental dysplasia	Active infections, unstable medical illness, any general condition incompatible with surgery or rehabilitation	2 hours, 500 mL acute blood loss, and slow blood loss postoperatively ↑ Risk for venous thromboembolism and fat emboli Infection rates < 1%	Regional anesthesia may be associated with better initial outcomes; hypotensive anesthesia associated with decreased intraoperative blood loss
Total hip resurfacing	Younger, high-demand patients	Active infections, unstable medical illness, general condition incompatible with surgery or rehabilitation	Increased blood loss and operative time expected but revision surgery likely less demanding than for total hip arthroplasty	Unique risks of femoral neck fracture and osteonecrosis of remaining femoral head
Revision total hip arthroplasty (18%)	Loosening, osteolysis, instability, infection, and periprosthetic fractures	Unstable medical illness, general condition incompatible with surgery or rehabilitation	Removal of components, reconstruction of bony defects, creation of a stable implant, and restoration of hip center Infection rates < 2%	Goal to increase mobility and reduce pain. Results usually inferior to those of primary total hip arthroplasty with higher costs and complication rates

achieves maximal stability within 24 hours. Generally recommended for physiologically younger patients, cementless fixation relies on an initial mechanical press fit, with subsequent osseous ingrowth into the prosthesis. Over millions of cycles, bone remodeling can occur around the prosthesis. This dynamic biologic fixation may provide a lifelong bond. Bearing surfaces have historically been metal (cobalt chrome) on plastic (polyethylene). This hard-on-soft bearing has been plagued by wear and osteolysis caused by the biologic reaction to wear debris. Improvements in polyethylene production, in particular cross-linking, have shown significant reduction in wear. Hard-on-hard bearings, that is, metal on metal or ceramic on ceramic, have also shown dramatic reductions in wear. Unique concerns such as elevated metal ion levels, ceramic fracture, and squeaking are under investigation. With stable fixation of the prosthesis and improved wear of the bearing surface, the longevity of current THAs should be improved.

A viable alternative to THA, total hip resurfacing is technically demanding and proper patient selection is crucial. Resurfacing involves removing only the diseased portion of the femoral head thereby conserving proximal femoral bone stock. The femoral component is cemented and coupled to an acetabular component with a metal-on-metal surface bearing.

Guidelines recommend 24 hours of prophylactic perioperative antibiotics and surgical wounds are monitored daily. Patients should receive both mechanical (sequential compression devices and early mobilization) and pharmacologic (aspirin, warfarin, or low-molecular-weight heparin) thromboembolic prophylaxis. Due to lack of consensus, the specific drug and duration of pharmacologic prophylaxis depends on surgeon preference or hospital protocols.

Although there is no universally accepted postoperative THA protocol, certain guidelines do exist. The surgeon determines weight bearing status usually full or partial. Assistive devices are recommended and discontinued at approximately 6 to 12 weeks. Hip precautions are taught to prevent dislocations. Hip abduction pillows may maintain a "safe" position for the hip. Pain control initially involves parenteral narcotic medications with early transition to enteral medications. Regional anesthesia and intraoperative capsular injections may decrease narcotic requirements. Hospital length of stay is typically 2 to 4 days postoperatively. Patients with poor mobility may require extended inpatient rehabilitation. External staples and sutures are removed at 2 weeks. Patients may typically resume their normal lifestyle at 3 months with subtle improvement noted for up to 1 to 2 years.

Efforts to prevent or minimize infections should focus on evidence-based use of perioperative antibiotics, surgical technique, and wound care. Early postoperative infections may be treated with an incision and drainage with component retention. Late infections often require a two-stage explant/replant. Dislocation rates are 1% to 5% lifetime for primary THA and may exceed 10% for revisions. Most dislocations may be managed with urgent reduction and nonoperative measures. Revision surgery is reserved for recurrent instability, particularly in the setting of implant malposition.

HIP FRACTURE

Treatment algorithms are based on patient age and fracture location (**Table 65-2**). The main anatomic subgroups are femoral neck and intertrochanteric fractures.

> **PRACTICE POINT**
>
> - Inpatient mortality rates from primary arthroplasty procedures are 0.16–0.5% with the most common cause being underlying cardiac disease followed by pulmonary embolism. Postoperatively, immediate mobilization is recommended with weight bearing as tolerated, if possible. With poor bone quality and less than optimal fracture reduction/fixation, limited weight bearing may be necessary. Unless a primary arthroplasty was performed, no dislocation precautions are necessary.

Femoral neck fractures

Femoral neck fractures occur between the distal extent of the femoral head articular surface to the most proximal extent of the intertrochanteric region. These intracapsular fractures are either nondisplaced (including valgus impacted patterns) or displaced.

TABLE 65-2 Hip Fractures

Hip Fracture	Timing	Complications	Comments
Displaced femoral neck fractures	Young (from high energy trauma): any surgical delays increase the risk of avascular necrosis Elderly (from low energy trauma): urgent but not emergent surgery	Deep vein thrombosis rates (20–50%) further increase with surgical delay >48 hours Risk of nonunion and osteonecrosis (30%)	Treatment depends on age of patient and stability of fracture pattern Elderly: 1-year mortality 30%. Highest in the first month of injury, returning to age adjusted norms at 6 months. Evaluation and treatment of osteoporosis
Nondisplaced femoral neck fractures	Urgent surgery as soon as patient medically optimized	Internal fixation: nonunion of the fracture and avascular necrosis of the femoral head (5%)	Evaluation and treatment of osteoporosis
Intertrochanteric fractures	Urgent surgery as soon as the patient medically optimized	Complication rates similar to femoral neck fractures. Mechanical failure from unstable fractures with poor bone quality, malreduction, and improper implant choice or position Osteonecrosis and nonunion much less common given the excellent blood supply	Surgical time and blood loss can vary widely depending on fracture pattern, body habitus, and bone quality Overall decline in hip function common Secondary reconstructive surgeries complex but rarely necessary Evaluation and treatment of osteoporosis

PRACTICE POINT

Timing of surgery for hip fractures

- Displaced femoral neck fractures in young patients are surgical emergencies. Coordinated trauma care is recommended. Displaced femoral neck fractures in elderly patients: surgery is urgent, but not emergent. Medical comorbidities should be optimized prior to surgery, particularly cardiopulmonary and fluid electrolyte imbalance.
- Surgery for intertrochanteric fractures should be performed as soon as the patient is medically optimized.
- If at all possible, weight bearing as tolerated should be allowed postoperatively.

Younger patients The blood supply to the femoral head is retrograde from the medial circumflex to the ascending lateral epiphyseal artery. Any surgical delays increase the risk of avascular necrosis. In this population, femoral neck fractures are treated with closed versus open reduction and internal fixation with multiple lag screws. Postoperative weight bearing is determined by the quality of fracture reduction and fixation. Femoral neck fractures in younger patients are high energy injuries with a 50 to 60% incidence of associated trauma elslewhere.

Older patients In older patients, nondisplaced or stable femoral neck fractures are treated with gentle fracture reduction and multiple lag screws placed percutaneously. This generally low-morbidity procedure has minimal blood loss and patients generally recover rapidly. Displaced fractures have a high incidence of nonunion and avascular necrosis; therefore, internal fixation with preservation of the femoral head is not recommended and hemiarthroplasty (partial hip replacement) is typically performed. Hemiarthroplasties may be cemented or noncemented. It is unclear whether a bipolar (ball within a ball) prosthesis provides any advantage over a unipolar prosthesis to justify the added expense. Total hip arthroplasty may provide improved function and pain relief in physiologically younger patients, but has a higher risk of dislocation.

Postoperatively, immediate mobilization is paramount. Elderly patients have difficulty complying with any weight-bearing restrictions, and nonweight bearing is associated with higher joint reactive forces than weight bearing. No dislocation precautions are necessary with internal fixation. Hemiarthroplasties are inherently stable given the large head size coupled with an intact labrum. However, dislocation precautions are still usually recommended given the high rate of cognitive impairments in this population. Patients should receive routine wound care with external staple or suture removal at 2 weeks. Guidelines recommend chemical and mechanical deep vein thrombosis (DVT) prophylaxis. Any sedating medications should be used judiciously due to the high incidence of delirium. Patients are typically discharged at 3 to 4 days postoperatively and often require prolonged inpatient rehabilitation.

Intertrochanteric fractures

Intertrochanteric hip fractures occur between the extracapsular distal aspect of the femoral neck to the lesser trochanter. This region of the femur is mainly cancellous bone with an excellent blood supply and therefore a low risk of nonunion. The posteromedial femoral calcar provides stress transfer from the hip to the femoral shaft. Any comminution or displacement in this area leads to an unstable pattern. Intertrochanteric fractures are classified as stable or unstable and require surgical management. Nonoperative treatment may be reserved for patients who are nonambulatory, confused, and/or medically unstable or for isolated nondisplaced and minimally displaced fractures of the greater trochanter. Imaging studies such as a CT scan or MRI are recommended for isolated, minimally displaced fractures of the greater trochanter to ensure there is no extension across the trochanteric area. Isolated lesser trochanteric fractures in the elderly should raise suspicion for a pathologic fracture. Treatment is based on the nature and extent of the pathologic process.

Initially a reduction is attempted using closed techniques but open reductions may be necessary. Internal fixation is achieved with either a sliding hip screw or an intramedullary device. These implants often allow for controlled collapse of the fracture to a stable construct. Intramedullary devices have biomechanical advantages and may be preferred in certain unstable fracture patterns. Higher surgical complication rates have been noted with intramedullary devices. Surgical time and blood loss can vary widely depending on the fracture pattern, body habitus, and bone quality. Outcomes are also dependent on the quality of the fracture reduction and optimal implant choice and position. Primary prosthetic replacement may be an option with certain unstable patterns, tumors, or preexisting arthritis, but is often a much more extensive procedure. Standard antibiotic and DVT prophylaxis are recommended. Wounds are monitored daily with staple or suture removal in 2 weeks. In the absence of complications, hospital length of stay is 3 to 4 days postoperatively. Debilitated patients often require prolonged inpatient rehabilitation.

THE KNEE

ANATOMY

The knee functions as a weight-bearing hinge; subtle rotation and translation predisposes this joint to injury. The anterior and posterior cruciate ligaments in the sagittal plane and medial and lateral collateral ligaments in the coronal plane provide primary stability. The traversing quadriceps and hamstring muscle groups provide secondary stability. Because the medial and lateral menisci are important in stress distribution, injury or removal of the menisci results in accelerated degeneration of the joint. The knee is divided into medial, lateral, and patellofemoral compartments. With malalignment, one compartment of the knee may receive excessive stress resulting in early degeneration. The synovial lining of the knee capsule produces synovial fluid, which provides lubrication and nutrition to the articular cartilage. The avascular articular cartilage has limited reparative potential in adults.

TOTAL KNEE ARTHROPLASTY

During total knee replacement, surgical goals are to restore mechanical alignment, balance the soft tissues, and obtain good fit and fixation of the prosthesis (**Table 65-3**). The patient is supine with compression devices on the nonoperative leg. Tourniquets are typically used; therefore, blood loss is minimal intraoperatively with postoperative blood loss typically 500 to 1000 mL. Lowering the transfusion threshold to a hemoglobin of <8.5 g/L decreases the rate of allogenic blood transfusions. An anterior midline skin incision followed by a medial parapatellar approach provides access to the deep structures of the knee. The surgeon removes the diseased surfaces of the distal femur and proximal tibia to restore alignment to the knee and make room for the prosthesis. Although press fit designs are available, usually the surgeon cements the appropriate size implants and places a polyethylene liner of appropriate thickness between the metallic femoral and tibial prosthetic components. Controversy exists regarding resurfacing the patella and also retaining or sacrificing the posterior cruciate ligament. Specific approaches, techniques, and implants are highly surgeon dependent. Regional anesthesia (epidural, spinal, or femoral and sciatic nerve blocks) as well as pericapsular knee injections may decrease postoperative pain and narcotic requirements.

PRACTICE POINT

- Following total knee replacement immediate mobilization is recommended with weight bearing as tolerated. Physical therapy assists with gait training and range of motion. Continuous passive motion machines are optional as they achieve increased early motion but do not improve long-term results.

Antibiotic prophylaxis is prescribed for 24 hours perioperatively. Antibiotics beyond 24 hours have not demonstrated any additional benefit. Both mechanical (sequential compression devices and active ankle pumps) and pharmacologic measures (aspirin, warfarin, or low-molecular-weight heparin) provide DVT prophylaxis. Choice and duration of chemical prophylaxis remain controversial and should be decided in advance by the surgical team. Warfarin and low-molecular-weight heparin have demonstrated a significant decrease in venogram documented thrombosis with a small increase in bleeding. Advocates of aspirin note comparable pulmonary embolism rates with decreased bleeding. Optimal pain management includes initial parenteral then oral narcotic medications, COX-2 inhibitors, regional anesthesia, peripheral nerve blocks, and capsular injections. Surgeons monitor the wound daily and remove external staples and sutures at 2 weeks. Any wound drainage past 3 to 4 days should be reported. Acute infections require irrigation and debridement with component retention. Chronic infections require a two-stage explant, followed by a replant. With all deep infections, a minimum of 6 weeks of intravenous antibiotics are recommended. Length of stay is typically 3 to 4 days postoperatively with a majority of patients being discharged to home.

THE CERVICAL SPINE

ANATOMY

The cervical spine has a lordotic curve consisting of the first seven vertebrae (C1–C7). The base of the skull (occiput) sits on top of C1, also called the atlas. Two thickened bony arches form a large hole through the center of the atlas. The large opening accommodates the spinal cord at its widest point where it first exits the brain and skull. Compared to other vertebrae, the atlas also has much wider bony projections pointing out to each side. The atlas sits on top of the C2 vertebra, also called the axis. The axis has a large bony protrusion on top, called the dens (or odontoid). The dens protrudes upward into a hole in the atlas. The articulation between the atlas and axis give the neck most of its ability to rotate side to side. C3 through C7 complete the cervical spine region.

Typical landmarks for the cervical vertebrae include base of nose and the hard palate corresponding to C1, teeth corresponding to C2, mandible and hyoid bone corresponding to C3, thyroid cartilage extending from C4 to C5 and the cricoid cartilage extending from C6 to C7.

Separating the vertebral bodies, the intervertebral disc contains an outer fibrous sheath, the annulus fibrosus, with obliquely oriented type I collagen fibers in alternating layers. In contrast, the disc center contains a soft, highly elastic amorphous substance composed of type II collagen and approximately 88% water. The discs and vertebral bodies support more than 80% of the axial load of the spine while the facet joints carry the remainder. The vertebrae articulate with each other via facet joints, which are synovial articulations with capsules and ligaments that are critical to spine stability.

Anteriorly, the anterior longitudinal ligament (anterior to body) and posterior longitudinal ligament (posterior to body) support the cervical spine. Posteriorly, the ligamentum flavum, the nuchal ligament, and the interspinous ligament provide strong structural support.

The spinal cord travels down from the brain posterior to the vertebral body and is surrounded by the bony arch of the pedicles and laminae. At each level, nerve roots branch off the spinal cord and pass through the neural foramina. These nerves innervate dermatomes of the head and upper extremities. In the cervical spine, the nerve roots exit above the pedicle of the same number. For example, the C5 nerve root exits at the C4-C5 interspace. This contrasts to the lumbar spine, where the nerve roots exit below the

TABLE 65-3 Knee Surgery

Procedure	Indications	Complications	Comments
Total knee replacement	For suitable patients with debilitating symptoms, failure of less invasive treatments, and radiographically confirmed advanced joint disease Contraindications include active joint infection and a nonfunctional extensor mechanism	Mortality < 0.5%, typically from cardiac disease Deep vein thrombosis rates without prophylaxis approach 40–50% with most clots being distal Infection rates 1% Immediate mechanical: neurovascular injury, compartment syndrome, hematomas, and skin necrosis Late mechanical: stiffness, instability, loosening, and wear	Total knee arthroplasty performed under general or regional anesthesia typically over 1–2 hours Most patients experience significant improvements by 3 months with continued improvements for up to 1 year Survivorship for a properly performed total knee arthroplasty 90% at 10 years and 75% at 20 years
Unicompartmental knee arthroplasty	For suitable patients with primarily one diseased compartment First arthroplasty for younger patients due to preservation of noninvolved compartments Last arthroplasty for older patients due to less surgical trauma, faster recovery	Failure requiring revision surgery most commonly for progression of arthritis in nonresurfaced compartments, loosening, polyethylene wear	Advantages: faster recovery, more normal knee kinematics, preservation of bone stock With appropriate patient selection and improved designs, survivorship approaching that of total knee arthroplasty
Osteotomy	Alternative for younger active patients with malalignment and unicompartment disease For varus (bow leg) deformity: valgus-producing osteotomy on proximal tibia by either closing wedge laterally or opening wedge medially For valgus (knock knee) deformity: varus-producing osteotomy of distal femur by either closing wedge medially, or opening wedge laterally	Nonunion, progression of arthritis, and neurovascular injury, particularly of the peroneal nerve	Osteotomy has distinct advantage of preserving native joint. After osteotomy has healed, there are no activity restrictions Usually a temporizing procedure prior to total knee arthroplasty, but lower knee scores commonly reported following conversion to total knee arthroplasty With appropriate patient selection and technique, 10 years survival rates approach 90%
Total knee replacement revisions (10% of knee arthroplasties)	Aseptic loosening, polyethylene wear, infection, instability, stiffness, and malalignment Surgical goals: to remove components, restore joint line, fill bone defects, balance the knee ligaments, and achieve stable fixation of final prosthesis	More demanding, longer procedures with increased blood loss, complications, and costs than for primary total knee arthroplasty Infection rates 2% for revision total knee arthroplasty	If the mode of failure of the initial total knee arthroplasty is identified and addressed, significant improvements in knee function and pain expected

pedicle of the same number. For example, the L4 nerve root exits at the L4–L5 interspace.

CERVICAL RADICULOPATHY AND MYELOPATHY

Often, both cervical radiculopathy and myelopathy result from a pathologic degeneration of the cervical spine that originates at the intervertebral disc. This may cause a domino effect resulting in compression of spinal elements at the root or cord level. The cervical intervertebral disc is composed of a firm fibrous ring, the annulus fibrosus, and a soft gelatinous interior, the nucleus pulposus. In the degenerative disc, the inner nucleus pulposus loses its water content as well as its shock absorbing capacity and becomes more fibrous in composition. Eventually, it becomes indistinguishable from its surrounding annulus. The disc eventually loses its height and structure, starts to bulge at the periphery, and allows settling and increased pathologic motion between its neighboring vertebraes. This process is thought to lead to a cascade of degeneration, including osteophyte formation and encroachment on traversing nerve root and the spinal canal. In the herniated disc, fissures develop in the outer annulus fibrosus with preservation of the integrity of the nucleus. These fissures allow the nucleus pulposus to herniate through the weakened portion of the outer ring. The nature and location of compression from these processes can lead to radiculopathy and/or myelopathy.

Cervical radiculopathy refers to symptoms in a dermatomal distribution in the upper extremity resulting from nerve root compression. Patients will often express significant unilateral sharp neck and shoulder girdle pain with a tingling sensation that travels down their arm. These symptoms make it difficult for them to find a comfortable sitting position. Patients often recollect that activities that demand extension of the neck and rotating of their head toward the symptomatic arm cause exacerbation of their symptoms. They may awkwardly tilt their head away from the painful side and hold the symptomatic extremity above their head. Certain dermatomal patterns commonly implicate the offending root level. The examiner may identify associated root level weakness and hyporeflexia.

Patients with myelopathy often represent a more diagnostic conundrum, because they present with more subtle complaints as a result of spinal cord compression. Patients typically express a vague history of clumsiness of the hands that make getting dressed in the morning or eating with utensils increasingly difficult. They also have increased difficulty with balance and gait that may have been ignored for some time and attributed to age. Family members are often the first ones to notice the patients' unsteady or awkward gait. The examiner may identify hyperreflexia and pathologic reflexes that point to an upper motor neuron lesion, motor weakness, and distal muscle wasting.

PRACTICE POINT

- The natural history for cervical radiculopathy is often favorable with conservative management. However, myelopathic patients typically go through a predictable step-wise progression over weeks to years unless successfully treated with surgical intervention.

Both radiculopathy and myelopathy can be successfully treated with either anterior or posterior surgical procedures depending on the location and extent of compression. Common surgical options include anterior cervical discectomy and fusion (ACDF), anterior cervical corpectomy and fusion, cervical laminectomy with fusion, or laminoplasty (**Table 65-4**).

ANTERIOR CERVICAL DISCECTOMY AND FUSION

The patient is positioned supine with the neck in slight extension. A transverse incision is placed within a neck skin crease. A longitudinal incision, although less cosmetically appealing, may be used for a more extensile approach. The surgeon continues dissection through the subcutaneous soft tissue to the platysma, divides the platysma in line with the incision, and bluntly dissects down medial to the sternocleidomastoid and the carotid artery and lateral to the esophagus through the pretracheal fascia to the anterior cervical spine. Intraoperative radiographs confirm appropriate level for decompression. After exposure of the appropriate disc level, the surgeon removes the entire disc and cartilage under magnification. A high-speed burr decorticates the endplates and creates a rectangular space for an appropriate-sized bone autograft or allograft. If preoperative imaging reveals evidence of foraminal impingement, the surgeon decompresses the impingement as well. The surgeon often places a deep drain in the retropharyngeal space to prevent hematoma formation.

ANTERIOR CORPECTOMY AND FUSION

Following exposure of the appropriate cervical vertebral body, removal of the cancellous bone of the vertebral body, and fine decompression, the surgeon removes more bone under direct visualization until a thin posterior shell of vertebral body remains. The posterior longitudinal ligament can also be removed as deemed necessary for adequate decompression along with neighboring discs and endplates. The removed portion of the vertebral body and discs are replaced with bone graft and stabilized with an anterior cervical plate construct. The surgeon often places a deep drain in the retropharyngeal space to prevent hematoma formation.

Bracing after ACDF or corpectomy and fusion is used at the surgeon's discretion. The deep drain is usually removed on the first postoperative day. Patients are encouraged to mobilize as tolerated.

CERVICAL LAMINECTOMY

Cervical laminectomy requires a midline incision between C2 and T1. After dissection of the ligamentum nuchae and the paracervical muscles from the spinous processes, the surgeon removes the spinous process and lamina and any neighboring bony or soft tissue structures that may be contributing to neural compression. Up to 25% to 50% of each facet can be removed before mechanical instability is likely to develop necessitating a concomitant fusion. When fusion is necessary to address potential instability, the surgeon may use several techniques, including posterior wiring, posterior plating, lateral mass screws, or pedicle screws and rods.

Postoperatively, a cervical collar is worn from 6 weeks to 3 months. Physical therapy is initiated in the hospital to encourage and assist with mobilization. Drains are used at the discretion of the surgeon.

CERVICAL LAMINOPLASTY

In general, a midline posterior cervical incision is made between the second and seventh cervical spinous processes. The dissection is continued subperiosteally, exposing the spinous process then both laminae at each level required for decompression, typically from C3 to C7. The opening is maintained using sutures, mini-plates, spacers, or bone grafts.

The length and type of postoperative immobilization may range from immediate mobilization with a soft collar for comfort to a hard collar for 4 to 8 weeks.

THE LUMBAR SPINE

ANATOMY

The lumbar spine contains five vertebrae (L1–L5) along with their intervening intervertebral discs and has an average of 55° to 60° of lordosis. Lumbar vertebrae have large bodies compared with their cervical and thoracic counterparts. Cephalad and caudad to the intervertebral foramina, stout pedicles project posteriorly from the body. Laminae extend further posteriorly and meet in the midline to complete the bony arch of the vertebral foramen, which encloses the spinal cord. Tranverse processes project laterally from the intersection of the pedicle and lamina. The spinous process extends posteriorly from the laminae at the midline. Barely medial to the pedicle, the pars interarticularis connects the superior and inferior articlar facets. "Posterior elements" describe all bony anatomy of a vertebra except the body.

The vertebral disc contains an outer fibrous sheath, the annulus fibrosus, with obliquely oriented type I collagen fibers in alternating layers. In contrast, the disc center contains a soft, highly elastic amorphous substance composed of type II collagen and is approximately 88% water. The discs and vertebral bodies support more than 80% of the axial load of the spine, and the remainder is carried by the facet joints. The vertebrae articulate with each other via facet joints, which are synovial articulations with capsules and ligaments that are critical to spine stability.

The anterior longitudinal ligament and posterior longitudinal ligament lay on their respective aspects of the vertebral bodies. The posterior elements are connected by several structures. Pairs of ligamentum flava connect the deep caudad margin of one lamina to the cephalad margin of the next. The supraspinal ligament is a longitudinal band attaching to the tips of all the spinous processes. The interspinous ligament extends from the supraspinal ligament and attaches to the deeper margins of adjacent spinous processes. Intertransverse ligaments connect adjacent transverse processes.

TABLE 65-4 Cervical Spine Surgery

Procedure	Indications	Technique	Complications	Comments
Anterior cervical discetomy and fusion	Disabling radicular pain or myopathic symptoms	Complete removal of cervical disc and fusion of neighboring vertebral bodies. Successful fusion rate 72–100% depending on number of levels and graft, instrumentation technique	Low incidence: transient dysphagia, dysphonia, hardware failure, nonunion; neurological, esophageal, or vertebral artery injury, and airway compromise from swelling or hematoma	Significant pain relief (80–90% of patients with radiculopathy) Significant prevention of progression of myopathic symptoms
Anterior cervical corpectomy and fusion	Disabling radicular pain or myopathic symptoms from thickening of posterior longitudinal ligament behind vertebrae, osteophytes, or kyphosis of vertebral column	Removal of portion of cervical vertebral body and its adjacent intervertebral discs and fusion of remnants of vertebral body to vertebrae above and below 72–100% successful fusion rate	Low incidence	Significant pain relief (80–90% of patients with radiculopathy) Significant prevention of progression of myopathic symptoms
Cervical laminectomy	Disabling radicular pain or myopathic symptoms due to single or multilevel spinal stenosis For patients with lordotic or neutral alignment of cervical spine to maximize decompression and drifting of spinal elements posteriorly	Indirect decompression of neural elements by providing increased space for spinal cord and nerve roots and direct decompression by removing any bony or soft tissue structures mechanically compressing them	Spinal cord and nerve root injuries (0–10%), dural tears With fusion: ↑ morbidity and risk for hardware and fusion-related complications; ↑ risk for neurological injury or failure if fusion not accomplished	If instability a concern, frequently combined with simultaneous posterior cervical fusion to avoid neurologic deterioration due to progressive postsurgical kyphosis
Cervical laminoplasty	Disabling radicular pain or myopathic symptoms due to multilevel spinal stenosis Severity of preoperative myelopathic symptoms is most important prognostic factor	Widening dimensions of spinal canal without permanently removing posterior elements Retaining posterior elements decreases risk of postoperative instability without requiring fusion procedure and thus, in theory, preserves motion	Axial neck pain and stiffness up to 1 year postop, nerve root injury at C5 level (2–11%), shoulder pain and weakness 1 to 3 days postop ≈ other cervical decompression procedures. Rarely failure of hardware or maintaining the posterior opening, hinge fracture	Compared with laminectomy or fusion, ≈ rates of neurological improvement (50–90%) Lower rates of complication and neurologic deterioration, less postop pain than with laminectomy Symptomatic improvement stable for up to10 years

When the spinal cord reaches L1, it tapers to the conus medularis. The filum terminale surrounded by nerve roots are termed the cauda equina and continue to the sacrum, providing segmental innervation. Nerve roots exit the spinal canal below their corresponding pedicle and through the intervertebral foramina. These nerves innervate dermatomes of the back and lower extremities. In the lumbar spine, the nerve roots exit below the pedicle of the same number. For example, the L4 nerve root exits at the L4–L5 interspace. This is in contrast to the cervical spine, where the nerve roots exit above the pedicle of the same number. For example, the C5 nerve root exits at the C4–C5 interspace.

The great radicular artery of Adamkiewicz provides the primary blood supply to the anterior two-thirds of the lumbar spine. It may originate from a superior lumbar artery or from an inferior intercostal artery. Aortic segmental vessels extend dorsocaudally giving lateral and intermediate branches to back muscles and medial branches that pass close to the pars and terminate posterior to the spinal process in an anastomosis with the contralateral vessel.

ANTERIOR LUMBAR INTERBODY FUSION

The anterior lumbosacral spine may be exposed via retroperitoneal or transperitoneal approaches. All spine surgeries in this review use positioning pads, urinary catheters, sequential compression devices, prophylactic antibiotics, spinal cord monitoring, and radiographic localization (**Table 65-5**).

For the retroperitoneal approach, a semilateral position, used with the body angled 45° to the horizontal supported by sand bags or a cushioned post, permits the peritoneal organs to fall away form the incision. With the left flank positioned upward, a standard oblique incision from the posterior half of the twelfth rib extending distally and anterior to point midway between the umbilicus and symphysis divides the muscles of the abdominal wall. More experienced

TABLE 65-5 Lumbar Spine Surgery

Procedure	Indications	Technique	Complications	Comments
Anterior lumbar interbody fusion	Degenerative disc disease, grade I spondylolisthesis (< 25% listhesis or "slippage" of 1 vertebral body on another), annular tears, and salvage of failed posterior fusion	May be used in concert with posterior decompression and fusion for primary symptomatic lumbar stenosis and revision procedures Solid fusion main predictor of improved outcomes	Vascular injuries at L4-L5 disc space: Venous lacerations (majority left iliac vein, inferior vena cava, and iliolumbar segmental inferior vena cava branch in descending order of frequency), rare arterial lacerations Graft dislodgement, injury to sympathetic chain or presacral plexus	Stand-alone contraindicated for patients with referred or radiating leg pain or objective neurologic compromise Following discectomy, recurrence at same or adjacent site in up to 10% with more advanced degenerative joint disease preoperatively or new injury
Lumbar decompression (laminectomy, laminotomy)	Lumbar spinal stenosis, herniated nucleus pulposus grade I degenerative spondylolisthesis and neoplastic or infectious pathology Laminotomy traditionally performed for herniated nucleus pulposus or lateral canal stenosis Cauda equina syndrome and progressive neurologic deficits are urgent indications for decompression	Laminotomy: only exposure of the involved side necessary Revision required in 3–5 years for back and leg symptoms in 10–15%	Laminectomy: pars interarticularis stress fracture, progressive instability (spondylolisthesis or kyphosis) and scarring Incidental durotomy with no ↑ morbidity if repaired during index surgery Rare vascular injury during posterior lumbar decompression	Flatback syndrome (loss of lumbar lordosis or frank lumbar kyphosis) caused by posterior distraction with fusion instrumentation, laminectomy, or disc space collapse
Lumbar decompression with fusion	Spinal instability	Incidental durotomy (3% of all lumbar spine surgeries, 8.1% in revision)		

surgeons may use smaller incisions. Deep to the transversalis fascia, blunt dissection develops a plane between the retroperitoneal fat and the psoas fascia. The peritoneal organs are swept medially, the left ureter loosely fixed to the peritoneum and mobilized accordingly. After confirming vertebral levels radiographically, the segmental arterial and venous connections to the vertebral bodies are ligated to mobilize the aorta and inferior vena cava. Care is taken to preserve the sympathetic chain at the lateral margin of the vertebral body and the genitofemoral nerve along the anterior surface of the psoas.

For the transperitoneal approach, the patient is positioned supine for a longitudinal midline incision. The rectus abdominis muscles may be divided bluntly after incision of the linea alba of the rectus sheath. The surgeon incises the peritoneum longitudinally taking care to protect the underlying viscera, and packs the bowels cephalad with the aid of moist surgical sponges and Trendelenburg. The posterior peritoneum is incised at the base of the sigmoid, allowing mobilization of the colon cephalad and rightward. The aortic bifurcation overlies L4 anteriorly. Ligation of the fourth and fifth segmental lumbar vessels permits mobilization of the aorta, inferior vena cava, and left common iliac vessels toward the right. The left ureter is retracted laterally. The L5-S1 disc space is distal to the great vessels and can be approached with a peritoneal incision. The middle sacral artery along the anterior sacral surface must be ligated and blunt dissection is used to preserve the branches of the presacral parasympathetic plexus.

Once the surgeon mobilizes the great vessels, he or she must visualize the midline and lateral margins of the disc spaces. An annulotomy is created adjacent to the inferior and superior vertebral endplates and extended to permit excision of the anterior longitudinal ligament and an anterior segment of the annulus. A complete discectomy is performed while the lateral segments of the annulus are preserved. The surgeon minimizes subsidence of the interbody fusion device by curetting the cartilaginous endplate without violating the bony endplate. Reaming the disc space forms parallel surfaces within the endplates. He may insert a variety of interbody fusion devices. Cancellous autograft, allograft, recombinant human bone morphogenic protein-2, or other biologics typically augment interbody fusion devices.

Regardless of the fusion device and graft choice, the principles of the technique are consistent. Expansion of the collapsed disc space to tension the annulus and adjacent ligamentous structures reduces deformity, restores lumbar lordosis, preloads and compresses the interbody device, and may indirectly decompress nerve roots. The interbody device should not penetrate beyond the posterior margins of the disc space. During closure, closed suction drains are often left in the retroperitoneal space. The abdominal wall is repaired meticulously to avoid an incisional hernia.

Postoperative care typically consists of patient-controlled anesthesia for 24 hours followed by oral medication with intravenous therapy for breakthrough pain only. Many surgeons will avoid nonsteroidal anti-inflammatory medications (NSAIDs) as they have been demonstrated to compromise spine fusion rates. A postoperative ileus may occur, so intravenous hydration and fasting may be required while awaiting the return of bowel function. Incentive spirometry is commonly prescribed and sequential compression devices provide venous thromboembolism prophylaxis. Anticoagulants and antiplatelet medications are held in the acute postoperative period unless the risk of cardiopulmonary compromise outweighs the risk of hematoma formation. Closed suction drains are typically maintained until the output declines below 30 cc for an 8-hour period, usually by the second postoperative day. The postoperative dressing is left in place for a minimum of 48 hours, but otherwise routine dressing management varies significantly. Prophylactic antibiotics are given for 24 hours. Postoperative casting and bracing regimens vary considerably, but postoperative physical therapy usually focuses on transfers and ambulation. Patients are discharged when they are hemodynamically stable, comfortable on oral pain medication, and ambulating adequately.

PRACTICE POINT

- Following anterior lumbar body, fusion patients are allowed to bear weight as tolerated, but are restricted to manually carrying less than 5 pounds.

Fusion rates are approximately 90% but vary from 43% to 95%. Surgical decompression and fusion for isthmic spondylolisthesis (due to pars interarticularis defect) usually yields 80% to 85% self-rated good to excellent results.

LUMBAR DECOMPRESSION

As in most spine surgery, physical examination findings should correlate with imaging studies, and an aggressive trial of nonoperative therapy should be exhausted.

Patients are intubated in the supine position, and transferred to the operating table prone. While a variety of surgical tables exist, the principles remain the same. The thorax and abdomen are maintained free to facilitate mechanical ventilation, reduce intra-abdominal and vena caval pressure and decrease the amount of blood in the epidural venous system. The legs are well padded and flexed slightly at the hips and knees

Laminectomy

A standard lumbar laminectomy is performed through a midline posterior incision. After incising the fascia, the paraspinal musculature is elevated subperiosteally from the spinous processes and laminae proceeding laterally to the facets. Meticulous hemostasis is maintained to enhance visualization, and vertebral levels are confirmed radiographically. Soft tissues are debrided from the interlaminar space. Next, the ligamentum flavum is excised taking care to protect the underlying dura.

Laminectomy for central lumbar stenosis is usually performed bilaterally. Care is taken not to compromise the facet joint or facet joint capsule. Partial facetectomy and pars resections may be necessary to decompress the nerve root. If more that 50% of either facet joint is compromised at a vertebral level or if discectomy is required in concert with laminectomy, the resulting instability should be managed with fusion at these levels.

When treating lateral canal stenosis, medial facetectomy, anterior facetectomy, or peridiscal osteophyte, debridement may be required depending on the level of pathology. More aggressively, total facetectomy and pars excision may also decompress the space, but the resulting instability will require fusion. A drain is typically placed deep to the fascial closure to decompress a potential postoperative hematoma and avoid cauda equina syndrome.

In the absence of instability, spinal stenosis can be treated with decompression alone, provided that the posterior elements are retained. When used to treated spondylolisthesis, 80% of laminectomy patients have excellent results provided the facets are preserved. Intertransverse or posterolateral fusions are recognized to improve these results.

Laminotomy

Laminotomy is traditionally performed for herniated nucleus pulposus or lateral canal stenosis and only the involved side needs to be exposed. The caudad edge of the lamina is progressively removed until there is sufficient exposure of the herniation and visualization lateral to the nerve root. As the nerve root is gently retracted toward the midline, the herniated material is debrided and a partial discectomy is performed. Closure is similar to a laminectomy but closed suction drainage is often not required.

Postoperative care is similar to that described for anterior lumbar interbody fusions, but without dietary restrictions.

LUMBAR DECOMPRESSION AND FUSION

Fusion is indicated for spinal instability, whether it is due to the primary pathology or when adequate decompression mandates compromising stability. Instability may be indicated by facet subluxation or spondylolisthesis greater than 25%.

If the same exposure can be used, most fusions will be performed during the same procedure following the decompression. Fusion methods are defined by the location of the fusion and the approach used to place the graft. Techniques include posterolateral fusion, posterior lumbar interbody fusion, transforaminal lumbar interbody fusion, extreme lateral interbody fusion, and anterior lumbar interbody fusion. Fusions may also be instrumented or uninstrumented. Instrumentation is usually segmental with pedicle screw and rod constructs and it has replaced historical nonsegmental hook/wire based fixation. Patient health notwithstanding, the foundation of successful fusion is preparation of the bony bed and mechanical stability.

Pedicle screw instrumentation has emerged as the most common spine fixation system. Screws are placed longitudinally within the pedicle with their sizes and trajectories selected to avoid perforation of the spinal canal and the anterior cortex of the vertebral body. Typically, the surgeon places a rigid rod longitudinally along each side of the spinous processes to connect all the screws along their respective sides. The rod and pedicle screws are fastened to together to create a fixed-angle construct. The two longitudinal rods may be connected with cross-links to improve torsional rigidity of the construct. If pedicle anatomy will not support screws, laminar hooks or sublaminar wires may be used to secure the rod to the spine. Bone graft is usually applied after instrumentation.

Pseudoarthrosis refers to the absence of bony bridging within the fusion mass or across vertebrae when evaluated with standard imaging modalities. The most common cause is smoking. Pseudoarthrosis rates vary widely, 3% to 68%, even when using the same technique. Many pseudoarthroses are asymptomatic, and others may be a source of persistent pain.

Adjacent segment degeneration remains a concern with any spine fusion construct. However, radiographic changes do not correlate with patient function. The relative contributions of natural lumbar degenerative changes and adjacent segment degeneration due to fusion remain undefined. Risk factors for adjacent segment degeneration include fusion instrumentation and length, sagittal malalignment, facet injury, age, and preexisting degenerative changes.

CONCLUSION

Hospitalists can play a critical role in the care of surgical patients, who often have significant comorbidities. Appropriate patient selection, surgical technique, and medical evaluation are critical to achieving successful results. Prophylaxis against infection and thromboembolic disease are routinely recommended. Early mobilization is essential and aided by anesthetic adjuncts and multimodal pain management. A multidisciplinary team approach requires effective and timely communication. Aggressive anticoagulation with intravenous heparin or therapeutic doses of low-molecular-weight heparin for suspected but not yet confirmed pulmonary embolism should be discussed with the orthopedic surgeon. In the absence of complications, significant improvements in quality of life are to be expected.

SUGGESTED READINGS

Hip and Knee

Guidelines on the prevention of symptomatic pulmonary embolism in patients undergoing hip or knee arthroplasty. American Academy of Orthopedic Surgeons. *Rosemont, IL:* 2007. Available at: http://www.aaos.org/research/guidelines/PEguide.asp. Accessed June 15, 2011.

Geerts WH, Berqqvist D, Pineo GF, et al. Prevention of venous thromboembolism: American College of Chest Physicians Evidence-Based Clinical Practice Guidelines. 8th ed. *Chest.* 2008;133 (suppl 6):381S–453S.

Cervical Spine

Bernhardt M, Hynes RA, Blume HW, AA White III. Current concepts review. Cervical spondylotic myelopathy. *J Bone Joint Surg Am.* 1993;75:119–128.

Clark CR. Cervical spondylotic myelopathy: history and physical findings. *Spine.* 1988;13:847–849.

Ferguson RJ, Caplan LR. Cervical spondylotic myelopathy. *Neurol Clin.* 1985;3:373–382.

Heller JG, Edwards CC II, Murakami H, Rodts GE. Laminoplasty versus laminectomy and fusion for multilevel cervical myelopathy: an independent matched cohort analysis. *Spine.* 2001;26:1330–1336.

Levine MJ, Albert TJ, Smith MD. Cervical radiculopathy: Diagnosis and nonoperative management. *J Am Acad Orthop Surg.* 1996;4: 305–316.

Rhee JM, Riew KD. Evaluation and management of neck pain, radiculopathy, and myelopathy. *Semin Spine Surg.* 2005;17: 174–185.

Sampath P, Bendebba M, Davis JD, Ducker TB. Outcome of patients treated for cervical myelopathy. A prospective, multicenter study with independent clinical review. *Spine.* 2000;25:670–676.

Lumbar Spine

Gibson JNA, G Waddell. Surgery for degenerative lumbar spondylosis [update of Cochrane Database Syst Rev. 2005;(2): CD001352]. Cochrane Database Syst Rev. 2005(4):CD001352.

Sengupta DK, HN Herkowitz. Lumbar spinal stenosis. Treatment strategies and indications for surgery. *Orthop Clin North Am.* 2003; 34(2):281–295.

Watters WC III, CM Bono, TJ Gilbert, et al. American Spine: 2009. An evidence-based clinical guideline for the diagnosis and treatment of degenerative lumbar spondylolisthesis. *Spine J.* 2009;9(7): 609–614.

CHAPTER 66

Rehabilitation of the Orthopedic Surgical Patient

Doris J. Armour, MD, MBA
John L. Lin, MD

INTRODUCTION

Acute rehabilitation tries to restore the premorbid physical and mental functioning of patients as much as possible by increasing muscle strength and patient endurance, improving muscular coordination and control, and providing adaptive equipment when necessary. Choosing the appropriate setting for provision of the needed services requires a working knowledge of the different levels of care available for rehabilitation services—acute inpatient rehabilitation, subacute rehabilitation, outpatient rehabilitation, and home health services. Determinants of the appropriate level of care include the functional limitations of the patient, the need for medical monitoring, social support, cognitive functioning, nursing needs, therapeutic disciplines required, and ability to tolerate three hours of therapy a day.

The Centers for Medicaid and Medicare Services recently instituted a prospective payment system for acute inpatient rehabilitation facilities. For Medicare approved facilities, a certain percentage of all admitted patients must have 1 of 13 diagnoses: stroke, brain injury, burns, SCI, neurological disorders, major multiple trauma, congenital abnormalities, inflammatory polyarthritis with impairments of ambulation and ADLs that have not responded to less intensive therapies, amputations, hip fractures, bilateral joint replacements, and unilateral joint replacements in individuals > 80 years old or the morbidly obese. Rehabilitation centers must provide, and patients admitted to the acute rehabilitation center must require, interdisciplinary, team-based care, 24-hour rehabilitation nursing, daily physician assessment, and three hours of therapy daily. The interdisciplinary team in acute rehabilitation facilities consists of a physician leader, registered nurse (RN) with rehabilitation certification or expertise, physical therapy, occupational therapy, speech therapy, therapeutic recreation, social work, nutrition, neuropsychology, and often psychology, an orthotist, prosthetist, and a chaplain. Patients receive therapy five to seven days a week (**Table 66-1**).

Long-term acute care (LTAC) facilities may also provide daily therapies using speech (ST), physical (PT), and occupational therapy (OT) but these facilities are best suited for patients whose medical needs, such as ventilatory support, telemetry, wound care, long-term IV antibiotics, and administration of chemotherapy, preclude their participation in rehabilitation at an intensive level. By providing highly concentrated medical and nursing services that exceed the level of medical care that can be delivered at a skilled nursing facility, LTAC is considered hospital-level care. The LTAC rehabilitation goals resemble that of the acute inpatient rehabilitation with the goal of establishing and maintaining medical stability. The length of hospitalization typically lasts longer, around 25 days. If they meet criteria, patients may be admitted to acute rehabilitation following a LTAC stay (**Table 66-2**).

At either type of facility, rehabilitation or LTAC, the rehabilitation professionals simultaneously provide care for cancer, cardiovascular, musculoskeletal, neurologic, pulmonary, organ transplantation, postoperative and trauma complication, and other medical comorbid conditions (**Table 66-3**).

This chapter will focus on rehabilitation of patients hospitalized for orthopedic problems affecting the spine or lower extremities. Typical conditions requiring hospital-level rehabilitation include: traumatic spinal cord injury, intervertebral disc prolapse, transverse myelitis; joint replacement surgery, particularly hip arthroplasty; spinal surgery, limb amputation, limb trauma, heterotopic ossification, and compartment syndromes.

TABLE 66-1 Criteria for Admission to Acute Rehabilitation

Preadmission assessment must include:

- Prior level of function
- Expected level of improvement
- Expected length of time to accomplish improvement
- Risk for clinical complications (ie, decubitus ulcer, UTI, etc.)
- Condition that caused need for rehabilitation (etiologic diagnosis, ie, stroke)
- The impairments necessitating rehabilitation (diagnosis, ie, hemiparesis, dysphagia)
- Combination of treatments needed (wound care, bowel/bladder training, antibiotics, therapies)
- Expected duration of rehabilitation
- Anticipated discharge destination (must be to community, SNF is not an acceptable discharge destination)
- Any anticipated post acute rehabilitation therapies needed (ie, HH, outpatient therapy)

Acute inpatient rehabilitation is deemed reasonable and necessary if:

- Multiple therapy disciplines are needed (PT, OT, and or ST) and PT/OT referral from the index hospital
- Intensive level of rehabilitation provided (three hours per day and at least five days a week)
- Ability to participate in intensive therapy and make reasonable improvement demonstrated
- MD supervision provided on a daily basis
- Interdisciplinary team approach utilized
- Insurance approval required prior to transfer

HH, home health aid; OT, occupational therapy; PT, physical therapy; SNF, skilled nursing facility; ST, speech therapy; UTI, urinary tract infection.

Optimal transitions to acute rehabilitation require a collaborative assessment with the multidisciplinary health care team to determine the therapeutic disciplines needed and the extent of recovery anticipated. The team should also identify any medical comorbidities such as cardiopulmonary disease, hospital-acquired complications such as delirium, and any unresolved issues that will impede the patient's ability to participate in rehabilitation activities. The rehabilitation plan must address any impairment of motor, sensory, cognitive, communication, and emotional functioning.

Patients should expect three hours of therapy daily in 30 to 90 minute sessions, at least five days a week. They should view acute inpatient rehabilitation as the initial phase of their rehabilitation program and anticipate continuing that program post discharge with home-based therapies or in outpatient facilities. Patients and their caretakers will be informed of their rehabilitation goals and their expected length of stay within a few days of admission, and receive weekly progress reports following weekly team meetings reviewing attainment of stated goals and any barriers to progress.

THERAPEUTIC MODALITIES

EXERCISE

Exercise, the cornerstone of rehabilitation, can be designed to improve strength, improve balance, and increase endurance and range of motion. Strength combats sarcopenia and imbalance. Strength training programs involve movement against resistance (typically with rubber bands or the body's own weight). Balance exercises, for those individuals at high risk for falling involve practicing standing on uneven surfaces, one extremity, or on the balance beam. Exercises to improve endurance involve continuous activity such as walking and swimming. Improved endurance increases capacity for activities of daily living (ADLs) and for ambulation. Prolonged, low-intensity stretching exercises may also improve range of motion and increase flexibility.

PHYSICAL MODALITIES

Physical modalities such as heat, cold, massage, electrotherapy, and phototherapy may be used in conjunction with exercise to decrease pain and improve range of motion. The most substantial evidence for the efficacy of these therapies supports the use of electrotherapy, particularly in wound healing. Thermal therapies

TABLE 66-2 Alternative Options to Acute Rehabilitation

	Services	Eligibility	Emphasis
Subacute rehabilitation	Requires assistance with wound care, IV medications, and PT, OT, and ST; up to 2 hours of therapy each day; seen by a physician weekly or monthly; in general, 1:1 sitters must not be required for 24 hours prior to transfer; requires a 3-day hospital stay for Medicare to approve; some facilities may provide hospice care for patients with life expectancy of less than 6 months	Patients who do not require, or who cannot tolerate the more aggressive pace of acute rehabilitation yet require supervision and/or support for ADLs not available in the community	Up to 2 hours of therapy a day up to 5 days a week
Home care	PT, OT, and ST in the home setting; hospice care including nursing care, pain control, spiritual or emotional counseling, symptom management	Patients who are homebound or who require assistance to get out of the home	Safe mobility and performance of activities of daily living (ADLs) in the home, generally 1 to 2 times a week over a period of a few weeks
Outpatient therapy (Some offer more comprehensive and intensive day programs similar in intensity to inpatient acute rehabilitation therapy).	PT/OT/ST/TR/SW and nursing as well as orthotists, prosthetists, and neuropsychology services	Patients who need and can tolerate more aggressive therapy and who can be safely cared for at home	Therapy 4 to 5 hours per day, 5 days a week

ADL, acitivity of daily living; OT, occupational therapy; PT, physical therapy; ST, speech therapy; SW, social worker; TR, therapeutic recreation.

TABLE 66-3 Acute Rehabilitation Providers

Provider	Methods of Evaluation and Treatment
Physical therapy	• Assess muscle strength, joint range of motion, gait, and mobility • Provide exercise training to improve strength, ROM, endurance, balance • Employ physical modalities (heat, ultrasound, electrical stimulation, massage) to treat lower body deficits
Occupational therapy	• Assess joint strength and range of motion • Assess self-care skills (grooming, bathing, eating, toileting) • Assess ability to perform ADLs (food preparation, household activities) • Provide self-care, ADL training, assistive devices • Assess home safety (such as assessing which bathroom aids such as grab bars, raised toilet seat, and shower chairs would most benefit the patient) • Provide physical modalities (heat, ultrasound, e-stim, massage) to treat upper extremity deficits • Fabricate splints
Speech therapy	• Treat dysphagia, recommend diet consistencies to accommodate impairments of swallow • Assess speech, comprehension, cognition, and treat communication deficits
Recreation therapist	• Assess leisure skills and interests • Increase social interaction, which may include horticultural, music, and dance therapies • Facilitate community reentry • Can also facilitate some vocational activities
Rehabilitation nurse	• Evaluate self-care needs • Evaluate family/caretaker and home factors • Provide self-care training including bowel, bladder, and wound care • Instruct how to administer and monitor medications
Social worker	• Evaluate family/caretaker and home factors • Provide counseling • Assess psychosocial factors • Arrange home heath or outpatient post discharge services and equipment • Coordinate team
Nutritionist	• Assess nutritional status • Recommend diet to optimize nutrition and compensate comorbidities • Assist with recommendations for enteral and parenteral feeds when necessary
Neuropsychologist	• Assess cognition: judgment, reasoning, insight, executive functioning, recall, learning • Provide recommendations to patient, team, and family for compensating for deficits in cognition • Provide assistance with coping
Orthotist	• Make and fit orthotics such as braces, ankle-foot orthotics
Prosthetist	• Make and fit prosthetic limbs

include superficial modalities such as paraffin, heat packs, heating pads, and whirlpool, and deep modalities such as ultrasound and acoustical energy, which after absorbed by tissues converts to heat. Thermal therapies help eliminate edema, decrease pain, and increase extensibility of connective tissues. Delivered by cold packs, ice massage, vasocoolant sprays, and cold water immersion, cryotherapies decrease pain, especially in spastic extremities, thereby allowing more painless movement. Electrotherapy can be used for wound care but also includes transcutaneous electrical nerve stimulation (TENS) for pain and neuromuscular stimulation to enhance functional movement patterns such as with foot drop. Delivered via pads that emit light energy, phototherapy may help manage pain and provide wound therapy by enhancing nitric oxide release from hemoglobin.

ADAPTIVE EQUIPMENT

Adaptive and assistive devices enable patients to engage in activities otherwise impeded by their impairments. Assistive devices for mobility include straight and quad canes, standard and forearm crutches, and walkers (standard, rolling, rollator, and platform) as well as standard, motorized wheelchairs, and scooters for nonambulatory patients. Aids also exist for daily living activities such as utensils with enlarged handles for eating and assistive devices for manipulating buttons, zippers, and donning socks and shoes.

Spinal orthoses allow for healing of the nonosseous structures and maturation of stabilization by restricting range of motion of the spine. The terminology used for spinal orthosis, that is, braces, is uniform across organizations such as the American Academy of Orthotists and Prosthetists, American Academy of Physical Medicine and Rehabilitation, and American Academy of Orthopedic Surgeons. The terminology extends superiorly and inferiorly, describing the contiguous spinal segments involved by the orthosis. For example, any neck collar may be described as cervical orthosis, whereas body braces involving the thorax and the abdomen may be described as thoracolumbar orthosis. Typical acronyms for these are CO and TLO, respectively. Commonly, a TLSO is ordered to minimize mobilization of the thoracic, lumbar, and sacral spinal segments. Different orthoses may allow different freedom of movement in different planes, such as flexion, extension, lateral flexion, or rotation.

THE HIP

Hip fractures are almost always the consequence of a ground-level fall of an osteoporotic patient. The precipitating trauma can, however, be minimal depending on the degree of osteoporosis. Hip fractures present with acute pain, inability to walk, or pain on ambulation. The affected limb will typically be externally rotated, abducted, and shortened. Patients with avascular necrosis of the hip will have pain or discomfort of the hip with internal rotation, external rotation, and abduction of the hip and an antalgic gait. Hip fractures are classified as intracapsular (displaced or undisplaced femoral neck fractures) or extracapsular (stable or unstable intertrochanteric). Broadly divided into two basic types, simple and complex, acetabular fractures are almost always caused by trauma. Hip dislocations occur anterior (femoral head rests anterior to coronal plane of acetabulum) or posterior (femoral head rests posterior to the coronal plane of the acetabulum) in location. Anteroposterior (AP) pelvis and frog lateral radiographs of the hip can often diagnose avascular necrosis of the hip. Sclerotic changes of the femoral head can be one of the earliest changes of avascular necrosis but collapse of the femoral head can be seen. AP pelvis and groin lateral plain radiographs are usually sufficient to diagnose fractures of the pelvis and hip joint. If radiographs are negative but symptoms and risk factors support the diagnosis of avascular necrosis of the hip, MRI imaging should be obtained.

Anterior and posterior hip dislocations can start touch down weight bearing (or toe touch weight bearing) with a walker and assisted range of motion (ROM) within two days of reduction with progression to partial weight bearing and active ROM within one week. Progression to weight bearing as tolerated with resistance exercise generally occurs by the sixth week post injury.

The initial phase of the operatively managed femur fracture as well as the total hip arthroplasty (THA) for arthritis begins in the immediate postoperative period. Hip precautions are designed to prevent dislocation of the prosthetic joint. Posterior precautions consist of avoiding hip flexion greater than 90°, hip adduction, and internal rotation past midline. Anterior precautions avoid hip extension and external rotation. Hip precautions are adhered to until week six. Following repairs entailing total or hemiarthroplasty, OT includes education about hip precautions and training in safely accomplishing ADLs with emphasis on transfers and on mobility with weight bearing precautions. Intertrochanteric hip fractures are generally weight bearing as tolerated (WBAT); intracapsular fractures are partial weight bearing (PWB) or touch down weight bearing (TDWB), THA are WBAT. Hip and weight bearing precautions are maintained until 6 to 12 weeks post surgery.

Exercise protocols during the immediate postoperative period vary somewhat from facility to facility but generally consist of ankle pumps, hip flexions, quadriceps, and gluteal sets and exercises to strengthen hip abductors. These exercises aim to maximize strength, mobility, flexibility, and minimize risk of dislocation and excessive wear on the prosthetic joint. There are no prospective randomized trials to determine which protocols are most effective. Patients then advance to ambulation with a cane and pursue more aggressive resistance exercises, increasing endurance and facilitating gait patterns, which permit greater mobility in the community.

THE PELVIS

The pelvis allows transfer of weight from the vertebral column to the acetabula and the hip joints transfer the weight down to the legs. Patients with pelvic fractures present with acute onset of pain, tenderness to palpation over the area of fracture, and pain with weight bearing. Despite the variability in different classification schema for acute pelvic fractures, management depends on the presence or absence of displacement and stability. Pelvic fractures are divided into two types depending on the severity of the injury to the pelvic ring:

1. Low-energy injuries are fractures of individual bones of the pelvis that do not disrupt the integrity of the ring. Usually ground-level falls, sports injuries, low velocity motor vehicle accidents (MVAs), or avulsion injuries (in skeletally immature patients) cause low energy injuries.
2. High-energy fractures, often associated with soft tissues and visceral injury, disrupt the integrity of the pelvic ring due to two or more pelvic bone fractures. Higher velocity MVAs, falls from a height, and crush injuries typically cause high energy injuries fractures.

Sacral fractures can result from trauma or occur as insufficiency fractures in patients with osteoporosis and minimal antecedent trauma. Most pelvic fractures can be managed conservatively but unstable fractures may require internal fixation.

Weight bearing status in the operatively managed patient depends on the stability of the pelvis. If there is posterior stability, full weight bearing is permitted. If there is posterior instability, touch down weight bearing on the affected side is advised. If there is bilateral disruption posteriorly, no weight bearing is permitted.

THE KNEE

The goal of postoperative rehabilitation of total knee replacement (TKR) is to restore mobility, strength, and flexibility and to minimize complications such as deep venous thrombosis (DVT) and infection. The rehabilitation team emphasizes adherence to precautions and exercise protocols to protect prosthetic joint integrity and optimize function. Most protocols advocate early out of bed with range of motion exercises of the knee progressing to both isotonic and isometric exercises of the knee and hip musculature by the fourth postoperative day. Supine knee extension is encouraged throughout. Manual knee flexion helps improve ROM. Gait training for patients who are able to handle assistive devices begins within a few postoperative days. Use of a continuous passive motion (CPM) machine following TKR has been shown in multiple studies to improve knee flexion earlier, decrease the need for manual mobilization, and lessen pain without a measurable difference in long-term outcomes.

AMPUTATIONS

The patient with an amputation requires, arguably, the most comprehensive skills and attention of the rehabilitation team. Loss of part or all of a limb and the associated impairment often causes significant psychological impact. Rehabilitation of the amputee begins early in the postoperative period with education on proper positioning, ROM, and mobilization of the hip and knee, and assessment of needs for durable medical equipment and adaptive equipment. Careful attention must be paid to wound care and control of edema in the residual wound, particularly since a large proportion of amputations occur in patients with some underlying vascular insufficiency. Compressive wraps and dressings, such as a stockinette, may promote wound healing and lessen pain by reducing edema. The team must inspect the wound daily, especially after weight bearing activity.

Knee and hip flexion contractures and hip abduction and external rotation are common consequences of below-the-knee and above-the-knee amputations respectively. The rehabilitation process, which begins in the hospital and continues in the rehabilitation facility includes:

- Critical education about proper positioning
- Extension exercises, including prone positioning and use of knee extension boards or knee immobilizers
- Strengthening of the hip and knee extenders, an important adjunct to proper positioning
- Exercises to improve arm strength and to increase endurance and conditioning
- Optimization of comorbid conditions such as diabetes

The social supports available to the amputee along with the home environment help guide treatment choices and can impact functional outcomes. Patients are generally fitted for a custom prosthesis after the wound is completely healed and postoperative pain and edema have resolved, typically two to six months post amputation.

THE SPINE

The anterior, middle, and posterior columns achieve the stability of the spine. Anterior longitudinal ligaments, the anterior half of vertebral body, and the anterior half of annulus fibrosus make up the anterior column. The posterior vertebral body, posterior annulus fibrosus, and the posterior longitudinal ligament form the middle column. All the spinal structures posterior to the apex of the spinous processes, inclusive of the pedicles, articular processes, the lamina, and the ligamental complex make up the posterior column. Trauma, spinal stenosis, osteophytes, foraminal stenosis, ligamental hypertrophy, ligamental ossification, disc herniation, or desiccations can encroach upon neural elements, thereby causing pain and sensory or motor deficits by encroaching upon neural elements. In traumatic spine injuries, the pathological process involves an unstable spine defined as disruption of the middle column or involvement of two columns. For the traumatic cervical spine, mechanisms of injuries include flexion, extension, or compressive forces, most commonly from motor vehicle crash, fall, and sports activity. Extra-osseous injuries, such as ligamental injuries, may also account for significant neurologic sequelae, especially in the upper cervical spine.

In the majority of cases a plain radiograph of the primary area will identify the injury, keeping in mind that approximately 5–20% of injuries may be seen in a different spinal segment. Because plain radiographs do not always identify structural deficits, a significant fracture identified by screening imaging or significant neurologic alteration should be further evaluated with advanced imaging by either computed tomography or MRI. Radiographic criteria for vertebral instability includes greater than 2 mm deviation of any of the following: displacement, interlaminar space widening, facet joint widening, vertebral canal enlargement, and posterior vertebral body line disruption.

Upon admission to the rehabilitation ward, a detailed examination of the post–spine stabilization patient should include examination of the integrity and stability of the spine and a neurological examination of the spinal cord function. Patients with disproportional increase in pain with motion need to have radiographic confirmation of spinal stability prior to further intervention. Although anteroposterior and lateral plain films of the spine suffice for the majority of the cases, pathology involving the C1 and C2 segments may require special studies, for example, open mouth odontoid views or computed tomography.

All surgical recommendations for orthotic wear should be strictly followed. If one is not prescribed, pain-limiting active range of motion by the patient should be performed in a supine position for lateral flexion and rotation, and in a lateral decubitus position for forward flexion and extension. Although operative stabilization is likely to restrict full range of motion, any instability or disproportional pain warrants further radiographic study.

The American Spinal Injury Association impairment rating examination should be performed to assess the spinal cord function. At a minimum the examiner should assess the function of the posterior column and the spinal-thalamic tracts by using a pin and a cotton swab to detect pin prick and light touch sensations. Manual muscle testing should be directed at the examinable spinal root levels, for example, C5-T1 and L2-S1:

- Biceps brachii in elbow flexion (C5)
- Extensor carpi radialis in wrist extension (C6)
- Triceps in elbow extension (C7)
- Flexor digitorum profundus in finger flexion of the distal interphalangeal joint of the middle finger (C8)
- Abductor digiti minimi in small finger abduction (T1)
- Iliopsoas in hip flexion (L2)
- Quadriceps in knee extension (L3)
- Tibialis anterior in ankle dorsiflexion (L4)
- Extensor hallucis longus in great toe extension (L5)
- Gastroc-soleus complex in ankle plantar flexion (S1)

In addition, a rectal examination should assess sensation and anal sphincter contraction for spinal root levels S4-5. These examinations serve the important function of establishing a baseline for all future sensory and motor changes.

A baseline plain radiograph of the spine is usually performed at the receiving rehabilitation facility for comparison prior to later discontinuation of an orthosis. The timing of poststabilization radiograph may vary widely from case to case, typically 4 to 12 weeks for maturation with limitation of external spinal orthosis. The following factors commonly prolong the length of time that orthosis should restrict range of motion: the mobility of the segment of instrumentation (longer with cervical or lumbar injury), osteopenia/osteoporosis, and more extensive spinal injuries.

In posttraumatic compression fracture, the principal therapeutic exercises avoid the flexion-based mechanics that initially led to the injury. Thus, a lumbar extension–based exercise should be prescribed for patients who have suffered a lumbar fracture.

In fractures of the posterior elements, extension-based exercises are restricted. The primary therapy goals are strengthening of the lumbar flexors and minimizing lumbar lordosis through stretching of the paraspinals.

MEDICAL COMPLICATIONS

Most patients admitted to hospital-level care have significant comorbid diseases that require skilled nursing care. Nursing care is integral to the inpatient's rehabilitative treatments as patients are often partially, if not at times completely, dependent, due to pain, orthotic restrictions, or neurologic impairments. Patients with ventilatory failure need respiratory therapy support. Patients with quadriplegia require frequent turns, usually every two hours, to prevent decubitus ulcers. More mobile patients may require assisted transfers out of bed to a mobility device, for example, to a walker or wheelchair.

Bladder dysfunction may result from multifactorial causes, including postoperative paralytic atony, narcotic use, neurogenic bowel and bladder, symptomatic urinary tract infections, and infrequently trigone irritation. For bladder care, discontinue the Foley catheter when patients have regained functional toiletry mobility or as soon as possible to avoid hospital-acquired urinary tract infections. Urinary retention may indicate persistent vesicular atony, which may require timed voiding or intermittent catheterization for postvoid residual volumes persistently greater than 150 ml. If bladder ultrasound scans are not readily available, direct catheterizations can assess postvoid residual volumes. Most of the patients with quadriparetic injuries safely continue Foley catheterizations during the hospitalization period.

Bowel function often parallels that of bladder function. Similar etiologies leading to bladder dysfunction (eg, postoperative paralytic atony, narcotic use, or neurogenic bowel) commonly cause constipation. Stool softeners are ineffective in the treatment of preexisting constipation, obstipation, or partial obstruction or in the setting of chronic opioid use. Laxatives such as magnesium citrate or enemas may be used for short-term relief but are not advocated for long-term bowel function. For patients with neurogenic bowel, long-term maintenance of bowel function requires a consistent bowel regimen. A crucial component of a functional bowel program starts with good diet with adequate dietary fiber and fluid intake, accompanied by maintenance of a soft stool consistency with additional stool softeners. However, the essential component to the long-term maintenance is the use of intrinsic colonic reflexes, for example, gastrocolic, rectocolic, or colo-colonic reflexes. Suppositories or digital rectal examination stimulate the rectum. Digital rectal stimulation, an example of the recto-colic reflex, differs from digital rectal disimpaction because the stimulation of the rectal mucosa continues even after the evacuation of bowel content from the rectum in order to trigger the massive colonic propulsive movement through the recto-colic reflex. Prolonged use of incontinence briefs and rectal tubes are discouraged due to perineal and anal irritations and injuries.

DISCHARGE PLANNING

Physical therapists should begin treatment before the patient leaves the hospital and they are required to make specific recommendations to the receiving facility. Physicians need to work with hospital discharge planners to plan for the expected discharge date, prepare the appropriate paperwork, communicate the discharge plan to the patient and family who must be in agreement, and ensure that appropriate medications and special equipment have been approved by insurance and will be available at the receiving facility. It is critically important to have an accurate discharge medication list.

A postdischarge phone call from the health care team to the receiving rehabilitation hospital may help ensure a safe transition, answer any questions about the transfer, and avoid any unnecessary transfers back to the index hospital.

PRACTICE POINT

Discharge information to rehabilitation

Detailed instructions for specific drugs in addition to an updated, reconciled discharge medication list:

1. Anticoagulation
   Warfarin: start date, recent dosage changes, target INR, duration of treatment, date of next scheduled INR, responsible clinic or physician for monitoring
   Low-molecular-weight heparin: duration of treatment, time of next scheduled dose, any insurance issues, as patients may not be able to afford medication after discharge from rehabilitation
2. Antibiotics
   Duration of treatment: presence of long line versus PICC line and documentation of placement of the line
   Indications for an extended course of antibiotics and identification of who should be consulted in case problems arise, and monitor therapy if continued post rehabilitation
   Any insurance issues: availability of coverage for IV medications once patient leaves rehabilitation
3. Narcotic/benzodiazepine dosing
   Indication, therapeutic endpoint, recent changes and reason
4. Insulin therapy
   Indicate exact doses, whether additional control was required by a sliding scale, and include amount of additional insulin in prior 24 hours as well as whether there were any issues relating to hypoglycemia
5. Oncology Medications
   Specify exact treatment with prescriptions at least 1–2 days before discharge

Nutrition

1. If total parenteral nutrition or tube feedings, include orders and prescriptions if required
2. Specify goal of therapy and who will follow-up

Supplemental Oxygen

Document O_2 saturation and requirement of O_2 to maintain O_2 saturation above 88%

Special Equipment (VAC dressings, pleurax catheters)

May or may not be covered by insurance and can take time to obtain

Monitoring

1. Document monitoring required for all drugs, TPN, and other Interventions and whether patient had developed any signs or symptoms of toxicities during hospitalization, what medications were used but discontinued with reason
2. Dry weight and diuresis goals
3. Wound
4. Blood pressure

Very brief description of reason for index admission, hospital course, complications of hospitalization, how the patient is at time of discharge (cognitive, cardiopulmonary, and functional status)

Consultation during prior hospitalization

1. Document final impression or send with patient consult note
2. Identify consultants by name and who to contact if a problem arises

Brief summary of relevant and abnormal test results and identification of person responsible for follow-up of abnormal or pending test findings and unresolved issues as well as follow-up appointments with consultants and primary care physician

Family spokesperson with numbers, code status, health care proxy

Goals for rehabilitation if not obvious and contingency planning if patient does not respond to treatment

CONCLUSION

The timing of the transition to acute rehabilitation is critical in order to restore the premorbid physical and mental functioning of patients as much as possible. Hospitalists can optimize care transitions by recommending the best setting for provision of the needed services, initiating appropriate inpatient consultation and screening. Planning discharge requires recognizing the functional limitations of the patient, the need for medical monitoring, social support, cognitive functioning, nursing needs, therapeutic disciplines required, and ability to tolerate 3 hours of therapy a day. It also requires effective communication with all members of the health care team, patients, and families, physicians who will care for the patient following transfer, and primary care physicians who will see the patient following discharge from rehabilitation. A discharge checklist may facilitate this process so that key information such as pending test results is not overlooked.

SUGGESTED READINGS

Brander V, Mullarkey C. Rehabilitation after Total Hip Replacement for Osteoarthritis. *Physical Medicine and Rehabilitation: State of the Art Reviews.* 2002;16(3):415–430.

Kaplan R, Gilbert A, Rehabilitation after Pelvic and Hip Fractures. *Physical Medicine and Rehabilitation: State of the Art Reviews.* 2002;16(3):389–414.

Kuiken T, Huang M, Harden N. Perioperative Rehabilitation of the Transtibial and Transfemoral Amputee. *Physical Medicine and Rehabilitation: State of the Art Reviews.* 2002;16(3):521–538.

Mullarkey C, Brander V. Rehabilitation after Total Knee Replacement for Osteoarthritis. *Physical Medicine and Rehabilitation: State of the Art Reviews.* 2002;16(3):415–430.

CHAPTER 67

Co-Management of Orthopedic Patients

Christopher Whinney, MD, FACP, FHM

INTRODUCTION

Musculoskeletal disorders and diseases are the leading cause of disability in the United States and account for more than one-half of all chronic conditions in people over 50 years of age in developed countries. More than one in four Americans have a musculoskeletal condition requiring medical attention. Annual direct and indirect costs for bone and joint health are $849 billion, 7.7% of the gross domestic product.

Based on this data it is little wonder that orthopedic surgery will have increasing volumes of patient visits and operative interventions in the coming years, especially in the setting of an aging population with increasing expectations for functional recovery and quality of life. The challenge associated with this growth will be the increasing number of medical comorbidities in these older patients and the need for a systematic evaluation of such comorbidities to optimize the perioperative course. It is estimated that surgery-related costs will rise 50% and surgical complications 100% in the United States in the next two decades.

From the beginning hospitalists have filled a collaborative role, assuming care of primary care physicians' patients in the hospital. Just as primary care physicians (PCPs) cannot feasibly be in two places at once (the office and the hospital), surgeons cannot simultaneously manage complex inpatients and perform surgeries. Combining limited surgical availability with restricted surgical resident work hours, which creates added pressure for surgical residents to maximize operating room time, the active involvement of a medical comanager makes great practical and economic sense if it is planned well and actively managed.

LITERATURE ON ORTHOPEDIC COMANAGEMENT

Early literature on orthopedic comanagement focused on geriatrician collaboration with surgeons. Despite inconsistent data on length of hospital stay and mortality, these studies and more recent ones demonstrate that systematic geriatric evaluation and management can decrease the incidence of common postoperative medical complications such as congestive heart failure, arrhythmias, venous thromboembolism (VTE), and delirium, and improve compliance with antiosteoporotic therapy and VTE prophylaxis. More recent literature has focused on hospitalist collaboration with orthopedics and has shown lower adjusted length of hospital stay and decreased complication rates in some studies, although mortality and readmission rates were not changed. In one study of hip fracture patients, delirium was diagnosed more often in the comanagement group, but this was associated with an earlier discharge after surgery. This may reflect greater attention to the presence of delirium, better documentation, and more prompt treatment.

In practice, comanagement is becoming a more prominent practice pattern especially as an integrated part of hospitalist practice. A recent retrospective study of Medicare beneficiaries has shown an 11.4% per year rise in comanagement practice by generalist physicians between 2001 and 2006. Thus, in all likelihood, the practice of comanagement by hospitalists will not wane, and more surgeons, especially orthopedists, will call on hospitalists in this collaborative spirit. The 2005–2006 Society of Hospital Medicine (SHM) survey indicated that 85% of Hospital Medicine groups did a form of comanagement.

PLANNING STAGES

Comanagement of surgical (and medical subspecialty) patients has rapidly evolved with much initial enthusiasm. However, when proposals do not clearly delineate the nature of these relationships, great potential for confusion of roles, miscommunication, suboptimal patient care, and dissatisfaction of both parties can result as the service expands and staffing becomes more of an issue.

Based on the author's experience and on other hospitalists' successful collaborations, this chapter will suggest specific steps that can be taken to initiate a potential orthopedic comanagement effort and avoid common pitfalls. Institutional support for this activity is paramount and the medical administration should be involved in these initial meetings from the outset. Initially, ask the following questions:

1. Why are we doing this?

To start out, it is best to clarify explicitly the motivation for starting such a program: Are the surgeons stretched thin between operating room (OR) time and patient care responsibilities on the floors and in the office? Are orthopedic residents more limited by duty hour restrictions and therefore less able to focus on patient care on the floors? Are there concerns with care quality within the standard structure of medical subspecialty consultation? Are nursing and ancillary staff having issues with access to practitioners for patient medical needs and issues? Do they want someone to take on the burden of doing histories and physicals and discharge notes and summaries? These are just a few questions that might help to focus the expectations of the proposing orthopedists.

2. Is the hospitalist service the best solution to this problem?

Once it becomes clear what your orthopedic colleagues desire, then clarify how hospitalist services and skills can (or should) address these issues. Is a hospitalist the best solution to this problem? Certainly hospitalists are adept at addressing medical issues in hospitalized patients as medical consultants, but to what degree should they assume the detailed minutia of patient care (ie, acetaminophen orders, renewing intravenous (IV) fluids)? This presents the potential to become a "glorified resident" in the care of these patients, which many hospitalists abhor. In addition, issues like surgical wound care and drain management may be pushed upon hospitalists despite concerns that their scope of practice exceeds their internal medicine training. Similar concerns have been raised when hospitalists assume primary responsibility for patients with intracranial bleeds for neurosurgeons.

3. What other solutions have been considered?

If the first call from nursing for a problem traditionally has gone to orthopedic residents and/or staff who now are tied up elsewhere, is the hospitalist the next logical call in an equitable "comanagement" relationship? Some newer hospitalists or hospitalist groups may accept this as part of their growth and cultivation of their practice; whereas others fear the mission creep to becoming a "glorified resident," as described previously. In our institution, nurses channel most first calls for a variety of issues to one nurse practitioner (NP) and one physician's assistant (PA), both stationed on the dedicated orthopedic ward. If relevant medical issues arise that require hospitalist involvement, they will find us on the ward and relay the information to us. This allows us as hospitalists to focus on the more sophisticated medical issues that are more consistent with our scope of practice; in addition, we can also serve as the gatekeeper to further subspecialty consultation when needed, avoiding superfluous consultations and testing.

4. Will a comanagement service jeopardize other relationships, such as with subspecialty consultants and with other medical groups in a community hospital setting?
5. Should the hospitalist service initially limit comanagement to specific patient demographics for the orthopedist, such as for certain PCPs who admit their patients?

ANALYZE THE CURRENT STRUCTURE

Analysis of the current structure of care delivery in orthopedics serves a useful measurement both as a baseline and after the intervention. In our analysis at the Cleveland Clinic, we found that there were significant differences in the delivery of care on medical services and on orthopedic services due to the following factors:

- Limited supervision of medical care provided by the NP and PA.
- Competing responsibilities of orthopedic residents providing backup for other providers or assisting in the OR.
- Lack of internal medicine training of orthopedic residents to address complicated medical issues.
- Significant medical comorbidities of patients requiring routine medical surveillance to prevent, detect, and intervene during their hospitalization.
- Limitations of general medical consultation service that typically "reacts" to consultation requests when problems have already been identified and lacks the capacity to prospectively affirm or develop a medical plan of care for high-risk or complicated medical patients.

CLARIFY ROLES AND EXPECTATIONS

At this point clarifying and documenting roles and expectations can avoid the potential for confusion and divisiveness. **Table 67-1** outlines our expectations for our hospitalist roles and responsibilities and the ongoing orthopedic roles and responsibilities. **Table 67-2** lists the conditions that should trigger referral to the hospitalist comanagement service.

These are not firm and inflexible rules; other comanagement relationships may opt to take on some of the responsibilities listed above in the orthopedic section, such as blood and fluid management, pain management, and family communication, all of which are in a reasonable scope of hospitalist practice. However, it is critical to delineate who will take on these tasks and to have a mechanism for resolution of disagreements.

Periodic meetings between hospitalist and orthopedic champions as well as nursing, other members of the comanagement team, and administration should review program functioning and processes of care; address specific problems in direct patient care; and further define roles and expectations. In addition, this group may assess the impact of the comanagement service on teaching of medical and surgical trainees and explore future directions. Our medicine housestaff now routinely rotate with our hospitalist comanager as part of an innovative medical consultation experience, and our relationship provides new opportunities for creating academic value such as the potential for publication of program outcomes, collaboration in research, and orthopedic quality improvement projects. **Table 67-3** delineates the development timeline of our comanagement service.

PATIENT SELECTION AND TRIAGE

Decisions about which patients should be followed by the comanager should be based on patient needs and provider capacity. Patients with minimal or no medical comorbidities rarely benefit from hospitalist input and may only serve to direct clinician

TABLE 67-1 **Delineation of Hospitalist versus Orthopedics Roles and Responsibilities**

Hospitalist	Orthopedics
Confer each morning with orthopedic providers and review outpatient preoperative assessment (done in our hospitalist-run preoperative clinic) or the medical comorbidities of nonelective admissions to identify suitable patients for comanagement.	Retain the appropriate clinical support infrastructure including residents and current physician's assistant and nurse practitioner positions.
Promptly evaluate and document findings on comanaged patients, and enter orders on these patients.	Perform daily rounding, assessments, and progress notes and orders for routine and stable medical issues including postoperative orders.
Follow-up on tests and studies ordered by the comanager.	Address the "first call" from nurses for questions and patient assessments, perform full and appropriate patient assessments prior to calling medical physicians for further support.
Provide formal and informal preoperative and postoperative medical consultation as requested.	Remain as primary service for patients without substantial medical complexity.
Provide teaching to orthopedic surgery service providers on medical issues.	Provide night, weekend, and holiday coverage of orthopedic patients with support by the medicine consult resident.
Participate in daily multidisciplinary rounds with nursing, nonphysician providers, and case management to identify patients with ongoing medical needs not otherwise captured by the mechanisms above.	Follow-up on studies and tests ordered by the orthopedic service.
	Address routine postoperative management orders including: Initiate and comply with orthopaedic protocols. Manage blood and fluids. Manage pain and routine prn medications. Order DVT prophylaxis and medications. Assess and care for wounds and order perioperative antibiotics. Admit and plan discharge, prepare forms, and provide discharge prescriptions. Communicate with families and facilitate discharge planning.

efforts away from the patients that need more intensive medical attention. Patients with acutely decompensated problems and/or multiple chronic comorbidities will more likely benefit from comanagement attention; in some circumstances admission to a medical service with orthopedic consultation may be the most appropriate path. **Figure 67-1** delineates the decision process for triage at our institution.

ROLE OF A PREOPERATIVE ASSESSMENT CLINIC

Some institutions (including ours) have an internist- or hospitalist-run preoperative assessment clinic that works in conjunction with the surgeon and anesthesiologist to provide a broad systematic evaluation of readiness for surgery and to facilitate optimization of key medical conditions. Instead of being seen in the hospital or by the patient's primary care provider, clinicians with more concentrated expertise in assessing and preparing patients for surgery see the patient in advance and then communicate their findings and recommendations to the surgeon and anesthesiologist. In our case, we also communicate with the orthopedic comanager via e-mail, page, or shared EMR patient list about planned admissions of surgical patients with relevant comorbidities. The preoperative clinic model may reduce cancellation rates and can identify decompensated medical problems that might lead to increased perioperative morbidity and mortality, as well as identify conditions that could easily decompensate if not scrutinized (eg, excessive intravenous fluids postoperatively in a patient with systolic heart failure).

MEASURING SUCCESS

Defining what constitutes success of the program in measurable terms is an essential piece of the puzzle, as it can provide information about practice changes, variability of practice patterns, outcome changes, and financial benefits or risks of the relationship.

Table 67-4 lists some suggested metrics to consider at the outset. It would also help to obtain data on these metrics prior to the initiation of comanagement to determine the influence of the program.

Especially challenging for the modern orthopedic surgeon is that in August 2008, the U.S. Centers for Medicare and Medicaid Services (CMS) added deep venous thrombosis and pulmonary embolism after total knee arthroplasty (TKA) and total hip arthroplasty (THA) to the list of never events. If a patient experiences deep venous thrombosis or pulmonary embolism following one of these procedures, a portion of the payment made by CMS to hospitals is withheld. While this decision has been criticized because prophylaxis is neither perfect nor risk free, it is a reality of practice, and the hospitalist comanager must be aware of this and engage the orthopedist regarding appropriate evidence-based prophylaxis methods.

One must keep in mind that not all metrics can be expected to improve in a "positive" way; in the study described previously about hip fractures, the rates of delirium were increased, which traditionally would be perceived as a negative result. However, this was due to increased recognition, documentation, and treatment

TABLE 67-2 Conditions Triggering Referral to Comanagement Service

Chronic Medical Conditions

- Stable or known coronary artery disease (chest pain, shortness of breath (SOB), electrocardiogram (ECG) changes)
- Congestive heart failure (SOB, pulmonary edema, edema, oxygen desaturation)
- Hypertension (especially if blood pressure > 160 systolic blood pressure or > 100 diastolic blood pressure)
- History of stroke
- Moderate/severe peripheral vascular disease
- Mild-moderate chronic obstructive pulmonary disease (COPD) (SOB, wheezing, oxygen desaturation)
- Mild-moderate/stable asthma (SOB, wheezing, oxygen desaturation)
- Current antibiotic treatment for pneumonia/acute bronchitis
- History of upper/lower GI bleed in the last three months (drop in Hgb/Hct, concern for active bleeding)
- Patients on chronic enteral tube feedings or hyperalimentation/total parenteral nutrition (TPN) (in addition to nutrition team/TPN consult)
- Diabetes mellitus type 1 or 2
- Stable psychiatric illnesses including affective disorders, dementias, bipolar disorder, schizophrenia (with additional psychiatry consultation for medication concerns or decompensation of psychiatric illness)
- Chronic anticoagulation (comanagement consultation on all patients)
- Recent anticoagulation for deep vein thrombosis (DVT) or pulmonary embolism (PE) within the last six months (comanagement consultation on all patients and possibly vascular medicine consultation)
- Chronic immunosuppression (prednisone, cyclosporine, methotrexate, FK 506, azathioprine, TNF-alpha blockers, etc)
- Physiologic glucocorticoid treatment within the last year (≥ 7.5 mg/day of prednisone, or the equivalent, for two or more weeks).
- Medical issues that require medical evaluation, monitoring, or treatment:
- Atypical chest pain without evidence of an acute coronary syndrome
- Shortness of breath
- Acute DVT or PE
- Baseline anemia or postoperative anemia
- Urinary tract infection with indwelling Foley catheter
- Acute delirium
- Electrolyte disorders
- Hyperglycemia without evidence of diabetic ketoacidosis (DKA) or non-ketotic/hyperosmolar state
- Acute renal failure
- Others

TABLE 67-3 CCF Program Timeline

December 2007	Presentation of the concept of the "embedded consultant" with a mini white paper summarizing the literature regarding benefits of comanagement by the department of orthopedics to the chairs of the Medicine Institute and department of Hospital Medicine
December 2007–March 2008	Draft proposal resulting from outreach to existing programs and internal multidisciplinary planning
March 2008	Acceptance of pilot program by departments of Hospital Medicine and orthopedics
March 2008	Presentation of proposed pilot to hospital operations committee and approval of the hiring of two additional full-time equivalent (FTE) for the program
April 2008–July 2008	Recruitment and finalization of pilot protocols with NPs
August 2008	Kickoff
Ongoing	Oversight with orthopedic champion Metrics collection Creation of a link with IMPACT (preoperative clinic)

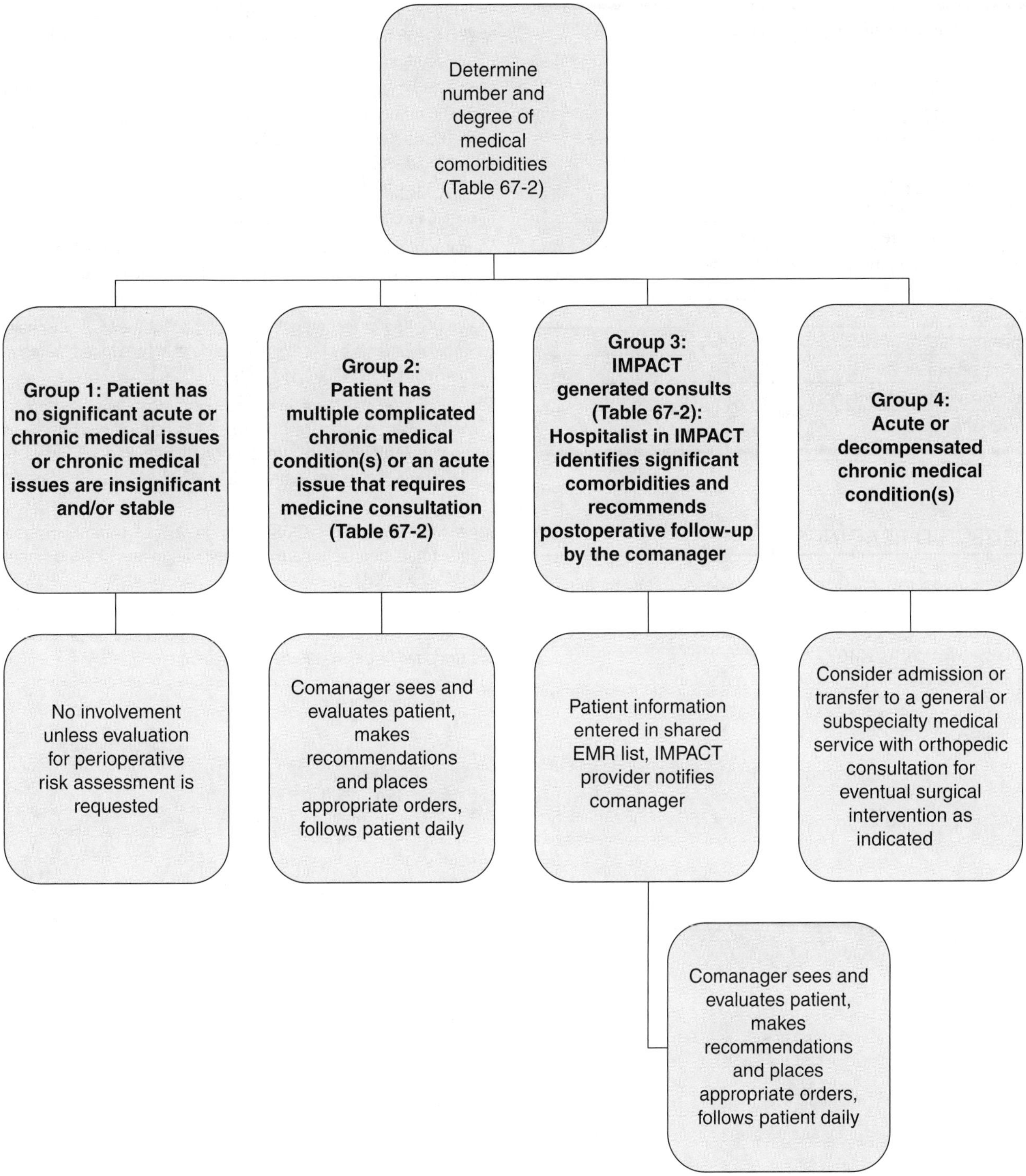

Figure 67-1 *Cleveland Clinic orthopedic comanagement triage algorithm.*

of delirium by physicians, which many would agree is a beneficial intervention. Also, these individual metrics are not in a vacuum; an increase in length of hospital stay coupled with decreased readmission rates might reflect the hospitalist taking an extra half to full day to optimize certain medical conditions, which results in fewer readmissions for decompensation.

Early results revealed that our program provided a net cost savings to the orthopedic department in terms of reduced surgical cancellations and improved patient satisfaction with care delivery.

CONCLUSION

Comanagement of orthopedic patients provides a novel diversity of practice to hospitalists and can be rewarding in that improved collegiality with surgical specialties can result. Engaging in a new comanagement relationship requires forethought and planning, and clarifying expectations, responsibilities, and metrics of success. However, when designed and managed well, a comanagement service can benefit hospitalists, orthopedists, and most importantly, the patients who trust us with their care.

TABLE 67-4 Proposed Program Metrics

Volume data
Case mix
Patient satisfaction
Length of stay
OR cancellation rates
Hospital cost and ancillary utilization
Productivity measures (RVUs and billing)
Provider satisfaction (hospitalist, orthopedist, nursing, residents)
Mortality
Unplanned ICU or medical service transfers
Readmission rates
Quality/patient safety metrics
JCAHO core measures

SUGGESTED READINGS

American Academy of Orthopedic Surgeons. The Burden of Musculoskeletal Diseases in the United States: Prevalence, Societal and Economic Cost. 2008; http://www.boneandjointburden.org/. Accessed March 10, 2010.

Deep vein thrombosis/pulmonary embolism. Fed Regist. 2008; 73(161):48480–48482. http://edocket.access.gpo.gov/2008/pdf/E8-17914.pdf. Accessed March 10, 2010.

Fisher AA, Davis MW, Rubenach SE, et al. Outcomes for older patients with hip fractures: the impact of orthopedic and geriatric medicine cocare. *J Orthopaed Trauma*. 2006;20(3):172–178; discussion 9–80.

Jaffer A, Michota F. Why perioperative medicine matters more than ever. *Clev Clin J Med*. 2006:73(suppl 1);2006:S1.

Marcantonio ER, Flacker JM, Wright RJ, et al. Reducing delirium after hip fracture: a randomized trial. *J Am Geriatr Soc*. 2001;49(5): 516–522.

Sharma G, Kuo Y, Freeman J, et al. Comanagement of Hospitalized Surgical Patients by Medicine Physicians in the United States. *Arch Intern Med*. 2010;170(4):363–368.

Society of Hospital Medicine. Measuring Hospitalist Performance: Metrics, Reports and Dashboards; 2006. http://www.hospitalmedicine.org/AM/Template.cfm?Section=White_Papers&Template=/CM/HTMLDisplay.cfm&ContentID=14632. Accessed March 10, 2010.

Streiff MB, Haut ER. The CMS ruling on venous thromboembolism after total knee or hip arthroplasty: weighing risks and benefits. *JAMA*. 2009;301(10):1063–1065.

Zuckerman JD, Sakales SR, Fabian DR, et al. Hip fractures in geriatric patients. Results of an interdisciplinary hospital care program. *Clin Orthopaed Relat Res*. 1992;274:213–225.

SECTION 8

Bariatric Surgery

CHAPTER 68

Common Surgical Options for the Treatment of Obesity

Jacqueline J. Wu, MD
Richard A. Perugini, MD

INTRODUCTION

Obesity has become a global problem. The definition and classification of obesity is based on the body mass index (BMI), which is calculated as weight in kilograms divided by height in meters squared. An estimated 1.7 billion adults worldwide are now considered overweight (BMI >25 kg/m^2). Of these, 300 million are obese (BMI >30 kg/m^2). In the United States, two-thirds of adults are overweight, one-third of adults are considered obese, and almost 5% are morbidly obese (BMI >40 kg/m^2). In addition, the number of obese children has more than doubled over the past 3 decades to 16%. The more than 50 million obese Americans are at risk of developing numerous obesity-related health problems, including hypertension, diabetes, and coronary artery disease, to name just a few (**Table 68-1**).

Currently, the annual cost for treating obesity and its related comorbid conditions is estimated at $100 billion. Obesity accounts for more than 100,000 premature deaths annually and is considered the second most preventable cause of death, after cigarette smoking.

EFFECTIVENESS OF AVAILABLE BARIATRIC SURGERY PROCEDURES

To date, surgery is the most effective means of achieving and maintaining long-term weight loss in obese patients. Weight loss, measured as percentage of excess body weight loss (EBWL is calculated as weight loss/excess weight x 100), and improvement in comorbid conditions varies with the different types of procedures. Maximum weight loss is most often seen in the first 1 to 2 years after surgery.

ROUX-EN-Y GASTRIC BYPASS

The Roux-en-Y gastric bypass (RYGB) is currently the most common bariatric procedure performed worldwide. Much of the popularity stems from the ability to perform the surgery laparoscopically and the significant weight loss that can be achieved by the patients. The Swedish Obese Subjects Study, the largest study on weight loss surgery to date and the study with the longest follow-up, reports a mean percent weight loss of 32.5% of total body weight (percent of total weight loss is roughly equal to half of EBWL) 1 to 2 years after gastric bypass and 25% 10 years post-bypass. A 2004 meta-analysis by Buchwald, et al, reported a mean EBWL of 61.6% after 1 to 2 years, which is comparable to the Swedish Obese Subjects Study.

Roux-en-Y gastric bypass also provides excellent improvement and even remission of comorbid conditions (**Table 68-2**).

More than 75% of patients with diabetes undergoing RYGB will have remission of their diabetes. Here remission is defined as discontinuation of all diabetes-related medications as well as the ability to maintain blood glucose levels within the normal range.

Roux-en-Y gastric bypass patients will likely also have remission of their hypertension. Multiple studies show improvement and even resolution of hypertension in approximately 65–85% of patients.

Hyperlipidemia, hypercholesterolemia, and hypertriglyceridemia are also greatly improved in more than 90% of patients after gastric bypass surgery. In Buchwald's meta-analysis, total cholesterol levels were seen to decrease by 0.96 mmol/L, LDL by 0.89 mmol/L, triglycerides by 1.07 mmol/L, and HDL was seen to increase by 0.05 mmol/L.

In addition to the comorbidities mentioned above, obstructive sleep apnea is reported to be improved or resolved in 80–90% of

TABLE 68-1 Obesity-related Comorbidities

Type 2 diabetes
Hyperlipidemia
Hypercholesterolemia
Hypertriglyceridemia
Coronary artery disease
Hypertension
Obstructive sleep apnea
Obesity hypoventilation syndrome
Asthma
Gastroesophageal reflux disease (GERD)
Depression
Pseudotumor cerebri
Cancer
Colon
Breast
Endometrium
Prostate
Sex hormone anomalies
Polycystic ovary disease
Gynecomastia
Hirsutism
Infertility
Stress urinary incontinence
Venous stasis disease
Deep venous thrombosis
Degenerative joint disease
Steatohepatitis
Abdominal wall hernias

patients after gastric bypass. Eighty-five percent of morbidly obese patients with gastroesophageal reflux disease (GERD) reported complete resolution of symptoms after RYGB. Although more difficult to quantify, patients have also reported improvements in depression, joint pain, stress incontinence, infertility, self-esteem, and overall quality of life.

LAPAROSCOPIC ADJUSTABLE GASTRIC BANDING

Laparoscopic adjustable gastric banding (LAGB) is another popular bariatric procedure both in the United States and worldwide. Although technically less challenging than RYGB, the LAGB requires frequent clinic visits in order to properly adjust the band and maintain the proper amount of gastric restriction and thereby weight loss. Studies have shown good weight loss results with LAGB. The Swedish Obese Subjects Study reports 20% total body weight loss 1 to 2 years after LAGB and 14% 10 years post-banding. Meta-analysis data shows a similar 47.5% EBWL after 1 to 2 years.

As with RYGB, LAGB also provides excellent remission or improvement in comorbidities. Multiple studies report remission of diabetes in 50–80%, lower than in patients undergoing RYGB. In addition, Abbatini, et al showed that time to remission is longer in patients with LAGB (12 months) when compared to patients who underwent RYGB (3 months).

Although LAGB provides improvement and remission of hypertension, the effect is not as great as after RYGB (45–70% vs. 65–85%). Lipid profiles are also improved after LAGB, but again, not as significantly as after RYGB. Hyperlipidemia, hypercholesterolemia, and hypertriglyceridemia improve in approximately 60%, 80%, and 75% respectively after LAGB. Based on meta-analysis data, total cholesterol, LDL, and triglyceride levels decrease by an average of 0.3 mmol/L, 0.11 mmol/L, and 0.76 mmol/L respectively, while HDL increased by an average of 0.12 mmol/L.

Symptoms of sleep apnea were reported to be improved in 95% of patients post-LAGB. Menstrual irregularities and GERD have also been reported to improve significantly after LAGB as well.

MALABSORPTIVE PROCEDURES

Malabsorptive procedures include jejunal-ileal bypass, which is now never performed, biliopancreatic diversion (BPD), and duodenal switch (DS). Many experts believe that DS provides greater early weight loss than RYGB; however, few studies comparing these two procedures are available. Skroubis, et al, in a randomized study of 160 morbidly obese adults, compared RYGB results to the results of their variation of BPD/DS. Eighty patients were randomized to undergo RYGB while the other 80 underwent BPD/DS. Their study showed that even after 2 years, 100% of the BPD/DS patients maintained a greater than 50% EBWL while only 88.7% of RYGB patients were able to maintain similar weight loss. These numbers are consistent with Buchwald's 2004 meta-analysis that found that average weight loss 1 to 2 years following BPD/DS was 70.1% EBWL, compared with 61.6% in the RYGB patients. In long-term follow-up, more calories lost in fecal fat are balanced by more calories eaten.

Although BPD/DS may be a more complex procedure, patients who undergo this procedure appear to have the best outcomes with regard to resolution of comorbidities. At the 2-year follow-up in the study by Skroubis et al, glucose intolerance, hypercholesterolemia, hypertriglyceridemia, and sleep apnea had completely resolved in both the BPD/DS and RYGB groups. However, while 100% of diabetic patients undergoing BPD/DS experienced remission of the disease, only 70% of RYGB patients with diabetes did so. Similarly, 81% of BPD/DS patients who had suffered from hypertension preoperatively were normotensive at 2-year follow-up, while only 63% of RYGB patients who were hypertensive reached a normotensive state. Lipid metabolism also followed the same pattern: both the BPD/DS and RYGB groups showed decreases in total cholesterol, triglycerides, LDL, and an increase in HDL; however, changes in total cholesterol, LDL, and HDL in the BPD/DS group were significantly ($p < 0.005$) greater than the RYGB group.

The data from Skroubis, et al's study is consistent with Buchwald's large meta-analysis that showed remission of diabetes in 97% of patients 1 to 2 years after BPD/DS. Hypertension is also shown to have resolved in a larger number of patients after this malabsorptive procedure (83%) when compared to RYGB. Hyperlipidemia, hypercholesterolemia, and hypertriglyceridemia showed vast improvement after BPD/DS according to Buchwald's analysis. Ninety-nine percent of those with hyperlipidemia, 87% of patients with hypercholesterolemia, and 100% of patients with hypertriglyceridemia have normal lipid profiles postoperatively. On average, total cholesterol, LDL, and triglycerides dropped by 1.97 mmol/L, 1.36 mmol/L, and 0.8 mmol/L respectively. HDL increased by 0.07 mmol/L.

Sleep apnea is also greatly improved after BPD/DS with reported improvement or remission in more than 85%. Additionally, although more difficult to quantify, patients have reported significant improvements in depression, joint pain, stress incontinence, infertility, self-esteem, and overall quality of life.

Although there is great improvement of comorbid conditions, the improved resolution of these conditions must be balanced against the increased likelihood for vitamin and nutritional deficiencies.

TABLE 68-2 Outcomes of Various Bariatric Surgeries

	Laparoscopic Adjustable Gastric Banding (LAGB)	Roux-en-Y Gastric Bypass (RYGB)	Biliopancreatic Bypass/Duodenal Switch (BPD/DS)	Sleeve Gastrectomy (SG)
Mean weight loss 1–2 years postoperatively (% EBWL)	40–50	60–65	65–75	40–80
Mortality (%)	0.1	0.5	1.1	0.5
Percentage of patients with diabetes remission	50–80	75–85	95–100	70–75
Percentage of patients with diabetes improvement	60–80	80–95	75–85	70–75
Percentage of patients with hypertension remission	45–70	65–85	80–85	60–65
Percentage of patients with hypertension improvement	60–70	65–85	80–90	60–65
Percentage of patients with hyperlipidemia improvement	58	>90	99	N/A
Percentage of patients with hypercholesterolemia improvement	78	>90	80–90	N/A
Percentage of patients with hypertriglyceridemia improvement	77	>90	90–100	N/A
Average change in total cholesterol (mmol/L)	-0.3	-0.96	-1.97	N/A
Average change in HDL (mmol/L)	0.12	0.05	0.07	N/A
Average change in LDL (mmol/L)	-0.11	-0.89	-1.36	N/A
Average change in triglycerides (mmol/L)	-0.76	-1.07	-0.8	N/A
Percentage of patients with obstructive sleep apnea remission	90–95	70–80	70–90	N/A
Percentage of patients with obstructive sleep apnea symptom improvement	90–95	80–95	70–90	N/A

SLEEVE GASTRECTOMY

Laparoscopic sleeve gastrectomy (SG) has recently gained popularity as a singular operation for weight loss. This procedure was initially used as the first stage of a 2-stage DS operation. Because a gastric tube of 100–150 ml is created, SG was originally thought to be a purely restrictive procedure. However, a recent study by Peterli, et al has shown a post-SG impact on incretin secretion similar to post-RYGB. Abbatini, et al have shown that remission of diabetes after SG occurs at the same early time course and in as high a percentage of patients as RYGB, and earlier and more frequently than in LAGB patients. The data from these studies suggest that although none of the intestine is bypassed, a hormonal change is still achievable.

In small, noncontrolled studies, weight loss results after SG rivaled that of RYGB. In some small series, weight loss after SG was similar to weight loss after adjustable gastric banding. Excess body weight loss has been reported anywhere from 40–80% after 1 year. Because sleeve gastrectomy on its own is a relatively new procedure, few long-term studies or randomized controlled trials are available. However, it is clear that sleeve gastrectomy is effective in achieving significant weight loss and remission of comorbidities and will likely have long-term results between that of RYGB and LAGB.

INDICATIONS FOR REFERRAL FOR BARIATRIC SURGERY

A healthy diet and exercise should be integral to any health care regimen. However, medical management alone for treatment of morbid obesity has a high failure rate. Long-term maintenance of more than 10% EBWL is extremely uncommon with medical management alone. Therefore, based on the 1991 consensus statement on bariatric surgery for morbid obesity issued by the NIH, it is recommended that patients with BMI greater than 40 kg/m^2 or 35 kg/m^2 with two or more significant obesity-related comorbidities (Table 68.1) who have failed other methods of weight loss be referred to a bariatric surgeon.

PRACTICE POINT

- Patients with BMI greater than 40 kg/m^2 or 35 kg/m^2 with two or more significant obesity-related comorbidities, who have failed other methods of weight loss, should be referred to a bariatric surgeon (1991 NIH consensus statement on bariatric surgery).

PREOPERATIVE RISK ASSESSMENT SPECIFIC TO BARIATRIC SURGERY

Once a patient has been referred for bariatric surgery, a thorough screening must be conducted by a multidisciplinary team. This team should include specialists from nutrition, bariatric medicine, bariatric surgery, and behavioral medicine.

Nutrition counseling is extremely important to educate the patient about healthy eating habits that lead to long-term success. These habits include regular eating patterns throughout the day (no skipping meals), intake of an adequate amount of protein at each meal so that total protein intake per day is 40–60 grams, avoidance of high carbohydrate snack foods that could lead to dumping syndrome after intestinal bypass procedures (RYGB, BPD/DS), and the need for lifetime vitamin supplementation. Patients are also taught that the intense effects of bariatric surgery such as repression of hunger and decreased appetite are time-limited to approximately 2 years after surgery. Therefore, long-term success requires permanent lifestyle changes, including modifications in eating habits, dietary changes, and increased exercise and physical activity.

In addition to being seen by a nutritionist, prospective patients are seen by a psychiatrist, psychologist, or social worker during the initial evaluation process to determine the patient's capacity to fully understand the risks and benefits of a life-changing operation. These patients are also counseled on mindful eating; that is, they need to understand whether they are eating to satisfy hunger or to satisfy an emotional need. Counseling may also include addressing the prospective patient's expectations for weight loss, health outcomes, as well as the psychosocial impact of bariatric surgery.

The psychiatrist/psychologist/social worker must also be able to identify if any overt psychoses or mental illnesses are present that would require treatment before surgery. Eating disorders, such as binge eating are screened for, since they are associated with poor outcomes after bariatric surgery. Also important is identification of any signs of substance abuse or severe situational stress that would adversely affect the patient after surgery and hinder compliance with strict dietary and lifestyle modifications. It is important that patients seriously considering bariatric surgery are evaluated to determine whether they would be able to comply with a strict postoperative diet and lifestyle change, whether they have a support system in place, and whether or not long-term follow-up is in place before surgery.

Since morbidly obese patients have had poor results and often negative experiences with exercise in the past, it is important that physical activity, both aerobic and strength training, be stressed. It is often extremely helpful for patients to be seen by a clinical exercise physiologist to receive advice on implementing an exercise regimen and the benefits of combining cardiovascular activity with strength training. In addition, a clinical exercise physiologist can offer strategies to compensate for weight bearing joint pain during physical activity. These referrals are often quite helpful in reducing barriers to adopting exercise programs, which have been shown to be necessary for long-term success after any bariatric procedure. Although the help of an exercise physiologist can be quite beneficial, not all bariatric programs have one in their multidisciplinary team, since it is not yet a requirement. When this is the case, it is important for the physician to refer a patient to a clinical exercise physiologist who is certified by the American College of Sports Medicine. Referrals are especially useful for patients with multiple medical problems. Often exercise physiologists working in the cardiac or pulmonary rehabilitation units within the same health care system can be helpful in guiding patients in their exercise regime. When severely overweight individuals begin an exercise program, early weight loss is often quite remarkable. This weight loss can be a strong positive reinforcement for an individual. After significant weight loss though, the effect of exercise becomes less impressive.

The remainder of the preoperative assessment focuses on factors that predispose the patient to increased surgical risk such as age, cardiovascular risk factors (coronary artery disease, congestive heart failure, cardiomyopathy, hypertension, pulmonary hypertension), pulmonary risk factors (asthma, obstructive pulmonary disease, obstructive sleep apnea, smoking), and vascular risk factors (venous stasis, hypercoaguable states secondary to obesity, prior deep venous thromboses, use of oral contraceptives) (**Table 68-3**).

EARLY POSTOPERATIVE COMPLICATIONS OF GASTRIC BYPASS

All bariatric surgery patients are at risk of developing the same postoperative complications as patients undergoing general surgery. These include surgical site infection, atelectasis, deep venous thrombosis, pulmonary embolus, MI, and stroke, among others. However, there are several postoperative complications specific to bariatric surgery.

TABLE 68-3 Preoperative Assessment

- History and physical
- ECG
- Cardiac stress test (if indicated by poor exercise tolerance, angina, or history of coronary artery disease)
- Laboratory tests
  - CBC
  - Basic metabolic panel
  - Liver function tests
  - Hemoglobin A1c
  - Albumin
  - Fasting lipid profile
  - Vitamin B12, folate, thiamine levels
  - Pregnancy test
- Abdominal ultrasound to rule out gallstones
- Upper GI series to check for hiatal hernia
- Pulmonary function tests
- Chest X-ray
- Sleep study
- Smoking sessation

ANASTOMOTIC LEAK

Anastomotic leak (leak at the gastrojejonostomy), although rare, is the most feared complication of bariatric surgery. Reported incidence of anastomotic leak after RYGB ranges from 0.5–5%. Several risk factors are associated with increased risk of anastomotic leak. Patient factors include multiple comorbid conditions, smoking, and poor glycemic control. Smokers are counseled to quit smoking preoperatively and diabetics must keep their HgA1c < 7 preoperatively. Technical factors of the surgery that increase risk of anastomotic leak include open gastric bypass technique, retrocolic anastomosis, single layer closure, and revisional surgery. Patients usually present in the first 3 days postoperatively with tachycardia, tachypnea, epigastric pain, and/or fevers. Tachycardia is an early sign, and often times the first sign of a leak. Diagnosis varies based on the institution, but usually includes UGI series and/or CT abdomen with orally contrast.

Based on the clinical status of the patient and the radiographic findings, surgeons may opt to treat the anastomotic leak conservatively (nonoperatively) or with reoperation. Conservative management includes keeping the patient nil per os (NPO), on intravenous fluids, and antibiotics. If a collection is found on CT scan, this may be drained percutaneouly. Operative intervention is rarely indicated; however, when deemed necessary, many bariatric surgeons recommend placement of a Graham patch over the anastomosis and keeping the patient NPO until the leak heals. Resection and reanastomosis in this urgent setting is usually an extensive operation that can lead to additional problems. A feeding gastrostomy tube may be placed into the remnant stomach at the time of reoperation if postoperative oral feeding is not anticipated for a prolonged period.

GASTROINTESTINAL BLEEDING

Gastrointestinal bleeding (GIB) is another complication that can occur early in the postoperative period. GIB during the first 72 hours is usually due to bleeding from the staple or suture lines. Risk factors include history of anticoagulation, history of antiplatelet therapy, thick, inflamed tissues, or thin tissues. Diagnosis of GIB in a postoperative RYGB patient is no different than diagnosis in any other patient; however, care must be taken in any invasive diagnostic technique performed including nasogastric lavage and endoscopy. These procedures can distend the newly created gastric pouch and disrupt the staple or suture line. Most staple/suture line bleeding can be treated nonoperatively by keeping the patient NPO, with fluid resuscitation, checking frequent hematocrits, reversing any anticoagulation, and monitoring urine output.

LATE POSTOPERATIVE COMPLICATIONS OF GASTRIC BYPASS

SMALL BOWEL OBSTRUCTION

Although rare, small bowel obstructions can occur after RYGB. The majority of intestinal obstructions after RYGB are due to adhesions, internal hernias, or kinking of the jejunojejunostomy. Symptoms are typical of small bowel obstructions: abdominal pain, nausea, vomiting, and/or obstipation. Clinical and laboratory findings are often nonspecific. Workup should consist of chemistries, complete blood count, radiologic tests including plain abdominal films, and CT scan of the abdomen, which is the gold standard. If a mesenteric swirl is found on CT scan, an internal hernia—a loop of bowel herniated through an iatrogenic defect in the mesentery—should be suspected. This finding should prompt *urgent* surgical exploration and reduction of the hernia. Delay in doing so can lead to necrotic bowel.

There should be a low threshold to surgically explore patients with previous RYGB who are suspected of having small bowel obstructions. Before an operative intervention is undertaken, however, it is important to have imaging studies as a guide (CT scan is gold standard for most). Laparoscopic exploration is feasible in the majority of these patients and a thorough exploration can be conducted to look for internal hernias or kinking of the jejunojejunostomy using this minimally invasive technique. Conversion to open surgery may occasionally be necessary. If an internal hernia or bowel kinking are found at the time of exploration, they can be fixed at that time. A revision of the RYGB can also be carried out as well in that setting if it is deemed necessary by the bariatric surgeon. If adhesions are present, they can be lysed at that time, if they have been documented to have been problematic.

STOMAL STENOSIS

Stomal stenosis is another potential late complication of RYGB. Stomal stenosis is an anastomotic stricture at the gastrojejunostomy. The reported incidence is between 3% and 15%, making it one of the most common complications of gastric bypass. There is no clear single etiology of stomal stenosis. Risk factors include the method of creation of the anastomosis (circular stapler vs. linear stapler vs. hand-sewn), ischemia to the anastomosis, and marginal ulcers (which will be discussed later). Symptoms of stomal stenosis include nausea, vomiting, dysphagia, and food intolerance.

The diagnosis of stomal stenosis can sometimes be made with history alone. However, it can be difficult to distinguish between someone who has stomal stenosis versus a patient who is eating too much, too quickly. Tests such as UGI or barium swallow may be of use to diagnose the condition; however, both tests lack sensitivity. Upper endoscopy can be both diagnostic and therapeutic and is a much more sensitive test.

Dilation of the stenosis using endoscopic balloon dilators remains the treatment of choice. Studies report 55–80% success. Complications such as perforation are uncommon and can be managed nonoperatively. Surgical repair or revision of the gastrojejunostomy is reserved for those who have complete obstruction or who have failed multiple attempts at endoscopic dilation. This is common when the stricture is due to ischemia or when long-term inflammation has been present, maturing the tissues into scar.

MARGINAL ULCER

Marginal ulcer, or ulcer at the gastrojejunostomy anastomosis, is also a potential complication of RYGB with rates ranging from 2–4% in recent studies. Marginal ulcers usually occur at the jejunal side of the gastrojejunostomy. These ulcers are thought to be due to exposure of gastric acid to the jejunal mucosa. Several factors are thought to contribute to the formation of marginal ulcers including NSAIDs, tobacco use, ischemia, H. pylori, alcohol, foreign body reaction, large gastric pouch, and gastrogastric fistula.

Treatment begins with acid suppression as well as treatment of the underlying cause, such as eradication of H. pylori, cessation of tobacco and alcohol, and starting an oral sucralfate slurry regimen. There is no definitive duration of such therapy, although studies have shown that 6 to 12 months appear to be adequate. Repeat upper endoscopy can help to guide therapy. If symptoms persist or if they become debilitating to the patient, surgical intervention may be warranted. Resection and revision of the gastrojejunostomy may be required to remove the ulcerated area. In the setting of an acute ulcer perforation, the patient should be taken to the operating room. Many bariatric surgeons opt for a Graham patch of the perforation in these cases. More extensive interventions are usually unnecessary and can potentially cause more problems.

GASTROGASTRIC FISTULA

The gastrogastric fistula (GGF) is a rare complication after RYGB. These are usually due to staple line disruptions and allow communication between the gastric pouch created for the RYGB and the excluded stomach. This communication allows gastric acid to flow from the excluded stomach to the gastric pouch and down into the jejunum. GGF are extremely rare, with a reported incidence ranging from 1–2%. Symptoms include heartburn, epigastric pain, nausea, and weight regain. Several options exist for the treatment of GGF including endoscopic injection of fibrin glue, endoscopic plication/suturing, and endoscopic clipping. Surgical interventions all start with resection of the fistula tract. Some surgeons separate the pouch from the excluded stomach via stapling or oversewing or resection. Others prefer to resect the excluded stomach all together to prevent any future GGF from forming.

POSTOPERATIVE COMPLICATIONS OF ADJUSTABLE GASTRIC BANDING

Several adjustable gastric band complications are possible and can either occur early or late. These complications include port or port-site infection, band infection, band slippage or gastric prolapse, hiatal hernia, and band erosion.

INFECTIONS

Port and port-site infections can initially be treated with antibiotics alone; however, if these infections occur in the late postoperative period, the surgeon should consider that the patient may actually be presenting with a gastric erosion. In this situation, a prompt upper endoscopy is indicated to rule out an erosion. For recurrent infections or infections that do not resolve with a course of antibiotics, the port should be removed and cultured. Patients should then be treated with the appropriate antibiotics for 7 to 10 days. After 2 to 3 months a new port can be placed in a fresh site.

The intra-abdominal portion of a band can also become infected both in the early and late postoperative period. Patients may initially present with port or port-site infections that do not resolve despite antibiotic treatment. As the infection progresses patients may develop fever, abdominal pain, abscesses, and peritonitis. Treatment is removal of the infected band. Patients should have intraoperative tests to determine whether there is a leak from the stomach or esophagus. Antibiotics are also warranted for 7–10 days postoperatively. Bands can usually be replaced after 3 months.

GASTRIC PROLAPSE OR BAND SLIPPAGE

Gastric prolapse or band slippage occurs in approximately 5% of patients. This phenomenon refers to the cephalad herniation of the gastric fundus through the band. Symptoms of band slippage are secondary to a gastric outlet-type obstruction and include nausea, heartburn or reflux, and the inability to swallow liquids. Some patients may complain of erratic function of the band; some days they feel no restriction, whereas other days they are unable to eat anything. These symptoms of gastric prolapse and/or band slippage can sometimes be relieved by removing some of the fluid from the band. In patients with worsening or persistent symptoms and in patients in whom removing fluid from the band does not improve symptoms, urgent surgery is required to either remove the band or move the band to the correct position on the stomach. After reduction of the prolapse, it is important to test the stomach and esophagus for evidence of leak.

HIATAL HERNIA

Hiatal hernias can be found preoperatively on UGI series. If found preoperatively, these hernias should be repaired at the time of placement of the adjustable gastric banding. Occasionally hiatal hernias are found intraoperatively at the time of the dissection performed to free the right crus. If hiatal hernias are not fixed at the time of band placement or develop after band placement, patients may have symptoms of heartburn and reflux when the band is tightened. These symptoms tend to be alleviated with loosening of the band. If symptoms are persistent or weight loss is suboptimal due to the small amount of fluid in the band, repair of the hernia is indicated. This often requires removal and replacement of the band in addition to repair of the hiatal hernia.

BAND EROSION

Erosion of the gastric wall by an adjustable gastric band can occur after the first few weeks of placement or after a prolonged period. Incidence of band erosion is reported to be between 0.5% and 1%. Early erosions are thought to be secondary to unrecognized operative trauma to the stomach and may be considered an intraoperative injury more than a true band erosion. These patients can present with peritonitis requiring emergent operation; however, the large majority of patients with band erosions have a silent, chronic course. A typical course of band erosion develops over months to years. As the gastric juices slowly leak out, the body develops a local inflammatory response. This response can be thought of as the body trying to exclude the infected band by extruding it into the gastrointestinal tract. The inflammation eventually tracks out to the subcutaneous port and skin via the tubing that connects the band and the port, leading to local port-site infection. The development of gastric ulcers can also lead to band erosion. Patients with band erosions often do not have overt symptoms; instead they often present with failure of the restrictive properties of the band and/or a nonfunctioning band.

Diagnosis of band erosion is best made with upper endoscopy. Most erosions occur between the gastric fundus anteriorly and the band at the location where the fundus has been plicated over the band. UGI series are rarely useful in diagnosing band erosion.

Treatment is removal of the gastric band and repair of any areas of perforation on the stomach. Intraoperative tests should be conducted to rule out the presence of a leak. If a leak is found, a drain should be placed. Some advocate an UGI series on the first postoperative day to rule out a persistent leak. Diets can usually be resumed after the UGI series, if no abnormalities are found. Most bariatric surgeons do not replace the band during removal of an eroded one given the degree of inflammation and contamination.

LATE COMPLICATIONS OF BARIATRIC SURGERY: NUTRITIONAL DEFICIENCIES

Despite having large stores of energy in the form of excess fat, morbidly obese patients usually have some underlying nutritional deficiencies, even preoperatively, due to poor dietary habits over a prolonged period of time. These deficiencies can be exacerbated postoperatively. The severity of these deficiencies is dependent on several factors: the patient's preoperative nutritional status, the type of bariatric surgery, the patient's compliance to the postoperative diet and vitamin supplement regimen, as well as routine follow-up with the bariatric surgeon, nutritionist, and primary care provider. All bariatric patients are instructed to take a multivitamin daily and undergo routine blood tests to check for any nutritional deficiencies.

Vitamin deficiencies are common after bariatric surgery. Vitamin B12 deficiency is common, especially after a RYGB. The parietal cells that secrete acid and intrinsic factor, and the chief cells that secrete pepsinogen are mainly located in the fundus and body of the stomach, which is excluded from the tiny pouch that is created in the RYGB. There is also no time for the intrinsic factor to mix with the vitamin B12 since the pylorus has been removed and can no longer slow gastric emptying. The small amount of acid secreted by the pouch combined with decreased production of intrinsic factor causes vitamin B12 to remain in the crystalline form, which is not readily absorbed in the terminal ileum.

The prevalence of vitamin B12 deficiency is approximately 15–30%. However, this number varies depending on compliance with supplementation. Because the body usually has large stores of vitamin B12, levels often do not drop significantly for 2–5 years after gastric bypass. For this reason, patients must continue to have vitamin B12 levels monitored long-term on a regular basis and continue with vitamin B12 supplementation. Routine vitamin B12 supplementation can lead to eventual supranormal levels and reduction of the amount of supplementation given.

Calcium deficiency can be seen after procedures such as RYGB and BPD in which the duodenum and proximal intestines are bypassed. Normally calcium absorption occurs in the duodenum. All patients who have undergone RYGB or BPD require a high daily intake of calcium (2 g/day) as well as calcium supplementation (1200–1500 mg calcium/day). A lack of calcium can lead to increased levels of parathyroid hormone (PTH), which can then lead to the release of calcium from bone. Therefore, after RYGB, BPD, or other procedures that bypass the duodenum, patients should have regular tests for serum calcium, ionized calcium, serum phosphorus, alkaline phosphatase, and PTH.

In addition to vitamin B12 and calcium deficiencies, patients who have had a malabsorptive procedure, such as BPD, will have malabsorption of fat-soluble vitamins (A, D, E, K). It is important for these patients to include supplementation of fat-soluble vitamins into their daily regimen and to be monitored for any deficiencies.

Mineral deficiencies are also common in bariatric patients. Iron deficiency and anemia occur frequently in both the preoperative and postoperative bariatric patient. Postoperative causes for iron deficiency include decreased absorption due to bypass of the duodenum, decreased gastric acid, which is needed to reduce iron to its more soluble form, and reduced iron intake. About 20–70% of patients develop iron deficiency after RYGB. Symptoms include fatigue, glossitis, stomatitis, and feeling cold due to impaired temperature regulation. Supplementation of ferrous sulfate 320 mg twice daily

Evidence

Abbatini F, Rizzello M, Casella G, et al. Long-term effects of laparoscopic sleeve gastrectomy, gastric bypass and adjustable gastric banding on type 2 diabetes. *Surg Endosc.* 2010;24:1005–1010.

Buchwald H, Avidor Y, Braunwald E, et al. Bariatric Surgery A Systematic Review and Meta-Analysis. *JAMA.* 2004;292(14):1724–1737.

Sjostrom L, Narbro K, Sjostrom D, et al. For the Swedish Obese Subjects Study. Effects of Bariatric Surgery on Mortality in Swedish Obese Subjects. *NEJM.* 2007;357(8):741–752.

Rosenthal RJ, Szomstein S, Kennedy CI, Soto FC, Zundel N. Laparoscopic Surgery for Morbid Obesity: 1,001 consecutive bariatric operations performed at the Bariatric Institute, Cleveland Clinic Florida. *Obes Surg.* 2006;16:119–124.

Schauer PR, Burguera B, Ikramuddin S, et al. Effect of Laparoscopic Roux-en-Y gastric bypass on type 2 diabetes mellitus. *Ann Surg.* 2003;238(4):467–485.

Sugerman HJ, Wolfe LG, Sica DA, Clore JN. Diabetes and hypertension in severe obesity and effects of gastric bypass-induced weight loss. *Ann Surg.* 2003;237(6):751–758.

Tataranni PA, Mingrone G, Raguso CA, et al. Twenty-four-hour energy and nutrient balance in weight stable postobese patients after biliopancreatic diversion. *Nutrition.* 1996;12(4):239–44.

is often sufficient. Vitamin C supplementation has been shown to improve absorption of iron.

CONCLUSION

The National Institutes of Health recommend that bariatric surgery be considered in patients with a BMI of ≥40 or if they have a BMI of ≥35 with high risk comorbid conditions after trying other nonsurgical approaches that augment weight loss. Surgical procedures are superior to alternative approaches in this patient population, and outcomes are related to the bariatric procedures. Surgical procedures accomplish weight loss by restriction as in gastric banding, or by malabsorption or a combination of the two as in gastric bypass. Although gastric bypass is more effective than gastric banding, it is also more invasive and associated with a different risk profile than gastric banding. Even a 10% weight loss accomplished by either method will reduce cardiovascular risk factors. Unfortunately, there are health care disparities with fewer eligible African American and Hispanic patients undergoing recommended surgery and overall, less than 1% of eligible patients actually undergo bariatric surgery. Hospitalists encounter many eligible patients during hospitalization and can play a role in appropriately referring these patients to surgeons after they recover from their illness.

SUGGESTED READINGS

Buchwald H. Consensus Conference Statement. Bariatric surgery for morbid obesity: Health implications for patients, health professionals, and third-party payers. *Surg Obes Rel Dis.* 2005;371–381.

Fontain KR, Redden DT, Wang C, Westfall AO, Allison DB. Years of life lost due to obesity. *JAMA.* 2003;289(2):187–193.

Jones DB, Jones S. Obesity Surgery: Patient Safety and Best Practices. Woodbury, CT: Cine-Inc; 2008.

Nguyen NT, DeMaria EJ, Ikramuddin S, Hutter MM. The SAGES Manual: A Practical Guide to Bariatric Surgery. New York, NY: Springer; 2008.

Pories WJ, Swanson MS, MacDonald KD, et al. Who would have thought it? An operation proves to be the most effective therapy for adult-onset diabetes mellitus. *Ann Surg.* 1995;222(5): 339–352.

Sjostrom L, Lindroos AK, Peltonen M, et al. For the Swedish Obese Subjects Study. Lifestyle, diabetes, and cardiovascular risk factors 10 years after bariatric surgery. *NEJM.* 2004;351(26): 2683–2693.

PART III

Clinical Problem-Solving in Hospital Medicine

CHAPTER 69

Principles of Evidence-Based Medicine

Jeffrey S. Ginsberg, MD, FRCP(C)

INTRODUCTION

Evidence-based medicine (EBM) is a juggernaut that has taken practitioners by storm. Over the last 20 years, my colleagues at McMaster University, as well as at other academic institutions, have spearheaded the EBM movement to the point where journal articles with "evidence-based" in the title are ubiquitous. While EBM is not perfect and is a continuing work in progress—qualitative levels of evidence seem to change definition regularly—the fundamental principles of EBM are unquestionably an advance in the management of patients.

As a rule, physicians are dedicated to their patients and usually convinced that they deliver the best possible care. It is difficult to accept the possibility that our patients might not be getting optimal care because of our decision-making processes. For decades, the main teaching methods in medical schools consisted of noninteractive didactic teaching sessions and rounds with attending physicians and senior residents where each would try to "out anecdote" the other. These rounds usually created a competitive environment, in which the primary focus was placed on cases we had never seen before and would never see again. From these "canaries," the words and experience of the senior attending, which were based on his "vast experience" of two or three patients, were gold nuggets. Nobody questioned, let alone challenged him. Over the last three or four decades, it has become clear that not everything in medicine is black or white and that disagreements among clinicians is quite common.

So how do we reconcile the "If I say it, it must be true" or the disagreements? In retrospect, the answer was so simple and yet until recently, the technology did not exist to make the transformation to evidence-based medicine. Since one of the main purposes of publishing papers is the dissemination of information, it seems only logical to use the Internet to perform a literature review and see not only the experience of others, but also if any well-designed studies had been done addressing the issue. Unfortunately, in the early to mid 1980s, computers were slow and the internet was still in its infancy, and so performing literature reviews for every clinical question was highly impractical.

Over the next 10 to 20 years remarkable advances have facilitated literature reviews and spawned a generation of practitioners who practice evidence-based medicine. The main advances included the vast expansion of the World Wide Web, the availability of portable and powerful computers to access the Internet, and the recognition that the uncritical acceptance of the professor's experience, while somewhat useful, was very limited and often wrong. In parallel, the National Library of Medicine simplified the performance of literature reviews within an enormous database and made it widely available and easily accessible.

EXPERIENCE: ASKING THE RIGHT QUESTIONS

It is difficult to justify the "professor's experience" approach to clinical decision making while ignoring the vast amount of relevant literature that is accessible in a handheld device or laptop computer. The fundamental principles of EBM include an approach to patients that identifies key issues, generating clinically important questions that address these issues, performing literature reviews that will identify papers that address the question, interpreting the quality, conclusions, and applicability of the literature, and finally applying the knowledge to patient management. Although many of us have considerable expertise at obtaining and refining "best available evidence," where some of my colleagues and I often fall down is the knowledge translation. This incorporates patient preferences and values into decision making about interventions. I am not very good at this critical aspect of EBM because it is usually very time consuming and can be mundane; my time is valuable, and I am always busy.

EBM: WHAT IT IS AND WHAT IT IS NOT

PRACTICE POINT

- EBM does not exclude the "professor's opinion" as evidence, but simply puts it into perspective as the lowest level of evidence.

EBM is here to stay. Despite passionate complaints about the arrogance of some proponents of EBM, continual debate about the relative strength of randomized trials versus observational studies and the lack of uniformity in grading levels of evidence in consensus conferences and guidelines, there is little doubt that EBM represents a significant advance in our approach to patients. EBM does not exclude the "professor's opinion" as evidence, but simply puts it into perspective as the lowest level of evidence. It is also critical to understand that EBM is in its infancy and is constantly evolving and adapting as problems arise.

In order to make individual decisions about health care (eg, performing or withholding an intervention), it is important to incorporate the best available evidence with patients' preferences. With few exceptions, patient preferences "trump" physician preferences. To a variable extent, the physician has several layers of responsibility. The first is to obtain the best available evidence in favor of (or against) an intervention (this will be further discussed later in the chapter). The second is communicating the evidence, in understandable terms, to the patient and/or their guardian. Finally, patient preference should be ascertained. In a perfect world, data providing evidence are clear and noncontroversial, patients understand the pros and cons of the intervention and the physician and patient have similar values and preferences. However, it is far more common than not that at least one of these criteria is not met and/or physicians fail to communicate effectively with their patients.

PRACTICE POINT

- In order to make individual decisions about health care (eg, performing or withholding an intervention), it is important to incorporate the best available evidence with patients' preferences. With few exceptions, patient preferences "trump" physician preferences.

FAILURE OF KNOWLEDGE TRANSLATION

During the first decade of the 21st century (and for years prior to 2000), there was incontrovertible evidence that warfarin was effective for the reduction of the incidence of embolic stroke in subjects with nonvalvular atrial fibrillation. Moreover, high-quality data were available on the relative and absolute risks of stroke and major bleeding in specific subpopulations. Consensus guidelines laid out specifics of who should be treated and the expected risks and benefits of warfarin. Despite the compelling information and recommendations, surveys consistently showed that less than 50% of subjects with nonvalvular atrial fibrillation who should have been treated with warfarin were actually treated. There were many reasons for this failure of "knowledge translation." First, not all primary care physicians were aware of the compelling evidence. There was the problem of the perception by patients that they were receiving "rat poison" that was inconvenient and meant regular blood sampling for INR results and adjustment of warfarin dosing, when appropriate. Many patients resented having their lifestyles infringed upon, typically involving dietary restrictions on intake of foods containing vitamin K, caution because of drug interactions, and some restriction of activities (eg, contact sports). There was also considerable inertia by primary care physicians who might only have a handful of patients taking warfarin and starting up and following warfarin therapy is onerous and not very lucrative. Finally, older patients, who are more likely to be unsteady on their feet, are often not put on warfarin because of the concern that they might fall and have a critical hemorrhage. Unfortunately, these patients are also the likeliest to benefit from warfarin, as the embolic stroke rate in elderly patients is often quite high.

PRACTICE POINT

The optimum use of EBM requires:

1. Gathering the best available evidence
2. Effectively communicating the evidence using understandable language
3. Elaborating on how relevant the available evidence is for the patient in front of you
4. Fairly and objectively discussing the pros and cons of the intervention

Thus, the optimum use of EBM is not simply gathering the best available evidence, but also includes effectively communicating the evidence using understandable language, elaborating on how relevant the available evidence is for the individual, and fairly and objectively discussing the pros and cons of the intervention. In addition, patients might have inaccurate or partially accurate preconceived ideas about the intervention and the expected benefits and side effects; best efforts should be made to correct obvious misconceptions. It seems that whereas much time, expense, and efforts are put into large randomized trials and systematic reviews in order to obtain high-quality evidence, fewer strides are being made in the area of knowledge translation where patient values and perceptions are incorporated into the decision-making process.

APPLYING EBM IN CLINICAL PRACTICE

GATHERING AND GRADING THE EVIDENCE

In determining available evidence, it is critically important to identify the question being asked.

CASE 69-1

You are asked by the emergency room physician to see a 64-year-old woman with a history of breast cancer with known metastases to her cervical and thoracic vertebrae. She presents with a three-day history of left leg swelling and pain. She undergoes duplex ultrasound, which shows noncompressibility in the femoral and popliteal veins, diagnostic of proximal deep vein thrombosis (DVT). She has been given a dose of dalteparin 100 U/kg and the nurse is processing an order for 10 mg of warfarin.

You remember reading about use of low-molecular-weight heparin (LMWH) instead of warfarin in the long-term management of DVT in cancer patients. You are also familiar with the regular guidelines compiled every three or four years by the American College of Chest Physicians (ACCP) on use of antithrombotic and thrombolytic therapy.

THE WELL-BUILT CLINICAL QUESTION

The question in this case is: What is the relative efficacy and safety of warfarin compared to LMWH for the long-term management of DVT in cancer patients? You look online for the most recent ACCP guidelines. You find the most recent edition, which was published in 2008, and note that there is a chapter that deals specifically with treatment of DVT. In this chapter, there is a strong recommendation for the use of LMWH for the secondary prevention of recurrent venous thromboembolism (VTE) in cancer patients with acute venous thromboembolism. The evidence is based primarily on the results of a large randomized trial comparing dalteparin (200 U/kg/day for 1 month followed by a decrease to ~75% of the daily dose after 1 month) to warfarin (target INR of 2.0–3.0) after initial treatment for at least 5 days with dalteparin. The study showed a significant reduction in the rate of recurrent VTE without an increase in bleeding in the group of patients who received dalteparin.

You then decide to scrutinize the trial that generated the strong recommendation for LMWH over warfarin. On review, you note that the trial was large (n > 600 or > 300 per arm), multicenter, and included patients with a variety of malignancies, including breast cancer. These factors increase the probability that the study can be generalized to your patient. The study is randomized with concealed treatment allocation and well-described, valid randomization procedures. The trial is not double-blind, but rather an open study. This has the potential to cause bias if some of the investigators had preconceived ideas about the relative efficacy and safety of one of the treatment arms. For example, if an investigator had a strong sense that dalteparin was more efficacious than warfarin, they might investigate patients with trivial symptoms more readily if the patient was allocated to warfarin than dalteparin. Given the difficulty that duplex ultrasound has in diagnosing recurrence (ie, extension), this potential bias could result in an overestimate of recurrence rates in the warfarin group. On careful reading of the manuscript, you are reassured by the efforts the investigators made to minimize the potential for bias by stating explicitly that all patients with symptoms consistent with new DVT or pulmonary embolism were investigated in a standardized way with diagnostic testing and that each suspected recurrence was adjudicated centrally by an independent panel of experts who were blinded to the patient's randomization arm. As with all randomized trials, there are exclusion criteria and potential confounders, such as different forms of chemotherapy and old age that might have an effect on the generalizeability of the study to these different subgroups of patients, but you note that your patient probably would have been eligible for the study. Therefore, the observed results can probably be extrapolated to your patient. You note that the study had virtually complete follow-up on all patients. Finally, the treatment effect showed a reduction in the recurrence rate from 17% to 9%, an absolute difference of 8% (number needed to treat to prevent one episode of recurrent VTE ~13). This would be considered a clinically important benefit by most experts in the field.

You update the literature review to see if other LMWHs have been evaluated for the treatment of VTE and come across a smaller (N = 146 patients) randomized study that used enoxaparin 1.5 mg/kg once daily instead of dalteparin and showed results similar to those with the dalteparin study. On further review of the literature you do not find anything else that would change your estimate of the benefit of LMWHs over warfarin and assume that there is probably a "class effect."

It is relatively uncommon that patients present to hospital where the evidence is as clear as it is in this woman; we have convincing data that LMWH reduces the risk of clinically important recurrence without an increase in bleeding or other adverse experiences. The other advantage of LMWH is that because of its short half-life, it can simply be withheld 12 to 24 hours prior to any invasive procedure and restarted when it is deemed safe to do so. On the other hand, because of its long half-life (~31 hours), warfarin should be withheld for 2 to 5 days before invasive procedures and simply restarting warfarin postprocedure means that there will be a relatively lengthy window during which she would be unprotected.

PATIENT PREFERENCES AND VALUES

As clinicians practicing EBM, our job is only partially completed once we obtain the best available evidence. We also need to consider how to convey the information to the patient.

CASE 69-2

You introduce yourself and explain to her about DVT and how there is strong evidence that patients like her are suitable candidates for out-of-hospital therapy with anticoagulants. You also explain that although the usual therapy is LMWH by injection once or twice daily for 5 to 7 days, followed by warfarin in doses adjusted to target an INR result to 2.0 to 3.0, patients with cancer benefit from long-term LMWH instead of warfarin.

She understands, but has two problems with LMWH; the first is the administration of injections and the second is the cost of the drug. She explains that she has had so many needles related to chemotherapy for her breast cancer that any therapy involving daily injections is very unappealing. She also inquires about who will administer the injections as she could not possibly self-administer. You explain to her that ideally patients and/or their families administer the LMWH and fortunately her daughter is a nurse who has agreed to give her the daily injections.

With respect to costs, it is clear in your mind that from a societal point of view, LMWH is cost-effective because the extra cost of the drug (~$1000 per month versus ~$50 per month for warfarin) is less than the additional costs of laboratory monitoring of warfarin, and the incremental costs to the health care system associated with the higher recurrence rates. However, what is less clear is the cost to the individual. This largely depends on what part of the cost of the patient's care is paid for by third-party payers, which varies among countries, states, and provinces and among individual patients, some of whom have independent insurance that pays for drug costs and a variety of other medical costs. In the province of Ontario, diagnostic testing, hospitalization, and most in-hospital medications are paid for by government insurance. Many individuals have "drug plans" that cover the cost of the drugs and fortunately your patient is one of those. However, it is easy to see how someone without a drug plan or who has a plan that will not cover LMWH might opt for the much more affordable warfarin and take their chances. After all, the costs of monitoring warfarin are insured services and many patients simply cannot afford the extra cost of LMWH.

CASE 69-3

Fortunately, your patient has the resources to pay for the LMWH and after a lengthy discussion with the patient and her family, she is sent home with dalteparin 200 U/kg once daily. You refer her back to her oncologist after informing him of this recent complication of her breast cancer. You also make a referral to a social worker and to home care to assist her with managing at home. Finally, while dictating your consultation note, you ensure that the family physician receives a copy so that she is "in the loop."

This patient represents a typical patient that a hospitalist might be consulted upon on a day when there are a dozen other patients waiting to see you in the emergency department and there are a dozen other ward patients who require attention. This begs the question: How do we assure that we practice fastidious EBM on the myriad of patients that we are asked to see on a daily basis? The answer is simple: We can't! After all, even the most dedicated physician needs a few hours of sleep, some nourishment, and some time for extracurricular activities. Although the case described above has the potential to be time consuming, so do most patients we see. Therefore, the goal of practicing evidence-based medicine is not perfection but progress.

TIPS

Some tips in practicing EBM include:

1. Ensure you have rapid, easy access to the Internet and the National Library of Medicine, so that literature reviews can be done quickly and at any time.
2. Use a portable (preferably handheld) device on which key articles/recommendations can be downloaded for rapid and easy access.
3. Practice performing literature reviews; this includes defining and refining the clinical question(s), identifying key words, identifying key papers, systematic reviews, and meta-analyses.
4. Learn how to carefully, quickly, and critically review abstracts so that you identify papers of the highest quality that are addressing your clinical question.
5. Let others do the work for you. Identify relevant evidence-based consensus guidelines. When performed properly, expert consensus guidelines can be a very useful addition to your clinical armamentarium. Journal clubs with like-minded EBM practitioners, which target clinical scenarios and/or key articles, can be useful and enjoyable.
6. Avoid unfocused clinical questions. Make the question as specific and as relevant to your patient as possible. This will reduce the tendency to get distracted and off-track. It will also result in fewer identified papers to scrutinize and decrease your workload.
7. Use validated care maps, protocols, algorithms, and clinical prediction rules developed for your institutions or (with care about copyright infringement) other institutions.
8. Be patient! The endpoint in practicing EBM should be an improvement in patient care and outcomes. For the many current practitioners of EBM, there is no diploma or finite endpoint. It is a gradual transition that at times can be frustrating (Internet access will continue to be unavailable at times, computers will continue to crash and become infected). The most useful ancillary equipment is an open mind and the willingness to change.

SUGGESTED READINGS

Choudhry NK, Fletcher RH, Soumerai SB. Systematic review: the relationship between clinical experience and quality of health care. *Ann Intern Med.* 2005;142:260–273.

Guyatt G, Rennie D, Meade MO, Cook D, eds. Users' Guides to the Medical Literature: A Manual for Evidence-based Clinical Practice. 2nd ed. New York: McGraw-Hill; 2002.

Lee AYY, Levine MN, Baker RI, et al. Low-molecular weight heparin versus a coumarin for the prevention of recurrent venous thromboembolism in patients with cancer. *N Engl J Med.* 2003;349: 146–153.

Meyer G, Marjanovic Z, Valcke J, et al. Comparison of low-molecular-weight heparin and warfarin for the secondary prevention of venous thromboembolism in patients with cancer. A randomized controlled study. *Arch Intern Med.* 2002;162:1729–1735.

CHAPTER 70

The Quality of Evidence

Jeremy Paikin, MD
Mark A. Crowther, MD, MSc, FRCPC

INTRODUCTION

In the past, physicians passively applied their knowledge of pathophysiology and pharmacology to treat their patients. While a keen understanding of human physiology (and disease processes) is crucial, several groundbreaking epidemiologists believed it was not enough for the care of patients. Especially in this modern era of explosive growth in technology and new drugs on the market, there is a surplus of information available to health care professionals.

In 1981, a group led by Dr. David Sackett introduced the concept of *critical appraisal*. Critical appraisal was a term that implied an ability to systematically scrutinize medical literature and apply the findings to patients. However, it was not until 1991 when Dr. Gordon Guyatt published an article in *ACP Journal Club* where he coined the now ubiquitous term *evidence-based medicine*. Sackett defines it as the "integration of the best research evidence with clinical expertise and patient values." Therefore, the practice of evidence-based medicine (EBM) does not blindly appraise the medical literature; nor does it absolve physicians from their duties to apply common sense and work closely with their patients to determine the best course of care. In fact, to practice EBM, physicians must adhere to two underlying principles:

1. "Best evidence" is determined using a rigorous process of data extraction and interpretation that weights some forms of evidence over others.
2. Evidence must be interpreted in the setting of the individual patient and his or her characteristics.

PRACTICE POINT

To practice evidence-based medicine, physicians must adhere to two underlying principles:

1. "Best evidence" is determined using a rigorous process of data extraction and interpretation that weights some forms of evidence over others.
2. Evidence must be interpreted in the setting of the individual patient and his or her characteristics.

Evidence-based medicine is vital to providing the best patient care. The focus of this chapter will be on evidence-based interpretation of the medical literature; however, other tenets of EBM should not be overlooked.

BASIC CONCEPTS

Assessing the quality of evidence and applying evidence-based principals requires familiarity with a number of "buzzwords" and basic concepts. This knowledge provides the foundation for a better understanding of the fundamentals of assessing the quality of medical literature.

COINTERVENTIONS

Cointerventions are treatments or interventions that may be differentially applied across experimental and/or control groups that may have an effect on the target outcome, and hence lead to biased results. For example, a study is designed to determine the impact of a novel chemotherapeutic agent to palliate patients with end-stage myeloma. This double-blind, randomized controlled trial (RCT) shows that patients receiving the experimental agent have less bony pain. However, after study completion and careful review, investigators discovered that the chemotherapeutic agent caused an intractable cough that could only be treated with a narcotic-containing syrup. Investigators are now unable to determine whether the reduction in bony pain was secondary to the experimental agent or to the narcotic.

CONFOUNDERS

Confounders are variables or characteristics of the enrolled patient population (that may be differentially distributed between the experimental and control group) that have an influence on the target outcome. For instance, a large RCT designed to test a new immunomodulatory therapy for patients with antiphospholipid syndrome allocates, by chance, more patients with systemic lupus erythematosus (SLE) to the placebo group as compared with the treatment group. If the results demonstrate the treatment leads to a reduction in the target outcome investigators would be unsure whether this observation was due to the therapy or because patients in the treatment group were less likely to have SLE (as the presence of the disease may have made the placebo group, on average, more likely to suffer study-relevant outcomes).

BIAS

Bias is a systematic error, which leads to a distortion of the results; as a result, bias and not treatment may be responsible for the observed treatment effect. Bias may occur at different points in a study and is often difficult to measure. There are many types of bias. To enumerate them all is beyond the scope of this chapter. However, a working knowledge of a few key types of bias is useful for the practicing clinician.

1. **Channeling bias:** Channeling bias occurs most frequently in observational studies. This bias occurs when patients with selected baseline or time-dependent characteristics are preferentially allocated to a therapy; if this occurs the differences in baseline characteristics (and not the treatment) explain the observed difference in outcome. An example would be a new test is made available at the same time as a new treatment; when compared with historical outcomes the patients getting the new drug do better compared with historical controls. However, one cannot conclude that the new intervention is "better"—rather, the improved outcome could be due to either the drug, or to better classification of patients leading to fewer patients who do not have the disease (and who therefore cannot respond to the treatment) being allocated to the treatment in more modern studies.
2. **Detection bias:** A detection bias is a bias caused by differing abilities to detect a disease or outcome. For example, rates of cardiovascular disease may appear to fall over time. Although this may be due to actual changes in disease prevalence, it may also be due to better diagnostic tests that more accurately assign patients to have, or not have, cardiovascular disease. As the number of false positive tests falls the prevalence of disease will fall; the fall is a result of better detection, not better treatments. A detection bias can lead to a channeling bias.
3. **Publication bias:** There are a variety of publication biases. The most prevalent is a propensity for negative studies in general, and small negative studies in particular, to not be published. During literature review (either systematically or nonsystematically), the small missing studies may lead to a misperception that an intervention works. However, and in fact, the intervention does not work—the observed effect is due to failure to include the results of small negative studies.

A list of several biases found in and/or mitigated by randomized controlled trials can be found in **Table 70-1**.

HOW DO WE MINIMIZE THESE EFFECTS?

Designing, analyzing, and reporting clinical trials can be challenging due to the aforementioned issues such as cointerventions,

TABLE 70-1 Biases That May Be Found and/or Mitigated by Well-done Randomized Controlled Trials

Types of Bias	Explanation of Bias	Strategy to Minimize Bias
Experimental and control groups differ in prognosis	Experimental and control groups must be balanced for known and unknown prognostic factors	Randomization
Selection bias	Preferential enrollment of patients into a study (knowingly or unknowingly) and/or preferential administration of a treatment of choice	Allocation concealment (investigators blinded to enrollment process and/or allocation of patients to treatment group)
Placebo effect bias	Positive effect on patients receiving "any therapy" irrespective of its physiologic value	Patient blinding (patient unaware of whether they are receiving the experimental or control therapy)
Cointervention bias	Interventions that may be differentially applied to patients across experimental or control groups that may change the target outcome	Careful record keeping of all treatments that patients receive/statistical adjustment
Ascertainment bias	Results of a study are distorted by knowledge of which treatment patients have received	Investigator blinding (investigators/assessors unaware of which treatment patients received)
Withdrawal bias	Experimental and control groups become prognostically imbalanced due to patient drop outs or those lost to follow	Careful follow-up and intention to treat analysis (analyze patients in the groups to which they were initially allocated)
Selective reporting bias	Reporting positive finding and/or findings that favor the intervention	Prespecify outcomes to be reported and list trial (with intended outcomes to be reported) in publically available database

confounders, and biases. How can we best mitigate these issues? There are a number of measures that investigators may take including: (a) randomization, (b) blinding, (c) concealed allocation, (d) uniform follow-up, (e) accurate accounting of cointerventions, and (f) full disclosure of the fate of all patients.

THE EVIDENCE-BASED MEDICINE PROCESS

In order to properly identify, evaluate, and apply medical literature, it is important to proceed systematically. The evidence-based medicine process includes: (1) formulating a focused clinical question, (2) finding the highest level of evidence, (3) critically appraise the evidence, and (4) apply the evidence to your patient. For the remainder of the chapter, we take you through these four critical steps to making evidence-based decisions for patient care.

PRACTICE POINT

The evidence-based medicine process includes:

1. Formulating a focused clinical question
2. Finding the highest level of evidence
3. Critically appraising the evidence
4. Applying the evidence to your patient

1. **Formulating a focused clinical question:** Asking a precise clinical question is a key first step in the EBM process. Without a clear question a clinician will not be able to find the appropriate medical literature. It is advisable to form a "well-built" question by separating it into four key parts; this helps to clarify the question and will facilitate the literature search. The acronym PICO has been suggested to aid in the development of a clear clinical question:

    Population/patients: Which patient population of interest?
    Intervention: What is the therapeutic intervention of interest?
    Comparator: What is the control intervention/exposure?
    Outcome: What are the important patient outcomes of interest in result of the exposure(s)/intervention(s)?

Now let's proceed to an example of how to properly formulate a clinical question based on a clinical scenario.

CASE 70-1

A 76-year-old gentleman with diabetes mellitus (type 2), hypertension and rate-controlled atrial fibrillation presents to your outpatient office. The patient's medications include metformin, hydrochlorothiazide, and bisoprolol. As the patient's physician you know the patient requires anticoagulation to prevent stroke. However, you are unsure as to whether you should initiate dabigatran etexilate or warfarin, based on the latest data.

You use the $CHADS_2$ risk stratification tool (C = congestive heart failure, H = hypertension, A = age > 75, D = diabetes mellitus, S = stroke/TIA) to predict the risk of stroke in patients with nonvalvular atrial fibrillation. His $CHADS_2$ score of 3 puts him in a high-risk category for stroke (Singer, et al, 2008).

P: Adult patients with atrial fibrillation at high risk of stroke
I: Dabigatran etexilate (150 mg twice a day)
C: Warfarin (as per INR)
O: Stroke or systemic embolism

Once these four elements have been identified, a well-structured and answerable clinical question can be asked as follows: "In adult patients with atrial fibrillation at high risk for stroke, is dabigatran etexilate more effective than warfarin in preventing strokes?"

Once a properly structured clinical question is created, one may then proceed to finding the highest level of evidence to answer the question.

2. **Finding the highest level of evidence:** We currently find ourselves in the midst of the Information Age which is allowing knowledge to be created, synthesized, disseminated, and made available to clinicians at more rapid rates than ever before. Although providing clinicians with vast amounts of information, the risk inherent in this flood of information is that clinicians will develop "information overload." In this setting, the quality of the information must be carefully interpreted—particularly, when the results are going to be directly translated to something as important as patient care.

A "hierarchy of evidence" has been proposed as a rough guide to assist clinicians in determining the believability of studies. The list in **Table 70-2** ranks the various types of medical literature based on their purported methodologic rigor.

TABLE 70-2 Types of Medical Literature

Systematic review of randomized controlled trials (RCTs)	Identification and systematic evaluation of literature (RCTs in this case) that has attempted to answer a particular question
Randomized controlled trials	Participants are randomly assigned to receive an experimental intervention or control, and they are followed along to determine the effect of the intervention on prespecified outcomes
Systematic reviews of cohort studies	Identification and evaluation of literature (cohort studies in this case) that has attempted to answer a particular question
Cohort studies	Prospective study where participants who are/who are not exposed to a proposed cause of a disease of interest are followed to compare the incidence of the outcome of interest
Systematic reviews of case controlled trials	Identification and evaluation of literature (case controlled studies in this case) that has attempted to answer a particular question
Case control studies	Study where patients with/without an outcome of interest are compared based on their exposure to a proposed cause of the outcome
Case series	A report of a collection of patient outcomes who were treated in a similar fashion (no control group)
Expert opinion (most textbooks)	Experiential report (in most cases) of anecdotes, clinical experience and nonsystemic literature review
Case reports, personal experience	Physicians experiential insight; documented formally or not

In addition to the hierarchy of evidence, several expert groups on EBM have created systems to assist clinicians in determining the validity of studies they read. Many such groups exist; a few include the U.S. Preventive Services Task Force, the U.K. National Health Service, and the Grade Working Group.

Despite the efforts of these working groups to simplify the process of ensuring that clinical studies are valid and can be relied upon physicians must continue to closely scrutinize individual studies.

HOW DO WE CRITICALLY APPRAISE RANDOMIZED CONTROLLED TRIALS ABOUT THERAPY?

The focus of the chapter will be on developing a systematic approach to critically appraising randomized controlled trials that set out to test a therapeutic intervention. The User's Guide to the Medical Literature has suggested three key questions to determine the believability of a randomized controlled trial:

1. Are the results valid?
2. What are the results?
3. How can I apply these results to my patient?

Are the results valid?

The initial goal in critically appraising a randomized controlled trial about therapy is to determine if the results are believable. Essentially, the reader must judge whether the research was carried out in a fashion whereby the stated results are unbiased, and are representative of the true treatment effect.

The Users' Guide to the Medical Literature has set out a number of questions to help one determine if a study's results are valid.

1. **Were the patients randomized?** Randomization in a clinical trial implies that no factor other than chance accounts for the group to which the patient is allocated. This reduces the likelihood that measured or unmeasured biases cause the observed outcome. Allowing patients or physicians to choose the treatment will lead to groups with dissimilar baseline characteristics (known or unknown prognostic factors that may have an influence on the outcomes of interest). If the groups are not evenly balanced prior to the initiation of the therapy, determining whether the intervention is responsible for observed results, or some other underlying patient characteristic, is impossible.
2. **Was randomization concealed?** A study has successfully concealed randomization when, at the end of the randomization process, no one involved in the study is aware what treatment the patient received. Awareness of patient allocation biases the study because knowledge of allocation may influence enrollment in the study or may modify subsequent treatments or efforts to detect outcomes of interest.
3. **Were patients analyzed in the groups to which they were randomized?** Patients in RCTs may not actually receive the intervention that they were intended to receive. Analyzing patients by the intervention they actually received introduces a bias that may explain an observed difference in treatment effect. Thus, in a hypothetical study of chemotherapy for lymphoma, patients might be allocated to receive a novel therapeutic agent; however, after randomization those patients who developed nausea after a "run-in period" were excluded from the analysis. In the final analysis it was noted that patients receiving the novel agent had a lower risk of gastric perforation. However, unbeknownst to the study designers, patients with gastric involvement with lymphoma were more likely to develop nausea in the run-in period after the novel agent than after placebo. Since such patients were preferentially excluded from the treatment group one cannot determine if the final observed effect was due to a true benefit of the novel agent or due to the fact that the placebo group included more patients with gastric involvement who are (presumably) at increased risk of gastric perforation. The process of analyzing patients in the group to which they were assigned (whether or not they received the intervention) is called an "intention-to-treat" analysis. The goal of intention-to-treat analysis is to preserve the integrity of randomization, and overcome the biases associated with participant crossover and dropout.
4. **Were patients in the treatment and control groups similar with respect to known prognostic factors?** As described earlier, the goal of randomization is to form experimental and control groups with similar baseline characteristics. More specifically, it is important to ensure that "prognostically important" characteristics (for the target outcome) are balanced between the groups. For example, if (by chance) sicker patients are allocated to a novel treatment, the true impact of the intervention may be underestimated (or vice versa). As investigators, we can never be sure about "unknown prognostic factors." In other words, there are bound to be relationships between some patient characteristics and target outcomes that have yet to be elucidated and therefore cannot be accounted for. However, we should be cognizant of known prognostic factors for our target outcome and ensure that they are balanced between the groups. The larger the sample, the less likely there will be imbalances. If there are significant imbalances there are statistical maneuvers to help overcome this potential bias. Data to guide the reviewer about the distribution of known biases are usually provided in the first table in most scientific publications.
5. **Were patients, clinicians, and/or outcome assessors aware of group allocation?** If patients, clinicians, or outcomes assessors are aware of group allocation bias may ensue. Patients' awareness may lead to the placebo effect. The placebo effect is defined as the effect of a treatment on patients irrespective of its biologic properties. Clinician awareness may lead to differences in medical care depending on whether the patient is known to be receiving the treatment or not. In essence, differences in clinical care can alter the clinical course of patients (change their prognosis), and therefore, make it difficult to determine whether it is the therapy that was responsible for the observed results, or the differences in clinical care. Outcome assessors ought to be blinded because knowledge of the group that a patient belongs to may influence their interpretation/reporting of target outcomes.
6. **Was follow-up complete?** Investigators must ensure that all participants are accounted for at the end of a study. Patients that drop out of studies are often a different patient population (from a prognosis standpoint) than those that remain until study completion. Often, those that dropout are a sicker patient population and therefore, the remaining patients in each group may be generally more well than at the beginning of the study and become prognostically dissimilar. Unfortunately, there is no "acceptable" dropout rate that can be applied across all clinical trials. A commonly employed technique to determine whether dropouts compromise a study's validity is to treat each patient that drops out as a worst-case scenario (ie, death). If the overall results of the study remain unchanged with the worst-case scenario, then validity is unlikely to be compromised by dropouts.

What are the results?

Once the results of a clinical study are deemed to be valid the reader should then look at the results and make a judgment regarding the magnitude and precision of the treatment effect.

1. **How large was the treatment effect?** A detailed explanation of the statistical methods used to describe the magnitude of treatment effect is beyond the scope of this chapter. However, two simple techniques that are used to determine magnitude of effect are calculating the absolute and relative risk reductions. The following example will help illustrate each of these concepts. Participants with atrial fibrillation at risk for cardioembolic stroke were randomized to receive a new oral anticoagulant or warfarin therapy. At the end of the study, 2% of those randomized to the new oral anticoagulant group suffered a stroke, whereas 4% of those randomized to warfarin had a stroke.

Relative risk reduction (RRR):

The RRR is defined as: (1 − [% of participants in treatment group suffering target outcome/% of participants in control group suffering target outcome]).

$$= \left(1 - \frac{2}{4}\right) = 0.50 = 50\%$$

Therefore, the new oral anticoagulant led to a 50% RRR of cardioembolic stroke as compared to warfarin.

Absolute risk reduction (ARR):

The ARR is as: % of participants in the control group suffering from the target outcome − % of participants in experimental group suffering from the target outcome.

$$= 4\% - 2\% = 2\%$$

Therefore, the new oral anticoagulant led to a 2% ARR as compared to warfarin.

2. **How precise was the treatment effect?** The simplest method to determine the precision of a treatment effect is to look at the confidence interval (CI). A CI is a simple representation of the best estimate of the treatment effect. Rather than stating the estimate as a simple value, a CI represents a range of values in which the "true" result will fall. The confidence coefficient represents the certainty that the "true" result will fall within the given CI. It is unlikely, but not impossible, that the true value is outside the range—the narrower the range the more precise the estimate and the more valuable the result.

HOW CAN I APPLY THE RESULTS TO PATIENT CARE?

Once the study has proved to be valid and has demonstrated an important treatment effect, the treating physician must then decide as to whether he can apply the findings to his patient.

1. **Were the study patients similar to the patient in my practice?** The most important considerations when determining whether the results are applicable to your patient is to ensure that your patient:
   (a) Meets the inclusion criteria of the study
   (b) Does not meet any of the exclusion criteria

However, difficulty may arise when the patient in your clinic does not meet the specific criteria of the study. In this case, the physician is left with a difficult to decision in trying to determine whether the results of the study are generalizeable. If faced with this difficult scenario, a general rule is to ask oneself if there is a good reason to disbelieve the applicability of the results (from a physiologic perspective or from prior studies with contradicting results).

2. **Were all clinically important outcomes considered?** Physicians must use their judgment to determine whether the outcomes of the trial are important to patients. For example, in trials that have been done to evaluate oral anticoagulants to prevent stroke in patients with atrial fibrillation, few would disagree that strokes and major bleeding events are important outcomes for patients. However, "softer" outcomes or "surrogate outcomes" are defined as outcomes that are *associated* with important outcomes for patients. There are many examples of this in medical practice. For instance, we know that the INR is a good marker of bleeding risk in the chronic setting; however, we know from RCTs that lowering INRs in supratherapeutic patients does not reduce bleeding events. This speaks to the importance of studying patient important outcomes.
3. **Are the likely treatment benefits worth the potential harms and costs?** It is always important to weigh benefits with the risks (or costs) prior to initiating therapy. An important concept known as the number needed to treat (NNT) helps one determine the magnitude of potential benefit for a given therapy. This is defined as the number of patients that need to be treated to prevent one event. The equation used to calculate the NNT is:

$$\text{NNT} = \frac{1}{\text{ARR}}$$

The NNT provides a good estimate of the treatment effect of a particular therapy. However, the economics of instituting therapy must also be considered, particularly within the financial constraints of health care systems. Quality-adjusted life years (QALY) is used to determine the value the health care provider is getting for a particular intervention. A rough guide for the model of cost-effectiveness is that 1 QALY = GDP of 1 individual in a given society.

ADDITIONAL CONSIDERATIONS: POST HOC ANALYSIS

Post hoc analysis involves examining the data after the clinical trial has been completed with the intention of finding patterns (from outcomes) that were not prespecified in the study design. Some investigators may look at the data and find subgroups in which the therapeutic intervention may have been much more effective. We encourage everyone to be skeptical of subgroup analyses. While these findings may be hypothesis generating, they should not be considered strong evidence for a therapeutic advantage in one group or another.

P VALUES

P values are defined as the percentage of time that we would be willing to accept that a treatment effect found (by a particular therapy) in an RCT is not due to chance. Conventionally, investigators have set the *P* value as $P = .05$. This can be interpreted as the following: the result of a clinical trial would be accepted as being "statistically significant" if there is less than a 5% chance that the difference between the experimental and control groups is due to chance (and not the treatment itself).

STOPPING TRIALS EARLY

Experimental therapies have the potential to cause harm to the participants. Therefore, investigators may set up interim analyses to ensure that patients are not being harmed. At these analyses, there is a tendency of investigators to celebrate an observed benefit (prior to study completion). Work done by Dr. Montori has shown that trials stopped for benefit should be looked at with skepticism because they may show implausibly large treatment effects, and fail to report the criteria used to stop the study early.

CONCLUSION

An understanding of how to systematically appraise RCTs and appropriately apply the results to patients is fundamental to providing the best care. Evidence-based medicine is about more than interpreting clinical trials—it is about using clinical trials to guide therapy within the framework of patients/physicians values and preferences. We hope that this introduction to EBM (while not comprehensive), will be a useful start in understanding the basic principles of practice.

SUGGESTED READINGS

Crowther MA, Ageno W, Garcia D, et al. Oral vitamin K versus placebo to correct excessive anticoagulation in patients receiving warfarin: a randomized trial. *Ann Intern Med.* 2009;150:293–300.

Guyatt GH, Sackett DL, Cook DJ. How to use an article about therapy or prevention. A. Are the results of the study valid? Evidence-based Medicine Working Group. *JAMA.* 1993;270:2598–2601.

Guyatt GH, Sackett DL, Cook DJ. How to use an article about therapy or prevention. B. What are the results and will they help me care for my patients? Evidence-based Medicine Working Group. *JAMA.* 1994;271:59–63.

Guyatt GH. Evidence-based medicine. *ACP Journal Club.* 1991;114:A-16.

Montori VM, Devereaux PJ, Adhikari NK, et al. Randomized trials stopped early for benefit: a systematic review. *JAMA.* 2005;294:2203–2209.

Singer DE, Albers GW, Dalen JE, et al. Antithrombotic therapy in atrial fibrillation: American College of Chest Physicians Evidence-Based Clinical Practice Guidelines (8th Edition). *Chest.* 2008;133:546S–592S.

CHAPTER 71

Role of Diagnostic Testing in Patient Care

Jeffrey S. Ginsberg, MD, FRCP(C)

INTRODUCTION

The scope of diagnostic tests ranges from signs and symptoms elicited during clinical examination, imaging tests, to biochemical, pathologic, and psychological tests. Tests that are capable of fully discriminating between the presence or absence of a disease are uncommon. Diagnostic testing is generally performed to screen for, detect, and monitor diseases. To optimize the use of diagnostic testing, clinicians should be aware of how the results of testing will affect determination of the probability of the presence of disease. To be useful, diagnostic tests should have the potential to change the pretest probability of disease into a post-test probability that is more definitive. The process of diagnostic testing should be based on a logical sequence that arrives at a sufficiently high probability of disease to make the diagnosis or a sufficiently low probability to exclude the diagnosis. These thresholds will vary from disease to disease; when the consequences of missing the disease (false-negative) have high potential to be disastrous, the threshold of post-test probability should be very low, whereas when the consequences of falsely making a diagnosis of the disease have the potential to be disastrous, the threshold of post-test probability should be very high. For example, when a patient has a suspected myocardial infarction (MI), clinicians require a combination of test results that has a very low (< 2%) post-test probability since the consequences of missing an MI and sending the patient home are potentially disastrous. On the other hand, when making a diagnosis of MI, clinicians need a high post-test probability because the consequences of treatment (thrombolytic therapy, invasive strategies) and on prognosis (life expectancy) can be serious.

PRACTICE POINT

- To optimize the use of diagnostic testing, clinicians should be aware of how the results of testing will affect determination of the probability of the presence of disease. To be useful, diagnostic tests should have the potential to change the pretest probability.

INTERPRETATION OF DIAGNOSTIC TESTING

The process of considering the diagnosis of a disease is often triggered by components of the history and physical examination, which lead the clinician to consider the presence of the disease. Other key components in considering a diagnosis include the experience and knowledge base of the diagnostician, the frequency of the disease, and the clinical importance of making or refuting a diagnosis.

Experience and knowledge base not only affect whether a disease shows up on the "radar screen," but can also influence the accuracy of assessment of the clinical pretest probability (PTP). Two ways of evaluating PTP are by using clinician's "gestalt" or by using validated clinical prediction rules. The former might be favored by clinicians experienced in the disease of interest (eg, cardiologists for diagnosing MI), particularly when there is some subjectivity in aspects of the diagnosis. For pulmonary embolism (PE), the challenge becomes the spectrum of disease (ranging from clinically silent to multiple clinical presentations often with nonspecific symptoms and signs to hemodynamic collapse), the limitations of the history and physical examination ("the great masquerader"), and the absence of a single effective noninvasive test. Despite this, clinicians can assign meaningful probabilities for acute PE. When PIOPED clinicians assigned a high probability of PE prior to V/Q scanning, 67% of patients had PE. When they assigned a low probability of PE, only 9% had acute PE. Among the PIOPED patients, 64% had intermediate probabilities for PE.

The main purpose of clinical prediction rules is to take components of the history and physical examination sometimes combined with simple widely available diagnostic tests (eg, oxygen saturation, electrocardiogram, chest radiography), and use them to estimate the PTP into clinically useful categories. With any clinical prediction rule, the simpler and more objective the rule, the more likely it is to be useful. Although beyond the scope of this textbook, validation of clinical prediction rules involves assessment at several institutions by a wide range of appropriate clinicians in methodologically sound studies. Ideally, this should involve careful evaluation of both intra- and interobserver variation. The rule should first be validated in accuracy studies where it is compared to the reference standard, and subsequently validated in management studies where it is used (often in conjunction with other tests) to make management decisions.

PRACTICE POINT

- The main purpose of clinical prediction rules is to take components of the history and physical examination sometimes combined with simple widely available diagnostic tests (eg, oxygen saturation, electrocardiogram, chest radiography), and use them to estimate the clinical pretest probability into clinically useful categories.

Diagnostic frequency is a key component in determining whether considering disease entities as a cause of symptoms. In developed countries, where both myocardial infarction and pulmonary embolism are common, these diagnoses must be considered in adults who present with chest pain. On the other hand, in North America, a diagnosis such as leprosy would be uncommon in a patient presenting with a skin rash.

Some diseases are important to diagnose or exclude because treatment is available for the disease that is specific and quite often (as in pulmonary embolism and meningococcal meningitis) required urgently to avoid a tragic outcome. These factors affect the approach to diagnosis because, even if the PTP is not high, the clinical consequences of missing the diagnosis or making a tardy diagnosis can be fatal. Therefore, even though musculoskeletal problems are a more common cause of pleuritic chest pain than pulmonary embolism in the community, the latter must be at least considered because not administering anticoagulants to a patient with pulmonary embolism can result in fatal recurrence.

Diagnostic testing and its interpretation are among the key elements to making or excluding the presence of a suspected disease. When first exposed to the concept of the accuracy of diagnostic testing, confusion often arises because of misunderstanding of some of the key accuracy indices, such as sensitivity, specificity, negative predictive value (NPV), positive predictive value (PPV), and likelihood ratios. The simplest way of depicting these characteristics is by first generating a 2 × 2 contingency table (**Table 71-1**).

Sensitivity is defined as the proportion of patients with a disease of interest who have an abnormal test result or A/A + C.

Specificity is defined as the proportion of patients without the disease of interest who have a normal test result or D/B + D.

The sensitivity and specificity alone do not give us the probability that the test will give us the correct answer. In addition to knowing the test's average sensitivity and specificity, the clinician must be aware of how the test performs in different segments of the population.

TABLE 71-1 2 × 2 Contingency Table

		Disease Present?	
		Yes	No
Diagnostic test result	Positive	A	B
	Negative	C	D

NPV is defined as the proportion of patients with a negative test result who do not have the disease of interest D/C + D.

PPV is defined as the proportion of patients with a positive test result who have the disease of interest A/A + B.

As the prevalence of disease falls, the PPV falls and the NPV rises. If the prevalence of disease is very low, the PPV will not be close to one even if the sensitivity and specificity are high. Therefore, in screening the general population, many people with positive test results will have false positives.

The ideal test has a sensitivity of 100% and a specificity of 100%. Such a test would be a gold standard diagnostic test for the disease of interest and in real life is rare for most diseases. In clinical practice, we intuitively think in terms of predictive values since we are often faced with a laboratory result and the clinical questions are whether a negative test result excludes the disease of interest and whether a positive test result diagnoses the disease of interest.

Not all tests are sensitive and specific, but rather have a high sensitivity or specificity. Such tests can still be highly useful provided they are interpreted correctly. One way to remember the effects of sensitivity and specificity are the acronyms "SpPin" and "SnNout," which refer to a highly specific test rules in a diagnosis when the results are positive, whereas a highly sensitive test rules out a diagnosis when the results are negative.

A somewhat different way of expressing the accuracy of diagnostic testing is by calculation of likelihood ratios. A likelihood ratio describes how many times someone with a disease is more likely to show a test result than someone without disease. Using the 2 × 2 table above, the negative likelihood ratio is calculated as 1-sensitivity/specificity, whereas the positive likelihood ratio is calculated as sensitivity/1−specificity. A likelihood ratio of > 1.0 is associated with the presence of disease, whereas a likelihood ratio of < 1.0 is associated with the absence of disease.

For example, using the "gold standard" of elevated cardiac enzymes for the diagnosis of MI, new ST-segment elevation has the highest LR (ranging from 5.7 to 54) and a normal ECG decreases the probability of MI. However, a "normal" ECG is not a substitute for clinical judgment and the ECG should be repeated for any patient with ongoing symptoms or as part of a "rule-out" protocol while cardiac enzymes are pending.

ODDS RATIOS AND RECEIVER OPERATING CHARACTERISTIC CURVES

A disadvantage of sensitivity, specificity, as well as positive and negative likelihood ratios is that they result in two or more parameters to describe the accuracy of a diagnostic test. Two relatively common methods of producing single parameters are odds ratios (OR) and receiver operating characteristics (ROC) curves. The OR is calculated as the positive likelihood ratio divided by the negative likelihood ratio. Using the 2 × 2 contingency table above, OR can be calculated as *ad/bc*. ROC curves simply plot (in graphic form), the sensitivity on the *y*-axis and 1−specificity on the *x*-axis using several different test results. The area under the ROC curve estimates the ability of the test to accurately classify patients as having or not having a disease. A test with 100% sensitivity and specificity has an area of 1.0, whereas a test that is no better than chance has an area of 0.5.

Major technologic advances permit faster diagnosis of treatable diseases such as appendicitis less invasively through imaging. The ROC plot of the appendiceal CT technique has positively affected use of resources by avoiding unnecessary hospitalizations for observation and appendectomy. The helical CT has a sensitivity of 100%, specificity of 95%, accuracy of 98%, PPV of 97%, NPV 100% for appendicitis using the diagnostic criteria of thickened appendix (>6 mm diameter), periappendicular stranding, focal thickening of the apex of the cecum, and appendicoliths.

PITFALLS OF DIAGNOSTIC TESTS

When evaluating the validity of a diagnostic test, clinicians should be aware of several key elements to the proper ascertainment of the accuracy of a diagnostic test. It is always useful to stay in touch with the laboratory and diagnostic imaging departments of your hospital. Examples of laboratory tests that have been used to make or exclude a diagnosis of disease in well-designed studies include D-dimer testing (for excluding a diagnosis of deep vein thrombosis and pulmonary embolism) and anticardiolipin antibody testing (for diagnosing antiphospholipid antibody syndrome).

Incredibly, despite a myriad of studies showing very high sensitivity (and therefore high negative predictive value) for deep vein thrombosis and pulmonary embolism, there has been little effort among manufacturers to standardize the kits. Consequently, because there are many different D-dimer kits available, the optimal cut point for different assays might not show the same accuracy indices among different kits. Additionally, the "absolute" values of D-dimer measured vary dramatically among different manufacturers. It is important for clinicians (and essential for laboratory heads) to be aware of the wide variety of D-dimer kits that are available, to choose the correct cut-point for the D-dimer used and even to test a number of samples to ensure that the published accuracy indices can be replicated. It is also important for the clinician to appreciate when to use this screening test which will be falsely positive in most hospitalized patients due to recent surgery, underlying diseases such as cancer, renal failure, and acute infection.

Anticardiolipin antibody testing is fraught with problems related to lack of a gold standard test and the large number of commercially available kits with poor inter-kit agreement. Commercially available kits are almost all ELISAs which have a cardiolipin "antigen" in the wells and provide a quantitative estimate of the titer of anticardiolipin antibody present. Abnormal results defined by a greater than a predefined cut-point are usually further subcategorized as low, intermediate, or high titer depending on the degree of elevation abnormal results. Because the antigen in wells for the ELISA varies substantially from kit to kit, the results of any given patient can vary tremendously and run the gamut from normal to high titer for the same patient sample. Compounding the problem of lack of standardization among assays is the fact that the titers of anticardiolipin antibodies can vary over time within a given patient. Why are all of these issues important? In the diagnosis of antiphospholipid antibody syndrome, a patient must have both a clinical complication (thrombotic event, recurrent pregnancy loss, or thrombocytopenia) and laboratory abnormalities (a positive lupus anticoagulant or anticardiolipin antibody assay on two separate occasions at least 6 weeks apart). Since thrombosis and pregnancy loss are both relatively common complications in an otherwise healthy population, errant anticardipolipin antibody assay results can lead to a false diagnosis of antiphospholipid antibody syndrome or result in a false negative diagnosis. Either problem can easily result in patient mismanagement.

CRITICAL EVALUATION OF THE QUALITY OF EVIDENCE FOR DIAGNOSTIC TESTING

Before integrating a diagnostic test into clinical practice it is important to be aware of the diagnostic standard(s) and its limitations. In general terms, there are three stages in evaluation of a diagnostic test. In the first phase, the "exploratory" phase, the inter- and intraobserver variabilities are estimated, as is the reproducibility of the test. This is generally the phase during which the "kinks" in the test are worked out and a "normal range" is established. The second or "accuracy" phase involves comparison of the test with a criterion standard. If no true gold standard exists, then a surrogate is used. This might include a single test or combination of tests to diagnose the condition of interest and either the same tests or some combination of tests to exclude the condition of interest. Ideally, this should provide accurate estimates of the sensitivity, specificity, positive predictive value, and negative predictive value, as well as the positive and negative likelihood ratios. Once these accuracy indices are determined, the third phase, or the "clinical management" phase, should be undertaken. In this phase, large, well-designed studies should be performed in which the consequences of patient management decisions based on the results of the test are formally evaluated.

Ideally, all diagnostic tests should undergo the rigorous evaluations described above. Unfortunately, most tests used in day-to-day practice do not undergo clinical management studies, but rather accuracy studies only.

Technical considerations that influence the specific test result include spectrum bias, reporting bias, and reproducibility. Spectrum bias refers to disease factors that affect the sensitivity and specificity of a diagnostic test—severity of disease, cyclic nature of disease activity, duration of disease, therapy, and control group composition. Reporting bias refers to the tendency to report strongly positive or negative results (and not to report results with weaker findings). Availability heuristic is a bias that makes noteworthy outcomes more likely such as a radiologist overestimating the likelihood of cancer in imaging findings. Reproducibility not only refers to the consistency of the test performance but also result interpretation. Interobserver agreement is expressed using the kappa statistic. A K value = 0 is the same as that by chance; 0.2–0.4, fair agreement; 0.4–0.6 moderate agreement; 0.6–0.8 substantial agreement; and 0.8–1.0 almost perfect agreement. For most of our diagnostic tests, K statistics not only reflect the specific study but also the examiner's experience. For CT imaging a negative result must be interpreted in the context of technical factors. For example, a head CT screen for subarachnoid hemorrhage may be negative, equivocal, or technically inadequate. Technical factors include variation in the thickness of slices taken at the base of the brain and motion artifact. The sensitivity also declines with increasing time between onset of headache and scanning and there may be false-negative results for bleeding if the patient has a Hct < 30% because blood with a Hg concentration below 10 g/dL may appear isodense. So in addition to understanding the test characteristics, clinicians need to apply the test to the patient in front of them. They have to ask what are the best tests to diagnose the problem and in what sequence.

NEW DIAGNOSTIC TESTS: MEETING A CLINICAL NEED

New technologies generate new diagnostic tests. To be clinically useful, a new diagnostic test should have one or more of the following characteristics:

1. It should fulfill an unmet clinical need.
2. It should improve diagnostic accuracy and result in improved patient outcomes.
3. It should reduce the risk of adverse experiences in the population of interest.

4. It should simplify the diagnostic process.
5. It should reduce the costs of the diagnostic process.

PRACTICE POINT

- When evaluating the validity of a diagnostic test, clinicians should be aware of several key elements to the proper ascertainment of the accuracy of a diagnostic test. It is always useful to stay in touch with the laboratory and diagnostic imaging departments of your hospital. Although newer imaging technologies have expanded our ability to define anatomic and physiological abnormalities, the frequency of misdiagnosis remains unchanged.

For example, when magnetic resonance imaging (MRI) was first developed for use in "medicine," it was heralded with tremendous optimism as a diagnostic test. In the United States, many private companies and laboratories purchased them, resulting in a "glut" of MRI units. The momentum for the development of MRI technology was driven to some extent by financial gain. Although most clinicians marvel over the incredible resolution of MRI for both soft tissue and bony structures and it was "obviously" destined to revolutionize diagnostic imaging, definitive indications for this technology have been limited. For example, although accurate for diagnosing deep vein thrombosis in symptomatic patients, MRI has not replaced far less expensive tests such as assessment of clinical pretest probability, D-dimer testing, and venous ultrasonography. In a sense, it was (and perhaps, still is) a technology looking for indications. Although newer imaging technologies have expanded our ability to define anatomic and physiological abnormalities, the frequency of misdiagnosis remains unchanged.

SUGGESTED READINGS

Edlow JA, Caplan LR. Avoiding pitfalls in the diagnosis of subarahnoid hemorrhage. *N Engl J Med.* 2000;342(1):29–36.

Guyatt G, Rennie D, Meade MO, Cook D, eds. Users' Guides to the *Medical Literature: A Manual for Evidence-based Clinical Practice.* 2nd ed. New York: McGraw-Hill; 2002.

Rao PM, Rhea JT, Novelline RA, et al. Helical CT technique for the diagnosis of appendicitis: prospective evaluation of a focused appendix CT examination. *Radiology.* 1997;202(1):139–144.

CHAPTER 72

Systematic Reviews and Meta-Analysis

Mark A. Crowther, MD, MSc, FRCPC
Mark Crowther, MD, ChB, MRCP, FRCPath

INTRODUCTION

With the continual increase in the volume of medical literature being produced health care providers are finding it increasingly difficult to keep up to date with the latest evidence. For example a search for "ACE inhibitors" in PubMed produced 1588 possible articles in 2009 alone. Traditionally, people referred to review articles in the hope that these will provide the latest evidence and hence reduce the need for them to perform exhaustive personal appraisal of the available literature. However, review articles are susceptible to bias as they (potentially) convey only the authors' views on the topic; furthermore, unless authors perform a comprehensive literature review, the article may not include contemporaneous, practice changing papers. Systemic reviews aim to reduce bias in review articles by providing readers with the best available information on the topic and, with meta-analysis, try to combine data from several studies to produce a single result. In this chapter we will describe how a systematic review is produced and how to critically appraise a systematic review. The systematic approach is also useful when trying to answer day-to-day clinical questions in your own clinical practice. Detailed guidance on producing a systematic review can be found at the Cochrane Collaboration's Website where their handbook can be downloaded. A checklist to ensure all important information is reported in a systematic review was produced by the QUOROM collaboration and provides a useful tool for guiding the appraisal of systematic reviews; a modified version is presented in **Table 72-1**.

THE CLINICAL QUESTION

What is the clinical question that needs to be answered? A careful articulation of the question is critical, as it provides the scope of the review. Thus, a systematic review on insulin treatment for type 2 diabetes will be a far greater undertaking than a systematic review of the best injection sites for insulin. When reading a systematic review, one must always ascertain that the reviewers are answering the question originally asked.

PRACTICE POINT

- When reading a systematic review one must always ascertain that the reviewers are answering the question originally asked.

SEARCH STRATEGY

The completeness of the search strategy will determine the completeness of review, although the more exhaustive the search the greater the effort will be of producing the systematic review. Usually the search for studies takes place in several areas:

- **Electronic databases.** There are a wide range of searchable electronic databases, often specific to a certain area of health care (ie, CINAHL for nursing and allied health care studies) but for medicine the common databases are Medline/PubMed, Embase, and the Cochrane Library. These databases display studies that meet the provided search strategy. Usually the search strategy uses Boolean language (AND, NOT, OR). It must be decided what databases are to be searched (this is often specific to the topic), the search strategy (the more general the search the more complete it will be, but the longer it will

TABLE 72-1 The QUORUM Statement on How to Report a Systematic Review

Heading	Subheading	Descriptor
Title		Can clearly determine that report is a systematic review.
Abstract		Uses a structured format.
	Objectives	Describes clinical question explicitly.
	Data sources	Lists the databases used and other sources of data.
	Review Methods	Describes how the data was selected, quality assessment, data extraction, and any meta-analysis performed.
	Results	Describes included and excluded studies and the results of any meta-analysis.
	Conclusion	Describes the main results.
Introduction		Discusses the clinical problem, why the intervention may work, and the reasons for performing the review.
Methods	Searching	Describes the data sources (eg, databases, handsearching, registers, researchers) and any search exclusions (date, language, etc).
	Selection	Inclusion and exclusion criteria.
	Validity assessment	Describes how any quality assessment was performed.
	Data abstraction	Discusses how data was extracted from studies.
	Quantitative data synthesis	Information on how data was combined (meta-analysis), including statistical methods used, measures of effect and any sensitivity, and subgroup analysis performed. Also what tests were performed looking for heterogeneity and publication bias.
Results	Trial flow	Provides a figure demonstrating number of studies screened, included and excluded at each step.
	Study characteristics	Each trial is described briefly, including participant demographics, number of participants, intervention, and follow-up.
	Quantitative data synthesis	Presents simple summary results for individual studies and any meta-analysis performed.
Discussion		Discusses the answer to the original question in the light of the best available evidence and any possible biases. Also suggested future research.

Data from Moher D, Cook DJ, Eastwood S, et al, for the QUOROM Group 1999. Improving the quality of reports of meta-analyses of randomized controlled trials: the QUOROM statement. *Lancet*. 1999;354(9193):1896–1900.

take as it will produce more results that need careful review) and the number of people who will perform the search (one person may make mistakes; therefore, it is better if the search is duplicated and the success of duplicate searching measured statistically, using correlation statistics). The search will produce a large quantity of results, many of which will not be relevant. For efficiency, many of these early results can be excluded on the basis of their title and abstract. However, more detailed review of individual papers is required for those papers passing the initial screen.

It is best to establish, a priori, criteria for accepting papers. These criteria should be explicit and the most rigorous reviews record the specific reasons for including or excluding all papers identified in the literature search. Specific recording for each paper not only reduces the risk of bias, it also allows rapid re-assessment should the rationale for exclusion of one or more papers be called into question.

When appraising a review you need to determine how complete the database search is. Are all relevant databases searched? Might the condition have more than one name or spelling (hemolytic anemia in the US/Canada and haemolytic anaemia in the UK)? Could the search strategy have excluded relevant papers by being too specific (eg, when determining the effect of beta-blockers on hypertension a search strategy might be "hypertension AND beta-blockers," but this may miss a paper which primarily looked at survival but reported hypertension in the text).

Consultation with a skilled librarian will almost always improve the quality and yield of a review. It should be strongly considered in all cases, particularly if the investigator is less experienced in systematic reviews.

- **Conference abstracts.** Searching conference abstracts may provide studies that have yet to be published in full. Hence it is useful to search the last few years for relevant conferences. Studies that demonstrate inconclusive results for an intervention are less likely to be published, but are still valuable evidence, and searching conference abstracts may find these. Care has to be taken when applying the results of conference abstracts to a systematic review, as the abstracts will not have not undergone the rigorous peer review of journal articles.
- **Handsearching.** As a final check, the reference lists of included studies should be checked for papers not found by other means. One can also search journals in which papers on the subject of the review are likely to be published.
- **Contacting researchers.** Writing to researchers active in the area may provide results of studies yet to be presented or published; however, care has to be taken with this information, as with conference abstracts, it has not undergone a rigorous peer review process. Furthermore, most investigators will be hesitant to provide unpublished information as its inclusion in a systematic review may hamper subsequent publication. Perhaps the greatest utility of inquiring with researchers is gaining knowledge of papers that are about to be published—delaying the review article will allow inclusion of these articles and thus make the review more timely.

INCLUDING AND EXCLUDING STUDIES

Deciding what studies to include or exclude in the review is very important. Inclusion or exclusion is usually based on different reasons:

- To improve the quality of studies, if it is known that there are randomized controlled trials (RCTs) in the area of the review, then the studies may be limited to RCTs, as these are the type of study which are less prone to bias.

- Limiting studies by language will reduce the number of studies needed to review, especially if there is difficulty in translating a paper. This may be acceptable for many reviews but in some areas (eg, hepatitis infections where it is endemic to certain countries), a large amount of information published in other languages needs to be reviewed. As a result, limiting publications to English is discouraged.
- Limiting studies by date; there is no point searching for studies in a topic if prior to a date it does not exist; therefore, searches may be limited by date (*Helicobacter pylori* was only described in the 1980s, hence there will be no papers on treatment published prior to that).
- Question-specific limitations; if the clinical questions are only for a subgroup of a disease (eg, acute rather than chronic otitis media), then studies can be excluded that don't meet the criteria set by the original question. The same is true for setting limits by patient demographics (age, sex, etc).

ASSESSING THE QUALITY OF STUDIES

Once all the relevant studies have been found, it is then important to determine how good quality the studies are. The quality of included studies determines the certainty with which you can make any conclusions based on the summation of the evidence. A formal quality assessment is particularly important if there is contradictory evidence. As assessment of quality can be subjective, more than one researcher should perform the quality assessment and the results compared using correlative statistics.

Generally, RCTs (studies where participants are randomly assigned an intervention) are intrinsically of better quality than nonrandomized studies (where participants are given an intervention and compared to another group who are similar but did not receive the intervention), that in turn is better than case reports or case series. The randomization process should equally distribute confounding factors between the two groups. As a result any difference observed over the course of the study should be due to the intervention. Given the reduced likelihood for bias many systematic reviews, only include RCTs; nonrandomized data is only included if randomized data is not available.

There are various tools designed for performing checklist-quality assessment of studies. Some are specific for certain types of studies. A modified example is seen in **Table 72-2** (Jadad score for RCTs). Other tools are available online (eg, the Newcastle-Ottowa score for nonrandomized studies). In general, however, the important points are as follows:

- The participants are similar to those found in normal clinical practice, not highly selected (content validity).
- Neither the participants nor the researchers are able to tell what the randomization result is before randomization (allocation concealment—eg, if sealed envelopes are used, can they be held up to light to tell what is in them?).
- Participants are followed up for an appropriate length of time (this can be shorter for conditions like bacterial infections which have a short time frame compared to the effects of a cholesterol-lowering drug which may take several years to have an effect). The follow-up should be as complete as possible, with as few participants as possible being lost to follow-up. Information should also be provided why patients dropped out or were lost in order that the reviewer can determine if these losses were due, in whole or in part, to side effects of the treatment.
- As many people as is feasible who are involved in the study are masked to treatment received—ideally, participants, care providers, those collecting data, and those adjudicating outcomes should be masked. In selected cases, the analyst can also be masked to the specific intervention.
- Ideally, the study should also report the results as intention-to-treat (all patients who underwent allocation are analyzed regardless of how long they stayed in the study; this provides the best "real world" estimate of the effect) and per-protocol (only patients who remained within the protocol for a predetermined period are analyzed, this gives the best safety data).

TABLE 72-2 The Modified Jadad Scoring System for RCTs

	Score
1. Was the study described as randomized? If yes, score 1 point.	
2. If yes to question 1, was an **appropriate** randomization sequence described and used (eg table of random numbers, computer generated, etc)? If yes, score 1 point.	
3. If yes to question 1, was an **inappropriate** method to generate the sequence of randomization used (patients were allocated alternately, or according to date of birth, hospital number, etc)? If yes, subtract 1 point.	
4. Was the study described as double blinded? If yes, score 1 point.	
5. If yes to question 4, was an appropriate method of blinding used (eg, identical placebo, active placebo, dummy, etc)? If yes, score 1 point.	
6. If yes to question 4, was an inappropriate method for blinding used (eg, comparison of tablet vs injection with no double dummy)? If yes, subtract 1 point.	
7. Were the withdrawals and dropouts described? If yes, score 1 point.	

When appraising a review the questions to ask are, has an appropriate quality assessment tool been used; did more than one researcher perform the quality assessment; and, if so, was there agreement; and are the quality assessment result reported in an appropriate way?

DATA EXTRACTION

The data from the papers can then be extracted, usually onto prepared data case report forms. Data extraction should be done in duplicate to reduce transcribing errors. The data to be extracted should be carefully considered before the start of the review as failure to do so can result in important data being "missed" requiring re-review. Again, data extraction can be done in duplicate to detect transcription errors. The degree of correlation between the results of the data extraction can be calculated and presented, if desired.

COMBINING THE DATA (META-ANALYSIS)

If suitable, data from several studies can be combined to give an overall result (usually, although not always, only data from RCTs are combined). This overall result, as produced from the results of a larger number participants than individual studies, may be more accurate and reduces the chances of a type 2 error (failing to detect a difference that exists between the two groups), hence

Study or Subgroup	Experimental Events	Experimental Total	Control Events	Control Total	Weight	Risk Ratio M-H, Fixed, 95% CI
Crippen 2009	10	27	15	25	13.6%	0.62 [0.34, 1.11]
Jeeves 2001	17	52	33	50	29.5%	0.50 [0.32, 0.77]
Jones 2005	10	20	16	21	13.7%	0.66 [0.40, 1.08]
Smith 2007	24	50	41	48	36.6%	0.56 [0.41, 0.77]
Wooster 2005	5	14	7	12	6.6%	0.61 [0.26, 1.43]
Total (95% CI)		**163**		**156**	**100.0%**	**0.57 [0.46, 0.70]**
Total events	66		112			

Heterogeneity: $Chi^2 = 0.81$, df = 4 (p = 0.94); I^2 0%
Test for overall effect Z = 5.36 (P < 0.00001)

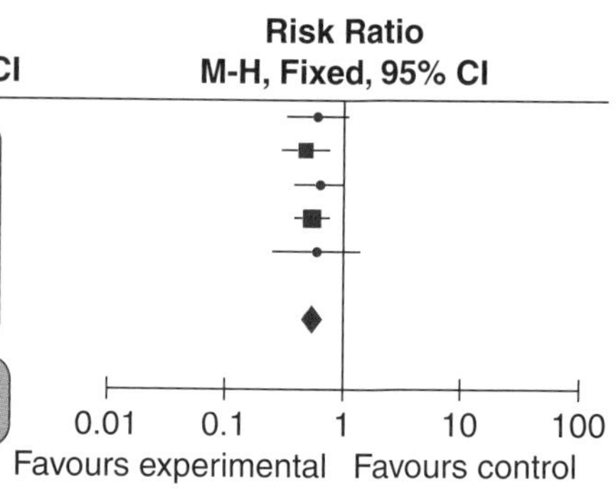

Figure 72-1 *An example of a Forest plot. The names of the individual studies are on the left, the individual studies results are seen in the blue boxes, and the overall result is seen in the red box. The green box shows the weighting (importance in the overall result) given to each study; this is based on the number of participants (the bigger the better) and with continuous data the spread of the results (the smaller the spread, ie, the smaller the standard deviation, the better as it is felt to be a better designed study which gives a more narrow spread of results). The orange box displays the statistics for the meta-analysis, including whether the overall result is statistically significant (test for overall effect) and two measures of heterogeneity (Chi² and I²). On the far right is the graphical representation of the results. Each study is represented by a blue box and a black line; the blue box represents the result of the study, with the larger the box the greater the weight of the study to the overall result, and the horizontal line the 95% confidence intervals for that study. If the box and the line lies to the left of the vertical line, then that study demonstrates that the intervention is statistically significantly better than the control; if the box and line all lie to the right of the vertical line, then the control is significantly better. If the box or line cross the vertical line, then the individual study is not statistically significant. The overall result is represented by a diamond, with the size being determined by the 95% confidence intervals. If the diamond does not touch the vertical line, then the overall result is statistically significant; to the left, the intervention is better than the control group and to the right the control group is better. If the diamond touches the line, then there is no statistical difference between the two groups.*

increasing the power of the analysis. One of the major criticisms of meta-analysis is that studies that are quite different have their results combined (combining apples and pears); therefore; when combining the results, it should be of studies with similar interventions/patients/measures of outcomes. For example, three studies which compare atenolol with placebo for blood pressure control and measure blood pressure at 3 months can have their results combined; however, care would have to be taken if one of the studies measures blood pressure at 1 week compared to 3 months, another compares atenolol to propranolol rather than placebo, while another study uses the average of 24-hours blood pressure compared to others which take a single measure of blood pressure.

The most commonly used meta-analysis software is RevMan, available for free from the Cochrane Collaboration. Data (either categorical, eg, number of deaths; or continuous, eg, length of hospital stay) is input into the program and it produces a Forest plot demonstrating the results of the data combination (explained in **Figure 72-1**). There are various statistical methods used for combining different types of data. The common methods are the Mantel-Haenszel method for categorical data that produces a risk ratio (or relative risk). The risk ratio expresses the chance that an event will occur if the patient receives the intervention compared to if they received the control. For continuous data, the inverse variance method is used, this produces the mean difference (the average difference that will be achieved by giving the patient the intervention rather than the control). The mean difference is used where the outcome that is measured is the same in all the studies, while the standard mean difference is used if the outcomes are measured slightly differently (eg, comparing studies looking at postoperative pain relief; if all the studies used the same pain scale, the mean difference can be used for meta-analysis; but if some of the studies use different pain scales, then standard mean difference should be used).

If there are enough studies, subgroup analysis may be performed. In such analyses, the researcher will examine results within individual clinical subgroups to determine the specific effect for those patients. Common subgroups may be based on age, sex, race, drug dosage, or other factors.

As discussed earlier, one of the major problems with meta-analysis is studies being combined that are too different (apples and pears), producing what is termed heterogeneity. There will always be some heterogeneity (difference) between studies due to chance; but when performing meta-analysis, this needs to be investigated to determine if the data can in fact be combined reliably. RevMan produces two measures of heterogeneity, the Chi^2 test and the I^2 test, and if these are either <0.10 and/or >40%, respectively, then heterogeneity may be present.

If heterogeneity is present, it needs to be investigated. Heterogeneity is investigated by removing studies/individual patients and seeing if that removes heterogeneity. Differences between studies in included patients may explain the heterogeneity (clinical heterogeneity); for example, do some studies have different age groups/different ethnic mixes/different drug doses? Do studies that are well performed have different results to those that are not performed well? Do commercial studies have different results from those that did not have commercial sponsorship? If after detailed investigation there is no obvious cause for the heterogeneity found, then it has to be accepted. In such cases, a more conservative overall result will be obtained if the analysis uses a random effect model, as compared with a fixed effect model.

Large poorly performed studies will have a greater weighting than smaller well-performed studies. As a result, sensitivity analysis is usually also performed. This involves the removal of studies that meet certain criteria (eg, poor quality, commercial sponsorship, conference abstract) to determine their effect on the overall result. For example, it must be made clear to the reader if a drug appears to have a positive effect but this effect disappears when commercial studies are removed then there may be bias in the result.

As mentioned earlier, studies that do not report a positive result are less likely to be published (publication bias); to check for this, a funnel plot can be produced. An example can be seen in

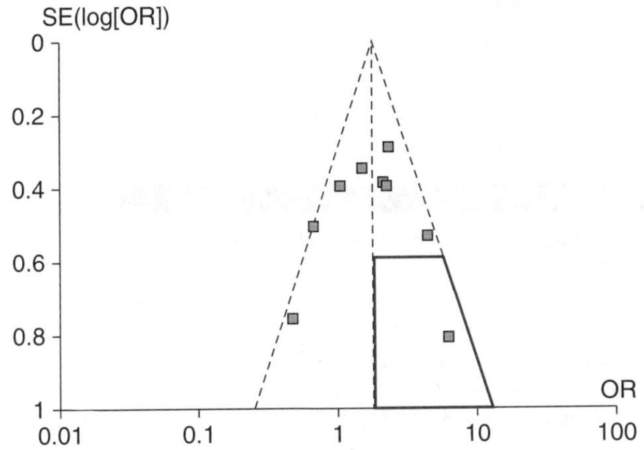

Figure 72-2 *A funnel plot; individual studies are represented by the small squares; if there is publication bias, the studies will not be equally distributed within the inverted V. The usual sign of publication bias is the absence of studies in the red box that represents where small negative studies lie.*

Figure 72-2. If there is no publication bias, all the studies should uniformly fall within the inverted V. If a section of the inverted V is devoid of studies, this indicates a publication bias (most often the failure of small negative studies to be published and thus included in the analysis).

ASSESSMENT OF STUDY CONCLUSIONS

PRACTICE POINT

When appraising a review the questions to ask are

1. Has an appropriate quality assessment tool been used?
2. Did more than one researcher perform the quality assessment and, if so, was there agreement?
3. Are the quality assessment result reported in an appropriate way?
4. Is the final conclusion based on the available evidence, not on personal opinion?

When all suitable studies have been collected, quality assessed, data extracted, and if possible meta-analysis performed, then conclusions need to be made. The authors must refer back to the original question and ask first if is there enough evidence to make any conclusions and, if so, how strong is the evidence. Discussions should include if there are any patient groups in which the evidence is stronger than in others. If meta-analysis has been performed, was there any heterogeneity or discrepancies when sensitivity analysis was performed? The most important factor in evaluating a systematic review is "Is the final conclusion based on the available evidence, not on personal opinion?"

PRACTICE POINT

When reviewing a systematic review you should consider the following:

1. Is the search strategy complete—could any studies have been missed?
2. Is the inclusion/exclusion criteria appropriate?
3. Has a quality assessment been performed, if so was it done in duplicate and does it present its findings?
4. If possible has meta-analysis been performed and is heterogeneity investigated and sensitivity analysis conducted?
5. Is the final conclusion based on the available evidence, not on personal opinion?

SUGGESTED READINGS

Cochrane Collaboration. http://www.cochrane.org. Cochrane Library. http://www.thecochranelibrary.com

Jadad AR, Moore RA, Carroll D, et al. Assessing the quality of reports of randomized clinical trials: Is blinding necessary? *Controlled Clin Trials*. 1996;17(1):1–12.

Moher D, Cook DJ, Eastwood S, et al, for the QUOROM Group 1999. Improving the quality of reports of meta-analyses of randomized controlled trials: the QUOROM statement. *Lancet*. 1999;354(9193):1896–1900.

Schulz KF, Chalmers I, Grimes DA, Altman DG. Assessing the quality of randomization from reports of controlled trials published in obstetrics and gynecology journals. *JAMA*. 1994;272(2):125–128.

Wells GA, Shea B, O'Connell D, et al. Ottawa Hospital Research Institute. The Newcastle-Ottowa score for non-randomized studies in meta-analyses. http://www.ohri.ca/programs/clinical_epidemiology/oxford.htm

CHAPTER 73

Knowledge Translations to Clinical Practice

Andrew Mente, PhD
Sonia Anand, MD, PhD, FRCP(c)

INTRODUCTION

A major aim of evidence-based medicine is to protect patients from ineffective or harmful treatments while ensuring that appropriate treatments are offered. In an ideal world, once a treatment is rigorously evaluated, results are incorporated into clinical guidelines which, in turn, inform health care delivery policies. However, the process that leads to effective sustainable solutions to health problems is in fact nonlinear, and different forms of evidence are needed at different stages by different parties. Knowledge translation is a complex and multidimensional concept that demands a comprehensive understanding of its mechanisms, methods, and measurements, as well as of its influencing factors at the individual and contextual levels—and the interaction between both those levels.

This chapter begins by presenting the definitions of knowledge translation and discussing the underlying basis for translational research under three often-cited phases. We outline the differences between these phases and illustrate that each step can generate new research questions which must be answered through a research continuum that requires different methods and constant two-way engagement with the global research community. Then the knowledge translation strategies and their applications are explored, drawn from specific examples from the field of cardiovascular disease. Finally, several methods and approaches to training in knowledge translation, types of studies, and funding issues will be presented.

DEFINITIONS AND CONCEPTS

Many terms have been used to describe the process of putting knowledge into action, from the term "implementation science" used in the United Kingdom and Europe to the terms "knowledge transfer and uptake" used in the United States. In Canada, however, the terms "knowledge transfer and exchange" and "knowledge translation" are commonly used. The common element among these different terms is a move beyond the simple dissemination of knowledge into actual use of knowledge. Knowledge translation is the process which leads from evidence based medicine to sustainable solutions for health problems.

PRACTICE POINT

- Essentially, knowledge translation is an interactive process underpinned by effective exchanges between researchers who create new knowledge and those who use it. As stated by the Canadian Institutes of Health Research, bringing users and creators of knowledge together during all stages of the research cycle is fundamental to successful knowledge transfer.

Knowledge translation is defined by the Canadian Institutes of Health Research as a dynamic and iterative process that includes the synthesis, dissemination, exchange and ethically sound application of knowledge to improve health, provide more effective health services and products, and strengthen the health care system. This definition has been adapted by others, including the United States National Center for Dissemination of Disability Research and the World Health Organization.

Most recently, the National Center for the Dissemination of Disability Research proposed another working definition of knowledge translation as "the collaborative and systematic review, assessment, identification, aggregation, and practical application of high-quality disability and rehabilitation research by key stakeholders (ie, consumers, researchers, practitioners, and policymakers) for the purpose of improving the lives of individuals with disabilities."

CHARACTERISTICS OF KNOWLEDGE TRANSLATION

Knowledge creation (ie, primary research), knowledge distillation (ie, the creation of systematic reviews and guidelines), and knowledge dissemination (ie, appearances in journals and presentations) are not enough on their own to ensure the use of knowledge in decision making. A key characteristic of knowledge translation is that it encompasses all steps between the creation of new knowledge and its application to yield beneficial outcomes for society. Essentially, knowledge translation is an interactive process underpinned by effective exchanges between researchers who create new knowledge and those who use it. As stated by Canadian Institutes of Health Research, bringing users and creators of knowledge together during all stages of the research cycle is fundamental to successful knowledge translation.

Knowledge translation strategies can help define research questions and hypotheses, select appropriate research methods, conduct the research itself, interpret and contextualize the research findings, and apply the findings to resolve practical issues and problems. Continuing dialogues, interactions, and partnerships within and between different groups of knowledge creators and users for all stages of the research process are integral parts of knowledge translation. For example, different interactive groups may include researchers within and across research disciplines; policymakers, planners, and managers throughout the health care, public health, and health public policy systems; health care providers in formal and informal systems of care; general public, patient groups, and those who help to shape their views and/or represent their interests, including the media, educators, nongovernmental organizations, and the voluntary sector; and the private sector, including venture capital firms, manufacturers, and distributors.

TRANSLATIONAL MEDICINE AND TRANSLATIONAL RESEARCH

Fulfilling the promise of knowledge translation for improving the health and longevity of the world's populations depends on developing broad-based teams of scientists and scholars who are able to focus their efforts to link basic scientific discoveries within the arena of clinical investigation, and translating the results of clinical trials into changes in clinical practice, informed by evidence from the social and political sciences. Thus translational research is the underlying basis for translational medicine and has three phases. The process is not necessarily linear, as each step can generate new research questions, which must be answered through a research continuum that requires different methods and constant two way engagement with the global research community (Lean, et al, 2008).

PHASE 1 RESEARCH (T1): "BENCH TO BEDSIDE"

Phase 1 translational research is the research process that explores needs, develops potential treatments in basic laboratory research, and tests safety and efficacy, principally in randomized clinical trials. The concept arose from research into pharmacotherapy and formed the initial basis for evidence-based practice and clinical guidelines, now incorporated into translational medicine. In the case of drug discovery and development, translational research typically refers to the translation of laboratory-based research into real therapies for real patients. This is often called the "bench to bedside" definition. Many pharmaceutical companies are building (phase 1) translational medicine groups to facilitate the interaction between basic research and clinical medicine, particularly in clinical trials. The clinical evaluation of therapies drawn from other disciplines (eg, psychology, physical activity, nutritional) can also be included within phase 1 translational research.

For this area of research, namely the interface between basic science and clinical medicine, the endpoint is the production of a promising new treatment that can be used clinically or commercialized ("brought to market"). This enterprise is vital for implementing new approaches for prevention, diagnosis, and treatment of disease is essential for improving health.

PHASE 2 RESEARCH (T2): FROM CLINICAL RESEARCH TO ROUTINE PRACTICE

Phase 2 translational research examines how findings from clinical science function when they are applied in routine clinical practice, as first described by Hiss in 2004. It thus addresses development and application of new technologies in a patient-driven environment where the emphasis is on real patients in real-life situations, where demographic factors and competing priorities modify clinical decisions, and treatment responses. Phase 2 translational research thus informs guidelines about needs, acceptability, effectiveness, and cost-efficiency in ecological settings and policies to promote uptake for optimal management and resource use.

Thus, phase 2 of translational research refers to translating clinical research into practice, ie, ensuring that new treatments and research knowledge actually reach the patients or populations for whom they are intended and are implemented correctly. As such, health services researchers and public health investigators whose studies focus on health care and health as the primary outcome play a prominent role in phase 2. The production of a new drug, an endpoint for "bench-to-bedside" translational research, is only the starting point for this second area of research. According to McGlynn et al (2003), US patients receive only half of recommended services. Phase 2 of translational research seeks to close that gap and improve quality by improving access, reorganizing and coordinating systems of care, helping clinicians and patients to change behaviors and make more informed choices, providing reminders and point-of-care decision support tools, and strengthening the patient-clinician relationship (Woolf, 2008).

Referring to T1 and T2 by the same name, knowledge translation, has become a source of some confusion. The two spheres are alike in name only. Their goals, settings, study designs, and investigators differ. T1 research requires mastery of molecular biology, genetics, and other basic sciences; appropriately trained clinical scientists working in strong laboratories and with cutting-edge technology; and a supportive infrastructure within the institution (Woolf, 2008).

In contrast, the "laboratory" for T2 research is the population and ambulatory care settings, where population-based interventions and practice-based research networks bring the results of T1 research to the public. T2 requires different research skills: mastery of the "implementation science" of fielding and evaluating interventions in real-world settings and of the disciplines that inform the design of those interventions, such as clinical epidemiology and evidence synthesis, communication theory, behavioral science, public policy, financing, organizational theory, system redesign, informatics, and mixed methods/qualitative research. T1 and T2 face different challenges. T1 struggles more with biological and technological mysteries, trial recruitment, and regulatory concerns. T2 struggles more with human behavior and organizational inertia, infrastructure and resource constraints, and the messiness of proving the effectiveness of "moving targets" under conditions that investigators cannot fully control (Woolf, 2008).

How attention and resources are apportioned to T1 and T2 matters because, for many diseases, T2 could save more lives than T1. The "bench-to-bedside" T1 enterprise occasionally yields breakthroughs that markedly improve the prognosis for a disease, but most new drugs and interventions produced by T1 only marginally improve efficacy. These incremental advances are certainly welcome, but patients might benefit even more—and more patients might benefit—if the health care system performed better in delivering existing treatments than in producing new ones. For example, increased administration of aspirin to eligible patients might prevent more strokes compared to the costs associated with developing a newer more potent antiplatelet agent. At a time when experts warn of the fragmented health care system and of a widening "chasm" in access, quality, and disparities, interventions to close these gaps—the work of T2—may do more to decrease morbidity and mortality than a new imaging device or class of drugs (Woolf, 2008).

PHASE 3 RESEARCH (T3): FROM EFFECTIVE TREATMENT/PREVENTION STRATEGIES TO SUSTAINABLE SOLUTIONS

Phase 3 translational research adds the necessary information to convert treatments and prevention strategies, shown to be effective and cost-effective in phase 2 translational research, into sustainable solutions. Thus, governments can generate enduring evidence-based policies. These require different types of research processes to evaluate the complex interacting environmental and policy measures that affect susceptibility to disease and the sustainability of clinical and public health management and prevention strategies (Lean, et al, 2008).

Achieving sustainability depends on evidence from two fronts. First, closed-loop audit approaches are needed within continuous improvement methodology to refine the intervention. Lessons can be learned from successful commercial and product developments, which use multidisciplinary nonexperimental research to inform incremental improvements. Continuous improvement methodology is known as *kaizen* in Japanese, where it originated. Second, research is needed to obtain evidence for making changes to multiple environmental and policy factors, which will reduce the need for funding to sustain the intervention.

Example of obesity

Controlling the mounting prevalence of obesity and its secondary diseases will require new multicomponent methods for effective treatments, based on randomized clinical trials and continuous improvements of community-based approaches, and also effective and sustainable approaches for prevention. This needs an integrated view of educational and environmental actions to facilitate greater physical activity, together with fiscal and regulatory changes to promote production, promotion, and delivery of healthier meals and total food supply. Practitioners, policy makers, and the public need sound evidence from different and new research methods, involving both experimental and nonexperimental methodologies that are sensitive to cultural and ethnic priorities.

Westfall, et al (2007) redrew the model to include a third step (T3), practice-based research, which is often necessary before distilled knowledge (eg, systematic reviews, guidelines) can be implemented in practice.

Even this expanded model is incomplete because it sees knowledge implementation only through the eyes of physicians, but practitioners other than health care professionals also translate research into practice. Science informs choices about health habits (eg, diet, smoking), environmental policy, injury prevention, parenting, healthy workplaces and schools, population health campaigns, and other interventions outside the clinic. The "practitioners" who apply evidence in these settings include patients, public health administrators, employers, school officials, regulators, product designers, the food industry, and other consumers of evidence. Trials that test the implementation of evidence in these settings can be just as vital as similar T2 work in clinical settings.

THE KNOWLEDGE-TO-ACTION FRAMEWORK

The knowledge-to-action framework is a conceptual framework developed by Graham and colleagues (2006) in order to illustrate an organic process with defined steps. It is a dynamic and complex process in which users may opt to use phases out of sequence. A process of knowledge creation was added to this model. It has been adopted by the Canadian Institutes of Health Research as the accepted model for promoting the application of research and for the process of knowledge translation.

The funnel of knowledge creation and the major action steps or stages comprising the model for translating knowledge to action are illustrated in **Figure 73-1**.

KNOWLEDGE CREATION

Knowledge creation, or the production of knowledge, is composed of three phases: knowledge inquiry, synthesis of knowledge, and creation of knowledge tools. The knowledge creation "funnel" conveys the idea that knowledge needs to be increasingly distilled before it is ready for application by end users. Knowledge inquiry includes the completion of primary research, while the knowledge synthesis stage brings together the different research findings that may exist globally on a topic and attempts to identify common patterns. Systematic reviews are the foundation of most activities related to knowledge translation, reflecting that the totality of the evidence should be considered rather than the results of individual studies. Quality of the evidence must also be considered. At the stage of development of tools and products, the best-quality knowledge is further synthesized and distilled into decision-making tools such as practice guidelines, aids for patient decisions or algorithms.

THE ACTION CYCLE

The seven action phases can occur sequentially or simultaneously, and the knowledge phases can influence the action phases at any point in the cycle. For example, as knowledge is updated, the need to reconsider barriers that exist to this knowledge arises. Included in the cycle are the processes needed to use knowledge in health care settings: identifying the problem; identifying, reviewing, and selecting the knowledge to implement; adapting or customizing the knowledge to the local context; assessing the determinants of knowledge use; selecting, tailoring, implementing, and monitoring interventions related to knowledge translation; evaluating outcomes or impacts of using the knowledge; and determining strategies for ensuring sustained use of knowledge. Integral to the framework is the need to consider the various stakeholders (including patients, clinicians, managers, or policy makers)—that is, who are the end users of the knowledge that is being implemented.

APPLICATION OF KNOWLEDGE TRANSLATION: SOME EXAMPLES

Knowledge translation and cardiovascular disease in Canada

Despite the advances in the field of cardiovascular medicine, knowledge gaps still exist. The knowledge gap is represented by the discrepancy between processes of care that are recognized as best practice and the care provided in clinical settings. Estimates of the size of the knowledge gap indicate that 30% to 40% of patients fail to receive treatments of proven effectiveness, and 20% to 25% of patients may receive care that is not needed or is potentially harmful.

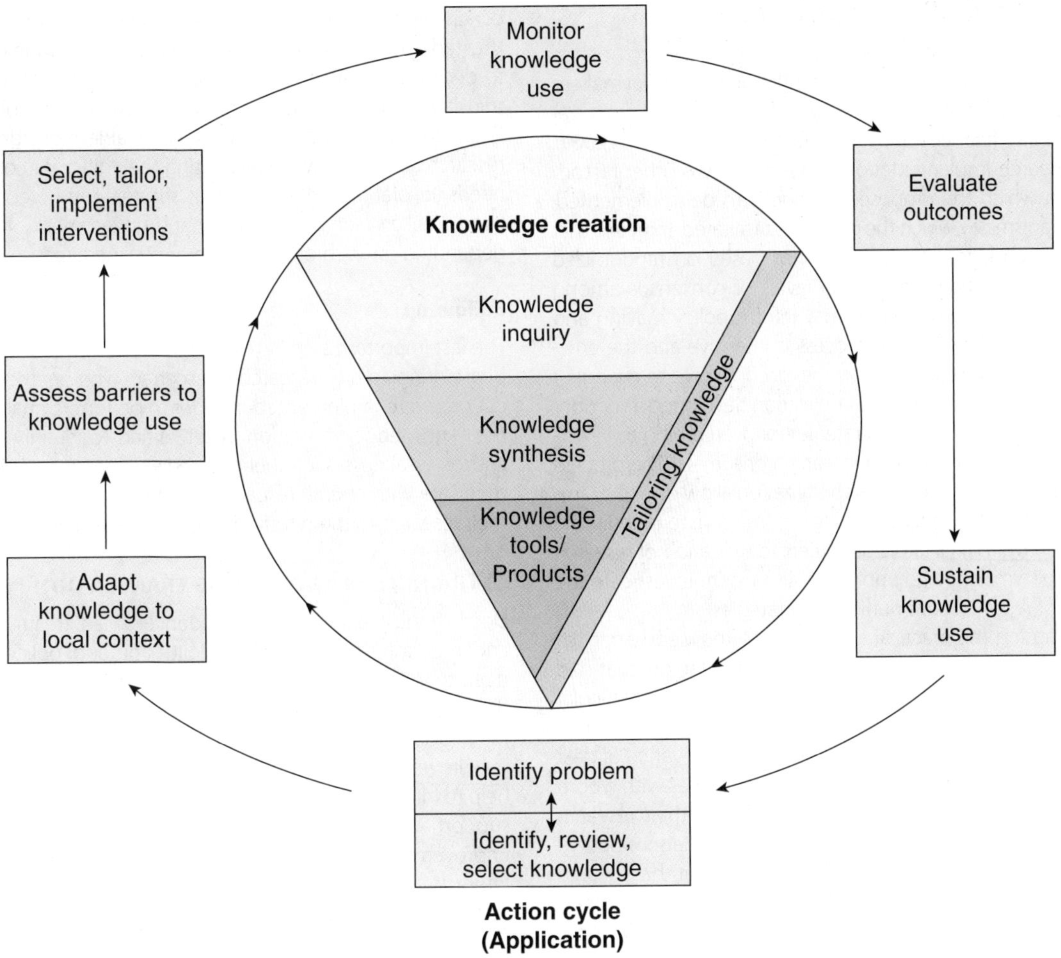

Figure 73-1 *The knowledge-to-action framework. (Reproduced, with permission, from Graham ID, Logan J, Harrison MB, et al. Lost in knowledge translation: time for a map? J Contin Educ Health Prof. 2006;26:13–24.)*

The Canadian Cardiovascular Society (CCS) is the national voice for cardiovascular physicians and scientists. The mission of the CCS is to promote health and care through knowledge translation, professional development and leadership in health policy. Currently, the CCS is taking a number of steps to improve its position in knowledge translation. For example, it is launching HeartStroke Canada, a computerized interactive tool for cardiovascular risk reduction and management. The expected effect of intervention is calculated from large, randomized controlled trials. At the end of a clinical consultation, the clinician can print out an individual's health advice based on their risk profile. Advice for the patient is compiled from endorsed Canadian professional sources. The program is flexible and can be updated as new evidence emerges.

Known gaps in the care of patients with the chronic conditions including diabetes, heart disease, stroke, and congestive heart failure highlight the need for improved practice and knowledge translation among primary care physicians. An integral component of translating research into efficacious prevention strategy is the development and use of innovative research tools and information technologies that promote application of new knowledge and techniques to patient care. For example, general practice electronic patient record systems as used now in several countries and which may include records of most modifiable cardiovascular risk factors and cardiovascular risk calculators embedded within them may facilitate the identification of people at increased risk for myocardial infarction and stroke (Debar, et al, 2010).

The recent launch of the National Institutes of Health's Clinical and Translational Science Award program in the United States is aimed at the translation of knowledge on cardiovascular health from epidemiological studies and clinical trials, particularly in women. The program offers opportunities to address these gaps and represents a unique opportunity to use innovative research tools and information technologies that promote application of new knowledge and techniques to patient care. The emphasis is on patient education and utilization of the recently published American Heart Association guidelines on "Evidence-Based Guidelines for Heart Disease Prevention in Women."

Effective approaches in translating nutritional research into beneficial diets is also an important challenge. It is becoming increasingly evident that poor nutrition plays an important role in inducing cardiovascular disease. Just as importantly, data now support the contention that appropriate nutritional interventions may have just as important an effect in preventing or delaying the appearance of cardiovascular disease. If this is indeed true, then it is critical that these advances in our knowledge of the effects of nutritional interventions be translated into effective strategies to combat cardiovascular disease. The translation of nutritional interventions can provide powerful approaches to alleviating the clinical challenges currently facing societies today in the cardiovascular field. Furthermore, the value-added economic advantages of translating nutritional strategies on a wide scale into the public become another intriguing argument to further support investigations in this growing field.

STRATEGIES FOR FACILITATING CHANGE

It is well documented that evidence-based health research per se currently does not have a large direct influence on policymakers, administrators, or clinicians, due to a variety of political, organizational, procedural, financial and other factors (Reitmanova, 2009). Successful research implementation depends on two other factors: the context in which the proposed change is to be implemented, and the mechanisms by which the change is facilitated. It means that even low research evidence (evidence not based on randomized control trials, systematic reviews, high levels of consensus among experts, and patients' involvement) may inform policy making and implementation if the facilitation process is intensive and the environment receiving the research outcomes is conducive to change.

Experts in the field of knowledge application developed a number of quality theories, methods, and strategies for overcoming the existing silos between researchers and research consumers. The process of knowledge translation and research utilization allow one to examine the role of research evidence in decision making, to identify the factors that behave as facilitators or barriers to utilization of research evidence in policymaking and implementation, or to investigate the effectiveness of research communication strategies.

In demonstrating the practical application of knowledge translation theory, Reitmanova et al (2009) identified the factors that had facilitated the utilization of previous research findings in a particular area of human health. As a first step, they suggest an environmental scan, which involves assessing the timeliness and relevance of past research results, and also identify the research audiences with whom they established active links in order to determine their research questions and research communication needs. They also assessed the culture of the receiving environment to ensure that the research would be in accordance with decision makers' values and to determine that there would be enough human, material, and financial resources available in order to facilitate a change. With the help of "trusted sources," they communicated their research through diverse communication channels, ensuring that the content and format were suitable for the varied needs of the research audiences. Finally, they followed up on the change implementation outcomes with several stakeholders. All of these strategies proved to be effective in facilitating the utilization of existing research.

Increasing awareness of research findings

Increasing awareness of the study is the first essential step toward an effective knowledge translation (Reitmanova, 2009). However, not all researchers are aware that the traditional one-way communication of research findings in journal publications and scientific conferences (called diffusion) does not prove effective in research uptake by policy makers and service providers. The other communication modes such as targeted mailing and presentations (called dissemination), and interactive workshops (called implementation) have much stronger impact on research utilization. Consequently, Reitmanova suggest that communication strategies should not be limited to journal publications and several presentations at local, national, and international conferences, but instead should include three separate seminars: one for policymakers and service providers in immigration; a second for policymakers and service providers in mental health; and a third for researchers, students, and faculty conducting research in public health.

Increasing research utilization

The use of diverse communication channels to disseminate research findings is merely part of a concerted effort to increase research utilization. Weiss (1979) suggested that communicated messages should be crafted as a narrative rather than a statistical summary. Moreover, factors such as content filled with actionable messages, a concise appealing format, and the involvement of opinion leaders or "trusted sources" to endorse the research or communicate it directly to decision makers are all very important facilitators of knowledge translation. Thus, during the research dissemination phase, one can focus on providing a package of actionable messages directed at research audiences while respecting their different communication needs (ie, oral presentation versus shorter written report for certain policy makers, service providers, and government office agencies, depending on each of their preferences and aims).

Follow-up

The last important step in research communication is the follow-up phase during which researchers ascertain whether their recommendations were implemented in order to perform a final evaluation of their knowledge translation initiative and to identify the strengths and/or weaknesses of their strategies. Therefore, one may communicate with several research stakeholders after they disseminate their research to them to find out how the research was used.

TRAINING IN KNOWLEDGE TRANSLATION

Doctors must already make evidence-based treatment decisions and monitor their outcomes. Politicians and policy makers also need to access best quality evidence and show how it informs the development of policies. Training in translational research methods for clinicians, guideline writers, grant awarding bodies, and policy makers would enable better assessment of complex evidence bases, help to integrate effective and culturally sensitive interventions with supporting environmental changes, and encourage continuous improvement of evidence-based public policies. It would be in the interest of all parties for such training programmes in translational research to be established (Lean, et al, 2008).

TYPES OF STUDIES IN KNOWLEDGE TRANSLATION

The concept of scientific evidence is fairly new. Some authorities maintain that randomized controlled trials form the only acceptable evidence of treatment efficacy and safety in health research and are the top of evidence hierarchies. While it is agreed that treatments based on anecdotal evidence should be rejected, some vital evidence from nonrandomized controlled trials has been devalued or dismissed. Diseases such as heart disease, cancer, and diabetes are seldom cured but may be modified and even prevented by improving diet and lifestyle. Controlled experimental approaches are sometimes possible but are slow and expensive, and they are often not best suited to testing multiple interventions alongside complex lifestyle changes over long time periods. Well-conducted prospective cohort studies, nonrandomized clinical trials, and pre-intervention or post-intervention prevalence studies are now beginning to be accepted as providing strong enough evidence to justify recommendations for action (Lean, et al, 2008).

EMERGENCE OF KNOWLEDGE TRANSLATION AND FUNDING

The National Institutes of Health (NIH) has made translational research a priority, forming centers of translational research at its institutes and launching the Clinical and Translational Science Award (CTSA) program in 2006. By 2012, the NIH expects to fund 60 CTSA centers with a budget of $500 million per year. Besides academic centers, foundations, industry, disease-related organizations, and individual hospitals and health systems have also established translational research programs, and at least two journals (*Translational Medicine* and the *Journal of Translational Medicine*) are devoted to the topic (Woolf, 2008).

While T1 and T2 research are both vital, T1 seems to overshadow T2 in North America. Most individuals associate T1 with the term translational research and T1 attracts more funding. As stated by Woolf (2008), the $22.1 billion NIH budget for 2002 included $9.1 billion for "applied and development research" ($13.0 billion for basic research) but only $787 million for health services research. The NIH maintains an active program in "dissemination" research, but across all funding sources in 2002 (ie, federal and foundations) spending on health services research represented only 1.5% of biomedical research funding. NIH leaders and the CTSA program advocate both T1 and T2, but the focus has been on T1 (Woolf, 2008). Adequate investment in T2 research is vital to fully salvage investments in T1 research. Bringing a drug to market without knowing how to bring it to patients undermines its larger purpose and can only diminish its profitability for investors (Woolf, 2008). A consequence of a stronger commitment to T2, especially outside clinical settings, is to expand the boundaries of basic science beyond the bench research that T1 typically showcases. Successful health interventions in hospitals, homes, and statehouses require the translation of other "basic sciences"—such as epidemiology, behavioral science, psychology, communication, cognition, social marketing, economics, political science—not only the translation of biotechnological insights and novel therapies. These disciplines deserve their place not only in definitions of basic science but also in funding priorities. Poverty matters as much as proteomics in understanding disease.

HEALTH ECONOMICS AND BIOMEDICAL RESEARCH: THE ROLE OF KNOWLEDGE TRANSLATION

The rapidly escalating costs of health care characterized by the shift from acute to chronic conditions, aging of the population, persistence of health disparities, and new public health challenges such as obesity call for the acceleration of our basic understanding of the complexity of biological systems and increase the need for more effective strategies for pursuing translational and clinical science.

Despite a steady increase in research funding over the last decade, a parallel increase in the development of new medical therapies has been absent. Translating investment in biomedical research into new therapies is becoming increasingly difficult across all areas of medicine. Identifying means to either decrease the cost of research or increase the output of new therapies will challenge all those who invest in research, and these challenges will only grow as funding constraints from industry and governments become more apparent. While funding is correlated with disease burden, it was not associated with an increase in new therapies, even when incorporating a lag of 8 years between funding and new drug approvals. Probable explanations are longer and more complex clinical trials and the associated additional cost of drug development, with current estimates in the United States ranging from $600 million to $1.2 billion.

In 2007, the FDA approved 19 new drugs, the fewest in 24 years. The increased funding and absent rise of new drugs in all therapeutic areas adds to the growing concerns about the productivity of biomedical research and underscores a need to examine noneconomic factors in the search for new treatments. Economists and historians of science stress that financial investment is but one of several elements that are necessary for scientific progress. Other requirements include the ready supply of talent (with relevant skill), favorable geography (proximity of universities and companies), and a culture that supports mobility between institutions (of people, ideas, and material). These factors have been recognized by the NIH, foundations, and companies as priorities equal to additional investment and nonfinancial factors, such as exploring partnerships between academia and industry, are receiving growing attention in the scientific press. The challenge is to increase productivity, which is not commonly the focus of scientists. Money, while necessary, is not sufficient to find new drugs. Possible solutions to improve research productivity have been offered and include decreasing the costs of clinical trials, modifying the economic incentives that pharmaceutical companies face (to favor high-impact/high-cost conditions), increasing the scale of research, open dissemination of negative results, and reorganizing research enterprises to bring talent, instrumentation, information, and material together in new ways. Importantly, as demonstrated by recent experience, further increases in the investment in research are probably inadequate, unless they are complemented by such nonfinancial factors.

CONCLUSIONS AND IMPLICATIONS

Discovering better ways to ensure that patients receive the care they need—safely, compassionately, and when they need it—is not easy and poses formidable methodologic challenges. Scientific discoveries and spectacular new devices are more fascinating to the public and more lucrative for industry. The betterment of health, however, should dictate priorities in health research. Funders should strike a balance between areas of research—T1 vs T2 vs T3, clinical vs population-based research vs sustainable evidence-based solutions—and emphasize each endeavor in proportion to its ability to improve health (Woolf, 2008).

Reliance on actions within health services will be insufficient to control rising obesity, diabetes, and associated diseases. Clinical science and ecological support from effective policies cannot continue to be regarded as independent disciplines. Integrated training in translational research methods is needed for clinicians, guideline writers, grant awarding bodies, and policy makers, in order to redress current biases in funding and research publications, in order to reflect better the balance of research efforts which are necessary for better assessment of complex evidence bases, to integrate effective and culturally sensitive interventions with supporting environmental changes, and to encourage continuous improvement of evidence-based public policies.

SUGGESTED READINGS

Debar S, Kumarapeli P, Kaski JC, de Lusignan S. Addressing modifiable risk factors for coronary heart disease in primary care: an evidence-base lost in translation. *Fam Pract.* 2010;27:370–378.

Graham ID, Logan J, Harrison MB, et al. Lost in knowledge translation: time for a map? *J Contin Educ Health Prof.* 2006;26:13–24.

Hiss RG. Fundamental issues in translational research. Translational research—two phases of a continuum. In: From clinical trials to community: the science of translating diabetes and obesity research. Natcher Conference Center, National Institutes of Health, Bethesda, Maryland, 2004:1–4.

Lean ME, Mann JI, Hoek JA, Elliot RM, Schofield G. Translational research. *BMJ.* 2008;337:a863.

McGlynn EA, Asch SM, Adams J, et al. The quality of health care delivered to adults in the United States. *N Engl J Med.* 2003;348: 2635–2645.

National Center for the Dissemination of Disability Research. What is Knowledge Translation? Technical Brief Number 10. Southwest Educational Development Laboratory, 2005. http://www.ncddr.org/kt/products/focus/focus10/. Accessed October 12, 2010.

Reitmanova S. Knowledge translation in health research: a novel approach to health sciences education. *Med Educ Online.* 2009;14:10.

Weiss CH. The many meanings of research utilization. *Public Adminn Rev.* 1979;39:426–431.

Westfall JM, Mold J, Fagnan L. Practice-based research–"Blue Highways" on the NIH roadmap. *JAMA.* 2007;297:403–406.

Woolf SH. The meaning of translational research and why it matters. *JAMA.* 2008;299:211–213.

PART IV

Approach to the Patient at the Bedside

CHAPTER 74

Acute Abdominal Pain

Norton J. Greenberger, MD, MACP

Key Clinical Questions

1. What are the important features in the history and physical examination that can help to determine the cause of acute abdominal pain?
2. What tests have the greatest impact in the diagnosis of patients with acute abdominal pain?
3. What are the important metabolic/endocrine disorders that cause acute abdominal pain simulating an acute abdomen?
4. What are the important hematologic/immunologic disorders that cause acute abdominal pain simulating an acute abdomen?

INTRODUCTION

Acute abdominal pain, particularly when severe, requires an expeditious evaluation because a missed or delayed diagnosis may lead to significant morbidity and mortality. The first step is to determine whether the patient has a life-threatening cause of acute abdominal pain. After the patient has been stabilized, the emergency physician or hospitalist must then determine whether the patient needs emergent surgery. The decision to obtain an emergency surgical consultation depends on the history and physical examination (with ancillary radiographic examinations of secondary importance), and when signs of an acute abdomen are present, a surgical consult should be requested, with concurrent diagnostic testing as appropriate. In other instances, a thorough history and physical examination is required with close observation and repeat examinations are often needed. Elderly patients and very young patients may present with atypical or nonspecific signs and symptoms that otherwise might be dismissed as insignificant.

Appendicitis, cholecystitis and choledocholithiasis, intestinal obstruction, pancreatitis, mesenteric ischemia, bowel perforation, and diverticulitis account for two-thirds of hospital admissions for acute abdominal pain and are associated with significant morbidity and mortality. In addition, physicians must be mindful of complications following procedures.

PATHOPHYSIOLOGY

Patients may experience visceral pain, parietal pain, and/or referred abdominal pain.

Visceral pain is typically dull or crampy in character. It is caused by stretching, torsion, distention, or contraction of organs. The visceral innervation of the gut and accessory organs comes via the anchoring mesentery, so pain does not always localize to the quadrant in which the pathology resides, and is often midline. Pain innervation corresponds to dermatomes that match the innervations of the injured organ. Epigastric visceral pain corresponds with

PRACTICE POINT

Acute cholecystitis

- Initially there is visceral pain in the epigastric region due to stretch and distention of the gallbladder.
- Then parietal pain develops due to direct irritation of the peritoneal lining in the right upper quadrant (location).
- Ultimately, referred pain develops in the right shoulder.

Splenic hematoma

- Initially there is visceral pain in the epigastric region due to stretch and distention of the spleen.
- Then parietal pain develops due to direct irritation of the peritoneal lining in the left upper quadrant (location).
- Ultimately, referred pain develops in the left shoulder.

Acute appendicitis

- Initially there is visceral pain in the periumbilical region due to stretch and distention of the appendix.
- Then parietal pain develops due to direct irritation of the peritoneal lining in the right lower quadrant (location).
- Ultimately, referred pain develops in the flank, depending on the location of the appendix.

organs proximal to the ligament of Treitz, including the hepatobiliary system and the spleen. Periumbilical visceral pain corresponds with injury to organs distal to the ligament of Treitz and the hepatic flexure of the colon. Lower abdominal visceral pain corresponds to injury to organs distal to the hepatic flexure.

Parietal pain is sharp in character and localized to the site of peritoneal inflammation or capsular. This pain is similar to skin and muscle pain and lateralization occurs due to unilateral parietal innervations.

Referred pain is typically well localized. It occurs because visceral afferent nerves carrying stimuli from an inflamed organ enter the spinal cord at the same level as somatic afferent nerves from remote locations.

THE HISTORY

DID THIS PATIENT'S ABDOMINAL PAIN OCCUR ABRUPTLY?

Pain that occurs suddenly increases the likelihood of intestinal, ureteral, or biliary obstruction, an acute vascular problem such as an aortic dissection or rupture or hemorrhage into the retroperitoneal space, or perforation of a viscus. Intermittent, colicky pain is more suggestive of obstruction of a viscus rather than the severe, persistent, or worsening pain of a perforation. The onset of pain associated with inflammation such as appendicitis is more gradual and in the early stages may not cause severe pain. Appendicitis should be considered in all patients with acute abdominal pain.

> **PRACTICE POINT**
>
> **The alvarado clinical decision rule for appendicitis (LR+ = 3.1)**
>
> ***Variable score***
>
> **M**igration = 1
> **A**norexia-acetone = 1
> **N**ausea-vomiting = 1
> **T**enderness in right lower quadrant = 2
> **R**ebound pain = 1
> **E**levation of temperature = 1
> **L**eukocytosis = 2
> Shift to the left = 1
> Maximum total score = 10
> Positive ≥7
>
> Data from does this patient have appendicitis? Wagner J. Simel DL, Rennie D, eds. The Rational Clinical Examination. New York: McGraw-Hill; 2008; page 63.

Women should always be asked about the menstrual cycle, possible pregnancy, and birth control pills.

DID THIS PATIENT'S ABDOMINAL PAIN LOCALIZE?

Localization of pain may be useful in determining its cause.

Diffuse pain may result from gastroenteritis, peritonitis, perforation, gastrointestinal hemorrhage, abdominal abscess, acute pancreatitis, intestinal obstruction, early appendicitis, ileocolitis, sigmoid diverticulitis, strangulated hernia, inflammatory bowel disease, mesenteric ischemia, aortic dissection or rupture, and traumatic injury. Angioedema of the bowel (hereditary, idiopathic or medication induced), familial Mediterranean fever, sickle cell crisis, acute porphyria, diabetic ketoacidosis, uremia, hypercalcemia, opiate withdrawal, and heavy metal intoxication may also cause diffuse pain.

Mid upper abdominal pain may be caused by peptic ulcer disease; pancreatic cancer, pancreatitis; biliary colic, cholecystitis, or ascending cholangits; esophagitis, gastroesophageal reflux disease, or pill-induced esophagitis, myocardial ischemia or pericarditis, mesenteric ischemia, rupture or dissection of the aorta, and traumatic injury.

Periumbilical pain may arise from early appendicitis, obstruction of the small bowel, gastroenteritis, mesenteric ischemia, aortic aneurysm rupture or dissection, and traumatic injury.

Right upper quadrant pain may result from acute cholecystitis, ascending cholangitis or biliary colic, acute hepatitis, hepatic abscess, hepatic congestion secondary to congestive heart failure, perforated duodenal ulcer, acute pancreatitis, retrocecal appendicitis, colitis, right-sided diverticulitis, myocardial ischemia, pericarditis, right lower lobe pneumonia, pulmonary embolism, subphrenic abscess, pyelonephritis, renal calculi, perinephric abscess, and traumatic injury.

Right lower quadrant pain suggests appendicitis, inflammatory bowel disease, right-sided diverticulitis, ileocolitis, ischemic colitis, gastroenteritis, hernia, Merckel diverticulosis, cecal diverticulosis, mesenteric adenitis, incarcerated strangulated groin hernia, leaking aneurysm, ruptured ectopic pregnancy, twisted ovarian cyst, pelvic inflammatory disease, salpingitis, Mittelschmerz, endometriosis, gynecologic cancer, pyelonephritis, renal calculi, prostatitis, seminal vesiculitis, psoas abscess, and traumatic injury.

Left upper quadrant pain may be caused by gastritis or peptic ulcer disease; acute pancreatitis or pancreatic cancer; splenic enlargement or infarction, rupture, infarction or aneurysm, myocardial ischemia, pulmonary embolism, subphrenic abscess, left lower lobe pneumonia, pyelonephritis, renal calculi, perinephric abscess, and traumatic injury.

Left lower quadrant pain may result from sigmoid diverticulitis, ischemic colitis, inflammatory bowel disease, ileocolitis, gastroenteritis, incarcerated or strangulated groin hernia, regional enteritis, leaking aneurysm, ruptured ectopic pregnancy, Mittelschmerz, twisted ovarian cyst or torsion, gynecologic cancer, salpingitis, pelvic inflammatory disease, endometriosis; pyelonephritis, perinephris abscess, ureteral calculi, seminal vesiculitis, prostatitis, psoas abscess, and traumatic injury.

With any lateralizing pain location (any of the four quadrants), particularly when there is a lack of clinical evidence for an intra-abdominal process, the physician should think about the possibility of herpes zoster (lateralizing sharp pain, classically band like along a dermatome, sometimes preceded by tingling), which may arise prior to development of the classic eruption. Abdominal wall processes and muscular processes (including hematoma, infection, and muscle strain) should also be considered in the appropriate setting.

DOES THIS PAIN RADIATE?

Gallbladder pain, liver disease, and referred pain from diaphragmatic irritation typically radiate to the back and/or shoulder. Liver disease and gallbladder disease may also radiate to the tip of the scapula. Pancreatitis, posterior perforation of an ulcer, kidney disease, and dissecting aneurysm can cause severe back pain due to inflammation in the retroperitoneum, occasionally with radiation to the shoulder. Other retroperitoneal structures such as kidney or ureter may also cause abdominal or flank pain that radiates to the back. Abdominal pain radiating to the groin/testicles may be due to an obstructing renal stone in the ureter.

WHAT IS THE SEVERITY OF THIS PATIENT'S PAIN NEAR THE TIME OF ONSET?

Although pain is experienced subjectively, there are certain types of pain that are classically intense within seconds or minutes of onset. Acute vascular insufficiency from torsion of a visceral structure or an acute embolic event (eg, in a patient with atrial fibrillation), perforation, hemorrhage, and dissection will often present with intense, acute pain. Renal colic also can present acutely, but waxes and wanes often with near-complete resolution between pain peaks.

HOW DOES THE PATIENT DESCRIBE THE QUALITY OF PAIN?

Abdominal pain in a patient with bowel obstruction is colicky in nature. Repeated episodes of colicky abdominal pain may suggest internal hernias as the cause of intermittent or acute intestinal obstruction. An intraabdominal hernia occurs when an anomalous fold or outpocketing of the peritoneum traps an intestinal loop. Acute strangulation of the intestinal loop may result in compression of the vasculature or gangrene of the bowel (50% of patients) or volvulus (14% of patients).

Biliary colic is a misnomer, the pain does not wax and wane but builds over 15 to 60 minutes, then is steady for several hours and dissipates slowly (visceral pain).

Pain in cholecystitis usually lasts longer than 6 hours and is located in the right upper quadrant due to progressive inflammation (parietal pain).

Although peptic ulcer disease may be asymptomatic and occasionally a patient may report crampy abdominal pain, most patients characterize the pain as burning/gnawing pain.

Visceral pain in diverticulitis is initially crampy in character, followed by parietal pain as the inflammation progresses.

Pain in acute mesenteric ischemia is acute in onset and severe. The patient reports periumbilical visceral pain out of proportion to the physical examination. Parietal pain and localizing exam findings are ominous findings in mesenteric ischemia, suggesting that the bowel may have infarcted or perforated. A dissecting aneurysm usually manifests with sudden severe pain, sometimes described as tearing/ripping sensation that radiates to the back. The onset may be in the epigastric region but then may progress to involve the lower quadrants as the dissection proceeds. Often the intense pain occurs intermittently as new tearing episodes occur.

HOW HAS THE PAIN PROGRESSED?

Has the patient experienced similar episodes in the past? If so, have the patient describe them, and determine what prior evaluation has been performed and what presumptive diagnoses were obtained.

WHAT ARE THE ASSOCIATED SIGNS AND SYMPTOMS?

Is there a history of systemic symptoms, such as fever, anorexia, weight loss? Acute inflammatory symptoms such as fever, particularly when infectious diarrhea is not suspected, may suggest the need for urgent imaging. Fever may be due to a loss of bowel wall integrity (perforation or severe mucosal injury) or due to infection in other abdominal structures (eg, cholecystitis). Weight loss may suggest a chronic inflammatory condition, mesenteric ischemia, malignancy, a problem with absorption, or a stricture. Sometimes food avoidance due to fear of pain may be the cause of weight loss.

Vomiting preceding the pain suggests the diagnosis of gastroenteritis, intestinal obstruction, biliary colic, or ureteral colic. Gastroenteritis, however, is usually associated with diarrhea. In appendicitis, vomiting rarely precedes pain. Bilious vomiting suggests mechanical obstruction.

Obstruction caused by a tumor, diverticulitis, stricture, or less commonly by a colonic volvulus, may have nausea, vomiting, abdominal distention, and pain.

Dark urine and pale stools suggest biliary obstruction. Be cautious in interpreting these complaints, however, since loose stools in general are often paler than formed stools, and truly acholic stools are uncommon. Further, dehydration—common with poor oral intake—leads to concentrated urine, so the clinician should specifically seek a history of brown or tea colored urine rather than simply asking if the urine is "dark." Jaundice is often not present early on after a biliary obstruction since scleral icterus reflects bilirubin levels from days earlier.

WHAT FACTORS EXACERBATE THE PAIN?

The examiner should specifically inquire whether eating exacerbates the pain. If so, it is important to clarify the time course of the pain, the associated symptoms (such as nausea and vomiting), and the types of food or drink that cause the symptoms. If pain occurs during swallowing or immediately afterward, an esophageal problem such as stricture or achalasia is likely. Although dysphagia usually presents with chest discomfort and not abdominal pain, some patients will have epigastric pain. If the pain is exacerbated by acid-containing foods (eg, citrus fruits or tomato sauce), caffeine, or alcohol, mucosal pain (esophagitis, gastritis, duodenitis, and possibly ulceration) should be considered. These symptoms can occur shortly after ingestion, but sometimes will not start for up to one to two hours later. If fatty foods in particular seem to be a culprit, consider gallbladder or biliary disease, or perhaps pancreatitis if the pain is severe. Postprandial pain may also suggest chronic mesenteric ischemia (ie, "mesenteric angina") due to a fixed vascular obstruction.

A patient with esophagitis/gastroesophageal reflux disease will often have increased pain when lying down. Patients with pancreatitis report steady, boring pain that makes them uncomfortable when lying supine.

A patient with a perinephric abscess may experience more pain with bending toward the uninvolved side.

Pain associated with salpingitis or endometriosis is worse before and during menstruation.

IS THERE A HISTORY OF PRIOR ABDOMINAL SURGERY?

Adhesions are almost exclusively seen in patients with prior abdominal surgeries—regardless of when the surgery occurred—and are the main causes of partial and complete obstructions of the small bowel. If the surgery was recent, then acute infections (eg, abscess) must be considered.

Even seemingly minor procedures may be associated with serious complications. For example, upper endoscopy may be complicated by esophageal perforation, aspiration pneumonia, or bleeding. Colonoscopy may cause abdominal bloating, lower gastrointestinal bleeding, perforation, or (rarely) splenic rupture. Cardiac catheterization and closed renal biopsy may lead to retroperitoneal bleeding. Interventions involving the biliary or pancreatic ducts (ie, endoscopic retrograde cholangiopancreatography) are commonly complicated by pain and transient elevations of pancreatic enzymes, even in the absence of overt pancreatitis, but if the pain persists or worsens, true pancreatitis should be considered.

WHEN WAS THE PATIENT'S LAST BOWEL MOVEMENT?

A constipated patient with abdominal pain may be developing a serious complication, such as obstruction, ischemia, or perforation. Obstruction may precipitate new onset constipation or exacerbate chronic constipation. Volvulus should be considered in any patient experiencing a sudden onset of constipation associated with abdominal pain, distention, and nausea and vomiting. Patients with small bowel obstruction will often evacuate their bowels shortly after the obstruction occurs, sometimes in parallel with the onset of vomiting, due to accelerated peristalsis throughout the gut. With prolonged obstruction, a lack of bowel movements is the norm. See Chapter 78 for a detailed discussion of constipation.

Likewise, the presence of diarrhea may provide clues to the cause of the abdominal pain. See Chapter 80 for a detailed discussion of diarrhea.

WHAT ARE THE PATIENT'S RISK FACTORS FOR GASTROINTESTINAL DISORDERS?

Is there a history of excessive alcohol use?

Injury to the lumen of the upper gastrointestinal tract (esophagitis, gastritis, or duodenitis, with or without ulceration) is common in this setting, as are pancreatitis and acute alcoholic hepatitis.

Is there accompanying iron deficiency anemia, weight loss, or a personal or family history for colorectal cancer?

Does the patient have a prior history of gastrointestinal disease or surgery?

A stricture should be considered on the differential diagnosis in any individual who has had prior colonic resection, a history of diverticulitis, peritonitis, or inflammatory bowel disease.

Does the patient have a systemic disorder that predisposes him to the development of acute abdominal pain?

Known cardiovascular, cerebrovascular, or peripheral vascular disease increases the risk of bowel ischemia or aortioiliac disease (**Table 74-1**). Regarding mesenteric ischemia, several historical features may suggest either an arterial or venous event as the cause of abdominal pain. Risk factors for either superior mesenteric arterial thrombosis due to atherosclerotic stenotic lesions or superior mesenteric arterial embolism of cardiac origin include the usual risk factors for cardiovascular disease and a history of vascular disease in several distributions (peripheral, cerebrovascular, cardiac). The examiner should specifically inquire about a history of intestinal angina suggested by postprandial pain and gut emptying, avoidance of food, and significant weight loss. Because collateral circulation will compensate for chronic occlusive disease of the superior, celiac, and inferior mesenteric arteries, mesenteric ischemia would not be expected to result unless one or two main vessels are thrombosed. When the third artery becomes occluded, the patient develops diffuse ischemia involving the liver, gallbladder, and much of the colon and associated metabolic abnormalities. Embolism of the superior mesenteric artery may also cause acute abdominal pain because of the lack of preexisting arterial collaterals. Risk factors include cardiac arrhythmia, recent myocardial infarction, or proximal aortic disease. These patients typically do not have a history of intestinal angina. Cholesterol embolism may affect branches and terminal arteries leading to segmental bowel involvement and abdominal pain without focal findings until necrosis of the entire bowel wall occurs.

Mesenteric ischemia of venous origin is characterized by acute and chronic forms. The chronic form causes abdominal pain

TABLE 74-1 Nonsurgical Disorders Causing Acute Abdominal Pain

Category	Key Diagnostic Feature
Metabolic/Endocrine	
Diabetic ketoacidosis	High serum glucose; ketoacidosis
Hyperthyroidism	High T4, low TSH
Hypercalcemia	High serum calcium
Hypokalemia	Low serum potassium
Hypophosphatemia	Low serum phosphate
Addison disease	Low serum cortisol, elevated ACTH
Porphyria	High prophobilinogen and delta ALA
Familial Mediterranean fever	Duration > 1–2 days; pleuritis and peritonitis
Vascular/Cardiopulmonary	
Myocardial ischemia/infarction	Abnormal ECG, high troponin
Aortic dissection	Widened mediastinum and diagnostic CT angiography
Median arcuate ligament syndrome	MRA or CTA
Pneumonia/pleurisy	Chest x-ray
Pulmonary embolus	Well's score, high D-dimer, CT-PA
Drug/Toxin	
Salicylate	Tinnitus, confusion, mixed respiratory alkalosis and metabolic acidosis
Anticholinergics	Confusion, dilated pupils, tachycardia, ileus, urinary retention
Tricyclic anti-depressants	Delirium, anticholinergic symptoms, ECG changes, serum/urine TCA level
Cocaine	Tachycardia, HTN, systemic end-organ ischemia, positive toxic screen
Heavy metals	Renal, neurological toxicity, 24 urine assay
Vasculitis/Connective Tissue	
Systemic lupus erythematosus (SLE)	> 4 of 11 SLE criteria are met
Systemic vasculitis	Multiorgan disease with + p-ANCA and ANA, low complement
Scleroderma	Skin changes, Raynaud's phenomenon and visceral disease
Hematologic/Immunologic	
Sickle cell crisis	History, periarticular pain, effusions
Henoch-Schoenlein purpura	Skin biopsy: leukocytoclastic vasculitis with IgA and C3 deposition
Hemolytic uremic syndrome	ARF with schistocytes on smear
Hereditary angioneurotic edema	Low C1 esterase inhibitor level
Systemic mast cell disease	High serum tryptase and urinary histamine; increased tissue mast cells
Thrombotic thrombocytopenic purpura	Fever, confusion, thrombocytopenia, schistocytes

(continued)

TABLE 74-1 Nonsurgical Disorders Causing Acute Abdominal Pain (*continued*)

Category	Key Diagnostic Feature
Infectious	
Staphylotoxin	Fever, hypotension, rash (CDC case definition)
Bornholm disease	Fever, rash, spasmodic pain, enterovirus (coxsackie/echo)
Yersinia enterocolitica	Diarrhea, fever, positive stool culture, ileal inflammation
Tuberculous mesenteritis	Fever, fatigue, diarrhea, right lower quadrant mass and ascites, positive biopsy
Dengue fever	Fever, HA, myalgias/arthralgias, low platelets, high LFTs, positive serology
Malaria	Fever, chill, diaphoresis, HA, myalgia, cough, multiorgan disease, red blood count smear
Musculoskeletal	
'Slipping rib' (lower rib margin) syndrome	Production of pain with rib compression only on affected side
Rectus sheath hematoma/neuroma	Carnett's sign
Chronic abdominal wall pain syndrome	Right upper quadrant (mainly) tenderness and positive Carnett sign
Neurologic/Psychiatric	
Herpes zoster	Unilateral, painful vesicular rash in dermatomal distribution, positive DFA of lesion or PCR of fluid
Abdominal migraine	Adolescents, cyclic occurrence
Temporal lobe seizures	Adolescents, aura, abnormal EEG
Radiculopathy	Mechanical pain in dermatomal distribution, positive MRI
Irritable bowel syndrome	Manning or Rome III criteria
Renal	
Nephro/ureterolithiasis	Hematuria and positive CT
Papillary necrosis	Hematuria, obstructive uropathy, diabetes, sickle cell disease

ACTH, adrenal corticotropin hormone; ALA, aminolevulinic acid; ANA, antinuclear antibody; ARF, acute renal failure; CDC, centers for disease control and prevention; CT, computed tomography; CT-PA, computed tomography-pulmonary angiography; CTA, CT angiography; DFA, direct fluorescent assay; ECG, electrocardiogram; EEG, electroencephalogram; HA, headache; HTN, hypertension; IgA, immunoglobulin A; LFT, liver function test; MRA, magnetic resonance angiography; MRI, magnetic resonance imaging; PCR, polymerase chain reaction; SLE, systemic lupus erythematosus; TCA, tricyclic antidepressants; TSH, thyroid stimulating hormone.

Data from Makrauer FL, Greenberger NJ. Acute abdominal pain: basic principles & current challenges. In: *Current Diagnosis & Treatment: Gastroenterology, Hepatology, & Endoscopy*. Greenberger NJ, Blumberg RS, Burakoff R, eds. New York: McGraw-Hill; 2009:1–10.

and diarrhea, but does not usually progress to acute abdominal findings. Risk factors include prior venous thromboembolism and primary hypercoagulable states, previous abdominal surgery, intraabdominal cancer, inflammatory bowel disease, and portal hypertension. The acute form is more likely to involve a major venous vessel such as the portal or superior mesenteric vein. The chronic forms may develop in small peripheral veins and progress proximally.

Elderly vasculopathic patients are particularly prone to developing ischemic colitis—a clinically distinct entity from mesenteric ischemia—in which small vessel insufficiency results in sloughing of the metabolically active mucosal lining of the colon. This condition is often confused with inflammatory or infectious colitis since it often presents with crampy pain and diarrhea (often positive for occult blood, and sometimes grossly bloody), and often with fever. Since this condition results from small vessel insufficiency, there is rarely any role for evaluation of mesenteric vessels.

THE PHYSICAL EXAMINATION

DOES THE PATIENT LOOK SICK?

A patient who lies still, has his knees flexed, and has a rigid abdomen most likely has peritoneal inflammation. Patients who are restless, unable to get comfortable, and pace may have renal colic. Patients with a perinephric abscess may bend over toward the involved side.

WHAT ARE THE VITAL SIGNS?

Although lack of fever does not rule out an inflammatory process, especially in immunocompromised hosts, patients with renal failure, or the elderly, its presence requires further evaluation. Tachycardia may result from pain from any source, fever, and dehydration. Hypertension can arise from any severe pain but may also predispose to vascular events. It is initially present in more than 70% of patients with acute aortic dissection. Hypotension in association with acute abdominal pain raises the possibility of aortic rupture or dissection, sepsis, gastrointestinal bleeding, dehydration, and pump failure (acute myocardial infarction, pulmonary embolism). Patients may also develop nonocclusive mesenteric ischemia associated with a low-output state related to septic shock, myocardial infarction, and other causes of hypotension. Patients with chronic adrenal insufficiency may experience nonspecific abdominal pain and have relatively low blood pressures but otherwise appear well.

Tachypnea may be associated with anxiety, severe pain, sepsis, acute pulmonary embolism, pneumothorax, and other respiratory causes.

ARE THERE ANY SIGNS OF SYSTEMIC ILLNESS?

A general physical examination should be performed to determine the presence of systemic illness that may be associated with abdominal pain.

PRACTICE POINT

- The abdominal examination may confirm the clinician's pretest suspicion of an underlying disorder. However, most signs are useful if present but not if absent.
- For example, elderly patients may have acute cholecystitis without any signs or symptoms in the right upper quadrant. The clinician's gestalt has a reported LR+ 25–30 compared with a positive Murphy sign, LR 2.8 (0.8–8.6) and right upper quadrant tenderness, LR 1.6 (1.0–2.5).
- The presence of ecchymoses, signifying subcutaneous blood from intraperitoneal or retroperitoneal hemorrhage dissecting the skin overlying the flanks (Turner sign), a periumbilical bruise (Cullen sign) or a green or jaundiced discoloration at the umbilicus (Ransohoff sign of a ruptured bile duct) is helpful only if present. Prominent venous patterns may suggest portal hypertension or inferior vena caval syndrome but are also seen in normal elderly patients.
- Regarding ascites, the presence of a fluid wave has a reported LR+ 6.0 (3.3–11) and shifting dullness LR+ 2.7 (1.9–3.9). The absence of a fluid wave or shifting dullness does not rule out the presence of significant ascites in the patient with risk factors or symptoms of ankle swelling, weight gain, and abdominal distention.
- Palpating a liver edge below the right costal margin may increase the patient's pain and correlates poorly with the actual liver span (LR+ 2.0). For patients with risk factors for splenomegaly, the reported LR+ for percussion of Traube space is 2.3 (1.8–2.9) and palpation 8.2 (5.8–12).
- The sensitivity of abdominal palpation in patients with a ruptured abdominal aneurysm, especially in obese patients or those who cannot relax their abdomen, is sufficiently low that emergent surgical consultation and imaging is required if the index of suspicion is sufficiently high. The LRs vary with the size of the aneurysm; for aneurysms > 4 cm the reported LR+ is 16 (8.6–29).

Data from Simel DL, Rennie D, eds. The Rational Clinical Examination. McGraw-Hill; 2008; pages 27, 73, 147, 300, 613.

THE ABDOMINAL EXAMINATION

Inspection

The abdominal examination must be performed gently and carefully to elicit localized and generalized peritoneal signs. The examiner should first inspect the abdomen at the foot of the bed to detect visible peristalsis, asymmetry suggesting hernias or masses, and distention. Unless there are surgical scars or a prior term pregnancy, the umbilicus should be within 1 cm of the midpoint between the xiphoid and the pubis. Organomegaly, masses, or ascites may cause displacement of the umbilicus. Eversion or outward protrusion of an inverted umbilicus is not a reliable sign for chronic ascites. In generalized peritonitis, respiratory motion is not associated with movement of the abdominal wall. The clinician should also note any changes in skin color, the presence of ecchymoses, and the presence of scars. The presence of surgical scars increases the likelihood that abdominal adhesions may be causing acute pain. If the patient can attempt a modified sit-up that contracts his rectus abdominal muscles, a ventral hernia may be more visible than palpable.

Ausculation

In general, auscultation for abnormal bowel sounds should be performed prior to performing percussion or palpation of the abdomen. Of note, the absence of bowel sounds may be normally present between episodes of normal bowel motility and, hence, is not specific by itself for advanced intestinal obstruction or secondary ileus from inflammatory conditions such as pancreatitis, pyelonephritis, or peritonitis. In fact, some experts believe that the examiner must listen for at least four minutes before concluding that the bowel sounds are in fact absent. However, it is worthwhile to listen for the very high-pitched tinkles and rushes characteristic of small bowel obstruction. A succession splash suggests gastric outlet obstruction. An epigastric bruit with a diastolic component may suggest hemodynamically significant stenoses of branches of the aorta including the celiac axis and superior mesenteric artery as well as in disease of the aorta, or the renal arteries. Friction rubs may rarely be appreciated over an inflamed gallbladder, splenic infarct, and in cases of hepatoma, cholangiocarcinoma, and metastatic carcinoma. A murmur due to compression of the splenic artery may be appreciated in patients with pancreatic carcinoma.

Percussion

Light percussion to estimate the liver span (with > 15 cm consistent with liver enlargement) is the most reliable method to check for the presence of hepatomegaly. If the patient's abdomen is distended, the examiner should look for signs of ascites (fluid wave, shifting dullness) or perhaps perform a bedside ultrasound. Likewise, the clinician should start with light percussion to determine whether splenomegaly is present. A full bladder is defined as at least 250 mL of urine. An enlarged bladder requires ultrasound confirmation due to the unreliability of the physical examination in detecting bladder distention.

Palpation

The examiner should always first explain to the patient what the examination will entail and examine the most painful area last. The patient should be asked to distinguish between pressure and pain during examination of all quadrants. During the abdominal examination the patient's hips and knees should be flexed to relax the abdominal musculature. Involuntary guarding and rebound tenderness may be an indication of parietal peritoneal (layer of the abdominal wall) involvement, a rough or cold examining hand, or due to patient apprehension. The examiner should ask the patient to point to the area of pain. A patient with appendicitis may be able to precisely localize the pain using one finger, especially after coughing or performing the Valsalva maneuver. A positive Murphy sign is elicited when the inflamed gallbladder descends to the examiner's thumb and causes pain sufficient to abruptly cease inspiration. The reported sensitivity of the Murphy sign is only 27% but increased with bedside ultrasound imaging the precise location of the gallbladder. Some experts do not recommend testing for rebound tenderness because the test is only useful if positive and it causes unnecessary pain. If the pain is significantly out of proportion to the physical findings, obstruction and ischemia should be suspected. Try to determine if abdominal pain is originating from interior abdomen or the anterior abdominal wall (Carnett sign—tense abdominal muscles increase pain if the source of pain originates from the anterior abdominal wall unlike intraabdominal etiologies of pain).

If the patient can relax, the abdomen should be deeply palpated a few centimeters above the umbilicus slightly left of midline to detect a widened aorta. A normal abdominal aorta is usually less than 3 cm wide. Obesity, voluntary guarding, firm musculature limit the sensitivity of the examination. Palpable kidneys are consistent with bilateral polycystic kidney disease or hydronephrosis. Pancreatic pseudocysts may also be palpable in approximately 50% of patients.

PRACTICE POINT

Findings	Systemic Disease that May be Associated with Abdominal Pain
Clubbing	Inflammatory bowel disease, pulmonary malignancy, cirrhosis, congenital heart disease, endocarditis (bacterial endocarditis), artrioventricular malformations, fistulas
Koilonychia	Iron deficiency anemia, systemic lupus erythematosus (SLE)
Onycholysis	Hyperthyroidism, amyloidosis, connective tissue disorders
Beau lines	Any severe systemic illness that disrupts nail growth
Yellow nail	Rheumatoid arthritis (RA), nephritic syndrome, tuberculosis, immunodeficiency
Terrys (white nails)	Hepatic failure, cirrhosis, diabetes, congestive heart failure (CHF), hyperthyroidism, malnutrition
Asure lunula	Wilson disease, silver poisoning
Half-and-half nails	Chronic renal failure, cirrhosis
Muehrckes lines	Hypoalbuminemia
Mee lines	Arsenic poisoning, Hodgkins disease, CHF, leprosy, malaria, carbon monoxide poisoning, other systemic insults
Splinter hemorrhage	Subacute bacterial endocarditis, SLE, RA, antiphospholipid syndrome, peptic ulcer disease, malignancies
Telangiectasis	RA, SLE, dermatomyositis, scleroderma
Skin lesions	Vasculitis, septic emboli
Gangrene, dependency rubor	Peripheral vascular disease
Pallor	Severe anemia (Hg < 7 g/dL)
Jaundice	Liver disease, biliary tract disease, biliary obstruction
Slate brown color	Addison disease
Rash and fever	Infection
Pyoderma gangrenosum	Inflammatory bowel disease
Bruits	Vascular disease
Heart murmurs, gallops	Significant heart disease
Pulmonary signs and symptoms	Pneumonia, pulmonary embolism, pneumothorax, empyema
Peripheral edema	CHF, ascites, deep venous thrombosis

The abdominal examination should include a rectal and genital examination.

CASE 74-1

A 57-year-old man developed acute right upper quadrant abdominal pain that radiated to his back. Similar to prior episodes, the pain was severe, abrupt onset, colicky in nature, lasting 45 to 60 minutes followed by an aching right upper quadrant discomfort lasting several hours. His laboratory tests, including CBC, comprehensive metabolic profile, serum amylase and lipase, urinalysis without the presence of bilirubin, and esophagogastroduodenoscopy, were all normal. Three ultrasound examinations obtained during three separate Emergency Department visits visualized the gallbladder but did not detect gallstones.

On physical examination the patient had normal vital signs and his blood pressure was equal in both arms. His heart and lung examination was normal. Examination of the abdomen revealed thump tenderness in the right upper quadrant but not the left upper quadrant, thump tenderness over the right lower anterior chest but not the left lower anterior chest, and a palpable liver that was tender to deep palpation. The gallbladder which is usually identified by the junction of the right lateral rectus muscle and the costal margin was not palpable.

Consistent with gallbladder disease but in the absence of stones, the clinical picture of this case is termed acalculous cholecystopathy. Delayed gastric emptying characterized by postprandial bloating and distention is less likely due to long intervals between acute attacks. A HIDA scan with injection of cholecystokinin would be the next test to perform. It should reproduce the patient's pain during his attacks and show a reduced gallbladder ejection fraction to less than 35%. If this test is positive it would obviate the need for further testing such as CT scan, MRI, CT angiogram, or MR angiogram.

The patient underwent a laparoscopic cholecystectomy from which pathologic specimens showed clear-cut evidence of chronic cholecystitis.

This case highlights that the finding of a normal ultrasound examination should not deter the clinician from seeking additional studies to help establish this diagnosis for patients who have symptoms clearly suggestive of gallbladder disease. Consultation with a radiologist about the bedside clinical information might have facilitated an earlier diagnosis.

ANCILLARY LABORATORY TESTS

Laboratory studies are often of limited value. A normal complete blood count (CBC) does not rule out appendicitis or other inflammatory processes. Complete blood count, liver enzymes, urinalysis, and pregnancy test are helpful when abnormal. A urinalysis may point to nephrolithiasis or urinary tract infection. Plain radiographs of the abdomen are not helpful in most cases of abdominal pain, but can be diagnostic in cases of small bowel obstruction or volvulus and when there is a perforated viscus. In patients with abdominal distention, pain and constipation, plain abdominal radiography can be helpful assessing the degree of constipation and ruling out obstruction. Abdominal radiographs may demonstrate a dilated colon or small bowel with air fluid levels indicative of obstruction. The presence of free air on plain abdominal radiograph would indicate perforated bowel. Calcifications in the pancreatic bed indicate the presence of chronic pancreatitis. (See Chapter 109.)

If abdominal radiography demonstrates colonic dilatation suggestive of an obstruction, additional imaging should be performed (**Table 74-2**). Computed tomography (CT) has led to the greatest improvement in the care of patients with acute abdominal pain, and is usually the next diagnostic test in a patient with unexplained pain symptoms and clinical suspicion of significant abdominal pathology. Ultrasound is often the best modality to image a fluid filled body such as a cyst or gallbladder but CT is usually diagnostic in these conditions as well. Ultrasound is the modality of choice in any woman who may be pregnant.

TABLE 74-2 Major Causes of Acute Abdominal Pain with Preferred Diagnostic Test for Each

Common Conditions	Key Diagnostic Test(s)
Acute appendicitis	CT scan
Acute cholecystitis, choledocholithiasis	Ultrasound
Acute diverticulitis	CT scan
Acute pancreatitis	Serum amylase/lipase, CT scan
Bowel perforation	CT scan
Acute mesenteric ischemia	CT angiogram, MRI
Ischemic colitis	Colonoscopy
Intestinal obstruction	Flat film, imaging study
Anterior abdominal wall pain (in rectus hematoma)	Carnett sign, Fothergill sign
Sigmoid volvulus	CT scan or Barium enema
Biliary duct or pancreatic duct rupture	MRCP, ERCP

CT, computed tomography; ERCP, endoscopic retrograde cholangiopancreatography; MRCP, magnetic resonance cholangiopancreatography; MRI, magnetic resonance imaging.

Data from Makrauer FL, Greenberger NJ. Acute abdominal pain: basic principles & current challenges. In: *Current Diagnosis & Treatment: Gastroenterology, Hepatology, & Endoscopy*. Greenberger NJ, Blumberg RS, Burakoff R, eds. New York: McGraw-Hill; 2009:1–10.

CASE 74-2

An 86-year-old woman with a prior history of coronary artery disease, hypertension, cholecystectomy, and renal artery stenosis presented to an outside hospital with worsening postprandial abdominal pain for over six months. There was no history of diarrhea, hematochezia, or reflux symptoms. Studies performed within the prior three months included an unrevealing esophagogastroduodenoscopy and a colonoscopy. At the outside hospital laboratory testing reported an elevated serum amylase and lipase, and a noncontrast enhanced CT scan identified a 15 mm by 7 mm hypoechoic mass in the head of the pancreas. She was transferred to a tertiary hospital for further evaluation of superimposed acute-on-chronic abdominal pain and the pancreatic lesion.

Key questions to ask include:

- Has the patient ever had an episode of acute pancreatitis?
- Is the pain she is experiencing similar to the pain she experienced prior to her cholecystectomy?
- Does the size of the meal that she eats influence the severity of her postprandial pain?
- If she eats smaller quantities of food, does she experience less pain?
- Has she lost weight and if so, how much?

This patient's vital signs were notable for temperature 97.1° F, pulse 107 and regular, blood pressure 126/70 mm Hg, respirations 18, SaO_2 98% on room air. Head/neck examination revealed no thyromegaly jugular venous distention or lymphadenopathy. Lungs were clear to auscultation and cardiac examination revealed a regular rate and rhythm without murmurs. Abdominal examination revealed a soft, nondistended abdomen. However, she was tender to palpation in the right upper quadrant, left upper quadrant, and the periumbilical area. The abdominal pain seemed out of proportion to the fairly benign examination of the abdomen. There was no mention of an abdominal bruit, which would have been an important physical finding. There was no shake tenderness. A rectal examination revealed hemoccult negative stool.

Laboratory data included white blood cell count 15,500/mm^3, hemoglobin 11.5 g/dL, hematocrit 33.6%, platelets 283,000. Metabolic profile sodium 140 mEq/L, potassium 3.8 mEq/L, chloride 105 mEq/L, and HCO_3 25 mEq/L, BUN 44 mg/dL, creatinine 0.8 mg/dL, and blood glucose 188 mg/dL. Liver tests revealed serum ALT 11 U/L, serum AST 14 U/L, serum alkaline phosphatase 101 U/L, total bilirubin 0.4 mg/dL, serum amylase 140 U/L (normal < 120 U/L), and serum lipase 190 U/L (normal < 60U/L).

A magnetic resonance cholangiopancreatography revealed subcentimeter ill-defined irregular areas of decreased enhancement of the pancreas consistent with either sidebranch intraductal papillary mucinous neoplasm or pancreatic cancer. There were also findings consistent with chronic pancreatitis with irregularity of the main pancreatic duct. An endoscopic ultrasound examination to clarify the lesion in the pancreas revealed congestion and edema in the stomach, along with several small areas of erosion and shallow ulcerations also in the stomach. Endosonographic findings revealed an irregular mass-like lesion in the pancreatic head. Biopsy of the 15 mm by 7 mm hypoechoic lesion revealed only pancreatic tissue. Before a decision was made about whether she should undergo a laparotomy with biopsy of the pancreatic mass, she developed increasingly severe abdominal pain and continued tenderness in the abdomen.

A MR angiogram of the abdomen without contrast revealed the superior mesenteric artery arising with the celiac artery. There was moderate-to high-grade stenosis at the ostium of the celiac axis. The superior mesenteric artery was considerably narrowed but still retained some patency.

Shortly after the completion of these studies, the patient became increasingly confused, tachycardic, and hypotensive. Laboratory studies at that time revealed serum amylase 334 U/L (normal 20–70 U/L), serum lipase 276 U/L (normal 3–60 U/L), a low arterial blood gas pH 7.29, and elevated serum lactate level 5.0 mg/L.

At this juncture it seemed clear that she had severe mesenteric vascular ischemia and that she probably had developed gut infarction. She underwent exploratory laparotomy. There was marked ischemia and some transmural necrosis of the small bowel, from approximately 30 cm from the ligament of Treitz to the distal ileum, which was resected. She developed ST-segment elevation consistent with acute myocardial infarction. Thereafter, the patient's family requested comfort measures only and she died shortly thereafter.

The diagnosis of mesenteric vascular ischemia clearly explained virtually all the findings, and the lesions in the pancreas, while of some interest, were not the most important issue to address in this patient after she presented. Clues that this patient had significant mesenteric vascular ischemia included:

- Risk factors (hypertension, coronary artery disease)
- Postprandial pain, worse with larger meals, somewhat better with smaller meals or without eating
- Weight loss
- Abdominal pain out of proportion to any physical findings

The physical examination did not document whether she had an abdominal bruit, the presence of which would have increased the likelihood of mesenteric ischemia as the cause of her symptoms. Her clinicians also overlooked the possibility that the abnormal pancreatic enzymes resulted from gut ischemia.

The findings in the pancreas obfuscated the very real danger of mesenteric vascular ischemia. By the time any patient develops lactic acidosis and elevated liver enzymes, frank gut infarction has usually developed. A cardinal rule is that once the diagnosis of mesenteric vascular insufficiency is entertained, determining the status of the mesenteric vasculature becomes of prime importance and overrides virtually all other diagnostic considerations. It would have been more appropriate to do a MR angiogram early in the course of this patient's illness and upon the demonstration of severe mesenteric vascular ischemia a decision should then have been made as to how to address this diagnosis.

CONCLUSION

The possibility of an intrathoracic lesion must be considered in every patient with abdominal pain, especially if pain is in the upper abdomen. An orderly, painstakingly detailed history is vital, especially the chronologic sequence of events. Careful pelvic and rectal examinations are *mandatory* on every patient with acute abdominal pain. Laboratory studies may be of considerable value, but they infrequently establish the diagnosis. Sometimes, even under the best of circumstances, a definitive diagnosis cannot be established at the time of the initial examination.

SUGGESTED READINGS

American Gastroenterological Association Medical Position Statement: Guidelines on Intestinal Ischemia. *Gastroenterology* 2000;118:951–953.

Greenberger NJ, Hinthorn DR. *The abdomen*. In: History Taking and Physical Examination: Essentials and Clinical Correlates. St. Louis, MO: Mosby-Year Book, Inc.; 1993:199–261.

Greenberger NJ, Paumgartner G. *Acalculous cholecystopathy. Diseases of the gallbladder and bile ducts*. In: Harrison's Principles of Internal Medicine. 17th ed. Fauci AS, Kasper DL, Longo DL, Braunwald E, Hauser SL, Jameson JL, Loscalzo J, eds. New York: McGraw-Hill; 2008:1996.

Greenberger NJ. Sorting through the nonsurgical causes of acute abdominal pain. *J Crit Illn*. 1992;7:1602–1604, 1609.

Greenberger NJ. Techniques for physical assessment of acute abdominal pain: getting the most out of the history and physical exam. *J Crit Illn*. 1994;9:397–404.

Grunkemeier DM, Cassara JE, Dalton CB, et al. The narcotic bowel syndrome: clinical features, pathophysiology, and management. *Clin Gastroenterol Hepatol*. 2007;5:1126–1139; quiz 1121–1122.

Lewis FR, Holcroft JW, Dunphy E. Appendicitis. A critical review of diagnosis and treatment in 1,000 cases. *Arch Surg*. 1975;110: 677–684.

Makrauer FL, Greenberger NJ. *Acute abdominal pain: basic principles & current challenges*. In: Current Diagnosis & Treatment: Gastroenterology, Hepatology, & Endoscopy. Greenberger NJ, Blumberg RS, Burakoff R, eds. New York: McGraw-Hill; 2009: 1–10.

Rettenbacher T, Hollerweger A, Gritzmann N, et al. Appendicitis: should diagnostic imaging be performed if the clinical presentation is highly suggestive of the disease? *Gastroenterology*. 2002;123:992–998.

Saito YA, Locke GR, Talley NJ, et al. A comparison of the Rome and Manning criteria for case identification in epidemiological investigations of irritable bowel syndrome. *Am J Gastroenterol*. 2000;95:2816–2824.

CHAPTER 75

Acute Back Pain

Marzouq Awni Qubti, MD
John A. Flynn, MD, MBA, FACP, FACR

Key Clinical Questions

1. What are the key questions that an examiner should ask when approaching a patient with acute back pain?
2. What should the examiner look for on physical examination?
3. What are "red flag" findings that should heighten your level of concern when approaching a patient with acute back pain?
4. What are some nonspinal etiologies of back pain?

INTRODUCTION

Back pain has a major impact on patient well-being and health care budgets in developed nations. It is the fifth leading cause of hospital admissions, and the third most common reason for surgical procedures. Back pain ranks second only to upper respiratory tract infections as a reason for primary care physician office visits. The annual prevalence of chronic low back pain ranges from 15% to 33%, and 7% of adult patients may have low back pain at any given time. In the United States, back pain, including chronic low back pain, is the leading cause of disability in subjects younger than 45 years of age. Individuals with back pain in the United States account for $90 billion in direct health care expenditures, and approximately 2% of the U.S. workforce is compensated for back injuries each year.

Roughly 95% of visits for back pain stem from benign causes. However, in hospitalized patients, the percentage with serious pathology may be higher, so clinicians to have to have a high index of suspicion. This chapter focuses on the initial evaluation of acute low back pain in patients admitted to the hospital, as well as patients hospitalized for other reasons who develop back pain as a complication of hospitalization.

PATHOPHYSIOLOGY

The function of the anterior spine is to absorb the shock of body movements such as walking and running. The function of the posterior spine is to protect the spinal cord and nerves, and to stabilize the spine by providing sites for attachment of muscles and ligaments. The normal alignment of the spine is notable for:

- Lumbar and cervical lordosis and thoracic kyphosis on lateral view
- Straight column on anterior view

Movements of the cervical and lumbar regions are greater than the thoracic regions during activity. The elasticity of vertebral disks—largest in the cervical and lumbar regions—allow the bony vertebrae of the spine to move easily upon one another. Elasticity declines with age.

CASE 75-1

ACUTE ABDOMINAL AND BACK PAIN IN AN EMERGENT SETTING

An 81-year-old man with a history of myocardial infarction 10 years ago presented with new-onset low back pain and crampy abdominal pain that had begun 2 hours prior. He had never had this type of back pain before. His exam revealed a blood pressure of 110/70 mm Hg. His creatinine was 2.5 mg/dL with a glomerular filtration rate (GFR) of < 35/mL/1.73 m^2 which is his baseline after his myocardial infarction 10 years ago. He had good pedal pulses, and his abdominal exam revealed a soft abdomen with diffuse tenderness without rebound or guarding and normal bowel sounds. The patient's back and abdominal pain improved after narcotic administration. A computed tomography (CT) scan without contrast showed an abdominal periaortic hematoma. A 2D echocardiogram did not identify a dissection in the ascending aorta or aortic arch. A stable descending abdominal dissection was diagnosed and a vascular surgery consultation obtained for further management.

Different types of pain suggest different etiologies.

VISCERAL OR REFERRED PAIN

Visceral pain is poorly localized pain that is usually bilateral. It may arise from distension of abdominal organs, torsion, or contraction. The pain radiates along the dermatomes that innervate the involved organ (**Figure 75-1**). For this reason, it is possible to have pain referred to the back (ie, the posterior portion of the spinal segment that innervates the diseased organ).

Because of visceral innervation, diseases involving the pelvic organs, kidneys, gastrointestinal (GI) tract, and thorax may initially cause isolated back pain.

In general, the referral patterns are as follows:

- Upper abdominal diseases: pain T8 to L1 or L2
- Lower abdominal diseases: L2 to L4
- Pelvic diseases to the sacral region

Usually the patient has associated thoracic, abdominal, or pelvic pain depending on the location of the diseased organ. For example, sudden lumbar pain in a patient with a coagulopathy may indicate retroperitoneal hemorrhage. Changes in position do not usually affect visceral pain (**Table 75-1**).

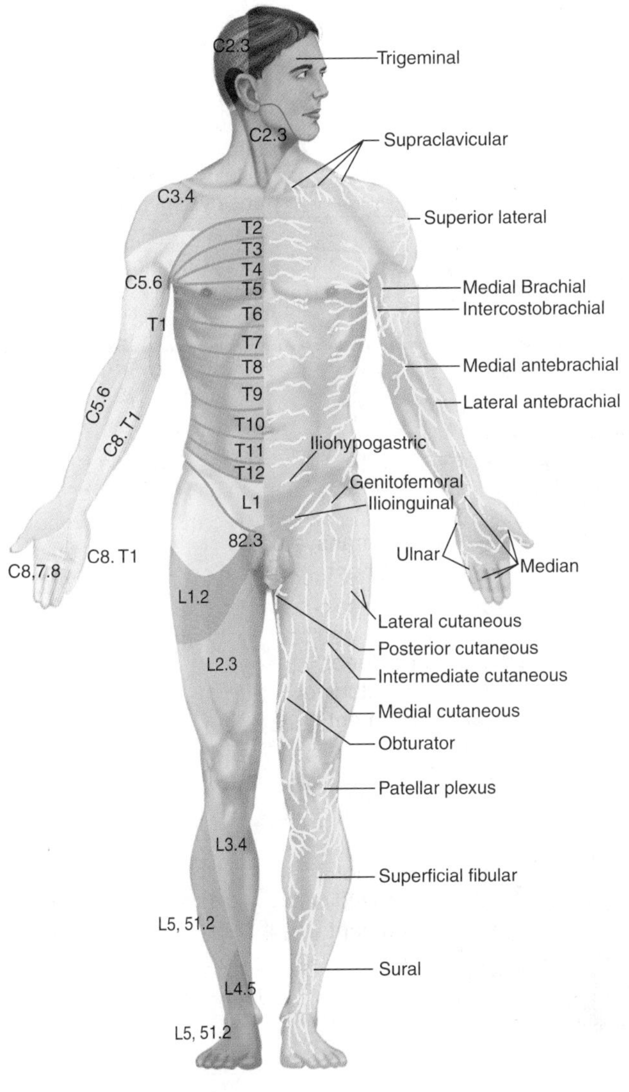

Figure 75-1 *Dermatomes.*

LOCALIZED PAIN

Back pain may be produced by irritation or compression of local sensory nerve endings. Diseases of any of the pain-sensitive structures of the back—periosteum of the vertebrae, dura, facet joints, annulus fibrosus, epidural veins, and the posterior longitudinal ligament—may cause back pain without nerve root compression (**Figure 75-2**).

Back pain may result from direct injuries (usually musculoligamentous, but sometimes fractures with or without spinal cord trauma) and degenerative processes (spinal stenosis, disk herniation, changes in the intervertebral disks and other structural abnormalities). Ordinarily, the nucleus pulposus and inner annulus fibrosus do not have innervation. However, inflammatory cytokines, ingrowth of pain nerve fibers into the damaged disks, and nerve root injury due to disk herniation have been hypothesized as possible mechanisms of pain related to disk disease. Substantial genetic influences rather than age-related changes determine the incidence of disk disease which recurs in 40% of patients within six months. Pain from the lumbar spine may be felt in the coccyx, hips or buttocks. The pain should not shoot down the posterior thighs without disk impingement on an exiting nerve root.

Structural abnormalities specific to the spine include congenital and acquired anomalies. Spondylolysis is a defect in the pars interarticularis leading to vertebral body instability of the lumbar vertebral bodies that may lead to bilateral stress fractures. In such cases, the activity related persistent back pain is the main feature of the disease.

Alterations of the microarchitecture of the vertebral body may lead to compression fractures and localized back pain (**Figure 75-3**). The pain may be exacerbated by movement, relieved by lying flat in bed, and may radiate to the extremities. Common underlying causes include immobilization, endocrine disorders (hyperparathyroidism, hyperthyroidism), malignancy (multiple myeloma, metastatic carcinoma), chronic glucocorticoid use, and osteoporosis and osteomalacia.

Bacteremia in the setting of endocarditis, pneumonia, or pyelonephritis may seed the vertebral bodies and disk, leading to osteomyelitis and diskitis. Less commonly, vertebral osteomyelitis may arise from local infection, such as postoperative infection after surgery. Extension of infection can lead to meningeal involvement, with an epidural or subdural abscess. The thoracolumbar vertebral bodies are the usual sites of involvement, but any area of the spine may be affected. After spinal surgery, reverse extension of the infection from the disk space to the endplates may occur. *Mycobacterium tuberculosis* of the spine, also known as Pott disease, is common in patients from endemic regions, and typically affects the lower thoracic spine.

Arthritic spine diseases include ankylosing spondylitis (AS), reactive arthritis, psoriatic arthritis, and inflammatory bowel disease associated spondyloarthritis and undifferentiated spondyloarthritis. Patients may report insidious onset of low back pain and buttock pain. A suggestive feature is worsening pain with rest, or back pain that awakens the patient at night. Patients with AS frequently report alternating upper buttock or lower lumbosacral pain, deep in nature, which worsens on long car rides or with prolonged sitting. The patient may improve on ambulation or exercise. Patients with psoriatic arthritis, as in reactive arthritis, have their spine involved much less frequently than in AS.

RADICULAR PAIN

Nerve roots exit from the vertebral bodies. They may be injured at any point along their intraspinal course to their exit at the intervertebral foramen. Facet joint hypertrophy can produce unilateral radicular symptoms due to bony compression of the nerve roots.

TABLE 75-1 Referred Pain

Visceral Disease	Referred Pain	Pathology	Comments
Peptic ulcers, tumors of posterior wall of stomach or duodenum	Midline back or paraspinal pain	Retroperitoneal extension	
Pancreatitis, pancreatic tumors	Back pain to the right or left of the spine	Involvement of head of pancreas (right sided); body or tail (left sided)	Chapter 156: Acute Pancreatitis
Retroperitoneal structures	Paraspinal pain that radiates to the lower abdomen, groin, or testicles	Hemorrhage, tumors, pyelonephritis	
Abdominal aortic aneurysm	Isolated LBP (15–20% of patients)	Contained rupture	Abdominal pain, shock, back pain < 20% of patients; hypotension 50%; 2 of 3 features in 66%; typical patient elderly male smoker
Iliopsoas mass or abscess	Unilateral lumbar pain to groin, labia or testicles		
Colitis, diverticulitis or colon cancer	Midlumbar pain ± beltline distribution around body	Lesion in transverse or proximal descending colon (mid or left L2–3); sigmoid (upper sacral)	Lower abdominal pain or isolated back pain or both
Endometriosis, uterine cancers, uterine malposition, menstrual pain, remote radiation therapy to pelvis	Sacral pain	Lower back pain rare except in disorders involving uterosacral ligaments	
Pregnancy	Lower back pain radiating to one or both thighs	Last weeks of pregnancy	
Chronic prostatitis; prostate cancer metastatic to spine; ureteral obstruction from stones	Lumbosacral back pain		
Infectious, inflammatory, or neoplastic renal disease; renal vein thrombosis	Ipsilateral lumbar sacral pain		Chapter 251: Kidney Stones; Chapter 205: Urinary Tract Infections and Pyelonephritis
Hip pain	May mimic lumbar spine disease		Patrick sign or heel percussion sign may help distinguish from spine etiologies

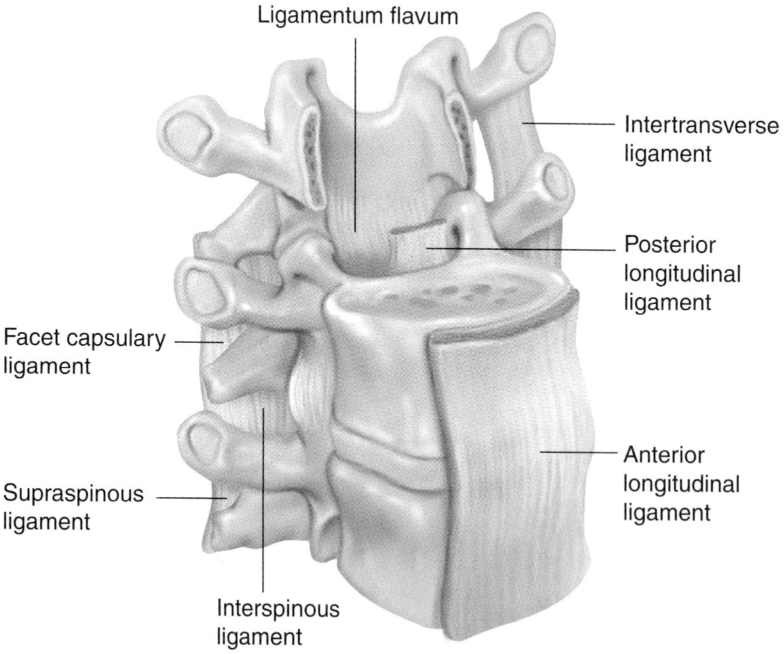

Figure 75-2 *Ligament structures in the lumbar spine.*

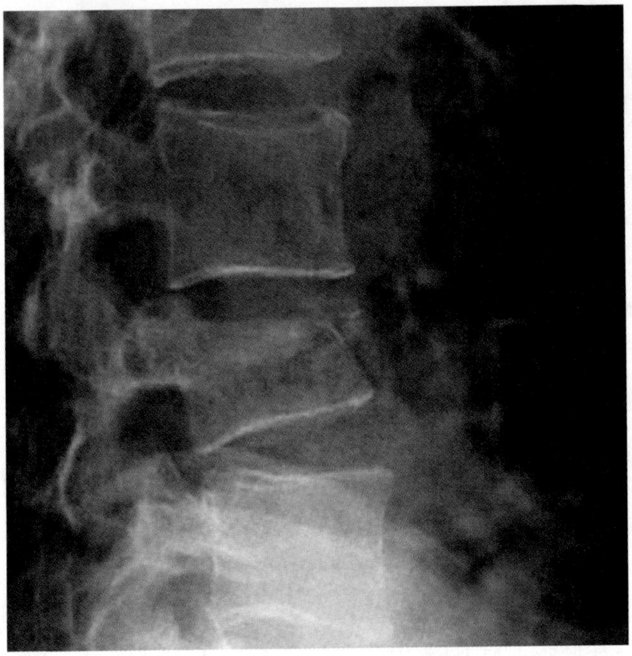

Figure 75-3 *Compression fracture on plain film.*

With worsening facet osteoarthritis, cysts may protrude, and cause further narrowing of the spinal canal. Referred pain can be associated with radicular pain. For example, a retroperitoneal bleed can cause neuropathic pain along the femoral nerve.

Pain originating from spinal nerve roots may be referred to the extremities. For example, pain originating from the lumbar region may be referred to the buttocks or legs, or localized to the lumbar region. Diseases of the upper lumbar spine may cause pain localized to the lumbar region, groin or anterior thighs. Diseases of the lower lumbar region may cause pain referred to the buttocks, posterior thighs, or rarely, the calves or feet.

Radicular pain is often aggravated by postures that stretch nerves and nerve roots. Because the sciatic nerve (L5 and S1 roots) passes posterior to the hip, sitting increases pain arising from stretching of the sciatic nerve. Pain arising from the femoral nerve (L2, L3, and L4 roots), however, will not be stretched from the sitting position because the femoral nerve passes anterior to the hip.

Disk herniations may impinge upon a nerve root, thereby causing radicular pain. The L5 and S1 nerve roots are involved in close to 95% of lumbar-disk herniations (**Figure 75-4**). These patients will describe a subacute to chronic, deep, burning, aching lower back pain that involves the buttocks and radiates down the posterior thigh to the posterolateral aspect of the calf.

Radiating pain may be elicited by lifting heavy objects, straining to have a bowel movement, coughing, or sneezing.

Spondylolisthesis or anterior slippage of one vertebral body, pedicles, and superior articular facets over another, may arise from congenital anomalies of the lumbosacral spine with one example being spondylolysis (**Figure 75-5**); other common causes include degeneration, osteoporosis, trauma, prior surgery, infection, and tumor. When symptomatic, it may cause low back pain, tightness of the hamstring muscles, and nerve root injury, most frequently of L5.

Lumbar adhesive arachnoiditis causes radicular pain due to injury of the subarachnoid space. Multiple lumbar operations, chronic spinal infections, spinal cord injury, intrathecal injection, demyelination polyneuropathies, or neoplastic infiltration can cause inflammation with subsequent fibrosis.

Lumbar spinal stenosis causes radicular pain due to a narrowed spinal canal that impinges on the spinal cord during certain postures.

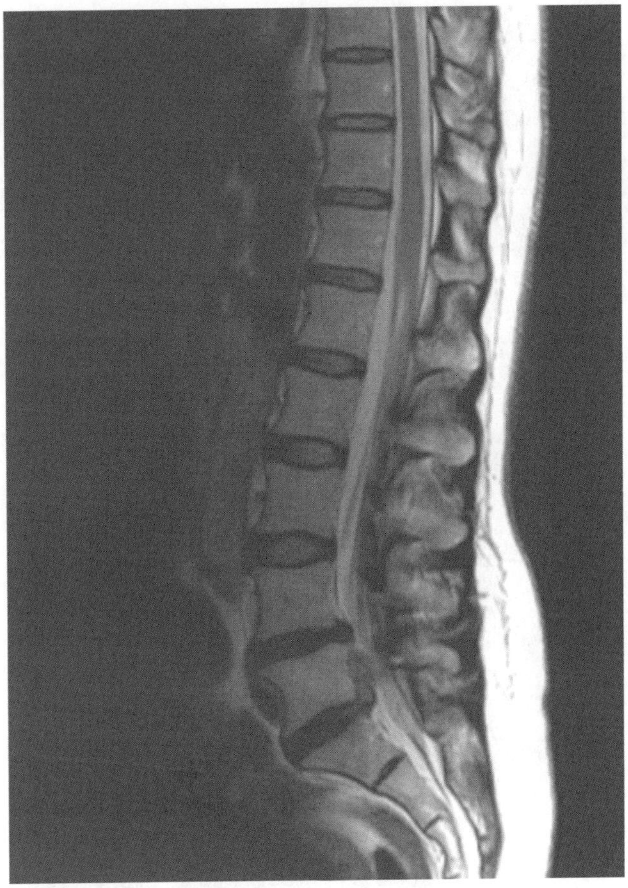

Figure 75-4 *MRI of L5-S1 disk herniation.*

Spinal stenosis may develop secondary to congenital defects such as spondylolysis and acquired causes such as spondylolisthesis or adjacent to prior sites of fusion surgery. The discomfort, commonly referred to as neurogenic claudication, radiates from the lower back to the buttock, and even down to the proximal legs (**Figure 75-6**). The pain is worse with prolonged walking and standing and much better on sitting or change in posture—a clear distinction from the inflammatory back pain syndromes.

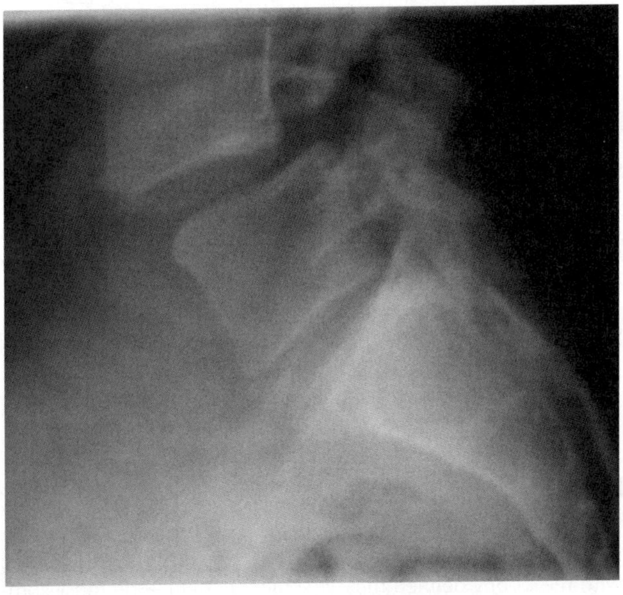

Figure 75-5 *Plain film showing spondylolisthesis.*

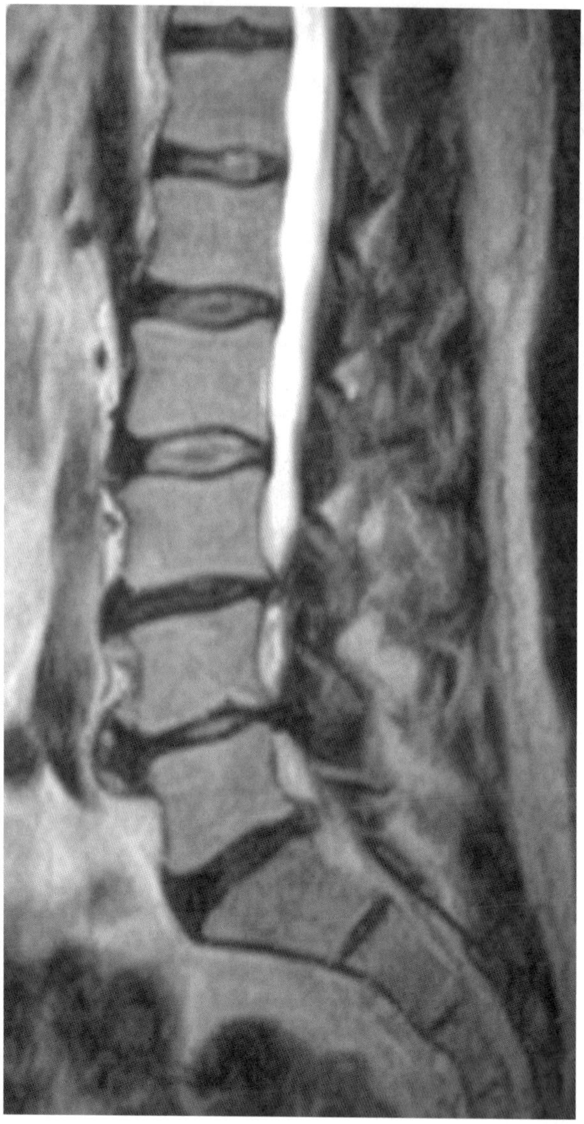

Figure 75-6 *MRI of a patient with lumbar spinal stenosis.*

Cauda equina syndrome (CES) can cause acute or subacute back pain. By definition, it is associated with serious neurologic deficits, such as impairment of bladder, bowel, or sexual function and perianal "saddle" numbness. A centrally herniated disk is the most common cause of this syndrome. Less common causes of the CES include spinal injury, spinal stenosis, neoplasms, abscesses, tuberculosis, AS, spinal anesthesia, back manipulation, or postoperative complications such as hematoma. CES can present acutely as the first symptom of lumbar disk herniation, or insidiously with slow progression to numbness and urinary symptoms. CES need not present with complete urinary retention and reduced urinary sensation. The loss of desire to void and a poor stream are symptoms of an "incomplete" CES. This condition requires a high index of suspicion to make the diagnosis, especially if the patient has preexisting urinary difficulties. In fact, patients have inappropriately undergone prostate surgery with no improvement in their symptoms prior to reaching the correct diagnosis of CES.

MUSCLE SPASM PAIN

Spasms of taut paraspinal muscles will produce nonspecific localized dull pain aggravated by abnormal posture. 90% of patients with the poorly defined muscle sprain or strain—the most common cause of nonemergent back pain—will recover within two weeks. Heavy lifting, pushing, pulling, prolonged walking and standing, and driving are associated with this type of back pain.

Systemic diseases such as primary or metastatic cancer, infection, or arthritic spine disease may cause back pain by multiple mechanisms, including stretching of the nerve fibers entering the spinal cord, disrupting bony structures, occupying space in the vertebral bodies, or referred pain from visceral structures. The most common malignancies that metastasize to the extradural space include breast, lung, prostate, thyroid, kidney, GI tract, multiple myeloma, and lymphomas. Primary tumors—chordomas, neurofibromas, osteoid osteomas, osteoblastomas, hemangiomas, and aneurysm bone cysts—rarely do this. Schwannomas, meningiomas, neurofibromas, and lipomas may grow in the intradural extramedullary space. Astrocytomas and ependymomas affect the intramedullary space. Leptomeningeal metastases, most commonly from leukemia, lymphoma, breast cancer and lung cancer, may initially present with back pain or postural headache, and signs or symptoms at multiple sites in the spinal cord, brain, and cranial nerves. Pelvic cancer may cause a lumbosacral plexopathy.

PRACTICE POINT

- Thoracic pain suggests metastatic cancer or possibly Pott disease.

CASE 75-2

ACUTE AND SUBACUTE FOCAL LESIONS INVOLVING THE VERTEBRAL COLUMN

A 60-year-old diabetic farmer with a history of prostate cancer and normal PSA on lupron after radiation therapy five years ago reported three months of low back pain without numbness or tingling, urinary or bladder retention, or lower extremity weakness. He mentioned low-grade fevers between 100.5°–102°F that had previously been treated with nonsteroidal anti-inflammatories. He reported a 5 lb weight loss in the past three months. He denied any recent trauma to his back but an episode of lower extremity cellulitis required oral antibiotics close to four months earlier. He was taking warfarin for stroke prophylaxis due to fibrillation and aspirin for cardiovascular protection given a strong family history of heart disease. His vital signs were normal and his examination significant for focal tenderness on palpating the spinous process of two vertebrae in the mid thoracic spine.

DIAGNOSIS

Acute back pain requires immediate assessment to avoid progressive morbidity and mortality that can arise from serious underlying causes. The challenge for the examiner at the bedside is identify those patients who require emergent consultation and/or imaging due to evidence of:

1. Systemic underlying disease such as metastatic cancer or bacteremia
2. Neurologic compromise
3. Complications of hospitalization that require intervention

The hospitalist should expeditiously review the reason for admission to the hospital, past medical history, and hospital course, ask about the quality of pain, and seek neurologic symptoms and signs that suggest a worrisome diagnosis. Chart review, including any consultant notes and prior physical therapy evaluations, may reveal important historical and physical findings that may suggest structural causes (**Table 75-2**).

TABLE 75-2 Chart Review Risk Factors for Serious Underlying Causes

History
• Age > 50 years • Reason for admission: intractable pain, worse at rest, worse at night, failed conservative management; metastatic cancer, bacteremia (lung, urinary tract, skin), trauma, progressive neurologic problem (falling, weakness, urinary retention, or incontinence) • Medication use: intravenous drug abuse, chronic steroids, immunosuppression • Past medical history: cancer, chronic infections, immunosuppression, known coagulopathy or thrombocytopenia, known abdominal aortic aneurysm or significant vascular disease, unexplained weight loss, prior procedures
Medications
• Glucocorticoids • Antibiotics that may not cover specific organisms likely to affect spine • Warfarin, antiplatelet agents
Hospital course
• Procedures (epidural anesthesia, spine surgery, lumbar puncture, central lines) • Unexplained fever
Physical examination
• Fever, hypotension • Progressive focal neurologic deficits (signs of spinal cord injury, focal weakness or muscle atrophy, reflex changes, diminished sensation in the extremities) • Percussion tenderness over spine • Abdominal, rectal, pelvic mass

PRACTICE POINT

- Back pain following any procedure requires immediate communication with the surgeon or proceduralist.

The patient's primary nurse, who has spent time with the patient, should be consulted.

Although more recent systematic reviews on screening red flag questions have warned against their false-positive rates, they provide a framework for the overall clinical assessment and triage process usually in the primary care setting. Recommendations regarding the use of red flags in assessing patients with acute low back pain are summarized in **Table 75-3**.

PRACTICE POINT

- The mere fact that a patient is hospitalized is a "red flag" that the patient is at risk for a serious underlying cause of back pain.

THE PHYSICAL EXAMINATION

The physical examination is helpful if it confirms the examiner's provisional diagnosis. However, the absence of neurologic signs does not rule out catastrophic etiologies of acute back pain. Therefore, clinicians need to synthesize risk factors, past medical history, quality of pain, acuity and severity of pain, as well as the physical examination, to determine whether emergent consultation and imaging are required.

Vital signs should be checked first. Hypotension, hypoxia, or fever point to systemic disease, such as ruptured aortic aneurysm or dissection, myocardial infarction, bacteremic seeding of the spine, retroperitoneal hemorrhage, perforated viscus, or injuries related to trauma. When there is hemodynamic instability, the focus should be on immediate stabilization and obtaining preliminary tests that do not require moving the patient, such as portable chest radiograph, electrocardiograph (ECG), blood work, and appropriate consultation and triage.

When vital signs are abnormal but stable, the examiner starts with a targeted examination for signs of systemic disease, as well as performing a neurologic examination. For example, a widened pulse pressure may suggest aortic insufficiency, and the examiner should carefully perform cardiac auscultation to appreciate an aortic regurgitant murmur. Fever in any patient with back or buttock pain should prompt the clinician to examine the skin for evidence of an embolic process, vasculitis, or infection, listen for new murmurs that may suggest endocarditis, examine the lungs to assess for pneumonia, solicit spine percussion tenderness, which may suggest vertebral osteomyelitis, spondylodiskitis, or epidural abscess, check for costovertebral tenderness that would suggest acute pyelonephritis or renal abscess, examine the abdomen, and to order blood and urine cultures and appropriate imaging.

The back examination begins with observation. Clues to a systemic process include an assessment of whether the patient appears acutely ill, in severe pain, confused, or has evidence of skin abnormalities. The curvature of the spine should be examined for changes in the normal alignment, scoliosis, and other structural abnormalities. Forward bending or asymmetry of the paraspinal muscles is most consistent with muscle spasm. The presence of an indwelling Foley requires a consideration of progressive cord lesions, in addition to the usual causes of acquired urinary retention during hospitalization, such as deconditioning and administration of narcotics and sedatives.

PRACTICE POINT

- In patients with cord lesions, the blood pressure can be very labile. Avoid overtreatment of the blood pressure.

Examination should proceed with palpation of the paraspinal muscles. Palpation and percussion over the spine may reproduce bony pain originating from the spine. The examiner should note whether motion exacerbates the pain during changes in position. Motion exacerbates the pain from vertebral osteomyelitis and mechanical back pain, but rest only relieves mechanical etiologies. Referred pain from visceral structures is unaffected by positional changes. Vertebral tenderness, particularly when elicited by percussion with a fist over the affected area, is a sensitive sign of infection, but it lacks specificity, also being seen in metastatic disease to the spine, vertebral compression fractures, and other causes of localized pain. The bedside examination cannot exclude osteomyelitis. Fever is present in fewer than 50% of patients, and only 15% have motor and sensory deficits.

PRACTICE POINT

- Most spine tumors compress rather than invade. In patients with a history of cancer and progressive spinal cord symptoms, especially involving bowel and bladder, assume that cord compression is the cause of their back pain until proven otherwise. Weakness usually affects the legs first, so be sure to check motor function of the lower extremities. Also check position and vibration sense, which are very sensitive for compression.

TABLE 75-3 Red Flags

Serious Considerations	Clinical Findings
Acute, severe back pain with associated chest or abdominal pain in the majority of patients • Note: specificity of additional features such as ripping or tearing pain or migrating pain in the diagnosis of aortic dissection is unknown Aortic dissection not only causes pain but may be associated with neurologic compromise if the false lumen is supplying the spinal cord.	Thoracic aortic dissection and myocardial infarction See Chapter 124: Acute Coronary Syndromes See Chapter 262: Diseases of the Aorta
Back pain that awakens the patient at night	Cancer, inflammatory back pain associated with ankylosing spondylitis (AS)
New-onset back pain in a patient age > 50 years, failure to improve with conservative therapy, pain > 1 month, previous history of cancer, insidious onset, systemically unwell Pain from bony metastatic disease becomes constant, dull, unrelieved by rest and worse at night unlike mechanical low back pain.	Bony metastatic disease See Chapter 182: Oncologic Emergencies
Risk factors • Recent epidural anesthesia, spine surgery, procedure such as intrathecal devices • Anticoagulant use or coagulation disorder, thrombocytopenia Symptoms • Sudden, severe back or neck pain around the involved vertebrae with radiating pain • Within hours to days, ascending numbness, radicular paresthesia, and progressive paraparesis may develop Treatment • Early decompressive laminectomy with hematoma evacuation is essential	Spinal hematoma See Chapter 64: Common Complications in Neurosurgery
Risk factors • IV drug use or longer term catheter placement, recent bacterial infection, immunosuppression from steroids, HIV, or organ transplantation Symptoms • Fever, neurologic symptoms	Osteomyelitis of the vertebral body or epidural abscess See Chapter 200: Osteomyelitis and Septic Arthritis
Risk factors • History of herniated disks Symptoms • Loss of bowel or bladder function, saddle anesthesia, widespread or progressive motor weakness	Cauda equina syndrome
Risk factors • Age > 70 years, significant trauma, prolonged use of corticosteroids, altered sensation from trunk down, diagnosis of fracture Symptoms • When symptomatic, the pain with a compression fracture may be sharp or dull, localized and may arise acutely or insidiously. Sitting or moving may aggravate the pain while laying supine is usually the most comfortable position	Vertebral compression fracture Vertebral osteomyelitis (spondylodiskitis)
Risk factors • Family history of AS, personal history of psoriasis, uveitis, inflammatory bowel disease, or recent infection Symptoms • Gradual onset before age 40 years • Worse with rest and improved with exercise • Morning stiffness ≥ 0.5–1.0 hours • Peripheral joint arthritis	Axial spondyloarthritis

A straight leg–raising (SLR) test is performed with the patient supine, and the examiner's hand holding the leg straight and cupping the heel. This maneuver stretches the L5 and S1 nerve roots and the sciatic nerve. Passive dorsiflexion of the foot further increases the stretch. Reproducing the patient's back or extremity pain with leg elevation to less than 60 degrees is considered a positive test. Tight hamstring muscles may limit the degree of elevation without pain but would not be expected to reproduce the patient's presenting pain. A positive crossed SLR test reproduces the patient's symptoms in the opposite leg from the flexed limb. This maneuver is less sensitive but more specific for lumbosacral radiculopathy. The examiner should also perform a hip examination, because hip pain can be confused with low back pain and any patient with bacteremia can seed the hip as well as the spine.

The purpose of the neurologic assessment is to identify deficits that would require emergent neurosurgical consultation and

TABLE 75-4 Neurologic Examination

	Examination Findings			
Lumbosacral Nerve Roots	**Reflex**	**Sensory**	**Motor**	**Pain Distribution**
L2*	—	Upper anterior thigh	Psoas (hip flexion)	Anterior thigh
L3*	—	Lower anterior thigh Anterior knee	Psoas (hip flexion) Quadriceps (knee extension) Thigh adduction	Anterior thigh, knee
L4*	Quadriceps (knee)	Medial calf	Quadriceps (knee extension)† Thigh adduction Tibialis anterior (foot dorsiflexion)	Knee, medial calf Anterolateral thigh
L5§	—	Dorsal surface—foot Lateral calf	Peroneii (foot eversion)† Tibialis anterior (foot dorsiflexion) Gluteus medius (hip abduction) Toe dorsiflexors	Lateral calf, dorsal foot, posterolateral thigh, buttocks
S1§	Gastrocnemius/ soleus (ankle)	Plantar surface—foot Lateral aspect—foot	Gastrocnemius/soleus (foot plantar flexion)† Abductor hallucis (toe flexors)† Gluteus maximus (hip extension)	Bottom foot, posterior calf, posterior thigh, buttocks

*Reverse straight leg–raising sign present—see "Examination of the Back."
†These muscles receive the majority of innervation from this root.
§Straight leg–raising sign present—see "Examination of the Back."
Reproduced, with permission, from Fauci AS, Braunwald E, Kasper DL, et al. Harrison's Principles of Internal Medicine. 17th ed. New York: McGraw-Hill; 2008, Table 16-2.

to document a baseline examination in the event that the patient goes to surgery (**Table 75-4**). Ask the patient to walk. If a patient is unable to walk due to weakness, the examiner should look for focal weakness that may suggest a cord compression or spinal hematoma. In patients with spinal stenosis, walking in a forward-hunched position may relieve the pain with ambulation (anthropoid posture). These patients may have a positive Romberg maneuver, a wide-based gait, and claudication on forced lumbar extension, but are unlikely to have motor signs or weakness (**Table 75-5**).

Asymmetric reflexes may assist in localization of the defect:

- Hyporeflexia of the patellar reflex: disk herniation at L4; Achilles reflex: disk herniation at S1
- Hyperreflexia below the lesion: spinal cord compression, spinal hematoma, spinal stenosis. Note whether clonus is present
- Absent perirectal tone and perineal sensation: cauda equina syndrome.

PRACTICE POINT

- The examiner should document the timing and nature of any bowel, bladder, motor, and sexual dysfunction once a diagnosis that may be associated with neurologic compromise is suspected. Be sure to record any deficits prior to surgical intervention.

USE OF IMAGING TO EVALUATE BACK PAIN IN HOSPITALIZED PATIENTS

Back pain is a common, often chronic, problem that may not require evaluation during hospitalization. Early magnetic resonance imaging (MRI) in outpatients without serious neurologic or systemic signs or symptoms does not alter treatment or overall quality of low back pain after 8 and 24 months. The presence of degenerative lumbar disk changes of herniation, degeneration, or an annular fissure do not correlate with symptoms, and are also seen in 14% to 50% of healthy volunteers. However, hospitalized patients are a different population. For patients with chronic pain in particular, it is important to determine whether the patient has had prior appropriate imaging, if the patient has had a procedure during or prior to hospitalization that might result in complications affecting the spine, and whether the patient's symptoms have changed or simply noted during review of symptoms.

The presence of additional signs, symptoms, and underlying chronic disease conditions determine the proper differential diagnosis and direct selection of imaging. New back pain demands careful consideration of causes for which prompt imaging will avoid catastrophic effects upon patient outcome. Aortic dissection is characterized by back pain and may be accompanied by chest pain or abdominal pain. Physical examination may reveal hypertension, differential blood pressures, pulsus paradoxus and possibly a pulsatile aorta in addition to evidence of organ compromise, depending on the location and extent of dissection or it may be unrevealing. Recent angiography or other vascular intervention may also increase concern. The diagnosis of dissection and determination of extent must be undertaken emergently. In this case, the rapidity with which the examination can be performed outweighs the imaging modality selected. CT and MRI are both widely used for evaluation of the entire aorta. Dissection may also be diagnosed on angiography and ultrasonography although the extent of dissection may be outside the imaging that is being performed for other purposes. The careful evaluation of images by the radiologist makes a critical difference in patient care, particularly when dissection is the cause of back pain for which a spine MRI has been ordered.

Any condition leading to impending cord compression is a reason for emergent MRI examination. There is one exception—trauma. In the setting of trauma, since the most helpful identifications are

TABLE 75-5 Targeted History and Physical Examination of the Spine

Symptoms including reported neurologic deficits
Onset including precipitating factors
Examples: cord contusion following hyperextension of the spine due to severe trauma with underlying pathology causing stenosis or instability or rarely, spontaneous epidural hematoma following valsalva maneuvers with coughing and sneezing, cocaine use, back manipulation, and even exercise.
Pain (mild, moderate, severe; bilateral versus unilateral; radiating)
Bladder/bowel
Sensory
Motor
Vital signs
Lability of BP (very labile with cord lesions, especially during pain)
Specifically note presence of hypotension, fever in last 24 hours
Cardiac examination
Murmurs (especially if fever present or known bacteremia)
Pulmonary
New signs suggestive of pneumonia (especially if fever or known bacteremia)
Abdomen
Bowel sounds
Check for tenderness, guarding, presence of pulsatile mass
Percussion of bladder if urinary retention suspected
Vascular
BP in both arms
Pulses, including examination of extremities for cyanosis
Bruits
Bowel/bladder
Presence of Foley catheter or diapers
Evidence of urinary retention
Spine
Alignment
Tenderness
Spasm
Deep tendon reflexes (biceps, triceps, brachioradialis, knee, ankle, Babinski)
If brisk, check clonus, spreading
If spine cord injury suspected, check abdominals, suprapubic, cremasteric, anal reflexes (place a gloved finger in the patient's anal canal to check the "anal wink" or contraction of external anal sphincter in response to noxious stimuli; place a finger on the perineum right behind the scrotum, pull on penis or bladder catheter to check the bulbocavernosus reflex or contraction of the cavernosus muscle).
Straight leg raise to reproduce patient's pain: L5, S1
Reverse straight leg raise: L3 or L4
Hip
FABER (put ankle on opposite knee; rotate knee towards examination table) positive for mechanical LBP or hip pathology but not for disk disease
Patrick sign (internal and external rotation at the hip with hip and knee in flexion)
Heel percussion sign (tapping heel when extremity extended)
Motor
Deficits (slow movements; fast but weak movements; arms compared to legs)
Atrophy
Fasciculations
Tone (rigidity, spasticity)
Gait
Sensory
Pin
Light touch
Temperature
Cranial nerves (if leptomeningeal metastases suspected)

of bone fragments, CT would be chosen over MRI for initial workup because calcium voids are a limitation of MRI. Regarding cancer and infection, it is the presence and degree of cord compression that is the real emergency issue, as opposed to whether the etiology is due to tumor or infection. Radiography, radionuclide bone scans, and CT scans are helpful for identifying musculoskeletal metastases from a wide variety of tumors but MRI allows identification of nerve roots and tumor extension into the thecal sac. If cancer is suspected, MRI imaging of the entire spine is indicated. Like cancer, epidural abscess usually requires rapid identification and treatment to prevent permanent neurologic deficit. CT may miss a significant epidural collection that could suddenly cause neurologic compromise; thus, MR is preferred. With concerns about the risks of IV contrast enhancement, higher field strengths may allow more alternatives to IV contrast enhancement of MR sequences.

PRACTICE POINT

- Consult with the radiologist at your institution to determine the best emergent imaging study and whether contrast is required to avoid unnecessary delays and to avoid imaging studies that do not rule out the condition you suspect.

In an elderly woman with known osteoporosis, back pain may arise from an acute compression fracture of a vertebra and be confirmed by chest radiographs or radiography of a single region of the spine. Osteoporosis is also associated with chronic disease and treatments, such as steroids making this an even more common possibility among hospitalized patients. Some conditions cause bone deformities that also increase potential for mild trauma to become devastating during a hospitalization. It is important to remember that endoscopic examinations and intubation can stress abnormal spines setting up catastrophic complications. In a patient with rheumatoid arthritis, new-onset neck pain may indicate a C1–C2 subluxation. In a patient with AS, new onset neck pain may indicate an unstable fracture of the fused cervical spine. In either case neck immobilization should precede cervical spine imaging.

MANAGEMENT

CASE 75-3

NONEMERGENT HOSPITALIST ADMISSION FOR BACK PAIN

A 35-year-old construction worker was evaluated in the emergency department with severe low back pain that had been ongoing for four days and has culminated in limiting his ability to walk. He had never had back pain before and the pain was described as dull and constant but markedly worse on ambulation. The pain did not arouse the patient once he was able to fall asleep. Acetaminophen and ibuprofen taken intermittently had not relieved the pain. He denied any pain in his lower extremities, numbness, tingling, or any bowel or bladder symptoms, sexual dysfunction, chest pain, shortness of breath, nausea, vomiting, or abdominal pain. There had been no fever or weight loss. His review of systems was otherwise unremarkable. He drank six to ten beers on a daily basis, and had been smoking a pack a day for seven years. He occasionally used intranasal cocaine on a recreational basis. He denied using intravenous illicit drugs and reported no HIV risk factors. He has recently started working in his current job, which involves heavy lifting. He reported that his mother has hypertension and his father has both hypertension and a prior history of a myocardial infarction. He also reported a younger brother who has psoriasis. On exam the patient was afebrile. His pulse was 88 beats per minute, and his blood pressure was 140/80 mm Hg. Respirations and pulse oximetry were normal while breathing ambient air. The examination was significant for a negative straight leg test. He had full range of motion of his cervical spine and tenderness to palpation of the paraspinal muscles at the lumbar and sacral spine. His upper extremity strength was 5/5 in all muscle groups but it was difficult to assess his lower extremity strength due to pain with any motion. His labs were significant for a white blood cell count of 9000/cu.mm, a normal erythrocyte sedimentation rate, and normal PA and lateral films of the thoracic and lumbar spine. His pain was mildly improved with intravenous hydromorphone at 2 mg every four hours, but he was still not able to walk. The hospitalist on duty was contacted to assess this patient for a possible admission.

What emergent causes of back pain will need to be ruled out prior to discharge? What are the more common nonemergent causes of this type of back pain? What are the next steps in this patient's management? How can this patient be safely transitioned to the outpatient setting?

The above case represents a patient who did not appear to have "red flags" that would suggest an emergent cause that would warrant any further testing in an inpatient hospital setting. The history and physical examination in the ED were consistent with acute low back pain that did not portend serious underlying pathology. His presentation was not consistent with a cardiopulmonary pathology. He had no worrisome lab values consistent with an infection or an inflammatory state. His neurologic review of systems and exam did not suggest an acute lumbar disk protrusion leading to the cauda equina syndrome. He was not presenting a history or exam consistent with inflammatory back pain and a spondyloarthritis.

If the patient continued to have difficulty ambulating, an admission for IV ketorolac followed by a transition to oral ibuprofen (with or without a proton pump inhibitor given his alcohol consumption) might be warranted. Based on the patient's wishes and ability to ambulate within the next 12 hours, a social work consultation as well as an inpatient physical therapy consultation was recommended. The patient might be prescribed ibuprofen at 1800–2400 mg in three divided doses for five days, with consideration of a proton pump inhibitor upon discharge. He should see his primary care physician within two weeks of his hospitalization. The patient might also be prescribed cyclobenzaprine at a dose of 10 mg orally at night for the first two weeks. It is vital that person to person communication between the inpatient team and the primary care physician be established in all cases where compliance is in question or when other specific case peculiarities have arisen during the hospital stay.

Initial management requires a decision about consultation. For inter-hospital transfers and patients admitted through the emergency department, it is very important to consider a wide range of diagnostic possibilities, in addition to the provisional diagnosis. When a patient is transferred from an outside hospital for intractable back pain, conservative management generally has failed, and emergent consultation with specialists, including neurosurgery, should be considered. The outside films should be reviewed with a radiologist to guide the need for additional imaging. Emergent imaging may be required if there are red flags suggestive of infection or other serious pathology, or technical limitations of the outside films.

See Chapter 96: Pain.

PRACTICE POINT

- Indications for emergent neurosurgical consultation include decompression of the spine in the setting of epidural abscess, tumor, or hematoma; urgent need for a tissue diagnosis; spinal instability, with displaced bone or ligaments; and metastatic disease that has recurred despite radiation therapy.

CONCLUSION

Clinicians need to assimilate the history and physical examination within the context of a new patient—one whose personality, pain tolerance, and unique qualities may not be apparent during a single encounter. Clinically excluding life-threatening and neurologically serious possibilities may require taking advantage of all the resources in the hospital including careful review of the chart, communication with caregivers who know the patient best, framing appropriate questions about risk factors and antecedent events, and emergent consultation and imaging. Although in general, hospitalists should avoid the temptation to pursue unnecessary and expensive diagnostic imaging when chronic conditions do not require inpatient workups such as spinal stenosis, it is also critical to advocate for appropriate and emergent imaging studies in selected patients based on rational choices. The responsible attending should always ask the question: What are the kinds of things that cannot be missed such as acute cord compression that may require emergent surgery and radiation therapy? In these instances, MRI may be the only imaging modality that will give you the information that you need. Although there is a vast literature about back pain in the outpatient setting, it is always important to remember that hospitalized patients are a different population.

SUGGESTED READINGS

Caragee E. Persistent low back pain. Clinical practice. *N Engl J Med.* 2005;352:1891–1898.

Chou R, Hoyt Huffman L. Medications for acute and chronic low back pain: a review of the evidence for an American Pain Society/ American College of Physicians Clinical Practice Guideline. *Ann Intern Med.* 2007;147:505–514.

Gilbert FJ, Grant AM, Gillan MG, et al. Low back pain: influence of early MR imaging or CT on treatment and outcome- multicenter randomized trial. *Radiology.* 2004;231:343–351.

Henschke M, Maher CG, Refshauge KM. A systematic review identifies five "red flags" to screen for vertebral fracture in patients with low back pain J Clin Epidemiol 2008;61(2):110–118.

Henschke N, Maher C, Refshauge K. Prevalence and screening for serious spinal pathology in patients presenting to primary care setting with acute low back pain. *Arthritis Rheum.* 2009;60: 3072–3080.

Henschke N, Maher CG, Refshauge KM. Screening for malignancy in low back pain patients: a systematic review. *Eur Spine J.* 2007;16: 1673–1679.

Katz JN, Harris MB. Lumbar spinal stenosis. *N Engl J Med.* 2008;358: 818–825.

Klinberg E, Mazanec D, Orr D, et al. Masquerade: medical causes of back pain. *Cleve Clinic J Med.* 2007;74:905–913.

Lavy C, James A, Wilson-MacDonald J, et al. Cauda equina syndrome. *BMJ.* 2009;338:881–884.

CHAPTER 76

Bleeding and Coagulopathy

Meridale V. Baggett, MD
Daniel P. Hunt, MD

Key Clinical Questions

1. What are the initial priorities for the patient with severe or life-threatening bleeding?
2. Is the bleeding medically remediable, or does it require structural intervention (interventional radiology or surgery)?
3. Does the patient have a coagulopathy or a platelet disorder based on history and examination?
4. What explains an elevated INR; an elevated PTT; a low platelet count?
5. How should coagulopathy be managed in the bleeding patient?
6. If a coagulopathy is present, what should be done to prepare a patient for an invasive procedure?

CASE 76-1

The orthopedic service requests Hospital Medicine consultation for bleeding from a wound site and for rapid drop in hematocrit. The patient is a 73-year-old woman admitted 2 weeks prior to consultation because of acetabular breakdown at the site of a previous left total hip replacement. On the day of admission, she underwent a revision of the left hip with bone grafting and trochanteric fixation. Because of substantial blood loss during the procedure, she required 4 units of packed red blood cells. Her postoperative course was complicated by transient hypoxemia related to volume overload and by delirium that gradually cleared by hospital day 7.

Unfortunately, while anticipating transfer to a rehabilitation facility, she experienced dislocation of the left hip. She returned to the operating room on hospital day 13 for complex revision of the left hip arthroplasty. Postoperatively, she had continuous oozing of blood from the left hip incision. On hospital day 15, her hematocrit dropped from 31 to 27 and she was noted to have a melenotic stool.

Her past medical history was notable for hypertension, and a history of peripheral vascular disease. She had a right carotid endarterectomy 6 years prior to admission and also had an emergent bowel resection about four years prior, due to intestinal ischemia. Other medical issues include degenerative joint disease of both hips and knees, gastroesophageal reflux, depression, fibromyalgia, and a history of a deep vein thrombosis following a right total knee replacement 1 year prior.

Her medications at the time of consultation included fluoxetine, lamotrigine, amitriptyline, fentanyl patch, morphine as needed for breakthrough pain, atenolol, furosemide, nifedipine, ranitidine, and cefazolin for "wound prophylaxis." She had been receiving enoxaparin for thrombosis prophylaxis but this was discontinued the day prior to consultation because of continued bleeding.

INITIAL BEDSIDE PRIORITIES

Initially, the goals for the hospitalist should be resuscitation of the unstable patient, control of bleeding, and prevention of further bleeding. Bedside evaluation of patients with apparent brisk bleeding (gastrointestinal, pulmonary, postpartum) includes vital sign measurement and assessment for adequate perfusion (mentation, capillary refill, urine output). Evidence of hemorrhagic shock mandates aggressive resuscitation using large bore intravenous access for intravenous fluids and blood products.

Life-threatening bleeding events may include intracranial hemorrhage (intracerebral, subdural, epidural, subarachnoid), gastrointestinal hemorrhage, massive hemoptysis, postpartum hemorrhage, and retroperitoneal hemorrhage. Spontaneous intracerebral hemorrhage portends a 25% to 30% in-hospital mortality. Upper gastrointestinal hemorrhage from varices predicts substantial in-hospital mortality.

Similar to management of severe traumatic hemorrhage, the bedside approach should minimize the time between recognition of severe or life-threatening bleeding and bleeding control. Each diagnostic intervention, including history, physical examination, laboratory testing, and radiographic testing should have the potential to lead directly to therapeutic intervention. The adage of the trauma surgeon that "the only diagnostic test that is absolutely

TABLE 76-1 Consultative Approach to Severe Bleeding

Bleeding Event	Urgent Consultation	Expected Intervention
Spontaneous intracerebral hemorrhage	Neurosurgery	*Assessment for surgical intervention**
Traumatic brain injury associated hemorrhage • Extradural hematoma • Subdural hematoma • Intracerebral hemorrhage	Neurosurgery Trauma surgery	*Assessment for surgical intervention**
Upper gastrointestinal hemorrhage • Esophageal variceal bleeding • Non-variceal bleeding • Bleeding peptic ulcer after endoscopic treatment	Gastroenterology General surgery Interventional radiology	*Upper gastrointestinal hemorrhage often amenable to endoscopic intervention.* *Surgery should be involved in most patients with substantial bleeding and should be consulted early.*
Lower gastrointestinal hemorrhage	Gastroenterology General surgery Interventional radiology	*Lower gastrointestinal hemorrhage may require angiography for localization and potential intervention*
Retroperitoneal hemorrhage	General surgery Interventional radiology (Urology)	*Although most patients are managed with conservative approaches and correction of coagulopathy/reversal of anticoagulation, surgical opinion should be obtained early.* *Ureteral compression may require urologic intervention.*
Postpartum hemorrhage	Obstetrics	*Assessment for surgical intervention**
Massive hemoptysis	Thoracic surgery Interventional radiology Pulmonary	*Bronchial artery embolization has a role in stabilizing patients and may be adequate primary treatment.*

*Surgery team may request assistance from Hospital Medicine in managing coexistent coagulopathy.

required before operating on the severely injured trauma patient is a type and cross for blood products" emphasizes the absolute focus on intervention that is required for acute, severe bleeding. In general, control of active bleeding requires a multidisciplinary approach that may involve surgery, interventional radiology, and/or endoscopy. **Table 76-1** provides guidance regarding the appropriate consultative services to engage urgently for each of the serious or life-threatening hemorrhagic problems along with the anticipated approach.

CASE 76-1 *(continued)*

What are the initial priorities for the patient with severe or life-threatening bleeding?

Is the bleeding medically remediable or does it require structural intervention (interventional radiology, endoscopy, or surgery)?

The patient is actively bleeding from the wound site, but the nursing staff reports that they are changing the dressing once a shift and feel the bleeding is manageable. The patient herself is disappointed at "another setback," but generally feels comfortable. She has not experienced shortness of breath, chest pain, abdominal pain, or nausea. She is thirsty. She noted that her bowel movement this morning was "very dark and smelly." The nurse confirms melena and reports that the hemoccult was positive.

Examination shows an older woman in no distress. She is alert and oriented. Blood pressure is 140/96 mm Hg, pulse 74 and regular. Mucous membranes are dry. Jugular venous pressure is estimated at 5 cm. Lungs are clear. Cardiac exam is normal. The abdomen is soft, with minimal tenderness over the epigastrium. The left hip wound is oozing blood and the thigh is swollen, somewhat indurated, and mildly tender.

Available labs include a hematocrit of 29.1%, platelets 401,000/mm^3. The INR is 1.9, and the aPTT is prolonged at 43 seconds (normal range, 22.1–34.0 sec). Creatinine is 0.7 mg/dL and BUN is 25 mg/dL.

Analysis: Although the melena is worrisome, the patient appears to be hemodynamically stable. She is mentating well. Her blood pressure is adequate and her pulse is normal. Bleeding from the wound is troublesome but controlled at present.

The hematocrit is adequate, but may not reflect acute bleeding.

PRACTICE POINT

- Initial Assessment: Beta-blockers or calcium channel blockers may blunt the usual heart rate response to severe bleeding.
- Among patients with chronic hypertension, a "normal" blood pressure may actually suggest relative hypotension.
- Bleeding from sites that cannot be directly visualized (gastrointestinal, intracerebral, bronchial tree) should prompt great wariness.

Initial interventions for this patient should be assurance of adequate intravenous access and alerting gastroenterology to the potential need for endoscopic evaluation. At this point, resuscitation is not an issue and it seems likely that there is time for assessment of medical issues that may be contributing to her bleeding.

SECONDARY HISTORY AND PHYSICAL EXAMINATION FOR BLEEDING DISORDERS

Systematic assessment of bleeding disorders requires a working knowledge of normal hemostasis. The two major mechanisms that contribute to clotting in distinctive but interrelated fashion are (1) platelet adhesion, activation, and plugging ("primary hemostasis") and (2) the coagulation cascade that generates a fibrin clot ("secondary hemostasis") with resultant consolidation of the platelet plug. Endothelial injury that exposes the circulating blood to subendothelial tissue factor and collagen activates both clotting

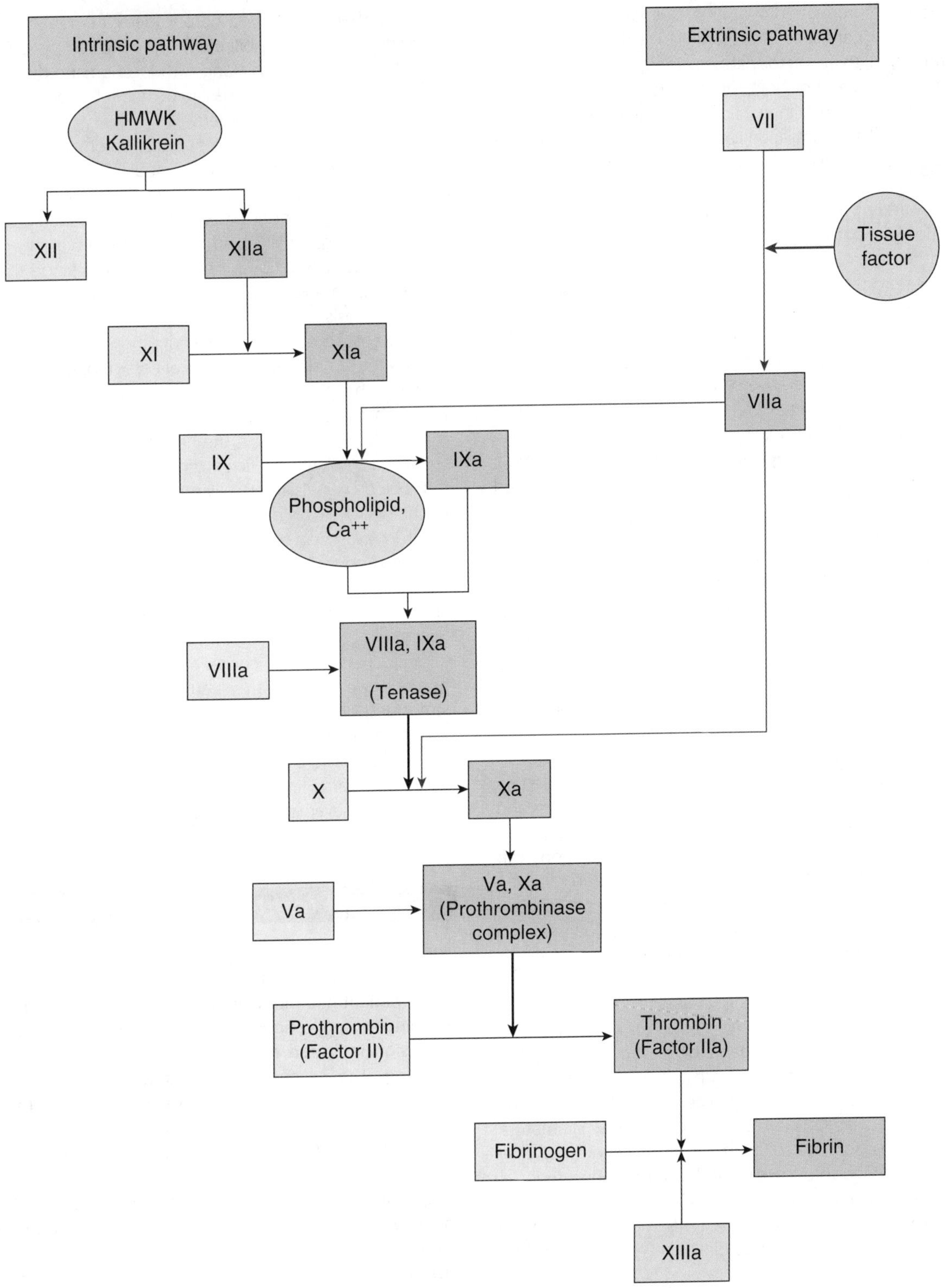

Figure 76-1 *Simplified Coagulation Cascade.*

mechanisms. Platelets adhere to exposed collagen and to exposed collagen-bound von Willebrand factor. Collagen exposure also activates the platelet, inducing a change in the shape of the platelet to a more irregular form that enhances adhesion and interaction with other platelets. Activated platelets discharge fibrinogen, fibronectin, von Willebrand factor, platelet factor 4, factor V, and factor VIII, promoting adhesion and aggregation of other platelets. In addition, activated platelets secrete adenosine diphosphate, adenosine triphosphate, and serotonin that also increase platelet activation. Thrombin generated by the coagulation cascade also aggressively activates platelets.

Exposure of blood to tissue factor in the subendothelium initiates the coagulation cascade, as depicted in **Figure 76-1**. This complex interaction of enzymes and cofactors generates fibrin clot that stabilizes the platelet plug. Deficiencies of components in the clotting cascade lead to bleeding disorders of varying severity depending on the qualitative and quantitative defect. Platelet adherence, activation, and aggregation in combination with the explosive production of a fibrin clot via the coagulation cascade has the potential to induce excessive thrombus formation. Antithrombin, tissue factor pathway inhibitor, and activated protein C limit the extent of clot propagation.

Clotting requires complex interaction of the injured endothelium with platelets and the coagulation cascade. Defects or deficiencies in any of these steps may lead to excessive bleeding or bleeding risk.

The history and physical examination are critical components in the evaluation of a patient with a suspected bleeding disorder. It is important to determine if the patient has had significant bleeding in response to past hemostatic challenges such as dental extractions, surgery, trauma, or childbirth. Ask about each previous surgery in detail, seeking surgical reports of bleeding, need for transfusion, repeated operations, or potential anatomic contributors to operative or perioperative bleeding. Immediate bleeding suggests primary hemostatic defects (ie, platelet abnormalities or vascular endothelial abnormalities, such as blood vessel fragility in senile purpura or scurvy), whereas secondary hemostatic defects (ie, clotting factor abnormalities) typically cause delayed bleeding.

Patients with defects in secondary hemostasis may report a history of hemarthosis or other deep tissue bleeding. A history of mucosal bleeding usually indicates a defect in primary hemostasis. Examples of mucosal bleeding include epistaxis, oral bleeding, gastrointestinal or genitourinary bleeding (without a local cause such as malignancy), hemoptysis, and protracted menstrual bleeding. Inquiring specifically about transfusion requirements, interventions such as suturing or packing, and the need for hospitalization allows estimation of bleeding severity.

A history of bleeding since infancy or early childhood suggests an inherited disorder. Eliciting a family history of abnormal bleeding can be helpful when considering inherited bleeding disorders and coagulopathies. Lack of such a history, however, is not sufficiently sensitive to exclude a hereditary process. Genetic mutations can arise de novo. Variable penetrance may mask disease in relatives. Recessive genetic defects will not be clinically apparent in relatives with one functional copy of the gene. Further, sometimes congenital coagulopathy may be inapparent until a major hemostatic challenge.

Review of a patient's medication list should include assessment of prescribed, over-the-counter, and herbal remedies. Warfarin and heparin products cause iatrogenic defects in secondary hemostasis. Platelet dysfunction induced by aspirin, clopidogrel, or nonsteroidal anti-inflammatory drugs can cause bleeding in the setting of normal platelet counts and coagulation parameters. Other medications, such as sulfonamides and vancomycin, may contribute to bleeding through drug-induced thrombocytopenia. Quinine-containing beverages (such as tonic water) or medications can also cause thrombocytopenia. Herbal agents (particularly the "g" herbs such as ginseng, garlic, ginko) have been linked with bleeding.

Patients with irregular dietary habits, such as hospitalized patients, alcoholics, those with mental illness, and the elderly, are at higher risk for nutrition-related bleeding disorders. Vitamin K deficiency can lead to bleeding through coagulation factor deficiencies. Vitamin C deficiency may manifest as perifollicular hemorrhages due to impaired collagen synthesis leading to blood vessel fragility. Altered bowel flora due to recent antibiotic use is another cause of vitamin K deficiency in hospitalized patients.

Examination of the skin and mucous membranes are of central importance in the bedside approach to bleeding disorders. Purpura is caused by the extravasation of blood through the vessel walls into subcutaneous or intracutaneous tissues, resulting in nonblanching skin lesions. Over time, these lesions evolve in color from red (hemoglobin) to purple (deoxyhemoglobin) to green (biliverdin) to orange (bilirubin). Purpuric lesions are classified according to size, which along with location and the presence or absence of preceding trauma can be helpful in identifying platelet disorders and clotting disorders.

Petechiae are nonpalpable purpuric lesions less than 3 mm in diameter. Petechiae should be distinguished from telangiectasias, which are blanchable. Petechiae are most commonly found in gravitationally dependent areas, so attention should be directed to the lower legs, ankles, and feet. Petechiae typically result from platelet deficiency or dysfunction, but can also be the result of increased intravascular pressure, inflammation of capillary beds, or venous stasis.

Ecchymoses are non-palpable purpuric lesions larger than 3 mm in diameter. The size and location of ecchymoses are helpful in determining the type of bleeding disorder causing them. Small, superficial ecchymoses are most commonly due to blood vessel fragility or multiple blood draws in the hospitalized patient, but may also be caused by platelet deficiency or dysfunction. Ecchymoses from fragile blood vessels are usually round or oval with smooth borders and no necrosis. This differs from the ecchymoses seen in disseminated intravascular coagulation (DIC), which often show central necrosis surrounded by stellate ecchymoses.

Lesions larger than 2 cm or evidence of deep tissue bleeding (eg, hematomas or hemarthroses) indicate a defect in secondary hemostasis. Large, spontaneous, and centrally-located ecchymoses or hematomas are more concerning for underlying pathology than the peripheral bruising after trauma seen in patients with normal hemostasis.

Mucosal bleeding is generally due to platelet deficiency or dysfunction. Epistaxis, conjunctival bleeding, or gingival bleeding may be seen on exam. Hemorrhagic mucosal bullae ("wet purpura") typically indicate severe platelet deficiency or dysfunction, and a higher risk for spontaneous intracranial bleeding.

CASE 76-1 *(continued)*

Does the patient have a coagulopathy or a platelet disorder based on history and examination?

The patient had multiple previous surgeries without apparent bleeding complications. The operative reports during this admission indicated no difficulties with hemostasis or diffuse bleeding. The secondary examination reveals no petechiae, purpura, or ecchymoses besides that noted around the left thigh wound site.

It is likely that if this patient has a bleeding diathesis, it is acquired and fairly recently acquired, given her uncomplicated surgical history. Delayed bleeding is consistent with a defect in secondary hemostasis. Her current medications included enoxaparin after surgery that may have contributed to bleeding. She has been eating poorly during the hospital stay and would be at risk for nutritional deficiencies. Antibiotics may be contributing to vitamin K deficiency.

PRACTICE POINT

- Secondary History and Examination: Aspirin or anti-platelet agents are the most common cause of petechiae in hospitalized patients.
- Bleeding from a wound that begins several days after the initial procedure suggests nutritional deficiency or medication-induced coagulopathy.

TABLE 76-2 Clinical Clues to Coagulation Defects

	Primary Hemostasis Defect	Secondary Hemostasis Defect
Etiology	Platelet deficiency or dysfunction Vascular endothelial abnormalities	Coagulation factor abnormalities
Timing of bleeding post trauma or surgery	Immediate	Delayed
Characteristic bleeding sites	Mucosal	Deep tissue or hemarthosis
Physical examination findings	Petechiae Epistaxis	Large, central, spontaneous ecchymosis Hemarthrosis

LABORATORY TESTING FOR BLEEDING DISORDERS

The most useful initial laboratory assessments for coagulation defects include the prothrombin time (PT) that is now most commonly reported as the International Normalized Ratio (INR), the activated partial thromboplastin time (aPTT), and the platelet count. These studies should be obtained in addition to the history and physical examination in an attempt to determine the presence of coagulopathy and to begin to define the specific cause of the defect.

CLOTTING ABNORMALITIES

Table 76-2 summarizes the common causes of elevated INR and/or prolonged aPTT. Prior to considering specific causes of abnormal INR or aPTT, the clinician should consider possible artifactual causes for these abnormalities. The aPTT and/or INR may be prolonged by incorrect collection of the blood specimen. Collection problems include an inadequate amount of blood in the specimen tube which results in elevated aPTT and INR. Additionally, obtaining the sample above or from a line that has been flushed with heparin can prolong not only the aPTT but also sometimes the INR. When artifactual elevation is suspected, the assays should be repeated on a specimen obtained by careful peripheral venipuncture. The measured aPTT may be artifactually prolonged in patients with polycythemia (hematocrit > 55), lipemia, icteric specimens, or hemolyzed specimens. In these situations, the clinical laboratory can be helpful in determining the appropriate approach.

To efficiently assess the etiology of an elevated INR or aPTT, the next step after exclusion of artifactual abnormality is to carefully review medications for the presence of anticoagulants (vitamin K antagonists including warfarin, heparins, or direct thrombin inhibitors). Systemic diseases that might prolong clotting time should be considered on the basis of the history and examination. For unexplained elevated INR or prolonged aPTT, a mixing study with normal plasma may help differentiate between a factor deficiency and the presence of an inhibitor. If the aPTT corrects in a mixing study, then specific assays for factors in the intrinsic pathway (Figure 76-1) are indicated. Correction of a prolonged prothrombin time in the mixing study implies deficiency of prothrombin, fibrinogen, or factors V, VII, or X. For a hospitalized patient with an elevated INR due to factor deficiencies, the most common causes are warfarin or vitamin K deficiency due to antibiotics and poor nutritional intake.

If the mixing study shows a persistent prolongation of aPTT, this implies the presence of an inhibitor of the aPTT assay system. These inhibitors include unfractionated heparin, direct thrombin inhibitors (lepirudin, argatroban), lupus anticoagulant, or specific factor inhibitors including inhibitors of factor VIII or factor V. Additional studies that allow the laboratory to determine the presence of heparin or a direct thrombin inhibitor include the thrombin time (TT) and reptilase time. Either class of drugs will prolong the TT, but demonstrate a normal reptilase time.

Persistent prolongation of the prothrombin time despite mixing with normal serum implies an inhibitor of the PT and generally is associated with prolongation and inhibition of the aPTT. These inhibitors include factor V inhibitors, direct thrombin inhibitors, excess heparin in the laboratory specimen, or, less commonly, a lupus anticoagulant.

If the examination demonstrates petechiae or there is significant mucosal bleeding, a quantitative or qualitative abnormality of platelets should be considered. There are many potential causes of thrombocytopenia in hospitalized patients. **Table 76-3** provides a framework for considering a low platelet count. Assessment of platelet function is more difficult, although the medication history is often revealing as the most common causes of petechiae or platelet dysfunction among hospitalized patients are antiplatelet medications.

The bleeding time has traditionally been used as an initial screening test for primary hemostasis, but recent guidelines argue against its use. The test requires a small incision of the skin followed be measurement of time to clot formation. Technical variables including direction of the incision, exercise, cuff pressure on the tested arm, previous testing, patient anxiety, local edema, and excessive wiping of the incision make reproducibility of the test challenging. Numerous medications (including aspirin, nonsteroidal anti-inflammatories, antibiotics, calcium channel blockers) and clinical conditions (including von Willebrand disease, uremia, liver disorders, paraproteinemias, chronic myeloproliferative disorders) may cause prolongation of the bleeding time (**Table 76-4**). A prolonged bleeding time, even assuming technical reliability, is a very nonspecific finding. Additionally, normal bleeding times do not assure hemostasis with invasive procedures, while prolonged bleeding times are not necessarily associated with excessive hemorrhage. A 1998 position statement from the College of American Pathologists and the American Society of Clinical Pathologists concluded that the bleeding time test failed as a screening test. Many hospital laboratories no longer offer the bleeding time test. Automated platelet function testing may provide better insight when patients are suspected to have defects in primary hemostasis, but have normal PT, PTT, and platelet count. The Platelet Function Analyzer (PFA-100) has been adopted by many laboratories and has received considerable attention in the literature. This test stimulates platelets through interaction with a membrane coated with collagen and either adenosine diphosphate or epinephrine and then measures the time required for the platelets to close an aperture of the membrane. This is thought to simulate the adhesion and aggregation of platelets in vivo. A systematic review found that the sensitivity of the PFA-100 system is 82% to 89%, while the specificity is 67% to 86% for detection of a defect in primary hemostasis as determined by more comprehensive platelet function testing. For patients who are highly suspected of having a disorder of platelet function, a negative PFA-100 test would not absolutely exclude a functional problem. In these cases, consultation with a hematologist and with the clinical laboratory is advisable.

CASE 76-1 *(continued)*

What explains an elevated INR; an elevated PTT; a low platelet count?

Both the INR and the aPTT are elevated. These elevations should be confirmed with a second laboratory draw. Assuming

TABLE 76-3 Causes of Abnormal INR or aPTT

Test Result		Causes	
INR	aPTT	Inherited	Acquired
Elevated	Normal	Factor VII deficiency	Warfarin or other coumarins (such as rat poison) Liver disease Vitamin K deficiency Acquired factor VII deficiency Inhibitor of factor VII
Normal	Prolonged	Deficiency of factors VIII, IX, or XI Deficiency of factor XII, prekallikrein, or high-molecular-weight kininogen (HMWK) (associated with abnormal labs but not bleeding) von Willebrand disease	Heparin Low-molecular-weight heparin (particularly when dosed excessively) Inhibitor of factors VIII, IX, XI, or XII Acquired von Willebrand disease Lupus anticoagulant
Elevated	Prolonged	Deficiency of prothrombin, fibrinogen, or factors V or X Dysfibrinogenemia Combined factor deficiencies	Liver disease Disseminated intravascular coagulation Heparin Supratherapeutic warfarin, or other coumarins (including rat poison) Vitamin K deficiency Combined warfarin and heparin Inhibitor of prothrombin, fibrinogen, or factors V or X Direct thrombin inhibitors Primary amyloidosis (factor X deficiency)

that the elevations are correct, this implies a defect in both the intrinsic or extrinsic coagulation pathways or in the common pathway (factor X, factor V, prothrombin, fibrinogen). The next diagnostic test would be a mixing study. Correction of the INR and aPTT in the mixing study would imply a deficiency of a factor or factors as outlined in Table 76-2. The available history allows a hypothesis for this patient that should lead directly to a therapeutic intervention. Given the patient's limited nutrition, exposure to broad spectrum antibiotics, and absence of findings to suggest liver disease, the most likely cause of her coagulopathy is vitamin K deficiency.

Additionally, enoxaparin elevates the aPTT; however, this anticoagulant was discontinued 24 hours before the consultation, making it unlikely to be a cause a persistent aPTT elevation.

Although this patient did not receive massive blood transfusion, patients who receive large volume RBC transfusions may develop low levels of remaining clotting proteins even if they receive concurrent FFP along with their RBC transfusions at the time of surgery. Each unit (250 ml) of packed RBCs transfused results in approximately a 5% decrease in the concentration of clotting proteins, and the half life of FFP is hours in contrast to RBCs which are in the order of weeks. For malnourished surgical patients who received significant transfusions, they may not make sufficent innate clotting factors quickly enough to make up for the recent blood loss.

The patient's platelet count is normal, excluding a quantitative platelet problem, although platelet dysfunction could still be considered. The absence of petechiae, the delayed nature of

TABLE 76-4 Causes of Thrombocytopenia

Decreased Platelet Production		Increased Platelet Destruction	
Marrow processes	Other processes affecting production	Immune-mediated processes	Consumptive processes
Myeloproliferative disorders Aplastic anemia Radiation	Drugs B12 or folate deficiency Infections (such as HIV or parvovirus) Cirrhosis (decreased thrombopoietin)	Immune Thrombocytopenia purpura Drugs (eg, heparin) Infections Post-transfusion	Thrombotic thrombocytopenia purpura Hemolytic uremic syndrome Sepsis Eclampsia/HELLP syndrome Disseminated intravascular coagulation Hypersplenism

TABLE 76-5 Management of Coagulopathy in the Bleeding Patient

Defect	Treatment	Suggested Initial Dose	Expected Response	Potential Complications
Primary Hemostasis				
Thrombocytopenia or platelet dysfunction (ie, NSAID use)	Platelet transfusion	6 pack (4–6 whole blood derived units pooled) or 1 apheresis unit	30–60,000/uL increase in platelet count; less response in hypersplenic patients	Infection Hemolytic transfusion reaction Transfusion-related acute lung injury (TRALI)
Secondary Hemostasis				
Elevated PTT with unknown factor deficiency	Fresh frozen plasma	10–15 mL/kg	Not well defined	Infection Hemolytic transfusion reaction TRALI Volume overload
Vitamin K deficiency (ie, nutritional deficiency or warfarin use)	Vitamin K*	10 mg IV	INR improvement within 4–6 hr	Anaphylaxis
	Fresh frozen plasma	10–15 mL/kg	Not well defined	Overcorrection and warfarin resistance
	Prothrombin complex concentrate	Dosage varies dependent on manufacturer	Emergent reversal of vitamin K antagonists	Potential risk of venous and arterial thrombosis

*For serious bleeding, administer fresh frozen plasma concurrently for immediate replacement of vitamin K–dependent coagulation factors.

the bleeding, and the absence of medications that would likely affect platelet function are reassuring. There is no clinical indication to assess platelet function in this patient.

PRACTICE POINT

- Laboratory Evaluation: If the INR and/or aPTT are unexpectedly elevated, the studies should be repeated to exclude artifact.
- Mixing studies are a key step in determining whether the apparent defect is a deficiency or an inhibitor of factor(s) in the coagulation pathway.
- Bleeding time is no longer used to assess platelet function.

TREATMENT OF COAGULOPATHY IN THE BLEEDING PATIENT

The bleeding patient should be assessed for concomitant acute or chronic defects in either primary or secondary hemostasis so that appropriate corrective treatment can be administered alongside hemodynamic support and transfusion of red blood cells in anticipation of any necessary structural interventions. **Table 76-5** summarizes treatment options to address hemostasis defects in bleeding patients.

It is useful to assess the degree of bleeding using the WHO bleeding grades when deciding interventions for coagulopathies. The grades are as follows: Grade 0 = no bleeding; Grade 1 = petechiae, ecchymosis, mucosal bleeding; Grade 2 = gross bleeding, including melena, hematemesis, hematuria, or hemoptysis; Grade 3 = bleeding that requires red blood cell transfusion; and Grade 4 = retinal bleeding with visual impairment, intracranial bleeds, and life-threatening bleeds (massive gastrointestinal hemorrhage, retroperitoneal hemorrhage, massive hemoptysis). For hemorrhage that is considered WHO Grade 2 or greater, platelet transfusions are indicated if thrombocytopenia is present although the specific threshold for transfusion should be individualized. In general, target for the platelet count after transfusion should be greater than 50,000. Transfusion of platelets for patients with suspected platelet dysfunction is reasonable in the setting of substantial bleeding, although there are no readily available laboratory parameters to guide management.

Fresh frozen plasma (FFP) contains plasma proteins including coagulation factors. It is indicated for bleeding patients with vitamin K deficiency or warfarin therapy, liver disease, acute DIC with a treatable trigger, massive transfusion, and acquired deficiencies of single coagulation factors. Laboratory parameters that would prompt use of FFP in any of these conditions include significantly increased prothrombin time, INR, or aPTT, although massive red blood cell transfusion of greater than one blood volume should prompt use of FFP even if coagulation parameters are unknown. FFP carries a substantial risk of transfusion-related acute lung injury (TRALI) and a number of studies caution about its overuse, particularly for patients with minimally elevated INR (up to 1.7) or aPTT.

CASE 76-1 *(continued)*

How is coagulopathy managed in the bleeding patient?

The options for management of the coagulopathy for this patient include vitamin K or fresh frozen plasma. She appears to be hemodynamically stable at this point which would argue against immediate use of FFP given the risk of TRALI. Oral vitamin K is the preferred route of administration for most patients with mildly elevated INR in the absence of life-threatening hemorrhage.

PRACTICE POINT

- Correction of Coagulopathy: Patients with severe bleeding and suspected platelet dysfunction (eg, from antiplatelet agents) should be considered for platelet transfusion despite normal platelet counts.
- FFP and platelet transfusions are associated with a higher risk of transfusion-related acute lung injury than red blood cell transfusions.

INVASIVE PROCEDURES IN THE COAGULOPATHIC PATIENT

Hospitalized patients are frequently subjected to invasive procedures for both diagnostic and therapeutic purposes, and hospitalists frequently consult on patients prior to surgical procedures. The potential for bleeding complications plays a central role in the discussion of risks and benefits of proposed procedures, and despite a lack of high-quality evidence to support indiscriminant preprocedural coagulation testing, it is common practice for patients to have coagulation testing in anticipation of most procedures. However, identifying patients at high risk for bleeding requires a clinical history, and should not rely on laboratory testing alone. PT and PTT tests may be insensitive to rare but clinically important bleeding disorders. For example, patients with factor XIII deficiency (who usually have a positive bleeding history) may have normal PT and PTT tests, but experience life threatening surgical bleeding. Current recommendations from the British Committee for Standards in Hematology are to obtain a bleeding history in all patients undergoing invasive procedures or surgery, including bleeding following prior trauma or surgery, a family history of bleeding, and the use of prescription and non-prescription medications that predispose to bleeding.

Selected patients should undergo coagulation testing. Patients who may benefit from coagulation testing include those with a positive bleeding history, evidence of systemic disease that may affect coagulation (eg, liver disease), or risk factors for malabsorption or malnutrition. Patients planned for procedures associated with a higher risk of morbidity and mortality from bleeding complications (eg, intracranial, neurosurgical) typically have preoperative coagulation testing.

Patients with abnormal bleeding histories or other clinical indications warrant directed diagnostic testing guided by their clinical features, and may require hematology consultation to help guide further work-up and the plan for correction prior to undergoing procedures.

If diagnostic testing reveals prolongation of the PT, options for correction will be dictated by the underlying etiology. Those with nutritional deficiencies typically respond to administration of vitamin K. While oral administration of vitamin K is slower to take effect, there is less risk of anaphylaxis which has been associated with intravenous administration of vitamin K. Subcutaneous vitamin K works more slowly than oral vitamin K, and in one meta-analysis was similar to placebo in treating excessive anticoagulation.

Although widely practiced, the prophylactic use of FFP for patients with prolonged PT undergoing procedures lacks sufficient evidence to support or refute its efficacy and the potential hazards of transfusion are well documented. In patients with minimally prolonged PT, transfusion of FFP may have little effect on the PT, and the effects may be transient if the patient is not provided with substrate (vitamin K) to generate more clotting factors. Many inpatient procedures are performed by specialists and interventional radiologists, and the preference and comfort of the operator will largely drive the pre-procedural testing and transfusion practice.

CASE 76-1 *(continued)*

If a coagulopathy is present, what should be done to prepare a patient for an invasive procedure?

If the patient required an invasive procedure, for example re-exploration of the left hip, the clinical assessment is similar to that for management of active bleeding. The platelet count is adequate and there are no historical concerns for platelet dysfunction. The INR of 1.9 is above a level of 1.5 at which most interventions could safely take place. If the procedure is urgent, FFP should be considered, realizing that it may require multiple units to normalize the INR. Although there is no randomized controlled trial evidence to support a reduction in bleeding risk through use of FFP in this situation, clinical reason suggests that there may be a benefit. This is a reasonable approach until there is better evidence on which to base this decision.

PRACTICE POINT

- Preprocedure Evaluation for Coagulopathy: Obtaining a bleeding history from a patient may help uncover coagulopathies not evident on routine testing.
- Oral vitamin K is the preferred treatment of nutrition related coagulopathy in patients planned for nonemergent procedures.

CONCLUSION

The approach to a bleeding patient starts with emergent resuscitation if required, identification of the bleeding site, evaluation for the presence of a coagulopathy (initially PT, INR, aPTT, and platelet count), and management of bleeding which may require specialty consultation. A stepwise approach begins with a focused history and physical examination. The cause of a surgical patient's elevated INR and bleeding are most likely due to a number of factors: 1) poor nutrition causing relative Vitamin K deficiency, 2) exposure to broad spectrum antibiotics, 3) exposure to anticoagulants, and/or 4) in cases of major trauma requiring recent large volume RBC transfusion, low levels of remaining clotting proteins. Other considerations for an elevated INR in the absence of warfarin include: severe liver disease (history of alcohol use, abnormal liver function tests, clinical signs of cirrhosis, preoperative elevation of INR), acquired Factor VIII inhibitors or Factor VIII deficiency, von Willebrand disease causing some degree of Factor VIII deficiency, DIC or significant renal or hepatic insufficiency resulting in supratherapeutic doses of low molecular weight heparin.

Evaluation of thrombocytopenia should include review of the peripheral smear. The timing of onset of thrombocytopenia is a valuable clue regarding its possible etiologies. In general, patients with low platelet counts or documented platelet function abnormalities who are bleeding are likely to benefit from platelet transfusions. However, unlike correction of anemia, not all causes of thrombocytopenia may be safely treated with the transfusion of platelet products. Conditions associated with immune destruction of platelets (such as immune thrombocytopenia or heparin induced thrombocytopenia) or microangiopathic hemolysis (thrombotic thrombocytopenic purpura) can be dangerously aggravated by platelet transfusions. See chapters 75 and 176.

SUGGESTED READINGS

Chee YL, Crawford JC, Watson HG, Greaves M. Guidelines on the assessment of bleeding risk prior to surgery or invasive procedures. British Committee for Standards in Haematology. *Br J Haematol.* 2008;140(5):496–504.

Eckman MH, Erban JK, Singh SK, Kao GS. Screening for the risk for bleeding or thrombosis. *Ann Intern Med.* 2003;138(3):W15–W24.

Kamal AH, Tefferi A, Pruthi RK. How to interpret and pursue an abnormal prothrombin time, activated partial thromboplastin time, and bleeding time in adults. *Mayo Clin Proc.* 2007;82(7):864–873.

Maltz GS, Siegel JE, Carson JL. Hematologic management of gastrointestinal bleeding. *Gastroenterol Clin North Am.* 2000;29(1):169–187, vii.

Rossaint R, Bouillon B, Cerny V, et al. Management of bleeding following major trauma: an updated European guideline. *Crit Care.* 2010;14(2):R52.

Rossaint R, Duranteau J, Stahel PF, Spahn DR. Nonsurgical treatment of major bleeding. *Anesthesiol Clin.* 2007;25(1):35–48, viii.

Slichter SJ. Platelet transfusion therapy. *Hematol Oncol Clin North Am.* 2007;21(4):697–729, vii.

Tanaka KA, Key NS, Levy JH. Blood coagulation: hemostasis and thrombin regulation. *Anesth Analg.* 2009;108(5):1433–1446.

Triplett DA. Coagulation and bleeding disorders: review and update. *Clin Chem.* 2000;46(8 Pt 2):1260–1269.

CHAPTER 77

Chest Pain

Mary C. Westergaard, MD
Arjun S. Chanmugam, MD, MBA

Key Clinical Questions

1. What signs and symptoms point to a serious cause of chest pain?
2. What key historical elements will help to narrow the differential diagnosis?
3. What studies should be ordered?

INTRODUCTION

According to the 2006 National Hospital Ambulatory Medical Care Survey, 6,392,000 patients presented to emergency departments with a chief complaint of chest pain or related symptoms. Of those, 1,976,000 patients were admitted to the hospital, with a mean length of stay of 3.7 days. Chest pain was the principal admitting diagnosis in 5.4% of all admitted patients.

Because the morbidity and mortality is high if clinicians "miss" a cardiac presentation of chest pain, a significant portion of these admissions are specifically for the purpose of ruling out myocardial infarction. In one study of patients presenting to an emergency department with complaints consistent with cardiac ischemia, 17% ultimately had cardiac ischemia, while 27% had stable angina or other cardiac conditions. Fifty-five percent had noncardiac conditions causing their symptoms. The wide differential diagnosis for this heterogeneous group of patients includes nonischemic life-threatening etiologies as well as more benign causes. Unfortunately, in this study, 2.1% of the patients with acute myocardial infarction were erroneously discharged; this figure plays prominently in the low threshold to admit patients with chest pain.

Chest pain also occurs in patients already admitted to the hospital for other reasons. These patients have already suffered some degree of physical decompensation and the occurrence of chest pain may indicate illness, a complication of hospitalization, or a patient's response to a very stressful situation. The hospitalist must evaluate the possibility of an immediate life-threatening event, consider the entire differential of possible etiologies, and integrate this information with the patient's prior clinical diagnoses and course.

BEDSIDE APPROACH

RAPID ASSESSMENT

The initial evaluation of a patient reporting chest pain requires the rapid identification and treatment of any life-threatening conditions. These include the five "do-not-miss" causes of chest pain: (1) aortic dissection, (2) acute myocardial infarction, (3) pulmonary embolism, (4) pneumothorax, and (5) esophageal rupture (**Table 77-1**). The electrocardiogram (ECG) is the most important screening intervention for early risk stratification and is often performed at the point of triage as one of the "vital signs."

All potentially unstable patients with chest pain should have an intravenous line, supplemental oxygen, and a cardiac monitor placed as soon as possible. This can be accomplished even before the arrival of the physician at the patient's bedside. The ECG, chest pain characteristics, prior history of coronary artery disease (CAD), and age are independent predictors of acute MI. Although the traditional risk factors for CAD predict long-term risk of disease, they are less helpful in predicting acute MI, and a primary focus on risk factors could be misleading for patients with ACS but with few risk factors. Therefore, an initial risk stratification assessment should include a review of the ECG, analysis of current vital signs, and a targeted history and physical examination. A stat portable chest radiograph should be ordered. With this information, patients can be assigned to one of four classes:

1. Those with new ST-segment elevations on initial ECG. (These patients should receive immediate consideration for emergent reperfusion therapy.)
2. Those without ST-segment elevation on initial ECG but who are at high risk on the basis of ECG findings, hemodynamic

TABLE 77-1 Life-Threatening Causes of Chest Pain

Diagnosis	Risk Factors	Characteristic Findings	Diagnostic Testing
Aortic Dissection	Hypertension, connective tissue disease, vasculitis, prior heart or valvular surgery, Turner syndrome, crack cocaine use, cardiac catheterization	New diastolic murmur, upper-extremity pulse deficit, neurologic complications of stroke	Computed tomography, magnetic resonance imaging, transesophageal echocardiography, angiography
Special considerations: Aortic dissection can be difficult to diagnose, but patients will most commonly present with chest pain; syncope may occur at the time of symptom onset. Dissections can be classified as Stanford type A (involving the ascending aorta) or type B (all others). In one study, 72.7% of patients reported chest pain, 90.6% reported severe or worst pain ever, and 84.8% had abrupt onset. Aortic insufficiency murmur was noted in 31.6% and pulse deficit was noted in 15.1 %. Chest radiograph showed widened mediastinum in 61.6%, and ECGs were less helpful, being normal in 31.3%.* Medical treatment is initially indicated for type B dissections with careful blood pressure control (beta-blockade and nitroprusside). Given the high risk for life-threatening complications such as tamponade, aortic regurgitation, and myocardial infarction, type A dissections are treated as surgical emergencies.			
Myocardial Infarction	Male sex, age over 55, tobacco use, family history of coronary artery disease, diabetes, hypercholesterolemia, hypertension	S_4 or S_3 gallop, vomiting, diaphoresis, Levine sign (fist over center chest, low predictive value)	Electrocardiography, cardiac biomarkers
Special considerations: The diagnosis of ST-segment elevation myocardial infarction should be readily made from a 12-lead ECG and requires urgent intervention to improve survival. These patients will benefit from standard medical therapy as well as reperfusion. According to the 2007 ACC/AHA focused update on the management of patients with ST-elevation myocardial infarction, patients with acute STEMI will benefit from primary percutaneous intervention with a goal door-to-balloon time of 90 minutes or less. Fibrinolytic therapy within 30 minutes is preferred if transfer to a PCI-capable facility will make door-to-balloon time greater than 90 minutes.† These guidelines are directed toward patients presenting to the hospital with STEMI, but may also help to decide when to transfer inpatients who develop STEMI.			
Pulmonary Embolism	Immobilization, recent surgery, stroke, paralysis, prior venous thromboembolism, malignancy, recent central venous instrumentation	Dyspnea, pleuritic pain, calf or leg pain or swelling, jugular venous distention	Computed tomography, ventilation-perfusion scan, pulmonary angiography
Special considerations: Thrombolytic therapy for submassive pulmonary embolism (PE) is a controversial treatment modality. It has been advocated for patients with evidence of right ventricular dilation or hypokinesis on echocardiography, but this indication for use is generally not widely accepted. Thrombolysis for cardiac arrest from PE has been successful in case reports, but does not seem to be helpful in cases of pulseless electrical activity.§ Thrombolytic regimens for PE range from 2–24 hour infusions. For imminent or actual cardiac arrest, a bolus therapy is indicated. One such regimen is tPA, 0.6 mg/kg over 2 minutes.			
Pneumothorax	*Pneumocystis jirovecii*, tuberculosis, chronic obstructive pulmonary disease, Marfans, familial, mechanical ventilation, smoking, cystic fibrosis	Decreased breath sounds, hyperresonant percussion, distended neck veins, tracheal deviation	Chest radiography, computed tomography
Special considerations: Of all emergency diagnoses, the only one that is immediately reversible is a tension pneumothorax. Needle decompression involves placing a 14-gauge angiocath in the second or third intercostal space in the midclavicular line. In a study of trauma patients with computed tomography scans of the chest, the mean chest wall thickness studied averaged 4.24 cm at this location, and almost a quarter of patients had chest walls thicker than 5 cm.¶ Therefore, one should use the longest catheter possible. Alternatives include using a spinal needle or rapid tube thoracostomy.			
Esophageal Rupture	Esophageal instrumentation, forceful emesis, ulcers or esophagitis	"Hammans sign" (mediastinal crunching sound), subcutaneous emphysema, odynophagia, hoarseness (cervical rupture)	Cervical and chest radiography, computed tomography, contrast esophagography
Special considerations: More than half of all cases of esophageal rupture occur as a complication of medical procedures that involve instrumentation of the esophagus, so knowledge of the inpatient course is paramount.** Spontaneous ruptures classically occur after forceful vomiting, but may also be associated with ingestion of caustic substances or pills, eosinophilic esophagitis, Barretts esophagitis, or ulcers.			

*Hagan PG, Nienaber CA, Isselbacher EM, et al. The International Registry of Acute Aortic Dissection (IRAD): new insights into an old disease. *JAMA.* 2000;283:897.

†Antman EM, Hand M, Armstrong PW, et al. 2007 focused update of the ACC/AHA 2004 Guidelines for the Management of Patients With ST-Elevation Myocardial Infarction: a report of the American College of Cardiology/American Heart Association Task Force on Practice Guidelines (Writing Group to Review New Evidence and Update the ACC/AHA 2004 Guidelines for the Management of Patients With ST-Elevation Myocardial Infarction). *J Am Coll Cardiol.* 2008;51:210–247.

§Abu-Laban RB, Christenson JM, Innes GD, et al. Tissue plasminogen activator in cardiac arrest with pulseless electrical activity. *N Engl J Med.* 2002;346:1522.

¶Givens ML, Ayotte K, Manifold C. Needle thoracostomy: implications of computed tomography chest wall thickness. *Academic Emergency Medicine.* 2004;11(2):211–213.

**Pasricha P, Fleischer D, Kalloo A. Endoscopic perforation of the upper digestive tract: A review of their pathogenesis, prevention and management. *Gastroenterology.* 1994;106:787.

TABLE 77-2 Differential Diagnosis of Chest Pain

Cardiac	Pulmonary	Other
Aortic dissection	Pneumothorax	Esophageal rupture
Myocardial infarction	Pulmonary embolism	Mallory-Weiss tear
Angina	Pleuritis/serositis	Esophageal spasm
Coronary spasm	Pneumonia	Pancreatitis
Pericarditis	Cancer	Biliary tract disease
Myocarditis	Sarcoidosis	Costochondritis
Valvular disease		Musculoskeletal injury
Stress-induced cardiomyopathy		Peptic ulcer disease
		Gastritis/esophagitis/reflux
		Herpes zoster
		Mediastinitis
		Psychogenic/psychosomatic

instability, or history. (These patients should be admitted and consideration should be given for immediate antiplatelet and antithrombotic treatment if no contraindications.)

3. Those who have no objective evidence of ACS but have symptoms that warrant evaluation. (These patients form the "low risk" chest pain cohort that constitutes the majority of patients undergoing ED evaluation for chest pain.)
4. Those who have an obvious noncardiac cause for symptoms.

Patients with hemodynamic instability, persistent ECG changes, or ongoing symptoms should be evaluated for emergent coronary angiography. Patients with an obvious noncardiac cause for symptoms would be managed, depending on the alternative diagnosis.

HISTORY

The history remains critically important in initial risk stratification because objective evidence including a diagnostic ECG is only present in a minority of patients. Once emergency conditions have been ruled out or stabilized, a targeted history should be used to identify and prioritize a list of differential possibilities (**Table 77-2**). The examiner needs to determine what portions of the history and physical examination are relevant to the clinical questions of whether the patient's symptoms and signs point to cardiac disease or to other serious causes requiring immediate intervention and, if the evaluation is taking place in the emergency department, whether the patient requires admission to the hospital. Coronary artery disease (CAD) is the leading cause of death for both men and women, and most patients with a prior history of CAD should be admitted to the hospital if they present with chest pain and have a clinical presentation that could be consistent for acute coronary syndrome. For this reason, in patients presenting with chest pain, obtaining a prior history of angina or known CAD is essential to determining if the patient's current symptoms suggest either an acute coronary syndrome (ACS) or unstable angina (USA).

More than 30 years ago, the Coronary Artery Surgery Study (CASS) enrolled 18,844 men and 6,097 women after coronary angiography. Using the reported chest pain characteristics, they classified patients as having definite angina, probable angina, probably not having angina, and definitely not having angina. Combining all patients classed as probably not and definitely not having angina as having nonischemic pain was subsequently shown to discriminate between patients with CAD and those with negative ETT and coronary angiograms. Even today, this scheme is used to facilitate decision making. Classic symptoms of angina include chest heaviness, pressure, tightness, or burning (sometimes with vigorous denial of pain), provocation by physical or emotional stress or cold, relief by rest, radiation to neck, jaw, or shoulder, duration >2 minutes and <20 minutes (unless MI), +/– dyspnea, nausea, and vomiting, diaphoresis, presyncope, and palpitations (**Table 77-3**).

Patients should be questioned regarding the nature of their "discomfort" (as some patients may not believe that they are experiencing chest pain). Additional questioning should include location, onset, character, severity, radiation, alleviating and exacerbating factors, time course, history of similar episodes, and associated symptoms such as diaphoresis, shortness of breath, and nausea and vomiting. Early questioning about prior experiences of identical symptoms may save considerable time and effort, but one must take care to avoid premature closure in diagnostic decision making, especially when myocardial ischemia is a possibility.

PAIN CHARACTERISTICS

The "PQRST" (provocative/palliative factors, quality, radiation, severity, timing) approach can be used to qualify the different aspects of the patient's pain and suggest likely etiologies. Physicians should be aware that differences in gender, culture, and underlying pathology may lead to differences in the experience and description of pain. Atypical presentations of ACS are more likely in the elderly and women, especially those over the age of 65, and include symptoms such as dyspnea, epigastric discomfort, and palpitations. In one study of patients with active cardiac ischemia, women reported pain in the neck area while men were more likely to feel pain in the shoulder. Women were more likely to describe their pain as sharp, hot, burning, throbbing, or pressing. In addition, women were more likely to experience various nonpain symptoms, such as trembling, upset stomach, shortness of breath, postprandial pain, palpitations, and neck or throat sensations. Despite anecdotal evidence, most studies have not found a significant increase in the prevalence of unrecognized or atypical presentations in diabetics.

TABLE 77-3 Prior Probability (%) of CAD According to Age, Gender, and Quality of Symptoms

Age, Year	Asymptomatic		Nonanginal CP		Atypical Angina		Typical Angina	
	Men	Women	Men	Women	Men	Women	Men	Women
30–39	1.9	0.3	5.2	0.8	21.9	4.3	69.7	25.8
40–49	5.5	1.0	14.1	2.8	46.1	13.3	87.3	55.2
50–59	9.7	3.2	21.5	8.4	58.9	32.4	92.0	79.4
60–69	12.3	7.5	28.1	18.6	67.1	54.4	94.3	90.6

Provocative and palliative factors

Pain associated with exertion (physical exercise, stress, or sexual intercourse) is often due to cardiac causes. Pain with swallowing suggests an esophageal disorder. Patients with pain that reliably occurs after eating likely have a gastrointestinal etiology; however, some patients with coronary disease have postprandial angina (typically after dinner) in addition to rest angina. One possible mechanism for postprandial angina involves increased myocardial oxygen demand after food intake, but studies suggest that a decrease in coronary blood flow (steal phenomenon) may play a role. In contrast, improvement with food or antacids suggests peptic ulcer disease or gastritis. Pleuritic pain is worst with deep inspiration and suggests pulmonary disease, pericarditis, or a musculoskeletal etiology. In one study, 47% of all patients who were evaluated for and ultimately found to have pulmonary embolism reported pleuritic pain. However, 17% of all patients found to have pulmonary embolism reported chest pain that was nonpleuritic.[3] Pain that is worse with exertion and better with rest is suggestive of cardiac ischemia or pulmonary embolism. More commonly pleuritic but sometimes severe, steady, and retrosternal, the pain of acute pericarditis is classically worst with lying flat and improved with leaning forward. Musculoskeletal pain will be reliably triggered by specific movements. An important consideration is that improvement with nitroglycerin or mucosal anesthesia ("GI cocktail") is not helpful for distinguishing cardiac from noncardiac causes of pain. Physicians should use these medicines as appropriate to relieve pain but avoid the error of using the patient's response to guide decision making. Likewise, pain with chest wall palpation should not be used to exclude a cardiac etiology for chest pain.

Quality

The patient's description of the quality of pain should be noted (**Table 77-4**). In the International Registry of Acute Aortic Dissection (IRAD) study, 50.6% of patients with aortic dissection described a ripping or tearing sensation. In contrast, the pain of myocardial ischemia is classically described as heavy, squeezing, crushing, or pressure. Sharp pain is most typical of pulmonary, musculoskeletal, or gastrointestinal causes; however, beware of the imprecision of the term *sharp*, which to some patients simply means *intense*. Burning pain can be seen in cardiac and gastrointestinal disease. Patients suffering from herpes zoster may also report a burning sensation. The nature of the chest pain does not definitely discriminate cardiac from noncardiac chest pain. Keep in mind that "atypical" descriptions of pain are quite common in patients with myocardial ischemia, including sharp, stabbing or, less commonly, pleuritic pain. For example, pain described as pressure-like or squeezing has a likelihood ratio (LR) of less than 2 and hence does not reliably distinguish cardiac disease from other causes of chest pain such as esophagitis. Likewise, a pleuritic, stabbing chest pain that has a LR of 0.2 – 0.3 may reduce the likelihood that the chest pain is cardiac in origin but it does not rule it out.

TABLE 77-4 Symptoms of Cardiac Chest Pain

Typical symptoms: pressure, tightness, squeezing, indigestion, or those similar to prior ACS events
Atypical symptoms: stabbing, pleuritic, pinprick discomfort
Associated symptoms with increased risk: nausea and vomiting
Associated symptoms not predictive of increased risk: symptoms relieved by rest or sublingual NTG

ACS, acute coronary syndrome; NTG, nitroglycerin.

Radiation

A description of pain radiation may be helpful. Patients suffering from cardiac ischemia will often describe radiation down the left arm or up into the neck or jaw. Interestingly, right arm radiation was also shown to have an increased predictive value for true myocardial ischemia in one study (radiation to the left arm LR 2.0; right arm LR 3.0; both arms LR 7.0). Aortic dissection should be suspected in patients complaining of pain radiating to the back, especially the interscapular area. This can also occur with posterior ulcers as well as with myocardial ischemia. Radiation to the trapezius ridge is a feature of pericarditis. Kehr's sign refers to pain felt at the tip of the scapula that is a referred symptom from diaphragmatic irritation due to intraabdominal pathology. Conditions causing this symptom are generally serious (ie, splenic rupture or acute cholecystitis), so a careful abdominal exam should be performed in all patients reporting shoulder pain without a clear thoracic etiology.

Severity

The severity of pain reported is dependent on each patient's pain tolerance. Very severe pain with signs of distress should bring to mind aortic dissection, acute myocardial infarction, acute pulmonary embolism, acute pericarditis, tension pneumothorax, or ruptured esophagus. Quantifying pain on a scale from 1 to 10 enables assessment of treatment response.

Timing

Pain from cardiac ischemia generally lasts minutes; myocardial infarction pain can last for hours. Pain lasting for seconds is not due to myocardial ischemia, and can be a helpful feature in narrowing the differential. Likewise, constant pain for days to weeks is very unlikely to be cardiac in nature. Myocardial infarction follows circadian rhythms and is more likely to occur in the morning. Pain that is maximal at sudden onset can be due to pneumothorax, pulmonary embolism, or aortic dissection. Patients with herpes zoster can have pain lasting for days before the rash appears.

ASSOCIATED SYMPTOMS

While taking the history, the physician should note associated symptoms volunteered by the patient, in addition to inquiring about the presence of others. Prominent dyspnea should raise concern for pulmonary or myocardial/pericardial etiology. Nausea and vomiting are associated with cardiac disease as well as gastrointestinal disease. Diaphoresis is also associated with cardiac disease but may simply be a marker of severe pain. Diaphoretic patients with chest pain should be assumed to have an emergency condition until proven otherwise. Belching or sour taste in the mouth often represents reflux, but nausea and belching may accompany cardiac ischemia, classically when the inferior myocardial wall is involved. Generalized fatigue with recent illness may indicate myocarditis or pericarditis. Severe emotional distress may trigger acute stress-induced or takotsubo cardiomyopathy, which can present with or without chest pain. Fever, night sweats, and weight loss should suggest cancer and possible complications. Syncope with chest pain could be due to ischemia-induced arrhythmia, severe aortic stenosis, aortic dissection, or massive pulmonary embolism. Stroke symptoms can occur in Type A aortic dissections when the carotid arteries are involved.

Risk factors

The presence or absence of risk factors for CAD does not change the likelihood of cardiac disease sufficiently to discriminate between those who might have the disease and those who do not require admission to the hospital. Although the presence of risk factors for CAD may change the prior probability of CAD and are useful in assessing the risk in populations, the absence of these risk factors alone does not sufficiently reduce the likelihood of

CAD in individual patients to allow discharge without considering other factors. The presence of chest pain as in this case and/or ECG changes remain predictive of cardiac ischemia in the acute setting, even in the absence of risk factors of CAD.

Male gender, age over 55 years, family history of CAD, known CAD, vascular disease (cerebrovascular, peripheral vascular disease), diabetes mellitus, hypercholesterolemia, hypertension, and tobacco use are recognized as risk factors for CAD. Cocaine is a risk factor for acute myocardial ischemia as well as atherosclerosis, and a history of recent cocaine use by a patient complaining of chest pain should prompt consideration of CAD work-up. As mentioned previously, the absence of these risk factors is not sufficient to exclude ACS. For example, in a 40-year-old patient with anginal chest pain the risk of CAD is roughly 6%; smoking increases this risk to 13%. However, physicians cannot afford to miss the 6% of patients who have significant CAD, so the absence of a smoking history or other risk factors should not remove consideration of ACS.

The symptoms and signs of chest pain in acute PE depend upon the size of embolism. Small to medium sized emboli may cause dyspnea, chest pain, cough, tachypnea, tachycardia, mild fever (<39 degrees), and wheezing in <5% of patients. Massive pulmonary emboli may cause syncope, chest pain, dyspnea, and signs of right ventricular (RV) dysfunction (RV heave, RV S_3, JVP, soft systolic murmur of tricuspid regurgitation). Because these symptoms are nonspecific for PE and are commonly associated with other potentially life-threatening causes of chest pain, risk factors for PE do help guide the clinical decision making process. A prior history of venous thromboembolism (VTE), known cancer, or known hypercoagulable states place the patient with dyspnea, pleuritic chest pain, apprehension, cough, diaphoresis, hemoptysis, or syncope into a high risk category. For patients that have never had a VTE, asking about risk factors can guide further testing and the decision to admit the patient to the hospital.

PRACTICE POINT

- The presence or absence of risk factors for coronary artery disease does not change the likelihood of cardiac disease sufficiently to differentiate between those who might have the disease and those who do not require admission to the hospital.

As most pulmonary emboli result from deep vein thrombosis, the risk factors are the same for both entities. Patients with pulmonary embolism will most often have at least one risk factor, and those who do not are often found later to have occult cancer or coagulation abnormalities. Common risk factors for deep vein thrombosis include immobilization (paresis, paralysis), institutionalization or hospitalization within the previous three months, recent surgery, central venous procedure, cancer, pregnancy, estrogen and progestin drugs, inherited thrombophilias, coagulation disorders, trauma, acute inflammatory diseases, acute infection, chronic obstructive pulmonary disease, certain renal diseases, and heart failure. A case-control study in Olmsted County, Minnesota, found the following risk factors most predictive for first-time VTE: hospital or nursing home residence, surgery, trauma, cancer, chemotherapy, neurologic disease with paresis, central venous catheter or pacemaker, varicose veins, and superficial vein thrombosis.

Results have been mixed in studies of smoking as a risk factor for pulmonary embolism. Obesity, heavy smoking, and hypertension were found to be risk factors for pulmonary embolism specifically in women in one study. Prolonged air travel increases risk, especially in flights lasting more than eight hours.

The most common risk factor for aortic dissection is systemic hypertension. Other recognized risk factors include history of connective tissue disease (such as Marfan syndrome or Elhers-Danlos syndrome), vasculitis, prior heart or valvular surgery, Turner syndrome, crack cocaine use, positive family history, and cardiac catheterization.

Risk factors for spontaneous pneumothorax include positive family history, chronic obstructive pulmonary disease, cystic fibrosis, Marfan syndrome, smoking, homocystinuria, and extrapelvic endometriosis. Occasionally, spontaneous pneumothorax occurs in otherwise healthy individuals, classically in tall young men. In addition, patients infected with the human immunodeficiency virus are at increased risk for pneumothorax resulting as a complication of *Pneumocystis jirovecii* or mycobacterial infection. Patients already hospitalized may develop pneumothorax as an iatrogenic complication of a procedure (thoracentesis or central line placement).

CASE 77-1

A 51-year-old male with newly diagnosed HIV has been admitted to the hospitalist service for treatment of presumed *Pneumocystis jiroveci* pneumonia. The diagnosis was made based upon classic radiographic and historical features, combined with a positive rapid HIV test done in the emergency department. After several hours on the floor, the patient alerted his nurse that he was experiencing chest pain with shortness of breath.

This case brings several differential possibilities to mind. As with any high-risk complaint, though, the bedside approach must begin with an assessment of the patient's overall stability. A quick look at the vital signs, monitor tracing (if available), and clinical appearance will alert the physician to the need for immediate action to stabilize the patient's condition. After this rapid assessment is complete, an organized approach should be employed to narrow the differential diagnosis and plan treatment. Specifically, one must decide which historical elements, diagnostic studies, and additional resources are necessary to diagnose and treat the patient successfully.

The physical examination

The physical examination is often normal in patients with chest pain, even when serious pathology is present. However, certain signs can be helpful for risk stratification and for determining symptom etiology. As mentioned above, overall appearance combined with vital signs including pulse oximetry should be noted early in the assessment. Tachycardia and hypotension are ominous signs in the patient with chest pain and may require intervention to prevent cardiovascular collapse. Tachypnea can be subtle; the clinician should measure this vital sign independently if suspicious despite a normal documented respiratory rate, as it is the most common sign of pulmonary embolism. New fever can direct the workup toward infectious etiologies but low-grade fever is a nonspecific finding and may also be associated with pulmonary embolism, myocardial infarction, pneumonia, and pericarditis. New hypoxia is a clue to either cardiac (pump failure with CHF) or serious pulmonary pathology. However, a normal oxygen saturation level or A-a gradient does not rule out PE. In one study of angiographically proven PE, 17% of patients had a pO_2 greater than 80 mm Hg and 5% had a pO_2 >100 mm Hg. The A-a gradient is no more accurate than the O_2 saturation and not all patients will be hypoxic or have tachypnea or tachycardia.

It is important to perform cardiac auscultation in a quiet room and ask the patient to lean forward. Using the diaphragm of the stethoscope, the examiner should listen for regurgitant murmurs and pericardial friction rubs. The finding of a new systolic mitral insufficiency murmur might indicate myocardial ischemia, a flail mitral leaflet, or decompensated heart failure and puts the patient in a high risk category. A new murmur of tricuspid insufficiency might signal right ventricular overload from PE. A diastolic murmur may reflect acute aortic insufficiency and aortic dissection. Any new murmur, especially in the presence of fever, may signify endocarditis. A pericardial friction rub classically occurs in three phases corresponding with atrial systole, ventricular systole, and ventricular diastole. However, it is uncommon to hear all three phases, and the rub may be transiently heard. The examiner is mostly likely to appreciate the friction rub by firmly placing the diaphragm of the stethoscope over the left lower sternal border with the patient leaning forward after an exhalation. The examiner should ask the patient to stop breathing for a few seconds to distinguish a pericardial from pleural rub. A pericardial friction rub does not always specify primary acute pericarditis. It may also be associated with a large transmural acute MI. A pleural rub may be present in patients with pulmonary embolism, effusion, pneumonia, or pleuritis. Hammon's sign (mediastinal crunch) is synchronous with the heartbeat and indicates mediastinal or pericardial air suggestive of ruptured esophagus, pneumothorax, or tracheobronchial tree injury. An S_3 or S_4 gallop could signal changes in ventricular compliance and function and an accentuated P_2 (second heart sound louder over the pulmonic area) is consistent with pulmonary hypertension.

Pulmonary examination may reveal unilateral absent or decreased breath sounds in patients with pneumothorax. Rales may indicate acute heart failure in the patient experiencing myocardial infarction, atelectasis (commonly seen with splinting from PE, trauma, or musculoskeletal pain), or pneumonia. Abdominal examination should focus on identifying potential abdominal causes of chest pain, such as biliary disease, pancreatitis, or trauma.

The musculoskeletal exam may reveal chest wall tenderness that exactly mimics the patient's symptoms. It is important to note that tenderness may be present along with myocardial ischemia in some patients. In fact, up to 15% of patients with chest wall tenderness on palpation that reproduces their pain will have an acute MI.

Lower extremities should be examined for signs of heart failure or deep vein thrombosis.

DIAGNOSTIC CONSIDERATIONS

ELECTROCARDIOGRAPHY

Myocardial ischemia

Inpatients reporting chest pain should have an ECG, and comparison with prior ECGs should be made to assess for dynamic changes.

ST-segment elevation: The ESC/ACCF/AHA/WHF committee for the definition of myocardial infarction established specific ECG criteria for ST-segment elevation myocardial infarction including 2 mm of ST segment elevation in the precordial leads for men (1.5 mm for women) and greater than 1 mm in other leads. The elevations must be present in at least two contiguous leads, corresponding to a specific arterial territory. A new left bundle branch block should be treated similarly to ST-segment elevation in the appropriate patient, with immediate reperfusion therapy.

Many patients will have alternate causes of ST-segment elevation (benign early repolarization, left ventricular aneurysm, pericarditis, hyperkalemia, bundle branch block, Prinzmetal's angina) so experience interpreting ECGs and comparison with old ECGs is critical.

Bundle branch block and paced rhythms make ECG interpretation challenging. The Sgarbossa criteria assign points to significant ECG findings in the presence of an old left bundle branch block: concordant ST-segment elevation of 1 mm or more in any lead (5 points), ST-segment depression of 1 mm or more in leads V1, V2, or V3 (3 points), discordant ST-segment elevation of 5 mm or more (2 points). A score of at least 3 is associated with high specificity for myocardial infarction but low sensitivity. In patients with LBBB or paced rhythms, the finding of ST-segment elevation ≥5 mm in leads with a negative QRS complex is highly specific for myocardial infarction.

Identification of inferior wall myocardial infarction should be followed by careful examination for evidence of posterior wall involvement (V_1 ST depression), conduction disturbance (Wenckebach, bradycardia, or complete heart block) and right ventricular infarction (right-sided ECG, lead rV_4).

ST-segment depression: ST-segment depression (0.5 mm or greater) predicts increased risk of myocardial ischemia. The greater the extent of depression, the higher the risk of MI and death. Posterior leads may help differentiate the patient with anterior ST-segment depression who has ischemia from the patient who has an acute posterior wall MI.

T-wave inversion: These indicate lower risk than ST depressions. Likewise, the presence of Q-waves is less predictive of adverse cardiac events than ST-segment depression or elevation.

Pulmonary embolism

The findings of right ventricular strain, $S_1Q_3T_3$, and new incomplete right bundle branch block may suggest pulmonary embolism but are not sensitive. Sinus tachycardia is the most common rhythm disturbance. Atrial fibrillation is seen in a small percentage of patients with pulmonary embolism but is rarely the only sign pointing to that diagnosis.

Although often abnormal in small- to medium-sized pulmonary emboli, the ECG is nonspecific and is normal in 23% of patients with submassive PE and 6% of patients with massive PE. For this reason, a normal ECG by itself cannot guide decision making relating to further diagnostic workup.

Pericarditis

Characteristic findings include diffuse ST-segment elevation that may be confused with acute MI or early repolarization. The lack of regional ischemic changes (ie, diffuse rather than localized ST elevations), as well as a suggestive history and cardiac examination will help distinguish this entity from acute MI.

Classic stages of ECG changes in pericarditis are:

Stage I (first few weeks of pericardial inflammation)

- Diffuse concave-upward ST-segment elevation with concordance of T waves
- ST-segment depression in aVR or V_1
- PR-segment depression in all leads except aVR and V_1
- Low voltage
- Absence of ST-segment changes

Stage II (days to several weeks)

- ST segments returning to baseline
- T-wave flattening

Stage III (end of second or third week)

- T-wave inversion

Stage IV (lasts up to three months)

- Gradual resolution of T-wave inversion

The classic four stages of ECG changes occur in only 50% of patients, and the ECG may be normal in 10% of patients. Some of the changes are nonspecific and may be confused with myocardial infarction or early repolarization.

Additional considerations

The findings of electrical alternans or low voltage in an ECG for a patient with chest pain should prompt consideration of pericardial effusion or hemorrhage. ECG abnormalities are common after stroke. Cerebral T waves (deep, symmetric T-wave inversions) are classically seen with subarachnoid hemorrhage. ST-segment deviations may occur in stroke patients as well, sometimes making differentiation between stroke and myocardial infarction challenging in difficult-to-assess patients.

Laboratory testing

Patients admitted to the hospital with chest pain or who develop chest pain while hospitalized should have basic laboratory tests performed, including a metabolic panel and complete blood count. Additional laboratory tests may be sent based upon clinical suspicion. Cardiac biomarkers and D-dimer assays are discussed below. Patients with possible intra-abdominal pathology should also have liver enzymes and a lipase ordered as well as appropriate imaging. Cardiac biomarkers should be drawn as a baseline but should not deter admission as they may initially be negative despite ischemia.

Cardiac biomarkers: A current definition of myocardial infarction involves typical rise and/or fall of cardiac biomarkers, along with ischemic symptoms, ischemic ECG findings (ST-segment deviation, Q waves), and/or coronary artery intervention. Thus, cardiac biomarkers are essential in the work-up of patients suspected of having cardiac etiology of their chest pain.

Creatine kinase (CK) and the CK-MB isoform (unique to the myocardium) have similar temporal patterns in cases of myocardial injury, rising within 4 to 8 hours and peaking between 12 and 24 hours (slightly earlier for CK-MB). CK-MB is cleared within 36 to 48 hours, and CK is cleared within 3 to 4 days. Troponin levels rise within 6 hours, peak after 12 hours, and are cleared after 7 to 14 days.

Troponins exhibit superior sensitivity and specificity when compared with CK and CK-MB for the diagnosis of myocardial infarction and help identify those patients at increased short- and long-term risk. Elevations identify patients who would benefit from aggressive treatment such as antithrombotic, antiplatelet, and coronary intervention. Cardiac troponin I has a higher specificity than cardiac troponin T, as it is not found in skeletal muscle. Some advisory groups argue for use of CK-MB to diagnose reinfarction, but others prefer troponin for this purpose as well.

Cutoff values for troponins, CK, and CK-MB vary by institutions. CK-MB in healthy patients generally ranges up to 5 microg/L or <3% of the total CK. Higher values are abnormal and may be due to myocardial injury or several other conditions generally easily differentiated based upon clinical grounds. There is ongoing debate regarding whether rises in serum biomarkers represent only irreversible or both reversible and irreversible injury, but rising cardiac biomarkers should be assumed to indicate at-risk myocardium. Likewise, the "normal range" of cardiac troponin is a troublesome concept, as any detectable troponin level has been shown to have prognostic significance and may be a marker of chronic as well as acute disease.

Troponins may be elevated in patients with renal failure who do not have evidence of myocardial damage. This is possibly due to decreased clearance as well as increased incidence of comorbid pathology (including pathology seen at the cellular level). These patients also have a high rate of coronary disease. Therefore, an appropriate serial rise in troponin is more helpful than an elevated, stable value for the diagnosis of myocardial infarction. Other conditions associated with increased troponin values include massive pulmonary embolism, myocarditis, cardiopulmonary resuscitation, cardioversion, heart failure, stroke, stress cardiomyopathy, and demand ischemia (**Table 77-5**).

A typical "rule-out" protocol after negative initial troponin often includes additional troponins at regular intervals (sometimes as frequently as every three hours) and a final troponin at the end of six to nine hours. Limitations: Although troponin is not detected in the blood of healthy people and is the standard criterion for the diagnosis of MI, the biomarker lacks sensitivity for USA.

TABLE 77-5 Differential Diagnosis of Elevated Troponin in the Absence of Acute Myocardial Infarction or Congestive Heart Failure

Cardiac and vascular disease	Aortic dissection, CVA
Respiratory disease	Acute PE, ARDS
Cardiac inflammation	Pericarditis, endocarditis, myocarditis
Muscular damage	Rhabdomyolysis
Infections	Sepsis, viral disease
Acute complications of inherited disorders	Neurofibromatosis, Duchenne muscular dystrophy, Klippel-Feil syndrome
Environmental exposure	Carbon monoxide, hydrogen sulfide, colchicine, evenomations (snake, jellyfish, spider, centipede, scorpion)
Chronic diseases	ESRD, cardiac infiltrative disorders (amyloidosis, sarcoidosis, hemochromatosis, scleroderma), HBP, diabetes, hypothyroidism
Iatrogenic disease	Invasive procedures (heart transplant, congenital defect repair, radiofrequency ablation, lung resection, ERCP), noninvasive procedures (cardioversion, lithotripsy), pharmacologic (chemotherapy)
Myocardial injury	Blunt chest trauma, endurance athletes
Miscellaneous	Kawasaki disease, stress cardiomyopathy, TTP, birth complications in infants, GI bleeding

ARDS, acute respiratory distress syndrome; CVA, cerebrovascular accident; ERCP; endoscopic retrograde, cholangiopancreatogram; ESRD, end-stage renal disease; GI, gastrointestinal; HBP, high blood pressure; PE, pulmonary embolism; TTP, thrombotic thrombocytopenic purpura.

Data from Kelley WE, Januzzi JL, Christenson RH. Increases in cardiac troponin in conditions other than ACS and HF. *Clin Chem*. 2009;55(12):2098.

D-dimer: The D-dimer is formed during breakdown of thrombi, occurring in cases of venous thromboembolism (VTE) but also as an integral part of the body's repair mechanism in other conditions (**Table 77-6**). The use of D-dimer in the appropriate patient can exclude pulmonary embolism as a cause of chest pain. The test demonstrates high sensitivity with poor specificity overall, but assays differ significantly in their sensitivities. ELISA assays are more sensitive than latex or erythrocyte agglutination assays for diagnosis of pulmonary embolism and are thus preferred. The Wells score

TABLE 77-6 Differential Diagnosis of Elevated D-Dimer

Infection	Stroke
Inflammation	ESRD
Cancer	Pregnancy
Surgery	DIC
Trauma	Aortic dissection
Ischemic heart disease	Advanced age

DIC, disseminated intravascular coagulopathy; ESRD, end-stage renal disease.

TABLE 77-7 Wells Score for Pulmonary Embolism

Variable	Points
Clinical signs and symptoms of deep vein thrombosis	3
Alternative diagnosis less likely than PE	3
Pulse greater than 100	1.5
Immobilization more than 3 days or surgery within prior 4 weeks	1.5
Previous PE or DVT	1.5
Hemoptysis	1
Malignancy (receiving treatment, treated within last 6 months or palliative)	1
Probability assessment	**Score**
Low	<2
Moderate	2 to 6
High	>6

DVT, deep venous thrombosis; PE, pulmonary embolism.
Data from Wells PS, Anderson DR, Rodger M, et al. Derivation of a simple clinical model to categorize patients probability of pulmonary embolism: increasing the models utility with the SimpliRED D-dimer. *Thromb Haemost.* 2000;83(3):416–420.

defines low, moderate, and high risk patients. Evidence suggests that a low Wells score combined with a negative D-dimer result (less than 500 ng/mL) is sufficient to exclude pulmonary embolism (**Table 77-7**).

The use of D-dimer testing may be of limited to no value in patients who are already hospitalized at the time of suspected pulmonary embolism, in contrast to those whose initial presentation is consistent with this diagnosis. Although the D-dimer has a very high negative predictive value, the test is not useful in cases of high pretest clinical probability. The usefulness of the test in patients with concomitant diseases is also limited. In pregnancy, not only are D-dimer levels typically elevated, but a negative D-dimer does not rule out VTE. The specificity of the D-dimer also decreases with increasing age. In 1 study, D-dimer allowed exclusion of VTE in roughly 52% of patients 40 years of age or less as compared to only 5% of those 80 years old. Hence, it should only be ordered in patients with a low clinical pretest probability of PE and does not add any additional diagnostic value in those patients who need to proceed directly to imaging.

Imaging

Patients reporting chest pain should have a chest radiograph taken. Lateral decubitus imaging is most sensitive for diagnosing pneumothorax (with the affected side positioned higher than the unaffected side), but pneumothoraces of at least 100 mL should be visible on upright films. Supine films may miss much larger pneumothoraces. Mediastinal air should raise concern for ruptured esophagus or airway. A widened mediastinum may be seen simply due to technique, but it is also associated with aortic dissection, seen in 61.6% of dissections in one study.

Computed tomography with contrast is commonly used to detect pulmonary embolism, and the historical gold standard, pulmonary angiography, is rarely needed. Studies have suggested a negative CT scan is sufficient in ruling out the diagnosis for patients with a low or moderate pretest probability, but high suspicion combined with a negative scan should prompt consideration of further workup. Further workup for high risk patients may include pulmonary angiography or lower-extremity venous ultrasound, the later only positive in 60% of patients with acute PE. Some institutions perform CT venography immediately after CT pulmonary angiography in order to increase sensitivity for thromboembolic disease but this requires an increased exposure to contrast.

Computed tomography is often the initial test for evaluation of aortic dissection, but transesophageal echocardiography is an excellent alternative and can be performed at the bedside. Magnetic resonance imaging is useful for imaging chronic dissections to determine whether an interval change has occurred.

Bedside echocardiography is a noninvasive imaging modality that can be rapidly performed to assist diagnosis and management of several conditions associated with chest pain. Specifically, its use should be considered for patients with suspected acute valvular disease, aortic dissection, pericardial effusion, or unexplained hemodynamic instability. It may also be helpful for distinguishing acute MI from pericarditis, with important treatment implications.

Stress testing

Hospitalists are increasingly asked to manage the workup of chest pain patients who are at low but not negligible risk for coronary disease. The admission status of these patients will vary by institution. Chest pain "observation units" are becoming more popular and may be staffed by emergency physicians, hospitalists, cardiologists, or nonphysician providers. The general goal of these units is to expedite the workup of patients at low risk for an acute coronary syndrome. After a negative evaluation with serial biomarkers and ECGs, further risk stratification with stress testing is often performed to identify patients with missed acute coronary syndrome and those at high risk for early adverse events.

Choosing which type of stress test to use will depend on the characteristics of the patient, resources available, and the policies of the institution, as well as the information desired. Exercise ECG testing without imaging is the preferred test in most patients with interpretable ECGs and adequate exercise capacity. Exercise testing with echocardiography or radionuclide myocardial perfusion imaging will allow localization of abnormalities. Patients who are unable to exercise can undergo pharmacologic stress testing with dipyridamole, adenosine, or dobutamine. Dobutamine echocardiography, however, should be avoided in patients who may be suffering from active or unstable ischemia.

In general, patients with ongoing chest pain should be managed as if they have unstable angina. However, low-risk patients with no prior history of myocardial infarction may have rest imaging performed with myocardial perfusion imaging or echocardiography. Coronary computed tomographic angiography shows promise in single-center studies for excluding acute coronary syndromes in patients with no history of myocardial infarction or known coronary disease, but this alternative to stress testing requires further validation of efficacy, cost effectiveness, and safety before widespread use can be endorsed.

Stress testing is useful both for diagnostic and prognostic purposes in patients suspected of having coronary heart disease, but due to the test characteristics, diagnostic testing should not be performed in patients with a very low pretest probability (based upon any of several validated decision aids) of having disease, as most positive tests in this setting represent false positives. Women have been noted to exhibit more false positives on stress testing, though current recommendations do not differ for men and women.

Some patients assessed to be at low risk for acute coronary syndrome may be safely discharged for outpatient stress testing within 72 hours in accordance with the 2007 ACC/AHA guidelines. Prior to discharge, these patients should have undergone at least a 6–12 hour observation period with two or three sets of negative cardiac enzymes and have normal or unchanged ECGs. One observational study found this to be a safe and feasible approach associated with a low risk of short-term adverse outcomes. Of 871 low risk patients undergoing outpatient stress testing, 2% had coronary artery disease requiring intervention and 0.3% had a myocardial infarction within six months. Importantly, the stress test appointment was made for the patient at the time of evaluation, and 92.2% of patients completed the outpatient stress test. Seventy-six did not have the test completed due to cancellation of the test or failure to keep the appointment. Available follow-up on 67 of these 76 patients showed no adverse cardiac events. This strategy is not appropriate for patients with questionable compliance with follow-up appointments. Direct scheduling and/or verbal communication with the primary care physician is advisable. Patients with a positive (and possibly indeterminate) stress test result should have a cardiology consultation while in the hospital. Those with negative results may be discharged.

IMPROVING QUALITY OF CARE FOR CHEST PAIN PATIENTS

As is true for many aspects of hospital-based medicine, hospitalists are uniquely positioned to enact quality improvement measures that will benefit chest pain patients. These measures will be institution specific, but several general considerations deserve attention. It is important to avoid the pitfall of placing too much diagnostic importance on an individual patient's response to therapy. However, treating pain adequately should be a primary goal implemented early in the evaluation of a chest pain patient, regardless of presumed etiology. The hospitalist is tasked with coordinating all aspects of a patient's care, and effective communication among health care workers is paramount. In addition, patient-centered care requires effective communication and understanding of the hospital experience from the patient perspective. Knowledge and respect for patients' needs and concerns can diminish the helplessness many feel during admission to the hospital. Standardizing chest pain algorithms, especially for acute coronary syndrome evaluation, can save considerable time and effort and if accepted institution-wide, may allow discharge of low-risk emergency department patients who would have otherwise been admitted. Lastly, taking time to communicate and coordinate with primary care physicians will enable earlier discharges and improve overall patient care.

CASE 77-2

The patient's primary nurse was asked to gather a complete set of vitals and ensure the patient had supplemental oxygen, IV access, and was on a cardiac monitor. Upon arrival to the patient's room, the clinician noted a thin man in moderate pain. A glance at the cardiac monitor showed a narrow-complex tachycardia. Vital signs were as follows: temperature 39 degrees Celsius, pulse 110, blood pressure 110/70, respiratory rate 26, room air saturation 90%, 100% on 2 L nasal cannula. A brief history from the patient revealed that his pain was right-sided and started suddenly about 10 minutes ago. He stated that it was sharp in nature and poorly localized without radiation; he rated his pain as 7 out of 10. Brief auscultation of the lungs revealed decreased breath sounds on the right but there was no apparent tracheal deviation. ECG showed sinus tachycardia without any ischemic changes. While the clinician remained at the bedside with the patient, the heart rate and blood pressure remained relatively constant. Imaging reveals a large right-sided pneumothorax and surgical consultation was requested for urgent tube thoracostomy.

The physician explained his proposed diagnosis and treatment in lay terms to the patient and ordered 4 mg of morphine IV for pain, with a repeat dose after 10 minutes if needed. He introduced the patient to the health care team members, including the surgical team who has just arrived, and explained each person's role in providing emergent care.

CONCLUSION

The symptom of chest pain suggests a wide differential diagnosis that can be narrowed by a careful history, physical examination, and appropriate testing to rule out life-threatening disorders. Most patients will turn out to have non-lifethreatening disorders. Although these patients likely do not require continued hospitalization, they should receive education about the most likely diagnosis, treatment, what symptoms would prompt a reassessment and where this should occur, and follow-up with their primary care physicians.

SUGGESTED READINGS

Berger JP, Buclin T, Haller E, et al. Right arm involvement and pain extension can help to differentiate coronary diseases from chest pain of other origin: a prospective emergency ward study of 278 consecutive patients admitted for chest pain. *J Intern Med.* 1990;227:165.

Hagan PG, Nienaber CA, Isselbacher EM, et al. The International Registry of Acute Aortic Dissection (IRAD): new insights into an old disease. *JAMA.* 2000;283:897.

Heit JA, Silverstein MD, Mohr DN, et al. Risk Factors for Deep Vein Thrombosis and Pulmonary Embolism. *Arch Intern Med.* 2000;160:809.

Meyer MC, Mooney RP, Sekera AK. A critical pathway for patients with acute chest pain and low risk for short-term adverse cardiac events: role of outpatient stress testing. *Ann Emerg Med.* 2006;47:435.

Pope JH, Aufderheide TP, Ruthazer R, et al. Missed diagnoses of acute cardiac ischemia in the emergency department. *N Engl J Med.* 2000;342:1163–1170.

Sgarbossa EB, Pinski SL, Barbagelata A, et al. Electrocardiographic diagnosis of evolving acute myocardial infarction in the presence of left bundle branch block. *N Engl J Med.* 1996;334:481.

Stein PD, Beemath A, Matta F, et al. Clinical characteristics of patients with acute pulmonary embolism: data from PIOPED II. *Am J Med.* 2007;120:871.

Weiner DA, Ryan TJ, McCabe CH, et al. Exercise stress testing. Correlations among history of angina, ST segment response and prevalence of CAD in the Coronary Artery Surgery Study. *N Engl J Med.* 1979;301:230.

CHAPTER 78

Constipation

Linda Lee, MD
Eugenie Shieh, MD

Key Clinical Questions

1. What are the risk factor(s) for developing constipation in the hospital?
2. How do you prevent constipation in a hospitalized patient with a history of constipation?
3. What are the likely causes of new constipation in a hospitalized patient?
4. What is the treatment of common causes of new constipation?

CASE 78-1

An 82-year-old man with relapsed diffuse large cell lymphoma presents with severe abdominal pain, distention, and vomiting beginning 24 hours ago. The pain is intermittent, crampy, and diffuse. He has not had a bowel movement in 7 days. He has been receiving rituximab for his lymphoma. He has no history of abdominal surgery. He does have a history of thyroid disease, atrial fibrillation, gout, and diabetes.

The patient has a long-standing history of chronic constipation, and has used polyethylene glycol (PEG) 3350 daily for 2 years. When he was hospitalized a week ago, he was given docusate sodium daily instead of his usual regimen. His other medications include warfarin, allopurinol, levothyroxine, glimepiride, and amlodipine.

His physical exam is remarkable for normal vital signs and a moderately protuberant abdomen. There are bowel sounds but no palpable masses. There is mild diffuse tenderness, but no rebound. The rectal exam reveals no stool in the vault. His laboratory tests are normal. An abdominal flat plate shows a large amount of stool in the right and transverse colon.

What are the causes of this man's constipation? What is the best way to manage his constipation acutely and chronically?

INTRODUCTION

Constipation has many meanings, but for the purposes of this chapter, the medical definition of constipation includes one or all of the following: fewer than three bowel movements per week; passing hard, lumpy stools; straining with defecation; or having a sense of incomplete evacuation. Constipation can newly arise in a patient hospitalized for other medical reasons, represent an exacerbation of a chronic problem, be the principal reason for hospitalization, or be a manifestation of an acute, possibly catastrophic, event.

Chronic constipation is a common complaint that compromises quality of life and frequently prompts use of health care services. Constipation results in 2.5 million physician visits and 92,000 hospitalizations per year in the United States. The prevalence of constipation in North America is estimated to range from 2% to 27%, with most studies citing a prevalence of 15%. This variation in prevalence reflects different diagnostic criteria for constipation and study design. The estimated prevalence of constipation in other developed countries is similar to that in North America at 17.1% in Europe, 14.3% in Hong Kong and 16.5% in South Korea. Constipation is reported more often by females (2-3:1 predominance), nonwhites, individuals of lower socioeconomic status, and the elderly (prevalence of 20–24%). The cumulative incidence of constipation over more than 1 decade is about 1 in 6. This incidence increases dramatically in the setting of certain comorbidities.

Although most individuals with constipation do not specifically seek medical care constipation contributes significantly to health care expenses. In the United States, the total health care cost of constipation diagnosis per patient exceeds $2500, and in 2001, $235 million dollars were spent for constipation, with more than half of the cost incurred from inpatient care. In the California Medicaid program, 0.6% of patients presenting to a physician with a medical complaint of constipation were admitted to a hospital, averaging almost $3000 per admission. This chapter will discuss how to distinguish, evaluate, and manage the conditions in which constipation occurs.

PATHOPHYSIOLOGY

The pathophysiology of constipation can be understood first by a very brief review of the elements required for normal colonic transit and defecation. Normal colonic transit requires segmental activity and propagated activity, which depends on both low-amplitude and high-amplitude propagated contractions. Normal defecation requires intact pelvic floor muscles and rectal compliance. The muscles of the pelvic floor include the internal anal sphincter, the external anal sphincter, and the puborectalis muscle. The internal sphincter muscle, which is tonically contracted, is innervated by the enteric nervous system. The external sphincter and puborectalis muscles are innervated by the pudendal nerves (S2, S3, and S4). During defecation, both must relax in order for normal defecation to occur. The puborectalis muscle forms a U-shaped sling around the rectum, and when contracted maintains the rectum at a 90 degree angle (that is, perpendicular) with respect to the anal canal. This muscle must relax with voluntary defecation so the angle can widen to 135 degrees to allow unobstructed passage of stool from the rectum to the anal canal. Medications, medical illness, prior surgery, and other factors can diminish colonic contractions, contribute to pelvic floor weakness, alter rectal compliance, or cause obstruction.

NEW CONSTIPATION IN THE HOSPITALIZED PATIENT

New constipation commonly arises in hospitalized patients and has been attributed to multiple causes (**Table 78-1**). Lack of physical activity, change in diet, electrolyte disturbances, use of anesthetics and narcotics, medication side effects, and failure to continue the home laxative regimen may precipitate constipation. In the elderly, acute hospitalization further increases the prevalence of constipation in an already susceptible age group, with one-third of hospitalized geriatric patients requiring laxatives 3 times daily. The incidence of new-onset constipation at 4 weeks after a first stroke exceeds 50%. The incidence of constipation among cancer patients is 60%, but increases to 87% in those using opioids. Constipation can also be part of a symptom complex representing a serious, acute event. If abdominal distention, high-pitched bowel sounds, and pain are present, then colonic obstruction must be considered. Accompanying fever and rebound tenderness should trigger an evaluation for perforation.

The patient's history is essential to identify the cause of constipation and its management. It is important to define the duration of constipation, the frequency of bowel movements, whether there is incomplete evacuation, straining, or passage of hard (scybalous) stool. Associated symptoms may suggest a cause for constipation. Blood or mucus in the stool may indicate an obstructive process, anal fissure, rectal prolapse, or hemorrhoids. Tenesmus suggests hard stool or possibly rectal obstruction. Overflow fecal incontinence or mental status changes can be presenting symptoms of fecal impaction in elderly patients.

Important elements of the past medical history include an obstetric and surgical history. A thorough review of all medications can reveal a drug-related cause of constipation. Common culprits of constipation-induced medications include prescription medications (opiates, anticholinergics, and calcium-channel blockers), over-the-counter drugs, and herbals (**Table 78-2**). In the elderly, home use of laxatives is the only identifiable risk factor for developing constipation in the hospital. A family history of bowel disorders should be sought. The social history should explore physical activity and dietary habits, including amount of fiber intake, fluid intake, number and timing of meals, and dehydration. Red flags for a serious underlying etiology of constipation include weight loss, abdominal pain, rectal bleeding, iron deficiency anemia, or a significant family history of colon cancer. Complaints of severe pain with abdominal distention could signal colonic obstruction or intestinal ischemia with potentially life-threatening complications.

A complete physical exam searching for signs of a systemic illness is essential, although it is often unrevealing. In particular, the abdominal exam should focus on palpating for stool in the left or right lower quadrant. Severe abdominal distention, high-pitched bowel sounds, and tenderness to palpation are suggestive of an obstructive etiology. Evaluation of the patient may sometimes reveal a fecolith palpable through the abdominal wall or on digital examination of the rectum. A complete neurologic examination may provide evidence of occult neurologic disease such as Parkinson disease. The anorectum should be inspected for hemorrhoids, anal fissures, skin tags, or rectal prolapse. If cauda equina syndrome is suspected, perineal sensation can be evaluated by

TABLE 78-1 Causes of New Constipation in the Hospitalized Patient

Drugs and supplements
Reduced physical activity
Bedridden for length of time more than 2 weeks
Postsurgical
Dietary change
Low fiber diet
Dehydration
Electrolyte disturbances: hypercalcemia, hyponatremia, hypokalemia, uremia
Paraneoplastic syndrome

TABLE 78-2 Drugs by Class that Cause Constipation

Anticholinergics
Antidepressants
Antiparkinsonian drugs
Antipsychotics
Antispasmodics
Analgesics
Nonsteroidal anti-inflammatory drugs
Neurally acting agents
Adrenergics
Anticonvulsants
Antihistamines
Antihypertensives
Calcium channel blockers
Opiates
Vinca alkaloids
Cation-containing agents
Aluminum
Barium sulfate
Calcium
Iron supplements

using a Q-tip or sharp point of a pin to gently stroke all quadrants. An anocutaneous reflex ("anal wink") can be elicited by stroking the perineal skin; the absence of reflex contraction of the external anal sphincter would suggest a neuropathy. The digital rectal examination can evaluate sphincter tone, the contents of the rectal vault, and allow detection of blood in the stool. Fever, tachycardia, and other signs of hemodynamic instability are clues to complications of perforation or ischemia.

Pertinent laboratory tests in the evaluation of constipation include a complete blood count, electrolytes, including calcium, phosphorous, and magnesium, blood urea nitrogen, creatinine, glucose, and thyroid function tests. Other laboratory tests, such as serum protein electrophoresis, urine porphyrins, serum parathyroid hormone, and evaluation for adrenal hypofunction should be considered, if indicated by history or physical exam.

Diagnostic imaging is not a necessary component of every evaluation of constipation, but can provide critical information in the right clinical scenario. In patients with abdominal distention, pain, and constipation, plain abdominal radiography can be helpful in assessing the degree of constipation and ruling out obstruction. Abdominal radiographs may demonstrate a dilated colon or small bowel with air fluid levels indicative of obstruction. Plain abdominal radiographs can also help diagnose a sigmoid or cecal volvulus. The presence of free air on plain abdominal radiograph would indicate perforated bowel (see Chapter 109 Basic Abdominal Imaging).

If abdominal radiography demonstrates colonic dilatation suggestive of an obstruction, additional imaging should be performed. A flexible sigmoidoscopy or colonoscopy, barium enema, or CT scan can help define a colonic obstruction. Flexible sigmoidoscopy and colonoscopy can also identify a mucosal lesion, such as a malignancy or stricture. The timing of the latter studies would depend on the risk of perforation from performing the study. For example, acute diverticulitis causing obstruction would require treatment prior to performing a colonoscopy to rule out the possibility of an occult cancer underlying the inflammation.

DIFFERENTIAL DIAGNOSIS OF ACUTE CONSTIPATION

Fecal impaction

Impaction of feces occurs in children, institutionalized individuals, and the elderly, and sometimes as a complication of opioid use. Large calcified fecoliths as well as seed bezoars have caused large bowel obstruction. Treatment of fecal impaction requires aggressive management since impaction may lead to urinary tract obstruction, perforation of the colon, dehydration, electrolyte imbalance, renal insufficiency, fecal incontinence, decubitus ulcers, stercoral ulcers, and rectal bleeding. Treatment of fecal impaction in part depends on where the impaction is located. Fecal impaction may require urgent manual disimpaction, especially in the elderly, a population in whom risk factors of immobility, dehydration, and multiple medications predispose it to complications of mental status changes, agitation, and worsening confusion.

In the left colon, manual disimpaction may be followed by enemas, which work primarily by stimulating rectal propulsion in this situation. Soapsuds enemas (composed of 6 grams castile soap/liter) are chemical irritants and promote intestinal fluid secretion. There are rare reports of colitis after administration of soapsuds enemas for more than 5 days in a row. Hypertonic solutions, like sodium phosphate, work by osmosis, drawing water into the lumen. Sodium phosphate enemas should be used with caution, because retention of the enema in the absence of defecation can lead to dehydration, hyperphosphatemia, and acute renal failure.

Large volume oral laxative solutions are often effective for the treatment of fecal impaction, particularly if the impaction is proximal to the sigmoid colon. Polyethylene glycol (PEG) 3350 with electrolytes has been shown to be effective monotherapy for the treatment of fecal impaction in children, and is superior to lactulose in preventing future episodes. Following disimpaction, all patients need preventative therapy, and maintenance with daily dosing with oral PEG 3350 (at least 17 grams daily) is highly recommended. Occasionally, twice daily dosing with PEG 3350 is required to prevent recurrent constipation.

Colonic obstruction due to tumor, stricture, or volvulus

PRACTICE POINT

- In any patient experiencing a sudden onset of constipation associated with abdominal pain, distention, and nausea and vomiting, volvulus should be considered.
- Consulting a gastroenterologist and surgeon is advised when volvulus is suspected, even in the absence of frank perforation.

Obstruction may precipitate new onset constipation or exacerbate chronic constipation. Obstruction may be caused by a tumor, stricture, or less commonly by a colonic volvulus, leading to nausea, vomiting, abdominal distention, and pain. Concern for a possible malignant growth would be heightened if there is accompanying iron deficiency anemia, weight loss, or a personal or family history raising the risk for colorectal cancer. A stricture should be considered in the differential diagnosis in any individual who has had prior colonic resection or history of diverticulitis.

Volvulus should be considered in the patient experiencing a sudden onset of constipation associated with abdominal pain, distention, and nausea and vomiting. A sigmoid volvulus caused by the twisting of the colon around the mesenteric axis accounts for up to 5% of colonic obstruction in the U.S. Cecal volvulus, which is rarer than sigmoid volvulus, occurs when there is a mobile cecum, and has been reported as a complication following left colectomy, cholecystectomy, and other laparoscopic procedures. It is thought that adhesions may serve as the fulcrum for torsion in some cases. Cecal volvulus has also been rarely reported following routine colonoscopy. Twenty-eight percent of patients with acute cecal volvulus occur in patients hospitalized for other medical reasons. Abdominal plain imaging may demonstrate marked distention of an ahaustral colon with an appearance of a large "coffee-bean" pointing toward the right upper quadrant (in the case of sigmoid colon) or left upper quadrant (in the case of cecal volvulus). However, this radiographic sign is not always present. If there is proximal bowel dilatation, the diagnosis of volvulus can be very difficult to make based on abdominal films alone. Computed tomography may demonstrate a "whirl sign," which represents a twisted loop of intestine and engorged mesenteric vessels. Another CT finding is a "bird's beak" appearance of dilated bowel tapering to a point at the site of torsion. CT signs of ischemia and/or perforation include circumferential wall thickening, pneumatosis intestinalis, increased density in the mesenteric fat, and pneumoperitoneum. If the diagnosis is suspected but remains uncertain, barium enema has been reported to be diagnostic in 88% of cases and even therapeutic. A barium enema should only be performed if there are no signs of ischemia or perforation. No colonic preparation is given for this test in this circumstance. Consulting a gastroenterologist and surgeon is advised when volvulus is suspected, even in the absence of frank perforation. Sigmoidoscopy may diagnose and treat a sigmoid volvulus, and is preferable to barium enema because of a lower risk of perforation.

Ogilvie syndrome/intestinal pseudoobstruction

PRACTICE POINT

- Laxatives should not be given, particularly those that can be fermented by colonic bacteria to produce gas, for patients with pseudoobstruction. Rare reports of colonic perforation exist when such patients are given lactulose. Endoscopic or pharmacologic decompression may be required if patients do not respond within 24–48 hours to supportive therapy or if the cecal diameter reaches 10 cm (thereby increasing the risk of perforation or ischemia).

Colonic dilatation without evidence of a mechanical obstruction may be due to intestinal pseudoobstruction or Ogilvie syndrome. First described in cancer patients with malignant infiltration of the celiac plexus, it is now known to arise in all types of patients, including those with trauma, cardiac disease, obstetrical or surgical conditions, or neurologic disease. The cause of Ogilvie syndrome has been attributed to imbalanced parasympathetic and sympathetic stimulation of the colon. Since the right colon receives its parasympathetic innervation by the vagus nerve and the left colon from S2-4, Ogilvie syndrome has been attributed to decreased colonic contractility of the left colon as a result of perturbed parasympathetic innervation. Other risk factors for Ogilvie syndrome include electrolyte disturbances and the use of opioids. Intestinal pseudoobstruction can be associated with collagen vascular disease, like scleroderma, or a paraneoplastic syndrome. Intestinal pneumatosis may be evident on abdominal films or CT. Serum antibodies (anti-Hu) directed against the myenteric plexus may be detectable in patients with some types of malignancies, especially small cell carcinoma.

In the absence of a definite obstructing lesion, the management of acute intestinal pseudoobstruction is supportive initially. Patients should be NPO and if vomiting, a nasogastric tube should be inserted and placed on low-intermittent suction. Laxatives should not be given, particularly those that can be fermented by colonic bacteria to produce gas. Rare reports of colonic perforation exist when such patients are given lactulose. Electrolyte abnormalities should be corrected and medications known to exacerbate constipation should be discontinued if possible.

Once the cecal diameter reaches 10 cm increasing the risk for ischemia or perforation, or when the patient continues to do poorly on supportive therapy for more than 24–48 hours, endoscopic or pharmacologic decompression may be required. The risk of colonic perforation is estimated to be at about 3% when the cecal diameter exceeds 12 cm. Neostigmine 2.0 mg administered intravenously can be used to decompress patients with acute intestinal pseudoobstruction. The response usually occurs rapidly after intravenous administration. The dose may be safely repeated if colonic dilatation recurs. In a small placebo-controlled randomized study, 91% of those receiving neostigmine experienced a reduction in abdominal distention. However, patients must undergo cardiac monitoring while receiving IV neostigmine, and atropine must be on hand in the event that severe bradycardia is induced. Contraindications to neostigmine use include ischemia, active bronchospasm, serum creatinine >3 mg/dL, cardiac arrhythmias, pregnancy, or bowel obstruction.

Alternatively, colonic decompression can be achieved endoscopically, recognizing the risk of perforation as a result of the procedure. A bowel prep should not be administered prior to this procedure. If there are concerns about recurrence, a colonic decompression tube can be left in place. This is preferred to a rectal tube, which succeeds mostly in decompressing the left colon.

MANAGING NEW CONSTIPATION IN THE HOSPITALIZED PATIENT

The management of acute constipation in the hospitalized patient has 2 arms: relieving the current discomfort associated with the constipation and preventing the situation from arising again. The treatment of acute constipation should be dictated by the severity of the patient's symptoms and the cause for the constipation. For example, a patient who typically had daily bowel movements but while hospitalized has had no bowel movement for several days and complains of abdominal discomfort, bloating, or distention, would probably achieve the most rapid releif by taking a stimulant laxative until a bowel movement is achieved. In patients with only mild symptoms of constipation, an osmotic laxative may achieve satisfactory results. Enemas may be helpful for helping to eliminate stool from the left side of the colon, particularly if the patient complains of a sense of rectal fullness. An abdominal flat plate can sometimes be helpful in determining the location and extent of fecal retention. In those patients who are severely constipated, right colonic stimulation may be required, and an oral stimulant laxative is suggested. Alternatively, oral lavage using large volume PEG 3350 solutions (as used for colonoscopy preparation) can be very effective, provided the patient is not experiencing nausea or vomiting. Reducing the amount of opioids and correcting electrolyte disturbances are paramount to the treatment and prevention of constipation.

In patients with symptoms of severe constipation, stool softeners are likely to be ineffective and add little to a preventative laxative regimen. Lactulose should also be avoided in this situation, since colonic fermentation of lactulose produces gas and increases distention and abdominal pain. Rare instances of colonic perforation have been reported when lactulose has been administered in this scenario. However, lactulose may be used later to prevent recurrent constipation.

PREVENTING RECURRENT CONSTIPATION IN THE HOSPITALIZED PATIENT

Once a satisfactory bowel movement has occurred, the patient should be placed on a laxative regimen to prevent constipation from occurring again. It is helpful to immediately start the patient on an osmotic laxative, such as lactulose or polyethylene glycol 3350, on a daily basis. Addition of a stimulant laxative may be required intermittently or daily, particularly in those individuals at high risk for recurrent constipation. This would include those who are immobile, have neurologic disease, or use opioids.

CHRONIC CONSTIPATION

Many patients who complain of constipation during their hospitalization have a history of chronic constipation prior to being hospitalized. It is important to recognize that the chronic constipation can be difficult to define due to differing patient and physician perceptions. Patients with chronic constipation often present with a variety of symptoms including hard or lumpy stools, infrequent stools, excessive straining, feeling of incomplete evacuation, and rectal fullness or discomfort. The Rome III classification accounts for this heterogeneity of symptoms by basing its criteria on symptoms. Using Rome III criteria, a diagnosis of functional constipation is made when 2 or more of the symptoms in **Table 78-3** are fulfilled, when loose stools are rarely present without laxative use, and when the criteria for irritable bowel syndrome with constipation (IBS-C) subtype in **Table 78-4** are not met. In addition, symptoms must have started ≥6 months ago and must have been present for the last 3 months.

■ TYPES OF CONSTIPATION

Constipation can be classified into three pathophysiologic subtypes: normal-transit, slow-transit, and pelvic outlet dysfunction. The

TABLE 78-3 Rome III Criteria for Functional Constipation*

1. Must include *2 or more* of the following:
   a. Straining during at least 25% of defecations
   b. Lumpy or hard stools in at least 25% of defecations
   c. Sensation of incomplete evacuation for at least 25% of defecations
   d. Sensation of anorectal obstruction/blockage for at least 25% of defecations
   e. Manual maneuvers to facilitate at least 25% of defecations (eg, digital evacuation, support of the pelvic floor)
   f. Fewer than 3 defecations per week
2. Loose stools are rarely present without the use of laxatives
3. There are insufficient criteria for IBS

**Criteria fulfilled for the last 3 months with symptom onset at least 6 months prior to diagnosis*

TABLE 78-4 Rome III Diagnostic Criteria for Irritable Bowel Syndrome with Constipation (IBS-C)*

Recurrent abdominal pain or discomfort† at least 3 days per month in the last 3 months associated with *2 or more* of the following:

1. Improvement with defecation
2. Onset associated with a change in frequency of stool
3. Onset associated with a change in form (appearance) of stool—hard or lumpy stools§ ≥25% and loose (mushy) or watery stools,¶ <25% of bowel movements**

*Criteria fulfilled for the last 3 months with symptom onset at least 6 months prior to diagnosis.
†Discomfort means an uncomfortable sensation not described as pain.
§Bristol Stool Form Scale 1–2 (separate hard lumps like nuts [difficult to pass] or sausage-shaped but lumpy).
¶Bristol Stool Form Scale 6–7 (fluffy pieces with ragged edges, a mushy stool or watery, no solid pieces, entirely liquid).
**In the absence of use of antidiarrheals or laxatives.

three subtypes can overlap. *Normal-transit constipation*, the most common subtype, is characterized by normal colonic transit time and normal defecatory function. A subset of these individuals has reduced colonic tone or compliance. *Slow-transit constipation* is characterized by delayed transit of stool through the colon due to a myopathy or neuropathy. Slowed colonic transit arises from diminished motor activity, such as reduced high-amplitude contractions. This type of constipation is moderately predicted by stool form (scybalous, or hard lumpy balls of stool). In contrast to slow transit constipation, *pelvic floor dysfunction*, the most common subtype among women, is characterized by difficulty or inability to evacuate stool from the anorectum. Pelvic floor dysfunction can be caused by failure of the internal anal sphincter or pelvic floor muscles to relax or paradoxical contraction of the external anal sphincter or puborectalis muscle while straining during defecation. Pelvic floor dysfunction is also referred to as defecatory disorder, anismus, pelvic-floor dyssynergia, paradoxical pelvic-floor contraction, obstructed constipation, functional rectosigmoid obstruction, spastic pelvic-floor syndrome, and functional fecal retention in childhood.

EVALUATION

The initial evaluation of a patient presenting with chronic constipation should consist of a careful history, physical examination, laboratory testing, and imaging to exclude secondary causes, prior to pursuing a diagnosis of functional constipation. Symptoms alone cannot distinguish between the subtypes of functional constipation. Certain historical clues, however, should generate a high index of suspicion for pelvic outlet dysfunction as a cause of constipation, including a sense of obstruction in the anal region, and manual maneuvers to facilitate stool evacuation, including unusual postures on the toilet, support of the perineum, digital manipulation of the rectum, and posterior vaginal pressure.

While a thorough examination of the abdomen, perineum, and anorectum should be performed, the physical exam should pay particular attention to pelvic floor motion. The examiner should inspect for perineal abnormalities while the patient bears down, including pulling forward of the anus. While performing the digital rectal exam, the examiner should assess sphincter tone by having the patient bear down to elicit perineal descent and relaxation of the sphincter. Abnormal findings on palpation include high resting anal-sphincter tone, descent of the perineum <1.0 cm or >3.5 cm while straining, posterior rectal wall tenderness, a palpable mucosal prolapse or defect in the anterior rectum. Physiologic testing for functional constipation should be performed only after excluding secondary causes of constipation in cases refractory to a high-fiber diet and laxatives. Colonic transit studies with radiopaque markers (Sitzmarks®) or scintigraphy are the initial tests of choice, allowing differentiation between normal transit, slow transit, and pelvic outlet obstruction. The patient ingests a capsule containing radiopaque markers and an abdominal flat plate is obtained 120 hours later. No markers will be retained in those with normal transit. However, markers retained throughout the colon are indicative of slow transit. Accumulation of markers in the left colon is suggestive of pelvic outlet obstruction, but could also be compounded by slow transit.

If the history and physical exam are suggestive of pelvic floor dysfunction, anorectal manometry, balloon expulsion testing, and defecography are useful tests. Anorectal manometry assesses rectal sensation and compliance, sphincter pressures, and anorectal reflexes. The test may suggest Hirschsprung disease. The balloon expulsion test can identify but cannot exclude dyssynergic defecation. As an adjunct to other testing, MRI or video defecography can be used to confirm or exclude pelvic floor dysfunction, and can identify a clinically significant rectocele, rectal intussusception, and rectal prolapse. Finally, electromyography of the anal sphincter muscles can evaluate for dysfunction of the striated pelvic floor muscles.

MANAGING CHRONIC CONSTIPATION

PRACTICE POINT

- No currently available stimulant laxatives have been associated with an increased risk for neoplasia. The evidence that chronic stimulant laxative use damages neurons and causes cathartic colon is very limited and remains controversial.

Understanding how each laxative type works is essential for proper management of acute and chronic constipation (**Table 78-5**). For those individuals with mild, intermittent constipation, use of an occasional stool softener or magnesium-based osmotic laxative can be effective. Nearly all patients can benefit somewhat from increasing daily fiber consumption to at least 30 grams per day. Daily fiber, be it insoluble or soluble, can be consumed in the diet or by use of one of numerous fiber supplements available over the counter. Patients should be encouraged to use the equivalent of 5 to 10 grams of fiber daily, be it in the form of a supplement or foods, such as a high fiber cereal that gives

TABLE 78-5 Pharmacologic Agents Used to Treat Constipation

Bulking agents containing psyllium.
Osmotic laxatives: these draw water into the intestinal lumen and are useful in those who report hard or scybalous stool that is unresponsive to dietary fiber
Polyethylene glycol
Lactulose
Magnesium and sulfate salts
Stimulant laxatives
Anthraquinones: senna, aloe, cascara, frangula
Polyphenolic (diphenylmethane) compounds: bisacodyl, sodium picosulfate
Detergents/stool softeners
Docusate sodium
Liquid paraffin
Prokinetic agents
Colchicines
Misoprostol
Chloride channel activator
Lubiprostone
Opioid antagonists
Methylnaltrexone
Alvimopan
Enemas and suppositories
Sodium lauryl sulphoacetate, osmotic agents, glycerol
Saline and water enema
Hypertonic sodium phosphate enemas
Glycerin suppositories, bisacodyl suppositories or enema, oxyphenisatin

10–13 grams per cup. When using fiber to manage constipation, patients must be informed before they become discouraged that they may not observe a change in their stool consistency for 7 to 14 days after initiating daily fiber supplementation. In addition, they may experience increased gassiness during this 2-week period as a result of increased bacterial fermentation. Patients with irritable bowel syndrome may be exquisitely sensitive to the gas produced by increased fiber intake, and may be intolerant of it.

In patients who report passage of hard, scybalous, stool with either normal- or slow-transit constipation, if fiber fails to alleviate the hard stool, addition of a daily osmotic laxative, such as lactulose or PEG 3350, is usually effective. Because osmotic laxatives are not the same as stimulant laxatives, patients must be told to assess the full impact of this regimen after 7 to 14 days have passed. After that, the dose and timing of the laxative can be adjusted to better suit the lifestyle and expectations of the patient. Lubiprostone, a calcium channel stimulator, draws water into the colon and can be used in patients with mild to moderate constipation. The advantage of lubiprostone is that it is available in pill form, but does cause nausea in a third of users, and therefore should be taken with food. In a clinical trial involving individuals with chronic constipation, the majority of individuals had a bowel movement within 24–48 hours of taking the medication. Lubiprostone has also been approved by the FDA for the treatment of IBS-constipation, but at a dose of 8 mcg bid as opposed to 24 mcg bid approved for functional constipation.

In patients with pelvic floor dysfunction, use of a suppository can be helpful if rectal stimulation is required to initiate the bowel movement. These patients frequently benefit from using a stimulant laxative, such as a sennasoide or bisacodyl, every day or every other day. Occasional enema use can also help address the left-sided fullness and stimulate defecation. Patients with pelvic floor dysfunction may also report hard stool, so a regimen using both an osmotic and stimulant laxative is sometimes required.

Patients frequently express concern about long-term stimulant laxative use. They fear chronic use causes "dependency" or a "lazy colon." Many health care providers share this concern because of early reports of a possible relationship between chronic stimulant laxative use and cathartic colon. However, the evidence that chronic stimulant laxative use damages neurons and causes cathartic colon is very limited and remains controversial. While it is true that chronic use of an anthraquinone may cause the diffuse colonic pigmentation known as melanosis coli, this is of no clinical significance. An additional concern was that use of stimulant laxatives could increase cancer risk. Most phenolphthalein-containing laxatives were withdrawn from the market when they were shown to increase ovarian, adrenal, renal, and hematopoietic neoplasms in rodents. No other stimulant laxatives have been associated with an increased risk for neoplasia.

TIMING OF CONSULTATION WITH A GASTROENTEROLOGIST OR A SURGEON

A GI and/or surgical consultation should be obtained for any constipated patient who has severe pain, pain out of proportion to exam, or who has signs suggesting development of a serious complication, such as ischemia, perforation, or obstruction.

A consultant can be particularly helpful in the management of suspected colonic obstruction. Treatment of sigmoid volvulus includes placement of a temporary rectal tube or endoscopic reduction as long as there are no clinical, radiological, or laboratory signs of ischemia or perforation. Barium enema can also be performed, but carries a higher risk of perforation than endoscopic decompression. Sigmoid volvulus is very amenable to initial endoscopic reduction, but recurrence rate may be as high as 70% so elective resection after decompression is recommended. Any sign of ischemia, such as bloody stool, during endoscopic reduction is an indication for urgent surgery. Endoscopic reduction of cecal volvulus is successful in only 30% of cases, so surgery is generally recommended as first-line treatment unless the patient is a poor surgical candidate. Benign or malignant colonic strictures can be diagnosed by colonoscopy and biopsy. Benign strictures can be dilated endoscopically using balloon dilators or colonic stents. Surgery may be necessary to resect benign or malignant colonic strictures.

PREVENTION

PRACTICE POINT

- Stool softeners are largely ineffective in patients who take opioids, have undergone surgery causing them to be bedridden, or have a history of chronic constipation. A major contributing factor to constipation emerging as an active issue in the hospitalized patient is the failure to (1) obtain an accurate history of chronic constipation and (2) continue the patient's home laxative regimen.

A major contributing factor to constipation emerging as an active issue in the hospitalized patient is the failure to obtain an accurate history of chronic constipation and not continuing the patient's home laxative regimen. In fact, it is very common for admitting orders on some services to ignore the patient's home laxatives and reflexively include an order for stool softeners. Stool softeners are largely ineffective in patients who take opioids, have undergone surgery causing them to be bedridden, or have a history of chronic constipation. In the acutely hospitalized older patient, the use of laxatives at home was a good predictor for constipation while in the hospital. There is also the mistaken impression that patients who are not eating will not have any bowel movements at all.

Identifying the risks for constipation, as well as a prior history of constipation, is essential for preventing constipation in the hospitalized patient. In those at high risk, starting a daily osmotic laxative can be highly effective, recognizing that their effectiveness may not be immediately apparent. In selecting an osmotic laxative, it is important to be aware that frequent administration of magnesium-based compounds raise serum magnesium levels in patients with chronic renal insufficiency. A daily stimulant laxative may be helpful in those at highest risk or in whom the history suggests pelvic floor dysfunction.

CONCLUSION

Constipation is a common problem in the hospitalized patient. New constipation may be precipitated by many factors associated with hospitalization. Recognizing the risks for constipation is the mainstay of managing and preventing constipation. The major risks are a prior history of chronic constipation, use of constipating medications, particularly opioids, and lack of physical activity due to medical illness or surgical recovery. Selecting the proper laxative for management or prevention of constipation requires familiarity with the different types of laxatives and educating patients about these differences to address their expectations about their efficacy. Finally, it is also essential for the hospitalist to recognize when constipation is actually a manifestation of an acute, possibly emergent event that requires immediate management by consultants.

SUGGESTED READINGS

American Gastroenterological Association Position Statement: Guidelines on Constipation. *Gastroenterology*. 2000;119: 1761–1778. Provides various treatment algorithms based upon type of constipation.

Constipation: evaluation and treatment of colonic and anorectal motility disorders. *Gastroenterol Clin North Am*. 2007;36:687–711. An excellent review on the pathophysiology of chronic constipation is provided by Rao.

Lal SK, Morgenstern R, Vinjirayer EP, Matin A. Sigmoid volvulus an update. *Gastrointest Endosc Clin N Am*. 2006;16:175–187.

Lembo A, Camilleri M. Chronic constipation. *N Engl J Med*. 2003;349:1360.

Managing Chronic Constipation GUIDELINES Pocketcard™. Constipation treatment algorithms on a pocket card. Available for $4.25 from the American Gastroenterological Association.

CHAPTER 79

Delirium

Karin J. Neufeld, MD, MPH
Amy Huberman, MD
Dale M. Needham, MD, PhD

Key Clinical Questions

1. What is the prevalence of delirium in hospitalized patient populations?
2. What are the most common causes of delirium?
3. Why is it important to detect delirium?
4. What are the symptoms of delirium?
5. How is delirium diagnosed?
6. How can delirium be prevented and treated?

CASE 79-1

A 56-year-old bank manager with a history of lumbar stenosis and major depression was admitted to the hospital five days ago with cellulitis of the left thigh. He was started empirically on intravenous cefazolin, and his fever (40° Celsius on admission) resolved over 96 hours. During his hospital stay, he was given his home dose of fluoxetine 30 mg daily. During preparation of discharge paperwork the medical team is informed that he is pulling at his intravenous line and threatening to leave against medical advice. Excitedly reaching into the air in front of him, he comments "I'm popping the bubbles." When no bubbles are observed, what should be the next steps?

CASE 79-2

A 73-year-old retired secretary with a history of hypertension, diabetes, and hypercholesterolemia, was readmitted from an acute rehabilitation facility for failure to thrive. She was discharged from the hospital one week ago, after having recovered uneventfully from a thoracoabdominal aortic aneurysm repair two weeks earlier. Her nurse at the rehabilitation facility informed the medical team that "she was just not motivated to get better—she refused physical therapy and would not eat her meals." Her daughter reports that "before her surgery she had all her marbles, but now she gets confused about where she is, and sometimes she doesn't even recognize me." During family visits she was unusually distractible and drowsy during the day. How should the health care team approach this problem?

INTRODUCTION

Delirium is common in hospitalized patients. The prevalence of delirium may be as high as 80% in mechanically ventilated patients in the intensive care unit (ICU), 50% in geriatric post-operative patients, and 10% to 40% in general medical patients. Patients who develop delirium frequently have multiple risk factors. These include nonmodifiable factors, such as increased age, preexisting cognitive impairment, and a history of prior stroke or brain injury. Important modifiable risk factors include (1) exposure to deliriogenic medications, (2) infection, (3) metabolic derangement, (4) organ failure, (5) dehydration, (6) malnutrition, (7) surgery, (8) immobility, (9) use of physical restraints, (10) sensory impairment, (11) sleep deprivation, (12) pain, and (13) drug withdrawal or intoxication.

PRACTICE POINT

Delirium as a red flag

- Think of delirium as a nonspecific warning sign, like fever or hypotension, that something serious may be wrong and requires further investigation. Thirty-nine percent of inpatients with delirium die within one year. *Don't ignore this red flag.*

Delirium is associated with increased mortality, morbidity, and length of stay. Estimates of annual U.S. health care costs attributed to delirium range from $40 billion to $150 billion. Delirious patients require extra care following discharge from acute inpatient units and are at increased risk of being discharged to a skilled nursing facility rather than an acute rehabilitation facility or directly home. Patients often suffer because of frightening memories from delirious episodes while hospitalized. Such experiences can result in appreciable anxiety and preoccupation long after delirium has cleared, significantly impacting the patient's quality of life for months to years. Family members are often distressed by the changed demeanor and behavior of their loved one, making care and support more challenging.

PATHOPHYSIOLOGY

The central feature of delirium is an acute disturbance of consciousness that is accompanied by altered cognition and/or perception. Disruptions in brain function occur in the brainstem, thalamus, prefrontal cortex, fusiform cortex, and parietal lobes. This widespread cortical dysfunction is typically associated with diffuse and symmetric slowing of electrical activity on electroencephalography (EEG), although fast electrical activity occurs in some cases, especially in alcohol or sedative withdrawal.

Figure 79-1 depicts numerous potential pathways to delirium and underscores its complex pathogenesis. Neurotransmitter imbalances, especially cholinergic deficiency and dopaminergic excess, may play a key role in the development of delirium. This

Diagnostic Criteria for Delirium*

All of the following are required:

1. Disturbance of consciousness (ie, reduced clarity of awareness of the environment) with reduced ability to focus, sustain, or shift attention.
2. A change in cognition (such as memory deficit, disorientation, language disturbance) or the development of a perceptual disturbance that is not better accounted for by a preexisting, established, or evolving dementia.
3. The disturbance develops over a short period of time (usually hours to days) and tends to fluctuate during the course of the day.

*The DSM-IV TR includes a fourth criterion that relates to etiology. For example, for Delirium Due to a General Medical Condition, criterion D states: "There is evidence from the history, physical examination, or laboratory findings that the disturbance is caused by the direct physiological consequences of a general medical condition." For Substance-Induced Delirium, Substance Withdrawal Delirium, and Delirium Due to Multiple Etiologies, criterion D is specific to etiology, while criteria A, B, and C remain constant. The DSM-IV TR also includes the diagnosis Delirium Not Otherwise Specified, which can be used when an etiology has not yet been identified, or if the delirium is due to causes other than those listed above, such as pain or sensory deprivation.

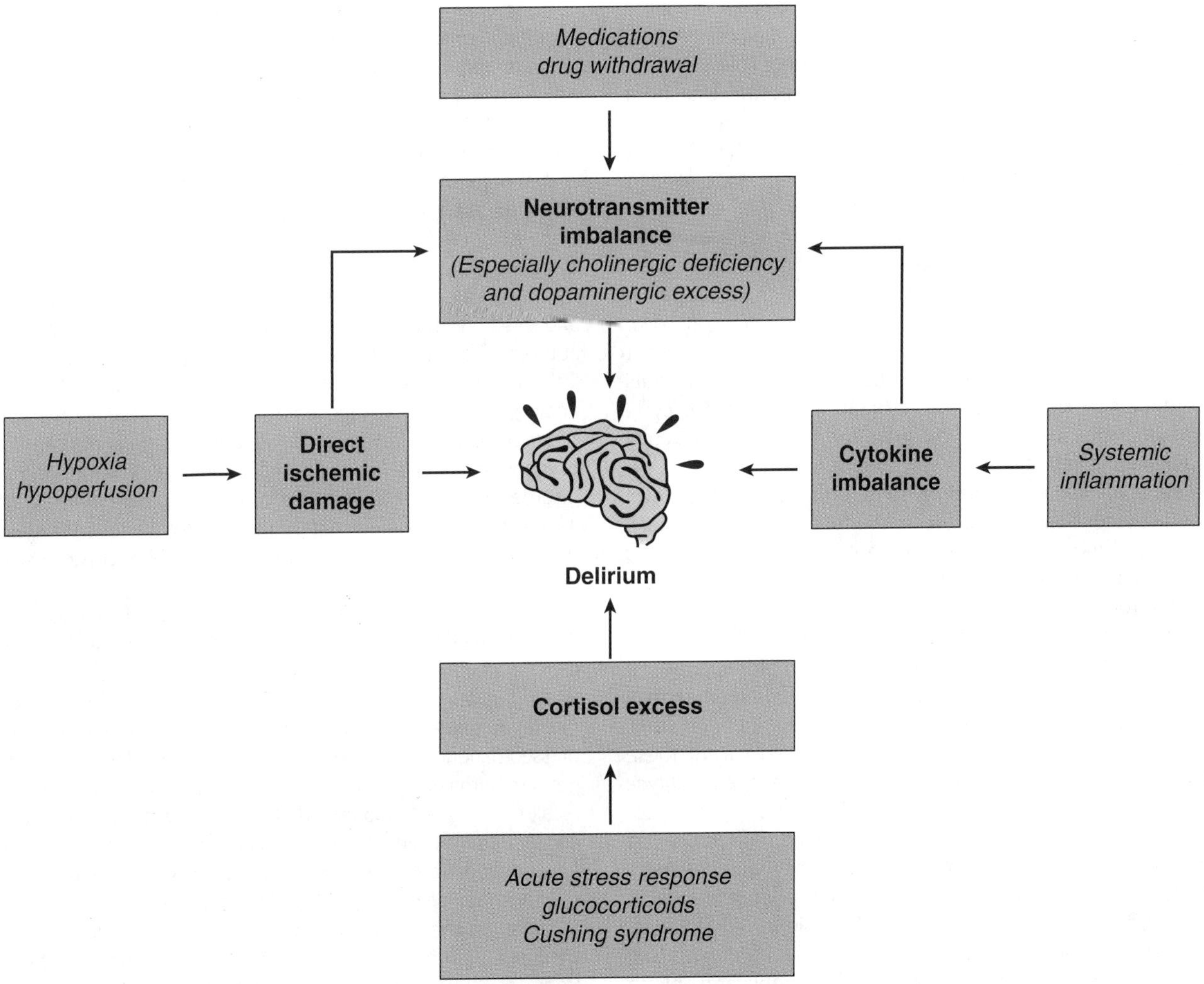

Figure 79-1 *Pathophysiology of delirium.*

hypothesis is supported by the observation that anticholinergic and dopaminergic drugs frequently precipitate delirium, whereas antidopaminergic drugs, such as antipsychotics, effectively treat the symptoms of delirium. Other neurotransmitters, such as glutamate, GABA, serotonin, norepinephrine, and histamine, have also been implicated in the pathogenesis of delirium (for example, norepinephrine and glutamate hyperactivity and GABA hypoactivity are associated with *delirium tremens,* while GABA hyperactivity is associated with hepatic encephalopathy).

Proinflammatory cytokines have a direct neurotoxic effect on the brain and affect the synthesis and release of neurotransmitters, thereby indirectly contributing to delirium. Finally, elevated cortisol levels and ischemic brain damage from hypoperfusion or hypoxia also have been linked to delirium. For a more detailed discussion see Chapter 26 in *Harrison's Principles of Internal Medicine, 17th edition,* Maldonado, 2008.

DIAGNOSIS OF DELIRIUM

The diagnosis of delirium is based on clinical observation of a relatively abrupt alteration in the level of consciousness, which often waxes and wanes over the course of a day, with associated inattention and changes in cognition and/or perception. Due to inattention, patients may ask the same question repeatedly or perseverate on an answer. Cognitive deficits may affect short-term and intermediate recall, word finding, orientation, and the ability to learn new information. Perceptual disturbances, such as illusions or hallucinations, are also common. Illusions are misinterpretations of stimuli (eg, mistaking an intravenous line for a snake), while hallucinations are perceptions without stimuli. Hallucinations are most frequently visual (eg, seeing bugs crawling on the walls), but can be auditory (eg, hearing voices), or tactile (eg, feeling bugs crawling on the skin). These disturbances arise as physiologic consequences of medical illness or from substance intoxication or withdrawal, rather than from an underlying psychiatric condition.

There are other common features of delirium that are not necessary for the diagnosis but are noteworthy because they often mimic mental illness. Patients may develop fixed, false, idiosyncratic beliefs (delusions), often persecutory in nature. For example, delirious patients commonly believe that their nurses or doctors intend to harm them. Other frequent findings include speech that is difficult to follow or that frequently wanders off topic (disorganized speech). Patients may also experience significant and rapid shifts in emotional tone (affective lability), with bouts of tearfulness, anxiety, or increased irritability. Sleep-wake cycle disruption, with increased napping during the day and difficulty with sustained sleep at night, is common.

Subtypes of delirium are distinguished by the predominant level of psychomotor activity. The *hypoactive subtype* is characterized by decreased motor activity and increased somnolence. Patients appear quietly indifferent to their surroundings and have great difficulty arousing and sustaining attention. Treating physicians may misattribute this presentation to a depressive disorder. The *hyperactive subtype* is associated with increased motor activity and agitation. Patients are restless, talkative, and aroused. They may pull at intravenous lines and indwelling catheters or even strike out against caregivers. Although they appear fully alert, these patients have trouble sustaining attention. The *mixed subtype* includes features of both increased and decreased psychomotor activity. While hyperactive behavior is easy for nurses and doctors to identify, hypoactive delirium is often overlooked because these patients are not demanding, and their cognitive limitations must be elicited through direct examination. To avoid missing hypoactive delirium, physicians must maintain a high index of suspicion and should expect all patients to be easily arousable and able to perform basic cognitive tasks at their preadmission level.

A number of screening tools for delirium have been developed. The Mini-Mental State Examination (MMSE) is a nonspecific but widely used tool that tests cognitive performance. Baseline scores vary widely, so it is most useful when performed upon hospital admission, if a patient is not delirious, and then repeated serially throughout the hospitalization. When using the MMSE, physicians should be aware that highly educated individuals may perform well even when frankly delirious. Examples of more specific screening tools include the Confusion Assessment Method (CAM) and the Delirium Rating Scale-Revised-98 (DRS-R-98), both of which have been validated in general medical or geriatric populations. For patients in the ICU setting, the CAM-ICU (a modified version of the CAM that can be administered to nonverbal, mechanically ventilated patients) has been demonstrated to be a valid and highly reliable screening tool that is easily administered by ICU nurses. Another validated instrument for the critical care setting is the Intensive Care Delirium Screening Checklist (ICDSC), a cumulative checklist that is completed during each nursing shift over a 24-hour period. Both the CAM-ICU and the ICDSC can be downloaded from the following Web site: http://www.icudelirium.org. Finally, the EEG, which typically reveals diffuse slowing in the setting of delirium (except in *delirium tremens,* which is associated with fast activity), may help support a diagnosis of delirium or rule out nonconvulsive seizure activity; however, its use as a primary diagnostic tool is not indicated, since it is neither sufficiently sensitive nor specific.

DIFFERENTIAL DIAGNOSIS

Physicians frequently misattribute signs and symptoms of delirium to psychiatric illness. For example, distinguishing delirium from dementia can be challenging. Both diagnoses are associated with cognitive impairment. However, dementia without superimposed delirium does not result in waxing and waning levels of consciousness. The patient's recent baseline physical and mental status, along with timing of onset, pattern of symptom fluctuation, and duration of symptoms will help to distinguish these two syndromes and should be carefully elicited from collateral informants (eg, family, bedside nurse). Delirium is rapid in onset over hours to days, while dementia involves a protracted decline over months to years. "Sundowning," variably defined in the literature, refers to an increase in confusion and agitation during late afternoon and evening among a subset of patients with dementia. Some authors regard this as a delirium-related phenomenon; however, little systematic research has been conducted, and multiple other etiologies have been proposed (for example, the phenomenon has been explained as a response to fatigue or to unmet physical or psychological needs, or as the consequence of underlying sleep disorders or inadequate light exposure during the day). In practice, it must be remembered that demented patients can also develop delirium. Whenever there is a fluctuating level of consciousness, a workup for delirium should be initiated.

Delirium, especially the hypoactive subtype, is also commonly confused with a depressive illness. Patients with either diagnosis may have significant psychomotor slowing, poor oral intake, and sleep disruption. They may appear withdrawn and sad, and they may even express a desire to die or end their lives. However, depressed patients do not experience alterations in level of consciousness. They may be inattentive and have problems with short-term recall, but they remain oriented. They also frequently have a personal and/or family history of depression and describe a gradual onset of symptoms, in contrast to the acute onset observed with delirium.

A number of other psychiatric disorders also may be misdiagnosed in the delirious patient. Hyperactive delirium may be confused with mania, and prominent hallucinations or delusions frequently raise concern for schizophrenia. Delirious patients who are anxious may be misdiagnosed with anxiety disorders.

Moreover, those who are irritable (such that they refuse medical care) or inattentive (such that they fail to follow nursing instructions) may be considered "difficult" or "noncompliant," even when their behaviors result from delirium and are not within their control. In all these cases, if there is a fluctuating level of consciousness or disorientation, delirium is a more likely diagnosis than any other psychiatric condition. The past psychiatric history and timing of symptom onset are also essential in making a diagnosis. Most psychiatric disorders present by early adulthood, although there are exceptions, such as depressive disorders. Nevertheless, if a geriatric patient is suddenly seeing rats scurrying across the room or is described by family members as "easy-going and slow-to-anger" but is observed to be "difficult," a new-onset psychiatric disorder is unlikely, and delirium should be high on the differential diagnosis.

Because delirium can masquerade as almost any psychiatric disorder, it is imperative that physicians avoid basing any new psychiatric diagnoses on a patient's mental status while he or she is still delirious. Even if history obtained from collateral informants suggests that there is an underlying anxiety disorder or major depressive disorder, pharmacologic treatment of these disorders should not be initiated until the patient's delirium has cleared, since new medications may worsen the delirium and response to a new medication cannot be properly assessed while a patient is still delirious. Physicians should also be wary of attributing psychiatric symptoms to a patient's known chronic psychiatric illness without thoroughly evaluating whether the symptoms are consistent with that illness. Just as demented patients can become delirious, so can patients with any other psychiatric disorder.

TREATMENT OF DELIRIUM

Delirium is a medically important indicator. It may be the first sign of a new medical condition that is life threatening, such as worsening organ failure, overdose, new infection, or a central nervous system (CNS) event (see **Table 79-1** for a list of common causes). The most important goal in treating delirium is to discover and correct the underlying cause(s). **Table 79-2** outlines considerations in the work-up of delirium. Start by reviewing the history, doing a physical exam, and performing basic laboratory investigations.

WITHDRAWAL-RELATED DELIRIUM

As a first step, determine whether alcohol, benzodiazepine, or barbiturate withdrawal is a cause of the delirium. Obtain a history from the patient and collateral informants (including outpatient health care providers) to determine the duration, pattern, and quantity of alcohol intake; the extent of any prescription or illicit use of benzodiazepines or barbiturates; and whether there are any prior episodes of withdrawal symptoms. Review the street names for readily available prescription drugs in your area. For example, "pins" can refer to Klonopin (clonazepam) tablets, and "bars" can refer to 2-mg Xanax (alprazolam) tablets, which are commonly sold in illicit settings.

If a patient is in withdrawal, physical examination will typically reveal autonomic arousal (hypertension, fever, tachycardia, tongue and extremity tremor, agitation) or pronounced instability of vital signs. Peak autonomic withdrawal from alcohol occurs 72 to 96 hours from the last drink, while withdrawal from long-acting benzodiazepines (eg, diazepam) may take up to one week to peak. Delirium may then extend several weeks beyond the presence of withdrawal signs. GABAergic agents such as chlordiazepoxide, diazepam, oxazepam, or lorazepam are the treatment of choice. One approach is to give a loading dose of a long-acting agent (eg, chlordiazepoxide 50–100 mg orally every 1–2 hours for mild to moderate withdrawal or diazepam 5–10 mg IV as frequently as every 5–10 minutes for severe withdrawal) until the patient is calm. The long half-life of these agents then allows for a smooth self taper. In the event of breakthrough withdrawal signs, additional medication (eg, chlordiazepoxide 25–50 mg orally or

TABLE 79-1 Causes of Delirium: "DELIRIVM"

D	Drugs/Poisons • *Medications* (see Table 79-3) • *Drugs of abuse* (eg, alcohol, cocaine, PCP, inhalants) • *Industrial poisons* (eg, organophosphates, heavy metals, organic solvents) • *Animal, plant, and mushroom toxins* • *Withdrawal* (from alcohol or sedatives/hypnotics)
E	External insults • *Closed-head injury* • *Heat stroke* • *Hypothermia* • *Electrocution*
L	Lesions from cancer • *Primary brain cancer* • *Meningeal carcinomatosis* • *Metastatic lesions* (especially from melanoma and lung, breast, colon, and kidney cancers)
I	Infections • *Intracranial* (bacterial/viral/fungal encephalitis or meningitis, brain/epidural/subdural abscess, trichinosis, cerebral malaria, fungal infections, Creutzfeld-Jakob disease, neurosyphilis; in HIV/AIDS: cytomegalovirus encephalitis; cryptococcal meningitis, progressive multifocal leukoencephalopathy, toxoplasmosis, tubercular meningitis) • *Systemic* (sepsis, pneumonia, subacute bacterial endocarditis, influenza, mononucleosis, mumps, typhoid fever, Lyme disease, Behcet disease, brucellosis, psittacosis, Rocky Mountain spotted fever, typhus; in HIV/AIDS: disseminated herpes zoster, candidiasis)
R	Remote effects of cancer (paraneoplastic syndromes) • *Paraneoplastic limbic encephalitis* (especially with lung, breast, or testicular cancers; paraneoplastic syndromes may occur before there are any signs of cancer on imaging)
I	Ictal/Interictal/Postictal (Seizures)
V	Vascular Causes • *Emboli from cardiac source* • *Intracranial bleed or thrombosis* • *Hypertensive encephalopathy* • *Autoimmune* (lupus cerebritis, sarcoid, polyarteritis nodosa, thrombotic thrombocytopenic purpura) • *Circulatory collapse* (shock)
M	Metabolic Causes • *Hypoxia* • *Hypoglycemia* • *Electrolyte imbalance* (hyponatremia, hypernatremia, hypercalcemia, hypocalcemia, hypokalemia, hyperkalemia, hypomagnesemia, hypermagnesemia, hypophosphatemia) • *Acidosis or alkalosis* • *Errors of metabolism* (porphyria) • *Vitamin deficiency* (vitamin B12, thiamine, nicotinic acid) • *Vitamin intoxication* (vitamin A, vitamin D) • *Organ failure* (kidney, liver, lungs, pancreas) • *Endocrinopathies* (hyperthyroidism, hypothyroidism, hyperparathyroidism, hypopituitarism, Addison disease, Cushing syndrome, insulinoma, diabetic ketoacidosis, hyperosmolar nonketotic hyperglycemia)

TABLE 79-2 A Delirium Checklist

✓ **Start with a history, physical exam, and targeted testing.**

- History should include a time-course of changes in behavior and cognition; a thorough substance abuse history; and a complete list of medications, including any recent changes.
- Physical exam should include a complete neurologic exam.
- Basic tests should include a CBC, CMP, Ca, Mg, phosphate, glucose, thyroid function tests, B12, ECG, CXR, oxygen saturation, urine toxicology screen, and urinalysis.

✓ **Consider withdrawal** as a possible cause of delirium, especially if the patient is agitated and has autonomic hyperactivity, with tachycardia, hypertension, fever and/or tremor. Obtain a detailed history of prior alcohol or benzodiazepine use. Treat with benzodiazepines using a loading method with long-acting benzodiazepines or a symptom-based approach with short-acting benzodiazepines. See the earlier section on Withdrawal-Related Delirium for more detailed guidelines.

✓ **Review medication list.**

Does the addition of a new medication coincide with the change in mental state?
Discontinue/replace offending drugs, such as:

- Benzodiazepines, propofol, nonbenzodiazepine hypnotics
- Anticholinergics, such as diphenhydramine, ranitidine, promethazine, atropine
- Corticosteroids
- Opioids
- Other known deliriogenic medications (see Table 79-3)

Obtain medication levels when relevant (for example, for cyclosporine, digoxin, lithium, phenobarbital, phenytoin, theophylline, valproic acid).

✓ **Ensure adequate analgesia,** but discontinue patient-controlled analgesia device (PCA).

✓ **Workup for new infection:** Review CBC, urinalysis, and CXR. Send urine for culture and sensitivity if urinalysis is abnormal. Obtain blood cultures if the patient is febrile. Get a head CT and lumbar puncture if headache or nuchal rigidity are present.

✓ **Consider worsening organ failure** (eg kidney, liver): Check labs and correct where possible.

✓ **Correct abnormal electrolytes**

- Aim for Na close to 140, especially in the elderly
- Treat hyper- and hypocalcemia
- Correct hypomagnesemia

✓ **Consider hypoxia or hypercarbia:** Get blood gas/pulse oximetry and CXR. If indicated, provide supplemental oxygen or noninvasive ventilation.

✓ **Consider the following tests if initial workup proves negative:**

- RPR, ANA, HIV, ammonia
- Brain MRI
- Heavy metal screen, urine porphyrins, paraneoplastic antibodies (anti-Hu, anti-Ma, anti-Ta)
- EEG (to rule out seizure activity or if the diagnosis of delirium is in doubt)

✓ **Ensure adequate nutrition and hydration, as well as regular bowel movements.**

✓ **Improve sleep-wake cycle.**

- Reorient patient to day/night (keep lights on and blinds open during day; keep room dimly lit and control noise at night).
- If sleep aid is needed, use haloperidol or an atypical antipsychotic agent.

✓ **Provide glasses and hearing aids,** if applicable.

✓ **Reorient the patient regularly.**

- Provide a board with the day's date, the name of the hospital, the patient's location within the hospital, and names of care team members.
- Avoid staff and room changes.
- Encourage family members to bring in photographs and familiar items from home, to visit frequently, and to stay overnight if possible.
- Verbally reorient and reassure the patient throughout the day.

✓ **Avoid restraints.**

- Obtain a 24-hour sitter or family member to redirect and reassure the patient.
- Turn off the TV, play soothing music, and speak calmly and softly to the patient.
- Treat agitation with neuroleptics if redirection and reassurance fail.
- Discontinue urinary catheters and intravenous lines as appropriate.

✓ **Mobilize the patient.**

- Get the patient out of bed and engaged in physical and occupational therapy.

ANA, antinuclear antibody; Ca, calcium; CBC, complete blood count; CMP, comprehensive metabolic panel; CT, computed tomography, CXR, chest radiography; ECG, electrocardiography; EEG, electroencephalogram; Mg, magnesium; MRI, magnetic resonance imaging; RPR, rapid plasma reagin.

diazepam 5–10 mg IV) can be given every 2 hours as needed. Another option is symptom-triggered dosing of a short-acting agent (eg, oxazepam 15–30 mg orally or lorazepam 1–2 mg IV every 2 hours as needed for symptoms of withdrawal, such as tremor, agitation, insomnia, elevated heart rate, or elevated blood pressure). Individuals with advanced liver disease should be treated with oxazepam or lorazepam preferentially, as these medications have shorter half-lives and no active metabolites. If the patient cannot be closely monitored for signs of withdrawal, then these short-acting agents should be given on a fixed schedule

TABLE 79-3 Common Medications Linked to Delirium

Antiarrhythmics	***Antidepressants***	Famotidine
Disopyramide	Tricyclics	Ranitidine
Lidocaine	Phenelzine	***Immunomodulators***
Procainamide	Trazodone	5-Fluorouracil
Quinidine	Paroxetine	Cyclosporine
Antibiotics	Fluoxetine	Chlorambucil
Acyclovir	Citalopram	Ifosfamide
Amphotericin B	Escitalopram	Interferon
Aminogylcosides	Mirtazapine	Interleukin-2
Cephalosporins	***Antihistamines***	Tacrolimus
Chloroquine	Diphenhydramine	Tamoxifen
Chloramphenicol	Hydroxyzine	Vinblastine
Ganciclovir	***Antihypertensives***	Vincristine
Isoniazid	Clonidine	***Muscle Relaxants***
Mefloquine	Nifedipine	Baclofen
Metronidazole	Methyldopa	Cyclobenzaprine
Rifampin	Propranolol	***Narcotics***
Sulfonamides	Timolol	All formulations
Tetracyclines	***Anti-inflammatory Agents***	***Other Medications***
Vancomycin	Corticosteroids	Digitalis preparations
Voriconazole	Ibuprofen	Dipyridamole
Anticholinergics	Indomethacin	Disulfiram
Atropine	Naproxen	TC
Benztropine	Sulindac	Lithium
Scopolamine	***Antipsychotics***	Pregabalin
Trihexyphenidyl	Clozaril	Propylthiouracil
Anticonvulsants	Low-potency typical antipsychotics	Sildenafil
Ethosuximide	Quetiapine	Timolol ophthalmic
Carbamazepine	Olanzapine	Tramadol
Gabapentin	***Dopamine Agonists***	Warfarin
Phenobarbital	Amantadine	***Sedatives***
Phenytoin	Bromocriptine	Barbiturates
Primidone	Levodopa	Benzodiazepines
Valproic acid	Selegiline	Nonbenzodiazepine hypnotics
Antiemetics	***HIV Medications***	***Sympathomimetics***
Chlorpromazine	Efavirenz	Amphetamine
Metoclopramide	Nevirapine	Ephedrine
Promethazine	Zidovudine	Phenylephrine
Prochlorperazine	***H2 Blockers***	Theophylline
	Cimetidine	

and tapered by 20–25% daily. Although symptom-triggered dosing has been associated with less total benzodiazepine administration and fewer days of delirium per patient than fixed schedule therapy, it is fully effective only when nurses have both the time and ability to monitor patients regularly and frequently.

If a patient's delirium worsens or fails to respond to treatment with benzodiazepines, the treating physician should consider alternative etiologies of the patient's continued delirium. For example, benzodiazepines may effectively treat *delirium tremens* while simultaneously precipitating hepatic encephalopathy. If a formerly agitated patient becomes sedated and confused, clinicians should consider both overuse of benzodiazepines and hepatic encephalopathy.

MEDICATION-RELATED DELIRIUM

It is important to review patients' medication lists, looking for any new medication that coincided with the onset of delirium. In the setting of worsening kidney or liver function, a previously well-tolerated medication may cause delirium due to decreased drug clearance. The addition of new medications may render an old medication newly deliriogenic by inhibiting its metabolism, or old medications may cause delirium in the setting of new neurologic insults. Review the medication list for anticholinergic and other frequently implicated agents (listed in **Table 79-3**) and discontinue or replace these medications.

If history and physical exam reveal little or no risk of withdrawal-related delirium, avoid using benzodiazepines (unless a patient was

TABLE 79-4 Guide to the Use of Antipsychotics in Treating Delirium*

1. **Obtain an ECG.** If QTc ≥ 450 msec, weigh the risks and benefits of available treatment options and carefully monitor the QTc interval if antipsychotic started.
2. **Check serum calcium, potassium, and magnesium.** Keep $K^+ > 4$ and $Mg^{++} > 2$ mEq/L[†]. Normalize serum calcium.
3. **Avoid use of other QTc-prolonging medications.** For a list of such medications, see http://www.long-qt-syndrome.com/lqts_drugs.html.
4. **Select antipsychotic** based on side effect profile, ease of administration, and cost.[§] Haloperidol is a good first choice, given its low cost, known efficacy, and ease of administration (it's available intravenously and intramuscularly). At low doses it is unlikely to cause extrapyramidal side effects such as acute dystonia, akathisia, or parkinsonism. If these do occur, risperidone or olanzapine can be tried.
5. **Titrate dosing of antipsychotic** to the patient's level of agitation:

Initial oral dosing of haloperidol[¶,**]

Level of agitation	*Young/healthy*	*Elderly/frail*
Mild	0.5–1.0 mg	0.25–0.5 mg (**start low**)
Moderate	2.0–5.0 mg	1.0 mg
Severe	5.0–10.0 mg	2.0 mg

Initial oral dosing of atypical antipsychotics

Antipsychotic	*Initial dose*	*As-needed dose*
Risperidone	0.25–0.5 mg twice daily	0.25–0.5 mg every 4 hours; up to 4 mg/day
Olanzapine	2.5–5.0 mg qhs	2.5–5 mg every 6 hours; up to 20 mg/day
Quetiapine	25–50 mg twice daily	25–50 mg every 4 hours; up to 600 mg/day

6. **Monitor for side effects.** Akathisia can be mistaken for worsening agitation. Examine patients daily for cogwheeling and stiffness. Follow QTc and consider alternative treatment options if ≥450 msec or > 25% above baseline. Keep $K^+ > 4$ and $Mg^{++} > 2$ mEq/L. Normalize serum calcium.
7. **Continue to search for causes of delirium.**
8. **Taper antipsychotic slowly,** over a period of days, once the patient's agitation and sleep disruption have fully resolved.

*Neuroleptics have consistently proven more efficacious than placebo in the treatment of delirium; however, the Federal Drug Administration has not approved any medication for the treatment of delirium.

[†]This recommendation comes from Huffman J, Stern T, Januzzi J. The Psychiatric Management of Patients with Cardiac Disease. In: Stern T, Fricchione G, Cassem N, et al (eds.). *Massachusetts General Hospital Handbook of General Hospital Psychiatry, 5th ed.* Philadelphia: Mosby, 2004, pp. 547–569. In our own experience, a magnesium level of > 2 mEq/L is hard to achieve. A more realistic goal may be to keep magnesium levels above the low end of normal (ie, > 1.3 mEq/L), aiming for the higher end of normal (ie, 2 mEq/L).

[§]Haloperidol is the most widely studied neuroleptic in the treatment of delirium. There have been few randomized controlled trials comparing the efficacy of individual neuroleptics. Several small studies have failed to demonstrate a difference in efficacy between haloperidol and risperidone or between haloperidol and olanzapine. Other atypicals have not been compared to haloperidol.

[¶]Intravenous and intramuscular haloperidol are twice as potent as oral haloperidol. Thus, 1 mg orally is equivalent to 0.5 mg IM/IV.

**May repeat as frequently as every 30 minutes, until agitation subsides. Standing doses can be given every 8–12 hours.

taking them prior to admission, in which case they should be continued at the preadmission dose). Avoid even the nonbenzodiazepine hypnotics, or "z" drugs used for sleep, such as zolpidem or zaleplon. These medications can also cause or contribute to delirium. Complaints of anxiety and agitation are common in delirious patients. Resist the urge to treat with benzodiazepines. If reassurance and redirection fail to calm a patient's agitation, try antipsychotics instead (See **Table 79-4**).

PRACTICE POINT

Beware of benzodiazepines

- Be wary of using benzodiazepines to treat agitation in a delirious patient who is not in alcohol or benzodiazepine withdrawal. Benzodiazepine use can be like **adding fuel to the fire.**

Opioids can also contribute to delirium. Reduce the dose of opioids and consider nonopioid methods of pain management. Tramadol should be used with caution, as this medication has also been associated with the development of delirium. If a patient with a patient-controlled analgesia (PCA) pump becomes delirious, discontinue its use promptly. Patients who have difficulty remembering and attending to their surroundings will often unintentionally overuse the PCA. In addition, mounting anxiety from delirium may result in frenetic use of the PCA, which, in turn, can worsen delirium. Use nurse-administered intravenous or oral agents instead. The management of pain in the delirious patient is a delicate balancing act; just as the overuse of opioids can cause delirium, so can pain itself precipitate or worsen delirium if it is poorly controlled. Careful assessment and treatment of the patient's pain are vital.

INFECTION, ELECTROLYTE IMBALANCE, AND ORGAN FAILURE

Look for new sources of infection and perform an appropriate workup. Include cultures and antibiotic treatment as indicated. A relatively minor urinary tract infection in a mildly demented elderly patient can trigger delirium. Electrolyte abnormalities such as hypo- and hypernatremia or hypo- and hypercalcemia are relatively common. Screen for these, and correct any imbalances. Organ failure, including pulmonary compromise (with hypoxia and hypercarbia), renal failure (with uremia), and hepatic failure (with hyperammonemia) are all potentially reversible causes of delirium. If history and physical examination are consistent with a neurologic condition (eg, the patient has a history of headache, head trauma, anticoagulation, fever, stiff neck, or focal neurologic findings on physical exam), consider CNS imaging and lumbar puncture.

NONPHARMACOLOGIC MANAGEMENT OF DELIRIUM

1. **Orient patients by providing environmental cues.** Delirious patients have great difficulty acquiring and retaining new information. Because disorientation is common, staff and family should regularly remind patients of where they are and why they are in the hospital. Provide glasses and hearing aids if patients suffer from visual or auditory impairment. Familiarize patients with their surroundings by placing family photos, clocks, and calendars within their view. Encourage family members to visit/and or stay with patients, and make every effort to provide delirious patients with private rooms so that family members can stay overnight. Limit room and staff changes as much as possible.
2. **Reduce overstimulation.** Reduce noise, loud talk, and laughter. Delirious, disoriented individuals can easily assign sinister meanings to these random stimuli. Urge staff to use a quiet voice and to interact calmly with the delirious patient. Turn off the TV if the patient is not attending to it. Try soothing music to calm the patient.
3. **Reduce restraint use.** The use of physical restraints can often worsen anxiety, increase delirious patients' misgivings about their safety, and contribute to delusional beliefs about persecution. Round the clock observation of the patient by staff, family, or friends can minimize the need for restraints, especially when an observer is skilled at redirecting and reassuring the patient. Remember that a wide variety of medical equipment, including catheters and intravenous lines, function as restraints and may exacerbate agitation. Avoid their use as much as possible.
4. **Improve sleep-wake cycle.** Strong circadian signals can help combat delirium-associated sleep disturbance. Thus, treatment of delirium should include opening window blinds during the day and shutting off or dimming lights at night. Instead of sedative medications, use back massage, warm milk or herbal tea, and relaxing music or "white noise" to help patients sleep at night.
5. **Mobilize early.** Get patients out of bed and involved in occupational and physical therapy as soon as possible. Studies in several ICUs in the United States have shown that decreased sedation and early mobilization protocols result in a dramatic reduction in the prevalence of delirium and a commensurate drop in length of stay, even among critically ill individuals.
6. **Maintain nutrition, hydration, and oxygenation.** Monitor nutrition and hydration status, and maintain adequate oxygenation. Dehydration and hypoxia are common contributors to delirium. Ensure regular bowel movements and monitor urinary output, as constipation and urinary retention can both lead to agitation.

PHARMACOLOGIC MANAGEMENT OF DELIRIUM

The treatment of an agitated and/or combative delirious patient is particularly challenging. Treatment of agitation should begin with nonpharmacologic measures, such as reassurance and redirection of the patient. Medications should be considered only if nonpharmacologic management fails to control agitation or if patients are experiencing delusions or perceptual disturbances. There are limited numbers of randomized clinical trials examining the pharmacologic management of delirium. While haloperidol is the most commonly used medication (see Table 79-4), it is important to stress that its use, as well as the use of other antipsychotic agents in this setting, has not been approved by the Food and Drug Administration and remains "off-label." Current evidence suggests that there is no significant difference between low-dose haloperidol (≤ 3 mg/day) and atypical antipsychotics (such as olanzapine and risperidone) in decreasing the severity of delirium symptoms or in the incidence of extrapyramidal side effects (EPS). Higher daily doses of haloperidol are associated with an increased risk of EPS, and this may be reason to consider an atypical agent instead. The main advantages of haloperidol are its availability in intravenous and intramuscular formulation, as well as its low cost.

Prolongation of the electrocardiographic QT interval leading to torsade de pointes is a rare but recognized complication of all antipsychotic agents and can be made more severe by intravenous administration of these drugs. Monitor the QTc regularly and titrate medications accordingly. Table 79-4 includes current guidelines for the use of antipsychotics in the delirious patient.

Benzodiazepines should be used as a first-line treatment in patients with GABAergic-withdrawal-related delirious states, as described above. Avoid the use of these agents in treating agitated delirium due to other causes. Benzodiazepines may make confusion and agitation much worse. The use of as-needed bolus, rather than continuous infusion, of sedation medications in the ICU has been associated with significantly fewer days of delirium.

Case studies have suggested that cholinesterase inhibitors may be effective in the treatment of delirium, but one small randomized controlled trial of donepezil versus placebo in postoperative patients showed no significant decrease in the incidence of delirium.

THE ROLE OF PSYCHIATRIC CONSULTATION

The hospital physician will invariably encounter cases in which the diagnosis and/or management of delirium are not straightforward, even after following the guidelines presented in this chapter. In such cases, psychiatric consultation should be obtained. The psychiatric consultant can help clarify an ambiguous diagnosis, recommend further diagnostic studies, or suggest alternative management strategies when those suggested above prove insufficient.

PRACTICE POINT

30–40% of delirium cases are preventable.

- It's easier to prevent than to treat delirium.
- Address modifiable risk factors in patients at high risk for delirium.

PRIMARY PREVENTION

Delirium is often preventable. The most effective way to "treat" delirium is to prevent its occurrence. The interventions described under Nonpharmacologic Management of Delirium have been demonstrated to decrease the incidence of delirium when used preventatively. In a landmark study of elderly patients admitted to a general medical service, a multicomponent intervention (including regular orientation and cognitive stimulation, use of nonpharmacologic methods to promote sleep, early mobilization, correction of dehydration, and proactive use of visual and auditory aids), significantly reduced the incidence of delirium to 9.9% in the intervention group (n = 429) compared to 15% in those who received usual care (n = 429). This striking reduction in the development of delirium suggests that these strategies should be considered a part of routine care for all high-risk hospitalized patients.

Other interventions have also been studied in randomized controlled trials. A study of mechanically ventilated patients in the ICU showed that early introduction (ie, within 72 hours) of routine, daily physical and occupational therapy reduced the median number of days of delirium per patient from 4 in control patients ($n = 55$) to 2 in study patients ($n = 49$). An Australian study demonstrated a decreased incidence of delirium when geriatric patients received rehabilitation services at home instead of in the hospital. Importantly, the patients who received home rehabilitation were followed by a team that included physicians who proactively assessed and treated medical conditions (eg, obtained cultures and started IV antibiotics) in order to avoid readmission to the hospital.

Other preventative strategies include avoiding exposure to known deliriogenic medicines, especially anticholinergics and benzodiazepines, in patients at high risk for delirium. See Table 79-3 for a list of medications that are associated with delirium. A detailed history of alcohol, benzodiazepine, and barbiturate use and prophylactic treatment with a benzodiazepine can also prevent withdrawal-related delirium in susceptible patients.

Several studies have suggested a role for oral haloperidol in delirium prophylaxis. While the use of haloperidol in a group of older patients presenting for elective hip surgery reduced the number of delirium days as well as the severity of delirium episodes, it did not reduce the overall incidence of delirium. Further study is needed before its use as a prophylactic agent becomes routine (**Table 79–5**).

Studies have also suggested a role for anticholinesterase inhibitors in delirium prophylaxis. A retrospective cohort study of hospitalized geriatric patients comparing the incidence of delirium in those who were on chronic rivastigmine therapy to controls found a delirium in 45.5% in the rivastigmine group ($n = 11$) compared to 88.9% in the control group ($n = 29$). This difference was statistically significant. An open-label 24-month prospective study of patients with vascular dementia found that 40% of those who received rivastigmine ($n = 115$) developed delirium, compared to 62% of control subjects ($n = 115$). The mean duration of delirium was also shorter in the rivastigmine group (4 vs. 7.86 days), and benzodiazepine or antipsychotic intake was less in the rivastigmine group, with all these differences of statistical significance. However, double-blind placebo-controlled studies in more generalizable populations are required before rivastigmine can be recommended for routine use in delirium prophylaxis.

COMPLICATIONS

Delirium is associated with significantly increased morbidity and mortality. It can lead to a host of complications, including aspiration pneumonia, pressure ulcers, trauma from accidental falls or removal of medical devices, and decreased oral intake, which may contribute to, and/or result from, an increased length of stay. The cumulative 1-year mortality rate for elderly patients with delirium ($n = 171$) has been reported to be 38%, compared to 21% for control subjects ($n = 95$) admitted to a community hospital. Studies have also found an association between delirium and subsequent long-term cognitive impairment. One study of nondemented patients aged 65 years and older reported that 18.1% of delirious patients ($n = 16$) were diagnosed with dementia by 3-year follow-up, compared to 5.6% of nondelirious patients ($n = 148$). As discussed previously, the presence of mild cognitive impairment is a known risk factor for the future development of delirium. Whether delirium actually causes long-term cognitive decline, or whether its association with cognitive decline can be attributed to preexisting subclinical neurologic pathology, is currently being investigated.

Research does demonstrate that delirium is associated with psychological sequelae, including anxiety disorders, related to the frightening nature of perceptual experiences during delirium. A systematic review of the literature reported that the rate of clinically significant PTSD symptoms up to 2 years after in-hospital delirium was 14%. Clinically significant depressive symptoms occurred in 31% of previously delirious patients.

DISCHARGE PLANNING

The goal in delirium management is to restore patients to their baseline mental state prior to discharge from the hospital by identifying and treating the underlying causes of delirium. Sometimes the underlying causes are not reversible. For example, the delirium seen in dementia with Lewy bodies seems to be caused directly by the dementing illness itself. In addition, in palliative care, up to 80% of patients may be delirious due to CNS involvement or end-stage organ failure. Adequate precautions should be taken for patients who remain delirious at the time of acute care discharge. These patients need 24-hour supervision. Staff or family caretakers should be educated in the management of the delirious patient.

QUALITY IMPROVEMENT TO ADDRESS PERFORMANCE GAPS

DELIRIUM AS AN INDICATOR OF HEALTH CARE QUALITY

The National Quality Measures Clearinghouse of the Agency for Health Care Research and Quality has identified delirium as a marker of quality of care and patient safety. Hospital-acquired delirium was proposed for the Medicare "no-pay list" but was eliminated during the public comment stage of this proposal. In part, this Medicare strategy would have inadvertently discouraged care providers from identifying and treating delirium during a hospital stay.

Timely identification of delirium is important in reducing poor outcomes; however, multiple studies suggest that physicians and nurses frequently miss this diagnosis. Medical education curricula often fail to emphasize that delirium is a medical emergency and offer little instruction regarding its diagnosis and management. A patient's cognition requires regular evaluation. This is particularly critical in the case of the quietly delirious patient (hypoactive subtype), who may utter few words and simply nod in the affirmative to leading questions. One approach to early detection of delirium is to screen all patients on units with a high prevalence of delirium, such as the ICU or geriatric units. Successful use of screening instruments depends on multidisciplinary education regarding the signs, symptoms, etiology, management, and adverse outcomes of delirium.

CASE 79-1 *(continued)*

This 56-year-old bank manager scores 23/30 on the Mini-Mental State Examination (MMSE), missing 1 point on short-term recall, 4 points on attention (spelling "WORLD" backwards), and 2 points on orientation (the day of the week and the date). His wife is alarmed by his performance and tells you that he would have "whipped through that test without any problem" at baseline. His sudden change in mental status, including changes in level of consciousness (new-onset hyperarousal), attention, cognition (disorientation and poor recall), and perceptual disturbances, is sufficient to make a diagnosis of delirium—but the cause of the delirium is unclear. This patient has a history of depression, but this would not explain his visual hallucinations and disorientation. Although cephalosporins can precipitate delirium, he did not develop signs of delirium until day five of cefazolin. On admission he reported consuming "no more than three drinks in a week—I don't like hangovers."

TABLE 79-5 Evidence-based Medicine: Key References for Delirium

Study	Methodology	Results	Limitations	Bottom Line
Inouye SK, et al. *N Engl J Med.* 1999; 340:669–676.	Prospective, individual-matched (ie, not randomized) controlled trial of a multicomponent strategy for primary prevention of delirium vs. usual care for geriatric patients on general medical units who were nondelirious at the time of admission	426 patients were assigned to each arm of the study; the incidence of delirium was lower in the intervention group (9.9% vs. 15.0%, $P = 0.02$), and the total number of days of delirium was also lower in the intervention group (105 vs. 161, $P = 0.02$), but in cases of delirium there was no difference in severity or rates of recurrence between the 2 groups.	The study was not randomized and may be subject to selection bias; a contamination effect in the usual-care group probably decreased the overall rates of delirium, which were substantially lower than anticipated on the basis of earlier studies in the same study population.	Management of delirium risk factors can be effective primary prevention of delirium in elderly patients on general medical units, but there's no evidence that it speeds the resolution of delirium or limits its severity in those who develop it.
Marcantonio E, et al. *J Am Geriatr Soc.* 2001;49: 516–522.	Prospective, randomized, blinded trial of proactive geriatrics consultation for primary prevention of delirium vs. usual care in geriatric patients admitted emergently for surgical repair of hip fracture	62 patients were randomized to geriatrics consultation and 64 to usual care; the incidence of delirium was lower in the intervention group (32% vs. 50%, $P = .04$), and especially decreased for severe delirium (12% vs. 29%), but the intervention showed little or no benefit in patients with prefracture dementia or activities of daily living (ADL) impairment.	Prefracture dementia and ADL impairment were greater in the usual-care group. When adjusted for this imbalance, effect sizes remained unchanged, but were no longer statistically significant.	Proactive geriatrics consultation involving targeted recommendations may play an important role in reducing delirium in elderly patients after hip-fracture repair, but there's no evidence that it's effective in patients with prefracture dementia or ADL impairment.
Skrobik Y, et al. *Intensive Care Med.* 2004;30: 444–449.	Prospective, randomized, nonblinded trial of oral haloperidol vs. oral olanzapine for treatment of acute delirium in ICU patients. This study was sponsored by Eli-Lilly, the manufacturer of Zyprexa.	45 patients received haloperidol and 28 patients received olanzapine; there was no difference between groups in reduction of delirium severity or in use of rescue haloperidol or benzodiazepines, but there were more extrapyramidal side effect in the haloperidol group.	High haloperidol dose (mean 6.5 mg/day vs. 4.5 mg/day of olanzapine). Similar benefit possibly achieved on lower dose haloperidol, with fewer side effects. Small sample size of patients on olanzapine reduced power to detect side effects.	Haloperidol and olanzapine appear to be equally effective at treating delirium in ICU patients, although haloperidol may be associated with more extrapyramidal side effects.
Kalisvaart K, et al. *J Am Geriatr Soc.* 2005;53:658–666.	Prospective, double-blind, randomized, placebo-controlled trial of haloperidol 1.5 mg/day started preoperatively and continued 3 days postoperatively to decrease incidence, severity, and duration of postoperative delirium in geriatric hip-surgery patients at intermediate or high risk for delirium.	212 patients received haloperidol and 218 received placebo; there was no significant difference in the incidence of delirium between the two groups, but mean delirium rating scale scores were lower with haloperidol than with placebo (14.4 vs. 18.5, $P = <.001$), mean delirium duration was shorter (5.4 vs. 11.8 days, $P = <.001$), and mean hospital stay was shorter (17.1 vs. 22.6 days, $P = <.001$) in those who developed delirium. No haloperidol-related side effects were noted.	The haloperidol dosage was low. A higher dosage could potentially allow for primary prevention of delirium but may result in more common and severe side effects.	Prophylactic use of low-dose haloperidol in orthopedic geriatric patients at intermediate or high risk for postoperative delirium did not decrease the incidence of delirium, but decreased both severity and duration of delirium, and duration of hospital stay.

His wife confirmed this pattern of drinking and denied any history of withdrawal symptoms. In response to subsequent questioning whether he takes any medicines "to help his nerves or to help him sleep," "Well, there's the Prozac for his nerves, and then there's that pill he takes at night," she replies. His wife does not recall the name of the medication, but she does remember the name of the pharmacy where her husband fills his prescriptions. The pharmacy reports a regularly filled prescription of diazepam 10 mg at bedtime. After delaying his discharge and administering diazepam 20 mg orally, the patient had a quiet night. The next morning he achieves a perfect score on the MMSE. He recalled a strange perceptual disturbance of seeing bubbles floating all around his room and even feeling a wet sensation when he popped them. Fortunately, he no longer sees them. The patient is discharged to home uneventfully on oral antibiotics, fluoxetine 30 mg daily, and diazepam 10 mg nightly.

CASE 79-2 *(continued)*

On exam, this retired 73-year-old secretary appears intermittently alert and drowsy. She is tearful and describes her mood as "sad and frustrated." She scores 19 out of 30 on the MMSE, missing 2 points for orientation (the date and the year), 5 points for attention (spelling "WORLD" backwards), 3 points for short-term recall, and 1 point for praxis (drawing interlocking pentagons). Her symptoms of tearfulness, lack of interest in meals, and her refusal to participate in physical therapy suggest the possibility of depression. However, this diagnosis does not explain her disorientation and drowsiness. Her change in mental status since the surgery, marked by drowsiness, inattention, and cognitive deficits (disorientation, poor recall, and poor praxis) is most consistent with a new diagnosis of delirium. Both she and her daughter deny any history of alcohol or sedative use, and an untreated alcohol or sedative withdrawal syndrome would not cause drowsiness. The results of basic tests recommended in Table 79-2 are only notable for a positive urinalysis. After empiric treatment with ciprofloxacin pending urine culture results, her scores on the MMSE trend slowly upwards, and she begins to eat meals and to engage in physical therapy. At the time of discharge 10 days after admission, this patient is fully alert, scores a 29 on the MMSE, and describes herself as "determined to get my independence back."

CONCLUSION

Delirium is a medical emergency that can often be prevented if at-risk patients are identified and specific interventions are put in place. Although it is common in hospital settings, it may be missed on morning rounds, as delirious patients are often quiet and withdrawn. In order to identify hypoactive delirious patients, the treatment team must maintain a high index of suspicion and actively look for deficits in attention and cognition. Once a diagnosis of delirium has been made, triggers and sustaining factors must be identified and reversed, and specific nonpharmacologic treatments should be administered. Antipsychotic medications may be indicated if agitation and sleep-wake reversal fail to respond to nonpharmacologic measures or if delusions or perceptual disturbances are present. In ambiguous or difficult cases, psychiatric consultation should be obtained. The prevention and prompt identification and management of delirium may significantly reduce length of stay, morbidity, mortality, and health care costs. It can also save patients, family members, and caretakers considerable suffering and distress.

SUGGESTED READINGS

Breitbart W, Alici Y. Agitation and delirium at the end of life. *JAMA.* 2008;300:2898–2910.

Campbell N, Boustani MA, Ayub A, et al. Pharmacological management of delirium in hospitalized adults—a systematic evidence review. *J Gen Int Med.* 2009;24:848–853.

Fong T, Tulebaev S, Inouye S. Delirium in elderly adults: diagnosis, prevention, and treatment. *Nat Rev Neurol.* 2009;5:210–220.

Maldonado JR. Pathoetiological model of delirium: a comprehensive understanding of the neurobiology of delirium and an evidence-based approach to prevention and treatment. *Crit Care Clin.* 2008;24:789–856.

Michaud L, Büla C, Berney A, et al. Delirium: guidelines for general hospitals. *J Psychosom Res.* 2007;62:371–383.

Slavney PR. Psychiatric Dimensions of Medical Practice: What Primary-Care Physicians Should Know about Delirium, Demoralization, Suicidal Thinking, and Competence to Refuse Medical Advice. Baltimore, *MD: The Johns Hopkins University Press;* 1998.

CHAPTER 80

Diarrhea

Danielle B. Scheurer, MD, MSc, FHM

Key Clinical Questions

1. What questions in the diarrhea history will guide the need for diagnostic testing?
2. What is the yield of commonly ordered diagnostic stool tests?
3. What is a practical algorithm to guide rational diagnostic stool testing?
4. What are practical supportive therapies for hospitalized patients with diarrhea?
5. What are the key preventative measures for preventing the spread of infectious diarrhea?

CASE 80-1

A previously healthy 45-year-old man sustained a motor vehicle accident resulting in multiple bony fractures and a traumatic brain injury. As such, he was admitted to the intensive care unit, intubated, sedated, and later taken to the operating room for repair of multiple fractures. On hospital day 3, the surgical team requested a medicine consultation for assessment and management of diarrhea. The patient had no history of diarrhea prior to admission, and his symptoms began on hospital day 2. The diarrhea was loose, semi-formed, 4–6 times a day, without blood, mucus, or pus. The patient remained intubated and sedated. His vital signs were stable, he was afebrile, and his abdominal exam was benign. He received feedings via a nasogastric tube, reaching nutritional goals. His medications included subcutaneous heparin prophylaxis, a proton-pump inhibitor, docusate, senna, intravenous propofol, and intravenous morphine. He had normal laboratory tests, including a white cell count of 8,000 per cubic millimeter.

INTRODUCTION

DEFINITION

The typical adult eating a western diet excretes 100–200 grams of fecal matter a day, which consists of water, electrolytes, indigestible matter, unabsorbed food, intestinal secretions, epithelial cells, and enteric bacteria. Diarrhea is defined as an abnormal increase in excretion of fecal matter to > 200 grams a day. Although no official definition for nosocomial diarrhea exists, if surmised from the definition of acute diarrhea, it is diarrhea of < 2 weeks duration that first presents during an inpatient stay.

The epidemiology of acute nosocomial and acute community-acquired diarrhea are quite disparate, and this chapter will focus on the former. The usual bacterial, viral, and protozoal suspects in community acquired diarrhea are rare culprits in nosocomial diarrhea. They will be mentioned in this chapter, to sufficiently discuss the differential diagnosis of acute diarrhea, but will be appropriately deemphasized as likely causes of diarrhea in hospitalized patients.

INCIDENCE

Diarrhea is 1 of the most common afflictions in hospitalized patients, occurring in 33–50% of inpatients. Patients who acquire diarrhea while in the hospital have longer lengths of stay and higher mortality than those who do not. Diarrhea also is associated with more diagnostic testing (stool studies, imaging exams, electrolyte monitoring), and interventions (intravenous fluids, electrolyte supplementation, and medication adjustments). It also creates issues for sanitation and quality of life, especially in patients that are not independent in mobility and self-care.

The differential diagnosis for diarrhea in hospitalized patients is extensive, but is most conveniently dichotomized into infectious and noninfectious etiologies.

INFECTIOUS DIARRHEAS

There are more than 200 million cases of infectious diarrhea in the U.S. each year, resulting in 1.8 million hospitalizations. Most infectious diarrheas are acquired by fecal-oral transmission, by

TABLE 80-1 Transmissibility of Bacterial Diarrheal Diseases

Organism	Usual Transmission	Inoculum Required to Cause Disease
Salmonella typhi	Person to person Food	High
Nontyphoidal Salmonella	Environmental animal reservoir	Low
Campylobacter	Food	Low
Escherichia coli 0157:H7	Food	Low
Shigella	Person to person Food	Low

person-to-person contact, or by food/liquids (although the latter is highly unusual in the hospital setting). Contagious spread by person-to-person contact also includes transmission through fomites, such as stethoscopes, bedside commodes, or other medical equipment. The vast majority of infectious diarrhea in inpatients is caused by *Clostridium difficile*. A full discussion of *Clostridium difficile*-associated diarrhea (CDAD) diagnosis, management, and prevention can be found in Chapter 188 *C difficile* colitis. However, a few other bacterial, viral, and protozoal agents can be acquired in the hospital setting, and these are discussed below.

BACTERIAL PATHOGENS

The bacterial pathogens that commonly cause community-acquired diarrhea are rarely a cause of diarrhea in the hospitalized patient. However, cases do arise. In the U.S., there are 5.2 million cases of bacterial diarrhea, 46,000 hospitalizations, and 1500 deaths annually. The majority of these occur in outpatients as a result of food-borne transmission. Person to person transmission is less common, and usually occurs with pathogens that only require a small inoculum to cause disease (**Table 80-1**). The usual bacterial suspects include *Salmonella spp, Shigella spp, Campylobacter spp, and Escherichia coli* 0157:H7.

Salmonella typhi is almost always acquired by person to person transmission, from an acutely infected or chronic carrier, but rarely can be transmitted through food or water. Such was the case of Mary Mallon "Typhoid Mary," a healthy Irish immigrant cook who, as an asymptomatic carrier, transmitted the infection to at least 22 people over 7 years before being identified as the source of the outbreaks. The rarity of *Salmonella typhi* outbreaks in the U.S. is a reflection of exemplary hygiene and sewage standards. Transmissibility of the organism depends on the density of the organism in the infected person, and the infectivity of the strain. Generally a high density of inoculum is required to result in clinical symptoms, based on voluntary experimental ingestions. Nontyphoidal *Salmonella spp*, on the other hand, are rarely transmitted person to person, usually derive from an environmental animal reservoir (farm animals), and require a much lower density of inoculum to cause clinical infection.

Campylobacter spp, similar to nontyphoidal *Salmonella spp*, is rarely transmitted person to person, and is usually linked to contaminated food sources (meat, dairy, or water). Although a small inoculum is required for infection, widespread outbreaks rarely occur, because most patients remain asymptomatic.

Escherichia coli 0157:H7 transmission also usually occurs through contaminated food (meats or fertilized fruits/vegetables), although secondary person-to-person transmission can subsequently occur. The infamous large outbreak in the early 1990s was linked to contaminated hamburger, and secondary infection was rampant, occurring in up to 20% of close contacts.

Shigella spp spreads from person to person or through contaminated food, but has no environmental reservoir (similar to *salmonella typhi*). It is highly contagious, with a low density of inoculum required to result in clinical infection. It therefore commonly causes outbreaks, usually within households and day care centers.

Other causes of bacterial diarrhea in hospitalized patients include *Klebsiella oxytoca, Klebsiella pneumonia, Staphylococcus aureus*, and Clostridium perfringens, all of which have been implicated in causing a toxin-associated diarrheal illness that can be clinically indistinguishable from CDAD. A small case series of patients with (non-*Clostridium difficile*) antibiotic-associated hemorrhagic colitis found that a majority of cases were caused by *Klebsiella oxytoca*, which produces a cytotoxin that causes epithelial cell death. Similarly there are strains of *Klebsiella pneumonia* that produce an enteropathogenic toxin that causes hemorrhagic diarrhea. There are also some strains of *Staphylococcus areus* that produce an enteropathogenic toxin, and may be the etiologic agent in patients with (non-*Clostridium difficile*) antibiotic-associated diarrhea. Enterotoxin producing *Clostridium perfringens* has also been suspected to be a causal agent in nosocomial diarrheas. Although there is still some disagreement about the role that these organisms play in non-*C difficile* toxigenic diarrheal syndromes, there does appear to be evidence of their existence.

Candida spp have also been implicated in nosocomial diarrhea. It is thought to cause a secretory diarrhea (without evidence of colitis) in critically ill or debilitated patients, but it is unclear how to treat or manage these patients.

VIRUSES/PROTOZOA

Viral outbreaks of diarrhea occur more commonly than bacterial outbreaks, both in the community and hospital setting. The most common viral causes of acute infectious diarrhea include the caliciviruses (Norwalk and Sapporo viruses), rotavirus (primarily in children), adenovirus, and astrovirus.

By far the most common are the caliciviruses, estimated to account for more than 90% of acute gastrointestinal outbreaks in the U.S. They are associated with a high infectivity rate (with attack rates reported to be as high as 50% in close contacts) and a low density of required inoculum. Cruise ships notoriously are headlined with these outbreaks, but they can (and have) occurred in medical environments, including nursing homes and hospitals. These viruses are transmitted both by infected food and water, and by secondary person-to-person spread. The viral particles are present in both the vomitus and the feces (as opposed to bacterial enteritis, in which the bacteria are present only in stool), increasing the likelihood of person-to-person transmission. Unfortunately, these viruses also persist on environmental surfaces and are resistant to ordinary cleaning agents (although are inactivated by household bleach).

Rotavirus infections tend to cause symptomatic disease only in children. Similar to the caliciviruses, the organism can remain in the environment for prolonged periods of time and are difficult to eradicate with routine cleaning agents. Enteric adenoviral strains also rarely produce symptomatic diarrheal disease in adults. Astroviral outbreaks spread from person to person and have occurred in the hospital setting. Although they much more commonly occur in pediatric populations, they also afflict the elderly, immunocompromised, and institutionalized.

Protozoal causes of acute diarrhea are most commonly caused by *Giardia lamblia*, cryptosporidium, and *Entamoeba histolytica*. These are usually connected with contaminated water sources, with secondary person-to-person transmission occurring via the fecal-oral route. They are transmitted via a very small inoculum and are therefore highly transmissible. These protozoa usually cause outbreaks in schools and daycare settings, and medical setting outbreaks are highly unusual.

Immunocompromised patients (especially HIV with CD4 < 50) clearly have a more extensive infectious differential diagnosis for nosocomial diarrhea. The additional organisms that should be considered include cryptosporidia, microsporidia, cyclospora, isospora, mycobacterium avium complex (MAC), and cytomegalovirus (CMV).

NONINFECTIOUS DIARRHEAS

Noninfectious nosocomial diarrhea can be due to a host of insults, including the introduction of new agents or therapies (medications, foods, additives, enteral feedings, contrast agents, radiation therapy), and new diagnoses (fecal impaction, inflammatory bowel disease, opiate withdrawal, transplant rejection, GI bleeding, fat malabsorption, and biliary obstruction).

NEW AGENTS OR THERAPIES

Medications are a common offender for noscomial diarrhea, and a careful review of medications is warranted (**Table 80-2**). Antibiotic-associated diarrhea is a common occurrence, the frequency of which depends on the antimicrobial agent, ranging from 2–25% (with no significant difference between intravenous and oral antibiotics). The spectrum of disease caused by antibiotic-associated diarrhea can range from uncomplicated loose stools to frank colitis. Antibiotics can result in diarrhea by two primary mechanisms. Erythromycin, which is a motilin receptor agonist, directly stimulates gut motility; clavulanate also can activate gut motility, albeit less dramatically. Virtually all antibiotics can indirectly impact gut motility by killing some of the fecal flora; this can reduce the metabolism of carbohydrates, resulting in an osmotic diarrhea.

TABLE 80-2 Medications Commonly Associated with Noscomial Diarrhea

Antibiotics	Clindamycin Erythromycin Cephalosporins Ampicillin
Gastrointestinal agents	H_2 blockers Proton pump inhibitors Antacids (magnesium-containing) Misoprostol
Cardiovascular agents	Digitalis Quinidine
NSAIDs	All types (including aspirin)
Supplements	Magnesium Phosphorus Elixir additives (sorbitol/lactose)
Immunosuppressive agents	HIV medications (protease inhibitors) Chemotherapeutic agents Tacrolimus Cyclosporin Azathioprine
Other agents	Colchicine (dose-limiting) Levothyroxine (dose-related) Theophylline

The introduction of new foods during the hospital stay can also result in diarrhea. Offending agents include sugar-free gum or candy, and any new foods with a higher than usual content of milk products in patients with previously unrecognized lactose intolerance. Medication elixirs often contain substances such as sorbitol, which cause an osmotic diarrhea. Enteral feedings are also a common cause of osmotic diarrhea, which occurs in 15% of patients upon initiation of enteral feedings (discussed more below).

Oral contrast agents used in imaging present an osmotic load to the intestinal system that can result in transient diarrhea. Radiation therapy in the abdominal and pelvic region can cause both acute and chronic diarrhea. The symptoms of acute radiation enteritis generally start during or shortly after radiation therapy, and usually improve within 2–6 weeks of cessation of the radiation, but occasionally can persist long-term.

NEW DIAGNOSES

A number of new diagnoses during the hospital stay can result in diarrhea. Fecal impaction, especially in the elderly, psychiatric patients, and in immobilized patients receiving high doses of opiates without an adequate bowel regimen, can present with diarrhea due to leakage around the impaction. New onset inflammatory bowel disease should be entertained in cases of inflammatory diarrhea for which infectious causes have been ruled out. In patients who were taking opiates before the hospital stay, a reduction or cessation of their usual amount can present with diarrhea as a symptom of a withdrawal syndrome. Since nausea and vomiting often accompany opiate withdrawal, vomiting up oral opiates may be an important exacerbating factor. Bone marrow transplant patients can present with diarrhea as a symptom of graft versus host disease. GI bleeding can present with diarrhea, although the color of the stool should trigger an evaluation for bleeding. Fat malabsorption resulting from a new small bowel or pancreatic dysfunction can result in steatorrheic diarrhea. Biliary tract obstruction can result in bile acid–associated diarrhea.

HISTORY

HISTORY OF THE DIARRHEA

A full history of the onset, duration, frequency, color, consistency, and character of the diarrhea, as well as associated symptoms can provide clues to the diagnostic testing required to determine the etiology. A history of the degree of volume depletion should be sought (thirst, urine color and amount, lethargy). Patients should be queried about their epidemiological risks for infectious diarrheas (health care/daycare attendance or employment, pet or farm contacts, eating unpasteurized or raw foods, or recent ill contacts). Infectious diarrhea is often accompanied by nausea, vomiting, fever, tenesmus, or abdominal pain, and the stool character can be watery, malabsorptive, or dysenteric. Black tarry stools usually indicate digested blood, usually from the upper GI tract, and maroon/red/pink stools indicate undigested blood, usually in the lower GI tract (or upper GI tract with rapid transit time). Greasy stools that float indicate fat malabsorption, and clay-colored stools can be indicative of biliary obstruction. Direct gross examination of the stool can be tremendously helpful in defining the differential diagnosis and determining the need for further diagnostic testing.

PHYSICAL EXAM

The physical exam should focus on the vital signs, general appearance, abdominal, and rectal exam. The patient should be assessed for fever, signs of dehydration, and hemodynamic instability. The abdominal exam should assess for pain, distention, and peritoneal signs. The rectal exam should include testing for gross or microscopic blood.

DIAGNOSTICS

DIAGNOSTIC TESTING OF THE STOOL

A number of diagnostic stool tests are available to help determine the etiology of diarrhea, most of which are discussed below. Physicians should adhere to the "3-day rule" of diagnostic testing for bacterial or protozoal pathogens, ie, that if the diarrhea developed after hospital day 3, it is unlikely due to these types of pathogens, and diagnostic testing for them is not cost effective.

A routine stool culture will usually yield *Shigella, Salmonella, Aeromonas*, and *Campylobacter*. Routine stool cultures will usually not identify *Escherichia coli* 0157:H7 (which requires sorbitol-MacConkey medium and Shiga-toxin testing), *Vibrio cholera*, and some *Yersinia* (which require cold enrichment). Generally, stool cultures should be ordered for patients with severe diarrhea (>6 stools/day), with fever or dysentery, or if there are clusters of patients with similar symptoms suggesting an outbreak. Stool cultures are not recommended in mild or watery diarrhea. A single specimen is sufficient in qualified laboratories. Stool cultures will usually not be able to distinguish colonization versus infection in toxin-mediated diarrhea secondary to *Staphylococcus aureus, Klebsiella spp, Clostridium perfringens*, or candidal spp.

A routine stool test for ova and parasites (O & P) consists of a gross and microscopic examination of the stool to look for parasites or their eggs. Direct antigen testing for *Giardia*, cryptosporidia, and *Entamoeba* have an excellent sensitivity of at least 95%. Acid-fast staining of the stool specimen can identify Cylclospora and isospora, but the test has a low sensitivity and low specificity (usually due to swallowed sputum of mycobacterial species that may or may not be pathogenic). In general, parasitic evaluations require multiple testing, due to the periodic nature of their fecal excretion.

Viral testing of the stool is rarely performed, outside of special testing by local, state, or federal labs for outbreaks. Viral cultures can yield CMV, enterovirusus, and adenoviruses, but are rarely performed and take up to 14 days to yield an organism. Rotaviral antigen tests are readily available, but are rarely performed in adults, as rotavirus rarely produces symptomatic illness in adults.

Testing the stool for occult blood can help to distinguish blood from food and dyes in stool specimens that are grossly red or pink. The most common assays utilize the pseudoperoxidase activity of hemoglobin reacting with hydrogen peroxide to convert a colorless compound to one of a blue color. False-positive testing occurs between 1–10%, and usually occurs in response to diets rich in meat or vegetable sources of peroxidase (turnips, horseradish, red meats, cauliflower, broccoli, cantaloupe, parsnips, mushrooms, apples, and bananas), and with some medications (including colchicine). False negatives are rare, but can be caused by foods and diets high in vitamin C.

Stool pH is rarely utilized as a diagnostic test for nosocomial diarrhea. Normal stool pH is about that of the body, with a normal range of 7.0–7.5. Conditions resulting in acidic pH often are malabsorption syndromes that allow for high rates of fermentation of undigested food by gut bacteria. Conditions resulting in alkaline pH include antibiotic use (due to impaired bacterial fermentation) and colonic inflammation.

PRACTICE POINT

Key historical points that might point to the need to perform an infectious workup include the presence of

1. Immunosuppression
   - IgA deficiency, common variable hypogammaglobulinemia, chronic granulomatous disease
   - AIDS (common enteric and opportunistic pathogens)
   - Medication related (chemotherapy, corticosteroids)
2. Malnutrition
3. Recent or current antibiotic use

Key historical points that might point to a specific cause of acute infectious diarrhea include

1. Travel history
   - Latin America, Africa, Asia (*Escherichia coli, Campylobacter, Shigella, Aeromona, Coronavirus, Salmonella,* norovirus)
   - Russia and wilderness areas (*Giardia*)
   - Cruise ships (Norwalk virus and other causes of infectious gastroenteritis)
2. Daycare exposure
   - *Shigella Giardia, Cryptosporidium*, rotavirus among others
3. Recent food ingestion
   - Chicken (*Salmonella, Campylobacter, Shigella*)
   - Eggs (*Salmonella*)
   - Mayonnaise or creams (*Staphylococcus aureus* or *Salmonella*)
   - Hamburger (hemorrhagic *E coli* 0157:H7)
   - Raw seafood (*Vibrio species, Salmonella*, or acute hepatitis A)
   - Fried rice (*Bacillus cereus*)
4. Recent or current hospitalization or nursing home (*C difficile*)
5. Recent or current antibiotic use (*C difficile*)
6. Diagnosis of hemochromatosis (*Vibrio species, Yersinia*)

Symptoms that may suggest an etiology include

1. Associated vomiting
   - Toxins
2. Abdominal pain and fever
   - *C difficile*, hemorrhagic *E coli*
   - Invasive organisms
3. Bloody diarrhea
   - *Salmonella, Shigella, Campylobacter*, enteroinvasive *E coli* (0157:H7), *Entamoeba histolytica*
   - *Aeromonas* species, *Vibrio parahaemolyticus, Yersinia* Immunosuppression
4. Profuse watery diarrhea
   - *Bacillus cereus, Staphylococcus aureus, Clostridium perfringens*
   - *Vibrio cholerae*, enterotoxigenic *E coli, Klebsiella pneumoniae, Aeromonas*
   - Enteropathogenic and enteroadherent *E coli, Giardia*, cryptosporidiosis, helminths

Stool leukocytes are not normally present in the stool, and their presence indicates infection (with invasion of the intestinal wall) or inflammation (such as inflammatory bowel disease). For that reason, stool leukocytes are more likely to be present in invasive bacterial infections (*Salmonella, Shigella, Campylobacter, Yersinia*, invasive *Escherichia coli*) but are unlikely to be present with a viral infection, parasitic infection, or toxigenic bacterial infection. The sensitivity and specificity of stool leukocytes is relatively low, so it is not a very useful diagnostic test. However, a less readily available test, the immunoassay for the neutrophil marker lactoferrin, has higher sensitivity and specificity.

PRACTICE POINT

Noninfectious etiologies of acute diarrhea in hospitalized patients include
1. Recent new medications or oral contrast
2. Toxin or radiation exposure prior to admission
3. Acute diverticulitis
4. Inflammatory bowel disease
5. Ischemic colitis
6. Graft-versus-host-disease

Fecal fat can be assessed by qualitative methods, which can be done on a random stool sample, with abnormal testing being > 50 fat globules per high power field. Qualitative testing correlates well with quantitative testing, which is rarely required in inpatients.

Stool osmolality can be performed on a random stool sample, and normal values range from 275–295 mosm/L. The measured stool osmolality can be compared to calculated stool osmolality (2 x [Na + K]) to determine if there is an osmolar gap. A gap (> 50) indicates an osmotic diarrhea, usually due to carbohydrates (sodium citrate, magnesium citrate, laxatives, lactulose, or sorbitol) or fat (mineral oil or castor oil). A stool osmolality > 500 mg/dL is highly suspicious for factitious diarrhea (usually due to laxative abuse).

PRACTICE POINT

Systemic manifestations associated with infectious diarrhea
1. Reiter syndrome (*Salmonella, campylobacter, Shigella, Yersinia*)
2. Hemolytic-uremic syndromes (*E coli* [0157:H7], *Shigella*)
3. Thyroiditis, pericarditis, acute glomerulonephritis (*Yersinia*)

APPROACH TO DIAGNOSTIC TESTING

An approach to rational diagnostic testing is presented in **Figure 80-1**.

TREATMENT

REMOVE THE OFFENDING AGENT/THERAPY

A careful review of new foods, additives, and medications may uncover an offending agent to be discontinued. Antibiotic-associated diarrhea usually responds to discontinuation of the agent. There is limited evidence that probiotics effectively treat antibiotic-associated diarrhea, but their use is widespread and there is little data suggesting harm (except in immunocompromised patients). Diarrhea related to new enteral feeds can be reduced by changing to a lower osmotic agent, reducing the rate, or adding antimotility agents (discussed below). Contrast-associated diarrhea is self-limited and should be given supportive care until resolution. Radiation-associated diarrhea should also be given supportive care, unless intolerable symptoms dictate temporary cessation of the treatment.

TREAT THE NEW DISEASE

A detailed outline of the specific therapies for the infectious diarrheas is not warranted, although a few deserve specific mention (**Table 80-3**).

Empiric treatment for suspected bacterial pathogens (with a quinolone) should be initiated in patients with acute febrile dysentery, but only after a fecal sample has been sent. In patients without fever or frank dysentery, empiric treatment is not warranted. For established diagnoses, patients should be treated according to Table 80-3. In patients with uncomplicated nontyphoidal *Salmonella* diarrhea, treatment with antibiotics does not reduce the duration of illness or fever, but does increase relapse rates and prolongs fecal shedding. However, patients with known or suspected bacteremia (toxic appearance or high fever), should be treated to prevent septicemia. Treatment of *Escherichia coli* 0157:H7 has also been shown to increase the risk of hemolytic uremic syndrome and is not currently recommended.

Diarrhea related to fecal impaction usually requires a combination of mechanical and medical disimpaction. See Chapter 78 Constipation. New symptomatic IBD usually requires immunosuppressive and/or antibacterial agents, and bowel rest to relieve symptoms. See Chapter 163 Inflammatory Bowel Disease. Treatment of withdrawal symptoms and transplant rejection are beyond the scope of this chapter. A new diagnosis of fat malabsorption warrants treatment of the underlying pancreatic or small bowel dysfunction, and usually requires enzymatic supplementation to correct. Similarly, a new diagnosis of biliary obstruction requires investigation and relief of the obstruction.

SUPPORTIVE THERAPIES

A trial of nothing by mouth for 24 hours is of reasonable diagnostic and therapeutic value, to distinguish osmotic from secretory etiologies. An oral diet can be initiated and advanced as tolerated. Use of a lactose-free diet (due to a transient lactase deficiency) is usually recommended, although data supporting its use are limited. Probiotics may have a role in the treatment of infectious diarrheas, as a Cochrane review found that probiotics reduced the mean duration of infectious diarrhea by 30 hours. There is not good evidence supporting their role in noninfectious diarrheas. Patients who cannot tolerate oral hydration will need intravenous hydration, of which iso-osmotic fluids are preferred, unless substantial sodium electrolyte abnormalities dictate otherwise. Supplementation of potassium (if warranted) can usually be accomplished orally (depending on the severity of the depletion), but magnesium or phosphorus supplementation are generally preferred intravenously, as they can be caustic to the gut and exacerbate diarrhea.

PRACTICE POINT

- In patients with uncomplicated nontyphoidal *Salmonella* diarrhea, treatment with antibiotics does not reduce the duration of illness or fever, but does increase relapse rates and prolongs fecal shedding. However, patients with known or suspected bacteremia (toxic appearance or high fever) should be treated to prevent septicemia.
- Treatment of *Escherichia coli* 0157:H7 has also been shown to increase the risk of hemolytic uremic syndrome and is not currently recommended.

ANTIDIARRHEAL AGENTS

Although hundreds of agents have reported effects for diarrhea, only 3 have FDA labeling to support their use. Antidiarrheal agents in general should be avoided in patients with any suspected inflammatory diarrhea. These agents have been associated with prolonged fever with *Shigella spp*, hemolytic uremic syndrome with *Escherichia coli* 0157:H7, and toxin megacolon with *Clostridium difficile*-associated diarrhea.

Loperamide (Imodium) inhibits peristalsis and has antisecretory effects. Bismuth subsalicylate reduces symptoms of nausea,

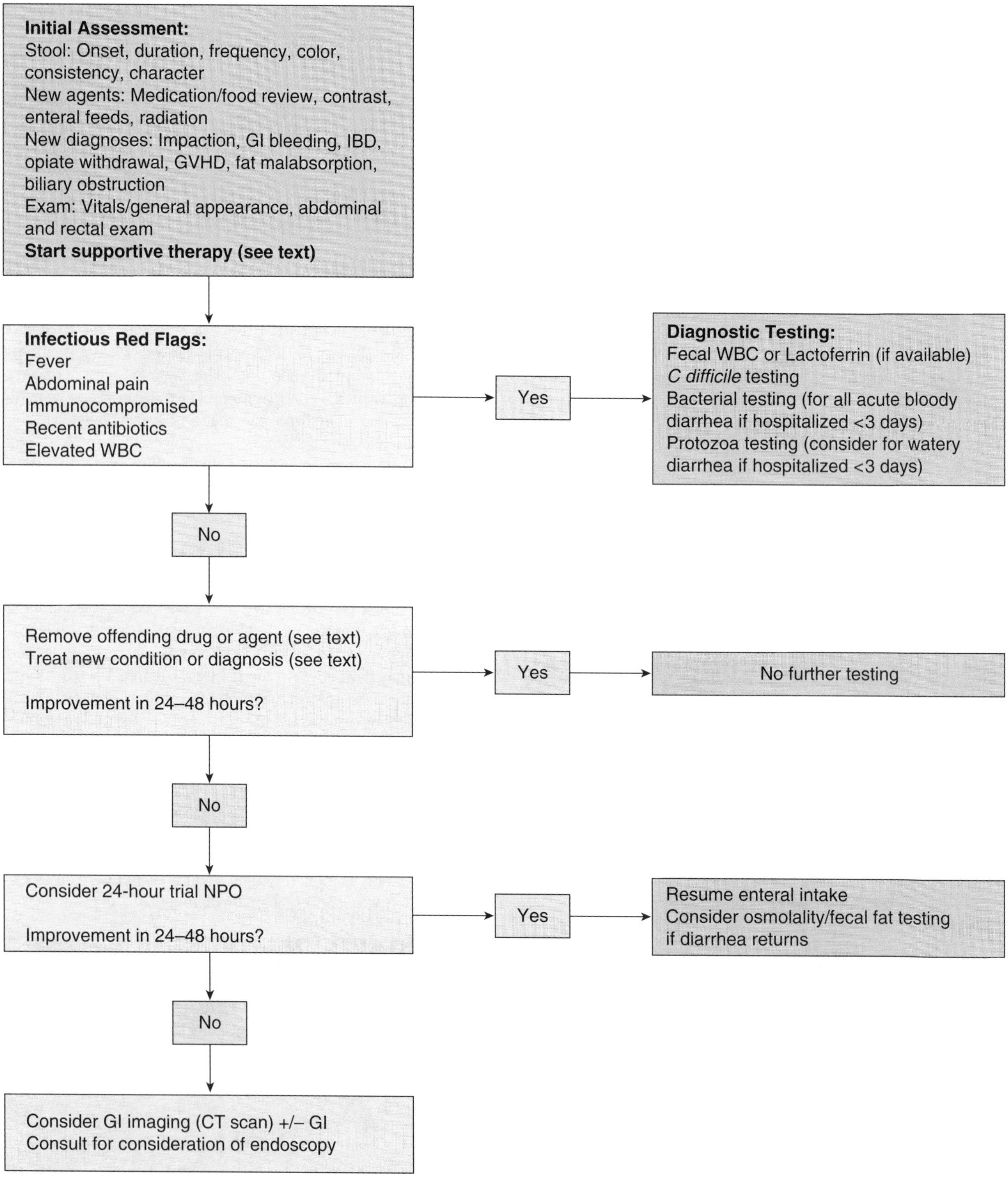

Figure 80-1 *Diagnostic approach to nosocomial diarrhea.*

diarrhea, and abdominal pain in patients with traveler's diarrhea, but its use in other types of diarrhea (especially nosocomial variants) is unstudied. Diphenoxylate (Lomotil) is an opiate agonist that is effective at reducing stool volume.

THE HOSPITAL OF THE FUTURE

As previously mentioned, diarrhea is one of the most common afflictions in hospitalized patients, and patients experiencing diarrhea have longer lengths of stay and higher mortality than those who do not. The condition is also associated with more diagnostic testing, monitoring, and interventions. As such, it can be a significant challenge to the delivery of high quality and safe care to hospitalized patients.

It is of paramount importance to prevent nosocomial diarrhea if possible. Prevention of infectious nosocomial diarrheas includes the usual hygiene provisions and universal precautions. Interventions promoting hand-washing have been proven to reduce diarrheal episodes among children in institutions by 30–40%.

TABLE 80-3 Treatment of Known or Suspected Bacterial Pathogens

Bacterial Pathogen	Antibiotic Options/Duration
Campylobacter jejuni	Azithromycin 500 mg 3 days Erythromycin 500 mg four times a day for 3 days
Vibrio cholera	Doxycycline 300 mg (single dose) Tetracycline 500 mg four times a day for 3 days Azithromycin 500 mg 3 days Erythromycin 250 mg three times a day for 3 days
Escherichia coli 0157:H7	Not recommended
Escherichia coli (enterotoxigenic, enteroaggregative, or traveler's diarrhea)	Ciprofloxacin 750 mg 1–3 days Azithromycin 1000 mg (single dose) Rifaximin 200 mg three times a day for 3 days
Salmonella (nontyphoid)* *Salmonella* (typhoid)	Levofloxacin 500 mg 7 days Azithromycin 500 mg 7 days Duration 14 days if immunocompromised
Shigellosis *Aeromonas* *Plesiomonas* *Escherichia coli* (enteroinvasive) Noncholeraic vibrios*	Ciprofloxacin 750 mg 3 days Azithromycin 500 mg 3 days

*Not recommended if uncomplicated

PRACTICE POINT

- It is of paramount importance to prevent nosocomial diarrhea if possible. Prevention of infectious nosocomial diarrheas includes the usual hygiene provisions and universal precautions. Alcohol-based solutions will not eliminate spores from *C difficile*, and practitioners should use soap to wash their hands. Consult your hospital infection control policies regarding which patients require isolation in private rooms.

A key strategy to the prevention of noninfectious nosocomial diarrheas includes a careful review of the patient's home diet and medications, which should be carefully re-reviewed upon each care transition. Cessation or initiation of new foods, additives, or medications should be done with a careful review of the risks and benefits. Routine use of stool softeners in hospitalized patients is often unnecessary and may lead to unnecessary diarrhea. In patients starting a course of antibiotics during their hospital stay, probiotics have shown some promise in reducing the incidence of antibiotic-associated diarrhea in adults, and are generally safe in immunocompetent patients, but may not be universally available.

If despite preventive interventions, a hospitalized patient does experience nosocomial diarrhea, a step-wise, rational approach to diagnostic testing should be initiated, as outlined in Figure 80-1. Therapeutic and supportive interventions should be initiated based on the diagnostic evaluation, in a timely and cost-efficient manner.

CASE 80-1 *(continued)*

Based on the algorithm outlined in Figure 80-1, the patient's diarrhea started in the hospital, had been present for 1 day, was occurring 4–6 times a day, was brown, and semi-formed. His medication list included docusate, senna, and a PPI, all of which can result in diarrhea. He had recently received perioperative antibiotics (for the prevention of surgical site infections), but was on no current antibiotic therapy and he was without any other infectious red flags. He had also recently been initiated on enteral feedings, and had received oral contrast 2 days ago for abdominal imaging. As such, we discontinued his PPI, colace, and senna, and reduced the rate of his enteral feeds. His diarrhea resolved within 48 hours and no further diagnostic testing was performed.

CONCLUSION

Diarrhea in hospitalized patients is a common occurrence, and can result in higher morbidity and mortality, and lower quality of life. Preventing nosocomial diarrhea by infection control standards and careful medication use is of paramount importance. For those afflicted despite preventive measures, a rational stepwise approach to diagnostic testing and treatment should be undertaken.

SUGGESTED READINGS

Allen SJ, Okoko B, Martinez EG, Gregorio GV, Dans LF. Probiotics for treating infectious diarrhoea. *Cochrane Database of Systematic Reviews.* 2003; Issue 4. Art. No.: CD003048. DOI: 10.1002/14651858.CD003048.pub2.

Bartlett JG. Antibiotic associated diarrhea. *N Engl J Med.* 2002;346:334–339.

Cunha BA. Nosocomial Diarrhea. *Critical Care Clinics.* 1998;14(2):329–338.

de Bruyn G, Hahn S, Borwick A. Antibiotic treatment for travellers' diarrhoea. *Cochrane Database of Systematic Reviews.* 2000; Issue 3. Art. No.: CD002242. DOI: 10.1002/14651858.CD002242.

Dupont HL. Bacterial diarrhea. *NEJM.* 2009;361:1560–1569.

Ejemot RI, Ehiri JE, Meremikwu MM, Critchley JA. Hand washing for preventing diarrhoea. *Cochrane Database of Systematic Reviews.* 2008; Issue 1. Art. No.: CD004265. DOI: 10.1002/14651858.CD004265.pub2.

Guerrant RL, Van Gilder T, Steiner TS, et al. Practice guidelines for the management of infectious diarrhea. *Clin Infect Dis.* 2001;32:331–350.

Musher DM, Musher BL. Contagious acute gastrointestinal infections. *N Engl J Med.* 2004;351:2417–2427.

Sirinavin S, Garner P. Antibiotics for treating salmonella gut infections. *Cochrane Database of Systematic Reviews.* 1999; Issue 1. Art. No.: CD001167. DOI: 10.1002/14651858.CD001167.

Thielman NM, Guerrant RL. Acute infectious diarrhea. *N Engl J Med.* 2004;350:38–47.

CHAPTER 81

Disorders of the Eye

Ala Moshiri, MD, PhD
Prem S. Subramanian, MD, PhD

Key Clinical Questions

1. Which conditions should prompt emergent ophthalmologic consultation?
2. Which conditions require prompt imaging and/or consultation with neurologists or neurosurgeons?
3. For hospital employees with viral conjunctivitis what are the recommendations to prevent nosocomial spread to hospitalized patients?
4. What are the risks of topical corticosteroids in patients with allergic conjunctivitis?

INTRODUCTION

Ophthalmologic concerns in the hospitalized patient fall into two broad categories: signs and symptoms of the systemic condition for which the patient has been admitted, and unrelated but potentially urgent disorders of the eye that may threaten vision. While some of the conditions discussed in this chapter may relate to the former issue, our approach will be to describe common ophthalmologic disorders for which inpatient consultation is often considered, and to provide information on appropriate triage and workup prior to obtaining the consultant's opinion. In many cases, outpatient evaluation after the acute illness has passed may be more useful, since the patient's cooperation with subjective testing methods is much more reliable. Symptoms that may prompt urgent evaluation include red eyes (with or without pain), double vision, and subjective loss of vision. There are a number of bedside examination techniques that do not require specialized equipment but can yield important information to narrow the differential diagnosis and help determine the urgency of further testing.

The consulting physician should perform a focused but detailed eye history and physical examination prior to consulting an ophthalmologist. Time of onset, monocular or binocular nature, duration, and associated neurologic symptoms are especially important. Past medical and ocular history are relevant, as are recent interventions during the current hospitalization that might contribute to the visual complaints. The examination should ideally include best corrected visual acuity (with glasses) measured for each eye, either with a near reading card or distance chart. It should be noted whether the pupils are equal in size and reactive to illumination. Abnormal extraocular movements may be seen with new binocular double vision. Peripheral vision testing with a small red object (pinhead, marker cap) can detect up to 75% of clinically relevant deficits. Finally, a hand-light examination should be done at the bedside to look for eyelid swelling or redness, conjunctival hyperemia and discharge, corneal clarity or haze, and gross iris and anterior segment abnormalities. If a direct ophthalmoscope is available, examination of the fundus should be attempted. This is best done in dim lighting so that the pupil is somewhat large. If a normal appearance of the optic nerves, retinal vessels, and maculae can be confirmed, this can be very helpful. This requires some level of practice and proficiency, but is within the scope of physical examination techniques of every physician.

PRACTICE POINT

Ophthalmologic consultation is required for any condition that may cause severe and permanent vision loss, including

- Corneal ulcers
- Iritis
- Acute angle glaucoma
- Sudden visual loss
- Orbital mass, including orbital abscess
- Stevens Johnson Syndrome with mucosal involvement.

TABLE 81-1 Differential Diagnosis of Common Red Eye Complaints

	Conjunctivitis	Iritis	Acute Glaucoma	Corneal Infection
Incidence	Very common	Common	Uncommon	Common
Discharge	Copious	None	None	Watery
Vision	Unaffected	Slightly blurred	Severely blurred	Usually blurred
Conjunctival injection	Diffuse	Circumcorneal	Circumcorneal	Circumcorneal
Pain	None	Moderate	Severe	Moderate to severe
Cornea	Clear	Usually clear	Steamy	Variable
Pupil size	Normal	Small	Mid-dilated	Normal
Pupillary light response	Normal	Sluggish	Fixed	Normal
IOP	Normal	Normal	Elevated	Normal

THE INFLAMED EYE

EMERGENT CONSIDERATIONS

In addition to the infections detailed below, loss of sympathetic innervation may give a mild red eye from vasodilation. When accompanied by ptosis (with or without miosis) as in Horner syndrome, this condition may be mistaken for ocular inflammation. Acute onset in a postpartum patient, with or without headache, may result from carotid artery dissection, and MR or CT angiography must be performed with consideration given to anticoagulation.

TEAR DYSFUNCTION SYNDROME (DRY EYE)

CASE 81-1

A 62-year-old woman is admitted for respiratory failure from a bacterial pneumonia. After 2 weeks of intubation in the intensive care unit on broad spectrum antibiotics, her condition improves. She is extubated and transferred to the medicine ward, where she reports eye irritation. Both eyes appear slightly red, and she reports some tearing and sensitivity to bright lights. Her vision is mildly blurred, and measures 20/25 in each eye with her reading glasses using a pocket visual acuity card. The remainder of her eye exam is essentially normal.

This patient is likely suffering from exposure keratopathy or corneal abrasion (**Table 81-1**). Under normal conditions, the ocular surface and eyelid glands produce aqueous, oily, and proteinaceous tear secretions essential for normal eye health. Insufficient lubrication is common in the setting of an intubated and sedated patient and can lead to breakdown of the surface of the cornea with subsequent corneal infection and ulceration. For this reason, in such patients ICU protocols commonly include frequent lubrication of the eyes with ointments to prevent ocular surface disease. Despite this effort, mild damage to the cornea and conjunctiva, especially in a long hospitalization, may occur. Dry eye symptoms frequently include eye irritation, blurry vision, foreign body sensation, and mild eye redness. Other patients at risk include those with known facial nerve paresis, recent anesthesia with insufficient eyelid taping during the procedure, and dementia. Reassurance and further lubrication are warranted to relieve symptoms.

In contrast, a corneal ulcer presents as an opaque area in the cornea that may appear hazy or even white. The ulcer may have a significant mucopurulent exudate and will likely be very painful. The conjunctiva will frequently be bright red (**Figure 81-1**). At the bedside, the physician may use fluorescein dye to look for an epithelial defect. If corneal staining occurs, then the potential for corneal ulceration is high, even if an infiltrate is not yet seen and pain is minimal. Ophthalmologic consultation is required. Corneal ulcers may cause severe and permanent vision loss. The patient must be seen by an ophthalmologist that same day for culture of the corneal surface and broad spectrum topical antibiotic therapy to prevent corneal perforation and endophthalmitis, which frequently will lead to loss of the eye. The ophthalmologist may prescribe fortified topical antibiotic drops to be applied every 30 to 60 minutes around the clock for the first 24 to 48 hours, and the nursing staff must be made aware of the importance of adherence to this very demanding but effective medical therapy.

CONJUNCTIVITIS

CASE 81-2

A 22-year-old man is admitted for respiratory distress attributed to an acute asthma attack. He is treated overnight with nebulized adrenergic agonists that are gradually weaned and

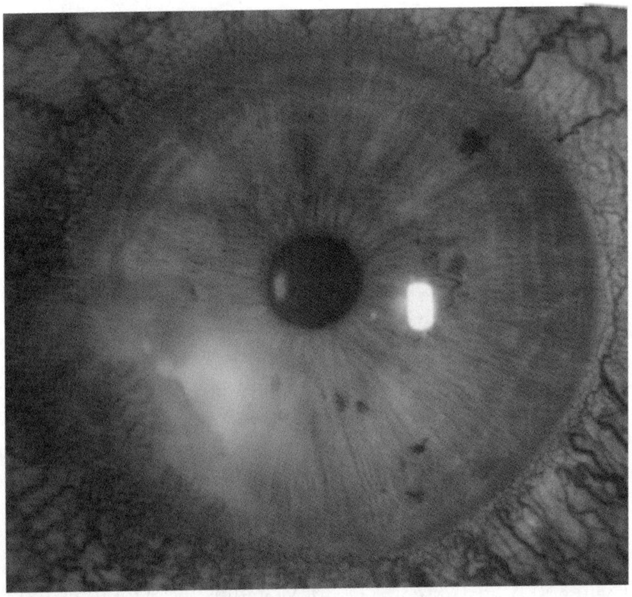

Figure 81-1 *Corneal ulcer with typical white exudate at the corneal limbus and severe conjunctival injection.*

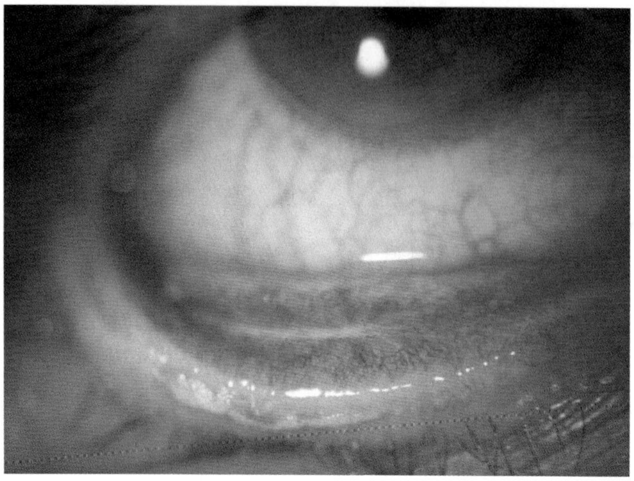

Figure 81-2 *Allergic conjunctivitis with formation of follicles in the inferior conjunctival fornix. Inspection alone does not allow differentiation from viral infection.*

prescribed systemic steroid therapy. It is also noted that he has mild eczematous changes on his hands that are not new. His roommate notes that he has had red eyes for the past 2 days, which have been itching and tearing as well. There has been no crusting of the eyelashes upon waking up and there is no frank pain. The eyes are mildly irritated, but itching has been the prominent feature. The skin beneath his eyelids is also slightly hyperpigmented. He has had similar episodes of red eyes before, which had resolved without serious complication.

This case illustrates a classic example of allergic conjunctivitis. Severe itching is the most prominent symptom. Frequently, there will be generalized hyperemia (redness) of the conjunctiva and mild to moderate tearing (**Figure 81-2**). Visual blurring, if present, is mild and attributable to the tearing. Eye rubbing is typical, and the patient may have symptoms of allergic rhinitis as well, with associated rubbing of the nose. This rubbing can sometimes lead to mild eyelid edema and temporary hyperpigmentation (a.k.a. allergic shiners, raccoon eyes) and a crease on the nose from manipulation as well. Common associations are with asthma, eczema, or history of other atopy. Symptoms can be managed with artificial tear lubricants and cool compresses if mild to moderate. If symptoms are severe or persistent, inpatient consultation with an ophthalmologist may be warranted, and treatment may require immune modulation with a topical antihistamine, mast cell stabilizer, or mild steroid. Topical corticosteroids should never be prescribed without active participation by the ophthalmologist, since untoward effects may include promoting viral infection (especially if there is a history of ocular herpes simplex) and intraocular pressure elevation.

VIRAL CONJUNCTIVITIS

Viral conjunctivitis also presents with bilateral red eyes. However, the symptoms will often have started in one eye 1 to 2 days prior to starting in the fellow eye. Often the eyes are very red with copious tearing, and the most prominent symptom is pain and burning. Mucous crusting of the eyelashes, especially in the morning, may be so copious as to preclude eyelid opening without manual assistance. A preauricular lymph node may also be palpated on exam and is relatively specific for viral etiology. Symptoms tend to worsen for the first few days of infection and generally resolve within 1 to 2 weeks. Household contacts may have had a recent URI or similar eye symptoms. Hand washing and contact precautions are crucial in preventing the spread of infection. If hospital workers become infected, they must be removed from patient contact for at least 7 days after symptoms start in the second eye to avoid nosocomial spread (spread to both eyes is very common even when infected persons are very cautious).

BACTERIAL CONJUNCTIVITIS

In contrast, bacterial conjunctivitis is often unilateral at presentation, which helps to distinguish it from allergic and viral etiologies, but it may spread to both eyes via the hands to become bilateral. Common organisms include Neisseria, pneumococcus, Staphylococcus, Haemophilus Influenzae, Moraxella, and others. Copious mucopurulent discharge is the most prominent feature. Pain and irritation with severe hyperemia may occur, but there should not be frank vision loss. Bilateral cases can be challenging to distinguish from viral conjunctivitis, and an ophthalmologist should make this distinction. Debilitated patients are most prone to bacterial conjunctivitis, and suspicion for this diagnosis will be higher in such individuals. Treatment is usually with topical antibiotic ointments or drops, and may require cultures to determine the causative organism if the symptoms and signs are anything other than mild. Otherwise immunocompetent patients with unilateral disease may be treated empirically with topical fluoroquinolones such as moxifloxacin or gatifloxicin, both of which have broad-spectrum activity against the common organisms. If improvement is not seen within 48 hours, then cultures should be repeated and ophthalmologic consultation requested.

PRACTICE POINT

Conjunctivitis

- Allergic Conjunctivitis: Topical corticosteroids should never be prescribed without active participation by the ophthalmologist, since untoward effects may include promoting viral infection and intraocular pressure elevation.
- Viral Conjunctivitis: If hospital workers become infected, they must be removed from patient contact for at least 7 days after symptoms start in the second eye to avoid nosocomial spread.
- Bacterial Conjunctivitis: Treatment is usually with topical antibiotic ointments or drops, and may require cultures to determine the causative organism if the symptoms and signs are anything other than mild. If improvement is not seen within 48 hrs, then cultures should be repeated and ophthalmologic consultation requested.

IRITIS

CASE 81-3

A 32-year-old man is admitted for acute persistent diarrhea leading to electrolyte imbalances. Workup of his gastrointestinal distress reveals abnormal ulcerations on colonoscopy consistent with inflammatory bowel disease. During the first hospital day, the patient reports blurry vision and photophobia in the left eye only, which had started several days ago and has been gradually worsening. The eye is slightly red on examination and visual acuity is reduced to 20/40. The right eye is normal.

This patient has anterior uveitis associated with inflammatory bowel disease, but many autoimmune conditions can be associated with inflammation of the eye. The most prominent feature is photophobia. Often, patients are extremely sensitive

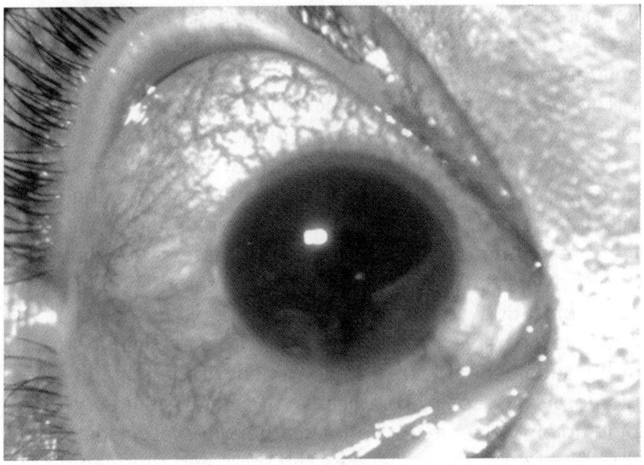

Figure 81-3 *Characteristic limbal flush (redness) seen in cases of acute iritis.*

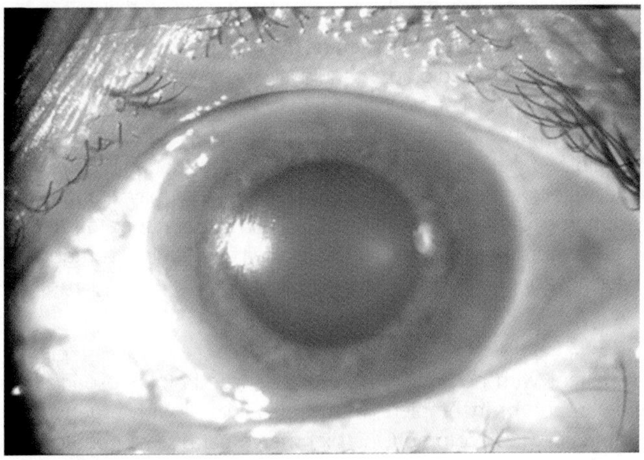

Figure 81-4 *Mid-dilated pupil and corneal clouding (seen as loss of typical corneal sheen and dulling of corneal light reflex) in a case of acute angle closure.*

to light; they may keep room lights off and blinds closed and even wear sunglasses indoors during an episode. Symptoms may be unilateral or bilateral, although the former is more common. Prior episodes also are common but vary in severity and laterality. Hyperemia is seen as a characteristic red ring of inflammation around the edges of the cornea called limbal flush (**Figure 81-3**). Diagnosis requires a slit lamp, as inflammation cannot be diagnosed accurately without sufficient magnification of the anterior segment. Diagnosis, therefore, requires consultation with an ophthalmologist. While ocular inflammation may be related to autoimmune conditions as in the case above, it may also be the result of infection, and this must be ruled out in every case. The ophthalmologist will direct the appropriate investigations for possible infectious etiologies. Serum tests for syphilis, Lyme disease, toxoplasmosis, and skin testing for tuberculosis exposure are commonly performed. In addition, the ophthalmologist may recommend chest imaging for sarcoidosis, and if the review of systems suggests a possible undiagnosed autoimmune disease, serum testing for HLA-B27 may be performed as well. Rheumatologic consultation also may be appropriate.

ANGLE CLOSURE GLAUCOMA

CASE 81-4

A 68-year-old Caucasian woman is hospitalized for workup of chest pain. Spending most of her day in a dimly lit hospital room watching TV, she suddenly develops a red, painful, blurry right eye. The pain and redness worsen over the next hour and do not remit. During this period of time, the vision is profoundly blurred. Visual acuity in the right eye is roughly 20/400, as she is able to only make out the largest letters on the pocket vision chart. The vision does not improve even with the use of her glasses, which are bifocals that are somewhat thick. The patient reports she is far-sighted and has been for many years. The patient also reports that she has had similar episodes in the past several years on occasion, sometimes in the left eye, other times in the right eye, but never at the same time. She has attributed her symptoms to headache, and she has seen her primary care provider who diagnosed her with mild migraines and recommended Excedrin.

Acute angle closure glaucoma is virtually always unilateral. It is a rare but vision-threatening condition and should not be missed. Prompt ophthalmology referral is required to prevent permanent vision loss. It can be recognized by a very painful and red eye with profoundly decreased vision. Patients commonly present with a severe headache on the affected side, sometimes with associated nausea and vomiting; symptoms typically last for minutes to hours, not days or weeks. Similar episodes may have occurred in the past in the same eye, or in the fellow eye, usually in dim lighting, such as a movie theatre, since pupillary dilatation bunches up the iris tissue in the angle. The pupil is usually slightly larger than the fellow eye and is unreactive. The cornea is often cloudy because the elevated pressure impairs corneal endothelial function, and this clouding makes it difficult to see the iris as clearly on the affected side in comparison to the fellow eye (**Figure 81-4**). There should be no discharge or exudate. This condition occurs more commonly in women and is associated with far-sightedness (hyperopia). The affected eye may feel much more hard (be difficult to indent) in comparison with the fellow eye when palpated through closed eyelids. This is indicative of a severely elevated intraocular pressure, which is the cause of the potential optic nerve damage in glaucoma. If this diagnosis is suspected, immediate ophthalmic consultation should be made for prompt reduction of the intraocular pressure, initially with topical agents. Ultimately this condition requires laser peripheral iridotomy in the affected eye as soon as possible, and in the fellow eye to prevent future episodes. Importantly, the vast majority of patients with glaucoma do not suffer from angle closure attacks, but rather primary open angle glaucoma, which is largely asymptomatic and has no commonality with an angle closure attack as described above. A patient with red eyes and a history of "glaucoma" for which they take eye drops on a regular basis is almost certainly not having an acute angle closure attack.

DIPLOPIA

EVALUATION

The evaluation of diplopia must begin with determination of whether or not the symptoms are binocular. Monocular diplopia, that is, double vision in one eye only, is virtually never an ophthalmic emergency. Many entities can cause double vision in one eye, such as cataract, corneal pathology, or incorrect spectacle prescription. Binocular diplopia, double vision due to misalignment of the eyes, virtually always requires ophthalmologic evaluation for proper diagnosis and treatment. Therefore, the first question to the patient who complains of diplopia should always be, "does the double vision go away when you cover either eye?" If the answer is yes, then the patient has binocular diplopia and an ophthalmologist should be called when the remainder of the evaluation is complete. The diplopia may be intermittent or constant and may change with position of gaze. Patients should be asked about associated neurologic symptoms such as headache, nausea or vomiting, vertigo, and weakness or tingling.

EMERGENT CONSIDERATIONS

A patient with new third nerve paresis (see below), especially if painful and/or incomplete, must be evaluated with urgent neuroimaging. Less commonly, a sixth nerve paresis may be accompanied by ipsilateral ptosis and miosis consistent with Horner syndrome, localizing the process to the cavernous sinus; acute onset can arise from cavernous sinus thrombosis or rapid tumor growth or hemorrhage.

SPECIFIC CAUSES OF DIPLOPIA

Cranial nerve paresis

CASE 81-5

A 73-year-old man is admitted with double vision that resolves upon covering either eye. He reports that his symptoms started that morning. He has also noticed the right eyelid drooping since this morning. He has not had any prior eye problems except for using reading glasses, and has had cataract surgery in both eyes 3 years ago. He has hypertension controlled with 2 oral antihypertensive medications, and no other chronic medical conditions. On examination, his visual acuity is 20/25 on the pocket visual acuity chart in each eye with his reading glasses on. The examination of the pupils reveals that the right pupil is larger than the left, and reacts more slowly than the left as well. He reports that no eye doctor has ever noted a pupillary abnormality before. His extraocular movements demonstrate limitation in elevation, depression, and adduction of the right eye. When he is looking straight, the right eye is misaligned downward and temporally. In addition, the right eyelid hangs lower than the left one (**Figure 81-5**). Visual fields tested by confrontation are grossly full. Hand light examination reveals normal-appearing anterior segments without hyperemia or opacity of the cornea. Direct ophthalmoscopy reveals normal-appearing optic nerves, retinal vessels, and maculae in each eye, though the view was easier in the right eye due to the enlarged pupil.

This patient has an acute oculomotor (third cranial nerve) palsy. This may be due to ischemia of the nerve itself secondary to chronic microvasculopathy related to hypertension and/or diabetes, a cerebral aneurysm, a mass impinging on the nerve, viral infection, or trauma. The most concerning and potentially life-threatening cause is aneurysmal compression. Aneurysms often arise at the junction of the internal carotid and posterior communicating arteries. Because the pupillary fibers of the oculomotor nerve run peripherally within the nerve fascicle in the subarachnoid space, involvement of the pupil in an oculomotor nerve palsy is indicative of a cerebral aneurysm impinging on the nerve until proven otherwise. Vascular insults to the third nerve generally spare the pupil and thus can be distinguished clinically from compressive lesions when the third nerve paresis is complete. An oculomotor nerve palsy affects the superior rectus, inferior rectus, medial rectus, and inferior oblique muscles, in addition to the iris and ciliary body. The lateral rectus and superior oblique muscles are intact, and hence the eye may rest in a "down and out" position. Limitations in elevation, depression, and adduction are typical but frequently are not complete, as some residual function may persist.

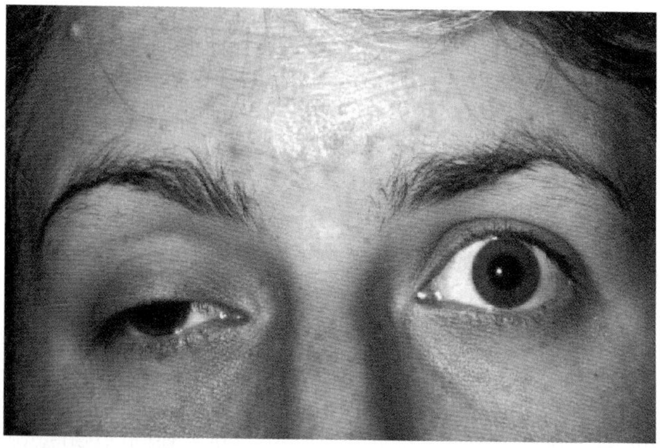

Figure 81-5 *Ptosis and ophthalmoparesis seen with third nerve palsy. Note dilation of the right pupil; this is not pharmacologic.*

Trochlear (fourth cranial nerve) palsy results in double vision with images appearing tilted with respect to one another. Diplopia with a torsional component should make the examiner suspicious of this diagnosis. On examination, the affected eye appears higher than the fellow eye (hypertropia). This hypertropia increases when the affected eye looks down or in toward the nose. Congenital partial trochlear nerve palsy is relatively common and often well-controlled until adulthood, when it may decompensate and cause manifest diplopia. The patient in this scenario will have a history of tilting the head toward the affected side. This can be confirmed by looking at old photographs. Acquired trochlear paresis is also common and may be seen with even mild head trauma. It may also occur due to microvascular disease or cranial surgery.

Abducens (sixth cranial nerve) palsy results in horizontal diplopia with images appearing side by side due to limitation or absence of abduction of the eye. When the patient is looking straight ahead, the affected side may be misaligned with the eye pointing inward (esotropia). The remainder of eye movements are normal. Frequently, the paresis is incomplete with some residual ability to abduct the affected eye. Most cases of abducens nerve palsy in older adults are related to microvascular disease from hypertension, diabetes, and hyperlipidemia, and these tend to resolve over weeks with no intervention. Careful ophthalmologic follow-up is required. If the abducens palsy does not resolve as expected, then tumor, arteriovenous fistulas, and other intracranial processes must be ruled out.

ORBITAL DISORDERS

Orbital masses may affect globe position and disturb normal extraocular muscle action with resulting binocular diplopia. Thyroid eye disease, most commonly associated with Graves disease but which can also be present in some hypothyroid and euthyroid states, is an infiltrative disease of the extraocular muscles and orbital fat that produces a congested orbit and proptosis. Unbalanced muscle involvement may lead to binocular diplopia. The diplopic patient must be asked about endocrine dysfunction. Orbital masses, in addition to causing double vision, frequently cause proptosis, which the astute observer will note even without exophthalmometry. If an orbital mass, including an orbital abscess, is suspected, prompt ophthalmic attention is required.

TABLE 81-2 Causes of Vision Loss in Hospitalized Patients

	Time of Onset	Severity	Unilateral vs. Bilateral	Treatment
Cataract	Gradual	Usually mild or moderate	Bilateral >> unilateral	Observation, refraction, surgery
Glaucoma	Gradual	Severe when noticed by patient	Bilateral >> unilateral	Medication vs. surgery
Macular degeneration	Gradual (dry) Rapid (wet)	Often severe	Bilateral >> unilateral	Intravitreal medication, laser therapy
Diabetic retinopathy	Gradual	Moderate to severe	Unilateral > bilateral	Laser therapy
Nonarteritic ischemic optic neuropathy	Sudden	Moderate to severe	Unilateral >> bilateral	Usually none
Arteritic ischemic optic neuropathy	Sudden	Severe	Unilateral >> bilateral	Immediate systemic corticosteroid therapy
Optic chiasm / postchiasmal disease	Sudden > gradual	Moderate to severe	Bilateral	Varies by underlying cause

Table 81-2 is meant to be representative and is not exhaustive. A comprehensive ophthalmology text should be consulted if necessary.

MYASTHENIA GRAVIS

Myasthenia gravis is a disease of the neuromuscular junction with antibodies against the nicotinic acetylcholine receptors on the motor end plate. It frequently presents (up to 75%) with ocular symptoms and may be limited to the eye. The most common presenting sign is ptosis, but any of the extraocular muscles may be involved. Therefore, ocular myasthenia gravis may mimic virtually any cranial neuropathy. The pupil is virtually never involved in myasthenia gravis. Thus, pupillary abnormalities are a helpful clinical sign that can distinguish this disease process from others. Diplopia in a patient with myasthenia typically waxes and wanes over the course of a day, improves with rest, and often has symptoms that have been occurring for the previous months of years. Ocular myasthenia may be unilateral or bilateral. If this disease is suspected, the ophthalmologist may use tests of fatigability or the ice test to help in diagnosis, in conjunction with short-acting acetylcholinesterase inhibitors.

PRACTICE POINT

Cranial Nerve Palsies

- CN III: A patient with new third nerve paresis, especially if painful and/or incomplete, must be evaluated with urgent neuroimaging.
- CN IV: Trochlear palsy results in double vision with images appearing tilted with respect to one another; it arises from microvascular disease or neurosurgery,
- CN VI: The Horner syndrome (a sixth nerve paresis accompanied by ipsilateral ptosis and miosis) localizes the process to the cavernous sinus; acute onset can arise from caversous sinus thrombosis or rapid tumor growth or hemorrhage.

Ocular myasthenia gravis may mimic virtually any cranial neuropathy but the pupil is virtually never involved.

SUDDEN VISION LOSS

Both visual acuity and confrontation visual field testing at the bedside must be performed and should help the clinician localize the vision loss to one eye or hemifield. If there is bilateral loss, then the degree of asymmetry is important to record. The presence of other ocular and orbital signs (redness, ocular motility disturbance, eyelid swelling, ptosis) should be noted, as they will assist in anatomic localization. Pupillary reactions provide objective evidence of afferent visual loss and may direct the workup even when other data are conflicting or unreliable.

If an obvious visual disturbance (severe unilateral vision loss with afferent pupillary defect, gross homonymous hemianopia) is not found, then further workup should be deferred and an ophthalmology consult obtained. Automated perimetric testing, dilated fundus examination, photography and advanced imaging of the retina and optic nerve, and even refraction performed by the ophthalmologist will allow for a much more directed investigation, and may reveal other benign causes of vision loss (**Table 81-2**)

CASE 81-6

A 76-year-old man with long-standing congestive heart failure is being treated with intravenous antibiotics for a community-acquired pneumonia. On hospital day 2, he complains of blurred vision in his left eye. He is unsure if it came on suddenly but notices it when he tries to read or watch television. There is no eye pain, and the eye and periorbital area are normal without erythema, warmth, or tenderness.

As in the assessment of diplopia, the first question to answer is whether the symptoms are monocular or binocular. Even very sophisticated patients may report vision loss in one eye when in fact they have a homonymous hemianopia on the side of reported monocular vision loss. Simple bedside testing with alternating eye occlusion is sufficient to get an answer. Most patients will have monocular symptoms. Painful vision loss often indicates a more acute process within the orbit, intracranial space, or systemically. Orbital or optic nerve infarction in giant cell arteritis is a rare but potentially life-threatening cause of severe, unilateral vision loss. Timing is the next crucial factor to determine. Vision loss may be discovered suddenly but be subacute in its true progression; the existence of an intercurrent acute illness may prompt attention to other organ systems as well. Finally, vision loss may be transient or fixed, and the differential diagnosis may be altered significantly (Table 81-2).

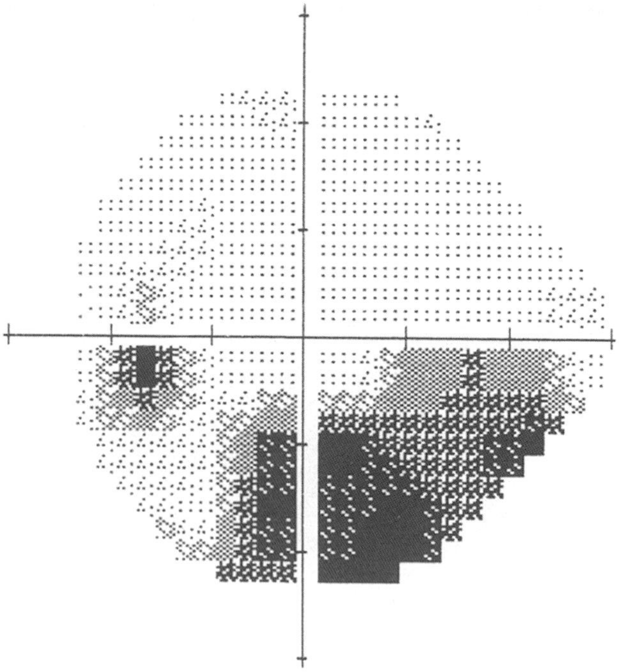

Figure 81-6 *Visual field testing showing loss of the inferior field of vision in a patient with superior branch retinal vein occlusion and retinal ischemia. The field defect respects the horizontal meridian, consistent with the distribution of the retinal vascular supply.*

Bedside visual acuity is 20/20 OD, 20/70 OS. It does not improve with use of a pinhole. There is no relative afferent pupillary defect, and the fundi are difficult to see without dilation. Upon dilation, the consultant reports that the left retina has hemorrhages and lipid deposition superiorly, matching an inferior defect on perimetry (**Figure 81-6**). Fluorescein angiography confirms a branch retinal vein occlusion. CBC and coagulation panel are unremarkable, and a TTE/TEE are also found to be normal. Carotid duplex scans show no hemodynamic abnormalities. The patient is scheduled for outpatient ophthalmology follow-up in 30 days to screen for possible retinal neovascularization and resolution of macular edema. He is advised to maintain good glycemic and blood pressure control as an outpatient.

Acute vision loss from retinal or optic nerve disease can be precipitated by hemodynamic shifts in acutely ill patients or from adverse effects (hypotension, direct toxicity) of new medications. A thorough review of the patient's medical risk factors for vision loss is required so that no possibilities are overlooked. The acute treatment of these patients addresses the underlying hemodynamic or coagulation disorders that may be present and the systemic illness that may have precipitated the visual loss event. Careful ophthalmologic follow-up is essential, especially in cases of central retinal vein occlusion (CRVO), in which there is a high risk of later retinal neovascularization and development of severe glaucoma. If giant cell arteritis

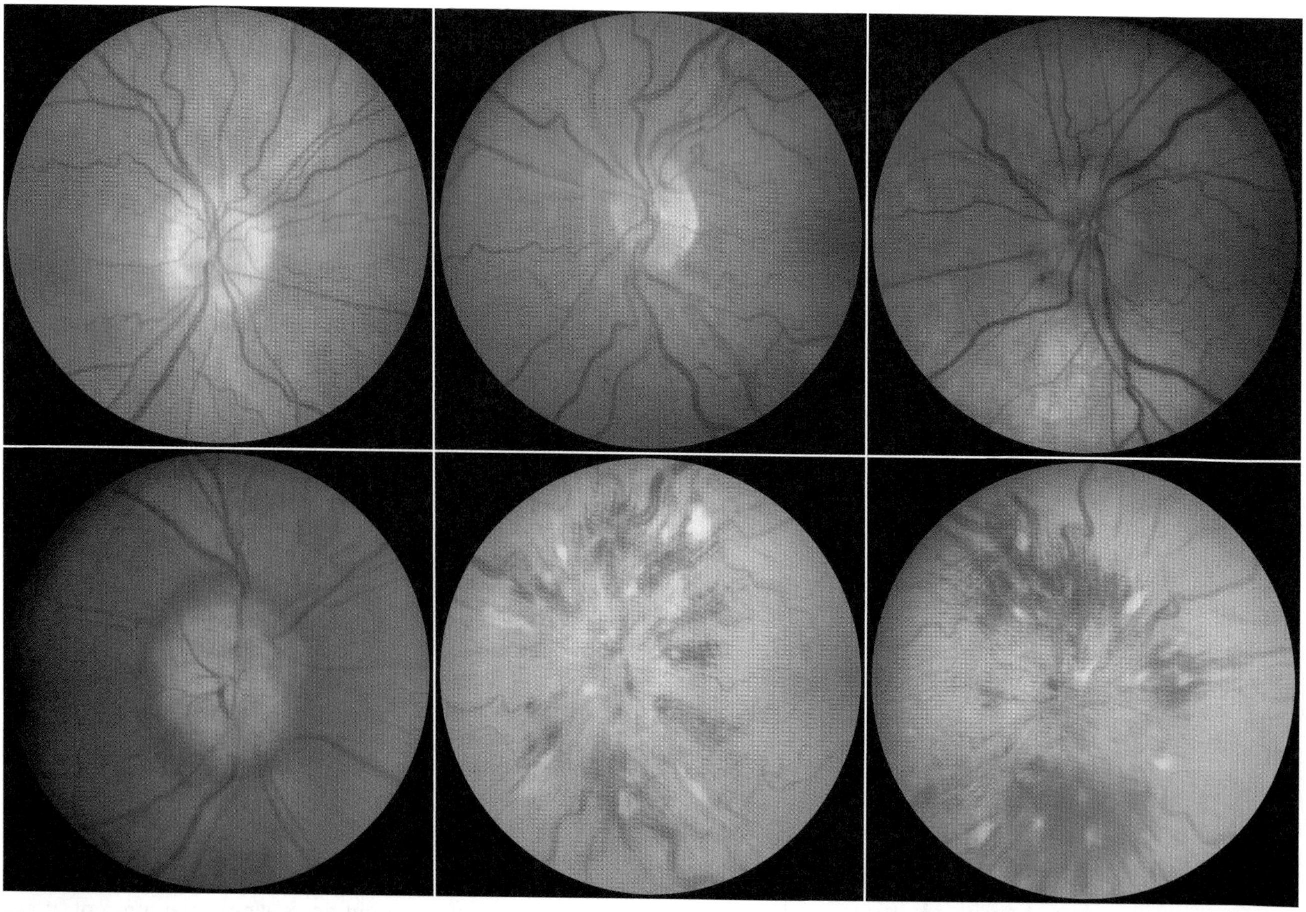

Figure 81-7 *Frisen Papilledema Scale, Grades 0–5.*

is suspected, then corticosteroids (preferably intravenous) should be started immediately. Waiting for an ophthalmology consultation and/or temporal artery biopsy is not necessary and may be harmful since it might delay treatment of a vision-threatening condition. While consultation and biopsy are necessary to confirm the diagnosis, they can be done after treatment begins and the patient is being protected from further events.

In the pregnant or immediate postpartum patient, hypertensive retinopathy with or without papilledema may occur at blood pressures below levels usually associated with malignant hypertension. Central vision loss is unusual except in severe or advanced disease; its presence should alert the clinician that urgent intervention is required to avoid permanent vision loss. Subtle optic disc swelling or hemorrhage may be difficult to appreciate with undilated fundoscopy, and ophthalmologic consultation should be obtained (inpatient if vision loss is present; otherwise, outpatient evaluation is indicated). The retinal changes should improve as better blood pressure control is obtained (**Figure 81-7**).

CONCLUSION

Hospitalized patients may develop a number of ocular disorders that will be brought to the attention of the treating physician. In many cases, the problems are simple and self-limited, especially when the patient's visual function is not impaired. Most of these issues are best managed in the outpatient setting, where the patient can see his/her general ophthalmologist. In more complex or concerning cases in which central or peripheral visual field loss is seen, or the patient reports severe pain, a basic bedside eye exam with attention to visual acuity ("the vital sign of the eye"), pupillary reaction, confrontational fields, and ocular motility will, along with basic inspection of the eye and adnexa, provide the ophthalmic consultant with invaluable information, allowing him or her to provide optimal care to the patient.

SUGGESTED READINGS

Dayan M, Turner B, McGhee C. Acute angle closure glaucoma masquerading as systemic illness. *Bmj.* 1996;313(7054):413–415.

Kerr NM, Chew SS, Danesh-Meyer HV. Non-arteritic anterior ischaemic optic neuropathy: a review and update. *J Clin Neurosci.* 2009;16(8)994–1000.

Prisco D, Marcucci R. Retinal vein thrombosis: risk factors, pathogenesis and therapeutic approach. *Pathophysiol Haemost Thromb.* 2002;32(5–6)308–311.

Sanders S, Kawasaki A, Purvin VA. Patterns of extraocular muscle weakness in vasculopathic pupil-sparing, incomplete third nerve palsy. *J Neuroophthalmol.* 2001;21(4):256–259.

Wilson LA. *Acute bacterial infection of the eye: bacterial keratitis and endophthalmitis. Trans Ophthalmol Soc U K.* 1986;105(1):43–60.

CHAPTER 82

Dizziness and Vertigo

Joseph M. Furman, MD, PhD

Key Clinical Questions

1. How do you determine whether a hospitalized patient has a benign cause of vertigo?
2. How might the physical examination confirm your suspicion of a benign cause of vertigo?
3. How do you treat vertigo?

INTRODUCTION

Dizziness and vertigo are common complaints and encompass a myriad of symptoms that may stem from many organ systems. A sensation of lightheadedness or faintness may relate to the presence of orthostatic hypotension, abnormalities of the cardiovascular system, altered ambulation as seen in patients with impaired vision and sensation of feet (multiple-sensory-defect dizziness), or decreased position sense and reduced vision commonly experienced by elderly patients (benign disequilibrium of aging). Many patients describe dizziness in reference to impaired ambulation and fear of falling or when they have blurred vision or feel confused. Hyperventilation may also cause symptoms of dizziness. These symptoms may be associated with significant disability and possibly mortality.

PRACTICE POINT

- A sensation of lightheadedness or faintness may relate to the presence of orthostatic hypotension, abnormalities of the cardiovascular system, hyperventilation, altered ambulation as seen in patients with impaired vision and sensation of feet (multiple-sensory-defect dizziness), or decreased position sense and reduced vision commonly experienced by elderly patients (benign disequilibrium of aging).

On the other hand, the sensation of vertigo defined as an illusion of movement of self or surroundings is much more likely to be a reflection of an abnormality of the peripheral or central vestibular system. It may be physiologic occurring with seasickness or after spinning or pathologic of central or peripheral origin. The misuse of the term *vertigo* as a diagnostic term rather than as a symptom should be eschewed in favor of a recognized diagnostic entity. Simply assigning a diagnosis of *vertigo* could prematurely terminate the evaluation and thereby miss an opportunity for accurate diagnosis followed by appropriate treatment. In some cases, the term *vertigo* is used as shorthand for benign paroxysmal positional vertigo. Because of the high prevalence of this disorder in the outpatient setting, these patients may receive proper treatment despite sloppy documentation and failure to convey accurate information to colleagues.

This chapter primarily focuses on the symptom of vertigo in patients admitted to the hospital. Chapter 99 includes cardiac causes of presyncope. Other medical illnesses, drug toxicity, and substance abuse that may produce symptoms of dizziness and vertigo are covered elsewhere in this book. The studies reviewing a systematic approach to the diagnosis and treatment of the symptom of vertigo relate to the outpatient or emergency room settings. Hospitalized patients are a different population. If symptoms of dizziness and vertigo are new experiences, the clinician should consider iatrogenic causes in addition to the usual suspects.

CASE 82-1

A 75-year-old woman with diabetes and hypertension underwent a total knee replacement. On the first postoperative day, she experienced vertigo when turning in her hospital bed. Each brief vertiginous episode was associated with mild nausea. The patient was essentially asymptomatic when sitting or lying still. She did not suffer any perioperative hypotension.

Physical and neurologic examinations revealed normal findings. What additional diagnostic testing should be considered?

THE VESTIBULAR SYSTEM

The vestibular system can be divided anatomically into the peripheral and central vestibular systems. The peripheral vestibular system consists of the left and right vestibular labyrinths and the eighth cranial nerve. The central vestibular system consists of the vestibular nuclei in the medulla and caudal pons and the pathways that subserve the vestibulo-ocular reflex, vestibulo-spinal reflexes, vestibular influences on spatial orientation, and the vestibulo-autonomic pathways that are important for the nausea and occasional vomiting that accompany vestibular system disease. Each vestibular labyrinth consists of three semicircular canals, which sense angular motion; and two otolithic organs, the utricle and saccule, which sense linear acceleration and orientation with respect to gravity. The vestibular labyrinth senses motion of the head. This signal is conveyed to the vestibular nuclei via the eighth nerve. At that site, vestibular signals are combined with signals from the visual and somatosensory systems to provide the central nervous system with an accurate representation of head orientation. With this information, the central nervous system can accurately control eye position and postural stability. Note that eighth nerve afferents have a nonzero tonic resting activity, which is illustrated diagrammatically in **Figure 82-1**.

Tonic signals from the left labyrinth drive the eyes and the body to the right, whereas signals from the right vestibular labyrinth drive the eyes and body to the left. At rest, these influences are balanced. During movement, the afferent activity from one labyrinth increases while the afferent activity from the opposite labyrinth decreases. This imbalance leads to movement of the eyes or the body as appropriate to maintain stable vision and upright posture.

PATHOPHYSIOLOGY OF THE VESTIBULAR SYSTEM

Vestibular disorders can be either peripheral or central. Most peripheral vestibular disorders affect only a single labyrinth. Damage to a single labyrinth causes a left-right vestibular imbalance. This imbalance is interpreted as intense movement toward the intact labyrinth, which leads to excessive eye movement in the form of nystagmus, gait instability, spatial disorientation, and autonomic symptoms such as nausea, vomiting, and, in some patients, changes in heart rate and blood pressure, (ie, either hypotension or hypertension). The effects of a unilateral vestibular loss are illustrated in **Figure 82-2**.

Over time, usually in a matter of days, central vestibular circuits rebalance despite the absence of a signal from one of the labyrinths. This process of rebalancing, known as *vestibular compensation*, leads to a gradual resolution of nystagmus and gait instability (see **Figure 82-3**).

Peripheral causes of vertigo include acoustic neuroma, aminoglycoside toxicity, benign positional vertigo, cholesteatoma, herpes zoster oticus, labyrinthine concussion related to head trauma, Ménière disease, perilymph fistula, otosclerosis, recurrent vestibulopathy, and vestibular neuronitis.

Central causes of vertigo include brain tumors, cerebellar or brainstem stroke, multiple sclerosis, vertebrobasilar transient ischemic attacks, and migraine-related dizziness.

HISTORY OF THE PATIENT WITH DIZZINESS OR VERTIGO

DOES THIS PATIENT HAVE VERTIGO?

The history is the most critical first step in distinguishing vertigo from other causes of dizziness and may pinpoint the etiology of the patient's symptoms in up to three-fourths of patients. The examiner should carefully ask the patient what is meant by these symptoms and what brings them on. Some patients may be unable to explain their symptoms at all and respond simply that "I'm just dizzy." Be sure to obtain an interpreter if English is not the primary language; do not make assumptions or characterize the symptoms for the patient in the interest of time. Most patients cannot adequately describe their symptoms because the sensation of dizziness and vertigo is not a normal sensation, and, unlike sensations such as vision and hearing, vestibular sensation does not have an associated vocabulary such as brightness, loudness,

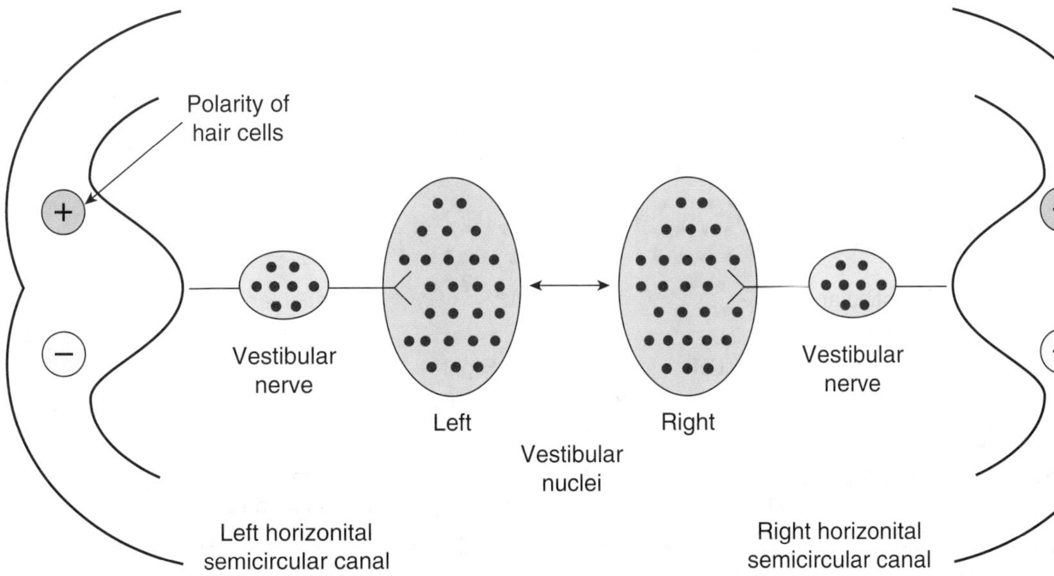

Figure 82-1 *Push–pull action of the horizontal vestibulo-ocular reflex, with no head movement, left and right vestibular influences are balanced.*

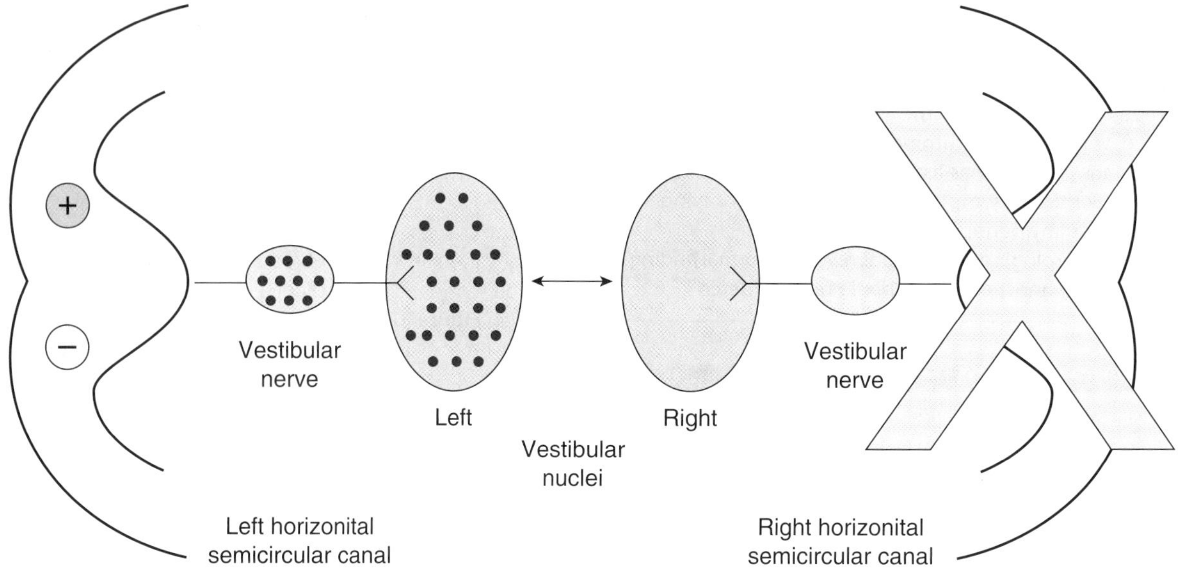

Figure 82-2 *The reciprocal push–pull interaction of the two labyrinths is disrupted after acute peripheral labyrinthine injury. For example, following the acute loss of right unilateral peripheral vestibular function, there is a loss of resting neural activity in the right vestibular nerve and right vestibular nuclei. Because the brain normally detects differences in activity between the two vestibular nuclear complexes, even when stationary the imbalance in neural activity is interpreted as a rapid head movement, in this case to the left.*

color, or pitch. Some patients complain of a head sensation such as light-headedness, heavy-headedness, foggy-headedness, or presyncope. These three general types of symptoms, namely a sense of motion, imbalance, and head sensations, are not mutually exclusive. A nonspecific complaint of a head sensation, especially light-headedness, does not exclude the possibility of a vestibular disorder whether peripheral or central, and it may result from a metabolic derangement, drug effect, or other organ system disease. In fact, dysequilibrium, reduced cerebral perfusion, and vertigo can all be associated with the symptom of dizziness with standing. Ask whether or not the dizziness is characterized by a sense of motion such as spinning, rocking or tilting, imbalance when walking, veering to the right or left, or if the patient fears falling or has fallen.

PRACTICE POINT

- The history is the most critical first step in distinguishing vertigo from other causes of dizziness, and may pinpoint the etiology of the patient's symptoms in up to three-fourths of patients. The sensation of vertigo, defined as an illusion of movement of self or surroundings, is much more likely to be a reflection of an abnormality of the peripheral or central vestibular system. The misuse of the term *vertigo* as a diagnostic term rather than as a symptom should be eschewed in favor of a recognized diagnostic entity. If the physical examination confirms the presence of benign positional vertigo and the rest of the examination is unrevealing, then no further evaluation is necessary.

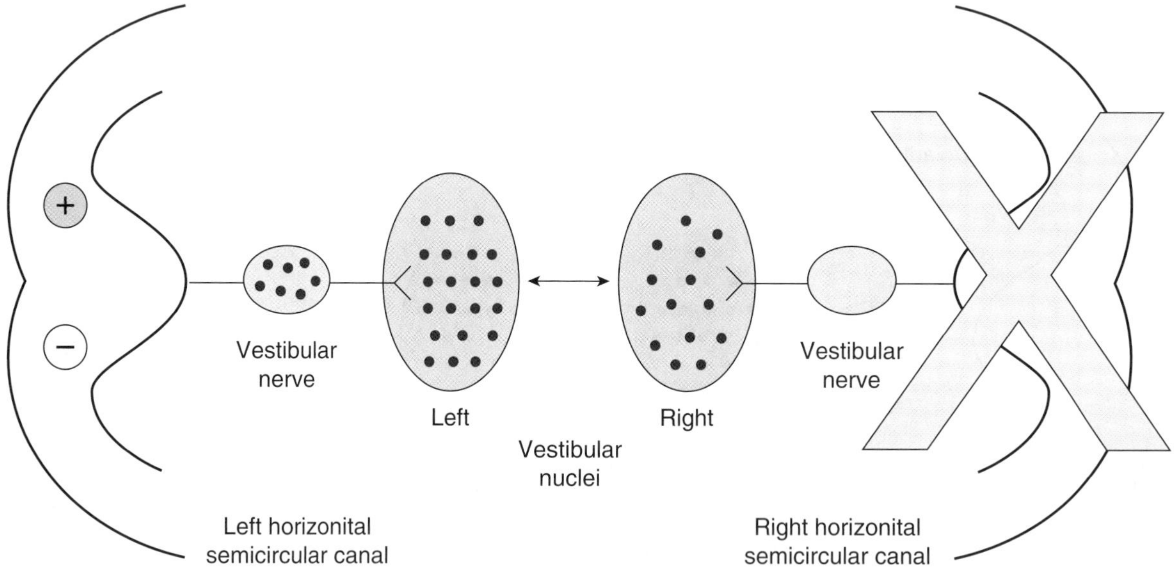

Figure 82-3 *When a peripheral vestibular injury is chronic, in this case on the right, the central nervous system is able, through vestibular compensation, to partially restore the lost resting activity within the deafferented vestibular nucleus, and thus reduce the asymmetry of neural activity between the vestibular nuclei at rest and partially restore the function of the vestibulo-ocular reflex.*

TABLE 82-1 Symptom Patterns of Vertigo

Benign paroxysmal positional vertigo (benign positional nystagmus, cupulolithiasis): Normal hearing, intermittent episodes of vertigo with head turning, the most common cause of vertigo
Vestibular neuronitis (vestibular neuritis, labyrinthitis): Normal hearing, sudden onset of severe, constant vertigo made worse by head movement that resolves over the course of days to weeks, second in frequency
Recurrent vestibulopathy: Normal hearing, intermittent episodes of constant vertigo lasting minutes or hours
Toxins (drugs such as aminoglycoside toxicity or alcohol): Vertigo with or without hearing loss, bilateral labyrinthine dysfunction
Central causes of vertigo: Vertigo with symptoms of neurologic dysfunction including weakness, impaired speech, diplopia

After giving the patient time to respond, sometimes asking about specific circumstances such as when the symptoms occur, other neurologic or otologic symptoms, and whether they are recurrent may help pinpoint the diagnosis more than the description of the dizziness. Associated symptoms should be specifically questioned: loss of consciousness, headache, tinnitus, decreased hearing, disturbance of other cranial nerves, trouble walking or controlling extremities, visual impairment, and nausea and vomiting. The examiner should determine whether the onset of dizziness or vertigo was sudden, how long it lasted, and whether worse when supine, standing, stooping, or turning the neck. Risk factors to consider include: antecedent head or neck trauma (such as hyperextension of the neck), episodes of low or high blood sugar, hypertension, prior stroke, and dehydration.

Medication review is essential. Many new medications and/or toxic levels of medications due to drug-drug interactions, changes in metabolism due to renal and/or liver derangements, or incorrect prescribing can cause dizziness. Typical examples include phenytoin toxicity and reactions to some antibiotics. Because nearly all medications can potentially cause "dizziness," clinicians should specifically inquire about new medications.

DOES THIS PATIENT HAVE A BENIGN CAUSE OF VERTIGO?

When formulating a differential diagnosis for a patient who presents with vertigo, consider whether the patient's abnormality is affecting the peripheral vestibular apparatus, the central vestibular system, or both and the nature of the disease process, (eg, inflammatory, vascular, or neurochemical derangements). Note that peripheral vestibular disorders often are associated with otologic complaints such as hearing loss, tinnitus, or ear fullness. Central vestibular disorders are more likely to include associated neurologic symptoms such as numbness, weakness, and incoordination. A common misconception when obtaining a history from patients with dizziness is to insist that patients with vertigo indicate whether they or the world around them appear to be moving. Although it is helpful to elicit a history of self-motion and/or motion of the surroundings versus simply lightheadedness, making a distinction between motion of self and motion of surround has no diagnostic utility (**Table 82-1**).

THE PHYSICAL EXAMINATION OF PATIENTS WITH VERTIGO

The medical history identifies patients who have true vertigo. These patients are most likely to have a peripheral vestibular etiology. Because true vertigo may be associated with other disorders, the evaluation of a patient complaining of vertigo should consist of a general physical examination, a neurologic examination, and, as appropriate, specialized bedside examination provocative tests. If the physical examination confirms the presence of benign positional vertigo and the rest of the examination is unrevealing, then no further evaluation is necessary. Hospitalized patients may be more likely to have multifactorial causes to their symptoms due to their medications, fluid and nutritional status, deconditioning, and other comorbid conditions (**Table 82-2**).

Hospitalized patients who are more likely to be hypovolemic may have the following: nausea and vomiting due to the vertigo, acute blood loss (surgical or medical), third spacing (severe liver disease), burns, or poor oral intake with limited fluid replacement. The first step is always to examine the patient's vital signs. The physical examination should include checking for orthostatic blood pressure changes, examining the tympanic membranes, and performing a cardiovascular examination along with listening for bruits. The criterion of a pulse increment of > 30 beats per minute from the supine to standing position may have limited utility in patients taking nodal blockers or with conduction system disease. Deconditioning can lead to orthostatic blood pressure changes as can autonomic nervous system dysfunction and medications. Hence, clinical judgment is required to assess abnormal vital signs.

The bedside neurologic examination should include performing an eye examination, testing for hearing loss and checking other cranial nerves, Romberg and postural reflexes, decreased sensation of the feet, and an assessment of gait and station; see Chapter 207. An abnormal neurologic examination will likely localize the illness and determine the need for imaging

SPONTANEOUS NYSTAGMUS

Vertical nystagmus is a central vestibular sign that usually warrants MRI specifically of the vestibular nuclei or of the cerebellar vermis. A unidirectional horizontal nystagmus that includes a slight torsional component is more likely caused by a peripheral abnormality. Upbeating nystagmus seen only on upward gaze is usually a benign finding akin to bidirectional horizontal gaze-evoked nystagmus.

If the patient does not have spontaneous nystagmus, the examiner should perform a provocative maneuver to test for positional nystagmus

Head-thrust test

To perform the head-thrust test, the patient's head is abruptly rotated to the right or left while the patient attempts to fixate on a distant stationary object. The examiner looks for a small rapid eye movement opposite to the direction of head movement that signifies an inadequate vestibulo-ocular reflex resulting from a disorder of the labyrinth toward which the head has been moved. Performing this test can be difficult in patients with an acute vestibular imbalance.

Dix-Hallpike maneuver

To perform the Dix-Hallpike maneuver, the examiner stands at the patient's side and rotates the patient's head 45 degrees to the nearside to align the ipsilateral posterior semicircular canal with the sagittal plane of the body. The patient is instructed to keep his or her eyes open, especially if he or she experiences vertigo. The examiner then moves the patient, whose eyes are open, from the seated to the supine ear-down position and then extends the patient's neck slightly so that the chin is pointed slightly upward. The latency, duration, and direction of nystagmus, if present, and the latency and duration of vertigo, if present, should be noted. A positive test produces a paroxysmal upbeating-torsional nystagmus. The examiner observes the patient's eyes for the characteristic nystagmus that generally lasts for the duration of the patient's vertigo.

TABLE 82-2 The Clinical History and Physical Examination

Does this dizzy patient have vertigo?
- True vertigo accounts for roughly half of the causes of dizziness.
- Sometimes asking about specific circumstances such as when the symptoms occur, other neurologic or otologic symptoms, and whether symptoms are recurrent may help pinpoint the diagnosis more than the description of the dizziness.

Ask the following questions:
- Are the symptoms characterized by a sense of motion such as spinning, rocking, or tilting?
- Is there a sense of imbalance when walking, veering to the right or left, or concern about falling? If so, inquire whether the patient does not have symptoms of dizziness when sitting or lying down. Dysequilibrium accounts for roughly 3% of causes of dizziness.

Does this patient have a benign cause of vertigo?
- Forty percent of dizzy patients will have peripheral vestibular disorders affecting the inner ear and cranial nerve VIII.
- Benign positional vertigo and vestibular neuronitis are most frequent diagnoses

Inquire about associated hearing loss.
- For patients without associated hearing loss, the likelihood of a cerebello pontine mass as the cause of vertigo is low (probability 1×10^{-4}).

Inquire about whether the vertigo is episodic or persistent.
- No hearing loss and episodic, brief, intense vertigo is likely benign positional vertigo.
- No hearing loss and persistent vertigo lasting hours to days with nausea is likely vestibular neuronitis.

Inquire about associated otologic complaints.
- Peripheral vestibular disorders are often associated with otologic complaints such as hearing loss, tinnitus, or ear fullness.
- Hearing loss and episodic vertigo lasting hours with tinnitus and a sensation of ear fullness is most consistent with Ménière disease.
- Hearing loss and severe persistent vertigo lasting hours to days with nausea is most consistent with labyrinthitis.

Does this patient have a central cause of vertigo?
- Roughly 10% of all dizziness may be central in origin.

Inquire about associated neurologic complaints.
- Central vestibular disorders are more likely to be associated with numbness, weakness, and incoordination.

Inquire about antecedent trauma and other risk factors.

Review medication list.

Is this patient orthostatic?

Does this patient have an abnormal neurologic examination?

Does this patient have an abnormal ear examination?
- Ear drainage is seen as a complication of chronic otitis media along with hearing loss and vertigo (cholesteatoma).
- Ramsay Hunt syndrome may be identified by the presence of vesicles along with hearing loss and facial palsy.

Does this patient have spontaneous nystagmus?
- Spontaneous horizontal nystagmus with or without torsional nystagmus is usually seen in patients with vestibular neuronitis or in other peripheral disorders.
- Vertical nystagmus is a central vestibular sign.
- Upbeating nystagmus only on upward gaze and bidirectional horizontal gaze–evoked nystagmus are usually benign findings.
- Absence of nystagmus during vertigo may suggest psychogenic vertigo.

Does this patient have positional nystagmus that reproduces the patient's symptoms?

COMMON VESTIBULAR DISORDERS IN THE HOSPITAL

Common vestibular disorders that may lead to a hospital admission or that may present once a patient has been admitted for an unrelated ailment involve peripheral disorders, including vestibular neuritis, benign paroxysmal positional vertigo, and Ménière disease, and central disorders, including migraine-related dizziness, medication-induced dizziness and vertigo, and posterior fossa stroke. Note that patients admitted following trauma may experience dizziness or vertigo on either a peripheral or central basis and that some psychiatric illnesses, notably panic disorder, may include dizziness.

BENIGN PAROXYSMAL POSITIONAL VERTIGO

Benign paroxysmal positional vertigo (BPPV) represents a very common vestibular disorder in the outpatient and emergency room setting. BPPV may be encountered in the hospital setting, especially in patients who have undergone a surgical procedure or who require prolonged bed rest. BPPV is characterized by brief periods, generally 10 to 20 seconds, of intense rotational vertigo that may or may not be associated with nausea. Aside from attacks of positional vertigo, patients with BPPV are often asymptomatic. A definitive diagnosis of benign paroxysmal positional vertigo can be made at the bedside using the Dix-Hallpike maneuver. The nystagmus may be complex with a mixture of both upbeating and torsional (rotary) eye movement. Physical examination will be normal otherwise.

Treatment for benign paroxysmal positional vertigo consists of a particle repositioning maneuver to relocate otolithic debris from the posterior semicircular channel to the vestibule. Patients may be referred to the following Web site regarding the Epley maneuver or referred to a physical therapist for instruction in how to perform these exercises: www.charite.de/ch/neuro/vertigo.html.

Patients with chronic vertigo of vestibular origin may benefit from a vestibular rehabilitation program designed to facilitate central compensation.

■ VESTIBULAR NEURITIS

Vestibular neuritis generally presents with the acute or subacute onset of severe vertigo, nausea, vomiting, and disequilibrium sometimes as the sequelae of a flu-like illness or an afebrile viral illness. Symptoms are present at rest and are exacerbated by any head movement. Certain head positions may exacerbate or reduce symptoms. Severe symptoms usually last for one to three days during which acute management is required. Then, symptoms gradually resolve over a period of days.

Physical examination generally reveals a unidirectional horizontal nystagmus that increases when the patient gazes in the direction of the quick component of the vestibular nystagmus. Gait instability is the rule. Note, however, that patients with vestibular neuritis are able to ambulate although they may require assistance. The head-thrust test is generally abnormal in patients with vestibular neuritis. Imaging in patients with vestibular neuritis is normal and usually not indicated. If there was something clinically that did not quite fit with this diagnosis and generates some concern on the physician's part, a definitive diagnosis of vestibular neuritis can be established by caloric testing in the vestibular laboratory indicating a markedly reduced or absent caloric response unilaterally.

It is the standard of practice to treat with corticosteroids although their benefit has not been consistently shown. Antiviral agents have not been shown to be effective. Supportive measures may include vestibular suppressants such as meclizine, tranquilizers, and bedrest for one to two days.

■ MÉNIÈRE DISEASE

Ménière disease is a term that should be reserved for patients who suffer from presumed endolymphatic hydrops, a pathophysiology that produces the triad of vertigo, unilateral hearing loss, and unilateral tinnitus, that is, the term should be reserved for the characteristic syndrome and should not be used to describe patients with presumed peripheral vestibular disease of uncertain etiology. These symptoms are frequently associated with unilateral ear fullness. Symptoms generally last from several minutes to several hours and occur in episodes; patients are usually asymptomatic between episodes. During episodes, patients may experience nausea, vomiting, and severe gait instability. They would be expected to exhibit a marked horizontal-torsional nystagmus independent of head position, worse with loss of visual fixation. Between episodes, patients may manifest unilateral low-frequency sensorineural hearing loss, which can be discovered using tuning forks and confirmed definitively with audiometry. Balance laboratory testing often reveals a reduced vestibular responsiveness on the same side as the patient's tinnitus and hearing loss. Treatment for Ménière disease consists of a reduction of dietary intake of sodium (2 g/day) and pharmacotherapy with a combination of hydrochlorothiazide and triamterene.

■ MEDICATION-INDUCED DIZZINESS

Patients with medication-induced dizziness generally do not experience vertigo, and the mechanism by which medications produce dizziness is unknown. Patients may experience nonspecific head sensations and gait instability. Medications that are especially likely to cause dizziness include centrally acting agents such as benzodiazepines, anticonvulsants, antidepressants, and antirejection medications such as tacrolimus. These patients may never experience vertigo and may not experience dizziness or imbalance until their vestibular loss is severe because of the symmetric damage. A special circumstance relates to known ototoxic medications such as aminoglycosides and cis platinum. These medications may produce bilateral peripheral vestibular loss via hair cell damage and lead to oscillopsia (jumbled vision) and gait ataxia. Patients with medication-induced dizziness may have postural hypotension and gait instability. Establishing a diagnosis of medication-induced dizziness may be challenging in that changing a patient's medication regimen may not be possible. Vestibular laboratory testing of such patients is generally unrevealing aside from nonspecific abnormalities of ocular motor function in patients receiving centrally acting drugs. Patients with ototoxicity will have decreased vestibular responses.

CEREBROVASCULAR DISEASES

Cerebrovascular accidents affecting the brainstem and cerebellum may present with dizziness and vertigo. The most commonly recognized conditions include Wallenberg syndrome, which is caused by ischemia in the territory supplied by the posterior inferior cerebellar artery, by ischemia in the territory supplied by the anterior inferior cerebellar artery, or by cerebellar hemorrhage. Symptoms and signs will of course depend upon the precise location of the central nervous system abnormality. In general, however, patients will present with definitive central nervous system symptoms and signs.

■ HEAD AND NECK TRAUMA

Patients admitted following traumatic injuries of the head and neck may experience dizziness. Diagnostic considerations include BPPV, which may be posttraumatic, and labyrinthine concussion. Some patients following trauma of the head and neck experience combined injury to the peripheral vestibular system and the central vestibular pathways. It is important to consider cervical injuries as exacerbating factors for dizziness because somatosensory neck muscles afferents that normally provide signals related to head position may be damaged. This damage can cause dizziness because of a mismatch between vestibular and somatosensory signals. Hyperextension of the neck as seen in motor vehicle accidents or during neck manipulation may result in injury of the vertebrobasilar system and subsequent dissection producing ischemic symptoms.

■ MIGRAINE-RELATED DIZZINESS

Migraine-related dizziness is an increasingly recognized disorder characterized by vestibular signs and symptoms in association with migrainous symptoms. Whereas patients with vestibular neuritis and benign paroxysmal positional vertigo experience clearly defined vestibular-related symptoms, patients with migraine-related dizziness often have more nonspecific symptoms, making diagnosis more challenging. Migraine-related dizziness should be considered especially in patients who have suffered from migraine headache over a span of many years and then begin to experience episodic attacks of vertigo and dizziness exacerbated by head movement. The duration of migraine-related dizziness episodes is highly variable; attacks can last for seconds, minutes, hours, or days. Examination is usually normal between attacks. During attacks, patients may manifest either peripheral vestibular signs, central vestibular signs, or both. Migraine-related dizziness remains a diagnosis of exclusion in that there are no pathognomonic signs or symptoms or laboratory test abnormalities to confirm this diagnosis. Approximately 25% of patients with migraine-related dizziness manifest a unilateral reduction of vestibular function when assessed in the vestibular laboratory. Treatment of migraine-related dizziness is similar to the treatment of migraine headache as treatment may be preventative, abortive, or symptomatic. Preventive medication may consist of antidepressants, beta-blocking agents, anticonvulsants, and calcium channel–blocking agents. Symptomatic treatment may include vestibular suppressants. Abortive treatments with triptans may be efficacious.

TABLE 82-3 Medications Commonly Used to Reduce Dizziness, Vertigo, and Associated Nausea

Drug (Brand Name)	Pharmacologic Class	Dose	Primary Use	Adverse Reactions
Meclizine (Antivert, Bonine)	Anticholinergic Antihistamine	25 mg every 4–6 hours orally	Dizziness	Drowsiness
Dimenhydrinate (Dramamine)	Anticholinergic Antihistamine	50 mg every 4–6 hours orally	Dizziness	Drowsiness
Cyclizine (Marezine)	Anticholinergic Antihistamine	50 mg every 4–6 hours orally or IM	Dizziness	Drowsiness
Diazepam (Valium)	Benzodiazepine	1–2 mg twice daily orally; 2–10 mg (1 dose) given acutely orally, IM or IV	Dizziness	Lethargy
Clonazepam (Klonopin)	Benzodiazepine	0.25–0.5 mg twice daily orally	Dizziness	Lethargy
Prochlorperazine (Compazine)	Phenothiazine	10 mg orally or IM every 6 hours or 25 mg rectally every 12 hours	Nausea	Extrapyramidal reactions, drowsiness, anticholinergic effects
Promethazine (Phenergan)	Phenothiazine	25 mg every 6–12 hours orally or rectally	Nausea	Extrapyramidal reactions, drowsiness, restlessness
Trimethobenzamine (Tigan)	Substituted ethanolamine	250 mg every 6–8 hours or 200 mg rectally or IM	Nausea	Extrapyramidal reaction (unusual)
Diphenhydramine (Benadryl)	Antihistamine	25–100 mg every 8 hours orally	Nausea	Drowsiness
Hydroxyzine (Vistaril, Atarax)	Piperazine derivative	25–50 mg every 8 hours orally	Nausea	Drowsiness

PSYCHIATRIC DIZZINESS

Psychiatric dizziness represents a diagnosis of exclusion and should be used with caution in that many patients with vestibular system abnormalities develop psychiatric manifestations, notably anxiety, including panic attacks. However, some patients with primary anxiety disorders can present with dizziness, especially in association with panic attacks. Although some of these patients will suffer from an underlying vestibular disorder, many will not. Treatment of psychiatric dizziness consists of identifying the psychiatric disorder and treating it appropriately. For dizziness associated with panic attacks, treatment with antidepressants and benzodiazepines should be considered.

NONSPECIFIC DIZZINESS

Unfortunately, for many patients who experience dizziness and vertigo, no definitive diagnosis can be reached. If worrisome disorders are not a consideration, empiric treatment can be safely recommended. When considering treatment options, it is important to understand that the compensation process can be slowed by vestibular suppressant medications, such as meclizine and benzodiazepines.

The table provides a list of medications that should be considered for the symptomatic treatment of dizziness, vertigo, and associated nausea (**Table 82-3**).

Note that vestibular suppressant medications should not be continued indefinitely. Thus, if a patient is provided with a prescription for a vestibular suppressant upon discharge from the hospital, arrangements should be made for follow-up care.

CASE 82-1 *(continued)*

The patient was found to be suffering from BPPV based on a positive Dix-Hallpike maneuver. The patient underwent particle repositioning appropriate for posterior semicircular canal BPPV, which lead to complete relief from positional vertigo. The patient continued to experience some gait instability, which was thought to be related to her orthopedic problem primarily with a history of BPPV as a secondary component. Additional physical therapy for balance rehabilitation was ordered.

CONCLUSION

The history is the most critical first step in distinguishing vertigo from other causes of dizziness, paying attention to underlying systemic diseases and risk factors as well as possible medication related dizziness and vertigo. The examiner should check for orthostatic vital signs, perform a cardiovascular and neurologic examination and make an assessment of the patient's overall health. If the patient appears to have vertigo, the clinician should try to pinpoint a precise etiology, consistent with symptom pattern of vertigo the patient is describing. If a central cause of vertigo is suspected, the patient should proceed directly to imaging. If a peripheral cause of vertigo is suspected, a physical examination should confirm the absence of impaired speech, weakness, numbness, incoordination or other neurologic signs suggesting a central etiology.

SUGGESTED READINGS

Baloh RW. Clinical practice. Vestibular neuritis. *N Engl J Med.* 2003;348(11):1027–1032.

Epley JM. The canalith repositioning procedure: for treatment of benign paroxysmal positional vertigo. *Otolaryngol Head Neck Surg.* 1992;107(3):399–404.

Furman JM, Cass SP. Benign paroxysmal positional vertigo. *N Engl J Med.* 1999;341(21):1590–1596.

Halmagyi GM, Curthoys IS. A clinical sign of canal paresis. *Arch Neurol.* 1988;45(7):737–739.

Shupak A, Issa A, Golz A, Margalit Kaminer, Braverman I., Prednisone treatment for vestibular neuritis. *Otol Neurotol*. 2008;29(3):368–374.

Strupp M, Zingler VC, Arbusow V, Niklas D, Maag KP, Dieterich M, Bense S, Theil D, Jahn K, Brandt T. Methylprednisolone, valacyclovir, or the combination for vestibular neuritis. *N Engl J Med*. 2004;351(4):354–361.

von Brevern M, Zeise D, Neuhauser H, Clarke AH, Lempert T. Acute migrainous vertigo: clinical and oculographic findings. *Brain*. 2005;128(Pt 2):365–374.

von Brevern M, Radtke A, Lezius F, Feldmann M, Ziese T, Lempert T, Neuhauser H. Epidemiology of benign paroxysmal positional vertigo: a population based study. *J Neurol Neurosurg Psychiatry*. 2007;78(7):710–715.

Wrisley DM, Sparto PJ, Whitney SL, Furman JM. Cervicogenic dizziness: a review of diagnosis and treatment. *J Orthop Sports Phys Ther*. 2000;30(12):755–766.

CHAPTER 83

Dyspnea

Tracy J. Wanner, MD
Richard M. Schwartzstein, MD

Key Clinical Questions

1. What are the underlying physiologic mechanisms that result in dyspnea?
2. How can a physician elicit a patient's personal description of shortness of breath in order to gain insight into the underlying diagnosis?
3. What physical exam findings are concerning for impending respiratory failure?
4. What are the key diagnostic studies a physician should order to further elucidate the cause of a patient's dyspnea?
5. How can the disease states associated with dyspnea be organized into a clinical framework?

CASE 83-1

INPATIENT ADMISSION

A 63-year-old woman describes shortness of breath on postoperative day 3 after a hip replacement. At 3 AM, the patient starts complaining that she "can't catch her breath" and feels as though she is suffocating. Sitting upright, she appears in acute distress with rapid, shallow breathing and expiratory grunting. Her blood pressure is 210/95 mm Hg with a heart rate of 120 beats per minute and an oxygen saturation of 92% while using supplemental oxygen at 6 liters/min by nasal cannula. On physical exam, auscultation of the lungs reveals rales over the lower one-third of the lung fields with dullness at the bases, as well as significant peripheral pitting edema. Since the patient has been receiving intravenous normal saline at 100 cc/hour since the surgery, she is likely suffering from pulmonary edema. A chest radiograph (CXR) demonstrates increased interstitial markings and bilateral costophrenic angle blunting, which explain her clinical presentation. Increased interstitial edema activates a variety of receptors that stimulate the respiratory controller and cause air hunger, while pleural eff usions cause an increase in work of breathing by affecting the body's ventilatory pump.

The history, exam findings of hypertension, orthopnea, and rales, and the CXR findings help to confirm the diagnosis of volume overload. Other potential causes of dyspnea in an older patient who has undergone major surgery include myocardial ischemia, aspiration, and pulmonary embolism. In addition to treating congestive heart failure (CHF), it is important to seek out any underlying error that may have caused the condition and effect a system change that can improve quality of care for future patients. In the above case, indiscriminant use of maintenance fluids was the culprit; focused provider education and adjustment of existing order sets may be needed.

PRACTICE POINT

- Indiscriminant use of maintenance fluids is a common and preventable cause of pulmonary edema in inpatients.

INTRODUCTION

Dyspnea, or "shortness of breath," is a common problem affecting up to half of patients in acute, tertiary care hospitals and one quarter of ambulatory outpatients. This sensation of breathlessness can be associated with anxiety, fear, or depression and, thereby, cause substantial disability. The American Thoracic Society consensus statement on dyspnea describes it as "an uncomfortable sensation of breathing," which encompasses several qualitatively distinct sensations that reflect the subjective nature of the experience as well as the psychological, social, and environmental factors that contribute to the symptoms. A solid understanding of these distinct sensations and the pathophysiologic mechanisms underlying them can help physicians better understand, diagnose, and treat their patients.

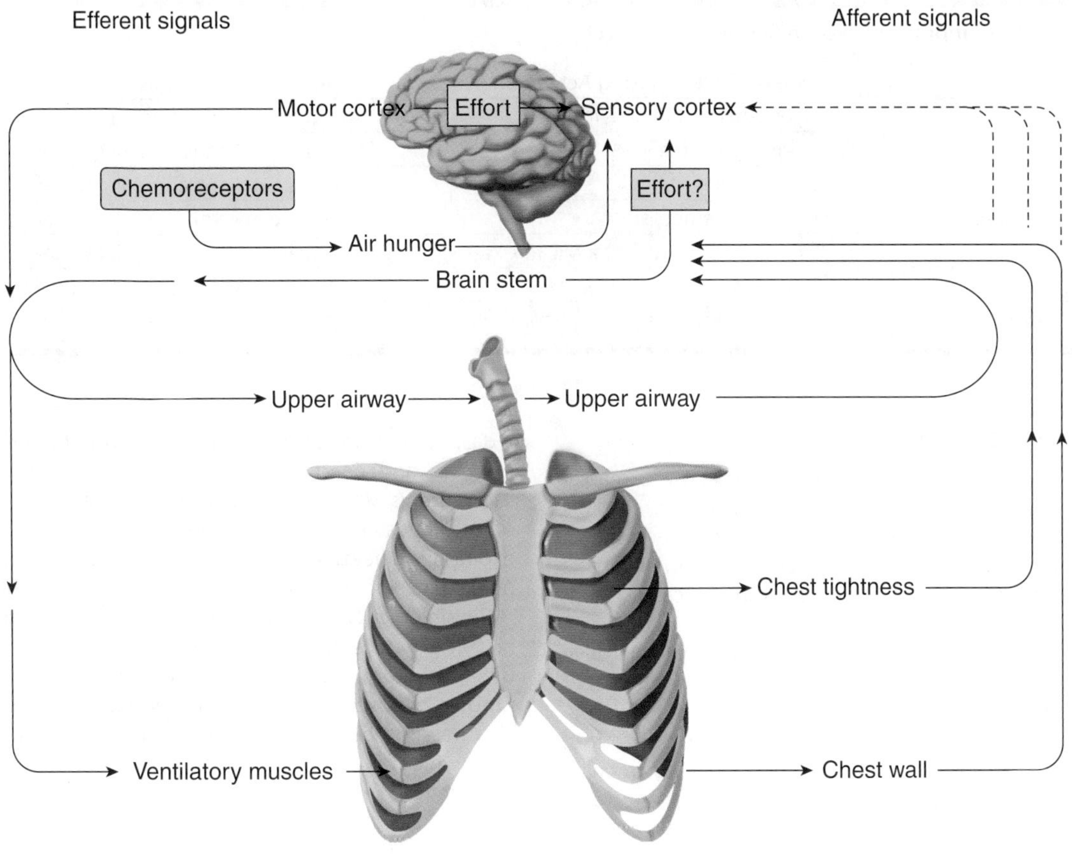

Figure 83-1 *The sense of respiratory effort is believed to arise from a signal transmitted from the motor cortex to the sensory cortex coincidently with the outgoing motor command to the ventilatory muscles. The arrow from the brain stem to the sensory cortex indicates that the motor output of the brain stem may also contribute to the sense of effort. The sense of air hunger is believed to arise, in part, from increased respiratory activity within the brain stem, and the sensation of chest tightness probably results from stimulation of vagal irritant receptors. Although afferent information from airway, lung, and chest-wall receptors most likely passes through the brain stem before reaching the sensory cortex, the dashed lines indicate uncertainty about whether some afferents bypass the brain stem and project directly to the sensory cortex.*

MECHANISMS OF DYSPNEA

Similar to the feelings of thirst or hunger, the complex sensation of dyspnea is a visceral experience that integrates information from a number of sensory receptors and, in the case of dyspnea, is the consequence of a variety of pathophysiologic mechanisms. Dyspnea begins with a physiological impairment or stimulus that activates a range of sensory receptors that transmit incoming or afferent information to the cerebral cortex and to respiratory centers in the brainstem. Together, all the elements of the system that alter rate and depth of breathing can be considered the "respiratory controller"—akin to a thermostat—whose function is to set the rate and depth of each breath. Additionally, the brain sends efferent or outgoing neural messages to the muscles of ventilation, activating the "ventilatory pump." Most often, a patient's dyspnea can be attributed to abnormalities in one or both of these components of the respiratory system, and any additional mismatch between this motor feed-forward message and sensory feedback (ie, unsatiated air-hunger) increases the intensity of dyspnea (**Figure 83-1**).

■ VENTILATORY PUMP

Patients with disorders that affect the ventilatory pump experience an increased sense of "effort to breathe" or "work of breathing." The ventilatory pump consists of peripheral nerves, muscles of ventilation, supporting skeleton, pleura, and airways; any disorder that affects these components can lead to an increased sense of the work of breathing. Hyperinflation causes dyspnea by placing the breathing muscles at a mechanical disadvantage and by forcing the patient to breathe at lung and chest wall volumes associated with reduced compliance, or greater stiffness of the respiratory system. The shortening of the inspiratory muscles that accompanies hyperinflation makes them less effective in generating tension. Furthermore, a change in the radius of the curvature of the diaphragm (it is relatively flat in patients who have hyperinflation) represents an additional load for the inspiratory muscles to overcome. In addition to hyperinflation, disorders such as chronic obstructive pulmonary disease (COPD) and asthma can also lead to increased airway resistance, further augmenting the work of breathing. Myopathies can cause muscular weakness, and kyphoscoliosis can lead to a stiff chest wall. Both of these conditions contribute to an increased sense of effort to breathe. Lastly, pleural effusions increase the work of breathing by expanding the chest wall and shortening inspiratory muscles, and may stimulate pulmonary receptors via associated atelectasis of regions of lung compressed by the fluid.

TABLE 83-1 Afferent Inputs Involved in Respiratory Control

Receptors	Disease States Causing Activation	Resulting Effect/Sensation
Chemoreceptors	Hypoxemia, acute hypercapnea, acidemia	Increase in ventilation; air hunger
J-receptors	Interstitial edema	Increase in ventilation; air hunger
C5 receptors	Inflammation	Increase in ventilation; air hunger
Pulmonary vascular receptors	Pulmonary embolism	Increase in ventilation; air hunger
Metaboreceptors	Exercise; increased metabolic rate	Increase in ventilation; air hunger
Mechanoreceptors Lung	Bronchospasm	Increase in ventilation; chest tightness
Mechanoreceptors Muscles	COPD, asthma, chest wall abnormalities	Sensation of increased work of breathing

RESPIRATORY CONTROLLER

Patients with disorders that stimulate the respiratory controller experience the sensation of "air hunger." Activation of receptors throughout the respiratory system—for example, irritant and stretch receptors in the airways and lung parenchyma, flow receptors in the central airways, and chemoreceptors in the carotid bodies and medulla—lead to stimulation of the control centers in the brainstem. We observe this as an increase in ventilatory drive (increased rate and depth of breathing, use of accessory muscles of ventilation, etc) and patients perceive a sense of an increased urge to breathe or air hunger. Interstitial edema activates J-receptors; inflammation activates C fibers; and acute changes in pulmonary artery pressure (eg, pulmonary emboli) activate C fibers in pulmonary vessels and pressure receptors in the pulmonary vasculature or right atrium. Changes in the metabolic rate during exercise affect metaboreceptors located in the skeletal muscle, which also contribute to uncomfortable breathing. Nondisease states, such as the hypoxemia associated with high altitude, pregnancy's high progesterone state, and drugs such as aspirin, can also stimulate the respiratory controller and cause dyspnea. Furthermore, some receptors provide afferent input that leads to other sensations that can be interpreted as dyspnea. For example, bronchospasm stimulates mechanoreceptors in the lungs, which we believe leads to a sensation of chest tightness, which is sensed through vagal afferents, and may act as another stimulus for dyspnea (**Table 83-1**).

Some disorders, such as pneumonia, pulmonary edema, aspiration, pulmonary embolism, asthma, and COPD, not only contribute to dyspnea by the mechanisms outlined above, but also result in abnormalities in gas exchange. The hypoxemia, acute hypercapnea, and subsequent acidemia associated with these conditions activate chemoreceptors in the carotid bodies and medulla and cause an increase in ventilation to compensate for the ventilation/perfusion abnormalities, thereby contributing to the sensation of dyspnea.

CASE 83-2

EMERGENCY ROOM

Recently diagnosed with asthma due complaints of intermittent dyspnea and occasional wheezing, a 54-year-old man presents with progressive shortness of breath for 2 days to the Emergency Department. He states that breathing is a lot of work, he feels an increased urge to breathe, and sometimes he cannot get a full breath. His symptoms are worse with exertion. He denies problems when he goes out in cold air, but does have a chronic cough productive of small amounts of gray sputum. Although he initially claimed to have quit smoking a year ago (he has a 30 pack-year history of cigarette smoking), further questioning reveals that he has continued to smoke up to 1 pack of cigarettes a day, but has been trying to hide this from his wife. His blood pressure and heart rate are unremarkable, but his oxygen saturation is 88% on room air. On physical exam, auscultation of the lungs reveals distant breath sounds and intermittent expiratory wheezing. A CXR demonstrates hyperinflation with no evidence of infiltrates or effusions; heart size is normal.

Physiologically, the patient is experiencing activation of his airway receptors and chemoreceptors, which stimulate the respiratory controller and increase his urge to breathe. Chronic hypoxemia, and potentially acute hypercapnea, may also be contributing to his sensation of dyspnea. Hyperinflation, which affects the efficacy of the ventilator pump and leads to reduced inspiratory capacity, contributes to the sensation of an unsatisfying breath (with increasing end-expiratory lung volume, the patient's inspiratory capacity may literally be constrained by the limits of his lungs and chest wall to expand, ie, total lung capacity). Lastly, this patient may have dynamic airway compression that is sensed through vagal afferents as another stimulus for dyspnea. These physiologic mechanisms, coupled with the physical exam and radiographic findings, are consistent with a diagnosis of COPD exacerbation. Additional potential etiologies of dyspnea and wheezing in an obese smoker include CHF/pulmonary edema, pulmonary embolism, and myocardial ischemia; acute onset of asthma in a 50-year-old patient would be unusual without an antecedent respiratory infection. This case highlights the risk of anchoring bias, or the tendency to place too much importance on one piece of information, eg, a prior diagnosis of asthma. It is important to know what history is available before you see the patient, but you must then be disciplined to evaluate the patient with fresh eyes.

PRACTICE POINT

- Adult onset asthma is unusual and generally does not result in resting hypoxemia unless the condition is severe.

APPROACH TO THE PATIENT WITH DYSPNEA

Dyspnea as a symptom must be differentiated from the physical signs associated with "respiratory distress," such as tachypnea, use of accessory muscles of respiration, or intercostal retractions. In describing a patient's dyspnea, one should be careful to elicit the patient's own qualitative descriptors of their dyspnea, rather than use general terms that reflect the physical signs observed, such as "labored breathing." Common to these individual descriptors is the concept of "discomfort in the act of breathing," but it is the subtle differences in a patient's descriptors that may help elucidate the underlying physiological mechanisms.

TABLE 83-2 Association of Qualitative Descriptors and Pathophysiologic Mechanism of Shortness of Breath

Qualitative Descriptor	Pathophysiologic Mechanism (Disease States)
Chest tightness or constriction	Bronchoconstriction (asthma), interstitial edema (myocardial infarction)
Increased work of breathing, effort to breathe	Airway obstruction (COPD, moderate to severe asthma), neuromuscular disease (myopathy), chest wall disease (kyphoscoliosis)
Air hunger, need to breathe, urge to breathe	Increased drive to breathe (CHF, PE), moderate to severe airway obstruction (COPD/asthma)
Cannot get a deep breath, unsatisfying breath	Hyperinflation (asthma, COPD), restricted tidal volume (pulmonary fibrosis, chest wall disorders), anxiety
Heavy breathing, rapid breathing, breathing more	Deconditioning

Data from Manning, et al, Simon, et al, and Elliott, et al.

QUALITATIVE DESCRIPTORS OF DYSPNEA

The descriptor, "shortness of breath," reflects different sensations in patients with differing etiologies and mechanisms of their discomfort. The varied and overlapping vocabulary chosen by patients to describe their dyspnea relate to the different physiologic factors that produce each particular form of dyspnea (**Table 83-2**).

Ongoing studies are looking into the sensitivity and specificity of these characteristic phrases, and of the potential use of a multidimensional dyspnea profile (MDP) to measure separate dimensions of dyspnea (for example, distinguishing the sensory quality from emotional content). It can be helpful for the physician to think of dyspnea as an all-encompassing descriptor, such as pain. Pain arises from numerous mechanisms and is experienced differently depending on the origin and the patient's perception. In taking a medical history, we typically elicit common descriptive qualities of pain and link them to the underlying pathology, such as the "burning" pain from acid reflux or the "crushing" pain of a myocardial infarction. One reason our interviewing techniques for patients with dyspnea have not evolved along the same lines is the fact that healthy physicians rarely experience dyspnea other than with exercise, whereas many physicians (and their patients) have had varying types of pain throughout their lives.

HISTORY

A good place to start is asking the patient to describe the sensation of dyspnea in his or her own words. If the patient finds this difficult, suggest phrases such as chest tightness, increased effort to breathe, urge to breathe, cannot get a deep breath, or rapid breathing; or using a dyspnea questionnaire may help the patient describe the sensation he/she is experiencing (**Table 83-3**).

These phrases may give the physician clues to the underlying diagnosis as certain qualitative descriptors are associated with specific pathophysiologic mechanisms of dyspnea. Additionally, one must not overlook special forms of dyspnea, such as the orthopnea associated with CHF, paroxysmal nocturnal dyspnea associated with peripheral edema, or platypnea associated with left atrial myxoma and hepatopulmonary syndrome.

Next, it is important to define the timing of and precipitating factors for the dyspnea. When did the dyspnea start? Was the onset sudden or gradual? Is it episodic or continuous? Does the dyspnea occur only with exertion, or at rest? Dyspnea on exertion can be a manifestation of underlying lung disease that becomes evident with the increased metabolic demands of activity, or it may reflect cardiovascular deconditioning. For example, patients with COPD or interstitial lung disease may experience an acute physiologic change while exerting themselves, such as hyperinflation, bronchospasm, or hypoxemia, or may be deconditioned due to the sedentary lifestyle that often accompanies chronic illness.

PRACTICE POINT

- Chronic dyspnea at rest usually indicates more severe underlying structural lung or heart disease than dyspnea present only with activity.

Precipitating factors associated with breathing discomfort are also important clues. For example, dyspnea that occurs following exposure to fumes or cigarette smoke may indicate a bronchospastic response typical of asthma or COPD. Worsening of symptoms when the patient is at home or at work followed by resolution of symptoms while on vacation suggests hypersensitivity pneumonitis, often due to an exposure at work. Dyspnea that primarily occurs when lying down or bending over can be suggestive of diaphragm paralysis, usually idiopathic or as a result of phrenic nerve injury, or moderate to severe abdominal obesity.

Lastly, the patient needs to be questioned regarding other factors associated with his or her respiratory symptoms. For example, fevers, upper respiratory symptoms, and pleuritic chest pain indicate a possible pulmonary infection. Risk factors for venous thromboembolism (VTE), antecedent calf pain, and pleuritic chest pain may suggest pulmonary embolism. Chest pressure, nausea, and diaphoresis may

TABLE 83-3 Breathlessness Descriptor Questionnaire

Breathlessness Descriptor Statements
I feel that I am smothering.
I feel that I am suffocating.
I cannot get enough air.
I feel out of breath.
I feel hunger for air.
My breathing requires work.
My breathing requires effort.
My chest is constricted.
My chest feels tight.
My breathing is heavy.
I feel that my breathing is rapid.
I feel that I am breathing more.
My breathing is shallow.
My breath does not go out all the way.
My breath does not go in all the way.

Patients select statements that describe qualities of their breathlessness from the 15-item questionnaire above.
Data from Mahler DA, et al.

indicate an acute coronary syndrome. Fatigue and muscle weakness could be symptoms of myasthenia gravis or amyotrophic lateral sclerosis. Rashes and joint symptoms may indicate a collagen-vascular disease and associated interstitial lung disease (ILD). It is important to remember that as the history is elicited, the physician must be aware of any concerning features that may indicate a life-threatening diagnosis requiring emergent intervention, such as pulmonary embolism, tension pneumothorax, pericardial tamponade, acute myocardial ischemia, anaphylaxis, upper airway obstruction, or impending respiratory failure from pulmonary edema, pneumonia, or obstructive lung disease.

PHYSICAL EXAM

The physical exam starts as soon as you enter the patient's room. A quick assessment of the patient's overall respiratory status and a review of the vital signs may alert the clinician to impending respiratory failure. Concerning signs include use of accessory muscles of respiration, supraclavicular retractions, sitting in a tripod position (leaning forward with hands braced on the knees), pursed lip breathing, cyanosis, tachypnea, the inability to speak in full sentences without stopping to take a breath, audible stridor, or general distress with increased effort to breathe. An elevated heart rate, elevated blood pressure, rapid respiratory rate, and an exaggerated pulsus paradoxus (a fall in the systolic blood pressure greater than 10 mm Hg with inspiration, which is indicative of large swings in pleural pressure during the respiratory cycle and is typically associated with moderate to severe airway obstruction) are all concerning vital signs. The oxygen saturation is another useful vital sign since the recognition of hypoxemia can be critical to a patient's evaluation. However, normal oxygen saturation does not exclude a gas exchange problem. Hyperventilation may mask a large arterial-alveolar gradient, which defines the presence of a problem with the gas exchanger; oximetry merely tells you about oxygen saturation.

Physical exam findings can help elucidate the underlying physiologic mechanism of the patient's dyspnea. Increased work of breathing, as evidenced by the use of accessory muscles of respiration, supraclavicular retractions, and tripod positioning, is indicative of increased airway resistance, decreased compliance of the lungs and chest wall, or other disorders of the ventilatory pump. Pursed lip breathing helps reduce hyperinflation by slowing the respiratory rate and is commonly seen in patients with COPD. Rounding of the abdomen during expiration with an associated end-expiratory grunt can be a fairly specific sign of congestive heart failure. Inability of the patient to speak in full sentences without taking a breath indicates stimulation of the respiratory controller or reduced vital capacity. The clinician should also look for paradoxical movement of the abdomen with breathing. If the abdomen appears to be "sucked in" during inspiration, this suggests diaphragmatic weakness due to paralysis or fatigue. Conversely, in patients with high-thoracic or low-cervical spinal cord injuries, there may be retraction of the thoracic wall with inspiration resulting from paralyzed intercostal muscles.

If the patient is stable, then the physician should proceed with a full physical exam, focusing on the evaluation of the chest (respiratory and cardiovascular status), and extremities. Examination of the chest should include the elements of inspection (symmetry, kyphoscoliosis), auscultation (crackles/rales, wheezes, rhonchi, diminished breath sounds, prolonged expiratory phase), and percussion (dullness, hyperresonance). A cardiac examination should look for elevated jugular venous pressure, a prominent S_2, S_3/S_4 gallop, or a murmur suggesting cardiovascular dyspnea; a right ventricular heave, an accentuated accentuated P_2, a new soft systolic murmur of tricuspid regurgitation, and a pusatile liver consistent with significant pulmonary hypertension. The extremities should be examined for clubbing or cyanosis indicating severe hypoxemia, edema suggesting congestive heart failure or VTE, or rashes and/or joint deformities suggestive of rheumatologic disease and associated ILD. If the patient is complaining of exertional dyspnea, you should consider walking with the patient while observing her performance and measuring her ambulatory oxygen saturation; both can provide very useful information. Normal oxygen saturation at rest with evidence of significant desaturation while walking is indicative of processes that destroy lung tissue (COPD, pulmonary fibrosis) or impair diffusion of oxygen from the alveolus into the pulmonary capillaries (eg, pulmonary vascular diseases, acute pulmonary edema, or interstitial pneumonia).

DIAGNOSTIC STUDIES

Further evaluation of the patient with unexplained dyspnea should begin with a CXR and an electrocardiogram (to rule out myocardial ischemia). Interpretation of the CXR should start with an evaluation of lung volumes. Decreased lung volumes can suggest pulmonary processes such as interstitial edema, fibrosis or atelectasis, or impaired chest wall or diaphragmatic motion, possibly from neuromuscular disease. Do not assume that low lung volumes are due to a "poor inspiration" by the patient! Unilateral elevation of the hemidiaphragm can point to diaphragmatic paralysis. Hyperinflation indicates obstructive lung disease. Next, one can evaluate the pulmonary parenchyma for evidence of emphysematous changes, bullae, or interstitial changes. Pleural effusions can be bilateral (suggestive of CHF) or unilateral (concerning for carcinoma, liver failure, PE, or other such processes). An effusion associated with an infiltrate raises the concern for a parapneumonic process that will need urgent sampling and possible chest tube placement. An enlarged cardiac silhouette and prominent pulmonary vasculature in the upper zones can point to mild CHF, while enlarged central pulmonary arteries suggest pulmonary arterial hypertension. The consideration of chest radiographic findings that support the diagnosis of a systemic disease almost always benefits from direct consultation with the radiologist.

Based on the CXR and suggestive elements of the history and physical, further testing modalities may include blood tests (CBC to assess for anemia, serum electrolytes to assess the acid-base status of the patient), a computed tomography angiogram (CTA), and/or transthoracic echocardiogram (TTE). An arterial blood gas can be particularly useful in assessing the degree of hypoxemia or hypercarbia, as well as impending respiratory failure and acidosis. If possible, always perform an arterial blood gas with the patient breathing room air, ie, no supplemental oxygen, to enable you to assess the alveolar to arterial oxygen gradient. This will help you determine the presence of a gas exchange problem in the setting of either hyperventilation or hypoventilation. If the patient is receiving supplemental oxygen and it is removed, make sure the patient has been off oxygen long enough for the alveolar gas to reflect atmospheric gas (up to 15–20 minutes in a patient with COPD) before the ABG is performed. Additional blood tests that may be useful include B-type natriuretic peptide (BNP or NT pro-BNP) to evaluate for volume overload and methemoglobin or carboxyhemeglobin levels if the patient has been on particular medications or has a history that suggests exposure to fumes from a fire or furnace. A D-dimer to assess for possible pulmonary embolus has low utility for acutely ill hospitalized patients. See Chapter 259. A CTA can evaluate for acute pulmonary emboli while providing a more detailed look at the interstitium of the lung. A TTE is useful in patients with suspected cardiovascular dyspnea, as it can provide evidence of systolic or diastolic dysfunction, as well as occult valvular disease. The diagnostic accuracy of TTE for pulmonary hypertension is unfortunately not as reliable as many believe, but the presence of right-heart dysfunction with dilatation strongly suggests pulmonary hypertension. A right heart catheterization would be the diagnostic modality of choice to confirm the diagnosis of pulmonary hypertension.

PRACTICE POINT

- Always perform an arterial blood gas with the patient off supplemental oxygen, if possible.

In patients with persistent unexplained dyspnea, more specialized pulmonary testing may need to be performed, including pulmonary function testing (PFT), a sniff test, a methacholine challenge, and/or exhaled nitric oxide level. Standard PFTs consist of 3 parts: spirometry, with pre- and postbronchodilator values to evaluate for obstructive lung disease and reactive airways disease, lung volumes to assess for restrictive lung disease and hyperinflation, and diffusing capacity to assess for interstitial disease, emphysema, or pulmonary vascular disease. A 6-minute walk test is performed with continuous oxygen saturation monitoring and is useful to get a quick evaluation of a patient's exercise capacity and possible gas exchange problems. Maximal inspiratory and expiratory pressures are useful in assessing neuromuscular or diaphragmatic weakness. If unilateral hemidiaphragm paralysis is suspected, a fluoroscopic sniff test may confirm the suspicion by demonstrating paradoxical elevation of the paralyzed diaphragm with inspiration, although this test is increasingly being replaced by ultrasound evaluation of diaphragm movement during normal breathing. If a diagnosis of asthma is suspected, PFT laboratories can also perform bronchoprovocation testing with methacholine or measure exhaled nitric oxide levels, elevation of which is indicative of airway inflammation.

When the diagnosis is still unclear, a cardiopulmonary exercise test (CPET) can be helpful, especially in patients with an exertional component to their dyspnea or concurrent pulmonary and cardiovascular disease. This test includes a graded exercise protocol during which frequent measurements of respiratory and cardiovascular system mechanics and gas exchange are made. Arterial and right heart catheters may be included in the protocol when there are particular concerns about pulmonary vascular or cardiac disease. The resulting data can help determine what is physiologically limiting the patient's ability to exercise by differentiating between deconditioning, cardiovascular diseases (myocardial ischemia, heart failure, exercise-induced pulmonary arterial hypertension), and underlying lung disease.

PRACTICE POINT

- Many of these specialized tests can be deferred to the outpatient setting, and may yield better results when the patient is at her baseline clinical status.

CLINICAL FRAMEWORK OF CARDIOPULMONARY DISEASES

A reasonable clinical framework for approaching the common disease states associated with dyspnea is to divide them into those diseases associated with disorders of the respiratory system or those associated with problems of the cardiovascular system. Key elements of the history and physical exam, coupled with the diagnostic studies discussed above, can help determine into which broad pathophysiologic category a patient's dyspnea can be classified.

RESPIRATORY SYSTEM

As discussed above, respiratory system dyspnea can be divided into disorders of the ventilatory pump, respiratory controller, or gas exchanger. Acute bronchitis and pneumonia are common causes of respiratory system dyspnea. Pathophysiologically, acute bronchitis increases airway resistance due to sputum production, and pneumonia further increases airway resistance due to airway edema. Both may impair gas exchange by disturbing ventilation-perfusion relationships, while some pneumonias are characterized by shunt physiology due to filling/collapse of alveoli with inflammatory material. Patients with acute bronchitis typically present with cough and sputum production and may have rhonchi on exam. In contrast, patients with pneumonia additionally will note fever, may complain of pleuritic chest pain, and have rales on exam. An infiltrate on CXR often confirms the diagnosis of pneumonia. Acute bronchitis is usually not treated with antibiotics unless the patient has preexisting lung disease such as COPD or bronchiectasis. The mainstays of treatment of pneumonia are antibiotics and supplemental oxygen. Aspiration pneumonitis has a very similar physiologic mechanism and clinical presentation to pneumonia, and should be suspected in patients who were obtunded or have swallowing difficulties due to a stroke or other neuromuscular problems. Although aspiration pneumonitis due to gastric acid does not need to be treated with antibiotics, most clinicians add antimicrobial coverage, particularly if there is an elevation in the patient's temperature or white blood cell count, as there may be an infectious component due to aspiration of oral or GI flora.

PRACTICE POINT

- It is important to protect patients against aspiration by elevating the head of the bed or by obtaining a formal swallowing evaluation if there is concern about the ability of the patient to protect her airway during eating.

Obstructive airway diseases, including asthma and COPD, are another common cause of dyspnea. Like COPD, asthma also affects the respiratory controller, ventilatory pump, and gas exchanger. Bronchoconstriction increases airway resistance, thereby overworking muscles of inspiration. The patient often develops hyperinflation (breathing at higher lung volumes than normal), which shortens the inspiratory muscles (including the diaphragm) and makes them less effective. This is often accompanied by auto-PEEP (the persistence of positive pressure at the end of exhalation due to the prolonged exhalation time), which further increases the mechanical load on the inspiratory muscles, thereby augmenting the work of breathing. Severe airway obstruction can lead to hypoxemia and hypercarbia, which may have an additive effect on the respiratory controller. Patients with acute bronchoconstriction characteristically have hypocapnia (ie, hyperventilation) even in the absence of frank hypoxemia. This is evidence of increased respiratory drive that is believed to result from stimulation of airway receptors secondary to bronchospasm and airway inflammation. Patients with asthma often present with complaints of "chest tightness," a sensation attributed to stimulation of airway receptors, and a sensation of an "inability to take a deep breath" and "air hunger," which likely arises from the increased drive to breathe and limited tidal volume resulting from hyperinflation.

On exam, these patients are found to be hyperinflated (low diaphragm on percussion, positive Hoover's sign [inward motion of the lower lateral rib cage on inspiration], increased antero-posterior diameter of the chest) with a prolonged expiratory phase and with polyphonic expiratory wheezing on auscultation. CXR often confirms hyperinflation. Treatment for both asthma and COPD

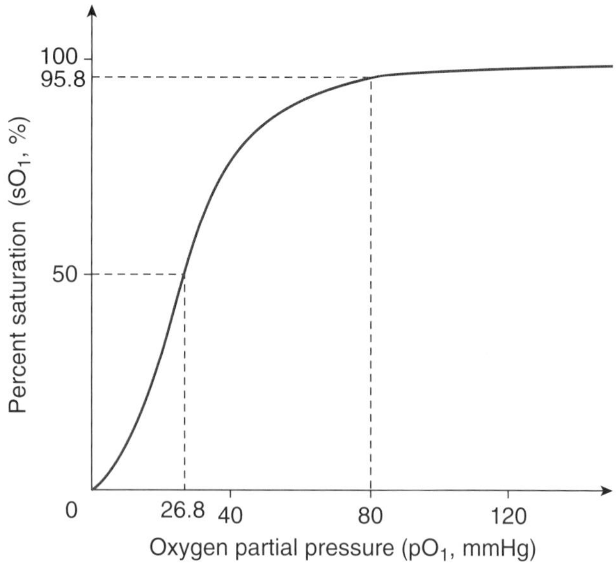

Figure 83-2 *Oxygen-hemoglobin Dissociation Curve.*

includes bronchodilators and steroids, although anticholinergic inhalers may be more effective in COPD than in asthma. A COPD exacerbation can further be treated with antibiotics if there has been a change in the quality or color of their sputum or evidence of pneumonia; antibiotics are not indicated in most acute asthma attacks. Judicious use of oxygen in patients with COPD is important because high concentrations of supplemental oxygen may worsen hypercarbia (largely due to worsening of ventilation/perfusion mismatch). Furthermore, excessive supplemental oxygen may mask hypoventilation by placing the patient far out on the plateau of the oxygen-hemoglobin association curve, rendering pulse oximetry insensitive to potentially dangerous increases in carbon dioxide tension (**Figure 83-2**).

PRACTICE POINT

- In most clinical situations, patients with COPD who need supplemental oxygen should have a target oxygen saturation of 89% to 92%.

Stridor (wheezing on inspiration, typically localized to the neck), often due to anaphylaxis or foreign body obstruction, is a special form of upper airway obstruction that causes acute respiratory distress. When severe, it is considered a medical emergency that may require emergent intubation or tracheostomy. Occasionally the patient can be temporized with administration of heliox as the inspirited gas. Inhalation of a mixture of helium and oxygen, which has a lower density than nitrogen and oxygen, lessens the work of breathing by reducing turbulent flow.

Pleural effusions can cause dyspnea by increasing the work of breathing due to alterations in the mechanics of the ventilatory pump and by activating pulmonary receptors if there is associated atelectasis. If the pleural effusions are associated with other conditions, such as pneumonia or pulmonary edema, the physiologic mechanisms of those disease states will also play a role in the sensation of dyspnea. Patients with pleural effusions usually present primarily with complaints of pleuritic chest pain or dyspnea as well as symptoms that relate to the underlying cause of the effusion, ie, cough and fever from pneumonia, abdominal pain, and distension from ascites in liver disease, anuria in renal disease, or cachexia from metastatic malignancy. A CXR may demonstrate blunting of the costophrenic angle and associated atelectasis. The first step in the evaluation of a patient with a pleural effusion of unknown etiology is to remove some of the fluid and determine whether it is exudative or transudative. Usually the fluid is analyzed for lactate dehydrogenase, protein, pH, glucose, cholesterol, microbiologic studies, and cytology. Any patient with an infiltrate and an effusion concerning for a parapneumonic effusion needs a diagnostic thoracentesis urgently to assess for evidence of a complicated parapneumonic effusion that would require early surgical drainage or chest tube placement. For simple effusions, treating the underlying condition usually leads to resolution of the effusion, but if it is recurrent, repeated thoracenteses, chest tube placement, pleurodesis, video-assisted thoracoscopy (VATs), and decortication are available options.

Neuromuscular diseases, such as myopathies, amyotrophic lateral sclerosis, or myasthenia gravis, can also lead to dyspnea. In these patients, the mechanics of the respiratory system are normal but the ventilatory muscles are weakened, so a greater neural drive is needed to move the chest wall. This heightened efferent output is sensed as increased effort or work of breathing. On exam, other findings consistent with muscular weakness are often seen. These patients usually require noninvasive ventilation or chronic tracheostomies to facilitate intermittent invasive ventilation to assist the weakened respiratory muscles. Chest wall diseases, such as kyphoscoliosis, result in a stiffened chest wall and are also associated with an increased effort to breathe.

CARDIOVASCULAR SYSTEM

Cardiovascular dyspnea can be subdivided into high cardiac output (anemia or shunt), normal cardiac output (diastolic dysfunction, myocardial ischemia, constrictive pericarditis, or deconditioning), or low cardiac output (congestive heart failure or pericardial effusions). Physiologically, high cardiac output dyspnea may result from reduced oxygen delivery to the tissues, as seen with severe anemia, or from the increased intracardiac pressures required to achieve the elevated cardiac output, as might occur with a large arteriovenous shunt. The exact mechanism by which anemia causes dyspnea, however, is unclear. These patients usually complain of dyspnea on exertion when an increased cardiac output is required to meet the demand of increased metabolic activity. Patients with diastolic dysfunction have normal cardiac output at rest, but their stiffened left ventricle is unable to dilate with exercise to accommodate greater stroke volume without significant increases in left ventricular end diastolic pressure (LVEDP), which leads to interstitial edema and stimulation of pulmonary receptors as well as stiffening of the lung and increased work of breathing.

Patients with diastolic dysfunction present with dyspnea on exertion and signs or symptoms of pulmonary edema. They may also have a history and physical exam findings suggestive of the cause of their diastolic dysfunction, such as a history of hypertension, the systolic ejection murmur of aortic stenosis, or an episode of syncope, which may be associated with hypertrophic cardiomyopathy. These patients require a TTE to aid diagnosis. However, the presence of impaired diastolic filling or left ventricular hypertrophy alone may not be diagnostic since these findings are common among asymptomatic patients. Another cause of normal cardiac output dyspnea is myocardial ischemia. In any patient with risk factors for coronary artery disease, dyspnea should be considered as a potential anginal equivalent. The pathophysiology of dyspnea in ischemia is likely related to high left ventricular filling pressure secondary to the impaired contractility of the ischemic region of the heart, which causes pulmonary edema. These patients often describe sensations of chest tightness or heaviness and chest pain, in addition to dyspnea.

In patients with low cardiac output dyspnea, CHF is the predominant etiology. In this cardiovascular disease state, the respiratory controller is stimulated by elevated vascular pressures as well as the resultant interstitial edema. Pulmonary edema affects both the respiratory controller, through activation of J receptors in the lung, as well as the gas exchanger. Patients with CHF often complain of air hunger, an increased urge to breathe, or a sensation of not being able to get enough air. Additional complaints of nocturnal dyspnea, dyspnea on exertion, and orthopnea are also suggestive of cardiac dyspnea. On exam, patients usually have peripheral edema, an elevated jugular venous pressure, an S_3 gallop, and bibasilar crackles on auscultation. An "expiratory grunt," or rounding of the abdomen during expiration, has been found to be a fairly specific physical finding in CHF. The CXR typically shows an enlarged cardiac silhouette, vascular cephalization, perihilar or bibasilar alveolar infiltrates, and bilateral pleural effusions. A TTE is also exceptionally helpful in this population to assess myocardial contractility and acute valvular dysfunction. An optimal cardiac regimen includes diuretics, medications to reduce afterload and, in select cases, to enhance contractility.

Pulmonary embolism is a unique cause of dyspnea. The mechanism leading to the symptom is complex and poorly understood and often the symptoms are out of proportion to the derangement in pulmonary mechanics or gas exchange. One possible mechanism contributing to the sensation of dyspnea is activation of C fibers in the pulmonary vasculature or stimulation of pressure receptors in the right atrium. Pulmonary emboli also cause hypoxemia and hypercarbia. Although this may contribute to the sensation of dyspnea, the dyspnea is largely independent of these gas transfer defects. The addition of supplemental oxygen to correct hypoxemia typically has little effect on the breathlessness associated with pulmonary embolism, and acute hypercarbia is unusual with small and medium size emboli. Clues to this diagnosis may include sudden onset of chest pain and dyspnea, possibly associated with unilateral lower extremity swelling. Hospitalization is a major risk factor for VTE for all patients irrespective of VTE prophylaxis, even in those receiving prophylaxis since none of the commonly used forms of DVT prophylaxis other than "therapeutic" anticoagulation prevents more than 75% of events.

PRACTICE POINT

- A pulmonary embolus caused by inadequate DVT prophylaxis is a partially preventable cause of dyspnea. All inpatients should be considered for DVT prophylaxis.

On exam, these patients are tachycardic and tachypneic, but their chest exam and CXR are relatively unremarkable. Pulse oximetry may remain normal despite the presence of a widened alveolar-arterial oxygen gradient because of the hyperventilation typical of acute pulmonary embolism. Usually the diagnosis is made with a PE-protocol CTA. Although a normal D-dimer has a high negative predictive value, its utility is limited for excluding clots in hospitalized patients who are usually high risk. See chapter 260 for treatment options.

PERSISTENTLY UNEXPLAINED DYSPNEA

Occasionally neither the diagnosis nor the physiologic mechanisms of dyspnea are clear. These patients often have normal physical examinations and diagnostic workups. CPETs are particularly helpful in this population to assess the patient for evidence of deconditioning as well as to look for findings consistent with malingering or hyperventilation syndrome. Patients with hyperventilation syndrome typically complain of a sensation of inability to get a deep breath despite breathing with very large tidal volumes. They often have a concomitant anxiety disorder. Anxiety can also explain dyspnea out of proportion to the underlying cause, as it can alter the perception of sensory data and lead to breathing patterns that worsen physiologic abnormalities. Anxiety is particularly troublesome in patients with hyperinflation since the behavioral issues lead to increased respiratory rate, which worsens hyperinflation and increases further the work of breathing in patients with expiratory airflow obstruction.

GOALS OF TREATMENT

Although not all dyspnea can be fully eliminated by efforts to correct the underlying disorder, there are ways to lessen the distress. For example, administration of oxygen can diminish the activation of chemoreceptors, pursed-lip breathing can lessen dynamic airway collapse, and inspiratory muscle training can strengthen the ventilatory pump. Many patients with chronic dyspnea, particularly those with COPD, can benefit from pulmonary rehabilitation to overcome the cardiovascular deconditioning that often accompanies chronic dyspnea.

CONCLUSION

Dyspnea is a complex symptom that encompasses many distinct sensations. Encouraging patients to choose their own qualitative descriptors can give the physician insight into the disease causing the dyspnea and its underlying physiologic mechanisms. This understanding, coupled with the physical exam and diagnostic data, can help the physician decide if the patient has dyspnea related to the respiratory or cardiovascular system and subsequently investigate the specific disease state responsible for the problem. The expectation is that this knowledge will help prevent common diagnostic errors, facilitate the correct management, and improve the quality of care of patients with dyspnea.

SUGGESTED READINGS

American Thoracic Society. Dyspnea: Mechanisms, Assessment, and Management: A Consensus Statement. *Am J Respir Crit Care Med.* 1999;159:321–340.

Berkman N, Avital A, Breuer R, et al. Exhaled nitric oxide in the diagnosis of asthma: comparison with bronchial provocation tests. *Thorax.* 2005;60(5):383–388.

Crapo RO, Casaburi R, Coates AL, et al. Guidelines for methacholine and exercise challenge testing-1999. This official statement of the American Thoracic Society was adopted by the ATS Board of Directors, July 1999. *Am J Respir Crit Care Med.* 2000;161:309.

Elliot MW, Adams L, Cockroft A, et al. The language of breathlessness: Use by patients of verbal descriptors. *Am Rev Respir Dis.* 1991;144:826–832.

Mahler DA, Harver A, Lentine T, et al. Descriptors of breathlessness in cardiorespiratory disease. *Am J Resp Crit Care Med.* 1996;154: 1357–1363.

Manning HL, Schwartzstein RM. Pathophysiology of dyspnea. *NEJM.* 1995;333:1547–1533.

Schwartzstein RM. Dyspnea and Pulmonary Edema. In: Fauci AS, ed. *Harrison's Principles of Internal Medicine.* 17th ed. New York, NY: McGraw-Hill: 2008.

Schwartzstein RM. The language of dyspnea. In: Mahler DA and O'Donnell DE, eds. *Dyspnea: Mechanisms, Measurement, and Management.* 2nd ed. Boca Raton, FL: Taylor & Francis:2005.

Simon PM, Schwartzstein RM, Weiss JW, et al. Distinguishable types of dyspnea in patients with shortness of breath. *Am Rev Respir Dis.* 1990;142:1009–1014.

CHAPTER 84

Edema

Teresa L. Carman, MD

Key Clinical Questions

1. How can the history and physical examination findings direct the evaluation of lower extremity edema?
2. What diagnostic or laboratory studies will help better delineate the differential diagnosis?
3. What therapeutic options may be beneficial in the management of edema?

CASE 84-1

A 42-year-old woman with a medical history of vascular disease presented to the emergency department with difficulty walking from painful leg and foot wounds present for 4 weeks. Her medical history included traditional vascular risk factors (hypertension, diabetes, hyperlipidemia), coronary artery disease (four myocardial infarctions, s/p stent placement, ischemic cardiomyopathy with ejection fraction of 25% of left apical thrombus), venous thromboembolism (deep venous thromboembolism, pulmonary embolism, s/p inferior vena caval filter placement), warfarin associated gastrointestinal bleeding, and status post partial amputation of her right foot due to osteomyelitis. She had not been taking her medications for two weeks. She complained of acute blisters of unknown etiology on her feet. The left was more involved than the right. She had previously been evaluated at an outside hospital for similar findings and a biopsy was done without defining an underlying etiology.

On examination vital signs included temperature 99.4 (F); heart rate 116; blood pressure 133/93 mm Hg, respiratory rate 20, with a room air pulse oximetry at 100%. Her neck veins were distended and elevated to 14 cm. She was tachycardic with a regular rate with a 3/6 systolic murmur at the apex. No gallop was noted. Her lungs were clear without wheezes or crackles. Her abdomen was soft. No abdominal bruits were noted. She was tender to palpation in the right upper quadrant. Lower extremity edema extended from the feet to the proximal hips and lower abdominal wall bilaterally. There were multiple punched-out fibrous-based wounds as well as intact fluid-filled blisters over the thighs and posterior knees. The left foot was completely involved with a partially hemorrhagic bulla. Pulses were not palpable.

Initial laboratory examination revealed a hemoglobin of 7.7 g/dl; hematocrit 26.1%. Albumin was 1.8 g/dl, prealbumin 5.0 mg/dl, and total protein was 6.5 g/dl. BUN and creatinine were 21 and 1.14 respectively. Glucose was elevated at 401 mg/dl. Urinalysis demonstrated 3+ protein, 2+ blood, and 1000 mg/dl glucose. Further workup during the admission was directed at identifying the etiology of her volume overload, managing her edema, and local wound care.

INTRODUCTION

Edema or lower extremity swelling is a common clinical complaint of both hospitalized and ambulatory patients. The differential diagnosis for lower extremity swelling is quite extensive. Despite the clinical frequency of the complaint, few clinical series address the etiology, evaluation, or diagnostic approach to lower extremity swelling. Clinically, edema and lymphedema are often mistakenly used interchangeably to refer to soft tissue fluid accumulation. However, these conditions are very different with respect to their pathophysiology and clinical implications.

All swelling results from an increase in interstitial or tissue fluid, which is mostly water. The transcapillary tissue fluid may be predominantly water (edema), the result of abnormal intravascular hydrostatic pressure or oncotic pressure, or may be due to the failure of the lymphatics to clear residual tissue fluid and proteinaceous material from the tissue space (lymphedema). Venous return is responsible for approximately 80% of tissue fluid drainage and transportation from the interstitial space. The lymphatic system accommodates the return of protein, cellular debris, and the remaining 20% of interstitial fluid. Therefore, lymphedema has a distinct pathophysiology resulting in regional increases in protein-rich fluid due to either decreased uptake or transport of tissue fluid. This will be discussed in more detail at the end of the chapter.

PATHOPHYSIOLOGY

Intravascular and extravascular fluid homeostasis requires stable capillary filtration supported by normal venous and lymphatic return to the systemic circulation. If the capillary fluid filtration rate exceeds the tissue drainage or transportation rate, fluid will accumulate within the extravascular space. Capillary filtration depends upon a normal, intact vascular endothelium and adequate serum oncotic pressure or protein/albumin content as well as equal ion distribution between the intravascular and extravascular compartments. In the most basic terms, if capillary filtration is adequately offset by vascular reabsorption, normal tissue fluid balance is maintained.

Maintaining endothelial integrity is the initial step in controlling edema. Vascular integrity is tightly regulated. As part of normal fluid homeostasis approximately 30% of post-capillary venule endothelial junctions are open and permeable. When regulation is disrupted, increased permeability may result in edema. This mechanism typically underlies the edema associated with inflammation, infection, trauma, or medications. Most stimuli that affect vascular integrity are reversible and do not cause permanent endothelial impairment.

Even when there is no disruption in vascular permeability, edema may be caused by increased capillary filtration with a shift of intravascular fluid from the vessels into the extravascular space. This is usually due to physiological changes in oncotic pressure, changes in hydrostatic pressure, or changes in intravascular fluid volume (**Table 84-1**). In this case, normal homeostasis and fluid balance between the intravascular and extravascular space is determined by hydrostatic pressure and oncotic gradients.

Intravascular oncotic pressure is influenced by protein and albumin content. If oncotic pressure within the vessels is decreased by nutritional depletion of albumin or protein, decreased synthesis as in cirrhosis, or by a loss of protein through the kidneys or the gastrointestinal tract, water will move from the vessels into the interstitium to maintain a constant oncotic pressure between the intravascular and extravascular compartments. Similarly, if the intravascular oncotic pressure is decreased due to intravascular fluid or volume accumulation this will also promote fluid shifts into the tissues and cause edema.

PRACTICE POINT

- The calf muscle pump is required to propel the column of venous blood back to the heart against a high pressure gradient along with competent venous valves to maintain normal venous return. Anything that disrupts or impairs the calf muscle pump may be associated with edema. Immobility, an impaired or shuffling gait frequently seen in the elderly or those with neurologic disorders, and paresis are common conditions that cause loss of the calf muscle pump.

A second important pressure gradient (hydrostatic pressure) occurs within the venous system. There is a static pressure within the veins that depends on the height of the column of blood. Any condition that raises the resting right heart pressures or intravenous pressure may cause edema (Table 84-1). Normal systemic venous return relies upon a normal cardiac pump, an intact calf muscle pump, intact venous valves to support antegrade venous return, and a pressure gradient between the ankle and the right heart. Chronic venous hypertension may result when any of these primary components are abnormal.

TABLE 84-1 Etiology of Tissue Edema

Capillary filtration
Inflammation or trauma
Vasodilation or increased permeability
Decreased intravascular oncotic forces
Hepatic insufficiency with hypoalbuminemia
Cirrhosis
Hypoalbuminemia due to nutritional deficiency
Low protein due to renal loss or protein-losing enteropathy
Increased intravascular volume (plasma volume)
Activation of the rennin-angiotensin-aldosterone system
Heart failure and relative volume retention
Decreased renal output/regulation of volume
Hormonally-related fluid retention
Medications causing volume/sodium retention
Changes in venous pressure
Elevated right heart pressures
Decreased left ventricular ejection fraction
Primary pulmonary hypertension or chronic thromboembolic disease
Post-thrombotic changes with venous obstruction
Valvular insufficiency with reflux
Chronic limb dependency
Gait abnormalities or immobilization with loss of the calf muscle pump

Venous valvular insufficiency due to loss of valve integrity or damage will frequently result in increased venous pressures, so-called venous hypertension. The loss of valve integrity may be primary, related to varicose veins and valve degeneration, or secondary, from trauma or injury to the valves usually associated with venous thrombosis. Regardless, loss of valve integrity may result in increased venous pressure due to the static column of blood within the vein and secondary increased capillary filtration along the pressure gradient.

The importance of the calf muscle pump, in conjunction with competent venous valves, must not be overlooked for normal venous return. Venous pressure at the ankle may be as high as 100 mm Hg in the standing position. The calf muscle pump is required to propel the column of venous blood back to the heart against this pressure gradient. Anything that disrupts or impairs the calf muscle pump may be associated with edema. Immobility, an impaired or shuffling gait frequently seen in the elderly or those with neurologic disorders, and paresis are common conditions that cause loss of the calf muscle pump.

A common cause of edema in hospitalized patients is an increase in plasma volume. Increased plasma volume caused by sodium and water retention results in secondary changes in both intravascular pressure as well as lowered oncotic forces. Plasma volume is maintained through intact renal excretion of ions followed by passive water excretion. Heart failure, renal disease, liver disease, medications, pregnancy, or any other condition that augments the neurohormonal reabsorption of sodium and water through activation of vasopressin or the renin-angiotensin-aldosterone system may result in secondary edema due to sodium and water retention. In reality, most edema is multifactorial and many variables and pathophysiologic mechanisms may be contributing. Clinical clues and historical elements may help focus your evaluation of the patient. A thorough evaluation of edema should focus on evaluating for underlying cardiopulmonary, kidney disease, liver disease, contributing medications, and venous disorders.

PRACTICE POINT

- The approach to bilateral lower extremity edema of an unclear etiology should focus on the most common clinical contributors. Testing should be used to evaluate the clinical conditions with the most significant impact. A thorough evaluation of edema should focus on evaluating for underlying cardiopulmonary disease, kidney disease, liver disease, contributing medications, and venous disorders.

The approach to lower extremity edema of an unclear etiology should focus on the most common clinical contributors. Testing should be used to evaluate the clinical conditions with the most significant impact. Edema is frequently considered cosmetic, but the underlying clinical contributors may indeed be life threatening. The most important clinical questions that may help evaluate edema are the following:

1. Is the swelling unilateral or bilateral?
2. What is the age of the patient?
3. Are there associated clinical symptoms of pain, erythema, fever, or systemic illness?
4. What are the onset, duration, and progression of the symptoms?
5. Are there associated clinical examination findings?
6. What exacerbates or relieves the edema?
7. Is there known coexisting medical illness, predisposing factors, or medications known to cause edema?

EVALUATION

UNILATERAL vs. BILATERAL EDEMA

The differential diagnosis of unilateral edema can be extensive (**Table 84-2**). Unilateral edema is typically due to a localized process as opposed to systemic factors. While it is common for patients with systemic illness, such as heart failure, to have a modest or moderate degree of asymmetry in their lower-extremity edema, complete sparing of one leg is not typical. In general, the initial evaluation of a patient with acute onset, unilateral edema should include testing to either diagnose or exclude deep venous thrombosis (DVT). The signs and symptoms of DVT are notoriously nonspecific and the consequences of venous thromboembolism may be severe. In addition, several clinical conditions have been associated with secondary DVT related to inflammation or venous compression, therefore evaluation to exclude the diagnosis of DVT should be pursued. This can be done using Well's criteria, D-dimer testing, and objective imaging. It is important to recognize that a patient with a high pretest probability on Well's criteria may require more than a simple venous duplex examination to exclude DVT. In particular, duplex ultrasound is often unable to diagnose or exclude common iliac or proximal external iliac vein DVT, so CT or MRI imaging may be needed if isolated proximal DVT is suspected (such as in a patient with recent pelvic or hip trauma). Once acute DVT has been excluded, other clinical or historical clues may lead one to suspect etiologies related to other clinical conditions (Table 84-2).

TABLE 84-2 Partial List of Differential Diagnoses Associated with Unilateral Limb Swelling. The Mnemonic VINDICATE may be Helpful to Expand Initial Considerations when Evaluating the Patient

Vascular: deep vein thrombosis, lymphedema, varicose veins, post-thrombotic syndrome, vascular compression (ie, May-Thurner syndrome)
Infectious/inflammatory: cellulitis, erysipelas, insect envenomation, inflammatory arthropathies
Neoplastic: soft tissue tumors may cause focal swelling or fullness, with compression of vascular structures, or lymphatics may also cause secondary edema, diffuse cutaneous tumor infiltration (while uncommon) may be perceived as edema
Drugs: unlikely to cause unilateral edema but a frequent case of bilateral swelling (Table 84-4)
Iatrogenic: disruption of lymphatics during surgery (ie, hernia or vein harvest), vascular intervention-related hemorrhage (ie, central line placement or cardiac catheterization)
Congenital/developmental/inherited: varicose veins, Klippel-Trenaunay syndrome, Parks-Weber syndrome, congenital or familial lymphedema
Anatomic: May-Thurner syndrome, popliteal vein entrapment
Trauma: sprain, strain, rupture of the medial gastrocnemius muscle, muscular hemorrhage, ruptured popliteal cyst, reflex sympathetic dystrophy/chronic regional pain syndrome
Environmental/endocrine: plant or insect exposure/hypersensitivity, myxedema

PRACTICE POINT

- The approach to unilateral edema should focus on a localized process as opposed to systemic factors. While it is common for patients with systemic illness, such as heart failure, to have a modest or moderate degree of asymmetry in their lower-extremity edema, complete sparing of one leg is not typical. In general, the initial evaluation of a patient with acute-onset, unilateral edema should include testing to either diagnose or exclude deep venous thrombosis (DVT).

Bilateral lower extremity edema suggests a more central or systemic etiology (**Table 84-3**) or central venous obstruction. In patients with new onset bilateral edema, the clinician should conduct a thorough evaluation for underlying cardiac conditions, hepatic or renal insufficiency, and if these conditions are absent, bilateral or central venous thrombosis. Evaluation for venous thromboembolism with venous duplex ultrasound is often still prudent, but of lower yield. Many common medications are associated with edema (**Table 84-4**) and should not be overlooked. Symmetric bilateral lower extremity swelling usually has a systemic predisposition (**Table 84-5**) whereas unilateral swelling will typically be related to a limb or localized body quadrant etiology. Bilateral swelling with an asymmetric characteristic may have an additional component of venous or lymphatic insufficiency in addition to the underlying systemic pathology.

AGE-RELATED EVALUATION

Evaluation of edema should be directed primarily by ancillary clinical clues since the differential diagnosis, which is quite broad, may change considerably. Edema in children is uncommon and

TABLE 84-3 Systemic Contributors to Bilateral Edema

Elevated right-heart pressure
Left or right ventricular failure
Tricuspid regurgitation
Pericardial constriction
Cor pulmonale
Pulmonary hypertension
Obstructive sleep apnea
Endocrine disorders
Myxedema (may be mistaken for edema)
Cushing syndrome
Medications (see Table 84-4)
Metabolic dysfunction
Protein imbalance
Decreased hepatic production
Excess protein losses
Malnutrition
Vascular
Varicose veins/venous insufficiency
Caval occlusion

should raise immediate clinical concern. Protein-losing enteropathy, malnutrition, nephrotic syndrome, medication-induced, trauma, injury, infection, and cardiac conditions prevail. Venous thromboembolism is less common but increasingly recognized in pediatric populations and should not be overlooked especially in chronically ill or hospitalized patients.

The most common cause of edema in the second or third decade of life is idiopathic edema, also referred to as cyclic edema. Patients may report associated facial and hand swelling. Other systemic causes for swelling should be excluded. Diuretic abuse is common with this disorder. In middle-aged patients, chronic venous insufficiency prevails as the most common diagnosis. However, patients with new onset edema after the age of 40 should be fully evaluated for underlying systemic causes.

Most chronic edema in the elderly is multifactorial. Gait and mobility assessment may be important since decreased ambulation is a frequent contributor to bilateral swelling. In addition, patients should be questioned regarding sleep habits. Due to physical disabilities or sleep irregularities many patients sleep in a chair leaving their legs chronically dependent. This will only be discovered by direct questioning. All of the aforementioned differential diagnoses must be considered. In addition, obstructive sleep apnea is frequently overlooked as a cause of edema.

TABLE 84-4 Pharmaceuticals Associated with Edema

Antidepressants
Antihypertensive agents
Calcium channel blockers
B-blockers
Direct vasodilators
Antisympathomimetics
Hormones
Oral contraceptives
Prednisone/Steroids
Estrogen replacement
Testosterone
Steroids
Nonsteroidal anti-inflammatory agents
Thiazolidinediones
Pioglitazone
Rosiglitazone
Antiepileptic drugs
Gabapentin
Pregabalin

TABLE 84-5 Partial List of Differential Diagnoses Associated with Bilateral Limb Swelling Using the Mnemonic VINDICATE

Vascular: bilateral deep vein thrombosis, acquired lymphedema, varicose veins, post-thrombotic syndrome, structural and hemodynamic cardiac conditions, obstructive sleep apnea
Infectious/inflammatory: cellulitis, erysipelas, inflammatory arthropathies, retroperitoneal fibrosis
Neoplastic: retroperitoneal tumors with compression of vascular structures or lymphatics, lymphoma, vascular invasion (ie, renal cell cancer)
Drugs: a frequent case of bilateral swelling (Table 84-4)
Iatrogenic: disruption of lymphatics during surgery (ie, hernia or vein harvest), vascular intervention-related thrombosis (ie, IVC* filters)
Congenital/developmental/inherited: congenital lymphedema
Anatomic: absent or atretic IVC
Trauma: IVC injury/ligation
Environmental/endocrine: myxedema, Cushing syndrome

*IVC, inferior vena cava.

CLINICAL FINDINGS

Physical examination findings may help support diagnostic suspicion. All patients should be thoroughly evaluated for signs of systemic processes contributing to edema. Examination should include an assessment for jugular venous distension, extra heart sounds including gallops or murmurs, truncal telangectasias, hepatojugular reflux, lung crackles, ascites, etc. Lower extremity tenderness, increased warmth, and pitting are nonspecific findings frequently associated with edema. Inflammation is frequently associated with edema and contributes to these clinical findings. Therefore, both acute and chronic conditions may present with this nonspecific constellation of symptoms. Soft doughy pitting in the absence of inflammation may be more consistent with hepatic dysfunction, renal protein losses or nephrotic syndrome, or acute/subacute cardiac etiologies; however, this can be quite variable. Chronic skin changes of hyperpigmentation or hemosiderin staining, eczema or dermatitis, and brawny skin thickening (called lipodermatosclerosis) are characteristic of chronic venous hypertension. Chronic venous insufficiency is a nonspecific term used to identify edema associated with varicose veins and chronic venous hypertension. The term varicose vein collectively includes typical large ropey varicosities, small 1–3 mm subcutaneous reticular veins, and even dermal telangectasias. The common clinical finding of clusters of small dilated veins at the ankles sometimes called corona phlebectatica is consistent with chronic venous stasis and chronic venous hypertension and frequently associated with edema.

Edema that terminates at the ankle and spares the foot may be consistent with lipoedema. Lipoedema is frequently mistaken for edema or lymphedema. This is typically identified in women. It may be considered a physiologic variant consisting of bilateral, symmetric deposition of adipose tissue.

ONSET, DURATION, EXACERBATING AND REMITTING FACTORS

Acute edema, especially when unilateral, is typically more concerning for a venous obstructive process and necessitates evaluation for DVT. Chronic, longstanding swelling is clinically relevant and certainly may impact the function and quality of life of the patient, thus evaluation and treatment is warranted. However, in most of these patients routine venous duplex is not indicated. In patients with long-standing swelling, a change in the characteristic or nature of the swelling, new onset pain or a change in pain quality, or other clinical findings may indeed provoke the need for VTE imaging.

Edema related to venous disease will frequently improve overnight or with elevation due to the decrease in venous pressure. During the day patients with underlying venous disease typically experience an increase in swelling due to the dependent nature of the legs and increased pressure-drive venous filtration. Patients with underlying cardiac, hepatic, or renal issues predisposing to edema are less likely to notice dramatic daily changes in their edema but there is often a modest degree of diurnal variation.

DIAGNOSTIC TOOLS

Duplex ultrasound is both sensitive and specific for the diagnosis of venous thromboembolism as well as venous reflux in the visualized segments. The testing uses both compression imaging as well as Doppler insonation of the vessels (**Figures 84-1** and **84-2**). Vessels from the common femoral vein or even the distal external iliac vein through the popliteal vein and into the calf are easily imaged. If a segment cannot be imaged adequately due to bandaging, dressings, patient comfort, patient positioning, patient cooperation, obesity, or extensive edema adding significant tissue depth, then DVT cannot be fully excluded. It is important to recognize that duplex sonography is less sensitive for calf vein thrombosis than for proximal DVT. Therefore calf vein DVT may be missed by venous duplex examination. In a patient with high clinical suspicion and negative initial imaging it may be prudent to repeat testing in 5–7 days to exclude DVT. In addition, some vascular laboratories and radiology departments do not routinely visualize calf veins and therefore cannot exclude DVT involving these segments.

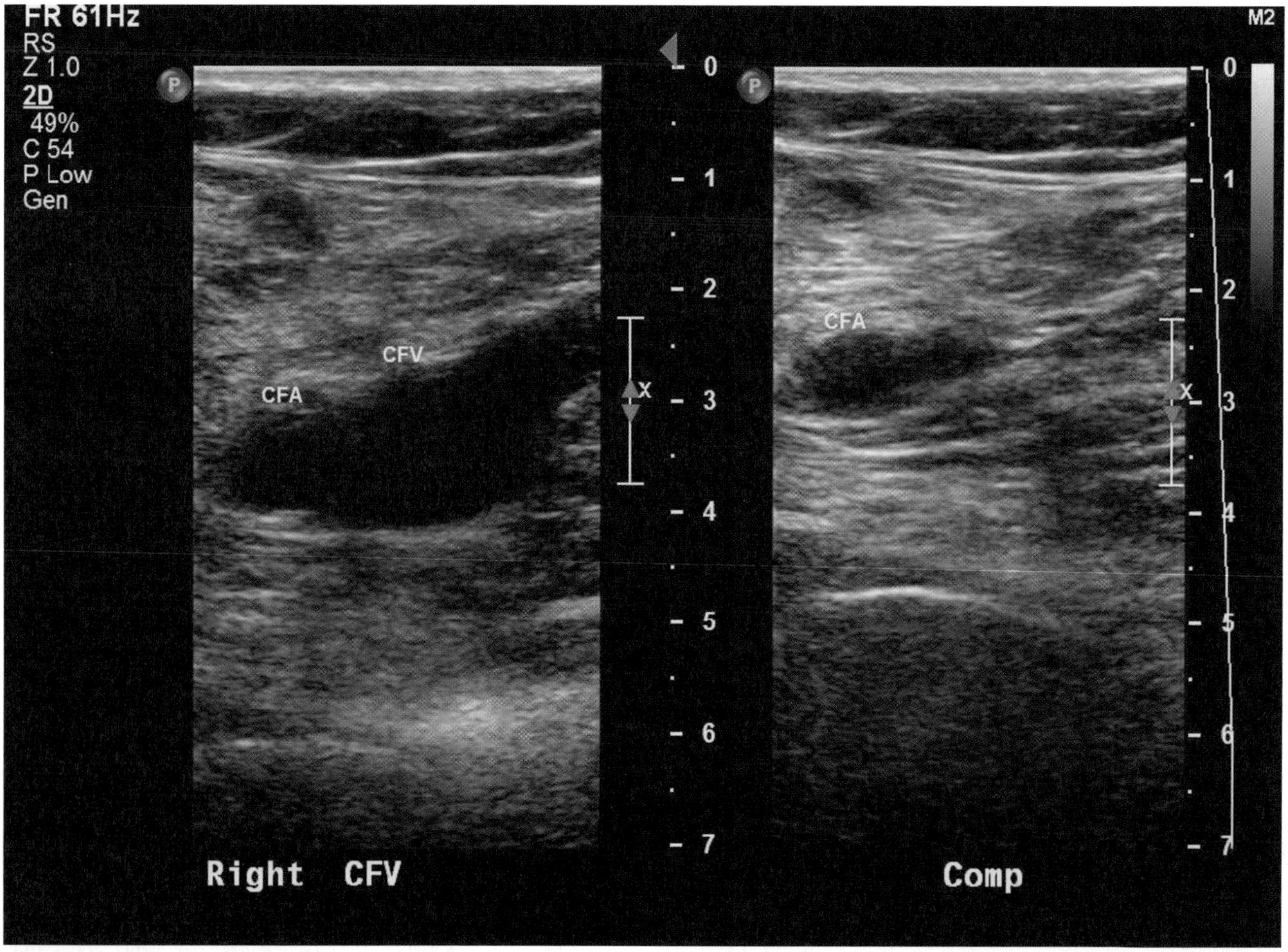

Figure 84-1 *Compression image of the artery and vein at the level of the groin demonstrating a normal common femoral artery (CFA) and vein (CFV). With compression over the vein, the walls of the vein coapt when the vein is free of thrombus.*

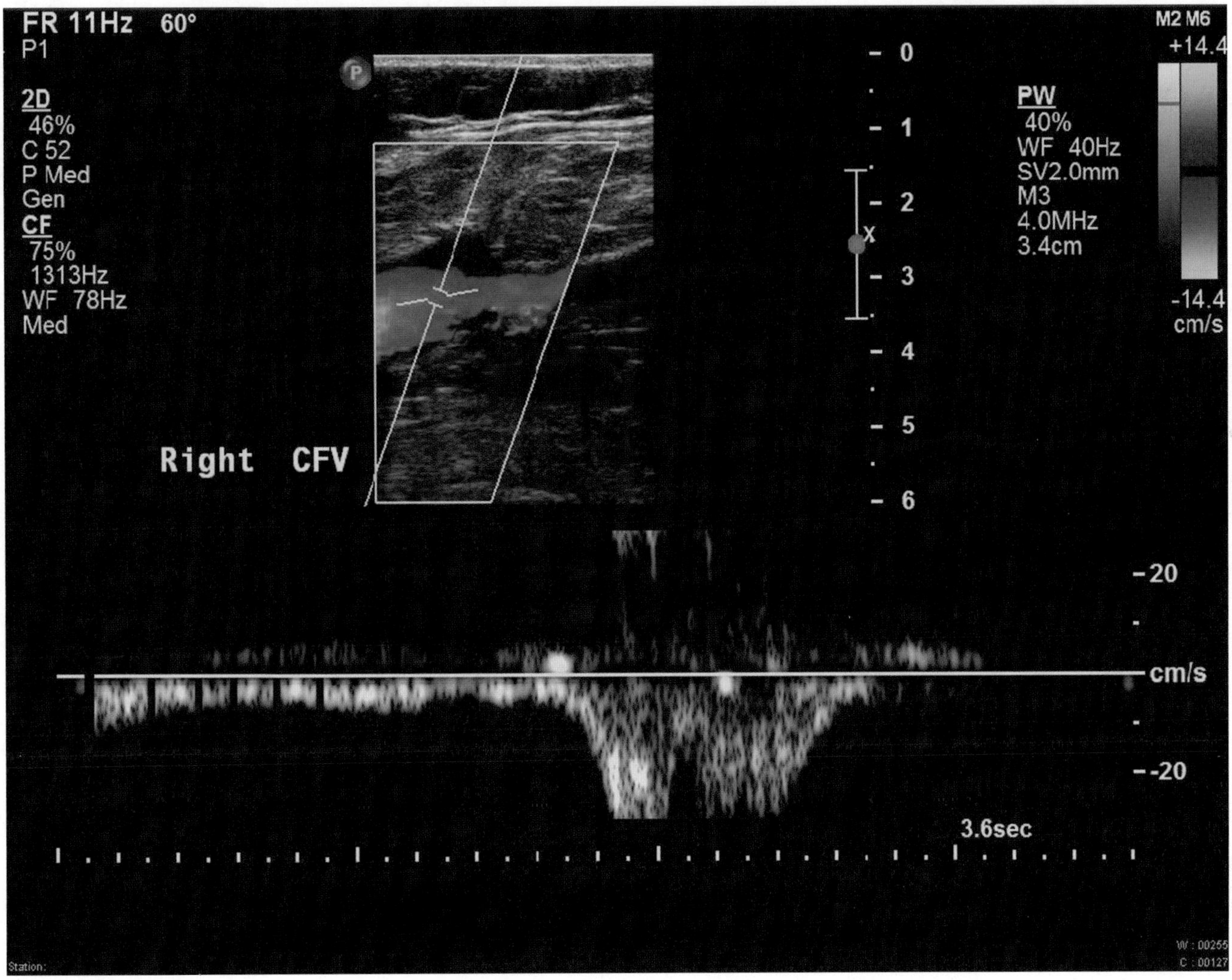

Figure 84-2 *A normal vein demonstrates spontaneous respirophasic flow and augmentation of venous return when the calf muscle is compressed.*

Subtle changes in the Doppler waveforms may suggest underlying conditions that require further evaluation. Pulsatile venous flow suggests elevated right-sided heart pressures, significant tricuspid regurgitation, or increased venous pressures (**Figure 84-3**). Monophasic flow, the absence of spontaneous respirophasic flow, or decreased return with distal augmentation suggests more proximal occlusion or obstruction and may require additional imaging (**Figure 84-4**). In this setting, further imaging with abdominal/pelvic computed tomography (CT), CT venography, or magnetic resonance (MR) venography may be helpful.

The ultrasound evaluation for venous insufficiency differs from venous duplex imaging for DVT. To evaluate for venous insufficiency, the patient is examined in a standing position with the index leg offloaded. The deep venous system is evaluated for evidence of DVT or venous reflux. In addition the technician spends considerable time evaluating all segments of the great and small saphenous veins for thrombosis as well as reflux with Valsalva or compression.

Abdomen and pelvis computed tomography (CT) with intravascular contrast may demonstrate obstruction or occlusion at the level of the inferior vena cava (IVC) or iliac veins as an etiology (**Figure 84-5**). The IVC may be visible on duplex ultrasound, but this is variable and not necessarily reliable. IVC and iliac imaging relies predominantly on Doppler insonation. Computed tomography (CT) venography, magnetic resonance (MR) venography, or conventional ascending contrast phlebography are the most reliable imaging for the IVC and iliac veins. They directly image veins for the presence of intraluminal thrombus or external compression as an etiology for edema. Intravascular pressure measurements or intravascular ultrasound combined with ascending phlebography may be required to evaluate subtle abnormalities to assure there is no hemodynamic significance to the changes. Typical limitations of CT and MR should be noted including the use of contrast, prolonged imaging times for MR, and the inability to image in the setting of some indwelling devices.

Patients with suspected cardiopulmonary etiology for their edema should have an ECG and chest X-ray as well as echocardiogram. Echocardiography can be used to assess hemodynamics including preload and afterload, ventricular function and contractility, pulmonary hypertension, or physiologic and anatomic valve abnormalities. Echocardiography should be included in the evaluation in patients with evidence of heart failure, unexplained volume overload, or murmurs on examination. In some cases central pressure monitoring or even right heart catheterization may be useful. Sleep apnea and associated heart failure and pulmonary hypertension is an under-recognized cause of lower extremity edema. Edema that is worse upon awakening is sometimes reported, and is a major clue to the diagnosis. Polysomnography testing may be helpful.

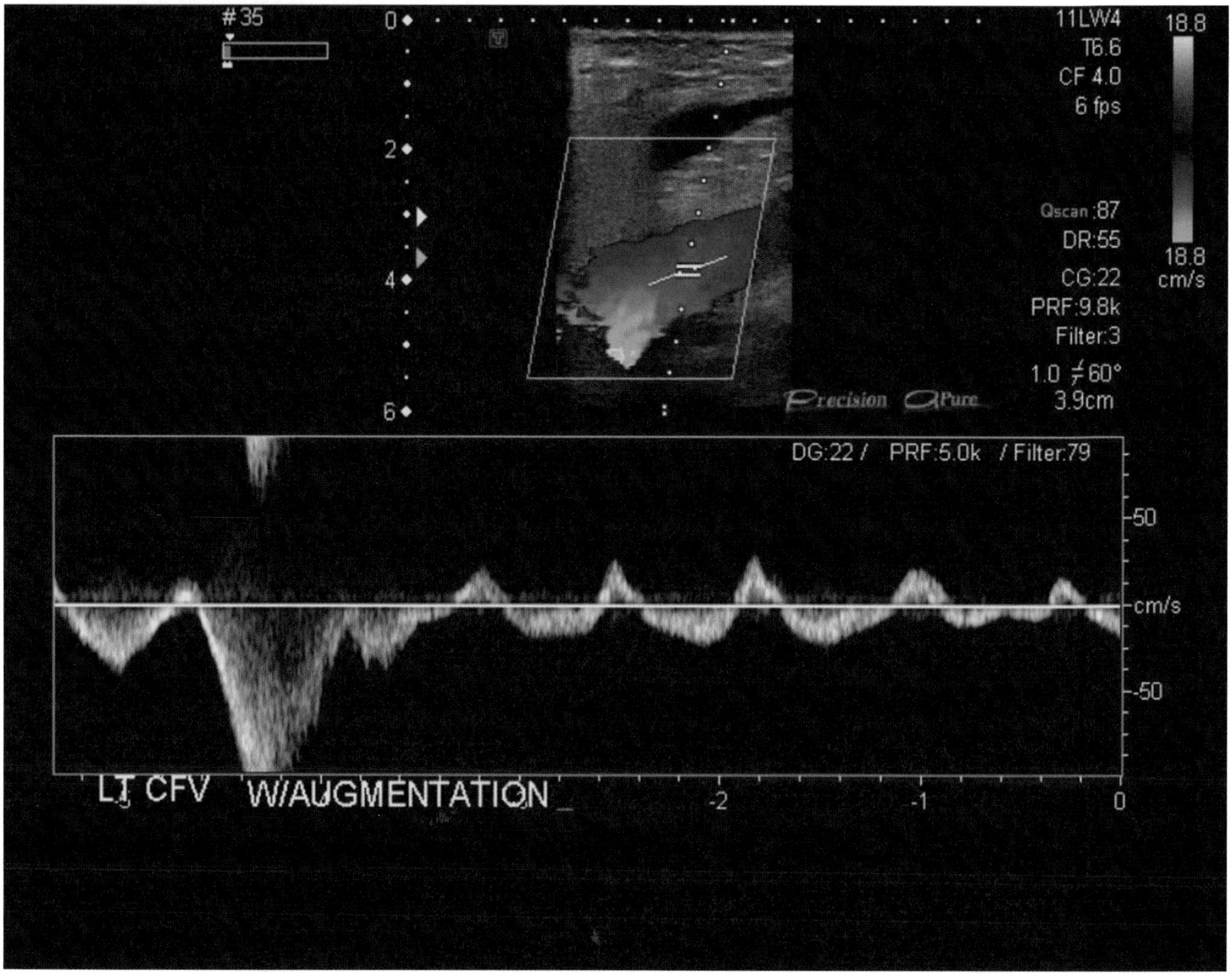

Figure 84-3 *Pulsatile venous waveforms are due to reflection of pressure down through the inferior vena cava. This is usually consistent with volume overload or elevated right heart pressures.*

LABORATORY EVALUATION

Further evaluation for a systemic etiology should include a basic laboratory evaluation. A complete metabolic panel will help exclude low protein or albumin states and provide a basic assessment of liver integrity, renal function, and ion balance. Urinalysis is useful to identify renal protein loss. Prothrombin time (PT), albumin, and prealbumin provide an assessment of the synthetic function of the liver. Urinalysis should be performed to exclude significant proteinuria. Prealbumin should be ordered when there is suspicion for significant hypoalbuminemia or malnutrition. Brain natriuretic peptide (BNP) or pro-BNP may be useful to exclude heart failure. Clinical clues suggestive of an underlying endocrinopathy such as Cushing syndrome or thyroid disease should prompt appropriate testing.

TREATMENT

Edema should be managed according to the underlying diagnosis. Venous thromboembolism should be treated with systemic anticoagulation. Consideration may be given to more aggressive management with pharmacomechanical thrombolysis in an effort to preserve venous valve function and minimize later effects of the post-thrombotic syndrome. Many practitioners treat edema with diuretics. However, in many cases edema is not due to excess intravascular volume and therefore diuretics are not indicated nor are they likely to be helpful. In cardiac conditions causing volume retention, and sometimes in liver disease or renally mediated volume retention, diuretics may be helpful. However, renal function and intravascular volume should be followed closely. Lifestyle modification and optimizing pharmacotherapy should be the primary focus.

Most patients benefit from an aggressive skin care regimen to prevent eczema and ulceration associated with increased tissue fluid. Decreasing edema through elevation and compression are mainstays of therapy. Elevating the foot of the bed by several inches will decrease the pressure gradient between the ankle and the right atrium and improve venous return. Combined elevation with active calf muscle exercise increases volume reduction when compared to elevation alone.

Patients with chronic venous insufficiency and lymphedema should wear compression stockings. Typically 20–30 mm Hg or even 30–40 mm Hg compression is required. However, the most important factor when prescribing compression therapy is to tailor the therapy to the ability of the patient to don and doff the garment. In many cases elderly patients are best served by a 15–20 mm Hg garment due to physical limitations of mobility, arthritis, and strength that may impede the use of a stronger compression. Thromboembolic deterrent (TED) hose may be helpful to decrease and control edema in hospitalized patients but these are typically not sufficient to control swelling in ambulatory patients. ACE wraps

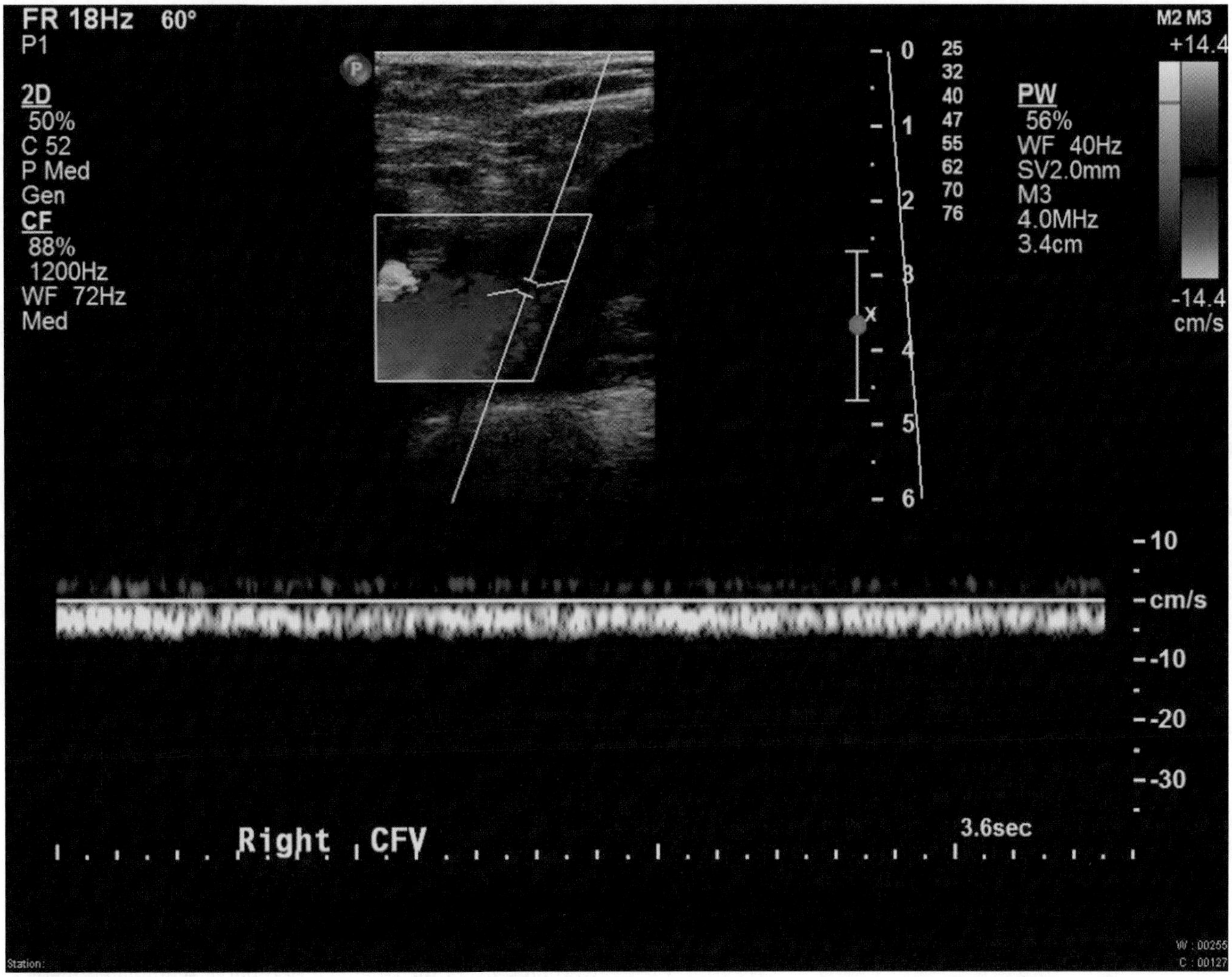

Figure 84-4 *Monophasic flow within the vein should raise concern for a more proximal obstruction within the venous system.*

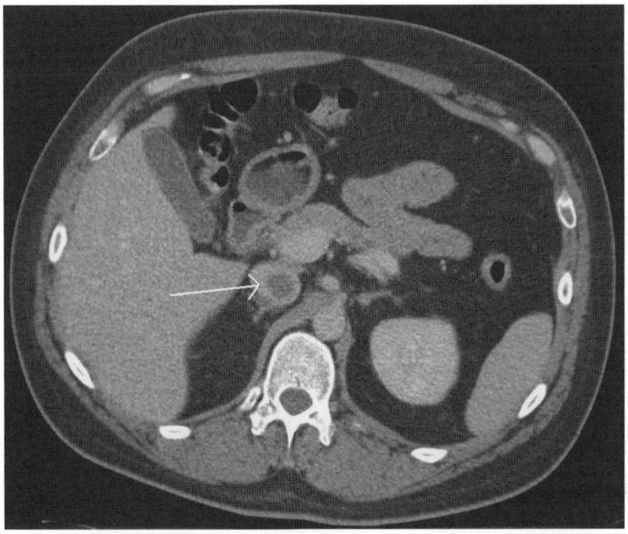

Figure 84-5 *Contrasted CT scan of the abdomen demonstrating partially occlusive thrombus within the inferior vena cava (arrow).*

may also be used to control edema. However, the elastic nature of the compression typically causes variable constriction and relaxation which limits their use in ambulatory patients, and, if misapplied or bunched up such that the proximal pressures are higher than distal pressures, venous return may actually be impaired.

Compression may cause significant volume mobilization and therefore, should be used cautiously in patients with underlying cardiac insufficiency or heart failure. Caution should also be used when applying compression to patients with underlying peripheral arterial disease (PAD). In general, compression stockings should not be recommended for patients with PAD and an ankle-brachial index < 0.5.

LYMPHEDEMA

Lymphedema is the accumulation of protein-rich interstitial fluid due to impaired lymphatic function. The lymphatics are responsible for collecting and transporting cellular debris as well as interstitial fluid and protein not returned to the circulation by the venules. The lymphatic vessels are small blind-end vessels that begin in the dermis as lymphatic capillaries. These join to form precollector vessels and collecting vessels that through one-way transport move the lymphatic fluid into the lymph nodes and major lymphatic channels to the thoracic duct. Lymphedema may be primary (ie, no underlying etiology for the lymphatic failure can be identified) or it may be secondary to a myriad of

TABLE 84-6 Classification of Lymphedema

Primary	
Congenital	Onset < 1 years of age
Preacox	Onset during adolescence or 20s
Tarde	Onset over age 40
Secondary	
Surgery	Lymph node dissection, hernia repair, vein harvest, groin exploration, any surgical disruption of lymphatic tissue
Malignancy	Tumor infiltration or related to treatment including radiation therapy
Infection/ Inflammation	Most commonly cellulites or chronic stasis inflammation as seen in phlebolymphedema
Trauma/injury	Burns, crush injury, any significant soft tissue trauma

acquired causes (**Table 84-6**). Lymphedema can be graded based on the clinical presentation (**Table 84-7**). Most patients present with painless swelling of the limb and dorsum of the foot. Clinically, squared, thickened, and edematous toes and a positive Stemmer sign—the inability to pinch a skin fold at the base of the second toe—are frequently present, especially with later presentations. When the clinical diagnosis is in doubt, lymphoscintigraphy can be used to evaluate the lymphatic function and when abnormal it is diagnostic. Patient education is paramount to successful management of lymphedema. This condition is not reversible and may indeed worsen if left untreated. Patients should be treated with an aggressive skin care regimen to prevent injury and secondary infection. Heavy emollients may help soften and even reverse the hyperkeratotic skin changes. Manual lymphatic drainage is therapist-directed lymphatic massage and limb wrapping designed to stimulate and drain the lymphatics. As a component of complex decongestive therapy manual lymphatic drainage should be used to decrease limb volume and help restore function. Chronic compression therapy provides the maintenance phase for maintaining the gains of manual lymphatic drainage.

Phlebolymphedema is an under-recognized condition with characteristics of both venous insufficiency and lymphedema. The venous and lymphatic systems are intimately related both anatomically and physiologically. The diagnosis of phlebolymphedema is primarily based on clinical history and examination. The patient will typically have evidence of chronic venous hypertension with varicose veins but will also have significant swelling of the dorsum of the foot, squared toes, and skin changes mimicking lymphedema. The underlying pathophysiology is related to the chronic venous hypertension with accumulation of interstitial fluid. When the increased fluid exceeds the capacity of the lymphatics transport capacity a low-protein edema results. Treatment should focus on managing the underlying chronic venous hypertension. Compression therapy is a mainstay, while surgical or endovascular procedures to manage venous reflux or obstruction may be prudent.

TABLE 84-7 Lymphedema Grading Based on Clinical Presentation

Grade 1
Extremity swelling that typically pits and will decrease with elevation of the limb
Grade 2
Frequently is nonpitting. Little improvement is seen with overnight elevation. The skin becomes thickened and fibrotic. Skin may begin to develop changes with hyperpigmentation.
Grade 3
Described as "elephantiasis." The edema is fixed and does not pit or change with elevation. The skin is brawny and thickened. The dermal elements may hypertrophy causing hyperkeratotic or verrucal changes to the skin.

CASE 84-1 *(continued)*

OUTCOME

A limited study due to her edema, Duplex ultrasound demonstrated normal compressibility in the visualized segments and the proximal waveforms were pulsatile bilaterally (see Figure 84-3), consistent with intravascular volume overload and elevated right heart pressures. On echocardiogram her left ventricle ejection fraction was 20–25% with global hypokinesis and a restrictive diastolic filling pattern. The right ventricle was moderately dilated with decreased systolic function and a calculated systolic pressure of 85 mm Hg. A 24-hour urine collection demonstrated protein loss of 2071 mg/24 hours. Under the direction of the heart failure service she was managed with aggressive diuresis, sodium and fluid restriction, and control of her diabetes with the addition of an ACE inhibitor for renal protection. Nutrition consultation provided recommendations to optimize her nutrition while strictly limiting her salt and carbohydrate intake. Her underlying edematous state was felt to be related to her heart failure, malnutrition, and renal protein losses. This patient demonstrates the multifactorial nature of edema that may be encountered in some acutely ill patients who present for management of otherwise unrelated medical concerns.

CONCLUSION

When confronted with a patient with lower extremity swelling it is necessary to determine what pathophysiology is underlying the condition. Successful management should be directed at the pathophysiology and not at the physical finding of swelling. Edema may be best managed by addressing the medical conditions related to the underlying volume retention and diuretic therapy may be helpful. In patients with chronic venous insufficiency and venous hypertension, diuretics have limited benefit. The mainstay of therapy should be directed toward managing the underlying venous hypertension using elevation and compression. Surgical management of venous reflux and incompetent perforators may be appropriate for some patients. Lymphedema is best managed by a combination of limb decongestion and maintenance with compression therapy. Attention to skin care and protection of the limb is also of paramount importance.

SUGGESTED READINGS

Blankfield RP, Finkelhor RS, Alexander JJ, et al. Etiology and diagnosis of bilateral leg edema in primary care. *Am J Med.* 1998;105:192–197.

Bunke N, Brown K, Bergan J. Phlebolymphedema: usually unrecognized, often poorly treated. *Perspect Vasc Surg Endovasc Ther.* 2009;21:65–68.

Ely JW, Osheroff JA, Chambliss ML, Ebell MH. Approach to leg edema of unclear etiology. *J Am Board Fam Med.* 2006;19: 148–160.

Felty CL, Rooke TW. Compression therapy for chronic venous insufficiency. *Semin Vasc Surg.* 2005;18:36–40.

Kerchner K, Fleischer A, Yosipovitch G. Lower extremity lymphedema update: pathophysiology, diagnosis and treatment guidelines. *J Am Acad Dermatol.* 2008;59:324–331.

Meissner M, Moneta G, Burnand K, et al. The hemodynamics and diagnosis of venous disease. *J Vasc Surg.* 2007;46:4S–24S.

Murakami M, Simons M. Regulation of vascular integrity. *J Mol Med.* 2009;87:571–582.

Schrier RW. Water and sodium retention in edematous disorders: role of vasopression and aldosterone. *Am J Med.* 2006;119(Suppl 1): S47–S53.

Tan M, van Rooden CJ, Westerbeek RE, Huisman MV. Diagnostic management of clinically suspected acute deep vein thrombosis. *Br J Haematol.* 2009;146:347–360.

Yale SH, Mazza JJ. Approach to diagnosing lower extremity edema. *Comp Ther.* 2001;27:242–252.

CHAPTER 85

Falls

Rollin M. Wright, MD, MA, MPH
Adrian Visoiu, MD
Robert M. Palmer, MD, MPH

Key Clinical Questions

1. For patients admitted to the hospital after a fall, what historical features are helpful in formulating a provisional diagnosis?
2. Which hospitalized patients are most at risk of an incident fall?
3. What bedside tools exist to identify potential fallers?
4. What interventions have been shown to reduce fall risk and prevent injurious falls?

CASE 85-1

An 85-year-old woman, admitted 2 days ago after a fall resulted in a left proximal humerus fracture, fell again in the hospital. After she stood from the bed and leaned forward to answer the phone located on the bedside table just out of her reach, she fell, struck her forehead on the corner of the bedside table, and twisted her right arm, which she was using to grasp the bedrail and steady herself.

Her medications included trimethoprim/sulfamethoxazole for a urinalysis suggestive of urinary tract infection; metoprolol for hypertension and irregular heart rhythm; calcium carbonate with vitamin D; subcutaneous enoxaparin for prophylaxis against thromboembolism; aspirin; hydrocodone for severe shoulder pain; and trazodone for sleep. The previous night she received 5 mg orally of haloperidol because of her restlessness and calling out for help.

Her past history included macular degeneration in the left eye, osteoporosis, hypertension, mild cognitive impairment, and recurrent falls. The nurses reported that she has been delirious, with episodes of restlessness and frequent attempts to get out of bed.

At the bedside, crying for help, she was lying prone on the floor by the bed and with her left arm in a sling under her. She had a bleeding laceration that will require suturing over the right zygomatic bone and a large hematoma forming over her right eye. She reported pain in her right hand and arm.

1. Using the NQF definitions of harm, what level or category of harm does the patient in the case suffer as a result of her fall?
2. Referring to the case study, how many predisposing risk factors for falling during her hospital stay does the patient have? What are her intrinsic and extrinsic risk factors?
3. What interventions might you consider implementing to prevent a patient with these risk factors from suffering an injurious fall in your hospital?
4. What diagnostic workup, if any, is warranted to assess this patient for any injuries that might have been sustained as a result of her fall?

INTRODUCTION

Falls are the leading cause of nonfatal injury in almost every age group in the United States, especially the elderly. Falls account for two-thirds of accidental deaths among older adults. About one-third of adults aged 65 years and older who live in the community (outside of assisted living or nursing facilities) fall at least once a year. This rate increases to 50% for those aged 80 years and older. Although most falls do not result in serious injury, about 5% of adults over 65 who fall experience a fracture or require hospitalization. Approximately 200,000 hip fractures occur annually in the United States, usually as the result of a fall.

Falls are the most common adverse event in hospitals and one of the most common causes of hospital-acquired injury reported. Accidental falls in hospitalized patients are associated with injuries, prolonged hospital stay, and poor clinical outcomes. Most falls in the hospital occur in patients' rooms and bathrooms during transfers between the bed and a chair or while using the toilet or shower. Hospitalized elderly patients fall at a rate of 3 to 17 falls per 1,000 patient days. About one-third of these falls result in an injury. Patient safety groups suggest a benchmark rate of 2.5–3.5 falls per 1,000 patient-days with a goal rate of no more than 0.1 injurious falls per 1,000 patient days. Considered preventable and costly to the health care system, fall-related injuries appear on the Centers for Medicare and Medicaid Services' (CMS) list of "hospital-acquired conditions" (HAC). As of October 1, 2008, CMS no longer pays hospitals for the costs of treatment of HACs such as injuries sustained from a fall in a hospital. The inclusion of falls-related injuries as a HAC creates for hospitalists an important opportunity to improve quality of patient care while simultaneously implementing everyday practices that could reduce financial losses related to falls in the hospital. Regulatory incentives create an opportunity for hospitalists to assume a medical leadership role with nursing and hospital administration to design processes of care that prevent injurious falls.

THE NORMAL GAIT

With understanding of the normal maintenance of balance and gait, clinicians should be able to identify patients at high risk for falls and prescribe preventative measures. A normal gait requires an adequate systolic pressure for a standing posture, normal motor function (locomotion), maintenance of the center of gravity (dynamic balance), sensory input from the visual and vestibular systems, proprioception, normal attention, and adequate cognitive function to avoid obstacles. If a slip does occur, the patient is equipped to compensate and avoid falling. The normal gait has the following features:

- An erect posture achieved by antigravity reflexes dependent on an intact spinal cord and brain stem connections to extend the spine.
- A forward step accomplished by hip flexion, knee flexion, and ankle dorsiflexion.
- Fluidity of movement tracing a straight path requiring coordination.

THE DEFINITION OF A FALL

The definition of a fall is any unplanned descent to the floor, the ground, or any lower level. Falls are further classified as injurious or noninjurious. **Table 85-1** gives examples of common injuries that occur as a result of falls and classifies injury according to the degree of harm incurred by the fallen individual.

A fall is a complex event that often results from an interaction between patient characteristics and the physical environment. Many underlying conditions may cause patients to fall. Most falls have a multifactorial etiology rather than a single cause. An elderly patient may be prone to falling due to mechanical locomotor problems such as an unsteady gait and/or cognitive impairment, reduced proprioception, and debility. Cognitive impairment (related to specific medications, polypharmacy, or substance abuse) coupled with an intercurrent illness may cause delirium or inattention to obstacles in the environment, thereby increasing the elder's risk of falling. Falls may also result from orthostatic hypotension, syncope, stroke, seizure, and neuromuscular weakness. The accompanying case illustrates the presence of several risk factors predisposing a patient to an in-hospital fall with injury. It also illustrates opportunities to implement interventions that might have prevented an injurious fall.

RISK FACTORS FOR FALLS

Common intrinsic and extrinsic risk factors for falls have been identified in studies of community-residing and hospitalized older patients. Intrinsic risk factors describe patient-specific and physiologic characteristics that increase risk of falling (**Table 85-2**). Some intrinsic risk factors, such as gait and balance abnormalities, may be modifiable. Patients with gait disorders are especially prone to falling. Approximately 15% of people older than 60 years of age and 25% of those 85 years of age or older have a history of gait disorder that predisposes them to fall.

TABLE 85-1 The National Quality Forum (NQF) Definitions of Harm and Examples of Common Injuries from Falls

Category	Action Required	Common Injuries
No harm	none	
Minor harm	Application of dressing, ice, topical medication Cleansing wound Leg elevation	Minor limb contusions Lacerations Minor sprains or strains Minor head injury
Moderate harm	Suturing, steri-strips, splinting	Lacerations of arms, legs, and head Sprained ankle, wrist Vertebral and rib fractures Minor traumatic brain injury and Small subdural hematoma
Major harm	Surgery, casting, traction ICU monitoring	Fractures of the hip, forearm, leg, ankle, pelvis, upper arm, hand, skull Traumatic brain injury such as a subdural hematoma or epidural hemorrhage
Death		Head and neck trauma Major internal organ damage and hemorrhage

TABLE 85-2 Risk Factors for Falls

Intrinsic risk factors:

- Lower extremity weakness
- Poor grip strength
- Gait and balance deficits
- History of falls
- Need for some help with daily activities
- Requires 1:1 supervision or assistance with bed transfers and walking
- Urinary incontinence
- Sensory (visual, auditory) impairment
- Cognitive impairment (delirium, dementia)
- Depression
- Orthostasis
- Age

Extrinsic risk factors:

- Use of four or more prescription drugs (polypharmacy)
- Use of high risk medications (benzodiazepines, antipsychotics)
- Environmental challenges (poor lighting, slippery floors, bed height, and absence of grab bars or assistive devices)
- Restraint use (wrist restraints, tubing for intravenous and bladder catheters)

TABLE 85-3 Gait Disorders

Gait Type	Gait Description
Age-related	A shorter and more broad-based stride due to a reduction in velocity, stride length, pelvic rotation, muscle strength, and joint movement. Cervical spondylosis, stroke, or peripheral neuropathy may further result in an ataxic gait. Usually due to multiple comorbidities rather than a single, specific cause.
Defensive posture	A forward posture, broad base, shortened stride, reduced cadence. Usually due to reduced confidence.
Hydrocephalus or cerebellar injury	Widely separated feet when standing or walking and unsure, jerky steps, varying in size, with trunk swaying forward. Mild deficits will cause the patient to fall to one or both sides during tandem walking. Visual input marginally compensates for cerebellar deficit so that stance is unsteady with eyes open and closed.
Parkinson disease	A slow, shuffling gait due to a flexed, stooping posture. The patient leans forward to initiate walking and then hurries to catch up.
Sensory ataxia	A normal stance with eyes open due to visual compensation for proprioceptive loss. Feet usually stamp on the ground; unsteady stance with eyes closed ("positive" Romberg). Patients will have impaired joint position sense. Examples include sensory peripheral neuropathy, spinal cord disease, primary sensory ganglionopathy due to interruption of afferents in peripheral nerves or posterior columns, spinocerebellar tracts of the spinal cord.
Spastic hemiparetic gait	Extended leg and the toes forced downward. Adduction and circumduction at the hip prevent the toes from catching on the ground. Mild weakness may not affect the gait, but excessive wear of the patient's shoe sole may be apparent at the outer front aspect.
Frontal lobe gait	A wide-based gait, with a tendency to fall backwards despite normal motor strength and sensation. Difficulty initiating a walk due to deficits involving connections between the frontal cortex, basal ganglia, and cerebellum. Feet may seem stuck on the floor.
Steppage gait	Lifts leg high so that the toes clear the ground. Due to lower motor neuron disorder causing weakness of pretibial and peroneal muscles.
Myopathic gait	A waddling gait with a sway-back, pot-bellied appearance. Due to trunk and pelvic muscle weakness.

In the hospital setting, the presence of cognitive impairment due to dementia or delirium poses the highest risk of falling. Patients who are immobile for medical reasons or who are mechanically restrained and confined to bed often become too physically deconditioned and unsteady to walk safely, placing them at risk of sustaining an injurious fall. Notably, detectable gait abnormalities (**Table 85-3**) affect 20% to 40% of community-dwelling individuals aged 65 and older and 40% to 50% of those aged 85 and older. Thus, predisposition to falling often exists in certain people, especially older patients, before they arrive at the hospital.

Extrinsic factors include the hazards imposed by the hospital's physical environment. For example, obstacles or clutter challenge the debilitated patient who tries to navigate a hospital room or hallway. Moreover, many older hospitalized patients take multiple medications, including some with potentially adverse effects on cognition and balance, which are implicated in falls. Examples of medications known to increase fall risk include those that cause orthostatic hypotension, loop diuretics, antihypertensive medications such as alpha-blockers, antidepressants, antipsychotics, nonsteroidal anti-inflammatory agents, and benzodiazepines. Most extrinsic risk factors are modifiable.

Certain factors place some hospitalized patients at a particularly high risk of suffering a fall-related injury. The patient populations at highest risk of a serious injury caused by a fall in the hospital include patients over the age of 85, those with osteoporosis and other bone diseases, patients receiving anticoagulation treatment or who have bleeding disorders, and patients with sutured wounds after a recent surgery (particularly amputation, abdominal, and thoracic surgeries). The presence of four or more risk factors also seems to confer a higher risk of injury after a fall. Not uncommonly, a confused patient on intravenous fluids and anticoagulation therapy falls while getting out of bed at night to go to the bathroom when lights are out and no one is around to assist him.

THE HISTORY: WHY DID THIS PATIENT FALL PRIOR TO ADMISSION?

If the patient is unable to provide a history due to cognitive impairment, the examiner should question family members or those involved in the patient's care to identify a history of impaired mobility and bed transfers that places the patient at high risk of falling in hospital and to identify the possibility of intercurrent illness that may underlie the increased risk of a fall due to myalgias, fatigue, or delirium.

Neuromuscular weakness may cause difficulty in motor performance. Neurologic causes of weakness include spasticity, myotonia, stiffness, rigidity, or a peripheral nerve deficit. Generalized weakness may result from deconditioning, disuse, and debility ("frailty"). In approaching a patient with possible weakness, the examiner should determine whether true weakness exists versus nonspecific generalized fatigue that may result from a systemic illness (infection, anemia, hypoxia, obstructive sleep apnea, congestive heart failure, hypotension, malignancy). Patients with chronic pain or other mechanical factors that limit movement may perceive their limited mobility as weakness but will have normal strength on physical examination. Stiffness or rigidity may also result from Parkinson disease. Episodic weakness may result from a transient ischemic attack and seizure as well as a variety of other neurologic syndromes and medical illnesses. The temporal profile—acute (hours to days), subacute (weeks), chronic (months to years), or relapsing (chronic inflammatory demyelinating polyneuropathy or vasculitis)—may provide critical clues to the most likely diagnosis. Collagen vascular diseases, endocrinologic disorders, infections such as HIV, Lyme disease, granulomatous disorders, malignancies, and drugs have all been associated with neuropathies.

If the patient describes true weakness, the examiner must characterize the pattern of weakness and determine whether there is a primary pathologic process (such as cord compression or acute stroke) that requires urgent intervention. Most patients with neuromuscular weakness do not refer to their symptoms as weakness but rather describe difficulty performing specific tasks. The most important first step in localizing the source of the weakness is to ask patients to describe the details of their weakness in terms of their daily life. Do they find that they fall and trip on stairs, curbs, edge of carpets? Do they have difficulty rising from sitting and climbing stairs? Do they need help with daily activities? Patients with myasthenia gravis describe significant weakness with repetitive maneuvers.

A complete history includes an assessment of sensory (visual, auditory) impairment and depression, both important risk factors for falling, and a detailed review of systems (with the caregiver if the patient cannot provide information) to inquire about recent events. Medication review may uncover additional risk factors for falling (Table 85-2).

The examiner should inquire about urinary incontinence. A risk factor for falling, chronic urinary incontinence commonly affects the elderly. Acute urinary incontinence may also be a symptom of a urinary tract infection or an impending cord compression. Falls can occur when incontinent patients slip on urine as they prepare to toilet in the bathroom.

PRACTICE POINT

- The importance of diagnosing incontinence is highlighted by the patient who has impaired bed transfers or generalized weakness. For him, assisted toileting by a nurse or the provision of a bedside commode might prevent a fall due to incontinence.

THE PHYSICAL EXAMINATION

The physical examination begins with the vital signs. The examiner should check the patient's blood pressure lying and then standing if possible. The presence of fever may be an important clue that the patient has an infection that may have resulted in dehydration, orthostasis, spinal cord dysfunction, or caused delirium.

The neurologic examination starts with an assessment to determine if the patient is cognitively impaired due to delirium. An acute change in cognition with inattention and fluctuation suggests the presence of delirium. Interpretation of the neurologic examination may be clouded by the patient's delirium. The workup of delirium is described in Chapter 79.

PRACTICE POINT

- Although falls may be due to locomotor problems, which are more common in the elderly, syncope, seizure, stroke, orthostatic hypotension, and any condition causing delirium may cause an elderly patient to fall. It is therefore important not to assume that an elderly patient admitted to the hospital due to increasing falls at home requires "placement." Clinicians should perform a history and physical examination so that they can recognize precipitating acute illness and modify, to the extent possible, each patient's intrinsic and extrinsic risk factors for falling and injurious falls.

If the patient is able to cooperate with a neurologic examination, the first step is to determine whether true weakness is present and localize the cause of weakness (central lesion(s), spinal cord disease, myopathic disease, neuropathy, neuromuscular junction, or anterior horn cells). The examiner should try to characterize the pattern of weakness: whether generalized symmetric weakness, generalized asymmetric weakness, multifocal weakness, predominantly proximal (myopathy or neuromuscular transmission disorder such as myasthenia gravis) or distal (a neuropathy), or predominantly upper or lower extremity weakness. If a central lesion is suspected, the examiner should check for signs of hemiparesis (acute stroke or hemorrhage, mass lesion if subacute) and quadriparesis (acute brainstem infarct, transverse myelitis, multiple sclerosis if subacute). Cranial nerve dysfunction is common in disorders of neuromuscular transmission (myasthenia gravis) and motor neuron disease (amyotrophic lateral sclerosis) or may signify a central lesion. A cervical cord process may be suggested by quadriparesis with hypertonicity and brisk reflexes if no cerebral signs or symptoms. A paraparesis sparing the arms with spasticity and brisk reflexes may suggest a disorder of the thoracic spinal cord. In general, paraparesis with flaccidity and hypoactive reflexes indicates a peripheral problem. Sensory loss or pain may result from spinal cord dysfunction (also associated with bowel and bladder dysfunction) or a neuropathy.

SCREENING FOR FALL RISK

Nursing staff in most hospitals conduct a routine fall risk assessment upon admission of a patient to the hospital. Fall risk assessment tools are divided into those that predict a probability of falling (risk screening tools) and those that assess factors that contribute to the patient's risk of falling (risk factor assessment tools). The most common, validated tools used for risk screening are summarized in **Table 85-4**. In general, fall risk screening tools are not very predictive of injurious falls in the hospital. They have high false-positive rates (low specificity) and low positive predictive value. Ultimately, risk screening tools in clinical trials have not proven effective at reducing the incidence of injurious falls in the hospital. Simple risk assessment, on the other hand, involves identifying all intrinsic and extrinsic risk factors for falling. Risk factors identified through risk assessment as modifiable may be the most appropriate targets for unifactorial and/or multifactorial interventions. In quality improvement studies, interventions designed to alter one or more modifiable risk factors (eg, reducing polypharmacy) are promising approaches to reduction of fall rates and fall-related injuries. At the bedside, the high risk patient is often identified as a cognitively impaired person (with delirium, dementia, or both) who is unable to transfer independently from bed to a chair or to stand up without assistance. The hospitalist who admits this patient could note modifiable risk factors, such as generalized weakness or potential medication side effects, and then address them with an intervention geared toward preventing an injurious fall.

STRATEGIES TO PREVENT FALLS AND FALL-RELATED INJURIES

Ideally, nursing staff and physicians assess all patients at admission for risk of falls and fall-related injuries. Patients considered at risk for falls receive universal and/or targeted interventions. Universal fall interventions are standard procedures applied to all patients admitted to the hospital, regardless of how many risk factors they may have. For example, nursing staff orient all patients to the hospital environment. All patients' possessions and a call bell are placed within easy reach. Floor surfaces in all patients' rooms are clean and dry, and all patients receive nonskid socks to wear. Nursing efforts are complemented by the physician's assessment of physical strength and mobility limitations during the initial history and physical exam.

Patients identified as having many fall risk factors or judged to be at particularly high risk of suffering a fall-related injury require additional, targeted interventions to reduce fall risk. These more aggressive interventions focus on modifiable risk factors including those listed in Table 85-4. Common interventions include 1:1 monitoring with a sitter or companion, use of bed and chair

TABLE 85-4 Falls Risk Screening Tools

Tool	Items Measured	Scoring	Comments
Morse Fall	• History of falling • Secondary diagnosis of falls • Use of ambulatory aid	• Yes/No responses for each item. • Each item is weighted	• Oldest of validated falls risk tools • Time consuming to complete
Scale*	• Intravenous therapy • Gait impaired • Mental status impaired	• Total score = 0–125 • Low risk = 0–24 • Medium risk = 25–44 • High risk = 45–100	• Low positive predictive value for incident falls • Low specificity
St. Thomas Risk Assessment Tool in Falling Elderly Inpatients (STRATIFY)†	• Fall on or during admission to hospital • Agitation present • Vision impaired • Need frequent toileting • Transfer/mobility impaired	• Yes/No responses for each item • Total score = 0–5 • Fall risk = ≥ 2	• Validated falls risk tool • Simple scoring • Low positive predictive value • The population and setting affect STRATIFY performance.
Hendrich II§	• Confusion/disorientation • Depression • Altered elimination • Dizziness/vertigo • Male gender • Administered antiepileptics • Administered benzodiazepines • Abnormal "Get up and Go" item #2 (rising from chair)	• Yes/No responses • Each item is weighted • Total score = 0–20 • High risk = ≥ 5	• Validated falls risk tool • Brief tool • Only tool that includes at-risk medications • Slightly higher specificity than the Morse scale • Low positive predictive value

Data from

*Morse JM, Morse RM, Tylko SJ. Development of a scale to indentify the fall-prone patient. *Canadian Journal of Aging.* 1989;8:366.

†Oliver D, Britton M, Seed P, Martin FC, Hopper AH. Development and evaluation of evidence based risk assessment tool (STRATIFY) to predict which elderly inpatients will fall: case-control and cohort studies. *BMJ.* 1997;315:1049.

§Hendrich AL, Bender PS, Nyhuis A. Validation of the Hendrich II fall risk model: a large concurrent case/control study of hospitalized patients. *Appl Nursing Res.* 2003;16:9.

alarms, physical therapy, supervised toileting, scheduled toileting, judicious review and modification of medication lists containing medications that increase risk of falls, or a combination of these in a multifactorial, patient-specific intervention. Though not specifically demonstrated as an intervention strategy in clinical trials, delirium prevention strategies could conceivably reduce the incidence of falls.

A handful of fall-prevention strategies have been studied specifically in the acute care hospital setting (**Table 85-5**). A recent Cochrane review found that studies using a single, unifactorial intervention did not yield significant change in fall or injury rates. However, a meta-analysis of several studies using multifactorial interventions in the hospital showed a significant reduction of 18% for falls but no significant effect on the number of fallers or fractures. Most of the interventions designed to reduce falls in the hospital either did not use rigorous methodology or did not include prevention of fall-related injuries as a primary outcome. Despite a paucity of evidence in the literature, the interventions listed in Table 85-5 demonstrate varying degrees of face validity, and they remain the mainstays of hospital fall prevention programs. The results of the available evidence to date on interventions to prevent falls and fall-related injuries in hospitals suggest that multifactorial strategies will likely be superior to single (unifactorial) interventions.

APPROACH TO THE PATIENT WHO HAS FALLEN IN THE HOSPITAL

Hospitalists are often called to the bedside to evaluate the fallen patient. **Table 85-6** offers suggestions for the hospitalist's workup of a fallen patient. A comprehensive approach to risk factor identification and possible injuries (Tables 85-1 and 85-2) is advisable and often informs clinical decision making. For example, patients with dementia, delirium, or altered mental status may not be able to provide accurate description of the fall and injury that occurred. They might not be able to verbalize or communicate important symptoms. Therefore, some detective work on the part of the hospitalist, along with a high index of suspicion for occult or serious injury, is required in order to avoid missing important injuries.

The assessment of a fallen patient begins with a documentation of the circumstances of the fall and the condition of the fallen patient. The examiner should obtain a set of vital signs followed by a physical examination looking for the presence of injury to the brain, spine, or other musculoskeletal site. The examining physician determines if the patient lost consciousness and whether a syncope workup is thereby indicated. A thorough pain assessment is warranted along with prompt and appropriate analgesia (ice, splinting, medication) for the fallen patient in pain. The remaining workup concentrates on specific sites of injury (Table 85-6).

When clinical suspicion is high, multiple X-ray views of all injured sites are obtained. A computed tomography (CT) scan is recommended when clinical suspicion is high and X-rays are negative (especially for hip and vertebral compression fractures), as some fractures might not be evident on plain films. Lacerations and ecchymoses on face or scalp prompt further evaluation for concussion and traumatic brain injury. For patients who have sustained blunt trauma to the head, even if no bruising or trauma is apparent on exam, neuroimaging should be considered in elderly patients, particularly if anticoagulated, to exclude subdural hematoma. In elderly or fragile patients a pelvic fracture can be sustained from low energy trauma such as a fall from a standing position. Such pelvic fractures should not be overlooked as they are associated with significant bleeding and concomitant injuries including muscle contusions and high mortality. Intra-abdominal organ injury is rare in falls, but is possible when the patient suffered blunt abdominal trauma.

TABLE 85-5 Interventions that May Potentially Prevent Falls and/or Fall-Related Injuries in Acute Care Hospitals*

Intervention Domain	Intervention Type	Fall Prevention	Injury Prevention	Supportive Evidence Base
Exercises	Physical, occupational therapy	X		X
	General physical activity	X		
Medication modification targets/ Nonpharmacologic treatment substitution targets	Antihypertensives	X	X	X
	Calcium	X	X	
	Vitamin D	X	X	
	Reduce burden of medications active on the central nervous system (benzodiazepines, sleep aids, narcotics, antipsychotics, antidepressants)	X	X	
	Anticoagulation therapy		X	
	Parkinson disease medications	X	X	
	Reduce polypharmacy	X	X	
Toileting and incontinence management	Scheduled toileting assistance	X	X	
	Bladder catheter need assessment	X		
Education and behavior change	Video, reading material	X	X	X
	Teach back	X	X	
Environmental modifications/ assistive techniques	Nursing assistance with daily activities	X	X	
	1:1 supervision by family member or caregiver	X	X	
	Hip protectors		X	
	Bedside floor mats		X	
	Adjustable-height beds		X	
	Bed and chair alarms	X	X	
	Location close to nurses station	X		
	Helmets		X	
	Removal of physical restraints	X	X	
	Brightly colored wrist bands, identifiers of risk	X		
	Sensory impairment aids (hearing aids, glasses)	X		
	Flooring modification	X	X	

*Data from Cameron ID, Murray GR, Gillespie LD, et al. Interventions for preventing falls in older people in nursing care facilities and hospitals. *Cochrane Database of Systematic Reviews.* 2010; Issue 1. Art. No.: CD005465.DOI: 10.1002/14651858.CD005465.pub2.

CASE 85-1 *(continued)*

Our patient suffered moderate harm from her injurious fall in the hospital and required five sutures for a laceration of her right cheek. On examination she was delirious (which limited her neurologic examination). She appeared to have sprained her right wrist, an injury that would further limit her ability to use a walker. She was not orthostatic. She had negative CT brain scan, negative imaging of the face, no new fractures of her left and right upper extremities.

Intrinsic risk factors for falling included a past history of falls, probable gait abnormality, visual impairment, cognitive impairment, and age. Extrinsic risk factors included polypharmacy, recent exposure to an antipsychotic (haloperidol), a table out of reach, a high bed, and possibly the bladder catheter.

The following steps were taken to reduce the risk of another injurious fall:

1. Improved medication safety
    - Use antipsychotics with caution. Require that a face-to-face physician assessment prior to administration of addition haloperidol. Use haloperidol only when the patient exhibits life-threatening or injurious behaviors. If haloperidol is required, start with the lower dose of 0.5 mg.
    - Discontinuation of trazodone (a sedative prescribed for sleep).
    - Elimination of aspirin while on enoxaparin to reduce bleeding risk.
    - Around-the-clock acetaminophen for analgesia with frequent pain assessments and a small dose of hydrocodone available for breakthrough pain.
2. Physical therapy consultation and bedside to chair transfers at least twice a day.
3. A toileting schedule with a bedside commode.
4. Low bed and floor mats, bed alarm.
5. Placement of her tray table with her phone, glasses, call bell, and a cup of water easily within her reach.
6. 1:1 sitter.

Two days later, this patient's delirium and pain control had improved. She was eating and sleeping on a more regular schedule. Given her overall deconditioning and mobility limitations, she was discharged to a skilled facility on hospital day 5 for rehabilitation.

TABLE 85-6 Suggested Workup of the Fallen Patient Based on Site-specific Injuries

Site of Injury	Type of Injury	Signs and Symptoms of Injury	Evaluation and Management Options
Head	Traumatic brain injury (concussion, subdural hematoma), stroke	Altered consciousness Acute/subacute confusion, headache, light-headedness, visual changes, focal neurologic deficit	Stop anticoagulation. If anticoagulated and bleeding, consider administration of vitamin K and fresh frozen plasma. Mental status assessment. Neurology, neurosurgery consultation. Perform neurologic assessments every 2 hours for 24 to 48 hours. Imaging.
Spinal column	Cord injury Vertebral fracture	Absence of sensation. Inability to move. Localized pain.	Immediate stabilization of spine and immobilization with backboard, rigid cervical collar, lateral head supports. Palpate entire spine. Consult spine surgery for assessment. Imaging with X-rays, CT scan. Analgesia.
Skin	Laceration	Bleeding Visible alteration of skin integrity	Hemostasis with pressure, ice. Cleansing, sterilization. Suturing, stapling. Pain management.
	Ecchymoses	Discoloration	Ice. Pain management.
Extremities	Fracture Dislocation	Pain Limb, joint deformity Inability to bear weight	Imaging of injury site. Check neurovascular integrity distal to injury site. Splint site. Consult orthopedics or reduce dislocation.
Abdominal and pelvic injuries	Blunt trauma Pelvic fracture	Pain	Physical exam. X-ray/CT

CONCLUSION

Falls are the leading cause of nonfatal injury in almost every age group in the United States, especially the elderly. Accidental falls in hospitalized patients are associated with injuries, prolonged hospital stay, and poor clinical outcomes. Key to prevention and assessment of falls once they have occurred is the hospital physician's ability to recognize and modify, to the extent possible, each patient's intrinsic and extrinsic risk factors for falling.

SUGGESTED READINGS

Cameron ID, Murray GR, Gillespie LD, et al. Interventions for preventing falls in older people in nursing care facilities and hospitals. *Cochrane Database of Systematic Reviews* 2010; Issue 1. Art. No.: CD005465.DOI: 10.1002/14651858.CD005465.pub2.

Comprehensive and evidence-based overview of risk factors and interventions to prevent falls in hospitalized patients. AGS Clinical Practice Guideline: *Prevention of Falls in Older Persons,* 2010. http://www.americangeriatrics.org/health_care_professionals/clinical_practice/clinical_guidelines_recommendations/2010/. Accessed October 14, 2010.

Institute for Clinical Systems Improvement (ICSI). Report: Health Care Protocol: Prevention of Falls (Acute Care). http://www.icsi.org/falls__acute_care___prevention_of__protocol_/falls__acute_care___prevention_of__protocol__24255.html. Accessed November 2009.

Lakatos BE, Capasso V, Mitchell MT, et al. Falls in the general hospital: association with delirium, advanced age, and specific surgical procedures. *Psychosomatics*. 2009;50:3.

National Quality Forum (NQF). A detailed guideline for the screening and detection of older patients at risk of falling. In: *Safe Practices for Better Healthcare–2010 Update: A Consensus Report.* Washington, DC: NQF; 2010. Accessed August 28, 2010.

Oliver D, Connelly JB, Victor CR, et al. Strategies to prevent falls and fractures in hospitals and care homes and effect of cognitive impairment: systematic review and meta-analyses. *BMJ*. 2007;334:82.

Quigley PA, Hahm B, Powell-Cope G, Sarduy I, Tyndal K, White SV. Reducing serious injury from falls in two Veterans' Hospital medical-surgical units. *J Nurs Care Qual*. 2009;24:33.

Woolcott JC, Richardson KJ, Wiens MO, et al. Meta-analysis of the impact of 9 medication classes on falls in elderly persons. *Arch Intern Med*. 2009;169:1952.

CHAPTER 86

Fever and Rash

Shanta M. Zimmer, MD

Key Clinical Questions

1. What are the most common causes of fever and rash in the hospitalized patient?
2. What is the pathophysiology of fever and rash?
3. What other clinical symptoms and findings are associated with fever and rash?
4. How can laboratory tests help with diagnosis of the etiology of rash?

CASE 86-1

A 25-year-old graduate student who living in student housing presented to the hospital complaining of a 4-day history of upper respiratory tract symptoms that have progressed to include fever and rash on his extremities. The rash began on his hands and feet as a pink, flat rash, but has progressed over the last several hours to be purplish in nature, and extends now to his trunk and face. He is admitted to your service for further evaluation and treatment.

The rapid progression of the patient's rash and the appearance of macular rash that progressed to petechiae and purpura raised immediate concern for meningococcemia. The patient was placed in droplet precautions, blood cultures were collected, and ceftriaxone therapy initiated. Vital signs revealed blood pressure of 110/60, pulse 118, respiratory rate 24, and temperature of 39.2. No nuchal rigidity was noted. The patient's respiratory status declined and he was admitted to the ICU and intubated. Blood cultures grew *Neisseria meningitidis* at 24 hours and laboratory findings were consistent with DIC. A lumbar puncture was not performed due to severe thrombocytopenia. Multisystem organ failure developed rapidly. In addition to inotropic support, the use of recombinant activated protein C was considered.

INTRODUCTION

The combination of fever and rash in the hospitalized patient has many different possible etiologies and the presentation can be varied, but an organized approach to the problem will alleviate some of the guesswork involved in diagnosing and treating these patients. This chapter will cover the presentation of rash plus fever and avoid a discussion of the causes of rash that are not typically associated with fever.

The clinical presentation of patients with rash and fever when they come to the hospital must be divided into categories of those who are critically ill vs. those who are not. Critically ill patients with rash often have fulminant onset of both the fever and the rash and must be diagnosed quickly to receive appropriate care. The timing of the rash is important for judging the severity of the disease with rapid onset often portending a more rapidly progressive course. The most worrisome cause of fulminant onset of rash is septicemia, especially purpura fulminans of meningococcemia, which can progress over hours or even minutes. More gradual or waxing and waning rash and fever suggest a more chronic process or one that may be noninfectious such as rheumatological disease or even a malignancy.

PRACTICE POINT

- Patients presenting in the hospital with rash and fever must be divided into two categories: those who are critically ill and those who are not. Causes of critical illness include hemorrhagic fever, meningococcemia, Rocky Mountain spotted fever, toxic shock syndrome, Stevens-Johnson syndrome, toxic epidermal necrolysis, and acute vasculitis.

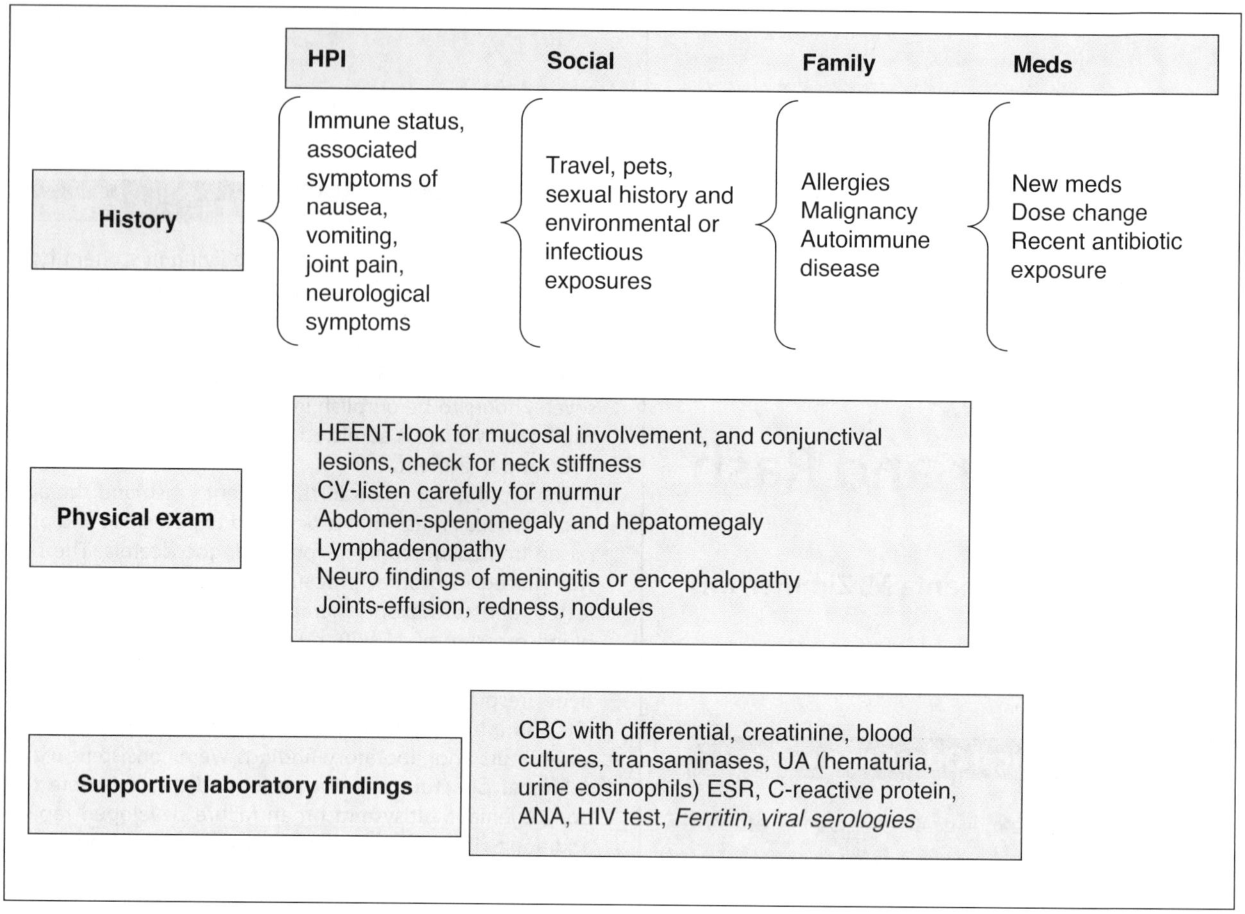

Figure 86-1 *History, physical, and laboratory tests in patients with fever and rash.*

APPROACH TO FEVER AND RASH AT THE BEDSIDE

Some acute rash and fever syndromes are caused by infectious diseases that can be spread by airborne or respiratory droplets. Therefore, before beginning the history and physical, if such a transmissible disease is suggested, appropriate precautions should be instituted (**Figure 86-1**).

> **PRACTICE POINT**
>
> - Some acute rash and fever syndromes are caused by infectious diseases that can be spread by airborne or respiratory droplets. Therefore, before beginning the history and physical, if such a transmissible disease is suggested, appropriate precautions should be instituted.

HISTORY

The age of the patient and the season of the year provide important epidemiologic clues to the differential diagnosis. Appropriate medical history that includes timing of the rash and fever and associated symptoms are important aspects of the initial evaluation. Specifically, patients should be asked about location of onset and timing of progression. Secondary changes to the rash such as those that might have occurred through self-treatments (lotions, over-the-counter ointments) or through excoriations or picking should be specifically asked about. In cases in which multiple lesions are present, in order to get a sense of how the rash has progressed, it may be helpful to ask the patient, "Can you show me an area that looks like how the rash started?" or "Are there any new lesions?" Associated symptoms of fever, sore throat, lymphadenopathy, and other systemic symptoms such as weight loss and joint pain should also be noted. Additionally, there are key aspects of each part of the history that should be explored. Medication lists should be scrutinized for new medications or changes in dosing of old medications. While many allergic reactions occur within the first several days or weeks of an exposure to a new drug, some reactions do not occur until after more prolonged exposure; in particular, antiepileptic drugs such as phenytoin are notorious for presenting with fever and rash after a few weeks of exposure, and only rarely within the first few days. Family and personal history of fever syndromes or allergies can also be a clue to the risk of drug allergy. Although often overlooked in adult patients, vaccination history and prior history of illnesses of childhood are important when evaluating some fever and rash presentations. Family history of rheumatologic diseases should also be specifically gathered, including history of lupus, vasculitis, or juvenile onset arthritis. Social, travel, and exposure histories are especially important when evaluating patients with fever and rash. Sexual history might suggest risk factors for acute HIV infection, syphilis, or gonococcal disease. Travel to endemic areas may suggest exposures to certain mosquito-borne illnesses such as dengue or malaria or tick-borne illnesses such as Rocky Mountain Spotted Fever (RMSF) or Lyme disease. Social history should include exposures to small children either through work (daycare, school teacher), or home.

PHYSICAL EXAM

As with all hospitalized patients, vitals signs and general appearance will contribute to the overall gestalt of the patient's condition and may suggest rapid intervention or therapy. In particular, pulse-temperature dissociation (elevated temperature without elevation in pulse) may be a clue to infection with an intracellular pathogen, including Rickettsial disease, and is often present with drug reactions. Careful evaluation of lymphadenopathy and tenderness should be noted. Localized, tender lymph nodes may point to infectious etiologies while more diffuse lymphadenopathy is more commonly associated with a disseminated viral infection such as EBV, or malignancy, especially lymphoma.

Mucosal involvement of rash or ulcers, including oral and genital membranes should be noted. Cardiac exam should include careful evaluation for a new murmur or evidence of congestive heart failure, which could point to endocarditis. Abdominal exam should include palpation for hepatosplenomegaly, which can be found in noninfectious causes of fever and rash or in viral illnesses such as EBV or CMV infection. Splenomegaly is also present in many patients with subacute bacterial endocarditis. Careful joint examination, noting effusions, tenderness, or signs of synovitis as well as assessment for neurological symptoms should be done. The rash itself should be characterized by the color and type of lesion (nodule, macule, or pustule); distribution of lesions (trunk, head, etc); palpation and associated findings such as scale, purulence, or secondary changes.

ASSOCIATED FINDINGS

Although most findings are nonspecific, laboratory clues to the etiology of fever and rash should be considered. The differential on the white blood cell count (WBC) may reveal eosinophilia, usually a clue to allergic reaction, but also seen with cholesterol emboli syndrome. Leukopenia is seen with viral illnesses including arboviral infections, CMV, measles, and dengue; leukocytosis with atypical lymphocytes is a hallmark of mononucleosis from Epstein-Barr virus (EBV). Leukopenia may also be a feature of systemic lupus erythematosus (SLE). Thrombocytopenia may be noted in severe sepsis, drug reaction, DIC, hematological malignancies, and some specific infections and should be looked for, especially if a rash is petechial. Similarly, assessment of coagulation should be done. Transaminases are often elevated in herpes virus infections (including CMV and EBV), in Rickettsial diseases, toxic shock, and sometimes in beta-lactam drug reactions. Urinalysis should be performed to look for hematuria and protein, which may be a clue to vasculitis or endocarditis. If drug allergy is suspected, consider checking for urinary eosinophils, which are sometimes seen in interstitial nephritis, classically caused by beta-lactam antibiotics, especially nafcillin. However, the absence of urinary eosinophils does not exclude the diagnosis, and renal biopsy may be needed if renal function is deteriorating.

THE RASH

Appearance of the lesions is critical to determining the differential diagnosis and also in communicating appropriately with consultants (**Table 86-1**). For a thorough description of all lesion types and associated differential diagnosis, a dermatology textbook should be consulted. Common lesions associated with fever and rash are limited and for the most part include macules, vesicles and bullae, papules, nodules, and sometimes plaques.

PRACTICE POINT

- Appearance of the lesions is critical to determining the differential diagnosis and also in communicating appropriately with consultants.

CRITICALLY ILL vs. NOT CRITICALLY ILL

Critically ill patients with fever and rash are usually suffering from a significant infectious process that could progress rapidly to shock. It is important to recognize diagnostic signs of these patients early so as to institute appropriate therapy rapidly. Blood cultures should be drawn and antibiotics initiated immediately upon presentation.

Consideration should also be made for isolation procedures if needed, especially in the case of hemorrhagic fever or meningococcemia.

Meningococcemia caused by the gram-negative diplococcus, *Neisseria meningitidis,* is a rapidly progressive, often fatal infection seen most commonly in adolescents and young adults. The rash and fever may be preceded by upper respiratory symptoms. The rash of meningococcemia may begin as pink macules and progress to purpura even bullous lesions. Meningitis may or may not be present in meningococcemia. Findings of leukocytosis, thrombocytopenia, and DIC are often present in laboratory evaluation.

Meningococcemia may be difficult to distinguish from Rocky Mountain Spotted Fever (RMSF), which also may progress to shock and multisystem organ failure, but a few important distinguishing features may help with the differential diagnosis. The rash of meningococcemia may present even before the patient feels ill, while the rash of RMSF usually occurs 3–5 days after onset of symptoms of fever and is most commonly distributed on the ankles and wrists. As noted above, pulse-temperature deficit is an important clue to the presence of RMSF. The WBC in RMSF may be decreased while it is usually elevated in meningococcemia.

Other causes of fever and rash in the critically ill patient include toxic shock syndrome due to the superantigens of either Group A streptococcal infection or *Staphylococcus aureus* infection. These syndromes present with diffuse erythroderma, hypotension, high fever, and sometimes are accompanied by nausea or vomiting. Blood cultures may be positive for the causative organism in staphylococcal infections but are often negative in streptococcal toxic shock syndrome. Treatment of the critically ill patient with

TABLE 86-1 Description of Common Types of Skin Lesions and Examples of Pathologic Causes

Macule	Papule	Nodule	Vesicle/Bulla	Pustule	Plaque
Flat, in the plane of the skin, nonpalpable	Small, solid, raised, palpable	Larger papule, solid	Fluid-filled blister, usually clear or bloody fluid	Small, blister filled with pus	Flat, like a macule, but palpable and usually larger; may have secondary changes such as scale or crusting
Drug rash, viral exanthema, syphilis, HIV	Viral, allergic reaction, stigmata of endocarditis	Erythema nodosum, fungal or atypical mycobacterial infections	Varicella, HSV, bullous diseases, drug eruptions	Bacterial infection or superinfection	Psoriasis, MCTD, syphilis, atypical drug eruption, malignancy

fever and rash is directed at the underlying illness and will often include empiric coverage for staphylococcal (both methicillin-sensitive and MRSA) and streptococcal infections. If toxic shock syndrome is suspected, an infectious disease specialist should be consulted for consideration of intravenous immunoglobulin infusion and appropriate antibiotic selection, including addition of clindamycin in streptococcal infections for its antitoxin effect. In some cases of toxic shock with skin and soft tissue involvement, surgical intervention is required as complications can include necrotizing fascitis and myonecrosis. Surgical consultation should be made early in the course of disease as rapid debridement of affected tissue can be life-saving.

CASE 86-2

A 57-year-old diabetic man with end-stage liver disease secondary to hepatitis C was admitted to the hospital for fevers and found to have methicillin-resistant *Staphylococcus aureus* (MRSA) bacteremia. He was started on vancomycin on admission, but fevers persisted for 3 days and on hospital day 4 he developed a diffuse macular rash on his abdomen, chest, arms, and legs as well as an increased temperature of 38.8°C.

The rash was most prominent on the trunk and had a macular appearance with irregular borders and areas of confluence. The erythema was blanching and seemed to be spreading. The patient was otherwise well-appearing, and complained of slight itchiness on his abdomen. Suspecting allergic drug eruption, his physicians checked carefully in the mouth and genital region for evidence of mucosal erythema, ulceration, or sloughing. Orders included repeat blood cultures, UA with micro, urinary eosinophils, CBC with differential, and a chemistry panel, including creatinine and transaminases. In the meantime, vancomycin was held.

Hypersensitivity to a medication is one of the most common causes of fever and rash in a hospitalized patient, and antibiotics are among the most often implicated as responsible for cutaneous adverse drug reactions (CADR). Several clinical clues suggest the medication as cause of the fever and rash. Timing of initiation of the drug is important but not always helpful since patients may develop allergy to a medication at any time during its use. Allergic reactions to antibiotics commonly occur after 7–10 days of therapy but may occur immediately or at a later time. Fever from drug rash is often very high (> 38.8°C) and not associated with other symptoms of toxicity such as tachycardia or hypotension. Skin findings usually include an erythematous macular rash that is sometimes papular and can involve any part of the body, including the palms and soles. Bullous lesions or mucosal ulceration are signs of severe disease and progression, so patients should be examined carefully for evidence of mucosal involvement, including oral, conjunctival, and genital areas. Laboratory findings of eosinophilia are supportive but not required to make the diagnosis of drug reaction. Severe drug toxicity may also include hepatitis or renal involvement. In hospitalized patients, polypharmacy may make the decision difficult about which drug is responsible. Certain medications are more frequent causes of this presentation and should be eliminated first. As always, patients' medication lists should be reviewed for new additions and unnecessary medications that can be eliminated or placed on hold.

The exanthematous drug eruption, often referred to as a morbilliform rash, following administration of a new medication is the most common CADR seen in hospitalized patients, accounting for 40–90% of all drug rashes seen. Antibiotics (including sulfonamides, penicillins, and cephalosporins), antiepileptic medications, and NSAIDs are among the most commonly implicated medications for this syndrome.

Vancomycin is not listed among the most commonly cited causes of fever and rash, but with the increased use of vancomycin in the setting of prevalent MRSA infections, this association may become more common seen. Another cutaneous reaction associated with vancomycin, "Red Man Syndrome" consists of flushing and warmth with erythema of the face, neck, and chest during infusion in between 4–50% of patients. This reaction can be ameliorated with slowing the infusion and sometimes with antihistamine medications. Patients may experience fever during the infusion, but prolonged fever in association with rash is more indicative of a true drug allergy.

More severe and rare forms of drug reactions include the spectrum of Stevens-Johnson syndrome (SJS) to toxic epidermal necrolysis (TEN). These syndromes can be life-threatening and may require ICU support. SJS presents as an inflammatory reaction with erythroderma, mucosal involvement, and systemic symptoms. Mucosal involvement is a hallmark feature and another diagnosis should be considered if this is not present. Immune mediated bullous diseases should be considered in the differential diagnosis. Although SJS/TEN can occur in response to a viral infection or idiopathically, drugs are implicated as the cause in approximately 70% of cases. A case-control study found increased risk of these rare adverse drug events with sulfonamides, oxicam NSAIDs, anticonvulsants, and allopurinol. Surprisingly, corticosteroids were also associated with an increased risk of SJS. In addition to the drug itself, coexisting conditions also increase the risk for SJS/TEN, especially HIV infection, systemic lupus erythematosus, and chronic Ebstein Barr virus infection.

Treatment of SJS, which may be fatal in 5–15% of cases, includes immediate cessation of the offending drug. Multidisciplinary care is often required and consultation with dermatology and burn unit teams should be made promptly. Mucosal involvement may necessitate consultation by ophthalmology and urology specialists. Supportive care is the mainstay of therapy, including fluid and nutritional support. Corticosteroids are not recommended, but a role for IVIG has been suggested and may be helpful.

CASE 86-3

A 37-year-old woman with 2 small children presented to the hospital complaining of fever associated with night sweats and sore throat for the past several weeks. Her only other symptoms were fatigue and knee pain. She denied travel, sick contacts, or exposure to unclean water or pets. She did not take any medications except ibuprofen, which seems to alleviate some of her symptoms. Physical examination was notable for fever of 40°C degrees and a macular rash over her chest, back, arms, and legs. The nonpalpable rash was lacy in appearance. Other notable findings include splenomegaly without other lymphadenopathy.

Her physicians are concerned about the possibility of lymphoma, mononucleosis-like illness, or a rheumatologic disease such as SLE or adult Still disease. Complement levels, ANA, ESR, ferritin level, blood cultures, and routine CBC are ordered as well as a heterophile antibody to look for mononucleosis due to EBV. Blood cultures remained negative and remaining labs revealed elevated WBC, slight elevation in transaminases, evidence of prior infection with both EBV and CMV, elevated ESR, and ferritin of 15,000 ng/mL. ANA and RF were negative and a CT scan of the chest, abdomen, and pelvis revealed splenomegaly and diffuse lymphadenopathy. Rheumatology was consulted for treatment of adult Still disease.

The broad differential diagnosis of fever and rash includes bacterial syndromes such as bacteremia and endocarditis, viral illnesses due to EBV or CMV, SLE, adult Still disease, Familial Mediterranean Fever, or others of the periodic fever syndromes, vasculitis, or malignancy, especially lymphoma. Adult Still disease is a diagnosis of exclusion because there is no gold standard and the overlap with rheumatologic and malignant diseases is great. After reasonable exclusion of illnesses listed above, the clinical criteria include arthralgias or arthritis, sore throat, and characteristic salmon-pink rash in an otherwise healthy patient with fever for greater than 2 weeks; additional laboratory features suggestive of this illness include a leukocytosis with a polymorphonuclear predominance and a markedly elevated ferritin level; nonbulky adenopathy is common.

OTHER CLINICAL SYNDROMES

A few other clinical syndromes warrant mention as causes of fever and rash in hospitalized patients. With thorough physical exam and careful history, a differential diagnosis is usually straightforward.

Viral illnesses in children are responsible for many macular rashes with fever in pediatrics, and in young adult patients or nonimmune adults, viral causes should still be considered, especially those due to EBV, CMV, or parvovirus B19. Although the rash of parvovirus usually follows the febrile illness, in immunocompromised patients, the timing of fever can coincide with the rash. Classic vesicular lesions of varicella should prompt concern in adult patients in which the disease is often more severe and can include pneumonia and respiratory failure, especially in immunocompromised or pregnant patients. Varicella zoster, on the other hand, represents reactivation rather than primary disease and is usually limited to one or two dermatomes. Again, these patients may have a more severe course if underlying immunodeficiency is present such as HIV, transplantation, or other immunosuppressant medications. HIV infection is another important cause of fever and rash in adult patients. Although many different rashes have been described in the acute seroconversion syndrome associated with HIV infection, the rash is *usually a diffuse, macular erythema typical of a viral exanthem*. Patients suspected of having acute HIV infection should undergo testing with an HIV viral load rather than an antibody test, which is often negative at the time of acute infection. HIV also increases the risk for drug reactions. In particular, allergic reactions to sulfa antibiotics are more commonly seen in this group of patients even those who tolerated these drugs prior to their HIV illness.

Syphilis, the "great imitator" is another cause of fever and rash, and while it does not usually require hospitalization, rash without a clear etiology should prompt an evaluation for syphilis with a treponemal antibody test. Vasculitis and mixed connective tissue disorders may cause fever and rash and consultation with dermatology and rheumatology should be considered if the appearance of the rash suggests a noninfectious purpura. These lesions often require biopsy for diagnosis and multisystem involvement is the rule.

Finally, some malignancies may present with fever and rash, especially the hematological malignancies such as lymphoma or some types of leukemia. Careful lymph node exam and examination of the peripheral blood smear are warranted in cases in which malignancy is considered. Skin and bone marrow biopsy may be required.

CONSULTATION

In general, all critically ill patients with fever and rash should be treated empirically with appropriate antibiotics, and consultation with an infectious diseases physician is usually prudent, due to the fact that the most common etiologies include severe sepsis syndromes. Issues surrounding infection control and postexposure prophylaxis in the setting of meningococcal infection can be facilitated by the hospital epidemiologist and/or infectious diseases consultant. For mild to moderate drug reactions due to antibiotics, infectious disease consultation can help in selecting an alternative therapy. In cases in which toxic shock is considered the etiology and necrotizing infection is suspected, timely surgical consultation is most important and should be done quickly as a life-saving and often limb-saving procedure may be needed. Dermatology consults are important in cases in which the diagnosis is unclear or in which a systemic or cutaneous vasculitis is suspected. Skin biopsy can be helpful to distinguish between drug reactions and viral illnesses or vasculitis and may be especially helpful in confirming diagnosis of SJS or TEN. Consultants can also be helpful in communicating the prognosis of certain illnesses with family members and in-hospital consultation may facilitate outpatient follow up for chronic conditions such as adult Still disease, vasculitis, or SLE.

RISK MANAGEMENT

In the case of drug-induced fever and rash, there may be questions of blame on the part of family members or patients. Although adverse drug events related to allergy are often not avoidable if no preexisting allergy is noted, the severity and suddenness of the disease can be alarming. Communication with the patient and family members about the harm done by the medication is important in an ethical, professional, and open manner.

CONCLUSION

The 3 case scenarios presented in the chapter comprise the most common presentations of fever and rash in hospitalized patients. Prompt recognition of rash and fever in critically ill patients with meningococcemia, toxic shock, or SJS/TEN can result in early institution of life-saving treatments. The skin is often a window to other systemic illnesses and the keys to diagnosis rest in careful history and physical examination of those other systems. In cases of fever and rash, always be willing to go back to the patient for additional details regarding the presentation. Revisiting the initial presentation for clues to new environmental, medication, travel, or infectious exposures (including sexual history) may often uncover a clue to the etiology. See chapters 142: Adverse Cutaneous Drug Reactions and 147: Dermatologic Findings in Systemic Disease for further management.

SUGGESTED READINGS

Bagnari V, Colina M, Ciancio G, Govoni M, Trotta F. Adult-onset Still's disease. *Rheumatol Int*. 2010;30:855–862.

Coco A, Kleinhans E. Prevalence of primary HIV infection in symptomatic ambulatory patients. *Ann Fam Med*. 2005;3:400–404.

Cunha BA. Rash and fever in the critical care unit. *Crit Care Clin*. 1998;14:35–53.

Gruchalla RS, Pirmohamed M. Clinical practice. Antibiotic allergy. *N Engl J Med*. 2006;354:601–609.

Hazin R, Ibrahimi OA, Hazin MI, Kimyai-Asadi A. Stevens-Johnson syndrome: pathogenesis, diagnosis, and management. *Ann Med*. 2008;40:129–138.

Ramdial PK, Naidoo DK. Drug-induced cutaneous pathology. *J Clin Pathol*. 2009;62:493–504.

Ramos-e-Silva M, Pereira AL. Life-threatening eruptions due to infectious agents. *Clin Dermatol*. 2005;23:148–156.

CHAPTER 87

Headache

Rafael H. Llinas, MD

Key Clinical Questions

1. Are there warning signs of a secondary headache that would require further imaging?
2. Is the headache new or different?
3. Is the headache brought on by exertion, sexual intercourse, coughing, or sneezing?
4. Is the onset of the headache sudden or severe?
5. Has the patient experienced antecedent head or neck trauma?
6. Does she have any neurologic symptoms other than visual symptoms occurring only at the beginning of the headache syndrome?
7. The patient described her typical migraine headaches.

CASE 87-1

A 25-year-old, right-handed woman with a 3-year history of headaches is admitted to the hospital for "pain control." In the emergency department she had a negative noncontrast head computed tomographic (CT) scan and was prescribed a hydromorphone (Dilaudid) drip.

Does the patient have any other medical problems or risk factors for intracranial pathology?

Her past medical history and review of systems is otherwise negative. Her family history is positive for migraine.

What factors worsen the headaches?

Tension and stress triggered her headaches, typically worse 2 or 3 days before her menstrual period begins. Alcohol, chocolates and peanuts may aggravate her headache. She tried stopping the oral contraceptive and noticed no improvement in her headaches. Social history reveals that she is single and disabled from her headaches.

What medications has she tried?

She has tried many different medications, including analgesics, antidepressants, calcium channel blockers, and ß-blockers. The only medications that help her are sumatriptan taken subcutaneously and narcotics, currently hydrocodone at least one tablet a day. She has been taking alprazolam 10 mg three times a day for a couple of years. She also uses promethazine for nausea. Recently she is beginning to have daily headaches and has to make trips to the emergency department to get shots of meperidine.

What has been her work-up to date?

She has seen multiple neurologists. She has been treated with biofeedback and has seen psychologists. She had multiple CT scans and magnetic resonance imaging (MRI) of her head.

INTRODUCTION

Complaints of headache represent a major health problem due to their prevalence, chronicity, and the cost of ruling out life-threatening or serious underlying pathology that may cause significant morbidity and mortality. Up to 4.5% of all emergency department visits may be attributed to symptoms of headache, and headache may be the fifth most common reason for primary care visits (following checkups, upper respiratory illnesses, back pain, and skin rashes). Loss of productivity due to headache is also substantial with an estimated cost of billions of dollars.

The International Headache Society classifies headache as primary and secondary. Primary headaches account for at least 90% of all headaches and have benign outcomes. Primary headaches include migraine with or without aura, tension type headache, and less commonly, cluster headache. Some patients with a history of primary headaches have significant risk factors for developing secondary headaches. This chapter focuses on the diagnostic approach for the patient with headache in the hospital, and the reader is referred to subsequent chapters for specific management.

PRACTICE POINT

Headache occurrence in the hospital may be the following:

1. An initial presenting symptom of a systemic disease precipitating admission
2. A complication of a diagnostic procedure or medical therapy acquired during hospitalization
3. Coexisting benign headache syndromes (primary headaches)

Secondary headaches may be either one of the presenting symptoms leading to admission or acquired secondary to a diagnostic or therapeutic intervention. Rarely, the initial presentation of a primary headache syndrome may occur in the hospital. For patients with preexisting headache syndromes, it is important to recognize that there may be significant drug interactions between medications used to treat chronic headache and those used to treat systemic disease, and there are also important contraindications to commonly used migraine medications that may limit the safety of these drugs in hospitalized patients.

PRIMARY HEADACHE

Elucidating the cause of a headache, particularly when severe, requires an understanding of the pathophysiology of the major headache types and recognizing the classic types of pain syndromes (and associated symptoms) they produce. Primary headaches should not cause focal neurologic signs and symptoms, except sometimes briefly during the aura phase of a complex migraine.

MIGRAINE

In general, migraine causes episodic severe headache pain associated with nausea, photophobia, and photophobia insensitivities to external stimuli. This disorder is typified as much by nausea and photophobia as it is by pain. Because of the severity of pain associated with migraines, it is the most common headache that leads patients to medical attention (even though it is not nearly as common as tension headaches). Environmental or physiologic stimuli trigger recurrent and stereotyped headache spells that may be associated with meningeal symptoms and signs. Many patients will describe an aura or warning beforehand. A history of recurrent headaches, similar in severity and character occurring with weather changes, the menstrual cycle, stress, sleep deprivation, excessive sleep, withdrawal from caffeine, or associated with ingestion of certain types of food are often migrainous headaches (**Table 87-1**). Migraine runs in families and can be associated with mitral valve prolapse. The precipitating etiology is probably electrical, much like seizures, rather than vasoconstriction followed by vasodilatation as previously thought.

In general, the most important question to answer when considering migraine is whether the patient has ever had a headache like this before. The classic question about the severity of headache—the worst headache ever—does not help distinguish between primary and secondary headache because every migraine sufferer will have the worst migraine of her life at some point, and the most severe headaches are more likely to trigger medical consultation. The evolution of symptoms may help distinguish migraine from other causes of neurologic deficit. Classically migraines begin mildly, following an aura, and worsen over minutes to hours to reach a pinnacle of pain. Patients can often predict when they are about to get a headache as they begin to feel ill or have mild photophobia as the symptoms begin to worsen over time. The pain is not maximal at onset.

TABLE 87-1 Diagnostic Criteria for Migraine

Migraine without aura

A. At least five attacks fulfilling criteria B–D below
B. Headache attacks lasting 4–72 hours (untreated or unsuccessfully treated)
C. Headache has at least two of the following characteristics:
   1. Unilateral location
   2. Pulsating quality
   3. Moderate or severe intensity (inhibiting or prohibits daily activities)
   4. Aggravation by walking stairs or similar routine physical activity
D. During headache at least one of the following:
   1. Nausea and/or vomiting
   2. Photophobia and phonophobia
E. No evidence of contributing underlying disorder

Migraine with aura

A. At least two attacks fulfilling B.
B. At least three of the following four characteristics:
   1. One or more fully reversible aura symptoms indicating focal cerebral cortical and/or brain stem dysfunction
   2. At least one aura symptom developing gradually over more than 4 minutes or two or more symptoms in succession
   3. No aura symptom lasting more than 60 minutes. If more than one aura symptom is present, accepted duration is proportionately increased
   4. Headache following aura with a free interval of less than 60 minutes. It may also begin before or simultaneously with the aura.
C. No evidence of contributing underlying disorder

Headache Classification Committee of the International Headache Society. Classification and diagnostic criteria for headache disorders, cranial neuralgias and facial pain. *Cephalalgia*. 1988;8(suppl 7):1–96.

PRACTICE POINT

Migraine

- Migraine sufferers usually experience positive phenomena (flashing lights) but complex migraine may be associated with speech or motor deficits. In contrast, more serious migraine mimics such as stroke or transient ischemic attacks usually present with loss of function (weakness, lack of sensation, impaired vision, and language dysfunction).

At the bedside patients will often exhibit significant photophobia and complain of nausea, although not always with vomiting. They will often have some neck stiffness. While it is true that migraines can occasionally present with focal neurological findings (termed complex migraines when such focal findings exist), it is best to assume that patients with severe headache and focal neurologic findings have something more ominous until proven otherwise.

TABLE 87-2 Diagnostic Criteria for Tension Type Headache

A. At least 10 episodes fulfilling criteria B–D below (< 180/year or < 15/month)
B. Headaches lasting from 30 minutes to 7 days
C. Headache has at least two of the following characteristics:
   1. Bilateral location
   2. Pressing/tightening (nonpulsatile) quality
   3. Mild or moderate intensity (may inhibit but does not prohibit activities)
   4. Not aggravated by routine physical activity such as walking or climbing stairs
D. Both of the following:
   1. No nausea or vomiting (anorexia may occur)
   2. Photophobia or phonophobia absent, or one but not the other present
E. No evidence of contributing underlying disorder

Data from Headache Classification Committee of the International Headache Society. Classification and diagnostic criteria for headache disorders, cranial neuralgias and facial pain. *Cephalalgia*. 1988;8 (suppl 7):1–96.

TENSION OR MUSCLE CONTRACTION HEADACHES

These are usually due to tension or a spasm within the pain-sensitive muscles of the neck or temples. Tension headaches are a muscular pain syndrome similar to a strained muscle in any other portion of the body (**Table 87-2**).

Patients with muscle contraction pain due to tight muscles in the neck, tension from grinding the jaw, or chronic stress can have a different history and physical than any other headache type. In general, tension headaches or muscle contraction headaches do not have associated photophobia, phonophobia, nausea, or vomiting. They tend to be unilateral or bilateral aching pain and worsen with stress. They are usually not disabling.

PRACTICE POINT

Tension headache

- The important thing to remember is that muscular pain localizes poorly, and neck pain can present in many patients with referred pain to the cranial region.
- Beware of typical-sounding tension headaches in the patient over the age of 60 or 65, particularly when the headaches are new, since giant cell arteritis can present in this fashion. The physical exam may reveal tenderness in the muscles of the shoulder as well the temples. There will almost always be an elevated erythrocyte sedimentation rate, typically above 65 mm/hr. There may be transient visual loss or visual changes, or jaw claudication.

CLUSTER HEADACHES

Cluster headaches abruptly reach maximum intensity on one side of the head, last 1 to 2 hours, and have associated ipsilateral autonomic signs such as tearing, miosis, ptosis, or rhinorrhea. Patients should not have focal neurologic signs or symptoms (**Table 87-3**).

TABLE 87-3 Diagnostic Criteria for Cluster Headache

A. At least five attacks fulfilling B–D
B. Severe unilateral orbital, supraorbital, and/or temporal pain lasting 15 to 180 minutes untreated
C. Headache associated with at least one of the following signs, which must be present on the pain side:
   1. Conjunctival lacrimation
   2. Lacrimation
   3. Nasal congestion
   4. Rhinorrhea
   5. Forehead and facial sweating
   6. Miosis
   7. Ptosis
   8. Eyelid edema
D. Frequency of attacks from one every other day to eight per day
E. No evidence of contributing underlying disorder

Data from Headache Classification Committee of the International Headache Society. Classification and diagnostic criteria for headache disorders, cranial neuralgias and facial pain. *Cephalalgia*. 1988;8(suppl 7):1–96.

SECONDARY HEADACHE

HISTORY

"Do not miss headaches"

While the vast majority of headache pain may have benign causes, a small percentage may be "sentinel events" heralding dangerous and life-threatening sequelae. Secondary headaches result from underlying diseases that require further evaluation and treatment on an emergent basis (**Table 87-4**).

The clinician should question patients with headache about high-risk historical features and risk factors. Many of the patients who present with acute and serious headache pathology will have had a prior history of primary headaches, so it is important not to assume that a headache is benign based on a known headache history.

Subarachnoid hemorrhage (SAH), carotid and vertebral artery dissections, venous sinus thrombosis, pituitary apoplexy, and hypertensive emergencies may present with the abrupt onset of excruciating pain. Cluster headaches may have a similar presentation, but tearing or rhinorrhea should be present, and the pain should remit within a couple of hours. Migraines gradually increase to a maximal level over 1 to 2 hours.

PRACTICE POINT

Intracranial hemorrhage

The headaches associated with intracranial hemorrhage come in two varieties:

1. Meningeal irritation headache secondary to blood in the subarachnoid space. This can present like migraine pain. There can be nausea, vomiting, photophobia, and phonophobia as well as unilateral or bilateral throbbing pain.
2. Intracerebral hemorrhage. This will tend to present with pain associated with increased intracranial pressure but more acute in onset than that associated with tumors.

Particular caution is indicated since pain medications can reduce arousal and may reduce ventilation, which can worsen the neurological status, as well as make following the neurologic exam difficult. Nonsteroidal anti-inflammatory drugs are unadvisable due to their effects on platelets.

TABLE 87-4 "Do Not Miss Headaches"

Disorder	Headache	Exam	Comment
Aneurysmal SAH ↑ risk factors: autosomal dominant polycystic kidney disease, coarctation of aorta, connective tissue disorders, neurofibromatosis, pituitary tumors, AVM, sympathomimetic drugs including cocaine **SAH from stroke** ↑ risk factors: stroke risk factors, cocaine 10% of strokes are associated with SAH	Prodrome of headache due to either a small, warning (sentinel) bleed or to aneurysmal dilation before rupture; unilateral in 30% Rupture when patient active, unusually severe or atypical H/A, especially if brief LOC, N/V, meningismus, or any focal findings Bleed → acute rise in intracranial pressure	Cushing sign (↑ BP, bradycardia, ↑ ICP); fever; nuchal rigidity, focal neurologic signs including ptosis of one eyelid with dilated, nonreactive pupil and impaired adduction and vertical movement of affected eye Tersen syndrome: preretinal hemorrhages and SAH	ECG changes, elevation of cardiac enzymes due to release of catecholamines; neurogenic pulmonary edema; hyponatremia probably mediated by hypothalamic injury
Intracerebral hemorrhage Risk factors: HBP, cerebral amyloid, stroke risk factors 10% of all strokes are associated with intracerebral hemorrhage	Usually no prodrome, typically H/A when patient active, maximum deficit minutes to hours	AVM rupture commonly associated with seizure; fever	Typically hemorrhage into subcortical regions (putamen, thalamus, caudate) or if AVM, in that location
Rupture of bacterial abscess	Severe, sudden pain, LOC	Fever, nuchal rigidity	Acute ventriculitis and meningitis
Raised ICP of any etiology	Unilateral or bilateral, a boring, aching pain typically without photophobia or phonophobia or environmental triggers; worse lying down; nocturnal awakening	Cushing sign; abducens paresis; papilledema may be present When SAH causes ↑ ICP, blood may extravasate into retina (subhyaloid hemorrhage); can be bilateral; nuchal rigidity; seizures; may have subtle focal signs	CN VI dysfunction "false localizing sign" as refers to diffuse ↑ ICP rather than localized to 6th CN or nucleus pathology
Meningitis	Often a throbbing component of the headache, hypersensitivity to sound and light, nausea and sometimes vomiting	Fever, photophobia, nuchal rigidity, obtundation	
Giant cell arteritis	Severe throbbing but also dull, sharp or burning headaches, localized to the temples (50%) or diffuse, acute onset	Usually associated with painful, stiff proximal extremities, myalgias, weight loss, and other systemic symptoms, jaw claudication, and visual disturbances (sudden monocular blindness or stuttering, visual loss, amaurosis fugax, diplopia, or field cut)	Asymmetric temporal arterial pulses, thickened or tender temporal arteries may be a clue
Trauma: **Status post (s/p) neck injuries with muscle spasm** **Dissection of great vessels** **Subdural hematoma** **Intracranial hemorrhage**	Tension-type or occipital headache	Neck or upper shoulder pain and palpation of affected muscles will exacerbate the pain syndrome; reduced range of motion of the neck LOC, focal signs should prompt further evaluation	Seemingly minor trauma may however be associated with dissection and subdural hematoma. Elderly patients receiving anticoagulants may suffer intracranial hemorrhage without severe headache
Carbon monoxide poisoning (or inhaled methyl chlorine)	Diffuse headache most common	Presentation highly variable and nonspecific (malaise, dizziness)	Suspect when multiple family members have headache; seasonal and regional variation; workers who use methyl chloride or inhale paint remover

AVM, arteriovenous malformation; BP, blood pressure; CN, cranial nerve; ECG, electrocardiogram; H/A, headache; HBP, high blood pressure; ICP, intracranial pressure; LOC, loss of consciousness; N/V, nausea and vomiting; SAH, subarachnoid hemorrhage.

Headache or migraine that coincides with stroke syndromes should raise the specter of hemorrhagic stroke. Twenty percent of strokes are associated with SAH (10%) and intracerebral hemorrhage (10%). Headache occurring at the onset of stroke should be assumed to signify SAH. In intracerebral hemorrhage, pain sometimes occurs acutely at the time of the hemorrhage but may be delayed until the hematoma expands and compresses pain-sensitive intracranial structures such as large arteries and meninges. In ischemic stroke involving large vessels, headache is usually not a feature but occasionally occurs prior to, during, or after the onset of stroke. Cerebrovascular dissection may cause both headache and stroke. Subcortical strokes (lacunar infarcts—pure motor, pure sensory, ataxic hemiparesis, clumsy hand dysarthria, sensorimotor where face, arm, leg more equally affected than in cortical infarcts) only rarely cause headache.

In general, space-occupying lesions in the brain tend not to cause pain unless they become large enough to compress pain-sensitive structures. The most common presenting symptom of brain tumors is seizure—not headache—although not infrequently patients with brain tumors will develop progressive headaches as the tumor becomes larger. They tend to be mild to moderate in intensity and unremitting. Patients often ignore these symptoms for some time since they tend not to interfere with activities of daily living and work. Increased intracranial pressure headaches can also occur from occlusion of the venous sinuses, which may present with severe headache, seizures, and bilateral papilledema. The most concerning symptom to suggest increased intracranial pressure is a history of worsening headache with lying down. Most migraine headaches are relieved somewhat by rest. Patients with increased intracranial pressure will classically awaken from sleep with a severe headache and may vomit due to slight hypoventilation during sleep, which leads to hypercarbic vasodilatation and increased intracranial pressure.

PRACTICE POINT

Increased intracranial pressure

- Intracranial pressure headaches typically occur as the meninges are stretched or the blood vessels are compressed. These are classically boring bilateral headaches that are worse when supine often with a history of nausea and vomiting only when lying flat. Focal neurologic signs are often present. Usually not acute in onset, they become slowly more severe over days to weeks to months.

Patients with chronic headaches and new seizures should always be considered for the possibility of an intracranial mass. Patients, particularly those in middle age, with chronic headaches that do not appear to be analgesic withdrawal headaches and that lack migrainous components should generally undergo brain imaging.

Underlying systemic illness

A new or change in headache in a patient with risk factors for intracranial illness (such as cancer, hematologic disorders, infection) should also alert the clinician to the possibility of a serious headache etiology (**Table 87-5**). The neurologic presentations of systemic diseases should help the clinician order the appropriate studies. For example, patients with AIDS have increased risk for toxoplasmosis, abscess, lymphoma, and meningitis and should undergo neuroimaging prior to analysis of the spinal fluid. Patients with HIV may first present with aseptic meningitis. Similarly, a new, progressively worsening headache in any patient with malignancy should prompt magnetic resonance imaging (MRI) of the intracranial venous channels.

Head and neck trauma is a risk factor for subdural hematoma (SDH) as well as SAH and intracerebral hemorrhage. Injuries caused by abrupt flexion and extension of the neck (as in boxing, motor vehicle accidents), patients with connective tissue disorders, and severe straining (by pregnant women during delivery) may be associated with dissection of the extracranial vessels.

A decrease or loss of vision with headache may result from temporal arteritis, carotid dissection, and acute narrow-angle glaucoma.

Nausea and vomiting are seen with SAH, intracranial hemorrhage, acute angle glaucoma (as well as migraine). Narrow-angle glaucoma headaches are typically centered over the affected eye.

Headache precipitated by cough or Valsalva may be associated with cerebrovascular disease or underlying malignancy.

PRACTICE POINT

Toxins

- Toxins may cause headache. If multiple family members present with headache, consider carbon monoxide poisoning.

Medications that increase bleeding risk include anticoagulants, nonsteroidal anti-inflammatory drugs (NSAIDs), and antiplatelet agents.

Acute sinusitis, seizure, temporomandibular joint syndrome, hypercalcemia and/or hyperviscosity, and glaucoma sometimes present with headache in the hospital setting.

Drugs

Medications are an especially common cause of headache (**Table 87-6**)

Analgesic withdrawal headaches

Patients with analgesic withdrawal headaches are usually easy to diagnose but can be a challenge to treat. In general, the worst actors for analgesic withdrawal headaches are any medications that have significant amounts of caffeine, particularly short-acting medications. Even ibuprofen or acetaminophen taken frequently can cause analgesic withdrawal headaches. Anyone who takes medications on a daily basis for headaches more than 15 times a month probably has at least a component of analgesic withdrawal headaches. These headaches tend not to have associated meningeal signs. Historical aspects to make one suspicious of analgesic withdrawal headaches include the following:

1. Pain medications on chronic daily basis for at least two to three weeks
2. Occurrence of headaches in the morning as soon as the previous dose of medication wears off
3. Taking medications first thing the morning every day for at least at least 2 to 3 weeks
4. Resistance on the patient's behalf to change or discontinue the chronic daily medications

The physical examination, including the neurological examination, should be normal.

PRACTICE POINT

Analgesic withdrawal headache

- Headache is probably one of the only pain disorders that will often become worse with ongoing treatment. The classical analgesic withdrawal headache is the caffeine withdrawal headache. As long as patients take caffeine, they do not have pain. Once they acutely discontinue caffeine, they begin having throbbing and severe headaches that are only made better with caffeine. Unfortunately withdrawal headaches can occur from almost any analgesic medication. Short-acting medications are more likely to cause analgesic withdrawal headaches once they are discontinued.

TABLE 87-5 Systemic Diseases and Headache

Disorder	Type of Headache	Symptoms and Signs	Pathophysiology
Cardiology			
Atrial fibrillation, atrial myxoma, ventricular aneurysm, severe dilated cardiomyopathies, valvular heart disease, and myocardial infarction	Sudden onset, severe	Focal symptoms and signs involving a vascular territory	Cerebral embolism from cardiac surgery or associated heart disease
Endocrinology			
Obesity, menstrual disorders, hypoparathyroidism, hypo- or hyperthyroidism, and adrenal insufficiency (either primary or secondary to steroid withdrawal)	Chronic, recurring diffuse headaches	With or without papilledema	Benign intracranial hypertension
Hypo- or hyperthyroidism, hyperparathyroidism, hyperaldosteronism, mineralocorticoid excess, steroid withdrawal, and hypoglycemia			Intracranial vasodilatation
Pheochromocytoma	Diffuse, throbbing headache	Excessive perspiration, tachycardia, and labile hypertension	
Some disorders of the urea cycle, acquired partial lipodystrophy	Migraine-like headaches		
Tumors of the hypophyseal–pituitary axis		Visual field cuts with the presenting endocrinopathy	
Gastroenterology			
Crohn disease and ulcerative colitis	Diffuse, sometimes hemicranial, recurrent headaches		Recurrence may be related to the severity of IBD
Hematology			
Underlying malignancy	A new progressively worsening headache		Hypercoagulable states causing intracranial venous thrombosis
Multiple myeloma, polycythemia vera, and other hematologic malignancies			Hyperviscosity due to paraproteinemias or marked leukocytosis or thrombocytosis causing vascular congestion or venous occlusion
Cerebellar hemangioblastomas	Diffuse pain, resulting from hyperviscosity or hydrocephalus, or localized posteriorly due to the location of the tumor		Tumor secretion of erythropoietin
Leukemias, lymphomas, and rarely multiple myeloma	Diffuse, progressively severe headache	Cranial nerve palsies, nuchal rigidity, papilledema, or hydrocephalus	Studding the cranial meninges
Thrombocytopenia related to idiopathic thrombocytopenic purpura (ITP), thrombotic thrombocytopenic purpura (TTP), and disseminated intravascular coagulation (DIC)	Focal or diffuse headache or recurrent headaches similar to migraine		Brain hemorrhage or infarction
Hemophilia and Christmas disease	Sudden onset, severe headache		Cerebral hemorrhage
Anemia (usually <8 g/dL)	Diffuse, throbbing headache that is worse with exertion		Rarely, iron deficiency anemia has been associated with benign intracranial hypertension
Sickle cell disease	Focal or diffuse	Focal findings of stroke	Cerebral infarction
	Rare syndrome of frontal headache, proptosis, and lid edema		Infarction of orbital bones

(continued)

TABLE 87-5 Systemic Diseases and Headache (*continued*)

Disorder	Type of Headache	Symptoms and Signs	Pathophysiology
Oncology			
Brain tumors	Nondescript pain, not necessarily more likely in the early morning, with straining or bending over, or accompanied by vomiting	Usually other neurologic symptoms predominate, such as weakness, confusion, seizures	Lack of pain due to location in cerebral hemisphere
Meningeal carcinomatosis	Diffuse, progressive, severe headache	Often with other symptoms such as vomiting, back pain, meningeal irritation, decreasing consciousness, cranial nerve palsies, papilledema, and diabetes insipidus	Breast, bronchial, gastrointestinal, and melanoma are the most common cancers, sometimes present for months or years
Lung cancer	Pain in the angle of the jaw or ear		Irritation of the pain fibers in the ipsilateral vagus nerve
Mediastinal tumor	Worsening headache	Cough, dyspnea, hoarseness, airway obstruction	Obstruction of the superior vena cava with death from increased intracranial pressure or cerebral hemorrhage
Infectious Disease			
Bacterial endocarditis			Septic cerebral embolism with resultant hemorrhage from a mycotic aneurysm
Brain abscess (bronchiectasis, empyema, TB)	Rupture of brain abscess may cause meningitis and sudden severe diffuse headache	Focal findings, seizure, altered mentation	Due to the mass effect symptoms analogous to brain tumor unless there is associated meningeal irritation
Meningitis		Focal cranial nerve dysfunction seen with Listeria, TB, and fungal meningitis	Due to affecting basal meninges
Infective enteritis (bacterial, viral, or parasitic)	Headache which subsides with resolution of the infection		
Many pneumonias, classically *Mycoplasma pneumoniae*	Diffuse headaches, which are worse with coughing		
Infection in the paranasal or mastoid sinuses or lungs (such as *M pneumoniae*) may serve as a nidus	Severe headache	Meningeal signs, fever	Meningeal spread or development of brain abscess
Pregnancy and postpartum period			
Intracranial venous thrombosis Benign intracranial hypertension Intracranial tumors			Growing
Pre-eclampsia in the last trimester of pregnancy	May have headache as a presenting symptom	In addition to hypertension, proteinuria, and edema	
Arteriovenous malformations (AVMs) and subarachnoid hemorrhage (SAH)	Sudden severe headache	Bleeding more likely in the 2nd trimester for AVMs and 3rd trimester for SAH	Bleeding
Carotid dissection during delivery		Horner's ± focal neurologic symptoms and signs	Straining during labor and delivery
Psychiatry			
Anxiety, depression, somatoform disorder	Nondescript, migraine or tension		
Intoxication	Severe diffuse headache	Signs of sympathetic over activity	Cocaine due to hypertension or cocaine-induced migraine or SAH or intracranial hemorrhage
Withdrawal syndromes	Severe diffuse headache	Signs of sympathetic overactivity	Alcohol or opiate withdrawal

(*continued*)

TABLE 87-5 Systemic Diseases and Headache *(continued)*

Disorder	Type of Headache	Symptoms and Signs	Pathophysiology
Pulmonary			
Acute respiratory failure or chronic disorders (eg, OSA or severe COPD)	Morning headaches worse with coughing	Low head position during sleep may increase cephalic congestion along with impaired respiratory efficiency	pCO_2 retention and hypoxia → Cerebral vasodilation, may have associated polycythemia
Renal			
Hyponatremia	Generalized headache		
Rarely, uremia	Diffuse and throbbing headaches that abate following dialysis or renal transplantation		Cerebral edema and increased pressure
Rheumatology			
	Migraine-like headaches, symptoms of meningitis, focal or localized headache	Focal neurologic defects (vasculitis)	Vasculitis, cranial arteritis Aseptic meningitis Pseudotumor cerebri Infiltration of meninges, arthritis of cervical spine
Surgery			
Acoustic neuroma	Dull headache in region of incision		Damage to regional nerves
Carotid endarterectomy	Vascular headache		Removal of stenosis distends already dilated poststenotic vessels
Lumbar puncture	Postural headache		

AVM, arteriovenous malformation; COPD, chronic obstructive pulmonary disease; DIC, disseminated intravascular coagulation; IBD, Inflammatory Bowel Disease; ITP, idiopathic thrombocytopenic purpura; OSA, Obstructive Sleep Apnea; SAH, subarachnoid hemorrhage; TB, tuberculosis; TTP, thrombotic thrombocytopenic purpura.

Data from Hospitalist Neurology edited by Samuels, M. Edmeads J. Chapter 1 Headache 25 Publisher Butterworth Heinman 199.

Low pressure headaches

Most common following lumbar puncture, low pressure within the cranial vault likely causes pain by traction or irritation of the meninges. Low pressure (LP) headaches can also be seen after neurosurgery or spontaneously after a particularly violent sneeze or cough, even with no significant trauma. The patient may experience positional bilateral throbbing, temporal, squeezing pain with photophobia and rarely phonophobia. However nausea and vomiting are generally absent for unknown reasons. The propensity for migraine headaches increases the likelihood of developing this type of headache as does younger age (due to less free space in the cranium). There should be no cranial nerve deficits as long as the intracranial hypotension is not severe. Classically, when patients lie flat, the pain becomes much improved as the pressure equalizes between the low back and the cranium. As patients sit or stand, particularly if they move quickly, the headache will begin again. Although most migraine headaches will also worsen as patients stand up, complete or near-complete relief with recumbence is not typical for migraines. In general there are no physical exam findings that are particularly helpful, and the neurologic exam is nonfocal.

Most post-LP headaches will resolve spontaneously over 1–5 days. Opiates are usually ineffective in the acute or chronic treatment of this disorder. In general, because there is some meningeal traction, these headaches can be treated using an acute migraine protocol, which can include caffeine and migraine-specific medications. Maintaining a recumbent position will often help to keep the pain from becoming severe, and abdominal binders can be tried to increase pressure in the cerebrospinal fluid (CSF). When conservative measures fail and symptoms persist for more than 2 days, the leak can be sealed. Evidence-based studies of post-LP headaches show that epidural blood patch is the most effective form of treatment; this is performed by injecting some of the patient's blood in the epidural space at the site of the prior LP and allowing it to thrombose and seal the area. It will ultimately be absorbed, and there is minimal risk of infection.

Neuropathic pain syndromes

In general, neuropathic pain syndromes involving the face and skull present with focal areas of extreme, lancinating, shooting, or stabbing pain in the face within any of the distributions of the trigeminal nerve, or on the back of the skull within the distribution of the occipital nerve. Sometimes the stabbing, lancinating pain occurs within the eye or in the posterior pharynx. Neuropathic pain syndromes may have an area of anesthesia that when touched or irritated elicits the paroxysm of pain. Patients will often point to one area that is exquisitely tender, and as you move to examine this area there is a certain amount of guarding. These pain

TABLE 87-6 Common Medical Interventions Associated with Headache

Cardiology
• Nitrates (diffuse throbbing headaches with initial use) and adrenergic inhibitors such as hydralazine, minoxidil, reserpine (vasodilators) • Some calcium channel blockers (diltiazem and dihydropyridines)
Endocrinology
• Withdrawal of glucocorticoids (new headache or triggering preexisting migraine)
Gastroenterology
• Ranitidine and famotidine • Sulfasalazine
Hematology
• Intravenous immune globulin (nondescript headache or trigger migraine in susceptible individuals)
Oncology
• Chemotherapy (nonspecific, sometimes change preexisting migraine pattern) • Intrathecal methotrexate (acute aseptic meningitis)
Infectious disease
• Antibiotics especially trimethoprim-sulfamethoxazole (direct vascular effect or aseptic meningitis) • Zidovudine (AZT) (unknown mechanism in first few weeks of treatment) • Interferon-alpha • Antimalarial drugs
Pregnancy
• Spinal headache (from epidural anesthesia that is actually a spinal tap)
Psychiatry
• Drug interactions (severe hypertension from sympathomimetic drugs such as meperidine or bronchodilators in patients already taking monoamine oxidase inhibitors) • Benzodiazepines (dull nondescript headache during initiation)
Pulmonary
• Theophylline, albuterol, terbutaline
Renal
• Hemodialysis (recurrent nondescript headache associated with hemodialysis or part of the "dialysis disequilibrium syndrome" more commonly at the end of hemodialysis due to osmotic shifts) • Central nervous system infections or lymphomas (from immunosuppression in renal transplant patients)
Rheumatology
• Nonsteroidal anti-inflammatory drugs (direct vascular effect, increased intracranial hypertension or aseptic meningitis)
Surgery
• Fasting prior to surgery especially in patients with preexisting migraines or unrecognized substance dependency

syndromes can be unremitting and severe. This syndrome can be precipitated by any etiology that leads to sensory nerve irritation such as viral infections, bony compression, demyelination, masses, or soft tissue compression. The clinician should recognize that herpes zoster can sometimes present with this type of pain before the vesicles appear.

In summary, warning signs for serious pathologies include the following:

- New headache with meningeal symptoms and signs that is maximal at the time of onset
- Any headache associated with alteration of mental status or new cranial nerve findings
- Chronic or subacute headache in patients over the age of 50, particularly worse at night, awakening patients from sleep, especially with focal neurologic deficits
- New headaches in patients over the age of 60 that are associated with elevated markers of inflammation, and pain within the back of the neck, shoulders, and arms

CASE 87-1 *(continued)*

Does she appear acutely ill?

On examination she is a well-developed, well-nourished, young woman in no acute distress with normal vital signs. Her general physical examination is normal and noncontributory.

Is she confused?

Her mental status is normal and she does not appear intoxicated.

Does she have a "non-focal" neurologic examination?

No bruits are heard over the orbits, cranial vessels, or temples. Cognitive function, language, and memory are all intact. Her cranial nerve examination is completely normal, including sharp optic discs and normal visual fields. She does not have meningeal signs. Her motor exam shows full and equal tone, power, and bulk in all four extremities. Her sensory exam is intact for all modalities, and the Romberg test is negative. Tests of coordination in the upper and lower extremities are all normal. There is no evidence of cerebellar dysfunction. Her gait and stance are normal, including tandem gait. Her reflexes are average in amplitude and equal bilaterally; both plantars are flexor. No pathological reflexes are elicited.

PHYSICAL EXAMINATION

DOES THE PATIENT APPEAR ACUTELY ILL?

If a patient appears toxic or hemodynamically unstable, the headache is more likely to have an underlying secondary cause. In severe meningitis, the patient may be sitting upright on the edge of the bed with knees and hips flexed, the neck extended with a lordotic curvature of the spine, and the arms brought back to support the thorax—the tripod position referred to as the Amoss or Hoyne sign.

WHAT ARE THE PATIENT'S VITAL SIGNS?

Does the patient have a fever? Fever may be associated with SAH, intracerebral hemorrhage, meningitis, encephalitis, rupture of brain abscess, septic cerebral emboli, or arterial dissection and may prompt the need for a spinal fluid examination, usually following neuroimaging to ensure the absence of serious mass effect. Of the classic clinical triad of fever, neck stiffness, and altered mental status, fever is the most sensitive sign of meningitis.

Does the patient have hypertension? Ordinarily, hypertension does not cause headache unless severe. However, hypertension and bradycardia may be a clue that the patient has increased intracranial pressure (Cushing sign).

> **PRACTICE POINT**
>
> **Hypertension**
>
> Hypertension does not usually cause headaches, unless severe. If a patient with hypertension is experiencing headache, consider medications being used to treat the hypertension. Headache may be observed when the patient has
>
> - chronic, severe hypertension (diastolic > 120 mm Hg) with early morning headaches;
> - acute hypertensive crisis (from catecholamine states such as acute cocaine intoxication, pheochromocytoma, or administration of sympathomimetic drugs with monoamine oxidase inhibitors);
> - hypertensive encephalopathy (patchy edema, hemorrhages, infarcts on brain imaging) with headaches along with seizures, multifocal deficits, and obtundation;
> - drug therapy (hydralazine, diltiazem, other vasodilators or reserpine, which can trigger migraine).

DOES THE PATIENT HAVE SIGNS OF MENINGEAL IRRITATION?

For patients with meningeal irritation headaches, the examiner should note any historical information, symptoms and signs that would indicate a need for head imaging prior to consideration of a lumbar puncture. These include age greater than 60, history of central nervous system disease or recent seizure, immunocompromised state, decreased level of consciousness, inability to answer questions or follow commands, abnormal language or motor function, the presence of a gaze or facial palsy, or abnormal visual fields. The examiner should also note the presence of fever and nuchal rigidity.

Although fever occurs in the majority of patients with meningitis, followed by neck stiffness, immunocompromised patients and the elderly are less likely to have fever or nuchal rigidity. The classic signs of meningeal irritation include positive Kernig, Brudzinski, and contralateral signs and worsening of headache with the Jolt maneuver. A positive Kernig sign occurs when extension of the knee causes resistance or pain in the lower back or posterior thigh in a supine patient with hips flexed at 90 degrees. A positive Brudzinski sign occurs when passive neck flexion causes flexion of the knees and hips in a supine patient. The contralateral reflex occurs when passive flexion of the hip and knee results in flexion of the opposite leg. A positive Jolt test causes worsening of headache when the patient turns the head horizontally at a frequency of two to three rotations per second. The absence of all three signs of fever, neck stiffness, and altered mental status makes the diagnosis of meningitis much less likely, but no constellation of symptoms or signs are sufficiently sensitive with low negative likelihood ratios to rule out meningitis. Cryptococcal meningitis and localized inflammatory processes involving the meninges such as a neurosurgical wound are not associated with positive stretch signs. Positive stretch signs may be associated with noninfectious causes such as musculoskeletal problems, tumors, carcinomatous meningitis, Mollaret's meningitis, SAH and other conditions. If meningitis is suspected, further diagnostic testing is required to confirm the diagnosis.

> **PRACTICE POINT**
>
> **Meningeal irritation**
>
> - There are very few structures within the brain that actually respond with pain when stimulated. In fact, not uncommonly, a patient will present with a large, slowly growing tumor without any headaches whatsoever. Pain-sensitive structures within the brain include the meninges, blood vessels, and the nasal sinuses. Unfortunately, meningeal irritation syndromes often present with pain that is very similar in quality and associated symptoms to migraine headaches. Patients with meningeal irritation headaches in the setting of fever, alteration of mental status, or focal neurologic findings should never be diagnosed with migraine without a detailed evaluation for life-threatening pathology.

The most concerning cause of meningeal irritation headaches is blood within the meninges, particularly from an SAH. But meningitis, encephalitis, or any type of central nervous system (CNS) infection/inflammation can present similarly. In general, SAH tends to be a meningeal-type headache that can resemble by history a migraine headache. Since some patients with SAH happen to be migraine sufferers, it is crucial not to assume that all headaches in a patient with a history of migraines are due to migraines. In general, migraine sufferers who present with a new type of headache, particularly if maximal at onset, should have an evaluation for another cause of headache pain. Classically a very stiff neck is more common with the meningitis or subarachnoid hemorrhage than with migraine, whereas photosensitivity and nausea tend to be more marked with migraine.

If SAH is strongly suspected and head imaging is negative, proceed with a lumbar puncture. The sensitivity of head computed tomography (CT) for identifying SAH depends on the size of the bleed (lower with minor bleeds) and timing relative to the rupture with the highest sensitivity in the first 12 hours after SAH (almost 100%).

PRACTICE POINT

Bloody spinal fluid

SAH	Traumatic tap
• ↑ RBC in both tubes 1 and 4 although unreliable sign by itself • ↑ WBC by 1 for ≈ every 500–700 RBC (if a normal WBC:RBC ratio in the peripheral blood) • Xanthochromia usually present (takes 2–4 hours to develop).	• Significant fall in RBC from tubes 1 to 4 • Mild increase in WBC explained by bloody contamination alone, with WBC:RBC ratio comparable to that observed in the patient's blood • Xanthochromia absent

If meningitis is suspected, but altered mental status, papilledema, or focal neurologic findings suggest the need for CT prior to lumbar puncture, antibiotics should not be delayed.

DOES THE PATIENT HAVE ALTERED MENTATION?

Acute meningitis, encephalitis, and SAH may cause confusion or obtundation. Alteration of the level of consciousness is extremely uncommon in migraine headaches unless the patient has been treated pharmacologically. Although assessing the patient's level of awareness involves determining whether the patient is oriented to person, place, and time, orientation is not sensitive enough to pick up confusion, and disorientation is nonspecific (and can be due to psychosis, aphasia, amnesia). Family members may be the first people to note altered mentation or a subtle personality change. It is essential to test attention before moving on to testing language, memory, calculation, construction, and abstraction, and looking for focal neurologic deficits by screening cranial nerve, reflex, motor, and sensory exams. If a patient cannot sustain attention or if he has an altered level of arousal, proceed with a workup which includes neuroimaging and possibly an examination of the spinal fluid.

DOES THE PATIENT HAVE FOCAL NEUROLOGIC SIGNS?

Abnormalities on neurologic examination are often diagnostic for intracranial pathology. A neurologic evaluation should include a detailed cranial nerve exam to look for dilated or unreactive pupils, limitation in range of motion of the eyes, facial droop, lateralizing weakness, sensory loss, or asymmetric deep tendon reflexes. None of these findings should really be seen in a migrainous disorder, except in the rare patient with complex migraines. Intra-axial (intraparenchymal) lesions cause conjugate eye deviation, visual field defects, asymmetrical motor tone, strength, reflexes, and Babinski signs. Focal neurologic findings are often, but not always, seen in SAH and meningitis.

If a dilated, nonreactive pupil is noted, consider the following diagnostic possibilities:

1. Eye drops containing anticholinergic medications, scopolamine patches, systemic atropine (patients are alert without focal neurologic symptoms or signs)
2. Holmes-Adie syndrome due to loss of parasympathetic neurons innervating the eye resulting in unopposed sympathetic dilation of the affected pupil (patients may have blurred vision, areflexia)
3. Aneurysmal cranial nerve compression leading to unilateral papillary dilation (patients may have associated oculomotor dysfunction and headache)
4. Uncal herniation due to large temporal lobe mass lesions (comatose patients)

If a Horner sign is appreciated in a patient with headache, carotid or vertebral dissection should be considered.

Focal findings along a vascular territory and headache should increase suspicion for extracranial large vessel disease (atherosclerosis, dissection, fibromuscular dysplasia, and aortic disease) and intracranial large vessel disease (inflammatory arteriopathies and atherosclerosis).

PRACTICE POINT

Vascular territory

Anterior circulation	Posterior circulation
• Motor dysfunction of contralateral extremity or face or both • Ipsilateral visual loss, homonymous hemianopia • Aphasia (dominant hemisphere) • Dysarthria • Sensory deficit of contralateral extremity or face or both Aphasia, cortical sensory loss or weakness • MCA—predominantly face and arm > leg • ACA—leg > arm or face	• Motor dysfunction of ipsilateral face and/or contralateral extremity • Loss of vision of one or both eyes, homonymous visual fields • Sensory deficit of ipsilateral face and/or contralateral extremity • Typical associated symptoms (not diagnostic in isolation) ▪ Ataxia ▪ Vertigo ▪ Diplopia ▪ Dysphagia ▪ Dysarthria

Cortical signs include aphasia, visual field defects, monoparesis (clumsy, weak, or flaccid), hemineglect, cortical sensory loss (numbness, paresthesias), and abulia.

If a patient has focal neurologic signs, proceed with neuroimaging and consider imaging of the large vessels at the same time, especially if the patient has signs and symptoms along a vascular territory. With CNS mass lesions, focal neurological deficits are usually present, although not invariably, and are often extremely subtle.

DOES THE PATIENT HAVE SIGNS OR SYMPTOMS OF INCREASED INTRACRANIAL PRESSURE?

Extra-axial processes (outside of brain tissue) commonly cause raised intracranial pressure and may cause the following signs to be present: evidence of raised intracranial pressure (Cushing reflex), ptosis of one eyelid (aneurysmal compression of the ipsilateral third cranial nerve), dilated nonreactive pupil (constriction controlled by ipsilateral third cranial nerve), impaired adduction and vertical movement of one eye (complete third cranial nerve compression), impaired lateral rectus muscle function (stretching of sixth cranial nerve from increased intracranial pressure), subhyaloid hemorrhage on retinal examination.

DOES THE PATIENT HAVE SIGNS OF AN UNDERLYING SYSTEMIC DISORDER?

A general physical examination should search for the source of any fever, with particular attention to the ears, sinuses, respiratory system, and skin due to the association with meningitis. Any infection may cause a toxic vascular headache characterized as bilateral throbbing headaches increased by exertion, bending, and straining or may trigger migrainous attacks. Like toxic vascular headache, bacterial, viral, fungal, or protozoal systemic infections may cause meningeal irritation.

A general physical examination may uncover a new diagnosis of cancer or evidence of metastatic disease. For example, approximately 50% of patients with meningeal carcinomatosis may have no history of systemic cancer. Patients with known cancer may develop headaches secondary to parenchymal or skull tumor metastases, carcinomatous meningitis, or intracranial venous thrombosis; however, they are more likely to have headaches from primary causes (migraine or tension headaches) or from fever and sepsis or from drug therapy. Because of the potentially subtle findings, new-onset headaches in older patients and headaches that fail to meet diagnostic criteria for primary functional headaches should prompt neuroimaging (see Tables 87-1, 87-2, and 87-3 for the diagnostic criteria by the International Headache Society).

Patients with rheumatologic disorders may have a number of different mechanisms for headaches, including recurrent headaches similar to migraine or chronic headaches due to vasculitis, pseudotumor cerebri, or aseptic meningitis. The signs and symptoms of cerebral vasculitis include multifocal neurologic deficits and headache, often associated with systemic inflammation and fever. Granulomata from Wegener disease, lymphomatoid granulomatosis, and sarcoidosis may infiltrate the meninges and produce headache and multiple cranial nerve deficits. Arthritis of the cervical spine may lead to neck stiffness and occipital headaches.

CASE 87-1 *(continued)*

NEUROLOGY CONSULTATION

Almost certainly too much medication has caused a syndrome of chronic daily headache superimposed on a history of migraine. The best course of action would be for her to

consult a headache expert, to help her get on a program that would allow her to taper alprazolam and hydrocodone with the goal of discontinuation and start a more rational, abortive treatment program for her headaches. The general rule is that oral medications do not help much during migraine because of atony of the stomach. Subcutaneous sumatriptan has helped her but is very expensive. It may be better to use rectal indomethacin at the first sign of the headaches. Cyproheptadine, a mild antiserotonin drug, may cause some sedation, which in her case may be useful since sleep and rest make the headaches better.

FOLLOW-UP

Instead, the patient consulted a pain clinic, which continued her narcotics and added a number of new medications. She continues to periodically visit emergency departments for pain relief.

CONCLUSION

The history and physical examination are the most important parts of the evaluation of headache at the bedside. Headache symptoms of concern include sudden rapid onset, occipitonuchal radiation, or association with focal neurologic symptoms or altered mental status. Patient-specific risk factors include older age, coexistent malignancy, infectious disease, coagulopathy, or underlying immunosuppression. Precipitating factors of concern include onset during exertion or antecedent head or neck trauma. Physical examination findings of concern include toxic appearance, fever, meningismus, papilledema, altered mental status, and focal neurologic signs. Unfortunately, it can sometimes be difficult to differentiate each form of headache type from another, and the neurologic examination may be normal. This is why imaging is so often needed.

SUGGESTED READINGS

Attia J, Hatala R, Cook DJ, Wong JG. In: Simel DL, Rennie D, eds. The Rational Clinical Examination. New York: McGraw-Hill; 2009:400:175–181.

Peter J. Goadsby, Richard B. Lipton, Michel D. Ferrari, et al. Migraine—the current understanding and treatment. *N Engl J Med*. 2002;346:257–270.

Rasmussen BK. Epidemiology of headache. *Cephalalgia*. 1995;15(1): 45–68.

Samuels MA, ed. Hospitalist Neurology, Butterworth/Heinemann; Waltham, Massachusetts; 1999.

Sapira JD. The Art and Science of Bedside Diagnosis. Baltimore, MD: Urban & Schwarzenberg; 1990:469–470.

Stephen D. Silberstein, Richard B. Lipton, Martin Sliwinski, et al. Classification of daily and near-daily headaches. *Neurology*. 1996;47:871–875.

Sun-Edelstein C, Bigal ME, Rapoport AM, et al. Chronic migraine and medication overuse headache: clarifying the current International Headache Society classification criteria. *Cephalalgia*. 2009;29:445.

CHAPTER 88

Hemoptysis

Margaret M. Hayes, MD
Christian A. Merlo, MD, MPH

Key Clinical Questions

1. What is the definition of hemoptysis and what is the difference between massive and nonmassive hemoptysis?
2. What are the initial assessments and diagnostic tests that should be performed when evaluating a patient with hemoptysis?
3. What are the most common causes of hemoptysis in the hospitalized patient?
4. What are the recommended management strategies for both massive and nonmassive hemoptysis?

CASE 88-1

A 24-year-old white male with cystic fibrosis presents to the emergency department with two weeks of daily hemoptysis. He states that he has been coughing up a half cup of blood daily and has had worsening dyspnea on exertion for the last week. His baseline cough is more frequent and his sputum has increased in production. He also denies fever, chills, chest pain, and abdominal pain. On exam, he is tachypneic and in mild distress, with an oxygen saturation of 95% on room air. His lungs have crackles bilaterally in the upper lung fields. He is admitted to the hospital for further workup of his hemoptysis. What are the next steps in the evaluation and treatment of this patient with hemoptysis?

INTRODUCTION

Hemoptysis (from the Latin *heme* meaning blood and the Greek *ptysis* meaning to spit) is defined as the coughing up of blood or blood-tinged sputum and can be further categorized as being massive or nonmassive based on the volume of blood that is expectorated. The definition of massive hemoptysis varies as it has been defined as anywhere from over 100 mL to 1000 mL of blood expectorated in a 24-hour period. The exact frequency with which hemoptysis occurs is not known, but it is estimated that 5% of all hemoptysis is massive, and the mortality rate of massive hemoptysis is estimated to approach 80%.

The first step in the assessment of a patient with reported hemoptysis is to make sure that the blood is coming from the respiratory tract. Pseudohemoptysis is the coughing up of blood that is not from a pulmonary source and hematemesis is bloody vomitus. Hematemesis can often be confused with hemoptysis because vomiting and retching are often accompanied by coughing and gagging. Patients are frequently unsure whether they coughed or vomited up blood. Bloody vomitus is often aspirated into the lungs and then coughed back up. Additionally, bleeding sites in the nose or pharynx can sometimes be confused with hemoptysis, particularly when this blood is aspirated. Another mimicker of hemoptysis is the pink frothy sputum that is often seen in massive pulmonary edema secondary to heart failure. This sputum is different from hemoptysis as it is not red and is typically light and frothy. A more detailed discussion of pseudohemoptysis and hematemesis is beyond the scope of this chapter; only true hemoptysis is discussed here.

PATHOPHYSIOLOGY AND CAUSES OF HEMOPTYSIS

To understand why the pulmonary system can bleed, it is best first to understand the pulmonary blood supply. Both pulmonary and bronchial arteries are possible culprits of bleeding. Although the pulmonary arteries have just about the entire cardiac output coursing through them (high volume), they are under low pressure. In contrast, the bronchial arteries receive much less blood (low volume) but are under high pressure because they are part of the systemic circulation. Because the bronchial arteries—which typically come off the aorta but occasionally come off the intercostal arteries—are under higher pressure, they are usually the source of bleeding, as opposed to the pulmonary arteries.

The exact pathophysiologic mechanism of bleeding is dependent upon the cause and source. For example, in bronchiectasis, bleeding occurs because the bronchial arteries become tortuous and

TABLE 88-1 Differential Diagnosis for Hemoptysis Broken Down by Category

Tumor
Bronchogenic carcinoma
Kaposi sarcoma
Lymphoma
Leukemia (post-Bone marrow transplant (BMT))
Melanoma
Infection
Bronchitis
Bronchiectasis
Tuberculosis
Angioinvasive organisms (aspergilloma)
Streptococcus pneumoniae infection
Klebsiella infection
Parasitic infections (*Ascaris, Paragonimus, Echinococcus*)
Lung abscess
Miscellaneous
Wegener granulomatosis
Goodpasture syndrome
Systemic lupus erythematosus with alveolar hemorrhage
Pulmonary hypertension
Pulmonary capillary hemangiomatosis (PCH)
Pulmonary embolus
Ruptured (Pulmonary Arteriovenous Malformations (PAVM))
Valvular heart disease

hyperplastic and are thus friable and easily disturbed. To identify the exact cause, it is best to think in general terms of what can bleed in the pulmonary system: airways, parenchyma, and vasculature. The most common causes of hemoptysis are bronchitis, bronchogenic carcinoma, bronchiectasis, and pneumonia, but there is a long list of causes as shown in **Table 88-1**.

In developing countries tuberculosis (TB) remains an important cause of hemoptysis. In the United States TB was a leading cause prior to 1960. Currently infection is the most common cause, accounting for 60–70% of cases of hemoptysis. Infection causes hemoptysis due to superficial bleeding from mucosal irritation and edema. Primary lung cancers have been implicated in about 20% of hemoptysis cases, with the most common cancer being bronchogenic carcinoma. Of note, metastatic lung cancers do not usually cause hemoptysis.

APPROACH TO THE PATIENT

The most important initial determination is the volume of hemoptysis. Massive hemoptysis is life threatening and needs emergent stabilization and then intervention to stop the bleeding (to be discussed further in the management section).

PRACTICE POINT

Definition of massive hemoptysis

- Although hemoptysis is usually not life threatening, massive hemoptysis may cause airway obstruction, which is more life threatening than shock from acute hemorrhage. Massive hemoptysis is defined as expectoration of 200 mL per cough, 400 mL per 24 hour, hemoptysis requiring transfusion to stabilize a hematocrit. Intrabronchial bleeding may rapidly cause death from "drowning" rather than from hypoxemia.

Patients with massive hemoptysis may describe a warm sensation in the chest or gurgling. For nonmassive hemoptysis, a good history and physical exam can often identify the cause of hemoptysis. It is first important to quantify the type, frequency, and duration of hemoptysis. Is it frank blood or blood-tinged sputum? Is it dark maroon or bright red? How many times a day is the hemoptysis occurring? See **Table 88-2** for helpful questions.

TABLE 88-2 Helpful Historical Questions to Assess Hemoptysis

1. Is the sputum frank blood or blood tinged?
2. How many teaspoons (or cupfuls) are being expectorated in 24 hours?
3. Is the blood bright red?
4. Are there clots?
5. Does the sputum have a foul smell?

Acute-onset hemoptysis may result from bronchitis or bronchiectasis. Fevers, night sweats, and weight loss are classic symptoms of tuberculosis. Bronchogenic carcinoma may present with change in chronic cough, anorexia, and weight loss in addition to hemoptysis. Patients with alveolar hemorrhage and renal disease may experience relatively minor hemoptysis despite significant dyspnea. Aspiration of a foreign body lodged in bronchi may result in repeated hemoptysis (and pulmonary infections) many years after the insult.

PRACTICE POINT

Clinical features

- A history of underlying lung disease is the most significant risk factor for hemoptysis.

Hemoptysis may also be a symptom of a parasitic disease (*Ascaris, Paragonimus, Echinococcus*). For example, over 3 million Americans are infected annually from *Ascaris lumbricoides*. In addition to hemoptysis, patients may experience cough, dyspnea, fever, and eosinophilia. Hemoptysis associated with valvular heart disease is typically frothy pink due to the association with pulmonary edema. However, if the patient suffering from pulmonary hypertension may develop frank hemoptysis from rupture of distended bronchial veins. The most common cause of hemoptysis from valvular heart disease, mitral stenosis, may lead to severe hemoptysis requiring transfusion and surgery.

How much blood is expectorated? Important historical questions to ask are smoking history, history of lung cancer, TB risk factors, HIV risk factors (as immunocompromised patients have higher incidence of fungal infections), constitutional and infectious symptoms, and history of rheumatologic disease (such as sarcoid, which is known to cause hemoptysis).

The physical exam should include vital signs, specifically looking for tachycardia and hypotension to give clues about blood loss, and respiratory rate and oxygen saturation to assess the patient's respiratory stability. The presence of fever may suggest an infectious etiology. The patient should not be hypotensive unless exsanguinating or septic. The exam should also include an inspection of the mouth and nose to look for bleeding. A lung exam may reveal fine inspiratory crackles associated with alveolar hemorrhage, inspiratory and expiratory crackles associated with blood or secretions in the airway, or wheezing associated with narrowing of the airway. A bruit appreciated during chest auscultation coupled with a prior history of chest trauma and symptoms and signs of hypoxemia would be consistent with pulmonary arteriovenous fistula. A comprehensive cardiovascular exam may uncover mitral stenosis or mitral regurgitation in the setting of pulmonary edema. A skin exam may identify rashes (suggesting vasculitis), purpura (suggesting a coagulopathy), and telangiectases (suggesting a ruptured pulmonary arterial venous malformation as seen in hereditary hemorrhagic telangiectasia). Clubbing of the extremities may be associated with bronchiectasis or some bronchogenic carcinomas. Cyanosis would indicate massive hemoptysis interfering with oxygen exchange.

PRACTICE POINT

The physical examination

- Although the physical examination cannot reliably localize the site of bleeding, it can be useful in assessing the cause (infection versus tumor versus miscellaneous) and severity of hemoptysis.

The initial laboratory evaluation should include a complete blood count and coagulation studies, arterial blood gases to look for hypoxia, and, if the cause is not readily apparent from the history, a urinalysis with urine microscopy and creatinine to rule out pulmonary-renal syndromes. Finally, a sputum culture is used to assess for infection. Depending upon the history and physical exam, laboratory studies looking for antineutrophil cytoplasmic antibodies (ANCAs) and anti-glomerular basement membrane (GBM) antibodies may be performed as well.

A screening chest radiograph may identify predisposing lung pathology such as masses suggestive of lung cancer, cavities, or evidence of trauma, and in the case of unilateral pulmonary hemorrhage, the affected side. Further studies should include high-resolution computed tomographic (CT) scan of the chest, which, if possible, should be done with contrast to evaluate for pulmonary embolism, and possibly bronchoscopic correlation of the likely source of bleeding.

PRACTICE POINT

Radiographic signs

- A screening chest X-ray may identify underlying lung pathology, the distribution of extravascular blood in the lungs, and conditions such as mycetomas, lung masses, or cavities that predispose to hemoptysis. Hemothorax is usually caused by bleeding from a lung injury such as a motor vehicle accident. Lung abscess from aspiration pneumonia may have signs of impending hemoptysis: (1) emptying and refilling of abscess cavity on serial films, (2) variations in lucency and height of air-fluid level, (3) variable parenchymal densities (blood clots) within the cavity.

Essential blood work includes a complete blood count, prothrombin time, partial thromboplastin time, and urinalysis. If a reduced oxygen saturation in the setting of hemoptysis suggested hypoxemia, an arterial blood gas should be obtained to determine whether hypercapnia is present.

MANAGEMENT OF HEMOPTYSIS

The initial management is dependent upon the amount of hemoptysis. If the hemoptysis is life threatening (ie, massive), the two urgent management goals are to (1) stabilize and (2) intervene. Stabilization includes the A, B, Cs, of advanced cardiac life support. Intravenous access, with two large-bore IVs should be obtained. Coagulopathy should be reversed and blood products should be given.

In general, a patient with massive hemoptysis will require endotracheal intubation to avoid asphyxiation, which is the most frequent cause of death in massive hemoptysis. Thus massive hemoptysis should be managed in conjunction with pulmonary/critical care physicians to help stabilize the patient. Interventional pulmonologists, interventional radiologists, and cardiothoracic surgeons may be needed to intervene. In massive hemoptysis, mortality ranges from 7% to 80%, but when the bleeding is >1L in 24 hours, the mortality rate is >50%. It is recommended that a patient be intubated with a large-bore endotracheal tube in the event that bronchoscopy needs to be performed. A double-lumen endotracheal tube can also be used to isolate the nonbleeding lung for better airway control. In the event of unilateral bleeding, the patient should be positioned with the bleeding lung down so that blood does not spill over into the nonbleeding lung

Bronchoscopy can be performed emergently in massive hemoptysis (after the patient is stabilized, as already described). Flexible bronchoscopy is most commonly performed but rigid bronchoscopy, if available, can also be performed when there is uncontrollable bleeding as it allows for better control of the airway. Bronchoscopy is both diagnostic, as it can identify the source of the bleeding, and therapeutic, as the bleeding can be stopped with topical thrombin or fibrinogen, balloon tamponade, epinephrine injections, or electrocautery. Although these therapies are available, limited data exist on their efficacy. The most widely accepted emergent intervention is bronchial artery embolization performed by interventional radiologists. Embolization works by stopping systemic arterial inflow to the bleeding vessels, thus reducing perfusion pressure and rebleeding.

If the bleeding is unable to be controlled by either endobronchial therapies or arterial embolization, then emergent surgical resection must be performed. In the emergent setting the mortality rate of surgery is about 40%.

In the setting of nonmassive hemoptysis, the same interventions can be performed but with less urgency. In this setting bronchoscopy is usually done so an airway inspection can be performed to look for evidence of bleeding. Biopsies can also be taken during bronchoscopy if cancer is suspected. Bronchial artery embolization can also be done, but if the bleeding is not brisk or active, it is often difficult to find the bleeding vessel and embolize it.

Patients with both massive and nonmassive hemoptysis should have serial hematocrits. After bleeding is controlled in massive hemoptysis and in all cases of nonmassive hemoptysis the cause must be found by sending off the aforementioned blood tests and imaging studies. Then treatment can be tailored to the exact cause of the hemoptysis.

CASE 88-2

Our patient was watched in the hospital for 48 hours with no evidence of active hemoptysis and stable blood cell counts. His CT scan showed evidence of worsening bronchiectasis. He underwent bronchoscopy during his admission, which did not show any signs of active bleeding. He was started on intravenous antibiotic therapy for a cystic fibrosis pulmonary exacerbation and was discharged home after 48 hours. He had nonmassive hemoptysis, which was monitored closely in the hospital while he was worked up for the cause of his hemoptysis.

CONCLUSION

In the case of this patient and all patients it is important first and foremost to determine whether the hemoptysis is massive or nonmassive. Once that determination is made, the patient is stabilized, and a workup and intervention can be performed as outlined here.

SUGGESTED READINGS

Bidwell JL, Pachner RW. Hemoptysis: diagnosis and management. *American Family Physician*. 2005;72(7):1253–1260.

Haponik EF, Fein A, Chin R. Managing life-threatening hemoptysis: has anything really changed? *Chest*. 2000;118:1431–1435.

Thomas NW, Puro HE, Arbula A. The significance of hemoptysis in lung abscess. *J Thorac Cardiovasc Surg*. 1970;59:617.

CHAPTER 89

Hypertension

Nicholas Tsapatsaris, MD
Durathun Farha, MD

Key Clinical Questions

1. What are the major causes of hypertension in hospitalized patients?
2. What are the common hospital-acquired or iatrogenic causes that induce hypertension?
3. What signs and symptoms should be assessed in the initial evaluation of a patient with reported hypertension?
4. When should you lower blood pressure acutely?
5. What are the risks associated with acutely lowering the blood pressure in the hospital?

INTRODUCTION

The lifetime risk for the development of high blood pressure (BP) (systolic BP > 140 mm Hg), is 90%; half of patients age 60–70, and three quarters age 70–80 have hypertension. The prevalence of hypertension in the hospital setting has been reported to range from 50.5% to 72%.

The decision about whether to treat high BP in the hospitalized patient with antihypertensive agents is an important one, but it is not always straightforward. The definition of hypertension, goals for treatment, and benefits of therapy in reduction of cardiovascular morbidity and mortality have been well established in numerous clinical trials and widely disseminated to practicing physicians in evidence-based consensus documents. Unfortunately these goals do not necessarily apply to acutely ill patients. Thus the management of hypertension in the hospitalized patient should be highly individualized. There are few if any prospective trials regarding choice of antihypertensive medications in this setting. Recommendations are generally based on consensus opinion, customary use, extrapolation from animal models, and commonsense application of physiologic principles.

CASE 89-1

A 75-year-old man admitted for renal colic was noted on routine vital signs to have a BP of 180/98 mm Hg and a regular pulse of 98. His BP since admission has been in the range of 160–170/85–95 mm Hg. He passed a kidney stone earlier in the evening and his pain was subsiding. He had received saline IV and morphine sulfate for pain earlier. He reported minimal flank pain. Otherwise he felt fine and denied shortness of breath, chest pain, or headache.

He was told years ago that he had high blood pressure and was given medication. He never took the medication and never returned to see a physician. His admission ECG showed nonspecific ST–T wave changes and evidence of a possible prior inferior myocardial infarction, his chemistry profile was notable for a normal potassium and creatinine. A urinalysis showed microscopic hematuria but no protein. His nonenhanced abdominopelvic CT scan showed symmetric, normal sized kidneys and there was no evidence of hydronephrosis.

The covering urology resident ordered topical nitroglycerin (Nitropaste), which reduced his BP to 150/95 mm Hg in 15 minutes.

Two hours later, the patient woke up with a headache and stood up to go to the bathroom. He fainted, fell, and could not stand up because of hip pain. Although he was alert, oriented, and had no focal findings on neurologic examination, he had intense left groin pain and a shortened and externally rotated left leg, suggesting a hip fracture. His heart rate was 90 and his BP was 110/70 mm Hg. Nitropaste was removed and his BP rose to 150/85 mm Hg. His syncope was attributed to postural hypotension precipitated by Nitropaste. A x-ray confirmed a left hip fracture.

It is crucial not to reflexively order antihypertensive medications in all hospitalized patients with high BP and to recognize precipitating factors that commonly augment BP in the acutely ill and require a different approach. When treatment is initiated, it is important for the clinician to choose appropriate agents and optimal BP targets

TABLE 89-1 Prevalence of Hypertension (HTN) in the Inpatient Settings

Clinical Question	Findings
Accuracy of routine inpatient BP measurements	56.4 to 72.6% of inpatients receiving 24-hour BP monitoring had hypertension 28 to 38% of patients had masked hypertension identified by 24-hour monitoring but not revealed by routine inpatient BP measures
Proportion of hypertensive patients uncontrolled on admission	86.9% of patients with previously documented hypertension were uncontrolled on admission
Proportion of hypertensive patients uncontrolled at discharge	37 to 77% of inpatients with hypertension still had BP > 140/90 mm Hg at the time of discharge
Proportion of hypertensive patients without a recorded diagnosis at discharge	8 to 44% of patients with elevated BP > 140/90 mm Hg were discharged without a documented diagnosis of hypertension
Proportion of uncontrolled hypertensive patients receiving intensification of therapy during index admission	53.1% of patients with uncontrolled BP received additional anti hypertensive medication upon discharge
Proportion of hypertensive patients with BP controlled at follow-up	50% of patients with hypertension were controlled to < 140/90 mm Hg at follow-up

based on the underlying pathophysiology, acuity of the problem, and target end-organ damage. It is also important to capitalize on the opportunity to modify this traditional cardiovascular risk factor for patients who will likely benefit and thus reduce disparities in health care (**Table 89-1**).

PATHOPHYSIOLOGY

Management of BP should take into consideration the basic principles:

- BP = cardiac output × vascular resistance.
- Cardiac output = heart rate × stroke volume.

The higher the heart rate (assuming no change in stroke volume, blood volume, blood viscosity, or peripheral resistance), the higher the BP. The autonomic nervous system predominantly mediates acute (instantaneous) changes in BP by inducing changes in heart rate, systemic vascular resistance, and venous tone. The feedback loop from mechanoreceptors in the carotid sinuses and aortic arch respond to acute fluctuations in BP, but in chronic essential hypertension, the set point rises, and a higher basal BP is tolerated. The renin-angiotensin-aldosterone system mediates chronic changes over days to weeks via the kidney. Low kidney perfusion, elevated sympathetic response, and other stimuli, common in the hospitalized patient, stimulate the release of renin. Angiotensin II increases both systolic and diastolic BP and signals the adrenal cortex to secrete aldosterone, which in turn increases the reabsorption of sodium from urine, sweat, saliva, and bowel. Catecholamines, especially epinephrine, from the sympathetic nervous system greatly affect BP. Binding of epinephrine to α_1 receptors leads to vasoconstriction and increased peripheral vascular resistance, causing BP to rise. Binding to β_1 receptors increases heart rate and cardiac output, which also raises BP. See Chapter 252, Hypertensive Urgencies.

TABLE 89-2 Factors Associated with Hypertension in Hospitalized Patients

Preexisting factors
- Advanced age
- Hypertension (especially if poorly controlled)
- Diabetes mellitus
- Renal disease

Hospital-related factors
- Pain, anxiety
- Postoperative state
- Hypoxia, hypercarbia, pulmonary embolism, chronic obstructive pulmonary disease exacerbation and other conditions that increase the work of breathing, bronchodilators
- Myocardial ischemia
- Increased intracranial hypertension
- Hypervolemia (saline, transfusion)
- Bladder distension
- Antihypertensive medication withdrawal
- Alcohol, narcotic, and anxiolytic/hypnotic drug withdrawal
- Drug interactions

A minority of patients may be admitted to the hospital with a primary diagnosis of hypertensive crisis. In a hypertensive emergency, a surge in BP is accompanied by end-organ damage. Hypertensive urgency, however, is an acute elevation in BP without end-organ damage. There is no BP threshold that defines a hypertensive crisis. Most patients have pressures that exceed 180/120 mm Hg, with diastolic BPs over 120 mm Hg being most strongly associated with end-organ damage. However, pregnant patients may develop target end-organ damage at significantly lower readings.

The hypertensive hospitalized patients have usually been admitted for other reasons and are incidentally noted to have hypertension due to monitoring of vital signs. There are many secondary factors that can acutely raise blood pressure in hospitalized patients (**Table 89-2**). The most common include stopping hypertensive medications because of failure to reconcile outpatient medications on admission, restriction of oral intake, volume expansion (often from crystalloid administration), the postoperative state, pain, anxiety, and withdrawal from alcohol, narcotics, or antianxiety/sedative drugs.

IS THE REPORTED BLOOD PRESSURE MEASUREMENT ACCURATE?

The first step is to determine whether the reported BP reading is a valid measure of intra-arterial BP. Many factors may affect the immediate accuracy of a BP measurement, including the device used (cuff size, leaky bulb, faulty aneroid device), the technique and bias of the examiner (positioning of the patient, placement of the cuff, inappropriately rapid deflation, excess bell pressure), and a noisy environment. Most errors overestimate the BP. In general, it is best to palpate the BP first to avoid underinflation in patients with an auscultatory gap. The BP should be checked in both arms.

IS THIS PATIENT EXPERIENCING SYMPTOMS AND SIGNS FROM THE BLOOD PRESSURE ELEVATION?

Deviations from "normal" BP must be considered in the context of the patient's chronic BP. A patient's BP normally varies depending on the time of day, even from minute to minute, and typically decreases during sleep. Arterial monitoring has shown that the systolic and diastolic BP also varies with the respiratory cycle and with each heartbeat. According to ambulatory BP monitoring, elderly patients are more likely to have wide fluctuations or lability of BP.

Patients with untreated or inadequately treated hypertension are prone to sudden elevations in BP and the development of hypertensive crises. Patients who develop a hypertensive crisis in settings other than chronic essential hypertension may develop end organ damage at lesser degrees of BP elevation, as they lack the vascular smooth muscle hypertrophy that provides some protection against the effects of uncontrolled hypertension. This is especially true for pregnant patients.

IS THIS PATIENT SUFFERING FROM A HYPERTENSIVE EMERGENCY?

The next step is to obtain a history and physical examination along with basic tests (**Table 89-3**) to determine whether the patient has evidence of a hypertensive emergency and to determine the acuity of this patient's hypertension and underlying precipitating factors.

Hypertensive emergencies are characterized by severe elevations complicated by evidence of impending or progressive target organ dysfunction. Examples include hypertensive encephalopathy, intracerebral hemorrhage, acute myocardial infarction (MI), acute left ventricular failure with pulmonary edema, unstable angina pectoris, dissecting aortic aneurysm, acute funduscopic changes and eclampsia.

Hypertensive urgencies are those situations associated with severe elevations in BP without progressive target organ dysfunction. Examples include upper levels of stage II hypertension associated with severe headache, shortness of breath, epistaxis, or severe anxiety. The majority of these patients present as noncompliant or inadequately treated hypertensive individuals, often with little or no evidence of acute target organ damage, although chronic target organ damage (such as S_4 gallop from left ventricular hypertrophy, chronic fundoscopic changes, or chronic renal insufficiency) is common.

Patients should be asked about their outpatient medications and substance abuse. Medication withdrawal (rebound hypertension) can be associated with acute severe elevation in BP. It is most common with abrupt withdrawal of beta-blockers or clonidine. It is less likely to happen with other antihypertensives. Medication withdrawal hypertension is best treated by reinstituting the same medication orally, intravenously (IV), or transdermally. Beta-blockers can be replaced with IV labetolol, esmolol, or metoprolol, and oral clonidine can be administered transdermally in patients who cannot tolerate oral medications. Transdermal patches may contain aluminum, so it is important to remove the patch prior to magnetic resonance imaging (MRI), and before cardioversion or defibrillation. Transdermal clonidine may take several days to achieve adequate drug levels.

It is important to review whether the patient has received any new medications, including medications as needed, over the previous 24 hours. Patients who take monoamine oxidase inhibitors (MAOIs), including the antibiotic linezolid and over-the-counter drugs with MAOI activity such as St. John's wort, are at risk for developing hypertensive crisis with confusion if they also ingest selective serotonin reuptake inhibitors, tricyclic antidepressants, meperidine, tramadol, methadone, dextromethorphan, or tyramine-containing foods. Bevacizumab, a monoclonal antibody against vascular endothelial growth factor that is approved for use in several advanced adenocarcinomas, may lead to hypertensive crisis.

Postoperative patients commonly have hypertension due to increases in sympathetic tone and vascular resistance. Postoperative hypertension is arbitrarily defined as systolic BP ≥ 190 mm Hg or diastolic BP ≥ 100 mm Hg on two consecutive readings following surgery. More than 50% of patients have a history of hypertension prior to surgery. In addition, acute pain, the presence of agitation associated with delirium, postoperative hypoxia, and anxiety may contribute to hypertension.

TABLE 89-3 Diagnostic Aids in the Assessment of Severe Hypertension

Complete set of vital signs including bilateral blood pressure assessment, pulse, and urine output
Cardiovascular, fundoscopic and neurologic examination to look for target end organ damage
Vascular examination (bruits, verification of brachial, femoral and carotid pulses)
Hematocrit
Serum electrolytes, blood urea nitrogen, serum creatinine
Urinalysis
Electrocardiogram
Troponin
B-type natriuretic peptide BNP test
Head computed tomography (if confusion, seizure, or signs and symptoms of neurologic disease)

For patients with significant heart disease, poorly controlled hypertension may precipitate symptoms and signs of demand myocardial ischemia or flash pulmonary edema. Chronic hypertension with resultant left ventricular hypertrophy is a major cause of heart failure (HF) with preserved ejection fraction. Elevations in systemic BP increase left ventricular wall stress and systolic load, which can impair myocardial relaxation in patients with diastolic HF. Diastolic function is often abnormal in patients with HF and reduced left ventricular ejection fraction (LVEF) as well. Patients with diastolic HF may not tolerate tachycardia since increases in heart rate shorten the duration of diastole and truncate the late phase of diastolic filling. Paradoxically, tachycardia may be important to preserve exercise tolerance when stroke volume is limited.

For patients with acute kidney injury (AKI) complicated by hypertension, it is important to determine whether the hypertension is the cause of the acute kidney failure (as in a hypertensive emergency) or secondary to inadequately treated chronic hypertension. An estimated 50–75% of patients with a glomerular filtration rate (GFR) < 60 mL/min/1.73 m^2 (chronic kidney disease stages 3–5) have hypertension, and as renal function declines, hypertension becomes increasingly prevalent.

Female patients of child-bearing age should be questioned about the possibility of pregnancy, which would have important ramifications for treatment.

In addition to checking the BP, the examiner should verify the brachial, femoral, and carotid pulses. A thorough cardiovascular and neurological examination should be conducted. Funduscopic examination should be done to detect any acute hypertensive changes (hemorrhages, exudates, or papilledema) and chronic changes (arteriovenous nicking, copper wiring). (See Chapter 81 Disorders of the Eye: Frisen Grades.) The abdomen should be auscultated for any renal bruits. This requires listening in a quiet room, applying adequate pressure with the diaphragm of the stethoscope, and simultaneously palpating the carotid artery during listening to see if the abdominal bruit extends beyond the carotid upstroke. According to the Rational Clinical Examination Series, the likelihood of renal artery stenosis increases in patients with refractory hypertension if the patient has a history of arterosclerotic disease (LR+ 2.2), systolic bruit (LR+ 4.3), systolic-diastolic bruit (LR+ 39).

The presence of vascular disease elsewhere would be another indicator that the patient requires aggressive secondary prevention.

TREATMENT OF PRECIPITATING FACTORS

The relief of pain and anxiety and the initiation of appropriate protocols and aggressive management of alcohol and drug withdrawal may be effective for BP reduction in many hospitalized patients.

In this case, pain and the anxiety of hospitalization likely increased his heart rate. In addition, volume expansion, intended to help with renal stone passage, may have increased intravascular volume thus increasing stroke volume and contributing to a rise in BP. One liter of normal saline contains 9 grams of sodium chloride, so patients in the hospital on "maintenance" fluids, are often receiving far more sodium than would be consumed on a regular diet.

PRACTICE POINT

- One liter of normal saline contains 9 grams of sodium chloride, so patients in the hospital on "maintenance" fluids are often receiving far more sodium than would be consumed on a regular diet.

ACUTELY LOWERING THE BLOOD PRESSURE

There are occasional situations, classified as hypertensive urgencies and emergencies, that mandate acute BP lowering in hospitalized patients. They require immediate BP reduction (not necessarily to normal) to prevent or limit target organ damage. Hypertensive emergencies, along with preferred drugs for their management, are listed in **Table 89-4**.

Some patients with hypertensive urgencies may benefit from treatment with an oral, short-acting agent such as captopril, labetalol, or clonidine followed by several hours of observation. However, there is no evidence to suggest that failure to aggressively lower BP in the hospital is associated with any increased short-term risk to the patient who presents with severe hypertension. Such patients may also benefit from adjustment in their antihypertensive therapy, particularly the use of combination drugs, or reinstitution of medications if noncompliance is a problem. Most importantly, patients should not leave the emergency department or hospital without a confirmed follow-up visit within several days.

TABLE 89-4 Treatment of Hypertensive Emergencies

Hypertensive Emergency	Preferred Drugs	Comments
ACS	Beta-blocker (esmolol, metoprolol, atenolol, propranolol) by decreasing double product Nitroglycerin by decreasing ventricular preload and increasing myocardial oxygen delivery Morphine (STEMI pain management class I) by relieving pain, anxiety, and possibly other beneficial effects in treating ACS	Standard therapy 5 mg IV metoprolol every 5 minutes, × 3 doses, followed by oral dose 25–50 mg every 6–8 hours Standard therapy intravenous nitroglycerin. started at an initial rate of 5–10 μg/min with increases of 10 μg/min every 3–5 minutes until the patient is pain free or the systolic BP falls below 100 mm Hg. Morphine may be associated with increased adverse events in UA/NSTEMI (class IIB) Avoid hydralazine, nitroprusside Goal to decrease BP by 25% within 15 minutes
Adrenergic crisis	Phentolamine Nitroprusside Labetalol	Use labetalol in cocaine crisis Use labetalol with caution in the setting of bradycardia, atrioventricular block, heart failure, and bronchospasm
Aortic dissection	Esmolol Labetalol Nitroprusside	Always prescribe a beta-blocker with nitroprusside Avoid hydralazine, nicardipine Goal to decrease BP by 25% within 15 minutes
CNS: acute stroke	In order of use: First, beta-blocker, then add calcium channel blocker, then ACE inhibitor, then nitrates, then hydralazine, then $alpha_1$-blocker Intravenous: labetalol → nicardipine → enalapril → nitroprusside → hydralazine Oral: metoprolol → diltiazem → captopril → isosorbide → hydralazine	The brain needs a higher perfusion pressure → maintain or even increase hypertension by holding routine BP medications Exceptions: ACS or severe CAD, aortic dissection, CHF, large stroke, hemorrhagic transformation, patients s/p tPA, thromborrhexis, CEA • In patients s/p procedure avoid SBP > 140 mm Hg (to prevent reperfuson syndrome) • In patients who have not received tPA, avoid SBP > 185 or DBP >110 mm Hg When HBP requires treatment, short-acting preferred: use IV Nimodipine may be preferred in SAH; it is associated with reflex tachycardia, headache, and flushing Avoid drugs that can make BP abruptly fall (nifedipine) Avoid drugs that directly dilate arteries (hydralazine, nitrates) as they may hinder cerebral autoregulation Avoid drugs that are sedating (clonidine) Avoid drugs that may increase intracranial pressure (nitroprusside) Goal is to decrease BP by 25% within 6–12 hours if cerebral hemorrhage present

(continued)

TABLE 89-4 Treatment of Hypertensive Emergencies *(continued)*

Hypertensive Emergency	Preferred Drugs	Comments
CNS: Hypertensive encephalopathy	Labetalol Nicardipine Nitroprusside Fenoldopam Enalaprilat	Usually SBP > 250 mm Hg or DBP > 130 mm Hg with evidence of end-organ damage (brain, eyes, heart, kidneys) Arterial line: IV labetalol first choice as IV nitroprusside contraindicated if cerebral edema or coronary ischemia Goal is to reduce BP by 25% within 3–6 hours if papilledema present; within 6-12 hours if cerebral hemorrhage; within 15 minutes if ACS or dissection. Fenoldopam, a selective dopamine receptor antagonist and short-acting vasodilator, seems as effective as sodium nitroprusside in hypertensive crisis, with the advantages of improved renal perfusion and promotion of diuresis. Tachyphylaxis develops after 48 hours.
Congestive heart failure	Nitroglycerin Loop diuretics Enalaprilat	Optimal management will depend on whether the patient has systolic or diastolic heart failure, severe congestion, and coexisting signs of reduced perfusion.
Postoperative	Nitroglycerin Nitroprusside Labetalol Nicardipine Fenoldopam	Postoperative hypertension is most common after cardiac surgery, major vascular surgery, such as carotid and aortic procedures, head and neck surgery, neurosurgery, trauma, and organ transplantation.
Preeclampsia or eclampsia	Labetalol Hydralazine	While still pregnant, blood pressure goals must minimize maternal hypertensive complications, which are more likely above 160 mm Hg systolic and 110 mm Hg diastolic, while maintaining sufficient uteroplacental flow. Blood pressure reduction should be attempted promptly with caution in pregnant women given the potential for impaired uteroplacental flow and fetal compromise. Options include IV labetalol or hydralazine, noting that hydralazine has been associated with greater hypotension in this setting. Indications for hemodynamic monitoring specific for obstetric patients include severe preeclampsia with either refractory hypertension, oliguric renal failure, or unclear intravascular volume status. Close collaboration with obstetrics is essential for optimal maternal (and fetal/neonatal) outcome. Although often maternal manifestations of preeclampsia are quickly reversible with delivery and judicious fluid and BP management, they may persist or even worsen in the postpartum period. Avoid nitroprusside, enalaprilat
Renal insufficiency	Nicardipine Fendolapam	Diuretics, particularly loop diuretics, can be particularly useful in optimizing BP. Loop diuretic doses should be titrated upward as tolerated until normalization of BP is achieved or the patient develops symptoms or signs of overly aggressive diuresis (eg, lightheadedness, hypotension, rising BUN and creatinine). Avoid hydralazine whose half-life is markedly increased in renal failure

ACE, angiotensin-converting enzyme; ACS, acute coronary syndrome; BUN, blood urea nitrogen; CEA, carotid endarterectomy; CNS, central nervous system; DBP, diastolic blood pressure; IV, intravenous; NSTEMI, non-ST-elevation myocardial infarction; SAH, subarachnoid hemorrhage; SBP, systolic blood pressure; STEMI, ST-elevation myocardial infarction; UA, unstable angina.

Unfortunately, the term *urgency* has led to overly aggressive management of many patients with severe, uncomplicated hypertension. Aggressive dosing with intravenous drugs or even oral agents, to rapidly lower BP is not without risk. Oral loading doses of antihypertensive agents can lead to cumulative effects causing hypotension, sometimes following discharge from the hospital. The lower limit of cerebral blood flow (CBF) autoregulation differs between hypertensive and normotensive patients. Hypertensive patients may show signs or symptoms of cerebral hypoxemia, including loss of consciousness, coma, or seizures, at mean arterial pressure (MAP) levels of 50 ± 5 mm Hg and below, whereas normotensive patients will show these symptoms at a MAP of 40 ± 5 mm Hg and below. This has important implications for the management of hypertensive emergencies and urgencies: too rapid lowering of BP in these patients poses a risk of cerebral hypoperfusion.

The decision to lower BP acutely should be made to reduce immediate risk for harm, a situation that is infrequent in the hospitalized patient.

PRACTICE POINT

- The decision to lower BP acutely should be made to reduce immediate risk for harm, a situation that is infrequent in the hospital patient.

PRACTICE POINT

- Hydralazine is currently less often used in the treatment of hypertensive crises because of its prolonged and unpredictable antihypertensive effects. In patients with renal insufficiency the half-life of hydralazine is markedly prolonged.

CASE 89-1 *(continued)*

The most important intervention for managing this patient's hypertension was the relief of pain and anxiety. If there had been clear evidence of volume overload then a loop diuretic might have been considered.

This patient likely had long-standing hypertension, and the reason to initiate treatment would be to lower long-term risk for stroke, MI, congestive heart failure (CHF), and renal insufficiency. He did not fulfill criteria for hypertensive urgency. Treatment did not need to be started in the middle of the night.

The following morning, the patient was seen by orthopedics and surgery was recommended.

The patient's pain was reasonably controlled. His BP was 176/104 mm Hg, and his heart rate was 60 bpm. The orthopedist asked whether his BP needs to be better controlled prior to surgery. Prior to admission, the patient had been active, able to walk up to 2 miles, and maintain a large yard without limitations. Should surgery be delayed? Should BP medications be started?

PRACTICE POINT

- Recognition of new hypertension or undertreated hypertension is a golden opportunity to educate the patient about risks of hypertension and to introduce appropriate strategies and medications to achieve control.

PREOPERATIVE RISK ASSESSMENT OF HYPERTENSIVE PATIENTS

PATIENTS WITH PREEXISTING HYPERTENSION

A systematic review and meta-analysis of 30 observational studies involving 12,995 patients with hypertension demonstrated an odds ratio for the association between hypertensive disease and perioperative cardiac outcomes to be 1.35. The authors felt this association, while statistically significant, was not clinically relevant because there is little evidence for an association between admission BPs of less than 180 mm Hg systolic or 110 mm Hg diastolic and perioperative complications. Patients with BP above this range may be more prone to perioperative ischemia, arrhythmias, and cardiovascular lability, but there is no clear evidence that deferring surgery reduces perioperative risk. The authors concluded that anesthesia and surgery should not be canceled on the grounds of elevated BP and that intraoperative BP should be maintained within 20% of the best estimate of preoperative BP, especially in patients with markedly elevated BPs.

The American College of Cardiology/American Heart Association guidelines comment that stage 1 or 2 hypertension is not an independent risk factor for perioperative complications. They do suggest that BP > 180/110 should be controlled before surgery. In the postoperative period, the clinician may expect significant lowering of BP as a nonspecific response to blood loss and bed rest if the patient does not have other factors that commonly augment BP. This lowering can persist for months but a gradual return to preoperative levels is expected. Chronic untreated hypertension alters the autoregulatory threshold so that higher mean arterial pressures are needed to maintain target organ blood flow. Since fluid shifts, blood loss, and medications used during the perioperative period may also contribute to suboptimal blood flow to target organs (brain and kidney in particular), it is prudent to avoid overcorrecting BP in the perioperative setting.

It is generally recommended that patients take most of their usual antihypertensive medications with sips of water the morning of surgery, although angiotensin receptor blockers (ARBs) have been associated with intraoperative hypotension and are usually held. Angiotensin-converting enzyme (ACE) inhibitors and diuretics are often held according to physician preference. If the patient cannot take oral medications after surgery, parenteral or transdermal equivalents can be administered. For example, patients prescribed diuretics may receive intravenous furosemide or bumetanide; those prescribed beta-blockers may be treated with esmolol, labetalol, or metoprolol; patients prescribed ACE inhibitors can receive enalaprilat; and those prescribed calcium channel blockers may receive nicardipine. If the patient is chronically treated with a beta-blocker, this drug should be maintained to avoid unmasking preexisting heart disease and to reduce the risk for postoperative atrial fibrillation. Clonidine should not be withheld in the perioperative setting due to the risk of rebound hypertension; a patch can be used to replace oral clonidine if needed, bearing in mind that it may take a day to achieve therapeutic blood levels with transdermal dosing.

The bottom line: it is safe to proceed to nonvascular surgery with this level of BP and avoid the morbidity of an unnecessary delay. If the patient becomes hypertensive in the perioperative period, selection of a short-acting beta-blocker would be reasonable given his baseline electrocardiogram (ECG).

CASE 89-1 *(continued)*

The patient went to surgery without hypertensive medication, did well, and did not suffer any perioperative complications. During his hospitalization, BP was maintained in 120–140/80–90 mm Hg range. The patient was sent to rehabilitation on no hypertension medications. Three days later the physiatrist called the discharging physician for advice regarding BP management since the patient as yet did not have a primary care physician and the BP was 165/95 mm Hg.

While it is possible BP elevations were situational, it was more likely he had long-standing hypertension, especially if there was evidence of target end-organ damage.

PRACTICE POINT

- It is not unusual for BP in patient with chronic hypertension to improve during hospitalization. BP usually returns to prehospital levels within weeks of discharge.

It is important that appropriate follow-up is made to monitor the patient for recurrent hypertension if BP medications are not resumed or to monitor the response to drug therapy if medications are initiated.

■ SHOULD BP MEDICATIONS BE STARTED AND IF SO WHICH ONE?

In most patients with stage I hypertension, therapy begins with lifestyle modification, and if the BP goal is not achieved, thiazide-type diuretics should be used as initial therapy for most patients, either alone or in combination with one of the other classes (ACE inhibitors, ARBs, beta-blockers, Calcium Channel Blockers, CCBs) that have also been shown to reduce one or more hypertensive complications in randomized controlled clinical trials. Selection of one of these other agents as initial therapy is recommended when a diuretic cannot be used or when a compelling indication is present that requires the use of a specific drug (such as beta-blockers and ACE-inhibitors for a patient with systolic heart failure). If the initial drug selected is not tolerated or is contraindicated, then a drug from one of the other classes proven to reduce cardiovascular events should be substituted.

Since most hypertensive patients will require two or more antihypertensive medications to achieve their BP goals, the addition of a second drug from a different class is often needed. When BP is >20 mm Hg above the systolic goal or 10 mm Hg above the diastolic goal, consideration should be given to initiate therapy with two drugs, either as separate prescriptions or in fixed-dose combinations.

CASE 89-1 *(continued)*

In retrospect, it would have been reasonable to begin an antihypertensive medication along with aspirin prior to discharge from the hospital, given evidence of target end-organ damage (possible inferior MI of indeterminate age on ECG) and to increase long-term compliance. Follow-up with a primary care provider is essential.

In this case, BP elevation by history was long-standing, and lifestyle modifications, which on average lower BP by only 5–10 mm Hg, will not likely be effective. A thiazide diuretic may be a good choice, particularly if the patient has calcium-oxalate nephrolithiasis and no evidence for hypercalcemia. Thiazides reduce urinary calcium excretion and can reduce the incidence of calcium stones. However, concurrent diuretic therapy and intravenous fluid should be avoided in hospitalized patients since saline hydration will tend to negate any antihypertensive benefit, yet the patient will still be at risk for electrolyte losses, particularly potassium. Alternatively, if this patient's ECG signifies the presence of coronary artery disease, agents that prevent secondary cardiac events should be considered.

PRACTICE POINT

- Concurrent diuretic therapy and intravenous fluid should be avoided in hospitalized patients since saline hydration will tend to negate any antihypertensive benefit, yet the patient will still be at risk for electrolyte losses, particularly potassium.

There may also be a role for using combination therapy (a beta-blocker and a thiazide) from the outset since this practice has been associated with more effective BP control. Clinical trial data demonstrate that it takes three or four BP medications on average to achieve excellent BP control. Optimal BP control resides in the outpatient setting.

CONCLUSION

Overtreatment of hypertension in the hospital setting without diligence in determining underlying precipitating factors may have serious consequences as in this case. Ideally, practitioners should initiate appropriate therapy in patients with evidence of target end-organ damage in the inpatient setting and arrange for close follow-up by a receiving physician to optimize BP when the patient is no longer acutely ill.

SUGGESTED READINGS

Axon RN, Cousineau L, Egan BM. Prevalence and management of hypertension in the inpatient setting: a systematic review. *J Hosp Med*. 2011;6:417–422.

Chobanian AV, Bakris GI, Black HR, Cushman WC, Izzo H. Seventh report of the Joint National Committee on Prevention, Detection, Evaluation and Treatment of High Blood Pressure. National High Blood Pressure Education Program Coordinating Committee. *Hypertension*. 2003;42:1206–1252.

Conen D, Martina B, Peruuchoud AP, Leimenstoll BM. High prevalence of newly detected hypertension in hospitalized patients: the value of inhospital 24-h blood pressure measurement. *J Hypertension*. 2006;24(2):301–306.

Herzog E, Frankenberger O, Aziz E, et al. A novel pathway for the management of hypertension for hospitalized patients. *Crit Path Cardiol*. 2007;6(4):150–160.

Simel DL, Orlando L. Is Listening for Abdominal Bruits Useful in the Evaluation of Hypertension? Update. page 35–37. The Rational Clinical Examination. Simel DL, Rennie DR, editors. McGraw-Hill. New York. 2009.

Tsapatsaris NT, Farha D. In: O'Donnell JM, Naquel PE, eds. *Surgical Intensive Care Medicine. Post Operative Hypertension*. 2nd ed. New York City: Springer; 2009:191–198.

CHAPTER 90

Hyperthermia and Fever

Chad S. Miller, MD, FACP, FHM
Jeffrey G. Wiese, MD, FACP, FSM, SFHM

Key Clinical Questions

1. What is the difference between hyperthermia and fever?
2. What are the underlying mechanisms of hyperthermia and fever?
3. What are the implications of treatment for hyperthermia and fever?
4. Who is at greatest risk of developing hyperthermia?
5. What are the lasting effects of prolonged hyperthermia?

CASE 90-1

An 82-year-old man was brought to the emergency department with altered mental status. His neighbor found him unresponsive in his apartment on an extremely hot, humid summer day. He has a history of poorly controlled type 2 diabetes, hypertension, benign prostatic hypertrophy, and urinary urgency. He was currently taking glipizide, lisinopril, hydrochlorothiazide (HCTZ), doxazosin, oxybutynin, and diphenhydramine.

His temperature was 40°C, a pulse of 120 beats per minute, a respiratory rate of 18 breaths per minute, a blood pressure of 90/60 mm Hg, and pulse oximetry of 98% on room air. He responds to a sternal rub, but is otherwise nonresponsive and does not follow commands. His skin is flushed, warm, and dry. His pupils are 4 mm and minimally responsive to light. Bowel sounds are present.

What is the most likely cause of this patient's altered mental status and hyperthermia?

This man most likely has heat stroke, but there are multiple contributing factors in this case. The ambient temperature is extremely hot significantly increasing the risk of heat stroke. Patients his age do not sense changes in temperature as well as younger adults. This man also takes oxybutynin and diphenhydramine, two medications with anticholinergic properties that make him susceptible to anticholinergic poisoning as well as lower his threshold for heat stroke. Although anticholinergic toxicity is possible, his lack of mydriasis and present bowel sounds suggest that this is not the primary contributing factor. Uncontrolled diabetes and HCTZ have also likely contributed to this man being chronically volume depleted, further lowering his threshold for heat stroke.

INTRODUCTION

Vital signs are routinely measured for all hospitalized patients on admission, during nursing shifts, and when infusions are being administered. Clinicians should be able to recognize when abnormal temperatures require immediate action to avoid adverse consequences that may be potentially life threatening.

The 99th percentile for healthy individuals defines the maximum oral temperature as 37.2°C (98.9°F) at 6 am and 37.7°C (99.9°F) at 4 PM. The normal daily temperature typically varies no more than 0.5°C (0.9°F). The hypothalamus thermoregulatory center maintains a normal temperature despite variations in environment causing heat dissipation from the skin and lungs balanced by metabolic activity from muscle and liver. The postprandial state, pregnancy, and endocrine disorders may affect body temperature. The morning temperature tends to be lower in the 2 weeks prior to ovulation in menstruating women and then rises by 0.6°C (1.6°F) with ovulation until the next period (**Table 90-1**).

HYPERTHERMIA AND FEVER PRESENTATIONS

HYPERTHERMIA

Hyperthermia is defined as an elevation in the body's temperature due to excess generation of heat, or the inability to eliminate heat. A fever is defined as a morning temperature > 37.2°C (98.9°F)

TABLE 90-1 Body Temperature Measurements

Type of reading	Normal 36.0°–38.0°C	Core body temperature is tightly regulated between a normal diurnal range of 36.0°C and 37.5°C.
Rectal	0.4°C (0.7°F) higher than oral readings	May be 0.2°–0.3°C higher than actual core body temperature
Oral	Lower readings due to mouth breathing	Influenced by eating, drinking, breathing devices, tachypnea, and mouth breathing
Tympanic membrane (TM)	Measures radiant heat from TM and nearby ear canal; more variable readings than oral or rectal modes	Preferred to oral measurements in patients with pulmonary disorders such as asthma or pneumonia
Axillary	Underestimates core body temperature	Not recommended

and an evening temperature >37.7°C (99.9°F). Fever is a subset of hyperthermia, and the two should be distinguished from each other because hyperthermia can rapidly cause death and does not respond to antipyretics.

Hyperthermia is the elevation of the body temperature due to imbalances in metabolic heat production and heat loss, or exposure to extreme environmental heat. This is not mediated by inflammatory cytokines. Body temperatures may rise to levels greater than 41.1°C. An infectious etiology rarely results in a fever this high unless the hypothalamic regulatory center has been damaged by the infection, as might occur with a brain abscess or severe meningitis. Other causes of hyperthermia include malignant hyperthermia, neuroleptic malignant syndrome, serotonin syndrome, anticholinergic drugs, sympathomimetic drugs, thyrotoxicosis, and heat stroke (**Table 90-2**).

The clinical presentation of the causes of hyperthermia is varied, but the most common presentation of anyone with hyperthermia is mental status changes or confusion. Hyperthermia can be difficult to distinguish from fever, but it should be considered in the presence of a high temperature and significant mental status changes, especially when infection has been excluded. Key historical clues such as exposure to extremely high ambient temperatures or to certain medications, anesthetics, or recreational drugs should guide the clinician's evaluation. Common offending agents include halothane, isoflurane, succinylcholine, and the recreational drugs cocaine, ecstasy, and amphetamines. An alteration in mental status is one of the earliest signs in 80% of patients with severe hyperthermia. Heat stroke is often preceded by symptoms of heat exhaustion such as fatigue, malaise, nausea, muscle cramping, and headache. The progression to mental status changes such as confusion or coma is consistent with heat stroke and the inability to dissipate excessive heat. The core temperature usually exceeds 40.0°C.

Certain populations are at greater risk for hyperthermia. The very young, very old, bedridden, and those confined to poorly ventilated areas without air conditioning are at significant risk for nonexertional heat stroke. Young men tend to be at greatest risk for exertional heat stroke, but anyone engaging in strenuous activity, especially in high ambient temperatures, is at risk. Outdoor athletes, especially football players, and military recruits have a higher incidence. Dehydration, medications with anticholinergic effects, and recreational drugs, may accelerate the time to heat stroke in susceptible populations.

PRACTICE POINT

- Hyperthermia can be difficult to distinguish from fever, but should be considered in the presence of a high temperature and significant mental status changes, especially when infection has been excluded. Key historical clues such as exposure to extremely high ambient temperatures or to certain medications, anesthetics, or recreational drugs should guide the clinician's evaluation.

Prolonged hyperthermia may result in irreversible neurologic damage. Severe morbidity and even death may result from disseminated intravascular coagulation, rhabdomyolysis, electrolyte disorders, and severe acid–base disturbances, often due to buildup of lactic acid, in the setting of sustained hyperthermia.

PRACTICE POINT

- Prolonged hyperthermia may result in irreversible neurologic damage. Severe morbidity and even death may result from disseminated intravascular coagulation, rhabdomyolysis, electrolyte disorders, and severe acid-base disturbances, often due to build-up of lactic acid, in the setting of sustained hyperthermia.

FEVER

Fever is the most common temperature disturbance in the hospital setting. Fever is the body's upregulation of the thermal set point, and it is mediated by the hypothalamus in response to cytokine activation. These cytokines include interleukin (IL)-1, IL-6, and tumor necrosis factor (TNF-α). Fever is defined as a core body temperature greater than 38.0°C. Because most microbial organisms have a defined thermal range for survival, it is theorized that fever is a teleological advantage in overcoming infection. However, there is no clinical evidence that fever hastens recovery from infection or that use of antipyretics delays recovery. While noninfectious causes of fever exist, the presumption should be that an infection is the cause of fever until excluded.

Many patients may be asymptomatic and have fever as the only sign of illness. In others, fever is one marker among a constellation of signs and symptoms. Symptoms that commonly accompany fever include diaphoresis, flushing, rigors, and chills. Rigors and chills are due to the quick alteration in the body's thermal set point, causing the sensation that the body's current temperature (under the newly elevated set point) is too low, thus inducing a sensation of chills. The rigors, isometric contraction of muscles, are an effort to elevate the body's core temperature to meet the new thermal set point.

In the elderly and residents of long-term-care facilities, a decline in functional status, confusion, incontinence, falling, deteriorating mobility, reduced food intake, or failure to cooperate with staff should prompt a temperature measurement and evaluation for potential infectious causes. Fever is less common in hemodialysis patients, as the core body temperature is lost with each dialysis episode; over time, the baseline thermal set point is adjusted to a value lower than normal. Elevations in temperate between 0.5°C and 1.0°C in dialysis patients should prompt evaluation for infection.

Infections are the most common cause of fever, but many noninfectious inflammatory conditions cause the release of proinflammatory cytokines with a febrile response. Noninfectious

TABLE 90-2 Common Causes of Hyperthermia

Malignant Hyperthermia
Mechanism: genetic disorder of calcium channels in skeletal muscle that allows an uncontrolled influx of calcium into the cell resulting in sustained muscle contraction and increased metabolism
Causes: inhalational anesthetics—halothane, enflurane, isoflurane; succinylcholine
When to suspect: hyperthermia in anyone receiving inhalational anesthetics or succinylcholine
Neuroleptic Malignant Syndrome (NMS)
Mechanism: unproven, but dopamine receptor blockade is thought to play a key role in precipitating NMS
Causes and examples:
1. Typical antipsychotic medications—haloperidol, chlorpromazine, loxapine
2. Atypical antipsychotic medications—aripiprazole, olanzapine, quetiapine, risperidone
3. Dopamine antagonists—metoclopramide, promethazine
When to suspect: hyperthermia, rigidity, altered mental status in a patient taking any of the classes of medications known to cause NMS
Serotonin Syndrome
Mechanism: overstimulation of 5-HT_{1A} receptors in the central grey nuclei and the medulla; 5-HT_2 receptors may also play a role
Causes and examples:
1. Excess precursors of serotonin or serotonin agonists—buspirone, L-dopa, lithium, LSD, L-tryptophan, trazodone
2. Increased release of serotonin—amphetamines, 3,4-Methylenedioxymethamphetamine (MDMA), cocaine, reserpine, fenfluramine
3. Reduced uptake of serotonin—Selective serotonin reuptake inhibitors (SSRIs), tricyclic antidepressants (TCAs), trazodone, venlafaxine, meperidine
4. Slowing of serotonin metabolism—monoamine oxidase inhibitors
When to suspect: hyperthermia, hyperhidrosis, confusion or agitation with significant autonomic and neurologic derangement
Sympathomimetic Poisoning/Overdose
Mechanism: central and peripheral disturbances in thermoregulation
Causes: amphetamines, methamphetamines, cocaine, MDMA or ectsasy
When to suspect: recreational drug users and other high-risk populations with hyperthermia, mental status changes, and evidence of adrenergic stimulus
Anticholinergic Poisoning/Exposure
Mechanism: central and peripheral muscarinic receptor blockade
Causes: antihistamines, atropine, belladonna alkaloids, carbamazepine, diphenhydramine, meclizine, phenothiazines
When to suspect: Hyperthermia, altered mental status, dry mouth, lack of perspiration, flushing, and urinary retention
Endocrine
Mechanism: elevated endogenous metabolism
Causes: thyrotoxicosis, pheochromocytoma
When to suspect: hyperthermia, adrenergic symptoms, hypertension, and no associated drug exposures or heat exposures
Heat Stroke
Mechanism: inability to dissipate heat
Causes: exposure to high ambient temperatures, strenuous exercise
When to suspect: hyperthermia, dry skin, delirium in a patient exposed to high temperatures or having undergone severe exercise
Central Nervous System Damage
Mechanism: damage of the hypothalamic regulatory center
Causes: subarachnoid hemorrhage, status epilepticus, hypothalamic injury
When to suspect: hyperthermia (> 104°F) with associated head trauma, central nervous system infection, or history of seizures

disorders rarely cause a fever greater than 38.9°C, although notable exceptions include adult Still disease, lymphoma, transfusion reactions, biologic cytokine therapy, as well as agents implicated in hyperthermia. Any temperature above this threshold should prompt an evaluation for infection, as well as consideration of hyperthermia (hyperpyrexia) not mediated by inflammatory cytokines, but by disrupted thermoregulation.

THE FIREPLACE METHOD APPROACH

HYPERTHERMIA

Hyperthermia is the result of a mismatch between heat production and heat loss, in the same way that overheating a home is due to a mismatch between heat production and heat loss from the home's fireplace. The resultant problems usually stem from one of three components: there is too much firewood being burned (too much fuel), too much fire (metabolism), or too much insulation (heat retention).

The fuel (firewood) for basal metabolism must be adequate in order to generate heat. This includes normoglycemia, adequate nutrition, and adequate muscle mass. Increased muscle mass is a risk factor for malignant hyperthermia, due to increased metabolic demands. The extra available fuel allows the body to reach the higher temperatures much more rapidly because the main source of increasing basal metabolism is through skeletal muscle.

Rarely, excessive fuel supplies the cause of hyperthermia; instead, the *body's metabolism* (fire) should be considered as a potential cause. Acute hyperthyroidism, malignant hyperthermia, neuroleptic malignant syndrome, and the serotonin syndrome are the common causes of acute elevations in metabolic rate. In these scenarios, the catalyst is endogenous (acute thyroid hormone elevations), or iatrogenic: anesthesia (in patients with a genetic predisposition), neuroleptics, or a combination of drugs that work on the serotonin receptors. The metabolism reaches levels far too great for the normal compensatory mechanisms of heat loss to handle.

Once fuel supplies and metabolism have been excluded, *causes of heat elimination/conservation* (insulation) should be considered. The vasoconstriction associated with cocaine, sympathomimetics, and anticholinergic drugs may result in hyperthermia due to the inability to expel heat. Although mortality from cocaine overdose increases substantially in hot weather due to the inability to dissipate heat, cocaine has not been shown to affect core temperature in the absence of external heat stress. Anticholinergics competitively antagonize muscarinic receptors in sweat glands, decreasing the body's ability to sweat, a phenomenon dependent on cholinergic nerve fibers.

If the foregoing categories have been excluded, *the mechanism for regulating the thermal set point* (uncontrollable fire) should be considered. Core body temperature is maintained through balancing the intrinsic mechanisms of heat production and heat loss. This equilibrium is rigorously managed by the hypothalamus, brain stem, and cervical spinal cord. While damage to any of these components may result in hyperthermia or hypothermia, the most common etiology is the administration of antipsychotic drugs. Barbiturates, opioids, tricyclic antidepressants, and benzodiazepines can cause central thermoregulatory failure resulting in either hypothermia or hyperthermia. Phenothiazines impair central thermoregulation and inhibit peripheral vasoconstriction.

Although usually obvious from the history, prolonged exposure to heat may cause hyperthermia. The history or manner in which the patient is brought into the hospital should provide the clinical clues.

FEVER

The approach to fever in the hospitalized patient should begin with the presumption that the fever is due to an infection, while simultaneously excluding noninfectious causes of fever and additional causes of hyperthermia.

Infectious causes

The approach to infectious causes of fever should begin with the most likely places for infection to reside. The lungs, blood, urine, skin, and sinuses are the most common sites of infection. Evaluation of all five is suggested unless the source is clinically apparent. The presenting symptoms should guide the evaluation, but where symptoms are not present, the hidden sources of infection should be considered (see Table 90-1). Based upon the Centers for Disease Control and Prevention's (CDC's) "opt out" recommendations, all patients with a reasonable possibility of having HIV should be tested unless the patient opts out of testing. HIV status should be determined early, as this may broaden the search for opportunistic infections. The role of atelectasis as a cause of fever is unclear; however, atelectasis probably does not cause fever in the absence of pulmonary infection.

Noninfectious causes

The noninfectious causes fall into three categories: vascular, inflammatory, autoimmune, and endocrine.

Vascular causes Any disruption in the vasculature is a potential cause of fever. The decreased blood supply from vascular compromise leads to tissue necrosis, which results in the release of inflammatory cytokines that may result in fever. Potential causes include cerebral infarction/hemorrhage, subarachnoid hemorrhage, myocardial infarction, ischemic bowel, fat emboli, deep venous thrombosis, pulmonary emboli, and gastrointestinal bleeding. It should be noted that hematomas may result in fever, not only from the underlying vascular injury but due to the immune activation during resorption, especially for a large hematoma.

Inflammatory causes Inflammatory causes of fever may be due to a cytokine response to noninfectious antigens. The body responds as if it is infected, even though the inflammatory response is to a noninfectious antigen. Examples are posttransfusion fever, drug fever, organ transplant rejection, and intravenous contrast dye reactions. Other inflammatory causes may be due to tissue injury or immune dysfunction. These include aspiration pneumonitis, acute respiratory distress syndrome (ARDS), gout, pseudogout, and neoplastic fevers. Treatment with organ-specific cytokine therapy (eg, interferon-γ, interleukin-2) usually results in fever through the same mechanisms, but, in contrast, the cytokines are introduced iatrogenically. It is important to note that after the age of 50, the incidence of fevers due to malignancy and autoimmune disease increase relative to infection.

Autoimmune causes Autoimmune disease overlaps the inflammatory and the vascular categories. By definition, autoimmune diseases have an inflammatory reaction to "self" antigens, and many autoimmune diseases have a concomitant vasculitis.

Endocrine causes Thyrotoxic storm and pheochromocytoma are rare causes of fever.

PREVALENCE AND ADJUSTMENTS

BASELINE PREVALENCE

Death from extreme temperatures remains relatively uncommon. Early diagnosis and treatment can often prevent mortality. In the United States a total of 3442 deaths from exposure to extreme heat were reported between 1999–2003. Of these deaths, 2239 (65%) were recorded as exposure to excessive heat and 1203 (35%) were due to nonexposure hyperthermia. From 2003 to 2005, the number of cases of malignant hyperthermia, related to anesthesia, increased from 372 to 521 per year in the United States.

FACTORS THAT IMPACT PREVALENCE

Age

There is a significant increased risk of dying from hyperthermia in adults over the age of 65. The ability to sense heat is reduced with age. The elderly have a higher threshold for sweating and cutaneous vasodilation. The use of medications, especially those with anticholinergic or diuretic effects, accentuate the risk of heat stroke in the elderly. Greater than 40% of all hypothermia- and hyperthermia-related deaths are in this age group.

Patients 65 years or older who are diabetic have a slightly higher risk of dying on hot days than other subjects [odds ratio (OR): 1.17; 95% confidence interval (CI) = 1.04–1.32].

Gender

Men have a twofold increased risk of death due to hyperthermia as compared to women. The discrepancy is likely explained by exertional heat illness that occurs in previously healthy young men during exercise. Men, on average, have a higher skeletal muscle mass for a given surface area. Therefore, the ability to dissipate heat is decreased compared to women. Typical scenarios include military exercises undertaken by personnel recently arrived in a hot country, and long-distance races that coincide with one of the first hot days of the year. The one exception to the male predominance is malignant hyperthermia. There is a slightly greater mortality risk for female patients.

Race, ethnicity

While there is a hereditary risk for malignant hyperthermia in the setting of anesthetics, it is not tightly associated with any one race. The better approach is to inquire as to a family history of problems following the administration of anesthetics.

THE HISTORY

HYPERTHERMIA

The causes of hyperthermia are often apparent from events immediately preceding the temperature elevation, such as severe heat exposure, exertion, or ingestion of drugs that affect thermoregulation.

MALIGNANT HYPERTHERMIA

- ***Has this patient recently been administered anesthetics or succinylcholine?*** If yes, this increases the likelihood of malignant hyperthermia; a positive family history of adverse reactions to anesthetics increases this possibility.

Neuroleptic malignant syndrome

- ***Is the patient taking neuroleptics?*** If yes, this increases the possibility of neuroleptic malignant syndrome (NMS). High-potency neuroleptic drugs with strong D2 receptor antagonism, such as haloperidol and thiothixene, are more likely to cause NMS than are lower-potency antipsychotics, such as chlorpromazine or thioridazine.
- ***Is this patient taking antipsychotic medications?*** If yes, this increases the likelihood of hypothalamic dysfunction resulting in extremes of temperature.

Serotonin syndrome

- ***Is this patient taking selective serotonin receptor inhibitors (SSRIs), monoamine oxidase inhibitors (MAOIs), meperidine, or linezolid, particularly in combination?*** If yes, this increases the possibility of serotonin syndrome. Linezolid has weak, reversible, competitive and noncompetitive MAOI activity.

Sympathomimetic

- ***Has this patient used cocaine or a sympathomimetic?*** Drugs with sympathomimetic properties include amphetamines, ephedrine/pseudoephedrine, which are present in over-the-counter decongestants and dietary agents (eg, Ma Huang). If yes, this increases the likelihood of heat illness due to inability to dissipate heat.

Anticholinergic

- ***Is this patient taking anticholinergic medication?*** Medications that have anticholinergic properties include antihistamines, parkinsonism medications, atropine/scopolamine, belladonna alkaloids such as phenobarbital, neuroleptics, antispasmodics, tricyclic antidepressants, and many species of plants, the most common being jimsonweed.

Endocrine

- ***Does this patient have a history of thyroid disease or is the patient currently taking thyroid medication?*** Thyroid disease is the most common endocrine disease that may manifest with elevated core body temperature.

Heat stroke

- ***Is the patient's temperature greater than 40°C?*** If yes, this increases the likelihood that this is hyperthermia and not mediated by inflammatory cytokines.
- ***Is it one of the hottest days of the year?*** If yes, the patient's heat dissipation mechanisms may be altered even if the patient is otherwise healthy.
- ***Has this patient recently undergone extreme exertion?*** If yes, the patient's heat dissipation mechanisms may be altered even if the patient is otherwise healthy.

CNS injury

- ***Does this patient have other signs of CNS infection?*** If yes, this may be the exception where both inflammatory mediators and hypothalamic derangement are contributing to the elevated temperature.
- ***Has this patient sustained recent head trauma?*** Intracranial hemorrhage may result in extremely high temperatures.
- ***Is this patient taking anticoagulants?*** Increases the potential for intracranial hemorrhage.

FEVER

Infectious causes

There are various risk factors for infection (**Table 90-3**).

- ***Does this patient note any potential infectious symptoms?*** If yes, the line of questioning should proceed as appropriate for the differential diagnosis in question (eg, if sputum production and cough are present, the line of questioning should address the diagnoses of pneumonia, bronchitis, etc). If the patient has none of these symptoms, subsequent questions should be directed at risk factors for infection and hidden sources of infection.

TABLE 90-3 Risk Factors for Infection

Exposure Risks
• Indwelling catheter (vascular or urinary)?
• Intravenous drug use?
• Open sores?
• Resides in long-term care facility?
• Sick contacts?
• Recent travel?
• Occupational exposures?
• Pets and/or animal contacts?
• Recent trauma or surgery?
• Recent hospitalization?
Innate Risks
• Is this patient HIV positive?
• Does this patient have diabetes?
• Is this patient on immunosuppressive medications?
• Is there a history of recurrent infections?

- ***Does this patient have any potential predisposing factors for infection?*** If yes, the line of questioning should proceed as appropriate for the risk factor being considered (eg, if there is a recent sick-contact exposure, the nature of the exposure and the symptoms of the index case should be explored). For all affirmative answers, the physical examination and laboratory/study examination should be directed to further evaluate the patient's risk.

  Because noninfectious causes of fever are usually less life threatening to the patient, the line of questioning for these diagnoses should proceed after the pretest probability for infection has been sufficiently reduced or excluded. Patients presenting to the hospital with fever on the day of admission are much more likely to have an infection than they are to have a noninfectious cause of their fever (90% vs 10%). As the hospitalization proceeds, however, the pretest probability for noninfectious causes increases (60% vs 40%), and this line of questioning should be routinely employed.

Vascular causes

- ***Does this patient have signs of focal neurologic deficits or increased intracranial pressure?*** If yes, evaluate for intracranial bleed.
- ***Does this patient complain of chest pain and have risk factors for atherosclerosis?*** If yes, consider myocardial infarction, especially if the fever is low grade.
- ***Has this patient sustained a severe fracture?*** If yes, the likelihood of fat emboli is increased.
- ***Is this patient in a hypercoagulable state?*** If yes, the likelihood of venous thromboembolism is increased.
- ***Does this patient have signs or a history of vascular stasis?*** If yes, the likelihood of venous thromboembolism is increased.
- ***Has this patient recently been hospitalized or had surgery?*** If yes, the likelihood of venous thromboembolism is increased.
- ***Does this patient have risks for endothelial damage (smoking, other inflammatory diseases, etc)?*** If yes, the likelihood of venous thromboembolism is increased.
- ***Does this patient have signs of bruising or bleeding?*** If yes, these could be signs of vascular damage and tissue necrosis.
- ***Does this patient have a large hematoma?*** If yes, large hematomas may cause fever from both vascular injury and immune activation during resorption.
- ***Has this patient recently had intravenous access or engaged in intravenous drug use?*** This increases the likelihood for thromboembolism or infection.

Antigen stimulation and inflammation causes

- ***Has this patient received a transfusion of blood products in the last 24 hours?*** If yes, this increases the likelihood of serum sickness or a reaction to blood products.
- ***Is the patient receiving a medication, especially intravenous, known to cause drug fever (eg, antibiotics)?*** If yes and infectious causes are unlikely, consider drug fever.
- ***Are routine cultures negative for infection?*** If yes, this decreases the pretest probability of common infections and must increase the likelihood of other causes, including noninfectious causes.
- ***Is this patient at risk for aspiration?*** If yes, consider aspiration pneumonitis.
- ***Does this patient have a transplanted organ?*** If yes, this increases the risk that the fever is from transplant rejection. However, unless there is a clear indication of transplant organ dysfunction, a thorough evaluation for infection must be completed before this etiology is pursued, because these individuals are on immunosuppressive medications.
- ***Is this patient maintaining proper oxygen saturation?*** If no, ARDS, could be considered. Although many underlying causes of ARDS are infectious, a significant number are noninfectious (eg, pancreatitis).
- ***Is this patient complaining of severe joint pain?*** If yes, consider potential for gout and pseudogout.
- ***Has this patient received intravenous contrast in the previous 24 hours?*** If yes, increase the risk for contrast dye reactions.
- ***Has this patient had routine cancer screening?*** If no, consider evaluating the patient for malignancy, based upon age and gender, among other factors.
- ***Does this patient have additional risk factors for malignancy?*** If yes, risk factors such as tobacco smoking, HIV, family history, should prompt additional evaluation if no other cause of fever is determined.

Inflammatory and vascular (autoimmune) causes

- ***Does this patient or a family member have a history of autoimmune disease or vasculitis?*** If yes, the likelihood of the patient having an autoimmune disease may increase.
- ***Does this patient have other complaints consistent with autoimmune disease such as arthralgias, arthritis, myalgias, rash, photosensitivity, Reynaud phenomenon, pulmonary/renal disease, or other signs of severe inflammation?*** If yes, this should prompt a further workup for autoimmune disease.

Endocrine causes

- ***Does this patient have a family history of thyroid disease, known thyroid disease, or symptoms suggesting hyperthyroidism?*** See Table 90-5.
- ***Does this patient have a family history of pheochromocytoma, known pheochromocytoma, or symptoms suggesting pheochromocytoma?***

THE EXAMINATION

HYPERTHERMIA

If the patient has a pontine hemorrhage, the temperature may have a significant role in prognosis (**Table 90-4**).

Although unusual to reach extremely high temperatures, thyrotoxicosis may cause elevated temperatures through significantly increasing the basal metabolism. **Table 90-5** lists physical exam findings that may be helpful in making the diagnosis of hyperthyroidism.

The diagnosis of NMS based upon Levenson and Sternbach requires meeting three major criteria, or two major and four minor criteria plus a supportive history (**Table 90-6**). Infection, metabolic disturbances, and substance abuse must be excluded.

The Hunter Serotonin Toxicity Criteria have replaced Sternbach's criteria for serotonin syndrome (**Table 90-7**). The Hunter criteria are

TABLE 90-4 Utility of Temperature Predicting Mortality in a Patient with a Pontine Hemorrhage

	+LR (95% CI)	−LR (95% CI)
Temp > 39°C predictive of mortality in a patient with a pontine hemorrhage	23.7 (1.5, 371)	0.4 (0.2, 0.6)

TABLE 90-5 Utility of Clinical Findings for Diagnosing Hyperthyroidism

	+LR (95% CI)	−LR (95% CI)
Pulse ≥ 90 beats/min	4.4 (3.8, 5.1)	0.2 (0.2, 0.3)
Skin moist and warm	6.7 (5.0, 9.1)	0.7 (0.7, 0.7)
Enlarged thyroid	2.3 (2.1, 2.5)	0.1 (0.1, 0.2)
Eyelid retraction	31.5 (16.6, 59.7)	0.7 (0.6, 0.7)
Eyelid lag	17.6 (9.2, 33.7)	0.8 (0.8, 0.8)
Fine finger tremor	11.4 (8.7, 14.8)	0.3 (0.3, 0.4)
Wayne index ≥ 20 points	18.2 (2.9, 113.5)	

TABLE 90-7 Hunter Serotonin Toxicity Criteria

Hunter Serotonin Toxicity Criteria:

In the presence of a serotonergic agent, must meet one of the five criteria below

1. Spontaneous clonus
2. Inducible clonus and agitation or diaphoresis
3. Ocular clonus and agitation or diaphoresis
4. Tremor and hyperreflexia
5. Hypertonic and temperature > 38°C and the presence of either ocular clonus or inducible clonus

84% sensitive and 97% specific for diagnosing serotonin toxicity. The positive likelihood ratio is 28.0 and the negative likelihood ratio is 0.16.

Distinguishing between serotonin syndrome and neuroleptic malignant syndrome is difficult. Some have suggested that patients with NMS demonstrate higher fevers and more pronounced extrapyramidal effects, while patients with serotonin syndrome have lower fevers, myoclonus, and gastrointestinal symptoms.

FEVER

When pursuing infectious etiologies, the physical exam should be directed by the presenting complaints but should still maintain a comprehensive evaluation of all organs, including all aspects of the skin. Because pneumonia and bacteremia are two of the most common diagnoses in the inpatient setting, it is important to fully evaluate for these possibilities.

The patient's perception of fever, or the examiner simply detecting an abnormally warm forehead, is associated with an increasing likelihood of fever before a fever has been objectively detected. The patient's perception carries a positive likelihood ratio of 2.9 (95% CI: 1.1–8.0) and the finding of a warm forehead carries a positive likelihood ratio of 2.9 (95% CI: 2.5–3.5).

Physical exam findings or maneuvers that may help with the diagnosis of bacteremia are listed in **Table 90-8**. The presence of hypotension is the most helpful for increasing the probability of bacteremia. Being below the age of 50 or having a temperature less than 38.5°C is the most helpful for ruling out bacteremia. This does not consider whether the patient is HIV positive.

Physical exam findings or maneuvers that may help with the diagnosis of pneumonia are listed in **Table 90-9**. The most helpful findings are diminished breath sounds, bronchial breath sounds, egophony, cachexia, percussion dullness, and Heckerling score of 4 or 5. The absence of any of the findings above is not helpful for ruling out pneumonia.

For diagnosing meningitis, nuchal rigidity assessment can be helpful (**Table 90-10**).

TABLE 90-6 Criteria for the Diagnosis of Neuroleptic Malignant Syndrome

Major Criteria for NMS	Minor Criteria for NMS
Fever	Tachycardia
Muscular rigidity	Labile blood pressure
Elevated creatinine phosphokinase (or aldolase, creatine kinase)	Tachypnea
	Altered consciousness
	Sweating
	Leukocytosis

For a few of the noninfectious causes of fever, there are significant physical exam findings that may aid in diagnosis. For example, **Table 90-11** shows findings helpful for diagnosing a pulmonary embolism. The most helpful findings are a high probability Wells score or unilateral calf pain. A temperature greater than 38°C suggests an alternative diagnosis.

The findings helpful for detecting deep vein thrombosis are provided in **Table 90-12**. The most helpful findings are a history of active cancer, asymmetric calf swelling, and high pretest probability Wells score.

THE LABORATORY APPROACH

HYPERTHERMIA

A creatine phosphokinase or aldolase evaluation should be ordered. These tests are usually highly elevated in malignant hyperthermia, NMS, or serotonin syndrome, but they may also be elevated in sympathomimetic overdose, anticholinergic overdose, and heat stroke. If infection remains likely, an evaluation of the central nervous system (CNS) is warranted, and a diagnostic lumbar puncture should be performed if there are no signs of increased intracranial pressure or focal neurologic deficits.

FEVER

The history and physical exam should guide the laboratory approach based upon the pretest probability for serious infection or underlying malignancy. If serious infection remains likely, the laboratory approach should include a complete blood count, complete metabolic panel, blood cultures, urinalysis, and chest X-ray. A left shift in the white blood cell count with bandemia, toxic granulations, and Dohle bodies suggests bacteremia (**Figure 90-1**). A C-reactive protein level may be helpful to screen for the presence of disease in patients with low-grade or borderline fever.

TABLE 90-8 Utility of Clinical Findings for Diagnosing Bacteremia

	+LR (95% CI)	−LR (95% CI)
Age 50 or greater	1.4 (1.2, 1.6)	0.3 (0.1, 0.8)
Temperature ≥ 38.5°C	1.2 (1.1, 1.3)	0.5 (0.2, 1.0)
Tachycardia	1.2 (1.1, 1.4)	0.7 (0.6, 0.9)
Respiratory rate > 20	0.9 (0.8, 1.1)	1.2 (0.8, 1.7)
Hypotension	2.6 (1.6, 4.4)	0.9 (0.9, 1.0)
Confusion or depressed sensorium	1.5 (1.3, 1.8)	0.9 (0.8, 1.0)

TABLE 90-9 Utility of Clinical Findings for Diagnosing Pneumonia

	+LR (95% CI)	−LR (95% CI)
Diminished breath sounds	2.3 (1.9, 2.8)	0.8 (0.7, 0.9)
Bronchial breath sounds	3.3 (2.0, 5.6)	0.9 (0.8, 1.0)
Egophony	4.1 (2.1, 7.8)	0.9 (0.9, 1.0)
Crackles in patients with cough and fever	1.8 (1.2, 2.7)	0.8 (0.7, 0.9)
Absence of sore throat	1.8 (1.3, 2.5)	0.7 (0.6, 0.9)
Absence of rhinorrhea	2.2 (1.5, 3.2)	0.8 (0.7, 0.9)
Cachexia	4.0 (1.7, 9.6)	0.9 (0.8, 1.0)
Abnormal mental status	1.9 (1.2, 3.0)	0.9 (0.9, 1.0)
Temperature > 37.8°C	2.0 (1.5, 2.6)	0.7 (0.6, 0.8)
Respiratory rate > 28/min	2.0 (1.4, 2.8)	0.8 (0.7, 0.9)
Heart rate > 100 beats/min	1.6 (1.4, 1.7)	0.8 (0.7, 0.9)
Percussion dullness	3.0 (1.7, 5.2)	0.9 (0.8, 1.0)
Heckerling score, 4 or 5 findings	8.2 (5.8, 11.5)	

If there is reversal of usual peak and trough temperatures, disseminated tuberculosis (TB) and typhoid fever could be considered. A temperature–pulse dissociation with relative bradycardia may be seen with typhoid fever, brucellosis, leptospirosis, babesiosis, malaria, legionella, viral hemorrhagic fevers, gram-negative invasive rods (eg, Escherichia coli, Salmonella, Shigella), factitious fever, and some drug-induced fevers. Relative bradycardia in an obscure febrile illness in the hospital, in the absence of pneumonia, suggests a drug fever–hypersensitivity reaction marked primarily by fever and a pulse–temperature deficit with no cutaneous manifestations. It is estimated that up to 10% of patients hospitalized in the United States have fevers due to drug hypersensitivity.

Fever patterns of hospitalized patients are often of limited utility, but characteristic tertian (every third day) or quotidian (every fourth day) fevers should prompt consideration of *Plasmodium vivax* or *Plasmodium malaria*, respectively. If exposure is likely, this would guide test ordering to include thick and thin blood smears.

Fevers that last for 3–10 days followed by similar afebrile periods (Pel-Ebstein fevers) are seen with lymphomas, including Hodgkin lymphoma. Fevers every 21 days accompanying neutropenia are associated with a condition termed cyclic neutropenia.

RARE CAUSES

Pheochromocytoma, a neuroendocrine tumor of the medulla of the adrenal glands, or thyrotoxic storm, may increase the metabolic rate to a point where the body generates heat faster than it can be dissipated.

TABLE 90-10 Utility of Nuchal Rigidity for Diagnosing Meningitis

	+LR (95% CI)	−LR (95% CI)
Nuchal rigidity	3.0 (2.1, 4.2)	0.1 (0, 2.0)

TABLE 90-11 Utility of Clinical Findings for Diagnosing Pulmonary Embolus

	+LR (95% CI)	−LR (95% CI)
Temperature > 38°C	0.4 (0.3, 0.7)	1.1 (1.0, 1.2)
Pulse > 100/min	1.2 (0.9, 1.5)	0.9 (0.8, 1.1)
Respiratory rate > 30/min	2.0 (1.5, 2.8)	0.9 (0.8, 0.9)
Systolic blood pressure < 100 mm Hg	1.9 (1.1, 3.0)	1.0 (0.9, 1.0)
Wheezes	0.2 (0.1, 0.4)	1.1 (1.1, 1.1)
Unilateral calf pain or swelling	2.3 (1.8, 3.0)	0.9 (0.8, 1.0)
Wells score, moderate probability, 2–6 points	1.7 (1.5, 2.0)	
Wells score, high probability, 7 or more points	5.0 (2.5, 10)	

Rare causes of fever are covered in Chapter 191, Fever of Unknown Origin (FUO).

TREATMENT

HYPERTHERMIA

Once the diagnosis of hyperthermia is established, any potential offending drugs should be discontinued. The central core temperature should be monitored continuously by rectal, esophageal, or tympanic probe. All vital signs should be closely monitored as well. Aggressive volume resuscitation is extremely important. If rhabdomyolysis is significant, intravenous fluids are essential to avoid the risks of myoglobinuria. Active measures should be taken to lower body temperature (**Table 90-13**). The best method is debated, but direct application of ice packs to the groin, axilla, and neck can be used. Evaporative cooling may be used where the naked patient is sprayed with alcohol and water and cooled with fans. Immersion in cool water is an option but may interfere with resuscitation and may have more complications from vasoconstriction. Other methods include extracorporeal bypass, cooling blankets, and iced peritoneal or gastric lavage. To prevent excessive cooling, these methods should be halted when core body temperature reaches 38.5°C.

Antipyretics, such as nonsteroidal anti-inflammatory drugs (NSAIDs) or acetaminophen, have no role in hyperthermia because the actions of these medications are distinct from the underlying mechanisms of hyperthermia. Acetaminophen can hasten hepatic damage, and salicylates can worsen existing coagulopathy.

TABLE 90-12 Utility of Clinical Findings for Diagnosing Deep Venous Thrombosis

	+LR (95% CI)	−LR (95% CI)
Active cancer	2.9 (2.4, 3.6)	0.9 (0.8, 0.9)
Recent immobilization	1.6 (1.3, 2.1)	0.9, (0.8, 0.9)
Recent surgery	1.6 (1.3, 1.9)	0.9 (0.9, 1.0)
Any calf or ankle swelling	1.2 (1.1, 1.3)	0.7 (0.6, 0.8)
Asymmetric calf swelling, ≥ 2 cm	2.1 (1.8, 2.5)	0.5 (0.4, 0.7)
Swelling of entire leg	1.5 (1.2, 1.8)	0.8 (0.6, 0.9)
Superficial venous dilation	1.6 (1.4, 1.9)	0.9 (0.8, 0.9)
Wells score, high pretest probability	5.2 (3.2, 8.5)	

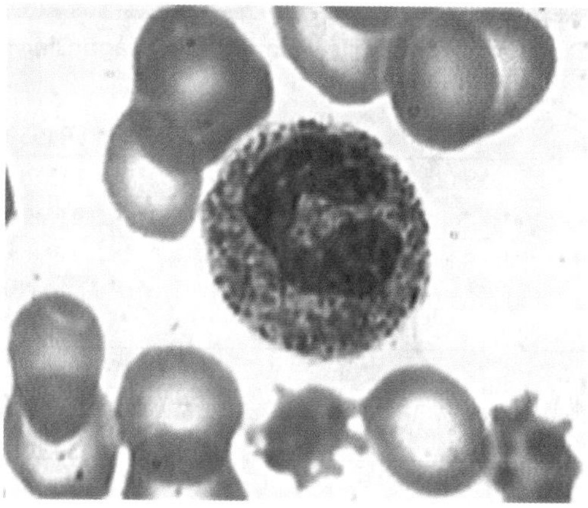

Figure 90-1 *Toxic granulations of a neutrophil.*

FEVER

NSAIDs and acetaminophen are useful for treating fever. In short, NSAIDs decrease prostaglandin E2 through inhibition of cyclooxygenase (COX)-1 and COX-2. Acetaminophen is a poor inhibitor of COX in the periphery and is thought to work as an inhibitor of COX-3, which is located in the CNS. There is no convincing evidence that treating a fever changes time to recovery from infection. Preexisting cardiac, cerebrovascular, or pulmonary disease is aggravated by fever, and aggressive treatment should be considered. Aspirin should not be used for patients with thyrotoxic storm; it can displace thyroid hormone from thyroid binding globulin and thereby increase free T4.

Ultimately, the underlying cause of the fever should be targeted, whether it is infectious, malignant, or autoimmune in nature.

TABLE 90-13 Additional Treatments for Specific Causes of Hyperthermia

Cause of Hyperthermia	Specific Additional Treatments
1. Malignant hyperthermia	Dantrolene, hyperventilation with 100% oxygen
2. Neuroleptic malignant syndrome	Bromocriptine, dantrolene, muscle relaxants
3. Serotonin syndrome	Serotonin antagonists, propranolol, benzodiazepines, cyproheptadine
4. Sympathomimetic	Sympatholytics, benzodiazepines
5. Anticholinergics	Physostigmine (rarely needed), sedatives
6. Endocrine	Propranolol, methimazole
7. Heat stroke	Supportive care
8. CNS injury/infection	Antibiotics

SUGGESTED READINGS

Cunha B. The clinical significance of fever patterns. *Inf Dis Clin N Am.* 1996;10:33–44.

Gruber MP. Diagnosing neuroleptic malignant syndrome. *Chest.* 2004;125:1960–1961.

Marik PE. Fever in the ICU. *Chest.* 2000;117:855–869.

Martinez M, Devenport L, Saussy J, Martinez J. Drug-associated heat stroke. *South Med J.* 2002;95:799–802.

McGee SR. *Evidence-Based Physical Diagnosis.* 2nd ed. St. Louis, MO: Saunders Elsevier; 2007.

CHAPTER 91

Hypotension

Danielle Jones, MD
Anna Kho, MD
Lorenzo Di Francesco, MD, FACP, FHM

Key Clinical Questions

1. What symptoms and signs should be assessed in the initial evaluation of a patient with reported hypotension?
2. What are the major categories of shock?
3. What are the common iatrogenic complications that produce hypotension in the hospital?

INTRODUCTION

According to the Agency for Health Care Research and Quality (AHRQ), as many as 52,000 patients experience hypotension while hospitalized, leading to 162 deaths and an average of 3.7 additional hospital days in the United States annually. Hypotension may be the presenting reason for hospital admission or it may develop during hospitalization, sometimes as an iatrogenic complication. Because patients with hypotension may decompensate quickly, suffer irreversible end-organ damage, and ultimately die, clinicians should be able to recognize the clinical presentation of patients with life-threatening or reversible causes of hypotension and appropriately intervene.

Deviations from "normal" blood pressure must be considered in the context of the patient's baseline blood pressure. A patient's blood pressure normally varies depending on the time of day, even from minute-to-minute, and typically decreases during sleep. Arterial monitoring has shown that the systolic and diastolic blood pressure also varies with the respiratory cycle and with each heartbeat. Although hypotension typically refers to blood pressure lower than 90/60 mm Hg, some patients may be completely asymptomatic at such readings, whereas other patients may develop clinically important hypotensive symptoms at much higher readings. A patient with advanced cirrhosis, for example, may have a chronic stable systolic blood pressure of 85–90 mm Hg that requires no intervention, whereas a severely hypertensive patient may experience a stroke, myocardial infarction, or renal insufficiency from relative hypotension with "normal" blood pressure readings. Acute decreases in mean arterial pressure (typically more than 25%), such as after receiving an antihypertensive medication, put patients at greatest risk for such end-organ damage.

CASE 91-1

The hospital's rapid response team was summoned to the bedside of an 87-year-old man who had recently undergone a total hip replacement after sustaining a hip fracture from a mechanical fall. His vital signs were notable for no discernible blood pressure, a heart rate of 110, respiratory rate of 20, O_2 saturation of 95% (2 liters via nasal cannula), and a temperature of 96° F. Telemetry review revealed sinus tachycardia. Postoperatively he had an agitated delirium, developed renal insufficiency, and became hypertensive. He had received 10 mg of intravenous (IV) hydralazine for a blood pressure of 180/100 mm Hg 30 minutes earlier.

His palpable systolic blood pressure after placement in the Trendelenburg position was noted to be 70 mm Hg. Rapid infusion of normal saline was ordered. His usual antihypertensive medications were held, and he was transferred to the intensive care unit.

Of note, a potent vasodilator like short-acting nifedipine, hydralazine use in acutely ill patients, especially the elderly, can be unpredictable. Renal insufficiency prolongs its half-life. Treatment of the underlying condition that caused this patient's hypertension (agitated delirium) is likely to be more effective and safer than using antihypertensive agents to treat the elevated blood pressure directly.

IS THE REPORTED BLOOD PRESSURE MEASUREMENT ACCURATE?

After quickly ensuring that the patient is alert and responsive and that ACLS does not need to be initiated, the first step is to determine whether the reported blood pressure reading is a valid measure of intraarterial blood pressure; this requires assessing the blood pressure manually. Many factors may affect the immediate accuracy of a blood pressure measurement, including the device used (cuff size, leaky bulb, faulty aneroid device), the technique or bias of the examiner (positioning of patient, placement of the cuff, inappropriately rapid deflation, excess bell pressure), and a noisy environment. Most errors overestimate the blood pressure, so a report of low blood pressure should alert the clinician to an impending emergency. In general, it is best to use the palpatory method first to avoid underinflation in patients with an auscultatory gap and overinflation in those with a very low blood pressure.

PRACTICE POINT

The palpatory method

- If the blood pressure cannot be appreciated by indirect blood pressure auscultation, systolic blood pressure can be determined by palpation to within 10 mm Hg.
  1. Rapidly inflate the blood pressure cuff to 70 mm Hg and increase by 10 mm Hg increments while palpating the radial pulse.
  2. Note the level of pressure when the pulse disappears and subsequently reappears during deflation.*
  3. Systolic blood pressures by the palpatory method measure approximately 7 mm Hg lower than by the auscultatory value.

*The patient's systolic blood pressure is identified when the radial pulse reappears.

When assessing a hypotensive patient, the examiner should obtain a blood pressure reading by inflating the bladder to a pressure 20–30 mm Hg above the level previously determined by palpation with a manual device. Interobserver variation increases when arrhythmias such as atrial fibrillation cause a variable cardiac output from beat to beat; examiners should ignore premature beats as well as the subsequent beat because they do not represent mean arterial pressure.

DOES THE BLOOD PRESSURE READING REFLECT CENTRAL ARTERIAL PRESSURE?

After a low blood pressure is confirmed, the next step is to determine whether the blood pressure reading reflects an acute drop in central arterial pressure. In general during their first encounters with patients, physicians should personally record blood pressure measurements in both arms and, depending on the reason for admission and comorbidities, obtain orthostatic blood pressure readings. In an asymptomatic patient who has a history of vascular disease, a targeted vascular examination should be performed. Any hemodynamically significant vascular stenosis will result in a systolic difference of at least 10 or 15 mm Hg. To perform an optimal assessment and control for normal variation in blood pressure and other factors such as impaired baroreceptors, two examiners should measure the upper extremity blood pressure at the same time, and then change sides. If there is a discrepancy in blood pressure readings, the higher of the two readings reflects the central blood pressure, and subsequent blood pressures should be checked in the higher arm. Uncommonly, patients may have bilateral stenoses in both subclavian arteries, resulting in low blood pressure in both arms, but in this setting a low blood pressure reading would be unlikely to cause symptoms of decreased perfusion unless accompanied by vascular disease elsewhere. If upper extremity vascular disease is suspected as the etiology for inaccurate upper extremity blood pressure readings, large thigh cuffs can sometimes be used (with the patient reclined), but the patient's body habitus and the presence of diffuse vascular disease may limit success (**Table 91-1**).

PRACTICE POINT

Postural hypotension

- Normally the diastolic pressure remains the same or rises slightly and the systolic pressure stays the same or drops slightly when a patient stands.
  - The diastolic pressure almost never drops, and when it does, the drop is small and the systolic pressure will rise so that mean arterial pressure (DBP + 0.4 [SBP – DBP]) does not change.
- Hypotension in the upright position compared with the recumbent position is caused by the following:
  - Volume depletion from hemorrhage, surgery, adrenal insufficiency, or diuretics
  - Neurogenic factors from some antihypertensive medications, autonomic dysfunction due to diabetes, Shy-Drager syndrome, prolonged bedrest, severe heart failure due to inability to increase cardiac output with standing
- Failure of the pulse rate to rise in response to an orthostatic drop in blood pressure suggests neurogenic factors rather than volume depletion.
  - Exceptions include patients receiving β-blockers or nondihydropyridine calcium channel blockers and patients with predominant vagal insufficiency (some diabetics, cardiac transplant and patients with Wernicke encephalopathy).
- Measure blood pressure and pulse after the patient has rested in the supine position for five minutes, then stand for two to three minutes.
  - Avoid the sitting position unless the patient is unable to stand due to partial equilibration prior to standing.
  - Postural hypotension is defined as a fall in systolic blood pressure of ≥ 20 mm Hg or < 90 mm Hg associated with symptoms.

DOES THE LOW BLOOD PRESSURE READING REFLECT THE PATIENT'S AVERAGE BLOOD PRESSURE?

The next step is to determine whether the patient is experiencing any symptoms related to low blood pressure. If the patient is asymptomatic, the clinician has more time to review the previous days' blood pressure measurements and hospital record with the goal to review and adjust any medications that may be contributing. Assuming a confirmed accurate low blood pressure reading, asymptomatic patients are more likely to be young and healthy, pregnant, or have systemic diseases such as severe hypothyroidism, chronic adrenal insufficiency, heart failure, cirrhosis, or vascular disease.

WHAT ARE THE SYMPTOMS AND SIGNS OF HYPOTENSION?

Symptoms and signs of hypotension relate to the underlying pathophysiology of low blood pressure. The mechanism of injury includes inadequate blood flow to tissues, leading to inability to meet nutritional requirements and clear toxic metabolites, resulting

TABLE 91-1 Etiologies and Classifications of Hypotension

Anaphylaxis/Anaphylactic Shock	Neurologic
Cardiogenic and obstructive	Age-related
Acute coronary syndrome	Central nervous system
Arrhythmias	Medullary stroke
Cardiomyopathy	Parkinsonism
Congestive heart failure	Shy-Drager syndrome
Valvulopathy	Wernicke syndrome
Pulmonary embolism	Dysautonomia
Pulmonary hypertension	Diabetes
Cardiac tumors	Postprandial
Cardiac tamponade	Peripheral neuropathy
Tension pneumothorax	Amyloidosis
Drug-Induced	HIV
Alcohol	Sensory
Anesthesia	Alcohol
Antidepressants	Syphilis
Antihypertensives	Vasomotor
Antipsychotics	Emotional
Anxiolytics	Micturition
General anesthesia	Orthostatic
Narcotics	Anemia
Endocrinologic	Dehydration
Adrenal insufficiency	Endocrine-mediated
Diabetes	Medication-induced
Hypothyroidism	Neurally mediated
Hypovolemia	Pregnancy
Hemorrhage	Structural
Dehydration	Pregnancy (pressure on the inferior vena cava)
Dialysis	Trauma
Infectious	Vascular
Septic shock	Aortic dissection or rupture
Measurement error	Peripheral vascular disease
	Pulmonary embolism

in the development of shock as the body attempts to increase vital organ perfusion to meet metabolic demands. Major components to consider when assessing hypotension and shock are (1) cardiac output (stroke volume multiplied by heart rate), (2) blood volume, and (3) systemic vascular resistance.

Symptoms and signs of hypotension depend on the mechanism of low blood pressure, the acuity of the drop, and the patient's overall health and age. Initially, patients may experience lightheadedness, dizziness, syncope, or even no symptoms. The examiner should assess the patient's hemodynamic stability by noting whether the patient appears acutely ill and obtain a complete set of vital signs. An abnormal heart rate may affirm that the hypotension is uncompensated and, therefore, unstable. Both bradycardia and tachycardia should prompt you to obtain an electrocardiogram (ECG). Pulsus paradoxus is by definition an exaggeration of the normal inspiratory respiratory fall in systolic blood pressure (>10 mm Hg). It is most commonly associated with cardiac tamponade and severe obstructive lung disease, but it can also be seen in tension pneumothorax, massive pulmonary embolism, severe mitral stenosis with right heart failure, cardiogenic shock, and/or severe hypovolemic shock.

The initial examination should include an assessment of volume status (by estimating central venous pressure and noting urine output), cardiac output (by examining heart and lungs), and perfusion of organs (by assessing the patient's mental status, the presence of pain, and the perfusion of the extremities). Skin pallor and the degree of diaphoresis should be examined, and recent administration of medications reviewed.

FRAMEWORK OF EVALUATION

Upon arrival, the examiner should manually confirm the low blood pressure, and then, if the patient appears unstable, lower the head of the bed, place the patient on a bedside monitor, and evaluate for the presence of a shockable tachyarrhythmia or evidence of severe bradyarrhythmia that might require administration of atropine and possibly pacing. If the patient is in extremis, advanced cardiac life support (ACLS) protocols should be followed. **Figure 91-1** provides the initial assessment and stabilization algorithm. The examiner should rapidly determine the likely mechanism of the patient's hypotension. Most causes of hypotension will respond to aggressive fluid resuscitation; however, excessive fluid expansion may worsen right and left ventricular failure. Treatment of cardiogenic hypotension, therefore, is directed at the underlying etiology.

While resuscitating a hypotensive patient, the clinician should communicate with the patient's bedside nurse and others familiar with the patient to help identify changes in mental status, and perform a focused chart review to assess vital signs, urine output, and risk factors for causes of hypotension. Always review the notes for the last 24 hours and the medications that have recently been administered (**Table 91-2**). Discontinue any medications that likely exacerbated or caused the hypotension. Order stat studies including 12-lead ECG, cardiac enzymes, complete blood count, comprehensive metabolic profile, coagulation profile, lactate, arterial blood gas, blood and urine cultures, and type and cross for possible blood transfusion.

HYPOVOLEMIC HYPOTENSION

The presentation of hypovolemic hypotension depends on the etiology, severity, and duration of the problem as well as the patient's age and underlying medical conditions. Patients typically have abnormal vital signs (tachycardia and tachypnea) and a narrow pulse pressure in addition to low blood pressure. Symptomatic patients appear pale with flattened neck veins and cool, clammy, or mottled extremities, poor capillary refill; diminished peripheral pulses; and altered mentation. Make note of any administrations of β-blockers and nondihydropyridine calcium channel blockers as they may mask some of the early symptoms and signs of acute blood loss and dehydration, particularly the reflex increase in heart rate. β-blockers can also mask other signs of increased adrenergic tone, such as diaphoresis.

Hypovolemia is characterized by reduced blood volume or central venous pressure (CVP) and increased systemic vascular resistance in an effort to maintain perfusion. Acute blood loss triggers cardiovascular, respiratory, renal, hematologic, and neuroendocrine responses to increase heart rate and contractility, conserve sodium and water, control blood loss at the source of bleeding, and redistribute blood flow to preserve vital organ function. With progressive hemorrhage without resuscitation, cardiac output can no longer compensate, leading to hypoperfusion.

If the examiner identifies symptoms and signs of hypovolemia, volume depletion and/or acute blood loss likely accounts for the hypotension. Dehydration in the hospital setting may result from decreased fluid intake or from increased fluid losses, especially seen with vomiting, nasogastric suction, drains, diarrhea, and intentional diuresis. Increased rates of insensible losses can be dramatic when the skin is damaged (burns, Stevens-Johnson syndrome) or when patients have a high fever and lose fluid via perspiration and a high respiratory rate.

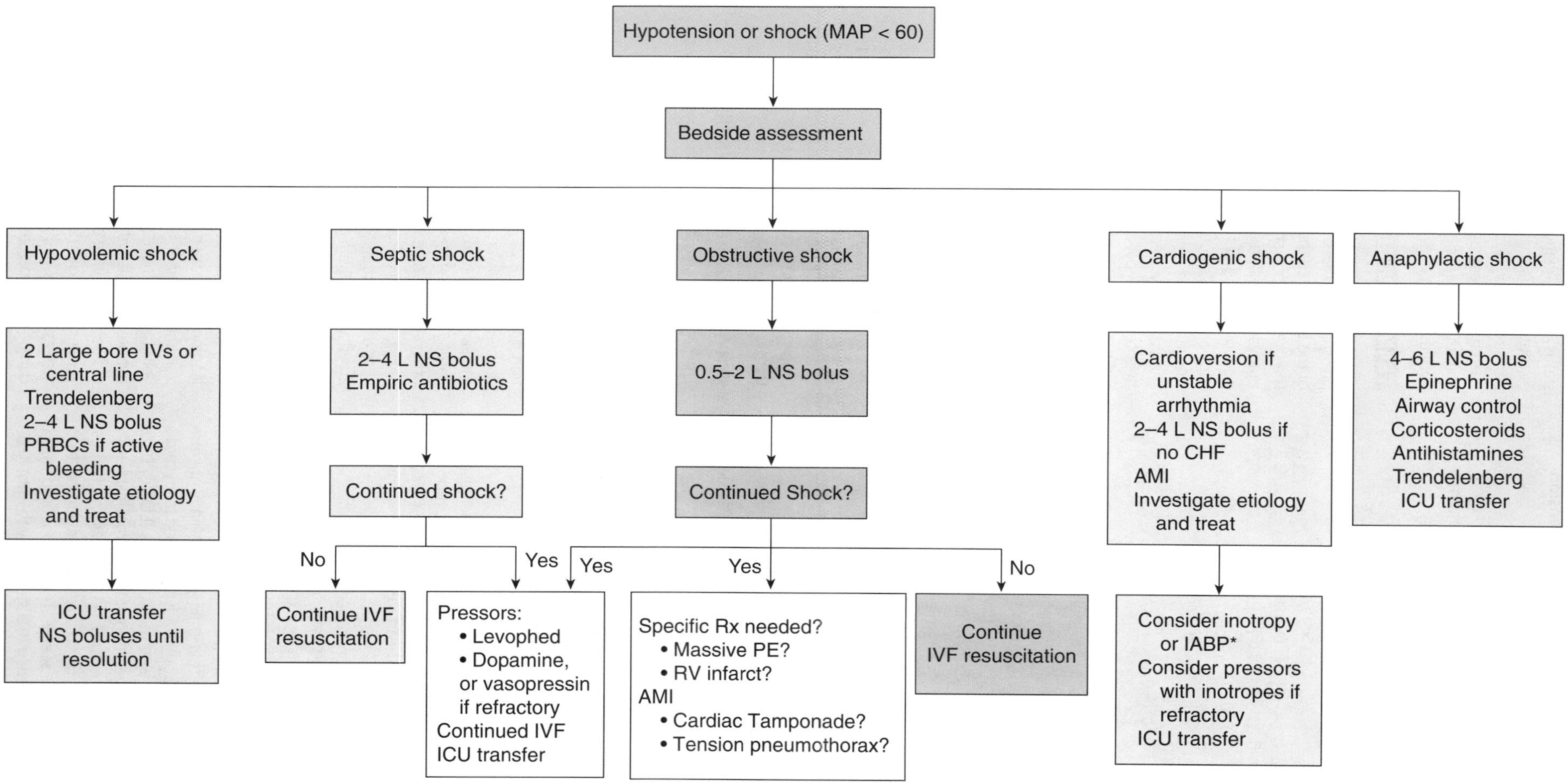

Figure 91-1 *Framework of Evaluation of Hypotension. (AMI, acute myocardial infarction; CHF, congestive heart failure; ICU, intensive care unit; IVF, IV fluids; MAP, mean arterial pressure; NS, normal saline; PE, pulmonary embolism; RV, right ventricle).*

TABLE 91-2 Common Hypotension-Inducing Drugs

Drug	Mechanism of Hypotension
Alcohol	Potentiation of orthostatic hypotension via impairment of vasoconstrictor response
Alpha blockers	Loss of reflex vasoconstriction upon standing
Anesthesia (general and regional)	Vasodilatation and decreased cardiac contractility
Antihypertensives (including beta blockers and nondihydropyridine calcium channel blockers)	Decreased cardiac output via heart rate depression and negative inotropy
Antidepressants (including monoamine oxydase inhibitors and tricyclics)	Orthostatic hypotension
Antipsychotics	Alpha-adrenergic blockade, calcium blockade, inhibition of centrally mediated pressor reflexes, and a negative inotropic effect especially in older, typical antipsychotics
Anxiolytics (including benzodiazepines)	Central inhibition of sympathetic outflow
Diuretics	Orthostasis via hypovolemia
Nitrates	Vasodilatation
Opiates	Increase in histamine release, direct vasodilatation, depression of the medullary vasomotor center
Phenothiazines	Alpha-adrenergic blockade
Sildenafil and other systemic drugs for erectile dysfunction	Vasodilation

Hemorrhage may result from trauma, bleeding from the genitourinary or gastrointestinal tracts, and vascular etiologies. Hospital-acquired etiologies include trauma from surgery or procedures and drug interactions relating to excessive anticoagulation. Retroperitoneal hemorrhage may occur following a closed renal biopsy, cardiac catheterization, and pancreatitis, and from fractures, especially involving long bones and pelvis. Splenic rupture has been reported following colonoscopy. In addition to vascular trauma, vascular etiologies include aneurysms, dissections, and arteriovenous malformations.

PRACTICE POINT

Hypovolemic hypotension

Blood Loss	Associated Signs
< 20% of circulating blood	Cool, clammy skin, decreased capillary refill, ↓ pulse pressure
20–40%	Tachycardia, tachypnea, postural blood pressure changes, confused or agitated; ongoing losses without resuscitation: hypotension, oliguria, deeper and faster respirations, mottling of skin
>40%	Tachycardia, profound hypotension, either tachypnea or irregular respirations, ↓↓ urine output, ↓ or absent pulses, pallor, lethargy, obtundation
Death from severe hemorrhage	Respiratory arrest prior to circulatory arrest due to fatigue of respiratory muscles and bradycardic or asystolic rhythms or pulseless electrical activity (PEA)

■ CARDIOGENIC SHOCK

Decreased cardiac output and systemic hypoperfusion may result from a variety of insults affecting the heart itself or affecting the blood flow to the left ventricle. The presentation depends on the etiology, severity, and duration of the problem as well as the patient's age and underlying medical conditions. Signs of cardiogenic shock include a narrowed pulse pressure, diaphoresis, elevated jugular venous pressure, rales, and cool and clammy extremities.

Obstructive hypotension occurs when left-sided cardiac output is impaired by a physiologic or anatomic limitation to flow, which may occur at any point in the circuit. In pericardial tamponade and tension pneumothorax and other causes of pericardial or superior vena caval compression, there is impaired filling of the right heart due to external compression. Pulmonary embolism, pulmonic stenosis, and decompensated severe pulmonary hypertension lead to impaired flow of blood from the right heart to the left heart. Left atrial myxoma (and other cardiac tumors) can impact flow through the heart itself. Mitral stenosis, aortic stenosis, and dynamic left ventricular outflow obstruction due to hypertrophic cardiomyopathy impair flow through and out of the left heart. Lung cancers may also impair left-sided cardiac output.

Primary myocardial dysfunction may occur in acute myocardial infarction and other acute cardiomyopathies (such as stress cardiomyopathy). With an acute right ventricular myocardial infarction, aggressive fluid resuscitation should complement standard treatment to passively get blood through the pulmonary circulation, whereas fluids are likely to exacerbate pulmonary edema in left ventricular failure. If the patient's heart rate is sufficiently slow (generally < 40 beats per minute) or fast (> 50 beats per minute), brady- or tachyarrhythmias may interfere with cardiac output leading to hypotension. In emergency situations, review of monitor strip lead V_1 may be sufficient to make a diagnosis and initiate appropriate treatment without wasting valuable time obtaining a 12-lead ECG and a right-sided 12-lead ECG.

Arrhythmias may precipitate heart cardiogenic hypotension by a variety of mechanisms. Bradycardia reduces cardiac output directly but may also be associated with atrioventricular dyssynchrony, as in complete heart block. Ineffective ventricular contractions may occur in ventricular tachycardias. In patients with acute hypotension due to bradyarrhythmias or tachyarrhythmias, ACLS protocols should be initiated immediately. In atrial fibrillation and flutter, some patients (particularly the elderly and other

PRACTICE POINT

Obstructive and cardiogenic hypotension

Clinical question	Pearls and signs	*The rational clinical exam reference*
Does this patient have abnormal central venous pressure?	• Use the abdominal pressure to identify the internal jugular vein. • A JVP > 3 cm above the sternal notch or a sustained JVP > with abdominal compression: three- to fourfold fold ↑ likelihood of ↑ JVP.*	Cook DJ, et al. *JAMA*. 1996;275(8):630–634, February 28, 1996, pp. 125–135.
Does this patient have left-sided heart failure?	• A pulse > 90–100/min and an SBP < 90 mm Hg is associated with ↓ EF. • The presence of an S3 (which may be easier to appreciate by palpation) likelihood ratio 57 for congestive heart failure.	Badgett RG, et al. *JAMA*. 277(21):1712–1719, June 4, 1997, pp. 183–207.
Does this patient have an abnormal systolic murmur?	• Absence of murmur radiation to the R clavicle makes moderate to severe. AS much less likely. • Presence of maximal murmur intensity in second R intercostal space or reduced carotid pulse volume or slow rate of increase of carotid pulse or reduced or absent S2 makes moderate-to severe. AS much more likely.	Etchells E, et al. JAMA. 277(7): 564–571, February 19, 1997, pp. 433–448.
Does this patient have aortic regurgitation?	• A wide pulse pressure is a clue to the presence of AR. • Typical early diastolic murmur appreciated in a quiet room with a comfortable, cooperative patient. • The presence of S3 in patients with isolated AR predicts severity.	Choudhry NK, et al. *JAMA*. 281(23):2231–2238, June 16, 1999, pp. 419–428.
Is this patient having a myocardial infarction?	• Patients presenting with chest pain and diaphoresis, third heart sound, or hypotension.	AA Panju, et al. *JAMA* 280(14): 1256–1263, October 14, 1998, pp. 461–470.
Does this patient have a pulmonary embolism?	• Tachypnea and tachycardia most common but nonspecific signs. • Use a structured model to assess pretest probability of pulmonary emboli (such as Wells scoring system); if a discrepancy is noted between clinician gestalt and a clinical prediction rule, assign the higher of the two pretest probabilities.	Chunilal SD, et al. *JAMA*. 290(21):2849–2858, December 3, 2003, pp. 561–575.
Does this patient have an acute thoracic aortic dissection?	• Associated signs ≤ one third of cases. • Pulse deficits, focal neurologic deficits ↑ likelihood in appropriate clinical setting. • The absence of a diastolic murmur is not useful.	Klompas M. *JAMA*. 287(17): 2262–2272, May 1, 2002, pp. 659–670.
Does this patient have cardiac tamponade?	• Acute surgical cardiac tamponade: hypotension, ↑JVP, and quiet heart sounds. • Medical patients with known pericardial effusion, pulsus paradoxus may support diagnosis, and occasionally pericardial friction rub. • Pulse oximeter may also display exaggerated decline in BP that occurs with inspiration.	Roy CL, et al. *JAMA*. 297(16): 1810–1818, April 25, 2007, pp. 1811–1818.
Does this patient have a tension pneumothorax?	• Clinical diagnosis based on symptoms of sudden severe ipsilateral pleuritic chest pain and signs of hypotension, diaphoresis, cyanosis, cardiovascular collapse, tracheal deviation. • Immediately place a 14- to 18-gauge angiocatheter in second intercostal space at midclavicular line or fourth or fifth intercostal space at anterior axillary line.	(Not from The Rational Clinical Exam Series)

AR, aortic regurgitation; AS, aortic stenosis; BP, blood pressure; JVP, jugular venous pressure; ↑ = increase; ↓ = decrease; ↑↑ = greatly increase.
*A SVP measured >8 cm or a sustain JVP of >3 cm measured vertically with abdominal compression suggests an elevated CVP.

patients with stiff ventricles) may experience a modest degree of hypotension or other pump failure symptoms due to a lack of atrial "kick," but this can be confounded by the difficulty in accurately determining blood pressure in the setting of an irregular rhythm with erratic stroke volumes.

VASOGENIC SHOCK

Sepsis, anaphylaxis, and neurogenic disorders may lead to vasogenic shock. The presentation of vasogenic hypotension depends on the etiology and severity of the underlying problem. Flushing, warm extremities, and a widened pulse pressure suggest vasogenic shock. Patients may also have signs of hyperthermia or hypothermia, tachycardia, tachypnea, and mental status changes.

PRACTICE POINT

Vasogenic shock

Type of Shock	Signs
Septic	• Hypothermia, hyperthermia, flushing, warm extremities, purpura, petechial rash as well as obtundation • Important clue: Acute hyperventilation with respiratory alkalosis (Pco_2 < 30 mm Hg)
Anaphylactic	• Urticaria; flushing or generalized erythema; tachypnea; angioedema most often involving head, neck, face, and upper airways; hoarseness; stridor; and wheezing • Vomiting and diarrhea • Cardiac dysrhythmias
Neurogenic	• Bradycardia and flaccid paralysis (lesions proximal to T4)

In the early stages of septic shock patients have warm extremities due to the predominance of vasodilatory mediators. There is an initial decrease in the right ventricular and left ventricular ejection fraction with an increase in both end-diastolic and end-systolic volume indices and normal stroke volume. Systemic vascular resistance and cardiac filling pressures decrease. When accompanied by the adult respiratory distress syndrome (ARDS), there is increased microvascular permeability in the lungs resulting in hypoxemia due to perfusion of underventilated alveoli and right-to-left shunting. Skin lesions associated with sepsis include primary infection (cellulitis, erysipelas, fasciitis), disseminated intravascular coagulation (acrocyanosis and necrosis of peripheral tissues), and lesions related to infective endocarditis (microemboli, immune complex vasculitis). Retinal hemorrhages, cotton wool spots, conjunctival petechiae, endophthalmitis, and panophthalmitis are ophthalmic manifestations of sepsis.

Anaphylaxis refers to the clinical syndrome of a severe hypersensitivity reaction characterized by cardiovascular collapse and respiratory compromise. Immediate hypersensitivity reactions occur within seconds or minutes after presentation of the antigen, most commonly antibiotics (penicillins or related antibiotics, trimethoprim-sulfamethoxazole, vancomycin), aspirin, or nonsteroidal anti-inflammatory agents. Iodinated vascular contrast may elicit a similar reaction (sometimes referred to as *anaphylactoid* since it does not involve antibodies, but has similar clinical presentation to true anaphylaxis). Anaphylaxis usually has characteristic symptoms and signs that include urticaria, flushing, tachypnea, hoarseness or throat tightness. The skin and gastrointestinal tract are most commonly affected, but multiorgan involvement and failure may be rapid in onset. Although the diagnosis may be clear at the time of presentation due to the presence of urticaria and/or stridor, the severity of the reaction may not initially be appreciated.

Neurologic causes of hypotension are often accompanied by abnormal heart rate. Although increases in intracerebral pressure lead to reflex hypertension, acutely subarachnoid hemorrhage may lead to hypotension with associated bradycardia. Loss of consciousness, focal neurologic deficits, and severe headache are common. Spinal cord injury disrupts sympathetic stimulation to vessels, and loss of sympathetic tone causes arterio- and vasodilatation, which may lead to reflex tachycardia. However, cardiac and thoracic vessel sympathetic innervation is from T1 to T8; lesions proximal to T4 may disrupt sympathetic, but spare vagal innervation, leading to bradycardia. Dysautonomia may also present as hypotension without the typical tachycardic response in patients with longstanding diabetes, amyloidosis, Parkinson disease and other forms of Parkinsonism (such as Shy-Drager syndrome), or other neurodegenerative diseases.

PHARMACOLOGIC SHOCK

Pharmacologic shock results from vasodilatation or myocardial depression. Medications are a leading cause of iatrogenic hypotension in hospitalized patients. Data from 2007 collected by AHRQ indicate a 0.7% national mortality rate associated with iatrogenic hypotension. Any medication that affects cardiac output, volume status, and/or systemic vascular resistance can cause pharmacologic shock (**Table 91-3**).

INITIAL MANAGEMENT

With few exceptions an unstable, hypotensive patient should receive a bolus of IV fluid (IVF), usually a liter of normal saline. In the absence of severe heart failure, many patients may in fact require very aggressive fluid resuscitation prior to the initiation of pressors (5–7 liters of crystalloid is not uncommon) if hypotension persists.

PREVENTION

Patient safety considerations include daily review and adjustment of all medications whose metabolism may become altered due to drug-drug interactions or the development of liver or renal insufficiency. Remember prompt removal of unnecessary lines and urinary catheters, and early recognition of impending problems. In elderly patients especially, pay attention to the initial dosages of medications and eliminate polypharmacy. Quality improvement initiatives may start with a review of all intensive care unit (ICU) transfers, and include information technology support to alert prescribers of drug-drug interactions and appropriate dosing.

CONCLUSION

This chapter provides a framework for the initial bedside assessment of the patient with hypotension. When a significant fall in mean arterial pressure occurs, the clinician must take steps to avoid end organ damage by directing immediate therapy, determining the need for emergent surgical and specialty consultation and ensuring appropriate level of care. In general, IVF administration will raise the blood pressure until specific measures can be undertaken, but it must be prescribed with care for some causes of obstructive hypotension. Given the demonstrated mortality benefit, early initiation of empiric broad-spectrum antimicrobials for suspected sepsis should be initiated pending culture

TABLE 91-3 Initial Management of Common Types of Hypotension

Type of Hypotension or Shock	Initial Management	Pearls and Pitfalls
Hypovolemic	Aggressive IV fluid resuscitation	Caution in patients with CHF who are hypotensive due to overdiuresis
Obstructive or Cardiogenic Hypotension		
Fulminant dilated cardiomyopathy or necrosis of > 40% of left ventricular mass	Inotropic and mechanical support with intraaortic balloon	Avoid fluid resuscitation
Right ventricular infarct	IV fluid volume load and dobutamine	Obtain right-sided electrocardiogram to diagnose; avoid diuretics that decrease preload and worsen already poor cardiac output; avoid dopamine, which increases pulmonary vascular resistance
Rupture of papillary muscles or the ventricular wall	Cardiac surgery	
Acute, massive pulmonary embolism	Thrombolysis and IV fluids as needed	
Tension pneumothorax	Needle aspiration, chest tube	Administer IV fluids carefully as excessive fluid expansion may worsen right ventricular failure
Pericardial tamponade (retrograde aortic dissection, constrictive pericarditis)	Aggressive fluid resuscitation	Removal of even a small amount of fluid can lead to dramatic improvement
Hypotension due to severe, decompensated pulmonary hypertension	Consider fluid retention if patient does not have neck vein distension; may need pressor support in an intensive care unit setting and urgent specialty consultation	Paradoxical worsening of hypotension may develop if right ventricle is severely dilated and septal bowing compromises left ventricular filling
Vasogenic shock		
Septic shock	Aggressive fluid administration, pressors, antibiotics	
Anaphylaxis	Stop drug, aggressive fluid administration, epinephrine	
Neurogenic	Fluid administration	
Pharmacologic	Administer IV fluids and discontinue precipitants See **Table 91-4** for anecdotes	Carefully review all medications, including as needed medications

TABLE 91-4 Agents Used to Reverse Medication-Induced Hypotension

Hypotension-Inducing Agent	Antidote	Antidote Dosing
Anticholinergics (eg, atropine)	Physostigmine	0.5–2 mg IV or IM (may repeat every 20 min until response occurs)
Benzodiazepines	Flumazenil	0.2 mg IV (may repeat)
Beta-blockers	Glucagon	5–10 mg IV
Calcium channel blockers	Atropine (if bradycardia present)	0.5–2 mg IV
	Calcium chloride (10%)	10 mL or 1–2 g IV (may repeat to max 10–12 g)
	Calcium gluconate (10%)	20 mL IV
Opiates	Nalmefene	Nonopioid-dependent: 0.5–1 mg/70 kg (may repeat)
	Naloxone	Opioid-dependent: 0.10.5 mg/70 kg (may repeat)
		0.4–2 mg IV (may repeat)
		IM and SQ available (longer onset to action)
Tricyclic antidepressants	Sodium bicarbonate	50–100 mEq IV bolus or norepinephrine 4–8 mcg/min IV infusion

Data from Olson K. Poisoning. In: McPhee SJ, Papdakis MA, eds. *Current Medical Diagnosis and Treatment* 2010. New York: The McGraw-Hill Companies; 2009: Chapter 38.

results. For medication-induced hypotension, the offending agent should be discontinued and if possible, reversed. Timely administration of epinephrine may be life saving in the treatment of anaphylaxis. The reader is referred to Part VI Clinical Conditions for a more detailed discussion of the management of specific causes of hypotension commonly encountered in the hospital setting.

SUGGESTED READINGS

Cook DJ, Simel DL. The rational clinical exam: does this patient have abnormal central venous pressure? *JAMA*. 1996;275(8):630–634.

Freeman MB. Neurogenic orthostatic hypotension. *N Engl J Med*. 2008;358:615–624.

Levy JH. Treating shock—old drugs, new ideas. *N Engl J Med*. 2010;362:841–843.

Luciano GL, Brennan MJ, Rothberg MB. Postprandial hypotension. *Am J Med*. 2010;123(3):281.e1–e6.

Pickering TG, Hall JE, Appel LJ, et al. Recommendations for blood pressure measurement in humans and experimental animals, I: Blood pressure measurement in humans: a statement for professionals from the Subcommittee of Professional and Public Education of the American Heart Association Council on High Blood Pressure Research. *Circ*. 2005;111:697–716.

CHAPTER 92

Hypothermia

Chad S. Miller, MD, FACP, FHM
Jeffrey G. Wiese, MD, FACP, FSM, SFHM

Key Clinical Questions

1. What are the signs and symptoms of hypothermia?
2. What are the most common causes of hypothermia?
3. Does intoxication associated with hypothermia suggest a better or worse prognosis?
4. What are the dangers associated with hypothermia?
5. Who is most likely to die from hypothermia?

CASE 92-1

A 54-year-old man was brought to the hospital after being found unresponsive in his apartment. His family noted that he had been recently hospitalized for pneumonia and had been released from the hospital 3 days earlier. The ambient temperature of the apartment was normal per the EMS report.

His temperature was 32°C, his heart rate was 50 beats per minute, his respiratory rate was 14 breaths per minute, and his blood pressure was 90/60 mm Hg. His head and neck, cardiovascular, and abdominal examinations were normal. His skin was cool but warmer than expected given his core temperature; pulses were present in all extremities. There were decreased breath sounds and egophony in the right lower lobe; the signs of consolidation were confirmed by chest X-ray.

What is the cause of this man's mental status changes and what is his prognosis?

INTRODUCTION

Vital signs are routinely measured for all hospitalized patients on admission, during nursing shifts and when infusions are being administered. Clinicians should be able to recognize when abnormal temperatures require immediate action to avoid adverse consequences that may be potentially life-threatening.

HYPOTHERMIA PRESENTAIONS

Core body temperature is tightly regulated between a normal diurnal range of 36.0°C and 37.5°C. Temperatures below 36.0°C are considered abnormal. Patients admitted to the inpatient service frequently have temperature abnormalities on admission or may develop them during the hospital stay.

Because of potential life-threatening causes, it is essential to obtain an accurate measurement of core body temperature. Although temperature is most accurately measured by the gold standard methods of intravascular, esophageal, or bladder thermistors, the most commonly used clinical methods are rectal, oral, and tympanic membrane measurements. Axillary measurement routinely underestimates core body temperature and lacks precision; therefore, it is not recommended. It should be noted that oral measurements can be influenced by eating, drinking, breathing devices, tachypnea, and mouth breathing. Rectal temperatures may be two to three tenths of a degree Celsius higher than actual core body temperature.

EXPOSURE HYPOTHERMIA

Exposure hypothermia is defined as an unintentional fall in core body temperature below 35.0°C from exposure to a cold environment. The most common cause is lack of shelter, warm clothing, or heat during the winter months. When environmental exposure to cold ambient temperatures is not obvious, making the diagnosis can be challenging because the presenting signs are often subtle and associated with numerous potential diagnoses. The initial phase of hypothermia usually consists of shivering, tachycardia, tachypnea, and peripheral vasoconstriction. Shivering

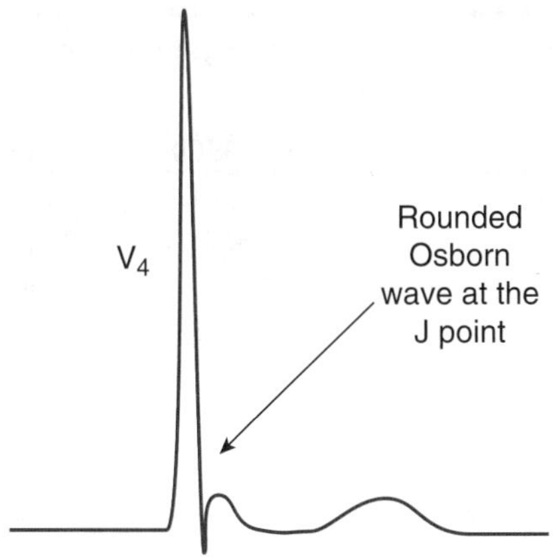

Figure 92-1 *Osborn wave.*

PRACTICE POINT

- Severe (< 28.0°C) hypothermia may result in coma, hypotension, extreme oliguria, and peripheral areflexia.

may disappear if hypothermia is prolonged or progresses to severe levels. Other signs include confusion, drowsiness, dysarthria, decreased coordination, and arrhythmias. In moderate hypothermia (28.0°C–32.0°C), pupillary dilatation, hallucinations, and the phenomenon of paradoxical undressing—the removal of clothes as core temperature drops—may be present. Cardiac manifestations such as bradycardia and arrhythmias begin to develop. Electrocardiographic (ECG) findings, such as a prolonged QT interval as well as an Osborn wave, sometimes referred to as a J wave, may be present (**Figure 92-1**). The Osborn wave is also seen in severe hypercalcemia, but the ECG is distinct from a patient with hypothermia. The QT interval is usually shorter in hypercalcemia, and the patient is more likely to be tachycardic from volume depletion. Movement artifact from shivering may also be present in patients with hypothermia, especially in the limb leads with relative sparing of the precordial leads.

Severe (< 28.0°C) hypothermia may result in coma, hypotension, extreme oliguria, and peripheral areflexia.

At any stage of hypothermia, the precapillary vascular resistance may fail, with resultant vasodilation. The increased blood that follows may cause sufficient warming to restore vascular function and reinstate local vasoconstriction. The oscillation between dilatation and constriction is known as the Lewis-Hunting reaction and occurs primarily on the fingertips, toes, ears, and face resulting in paroxysms of flushing.

Finally, there are hematologic changes associated with hypothermia that are important. Cold directly inhibits the enzymatic reactions of both the intrinsic and extrinsic pathways of the clotting cascade. At low temperatures, patients may have significant bleeding or hemorrhage.

NONEXPOSURE HYPOTHERMIA

Nonexposure hypothermia should be considered sepsis until proven otherwise. The peripheral vasodilatation associated with progressive sepsis results in the inappropriate liberation of body heat, lowering the body's temperature. Unusual causes of nonexposure hypothermia include metabolic disturbances that result in downregulation of the body's metabolic rate. Euthyroid sick syndrome, hypothyroidism, and adrenal insufficiency are the most common.

THE FIREPLACE APPROACH

Approach to hypothermia

Hypothermia is ultimately the result of a mismatch between heat production and heat loss, in the same way that underheating a home is due to a mismatch between heat production from the home's fireplace and heat loss from the home's insulation, or lack thereof. The resultant problems stem from three components: There is not enough wood (fuel), not enough fire (metabolism), or not enough insulation (heat loss).

The *fuel* (wood) for basal metabolism must be adequate in order to generate heat. Hypoglycemia, malnourishment, and decreased muscle mass contribute to hypothermia as the patient has too little fuel to generate heat. The hypothermia of hypoglycemia is a result of glucopenia in the hypothalamus, resulting in a down-adjustment of the thermal set point that is presumptively to reduce metabolic rate in the setting of inadequate fuel supply. The chronic malnourishment of alcohol abuse places alcoholics at even greater risk of hypothermia.

If fuel supplies are adequate, the *body's metabolism* (fire) should be evaluated as a potential cause of the hypothermia. Hypothermia from inadequate metabolism may be caused by hypothyroidism, adrenal insufficiency, and hypopituitarism. The body simply cannot generate enough heat to keep up with the heat loss.

Once fuel supplies and metabolism have been excluded, *causes of heat elimination/conservation* (insulation) should be considered. Hypothermia may result from induced vasodilation. This results in a greater amount of warm blood in the periphery, which allows a greater amount of heat to be lost to the environment. Acute alcohol consumption, vasodilatory medications, infections, and toxins are the common causes. Although usually obvious from history, prolonged exposure to cold (exposure hypothermia) results in too much heat lost to the environment.

PRACTICE POINT

- Non-exposure hypothermia should be considered sepsis until proven otherwise. The peripheral vasodilatation associated with progressive sepsis results in the inappropriate liberation of body heat, lowering the body's temperature.

PREVALENCE AND ADJUSTMENTS

Baseline prevalence

Death from extreme temperatures remains relatively uncommon. Early diagnosis and treatment can often prevent mortality. Between 1999 and 2002, 4607 deaths in the United States were due to hypothermia-related diagnoses. Exposure to excessive natural cold was the underlying cause in 2622 deaths, and 1985 hypothermic deaths were from causes other than exposure. The overall rate of deaths related to hypothermia tends to be higher in the northern and western states, in particular, Montana, Wyoming, and Alaska.

Those at greatest risk for exposure hypothermia are the elderly, alcoholics, persons with psychiatric conditions, and the physically impaired. Aging results in a delayed vasoconstrictor response to cold as well as a decreased perception of cold. Although temperature homeostasis declines with age, of greater relevance to hypothermia are poor social circumstances, comorbidities, and the drugs used in treating these. Patients hospitalized for hypothermia and acute intoxication have a far better prognosis than patients found at home whose hypothermia was not linked to intoxication. Hypothermia portends a poor prognosis in sepsis as well as congestive heart failure. Patients over the age of 65 years admitted for congestive heart failure with a temperature below 35.2°C (< 95.5°F) were found to have an odds ratio of death of 4.46 [95% confidence interval (CI): 1.38–14.3] compared to normothermic patients with congestive heart failure.

How prevalence changes with age

There is a significant increased risk of dying from hypothermia in adults over the age of 65. Greater than 40% of all hypothermia-related deaths are in this age group. The rate of death from hypothermia of individuals greater than 75 approaches six per 100,000 population, compared to less than three per 100,000 in individuals younger than 65 years.

Patients 65 years or older with chronic obstructive pulmonary disease (COPD) have a slightly higher risk of dying on cold days [odds ratio (OR): 1.19; 95% CI: 1.07–1.33].

Gender

Men have a threefold increased mortality from hypothermia as compared to women.

Race, ethnicity

While mortality from hypothermia is lower in Caucasians, the discrepancy is likely due to social as opposed to physiologic reasons.

THE HISTORY

- **Was this patient brought in from home?** If yes, the prognosis is worse.
- **Was this patient found outside?** If yes, prognosis is better.
- **Does this patient drink excessive amounts of alcohol or engage in recreational drug use?** If yes, prognosis is better.
- **Is it winter, or one of the coldest days of the year?** If yes, the likelihood of cold ambient temperatures contributing to pathology increases.
- **Is the patient greater than 65 years?** Increased age increases risk of hypothermia.
- **Has the patient recently had a fever? Is this patient at risk for infection? Does this patient have other signs or symptoms of infection or sepsis?** If yes, an infection is more likely.
- **Has the patient recently undergone extreme exertion under very cold conditions?** If yes, the patient may have exposure hypothermia.
- **Is the patient malnourished?** If yes, this decreases the patient's ability to increase basal metabolism.
- **Is the patient taking hypoglycemic medications?** If yes, the patient may have become unconscious and unable to avoid excessive cold.
- **Is the patient elderly or frail?** If yes, this decreases the patient's ability to increase basal metabolism.
- **Does this patient have a history of adrenal, thyroid, or pituitary disease?** If yes, this places the patient at greater risk because he or she cannot increase basal metabolism.
- **Is this patient taking medications that cause peripheral vasodilation?** If yes, this puts patient at risk for excessive heat loss.
- **Does this patient have signs of vascular insufficiency?**
- **Is this patient taking antipsychotics?** If yes, may cause significant temperature dysregulation.
- **Does this patient have a history of congestive heart failure?** If yes, portends a worse prognosis.

TABLE 92-1 Utility of Clinical Findings for Diagnosing Hypothyroidism

	+LR (95% CI)	–LR (95% CI)
Cool and dry skin	4.7 (3.1, 7.1)	0.9 (0.8, 0.9)
Coarse skin	3.4 (1.4, 8.0)	0.7 (0.5, 0.9)
Dry palms	1.5 (1.0, 2.4)	0.8 (0.6, 1.1)
Hair loss of eyebrows	1.9 (1.1, 3.6)	0.8 (0.7, 1.0)
Slow pulse rate	4.1 (3.2, 5.3)	0.8 (0.7, 0.8)
Hypothyroid speech	5.4 (2.7, 10.7)	0.7 (0.5, 0.9)
Enlarged thyroid	2.8 (2.3, 3.4)	0.6 (0.6, 0.7)
Delayed ankle reflexes	3.4 (1.8, 6.4)	0.6 (0.4, 0.9)
Billewicz score +30 point or more	18.8 (1.2, 300.5)	

THE EXAMINATION

Hypothyroidism is a common underlying cause of hypothermia. The findings in **Table 92-1** can help make the diagnosis.

If a hypothyroid patient becomes hypothermic and develops myxedema coma, the clinician should search for an underlying precipitant such as infection. It is critically important to diagnose this condition, because of the significant mortality, especially if the diagnosis is overlooked and because the treatment of hyperthermia differs from other causes.

The signs of adrenal insufficiency are often subtle and present insidiously. A high suspicion must be maintained in the setting of hypothermia, especially if there is not a likely alternative explanation. The physical exam should note the patient's general nutritional status as malnutrition is associated with hypothermia. Age and decreased muscle mass should be noted. Evidence of vascular insufficiency such as varicose veins, lower extremity edema, and stasis ulcers should be noted.

The patient must undergo a thorough evaluation for sepsis. Blood pressure should be documented. Intravenous lines or indwelling catheters should be considered as potential sources and removed if indicated. The physical exam should specifically note common sites of infection including the lungs, skin, genitourinary system, oropharynx, and sinuses.

Physical exam findings or maneuvers that may help with the diagnosis of bacteremia are shown in **Table 92-2**.

THE LABORATORY APPROACH

Patients should be evaluated for infection as well as endocrine disturbances. A complete blood count, blood cultures, urinalysis, and chest X-ray are all potentially indicated. A thyroid-stimulating

TABLE 92-2 Utility of Clinical Findings for Diagnosing Bacteremia

	+LR (95% CI)	–LR (95% CI)
Age 50 or greater	1.4 (1.2, 1.6)	0.3 (0.1, 0.8)
Tachycardia	1.2 (1.1, 1.4)	0.7 (0.6, 0.9)
Respiratory rate > 20	0.9 (0.8, 1.1)	1.2 (0.8, 1.7)
Hypotension	2.6 (1.6, 4.4)	0.9 (0.9, 1.0)
Confusion or depressed sensorium	1.5 (1.3, 1.8)	0.9 (0.8, 1.0)

hormone (TSH) and a cosyntropin stimulation test should be considered. If there is a possibility of adrenal crisis, do not withhold corticosteroids for fear of interfering with the stimulation test.

An ECG should be performed. Supraventricular arrhythmias occur frequently in hypothermic individuals, and atrial fibrillation is the most common. Cardiac arrhythmias usually resolve spontaneously after rewarming.

DESIGNING MANAGEMENT WHILE THE DIAGNOSIS IS PENDING

An exposure hypothermia patient may recover neurologically intact after prolonged cardiac arrest. There have been reports of young adults with rectal or esophageal temperatures as low as 17.5°C. There are also reports of neurologically intact survival despite documented cardiac arrests of 4.5 hours at extremely low temperatures. Resuscitation efforts are recommended until arrest persists after a 35°C core temperature has been reached.

Patients who are malnourished or alcoholic may develop Wernicke encephalopathy on rewarming due to thiamine deficiency. Any patient that is malnourished or has a history of alcohol abuse should receive intravenous thiamine.

If myxedema coma is being considered, immediate administration of intravenous triiodothyronine is recommended. Recognize that this may precipitate adrenal crisis if adrenal insufficiency coexists; it is prudent to give intravenous corticosteroids. Because sepsis is common in patients with hypothermia but can be difficult to detect because classic features may not be present, broad-spectrum antibiotics may be indicated if you suspect sepsis, even if it is not clinically obvious. Although hypothermia in myxedema coma should be treated, active rewarming methods and direct heat should be avoided as this may lead to peripheral vasodilatation and worsen hypotension and shock. Passive rewarming with blankets and other methods is preferred.

For mild hypothermia (34°C–35°C) in patients not in cardiac arrest begin passive rewarming. Congestive heart failure patients frequently have mild hypothermia, and isolated reports have shown that warming improves symptoms and hemodynamic variables. Mortality was not investigated.

For moderate (30°C–34°C) hypothermia, begin active external rewarming. For severe (< 30°C) hypothermia, begin active internal rewarming; consider extracorporeal membrane oxygenation. If the patient has cardiac arrest, begin cardiopulmonary resuscitation (CPR). For moderate hypothermia and cardiac arrest, defibrillation for ventricular tachycardia or fibrillation may be attempted per advanced cardiac life support (ACLS) protocol. Space intravenous medications at longer intervals and provide active internal rewarming.

For severe hypothermia and cardiac arrest, begin CPR, attempt defibrillation only once, and withhold medications until temperature is > 30°C. Cardioactive medications may accumulate to toxic levels if given repeatedly. Provide active internal rewarming. Overall, ACLS management of cardiac arrest in hypothermia should focus more aggressively on core rewarming as the hypothermic heart may be unresponsive to cardiovascular drugs, pacemaker stimulation, and defibrillation.

Routine administration of corticosteroids, barbiturates, and antibiotics has not been documented to increase survival rates or decrease postresuscitation damage.

RARE CAUSES

There are only a handful of reports of recurrent episodic hypothermia associated with pathology of the hypothalamus. These include stroke, multiple sclerosis, brain tumors, and traumatic brain injury. Two specific syndromes of episodic hypothermia have been described. The first is Shapiro syndrome, with approximately 50 cases reported, comprising recurrent hypothermia and hyperhidrosis associated with agenesis of the corpus callosum. A second rare syndrome is called spontaneous periodic hypothermia. Patients present with cyclical hypothermia associated with hyperhidrosis, headache, vomiting, and abdominal pain. Neurological examination, endocrine studies, and imaging are all normal, and some speculate that it may be a migraine variant.

SUGGESTED READINGS

Epstein E, Anna K. Accidental hypothermia. *BMJ*. 2006;332:706–709.

Mallet ML. Pathophysiology of accidental hypothermia. *QJM*. 2002;95:775–785.

O'Neill P. Aging homeostasis. *Rev Clin Gerontol*. 1997;7:199–211.

O'Grady NP, Barie PS, Bartlett JG, et al. Guidelines for evaluation of new fever in critically ill adult patients: 2008 update from the American College of Critical Care Medicine and the Infectious Diseases Society of America. *Crit Care Med*. 2008;36:1330–1349.

Vassal T, Benoit-Gonin B, Carrat F, Guidet B, Maury E, Offenstadt G. Severe accidental hypothermia treated in an ICU: prognosis and outcome. *Chest*. 2001;120:1998–2003.

CHAPTER 93

Hypoxia

Natalie E. West, MD, MHS
Noah Lechtzin, MD, MHS

Key Clinical Questions

1. What key clinical entities must be considered in the initial assessment of a hospitalized patient with hypoxemia?
2. What are initial diagnostic tests and assessments that should be obtained in the hypoxemic patient?
3. What are the potential pitfalls of reliance on pulse oximetry to define hypoxemia, and how are these avoided?
4. How should supplemental oxygen be delivered in the hypoxemic hospitalized patient?

CASE 93-1

A 63-year-old white female with a history of chronic obstructive pulmonary disease (COPD), coronary artery disease with three stents, hypertension, obesity, diabetes mellitus (DM), and lung cancer was admitted to the hospital from clinic with worsening shortness of breath over the last 2 months, requiring oxygen supplementation. She had been on 2 liters per minute (LPM) of oxygen via nasal cannula for the past 3 years for COPD, but in the past few months has experienced worsening shortness of breath and dyspnea on exertion. At this point she cannot walk to the bathroom in her house without getting short of breath. She admited to orthopnea, lower extremity edema, fatigue, and chest pain as well. She now required 4–8 LPM of oxygen in order to maintain an oxygen saturation > 89%.

Her COPD was diagnosed in 2005, and she has been on supplemental oxygen since then. She had lung cancer in 1996, which was treated with lobectomy and radiation therapy. She had a 50 pack-year tobacco history but quit smoking 12 years ago. Pertinent medications included hydrochlorothiazide, simvastatin, pioglitazone, fluticasone/salmeterol inhaler, and tiotropium inhaler.

Her physical exam was notable for an oxygen saturation of 94% on 4 liters, but she desaturated to 81% when semirecumbent. Crackles were heard in the left lung base, and she became quite dyspneic and tachypneic upon minimal effort. A 1/6 systolic ejection murmur was heard, along with a loud P2 and paradoxical splitting of S2. Lower extremities had +1 pitting edema, and she had mild digital clubbing

What were the next steps needed to appropriately evaluate and treat this patient's hypoxia?

INTRODUCTION

Hypoxia is defined by an abnormally low arterial oxygen tension. A PaO_2 of 60 mm Hg generally corresponds with the point on the oxygen–hemoglobin dissociation curve in which hemoglobin is 90% saturated. The curve is steep at this point, and further decreases in oxygen tension correspond with dramatic falls in hemoglobin saturation and resultant inadequate oxygen delivery to tissues (**Figure 93-1**). Oxygen affinity can be affected by pH, carbon dioxide (CO_2), 2,3-diphosphoglycerate (2,3-DPG), and temperature. As pH decreases and CO_2 increases, oxygen is more readily released, shifting the oxyhemoglobin curve to the right, increasing delivery of oxygen to the tissues. Red blood cells contain 2,3-DPG, which helps modulate oxygen affinity. Increasing levels of 2,3-DPG decrease the oxygen affinity, also shifting the dissociation curve to the right. Elevated body temperature shifts the dissociation curve to the right, helping to unload oxygen at a time when additional oxygen to tissues may be needed.

HYPOXIA IN THE INPATIENT SETTING

Hypoxia is a common and an important cause of mortality and morbidity in the hospital. Therefore, rapid evaluation and treatment is critical to avoid serious complications resulting from hypoxia. History and physical exam alone is not sufficient to rapidly detect hypoxia, and other measurements should be used to accurately and efficiently detect hypoxia, including pulse oximetry and blood gas

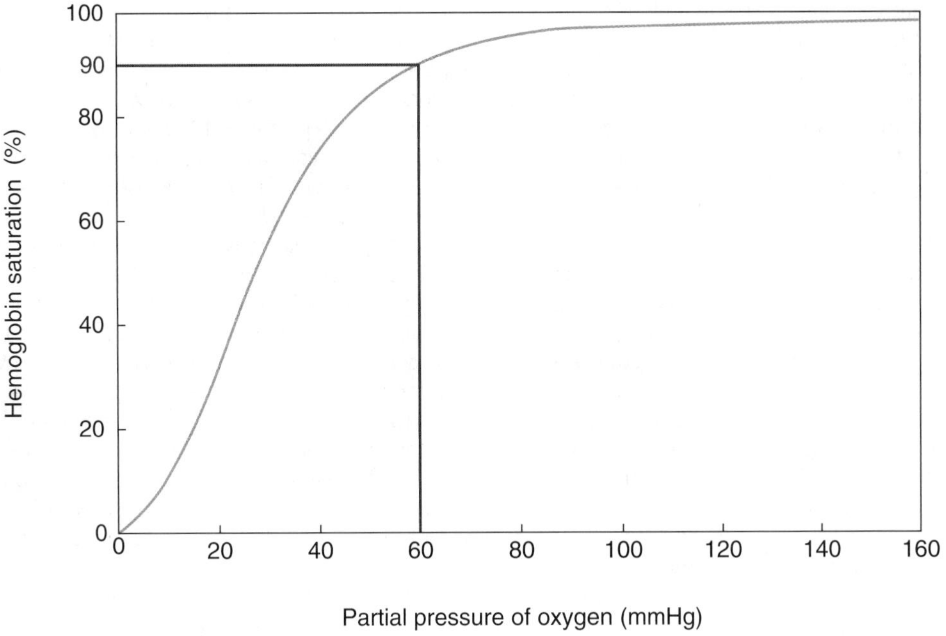

Figure 93-1 *The oxyhemoglobin dissociation curve. (Levitzky MG: Pulmonary Physiology, 7th Edition: http://www.accessmedicine.com).*

analysis. This chapter will cover the etiology and pathophysiology of hypoxia, considerations for diagnosis of hypoxia, common pitfalls, and treatment options to correct hypoxia.

PATHOPHYSIOLOGY AND MECHANISMS OF HYPOXIA

There are five general mechanisms that cause hypoxia: ventilation/perfusion (V/Q) mismatch, right to left shunt, hypoventilation, diffusion abnormalities, and reduced inspired oxygen tension (**Table 93-1**). Only the first four of these are clinically relevant, and only the first three generally cause hypoxia at rest. It is important for the clinician at the bedside to be familiar with these mechanisms and common disease states responsible for them. This will allow for more accurate diagnoses and will facilitate appropriate therapy. The underlying cause of hypoxia can often be elucidated with simple tests such as arterial blood gas (ABG) assessment and chest radiographs. Additionally, knowing how much the PaO_2 increases with oxygen supplementation can help differentiate shunt from other causes of hypoxia.

The most common cause of hypoxia is V/Q mismatch. Areas of the lung with low ratios of ventilation to perfusion result in low alveolar oxygen (O_2) tension. In most situations of V/Q mismatch, there are

TABLE 93-1 Mechanisms of Hypoxia

Mechanism	Example	Diagnostic Clues
Hypoventilation	• Central nervous system depression • Narcotic analgesics • Obesity hypoventilation syndrome • Chest wall disorders (ie, kyphoscoliosis) • Respiratory muscle weakness (ie, myasthenia gravis)	• Normal A-a gradient • Elevated CO_2 • Readily corrected by oxygen supplementation
Ventilation/perfusion (V/Q) mismatch	• COPD • Asthma • Pulmonary embolism • Interstitial lung disease	• Increased A-a gradient • Hypoxia improved by relatively low levels of oxygen
Right to left shunt	• Anatomic shunts ▪ Intracardiac shunt ▪ Arteriovenous malformation • Physiologic shunts ▪ Pneumonia ▪ Adult Respiratory Distress Syndrome ▪ Atelectasis	• Difficult to correct with oxygen supplementation
Diffusion impairment	• Pulmonary fibrosis • Pneumocystis pneumonia • Emphysema	• Hypoxia worsens with activity • Hypoxia corrects relatively easy with oxygen supplementation
Reduced inspired oxygen tension	• High altitude	• Hypoxia corrects relatively easy with oxygen supplementation

areas with low V/Q ratios, normal V/Q ratios, and high V/Q ratios. While areas of high V/Q ratio will have a higher alveolar oxygen tension, this will not offset the low PaO_2 from low V/Q areas. This is because the hemoglobin saturation does not change very much from normal V/Q areas to high V/Q areas; therefore the increase in arterial oxygen content from these areas is small and does not offset the decrement in oxygen content from the low V/Q areas.

Common causes of V/Q mismatch include obstructive lung diseases such as asthma and chronic obstructive pulmonary disease (COPD), but V/Q mismatch is seen in many other lung diseases, including pulmonary embolism, pulmonary vascular diseases, and interstitial lung diseases. In a pulmonary embolism, gas exchange abnormalities occur from increased alveolar dead space, but hypoxia can also occur due to V/Q mismatch, right to left shunting, and a low mixed venous O_2 level. Low V/Q ratios develop because blood flow is redistributed away from the obstructed vessel, resulting in overperfusion of normal lung regions. Humoral mediators released by platelets stimulate bronchoconstriction, causing atelectasis, which complicates hypoxia. In addition, physiologic shunting occurs because of increased flow through some areas of low V/Q ratios. V/Q mismatch is characterized by an increased alveolar-arterial (A-a) gradient. The A-a gradient is the difference in PaO_2 between the alveoli and arterial blood (see later discussion for additional information).

Hypoxia caused by V/Q mismatch is improved by relatively low levels of supplemental oxygen, which helps differentiate V/Q mismatch from hypoxia caused by a shunt (see later discussion), as a shunt is not readily corrected by increasing levels of FiO_2. Even with supplemental oxygen, shunted blood does not come into contact with alveoli with a higher PO_2. However, with supplemental oxygen in V/Q mismatch, in the low V/Q regions, the PaO_2 increases with a higher FiO_2, and the blood flow to these regions will have a higher capillary oxygen content, therefore producing a higher PaO_2.

Right to left shunt refers to conditions in which deoxygenated blood from the right side of the heart bypasses oxygenation in the lungs and goes to the left side of the heart. One way to consider shunt is in terms of V/Q ratios. The extreme case of V/Q ratio in which there is perfusion but no ventilation is synonymous with shunt. Shunt can occur due to anatomic abnormalities such as intracardiac shunts or arteriovenous malformations. Shunt also occurs due to alveolar filling processes such as pneumonia, acute respiratory distress syndrome, or alveolar collapse (ie, atelectasis). As already noted, shunt is less responsive to supplemental oxygen than other causes of hypoxia. This can be helpful in diagnosing shunt.

In hypoventilation, alveolar CO_2 increases; as a result alveolar O_2 must decrease. Alveolar hypoventilation is a common occurrence in hospitalized patients. It can be caused by narcotic analgesics and other central nervous system depressants. There are also central hypoventilation syndromes such as obesity-hypoventilation syndrome. Conditions that cause weakness of the respiratory muscles such as Guillain-Barré syndrome, amyotrophic lateral sclerosis, and myasthenia gravis may result in hypoventilation, as will disorders of the chest wall such as kyphoscoliosis. An ABG taken in the setting of hypoventilation will reveal an elevated CO_2 but will have a normal A-a gradient. The latter may be increased if hypoventilation is coupled with atelectasis, as it frequently is. Furthermore, hypoxemia due to hypoventilation is readily corrected by an increase in fraction of inspired oxygen (FiO_2). However, one should use caution in patients with hypoxia due to hypoventilation. It is critical to treat the hypoxia, but patients with hypoventilation syndromes may have a blunted respiratory response to hypercarbia and may depend on their hypoxic respiratory drive. Their hypoventilation and CO_2 retention may worsen in response to supplemental oxygen, and CO_2 narcosis can ensue. Additionally, increasing PaO_2 without improving hypoventilation will mask the ability to detect ongoing hypoventilation with pulse oximetry. In other words, hypoventilation and hypercarbic respiratory failure may continue and worsen, but oxygen saturations will remain above 90%. Ventilatory assistance, frequently with noninvasive ventilation, is often necessary to treat hypoxia due to hypoventilation.

Lung diseases that impair diffusion of oxygen across the alveolar capillaries and into the bloodstream can result in hypoxia. However, at rest, gas exchange is completed by the time blood has moved a third of the way through the alveolar capillaries. Therefore, even in the setting of severe decrements in diffusing capacity, there is usually enough time in the alveolar capillaries for gas exchange to be completed, and hypoxia does not occur. However, exercise and other conditions that decrease the transit time of blood in alveolar capillaries will lead to hypoxia in the setting of impaired diffusion. Common conditions that cause impaired diffusion are disorders of interstitial inflammation such as idiopathic pulmonary fibrosis or pneumocystis pneumonia. Diseases that result in loss of alveolar surface area, such as emphysema, will also lead to impaired diffusion. Furthermore, these diseases may also be associated with V/Q mismatch and have mixed etiologies for hypoxia. Hypoxia from impaired diffusion is often associated with desaturation with activity and corrects relatively easily with supplemental oxygen.

Hypoxia will occur if the inspired oxygen tension is reduced. Fortunately this does not occur in hospitals but is an important phenomenon in mountaineers. Compensatory mechanisms cause hyperventilation and the ABG value shows a low $PaCO_2$ and a low PaO_2. This condition also improves with supplemental oxygen.

CONFIRMING HYPOXEMIA AT THE BEDSIDE: MEASURES OF OXYGENATION

■ PULSE OXIMETRY

The use of pulse oximetry is ubiquitous in the hospital setting and provides valuable information quickly and noninvasively. Pulse oximetry is based on differences in the absorption of light by oxygenated hemoglobin and deoxygenated hemoglobin. Oxygenated hemoglobin reflects light more effectively than deoxygenated at 660 nm, whereas the reverse is true at 940 nm. Pulse oximeters calculate the relative amounts of oxygenated and deoxygenated hemoglobin based on the reflection of light at these two wavelengths. Pulse oximeters do not account for the presence of methemoglobin or carboxyhemoglobin. If significant amounts of abnormal hemoglobin are present the oximetry reading will be falsely elevated. Pulse oximetry is very useful in that it can provide rapid and continuous information about arterial oxygen tension. Pulse oximetry results are inaccurate in the setting of methemoglobinemia and carbon monoxide poisoning. In carboxyhemoglobinemia, the pulse oximeter recognizes oxyhemoglobin and carboxyhemoglobin as identical because of similar wavelengths, and therefore overestimates the oxyhemoglobin concentration (and therefore the oxygen saturation is incorrectly reported as high). Methemoglobinemia registers at both frequencies of the pulse oximeter and therefore tends to result in a reading that is close to an 85% saturation, which fails to respond normally to changes in oxygen levels. Individuals with very dark skin pigmentation may have artificially low readings, and dark nail polish may also affect results (**Table 93-2**).

Co-oximetry can be performed to measure accurate levels of methemoglobin and carboxyhemoglobin. A co-oximeter measures absorption of different wavelengths, and the proportions of oxyhemoglobin, carboxyhemoglobin, and methemoglobin can be readily distinguished. When a patient presents with carbon monoxide poisoning, for instance, a co-oximeter can detect the carboxyhemoglobin and therefore report the oxyhemoglobin (and oxygen saturation) as markedly reduced.

TABLE 93-2 Pitfalls of Pulse Oximetry Interpretation

Mechanism	Result	Management
• Methemoglobinemia ▪ Hereditary Methemoglobinemia ▪ Drugs (anesthesia)	• Pulse oximetry shows a result ~85% • Oxygen supplementation does not raise O_2 saturation	• Place a co-oximeter to confirm presence of methemoglobinemia
• Carboxyhemoglobinemia ▪ Carbon monoxide poisoning	• Falsely high saturation	• Place a co-oximeter to confirm presence of carboxyhemoglobinemia
• Dark skin pigmentation	• Artificially low readings	• Confirm hypoxemia with arterial blood gas (ABG)
• Dark nail polish	• Artificially low readings	• Confirm hypoxemia with ABG
• Bilirubin	• Falsely low saturation	• Use ABG to guide management
• Poor peripheral perfusion	• Low signal, unreliable results	• Use ABG to guide management

PRACTICE POINT

Oximetry pitfalls

- Pulse oximetry is a valuable tool but can occasionally be inaccurate. One should make sure the pulse tracing is accurate and matches with the cardiac monitor. Patients with poor peripheral circulation such as those with systemic sclerosis or severe hypotension and shock frequently have inaccurate or unobtainable pulse oximetry. Patients with very dark skin pigmentation or dark nail polish may also have inaccurate pulse oximetry. Lastly, pulse oximetry is falsely elevated in patients with methemoglobinemia and carboxyhemoglobinemia.

PRACTICE POINT

- When an individual is on supplemental oxygen, the actual FiO_2 depends on minute ventilation and respiratory patterns. More room air (PO_2 of ~21%) can be mixed in with delivered O_2, and it is difficult to determine the actual FiO_2 the patient is receiving. For example, 4 liters of oxygen deliver approximately 36% FiO_2. Yet, in a patient with chronic obstructive pulmonary disease (COPD) with a high minute ventilation and prolonged expiratory phase (who entrains more ambient air), the FiO_2 actually delivered may be 28%. Every 0.05 increase in the FiO_2 will decrease the calculated A-a gradient by 35 mm Hg. Therefore, in the COPD patient example, the calculated A-a gradient may be incorrectly high. We recommend always calculating the A-a gradient on room air.

ARTERIAL BLOOD GAS

Direct sampling of arterial blood provides the ability to measure arterial tensions of oxygen and CO_2 and arterial pH. The greatest advantage measuring ABGs has over pulse oximetry is that $PaCO_2$ can be accurately measured. This allows one to determine whether hypoventilation is present, and one can calculate the A-a oxygen gradient. The A-a gradient is the difference in PaO_2 between the alveoli and arterial blood. To calculate the A-a gradient one must first use the alveolar gas equation to estimate the alveolar oxygen tension. The alveolar gas equation is: $P_AO_2 = FiO_2(P_B - P_{H2O}) - (Pa_{CO2}/R)$, where FiO_2 is the fraction of inspired oxygen, PB is the barometric pressure, P_{H2O} is the vapor pressure of water, and R is the respiratory quotient. If a patient is breathing room air and is near sea level the equation simplifies to $PaO_2 = 150 - (Pa_{CO2}/0.8)$. To calculate the A-a gradient one simply subtracts the measured PaO_2 from the calculated P_AO_2. A normal A-a gradient for a 20-year-old ranges from 4 to 17 mm Hg and increases by 3–4 mm Hg per decade of age. The A-a gradient will also normally increase with increasing levels of inspired oxygen. Therefore, it is best to calculate the A-a gradient on room air.

APPROACH TO HYPOXIA AT THE BEDSIDE

Hypoxia can be acute or chronic. For the purposes of this chapter we will focus on the acute syndrome as is typically seen in the hospital setting. It is important to recognize signs and symptoms of hypoxia, differentiate between a pulmonary etiology and other causes, and treat quickly and appropriately. The principles of management of acute hypoxia include identifying the correct clinical setting for the patient, airway management, correction of hypoxemia, and treatment of the underlying cause.

There are circumstances when acute hypoxia is considered a life-threatening condition, necessitating immediate action. Fulminant hypoxic respiratory failure and cardiopulmonary arrest are indications for emergent intubation and mechanical ventilation. In these situations, it is necessary to secure the airway first, attempt to correct the hypoxemia, and then work up the potential cause for the respiratory arrest.

There are many different reasons an individual may become hypoxic. Abnormalities of the central nervous system can cause suppression of the neural drive to breathe, resulting in hypoventilation and hypercapnia. Examples include overdose of narcotic or sedative drugs, meningoencephalitis, localized tumors of the medulla, strokes affecting the medulla, hepatic failure, and uremia. Drugs can particularly negatively affect individuals whose respiratory center is already desensitized by hypoventilation syndromes, such as obstructive sleep apnea or obesity hypoventilation. Disorders of the peripheral nervous system or muscles can cause hypoventilation and hypoxemic respiratory failure, including Guillain-Barré, myasthenia gravis, muscular dystrophies, and disorders of the chest wall (kyphoscoliosis). Obstruction of the airways is a common cause of hypoxemia, especially in pediatric populations. Upper airway examples include acute epiglottitis, foreign body aspiration, and tumors. Lower airway obstruction can be caused by COPD, asthma, and cystic fibrosis. Disorders of the alveoli themselves can result in hypoxemia, characterized by diffuse alveolar filling. This most commonly occurs in pulmonary edema, pneumonia, pulmonary hemorrhage, and aspiration.

After ensuring that the patient is not acutely decompensating, a comprehensive history should be obtained to help elucidate the possible cause of hypoxemia. Smoking status, possible occupational exposures, sick contacts, recent travel, and personal medical history may give diagnostic clues to the etiology of the hypoxemia. For instance, a history of COPD, coronary artery disease, cystic fibrosis, neuromuscular disorder, or stroke can give an indication of the cause of hypoxia.

An individual may display signs and symptoms of hypoxia in a variety of different ways. Pulmonary signs include tachypnea, dyspnea, and cyanosis. Cardiac manifestations include tachycardia, palpitations, arrhythmias, hypotension, chest pain, diaphoresis, and shock. Hypoxia may be evident by the presence of altered mental status, delirium, headache, seizures, obtundation, and tremors. It is important to thoroughly look for these signs and symptoms, and initiate the appropriate workup for the etiology of hypoxia.

The initial goal of treatment of hypoxemia is to provide adequate oxygen delivery to organs and tissues, keeping the $PaO_2 \geq 60$ mm Hg. Supplemental oxygen is supplied by low-flow or high-flow systems, based on the clinical circumstances. In more severe cases of hypoxemia, continuous positive airway pressure (CPAP) or bilevel positive airway pressure (BiPAP) is necessary to provide sufficient oxygen delivery. However, if an acceptable PaO_2 can't be obtained by these means, intubation is required.

Confirmation of the diagnosis of suspected hypoxia is based on arterial blood analysis. Evaluation must be initiated early, concurrent with the treatment of acute respiratory failure and/or hypoxia. The ABG value is used to assist in the diagnosis of hypoxia, differentiate between acute and chronic forms, and help guide treatment.

A chest X-ray (CXR) should be obtained to look for causes of hypoxia such as pneumonia, pneumothorax, pulmonary edema, or masses that can be further evaluated and treated. A computed tomographic (CT) scan of the chest may also be warranted to follow up an abnormal CXR. Consideration should be given to a possible pulmonary embolus as an etiology for acute hypoxia and can be evaluated with lower-extremity Doppler ultrasound, V/Q scan, CT scan of the chest, and/or echocardiogram.

HYPOXIA WITH A CLEAR CHEST X-RAY

One situation that is commonly faced in the hospital is a patient that presents with hypoxia but has a clear chest radiograph. Fortunately, the differential diagnosis is relatively limited, and the etiology can generally be discerned with a thorough history and readily available tests. Potential causes include pulmonary embolism, bronchospasm from obstructive lung disease such as asthma, early pneumonia (especially pneumocystic carinii pneumonia (PCP)), early interstitial lung disease, shunt due to intracardiac causes or arteriovenous malformations, hypoventilation, and lastly microatelectasis. It should be apparent that a history and physical exam can help narrow the etiology. Patients with asthma will often wheeze and have a history of asthma. Additionally they should respond to appropriate therapy such as bronchodilators and steroids. While the diagnosis of pulmonary embolism can be challenging, there are items on the history that should make one suspicious. These include risk factors for deep venous thrombosis (DVT), and the acute onset of dyspnea and/or chest pain. Patients with early pneumonia will frequently have fever, cough, and sputum production.

Microatelectasis needs to be thought of if no other causes are found. Even relatively small amounts of atelectasis can cause significant shunt physiology and hypoxia. Atelectasis should be identifiable on CT scan.

Hypoventilation will be detected with the correct clinical scenario and an ABG value showing an elevation in $PaCO_2$ without an increased A-a gradient.

TREATMENT CONSIDERATIONS

Oxygen supplementation can be given in a variety of ways, depending on how hypoxic an individual is and the underlying reason for being hypoxic. Indications for acute oxygen therapy include hypoxemia [PaO_2 < 60 mm Hg or oxygen saturation (SaO_2) < 90%] or tachypnea with a respiratory rate > 24 breaths/minute. Indications for long-term oxygen therapy are PaO_2 < 55 or an SaO_2 < 88% at rest. During oxygen supplementation, it is important to remember that a PaO_2 of 60 mm Hg is approximately equal to an SaO_2 of 90%. It is reasonable to aim for a goal of PaO_2 of 60 mm Hg in initial treatment of hypoxia, although in certain situations the acceptable threshold level may be adjusted up or down. For instance, in sickle cell anemia, hypoxia associated with cardiac disease, or chest pain, increases above a PaO_2 of 60 mm Hg may be important. Those with chronic CO_2 retention may need to have a lower goal because of abnormal control of respiration.

There are two main oxygen delivery systems: low flow and high flow delivery systems. Low-flow systems include oxygen delivery by nasal cannula (NC), simple mask, and reservoir mask (partial rebreather and nonrebreather). Low flow systems do not deliver a constant inspired oxygen concentration since there is room air entrained into the NC or mask. Changes in inspiratory flow rate and tidal volumes will entrain more or less room air, changing the actual FiO_2 received. High flow oxygen delivery systems (eg, venturi masks) maintain the selected FiO_2 by using an oxygen flow rate that is higher than typical inspiratory flows or a reservoir bag.

Nasal cannulas can deliver up to 6 LPM of oxygen. Higher flow rates become uncomfortable for patients. One liter per minute of oxygen delivers approximately 24% oxygen (FiO_2 0.24), with each additional liter adding approximately 3–4% of oxygen (**Table 93-3**). However, these estimates are very crude and can vary greatly. Different respiratory patterns can affect how much room air is entrained into the mask, therefore mixing room air with delivered O_2, resulting in a lower or higher inspired PO_2. Low minute ventilation and hypoventilation will increase the actual inspired FiO_2. Prolonged expiratory phase, increased metabolic rate associated with sepsis, and hyperventilation from exercise will decrease the actual FiO_2. Therefore, the percent of oxygen supplied by each liter is a rough estimate, and breathing patterns can alter the amount of oxygen actually delivered. Simple masks can deliver up to 50–60% oxygen, and require a 5–6 LPM flow rate to avoid buildup of carbon dioxide (CO_2) in the mask. A reservoir bag can be attached to a simple face mask to increase the delivered oxygen to 80–85%. A flow rate of at least 5–8 LPM is needed to ensure distention of the mask and to keep CO_2 out of the mask. A nonrebreather mask can deliver nearly 100% FiO_2, by keeping inspiratory gases separate from expiratory gases by means of a one-way valve.

Air entrapment masks, which are frequently called venturi masks, can deliver up to 50% FiO_2 but are able to supply a constant FiO_2. Oxygen (100%) flows through a one-way valve and passes by two open ports, incorporating room air. The amount of air entrained depends on the flow rate and size of the two open ports, and as the inflow rate increases, less entrained room air is included. Therefore, the resultant FiO_2 remains constant, which is the main advantage to the venturi mask over simple masks. The venturi mask is ideal in treatment of hypoxia caused by COPD or chronic respiratory failure typified by hypercarbia because the FiO_2 can be accurately controlled, and a goal PaO_2 around 60 mm Hg (SaO_2 ~90%) can be obtained while decreasing the risk of worsening hypercarbia and acidosis. Nasal cannula or simple masks cannot accurately control the level of FiO_2 delivered, as already described; therefore giving too much oxygenation can decrease respiratory drive, increasing CO_2 retention.

TABLE 93-3 FiO_2 of Oxygen Delivery Devices

Oxygen Device	Approximate FiO_2 %
Nasal cannula	
1 liter	24
2 liters	28
3 liters	32
4 liters	36
5 liters	40
6 liters	44
Simple oxygen mask	
5–6 liters	40
6–7 liters	50
7–8 liters	60
Simple mask with reservoir	
6 liters	60
7 liters	70
8 liters	80
9 liters	90
10 liters	>99
Nonrebreather	100
Venturi masks	
3 liters	24
6 liters	28
9 liters	40
12 liters	40
15 liters	50

Low minute ventilation, hypoventilation will increase the actual inspired FiO_2. Prolonged expiratory phase, increased metabolic rate associated with sepsis, and hyperventilation from exercise will decrease the actual inspired FiO_2. Therefore, the amount of oxygen delivered by each device is a rough estimate of the actual amount.

Noninvasive positive pressure ventilation (NIPPV) can be employed in certain types of respiratory failure to avoid the complications of mechanical ventilation such as airway trauma and pneumonia. NIPPV is beneficial in patients with COPD, congestive heart failure, chest wall disorders, obstructive sleep apnea, and neuromuscular disorders. NIPPV allows the patient to be awake and interactive and allows swallowing to take place. Treating appropriate patients with NIPPV helps to avoid endotracheal intubation and the associated risk of ventilator-associated pneumonia. However, NIPPV should be avoided in patients with altered mental status, respiratory or cardiac arrest, and aspiration risk. Mask options include nasal masks or full-face masks. Nasal masks tend to be more comfortable, cause less claustrophobia, and create less dead space. However, acutely dyspneic patients tend to breathe through their mouth; therefore full face masks are generally the better option in the acute setting.

More severe hypoxemia may require intubation and treatment with mechanical ventilation, ensuring delivery of required FiO_2. Some patients who require mechanical ventilation may have relatively normal ABG values but have signs of increased work of breathing with accessory muscle use, nasal flaring, paradoxical movement of the abdomen, and supraclavicular and intercostal retraction. These are all signs of respiratory fatigue and impending respiratory failure. In these cases it would be prudent to intubate early rather than later. Mechanical ventilation relieves respiratory distress by improving gas exchange, decreasing the work of breathing, and reversing respiratory muscle fatigue, while allowing treatment of and recovery from the process that incited respiratory failure.

There are several different modes of mechanical ventilation, but the mode that is used most frequently initially is assist/control (A/C) ventilation. In A/C mode the ventilator delivers a preset tidal volume both at a set rate and when triggered by a patient's inspiratory effort. This mode allows patients to breathe above the ventilator's set rate but also gives them full support when they do so, allowing respiratory muscles to rest. Initial parameters to set include respiratory rate, tidal volume (Vt), FiO_2, and positive end-expiratory pressure (PEEP). Respiratory rate can be set at 10–12 if pH and CO_2 are normal, but higher rates are required to help correct acidosis. A good place to start may be 75% of the patient's respiratory rate before intubation. Tidal volume was traditionally set at 10–12 mL/kg, but more recent work over the past decade has shown that 6 mL/kg has a mortality benefit over the traditional approach in acute lung injury (ALI) and acute respiratory distress syndrome (ARDS). Many physicians now use the 6 mL/kg in patients with these syndromes and even in individuals without ALI or ARDS due to concerns about ventilator-induced lung injury. FiO_2 should initially be set at 100% and titrated down to keep $PaO_2 > 60$ mm Hg or $SaO_2 > 90\%$. Pulmonary toxicity can occur at higher FiO_2 levels, and the goal should be to titrate down to 60% FiO_2 and below as tolerated. PEEP is normally set at 5 cm H_2O unless the patient has ALI or ARDS, which require higher levels of PEEP. Methods to increase oxygenation (improve PaO_2) include increasing FiO_2 and PEEP. Techniques to decrease partial pressure of carbon dioxide ($PaCO_2$) include increasing the respiratory rate or increasing Vt.

PULMONARY CONSULTATION

Frequently the cause of hypoxemia can be determined and treated without need for pulmonary consultation. However, in complicated cases, or cases in which a patient is unstable, or when considering invasive or expensive testing, a pulmonary consultation can be valuable. The pulmonary consultant should provide a reasonably complete but focused differential diagnosis for the patient's hypoxia, can assist in selecting the appropriate diagnostic tests to confirm the diagnosis, and should also assist in guiding appropriate therapy to correct the hypoxia and the underlying cause of hypoxia.

CASE 93-2

Our patient's initial workup included pulmonary function tests, chest CT, echocardiogram, and arterial blood gas. Pulmonary function tests show a moderate obstructive defect, a moderate restrictive defect, and a severe gas transfer defect. A CT scan of the chest showed patchy interstitial thickening bilaterally, mild emphysematous changes, cardiomegaly, and a pericardial effusion.

ABG on 4 liters of oxygen revealed a pH of 7.49, $PaCO_2$ of 35 mm Hg, PaO_2 of 71 mm Hg, and bicarbonate of 26. Initial bloodwork was significant for a creatinine level of 1.4 (reference range 0.6–1.2 mg/dL). Antinuclear antibody (ANA) was positive, with a titer of 1:80 in a speckled pattern. B-natriuretic peptide (BNP) was 4347 (reference range 0–125 pg/mL). Echocardiogram showed a massively dilated right ventricle with evidence of pressure and volume overload. A bubble study was positive for a patent foramen ovale with right to left shunting. Severe pulmonary hypertension was also suggested on echocardiogram with a right ventricular systolic pressure of 78 mm Hg. Right heart

catheterization confirmed pulmonary hypertension, showing a mean pulmonary artery pressure of 58 mm Hg.

The etiology of her hypoxemia was thought to be secondary to pulmonary hypertension, which was multifactorial in nature. Causes included COPD, interstitial disease from radiation, and obstructive sleep apnea. She was aggressively diuresed, and discharged on diuretic therapy with spironolactone and furosemide. She was then started on sildenafil, a phosphodiesterase-5 inhibitor, as an outpatient in a pulmonary hypertension specialty clinic. Her oxygenation and symptoms improved with this treatment, and she has noticed improvement in her functional capacity. This patient is now able to leave the house to attend church, run errands, and participate in daily activities, which she was unable to do previously. This case highlights multiple possible causes of hypoxia and the many diagnostic tools available to evaluate hypoxia.

CONCLUSION

In summary, hypoxia is common in the hospital setting and requires close monitoring and treatment. It is important to recognize signs and symptoms of hypoxia, differentiate between a pulmonary etiology and other causes, and treat quickly and appropriately.

SUGGESTED READINGS

Branson RD. The nuts and bolts of increasing arterial oxygenation: devices and techniques. *Respir Care*. 1993;38:672–686.

George RB. Ventilation, gas exchange, and oxygen delivery. In: George RB, Light RW, Matthay MA, Matthay RA, eds. *Chest Medicine: Essentials of Pulmonary and Critical Care Medicine*. 3rd ed. Baltimore: Williams and Wilikins; 1995;63–78.

Glenny RW. Teaching ventilation/perfusion relationships in the lung. *Adv Physiol Educ*. 2008;32:192–195.

Grippi MA. Respiratory failure: an overview. In: Fishman AP, Elias JA, Fishman JA, Grippi MA, Kaiser LR, Senior RM, eds. *Fishman's Pulmonary Diseases and Disorders*. 3rd ed. New York: McGraw-Hill; 1998;2525–2535.

Hall JB, Schmidt GA, Wood LDH. Acute hypoxemic respiratory failure. In: Murray JF, Nadel JA, eds. *Textbook of Respiratory Medicine*. 2nd ed. Philadelphia: WB Saunders; 1994;2589–2613.

Ventilation with lower tidal volumes as compared with traditional tidal volumes for acute lung injury and the acute respiratory distress syndrome. The Acute Respiratory Distress Syndrome Network. *N Engl J Med*. 2000;342:1301–1308.

Wahr JA, Tremper KK. Noninvasive oxygen monitoring techniques. *Crit Care Clin*. 1995;11:199–217.

West JB. Ventilation-perfusion relationships. In: Patricia A. Coryell. *Respiratory Physiology: The Essentials*. 5th ed. Baltimore: Williams and Wilkins; 1995:51–69.

Williams AJ. ABC of oxygen: assessing and interpreting arterial blood gases and acid-base balance. *BMJ*. 1998;317:1213–1216.

Wood KE. Major pulmonary embolism: review of a pathophysiologic approach to the golden hour of hemodynamically significant pulmonary embolism. *Chest*. 2002;121:877–905.

CHAPTER 94

Insomnia: Assessment and Management of Sleep Disorders

Kimberly A. Hardin, MD, MS, FAASM
Kristina Antonson, MD, PhD
Anne B. McBride, MD
Julie S. Young, MD, MS

Key Clinical Questions

1. Why is it important to understand the regulation of normal sleep?
2. What are the most common causes of disrupted sleep in hospitalized patients?
3. What are the consequences of sleep deprivation?
4. What are the key questions that an examiner should ask when approaching a patient with impaired sleep?
5. What are nonpharmacologic and pharmacologic modalities for preventing and treating sleep problems in hospitalized patients?

CASE 94-1

A 59-year-old retired school teacher with a history of advanced ovarian cancer has been admitted for community-acquired pneumonia, responding well to appropriate antibiotic treatment. She had lost 10 pounds since her last clinic visit, and she revealed that she was having a difficult time sleeping during the night. Her husband was concerned that she had been "pretty down" recently. How should this problem be addressed?

CASE 94-2

A 48-year-old woman with obesity, hypertension, depression, and asthma, was admitted to the hospital for treatment of an exacerbation of her multiple sclerosis. Her physicians continued her home medications including lisinopril, hydrochlorothiazide, bupropion, and interferon beta. After 48 hours, her weakness improved in response to intravenous high-dose methylprednisolone, but the doctor on call has been called every night for a "sleeper." The patient stated: "I cannot sleep at all! I feel worse than when I came in! I just feel so anxious; this happens every time I have a flare." She has also been having trouble staying asleep because she needs to get up multiple times each night to urinate, a nurse interrupted her sleep at 2 AM every night to take her blood pressure, and her roommate has been watching TV all night. Although she uses continuous positive airway pressure (CPAP) at home, she forgot to bring the machine to the hospital. What adjustments can be made to improve the sleep of patients like her?

INTRODUCTION

Sleep disruption is a common problem among hospitalized patients. Patients frequently report disturbed sleep not only during their hospital stay but also prior to and after discharge. Approximately one-third of hospitalized patients have insomnia at the time of admission. Additionally, up to 69% of postsurgical patients continue to complain of prolonged sleep problems after hospital discharge. The high prevalence of sleep disturbance among this population warrants clinicians to incorporate the evaluation and treatment of sleep problems as part of routine hospital care. In order to effectively treat sleep complaints, one has to understand the regulation of normal sleep and how various disorders may influence or impair this process. Early recognition and treatment of sleep complaints can improve recovery among hospitalized patients.

PRACTICE POINT

- Sleep deprivation is associated with physiologic and psychological sequelae that may impair recovery from acute illness. Screening patients for sleep problems is the "new" sixth vital sign.

PATHOPHYSIOLOGY

Even in healthy individuals, partial and total sleep deprivation significantly impacts sleep architecture and sleep quality.

Evidence supports that persistent lack of sleep can impair physiologic processes and could potentially affect recovery from acute illness or injury. Sleep duration, architecture, and the sleep–wake cycle are closely associated with many metabolic and regulatory processes. Sleep deprivation can result in detrimental physiologic and psychological sequelae. Sleep deprivation has been associated with insulin resistance, impaired postural control, decreased ventilatory drive, increased sympathetic cardiovascular activation, blunted hypothalamic–pituitary–adrenal axis responsiveness, and impaired host defenses. The lack of restorative sleep increases the risk of developing anxiety, mood disorders, and delirium, especially in acutely ill older patients. In the presence of acute physical infirmity, inadequate sleep may further compound illness and recovery.

Sleep architecture refers to a characteristic pattern of sleep and includes two major stages: non–rapid eye movement (NREM) and rapid eye movement (REM) sleep. Normal sleep latency, or time to fall asleep, is usually 10 to 20 minutes, and total sleep time ranges from 6 to 9 hours per 24 hours. NREM sleep consists of three stages (S1–S3), with each stage leading to a progressively deeper level of sleep. S3 is known as deep sleep or slow-wave sleep (SWS), is predominant during the first third of the sleep period, and is believed to be necessary for physiologic restoration. SWS is associated with a decrease in metabolic rate, heart rate, and oxygen consumption and is anabolic in protein and hormone synthesis. REM sleep follows SWS and is characterized by an activated brainwave pattern seen with electroencephalography (EEG), muscle paralysis (atonia), and periodic bursts of rapid eye movements. Dreaming occurs during REM sleep and is hypothesized to be essential for emotional and cognitive well-being. REM sleep is a catabolic phase and can be associated with cardiovascular and respiratory instability. REM sleep occurs predominantly in the later period of sleep. Additionally, the ability to consolidate sleep declines with age, requiring most elderly persons to nap during the day in order to achieve a normal total amount of sleep.

Sleep disruption may also occur when regulatory processes are impaired or altered. Sleep regulation is a balance between a homeostatic or biologic need for sleep or "sleep debt" and the intrinsic body clock, or circadian pacemaker. Homeostatic mechanisms are regulated in the preoptic area in the brain, while circadian systems are governed by the suprachiasmatic nucleus (SCN) of the hypothalamus. Melatonin, a hormone produced by the pineal gland, is associated with sleep induction. It builds up as darkness increases and is inhibited by ambient light. The adrenal secretion of cortisol follows a circadian pattern and peaks in the early morning hours in preparation for the increased metabolic demands during wakefulness. Neurotransmitters are intrinsically involved in sleep regulation and include gamma-aminobutyric acid (GABA), serotonin, histamine, norepinephrine, acetylcholine, hypocretin, glutamate, and glycine. REM sleep is promoted by acetylcholine. SWS is induced primarily by GABA. Neurotransmitters that promote wakefulness include acetylcholine, histamine, noradrenaline (norepinephrine), serotonin, dopamine, and hypocretin (orexin). Many of the drugs that are commonly prescribed in hospitalized patients affect one or more of these neurotransmitters, thus promoting sedation (antihistamine) or activating effects (dopamine) such as wakefulness, and, in vulnerable patients, delirium.

ETIOLOGY AND DIFFERENTIAL DIAGNOSIS OF SLEEP COMPLAINTS

There are numerous factors that may contribute to disturbed sleep in hospitalized patients, including primary sleep disorders, medical illnesses, psychiatric illness, drugs, and the hospital environment. Additionally, the manifestations of sleep disruption and/or sleep deprivation will vary depending on the individual.

COMMON SLEEP DISORDERS

By far, insomnia is the most common sleep complaint among patients in both ambulatory and hospital settings. The prevalence of chronic insomnia is high, with approximately 20–30% of the general population reporting ongoing symptoms. Chronic insomnia is associated with decreased quality of life, daytime functional limitations, chronic pain, increased risk of medical and psychiatric illnesses, substance abuse, increased utilization of health services, and increased risk of death.

Insomnia can manifest in several ways. The *International Classification of Sleep Disorders* (ICSD-2), published by the American Academy of Sleep Medicine (AASM), defines insomnia as difficulty initiating or maintaining sleep, waking up too early, or sleep that is chronically nonrestorative or perceived to be poor in quality. To meet diagnostic criteria for insomnia, these symptoms *must* be associated with daytime mental or physical sequelae that impair the functional status of the individual. Insomnia may be a primary disorder or may be comorbid with another physical or mental illness.

In the landmark Sleep Heart Health Study, population subgroups were identified who were at increased risk for poor sleep. Older individuals (>60 years old) were shown to have a lower arousal threshold associated with increased awakenings at night, decreased sleep efficiency, and decreased REM quantity. Each of these changes contributes to poor sleep quality and can result in poor daytime functioning, excessive sleepiness, or cognitive changes, which are commonly noted in the elderly. Although women demonstrated increased SWS compared to men, they had more complaints of poor sleep quality associated with worsening daytime functioning. The precise reason for this is unknown but is speculated to involve hormonal influence as well as greater prevalence of comorbid conditions associated with insomnia, such as depression.

Other common primary sleep disorders that frequently coexist with medical illnesses include obstructive sleep apnea (OSA), restless leg syndrome (RLS), and periodic limb movement disorder (PLMD). **Table 94-1** describes these common sleep disorders and provides differential diagnoses to consider. These disorders may present with a variety of symptoms.

OSA affects approximately 24% of men and 9% of women in the United States and is associated with substantial mental and physical morbidity. Untreated OSA likely contributes to a significant proportion of acute hospital admissions, particularly for heart or respiratory failure. OSA may go unrecognized until a patient is incidentally hospitalized and observed to have difficulty breathing, paradoxical breathing, or oxygen desaturation. Risk factors for OSA include obesity, hypothyroidism, male gender, family history, African American race, and certain craniofacial characteristics: acromegaly, micrognathia or retrognathia, large tongue, or Mallampati class 3–4. OSA is characterized by episodes of complete or partial pharyngeal obstruction during sleep that causes snoring, apneic episodes, choking, dyspnea, and restlessness. These episodes are associated with intermittent nocturnal sympathetic activation leading to nocturnal awakenings and cortical arousals, all of which lead to daytime symptoms of fatigue, sleepiness, and cognitive impairment. Chronic sympathetic activation and intermittent hypoxemia are associated with increased vascular injury and inflammation that are known to occur in cardiovascular disease. Treatment of OSA with positive airway pressure (PAP) is shown to improve control of hypertension, diabetes, pulmonary hypertension, atrial fibrillation, and mortality.

Approximately 20% of patients with OSA have concomitant RLS or PLMD, which are distinct problems and need to be differentiated from peripheral neuropathy and positional or nocturnal leg cramps. RLS is thought to affect as much as 40% of the population and is characterized by an unpleasant crampy, "creeping" or "crawling" sensation in the lower extremities that is relieved by persistently moving the legs. RLS frequently starts in the late evening or before

TABLE 94-1 Clinical Features and Differential Diagnoses of Common Primary Sleep Disorders

Sleep Disorder	Clinical Features	Differential Diagnosis
Obstructive sleep apnea (OSA)	Repetitive episodes of upper airway obstruction that occur during sleep, usually associated with oxygen desaturation. Episodes include loud snoring or gasps lasting 20–30 seconds. Associated with morning headaches and dry mouth.	Sleep-related laryngospasm, nocturnal gastroesophageal reflux, narcolepsy, hypersomnia, PLMD, central alveolar hypoventilation, paroxysmal nocturnal dyspnea, primary snoring, Cheyne-Stokes ventilation, nocturnal asthma.
Periodic limb movement disorder (PLMD)	Periodic episodes of repetitive and stereotyped limb movements: extension of the big toe with partial flexion of the ankles, knees, or hips. Muscle contractions last 0.5 to 5 seconds, with 20- to 40-second intervals between them.	Sleep starts (occurs just prior to, not during, sleep, and does not have a regular periodicity like PLMD), nocturnal epileptic seizures, myoclonic epilepsy.
Restless leg syndrome (RLS)	Uncomfortable leg sensations that occur prior to sleep onset that leads to an irresistible urge to move the legs. Described as "achy," "crawling," "pulling," "prickling," or "tingling," and disrupts sleep onset.	Chronic myelopathy, peripheral neuropathy, akathisia, fasciculation syndromes. RLS may be triggred by iron deficiency anemia, so consider iron studies.
Sleep starts	Sudden, brief contraction of the legs that occurs at sleep onset. Usually benign, but may worsen during hospitalization, and interfere with sleep.	PLMD, RLS, hyperexplexia syndrome in which generalized myoclonus is readily elicited by stimuli.

OSA, obstructive sleep apnea; PLMD, periodic limb movement disorder; RLS, restless leg syndrome.
Data from American Academy of Sleep Medicine. International *Classification of Sleep Disorders, Revised: Diagnostic and Coding Manual*. Chicago, IL: American Academy of Sleep Medicine; 2001.

bedtime, and often is a major cause of sleep-onset insomnia. The requisite bed rest during hospitalization can worsen RLS, further exacerbating sleep problems. It is also associated with many metabolic disorders, particularly renal disease, iron deficiency, and diabetes. Other conditions associated with RLS include pregnancy, rheumatoid arthritis, fibromyalgia, multiple sclerosis, and Parkinson disease. The etiology of RLS is not completely understood, but it may relate to inadequate generation or transport of dopamine due to iron deficiency or other metabolic disturbances. Serum iron and ferritin levels should be evaluated and treated if ferritin levels are <75 μg. Aggressive treatment of other underlying diseases should be considered as first-line therapy. Selective serotonin uptake inhibitors (SSRIs) and alcohol may exacerbate RLS and should be avoided, if possible. Additional treatment includes the use of a dopaminergic agent at bedtime, such as ropinirole (Requip). Other agents that are effective, particularly in individuals with neuropathy, are gabapentin, narcotics, and benzodiazepines.

PLMD occurs in about 80% of those with RLS and is characterized by stereotyped involuntary limb movements that occur every 20 to 40 seconds during sleep. These can result in frequent cortical arousals, daytime somnolence, and fatigue. PLMD is found at higher frequency in several medical conditions, including hypertension, renal disease, and alcohol dependence. PLMD can be treated with longer-acting benzodiazepines such as clonazepam, and with dopaminergic agents.

GENERAL MEDICAL DISORDERS

Numerous medical illnesses can directly impair sleep physiology, leading to a cyclical interaction in which impaired sleep impedes recovery (**Figure 94-1**). **Table 94-2** lists selected medical and neurologic conditions, their associated sleep-related problems, and suggestions on how to alleviate these problems.

A recent study examined risk factors for sleep disturbance during hospitalization and found that the severity of comorbid conditions and poor performance of activities of daily living (ADL) predicted sleep complaints during admission. Physician awareness of the impact of sleep disturbance in hospitalized patients is vital since about half of patients admitted on general medical wards will complain of sleep disruption.

PRACTICE POINT

"Red flag"

- Poor performance of ADLs heralds a red flag for increased sleep disturbance while hospitalized.

Patients with pulmonary disorders and OSA can be profoundly affected by the normal physiologic changes that occur during sleep, particularly in REM sleep. REM sleep is associated with increased upper airway collapsibility and accessory muscle atonia (causing decreased muscle strength), which can result in episodes of marked oxygen desaturation. Patients with chronic obstructive pulmonary disease (COPD) demonstrate decreased total sleep time (TST), SWS, and REM sleep due to shortness of breath, nocturnal cough, and

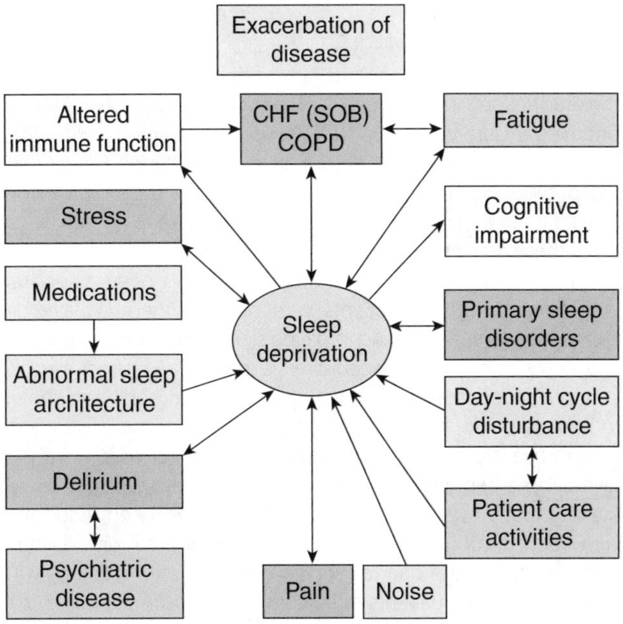

Figure 94-1 *Factors related to sleep deprivation and illness.*

TABLE 94-2 Common Chronic Diseases, Potential Effect on Sleep, and Suggested Interventions to Optimize Sleep

Disease	Effect on Sleep	Interventions to Improve Sleep
CHF	Orthopnea, paroxysmal nocturnal dyspnea, sleep-disordered breathing, increased sympathetic tone, nighttime diuresis, Cheyne-Stokes respiration.	Keep the head of bed elevated ≥ 30 degrees. Nocturnal O_2 to keep O_2 saturation > 88%. Daytime diuresis. Optimize cardiac function to treat Cheyne-Stokes respiration. Consider CPAP for CHF.
COPD	Persistent nocturnal hypoxemia with complications (eg, cor pulmonale, polycythemia).	O_2 for COPD and persistent hypoxemia (PaO_2 55–60 mm Hg).
	Sporadic nighttime desaturations.	PaO_2 ≤ 55 mm Hg → monitor O_2 saturation by pulse oximetry. If patient desaturates to ≤ 88% at night consistently, start nocturnal O_2. For hypercapnea, adjust O_2 to maintain O_2 saturation at 88–90%.
	Increased risk of airflow obstruction during REM.	Consider bedtime tiotropium and inhaled long-acting beta-adrenergic agonist agents.
	Inhibition of respiratory muscles in REM.	Avoid sedative-hypnotics that cause respiratory depression.
	Decreased functional residual capacity from recumbent position during sleep.	Keep the head of bed elevated > 30 degrees.
ESRD	Pruritus, nausea; increased risk of RLS and PLMD in patients with ESRD.	Consider ropinirole and pramipexole if RLS; if medications contraindicated, massage or walking will relieve discomfort. Correct hyperphosphatemia and uremia. Consider antipruritic and antiemetic agents.
Thyroid Disorders	Hypothyroidism—daytime hypersomnolence.	Treat underlying thyroid dysfunction. Discourage naps during the day, keep lights on during the day, and off during the night.
	Hyperthyroidism—hyperarousal symptoms (restlessness, tachycardia, diaphoresis, anxiety).	Treat underlying thyroid dysfunction. Low-dose beta-blocker (eg, propranolol, atenolol) for symptomatic relief.
Diabetes	Bedtime *hyperglycemia* → polydipsia, polyuria → frequent awakenings; or unnecessary nighttime monitoring of glucose levels. Inadequate scheduled or as needed insulin doses? High carbohydrate intake at bedtime?	Optimize blood glucose control. Increase scheduled or as needed insulin doses; consider consulting a dietitian to assess actual carbohydrate intake in the evening. Once bedtime glucose levels consistently ≤ 200 mg/dL, and no overnight hypoglycemic episodes, consider decreasing frequency of glucose monitoring at night.
	Early morning (eg, 0200–0400) *hypoglycemic* episodes → symptoms awaken patient, or lead to frequent routine glucose monitoring overnight.	Optimize blood glucose control. Once bedtime glucose levels consistently ≤ 200 mg/dL, and no overnight hypoglycemic episodes, consider decreasing frequency of glucose monitoring at night (eg, if currently checking every 2 hours → every 4 hours or more appropriate?)
Stroke	Focal neurologic deficits (eg, dysphagia, weakness or paralysis).	Keep the head of bed elevated > 30 degrees. Regularly suction secretions. Poststroke patients have an increased risk of hypersomnia, insomnia, and/or OSA.

CHF, congestive heart failure; CNS, central nervous system; COPD, chronic obstructive pulmonary disease; CPAP, continuous positive airway pressure; ESRD, end-stage renal disease; h, hours; OSA, obstructive sleep apnea; PLMD, periodic limb movement disorder; RLS, restless leg syndrome.

wheezing that impair sleep quality and duration. Sleep deprivation then further negatively impacts the work of breathing. Noninvasive positive pressure ventilation (NPPV) improves sleep efficiency, total sleep time, and quality of life in patients with hypercapnic COPD without significantly improving gas exchange and should be considered as an adjunctive therapy for improving sleep and quality of life in these patients.

Endocrine and metabolic disorders have also been associated with sleep disruption. Patients with diabetes mellitus have decreased total sleep time and impaired sleep quality due to nocturia and neuropathic pain. Inadequate sleep may also affect glucose control. Inadequate quality or quantity of sleep has been shown to be a risk factor for developing type 2 diabetes mellitus in large prospective studies and is associated with increased levels of glycosylated hemoglobin (HbA1c) in patients with type 2 diabetes mellitus. Both hypo- and hyperthyroidism have been associated with sleep disruption. Hypothyroidism is associated with daytime somnolence, fatigue due to reduced SWS and often coexists with OSA. Hyperthyroid patients often complain of insomnia, which has been attributed to a hypermetabolic state.

NEUROLOGIC AND PSYCHIATRIC CONDITIONS

Since the brain and its various neurotransmitter systems are critical in regulating sleep and wakefulness, patients with neurologic disorders have an increased risk of developing sleep disorders. Common problems include increased sleep fragmentation and wakefulness, with increases of stage 1 sleep and reductions of SWS and REM. Patients with neurodegenerative disorders have an increased risk of REM sleep behavior disorder characterized by vivid and unusual dreams with physically vigorous, violent-type behaviors that may appear as acute delirium and result in patient injury. About half of hospitalized patients with traumatic brain injury report insomnia and may develop circadian rhythm disturbances. Poststroke patients can develop insomnia or hypersomnia and are at higher risk for developing OSA in the first several months.

Fifty-seven percent of patients with chronic pain also complain of impaired sleep. Sleep disruption is so common in fibromyalgia (75%) that it is considered to be a key diagnostic symptom. Poor nighttime sleep is associated with decreased pain tolerance and greater pain intensity the following day. Pain causes sleep fragmentation by increasing cortical arousals; in turn, sleep deprivation may increase pain sensitivity by inhibiting opioid protein synthesis or reducing opioid receptor affinity.

PRACTICE POINT

- It is important to note that sleep is a biological necessity and will occur, albeit poorly, even among patients with intense pain; physicians must avoid the cognitive trap of assuming that a patient must not be having severe pain if he or she is able to sleep.

Sleep disturbance is a diagnostic criterion for mood, anxiety, substance abuse, and psychotic disorders. Thus, comorbid psychiatric disorders must be considered in hospitalized patients with sleep complaints, even if not previously diagnosed. Major depression is particularly common in hospitalized patients with early morning insomnia. Longitudinal studies have found that prior insomnia was associated with two- to fivefold increase in the odds of mood and anxiety disorders and suicide. Often, sleep disorders precede the onset of clinical depression, supporting the importance of assessing patient sleep quality during hospitalization.

Substance abuse disorders are also associated with sleep problems. Over half of patients undergoing alcohol rehabilitation exhibit symptoms of insomnia, such as increased sleep latency during the six months prior to entering treatment, and many report using alcohol for the purpose of initiating sleep. Indeed, untreated insomnia and other sleep problems may increase the risk of developing substance abuse problems due to "self-medicating" with alcohol and other substances to help with sleep. While alcohol and illicit substance intoxication and withdrawal are known to disrupt sleep directly, sleep disturbances may persist long after withdrawal symptoms have abated, sometimes years later.

DRUGS THAT AFFECT SLEEP

Many drugs used during hospitalization, such as antidepressants, anxiolytics, and narcotics, are well known to affect sleep. **Table 94-3** depicts commonly used drugs and their effect on sleep architecture.

A common misperception is that sedatives promote quality sleep. Sedatives may initially help with sleep onset, but they actually diminish SWS and enhance stage 2 sleep, causing nonrestorative sleep. This may manifest as next day "hangover," fatigue, irritability, and poor function. Additionally, routine medications used to treat medical illnesses also disrupt sleep. The most common agents that impair sleep include antiepileptic drugs (AEDs), tricyclic antidepressants (TCAs), antihypertensives, antihistamines, and corticosteroids. Lipophilic beta-antagonists such as propranolol and timolol can increase total wake time, decrease REM sleep, and increase the incidence of nightmares and insomnia. Hydrophilic beta-antagonists such as atenolol and sotalol do not have these effects. Anabolic steroids and beta-agonist bronchodilator therapy can cause severe anxiety, sleeplessness, and even psychosis. Vasopressor agents such as dopamine can cause cortical activation, leading to increased arousal and reduced SWS.

PRACTICE POINT

Beware

- Sedation with hypnotics results in *nonrestorative* sleep.

Medication dosing regimens used in the hospital can also impact sleep. For example, giving diuretics in the evening will result in nighttime polyuria, and dosing activating antidepressants in the late afternoon or evening can result in sleep-onset insomnia. Withdrawal from narcotics or alcohol or use of venlafaxine may cause severe REM intrusion associated with vivid dreams, nightmares, and exacerbation of underlying stress disorders. Carefully evaluate the medication regimens of elderly patients who develop sleep problems during a hospitalization, since these patients are especially vulnerable to drug-drug interactions, and paradoxical drug effects.

HOSPITAL ENVIRONMENT

Sleeping in an unfamiliar environment is likely to negatively impact sleep, but the hospital environment has many additional disruptions, particularly in high-acuity settings. Environmental noise and patient care activities account for about 30% of patient awakenings in intensive care unit (ICU) patients. Peak noise levels in the ICU have average sound peaks of over 150 dB and often exceed 80 dB between midnight and 6 am. By comparison, a lawn mower or truck traffic has a sound level of 90 dB. The high noise level in hospitals has long been implicated as the major sleep disruptor, but studies in the past decade have found that patient care activities also cause a substantial disruption in sleep. This is in part due to routine activities, such as bathing, vital sign monitoring, radiologic studies, and phlebotomy that are conducted at night or early morning due to scheduling constraints.

Understanding that numerous factors may impair sleep during hospitalization allows clinicians to systemically evaluate and treat sleep problems. More than just prescribing sedative/hypnotic agents, the treatment for sleep disruption includes addressing multiple medical, behavioral, and environmental factors.

EVALUATION OF SLEEP COMPLAINTS AND NONPHARMACOLOGIC MANAGEMENT

Assessment and evaluation of any sleep problem begins with an initial interview of the patient and family, as well as a review of the medical record for documentation of preexisting primary sleep disorders and any factor that could exacerbate or contribute to the current situation. Obtain a focused history by using questions listed in **Table 94-4** to characterize the onset, duration, frequency, and specific characteristics of the patient's current sleep patterns. Next, establish whether the onset of the patient's sleep complaint began at the time of hospitalization. If the sleep disruption began with hospitalization, subsequent questions can then focus on hospital factors that may be impairing sleep, such as altered sleep hygiene behaviors. Inquire about the use or abuse of substances such as sedatives, antidepressants, AEDs, and opioids. Ask questions about the presence of pain syndromes, nocturnal gastroesophageal reflux, and other symptoms that often impact sleep.

The next step is to assess for preexisting mood, anxiety, psychotic, and substance use disorders, all of which may be exacerbated during an acute hospitalization. It is also important to rule out delirium. The nighttime awakenings and behavioral disturbances associated with delirium should not be mistaken for "insomnia." This mistake can lead to delirious patients being treated with medications such as benzodiazepines or antihistamines, which can worsen the delirium. Before prescribing a sleep agent, assess for the presence of suboptimally treated medical, neurologic, psychiatric condition, or a primary sleep disorder (see Tables 94-1 and 94-2). Care should be taken to rely only on sound, documented evidence or a confirmatory medical history when formulating the diagnosis. For example, a patient may state that he has "apnea" because his wife speculates this, but he has never had a formal evaluation for OSA.

TABLE 94-3 Selected Drugs, Their Effects on Sleep Architecture, and Clinical Implications

Drug Class	Examples of Drugs	Sleep Architecture	Clinical Implications
CNS			
TCAs	Amoxapine, amitriptyline, imipramine, nortriptyline, desipramine, doxepin, clomipramine	Suppresses REM sleep, ↑ TST, ↑ stage 2 sleep	*Very sedating*. Can cause restlessness, psychomotor agitation during sleep, subjectively poorer sleep quality, and daytime sedation.
SSRIs	Fluoxetine, sertraline, citalopram, escitalopram, paroxetine	SSRIs ↑ TST, are less sedating than TCAs and MAOIs. May ↓ REM, ↑ TWT, ↑ TST, ↓ SE	Some patients experience activation rather than sedation.
SNRI	Venlafaxine, duloxetine	Varies. ↓ TST.	*Activating* in some patients; *sedating* in 12–31%. If keeps patient *awake*, switch to AM dosing. If *sedating*, switch to PM dosing. May cause vivid dreams or nightmares, and exacerbate underlying anxiety disorders such as posttraumatic stress disorder.
Stimulants	Ephedrine, pseudoephedrine, modafinil	↓ TST, ↓ SWS, ↑ sleep latency.	*Activating*. Avoid after 6 PM.
Cardiovascular			
Lipophilic beta-blockers	Propranolol, pindolol, metoprolol, timolol	↑ Awakenings, ↑ TWT, ↓ REM,	*Activating. Lipophilic* beta-blockers → ↑ daytime sleep when dosed in morning. Induce nightmares.
CNS Agents	Norepinephrine, epinephrine	*Activating*. ↓ REM, ↓ SWS.	Minimize use at night.
	Dopamine	*Activating*. ↓ REM, ↓ SWS.	Minimize use at night.
Ca^{++} channel blockers	Amlodipine, verapamil, nifedipine	Exacerbate underlying medical condition.	↓ Lower esophageal sphincter tone → nocturnal gastroesophageal reflux → sleep disturbance.
Diuretics	HCTZ, furosemide		Nighttime diuresis → frequent awakenings → ↓ sleep.
Other			
Opioids	Codeine, morphine.	*Sedating*. ↓ SWS, ↓ REM.	Minimize use at night.
NSAIDs	Ibuprofen, indomethacin, celecoxib	↓ TST, ↓ SE.	Minimize use at night.
Methyl xanthine	Theophylline	*Activating*. ↑ stage 1, ↓ REM.	Causes less restful sleep.
Antihistamines	Diphenhydramine, promethazine	*Sedating*	May have paradoxical effect on children. Can disrupt sleep if associated with delirium.
Corticosteroids	Dexamethasone, prednisone	*Activating*. ↓ REM, ↓ SWS, nightmares.	Can disrupt sleep, ↑ anxiety, induce mania or psychosis.
Quinolone	Ciprofloxacin, sparfloxacin, ofloxacin, grepafloxacin, levofloxacin	*Activating*.	Consider sleep agent after maximizing sleep hygiene. Linezolid rarely causes sleep disturbances.

CNS, central nervous system; HCTZ, hydrochlorothiazide; MAOIs, monoamine oxidase inhibitors; NSAIDs, nonsteroidal anti-inflammatory drugs; REM, rapid eye movement; SE, sleep efficiency; SNRI, serotonin norepinephrine reuptake inhibitor; SSRIs, selective serotonin reuptake inhibitors; SWS, slow wave sleep (stage 3 and 4, or deep sleep); TCA, tricyclic and tetracyclic antidepressants; TST, total sleep time; TWT, total wake time; →, leads to or causes; ↑, increase; ↓, decrease or reduce.

Lastly, evaluate the extent to which environmental factors such as noise level, various therapies, and hospital routines may be impairing sleep. Discuss the importance of maintaining a quieter environment with key staff members. When available, relaxation tapes, massage, and warm (noncaffeinated) beverages are preferable to pharmacologic strategies, as shown in **Table 94-5**.

In addition, limit potential iatrogenic causes of disrupted sleep by using alternative drugs or drug regimens, and consider altering evaluation and treatment interventions to promote uninterrupted sleep at night. Carefully review the medication list and consider whether the drugs themselves, the dosing regimens, or the methods of administration are disrupting sleep. If possible consider changing drugs or altering the timing of administration. An algorithm for diagnosing and treating sleep problems in hospitalized patients is outlined in **Figure 94-2**. By following these steps, the provider can develop a treatment plan that addresses primary sleep disorders, untreated comorbidities, and iatrogenic causes of poor sleep.

PHARMACOLOGIC MANAGEMENT OF SLEEP COMPLAINTS

Although nonpharmacologic therapies are ideal, it may be difficult to provide these in the hospital setting, or they may be only partially effective in resolving the sleep problem. In these instances, pharmacologic strategies may be needed. Care must be taken in choosing the appropriate drug due to increased risk of side effects and drug–drug interactions in sick patients. To

TABLE 94-4 Summary of Questions in a Focused Sleep History of Hospitalized Patients

Focus	Examples of Questions
Sleep pattern	When did the sleep problem start? What time do you try go to sleep? How long does it take you to fall asleep? How often do you wake up during the night? What wakes you up at night? How long does it take you to fall back asleep? What time do you wake up? What wakes you up in the morning? How long are you sleeping during the day (naps)?
Behavioral factors	How does your sleep at home compare with your sleep in the hospital?
Environment	Does the lighting or noise level in the hospital disrupt your sleep? How so? Are you awakened from sleep for tests, monitoring, bathing, or other nursing/medical procedures?
Patient comfort	Is your pain adequately controlled at night? If not, are you on a scheduled analgesic regimen, or do you have to ask for pain medications? Do you have breathing problems, gastroesophageal reflux, or some other type of discomfort that keeps you from sleeping well?
Substances	Do you drink alcohol? How much, and how often? When was your last alcoholic beverage? Do you use cocaine, methamphetamine, marijuana, or other substances? When was your last use?
Psychosocial	How was your mood just prior to being hospitalized? How has your mood been since you were admitted? Have you experienced any emotionally or physically traumatic event just prior to your hospitalization? Have you had any treatments or procedures during this hospitalization that were particularly bothersome to you (eg, intubation, resuscitation, surgery, blood draws, magnetic resonance imaging scan)?

TABLE 94-5 Common Sleep Barriers in the Hospital and Potential Solutions

Barriers	Strategies to Optimize Sleep in the Hospital
Noise and lighting	Limit the volume level of audiovisual and other electronic equipment (eg, televisions, radios, handheld games). Promptly respond to alarm monitors; consider liberalizing the monitor alarm setting. Keep patients' doors closed, if appropriate. Post signs to remind staff to minimize conversations at or near the bedside. Switch beepers and other electronic devices to "vibrate" at night. Offer earplugs and eye masks. Encourage exposure to brighter light during the day (turn on the lights, open the curtains), and turn off the lights by 8 PM.
Visitors	In shared hospital rooms, have patients and their visitors meet in another location (eg, conference room, cafeteria) Request that patients and their visitors turn off the ringer on their cell phones. Adhere strictly to visiting hours. Encourage visitors to minimize discussing emotionally difficult topics with patients near bedtime. Encourage patients to limit contact with anxiety-provoking individuals, especially in the evening.
Substances	Minimize use of benzodiazepines for sleep. Try to wean patients off benzodiazepines prior to discharge. Avoid starting multiple medications at one time. Minimize use of sleep-disrupting medications. Change medication regimens to promote sleep (eg, avoid night-time diuretics if possible). No caffeine or cigarette smoking after 6 PM.
Routines	Encourage regular nocturnal sleep time, and discourage lengthy naps during the day. Minimize bathing, dressing changes, room switches, and other activities at night. Regularly review nighttime orders to see if you could decrease the frequency of overnight monitoring.
Delirium	Provide an updated calendar to facilitate cognitive orientation. Discontinue nonessential medications. Minimize use of benzodiazepines, barbiturates, opiates, antihistamines, and anticholinergic agents. Regularly provide verbal and other cues to orient patients to the date, time, location, and circumstances.
Nocturnal discomfort	Optimize nighttime glycemic control and maximize pain management. For patients with reflux: No oral intake after 8 PM, and keep head of bed elevated ≥ 30 degrees. Provide nocturnal O_2, CPAP, and/or other medications, as appropriate. If patient is on CPAP, assess the mask's fit and comfort.

BzRAs, benzodiazepines; CPAP, continuous positive airway pressure.

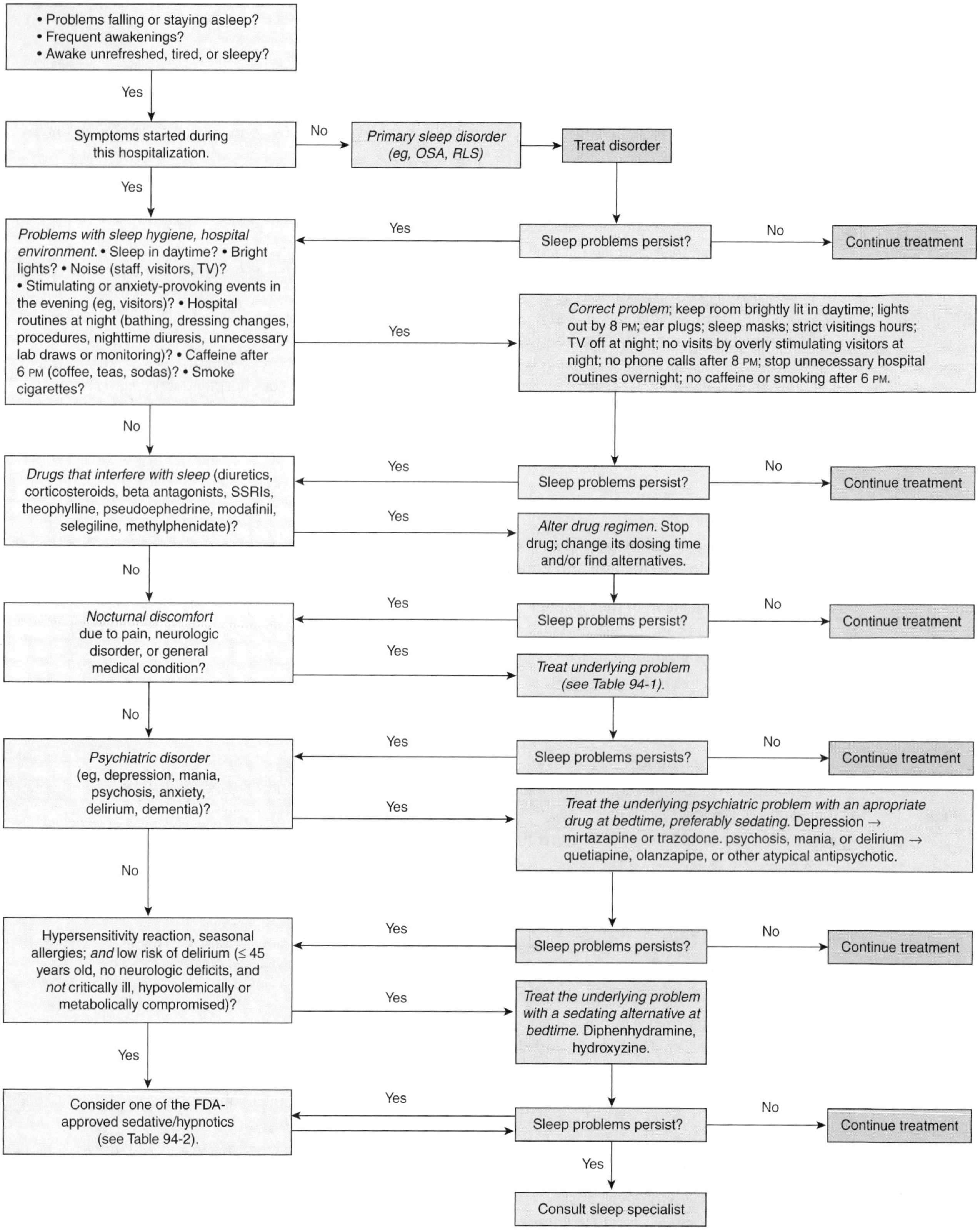

Figure 94-2 *A diagnostic and treatment algorithm for promoting sleep in hospitalized medical patients. OSA, obstructive sleep apnea; RLS, restless leg syndrome; SSRIs, selective serotonin reuptake inhibitors; FDA, food and drug administration. Data from Young JS, Bourgeois JM, Hilty DH, Hardin KA. Sleep in hospitalized medical patients, Part 2: Behavioral and pharmacological management of sleep disturbances. Journal of Hospital Medicine. 2009;4(1):50–59.*

TABLE 94-6 Food and Drug Administration-approved drugs for insomnia

Drugs	Adult Dose (mg)	Half-Life (minutes)	Onset(min)	Time to Peak Effect (Hours)	Major Effects/Clinical Comments
Benzodiazepine					***Caution** in elderly patients.* **Tolerance develops to the sedative, hypnotic, anticonvulsant effects.**
Estazolam (ProSom)	1–2	10–24	60	½–1½	Short-term (7–10 days) treatment for frequent arousals, early morning awakening. Not as useful for sleep onset. Avoid in patients with OSA. ***Caution** in elderly patients*, liver disease. High doses can cause respiratory depression.
Flurazepam (Dalmane)	15–30	47–100	15–20	3–6	In general, avoid in hospitalized medical patients, especially elderly patients.
Quazepam (Doral)	7.5–15	25–114		1½	In general, avoid in hospitalized medical patients, especially elderly patients.
Temazepam (Restoril)	15–30	6–16		2–3	Short-term (7–10 days) treatment for sleep onset and maintenance. Doses ≥ 30 mg/day: morning grogginess, nausea, headache, and vivid dreaming.
Triazolam (Halcion)	0.125–0.25	1.5–5.5	15–30	1.7–5	Maximum dose is 0.5 mg. Short-term (7–10 days) treatment. Rapid onset; should be in bed when taking medication. **Contraindicated** with atazanavir, ketoconazole, itraconazole, nefazodone, ritonavir.
Non-BzRAs					
Eszopiclone (Lunesta)	2–3	6–9		1	In elderly: difficulty *falling* asleep: initially 1 mg; maximum 2 mg. Difficulty *staying* asleep: 2 mg. Rapid onset; should be in bed when taking medication. For faster sleep onset, do not ingest with high-fat foods. No tolerance after 6 months.
Zaleplon (Sonata)	5–20	1	Rapid	1	Short-term (7–10 days) treatment for falling asleep and/or next-day wakefulness is crucial (eg, shift workers).
Zopiclone (Imovane)	5–15	3.8–6.5 (5–10 in elderly)	30	<2	Transient and short-term (7–10 days) treatment. **Contraindicated** in severe respiratory impairment. **Caution** in liver disease and depression; elderly prone to side effects. Anticholinergic agents may ↓ plasma level.
Zolpidem (Ambien)	5–20	1.4–4.5	30	2	Short-term (7–10 days) treatment for sleep onset and maintenance. Rapid onset; should be in bed when taking medication. For faster sleep onset, do not ingest with food. No tolerance after 50 weeks.
Melatonin agonist					
Ramelton (Rozerem)	8	1–2	30	1–1.5	For sleep *onset*. For faster sleep onset, do not ingest with high-fat foods. No tolerance. **Contraindicated** with fluvoxamine.

BzRAs, benzodiazepines; OSA, obstructive sleep apnea.

choose an appropriate sleep agent, evaluate the drug's efficacy, mechanism of action, and side-effect profile. Then match these characteristics with the patient's clinical condition(s). In patients with comorbid sleep and psychiatric problems, consider using a sedating psychotropic at bedtime to promote sleep.

The U.S. Food and Drug Administration (FDA) has approved three classes of medications for the treatment of insomnia: benzodiazepine $GABA_A$ receptor agonists, nonbenzodiazepine $GABA_A$ receptor agonists (non-BzRAs), and melatonin-receptor agonists (**Table 94-6**). Benzodiazepines include estazolam (ProSom), flurazepam (Dalmane), quazepam (Doral), temazepam (Restoril), and triazolam (Halcion). Flurazepam and quazepam have long half-lives, increasing the risks of side effects and drug interactions, and should generally be avoided in hospitalized patients. For similar reasons, it is prudent to avoid use of other long-acting benzodiazepines such as clonazepam (Klonopin) and diazepam (Valium), unless there is a specific indication such as RLS. All benzodiazepines except lorazepam, oxazepam, and temazepam have significant hepatic metabolism and should be used with caution in patients with liver disease.

Although non-BzRAs are structurally unrelated to benzodiazepines, they also act at the $GABA_A$ receptor, and have many similar characteristics and risks. These agents include eszopiclone (Lunesta), zaleplon (Sonata), zolpidem (Ambien), and zolpidem extended-release (Ambien CR). Both benzodiazepines and non-BzRAs have a risk for abuse and dependence. Although there is much less risk of dependence with the nonbenzodiazepines, it appears prudent to avoid using all of these agents to treat insomnia in patients with a prior history of sedative-hypnotic or alcohol dependence.

Side effects of benzodiazepines include daytime sedation, anterograde amnesia, cognitive impairment, incoordination, dependence, tolerance, rebound insomnia, and, importantly, respiratory depression. The side-effect profile of non-BzRAs is generally similar but appears to be less severe. Additionally, zolpidem and eszopiclone have been associated with delirium-like episodes, hallucinations, and sleepwalking, which can be exacerbated in the hospital setting. Long-acting agents should not be used in the elderly due to increased risk of falls, daytime sedation, and adverse cognitive effect. Ideally, both classes of drugs should

TABLE 94-7 Alternatives to FDA-Approved Drugs for Insomnia

Drug	Pertinent Side Wffects	Comments
Antidepressants		
Mirtazapine (Remeron)	Somnolence, $\uparrow$ appetite, $\uparrow$ weight, dry mouth	May be beneficial for comorbid depression and insomnia. Lower doses ($\leq$ 15 mg) increase sedation, but not effective for antidepressant action.
Trazodone	Residual daytime sedation, headache, orthostatic hypotension, priapism, cardiac arrhythmias	May be beneficial for comorbid depression and insomnia. Not recommended as first-line agent for insomnia. May be an alternative if benzodiazepines are contraindicated (severe hypercapnea or hypoxemia or history of substance abuse). Tolerance usually develops within two weeks. Lower doses (50–100 mg) than when used for depression (400 mg).
TCAs	Delirium, $\downarrow$ cognition, $\downarrow$ seizure threshold, orthostatic hypotension, tachycardia, acquired prolonged QT syndrome, heart block, acute hepatitis	**Avoid** in hospitalized patients due to their anticholinergic, antihistaminic, and cardiovascular side effects. May be beneficial for comorbid depression and insomnia.
Antihistamines		
Diphenhydramine (Benadryl)	Residual daytime sedation, delirium, orthostatic hypotension, $\downarrow$ psychomotor function, prolonged QT syndrome, blurred vision, urinary retention.	Better than placebo to treat insomnia, but data are lacking to definitively endorse diphenhydramine for insomnia. Tolerance to antihistamines develops within a few days. **Avoid** in patients > 60 years old.
Hydroxyzine	Drowsiness, dry mouth, dizziness, agitation, $\downarrow$ cognitive function	Efficacy as anxiolytic for > 4 months use not established. Not FDA-approved for insomnia. **Avoid** in patients > 60 years old, closed-angle glaucoma, prostatic hypertrophy, severe asthma, and COPD.
Antipsychotics		
Quetiapine (Seroquel)	Sedation, orthostatic hypotension, hyperglycemia, $\uparrow$ appetite, $\uparrow$ weight, hyperlipidemia	The most sedating of the atypical antipsychotics, it is frequently used as a sleep aid. Not recommended for insomnia or other sleep problems unless there is a comorbid psychiatric disorder. Dosed lower (25–100 mg) when used for insomnia versus for FDA-approved indications (600–800 mg).
Olanzapine (Zyprexa)	Sedation, hyperglycemia, $\uparrow$ appetite, $\uparrow$ weight, hyperlipidemia, prolonged QTc.	Of atypical antipsychotics, olanzapine is the most likely to cause metabolic complications. **Should not** be used solely for insomnia.
Haloperidol	Sedation, weight gain, prolonged QTc	Atypical antipsychotics should not be used in the elderly due to increased risk of death associated with atypicals. Haloperidol, a conventional antipsychotic can be given in low dose.
Barbiturate		
Chloral hydrate	Oversedation, respiratory depression, nausea, vomiting, diarrhea, drowsiness, $\downarrow$ cognitive function, psychotic symptoms (paranoia, hallucinations), vertigo, dizziness, headache	Chloral hydrate has been used for the short-term (< 2 weeks) treatment of insomnia, but is currently not FDA-approved for that indication. Additive CNS depression may occur if given with other sedative-hypnotics. **Comes in liquid form and has high abuse potential.** Highly lethal in overdose and should be avoided in patients with risk of suicide.

COPD, chronic obstructive pulmonary disease; FDA, U.S. Food and Drug Administration; TCAs, tri- and tetracyclic antidepressants (trimipramine, doxepin, amitriptyline, imipramine, nortriptyline, desipramine); $\uparrow$, increase; $\downarrow$, decrease.

be completely avoided in the elderly, but if absolutely needed, the lowest possible dose should be used.

Ramelteon (Rozerem) is a synthetic melatonin analogue with a longer half-life than natural melatonin. Ramelteon has demonstrated efficacy in decreasing sleep latency, as well as increasing total sleep time, but does not cause drowsiness the next day. Because ramelteon is not a general central nervous system (CNS) depressant, it would not be expected to decrease respiratory drive, and it appears safe in patients with COPD. Furthermore ramelteon has been shown to lack abuse potential. Interestingly, despite facilitating sleep, ramelteon does not make patients feel sedated, and some patients who expect to feel sedated prior to sleep (based on experience with other drugs) may believe that ramelteon is not working. Patient education may help ameliorate this problem.

Limited data exist on the efficacy of non-FDA-approved medications for insomnia, such as antihistamines, antidepressants, and conventional and atypical antipsychotics, examples of which are listed in **Table 94-7**.

The administration of antihistamines, barbiturates, chloral hydrate, and alternative/herbal therapies has been discouraged because the benefits rarely outweigh the risks associated with their use. Antihistamines are the most commonly used over-the-counter agents for chronic insomnia. Diphenhydramine (Benadryl) has been shown to be better than placebo to treat insomnia, but data are lacking to definitively endorse its use to promote sleep. Selecting a non-FDA-approved medication with a sedative effect can be appropriate when the patient has a concomitant illness that also requires treatment, such as a sedating antihistamine (diphenhydramine) in an individual with asthma who is also experiencing insomnia. The anticholinergic action of antihistamines may lead to orthostatic hypotension, urinary retention, or delirium in vulnerable patients. Therefore, diphenhydramine should probably be avoided in hospitalized patients.

Trazodone is the most commonly prescribed antidepressant for the treatment of insomnia. Trazodone is popular among prescribers because, unlike most benzodiazepines, trazodone does not have a recommended limited duration of use and is perceived as being "safer." However, with long-term use, the hypnotic effects of trazodone diminish. In addition, trazodone has been associated with arrhythmias in patients with preexisting cardiac conduction system disease. For this reason, we recommend that trazodone be used as a short-term alternative to benzodiazepines for patients with hypercapnia or hypoxemia, and in those with a history of drug abuse or dependence, but should not generally be prescribed for most patients with sleep disturbances who do not require treatment of depression. Mirtazapine, a newer antidepressant, which promotes both sleep and appetite, may be particularly helpful for patients with cancer, acquired immunodeficiency syndrome (AIDS), and other conditions in which the triad of poor sleep, anorexia, and depression is common. Mirtazapine is a noradrenergic and specific serotonergic agent that causes inverse, dose-dependent sedation (15 mg doses are less sedating). To target sleeplessness, start with a dose between 7.5 and 15 mg. If this dose is ineffective, it is unlikely that increasing the dose will be of benefit for sleep. Interestingly, some patients with OSA appear to exhibit a reduction in the apnea-hypopnea index with this drug, but mirtazapine's tendency to cause weight gain may limit its utility in this patient population.

TCAs are sedating and useful in a select population of patients who having underlying neuropathy or chronic pain syndromes. Otherwise, these should not be used as first-line agents to promote sleep in hospitalized patients. TCAs increase the risk of cardiac conduction abnormalities, decrease seizure threshold, and have significant anticholinergic and anti-alpha-adrenergic effects. In patients with dementia, the anticholinergic effect of TCAs may precipitate delirium. Also, conventional and atypical antipsychotics have a similar side-effect profile and should not be used routinely as first-line agents for insomnia, except in patients who have a psychiatric history where agitation may coexist or be precipitated by hospitalization, and in acute delirium. Atypical antipsychotics should be used cautiously in the elderly due to increased risk of death associated with them. Haloperidol, a conventional antipsychotic, may alternatively be given in a low dose. Electrocardiograms should be followed, particularly in patients with structural heart disease and those on medications that may prolong the QT interval. Lastly, chloral hydrate, the oldest hypnotic, has been displaced by barbiturates and subsequently benzodiazepines. However, it can still be useful in select circumstances. It comes in liquid or pill form and does not suppress epileptiform discharges; therefore, it is useful in patients where sedation may be masking seizure activity. Due to its high abuse potential, potential for lethal overdose, and hepatic and renal toxicity, it is essentially obsolete in the United States today.

CASE 94-1 *(continued)*

A more thorough sleep history of the 59-year-old retired school teacher with Stage IV ovarian cancer was consistent with comorbid depression. The patient noted the onset of her sleep problems about 2 months prior to admission characterized by difficulty with staying asleep and waking up too early. She had not had any recent change in medications or pain from her ovarian cancer which was adequately controlled by pain medications. There was no history of alcohol or any use of illicit substances. The patient reported a depressed mood over the past month, particularly a hopeless feeling about her future due to her cancer, loss of appetite and energy. She denied having any suicidal thoughts. Her physicians prescribed mirtazapine (Remeron), 15 mg nightly, because this particular antidepressant may be helpful for the triad of depression, insomnia, and poor appetite. The patient's mood, appetite and energy subsequently improved.

CASE 94-2 *(continued)*

Review of the medications of the 48-year-old patient with multiple sclerosis revealed that the timing of her medications were likely factors in her disordered sleep:

1. **Late afternoon methylprednisolone infusion with possibly increased anxiety at bedtime)**
2. **Afternoon hydrochorothiazide with resulting nocturia**
3. **Bupropion at bedtime due to its stimulant properties.**

Her physicians changed the medication administration times so that she received them in the morning. The order for routine vital signs was changed to once a shift with instructions not to disrupt her sleep. Due to staffing issues and lack of bed availability, she was not moved to another room. Her husband was advised to provide earplugs, a sleep mask, and her home CPAP machine to promote sleep. Although she reported that she did not sleep as well as she did at home, she was able to get a solid six hours of sleep without a pharmaceutical sleep aid.

CONCLUSION

Sleep disruption is extremely common among hospitalized medical patients, negatively impacting patient satisfaction and potentially delaying recovery. Sleep complaints can be addressed by identifying the cause or causes of poor sleep through a systematic evaluation. Treating the underlying factors first before prescribing sleeping aids is paramount and may include modifying treatment modalities and the hospital environment. Finally, pharmacologic sleep aids should be considered, but care needs to be taken to choose an appropriate drug based on the patient's age and medical comorbidities and the specific nature of their sleep problem.

SUGGESTED READINGS

Barczi SR, Juergens TM. Comorbidities: psychiatric, medical, medications, and substances. *Sleep Med Clin.* 2006;1(2):231–245.

Berry RB, Harding SM. Sleep and medical disorders. *Med Clin North Am.* 2004;88:679–703.

Colten HR, Altevogt BM. *Sleep Disorders and Sleep Deprivation: An Unmet Public Health Problem.* Washington, DC: Institute of Medicine; 2006.

Curry DT, Eisenstein RD, Walsh JK. Pharmacologic management of insomnia: past, present, and future. *Psychiatr Clin North Am.* 2006;29:871–893.

International Classification of Sleep Disorders: Diagnostic and Coding Manual. 2nd ed. Westchester, IL: American Academy of Sleep Medicine; 2005.

Kryger MH, Roth T, Dement WC. *Principles and Practice of Sleep Medicine.* 5th ed. Philadelphia, PA: Elsevier/Saunders; 2011.

Lautenbader S, Kundermann B, Krieg J-C. Sleep deprivation and pain perception. *Sleep Med Rev.* 2006;10:357–369.

Phillips BA, Collop NA, Drake C, Consens F, Vgontzas AN, Weaver TE. Sleep disorders and medical conditions in women. Proceedings of the Women and Sleep Workshop, National Sleep Foundation, Washington, DC, March 5–6, 2007. *J Womens Health.* 2008;17:1191–1199.

Schatzberg AF, Nemeroff CB. *The American Psychiatric Publishing Textbook of Psychopharmacology.* 4th ed. Washington, DC: American Psychiatric Publishing; 2009.

Shahar E, Whitney CW, Redline S, et al. Sleep-disordered breathing and cardiovascular disease: cross-sectional results of the Sleep Heart Health Study. *Am J Respir Crit Care Med.* 2001;163:19–25.

CHAPTER 95

Nausea and Vomiting

Susan Y. Quan, MD
John O. Clarke, MD

Key Clinical Questions

1. What key clinical entities must be considered in the initial assessment of a hospitalized patient with acute nausea and vomiting?
2. What is the clinical diagnostic approach to the inpatient with nausea and vomiting?
3. How should patients with nausea and vomiting in the hospital setting be treated?

CASE 95-1

A 28-year-old woman was admitted from clinic with refractory nausea and vomiting. She has a history of long standing type 1 diabetes mellitus, which has been complicated by retinopathy and neuropathy. From a gastrointestinal standpoint, symptoms began 3 years ago with the onset of early satiety, nausea, and vomiting. This has progressively worsened despite decent glycemic control and aggressive lifestyle modification. She reports constant nausea, which is worse with food, but present to some extent even if she has had nothing to eat. She also reports vomiting after most meals—this can be as soon as minutes after eating or as long as hours. Symptoms are present with both liquids and solids and may even be worse with liquid intake. She is taking ondansetron every 8 hours and promethazine as needed in between ondansetron doses. She has attempted therapy with metoclopramide in the past but did not feel any improvement and also developed a tremor (which reversed upon stopping metoclopramide). She had an attempted solid gastric emptying study but vomited the eggs shortly after ingestion. Her liquid emptying study was markedly abnormal. Prior endoscopy showed no evidence of gastritis, peptic ulcer disease, or gastric outlet obstruction. An upper gastrointestinal (GI) series with small bowel follow-through showed delayed gastric emptying, no abnormal distention, and apparently normal small bowel transit. She has now lost 70 pounds over the past year and was admitted for evaluation, rehydration, and further management.

INTRODUCTION

Nausea and vomiting are common and uncomfortable symptoms with a large number of underlying causes. Nausea is a subjective sensation, usually experienced in the epigastrium or throat when vomiting is imminent (although vomiting may or may not occur). Nausea may be followed by retching, which is repetitive active contraction of the abdominal musculature. Retching may occur in isolation without the forceful expulsion of gastric contents. In contrast, vomiting is a highly physical event that results in the evacuation of gastric contents. This should be distinguished from regurgitation, which is the effortless reflux of gastric or esophageal contents to the hypopharynx.

PATHOPHYSIOLOGY

Studies have suggested that the act of vomiting is controlled by a central neurologic center. Borison and colleagues have studied the mechanism of vomiting in cats and found that vomiting can be induced by electrical stimulation of a "vomiting center" located in the dorsal portion of the medulla. These studies, however, have not yet been repeated in human subjects. Experimental studies have also suggested that a chemoreceptor trigger zone (CTZ) activates the vomiting center when stimulated.

Emetic stimuli can cause vomiting by one of two mechanisms. One mechanism is by activation of afferent vagal and sympathetic neural pathways within the gastrointestinal tract that act directly on the vomiting center. Ablation of these pathways in experimental animals prevents vomiting induced by copper sulfate, which is known to cause vomiting. The second mechanism by which emetic stimuli can cause vomiting is via the CTZ. Unlike the vomiting center, the CTZ is not responsive to electrical stimuli, but only to chemical stimuli from the circulation that crosses the blood–brain barrier. These stimuli include drugs, uremia, diabetic ketoacidosis, and toxins derived from gram-positive bacteria. The exact neurotransmitters that are involved are not known, but there is strong evidence that both dopamine and serotonin may mediate vomiting.

Regardless of the emetic stimulus or the mechanism by which the vomiting center is activated, the act of vomiting is initiated from the vomiting center. The efferent pathways are primarily somatic and involve the vagus, phrenic, and spinal nerves that supply the abdominal musculature.

APPROACH TO NAUSEA AND VOMITING

Three steps should be considered in approaching nausea and vomiting:

1. What is the etiology?
2. What are the consequences and/or complications that need to identified and corrected?
3. What therapy can be provided?

There are a vast number of causes of nausea and vomiting (**Tables 95-1** and **95-2**). The differential diagnosis can be approached with a careful history and physical examination. The acuity of symptoms should first be addressed. Acute nausea and vomiting are usually associated with acute infection (especially

TABLE 95-1 Differential Diagnosis of Nausea and Vomiting

Abdominal Causes	**Nervous System Causes**
Mechanical obstruction	Autonomic system disorders
Gastric outlet obstruction	Demyelinating disorders
Small bowel obstruction	Hydrocephalus
Motility disorders	Congenital malformations
Chronic intestinal pseudoobstruction	High intracranial pressure
Functional dyspepsia	Low pressure hydrocephalus
Gastroparesis	Intracerebral lesions with edema
Irritable bowel syndrome	Labyrinthine disorders
Organic disorders	Labyrinthitis
Acute appendicitis	Meniere disease
Acute cholecystitis	Motion sickness
Acute hepatitis	Meningitis
Crohn disease	Migraine headaches
Inflammatory intraperitoneal disease	Seizure disorders
Mesenteric ischemia	Visceral neuropathy
Mucosal metastases	**Other Causes**
Pancreatic cancer	Alcohol abuse
Pancreatitis	Anxiety and depression
Peptic ulcer disease	Cardiac disease
Retroperitoneal fibrosis	Congestive heart failure
Drugs (See Table 95-2)	Myocardial ischemia
Infectious Causes	Radiofrequency ablation
Acute gastroenteritis	Cyclic vomiting syndrome
Bacterial	Eating disorders
Viral	Functional disorders
Nongastrointestinal infectious	Hypervitaminosis A
Otitis media	Intense pain
Systemic	Paraneoplastic syndrome
Metabolic and Endocrine Causes	Postoperative state
Acute intermittent porphyria	Postvagotomy
Addison disease	Radiation therapy
Diabetes mellitus	Rheumatologic disorders
Hypercalcemia	Scleroderma
Hyperparathyroidism	Sjögren syndrome
Hyperthyroidism	Systemic lupus erythematosis
Hyponatremia	Rumination syndrome
Hypoparathyroidism	Starvation
Pregnancy	
Uremia	

TABLE 95-2 Common Medications Associated with Nausea and Vomiting

Antibiotics	Cardiovascular drugs
Acyclovir	Antiarrhythmics
Antituberculosis drugs	Antihypertensives
Erythromycin	Beta-blockers
Sulfonamides	Calcium channel antagonists
Tetracycline	Digoxin
Antidiabetic agents	Central nervous system drugs
Antigout agents	Antiparkinsonian drugs
Aspirin	Anticonvulsants
Cancer chemotherapy	Diuretics
Cis-platinum	Gastrointestinal medications
Cytarabine	Azathioprine
Dacarbazine	Lubiprostone
Etoposide	Sulfasalazine
5-Fluorouracil	Narcotics
Methotrexate	Nicotine
Nitrogen mustard	Nonsteroidal antiinflammatory drugs
Tamoxifen	Oral contraceptives
Vinblastine	Theophylline

of the gastrointestinal tract), ingestion of toxins, gastrointestinal obstruction or ischemia, new medication, pregnancy, or head trauma/increased intracranial pressure. Chronic nausea and vomiting, which are usually defined as the persistence of symptoms for more than 1 month, suggest partial mechanical obstruction, intracranial pathology, motility disturbance as in gastroparesis, metabolic or endocrine etiology, or a psychologic disturbance.

The timing of vomiting in relation to meals can also be important in elucidating the etiology of symptoms. Patients with a pyloric peptic ulcer or psychogenic vomiting may present with vomiting during or soon after a meal. Patients with gastric outlet obstruction as in diabetic or postvagotomy gastroparesis are more likely to experience delayed vomiting of more than 1 hour after eating. The content of the vomitus can further provide important information. Old food in the vomitus may suggest gastroparesis, gastric outlet obstruction, or a proximal small bowel obstruction, while presence of bile indicates patency between the stomach and proximal duodenum.

The physical examination may be helpful in determining the underlying etiology and is important in assessing the consequences of nausea and vomiting. The general examination can detect important findings such as increase in pulse rate or postural decrease in blood pressure, which would suggest dehydration. Examination may also reveal jaundice, abdominal masses, or features suggestive of an endocrinologic process like thyrotoxicosis or Addison disease. Abdominal examination should focus on presence or absence of bowel sounds, tenderness, distention, as well as evidence of masses, hernias, or prior surgical procedures.

The history and physical examination should direct which lab tests and radiologic studies to order. Basic laboratory testing includes a complete blood count and electrolyte panel. Sustained vomiting resulting in loss of water and electrolytes may lead to dehydration and a hypokalemic metabolic alkalosis. In women, a pregnancy test should be obtained not only to determine if pregnancy is the cause of vomiting, but also as a prerequisite for any radiologic studies. Further laboratory testing may include serum drug levels in patients who are taking certain medications, as well as thyroid function tests.

Flat radiographs of the abdomen or a computed tomographic (CT) scan may reveal mechanical obstruction. An upper gastrointestinal series or endoscopy is particularly helpful in making the diagnosis when the history and physical examination suggest that peptic ulcer disease or gastric outlet obstruction is likely. It is important to recognize that the serial imaging included with a small bowel series adds important diagnostic information that a single image obtained during a CT scan may not. The absence of obvious obstructive pathology on a CT scan should not dissuade the clinician from obtaining a small bowel series. In patients with chronic nausea and vomiting who have a normal upper gastrointestinal series and endoscopy, further evaluation with a radionuclide gastric emptying study can be considered. Electrogastrography and antroduodenal manometry can also be considered if available; however, the clinical utility of these studies in most patients with chronic nausea is not well established, and these procedures are not offered at most facilities. In patients with normal gastric emptying and motility studies, evaluation with CT or ultrasonography may provide valuable information if a gallbladder, pancreatic, or hepatobiliary etiology is suspected. In addition, given that central nervous system processes can result in nausea, one should have a low threshold to perform neurologic imaging in the appropriate clinical context. Finally, a psychiatric consultation should also be considered if studies do not indicate any organic pathology.

When vomiting arises in the hospital, often it is medications that are to blame. Opiates, in particular, slow gastrointestinal transit and have additional direct emetogenic effects in some patients. Chemotherapeutic medications, antibiotics, and general anesthesia are also common precipitants of nausea in hospitalized patients. Abdominal procedures are also well known to result in nausea and delayed gut motility, independent of the anesthesia received. In many instances in which a clear precipitant is apparent, there is not a need to pursue aggressive diagnostic interventions; supportive care is adequate. However, if the symptoms are out of proportion to the clinical scenario or unusually prolonged (eg, persistent nausea and vomiting 4 days after general anesthesia for a nonabdominal procedure), diagnostic evaluation is wise. Additionally, other signs and symptoms such as fever or focal neurologic deficits should be sought out, and if present, should lead to prompt diagnostic evaluation. Finally, myocardial ischemia (particularly right-sided myocardial infarction) should be considered in hospitalized patients with cardiovascular risk factors. Diaphoresis, dyspnea, and changes in heart rate or blood pressure may suggest a cardiac etiology.

PRACTICE POINT

- In many instances in which a clear precipitant is apparent, there is no need to pursue aggressive diagnostic interventions; supportive care is adequate. However, if the symptoms are out of proportion to the clinical scenario or unusually prolonged (eg, persistent nausea and vomiting 4 days after general anesthesia for a nonabdominal procedure), diagnostic evaluation is wise.

TREATMENT

Treatment of nausea and vomiting involves correction of fluid and electrolyte imbalance if present, identification and treatment of the underlying cause if one exists, and relief of symptoms either by suppression or by elimination if the primary cause cannot be promptly identified and removed. Patients with long-standing chronic nausea and vomiting are at risk for developing malnutrition, and it is important to monitor for this in the hospital setting. If a patient is not able to tolerate adequate oral caloric intake after a 5-day period, consideration should be given for enteral or parenteral feeding.

Enteral feeding is usually the first option; however, dislodgment of enteral feeds with acute vomiting is not uncommon and occasionally parenteral feeding may be required.

Pharmacologic treatment

There are many commonly employed antiemetic agents, and these medications can be divided into two main categories: central antiemetic agents and peripheral prokinetic agents. In practice, many drugs employ both mechanisms and many of the specific pathways by which these medications exert benefit are still being elucidated. The main antiemetics are detailed in the next sections.

Dopamine D2 receptor antagonists Metoclopramide is the classic agent in this category and exerts a central antiemetic effect through antagonism of dopamine D2 receptors as well as a peripheral prokinetic effect through stimulation of peripheral 5-HT_4 receptors. Common indications include postoperative nausea and vomiting, chemotherapy and radiation therapy-induced nausea, and gastroparesis. The standard dose is 5–10 mg orally or intravenously three to four times daily. Metoclopramide is associated with significant side effects, including restlessness, anxiety, somnolence, extrapyramidal effects, QT interval prolongation, and, if used for a month or more, tardive dyskinesia (which in some cases is irreversible). Metoclopramide is currently the only U.S. Food and Drug Administration (FDA)-approved medication for gastroparesis; however, due to side effects it has a black box warning against use of greater than 12 weeks based on the risk of tardive dyskinesia.

Domperidone is a second agent in this category that crosses the blood–brain barrier poorly and is believed to act primarily through prokinetic function as a peripheral D2 receptor antagonist. Domperidone is a weaker antiemetic than metoclopramide, but as it is better tolerated, higher doses can be employed and the risk of anxiety and dystonia is significantly reduced. Domperidone is not approved for use in the United States; however, it can be obtained by filing an investigational new drug application with the FDA.

Phenothiazines Phenothiazines (chlorpromazine, promethazine) block D2 dopaminergic receptors in addition to muscarinic M1 receptors and histamine H1 receptors. These drugs induce relaxation and somnolence and are generally used parenterally or as suppositories in patients with acute intense vomiting of central origin (such as with migraine headaches and motion sickness). Although effective, side effects can be significant and often limit use. Of note, promethazine does have a black box warning from the FDA due to severe tissue injury; as a vesicant, if promethazine extravasates into subcutaneous tissues or is accidentally infused intra-arterially, severe local necrosis may occur.

Butyrophenones Butyrophenones block D2 dopaminergic receptors and muscarinic M1 receptors and are believed to affect nausea through central antiemetic effects. Commonly used agents in this category include droperidol and haloperidol. As with the phenothiazines already mentioned, side effects and safety concerns have limited routine use of these agents, although they may be of benefit on an adjunct basis.

Antihistamines and antimuscarinic agents These agents work primarily through blockage of histamine H1 receptors and muscarinic M1 receptors at a central level. Commonly used antihistamines are diphenhydramine, meclizine, and cyclizine. The most commonly used antimuscarinic agent is scopolamine. In addition, promethazine also has both antihistamine and antimuscarinic effects. Somnolence and drowsiness are the main limiting factors with these agents; however, anticholinergic effects can also be problematic—particularly for older patients. These agents are commonly used for treatment of motion sickness and nausea associated with vestibular disease.

Serotonin antagonists Serotonin 5-HT_3 receptors seem to play a key role in nausea, and selective antagonists (such as ondansetron) are particularly effective through central nausea mediation. In addition, these agents may have a mild gastric prokinetic function. These agents are primarily used for postoperative nausea and after chemotherapy and radiation therapy; however, given their efficacy they are often used for refractory nausea related to other conditions. Of note, headache is a common side effect.

Serotonin agonists Serotonin 5-HT_4 receptors seem to play a key role in gastric motility, and agonists of these receptors (such as metoclopramide, cisapride, and tegaserod) have significant prokinetic capabilities. Of these agents, cisapride has the most potent function and demonstrated efficacy for nausea associated with gastroparesis, pseudoobstruction, or other motility cause; however, cisapride was removed from the market due to QT-prolongation complicated by the risk of lethal ventricular arrhythmias. Tegaserod was also removed from the market due to increased associated cardiac events. At the moment, the only medication available in the United States that works through this mechanism is believed to be metoclopramide, and, as detailed earlier, this is but one mechanism by which metoclopramide is believed to exert benefit.

Motilin receptor agonists The classic motilin receptor agonist is the antibiotic erythromycin, which acts as a motilin receptor ligand on smooth muscle cells and enteric nerves, increasing gastric and intestinal peristaltic motor activity. In clinical practice, erythromycin may be used to treat acute nausea and vomiting associated with delayed gastric emptying and is also used to clear the stomach of retained food and blood prior to endoscopy. Erythromycin is best used acutely and is, unfortunately, not a good agent for chronic use in most patients as it is associated with tachyphylaxis. Erythromycin also induces nausea in a significant subset of patients and is associated with QT interval prolongation. New synthetic motilin agonists devoid of antibacterial activity are in development; however, none are ready for clinical use at the present time.

Ghrelin is a peptic structurally similar to motilin that also accelerates gastric emptying. Ghrelin receptor agonists are under development and may play a role in the future; however, they are not available at present for clinical use.

Glucocorticoids The antiemetic mechanism of glucocorticoids is not clear and numerous hypotheses have been raised, including inhibition of central prostaglandin synthesis, altered serotonin processing, and enhanced endorphin release. Regardless, glucocorticoids do appear to have an antiemetic effect and are often used for postoperative nausea or for treatment of nausea in the context of chemotherapy or radiation. In most cases, this use is as an adjunct therapy in combination with other agents rather than as a sole treatment modality.

Cannabinoids Synthetic cannabinoids have entered the therapeutic armamentarium for treatment of nausea. Two oral formulations, dronabinol and nabilone, are approved by the FDA for chemotherapy-induced nausea and vomiting refractory to conventional antiemetic therapy. While attractive to many patients, use of these agents is often limited by hypotension and psychotropic reactions.

Neurokinin-1 receptor antagonists Neurokinin-1 (NK) receptor antagonists inhibit substance P/NK-1 and are potent antiemetics. These agents (aprepitant, fosaprepitant) appear to be particularly effective for treatment of postoperative vomiting and may be used as adjunct therapy for patients not responding to the foregoing measures.

Benzodiazepines Although not proven nor approved as therapy for nausea, anecdotal experience supports the use of benzodiazepines in patients with refractory nausea, particularly when there appears to be a psychological or anticipatory component (ie, the patient reports nausea at the smell or sight of food prior to ingestion).

Alternative and surgical treatment

For patients with refractory nausea despite the pharmacologic options already detailed, it is occasionally necessary to explore alternative and surgical options. Acupuncture has been studied for treatment of nausea in select clinical situations and has shown benefit. Gastric electrical stimulation has also been explored for chronic nausea associated with gastroparesis. The concept is that an implantable neurostimulator delivers brief, low-energy impulses to the stomach, which alters afferent sensation, particularly with regard to nausea. This is approved for humanitarian use by the FDA; however, the procedure is not without risk, and clinical improvement is not universal—with most studies suggesting approximately a 40% response rate. At the moment, this is only approved for chronic nausea in the context of gastroparesis; however, studies are ongoing that may broaden this indication. Other surgical options for chronic nausea do not appear to have sufficient data to pursue further at the present time, except for perhaps completion gastrectomy in patients with nausea in the context of postsurgical gastroparesis.

CASE 95-1 *(continued)*

The patient was admitted for intravenous fluids and started on erythromycin, while being continued on the remainder of her regimen. She declined supplemental enteral or parenteral nutrition and after stabilization was discharged home. As an outpatient she was started on domperidone and seen in consultation by surgery for gastric stimulator placement, which she underwent later that year. Following gastric stimulator placement, she had a difficult postoperative recovery period and was discharged home on parenteral nutrition, which she was able to eventually taper off. She did well for a period of 3 months with marked improvement in nausea and significant weight gain, but unfortunately developed recurrent debilitating nausea and progressive weight loss, leading to a jejunal tube placement for enteral nutrition. At present, nausea remains a significant ongoing issue despite the efforts detailed here.

CONCLUSION

Nausea and vomiting are common in hospitalized patients and can occur due to a wide variety of causes. The initial step should be identifying whether the symptoms are acute or chronic. If acute, the differential diagnosis is somewhat more limited, and it is important to exclude life-threatening issues that require emergent action (shock, hypokalemia, perforation, cerebral edema, organ infarction, poisoning), and pregnancy. If chronic, the differential diagnosis is quite broad; however, by evaluating the patient's history, examination, and basic test results it is often possible to arrive at the etiology. The best treatment is removal of the causative factor. If this is not possible then there is a wide array of treatment options available from a pharmacologic standpoint to at least ameliorate the symptoms. The choice of which pharmacologic agent to use is an individual decision based on the suspected etiology of nausea and concern for side effects.

SUGGESTED READINGS

Carlisle JB, Stevenson CA. Drugs for preventing postoperative nausea and vomiting. *Cochrane Database Syst Rev*. 2006;(3)CD004125.

Chepyala P, Olden KW. Nausea and vomiting. *Curr Treat Options Gastroenterol*. 2008;5:202–208.

Hasler WL, Chey WD. Nausea and vomiting. *Gastroenterology*. 2003; 125:1860–1867.

Malagelada J, Malagelada C. *Nausea and Vomiting. Sleisenger and Fordtran's Gastrointestinal and Liver Disease*. 9th ed. Philadelphia, PA: Saunders Elsevier; 2010:197–209.

Matthews A, Dowswell T, Haas DM, et al. Interventions for nausea and vomiting in early pregnancy. *Cochrane Database Syst Rev*. 2010;(9)CD007575.

Quigley EM, Hasler WL, Parkman HP. AGA technical review on nausea and vomiting. *Gastroenterology*. 2001;120:263–286.

Soffer E, Abell T, Lin Z, et al. Review article: gastric electrical stimulation for gastroparesis—physiologic foundations, technical aspects and clinical considerations. *Aliment Pharmacol Ther*. 2009; 30:681–694.

CHAPTER 96

Pain

Meredith C.B. Adams, MD
Patrick J. Tighe, MD
Robert W. Hurley, MD, PhD

Key Clinical Questions

1. What are the goals of pain therapy?
2. How is the sensation of pain measured?
3. What are the types of pain?
4. How does patient comorbidities affect pain management?
5. What are the most appropriate and effective pain Treatment options available.

CASE 96-1

An 84-year-old female with a history of dementia, hypertension, hypercholesterolemia, coronary artery disease, chronic obstructive pulmonary disease, and chronic low back pain suffered a lower extremity fracture. The orthopedic surgery service has surgically repaired her leg and transferred her back to the primary service for management of multiple medical problems. On the postoperative day two pain has limited her movement and she has not been able to work with physical therapy or use the bathroom facilities. Home medications include atorvastatin, metoprolol, ramipril, hydrochlorothiazide, ipratropium, albuterol metereddose inhaler, and oxycodone sustained-release 20 mg twice a day. Her vital signs were: heart rate is 120 beats per minute, blood pressure 150/95 mm Hg, SpO_2 95% on 2 L of oxygen, and temperature 37.2°C. Laboratory results were notable for a glucose level of 212. Despite an order for 2 mg of intravenous (IV) morphine "as needed" every 2–4 hours, the patient reports "a lot" of pain "not coming down with the morphine."

INTRODUCTION

TAXONOMY

Any discussion on the diagnosis and treatment of pain must start with the definition of pain. The International Association for the Study of Pain defines *pain* as an unpleasant sensory and emotional experience associated with actual or potential tissue damage, or described in terms of such damage.

Pain can be classified in multiple domains. The first is the classification based on the underlying etiology of the pain. Nociceptive pain refers to the direct tissue injury from a noxious stimulus. Inflammatory pain refers to the release of inflammatory mediators that perpetuate and modulate nociceptive input. Direct injury to nerves results in a third type of pain, neuropathic pain, whereby the nature of sensory transmission is altered and accompanied by pain frequently described as a burning type of pain. Although these are described as discrete types of pain, they more often represent a continuum of the same injury. Surgical incision is a model of nociceptive injury that produces an inflammatory response. Incising the primary nociceptors in the skin with subsequent development of inflammatory neuritis can result in neuropathic pain.

The second domain of classification refers to the anatomic location of pain. In this category, pain can be described as either somatic or visceral. Somatic pain refers to a well-localized sensation related to skin, muscle, and bone, whereby visceral pain is poorly localized and is usually in response to distention of the internal organs such as the colon or small bowel, or compression or inflammatory injury, which occurs in pancreatic cancer or pancreatitis.

The final domain classifies pain based on the temporal nature of the pain. Acute pain usually refers to a neurophysiologic response to a noxious stimulus, a response expected to resolve with completion of wound healing. In contrast, chronic pain persists beyond the expected time course of an acute injury and its repair process. Chronic or persistent pain does not simply suggest that a given time interval has passed. Rather, such a diagnosis implies development of multiple neurophysiologic changes that alter the fundamental balance between noxious stimuli and their inhibitory mechanisms.

Such changes occur from the peripheral nerve to the dorsal horn of the spinal column, interneurons throughout the spinal cord, to the thalamus and cortical circuits. These changes ultimately result in remodeling in the organization of the central nervous system.

PRACTICE POINT

- Although the practitioner must be aware that the patient can manipulate the pain report, it is imperative to first validate the patient's understanding of his or her pain by receiving his or her report with an unbiased view.

EVALUATION OF PAIN

Pain is a subjective phenomenon and results from a patient's understanding of the physical and affective impact the sensation has had on them. There are multiple quantitative pain evaluation scales. Although these are subjective reports with no way to verify the answer's "truth," these scales have been used for decades and correlate well to experimental and clinical pain responsiveness. Although the practitioner must be aware that the patient can manipulate the pain report, it is imperative to first validate the patient's understanding of his or her pain by receiving his or her report with an unbiased view.

PRACTICE POINT

- Poorly controlled pain can present through multiple parameters including vital signs and laboratory values, reinforcing the impact of a patient under significant physiologic and psychological stress. Manifestations of this stress can include myocardial ischemia, immunosuppression, impaired wound healing, and thromboembolic events.

The numerical rating scale (NRS) may be the most commonly used tool for the evaluation of pain intensity. Patients are asked to rate their pain on a scale of 0 to10, with 0 translated as "no pain" and 10 the "worst pain imaginable." Similarly, the visual analog scale (VAS) allows patients to mark a point on a 10-cm line that corresponds to the level of their pain. The 4-point verbal rating scale (VRS) asks patients to categorize their pain as none, mild, moderate, or severe. The VAS and NRS demonstrate excellent agreement, and both offer superior discriminating ability to the categorical VRS.

The above case study involves a patient with dementia, which can pose additional challenges for the evaluation of her pain. Standard pain reporting scales are ineffective for patients who suffer from dementia, who are unconscious, or who are unable to communicate. Pain scales such as MOBID-2, Checklist of Nonverbal Pain Indicators, and Doloplus 2 have each been designed for the patient with dementia or in an assisted living facility. These scales have strong conceptual and psychometric support, however they are an indirect measure of the patient's pain and therefore at risk of the health care providers' intrinsic biases.

Timing and activity are relevant to the interpretation of pain scores. Reported pain scores may refer to the past hour, 24 hours, week, or month. Average, maximum, and minimum pain scores help ascertain the patient's range of pain. Pain scores may also be described as rest or static versus active or dynamic to correlate the given score with activity level. Pain scores reported by the patient when resting may not reflect pain-based limitations on activity. Because the goal of pain treatment usually includes improvement in mobility or function to decrease thromboembolic and pulmonary complications, addressing only rest/static pain may result in a failure to maximize the benefit of pain control.

The above scales are applied to all types of pain: acute, chronic/persistent, and cancer pain. The added complexity of chronic/persistent or cancer pain can require more multifaceted evaluation tools. Additional pain scales can be administered to these patients to better deliver more targeted pain care, but they will not be discussed as they are beyond the scope of this chapter.

Poorly controlled pain can present through multiple parameters including vital signs and laboratory values, reinforcing the impact of a patient under significant physiologic and psychological stress. Manifestations of this stress can include myocardial ischemia, immunosuppression, impaired wound healing, and thromboembolic events.

TREATMENT OF PAIN

Treatment of pain can utilize four primary modalities. These include medications, interventions, behavioral therapies and physical therapy/complementary treatments. This review will focus on the medical and interventional management of pain, although behavior and complementary treatments are essential components of improving the overall pain state in patients with persistent pain.

SYSTEMIC ANALGESIA

Opioids

Opioid medications remain the most common treatment for both acute and chronic/persistent pain. By activating the *mu* opioid receptor throughout the CNS, opioids modulate the perception and transmission of painful stimuli. Opioid-based therapies are not limited by a ceiling effect; increasing doses will theoretically yield increasing analgesic effects even at extremely high doses. However, increasing doses of opioids are functionally limited by side effects such as nausea, vomiting, constipation, sedation, and respiratory depression.

When used for acute pain, the most common routes of systemic opioid administration include intravenous (IV), intramuscular (IM), and per os (by mouth) (PO). Parenteral routes may also include transdermal (TD), subcutaneous (SC), transmucosal (TM), or iontophoretic transdermal (ITD). Epidural and intrathecal administration is also used in a variety of settings.

Intravenous administration of opioids ensures a rapid, predictable onset and distribution of analgesic functioning, making this the favored route for the initial treatment of severe acute pain. Intramuscular and enteral routes may result in delayed onset of effects, limiting their effectiveness in the acute pain setting. Similarly, TD (ITD excepted) and SC routes of administration have considerably delayed onset and are more often appropriate for long-term use such as in chronic pain or palliative care settings.

Table 96-1 lists several opioids commonly prescribed for acute and chronic pain medicine. Commonly, patients will experience excellent pain relief following administration of opioids. However, there can be a variable response to different formulations and pharmacologic compounds resulting from genetic polymorphisms involving *mu*-opioid receptor activation, receptor distribution, opioid metabolism, and the type of pain. Opioids are often best at treating static, nociceptive pain such as postsurgical pain; however they are less eff ective for dynamic or movement-related pain or neuropathic pain. Further, opioids are often ineffective in the treatment of bone fracture pain such as the pain experienced by the patient in the case study.

Opioid conversion: In the course of transitioning from severe acute pain to moderate, subacute pain, physicians will frequently transition the patient from parenteral to oral opioid administration.

1. Calculate the patient's 24-hour opioid use.
2. Convert this to "parenteral morphine equivalent" (PME).

TABLE 96-1 Common Opioid Medications Prescribed for Pain

Opioid	Starting Dose	Dose Interval	Metabolism and Excretion	Morphine Equivalent*
Morphine (IR)	10–15 mg	every 4 to 6 hours/as needed	H/R	
Morphine (SR)	15–30 mg	2 to 3 times a day		
Oxycodone (IR)	5–10 mg	every 4 to 6 hours/as needed	H/R	0.7 mg
Oxycodone (SR)	15–20 mg	2 to 3 times a day		
Oxymorphone (IR)	5–10 mg	every 4 to 6 hours/as needed	H/R	0.33 mg
Oxymorphone (SR)	5–10 mg	2 times a day		
Hydromorphone	2–4 mg	every 3 to 4 hours/as needed	R/H	0.2 mg
Fentanyl transdermal	12 mcg/hr	every 72 hours	H/R	0.6 mcg/hr
Methadone	2.5–5 mg	3 times a day	H/R	0.3 mg
Hydrocodone/Acetaminophen	5/325 mg	every 4 to 6 hours/as needed	H	10
Codeine	15–60 mg	every 4 to 6 hours/as needed	H/R	6.6 mg
Tramadol	50–100 mg	every 4 to 6 hours/as needed	H/R	5 mg

H, hepatic; IR, intermediate release; R, renal; SR, sustained release.
* This dose is based on the assumption of morphine 1 mg orally every 24 hours.

3. The total oral dose prescribed to the patient is commonly less than 100% of the parenteral dose equivalent; this decision is guided by the clinical milieu of the patient including "the patient's recovery from his or her pain."
4. Consider the division of this requirement into short- and/or long-acting opioids. This decision depends greatly upon the patient, the timing of his or her pain, and the nature of his or her pain.
5. Fifty percent of the 24-hour PME can be given as a sustained preparation, and 50% as shorter-acting, immediate-release medications ordered as needed.
6. To assist the physician with opioid conversion, numerous conversion tables and calculators are available (see www.hopweb.org).

Nonsteroidal anti-inflammatory agents (NSAIDs)

NSAIDs exert their analgesic effect via inhibition of the cyclooxygenase (COX) enzyme, thus interfering with prostaglandin (PG) production. Prostaglandins modify nociceptive thresholds at both peripheral and central sites. By limiting production of PG from COX-1 and COX-2, NSAIDs offer effective analgesia for mild to moderate pain. Further, this mechanism of action apart from the *mu*-opioid receptor provides a strong supplement to opioids during treatment of moderate to severe pain. Although opioid sparing, NSAIDs do have a ceiling effect, beyond which increasing doses will yield no increase in analgesia. Clinically, NSAIDs decrease pain associated with orthopedic injuries, and those with extensive prostaglandin involvement such as pain from uterine contraction and muscle inflammation. However, the risk of bleeding and mixed evidence regarding interference with union of fractures and spinal surgery necessitates involvement of the operative team in the decision to add NSAIDs.

Traditionally, NSAIDs were nonspecific for the isoforms of cyclooxygenase, COX-1 and COX-2. COX-1 is constitutively expressed in nearly all human tissues, while COX-2 is focally expressed with inflammation. Blockade of COX-1 may promote development of gastrointestinal irritation and bleeding. NSAIDs as a class may also interfere with autoregulation of renal perfusion. To minimize the effects of gastrointestinal irritation and bleeding, drug development turned to selective COX-2 inhibitors. Although effective in minimizing gastrointestinal bleeding, selective COX-2 inhibitors may result in a prothrombotic milieu that may increase the risk of myocardial infarction.

Acetaminophen may represent a special class of NSAIDs. While its mechanism of action is not completely understood, there is evidence of antagonistic activity against COX-2, and a splice variant of COX-1 named COX-3. Notably, acetaminophen appears to not inhibit peripheral COX-1, which may explain its favorable safety profile in regards to gastrointestinal, hematological, cardiovascular, and renal effects seen with other NSAIDs and selective COX-2 inhibitors.

In assessing comparative efficacy, the number of patients needed to treat (NNT) for at least a 50% reduction in pain after 4–6 hours for 1 g of acetaminophen is 4.4, which compares favorably to 650 mg of aspirin or 100 mg of ibuprofen. A more typical dose of ibuprofen, 400 mg, however, had an NNT of only 2.3. Celecoxib, a selective COX-2 inhibitor, has a NNT of 4.5 at 200 mg when compared with placebo for postoperative pain.

Ca-channel antagonists (anticonvulsants) and tricyclic antidepressants

Anticonvulsants such as gabapentin and pregabalin have found an increasing role in the treatment of chronic pain stemming from neuropathy. While designed to mimic the structure of gamma-aminobutyric acid (GABA), gabapentin does not actually bind to GABA receptors. Instead, its antihyperalgesic/antiallodynic effect likely stems from binding to the of alpha$_2$delta$_1$ accessory unit of voltage-dependent Ca_2 channels within the dorsal root ganglia of the spinal cord, which are upregulated following peripheral nerve injury. By inhibiting these calcium channels, gabapentin and pregabalin my inhibit glutamate release from primary afferent nerve fibers, which activate pain responsive neurons within the spinal cord. Although gabapentin and pregabalin are effective for a myriad of chronic pain conditions, their role in acute pain management is less clear. The gabapentinoids have a clear role in the treatment of postoperative pain when given in the perioperative period (pre- and postoperatively) in a number of major orthopedic and gastrointestinal surgeries. In the acute and chronic pain setting, they have been shown to be opioid sparing and show promise as successful adjuvant analgesics.

TABLE 96-2 Intravenous Patient-Controlled Analgesia Initial Settings

Opioid	Demand Dose	Lockout (Range)	Continuous Basal Infusion Rate*
Morphine	1–2 mg	10 min (6–10 min)	1–2 mg/hr
Hydromorphone	0.2–0.4 mg	10 min (6–10 min)	0.2–0.4 mg/hr
Fentanyl	20–50 mcg	5 min (5–10 min)	10–60 mcg/hr
Sufentanil	4–6 mcg	5 min (5–10 min)	2–8 mcg/hr
Tramadol†	10–20 mg	10 min (6–10 min)	10–20 mcg/hr
Meperidine§	10–20 mg	10 min (6–10 min)	10–20 mg/hr

*Continuous infusion of opioids is not recommended in the opioid-naïve patient.
In patients already receiving opioid medications:
a) If the patient is hospitalized, calculate the patient's 24-hour opioid use and convert this into the IV opioid equivalent, and give 50–75% of the total dose as the continuous infusion delivered over 24 hours and the remaining 25–50% as demand doses.
b) If the patient is on home oral opioid or transdermal regimen, calculate the patient's 24-hour baseline home regimen into the IV opioid equivalent and administer 75% of this as a continuous infusion and supplement with appropriate demand dose using the initial settings.
†Currently not available in North America.
§Meperidine is not recommended because of the significant side effects associated with its administration. Its use should be reserved for when no other opioid is available for PCA use.

CASE 96-1 *(continued)*

In managing the postoperative patient with dementia the goal is to minimize her opioid requirement (and side effect burden) by using NSAIDs and gabapentinoids as adjuncts. The patient has no history of renal insufficiency or gastric ulceration, and scheduled doses of ketorolac, ibuprofen, or celecoxib may be appropriate. However, this would require consultation with the operative surgeon due to associated bleeding risk and the possibility of impaired bone healing. In the absence of hepatic insufficiency, scheduled acetaminophen would also be appropriate. One may also consider starting low doses of pregabalin or gabapentin. When planning a multimodal approach, the physician should recognize that the synergy of potential side effects from several different medications might be greater than those from opioids alone.

Although developed initially for the treatment of depression, low-dose tricyclic antidepressants (TCA) are a mainstay of treatment for many chronic pain states, especially those involving neuropathic pain. Even though their mechanism of action remains unclear, TCAs may augment descending serotonergic and noradrenergic bulbospinal pathways on the dorsal horn of the spinal cord. This class of drugs has significant anticholinergic side effects, so in this case study (elderly and history of dementia), it would be contraindicated to use TCAs. They are titrated to goal dosing to gain benefit while decreasing the side effect profile. One advantageous side effect is somnolence, which is utilized by evening dosing and can facilitate sleep and decrease pain.

Patient-controlled analgesia

When compared to intermittent bolus dosing of opioids, IV patient-controlled analgesia (PCA) offers significantly greater analgesia and satisfaction. Both the strengths and risks of PCA systems depend upon a negative feedback loop: when in pain, the patient self-administers potent analgesics leading to pain relief, therefore limiting further opioid demands. An additional benefit of PCA dosing is that the patient is not dependent upon administration variables and has constant access to the prescribed dosing.

PCA systems allow for a continuous and demand dosing. Demand dosing is a preset amount that can be accessed at regulated intervals. This dosing also has an hourly maximum dose with lockout to prevent overmedication. **Table 96-2** lists common IV PCA programs for initial use with a variety of opioids.

As with any opioid-based therapy, PCA use may result in respiratory depression. If there is discordance between nociception (pain) and antinociception (opioid), a relative decrease in pain input or increase in opioid-based inhibition may each result in respiratory depression in the presence of opioids. However, minimizing the use of background infusions in opioid-naïve patients mitigates this risk. The incidence of respiratory depression is then decreased below the rate associated with provider-administered intermittent boluses. Background infusions are best used on an individual basis, but can be a method to incorporate a home opioid regimen to better control the overall pain state. Home opioid dosing can be converted to background infusion dosing with the addition of patient controlled dosing to assess and treat in the acute pain phase. Once on a stable regimen that adequately controls the patient's pain, this dosing requirement information can be used to transition to an oral regimen that will reflect the patient's requirements. Some institutions use pulse oximetry monitoring to assess the respiratory depression associated with opioid administration. Unfortunately, this monitoring is not appropriately sensitive, nor is it in any way specific enough to capture the relationship between respiratory depression and opioid administration when it is used concomitantly with supplemental oxygen. Pulse oximetry then lends a false sense of security in addition to monitoring and administrative burden without the benefit of providing predictive value. Capnography is a much more specific correlate of respiratory depression. However, capnography is not readily available in all institutions, nor is it appropriate to apply this universally to patients receiving opioid therapy. Its use would be best reserved for those patients who have substantial comorbidities that elevate the risks associated with opioid therapy.

INTERVENTIONAL TECHNIQUES

Peripheral nerve blocks

The use of peripheral nerve blocks, either as single injections or continuous infusions of local anesthetic, allows analgesia and anesthesia to be focused toward the locus of pain. Peripheral nerve blocks may offer superior analgesia, decreased opioid consumption, improved pharmacokinetic titration, and increased patient satisfaction when compared with systemic analgesic techniques or placebo.

Anesthetizing a targeted peripheral nerve or nerve plexus using anatomic landmarks, ultrasound, or nerve stimulation performs peripheral nerve blocks. Although single injections of local anesthetic can provide anesthesia and analgesia lasting up to 24 hours, placement of a perineural catheter through the needle allows the therapy to be extended for up to several weeks. Anesthesiologists can customize the regional anesthetic regimen to reflect each patient's surgical, perioperative, and rehabilitation requirements. Multiple injections and/or catheters may be needed to adequately anesthetize pertinent nerve distributions.

Neuraxial anesthesia

Neuraxial anesthesia refers to injections of local anesthetic and/or opioids into the epidural or intrathecal space, either through a needle as a single-injection or through an indwelling catheter.

Epidural anesthesia: Epidural anesthesia commonly refers to infusion of solutions containing local anesthetic and opioids through a catheter within the epidural space. As the solution infiltrates this potential space, it spreads superiorly and inferiorly within the spinal canal. This spread gives coverage along dermatomal distribution congruent with the level of the catheter or injectate. This spread is slightly affected by gravity and patient positioning; thus, patients may notice epidural effects predominating upon dependent locations when laterally positioned.

Epidural solutions commonly contain mixtures of local anesthetic and opioids. High local anesthetic concentrations will result in sympathectomy, sensory loss, and motor block depending upon the required dose for analgesia. In general, the low concentrations of local anesthetic used for analgesia offer a discriminatory block providing excellent analgesia, minimal sensory inhibition and nearly absent motor block. Opioid-only solutions avoid some side effects such as sympathectomy and motor block, but at the cost of nausea, pruritus, and less-potent analgesia. Solutions combining local anesthetic with opioids provide superior dynamic pain relief, decreased sensory block regression, and decreased local anesthetic dose requirement.

Epidural solutions are commonly delivered through continuous infusions rather than single shot administration. While effective, such infusions fail to account for the dynamic nature of painful conditions. The administration of epidural analgesia using patient-controlled epidural analgesia (PCEA) systems has become more common. The PCEA system allows the patient to self-administer an epidural bolus at a dose and schedule ordered by the physician, while providing continuous background infusion. Such systems allow for patient-controlled individualization of analgesic regimens. When compared with continual infusion-only regimens, PCEA systems offer lower drug use yet greater patient satisfaction.

Epidural side effects: As with all types of medications, epidural analgesia is not without side effects. Local anesthetics can result in anesthesia, motor blockade, and hypotension from sympathectomy. When placed in the lumbar and sacral epidural space, local anesthetics or opioids may result in urinary retention necessitating either bladder catheterization or frequent bladder scans. The lower extremity weakness, and potential orthostatic hypotension associated with epidural analgesia, make appropriate fall precautions necessary.

Sympathectomies due to epidural analgesia can result in profound hypotension, although the incidence with postoperative epidural analgesia averages 0.7–3.0%. If the epidural is dosed to the upper thoracic dermatomes, blockade of the cardiac accelerator fibers may also lead to severe bradycardia. Frequent hemodynamic monitoring is therefore essential during initiation and modification of epidural analgesia involving local anesthetics.

Epidural opioid administration is generally devoid of the hemodynamic perturbations seen with epidural local anesthetics. Side effects are usually those also seen with systemic administration, such as nausea, vomiting, pruritus, and respiratory depression. Pruritus due to neuraxial opioids appears to be related to central activation of "pruritus pathways" that mediate nonhistamine itch. Intravenous naloxone, naltrexone, and nalbuphine each appear efficacious for treatment of opioid-induced pruritus without affecting analgesia when dosed appropriately.

The rate of respiratory depression from neuraxial opioids does not appear to differ from that of systemic opioid administration, ranging from 0.1–0.9%. The concern for respiratory depression stems from the cephalic spread and systemic distribution of neuraxial opioids. Respiratory depression appears early after bolus with lipophilic opioids such as fentanyl or sufentanil, and may be delayed up to 12 hours with hydrophilic opioids such as morphine. Risk factors include increasing dose, age, concomitant systemic opioid or sedative use, thoracic surgery, prolonged or extensive surgery, and the presence of applicable comorbidities.

Paravertebral anesthesia: Occasionally, situations arise in which a patient would benefit from epidural analgesia confined to a single side of the body, or in which an avoidance of large-segment sympatholysis becomes critical. This can be accomplished by delivering local anesthetics to the paravertebral compartment either through a single injection or via continual infusion via catheter. Such techniques are finding increasing use for unilateral thoracic, breast, abdominal, and hip surgery, and for pain from rib fractures.

Risks of regional anesthesia

As with all medical and surgical therapies, the risk-to-benefit ratios of regional anesthesia should be thoroughly discussed with patients prior to implementation. Because regional anesthesia requires apposition of sharp instruments very near the spinal cord or peripheral nerves, there is a rare but catastrophic risk of direct mechanical injury to these structures. Bleeding and infection are likewise possible with any regional anesthetic, especially those related to the central nervous system. With regard to neuraxial and paravertebral analgesia, development of an epidural hematoma may result in spinal cord hypoperfusion, injury, and subsequent permanent paralysis. Epidural hematoma formation may occur during needle or catheter placement, and during catheter removal. Concurrent use of neuraxial or paravertebral analgesia with systemic anticoagulation requires exceptional vigilance to prevent or minimize complications involving epidural hematomas.

Infection represents another major concern, especially with neuraxial analgesia. Serious infections resulting in epidural abscess or meningitis following epidural analgesia are thankfully quite rare (< 1/1000 and < 1/50,000, respectively), although catheter colonization rates may approach 35%.

CASE 96-1 *(continued)*

In evaluating the case study patient with her associated comorbidities, one could consider a peripheral nerve block. A femoral nerve catheter would represent a relatively low-risk intervention, which may alleviate much, but not all, of her pain. The patient could also receive systemic anticoagulation with low-molecular-weight heparin without risk of an epidural hematoma. If a femoral nerve catheter does not suffi ciently control her pain, an epidural could be placed in the low lumbar region. This would require urinary catheterization, and appropriate precautions regarding anticoagulation, but may off er superior pain relief. Such interventions may decrease or obviate the need for supplemental opioids. The counterpoint to this treatment plan is that the ultimate goal with this patient is to improve functionality and have her out of bed and working with physical therapy. To achieve this, it is important to achieve a sensory blockade while maintaining motor function, decreasing her fall risk and improving her ability to work with physical therapy.

SPECIAL POPULATIONS

MEDICAL COMORBIDITIES

Elderly/dementia/delirium

Treatment goals:

- Maximizing functionality and pain control while minimizing cognitive side effects.

Treatment modalities:

- Oral medications, topical medications, and interventional therapies.

Special Considerations:

- Elderly patients have both multiple comorbidities and altered liver and kidney physiology, which impact their drug metabolism and clearance. Hepatic drug clearance can be reduced by 30% and renal clearance is decreased by 50% in two-thirds of elderly patients. This makes elderly patients particularly sensitive to many of the pain medications with subsequent CNS effects. Opioids, with the exception of buprenorphine, have increased active half-lives and metabolites. This requires decreased dosing and longer dosing intervals to minimize adverse events. Long-acting opioids can be beneficial due to improved compliance with dosing regimens, particularly transdermal fentanyl. Transdermal fentanyl is best used for patients with chronic pain, not acute or postoperative pain due to the risk of respiratory depression. Cognitive impairment is still a recognized sequelae and titration should be slow and gradual.
- Beers criteria for institutionalized elderly patients include 3-tiered recommendations for medications to avoid. Medications considered inappropriate include flurazepam, pentazocine, and meperidine. Risky medications include long-acting benzodiazepines such as diazepam. A more effective or better alternative medication includes ketorolac. Gurwitz and colleagues evaluated medication use in Medicare beneficiaries and found that 20.1% were on opioids and 19.8% were on nonopioid analgesics in outpatient settings, which resulted in a preventable adverse effect rate of 6.7% and 15.4% respectively.

Obstructive sleep apnea

Treatment goals:

- Optimize pain control while minimizing detrimental effects of treatment on respiratory mechanics.

Treatment modalities:

- Avoid opioid and centrally acting agents that suppress respiratory drive as much as possible. These can include adjuvants, NSAIDs, tramadol, regional anesthetics, and the use of home CPAP.

Special considerations:

- One of the most important factors in management is recognition of the disease to employ risk minimization strategies. This has been best evaluated with regard to the perioperative period. Proposed mechanisms for airway obstruction during sedation and anesthesia include factors that impact closing pressure and airway muscle activity leaving these patients more vulnerable to the effects of sedation. Sedatives, anesthetics, and analgesics appear to selectively compromise patients with obstructive sleep apnea (OSA) compared to unaffected individuals. Efficacy of CPAP has not been evaluated in the perioperative period or with concomitant use of analgesics or opioids. Treatment strategies can include minimization of centrally acting respiratory depressants such as opioids and reliance upon nonopioid therapies.

Peripheral vascular disease

Treatment goals:

- Peripheral arterial disease is present in 12–20% of Americans over age 65 with the majority of these patients having asymptomatic disease. Critical limb ischemia is defined as greater than two weeks of rest pain, ulcers, or tissue loss attributed to arterial occlusive disease. The primary mainstay of treatment is evaluation and possible interventional treatment by vascular surgery. Primary treatment modalities include medical therapy, revascularization, or amputation. Increasing numbers of patients are able to undergo revascularization because of developing endovascular strategies. Patients with disease and comorbidities that are not amenable to operable repair are left with medical analgesic therapy or spinal cord stimulation. Spinal cord stimulators are used extensively in Europe for this indication.

Treatment modalities:

- Oral medications, topical medications, and interventional therapies (spinal cord stimulation)

Special considerations:

- Spinal cord stimulator treatment has been found to improve 12-month limb salvage and lower analgesic use in nonoperable patients compared with conservative therapy. Conservative medication therapy can control pain in these patients, but spinal cord stimulation may provide analgesic benefit and facilitate wound healing.

Hepatic disease/failure

Treatment goals:

- Hepatic disease can be associated with dysfunction in several pathways that impede pain control strategies. Coagulation issues can preclude interventional management techniques including regional anesthesia, nerve blocks, and other injections. Liver dysfunction can affect opioid metabolism and preclude the use of medications containing acetaminophen.

Treatment modalities:

- Oral and transdermal therapy including opioids that do not have significant disruption of metabolism and additional adjuvants that are comorbidity appropriate.

Special considerations:

- Opioid metabolism can be significantly affected by hepatic insufficiency. Drugs with decreased clearance include meperidine, dextropropoxyphene, pentazocine, tramadol, and alfentanil. Morphine also has decreased clearance and increased oral bioavailability. These drugs can be used but would require a decreased dose or increased dosing interval. Meperidine can be metabolized to normeperidine, an active metabolite that can cause seizures. Fentanyl, sufentanil, and remifentanil metabolism do not appear to be altered.

Renal disease/failure

Treatment goals:

- Optimize pain control while minimizing impact upon renal function and adjust medications that are affected by impaired renal function.

Treatment modalities:

- Oral and transdermal analgesics, topical NSAIDs (minimizing systemic absorption), interventional therapies (pain-state specific).

Special considerations:

- Dialysis patients have significant pain that can be undertreated. Barakzoy and colleagues developed a modified WHO ladder paradigm to treat nociceptive and neuropathic pain in end-stage renal disease (ESRD) patients. These modifications include acetaminophen and adjuvants for mild pain; tramadol, hydrocodone, oxycodone, nonopioid analgesics, and adjuvants. Severe pain responded to the addition of hydromorphone, fentanyl, and methadone in addition to the lower-tier recommendations. Patients tolerated these medications well with the most challenging population being elderly patients on dialysis, although pharmacokinetics and side effect profiles are an issue in healthier patients in this age group.
- The use of NSAIDs is associated with an increased rate and severity of side effects in patients with renal dysfunction. These effects can range from electrolyte abnormalities to chronic renal failure on a dose and exposure basis. This relationship is best correlated with the plasma concentration of the NSAIDs, which does not eliminate their usage entirely, but requires caution. Diclofenac is a topical nonsteroidal that has demonstrated benefit in the patch and gel format for osteoarthritis, but has only 2% renal clearance, decreasing that concern in patients with renal insufficiency/failure.

SPECIFIC PAIN CONDITIONS

Postoperative: peripheral (orthopedic)

Treatment goals:

- Improved pain control to improve functionality and work with physical therapy.

Treatment modalities (as per detailed explanation above):

- Catheters and neuraxial blocks, adjunctive agents: neuropathic medications, NSAIDs, opioids: transitioning to oral medications from the PCA.

Special considerations:

- Hip and knee arthroplasty patients are stratified into highest-risk categories for thromboembolic events. Anticoagulation in these patients may direct therapeutic strategies for pain control and require special considerations when working with catheters and neuraxial blocks. NSAIDs use in postspine fusion has mixed evidence and will be dependent upon the individual surgeon's management preferences.

Postoperative: abdominal/thoracic

Treatment goals:

- Pain control to improve respiratory status.

Treatment modalities:

- Regional anesthesia has excellent benefits for the postoperative patient. Thoracic epidural for improved pain control without additional respiratory depression. While IV PCA is safe, epidural analgesia allows for superior pain control with an improved side effect profile. Patient satisfaction and surgical outcomes are also improved with the use of epidurals for the first 72 hours postoperatively; however, pruritus can be an issue.
- NPO status can be a directing factor in the pain regimen with these patients. Transitioning these patients from an epidural or IV PCA can be challenging due to limitations in oral dosing because of concerns about absorption issues and opioid-induced bowel dysfunction. Transdermal fentanyl can be a viable option, but is not a first-line choice in postoperative patients without a history of chronic pain because of the risk of respiratory depression.

Chest tube pain/thoracotomy

- Best managed by thoracic epidural, but once the epidural is removed, lidocaine patch can be a useful option.

Special considerations:

- Opioids have the undesirable side effects of respiratory depression and action on the gastrointestinal system as detailed later.

Ophthalmic pain

Treatment goals:

- Determining when to consult ophthalmology versus conservative management. Eye pain can be grossly divided into three categories:
  1. Ocular and orbital disorders with or without visible pathology of the eye (eg, redness, corneal opacity, or proptosis)
  2. Ophthalmologic syndromes associated with headache
  3. Headache syndromes associated with ophthalmologic findings.

Treatment modalities:

- Conservative management primarily consists of observation with no active intervention necessary.

Special Considerations:

- Red flags for ophthalmic pain necessitating consultation include:

New visual acuity defect	Color vision defect
Relative afferent pupillary defect	Visual field loss
Extraocular muscle abnormality	Ocular misalignment
Conjunctival chemosis, injection, or redness	Diplopia
Iris irregularity or nonreactive pupil	Proptosis
Recent intraocular surgery (within three months)	Corneal opacity
Fundus abnormality (eg, retinal hemorrhages, optic disc edema, or optic atrophy)	Hyphema or hypopyon
Iris irregularity or nonreactive pupil	Recent ocular trauma
	Lid retraction or ptosis

Stroke pain: central stroke pain

Treatment goals:

- Central stroke pain is disabling sequelae of stroke in 8–14% of patients.

Treatment modalities:

- First-line drugs include tricyclic antidepressants and neuropathic agents including pregabalin and gabapentin. Second-line drugs would include selective serotonin–norepinephrine reuptake inhibitors, lamotrigine, opioids, and drug combinations.

Special considerations:

- Diagnosis is made by exclusion of other likely causes of pain in the presence of a history consistent with stroke and pain in a distinct neuroanatomically plausible distribution supported by clinical

TABLE 96-3 Neuropathic Pain Medication Guidelines

Drug	Start Dose	Maximum Dose	Documented Effect	Side Effects
Gabapentin	300 mg/day	3600 mg/day	PHN, PDN, mixed neuropathic pain	Sedation, dizziness, edema
Pregabalin	25 mg/day	600 mg/day	PHN, PDN, mixed neuropathic pain, central pain	Sedation, dizziness edema
Tricyclic antidepressants	25 mg/day (NB: plasma level)	75–150 mg/day (NB: plasma level)	PHN, PDN, central pain, mixed neuropathic pain	Cardiac, anticholinergic, sedation
Specific serotonergic and noradrenergic reuptake inhibitors			Painful neuropathy	Sedation
Venlafaxine	37.5 mg/day	25–375 mg/day		
Duloxetine	60 mg/day			
Carbamazepine (oxcarbazepine)	300 mg/day (NB: plasma level)	1200–1800 mg (1/3 higher dose for oxcarbazepine) (NB: plasma level)	Trigeminal neuralgia	Sedation, dizziness, ataxia
Tramadol	50 mg/day	400 mg/day	Painful neuropathies	Sedation, dizziness, obstipation
Lamotrigine	25 mg/day* (NB: plasma level)	400–600 mg/day (NB: plasma level)	Trigeminal neuralgia, poststroke central pain	Sedation, tremor, rash
Opioids	5–10 mg/day, titrate substitute with long-acting opioids	Variable	PHN, PDN, postamputation pain	Sedation, dizziness, tolerance, drug abuse
Lidocaine patch			PHN, traumatic nerve injury	Allergic reaction
Capsaicin cream	4x/day for 8wks		PHN, PDN, HIV	

PDN, peripheral diabetic neuropathy; PHN, postherpetic neuralgia.
*To be titrated slowly.
Reproduced, with permission, from Jensen TS, et al. Pharmacology and treatment of neuropathic pains. *Current Opinion in Neurology*. 2009;22:467–474.

neurologic examination. This diagnosis is strengthened by indication of a concordant vascular lesion using imaging study.

Neuropathic pain

Treatment goals:

- Diagnosis of the cause of the neuropathy (ie diabetes mellitus, HIV, chemotherapy-induced peripheral neuropathy) should guide the management to prevent worsening of the neuropathy.

Treatment modalities:

- Oral and transdermal therapies are the primary modalities; spinal cord stimulation can be beneficial for some patients that are refractory to these therapies. First-line medications include tricyclic antidepressants, selective serotonergic and noradrenergic reuptake inhibitors, calcium channel alpha 2-delta ligands (pregabalin and gabapentin), and topical lidocaine. Opioid analgesics and tramadol are considered second-line agents that can be used as first-line treatments in certain patients. Third-line agents include other anticonvulsants, antidepressants, mexiletine, *N*-Methyl-D-aspartate (NMDA) receptors, and topical capsaicin (**Table 96-3**).

Special considerations:

- Herpes zoster vaccination should be considered in appropriate patient populations as one of the only preventative measures for neuropathic pain. Interventional therapies can include spinal cord stimulation.

Phantom limb pain

Treatment goals:

- Phantom limb pain occurs in 50–80% of both traumatic and operative amputees. The prevailing theory is based on central changes with some peripheral and psychological components involved in the development. Cortical reorganization seems to be the primary mechanism with peripheral sensitization, but the developmental mechanism is still unknown. Pain and sensory alterations at the site of amputation predominate in the initial postoperative and posttraumatic period. Phantom limb sensations and pain generally develop within one month of the amputation with a second peak of development approximately 12 months postamputation. Preoperative analgesia has been evaluated as a possibility to improve outcomes, but neither regional anesthetic techniques nor oral regimens have been found to decrease incidence of the development of phantom limb pain.

Treatment modalities:

- Treatment of phantom limb pain may require a multimodal therapeutic regimen. First-line therapies include transcutaneous electrical nerve stimulation (TENS) and biofeedback. Medication options include anticonvulsants (gabapentin), opioids, and NSAIDs. Other treatment modalities that have not been investigated fully but have benefitted some patients include: acupuncture, mirror-box therapy, NMDA, and calcitonin receptor agonists.

Special considerations:

- Psychological components, including coping mechanisms, appear to be a component in the development of phantom limb pain. Patients should be evaluated for the need to adjust prosthesis, stump neuroma, referred pain, and care of the residual limb.

Chronic abdominal pain/distention

Treatment goals:

- Minimizing opioids and maintaining motility. Evaluating patients for a correctable pathology is the primary step. This may involve evaluation by the gastroenterology or gynecology service.

Treatment modalities:

- NSAIDs, adjuvant medications, treatment of primary pathology, and interventional strategies.

Special Considerations:

- Opioid-induced constipation is a common side effect that limits the efficacy of this drug class for patients with abdominal pathology. Opioid use also can promote the development of narcotic bowel syndrome (NBS), which is the aggravation of chronic abdominal pain by opioid usage. Exposing patients to opioids for nonmalignant pain puts them at higher risk for developing aberrant drug-related behaviors and illicit drug use. Narcotic bowel syndrome can actually be the etiology of an acute abdominal pain exacerbation, as a diagnosis of exclusion with evaluation that is negative for pathology, moderate opioid usage greater than two weeks, and clinical history. Treatment of this NBS involves several factors including recognition of the syndrome, developing a relationship with the patient to facilitate this process, graded withdrawal of the narcotic according to a specified withdrawal program, and the institution of medications to reduce withdrawal effects.
- Methylnaltrexone is a newer agent that can be used to counteract opioid-induced constipation with minimal central effects and lack of withdrawal potential. These patients should be screened for ileus or other obstructive causes of constipation prior to administration.
- Epidural analgesia can be used for treatment and management of chronic abdominal pain of multifactorial origin. The management is similar to that of postoperative abdominal pain as above.
- Chronic pancreatitis may develop as part of an increased neural density and hypertrophy resulting in a neuropathic pain state, similar to the state that develops in pancreatic adenocarcinoma. Chronic pancreatitis treatment can use the neuropathic pain treatment paradigm as above. The limitation of this therapy is that the NMDA antagonists and tricyclic antidepressants can result in decreased gastrointestinal motility. Lifestyle modifications and analgesics are the mainstay of outpatient treatment. The addition of pancrease can be started under the guidance of gastroenterology and patients may have a reduction in pain associated with this. Tramadol can also be a useful alternative to stronger opioids with regard to pain control and GI motility side effects.
- Oral medications are the mainstay of treatment for this, but some providers will perform celiac plexus blocks/neurolysis. However, these are not permanent procedures with nerve regrowth within three to six months. This is not an entirely benign procedure with complication risks including paralysis. Spinal cord stimulation may prove to be a treatment strategy for refractory severe abdominal visceral pain.

TABLE 96-4 WHO (Modified) Analgesic Ladder

Step 1	Nonopioid analgesics Eg, acetaminophen, NSAIDs (OTC and Rx), adjuvants, antidepressants, membrane stabilizers, local anesthetics (topical and enteral), bisphosphonates, and steroids Pain procedural interventions
Step 2	Nonopioid and "weak" opioid analgesics Eg, codeine, hydrocodone, and tramadol Pain procedural interventions
Step 3	Nonopioid and "strong" opioid analgesics Eg, morphine, hydromorphone, fentanyl, methadone, and oxycodone Pain procedural interventions

Cancer pain

Treatment goals:

- Maximizing function and quality of life.

Treatment modalities:

- Oral medication including NSAIDs, opioids, and neuropathic agents, nerve blocks and neurolysis, spinal cord stimulators, and intrathecal therapy.

Special considerations:

- Cancer pain is globally undertreated, with significant impact on quality of life. The World Health Organization developed its "ladder" for treatment of malignant pain (**Table 96-4**). A major barrier to this is usage, but when implemented, significant proportions receive pain relief.
- Elderly patients dealing with malignant pain are particularly vulnerable to subtherapeutic treatment. In patients with comorbidities, interventional therapies can prove beneficial. These can include somatic/sympathetic blockades, intrathecal therapy, and spinal cord stimulation. Sympathetic blockade/neurolysis can be beneficial for certain pain states; one of the most commonly utilized is the celiac plexus block/neurolysis for pancreatic cancer. This procedure is primarily used for malignant pain due to associated risks, but a large component of efficacy is dependent on the location of the tumor. Neuraxial medication administration (epidural/intrathecal) has been found to be beneficial for both pain control and minimization of side effects. This is usually reserved for pain that is refractory to the WHO paradigm or limited by the side effect profile. This conservative practice of waiting until the cancer pain patient fails other therapies may extend the patients discomfort unnecessarily.

CONCLUSION

The evaluation and treatment of pain begins with an unbiased assessment of the patient's symptoms, individualized treatment plans that reflect the patient's comorbidities and types of pain, and a reassessment of treatment changes at appropriate intervals so that patients do not suffer needlessly. Hospitalists can improve patient care as they address pain issues across specialties on comanagement and medical services by frequently assessing and effectively communicating with patients as well as being readily available as problems arise. Appropriately converting different opioids and addressing pain issues will not only promote patient safety but patient satisfaction as well.

SUGGESTED READINGS

Breivik H, Borchgrevink PC, Allen SM, et al. Assessment of pain. *Br J Anaesth.* 2008;101:17.

Gachago C, Draganov PV. Pain management in chronic pancreatitis. *World J Gastroenterol.* 2008;14:3137.

Grunkemeier DM, Cassara JE, Dalton CB, et al. The narcotic bowel syndrome: clinical features, pathophysiology, and management. *Clin Gastroenterol Hepatol.* 2007;5:1126.

Hudcova J, McNicol E, Quah C, et al. Patient controlled opioid analgesia versus conventional opioid analgesia for postoperative pain. *Cochrane Database Syst Rev.* 2006;CD003348.

Hurley RW, Cohen SP, Williams KA, et al. The analgesic effects of perioperative gabapentin on postoperative pain: a meta-analysis. *Reg Anesth Pain Med.* 2006;31:237.

Kehlet H, Jensen TS, Woolf CJ. Persistent postsurgical pain: risk factors and prevention. *Lancet.* 2006;367:1618.

Nikolajsen L, Ilkjaer S, Christensen JH, et al. Randomised trial of epidural bupivacaine and morphine in prevention of stump and phantom pain in lower-limb amputation. *Lancet.* 1997; 350:1353.

Ritter JM, Harding I, Warren JB. Precaution, cyclooxygenase inhibition, and cardiovascular risk. *Trends Pharmacol Sci.* 2009;30:503.

Thomas J, Karver S, Cooney GA, et al. Methylnaltrexone for opioid-induced constipation in advanced illness. *N Engl J Med.* 2008;358:2332.

Werawatganon T, Charuluxanun S. Patient controlled intravenous opioid analgesia versus continuous epidural analgesia for pain after intra-abdominal surgery. *Cochrane Database Syst Rev.* 2005;CD004088.

CHAPTER 97

Significant Co-Morbid Disease

Rachelle E. Bernacki, MD, MS

Key Clinical Questions

1. How does the physician approach a patient with multiple comorbidities? How are they different than other patients?
2. How do multiple comorbidities affect a patient's prognosis?
3. How does the physician take prognosis into account when formulating treatment plans for patients?

CASE 97-1

A 79-year-old woman with moderately severe chronic diseases (obstructive pulmonary disease, osteoporosis, osteoarthritis, type 2 diabetes mellitus, and hypertension) was admitted to the hospital for a complicated urinary tract infection. She had recently moved to the area and needed to establish primary care following discharge. Her newly assigned primary care physician requested that "good maintenance medications" be prescribed for her chronic diseases prior to discharge. However, if the relevant clinical practice guidelines were followed, the patient would be prescribed 12 medications (her cost $406 per month) along with a complicated nonpharmacological regimen (see **Table 97-1**). The patient did not find these recommendations to be practical.

INTRODUCTION

The remarkable success of medicine combined with improved living conditions in the last century has led to an increase in life expectancy in the United States. In the 21st century, a 70-year-old woman in the top 25% percentile of health can expect to live an additional 21.3 years (see **Figure 97-1**). However, the medical successes that led to this dramatic increase in life expectancy have also created medical challenges. As more people are living into old age, the numbers of patients with multiple comorbitites are rising. In fact, very few patients have only hypertension or simply diabetes; many patients with chronic diseases have multiple comorbidities. In 1999, 48% of Medicare beneficiaries aged 65 years or older had at least three chronic medical conditions and 21% had five or more. Health care costs for individuals with at least three chronic conditions accounted for 89% of Medicare's annual budget. Comorbidity is associated with higher health care use, physical disability, polypharmacy/adverse drug events, poor quality of life, and increased mortality. Improving care for this population is clearly important, but it is a challenge for physicians, including hospitalists, who need to balance and prioritize treatment of the acute conditions requiring hospitalization with the chronic morbidities that may complicate treatment.

Until recently there have been few guidelines on how to account for patients' comorbidities and formulate reasonable treatment plans. Many physicians encounter patients as in Case 97-1—a 79-year-old for whom guideline concordance would result in expensive polypharmacy and potential noncompliance—and might struggle with how to proceed. Consequently, care can be haphazard, scattered, and costly for the patient, provider and health care system. Some argue that the best way to approach the above patient is to consider her prognosis in making recommendations on how to treat her various conditions and take patient preferences into account.

To a large degree, how a medical team decides to treat a patient's particular condition or comorbidity depends on the patient's prognosis. *"How long do I have?"* is among the most common questions asked by patients. Prognosis is defined as "a prediction of the probable course and outcome of a disease" or alternatively, "the likelihood of recovery from a disease." Current textbooks of internal medicine often give little attention to the prognosis of diseases. The 'ellipsis of prognosis' is described by Christakis: "concurrent with a shift in clinical thought from an individual-based to a

TABLE 97-1 Treatment Regimen Based on Clinical Practice Guidelines for a Hypothetical 79-Year-Old Woman with Hypertension, Diabetes Mellitus, Osteoporosis, Osteoarthritis, and COPD*

Time	Medications†	Other
7:00 AM	Ipratropium metered dose inhaler 70 mg/wk of alendronate	Check feet Sit upright for 30 min on day when alendronate is taken Check blood sugar
8:00 AM	500 mg of calcium and 200 IU of vitamin D 12.5 mg of hydrochlorothiazide 40 mg of lisinopril 10 mg of glyburide 81 mg of aspirin 850 mg of metformin 250 mg of naproxen 20 mg of omeprazole	Eat breakfast 2.4 g/d of sodium 90 mmol/d of potassium Low intake of dietary saturated fat and cholesterol Adequate intake of magnesium and calcium Medical nutrition therapy for diabetes§ DASH§
12:00 PM		Eat lunch 2.4 g/d of sodium 90 mmol/d of potassium Low intake of dietary saturated fat and cholesterol Adequate intake of magnesium and calcium Medical nutrition therapy for diabetes§ DASH§
1:00 PM	Ipratropium metered dose inhaler 500 mg of calcium and 200 IU of vitamin D	
7:00 PM	Ipratropium metered dose inhaler 850 mg of metformin 500 mg of calcium and 200 IU of vitamin D 40 mg of lovastatin 250 mg of naproxen	Eat dinner 2.4 g/d of sodium 90 mmol/d of potassium Low intake of dietary saturated fat and cholesterol Adequate intake of magnesium and calcium Medical nutrition therapy for diabetes§ DASH§
11:00 PM	Ipratropium metered dose inhaler	
As needed	Albuterol metered dose inhaler	

Abbreviations: ADA, American Diabetes Association; COPD, chronic obstructive pulmonary disease: DASH; Dietary Approaches to Stop Hypertension.

*Clinical practice guidelines used: (1) Joint National Committee on Prevention, Detection. Evaluation, and Treatment of High Blood Pressure VII. (2) ADA ; glycemic control is recommended; however, specific medicines are not described. (3) American College of Rheumatology; recent evidence about the safety and appropriateness of cyclooxygenase inhibitors, particularly in individuals with comorbid cardiovascular disease, led us to omit them from the list of medication options, although they are discussed in the reviewed clinical practice guidelines. (4) National Osteoporosis Foundation; this regimen assumes dietary intake of 200 IU of vitamin D. (5) National Heart, Lung, and Blood Institute and World Health Organization.

†Taken orally unless otherwise indicated. The medication complexity score of the regimen for this hypothetical woman is 14 with 19 doses of medications per day, assuming 2 as needed doses of albuterol metered dose inhaler plus 70 mg/wk of alendronate.

§Dash and ADA dietary guidelines may be synthesized, but the help of a registered dietitian is specifically recommended. Eat foods containing carbohydrate from whole grains, fruits, vegetables, and low-fat milk. Avoid protein intake of more than 20% of total daily energy; lower protein intake to about 10% of daily calories if overt nephropathy is present. Limit intake of saturated fat (< 10% of total daily energy) and dietary cholesterol (< 200–300 mg). Limit intake of trans unsaturated fatty acids. Eat 2 to 3 servings of fish per week. Intake of polyunsaturated fat should be about 10% of total daily energy.

(Reproduced, with permission, from Boyd CM, Darer JD, Boult C, et al. Clinical practice guidelines and quality of care for older patients with multiple comorbid diseases: implications for pay for performance. *JAMA*. 2005;10:294(6):716–724.)

diagnosis-based conceptualization of disease, prognosis came to be seen as intrinsic to diagnosis and therapy, and explicit attention to prognosis consequently diminished."

Prognosis guides individualized clinical decisions such as cancer screening or hospice, and identifies groups at high risk for poor outcomes in whom targeted interventions may be most useful. Importantly, prognosis can provide foundation for discussing goals of care. Many patients want to discuss prognosis with physicians, and inadequacy of prognostic information is often the greatest complaint patients/families have about end of life care.

PRACTICE POINT

- Inadequacy of prognostic information is often the greatest complaint patients/families have about end of life care.

Despite the importance of prognosis, physicians are often reluctant to prognosticate. In a national survey of physicians, 90% felt they should avoid being specific about prognosis. Furthermore, 57% felt inadequately trained in prognostication. In another study

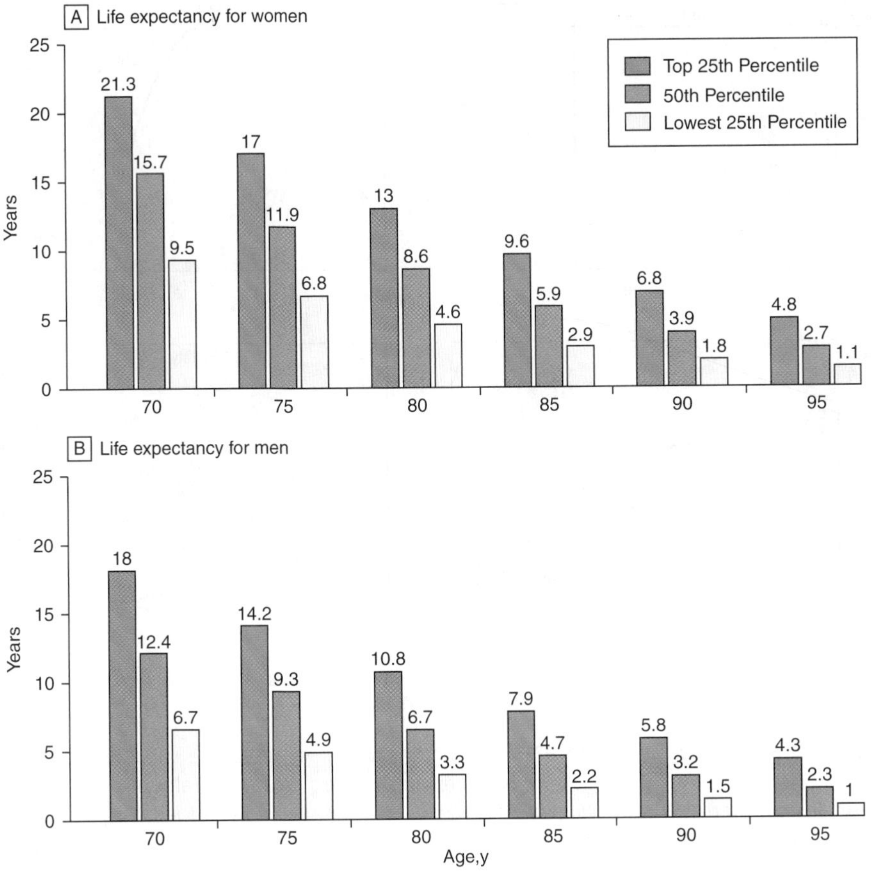

Figure 97-1 *Upper, Middle, and Lower Quartiles of Life Expectancy for Women and Men at Selected Ages. (Reproduced, with permission, from Walter LC, Covinsky KE. Cancer screening in elderly patients: a framework for individualized decision making. JAMA. 2001;285:2750–2756.)*

looking at the accuracy of physician prognostic skill, physicians were asked to provide survival estimates of terminally ill patients at the time of hospice referral. Physicians were accurate 20% of the time and overestimated survival time by a factor of 5.3. In addition, if the duration of the physician-patient relationship increased, prognostic accuracy decreased, suggesting that physician feelings toward patients may alter their ability to prognosticate. In part for this reason, but also because hospitalists often see patients in the midst of a clinical deterioration, it is crucial that hospitalists do not defer prognostication and end-of-life decision making to the outpatient provider.

PROGNOSTIC MODELS

Prognostication can be difficult, as there are many different pathways to death (see **Figure 97-2**). Certain diagnoses, like metastatic cancer, have a more predictable terminal period. However, only 21% of Medicare beneficiaries die of cancer and less than 16% will die suddenly. Many die of acute complications of a chronic condition in which the terminal period is much more uncertain, such as organ failure (20%). Patients who die from dementia or frailty (20%) may have long periods of debility with less predictable courses.

PRACTICE POINT

- There are four trajectories to death: sudden death, terminal disease, organ failure, and frailty. Determining which pathway your patient follows can help you prognosticate and communicate with patients and families.

Life expectancy tables can give rough estimates of prognosis (see Figure 97-1). Those at or above the top 25th percentile at each age are active patients with no significant comorbid illnesses; the 50th percentile is the median life expectancy at each age; and below the lowest 25th percentile at each age are patients with severe comorbid illnesses like dementia or congestive heart failure. Most hospitalized patients fall into the bottom of this latter group and the 25th percentile, therefore, can be used as an estimate for the "best" possible life expectancy for the typical hospitalized patient.

A prognostic index is a clinical tool that quantifies the contributions that various components of the history, physical exam, and laboratory findings make toward a diagnosis, prognosis, or likely response to treatment. Physicians can use prognostic indices to lend confidence to their judgments about prognosis and these indices provide an objective measure to support clinical intuition. Combining clinical estimates with prognostic indices results in more accurate estimates than either alone. Prognostic indices have many different names such as clinical prediction rules, decision rules, and staging systems (eg, Goldman Index, Dukes staging system for colorectal cancer, NYHA congestive heart failure class).

PRACTICE POINT

- Prognostic indices can be used to support clinical judgment and lend confidence to prognostic estimates.

CASE 97-2

An 81-year-old man with a history of mild congestive heart failure was admitted from home for nausea, vomiting, and lethargy. He improved with antibiotics prescribed for cholecystitis. During his hospitalization an echocardiogram reported an

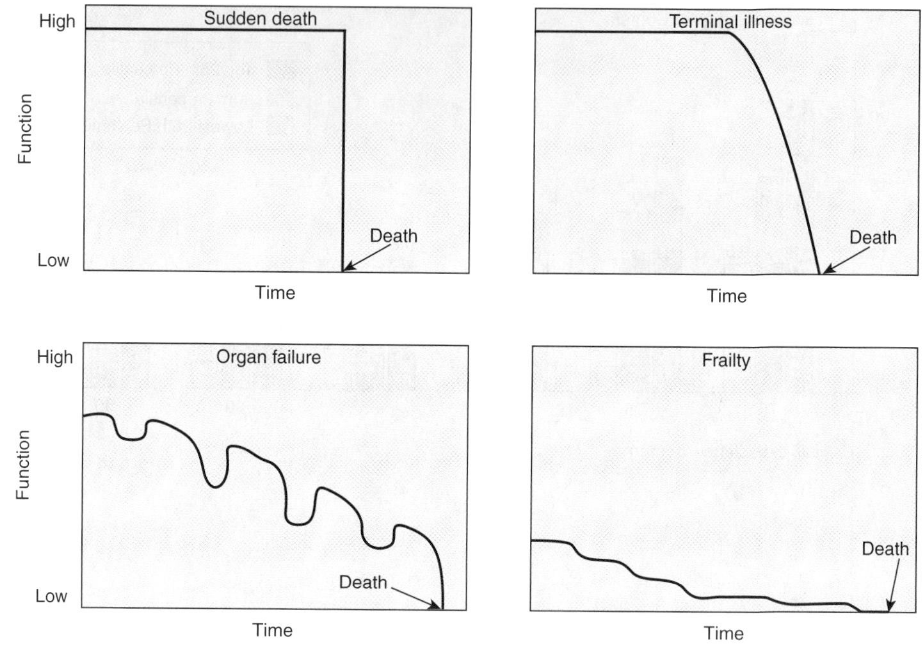

Figure 97-2 *Theoretical Trajectories of Disease. (Reproduced, with permission, from Lunney. JAMA. 2003;289(18): 2387–2392.)*

ejection fraction was 45%. An albumin of 2.9 g/dl prompted nutrition consultation which noted adequate caloric intake by the time he was ready for discharge. His physicians decided to transition him to a nursing home for assistance with activities of daily living (ADLs: bathing, dressing, and toileting). When asked by family members about his prognosis, how should his physicians respond?

Hospitalization is often a major health transition for elders and is often a time to reassess goals of care. Walter, et al, developed an accurate and easy-to-use index to stratify older adults into groups by their risk for one-year mortality after hospital discharge. The index was developed in a large heterogeneous group of patients aged 70+ admitted to a general medical service by identifying risk factors for mortality from multiple domains including demographics, comorbitites, laboratory findings, and functional status. Kaplan Meier survival curves of the four risk groups demonstrate that the groups have markedly different survival trajectories (see **Figure 97-3**). Using only using six accessible variables, (gender, congestive heart failure, cancer, creatinine, albumin, and ADL-*Activities of Daily Living* dependency at discharge), this prognostic index stratifies older adults according to one-year mortality after hospitalization. For example, our patient in Case 97-2 would receive 1 point for being male, 2 points for a history of congestive heart failure, 2 points for being discharged to a skilled nursing facility, and 2 points for poor nutritional status (albumin 2.9) for a total of 7 points (a patient with metastatic cancer receives 8 points). His one-year mortality is estimated at 68%. This study emphasizes the importance of considering multiple domains when assessing prognosis in older adults. Some hospices use the Walter criteria (> 6 points) to enroll patients.

IMPORTANCE OF FUNCTIONAL STATUS

Functional status is of utmost importance when estimating prognosis in older adults. In the Walter index (see Figure 97-3), measures of functional status added important information about risk for one-year mortality beyond that provided by medical

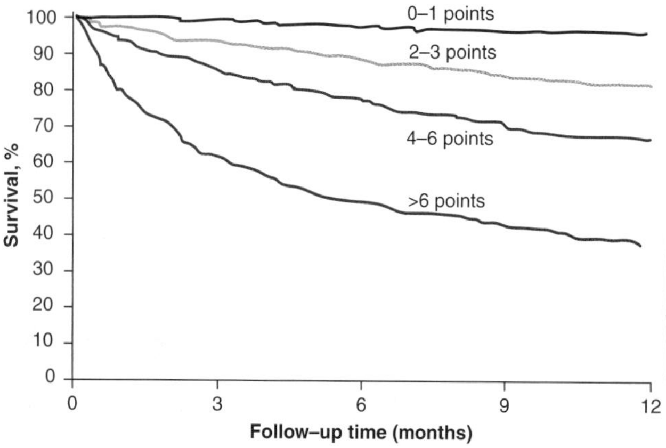

Characteristic	Points
Gender	
Male	1
ADL dependencies at discharge	
Partial dependence	2
Total dependence	5
Comorbid conditions	
CHF	2
Cancer (solitary)	3
Cancer (metastatic)	8
Lab abnormalities	
Creatinine > 3.0 mg/dL	2
Albumin 3.0-3.4 g/dL	1
Albumin < 3.0 g/dL	2

Figure 97-3 *Mortality at One Year Post Discharge. (Reproduced, with permission, from Walter LC, Covinsky KE. Cancer screening in elderly patients: a framework for individualized decision making. JAMA. 2001;285:2750–2756.)*

diagnoses or physiologic measures. Functional status reflects the severity and end-result of many different illnesses and psychosocial factors. Hospitalists do not routinely record functional status for their patients, but it is important for considering a patient's prognosis.

> **PRACTICE POINT**
>
> - Functional status reflects the severity and end-result of many different illnesses and psychosocial factors and is the best prognostic tool available.

Estimating prognosis based on functional status began with oncology patients; the Karnofsky Index (100 = normal; 0 = dead) and the ECOG scale (Eastern Cooperative Oncology Group), (0 = normal; 5 = dead) are the most commonly used scales. A median survival of three months roughly correlates with a Karnofsky score <40 or ECOG >3. Newer prognostic scales have also been developed. The simplest method to assess functional ability is to ask patients: *"How do you spend your time? How much time do you spend in bed or lying down?"* If the response is >50% of the time and this is increasing, estimate the cancer patients' prognosis at three months or less. An increasing number of physical symptoms, especially dyspnea, are also a good indication that time is short. The Palliative Performance Scale (PPS) uses five observer-rated domains correlated to the Karnofsky Performance Scale, commonly used to estimate prognosis in patients with cancer. The PPS is a reliable and valid tool and correlates well with actual survival and median survival time for patients. It has been found useful for purposes of identifying and tracking potential care needs of palliative care patients, particularly as these needs change with disease progression.

SPECIFIC CIRCUMSTANCES OR DISEASES

CARDIOPULMONARY RESUSCITATION

Survival to discharge following cardiac arrest occurring in the hospital is infrequent. In a recent study examining 433,985 Medicare patients who underwent in-hospital CPR, 18.3% of patients survived to discharge. For some diseases such as cancer, the prognosis is poorer; a meta analysis of survival rates for CPR revealed that 6.7% of cancer patients survived to discharge. Survival to discharge for ward cancer patients was better than ICU cancer patients: 10.1% versus 2.2%. CPR for hospitalized patients is associated with poor outcomes, as the cause of arrest is related to advanced life-threatening illness rather than a reversible acute cardiopulmonary event (eg arrhythmia). Even if the patient survives, he or she may then have significant morbidity including permanent neurological and functional impairment, a fact that should be included when having discussions about preferences for CPR. The actual statistics about survival of CPR are in sharp contrast to what the general public sees. In a study of survival of CPR depicted on television, 75% of the patients survived the immediate arrest, and 67% appeared to have survived to hospital discharge. Thus, the portrayal of CPR on television may lead the public to have an unrealistic idea of CPR and its chances for success. Physicians should be aware of the images of CPR depicted on television and the confusion these images may create when discussing preferences about CPR with patients and families.

Not only is prognosis important for planning, but patients may change decisions based on perception of prognosis. In a study of older adults, subjects were asked about preferences for cardiopulmonary resuscitation (CPR). Before learning the true probability of survival, 41% of subjects wanted CPR. After learning the true probability of CPR, 22% of subjects wanted CPR. If life expectancy was less than one year 5% of subjects wanted CPR.

CANCER

Cancer follows the terminal disease model (see Figure 97-2), a more predictable disease trajectory. Determining functional status is critical when estimating prognosis for cancer in older adults. In addition, some cancer syndromes have well-documented short median survival times:

- Malignant hypercalcemia: eight weeks (except newly diagnosed breast cancer or myeloma)
- Malignant pericardial effusion: eight weeks
- Carcinomatous meningitis: eight to twelve weeks
- Multiple brain metastases: one to two months without radiation; three to six months with radiation
- Malignant ascites, malignant pleural effusion, or malignant bowel obstruction: less than six months

Metastatic breast or prostate cancer patients with good performance status are exceptions to these, as these cancers may have an indolent course and have better treatment options.

CHRONIC OBSTRUCTIVE PULMONARY DISEASE (COPD)

Prognosis for patients with chronic obstructive pulmonary disease (COPD) is difficult to determine, and prognostic indicators are not well described. COPD follows the organ failure model (see Figure 97-2), an unpredictable disease trajectory. The forced expiratory volume in one second (FEV1) is one marker that is often used to grade severity of COPD, but a multidimensional grading system may better predict survival. The Bode index uses four factors to predict the risk of death: the body-mass index (B), the degree of airflow obstruction (O), dyspnea (D), and exercise capacity (E), measured by the six-minute–walk test. Comorbidity is also important in COPD; in one study of patients that required mechanical ventilation, the in-hospital mortality rate for the entire cohort was 28% but fell to 12% for patients with a COPD exacerbation but without a comorbid illness. In another study, patients ventilated more than 48 hours had a 50% one-year survival. Severity of illness and functional status were associated with short-term mortality while comorbidity and age were associated with one-year mortality.

CONGESTIVE HEART FAILURE (CHF)

Recently, the use of device therapies, beta-blockers, and ACE inhibitors has changed survival statistics for patients with congestive heart failure (CHF). CHF follows the organ failure model (see Figure 97-2), an unpredictable disease trajectory, and is modifiable by use of medications but is nevertheless subject to a high incidence of sudden death. These indicators have been associated with a limited prognosis in CHF:

- Cachexia
- Reduced functional capacity
- Comorbidities: diabetes, depression, COPD, cirrhosis, cerebrovascular disease, cancer, and HIV-associated cardiomyopathy
- Recent cardiac hospitalization (triples one-year mortality)
- Elevated BUN (defined by upper limit of normal) and/or creatinine ≥1.4 mg/dl
- Systolic blood pressure <100 mm Hg and/or pulse >100 bpm (each doubles one-year mortality)
- Decreased left ventricular ejection fraction (linearly correlated with survival at LVEF ≤45%)
- Ventricular dysrhythmias, treatment resistant
- Anemia (each 1 g/dl reduction in hemoglobin is associated with a 16% increase in mortality)
- Hyponatremia (serum sodium ≤135–137 mEq/l)

Several models have recently been developed to help in determining mortality in heart failure patients. The Seattle Heart Failure model is a 24-variable risk model and estimates mean one-, two-, and three-year survival and, importantly, incorporates clinical and laboratory variables, CHF medications, and device therapies. It awaits independent, prospective evaluation in unselected CHF patients. These prognostic indices require frequent updating for changing standards of CHF care and this makes accurate prognostication for patients with heart failure challenging.

DEMENTIA

Dementia is a syndrome of impaired cognition affecting memory, language, and problem solving. Depending on the cause, dementia can be irreversible, leading to progressive brain failure and death. Prognostication in dementia is difficult because it follows the frailty trajectory (see Figure 97-2) and progression is difficult to predict. The following factors have been associated with poorer prognosis: older age, male gender, comorbidity (including cancer, CHF, COPD, and diabetes mellitus), aspiration, bowel incontinence, recent weight loss, dehydration, fever, pressure ulcers, shortness of breath, dysphagia, poor oral intake, sleeping most of the day, and low BMI (body mass index). Hospitalized patients with end-stage dementia that reside in nursing homes have a particularly poor prognosis.

Functional Assessment Staging (FAST) identifies progressive steps of functional decline. Hospice guidelines state that a FAST stage 7A, ability to speak limited to six words, is appropriate for hospice enrollment if the patient also exhibits dementia-related comorbidities (aspiration, upper urinary tract infection, sepsis, multiple stage 3–4 ulcers, persistent fever, or weight loss > 10% within six months). The FAST scoring system is widely used; however its reliability in prognostication is limited. Also, many patients with dementia do not follow the stages sequentially, posing further challenges to accurate prognostication. Mitchell, et al, described the Mortality Risk Index (MRI), a score based on 12 risk factors from the MDS (Minimum Data Set), and is an alternative to FAST staging. Among patients with an MRI score of ≥ 12, 70% died within six months. Compared to FAST Stage 7C, the MRI had greater predictive value of six month prognosis. However, the MRI as only been evaluated in newly admitted nursing home residents and thus usefulness in community dwelling elders with dementia and in those who are hospitalized has not yet been determined. Estimation of prognosis in terminal dementia is in part dependent on the goals of care and decisions regarding the level of intervention that will be provided to treat acute medical problems such as urosepsis.

QUALITY IMPROVEMENT

Clinical practice guidelines, based on evidence and expert consensus, aid in defining standards of care and focus efforts to improve quality. Most guidelines address single diseases; however, physicians caring for patients with multiple comorbidites have to balance following guidelines and modifying recommendations for individual patients. Difficulties escalate with the number of diseases the patient has. Pay-for-performance (P4P) initiatives, which reward practitioners for providing specific elements of care, are usually based on single disease guidelines. These P4P programs may create incentives for disregarding the complexity of multiple comorbid chronic diseases and deter physicians from caring for individuals with multiple comorbid diseases for fear that they may be penalized for withholding care for a P4P-associated condition, when in fact avoiding polypharmacy might be in the patient's best interest. Boyd's example in Case 97-1 illustrates that better guidelines for patients with comorbidity are needed. Guided Care is a new, interdisciplinary model of health care designed by Johns Hopkins, which aims to improve efficiency of resource use for persons with medically complex health conditions.

DISCHARGE CONSIDERATIONS

One in five patients enrolled in Medicare is readmitted within 30 days. With readmissions being scrutinized, hospitalists' discharge plans for their patients need to be realistic. Improved prognostic skill allows physicians to discharge patients to appropriate settings, including home, skilled nursing facilities, and hospice. A frank and honest conversation about prognosis with the patient and family may save multiple frustrating readmissions in which little is accomplished. Hospitalists are in a unique position to spur these conversations, including prognostic disclosure, with patients and formulate discharge plans that are practical and sensible.

CASE 97-1 *(continued)*

The patient with moderately severe chronic diseases expressed her wishes to keep her medications to a minimum. She did not want to spend the rest of her life eating bland food. She worried about a low blood sugar (HgA1c is 7.3%), particularly since she had been living alone since the death of her husband. Her physicians reduced her glyburide dose to 5 mg, a change likely to be associated with a slightly higher HgA1c. According to the life expectancy tables, she had 4.6 years of life left. A nutritionist educated her how to liberalize her diet to her satisfaction. Her wishes were communicated to her new primary physician who will periodically reevaluate the changes.

CASE 97-2 *(continued)*

A family meeting was arranged with the 81-year-old patient admitted with cholecystitis, his niece, and the medical team. After introductions, the patient and family were queried about their understanding of his hospitalization, his progress, and likely prognosis. His physicians reviewed his improvement in the hospital and recommended a discussion about the future. His niece asked them to explain this recommendation. The physicians explicitly responded that while they saw no immediate concerns, they would not be surprised if he became significantly more ill or died within the next year. This hospitalization identified congestive heart failure, poor nutritional status, and need for discharge to a skilled nursing facility for help with ADLs. The patient responded that while he was feeling better, he was not surprised and found the opportunity for a discussion a "relief." After determining that the patient had not specified advance directives, the discussion shifted to an explanation of why this was important. Subsequent family meetings gave the patient the opportunity to appoint his niece as his health care proxy and outline his wishes if he were to become more ill and unable to speak for himself.

CONCLUSION

The number of patients with multiple comorbidities is rising and comorbidity is associated with higher health care use, physical disability, polypharmacy/adverse drug events, poor quality of life, and increased mortality. Improving care for this population is clearly important, but it is a challenge for physicians, particularly hospitalists. Prognostic skills of physicians vary, but indices are available and can aid in formulating prognoses. Evaluating comorbidity and estimating prognosis is a responsibility of clinicians, is important to patients, and is intimately linked to good individualized clinical decision making.

> It takes courage to make a prognosis. Fullness of knowledge does not always bring confidence; the more one knows the more timidity may grow. The faculty which enables a man to look all around a question, to take a philosophical view of it, may be tempered with doubt, and an inability to reach a conclusion. A cocksure diagnosis and a positive prognosis may express the assurance of ignorance.
>
> *Sir William Osler.*
> *Lancet. 1910;1:973–977.*

SUGGESTED READINGS

Anderson FF, Downing GM, Hill J, et al. Palliative performance scale (PPS): a new tool. *J Palliat Care*. 1996;12(1):5–11.

Boyd CM, Darer J, Boult C, et al. Clinical practice guidelines and quality of care for older patients with multiple comorbid diseases: implications for pay for performance. *JAMA*. 2005;294(6):716–724.

Celli BR, Cote CG, Marin JM, et al. The body-mass index, airflow obstruction, dyspnea, and exercise capacity index in chronic obstructive pulmonary disease. *N Engl J Med*. 2004;350(10):1005–1012.

Christakis NA. The ellipsis of prognosis in modern medical thought. *Soc Sci Med*. 1997;44(3):301–315.

Ehlenbach WJ, Barnato AE, Curtis JR, et al. Epidemiologic study of in-hospital cardiopulmonary resuscitation in the elderly. *N Engl J Med*. 2009;361(1):22–31.

Lamont EB, Christakis NA. Complexities in prognostication in advanced cancer: "to help them live their lives the way they want to." *JAMA*. 2003;290(1):98–104.

Leff B, Reider L, Frick KD, et al. Guided care and the cost of complex healthcare: a preliminary report. *Am J Manag Care*. 2009;15(8):555–559.

Levy WC, Mozafarrian D, Linker DT, et al. The Seattle Heart Failure Model: prediction of survival in heart failure. *Circulation*. 2006;113(11):1424–1433.

Mitchell SL, Teno JM, Kiely DK, et al. The clinical course of advanced dementia. *N Engl J Med*. 2009;361(16):1529–1538.

CHAPTER 98

Suspected Intoxication and Overdose

Carson R. Harris, MD
Samuel J. Stellpflug, MD

Key Clinical Questions

1. What information is important in the history to define a toxidrome?
2. What are the key areas of focus for the physical examination in the unknown poison/overdosed patient?
3. What are common toxidromes to consider?
4. What are the effective decontamination procedures to consider?
5. How do you determine appropriate disposition of the poisoned/overdosed patient?
6. When should you be concerned about delayed toxicity?
7. What is the role of a poison center and poison information specialist?

CASE 98-1

A 27-year-old man was observed stumbling in a local park. The police brought him to the emergency department (ED) for evaluation of his altered mental status and possible drug intoxication. A history was difficult to obtain because he was mumbling incoherently, hallucinating, and extremely agitated. It was unknown whether the patient had an underlying psychiatric disorder.

Due to increasing agitation and combativeness, the patient was placed in physical restraints. Initial vital signs included a BP 158/94 mm Hg, HR 133 beats per minute (bpm), RR 20, T101.5 F, and O_2 saturation 98%. Pupils were symmetric and approximately 6 mm. They reacted poorly to light. A limited physical examination was notable for dry oropharynx, absence of cardiac murmurs, clear lungs, and a soft, nontender abdomen. Bowel sounds were present but very infrequent. Neurologically he was confused and combative but moving all extremities with good strength equal bilaterally. Occasional myoclonic jerks of the upper and lower extremities were noted. The skin was warm and dry, and flushing noted at the face and neck.

A finger stick glucose was 100 mg/dL. Cardiac monitor revealed sinus tachycardia. Complete blood cell count, kidney function, and electrolytes were within normal limits. He received a normal saline fluid bolus and required a total of 4 milligrams of midazolam for sedation. The patient continued to be tachycardic and combative. He was admitted to the telemetry unit for monitoring and further treatment.

How would you further manage this patient?

INTRODUCTION

Nearly 2.5 million human exposures were reported in 2007 to U.S. poison control centers. The majority of these exposures involved analgesics, sedative-hypnotics, and antipsychotics. Substances more frequently involved in fatalities of adults include sedative/hypnotics/antipsychotics, opioids, antidepressants, acetaminophen in combination, cardiovascular drugs, stimulants, and street drugs. As this database is dependent upon calls to the poison center, the incidence of poisonings by overdose and deaths due to overdose and exposures are likely underestimated, since not all exposures are reported.

Of cases reported to the poison center, approximately 1.8 million (73%) are managed at the site of exposure, 15% are treated and released from the health care facility, but 5.7% are admitted for medical care. Many of these patients will be managed and stabilized by hospitalists. A systematic approach to overdosed and poisoned patients is needed to provide effective and efficient care. In most cases the basic stabilization measures involving airway, breathing, and circulation will have occurred in the emergency department. However, continued supportive care is required until each patient is medically stable and ready for discharge or transfer to psychiatry. Supportive care of the overdosed patient may involve administering oxygen, intravenous fluids, antidotes, vasopressor, anticonvulsants, or continuing decontamination of the gut.

TABLE 98-1 Identifying Common Toxidromes

	Mental Status	Vital Signs	Pupils	Skin
Sympathomimetic	Increased	Increased	Enlarged	Wet
Anticholinergic	Increased	Increased	Enlarged	Dry
Opiate	Decreased	Decreased	Small	
Sedative-hypnotic	Decreased	Decreased	Small	
Cardiovascular	Decreased	Decreased	Midsize	
Serotonin	Increased/Decreased	Increased/Decreased	Enlarged	Wet

THE INITIAL EVALUATION

TOXIDROMES

Toxidromes are defined as signs and symptoms associated with toxicity from a class of drugs (eg, opiate, cholinergic, etc). When assessing the unknown overdose patient, a common challenge is obtaining a coherent history either from the patient, his or her relatives, or from first responders. The key elements in the toxicology history include what medications or substances were ingested; the amount ingested, and/or the concentration if applicable; the time of ingestion; whether emesis occurred and if pill fragments were noted by the patient or other persons at the scene; and the reasons why the patient ingested the substance. Was this a suicide attempt, recreational use, accidental, or malicious?

Determining the patient's current symptoms is also helpful in defining a possible toxidrome and assists in management. Common toxidromes to consider include opiate, sympathomimetic, anticholinergic, cardiovascular, and anticholinergic (See **Table 98-1**). Looking for signs and symptoms of serotonin and neuroleptic malignant syndromes is also important in the management and disposition of these patients.

PRACTICE POINT

Key points in the toxicology history of ingestions

The toxicology history "MATTERS"

- Medication or substances ingested
- Amount ingested
- Time the medication was taken
- Toxicology of drug
- Emesis and presence of pill fragments
- Reasons for injestion
- Signs and Symptoms

PHYSICAL EXAMINATION

The physical examination findings in overdosed and poisoned patients may rapidly change. The mental status, vital signs, pupil size, and skin are important; and in some cases, odors can point to the diagnosis. The mental status may range from severe somnolence to extreme agitation or hallucinations. It is important to note whether the vital signs are elevated, normal, or depressed. Pupils are typically reported as "Pupils Equal Round Reactive Light Accommodation (PERRLA)" without reporting size. Whether the pupils are pinpoint, mid-size, or large may help with distinguishing the toxidrome. Skin changes may not be immediately noted, but specifically look for findings such as flushing or cyanosis, diaphoresis or dryness, needle track marks or bullous lesions, and note whether the skin is hot or cool to touch.

Several toxins may have a characteristic odor and will alert the provider to a possible diagnosis. Garlic odor in the breath of a patient with an unknown overdose may indicate thallium, organophosphate, arsenic, dimethyl-sulfoxide, selenium, or a phosphide ingestion; the odor of wintergreen is highly suspicious of a methylsalicylate ingestion; and, of course, the odor of distilled spirits may indicate an ethanol-containing beverage or substance. The odor of bitter almonds signifies the presence of cyanide; unfortunately only about 50% of people can detect this odor.

DIFFERENTIATING TOXIC VERSUS NONTOXIC CAUSES FOR ADMISSION

It is important not to get anchored to the initial one or two aspects of the patient's presentation (anchoring bias). There are numerous medical conditions that can mimic an overdose and vice versa. When the history is unclear, unreliable, or simply unknown, one must consider medical or traumatic causes for the patient's altered state. Attempt to obtain collateral history from relatives, medics, or others who may know the patient or found him unresponsive. Computerized tomography of the head may be needed to rule out intracranial hemorrhage or mass lesions. Chest or abdominal radiographs should be considered based on the clinical scenario and physical findings. Laboratory tests to consider based on clinical presentation include thyroid stimulating hormone, blood cultures, arterial or venous blood gases, salicylate level, hepatic function tests, pregnancy test, lactate, and creatinine kinase (CK).

Laboratory monitoring

Laboratory tests important in the evaluation of the unknown overdose patient include basic metabolic panel, acetaminophen level, serum osmolality, hepatic function tests, and urinalysis. Monitoring organ function by periodically assessing liver and renal laboratory values, CK, and possibly serial electrocardiograms may allow early detection of the delayed toxidrome and assist in providing expeditious management. A pregnancy test is routinely obtained in the altered female of childbearing age.

One issue that has been a source of controversy is the utility of toxicology screening tests or the urine drug screens. Kellerman, et al, conducted a prospective study of 582 consecutive emergency department patients with suspected drug overdose and found that more than 95% of cases had no significant change in treatment or disposition in response to routine toxicologic screening. Another test that is typically ordered indiscriminately is the salicylate concentration. In a retrospective case review of patients with salicylate concentrations obtained, and the presence of salicylates, Wood and colleagues concluded that "routine measurement of plasma salicylate concentrations is not required" unless there is a history of salicylate ingestion or the history and physical are unreliable and the patient has clinical features of salicylate poisoning. Knowing the patient's past medical history and

TABLE 98-2 Tests to Consider in the Unknown Poisoned Patient

Tests	Diagnoses to Consider
Rapid glucose test	Hypoglycemia, hyperglycemia, DKA
BUN/Creatinine	Overdose leading to acute renal insufficiency
Complete blood cell count	Anemia, leukocytosis, leukopenia, blood dyscrasias
Electrolytes	Electrolyte abnormalities
Acetaminophen	Acetaminophen overdose with potential hepatotoxicity
Serum osmolality	Toxic alcohol (ie, volatile) ingestion (calculate osmolal gap)
Urinalysis	Crystaluria (may indicate ethylene glycol ingestion)
Ethanol	Ethanol intoxication
Electrocardiogram	Cardiotoxic effects of cardiovascular or psychotropic drugs (QRS widening and QTc prolongation)
Computerized tomography	Intracranial process, (mass, hemorrhage, other)
Electroencephalogram	Seizure disorder

noting whether there are stigmata of a chronic disease process may prompt specific drug levels to be ordered. In patients with a history of seizure disorder who present with altered mental status, a postictal state or toxicity from anticonvulsive therapy should be considered. Similarly, a patient with a history or clinical evidence of congestive heart failure (CHF) or atrial fibrillation may have digitalis toxicity. Most hospital laboratories can perform serum levels of anticonvulsive medications (eg, phenytoin, phenobarbital, or carbamazepine) or digoxin. Although ethanol levels can be done in the hospital chemistry laboratory, determination of the presence of other toxic alcohols typically require the toxicology laboratory. Sending the specimen to a more sophisticated laboratory. This will take time and may not assist in management decisions. In such cases, hospitalists must rely on clinical presentation and application of supportive care. See **Table 98-2** for tests to consider in ruling out other diagnoses that may be confused with ingestion and vice versa.

DECONTAMINATION

The options for decontamination have been systematically reviewed by several toxicology societies and expert consensus has been issued on each of the common techniques. Syrup of ipecac is essentially inefficient and ineffective in decontaminating the gut and is no longer recommended for acute or chronic ingestions presenting to the emergency department. Circumstances in which ipecac may be of benefit are indeed rare. If considered, its use should be discussed with the local poison center or medical toxicologist.

Activated charcoal has limited use for ingestions and is only recommended when the patient presents within one hour after taking a potentially toxic overdose, the airway is intact and protected, and the product can be adsorbed by activated charcoal. Remember, caustics, alcohols, and metals have very little to no adsorption by activated charcoal. Routine administration of activated charcoal in managing oral overdoses has little to no significant impact on hospital length of stay or patient outcomes. Multiple doses of activated charcoal may impart some benefit for significant or life-threatening ingestions of carbamazepine, theophylline, phenobarbital, dapsone, and quinine. Volunteer studies have shown increase elimination of amitriptyline, digoxin, phenytoin, salicylates, and sotalol; however, there is insufficient research to support a recommendation for use of multidose activated charcoal in these overdoses.

Gastric lavage is indicated when the patient has ingested a potentially lethal amount of a drug and presents within one hour of the ingestion. This procedure carries high morbidity and should not be performed in any patient with an unprotected airway, those who have ingested caustics or hydrocarbons (which may render the gut vulnerable to perforation), or those who are at risk of perforation due to an underlying medical or surgical condition. Intuitively, removing the pills or substance from the stomach affords less material to be absorbed. However, clinical and experimental trials have failed to support a significant benefit. When weighing the advantages and potential complications, this procedure is seldom done. The overall benefit of gastric lavage is questionable at best and generally does not offer any more advantage over activated charcoal.

In some cases, efforts to increase elimination are used. This typically involves the use of whole bowel irrigation (WBI), hemodialysis, or pH manipulation. Although theoretically, WBI seems an ideal option for certain ingestions, a critical review of the scientific literature revealed insufficient evidence to support or exclude its use for potentially toxic ingestions of drug packets, iron, zinc, or lead. WBI involves using a polyethylene glycol-electrolyte solution (eg, GoLytely [r]) as a volume cathartic administering this solution at a rate of 1500–2000 mL per hour via orgogastric or nasogastric tube. Volunteer studies seem to show some benefit when this is used to manage significant ingestions involving enteric-coated or sustained-release products. Patients with renal insufficiency from drug overdose, or who have evidence of ingesting a toxic alcohol (ethylene glycol, methanol-containing products) may be candidates for hemodialysis to increase clearance and correct metabolic disturbances. Significant ingestions of salicylates, lithium, theophylline, long-acting barbiturates, and carbamazepine may also be treated with hemodialysis.

TRIAGE CONSIDERATIONS FOR PATIENTS WITH UNKNOWN DRUG INGESTIONS

ICU versus monitored general bed

It is not uncommon for an overdosed patient to be mistriaged or admitted to an inappropriate level of care. In the majority of cases, the patient will have signs and symptoms that predict potential deterioration. Hospitalists must pay close attention to mental status, hemodynamics, and any ancillary test results obtained in the ED. **Table 98-3** offers some broad guidelines in regard to admitting the overdose patient to an intensive care versus monitored bed. Consultation with the medical toxicologist or poison control center can help in making this decision. Of course, when in doubt, one must err on the side of the patient by placing him or her at the higher level of care until an adequate period of observation can be achieved.

POSTADMISSION CONCERNS

While the patient is on the ward, he or she may exhibit delayed toxic effects of the ingestion. Hospitalists must be aware of danger signs and symptoms occurring late that will need immediate attention. Do not overlook the possibility of acetaminophen toxicity, ingestion of illicit drugs, and withdrawal syndromes. Acetaminophen ingestion may present fairly benignly initially

TABLE 98-3 Triage Algorithm to ICU of Patients with Unknown Drug Overdose

Does this patient have hemodynamic instability? Yes
- Hypotension
- Non sinus cardiac rhythm
- Hypothermia
- Malignant hyperthermia (neuroleptic malignant syndrome)
- Hypoxia

Does this patient have evidence of end-organ damage? Yes
- Unable to respond to verbal stimuli, GCS < 13, unable to protect airway
- Confusion requiring monitoring for respiratory depression, withdrawal states
- Renal failure or possibly requiring emergency dialysis for removal of toxin(s) or metabolites
- Hypertensive emergency
- Respiratory failure
- Heart block other than 1st degree AV block, QTc > 500 ms, Osborn wave
- Life-threatening electrolyte disturbances or hypoglycemia that requires ongoing frequent monitoring and treatment
- Rhabdomyolysis
- Disseminated intravascular coagulation (DIC)
- Seizures or other neurologic conditions requiring ICU care
- Impending multisystem failure

Are there nursing requirements or other issues requiring ICU care? Yes
- 1:1 ICU nursing required to monitor and administer therapy
- Higher level of care due to limited resources on general medical floor

Clinical judgment that higher level of care required? Yes

and turn acutely worse after 24 hours postingestion due to the production of a toxic metabolite. At this point, the antidote, N-acetylcysteine, is less effective and the patient will sustain added morbidity and possibly die from hepatic failure. Thus, it is extremely important to detect acetaminophen poisoning early rather than late.

In addition to acetaminophen, there are several agents that could lead to a delayed toxic syndrome if a significant overdose has occurred. These include oral hypoglycemics (sulfonylureas), insulin, tricyclic antidepressants, iron, thyroid hormone, and toxic mushrooms. Another example might be methanol, ethylene glycol, isopropyl alcohol. Symptoms from these products may not appear for more than six hours post ingestion, and in the case of thyroid hormone overdose, several days after the ingestion. While the patient is on the ward or intensive care unit, he must be reassessed for any changes in mental status and vital signs.

Additionally, patients may have ingested packets of a drug (usually illicit) that rupture and lead to significant toxicity and death. This could be the case for the patient presenting above, in which the history is unknown and the clinician must rely upon physical findings and rational use of the laboratory and antidotes.

Another concern for the admitted patient is the development of withdrawal syndrome. Benzodiazepine and alcohol withdrawal can lead to seizures. Therefore, the patient with unknown history and altered mental status should be carefully monitored for signs and symptoms of drug withdrawal. Patients who are admitted with abnormal vital signs and altered mentation must be carefully monitored for deterioration. Agitated patients may subsequently develop elevation in creatinine kinase (CK) and if poorly monitored, may be at risk for acute renal failure, self-injury, or injury to staff. Hospitalists need to be very careful about prescribing medications to control agitation that might interact with substances ingested or delay clearance.

The ability to protect the airway of patients with severe central nervous system depression must be assessed. It is in the patient's best interest to be triaged to a higher level of care early in the course of inpatient management, rather than later.

Further decontamination and supportive care of the overdose patient

It is important to assess the need for further decontamination management. Although the majority of patients are stabilized in the emergency department prior to arriving on the ward, some may need continued decontamination. Continued gastric lavage may be needed if this was initiated in the ED. Patients who have had whole bowel irrigation initiated for appropriate reasons may need to have this continued until the effluent is clear. Likewise, if an infusion of an antidote (eg, naloxone, sodium bicarbonate, deferoxamine, insulin, pressors) was started prior to arrival to the ward, the effect will need to be assessed and reassessed during the initial management phase, particularly if the duration of action of the antidote may be shorter than the duration of action of the toxin (eg, naloxone treatment for methadone overdose). In the intentional overdose patient, flumazenil is not typically recommended due to risk of seizures from acute benzodiazepine withdrawal or coingestion of a proconvulsive drug. **Table 98-4** describes common antidotes and their uses. In cases of impaired renal function, the on-call nephrologist must be notified early in event of further deterioration and a need for hemodialysis.

TABLE 98-4 Common Antidotes

Toxin/Drug	Antidote
Carbon monoxide	Oxygen
Opiates/Narcotics	Naloxone
N-Acetylcysteine	Acetaminophen, carbon tetrachloride
Organophosphates	Atropine, pralidoxime
Hydrofluoric acid (rust removers and glass etching)	Calcium gluconate
Cyclic antidepressant—sodium channel antagonists	Sodium bicarbonate
Lead, arsenic, mercury	Dimercapto-succinic acid (Succimer)
Ethylene glycol, methanol	Ethanol, 4- methypyrizole (fomepizole)
Digoxin, cardiac glycosides	Digoxin-specific Fab
Insulin	Glucose/dextrose
Anticholinergic drugs	Physostigmine
Cyanide	Cyanide antidote kit (sodium nitrite, sodium thiosulfate), hydroxocobalamin
Isoniazid, hydrazines	Pyridoxine
Beta adrenergic antagonist	Glucagon, high-dose insulin/euglycemia
Calcium channel antagonist	Calcium chloride, high-dose insulin/euglycemia

Consulting the poison control center and medical toxicologist

Occasionally the provider's existing toxicology knowledge and the above provided information will not be enough to take the necessary steps. Knowing when and how to solicit the proper help is important. Texts, journals, and online sources can be very helpful, but gaining appropriate information to apply clinically can be time intensive and sometimes fruitless. There are ways to obtain easy access to poison specialists, no matter your location and the time of day, as long as you have access to a telephone. The United States poison center system, or poison control center system, includes 60 poison centers. By dialing 1-800-222-1222, anyone can gain access to the local poison center and speak with toxicology-trained poison specialists. Poison centers serve multiple functions for the medical community. They provide education and educational resources, and reduce the number of unnecessary hospital visits after poison exposures. More than 70% of the calls are managed at the site of the exposure and required no further medical attention. Most of the other 30% of the calls are from health care facilities.

The specialists in poison information are trained in poisoning management and triage, and this group includes physicians, pharmacists, nurses, and other poison information providers. Through a combination of local management protocols, specific online and text resources, and quick access to medical toxicologists, the poison information specialists provide the necessary advice to guide the management of the patient at hand. Medical toxicologists provide support for the providers answering the calls, and are on call in case the need for further expertise arises. When calling the poison center, specific information needed includes the patient's age, weight, substance to which the patient was exposed, time of exposure, up-to-date clinical picture including vital signs, laboratory studies, and ECG results if applicable, treatments administered thus far, and any particular questions you may have regarding management. With that information they can quickly provide advice about management, or if necessary, solicit the help of the medical toxicologist.

When do you need involvement of a medical toxicologist?

Often the toxicologist is involved in discussions of complicated or controversial management, or if the caller has questions that are beyond the scope of practice of the poison specialist fielding the call. Of note, since each poison center has toxicologists on call, callers can request to speak directly with that physician. This can be particularly useful in cases in which direct and immediate feedback is crucial for complex medical cases that involve poisons and toxins. Some cases may require multiple conversations between the hospital provider and the toxicologist due to changes in management based on a dynamic clinical course and/or updated results of testing. In cases in which patients are in any sort of extremis due to poisoning, early involvement of a medical toxicologist is recommended.

Another important role of the poison center, the poison center specialist, and the medical toxicologist is to help assess the patient's stability and appropriateness for various disposition options. The poison center information specialist and medical toxicologist can assist the hospitalist in determining the need for appropriate transfer depending on capabilites of the treating facility and nearby facilities. Using poison centers or hospital-based toxicologists can result in better management and disposition of poisoned patients resulting in more efficient use of the health care system and reduced morbidity for poisoned or overdosed patients (**Table 98-5**).

TABLE 98-5 Toxicology Resources for Hospitalists

Toxicology Resources for Hospitalists
Poison Center Hotline: 1-800-222-1222
Textbooks • Goldfrank's Toxicologic Emergencies (Flomenbaum N, et al (eds) 8th ed) • Critical Care Toxicology: Diagnosis and Management of the Critically Poisoned Patient (Brent J, et al (eds)) • Poisonings and Drug Overdose (Olson K, et al (eds) 5th ed) • Handbook of Poisonous and Injurious Plants (Nelson LS, et al (eds))
Online Resources • www.erowid.org - Erowid • www.acmt.net - American College of Medical Toxicology • www.clintox.org - American Academy of Clinical Toxicology • www.aapcc.org - American Association of Poison Control Centers • www.thepoisonreview.com - The Poison Review

CASE 98-2

During the night, the patient received an additional 6 milligrams of midazolam for agitation and experienced intermittent visual hallucinations. Approximately 24 hours after being admitted, he was awake and oriented to person, place, and time. His pupils remained dilated and he remained amnestic to the previous day's events. He admitted to being homeless, having a history of depression and noncompliance with his antidepressant medications. Prior to being found in the park, he had ingested an unknown amount of over-the-counter sleeping pills. The pills contained an anticholinergic agent that caused the patient's toxidrome. He was subsequently evaluated by psychiatry and transferred to an inpatient mental health ward.

CONCLUSION

The focus of this chapter has been on the approach to patients admitted from the ED for observation and management of suspected intoxication and overdose. In addition, the acutely ill hospitalized patient, especially the elderly, are vulnerable to adverse drug events due to polypharmacy, changing liver and kidney function, and exposure to new drugs that may interact with other medications. Physicians should be able to recognize the signs and symptoms associated with toxicity from different classes of drugs, obtain a focused toxicology history, and when necessary, request timely consultation of experts in critical care, nephrology, and/or poison control. There are many exposures in which serious morbidity and potential mortality can be prevented with appropriate early management. The medical toxicologist can offer recommendations by telephone or in some institutions, on site as a bedside toxicology consultant. In some scenarios of ingestion the patient may experience a change or deterioration; involving a toxicologist can help tremendously when dealing with complex decisions.

SUGGESTED READINGS

American Academy of Clinical Toxicology and European Association of Poison Centres and Clinical Toxicologists. Position statement and practice guidelines on the use of multi-dose activated charcoal in the treatment of acute poisoning. *J Toxicol Clin Toxicol.* 1999;37:731–751.

Bosse GM, Matyunas NJ. Delayed toxidromes. *J Emerg Med.* 1999; 17(4):679–690.

Bronstein AC, Spyker DA, Cantilena LR Jr, et al. 2007 Annual Report of the American Association of Poison Control Centers' National Poison Data System (NPDS): 25th Annual Report. *Clin Toxicol.* 2008; 46(10):927–1057.

Cooper GM, Le Couteur DG, Richardson D, et al. A randomized clinical trial of activated charcoal for the routine management of oral drug overdose. *Q J Med.* 2005;98:655–660.

Holubek WJ, Hoffman RS, Goldfarb DS, et al. Use of hemodialysis and hemoperfusion in poisoned patients. *Kidney Int.* 2008;74 (10):1327–1334.

Kellerman AL, Finn SD, LoGerfo JP, et al. Impact of drug screening in suspected overdose. *Ann Emerg Med.* November 1987;16: 1206–1216.

Sztajnkrycer MD, Mell HK, Melin GJ. Development and implementation of an emergency department observation unit protocol for deliberate drug ingestion in adults—preliminary results. *Clin Toxicol.* 2007;45(5):499–504.

Tenenbein M. Position statement: whole bowel irrigation. *J Toxicol Clin Toxicol.* 1997;35(7):753–762.

Vale JA, Kulig K. Position paper: gastric lavage. *J Toxicol Clin Toxicol.* 2004;42(7):933–943.

Wood DM, Dargan PI, Jones AL. Measuring plasma salicylate concentrations in all patients with drug overdose or altered consciousness: is it necessary? *Emerg Med J.* 2005;22:401–403.

CHAPTER 99

Syncope

Kush Agrawal, MD
Robert Young, MD
Daniel D. Dressler, MD, MSc, SFHM

Key Clinical Questions

1. What diagnostic testing should be considered for common causes of syncope?
2. When do clinicians need to rule out arrhythmias and how is this done?
3. What are the diagnostic criteria for neurocardiogenic syncope?
4. When do patients require hospital admission?
5. How do elderly patients differ from younger patients?
6. How should the history and physical examination be utilized to direct further testing or limit further testing in the evaluation of syncope?
7. What are the indications for advanced noninvasive or invasive tests in the evaluation of syncope?

INTRODUCTION

DEFINITION

Syncope is defined as a sudden, transient *loss of consciousness and postural tone* with rapid spontaneous recovery. Syncope results from *cerebral hypoperfusion* to the reticular activating system in the brain stem. Any condition that does not result from cerebral hypoperfusion should not be classified as syncope.

CASE 99-1

A 74-year-old female with early Parkinson disease presented to the Emergency Department with loss of consciousness while standing in the sun. She thought that she did not drink enough water during the day. She initially felt bilateral shoulder pain followed by dizziness, and then recalled awakening on her porch. She injured her forearm, but recovered fully within one minute. A witness described some brief jerking movements in her arms (lasted a few seconds). Blood pressure lying and standing were 130/80 mm Hg and 90/48 mm Hg respectively. Pulse was 86 beats per minute (bpm) lying and 88 bpm standing. Other vital signs, cardiac, and neurologic examination were all normal. An electrocardiogram (ECG) showed normal sinus rhythm with a heart rate of 88 bpm.

What is the approach to the patient? What further testing is indicated? What is the diagnosis? What is her overall prognosis following this syncopal event?

CASE 99-2

A 62-year-old male passed out while voiding just after awakening from sleep. He denied symptoms beforehand and awakened promptly. On further history, he did not report prior cardiovascular symptoms. His past medical history includes long-standing hypertension and he has a 40-pack-per-year tobacco history. Cardiovascular and neurologic examination was normal. Breath sounds were distant. His ECG is shown in **Figure 99-1**.

What is the best approach to this patient? What further testing is indicated? What is the diagnosis? What is his prognosis if left untreated?

EPIDEMIOLOGY

Syncope has a 3% incidence in the general population and 6% incidence in persons over age 75 years. It is responsible for up to 5% of emergency department (ED) visits and up to 3% of hospital admissions. The median cost of hospitalization of patients with syncope is approximately $8500, and many (up to 50%) may be discharged from the hospital without a clear or specific diagnosis that caused the syncopal episode.

Syncope can present various diagnostic challenges, as many episodes of transient loss of consciousness may occur as unwitnessed events and with limited available history. Furthermore, while the vast majority of syncope etiology is benign, a sizable minority of patients have etiologies with high risk of mortality (ie, patients with cardiac causes). Many testing modalities are also available in the evaluation

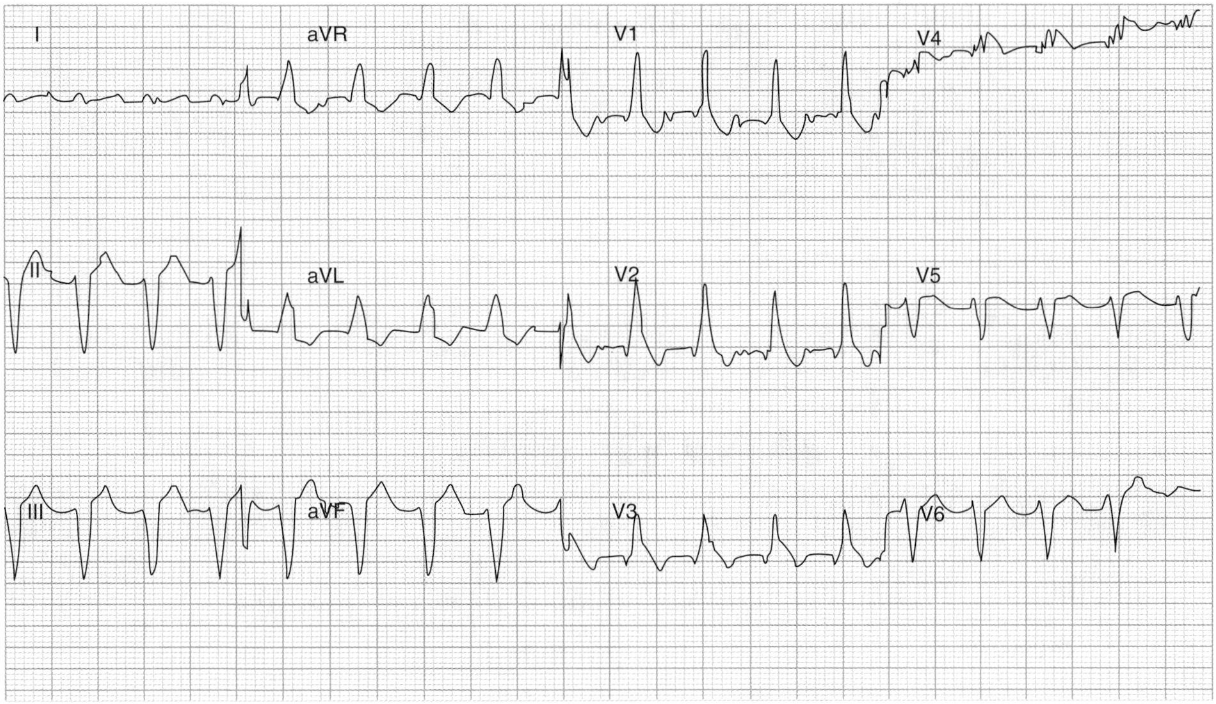

Figure 99-1 *ECG, First-degree atrioventricular (AV) block with right bundle branch block (RBBB) and left anterior fascicular block (LAFB).*

of syncope, and judicious selection as well as timing and order of the most appropriate modalities can be challenging. Finally, while many patients are admitted to the hospital, up to 40% of patients are discharged without a clear, well-delineated diagnosis following initial workup. However, following extended systematic evaluation (including outpatient evaluation when indicated), less than 20% of patients diagnosed with syncope will remain with a final diagnosis of unknown cause.

Estimates of syncope *recurrence* suggest that prior syncope, psychiatric illness, and age less than 45 years confer a higher risk of recurrent syncope. Surprisingly, severities of presentation, structural heart disease, and tilt test response have no predictive value on syncope recurrence. Carotid sinus syndrome (CSS), the association of a syncopal event or events with carotid sinus hypersensitivity, has the highest prevalence (43%) in a population of patients presenting with recurrent syncope to the ED. Approximately 12% of patients with recurrent syncope presenting to an ED have associated soft-tissue injury or fracture.

PATHOPHYSIOLOGY

Transient hypoperfusion of the brainstem or both cerebral hemispheres can result from either decreased cardiac output or significant decrease in peripheral vascular resistance. These two mechanisms form the basis of the pathophysiology behind all syncopal events (**Figure 99-2**). Specific diagnoses (or etiologies of the syncopal episode) may then be derived based on symptoms, signs, and additional testing that lead to their likely pathophysiologic origin.

In patients with traumatic injury (eg, coup-contracoup or concussion injury), transient LOC is not associated with decreased blood flow. In nontraumatic transient LOC, clinicians should consider seizure and psychogenic etiologies. Rarer causes of transient LOC without syncope include tumor, metabolic etiologies, or intoxications. Several conditions may be incorrectly diagnosed as syncope, (ie, "nonsyncope") (**Table 99-1**). Clinicians should consider anemia or pregnancy in the appropriate clinical setting.

DIFFERENTIAL DIAGNOSIS

Syncope etiologies (and relative frequencies) are broadly divided into four major categories (reflex syncope, orthostatic, cardiac, and neurologic) in addition to unknown etiology (**Table 99-2**). Reflex (most commonly vasovagal) syncope occurs most commonly, followed by cardiac etiologies. More than 70% of cardiac causes are due to arrhythmia, while the remainder is due to various types of structural heart disease.

Following identification of true syncope (ie, excluding nonsyncope based on history, physical exam, and initial testing), narrowing the differential diagnosis should be accomplished based on suggestive clinical features and appropriate diagnostic testing (**Table 99-3**). The relative yield and contribution of advanced diagnostic modalities in syncope should be considered when selecting modalities in the diagnosis of syncope patients.

DIAGNOSIS

HISTORY

The relevant aspects of the history include the patient's symptoms experienced *prior to and following* loss of consciousness, the setting in which syncope occurred, the patient's past medical and psychiatric history, medications, and social history. Prior episodes and frequency of syncope episodes may also potentially help guide diagnosis and/or testing.

Determination if the event is truly syncope, rather than nonsyncope, can help include or exclude items within the differential diagnosis (Table 99-1). This initial evaluation incorporates a careful history of events before and after the LOC, a thorough assessment of past medical history, a complete medication and allergy review, and assessment of family history (including sudden death) and social history (**Table 99-4**).

Did the patient actually experience a sudden, transient LOC? Was there spontaneous recovery without resuscitation?

Certain historical features may point toward a nonsyncopal event (Table 99-1). History should delineate if there was actual loss of

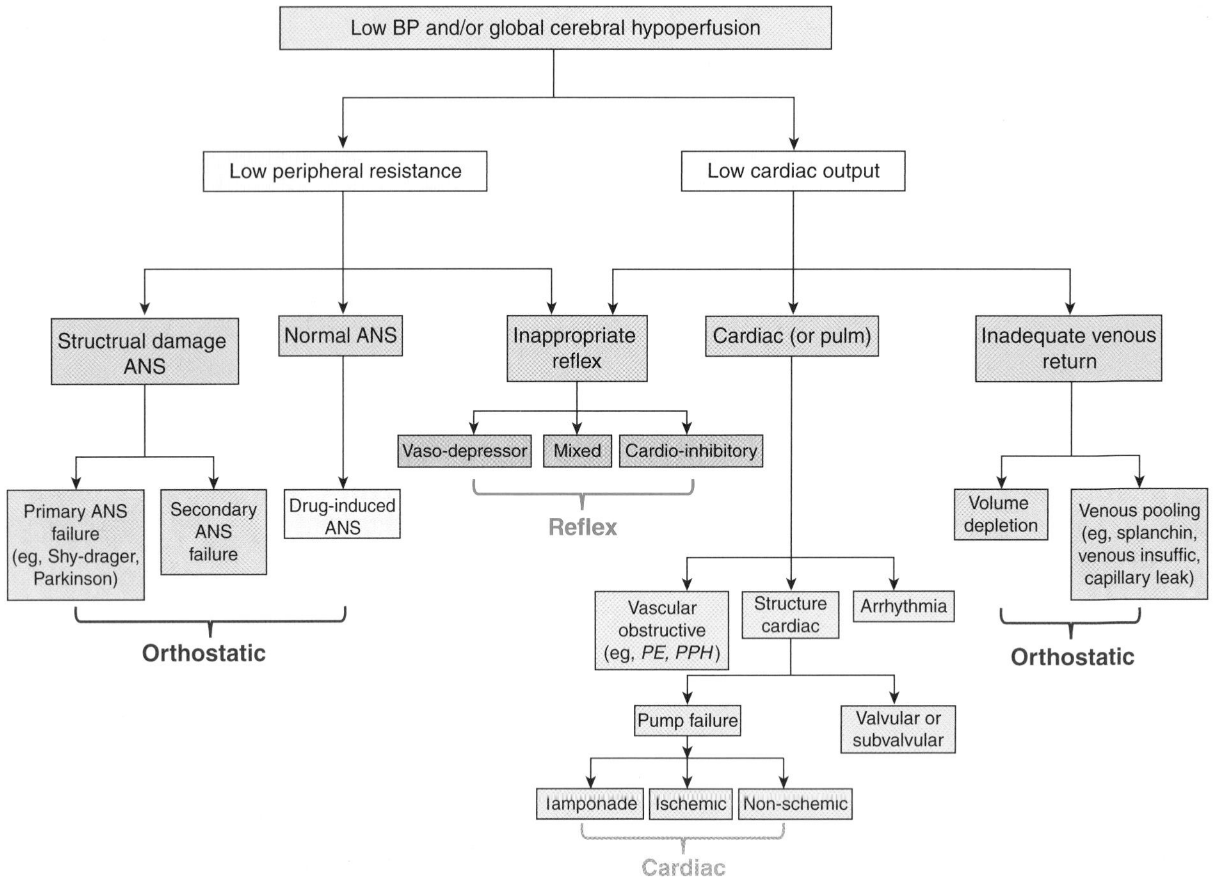

Figure 99-2 *Pathophysiologic basis of syncope. ANS, autonomic nervous system; BP, blood pressure; PE, pulmonary embolus; PPH, primary pulmonary hypertension.*

consciousness. A mechanical fall or confusion (altered consciousness) would not be termed syncope or even LOC.

If the patient did actually lose consciousness, consideration of nonsyncopal etiologies of transient LOC including intoxications, hypoglycemia, hypoxia, or severe anemia may be appropriate even though these rarely lead to LOC. These patients may have more gradual development of symptoms prior to a syncopal episode and/or delayed recovery (many minutes to hours) compared with true syncope.

When LOC was witnessed, description of tonic-clonic activity obviously points toward seizure as a nonsyncopal etiology of transient LOC; however, lay person witnesses of seizure activity may not be reliable in description. When a seizure is not witnessed, historical features that may point toward seizure as an etiology include lateral tongue biting or laceration (reasonably specific for seizure), pre-LOC aura, and bowel or bladder incontinence (the latter, a nonspecific finding that may occur in syncope as well). Prolonged recovery (more than one or a few minutes) to normal mentation is another hallmark of seizure, and differs significantly compared to true syncope.

Importantly, many patients with syncope are misdiagnosed as seizure due to misperception of witnesses or misinterpretation of body movement descriptions from bystanders. Any syncopal episode can lead to brief myoclonic activity (occurs in up to 10% of patients with vasovagal syncope and other types of syncope), and up to 1% of syncope patients can have benign brief (lasting one or a few seconds) "full body stiffening" prior to awakening. Many may misinterpret this as seizure activity (which alternately should last minutes or longer rather than seconds).

Extended duration of actual LOC is referred to as coma rather than syncope (which is transient). LOC that required resuscitation or defibrillation to return a pulse and consciousness is referred to as sudden cardiac death and not syncope.

Cardiac syncope (inadequate cardiac output, arrhythmias)

Historical features suggesting cardiac etiologies of syncope include chest pain prior to syncope, syncope during exertion, and syncope while supine. In ventricular tachycardia, patients may present with syncope that has no prodrome. Often those patients recall no specific symptoms prior to the syncopal episode, only recall awakening, and are often injured from a fall.

Pump failure:

Is this patient having an acute MI?

Up to 10% of patients with acute myocardial infarction (MI) present with syncope. Similarly, up to 7% of patients who present with syncope and no chest pain may have ischemia as the cause of their syncopal event. Please refer to Chapter 124 on Acute Coronary Syndromes (ACS) for relevant aspects of history and examination presentation of patients with acute MI or unstable angina. Any patient who presents with syncope who also had chest pain either before or after the syncopal episode needs to be evaluated for possible ACS with cardiac enzymes, telemetry monitoring, serial ECGs, and stress testing if indicated. In patients who have *syncope but no chest pain,* four factors are predictive of ACS as the etiology of the syncope: (1) arm, neck, shoulder, and throat pain, (2) history of stable angina (provoked by exercise), (3) the presence of rales on physical examination, and (4) electrocardiographic ischemic abnormalities.

TABLE 99-1 Nonsyncope: Conditions Misdiagnosed as Syncope

Conditions with LOC but no global cerebral hypoperfusion
1. Seizure
a. Tonic-clonic seizure (not witnessed)
b. Absence or partial complex seizure (LOC but no loss of postural tone)
2. Metabolic derangements
a. Hypocapneic hyperventilation
b. Hypoglycemia
c. Hypoxemia
d. Hyponatremia
e. Severe anemia
3. Acute alcohol or other drug intoxication
4. TIA or stroke of *vertebrobasilar* origin
5. Increased intracranial pressure
a. Tumor
b. Edema
c. Cough-induced
6. Narcolepsy
Conditions without LOC
1. Cataplexy
2. TIA or stroke of *carotid* origin
3. Falls
4. Drop attacks
5. Psychogenic pseudosyncope
a. Conversion or somatization disorders
b. Panic disorder, major depressive disorder (MDD), or anxiety disorder
c. Malingering, factitious disorder, or Munchausen syndrome
Conditions of cardiac arrest
1. Intervention, such as closed-chest compressions, medication, or defibrillation was required to regain a pulse and/or consciousness

LOC, loss of consciousness; TIA, transient ischemic attack.

TABLE 99-2 Syncope Differential Diagnosis

Syncope Category	Approximate Frequency	Specific Etiologies
Reflex Syncope (ie, nerually-mediated, neurogenic, or neurocardiogenic)	35–40%	Vasovagal
		Situational (micturition, defecation, cough, valsalva, mobilization after prolonged bed rest, etc) Carotid sinus hypersensitivity
Cardiac	20–25%	
Arrhythmia		• Tachyarrhythmias (eg, VT, SVT, torsades de pointe) • Bradyarrhythmias (third degree AVB, SSS, pacer malfunction)
Structural		• Valvular (aortic stenosis, mitral stenosis) • Obstructive (hypertrophic obstructive cardiomyopathy [HOCM], atrial myxoma) • Pump failure (large acute MI, cardiac tamponade) • Vascular (PE, PPH, subclavian steal, dissection)
Orthostatic	5–15%	• Drug-induced ANS failure (eg, beta-blocker, calcium channel blocker, digoxin)* • Primary ANS failure (eg, Parkinson disease, Shy-Drager syndrome) • Secondary ANS failure (eg, diabetes mellitus, HIV, renal failure, collagen vascular disease)
Neurologic	10–15%	• Vertebrobasilar TIA or stroke • Rare: SAH, migraine
Unknown	15–25%	

ANS, autonomic nervous system; AVB, atrioventricular block; HIV, human immunodeficiency virus; MI, myocardial infarction; PE, pulmonary embolus; PPH, primary pulmonary hypertension; SAH: subarachnoid hemorrhage; SSS, sick sinus syndrome (tach-brady syndrome); SVT, supraventricular tachycardia; VT, ventricular tachycardia.

Patients without ischemic abnormalities on ECG are not at risk for an acute ischemic event compared to those with ischemic abnormalities on ECG.

Obstruction:

Is there obstruction to flow resulting in inadequate cardiac output?

Patients may have valvular, subvalvular, or vascular obstruction leading to reduced or transiently blocked cardiac output and a syncopal event. Valvular causes include aortic stenosis (AS), mitral stenosis, pulmonic stenosis (PS), or prosthetic valve malfunction. Historical features may include exertional syncope.

Subvalvular cardiac causes include hypertrophic obstructive cardiomyopathy (HOCM) and atrial myxoma. Classic symptoms in HOCM include postexertional syncope. Vascular obstruction can occur due to pulmonary embolus (PE) or significant pulmonary hypertension. Of all patients admitted to the hospital with syncope, less than 1% are due to PE. However, despite occurring uncommonly clinicians should consider the diagnosis in patients with pleuritic chest pain, shortness of breath or symptoms to suggest lower-extremity venous thromboembolism.

Are ventricular arrhythmias suspected as the cause of syncope?

Risk factors include CAD, valvular AS, cardiomyopathy, congenital heart disease, prolonged QT interval on ECG, use of antiarrhythmic drugs especially in patients with reduced LV function, hypo- or hyperkalemia, and hypomagnesemia. History may include palpitations, chest pain, or syncope in association with exercise. However, classically patients with ventricular arrhythmia causing syncope present with no symptoms at all prior to the syncopal event, and injury can occur commonly. Syncope while supine is also concerning for possible ventricular arrhythmia. Finally, a variety of drugs may prolong the QT interval (www.qtdrugs.org), and place patients at risk for torsades de pointe.

Are supraventricular arrhythmias or bradyarrhythmias suspected as a cause of syncope?

TABLE 99-3 Major Causes of Syncope, Suggestive Clinical Features, and Relevant Further Testing

Pathophysiologic Mechanism	Subtypes/Specific Etiology	Examples	Suggestive Clinical/ Historical Features	Further Diagnostic Testing to Consider
1. Reflex Syncope (vasodepressor or cardioinhibitory)	Vasovagal, from a stress on the orthostatic regulatory system	Emotional hyperactivity, pain, fear of blood.	Precipitating event; nausea, diaphoresis, palpitation, bowel or bladder incontinence prior to attack; eyewitness account; abdominal discomfort; post-prandial; recurrent nature.	ECG Stress test or echocardiogram if history of cardiac disease. If negative, no further testing is needed
	Carotid sinus hypersensitivity/ syndrome		Neck movement; shoulder pain; age >40; neck tumor, syncope during shaving, due to tight shirt collars.	Carotid sinus massage
	Situational	Valsalva due to cough, micturition, defacation, vomiting.	See examples	None, if heart disease reasonably excluded
2. Orthostatic Hypotension	Primary ANF	Shy-Drager, Lewy body dementia, multisystem atrophy.	History of neurologic disease.	Orthostatic challenge
	Secondary ANF	Diabetes, uremia, spinal cord transection/injury, amyloidosis, HIV disease.	History of diabetes, HIV, rheumatologic, oncologic or neurologic disease.	Orthostatic challenge Neurologic testing to establish Dx, as needed
	Drug-induced OH	EtOH, diuretics, TCAs, SSRIs, vasodilators	Thorough medication review, including temporal relationship to fall.	Orthostatic challenge.
	Volume depletion	Hemorrhage, diarrhea, emesis, iatrogenic	Postural change; timing of standing to falling; prolonged standing; recent alpha-blocker or diuretic.	Orthostatic challenge, volume challenge and retest
	Venous Pooling	Postprandial, venous insufficiency	History of timing of syncope; varicosities or peripheral edema on examination.	Orthostatic challenge
3. Cardiovascular Syncope	Arrhythmia A. Bradyarrhythmia B. Tachyarrhythmia	Bradyarrhythmia: SSS, AV conduction disease, pacer malfunction Tachyarrhythmia: Atrial: SVT, Afib, MAT, WPW Ventricular: VTach, torsades, ICD malfunction	Family history of SCD, congenital heart disease such as channelopathy; QT-prolonging agents; palpitations; antiarrhythmic; ECG findings such as bifascicular block, AV conduction abnormality, sinoatrial block or inappropriate bradycardia, VT, WPW, LQTS, Brugada pattern, ARVC pattern, Q waves suggestive of MI. VT classically will have no prodrome	ECG, telemetry, outpatient monitoring (Holter, ILR), EP study
	Structural Cause A. Valvular B. Subvalvular C. Pump Failure	Valvular: AS, MR Subvalvular: HOCM, atrial myxoma Pump Failure: Ischemic CM (acute MI), DCM, Restrictive CM, Constrictive CM, tamponade.	Exertional syncope; angina; palpitations; Q wave suggestive of MI	Echo, stress test
	Pulmonary Vascular Cause	Pulmonary HTN, PE, dissection	Exertional syncope; dyspnea; pleuritic CP, tearing CP	Echo, ECG, diagnostic cath if indicated, CT chest if indicated

Afib, atrial fibrillation; ANF, autonomic nervous system failure; ARVC, arrhythmogenic right ventricular cardiomyopathy; AS, aortic stenosis; AV, atrioventricular; CM, cardiomyopathy; CP, chest pain; CT, computed tomography; DCM, dilated cardiomyopathy; Dx, diagnosis; ECG, electrocardiogram; EP, electrophysiology; EtOH, alcohol; HIV, human immunodeficiency virus; HOCM, hypertrophic obstructive cardiomyopathy; HTN, hypertension; ICD, implantable cardioverter-defibrillator; ILR, implantable loop recorder; LQTS, long QT syndrome; MAT, multifocal atrial tachycardia; MI, myocardial infarction; MR, mitral regurgitation; PE, pulmonary embolus; SCD, sudden cardiac death; SSRI, selective serotonin reuptake inhibitors; SSS, sick sinus syndrome; SVT, supraventricular tachycardia; TCAs, tricyclic antidepressants; VT, ventricular tachycardia; WPW, Wolff-Parkinson-White syndrome.

TABLE 99-4 Key Historical Points in the Evaluation of Syncope

History
Sudden standing or sitting (suggests orthostatic etiology)
Prodrome: palpitations, lightheadedness, anxiety, sweating, piloerection, nausea, warmth (suggests vasovagal syncope)
Severe pain, fear, instrumentation (suggests vasovagal syncope, unless there is concurrent structural or congenital heart disease, in which case adrenergic-mediated dysrhythmia should be considered)
Situation: micturition, defecation, coughing (suggests vasomotor syncope)
During or immediately following exertion (suggests cardiogenic syncope)
Chest pain, shortness of breath (suggests possible cardiopulmonary etiology)
Focal neurologic symptoms: headache, diplopia, dysarthria, weakness (suggests a neurological cause of syncope such as intracranial hemorrhage, vertebrobasilar ischemic event, or tumor)
Symptoms suggestive of seizure rather than syncope: tonic-clonic activity, bowel or bladder incontinence, lateral tongue biting
Postsyncope symptoms (eg, confusion) and duration of recovery (most true syncope should have recovery duration of less than a few minutes)
Poor oral intake, dehydration, GI bleed symptoms (suggests hypovolemic etiology)
Injury from fall
Family history of sudden death or arrhythmia (consider long QT syndrome or other congenital cardiac disease)
Past Medical History
Prior syncopal episodes: number, frequency, and surrounding history
Coronary heart disease, heart failure, arrhythmias
Psychiatric disease
CVA, TIA
Pulmonary hypertension
Medications or Drugs
Antihypertensives, antianginals, antidepressants, QT-prolonging drugs, CNS depressants (eg, opioids, sedatives), others (vincristine, digoxin, insulin, marijuana, alcohol, cocaine)

CNS, central nervous system; CVA, cerebrovascular accident; GI, gastrointestinal; TIA, transient ischemic attack.

While syncope occurs uncommonly in supraventricular tachyarrhythmias, risk factors may include prior history or risk of atrial fibrillation, atrial flutter, multifocal atrial tachycardia, and AV node reentrant tachycardia. Malignant bradyarrhythmias can lead to syncopal events, and may be due to conduction system disease, especially with AV nodal blocking agents, pacemaker malfunction, bundle branch blocks (BBB), or bifascicular block.

Reflex syncope

Is the patient having a benign vasovagal episode?

Reflex syncope, also known as vasodepressor syncope, vasovagal syncope, neurocardiogenic syncope, or the "common faint," is the most common cause of syncope. Reflex syncope is mediated by inappropriate vasodepressor (ie, loss of vasoconstriction during standing) or cardioinhibitory (ie, reflex reaction characterized by bradycardia and/or asystole) responses to orthostatic challenge or emotional stress. It may also be precipitated by Valsalva (eg, micturition, defecation, swallowing) or mobilization after prolonged bed rest.

Diagnosis is clinical by eliciting classic symptoms. The *classic prodrome,* exhibited by a *sympathetic response*—diaphoresis, palpitations/tachycardia, piloerection, anxiety, pallor—followed by a *parasympathetic* response—nausea and/or vomiting, warmth/venodilation, low heart rate—can help correctly diagnose the condition. Obviously, individual patients may exhibit only a portion of the classic symptoms.

In reflex syncope related to carotid sinus hypersensitivity, classically there is no mechanical trigger leading to syncope, and it should be diagnosed by provocation through carotid sinus massage. Occasionally, these patients may describe syncope after rapid head or neck movements.

Sometimes, reflex syncope can occur in response to serious vascular events, particularly subarachnoid hemorrhage or aortic dissection. In these cases, the syncope itself may be a benign reflex event, but the underlying precipitant is life threatening and must be identified through additional historical clues such as severe headache or intense chest and back pain.

Orthostatic hypotension

Is orthostasis causing the patient's syncope?

Syncope due to orthostatic hypotension (OH) can occur with (1) inadequate venous return (low cardiac output), (2) structural damage to the autonomic nervous system (ANS), or (3) transient impairment of normal autonomic nervous system function. The latter may occur with medications that block the normal autonomic responses of the heart (eg, beta-blockers or nonselective calcium channel blockers [CCBs]), or with medications that block the normal autonomic responses of the vasculature (eg, peripherally-acting CCBs or alpha-blockers).

Inadequate venous return may be caused by volume depletion due to inadequate intake or excess losses through the gastrointestinal track, kidneys, or insensible losses (skin, lungs). Low venous return due to venous pooling can occur within the splanchnic system following a meal or in the peripheral venous system (eg, venous insufficiency).

Low peripheral resistance can result from primary or secondary autonomic nervous system (ANS) failure (Figure 99-2). With an intact ANS, drug-induced ANS failure or inappropriate vasodepression during a reflex response can cause syncope. These etiologies can be categorized as syncope due to orthostatic intolerance or orthostatic hypotension (OH). Vasovagal syncope occurs when the initial adaptation reflex is appropriate with orthostatic challenge, but eventually venous return falls and there is an inappropriate cardioinhibitory response, leading to bradycardia (and low cardiac output) while blood pressure (peripheral vascular resistance) is already low.

Finally, postural orthostatic tachycardia syndrome (POTS) is a poorly understood entity believed to occur due to autonomic dysfunction that can be exacerbated by deconditioning. It is manifested by a pathologic excess of venous pooling, early palpitations (in which HR increases by 30 bpm, or up to 120 bpm with standing) and BP instability in response to the venous pooling. It may be associated with chronic fatigue syndrome.

In the elderly, in addition to drug-induced OH, there are two predominant forms of OH: classical OH and delayed OH. In classical OH, chronic ANS failure impairs sympathetic vasoconstriction leading to low systemic vascular resistance in an orthostatic challenge. systemic vascular resistance (SVR) in an orthostatic challenge. In delayed OH, a decline in venous return is coupled with inappropriately low CO and impaired vasoconstriction, leading to syncope.

PHYSICAL EXAMINATION

Initial physical examination should focus on vital signs, including orthostatic assessment and thorough cardiac and neurologic evaluations. At least two retrospective studies (including more than 2700 patients) have shown that orthostatic evaluation is documented in less than 40% of patients admitted to the hospital with syncope. The orthostatic evaluation is a critical piece of information (irrespective of having received intravenous fluids in the emergency department), and should always include heart rate in addition to pulse. Supine parameters should be obtained after the patient has been resting quietly for a few minutes, followed by having the patient stand upright if possible. Obtain and record blood pressure immediately upon standing, then repeat the process in the next two to three minutes, with a pulse rate obtained at the end of the standing period. Cardiac examination should include inspection, evaluation of arterial and venous pulsations and bruits (especially carotid auscultation), and cardiac palpation and auscultation. Evaluation for rales, jugular venous distention, any displacement of the apical impulse, and S_3 can aid in the diagnosis. A neurologic examination should include level of consciousness and orientation, cranial nerves, motor, sensory, cerebellar, and gait evaluations.

CLINICAL DIAGNOSIS AND RISK STRATIFICATION: ECG AND OTHER TESTING

Key historical features and physical examination should guide appropriate diagnostic direction (Table 99-4). The history and physical examination aid with rapid recognition of life-threatening etiologies and are critical for clinicians to make appropriate decisions regarding discharge versus further triage and management.

SIGNIFICANCE OF THE ECG

The ECG plays a critical role in the initial evaluation, risk stratification, and treatment course related to a syncopal event. An ECG should be obtained in all patients who present to the ED, clinic, or hospital following a syncopal episode. The ECG is abnormal in 50% of patients who present with syncope. However, the ECG is diagnostic in only approximately 5% of patients. An ECG can reveal ischemia, rhythm abnormalities, atrioventricular (AV) conduction abnormalities, preexcitation (Wolff-Parkinson-White, WPW), Brugada pattern (ST elevation in V_1-V_3 with right bundle branch pattern), long QT syndrome (LQTS), and arrhythmogenic right ventricular cardiomyopathy (V_1-V_2 negative T waves, epsilon waves, and delayed ventricular potential, ARVC). Please refer to the chapters on Supraventricular Tachyarrhythmias, Chapter 126, and Ventricular Arrhythmias, Chapter 128, for more information.

Findings considered *diagnostic* of syncope at the time of an event include high-grade AV block such as Mobitz type II second degree AV block or complete heart block, symptomatic sinus bradycardia (< 50 bpm), sinoatrial exit block, alternating RBBB and LBBB, rapid paroxysmal SVT or VT, sinus pause greater than three seconds, and pacemaker malfunction. ECG monitoring during inpatient telemetry is diagnostic when a syncopal event can be correlated to an ECG abnormality. However, inpatient telemetry is diagnostic for syncope etiology in only about 1% of inpatients admitted with a syncopal event.

Identification of lower-risk patients based on ECG

Relevant studies help clinicians utilize the ECG to identify patients at lower risk for ischemia or ventricular arrhythmias following a syncopal episode. The greatest predictors to identify patients with ischemia or ACS leading to syncope include ischemic abnormalities on ECG; history of arm, neck, or shoulder pain; rales on pulmonary exam; and history of stable angina.

Clinical predictors of ventricular arrhythmia or death within one year include abnormal ECG, history of ventricular arrhythmia, history of heart failure, and older age. Patients with none of these risk factors have < 1% risk of death or ventricular arrhythmia at one year; compared to >10% risk in those with two or more of the risk factors present.

A reassuring ECG coupled with a history suggestive of a benign syncopal etiology can help to identify low-risk patients who may be safe to discharge from an ED or hospital early in the evaluation process.

RISK STRATIFICATION

When the etiology of syncope remains uncertain after initial evaluation (history, physical examination, and ECG), risk stratification helps determine who deserves further immediate inpatient evaluation, and who can be safely discharged home for either no further evaluation or outpatient evaluation. Several risk stratification algorithms or "rules" have undergone prospective validation and can be used to identify short-term or longer-term risk (**Table 99-5**). These tools can help clinicians stratify patients for possible early discharge from the ED or hospital versus continued evaluation based on estimated risk of adverse outcome.

FURTHER EVALUATION IN THE HOSPITALIZED PATIENT

Reasons for hospital admission include suspicion of a neurologic or cardiac cause of syncope, frequent or recurrent symptoms, and/or documented injury or high estimated risk for injury. Clinicians should strongly consider hospital admission and evaluation of syncope patients with structural heart disease or coronary atherosclerotic heart disease, those with ECG or clinical findings suggestive of syncope due to arrhythmia or ischemia, and those with important comorbidities such as culprit electrolyte deficiencies (magnesium, potassium, calcium) or significant/symptomatic anemia.

Syncope guidelines suggest clinical criteria for admission of patients presenting with syncope (see **Table 99-6**).

INPATIENT ADMISSION VERSUS 24-HOUR OBSERVATION

Patients with syncope should be admitted under observation status unless there is a clear etiology identified or significant risk of bodily injury, recurrent syncope, or high mortality risk.

Figure 99-3 outlines a proposed algorithm for initial hospital evaluation of the patient and provides direction for further consultation and testing. In the patient without a clear cause of syncope, if historical features suggest a vasovagal cause or suspicion is low for cardiogenic syncope, the patient can be safely discharged with close follow-up.

OTHER INPATIENT TESTING

The following sections highlight key points of ancillary testing for inpatients and outpatients presenting with syncope (**Table 99-7**).

Telemetry monitoring

Although telemetry—inpatient continuous electrocardiographic monitoring—has been shown to have a poor diagnostic yield (1–16%) in the evaluation of syncope, it should be employed for patients with a high pretest probability of arrhythmia as the syncope etiology to avoid incurring further morbidity or short-term mortality. Telemetry monitoring during a hospitalization for syncope only occasionally identifies arrhythmia as syncope etiology, but also may help document absence of arrhythmia during a witnessed syncopal event, if that occurs during the monitoring.

TABLE 99-5 Risk Stratification of Syncope Patients at Initial Evaluation Based on Prospective Cohort Studies

Study	Risk Factor	Score	Endpoints	Results
San Francisco Syncope Rule	• Abnormal ECG • CHF • SOB • Hematocrit < 30% • SBP < 90 mm Hg	No risk = 0 items Risk = ≥ 1 item	**7-day** serious events	Validation cohort: Sensitivity: 98%, Specificity 56% LR(+) 2.5, LR(–) 0.06 (validation cohort); however, sensitivity may be as low as 74% and LR(–) as high as 0.46 in some settings (based on other reported cohorts)
ROSE Score (BRACES)	• **B**NP level ≥ 300 pg/ml • **B**radycardia ≤ 50 in Emergency Department or pre-hospital • **R**ectal examination showing fecal occult blood (if suspicion of gastrointestinal bleed) • **A**nemia—hemoglobin ≤ 90 g/l • **C**hest pain associated with syncope • **E**CG showing Q wave (not in lead III) • **S**aturation ≤ 94% on room air	No risk = 0 items Risk = ≥ 1 item	**1-month** serious outcome or all cause death	Sensitivity: 87% Specificity: 65% NPV: 98% LR (+): 2.5, LR (–) 0.2
Martin study	• Abnormal ECG • History of ventricular arrhythmia • History of CHF • Age > 45 years	0 to 4 (1 point each item)	**1-year** severe arrhythmias or death	Score 0: 0% Score 1: 5% Score 2: 16% Score 3 or 4: 27%
OESIL Score	• Abnormal ECG • History of cardiovascular disease • Lack of prodrome • Age > 65 years	0 to 4 (1 point each item)	**1-year** mortality	Score 0: 0% Score 1: 0.6% Score 2: 14% Score 3: 29% Score 4: 53%
EGYSIS Score	• Palpitations before syncope (+4) • Abnormal ECG and/or heart disease (+3) • Syncope while supine (+2) • Autonomic prodrome (–1) • Predisposing and/or precipitating factors (–1)	Sum of + and – points	**2-year** mortality	< 3: 2% ≥ 3: 21%

BNP, beta natriuretic peptide; CHF, congestive heart failure; ECG, electrocardiogram; LR, likelihood ratio; NPV, negative predictive value; SBP, systolic blood pressure; SOB, shortness of breath.

TABLE 99-6 Indications for Hospital Admission in Syncope

Hospital Admission Indicated
• History, physical examination, or ECG suggestive of: a. cardiac disease (eg CAD/ischemia, CHF, arrhythmia, valvular disease, prolonged QT) or, b. neurologic disease
Hospital Admission Possibly Indicated
• History suggesting: a. Sudden LOC with injury and no prodrome (may suggest ventricular tachycardia), b. exertional syncope (may suggest HOCM or exertion induced high grade atrioventricular [AV] block) c. medications likely to prolong QT (may increase risk for torsades de pointes) d. frequent unexplained episodes e. Older age • Physical Examination suggesting: ▪ Moderate to severe orthostatic hypotension

BBB, bundle branch block; CAD, coronary artery disease; CHF, chronic heart failure; CVA, cerebrovascular accident; ECG, electrocardiogram; HOCM, hypertrophic obstructive cardiomyopathy; LOC, loss of consciousness.

Echocardiography and cardiac imaging

While seldom diagnostic of syncope in the absence of severe aortic stenosis, atrial myxoma, or tamponade, echocardiography is a valuable tool in assessing cardiac structure and function. The echocardiogram can rapidly identify structural abnormalities including left ventricular dysfunction, hypertrophic cardiomyopathy with or without outflow tract obstruction, right ventricular strain or dysfunction in the setting of PE or moderate to severe pulmonary hypertension, and pericardial effusions or thickening in the setting of constrictive cardiomyopathy or cardiac tamponade.

In a patient with unexplained syncope, abnormal ECG, or history of cardiac disease, an echocardiogram helps risk stratify patients by ejection fraction and can help identify a subset of patients who may benefit from implantable cardioverter-defibrillator (ICD) placement for the primary prevention of sudden cardiac death (SCD). However, one study showed that *patients with an unremarkable cardiac history and normal ECG* do not benefit from echocardiography in the evaluation of syncope.

The use of CT, MRI, and transesophageal echocardiography (TEE) are limited to more specific situations, such as in the evaluation of aortic dissection, cardiac masses seen on transthoracic echocardiography, pulmonary embolism, diseases of the pericardium/myocardium predisposing to restrictive/constrictive cardiomyopathy, and congenital coronary artery anomalies.

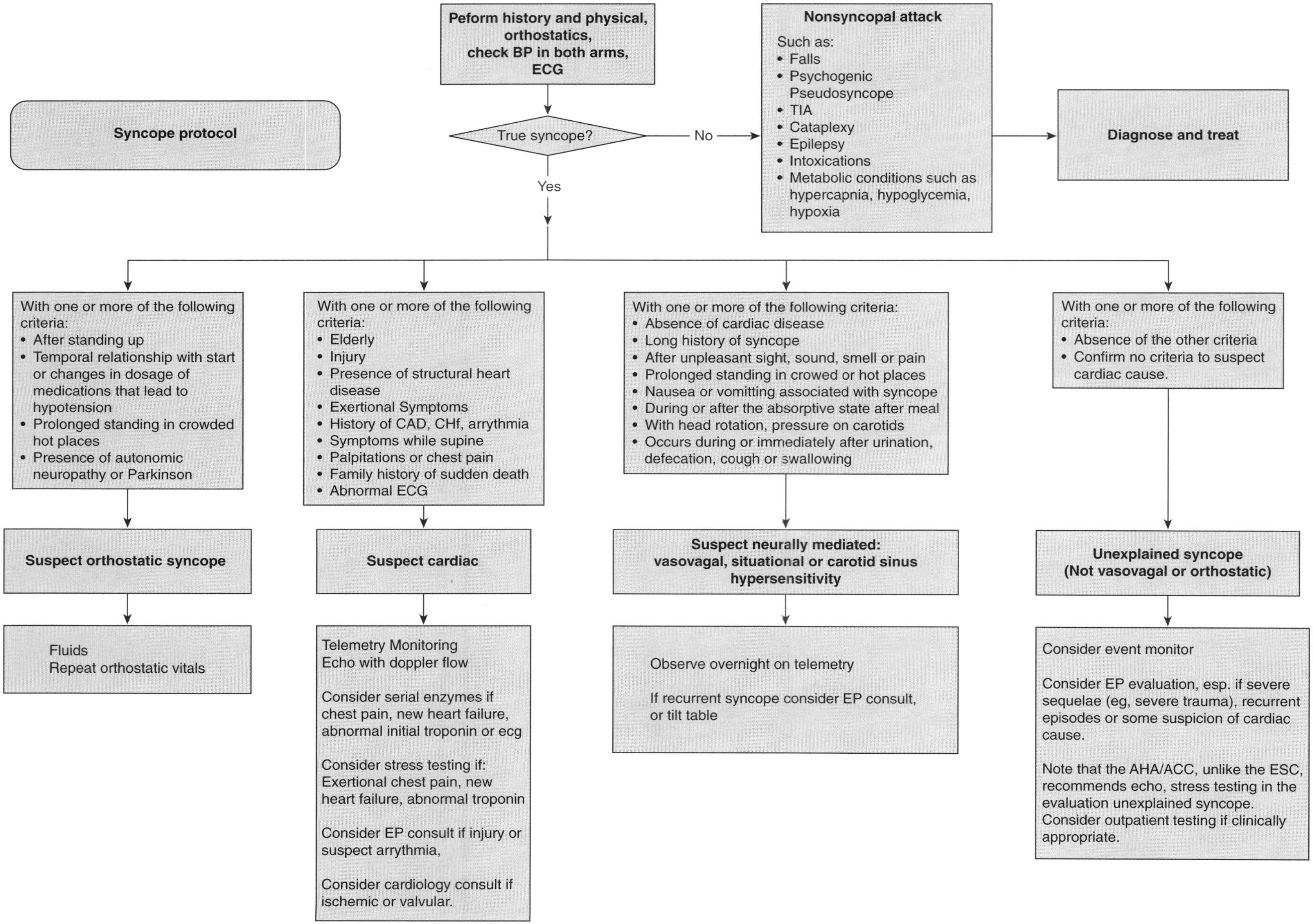

Figure 99-3 *Overview of syncope evaluation. CAD, coronary artery disease; CHF, chronic heart failure; ECG, electrocardiogram; EP, electrophysiology; TIA, transient ischemic attack.*

TABLE 99-7 Diagnostic Testing Modalities in Syncope and Estimated Yield

Test	Diagnostic Yield	Indication/Relevant Etiology of Syncope
Echocardiography	5–10%	Known or suspected structural heart disease
Exercise stress test	1%	Suspected coronary artery disease or exertional syncope
Carotid sinus massage	45% in selective monitored population	Elderly patients with unexplained syncope or suggestive history
Tilt-table testing	49% in those without isoproterenol testing	Recurrent unexplained syncope after structural heart disease excluded or not suspected
Signal-averaged ECG	Unknown positive yield, but 90% negative predictive value	When negative in patients with low to moderate risk for ventricular arrhythmia, helps exclude this condition in patients with unexplained syncope. Ideal candidates for this test are patients with normal heart structurally, but who unexplained syncope without a prodrome
Electrophysiological study	60%	High risk for arrhythmia (frail, elderly, risk of injury/fall), high suspicion for arrhythmia, or structural heart disease with negative initial workup
Holter Monitoring (24–72 hours)	19% (4% positive, 15% negative)	High suspicion for frequent arrhythmia, abnormal ECG, or structural heart disease
External loop recorder (3–4 weeks, or up to 2–3 months)	34% (13% positive, 21% negative)	Frequent syncope (> 1 episode/month) with suspicion for arrhythmia or abnormal ECG/structural heart disease with negative cardiac workup
Implantable loop recorder (ILR, 36 months)	59% (27% positive, 32% negative)	Negative cardiac workup, infrequent syncope, negative tilt examination, negative psychiatric examination. Some role for ILR use after initial negative workup.
Psychiatric evaluation	21%	Recurrent unexplained syncope without evidence of structural heart disease or negative cardiac workup, especially with suggestive history
Electroencephalogram (EEG)	1–2%	Witnessed seizure, postictal state, history of seizure, focal neurologic signs or symptoms
Head computed tomography (CT)	4% in patients with focal neurologic findings or witnessed seizure	History of head trauma, focal neurologic findings, or history consistent with seizure
Neurovascular imaging studies (eg, carotid ultrasound)	Unknown	Signs or symptoms suggestive of transient ischemic attack/stroke; at present no substantial evidence for use of carotid ultrasound or transcranial Doppler in syncope setting

Reproduced, with permission, from Fuster V, O'Rourke RA, Walsh RA, et al. Hurst's the Heart. 12th ed. New York: McGraw-Hill, 2008. Table 48-5.

Cardiac enzymes

Cardiac enzymes have relatively low yield if ordered in unselected patients presenting with syncope, and can lead to additional significant health care costs with the average cost effectiveness (ie, total screening cost of syncope patients per number of diagnoses yielded by screening) of indiscriminate screening equal to >$22,000 per diagnosis. However, at least one retrospective study suggested that up to 7% of patients with syncope and without chest pain had acute coronary syndrome as the etiology of the syncope. It is appropriate to order cardiac enzymes in syncope patients who present with signs or symptoms suggestive of cardiac-related syncope (eg, exertional syncope or syncope associated with chest pain, neck or arm pain, or shortness of breath), and in those with known or suspected coronary disease

Exercise stress testing

While exercise testing for syncope evaluation has very low diagnostic yield, such testing can provide value when ordered for specific indications (see **Table 99-8**). The 2006 ACC/AHA guidelines on syncope management recommend exercise testing in patients with history of coronary artery disease, after echocardiography has been completed to rule out outflow tract obstruction or other contraindication to exercise stress.

Syncope after exercise can be reflex-mediated, whereby tachycardia induces a high-grade AV block distal to the AV node; this finding is associated with underlying conduction disease and a risk for permanent AV block. Exercise stress testing is diagnostic when syncope and hemodynamic changes consistent with a syncopal state are reproduced and documented during exercise or when Mobitz II second degree or third degree AV block develop during exercise even without syncope.

TABLE 99-8 Indications for Exercise Stress Testing in the Setting of Syncope

- Indications
  1. Suspected ischemia
  2. Exertion-related syncope
  3. Exertion-induced tachyarrhythmias
  4. AVB w/ BBB (AVB can worsen w/exercise)
- **Yield:** 1%
- Echo may be necessary prior to stress testing to exclude structural heart disease (eg, AS, HOCM)

AVB, Atrioventricular block; AS, aortic stenosis; BBB, bundle branch block; HOCM, hypertrophic cardiomyopathy.

Carotid sinus hypersensitivity/syndrome (CSH/CSS) testing

At the bifurcation of the common carotid artery lies the carotid body baroreceptor, compression of which can lead to a slowing of heart rate and fall in blood pressure. CSH is defined as: carotid sinus massage (CSM) leading to a ventricular pause of greater than three seconds and/or a drop in systolic BP of 50 mm Hg or more without symptoms (or a SBP drop of 30 mm Hg or more with symptoms). CSH that produces syncope is classified as CSS.

CSS occurs more frequently in patients above 40 years old, and much more so in elderly patients (>70 years). The majority of patients with CSH do not present with a classic history of neck rotation or neck constriction leading to syncope. In those patients over age 40 without clear etiology of syncope after initial thorough workup, CSH should be evaluated with carotid sinus massage (CSM).

CSM should be conducted in a structured manner (**Figure 99-4**). Neurologic complications estimated from a compilation of over 7000 patients in three studies indicates a complication rate of 0.29%, suggesting this is a safe procedure with appropriate patient selection. CSM is recommended for elderly patients with unclear etiology of syncope.

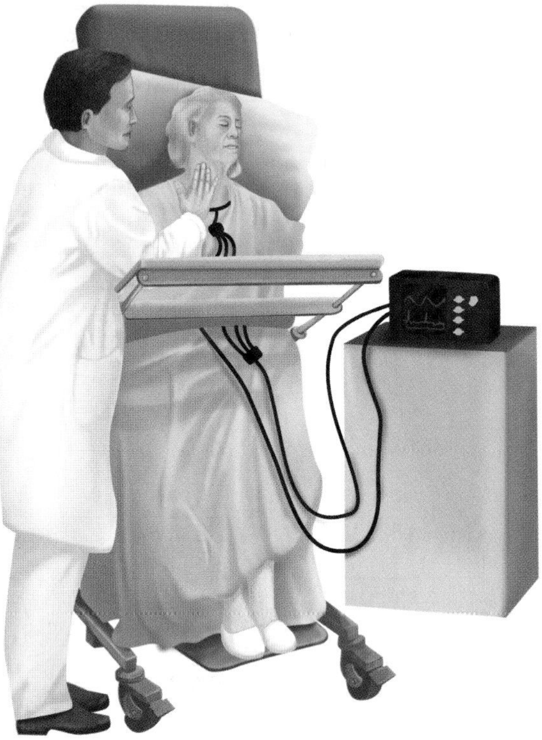

Figure 99-4 *Carotid sinus massage methodology.*

A. Contraindications: MI, TIA, or CVA in the past three months; history of VT or VF, or previous adverse reaction to carotid sinus massage (CSM).

B. Relative contraindications: carotid bruits require carotid ultrasound; if significant stenosis is present some recommend performing the CSM while the patient is supine. Others recommend against performing it.

C. With the patient supine (at least five minutes),

1. *Record baseline ECG, SBP, DBP, HR.*
2. *Perform CSM on the right side while patient is supine. Another operator should record hemodynamic variable changes. Carotid sinus is located midway between the thyroid cartilage and angle of mandible; firm longitudinal massage on area of maximal carotid artery pulsation is carried out for at least five seconds.*
3. *During CSM for five seconds, the operator performing massage should indicate "CSM ON" and "CSM OFF" to indicate those time points on continuous ECG recording, done by the second operator.*
4. *Nadir SBP and DBP occur typically 15 sec after stopping CSM. CSM should be discontinued if a sinus pause >3 sec occurs. In the case of prolonged asystole, a precordial "thump" is advised.*
5. *Repeat the procedure in the left supine, right erect, and left erect, only after patient's HR has reached pre-CSM levels in each case. Upright position CSM has an additional 30% diagnostic yield.*
6. *If neurological complications arise, lay the patient supine, ensure BP is returned to baseline as soon as possible, give aspirin 325 mg if not contraindicated, and admit for observation.*

CSM, carotid sinus massage; CVA, cerebrovascular accident; DBP, diastolic blood pressure; ECG, electrocardiogram; HR, heart rate; MI, myocardial infarction; SBP, systolic blood pressure; TIA, transient ischemic attach; VF, ventricular fibrillation; VT, ventricular tachycardia. (Reproduced, with permission, from Halter JB, Ouslander JG, Tinetti ME, et al. Hazzard's Geriatric Medicine and Gerontology. 6th ed. New York: McGraw-Hill, 2009. Fig. 57-4.)

Neurologic evaluation

Well-performed retrospective observational studies have demonstrated that indiscriminate ordering of neurologic testing (brain imaging, electroencephalogram [EEG], or carotid ultrasound) in patients with syncope has very low yield (1–2%) to find a neurologic cause of syncope, and is fraught with false-positive tests, particularly when carotid disease is identified, which is a common condition that almost never causes syncope absent a clinical stroke. Ordering neurological studies only when the history or physical examination suggests a neurologic etiology for syncope improves the yield of testing to 30–35%. Therefore, brain imaging, EEG, and carotid ultrasonography are not part of the routine evaluation of patients with syncope and should be reserved for patients with neurologic symptoms and/or signs.

Neurologic causes of syncope are rare and a more thorough evaluation should be pursued if the initial assessment is suggestive of such an etiology. Dysautonomia can lead to autonomic nervous system failure (ANF) in the elderly and should be evaluated as part of the orthostatic hypotension workup (Table 99-3).

Trauma and elevated intracranial pressure: While head trauma and conditions predisposing to increased intracranial pressure (eg subarachnoid hemorrhage and intracranial neoplasm) can cause transient loss of consciousness the patient's history and physical exam will generally identify neurologic findings such as headache, meningismus, pupil defect, and sensorimotor or cranial nerve defect. In these cases, it is appropriate to pursue further workup with head imaging such as computerized tomography or magnetic resonance imaging.

Cerebrovascular event: Cerebrovascular disorders can rarely lead to syncope. Subclavian "steal" phenomenon is seen when there is retrograde blood flow in a vertebral artery in the setting of a proximally stenosed left subclavian artery. Blood is, effectively, rerouted from the posterior cerebral circulation to supply the arm, and this may lead to syncope or other symptoms of posterior cerebral ischemia during asymmetric arm exercise.

A transient ischemia attack (TIA) or stroke of the carotid artery does not cause transient loss of consciousness, but global cerebral ischemia from chronic diffuse intracranial vascular disease can lead to syncope if the vertebrobasilar circulation is involved; however, focal neurologic deficit such as limb weakness, ataxia, or cranial nerve deficit would also be present.

The role of carotid ultrasound in the routine evaluation of syncope has not been established. However, carotid ultrasound in patients at high risk of carotid disease may be appropriate prior to carotid sinus massage (Figure 99-4). Finally, in the absence of focal neurologic deficit, the diagnostic yield of this test is demonstrably poor.

Seizure: Active seizures can predispose to transient loss of consciousness, and up to 5–10% of all events described as syncope may be due to seizures. Some cases of syncope are misdiagnosed as seizure because cerebral hypoxia from any cause can lead to myoclonic jerking motions or involuntary movement misrepresented by onlookers as a tonic-clonic or generalized seizure. The history is the most useful tool in distinguishing seizure from true syncope; seizure is more likely if an aura phenomenon is described preceding the event, classic automatisms (lip smacking, frothy oral secretions) are involved, postrecovery myalgia and fatigue are seen, or if recovery is prolonged more than seconds to a minute. Importantly, a postictal, prolonged (usually more than one minute) recovery state is suggestive of seizure rather than syncope.

If seizure is suspected as the most likely diagnosis or if there is a provoked attack resulting in a suspected case of psychogenic pseudosyncope or pseudoseizure, an electroencephalogram (EEG) is an important diagnostic tool. When syncope is the most likely cause, an EEG is usually inappropriate, because interictal EEGs often are usually normal and cannot rule out seizure, and because a small subset of patients without any clinical seizures have asymptomatic epileptiform spikes on EEG.

ADDITIONAL OUTPATIENT TESTING FOR SYNCOPE

Syncope that is recurrent or which is not considered life threatening after 24–48 hours of inpatient monitoring can be evaluated safely in an outpatient setting.

Electrophysiological study

Electrophysiologic (EP) studies evaluate patients for an abnormal cardiac electrical system that might lead to tachyarrhythmias or bradyarrhythmias as a cause of syncope. EP studies can be used to identify intermittent significant AV nodal block that is not caught on ECG in patients at risk (eg, patients with bifascicular block on ECG). It can also be used to identify inducible ventricular arrhythmias in patients with structurally abnormal hearts or those with other symptoms, signs, or testing to suggest ventricular arrhythmia risk. EP studies may also identify supraventricular tachyarrhythmias (SVTs), but most SVTs do not require invasive diagnostic modalities. However, it is sometimes used for treatment (eg, catheter ablation) of SVTs that cause symptoms, including recurrent syncope.

Head up tilt table testing

Introduced in 1986, head-up tilt-table testing (HUTT) can be utilized to establish the diagnosis of reflex syncope when the diagnosis is not obvious or clear based on the patient's history, physical examination (including orthostatic vital sign measurements), or other basic testing. Its greatest utility is in patients with *recurrent* episodes in which reflex syncope is suspected. Unless there are occupational hazards or a high risk of injury associated with syncope, testing for a single or rare event is not indicated. Furthermore, tilt testing can be used to help distinguish syncope from epilepsy (when the patient presents with jerking movements and seizure disorder is in doubt) or to help identify the cause of syncope in the elderly with multiple falls. Some protocols with HUTT use provocative agents (eg, isoproterenol or sublingual nitroglycerin) to decrease vascular tone or increase heart rate. These agents, when used, increase the test's sensitivity, but reduce specificity and reproducibility (**Table 99-9**).

TABLE 99-9 Head-up Tilt-table Test Protocol

- Performed in an electrophysiology lab under continuous ECG, BP, and HR monitoring.
- Patient is placed supine on a hydraulic table equipped with footboard and safety restraints, and capable of producing a tilt of 60–90 degrees of head-up from supine in less than 10 seconds.
- Baseline hemodynamic and ECG data should be obtained while supine for 5 minutes if nitroglycerin is used without establishing intravenous access and for 20 minutes if isoproterenol and consequent venous access are needed.
- Every 3–5 minutes, heart rate and symptoms are monitored; noninvasive BP is measured using finger arterial monitoring and beat-to-beat measurement or cuff inflation every 3–5 minutes. While the test is carried out for 20–45 minutes, it is interrupted if syncope is documented with a significant drop in HR and BP.
- The goal of isoproterenol is to increase HR to around 20–25% over baseline. Contraindications to isoproterenol use include ischemic heart disease, uncontrolled hypertension, significant aortic stenosis, and left ventricular outflow tract obstruction.
- Resuscitation equipment must be available, as atrial fibrillation and cardiopulmonary arrest have occurred in rare instances.

When the patient undergoes head-up tilt, venous pooling is the norm, but impaired cardiac output without an appropriate vasoconstriction response is seen in patients with reflex syncope. A positive response to tilt testing is documented when syncope occurs in the setting of hypotension preceding either a mixed *cardioinhibitory/vasodepressor response* (ie, HR falls to less than 40 bpm for 10 seconds or less), *cardioinhibitory response* (HR < 40 for > 10 sec, with or without asystole), or *vasodepressor response* (HR does not fall more than 10% from its peak). Exceptions to the diagnosis of vasodepressor response include chronotropic incompetence, in which the HR does not rise more than 10% above baseline at any time, and POTS, in which an excessive HR rise (defined as HR > 130 bpm) is seen at the onset of tilt and for the duration of the entire procedure.

Holter monitoring, external loop recorders and implantable loop recorders

Short-term or long-term electrocardiographic monitoring can help establish the diagnosis of arrhythmia as the cause of syncope or help in ruling out arrhythmia. In the patient whose syncope is not life threatening and in whom a definitive diagnosis has not been established, outpatient telemetry via Holter monitoring or loop recorders should be considered. In general, Holter recordings are most useful in patients with daily symptoms of lightheadedness or palpitations, whereas loop recorders are indicated for patients with less frequent symptoms.

Holter monitoring: Holter monitoring provides 24–72 hours (rarely a few days longer) of continuous ECG monitoring via surface electrodes and a portable battery pack/recording device at a cost of roughly $1000 per device and associated servicing costs. Patients who may benefit include those with a high suspicion of arrhythmia, structural heart disease, or an abnormal ECG without meeting inpatient criteria for syncope; or in the evaluation of the discharged patient without a definitive diagnosis. The yield for a diagnosis of syncope is from 1–4% and negative yield (ie, patients in whom an arrhythmia was not detected during a syncopal event, effectively ruling out arrhythmia) is near 15%. Holter monitoring carries a very high cost-per diagnosis ratio due to the infrequency of arrhythmic events in most patients with syncope of unknown etiology.

External loop recorder: An external loop recorder, also a portable system with cutaneous electrodes, can be worn and used to retrieve data generated over 3–4 weeks and up to 2–3 months if there is a history of syncope or symptoms suspicious for arrhythmia. Indications are similar to those for Holter monitoring. The loop recorder continually stores and deletes ECG data. At the time of patient manual activation of the recorder, 5–15 minutes of preactivation ECG data is stored for analysis. From prospective studies, at best the positive yield to achieve diagnosis is approximately 15–25%, and the negative yield is approximately 20%, giving this modality also a high cost-per-diagnosis ratio. Patient compliance beyond three weeks is unusual and further limits the usefulness of this test.

Implantable loop recorders: Implantable loop recorders (ILRs) can provide ECG data up to 36 months and obtain higher diagnostic yield per device than other recording modalities such as the Holter monitor. In selected populations, ILRs yield a diagnosis in 50–90% of patients, but come with an initial high cost (~$10,000 or more) and the requirement of implantation during a minor surgical procedure (similar to pacemaker placement).

The majority of patients evaluated in studies of ILR do not have an initial presentation consistent with reflex syncope or evidence of structural heart disease. Investigators in the International Study on Syncope of Unknown Etiology (ISSUE) group have proposed classification of ILR data into four broad groups: asystole, bradycardia, no/minimal rhythm disturbance, and tachycardia for standardization of patient data. ISSUE2 reported lower recurrent syncope rates in patients given therapy specific to their arrhythmia (ICD, pacemaker, catheter ablation, antiarrhythmic) in comparison to those who were given no specific therapy after patients in both treatment groups suffered from a vasovagal event. ISSUE3 will conduct a randomized placebo-controlled trial to test the efficacy of pacing for reflex syncope.

Syncope in the patient with psychiatric illness

Antipsychotic medications and side effects from chronic use can lead to orthostatic hypotension or QT interval prolongation, either of which may result in syncope. Key medications to inquire about include benzodiazepines, SSRI or MAOI antidepressants, barbiturates, neuroleptics and tricyclic antidepressants, as well as drugs of abuse such as ethanol.

In the evaluation of transient loss of consciousness (T-LOC), an EEG can be valuable in diagnosing pseudoepilepsy (ie, nonepileptic seizures or nonepileptic attack disorder), in which gross limb movements accompany T-LOC but an EEG shows no epileptiform activity. Furthermore, if the patient should lose postural tone, suffer a T-LOC, but show no signs of limb movement or epileptiform attack, a negative EEG and normal BP/HR during a positive tilt-table test help to effectively diagnose a condition referred to as pseudosyncope. In pseudosyncope, the patient history does not usually identify a trigger to the event. Attacks occur frequently and can last for several minutes—in contrast to only several seconds of T-LOC seen in true syncope. While pseudosyncopal events are believed to be involuntary just as syncopal events, suggestion by the clinician can potentially trigger a syncopal event in this functional disorder.

Psychiatric testing can be valuable and indicated in patients with multiple or frequent episodes of syncope without injury, or in recurrent syncope when other exhaustive workup or evaluation has not yielded any certain diagnosis.

SPECIAL CASE: RECURRENT SYNCOPE

Regardless of etiology, syncope recurs in approximately 30–40% of patients followed for three years after the diagnosis. In patients with vasovagal syncope, prognosis is generally excellent, but recurrence occurs in approximately 30% of patients followed from seven months up to five years. While age is not predictive of future risk of recurrence, shortened time to recurrence after diagnosis and number of previous syncopal episodes increase recurrence risk. While recurrent syncope does not confer a higher mortality risk than an isolated syncopal episode, the morbidity incurred via injury and trauma with recurrent episodes does impose restrictions on patient quality of life and well-being.

SPECIAL CASE: ELDERLY PATIENTS WITH SYNCOPE

Elderly patients often have coexistence of many predisposing medical conditions that can lead to syncope. Common causes in the elderly population include orthostatic hypotension, reflex syncope, and arrhythmias. Syncope of cardiac origin carries a similar mortality risk in both young and old.

As in all patients, a detailed but focused history and physical examination can yield a diagnosis in the great majority of initial evaluations. A comprehensive medication history focusing on temporal relationships between the falls/syncope and initiation of new medications or dosing changes is critical, as is consideration of changing drug levels due to dynamic renal or hepatic function. Any associated comorbidities such as deconditioning, dependence for activities of daily living, cognitive impairment, and performance status can also increase risk. A focused neurologic examination should be complemented by assessment of gait instability, orthostatic challenge, and balance. *Routine carotid sinus massage* is recommended for elderly patients presenting with syncope (who do not have contraindications to the test) in addition to the thorough initial assessment as used for younger patients (see Figure 99-4).

PRACTICE POINT

- A high-yield approach at initial evaluation involves a thorough history; medication review; physical examination focused on postural blood pressure measurement, cardiac, and neurologic examinations; and electrocardiogram. In those with an unclear etiology, further testing should be done with a focus on efficiency and high-yield tools based on the thorough history and physical examination. Risk stratification should be carried out on initial evaluation in accordance with well-validated risk-scoring tools.

TREATMENT AND PRIMARY PREVENTION OF SYNCOPE

TREATMENT OVERVIEW

Irrespective of establishing an etiology for syncope, the primary goals in the treatment of syncope are to reduce the risk of injury/trauma, improve survival, and evaluate and prevent recurrent syncopal events. At the time of initial evaluation, an etiology and mechanism of syncope is pursued. Treatment is aimed at an underlying cause if one can be identified (**Figure 99-5**).

REFLEX SYNCOPE, AUTONOMIC DYSFUNCTION, AND ORTHOSTATIC HYPOTENSION/INTOLERANCE

In autonomic dysfunction and consequent orthostatic hypotension (OH) or reflex/vasovagal syncope, the aim is to prevent syncope recurrence and limit risk of bodily injury or harm to the patient. Treatment of reflex syncope includes patient education, reassurance, and avoidance of triggers. Recognition of triggers and recognition of a prodrome warning period, such as nausea, lightheadedness, and sense of impending fall or loss of balance can help abort a syncopal event.

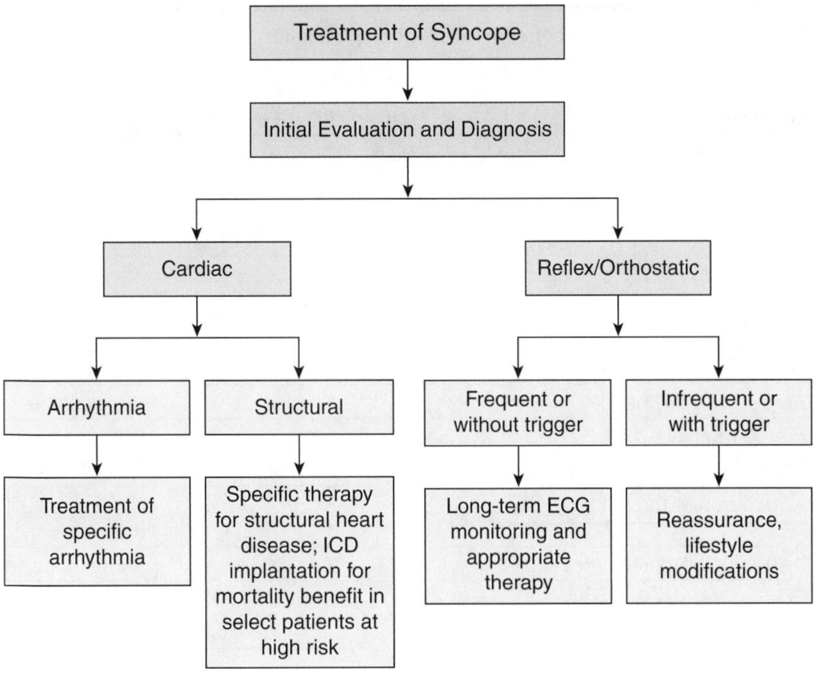

Figure 99-5 *Proposed inpatient algorithm for hospitalist management of syncope.*

Physical counter-pressure maneuvers (PCMS) to increase venous return can be instituted with success if done in a timely manner during prodrome or trigger recognition. These maneuvers involve causing a rapid increase in systolic and diastolic blood pressure through the timely initiation of either gluteal muscle tightening with concomitant leg crossing or arm tensing through interlocking handgrip and isometric contraction. In a multicenter, prospective trial, the burden of recurrent syncope enjoyed a relative risk reduction of near 40% when comparing patients who had received physical counter-pressure maneuver training with those who did not.

Pharmacologic therapy for prevention and treatment of reflex syncope address peripheral vasoconstriction, volume expansion, prevention of paradoxical bradycardia and excess vagal activity, and treatment of anxiety (**Table 99-10**). No randomized controlled trial evidence establishes benefit of these therapies. Acute reflex syncope during tilt testing is modestly improved with midodrine, but long-term studies are lacking. While a "pill-in-the-pocket" strategy for impending syncope along with counter-pressure maneuvers may benefit some patients taking midodrine, its frequent dosing and urinary retention limit its effectiveness. Randomized, placebo-controlled trials with beta-blockers to prevent reflex syncope show no long-term risk reduction from future syncopal events. A short-term follow-up study in a small number of patients showed modest benefit for paroxetine in preventing recurrent syncope in patients who did not tolerate beta-blockers, mineralocorticoids, and vagolytics. Fludrocortisone has not been proven effective in syncope prevention. None of the medications commonly used for reflex syncope has Food and Drug Administration approval for this indication.

Cardiac pacing and device therapy has shown no significant aggregate benefit in syncope based on meta-analysis of five large trials. The development of autonomic dysfunction and failure (ANF) is manifested by an inappropriate sympathetic nervous system response to orthostatic challenge and can be due to medications, underlying systemic illness, or primary systemic illness (Table 99-3). Volume depletion from dehydration and blood loss should be ruled out initially in the evaluation of these patients. A thorough medication history should rule out medication as the cause; common culprit medications include nitrates, alpha-blockers, calcium channel blockers, beta-blockers, anti-Parkinson medications, antipsychotics, and diuretics.

Treatment of orthostatic hypotension (OH) and intolerance should first seek to employ nonpharmacologic measures. Patients should change posture slowly, increase fluid and salt intake to 3 liters and up to 10 grams sodium per day if supine hypertension is not a comorbid illness, seek adjustment of antihypertensives with physician guidance, and avoid excessive durations of recumbency and sleep, while maintaining the head of the bed at 10–20 degrees. Avoiding the rapid ingestion of cold water, limiting the size of meals and carbohydrate intake, and avoidance of alcohol help reduce postprandial hypotension. The use of tight lower-extremity elastic stockings and occasionally abdominal binders can help maintain venous return while standing. Finally, as in reflex syncope, all patients should be counseled on anticipatory physical counter-pressure maneuvers (PCMs).

Pharmacologic measures for OH treatment are aimed at expanding central volume, improving vasoconstriction, and mitigating various factors such as anemia of chronic inflammation, nocturnal diuresis, and poor sympathetic tone. In those with insufficient plasma volume despite increased salt and water intake, fludrocortisone can be used to enhance distal tubular sodium absorption. Adverse effects include supine hypertension, hypokalemia, and headache. Midodrine, a direct alpha1-receptor agonist, is approved by the FDA for OH. Adverse effects include supine hypertension, bradycardia, and urinary retention. An adjunct therapy in select patients taking or having failed midodrine is the use of pseudoephedrine/ephedrine, direct and indirect alpha-receptor agonists. Adverse effects include tachycardia, central sympathomimesis, and worsening supine hypertension. Finally, adjunct therapies in special situations include desmopressin (DDAVP) to reduce nocturnal diuresis, erythropoietin to correct anemia of chronic inflammation or renal insufficiency, and pyridostigmine to enhance sympathetic nervous system transmission.

TABLE 99-10 Selected Therapies for Reflex Syncope/Orthostatic Hypotension

Treatment	Application	Form Effective in				Problems
		NCS	PD	HA	OH	
Reconditioning	Aerobic exercise 20 min 3 times/wk	X	X	X	X	If done too vigorously may worsen symptoms
Physical maneuvers (tilt training, etc)	30 min 3 times per day	X				Noncompliance is common
Sleeping with head tilted upright	During sleep	X		X	X	
Hydration	2 L orally per day	X	X		X	Edema
Salt	2–4 g/d	X	X		X	Edema
Fludrocortisone	0.1–0.2 mg orally per day	X	X		X	Hypokalemia, hypomagnesemia, edema
Metoprolol	25–100 mg twice a day			X		Fatigue
Labetalol	100–200 mg orally twice a day			X		Fatigue
Midodrine	5–10 mg orally three times a day	X	X		X	Nausea, scalp itching, supine hypertension
Methylphenidate	5–10 mg orally three times a day	X	X	X		Anorexia, insomnia, dependency
Bupropion	150–300 mg XL every day		X	X	X	Tremor, agitation, insomnia
Clonidine	0.1–0.3 mg orally twice a day			X		Dry mouth, blurred vision
Pyridostigmine	30–60 mg orally per day		X		X	Nausea, diarrhea
SSRI-escitalopram	10 mg orally per day	X	X		X	Tremor, agitation, sexual problems
Erythropoietin	10,000–20,000 g subcutaneously every week	X	X		X	Pain at injection site, expensive
Octreotide	50–200 micrograms SC three times a day		X	X	X	Nausea, diarrhea, gallstone
Permanent pacing		X				

HA, hyperadrenic postural orthostatic tachycardia syndrome; NCS, neurocardiogenic syncope; OH, orthostatic hypotension; PD, partial dysautonomia postural orthostatic tachycardia syndrome; SSRI, selective serotonin reuptake inhibitor.

ARRHYTHMIAS

Specific to the nature of the arrhythmia, treatment of syncope due to arrhythmia varies from medication discontinuation to ICD placement and radiofrequency catheter ablation (RFCA). The choice of therapy is influenced by systolic function and the presence or absence of a vasodepressor component to syncope. See Chapter 126 for more detailed information about Supraventricular Tachycarrhythmias, Chapter 127 for Bradyarrhythmias, and Chapter 128 for Ventricular Arrhythmias.

For sinus node dysfunction manifested primarily with bradycardia, if syncope is documented during a bradyarrhythmia, cardiac pacing has class I indications for the following situations, according to the European Society of Cardiology 2009 syncope guidelines: sinus arrest without a correctable cause, sinus node disease and evident abnormal corrected sinus node recovery time (CSNRT), and syncope with asymptomatic sinus pauses greater than three seconds. Presence of a vasodepressor component to sinus node dysfunction is an unfortunate cause of syncope recurrence in up to 20% of patients treated with pacing. Atrial tachyarrhythmias, especially as a manifestation of the sick sinus syndrome (SSS), can be effectively treated with RFCA.

For atrioventricular (AV) nodal conduction disease, there are only two class I indications for pacing: (1) syncope with second degree type II (Mobitz) block, complete AV block or advanced AV block; and (2) syncope with bundle branch block and inducible high-degree AV block on EPS.

For patients suffering from paroxysmal supraventricular tachyarrhythmias (pSVT) such as AV nodal reentrant tachycardia (AVNRT), AV reentrant tachycardia (AVRT), and typical atrial flutter (AFL), the availability, safety, and high efficacy of RFCA make this the preferred treatment of choice for syncopal episodes attributable to pSVTs. Syncope due to atrial fibrillation can be managed with RFCA or with pharmacologic therapy aimed at rate or rhythm control. In patients with refractory symptomatic atrial fibrillation producing rapid ventricular response and a predisposition to syncopal events, ablation of the bundle of His with subsequent pacemaker implantation can be considered a safe and effective therapy. Please see Chapter 126 on Supraventricular Tachyarrhythmias for further details about SVT management.

Rarely, ICD or pacemaker device malfunction can lead to syncope. Usually, this is manifested as retrograde conduction in a pacemaker. Device reprogramming or conversion of a single ventricular lead to dual chamber pacing can effectively resolve the problem. In battery/pulse generator failure or in lead fracture/dislodgement/conduction failure, device replacement is necessary and effective.

STRUCTURAL HEART DISEASE MANAGEMENT

The primary aim in treating patients with syncope due to structural heart disease is to identify the causative factor contributing to syncope and treat the primary process. An important aim also is to prevent sudden cardiac death (SCD). Structural heart disease such as aortic stenosis, hypertrophic obstructive cardiomyopathy (HoCM), inferior segment myocardial infarction, and cardiac tamponade can directly cause syncope, whereas conditions such as severely impaired systolic function from ischemic cardiomyopathy can lead to macro-reentrant ventricular tachycardia (VT), and predispose to syncope. Treatment is aimed at the underlying process believed to be causing syncope. Placement of an ICD has been established solely to improve mortality risk (not as a means to treat syncope) in patients with a) severe systolic heart failure (with an ejection fraction < 35%), b) HoCM with outflow tract obstruction, and c) patients with a specific predisposition to malignant ventricular arrhythmia (eg, arrhythmogenic right ventricular cardiomyopathy).

CONSULTATION

Hospitalists should rely on their consultant colleagues when there is a specific question or therapeutic aim to address by the approached specialty. A particularly useful result of the frugal use of consultation is deciding with the consultant whether the patient needs further inpatient testing or treatment and whether outpatient follow-up is sufficient for an otherwise stable condition.

CARDIOLOGY

In cases of syncope due to structural heart disease in which a link between the two conditions is relevant and clear, such as in moderate to severe aortic stenosis and exertional syncope, consultation with a cardiologist is valuable and necessary. When an outcome can be improved, such as in ICD placement for a syncopal patient presenting with VT and severely depressed ejection fraction, consultation for further treatment is also necessary and straightforward. Where outcome or causal relationship cannot be entirely established, as in a case of longstanding moderate to severe pulmonary hypertension with syncope, consultation can bring about a second opinion regarding advanced therapeutics.

Inpatient consultation for diagnostic or therapeutic catheterization, tilt-table carotid sinus massage (in elderly patients with recurrent symptomatic syncope of unclear origin), and EPS/pacemaker issues/ICD implantation are all appropriate. The presence of structural heart disease does not mean another noncardiac cause of syncope is less likely.

NEUROLOGY

It is rare for syncope to be due directly to neurologic causes. The routine use of brain computed tomography or carotid artery Doppler ultrasound in the initial evaluation of syncope does not have diagnostic value or cost effectiveness when active neurologic symptoms or findings are absent. Syncope can occur from vertebrobasilar insufficiency and associated "steal" syndrome, and a presentation that suggests vertebrobasilar insufficiency may be a rare instance in which neurology consultation is justified.

In the clarification of the patient's initial presentation with loss of consciousness, an EEG can be useful if the history and physical exam indicate seizure disorder or epilepsy in the differential diagnosis. Video-monitored 24-hour EEG can be undertaken if necessary with the help of a neurologic consultation.

PSYCHIATRY

Consultation with a psychiatrist in the evaluation of syncope is done rarely. Indications include identification of psychosomatic conditions predisposing to syncope, such as conversion, somatoform, or factitious disorder. Establishing a psychiatric diagnosis may be useful in patients with recurrent symptomatic syncope who have undergone a thorough negative workup for cardiac, reflex, and orthostatic syncope as appropriate. These patients, prone to suggestion, can be diagnosed with the assistance of a psychiatric consultation as having psychogenic pseudosyncope. Outpatient treatment may include SSRIs, cognitive behavioral therapy, and psychiatric outpatient follow-up.

DISCHARGE PLANNING

Prior to discharge, patients should be educated on measures to prevent recurrent reflex syncope, recognition of prodromal symptoms, and warning signs that warrant emergency care. Of particular concern to patients is the fear of syncope recurrence while driving. Driving following a syncopal episode is regulated by individual states, and clinicians should refer to their specific state laws when making recommendations. However, in general, private drivers have no restrictions on driving independent of those imposed by having an ICD according to current society guidelines. If, however, unexplained syncope occurs while driving and/or in the presence of structural heart disease, driving may be prohibited. For professional drivers, permanent restrictions are recommended if an ICD has been implanted, occasional syncope occurs during high-risk activity, syncope is recurrent and severe and treatment has not been established, and in unexplained syncope if treatment has not been established. Long-term accident and insurance data indicate, reassuringly, that rates of vehicular accidents are no higher than in the general population without syncope. Timely follow-up with appropriate outpatient physicians (primary care physicians, cardiologists, neurologists, as indicated) should occur within two to four weeks of hospital discharge.

QUALITY IMPROVEMENT TO ADDRESS PERFORMANCE GAPS

One of the major areas of practice improvement related to syncope (ICD-9 780.2) is resource utilization. Patients with syncope require a multidisciplinary approach in some cases and in other instances can be discharged safely from the emergency department with close follow-up.

In the United States, up to 5% of all ED patients present with syncope. This equates to approximately 500,000 visits per year. In addition, 3% or approximately 150,000 of all inpatient admissions per year are for syncope. With the cost of each admission ranging from $8000 to $75,000, it comes as no surprise that our annual expenditure for syncope is approximately $2 billion.

Hospitalists are keenly positioned to appreciate costs associated with syncope admissions and the benefits reaped by thoughtful resource utilization. Patients should be risk stratified using well-validated criteria, and further testing carried out to assess posthospital risk of injury and mortality.

Testing should be limited to that necessary for immediate risk stratification and/or diagnosis confirmation or treatments of the syncopal event. In a retrospective analysis of costs associated with inpatient admission of syncope in elderly patients, researchers found that postural blood pressure recording (ie, orthostatics measurement) costs $17 per test affecting the diagnosis or management of a case of syncope. In contrast, the cost effectiveness of cardiac enzyme measurement was $22,397, head CT $24,881, ECG $1020, and telemetry $710 per clinically relevant finding affecting diagnosis or treatment.

Admission for the syncopal patient should not be unnecessarily prolonged. On the part of the hospitalist as coordinator of care, this may require earlier consultation with specialists to plan earlier testing, discharge, and follow-up. In prospective, randomized controlled trials incorporating strict adherence to syncope criteria for admission and utilization of Syncope Management Units (SMU) in the ED to triage syncope patients, there is a marked reduction of hospital length-of-stay, number of tests conducted per patient, and associated lower costs. SMUs involve staffing by ED physicians, cardiologists, and/or neurologists and ready access to echocardiogram, tilt testing, beat-to-beat blood pressure, and continuous telemetry monitoring for up to six hours with a decision reached to admit or discharge in that timeframe. Long-term follow-up to two years has shown no difference in morbidity and mortality in these patients. With careful selection, triage, and early discharge, hospitalists can make a lasting impact on the resources utilized in the management of syncope.

CASE 99-1 *(continued)*

This 74-year-old woman suffered a syncopal event due to autonomic dysfunction related to her Parkinson disease. While the onlooker witnessed postevent jerking movements, these lasted only a few seconds and her recovery was spontaneous and complete. Her brief myoclonic jerking movement was likely secondary to transient cerebral hypoperfusion that accompanied her loss of postural tone. Her prognosis is likely unchanged from that of the general population and no further testing or treatment is indicated. Rather, the patient should be reassured and should receive education about autonomic dysfunction and how to reduce symptoms (eg, elevate head of bed a four to six inches; rise from lying or sitting slowly; increase daily salt and fluid intake, eat smaller and more frequent meals during the day, plan daily activities later in the day, and if possible, perform lower body resistance isometric training exercises to improve conditioning). If syncope recurs or significant injury results, patient may deserve medications (eg, fludrocortisone, midodrine) to reduce likelihood of syncope related to autonomic dysfunction.

CASE 99-2 *(continued)*

The ECG of this 62-year-old patient who passed out without warning is concerning for a "trifascicular" block, with first-degree atrioventricular block (AV), left anterior fascicular block, and right bundle branch block. His condition is likely due to age-related fibrotic changes in the nodal conductive tissue within the myocardium. EP study is likely necessary to confirm whether the first degree block is AV or sinoatrial in origin; the treatment may require permanent pacemaker insertion. He should be admitted to telemetry and cardiology consulted for consideration of EP study and permanent pacemaker insertion during this hospitalization.

CONCLUSION

Syncope is characterized by sudden, transient, reversible loss of consciousness with prompt recovery. Recurrent syncope can be distressing to the patient, carries a serious risk of bodily injury and harm, and can lead to significant lifestyle changes including loss of gainful employment. Diagnosis should occur in a timely, cost-efficient manner. At the time of discharge, the goal is to provide the patient with a reasonably confident estimate of prognosis, risk of recurrence, and goals and timing of further diagnostic studies and therapy.

A high-yield approach at initial evaluation involves a thorough history; medication review; physical examination focused on postural blood pressure measurement, cardiac, and neurologic examinations; and electrocardiogram. In those with an unclear etiology, further testing should be done with a focus on efficiency and high-yield tools based on the thorough history and physical examination. Risk stratification should be carried out on initial evaluation in accordance with well-validated risk scoring tools. (see Table 99-5)

Specific causes of syncope such as arrhythmias and structural cardiopulmonary disease should be quickly identified and treated in consultation with a specialist to expedite care as well as to establish adequate, timely follow-up after hospital discharge.

Finally, an area of active research in syncope is the use of syncope management units (SMUs), primarily in emergency departments. Success in Europe is the basis for ongoing investment of this concept in the United States. SMUs can help identify patients who would otherwise be deemed low risk by standardized triage protocols and discharged from the emergency department for rapid follow-up (**Table 99-11**).

TABLE 99-11 Evidence-based Medicine Key References for Syncope

Study	Methodology	Results	Limitations	Bottom Line
Soteriades, et al. *N Engl J Med.* 2002;347:878–885.	Cohort study of Framingham Heart Study (1971–1998) of patients with syncope and delineation of epidemiology and prognosis in a general population.	822 patients with syncope. Incidence of syncope 6.2 per 1000 person-years. Patients with cardiac syncope have higher risk of mortality (HR 2.01) compared with patients without syncope. Vasovagal syncope confers no additional mortality risk.	Lack of syncope was defined as not having had a clinical examination in four years. This confers a recall bias. Study composed of middle-age to elderly white men and women, thus not generalizable.	Cardiac syncope patients are at an increased risk of death from any cause. Patients with unknown syncope still have a higher mortality risk than those without syncope or those with vasovagal syncope.
Linzer, et al. *Ann Intern Med.* 1997;126:989–996. and Linzer, et al. *Ann Intern Med.* 1997;127: 76–86.	Clinical guideline paper, literature review using MEDLINE (1980 to 1997) of randomized trials, observational studies, cohort studies, case series with > 10 patients each.	History, physical exam, ECG are core of the syncope workup, > 50% diagnostic yield. Neurologic testing rarely helpful in absence of focal findings. Known or suspected heart disease should be hospitalized and cardiac causes ruled out as an etiology. Loop recording and tilt testing helpful in recurrent, noncardiac syncope. Psychiatric evaluation is an important adjunct for diagnosis in 25% of cases.	Review composed of case series, population studies, and referral series. No RCT data available for review. This review did not focus on a specific therapy. There is no gold standard for diagnosing syncope.	History, physical exam, and ECG have > 50% diagnostic yield. History alone has an approximate 45% diagnostic yield. Neurologic testing is low yield in absence of focal neurologic findings. Suspected or known cardiac disease in setting of syncope should warrant hospitalization.

(continued)

TABLE 99-11 Evidence-based Medicine Key References for Syncope *(continued)*

Study	Methodology	Results	Limitations	Bottom Line
Quinn, et al. (San Francisco Syncope Rule). *Ann Emerg Med.* 2004;43(2):224–232.	Prospective cohort study at a university hospital and ED of patients with syncope and presyncope, 7-day follow-up to establish risk factors associated with a predefined serious outcome (death, MI, PE, stroke, SAH, related ED return).	Of 684 syncope visits, 79 with serious outcomes, 50 predictor variables considered, 5 factors found to have 96% sensitivity, 62% specificity of predicting occurrence of the predefined serious outcome at 7 days.	In forming this prediction rule, 100% sensitivity not attained because of desire to maximize specificity. The predefined "serious outcome" was a consensus opinion, heavily focused on cardiac outcomes.	Upon derivation, the following 5 factors have a 96% sensitivity, 62% specificity: abnormal ECG, SOB, Hct < 30%, SBP < 90 mm Hg, history of CHF. Further studies with validation cohorts (n = 791; Ann Emerg Med. 2006;47(5):448–54. Epub 2006 Jan 18) confirm this predictive ability. Application of the SFSR in the ED can reduce hospitalization for syncope from 10–24%.
Brignole, et al. (ISSUE2 Study) *Eur Heart J.* 2006; 27(9):1085–1092.	Prospective, multicenter, observational study following pts with > 2 severe syncopal episodes who received an implantable loop recorder for neurally mediated syncope (NMS) and in whom orthostasis, carotid sinus, and cardiac syncope were excluded.	33% recurrent syncope rate after ILR implantation. Of 103 pts with recurrence, 53 received therapy specific to the documented culprit finding: pacemaker for asystole and antiarrhythmic therapy for tachyarrhythmia. In the other 50 patients, therapy was not tailored to the ILR findings at time of syncope. In comparison, the group receiving ILR-tailored therapy had 10% recurrence of syncope at 1 year vs. 40% in nontailored group; a RRR of 80%.	Excellent comparison of groups prior to first recurrent syncope, but this was NOT a blinded controlled study. ISSUE3 is a randomized, controlled study with results expected in 2011.	For patients with NMS who have received an ILR, therapy should be tailored to culprit arrhythmias, whether asystole or tachyarrhythmia. ISSUE3, a RCT, will focus on head-to-head comparison of these two groups (tailored vs. nontailored).
Brignole, et al. (EGSYS-2 Study group). *Europace.* 2006;8,644–650.	Prospective, controlled multicenter Italian study to assess efficacy of adherence to syncope guidelines in improving diagnostic yield and reducing costs associated with syncope.	Consecutive syncope patients presenting to Italian EDs were compared in two groups: all-comers during 1 month in 2001 (n = 929) given usual care vs. all-comers during 1 month in 2004 given ESC guideline-based care (n = 745). Patients in the guideline-based group had, on average, 8% less hospitalization, 1 lower day LOS, and 1 less test performed per patient; 20% more diagnoses of NMS were made with less diagnosed as pseudosyncope or idiopathic.	No follow-up or prognosis data were collected, being out of the scope of this hypothesis. A potential bias could have been introduced from the different management styles from different hospitals involved in the study. The two groups were not randomized.	Strict adherence to society guidelines at point of care is necessary in this era of skyrocketing syncope costs, most of which are associated with hospitalization. Fewer tests, less LOS, and more diagnoses can thus be achieved.
Shen, et al. (SEEDS Study). *Circulation.* 2004;110:3636–3645.	Prospective, single-center RCT comparing patients evaluated in a syncope management unit (SMU) vs. standard care. The SMU provided 6 hours of telemetry, hourly vital signs and orthostatics, echocardiogram for abnormal exam or ECG, 45-minute tilt testing as indicated, carotid sinus massage was performed supine and upright during tilt testing. Finally, beat-to-beat HR and BP were continuously monitored.	51 patients evaluated in the SMU group, 52 in the standard care group; of the SMU group, a diagnosis was established in 67% vs. 10% in standard care; hospitalization was required for 43% in SMU group vs. 98% in standard care; finally, total patient hospital days were reduced from 140 to 64 using an SMU. Two-year survival was 97% in the SMU group and 90% in the standard care group; survival from recurrent syncope was identical.	Subjects and physicians were unblinded to the two treatment arms. A large number of patients declined to participate in the study and the study consequently was not powered to detect the original planned difference between groups. Cost-benefit analysis was not performed on this data.	A dedicated SMU is cost effective, safe, and a good consideration for large referral centers that can accommodate the concept, especially in evaluating intermediate-risk profile patients.

(continued)

TABLE 99-11 Evidence-based Medicine Key References for Syncope *(continued)*

Study	Methodology	Results	Limitations	Bottom Line
Mendu, et al. *Arch Intern Med.* 2009;169(14): 1299–1305.	Review of 2106 admissions for syncope at an acute care hospital from 2002–2006 was performed to determine what tests and how frequently they were done, what the associated costs were, and a calculation was performed to estimate the cost of each test per diagnosis obtained.	EEG had the highest cost per test affecting the diagnosis at $32,973. CT scan of the head cost $24,881, cardiac enzymes cost $22,397, and finally postural BP recording cost $17 per test affecting the diagnosis of syncope. Among patients meeting SFSR criteria (as above), yield and cost for cardiac tests were better, overall.	This is a retrospective analysis of data from a single center. Secondly, post-discharge tests such as ILR and tilt testing were not evaluated. The cost of hospitalization was not added to cost calculations in this study.	Careful selection of tests is imperative for the hospitalist managing syncope, given the often low diagnostic yield and ongoing financial burden of the U.S. health care system. Postural BP recording is the most cost-effective test available.

CHF, chronic heart failure; ECG, electrocardiogram; ED, emergency department; Hct, hematocrit; ILR, implantable loop recorder; MI, myocardial infarction; NMS, neuroleptic malignant syndrome; PE, pulmonary embolism; SAH, subarachnoid hemorrhage; SBP, systolic blood pressure; SFSR, San Francisco syncope rule.

SUGGESTED READINGS

Brignole M, Sutton R, Menozzi C, et al. International Study on Syncope of Uncertain Etiology (ISSUE 2) Group. Early application of an implantable loop recorder allows effective specific therapy in patients with recurrent suspected neurally mediated syncope. *Eur Heart J.* 2006;27(9):1085–1092.

Chen LY, Benditt DG, Shen WK. Management of Syncope in Adults: An Update. *Mayo Clin Proc.* 2008;83(11):1280–1293.

Mendu ML, McAvay G, Lampert R, Stoehr J, Tinetti ME. Yield of diagnostic tests in evaluating syncopal episodes in older patients. *Arch Intern Med.* 2009;169(14):1299–1305.

Moya A, Sutton R, Ammirati F. Guidelines for the diagnosis and management of syncope (version 2009). The Task Force for the Diagnosis and Management of Syncope of the European Society of Cardiology (ESC). *European Heart Journal.* 2009;30: 2631–2671.

Reed MJ, Newby DE, Coull AJ, Prescott RJ, Jacques KG, Gray AJ. The ROSE (Risk Stratification of Syncope in the Emergency Department) study. *J Am Coll Cardiol.* 2010;55:713–721.

Sarasin FP, Junod AF, Carballo D, et al. Role of echocardiography in the evaluation of syncope: a prospective study. *Heart.* 2002;88:363–367.

Schnipper J, Kapoor W. Diagnostic Evaluation and Management of Patients with Syncope. *Med Clin N Amer.* 2001;85(2):423–456.

Shen WK, Decker WW, Smars PA, et al. Syncope Evaluation in the Emergency Department Study (SEEDS): a multidisciplinary approach to syncope management. *Circulation.* 2004;110(24): 3636–3645.

Soteriades ES, Evans JC, Larson MG, et al. Incidence and prognosis of syncope. *N Engl J Med.* 2002;347:878–885.

CHAPTER 100

Tachyarrthymias

Sylvia C. McKean, MD, SFHM, FACP

Key Clinical Questions

1. How do you initially manage a patient with a hemodynamically unstable wide complex tachyarrhythmia?
2. What are the electrocardiographic features that suggest that a wide complex tachyarrhythmia is of ventricular origin?
3. What are the electrocardiographic features that suggest that a wide complex tachyarrhythmia is of supraventricular origin?
4. What is the differential diagnosis for short RP tachycardia? What is the differential diagnosis for long RP tachycardia?
5. Radiofrequency ablation often cures which tachycardias?

INTRODUCTION

This chapter will review the initial bedside approach to a hospitalized patient with a new, potentially life-threatening tachycardia, defined as a heart rate ≥ 100 beats per minute (bpm). The reader is then referred to the cardiology chapters for definitive management of specific arrhythmias.

Normally, the sinoatrial node spontaneously activates the right atrium, then the interatrial septum, and then the left atrium. The initial portion of the P wave represents depolarization of the right atrium and the last portion depolarization of the left atrium. Normally, the atrioventricular (AV) node, His bundle, and bundle branches transmit impulses anterogradely from the atria to the ventricles. The QRS complex represents ventricular depolarization and the ST-T-U complex represents repolarization (**Figure 100-1**).

Unlike the normal AV conducting pathway, anomalous bands of tissue—accessory pathways—may be able to conduct in both directions between the atria and ventricles in a retrograde and antegrade fashion. Some anomalous bands of tissue, concealed bypass tracts, can conduct in a retrograde direction only from the ventricles to the atria.

Supraventricular tachycardias (SVTs) include all tachycardias that arise above the bifurcation of the bundle of His or that have mechanisms depending on the bundle of His.

Paroxysmal supraventricular tachycardias usually have narrow complexes with a normal QRS duration of < 90 ms; some, however, may have aberrant conduction notable for a different QRS configuration from the baseline ECG. Intraventricular conduction disturbances may be incomplete (100–120 ms) or complete bundle branch blocks (QRS ≥ 120 ms in duration) and may be rate related. A right bundle branch block (RBBB) configuration is more common than a left bundle branch block (LBBB) aberrant pattern. The altered depolarization causes secondary repolarization ST-T abnormalities, discordance of QRS-T wave vectors. Ischemia, electrolyte disturbances, and digitalis cause primary depolarization ST-T abnormalities independent of the QRS vector. Sudden death from SVT is rare.

Ventricular tachycardia (VT) arises from the ventricles and is more likely to cause cardiac compromise and sudden death.

INITIAL APPROACH

CASE 100-1

POSTOPERATIVE TACHYCARDIA

A 65-year-old female with past medical history of hypertension, rheumatoid arthritis, osteoarthritis, and GERD underwent elective left total hip replacement.

After transfer to the floor, at 11:00 PM she had an asymptomatic 15-beat run of wide-complex tachycardia with a variable heart rate ranging from 60–120 beats per minute (bpm).

Initial data: Telemetry (**Figure 100-2**) showed a wide-complex tachycardia at a heart rate of 120.

Vital signs: Systolic blood pressure was 110–140 mm Hg, O_2 saturation 98–100% shovel mask, afebrile.

Is this patient hemodynamically stable?

Critical assessment of a tachyarrhythmia requires a determination of whether the patient has a potentially life-threatening arrhythmia.

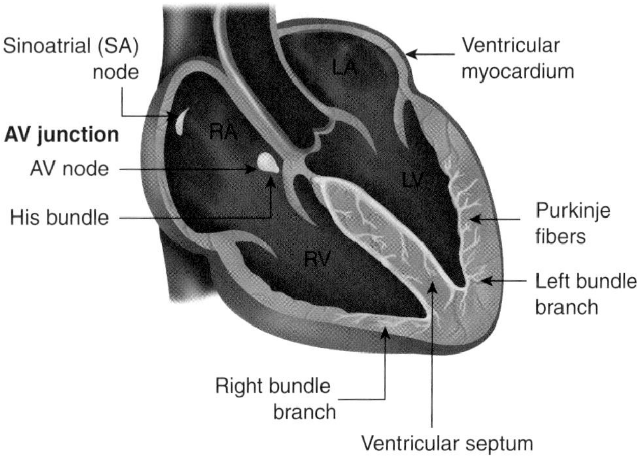

Figure 100-1 *Cardiac conduction system.*

The first step always begins with reviewing the patient's vital signs and identifying any artifacts that may have produced ECG findings mimicking cardiac arrhythmias. For example, motion artifact from muscle tremors or rigors may produce ECG changes that simulate cardiac tachyarrhythmias on a cardiac monitor tracing. When hemodynamic instability exists, VT is assumed as the cause of the wide-complex tachycardia, and clinicians should proceed promptly to direct-current cardioversion according to ACLS protocols (**Figure 100-3**).

PRACTICE POINT

- Critical assessment of a tachyarrhythmia requires a determination of whether the patient has a potentially life-threatening arrhythmia. The first step always begins with reviewing the patient's vital signs and identifying any artifacts that may have produced ECG findings mimicking cardiac arrhythmias. When hemodynamic instability exists, ventricular tachycardia is assumed as the cause of the wide-complex tachycardia, and clinicians should proceed directly to direct-current cardioversion according to advanced cardiac life support protocols.

In hemodynamically stable patients with sustained SVT, clinicians should try to determine the mechanism of the tachycardia before initiating treatment.

ECG INTERPRETATION

The goal of ECG interpretation is to identify the location of the ectopic impulse formation and to look for evidence of myocardial ischemia. (See Chapter 102: The Resting Electrocardiogram).

PRACTICE POINT

- The goal of ECG interpretation is to identify the location of the ectopic impulse formation and to look for evidence of myocardial ischemia.

Are the QRS complexes narrow or wide?

During the assessment of hemodynamic stability, clinicians examine the monitor strip to determine whether the QRS complex is narrow (<90 ms) or wide (> 90 ms). A SVT with intraventricular aberrant conduction, a SVT conducting to the ventricles over an accessory pathway, and a VT can all produce wide complex regular tachycardia. Distinguishing VT from SVT with aberrancy or SVT over an accessory pathway has important management implications.

Until proven otherwise, patients who have a wide QRS complex tachycardia and a history of structural heart disease (coronary artery disease or cardiomyopathy) are assumed to have VT. Application of the Brugada criteria may help differentiate VT from SVT with aberrant conduction, but requires interpretation of a 12-lead ECG.

PRACTICE POINT

Brugada criteria

- Using this criteria, VT is diagnosed on the basis of (1) absence of RS complex in all leads V_1–V_6; (2) the interval from the beginning of the R wave to the nadir of the S wave >0.1s in any RS lead; (3) presence of AV dissociation, fusion, or capture beats; and (4) morphology criteria for VT present in both leads V_1 and V_6.
- If none of these criteria are met, the diagnosis favors supraventricular tachycardia with aberration.

The presence of atrioventricular (AV) dissociation, fusion beats, and capture complexes generally favor the diagnosis of VT. AV dissociation, when the atrial and ventricular rhythms are independent of each other, is present when the P waves "march" through the tachycardic sequence and surface at the appropriate time interval after the last QRS complex of the tachycardia. The ventricular rate is greater than or equal to the atrial rate. The absence of P waves in up to 70% of the VT cases, should not, therefore, reassure the examiner that the arrhythmia is supraventricular in origin. In addition, AV dissociation may occur in the presence of an accelerated junctional rhythm that is faster than sinus rhythm and hence is not specific for VT (**Figure 100-4**).

Fusion beats, arising from simultaneous activation of the ventricle from two sources, have a QRS configuration that is intermediate between supraventricular and ventricular complexes, and arise when the ventricle is depolarized simultaneously via the normal conduction system and a ventricular focus (**Figure 100-5**).

A markedly widened QRS > 140 ms supports the diagnosis of VT, especially if associated with a left axis of the QRS complex in the

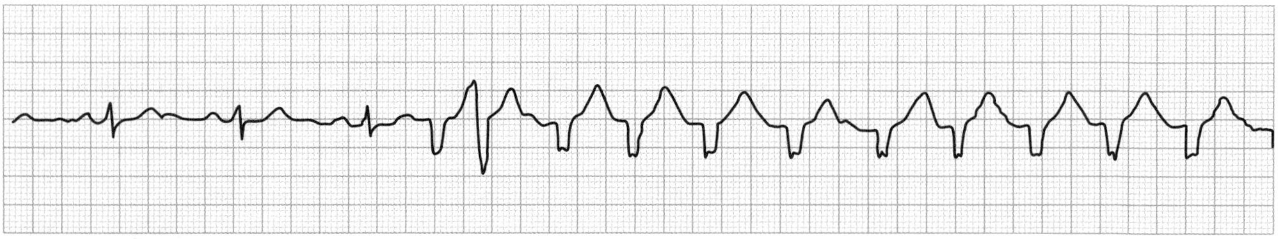

Figure 100-2 *Monitor tracing of the patient's heart rhythm showing wide complex tachycardia.*

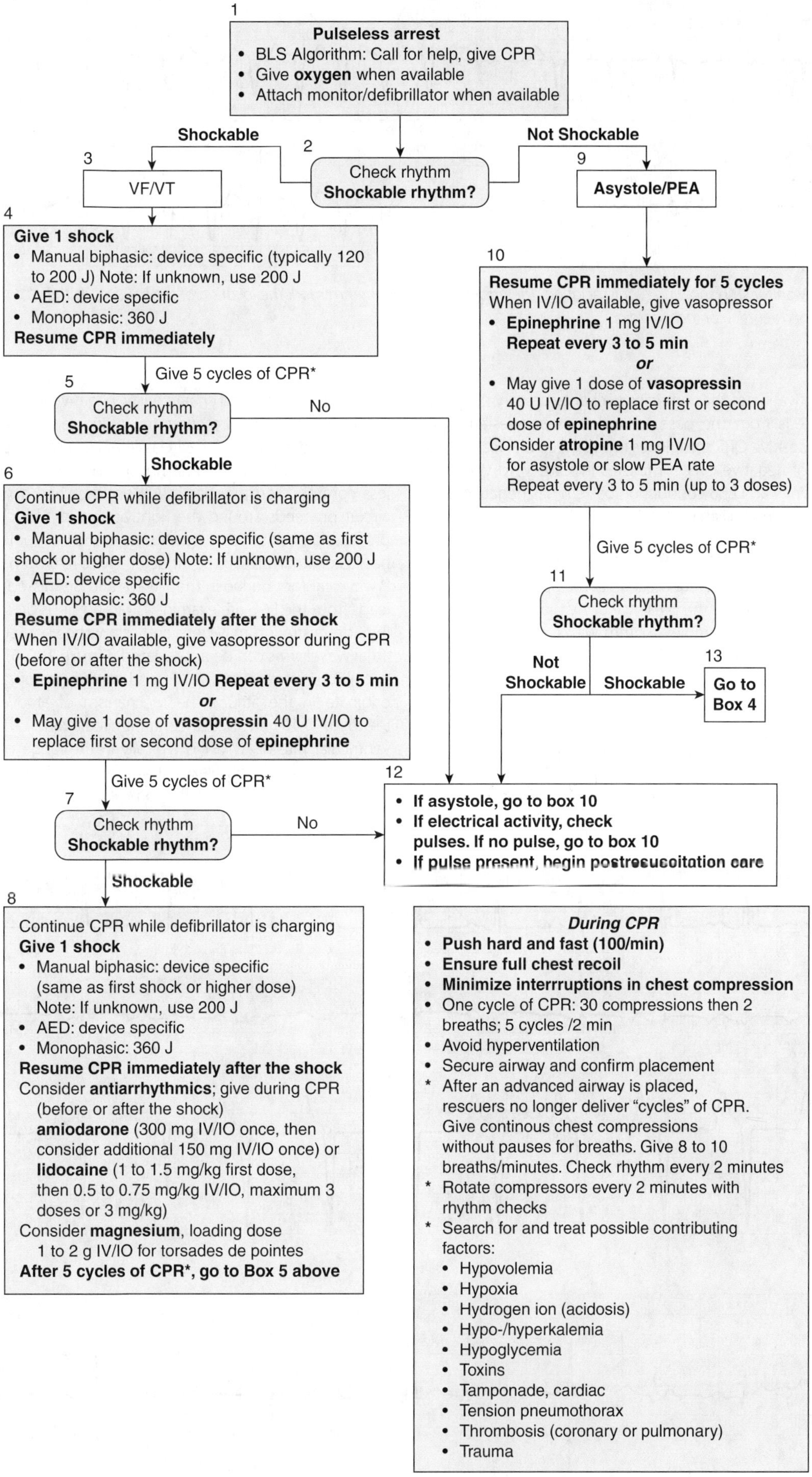

Figure 100-3 *ACLS algorithm for Ventricular Tachycardia.*

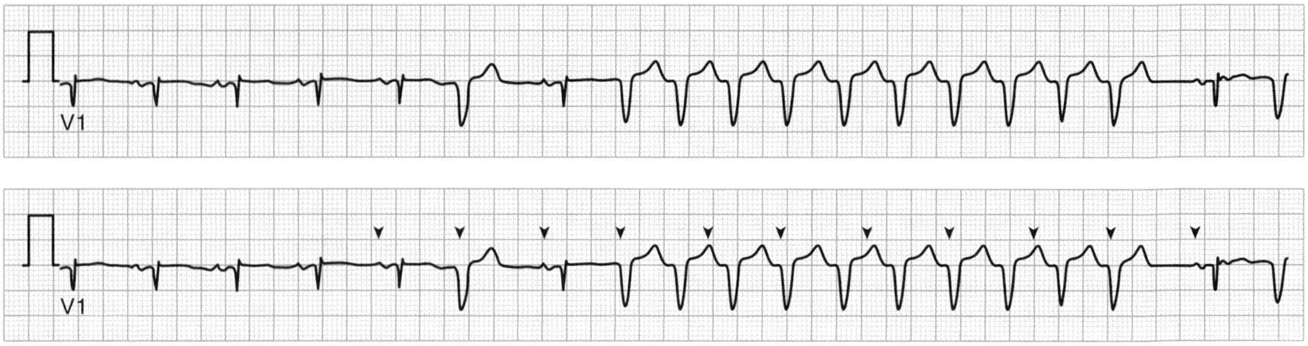

Figure 100-4 *Monitor strip showing AV dissociation. The arrows above the rhythm mark the location of the P waves as they "march" through the run of nonsustained ventricular tachycardia.*

frontal plane. Activation of the ventricles over an accessory pathway generally proceeds from the base toward the apex resulting in predominantly positive QRS complexes in the precordial leads V_4 to V_6. The finding of negative QRS complexes in leads V_4 to V_6 makes VT more likely, since an LBBB conduction pattern has negative QRS complexes in these leads (**Table 100-1**).

What is the rate of the tachycardia based on the R-R interval?

In patients with SVT, the heart rate must be ≥ 100 bpm but ventricular rates can be lower due to the presence of AV block. Sinus tachycardia is a regular narrow complex rhythm with a rate > 100 bpm. P waves are usually visible unless the rate is so rapid that they are buried in the T waves. Physiologic stress commonly causes sinus tachycardia, which should lessen with treatment of the underlying problem (such as postoperative pain, hypovolemia from blood loss or insufficient oral intake, sepsis, or withdrawal states).

Most patients with atrial flutter (AFl) have an atrial rate around 300 beats per minute, so with 2:1 conduction, the ventricular rate will be about 150 bpm and characteristic negatively directed "sawtooth" atrial waveforms are present in the inferior leads. The mechanism of this common form of Type I classic AFl is a macro reentrant circuit around the entire right atrium in a counterclockwise direction. A less common form of classic AFl occurs when a macro reentrant circuit proceeds around the right atrium in a clockwise direction, producing positive atrial waveforms in the inferior leads. Type II AFl has faster atrial rates in the range of 340 to 440 bpm. Sometimes the P wave can get buried in the T wave and be missed unless multiple leads from the ECG are examined. Carotid sinus pressure or adenosine administration may transiently slow the ventricular rate so that atrial waveforms can be appreciated (**Figure 100-6**).

Unlike sinus tachycardia, AFl, and other types of tachycardias that originate in the atrium, the mechanism of atrioventricular nodal reentry (AVNRT) involves a reentrant circuit within the AV node. The ventricular rate of AVNRT is typically in the range of 150–250 bpm with narrow QRS complexes. If visible, the P wave appears at the terminal portion of the QRS complex, reflecting retrograde atrial

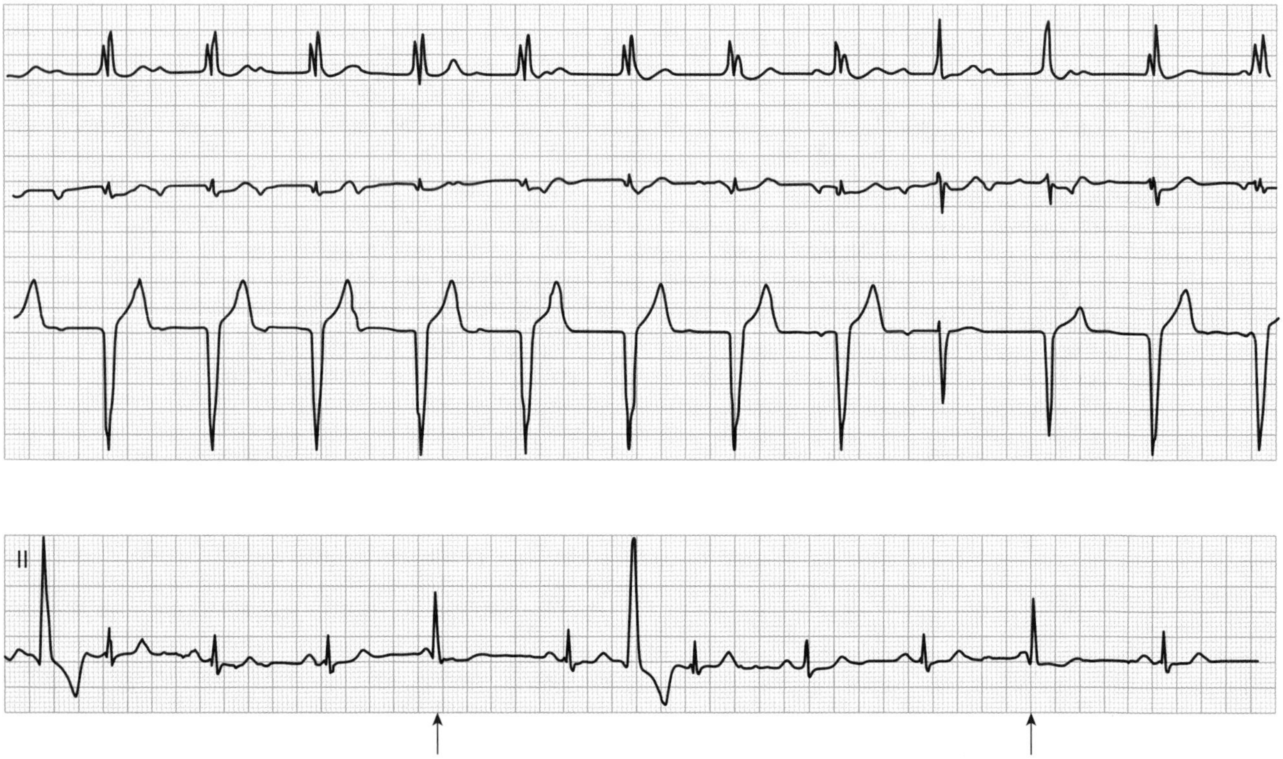

Figure 100-5 *Fusion beats and capture complexes.*

TABLE 100-1 Likelihood of VT Versus SVT with Aberrancy

Ventricular Tachycardia More Likely...	SVT with Aberrancy More Likely...
Hemodynamic instability or cardiac compromise	Hemodynamic stability
Structural heart disease	Patients with normal hearts
Wide complex tachycardia > 0.14 s in duration AV dissociation, capture, and/or fusion beats	Narrow QRS
Extreme axis deviation (leftward or northwest)	Similar QRS morphology to QRS during normal sinus rhythm or during an aberrantly conducted APC
Atypical bundle branch block	Presence of P waves
Ventricular concordance	Typical bundle branch block (<0.14 sec if RBBB; <0.16 sec if LBBB) if narrow QRS during sinus rhythm
Prolonged QT interval Tachyarrhythmia initiated by a VPC	Ventricular discordance (some QRS deflections in precordial leads positive, some negative)
	Tachyarrhythmia initiated by an APC
VPC	APC
QRS duration is almost always > 0.12 sec	Premature P wave relative to the normal PP interval with different morphology from sinus P wave.
No P waves precede the complex, which is premature relative to the normal RR interval; retrograde capture of the atria may occur.	QRS morphology similar to QRS complex in sinus rhythm or may be aberrant (most often RBBB pattern).
Initial direction of QRS often different from the QRS during sinus rhythm.	Typically the postextrasystolic pause noncompensatory (premature P to subsequent P wave interval < two PP intervals).
Secondary ST T wave changes in opposite direction of major deflection of QRS.	
May be associated with complete, incomplete, or no compensatory pause if VPC interpolated. A compensatory pause is defined as the RR interval containing the VPC = 2x the normal RR interval.	
Supraventricular beats with aberrancy less likely if	
... No P waves precede QRS	
... An LBBB pattern in V_1	
... A compensatory pause	
... RP interval > 0.20 seconds when there is retrograde atrial activation	

depolarization. In atrioventricular reentrant tachycardia (AVRT) atrial depolarization occurs later than in AVNRT so that the P waves may appear superimposed on the ST segment or T wave. Atrial tachycardia or AVRT is much less common than AVNRT (**Figure 100-7**).

Is the rhythm regular or irregular based on the R-R interval?

Sinus tachycardia, AFl with consistent AV conduction such as 2:1 block, AVNRT, AVRT, and atrial tachycardia cause regular tachyarrythmias. Atrial fibrillation (AF), multifocal atrial tachycardia (MAT), and tachyarrythmias due to multiple anterograde AV nodal pathways cause irregularly irregular rhythms (**Figures 100-8** to **100-10**). MAT may be distinguished from sinus tachycardia with frequent multifocal atrial premature complexes because it does not have one dominant atrial pacemaker. MAT may be identified by ectopic P waves of at least three morphologies best seen in leads II, III, and V_1, a ventricular rate of > 100 bpm, isoelectric baseline

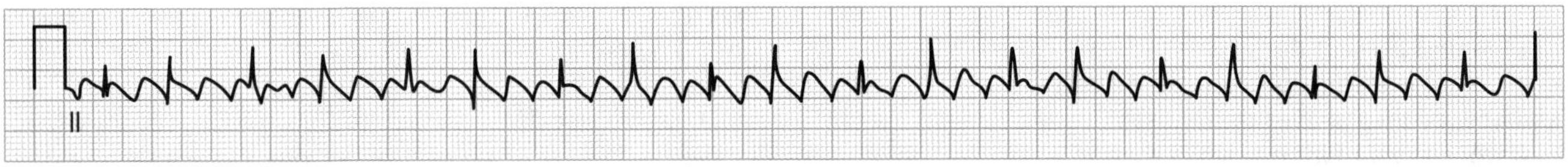

Figure 100-6 *A macroreentrant circuit in the right atrium causes atrial flutter "sawtooth" waveforms accompanied by an atrial rate that varies between 280 and 340 beat/minutes.*

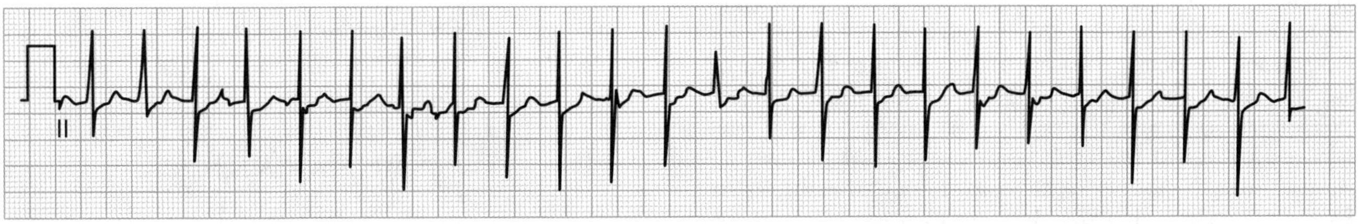

Figure 100-7 *A narrow QRS complex tachycardia in the range of 150 to 250 beats/min, often with P waves inscribed at the terminal portion of the QRS complex and reflecting retrograde atrial depolarization.*

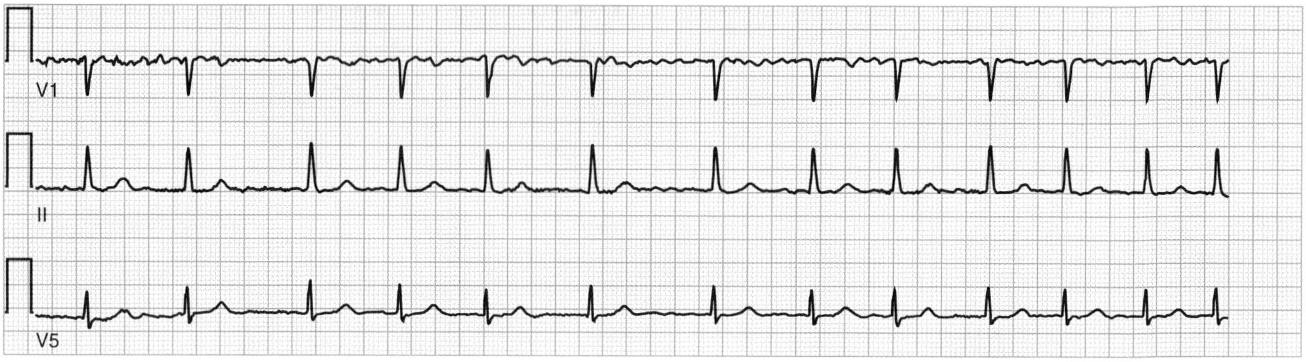

Figure 100-8 *An irregularly irregularly narrow complex tachycardia consistent with atrial fibrillation often associated with physiologic stress.*

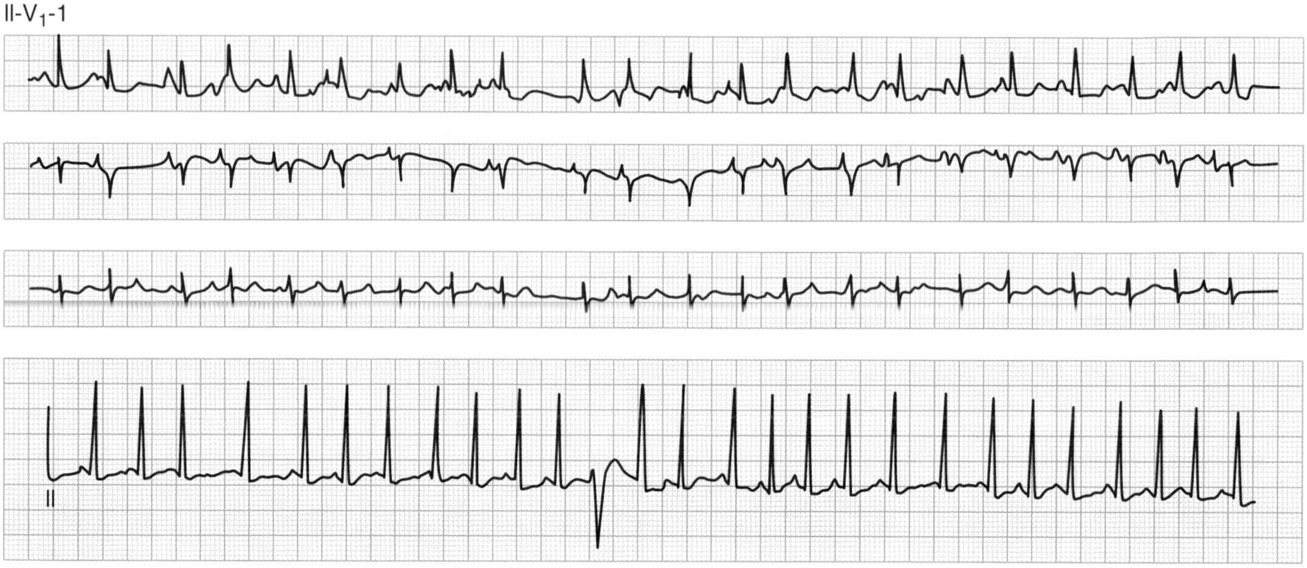

Figure 100-9 *MAT.*

between P waves, and varying PP, PR, and RR intervals. Some P waves may be blocked due to their rapid rate. Atrial tachycardias with variable AV block may also appear irregular. It is sometimes helpful to look for discrete RR intervals that have a common divisor, as for example, a rate of 150 bpm for some sequences and 100 bpm for others consistent with AFl with variable block (2:1 and 3:1 with a stable atrial rate of 300 bpm) (**Table 100-2**).

Are P waves present during the tachyarrhythmia? If yes, what is the morphology of the P waves and how do the P waves compare to the baseline ECG when the patient is in sinus rhythm?

The next step is to identify the presence of atrial activity and to examine the relationship between the P wave and the QRS complex. The P waves may be embedded at the end of the QRS complexes or within the T wave; therefore, it is important to compare the tracing to prior ECGs to examine for changes in the QRS and T wave morphology. The normal P wave is 0.08 to 0.11 seconds in duration and is always upright in leads I and II and always negative in lead aVR. It is usually upright in lead aVF. In lead III the normal P wave may be positive, negative, or biphasic and in lead aVL the normal P wave is usually negative or biphasic. In leads V_1 and V_2 the normal P wave is often biphasic and is always positive in leads V_3 to V_6.

Inferior leads, especially lead II and lead V_1 are most helpful places to start although all leads should be examined for P waves. Ectopic atrial rhythms may have upright P waves arising from an atrial focus near the sinus node or inverted arising from an ectopic focus in the lower atrium. The location of the ectopic focus relative to the AV conduction system and the presence or absence of delay in this system determines the duration of the PR interval (whether short, normal, or prolonged). The QT interval (representing the duration of ventricular depolarization and repolarization) is typically normal in ectopic rhythms. Ectopic P waves will have a different morphology from sinus P waves and may be easier to identify if there is an earlier ECG tracing of sinus rhythm used as a reference. If the right atrium is activated first, as in sinus rhythm, the P wave is positive or biphasic in lead aVL and negative or biphasic in lead V_1. If the left atrium is activated first, the P wave is negative or isoelectric in lead

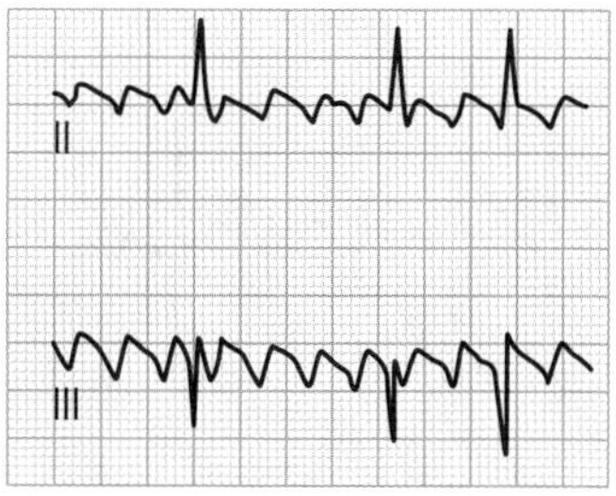

Figure 100-10 *Type 1 Aflutter with variable block.*

TABLE 100-2 Tachyarrythmias

Rhythm	Typical Rate	Predisposing Conditions	Electrical Physiology	Initial Management
Sinus tachycardia	Regular Normal p wave axis; P wave amplitude often increases and PR interval often shortens with increasing heart rate; Ventricular rate > 100 bpm; Narrow complex	Underlying disorder, hypermetabolic state or systemic stressor (anemia, fever, hypovolemia), drug effect	Sinus node the one dominant atrial pacemaker; Rapid narrow complexes usually similar to patient's baseline; PR interval may be short, normal, or prolonged	Treat underlying problem
Sinus node reentrant tachycardia (identical P waves to sinus P waves)	Regular ventricular rate > 100 bpm; abrupt onset and end; narrow complex	Rare	Reentry circuit involving sinoatrial node	
Unifocal atrial tachycardia	Regular rhythm with atrial rate usually < 250 and typically 150–240 bpm unlike AFl; Single P wave morphology; P wave axis or morphology different from the sinus node; Isoelectric intervals in all leads; Ventricular rate > 100 bpm.	Rare; structural heart disease may cause abnormal atrial refractoriness and conduction if reentry; digitalis intoxication	Arises from atria excluding SA node—either from enhanced automaticity or reentry; Paroxysmal if reentrant mechanism; incessant if enhanced automaticity.	
Multifocal atrial tachycardia (MAT)	Atrial rate at least 100 bpm; P waves with > three different morphologies; varying PR, RR, RP intervals; isoelectric baseline between P waves unlike AF	Acutely ill, with severe pulmonary or cardiac disease or postoperative state, infected, diabetic; very low K^+ and Mg^{+++}	Likely enhanced automaticity; MAT does not require AV conduction and may persist during AV block.	Treat underlying illness; replete K^+ and Mg^{+++}; rate control; digoxin of no value; cardioversion ineffective
Atrial flutter	Atrial rate of 240–340 bpm usually with 2:1 AV block; QRS may be normal or aberrant; rate and regularity depend on AV conduction; absent distinct isoelectric baseline (except V_1)	Usually underlying disease present (heart or lung); if no underlying cardiopulmonary disease, rule out PE and thyroid disease	Usually due to reentry around tricuspid valve in the right atrium; unstable rhythm	Low energy electrical cardioversion if patient hemodynamically unstable; vagal maneuvers slow rate
Atrial fibrillation	Absent P waves; Atrial activity irregular with fibrillatory waves of varying amplitude, duration, morphology causing random baseline oscillation; Ventricular rate of 130–200 bpm with an irregularly irregular rhythm If rate > 200 bpm & QRS > 0.12 s varying in width, consider WPW	Atrial enlargement due to any cause including mitral valve disease, dilated cardiomyopathy, hypertrophic cardiomyopathy, CAD; lung disease, hyperthyroidism, low Mg^{+++}, alcoholism, cocaine, physiologic stress	Likely increased automaticity and multiple reentrant wavelets predominantly in the left atrium around the pulmonary veins; ventricular rate may regularize in digitalis toxicity but atrial activity remains totally irregular	Rate control; electrical cardioversion if unstable
Ashman phenomenon	AF with a run of wide complex beats beginning with the shortest RR interval seen following a narrow complex; may be difficult to distinguish from VT Short R-R following a longer R-R		Conduction of the atrial impulse during relative refractoriness of the ventricular fascicles. Aberrancy common due to variable ventricular cycle lengths.	
WPW	Most asymptomatic with no dysrhythmias; ventricular rate usually ≈190 bpm when WPW and narrow complex tachycardia; may be associated with AFl and AF; interval from beginning of the P wave to end of QRS constant	Congenital – Ebstein anomaly – and acquired.	Bypass tract (Kent bundle) faster than AV node, a portion of electrical current reaches ventricle sooner (delta wave). PR interval < 0.12 s due to delta wave; delta wave may not be visible if accessory pathway concealed. QRS > 0.12 s due to fusion of normal QRS and bypass current	Electrical cardioversion if hemodynamic instability; ventricular rates > 285 at greatest risk of degenerating to VF

(continued)

TABLE 100-2 Tachyarrythmias (*continued*)

Rhythm	Typical Rate	Predisposing Conditions	Electrical Physiology	Initial Management
Junctional tachycardia	Rates usually between 100–120 bpm; nonparoxysmal; regular narrow QRS complex with either AV dissociation or 1:1 ventriculoatrial activation	Acute MI, after cardiac surgery, critically ill receiving pressors; digitalis intoxication, acute rheumatic fever	Enhanced impulse formation in the region of the lower AV nodal His bundle junction.	
Ventricular tachycardia	Three or more premature ventricular beats at a rate > 100 per minute in rapid succession; RR intervals usually regular but can be irregular; AV dissociation, capture and fusion beats, extreme axis deviation, atypical bundle branch block, prolonged QT interval; abrupt onset and end	Structural heart disease; hemodynamic instability or cardiac compromise	Brugada criteria: AV dissociation; RS complex absent in V_1–V_6; R to S interval >100 ms in any precordial lead; morphology criteria for VT in V_1–V_2 & V_6	

aVL and lead V_1. Negative P waves in the inferior leads are seen in AVNRT and AVRT and atrial tachycardias that originate in the lower atrium.

When ectopic P waves precede the QRS complex, even if the QRS complex is wide, the tachycardia is supraventricular. If retrograde P waves (inverted in lead II and upright in lead aVR) precede the QRS complex, even if the QRS complex is wide, the tachycardia is also supraventricular in origin. When ectopic P waves follow the QRS complexes, the origin of the tachyarrhythmia may be either supraventricular from the AV junction or ventricular. Tachycardia arising from the AV node more commonly has narrow QRS complexes. However, AV junctional tachycardia may be associated with aberrant conduction causing a wide QRS complex tachycardia.

If P waves are present, what is the R-P interval?

This requires examination of the ECG waveform and intervals to identify the presence of P waves that may be superimposed on the QRS complex or on the ST segment. If the rhythm strip is V_1 for example, it may show both P waves and R waves and is therefore sufficient to determine the R-P interval. If retrograde P waves are located farther from the preceding QRS complex than the following QRS complex, then the tachycardia is a long R-P tachycardia. Sinus tachycardia is a long R-P tachycardia. Sinus tachycardia can be difficult to identify when the P wave fuses with the T wave of the preceding QRS complex. This situation usually occurs in critically ill patients with heart rates greater than 180 bpm, patients receiving pressors, or when there has been significant volume loss. Visible P waves would be expected to be upright in ECG leads I, II, III, and aVF (**Table 100-3**).

Sinus nodal reentrant tachycardia appears identical to sinus tachycardia with the exception that the initiation and termination of the rapid rhythm is abrupt. The mean heart rate is typically 130–140 bpm. Carotid sinus massage or valsalva may terminate sinus nodal reentrant tachycardia and gradual slowing may precede termination.

Other than sinus tachycardia, atrial tachycardia is the most common long R-P tachycardia. AV block may occur without interrupting the tachycardia because the AV node is not an integral part of the arrhythmia circuit. An ectopic atrial tachycardia with 2:1 block may be identified by finding a second P wave buried in the terminal portion of the QRS complex in the inferior leads. In this case measurement of the timing of deflections will demonstrate that they occur exactly halfway between the more visible P waves (**Figure 100-11**).

Suspect digitalis intoxication if paroxysmal tachycardia is associated with AV block.

CASE 100-1 *(continued)*

POSTOPERATIVE TACHYCARDIA

Per OR notes: In the operating room this patient received 4 liters of IV fluids with no intraoperative hypotension or tachycardia. Estimated blood loss was approximately 1 liter. Subsequently, in the recovery room she was noted to be hypoxic as O_2 sat declined to 70% while receiving 4 liters of nasal oxygen while sleeping and was administered 100% NRB mask with improvement of her oxygenation level to ≥ 96%.

The covering team rapidly assessed the patient's airway, breathing and circulation, placed pads on the patient and brought a defibrillator to the bedside.

Her baseline ECG (**Figure 100-12**) was notable for sinus bradycardia, heart rate 54 beats per minute, normal intervals, normal axis, normal R wave progression, and no ST-T abnormalities. There may have been some slight slurring of the QRS in the precordial leads but normal PR interval and QRS duration. The baseline ECG was officially read by a cardiologist as normal.

History of present illness: She did not have a prior history of arrhythmia, coronary artery disease, or cardiomyopathy. She denied any chest pain, palpitations, shortness of breath, lightheadedness, dizziness, syncope, or diaphoresis. She had no history of substance abuse, including alcohol.

On review of systems her only complaints related to her recent hip surgery. She had no history of vascular disease.

Review of her home medications and her current medications were notable for her blood pressure medications (atenolol, lisinopril, and hydrochlorothiazide), extended release bupropion, calcium, vitamin D, omeprazole with new medications including enoxaparin, warfarin, ciprofloxacin, and hydromorphone via a patient controlled analgesia (PCA).

TABLE 100-3 RP Intervals

SHORT RP tachycardia (RP interval < ½ the RR interval)
Typical AVNRT (AV nodal reentry tachycardia)
… a reentrant circuit that goes down the slow conduction pathway of the AV node and up the fast conduction pathway
… retrograde P wave results after impulse travels up fast pathway typically at terminal portion of QRS complex.
Orthodromic AVRT (Atrioventricular reentrant tachycardia)
… a circuit that goes down the AV node to the His-purkinje system to the ventricles and then retrograde up the accessory pathway to the atria
… retrograde p wave more likely embedded within ST-T wave segment due to longer time it takes to complete the longer circuit than typical AVNRT circuit
Atrial tachycardia with first degree AV delay Junctional tachycardia
If no P wave seen, likely embedded within QRS complex and therefore Short RP tachycardia
Long RP tachycardia (RP interval > ½ the RR interval)
Sinus tachycardia
Atypical AVNRT
… a reentrant circuit that goes down the fast conduction pathway and up the slow pathway
… longer RP interval due to longer time it takes for p wave to form relative to ventricular depolarization
Atrial tachycardia
PJRT (permanent junctional reciprocating tachycardia)
… a reentrant circuit that involves atria, AV node and His-Purkinje system, ventricles, and a serpiginous posteroseptal accessory pathway
… retrograde conduction delayed sufficiently to produce long RP tachycardia
Sinus node reentry tachycardia
Treatment
Maneuvers (vagal, adenosine or other nodal blocking agents)
… any tachycardia involving a reentrant circuit through AV node
Radiofrequency ablation to break abnormal conduction
… slow pathway of the AV node (AVNRT)
… accessory pathway (AVRT)
… slow conducting isthmus of atrial tissue between the IVC and tricuspid annulus (AFl)
… posteroseptal accessory pathway (PJRT)

Physical examination: The patient was alert, oriented, and able to respond appropriately to questioning. The rest of her exam was notable for a difficult -to- assess JVP, distant heart sounds, absence of murmur, and clear lungs. No bruits were appreciated.

Is the mode of onset and termination of the tachycardia captured on the ECG?

Premature atrial complexes (PAC) trigger most paroxysmal supraventricular tachycardias. Ventricular premature complexes (VPC) usually trigger AV node-dependent tachycardias.

Is there a baseline ECG?

If the patient is stable, obtain a 12-lead ECG to look for any changes from the baseline ECG that might suggest cardiac ischemia and for the presence of preexisting bundle block (Figure 100-12). Is there evidence of a prolonged QT interval, AV dissociation, capture and fusion beats, extreme axis deviation, atypical bundle branch block that might suggest preexisting structural heart disease increasing the likelihood of a ventricular origin to the tachycardia? Although uncommon, ECG changes suggestive of Wolf-Parkinson-White (WPW), prolonged or shortened QT interval, R precordial ST abnormalities characteristic of the Brugada syndrome, and epsilon waves seen in arrhythmogenic RV dysplasia in the baseline ECG have important management implications.

A baseline ECG may allow for comparison of the QRS complexes during the tachycardia with the configuration of isolated ectopic beats preceding the tachycardia. If preexcitation is apparent during normal sinus rhythm, the tachycardia is preexcited. Isolated atrial premature beats may lead to atrial group beats, atrial tachycardia, atrial fibrillation (AF), or atrial flutter (AFl). When the atrial tachyarrhythmias terminate, isolated atrial premature contractions may follow. Likewise, when the QRS configuration during isolated ventricular premature contractions before and after the tachycardia is identical to that present during the tachycardia, the origin of the tachycardia is ventricular.

NEXT STEPS

ADDITIONAL DATA

For hemodynamically stable patients, physicians should perform a targeted history and physical examination specifically looking for signs and symptoms of significant heart and lung disease as well as vascular disease. Symptoms are more common in patients with structural heart disease. The neck veins should be examined for the presence of cannon A-waves that match the rate of tachycardia due to atrial contraction during ventricular systole when

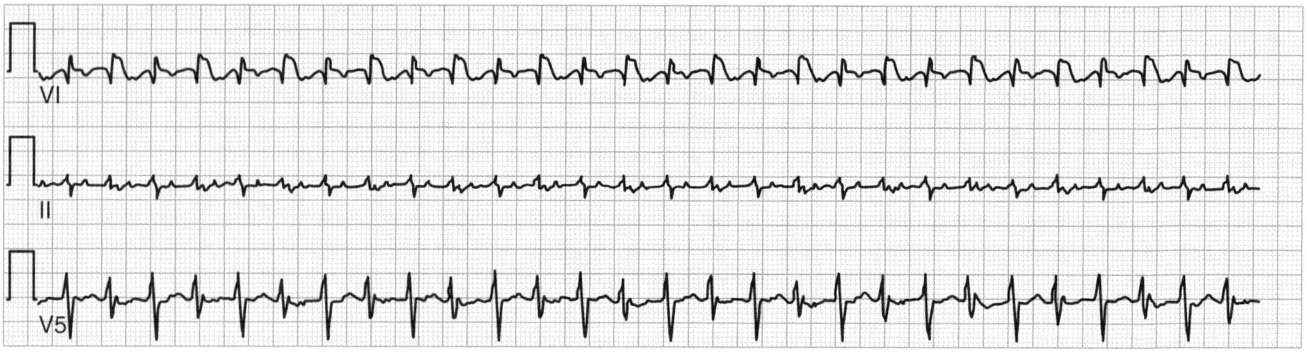

Figure 100-11 *Atrial tachycardia is characterized by a P-wave axis or morphology that is distinct from that of sinus rhythm, generally 150 to 250 beats/minute, characteristically slower than that of atrial flutter.*

the tricuspid valve is closed. Canon A-waves would not occur in sinus tachycardia, ectopic atrial tachycardia, or atrial flutter. Their presence does not differentiate the two principal types of AV reentrant tachycardia. Less commonly, cannon A-waves may occur in VT when retrograde AV conduction depolarizes the atria during ventricular systole.

For the postoperative patient, electrolytes, cardiac enzymes, and complete blood count should be obtained in addition to a resting ECG. Oxygen should be administered as necessary and continuous ECG monitoring should be provided (**Figure 100-13**).

CASE 100-1 *(continued)*

POSTOPERATIVE TACHYCARDIA

Initial intervention: Ventricular tachycardia (VT) is the most common cause of a wide-complex tachycardia and initial assessment included evaluation of hemodynamic stability and examining the 12-lead ECG for hallmarks of VT. Given the absence of known structural heart disease, stable vital signs, and absence of characteristic ECG features of VT, the clinicians felt that she most likely had a SVT with aberrant conduction.

Although she had no hallmarks suggestive of ventricular tachycardia seen on 12-lead ECG and her QT-interval was normal, upon arrival to the floor the consultant administered magnesium 2 gm IV as a one time dose just in case her arrhythmia was ventricular in origin. The patient received pain medication and also aspirin 325 mg in case the LBBB configuration signified occult coronary artery disease. This patient denied any history of vascular disease, and on physical examination she did not have a carotid bruit on either side. Maneuvers were attempted to prolong AV nodal refractoriness to the point of AV block.

Attempt to elucidate the underlying mechanism by slowing or terminating the tachycardia

The treatment options for tachycardia depend on identification of the underlying mechanism. An acutely ill patient may have difficulty performing the Valsalva maneuver, a maintained forced expiratory effort against a closed glottis, correctly. The examiner may give the patient simple instructions to insert his index finger in his mouth, close his mouth around his finger, and exhale into a closed space. Ausculation for carotid bruits prior to performing carotid massage is a reasonable but very imprecise way to determine whether cerebrovascular disease is present, but most experts would avoid carotid massage if they identified a cervical bruit. The Valsalva maneuver, carotid sinus massage, and facial immersion in cold water did not slow down or terminate the tachycardia in this patient.

Adenosine potently blocks AV conduction transiently and would be expected to terminate AVNRT but not sinus tachycardia, atrial tachycardia, atrial flutter, or nonparoxysmal junctional tachycardia. Before administering adenosine, physicians should specifically inquire about a history of asthma or reversible COPD and whether the patient is receiving dipyridamole. Adenosine can trigger acute

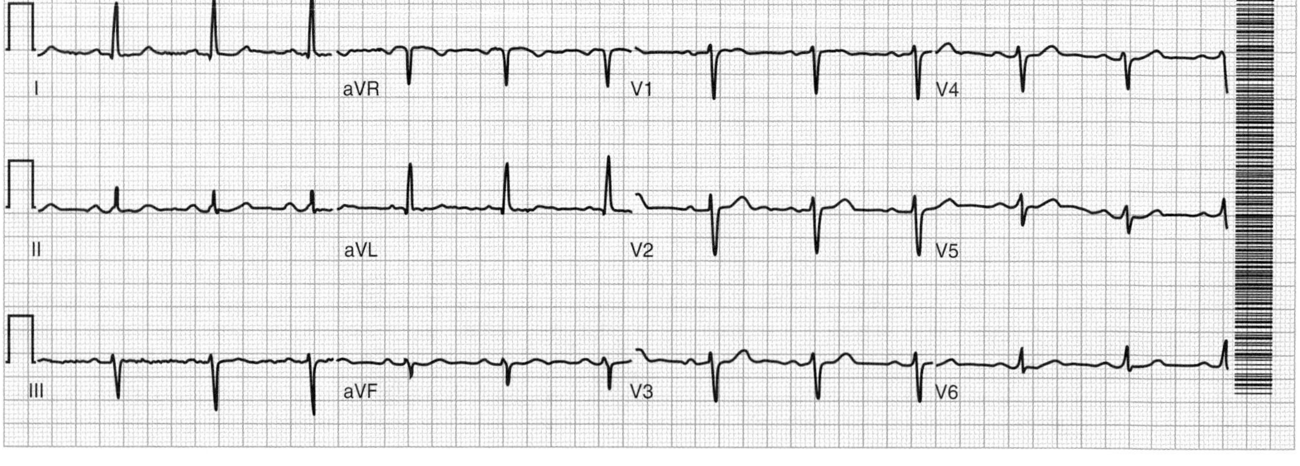

Figure 100-12 *Baseline ECG.*

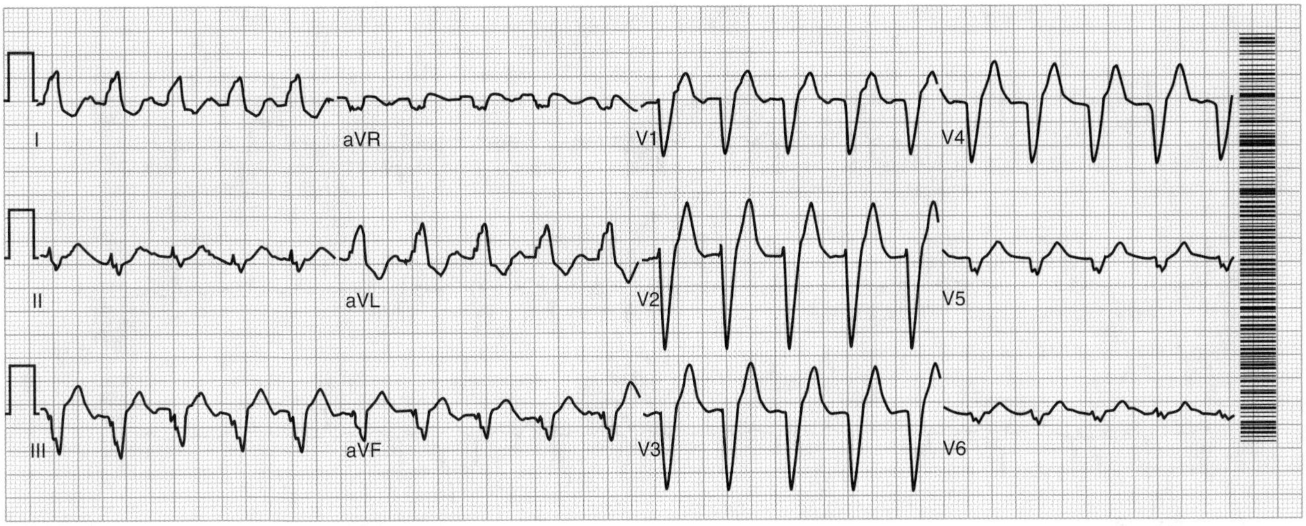

Figure 100-13 *Postoperative Sinus Tachycardia.*

bronchospasm in vulnerable patients and dipyridamole can potentiate AV block. At the time of administration, they should also warn the patient about transient sensations of chest tightness, nausea, and flushing.

CASE 100-1 *(continued)*

POSTOPERATIVE TACHYCARDIA

The wide complex tachycardia on 12-lead ECG was notable for a regular heart rate of 118, a wide complex QRS with LBBB morphology, left axis deviation, with no visible P waves and no ST-T abnormalities. Neither her baseline ECG nor this ECG demonstrated the hallmarks of WPW. A new small R wave in lead V_1 in the ECG with wide complex tachycardia but not present in the V_1 lead in the same patient in sinus rhythm would suggest atrial activation that occurs at the same time as the last portion of the QRS and extends into the ST segment. Such a pseudo-R would suggest AVNRT as the most likely diagnosis. It was not present in this case. Because this patient did not appear to have an AVNRT as the explanation of her wide-complex tachycardia, adenosine was not administered.

The clinician decided to initially administer a β-blocker to control this patient's heart rate. If there was any concern as to whether she would tolerate β-blockers, esmolol could be used. The patient received metoprolol 5 mg IV, three doses with some improvement in her heart rate (down to the 110 range) without a detrimental effect on blood pressure. She then received a calcium channel blocker, diltiazem 10 mg IV, which further slowed her heart rate to 100. Although the wide complex tachycardia persisted, P waves became visible at the slower rate before every QRS complex consistent with a SVT. She soon converted to sinus rhythm in the 50–60 beats per minute range (**Figure 100-14**).

Her 12-lead ECG (**Figure 100-15**) showed narrow QRS complexes, normal axis and intervals, without ST-T wave changes. The only change was poor R-wave progression through the precordial leads from her preoperative ECG. Her laboratory tests revealed a normal potassium of 4.1 mEq/L, magnesium of 1.5 mEq/L, negative troponin, and stable hematocrit of 28.9%. Her CPK was 655 U/L with a CKMB of 6.3%. Arterial blood gas on 40% shovel mask was reported as pH 7.38, pCO_2 45 mm Hg, pO_2 81 mm Hg.

Intravenous administration of nodal blockers may reduce the ventricular rate and alleviate distressing symptoms despite persistence of the tachycardia. Nondihydropyridine calcium-channel blockers are preferable to adenosine in patients with atrial tachycardia. However, adenosine and calcium-channel blockers should be avoided in patients who have AF with an anterogradely conducting accessory pathway since slowing the native pathway may precipitate conduction down the accessory pathway, thereby increasing the ventricular rate. For surgical patients already taking a beta-blocker, the negative inotropic effects of calcium channel blockers may be accentuated.

ASSESSMENT OF THE POSTOPERATIVE PATIENT WITH TACHYCARDIA

In a postoperative patient, sinus tachycardia is common due to the adrenergic drive that develops as a result of hypotension, volume shifts, acute blood loss, pain and/or anxiety.

AVNRT typically occurs in otherwise healthy patients without valvular heart disease or organic heart disease. However, it may occur slightly more often in patients when underlying structural heart disease is present, possibly because these patients are more likely

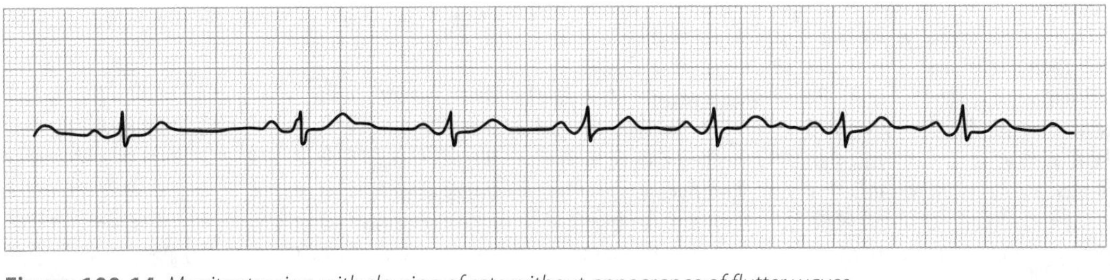

Figure 100-14 *Monitor tracing with slowing of rate without appearance of flutter waves.*

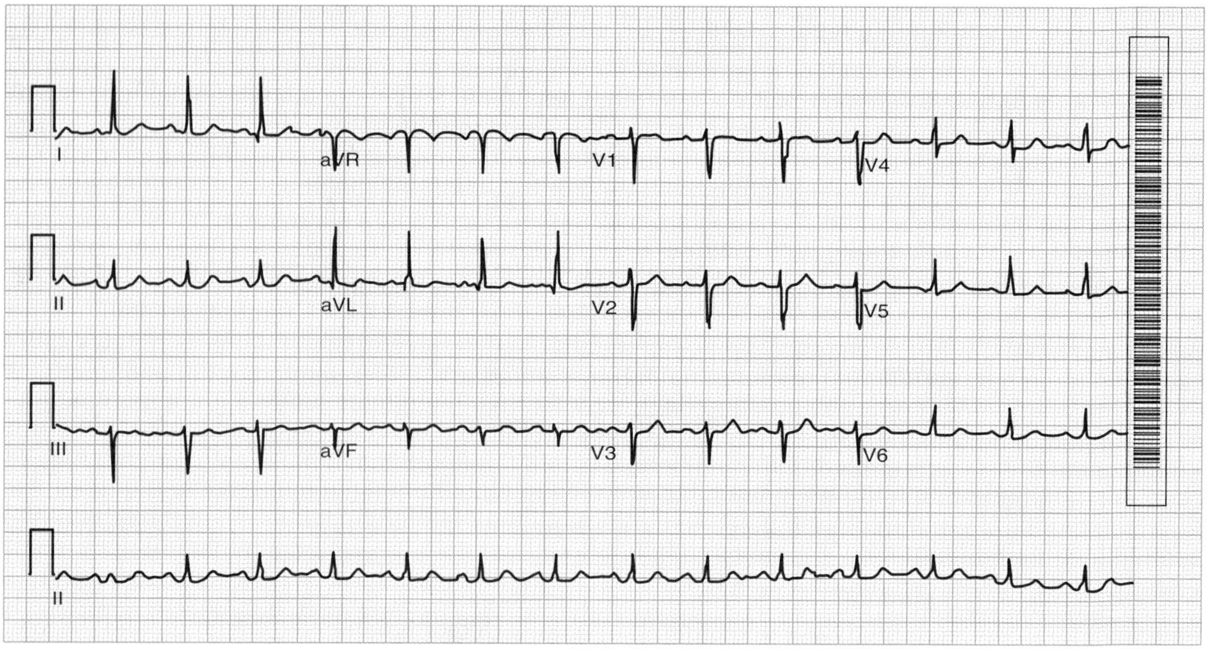

Figure 100-15 *ECG prior to discharge with resolution of rate related LBBB pattern.*

to have atrial or ventricular premature beats that can precipitate individual episodes of tachycardia.

In this patient, the tachycardia was mostly regular although at times appeared slightly irregular as well. The cycle length in most cases of paroxysmal SVT is regular although it may vary in a patient with more than one anterograde AV nodal pathway. Variable block in the AV node can produce a notably irregular ventricular rate in patients with atrial tachycardias.

Tachycardia-contingent bundle branch block may occur if either the right- or left-sided bundle branch reaches its effective refractory period and cannot conduct impulses to match the rapid rate of the tachycardia. In a patient with paroxysmal SVT-related wide complex tachycardia and a structurally normal heart, the bundle branch pattern will usually have a typical appearance, identical to conventional bundle branch morphology.

A change in AV rate with the development of bundle branch block aberration can only mean that the bundle branch block is part of the tachycardia circuit. This feature excludes every SVT mechanism except AV reentry. If there is no change in the AV rate with the development of bundle branch block aberration, AVNRT or atrial tachycardia is suggested because the bundle branches are not integral parts of these tachycardia mechanisms.

The presence of P-waves eliminated the possibility of atrial fibrillation in this postoperative patient, and no flutter waves were appreciated with slowing of the rhythm in response to vagal maneuvers. In addition to atrial fibrillation, preexcitation or conduction over an accessory pathway may cause the QRS morphology to be wide during SVT. Although this patient may have had some subtle slurring of the QRS in the precordial leads (ie, delta waves) on her baseline ECG, she did not have a short PR or wide QRS complex so WPW with a reentrant circuit seemed unlikely. She was also taking bupropion, which can cause tachycardia and arrhythmia. Her magnesium level was low and this may have contributed. Rheumatoid arthritis has been associated with conduction system disease. Comparison of P-wave morphology during sinus rhythm and during the tachycardia helped differentiate sinus tachycardia from atrial tachycardia.

In summary, the most likely etiology of the SVT was postoperative stress and hypoxia. Postoperative ischemia is also possible but less likely.

CONCLUSION

A stepwise approach to a hospitalized patient with a tachyarrhythmia should begin with asking the following questions:

1. Is this patient hemodynamically stable?
2. Are the QRS complexes narrow or wide?
3. Is the rhythm more likely to be ventricular in origin?
4. If the origin of the rhythm is likely supraventricular, what is the rate of the tachycardia based on the R-R interval? Is the rhythm regular? Are P waves present and if so, is their morphology the same as the baseline ECG when the patient is in NSR? What is the R-P interval?

Treatment of the rhythm will hinge on whether the patient has underlying structural heart disease, is hemodynamically unstable or in distress, and the likely mechanism. For all patients, electrolytes, cardiac enzymes, and a complete blood count should be obtained in addition to a resting ECG if possible. Oxygen should be administered as necessary and continuous ECG monitoring should be provided. Serum K^+ and Mg^{+++} should be repleted, hypoxia corrected, underlying precipitants such as failure to administer home medications, pain and withdrawal states identified and treated. Persistent tachycardias unresponsive to the usual measures or clinical deterioration should prompt emergent specialty consultation.

SUGGESTED READINGS

Brugada P, Brugada J, Mont L, et al. A new approach to the differential diagnosis of a regular tachycardia with a wide QRS complex. *Circulation*. 1991;83:1649–1659.

Ganz LI, Friedman PL. Supraventricular tachycardia. *NEJM*. 1995; 332(3):162–173.

Kalbfleisch SJ, El-Atassi R, Calkins H, et al. Differentiation of paroxysmal narrow QRS complex tachycardias using the 12-lead electrocardiogram. *J Am Coll Cardiol*. 1993;21:85–89.

Sauve JS, Laupacis A, Ostbye T, et al. Does this patient have a clinically important carotid bruit? *The Rational Clinical Examination*. David L. Simel and Drummond Rennie, editors. New York, NY: McGraw-Hill; 2009.

PART V

Hospitalist Skills

SECTION 1 Interpretation of Common Tests

SECTION 2 Optimizing Utilization of Radiology Services

SECTION 3 Procedures

SECTION 1

Interpretation of Common Tests

CHAPTER 101

The Simplest Diagnostic Tests

Sylvia C. McKean, MD, SFHM, FACP
Francine L. Jacobson, MD, MPH

Key Clinical Questions

1. What are the causes of inappropriate test ordering?
2. Why is it important to address the problem of inappropriate test ordering?
3. How do you quantify the diagnostic accuracy of a test?
4. With any procedure that entails more than negligible risk, the decision to perform the study must take into account what factors?

INTRODUCTION

Each field of medicine challenges clinicians to recommend a course of action for a specific patient at a particular time. To efficiently and safely obtain the right information through testing, physicians need to ask the right questions. Clinical expertise assumes that the physician has the ability to

- Comprehend the information that the test will provide relevant to the decision at hand.
- Appreciate the situation and consequences of each approach.
- Utilize the information rationally in the context of a coherent set of care goals and ethical values.
- Explicitly communicate choices regarding care to the patient or surrogate so that there is informed consent.

Prior to ordering any examination, clinicians should first question whether they require additional data collection to optimize medical decision-making. Clinicians need to weigh (1) medical indications, (2) patient preferences, (3) quality of life, and (4) contextual features to reach a decision that is right for the patient. Deciding whether or not to perform a diagnostic study involves balancing its risks and costs versus the information it could provide and the benefits and costs of having that information. As a general principle, clinicians should select the least invasive imaging examination that provides the needed information with the least amount of risk, including the smallest dose of ionizing radiation, and at the least cost.

PRACTICE POINT

- Diagnostic testing is rarely without risk or financial cost and almost never completely accurate. The pursuit of diagnostic tests may also delay much needed treatment; thus physicians cannot pursue every diagnostic avenue, even if patients want all the information.

There are times when the physician's most important job is to know when to ask for assistance and where to go to get that assistance. Initial decisions regarding the care of an acutely ill hospitalized patient must be continually reassessed in light of both new data and the patient's ongoing course.

THE PROCESS OF CLINICAL REASONING

The process of clinical reasoning—data collection, problem formulation, and the generation of a hypothesis—ideally results in pursuing the most viable hypotheses. One of the most important first steps in approaching a patient is to frame the problem either in term of a diagnosis or syndrome. The process of weighing the probability of one disease versus that of other diseases possibly accounting for a patient's illness leads to the creation of a differential diagnosis. This process requires both a pathophysiologic knowledge of the potential causes of a problem and an understanding of the effect of new data on the probability of each potential cause. It is important to consider all possible diagnoses but especially those that are either life-threatening or for which effective treatment exists.

Physicians generally develop a working hypothesis that is based on partial information. This is particularly true in the hospital when the patient is acutely ill and urgent decisions must be efficiently made, often without access to outside ambulatory records. Furthermore, elderly patients commonly have multiple comorbidities and their

TABLE 101-1 Common Presentations in the Elderly

Painless MI
Apathetic hyperthyroidism
Pneumonia without cough
TB as a change in mental status, gradual debilitation and nonspecific symptoms, and negative PPD due to declining delayed hypersensitivity reactions
Depression masquerading as dementia

admission may be precipitated by a decreased ability to perform ADLs or nonspecific symptoms such as lethargy, confusion, incontinence, or falls (**Table 101-1**). Physicians must be willing to reassess initial decisions when there is new data and the patient's ongoing course runs counter to expectations.

INAPPROPRIATE TEST ORDERING

Inappropriate test ordering refers to both under and over utilization. Physicians commonly repeat studies due to failure to properly review the medical record or because these tests are readily available and easier to obtain than outside information. We hope that these chapters will help the clinician avoid inappropriate testing due to not requesting the best test, underestimating the risk of testing, ordering tests "too soon" after the initial test, or ordering tests that are unlikely to affect patient management (**Table 101-2**).

It is important to fix this problem due to limited resources, patient safety issues, and patient discomfort. To do this, we need to take the time to do appropriate targeted history and physical examinations, know what the symptoms and signs mean, and most importantly, make sure that each test is preceded by a conscious decision that the test is indicated based on best practice whenever possible. Will the test increase the pretest probability sufficiently to alter patient management? The whole point of a diagnostic test is to use it to make a diagnosis, so we need to know the probability that the test will give the correct diagnosis. Will the test accurately distinguish between patients who do and do not have the disorder?

The simplest diagnostic test is one in which the results of an investigation such as a physical finding, blood test, or radiographic study are used to classify patients into two groups according to the presence or absence of a symptom or sign. The terms positive and negative are used to refer to the presence or absence of the condition of interest.

Sensitivity and specificity is one approach for quantifying the diagnostic accuracy of a test. In clinical practice, however, the test result is all that is known. We want to know how good the test is at predicting an abnormality. How many patients with abnormal test results are truly abnormal? The sensitivity and specificity do not answer this question. Values of test sensitivity and specificity derived in one clinical population cannot necessarily be used to make predictions about a different population. Test sensitivity increases with increasing severity of disease. What this means is that there is a distribution of sensitivities and specificities across the spectrum of patients. The values of sensitivity and specificity are actually average values across the population. In addition to knowing the test's average sensitivity and specificity, the clinician must be aware of how the test performs in different segments of the population. As the prevalence falls, the positive predictive value falls and the negative predictive value rises. Clinicians will, on average, learn the most from a clinical sign, symptom, or laboratory test when the likelihood of disease is 40–60%. If the prevalence of disease is very low, the positive predictive value will not be close to one even if the sensitivity and specificity are high. Thus, in screening the general population, it is inevitable that many people with positive test results will not have the disease.

TABLE 101-2 Examples of Inappropriate Test Ordering in the Hospital

Common examples • Under and over utilization • Unlikely to affect patient management • Repeat studies • Not requesting the best test • Inadequate clinical information • Underestimation of risk of testing • Short interval of follow-up studies
Factors that lead to inappropriate testing include • Time constraints that limit the physician's willingness to contemplate data before ordering a test or to obtain "outside" information • Diagnostic uncertainty, fear of missing a crucial diagnosis, concern about medical malpractice • The availability of sophisticated technology and support services • Pressure from patients and families • Risk of treating without an established diagnosis • Testing habits
Over utilization • Failure to examine the primary data when a patient has been hospitalized elsewhere and treatment may have impacted course of illness (fever of unknown illness): time constraints • "Ruling out" unlikely diagnoses (inappropriate ordering of D-dimer tests leading to unnecessary PE-protocol CT): fear of missing a crucial diagnosis • The availability of sophisticated technology and support services in the hospital • Pressure from patients and families • Risk of treating without an established diagnosis • Testing habits • Financial incentives
Under utilization • Disparities of health care for minorities: see chapter 3 • Financial incentives

Data from Clinical Problem Solving, Putterman, et al. *NEJM*. Nov 2, 1995.

The likelihood ratio (LR) represents the likelihood that a test result would be expected in a patient with the target disorder compared with the likelihood that the same result would be expected in a patient without the target disorder. The LR indicates the value of the test for increasing certainty about a positive diagnosis. A high LR may show that the test is useful, but it does not necessarily follow that the test is a good indicator of the presence of disease. For LR > 1, the probability of disease goes up; for LR < 1, the probability of disease goes down. When the LR is close to 1, the probability of disease is unchanged because the finding is equally likely in patients with and without the disorder.

The LR is more stable than sensitivity and specificity when the prevalence of disease changes because the direction of change is the same for the numerator and denominator of the LR. Unlike sensitivity and specificity (which limit the number of test results to just two levels, "positive" and "negative"), a LR can be generated for multiple levels of the diagnostic test result. The LR can be used to calculate the increase in probability of disease from baseline prevalence with positive test (LR positive) and decrease in probability of disease from baseline prevalence with negative test (using alternative LR negative) for any level of disease prevalence. The likelihood ratio can be used to shorten a list of diagnostic hypotheses because the pretest "odds" (the ratio of the probabilities for and against a diagnosis) of the target disorder multiplied by the likelihood ratio for the diagnostic test result equals the posttest odds for the target disorder. The LR allows you to carry out sequences of diagnostic tests. The posttest probability for one test becomes the pretest probability for a second, independent test with a distinct pathophysiology. For example, a result whose likelihood ratio is 2 increases the probability about 15%, 5 about 30%, and 10 about 45%. Likelihood ratios of 0.5 decrease the probability about 15%, 0.2 about 30%, and 0.1 about 45%. For diagnostic tests to be meaningful, they should increase or decrease probability by at least 20% to 25% (corresponding to likelihood ratios with values > 3 or < 0.3. Although the posttest probability can be calculated by a series of equations, they are at most only approximations in clinical medicine.

The past two decades have produced major technologic innovations that permit faster diagnosis of treatable diseases less invasively, such as appendicitis by CT imaging.

PRACTICE POINT

- Newer diagnostic technologies that have expanded our ability to define anatomic and physiological abnormalities have not reduced the frequency of misdiagnosis.

Spectrum bias refers to disease factors that affect the sensitivity and specificity of a diagnostic test. The following factors may affect the sensitivity or specificity of a diagnostic test:

- Severity of disease
- Cyclic nature of disease activity
- Duration of disease
- Therapy
- Control group composition

Reporting bias refers to the tendency to report strongly positive (or negative) results and not report results that are not clinically relevant at that time. Availability heuristic is a bias that makes noteworthy outcomes more likely (eg, a radiologist overestimating the likelihood of cancer in abnormalities seen on Chest CT so as to not miss a malignant tumor).

Reproducibility refers to the consistency of test performance and result interpretation. Interobserver agreement is expressed using the kappa statistic. A κ-value =

- 0 is the same as that by chance
- 0.2 – 0.4, fair agreement
- 0.4 – 0.6, moderate agreement
- 0.6 – 0.8, substantial agreement
- 0.8 – 1.0, almost perfect agreement

For most diagnostic tests, interobserver agreement is less than perfect, with κ statistics over a wide range depending on the diagnostic study or physical sign. Interobserver disagreement commonly relates to interpretation of the test's significance but also to the specific study and the examiner's experience. Abdominal ultrasound examinations are more subjective and require more expertise than CT.

PRACTICE POINT

- The link between communication and accuracy can change the pretest probability. Radiologists can only refine the differential diagnosis with the collaboration of the physician caring for the patient.
- For example, a 28-year-old man had a low probability but not Normal VQ scan. He is not from the population in which this is a typical finding in a normal patient and the presentation was compelling so additional imaging was ordered and indeed, the patient had clinically significant PE.

ASSESSMENT OF THE DATA

For each test, the examiner should take a systematic approach in assessment. The first step relates to the history and physical examination. What is the patient telling us? Does the physical examination confirm our suspicions? The second step is to examine the admission data in the context of the patient in front of us including the diagnostic quality of the study. For plain films, alignment of bones will provide information of whether the patient is properly positioned. Then the reviewer should have a mental checklist so that all aspects of the film are reviewed, not just the one area of concern. The third step starts with asking the question of whether additional testing is required prior to treatment. With any procedure that entails more than negligible risk, the decision to perform the study must take into account the following factors:

- The risk to the patient inherent in the procedure with the patient's comorbidity factored into the risk assessment
- The risk associated with missing a potentially dire diagnosis
- The likelihood that the procedure will result in a diagnosis relevant to the patient's care
- The cost of the procedure

PRACTICE POINT

- A first principle for chest radiography: If the pathology is where you think it is, the localization of it should be correct on both frontal and lateral views. If not, the localization is incorrect and a new hypothesis is needed. So, the fit between the data and the disease is something that reveals itself over time and dialogue.

Subsequent steps require informed consent. Is additional testing in accordance with the patient's goals and values? Never leave the patient out of the equation.

PRACTICE POINT

- Many tests are performed to "rule out" a particular problem. Beware of sign-out or progress note communication that states "negative" without looking at the final report.
- For example, a patient who suffered a ruptured uterus postpartum was noted to be dyspneic and tachycardic and underwent a PE-protocol CT to rule out a PE. The study was negative for a PE but showed a massive right-sided effusion. Cardiology consultation recommended a hypercoagulable workup for pulmonary hypertension noted by 2-D echo. No one acted on the effusion and the patient ultimately required a Video-Assisted Thoracic Surgery (VATS) procedure. Progress notes and sign-out failed to document the abnormality that was discovered during a change in coverage.

COMMUNICATION

Optimal use of consultants, including radiologists, requires effective communication so that key questions are answered. The most crucial clinical information for radiologists is the location of symptoms. One example, CT, contains complex information about multiple organ systems and anatomy. Clinical information directs the radiologist's attention to a specific problem. Interpretation attributes the observed abnormalities to a disease process. Accuracy is improved by improving sensitivity (perception) without affecting specificity. Clinical information improves accuracy with respect to diagnostic imaging, including radiography, CT, MR, and mammography by refining the pretest probability for the radiologist. In the absence of effective communication, the radiologist cannot be expected to be right more than 70% of the time.

PRACTICE POINT

- Radiology does not negate or trump physical exam findings and the creation of the differential diagnosis. If the patient is presented as "normal", the potentially ambiguous radiographic finding is overwhelmingly "normal". If the story changes as so often happens during the course of hospitalization, the study should be reread with the new defining information that would place the patient in a different population. A potentially different pretest probability might completely change the proper interpretation of the same potentially ambiguous finding. This holds for pneumonia, heart disease, and a large variety of tumors. It can be as basic as the significance of atelectasis when patient spikes a fever.

Hospital care requires teamwork and effective communication, often through progress notes in the medical record. From hospital day one a patient should have an accurate problem list that reflects a formulation of the care plan and promotes clear decision making. Although the practice of "cutting and pasting" computer generated progress notes improves efficiency of documentation for billing and other purposes, failure to synthesize the information in a concise and up-to-date problem list may impede the transfer of necessary information and impact the recommendations of consultants who may not review the primary data.

CONCLUSION

An admitting diagnosis is not absolute and is still inferential. The sequential acquisition of partial data is a multistep process. Refinement of the hypothesis usually requires additional diagnostic testing to verify the diagnosis. Deciding whether or not to perform a diagnostic study involves balancing its risks and costs versus the information that the test could provide and the benefits and costs of having that information for your patient.

The first section of this part if the book, Interpretation of Common Tests, will focus on the "low tech" tests that are routinely available on admission such as the ECG and urinalysis. The second section, Optimizing Utilization of Radiology Services, will address the selection of imaging tests, some of which carry significant risk and cost.

SUGGESTED READINGS

Berbaum KS, el-Khoury GY, Franken EA Jr, Kathol M, Montgomery WJ, Hesson W. Impact of clinical history on fracture detection with radiography. *Radiology*. 1988;168:507–511.

Berlin L. Accuracy of P\procedures: Has it improved over the last five decades? http://www.ajronline.org/cgi/content/full/188/5/1173.

Halkin A, Reishman J, Scaber M, et al. Likelihood ratios: getting diagnostic testing into perspective. http://qjmed.oxfordjournals.org/content/91/4/247.short.

Houssami N, Irwig L, Simpson JM, et al. The influence of clinical information on the accuracy of diagnostic mammography. *Breast Cancer Research and Treatment*. 2004;85(3):223–228.

Kaplan DM. Clear writing, clear thinking, and the disappearing art of the problem list. *Journal of Hospital Medicine*. July/August 2007;2(4):201–202.

Leslie A, Jones AJ, Goddard PR. The influence of clinical information on the reporting of CT by radiologists. *British Journal of Radiology*. 2000;73:1052–1055.

Loy C, Irwig L. Accuracy of diagnostic tests read with and without clinical information. *JAMA*. 2004;292:1602–1609.

Nancy L. Wilczynski. Quality of reporting of diagnostic accuracy studies: No change since STARD statement publication—Before-and-after Study. http://radiology.rsna.org/content/248/3/817.

Sackett DL, Richardson WS, Rosenberg W, et al. *Evidence-Based Medicine: How to Practice and Teach EBM*. 2nd edition. Edinburg, Scotland: Churchill Livingstone; 1997.

CHAPTER 102

The Resting Electrocardiogram

Prashant Vaishnava, MD
Sylvia C. McKean, MD, SFHM, FACP
Marc Miller, MD

Key Clinical Questions

1. How does the resting electrocardiogram (ECG) assist in the diagnosis and management of acute coronary syndrome (ACS)?
2. What are the key differentiating electrocardiographic features of ACS versus acute pericarditis and versus early repolarization?
3. How does the ECG assist in the diagnosis of acute pulmonary embolism?
4. How does the ECG assist in determining the cause of syncope?
5. What are the characteristic ECG findings of electrolyte disturbances?
6. What are the characteristic ECG findings of hypothyroidism, stroke, and drug effects?

INTRODUCTION

A graphic recording of electrical potentials generated by the heart, the electrocardiogram (ECG) is the most commonly performed cardiovascular laboratory procedure in the United States. As a noninvasive, versatile, reproducible, and inexpensive test, the ECG has utility in the evaluation of a range of signs and symptoms encountered by the hospitalist, including acute chest discomfort, breathlessness, syncope, and palpitations. While the ECG is useful in the detection of myocardial ischemia, arrhythmias, structural changes of the myocardium, and conduction system disease, clinicians should also be able hyperkalemia to recognize normal variants that may mimic cardiac disease and electrocardiographic manifestations of noncardiac illness. Guidelines for the use of electrocardiograms in patients with and without preexisting heart disease have been published by the American College of Cardiology and American Heart Association (ACC/AHA) and have changed little in recent years. An understanding of the clinical context and availability of prior electrocardiograms for comparison improves diagnostic accuracy when interpreting electrocardiograms.

THE NORMAL RESTING ELECTROCARDIOGRAM

The electrocardiogram is a graphical recording of the difference in potential between electrodes placed on the body surface. Twelve conventional leads that generate such a recording include the six extremity (limb) and six chest (precordial) leads. The chest leads (V_1–V_6) record electrical activity in a horizontal plane, and the limb leads (bipolar leads I, II, and III; and unipolar leads aVR, aVL, and aVF) record potentials transmitted on the frontal plane. Right-sided precordial leads (V_1R–V_6R) and electrode locations posterior to V_6 (V_7–V_9) may be useful in the assessment of right ventricular and posterior-lateral infarctions, respectively. If a wave of depolarization spreads toward the positive pole of a lead, a positive deflection is recorded in that lead. Conversely, if a wave of depolarization spreads toward the negative pole of a lead, a negative deflection is recorded in that lead. The components of the normal resting electrocardiogram are the P wave, generated by atrial contraction; the PR interval, representing conduction through the AV node; the QRS complex, generated by biventricular contraction; and the ST-T wave, reflecting biventricular recovery.

ACUTE CHEST DISCOMFORT

The initial diagnostic evaluation of the patient with acute chest discomfort centers on the recognition of life-threatening conditions, including acute coronary syndrome and pulmonary embolism.

ACUTE CORONARY SYNDROME

Electrocardiography is an indispensable tool in the diagnosis and management of acute coronary syndromes (ACS). Deviation of the ST-segment is generally the earliest electrocardiographic manifestation of myocardial injury. Elevation of the ST-segment is produced over the ischemic zone when acute ischemia is transmural and may be preceded by the appearance of tall, positive, hyperacute T waves and accompanied by often prominent reciprocal ST-segment depressions on leads overlying the contralateral surface of the heart. Within a period of hours to days, electrocardiographic changes evolve with T-wave inversions and Q-wave formation in the leads that demonstrated ST-segment elevations (**Figures 102-1, 102-2,** and **102-3**).

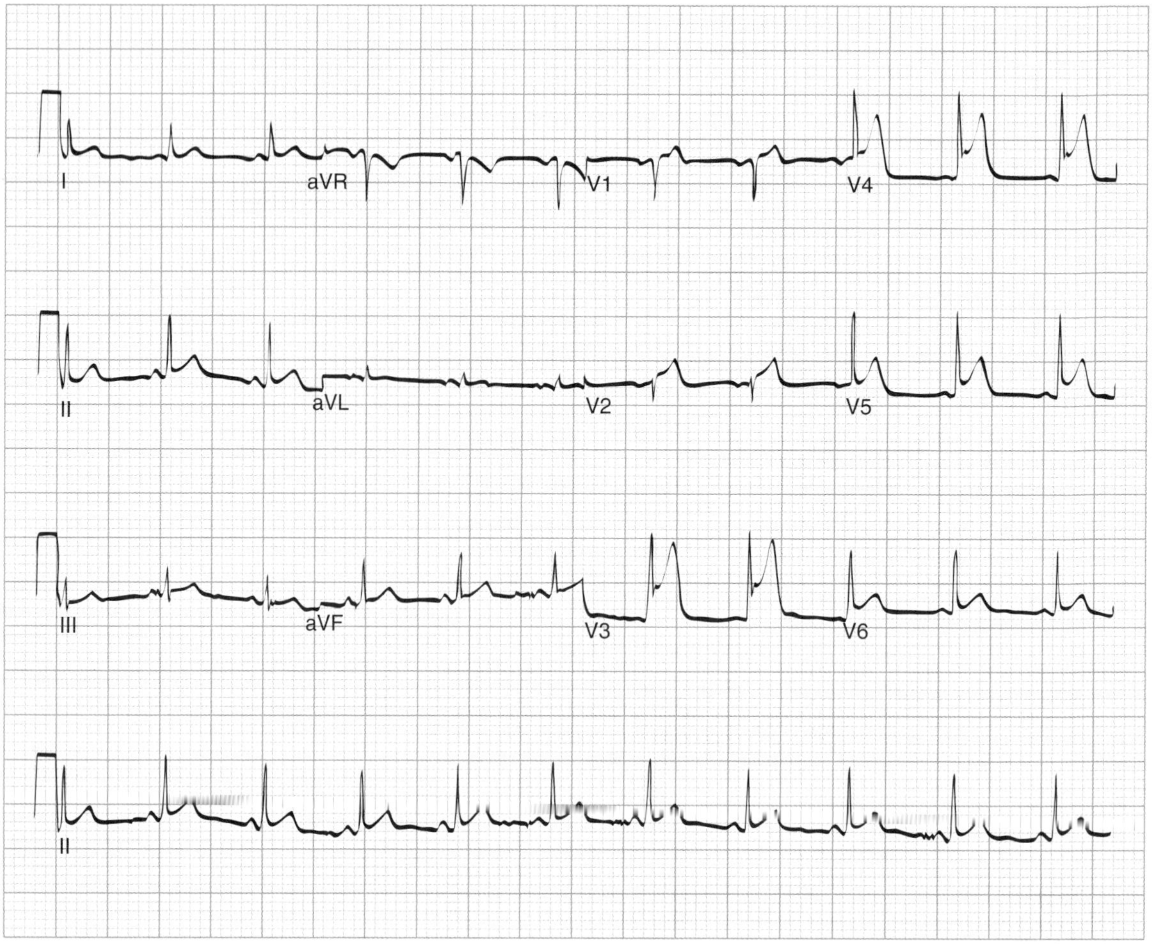

Figure 102-1 *Electrocardiogram reveals prominent anteroseptal and lateral ST-segment elevations, consistent with the thrombotic lesion visualized within the proximal left anterior descending artery and intervened upon during coronary angiography.*

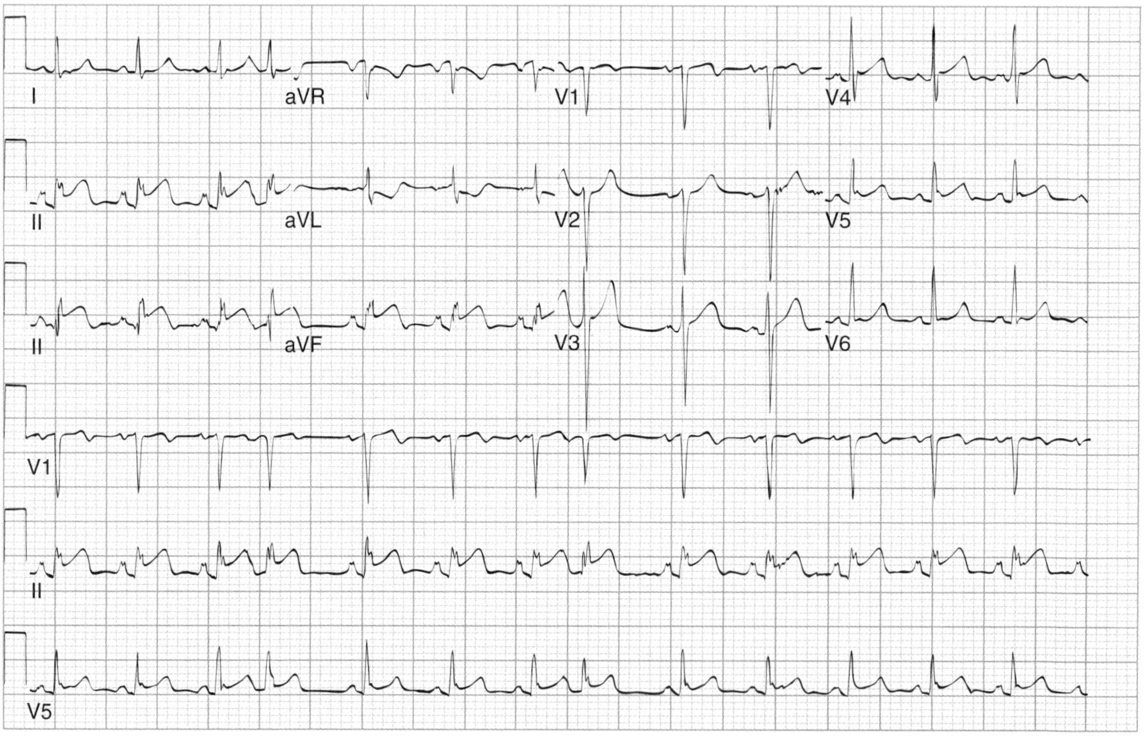

Figure 102-2 *59-year-old gentleman presenting with chest pain and prominent inferolateral ST-segment elevations. He underwent successful deployment of bare-metal stents to the mid- and distal-right coronary artery.*

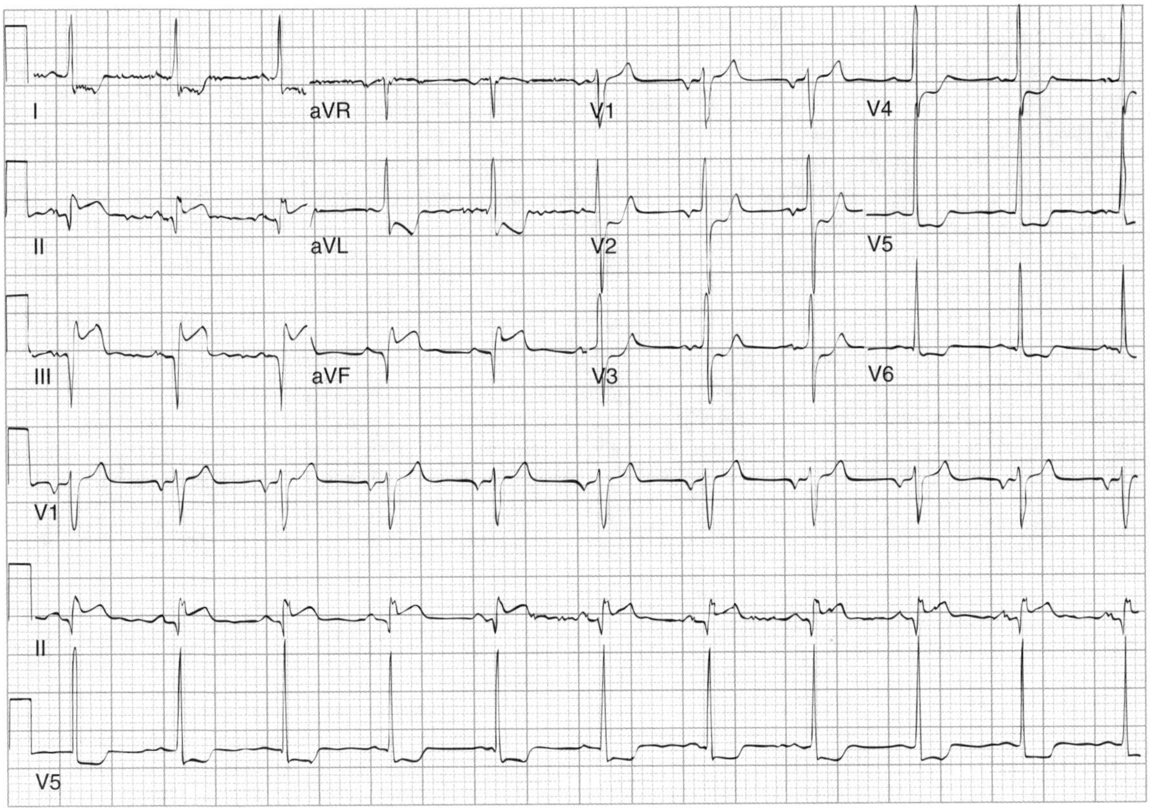

Figure 102-3 *Elevations of the ST-segment in the inferior leads is suggestive of a thrombotic lesion within the right coronary artery. Reciprocal changes are apparent in the lateral limb and precordial leads. ST-segment depressions in leads V_1 and V_2 suggest posterior involvement.*

PRACTICE POINT

Chest pain

Acute Myocardial infarction

- Epicardial injury or transmural ischemia is manifested by ST-segment deviation toward the ischemic zone, manifested by ST-segment depression or elevation.
- Reciprocal ST-segment depressions in other leads support a diagnosis of ischemia rather than early repolarization.

Prior Myocardial infarction

- < 1 mm ST-segment elevation in any lead and T waves upright in the leads with pathological Q waves (> 1/3 of the R-wave amplitude with duration of > 0.04 seconds).
- Suspect aneurysm or large akinetic region if wide deep Q waves across the precordial leads in a stable pattern.

Early repolarization syndrome

- Most clinically urgent problem—distinguish between early repolarization and ischemia.
- Diagnostic criteria:
  - Concave ST-segment elevation < 5 mm and most prominent in the precordial leads.
  - Reciprocal ST depression usually seen in AVR.
  - T waves usually asymmetric.
  - Notching of the R wave at its junction with ST-segment (≥ 50% of cases).
- During exercise the ST-segment elevation of early repolarization may return to baseline.

Acute pericarditis

- Depression of the PQ segment, reflecting atrial injury, early in course.
- Commonly, ST-segment elevation in all leads, except aVR, which has ST-segment depression.
- Other leads, often V_1 and aVL, sometimes lead III, in which the QRS complexes are predominantly negative, may not show ST-segment elevation.
- A relatively slow sinus rate is frequent with early repolarization and infrequent with acute pericarditis.
- Almost exclusively in pericarditis:
  - T wave amplitude ≤ 3 mm in V_6.
  - Ratio of height of the onset of the ST-segment to the amplitude of the T wave in V_6 ≥ 0.25.

(continued)

Pericardial effusion

- Low voltage, defined as limb leads < 5 mm peak to peak and precordial leads < 10 mm peak to peak, is seen in less that 1% of normal people.
  - Isolated low voltage in limb leads has no clinical significance.
- Low specificity of low voltage for pericardial effusion.
  - Any process that reduces the mass of electrically active myocardium (eg, MI, myocardial diseases, cardiac amyloidosis).
  - Interposition of air or tissue between the heart and surface electrodes.
    - Lung disease—pleural effusion, pneumothorax, emphysema.
    - Obesity, myxedema, as well as pericardial effusion.
- Abnormal position of heart within pericardial cavity may result in lack of normal R-wave progression in anterior leads.
- Beat-to-beat alternation of amplitude and direction of QRS (electrical alternans) seen in cardiac tamponade.
- Flattening of T waves and sinus tachycardia (large pericardial effusions with tamponade physiology).
- The slow or normal heart rate seen in myxedema is not present with other etiologies. Even though myxedema may produce large pericardial effusions, cardiac tamponade (electrical alternans) is not seen. Inflammatory changes, such as those of acute pericarditis, depend on the etiology. Idiopathic and neoplastic effusions are not associated with inflammation.

Patterns of ST-segment elevations may be useful in localizing the region of involved myocardium and may suggest the site of occlusion within the coronary arterial tree (**Table 102-1**).

Pathophysiologically, ST-segment elevations do not necessarily signify atherosclerotic plaque rupture and occlusive intraluminal thrombus formation. In fact, transient ST-segment elevations may indicate vasospasm from sympathomimetic effects (**Figure 102-4**).

When ischemia is primarily subendocardial, ST-segment depressions appear in the overlying leads (**Figure 102-5**).

Although hyperacute T waves may precede or accompany ST-segment elevations, inversion of the T wave or pseudonormalization of previously inverted T waves may also indicate ischemia. Deep and symmetrically inverted T waves in the anterior precordial leads, in particular, may indicate high-grade stenosis in the proximal left anterior descending artery, an exception to the rule that leads in which T-wave inversions are present do not correlate with the location of coronary stenoses (in contrast to localization allowed by ST-segment elevations or pathologic Q waves) (**Figure 102-6**).

Symmetric giant T waves (amplitude >10 mm in two or more leads) may be associated with pericarditis, pheochromocytoma, severe aortic insufficiency, myocarditis, and cerebrovascular disease. Commonly inverted in all precordial leads at birth, T waves may remain inverted in the right precordial leads in normal persons in a persistent juvenile pattern. Inversion of the T waves may also be normal in leads III, aVR, and V_1.

While a normal ECG throughout the course of an acute infarct is uncommon, the ECG has limited sensitivity and specificity in the diagnosis of acute coronary syndromes. Clinicians should recognize that changes in the ST-segment and T wave are not specific for myocardial ischemia and/or infarction and should, in particular, distinguish the changes associated with acute pericarditis and the normal variant of early repolarization from those seen with myocardial ischemia and infarction. In contrast to the regional ST-segment elevations created by myocardial infarction,

TABLE 102-1 Electrocardiographic Changes and Localization of Lesions

Region(s) of Myocardium Affected	Location of Culprit Stenosis or Lesion(s)	Electrocardiographic Changes
Anterolateral wall and septum	Proximal left anterior descending artery	ST-segment elevations in leads V_1–V_6 and limb leads I and aVL with reciprocal ST-segment depressions in limb leads III and aVF
Anterior and inferior walls	"Wrap around" left anterior descending artery that extends onto the inferior wall or multivessel disease	ST-segment elevations in leads V_1–V_6, accompanied by ST elevations in limbs leads II, III, and aVF
Inferior	Right coronary or circumflex arteries	ST-segment elevations in limb leads II, III, and aVF (and greater in lead III than lead II), along with elevation in lead V_1 suggestive of occlusion of proximal or mid-right coronary artery.
Posterior wall	Right coronary or circumflex arteries	ST-segment depressions in leads V_1 and V_2 with eventual appearance of prominent R waves. Posterior leads V_7–V_9 (V_7, posterior axillary line; V_8, posterior scapular line; and V_9, left border of spine) may show ST-segment elevations.
Right ventricle	Right coronary artery	ST-segment elevations in V_1R–V_6R (particularly V_4R) and limb leads II, III, and aVF, along with reciprocal ST-segment depressions in limb leads I and aVL

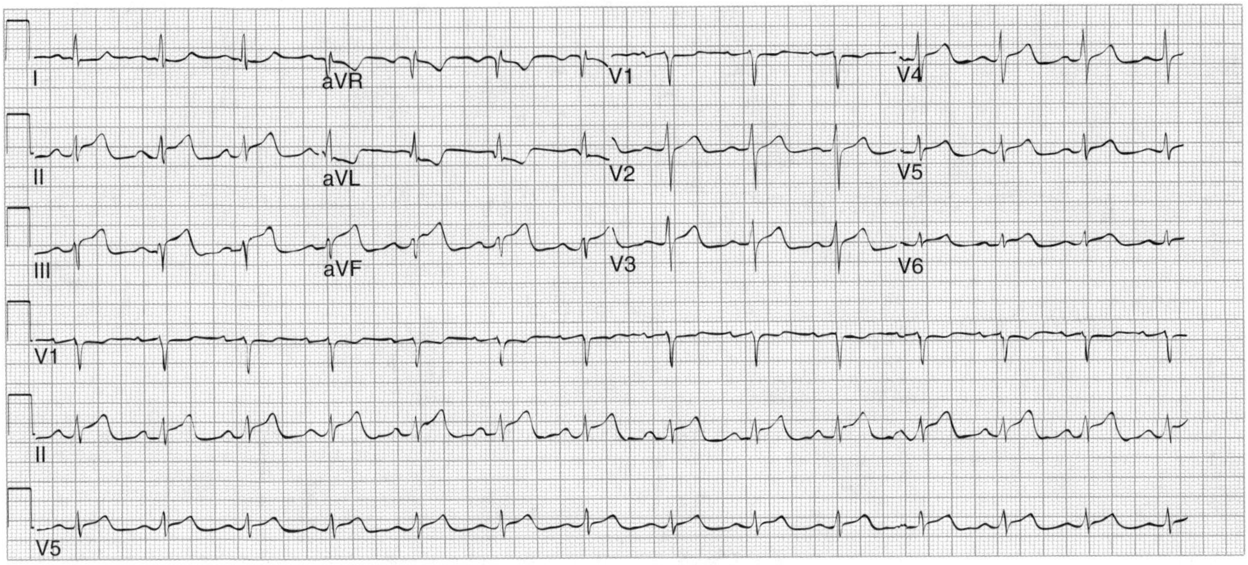

Figure 102-4 *55-year-old gentleman with nonobstructive coronary artery disease. Electrocardiogram reveals prominent inferolateral ST-segment elevations, attributed to coronary vasospasm and successfully treated with nitrates and calcium-channel blockade.*

acute pericarditis creates diffuse ST-segment elevations, often in the presence of PR segment elevation in aVR and reciprocal PR segment depressions in the other leads (**Figure 102-7**).

Also in contrast to the appearance of T-wave inversions while the ST-segments remain elevated, T-wave inversions in acute pericarditis generally do not develop until the ST-segments have returned to isoelectric baseline. The electrocardiographic signature of early repolarization is ST-segment elevation, especially in the midprecordial leads and more commonly at slow heart rates and among young adult men (**Figure 102-8**).

In contrast to the convexity seen in ST-segment elevations associated with myocardial ischemia, those seen with early repolarization are generally concave in form and associated with notching of the R wave at its junction with the QRS complex. Biphasic T-wave

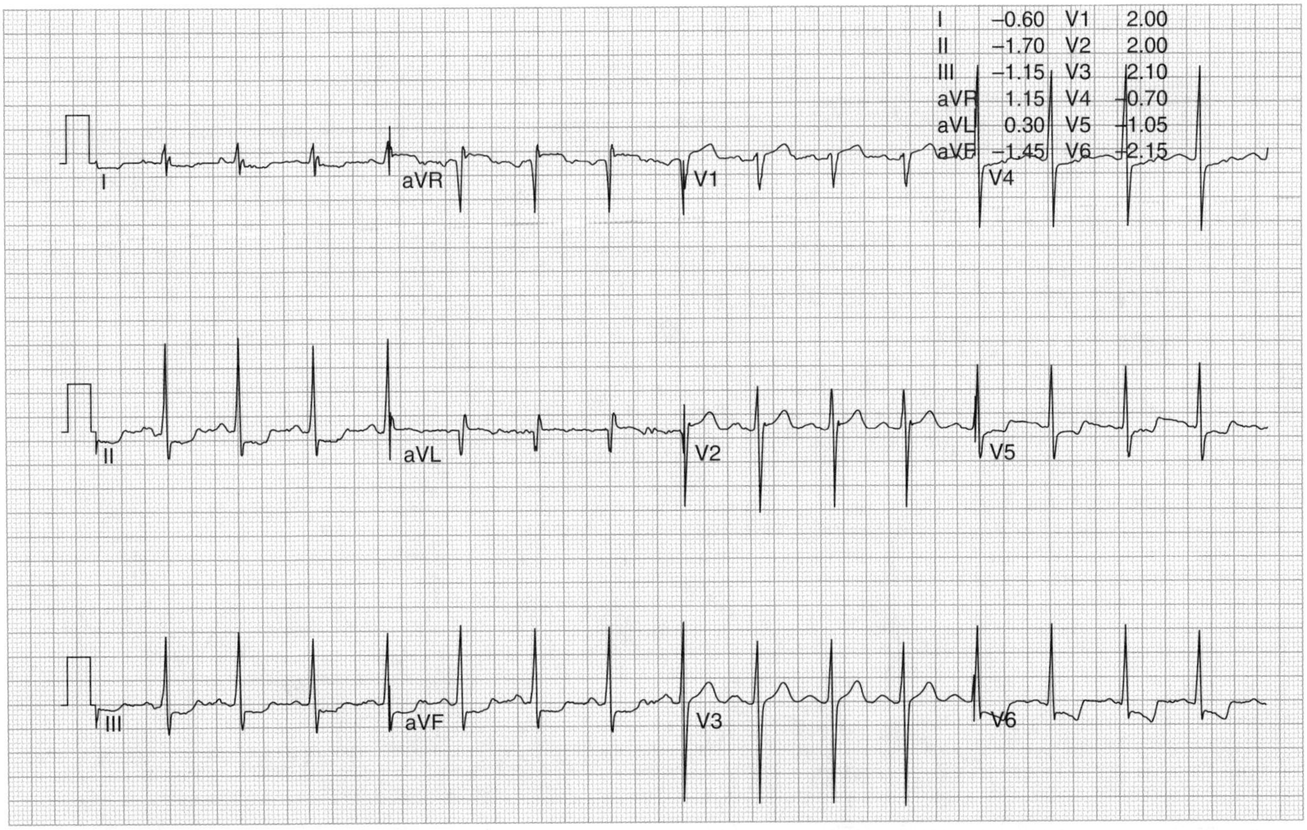

Figure 102-5 *When ischemia is subendocardial, ST-segment depressions with or without T-wave inversions may appear, as in this electrocardiogram of a 44-year-old gentleman with obstructive stenoses within the left anterior descending and left circumflex arteries on coronary angiography.*

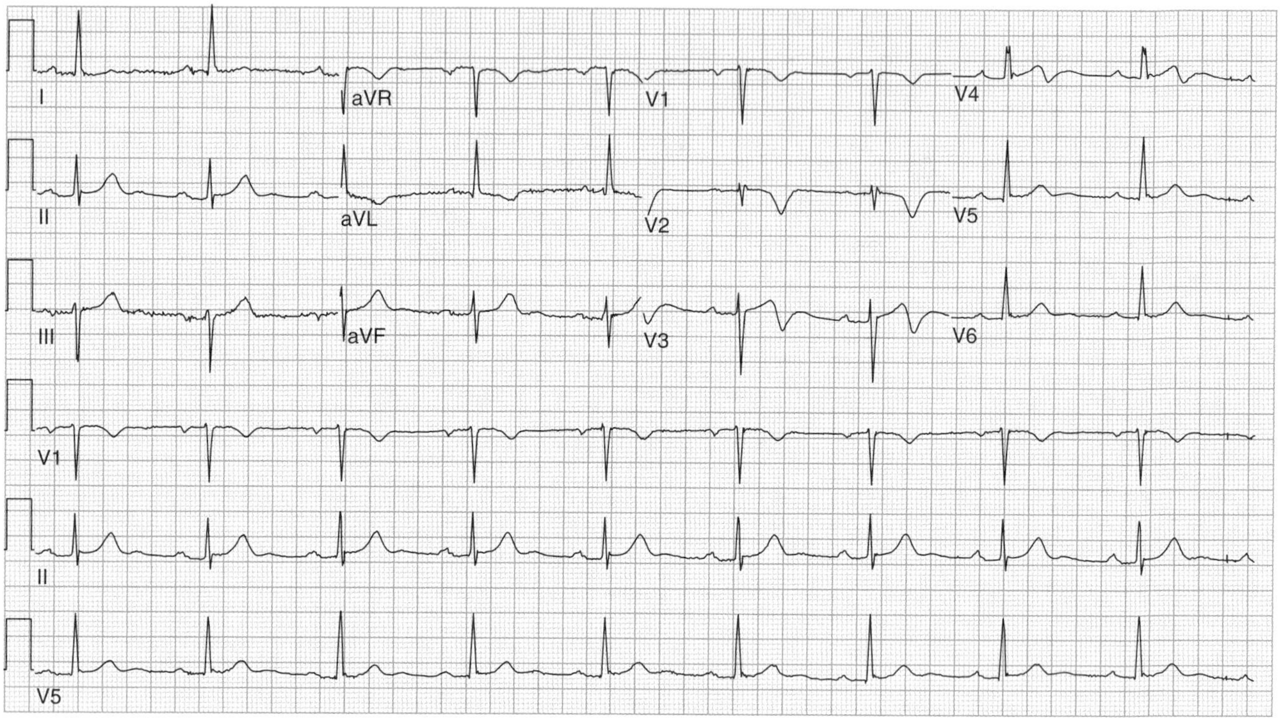

Figure 102-6 *Prominent and new T-wave inversions in the anterior precordial leads (a.k.a. Wellen sign) may indicate a high-grade proximal stenosis within the left anterior descending artery. This 70-year-old gentleman had a 90–95% thrombotic and ulcerated obstructive lesion within the left anterior descending artery.*

inversions may also accompany the ST-segment elevations seen with early repolarization.

Among patients with acute coronary syndrome, the electrocardiogram also offers utility in the recognition of ischemia-related benign and malignant arrhythmias and postinfarct complications. Accelerated idioventricular rhythm (AIVR) is a regular wide-complex ventricular rhythm, generally at a rate of 50–100.

Ventricular aneurysm may be suggested by ST-segment elevations that persist despite reperfusion.

New left bundle branch block (LBBB) in the setting of symptoms consistent with acute MI may indicate a large, anterior wall acute MI (**Figure 102-9**).

With preexisting LBBB, the diagnosis of acute STEMI may be obscured, but the presence of the following may be suggestive

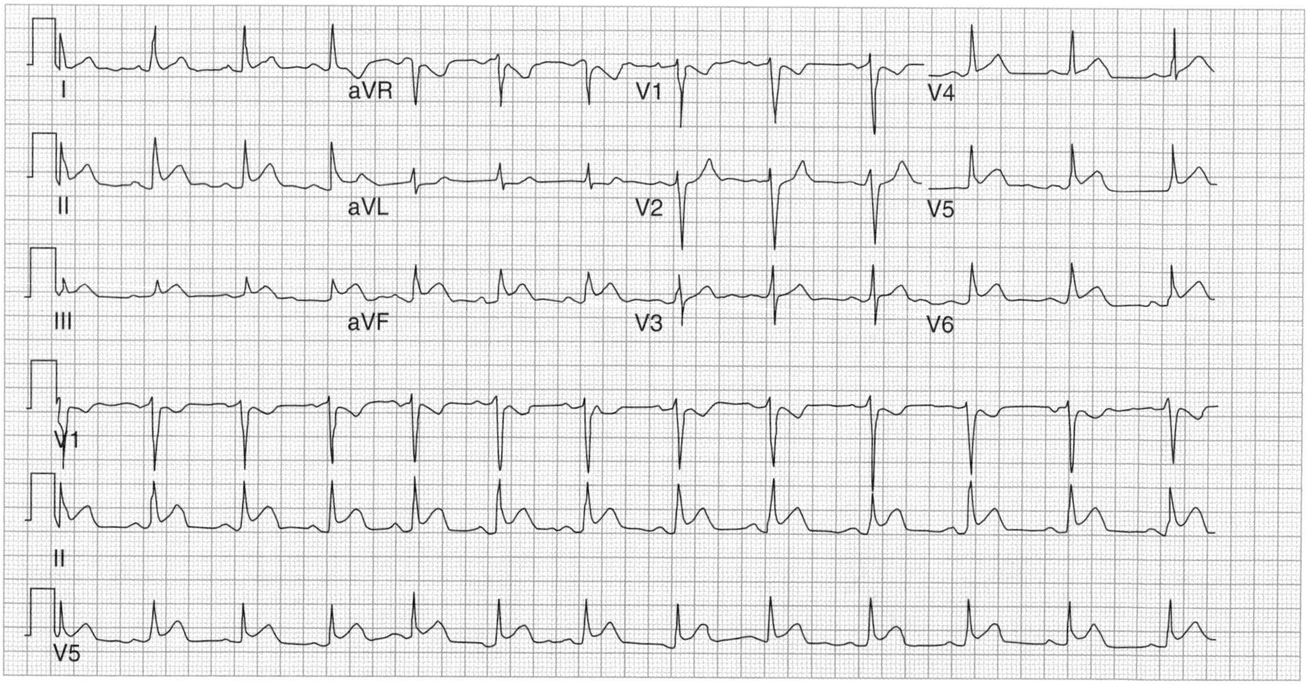

Figure 102-7 *Acute pericarditis creates diffuse ST-segment elevations, often in the presence of PR-segment elevation in aVR and reciprocal PR-segment depressions in the other leads.*

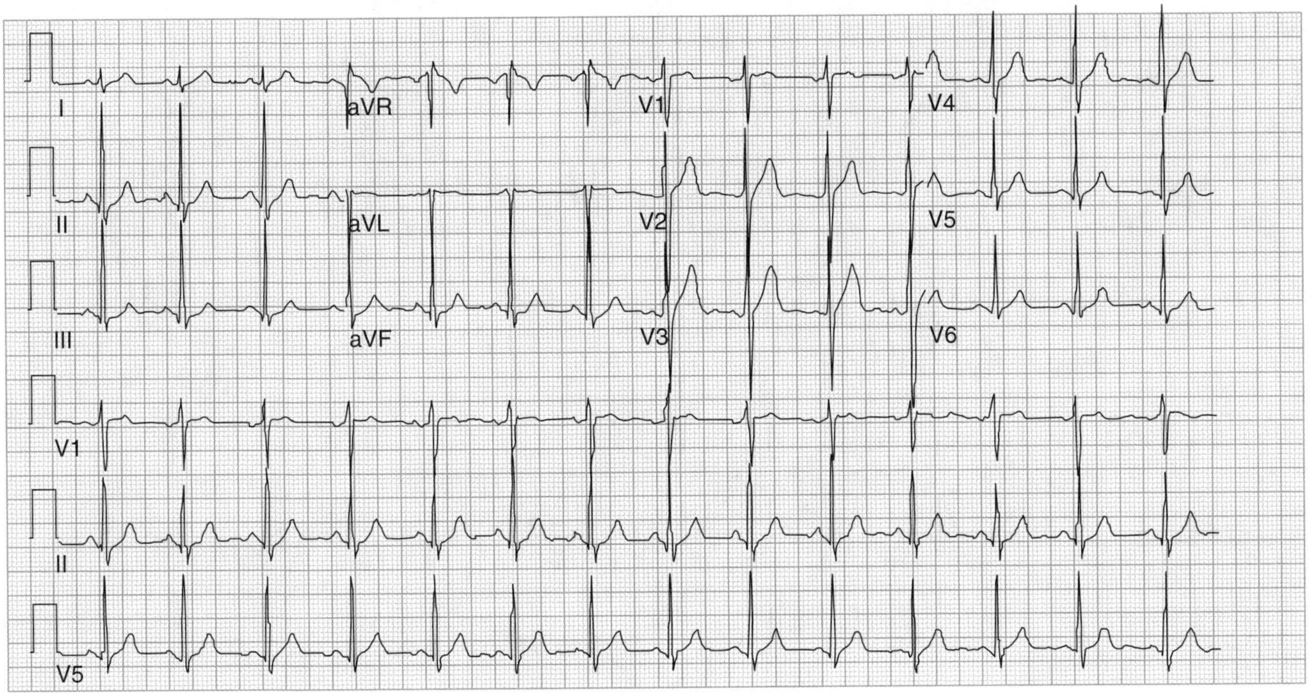

Figure 102-8 *The ST-segment elevation of early repolarization may mimic acute ischemia. In contrast to the convexity seen in ST-segment elevations associated with myocardial ischemia, ST-elevations seen with early repolarization are generally concave in form and associated with notching of the R wave at its junction with the QRS complex, as in this tracing from a healthy 23-year-old gentleman. During exercise, the ST-segment elevations of early repolarization may return to baseline.*

of acute ischemia: ST-segment elevation ≥ 1 mm concordant with the QRS complex; ST-segment depression ≥ mm in lead V_1, V_2, or V_3; or ST-segment elevation ≥ 5 mm discordant with the QRS. Right bundle branch block (RBBB) may obscure the diagnosis of an acute anterior MI by interfering with the interpretation of ST-segment elevations in leads V_{1-3}, but the pseudonormalization of the normally discordant T waves (ie, normally opposite the terminal deflection of the QRS complex) may suggest acute ischemia. Because RBBB itself may produce a large R wave in V_1, it is generally difficult to diagnose a posterior infarct in the presence of a RBBB.

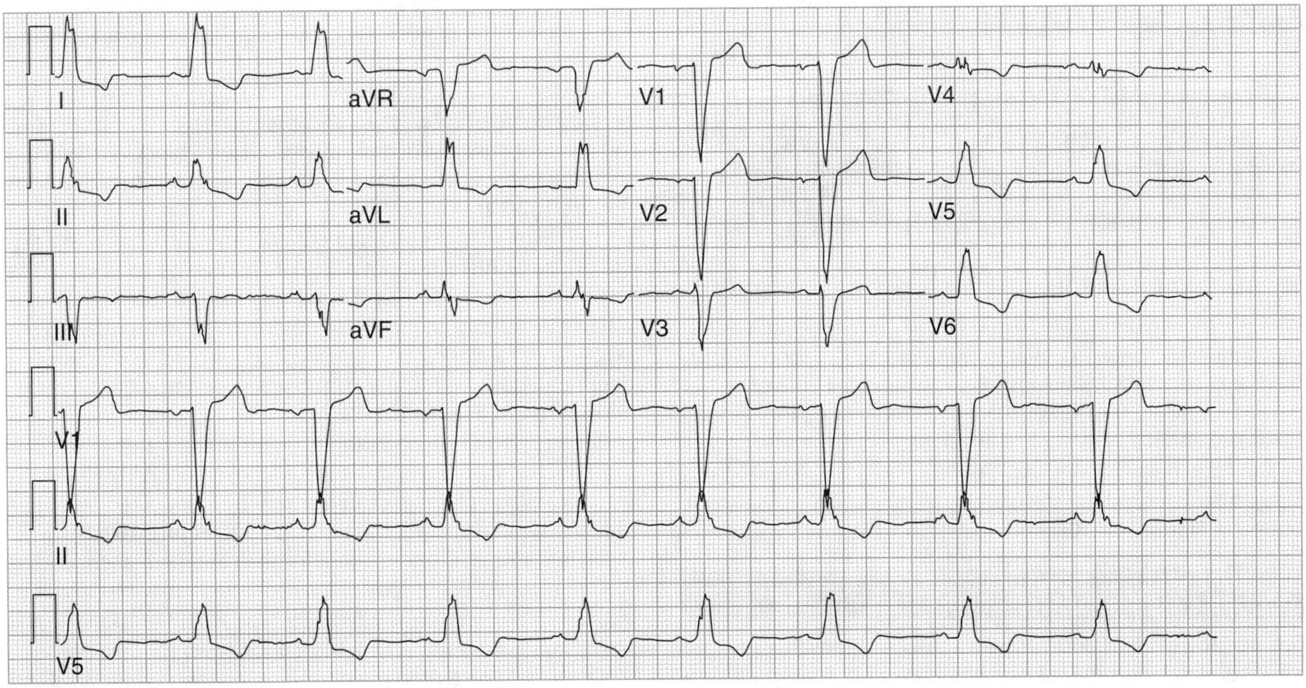

Figure 102-9 *New left bundle branch block, as shown in this electrocardiogram, may indicate a large, anterior wall acute MI in the appropriate clinical setting.*

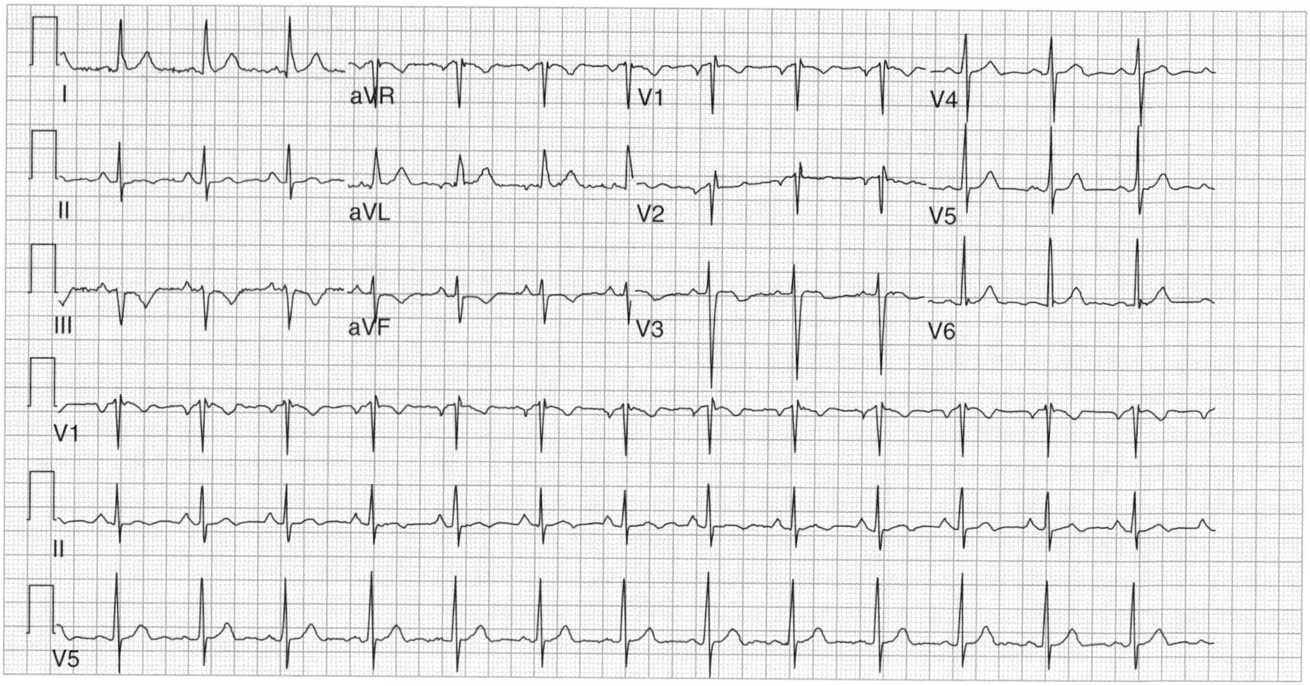

Figure 102-10 *This 47-year-old gentleman presented with dyspnea and had multiple filling defects on contrast-enhanced computed tomography of the chest, consistent with pulmonary emboli. T-wave inversions in the anterior precordial leads are suggestive of right-sided dysfunction, as was confirmed echocardiographically.*

> **PRACTICE POINT**
>
> **Pulmonary embolism**
>
> ECG in pulmonary embolism is clinically helpful mainly in patients with no history of heart or lung disease.
>
> - Sinus tachycardia
> - $S_1Q_3T_3$ pattern
> - Right atrial abnormality, right axis deviation, complete or incomplete RBBB
> - Left axis deviation, indeterminate axis, $S_1S_2S_3$, late precordial transition, low-voltage, nonspecific ST-T abnormalities
>
> Negative T waves in precordial leads in an anterior subepicardial ischemic pattern is the most frequent ECG abnormality of massive PE.

PULMONARY EMBOLISM

While pulmonary embolism frequently may not generate electrocardiographic changes or only subtle nonspecific abnormalities, there are characteristic findings that may indicate right ventricular pressure overload. These electrocardiographic findings may include T wave inversion in V_1–V_3 or a characteristic $S_1Q_3T_3$ with an S wave in lead I and new Q waves and T-wave inversions in lead III. Sinus tachycardia is frequently seen, and atrial fibrillation may also be observed (**Figure 102-10**).

SYNCOPE, PALPITATIONS, AND SUDDEN CARDIAC DEATH

Syncope, the sudden transient loss of consciousness with associated loss of postural tone, may be arrhythmic in origin. Sinus node dysfunction, atrioventricular block, and ventricular tachycardia need to be considered in the evaluation of arrhythmic syncope. Sinus arrest, or sinus pause, is a form of sinus node dysfunction that occurs when the sinus node fails to depolarize on time and manifests as pauses that may be last longer than three seconds. Pauses may also represent atrioventricular block (**Figure 102-11**).

Tachycardia-bradycardia syndrome, also referred to as sick sinus syndrome, presents as episodes of sinus or junctional bradycardia alternating with an atrial tachycardia. Sinus node dysfunction, documented in association with symptomatic bradycardia and due to factors that are irreversible or due to essential drug therapy, and symptomatic chronotropic incompetence are established indications for permanent pacing.

Atrioventricular disturbances are classified as first-, second-, or third-degree block. Often a consequence of AV-nodal slowing medications, first-degree atrioventricular block is characterized by prolongation of the PR interval beyond 200 milliseconds (**Figure 102-12**).

The hallmark of second-degree atrioventricular block is a failure of one or more, but not all, atrial impulses to conduct to the ventricles. Mobitz type I (or Wenkebach) block, characterized by a variable PR interval prior to a nonconducted atrial impulse, is often secondary to a block at a level above the His bundle and generally does not require permanent pacing unless symptomatic bradycardia is observed (**Figure 102-13**).

Generally, more pathologic, high-grade atrioventricular block is described as Mobitz type II atrioventricular block and is electrocardiographically characterized by conducted impulses that are preceded by a constant PR interval (**Figure 102-14**).

The site of block is generally infrahisian and permanent pacing is often required. For 2:1 conduction patterns, it may be difficult to distinguish between Mobitz type I or type II atrioventricular block. Third-degree atrioventricular block is also known as complete heart block and is characterized by complete dissociation of the atrial and ventricular electrical activity (**Figure 102-15**).

Electrocardiographically, atrial activity is more rapid than ventricular activity in complete heart block.

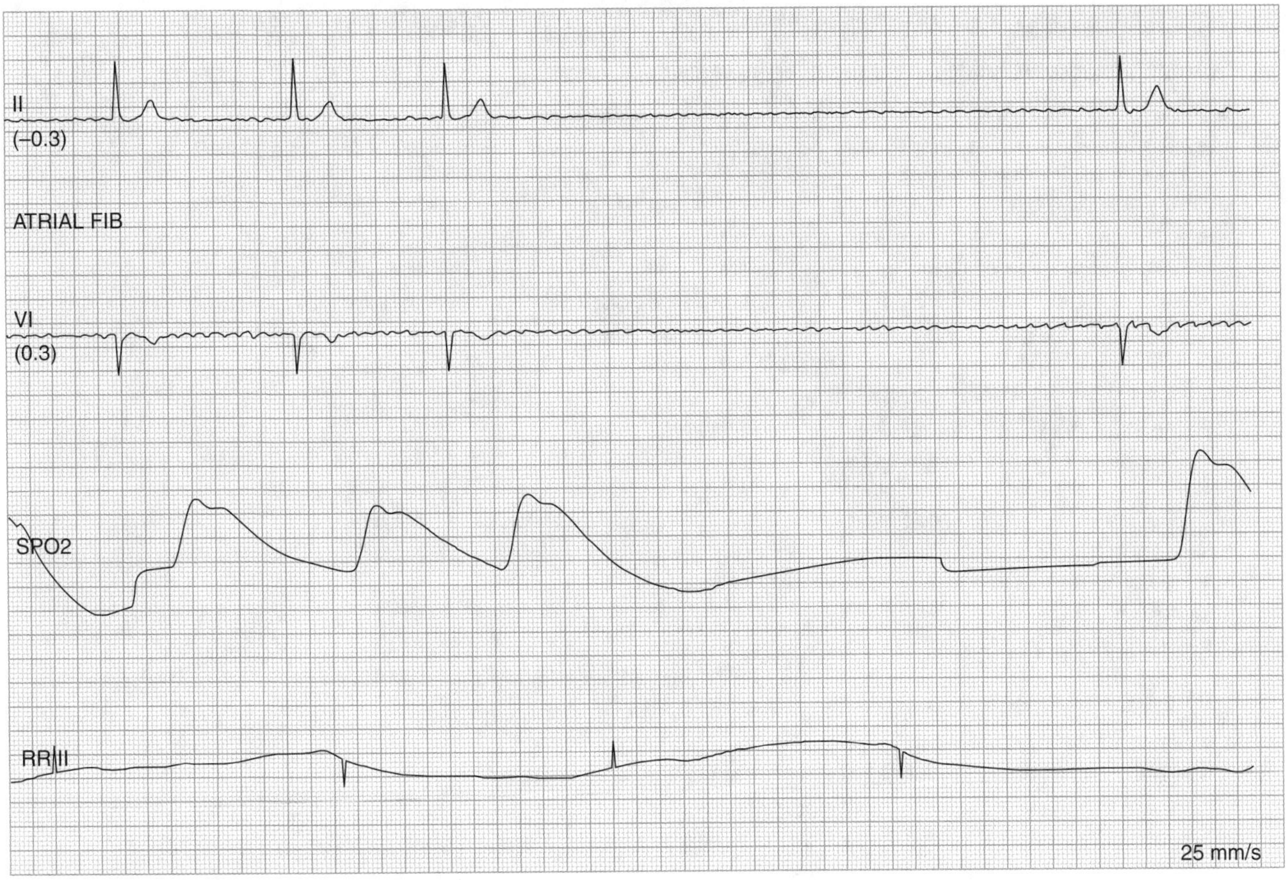

Figure 102-11 *A prolonged pause, as in this gentleman's electrocardiogram with underlying atrial fibrillation, signifies AV block and is generally an indication for permanent pacing.*

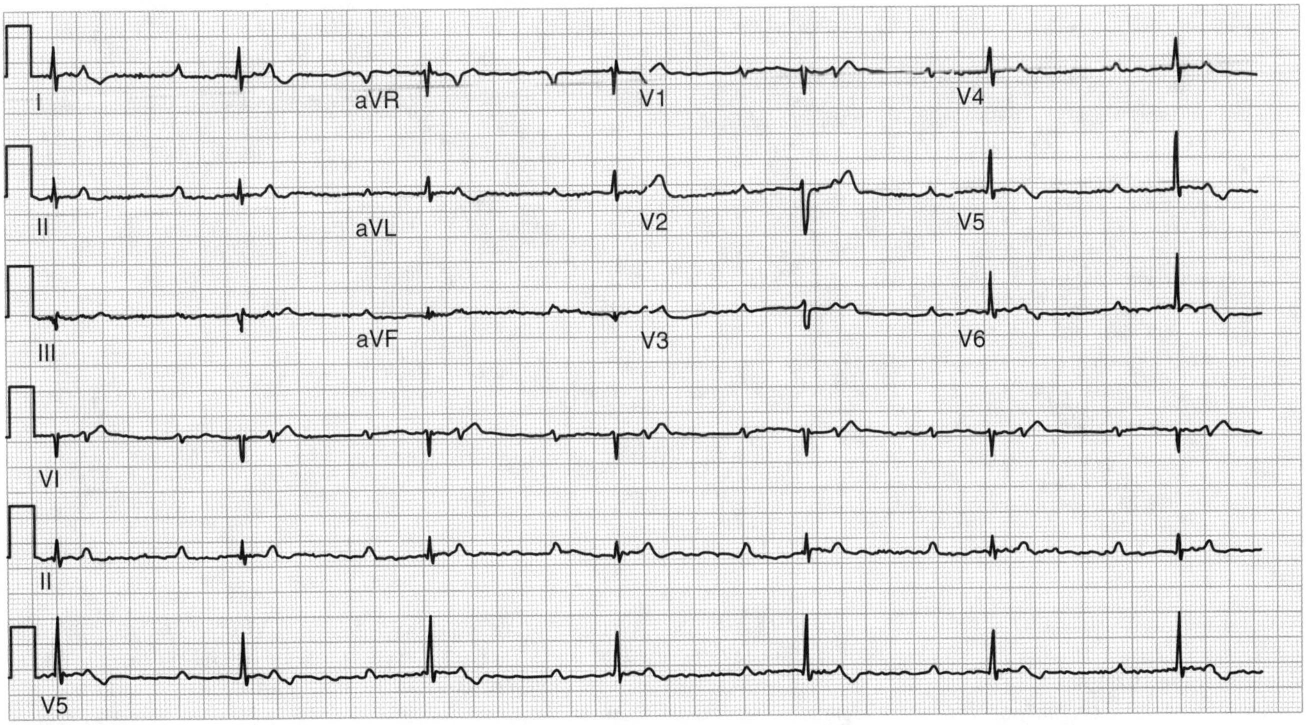

Figure 102-12 *First-degree atrioventricular block is characterized by prolongation of the PR interval beyond 200 milliseconds, as seen in this electrocardiogram from a 39-year-old gentleman on AV nodal–slowing medication.*

PART V

Hospitalist Skills

PRACTICE POINT

Syncope, presyncope, sudden death secondary to cardiac arrhythmias

- Sinoatrial exit block—long pauses and sinus arrest (sick sinus syndrome)
- AV nodal escape rhythm as a result of the depression of the sinus node, a consequence of inferior infarction. May also result from other arrhythmias.
- Stokes-Adams attacks—RBBB and LAFB
  - LAFB—frontal plane QRS axis is -30 to -90 degrees and an initial R wave is present in inferior leads. A qR complex is usually present in leads I and aVL.
  - Anterior MI, aortic valve disease, myocardial disease, including Lev disease or Lenegre disease (degenerative disease of the conduction system).
  - RBBB and LAFB or LPFB may precede complete heart block.
- Complete heart block
  - Independence of atrial and ventricular depolarizations.
  - The atrial rate is > ventricular rate, unlike other forms of AV dissociation in which the ventricular rate is > atrial rate.
  - Usual rate is 40–60 beats per minute. With blocks below the bifurcation of the bundle of His, the escape rhythm is idioventricular with a wide QRS and a rate of 30–40 beats per minute or slower.
- Wenckebach block
  - Inferior MI, digitalis toxicity, AV nodal disease.
- Ventricular tachycardia
  - Repetitive monomorphic ventricular tachycardia (VT)
    - Exercise-induced VT or catecholamine-induced VT in the absence of structural heart disease.
    - Rates of 130–180 beats per minute often nonsustained with runs of sinus rhythm.
  - Right ventricular outflow tract VT
    - Arrhythmogenic right ventricular dysplasia (ARVD).
    - LBBB VT and may have two or more morphologies of VT.
    - May have inverted T waves in leads V_1–V_4 and/or epsilon waves (in the terminal portion of the QRS complex).
    - Distortions of the ST-segment.
    - Associated with sudden death.
  - Bundle branch reentry tachycardia seen in dilated cardiomyopathy
  - Ischemic VT
    - AV dissociation due to an accelerated idioventricular rhythm at a rate of 60 beats per minute in s etting of acute MI.
    - Look for fusion beats (QRS complex displays characteristics of atrial and ventricular activation) following a run of VT.
  - Torsades de pointes
    - Appears as a polymorphic ventricular tachycardia
    - May be secondary to prolongation of the QT interval, measured from onset of the QRS complex to the end of the T wave
    - Prolonged QT may be acquired or congenital
    - Acquired QT syndrome generally related to ingestion of offending medications that disrupt one or more of the repolarizing cardiac potassium currents (eg, methadone, levofloxacin, macrolide antibiotics, metoclopramide, etc) or combination of medications that may act synergistically to prolong the QT interval (eg, macrolide antibiotic or cimetidine)
    - Congential QT syndrome may be provoked by a variety of stimuli (eg, swimming, other forms of exertion, auditory stimuli) and may be associated with deafness
  - Brugada syndrome
    - Intermittent RBBB pattern and/or upwardly coved ST elevation associated with recurrent VT in patients with no structural heart disease.

Ventricular tachycardia (VT) is defined as three or more QRS complexes of ventricular origin at a rate exceeding 100 beats per minute (**Figure 102-16**).

Nonsustained VT is generally defined as VT of duration of less than 30 seconds. Though frequently regular in rate and appearance, VT may be irregular and may be polymorphic. It may be difficult to discriminate VT from a supraventricular tachyarrythmia with aberrant intraventricular conduction. A good rule of thumb is to remember the substrate and regard any wide complex tachycardia in a patient with known ischemic heart disease as VT unless proven otherwise. And, while the Brugada criteria may be helpful in differentiating VT from supraventricular tachycardia with aberrant conduction, the presence of atrioventricular dissociation, fusion beats, and capture complexes generally favors VT. Ventricular fibrillation, a chaotic ventricular rhythm that reflects no organized electrical activity, is uniformly fatal without advanced cardiac life support (**Figure 102-17**).

The seasoned clinician should also be able to recognize motion artifacts simulating serious arrhythmias (**Figure 102-18**).

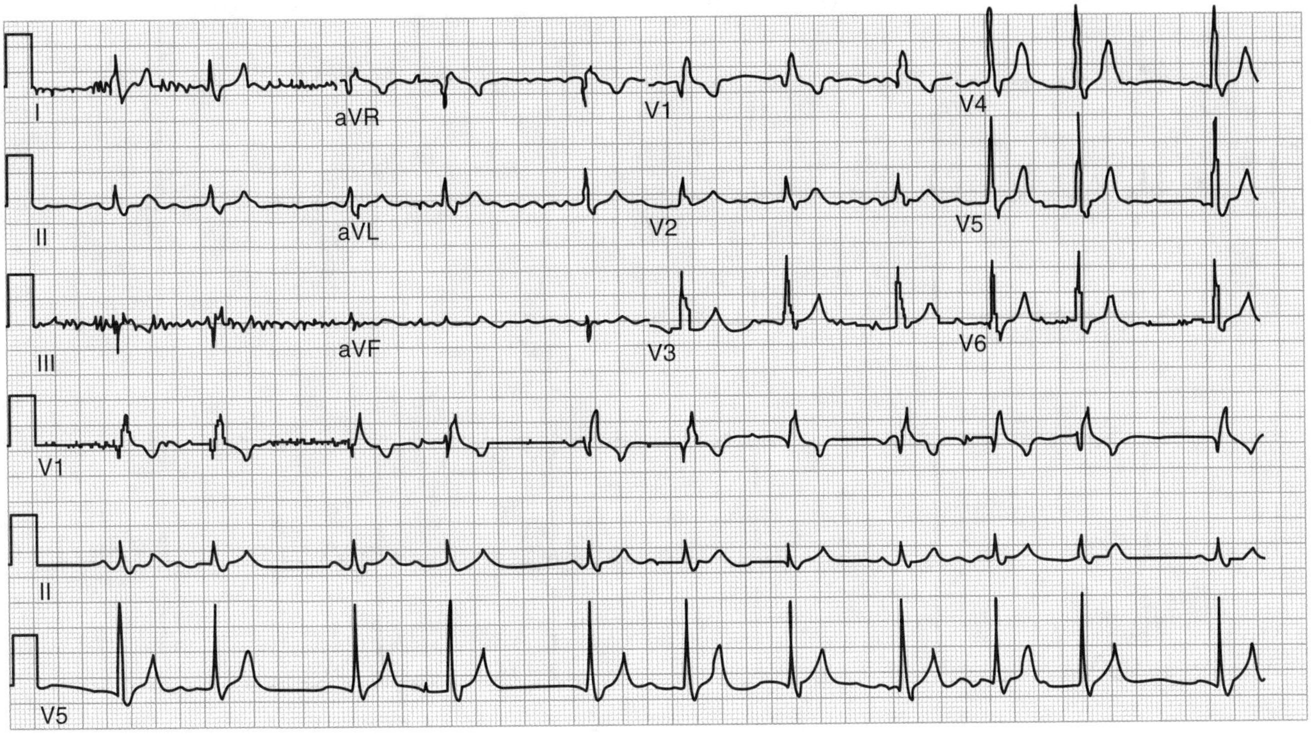

Figure 102-13 *Mobitz type I (or Wenkebach) block, characterized by a variable PR interval prior to a nonconducted atrial impulse, is often secondary to a block at a level above the His bundle. This electrocardiogram is from a 68-year-old gentleman who presented with unstable angina and underwent percutaneous coronary intervention to his left circumflex. The tracing also shows a right bundle branch block, which, together with atrioventricular block, suggests underlying conduction system disease.*

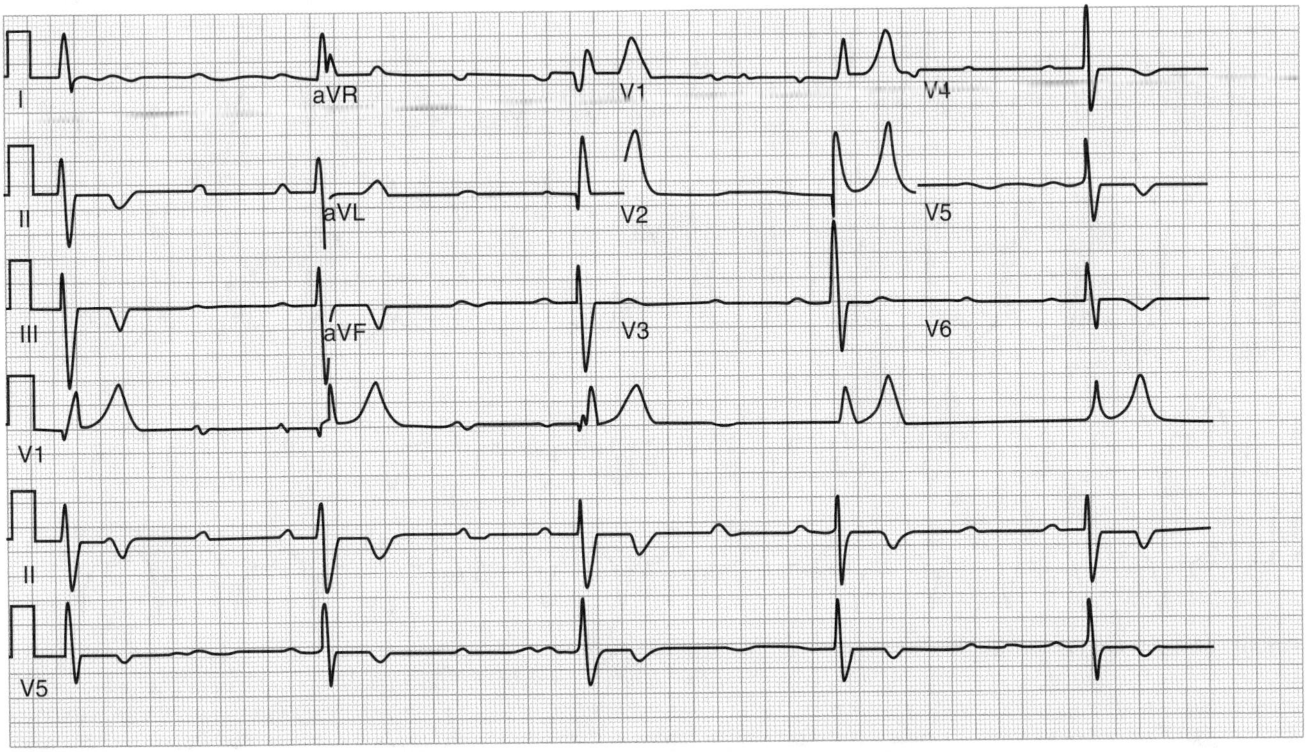

Figure 102-14 *Atrioventricular blood with 2:1 conduction. An Infra-Hisian origin of the conduction delay is suggested by the abnormal and prolonged QRS complex.*

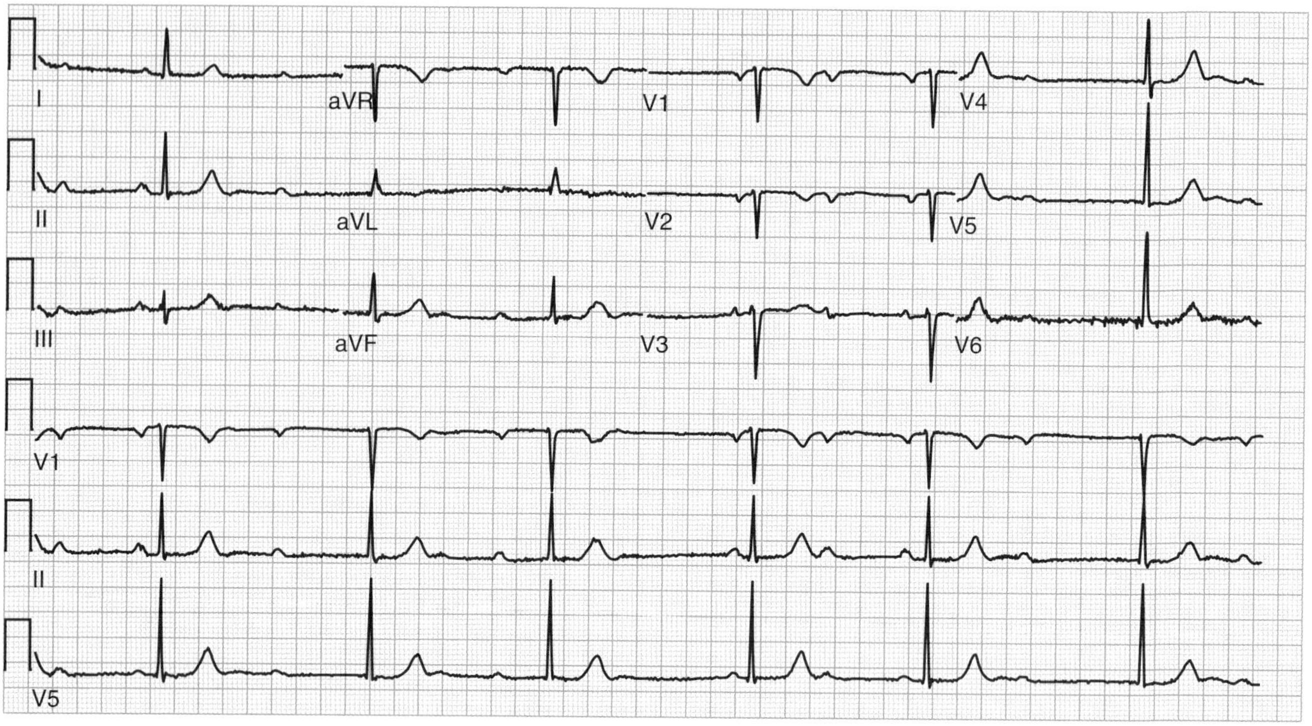

Figure 102-15 *Complete, or third-degree heart block, is characterized by atrioventricular dissociation, as seen in this electrocardiogram from a 78-year-old woman who presented with syncope and underwent successful placement of a dual-chamber permanent pacemaker. Sinus arrhythmia is also seen.*

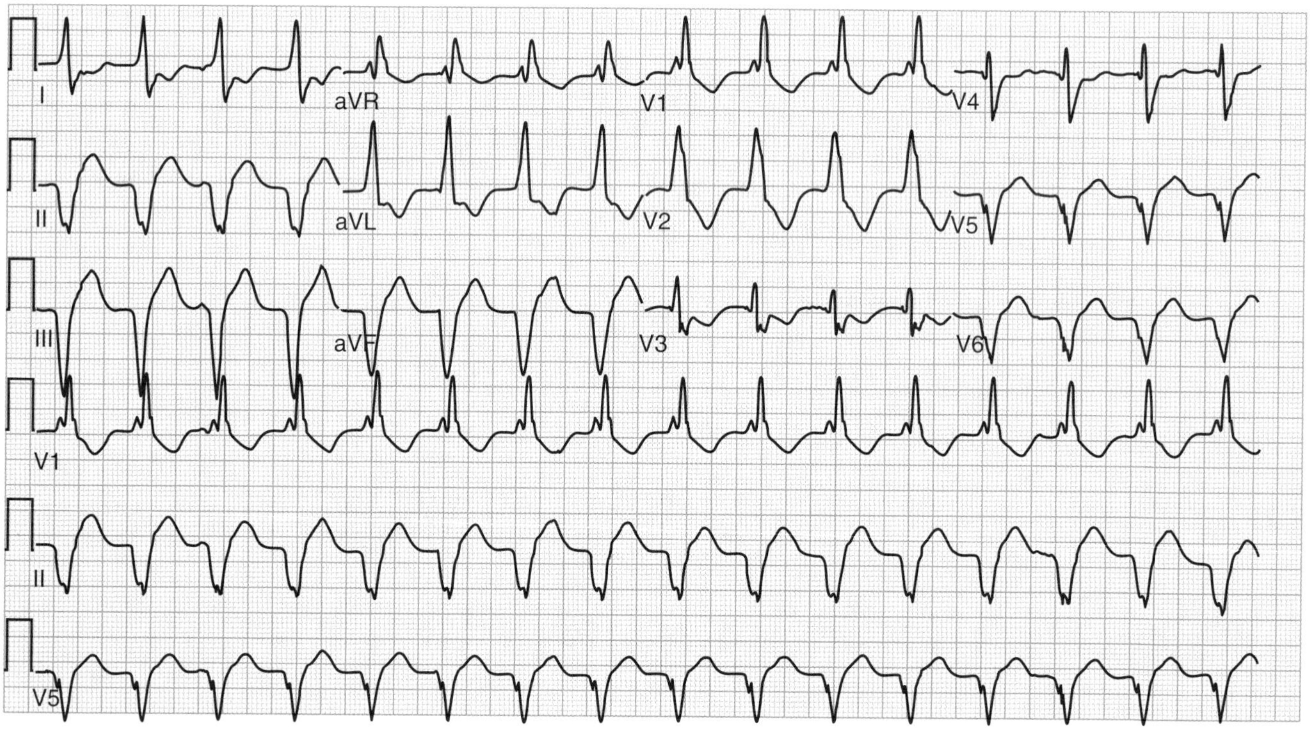

Figure 102-16 *Ventricular tachycardia is defined as three or more QRS complexes of ventricular origin at a rate exceeding 100 beats per minute. This electrocardiogram is from a 61-year-old gentleman with extensive ischemic heart disease status postsurgical and percutaneous revascularization. His ischemic substrate, as well as atrioventricular dissociation (with P waves inscribed within the QRS complex), is suggestive of scar-related ventricular tachycardia. He continued to have ventricular tachycardia despite intravenous amiodarone and required substrate modification with combined epicardial and endocardial ablation of his ventricular tachycardia.*

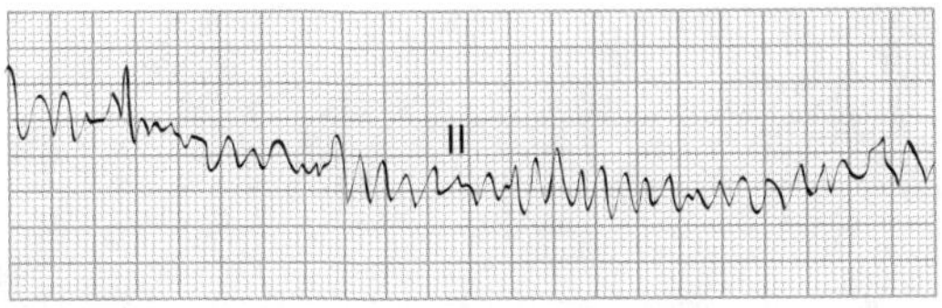

Figure 102-17 *Ventricular fibrillation, a chaotic nonperfusing ventricular rhythm that reflects no organized electrical activity, is uniformly fatal without advanced cardiac life support.*

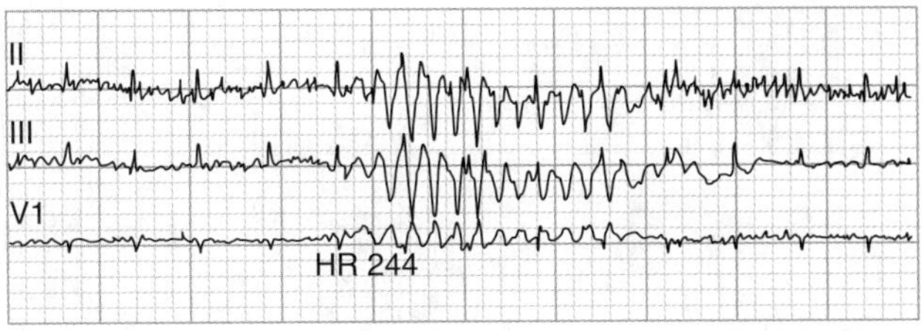

Figure 102-18 *Motion artifact should be distinguished from tachyarrhythmias. In this tracing, QRS deflections are visible at regular intervals throughout the region of artifact, making a ventricular arrhythmia much less likely.*

PALPITATIONS

Supraventricular tachyarrhythmias may account for the subjective perception of palpitations and include narrow-complex rhythms with a ventricular rate exceeding 100 beats per minute. Such tachyarrhythmias, which may be regular or irregular in appearance, commonly occur in the hospital setting. When regular, the following need to be considered: sinus tachycardia, atrial flutter with consistent atrioventricular conduction, atrioventricular node reentrant tachycardia (AVNRT), atrioventricular reentrant tachycardia, and atrial tachycardia. Multifocal tachycardia and atrial fibrillation account for irregular narrow-complex tachyarrhythmias.

Sinus tachycardia manifests as a sinus rhythm with a rate above 100 beats per minute and generally reflects a medication effect, a metabolic state, or an underlying process, such as fever, hypovolemia, or anemia (**Figure 102-19**).

Typical atrial flutter, characteristically the result of a macroreentrant circuit in the right atrium, is easily recognizable by the appearance of negatively directed "sawtooth" waveforms in the inferior leads accompanied by an atrial rate that varies between 280 and 340 beats per minute (**Figure 102-20**).

The mechanism of AVNRT involves a reentrant circuit within the AV node that generates a narrow QRS complex tachycardia in the range of 150 to 250 beats per minute, often with P waves inscribed at the terminal portion of the QRS complex (reflecting retrograde atrial depolarization) (**Figure 102-21**).

Similarly, AVRT relies on a reentrant circuit composed of an accessory pathway and the AV node. As atrial depolarization occurs after ventricular depolarization in AVRT, the P waves of AVRT are often inscribed later than in AVNRT, appearing superimposed on the ST-segment or T wave. Ventricular preexcitation, any condition in which anterograde ventricular or retrograde atrial activation occurs partially or totally via an anomalous pathway, may lead to AVRT. Wolff-Parkinson-White (WPW) syndrome is a form of ventricular preexcitation and electrocardiographically produces a short PR interval and QRS prolongation with a delta wave, an initial slurring of the QRS complex signifying ventricular activation by the accessory pathway (**Figure 102-22**).

Characteristically, both AVNRT and AVRT may be terminated with adenosine, which suppresses AV-node conduction. Atrial tachycardia, in contrast, generally does not terminate with adenosine and is characterized by a P-wave axis or morphology that is distinct from that of sinus rhythm (**Figure 102-23**).

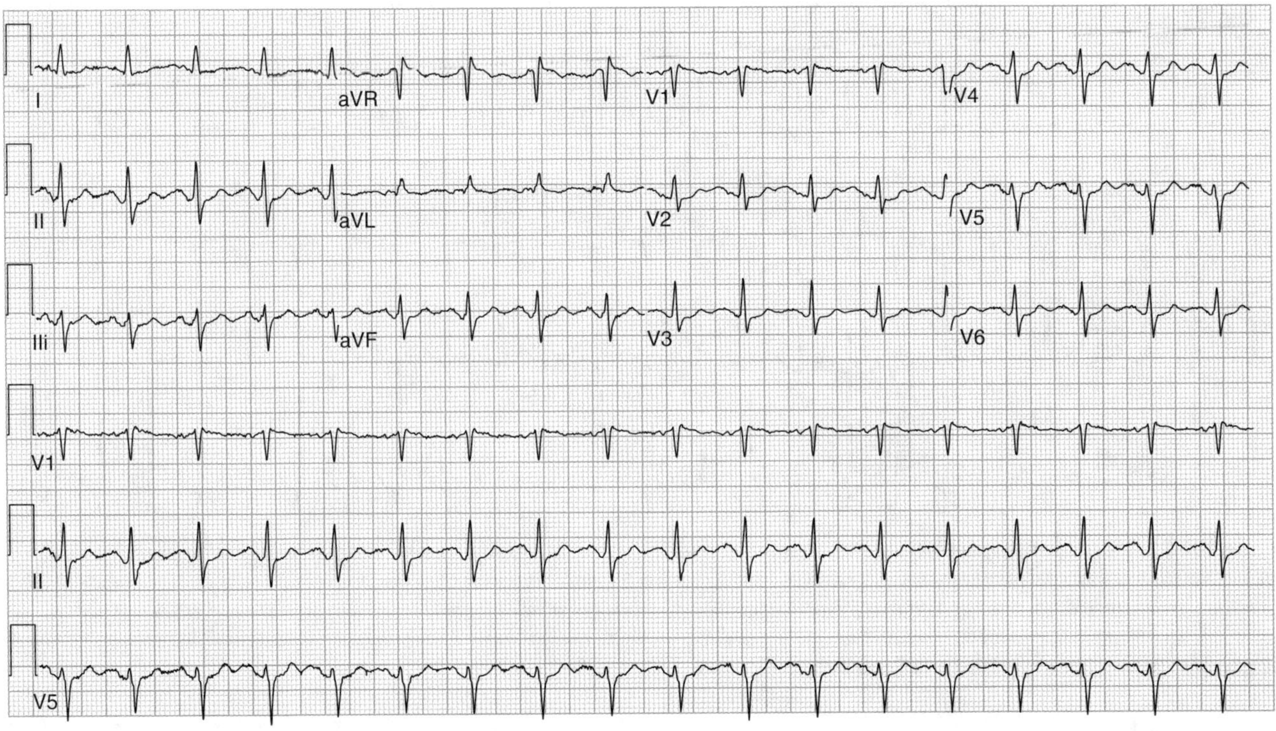

Figure 102-19 *Sinus tachycardia manifests as a sinus rhythm with a rate above 100 beats per minute and generally reflects an underlying process (eg, fever, hypovolemia, or anemia), metabolic state, or medication effect. This electrocardiogram is from a 54-year-old woman affected by opioid withdrawal and unresolved pain.*

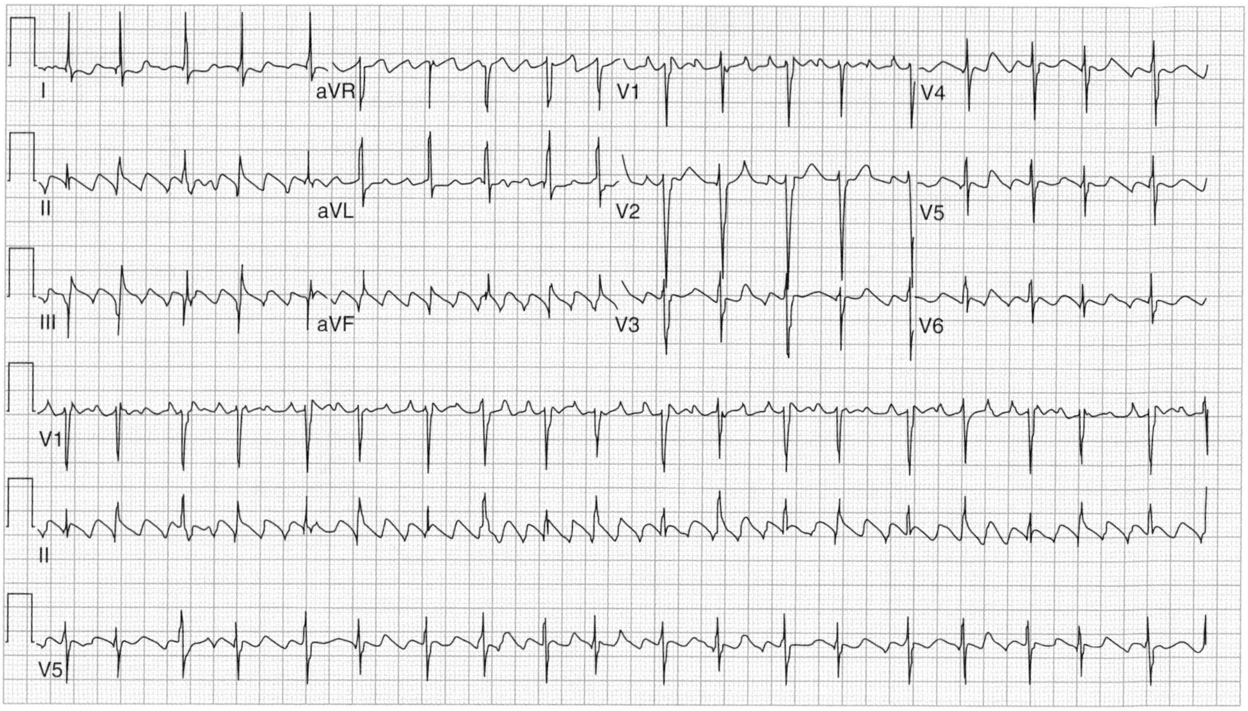

Figure 102-20 *Atrial flutter, characteristically the result of a macroreentrant circuit in the right atrium, is easily recognizable by the appearance of "sawtooth" waveforms accompanied by an atrial rate that varies between 280 and 340 beats per minute.*

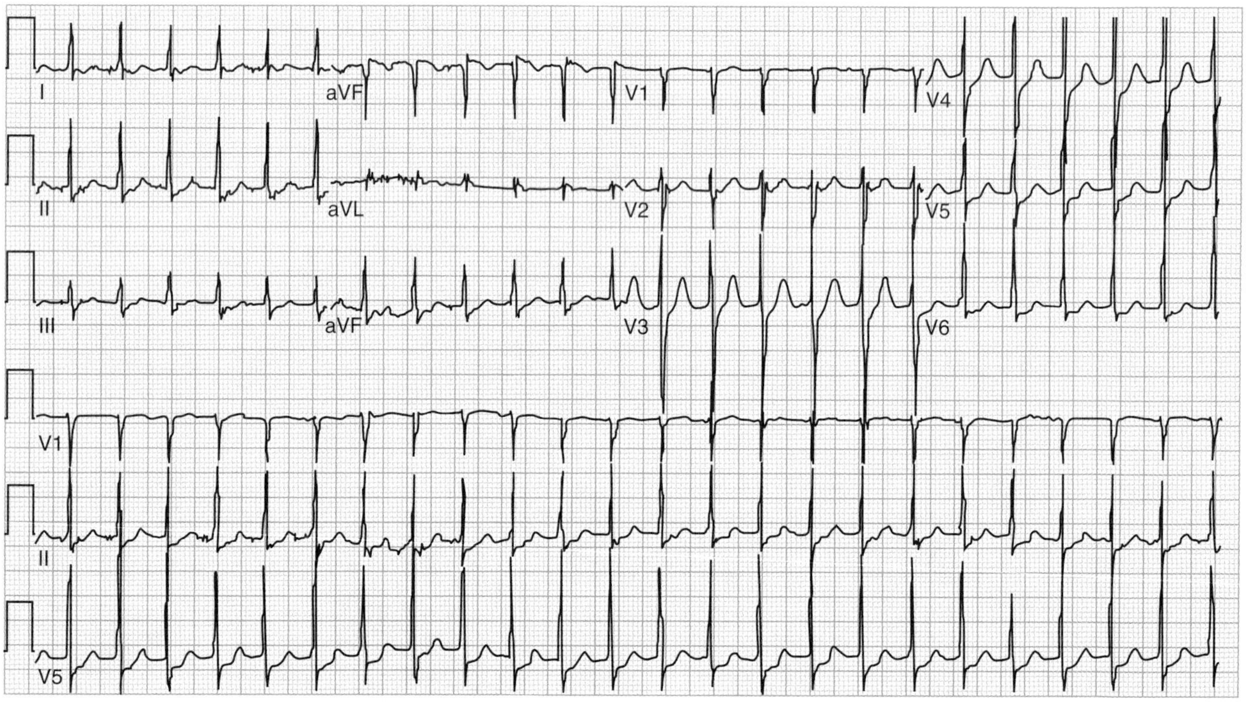

Figure 102-21 *The mechanism of AVNRT involves a reentrant circuit within the AV node that generates a narrow QRS-complex tachycardia in the range of 150 to 250 beats per minute, often with P waves inscribed at the terminal portion of the QRS complex and reflecting retrograde atrial depolarization, as in this electrocardiogram from a 66-year-old gentleman who presented with palpitations. Regional ST-segment depressions are also seen, suggestive of rate-related subendocardial injury. During electrophysiologic testing, dual AV node physiology was confirmed and radiofrequency ablation of the slow pathway was successfully performed.*

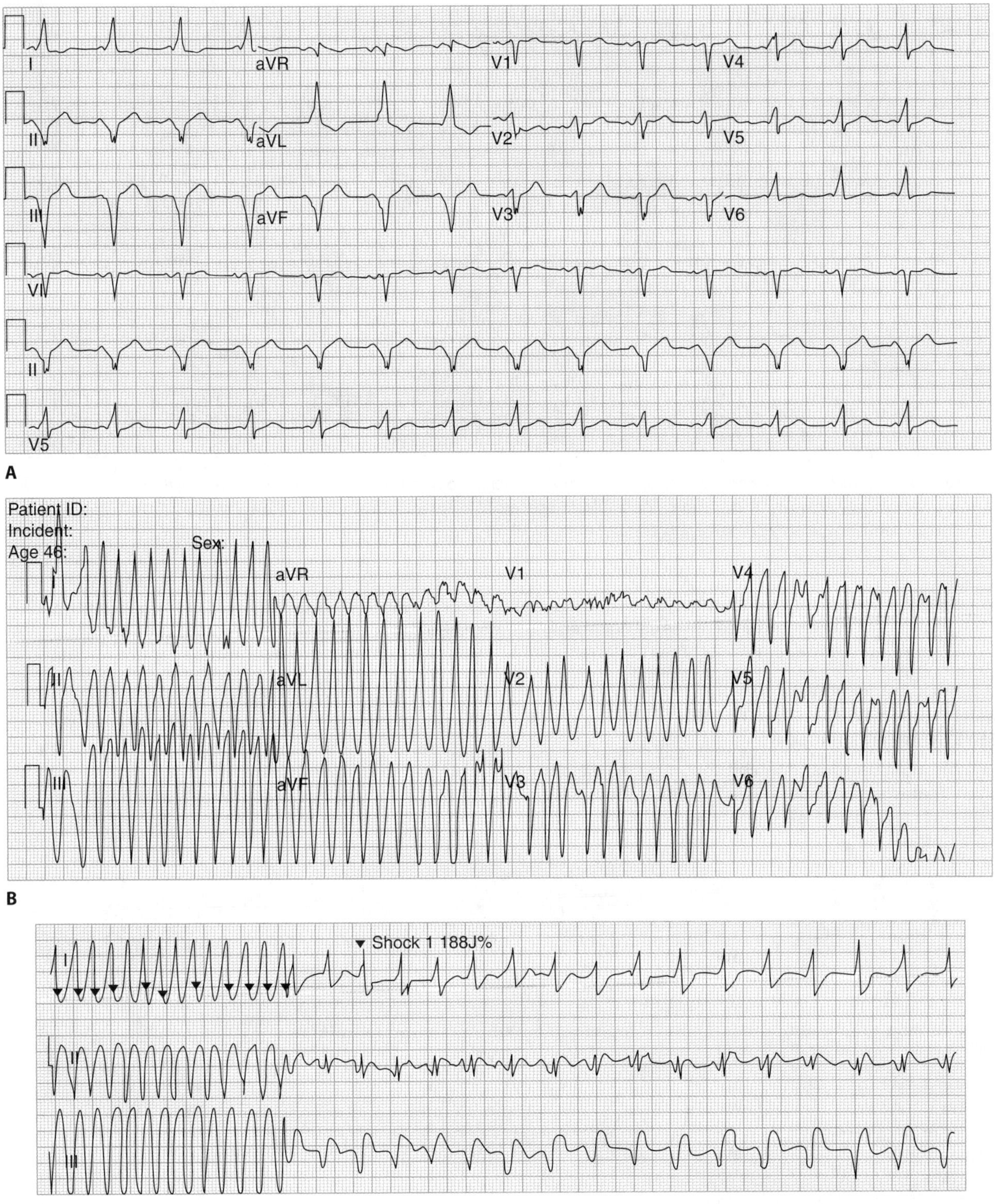

Figure 102-22 *Wolff-Parkinson-White (WPW) syndrome is a form of ventricular preexcitation and electrocardiographically produces a short PR interval and QRS prolongation with a delta wave, an initial slurring of the QRS complex signifying ventricular activation by the accessory pathway, as seen in (A) from an initially asymptomatic 48-year-old woman. After a year of close follow-up, she developed near syncope with hemodynamic instability, presenting with the irregularly irregular wide complex tachycardia seen in (B) and representing atrial fibrillation with rapid conduction through the accessory pathway. She underwent direct current cardioversion (C), followed by successful ablation of a postero-septal accessory pathway.*

Atrial tachycardia with atrioventricular block is typically seen with digoxin toxicity. Multifocal atrial tachycardia, an irregular arrhythmia, is characterized by an atrial rate greater than 100 beats per minute and P waves with three or more different lengths. It is frequently associated with concurrent pulmonary disease. A discussion of atrial fibrillation, the most common sustained tachyarrhythmia, is found elsewhere (**Figure 102-24**).

Often associated with physiologic stress, drugs, or chronic lung disease, atrial fibrillation may produce an irregularly narrow complex tachycardia that likely represents increased automaticity and multiple

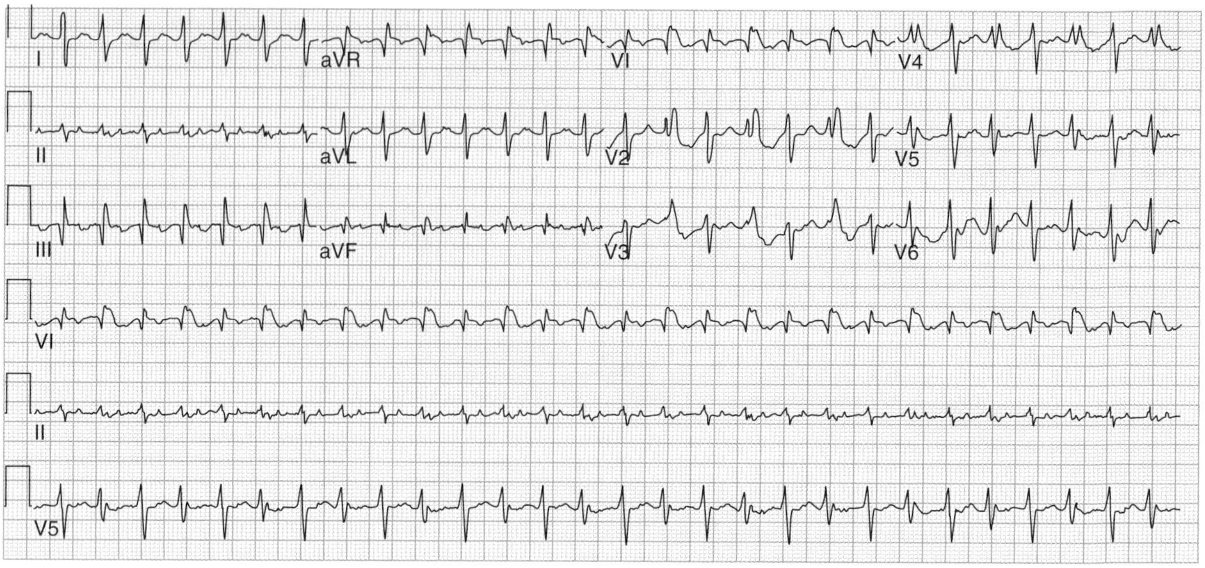

Figure 102-23 *Atrial tachycardia is characterized by a P-wave axis or morphology that is distinct from that of sinus rhythm, as in this electrocardiogram from a 64-year-old woman with palpitations. The atrial rate is generally 150 to 250 beats per minute, characteristically slower than that of atrial flutter. Right axis deviation and an incomplete right bundle branch block are also seen in this tracing.*

reentrant wavelets predominantly in the left atrium around the pulmonary veins. Multifocal atrial tachycardia can be distinguished from atrial fibrillation by an isoelectric baseline between the P waves.

ELECTROCARDIOGRAPHIC ASSOCIATIONS WITH SUDDEN CARDIAC DEATH AND GENETIC ARRHYTHMOLOGY

The seasoned clinician should be able to identify the electrocardiographic pattern associated with the Brugada and long QT syndromes. Brugada syndrome is a condition associated with sudden cardiac death and mutations linked to the *SCN5A* gene, encoding a cardiac sodium channel. Electrocardiographically, it is associated with right bundle branch block with ST-segment elevation in leads V_1–V_3 (**Figure 102-25**).

Prolongation of the QT interval may be congenital or, more frequently, acquired, as following ingestion of offending medications (eg, macrolides, fluoroquinolones, or antipsychotic drugs in a dose-relate manner) (**Figure 102-26**).

The QT interval, measured from the beginning of the QRS complex to the end of the T wave in the lead with the longest

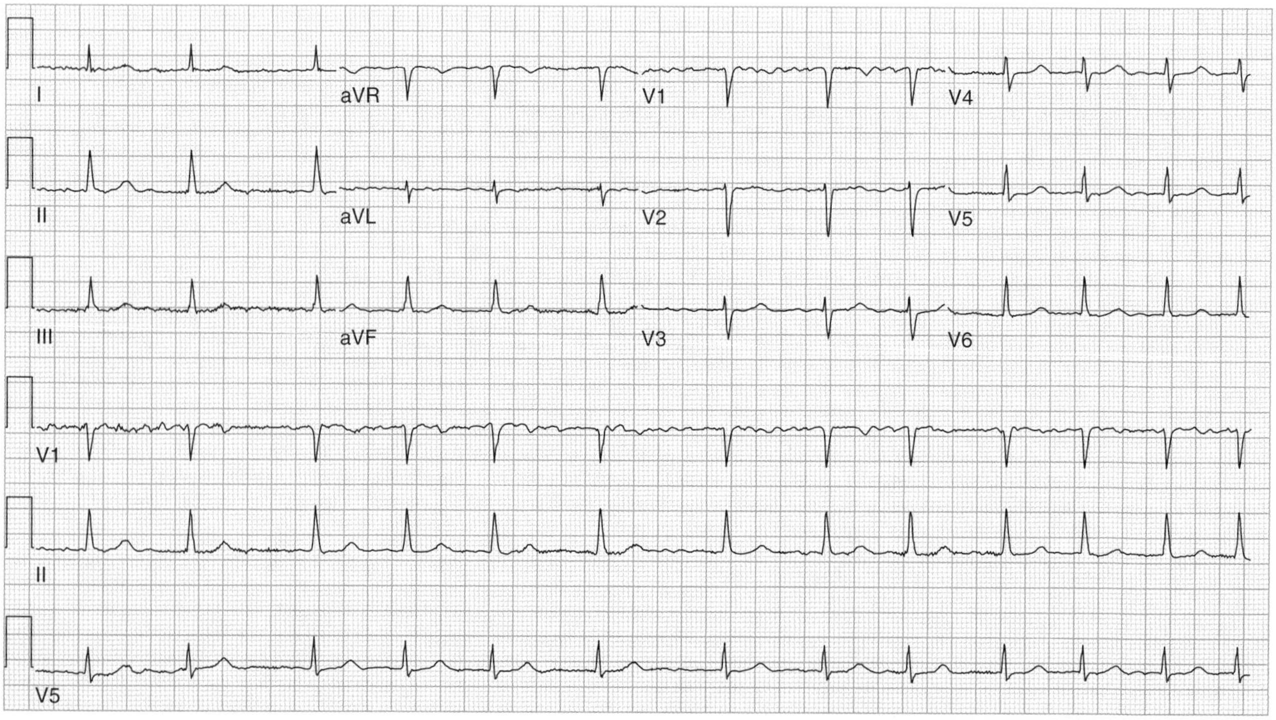

Figure 102-24 *Often associated with physiologic stress, sympathomimetic drugs, or chronic lung disease, atrial fibrillation may produce an irregularly narrow complex tachycardia. This electrocardiogram is from an 88-year-old gentleman with obesity-hypoventilation syndrome and advanced sleep apnea, ultimately requiring tracheostomy.*

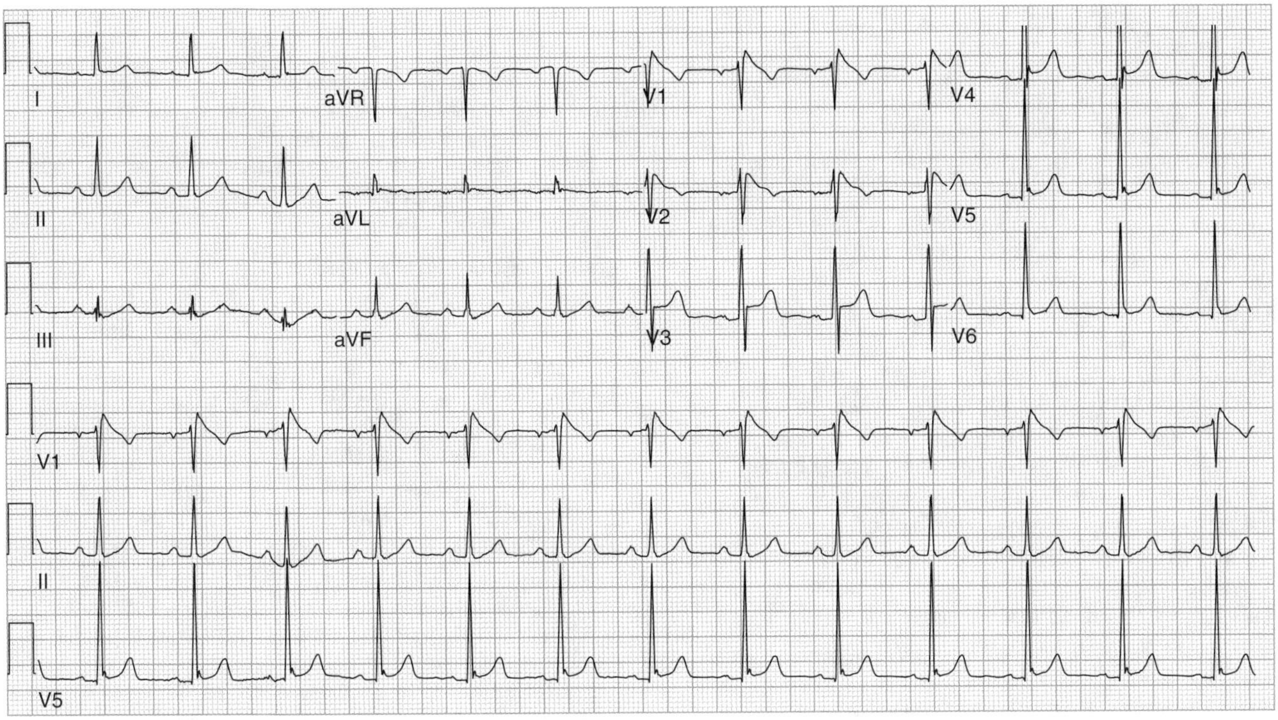

Figure 102-25 *Brugada syndrome is a condition associated with sudden cardiac death and mutations linked to the SCN5A gene, encoding a cardiac sodium channel. This electrocardiogram is from a 54 year-old gentleman with a syncopal episode. Coronary angiography revealed normal coronaries and the ST-segment elevations with biphasic T-wave inversions in V_1–V_3, along with his syncopal episode, implicated Brugada syndrome. He received a single-chamber implantable cardioverter-defibrillator (ICD) for secondary prevention.*

PRACTICE POINT

Medical illness

Hyperkalemia

- Sensitivity of the ECG for detecting hyperkalemia depends on the chronicity of the derangement. Patients with chronic hyperkalemia may have relatively minor ECG changes such as peaked T waves despite severe hyperkalemia whereas other patients may be at risk of unstable cardiac rhythms at lower serum potassium levels.
- Specificity of ECG pattern of hyperkalemia 0.85.
- Peaked T waves usually at K^+ levels >6.5 mEq/L.
- QRS widening usually at K^+ levels >7 mEq/L with higher levels causing wider complexes.
- Sinoventricular conduction—invisible P waves at K^+ levels >8.5 mEq/L—due to profound slowing of intra-atrial conduction, though the rhythm is still under control of SA node.
- Left and right axis deviation and RBBB and LBBB patterns may be seen secondary to AV conduction disturbances, but complete heart block rare.
- QT intervals normal or short unless concomitant hypocalcemia in which the QT prolongation is mainly due to prolongation of the ST-segment.

Hypokalemia

- Marked QT prolongation with or without a prominent U wave.
- Reduced amplitude of T waves and ventricular arrhythmias in severe hypokalemia.

Hypothermia

- Osborn waves, deflections at the junction of the QRS and the ST-segments, which are positive in leads over the LV, seen in leads V_2–V_6.
- Prolonged PR and QRS.
- Prolonged QT.
- Sinus tachycardia followed by bradycardia, atrial fibrillation, other atrial and ventricular arrhythmias.
- Limb leads obscured by movement artifact from shivering.

Hypothyroidism

- Reduced cardiac adrenergic activity, myocardial edema, pericardial effusion.
- Bradycardia (rarely severe).
- Reduced amplitude of all ECG waveforms.
- Increase in PR interval (due to sympathetic withdrawal and slower AV nodal transmission).
- Prolonged QT, QTc with accompanying T-wave inversion.

Stroke

- ST-segment depression or elevation, abnormal T and U waves, and/or prolongation of the QT interval in up to 75% of patients with subarachnoid hemorrhage and >90% of unselected patients with either ischemic stroke or intracerebral hemorrhage.
- All kinds of ECG changes including heart block (left) and supraventricular tachycardia (right side) can be seen with insular cortex infarcts.

(continued)

Drug therapy

- Digitalis Intoxication: atrial tachycardia with changing block, nonparoxysmal junctional tachycardias, second and third degree AV block, sinoatrial block and ventricular arrhythmias (including bidirectional ventricular tachycardia).
  - Near regularization of the ventricular rate in the presence of atrial fibrillation suggests digitalis intoxication.
  - Hypokalemia facilitates digitalis toxicity.
- Class IC agents (flecainide, propafenone): widening of the QRS and lengthening of the QTc interval due to QRS prolongation at normal doses (due to effects on conduction in the His-Purkinje system and the ventricular myocardium).
- Class IA agents (quinidine, procainamide, disopyramide): slight widening of the QRS at normal doses.
  - Prolongation of QT interval by quinidine may result in polymorphic ventricular tachycardia in the setting of hypokalemia and bradycardia.
- Class IIB agents (lidocaine, mexiletine, tocainide) and betablockers (including sotalol): do not effect QRS duration in therapeutic doses.
- SSRI in a dose related manner: prolonged QT.
- Lithium: prolonged QT and T-wave abnormalities.
- Tricyclic Antidepressants: nonspecific ST and T wave changes, prolonged QRS duration, PR and QT segment prolongation.
  - Toxicity: sinus tachycardia, prolonged QRS complex, first degree AV block, prolonged QT interval, prominent R wave in aVR.
    - A QRS duration < 100 ms favorable prognosis.
    - A QRS duration 100–60 ms moderate risk.
    - A QRS duration > 160 ms high risk of seizures and ventricular arrhythmias.
- Carbamezepine: sinus tachycardia in massive overdose; bradyarrythmias or AV conduction delay in elderly women with therapeutic or slightly elevated levels and abnormal renal function.

Chronic obstructive pulmonary disease pattern

- Pseudoinfarct pattern: right atrial abnormality, vertical P and QRS axes, dominant S waves across precordium, low voltage of R wave in V_6.
- Features that specifically suggest the presence of chronic obstructive pulmonary disease pattern disease if all present (> 90% specificity and > 50% sensitivity):
  1. P waves show a rightward axis in the range of +70° to +90° (ie, negative P wave in aVL). This reflects that atrial activation is directed more inferiorly than usual while the ventricular activation is more superiorly and posteriorly than normal due to the vertical suspension of the heart in the midline.
  2. The QRS complexes show low voltage in limb leads and precordial leads. This reflects the increased lung volume.
  3. The QRS axis is superior with negative complexes (QS or rS) in inferior leads.
  4. The precordial leads show predominant S waves through V_6.
  5. The R wave in V_6 is < 5 mm in amplitude.
- P-pulmonale from pulmonary hypertension is not required for the diagnosis.

interval, decreases as heart rate increases. The Bazett formula offers a mathematical means for relating the QT interval to heart rate as follows:

$$QT_{Corrected} = QT/(RR)^{1/2}$$

A prolonged QT interval may predispose to torsades de pointes, a type of polymorphic VT characterized by a typical "twisting of the points."

ELECTROCARDIOGRAPHIC MANIFESTATIONS OF NONCARDIAC ILLNESS AND METABOLIC DISTURBANCES

Electrolyte abnormalities, acid-base disturbances, and systemic hypothermia may produce characteristic electrocardiographic changes. Changes in extracellular potassium balance, in particular, are associated with a distinctive sequence of electrocardiographic changes. Hyperkalemia may initially produce narrowing and peaking of the T-waves, followed by widening of the QRS complex and decrement in P-wave amplitude (**Figure 102-27**).

With increasing severity of hyperkalemia, there may be loss of P waves, generating a sino-ventricular junctional escape rhythm. Hypokalemia, associated with myocardial hyperpolarization, leads to ST-segment depressions, T-wave flattening, increased U-wave prominence, and QT prolongation predisposing to torsades de pointes (**Figure 102-28**).

Changes in extracellular calcium content generally affect the action potential duration, with hypercalcemia and hypokalemia producing shortening and prolongation of the QT interval, respectively (**Figure 102-29**).

A late potential, the Osborn wave or convex elevation at the junction (J point of the ST-segment), may be associated with severe hypercalcemia and disappear with appropriate treatment. The Osborn wave is also seen in about one-third of hypothermic patients (**Figure 102-30**).

Hypothyroidism, related to decreased adrenergic activity, may produce bradycardia, prolongation of the PR interval, and reduced amplitude of all electrocardiographic waveforms (**Figure 102-31**).

This metabolic disturbance may also be associated with pericardial effusion, which, in addition to producing reduction of electrocardiographic waveforms, may produce electrical alternans (**Figure 102-32**).

Repolarization abnormalities in arrhythmias may occur in up to 70% of stroke patients. Prominent T-wave inversions, characteristically diffuse and often associated with changes in the ST-segment and/or QT prolongation, are often an electrocardiographic feature of a cerebrovascular accident, especially larger infarcts and hemorrhages. The insula in particular appears to effect heart rate and blood pressure. The right insula, as may be affected following a right middle cerebral artery infarct, may lead to tachyarrhythmias and hypertension. Bradycardia and vasodepression often occur in the setting of left insular injury. Among patients with cerebrovascular accidents, those presenting with electrocardiographic changes have a higher 6-month mortality.

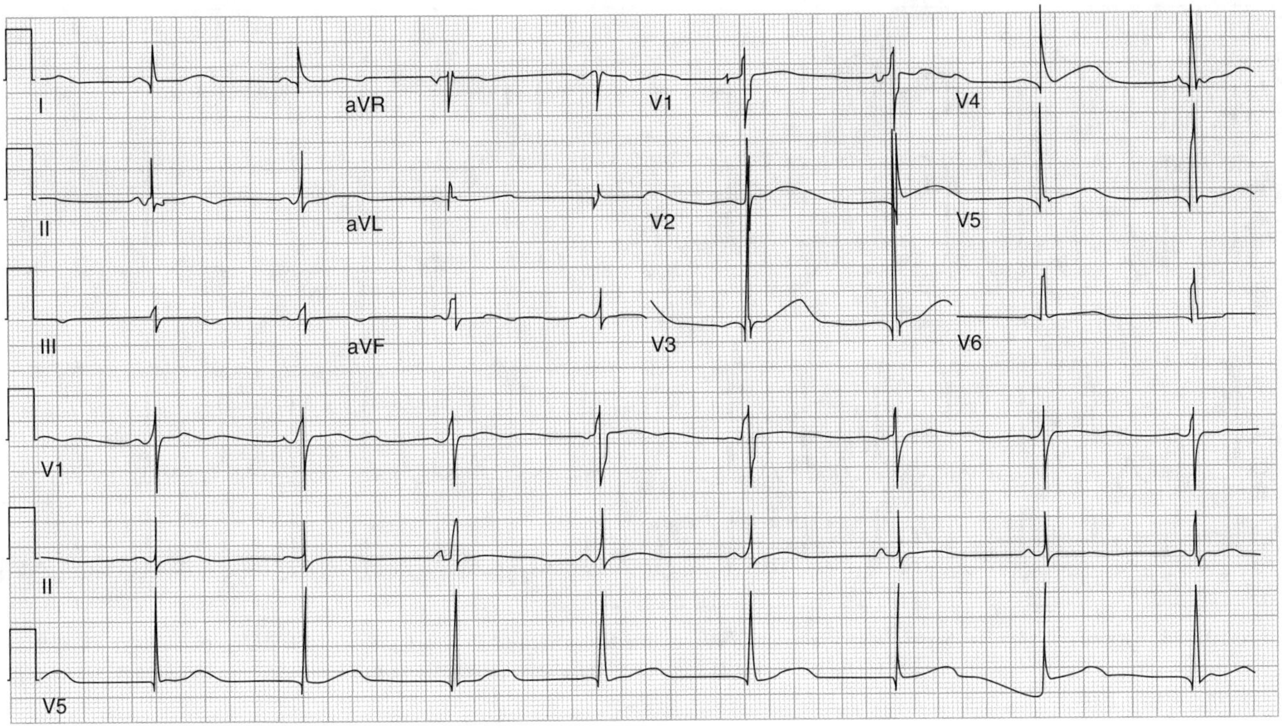

A

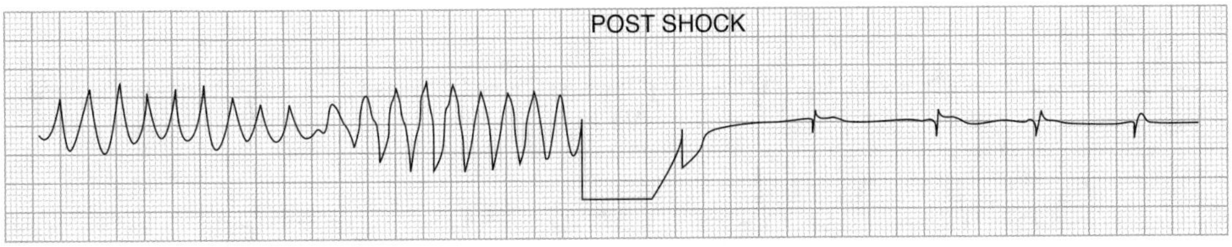

B

Figure 102-26 *Prolongation of the QT interval may be congenital or, more frequently, acquired, as following ingestion of offending medications. This electrocardiogram is from a gentleman who recently escalated the dose of his methadone. Prolongation of the QT interval is seen in (A). He developed torsades de pointes (B) A polymorphic ventricular tachycardia, requiring defibrillation.*

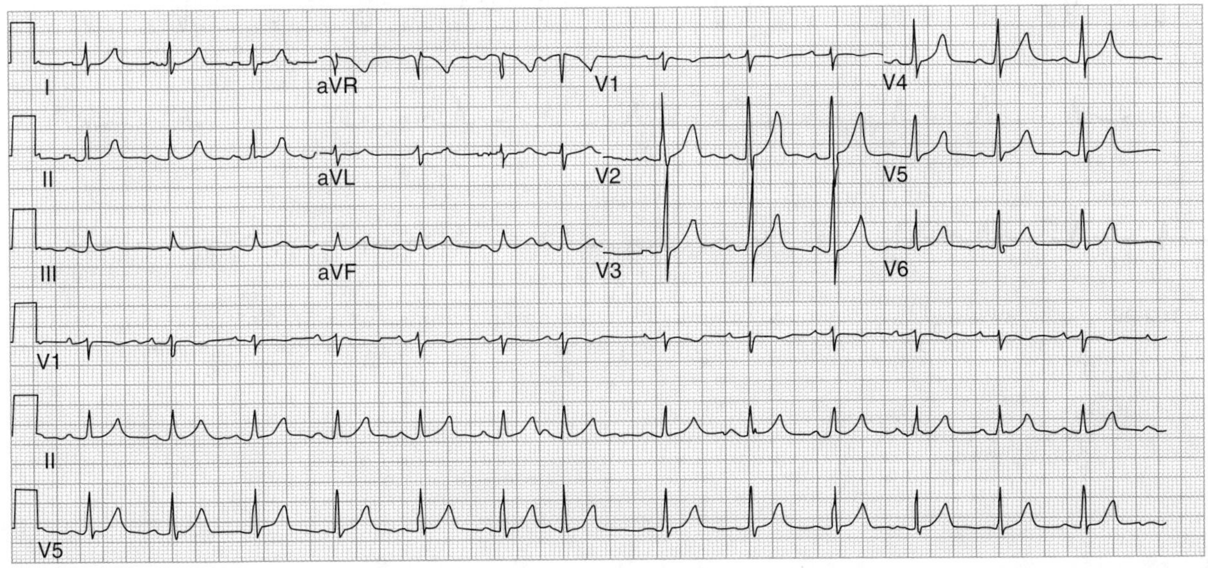

Figure 102-27 *Hyperkalemia may initially produce narrowing and peaking of the T waves, followed by widening of the QRS complex and decrement in P-wave amplitude. This electrocardiogram is from a 68-year-old gentleman with end-stage renal disease on hemodialysis; his serum potassium was 6.8 mg/dL.*

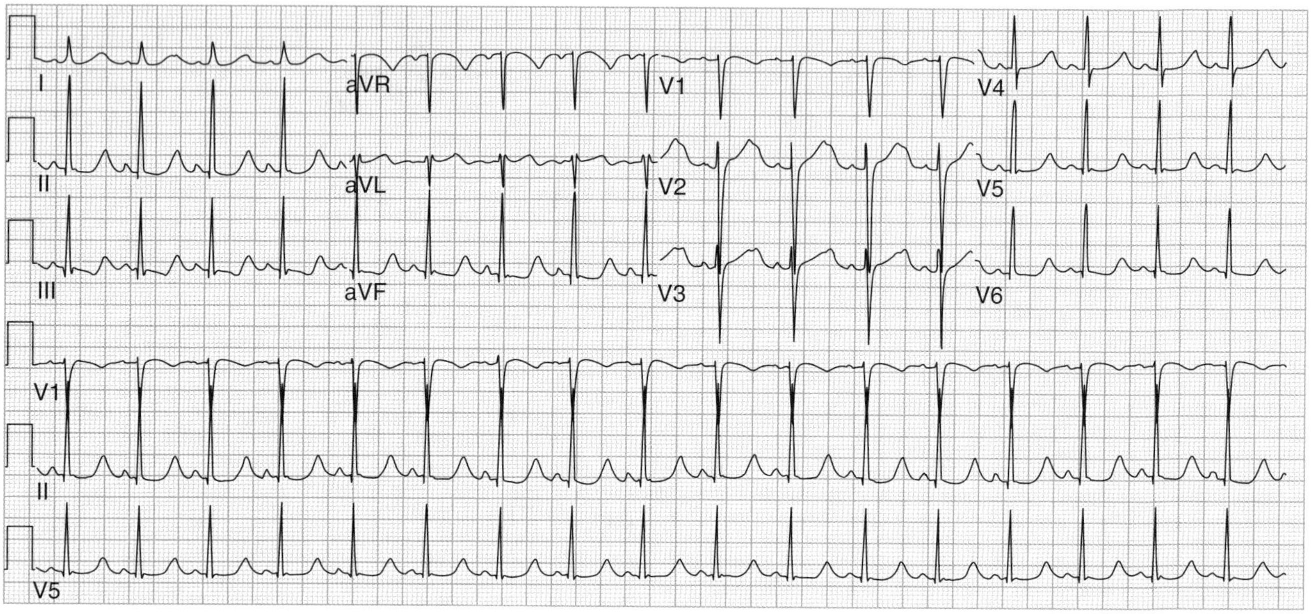

Figure 102-28 *Hypokalemia leads to ST-segment depressions, T-wave flattening, increased U-wave prominence, and QT prolongation. This electrocardiogram is from a 20-year-old woman with severe hypokalemia secondary to hyperemesis gravidarum. Resolution of QT prolongation was seen with electrolyte repletion.*

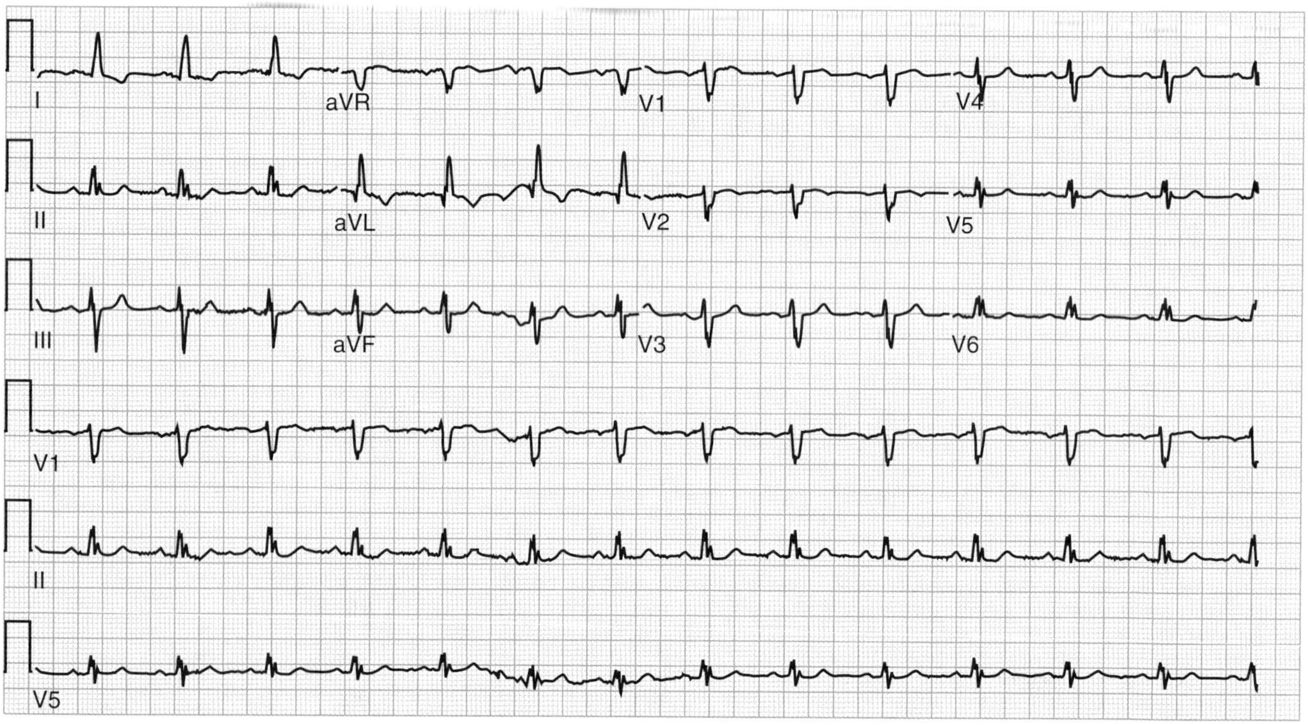

Figure 102-29 *Changes in extracellular calcium content generally affect the action potential duration, with hypercalcemia producing shortening of the QT interval, as in this electrocardiogram from a 58-year-old woman with excessive exogenous calcium intake and on antihypertensive treatment with hydrochlorothiazide.*

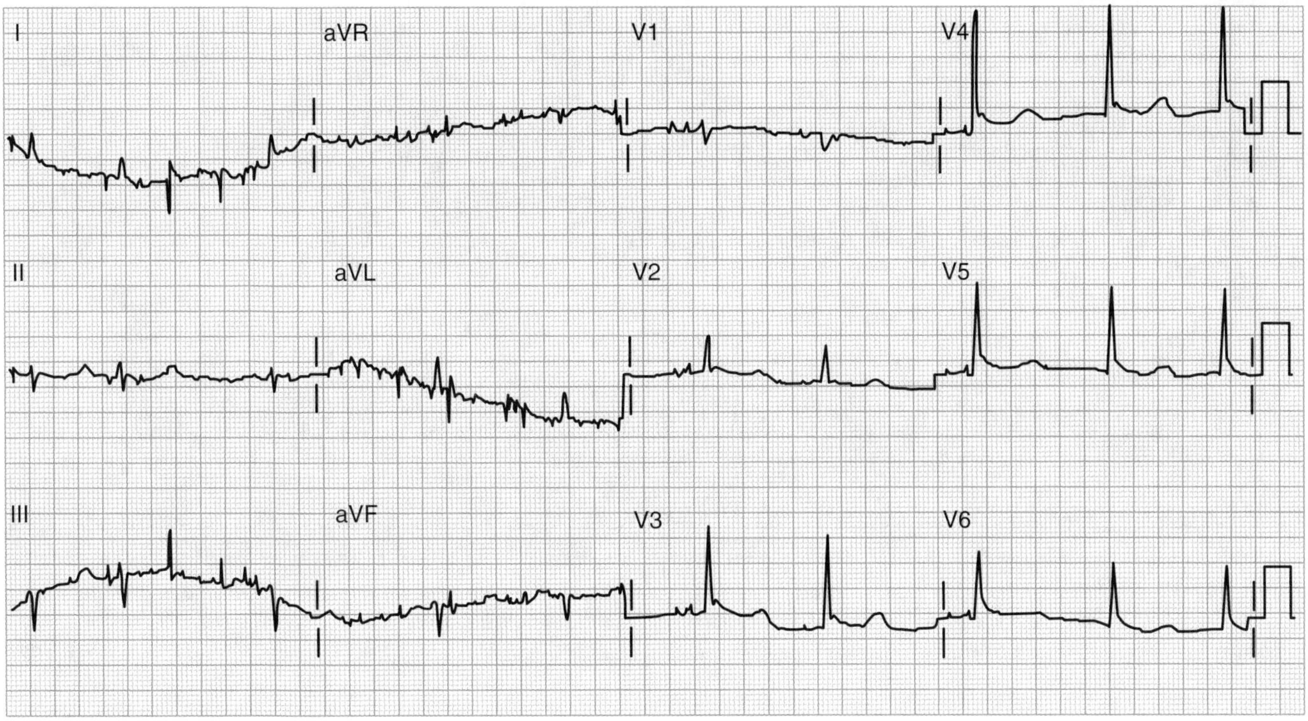

Figure 102-30 *Systemic hypothermia may generate a distinctive Osborn wave, or convex elevation at the junction (J point) of the ST-segment. This electrocardiogram is from a 90 year-old gentleman who was found unresponsive. Prominent artifact from his shivering is seen in the limb leads.*

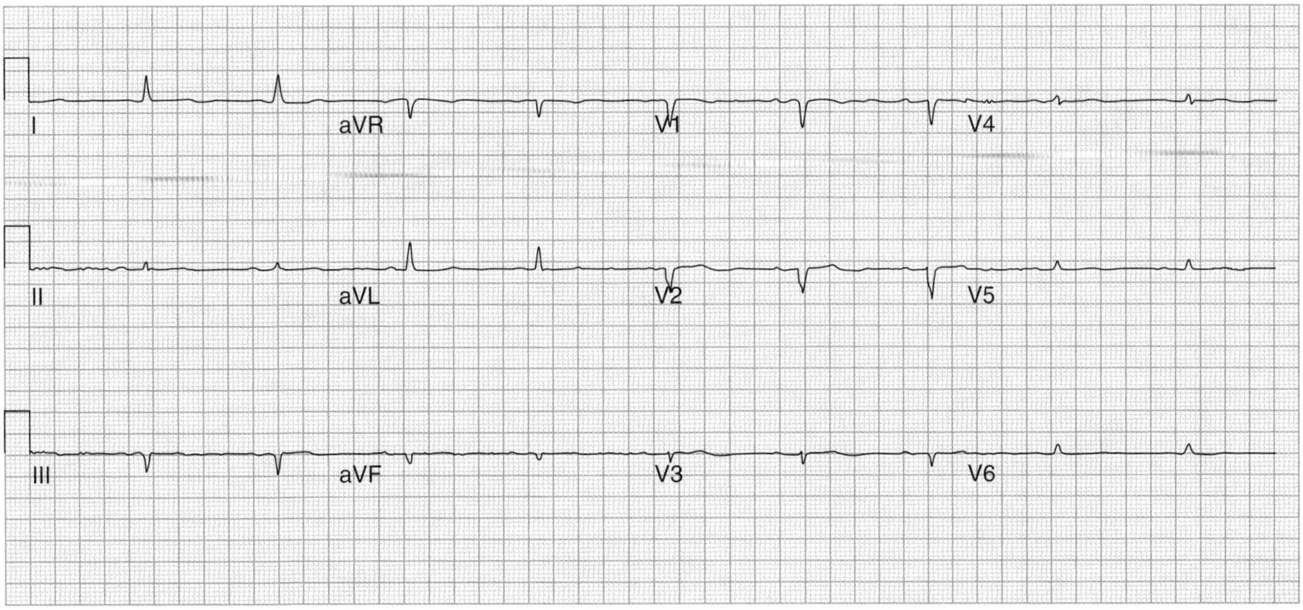

Figure 102-31 *Hypothyroidism, related to decreased adrenergic activity, may produce bradycardia, prolongation of the PR interval, and reduced amplitude of all electrocardiographic waveforms, as in this tracing from a woman with myxedema coma.*

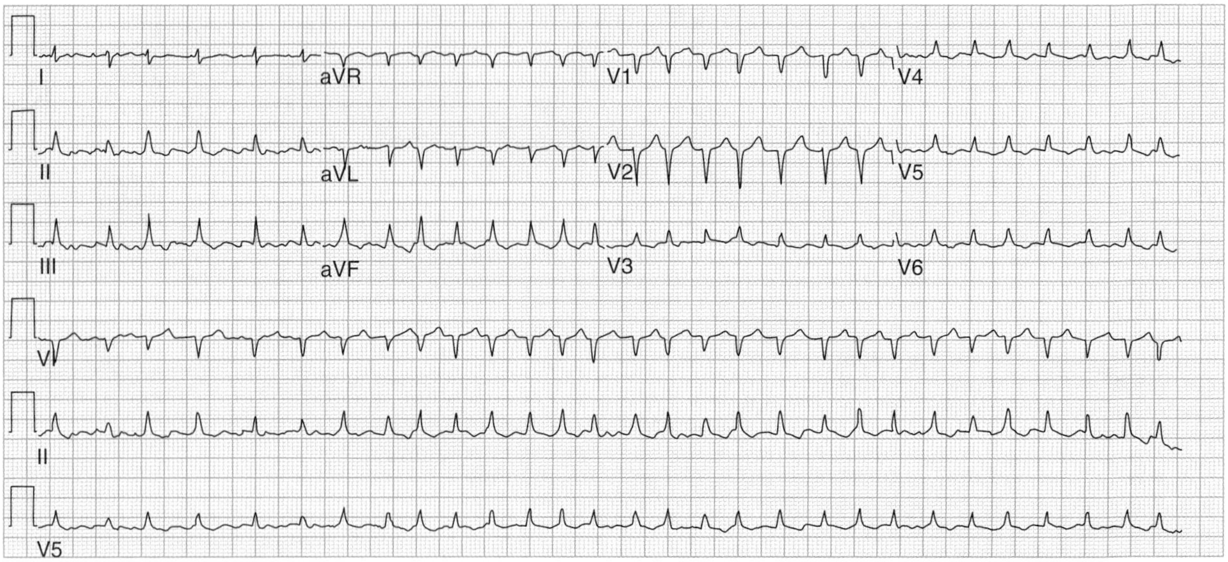

Figure 102-32 *Pericardial effusion may produce reduction in electrocardiographic waveforms, along with electrical alternans, as in this tracing from a 65-year-old woman with known lung cancer who presented with dyspnea and hemodynamic instability. Nearly 2 liters of hemorrhagic pericardial fluid were withdrawn emergently; cytology revealed malignant cells consistent with lung adenocarcinoma. Atrial fibrillation with rapid ventricular response is also seen.*

CONCLUSION

The electrocardiogram quickly provides valuable information that may suggest acute life-threatening illness and/or underlying medical illness. It is a valuable bedside tool when properly interpreted in the clinical context of the patient's presentation.

SUGGESTED READINGS

Channer K, Morris F. ABC of clinical electrocardiography: myocardial ischemia. *BMJ*. 2002;324:1023–1026.

Goldberger AL. Myocardial infarction: Electrocardiographic differential diagnosis. 4th ed. St. Louis, MO: Mosby-Year Book; 1991.

Klatsky AL, Oehm R, Cooper RA, et al. The early repolarization normal variant electrocardiogram: correlates and consequences. *Am J Med*. 2003;115:171.

Schlant RC, Adolph RJ, DiMarco JP, et al. Guidelines for electrocardiography. A report of the American College of Cardiology/American Heart Association Task Force on Assessment of Diagnostic and Therapeutic Cardiovascular Procedures (Committee on Electrocardiography). *J Am Coll Cardiol*. 1992;19:473.

Surawicz B, Parikh SR. Prevalence of male and female patterns of early repolarization in the normal ECG of males and females from childhood to old age. *J Am Coll Cardiol*. 2002;40:1870.

Wellens HJJ, Gorgels AP. The electrocardiogram 102 years after Einthoven. *Circulation*. 2004;109:562–564.

Zimetbaum PJ, Josephson ME. Use of the electrocardiogram in acute myocardial infarction. *NEJM*. 2003;348:933–940.

CHAPTER 103

Pulmonary Function Testing

Joseph J. Miaskiewicz, MD, FHM

Key Clinical Questions

1. What information do pulmonary function tests provide in addition to the history and physical examination?
2. What specific tests might you order to evaluate the acutely ill hospitalized patient and how does each test influence diagnostic evaluation or management?
3. What operations require preoperative pulmonary function tests as part of the preoperative evaluation?
4. What are the predictors of increased postoperative risk?

INTRODUCTION

Pulmonary function tests (PFTs) objectively assess lung function. Along with measurement of arterial blood gases, PFTs are used to evaluate how much a patient's symptoms or known lung disease impairs daily activities and the tests are helpful in management, such as when to treat a patient and in what setting. The purpose of PFTs is to evaluate dyspnea by assessing the mechanical function of the respiratory system, to quantitate the loss of lung function, and to monitor disease progression and response to treatment. PFTs also predict postoperative risk of pulmonary complications and which patients will likely have adequate pulmonary function after lung resection. Serial evaluations monitor respiratory muscular strength in progressive neuromuscular diseases such as Guillain Barre, myasthenia gravis, and muscular dystrophy.

PFTs estimate the following:

1. Volumes or the ability of the lungs to fully expand (TLC, FRC, RV)
2. Flow rates or the rate of inflow and outflow of air (FEV1, forced expiratory flow [25–75%])
3. Maximum voluntary ventilation or airflow through major airways by rapid inspiration and expiration maneuvers (MVV)
4. Maximum inspiratory and expiratory pressure, a measure of respiratory muscle strength (Pi[max], Pe[max])
5. Diffusing capacity (DLCO) or measurement of the ability of oxygen to get into the blood.

Interpretation will be (1) normal, (2) obstructive, (3) restrictive, or (4) combined obstructive and restrictive. For the majority of PFTs to be meaningful, patients must be able to physically perform the tests and to follow instructions. With the exception of oximetry, arterial blood gases (ABGs), and simple spirometry, PFTs are usually performed in the outpatient setting. Hospitalists should be able to (1) recognize patterns of pulmonary involvement when they review outside medical records, (2) know when to order specific tests to evaluate acutely ill patients, and (3) avoid unnecessary ordering of PFTs when they are of limited utility in hospitalized patients.

COMPONENTS OF TESTING

PFTs will detect significant increased resistance to airflow (airway obstruction) and increased resistance to expansion (parenchymal disease, weakness of respiratory muscles or abnormalities of the chest wall or diaphragm). ABGs supplement PFTs by measuring the effect of pulmonary and other illnesses on oxygenation and ventilation (**Figure 103-1**).

VOLUMES

TLC = Total lung capacity or the total volume of gas within the lungs after a maximal inspiration

RV = Residual volume or the volume of gas remaining in the lungs after a maximal expiration

VC = Vital capacity or the volume of gas expired after a maximal inspiration followed by a maximal expiration

FRC = Functional residual capacity or the volume of gas within the lungs at the end of expiration during normal tidal breathing at rest

To quantitate VC, ask the patient to breathe into a spirometer and obtain a spirometric tracing. To quantitate RV, FRC, and TLC, other methods such as dilution tests or body plethysmography are needed to measure the amount of air left in the lungs. These

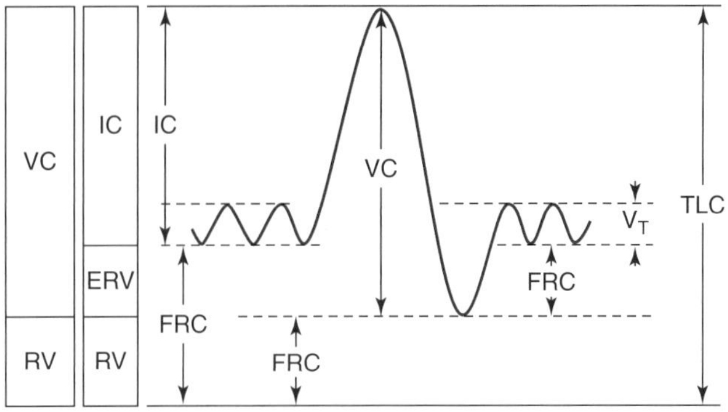

Figure 103-1 *Lung Volumes. (Reproduced, with permission, from Weinberger SE: Principles of Pulmonary Medicine, 4th ed. Philadelphia, Saunders, 2004.)*

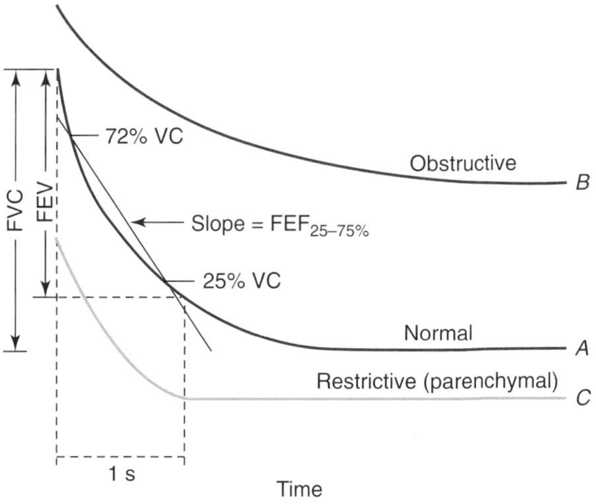

Figure 103-2 *Volume versus time. (Reproduced, with permission, from Fauci AS, Braunwald E, Kasper DL, et al. Harrison's Principles of Internal Medicine. 17th ed. New York: McGraw-Hill, 2008. Figure 246-2, p. 1586.)*

measurements require significant expertise on the part of the respiratory therapist in the PFT laboratory and maximal patient cooperation and ability to follow instructions. Inert gas dilution may underestimate lung volumes when there is airflow obstruction in patients who have air spaces such as bullae within the lung that do not communicate with the bronchial tree. Body plethysmography may overestimate lung volumes in airflow obstruction but may provide a more accurate measurement of intrathroacic gas volume in patients with noncommunicating airspaces within the lung.

Most diffuse lung disease is associated with decreased lung volumes. Restrictive PFTs means limitation to full expansion of the lungs. Volumes are decreased but flow rates are normal. Interstitial lung disease has reduced lung compliance and a restrictive defect. PFTs will reveal a decreased TLC, FRC, and RV. Although FEV1 and FVC may be decreased secondary to decreased volumes, the FEV1/FVC ratio is normal or increased. When the TLC and VC are decreased, the differential diagnosis includes restrictive lung disease (pulmonary fibrosis) or loss of lung volume (surgery, diaphragmatic paralysis, or skeletal problems). Decreases in the TLC, RV, and FRC can be interpreted as mild (60% to 80% reduction), moderate (40% to 60% reduction) or severe (<40% reduction). Marked decreases in the VC may also occur in certain neuromuscular diseases, and serial testing may be used to monitor disease progression in Guillain Barre Syndrome, myasthenia gravis, and muscular dystrophy.

FLOW RATES

Measurement of flow rates requires that the patient breathe into a spirometer as hard and as fast as possible from TLC down to RV. The information can be displayed as a flow versus volume graph or a volume versus time graph. The volume expired during this test is the forced vital capacity or FVC. The amount expired during the first second is the forced expiratory volume in 1 second, or FEV1. This maneuver also reports the forced expiratory flow between 25% and 75% of VC (FEF 25–75%), also referred to as the maximum midexpiratory flow rate (MMEFE or MMFR), which is the rate of airflow during the middle one-half of the expiration capacity. It is not effort or technique dependent (**Figure 103-2**).

Obstructive lung disease such as chronic obstructive pulmonary disease (COPD) is a spectrum of disorders that have in common impairment in expiratory flow. Diagnosis is made by spirometry showing a permanent reduction in FEV1/FVC ratio below 75%. The slow vital capacity or SVC will be greater than the FVC when the FVC is decreased in the setting of obstruction. Decreases in both FEV1 and FVC and a normal FEV1/FVC would suggest restrictive disease. Spirometry can be used to determine the degree of reversibility of the airways to bronchodilators and adequacy of treatment of obstructive airway disease. An increase in FEV1 of 200 cc or 12% is considered a significant response to bronchodilators and inadequately treated obstructive lung disease.

In addition to spirometry, flow rates may be measured using peak flow meters. Peak flow rates usually occur in the very early stages of the FVC maneuver and may be useful in measuring obstructive airway disease. Although a very simple test easily performed without too much training on the part of the operator or the patient, measuring the peak flow is very effort dependent and is not accurate enough to replace spirometry. The predicted values are rather nonspecific and the previously described prediction of severity of disease does not apply to these values. However, in the hospital it allows for a very simple, objective way of monitoring a patient´s obstructive airway disease and response to therapy. Measuring the peak flow is a simple way for patients with asthma to objectively measure the degree of obstruction, starting in the hospital in preparation for discharge home when patients should monitor their peak flow and understand when they need to return for medical evaluation before they are so ill that they need to be rehospitalized. A peak expiratory flow calculator using age, sex, and height may be found at the link http://www.dynamicmt.com/PEFform.html.

THE FLOW VOLUME LOOP

The flow volume loop graphically records the maximal inspiratory and maximal expiratory maneuvers with flow on the Y axis and volume on the X axis. The patterns of the flow volume loops can be diagnostic of various types of obstruction including intra- and extrathoracic obstruction, or fixed or variable obstruction. Although the beginning of a forced expiratory maneuver depends on effort, the latter part of forced expiration primarily reflects the mechanical properties of the lung and the resistance to airflow. The evaluation of the flow volume loop may be a qualitative visual analysis of the shape and concavity of the expiratory portion of the curve or a quantitative analysis comparing observed flow rates at specified volumes with predicted values.

In a fixed obstruction, changes in pleural pressure do not affect the degree of obstruction, and the inspiratory and expiratory portions of the curve reveal a plateau, reflecting a limitation in peak airflow of both inspiration and expiration.

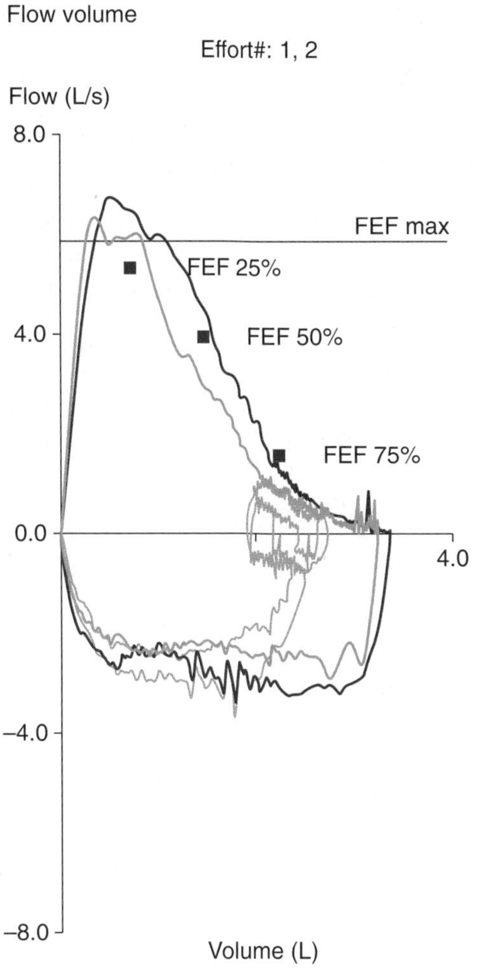

	Predrug reported	Predrug predicted	% Predicted	Postdrug reported	% Predicted	% Change
FVC	3.26	3.00	109	3.38	113	4
FEV1	2.39	2.19	110	2.62	120	9
FEF 25–75%	1.75	2.50	70	2.27	91	30
FEV1/FVC	73.49	72.79	101	77.48	106	5
MVV	73.93	88.87	83			
TLC	5.37	4.87	110			
RV	2.23	1.87	119			
RV/TLC	41.60	38.39	108			
DLCO	4.41	3.80	116			

Figure 103-3 *Normal flow volume loop, spirometry, and DLCO.*

In a variable obstruction the location of the lesion and the effect of alterations in pleural and airway pressure with inspiration and expiration determine the amount of obstruction. If the lesion is intrathoracic, the flow volume loop will demonstrate airflow limitation during expiration. If the lesion is extrathoracic, the flow volume loop will demonstrate airflow limitation during inspiration (**Figure 103-3**).

In obstructive disease the flow volume loop demonstrates a decrease in the expiratory loop, especially at the later part of the expiration (**Figure 103-4**).

MAXIMUM VOLUNTARY VENTILATION

This is the measurement of the maximum amount of air a patient can move in 12–15 seconds, using a spirometer. The results are expressed in liters/min. Because MVV tests airflow through major airways and muscle strength, consider weakness of respiratory muscles, especially the diaphragm, if MVV is low and flow rates are normal. Major airway lesions and neuromuscular disease result in a decreased MVV. Obstructive disease may also have a low MVV (MVV = FEV1 × 33). In theory, isolated restrictive disease should have a normal MVV; however, it is a nonspecific test

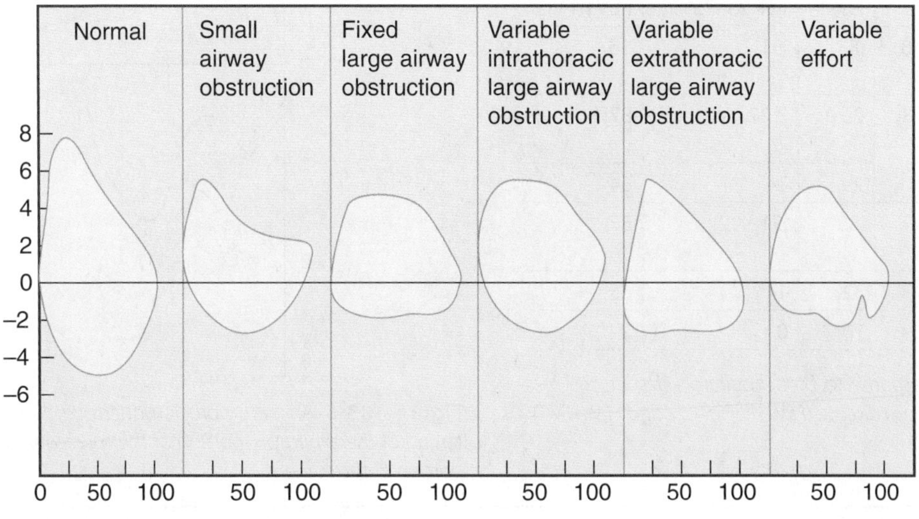

Figure 103-4 *Flow volume loop patterns.*

and reductions are seen in pulmonary diseases (restrictive and airway obstruction) and in neuromuscular disease (loss of coordination, diminished cognitive function, and overall deconditioning).

Between 10% and 30% of patients with Gullian Barre Syndrome will require ventilatory support. Patients most likely requiring mechanical ventilation present within 7 days of onset of symptoms, FVC < 60% predicted, maximal inspiratory pressure (MIP) < 30 cm H_2O, or an expiratory pressure < 40 cm H_2O. These patients are at great risk of requiring mechanical ventilation and should be monitored carefully with serial FVC and inspiratory pressure measurements.

MAXIMUM INSPIRATORY AND EXPIRATORY PRESSURE

This is a good estimate of muscle strength, which would be presumed to be normal with a normal maximum inspiratory and expiratory pressure. Patients must be able to cooperate with the test.

DIFFUSING CAPACITY (DLCO)

Usually measured as DLCO, diffusing capacity is the measurement of the rate of gas transfer from the alveolus to the capillary measured in relation to the driving pressure of CO across the alveolar-capillary membrane. It is reported as ml of CO/minute/mm Hg. The CO behaves like O_2 and is usually measured in a single breath. The diffusing capacity is most dependent on the surface area available for gas exchange and the volume of blood or hemoglobin in the pulmonary capillaries available to bind to CO. The observed value of the diffusing capacity is corrected for the patient's hemoglobin level. The diffusing capacity should be normal in diseases that only affect the airway such as asthma and chronic bronchitis and not pulmonary parenchymal disease, such as interstitial lung disease or emphysema.

The DLCO does not correlate with disease severity due to dependence on the Hgb level, pulmonary capillary volume, and thickness of the alveolocapillary membrane. Conditions that decrease the DLCO include:

1. Anemia, in which a decrease of 1 gm of Hg will decrease the DLCO by 7%
2. Anatomical emphysema, pneumonectomy, pulmonary hypertension, and recurrent pulmonary emboli due to decreased pulmonary capillary volume
3. Restrictive lung diseases such as interstitial lung disease due to increased thickness of the alveolar capillary membrane.

In the setting of obstructive disease, the DLCO helps distinguish between emphysema (decreased DLCO) and other causes of chronic airway obstruction such as asthma (normal DLCO). In the setting of restrictive disease, the diffusing capacity helps distinguish between intrinsic (or interstitial) lung diseases, in which DLCO is usually reduced, from other causes of restriction, in which DLCO is usually normal. Conditions that increase the DLCO include:

1. Alveolar hemorrhage, polycythemia, left to right shunt, and in some asthmatics due to increased pulmonary capillary volume
2. The supine posture, after exercise, high cardiac output states
3. Obesity.

The DLCO can be useful in the evaluation of diffuse pulmonary infiltrates when there is a large differential diagnosis.

HYPOXIA ALTITUDE SIMULATION TEST (HAST)

The purpose of the HAST is to simulate the oxygen tension while traveling by commercial airline flight. Aircraft pressure is maintained at an altitude of 8,000 feet. The pO_2 at this level is approximately 55 mm Hg. If the pO_2 falls below 50 mm Hg, supplemental oxygen is supplied and the test repeated. Predictive of the risk of

CASE 103-1

INTRATHORACIC OBSTRUCTION

This case demonstrates the PFT findings of a patient with a tracheal tumor. At the bedside the patient with a presumptive diagnosis of COPD exacerbation was found to have disproportionate upper airway wheezing.

	FVC	FEV1	FEF 25–75%	FEV1/FVC
Predrug reported	1.48	.83	.51	56
Predrug predicted	3.13	2.70	3.22	87
% Predicted	47	29	14	64
Postdrug reported	1.52	.88	.51	57
% Predicted	48	32	14	65
% change	2	10	0	2

Figure 103-5 *No response to bronchodilators despite the presence of severe obstructive disease (FEV1, FEF25–75, and FEV1/FVC).*

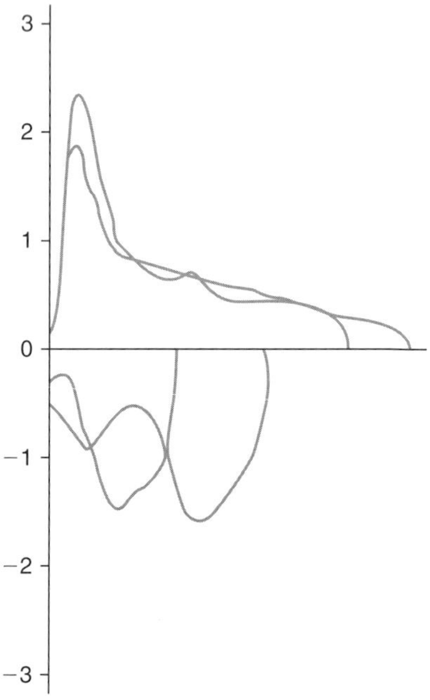

Figure 103-6 *An intrathoracic pattern by flow volume curve (a flattening of the expiratory portion of the curve with a preserved inspiratory portion of the curve).*

hypoxemia seen in flight, the HAST test identifies patients in need of supplemental oxygen when flying. Through a tight fitting mask the patient inspires air with 15.1% oxygen content. An ABG is obtained prior to the test and at 20 minutes. Continuous oxygen saturation and ECG monitoring is conducted. Symptoms are monitored.

INPATIENT PULMONARY COMPLIANCE STUDY

For intubated, mechanically ventilated patients, inpatient pulmonary compliance studies assess pulmonary mechanics by esophageal balloon. Esophageal balloon manometry provides an estimate of pleural pressure and lung compliance. Transpulmonary pressure can be recorded with PEEP and tidal volume titration. This information can be effectively used to improve oxygenation and respiratory system compliance in ventilated ARDS patients by identifying patients who derive benefit from higher levels of PEEP than would ordinarily be used.

PATTERNS OF PFT ABNORMALITIES

The obstructive pattern

Patients with asthma, chronic bronchitis, or emphysema typically have an obstructive pattern: decreased FEV1 with normal or decreased FVC.

The FEV1/FVC is normally decreased in obstructive lung disease, but may be near normal when the FVC is at very low volumes. The FEF 25–75% is usually quite low. The flow volume loop will be abnormal when flow rates measured by spirometry are reduced.

In addition to asthma syndromes and COPD, wheezing may be caused by tumors, laryngeal or vocal cord dysfunction due to GERD, postnasal drip or psychological states, allergic reactions, CHF, vasculitis, aspiration, and other pulmonary causes such as pulmonary embolism, bronchiectasis, sarcoidosis, and interstitial lung disease. Decreased FEV1 and FEV1/FVC are the hallmarks of obstructive disease. Flow volume loops can help identify if wheezing is originating from an intrathoracic or extrathoracic source and they can help identify if the obstructing lesion is fixed or variable. Measurement of the DLCO can be helpful in differentiating obstruction due to chronic bronchitis, emphysema, and asthma. The DLCO is lower in emphysema and is usually not affected in other forms of airway obstruction that cause wheezing. The presence of reversibility of airway obstruction suggests asthma or COPD requiring intensification of bronchodilator therapy. Measurements of arterial blood gases can be obtained to evaluate severity of illness and need for home O_2 therapy (**Figures 103-5** to **103-8**).

CASE 103-2

SEVERE OBSTRUCTIVE LUNG DISEASE

This case demonstrates the PFT findings of a patient with progressive and persistent obstructive symptoms; he would likely benefit from more intense therapy and pulmonary rehabilitation.

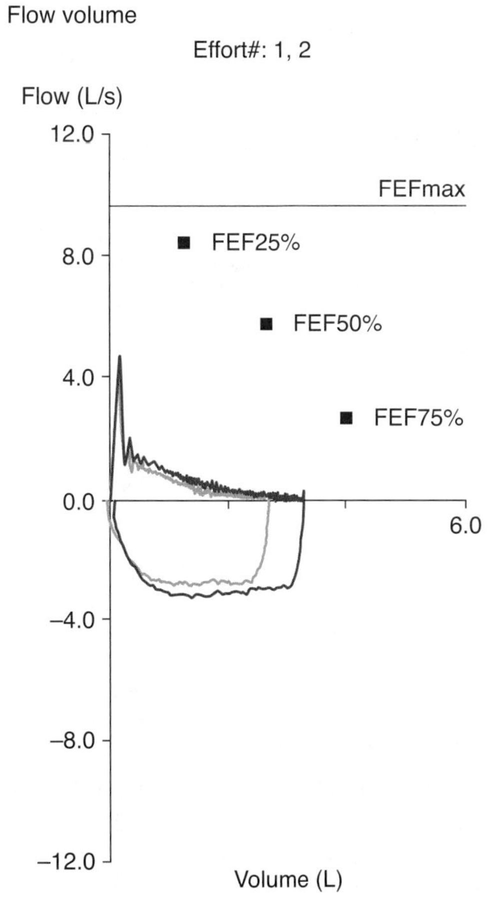

Figure 103-7 *A typical pattern of severe obstruction with a scooped terminal portion of the expiratory loop.*

	Predrug reported	Predrug predicted	% Predicted	Postdrug reported	% Predicted	% Change
FVC	2.69	5.42	50	3.30	61	23
FEV1	1.17	3.96	29	1.34	34	15
FEF 25–75%	.50	3.87	13	.54	14	8
FEV1/FVC	43.55	73.45	59	40.63	55	–7
MVV	51.39	145.61	35			
TLC	7.72	776	99			
RV	5.31	2.34	227			
RV/TLC	68.80	30.17	228			
DLCO	2.97	3.87	77			

Figure 103-8 *A markedly decreased FEV1, FEF 25–75, and FEV1/FVC with a significant response to bronchodilators consistent with severe COPD. The lung volumes suggest air trapping and the decreased DLCO the presence of emphysema.*

The restrictive pattern

Patients with severe skeletal deformities, diaphragmatic paralysis, s/p surgical repair, or pulmonary fibrosis typically have a restrictive pattern. A low TLC, a decrease in FEV1 and FVC with a normal FEV1/FVC, a normal or super-normal FEF 25–75%, and a low DLCO would suggest restrictive lung disease. The flow volume loop usually is normal in configuration but has low lung volumes (**Figures 103-9** and **103-10**).

The combined obstructive and restrictive pattern

Patients with cystic fibrosis, bronchiolitis obliterans, chronic obstructive lung disease (COPD) and congestive heart failure, COPD and pneumonia, or COPD with obesity typically have a combined obstructive and restrictive pattern (**Table 103-1**).

ANCILLARY TESTS

OXIMETRY

Reflective of the percentage of hemoglobin molecules occupied by oxygen, oximetry can be used to continuously monitor oxygen saturation. Oximeters transmit light at different wavelengths. The light absorption of oxyhemoglobin is different from reduced hemoglobin. A photo detector usually placed on a finger or ear compares pulsatile and baseline light absorption at the different wavelengths of light to calculate the oxygen saturation. The results may be falsely low when there is poor blood flow and perfusion to the fingertips, vasoconstriction due to hypothermia or sepsis, anemia, dark skin pigmentation, obscuring nail polish, and vital dyes. In certain circumstances the concentration of carboxyhemoglobin, such as in smoke inhalation, can significantly affect the results, falsely elevating the values. Oximetry does not take into consideration the pCO_2 and therefore, does not reflect ventilation or acid-base status.

ARTERIAL BLOOD GASES (ABGs)

While PFTs objectively assess lung function, ABGs assess the effects of the cardiopulmonary system on oxygen delivery by measuring both oxygenation and ventilation. ABGs directly measure the pO_2, pCO_2, and pH. Below a pO_2 of 60 mm Hg corresponding to an O_2 saturation of 80%, the oxyhemoglobin saturation curve is steep, and large changes in oximetry can mean small changes in oxygenation. Below this level oximetry may not correlate with oxygenation, and an arterial blood gas should be obtained (**Figure 103-11**).

The normal range for the pH is between 7.36 and 7.44 corresponding to a normal range of 36–44 torr for the pCO_2. Respiratory function and acid-base status determine the pCO_2 and pH. (See Chapter 245 Acid-base Disorders.) The normal range for the pO_2 is between 80 and 100 torr. Age and the pCO_2 determine alveolar O_2.

In hospitalized patients, ABGs are primarily obtained to assess ventilation. A high oxygen saturation may be falsely reassuring in patients whose respiratory drive is compromised by an increase of oxygenation in the hospital and retention of pCO_2. For patients with known severe lung disease, such as a history of oxygen-dependent O_2, an elevated serum bicarbonate may be a clue of chronic CO_2 retention and the ABG will confirm CO_2 retention. Neither oximetry nor ABGs will detect the presence of a reduced O_2 carrying capacity. This is because anemia, carbon monoxide poisoning, and methemoglobinemia do not affect the alveolar pO_2. An elevated carboxyhemoglobin will be required to make the diagnosis in carbon monoxide (CO) poisoning with levels above 20 diagnostic. Nonsmokers may have levels up to 3, smokers 10–15, and CO poisoning levels above 15. When there is CO poisoning, the oximeter will report normal O_2 saturation. This is due to the inability to differentiate between hemoglobin molecules with CO attached and those with O_2 attached. ABGs will also report normal values because the PaO_2 is a measurement of the oxygen dissolved in the blood and not the number of O_2 molecules attached to hemoglobin molecules. Likewise, the presence of abnormal hemoglobins, such as sickle cell, fetal hemoglobin, and methemoglobin will not affect the ABG results.

A-A GRADIENT

The A-a gradient is the difference between the oxygen in the alveoli (PAO_2) and the oxygen dissolved in the blood (PaO_2).

A normal A-a gradient is around 10–15 torr. An increase in the A-a gradient represents increased difficulty in getting O_2 from the alveoli to the blood. The A-a gradient may normally increase in the absence of underlying lung disease due

- Advancing age. A normal A-a gradient = 2.5 + 0.21 × age in years.
- Higher FiO_2 which disproportionately causes the PAO_2 to increase more than the PaO_2. When breathing 100% oxygen, older patients may normally have an A-a gradient as high as 80 torr and younger patients as high as 120 torr. It is best to calculate the A-a gradient on room air if possible.

The A-a gradient will also abnormally increase in the presence of

- Diseases that affect the pulmonary interstitium, such as interstitial lung disease, pneumonia, and CHF
- Pulmonary vascular disease, such as pulmonary emboli, shunts, pulmonary hypertension

CASE 103-3

RESTRICTIVE LUNG DISEASE

This case demonstrates the PFT findings of a patient with restrictive lung disease who failed to improve when treated for presumptive congestive heart failure.

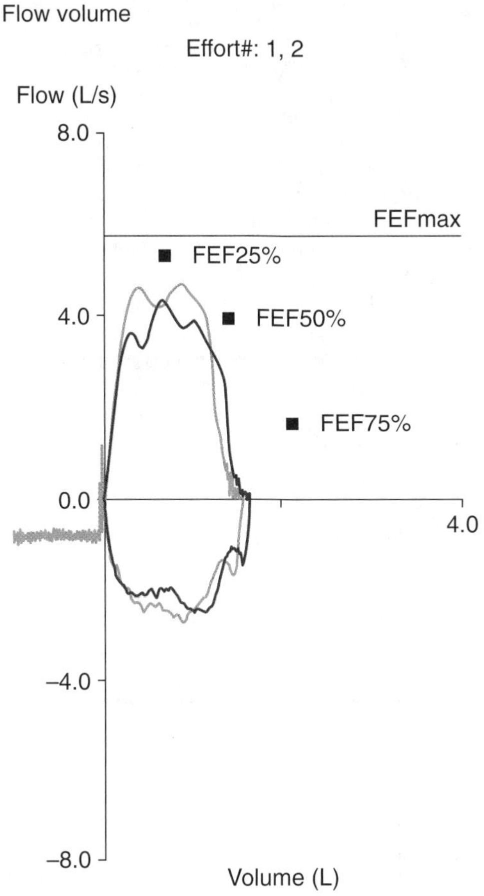

Figure 103-9 *The flow volume loop with a normal configuration but low lung volumes.*

	Predrug reported	Predrug predicted	% Predicted	Postdrug reported	% Predicted	% Change
FVC	1.59	2.84	56	1.67	59	5
FEV1	1.48	2.08	71	1.57	75	6
FEF 25–75%	4.29	2.47	174	3.79	153	−12
FEV1/FVC	92.96	73.22	127	94.27	129	1
MVV	75.33	86.63	87			
TLC	2.26	4.52	50			
RV	.66	1.68	39			
RV/TLC	29.12	37.15	78			
DLCO	1.63	4.05	40			

Figure 103-10 *A decreased FEV1 and FVC, an increased FEV1/FVC and FEF 25–75%, and a decreased DLCO consistent with parenchymal disease.*

TABLE 103-1 Summary of Pulmonary Function Findings in Certain Diseases

Pattern	FVC	FEV1	FEV1/FVC	TLC	RV	DLCO
Normal	Normal	Normal	Normal	Normal	Normal	Normal
Obstructive	Normal ↑or ↓	↓	Normal or ↓	Normal or ↑	Normal or ↑	Normal or ↓
Restrictive	↓	Normal or ↑	Normal or ↑	↓	Normal or ↓	↓
Neuromuscular	↓	↓	Normal or ↓	↓	Normal or ↑	Normal

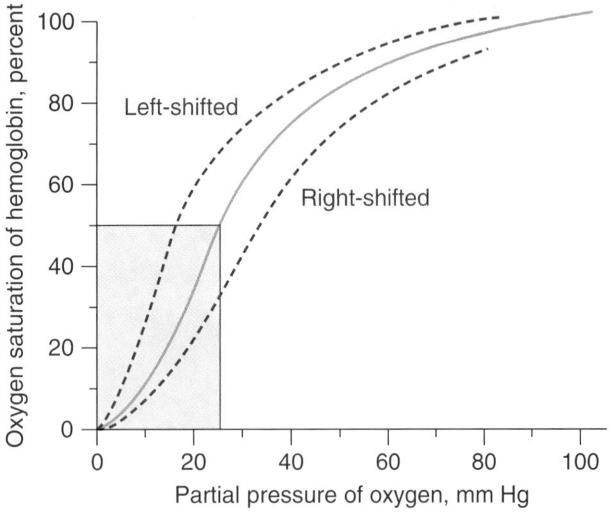

Figure 103-11 *Oxyhemoglobin dissociation curve.*

- Ventilation/perfusion mismatches of large vessels such as pulmonary or tumor emboli and of small vessels such as pulmonary hypertension, vasculitis, interstitial lung disease, and emphysema (**Table 103-2**). The following link may be useful for calculating the A-a gradient: http://www.mdcalc.com/a-a-o2-gradient.

Calculating the A-a gradient is most useful for determining the severity of the underlying disorder and whether there is a component of hypoventilation. Especially for hospitalized patients

TABLE 103-2 Causes of Hypoxemia

	ABG	A-a gradient
Hypoventilation	Elevated pCO_2 and decreased PAO_2.	A-a gradient is normal. The hypoxemia can be easily corrected with small amounts of O_2.
V/Q mismatch	Occurs normally and as part of many disease processes. The PAO_2 is decreased. The pCO_2 can be normal, low, or elevated.	The A-a gradient is increased and only a small to moderate amount of O_2 will correct the hypoxemia
Right to left shunt	Anatomic and physiologic. The PAO_2 is decreased. The pCO_2 can be normal, low, or elevated.	The A-a gradient is increased. The hypoxia can be difficult to correct with O_2.
Diffusion limited	Interstitial disease. The PAO_2 is decreased. The pCO_2 can be normal, low, or elevated.	The A-a gradient is increased.

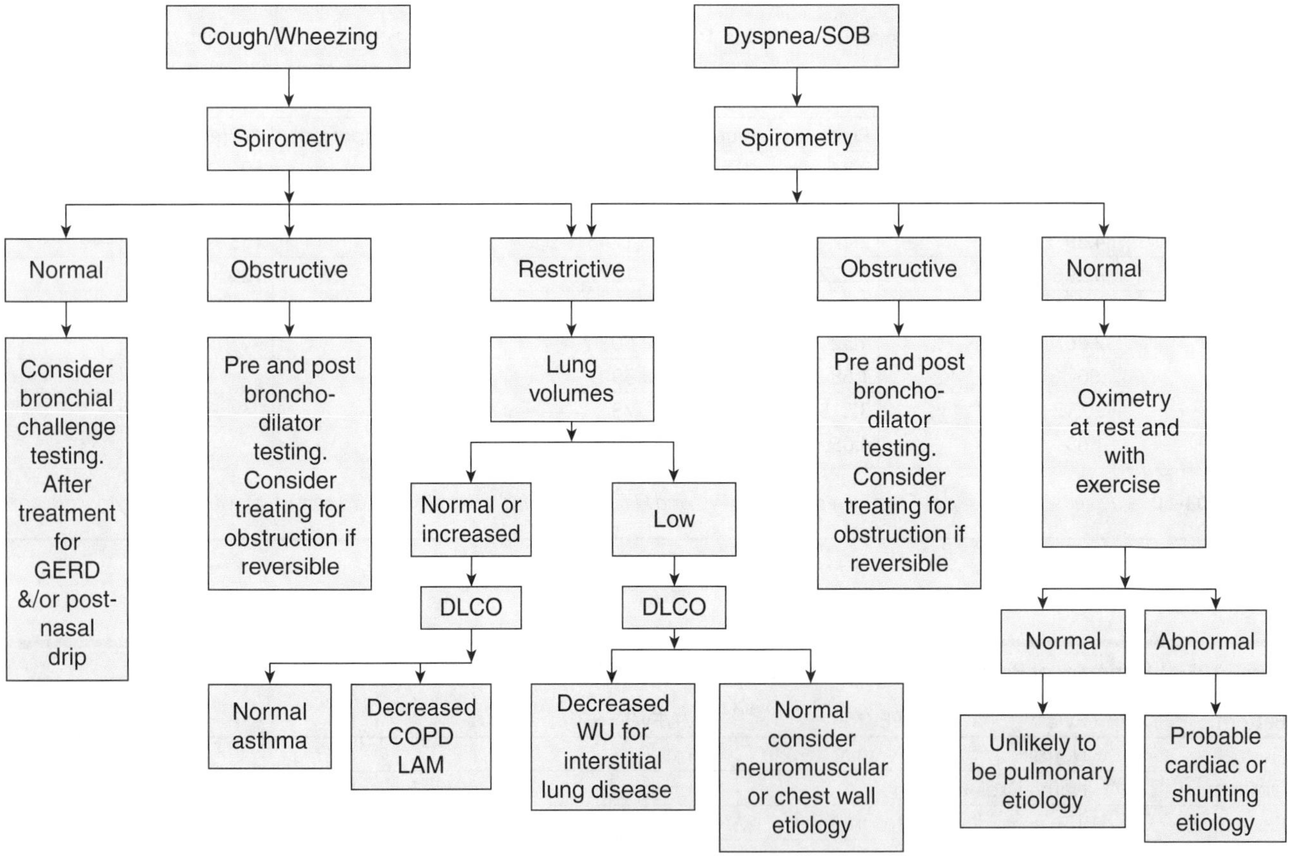

Figure 103-12 *Assessment of symptoms.*

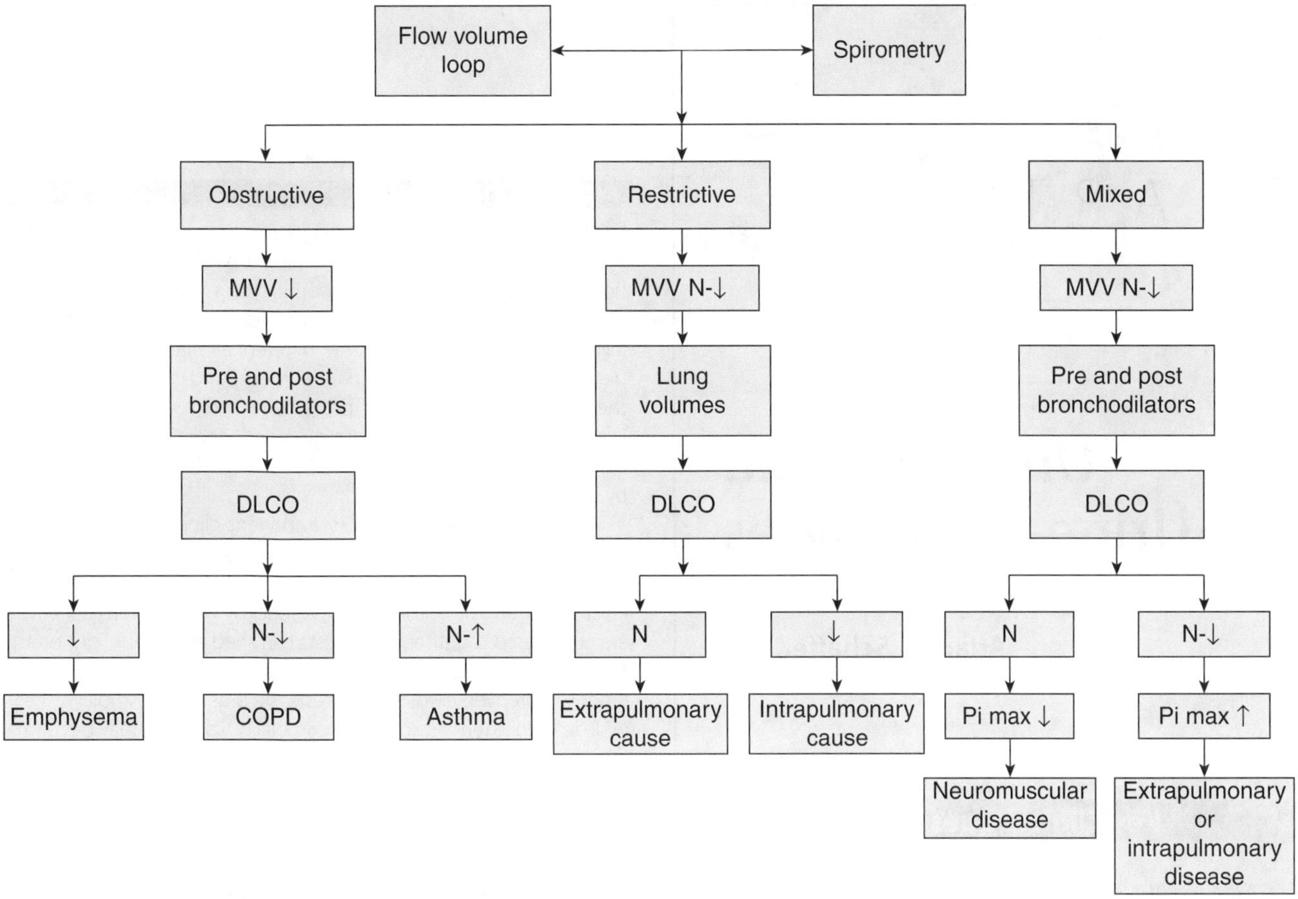

Figure 103-13 *Evaluation of abnormal PFTs.*

who have been prescribed medications which may suppress respiration, the A-a gradient is used to determine the relative contribution of hypoventilation to hypoxia due to underlying lung disease. If the A-a gradiant is normal, the ABG abnormality is all due to hypoventilation.

CALCULATION OF THE A-a OXYGEN GRADIENT FROM ABG

The A-a oxygen gradient = $PAO_2 - PaO_2$

A-a O_2 Gradient = [(FiO_2) * (Atmospheric Pressure – H_2O Pressure) – ($PaCO_2$ / Respiratory quotient] – PaO_2

Inspired air at sea level, the FiO_2 of room air = 0.21

Atmospheric pressure = 760 mm Hg

PH_2O at 37 F = 47 mm Hg

Respiratory quotient = 0.8

Normal Gradient Estimate = (Age/4) + 4

PREOPERATIVE PULMONARY FUNCTION TESTING

Pulmonary function testing is indicated for patients before undergoing lung resection, surgical coronary revascularization, and to evaluate optimization of medical management of respiratory obstruction or assessment of unclear respiratory symptoms. For patients scheduled for lung resection, combining the results of spirometry with radioisotope or CT lung scans predicts whether remaining lung function following lobectomy or pneumonectomy will be greater than 1 L. For patients scheduled for upper abdominal surgery, pulmonary function testing is important to evaluate respiratory obstruction to document optimization of medical management (**Figures 103-12** and **103-13**).

CONCLUSION

PFTs are usually deferred to the outpatient setting, when the acutely hospitalized patient has recovered sufficiently to be able to optimally perform the test. Review of outside records, including PFTs, may provide valuable information that cannot be obtained during acute illness, may point to an alternative diagnosis when a patient is not improving as expected, or provide important prognostic information. Interpretation of PFTs assumes "normal standards" based on nonsmoking control subjects based on age, height, and gender. The standards may vary from laboratory to laboratory. Most "normal" values are greater than 80% with the exception of the FEV1/FVC ratio, which is normally predicted to be around 75–80%. There is no specific spirometric or lung volume pattern associated with pulmonary vascular disease; hence, in general, no matter what criteria are used to define normal lung function, it is important to take all of the data into account to determine if a pattern is consistently present.

SUGGESTED READINGS

Crapo RO, Morris AH, Gardner RM. Reference spirometric values using techniques and equipment that meet ATS recommendations. *Am Rev Respir Dis.* 1981;123:659.

Crapo RO. Pulmonary function testing. *N Engl J Med.* 1994;331:25.

Gass GD, Olsen GN. Preoperative pulmonary function testing to predict postoperative morbidity and mortality. *Chest.* 1986; 89:127.

Guntupalli KK, Bandi V, Sirgi C, et al. Usefulness of flow volume loops in emergency center and ICU settings. *Chest.* 1997;111:481.

Hansen JE. Arterial blood gases. *Clin Chest Med.* 1989;10:227.

CHAPTER 104

Urinalysis and Urine Electrolytes

Adam C. Schaffer, MD

Key Clinical Questions

1. What useful clinical information can urinalysis provide?
2. What is the diagnostic significance of different urinary casts?
3. What are the appropriate clinical settings in which to measure the fractional excretion of sodium and the fractional excretion of urea?
4. What are the limitations of the different urinary tests?
5. How can the different pieces of information provided by various urinary tests be integrated to assist in making an accurate diagnosis?

INTRODUCTION

Urine tests can be a valuable diagnostic tool, especially since they are easily obtained and can provide a wide range of information. When interpreted in the context of a thorough history and physical examination, the clinician can use the information obtained from urinalysis to narrow the differential diagnosis and guide treatment. For example, in a patient presenting with kidney disease, the presence of significant proteinuria and red blood cell casts in the urine strongly suggests glomerulonephritis as a diagnosis. Unlike most blood tests, basic urinalysis can be performed rapidly by the examining physician.

This chapter will review how important clinical information can be obtained from various attributes of the urine—such as the appearance of the urine, urine specific gravity and osmolality, urine electrolytes, and urine microscopy. Especially when various urine tests are considered together, these tests can shed significant light on the patient's clinical status. However, all urine tests have significant limitations. Moreover, certain urine tests, such as urine osmolality, have wide reference ranges, so a urine osmolality value that may be normal in one patient could be abnormal in another patient. For example, a relatively low urine osmolality of 100 mOsmol/kg may be normal in a patient who takes in a large volume of water, but could suggest diabetes insipidus in a patient who is hypernatremic with polyruia.

URINE COLOR AND APPEARANCE

Even before any official urinalysis results are available, inspection of the urine can be revealing (see **Table 104-1**). For instance, urine may be pale yellow or clear in a patient who is well hydrated, whereas dark yellow urine can suggest a patient who is volume depleted. Urine may have a reddish hue in cases of significant hematuria, though a vaginal source or other perineal source needs to be considered. Myoglobinuria and hemoglobinuria, from rhabdomyolysis and hemolysis, respectively, can also cause red urine. Red urine can also result from the ingestion of certain foods, such as beets and rhubarb, and medications, such as senna and doxorubicin. Centrifugation of the urine can help distinguish hematuria from myoglobinuria and hemoglobinuria. Upon urine centrifugation, with hematuria the intact red blood cells (RBCs) should form a red-colored sediment only, whereas if the supernatant is red, that suggests the presence of myoglobinuria or hemoglobinuria. Foamy urine may be seen in patients with significant proteinuria.

Medications can account for other color changes in urine, including milky urine with propofol; dark brown urine with metronidazole (or povidone-iodine contamination); orange with rifampin; and blue-green with indomethacin, amitriptyline, triamterene, and propofol (depending on pH). Patients who are jaundiced can have dark yellow or brown urine, and patients with porphyria can have urine that is red or brown. The odor of the urine can also be diagnostically useful, with a foul-smelling urine suggesting infection and sweet-smelling urine raising the possibility of ketonuria.

URINALYSIS AND URINE DIPSTICK TESTING

SPECIFIC GRAVITY AND URINE OSMOLALITY

Urinalysis provides information about a number of different properties of the urine. Two related properties of the urine are urine osmolality and urine specific gravity. Clinical settings in which measuring urine osmolality can be useful include diagnosing

TABLE 104-1 Urine Appearance and Associated Medications and Conditions

Appearance of Urine	Associated Medications	Associated Conditions
Pale yellow		Volume replete
Dark yellow		Volume depleted Jaundice
Orange	Rifampin Phenazopyridine (Pyridium)	
Red	Senna Doxorubicin Phenytoin	Hematuria (sediment*) Hemoglobinuria (supernatant*) Myoglobinuria (supernatant*) Porphyrins Ingestion of beets Ingestion of rhubarb Ingestion of blackberries
Brown	Metronidazole Levodopa	Povidone-iodine contamination
Blue-green	Indomethacin Amitriptyline Triamterene Propofol (depending on pH)	*Pseudomonas aeruginosa* urinary tract infection
Milky	Propofol (depending on pH)	Lipiduria Chyluria
Foamy		Proteinuria

*Upon centrifugation.

Data from Foot CL, Fraser JF. Uroscopic rainbow: modern matula medicine. *Postgrad Med J.* 2006;82:126–129; Fogazzi GB, Verdesca S, Garigali G. Urinalysis: core curriculum 2008. *Am J Kidney Dis.* 2008;51:1052–1067; and Raymond JR, Yarger WE. Abnormal urine color: differential diagnosis. *South Med J.* 1988;81:837–841.

primary polydipsia as the cause of hyponatremia and evaluating a patient with polyuria. Urine osmolality is the concentration of particles per kilogram of solution. The usual physiologic range of urine osmolality is 50 to 1200 mOsmol/kg. Specific gravity is the density of the urine relative to the density of water. Unlike osmolality, which measures the solute concentration and is not a function of the size of the particles in solution, specific gravity is affected by the mass of the particles in the urine. Therefore, large particles that are excreted in the urine, such as radiocontrast material, can cause an increase in the specific gravity. Nonetheless, under most conditions, urine specific gravity usually correlates fairly well with osmolality. Urine specific gravities of 1.001, 1.010, and 1.030 are approximately equal to a urine osmolality of 40, 320, and 1200 mOsmol/Kg, respectively. In addition to the presence of radiocontrast in the urine, glucose and protein in the urine can also elevate the specific gravity. Urine osmolality is determined by a laboratory, whereas specific gravity is usually determined using a urine reagent strip (urine "dipstick").

Clinically, urine osmolality—and so also urine specific gravity—will be elevated in cases in which antidiuretic hormone (ADH) is elevated. ADH can be elevated appropriately in cases of hypovolemia, or inappropriately, as in cases of the syndrome of inappropriate antidiuretic hormone secretion (SIADH). Of note, in SIADH, the urine osmolality may not be absolutely high, but it is inappropriately high relatively speaking, given that the adaptive response to hyponatremia is to excrete free water. A urine osmolality >100 mOsm/kg is inappropriate in SIADH, although the urine osmolality frequently will be higher than this, typically higher than the serum osmolality. A urine osmolality <100 mOsm/kg in a hyponatremic patient suggests primary polydipsia. Patients with acute kidney injury (AKI) from acute tubular necrosis (ATN) will usually have a urine osmolality <400 mOsm/kg due to compromise of the kidney's urinary concentrating ability. In contrast, patients with prerenal azotemia will usually have a urine osmolality that is >500 mOsm/kg. In cases of polyuria, the urine osmolality can help distinguish a water diuresis from a solute diuresis. A urine osmolality >300 mOsm/kg is consistent with a solute diuresis, whereas a urine osmolality <150 mOsm/kg is suggestive of a water diuresis. In cases of a higher urine osmolality (>300 mOsm/kg) suggestive of a solute diuresis, possible causes include high salt intake, glucosuria, or mannitol. In cases of low urine osmolality (<150 mOsm/kg) suggesting a water diuresis, possible causes include diabetes insipidus or excessive water intake, as with primary polydipsia.

HEMATURIA

The initial test commonly used to evaluate for hematuria is the urine dipstick. Urine dipsticks have sensitivities of 91% to 100%, using 2 to > 5 RBCs per high power field (HPF) on sediment microscopy as the reference standard. Urine dipsticks have specificities in the 65% to 99% range, using microscopy as the reference standard. There are a number of conditions that can cause false positive results for hematuria on urine dipsticks. Myoglobinuria and hemoglobinuria, from rhabdomyolysis and hemolysis, respectively, cause urine dipsticks to read positive for heme. The absence of RBCs on urine microscopy in the setting of a urine dipstick positive for heme suggests the possibility of rhabdomyolysis or hemolysis. In one series by Grover, et al, examining patients with rhabdomyolysis, a urine dipstick showing moderate or large urine heme in the absence of hematuria had a sensitivity of 81% for detecting creatine kinase levels greater than 10,000 U/l. As noted above, centrifugation of the urine can be useful in this setting, because with myoglobinuria and hemoglobinuria the supernatant only should be red, whereas in true hematuria the sediment should consist of a pellet of RBCs. Another condition that can lead to false positives for heme on urine dipsticks includes some bacteria with pseudoperoxidase activity, such as certain species of staphylococci and streptococci. Ascorbic acid can result in false negative results for hematuria (and glucosuria).

Urine microscopy is important because a heme-positive dipstick result can occur in the absence of any RBCs in the urine. The conventional definition of hematuria on urine microscopy is greater than 3 RBCs/HPF or 1000 RBCs/ml. When reported, the morphology of any RBCs seen on microscopy can be helpful, as the presence of RBC casts and dysmorphic RBCs—particularly acanthocytes (ringform RBCs with blebs protruding off of it)—suggest the hematuria is glomerular in origin.

It is important to consider that urine dipsticks and microscopy signal hematuria, not necessarily disease. Epidemiological studies looking at the proportion of patients with hematuria who have serious disease have yielded inconsistent results, with rates of significant urologic disease among patients with microscopic hematuria varying from 17% to 56% in different studies. Mariani, et al, evaluated 1000 consecutive adults with asymptomatic hematuria (microscopic or macroscopic). Of these patients, 9.1% had what was deemed a life-threatening condition, most commonly bladder transitional cell cancer or renal adenocarcinoma. Significant findings, such as nephrolithiasis or cystitis, occurred in 22.8% of patients. In 56.4% of patients, only insignificant findings resulted from the evaluation of their hematuria, and in the remaining 11.7% of patients, no diagnosis to explain the hematuria was obtained. The authors of this study assert that there is no lower limit to the number of RBCs in the urine that rules out serious underlying disease, given that 18.6% of patients with life-threatening conditions produced a urinalysis with fewer than 3 RBCs/HPF within 6 months of the cancer diagnosis.

Unexplained hematuria requires further evaluation. The most important goal of this further evaluation is to assess for the presence of cancer affecting the kidney or urinary tract. In general, patients with unexplained hematuria should undergo imaging, such as a CT scan, urine cytology testing, and also be referred to a urologist for cystoscopy.

PROTEINURIA

Measuring proteinuria is an important part of evaluating any patient with known or suspected renal disease, as heavy proteinuria can signal significant glomerular disease, or can be a consequence of renal involvement in a systemic disease, such as multiple myeloma. Proteinuria >150 mg/day is considered abnormal. Microalbuminuria refers to urinary albumin excretion of 30–300 mg/day. Microalbuminuria is commonly used to detect early renal disease in diabetic patients, and so is mainly used in the primary care setting rather than the inpatient setting. When proteinuria exceeds 3.5 g/day, it is in the nephrotic range, and when accompanied by hypoalbuminemia, edema, and hyperlipidemia, full-blown nephrotic syndrome is present. Not only is the level of proteinuria diagnostically useful, but it is also a risk factor for progression of chronic kidney disease in both diabetic and nondiabetic patients.

There are 3 different methods of assessing for proteinuria: (1) a 24-hour urine collection for protein excretion; (2) a spot (ie, untimed) urine protein-to-creatinine ratio; and (3) a urine dipstick. The 24-hour urine collection, while often used as a reference standard, has a limited role in routine inpatient clinical practice. The 24-hour urine collection is inconvenient. Incomplete collections—which compromise the accuracy of this method—are common, and other methods will often provide the necessary clinical information. Under most circumstances, a spot urine can be obtained for a protein-to-creatinine ratio, which gives an estimate of the 24-hour protein excretion in the urine.

One study by Lane, et al, which looked at 103 patients in a renal and hypertension clinic, concluded that as the level of proteinuria increased, the accuracy of the spot urine protein-to-creatinine ratio decreased, and that at levels of proteinuria above 1 g/24 h, the spot measurement was inadequately accurate, and a 24-hour collection should be used instead. The authors argue that the spot measurement is helpful in answering whether the patient has significant proteinuria, but if the exact amount of that significant proteinuria needs to be known (such as for following the effect of treatment), then a 24-hour urine collection should be used. Nonetheless, in the inpatient setting, a spot urine protein-to-creatinine ratio will in most cases provide the necessary information.

Most urine dipsticks can detect albumin concentrations of 200–300 mg/L. There are semiquantitative assays, usually reporting the amount of proteinuria as 1+ to 3+ or 4+. Importantly, most dipsticks are insensitive for nonalbumin proteinuria, such as the light chains that may occur in the setting of myeloma kidney (Bence Jones proteins). Therefore, when there is a suspicion of nonalbumin proteinuria, other methods of assessing for proteinuria besides a dipstick should be used, such as a spot urine protein-to-creatinine ratio performed by the clinical laboratory. Sulfosalicylic acid, when added to a urine sample, will cause turbidity in the presence of protein in the urine (both albumin and nonalbumin protein) and so can be used as a point-of-care test to detect nonalbumin proteinuria (with a reported sensitivity of 76.7% and specificity of 75.4%). Another limitation of urine dipstick testing for proteinuria is that it is affected by the concentration of the urine sample being used. Using the albumin-to-creatinine ratio as the reference standard, a study of 310 general hospitalized patients by Pugia, et al, found that dipstick assessment for albuminuria had a positive predictive value of 82% and a negative predictive value of 99%. The authors concluded dipstick testing had good agreement with the quantitative albumin to-creatinine ratio.

LEUKOCYTE ESTERASE, NITRITE, AND THE DETECTION OF INFECTION IN THE URINE

The urine dipstick features used to diagnose a urinary tract infection (UTI) include the presence of leukocyte esterase and nitrites. White blood cells (WBCs) on urine microscopy and an organism isolated on urine culture help confirm the diagnosis. Leukocyte esterase is an enzyme contained in WBCs, while nitrites are a product resulting from the metabolism of nitrates by certain bacteria. Bacteria that can convert nitrates to nitrites include *E coli* and other bacteria in the family *Enterobacteriaceae*. However, a number of important urinary pathogens do not produce nitrites, including *S. saprophyticus, Pseudomonas,* and enterococci. Certain factors can cause a false negative nitrite test on dipstick testing, including insufficient nitrates in the diet to be converted by the bacteria and a dipstick that has been exposed to the air for a prolonged period. It takes at least 4 hours for bacteria to convert nitrates to detectable levels of nitrite, and so this test may be negative in patients with UTIs whose urinary frequency does not provide adequate time for bacterial conversion of nitrates to nitrites. The presence of urine eosinophils or *Trichomonas* in the urine can lead to false positive results. Factors that can lead to false negative results include the presence of ascorbic acid, high levels of glucose or protein, and certain antibiotics, including cephalexin and tetracycline.

A systematic review by Hurlbut, et al, of the test characteristics of dipstick leukocyte esterase and nitrite to detect UTI, which used >100,000 cfu/ml on the urine culture as the reference standard, found that considering either positive leukocyte esterase or positive nitrite to denote a positive test for UTI yielded the greatest area under the ROC curve. Considering either leukocyte esterase positive or nitrite positive to be a positive result for UTI yielded a sensitivity of 75% and a specificity of 82%. This review and other reviews concluded that in the setting of a high clinical suspicion, a dipstick negative for both leukocyte esterase and nitrite is not sufficient to exclude a UTI. A recent study of 408 women by Little, et al, found similar results. Using either a dipstick positive for nitrite or positive for both leucocytes and blood to be a positive test yielded a sensitivity of 77% and a specificity of 70%, using culture data as the reference standard.

In assessing the relationship between the degree of pyuria and likelihood of bacteriuria, measuring the leukocyte excretion rate is the most diagnostically useful. However, this method is cumbersome, and so the method employed in most clinical laboratories to measure pyuria is counting the number of WBCs per HPF in the centrifuged urine sample. A common break point used by clinical laboratories is ≥5 WBCs/HPF as being abnormal pyuria, though the break points used by clinical laboratories vary. In general, the higher the number of WBCs, the more likely there is to be significant bacteriuria. One older study by Holm, et al, found that among patients with 0–1 WBCs/HPF, 3% of patients had urine cultures with $>10^3$ bacteria/ml, whereas among patients with >9 WBCs/HPF, 87% had $>10^3$ bacteria/ml urine. A more recent study by Al-Daghistani, et al, examining the diagnostic characteristics of pyruia, using >50,000 cfu/ml as representing a true UTI, found that of ≥ 10 WBCs/HPF has a sensitivity of 34% and a specificity of 86.5%. Thus pyuria on microscopy, as currently performed by most clinical laboratories, cannot by itself be used to make the diagnosis of a UTI, and must be used in conjunction with other diagnostic information. Pyuria with a negative urine culture ("sterile pyuria") can be seen in the setting of partially treated UTIs and UTIs due to *Chlamydia trachomatis, Ureaplasma urealyticum,* and *Mycobacterium tuberculosis.* Other settings in which sterile pyuria can be seen include polycystic kidney disease, urolithiasis, papillary necrosis, Kawasaki disease, and tubulointerstitial diseases.

The most commonly used break point for the diagnosis of bacteriuria is $\geq 10^5$ cfu/ml of urine. Some authors have suggested that it would be preferable to use a lower threshold, such as $\geq 10^4$ cfu/ml of urine to define significant bacteriuria, with other authors suggesting thresholds as low as $\geq 10^2$ cfu/ml of urine. Three or more isolates each present in quantities of $\geq 10^5$ cfu/ml suggest contamination. A single isolate present in quantities of $<10^2$ cfu/ml is also a probable contaminant. Squamous epithelial cells seen on urine microscopy should raise suspicion of contamination.

The diagnosis of a UTI in patients with indwelling urinary catheters (Foley catheters) presents a challenge. In patients with indwelling urinary catheters, the association between pyruia and actual UTIs is weaker than in patients without such catheters. Therefore, in patients with indwelling urinary catheters, pyuria cannot be used to reliably diagnose a UTI. Moreover, many patients with indwelling urinary catheters who have UTIs may have minimal symptoms or be asymptomatic. According to a 2009 Infectious Diseases Society of America clinical practice guideline on catheter-associated UTIs by Hooton, et al, a catheter-associated UTI is "defined by the presence of symptoms or signs compatible with UTI with no other identified source of infection along with $\geq 10^3$ colony forming units (cfu)/mL of ≥1 bacterial species in a single catheter urine specimen or in a midstream voided urine specimen from a patient whose urethral, suprapubic, or condom catheter has been removed within the previous 48 hours."

■ GLUCOSURIA

Once serum glucose levels increase above about 200 mg/dL, glucose will start to appear in the urine. The presence of ascorbic acid and bacteria may cause false negative glucosuria readings on dipsticks. Dipsticks that are left uncapped and so exposed to the air for extended periods may provide false positive glucosuria results. Glucosuria may occur in the absence of hyperglycemia (known as renal glucosuria) in certain inherited disorders and in patients with Fanconi syndrome, which is a syndrome of renal proximal tubular dysfunction. Causes of Fanconi syndrome include medications—such as antiretroviral drugs (especially tenofovir), aminoglycosides, ifosfamide, and cisplatin. As part of the syndrome of proximal tubular dysfunction, wasting of bicarbonate, phosphate, calcium, and amino acids also occurs. Elevated levels of these substances in the urine support the diagnosis of Fanconi syndrome.

Case 104-1 shows how urine dipstick and urine microscopy testing can be used together to help arrive at a diagnosis.

CASE 104-1

USING URINE DIPSTICK AND URINE MICROSCOPY RESULTS TO SUGGEST A DIAGNOSIS

A 68-year-old female with a history of coronary artery disease, hypertension, and hyperlipidemia presents with malaise, weakness, and diffuse muscle aches that have been present for the past 3 days. Medications the patient is taking include metoprolol, aspirin, atorvastatin, and gemfibrozil. She notes that her urine has seemed darker than usual, but she denies any dysuria, urinary hesitancy, or foul-smelling urine. She also denies any fevers. Her urinalysis shows a specific gravity of 1.014, and is negative for glucose, protein, leukocyte esterase, and nitrites. The urinalysis is positive for hematuria. Urine microscopy detects no RBCs or WBCs.

A urinalysis positive for hematuria with no RBCs found on urine microscopy raises the possibility of myoglobinuria from rhabdomyolysis or hemoglobinuria from hemolysis. In this patient with muscle aches who is on atorvastatin and gemfibrozil, a drug combination that is a known cause of rhabdomyolysis, this is the most likely diagnosis. It would be appropriate to start IV hydration with isotonic fluids while awaiting the results of serum tests, which can confirm the suspected diagnosis. This patient's serum tests showed a creatine kinase level of 15,125 U/L, confirming the diagnosis of rhabdomyolysis.

URINE CASTS

Urinary casts can provide important information corroborating a suspected diagnosis. In some cases, a careful examination of the urine sediment can point to a possible diagnosis that may not have initially been given prominent consideration. Urine that is to be examined for casts and other urinary elements should be fresh and should be examined as soon as possible after it is obtained. **The procedure for preparing urine for examination is as follows. Ten milliliters of urine is centrifuged at 1500–2000 rpm for 5 to 10 minutes. Suction is used to remove 9.5 ml of the supernatant. The sediment at the bottom of the tube is resuspended in the remaining 0.5 ml of supernatant by tapping on the tube. Using a pipette, a single drop of the resuspended urine is placed on a slide and then a coverslip is placed on the urine drop. The sample should be examined under the low-power objective and the high-power objective of the microscope.**

Not all casts are pathologic. For instance, hyaline casts can be a normal finding. The presence of most casts, however, suggests renal disease. The absence of casts cannot be used to exclude a diagnosis, as casts may be missed or may degrade due to specimen processing. In general, casts are composed of the diagnostic element within a matrix of Tamm-Horsfall glycoprotein. Hyaline casts, which are composed primarily of Tamm-Horsfall glycoprotein, are faint, nearly colorless casts that can be seen in patients without renal disease. Renal tubular epithelial cell casts, which are composed of renal tubular epithelial cells shed in the setting of tubular injury, are most commonly seen in patients with ATN. Granular casts represent a degradation product that can contain broken down renal tubular epithelial cells and also other cellular elements. Thus granular casts may be seen in ATN, but are nonspecific and may also be seen in other types of renal disease. A scoring system by Perazella, et al, based on the number of renal tubular epithelial cells and granular casts was found to be useful in distinguishing prerenal AKI from ATN, as well as in predicting the worsening of either prerenal AKI or ATN. RBC casts are seen in pathologic states in which there is blood of glomerular origin, such as glomerulonephritis or vasculitis affecting the kidney. Leukocyte casts occur in pyelonephritis and acute interstitial nephritis, as well as in glomerulonephritis. Fatty casts, which contain lipid droplets and have a "Maltese cross" appearance under polarized light, may be seen in the setting of lipiduria, such as in patients with nephrotic syndrome. **Table 104-2** summarizes different casts and their clinical significance.

An important limitation in the use of casts as a diagnostic tool relates to the skill it takes to correctly identify urinary casts. One study by Tsai, et al, comparing the performance of nephrologists with that of the clinical laboratory found that the nephrologists were more likely to identify renal tubular epithelial cells, granular casts, renal tubular epithelial cell casts, and dysmorphic RBCs, as compared to the clinical laboratory. The clinical laboratory identified more squamous epithelial cells than the nephrologists, raising the possibility that the clinical lab was incorrectly identifying other urinary elements, such as renal tubular epithelial cells, as squamous epithelial cells. Overall, the nephrologists performed better than the clinical laboratory in deriving information from the urinalysis. Therefore, it is advisable to review a urinary sediment with a nephrologist, rather than relying on the clinical laboratory, if the results of the sediment examination are crucial.

URINE EOSINOPHILS

Testing for urine eosinophils is frequently used to aid in the diagnosis of acute interstitial nephritis (AIN). Older data supporting the use of urine eosinophils in diagnosing AIN have not been borne out by more recent reports. A 1986 study by Nolan, et al, of 92 patients, focusing on the technical advantages of using Hansel stain rather than Wright stain to detect urine eosinophils, found that 10 of 11 patients with AIN were positive for urine eosinophils using Wright stain. Notably, however, eosinophiluria was also seen in cases of acute prostatitis, rapidly progressive glomerulonephritis, postinfectious glomerulonephritis, and acute cystitis. No eosinophiluria was detected among patients with ATN or acute pyelonephritis. Corwin, et al, in 1989 reviewed 183 patients who had been tested for eosinophiluria, to evaluate the test characteristics of eosinophiluria in diagnosing AIN. The sensitivity (using Hansel stain) was 63% and the specificity was 93%. Eosinophiluria was also seen in two patients with UTIs, one patient with membranoproliferative glomerulonephritis, and in one patient with no diagnosis. The authors concluded that eosinophiluria was a good test for AIN.

Arriving at a different conclusion, a 1994 study by Ruffing, et al, tested 148 patients with pyuria for eosinophiluria. Considering only those patients in whom testing for urine eosinophils had been recommended by a nephrologist because of a suspicion of AIN, the authors found eosinophiluria had a sensitivity of 40% and a specificity of 72%. Conditions beside AIN in which eosinophiluria was detected included glomerulonephritis and chronic renal failure. The conclusion from this study was that eosinophiluria alone was inadequate to make the diagnosis of AIN, and that both false positive and false negative test results are a problem. An influential 2008 study of the value of eosinophiluria in diagnosing AIN by Fletcher included 534 quantitative urinary eosinophil tests and reported a sensitivity of 25% and a positive predictive value of 3%. A common methodological problem in studies assessing the test characteristics of eosinophiluria for diagnosing AIN is that many of the cases of AIN were established based on clinical criteria, not using the gold standard of renal biopsy.

The bottom line is that testing for eosinophiluria as a means of diagnosing AIN needs to be done with extreme caution, as its utility in diagnosing AIN is very limited. The presence or absence of eosinophiluria is not adequate to either establish or exclude the diagnosis of AIN. The results of testing for urine eosinophils must be viewed in the larger clinical context, and the presence of other clinical features typical of AIN, such as, in addition to kidney injury, fever, rash, eosinophilia, and arthralgias, need to be considered. Renal biopsy remains the gold standard for diagnosing AIN.

URINE SODIUM AND OTHER URINE ELECTROLYTES

URINE SODIUM

The urine sodium and fractional excretion of sodium (FE_{Na}) are of particular value in helping to determine the etiology of oliguric AKI and in assessing a patient's volume status, such as in a patient with hyponatremia. However, as will be discussed below, these indices have a number of important limitations.

In oliguric patients, a urine sodium <20 mEq/L suggests renal hypoperfusion, as can occur with intravascular volume depletion. This condition is what is commonly referred to as a "prerenal" state. The low urine sodium results from the hypoperfused kidney responding by retaining sodium, so as to maximize intravascular volume. In the setting of ATN, the renal tubular cells are damaged, and so are unable to retain sodium, resulting in a higher urine sodium, usually > 40 mEq/L. Urine sodium values between 20 and 40 mEq/L are indeterminate.

FRACTIONAL EXCRETION OF SODIUM

One limitation of the urine sodium is that it reflects free water handling in addition to sodium handling. The FE_{Na} (%), calculated as [(urine sodium x plasma creatinine)/(plasma sodium x urine creatinine)] × 100, takes into account both filtration and reabsorption of sodium. In the setting of AKI, a FE_{Na} < 1% suggests renal hypoperfusion (analogous to a urine sodium < 20 mEq/L), whereas a FE_{Na} > 2% suggests ATN (analogous to a urine sodium > 40 mEq/L).

The FE_{Na} has a number of limitations. For one thing, in patients with normal renal function with a moderate salt diet, a FE_{Na} < 1% may be normal because, with a normal GFR, a large amount of sodium is filtered, and a FE_{Na} < 1% may reflect the moderate sodium intake of the patient. Importantly, prolonged hypoperfusion itself may lead to ATN, and so a higher urine sodium. Thus an elevated FE_{Na} may represent a late consequence of renal hypoperfusion prolonged and severe enough to result in hypotension and ATN. There are certain clinical situations that are thought to be due to ATN, but when a low FE_{Na} often exists—including contrast induced nephropathy, acute kidney injury from myoglobinuria or hemoglobinuria, and glomerulonephritis. In patients with decreased effective circulating volume such as those with cirrhosis, congestive heart failure, and sepsis, the FE_{Na} may be low, as the kidney perceives hypoperfusion.

Another major limitation in using the FE_{Na} is that its accuracy diminishes in patients receiving diuretics, a treatment commonly used in hospitalized patients. A relatively recent study of 99 patients by Pepin, et al, looked at the performance of the FE_{Na} in predicting which cases of AKI were transient (<7 days, and so likely the result of renal hypoperfusion), as opposed to prolonged AKI (which is more likely the result of ATN) in patients on diuretics and in patients not on diuretics. The sensitivity and specificity of the FE_{Na} in predicting transient AKI in patients not on diuretics was

TABLE 104-2 Urinary Casts

Cast		Clinical Significance
Hyaline*	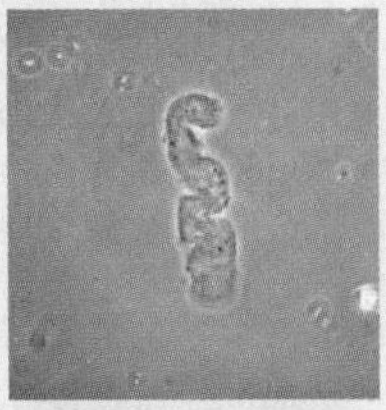	Nonspecific, may be seen in patients without renal disease
Renal tubular epithelial cell†	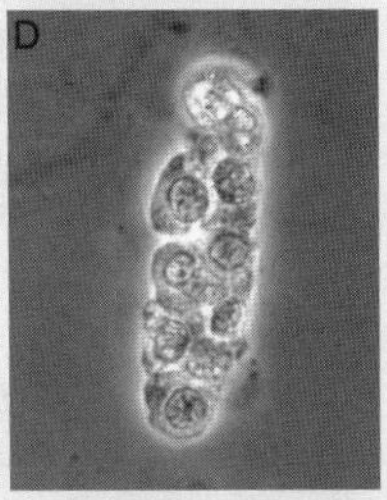	Seen in cases of acute tubular necrosis
Granular (fine)*	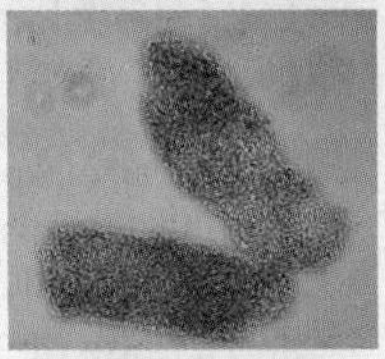	May represent degenerating renal tubular epithelial cell casts and so can be seen in cases of acute tubular necrosis. Also can represent other disintegrating cellular elements and proteins and so can be seen in a variety of renal diseases.
Granular (coarse)*	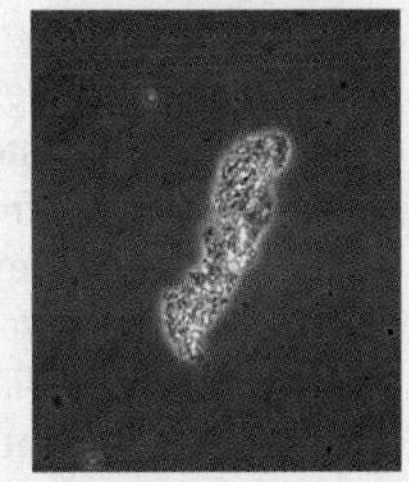	
Red blood cell*	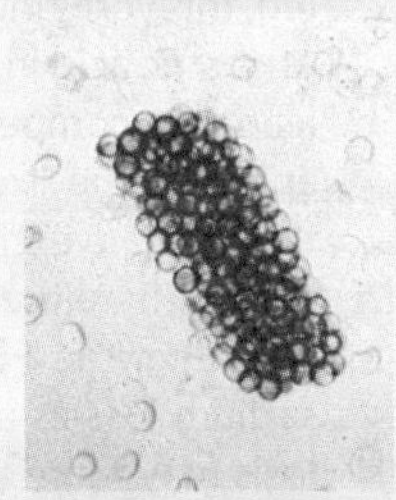	Seen in cases of bleeding that are glomerular in origin, such as glomerulonephritis or vasculitis affecting the kidney.
Leukocyte*	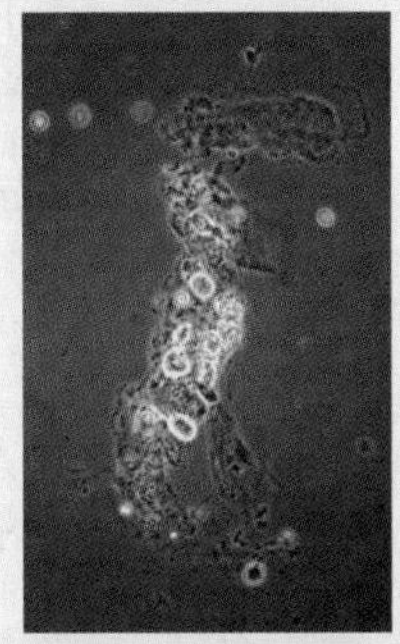	Seen in pyelonephritis, acute interstitial nephritis, and glomerulonephritis.
Fatty*	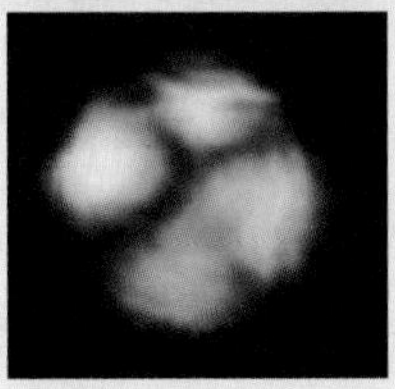	Seen in cases of lipiduria, such as nephrotic syndrome. Has Maltese cross appearance under polarized light.

*Images courtesy of Agnes B. Fogo, Vanderbilt Collection.

†Image reprinted, with permission, from Fogazzi GB, Verdesca S, Garigali G. Urinalysis: core curriculum 2008. *Am J Kidney Dis.* 2008;51:1052–1067, copyright 2008, Elsevier.

78% and 75%, respectively. On diuretics, the sensitivity of the FE_{Na} goes down to 58%, but the specificity is not markedly changed at 81%. The area under the curve (AUC) for the FE_{Na} in patients without diuretics is 0.83, whereas in patients with diuretics, the AUC falls to 0.75. It is worth noting that in patients receiving diuretics, a low FE_{Na} can be helpful, because patients with a low FE_{Na} despite receiving diuretics clearly have kidneys that are sodium avid, and so likely have renal hypoperfusion. However, in patients receiving diuretics, a FE_{Na} that is high is unhelpful, because it is impossible to distinguish whether the high FE_{Na} reflects the effect of the diuretics or the actual lack of sodium avidity by the injured renal tubules (as would be expected in ATN).

FRACTIONAL EXCRETION OF UREA

In response to the problem with using the FE_{Na} in patients on diuretics, the fractional excretion of urea (FE_{urea}) has been proposed as an alternative. Using the FE_{urea} is physiologically appealing in this setting, because urea is reabsorbed primarily in the proximal portion of the nephron, and so urea handling by the kidney would be expected to be less affected by diuretic administration than would salt handling. The FE_{urea} is calculated by the same method as the FE_{Na}, with the urine urea substituting for the urine sodium, and the plasma urea (blood urea nitrogen) substituting for the plasma sodium. The breakpoint used for the FE_{urea} is < 35%, which, analogous to the < 1% breakpoint used with the FE_{Na}, suggests an avid kidney responding to renal hypoperfusion. Pepin, et al, also examined the performance of the FE_{urea} in distinguishing between transient and prolonged AKI. This study found that the FE_{urea} did not perform well, even in patients on diuretics. The sensitivity of FE_{urea} for predicting transient AKI in patients on diuretics was 79% and the specificity was 33%. In patients not on diuretics, the FE_{urea} had a sensitivity of 48% and a specificity of 75%. Overall, the test characteristics were less favorable for FE_{urea}, which has an AUC of 0.56 for patients not on diuretics and 0.57 for patients on diuretics. This compares to an AUC for FE_{Na} of 0.83 in patients not on diuretics and 0.75 for patients on diuretics.

In contrast to the findings by Pepin, et al, a study by Carvounis, et al, supports the utility of the FE_{urea} in the setting of diuretic use. In this study, 102 episodes of AKI were categorized as being due to either prerenal azotemia in patients who were not treated with diuretics, prerenal azotemia in patients who were treated with diuretics, or due to ATN. FE_{urea} performed the best overall, with a sensitivity of 85% and a specificity of 92%. The AUC for FE_{urea} was 0.972, while the AUC for FE_{Na} was 0.889. Among prerenal patients on diuretics, 89% of them had a FE_{urea} < 35%, whereas only 48% of them had a FE_{Na} < 1%. FE_{urea} and FE_{Na} performed similarly in prerenal patients not on diuretics, with 90% of them having a FE_{urea} < 35% and 92% having a FE_{Na} < 1%.

Given these conflicting data, the FE_{urea} should be used as a diagnostic tool with caution. Outside of the setting of diuretic use, the FE_{Na} is preferred. In the setting of diuretic use, the available data do not clearly support using one over the other. One approach is to use both and to obtain urine electrolytes at multiple time points, and see if this larger pool of data is congruent so as to support a diagnosis of renal hypoperfusion or ATN.

URINE ELECTROLYTES IN ACID-BASE DISTURBANCES

Urine sodium is more commonly checked than urine chloride. Urine sodium and urine chloride should, in theory, correlate fairly closely with each other, though one report by Sherman, et al, found that a dissociation between urine sodium and urine chloride >15 mEq/L occurred in 30% of patients. One clinically important situation in which urine sodium and urine chloride will diverge is in acute acid-base disturbances. In the setting of an alkalosis, a normal kidney will excrete the excess bicarbonate. In order to maintain electroneutrality, the anionic bicarbonate excreted in the urine by the kidney will be accompanied by cations, such as sodium. Therefore, in the setting of an alkalosis, an elevated urine sodium may be a reflection of the renal compensation for the alkalosis, rather than the volume status. With an acidosis, a functioning kidney should respond by eliminating excess protons in the urine, which it does by excreting ammonium. For electroneutrality, the cationic ammonium is accompanied by anionic chloride. Thus in this setting, the urine chloride may be elevated primarily as a reflection of the kidney's effort to compensate for the acidosis, rather than the volume status. Case 104-2 shows the use of urine electrolytes in a patient having episodes of emesis.

CASE 104-2

URINE ELECTROLYTES IN A VOMITING PATIENT

A 45-year-old patient, reported by A.J. Nanji, with a history of alcoholic liver disease, presented with multiple episodes of vomiting. Initial vitals signs included a blood pressure of 100/80 mm Hg and a pulse of 90 beats/min. Serum electrolytes were notable for a blood urea nitrogen of 53 mg/dl and a creatinine of 7.0 mg/dl. Urine electrolytes showed a FE_{Na} of 2.4%.

Given the history of vomiting, intravascular volume depletion leading to AKI from a prerenal state would seem to be a leading diagnosis. However, the FE_{Na} of 2.4% suggests ATN as a cause of the AKI. This case illustrates a limitation of the FE_{Na} and how it can potentially be diagnostically misleading. In this patient, even if he does become intravascularly volume depleted because of vomiting, this vomiting will lead to a metabolic alkalosis due to the loss of gastric acid in the emesis. The resulting metabolic alkalosis will lead to a compensatory excretion of bicarbonate by the kidney, and with the excretion of bicarbonate in the urine, there will be the obligate excretion of sodium in order to maintain electroneutrality. Therefore, in this patient who is volume depleted due to vomiting, the FE_{Na} may be high because the increased urinary sodium loss as a result of compensation for the metabolic alkalosis may more than offset the sodium avidity that would be expected due to the intravascular volume depletion. In a case such as this, the urine chloride may be a more helpful guide. The urine chloride in this patient was low (<10 mmol/L), consistent with intravascular volume depletion. The patient's AKI improved with IV isotonic fluids.

THE URINE ANION GAP

These same principles described above underlie the urine anion gap, which is calculated as urine ($Na^+ + K^+ - Cl^-$). The urine anion gap is an indirect measure of urinary ammonium excretion, since urinary ammonium is an unmeasured cation, and increased ammonium excretion in the urine is accompanied by increased chloride excretion in the urine. Therefore, as urinary ammonium excretion is increased, urinary chloride is also increased, and so the urine anion gap decreases, and will often become negative. One of the main clinical situations in which the urine anion gap may be useful is in a nonanion gap (hyperchloremic) metabolic acidosis, in which one wants to help distinguish whether the nonanion gap metabolic acidosis is from diarrhea or either a type 1 (distal) or type

TABLE 104-3 Urinalysis and Urine Electrolyte Findings in AKI

Etiology of ARF	Urine Na (mEq/L)	FE_{Na}	FE_{Urea}	Proteinuria	Urine Sediment
Prerenal	<20	<1%	<35%	Minimal	Bland
Intrarenal					
ATN	>40	>2%	>50%	Minimal	Granular casts
AIN	Variable	Variable	Variable	Variable	Eosinophils
GN	<20	<1%	<35%	>150 mg/d	RBC casts
Postrenal	Variable	Variable	Variable	Minimal	Bland or RBCs

AIN, acute interstitial nephritis; AKI, acute kidney injury; ATN, acute tubular necrosis; GN, glomerulonephritis.
Adapted from Albright RC Jr. Acute renal failure: a practical update. *Mayo Clin Proc.* 2001;76:67–74; Singri N, Ahya SN, Levin ML. Acute renal failure. *JAMA.* 2003;289:747–751; Weisbord SD, Palevsky PM. Acute renal failure in the intensive care unit. *Semin in Resp and Crit Care Med.* 2006;27:262–273; and Michel DM, Kelly CJ. Acute interstitial nephritis. *J Am Soc Nephrol.* 1998;9:506–515.

4 (hyperkalemic) renal tubular acidosis (RTA). In a nonanion gap metabolic acidosis in which the kidney is functioning normally, such as in a patient with diarrhea, the kidney will respond by increasing ammonium production, and so the urine anion gap will be negative. In one series of patients with diarrhea described by Batlle, et al, the average urine anion gap was −20. In a nonanion gap metabolic acidosis caused by either a type 1 or type 4 RTA, the defect is in the kidney, and so it will not be able to mount an appropriate increase in ammonium excretion in response to the acidosis, and so the urine anion gap will be positive. Conditions that can render the urine anion gap less reliable include excretion of other unmeasured anions in the urine, such as ketoacids or lactic acid, and in certain types of dietary intake, such as cereals that provide chloride without Na^+ or K^+.

USE OF URINALYSIS AND URINE TESTING IN THE DIFFERENTIAL DIAGNOSIS OF ACUTE KIDNEY INJURY

In approaching the hospitalized patient with AKI, the results of the urinalysis and other urine testing can, in conjunction with the clinical picture, help elucidate the cause of the AKI. Particularly in cases in which both prerenal and postrenal causes of AKI have been determined to be less likely, the results of urine tests can help distinguish among intrarenal causes of AKI—such as ATN, AIN, and glomerulonephritis. In ATN, the tubular cells are damaged and so are unable to reabsorb sodium, so a $FE_{Na} > 2\%$ (and a $FE_{urea} > 50\%$) would be expected, along with minimal proteinuria and muddy brown casts in the urine sediment. In cases in which AIN is the cause of the AKI, one can consider looking for eosinophiluria (with the caveats discussed above). Most cases of AIN have only low-level proteinuria, except in cases of NSAID-induced AIN, which commonly involves nephrotic-range proteinuria. AKI from glomerulonephritis is characterized by elevated levels of proteinuria, RBC casts, and a FE_{Na} that is typically low. The use of urinary parameters in diagnosing AKI is summarized in **Table 104-3**.

CONCLUSION

All the urinary parameters discussed in this chapter have limitations. However, especially when taken together, these parameters can be very useful in arriving at a diagnosis. Appropriately, one of the most prominent uses of urinary tests is in determining the cause of AKI, as detailed in the section above. Beyond this use, urinary tests can also assist in identifying the cause of hyponatremia, diagnosing rhabdomyolysis, and determining the etiology of an acid-base disturbance. Considering the relatively low cost and ease of obtaining most urinary tests, they are an important, and often overlooked, means to obtain important diagnostic information.

Evidence Base and Literature

Hematuria and Myoglobinuria

Grover DS, Atta MG, Eustace JA, Kickler TS, Fine DM. Lack of clinical utility of urine myoglobin detection by microconcentrator ultrafiltration in the diagnosis of rhabdomyolysis. *Nephrol Dialysis Transplant.* Oct 2004; 19(10):2634–2638.

Mariani AJ, Mariani MC, Macchioni C, Stams UK, Hariharan A, Moriera A. The significance of adult hematuria: 1,000 hematuria evaluations including a risk-benefit and cost-effectiveness analysis. *J Urol.* Feb 1989;141(2): 350–355.

Proteinuria

Lane C, Brown M, Dunsmuir W, Kelly J, Mangos G. Can spot urine protein/creatinine ratio replace 24 h urine protein in usual clinical nephrology? *Nephrology.* Jun 2006;11(3):245–249.

Pugia MJ, Wallace JF, Lott JA, et al. Albuminuria and proteinuria in hospitalized patients as measured by quantitative and dipstick methods. *J Clin Lab Anal.* 2001;15(5):295–300.

(continued)

Evidence Base and Literature (*continued*)

Urine Dipsticks and UTI Diagnosis

Al-Daghistani HI, Abdel-Dayem M. Diagnostic value of various urine tests in the Jordanian population with urinary tract infection. *Clin Chem Lab Med.* Oct 2002;40(10):1048–1051.

Holm S, Wahlin A, Wahlqvist L, Wedren H, Lundgren B. Urine microscopy as screening method for bacteriuria. *Acta Med Scand.* May 1982;211(3):209–212.

Hooton TM, Bradley SF, Cardenas DD, et al. Diagnosis, prevention, and treatment of catheter-associated urinary tract infection in adults: 2009. International Clinical Practice Guidelines from the Infectious Diseases Society of America. *Clin Infect Dis.* Mar 1, 2010;50(5):625–663.

Hurlbut TA, Littenberg B. The diagnostic accuracy of rapid dipstick tests to predict urinary tract infection. *Amer J Clin Pathol.* Nov 1991;96(5):582–588.

Little P, Turner S, Rumsby K, et al. Dipsticks and diagnostic algorithms in urinary tract infection: development and validation, randomised trial, economic analysis, observational cohort and qualitative study. *Health Technol Assessment (Winchester, England).* Mar 2009;13(19):iii–iv, ix–xi, 1–73.

Urinalysis and Acute Kidney Injury

Perazella MA, Coca SG, Hall IE, Iyanam U, Koraishy M, Parikh CR. Urine microscopy is associated with severity and worsening of acute kidney injury in hospitalized patients. *Clin J Amer Soc Nephrol.* 2010;5(3):402–408.

Perazella MA, Coca SG, Kanbay M, Brewster UC, Parikh CR. Diagnostic value of urine microscopy for differential diagnosis of acute kidney injury in hospitalized patients. *Clin J Amer Soc Nephrol.* Nov 2008;3(6):1615–1619.

Tsai JJ, Yeun JY, Kumar VA, Don BR. Comparison and interpretation of urinalysis performed by a nephrologist versus a hospital-based clinical laboratory. *Amer J Kidney Dis.* Nov 2005;46(5):820–829.

Eosinophiluria

Corwin HL, Bray RA, Haber MH. The detection and interpretation of urinary eosinophils. *Arch Pathol Lab Med.* Nov 1989;113(11):1256–1258.

Fletcher A. Eosinophiluria and acute interstitial nephritis. *N Engl J Med.* Apr 17, 2008;358(16):1760–1761.

Nolan CR, 3rd, Anger MS, Kelleher SP. Eosinophiluria—a new method of detection and definition of the clinical spectrum. *N Engl J Med.* Dec 11, 1986;315(24):1516–1519.

Ruffing KA, Hoppes P, Blend D, Cugino A, Jarjoura D, Whittier FC. Eosinophils in urine revisited. *Clin Nephrol.* Mar 1994;41(3):163–166.

Fractional Excretion of Sodium and Urea

Carvounis CP, Nisar S, Guro-Razuman S. Significance of the fractional excretion of urea in the differential diagnosis of acute renal failure. *Kidney Int.* Dec 2002;62(6):2223–2229.

Pepin MN, Bouchard J, Legault L, et al. Diagnostic performance of fractional excretion of urea and fractional excretion of sodium in the evaluations of patients with acute kidney injury with or without diuretic treatment. *Amer J Kidney Dis.* Oct 2007;50(4):566–573.

Urine Electrolytes

Batlle DC, Hizon M, Cohen E, Gutterman C, Gupta R. The use of the urinary anion gap in the diagnosis of hyperchloremic metabolic acidosis. *N Engl J Med.* Mar 10, 1988;318(10):594–599.

Nanji AJ. Increased fractional excretion of sodium in prerenal azotemia: need for careful interpretation. *Clin Chem.* Jul 1981;27(7):1314–1315.

Sherman RA, Eisinger RP. The use (and misuse) of urinary sodium and chloride measurements. *JAMA.* Jun 11, 1982;247(22):3121–3124.

SUGGESTED READINGS

Espinel CH. The FE_{Na} test. Use in the differential diagnosis of acute renal failure. *JAMA.* 1976;236:579–581.

Fletcher A. Eosinophiluria and acute interstitial nephritis. *N Engl J Med.* 2008;358:1760–1761.

Fogazzi GB, Verdesca S, Garigali G. Urinalysis: core curriculum 2008. *Am J Kidney Dis.* 2008;51:1052–1067.

Kamel KS, Ethier JH, Richardson RM, Bear RA, Halperin ML. Urine electrolytes and osmolality: when and how to use them. *Am J Nephrol.* 1990;10:89–102.

Perazella MA, Coca SG, Kanbay M, Brewster UC, Parikh CR. Diagnostic value of urine microscopy for differential diagnosis of acute kidney injury in hospitalized patients. *Clin J Am Soc Nephrol.* 2008;3:1615–1619.

Sherman RA, Eisinger RP. The use (and misuse) of urinary sodium and chloride measurements. *JAMA.* 1982;247:3121–3124.

Wilson ML, Gaido L. Laboratory diagnosis of urinary tract infections in adult patients. *Clin Infect Dis.* 2004;38:1150–1158.

SECTION 2

Optimizing Utilization of Radiology Services

CHAPTER 105

Introduction to Radiology

Francine L. Jacobson, MD, MPH
Sylvia C. McKean, MD, SFHM, FACP

Key Clinical Questions

1. What determines the ability of plain films to differentiate between various substances and tissues? What are the limitations of a single radiographic view?
2. What are the limitations of ultrasound?
3. In addition to the five categories of density, computed tomography (CT) technology is able to detect what differences? What are Hounsfield units?
4. What are the limitations of magnetic resonance imaging (MRI)?
5. What are the advantages of nuclear imaging?

INTRODUCTION

The radiology examination that provides the required data with the least amount of radiation, expense, and need for extraneous follow-up supports the best practices of patient care. Although radiologic examinations have become vital adjuncts to clinical problem-solving, they should not replace the process of developing a coherent problem list generated by the patient's concerns, medical history, and physical examination. The ordering physician critically contributes to the process of radiology interpretation not only by asking the right questions of individual patients, but by selecting the right examination and effectively communicating the questions that need to be answered by imaging to patients, technologists, and radiologists. The physician should request only those studies that will influence management, continually filter the results in the context of the patient, and ensure appropriate follow-up of abnormal and incidental findings. Practitioners must not only balance risks and benefits of a specific study for an individual patient but also be mindful of the impact of clinical decision-making on populations of patients even if the test is readily available.

Ever-expanding technologies will always require the expertise of radiologists in interpretation; however, physicians must have a basic understanding of various imaging modalities, their limitations, risks, and relative costs in order to select the right examination for a specific patient.

PRACTICE POINT

Framework for utilization of radiology

A golden rule for ordering imaging tests:

- Avoid ordering tests when the results will not impact patient care.
- Review tests previously performed to answer current questions.
- Order the best test to maximize quality, efficiency, and cost-effectiveness.
- Prepare your patient to minimize delays in getting studies done; in general, patients should be hemodynamically stable and able to cooperate as active participants in creating optimal images.
- Provide the necessary clinical information to radiology technicians to answer the question,
- Consult your radiologist when unsure about next imaging steps, the meaning of a radiology report, or the significance of a negative or incidental finding.
- Provide patient-centered care: inform, consent, educate.

This chapter will introduce general concepts for different imaging modalities, how to "interpret" the radiology report, and what to do about "incidental findings" in the context of care transitions and handoffs. Chapter 106 will review principles of patient safety—risks of contrast, radiation exposure, and gadolinium. Subsequent chapters will cover the application of specific imaging modalities.

CASE 105-1

ORDERING THE RIGHT IMAGING STUDY

A 64-year-old male with a past medical history of multiple myeloma, status post bone marrow transplant, and recent extraction of a molar heard a crack on the left side of his mandible accompanied by pain while eating. On physical examination, the patient had fever, moderate swelling, and tenderness of the left angle of the mandible.

A maxillofacial CT scan revealed a lytic lesion with a nondisplaced pathologic fracture at the site of the left posterior mandible in the area where the molar had been extracted. The differential diagnosis included osteomyelitis and multiple myeloma. A whole body bone scan did not show an area of metastasis or obvious involvement by multiple myeloma, nor was there evidence of osteomyelitis.

Would this second imaging study provide any new information that could guide management? Or how good is this second imaging study at identifying an abnormality?

To answer this question, the ordering clinicians need to select imaging studies in the context of the uncertainty that needs to be resolved in the patient in front of them and then integrate the clinical presentation with the reported new data. This process requires both a pathophysiologic knowledge of the potential causes of a problem and an understanding of the effect of new data on the probability of each potential cause. In this case the clinicians should weigh the high likelihood of osteomyelitis (given the presentation and risk factors for infection) versus the much lower likelihood of recurrence of a previously treated multiple myeloma. Prior to ordering a specific imaging study, they should know the value of a positive test for increasing certainty about a diagnosis and likewise, the value of a negative test for decreasing probability of disease.

1. *What is the likelihood that a whole body bone scan will diagnose multiple myeloma?*

Even when lucencies within the bones are readily visualized by CT, a radionuclide bone scan may not identify multiple myeloma. A skeletal survey, which images most of the bones in the body while conserving radiation dose, is a better study to diagnose lytic lesions and other bone abnormalities. However, a bone scan can image metastases from solid tumors.

2. *What is the likelihood that a whole body bone scan will diagnose osteomyelitis?*

In this patient the bone scan imaging was performed only 3–4 hours following injection of radiotracer. This approach is insensitive for the diagnosis of osteomyelitis.

The bottom line: for either diagnosis—multiple myeloma or osteomyelitis—a negative whole body scan would not change the likelihood of disease or put another way, resolve the uncertainty raised by the abnormal maxillofacial CT scan. Failure to understand this concept (which also applies to the use of blood cultures to diagnose osteomyelitis) resulted in overreliance on negative imaging and treatment delays.

On the sixth hospital day a positive WBC study in nuclear medicine led to surgical repair of the mandible. Pathologic examination of the resected pathologic fracture revealed actinomycosis osteomyelitis. A soil organism that is radiographically important to diagnose, actinomycosis is easily treated with penicillin. The extension across bone, and through to the chest wall is also characteristic in other locations, such as the chest.

Given the high probability of osteomyelitis in this patient, what study should have been performed to confirm the diagnosis?

Three-phase bone scan augments the conventional radionuclide bone scan imaging at 3–4 hours with sequential images during and immediately following the injection to follow the tracer distribution in the soft tissues. The first "flow" phase provides a nuclear angiogram using 2–5 second images of a focal area of concern. The second phase "blood-pool" image is obtained approximately 5 minutes following injection. The third "bone image" phase is obtained after urinary excretion has decreased the amount of radionuclide in soft tissues.

Three-phase Radionuclide Bone Scan

Phase	Phase 1 Flow	Phase 2 Blood Pool	Phase 3 Bone Image
Cellulitis	Increased uptake	Increased uptake	Normal or diffusely increased
Osteomyelitis	Increased uptake	Increased uptake	Increased uptake

Field of view for phases 1 and 2 will be restricted to the predetermined area of specific interest.

Through comparison of radioisotope distribution in soft tissue and bone over time, it is possible to differentiate cellulitis from osteomyelitis that can be very difficult to diagnose. When clinical suspicion of osteomyelitis is high but 3-phase bone scan is normal, a gallium scan may be considered. It is important to consult directly with the radiologist or nuclear medicine physician to correctly tailor the examination.

BASIC RADIOLOGY

Projection radiographs are viewed as the radiologist looks at the patient, placing the patient's right side at his own left side. Coronal cross-sectional images use the same orientation, generally presented, from anterior to posterior. Axial images are viewed from the perspective of standing at the supine patient's feet, again placing the patient's right side at the radiologist's own left side. Sagittal images are generally presented from the patient's left side to the right side, although this convention is not always applicable to all studies, particularly MRI. It is helpful to reconcile the position of the heart in determining whether sagittal images are on the right or left side of the patient's body. The Visible Human Project and the proliferation of Web-based medical education materials now allow easy access to comparison images for anatomic identification in all three of these planes. Sophisticated image processing of volumetric CT data sets increasingly enables radiologists to provide data for surgery in the perspective of the surgeon. Surgeons have also learned to use conventional axial CT images to determine operability and plan specific surgeries.

The manner in which a standard radiological examination is performed may be modified to accommodate the inability of a hospitalized patient to have a more standard examination. Thus, a frontal chest radiograph may be made with the patient sitting up on a stretcher, sitting in a wheelchair, or lying in bed. In these instances, the radiograph will be made with projection from anterior to posterior rather than the standard erect imaging approach from posterior to anterior. The standing position facilitates obtaining radiographs in maximum inspiration. Gravitational effects are not as favorable in the supine position and other positions introduce a variety of variable complications. At minimum on an AP radiograph, the heart will appear larger due to magnification that varies with the inverse square law, whereby increasing the distance of the heart by a factor of 2 will increase the magnification by a factor of 4. This effect increases with increasing size of the patient, being particularly prominent when imaging an obese patient.

For a radiology examination to have maximal benefit in patient care, it should be performed at the right time. Sedation decreases cooperation and depth of respiration. Likewise, it may be better to presumptively treat an acutely tachypneic patient and obtain the diagnostic study after the patient is hemodynamically stable, able to lie flat, and breathe less rapidly for image acquisition.

The acute hospitalization may not be the right time for obtaining many important radiologic examinations. The patient participates in most imaging, whether by staying still, following breathing instructions, or moving through a series of positions. CT, MR, and fluoroscopic examinations that are not essential to address the immediate treatment of the acute process should not be performed when the images will most certainly be limited by uncontrolled respiration and superimposed acute processes. Thus, clinicians rarely help patients by obtaining an inpatient CT or MR to either spare the patient the outpatient trip or to work up a nonacute incidental finding, such as an indeterminate subcentimeter pulmonary nodule.

PLAIN FILMS

The most fundamental undertaking of all radiology examinations is the largely noninvasive visualization of tissues that make up the body, with differentiation of normal structures from pathology. Projection radiographs detect five categories of density: air, fat, water (including soft tissue and muscle), calcium, and metal. The relative radiodensities of various substances and tissues will determine the ability of plain films to differentiate between them. For example, blood, muscle, and liver will have an almost identical medium gray appearance as will most solid or fluid filled organs and tissue masses, greater than air, but less than bone or metal. The muscular heart filled with blood will appear homogeneous relative to the air-filled lungs on both sides of it.

The radiologist is able to process 2-dimensional data in 3 dimensions; focusing through various layers, perhaps starting with the posterior portions of the ribs and then the anterior, thinking about superimposed masses and the anatomic structures responsible for them. The lung is much thicker medially where it borders the mediastinum and inferiorly. There are more vessels superimposed on each other in the medial half of the lung field and in the lower half of the lung than the upper half. The radiologist notes an abnormal shadow by its proximity to a particular rib or interspace. "Fool's triangle" refers to the right cardiophrenic angle where many vascular trunks overlap due to the anterioriorly placed middle lobe superimposed on the vessels of the posterior lower lobe. Novices in radiology interpretation may overread infiltrates in this area or note the most obvious abnormality, whereas radiologists systematically study each film looking at various structures in a deliberate order, concentrating on the anatomy of each, while excluding superimposed shadows of other structures. The integration of two orthogonal views provides the maximal localization of individual structures and abnormalities. A single radiograph will not be able to precisely locate a foreign body or support line. Bony fractures may not be apparent with a single film and a second film at right angles should be ordered to identify the lack of alignment and possible fragments.

Serial radiographs may be more helpful than more sophisticated imaging through the introduction of the fourth dimension, following the course of disease and physiology over time. Radiography can be performed at the bedside when the patient is unable to travel to the radiology department and can be made available very rapidly.

ULTRASOUND (US)

US imaging takes advantage of sonographic properties such as augmented transmission through fluid and textures that may be influenced by fat, blood vessels, and other structures. However, there are important limitations because ultrasound is stopped by air, limiting its utility in lungs and in the setting of gas collection throughout the body. Ultrasound cannot penetrate bone and many medical devices (such as joint replacement).

The Doppler shift refers to the change in frequency that occurs when a sound wave is reflected by moving blood. This change in frequency is proportional to the velocity of the blood flow in the vessel being sampled. Since World War II Doppler technology has evolved from crude, continuous-wave Doppler flow detectors blindly applied to the skin surface to color flow mapping systems. Duplex instruments combine pulsed Doppler techniques with real-time ultrasound imaging, made possible through the introduction of electronically steered, phased array transducer systems and the application of signal processing and display techniques for analyzing ultrasound echoes.

Duplex Doppler imaging with 2-dimentional US provides anatomic information with pulsed-wave Doppler analysis to calculate a color overlay containing information about the direction and velocity of blood flow. Pulsed Doppler permits a smaller sample size, thereby permitting analysis of the arterial lumen without the associated vein. The spectral tracing is a quantitative depiction of red blood cell movement within a sample volume. A semiquantitative color encoding of the Doppler information is superimposed on the gray-scale, real-time image providing color Doppler imaging. The color depends on the mean velocity of flow and the direction of flow. Blue does not necessarily mean venous flow as seen in the reverse component of triphasic flow characteristic of normal arterial flow. Red does not necessarily mean arterial flow as seen in reflux of venous flow in incompetent veins. The hue reflects the relative blood velocity, so that fast flow just proximal to a critical stenosis may appear white whereas slow flow beyond the stenosis would have a deeper hue. Color duplex imaging increases the sensitivity of duplex imaging. Color Doppler imaging makes it easier to evaluate deep veins in obese or edematous individuals and to identify flow around a thrombus.

Doppler technology has largely replaced venography in the diagnosis of venous thrombosis involving the legs. Although noninvasive, safe, and less expensive, US may not always be able to image vessels for the following reasons: (1) the vessels too deep to be imaged due to overlying fat or edema using the 5 megahertz probe, (2) iliac veins and the inferior vena cava not typically imaged due to overlying bowel gas and depth of vessels, (3) a segment of the distal superficial femoral vein not visualized in the adductor canal (isolated clot in this area unlikely), (4) the small caliber and multiple branches of the calf veins, (5) limitations in distinguishing between acute and chronic thrombus in a patient with the postthrombotic syndrome, and (6) limited expertise of operator.

Duplex or color flow Doppler US may be used to confirm arterial perfusion of organ transplants and exclude venous thrombosis in portal, splenic, and renal veins. Doppler US indicates the direction of blood flow, which may be helpful in diagnosing subclavian steel or portal hypertension with altered hemodynamics or in the diagnosis of pseudoaneurysms or mesenteric ischemia. Doppler US may be used to characterize tumors, varices, or ectopic pregnancies that have characteristic flow patterns.

Pulse Doppler quantitates the degree of arterial stenosis. Real-time US may be able to characterize arterial plaque as calcified or soft. The reliability depends on whether the vessel can be imaged adequately, whether the vessel is straight or tortuous, whether there are tandem lesions, and on the skill of the sonographer. For vessels that can be imaged easily, the reliability of US is excellent. If the vessel is not well suited to imaging, the anatomic and hemodynamic information is unreliable, especially in inexperienced hands. The mere presence of a hemodynamically significant vascular lesion does not reliably prove that it is the cause of a particular symptom or that it is otherwise functionally significant.

Ultrasound guidance is being used with increasing frequency for central venous catheter placement, thoracentesis, and paracentesis.

Owing to increased concerns about patient exposure to ionizing radiation, ultrasound is being used increasingly for novel applications including joint examination. It is actively being explored as an adjunct for bedside physical examination in ICU settings.

COMPUTED TOMOGRAPHY (CT) SCANS

In addition to the 5 categories of density, air, fat, water (includes soft tissue and muscle), calcium, and metal detected by plain films, CT scans are able to detect the differences between water and a variety of specific soft tissues including liver and kidneys and in the case of the brain, between white and gray matter. CT provides detailed anatomic images in which a variety of soft tissues can be recognized; the resulting basic transaxial images are the in vivo equivalent of transaxial anatomic pictures of a cadaver. State-of-the-art multidetector CT scanners are capable of acquiring ever-increasing numbers of individual slices of data at one time. Four-detector scanners scan the chest in approximately 20 seconds, a practical time for patient breath holding. Readily available clinical models with the capability of producing 16 to 64 slices at one time can scan the chest in 10 seconds or less. Alternatively, very small structures can be studied using ever-smaller slice thickness. Development currently focuses on providing up to 320 slices at one time. Along with cardiac gating, this technology permits unprecedented in vivo evaluation of ultrastructure in lungs as well as the heart. Specialized CT examinations are performed according to disease-specific algorithms. The reconstructed image thickness of the CT determine its sensitivity and specificity for identifying certain underlying conditions, based primarily on the size of the structure being assessed. For example, a PE-protocol CT requires thinner images than a venous-CT of the lower extremities.

Hounsfield units derive their name from the developer of the CT scanner, Nobel Laureate Sir Godfrey N. Hounsfield. The scale arbitrarily assigns water the attenuation value of zero, and air -1000, with the attenuation of other materials defined in relation to these set points. These numerical values of normalized X-ray attenuation define the gray scale of all CT images. The display windows highlight various structures based on the relationships between the underlying fundamental gray scale and the composition of various tissues in the body.

Intravenous iodinated contrast material is commonly used to provide optimum delineation of vascular structures, particularly when they lie in close proximity to the pathologic entity. Thus, lung cancer staging is most often performed with IV contrast. Oral contrast is used to aid delineation of gastrointestinal (GI) tract structures. A routine abdomen/pelvis CT performed for nonspecific abdominal pain or cancer restaging typically employs both intravenous and oral contrast for optimal tissue characterization. Alternative routes of contrast material administration are also used for nonvascular examinations such as cystography and myelography. Nonionic contrast agents have replaced older ionic contrast agents as they produce fewer side effects. The use of well-functioning 20-gauge or larger peripheral IV is required for administration of iodinated contrast agents for optimal imaging, particularly for vascular CT applications that require high contrast flow rates. Whether in the GI fluoroscopy suite, CT fluoroscopy suite, or angiography suite, fluoroscopy provides physiologic information along with anatomic information but they are invasive tests, best preceded by appropriate subspecialty consultation.

Not all CT scans require IV or oral contrast material. For example, to diagnose the presence of a renal stone, a dedicated renal stone CT would not use intravenous or oral contrast as neither is needed to detect a high density renal stone. High resolution CT to assess interstitial lung disease is generally performed without contrast. Follow-up CT scans can be performed without contrast materials depending upon the tissue contrast between the structures of continuing interest.

PRACTICE POINT

CT

- CT scans of contiguous body parts such as chest, abdomen, and pelvis are frequently performed together. The sequence of scanning and the volume of contrast material utilized will be selected to maximize scanning efficiency and answer the clinical questions posed.
- Separate doses of IV contrast material are generally not required. The same bolus of contrast material may be followed through the body with attention to circulation time and distribution of contrast material within organs to optimize imaging. Bolus tracking methods in modern scanners provide individualized selection of delay. The chest can easily be imaged during the delay required for liver enhancement on an abdomen CT scan. In many instances, the chest portion of the CT scan will be equally diagnostic with or without IV contrast enhancement. The chest portion of the CT scan should be performed prior to contrast administration to assess interstitial lung disease or detect calcification in very small lung nodules. Chest CT scanning may also be performed during the administration of IV contrast material for some contrast enhanced head CT scans.

To ensure that the CT scan is tailored to the clinical questions and patient-specific needs, speak directly to the radiologist before ordering the CT scan. This will allow the radiologist to suggest potentially valuable alternatives and prevent waiting for test results from the wrong test that cannot further clinical decision-making.

PET-CT is a lengthy examination that is often better suited to outpatient follow-up. Patients are asked to avoid strenuous activities the day before the examination and may be given special preparatory dietary instructions to consume a fatty meal the evening before the examination, which is performed after the patient has been NPO for at least 4–6 hours. While PET-CT has become a central tool for the staging of malignancies, significant overlap in results between neoplastic and inflammatory processes limits the value of the study during hospitalization for acute illness.

MAGNETIC RESONANCE IMAGING (MRI)

MR uses very specific depolarizing pulse sequences to detect tiny differences in signal from soft tissues that may be otherwise indistinguishable. Gadolinium has paramagnetic properties that make it the most common contrast agent used for MR examinations. While inert, gadolinium does pose potential risk for nephrogenic systemic sclerosis (NSF), particularly in the setting of renal failure. MRI examinations are customized to the problem being evaluated. Coils used to perform the examination not only provide improved imaging but also control technical parameters such as field of view. The bore of the available MRI scanner, itself, may limit the size of patients who can have MRI. Larger bore and open scanners have decreased this limitation, but a patient may have to go to a special location to have such an examination.

Hospitalized patients are often unable to cooperate adequately to allow the full benefit of the MRI technology in their care. MRI examinations do not use ionizing radiation but can be quite lengthy, lasting one hour or more in duration. The request for wider coverage such as adjacent body parts is not easily accommodated in the same scanning session. It is therefore imperative to have a specific goal for the MRI from the outset. MRI and CT are equivalent for imaging lymphadenopathy. MRI imaging is by nature less than contiguous and should otherwise be viewed as complementary to CT imaging. In many instances, the patient will be better served by MRI as part of outpatient follow-up following recovery from the acute illness requiring hospitalization. The need for the information is a critical point in this decision as MRI/MRA can be valuable and rapid compared with conventional angiography for diagnosis of potentially surgical aortic disease such as aortic dissection. Selected for the wrong reason, MRI will increase the stress on the acutely ill patient and delay institution of needed therapy.

It is helpful to ask about patient claustrophobia before ordering the examination. Patients who are concerned about having the examination often benefit from oral premedication; those with severe claustrophobia or difficulty remaining still in the confines of the scanner may require sedation with an anesthesiologist present during the scan. Contraindications to an MRI include aneurysm clip, recent surgery (generally within 10 days) and noncompatible cardiac pacing devices. Some patients who have metallic implants such as joint prostheses will experience unacceptable heating of the region that will prevent completion of the examination. This is sometimes quite specific to the location of scanning relative to the location of the implant. These effects vary also with the field strength of the MRI unit. Relative contraindications can also include cochlear implants and neurostimulators. All patients should be screened for possible contraindications prior to scanning as routine practice in radiology. In addition, patients who have potential to have a metallic foreign body in an eye, typically due to occupational or other machine shop exposure, may need to have radiographs or even CT scanning of the orbits prior to MRI. There is not a known adverse effect of MRI on the fetus but the decision to scan during pregnancy should be made on an individual basis.

MRI exceeds CT for the multifactorial differentiation of fat and other tissue planes, properties that are particularly useful when studying the musculoskeletal system and in localizing boundaries of pathology, and fluids, including the differentiation of the various states of hemoglobin. In the brain, MRI images provide significantly more information that CT images, resulting in greater sensitivity for small and subtle lesions such as early brain metastases. The use of MRI for clinical problem solving is more apt to reflect the problem under consideration than a standardized approach. MR angiography (MRA) may provide high quality images of many parts of the body often adequate to replace conventional angiography.

The use of MRI for direct acquisition of multiplanar, sagittal, coronal, and axial images had diminished with increasing availability of PET-CT as well as multidetector CT scanners that permit data to be acquired with voxels of equal dimension in all three planes, thus providing high quality sagittal and coronal reformatted CT images. MRI imaging of calcium as a signal void is a particular pitfall in MRI imaging that highlights the complementary nature of CT for the study of bones and potentially calcified pathology.

NUCLEAR MEDICINE

Nuclear medicine images reflect the movement of tracer in the body as it travels and/or interacts with variably specific cells. Radiotracer can prove patency of central venous catheters, detect the spleen when present in the pleural space, identify low level bleeding otherwise difficult to localize, and evaluate function. For a patient with a normal chest X-ray, a normal perfusion scan alone still provides the finest exclusion of PE.

PRACTICE POINT

- Perfusion scan should be considered for exclusion of PE in a pregnant patient with a normal chest X-ray. With hydration and frequent voiding, the dose of ionizing radiation to the fetus can be lower level than from scattered radiation during a PE-CT of the chest.

Nuclear medicine is also used extensively for cardiac evaluation, even in the acutely ill. Tagged white blood cell scans may localize elusive infection in patients with unexplained fever. Likewise, 3-phase bone scanning may pinpoint osteomyelitis. These are very worthwhile tests when chosen for the correct reason. Consultation with the nuclear medicine physician can result in performance of examination tailored to the specific pathophysiologic question, beyond the most exhaustive list of nuclear medicine studies. PET-CT has been adopted in many institutions as a nearly universal substitute despite availability of more specific physiologically-oriented nuclear medicine studies.

Radionuclide substances can increase the radiation dose received due to their persistence within the body following the imaging. Depending on the radioisotope, the clearance may range between hours and days with most eliminated via urine. Encouraging fluids and frequent emptying of the bladder are important ways in which the radiation dose can be controlled. Allergic reactions have not been described and patients with renal failure can safely undergo nuclear medicine examinations.

PATIENT PREPARATION

Fasting is required for safe performance of many imaging procedures. Overnight fasting is required for proper adhesion of fluoroscopically administered oral contrast agents for barium swallow and upper GI series examinations. Fasting is also required for interventional procedures. Common contrast agents require specific preparations. For iodinated intravenous contrast material, 4 hours of pretest fasting is preferred to minimize risk of aspiration because administration of contrast material on a full stomach significantly increases the probability that a patient will become nauseated and vomit while lying down in a scanner. In a true emergency, this requirement for fasting may be modified or waived.

Dietary changes and careful timing in the administration of oral contrast agents can significantly improve the value of radiology examinations, most particularly for patients who are ill enough to require hospitalization. Contrast agents are the drugs most frequently ordered by radiologists. These may be administered by mouth, feeding tube, intravascular catheter, or rectal tube. More than one may be used for the same examination. Oral contrast agents are selected for consistency and risk of leakage into lungs, mediastinum, and peritoneal cavity. Radiologists may also order or recommend hormones, beta-blockers, or steroids largely to support the use of contrast agents in specific radiology examinations. On occasion, particularly in ultrasound, water will be administered as an oral contrast agent to increase through transmission to the pancreas that is located behind the stomach.

COST

With limited resources and decreasing reimbursements of imaging, all physicians must consider not only the clinical value of tests they order in terms of efficacy and safety, but also cost. It may not be possible to determine the actual cost and charges for medical imaging due to differences in reimbursement based on separate contractual agreements, insurance policies limiting the number of reimbursable radiologic examinations to one each day, and bundling of inpatient costs under disease related groups (DRGs). Intensive labor by billing experts to capture reimbursement for the most expensive test performed each day and prolonged hospitalization due to test ordering or complications from imaging add to the costs of medical imaging. Although inpatient reimbursement will differ from patient to patient, nevertheless, clinicians should have a general awareness of relative costs of different radiologic tests. For example, automatic ordering of costly imaging studies such as MRI often fail to offer significant additional information that influences clinical management.

Cost-effectiveness analysis, which compares the clinical benefit a patient receives from an intervention compared to the cost of the intervention, is increasingly being applied to radiology testing.

RADIOLOGY REPORTS

Radiology reports provide the reason given for the examination, the technique with comments about limitations, findings, and an impression or conclusion. Increasingly, radiologists will communicate directly with the physician about significant findings and document this communication within the report. At the physician's request, a radiology report can also be sent to the patient's primary care physician but this should not be relied upon as the primary documentation of communication with the primary care provider.

Maximizing the value of radiology examinations to acute patient care begins with consideration of prior radiology examinations. In an ideal world, the examinations would be reviewed directly within the new clinical context. Reading the reports, and even just recognizing what examinations have been performed, particularly the most recent prior radiology examinations can propel patient care forward without waste in time, resources, health care dollars, or patient radiation exposure. Many sophisticated and expensive radiology examinations have utility long after the original reason for performing the examination. This is especially true for cross-sectional imaging such as CT and MRI in which a single examination can serve as a permanent reference for anatomic variants that become confusing on projection radiographs in the course of acute care.

The review of as series of plain images over time with the radiologist may provide the most valuable pathophysiological data with the least amount of incidental findings for follow-up after hospitalization. The transfer of responsibility for follow-up of incidental findings unrelated to the admission is a crucial and often burdensome requirement for the physician who orders the radiology examination. It is important to document all such communication as directly as possible to avoid medico-legal disasters arising from lack of communication of findings such as potential lung cancer that could be treated successfully with prompt follow-up.

The busy clinician must always critically assess the data in the context of the patient. If the radiology report does not provide the best explanation for each constellation of symptoms and signs, the practitioner should consult the radiologist for a second look, perhaps to gain greater understanding for why a "false" diagnosis may be incorrect. In many instances this may require reviewing prior films whose interpretation may be altered by more recent events. In addition, without the proper clinical context, the practitioner may attach too much significance to incidental findings reported by radiologists who may not have received adequate clinical information to focus on a specific area or who do not want to overlook a potential malignancy.

A negative imaging examination in a patient with a compelling story and physical examination may not mean that a patient does not have the disease. The timing of the imaging study in the course of the disease and the limitations of the imaging study remind us that while positive X-ray findings may point to the diagnosis, incidental findings may mislead, and a negative study may prove less helpful. For example, the patient with military tuberculosis may not show the characteristic minute military densities in the lung parenchyma until several weeks after a presumptive clinical diagnosis has been made. An incidental pulmonary nodule may mislead the clinician into thinking that the underlying process for acute illness is lung cancer. Likewise, a PE-protocol CT may fail to reveal a pulmonary embolism if obtained weeks after the primary event or if there are technical limitations to the study. Yet concurrent illness may fail to explain the coexistence of pulmonary hypertension. At the same time, the clinician in consultation with the radiologist must be aware of the fallibilities of the imaging method for that same disease.

PRACTICE POINT

An important component of appropriate care in the 21st century

- Hospitalists can play a central role in balancing the well-being of patients through their lifetimes (direct patient care) with prudent resource allocation. More judicious use of imaging studies that do not meaningfully contribute to patient management decisions is the responsibility of all physicians. The majority of interventions in patient care can be replaced by evidence-based strategies that are far more cost effective without diminishing quality of care. The ethical mandate is to ensure equally high quality, affordable health services for all citizens.

CONCLUSION

The radiology chapters in this text are intended to provide the reader with a framework that can be applied over time, even as technology evolves, to clinical problem-solving relating to the diagnosis and treatment of the subpopulation of hospitalized ill patients. The results of any diagnostic imaging examination should always be germane to the patient's care during admission. Less expensive "low-tech" testing may provide valuable information regarding the next best imaging step to pursue. However, simple radiology films may falsely reassure the clinician that all is normal and may identify incidental findings that lead to more expensive testing. Ultrasound, MR, and nuclear medicine tests are more able to reveal physiologic function than CT and plain radiography. Optimal test ordering, therefore, requires asking the right question combined with an appreciation of the indications of a specific imaging test, the likelihood that a specific test will diagnose certain conditions depending on the patient population studied, the relative risks of different imaging modalities, absolute contraindications, and the inherent limitations of the testing, including impact of timing, body habitus, and observer variation among radiologists interpreting the same film. Clinicians should be able to inform patients about the indications, relative costs, preparation required, and risks. The input of radiologists will increase the value of the interpretation and often the rapidity with which the study will be interpreted.

SUGGESTED READINGS

Elgazzar, A. *Concise Guide to Nuclear Medicine*. New York, NY: Springer Publishing; 2011.

Hofer, M. *CT Teaching Manual: A Systematic Approach to CT Reading*. Fourth edition. New York, NY: Thieme Medical Publishers; 2011.

Hofer, M. *Ultrasound Teaching Manual: The Basics of Performing and Interpreting Ultrasound Scans*. Second edition. New York, NY: Thieme Medical Publishers; 2005.

Wetbrook, C. *MRI at a Glance*. Second edition. Hoboken, NJ: Wiley-Blackwell; 2010.

CHAPTER 106

Patient Safety Issues in Radiology

Aaron Sodickson, MD, PhD
Francine L. Jacobson, MD, MPH

Key Clinical Questions

1. How can cumulative radiation dose be estimated?
2. What commonly ordered CT scan delivers the highest dose of ionizing radiation?
3. What are the risk factors for contrast-related allergic reactions?
4. How can the potential for contrast-induced nephropathy be minimized?

INTRODUCTION

For an acutely ill patient whose illness is one snapshot in time, one must not lose sight of the cumulative risks of short- and long-term adverse effects of modern imaging. These may be due to contrast administration, ionizing radiation, and the possibility of incidental findings generating additional studies.

CONTRAST MATERIALS

ORAL CONTRAST

Contrast materials may be administered intravenously, orally, rectally, and for problem solving, through a variety of support lines and tubes. The selection of a specific oral contrast agent is based on the risk for aspiration versus the risk for extravasation of the contrast material. Catastrophic aspiration requiring ICU admission can occur when oral contrast material is administered to a patient with achalasia or other significant risk factors for aspiration, especially when contrast material is administered while the patient is supine. Although inert, when aspirated into the lungs, barium is permanent. Barium becomes concentrated as it passes through the GI tract and can contribute to constipation and obstipation, particularly at the concentrations administered for X-ray and fluoroscopic examinations. Gastrografin is more commonly used when there is concern for extravasation into mediastinum or peritoneal cavity. It is important to remember that although gastrografin will be reabsorbed, it can cause pulmonary edema due to its hypertonicity. Gastrografin contains iodine, and should not be used in patients with a known iodine allergy, as a small amount is absorbed in the GI tract. Specialized contrast agents may also be used for purposes such as distending the bowel without obscuring mucosal enhancement.

IODINATED INTRAVENOUS CONTRAST

Low osmolar nonionic contrast agents are almost universally used in current practice due to their reduced risk of fluid shifts and allergic reaction. In a labile patient, these risks may not be warranted for the increase in diagnostic information provided by the contrast enhancement. This is best determined in consultation with the radiologist, to explore how crucial the intravenous contrast is for the clinical question at hand (**Tables 106-1** and **106-2**).

RISK OF CONTRAST-INDUCED RENAL FAILURE

It is best to avoid ordering multiple contrast studies in rapid succession and seek alternative imaging modalities whenever possible because contrast-induced renal failure is associated with higher morbidity and mortality as well as longer length of hospitalization. Based on a generally accepted definition of contrast-induced renal failure, administration of contrast material causes renal failure in 0.1% to 13% of patients who receive it and it is responsible for 12% of cases of hospital-acquired renal failure. How contrast materials cause renal failure is unclear, but it is likely due to direct cellular toxicity and intrarenal vasoconstriction. If a patient has an estimated glomerular filtration rate < 60 ml/minute/1.73 m^2, the patient is at increased risk; the risk is much higher if there are other contrast-induced nephropathy risk factors, or if the patient has an acutely rising creatinine, even if below 1.5 mg/dL.

TABLE 106-1 Conditions Associated with Adverse Reactions to Contrast Material

Risk factors for contrast-acquired renal failure

- Preexisting renal insufficiency
- Diabetes alone, and diabetic nephropathy, especially > Cr 1.5 mg/dL, or 60 ml/minute/1.73 m^2
- Acutely rising Cr
- Concurrent use of vasoconstrictive (nonsteroidal anti-inflammatory medications), nephrotoxic medications (aminoglycosides), and volume-depleting agents such as diuretics
- States of reduced perfusion such as hypotension, hypovolemia, cirrhosis, and congestive heart failure
- Age > 70, hypertension, anemia, female gender, multiple comorbidities
- Urgent procedures
- Large volume contrast load

Risk factors for contrast-related allergy reactions

- Previous anaphylaxis to contrast material
- Asthma
- Multiple medication allergies, including food or medication

The risk of renal failure following contrast administration is dose dependent and occurs most frequently in patients with already diminished renal function, particularly diabetic nephropathy. A patient with preexisting renal insufficiency is 5 to 10 times more likely to develop contrast-induced renal failure than the general population. The risk of further renal injury may be decreased by hydration. Radiologists typically avoid administering iodine contrast agents to patients with multiple myeloma, especially if they are dehydrated, but it can be used when absolutely necessary. The risk of renal failure in patients with multiple myeloma is caused by an interaction of light chains and contrast material. Due to the decline of renal function with age, elderly patients are at increased risk of developing renal insufficiency from contrast. Institutional guidelines may include renal function testing prior to contrast administration based on patient age.

TABLE 106-2 Patient Safety Measures for All Patients About to Receive Contrast

1. Is the study necessary? How important is the study? If contrast is not administered, will you obtain the information you need to make a clinical decision?
2. Does the patient have risk factors for contrast-induced nephropathy?
3. Does the patient have allergy to contrast and if so, which type?
4. Is there an alternative study that does not involve contrast?
5. Are there any modifiable risk factors?
   - Discontinue NSAIDS at least 24 hours prior to the administration of contrast, particularly in patients at increased risk.
   - Discontinue metformin for 48 hours prior to the administration of contrast if the creatinine is abnormal; if normal, discontinue and perform the study, if required, without delay.
   - Consider holding oral hypoglycemics on the day of the study as most patients will be npo, and prescribe replacement insulin as needed.
   - Hold diuretics on the day of the study.
   - Regarding ACE inhibitors, the data is mixed because there is increased risk as well as protective effects. Do not start ACE inhibitors on the day of the procedure.
   - Optimize volume status prior to the procedure.
6. Will the patient require another contrast study within 72 hours?
7. If the patient is at increased risk for an ADE, has a discussion occurred with radiology to either reduce the risk or to consider an alternative study?

Patients treated with nephrotoxic medications (eg, aminoglycosides and nonsteroidal anti-inflammatory agents) and those who have recently received iodinated contrast material are at greater risk for acquiring renal failure. Metformin (Glucophage), frequently used to treat type II diabetes, may cause severe lactic acidosis following administration of intravenous contrast media. Metformin therapy may be suspended for at least 48 hours following the administration of iodine contrast material and resumed after the patient's renal function has returned to baseline serum creatinine level. Adjustment of medications that are excreted by the kidneys may also be helpful.

Patients with eGFR > 60 are considered by radiologists to have normal renal function for routine prescription of IV contrast. For eGFR between 30 and 60, the dose of contrast material may be reduced if the diagnostic quality of the scan may be preserved at lower contrast doses. If not, alternative diagnostic strategies should be pursued. When eGFR is less than 30, IV contrast material should be avoided. Patients with end stage renal failure on dialysis may receive IV contrast material when necessary if prior discussion with their nephrologists has taken place.

CASE 106-1

WEIGHING THE RISK OF CONTRAST

A 61-year-old female mentioned transient right-sided pleuritic chest pain to her nephrologist. When a CXR revealed a new moderate right-sided pleural effusion, he recommended a V/Q scan. Her glomerular filtration rate (eGFR) estimated at 32 ml/minute might not preclude a contrast study according to hospital protocols but she had only one functioning kidney. Extensive changes of intersitital lung disease were also reported on CXR. Lower extremity ultrasound did not reveal deep venous thrombosis.

Key question:

1. ***Would a V/Q scan provide any meaningful information given her extensive interstitial lung disease, bronchiectasis, and bullous emphysema?***
   This patient would most likely have an indeterminate or, perhaps, an intermediate probability scan. In a landmark PIOPED study, more than half of individuals with intermediate probability and indeterminate studies were found to actually have PE (pulmonary embolism).
2. ***Would hydration and mucomist provide suitable protection for PE protocol imaging?***
   Although hydration is definitely helpful, it may not provide adequate protection in patients with markedly compromised renal function. It is debatable whether mucomist would provide any additive benefit.
3. ***Should such a patient receive hemodialysis following administration of IV contrast for CT if required for adequate diagnosis or selection of treatment?***
   Hemodialysis will not adequately remove contrast material to conserve renal function.

4. ***What are the risks of gadolinium in patients with compromised renal function?***
   Gadolinium can no longer be recommended due to high risk of NSF.
5. ***Would there be any utility to performing MR without gadolinium?***
   MRI is infrequently used to address PE, and then almost always with gadolinium enhancement of vessels. MRI does not offer a practical solution for obtaining a diagnostic quality examination of pulmonary vessels in an acutely ill, dyspneic patient.
6. ***What if this patient had pleuritic chest pain from active SLE?***
   If the patient has active SLE, it is possible that her renal insufficiency might become unstable, thereby further increasing her risk. This patient also had light chains in her urine consistent with multiple myeloma.

The bottom line: Standard hospital protocols would not have prevented this patient from undergoing a contrast study given her estimated GFR > 30 ml/min. Yet, the best balance of risk and benefit may preclude a valuable frequently performed imaging test. A search for diagnostic precision may subject the patient to risks she would find unacceptable.

ADVERSE REACTIONS TO CONTRAST ADMINISTRATION

Immediate reactions

Dose-dependent, systemic adverse reactions to contrast material include generalized warmth or flushing, a metallic taste in the mouth, and nausea and vomiting. These reactions are usually non life-threatening, self-limited problems. The risk of vomiting in the supine position with a high probability of associated aspiration is the primary reason for fasting 4 hours prior to contrast administration. When this risk is less than the potential benefit, such as the finding of acute life-threatening injuries due to trauma, the examination will be performed without fasting.

Contrast reactions most frequently occur while the patient is having the examination. Acute bronchospasm, profound hypotension, and severe urticaria may occur during injection or within minutes of administration of contrast material and can occur in patients who have not been exposed to contrast material previously. The etiology of these reactions is unclear.

Mild iodine contrast reactions present with signs and symptoms and are self-limited, without evidence of progression. Limited urticaria with mild pruritis and transient nausea with not more than one episode of emesis are most common. A variety of sensations may be reported by the patient. Rash, hives, nasal and facial swelling, and anxiety may be present. Treatment is limited to observation to confirm resolution or lack of progression. Patient reassurance is usually helpful. Hives may develop shortly following the examination and increase over the next 15 minutes. Observation or treatment with 25 to 50 mg of intravenous diphenhydramine may be indicated. Some centers include a dose of diphenhydramine 1 hour before CT scan in the pretreatment protocol for patients who have had contrast reactions.

Moderate signs and symptoms of contrast reaction are more pronounced and may include tachycardia or bradycardia, hypertention, generalized erythema, dyspnea, wheezing, bronchospasm, laryngeal edema, and hypotension. The clinical findings may require prompt treatment and careful observation for progression to a life-threatening event.

Severe signs and symptoms of contrast reaction are often life-threatening and may include severe or rapidly progressive laryngeal edema, convulsions, unresponsiveness, cardiopulmonary arrest, profound hypotention, and cardiac arhythmias. Prompt recognition and aggressive treatment are required. Patients who have had such reactions should not again receive iodine contrast agents even following pretreatment.

Delayed reactions

Delayed adverse reactions occurring 30 minutes or more after the administration of contrast material are more likely following administration of an ionic contrast agent. Up to 30% of patients receiving ionic contrast materials develop delayed reactions whereas administration of nonionic agents is associated with delayed reactions in only 10% of patients. The symptoms of delayed reactions resemble a flu-like syndrome and include fever, chills, nausea, vomiting, abdominal pain, fatigue, and congestion. Recognizing these symptoms as a delayed reaction to contrast administration for CT or angiography may help limit the workup of the new symptoms in the hospitalized patient.

Extravasation of contrast

Extravasated contrast material causes direct toxic effects that can lead to a compartment syndrome if enough contrast material leaks into surrounding tissue. The use of well-functioning 20-gauge or larger peripheral IV for administration of iodinated contrast agents decreases the potential for extravasation of contrast material at the high injection rates required for optimum imaging, ranging up to 4–6 cc/second for vascular examinations. Immediate treatment includes milking contrast material out of the site and ice packs. Plastic surgery consultation should be sought, and may be initiated by the radiologist.

PRETREATMENT FOR CONTRAST ALLERGY

Consulting with the radiologist prior to ordering examinations that may require iodine contrast agents is most imperative when the patient has previously had an adverse reaction to iodine contrast material. Anaphylactic reactions are the most serious and potentially life-threatening allergic reactions associated with the administration of contrast material. Patients with a history of anaphylactic reactions to contrast material are more likely to have a similar reaction on repeat exposure. Patients with a history of multiple food and medication allergies or asthma have double the risk of developing adverse reactions compared to the general population. No substantive data support the myth that patients with seafood allergy are at higher risk of developing allergic reactions to contrast media.

Patients who have previously had mild to moderate contrast reactions can be pretreated with steroids in order to perform necessary iodine contrast enhanced CT scan. Pretreatment regimens vary, therefore specific guidance should be sought from the radiologist in your institution. Thinking ahead is important to allow time for 2 doses of steroid such as prednisone beginning 12 or more hours before the examination. It is important to provide the doses in addition to steroids being given for any other reason; 25–50 mg of diphenhydramine may be administered 1–2 hours prior to the scan. Coordination with the CT technologists should be started at the time of CT ordering in order to perform the scan at the prescribed interval after pretreatment (**Table 106-3**).

USE OF IODINE CONTRAST MATERIAL DURING PREGNANCY

The extent of potential mutagenesis of fetal tissue due to iodine contrast material is not known. It is paramount when balancing the risks and benefits of any imaging procedure performed during pregnancy to carefully consider the value of the procedure and need for contrast materials to safeguard the health care of the mother.

TABLE 106-3 Pretreatment Steroid Comparisons

Corticosteroid	Route of Administration	Equivalent Strength Dosage	Premedication for Iodine Contrast
Prednisone	p.o.	5 mg	40–50 mg
Methylprenisolone		4 mg	32–40 mg
Medrol	p.o.		
Solu-Medrol	i.v.		
Hydrocortisone		20 mg	200 mg
Cortef	p.o.		
Solu-Cortef	i.v.		
Dexamethasone	i.v., i.m., p.o.	0.75 mg	7.5 mg

PRACTICE POINT

A general rule for pregnant patients:

- The clinical needs of the mother should take precedence in determining the diagnostic approach.
- X-ray exposure to less than 5 rads has not been associated with fetal anomalies or pregnancy loss, but is thought to increase risk of childhood leukemia.
- Contrast material and radiation should be avoided when possible in pregnant women.
- There are no known associations of MRI with fetal abnormalities. Gadolinium administration is typically avoided in pregnancy.
- Ultrasound is the best imaging modality to use, when possible, for pregnant patients.

GADOLINIUM

While anaphylactic reactions are rare, nephrogenic systemic fibrosis (NFS) has been linked to administration of gadolinium contrast agents as a rare complication in patients with impaired renal function. Increasing concern for nephrogenic systemic fibrosis (NSF) has led to the institution of reduced-dose regimens for patients with impaired renal function. It is best to consult the radiologist beforehand to maximize the value of the MRI examination as special scanning sequences can sometimes be used to provide the needed information without any contrast agent.

RADIATION EXPOSURE

Much of what we know about radiation biology comes from long-term follow-up of atomic bomb survivors, and relatively small studies of medical or occupational exposure. These studies have demonstrated increases in cancer incidence for exposures on the order of 50–100 mSv, but controversy persists about the shape of the dose-response curve from smaller exposures or from fractionated or prolonged exposures. Until more data become available that directly explores risk models in these lower-dose regimes, radiation risk estimation will typically be performed using a linear-no-threshold (LNT) model in which cancer risk is assumed to rise linearly as a function of exposure.

Figure 106-1 shows results from the widely used BEIR-VII (Biological Effects of Ionizing Radiation) report that uses an LNT model. For a given exposure, female patients are at higher risk than male patients, and risk per dose increases at younger ages, due both to the increased radiation sensitivity of younger tissues, and the longer timeline remaining in which a radiation-induced cancer may develop. The lifetime attributable risk (LAR) represents an additive risk above baseline cancer rates (42% in the U.S. population).

These curves may be used for rough estimates of risk levels, based on the patient's age, gender, and level of exposure. However, it is important to realize that these models assume standardized U.S. life expectancies. Radiation-induced cancers typically have a 10–20 year latency (depending on the organ), so patients with short remaining life expectancy have very little associated risk from radiation exposure.

Radiation risks have been alternately downplayed and exaggerated in the literature and lay media, resulting in great confusion about the magnitude of these risks. While conventional X-ray, fluoroscopy, and nuclear medicine studies also expose patients to ionizing radiation, CT has appropriately received the greatest scrutiny because of the relatively high radiation dose per exam. Although it comprises about 15% of all medical imaging procedures, it produces approximately half of the population's medical radiation exposure. It is therefore most valuable to consider the approximate levels of risk imparted by CT, and the factors influencing these risks, to encourage a more rational decision making process by enabling risk estimates to be weighed against the perceived benefits of imaging. The continuing evolution of CT technology is now directed at strategies to reduce dose to the patient. Patient size may limit

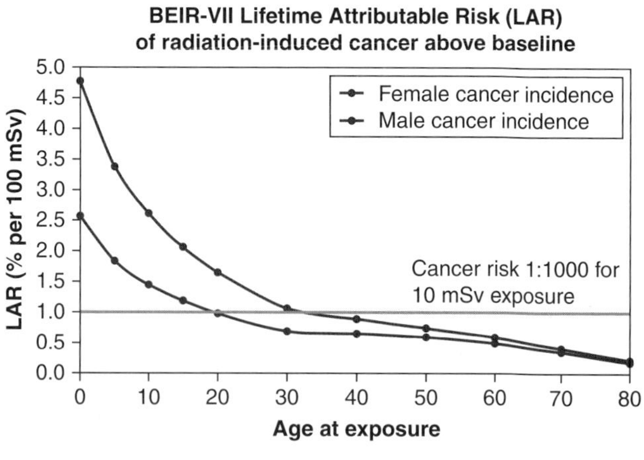

Figure 106-1 *Expected Lifetime Attributable Risk of radiation-induced cancer (data extracted from table 12D of BEIR-VII). For a 10 mSv exposure (solid horizontal line), approximate cancer risk is 1 in 1000 for a 33-year-old woman, or a 19-year-old man.*

TABLE 106-4 Approximate Effective Doses from Common Imaging Procedures

Imaging Study	Approximate Effective Dose per CT (mSv)
X-Ray: PA and lat chest	0.1
X-Ray: abdomen	0.7
X-Ray: lumbar spine	1.5
X-Ray: hip	0.7
Mammography	0.4
CT: head, face	2
CT: C-spine, neck	2
CT: chest, PE, T-Spine	8
CT: abdomen/Pelvis, L-Spine	15
CT: abdomen or Pelvis alone	7.5
Nucs: cardiac rest-stress MIBI	12
Nucs: cardiac stress-rest thallium	40
Nucs: V/Q	2.5
Nucs: FDG PET	14

the reduction of dose in extremely large patients. Small adults may be expected to receive smaller doses than the "typical" values in **Table 106-4**.

CUMULATIVE RISK

The risk from most individual CT scans is small, but many patients undergo large numbers of imaging studies over time. As radiation risks are generally believed to accumulate additively, recurrent imaging can lead to large cumulative risks over time. One can make a rough estimate of a patient's cumulative risk. Regardless of the estimation of cumulative risk, clinicians can take steps to reduce the cumulative risk (**Tables 106-5** and **106-6**).

PRACTICE POINT

The most important guiding principles:

- Focus imaging on the acute problem and limit the gathering of data that is outside the scope of the current illness.
- Use prior imaging in clinical context to provide additional/new information.
- Minimize radiation and contrast exposure when diagnostic quality of the exam can be preserved.
- Even with normal renal function, it is advisable to separate examinations that require administration of intravenous contrast material by at least 24 hours.
- Consult radiology prior to ordering invasive radiologic procedures.
- Responsibly handle incidental and nonemergent findings.

CONCLUSION

The balancing of risk and benefit requires the general understanding of patient risks from radiology tests presented in this chapter. Understanding the risks is helpful for minimizing them. The temporary discontinuance or delay in starting of a particular medication that will adversely affect patient hydration at the time of iodinated intravenous iodine contrast administration is a prime example of how the clinician can attenuate risk for a specific patient. The general discussions presented in this chapter should not substitute for direct consultation with the radiologist in choosing and scheduling the optimal imaging test for any particular patient. Although radiology imaging studies can provide more extensive and valuable information, it is important to focus on the acute illness and the guiding principle to order only the tests necessary for the selection of proper treatment of the acute illness.

TABLE 106-5 Estimation of Cumulative Risk

Approach for rough estimation of cumulative risk:

1. Count all prior chest and abdomen/pelvis CT scans.
2. Divide by 10. The result is the approximate LAR in percent above baseline.

To incrementally improve these estimates:

3. Adjust for scan type. The simplified approach above assumes that each CT scan imparted a 10 mSv effective dose. If all the scans were abdomen/pelvis, increase by 50% (see Table 106-1). If there are many head CTs, these can be included by adding 1/5 of them to the "scan count" of step 1.
4. Adjust for patient size. Assuming appropriate dose modulation techniques, increase by a factor of 2 for extremely obese patients, decrease by a factor of 2 for very small patients.
5. Adjust for age and gender. Multiply by the appropriate y-axis value from Figure 106-1.
6. Understand that these estimates are high for patients with life expectancy substantially shorter than age and sex-matched peers.

Example:

1. A moderately obese 60-year-old man has had 40 CT scans of the abdomen/pelvis.
2. The crude LAR estimate is 4% above baseline.
3. As all of these scans are relatively higher dose abdomen/pelvis scans, adjust to 6%.
4. Then adjust to 9% for moderate obesity.
5. Finally, multiply by .5 from Figure 106-1 to adjust for his gender and age.

The result is a LAR estimate of 4.5% above baseline, increasing his expected lifetime cancer risk from 42% to 46.5%.

6. If the patient is unlikely to survive this hospital admission, radiation risk estimation is irrelevant (Step 6).

In the future these types of calculations will likely be performed with appropriate extraction of relevant information from the electronic medical record.

TABLE 106-6 Patient Safety: Reduce Radiation Exposure

Methods to reduce radiation risk:

- Only order scans that will impact management.
- Review the patient's prior imaging history as thoroughly as possible, not just the last one or two studies.
- Move beyond the incremental risks of the single scan being considered at present, and balance the benefits of recurrent imaging against cumulative radiation risks.
- Take a longitudinal view of the patient. If numerous prior scans for the same complaint have been unrevealing, a new approach may well be warranted.
- Consider other imaging or diagnostic alternatives for focused questions, if the desired information is available by other means.
- Increase spacing between scans when possible.

Evidence

Allergic Reactions

Beaty AD, Lieberman PL, Slavin RG. Seafood allergy and radiocontrast media: are physicians propagating a myth? *Am J Med.* 2008;121(2):158.e1–e158.

Contrast Nephropathy

Harjai KJ, Raizada A, Shenoy C, et al. A comparison of contemporary definitions of contrast nephropathy in patients undergoing percutaneous coronary intervention and a proposal for a novel nephropathy grading system. *Am J Cardiol.* 2008;101(6):812.

Pannu N, Wiebe N, Tonelli M. Prophylaxis strategies for contrastinduced nephropathy. *JAMA.* 2006;295(23):2765–2779.

Scanlon PJ, Faxon DP, Audet AM, et al. ACC/AHA guidelines for coronary angiography. A report of the American College of Cardiology/American Heart Association Task Force on practice guidelines (Committee on Coronary Angiography). Developed in collaboration with the Society for Cardiac Angiography and Interventions. *J Am Coll Cardiol.* 1999;33(6):1756–1824.

Sinert R, Doty CI. Evidence-based Emergency Medicine review. Prevention of contrast-induced nephropathy in the emergency department. *Annals of Emergency Medicine.* 2007;50(3):335–345, 345.e1–e2.

Tramèr MR, von Elm E, Loubeyre P, Hauser C. Pharmacological prevention of serious anaphylactic reactions due to iodinated contrast media: systematic review. *BMJ.* 2006;333(7570):675.

Radiation

Amis ES Jr., Butler PF, Applegate KE, et al. American College of Radiology white paper on radiation dose in medicine. *J Am Coll Radiol.* 2007;4(5):272–284.

Mettler FA Jr., Bhargavan M, Faulkner K, et al. Radiologic and nuclear medicine studies in the United States and worldwide: frequency, radiation dose, and comparison with other radiation sources—1950–2007. *Radiology.* 2009;253(2):520–531.

Mettler FA Jr., Huda W, Yoshizumi TT, Mahesh M. Effective doses in radiology and diagnostic nuclear medicine: a catalog. *Radiology.* 2008;248(1):254–263.

National Research Council (U.S.). Committee to Assess Health Risks from Exposure to Low Level of Ionizing Radiation. Health risks from exposure to low levels of ionizing radiation: BEIR VII, Phase 2. Washington, D.C.: National Academies Press; 2006.

Sodickson A, Baeyens PF, Andriole KP, et al. Recurrent CT, cumulative radiation exposure, and associated radiation-induced cancer risks from CT of adults. *Radiology.* 2009;251(1):175–184.

Web-based Resource

http://www.acr.org/contrast-manual Manual on contrast media Version 6, 2008.

SUGGESTED READINGS

Bettman MA. Frequently asked questions: Iodinated contrast agents. *Radiographics.* 2004;24:S3–S10.

Davenport MS, Cohan RH, Caoili EM, Ellis JH. Repeat contrast medium reactions in premedicated patients: Frequency and severity. *Radiology.* 2009;253:372–379.

Greenberger PA, Halwig JM, Patterson R, Wallemark CB. Emergency administration of radiocontrast media in high-risk patients. *J Allergy Clin Immunol.* 1986;77(4):630–634.

Greenberger PA, Patterson R, Radin RC. Two pretreatment regimens for high-risk patients receiving radiographic contrast media. *J Allergy Clin Immunol.* 1984;74(4 pt 1):540–543.

CHAPTER 107

Basic Chest Radiography (CXR)

Francine L. Jacobson, MD, MPH
Sylvia C. McKean, MD, SFHM, FACP

Key Clinical Questions

1. What are the different types of plain chest radiographs and when would you order them?
2. What are the limitations of the anteroposterior (AP) film?
3. How does the chest radiography differentiate between different types of pneumonia from atelectasis?
4. What are the radiographic changes you should look for when considering acute, potentially life-threatening causes of chest pain?
5. What radiographic abnormalities require follow-up?

INTRODUCTION

Chest radiographs provide a snapshot of the patient's physiologic health and insights into a wide variety of systemic diseases. This chapter, as well as Chapter 108 on advanced chest imaging, provide the clinician with a systematic framework for ordering, interpreting films and reports, and consulting the expertise of radiologists.

The majority of hospitalized patients routinely have chest radiographs on admission or prior to surgery; they are also obtained to evaluate acute signs and symptoms, and to assess the possibility of a complication following a procedure. Chest X-rays are also used to monitor critical illness in the intensive care unit (ICU), response to therapy as in congestive heart failure or pneumonia, and stability of pulmonary nodules. Clinicians should always provide radiologists with sufficient information to interpret a radiograph in the clinical context of the patient. Otherwise, the radiologist may generate a wide differential diagnosis that may lead to unnecessary additional imaging or overlook subtle signs of infection in an immune compromised host. Consideration of chest radiographic findings that support the new diagnosis of a systemic disease almost always benefits from direct consultation with the radiologist; a study requisition does not allow an interchange of specific clinical information that can alert the radiologist to findings that might otherwise be ignored. **Figures 107-1** and **107-2** show the normal structures that contribute to the radiographic appearance of the chest.

PRACTICE POINT

Baseline radiographs

- When looking at radiographs without a radiologist, comparison with prior radiographs that look like the current examination can be most helpful. This is analogous to comparing a current ECG to a baseline ECG in a patient with possible cardiac ischemia.
- The degree of inspiration affects the appearance of the lower zone vessels. Hesitate to diagnose basilar pneumonia or cardiomegaly if the radiograph has the domes of the diaphragms at the posterior end of seventh ribs or higher.

The clinician can minimize unnecessary test ordering and delays in diagnosis by recognizing the indications for different types of radiographs and their limitations. The interpretation of any radiographic test begins with assessing the adequacy and technical quality of the film(s) in view. The degree of inspiration affects the appearance of the lower-zone vessels that seem more prominent with poor inspiration. The right hemidiaphragm should reach the anterior end of the right sixth or seventh rib or the posterior end of the ninth rib on full inspiration. Then the examiner should carefully inspect the heart, lungs, mediastinum, and chest wall and, whenever possible, compare the current radiograph with prior images. The bones should be examined for fracture and metastatic disease. Rib fractures in particular may indicate more severe pulmonary injury than is readily apparent from the plain film. Although the standard chest radiograph may provide information about the overall health of the bones, special views should be obtained to properly assess the thoracic spine and shoulder joints in cases of trauma or infection. **Table 107-1** summarizes the different types of chest projections, indications, and technical considerations. Although a posteroanterior

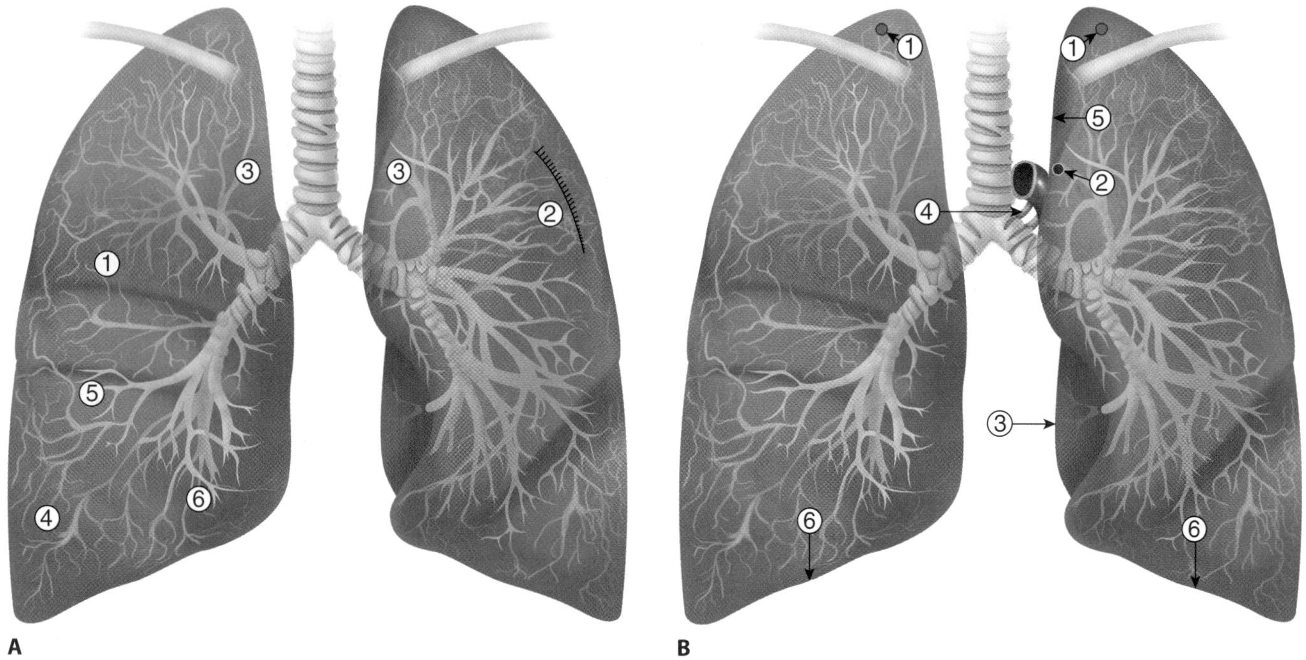

Figure 107-1 *(A) Normal chest radiograph anatomic schematic drawing of fissures on PA radiograph. 1, minor fissure; 2–4, major fissure; 5, superior accessory fissure; 6, inferior accessory fissure. (B) Normal chest radiograph anatomy schematic drawing of structures on PA radiograph 1, normal apical opacity; 2, aortic nipple; 3, descending aortic interface; 4, air in esophagus; 5, aortic pulmonary stripe; 6, diaphragm.*

(PA) radiograph provides more information than an anteroposterior (AP) projection, the patient must be able to cooperate and be clinically stable in order to be transported to another area in the hospital for acquisition. Due to magnification based on distance from the image data collector or film, the heart will appear larger on bedside AP chest radiographs and also in obese individuals. Hence, an AP image may suggest heart failure (upper lobe diversion, cardiomegaly, wide mediastinum, and high hemidiaphragms) in patients without fluid overload and significant pulmonary pathology may not be obscured. An AP film is also more likely to miss a small pneumothorax due to anterior collection of air, and diffuse shadowing may signify either poor inspiration or a posterior pleural effusion. Therefore, a PA radiograph may be required for more definitive diagnosis and is the preferred initial study.

The examiner should also routinely check for the presence and position of any invasive medical equipment such as central lines, feeding tubes, or endotracheal tubes (**Table 107-2** and **Figure 107-3**).

CHEST RADIOGRAPHIC TERMINOLOGY

The Fleischner Society Lexicon (Tuddenham, 1984) is the standard reference resource for chest radiographic terminology (**Table 107-3**). The term opacity is used to describe the addition of substances to lungs that results in lighter gray to white appearance of normally dark gray lungs. The term density is not used because density is a photographic term for increasing blackness in the image.

THE HEART

The simplest measurement of the cardiac silhouette, the transverse diameter of the heart, compares the measurements of the widest width of the heart with the widest width of the thorax on standard PA chest radiographs. Cardiomegaly is a nonspecific finding in fluid overload states. The heart may enlarge from baseline without meeting criteria for cardiomegaly, be normal in the setting of acute lung injury, or enlarged for other reasons. Viewing images with prior plain films provides a more reliable assessment of the presence of cardiomegaly due to a wide range of normal and abnormal heart sizes. An important sign of a possible pericardial effusion, separation of epicardial and pericardial fat, should prompt comparison with prior films to determine if there has been rapid enlargement and development of a globular configuration. A characteristic cardiac contour may suggest left ventricular enlargement, but right ventricular enlargement will, for the most part, be indistinguishable from right ventricular displacement in an enlarged heart. It takes at least two years of untreated hypertension to result in a hypertensive cardiovascular silhouette with ectasia of the aorta and more horizontal axis of the heart on PA chest radiograph. For patients with "labile" hypertension, the presence of target end organ damage would be an indication for treatment. Calcification and a change in contour may suggest left ventricular aneurysm, and bulging of the lower third of the left cardiac border may signify aortic valve disease. Prominence of left heart boarder or posterior enlargement of the left atrium may suggest the possibility of mitral stenosis.

PRACTICE POINT

Pericarditis

Compare current chest radiograph with prior chest radiographs to determine if there is

- A new separation of epicardial and pericardial fat
- Oligemic appearance of lungs

Anatomic landmarks within the heart are only identified if they are calcified or associated with radiopaque markers, such as coronary stents, prosthetic valves, and closure devices for patent foramen ovale (PFO).

THE LUNGS

Forty percent of the lung area and 25% of the lung volume may be obscured by the heart and mediastinum on a PA or AP chest radiograph. Both lungs should be equal in size. Fissures should

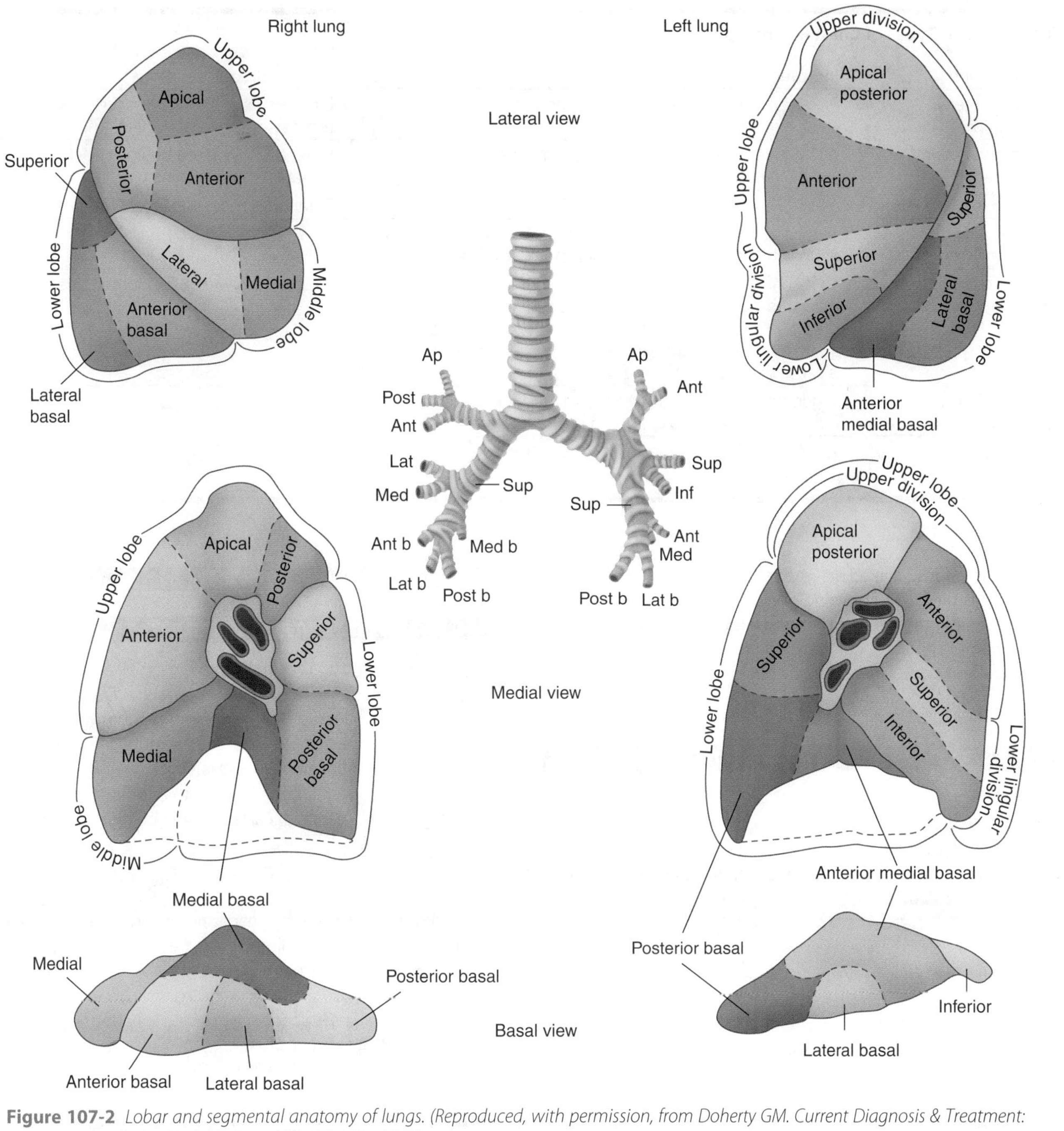

Figure 107-2 *Lobar and segmental anatomy of lungs. (Reproduced, with permission, from Doherty GM. Current Diagnosis & Treatment: Surgery. 13th ed. New York: McGraw-Hill, 2010. Fig. 18-7.)*

not be wider than hairline. The outline of the hemidiaphragms is usually smooth, arcuate, with the highest point medial to the midline of the hemithorax. Normally, airways are invisible unless they are abnormally thickened or pass through an area of consolidation. Consolidation is the hallmark of airspace disease. Air bronchograms are seen on projection radiographs as lucent tubular branching structures within a larger opacity produced by confluent filling of airspaces by fluid and other substances (Figure 107-3). Volume loss in the region may also contribute to the opacity.

Some terms suggest a broad differential diagnosis that can be considerably narrowed by the clinical context. Large irregular opacities may result from consolidation, lobar collapse, carcinoma, pleural abnormalities, or chest wall lesions. Single or multiple nodular opacities may reflect malignant causes (primary bronchogenic carcinoma, solitary or multiple metastasis) and benign causes (granulomas, atriovenous malformations (AVMs), intrapulmonary bronchogenic cysts, bronchial atresia, and traumatic hematomas. Collapse is often reserved for lobar collapse but by definition, atelectasis is correct at all levels whether a subsegment, segment, lobe or complete atelectasis of the entire lung. The differential diagnosis for collapse is most importantly an obstructing lesion -endobronchial tumor can be lung cancer (including carcinoid that has recently been reclassified as a flavor of lung cancer); endobronchial metastasis (particularly breast, GI tract and renal cell carcinoma); foreign bodies (for example, a peanut); and secretions as mucoid impaction (particularly important in an intubated patient). Pneumonia can occur with collapse related to secretions and particular pneumonias may be more likely to be associated with atelectasis—especially aspiration pneumonia. Atelectasis commonly occurs in the postoperative setting due to low lung volumes. In babies, atelectasis can also reflect decreased

TABLE 107-1 Types of Chest Radiographs

Type of Film	Indications	Technical Considerations
Posteroanterior radiograph	Preferred image unless patient unstable to evaluate acute signs and symptoms of the chest	Patient stands with anterior chest against film cassette; exposure is full inspiration.
Anteroposterior radiograph	Alternative to PA chest for unstable patients	Film cassette placed behind patient, portable X-ray machine used. Rotation is more likely than with a PA film.
Lateral view	To localize an abnormality seen in another view; to identify abnormalities obscured by the heart or costophrenic recess	
Lateral decubitus view	To identify a small pleural effusion or to distinguish from pleural thickening; to determine if raised hemidiaphragm due to subpulmonary hemothorax; to confirm clinical impression that pectus excavatum with depressed sternum is cause of unusual cardiac contour or cardiomegaly	Patient lying with his abnormal side down
PA inspiration-expiration views	To identify pneumothorax; expiration to identify inhaled foreign body when gas trapping is evident	
Apical lordotic views	To examine the lung apex usually obscured by clavicle and upper ribs	

surfactant—unusual in adults. Radiographic clues to the presence of atelectasis include: crowding of airways and vessels within the lobe, crowding of ribs shift of mediastinum and other structures, raised hemidiaphragm, compensatory hyperexpansion of ipsilateral lobe and contralateral lung. Additional terms are presented in Table 107-3.

PRACTICE POINT

- Acute airspace disease = water, pus, blood.
- Bilateral symmetric disease favors water. Focal air space disease favors pneumonia.
- Bilateral asymmetric and sparing of periphery are associated with hemorrhage.

Normally, blood vessels should be much more apparent in the lower lung zones than in the upper lung zones. Lines seen within 2 cm of the chest wall probably represent interstitial abnormalities such as edema, fibrosis, or metastatic disease.

THE MEDIASTINUM

PRACTICE POINT

Mediastinal contour anormalities

- Lymphoma: Typically a lobulated anterior mediastinal mass that most likely represents matted lymph nodes with associated mediastinal lymph nodes. Lymphadenopathy can also occur in sarcoidosis and infection.
- Thymoma: More focal and unilateral than lymphoma, not associated with paratracheal lymphadenopathy, seen in older patients.
- Germ cell tumor: Characteristic fat and calcification particularly in young patient.
- Metastatic disease: Middle mediastinum more likely to be involved by metastatic disease from testicular germ cell tumors, renal cell carcinoma, or melanoma.
- Vascular congenital anomaly or in a patient who has had cardiac surgery pseudoaneurysm at bypass pump cannulation site.

TABLE 107-2 Support Lines

Support Device	Optimum Placement	Proximal Limit	Distal Limit	Common Malposition
Endotracheal tube	Middle of intrathoracic trachea	Tip even with top of clavicle	Tip 2 cm from carina	Tip in right mainstem bronchus
Central venous catheter	Superior vena cava	Brachiocephalic vein	Cavoatrial junction	Right atrium; interrior vena cava; azygous vein following arch posteriorly; internal mammary vein with slight lateral direction; persistent left superior vena cava can be acceptable depending on vessel size
Peripherally inserted central catheter	Depends on use; localization will change with arm position	Arm for long term peripheral access	Cavoatrial junction	Visiting Nurse Association (VNA) service may require superior vena cava
Swan-Ganz catheter	Right or left main pulmonary artery	Right ventricle	Interlobar descending pulmonary artery	Distal placement only when wedged
Nasogastric tube	Stomach			Side vent marker needs to be distal to gastroesophogeal junction

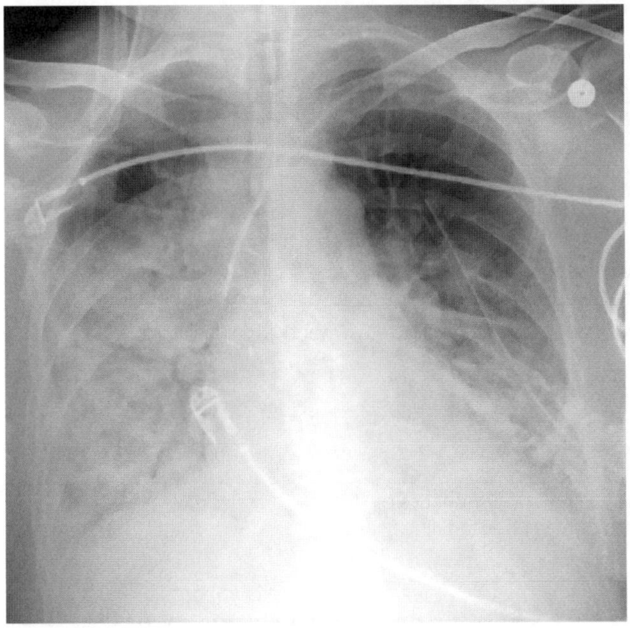

Figure 107-3 *ICU patient with dense consolidation and air bronchograms well seen in right lung base corresponding with pneumonia. Support lines include endotracheal tube, left subclavian central venous catheter and left chest tube placed for pneumothorax that may be due to line placement or barotrauma in setting of multi-organ system failure with injury pulmonary edema present.*

ANATOMY

The mediastinum is divided into radiographic compartments that differ somewhat from the anatomic divisions of the mediastinum.

1. The anterior mediastinum includes the retrosternal clear space seen on lateral chest radiograph. Radiologists may use either the anterior surface of the aorta or the anterior wall of the trachea as the posterior boundary of this compartment.
2. The middle mediastinum extends from this boundary to 1 cm behind the anterior surface of the vertebral bodies on the lateral view.
3. The posterior mediastinum extends posteriorly from the middle mediastinum to the posterior chest wall. The structures in this region all lie posterior to the mediastinum.

Although not a compartment, it is sometimes useful to apply the term superior mediastinum to the region above the aortic arch. The vascular pedicle can be clinically important, especially in the setting of congestive heart failure. It is assessed on the frontal view with greater magnification expected on bedside anteroposterior radiographs than standard posteroanterior radiographs. Distention of the azygous vein to greater than 11 mm in diameter along right side of trachea just above bifurcation signifies pulmonary vascular engorgement.

The hila are often considered with the mediastinal structures. The border-forming structures are the pulmonary arteries. The left pulmonary artery is approximately 2 cm higher than the right pulmonary artery. This slope is sometimes referred to as the hilar angle. It may be altered as in the case of right upper lobe volume loss

TABLE 107-3 Glossary of Terms

Descriptive Term	Differential Diagnosis
Infiltrate pathologic term often used clinically but not radiographically)	A relatively acute development of a diffuse process that includes little if any consolidation, corresponds with acute interstitial pneumonia (AIP), injury pulmonary edema, corresponding to clinical diagnosis of adult respiratory distress syndrome (ARDS)
Solitary pulmonary nodule • Typically homogeneous parenchymal lesion with sharply defined margins, ≤ 3 cm • Usually standard chest radiograph will not detect nodules < 1 cm • Nodules between 1 and 2 cm in size may be missed due to overlapping bones or vascular structures	Malignant nodules • Primary bronchogenic carcinoma • Solitary metastasis • Clues to origin: ▪ Smoker, past medical history (PMH) of head & neck cancer (lung) ▪ PMH extrathoracic cancer (metastasis from original site) Benign Diseases • Benign tumors ▪ Hamartomas, bronchial adenomas • Nonneoplastic processes ▪ Granulomas, intrapulmonary bronchogenic cysts, bronchial atresia, traumatic hematomas, AVMs • Clues to benign (as opposed to malignant) ▪ Calcification in a typical benign pattern ▪ No growth on serial chest radiograph over 2-year period ▪ Nonsmoker < 35 years old
Atelectasis • Decreases lung volume, at any level of lung organization • May be associated with other signs of volume loss in the hemithorax (ipsilateral shift of the mediastinum, decreased spacing of ribs and elevation of the diaphragm). • Collapse refers to complete lung atelectasis. • Subsegmental and segmental atelectasis refer to discoid or plate-like atelectasis based on projection	Pneumonia, pulmonary embolism, and abdominal fluid or pain that causes splinting. Mucoid impaction at the level of any bronchus, leading to collapse patterns that are specific for each lobe. In the case of the bronchus intermedius, atelectasis may involve both the right middle and right lower lobes. • Atelectasis of both right middle and lower lobes (bronchus intermedius) • Irregular bands of atelectasis (adhesion of airways possibly related to mucus) Low lung volumes and expiration (focal atelectasis)

(continued)

TABLE 107-3 Glossary of Terms (*continued*)

Descriptive Term	Differential Diagnosis
Kerley A lines • Longer (at least 2 cm) unbranching lines coursing diagonally from the periphery toward the hila in the inner half of the lungs • Never seen without Kerley B or C lines also present.	Distension of anastomotic channels between peripheral and central lymphatics of the lungs.
Kerley B lines • Short (< 2 cm long), straight, horizontal parallel lines (< 1 mm thick) at the lung periphery that end at right angles against the pleura • Generally absent along fissural surfaces in any zone but most frequently observed at the lung bases at the costophrenic angles on the PA radiograph, and in the substernal region on lateral radiographs	Fluid in interlobular septa, or dilated lymphatic channels visible with elevation of the pulmonary capillary wedge pressure (usually 25 mm Hg or higher). Associated with congestive heart failure (CHF) and interstitial lung diseases (ILD).
Kerley C lines • Short, fine lines throughout the lungs, with a reticular appearance • Least common of Kerley lines	Thickening of anastomotic lymphatics or superimposition of many Kerley B lines.

elevating the right hilum. The direction of the right and left central pulmonary artery differs resulting in expected mild asymmetry. The upper limit of normal currently used on CT scans for the main pulmonary artery is 24 mm with borderline to 29 mm. The upper limit of the normal range in size of the right interlobar descending pulmonary artery most easily measured on chest radiographs is 16 mm for a man and 14 mm for a woman. Increased intravascular pressure can be temporary as in the case of pulmonary edema or long-standing as in the case of pulmonary artery hypertension.

MEDIASTINAL MASSES

A mediastinal mass in the anterior mediastinum may be a thyroid mass (continuous with the thyroid gland causing deviation of the trachea), a thymoma or thymic cyst (typically marginated and sometimes lobulated), lymphoma and small-cell lung cancer (which may involve multiple lymph note groups), or a germ cell tumor (sometimes evidenced by fat, hair, and teeth). Middle mediastinal masses include tumors involving the esophagus, thyroid, and lymph nodes, duplication cysts including bronchogenic cysts (most frequently at the bifurcation of trachea and central airways, sometimes paraesophageal or intraparenchymal), lymphadenopathy, pericardial cysts (characteristically adjacent to the heart, especially in the cardiophrenic sulcus and smoothly marginated), intrathoracic goiter (with heterogeneous tissue), tracheal tumors, and vascular variants. Posterior mediastinal masses may represent neurogenic tumors and extramedullary hematopoiesis, esophageal abnormalities, and neurogenetic tumors.

HILAR ADENOPATHY

In an otherwise healthy adult, bilateral, noncalcified hilar adenopathy suggests sarcoid. In a patient with a prior history of malignancy, the presumption has to be malignancy. Most common malignancies that cause hilar adenopathy include bronchogenic carcinoma, lymphoma, bronchial carcinoid, and extrathoracic primary tumors metastasizing to the chest. Nonmalignant causes include pulmonary arterial or venous dilation or tortuosity, cysts, granulomatous adenopathy, and benign tumors. Reactive and malignant adenopathy may be radiographically indistinguishable unless there is obvious calcification. Vascular abnormalities are often asymmetric and can simulate adenopathy. The first step is to compare with prior films. Consultation with a radiologist and serial review of images will facilitate differentiation of hilar lymphadepathy from pulmonary artery enlargement.

MEDIASTINAL SHIFT

Since whole lung atelectasis and pleural effusion can both cause complete whiteout of a hemithorax, it can be most important to observe the direction of mediastinal shift. When the lung collapses, the shift will be toward the opaque hemithorax. Pleural effusion on the other hand occupies space and can cause contralateral shift of the mediastinum. Since both can be present at the same time, it is possible for the mediastinum to be midline with balanced volume loss due to atelectasis and pleural effusion. A low diaphragm will cause a right shift of the mediastinum, and a high diaphragm will cause a left shift.

FLUID OVERLOAD

Fluid overload, whether an initial presentation or an iatrogenic complication of hospitalization, typically has characteristic radiographic signs that can be correlated with the severity of the process. Early changes include minimal cardiomegaly and equalization of flow to upper and lower zones corresponding to pulmonary capillary wedge pressure of 15–25 mm Hg. The diameter of the upper lobe vessels is less than or equal to the lower lobe vessels at the same distance from the hilum, and pulmonary vessels in the first intercostal space are greater than 3 cm. As congestive heart failure (CHF) worsens, Kerley B lines are present at the basal aspects of the lung. These cannot be blood vessels because vessels are not normally seen as lung markings in the peripheral quarter of the lungs. Frank pulmonary edema (fluid accumulation in the alveolar spaces) becomes evident radiographically when bilateral, predominantly basilar and perihilar alveolar infiltrates are seen, and vessels near the hila become indistinct due to interstitial fluid accumulation.

It is important to remember the limitations of the chest X-ray. Poor inspiration (less than the 7th rib) make the lower zone vessels appear more prominent. Patients with severe parenchymal lung disease may have atypical radiographic changes for edema. The AP chest film may be misleading regarding cephalization and heart size.

Pulmonary edema may occur under special circumstances. Up to one-third of opiate overdoses develop pulmonary edema.

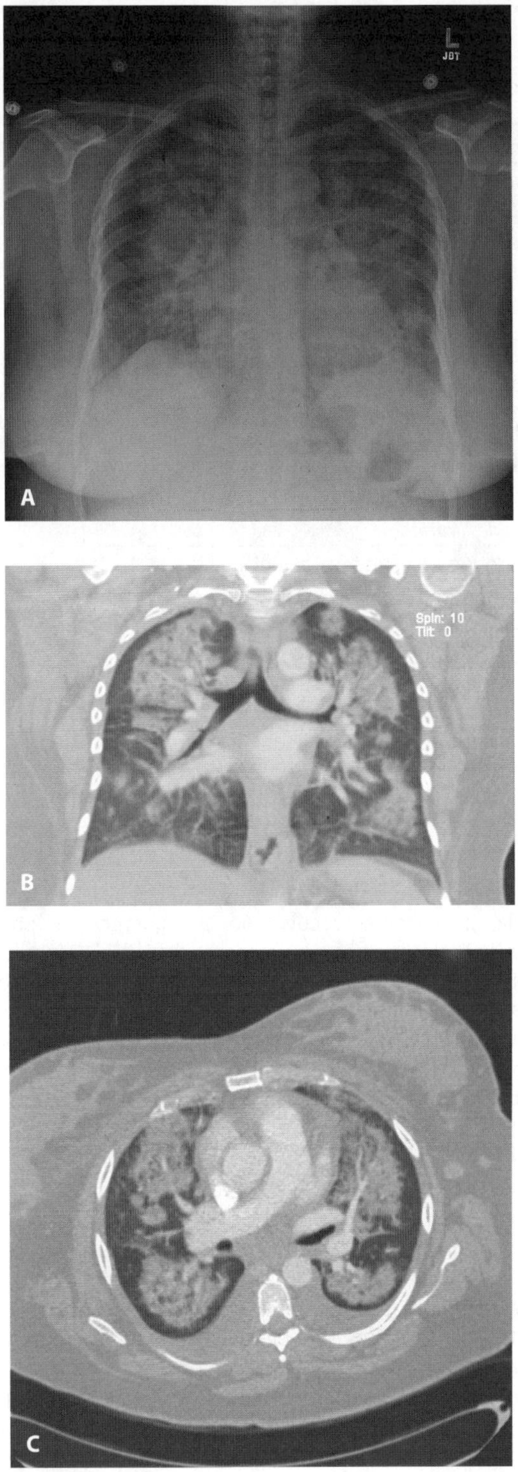

Figure 107-4 *(A) Perihilar airspace opacities are consistent with noncardiogenic pulmonary edema. Note sparing of lung bases and normal size of heart. (B) Coronal chest CT in the same patient with pulmonary edema. (C) Axial chest CT.*

Pulmonary edema due to inhaled or intravenous opiate abuse or inhalation of solvents or "crack" cocaine may have permeability edema with normal cardiomediastinal silhouette. Rapid clearing of edema is typical and pneumomediastinum or pneumothorax is occasionally associated.

Figure 107-4 demonstrates fluid overload. A chest X-ray was obtained to evaluate dyspnea in a postpartum patient who had received 5 liters of fluid resuscitation during delivery. The requisition order provided minimal clinical information—acute shortness of breath. The radiology report raised the possibility of pulmonary hemorrhage in addition to fluid overload. Despite no risk factors for pulmonary hemorrhage, on the same day this patient had an unnecessary computed tomography (CT) scan of the chest. It confirmed what was readily apparent from her physical examination (clear evidence of fluid overload). Pulmonary hemorrhage may produce similar acute radiographic signs but the patient should have risk factors for pulmonary hemorrhage, should not be have signs of fluid overload on exam, and the changes would resolve over a few days into a coarse interstitial pattern. Iatrogenic acute fluid overload would be expected to resolve very quickly with appropriate treatment.

PRACTICE POINT

Radiographic criteria of pulmonary edema
- Any fissure wider than hairline

Pulmonary vascular redistribution
- Cephalization in upright patient
- Lateralization in dependent lung of patient lying primarily on one side
- Equalization when neither upper or lower lobe vessels predominate
- Perihilar "bat-wing" pulmonary edema
- Kerley B lines in lower zones

Enlargement of hilar pulmonary vessels
- Cardiomegaly a nonspecific and not invariably present radiographic finding.

PNEUMONIA

The diagnosis of pneumonia hinges on the chest radiograph. It is mandatory for patients suspected of pneumonia, for acutely ill patients with new respiratory complaints or hypoxia, for patients with a exacerbation of chronic obstructive pulmonary disease (COPD), for immunocompromised patients with fever, and for elderly patients with confusion.

The diagnosis of pneumonia can only be made through radiographic imaging, but a chest film cannot definitively identify the causative pathogen or rule out noninfectious causes (**Table 107-4**). Clinical pneumonia in the immune-compromised host can present with a normal chest radiograph, as classically seen with *Pneumocystis jiroveci* (formerly PCP). Unlike a normal host, patients with neutropenic fever may have only subsegmental atelectasis or focal peribronchial thickening in the presence of a bacterial infection. Hence, with the knowledge of the patient's immune status and exposure history the radiologist will lower the threshold for detection of subtle abnormalities and compare with a baseline study whenever possible.

A patient who is dehydrated will have decreased pulmonary vessel sizes with resulting overall decrease in vascularity on chest radiography. After rehydration signs of pneumonia may "bloom."

ASPIRATION PNEUMONIA

Inhaled food is usually translucent, but if the inhalation has occurred some time previously, there may be segmental or lobar collapse. It is also possible for as little as 25 mm of sterile gastric contents to be aspirated more widely, resulting in Mendelson syndrome with visual appearance on chest radiograph that may be indistinguishable from pulmonary edema, although

TABLE 107-4 Typical Pneumonia Patterns

Multilobar pneumonia	*S pneumoniae* and *L pneumophilia* more common
Bilateral diffuse pulmonary infiltrates in a immunocompetent patient	More likely due to congestive heart failure or inhalation of a toxin or allergen than to a pneumonia caused by an atypical pneumonia
Community-acquired pneumonia due to methicillin-reistant staphylococcus aureus	Often bilateral cavitary lesions
Aspiration pneumonia	In a supine patient: left lower lobe (LLL) due to more posteriorly directed left mainstem bronchus Time course: More homogeneous consolidation within two days of aspiration • Necrotizing pneumonia (gram-negative and anaerobic organisms) • Cavities sometimes becoming thick walled over a period of a few weeks, thereby mimicking tuberculosis (TB). Unlike TB, lymphadenopathy is uncommonly associated.
Cavitary lesions	*S aureus*, *Pseudomonas*; TB; *Aspergillus* infections (pulmonary infarct picture) Mixed flora including anaerobes, aspiration (along with empyema) *Klebsiella* (may have a bulging fissure sign), *E coli* Thin-walled cavities: *Coccidioides immitis*
Mass-like lesions	Acute histoplasmosis: Hilar adenopathy and focal alveolar infiltrates Disseminating form: Multiple nodules and hilar adenopathy Blastomycosis: Mass-like opacities

pulmonary vasculature is unlikely to be engorged by this process. Gravity directs the location, and underlying bronchiectasis may increase the likelihood of developing active infection. Patient position at the time of aspiration may lead to logical patterns besides the classically described pattern, involving the superior segments of the lower lobes and posterior bacillar segments of the lower lobes.

FUNGAL PNEUMONIA

Fungal infections in healthy individuals are most frequently due to endemic species in particular locations. Travel history can be vital to the radiologist in identifying the likely organism and decreasing the number of serologic tests required to confirm the specific diagnosis. The size, number of nodules, and associated findings, including more chronic calcification from reactivation of prior infection, may help distinguish histoplasmosis from coccidiomycosis. Small, numerous nodules associated with mediastinitis (evidenced by linear calcifications), large calcified lymph nodes, and tiny calcifications in the spleen suggest an infection with histoplasmosis. The largest calcified lymph nodes, often referred to as histoplasmomas, may, for technical radiologic reasons, not appear calcified on standard chest radiographs with the high kilovolt techniques that decrease conspicuity of bones. Fewer large nodules with associated adjacent pleural thickening suggest coccidiomycosis.

PRACTICE POINT

Radiographic signs of pneumonia

- Consolidation from pneumonia may maintain, increase, or decrease the volume of the affected lung with air bronchograms present.
- Atelectasis, irregular aeration, peribronchial thickening and interstitial prominence may characterize more subtle pulmonary infections.
- Reactive lymphadenopathy is most common in ipsilateral hilum.
- Infection and infarction can have identical appearances on imaging studies.

Actinomycosis is the most frequent pneumonia to extend through the chest wall, characterized by suppurative and granulomatous inflammation that can lead to abscess formation and even sinus tracts through the skin that may be found on physical examination.

VARICELLA PNEUMONIA

Varicella pneumonia occurs most frequently in pregnant women. Varicella pneumonia presents as diffuse, 5–10 mm nodular opacities that are poorly defined and may coalesce as the nodules increase in size. Although hilar lymph nodes may enlarge, they do not usually calcify. Healing can result in small calcific opacities throughout the lungs that are smaller in size and less uniform than that observed with prior histoplasmosis (**Table 107-5**).

TUBERCULOSIS (TB)

The hematogenous spread of primary TB infection is radiographically inapparent in normal hosts. Miliary TB can be associated with primary progressive and reactivation of TB, particularly in immune compromised patients. The visualization of micronodules on radiographs represents superimposition of multiple such shadows most likely seen at lung bases. Late presentation of miliary TB may result in greater visibility of nodules in lung apices due to the oxygen rich environment favored by TB. Postprimary TB initially images as heterogeneous, poorly marginated opacities in the apical or posterior segments of the upper lobes or in the superior segments of the lower lobes; and later forms reticular and nodular opacities. Cavitation typically occurs within an area of consolidation and may result in endobronchial spread. Scarring, atelectasis, traction bronchiectasis, nodules, and calcification characterize healing. The presence of back or neck pain should be communicated to the radiologist to insure maximal study of the spine for osteomyelitis. The most frequently visible sign of Potts Disease is verge rum planum representing complete collapse of the affected vertebral body.

PULMONARY DISEASES

SCATTERED OPACITIES

Usual interstitial pneumonia (UIP), rheumatoid lung, scleroderma lung, chronic hypersensitivity pneumonitis, asbestosis, and pulmonary drug toxicity may all produce similar radiographic

TABLE 107-5 Classic Presentations of Pneumonia

Organism	Primary Finding	Secondary Findings	Evolution
Strep pneumoniae	Consolidation with air bronchograms that begins at the periphery and spreads to involve the entire segment or lobe; less likely with early appropriate treatment	Small pleural effusion (50%) Possible hilar adenopathy; air bronchograms Cavitation unusual for most serotypes but lymphadenopathy rare	Transient round pneumonia 24–48 hours, progresses to lobar consolidation, resolves by fading slowly
Mycoplasma pneumoniae	Bronchial wall thickening	May have focal opacities Nonspecific findings	Subtle persistent symptoms more prominent than radiographic findings
Legionella pneumophila	A focal homogeneous opacity that may mimic a tumor followed by rapid progression to bilateral parenchymal involvement with associated pleural effusions without evidence of lymphadenopathy	Sharply demarcated peribronchovascular opacity. Cavity formation may occur in immunocompramised patients but is uncommon in normal hosts.	Bilateral asymmetric opacities may range from ground-glass to dense consolidation.
Staph aureus *Klebsiella pneumoniae* *Pseudomans aeruginosa*	Consolidation with cavitation	Reactive lymphadenopathy May have sympathetic effusion	*Staph* may develop thin-walled cyst called a pneumatocele. *Klebsiella* may appear as enlarged, consolidated lobe
Pneumocystis (carinii) jiroveci	Diffuse bilateral, fine to medium reticulonodular subtle opacities that could easily be overlooked. Chest radiograph may be normal (10%).	Pneumatoceles (10%) Pneumothoraces (5–6%) No pleural effusion	Insidious can lead to consolidation.
Aspergillus	Nodular opacities with ground-glass halo	May be solitary or multiple May also have consolidation	Solid opacity that cavitates
Mucormycosis (Zygomycetes)	Nodular opacity with ground-glass center	May be solitary or multiple	Evolves as infarction
Mycobacterium avium-intracellulare (MAI) and mycobacterium avium-complex (MAC)	Bronchiectasis with tree-in-bud opacities	Lymphadenopathy may be present.	Chronic colonization may not progress without treatment.
M Tuberculosis			
Primary infection	Unilateral hilar lymphadenopathy and ipsilateral pleural effusion	Ipsilateral mediastinal lymphadenopathy Consolidation may be radiographically absent.	Develop Ghon complex with granulomas that calcify within two years.
	Miliary opacities of hematogenous TB become visible.	Lymphadenopathy and pleural effusion may be present or absent.	Primary progressive TB
Reactivation TB	Bronchiectasis and cavity particularly in upper lobe	Upper lobe volume loss	Development of new opacities

abnormalities. Typically, UIP shows a pattern of bibasilar irregular linear opacities, which on high-resolution CT appear as ground-glass opacities, traction bronchiectasis, and honeycomb cysts in the periphery without associated adenopathy or pleural effusions. The presence of rheumatoid nodules and pleural effusion may help to radiographically distinguish rheumatoid lung from UIP. Small nodules or an upper lobe predominance may suggest chronic hypersensitivity pneumonitis. Pleural effusion or pleural plaques are a clue to the diagnosis of asbestosis. Pulmonary drug toxicity (amiodarone, bleomycin, methotrexate, nitrofurantoin) may also produce fibrosis (honeycomb cysts, architectural distortion, traction bronchiectasis).

Bronchiolitis obliterans (BO) typically appears as scattered air space consolidations (or as ground-glass opacities and consolidations without evidence of fibrosis on CT) in a peripheral and subpleural distribution with slightly reduced lung volumes. Bronchial wall thickening or bronchiectasis is commonly present. BO may have associated pleural effusions, nodules, or irregular linear opacities in a smaller number of patients. When parenchymal opacities are present, it is considered part of cryptogenic organizing pneumonia (COP, formerly BOOP). Pulmonary lymphoma and multifocal bronchioalveolar carcinoma may have a similar radiologic appearance to COP on plain imaging.

Eosinophilic pneumonia from alveolar and interstitial infiltration by eosinophils and other inflammatory cells classically has peripheral and upper lobe opacities. The classic "reverse pulmonary edema" occurs in less than 50% of cases. Etiologies include pulmonary vasculitis (Churg-Strauss syndrome), allergic bronchopulmonary aspergillosis (ABPA), and drug reactions.

EMPHYSEMA

Panlobular emphysema typically has regional or generalized decreased lung attenuation preferentially affecting the lung bases. Initially, centrilobular emphysema preferentially affects the apices as 2–10 mm lucencies without walls that later form large regions of decreased lung attenuation.

BRONCHIECTASIS

Parallel lines (tram tracks), ring shadows, and mucus plugs are characteristic images of bronchiectasis. Basilar bronchiectasis may result from viral pneumonia (such as adenovirus or measles in childhood), repeated aspiration, or prior bronchiectasis. Cystic fibrosis typically involves the upper lobes more than the lower lobes. ABPA may show cylindrical or saccular central, but not peripheral, bronchiectasis and preferentially involves the upper lobes.

SARCOID

Up to 90% of patients will have abnormality on chest radiographs at some time over the course of their illness. Tissue diagnosis showing microscopic noncaseating granulomas present in lungs, even when the radiographic appearance of the chest is normal, establishes the diagnosis. The most classic radiographic presentation includes bilateral symmetric hilar and mediastinal lymphadenopathy, particularly in subcarinal and right paratracheal regions. Differential diagnosis includes lymphoma. Less common, asymmetric hilar lymphadenopathy may result from sarcoid. Metastatic disease, TB, and other infections are unlikely to produce symmetric hilar lymphadenopathy. Irreversible end-stage lung disease seen in stage IV sarcoid has the greatest correlation between imaging findings and symptoms (**Table 107-6**).

TABLE 107-6 Staging of Sarcoidosis

Stage	Findings	Location
0	Normal chest radiograph	
I	Lymphadenopathy	Bilateral hilar, subcarinal, right paratracheal regions
II	Lymphadenopathy and pulmonary parenchymal opacities	Opacities along bronchovascular bundles, particularly in upper lobes Small nodules that may also be seen peripherally
III	Pulmonary parenchymal opacities *without* lymphadenopathy	Peribronchial thickening, small nodules
IV	Honeycombing and traction bronchiectasis	Subpleural fibrosis accompanied by bronchiectasis Lung opacities seen in stages II and III may also be present.
	Alveolar sarcoid (stages II to IV)	Consolidation due to interstitial granulomas filling alveoli.

TABLE 107-7 Interstitial Lung Disease

Cause	Radiographic Finding
Asbestosis (prolonged exposure to asbestosis)	Lower-lung field predominance of infiltrates, pleural calcification, plaques
Silicosis	Hilar egg-shell calcifications
Sarcoidosis	Bilateral symmetrical hilar and paratracheal lymphadenopathy
Lymphagioleiomyomatosis (LAM)	Pneumothorax in a premenopausal woman, chylous effusions

INTERSTITIAL LUNG DISEASE OR DIFFUSE PARENCHYMAL LUNG DISEASE

The interstitium is the potential space between the alveoli and capillaries. Collagen deposition in the interstitium produces a radiographic appearance of diffuse interstitial opacification.

It is difficult and usually unnecessary to work up chronic interstitial lung disease during hospitalization for an unrelated acute illness. Fluid overload states cause pulmonary vascular engorgement from interstitial pulmonary edema producing thickening of interlobular septae on plain imaging. Repeated episodes of interstitial edema can lead to hemosiderin deposition, creating permanent visualization of interlobular septae even without pulmonary vascular engorgement or intrinsic interstitial lung disease. A nodular form of interstitial pulmonary edema may be reported as tiny nodular opacities or micronodules due to superimposed shadows. The clinical context is critical because micronodules may also represent hematogenous dissemination of infection (military TB or other fungal infections) or tumor. Visualization over time may help to avoid unnecessary evaluations for potential cancer. Unless directly related to the reason for admission, postdischarge follow-up after recovery of the acute illness would be advisable. See **Table 107-7** for examples of common radiographic findings that may suggest an underlying chronic disease process or exposure.

PULMONARY NODULES

Admission chest radiographs frequently identify incidental pulmonary nodules. By definition, a lung nodule measures up to 3 cm in diameter while a lung mass measures more than 3 cm in diameter. In clinical practice, these terms are not always used correctly. Doubling in less than 30 days generally indicates benign disease even when a lesion is large. Features of a nodular lesion and accompanying findings help to create a patient-specific differential diagnosis. Miliary TB, for example, may show diffuse 1–3 mm nodules that represent superimposition of micronodules not individualy resolved by radiography. The larger volume of lung in the lung bases usually makes it more apparent in the bases than the apices, although a patient with a late presentation of military TB can have larger, and therefore more easily seen, tiny nodules in the lung apices due to the affinity of TB for the oxygen-enriched apical regions of the lungs.

When one pulmonary nodule is noted, the answer may be "in the jacket" (ie, two years of radiographic stability ensures that the nodule is benign). When multiple pulmonary nodules are present, necessary workup may be limited to explaining a prior infection. Nodules measuring less than 5 mm in diameter that are very well seen on chest radiographs represent sequel of prior infection and require no further workup. Serial radiographs six months apart establish baseline when the patient has a positive PPD associated with scarring.

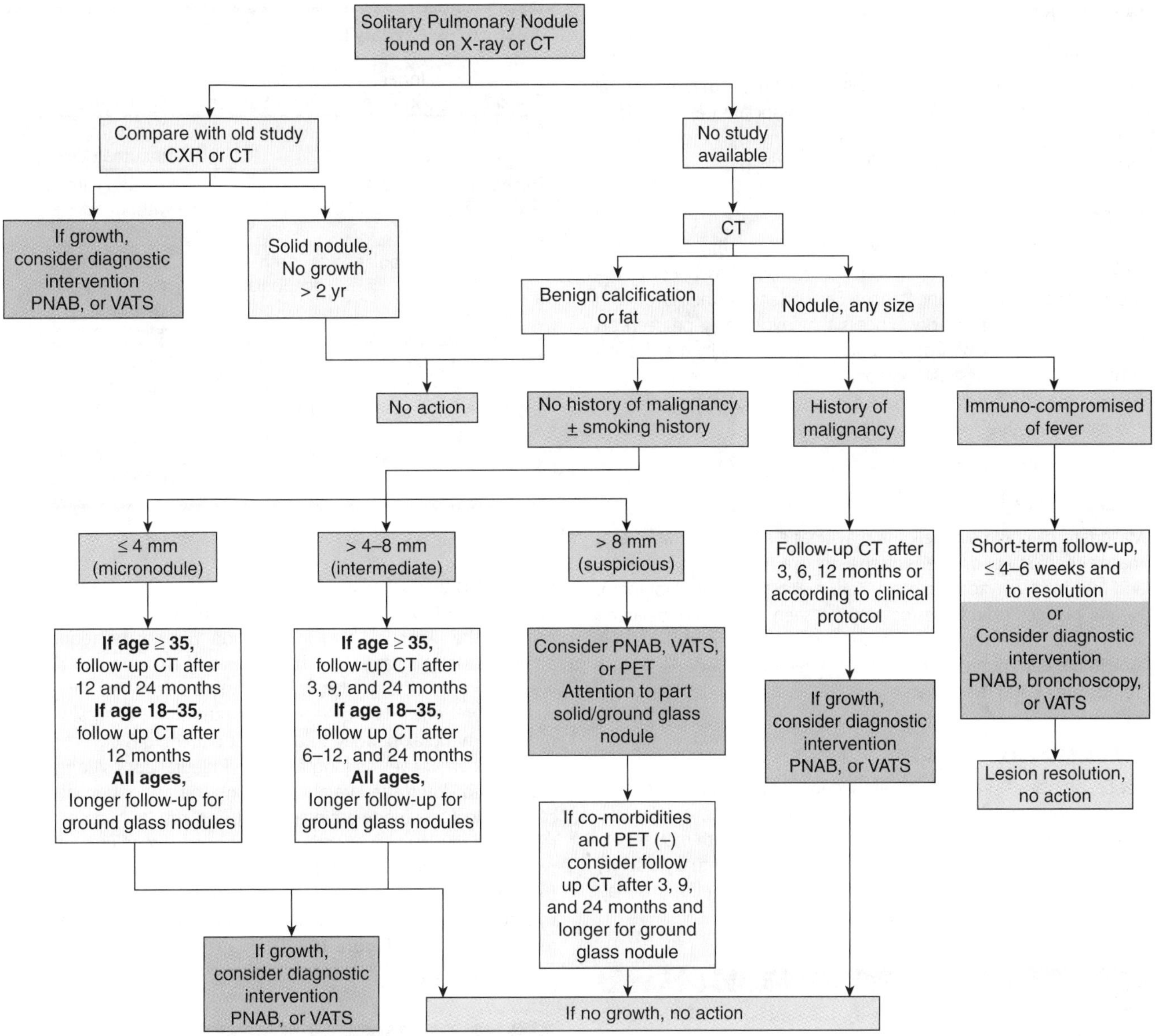

Figure 107-5 *Workup of Solitary Pulmonary Nodule.*

New nodules, nodules that increase in size, or nodules that have worrisome features should be evaluated by CT but not necessarily during the current hospitalization. Acute findings, such as atelectasis, pneumonia, pulmonary edema, and pleural effusions, often obscure important parenchymal findings. It can take two months or more for the appearance of the lung parenchyma following acute pneumonia to reach a new baseline. A plain film at that time may be sufficient to document complete clearing and the absence of an underlying nodule or central lesion causing a postobstructive pneumonia. The probability of cancer increases with the size of the nodule, although the size required for detection on chest radiographs varies with location. The best quality chest CT scan requires the patient to be able to perform the breath-hold maneuvers. **Figure 107-5** provides an algorithm for further evaluation. CT-based evaluation strategy is presented in Chapter 108.

BENIGN TUMORS

Arteriovenous malformation

Typically, atriovenous malformations (AVMs) appear as round, lobulated, well-defined masses ranging in size from less than one to several centimeters in diameter in the medial third of the lung. A chest radiograph may identify the enlarged feeding artery and draining vein, and a change in size may be apparent when erect versus supine radiographs are compared. Feeding vessels leading to the pulmonary nodule are prominent, enlarging rather than tapering along their often tortuous course. Small AVMs may require echocardiographic bubble study for detection. Radiographs may underdiagnose the number of AVMs present. It is therefore important to look for telangiectasias. Osler-Weber-Rendu syndrome is also known as hereditary hemorrhagic telangiectasia (HHT).

Hamartoma

Hamartomas are solitary nodules usually less than 4 cm in diameter located peripherally in 90% of cases and may have a "popcorn-like" appearance due to calcification.

Granuloma

Granulomas form in response to inflammatory processes including TB and sarcoidosis. Radiographic confirmation of calcification, often possible for nodules measuring less than 5 mm in diameter, confirms the benign nature of the nodule.

MALIGNANT TUMORS

Carcinoid

Bronchial carcinoid tumors occur 85% of the time within the central bronchi as hilar masses with or without associated atelectasis or obstructive pneumonia. The other 15% of tumors arise peripherally as solitary, well-circumscribed pulmonary nodules.

Bronchogenic carcinoma

Bronchogenic carcinoma may present as a smoothly marginated or spiculated nodule or mass. Adenocarcinoma has become the most frequent type of lung cancer. Early adenocarcinoma of lung can mimic an inflammatory process that might only be seen on CT scan. Even a very well-defined ground-glass opacity may be too subtle to see on chest radiographs because it does not obscure vessels. Adenocarcinoma in situ (AIS) has replaced bronchioalveolar cell carcinoma (BAC) as the pathologic term for this type of lung cancer.

Pleural tumors

Malignant pleural mesothelioma may image as a unilateral pleural mass, either focal or diffuse, is often associated with pleural effusion, and may locally invade the chest wall, mediastinum, or diaphragm. Pleural plaques from asbestos may be seen on the contralateral side, and are usually larger and more numerous in the mid to lower lung. More commonly encountered pleural tumors include solitary fibrous tumor and metastases.

PULMONARY INFARCT

Septic or bland infarcts, typically wedge-shaped and peripheral, are more numerous in the lung bases. Septic infarcts, usually 1 to 2 cm in diameter, cavitate in about 50% of nodules with moderately thick and irregular walls that decrease in size and eventually resolve, leaving in some cases a peripheral linear scar. Pleural effusions may be associated with septic or bland infarcts.

PULMONARY CAVITIES

When the lesion has a central cavity, the description of the wall is most valuable. The course over time is also helpful. One-third to one-half of Wegener granulomatosis lesions progress from solid nodules to thick-walled cavities, to thin-walled cavities, and finally resolve without necessarily leaving a scar. Ten percent of patients may also develop diffuse pulmonary hemorrhage. An individual patient may have a mixture of these findings at the same time or over time. The presence of a fluid level in a cavity indicates communication with the tracheobronchial tree. It does not necessarily mean the cavity is infected. Cavitation is not always obvious on chest radiographs and superimposition of small and coalescing opacities may simulate a cavity without one being present. CT scanning is most reliable for identification and description of a cavitary lesion. Large cavitary lesions will also be apparent on magnetic resonance imaging (MRI) (**Table 107-8** and **Figure 107-6**).

TABLE 107-8 Cavitary Lesions

Wall Thickness	Inner Surface	Outer Surface	Significance
Thin wall	Smooth	Smooth	Cyst, bulla, pneumatocele
Thick wall	Smooth	Irregular	Abscess with or without adjacent pneumonia
Thick wall	Irregular	Smooth, may be lobulated	Malignant lesion particularly squamous cell carcinoma
Air-crescent	Smooth	Well-defined, may have ground-glass halo	Invasive aspergillosis (occurs in immune-compromised host)

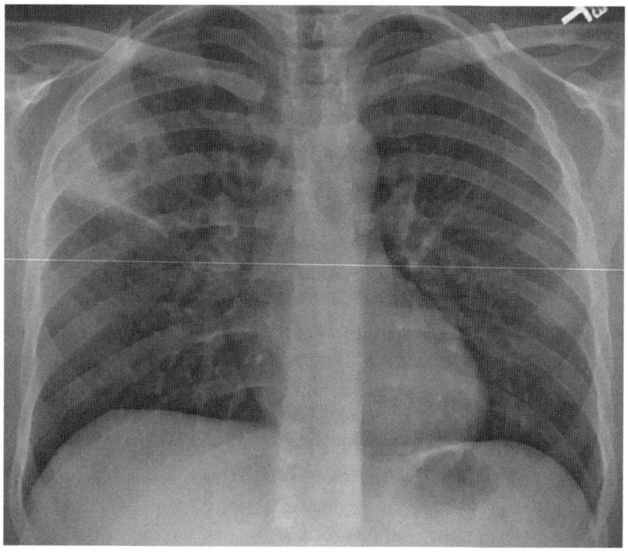

Figure 107-6 *Right upper lobe opacity with volume loss elevating the lateral aspect of the minor fissure contains a large central cavity due to necrosis. Gram negative bacteria, such as Pseudomonas aeruginosa or anaerobic bacteria from oral flora is likely cause of this necrotizing pneumonia that has resulted from aspiration.*

PNEUMOTHORAX

To identify a pneumothorax, first look at the boundary of a pneumothorax, which remains a thin white line parallel to the chest wall, in locations where it will be oblique to the ribs. Extensive lung opacities may obscure the thin white line, thereby creating a smooth boundary. Large bullae may be distinguished radiographically from a pneumothorax by their ring shadow or capsule. The sizing of a pneumothorax is often more reliable on chest radiographs than CT scans. Although symptoms dictate treatment of a pneumothorax rather than size, a reference for size ranges predicts the likelihood that intervention will not be required in an asymptomatic patient. In the absence of a continuing air leak, a small pneumothorax that is only visible above the lung apex will resolve in five days or less, at the rate of 1% of total volume of the hemithorax per day. In the erect patient, gas collection will only be seen above the lung apex, and pleural apposition will be maintained down the lateral chest wall. The apposition of lateral pleura is lost in a moderate pleural effusion, resulting in decreased resorption of pleural fluid and greater chance of requiring intervention. Large pneumothoraces allow separate visualization of lobes of the lung and may be associated with tension physiology including hypotension due to a potentially catastrophic decrease in venous return to the heart (**Figure 107-7**).

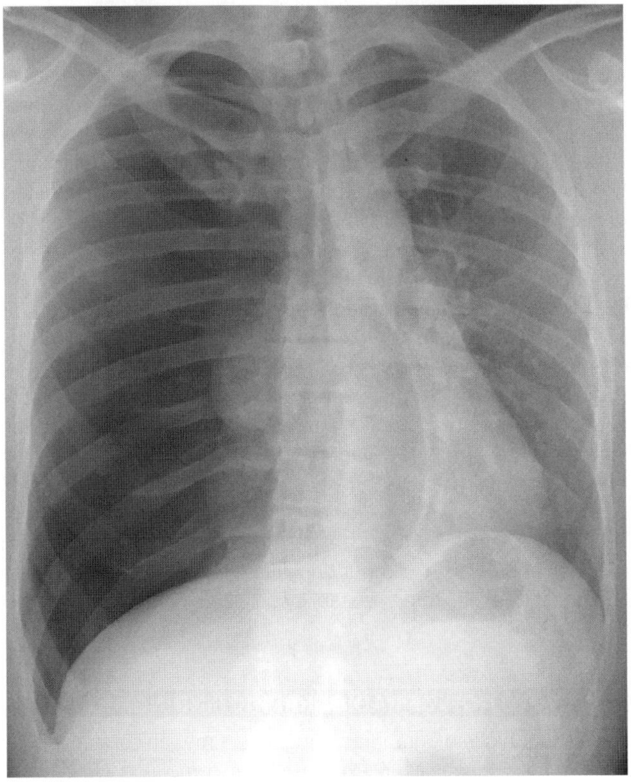

Figure 107-7 *Tension pneumothorax. Expiratory radiograph of right tension pneumothorax increases the apparent shift of midline structures including the azygoesophageal line, seen here behind the heart, to the left of the spine. The three lobes of the right lung are seen separating from each other centrally with complete absence of lung markings peripherally. Increased space between ribs and depression of the right hemidiaphragm also indicate expansion of the space occupied by the pneumothorax.*

PRACTICE POINT

Pneumothorax

- On the supine AP chest radiograph in the adult, one of the most reliable signs of pneumothorax is the deep sulcus sign. If air is in the pleural space, it can easily track down making the costophrenic angle deeper and more acute.
- Quantitative measurements, whether percentage pneumothorax or centimeters of displacement from the chest wall, are less useful than expert radiologic consultation, particularly when chest radiographs are obtained at the bedside.
- The sizing of pneumothoraces and pleural effusions is often more reliable on chest radiographs than CT scans.
- When a patient also has significant pleural effusion providing opacity outside the lung, it may become nearly impossible to detect the pneumothorax on a supine bedside chest radiograph.

PLEURAL EFFUSION

Normally, a thin white line represents the apposition of the parietal and visceral surfaces. Pleural disease, however, may cause expansion of the pleural space along with lobar collapse. Plain chest radiographs, rather than chest CT scans, may provide more reliable sizing of pleural effusions. An average of 300 cc of fluid is required to completely blunt a posterior costophrenic sulcus on a lateral chest radiograph. A *small pleural effusion* may not be visible on PA chest radiograph. A *moderate pleural effusion* is well seen on both PA and lateral views, and the distance between the stomach bubble and lung base may be increased. Subpulmonic collections may laterally displace the hemidiaphragmatic peak on the PA view. This does not in itself mean that the collection is trapped or loculated. Loculation may be associated with empyema, especially when it occurs in a patient who becomes increasingly ill despite improvement in treated pneumonia. A *large pleural effusion* severely restricts lung expansion, but retains visible lung on chest radiographs. A *very large pleural effusion* may result in complete whiteout of the hemithorax (**Figure 107-8**).

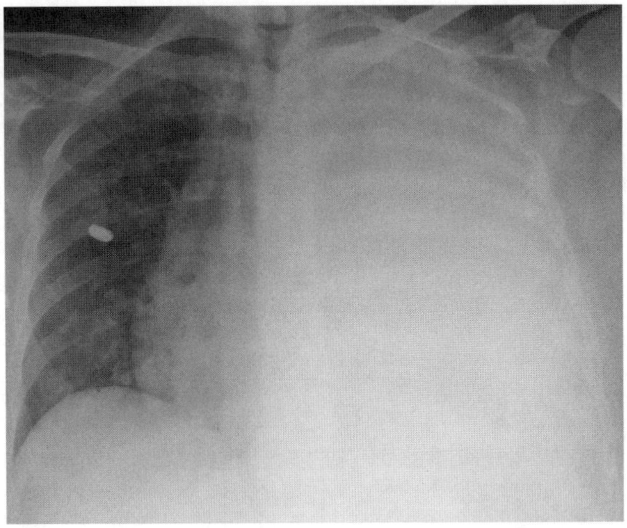

Figure 107-8 *A very large pleural effusion can also cause tension physiology. Note contralateral shift of the mediastinum.*

When a patient has a significant pleural effusion providing opacity outside the lung, it may become nearly impossible to detect the pneumothorax on a supine bedside chest radiograph. In this case, usually from barotraumas or line placement, the abnormal gas collection may take up to five days to become apparent, at which time the patient will have developed a pneumoperitoneum from a pneumomediastinum that communicated through the tight retroperitoneal cavity and dissected through the mesentery. Pneumoperitoneum has to be attributed to rupture of a hollow viscus until proven otherwise. For intubated patients who cannot be examined for an acute abdomen, this requires consultation with radiologists and other specialists and correlating with instrumentation.

EVALUATION OF CHEST PAIN AND/OR DYSPNEA

Commonly, chest radiographs are urgently ordered to evaluate causes of chest pain and to look for complications such as asymptomatic pulmonary edema in the setting of myocardial ischemia. Although the chest radiograph may be normal despite a life-threatening condition, such as an aortic dissection or pulmonary embolism (PE), plain chest radiographs may facilitate immediate identification if abnormal signs are present in addition to expediting management and further investigation.

PRACTICE POINT

Thoracic dissection: radiographic clues that should prompt advanced imaging

- Widening of superior mediastinum > 8 cm
- Blurring of the aortic contour
- Opacification of the angle between the aorta and the left pulmonary artery
- Tracheal shift to the right
- Depression of the left main bronchus to an angle < 40° with the trachea

Note: Aneurysms of the aorta are defined by the following measurements:

- > 3.5 cm aortic arch
- > 5 cm ascending thoracic arch
- > 3 cm abdominal aorta

PRACTICE POINT

Nonspecific radiographic findings associated with pulmonary embolism

- A normal chest radiograph
- Atelectasis the most common nonspecific finding associated with PE
- Small pleural effusions
- Elevated hemidiaphragm
- Abnormally increased lung lucency due to reduced pulmonary vessels distal to embolism (asymmetry of vessels)
- Abrupt cutoff or rat-tail appearance of pulmonary vessels
- More common than early features, later findings of pleural effusion, linear or wedge shaped opacities due to infarction, cavitation of infarction.

PRACTICE POINT

Flail chest

Look for rib fractures that may indicate more serious thoracic injuries.

- Two or more rib fractures in two or more places or when the clavicle and first rib are fractured indicates a flail segment, which is associated with pulmonary contusion and respiratory failure.
- Patchy consolidation, although an early finding, may underestimate the severity of the injury.

PRACTICE POINT

Ruptured esophagus

In the patient with severe central chest pain after vomiting, look for

- Pneumomediastinum suggested by a double outline
- Increasing left-sided pleural effusion

Typical life-threatening disorders that can alter the contour of the cardiomediastinal silhouette are acute vascular emergencies (ie, leaking thoracic aortic aneurysm or aortic dissection). If prior films are available for comparison, changes in aortic vessel diameter between two films are likely to be significant. For a stable patient, differentiating great vessel pathology from mediastinal disease requires advanced imaging unless there are prior images for comparison. If the plain chest imaging shows an abnormality of the mediastinum (eg, widening or distorted contour) or a displacement or narrowing of the trachea, the following potentially life-threatening diagnoses should be considered: primary and metastatic malignancy (bronchogenic and esophageal carcinoma, germ cell tumors, lymphoma, and thymoma), aortic disease (aneurysm, coarctation, dissection), congenital cysts, and vascular abnormalities. Benign diagnoses include asymmetric fat deposition, intrathoracic goiter, esophageal hernia, and vascular tortuosity.

Although a chest radiograph lacks specificity in the diagnosis of PE, it provides valuable data to use in the selection of further imaging to evaluate for PE, especially when pretest probability of PE is low. A chest film may identify abnormalities that explain the patient's symptoms or make interpretation of a ventilation scan indeterminate. If the chest radiograph is normal, a normal nuclear medicine perfusion study provides the best possible exclusion of PE. The patient with normal radiography will have an unambiguous ventilation/perfusion (VQ) scan, and the normal CT will only add radiation and contrast without benefit as well as potentially lead to additional CT scans to prove stability of incidentally identified small lung nodules.

THE EVOLUTION OF RADIOGRAPHIC FINDINGS

The evolution of radiographic findings over time can correctly single out the likely diagnosis to explain a chief complaint. While acute consolidation of lung can be due to hemorrhage, pneumonia, or pulmonary edema, each of these processes undergoes a different evolution over time. The clinical presentation provides supporting data, including suggestive symptoms in the setting of known risk factors such as anticoagulation or heart disease, abnormal vital signs, or confirmatory physical signs. Hemorrhage occurs suddenly and resolves over several days with a coarse interstitial pattern as it resolves. The radiographic features of pulmonary edema depend upon the rapidity of onset; an interstitial pattern that may be accompanied by small pleural effusions may be seen when symptoms have a gradual onset, whereas perihilar consolidation is more commonly seen with symptoms that arise suddenly. Both forms can clear quite quickly, often within 24 hours, especially in patients on dialysis who can have wide fluctuations in fluid status. Pneumonia will cause increasing opacity; as it resolves, it will fade slowly, often over a prolonged period of time, well beyond the hospitalization.

PRACTICE POINT

The rate of radiographic improvement of pneumonia

- The rate of radiographic improvement is directly related to age and, to a lesser degree, to the extent of radiographic involvement and to underlying chronic disease and alcoholism.
- 80% of patients less than or equal to 40 years of age with pneumonia will have complete resolution within six weeks after the initial diagnosis.
- Only 20% of patients 80 years of age will have complete resolution during this time period.
- Only about 67% of patients with community acquired pneumonia (CAP) will have clearing of pneumonia on chest imaging by the fourth week following initiation of treatment.

The evolution of these processes suggests the optimum time for follow-up imaging. For example, an elderly patient with pneumonia would not be expected to have radiographic resolution of a significant pneumonia at the time of his first follow-up appointment with his primary care physician in a week's time. The timing of follow-up films should depend on the need to confirm a diagnosis or to assess response to treatment. One film obtained after the acute illness has likely resolved may be all that is necessary as a new baseline for future patient care. The timing of a chest radiograph to check for resolution of pneumonia depends on the age of the patient, the severity of the pulmonic process, and whether there is a high likelihood of a postobstrutive pneumonia (lobar collapse).

FINDINGS THAT REQUIRE FURTHER FOLLOW-UP IMAGING

It may be useful to divide such findings into two broad categories: (1) follow-up is needed to ensure the chest has returned to normal and (2) follow-up is needed to evaluate a previously unknown finding of potential significance, such as a lung nodule. The further workup of incidental nodules that require CT scanning is best deferred until the patient has recovered and the appearance of the chest has otherwise returned to normal. This is also true of investigations for interstitial lung disease. The central question regarding pulmonary nodules is whether the nodule is likely to be benign or malignant. Solitary pulmonary nodules may be an early manifestation of lung cancer. In one study, 40% of lung cancers were originally detected as a solitary pulmonary nodule. Opacification and consolidation with radiodense bone lesions in multiple ribs would suggest that disease has already become metastatic. It is also important to examine the hilum and mediastinum, especially in patients with a prior history of cancer. Variations of appearance based on visual features about margins, calcification, cavitation, and wall thickness may evolve over time. The presence of a mixture of solid, thick-walled cavities, thin-walled cavities, and resolution of prior nodules without scarring is far more specific for Wegener granulomatosis when these features are all seen in the same patient over time (Figure 107-8).

CONCLUSION

Chest radiographs are the most frequently obtained medical imaging during acute illness. The radiographs can provide physiologic as well as anatomic data. A baseline followup examination following resolution of the acute abnormality is mandatory for the care of patients with pneumonia and extremely helpful for the care of patients who have episodes of CHF, exacerbations of COPD, or a tendency to development acute abnormalities superimposed on chronic changes. As more data is accumulated during the workup of the acute illness, reconsideration of prior chest radiographs may rapidly provide additional information without additional radiography or more advanced imaging. Increasing the clinical information provided to the interpreting radiologist will result in more specific answers to clinical questions. The radiologic differential diagnosis will also be reduced through consideration of the evolution of the radiographic findings over time.

SUGGESTED READINGS

Austin J, Simon M, Trapnell D, Fraser RG. The Fleishner Society glossary: critique and revisions. *AJR*. 1985;145:1096–1098.

de Lacey G, Morley S, Berman L. The Chest X-Ray: A Survival Guide. Philadelphia: Saunders, 2008.

Hall, FM. Language of the radiology report: primer for residents and wayward radiologists. *AJR*. 2000;175:1239–1242.

Ketai L, Meholic A, Fofgren R. Fundamentals of Chest Radiology, 2nd Edition. Philadelphia: Elseveir Saunders, 2006, p. 304.

Khan AN, Al-Jahdali H, AL-Ghanem S, Gouda A. Reading chest radiographs in the critically ill (Part I): Normal chest radiographic appearance, instrumentation, and complications from instrumentation. *Ann Thorac Med*. 2009;4(2):75–87.

Khan AN, Al-Jahdali H, AL-Ghanem S, Gouda A. Reading chest radiographs in the critically ill (part II): radiography of lung pathologies common in the ICU patient. *Ann Thorac Med*. 2009;4(3): 149–157.

MacMahon, Heber, Austin JHM, et al. Guidelines for management of small pulmonary nodules detected on CT scans: a statement from the Fleischner Society. *Radiology*. 2005;237:395–400.

Martin GS, Ely EW, Carroll FE, et al. Findings on the portable chest radiograph correlate with fluid balance in critically ill patients. *Chest*. 2002;122:2087–2095.

Miller JC. Evaluating pulmonary nodules. MGH Radiology Round Volume 4, Issue 8, August 2006. Available at http://www.mghradrounds.org/index.php?src=gendocs&link=2006_august.

Mittl RL Jr, Scwab RJ, Duchin JS, et al. Radiographic resolution of community-acquired pneumonia. *Am J Respir Crit Care Med*. 1994;149:630–635.

Tuddenham WJ. Glossary of terms for thoracic radiology: recommendations of the Nomenclature Committee of the Fleishner Society. *AJR*. 1984;143:509–517.

CHAPTER 108

Advanced Cardiothoracic Imaging

Francine L. Jacobson, MD, MPH
Sylvia C. McKean, MD, SFHM, FACP

Key Clinical Questions

1. What are the advantages of noncontrast computed tomography (CT) compared with other CT studies?
2. What are the indications for noncontrast CT with thin-section reconstruction?
3. When is the use of IV contrast with CT imaging mandatory?
4. What are the limitations of positron emission tomography (PET)-CT?
5. What are the main indications for cardiac-CT?
6. What are the Fleischner Society Guidelines recommendations concerning follow-up of incidental solid pulmonary nodules?
7. What are the disadvantages of cardiac magnetic resonance with late gadolinium enhancement?
8. Complementary to two-dimensional echocardiography, transesophageal echocardiography (TEE) is able to provide superior visualization of what cardiac structures?
9. What calcium score would preclude contrast computed tomography angiography (CTA)?

INTRODUCTION

The overwhelming majority of advanced chest imaging for hospitalized patients is performed by CT, with ultrasound, MRI, and nuclear medicine reserved for specific situations. The evolution of disease processes in the chest over time is central to the diagnostic process necessitating integration between modalities in choosing comparison studies. With the assistance of an experienced radiologist, serial bedside chest radiographs can provide physiologic and pathologic information that may not be available from more advanced imaging that reflects only a single moment in time.

The chief complaint should guide decisions about the extent of medical imaging necessary for the proper diagnosis and treatment of the acute illness. The radiologist reads the patient's body and disease processes much as the clinician completes the history and physical examination with a checklist that will identify both the truly incidental and unrelated findings as well as separate seemingly unrelated findings that complete the picture of the acute illness.

Many patients who require hospitalization for successful care of their acute illness have underlying medical conditions and chronic disease processes. Preexisting heart disease, lung disease, and systemic disease findings help to develop the personalized differential diagnosis for the reporting of the imaging studies whether obtained as radiographs, CT, MRI or any other modality. Diabetes, collagen vascular diseases, chronic obstructive pulmonary disease, atherosclerosis, and suppression of the immune system can lead the radiologist to different conclusions about the significance of particular findings in an individual patient.

Advanced imaging during hospitalization that risks complications in an acutely ill patient, provides suboptimal imaging requiring additional studies, and unnecessarily increases length of stay should be minimized. This chapter will focus on the abnormalities that most frequently require advanced imaging for diagnosis and the common incidental findings that require mandatory follow-up post discharge.

NORMAL VERSUS ABNORMAL FUNCTION OF LUNGS

Chest radiography images how lung function (gas exchange and perfusion of oxygenated blood) changes over time. Blood flow is greater to the lower lobes than the upper lobes, and greatest in the right lower lobe, while oxygenation is greater in the upper lobes. Because blood flow is greater to the lung bases, particularly the right lower lobe, hematogenous spread of infection and tumor likely begin in the lung bases. Pulmonary emboli also occur more often in lower lobes. Oxygen-loving mycobacterium organisms prefer the lung apices. Warm cigarette smoke rises most directly to the apical segment of the right upper lobe, not surprisingly causing the right upper lobe to be the most frequent site of primary lung cancer.

The deposition of calcium in lung parenchyma is also based upon physiology stemming from the diametrically opposed oxygenation of the apices and perfusion of the bases that result in a pH gradient from 7.52 in the lung apices to 7.39 in the lung bases. In the setting of hypercalcemia, as in renal failure, serum calcium will be precipitated in the lung apices. This abnormal "metastatic" deposition of calcium into normal tissues, reversible with correction of the hypercalcemia, only occurs in a base environment.

CT SCANNING

NONCONTRAST CHEST CT

The most basic noncontrast enhanced chest CT scan is performed with breath-holding in inspiration without oral or intravenous contrast material and requires no special patient preparation. Preferred for the acutely ill patient when CT scanning is indicated, multidetector CT scanners in current use can rapidly provide many images without respiratory motion artifacts despite continuous patient breathing. The scanning room can generally accommodate ventilators and extensive support devices. The aerated lung parenchyma provides exquisite contrast for branches of the pulmonary arteries and pulmonary veins without requiring the addition of oral contrast agents. In the absence of IV contrast material, visualization of great vessels is generally adequate due to the presence of fat in the mediastinum. The noncontrast chest CT should not be used to assess hilar lymph nodes, particularly when small to borderline in size, pulmonary emboli (PE), and acute cardiovascular disease.

NONCONTRAST ENHANCED CHEST CT WITH THIN SECTION RECONSTRUCTION

Noncontrast enhanced chest CT with thin section reconstruction is the standard imaging study of intrinsic, interstitial lung disease. Expiratory scans can be added to evaluate air-trapping. A second scan during forcible expiration will best demonstrate central airway narrowing and thereby identify tracheobronchial malacia, a potential cause of difficulty weaning a patient from ventilatory support. At end-expiration, thin section reconstruction will clearly image lung parenchyma and air-trapping in small airways. Prone images to more completely evaluate the extent of interstitial lung disease are more easily performed following resolution of the acute illness.

High Resolution Computed Tomography (HRCT) uses slice thickness ≤ 2 mm with high spatial frequency reconstruction to image lung structure distal to all but the most peripheral vasculature (the secondary pulmonary lobule). HRCT images do not require contrast enhancement, which can actually confound the findings (see **Table 108-1**).

CONTRAST-ENHANCED CHEST CT

Contrast-enhanced chest CT examinations differ by rate of injection and delay before imaging. The delay will be slightly longer when the primary concern is for aortic dissection. Cardiac gating is also possible, and may be used in some institutions to provide a triple-rule-out scan for coronary arteries, and aorta and pulmonary arteries.

The use of IV contrast material is mandatory for CT pulmonary angiography (CT-PA). Patients who have previously had mild to moderate contrast allergy reactions can be premedicated over approximately 12 hours prior to CT-PA (See Chapter 106 Patient Safety Issues in Radiology). If the history of allergic reaction is severe, select an alternative test. Ideally, the patient should be fasting for four hours prior to the administration of IV contrast material but a nonfasting patient may have CT-PA without delay when necessary. In order to adequately opacify pulmonary arteries, the contrast material should be injected at a high velocity of approximately four cc per second, which requires a large bore, minimum 20-gauge catheter. Using a tenuous or smaller IV for the study will almost certainly result in a nondiagnostic study. PE may be seen

TABLE 108-1 Radiologic Features and Differential Diagnosis of Idiopathic Interstitial Pneumonias

Histologic Pattern	Radiographic Features	Distribution on CT	HRCT Features	Differential Diagnosis
AIP [DAD]	Progressive diffuse ground-glass opacity leading to consolidation ARDS	Diffuse	Early: lobular sparing Late: traction bronchiectasis	Hydrostatic edema Pneumonia Acute eosinophilic pneumonia
COP [BOOP]	Patchy bilateral consolidation	Subpleural	Consolidation Nodules (small or large)	Infection, vasculitis, sarcoidosis, BAC, lymphoma, pneumonia, NSIP
RB-ILD	Bronchial wall thickening Ground-glass opacity Normal in 14%	Diffuse	Bronchial wall thickening Centrilobular nodules Patchy ground-glass opacity Emphysema	DIP NSIP Hypersensitivity pneumonitis
NSIP	Nonspecific Normal in 7%	Peripheral, subpleural, bases, symmetric	Centrilobular opacities Irregular lines Microcystic honeycombing	UIP DIP OP Hypersensitivity pneumonitis
DIP	Ground-glass opacity Normal in 3–22%	Peripheral bases Diffuse in 18%	Ground-glass attenuation Reticular lines Honeycombing	RB-ILD Hypersensitivity pneumonitis Sarcoidosis PCP
IPF [UIP]	Basal predominant reticular abnormality with volume loss Normal in 10–15%	Peripheral bases Subpleural	Reticular Honeycombing Traction bronchiectasis Bronchiectasis Architectural distortion Focal ground-glass	Asbestosis Collagen vascular disease Hypersensitivity pneumonitis Sarcoidosis

on standard contrast-enhanced chest CT scans, so clinicians should review any recent prior CT scans with the radiologist in light of new suspicion for PE.

THORACIC PET-CT

Thoracic PET-CT uses a radionuclide that binds to a D-glucose analogue to produce FDG. Because glycolysis is up-regulated in tumor cells as well as in normal cells during anaerobic conditions, PET-CT can identify tumors when other imaging is indeterminate. PET-CT identifies tumor through inflammatory characteristics; hence, high uptake of FDG may falsely suggest malignancy in metabolically active infections and inflammatory conditions. Originally, PET-CT was used to evaluate solitary pulmonary lesions that may be cancerous. However, TB or fungal granulomas, hyperplastic normal thymic tissue in the anterior mediastinum, and brown adipose tissue at the base of the neck, supraclavicular area, or superior mediastinum in adults may avidly take up FDG. Because FDG and glucose compete for the same receptor, decreased FDG uptake may occur when there is acute hyperglycemia. It can reliably evaluate 8 mm pulmonary nodules of unclear etiology, but some well-differentiated adenocarcinomas of the lung can be very slow growing and, therefore, reveal little or no FDG-glucose avidity.

Although PET-CT does not require contrast, the dose of ionizing radiation that the patient receives from the CT scan for attenuation correction is not negligible. The CT scan performed for attenuation correction of the PET scan is not a diagnostic quality CT scan. The uncertain and incidental findings will also lead to significant additional imaging.

PET-CT is usually used for staging *known* cancer. This long and very expensive examination should not be undertaken when the patient cannot adequately cooperate or has acute processes that will resolve in a short interval of time.

CARDIAC COMPUTED TOMOGRAPHY (CCT)

Cardiac-computed tomography (CCT) visualizes nonstenotic calcified and noncalcified coronary plaques with a very high negative predictive value (91–100%) to rule out the presence of coronary artery disease (CAD). Excellent images may be obtained within five minutes, thereby facilitating rapid triage from the emergency department in some institutions. Its primary use in acute chest pain should be reserved for patients with an intermediate pretest probability of coronary artery disease or for those patients at increased risk for aortic dissection and segmental pulmonary embolism that may be visualized at the same time. Patients with a low pretest probability should not be subjected to the risk of radiation; patients with a high pretest probability of CAD and suspected Non-ST Elevation Myocardial Infarction (NSTEMI) or Unstable Angina (UA) would not benefit because a negative CCT would not alter the pretest probability. Cardiac CT requires the administration of contrast.

DIAGNOSIS DRIVEN IMAGING

PULMONARY EMBOLISM

The diagnosis of PE has remained difficult despite successive improvements and refinements in imaging modalities. Patients who require hospitalization for acute care, particularly with advancing age, have comorbidities that increase the pretest probability of PE. Evaluation of ventilation-perfusion scanning by PIOPED investigators suggests that more than 50% of patients who are likely to be seen by hospitalists will fall into the category most at risk for actually having PE when the result is intermediate or indeterminate. As a result, CT-PA has been widely adopted as the primary diagnostic test for PE *although a normal perfusion scan still provides greater exclusion of PE.*

Pulmonary emboli can be hard to detect even in lobar arteries and the detection of the smallest peripheral emboli can be difficult to put in clinical perspective. The number of vessels present in each lung and each segment within each lung is daunting for complete assessment by conventional angiography. Pulmonary emboli are easier to identify in the larger vessels in the lower lobes that are also more readily examined in the axial plane. With increasing use of coronal and sagittal reformatted images and advanced image processing, the detection of upper lobe pulmonary emboli and smaller vessels will continue to improve. An important normal function of the lungs is to trap and make harmless the much more frequently occurring subclinical microemboli that fail to pass through the capillaries in the lungs, thereby not reaching other organs, particularly the brain. At what point should this normal function be deemed clinically significant pathology requiring treatment? The existence of significant sources of additional clot may inform the decision-making process more than the current miniscule burden of clot.

The evaluation of potential PE by CT initially included pelvic and lower extremity imaging to assess for DVT. This portion of the CT-PA examination is now largely historical as it required significant additional radiation and was rarely helpful. When the value of identifying DVT as a source for future PE is important, lower extremity noninvasive imaging (LENI) with ultrasound is preferred and may also obviate the need for CT-PA in the pregnant patient. The absence of clot is less helpful in the diagnosis of acute PE because one-third or more patients will have no evidence of clot in their lower extremities despite acute PE. The normal perfusion scan remains the single best test to exclude PE when the CXR is normal.

PRACTICE POINT

Pulmonary embolism (PE)

If the result of a "negative" PE-protocol CT does not support the clinical pretest probability and the lungs are not normal for a perfusion strategy, the options in order of descending preference are as follows:

1. Consult with your chest radiologist to obtain a "second opinion" about the original CT.
2. Consider an MRA versus a conventional pulmonary angiogram to address the areas in question on CT. The choice will vary depending on institutional resources.
3. Consider repeating the CT-PA; however, the yield is likely to be low unless there was a quality issue with the first scan (such as timing or velocity of administration of contrast bolus, respiratory motion).

As always, the result must be interpreted in the context of the patient sitting in front of you, including weighing the risk of empiric anticoagulation for a defined period of time. For example, if a patient had severe acute airspace disease or severe end-stage lung disease, a significant PE would likely lead to intubation. Of course the patient may have a real but tiny left lower lobe PE (LLL PE). In the setting of all the rest, it is not the problem.

The radiographic evolution between acute PE and infarction occurs over several days. It is not infrequent for pulmonary emboli to no longer be visible, particularly when peripheral, so that multiple subsegmental defects may elude detection several days after the acute symptoms such as pleuritic chest pain occur. It then becomes more important to consider whether any secondary signs of PE or right heart strain are present on the scan already obtained. Chronic changes that may result from prior PE include pulmonary artery wall thickening and segmental bronchiolitis obliterans with marked diminution of pulmonary vessels.

The detection of pulmonary emboli also varies due to patient factors, including respiratory factors and artifacts that can be minimized by relocating foreign bodies such ECG leads for the test. A shallower inspiratory breath-hold will maximize vessel opacification particularly in young and relatively healthy patients. Clinicians should prepare patients to expect to raise their arms and to hold their breath for the study. Respiratory motion and bolus quality often conspire to limit the exclusion of PE to central PA branches in the acutely ill patient. The interpreting radiologist should report the bolus quality and use variable display window and level settings to better visualize emboli.

CHEST PAIN OF UNCLEAR ETIOLOGY

In some institutions, patients with chest pain of less clear etiology may receive CT scans even while still in the emergency department. IV contrast material will be used to provide greatest opacification of the primary region suspected to be the cause of a particular patient's chest pain. Thus, a longer delay will be needed for contrast enhancement of the aorta than the pulmonary arteries. In fact, by the time the aorta is well-opacified, the standard bolus of contrast material may no longer be visible in the pulmonary arteries. In a patient who may suffer from an aortic dissection that may decrease perfusion of the kidneys, it is not advisable to increase the dose of IV contrast material to maintain contrast enhancement through pulmonary and systemic circulation simultaneously (**Figure 108-1** and **Table 108-2**).

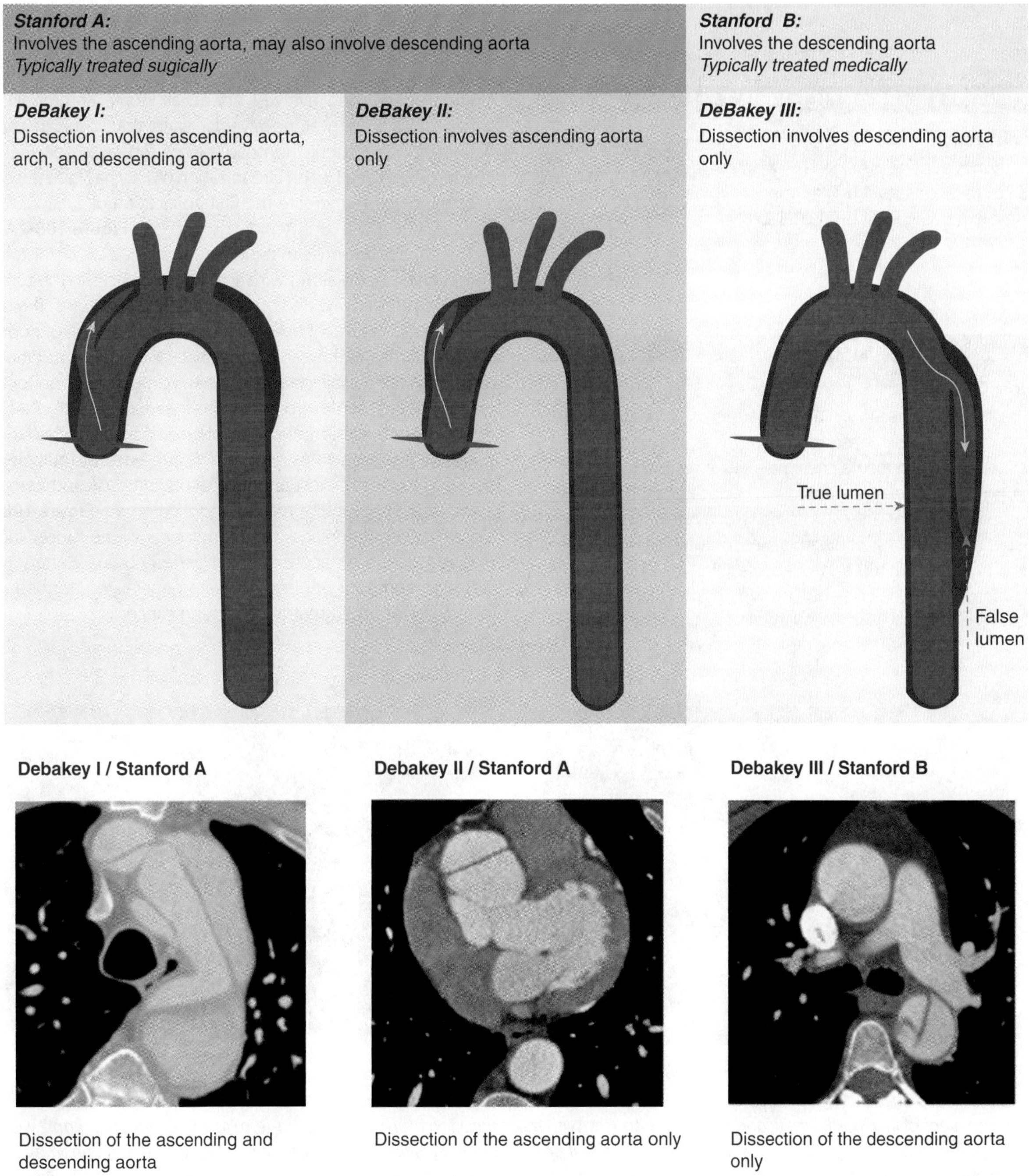

Figure 108-1 *Aortic images – Dissection. (Reproduced, with permission, from Jacob C. Mandell, MD, Brigham and Women's Radiology.)*

TABLE 108-2 Acute Chest Pain, Suspected Aortic Dissection

Radiologic Procedure	Appropriateness	Radiation Level
X-ray chest—do not expect to be definitive	9	☢
CTA chest and abdomen	9	☢ ☢ ☢ ☢
MRA chest and abdomen	8	☢ ☢ ☢ ☢
US echocardiography transesophageal	8	☢ ☢
Aortography thoracic	5	☢ ☢ ☢
US echocardiography transthoracic	4	

Appropriateness rating scale: 1, 2, 3 usually not appropriate; 4, 5, 6 may be appropriate; 7, 8, 9 usually appropriate. Relative radiation level: 0–4 (Data from http://www.acr.org/SecondaryMainMenuCategories/quality_safety/app_criteria.aspx).

PRACTICE POINT

Aortic dissection

- Dissection is generally imaged by the most rapidly available modality in the institution. The urgency will also lead to the greatest expertise using the most rapidly available imaging.

PRACTICE POINT

The triple CT scan

- The best quality CT scan will be achieved through careful pretest consideration of probability as well as a more complete description of the patient's chest pain, whether pleuritic, radiating to the neck, radiating to the back, or crushing. Accompanying signs and symptoms, such as elevated blood pressure and shortness of breath also contribute to the decision-making process and, of course, CT should not be used as a substitute for complete history and physical examination.

PERICARDIAL DISEASE

Visibility on chest radiographs of the separation of epicardial and pericardial fat depends upon a fortuitous relationship to the diverging X-ray beam. The shape or sudden increase in size of the cardiac silhouette requires confirmation with echocardiography. It is quite common to have discrepancy in reporting of pericardial effusion between CT scans and echocardiography, particularly when the anterior pericardial recess is used as an acoustical window in the course of transthoracic echocardiography. The recess itself may give the impression of being part of a more generalized effusion. Measured in millimeters on CT scans, a 1 cm pericardial effusion is comparatively large.

Calcification associated with constrictive pericarditis will be seen on plain radiographs and CT scans. On MRI it will appear as a signal void. However, MRA can demonstrate the altered function quite elegantly.

LUNG CANCER

Nonsolid and part solid adenocarcinoma of lung

The lung cancer CT screening trials begun more than 15 years ago have tremendously increased our understanding of how adenocarcinoma of the lung evolves. Adenocarcinoma commonly begins with lepidic growth along alveolar walls that result in very well-defined though subtle nonsolid, or ground-glass opacities on CT images. The World Health Organization (WHO) has initiated changes in terminology that create the first application of carcinoma in situ to lung cancer with only lepidic growth (see **Figure 108-2A**).

The bar-like opacities that indicate focal invasion on histology are visible on CT scans along with small cystic spaces in the tumor that may resemble airways and other parenchymal features. The progressive evolution of solid components leads to the type of nodule that is most worrisome for cancer, the part-solid nodule. Additional features may raise suspicion even higher, particularly when focal linear extensions are seen to cross the lung to pleural surfaces that may be remote from the lesion, and focal pleural thickening when the lesion is closely applied to the nodule. The presence of multiple lesions does not exclude cancer although acute infection and hemorrhage associated with nodules may be more common (**Figure 108-2B**).

Further evaluation and treatment for early lung cancer should be deferred during an acute illness. Needed coronary artery revascularization and valve replacement are generally performed prior to lobectomy or other treatment for lung cancer.

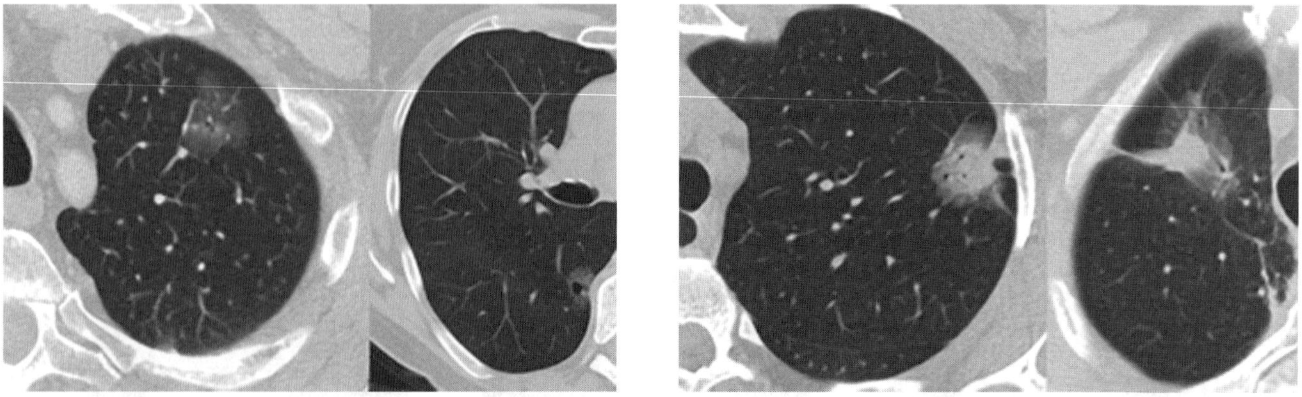

A B

Figure 108-2 *(A) Images of early adenocarcinoma of lung demonstrating well-defined ground-glass opacity without additional distinguishing features (left), and areas of increased density and small cystic spaces, with more specific features (right). Long-term follow-up (greater than 2 years) often required for confident diagnosis, as PET-CT will demonstrate little, if any, FDG-glucose avidity. (B) Images of progressive adenocarcinoma of the lung with thin extensions to distant pleura, focal pleural thickening, and sharp demarcation between the ground-glass opacity and the adjacent normal lung, unlike inflammatory lesions such as pneumonia.*

Lymphangitis carcinomatosis

Lymphangitis carcinomatosis most commonly represents the end process of hematogenous dissemination of a tumor with tumor cells in the lymphatics that course along with the pulmonary venous structures in the septae of the secondary pulmonary lobule. To differentiate from interstitial edema, it is helpful to look for pulmonary nodules, even micronodules, and nodular thickening of the fissures. The findings will not abate with diuresis. The finding no longer signifies imminent death within six months as patients often live three or more years with treatment. Twenty percent of lymphangitis is due to obstruction of central lymphatics rather than actual tumor. This is particularly likely when a central hilar mass such as a lung cancer obstructs the lymphatics. In this case, lymphangitis will generally be unilateral instead of bilateral as it is when due to hematogenous dissemination of tumor. Breast cancer can also be associated with unilateral lymphangitis carcinomatosis.

INCIDENTIAL CT FINDINGS

Incidental CT findings can pose a severe threat of future morbidity and mortality.

INCIDENTAL PULMONARY NODULES

Contrast enhancement of nodules to identify malignancy is infrequently performed in most centers that have PET-CT scanning readily available. The most reliable sign of benign disease in a pulmonary nodule is solid or central calcification. The presence of contrast material, regardless of timing, may limit the detection of calcium in a nodule. The Fleischner Society 2005 Recommendations and other guidelines to address indeterminate incidental pulmonary nodules found on chest CT scans will undoubtedly evolve to better serve patients (see **Table 108-3**).

The Fleischner Society Guidelines recommend follow-up of incidental solid pulmonary nodules based on size and features of the nodule but do not apply to patients less than 35 years of age or to patients who have a known malignancy. It is extremely unusual for incidentally-found, tiny, less than 4 mm average diameter nodules to be due to lung cancer so they do not require follow-up in patients at low risk for lung cancer. Assessment of risk, even known cigarette smoking, is difficult and in some centers nearly all patients will be considered high risk. Guidelines will always need to be interpreted in light of the clinical context of the patient in front of you. Not large enough for transthoracic needle biopsy or reliable PET scan, the 4–6 mm size category should be followed unless complete resection is performed. It is appropriate to refer the recommended follow-up to either a pulmonologist or thoracic surgeon who is accustomed to following these lesions and promptly acting upon the results when necessary. Pulmonary nodules require direct communication with the patient and the patient's primary care physician (PCP) to make certain the findings are not overlooked after the acute illness resolves.

TABLE 108-3 Fleischner Society Small Nodule Follow-up Recommendations

Nodule Size	Low Risk Patient	High Risk Patient
≤4 mm	None	12 month If no change, stop
4–6 mm	12 month follow-up If no change, stop	6–12 month follow-up If no change, 18–24 month follow-up
6–8 mm	6–12 month follow-up If no change, 18–24 month follow-up	3–6 month follow-up If no change, 18–24 month follow-up
>8 mm	CT scan at 3, 9, 24 months Consider PET-CT (in some centers also nodule enhancement chest CT) or biopsy	

PRACTICE POINT

Pulmonary nodules

- It is not appropriate to follow up previously identified nodules during acute pulmonary processes just because the patient is in the hospital.

Transthoracic CT-guided biopsy may be performed for actionable lesions in the 1 cm range.

Tiny, indeterminate pulmonary nodules

Multidetector CT scans are exquisitely sensitive for detection of solid nodules measuring 2–3 mm in diameter. These are seen in more than 50% of patients and will be overwhelmingly benign. In populations with high rates of endemic granulomatous infections, 90% or more of patients cared for by hospitalist physicians will have tiny indeterminate nodules. Through studies in Japan and the Early Lung Cancer Action Project, follow-up of thousands of such nodules reveals an extremely low rate of cancer in these tiny nodules that most often represent granulomas and intrapulmonary lymph nodes. In the lung cancer screening CT trials, the rare cancer identified at a site of indeterminate tiny nodule on a prior CT was so low that such nodules receive at most one follow-up CT scan. The rare nodule of this type that becomes a lung cancer generally grows in a short amount of time. A solitary pulmonary nodule identified on chest radiographs may prove to be one of multiple pulmonary nodules by CT. The primary purpose for CT scanning of a dominant pulmonary nodule with significant probability of malignancy is to stage lung cancer (see **Table 108-4**).

The most conservative approach to an incidental pulmonary nodule seen on abdominal CT is to obtain a chest CT to identify all

TABLE 108-4 Differential Diagnosis of Solitary Pulmonary Nodule

Primary considerations:
Lung cancer, including all neuroendocrine lung tumors (carcinoid-small cell)
Hamartoma
Granuloma
AVM
Solitary pulmonary metastasis
Specialized considerations:
Hematoma following trauma with laceration to lung parenchyma
Infection due to fungus, parasite, or atypical organism
Infarction, particularly from Swan-Ganz catheter
Noninfectious inflammatory process such as Wegeners granulomatosis
Vasculitis
Primary pulmonary lymphoma

lung nodules that might be present. This follow-up CT scan may be deferred when the incidental finding will not affect immediate treatment decisions.

INCIDENTAL FINDINGS OUTSIDE THE LUNG PARENCHYMA

Incidental findings of the aorta, kidneys, liver, and gallbladder will be frequently encountered on chest CT scans. When the finding is in the upper abdomen or lower neck, the follow-up will be with the more appropriate focal examination. Follow-up of findings with potential for imminent catastrophe, such as aortic rupture, and findings that might completely change the immediate decisions about the course of therapy should be worked up promptly during the hospitalization. Otherwise, it is appropriate to defer the workup until the patient is well and transient acute findings such as pleural effusion have resolved. For example, an aberrant right coronary artery arising from the left aortic leaflet is at risk for obstruction by adjacent structures, but it is unlikely to suddenly become symptomatic while the patient is acutely ill, although it makes the radiologist reporting the study uncomfortable. Management of incidental findings in the abdomen can be addressed through the recommendations of the American College of Radiology (ACR). Complete communication with the patient's PCP includes communication of findings. That are currently incidental to minimize future repetition of imaging when an incidental finding may become more meaningful in the context of the patient's overall health (**Figure 108-3**).

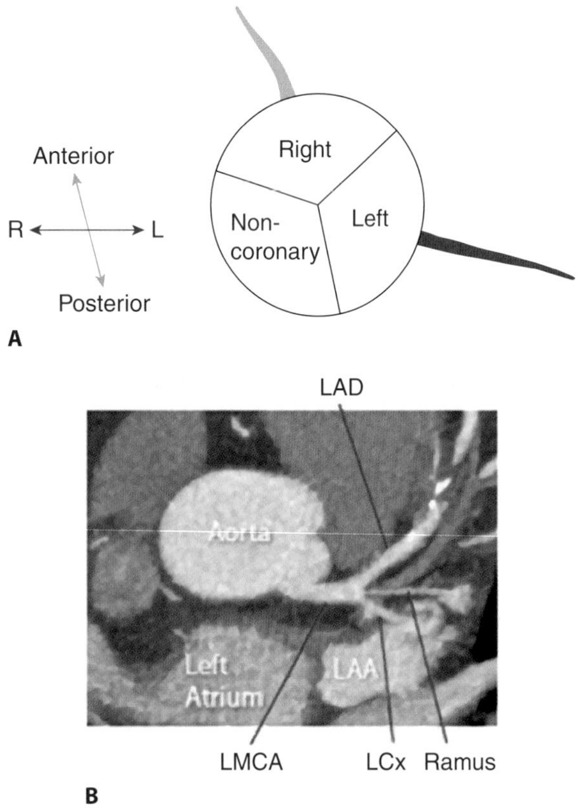

Figure 108-3 *There are most commonly two coronary artery origins from the proximal aorta, at the junction between the sinuses of valsalva and the aorta. The right coronary artery arises from the anterior right coronary cusp and the left coronary artery arises from the posterior left coronary cusp. Drawing (A) and CT scan image (B) provide axial image orientation. (Reproduced, with permission, from Jacob C. Mandell, MD, Brigham and Women's Radiology.)*

MAGNETIC RESONANCE IMAGING (MRI)

MRI can be very helpful for solving specific problems but should not be entertained lightly in an acutely ill patient. Organizing an MRI for a hospitalized patient is not a simple undertaking and examinations are frequently suboptimal when patients are acutely ill. All support lines and tubes must be specifically approved for imaging by MRI. In rare cases, the examination will require general anesthesia. In centers that can perform the examination under anesthesia, a radiologist and an anesthesiologist will generally both be required continually throughout the procedure, lasting on average one hour. See Chapter 105 Introduction to Radiology regarding contraindications to MRI.

MRI examinations in the chest are most frequently performed with a gadolinium-based contrast agent. Gadolinium is no longer considered inert and without risk. When used, the dose of gadolinium will be adjusted based on the patient's weight to minimize the risk of nephrogenic systemic fibrosis (NSF). If a patient has had a severe allergic reaction to iodinated contrast material used for CT, consultation with a radiologist will facilitate a decision between choosing noncontrast enhanced chest CT and MRI. MRI and CT can provide equivalent information regarding the mediastinum and the presence of lymphadenopathy. MRI can be superior to CT in examination of pleural fluid and pleural masses and confirm the presence of blood despite a mass-like appearance. The degradation of red blood cells provides changes in appearance of extravascular blood over time that can estimate the duration of the abnormality. MRI provides greater definition of fat planes and chest wall masses. MR angiography (MRA), coupled with cardiac gating, can provide high quality images in place of conventional angiography. CT may complement MRI for the study of bones due to the signal void on an MRI examination caused by calcification. Without correlative imaging, whether chest radiographs or CT scan, such signal voids can cause confusion. Any outside imaging that might bear on this issue should be brought to the attention of the interpreting radiologist.

Cardiac magnetic resonance (CMR) with late gadolinium enhancement may provide information about proximal coronary anatomy, myocardial perfusion, myocardial viability, acute versus chronic changes, and global and regional cardiac function. It may identify specific myocardial regions at risk and thereby provide additive information not only pertinent to risk stratification but also help target revascularization in patients with UA/NSTEMI. CMR is a rapidly evolving technology and the reported specificity, positive predictive value, and overall accuracy is likely to reflect expanded protocols. The disadvantages of CMR include cost, length of time required for scanning, the use of gadolinium in patients with reduced renal function, and contraindications (implanted pacemakers and defibrillators).

ULTRASOUND (US)

ADVANTAGES

Ultrasound can be brought to the patient at the bedside or performed in the radiology department. Ultrasound of the chest requires no special preparation, can be done in a variety of positions, and does not expose the patient to ionizing radiation.

LIMITATIONS

Patient body habitus and comorbidities may become limiting for ultrasound examinations, including echocardiography. Adipose tissue attenuates ultrasound and decreases the penetration, limiting the depth that can be examined. Since air stops the transmission of ultrasound, it is not routinely used to image lung parenchyma and the presence of an overlying lung can limit visualization even in normal individuals. This is of greater concern with destructive lung disease such as emphysema that also causes greater obscuration due to increased anterior extension of lung.

ULTRASOUND OF THE CHEST

The most frequent use of noncardiac ultrasound of the chest is for the planning and, if necessary, the performance of thoracentesis. US can differentiate complex fluid and pus from free fluid. The detection of septal structures that become dilated due to interstitial pulmonary edema by ultrasound is being studied to provide information about this physiology without ionizing radiation. Ultrasound lung comets (ULC), an echographic sign of extravascular lung water, originate from water-thickened interlobular septa. US may occasionally image extrathoracic soft tissues and accessible vascular structures.

Cardiac ultrasound 2-D echocardiography with color Doppler is frequently the first imaging acquired for the internal structure and functional evaluation of the heart, including ejection fraction. It may be ordered without prior chest radiographs for a young patient with a heart murmur. Coupling anatomic detail with physiologic function, it can assess a wide range of abnormalities from mitral valve prolapse to pulmonary artery hypertension and critical aortic stenosis. A bedside two-dimensional echocardiography will detect abnormalities of wall motion in all cases of STEMI and hence, may be indicated when there is uncertainty about the diagnosis (pericardial effusion, RV infarction, ventricular aneurysm, or LV thrombus), the need for emergent reperfusion therapy, or prognosis (reduced left ventricular function) (**Figure 108-4**).

Complementary to 2D-echocardiography, transesophageal echocardiography (TEE) is able to provide superior visualization of the posterior cardiac structures. The acoustical window provided by the esophagus allows excellent evaluation of the ascending aorta and a significant portion of the heart and descending thoracic aorta without intervening lung and bone. In institutions where transesophageal echocardiography (TEE) is readily available with high level of skill at the bedside, it may be used as the first, and potentially only, diagnostic test for aortic dissection that requires emergent surgical intervention. Since air stops sound waves, the region of the aortic arch is not completely imaged with this modality. Extension into great vessels is better assessed by CT or MRI.

In addition to suspected aortic dissection, TEE may be used as an initial test to guide percutaneous interventions for structural heart disease, assess the cause of fever in patients with intracardiac devices, and to evaluate the possibility of left atrial thrombus prior to cardioversion or radiofrequency ablation. Contraindications include esophageal problems and poor cooperation due to delirium or other causes of altered mental status. Patients with coagulopathy may have increased risk of bleeding. Complications are usually minor such as transient bronchospasm, hypoxia, nonsustained ventricular tachycardia, atrial fibrillation, hemoptysis, vomiting, or hematoma. Patients should fast for 4–6 hours prior to the procedure.

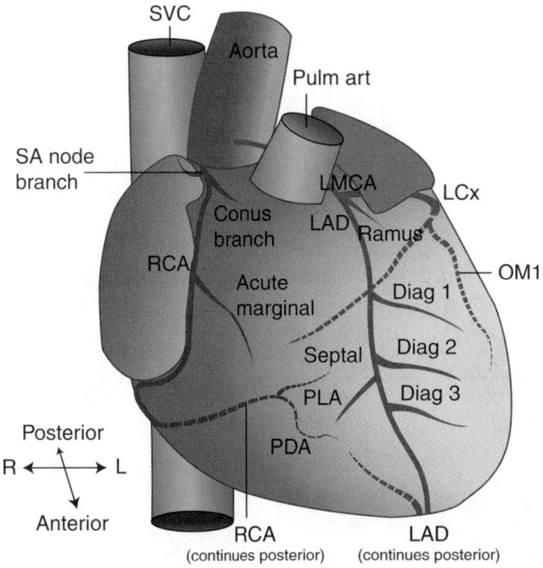

Figure 108-4 *Normal coronary anatomy.*

NUCLEAR MEDICINE

Nuclear medicine can provide powerful problem-solving information in tailored examinations. Radiotracer can prove patency of central venous catheters, identify spleen when present in the pleural space, and as in other organ systems, identify low level bleeding that is difficult to localize and evaluate function. For a patient with a normal chest X-ray, a normal perfusion scan alone still provides the finest exclusion of PE.

Nuclear medicine is also used extensively for cardiac evaluation, even in the acutely ill where pharmacologic stress can safely evaluate the heart muscle (**Table 108-5**).

PRACTICE POINT

Cardiac testing options

Exercise stress test: sensitivity 68%, specificity 77%

- No need to be fasting
- Still the best test for women with low pretest clinical probability even if more false positives
- Low risk (< 1% annual cardiac mortality) clinical patients without ETT abnormalities do not benefit from further imaging
- Intermediate risk (2–3% annual cardiac mortality)
- High risk (4% annual cardiac mortality) clinical patients should proceed directly to the cardiac catheterization laboratory without further imaging

Pharmacologic agents

- Dobutamine (broad adrenergic receptor agonist, titrated to heart rate response)
  - Contraindicated if ACS, VT, afibrillation with RVR
  - Fasting at least 4 hours
  - Can use with atropine
- Vasodilators (stimulate adenosine A2a receptors): adenosine, persantine (dipyramidole), regadenoson (Lexiscan)
  - Contraindicated if bronchospasm, AV block
  - Fasting at least 4 hours, no caffeine for 24 hours
  - No aggrenox

SPECT reported: sensitivity 88%, specificity 77%

- May be exercise or pharmacologic
- Total time 2–4 hours

ECHO reported: sensitivity 76%, specificity 77%

- May be exercise or pharmacologic
- Requires good US windows and can be enhanced by contrast

CT

- Requires contrast
- Must be pharmacologic
- Patient must be supine
- Total time 30 minutes

In general, exercise is preferred if patients can walk as long as they do not have contraindications. Absolute contraindications include Acute Coronary Syndrome (ACS), myocardial infarction within the previous 48 hours, unstable arrhythmias, decompensated congestive heart failure, symptomatic severe aortic stenosis, acute pulmonary embolism, acute myocarditis or pericarditis, aortic dissection,

TABLE 108-5 Radioactive Tracer Material

MIBI
• Technetium-99m (99mTc) labeled methoxy-isobutyl- isonitrile, aka 99mTc-sestamibi • T1/2 = 6 hours • Lipophilic molecule that passively diffuses through myocyte membrane • Higher photon energy • Minimal redistribution, stays fixed in myocyte, giving a snapshot at time of injection
Thallium (Tl-201)
• T1/2 = 73 hours • Low photon energy • Potassium analogue that enters normal myocytes • Peak myocardial activity occurs 5–15 min after injection • Intracellular concentration of thallium depends on vascular supply and membrane function • Does not remain fixed in myocyte, redistributes

and acute pulmonary embolism. Relative contraindications include left main stenosis, uncontrolled hypertension, tachy- or bradyarrhythmia, left ventricular outflow obstruction, inability to exercise adequately, ventricular pacing, and Left Bundle Branch Block (LBBB). Perfusion imaging is preferred for patients whose baseline ECG has ST-segment abnormalities, digitalis therapy, LBBB, or pacing, and for those who have a significant pretest likelihood for coronary artery disease (CAD) or a history of previous revascularization to determine extent of ischemia. If they can exercise safely, they should have an exercise imaging study. Pharmacologic stress imaging is indicated for those patients who cannot exercise and do not have contraindications to the agent such as severe hypertension (dobutamine) or acute bronchospasm or hypotension (adenosine).

The selection of imaging modality for the heart will vary with expertise and availability of services in each institution. Stress echocardiography can be performed with exercise or pharmacologic agents. In nuclear medicine, myocardial perfusion imaging is commonly performed with thallium (Tl-201) or sestamibi, creating planar or SPECT images. The nuclear medicine physician or radiologist who performs nuclear medicine studies can provide guidance in selection of pharmacologic stress testing. Both agents are highly sensitive in detecting ischemia and scarred myocardium. Thallium is better for detecting viable myocardium, particularly "hibernating myocardium" because of its redistribution. Since SestaMIBI is used in larger doses, image quality will be higher and there will be more flexibility in the imaging protocol because the radioisotope does not redistribute in tissue over time. Preparation for these examinations includes abstaining from caffeine for 12 hours prior to the test and abstaining from food and tobacco for two hours prior to the test. The test itself may take two or more hours. SPECT images are obtained in the cardiac axes, short, long, and vertical. Normal myocardial perfusion imaging is associated with < 1% annual mortality while abnormal high risk findings predict 3% annual mortality and should be evaluated for coronary revascularization.

In some centers, cardiac PET-CT may be performed with rubidium-82, nitrogen-13 ammonia, or F-18 fluorodeoxyglucose. It can be performed with or without stress, particularly if the SPECT study is inconclusive or there is discordance between prior cardiac imaging tests. It may be helpful in determining the significance of an anatomic abnormality or coronary stenosis.

SCREENING FOR CORONARY ARTERY CALCIUM

At the initiation and progression of an atherosclerotic plaque, active processes cause calcium deposition in the coronary arteries. Best seen on cardiac-gated noncontrast CT, coronary calcification independently predicts cardiovascular events in intermediate risk patients and therefore provides additional prognostic data beyond traditional risk factors of age, diabetes, smoking, hyperlipidemia, and family history (**Table 108-6**). Calcium screening may be more beneficial in women than in men because traditional risk factors

TABLE 108-6 Coronary Calcium (CAC) Scores, a Surrogate of Total Atheroma Burden Independent of Pretest Relative Risk of MI or Cardiac Death

CAC Score: Lifetime Impact of All Atherosclerotic Risk Factors, Known & Unknown	Relative CAD Risk Proportional to Score based on Population Studies	Comments: Not a Functional Test, Does Not Signify Location or Severity of Blockage	Next Steps
0	Excludes most clinically relevant CAD	Even in high-risk asymptomatic or symptomatic populations	Healthy lifestyle and guideline-based treatment of individual risk factors; consider other diagnoses if symptomatic
≤10	Very low likelihood of CAD (<1%)	Considered a negative test	Healthy lifestyle and guideline-based treatment of individual risk factors; consider other diagnoses if symptomatic
11–100	2:1	Score 11–400 high risk > 2% risk of future cardiac events; future risk of score higher if younger	Consider functional study along with intensive risk factor modification
100–400	3-6:1	Test + for atherosclerosis & ↑ risk	Intensive risk factor modification; further cardiac testing
400–1000	5–10:1 Majority of coronary events in people with high calcium scores & scores > 75th percentile relative to age- & sex-matched controls	> 400 indicate extensive coronary artery disease with 90% probability of > 70% stenosis of a coronary artery; ≈ 5% per year risk of developing symptomatic heart disease.	Intensive risk factor modification; further cardiac testing
>1000	10–30:1	Very high risk	Intensive risk factor modification

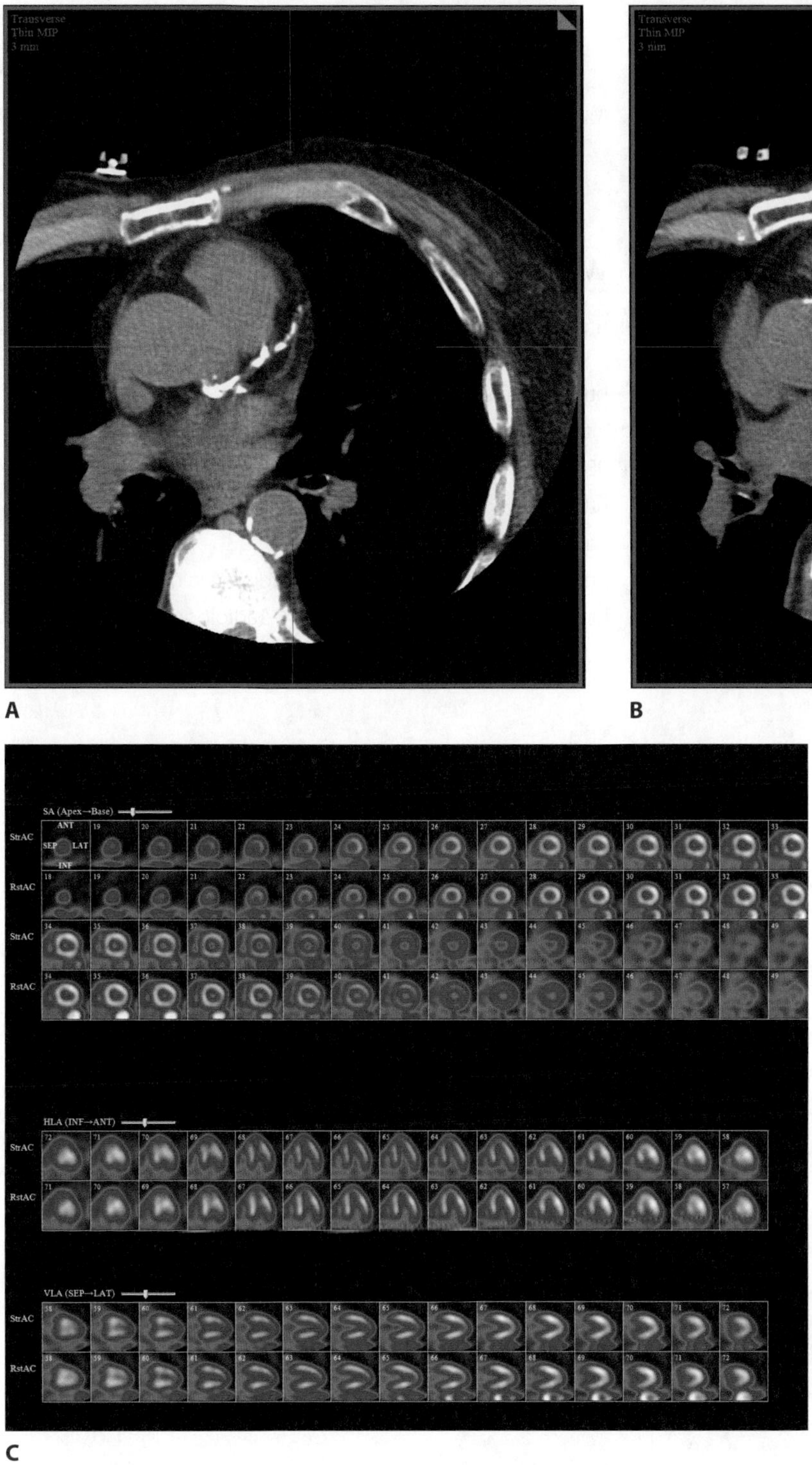

Figure 108-5 *Calcium score high, >3000; normal Rubidium-82 PET scan. (A and B) Calcification in left main coronary artery (left) continues in branches (right) seen on axial images from non-contrast enhanced cardiac-gated coronary CT scan. (C) Coronary artery calcifications not always indicative of obstructive CAD as in the same patient with no demonstrated functional impairment. Calcium scoring in a young patient more predictive of future risk.*

less accurately predict the presence of coronary artery disease in this population. Although there is no data supporting imaging for coronary calcification in low risk patients, it may be useful in asymptomatic intermediate risk patients to identify those patients who might benefit from the most aggressive risk factor modification or for imaging stable patients with chest discomfort to exclude obstructive coronary artery disease. The total (Agatson) score is based on the deposition of calcium in the left main, left anterior descending, left circumflex, and right coronary artery. A calcium score of more than 400 would preclude a contrast CTA given the significant decrease in PPV (**Figure 108-5**).

CONCLUSION

CT scanning is the primary advanced imaging for the chest in hospitalized patients. Through augmentation of chest radiographic data, the CT scan may answer questions that arise long after it is obtained. Accepting a negative result for definitive patient management is not appropriate when it is at odds with the pretest probability of the abnormality being present, particularly when the abnormality is one that cannot be missed, such as PE. In that situation, reviewing the images together with the radiologist may bring the report into agreement with the clinical impression that the likely abnormality is actually present. This process will also clarify the next steps, whether to treat the patient without further workup or order a different specific test. In the case of potential PE and other life-threatening possibilities, it is usually better to select a different modality. It is also important to consider the probability that the test will be adequate in relation to the interval since an acute event, particularly in the case of PE.

SUGGESTED READINGS

American Thoracic Society/European Respiratory Society International Multidisciplinary Consensus Classification of the Idiopathic Interstitial Pneumonias. *American Journal of Respiratory and Critical Care Medicine.* 2002;165(2):227–304.

Berland LL, Silverman SG, Gore RM, et al. Managing incidental findings on Abdominal CT: White paper of the ACR incidental findings committee. *Journal of the American College of Radiology.* 2010;7(10):754–773.

Robyn L. McClelland, Hyoju Chung, Robert Detrano, Wendy Post, Richard A. Distribution of Coronary Artery Calcium by Race, Gender, and Age: Results from the Multi-Ethnic Study of Atherosclerosis (MESA). *Kronmal Circulation*. 2006;113(1):30–37.

MacMahon H, Austin JH, Gamsu G, et al. Guidelines for management of small pulmonary nodules detected on CT scans: a statement from the Fleischner Society. *Radiology*. 2005;237:395–400

Mueller-Mang C, Grosse C, Schmid K, Stebellehener L, Bankier AA. What every radiologist should know about idiopathic interstitial pneumonias. *Radiographics*. 2007;27(3):595–615.

WEB RESOURCES

http://www.acr.org/SecondaryMainMenuCategories/quality_safety/app_criteria.aspx

http://jakemandell.com/iip/

interactive medical education

PE algorithm

http://www.guideline.gov/algorithm/5885/NGC-5885_2.pdf

Cardiac imaging

http://info.med.yale.edu/intmed/cardio/imaging/

http://www.ccsnm.org/pdfs/2010/radiologist-help-info/CardiacPracticeGuidelinesSummary.pdf

CHAPTER 109

Basic Abdominal Imaging

Francine L. Jacobson, MD, MPH
John M. Braver, MD
Sylvia C. McKean, MD, SFHM, FACP

Key Clinical Questions

1. What views are standard to evaluate the acute abdomen?
2. Which radiograph view is the most sensitive for detecting a small pneumoperitoneum?
3. What are the conditions simulating air under the diaphragm?
4. What are the causes of air-fluid levels on an erect abdominal image?
5. How do you quantify the amount of gas normally seen in the bowel?
6. What are the radiologic signs of bowel ischemia?
7. What are the most common abnormalities associated with acute pancreatitis?

INTRODUCTION

Despite the availability of newer imaging modalities to look for intestinal obstruction or perforation, the supine abdominal radiograph (KUB) remains indispensible for evaluating a patient with abdominal pain due to the ease and ready availability for rapidly screening patients with abdominal pain. The standard field of view extends from the lung bases to the pubic symphysis, thereby framing the genitourinary system, imaging kidneys, ureters, and bladder. Additional views include an erect chest radiograph, erect abdominal view, and left lateral decubitus.

Figure 109-1 is a line diagram pointing out the twelfth ribs, lumbar transverse process, kidneys, psoas line, inferior liver edge, terminal ileum, sacroiliac spine, gas in the ileum and jejunum, gas and feces in the transverse colon, haustral folds, and descending colon. A thin layer of adipose tissue should be visible as a lucent line between the transverse abdominal muscle and the peritoneum extending from above the lateral margin of the liver to below the iliac crest and between the dome of the bladder and the pelvic peritoneum.

The abdominal radiograph is not symmetric and in fact there is significant variation in a "normal" KUB as seen in **Figure 109-2**. Systematic review of examinations may be facilitated by use of a checklist (see **Table 109-1**).

In order to better perceive structures on abdominal radiographs and to better correlate physical exam and imaging findings, it can be helpful to study coronal anatomy images of computed tomography (CT) or magnetic resonance imaging (MRI) (see Chapter 110, **Table 109-2**).

Air helps to identify hollow viscous structures on radiographs. The anatomic rendering reveals the colon coursing from the right side of the pelvis, up to the liver, across to the spleen, and then down to the rectum. The presence of adipose tissue may assist interpretation. For example, a thin layer of fat is often seen between the dome of the bladder and the pelvic peritoneum as a lucent line. Location of this layer may be an important clue signifying an enlarged bladder (or urinary retention) as the cause of the patient's abdominal pain. Tissue-fat interfaces with the adjacent bowel facilitate assessment of organ size.

The erect chest radiograph is used to detect pneumoperitoneum, but it may also provide important clues to other causes from the chest that mimic an acute abdomen, including congestive heart failure from acute myocardial infarction, widened aorta seen in aortic dissection, pneumothorax, pneumomediastinum, pneumonia, and pleural fluid collections. The erect abdominal radiograph does not provide additional information to the standard KUB and erect chest film.

Working films may also be obtained for the management of support lines and tubes. The placement of tubes into the stomach and small bowel may be confirmed using a somewhat hybridized view of lower chest and upper abdomen.

RADIATION EXPOSURE

The KUB delivers a higher dose of ionizing radiation than a posteroanterior (PA) chest radiograph because the abdomen is almost always a thicker body part. The greater penetration provides enhanced visualization of lung bases and may identify lower lobe lung processes or pleural effusions associated with abdominal pain. It is particularly important to communicate with

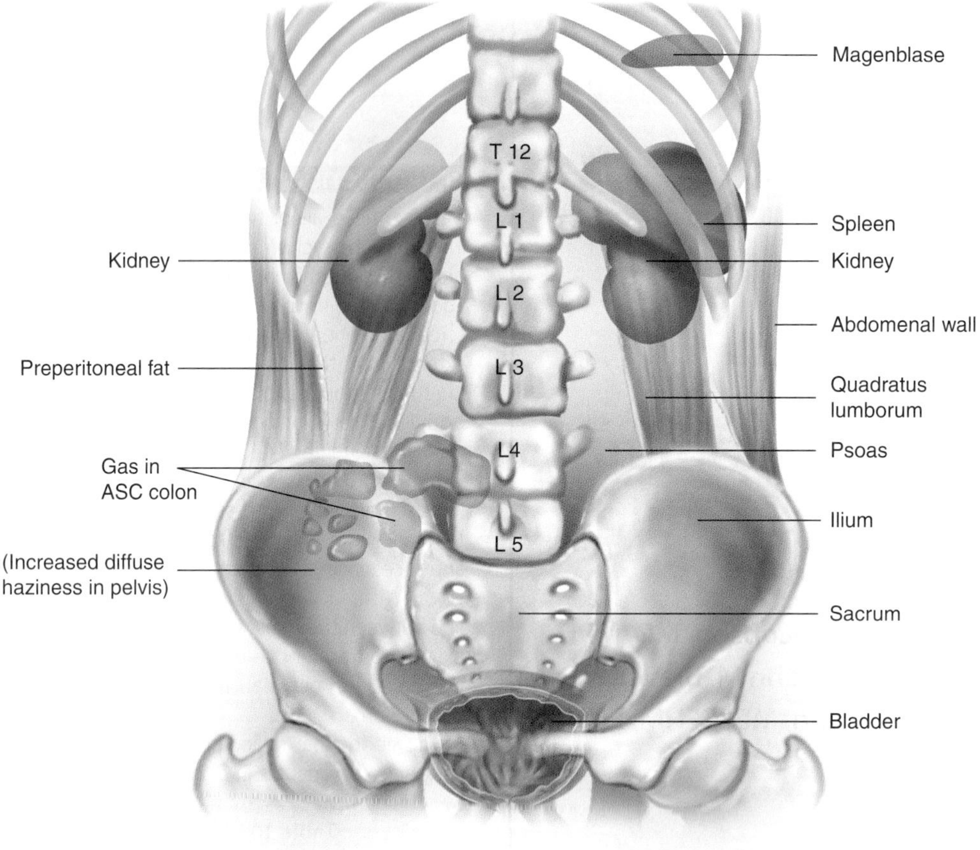

Figure 109-1 *Anatomic line drawing (including right kidney, psoas line, properitoneal fat line, inferior liver edge, terminal ileum, sacroiliac joint; twelfth rib, left psoas, haustral folds, lumbar transfer process, gas and feces in transverse colon, gas in jejunum, descending colon, gas in ileum).*

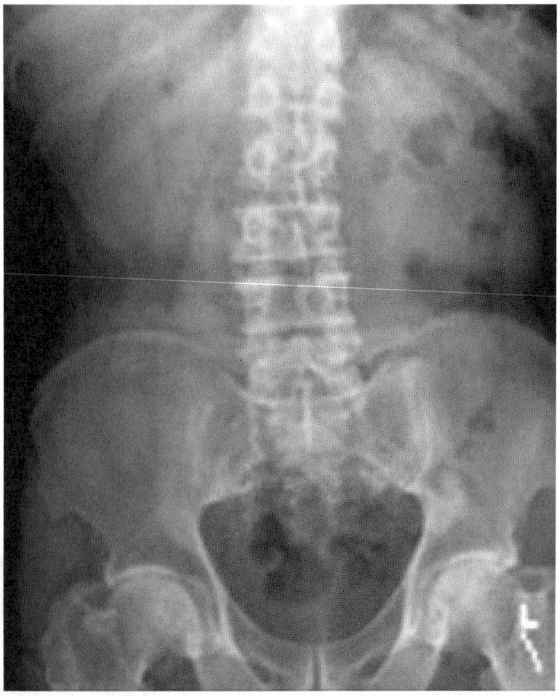

Figure 109-2 *Normal supine abdominal radiograph.*

the radiologic technologist regarding the priority areas for imaging when the patient is too large for a single 14 × 17 inch image. This can decrease duplication of exposure for completion of examination and repeated examinations that delay patient care.

PRACTICE POINT

Communication

- Provide specific localizing clinical information. This facilitates radiograph interpretation and limits radiation exposure when the patient is too large for a single 14 × 17 inch image.

SCREENING PLAIN FILMS

BONES

Plain films readily image ribs; lumbar vertebrae and appendages, especially transverse processes; sacrum; pelvis (iliac crests, acetabula, pubis); femoral head; and neck and may provide important clues to the patient's overall health. Patients with end-stage renal disease or endocrine disorders have characteristic bony changes and a screening plain film may uncover an underlying malignancy that has a prediction to bony metastasis.

Ribs, spine, and pelvic fractures can suggest location of soft tissue injury. If fractures are identified in the lower ribs and lumbar

TABLE 109-1 Checklist for Interpretation

- Diagnostic quality: Does the radiograph include the area from the diaphragm to the hernia orifices? Is the properitoneal lucency (flank stripe) separating the transverse abdominal muscle and parietal peritoneum visible?
- Alignment and integrity of bones, bone margins, joints: Are there any fractures of the lower ribs? Lumbar transverse processes? If so, worry about soft tissue injury to liver, spleen, and kidney. Is the acetabulum intact bilaterally?
- Soft tissues, fat-tissue interfaces.
- Air patterns: Look for pneumoperitoneum, abnormal bowel gas patterns, and air in biliary tree or portal vein.
- Size of organs.
- Calcification: Check for abnormal calcification (kidney stones, gall stones, pancreatic or splenic calcifications).

transverse processes, consider soft tissue injury to the liver, spleen, or kidney. Spine and sacroilliac (SI) joints may indicate chronic arthritic changes.

GAS PATTERNS

Normal

Air and fluid are both normally present in the gastrointestinal (GI) tract. Fluid is secreted into the GI tract even when a patient has no oral intake. The movement of gas through the system over time is valuable data for functional evaluation even from a single radiograph. The stomach and small and large bowels will normally distend to accommodate gas. The amount of gas normally seen in the small bowel is <2.5 cm in diameter and <5.5 cm in diameter for the colon. The cecum can normally be somewhat larger, up to 8 cm (**Table 109-3**).

TABLE 109-2 Visibility of Structures on KUB

Organ	Usually Seen	Potentially Seen	Not Seen
Liver	X		
Spleen	X		
Kidneys	X		
Stomach	X		
Duodenum		X	
Small intestine	X		
Cecum		X	
Colon	X		
Bladder	X		
Prostate		X	
Retroperitoneal fat	X		
Gallbladder			X
Pancreas			X
Adrenal glands			X
Ovaries			X
Uterus		X	
Ureters		X	
Lymph nodes			X
Mesentery			X
Vasculature			X

Calcification may localize otherwise inapparent organs.

TABLE 109-3 Bowel Gas Patterns

Ileus versus obstruction: air-fluid levels, distention of small and large bowels

Obstruction

- Small bowel obstruction: 3–5 hours after onset of complete obstruction, progression marked by collapse of distal bowel and absence of air in colon; central distribution, absence of feces, close valvulae conniventes extending across entire diameter of bowel, string of pearl sign.
- Large bowel obstruction: Peripheral distribution, haustral sacculations, presence of feces.
- Pseudoobstruction: Diffuse dilation of small and large bowel, often with prominent gastric distension.
- Volvulus: Closed obstruction of loops, leading to proximal and distal occlusion of portions of bowel, most commonly cecum (haustral sacculations present) and sigmoid colon.

Ileus

- Postoperative ileus.
- Sentinal loop sign focal adynamic ileus as in duodenum adjacent to inflamed pancreas.

Pneumoperitoneum

The acute abdomen is assessed by two types of radiographs, the abdominal flat plate "KUB" with the patient in the supine position, and at least one more radiograph of either the chest or abdomen in the erect or decubitus position in order to look for gravitational effects and, in particular, the abnormal gas pattern of pneumoperitoneum. In many institutions, an acute abdomen series will include a PA view of the chest, supine view of the abdomen, and an erect view of the abdomen. The erect chest radiograph is the most sensitive for detecting a small pneumoperitoneum; however, the best gravity view is the left lateral decubitus view for patients unable to stand. The patient should be placed in position for a minimum of 10 minutes prior to obtaining this view to allow air to rise above the liver where it will become radiographically apparent.

Although the 2–3 mm thick diaphragm provides a useful silhouette for free intraperitoneal air, both benign and pathologic conditions can mimic pneumoperitoneum. Distention of the stomach thin walls may cause concern for pneumoperitoneum actually due to air in a distended or overdistended stomach. Interposition of the colon between the right hemidiaphragm and liver, called Chilaiditis Syndrome, may raise concern for free air when the air is actually contained within the colon. Basilar pneumothorax causes thickening of the pleura or subsegmental atelectasis when parallel to the hemidiaphragm. The presence of gas within the bowel wall itself, pneumotosis coli, can also raise concern for pneumoperitoneum even when it is a benign finding.

Air-fluid levels and dilatation

Pain anywhere in the body can cause increased gas due to swallowed air. Abnormal gas patterns may suggest acute perforation, gastroparesis, adynamic ileus, small bowel obstruction, large bowel

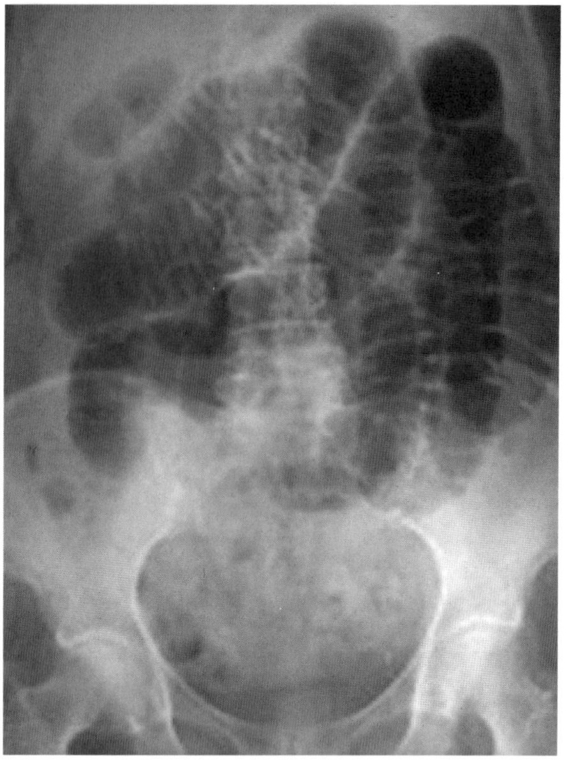

Figure 109-3 *Small bowel dilatation.*

obstruction, and toxic megacolon. However, fluid levels are not pathognomic of obstruction. In addition to ileus and obstruction, air-fluid levels on erect abdominal plain film may normally be seen (if < 2.5 cm in length) or related to gastroenteritis, electrolyte disturbances (hypokalemia), uremia, and ischemia. If on plain film of the abdomen the diameter of the small bowel exceeds 3 cm, it suggests either an obstruction or an ileus. If the small bowel dilatation is > 4 cm, an obstruction is more likely. The key to the differentiation of colonic obstruction and paralytic ileus on plain film is whether there is dilation of the cecum. If the transverse colon is more dilated than the cecum, a diagnosis of ileus is most likely. The cecum is the most dilated segment of the colon in obstruction. Megacolon refers to a dilation of the transverse colon > 5.0–6 cm. The cutoff is not precise because it depends on the clinical context. For example, as patient size increases, magnification increases so that a normal looking large colon that shill has haustration may be read as normal in an asymptomatic obese individual. When there is acute colonic distention with the cecum > 9 cm, there is an emergent risk of perforation (**Figure 109-3**).

The distribution of distension may localize the obstruction, which may be partial or complete. Small bowel dilated loops (central location and close valvulae across entire diameter) are usually evident within three to five hours after complete obstruction. Proximal to an obstruction, peristalsis increases as an attempt to move the bowel contents beyond a site of mechanical obstruction. The hyperperistalsis continues beyond the obstruction resulting in the clearing of the GI tract distal to the point of obstruction. These correlate with tinkles and rushes heard through the stethoscope. If dilated small bowel extends to the lower portion of the abdomen, it indicates that the obstruction is at least in the distal small bowel or perhaps in the proximal colon. Small bowel obstruction (SBO) will result in an emptied colon and central stair-step configuration of fluid levels in the small bowel. If air is seen distally in the colon or rectum, either a partial small bowel obstruction or an acute complete small bowel obstruction may be present (as some of the air distal to the obstruction site has not yet been expelled). Gallstone ileus from the passage of a gallstone into the GI tract infrequently produces signs of small bowel obstruction or gas in the biliary tree.

PRACTICE POINT

Guiding principles

Ensure that a patient receives the least radiation during imaging.

- Make sure that the study is necessary.
  - Do you need an initial KUB if you are planning to order an abdominal CT anyway?
  - Do you need an erect abdominal radiograph? The erect abdominal radiograph does not provide additional information to the standard supine abdominal radiograph and erect chest radiographs.
- You can save repeated examinations with consequent expense, added radiation, and attendant delay of clinical care by communicating your clinical concerns that the examination will address.
  - The size of a patient's abdomen is frequently larger than what can be captured by a single view.
  - The technologist performing the examination will need to cut off the anatomy depending on the clinical information provided.
  - To ensure that a patient receives the least radiation in the course of abdominal imaging, the order must include the clinical concern that the examination is supposed to address.
- When in doubt about the utility of an additional test, consult your radiology team.

Radiographic features of large bowel obstruction include peripheral location of dilatation, thick haustral sacculations that do not extend across the entire diameter, and the presence of feces. If the ileocecal valve is competent, there is a greater risk of cecal perforation. Pseudoobstruction may involve diffuse dilatation of both the small and large bowel as well as the stomach.

PRACTICE POINT

Obstruction

- If the small bowel dilatation is > 4 cm an obstruction is more likely. The key to the differentiation of colonic obstruction and paralytic ileus on plain film is whether there is dilation of the cecum. If the transverse colon is more dilated than the cecum, a diagnosis of ileus is most likely. The cecum is the most dilated segment of the colon in obstruction. Megacolon refers to a dilation of the transverse colon > 6 cm.

Adynamic ileus, most often seen in postoperative patients on large doses of pain medications, differs from the appearance of SBO because the small bowel and colon dilate to accommodate the large amounts of swallowed gas that is able to move freely within the bowel, even without the patient being able to pass gas.

Other abnormal gas patterns include "a string of pearls" sign, sentinel loop sign, and omega loop. As the lumen of an obstructed small bowel fills with fluid, small bubbles of air are trapped in most of the superior aspect of the lumen between the valvulae conniventes, looking like "a string of pearls." The sentinel loop sign refers to an ileus localized to a segment of bowel from a focal inflammatory process such as appendicitis, cholecystitis, or pancreatitis. The omega loop sign, referring to a massively dilated loop of colon that looks like an inverted U projecting out of the pelvis toward the right upper quadrant, suggests sigmoid volvulus (which is three times more common than cecal volvulus). Here there is a closed obstruction of loops resulting in complete occlusion of both the proximal and distal portions of the involved bowel.

An abdominal radiograph may also reveal emphysematous collections (typically in diabetics) referring to air outlining the gall bladder or urinary bladder. Pneumatosis coli is a benign condition presenting radiographically as intramural gas limited to the colon.

ABDOMINAL ORGANS

Differentiation between various soft tissue structures on radiographs is largely based on relationships between organs, adjacent gas-containing bowel, and fat planes. The soft tissue densities of the liver, spleen, and kidneys can be measured to determine their size.The liver typically measures 21–22.5 cm across the widest point, 15–17.5 cm in cranial-caudal extent, 10–12.5 cm from front to back. The size and shape of the liver, however, varies. Riedel lobe refers to its posterior edge, extending downward to the iliac crest. The spleen measures approximately 11 cm; autosplenectomy is common in sickle cell disease. The kidneys normally measure 12–14 cm. Asymmetry in kidney size may be an important clue to the presence of significant underlying kidney disease. In some instances the kidney size may be increased as in polycystic renal disease. The aorta normally measures 3 cm in diameter. Unless calcified, the pancreas will not be visualized on plain film.

CALCIFICATIONS

Pelvic phleboliths due to pelvic vein thrombosis and lymph nodes are the most common calcifications seen on KUB. Approximately 15% of gallstones and 85% of kidney stones appear radio-opaque and radiographs can reveal a staghorn calculus filling the intrarenal collecting system or the tiniest calcification at the ureteropelvic junction responsible for producing renal colic.

DO NOT MISS DIAGNOSES

With the exception of free peritoneal air, the diagnosis of most life-threatening disorders relies upon nonspecific radiographic signs in the clinical context of the patient. Concern about any of these possibilities should prompt further imaging or life-saving surgical exploration.

Pneumoperitoneum

A supine radiograph may reveal intraperitoneal air under the inferior aspect of the liver or hepatorenal recess (Morrison pouch). Air may be evident between adjacent loops of bowel such that air is seen on both sides of the bowel wall (Rigler sign). The Cupula sign refers to larger air collections under the central tendon of the diaphragm creating a central crescentic lucency. Following abdominal surgery, a pneumoperitoneum may be visible for up to a week or more, depending on the amount of gas and the body habitus of the patient. Pneumoperitoneum may be continually seen in the presence of a percutaneous gastrostomy.

Splenic injury

Risk factors for splenic injury include trauma, domestic violence, and complications from procedures. Splenic injury cannot be excluded by a normal abdominal or chest radiograph. Possible nonspecific clues to splenic injury may be found in the erect chest radiograph, such as raised left hemidiaphragm, pleural effusion, basal atelectasis, and lower rib fracture. The KUB may reveal a left upper quadrant mass and medial displacement of gastric air bubble, inferomedial displacement of splenic flexure, splenic enlargement due to subcapsular hemorrhage, or signs of hemoperitoneum.

Retroperitoneal hemorrhage

Risk factors for retroperitoneal hemorrhage include spontaneous bleeding due to a coagulopathy and procedure-related complications. Absence of a right psoas shadow may be normal in one-fifth of the population due to superimposed bowel contents or may be a clue to retroperitoneal hemorrhage due to free blood, psoas hematoma, or fractures of the vertebral spinous process. Other clues to retroperitoneal hemorrhage include bulging of the lateral margin of psoas shadow due to bleeding into the muscle fascia, loss of definition of the ipsilateral kidney, and ipsilateral fractures of the lower ribs or lumbar transverse processes.

Aortic dissection

Calcifications associated with an abdominal aortic aneurysm may increase suspicion for a leaking aneurysm and prompt scrutiny of surrounding soft tissues, which may be more prominent due to associated inflammation from blood. An increased soft tissue density between the descending colon and properitoneal line may signify blood in the left paracolic gutter (which may result from procedures, dissection, and splenic rupture).

Hepatic injury

Fracture of the right lower rib and a subphrenic fluid collection are nonspecific signs that may prompt additional imaging.

SEVERE ABDOMINAL PAIN

The more severe the abdominal pain, the greater the likelihood that the initial plain film will be abnormal. By screening for abnormal gas patterns, distention of bowel loops, organomegaly, calcification, and masses, the KUB and upright may indicate the need for additional imaging of a specific location.

Acute pancreatitis

Acute pancreatitis usually is associated with normal plain films, and less commonly with dilated duodenal sentinel loop surrounding the inflamed pancreas, loss of left psoas sign, signs of gastric outlet obstruction, and left-sided pleural effusion. The colon may appear distended by gas through the transverse segment with a "colon cutoff sign" with absence of gas in colon distal to the splenic flexure. Additional clues include sympathetic pleural effusion and the presence of radio-opaque gallstones (gallstone pancreatitis). Evidence of prior episodes of acute pancreatitis include loss of fat planes and masses that might represent pseudocysts and punctuate pancreatic calcifications.

Bowel ischemia

Bowel ischemia does not necessarily produce radiographic abnormality until late in the clinical course and it can also be intermittent. Nonspecific signs include bowel wall thickening and bowel wall dilatation. Pneumotosis intestinalis may be present. Bowel

TABLE 109-4 Suspected Diagnoses Not Requiring the KUB Before Going Directly to Advanced Imaging

- Appendicitis: Skip KUB and go directly to CT (specifying appendix).
- Biliary colic, acute choleycystitis, cholangitis: Skip KUB and go directly to right upper quadrant ultrasound.
- Diverticulitis: Skip KUB and go directly to CT abdomen
- Gastric or duodenal ulcer: Esophagogastroduodenoscopy; the erect chest radiograph is the most sensitive X-ray for detecting a small pneumoperitoneum.
- Intestinal obstruction if abdominal CT planned anyway.
- Pancreatitis: Skip KUB and go directly to right upper quadrant ultrasound to rule out gallstone pancreatitis.
- Abdominal CT in selected circumstances (see Chapter 110).

ischemia initially mimics mechanical obstruction, but with progression the bowel wall becomes severely thickened due to edema and necrosis. Ischemic colitis usually affects splenic flexure and descending colon imaged as thumb printing due to submucosal hemorrhage, with progressive linear gas in the bowel wall due to necrosis, and free air from perforation. Gas in the portal vein is a poor prognostic sign.

Acute inflammatory colitis

Initially, in ulcerative colitis the distribution of feces may indicate the extent of inflammation, where there is usually an abrupt cut off from normal bowel. With progression, there may be pseudopolyps, which represent extensive mucosal ulceration leaving small mucosal islands, a gasless colon, and finally, toxic megacolon when the transfer colonic diameter exceeds 5.5 cm.

SELECTION OF MORE SPECIFIC ABDOMINAL IMAGING

Specific diagnoses may require advanced imaging without a prior screening KUB (**Table 109-4**).

The KUB may be used to select more specific abdominal imaging. Ultrasound examination may be directed to the kidneys or the gallbladder based on history and physical examination as well as KUB. CT scanning is commonly used to image a larger area, typically including the pelvis with the abdomen, although the radiation dose required is relatively large (approximately 25 mSv). MRI is not commonly chosen based on KUB but can be valuable for assessment of specific organs and for patients who are allergic to the iodinated intravenous contrast material required for CT examination of vascular structures in the abdomen. Nuclear medicine is useful for investigation of gastric emptying and gastrointestinal bleeding.

Even a completely normal KUB may be helpful in patients with severe abdominal pain by directing additional testing. Ischemic bowel may have a grave prognosis, in part due to the discordance between signs and symptoms if the diagnosis is not suspected. These patients may not be further evaluated until the bowel is gangrenous and has perforated. (See Chapter 110).

ALTERNATIVE ABDOMINAL SCREENING

Depending upon presentation of the current illness, initial imaging of the abdomen may be directed to a more specific organ system leading to appropriate selection of an alternative screening examination. The ability of ultrasound (US) to study physiologic effects and localize symptoms is also valuable when screening the abdomen. Even without signs and symptoms specific to the GU or GI tract, screening of the abdomen can be performed with abdominal ultrasound examination. Although US does not image gas patterns well due to US properties, it provides superior information regarding solid organs and can assist the performance of paracentesis. Readily available, it can be performed at the patient's bedside, it costs less than CT and MRI examinations, and it limits patient exposure to ionizing radiation, particularly during pregnancy.

SERIAL FILMS

Although a change in patient condition is the best indication of when to order a follow-up KUB, serial abdominal films will demonstrate worsening GI tract dismotility that might require emergent surgical consultation to avoid acute perforation. When doubt exists, follow-up studies will demonstrate the resolution of GI tract dismotility from gastroparesis, small bowel obstruction, and adynamic ileus or the passage of kidney stones. Serial films over time monitor the evolution of such processes without more direct abdominal or GI tract imaging. This approach minimizes radiation both by decreasing the number of images and also because of the lower radiation dose.

Serial abdominal films can be very useful during hospitalization. The resolution of GI tract dismotility and restoration of normal bowel gas pattern are reassuringly demonstrated on follow-up studies. Progress of renal calculi through the ureter may be evaluated on follow-up studies as well. Change in patient condition is the best indicator of when to order a follow-up KUB. Bleeding with mass-like hematoma formation, bowel perforation due to stress, and return of abdominal pain related to adhesions from prior surgery are examples of situations in which working abdominal radiographs can quickly and inexpensively provide the information to optimize health care and minimize length of stay.

Serial working chest radiographs over time may monitor abdominal gastrointestinal disease processes such as gastroparesis, small bowel obstruction, and adynamic ileus without more direct abdominal or GI tract imaging. This is helpful for minimizing radiation both by decreasing the number of images and also because the radiation dose for the chest radiograph is less than for the KUB.

CONCLUSION

This chapter presents a framework for ordering plain abdominal imaging and stresses the importance of providing key clinical information and asking the right questions to get the most out of a radiologist's interpretation. The KUB most frequently identifies the presence of obstruction, calculi, gallstones, or ileus for patients with acute abdominal pain. Working with abdominal radiographs can quickly and inexpensively provide actionable information in acute abdominal pain related to surgical adhesions, bleeding with mass-like hematoma formation, and bowel perforation. The KUB may be used to select more specific abdominal imaging. Modalities used to image the abdomen include Ultrasound, CT, nuclear medicine, and MRI.

SUGGESTED READING

Begg JD. *Abdominal X-Rays Made Easy,* 2nd ed. London, England: Churchill Livingston Elsevier; 2006.

CHAPTER 110

Advanced Abdominal Imaging

Francine L. Jacobson, MD, MPH
Cheryl A. Sadow, MD
John M. Braver, MD

Key Clinical Questions

1. What are the advantages and limitations of abdominal ultrasound?
2. What are the indications for gastrointestinal (GI) fluoroscopy?
3. What are the advantages of computed tomography (CT) when compared with magnetic resonance imaging (MRI) for imaging abdominal structures?
4. What are the indications for nuclear medicine imaging studies?

INTRODUCTION

Radiologists expect to provide guidance in the use of advanced medical imaging tests in the care of acutely ill patients requiring hospitalization. This chapter is intended to present the thought processes that radiologists commonly use rather than dictate a particular test for a particular patient or situation.

Before ordering advanced imaging, it is always important to consider whether the information may be provided by prior studies. The kidneys ureter and bladder (KUB) is often ordered as a screening examination but also serves as the initial default imaging examination when selection of a more specific test cannot be made, as when a patient has diffuse abdominal pain without any localizing signs. No preparation is required. The radiation exposure is slightly higher than a chest radiograph. Although originally IV and orally contrast material was administered in conjunction with plain film radiography, this is no longer common practice. However, in the acutely ill patient who has received one or more contrast agents for a prior study, the KUB can provide additional information without readministration of contrast material, especially for patients with abdominal pain occurring during or shortly after imaging of a different region of the body. A rudimentary intravenous pyelogram (IVP) can be obtained following contrast-enhanced head or chest CT or even cardiac catheterization. The period of time over which the visualization persists will be inversely proportional to the patient's estimated glomerular filtration rate (eGFR) over several hours. The oral contrast material administered for an abdominal CT scan will be concentrated within the colon and often remain visible for several days.

ULTRASOUND OF THE ABDOMEN

Ultrasound can be the best possible examination for the acutely ill hospitalized patient. It is relatively inexpensive, uses no ionizing radiation, and tailored examinations can be performed at the patient's bedside if necessary. Ultrasound is enhanced by passage through water and stopped by air and bone. It is therefore able to detect a pleural effusion and guide thoracentesis of small to moderate pleural effusions. The information provided depends very much on the operator even with complete video recording. Ultrasound is a very useful tool for the interventional radiologist and may be chosen by the radiologist for a variety of biopsies including liver and prostate.

ABDOMINAL US

In the abdomen, renal and gallbladder ultrasounds are standard examinations. A screening abdominal ultrasound will also include images of the liver, spleen, and pancreas. The confirmation of a simple cyst can exclude more significant pathology in many organs, including ovaries, kidneys, and liver. In order to visualize the pancreas, the ultrasonographer will either compress the air out of the stomach or have the patient drink water to allow the stomach to act as an acoustical window, enhancing the through transmission of the sound waves to the pancreas behind the stomach. The tail of the pancreas may be inadequately examined due to air in the adjacent small bowel.

PELVIC US

Pelvic ultrasound imaging may be performed transabdominally through a full urinary bladder to provide an acoustical window or transvaginally for imaging ovaries. Ultrasound routinely evaluates pregnancies for diagnosis, prognosis, and on occasion, treatment of fetal disease.

VASCULAR US

Vascular ultrasound can identify DVT that prevents veins from collapsing when compressed. This is most helpful in the lower extremities and cannot be performed in regions, such as the pelvis, in which the veins cannot be directly compressed.

GASTROINTESTINAL (GI) FLUOROSCOPY

Limited GI fluoroscopy involves contrast administration followed by obtaining a KUB. A full fluoroscopic examination includes a physical examination by the radiologist to localize the patient's pain with palpation of the opacified structures of the gastrointestinal tract. During fluoroscopy, X-rays strike a fluorescent screen on which an image can be simultaneously formed and viewed. In early fluoroscopy units, the image was inferior, especially with larger patients, and the examination had to be performed in the dark (always literally, sometimes figuratively!) after the radiologist had first adapted his eyes to the dark by wearing red goggles. With modern equipment, which incorporates an image intensification system, the images can be viewed on a television monitor in comfortably subdued light.

The nature of the fluoroscopic examination provides physiologic as well as anatomic and pathologic information. The patient's position or physiologic state may be changed to provoke the chief complaint. The study begins with a supine view of the abdomen and continues with the radiologist at the bedside during the administration of contrast. With fluoroscopy, the radiologist can view the image directly on a television screen in real time without exposing an image and waiting for it to be processed. This "real-time" evaluation is especially useful for studying a dynamic, constantly changing system such as inducing gastroesophageal reflux. Attached to the image intensification tower is a device for making and transferring digital images to a picture archiving and storage system (PACS). During the examination, the radiologist will "spot image" areas of interest that he or she discovers fluoroscopically, and areas not optimally demonstrated on the overhead images, such as the convolutions of the sigmoid colon and the duodenal bulb. The spot images are not meant to replace or necessarily duplicate the overhead images the technologist takes. Many areas need to be "unfolded" and will be seen well only on adequately positioned spot images. The advantage of this system is that a permanent record can be made when the patient is perfectly positioned; otherwise one runs the risk of missing the abnormality on the overheads, which are exposed according to a set routine. Movie cameras (cine) and magnetic tape or computer-based recorders can be adapted to the basic system; the advance allows a dynamic recording of the constantly-in-motion GI tract for later review, and permanent storage if desired. This advance is particularly useful for interpreting and storing a videofluoroscopic study of the swallowing mechanism.

PATIENT PREPARATION

Patient preparation varies from no preparation, to nothing orally and full bowel preparation, depending on the examination. Patient preparation should also include planning for the excretion of contrast material that will be concentrated in the colon and potentially cause severe constipation. Fluid and physical movement, such as walking, are most helpful. Should follow-up working images of the abdomen or chest be obtained, one should pay attention to whether retained barium is present.

It is useful to watch several of these studies being performed in order to realize the best studies require active participation by the patient, moving through a series of positions that may include prone and every angle between prone and supine. GI fluoroscopy exams that require fasting are generally scheduled in the morning. In the afternoon, the same fluoroscopy suite may be used to study swallowing function in patients who are at risk for aspiration. Non-GI fluoroscopic examinations including retrograde cystography and joint arthroscopy, and chest fluoroscopy will also generally be scheduled after the completion of the GI fluoroscopy schedule.

ADVANCE COMMUNICATION WITH RADIOLOGIST TO TAILOR STUDY TO THE PATIENT

Examinations can be tailored to the specific needs and issues of the patient. Discussion in advance with the radiologist allows for more input than generally conveyed when ordering the examination. The examination types are used as starting points. A video swallow examination of the oropharynx is performed with a variety of liquid and solid contrast materials to determine risk for aspiration and identify protective positions in which a patient may swallow particular types of food safely. A barium swallow examination will briefly study the oropharynx and then focus on the esophagus itself in the erect position followed by the supine position. The stomach may be incompletely studied although the term "barium swallow" is also sometimes used as a synonym for the upper GI examination that includes the barium swallow with detailed examination of the stomach and duodenum. Delayed images to follow oral contrast material through the small bowel add the element of a small bowel follow-through to the upper GI examination.

The small bowel can be difficult to completely image and specialized small bowel enema, or enteroclysis, can be performed to identify rare small bowel lesions. For this examination, a feeding tube is placed through the nose to allow the contrast material to be delivered directly into the duodenum. The preparation may involve laxatives as well as a liquid diet for 24 hours or more prior to the enteroclysis. Medications that slow transit through the GI tract may need to be discontinued prior to the examination. Barium enema examinations may be performed with single or double contrast material. A limited study may be adequate to localize colonic obstruction such as seen with apple core colon cancer lesions in the sigmoid colon. Retained fecal material can interfere with the detection of polyps. Barium enema may be performed following incomplete colonoscopy to supplement the examination without repeating the preparation. The appendix and terminal ileum may be filled by the retrograde flow of contrast material.

CT SCAN OF THE ABDOMEN

Abdominal CT scanning may be performed as a screening examination or with a very specific protocol focusing on a single region or physiologic process. Thus it is very important to convey the reason for the examination to the radiologist in order for the examination to provide the needed diagnostic information. The information provided to the radiologist will determine the suitability of the examination performed to answer clinical questions at the time of examination and later on during the course of patient hospitalization. In many institutions, the pelvis will be included in a complete abdomen CT, while in some institutions a specific order may be required to include the pelvis. Pelvic CT can generally be ordered without an abdominal CT although this is most commonly done for pelvic fractures and on occasion for gynecological disease.

ABDOMINAL PAIN

Scanning is generally performed at least 70 seconds following the initial administration of IV contrast material. Such a scan will provide contrast enhancement of the liver, spleen, adrenal glands, kidneys, and if preceded by oral contrast administration, the GI tract including stomach, small bowel, and colon. This type of study is performed for the evaluation of abdominal pain and will allow detection of a wide variety of pathology, including abscesses, organ-specific masses, selected functional abnormalities and metastases, especially to liver and bones. It should be noted that on occasion, iodinated contrast material will decrease the visibility of liver metastases. This is particularly true of breast cancer metastases. In oncology centers, the liver may be imaged before and after the administration of IV contrast material to evaluate for potential breast cancer metastases.

Flank pain is most often addressed with CT performed without oral or intravenous contrast material. Intravenous contrast material is unnecessary for the detection of potentially calcified stones. In this setting, following of the ureter is generally facilitated by ureteral obstruction causing the renal colic.

Obstruction of hepatic ducts and pancreatic ducts also makes these structures more apparent and more easily measured. In the liver, the basic examination is generally adequate. The smaller pancreas benefits from a thin section examination with optimal parenchymal enhancement at 45 seconds after contrast material administration, earlier than that of the liver.

The gastrointestinal tract is increasingly imaged with CT, particularly for abnormalities that can also involve lymph nodes, such as lymphoma, and for abnormalities that lead to fistulae as a complication, such as Crohn disease. Intermittent symptoms may be due to intussusception or internal hernia. The identification of these abnormalities may be less straightforward and benefit from direct consultation with the radiologist. Appendicitis can be diagnosed on CT although the increasing concern to limit patient exposure to ionizing radiation may increase the use of ultrasound in the future.

HEMANGIOMAS

Sometimes focused CT scanning is performed to differentiate hemangiomas from metastases or from simple cysts. Hemangiomas in the liver are most often an incidental finding because they do not cause symptoms until very large. They have a greater tendency to lobulation and can overlap in appearance to metastases. In order to confirm the identity of a hepatic hemangioma, the lesion is localized prior to administration of IV contrast material, after which the same region is repeatedly scanned over time to document the characteristic filling in of the lesion by contrast material. When the differentiation appropriately can be delayed until the patient is an outpatient, MRI or nuclear medicine scintigraphy may be used for this purpose.

PRACTICE POINT

- When an "incidental" finding suggests the possibility of a malignancy or the need for follow-up studies, always review prior films. Imaging studies obtained for other reasons sometimes years earlier are often helpful and may reveal preexisting "stable" abnormalities. Any prior noted abnormalities should be clearly documented, added to the patient's current problem list, and include an assessment and follow-up plan based on radiologic consultation and communication with the patient's primary care physician.

ADRENAL GLAND

The adrenal gland is seen on upper abdominal CT. The most common lesion, often an incidental finding, is an adrenal adenoma. These are characterized by low attenuation on scans without intravenous contrast enhancement. Contrast can interfere with this determination, although the distinct smooth margin can make this the most likely lesion present. Adrenal metastases, most associated with lung cancer, generally have poorly defined margins and may infiltrate surrounding fat. The adrenal glands are generally included and reported specifically on chest CT scans. Functional tumors such as a pheochromocytoma may not be identified by CT when their physiologic effect is far greater than their size. Pheochromocytoma can also occur in the mediastinum, increasing the region of concern.

CT ANGIOGRAPHY

CT angiography is used increasingly to spare patients the invasiveness and radiation exposure of conventional angiography. It is particularly useful when vascular disease is part of a larger differential diagnosis. Pain out of proportion to findings on examination is a classic presentation of mesenteric ischemia. This can be difficult to assess in the acutely ill patient and may need to be considered in the planning of an abdominal CT scan.

PATIENT PREPARATION

Patient preparation most frequently involves fasting followed by oral administration of contrast material prior to the scan. Iodinated intravenous contrast material is frequently used, although different timing is selected for different purposes. Renal function testing is generally required prior to contrast administration in order to safeguard renal function that may be diminished, particularly in acutely ill patients.

MRI OF THE ABDOMEN

Most alternatives are preferable for hospitalized patients. MRI can be a very difficult examination for the acutely ill patient due to the length of the procedure, confinement, and noise. When the patient is unable to lie still, follow commands, and perform repeated breath-holds, the sought-after benefit will be elusive. For a patient who has had anaphylaxis in response to iodinated contrast material, MRI can be used in lieu of CT, particularly when vascular structures must be evaluated. MRI provides the highest possible level of tissue characterization and can identify each and every specific hemoglobin degradation product. MRI is relied upon for characterization of tissue in the adrenal gland and prostate gland. When pathology is identified on female pelvic ultrasound, the next examination may be MRI rather than CT. MRI is inferior to CT for characterization of calcification, which appears on MRI only as a signal void. The data from CT and MR are often complementary, with greater soft tissue characterization and fascial plane discrimination by MRI while CT has higher spatial resolution as well as visualizing calcifications.

MRI cannot be performed for patients who have just had surgery. Most MRI facilities are unable to offer MRI to a patient who has a pacemaker. Cerebral aneurysm clips placed many years ago are not safe in MRI. Patients who have worked with metals or could, for any other reason, have metal foreign bodies in their eyes must have screening radiographs of the orbits. Most patients with indwelling orthopedic hardware can have MR examination as long as the heating of the metal during the MRI is not excessive. MRI technologists will screen patients to ensure patient safety. In cases in which the patient is unable to communicate adequately with the technologist, it is important to enlist the aid of a family member or advocate. This person can safely remain in the imaging suite if that increases the ability of the patient to undergo the MRI examination.

MRI examinations are performed using surface coils that have finite sizes. The imaging range may need to be adapted to make sure the area of greatest interest is imaged. The use of Vitamin E capsules can be helpful when a palpable mass is present or the patient can point to a specific painful location. Unlike CT, in which extending the examination of the abdomen to include the pelvis is easily done, each type of MRI examination will require a separate set-up and imaging sequence. The abdomen and pelvis are separate examinations, as is the lumbar spine, which would each constitute a separate MRI examination with each requiring the full time for a MRI. Above all else, MRI is not a screening examination but rather an examination to solve a very specific problem.

Gadolinium contrast material is used for most but not all MRI examinations. Sliding scales have been introduced to decrease patient dose and the resulting risk of developing nephrogenic systemic fibrosis (NSF). Allergic reactions to gadolinium-based contrast agents are less common than to iodinated contrast agents but are not rare as previously thought based upon the inert nature of gadolinium.

NUCLEAR MEDICINE

The three most basic abdominal examinations for hospitalized patients are HIDA, GI bleeding, and gastric emptying studies. Specialized functional studies can be performed to identify endocrine tumors.

The radiotracer, most commonly technetium 99-m, is attached to an appropriate ligand to demonstrate the physiology of interest and is administered intravenously. While the radiation dose is small, the duration of exposure is most significant. The half-life of technetium 99-m is six hours. Other radiotracers used in nuclear medicine studies imaged with gamma camera have generally longer half-lives. New ultra-short half-life radiotracers are emerging for PET-CT scanning and will be used more extensively over time as molecular imaging agents. Patients should be instructed to drink freely and void often following the examination.

SELECTION OF ADVANCED IMAGING STUDIES

FIRST, REVIEW PRIOR FILMS

Adequate diagnostic information is often available from multiple modalities when imaging the abdomen and pelvis. Reviewing any preexisting imaging with the radiologist does not add expense or risk of radiation or contrast and may save time. Review of imaging studies obtained for other reasons may identify preexisting calcifications and small caliber of vessels that would put an elderly patient at greater risk for developing mesenteric ischemia as the cause of pain. In general, a tailored study to address specific questions will provide the best study possible (see **Tables 110-1** and **110-2**).

TABLE 110-1 Specific Abdomen Imaging Examinations

Organ System	Preferred Initial Examination	Alternate Examination
Gallbladder	US	HIDA, MR, ERCP
Liver	US	CT or MR
Pancreas	CT	US, MR, ERCP
Kidneys	US	CT
GYN	US, transvaginal	MR or CT
Small bowel	UGI-Small bowel follow through	CT enterography, small bowel enema
Colon	Colonoscopy, BE	CT
Vascular	US or CT	MR or angio

PRACTICE POINT

- While modern CT scanners make it easy to perform CT scan of the complete abdomen and pelvis, it should not be used as a replacement for the bedside physical examination. The localization of abdominal pain is crucial to the correct selection of imaging and optimal interpretation of images.

TABLE 110-2 Patient Preparation

Radiologic Procedure	Purpose	Preparation	What to Expect
Abdominal radiographs: KUB Acute Abdomen	Screen abdomen	None	Breathing instructions, expiration may need to stand or lie on left side
US examinations: tailored to region physiology anatomy	Examine: gallbladder kidneys pelvis vascular structures	NPO for gallbladder Full bladder for pelvis	Patient may be asked to drink water to facilitate imaging of organ such as pancreas through an acoustical window
CT abdomen: oral contrast IV contrast	Examine abdomen, multiple organ systems; pelvis may be included	NPO prior to oral contrast material steadily consumed for 1–2 hours	IV contrast material causes warmth
MRI: liver vascular pelvic	Problem solving: liver vasculature pelvis	Exclusions: foreign body metal in eyes pacemaker aneurysm clip; remove watch and metal jewelry; fasting may be required	Long examination, confined space, and loud noises; can be provided with earplugs
Nuclear medicine: HIDA bleeding infection gastric emptying	Specific physiologic tests	Dependent upon examination	Scanning may be performed over an extended period of time; most imaging agents are excreted by kidney—helpful to increase fluids and void frequently after the exam

IV contrast administration: NPO for 2–4 hours prior to exam decreases risk of aspiration.

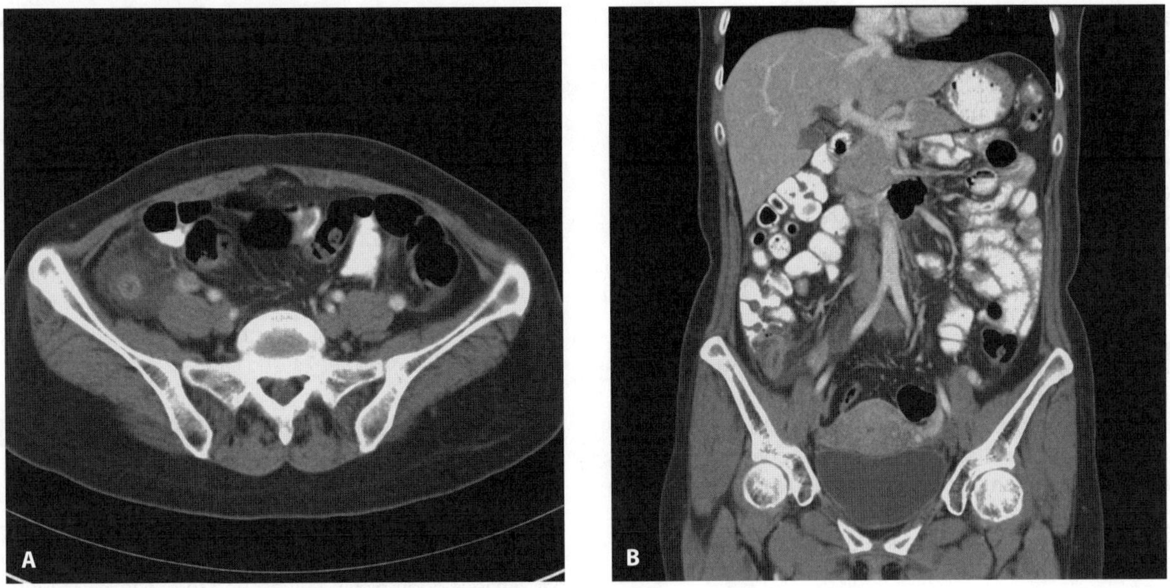

Figure 110-1 *(A) Appendicitis on axial CT image. Compare the dark gray, nearly black fat in left side of pelvis with irregular and lighter gray fat surrounding appendix, identified by its caliber and often also by its relationship to the ileocecal valve that may contain well-seen fat. (B) Appendicitis on coronal CT image. The infiltration of fat may seem less apparent on this image from the same CT scan, but it is useful also for orientation and correlation with physical examination. This scan has been performed with oral and IV contrast material maximizing the identification of GI tract and vascular structures.*

SECOND, TRY TO LOCALIZE THE ABDOMINAL PAIN

While modern CT scanners make it easy to perform CT scan of the complete abdomen and pelvis, it should not be used as a replacement for the bedside physical examination. The localization of abdominal pain is crucial to the correct selection of imaging. While true throughout the abdomen, it is particularly helpful in localizing disease affecting the GI tract that might not otherwise be apparent on CT scans. As the patient's experience of pain guides the examiner's hand to the location of pain, critical communication of this information guides the radiologist's eye to specific sites of active clinical disease (see **Figure 110-1A** and **110-1B**).

THIRD, CONSIDER THE CHARACTER OF THE PAIN AND HOW IT IS EVOLVING OVER TIME

The characterization is also very important, as different causes of abdominal pain will evolve differently over time. Serial examinations of the abdomen at the bedside are most helpful in this regard. Radiology tests are not continually needed to document the evolution whether from periumbilical pain to pain over McBurney point or intermittent symptoms from ureteral stone that will cause different descriptions of pain by the patient over time, perhaps moving from flank and nausea early in the course of the acute episode followed by groin pain and diarrhea when the stone approaches the ureteral vesicular junction (UVJ) (see **Table 110-3**).

CASE 110-1

FLANK PAIN IN A YOUNG WOMAN

An adolescent female with a negative past medical history developed sharp, severe pain in her lower back over a two week period.

Associated symptoms included a couple of days of abdominal pain and nausea, most recently with two episodes of vomiting. She also described premenstrual cramps (LMP four weeks ago), perhaps with some urgency but without dysuria, fever or chills.

Acetaminophen may have provided minimal relief. Her mother reported no family history of kidney stones and the patient was not sexually active. The patient was alert and able to cooperate with her examiners. On examination, she had normal vital signs.

Pertinent findings included a soft, nontender abdomen with normal bowel sounds and significant midlumbar spine tenderness, somewhat worse over the right flank.

TABLE 110-3 Localization of Acute Abdominal Pain

	Imaging Modality					
Site of Pain	KUB	US	GI fluoro	CT	Nucs	MRI
Diffuse	X			X		
RUQ		X			X	
LUQ				X		
Flank		X		X		
Epigastrium			X	X	X	
RLQ			X	X		
Pelvis		X	X	X		X

Negative laboratory tests included a complete blood count, metabolic profile, and pregnancy test. The only positive findings was a urinalysis (5019 WBC and 50–100 RBC/hpf)

Plain abdominal radiographs revealed a calcified structure in the right lower quadrant just caudal to the right side of the sacrum measuring approximately 5 mm x 10 mm. A nondiagnostic abdominal ultrasound reported the presence of mild hydronephrosis of her right kidney. An intravenous urography (IVP) revealed prompt excretion of contrast from the left kidney with delayed excretion of contrast from the right kidney.

Oblique radiograph with contrast in right ureter, however, did not coincide with the calcification. The medical team consulted an urologist regarding the ureteral obstruction and a general surgeon regarding the possibility of appendicitis. An abdominal CT scan was ordered but not performed due to the radiologist's reticence to administer a second dose of IV contrast material. Passage of a small amount of tissue containing a tiny stone in her urine did not relieve her worsening abdominal pain. The patient underwent surgical exploration which identified the cause of her symptoms—early appendicitis caused by an appendicolith.

SYNTHESIS

The stone was rather large for a ureteral stone raising the possibility of other causes of obstruction and calcifications in the right lower quadrant such as an appendicolith. Types of calcifications that can be present in the pelvis include very common vascular calcifications in veins and arteries and reproductive system calcifications frequently seen in middle-aged and older individuals.

RADIOLOGY PRACTICE POINT

Initial imaging with CT scanning both before and after administration of contrast material has largely replaced IVP in most institutions so that more information is acquired with the single dose of contrast material. The CT dose is relatively high so it is appropriate to also consider ultrasound, particularly in patients of child-bearing age, as long as the patient can cooperate adequately for complete examination.

The source for this case is Yamamoto LG. A Large Calcified Kidney Stone. Radiology Cases in Pediatric Emergency Medicine. Volume 7, Case 6. From the Kapiolani Medical Center for Women and Children, University of Hawaii John A Burns School of Medicine.

Available at http://www.hawaii.edu/medicine/pediatrics/pemxray/v7c06.html.

IS THE PAIN OUT OF PROPORTION TO PHYSICAL EXAMINATION?

Strong discordance between the patient's complaint of pain and findings on physical examination that are not due to medication raise concern for potentially catastrophic mesenteric ischemia in the right setting. (See Chapter 74, 2nd case).

CONCLUSION

The selection of modality will vary with availability of testing and other local factors, especially where multiple modalities can provide the needed diagnostic evaluation. Sometimes patients can be spared the risk of contrast and radiation simply by reviewing past images or employing ultrasound to dynamically augment the physical examination. For example, depending on the physcian's gestalt and skill at performing ultrasound, bedside ultrasongoraphic evidence of gallstones and a positive sonographic Murphy sign increases the likelihood of acute cholecystitis as the cause of pain. In addition, when the results are not as expected, nuclear medicine employs a small amount of radiation to provide functional information and allows imaging over time without added radiation exposure (See Chapter 74, 1st case).

Imaging compliments but must never replace the history and physical examination. Despite technologic advances the localization of abdominal pain at the bedside will remain crucial to the correct selection of imaging and optimal interpretation of images and should always be communicated to the radiologist.

SUGGESTED READING

Berland LL, Silverman SG, Gore RM, et al. Managing incidental findings on Abdominal CT: White paper of the ACR incidental findings committee. *Journal of the American College of Radiology.* 2010;7(10):754–773.

CHAPTER 111

Neurologic Imaging

Francine L. Jacobson, MD, MPH
Liangge Hsu, MD

Key Clinical Questions

1. What are the indications for a noncontrast head CT?
2. What are the indications for a contrast head CT?
3. What are the limitations of CT neuro imaging?
4. What are the indications for MRI neuro imaging?
5. What are the limitations for MRI imaging in the hospital setting?

INTRODUCTION

This chapter will present the thought processes behind general guiding principles for neurologic imaging. This chapter does not provide an exhaustive array of images because the goal is not to train hospitalists to interpret medical images but rather to provide a framework so that they can more effectively communicate with radiologists and order the most appropriate imaging modality to optimize timely evaluation and treatment. It will always be the responsibility of practitioners to provide radiologists with relevant clinical information so that recommendations regarding specific imaging and the actual interpretation are made in the context of the patient. A number of cases will be presented that highlight the limitations of imaging when this process does not occur.

Any patient with new neurologic symptoms and signs requires prompt imaging and appropriate specialty consultation to avoid catastrophic effects upon patient outcome. This is particularly true for processes that profoundly affect the homeostasis of anatomy and physiology with or without preexisting abnormality. Therefore, this chapter will review the characteristic findings to be expected for key "do-not-miss" diagnoses that would require the practitioner to contact the appropriate specialty services for emergent consultation and/or initiate steps for transfer to a tertiary care facility.

CORELATION OF NEUROLOGICAL EXAMINATION WITH IMAGING

Correlation of the neurological examination with any imaging study obtained is of paramount importance. Anatomic references may help clinicians localize abnormalities. When subtle, as at the onset of a stroke syndrome, the conviction that a potential finding is in the precise location indicated by the focal neurological deficit can make the difference between the radiologist overlooking the possibility and confidently confirming the abnormality. In turn, this approach leads to decreased imaging during the acute illness. The workup of incidental findings can also then be deferred for outpatient workup when the imaging study will often be of higher quality due to the greater ability of the recuperated patient to understand and cooperate for the imaging study.

Several drawings accompany this text to refresh memory of neuroanatomy. It can be invaluable to consult an interactive Internet atlas, especially when immediate radiologic consultation is not available, and particularly in situations in which the patient condition evolves during the hospitalization. The clarity of anatomy is greater on MRI than CT so it may prove most helpful to use an MRI reference atlas, even for looking at the more commonly obtained in the acute care setting CT scan (**Figure 111-1**).

SELECTION OF IMAGING MODALITY

Neurologic imaging requires considerations of anatomy and function and an appreciation for the limitations of each imaging modality. CT has the highest spatial resolution; however, the superior tissue characterization of MRI allows the most exquisite demonstration of neuroanatomy in a physiologically relevant manner. CT images lesions by the degree of hyperdensity in the following decreasing order of density: bone (the highest density); clotted blood; liquid blood; subacute or approximately two

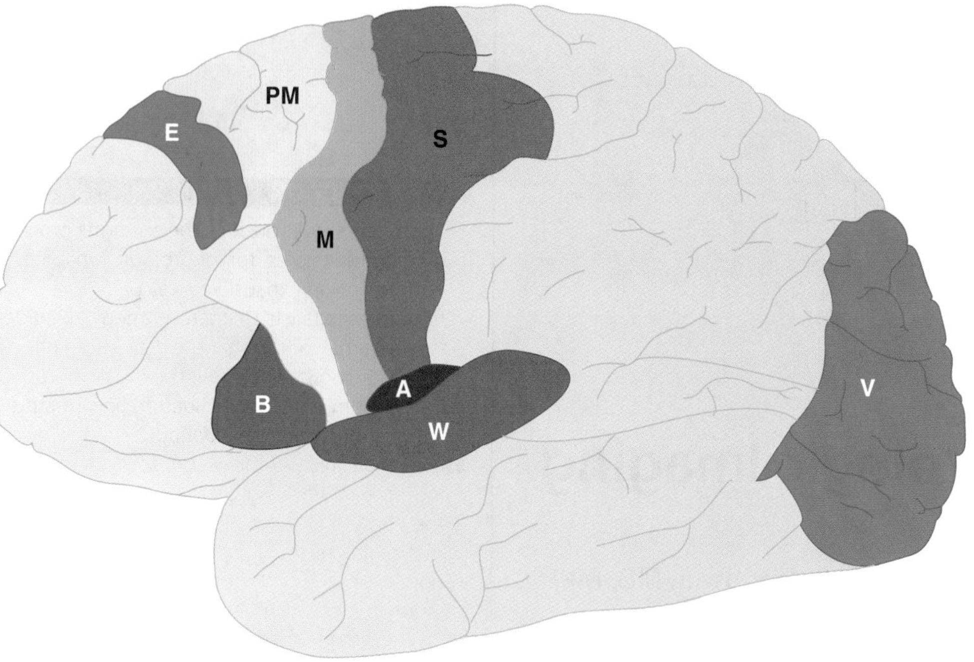

Figure 111-1 *Brain areas commonly resulting in stroke syndrome deficits: E is frontal eye field, PM is premotor, M is primary motor, S is primary sensory, V is visual, B is Broca's, W is Wernicke's and A is primary auditory.*

weeks of blood similar to brain tissue; CSF equal to the density of water (0–10 HU), and fat the least dense (a negative HU value). This means that a resolving phase of hemorrhage may have a density equal to brain tissue, making it inapparent. Hyperdense lesions suggest recent blood, hemorrhagic lesions such as metastases, hypercellular lesions like lymphoma, and meningioma, calcification, and bone. Hypodense abnormalities include infarcts greater than 12 hours, brain tumors, inflammation, old blood, edema, traumatic changes, fat, cysts, and air. Enlargement of the ventricles suggests atrophy, obstruction, or NPH. MRI can identify ring-enhancing lesions (abscess, partially thrombosed aneurysm, resolving stroke or infection, metastatic lesions, active demyelination, and radiation necrosis), amyloid angiography, arteriovenous malformations, brainstem lesions (especially if thin cuts obtained), dissection of cranial vessels, edema, hemorrhage (although in general not as well as CT in the acute setting), and tumor (with characteristic T1 and T2 densities for each type, location, presence, or absence of hemorrhage, edema, calcification) (**Tables 111-1** to **111-3**).

Nuclear medicine tests such as SPECT brain scan can provide functional information regarding Alzheimer's and other neurodedenerative diseases, stroke and seizure. PET-CT scans, increasingly being used to provide global assessment for metastases in patients with known cancer, have important limitations. The total body PET-CT does not provide adequate screening for brain metastases. In many centers, the application of this to the head is regarded as a separate examination. Centers that include the head on total body PET-CT scans may be doing so primarily to compare foci of increased activity with brain activity as a standardization procedure.

CT and MRI are both utilized for a wide variety of increasingly specific examinations, although the choice of CT or MRI may not be based upon the small differences in the value of the data obtained. One primary issue is the rapidity with which the examination can be obtained and interpreted. In acute neurological disease changes, time is of the essence, negating any benefit of more sophisticated imaging even if it would result in less ionizing radiation or possibly provide further information or a specific diagnosis that could effect less urgent treatment decisions.

It is extremely important to consider the effect the neurological event is having upon the patient. The ability of the patient to tolerate the examination may be diminished by the neurological event even as it is evolving. A CT scan is a significantly shorter examination than a MRI. The value that might be added by MRI can easily be negated by patient motion during the lengthy data acquisition sequences; thus the additional information that is often obtained from MR needs to be balanced by the logistics and added time for MR exam on a case by case basis. *The one exception is in acute stroke in which a fast diffusion sequence (a minute and half) can provide a definitive answer, especially when the CT is negative.* Neurologic imaging for chronic neurological findings may be deferred and performed on an elective basis following discharge.

PRACTICE POINT

- Neuroimaging screening in the acute setting may be helpful in a patient who is unable to cooperate for a neurologic examination due to altered consciousness, agitation, or other factors. However, the images may be suboptimal and a high index of suspicion of an underlying disorder or identification of an acute focal neurologic defect based on a thorough history and physical examination of the patient is critical to the selection of appropriate studies.

ABNORMALITIES ON NEUROIMAGING

Visualization of brain structure on imaging is generally based upon differences in gray and white matter and upon alterations of CSF spaces. Some disease processes are diffuse and others are

TABLE 111-1 CT Images of Common Abnormalities

Infarct	Acute 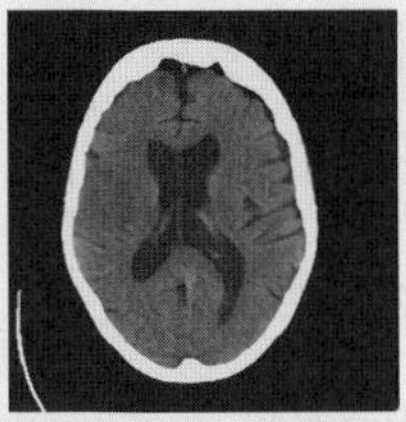	Subacute 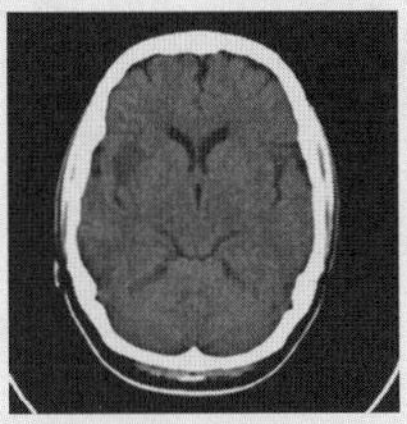	Chronic 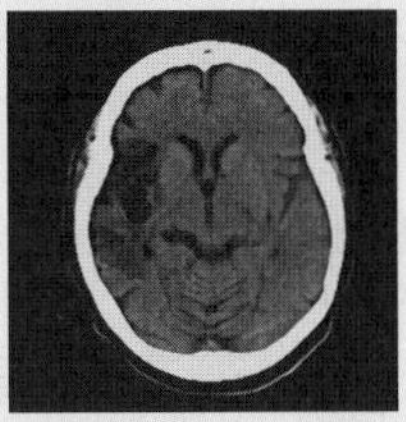	Lacune 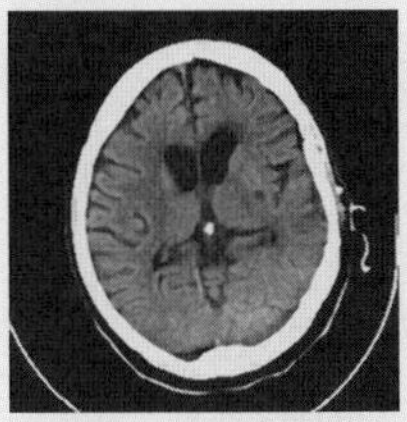
Intracranial Hemorrhage	Subarachnoid 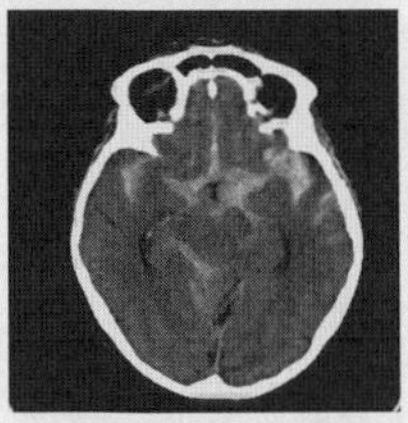	Intracerebral 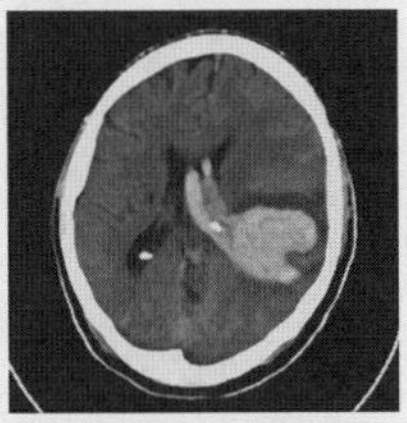	Epidural 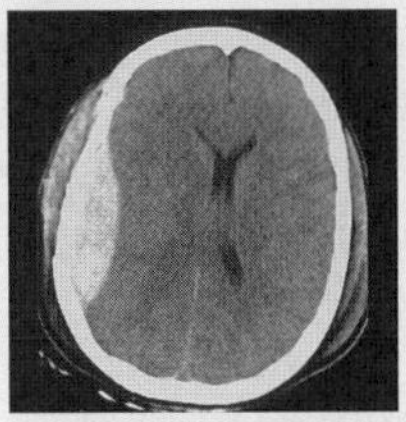	Subdural 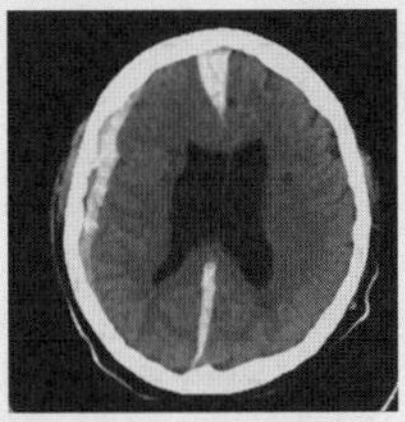
Mass effect	Edema 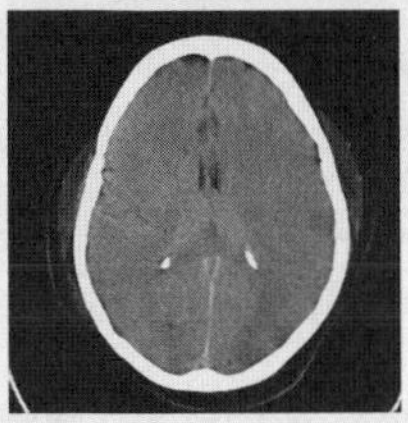	Effacement 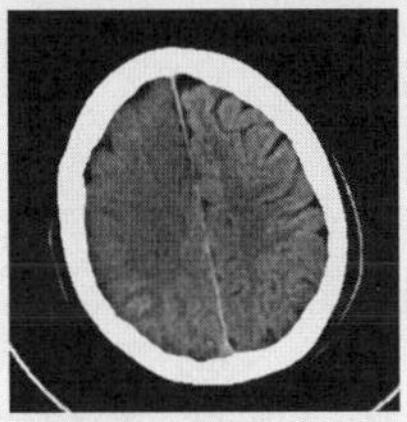	Herniation 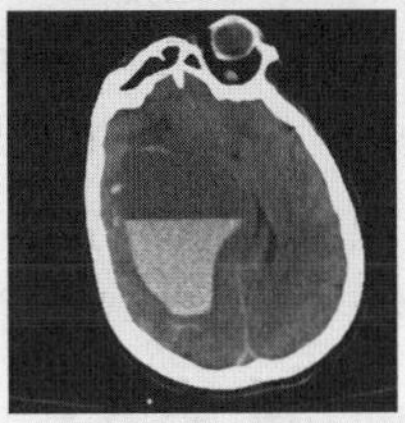	Hydrocephalus 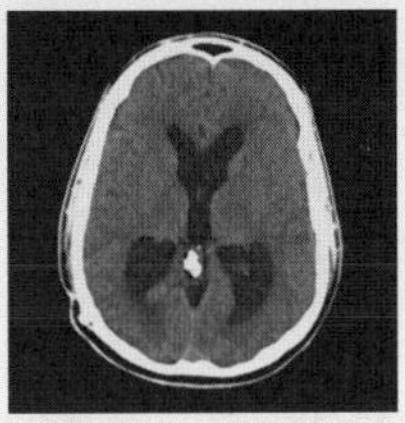

focal. Focal abnormalities may be accompanied by changes in surrounding tissue. The importance of the identification of blood cannot be overstated, whether in an extra-axial collection, subarachnoid hemorrhage, or hemorrhage into brain tissue itself. Blood degradation over time leads to different MRI signal characteristics that identify blood and provide a timeline (**Tables 111-4** and **111-5**).

STROKE SYNDROMES

In the setting of stroke, the exclusion of blood can be the most valuable outcome of the noncontrast enhanced screening head CT, allowing prompt thrombolytic therapy.

CASE 111-1

CONFUSION

A 57-year-old female with prior medical history (PMH) of panic attacks and recent diagnosis of cardiomyopathy was admitted to the hospital with the provisional diagnosis of confusion. Neighbors observed this previously independent woman having difficulty parallel parking her car and subsequently wandering in her backyard. Emergency department notes referred to her being covered in feces and having a "nonfocal" neurologic examination. Screening head CT was reportedly negative. The admitting hospitalist also documented a "nonfocal" neurologic

TABLE 111-2 MRI Techniques

Commonly used MR imaging techniques are the following:

- **T1-weighted imaging (T1-WI):** Cerebrospinal fluid (CSF) is dark due to *long relaxation time.*
- **T2-weighted imaging (T2-WI):** CSF is bright due to *long relaxation time.*
- **Proton density–weighted imaging:** CSF has a signal similar to brain tissue *as it is neither T1 nor T2 weighted.*
- **Gradient echo imaging:** has high sensitivity in detecting *hemorrhage or mineralization that appear as low intensity.*
- **Diffusion-weighted imaging (DWI):** images *reflect relative flow of water molecules.*
- **Perfusion-weighted imaging (PWI):** fast gradient weighted MR sequences are based on passage of MR contrast through brain tissue.

TABLE 111-3 Signal Characteristics of Blood on MRI with Time

Mnemonic	George Washington Bridge	The layers of an Oreo[R] cookie
Time	T1WI	T2WI
Acute	Gray	Black
Subacute	White	White
Chronic	Black	Black

Blood, hemosiderin, and calcium are dark on gradient echo images. FLAIR is helpful for detection of subarachnoid hemorrhage. DWI detects ischemia immediately and may be abnormal in TIA. ADC is decreased when ischemic tissue may still be viable. Diffusion restriction considers DWI and ADC together—bright on DWI and dark on ADC map.

TABLE 111-4 Neuroimaging Abnormalities

Disease Process	Findings on CT and MR	Clinical Information
Acute ischemic stroke	Diffusion MR + in 30 min-hrs CT Normal for up to 6 hours	
Early evolution of ischemic stroke	Decrease gray-white differentiation, effacement of sulci, increasing *swelling* of gray matter	Cytotoxic edema
Continued evolution of stroke 24–48 hours	Edema results in hypodense region may have mass effect	Mass effect on midline structures can lead to herniation
Extra-axial bleed	Crescentic collection that crosses	Subdural hematoma
Extra-axial bleed	Lentiform between sutures	Epidural hematoma requires emergency evacuation
Toxoplasmosis	Ring enhancing lesions better seen on MRI CT dDX abscess or tumor	MRI is more sensitive CT dDX abscess or tumor
Lymphoma	Periventricular enhancing lesions for primary lymphoma	Higher glucose utilization on PET-CT than toxoplasmosis
Astrocytoma/Glioma	Variable depending on grade, location and size	Variable presentation
Metastases	Can be solitary of multiple with no or extensive edema	Lung, breast, kidney, GI tract, melanoma
Leukoencephalopathy	Subcortical involvement Atrophy and white matter changes	AIDS dementia complex Impaired memory and slowing of motor skills, ataxia, hyperreflexia
Central pontine myelinolysis	Abnormal symmetric signal in central pons on MRI Widespread destruction of myelin pattern reverse of infarction	Coma, facial diplegia, spastic quadriparesis after rapid correction of hyponatremia

TABLE 111-5 Incidental Findings

Virchow-Robin space: Enlarged perivascular spaces (EPVS) surround blood vessels and serve as pathways for drainage of interstitial fluid; may be incidental in older patients but are likely to be abnormal in young adults.

Empty Sella Syndrome (ESS): Primary ESS is caused by CSF pressure flattening the pituitary and it is associated with obesity and high blood pressure in women. Secondary ESS is due to regression of the pituitary gland after trauma, surgery, or radiation therapy with destruction of the pituitary gland affecting fertility and menstrual periods.

Lacunes: Evidence of prior strokes usually due to atherosclerosis of deep penetrating arteries. These minute holes can be caused by a succession of transient ischemic attacks and over the years can lead to dementia.

Subcortical Arteriosclerotic Encephalopathy (SAE): Disease process in deep white matter that causes periventricular lucency and dementia.

PCOM and ACOM aneurysms: Small aneurysms of the anterior and posterior communicating arteries can be incidental findings during acute hospitalization.

Meningioma: Small meningiomas that are asymptomatic may be incidental findings in acute clinical context, particularly in elderly patients.

Calcifications: Basal ganglia calcifications are frequent incidental findings. They are easier to detect on CT, although characteristic signal voids are seen on MRI.

Normal pressure hydrocephalus (NPH): Chronic communicating hydrocephalus in which intracranial pressure is stable with mild elevation due to equilibration between formation of CSF and absorption. Triad: gait difficulty, urinary incontinence, and mental decline. NPH is a cause of potentially reversible dementia.

examination. The next day she was discharged by another hospitalist who tested her orientation and ability to pay attention and documented that she was no longer confused. Her family brought her back to the emergency department and a repeat Head CT confirmed a MCA-PCA watershed parietal stroke.

Synthesis

The mechanism of her stroke was likely cardioembolic given her known ischemic cardiomyopathy. In retrospect, she had standard risk factors for stroke, her presentation (inability to park a car) suggested a focal neurologic deficit, and she had stepped in dog feces in her backyard (due to neglect). The acute onset of a focal neurologic deficit during the prior week without preceding head trauma increased the odds of stroke greater than 90-fold. A focused neurologic examination (for example, asking her to bisect a straight line and testing for neglect) would likely have identified her parietal deficit at the time of her first hospitalization.

Radiology Practice Point

It is important to remember that CT imaging is often normal in patients with acute ischemic symptoms and may not become abnormal for 6 to 48 hours, even in those with persistent symptoms. (Table 111-1, evolving stroke). New clinical information – focal abnormalities rather than confusion – should be brought to the attention of the radiologist who would then take another look at the right parietal region. Retrospective review of the first CT did in fact identify subtle abnormalities in this region.

The head CT must be obtained to rule out the presence of bleeding prior to consideration of reperfusion therapy. The evolution of a clinical stroke syndrome may begin with the most severe deficit at the time of a completely normal head CT scan. Even without reperfusion therapy, patients may often improve over the first several days. This may be due to the salvaging of neurons through the luxury perfusion that is seen in the periphery of the affected brain territory, limiting the ultimate extent of abnormality and corresponding defect. Over time, the transfer of function to other neurons will also augment the improvement, although much of this occurs over a longer period of time with rehabilitation in the nonacute care setting. Hence, the CT complements the neurologic examination rather than replaces it. A "normal" CT report should not mislead clinicians into assuming that a patient does not have a focal neurologic deficit. Correlation of clinical findings from an in-depth neurological examination and study of CT scans may also identify evidence of chronic as well as acute stroke. The pattern of strokes can often point to more central vascular abnormalities, both in the brain, the great vessels and heart that require intervention to prevent additional strokes in the future.

CASE 111-2

STEREOTYPED "SPELLS"

A 65-year-old man with a PMH of hypertension and hyperlipidemia developed a five-minute spell of heaviness of the right side of his face and right arm. One hour later he experienced another spell, this time with word finding difficulty, lasting five minutes with complete resolution. He then experienced a third stereotyped episode during his examination in the emergency department. ECG and initial laboratory tests were normal.

Synthesis

This patient had experienced sudden symptoms in a vascular territory involving the anterior circulation of the left hemisphere. Three stereotyped spells in one vascular territory suggested an increased likelihood of a stenosis of the MCA or extracranial ICA. The pretest probability of extracranial internal carotid stenosis is 15–20%. For secondary stroke prevention this patient might benefit from a carotid endartectomy if he had, for example, a stenosis > 70%.

Radiology Practice Point

Screening CT radiography would not routinely image the carotid circulation unless specified by the examiner. Therefore, a CT angiogram would be appropriate as the initial test.

Any patient with symptoms of anterior circulation transient ischemic attacks (TIAs) as suggested in this patient who had motor dysfunction of the contralateral extremity and face, followed by difficulty word finding, would require an evaluation of his carotid circulation as the first step.

CASE 111-3

MOTOR VEHICLE ACCIDENT (MVA)

A 45-year-old female with a PMH notable for three successful pregnancies and one miscarriage sustained a MVA. She was hit from behind, leaving her with a stiff, sore neck. Three days later she suddenly developed unsteady walking, numbness on the right side of her face, and in her left hand and leg. Her voice became hoarse and she choked while drinking water. Initial laboratory tests were normal including initial head CT, CBC, INR, ESR, electrolytes, antiphospholipid antibodies, and ECG.

Synthesis

This patient had experienced sudden symptoms in a vascular territory involving the posterior circulation of the right hemisphere: motor dysfunction of ipsilateral face and contralateral extremity with associated symptoms of ataxia and dysphagia. Her neurologic examination would be expected to show sensory loss on the right side of her face, left hand and leg, reduced palatal elevation on the right, smaller pupil on the right with mild right ptosis, and hemitaxia on the right. Given a likely flexion-extension injury during a recent MVA, a posterior circulation dissection was the most likely cause of her deficits. Other less likely possibilities in a younger patient include PFO and antiphospholipid antibody syndrome.

Radiology Practice Point

Suspicion of localization to the posterior circulation is valuable information to share with the radiologist. Screening CT would not ordinarily include imaging of the right vertebral artery. In some institutions, a separate request for a neck CT or CT angiogram would be required. Tailoring the imaging to the specific patient avoids diagnostic delays, increased risk, and costs from performing multiple examinations.

The clinical information of a flexion-extension injury should be conveyed to the radiologist who would recommend imaging of the extra-cranial vessels in addition to the brain, and then specifically look at areas of the brain likely to be affected.

These cases highlight the importance of answering the following questions when a patient presents with neurologic symptoms and signs.

1. Are the symptoms consistent with stroke or TIA?
2. Where does the ischemic event localize (anterior circulation, posterior circulation, cortical versus subcortical)?
3. What is the mechanism of the ischemic event, cardioembolism, extracranial carotid stenosis, dissection (anterior or posterior circulation), septic emboli, hypercoagulable states, giant cell arteritis, among other possibilities?

Only by asking the right questions can the practitioner determine what tests are needed and how urgently.

Serial CT scans may be obtained as working films, much as serial chest radiographs are obtained in acutely ill patients. A patient who has an acute nonhemorrhagic infarction of the brain will acutely have a normal or nearly normal head CT. Several days later, the evolving infarction may be identified by "luxury perfusion" resulting in greater enhancement of the affected area on a contrast-enhanced head CT. In patients who are known to have a subacute stroke by history, contrast may not be required to document the extent of the infarction because it will become more apparent even on noncontrast enhanced CT. Remote infarctions may be recognized by the prominence of CSF spaces and changes of encephalomalacia. This may be seen as dilatation of the lateral ventricles or cortical sulci or as one or more small lucencies within the brain parenchyma, particularly in putamen, caudate, thalamus, pons, internal capsule, and corona radiate. Hypertensive lipohyalinosis may be the underlying cause of such lacunar infarcts that are best managed medically with optimization of blood pressure.

Cerebellar strokes may present with vertigo, nausea and vomiting, ataxia, and frequently with brainstem signs. Patients often complain of headache. Large cerebellar strokes (>3 cm) are a neurosurgical emergency due to the risk of herniation, which may occur within hours of presentation.

CASE 111-4

VERTIGO

A 51-year-old right-handed man with a PMH of high blood pressure was conducting a business meeting when he suddenly developed severe vertigo, a feeling of imbalance while standing, and nausea. He vomited while calling 911. He did not have a PMH of other traditional vascular risk factors (diabetes mellitus, smoking, known occlusive vascular disease, structural heart disease, or atrial fibrillation). He did not have a history of neurologic disease (multiple sclerosis), or migraine headache. He denied recent head trauma, flexion-extension injury or headache. He also denied symptoms of diplopia, reduced vision, dysarthria, dysphagia, or focal sensory or motor deficits that might be expected with acute vertigo and brainstem stroke. He did not have antecedent hearing loss, a pressure sensation in either ear, or a history of Meniere syndrome. He experienced no antecedent viral symptoms to suggest acute labrynthitis. He did have a history of bilateral tinnitus with normal audiograms in the past. His physical examination in the emergency department was notable for a middle-aged man who appeared extremely uncomfortable and reluctant to move. Horizontal nystagmus remained in the same direction when his gaze changed and was suppressed with visual fixation. He was able to walk without falling although he veered to his left. His neurologic examination was normal, including motor strength, the absence of dysmetria or sensory changes, and he had normal reflexes. Head CT imaging did not reveal any abnormalities of the cerebellum and fourth ventricle or the presence of multiple white matter lesions. The patient was admitted to the hospital for observation. The next morning he denied any symptoms of vertigo to the medical and neurology teams. His neurologic examination was completely normal and nystagmus was no longer present. At the recommendation of the neurology attending he underwent CT angiography which was negative. He was discharged home.

Synthesis

His history and normal neurologic examination did not suggest the possibility of dissection and he underwent an unnecessary CT angiography with its attendant risks of contrast and radiation exposure. If his 1st head CT had revealed a cerebellar infarction, emergent neurosurgical consultation and triage to an intensive care unit or to a stroke center would have been necessary.

Radiology Practice Point

CT scans of the cerebellum are usually normal in the first few hours following a cerebellar infarction; hence, the importance of a focused neurologic history and examination looking for cerebellar symptoms and signs, none of which were identified by multiple examiners over a 24 hour period of observation. If there were concern about cerebellar infarction or hemorrhage despite a "negative" CT, the clinician should consult with the radiologist. Routine MR imaging will likely detect an inferior cerebellar infarction but it is less sensitive for identifying a hemorrhage. The radiologist can arrange for MR sequences that would maximize identification of infarction and hemorrhage in the posterior fossa.

The mechanism of the stroke depends on the artery involved: superior cerebellar artery strokes are usually embolic but rarely cause hydrocephalus, posterior cerebellar artery strokes are equally likely to arise from stenosis or embolism, and anterior inferior cerebellar artery strokes are rare, and usually thrombotic with associated brainstem infarct.

ACUTE IMAGING OF BRAIN

Neuroimaging in the acute care setting relies on noncontrast enhanced head CT scanning both as the screening and, often, the definitive examination. For acute neurologic symptoms and signs and following trauma, timely initiation of the appropriate treatment requires identification of the presence and location of blood and/or mass effect. In many cases, this may be the only imaging required for the care of the patient.

Noncontrast enhanced CT scan is also the most important imaging to obtain when a patient presents with sudden onset of severe headache without any focal signs (assuming a complete neurologic examination) or symptoms suggesting focality. Most scans performed for this presentation will be negative.

Blood identified on noncontrast enhanced head CT scan must be localized to direct further workup and treatment of primary and secondary neurological disease. Subarachnoid hemorrhage indicates bleeding from within the brain parenchyma or a vessel within CSF containing subarachnoid space. Subarachnoid hemorrhage is most commonly associated with bleeding intracranial aneurysms (75% of cases) or arteriovenous malformation AVM (10% of cases). The finding of edema in addition to blood may reflect metastasis of tumor from another organ, such as lung or breast. The specialized team providing care for the individual patient may involve interventional radiology or surgery to select further imaging and plan for treatment.

On occasion, a patient with or without a previously known tumor may present with new onset seizure due to a brain lesion (mass effect or bleeding) or with new cranial nerve findings due to involvement of the leptomeninges. When no more specific reason for seizure is known, a screening head CT potentially followed by contrast enhanced CT or MRI examination should be considered.

CASE 111-5

SEIZURE

A 42-year-old female with a history of hypertension suddenly developed a severe headache and suffered a seizure. She had no history of substance abuse or known vascular disease. In the emergency department her blood pressure was initially 260/140 mm Hg. Screening head CT was negative for blood. Fundoscopic examination was not documented. Her neurologic examination was notable for altered mental status attributed to her seizure. The covering neurologist was concerned about subtle occipital changes appreciated on subsequent MRI and worried about the possibility of the basilar scrape syndrome. Anticoagulation was recommended, initially with heparin as a bridge to therapeutic warfarin. Her blood pressure normalized with treatment consisting of lisinopril and hydrochlorothiazide and her clinicians attributed the initial high blood pressure elevation to her having suffered a seizure and possible noncompliance with her outpatient regimen. After her discharge to home, she collapsed, and reimaging revealed a large hemorrhage with evidence of transtentorial uncal herniation.

Synthesis

In retrospect, her diagnosis was hypertensive crisis complicated by seizure. A fundoscopic examination might have revealed exudates, hemorrhages, and papilledema.

Radiology Practice Point

Subtle occipital changes appreciated on MRI likely reflected hypertensive changes. Diffusion-weighted MR imaging may reveal vasogenic edema in hypertensive encephalopathy without ischemia or infarction. This finding may have therapeutic implications.

Head trauma can occur in the elderly from a fall with or without direct impact upon the skull. Extra-axial collection of blood forming a lentiform-shaped epidural hematoma that is confined between adjacent sutures can accumulate quickly and cause life-threatening mass effect requiring prompt surgical drainage. The longer more crescentic collection that crosses the adjacent suture is usually a more slowly accumulating subdural collection adjacent to torn bridging vessels that may be watched if small. Such a collection will sometimes go undiagnosed until other indications require a head CT scan. In the chronic phase, it will appear as a subdural hygroma filled with CSF fluid. The head CT scan may thus also provide additional history such as prior strokes and prior falls and other trauma, particularly when a patient is unable to speak. In the elderly, these processes can be interrelated as the patient with a preexisting motor- or balance-affecting deficit will also be at greater risk of falling. A patient who has had a stroke that affects his or her ability to communicate may also be less able to describe the present illness. Complete bedside examination for coincidental trauma can be helpful in reconstructing the series of events leading to the hospitalization. A patient fall while in the hospital requires much the same attention to neurological and total body surface examination for correct treatment.

NEUROIMAGING OF THE SPINE

Radiographs of the chest, abdomen, and pelvis may provide the initial screening examination of the spine. The appearance of the spine can remain normal until loss of 40% of the bone mineralization. The spine may not be studied in depth or specifically reported by the radiologist when the patient has imaging for other indications. It is very helpful to inquire specifically about the possibility of lesions when signs and symptoms suggest their presence. A comparison with prior studies that image the region of abnormality are very helpful for the assessment of acuity and potential significance that may range from a benign osteoporotic fracture to osseous metastasis. The spinal cord itself will not be imaged. Spine MRI is the imaging modality of choice when looking for impending cord compression and it is a widely recognized reason for emergent MRI examination. CT is an alternative choice if MRI is contraindicated. Radiography, radionuclide bone scans, and CT scans are helpful for identifying musculoskeletal metastases from a wide variety of tumors. MRI allows identification nerve roots and tumor extension into the thecal sac. Radiographs, even when not specifically obtained for the bones, can be particularly helpful adjuncts in the evaluation of MRI and radionuclide bone scans. In patients who have had previous back surgery, intrathecal contrast material may be required for adequate CT examination. In cases in which hardware has been placed, artifacts can limit both CT and MR imaging. Such patients may not benefit from MRI due to artifacts, even if they tolerate the adjacent tissue heating that is likely to occur during the examination.

Oncologic patients often require specialized neurological imaging. The need may be less quickly recognized as part of the initial diagnosis. This is particularly true for back pain due to osseous metastases. If a patient has a known or suspected tumor, suspicion for cord compression requires prompt imaging to diagnose and intervene in order to preserve neurological function. Subtle presentation of impending cord compression is best addressed with outpatient MRI. While MRI is a standard examination for this indication, the hospitalized patient may not be able to adequately cooperate with the lengthy, complete spine MRI usually performed. A more limited examination may be considered based upon clinical examination. Very extensive bone destruction may be adequately studied for urgent treatment planning with CT scanning.

CASE 111-6

SEPSIS

A 51-year-old female with a PMH of a remote gastric bypass and a recent outside hospitalization for pneumonia was referred from an outside hospital (OSH) for MRI imaging of her spine. For the last couple of days she had been bedridden in her apartment and her family reported confusion. At the OSH her vital signs were notable for a BP of 90/55 mm Hg, pulse 110, regular, RR 24, T 100. She appeared acutely uncomfortable and described severe myalgias. A black eschar was noted on her fifth digit, which was attributed to trauma. At the tertiary hospital she was admitted for pain control after having a reportedly negative MRI of her spine in the ED. She had an aortic murmur, which had not been described previously. She was unable to externally rotate her right hip secondary to severe pain. Her multiple blood cultures revealed Staph aureus. Interventional radiology drained 5 cc of pus from her right hip, which required debridement in the operating room. She subsequently underwent an aortic valve replacement.

Synthesis

This case highlights the importance of performing a physical examination to direct imaging. MRI of her back was negative because she did not have an epidural abscess. In this case relying on the provisional diagnosis from the Emergency Department and performing a limited history and physical examination lead to performing the wrong test and delays in diagnosis and treatment. In retrospect, she was septic; the black eschar was due to a septic embolism.

Radiology Practice Point

Hospitalized patients are often unable to cooperate adequately to allow the full benefit of the MRI technology in their care. MRI examinations do not use ionizing radiation but can be quite lengthy, lasting an hour or more in duration. The request for wider coverage such as adjacent body parts is not easily accommodated in the same scanning session. It is therefore imperative to have a specific goal for the MRI from the outset.

CASE 111-7

READMISSION FROM REHABILITATION FACILITY

A 68-year-old female with PMH notable most recently for hiatal hernia repair with multiple postoperative complications, hypertension, and right breast carcinoma was transferred from acute rehabilitation to the medical service. She has been either at rehabilitation or in the hospital for most of the past year and returned from rehabilitation with a cough, bilateral sacral and sciatic pain, decreased ability to ambulate, and complaints of bilateral leg weakness. Pain was present only with movement, especially with attempts to ambulate; she described this pain as a "cramping" or "tightness" in the back of her thighs that ached increasingly with movement. She denied saddle anesthesia, change in bowel or bladder function or sensation, or leg numbness or tingling. The patient has been on multiple antibiotics for hospital-acquired infections. She currently had chest tube, J tube, and G tube in place. Examination was notable for a fully alert and appropriately interactive female. Her vital signs were normal. Her neurologic examination was diffusely abnormal including tongue fasciculation, motor weakness with fasciculations in her lower extremities, hypertonic reflexes with spasticity, clonus, bilateral Babinski signs. Rectal tone was normal. A STAT MRI of the L-spine was obtained and was reportedly negative. Patient was given 1 mg of lorazepam prior to a MRI of her cervical and thoracic spine but her coughing in the supine position precluded the examination. She was subsequently transferred to the intensive care unit after elective intubation.

Synthesis

The differential diagnosis for a causative lesion in the spine is quite broad and spans infection, structural, neoplastic, and vascular. Her examination suggested a myelopathic process involving the upper motor neurons of both legs. The lack of bowel, bladder, or saddle anesthesia symptoms made a full cauda equine syndrome less likely. As the patient has been NPO for some time, and has had many interruptions in her nutrition, a metabolic cause of her myelopathic picture should also be considered.

Radiology Practice Point

Selected for the wrong reason, MRI will increase the stress on the acutely ill patient and delay institution of needed therapy. In this case, the already debilitated patient likely required intubation due to respiratory suppression from lorazepam administration, deconditioning, and aspiration.

CONCLUSION

The scope of neuroradiology varies between institutions. In some centers, spine services are separately organized within neuroradiology or musculoskeletal radiology. Consulting the radiologists in your institution is important for understanding the availability and expertise in a variety of specialized examinations that might be available. The evolution of neurological findings over time can be very dynamic and inadequately conveyed on an imaging requisition. Continuing consultation during admission will provide the most clinical relevant data for patient treatment using the smallest number of scans and the least amount of contrast material possible.

SUGGESTED READINGS

Arslan A, Karaarslan E. Diffusion weighted MR imaging in non-infarct lesions of the brain. *EJR*. 2008;65:402–416.

Orrison WW Jr. *Atlas of Brain Function*. 2nd ed. New York, New York: Thieme; 2008.

Scarabino T, Salvolini U, Jinkins JR, eds. *Emergency Neuroradiology*. Published by arrangement with Casa Editrice Idelson-Gnocchi srl, Naples, Italy. Heidelberg: Springer Science+Business Media, Springer Berlin; 2006.

WEB RESOURCES

1. http://headneckbrainspine.com/
2. http://jakemandell.com
   http://www.lesionlocalizer.com
   http://jakemandell.com/headct/
3. The Whole Brain Atlas MRI views of the normal and diseased human brain. Collaboration of MIT and Harvard University. www.med.harvard.edu/aanlib/
4. http://www.neuroanatomy.ca/stroke_model/cross_section_anatomy.html.

CHAPTER 112

Critical Thinking

Francine L. Jacobson, MD, MPH
Sylvia C. McKean, MD, SFHM, FACP

Key Clinical Questions

1. What are the three domains of outcomes regarding competencies in Hospital Medicine?
2. What is meant by "critical thinking" in the ordering of imaging studies?

INTRODUCTION

Competencies in Hospital Medicine are classified within three domains of outcomes: cognitive (knowledge), psychomotor (skills), and affective (attitudes). Critical thinkers must have a basic knowledge about the methods of logical inquiry and reasoning (cognitive), some skill in applying these methods (psychomotor), and an attitude predisposed to thoughtful consideration of the problems and subjects that come within the range of one's experiences (affective). They must recognize the problems confronting patients; ask the right questions to address those problems; gather pertinent data from many sources; efficiently, logically, and resourcefully sort through complex information; acknowledge personal biases that may hinder analysis; interpret data in the context of each patient before them; and expediently reach trustworthy conclusions that form the basis of therapeutic approaches (**Tables 112-1** and **112-2**).

This chapter will draw upon a few cases to highlight basic concepts in critical thinking when ordering imaging studies. In the first case, overutilization of imaging studies subjected the patient to unnecessary risks of radiation and contrast and significantly prolonged length of hospital stay without altering management. In the second case, underutilization of imaging studies despite hospitalization resulted in diagnostic failure relating to a potentially life-threatening illness. In the third case, studies performed at the end of life were irrelevant to the patient's futile care.

ASKING THE RIGHT QUESTIONS

"The question is not what you look at, but what you see." Henry David Thoreau

The hallmark of critical thinking requires asking the right questions to obtain the right information. Without the right information, we cannot make the correct diagnosis or order the correct treatment. A thorough history and physical examination will in fact usually lead to the correct diagnosis, especially in complex or perplexing cases. During emergency medical conditions, clinicians, however, tend to order tests first and clinical problem solve after the results are known, especially with imaging studies. With this approach clinicians will not find out information if they skip the step of asking pertinent questions.

The evidence-based medicine (EBM) approach requires a series of steps, the first of which is to ask a clinical question that can be answered. Failure to follow the first step will result in an unproductive search that cannot be applied to the patient in front of you (**Table 112-3**).

OVERUTILIZATION

CASE 112-1

ACUTE DYSPNEA AND CHEST PAIN

A 59-year-old female with a past medical history of asthma and hypertension was admitted for surgery. The patient had no history of cardiac disease or pulmonary hypertension. A preoperative abdominal CT reported findings consistent with endometrial cancer. A preoperative CXR (PA and lateral) was normal. On postoperative day two, she developed chest tightness and shortness of breath. Her examination was notable for a blood pressure (BP) of 106/60 mm Hg, a pulse of 91 beats per minute (bpm), room air O_2 saturation of 92–95%, and a normal temperature of 97.9°F. Her physicians ordered chest physical therapy, furosemide, and nebulizer treatments, none of which relieved her symptoms. The patient subsequently developed severe 6–7/10 chest pain.

WHAT IS THE CLINICAL PROBLEM OR CHIEF COMPLAINT?

The patient developed chest tightness and shortness of breath on postoperative day #2. A skilled clinician would be able to quickly identify a pattern suggesting a specific diagnosis (such as postoperative pulmonary embolism) when presented with this clinical scenario. This patient had received no pharmacologic venous thromboembolism (VTE) prophylaxis despite high risk surgery (TAH BSO) along with other risk factors of cancer, obesity, and continued immobility. Crucial to the clinician's ability to limit the differential diagnosis would be recognition of the significance of the patient's risk factors for VTE. The absence of physical signs of pulmonary embolism should not dissuade him or her of this possibility. The clinician has now generated a hypothesis based on partial information that might lead him or her to order the appropriate imaging study.

Although the diagnosis is highly likely, does the diagnosis adequately explain this patient's symptoms? Or even if less frequent, what might cause her death?

TABLE 112-1 Critical Thinking Sidebar

Critical Thinking Defined by Edward Glaser

In a seminal study on critical thinking and education in 1941, Edward Glaser defined critical thinking as follows: "The ability to think critically, as conceived in this volume, involves three things:

1. An attitude of being disposed to consider in a thoughtful way the problems and subjects that come within the range of one's experiences,
2. Knowledge of the methods of logical inquiry and reasoning, and
3. Some skill in applying those methods.

Critical thinking calls for a persistent effort to examine any belief or supposed form of knowledge in the light of the evidence that supports it and the further conclusions to which it tends. It also generally requires ability to recognize problems, to find workable means for meeting those problems, to gather and marshal pertinent information, to recognize unstated assumptions and values, to comprehend and use language with accuracy, clarity, and discrimination, to interpret data, to appraise evidence and evaluate arguments, to recognize the existence (or nonexistence) of logical relationships between propositions, to draw warranted conclusions and generalizations, to put to test the conclusions and generalizations at which one arrives, to reconstruct one's patterns of beliefs on the basis of wider experience, and to render accurate judgments about specific things and qualities in everyday life."

Data from Glaser EM. An Experiment in the Development of Critical Thinking. Teacher's College, Columbia University. New York, NY; 1941.

TABLE 112-2 Clinical Problem Solving

1. Frame a question to answer a problem.
2. Formulate a concise and coherent hypothesis devoid of irrelevant information.
   - Organize thoughts and articulate them concisely and coherently.
   - Strip a verbal argument of irrelevancies and phrase it in its essential terms.
3. Seek and gather critical data to test and evaluate hypothesis.
   - Use evidence skillfully and impartially.
   - Distinguish between logically valid and invalid inferences.
4. Draw reliable conclusions from the result.
   - Suspend judgment in the absence of sufficient evidence to support a decision.
5. Habitually question one's own views and attempt to understand both the assumptions that are critical to those views and the implications of the views.
6. Reassess a hypothesis when data does not support that approach.

The broad differential diagnosis in the hospital setting includes

- Acute coronary syndrome (ACS)
- Demand ischemia
- Congestive heart failure or fluid overload disorder
- Aortic dissection
- Acute pulmonary embolism (PE)
- Aspiration pneumonitis
- Hospital acquired pneumonia
- Mucous plugging
- Pneumothorax (if a central line was placed)
- Bronchospasm
- Sepsis
- Musculoskeletal pain and splinting from postsurgical pain
- Anxiety

Critical thinking would rank these possibilities according to pretest likelihood based on symptoms, signs, risk factors, and simple tests. A screening CXR and ECG did not rule in or out any of these diagnoses. The patient's CBC showing an elevated WBC count of 14,000/mm^3 could simply reflect the stress of recent surgery.

Acute PE

This patient had major risk factors for PE. In the hospital setting, acute VTE may in fact account for 10% of hospital deaths. The clinicians caring for her appropriately ordered a PE-protocol CT.

TABLE 112-3 Evidence-based Patient Care (the PICO Question)

1. Ask questions specific to your Patient that can be answered.
2. Search for evidence to support an Intervention.
3. Assess the evidence for its validity and relevance and Compare to other interventions.
4. Integrate the evidence with clinical expertise and the patient's values.
5. Evaluate Outcomes.

Demand ischemia

Although the patient had no traditional risk factors or history of coronary artery disease (CAD), surgical stress (severe anemia, hypotension, hypoxia) can result in ischemia without the presence of hemodynamically significant CAD. She was not hypotensive during anesthesia and her blood loss was minimal. An electrocardiogram and cardiac enzymes were, however, reasonable due to her symptoms of shortness of breath and chest tightness.

ACS

This patient had no clinical risk predictors of postoperative cardiac events (prior MI, angina, CHF, vascular disease, diabetes, renal failure, or stroke); she underwent an intermediate risk procedure, and her self-reported functional activity was excellent. ACS, therefore, was unlikely (< 1%) but not a diagnosis that her clinicians would want to miss.

Aspiration pneumonitis

Aspiration of stomach contents commonly occurs even in healthy people but may occur in the perioperative period. Chemical pneumonitis or an inflammatory reaction to gastric acid (pH < 2.5) reportedly results from aspiration of a large volume of sterile gastric contents (>4 mL/kg) into the lower airways. The patient may remain asymptomatic or develop severe dyspnea, hypoxia, cough, and low-grade fever over minutes to hours after a witnessed or suspected episode of aspiration. If the patient is standing or upright, the basal segments of the lower lobes are usually affected. If the patient is supine, as this patient was in the scanner, the posterior segments of the upper lobes and the apical segments of the lower lobes are usually affected. Empiric antibiotic treatment is controversial. The lung infiltrates resolve over two to four days in about 60% of patients. However, about 15% of patients deteriorate within 24 to 36 hours and progress to hypoxic respiratory failure. Approximately 25% of patients will improve initially, and then show signs and symptoms consistent with bacterial superimposed infection and worsening of initial infiltrates and/or development infiltrates.

The signs of primary bacterial aspiration pneumonia seen in patients with risk factors (altered mental status, stroke, alcoholism, poor dentition, tube feedings) tend to be more indolent than chemical pneumonitis and would not apply to this patient who abruptly developed significant symptoms and signs. Characteristically, these patients have infiltrates involving mainly the lung bases (the right more than the left) and when inadequately treated develop complications such as lung abscess, empyema, bronchiectasis, and broncopleural fistula.

This patient certainly could have aspirated in the setting of vomiting from an abdominal ileus, perhaps exacerbated by narcotics. Her well-controlled asthma was not a predictor of postoperative pulmonary complications, nor did the surgical site put her at increased risk. Serial chest radiography (CXRs) would clarify whether a pneumonitis or pneumonia was the cause of her symptoms.

Bronchospasm

Given her prior history of asthma, bronchospasm may be more likely, especially if her preadmission medical regimen had been discontinued in the perioperative period. The examiner may ask her if her symptoms were similar to her usual asthma exacerbations; try to determine whether her asthma had been well-controlled prior to admission, and listen for signs of airflow limitation.

Fluid overload

Fluid overload is very common in the postoperative period. One liter of normal saline contains nine grams of sodium. "Maintenance" fluids for patients unable to drink may provide far more sodium than would be consumed on a regular diet. A screening CXR would likely identify congestive heart failure.

CASE 112-1 *(continued)*

The patient underwent a chest CT-PE protocol read as showing no evidence of pulmonary embolism (PE) or deep venous thrombosis (DVT). The report noted bibasilar subsegmental atelectasis, a common finding after surgery, and evidence of aspiration pneumonitis of right lower lobe (RLL). It is possible that she aspirated during the scan which revealed food in her esophagus.

Should the "negative" chest CT-PE protocol cause the clinician to discard his hypothesis that this postoperative patient likely had a PE?

At this point, the examiner may reconsider his hypothesis that this patient likely had a PE in light of discordant data. However, no test is infallible, including the most recent CT scanners due to

- technical limitations relating to body size, timing of contrast bolus;
- timing relative to onset of symptoms;
- the human factor in interpretation; and
- significance of other findings.

This chest CT, read at night, was of good diagnostic quality and the timing appropriate to diagnose PE relative to onset of symptoms (within four days).

Physicians often seek a unifying diagnosis to explain all of a patient's symptoms. A critical thinker might ask whether alternative diagnoses are plausible, especially the possibility of aspiration pneumonitis. If she first aspirated in the scanner, the time course of her symptoms did not actually support this diagnosis. In addition, it is not clear that aspiration of the RLL would cause 6-7/10 substernal chest pain and ongoing shortness of breath that was not relieved with nebulizer treatment.

Optimal evaluation would include reexamining the data with a chest radiologist who would be provided with specific patient information that might improve the diagnostic yield; and to examine the size of the right atrium and ventricle, not included in the overnight report.

CASE 112-1 *(continued)*

This step did not occur and the patient continued to deteriorate. On postoperative day three at 10 PM she became anxious that "something is wrong." Her dyspnea persisted, unchanged. Her vital signs revealed a BP of 100/60 mm Hg, heart rate 125 bpm, O_2 saturation 82% on room air, increasing to 97% on 4 L of supplemental oxygen, a temperature of 102°F. A cross-coverage note documented "flat" jugular venous pressure, coarse breath sounds, decreased at her lung bases, and decreased abdominal bowel sounds. Pertinent laboratory tests included a WBC 5,900/mm^3 with 51% bands, BUN 35 mg/dL, creatinine 2.9 mg/dL (previously 0.8 mg/dL), and normal cardiac enzymes. ECG revealed changes suggestive of right ventricular overload and bigeminy. Portable CXR reported low lung volumes, no edema, and small left effusion. Overnight she received two fluid boluses of 500 cc for systolic BP in the 70 s, and her O_2 requirement increased to 6 L. Arterial blood gas reported pH 7.31, pCO_2 52, pO_2 73 on face mask with 10 L supplemental O_2. At 3 AM she complained of severe shortness of breath; her blood pressure was 60/30, her pulse 125 beats per minute, her temperature 99.1°F.

How does the data help the clinician formulate a hypothesis? Does the screening CXR support the conclusion that presumed aspiration caused this patient's worsening hypoxia when no infiltrates were seen? Should her clinicians discard PE from the differential diagnosis? Is the patient now septic?

On one level this case appears to be straightforward. New clinical data suggested that this critically ill patient had an explanation for vomiting (the usual post-general anesthesia nausea or post-operative ileus), likely bacterial aspiration pneumonitis and sepsis. However, new clinical data should be interpreted in the context of the original working hypothesis of PE. As an increase in the number of chronic and acute illnesses in one patient increase, parsimony of diagnosis—Occam's razor—can fail. Hickam dictum: "A patient can have as many diagnoses as he darn well pleases," applies to this case.

CASE 112-1 *(continued)*

On postoperative day five, the patient still complained of shortness of breath, pleuritic chest pain, and ongoing nausea. Her vital signs were notable for a BP of 90–130/50–70 mm Hg, a heart rate 96–116 bpm, and O_2 saturation 97% (3L). Wheezing, diffuse rhonchi, and a tender right lower quadrant were now noted on physical examination.

Abdominal CT with contrast

Small bowel obstruction secondary to herniation between layers of anterior abdominal wall (Spigelian hernia).

Chest CT (without contrast)

New multifocal aspiration pneumonia with secretions or aspirated material in the right main stem bronchus.

On postoperative day six, this patient underwent repair of an incarcerated hernia. There was no evidence of ischemic bowel. Her laboratory tests revealed a Cr 0.7 mg/dL and an elevated troponin 0.16. Although she felt less short of breath and described nasal and chest congestion similar to her allergies, she now was coughing up blood-tinged sputum. A monitor strip showing bigeminy and she was transferred to medicine under the care of another clinician with the presumptive diagnosis of submassive PE.

Work-up on the medical service

An ECG did not show signs of right heart strain (negative T waves in the precordial leads, a new RBBB, classic S1Q3T3, and Qr in lead V_1), but a new Q in lead III was interpreted as consistent with an inferior myocardial infarction of indeterminate age. An echocardiogram did not confirm inferior segmental wall abnormalities, but reported moderately severe pulmonary hypertension and an enlarged right ventricle. Her troponin peaked at 0.44. The patient underwent an extensive evaluation for secondary causes of pulmonary hypertension including additional imaging (**Table 112-4**). All studies were unrevealing and she was empirically discharged on warfarin.

■ HOSPITAL-ACQUIRED PULMONARY HYPERTENSION

The most likely causes of hospital-acquired pulmonary hypertension are either massive fluid overload from fluid resuscitation, which should resolve with diuresis, or right ventricular overload from massive or submassive pulmonary embolism.

Cognitive factors unrelated to true prevalence such as the desire of a specialist not to miss anything in his or her specialty and the common situation of a generalist not questioning the consultant's recommendations probably drove the recommendation to perform additional testing. ***However, the medical team failed to revisit the primary data obtained by the surgeons.*** After the patient was discharged, a chest radiologist retrospectively reviewed the original chest PE protocol CT and noted an acute right interlobar descending pulmonary artery embolism, an enlarged right atrium and ventricle, once again highlighting the benefit of consulting radiology early when there is a diagnostic quandary. The clot (as they usually are when poorly seen) was initially surprisingly central. By the time the patient had the subsequent chest CT, the clot was no longer visible. The primary impediment to a more timely diagnosis was an excessive reliance on repeated testing long after the PE had occurred.

UNDERUTILIZATION

CASE 112-2

ACUTE ABDOMINAL PAIN

A 48-year-old African American male went to a local emergency room for acute abdominal pain, which developed suddenly four hours after eating pork ribs with his wife on a Sunday night. He characterized the pain as severe, sudden, epigastric in location. The pain was accompanied by an episode of nausea, vomiting, and diarrhea; he had no prodrome. His wife was not sick. His past medical history was notable for untreated labile hypertension. He did not drink alcohol or take illicit substances, nor did he smoke cigarettes.

Physical examination

BP 160/100 mm Hg, pulse 96 bpm, regular, temperature 99.6, room air O_2 sat 100%.

Healthy appearing male with a "benign" physical examination.

Laboratory tests

Standard plain imaging of his abdomen and chest: no free air, normal gas pattern.

CBC: WBC 13,768/μL Hct 48%, platelet count 92,000/μL

BUN 20 mg/dL; creatinine 2.1 mg/dL; total bilirubin 2.1 mg/dL, SGOT 98 mg/dL

He was discharged from the emergency department after six hours of observation during which time he became pain free. He was given the provisional diagnosis of food poisoning and was advised to see his primary care physician the next day for treatment of his hypertension and to follow up the laboratory test abnormalities.

His primary care physician was unavailable so he was seen by another physician who repeated his blood work, confirmed his hypertension, which was treated with nifedipine, and ordered a general ultrasound of his abdomen. The patient's symptoms had resolved.

Three days later he saw another physician in the primary care office. A complete physical examination was notable for BP 140/90 mm Hg in both arms, pulse of 72 bpm, temperature 98.8, A-V nicking on fundoscopic examination, a laterally displaced dynamic PMI, and a loud S4 heart sound. His abdominal examination was benign and no bruits were appreciated. He was a robust six-foot-four muscular gentleman and organomegaly was not possible to assess.

TABLE 112-4 Overutilization in Complex Illness (Case 112-1)

Imaging	Comments
Preadmission abdominal/pelvic CT: endometrial cancer	
Normal admission CXR(PA) and subsequent CXR (PA and lateral): atelectasis, low lung volumes, trace left effusion, retrocardiac density	
Chest CT PE protocol with contrast: aspiration RLL, bibasilar subsegmental atelectasis, no PE or DVT Chest CT- PE protocol	High pretest probability of PE with a "negative study" BUN 35 mg/dL, Cr 2.9 mg/dL (previously, Cr 0.8 mg/dL)
Repeat CXR (portable): to evaluate ongoing symptoms, now with hypotension, tachycardia, and worsening hypoxia: low lung volumes, no edema, small left pleural effusion	
CXR to evaluate chest pain, hypotension (BP 72/50, Pulse 125, 98% 2L): low lung volumes, no pulmonary edema, small left effusion	
Abdominal CT with contrast to evaluate RLQ pain, bilious vomiting, 57% bandemia: SBO secondary to Spigelian hernia	
Third chest CT PE protocol more than four days after the initial event to evaluate increasing hypoxia, 51% bands: multifocal aspiration pneumonia, secretions or aspirated material in right main bronchus, new pleural effusions	Likely to miss a PE four days after the event
ECHO: RV dilation on ECHO	An echo will rarely visualize a PE, and is usually normal despite PE. It is most useful for risk stratification and prognostication after the diagnosis of PE has been established.
Ultrasound of lower extremities: negative for DVT	40% of patients with acute PE are likely to have a negative ultrasound of the lower extremities
Persantine PET scan	
Cardiac MRI	
Right heart catheterization	
Hospital length of stay (LOS)	LOS (if the diagnosis of acute PE had been made at the time of the 1st chest CT) versus actual (to accommodate testing) a surrogate for increased cost
Risks of imaging	Cumulative radiation exposure, contrast

The abdominal ultrasound performed at a local imaging facility was reported as negative. His laboratory tests from the previous Monday were unchanged from the emergency department visit with a WBC count of 11,988 μL (85% polys), platelet count of 88,000 μL, mild elevation of transaminases, bilirubin, and creatinine of 1.9 mg/dL. An ECG revealed left ventricular hypertrophy. There was no prior ECG for comparison, nor was there a prior creatinine. Urine dipstick was positive for blood and protein. Microscopic examination revealed sheets of red blood cells without casts.

WHAT IS THE CLINICAL PROBLEM OR CHIEF COMPLAINT?

This hypertensive patient developed sudden, severe, abdominal pain. The emergency physician attributed this problem to food poisoning.

Does the diagnosis adequately explain this patient's symptoms? Or even if less frequent, what might cause his death?

The first step in making any diagnosis is to think of it. Although the differential diagnosis is broad, sudden severe abdominal pain would cause concern for acute perforation, acute bleeding, or aortic dissection. A KUB "ruled out" free air and his blood work did not suggest bleeding. Hypertension was noted but not identified as a risk factor for the cause of his abdominal pain.

A hypothesis generated by partial information requires diagnostic adequacy. Does the principle diagnosis explain all of the positive and negative findings? Are there no convincing alternative diagnoses? At each step in the process as more data becomes available, certain hypotheses can be eliminated. Overlooking discordant data as in this case resulted in failure to order appropriate imaging. Although highly likely based on prevalence in the community, the diagnosis of acute food poisoning would not explain the associated laboratory abnormalities. This diagnosis should have been rejected as implausible.

The patient was subsequently admitted to a tertiary care hospital for evaluation of what appeared to be multisystem disease of unclear etiology but with worrisome features.

This hospitalization presented another opportunity to generate an alternative hypothesis. The physicians had time to formulate an adequate and coherent diagnosis that could be verified with appropriate imaging. Instead, ECG findings of left ventricular hypertrophy (LVH) prompted a "rule out MI protocol" and then the patient was discharged to home without an explanation of the persistently abnormal blood work. In addition, no one appreciated the significance of the abnormal contour of the thoracic aorta, misread as tortuous.

This case highlights the importance at each step to test a limited number of hypotheses, not just ruling out one, to see whether the specific diagnoses fit the available information. This requires keeping an open mind until sufficient clinical data is obtained to favor one hypothesis over another, constantly reassessing the validity of the favored hypothesis in light of new data, and reexamining all data for any "minor" detail that might have been overlooked or in this case misinterpreted. A challenge physicians face on a daily basis is deciding when there is sufficient information to make a diagnosis, order appropriate treatment, and transition a patient to home. The sentinel clue in this case was the "tortuous aorta" reported on the CXR.

CASE 112-2 *(continued)*

Persistence of unexplained laboratory abnormalities prompted hospital admission. A CXR was read as showing a "tortuous aorta." An echocardiogram was reportedly unremarkable other than the presence of LVH, and he ruled out for a myocardial infarction. His laboratory blood work remained unchanged. He was discharged on Bactrim, Lisinopril, and hydrochlorothiazide and instructed to follow up with his receiving primary care physician.

At the first outpatient follow-up visit, the patient felt that his medications were making him sick, he wanted to discontinue them, and he was angry. His BP was 140/90 mm Hg and his examination unchanged. A urine sample was examined and revealed persistent sheets of red blood cells.

The patient initially refused additional imaging but agreed to a blood test as long as it had not been done previously. An erythrocyte sedimentation rate was 110. The primary care physician then called his wife to involve her in the decision-making process. Ultimately, three weeks after the initial presentation for abdominal pain the patient agreed to a CT of his abdomen and chest.

The chest and abdominal CT revealed a dissection of this patient's aorta originating just distal of the left subclavian artery and extending down to his iliacs. The false lumen was supplying blood to his spinal cord and to his left kidney.

The patient underwent successful aortic grafting at another tertiary facility. At the origin of the dissection the aorta was noted to be very friable, an area of lung consolidation was compressing this area, and sutures were placed more proximally. Postoperatively, his renal function normalized, and after a period of rehabilitation, he was discharged with only a slight limp.

END OF LIFE CARE

CASE 112-3

A 96-year-old man s/p PEG, tracheostomy in the setting of having suffered a massive stroke was transferred from rehabilitation for high fever, a rising WBC, and agitation.

In this case, a 96-year-old patient who had suffered a massive stroke, s/p tracheostomy, and PEG placement, was dying of a *Clostridium difficile* infection. Despite receiving maximal medical treatment, his WBC continued to climb to a peak of 83,000/mm^3 and he died in the intensive care unit. Despite his grave prognosis, he continued to undergo imaging that would not influence management. Given his comorbidities, he would not survive a surgical procedure. Instead he was admitted to the intensive care unit. The focus should have shifted to comfort concurrent with medical treatment.

Hospitalized dying patients frequently receive fully aggressive care up to and including life-sustaining treatment and resuscitation. Although distraught families sometimes drive this care, the critical core of the doctor-patient relationship requires the need for guidance and direction from the clinician for these families. The patient's surrogate can fire you and go elsewhere, but he or she cannot determine evaluation and/or treatment if it serves no meaningful purpose for the patient or may even contribute to distress.

QUALITY IMPROVEMENT

Is the average inpatient getting a body CT approximately every four days? How much is too much?

To answer what may seem at first glance an appalling question, clinicians may need to review how much imaging their patients are actually receiving, including any films prior to CT scans. The process of critical thinking would avoid collecting more information than is necessary (as was done in Cases 112-1 and 112-3) to reach a desired level of diagnostic certainty or treatment threshold. Refinement of a diagnostic hypothesis requires appropriate interpretation of test results, which did not happen in either Case 112-1 or 112-2.

Focused and deliberately considered ordering of medical tests can also benefit from the review of previous examinations. Newer imaging is not always better for hospitalized patients. The maxim, "The answer is in the jacket," provides power and rapid answer to a myriad of carefully framed specific questions. An old CT will frequently answer the question raised by subsequent health care teams as in Case 112-1. During the hospitalization, comparison of serial films, even bedside chest radiographs, may provide more information than can be derived over time than by more sophisticated imaging. The rate of evolution of abnormalities, both regarding progression and resolution, can separate many abnormalities that have the same potential appearance at a particular moment in time.

With computerized order entry, data on individual ordering of imaging studies will become readily available and increasingly, imaging guidelines will be developed along with performance measures to define and measure quality. Built on consensus, guidelines are typically evolving documents developed to answer important questions. However, they may not reflect evolving technology and/or conflicting recommendations from different societies in the ordering of imaging studies. They also may not be applicable to the acutely ill patient before you. Critical decision-making will therefore remain central to the privilege of caring for sick persons.

PRACTICE POINT

- Order as few examinations as necessary to guide management.
- Use prior imaging in clinical context to provide additional information.
- Minimize radiation.
- Consult radiology to reexamine original data if one imaging modality fails to reveal the expected result.
- Responsibility includes communication regarding incidental and nonemergent findings.

CONCLUSION

Critical decision-making rests upon the foundation of common sense, informed and experienced clinical judgment, and one of the old medical virtues, humility. An unflinching self-awareness recognizes that subjective assessments of events are often affected by factors unrelated to true prevalence, errors in assessing diagnostic value of clinical evidence, and errors in revision of probability.

Clinical problem solving relies upon inferential diagnosis to guide further action, whether in the selection of further testing or treatment. Experience provides a context for anticipating diagnoses and interpreting clinical events. Specialists may provide the necessary expertise to improve diagnostic accuracy but specialty focus may limit the categories of illness considered. Therefore, it will always be the responsibility of generalists to know when to ask for help and where to go for that help. The first step may be consultation with the radiologists in the interpretation of the data at hand.

SUGGESTED READINGS

Alpert JS. A review of clinical guidelines with some thoughts about their utility and appropriate use. *Am J Med.* 2010;123(7):573–576.

Coulehan MPH. On Humility. *Ann Intern Med.* 2010;153(3):200–201.

Kaplan DM. Clear writing, clear thinking, and the disappearing art of the problem list. *J of Hospital Medicine.* 2007;2(4):199–202.

Peterson MC, Holbrook JH, Von Hales D, et al. Contributions of the history, physical examination, and laboratory investigation in making medical diagnoses. *West J Med.* 1992;156:163–165.

Richardson W, Wilson M, Nishikawa J, et al. The well-built clinical question: a key to evidence-based decisions (editorial). *ACP J Club.* 1995;123:A12–A13.

Sackett DL, Rosenberg WMC, Gray JAM, et al. Evidence based medicine: what it is and what it isn't. *Br Med J.* 1996;312:71–72.

Warner MA, Warner ME, Weber JG. Clinical significance of pulmonary aspiration during the perioperative period. *Anesthesiology.* 1993;78:56–62.

SECTION 3
Procedures

CHAPTER 113

Introduction to Procedures

Grace C. Huang, MD

Key Clinical Questions

1. How can hospitalists be frontline defenders of procedural patient safety?
2. What should hospitalists ask themselves before performing any procedure safely?
3. What are additional considerations for training and supervising trainees? What is the role of simulation?
4. What is state of the art in procedural competence assessment?
5. How can hospitalists have an impact on an institutional policy and practice in procedures?

INTRODUCTION

Though traditionally considered a nontechnical role, hospitalists are increasingly performing procedures. In small hospitals without extensive specialty resources, hospitalists are often firstline operators of procedures. Continuing medical education courses on common procedures are being geared toward hospitalists. Procedure services staffed by hospitalists are emerging around the country, leading some hospitalists to call themselves proceduralists. In light of the fact that technical errors are a common cause of inpatient morbidity and mortality, hospitalists are well positioned to improve patient safety.

PREPARATION

Before performing any procedure, a hospitalist must ask him- or herself the following questions to reduce potential procedural errors (**Table 113-1**).

Considerations for using interventional radiology even before attempting at the bedside include: distorted anatomy due to prior surgeries (eg, posterior spinal fusion for lumbar punctures), small fluid volumes, previous failed attempts, and a narrow window for tolerating complications (eg, central lines in patients on positive-pressure ventilation).

PROCEDURES AND MEDICAL EDUCATION

For the hospitalist working in a teaching hospital, there are additional considerations when supervising an individual trainee performing a procedure. He or she should perform a needs assessment first to get a sense of the trainee's experience, known areas of weakness, and history of complications. The hospitalist should provide education tailored to the individual, which should include the elements of the preparation checklist (Table 113-1). The hospitalist should then establish expectations of his or her role beforehand. At what point should the hospitalist take over? How will the trainee communicate the need for help without alarming the patient? Next, the hospitalist should be purposeful in checking in with the trainee to see if there are remaining questions, steps to be reviewed again, or general concerns. Prior to the procedure, the hospitalist should introduce and describe his or her role as supervisor to the patient, if meeting the patient for the first time. During the procedure, the hospitalist should be attentive to the physical and emotional welfare of the patient and the educational, psychological, and material needs of the trainee. After the procedure, the hospitalist should initiate a debriefing session, beginning with the trainee's perceptions, a review of what went well and what went poorly during the procedure, general feedback, and a learning plan for addressing areas of needed improvement.

Institutions are increasingly developing educational programs to teach trainees or faculty to perform procedures, to address the inadequacy of the "see one, do one, teach one" tradition. Web-based educational materials on procedures, such as the New England Journal of Medicine Videos of Clinical Medicine series, and published literature are readily available for individual review. Procedure services at teaching hospitals can provide a mechanism for formal supervision, practice, and evaluation. Competency assessment of trainees remains an important area of investigation. Previous studies have used procedural comfort or confidence as a proxy for competence, but the research has evolved to routinely include patient-level measures.

TABLE 113-1 Preparation

Cognitive review	1. Is the procedure indicated? 2. Have I considered any possible contraindications for the procedure? 3. Have I mentally rehearsed the steps of the procedure?
Procedural issues	1. Have I obtained consent from the patient or the appropriate designee? 2. Are the coagulation parameters within acceptable limits (as deemed by clinical policies and/or according to the literature)? 3. Are any imaging studies necessary to confirm the anatomy or the location of the fluid? 4. Have I performed a preprocedural time-out?
Material issues	1. What is the level of contact precautions required for this procedure? 2. Have I familiarized myself with the kit? 3. Will I need extra antiseptic? 4. Will I need extra lidocaine? 5. Will I need extra collection tubes? 6. Is a bedside ultrasound available?
Logistical issues	1. Who is available to help in case I need additional materials? How will I contact them? 2. Have I set up the room in a way that will allow me to access my materials safely? 3. Have I identified the locations of the sharps container and the trash can? 4. What will I do with my pager and/or cell phone?
Contingency planning	1. Who is available for backup if I do not succeed? 2. Which other consultation services can I contact if the procedure cannot be done at the bedside?
Postprocedural issues	3. Immediate complications—what can I anticipate and how long should I monitor for them? 4. Delayed complications—what potential problems exist and how will I monitor for them?

The most promising development in procedural training is the availability of high-fidelity procedural models for common bedside procedures. These task trainers have widely become accepted as a safe alternative to practicing procedural skills on patients. They offer an opportunity for learners to practice skills deliberately in a controlled setting until a predefined threshold of skill is achieved. In addition, simulation allows exposure to scenarios that occur infrequently in clinical practice, such as simulated complications. Procedural models can be used in isolation for pure psychomotor learning or can be combined with standardized patients or Web-based patients to integrate tasks of communication and professionalism. Simulation-based training, in particular related to central venous catheterization, has demonstrated a benefit on procedural comfort, increased knowledge, and clinical outcomes such as decreased infection rates and decreased arterial sticks.

PROCEDURES AND QUALITY IMPROVEMENT

From an institutional perspective, hospitalists can positively influence the work flow. One study discussed the successful training of hospitalists to perform peripherally inserted central venous catheters (PICCs), which is of benefit because PICCs are associated with decreased risks of significant morbidity (Giuffrida, 1986). Procedural centers concentrate expertise and provide an infrastructure for managing procedural complications.

Research and quality improvement in procedures must have an infrastructure for ongoing data collection. Adverse events stemming from procedures should be included in case logs for medical peer review and should inform workgroups, which should convene regularly to revise kit contents, preparation checklists, or educational approaches.

CONCLUSION

Hospitalists can help minimize technical complications by taking a comprehensive approach to mental and physical preparation, complying with institutional guidelines, and becoming involved in systems-related efforts to decrease procedural harm. Trainee education should be tailored to individual experience but standardized across the training or curricular program, and simulation holds significant promise as an instructional approach to teaching procedures.

SUGGESTED READINGS

Akers AS, Chelluri L. Peripherally inserted central catheter use in the hospitalized patient: is there a role for the hospitalist? *J Hosp Med.* 2009;4(6):E1–E4.

Barsuk JH, McGaghie WC, Cohen ER, et al. Simulation-based mastery learning reduces complications during central venous catheter insertion in a medical intensive care unit. *Crit Care Med.* 2009;37(10):2697–2701.

Giuffrida DJ, Bryan-Brown CW, Lumb PD, et al. Central vs peripheral venous catheters in critically ill patients. *Chest.* 1986;90(6):806–809.

New England Journal of Medicine. *Videos in Clinical Medicine.* Available at http://content.nejm.org/misc/videos.dtl

Smith CC, Gordon CE, Feller-Kopman D, et al. Creation of an innovative inpatient medical procedure service and a method to evaluate house staff competency. *J Gen Intern Med.* 2004;19(5 Pt 2):510–513.

CHAPTER 114

Lumbar Puncture

Claude Killu, MD
Mark Ault, MD

Key Clinical Questions

1. What is the role of brain CAT scan imaging prior to lumbar puncture?
2. What is the best patient positioning to perform lumbar puncture?
3. What are important factors to consider in preventing post dural puncture headache?

CASE 114-1

A 54-year-old morbidly obese man described the "worst headache" of his life and mild photophobia to an examining physician. His medical history did not reveal any risk factors for increased intracranial pressure (age > 60 years, immune-compromised state, presence of CNS disease, new onset of seizure, confusion, or symptoms suggestive of focal neurologic abnormalities). His physical examination was notable for a temperature of 100.5°F, alert and appropriate mental status, supple neck examination, and the absence of focal neurologic findings (hemiparesis, aphasia, visual field cuts, or cranial nerve palsies). His physician ordered immediate empiric antibiotics prior to a head CT scan. A proceduralist performed an ocular ultrasound which demonstrated an optic nerve sheath diameter (ONSD) of 5.8 mm in the left eye and 6.0 mm in the right eye. Because the ONSD was elevated, a CT scan of his brain without contrast was obtained and reported no acute bleed, midline shift, or mass effect.

Using ultrasound guidance and a 22 g × 124 mm Gertie Marx needle, a lumbar puncture was performed to rule out subarachnoid hemorrhage and meningitis. Because of his girth, the patient sat upright during the procedure. After return of fluid was noted, the proceduralist replaced the stylet and gently lowered the patient to the left lateral position. The proceduralist documented an opening pressure of 380 mm Hg with the patient relaxed and breathing comfortably and the presence of respiratory variation in the manometer. He removed 40 cc of colorless CSF for diagnostic evaluation and recorded a closing pressure of 170 mm Hg. The WBC count was 300 with predominant neutrophils and the RBC count was zero. The results of the spinal tap (300 WBCs/hpf with predominant neutrophils and zero RBCs/hpf) were consistent with the diagnosis of acute meningitis and the patient was admitted for continued intravenous antibiotic therapy.

INTRODUCTION

Lumbar puncture (LP) is a procedure to sample the cerebrospinal fluid (CSF) surrounding the brain and spinal cord. It can be performed on an inpatient or outpatient basis using local anesthesia. Individuals trained to perform this procedure generally include hospitalists and other internists, proceduralists, emergency physicians, pediatricians, neurologists, and radiologists. It has been estimated that 400,000 diagnostic lumbar punctures are performed in the United States annually with charges estimated between $2000 to $3000 for each uncomplicated procedure.

PHYSIOLOGY

The majority of the CSF is in the subarachnoid space, where the arachnoid membranes bridge the sulci of the brain, in the basal cisterns and around the spinal cord. CSF moves within the ventricles and subarachnoid spaces under the influence of hydrostatic pressure generated by the production of CSF by the choroid plexus of the lateral third and fourth ventricles. The volume of CSF in humans is 140 to 150 ml, constituting 10% to 20% of brain weight. Only 30 to 40 mL is actually in the ventricular system, with a production rate of 21 mL/hr. The turnover rate of total CSF is about 5 hours for an average sized human.

CSF cushions the brain, regulates brain extracellular fluid, allows for distribution of neuroactive substances, and collects the waste products produced by the brain.

INDICATIONS

CSF may be collected for both diagnostic and therapeutic purposes. Diagnostically, emergent examination of the CSF provides essential information in many clinical situations:

1. Suspected central nervous system (CNS) bacterial, fungal, and viral infections. Lumbar puncture is most commonly performed to diagnose or exclude meningitis in patients presenting with fever, altered mental status, and headache with or without meningeal signs. CSF examination is highly sensitive and specific for determining the presence of bacterial and fungal meningitis.
2. Suspected subarachnoid hemorrhage when brain computerized tomography (CT) is negative. Now that brain CT scanning is more readily available and more technologically sophisticated, there may be a tendency to omit the LP from the workup in the setting of a normal CT scan. It is important to remember that the sensitivity of the CT scan for determining the presence of subarachnoid blood is less than 100% mandating the need in situations with a moderate to high clinical suspicion to perform an LP prior to eliminating this possibility.

A nonemergency LP is indicated to diagnose of the following conditions: pseudotumor cerebri, carcinomatous meningitis, tuberculous meningitis, normal pressure hydrocephalus, neurosyphilis, and vasculitis. LP is also useful but not diagnostic in multiple sclerosis and Guillain-Barré syndrome.

Therapeutically, an LP may be performed to remove excessive fluid or to lower intrathecal pressure as in cryptococcal meningitis or pseudotumor cerebri. It may also be performed to administer medication such as intrathecal chemotherapy, intrathecal antibiotics or for injection of contrast media for myelography and cisternography.

CONTRAINDICATIONS

The primary contraindication to performing LP is elevated intracranial pressure (ICP) from a mass lesion or massive cerebral edema. A continued CSF leak leading to fatal herniation can occur as a result; therefore, in general, patients with papilledema or focal neurological deficit must have a CT scan to rule out a mass lesion. If bacterial meningitis is strongly suspected clinically, appropriate antibiotics should be initiated and LP should not be deferred. Relative contraindications may be considered in patients with coagulopathy where caution should be used. The clinician must weigh the risks of the procedure on an individual basis versus the clinical need to obtain CSF. It is our observation that the risks tend to be overestimated and that close attention to needle size, choice of local anesthetic and the experience of the operator can often allow for safe collection of fluid in less than ideal situations.

INDICATIONS FOR IMAGING

Many emergency departments and health care professionals practice routine CT scanning prior to LP as the standard of care due to the concern about cerebral herniation. It seems though that the evidence to support this practice is lacking. Routine CT scanning is not necessary in all patients prior to LP and may not be adequate to exclude elevated intracranial pressure in others. Studies suggest that high-risk patients can be identified, allowing the majority of patients to safely undergo LP without screening CT.

In a prospective study of 301 adult patients with suspected meningitis by Hasbun, et al (2001), 235 patients had a CT scan before LP and only 5% (11 patients) had a mass effect. The risk of an abnormal CT scan was related to a history of previous CNS disease, seizure within 1 week and abnormal neurological findings such as decreased level of consciousness and focal motor deficit. This study also showed that patients who underwent CT scan before LP experienced an average of 2 hours delay in diagnosis and 1 hour delay in treatment.

Therefore, CT scan performance before an LP in cases of suspected meningitis is not warranted or recommended unless the patient has grossly altered mental status, active and recent seizures, focal neurologic signs, or papilledema. Patients with these findings or clinical risk factors should have a CT scan to identify mass lesions and other causes of increased ICP.

PRACTICE POINT

- Given concerns about cost-effective medical practice and emerging risks or radiation exposure, judicious use of CT scanning is prudent.

Other imaging modalities may be used during the actual performance of the procedure. The use of ultrasound has become particularly valuable as the emergence of portable ultrasound machines allows this technology with high-quality image capability to be taken to the bedside. We now routinely use ultrasound to map the anatomic landmarks prior to virtually all LP attempts.

Fluoroscopy-guided LP may be an invaluable adjunct for the extremely challenging patient in which bedside LP has failed. It shows the bony structures of the lumbar spine and provides real-time information about the position of the needle as it is being inserted. To avoid trauma and RBC in CSF, fluoroscopy-guided LP may be best used in cases of suspected subarachnoid hemorrhage with a negative brain CT if an experienced operator is not available. However, fluoroscopy-guided LP requires the availability of interventional radiologist and mobilizing the patient to the radiology suite when a mobile C-arm unit is not available at the bedside. Use of fluoroscopy requires the patient to lie in the prone position which may be uncomfortable and makes the measurement of opening pressures more challenging. Additionally, it results in greater patient charges: $160 for each LP performed and it does require exposure to radiation.

As an adjunct to risk assessment, measurement of optic nerve sheath diameter (ONSD) using ultrasound has been advocated as an additional parameter for the determination of elevated ICP. Using the high frequency linear ultrasound probe, the operator places the probe gently over the closed upper eyelids of the patient until the optic nerve is seen behind the globe (**Figure 114-1A, B**). Optic nerve sheath diameter is determined by drawing a vertical line from the infundibulum of the optic nerve to a distance of 3 mm and measuring the diameter of the optic nerve sheath at that point. A value of 5 mm or less is believed to correlate with a normal ICP. This technique, if validated, could be invaluable as a rapid method to determine at the bedside the need for CT scanning. In the original study by Blaivas, et al, ONSD was used as an assessment of intracranial injury due to trauma. Furthermore, it could be used to follow patients with anticipated elevations in ICP that would require a repeat LP for therapeutic purposes as in patients with cryptococcal meningitis. At present, confirmatory data is lacking and the procedure is operator dependent but may prove to be useful in the future.

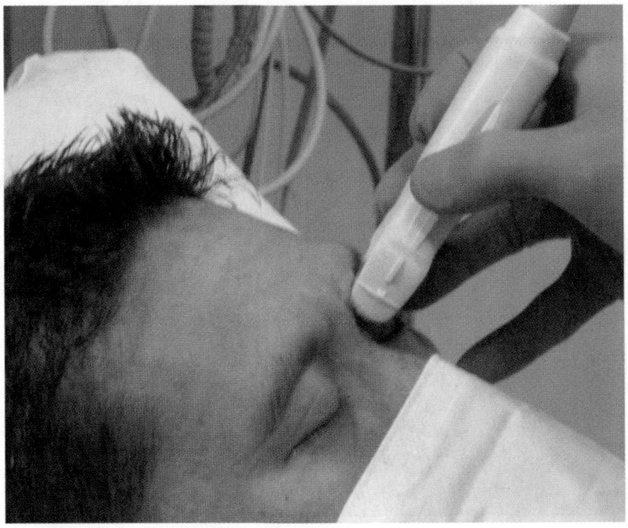

A

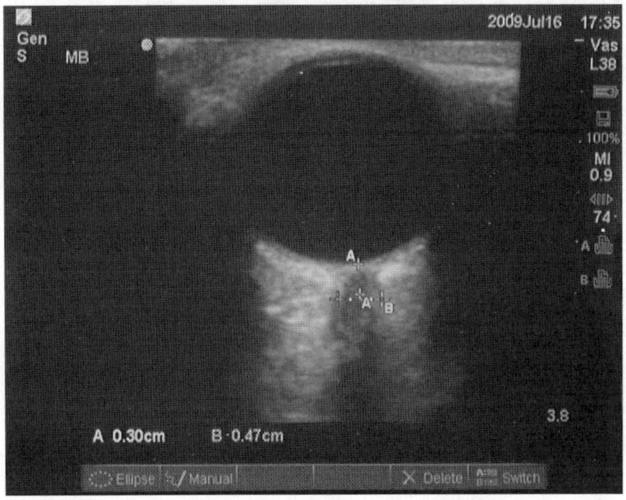

B

Figure 114-1 *(A) A high frequency ultrasound probe placed over a closed eyelid. (B) A vertical line (line a) is drawn from the infundibulum of the optic nerve to measure nerve SG = heath diameter.*

ANATOMY/SITES OF ENTRY

See below, How to Perform the Procedure.

PREPROCEDURE CHECKLIST

An informed consent prior to the procedure is preferred. LP is often considered an emergency diagnostic and life-saving procedure, and it should not be delayed for lack of consent in an unconscious patient or patients with altered mental status without immediate family available for consenting.

A formal "time-out" must be taken to properly identify the correct patient and to review any major concern such as severe coagulopathy or the presence of intracranial mass effect.

HOW TO PERFORM THE PROCEDURE

The lateral (right or left) recumbent position is the preferred position for the patient to yield an accurate measurement of the opening pressure. Although the procedure can be performed in the sitting upright position, and is often technically easier in this position, it makes measurement of the opening pressure somewhat more cumbersome.

Correct positioning of the patient determines success in obtaining CSF. The patient must remain in a "fetal position" where the neck, back, and limbs are held in flexion. The lower lumbar spine should be flexed with the back perfectly perpendicular to the edge of a bed. The hips and legs should be parallel to each other and perpendicular to the table. The procedure may be performed with the operator either sitting or standing behind the patient

> **PRACTICE POINT**
>
> - Correct patient positioning is key to the success of the procedure, and we prefer taking a little extra time to get both the patient and the operator comfortable before proceeding.

The spinal needle can be safely inserted into the subarachnoid space at the L3/4 or L4/5 interspaces, since this is well below the termination of the spinal cord. The precise level of entry of the spinal needle is most easily determined by identifying the highest points of the iliac crests visually and confirmed by palpation; and a direct line joining these is a guide to the fourth lumbar vertebral body. The spinous processes of L3, L4, and L5, and the interspaces between can usually be directly identified by palpation.

We routinely use ultrasound to define the anatomy. Using a high-frequency linear transducer the spinous processes may be identified in the transverse plane to establish the midline. This spot is marked on the patient's back (**Figure 114-2A, B**). The probe is then turned to the longitudinal position allowing identification of two spinous processes and the interspinous space (**Figure 114-3A, B**). This landmark is also marked on the back and the convergence of these two lines represents the optimal point of entry (**Figure 114-4**).

> **PRACTICE POINT**
>
> - Learn to use ultrasound. It will make the easy taps easier and difficult taps feasible.

The overlying skin must be cleaned and disinfected with chlorhexidine and alcohol containing sponges. A sterile barrier (drape) with an opening over the lumbar spine is then placed over the skin. Local anesthesia (1% lidocaine with or without epinephrine) is infiltrated with a 25-gauge needle into the previously identified lumbar intervertebral space and a 22-gauge spinal needle (or smaller) containing a stylet is inserted into the lumbar intervertebral space.

The spinal needle, preferably an atraumatic needle, should be advanced slowly, angling slightly cephalic. It is important, if a Quinke needle is being used, that the flat surface of the bevel of the needle should be positioned to face the patient's flanks to allow the needle to spread rather than cut the dural sac (the fibers of which run parallel to the spinal axis). When the subarachnoid space is entered, the stylet should be transiently removed to confirm the flow of CSF. It is worth noting that the design of the atraumatic needle necessitates only slight withdrawal of the stylet—not complete removal—making repositioning of the stylet easier.

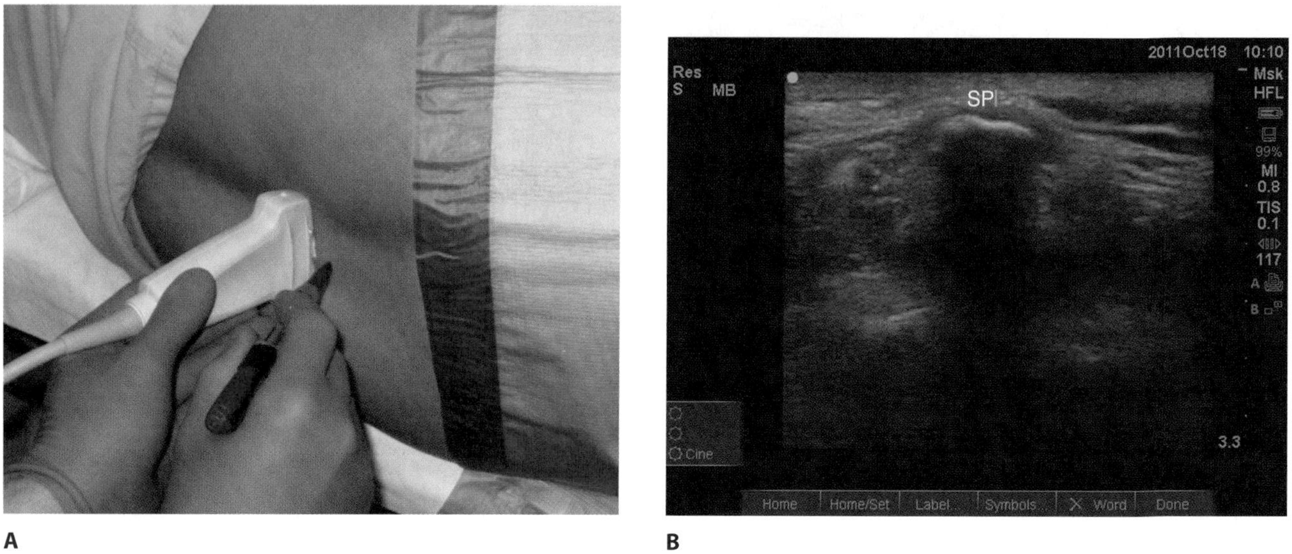

Figure 114-2 *(A) A high frequency ultrasound probe placed in the transverse plane. (B) Ultrasound image identifying the spinous processes. SP, spinous processes.*

When CSF appears and begins to flow through the needle, the patient's legs may be gently extended to allow free flow of CSF within the subarachnoid space and more accurate measurement of the opening pressure. A manometer should then be placed over the hub of the needle, stabilized during the procedure by an assistant and the opening pressure should be measured with the patient relaxed and breathing comfortably (**Figure 114-5**). Fluid is then serially collected in sterile plastic tubes. A total of 15 to 20 mL of CSF is typically removed during routine LP. However, when special studies are required, such as cytology or cultures for organisms that grow less readily (for example, fungi or mycobacterium), 40 mL of fluid can safely be removed. The fluid may be allowed to drip into the collection tubes; however, especially for larger volume fluid removal, a 3-cc syringe may be used to gently remove fluid taking care not to generate any significant amount of negative pressure.

A closing pressure may be obtained and is a useful parameter to follow when removing fluid for therapeutic purposes and may be used to calculate a pressure volumae index (PVI) as a quantitative estimate of central nervous system compliance in the setting of increased intracranial pressure. Using the formula described by G.S.U. Rao:

$$PVI = dV/\log(Pi - Pf)$$

Where dV = volume removed in milliliters, Pi is the initial pressure, and Pf is the final pressure.

Lower values of PVI correlate with decreased compliance and poorer outcomes. On a practical basis, routine measurement of both opening and closing pressures gives the operator a reasonable clinical feel for values to expect in the majority of situations.

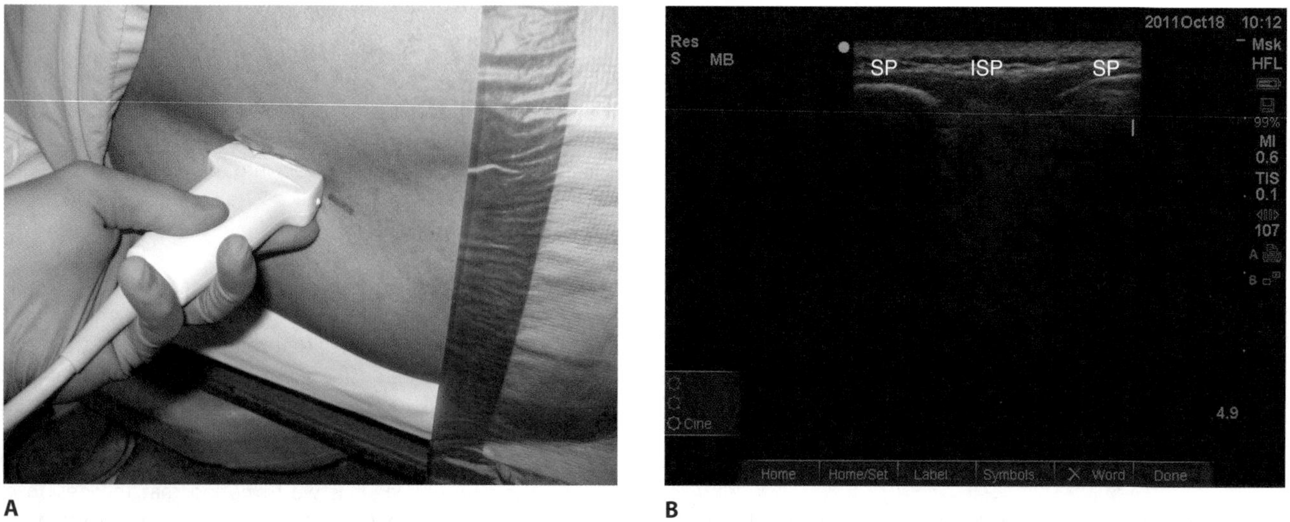

Figure 114-3 *(A) A high frequency ultrasound probe placed in the vertical plane. (B) Ultrasound image identifying two spinous processes and interspinous space. SP, Spinous process; ISP, Interspinous space.*

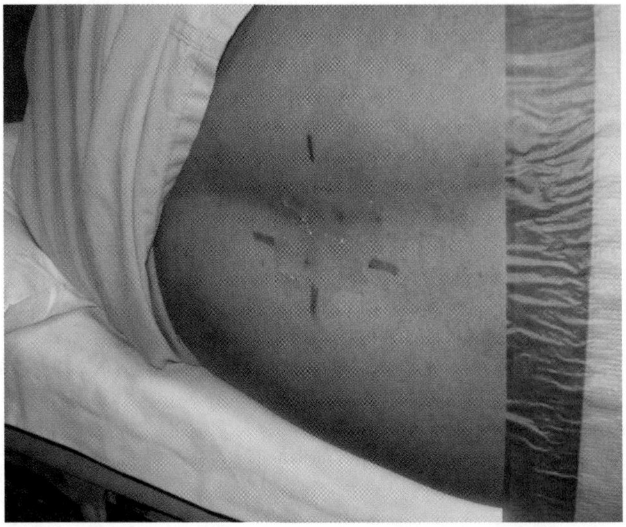

Figure 114-4 *Optimal point of entery is the convergence of the two lines.*

PRACTICE POINT

- Always measure a pressure. It is the only way to make some diagnoses (and it is inexpensive).

The choice of needle type (cutting vs atraumatic) and bore size can influence the risk of a post-dural puncture headache (PDPH). There is a large amount of convincing evidence, through several studies, that atraumatic spinal needles cause fewer PDPHs. However, adaption of these needles has been slow possibly because operators perceive increased difficulty with usage. Nevertheless, a type A recommendation with class I evidence has been adapted by the American Academy of Neurology for patients undergoing LPs supporting the use of atraumatic spinal needle to reduce the frequency of PDPH. Type A recommendation indicates strong positive recommendation, based on class I evidence which is provided by one or more well-designed, prospective, blinded controlled studies.

PRACTICE POINT

- The use of atraumatic needles whenever possible has become the standard of care. You may need the Quinke (traumatic) needle in some cases, but you are obliged to start with the atraumatic needle.

It is critical for all practitioners performing procedures to keep track of their data as a quality assurance measure. We routinely maintain a record of all of our cases with their successful completion rates and complication rates. Additionally, we maintain a record of parameters of quality outcomes we developed at our institution. The atraumatic index (ATI) as a measure of the quality of our taps, and the traumatic index (TI) as a surrogate marker for the proficiency of the tap. Both indices are easily determined as it requires knowledge only of the lowest red cell count in the spinal fluid. The ATI is determined by noting the percentage of taps that have zero red cells. We have found that it is possible to maintain an ATI of 30%. The TI is calculated by determining the number of LPs resulting in blood tinged or bloody taps representing excessively traumatic LP. We have found that a rate of blood tinged samples of

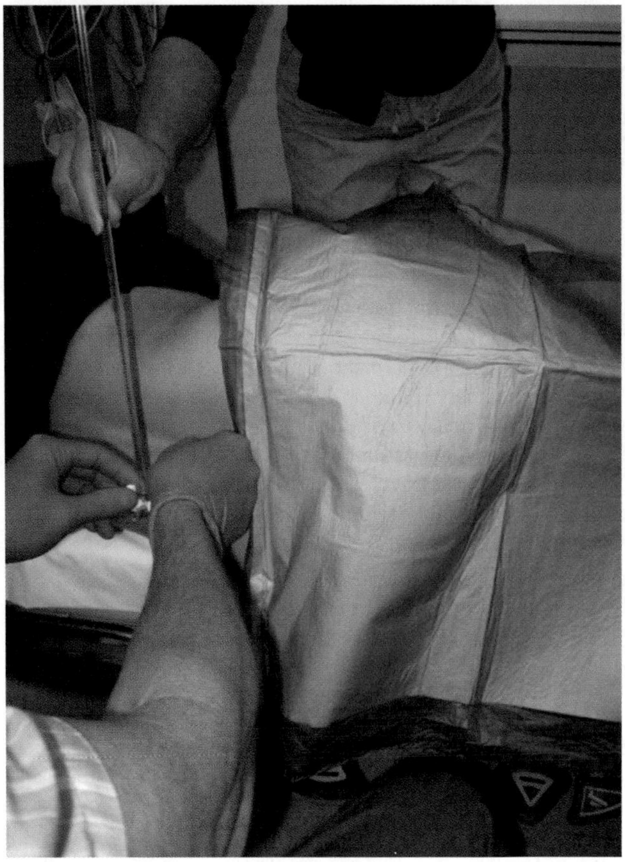

Figure 114-5 *Positioning and stabilizing of a manometer.*

3% and a rate of bloody samples of 0.2% is achievable (see sample data base report).

PRACTICE POINT

- Keep track of your data and quality indicators. You are responsible for monitoring both the quality and safety of your procedures.

DIAGNOSTIC CRITERIA

A minimum CSF sample of 15 to 20 mL must be collected for routine and basic testing and must include cell count, culture and sensitivity, total protein, and glucose. An extra tube of 3 to 5 mL is recommended to be collected if additional studies are warranted, for example, rapid plasma reagin, cryptococcal antigen, polymerase chain reaction for herpes simplex virus, etc.

Color

CSF appears normally colorless and clear. The presence of a couple hundred white blood cells (WBCs) or approximately 400 red blood cells (RBCs)/microL as a result of infectious or noninfectious diseases can change CSF appearance to turbid. CSF will appear grossly bloody if ≥6000 RBCs/microL are present (Scheld, et al, 1997).

The RBC hemoglobin breaks down in the CSF to oxyhemoglobin first (pink) and later to bilirubin (yellow) leading to a yellow-pink discoloration of the CSF called xanthochromia. In 90% of patients with a subarachnoid hemorrhage, xanthochromia appears within 12 hours after RBCs enter the subarachnoid space and persists for 2 to 4 weeks.

Xanthochromia is a result of hemoglobin degradation and indicates the presence of blood in the CSF for more than 2 hours. An LP performed earlier than this time can miss xanthochromia. This is an important consideration in the setting of suspected subarachnoid hemorrhage in patients with a negative CT scan where LP is often indicated. Repeating LP in those patients within 12 hours may reveal the presence of xanthochromia and help establish the diagnosis. Other causes of xanthochromia include increased protein concentration in the CSF (150 mg/dL or more), hyperbilirubinemia when serum bilirubin is greater than 10 to 15 mg/dL (Scheld, et al, 1997) and traumatic LP (100,000 RBC/microL or more). Xanthochromia is usually confirmed visually. More sensitive than visual confirmation, laboratory spectrometry is used to rule out traumatic LP by analyzing blood breakdown products as they progress finally to bilirubin.

The decrease in RBC count in each successive tube collected has been applied clinically to distinguish traumatic LP from subarachnoid hemorrhage (SAH), although the reliability of this parameter has been questioned.

For scenarios where the presence of xanthochromia is less clear or a traumatic tap cannot be excluded, a D-dimer assay may be useful. It does not require special handling and can be performed relatively quickly by the laboratory. Additionally, it is not affected by length of time from collection so that it can be added on at a later time. A positive value of greater than 400 confirms the presence of red blood cells that have been in the CSF long enough to be subjected to degradation. A normal D-dimer test virtually ensures the likelihood of a traumatic tap.

Cells

Normally there are zero cells present in the CSF obtained by LP, even though some indicate that 3 to 5 RBCs and 3 to 5 WBCs are considered normal in adults. The presence of an elevated WBC in the CSF must be interpreted carefully taking into consideration the following:

1. An increased WBC in CSF occurs in infectious but also inflammatory noninfectious causes.
2. Polymorphonuclear cells increase in the CSF of patients with meningitis; lymphocytes, for example, predominate in viral meningitis but rarely in bacterial meningitis.
3. Eosinophils may indicate either parasitic (mycoplasma, rickettsia) or fungal infections, and inflammatory processes such as leukemias, SAH, and obstructive hydrocephalus.
4. When different cells in the CSF can settle down and adhere to plastic tubes over time (>60 minutes), the cell count would be falsely low.

Typically, a CSF WBC count rises above 1000/microL, predominantly neutrophils, in bacterial meningitis and is usually less than 250/microL, and almost always less than 2,000/microL with predominance of lymphocytes in viral meningitis. In viral meningitis the differential typically shows lymphocyte predominance, although early infection may reveal a predominance of neutrophils which, within the next 24 hours, generally shows a shift from neutrophils to lymphocytes. Additionally, care must be taken when evaluating CSF in the setting of prior antibiotic treatment. While clearly ineffective for treating meningitis, even oral antibiotics may change the cellular content of the CSF enough to be misleading.

A "traumatic tap" refers to the increased number of RBCs and WBCs in the CSF as a result of trauma to capillaries during the procedure. When the peripheral WBC count is normal and a traumatic tap is suspected, it is safe to correct the observed WBC count by subtracting one WBC for every 500 to 700 RBCs to better assess the significance of the observed WBC count in the CSF.

Mayefsky, et al (1987) developed a formula to calculate the predicted WBC count, where

predicted CSF WBC count/microL = CSF RBC count × (peripheral blood WBC count ÷ peripheral blood RBC count).

The utility of this approach was illustrated in a report of 720 traumatic LPs in which approximately one-half of the CSF samples obtained from patients without meningitis had more white cells than could be accounted for by the proportionate number of red cells. A CSF WBC count that was more than 10 times the predicted value had a 48% positive predictive value for bacterial meningitis, while a value less than 10 times the predicted value had a 99% negative predictive value for meningitis. Bonadio, et al (1990) were able to show similar results in children, where 92 children had a traumatic tap and 93% had bacterial meningitis when their WBC count in the CSF was more than 10 times the predicted value.

Glucose

The CSF to serum glucose ratio is normally 0.6. This ratio is altered and has limited application in severe hyperglycemia. The glucose is used by cells lining the ventricles and removed by arachnoid villi. The equilibrium between the CSF and serum is maintained by simple diffusion and facilitated transport which takes several hours.

A variety of infections can lower CSF glucose concentration like bacterial or fungal CNS infections as well as noninfectious processes such as SAH, CNS sarcoidosis and cancer involving meninges. Typically CSF glucose concentration drops below 45 mg/dL (2.5 mmol/L) in bacterial meningitis and most viral CNS infections do not lower CSF glucose where it is usually more than 50% of serum concentration. CSF glucose concentration below 18 mg/dL highly suggests bacterial meningitis. Determination of this value may be particularly valuable in the neutropenic patient where and elevated WBC would not be anticipated.

Protein

Proteins enter the CSF via pinocytic vesicles transported across the capillary endothelial cells. Normal CSF concentration range in adults is 23 to 38 mg/dL and in neonates the range is higher.

The presence of RBCs in cases of traumatic LP or SAH can falsely increase CSF protein by approximately 1 mg of protein/dL for each 1000 RBCs/microL. It is therefore recommended that the CSF protein concentration and RBC count should be performed on the same tube of CSF.

CSF protein can be elevated in bacterial meningitis to concentration above 250 mg/dL and typically less than 150 mg/dL in viral meningitis. Values above 200 mg/dl strongly argue against a viral etiology.

Cytology

When looking at a CSF sample to examine cancerous cells and detect malignancy, a larger sample should be collected, usually about 10 mL, and may require three sequentially negative taps to exclude malignancy.

■ COMPLICATIONS

Lumbar puncture is a relatively safe procedure and the complication rate is low. Post dural puncture headache may be the most common significant complication and while its occurrence can not be completely eliminated, attention to needle choice and technique may mitigate many unnecessary headaches. Prevention is clearly the key as PDPH can be the cause of significant patient morbidity requiring prolonged bed rest or potentially a blood patch for symptom relief. In addition to needle type, factors leading to PDPH include needle size and replacement of the stylet prior to withdrawing the spinal needle. Smaller needle size has been positively linked to reduce PDPH and use of a 24-guage needle has been shown to significantly reduce this complication. The need to ensure adequate fluid collection and the possibility that pressure measurement may be less accurate with a 24-guage needle has led to the recommendation of a 22-guage needle in most clinical scenarios.

With regard stylet replacement, it had been argued that replacement was unnecessary and potentially increased the risk of nosocomial contamination. It has been clearly shown that failure to replace the stylet leads to an increase in PDPH and is now recommended before withdrawal of the spinal needle.

Other commonly touted factors to reduce the incidence of PDPH, including prolonged bed rest, fluid loading, and caffeine, have not been demonstrated to be beneficial. In the outpatient setting, we routinely discharge the patient immediately after the procedure. We recommend limitation of physical activity to include only avoidance of significant exertion and prolonged standing or lifting of heavy objects.

Other complications would include infection, which should be negligible, local bleeding, and minor neurologic symptoms such as radicular pain or numbness. Cerebral herniation is an unusual complication and can be eliminated by appropriate patient screening and selection. Similarly late onset epidermoid tumors of the thecal sac have been reported. This is extremely rare and has been reported in the context of patients receiving multiple therapeutic lumbar punctures.

CONCLUSION

Lumbar puncture is a relatively safe procedure performed potentially by both primary care and subspecialty physicians. Information provided by the lumbar puncture may be invaluable and unobtainable by other testing modalities. Attention to needle type and size and adjunctive use of ultrasound may improve individual success rates of the procedure and the comfort level for the patient. It is paramount to maintain ongoing quality assurance data to monitor quality and safety outcomes.

SUGGESTED READINGS

Armon C, Evans RW, Therapeutic and Technology Assessment Subcommittee of the American Academy of Neurology. Addendum to assessment: Prevention of post-lumbar puncture headaches: report of the Therapeutic and Technology Assessment Subcommittee of the American Academy of Neurology. *Neurology.* 2005;65:510–512.

Blaivas M, Theodoro D, Sierzenski PR. Elevated intracranial pressure detected by bedside emergency ultrasonography of the optic nerve sheath. *Ann Emerg Med.* 2005;45(3):336–337.

Bonadio WA, Smith DS, Goddard S, et al. Distinguishing cerebrospinal fluid abnormalities in children with bacterial meningitis and traumatic lumbar puncture. *J Infect Dis.* 1990;162:251.

Fishman RA. Cerebrospinal fluid in diseases of the nervous system. 2nd ed. Philadelphia: Saunders; 1992.

Hasbun R, Abrahams J, Jekel J, Quagliarello VJ. Computed tomography of the head before lumbar puncture in adults with suspected meningitis. *N Engl J Med.* 2001;345:1727.

Mayefsky JH, Roghmann KJ. Determination of leukocytosis in traumatic spinal fluid tap specimens. *Am J Med.* 1987;82:1175.

National guidelines for analysis of cerebrospinal fluid for bilirubin in suspected subarachnoid haemorrhage. *Ann Clin Biochem.* 2003;40:481.

Rao GSU. Neurological monitoring. *Indian J Anaesth.* 2002;46(4): 304–314.

Scheld WM, Whitley RJ, Durack DT. Infections of the Central Nervous System. 2nd edition. Philadelphia: Lippincott-Raven; 1997.

Spanos A, Harrell FE, Durack DT. Differential diagnosis of acute meningitis, an analysis of the predictive value of initial observations. *JAMA.* 1989;262:2700.

CHAPTER 115

Central Line Placement

Bradley T. Rosen, MD, MBA, FHM
Karl Wittnebel, MD, MPH

Key Clinical Questions

1. How many different types of central lines exist?
2. What is the role for using ultrasound in the placement of central lines?
3. Is there a preferred vein for the placement of a central line?
4. Are there any absolute contraindications to central line placement?
5. What is considered to be the best "skin prep" for site sterilization in preparation for central line insertion?
6. What are the three critical elements of proper sharps safety?

INTRODUCTION

The practice of hospital-based internal medicine has traditionally required proficiency in the insertion of central venous catheters (CVCs) for intravenous access. Athough the requirement that physicians-in-training become proficient in the placement of CVCs has been questioned by some, the fact remains that CVCs are a mainstay of inpatient medical care and many hospitals in the United States frequently rely on residents and hospitalists to place CVCs. This chapter reviews a number of key elements related to CVC placement, maintenance, and removal; indications and contraindications for CVC placement, procedure set-up and insertion techniques, and potential complications of CVCs. Lastly, we will comment on the essential nature of using real-time ultrasound guidance for optimal CVC placement.

WHAT IS A CENTRAL LINE?

A central line, or central venous catheter, is any vascular access device whose tip terminates in a large blood vessel of the body (most commonly the superior vena cava or inferior vena cava). On rare occasions (due to proximal thrombosis or stenosis) central lines will terminate in the subclavian vein; these "midline" catheters are also considered to be CVCs.

Almost any peripheral or central vessel can be the entry point for a CVC; the most commonly used veins for the insertion of CVCs include the internal jugular (IJ), subclavian (SC), and femoral veins. PICCs (peripherally inserted central catheters) are also considered to be CVCs and are inserted into a peripheral mid-arm vein such as the basilic vein or cephalic vein.

CVCs are made of either polyurethane or silicone. Some CVCs are designed to withstand the pressures required for the power injection of IV contrast for CT scans, and others have been impregnated with antibiotics (either chlorhexidine/silver sulfadiazine or rifampin/minocycline) in order to prevent catheter-related bloodstream infection (CR-BSI). CVCs range widely in diameter, from 3-Fr single lumen PICCs to 7-Fr 5-lumen CVCs to 15-Fr double-lumen dialysis catheters. The required diameter depends in part on the desired flow rate, which varies based on the indication, eg, 3 cc/min for CT contrast infusion, 70 cc/min for pheresis, or >300 cc/min for hemodialysis. Some CVCs have a natural safety lifespan of 10 to 14 days, while others can safely remain in place for years.

PORTS

Ports are a unique type of CVC. Ports are canisters (made of plastic or metal) that are implanted into a subcutaneous pocket in either the chest (Port-a-cath) or arm (PAS-port). The canister is attached to a polyurethane catheter which is inserted into the vascular space; the internal jugular, subclavian, or basilic veins are most commonly utilized for this purpose. Because the device is implanted and the catheter cut to length, fluoroscopic guidance is used to ensure proper positioning at the time of insertion. In order to infuse or draw blood through a port, the canister is accessed using a special, noncoring needle (Huber) that extends the life of the canister and reservoir. The main advantage of ports is that all elements of the device are buried underneath the skin, such that no dressing or covering is required when the device is not being used. This configuration minimizes the risk of infection, thereby distinguishing it from PICCs, nontunneled central lines, or tunneled catheters (discussed below), all of which protrude from the skin and have greater risk of infection from skin flora and require a sterile, occlusive dressing. Ports are typically used in patients who will need intermittent but recurrent, long-term (> 3 months) vascular access for infusion and/or phlebotomy, such as chemotherapy for cancer patients. More frequent port access increases the risk of port site infection, as the skin overlying the port is limited in its ability to tolerate repeated (or continuous) access while retaining integrity as a barrier to infection.

TUNNELED VS NONTUNNELED CATHETERS

Virtually any central line can be tunneled or nontunneled. Nontunneled central lines are commonly placed in intensive care units, operating rooms, and emergency departments. These lines (for example, a 7-Fr triple-lumen catheter) are designed for short-term access and involve the insertion of a catheter directly from the skin into a vessel below. A tunneled central line, by contrast, exits the skin at a site distant from where it enters the vascular space, traveling through a subcutaneous "tunnel" from venotomy to skin exit.

Tunneled catheters are typically used for longer-term access (> 2 weeks). The insertion procedure, similar to port implantation, is usually aided by real-time fluoroscopic guidance. Most tunneled CVCs are inserted into the internal jugular or subclavian veins and are routed through a subcutaneous tunnel 8 to 10 cm long on the chest wall, resulting in an exit site on the anterior chest. They characteristically possess a dacron cuff on the distal aspect of the catheter that is positioned within the tunnel. This cuff scars into the subcutaneous tissue over time and functions both to secure the catheter in place and as a mechanical barrier to bacterial migration. Insertion and removal of tunneled catheters are inherently more invasive than for nontunneled CVCs. Because of this, and due to their suitability for long-term use, the insertion of tunneled CVCs should be performed in patients who are free from active infections so as to minimize the chances that they become seeded with bacteria and require early removal.

Patients can be safely discharged from the hospital and live for extended periods with tunneled CVCs in place—another important difference between tunneled and many nontunneled CVCs. Outpatient hemodialysis is the most common use for these catheters, and various brand names are associated with them (Hickman, Quinton, or Permacath). Groshong catheters are of smaller diameter than dialysis catheters, but are otherwise similar. In addition, cuffed PICCs (usually < 7-Fr) can either be tunneled from the IJ or SC to the anterior chest or from the axilla to the mid-arm; these latter two tunneled CVCs are designed to meet long-term infusion and phlebotomy needs if arm veins are no longer usable.

INDICATIONS AND CONTRAINDICATIONS FOR CVC PLACEMENT

Common indications for central line placement include

1. Infusion of medications that would otherwise be caustic, toxic, or cause sclerosis of peripheral vessels if given through a peripheral IV. Common examples include chemotherapy, vasoactive medications, and some antibiotics (ie, vancomycin)
2. Recurrent and/or difficult phlebotomy, typically in hospitalized patients or for patients requiring frequent outpatient lab draws over extended periods
3. Performing ultrafiltration, hemodialysis, plasmapheresis, or any other blood filtering process
4. A need for long-term vascular access (PICC lines, ports, and tunneled catheters)
5. Infusing IV medications for patients in whom peripheral IV access is difficult or impossible to obtain
6. Hemodynamic monitoring, ie, pulmonary artery (Swan-Ganz) catheters for left ventricular end diastolic pressure and cardiac output monitoring

Given the severity of illness generally associated with the requirement for a CVC, establishing adequate venous access is frequently a matter of life and death. An actively hemorrhaging gastrointestinal bleed, for example, may require immediate placement of a large bore catheter regardless of INR or platelet levels. Similarly, a patient in intensive care may need immediate central access for antibiotics, vasoactive medications, and/or blood products, despite being severely coagulopathic and at high risk of internal or external bleeding from invasive procedures. In essence, there are no absolute contraindications to CVC placement provided that the likelihood and severity of potential complications are outweighed by the benefits of immediate venous access.

In less urgent situations, it is common practice to evaluate coagulation parameters (INR, PTT, platelets) and correct abnormalities (target INR < 1.5, PTT < 40, platelets > 50,000) prior to line insertion, although no randomized studies exist to support this approach. In reality, many CVCs can be safely placed in coagulopathic patients, and the likelihood of mechanical complication depends more upon the skill and experience of the operator in using ultrasound for guidance (discussed below) than it does on any single laboratory value. In experienced hands, the use of ultrasound guidance may be a more reliable predictor of complications than coagulopathy.

Bacteremic patients present a unique dilemma in that IV access is required for parenteral antibiotics, yet these patients are at high risk for developing secondary CR-BSI due to the seeding of the central line from circulating bacteria. In ideal circumstances bacteremic patients should be kept "line-free" (without any central lines) for at least 48 hours and/or until the bacteremia clears prior to placing a new central line. During this period, clinicians should rely on peripheral IV access for parenteral antibiotics. However, some patients inevitably will require central venous access during their bacteremic phase, and in those cases it is still acceptable to place a CVC in order to ensure the patient receives proper treatment and/or monitoring. In these patients, antibiotic-impregnated catheters are highly recommended along with the prompt removal of the CVC as soon as it is no longer required.

In summary, the indications and necessity for central venous access in all patients must be reviewed critically before proceeding with a CVC insertion. Indwelling lines pose definite risks to patients, and once inserted, the CVC should be regularly assessed for ongoing necessity with the goal of prompt CVC removal as soon as the risks eclipse the benefits. A broad assessment of a patient's clinical status, planned future interventions, operator expertise, and the appropriateness of the overall treatment plan should be considered in all patients prior to line insertion, as these risks and needs determine the optimal procedure for any given patient.

CVC COMPLICATIONS

Central line complications can be divided into three categories spanning the life of the catheter (from insertion to removal): insertion complications; persistence-related complications; and removal complications. During the insertion of a CVC, potential complications include the following:

- Arterial puncture and/or arterial cannulation
- Arteriovenous (AV) fistula creation
- Bleeding
- Hematoma
- Pneumothorax
- Hemothorax
- Bladder injury
- Nerve injury
- Introduction of bacteria to the circulation, with resultant bacteremia
- Retained foreign object (most commonly a guidewire)

- Operator needle stick injury
- Line malposition (eg, incorrect length, or tip placement in a vessel other than the SVC)

Complications related to the persistence of an indwelling CVC include

- Line dislodgement
- Line associated deep venous thrombosis (DVT)
- Rash or allergic reaction to dressing adhesive
- Catheter-related bloodstream infection

Complications associated with the removal of a CVC include

- Bleeding
- Air embolism
- Catheter fracture, with or without embolism of the retained fragment

A CRITICAL TOOL: PORTABLE ULTRASOUND

The single most important technique a clinician can utilize for a successful CVC placement and prevent insertion-related complications is real-time 2D ultrasound. Ultrasound uses high frequency sound waves (for vascular access, the probe operates at 5–10 MHz) which provide excellent axial resolution. The position of vessels can be determined because the speed of sound in soft tissue is relatively constant (1540 m/sec). The main advantages of ultrasound over other imaging modalities are images acquired in real time at the bedside allowing visualization of needle and wire placement during the procedure, and the biologic safety of ultrasound waves.

Ultrasound machines have become smaller and less expensive over the years, and the image quality of portable ultrasounds now rivals that of larger machines. Multiple studies have evaluated and confirmed the patient safety benefits resulting from the use of portable ultrasound for the placement of CVCs. Despite this preponderance of evidence, clinicians have been slow to adopt routine use of portable ultrasound in the United States. This inertia is likely the result of two independent obstacles: up-front cost and operator comfort. On the cost side, a single fully functional portable ultrasound package can cost well over $20,000, and more than one machine is usually required if physicians are going to have an ultrasound machine readily available for use. Unfortunately, this type of capital expense is not easily bankrolled by most hospitalist groups, which then must turn to their hospital administration to make the investment. To date, enthusiasm for this type of purchase has been tepid at best, and this is at least partially due to a failure of the medical community to convince hospital leadership of the essential nature of portable ultrasound for procedural guidance.

Even if purchased, the machines may end up sitting in the corner if two important realities related to operator comfort are not addressed: physicians are slow to change practice; and ultrasound-guided procedural techniques require **training** and **practice** in order to achieve comfort and proficiency. Portable ultrasound, while potentially transformative in its potential, is not a magic wand that need only be waved over a patient to reap its benefits. Rather, physicians must learn an entirely different insertion technique that involves a greater level of hand-eye coordination and translation of the three-dimensional world into two dimensions. In so doing, clinicians must shed the time-tested "landmark technique" in favor of an approach which has videogame-type qualities. To achieve critical mass for such a change requires opinion leaders within physician networks to learn, lead, and encourage their colleagues to do the same. Ample practice opportunities must also be readily available (ideally with simulators), with good behavior rewarded and bad practice patterns discouraged. Outcomes-based reimbursement may eventually force this type of best practice to the forefront by holding clinicians accountable on both ethical and financial grounds for their performance.

CVC SITE SELECTION

Site selection can sometimes be challenging. The operator should strive to avoid surgical or traumatic wounds, skin and soft tissue infections, or known intravascular thromboses. The Institute for Health care Improvement (IHI) recommends placement of CVCs in the subclavian (rather than the internal jugular or femoral vein sites) whenever possible in order to minimize CR-BSI. While we consider this a reasonable recommendation, it does not address the totality of considerations related to central line placement and maintenance. Downsides to SC placement include the following:

- Difficulty with visualization under ultrasound guidance (although ultrasound does reveal the location of the extra-thoracic subclavian vein as a viable target)
- Higher procedural complication rates (pneumothorax or hemothorax), given the vessel's proximity to the lung
- Inability to compress the subclavian vessels in the event of arterial puncture or failed CVC placement
- The development of catheter-induced subclavian vein stenosis, a poorly understood process likely exacerbated by a larger catheter size and/or long catheterization periods

Subclavian stenosis in renal failure patients presents a particularly difficult dilemma, because a stenotic subclavian leads to decreased venous flow rates and can render the ipsilateral arm useless for eventual arteriovenous fistula creation in current or future dialysis patients. For that reason, we recommend avoiding the subclavian veins in patients who are receiving (or are likely to receive) hemodialysis via an arm fistula or AV graft. On the other hand, in intubated or trached patients receiving mechanical ventilation, placement of CVCs in the IJ are at higher risk for infection from nearby oropharyngeal secretions, and significant bleeding complications from IJ or carotid punctures can lead to soft tissue swelling that can cause airway compromise. Femoral veins are often selected in urgent or emergent settings to facilitate airway and C-spine management, but are frowned upon due to their geographic proximity to the less hygienic groin area. They also have the risk of causing traumatic complications to the femoral artery or bladder. In summary, all insertion sites for central venous access have advantages and disadvantages, and we recommend a tailored approach to site selection that takes each patient's active medical issues and anatomic factors into consideration.

CVC INSERTION COMPLICATIONS

Every procedural complication must be managed calmly, promptly, and correctly in order to avoid turning a small error into a larger one. As discussed previously, many of these are nearly completely avoidable with the use of ultrasound and proper technique. Nonetheless, errors do occur even with the most experienced operators. Arterial puncture or cannulation or significant postprocedure hematomas require direct manual pressure for at least 10 minutes (without peeking). Occasionally, blood products such as plasma, platelets, or 1-deamino-8-D-arginine vasopressin (DDAVP) are required to control bleeding, and one should not hesitate to order them if clinical conditions warrant. As mentioned, significant bleeding from the IJ can lead to airway compromise requiring close respiratory monitoring in the ICU and/or intubation. Pneumothorax or hemothorax, if large and/or clinically symptomatic, may require the prompt placement of a chest tube. AV fistula formation (again, largely avoidable with the proper use of ultrasound) is not readily apparent at the time of insertion, but once it is identified requires a timely vascular surgery consultation.

If suspicion of arterial catheter placement is high due to the location of the CVC tip on a postplacement chest x-ray, or based on the color or briskness of blood return, a blood sample can be sent for pH, pCO_2, and pO_2 measurement to gather more definitive information. Immediate confirmation of venous placement may also be obtained at the bedside with a simple manometer made from IV tubing connected to a port on the newly inserted line. An arterial pressure of 70 mm Hg is equivalent to 950 mm H_2O, whereas typical venous pressures in a supine patient are generally less than 200 mm H_2O. Therefore, if the vertical blood column in a length of connected IV tubing climbs more than 20 cm above the midaxillary line or has large pulsations, the line should be assumed to be arterial and be removed at the earliest practical time. Given the potentially devastating (embolic) complications from a CR-arterial thrombus, the responsible action is to remove (and replace, if necessary) the device in question if one has reasonable doubt. Timely consultation with the interventional radiology service may be required if there is uncertainly about the location of the line prior to its removal.

PROPER CVC MAINTENANCE

After CVC insertion, the proper care and maintenance of central lines can make the difference between a long, uneventful catheter life and costly complications such as CR-BSI, symptomatic CR-DVT requiring anticoagulation, and/or line dislodgment resulting in a repeated insertion procedure. Key elements to routine CVC care include

- Regular dressing changes with chlorhexidine cleansing
- The use of topical antibiotic devices such as the Biopatch or equivalent
- Routine alcohol swabbing of valve hubs prior to connecting IV tubing or other devices
- Ensuring that dressings are kept clean, dry, and occlusive
- Use of proper securing devices to prevent dislodgement

One of the most serious maintenance-related CVC complications is the development of a CR-BSI. If present, these infections usually manifest >72 hours after insertion. Mechanisms are thought to involve (a) a breach in sterile technique during the procedure, (b) the migration of skin pathogens down the outside of the catheter into the vascular space, and/or (c) the contamination of the catheter hubs or valves during catheter use, causing subsequent infection of the fibrin sheath surrounding the catheter tip ("biofilm"). Seeding of a CVC during bacteremia from another anatomic source is another potential concern, and frequently this will be clinically indistinguishable from infections contracted from hub contamination. If there is reasonable suspicion for a CR-BSI, obtaining blood cultures and empirically starting antibiotics are prudent first steps. The decision to remove a CVC suspected to be infected should be based on the available evidence, clinical judgment, and an assessment of how difficult (and necessary) future vascular access will be to obtain. The use of antibiotic-impregnated (or coated) catheters has been shown to decrease the incidence of CR-BSI, is recommended by the Agency for Health care Research and Quality and IHI, and should be used whenever possible.

Catheter-related thrombosis, another unfortunate complication, is thought to be a function of catheter size relative to the vessel lumen and a patient's underlying clotting predisposition. Conflicting evidence exists in terms of the incidence of embolization of upper extremity or IJ thrombi, the risks and benefits of removing catheters for treatment, and the benefit of prophylactic anticoagulation. Traditional teaching is that upper extremity thrombi have a much lower risk of embolizing than do lower extremity clots, although this point is more dogmatic than evidence based.

If a catheter-related thrombus is identified in a symptomatic patient, we recommend full-dose anticoagulation if no contraindications exist. However, one should avoid the common mistake of removing an otherwise functioning CVC simply because a thrombus is identified. As with all CVCs, the line should be removed at the earliest possible convenience, *but not if ongoing vascular access is required.* To be clear, the identification of a thrombus does *not* mandate its prompt removal—in fact, removal and subsequent insertion of another CVC at another site simply subjects the patient to an additional procedure and the risk of causing another thrombus at the new insertion site. Once the catheter has been removed, a catheter-related DVT can be treated for 2 to 4 weeks (rather than a complete 3 month or longer course for other hospital-acquired DVTs) and the patient should be monitored clinically, with or without serial ultrasound exams.

In terms of prophylaxis, some studies have shown a benefit to prophylactic low-dose warfarin while other studies reveal no benefit. Current CHEST guidelines do not recommend routine thromboprophylaxis, but very little (if any) harm comes from low-dose (eg, 1 mg/day) warfarin administration, and several studies have shown clinical benefit. Further, given the high prevalence of catheter-associated thrombosis in certain patient populations (eg, oncology patients) especially when long-term devices such as PICCs and ports are involved, we consider low-dose warfarin prophylaxis to be a reasonable intervention with very little risk.

PROPER CVC REMOVAL

Complications to watch for at the time of catheter removal include air embolism, bleeding, and catheter fracture with resultant remnant embolus. These are all readily preventable through proper patient positioning, application of direct manual pressure, and careful removal technique. To minimize bleeding risk, for example, consideration should be given to correcting coagulopathies prior to removing CVCs such as tunneled catheters or ports. Air embolism can occur when the intravenous pressure drops below ambient air pressure; this is commonly the case in the superior vena cava, where most central lines by definition terminate. As little as 100 mL of air can induce circulatory collapse if introduced sufficiently rapidly, and this amount of air can flow through a 16-gauge catheter at ambient air pressure in a matter of seconds. Maneuvers designed to increase intrathoracic venous pressure prior to removing intrathoracic catheters such as Trendelenburg, bearing down, or fully exhaling during removal are all effective. At a minimum, patients should be placed supine in a flat position during line removal from the upper body. After removal, immediate manual pressure should be applied to the skin exit site and maintained for a period of 5 to 10 minutes (depending on insertion site and any underlying coagulopathy). Continued brisk bleeding after this initial pressure application requires an additional cycle of manual pressure for another ten minutes (or longer) until meticulous hemostasis is achieved. An occlusive dressing should be placed over thoracic sites following line removal to prevent air entry after manual pressure is released, and the patient returns to a more upright position.

PROPER INSERTION TECHNIQUE

As mentioned, a large body of evidence and professional opinion now support the use of real-time ultrasound guidance for CVC insertion. Operator experience with both line insertion and ultrasound use is correlated with lower complication rates, and the optimal training methods for new providers are still being refined at academic centers throughout the country. Further, many ultrasound-compatible simulators are now available to teach the eye-hand coordination required for the procedure, and these should be utilized to the extent practicable before moving to live patients.

Detailed directions for CVC insertion can be found on the New England Journal of Medicine website, including an instructional video which serves as a useful adjunct to hands-on training and practice. The following steps should generally be followed when placing a CVC. Note: These steps assume the use of real-time ultrasound guidance and follow traditional Seldinger technique. Also note that instructions for PICC placement will differ slightly than steps below due to the "modified" Seldinger technique employed with the "introducer-dilator" device used for PICC placement.

Pre-procedure checklist

1. Review relevant laboratory, imaging, and clinical information to best understand the indication for, and possible risks of, the planned procedure.
2. Scout potential insertion sites with ultrasound; confirm vessel patency using compression, and optimize ultrasound settings (gain, depth, etc).

   TIP: *IHI recommends SC insertion and avoiding the femoral sites to minimize the risk of developing a CR-BSI. However, clinical judgment should determine the safest and most appropriate insertion site for each patient.*

   Note: *Noncompressible vessels on ultrasound indicate possible thrombosis, and pulsatile vessels are likely to be arteries.*
3. Obtain informed consent (if nonemergent).
4. Perform a ***Universal Time-Out*** (including verification of correct patient, a physician order for procedure, indication for procedure, selection of correct site and desired catheter, and the presence of informed consent)
5. Check for allergies to tape, latex, and medications.
6. Position patient for the procedure and consider use of absorbent pads under the patient to avoid soiling bed sheets. Remember: the operator's comfort is paramount.

   TIP. *The use of silk tape is recommended to assist with pannus retraction when placing a femoral CVC in an obese patient*
7. Position the ultrasound machine on the opposite side of bed, facing the operator.

Wide sterile barrier setup

1. Place a hat and mask on every person in the room (including the patient).
2. Sterilize hands with appropriate surgical scrub.
3. Don sterile gown and sterile gloves (assistance from a nonsterile party is useful but not mandatory).
4. Prepare the procedure tray and supplies, organizing items on the tray in anticipated order of use.
5. Prepare and flush CVC.
6. Prepare the skin using **chlorhexidine** scrub for at least 30 seconds of continuous scrubbing and allow to fully dry, taking care to not touch non-sterile surfaces or patient with sterile gloves or gown.

   TIP: *Iodine is no longer considered the standard of care for skin prep.*
7. Apply **wide** sterile barriers using fenestrated drapes and sterile towels.

   TIP: *There is **no such thing** as **too** wide a sterile barrier. Proper draping should cover the majority of the patient, and the drape should ideally hang over the operator's side of the bed to ensure sterility.*
8. Apply sterile ultrasound sleeve to probe and cord (put gel inside sleeve).
9. Place absorbent sterile gauze on the sterile field at the anticipated insertion site.

Insertion steps

1. Hold the ultrasound probe in nondominant hand.
2. Reacquire vascular target in a transverse plane, using the sterile ultrasound probe, in newly created sterile field.
3. Holding the lidocaine syringe (attached to a 25-guage needle) with the dominant hand, infiltrate cutaneous and subcutaneous structures under direct ultrasound visualization at the site of anticipated cannulation. Anesthetic should be applied down to the superficial vessel wall, taking care to avoid injecting the vessel itself as this may cause venospasm and needlessly complicate the remainder of the procedure.

   TIP: *With ultrasound (and sufficient skill), the vessel wall itself can be infiltrated for maximum anesthetic effect.*
4. Using a large bore needle, penetrate the skin at ~45° angle through the lidocaine infiltration.
5. Under direct ultrasound visualization, follow the needle tip down to the vessel wall and pop through, confirming vascular access with ultrasound visualization of tip in vessel and with blood flashback.

   TIP: *Tracking the tip of the needle requires close coordination of movement between both hands. Learning this skill takes considerable practice. The ultrasound probe must be rocked back and forth to track the needle tip as it advances downward on an angle. Alternatively, the ultrasound probe may be moved translationally along the skin surface to maintain good visualization of the needle tip. Most importantly, one must strive to never lose site of the needle tip—it should be followed all the way into the vessel lumen. If you lose track of the tip, hold the needle still and move the ultrasound probe until the tip is reidentified. Subtle movements of the needle tip may oscillate surrounding tissues and help to reacquire the tip.*
6. Drop the ultrasound probe from nondominant hand and firmly grip and stabilize the needle by grasping the needle hub with thumb and forefinger; brace the palm and/or other digits of the same hand against the patient's body to maintain precise needle position.

   TIP: *For billing purposes, take a picture of the needle tip in the lumen of the target vessel and store the image in the patient's medical record.*
7. Lower the needle angle and disconnect the syringe from the needle with dominant hand—a flash should be visible in the hub of the needle (assuming sufficient intravascular pressure).

   TIP: *If blood is not seen issuing from the hub of a large-bore needle during an IJ or subclavian placement (in a nonhypotensive patient) after disconnecting the syringe, reconnect syringe immediately and aspirate to ensure proper needle placement. Then increase Trendelenburg, disconnect syringe, and look again for blood return.*
8. Grab the guidewire, and thread it through the needle.

   Note: *The guidewire should thread smoothly and easily, J-tip first—do not force. And **never** let go of the wire!*
9. Withdraw the needle over the wire and safely place onto procedure tray.

   TIP: Sharps safety *is of paramount importance. Key aspects include*
   a. Removing all sharps from the operative field while working
   b. Looking directly at all sharps when reaching for them
   c. Pointing the dull end toward the direction of movement when putting down a sharp. Avoid harpooning your assistant!
10. Make an adequate skin nick with scalpel, running the blade tip along the wire axially into the skin.
11. Slide and twist dilator ***smoothly*** over the wire, through the tissue, and into the vessel.

   Note: *While advancing dilator and catheter over wire, test the guide wire frequently to ensure that it glides smoothly in and out of the vessel while the dilator (or catheter) is held stationary. Resistance to wire movement may indicate wire kinking at the tip of the device in the subcutaneous space; this may lead to eventual misplacement of the CVC in a location other than the target vessel.*

   Note: *Take care to avoid over-insertion of the dilator. Most veins are no more than 5 cm from the skin surface, and the IJ in* *particular is usually within 2 cm of the skin surface. Overly aggressive insertion of the dilator in the IJ position may drive the dilator through the subclavian vein wall into the pleural space or artery. The risk of this occurrence is greater on the left than the right. The right IJ is preferred over the left IJ for central line insertion because of its "straight shot" to the SVC and right atrium.*

12. While leaving the guidewire in place, remove the dilator, taking care to hold pressure on the site until the catheter is inserted (now that the vessel is dilated it will ooze freely).
13. Slide CVC over the wire, through the dilated tissue, and into the vessel.
    Note: *Approximate lengths for CVCs depend on the site of insertion and the size of the patient. The following is a rough guide to follow for an average-sized adult patient, with the goal for the tip of the CVC to site in the mid SVC/IVC:*
    - RIJ = 13 cm
    - LIJ = 18–20 cm
    - RSC = 15 cm
    - LSC = 18 cm
    - Femoral = 20 cm or longer
14. Remove the wire.
15. Apply valves, draw, and flush each lumen.
16. Secure CVC to skin.
    TIP: *Do* ***not*** *overtighten sutures—this can lead to skin necrosis, causing sutures (and the catheter) to come out prematurely.*
17. Remove sterile drape(s) from site, taking care not to inadvertently dislodge the newly placed CVC.
18. Clean the insertion site, ensure hemostasis, and apply a sterile dressing (Tegaderm or Primapore) with adjunctive skin adhesive such as benzoin or mastisol.

Post-procedure clean-up and orders

1. Perform a thorough accounting of needles and wires.
2. Carefully dispose of all sharps in sharps containers.
3. Instruct nurses as to whether the line is ready for use or if a chest x-ray is required.
4. Clarify the flushing orders: saline, heparin?

Documentation

The operative note should contain

1. Procedure performed
2. Date of procedure
3. Indication for procedure
4. Name of clinician(s) involved
5. Completion of informed consent and Universal Time-Out
6. Use of wide sterile barriers and proper hand hygiene
7. Use of ultrasound (if applicable)
8. Vessel cannulated
9. Type of catheter used, including number of lumens
10. Catheter length
11. Any complications and patient's status during and after the procedure
12. Whether a post-procedure chest x-ray was ordered
13. Any other relevant findings or events during the procedure

SUGGESTED READINGS

Ely EW, Hite RD, Baker AM, et al. Venous air embolism from central venous catheterization: A need for increased physician awareness. *Crit Care Med.* 1999;27:2113–2117.

Hind D, Calvert N, McWilliams R, et al. Ultrasonic locating devices for central venous cannulation: meta-analysis. *BMJ.* 2003;327:1–7.

Lobo BL, Vaidean G, Broyles J, et al. Risk of venous thromboembolism in hospitalized patients with peripherally inserted central catheters. *J Hosp Med.* 2009;4:417–422.

Merrer J, De Jonghe B, Golliot F, et al. Complications of femoral and subclavian venous catheterization in critically ill patients: A randomized controlled trial. *JAMA.* 2001;286:700–701.

National Institute for Clinical Excellence (NICE) report: Guidance on the Use of Ultrasound Locating Devices for Placing Central Venous Catheters; 2002.

Taylor RW, Palagiri AV. Central venous catheterization. *Crit Care Med.* 2007;35(5):1390–1396.

WEB-BASED RESOURCES

http://content.nejm.org/cgi/content/short/356/21/e21

CVL placement video that requires subscription

http://www.sonoguide.com/line_placement.html

CHAPTER 116

Paracentesis

Sally Wang, MD, FHM

Key Clinical Questions

1. What are the indications for a paracentesis?
2. When should you use ultrasound guidance or involve interventional radiology?
3. When should you correct a coagulopathy?
4. What is the role of albumin administration?
5. What is the best site location to enter to reduce the risk of complications?

INTRODUCTION

Paracentesis is a procedure that involves removing ascitic fluid from the abdominal cavity with a needle or catheter. Using local anesthesia, hospitalists, other internists, Emergency Medicine physicians, proceduralists, and radiologists perform this procedure in either an outpatient or inpatient setting. A diagnostic paracentesis can determine the cause of ascites and rule out spontaneous bacterial peritonitis. A therapeutic paracentesis will remove excess fluid.

Dating back to the time of Hippocrates, paracentesis using large bore catheters was the only available option to remove ascitic fluid. In the 1950s, oral diuretics and sodium restriction were introduced as a safer alternative, typically requiring an extended hospital stay. In the mid 1980s, large-volume paracentesis was reintroduced without plasma expanders and was once again deemed a safe practice that would not cause a change in plasma volume. Abdominal imaging has replaced the practice of evaluating abdominal trauma by performing a diagnostic paracentesis.

PATHOPHYSIOLOGY

The mechanism for the development of ascites (excess fluid accumulation in the peritoneal space) is not well understood. Cirrhosis is the leading cause of ascites in the setting of portal hypertension. Capillary pressure increases with obstruction of venous blood flow through the damaged liver. Failure of the liver to metabolize aldosterone increases sodium and water retention through the kidney. Failure of the liver to produce albumin contributes to fluid moving from the vascular space into the peritoneal space.

In addition to cirrhosis, other causes of portal hypertension include right heart failure, portal vein thrombosis, Budd-Chiari syndrome, and liver metastases.

Pancreatitis, chylous fluid accumulation, nephritic syndrome, serositis, colitis, peritoneal carcinomatosis, tuberculous peritonitis, and peritonitis may cause ascites through a different mechanism.

CASE 116-1

A 55-year-old woman with hypertension and atrial fibrillation presented to the emergency department with an increase in abdominal girth, weight gain, shortness of breath and lower extremity edema over the last several months. She denied alcohol consumption and intravenous drug use. Her medications included metoprolol and warfarin. Her vital signs revealed that she was afebrile with an oxygen saturation of 92% on room air. Her physical examination was notable for tachypnea, significant ascites, and pitting edema. Her laboratory values significant for a normal white blood cell count, an INR of 2.6 and a platelet count of 125,000/mm^3. A paracentesis was performed.

- Indications: Any new onset ascites of unclear etiology needs to be tapped to determine etiology.
- Pre- procedure individual risk assessment of bleeding: Her warfarin was held and fresh frozen plasma was given. No platelets were administered as there is no evidence of a platelet cutoff in the literature.
- Procedure: A diagnostic and therapeutic paracentesis was performed under ultrasound guidance at the right lower quadrant. Ultrasound guidance was used as it was readily available and the largest pocket of fluid was in the right lower quadrant.

A therapeutic volume of six liters was removed to relieve her symptoms.
- Postprocedure: Albumin was given because greater than 4 to 5 liters of ascitic fluid was removed.
- Testing: Her fluid was sent for cell count and differential, gram stain and culture, albumin, and cytology.

INDICATIONS FOR THE PROCEDURE

Ascitic fluid may be collected for both diagnostic and therapeutic purposes. Diagnostically, emergent examination of the ascitic fluid provides essential information in many clinical situations:

1. New-onset ascites of unclear etiology. Evaluation of the fluid can help classify the cause into portal hypertensive causes (liver disease and congestive heart failure) or nonportal hypertensive causes (malignancy, pancreatitis, and malnutrition/protein wasting).
2. Any change in clinical status of a known cirrhotic including a hospital admission. A diagnostic paracentesis should be performed to rule out spontaneous bacterial peritonitis even if no signs of infection are apparent.
3. Suspected peritonitis relating to peritoneal dialysis.

Therapeutic paracentesis is performed to help relieve abdominal discomfort and dyspnea for symptomatic patients.

CASE 116-2

A 58-year-old man with known alcoholic cirrhosis presented to the emergency department with increased abdominal girth and shortness of breath. His physical examination was notable for tachypnea and tense ascites. His laboratory values were significant for a normal white blood cell count, platelet count of 75,000/mm^3, INR of 2.8, and creatinine of 3.0 mg/dL. A paracentesis was performed.

- Indications: Patient had deteriorated clinically.
- Preprocedure individual risk assessment of bleeding: There was no indication for FFP or platelets.
- Procedure: A diagnostic and therapeutic paracentesis was performed without ultrasound guidance in the left lower quadrant. No ultrasound (US) was readily available. The left lower quadrant is recommended when the tap is blind and there is tense ascites. Ten liters of straw colored fluid was removed from the left lower quadrant, the preferred location in this setting.
- Postprocedure: Albumin was given due to the possibility of hepatorenal syndrome and greater than 4 to 5 liters of fluid removal.
- Testing: His ascitic fluid was sent for cell count and differential, gram stain, culture, and albumin.

CONTRAINDICATIONS

Paracentesis is a relatively benign procedure even though contraindications do exist. Absolute contraindications include an acute abdomen, an uncooperative patient, and disseminated intravascular coagulopathy. Relative contraindications include coagulopathy, abdominal adhesions, infected abdominal wall at entry site, distended bowel or bladder, and pregnancy.

The American Association for the Study of Liver Diseases (AASLD) has not recommended reversing the INR or administering platelets in patients who have liver disease–induced coagulopathy or thrombocytopenia. Proceduralists should be cautious of performing paracentesis without reversing the coagulopathy on patients receiving anticoagulants. Although there is no recommended guideline, a generally accepted practice is to reverse the INR to less than 1.5 if the patient is receiving warfarin. There is inadequate data to guide proceduralists at this time relating to antiplatelet agents. Each patient should be evaluated individually to determine the risk of bleeding complications.

PRACTICE POINT

- There is no recommendation of INR or platelet cutoffs for patients with liver disease.
- It is generally accepted to reverse the coagulopathy to INR < 1.5 for patients receiving warfarin.
- Evaluate each patient for risk of bleeding.

COMPLICATIONS

Paracentesis is a relatively safe procedure with complications occuring in less than 1 in 1000 procedures. Complications include hypotension, infection, bowel perforation, sheared-off catheter fragments, persistent leak of ascitic fluid, hemoperitoneum, hematoma, and patient discomfort. The incidence of clinically significant bleeding with paracentesis is very low. In a retrospective study of more than 4700 patients, patients with elevated creatinines had an increased risk of bleeding that was not statistically significant.

Steps to minimize the complication rate include:

1. Check coagulation status prior to performing the procedure and reverse as appropriate.
2. Make sure that the patient does indeed have enough ascites that can be tapped. Ultrasound can be very useful to help confirm fluid location and amount.
3. Make sure the patient is not already hypovolemic.
4. Follow procedure protocols at your institution.
5. Ensure competency in performance or seek adequate supervision.
6. Intervene in a timely manner when a complication develops.

Action steps postprocedure include:

1. For hypotension, place the patient in the Trendelenburg position and administer appropriate fluids.
2. For suspected bowel perforation, initiate broad spectrum antibiotics, perform frequent serial abdominal examinations, and obtain emergent imaging and surgical consultation.
3. For sheared-off catheter fragments, request that interventional radiology or surgery retrieve the fragment.
4. For a persistent leak of ascitic fluid, place a temporary ostomy bag, repeat therapeutic paracentesis, or suture the opening.
5. For hemoperitoneums and hematomas, obtain emergent imaging to determine the severity and location of the complication which may be life threatening. Apply pressure over the site, consult surgery, check serial hematocrits, and transfuse as needed.

INDICATIONS FOR IMAGING

With the technical advances of portable ultrasound machines, it can be advantageous to confirm that there is fluid available to tap and directly visualize structures to be avoided. A small prospective study showed that there is a trend toward improvement in the success rate, reduction in time to completion and number of attempts, and lowering of the rates of complications. Although there is very little data supporting ultrasound use for paracentesis, ultrasound imaging as a bedside or interventional radiology procedure may be useful when there is:

- Very small amount of fluid or fluid primarily localized to key structures such as the liver

- History of abdominal adhesions or scars
- Suspected widely metastatic disease
- Prior failed blind attempts at the bedside
- Significant obesity

PRACTICE POINT

- Consider ultrasound-guided paracentesis if ultrasound is available. Ultrasound usage in bedside procedures is becoming standard of care.

PLASMA EXPANDERS (ALBUMIN) IN PARACENTESIS

The use of a plasma expanders such as albumin to try to mobilize fluid into the vascular space during paracentesis continues to be controversial. It is not readily available, can be quite expensive, poses an infectious risk, and can cause allergic reactions or anaphylaxis. To date, statistically significant differences in the use of albumin versus placebo have not demonstrated a reduced risk of death. However, the American Association for the Study of Liver Diseases (AASLD) states that it is not unreasonable to use a plasma expander such as albumin after a large-volume paracentesis of greater than 4 to 5 liters of ascitic fluid removal. They recommend 8 to 10 grams of albumin per liter of fluid removed. A patient diagnosed with spontaneous bacterial peritonitis should be treated with albumin in addition to antibiotics on day 1 with 1.5 grams of albumin per kilogram of body weight and on day 3 with 1.0 grams of albumin per kilogram of body weight. Albumin is also administered when the hepatorenal syndrome is suspected.

THE PROCEDURE

ANATOMY—SITES OF ENTRY

The operator should choose the best site based upon multiple factors including fluid presence, comfort, and least chance of complications. According to one study the left lower quadrant (LLQ) is likely the preferred site due to the LLQ location of the deepest pocket of fluid and smaller thickness of the subcutaneous tissue. The midline location is usually avascular; however, patients with significant portal hypertension may have varices in that region. The right lower quadrant entry site is associated with a higher risk of bowel perforation in those patients with cecal dilation from lactulose or other conditions or if they have adhesions from prior surgery. If the left or right lower quadrant is used, it is important to avoid the inferior epigastric vessels that run over the rectus abdominus muscles.

HOW TO PERFORM THE PROCEDURE

A preprocedure checklist (Table 116-1, Table 116-2)

1. Take a time-out to verify correct patient, procedure, location, and consent.
2. Properly position patient: supine with the head of bed elevated to 30°–40° (**Figure 116-1**).
3. Determine optimal site by either percussing fluid level, previously marking the area by ultrasound insonation, or using ultrasound in real time. Usually, the best site is several centimeters below the level of percussed dullness. Mark the best site (**Figure 116-2**).

PRACTICE POINT

- Avoid the inferior epigastric vessels, tap lateral to the rectus abdominus muscle.

TABLE 116-1 Preprocedure Checklist

1. Review indications
   - Up-to-date coagulation studies preprocedure (INR, platelet count, creatinine)
   - Tests to be obtained (cell count and differential, Gram stain and culture, cytology, albumin to determine the serum ascitic albumin gradient)
   - Whether ultrasound guidance is required to confirm presence of ascites
2. Review contraindications
   - Patient hemodynamically unstable or unable to cooperate
   - Acute abdomen, septic shock, disseminated intravascular coagulopathy
   - Absence of ascitic fluid
   - Coagulopathy from anticoagulants
3. Obtain informed consent that includes a discussion of complication rate in a language that the patient and/or family can understand
4. Ensure working intravenous line
5. Obtain paracentesis kit and supplies

INR, international normalized ratio.

Option 1: Select *left* or *right lower quadrants*, 2 to 4 cm medial and superior to the anterior superior iliac spine. The left is preferred over right if there is no relative contraindication. The advantages to the left lateral approach are a thinner abdominal wall and greater depth of ascitic fluid. Insertion must be lateral to the rectus sheath to avoid injury to the inferior epigastric vessels.

Option 2: Select *midline*, 2 cm below umbilicus. The advantage to this approach is that the linea alba is generally avascular. Adipose tissue is often greatest at this level, making it difficult

TABLE 116-2 Supplies

Sterile skin prep
Gauze
Sterile draping and nonsterile gloves
Sterile gown, sterile gloves, eye protection, facial shield, and bouffant (optional)
Lidocaine
Syringe (5 or 10 cc) with 25-gauge needle for lidocaine
22-gauge 1.5″ needle for deeper lidocaine infiltration (if necessary)
Lidocaine filter straw
14- to 18-gauge angiocatheter/needle or commercial catheter/needle system
60-cc syringe
Scalpel (optional)
Stopcock (optional)
Blood collection tubing or intravenous tubing
Collection container
16-gauge or larger needle
Bandage or Tegaderm
Collection tubes for samples: cell count and differential, albumin, Gram stain, cytology, other studies
Blood culture bottles (anaerobic and aerobic)
Transfer fluid adapter

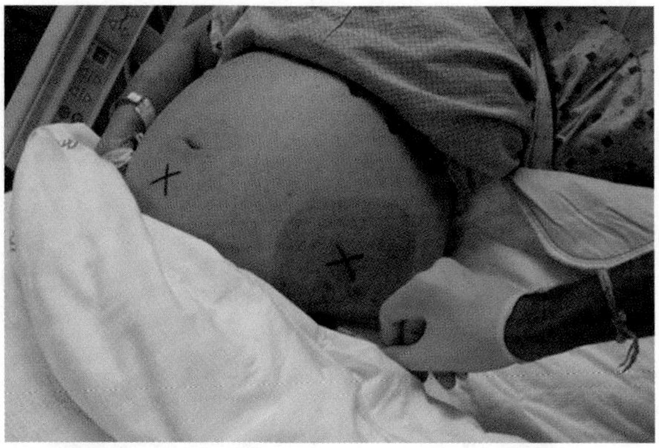

Figure 116-1 *Patient position.*

to obtain ascitic fluid, especially when using a shorter needle for a diagnostic tap.

4. Position chucks on bed, open paracentesis kit (if performing therapeutic tap).

Sterile setup

1. Don hat, mask, and eyewear. Sterilize area.
2. Discard those gloves, and don sterile gown and sterile gloves.
3. Place sterile drape around site providing a larger sterile field (**Figure 116-3**).

PRACTICE POINT

- With tense ascites, consider tapping left lower quadrant, followed by the midline, then the right lower quadrant. Go for where the fluid is located.

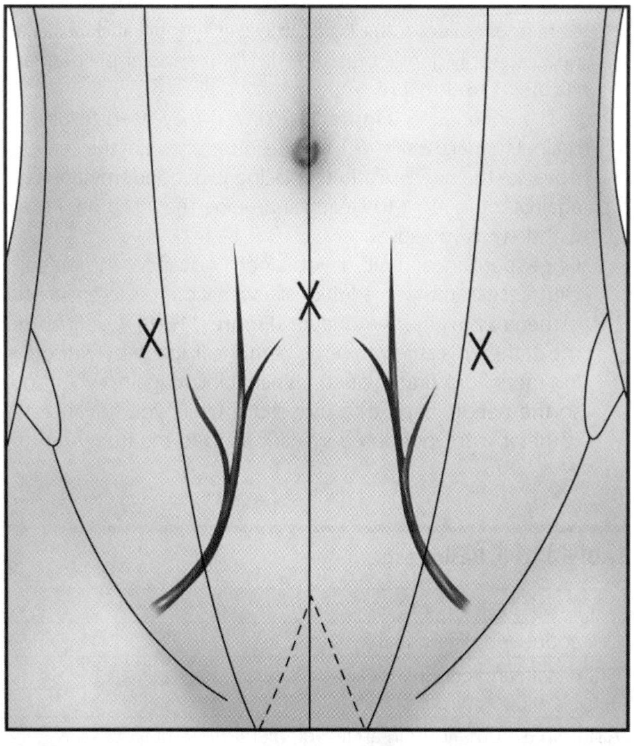

Figure 116-2 *Diagram of different sites. (Courtesy of Gil Z. Shlamovitz, MD.)*

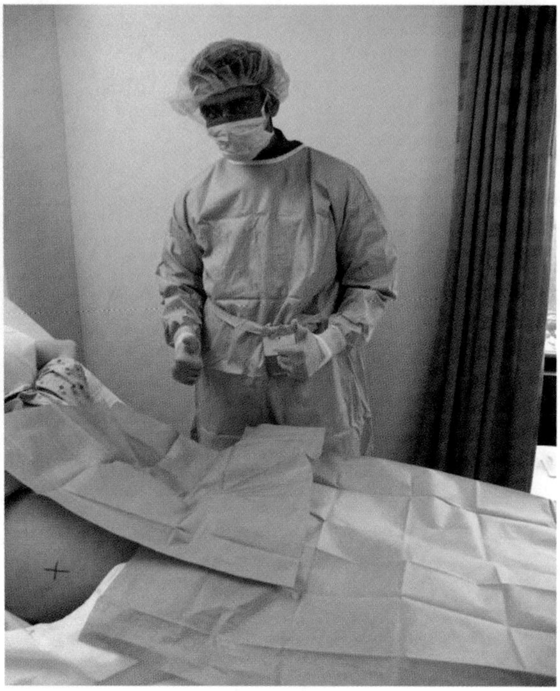

Figure 116-3 *Patient in position with sterile field.*

Insertion steps

1. Draw up lidocaine with a filter straw or needle in a small syringe. Gauze should be used to minimize the risk of injury when opening the glass vials of lidocaine.
2. Use a 25-gauge needle to create a wheal to anesthetize the skin and immediate subcutaneous tissue.
3. If necessary, you can provide further infiltration with local anesthetic with a 22-gauge, 1.5″ needle. Enter the skin through the wheal, aspirating while advancing to avoid injecting into a vessel. The ideal angle of entry should be perpendicular to the skin (**Figure 116-4**).
4. "Z-track-technique." There are two methods of creating the "Z" (**Figure 116-5**):
   - Enter through the skin at a 45° angle directed caudad, such that the skin and peritoneum create the horizontal top and bottom of the "Z," respectively.

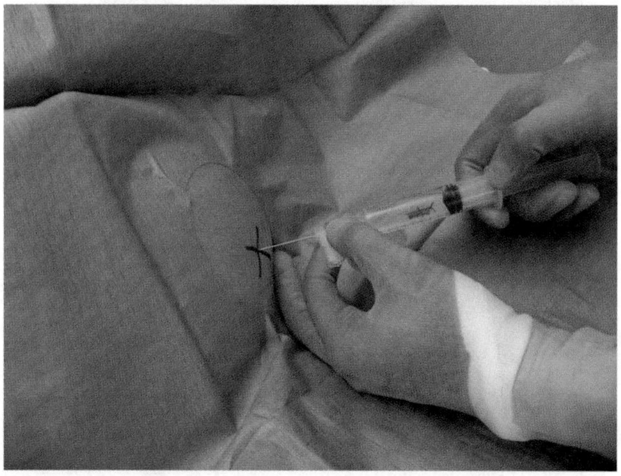

Figure 116-4 *Local anesthesia.*

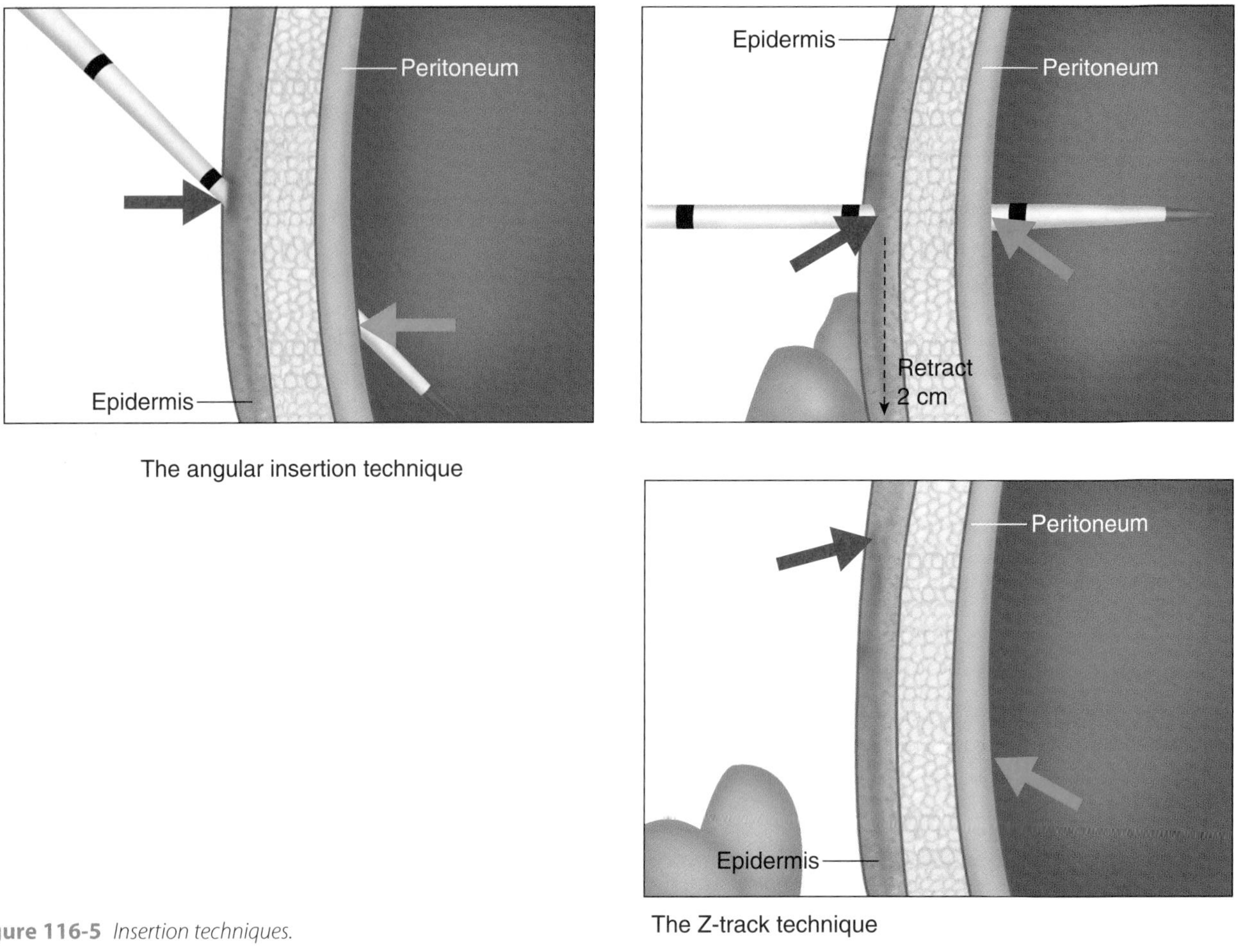

Figure 116-5 *Insertion techniques.*

- Place traction on the skin and enter straight, releasing traction after entering the peritoneum. When the tissue relaxes the path of the needle will be similar to that of the above technique, but in this way you maintain improved control over the trajectory of the needle tip.

5. Diagnostic tap (**Figure 116-6**): Use an 18-gauge needle or angiocatheter and attach a 60-cc syringe. Make sure the needle or angiocatheter is long enough to reach the peritoneum. You can use a spinal needle if you need more length. Aspirate while advancing. Once peritoneal fluid is obtained, collect a full 60 cc into the syringe and withdraw needle. Apply gentle pressure with gauze and apply bandage (**Tables 116-3** to **116-6**).

   Therapeutic tap (**Figure 116-7**): You may need to use the scalpel to make a skin nick to ease introduction of the catheter. Advance the needle/catheter placing your nondominant hand against the patient to steady and guide the insertion. Always withdraw as you advance.

6. Once peritoneal fluid is obtained, advance the needle/catheter assembly an additional few millimeters to ensure the catheter is in the peritoneum (**Figure 116-8**). Confirm that the catheter is still within the peritoneal space by withdrawing more fluid. Brace your dominant elbow against your body so the needle hand does not move while you advance the catheter with your non dominant hand to the hub. After the

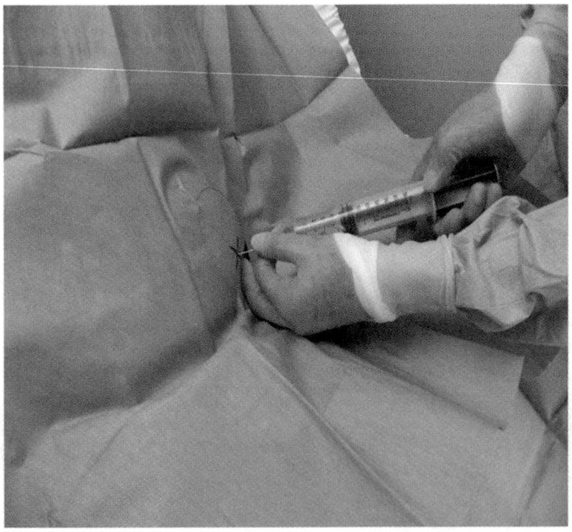

Figure 116-6 *Diagnostic tap: always withdraw as you advance.*

TABLE 116-3 Basic Tests

Diagnostic test: 60 cc of ascitic fluid
Cell count and differential (few mL)
Gram stain and culture (ideally 5 mL in an anaerobic and aerobic blood culture bottle)
Albumin (serum albumin ascites gradient) (few mL)
Cytology (the more, the greater the yield)

TABLE 116-4 Special Tests
Red cell count > 50,000 hemorrhagic ascites due to malignancy, tuberculosis, trauma
Amylase—pancreatitis
Triglyceride—chylous ascites
Acid fast bacillus, adenosine deaminase—tuberculosis

TABLE 116-6 Spontaneous Bacterial Peritonitis
> 250 polymorphonuclear cells/hpf
Treat with third-generation cephalosporin
Treat with intravenous albumin: • Day 1: 1.5 g/kg • Day 3: 1 g/kg

catheter has been advanced to the hub, withdraw the needle. Never pull back catheter over the needle as this can shear the catheter off. Remove them as a unit if there is problem with removal of fluid. Never withdraw needle before the catheter is fully into the peritoneal space.

7. Obtain fluid for analysis. A 60-cc syringe can be attached directly to the catheter at this point. The stopcock is not absolutely necessary but it can prevent leakage of ascitic fluid when changing from syringe to tubing.
8. If using the stopcock, attach to the end of the catheter. Withdraw an adequate volume, and close the stopcock by turning the handle (OFF position) to point in the direction of the patient. Remove the syringe and set aside.
9. Large-volume removal: of more than 4 to 5 liters of fluid: 8 to 10 g/L albumin may be administered.
   a. *To withdraw fluid using vacuum bottles* (**Figure 116-9**): Attach tubing to the catheter and attach a 14- to 16-gauge needle on the other end of tubing and insert into the vacuum bottle.
   b. *To withdraw fluid using gravity/suction tubing*: Attach Luer-Lock end of the stepped connector to distal or side port. Firmly introduce the distal, graduated end of stepped connector into the large bore suction tubing provided. A nonsterile assistant should affix the other end to a collection source—fluid will drain by gravity alone. Open stopcock, if using. Note: this tubing can be attached to a source of vacuum suction, but this can cause the bowel to be suctioned up against the catheter.
   c. *To withdraw fluid using pumping method:* Attach 60-cc syringe to Luer-Lock end of stop cock. Attach tubing with foley bag to side port of stop cock. Turn stopcock so that fluid can flow into the 60-cc syringe. Withdraw 60 cc of fluid into syringe and push into Foley bag (one-way valve). This method has been largely replaced by vaccum bottles or gravity collection.
10. Remove catheter, briefly apply gentle pressure with gauze and apply bandage or Tegaderm to site. For continued leakage, you can attach a colostomy bag to the site, place a stitch in the catheter hole or undergo an additional therapeutic paracentesis.

TABLE 116-5 Diagnostic Criteria
SAAG (serum albumin ascites gradient) for etiology of ascites
SAAG > 1.1 g/dL
Portal Hypertensive Causes (SAAG > 1.1 g/dL) • Cirrhosis • Portal vein thrombosis • Congestive heart failure • Budd-Chiari syndrome • Liver metastases
Nonportal Hypertensive Causes (SAAG < 1.1 g/dL) • Peritoneal carcinomatosis • Peritoneal tuberculosis • Pancreatic ascites • Nephrotic syndrome • Serositis

Postprocedure clean-up and orders

1. Dispose of all sharps in sharps container and any kit contents soiled with bodily fluids in the biohazard receptacle.
2. Administer albumin if deemed necessary.
3. Send fluid for studies.

Documentation

The procedure note should contain:

1. Procedure performed
2. Date of procedure
3. Indication for procedure
4. Name of clinician(s) involved
5. Completion of informed consent and universal timeout
6. Use of wide sterile barriers and proper hand hygiene
7. Location of paracentesis
8. Amount of peritoneal fluid removed, color of fluid
9. Administration of any IV fluids, colloid
10. Any complications and patient's status during and after the procedure
11. Any other relevant findings or events during the procedure

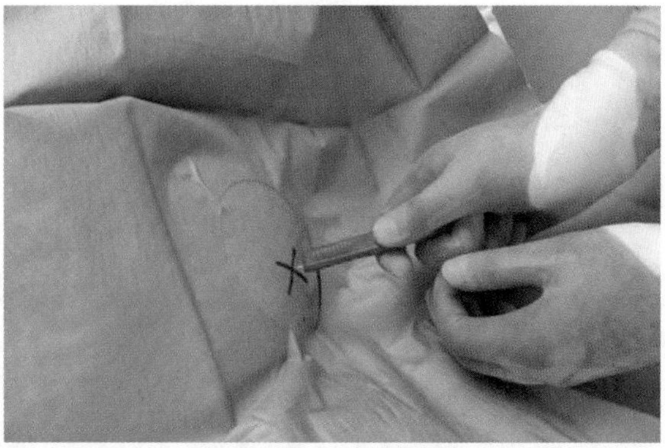

Figure 116-7 *Scalpel nick prior to therapeutic tap.*

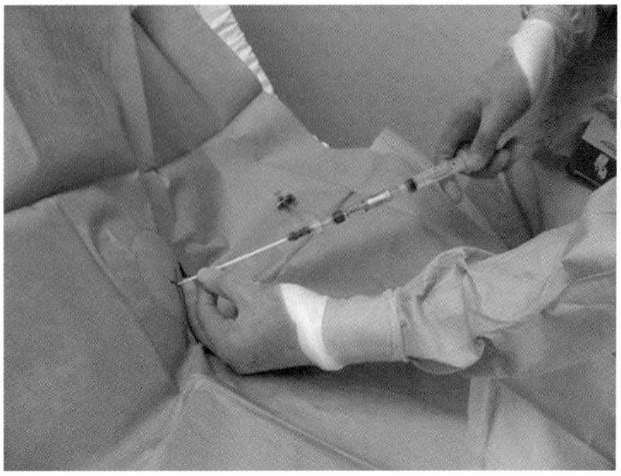

Figure 116-8 *Needle/catheter system.*

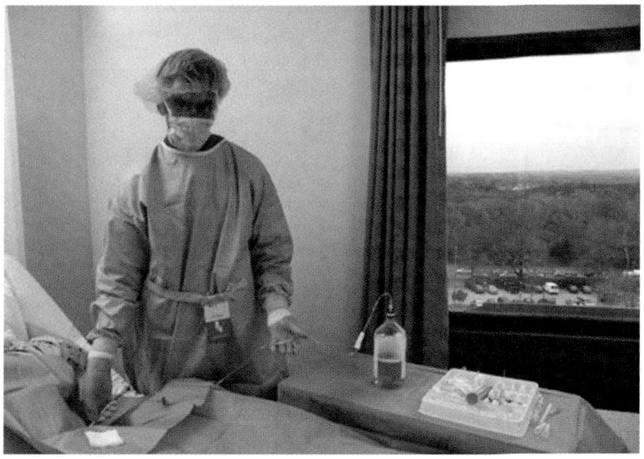

Figure 116-9 *Therapeutic paracentesis: Setup with catheter/tubing/vacuum bottles method.*

SUGGESTED READINGS

Ginès P, Tító L, Arroyo V, et al. Randomized comparative study of therapeutic paracentesis with and without intravenous albumin in cirrhosis. *Gastroenterology*. 1988;94:1493–1502.

Grabau C, Crago SF, Hoff LK, et al. Performance standards for therapeutic abdominal paracentesis. *Hepatology*. 2004;40(2):484–488.

Lin CH, Shih FY, Ma MH, et al. Should bleeding tendency deter abdominal paracentesis? *Dig Liver Dis*. 2005;37(12):946–951.

McVay PA, Toy PT. Lack of increased bleeding after paracentesis and thoracentesis in patients with mild coagulation abnormalities. *Transfusion*. 1991;31(2):164–171.

Nazeer SR, Dewbre H, Miller AH. Ultrasound-assisted paracentesis performed by emergency physicians vs the traditional technique: a prospective, randomized study. *Am J Emerg Med*. 2005;23(3):363–367.

Pache I, Bilodeau M. Severe haemorrhage following abdominal paracentesis for ascites in patients with liver disease. *Aliment Pharmacol Ther*. 2005;21(5):525–529.

Runyon BA; Practice Guidelines Committee, American Association for the Study of Liver Diseases (AASLD). Management of adult patients with ascites due to cirrhosis. *Hepatology*. 2004;39:841–856.

Sakai H, Sheer TA, Mendler MH, Runyon BA. Choosing the location for non-image guided abdominal paracentesis. *Liver Int*. 2005;25:984–986.

Sort P, Navasa M, Arroyo V, et al. Effect of intravenous albumin on renal impairment and mortality in patients with cirrhosis and spontaneous bacterial peritonitis. *N Engl J Med*. 1999;341:403–409.

CHAPTER 117

Thoracentesis

Christopher Parks, MD
Rabih Bechara, MD

Key Clinical Questions

1. What are the indications for performing a thoracentesis?
2. What steps should be taken to reduce the likelihood of complications?
3. What diagnostic criteria differentiate the three types of pleural effusions, namely, transudates, exudatives, and empyema?

INTRODUCTION

Physicians or other providers perform an estimated 173,000 thoracenteses in the United States every year. In general, the procedure is usually safe and well tolerated. However, when iatrogenic pneumothorax does occur, chest tube insertion may be required for up to 50% of the patients with an increased average length of stay of approximately four days. This complication not only incurs substantial increase in cost, but also increases morbidity and mortality.

PATHOPHYSIOLOGY

Pleural effusions develop secondarily to systemic changes (transudates) or to local causes (exudates). Systemic causes that lead to the formation and absorption of pleural fluid most commonly include left ventricular heart failure, pulmonary embolism, cirrhosis, and renal disease. Acute pancreatitis may cause a left-sided pleural effusion. Pleural effusions commonly occur after abdominal surgery due to the porous diaphragm and are usually benign. Renal diseases that can cause pleural effusion include the nephrotic syndrome and urinothorax from hydronephrosis. Myxedema and cerebrospinal fluid leak to the pleura are other causes of transudates.

Local causes (exudates) are most commonly bacterial pneumonia, viral infection, malignancy, and pulmonary embolism. Approximately 40% of patients with community-acquired pneumonia will develop pleural effusions, and approximately 10% of these will be complicated parapneumonic effusions or empyema. Parapneumonic effusions start out as sterile, reactive effusions and can rapidly progress to loculated empyema in immunocompromised patients or when there is a delay in administration of appropriate antibiotics. Other infectious causes include viral or fungal disease and tuberculosis. Failure to identify those patients with empyema or significant inflammation necessitating pleural drainage can result in trapped lung. Pancreatic pseudocyst, intraabdominal abscess, post–coronary artery bypass grafting or cardiac contusion, pericardial disease, drug-induced pleuritis, rheumatologic disease, uremia, and gynecologic disorders may also cause exudates.

The most common causes of malignant pleural effusions in descending order of frequency are lung cancer, breast cancer, and lymphoma. In a patient with a prior history of asbestos exposure, mesothelioma should be suspected, especially if the pleural effusion is grossly hemorrhagic. While dullness to percussion and reduced tactile fremitus are valuable findings to help identify a pleural effusion (positive likelihood ratio [LR+], 8.7 and 5.7, respectively)[1], the physical examination is usually not helpful in diagnosing the cause of the pleural effusion. If a patient has yellow, dystrophic nails, chronic peripheral edema, and chronic exudative effusions, the yellow nail syndrome should be suspected (Moldonado, and Ryu, 2009).

INDICATIONS

Thoracentesis is performed for diagnostic or therapeutic purposes. The strict indications for thoracentesis are the presence of pleural fluid of unknown etiology where the physician cannot initiate care prior to diagnosis, and severe dyspnea. The first step is to determine whether there is fluid by radiographic imaging. On chest X-ray (CXR), a pleural effusion will characteristically push the heart to the opposite side. If, however, the opacified space does not shift the heart, it is possible that the patient has significant atelectasis as the cause.

A lateral decubitus film should reveal whether there is free flowing fluid, and should be ordered to document free flow in most patients prior to thoracentesis procedure. If there is doubt, ultrasonography can identify solid from liquid pleural effusions with 98% accuracy when combined with CXR. Computed tomography (CT) imaging may be indicated prior to definitive drainage in some instances, and CT-PE protocol imaging should be performed if pulmonary embolism is suspected (See Chapters 107: Basic Chest Radiography and 108: Advanced Cardiothoracic Imaging).

For some patients, initiating treatment directed at the systemic cause (congestive heart disease, kidney disease, and cirrhosis) may be most appropriate. However, a diagnostic thoracentesis should be performed if the patient has an unexplained pleural effusion or fails to respond to treatment

In the setting of pneumonia, clinical judgment is neither sensitive nor specific in distinguishing between those patients who will require complete drainage of the pleural space due to empyema or significant inflammation. Hence, there are specific indications for a diagnostic thoracentesis as follows:

- Effusions > 1 cm in depth on a lateral decubitus chest film
- Increasing effusions despite appropriate antibiotic treatment
- Persistent unilateral effusion with persistent fever and tachycardia despite appropriate antibiotic treatment
- Imaging findings—pleural-based opacity with an abnormal contour on CXR or thickened parietal pleura on CT—that raise the possibility of a loculated effusion or empyema.

Therapeutic indications are usually for symptomatic relief. Most of the volume a pleural effusion occupies is by distending the diaphragm, thereby causing dyspnea. A therapeutic thoracentesis of a large pleural effusion will decrease intrathoracic volume.

It is usually prudent to perform a diagnostic thoracentesis prior to putting in a chest tube, but in situations with a very high likelihood of hemothorax such as trauma or when the lung has a large pleural effusion more than 50% of the thorax, this step may be bypassed.

CASE 117-1

A 58-year-old female with a history of multiple sclerosis and Parkinson disease was admitted after noted to be crying in pain. She had significant dysarthria limiting her history. She mentioned cough, right-sided pleuritic pain, and some shortness of breath for the past 22 weeks. She had no subjective fevers, chills, or night sweats.

CXR revealed a new, large, right pleural effusion occupying at least 60% of the right hemithorax with confluent airspace opacities in the right lower lobe.

CBC WBC 20.6 (87% PMN)

CRP 195 (0–3)

What is the next step?

Thoracic surgical consultation should be requested for patients with loculated effusions or effusions >50% of the hemithorax. Instead a thoracentesis was attempted.

US of the chest—unable to mark due to atelectatic lung and patient's inability to sit.

15 cc of orange cloudy pleural fluid removed with the following results:

- WBC 9700 (70 PMN, 0 B, 23 L, 4 M, 3 E)
- pH 7.47; glucose 106; TP 4.5; albumin 2.5; amylase 25; LDH 349; serum glucose 133; TP 6.2; albumin 3; CRP 195 (0–3)
- Culture negative
- Pathology: acute inflammatory histiocytes and rare reactive mesothelial cells

What is the interpretation of the fluid?

Chest CT revealed a large, loculated, right sided effusion with some anterior pneumothorax and compressive atelectasis of lung

Patient underwent right VATS drainage and decortication.

What do you think was found?

The patient had a lung abscess, presumably from aspiration given her impaired neurologic status.

Culture: abscess of right lung and bronchial washings: *Streptococcus intermedius*

Pathology:

- RUL wedge resection: subpleural scar consistent with apical cap, focal acute fibrinous pleuritis
- RLL wedge resection: necroinflammatory debris, acute fibrinous pleuritis with extensive necrosis

CONTRAINDICATIONS

Contraindications to thoracentesis include a hemodynamically unstable patient who cannot be positioned properly due to severe tachypnea or hypotension and skin infection over the proposed entry site. Relative contraindications include a coagulopathy that increases the risk of bleeding. While there is little data to support a platelet count threshold, in practice a platelet count of greater than 50,000/mm^3 is generally accepted as the safe level. For patients receiving antiplatelet therapy (eg, aspirin or clopidogrel), some authorities suggest that those agents should be discontinued five days prior to thoracentesis procedure, but recent expert opinion based guidelines by the American College of Radiology state that no waiting time is necessary. Similarly, an INR of < 1.5 is used as a cutoff for safely performing thoracentesis, but little data to supports this cutoff. Some studies suggest that thoracentesis can be safely performed in fully anticoagulated patients.

POTENTIAL COMPLICATIONS

Notable complications from the procedure itself have been reported in the following order of decreasing frequency: pneumothorax (3–30%), infection, hemorrhage, hypotension due to a vasovagal response, reexpansion pulmonary edema, and injury to liver or spleen (**Table 117-1**).

One study[2] found no association between postprocedure pneumothorax and a variety of possible risk factors, including size of the effusion, the presence of loculations, the needle type, operator characteristics, or the amount of fluid withdrawn. The only variable that correlated with the development of pneumothorax was the performance of multiple taps.

REAL-TIME ULTRASONOGRAPHY

Ultrasound guidance has long been used in the evaluation of loculated pleural effusions and more recent data suggests that it should be the standard of care for the evaluation of free-flowing effusions. Real-time ultrasonography is helpful in delineating the potential characteristics of the pleural effusion, the potential of a complicated effusion, and the presence of adhesions and septations (**Figures 117-1**). These findings may be crucial in the management of pleural effusions and the potential need for a more invasive approach than a simple thoracentesis in patients with pleural effusions. In a recent study the mandatory use of ultrasound decreased the pneumothorax rate from 8.8% to 1.1%. The number of dry taps with no fluid obtained was reduced from 15% to 0% because no tap is attempted if no fluid is seen. The number of complications decreased from 50% (including dry taps) to 0%. The bottom line: only attempt blind taps when ultrasound guidance is not available.

TABLE 117-1 Potential Complications of Thoracentesis

Complication	Risk Factors	Suspect When...	Imaging	Comments
Pneumothorax	Multiple thoracentesis procedures (also called "taps") "Blind" taps (or those attempted without the benefit of ultrasound guidance) Operator inexperience	Chest pain or shortness of breath ↓ O_2 saturation or hypotension	Plain chest X-ray	Air bubbles in the withdrawn fluid may be a sign of iatrogenic pneumothorax or trapped lung
Infection	Multiple taps and immunosuppressed states	Local pain at site Fever, redness or purulent drainage	Chest CT may be required	
Hemorrhage	Multiple taps Operator inexperience	Hypotension or change in the color or consistency of the withdrawn fluid.	Plain chest film	Reverse any coagulopathy or thrombocytopenia
Vasovagal		Sudden loss of consciousness with spontaneous recovery	Plain chest film to rule out other etiologies	Clinicians must rule out more serious conditions such as pneumothorax or hemorrhage
Reexpansion pulmonary edema	Removal of >2 L of pleural fluid	Cough	Plain chest film	
Injury to liver or spleen	Operator inexperience Blind taps	Bloody and dry tap	Abdominal CT	

In this case consider the next best alternative of ultrasound marking in the radiology department. During radiology ultrasound marking, the patient must be placed in the same position that the thoracentesis will be performed.

PRACTICE POINT

- Only attempt blind taps when ultrasound guidance is not available. In this case consider the next best alternative of ultrasound marking in the radiology department. During radiology ultrasound marking, the patient must be placed in the same position in which the thoracentesis will be performed.

PROCEDURE SET-UP AND INSERTION TECHNIQUES

PreProcedure checklist

1. Review relevant laboratory, imaging, and clinical information to best understand the indication for, and possible risks of, the planned procedure, and what equipment will be needed.
2. Obtain informed consent, including an explanation of the risks of the procedure and the alternative of not performing the procedure.
3. Perform a Universal Time-Out (to verify correct patient, a physician order for procedure, indication for procedure, selection of correct site, correct tubes for specimen collection, and the presence of informed consent).
4. Check for allergies to tape, latex, and medications.
5. Make sure to have the equipment you need and prepare the procedure tray and supplies, organizing the tray in anticipated order of use (**Figure 117-2**): chlorhexadine skin preps, sterile drape, hat, gloves, mask, 2% lidocaine, 3-cc syringe with 25-gauge needle for skin infiltration, 12-cc syringe with 18-gauge 1.5" needle, and specimen tubes.

   Note: Large-volume removal without a flexible catheter is not recommended due to the risk of lung puncture during reexpansion, and potential pneumothorax or bleeding.
6. Position patient for the procedure. Patient and operator comfort are paramount. The best patient position is seated at the side of the bed leaning forward with her/his head resting on a table (**Figure 117-3**).
7. Locate the appropriate site, preferably using ultrasound-guidance or marking prior to the procedure.

The bedside ultrasound-guided procedure avoids discrepancies in patient positioning if the site is marked by a radiologist or another provider. However, if real-time ultrasound guidance is not available, or if the effusion is small or loculated, radiologists should be consulted to safely perform a successful tap.

If no ultrasound-guidance is available, a moderately large effusion may be tapped blindly by performing percussion in the mid scapular line; when the upper limit is detected, select a site two rib spaces below just above the rib to avoid the neurovascular bundle.

Sterile barrier set-up

1. Sterilize hands with appropriate surgical scrub.
2. Don sterile gloves.
3. Clean the area broadly with chlorhexidine or betadine swabs, preferably three times.

Insertion

1. **Local anesthesia:** Using a 25-gauge needle place a wheel of lidocaine subdermally. Then at a 90° angle locally anesthetize deeper tissue layers all the way to the pleura. Lidocaine injected unintentionally into the pleura will cause no harm. Ideally, access the fluid with the 25-gauge needle to confirm proper position. If the patient's size does not permit this approach, then use continued anesthesia with the 18-gauge 1.5 inch needle.

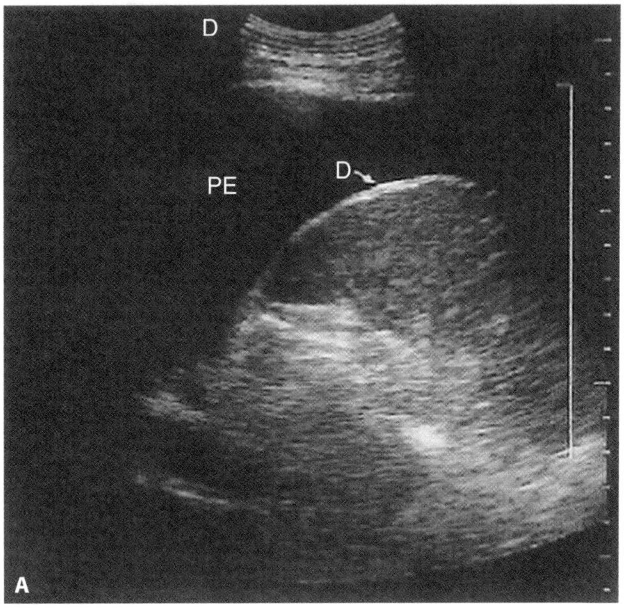

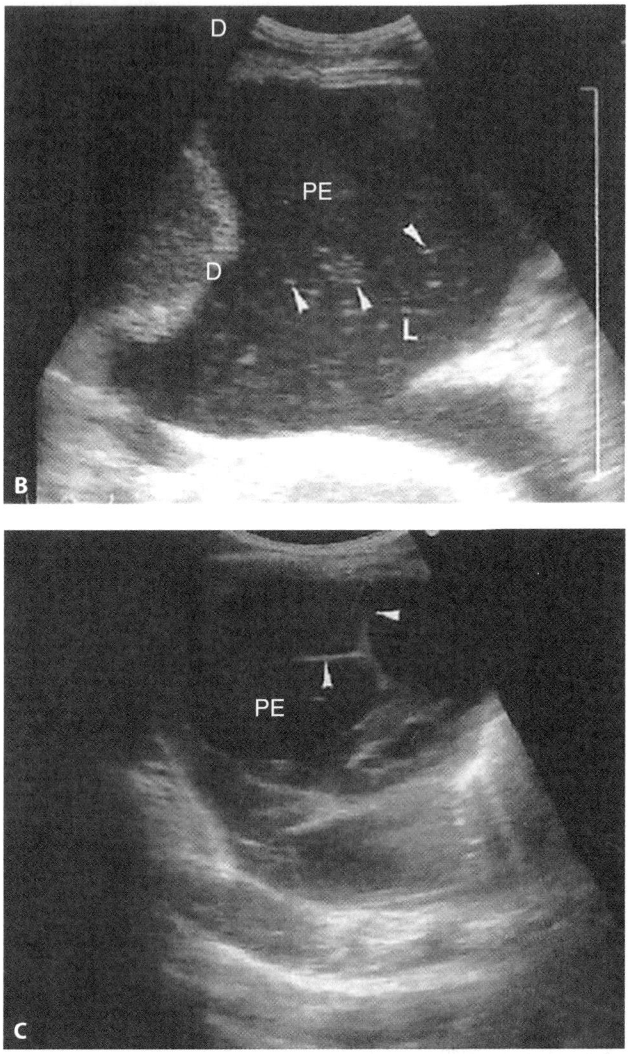

Figure 117-1 *(A) Pleural effusion is represented by an echo-free space (D, diaphragm; PE, pleural effusion). (B) Complex nonseptated effusion suggesting a transudate (arrows show echogenic foci in the pleural effusion). (C) Complex septated effusion (arrows indicate septations and potential need for surgical approach).*

2. **Entering the pleural space:** Once the skin and pleura are locally anesthetized and proper placement has been confirmed with the finder needle, the proceduralist uses a #11 blade scalpel to make a small incision through which the catheter can pass. The incision should be approximately 0.5 cm long and deep enough to penetrate the skin.

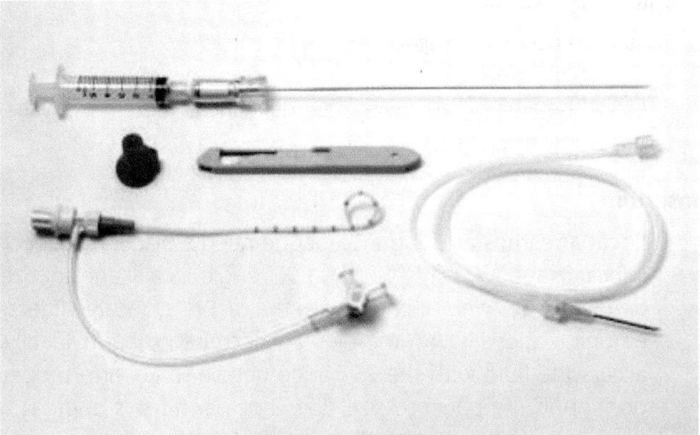

Figure 117-2 *Thoracentesis procedure equipment.*

3. **Catheter insertion:** Load the catheter onto the introducer needle. At a 90° angle slowly introduce the catheter until pleural fluid is obtained. Advance the needle another 1 to 2 cm to allow the catheter tip to enter the chest cavity. Then, holding the needle steady, slide the catheter over the needle into the chest cavity and remove the needle.
4. **Fluid removal:** Attach a three-way stopcock and tubing and use a 60-cc syringe to remove fluid. Do not collect fluid in vacuum bottles due to potentially high negative intrapleural pressures. Current guidelines state no more than 2 liters of fluid should be removed at one time. Fluid removal should be stopped early if the patient experiences chest pain or any concerning changes in vital signs. Cough is a sign of reexpanding lung and does not require procedure termination. Troubleshooting problems with fluid removal can be done quickly and easily at the bedside (**Table 117-2**).
5. **Catheter removal:** After the desired amount of fluid has been removed, the catheter is withdrawn while the patient actively increases intrapleural pressure. Asking the patient to hum while the catheter is removed will prevent the patient from taking a breath in and creating negative intrathoracic pressure and possibly entraining air into the pleural space after the procedure. A simple bandage is placed over the site following catheter removal.

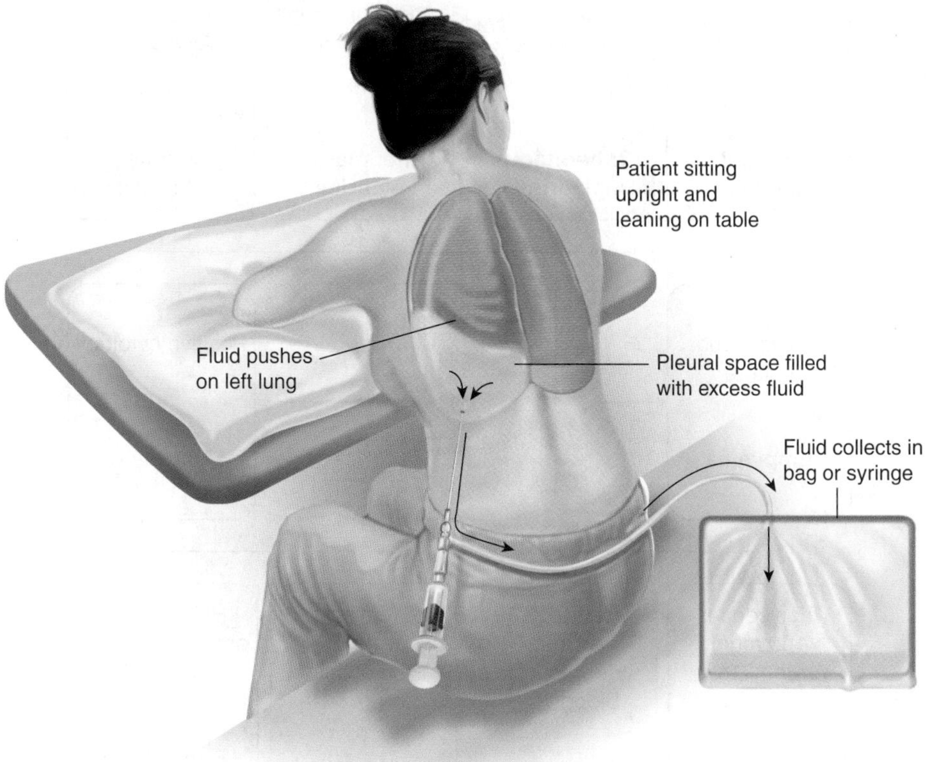

Figure 117-3 *Correct positioning of patient.*

TABLE 117-2 Trouble Shooting

Problem 1: No fluid
This is particularly common when ultrasound is not used but will happen occasionally with ultrasound guidance. Reconfirm position with ultrasound. If ultrasound is not available, consider going one rib space lower.
Problem 2: Fluid stops flowing
This happens particularly toward the end of the procedure as the end of the catheter abuts the pleura. Remove suction and withdraw slightly and try again. The catheter can become occluded with either very viscous effusions or effusions with large amounts of debris. If this happens, try flushing with 5 cc of saline and reapplying suction.
Problem 3: Bubbles in the fluid
When high negative pressure is applied to pleural fluid, oxygen is pulled out of solution and can be mistaken for a pneumothorax. When the negative pressure is released, the bubbles should disappear. If they do not, a pneumothrax may have occurred. If the patient is stable, a chest X-ray can be obtained for decisions of further management. If the patient is unstable and a tension pneumothorax is suspected, a chest tube should be placed empirically on the side of the thoracentesis prior to obtaining radiography.
Problem 4: Blood in the fluid
Many effusions especially those related to cancer can appear as blood. Also conditions such as trauma or surgery can leave blood in the chest. These can be difficult to tell from injury from thoracentesis. If there is concern for active bleeding, vital signs and serial hematocrits should be monitored and any coagulopathy reversed.

Testing postprocedure

1. **Imaging:** Valid evidence supports that a routine post procedure CXR is not necessary for uncomplicated thoracentesis. A CXR should be obtained if any procedural complications occur such as air or blood in the removed fluid or multiple "dry" taps. A CXR should also be obtained if there is any unusual patient symptomatology such as chest pain or shortness of breath or change in vital signs. Instances when pneumothorax is more likely—small effusions, multiple needle sticks or passes to obtain fluid, therapeutic taps, or blind taps—might also warrant a postprocedure CXR.
2. **Laboratory testing:** Clinicians should order appropriate serum testing and pleural fluid analysis. *Serum testing* should include: complete blood count, lactate dehydrogenase (LDH), total protein, glucose, blood cultures (if indicated). Routine pleural fluid analysis should include: cell count and differential, Gram stain, culture, LDH, protein, glucose. Other tests are required under specific circumstances (**Figure 117-4**):
   - Amylase (suspected pancreatitis, esophageal rupture, local malignancy)
   - pH (suspected primarily parapneumonic effusion or empyema)
   - Triglycerides (white pleural fluid samples for thoracic duct injury vs pseudochylous effusions associated with chronic inflammation)
   - Antinuclear antibody (drug induced lupus, systemic lupus erythematosus)
   - Pleural biopsy (suspected tuberculosis)
   - Hematocrit (if significantly bloody fluid)
   - Cytology (if malignant effusion suspected)
3. **Test interpretation:** Pleural fluid can be either transudative or exudative. Characteristics of either are defined by Light's

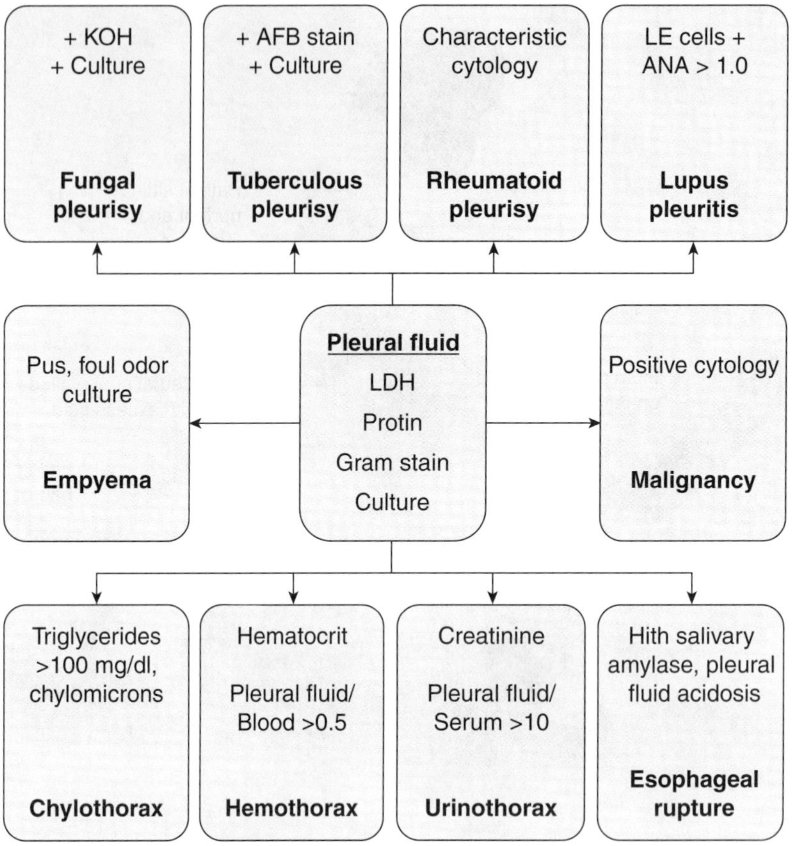

Figure 117-4 *Algorithm for pleural fluid analysis based on suspected etiology.*

criteria (see list below). Meeting any of these criteria is more consistent with an exudative process. A transudate usually occurs in the absence of pleural pathology while an exudate usually indicates pleural involvement with disease. Empyema is the presence of pus in the pleural cavity. The color and consistency may provide clues as to the diagnosis such as purulent material being consistent with empyema. Please see Chapter 243 for a more complete discussion of individual conditions.

Light's criteria for an exudate are as follows:

1. Pleural fluid protein/serum protein > 0.5
2. Pleural fluid LDH/serum LDH > 0.6
3. Pleural fluid LDH > 200 U/L

Postprocedure clean-up and orders

1. Perform a thorough accounting of needles.
2. Carefully dispose of all sharps in sharps containers.
3. Remove sterile drapes.

Documentation

1. Procedure performed
2. Date of procedure
3. Indication for procedure
4. Name of clinician(s) involved
5. Completion of informed consent and Universal Time-Out
6. Note the amount of fluid removed and appearance
7. Tests sent
8. Any complications and patient's status during and after the procedure
9. Any other relevant findings or events during the procedure
10. Results of examination

CASE 117-2

A 40-year-old female with an aggressive lymphoma is admitted to the oncology service with shortness of breath. CXR reveals complete opacification of her right hemithorax secondary to massive pleural effusion with complete collapse of her right lung and some mild mediastinal shift.

A thoracentesis is performed in order to send for cytology and culture and to provide some relief for her symptoms. She subsequently developed acute respiratory distress attributed to re-expansion pulmonary.

What is re-expansion pulmonary edema?

Re-expansion pulmonary edema is a syndrome of acute lung injury that occurs soon after a partially or completely collapsed lung is re-expanded. Typically, the patient complains of acute shortness of breath and cough typically within one hour following either thoracentesis or chest tube placement. The patient may become severely hypoxic, with cough and sometimes frothy sputum, and have crackles on pulmonary auscultation.

What is the risk of re-expansion pulmonary edema?

Re-expansion pulmonary edema is extremely uncommon. Patients may be at higher risk under the following conditions:

- Complete lung collapse from pleural effusion, airway compression or obstruction from a mass, or pneumothorax compared to those with partial collapse
- Duration of the collapse more than 3 days
- Removal of large volumes (> 1–1.5 liters) of fluid
- Rapid removal.

She required supportive care with intubation to achieve adequate oxygenation.

SUGGESTED READINGS

Feller-Kopman D. Ultrasound-guided thoracentesis. *Chest*. 2006; 129(6):1709–1714.

Gordon CE, Feller-Kopman D, Balk EM, Smetana GW. Pneumothorax following thoracentesis: a systematic review and meta-analysis. *Arch Intern Med*. 2010;170(4):332–339.

Heffner JE, Klein JS, Hampson C. Diagnostic utility and clinical application of imaging for pleural space infections. *Chest*. 2010;137(2):467–479.

Moldonado F, Ryu J. Yellow nail syndrome. *Curr Opin Pulm Med*. 2009;15(4):371–375.

Schoonover GA. Risk of bleeding during thoracentesis in anticoagulated patients. *Chest*. 2006;130(4 Suppl):141S–1142S.

Soubani AO, Valdivieso M. Complications of thoracentesis. *Intern Med J*. 2009;39(9):628.

Thompson TW, Delapena J, Setnik GS. Thoracentesis (Videos in Clinical Medicine). *N Engl J Med*. 2006;355:e16.

REFERENCES

1. Duncan DR, Morgenthaler TI, Ryu JH, Daniels CE. Reducing iatrogenic risk in thoracentesis: establishing best practice via experiential training in a zero-risk environment. *Chest*. 2009;135(5): 1315–1320.
2. Wong CL, Holroyd-Leduc J, Straus SE. Does this patient have a pleural effusion? (Rational Clinical Exam). *JAMA*. 2009;301(3): 309–317.

WEB-BASED RESOURCES

http://www.nejm.org/doi/pdf/10.1056/NEJMvcm053812

Excellent descriptions and an illustrated step by step guide of thoracentesis procedure

http://www.nlm.nih.gov/research/visible/visible_human.html

Pulmonary anatomy overview.

http://www.youtube.com/watch?v=6-9W-Y2dbpc

New England Journal Video on proper thoracentesis

http://www.youtube.com/watch?v=6ThpUpgjSiM

Sonosite corporation video depicting the use of chest ultrasound

CHAPTER 118

Arthrocentesis

Elinor Mody, MD

Key Clinical Questions

1. What are the indications for arthrocentesis?
2. When do you need to reverse a coagulopathy?
3. What is the best site to reduce the likelihood of complications?
4. What are the diagnostic criteria for a septic effusion? For gout?

INTRODUCTION

In the hospital setting, arthrocentesis is usually performed to diagnose whether a patient has a septic joint and to narrow antibiotic therapy once the cultures are known. Although bacterial infections may affect less than 20% of all cases of acute arthritis, failure to diagnose bacterial infection may lead to permanent cartilage damage, destruction of bone, loss of joint function, and, in extreme cases, loss of limb and death. Aspiration almost always yields a diagnosis, and in the case of the septic joint, is akin to draining an abscess. Luckily, in the vast majority of cases, aspirating a joint is a simple and safe procedure rarely complicated by infection. This chapter reviews a number of key elements related to arthrocentesis, including the indications and contraindications, procedure set-up and insertion techniques, and testing.

PATHOPHYSIOLOGY

In the vast majority of cases, septic joints are a result of hematogenous seeding. Inflamed and artificial joints have an increased risk of being seeded by bacteria. The vasculature of the synovium does not have a basement membrane, thereby allowing bacteria to enter the joint space. Direct trauma to the joint such as an animal bite is a much rarer cause of joint infection. Polyarticular involvement is uncommon, but is sometimes seen in patients with rheumatoid arthritis. Other risk factors for septic arthritis include age older than 80, immunosuppression, sexually transmitted diseases, diabetes mellitus, and HIV infection. Bacterial arthritis is most often caused by typical gram-positive bacteria, but there is an increasing incidence of gram-negative septic arthritis. Gonococcal arthritis remains the most common cause of bacterial arthritis in sexually active adults.

Crystal-induced arthritis, gout, and pseudogout may mimic septic arthritis, and may coexist with septic arthritis. They are an underrecognized cause of postoperative fever. Pseudogout is caused by the deposition of calcium pyrophosphate in the joint milieu resulting in an inflammatory response. Risk factors for pseudogout include older age, diabetes, hypothyroidism, hemochromatosis, abnormalities of calcium homeostasis, and endstage renal disease. Patients often have normal calcium levels despite the presence of pseudogout. Gout or monosodium urate–induced arthritis is caused by an inflammatory reaction to monosodium urate deposition in synovial tissue, bursae, and tendon sheaths. Gouty attacks occur when urate crystals are released from preexisting tissue deposits. Risk factors for gout include hyperuricemia; postmenopausal state, especially for those women taking thiazide diuretics; chronic renal insufficiency; immunosuppressives, such as cyclosporine; and sickle cell and other hematologic disease. Nevertheless, the factors responsible for the development of gout are not well understood. Although hyperuricemia is associated with an increased risk of gout and the higher the level the greater the risk, levels do not correlate with severity of disease. An acute elevation of uric acid as seen in the tumor lysis syndrome does not usually provoke gouty attacks, and gout is less common in endstage renal disease and rheumatoid arthritis than expected. In addition, the presence of urate crystals in synovial fluid is not always sufficient to produce an attack and many people have asymptomatic chronic hyperuricemia. Serum urate levels at the time of an acute gouty attack may in fact be in the normal range for the general population in as many as 40% of affected patients.

TABLE 118-1 Indications for Diagnostic Arthrocentesis

Monoarthritis
Trauma with joint effusion
Monoarthritis in a patient with chronic polyarthritis
Suspected septic arthritis, pseudogout, gout, or hemarthrosis

INDICATIONS

Excluding cases of trauma, pain with passive motion of a joint or palpation of the joint capsule suggests synovitis and requires further investigation.

A diagnostic arthrocentesis is indicated for patients with acute articular or periarticular pain and risk factors (**Table 118-1**). Patients with a sudden increase in pain in a previously damaged joint may have a bacterial infection but not necessarily have prodromal symptoms or fever. Fever may not be associated with bacterial infection in greater than 40% of patients and fever may be associated with other conditions that cause joint pain, including gout, especially when polyarticular. Hence, synovial fluid analysis is required to exclude the diagnosis.

Although radiography is essential in the diagnosis of trauma, it has no role in the early diagnosis of a joint infection. Neither CT or MRI or radionuclide scanning can distinguish between septic and noninfectious causes of inflammatory synovitis. Imaging is indicated, however, in the following patients with suspected

- Sternoclavicular joint infection: to look for mediastinal extension
- Sacroiliac joint infection: to look for pelvic involvement
- Osteomyelitis.

PRACTICE POINT

- Neither CT or MRI or radionuclide scanning can distinguish between septic and noninfectious causes of inflammatory synovitis. Only arthrocentesis will be able to guide therapy to avoid progressive joint damage. In addition, arthrocentesis should be performed before initiating chronic hypouricemic therapy indicated for gout but not for pseudogout.

Arthrocentesis or aspiration of tophi is needed to establish the diagnosis of crystal deposition disease and to distinguish between pseudogout and gout. Arthrocentesis should be performed before initiating chronic hypouricemic therapy indicated for gout but not for pseudogout.

Classic radiographic findings of gout occur only very late in the disease. Likewise, radiographic findings of chondrocalcinosis and cystic erosions without marked joint space narrowing may suggest pseudogout but cannot confirm that the patient's sudden increase in pain is caused by this disease and not by coexisting bacterial infection.

CONTRAINDICATIONS

There are very few contraindications to aspiration, and the ones that exist are only relative ones. Let's start with some "myths."

- Myth 1. Aspirating through a cellulitis can seed the joint. There is no literature to support this theory. Additionally, the risk of not aspirating a septic joint far outweighs any theoretical risk of seeding joints.
- Myth 2. Aspiration should not be performed if the patient is anticoagulated. This is a relative contraindication. If the joint is small, there is not much space to bleed into. Severe thrombocytopenia is the most worrisome scenario.
- Myth 3. Aspiration rarely leads to a diagnosis. This is not true; this is the only way to make a crystal proven diagnosis of gout or pseudogout, a diagnosis of septic joint, and can be very helpful in making the diagnosis of an inflammatory arthritis.

Injection of cortisone is a bit more complicated. Injecting an already septic joint can have truly disastrous results, and should be completely avoided. Even the small dose of cortisone that is in most injections can exacerbate glaucoma, and raise blood sugars transiently in diabetics; these patients and their other doctors need to be alerted to this potential complication.

Most joints can be aspirated safely even in the setting of clotting diathesis and warfarin therapy. However, if the INR is excessive, or the patient has hemophilia, partial correction may be appropriate prior to an arthrocentesis.

Orthopedic consultation is mandatory for joints that can not be adequately drained, especially the hip and shoulder, if percutaneous drainage is unsuccessful, and in the case of replaced joints.

STEROID INJECTIONS

Injecting a joint, tendon sheath, or bursa with a small amount of steroid is often a very useful procedure, giving the patient a tremendous amount of pain relief, without significant systemic side effects. While in general steroid injections will not fall within the prevue of the hospitalist, it is useful for the hospitalist to be aware of the possibilities, as resolving joint, tendon, or bursal pain with a steroid injection often can lead to shorter hospitalizations. The most common areas for steroid injection are the shoulder, trochanteric bursa, and knee. The shoulder is most typically injected due to adhesive capsulitis. While the definitive treatment for adhesive capsulitis is vigorous physical therapy, a steroid injection provides enough pain relief to allow the patient to undergo the necessary physical therapy. Trochanteric bursitis is a very common cause of pain, and can be extremely severe. It is often confused for pain of the true hip (which is usually in the groin), or sciatica. As they can coexist, injecting this bursa can help clarify the situation. Knees are usually injected due to inflammatory arthritis or osteoarthritis. The knee should not be injected if there is a concern for internal derangement, as steroids can impair healing.

POTENTIAL COMPLICATIONS

Although rare, potential complications include infection, bleeding, and pain. Skin atrophy may result from injecting corticosteroids.

PROCEDURE SET-UP AND INSERTION TECHNIQUES

Preprocedure checklist

1. Review relevant laboratory, imaging, and clinical information to best understand the indication for, and possible risks of, the planned procedure.
2. Obtain informed consent, with risks of bleeding, infection, and pain explained. If injecting corticosteroids, the risk of skin atrophy must also be explained.
3. Perform a ***Universal Time-Out*** (including verification of correct patient, a physician order for procedure, indication for procedure, selection of correct site, correct tubes for specimen collection, and the presence of informed consent).
4. Check for allergies to tape, latex, and medications.
5. Position patient for the procedure (remember: the operator's comfort is paramount) (**Figures 118-1** to **118-4**).

Sterile barrier setup

1. Sterilize hands with appropriate surgical scrub.
2. Don gloves.

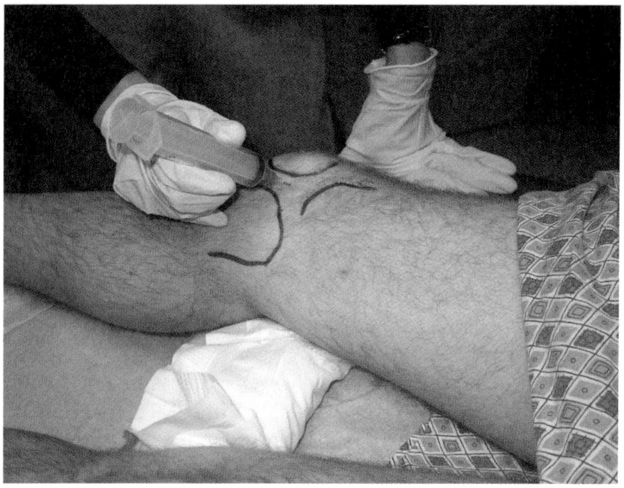

Figure 118-1 *Knee aspiration: Position the patient lying down on his/her back, with the affected knee in very slight passive flexion; this can be obtained by putting a rolled towel or sheet under the knee. The joint can be approached medially or laterally. In either case, aim the needle parallel to and just inferior to the patella, so that it slips in just underneath, into the joint itself.*

3. Prepare the procedure tray and supplies, organizing the tray in anticipated order of use.
4. A mark at the expected site of puncture can be made with the tip of the needle cap; this indentation can be seen after the area is sterile.
5. Clean the area broadly with betadine swabs, preferably three times.

Insertion steps

1. Local anesthesia can be used, either ethyl chloride spray, lidocaine, or both.

Testing

The clinician should order

- Cultures of blood and other potential extra-articular sources of infection

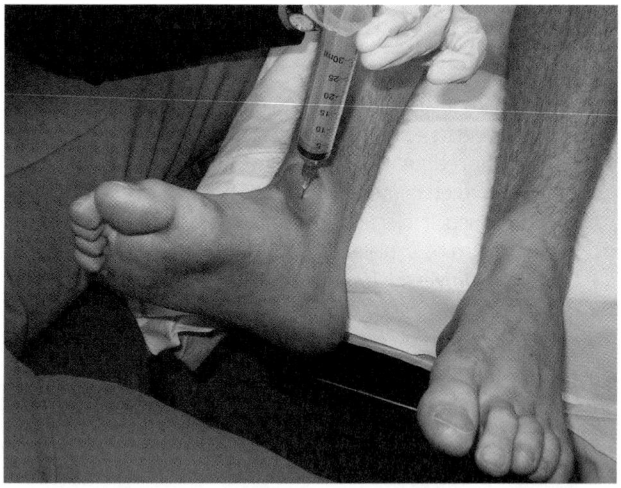

Figure 118-3 *Ankle aspiration: Position the joint in dorsiflexion. The needle should be aimed between the extensor hallicus longus and the medial malleolus.*

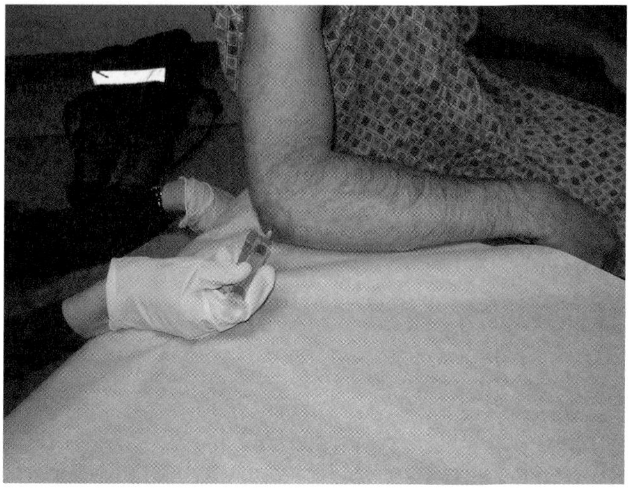

Figure 118-2 *Elbow aspiration: The patient should be positioned with the elbow at a 90° angle to assure maximum opening of the joint. The needle should be positioned lateral and slightly distal to the olecranon, and aimed toward the shoulder.*

- Culture and Gram stain of suspicious skin lesions
- Rectal, cervical, urethral and pharyngeal cultures for *Neisseria gonorrhoeae* if suspected
- C-reactive protein to monitor treatment response

Synovial fluid analysis:

- Leukocyte count
- Gram stain
- Culture–immediate plating on appropriate culture medium if gonorrhea culture suspected
- Polarized light microscopy examination

Synovial fluid glucose, protein, lactate dehydrogenase, lactic acid, autoantibodies and acute phase reactants are not recommended to confirm or exclude a diagnosis of septic arthritis. The following diagnoses may be suggested by synovial fluid analysis:

- Fracture involving the marrow space—large fat droplets or small lipid droplets

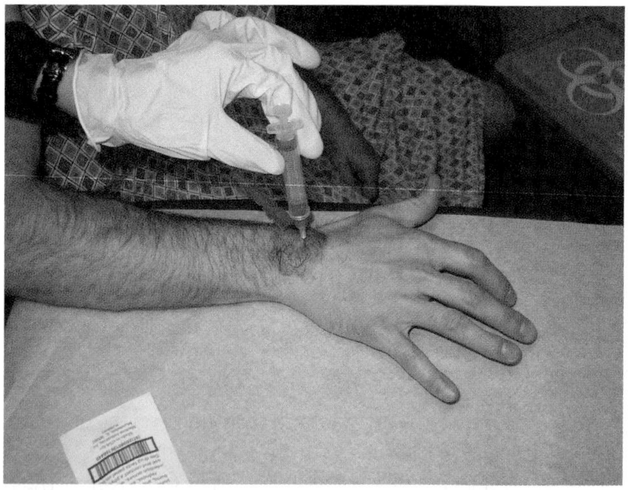

Figure 118-4 *Wrist aspiration: Position the patient's wrist over a rolled-up sheet or towel so that the hand and forearm are relaxed. Have the patient extend his thumb to accentuate the tendon. Palpate for the hollow medial to this tendon, and lateral to the extensor tendon of the index finger. Direct the needle straight in at a 90° angle.*

- Gout—brightly birefringent needles (by polarized microscopy); monosodium urate crystals (by normal light microscopy)
- Pseudogout (calcium pyrophosphate dihydrate deposition)—less intensely birefringent crystals than monosodium urate crystals; more rod shaped or rhomboid than needles as seen in gout with birefringence or weakly birefringent (by polarized light microscopy); small and difficult to see crystals (by normal light microscopy)
- Renal dialysis patients—bipyramidal oxalate crystals

Post-procedure clean-up and orders

1. Perform a thorough accounting of needles.
2. Carefully dispose of all sharps in sharps containers.
3. Remove sterile drapes.

Documentation

The procedure note should contain

1. Procedure performed
2. Date of procedure
3. Indication for procedure
4. Name of clinician(s) involved
5. Completion of informed consent and Universal Time-Out
6. Note the amount of fluid removed and appearance (Is the fluid clear or pale straw colored? Turbid and yellow? Opaque and purulent? Hemorrhagic? Viscous?) (**Table 118-2**)
7. Tests sent
8. Any complications and patient's status during and after the procedure
9. Any other relevant findings or events during the procedure
10. Results of crystal examination

TABLE 118-2 Characteristics of Joint Fluid

	Color	Turbidity	Crystals
Septic	Yellow	Very	–
Inflammatory	Yellow	Very	–
Crystal	Yellow	Very	+
Osteoarthritis	Yellow	No	–

SUGGESTED READINGS

Chui CH, Lee JY. Diagnostic dilemmas in unusual presentations of gout. *Aust Fam Physician.* 2007;36(11):931–934.

Goldenberg DL. Bacterial arthritis. *Curr Opin Rheumatol.* 1995;7(4):310–314.

Margues AR. Lyme disease: a review. *Curr Allergy Asthma Rep.* 2010;10(1):13–20.

Schumacher HR Jr. The pathogenesis of gout. *Cleve Clin J Med.* 2008;75(Suppl 5):S2–S4.

Tung CH, Chen YH, Lan HH, Hsieh TY, Chen DY, Lan JL. Diagnosis of plant-thorn synovitis by high-resolution ultrasonography: a case report and literature review. *Clin Rheumatol.* 2007;26(5):849–851.

CHAPTER 119

Placement of Nasogastric Tube

Ruma Rajbhandari, MD, MPH
Stephen C. Wright, MD

Key Clinical Questions

1. What are the indications for nasogastric tube (NGT) placement?
2. What are the contraindications to NGT insertion?
3. What are the immediate and long-term complications associated with NGT insertion?
4. What is the best method for insertion of an NGT to minimize complications?
5. What are the standards of care for postinsertion confirmation of position of an NGT?

CASE 119-1

A 69-year-old woman with a past medical history of diabetes mellitus type II, hypertension, and colon cancer, status post remote partial colectomy, developed abdominal pain, nausea, and bilious vomiting for the past twelve hours. Her vital signs were within normal limits with the exception of a heart rate of 110 beats per minute (bpm). She appeared uncomfortable, and her abdominal examination was notable for decreased bowel sounds with a succussion splash, mild guarding, and tenderness to palpation of the left and right lower quadrants without rebound. A CT scan of the abdomen reported a small bowel obstruction with a transition point in the distal ileum.

A nasogastric tube (NGT) was inserted through her nose with appropriate analgesia—auscultation of bubbling sounds in the epigastrium suggested correct placement in the stomach which was confirmed by chest x-ray. The NGT, which suctioned approximately 500 cc of yellowish-green bilious material, was subsequently attached to wall suction. Due to minimal drainage and resolution of her pain over the ensuing 3 days, her inpatient physicians removed the tube from her stomach and successfully advanced her diet.

INTRODUCTION

Nasogastric tube (NGT) insertion is a relatively common procedure performed in the hospital setting for a wide variety of indications, including enteral feeding, administration of drugs and other agents and gastric decompression after trauma or intestinal obstruction. The first use of a nasogastric tube is attributed to a 16th-century Italian professor of anatomy and surgery, Hieronymus Fabircius ab Aquapendent who used a silver tube for enteral feeding. Usually inserted at bedside, NGT placement enables early commencement of enteral feeding, thereby maintaining intestinal function even in critically ill patients. Traditionally, the nasogastric tube is a large tube that is inserted blindly through the patient's nose until its tip lies approximately 10 cm below the gastroesophageal junction. For patients in whom feeding beyond the ampulla of Vater is preferable (eg, pancreatitis, gastroparesis), small-bore postpyloric feeding tubes are also available. Recent advances in endoscopic and feeding tube technology allow postpyloric tube placement, with simultaneous gastric decompression, via double-lumen nasogastric decompression and jejunal feeding tubes. These are placed using flexible transnasal endoscopes that can pass small-diameter (5–6 mm) feeding tubes over a guidewire.

PHYSIOLOGY

Nasogastric tubes have been used for decades in chronically ill patients to provide bolus enteral feeds on a temporary basis until a more permanent surgical gastrostomy can be carried out. In the 1960s, the invention of total parenteral nutrition (TPN) allowed another method of providing nutrition to critically ill patients. However, a growing body of literature supports the view that patient outcomes are better with enteral feeding than with TPN, with regard to infection rates, multiorgan failure, and mortality. Although the exact mechanism for reduced complications and

TABLE 119-1 Evidence-based Medicine: Key References for Proven Benefits of Enteral Feeding

Study	Methodology	Results	Limitations	Bottom Line
Lewis SJ, Egger M, Sylvester PA, Thomas S. Early enteral feeding versus "nil by mouth" after gastrointestinal surgery: systematic review and meta-analysis of controlled trials. *BMJ.* 2001;323:773.	Meta-analysis of RCTs comparing any type of enteral feeding started within 24 hours after surgery with nothing by mouth in elective gastrointestinal surgery.	11 studies with 837 patients. Early feeding reduced the risk of any type of infection (RR, 0.72; $P = 0.036$) and mean length of stay in hospital (number of days reduced by 0.84; $P = 0.001$).	Meta-analysis of 11 small, clinically heterogeneous, randomized trials of varying quality.	No clear advantage to keeping patients NPO after elective gastrointestinal resection. Early feeding may be of benefit.
Kudsk KA, Croce MA, Fabian TC, et al. Enteral vs parenteral feeding: Effects on septic morbidity following blunt and penetrating trauma. *Ann Surg.* 1992;215:503–513.	RCT of enteral vs parenteral feeding after blunt and penetrating trauma looking at effects on septic complications.	98 patients enrolled. Enteral group had fewer pneumonias, intra-abdominal abscesses, and line sepsis; and sustained significantly fewer infections per patient. Significantly fewer infections in patients with injury severity score > 20 and abdominal trauma index > 24.	Small study	Significantly lower septic morbidity in patients fed enterally after blunt and penetrating trauma; most significant benefit seen in the more severely injured patients.
Gramlich L, Kichian K, Pinilla J, et al. Does enteral nutrition compared to parenteral nutrition result in better outcomes in critically ill patients? A systematic review of the literature. *Nutrition.* 2004;20(10):843–848.	Meta-analysis of RCTs comparing enteral nutrition with parenteral nutrition in critically ill patients with respect to clinically important outcomes.	13 studies included. EN was associated with a significant decrease in infectious complications but not with any difference in mortality compared to PN. No difference in number of days on ventilator or length of hospital stay. Some cost-savings with enteral nutrition.	Meta-analysis of small trials	Use of EN as opposed to PN results in an important decrease in the incidence of infectious complications in the critically ill and may be less costly. EN should be the first choice for nutritional support in critically ill.
McClave SA, Chang W-K, Dhaliwal R, Heyland, DK. Nutrition Support in acute pancreatitis: a systematic review of the literature. *J Parent Enter Nutr.* 2006;30(2):143–156.	Meta-analysis of 27 RCTs of adult patients with acute pancreatitis.	Use of EN was associated with significant reduction in infectious morbidity and hospital length of stay but had no effect on mortality when compared with PN.	Meta-analysis of small, diverse trials.	Patients with acute severe pancreatitis should begin enteral nutrition early—this is new gold standard therapy. When PN is used, it should be initiated after 5 days.

EN, enteral nutrition; PN, parenteral nutrition; RCT, randomized controlled trial; RR, relative risk.

associated benefits of enteral feeding are not completely understood, mucosal vulnerability induced by histologic changes in the intestinal mucosa (eg, atrophy of intestinal villi in parenterally fed rats) is considered to play a major role. Furthermore, there is evidence that the enteric nervous system and antigen stimulation of mucosal surfaces drives IgA defense. The actual processing of nutrients via the gastrointestinal tract appears to stimulate a complex series of responses which affect immunologic integrity. Please see **Table 119-1** for key evidence based references for the proven benefits of enteral feeding.

Despite all of the beneficial effects of enteral feeding, it is important to remember that enteral feeding has its limitations. For example, it does not prevent microaspiration from oropharyngeal contents in the cognitively impaired patient. It is also associated with an increased risk of gastroesophageal reflux.

INDICATIONS FOR THE PROCEDURE

Nasogastric tubes may be placed for both diagnostic and therapeutic purposes (**Table 119-2**). Diagnostically, emergent examination of gastric aspirate provides essential information in clinical situations such as the source and severity of upper gastrointestinal bleeding and in poisoning when undigested tablets are identified.

TABLE 119-2 Indications for Nasogastric Tubes

Nasogastric Tubes Diagnostic indications: • Sample gastric contents, especially in the assessment of GI bleeding Therapeutic indications: • Prevent vomiting and aspiration, especially in trauma settings • Provide drainage and/or lavage in drug overdose or poisoning • Drain gastric contents and decompress the stomach (gastric motor failure, partial small bowel obstruction, postoperative ileus, palliation in metastatic cancer) • Introduce a passage into the GI tract for initial, less than 1 month, of enteral feeding
Post-pyloric Tubes Enteral feeding in the setting of: • Poor gastric emptying due to critical illness or from gastric motor failure • Severe acute pancreatitis and other states where nasojejunal feeding tube positioning is required

Therapeutically, in severe upper gastrointestinal bleeding, nasogastric intubation and suctioning can provide symptomatic relief and prepare for endoscopic visualization of the gastric and duodenal mucosa. In trauma settings, NGTs may prevent vomiting and aspiration and in cases of drug overdose, they are used to lavage or drain stomach contents. In small bowel obstruction, NGT placement will decompress the gastrointestinal tract proximal to the obstruction; however, NGTs should not be used for enteral feeding in complete obstruction. NGTs are commonly employed when patients are NPO due to temporary aspiration risk following stroke, and other neurologic states, for the purposes of administering medications as well as enteral feeding.

An alternative method to the NGT of enteral feeding is the nasoduodenal/nasojejunal (postpyloric) tubes. Postpyloric feeding tubes are used in settings where it is desirable to feed beyond the ampulla of Vater. The main benefit of postpyloric tube placement is it bypasses the stomach, thereby, providing a large feeding capacity with less of a concern for aspiration in patients with poor gastric emptying. If the nasoenteric tube is placed more than 40 cm into the jejunum, past the ligament of Treitz, enteral feeding can be given without pancreatic stimulation which makes it useful in the management of severe acute pancreatitis. At the bedside, experienced personnel can place postpyloric tubes using bent guide wires in conjunction with a standard feeding tube. However, such techniques are less successful in critically ill patients and those with disturbed upper gastrointestinal motility and function in whom the feeding tube usually fails to pass beyond the ligament of Treitz. In such cases, an interventional radiologist or gastroenterologist can place a tube beyond the pyloris under radiographic guidance or endoscopically with guidewire exchange. Fully transnasal endoscopic procedures as well as double-lumen tube systems that include a proximal port for gastric decompression and a distal port for jejunal feeding have been developed.

More long-term feeding is accomplished by G-tube or J-tube. Please see **Table 119-3** for a summary of various options available for enteral feeding. If the patient does not recover sufficient function to allow for oral feedings, there are guidelines that can assist the clinician and family in the decision-making process.

TABLE 119-3 Options for Enteral Feeding

Type of Feeding Tube	Summary
Nasogastric	For patients with intact gag reflex, normal gastric emptying. Easy bedside insertion but highest risk of pulmonary aspiration.
Nasoduodenal/nasojejunal (postpyloric/Dobhoff tubes)	For patients with gastroparesis or gastric dysfunction. Reduced aspiration but potential for GI intolerance to goal tube feed rate. May require endoscopic placement for tube to go beyond pylorus; tube misplacement is a concern if proper procedure is not followed for insertion and confirmation.
Gastrostomy (G-tube)	For long-term feeding (>4 weeks) in patients with normal gastric emptying. Can be placed surgically or percutaneously. Needs stoma care and there is potential for fistula after the tube is removed.
Jejunostomy (J-tube)	Long-term feeding in patients at high risk of aspiration with impaired gastric emptying. Reduced risk of aspiration, can be placed endoscopically. Similar disadvantages as G-tube.

CONTRAINDICATIONS TO NASOGASTRIC TUBES

Nasogastric tubes are contraindicated in the presence of severe facial trauma (cribiform plate disruption), due to the possibility of inserting the tube intracranially. In this instance, an orogastric tube may be inserted. Esophageal abnormalities are also considered a relative contraindication to nasogastric tube insertion. For example, the risk of esophageal perforation is high in patients with a recent history of ingestion of caustic substances and in those with esophageal strictures or diverticula. However, nasogastric intubation may be performed safely in most patients with esophageal varices. Patients who are comatose should undergo endotracheal intubation prior to nasogastric intubation, because the procedure may precipitate vomiting and aspiration in such patients.

Risk factors for misplacement of nasogastric tubes, particularly into the tracheobronchial tree, include altered mental status, sedation, advanced age and recent prolonged endotracheal intubation, all of which are thought to decrease airway reflexes. Furthermore, nasogastric intubation in head and neck cancer patients may be especially difficult after radiation therapy due to difficulties in swallowing secondary to edema, mucositis, abnormal anatomy and sensation. All of these categories of patients, as well as patients who have had complications with NGT placement in the past and patients status post lung transplantation, would benefit from gastroenterology consultation for nasoendoscopic placement of nasogastric tubes (**Table 119-4**).

COMPLICATIONS

Complications of NGT placement can range from relatively minor events such as epistaxis and sore throat, to potentially lethal complications like misplacement (eg, in the trachea or bronchial tree), and direct mucosal injury with bleeding and/or perforation (**Figure 119-1**).

Tracheobronchopleural complications include bronchial placement leading to atelectasis, pneumonia and lung abscess; bronchial perforation and pleural cavity penetration leading to pneumothorax, enteral feeding hydrothorax, empyema and sepsis and

TABLE 119-4 Contraindications to Nasogastric Tubes

Absolute contraindications in the following conditions:

- Severe maxillofacial trauma
- Repair of choanal atresia and transnasal transphenoidal surgery

Relative contraindications in patients who have:

- Increased risk of perforation due to esophageal abnormalities (recent ingestion of caustic substances, strictures, diverticula)
- Undergone lung transplantation
- Prior pulmonary complication from nasogastric tube placement
- Altered mental status states and/or sedation

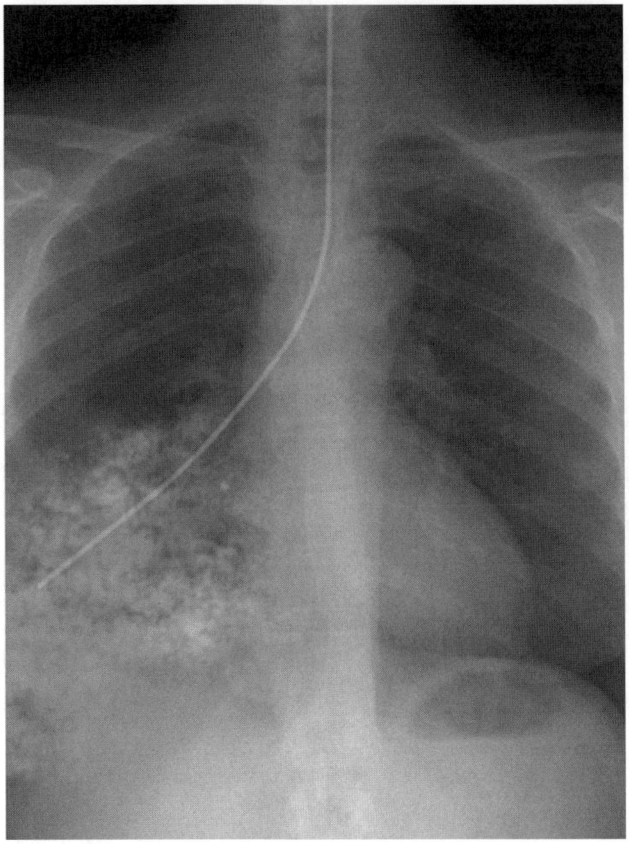

Figure 119-1 *Chest radiograph showing nasogastric feeding tube in the right lower lobe of the lung with infiltrate.*

possible pulmonary hemorrhage (**Table 119-5**). Pneumothoraces may account for approximately 60% of complications and half of these may require draining by chest tube. Rarely, a thoracotomy may be required to withdraw the tube. Enteral complications include bleeding, esophageal, gastric, or intestinal perforation, tube knotting and impaction, tube double backing and kinking, and tube breakage. Intravascular penetration includes erosion into a retroesophageal aberrant right subclavian artery, right internal jugular vein to right atrium. Intracranial injury is more likely following surgical repair such as transnasal transphenoidal surgery and in the setting of maxillofacial trauma.

Since misplacement can have such serious consequences, confirmation of placement is one of the most important parts of the NGT insertion procedure. If misplaced, the NGT should be removed as quickly as possible. No medications or feeding should proceed via the NGT without first confirming correct placement by CXR. Also, placement of the tube can induce gagging or vomiting; therefore, clinicians should be prepared to perform emergent suctioning.

TABLE 119-5 Complications Associated with Nasogastric Tubes

- Sinusitis, epistaxis, sore throat
- Tracheobronchopleural complications (2% incidence, 0.3% mortality)
- Intravascular penetration
- Esophageal trauma
- Intracranial injury
- Nasogastric tube syndrome

When nasogastric tubes are used for a prolonged period, the ciliary epithelium of the nasal mucosa can be damaged and this may lead to sinusitis. NGTs should be removed as soon as feasible, and frequent monitoring of the patient's dysphagia should be carried out by the speech and swallowing service.

A rare complication of NGT placement is the NGT syndrome. When postcricoid ulceration occurs, the posterior cricoarytenoid muscles are affected, leading to vocal cord abduction paralysis and upper airway obstruction. This syndrome can lead to life-threatening laryngeal obstruction.

HOW TO PERFORM THE PROCEDURE

A formal "time-out" must be taken to properly identify the correct patient and to review any major concerns and how to minimize patient discomfort during the procedure (**Table 119-6**).

1. Explain the procedure to the patient, including risks and benefits.
2. Examine the patient's nasal passageway to identify septal deviation or other anatomical restrictions in order to determine which naris might be most appropriate for insertion. If the nostrils are of unequal size, the wider one should be used.
3. The nasal passageways may be pretreated with oxymetozalone or phenylephrine to constrict the blood vessels of the nasal mucosa, thereby reducing the risk of epistaxis.
4. In order to reduce pain during the procedure, the nasal mucosa and the posterior oropharynx may be anesthetized topically with 4% lidocaine delivered with an atomizer or with viscous lidocaine applied directly. Alternatively, 4% lidocaine delivered with a nebulizer provides excellent anesthesia of both the nasal and the oral mucosa.

TABLE 119-6 The Procedure

Checklist for Procedure
1. Indications
2. Contraindications (review absolute vs relative contraindications)
3. Formal consent need not be obtained but inform patient/family about indications and incidence of complications.
4. Working IV
5. Equipment in room
• Personal protective equipment (gloves, gown, face shield)
• Nasogastric tube
• Catheter tip irrigation syringe (60 mL)
• Water-soluble lubricant, preferably viscous lidocaine
• Vasoconstrictor spray (eg, oxymetolazone)
• Topical anesthetic
• Atomized 4% lidocaine
• Adhesive tape
• Low powered suction device
• Stethoscope
• Cup of water (if necessary)/ice chips/straw
• Emesis basin
• Absorbent towels or pads
6. Collection of any specimens (if sampling gastric fluid to guaiac, or to check pH and presence of bile)
7. Action plan in case a complication results (such as an aspiration event, unexpected bloody aspirate, resistance to advancing tube)
8. Postprocedure chest x-ray, including identifying who is responsible for reviewing film

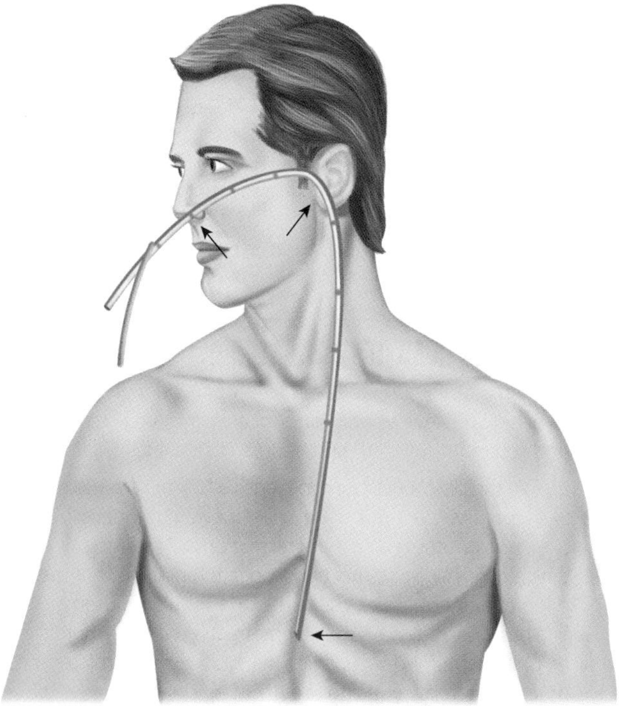

Figure 119-2 *Estimating the length of the nasogastric tube.*

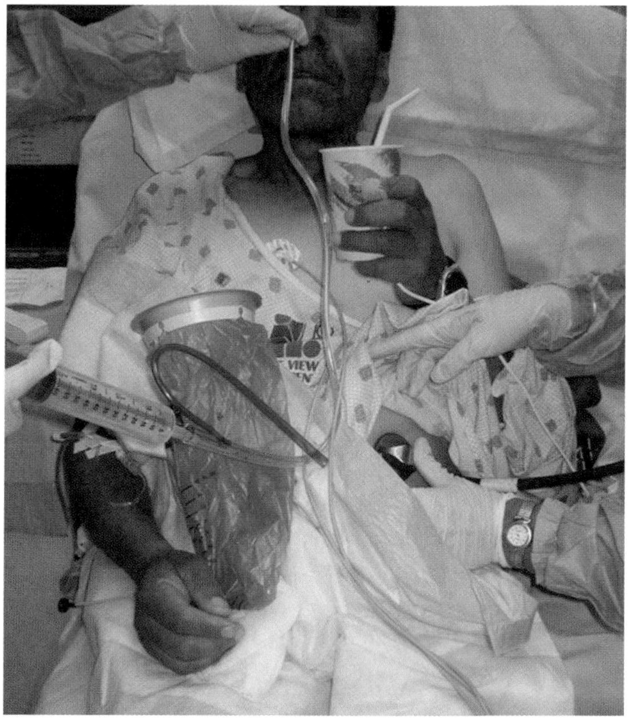

Figure 119-3 *Injecting air into the nasogastric tube via a syringe and auscultating over the epigastrium. (Courtesy of Gil Z. Shlamovitz, MD.)*

5. The length of tube that needs to be inserted can be estimated by measuring the distance from the xiphoid process to the angle of the mandible and then to the nostril (**Figure 119-2**). Mark this point on the nasogastric tube with a pen.
6. Lubricate 2 to 4 inches of the end of the nasogastric tube with viscous lidocaine after it has been cooled in an ice bath.
7. Position the patient upright in the "sniffing" position and insert the NGT approximately 15 to 20 cm.

PRACTICE POINT

- Flexion of the patient's head to his chest (the chin-tuck) narrows the trachea and opens to esophagus. In addition, rotating the patient's head toward the right or left shoulder may accomplish deviation of the tube tip away from the midline laryngeal opening.

8. Insert the tube into the nasal cavity, slowly passing it posteriorly along the floor of the nasal canal into the posterior oropharynx. Aim for a line that connects the earlobes, ie, straight back. The patient may start to gag and there might be resistance to passage of the tube as it encounters the posterior pharynx. If this happens, stop advancing the tube and ask the patient to sip ice water through the straw. As the patient swallows, the epiglottis will cover the trachea and you may advance the tube further. Once the tube is past the larynx, it can be guided rapidly down until the marked point is reached. Watch expectantly for the patient to initiate a swallow, and advance the tube when you see this happening. Do not advance against resistance because this may mean that you are in the wrong location or that the tube has coiled.
9. Withdraw the tube immediately if changes occur in patient's respiratory status or if he/she is unable to talk or if respirations can be heard through the nasogastric tube.
10. When the 50- to 60-cm mark is reached, secure the tube with a short length of tape (approximately 5–7 cm, 1" wide) cut halfway down vertically. Apply the wide end of the tape to the patient's nose, and wrap the two tails around the tube.
11. Aspirate to assess for the presence of gastric contents. Then use the catheter tip syringe to inject air into the tube while listening for borborygmus (bubbling sounds) over the epigastrium, which suggests proper placement of the tube in the stomach (**Figure 119-3**).

PRACTICE POINT

- Signs suggestive of correct tube placement such as absence of coughing, facile placement of tube to 60 cm, inspection of NGT aspirate, and epigastric auscultation may be misleading. Likewise, bubbling of the tube under water to suggest pulmonary misplacement can be falsely negative when the portholes of the NGT are plugged. Even phonation may be unaffected if a small fine bore tube in the bronchus has not interfered with the vocal cords.

12. A CXR should be obtained to confirm proper placement prior to instillation of activated charcoal, medications, or feedings through the tube. An abdominal x-ray (KUB) usually is not used to confirm placement of an NGT because most of the important complications of NGT placement are related to penetrating the esophagus or passing the tube in the trachea and bronchus. These misplacements will not be shown on a KUB (**Figure 119-4**).
13. For patients who require decompression, attach the nasogastric tube to low wall suction. Monitoring of ongoing volume outputs will help assess resolution of or persistence of the obstructing process.

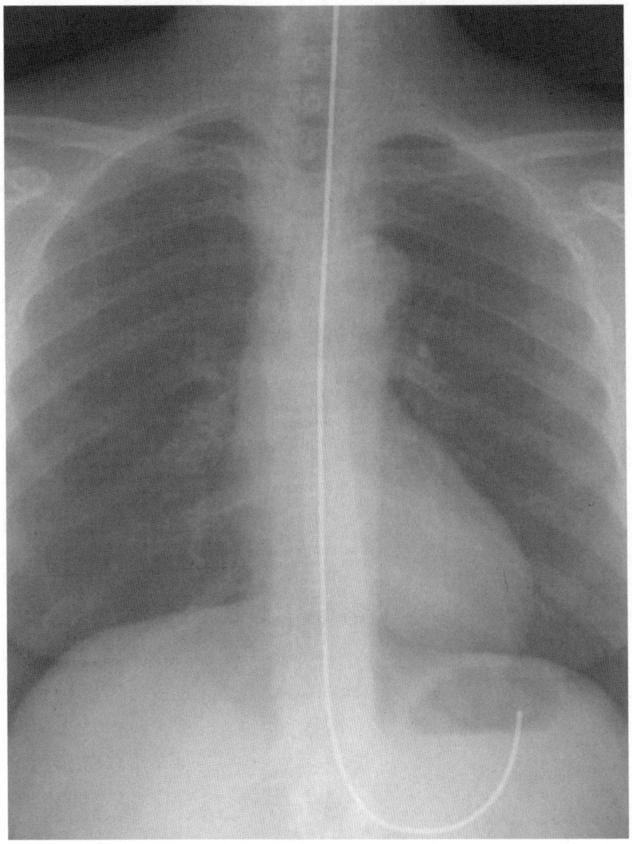

Figure 119-4 *Chest radiograph showing properly placed nasogastric feeding tube with tip visible below the diaphragm.*

PRACTICE POINT

- Partially cooling the tube can aid in easy and comfortable passage, particularly in the case of small bore tubes.
- 4% lidocaine delivered with a nebulizer provides excellent anesthesia of both nasal and oral mucosa, ensuring relatively pain-free passage of the tube.
- If resistance is felt, the tube should not be advanced.
- Always use chest x-ray to confirm placement of tube in all patients, including intubated patients.
- Never assume that cuffed endotracheal tube will always prevent inadvertent passage into trachea.

MAINTENANCE AND REMOVAL OF THE NASOGASTRIC TUBE

When the nasogastric tube is used for enteral feeding, a few simple measures can reduce the aspiration risk in critically ill patients. For example, the head of the bed should always be elevated by 30 to 40 degrees; feedings should be started slowly (eg, 25 mL/hr) and increased according to the patient's tolerance. Feeding should be given continuously without bolus feeding and gastric residual volumes should be checked every 4 hours to ensure that it is < 400 mL. If gastric residual volume continues to be high, a prokinetic drug like metoclopramide or a proton pump inhibitor to reduce gastric acid secretion can be used.

Nasogastric or nasoenteric feeding tubes should not be used for more than 4 weeks because of the discomfort to the patient and the risks of sinusitis and nasal injury. If enteral feeding is required for more than 4 weeks, a percutaneous endoscopic gastrotomy tube should be carried out.

When the indication for nasogastric tube placement is gastric decompression such as with small bowel obstruction, the NGT is usually placed at low wall suction, either continuous or intermittent. Once the patient's bowel function returns as manifested by the presence of bowel sounds, flatus, and lack of abdominal pain, the NGT can be clamped for a few hours to an entire day, then removed completely once residual volumes are shown to be minimal.

CONCLUSION

Nasogastric tube insertion is a relatively common procedure performed in the hospital setting for a variety of indications, including enteral feeding, gastric decompression, and sampling of gastric contents. Although relatively simple to perform, it is probably one of the most uncomfortable procedures for the hospitalized patient and carries with it the risk of life-threatening complications such as inadvertent and unrecognized passage of the tube into the tracheobronchial tree. For this reason, it is crucial to take the necessary steps to ensure patient comfort and to obtain a CXR for confirmation of placement of the tube.

SUGGESTED READINGS

Bankhead R, Boullata J, Brantley S, et al. Enteral nutrition practice recommendations. *J Parenter Enteral Nutr.* 2009;33(2):122–167.

Clarke JR. Confirming feeding tube placement: old habits die hard. *PA-PSRS Patient Safety Advisory.* December 2006;3(4):23–30.

Foley N, Teasell R, Salter K, Kruger E, Martino R. Dysphagia treatment post stroke: as systematic review of randomized controlled trials. *Age Ageing.* 2008;37:258–264.

Jian K, Chen XZ, Xia Q, Tang WF, Wang L. Early nasogastric enteral nutrition for severe acute pancreatitis: A systematic review. *World J Gastroenterol.* 2007;13(39):5253–5260.

Kudsk KA. Beneficial effects of enteral feeding. *Gastrointest Endosc Clin N Am.* 2007;17(4):647–662.

O'Keefe SJD. A guide to enteral access procedures and enteral nutrition. *Nat Rev Gastroeneterol Hepatol.* 2009;6:207–215.

Pearce CB, Duncan HD. Enteral feeding: Nasograstric, nasojejunal, percutaneous endoscopic gastrotomy, or jejunostomy: its indications and limitations. *Postgrad Med J.* 2002;78:198–204.

Pillai JB. Thoracic complications of nasogastric tube: review of safe practice. *Interact Cardiovasc Thorac Surg.* 2005;4:429–433.

Shlamovitz GZ, Shah NR. Nasogastric tube: treatment & medication. eMedicine Specialties from WebMD. http://emedicine.medscape.com/article/80925-treatment.

Thomsen TW, Shaffer RW, Setnik G. Nasogastric intubation. *N Engl J Med.* 2006;354:e16.

PART VI
Clinical Conditions

SECTION 17 Renal

SECTION 18 Rheumatology

SECTION 19 Vascular Medicine

SECTION 20 Wartime Medicine

SECTION 1

Emergency Medicine

CHAPTER 120

The Principles and Practice of Emergency Medicine

Todd L. Berger, MD, FACEP
Philip Shayne, MD, FACEP
Katherine L. Heilpern, MD

Key Clinical Questions

1. What performance gaps led to the emergence of Emergency Medicine (EM) as an independent specialty?
2. What training do emergency physicians receive during residency, and what subspecialties are available after training?
3. In what ways do Emergency Medicine and Hospital Medicine interact with respect to triage, patient flow, performance measures, comanagement, and care transitions?
4. What is the Emergency Medical Treatment and Active Labor Act (EMTALA), and how does it govern aspects of Emergency Medicine and Hospital Medicine practice?

INTRODUCTION

The American Board of Medical Specialties describes the practice of Emergency Medicine as focusing on the immediate decision making and action necessary to prevent death or any further disability both in the prehospital setting and in the emergency department (ED) by providing immediate recognition, evaluation, care, stabilization, and disposition of a generally diverse population of adult and pediatric patients in response to acute or episodic illness and injury. Emergency Medicine and Hospital Medicine share many common aspects, and, because many of the patients who will be admitted to the hospitalist service will begin their inpatient care from the ED, it is important for both specialties to have an in-depth understanding of each other's domain, scope of practice, areas of expertise, and foundation in order to provide seamless and integrated patent care.

EVOLUTION OF THE PRACTICE OF EMERGENCY MEDICINE

Emergency Medicine, much like Hospital Medicine, is a specialty that has significant overlap with many other specialties in that it is not a system or procedure-specific specialty but one that specializes in situational presentation of disease. Emergency Medicine is the initial management of any disease that may present in an acute or episodic manner, including acute manifestations of chronic diseases. The value of having a specific specialist available to care for patients emergently during the crucial "golden hour" of injury was first envisioned during the Korean War in the 1950s. Although it is difficult to envision a time when EDs were staffed by junior, untrained, rotating physicians, this was the case as recently as the 1960s and '70s and still persists in other countries. Prior to the 1960s and '70s, any manner of specialty would be assigned to "cover" the ED on a rotational basis as part of a physician's obligation to a hospital. In teaching hospitals, this rotation was often relegated to very junior trainees who would then contact more senior trainees depending on their perceived need.

Beginning in the early 1970s, groups of physicians began to leave private practice to devote all of their clinical work to the ED. The first of these groups was based in Alexandria, Virginia, and their plan, known as the Alexandria Plan, was to provide consistent attending-level emergency care 24/7 year-round by physicians whose only practice was Emergency Medicine. Soon after, the first Emergency Medicine training program was established at Cincinnati General Hospital in 1970, with several other residency programs following suit. With the establishment of the American College of Emergency Physicians (ACEP) there was recognition of Emergency Medicine training programs by the American Medical Association (AMA) and the American Osteopathic Association (AOA). In 1979 the American Board of Medical Specialties recognized Emergency Medicine as a specialty, and the American Board of Emergency Medicine was formed. Initially, there were two paths to board certification in Emergency Medicine; the practice path, which allowed physicians with significant experience in Emergency Medicine to sit for the boards, and residency training in Emergency Medicine. The practice pathway closed in 1990. Approximately 40,000 physicians currently practice Emergency Medicine in the United States, with 152 Emergency Medicine residencies graduating 1500 emergency physicians per year.

In 1975, the American College of Emergency Physicians and the University Association for Emergency Medicine, now the Society for Academic Emergency Medicine (SAEM), conducted a practice analysis of the emerging field of Emergency Medicine essentially

TABLE 120-1 Major Organizations in Emergency Medicine that Contributed to the Core Content of Emergency Medicine (2001)

- American Board of Emergency Medicine (ABEM)
- American College of Emergency Physicians (ACEP)
- Council of Emergency Medicine Residency Directors (CORD)
- Emergency Medicine Residents' Association (EMRA)
- Residency Review Committee for Emergency Medicine (RRC-EM)
- Society for Academic Emergency Medicine (SAEM)

producing an overview of common conditions, symptoms, and diseases that present to EDs. After multiple revisions and reorganizations, this initiative become the core content task force, culminating in an in-depth analysis of the clinical practice of Emergency Medicine and producing Core Content of Emergency Medicine—the Model of the Clinical Practice of Emergency Medicine (EM Model) (**Table 120-1**).

The most recent (2009) model of Emergency Medicine practice delineates (1) an assessment of patient acuity, (2) a description of the tasks that must be performed to provide appropriate emergency medical care, and (3) a listing of common conditions, symptoms, and disease presentations. This model represents the essential information and skills necessary for the clinical practice of Emergency Medicine by board-certified emergency physicians.

EMERGENCY MEDICINE RESIDENCY TRAINING AND FELLOWSHIPS

Three formats of Emergency Medicine residency training are available: a) 3 years of Emergency Medicine, b) 1 year preliminary or transitional internship followed by 3 years of Emergency Medicine, and c) 4 years of Emergency Medicine. The American Board of Emergency Medicine requires a minimum of 3 years of training to qualify candidates to sit for the board examination process, and the 3-year training program format remains the most common. This is consistent with the Centers for Medicare and Medicaid Services (CMS) funding for graduate medical education (GME) programs in Emergency Medicine. Some institutions offer a 5-year dual training program of Emergency Medicine/internal medicine, Emergency Medicine/Family Medicine or Emergency Medicine/Pediatrics. Wide curricular variation exists among Emergency Medicine residency programs, although most have a high concentration of intensive care unit and trauma rotations in addition to Emergency Medicine, with some programs sending their residents to train within a variety of off-service rotations (including inpatient internal medicine wards), whereas others train their residents in the ED for the majority of their residency. The Accreditation Council for Graduate Medical Education (ACGME) Residency Review Committee for Emergency Medicine (RRC-EM) does not require experience in inpatient internal medicine wards curriculum (**Table 120-2**).

TABLE 120-2 Residency Review Committee for Emergency Medicine (RRC-EM) Program Curricular Requirements (Minimums)

Minimum of 50% of their clinical experience in the emergency department (ED) (or supervised by Emergency Medicine faculty)
2 months of inpatient critical care
4 months of pediatrics (50% in the ED), or 16% of ED patients (under age 18)
Some out-of-hospital care (emergency medical services, disaster planning, etc)

TABLE 120-3 Emergency Medicine Fellowship Training Opportunities

ACGME Accredited Fellowships	
Critical care (7)	Hyperbaric and undersea medicine (6)
Medical toxicology (29)	Palliative care medicine (1)
Pediatric Emergency Medicine (48)	Sports medicine (10)
Nonaccredited Fellowships	
Administration (6)	Cardiovascular emergencies (3)
Clinical forensic medicine (2)	Clinical pharmacology (2)
Clinical research (10)	Disaster medicine (11)
Emergency medical services (52)	Environmental health (1)
Faculty development (5)	Geriatric Emergency Medicine (2)
Health policy (3)	Injury control (3)
International Emergency Medicine (25)	Legal medicine (1)
Medical education (4)	Medical informatics (3)
Neurologic/neurovascular (2)	Observation medicine (1)
Research (27)	Simulation (4)
Transport medicine (4)	Trauma/critical care (7)
Ultrasonography (46)	Wilderness medicine (5)

All fellowships listed are 1 to 2 years, except for some 3-year pediatric Emergency Medicine and research programs.

Emergency Medicine has become a competitive specialty in the National Residency Match Program (NRMP), with a >99% fill rate every year since 1995. A number of ACGME-accredited and nonaccredited subspecialty fellowships are available for candidates who have completed Emergency Medicine residency training (**Table 120-3**). Some graduates of these programs go on to practice in both fields, splitting their time between Emergency Medicine and their subspecialty, but they all have the opportunity to bring their newfound expertise and perspective back to their practice of Emergency Medicine. This is especially advantageous for dual-trained physicians who have the opportunity to practice both Emergency Medicine and Hospital Medicine, further bridging the two specialties and extending collaboration.

SCOPE OF CARE—CLINICAL PRACTICE IN THE EMERGENCY DEPARTMENT

RESUSCITATION

The practice of Emergency Medicine is broad and requires an expansive understanding of the emergent and urgent presentations of many disease processes, central to which is recognizing and stabilizing acute life-threatening conditions. Despite the public perception that the many patients who present to an ED are nonurgent, recent publications have described that less than 15% of ED patients are actually nonurgent. As a group, ED patients have higher acuity and greater potential for morbidity and poor prognosis than patients presenting to other outpatient settings.

EVALUATION OF THE UNDIFFERENTIATED PATIENT

Almost by definition, patients who present for emergency care are undifferentiated, and emergency physicians must be prepared to assess and initiate care for patients presenting with pathology from every organ system, and medical specialty. An emergency physician's approach to patient care begins with the recognition of constellations of symptoms that may represent distinct patterns that lead to a specific diagnosis or diagnoses. Like many other specialties, this pattern recognition is central to the practice of Emergency Medicine and guides both diagnostic testing and therapeutic interventions.

RISK ASSESSMENT AND DISPOSITION

Central to the practice of Emergency Medicine is the assessment of life-threatening risk to a specific presentation. Integral to this risk assessment is the development of a differential diagnosis and the way in which the differential diagnosis is ordered. In Emergency Medicine, the highest-risk diagnoses (as opposed to the most likely diagnosis) often lead the differential. Also core to the practice of Emergency Medicine are the ability and facility to make decisions and initiate empiric treatment for potentially serious illness and injury with very limited information and prior to securing a definitive diagnosis.

SOCIAL ASPECTS OF CARE

Because EDs often serve as the safety net for a certain segment of the population, caring for patients who are homeless, addicted, or otherwise disadvantaged is a common challenge. Also, both emergency physicians and hospitalists frequently manage patients who present with end-stage or terminal disease are must assist patients and families with end-of-life decisions, including hospice, living wills, and other palliative care options.

PREHOSPITAL MEDICAL DIRECTION AND INTEGRATION OF CARE

Very often, Emergency Medicine serves as the interface between the hospital and public health, fire, police, and emergency medical services. Although usually considered only working with ambulance services, emergency medical services (EMS) essentially includes any provision for acute medical care in the out of hospital or prehospital setting. This includes ambulance services, fire department first response, mass casualty and disaster preparedness, mass gatherings, and other venues and services, including air medical transports. All EMS systems require the provision for both medical control and direction. Medical direction usually describes the off-line activities of a medical director, including educating prehospital providers; developing policies, procedures, and protocols; as well as developing a comprehensive quality assurance and improvement program. Medical control describes the actual "controlling" or giving real-time direction to prehospital providers using one of many communication tools.

EMERGENCY DEPARTMENT FLOW AND QUALITY OF CARE

TRIAGE AND PATIENT FLOW

The provision for emergency care requires complex integration of tasks and services. Although beyond the scope of this chapter, most modern EDs are redesigning the process by which patients are cared for in the ED. Traditionally, patients typically arrive in an ED by either emergency or private transport and then encounter a member of the ED care team. After an initial encounter with a greeter, most EDs will do an initial triage usually performed by a specifically trained registered nurse. At triage, the ED staff determines the patient's level of acuity, and patients are seen in the order of acuity and not the time of arrival. In the interest of patient safety, patients with the highest acuity are seen and evaluated first, necessitating that some or many lower-acuity patients wait longer. The most commonly used system of triage is the Emergency Severity Index (ESI), which assigns a level (1–5) based on a basic, codified patient assessment. The assigned number correlates to both acuity and anticipated resource needs. Patients are then brought into the ED and encounter a nurse who performs an assessment followed by an emergency physician. In academic EDs, patients may also encounter trainees and students in serial fashion. Modern ED practice has eliminated this serial process, which dates back to the 1800s, and has instituted team-based care with parallel processing eliminating islands of waiting at the beginning of the encounter and decreasing the number of times patients must retell their tale.

TABLE 120-4 Emergency Department Outcomes Report Card

Census
Total ED patient visits
Total emergency department (ED) observation unit patients
ED patient admission percentage
Total time of ED emergency medical services (EMS) diversion
Average Length of Stay (ALOS)
Median time from arrival to provider
Average length of stay: all ED patients
Average length of stay: admitted patients
Average length of stay: discharged patients
Average length of stay: observation unit patients
Performance Measures
Door to needle time (Angioplasty vs thrombolytics)
Door to antibiotics time (pneumonia)
Patient Satisfaction
Third party patient satisfaction surveys

MONITORING OF OUTCOMES: PERFORMANCE MEASURES IN THE EMERGENCY DEPARTMENT

Performance outcomes monitored in the ED by hospital administration include various patient flow, patient safety, and patient satisfaction outcomes (**Table 120-4**).

INTERSECTION OF EMERGENCY MEDICINE AND HOSPITAL MEDICINE

COMANAGEMENT IN THE EMERGENCY DEPARTMENT

With the advent of Hospital Medicine and the availability of 24-hour inpatient physician coverage, there is significant opportunity for co-management of patients who require hospital admission.

OBSERVATION MEDICINE

Many large EDs contain an ED-based observation unit, and observation medicine is rapidly developing into a subspecialty within Emergency Medicine (see Chapter 123, Co-management of Patients in the Emergency Department). As Emergency Medicine evolves to become the interface and fulcrum between outpatient and inpatient medicine and as more care, diagnostics, and therapeutics are shifted to the outpatient arena, many patients may need more than a brief ED visit without needing a full admission. Most ED-based observation units are protocol based and designed for patients who will have an anticipated length of stay of less then 24 hours, although some observation units will function similarly to short-stay units and accommodate patients up to 72 hours. Staffing is variable and usually includes nurses as well as physician extenders. CMS has developed guidelines for reimbursement within short-stay observation units and approved four diagnoses for reimbursement for observation unit admissions: chest pain, heart failure exacerbation, asthma exacerbation, and nonketotic hyperglycemia, although most observation units will treat far more diagnostic categories.

TRANSITION OF CARE

A 2007 Institute of Medicine report focused on the critical issue of ED overcrowding. The report described the rapidly increasing number of ED visits (up 32% between 1996 and 2006), which directly correlated with increased ED wait times and an associated increase in untoward events and decreased compliance with certain specific quality metrics. As both emergency physicians and hospitalists are increasingly striving to reduce length of stay while meeting specific quality and safety metrics, seamless transitions in care as patients transition from the ED to inpatient environment are paramount. Transfers in care among providers are potential sources of error, and the use of structured, codified mechanisms and processes for transfers in care can reduce error. In order to effectively and safely manage transitions in care, strong communication and teamwork as well as mutually agreed upon structure are required.

> **PRACTICE POINT**
>
> - In order to optimize safe handoffs and care transitions, unambiguous accountability is paramount to achieve the safest possible care, keeping in mind that a rapidly decompensating patient may require personal attention by the most immediately available clinician. For patients already admitted to the hospital but still residing in the Emergency Department, first responders will likely be ED staff given their availability and proximity. In all instances there should be clear documentation of all medication and fluid administration; and interpretation of laboratory tests and resultant decision-making, orders, and pending test results. Medication reconciliation should occur at ED-to-inpatient transition so that patients receive appropriate home medications.

In order to optimize safe handoffs and care transitions, unambiguous accountability is paramount to achieve the safest possible care, keeping in mind that a rapidly decompensating patient may require personal attention by the most immediately available clinician. Clear, direct, and timely communication from one care provider to another will facilitate safe handoff. The ED physician should concisely report the patient's presentation, evaluation, ED management, pending results, and expected plan of continued care, including ongoing medical concerns, risk assessment, and social aspects of care. The hospitalist should clearly ask questions and share thoughts and recommendations regarding the next steps in care, including the initiation of any urgent orders and communication with other physicians involved in the patient's care. Interactive collegial communication between clinicians along with respectful feedback will facilitate the optimal care of patients individually and globally. Patients and families should take an active role in all aspects of care, especially during the time of handoff. They should receive clear information about care transfer and the new inpatient clinicians responsible for their care.

PUBLIC HEALTH AND PUBLIC POLICY

DISASTER PLANNING AND MASS CASUALTY INCIDENTS

Emergency preparedness (disaster planning) often falls within the bailiwick of Emergency Medicine. Most planning is in the context of contingency planning for mass care or mass casualty incidents, which may include epidemics, natural or humanmade disasters, terrorism, war, and weapons of mass destruction. (See Chapter 265, Hospital Disaster Emergency Preparedness). This planning often addresses both internal and external types of events and includes planning for preparedness, mitigation, response, and recovery. Emergency planners establish plans and protocols and set up effective communication with the medical facilities via the ED. Emergency physicians provide triage and medical support as patients arrive in the ED. Some situations require an emergency physician to go into the field to serve as an incident commander and coordinate triage, transportation decisions, resource utilization, and communication. In other situations, the emergency physician may serve in this role remotely while remaining in the hospital ED.

U.S. LAWS GOVERNING EMERGENCY DEPARTMENT CARE

The Emergency Medical Treatment and Active Labor Act (EMTALA, http://www.cms.hhs.gov/emtala), passed in 1986, is a federal law that dictates certain specific responsibilities of EDs and patient's rights (**Table 120-5**). It requires EDs to evaluate and treat any patient presenting to an ED, regardless of the patient's ability to pay for care. By EMTALA regulations, all patients must be offered

TABLE 120-5 Provisions of EMTALA, the Federal Emergency Medical Treatment and Labor Act

Any patient who "comes to the emergency department" requesting "examination or treatment for a medical condition" must be provided with "an appropriate medical screening examination" to determine if he is suffering from an "emergency medical condition." If so, then the hospital is obligated either to provide him with treatment until he is stable or to transfer him to another hospital in conformance with the statute's directives.

- Imposes no further obligation on the hospital if the patient does not have an "emergency medical condition".
- Requires admission and treatment of pregnant patients who present in active labor until delivery is completed, unless a transfer under the statute is appropriate. The statute explicitly provides that this must include delivery of the placenta.
- Imposes an affirmative obligation on the part of the hospital to provide a medical screening examination to determine whether an "emergency medical condition" exists
- Imposes restrictions on transfers of persons who exhibit an "emergency medical condition" or are in active labor, which restrictions may or may not be limited to transfers made for economic reasons
- Imposes an affirmative duty to institute treatment if an "emergency medical condition" does exist. The person who does the examination must be specifically determined to be a "qualified medical person" by the hospital bylaws.
- Requires that the hospital post a conspicuous sign that notifies patients and visitors of the right to be examined and to receive treatment.
- Defines a "dedicated emergency department" as a state-licensed emergency room or a place where medical services are provided on an urgent basis, without the need for an appointment, including (significantly) hospital-based ambulatory care centers
- Permits an abbreviated assessment by a qualified medical person for patients not presenting for examination or treatment, whose presentation is not likely to involve an emergency medical condition
- Requires evaluation of a person presenting for the dispensation of medications at a physician's direction in accordance with EMTALA obligations, because the person may have a medical condition that needs evaluation. A person being brought in by law enforcement personnel for blood alcohol testing may or may not trigger the obligation, depending on the circumstances.

a physician screening examination, and any identified emergent condition must be stabilized. The purpose of this federal mandate is to prevent hospitals from refusing care to ill patients, or transferring them ("dumping") to other hospitals based on a patient's inability to pay for care. This law operates under the presumption that in time of acute illness, injury, or active labor, all patients deserve potentially life-saving health care regardless of their ability to pay. The specific tenets of EMTALA are beyond the scope of this text, and it behooves every physician actively engaged in acute inpatient care or those who transfer or accept transfers to have a detailed understanding of their obligation under EMTALA legislation.

PUBLIC HEALTH/ADVOCACY

EDs are the safety net for health care, and as such, public health issues are magnified and advocacy goes hand in hand with clinical practice. On the front line, emergency physicians see the consequences of the uninsured and underinsured public, the lack of access to primary care, on-call specialist shortages, and ED crowding and surges on capacity. By becoming involved through local and national organizations and contacting policy makers, emergency physicians help create legislative policy to address the public's health care needs.

Additionally, emergency physicians see firsthand the effects of preventable health threats in a very personal way. The effects of poor and ineffective gun control laws, seat belt use, smoking cessation programs, community cardiopulmonary resuscitation (CPR) education, driving under the influence (DUI) laws, motorcycle helmet use, and the like, are apparent every day in the ED. The stories of the individual patients and families whose lives have been shattered by poor public policies are far more compelling for lawmakers than impersonal statistics they read in a report. The emergency physician has an obligation to those patients to assure that their voices are heard, and to impact change to protect patients from future preventable illnesses and injuries.

PUBLIC POLICY AND EMERGENCY MEDICINE PRACTICE

EMTALA clearly changed the role and mission of the ED. In 2007, the Institute of Medicine published a study of emergency care in America detailing the challenges of a high demand and inadequate system capacity, and offering recommendations to improve ED efficiency, organization, care access, and care delivery (**Table 120-6**). The report notes that from 1993 to 2003 the U.S. population grew by 12%, hospital admissions increased by 13%, and annual ED visits rose from 90.3 to 113.9 million patients. During that time period there was a net loss of 425 EDs, creating the challenges common to all EDs today. The report describes the aggregate result of this imbalance between public demand and hospital capacity as an epidemic of overcrowded EDs, patients frequently waiting in the halls of the ED for an inpatient bed ("boarding"), and ambulance diversion. Another study demonstrated an increase of 16% in the average length of stay in the ED between 2001 and 2005 for all patients, with a 37% increase (79 minutes) in the average wait in the ED for critically ill patients. Since the release of the report with the subsequent downturn of the U.S. economy starting in 2008, the issues have become even more pervasive and acute. A 2009 report by the Government Accountability Office (GAO), Congress's investigative arm, found that emergency patients who should have been seen immediately waited nearly half an hour. Subsequent studies have demonstrated that ED crowding leads to adverse patient outcomes and contributes to racial disparities in care. Health care reform in the future will likely affect health care coverage and ED crowding. Likely, more patients will have insurance coverage in the future, and insured patients utilize EDs more frequently than the uninsured.

TABLE 120-6 Recommendations from the 2007 IOM Report, *Hospital-Based Emergency Care at the Breaking Point*

Enhanced operational efficiencies
Incentives to reduce crowding and boarding
Leadership in improving hospital efficiency
Use of informational technology
Funding of uncompensated emergency care
Address inadequate disaster response
Surge capacity
Training
Protection of hospitals and staff
Approaches to improve disaster preparedness
The emergency care workforce
Regionalize critical specialty on-call services
Mitigate the adverse impact of *the exposure of emergency* Providers to medical malpractice claims
Link rural hospitals to academic medical centers
Optimize the organization and funding for emergency care
Research

TABLE 120-7 Web References

www.acep.org for clinical policy statements including the Model of Clinical Practice, and advocacy papers
www.saem.org for residency and fellowship catalogs, and research, academic, and advocacy papers
www.acgme.org for Residency Review Committee for Emergency Medicine (RRC EM) program requirements
www.abem.org for Emergency Medicine board certification requirements
www.emtala.com for current information about the Federal Emergency Medical Treatment and Labor Act

CONCLUSION

Hospital Medicine physicians and Emergency Medicine physicians collaborate in the care of the many admitted patients who enter the hospital through the ED. As ED visits and overcrowding increase, the proportion is likely to grow. Collaborative efforts and policies among the two groups have begun to create seamless and safe transitions of patient care between multiple hospital environments, but more work still needs to be done to optimize care during that vulnerable transition period. Additionally, sharing the constraints of the hospital walls allows these two specialties to collaborate to support and augment new models of patient-centered care. Hospital Medicine and Emergency Medicine should continue to foster these natural alliances to promote best practices, patient safety, and efficiency as patients transition from the ED to other settings (**Table 120-7**).

SUGGESTED READINGS

Cyuldka R, Korte R. Career satisfaction in Emergency Medicine: The ABEM longitudinal study of emergency physicians. *Ann Emerg Med.* 2008;51:714–722.

Ginde AA, Sullivan AF, Camargo CA. National study of the Emergency Physician Workforce, 2008. *Ann Emerg Med.* 2009;54:349–359.

Goldberg R, Boss RW, Chan L, et al. Burnout and its correlates in emergency physicians: four years' experience with a wellness booth. *Acad Emerg Med.* 1996;3:1156–1164.

Herring A, Wilper A, Himmelstein DU, et al. Increasing length of stay among adult visits to U.S. emergency departments. *Acad Emerg Med.* 2001–2005;16:609–616.

Horwitz LI, Meredith T, Schuur JD, et al. Dropping the baton: a qualitative analysis of failures during the transition from emergency department to inpatient care. *Ann Emerg Med.* 2009;53(6): 701–710e1.

Institute of Medicine. *Hospital-Based Emergency Care at the Breaking Point.* Washington DC: *National Academies Press*; 2007.

Kulstad EB, Kelley KM. Overcrowding is associated with delays in percutaneous coronary intervention for acute myocardial infarction. *Int J Emerg Med.* 2009;2:149–154.

Pines JM, Localio AR, Hollander JE. Racial disparities in emergency department length of stay for admitted patients in the United States. *Acad Emerg Med.* 2009;16:403–410.

Pines JM, Pollack CV, Diercks DB, et al. The association between emergency department crowding and adverse cardiovascular outcomes in patients with chest pain. *Acad Emerg Med.* 2009;16: 617–625.

U.S. Government Accountability Office. *Hospital Emergency Departments: Crowding Continues to Occur, and Some Patients Wait Longer than Recommended Time Frames.* GAO-09–347;2009.

CHAPTER 121

Inpatient Cardiac Arrest and Cardiopulmonary Resuscitation

John E. Moss, MD
Jason Persoff, MD, FHM

Key Clinical Questions

1. What are the fundamental goals of cardiopulmonary resuscitation?
2. Which components of resuscitation are considered vital to success?
3. How can the common pitfalls of resuscitation be surmounted?
4. What treatments should be instituted immediately upon successful resuscitation?
5. How should outcomes in resuscitation shape the discussion of advanced directives?

INTRODUCTION

This chapter focuses on cardiopulmonary arrest and the events immediately antecedent to this life-threatening event. Cardiopulmonary resuscitation is a *time-dependent, team-based effort* to reverse physiologic events that may culminate in a patient's imminent death. Biblical and ancient Egyptian hieroglyphic texts allude to mouth-to-mouth ventilation in divine contexts, but other texts indicate Jewish midwives used mouth-to-mouth resuscitation as early as 3300 years ago to revive stillborn children.

Since standardization of closed chest cardiac massage was first described systematically in the medical literature in 1960, *chest compressions have remained the only reliable means of reviving a patient in cardiopulmonary collapse.*

In the United States an estimated 375,000 to 750,000 hospitalized patients suffer in-hospital cardiac arrest (IHCA) requiring advanced cardiac life support (ACLS) annually. The incidence of IHCA is estimated to be as high as 1–2% of all patients admitted to academic hospitals with a prevalence of approximately 65 people per 100,000 nationally.

IHCA encompasses a spectrum of disorders, from insufficient cardiac output to generate appreciable cerebral perfusion, including arrhythmia or shock, to complete cessation of cardiac activity. Vital sign anomalies can often herald impending inpatient cardiac arrest by minutes to hours, but many cardiac arrests occur suddenly and without warning. Acute pulmonary arrest may precede IHCA and can occur iatrogenically related to sedative or opiate analgesics overdose.

TRIAGE

Since standardization of closed chest cardiac massage (CCCM) was first described systematically in the medical literature in 1960, *CCCM has remained the only reliable means of reviving a patient in cardiopulmonary collapse.* It is an effective and powerful intervention that, when unnecessarily delayed, can lead to poor patient outcomes. In one study, survival dropped from 34% to 14% if CCCM was delayed even as little as 60–120 seconds from the time the patient collapsed. Therefore, clinicians must recognize and respond to cardiac arrest immediately for resuscitation measures to be effective.

Advanced cardiac life support (ACLS) combines basic life support (BLS) measures with specific interventions such as medication, defibrillation, transthoracic pacing, and advanced airway management. This chapter focuses on (1) the techniques that are essential to successful cardiopulmonary resuscitation, neurologic recovery (as defined by the cerebral performance category 0–1), and (2) decision making based on patient resuscitation status.

While often considered adequate for credentialing purposes, completion of American Heart Association courses fails to result in long-term meaningful skill performance. Health care providers' capabilities to demonstrate appropriate technique for CCCM and capabilities to successfully navigate the steps of cardiopulmonary resuscitation begin to degrade just weeks following course completion. Therefore, for the whole medical team to respond concisely and in a coordinated fashion, clinicians must have extensive medical knowledge, training, drilling practice, continued education, and feedback.

Many providers are reluctant to initiate CCCM without complete assurance that the patient is truly in cardiopulmonary arrest (confirmed by vital signs or electrocardiographic rhythm), often leading to unnecessary delays in initiation of potentially life-saving treatment. Furthermore, fundamental pulse assessment, even in nonemergency situations, is not consistently accurately evaluated by clinicians. One study tasked providers to determine whether or not patients had palpable pulses during elective cardiopulmonary bypass surgery. Ultimately providers took around 20 seconds to assess the pulse and were less than 70% accurate.

Time spent gathering cardiac monitoring, attaching leads, and setting up equipment can further delay promptly needed interventions to prevent death. In fact, clinicians may need to initiate CCCM prior to confirming cardiopulmonary arrest. Prompt initiation of CCCM for any patient who appears to be in extremis (ie, unarousable, or clinically unstable with suspicion of cardiopulmonary arrest) should occur until confirmatory evaluation, often by a multispecialty resuscitation team, offers a high degree of confidence that CCCM can be discontinued. Providers should share a culture of support that accentuates that the greater harm to patients is in failing to initiate CCCM in contrast to the potential harms of CCCM (rib fracture, pneumothorax, organ perforation, etc).

PRACTICE POINT

- Providers should initiate closed chest cardiac massage (CCCM) to any patient who appears in extremis without awaiting 100% confirmation that the patient is in cardiopulmonary arrest. Even delaying CCCM by as little as 30 seconds confers worse survival outcomes for patients in cardiopulmonary arrest.

PATHOPHYSIOLOGY

Cardiopulmonary arrest heralds death and may be an expected outcome in many hospitalized patients. However, rarely is cardiopulmonary arrest the first manifestation of physiologic events that ultimately culminate in collapse: patients frequently have alteration in mental status or significant vital sign changes (pyrexia, hypotension, bradycardia, decrease in oxygen saturation, change in respiratory rate, etc), often hours before developing cardiac arrest. Intervention during this pre-arrest period may prevent cardiac arrest altogether. Alternatively, health care personnel may identify patients who are at the end of life and may thus benefit from a meaningful discussion about limiting resuscitative measures, including offering "Do Not Resuscitate" or "Allow Natural Death" orders. Many patients are not well informed about the resuscitative process and may have inflated images of routine successful resuscitation shaped from popular culture embodied by television and film. Clinicians often perform cardiopulmonary resuscitation on patients without informed consent—a discussion of the relevant risks, benefits, and alternatives to therapy along with the clinicians' recommendations. Thus the pre-arrest period may offer an unparalleled opportunity to give patients an active role in deciding whether resuscitation is desired.

While no one specific condition results in cardiopulmonary collapse, many health care–associated interventions predispose patients to arrest and often require minimal intervention early on to alter the course of catastrophe (**Table 121-1**). Intervention during impending cardiac arrest requires a detailed history of recent interventions ranging from invasive procedures to recent sedation or anesthesia.

Responses to inpatient emergencies require multiple individuals who take on individual roles and integrate as a team. For care to function effectively and seamlessly during health care emergencies, each clinician must assume a narrowly focused essential function or task (such as assessing a patient's airway, recording data in a flowsheet, or ensuring chest compressions are adequate) and perform the task with high quality to facilitate the best possible patient outcome engendered by the team as a whole.

TABLE 121-1 Interventions to Specific Conditions that may Prevent Evolution to Cardiopulmonary Arrest in Hospitalized Patients

Cause	Intervention
Hypoxia due to medication or anesthesia	Supportive oxygen, reversal agents (naloxone for opiates, flumazenil for benzodiazepines)
Acidemia due to hypercapnic respiratory failure from medication or obstructive sleep apnea	Ventilation support (noninvasive or mechanical ventilation)
Pulmonary embolism	Appropriate VTE prophylaxis (pharmacologic unless significant contraindication); high index of suspicion and timely treatment
Cardiac arrhythmia due to acute coronary syndrome	Appropriate early intervention including antiplatelet therapy, beta-blockers, anticoagulation and early percutaneous coronary intervention (PCI)
Hyperkalemia	Calcium, sodium bicarbonate, insulin with dextrose, consideration of early hemodialysis; check for acid–base derangements
Hypokalemia	Correction of magnesium (first) followed by potassium; check for acid–base derangements
QT prolongation	Attention to medications known to prolong the QT interval (such as fluoroquinolones) and consideration of cardiac monitoring
Hypotension from severe sepsis	Early massive volume resuscitation with consideration of inotropes
Anticipated end-of-life care	Discussion of appropriate "Do Not Resuscitate" or "Allow Natural Death" orders and palliative care in appropriate patients

RAPID RESPONSE TEAMS AND THE PRE-ARREST PERIOD

Recognizing that early intervention in impending cardiopulmonary arrest may prevent the arrest altogether, many hospitals have implemented rapid response teams (RRTs), consisting of any combination of critical care nurses, respiratory therapists, pharmacists, and/or physicians to attend to patients who have some parameters of clinical instability but are not yet in extremis. While data remain mixed about the success of RRTs to stave off cardiopulmonary arrest, most data suggest RRTs facilitate earlier discussion of patient advanced directives and improve communication with critical care teams and intensivists, potentially reducing mortality and need for crisis activation of cardiopulmonary arrest teams (ie, code teams). Speculation exists that RRTs have not yet realize their full outcome potential because some staff still hesitate to call an RRT when indications to do so are present.

PRACTICE POINT

- Rapid response teams facilitate earlier discussion of patient advanced directives and improve communication between critical care team members, potentially reducing mortality and the need for crisis activation of cardiopulmonary arrest teams.

Computerized medical records with "involuntary" initiation of an RRT due to deviations in certain predefined criteria (heart rate or blood pressure instability, depression of mental status, or decrease in oxygen saturation) may allow RRTs to fulfill their full potential and may reduce code team activation and improve patient outcomes. In the interim, hospitalists must foster a culture of safety where any provider can initiate an RRT for any reason without fear of reprisal or judgment. Hospitalists should always thank other clinicians for calling RRTs and keeping the patients' safety of the utmost concern.

RESPIRATORY ARREST

Respiratory arrest from medications (anesthesia, benzodiazepines, or opiates) can lead to cardiac arrest through hypoxia and changes in the pH due to combined metabolic and respiratory acidosis. Respiratory arrest is often masked for some time due to the ubiquity of oxygen administration in hospitalized patients, which can lead to a prolonged period of hemoglobin oxygenation while ventilation may have already stopped. *Overreliance on pulse oximetry as a sole source of interpreting ventilation effort may delay response to respiratory arrest until the patient is hypoxic and profoundly acidemic.* Systemic hypoxia causes pulmonary artery constriction, right ventricular failure, and systemic hypotension from poor right heart output coupled with loss of vascular tone from hypoxia (circulatory shock).

GASPING

Gasping is a powerful agonal respiration that improves patient survival through increased cardiac output, improved oxygenation, improved ventilation, and improved cerebral blood flow. Positive pressure bag-valve-mask (BVM) ventilations may confer a negative effect on the ability of patients to gasp suggesting a role for delaying aggressive airway management until later on in a cardiac resuscitation. Conversely, in pure respiratory arrest, early aggressive airway management to prevent deterioration into cardiac arrest may be warranted.

PRACTICE POINT

- Gasping is a powerful agonal respiration that augments cerebral blood flow and serves as a surrogate marker of relatively good prognosis.

CARDIAC ARREST

Cardiac arrest can occur from multiple distinct mechanisms. True cardiac arrest (cardiac standstill) occurs either as a primary mechanism (from arrhythmias like ventricular fibrillation that prevent normal cardiac function) or as a secondary mechanism (from asystole or from an extended period of failed resuscitation and cardiac myocyte death). Most cardiopulmonary arrest episodes do not occur due to true cardiac standstill but rather from marked impairment in cardiac output resulting in systemic arterial hypotension, tissue hypoxia, and organ failure. Precardiac, intracardiac, or postcardiac mechanisms may independently or in combination result in cardiopulmonary arrest (**Table 121-2**).

TABLE 121-2 Cardiac Arrest Etiology by Anatomic Location

Precardiac	Intracardiac/ intrapulmonary	Postcardiac
• Hypovolemia • Shock (septic, distributive) • Pericardial Tamponade • Pneumothorax • Hypoxia	• Pulmonary embolism • Myocardial infarction • Shock (cardiac) • Cardiac arrhythmia (ventricular or atrial) • Left ventricular rupture • Hypertrophic cardiomyopathy	• Aortic dissection • Hemorrhage • Postcardiac

SUBTYPES OF CARDIAC ARREST

Once appropriate resuscitation equipment has arrived, clinicians can begin to differentiate whether the cardiac arrest is due to a "shockable" or "nonshockable" cardiac rhythm.

Shockable rhythms

Transthoracic electrical shocks can terminate some pathological cardiac rhythms that inhibit normal cardiac function. These can include *ventricular fibrillation, ventricular tachycardia, AV nodal reentrant tachycardia, atrial fibrillation, and atrial flutter.* While ventricular fibrillation has a very characteristic pattern, the other rhythms may be difficult to differentiate during an emergency and in the absence of 12-lead electrocardiography. In the setting of an unconscious patient in extremis, all of these rhythms are considered pathologic and warrant immediate electrical shock.

Despite recommendations by the International Liaison Committee of Resuscitation (ILCOR) (the subsection of the American Heart Association responsible for publication of the ACLS guidelines) that differentiation of the exact cardiac arrhythmia may dictate very different types of cardiac intervention, ranging from dose (in joules) of electrical therapy to medication selection, confirming an exact rhythm diagnosis may not be practical. Thus it is reasonable to treat all of these rhythms similarly in a cardiopulmonary arrest in the event of clinical uncertainty. Fundamentally similar to administration of CCCM, delays in electrical therapy can significantly negatively impact patient outcomes with even minimal delays. If a patient is not critically ill, then time allows for conscientious assessment of cardiac rhythm via 12-lead electrocardiogram (ECG) with appropriately targeted therapies for the underlying arrhythmia (see Chapters 126 and 128 on supraventricular tachyarrhythmias and ventricular arrythmias).

PRACTICE POINT

- Precise differentiation between *ventricular fibrillation, ventricular tachycardia, AV nodal reentrant tachycardia, atrial fibrillation, and atrial flutter* may not be practical when a patient is in extremis. Thus it is reasonable to treat all of these rhythms similarly in a cardiopulmonary arrest in the event of clinical uncertainty.

Ventricular fibrillation results from disorganized myocardial electrical activity, and the heart is unable to generate a contraction to produce cardiac output. Hospitalists should be able to identify ventricular fibrillation confidently on rhythm strip (**Figure 121-1**).

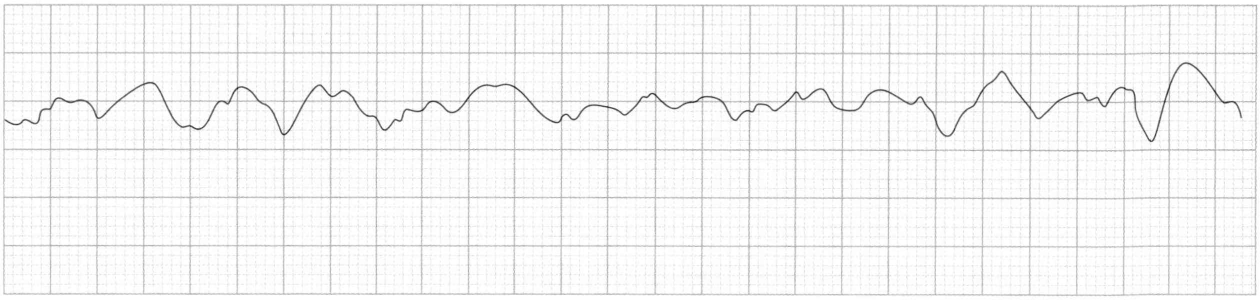

Figure 121-1 *Rhythm strip of a patient with ventricular fibrillation.*

The characteristic physiologic phases of ventricular fibrillation arrest underscore the importance of rapid electrical therapy. During the first few minutes of ventricular fibrillation (reflecting the combination of the "acute" and "electrical" phases of arrest, lasting up to 5–6 minutes), the myocardium is highly responsive to counter shock. This explains in part why successful defibrillation is so common on commercial airlines and in casinos where employees are trained to rapidly attach and initiate automated external defibrillators (AEDs). The acute and electrical phases can be extended when CCCM is initiated promptly, thus underscoring how critical CCCM is as an immediate therapy while definitive defibrillation equipment is located, attached, and initiated.

In the absence of CCCM, patients will degenerate into the "circulatory" phase where electrical therapies are less effective due to progressive tissue hypoxia and myocyte death. During this phase, CCCM must be performed for several minutes antecedent to attempts at defibrillation.

Unchecked, patients will eventually enter the "metabolic" phase of ventricular fibrillation starting around the tenth minute of cardiac arrest. While there remains a slim hope of successful cardiac resuscitation at this point, in the absence of effective CCCM irreversible brain damage occurs and survival to hospital discharge rapidly becomes improbable.

Ventricular tachycardia resulting in cardiopulmonary arrest fundamentally is identical to ventricular fibrillation in treatment: CCCM and early electrical shock are indicated.

Perhaps the most overwhelming change to resuscitation in recent years is the acknowledgment of severe ventricular stunning following electrical shock. For several minutes following defibrillation—and extending for a variable duration thereafter—the heart is mechanically dysfunctional and unable to generate an adequate cardiac output for organ perfusion or brain function. Consequently, it is absolutely critical to reinitiate CCCM for 1–2 minutes after defibrillation whether or not the shock is successful at aborting the ventricular arrhythmia.

PRACTICE POINT

- Even when defibrillation is successful, patients require at least 1–2 minutes of CCCM immediately following the shock due to stunning of the left ventricle. Resumption of a sinus rhythm does *not* equate to resumption of normal mechanical heart function.

Nonshockable rhythms

Nonshockable rhythms (characterized by bradycardia, asystole, and pulseless electrical activity) constitute the majority of inpatient cardiac arrests. Deterioration in clinical status signified by deviations in mental status or marked changes in vital signs often foreshadows these types of cardiopulmonary arrests, and they may be preventable.

Bradycardia may be due to a primary arrhythmia (such as sick sinus syndrome or arterioventricular block), or may be due to a secondary cause such as medications (particular arterioventricular [AV] nodal blocking agents) or excessive vagal tone (due pain or nausea). Bradycardia severe enough to cause hemodynamic instability warrants immediate correction and treatment of the underlying cause. Atropine is a vagolytic that can potently reverse excessive vagally mediated bradycardia. However, with unpredictable effects and a narrow therapeutic window (too high or too low a dose of atropine can potentially paradoxically worsen bradycardia), its use is confined to select patients and only for short-term use. Chronotropic agents such as dopamine can be administered if time allows setup of an intravenous drip.

Bradycardia and asystole may respond to transcutaneous pacing, but this must be instituted very early on to be successful. In conscious bradycardic patients transcutaneous pacing can prove to be exceptionally uncomfortable but should be used to bridge to transvenous pacing. Patients may require analgesia or sedation during transcutaneous pacing while awake.

Asystole as a primary cause of cardiac arrest is uncommon. Asystole typically is the end result of another pathophysiologic process, such as sustained hypoxia or coronary thrombosis. As such, asystole is a fairly late finding. Fine ventricular fibrillation looks electrocardiographically similar to asystole, but, whereas defibrillation is likely to benefit a patient in ventricular fibrillation (and is necessary to terminate the rhythm), shocking a patient in asystole may result in depleting the heart of any remaining adenosine triphosphate (ATP) and with it any chance of successful resuscitation. In general, if clinicians aren't certain whether asystole or ventricular fibrillation is the underlying rhythm, defibrillation is favored due to the overwhelming benefit patients with ventricular fibrillation receive from defibrillation compared to the minimal excess risk posed to those already in asystole.

Pulseless electrical activity (PEA) represents a complex spectrum of disorders where patients appear to have an electrocardiographic rhythm that would be anticipated sufficient to generate a cardiac output, but clinical examination reveals no evidence of a palpable pulse. *By definition, PEA is not a rhythm derangement, and therefore will not respond to any form of electrical shock.* PEA is a problem with either too little cardiac preload (vasodilation, pulmonary embolism, or profound volume depletion), ineffective cardiac output (due to cardiac failure or stunning), or extrinsic compression of the heart muscle (tension pneumothorax, severe airway obstruction, or pericardial tamponade). While seeking a cause, clinicians must pursue concomitant treatment with CCCM in spite of the apparently normal-appearing cardiac rhythm. Clinicians should use epinephrine and intravenous fluids along with the goal to furnish targeted treatment of the apparent cause of PEA (fibrinolytics for pulmonary embolism or myocardial infarction, intubation for hypoxia or respiratory distress, chest tube insertion for tension pneumothorax, pericardiocentesis for tamponade, etc).

MANAGEMENT

While the approach to cardiac arrest has changed considerably over the past 5 decades, survival has not improved at all the since initial reports on CCCM in 1960. ILCOR has published basic and advanced cardiac life support guidelines every 5 years, becoming the de facto standard-of-care in the United States and internationally. Despite their evidence base, criticism exists that many find the guidelines to be too complex and difficult to remember weeks to years following completing a course in life support. Also discordantly, the single most effective stratagem in resuscitation—effective chest compressions—frequently is not taught well or performed well during or following courses, with a time-dependent loss of skill following course completion.

While many providers learned that resuscitation begins with the "ABCs," increasing evidence suggests that establishing an airway and initiating rescue breathing (accomplished in most hospitals via BVM ventilations) are not nearly as important as CCCM during the early phases of most adult inpatient cardiac arrests (**Figure 121-2**). Certainly, in primary respiratory arrest (such as from medications) and in children (in whom respiratory arrest is much more common than cardiac arrest), management of airway and respiration must occur rapidly (see Figure 121-2).

CHEST COMPRESSIONS (CLOSED CHEST CARDIAC MASSAGE)

When a patient appears to be unconscious and is unarousable, clinicians should assume that the patient might be in cardiopulmonary arrest and should institute chest compressions without delay. The mantra for quality chest compressions is push hard, pump fast, and allow good chest recoil.

PRACTICE POINT

- Good chest compression technique requires pushing hard, pumping fast, and allowing adequate chest recoil.

Push hard

Many providers are concerned with pushing down on the sternum too hard; however, this occurs rarely, and evidence does not support the assertion that pushing too hard occurs. Current recommendations suggest a compression depth of about 1.5–2 inches, but that measurement is very difficult to extrapolate in clinical terms during a resuscitation. The best advice is for rescuers to push as deeply as possible with arms locked and with the rescuer's shoulders directly over the patient's sternum with the rescuer using his or her body weight and waist flexion to deliver the compression.

Because most patients go into cardiopulmonary arrest in hospital beds, achieving proper positioning can be difficult, particularly when a patient is obese or the rescuer's arm length is short; a stool or other lift may prove critical for proper hand positioning. Compressing the chest solely with the force of the rescuer's arms may be highly kinetic in appearance but will offer virtually no benefit to the patient.

Compressions must be done on a hard surface, something a hospital mattress does not offer. As soon as possible, a backboard should be inserted behind the patient. Real-time feedback devices, such as accelerometers, may offer the best opportunity for ensuring adequate compression depth; however, these devices have technological limitations. Frequently the devices interpret total patient motion as compression depth when in fact a substantial amount of the compression is expended compressing the mattress and not the patient's chest. Compression depth indirectly correlates with patient survival.

Pump fast

Since ideal chest compressions result in only one-third normal cardiac output, about 10% of normal cerebral blood flow, and < 5% of normal cardiac blood flow, compression rate has a substantial effect on tissue perfusion. Target compression rate of 100 compressions per minute should be instituted, but interruptions in chest compressions during change of rescuers, intubation, or rhythm analysis all result in a markedly lower total number of compressions over time. Studies consistently show that compressions are almost uniformly lower than 100 per minute, underscoring the need for practice, simulation, and feedback for all rescuers on a regular basis following completion of chest compression training.

Good compressions require a high degree of physical ability, but frequent rescuer rotation must be balanced with the need for uninterrupted compressions. While automated solutions (such as mechanical compression devices) will certainly eventually replace most rescuer-performed compressions in inpatients, current devices are unwieldy or have failed to show noninferiority to manual chest compressions.

Some aspects of resuscitation are incompatible with ongoing chest compressions (such as rhythm analysis and intubation). In these situations, rescuers must limit the duration of the interruption as return of spontaneous circulation and neurologically intact survival are directly tied to chest compression rate. Furthermore, current evidence suggests it is essential to resume chest compressions immediately following a defibrillation attempt independent of the rhythm due to left ventricular stunning with resultant highly impaired cardiac output.

Lastly, the beneficial effects of chest compressions are lost within seconds of discontinuation. Chest compressions' benefits appear to be additive to one another over time with subsequent compressions improving circulation and perfusion pressures; if compressions are widely spaced or stopped for any length of time, the benefits of the previous compressions' vascular effects are lost. Defibrillation success also depends on short "hands off" intervals (time when no compressions occur) as the chances of successful defibrillation diminish within seconds. This latter finding suggests that there is very little latitude for prolonged rhythm analysis during a cardiac arrest.

Good chest recoil

At the completion of a chest compression, rescuers must extend at the waist allowing the patient's chest to rise back to its rest position. The mechanisms by which compressions exert their physiologic effect appear to be a combination of increased intrathoracic pressure leading to compression of the great vessels and direct pumping of the heart through reduction of the anterior-posterior diameter of the chest. The recoil phase is effectively "diastole," and incomplete recoil of the chest thus results in impaired blood return to the great vessels and heart resulting in further impairment in circulation in an already desperate perfusion environment. If recoil is consistently poor, rescuers will be incapable of surmounting this critical phase of circulation with adequate or consistent depth of compressions.

ELECTRICAL THERAPY

Defibrillation is used to depolarize all myocytes simultaneously in order to achieve a uniform repolarization period whereby the sinoatrial node theoretically resumes the pacemaking role of the heart, thus restoring normal cardiac function. The standard dose for defibrillation is 360 joules for monophasic defibrillators and 150 joules for biphasic defibrillators.

Caregivers will be unlikely to divine the workings of a defibrillator in a crisis without copious practice beforehand. Automated external defibrillators are ubiquitous even in nonhospital settings, but even their setup can prove to be puzzling during a crisis if providers have not practiced using them.

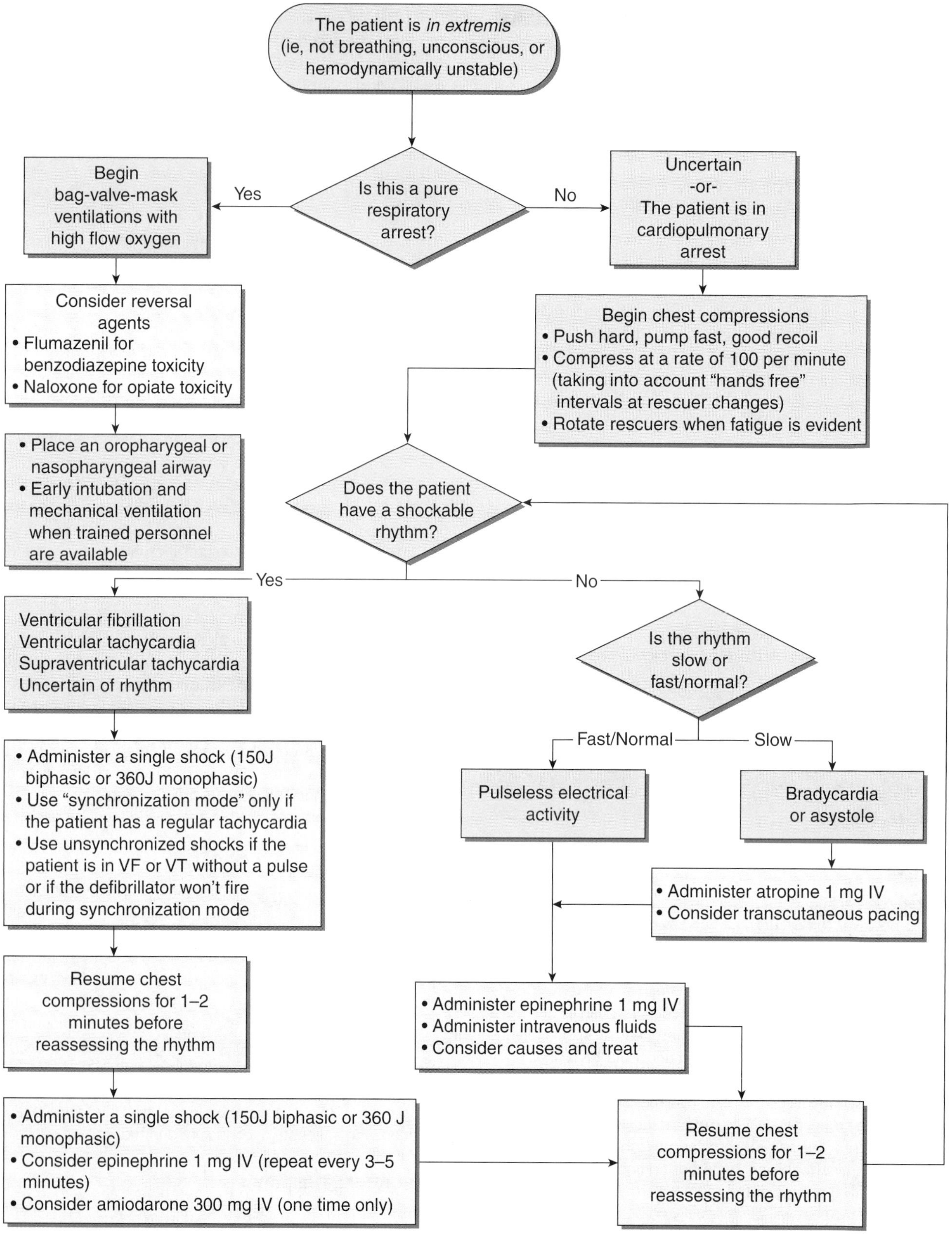

Figure 121-2 *Flow diagram of assessment and treatment of during cardiac or pulmonary arrest.*

Most manual defibrillators have paddles that are applied to the sternum and the left midaxillary line (about the location of the cardiac apex) to deliver shocks. The paddles can concomitantly offer a "quick look" mode, displaying the patient's cardiac rhythm independent of cardiac leads. This means rescuers can simultaneously identify a patient's cardiac rhythm while charging the paddles, and then deliver a shock without ever lifting the paddles up off the chest.

Automated external defibrillators utilize self-adhesive pads in place of paddles but require a period of up to 20 seconds for computer rhythm analysis, during which time rescuers are not performing CCCM. Manual defibrillators can also use these self-adhesive pads, but they often require a change in cables that can take time. After an initial defibrillation, all patients should have self-adhesive defibrillator pads attached as these offer continuous monitoring and allow rescuers to deliver shocks or to pace the patient. Newer models also offer real-time feedback to compression depth, recoil quality, and compression rate.

All shocks need to overcome the inherently high resistance of the chest wall (skin, muscle, bone, and pericardium), which is accomplished through pressure (using paddles), area (using the pads), and transducing gel (applied to the paddles, applied to the patient, or already adherent to the pads).

Most defibrillators in clinical use employ either a monophasic waveform, in which polarity during the shock travels from one paddle unidirectionally to the other paddle, or a biphasic waveform, in which polarity reverses during the shock. Biphasic devices are becoming more common and appear to confer better neurological outcomes. Defibrillators can deliver shocks that are synchronized to patients' cardiac rhythms to prevent administration of a shock during the critical repolarization phase represented by the T-wave (resulting in the "R on T" phenomenon and concomitant risk for precipitation refractory arrhythmias). Since ventricular fibrillation is a disorganized cardiac rhythm where no discrete T-waves exist, defibrillators set to "synchronization mode" may not delineate a safe period to deliver a shock and therefore may not fire at all. Most defibrillators will not have synchronization enabled when turned on without a clinician specifically enabling it. Nevertheless, clinicians must have good familiarity with the location of the synchronization button along with all functions on their hospitals' defibrillators so that when a defibrillator fails to fire, clinicians know where and how to deactivate synchronization prior to another attempt at defibrillation.

Increasing data suggest that the risk of shock to caregivers during a defibrillation is considerably lower than previously posited, even when a rescuer comes into contact with the patient. With escalating evidence supporting the importance of uninterrupted chest compressions, including the resumption of compressions immediately postshock, possible future directions in resuscitation are likely to include shocking the patient while CCCM is in progress.

Rescuers should attempt to defibrillate a patient as soon as the code cart arrives and the defibrillator is fully set up and ready to deliver a shock. Compressions should continue unabated until the defibrillator is fully prepared, otherwise unnecessary hands-off intervals will result in poorer patient outcomes. Early defibrillation is critical as soon as a shockable rhythm is diagnosed or suspected clinically since the window for successful defibrillation decreases as patients progress from the electrical phase of ventricular fibrillation into the circulatory and metabolic phases. Chest compressions extend this window for a limited period of time, maintaining patients' responses to defibrillation.

RESPIRATORY THERAPY

Positive pressure ventilation via BVM provides oxygenation and ventilation. *Ideally, the technique for using a BVM involves three hands: two to properly seal the mask over the patient's mouth and nose while tilting the head back to move the tongue away from the back of the throat, and one hand (from a second rescuer) to squeeze the bag.* The design of the BVM is such that a one-handed squeeze provides the appropriate tidal volume for most adults in cardiopulmonary collapse: roughly 750 mL. Often, however, rescuers will use two hands to squeeze the bag, resulting in larger tidal volumes that may exceed 1000 mL. Data suggest that rescuers often deliver BVM ventilations at rates well beyond the recommended 1 ventilation every 5 seconds, with at least one report where ventilation rate exceeded the chest compression rate.

PRACTICE POINT

- The ideal technique for bag-valve-mask (BVM) use involves three hands: two to properly seal the mask over the patient's mouth and nose while tilting the head back, and one hand (from a second rescuer) to squeeze the bag. The BVM is designed for a one-handed squeeze, which provides the appropriate tidal volume (750 mL) for most adults in cardiopulmonary collapse. Two-hand BVM squeeze results in larger tidal volumes that may exceed 1000 mL, potentially leading to hyperventilation and auto-positive end-expiratory pressure. Recommended BVM ventilations rate is one ventilation every 5 seconds.

Well-intentioned rescuers often believe that hyperventilation will result in improved oxygenation, improved carbon dioxide levels, and improved acid–base balance, but in fact hyperventilation sets off a cascade of pathophysiologic changes that culminate in very high intrathoracic pressures, decreased cerebral and coronary circulation, and decreased survival. Since tissue perfusion (and by convention intact circulation) is a prerequisite to oxygenation, hyperventilating a patient without attending to proper chest compressions fails to bolster tissue oxygen levels. While carbon dioxide levels rise rapidly in circulatory collapse, carbon dioxide can only be off-gassed via ventilation if venous blood flow is able to enter the thorax and thereby the lungs. Last, the single most effective treatment for the combined respiratory and metabolic acidosis uniform in cardiopulmonary arrest is resumption of physiologically normal circulation. Therefore, the proper route to achieve rescuers' intents is via high-quality chest compressions with supplemental oxygen administered via BVM ventilations (if rescuers are competent in its use) or via passive "blow-by" oxygen administered from a nonrebreather mask (if rescuers' skills are in doubt).

During cardiopulmonary arrest, the upper airway musculature can become lax, resulting in the tongue and jaw occluding the airway. Proper head positioning during ventilations will help decrease the risk of airway obstruction, but frequently other measures are required. Placement of either an oropharyngeal or nasopharyngeal airway requires little training and can help stabilize the upper airway sufficiently to provide effective BVM ventilations. Nevertheless, rescuers may need to obtain an invasive airway (via laryngeal mask, endotracheal tube, or tracheostomy) in order to properly ventilate the patient. Only medical personnel with considerable training and experience in advanced airways should attempt to place an invasive airway. Experience is necessary in part to limit the duration of time needed to achieve the airway (during which CCCM frequently is halted) and to minimize the risk of complications (laryngeal spasm, esophageal intubation, induction of vomiting, etc).

Almost all patients who suffer cardiopulmonary arrest will require an invasive airway to allow for ventilation in the postresuscitation period, but controversy exists as to the ideal timing to attempt airway stabilization. The airway is the key focus in patients in pure respiratory arrest, but increasingly it appears that CCCM and initial defibrillation attempts should supersede airway priority in patients in cardiac arrest. In fact, recently ILCOR removed ventilation as a component of layperson adult resuscitation to further emphasize the importance of chest compressions as the single most important intervention during cardiopulmonary collapse.

MEDICATIONS

Vasoactive medications have traditionally played a large role in treatment of cardiac arrest care. Two vasoactive medications, epinephrine and vasopressin, are guideline recommended for use during cardiac arrest. Epinephrine is a sympathomimetic agent with beta-1, beta-2, and alpha-1 agonist properties. Beta-1 stimulation increases heart rate (chronotropy) and also increases contractility (inotropy), allowing for increased cardiac output secondary to higher heart rate and stroke volume. Beta-2 stimulation causes arterial vasodilation, yet its effect is mostly countered by the alpha-1 stimulation, which causes arterial vasoconstriction. Epinephrine continues to be the primary adrenergic agent used during resuscitation care. The alpha-adrenergic stimulating properties of epinephrine have been found to increase coronary perfusion pressure, but its beta-adrenergic effects are potentially detrimental, having been found to increase postresuscitation myocardial dysfunction and possibly worsen reperfusion injury. High-dose epinephrine (1 mg followed by 3 mg and then 5 mg of epinephrine depending on response) is definitely injurious, resulting in higher rates of successful *cardiac* resuscitation but disproportionately *higher rates of poor neurologic outcomes.*

One milligram of epinephrine should be administered intravenously after the rescuers deliver the first defibrillation and then every 3–5 minutes thereafter. Interruption of chest compressions to place a central line is not acceptable, especially if the femoral vein is accessible. If no intravenous access is available, double-dose epinephrine may be administered down an endotracheal tube. Other medications that may be administered via endotracheal tube if indicated include naloxone, atropine, vasopressin, epinephrine, and lidocaine (NAVEL).

Forty units of intravenous vasopressin may be used instead of epinephrine initially as a one-time dose. Clinical studies on vasopressin generally fail to demonstrate significantly improved outcomes over epinephrine, however.

Atropine is an anticholinergic medication that increases heart rate via blockade of acetylcholine-mediated bradycardia. Data suggest that atropine use be confined to symptomatic bradycardia, PEA *with bradycardia*, and asystole as this medication has no role in other forms of cardiopulmonary arrest. Atropine has a narrow therapeutic window requiring at least 0.5 mg, and not exceeding 3 mg total dose, and may paradoxically worsen bradycardia at either extreme. The dose of atropine is 1 mg intravenously during cardiac arrest, and this may be repeated up to two times in 24 hours if needed.

The 2010 ACLS guidelines recommend use of antiarrhythmic therapy for patients suffering cardiac arrest due to ventricular fibrillation or pulseless ventricular tachycardia. Whereas lidocaine used to be the favored antiarrhythmic medication in cardiopulmonary arrest, amiodarone (300 mg delivered as an intravenous bolus) has proven to be superior to lidocaine based largely on out-of-hospital data showing improved rates of return of spontaneous circulation. No studies demonstrate that neurologic outcomes or survival to hospital discharge are better in patients receiving antiarrhythmic therapy, however.

Other medications, including sodium bicarbonate, calcium, and magnesium, have very specific roles in resuscitation, but their use is beyond the scope of this chapter. None of these medications is indicated routinely, and all have been associated with worse overall outcomes in nonselected patients in cardiopulmonary arrest.

■ RECOMMENDED APPROACH TO THE PATIENT IN CARDIOPULMONARY ARREST

The patient in apparent cardiopulmonary arrest requires prompt initiation of CCCM with very close attention to proper rate, depth, and recoil of compressions. Concomitantly the patient should be placed on a nonrebreather at > 15 liters per minute of oxygen until adequate personnel are available to initiate stabilization of the airway.

Electrical shock serves as the penultimate goal in patients suffering from a shockable arrhythmia and in those in whom certainty of the underlying rhythm is not possible. Rescuers should attempt an initial "quick look" using manual defibrillator paddles while charging the paddles (360 J with a monophasic defibrillator or 150 J with a biphasic defibrillator). If indicated, personnel should deliver the shock and then begin to connect the self-adhesive defibrillator pads to the patient for downstream intervention.

CCCM should continue with minimal interruption (5–15 seconds) for rhythm analysis and shock delivery. Following the shock, CCCM should resume immediately without further rhythm analysis until at least an additional 150 compressions are delivered over the next 60–90 seconds due to the possibility of postshock ventricular stunning. After the first shock is delivered, rescuers need to embark on securing intravenous access and managing the patient's airway and breathing.

Initial airway maneuvers should focus solely on oxygen delivery and alleviating any upper airway flow resistance with temporary placement of an oropharyngeal or nasopharyngeal airway. If personnel with adequate training, practice, and experience respond to the cardiopulmonary arrest, BVM ventilations can be initiated at a rate of 5 ventilations per minute. An invasive airway should not be placed until the patient has received adequate chest compressions and an initial shock.

Once the rhythm is reassessed, if the patient remains in a shockable rhythm, epinephrine 1 mg or vasopressin 40 IU should be administered intravenously followed by another 1–2 minutes of compressions to allow for adequate circulation of the medication. The rhythm is then reassessed and another shock (at higher dose if appropriate) delivered if the arrhythmia is still present once again with a focus on resumption of chest compressions as soon as the shock is completed.

Clinicians should administer amiodarone 300 mg as an intravenous bolus if the arrhythmia continues followed by an additional shock 1 minute later. By this point in the cardiopulmonary collapse, clinicians with specialty training in Hospital Medicine, intensive care medicine, or Emergency Medicine should determine the next steps, if any, at ongoing resuscitation attempts.

In the case of a nonshockable rhythm, the defibrillation attempts and antiarrhythmic therapy would not be warranted, but otherwise the resuscitation should proceed in a similar manner.

In all cases of resuscitation, clinicians should attempt to determine the underlying cause while avoiding the pitfall of inaction (**Table 121-3**).

■ POSTRESUSCITATION CARE AND TERMINATING THE RESUSCITATION

No criteria exist to guide clinicians when resuscitation is futile save in cases of obvious rigor mortis, evidence of decapitation, or evidence of decomposition. Complicating matters further, most resuscitation research confines its reach to the first minutes of resuscitation, leaving clinicians to use their best judgment as to whether resuscitative measures should continue. In general, clinicians should factor in the length of time the brain has been exposed to hypoxia and inadequate perfusion in deciding whether or not the hallmark of successful resuscitation—neurologically intact survival—is likely.

PRACTICE POINT

- The decision to forgo further resuscitation efforts should be made by the entire resuscitative team in a manner that considers premorbid level of function, duration of the resuscitative effort, and other team members' opinions and suggestions.

When deciding to forgo further resuscitation efforts, the decision should be made by the entire resuscitative team in a manner that considers premorbid level of function, duration of the

TABLE 121-3 Pitfalls in Cardiopulmonary Resuscitation and High-impact Countermeasures to Abrogate Them

Pitfall	Cause	Countermeasure
• Failure to initiate closed chest cardiac massage (CCCM)	• Concern about potentially causing harm (rib fractures, organ perforation, pain, etc) • Uncertainty about whether the patient is truly in cardiopulmonary arrest	• Initiate CCCM immediately as the greater harm is in delaying treatment
• Focusing on airway and bag-valve ventilation preferentially to CCCM	• Possibility of improving oxygenation and ventilation	• Place the patient on a nonrebreather with oxygen delivery > 15 liters per minute • Consider placing an oropharyngeal or nasopharyngeal airway
• Incorrect CCCM technique	• Providers pushing too shallowly, too slowly, or failing to release compression adequately	• Remember the adage: "Push Hard, Pump Fast, Good Recoil"
• Delay in transthoracic shock due to uncertainty in cardiac rhythm	• Concern about causing torsades-de-pointes or ventricular fibrillation • Concern about misidentification of a benign rhythm for a malignant one • Lack of familiarity with equipment and its use	• Transthoracic shocks are the only intervention, other than CCCM, that have meaningfully valuable impacts on patient survival, but survival begins to decrease every second a patient remains in a shockable rhythm. Early shocks lead to improved outcomes. • Torsades-de-pointes and ventricular fibrillation are themselves shockable rhythms • Recognize that correct rhythm diagnosis may not be possible early on in a resuscitation • Recurrent training, practice, simulation, and feedback are essential to educate those who are expected to use resuscitation equipment in an emergency

resuscitative effort, and other team members' opinions and suggestions. Pediatric literature supports allowing family members the decision to view the resuscitation prior to termination of efforts (with evidence suggesting that family members who witness the resuscitation have lower incidences of pathological mourning 1 year after the patient's death), though clinician comfort with this approach is low.

Postresuscitation hypothermia

In those in whom resuscitation appears successful, clinicians should consider initiation of therapeutic hypothermia. Hypothermia after cardiac arrest was first described in ancient Russian times, but was rediscovered in the 1950s. It was abandoned at that time due to uncertain benefit and difficulty with use.

Interest resurged in the 1990s based on sound basic science suggesting that induced hypothermia reduces oxidative and reperfusion neuronal injury. Extensive research subsequently has demonstrated that inducing hypothermia following cardiac arrest improves neurologic outcomes (as defined by Cerebral Performance Category) when patients develop cardiopulmonary arrest due to a shockable rhythm. The data for improved neurologic recovery are not as strong in PEA or asystole, however.

Therapeutic hypothermia requires continuous central temperature monitoring via specialized equipment such as bladder thermography. The goal of therapeutic hypothermia is rapid cooling of the patient's core temperature to 32–34°C via external cooling devices (ice packs can be used, but become a significant issue as melting ensues), internal cooling (utilizing chilled saline), or a combination of both. Since human physiology abhors hypothermia and will attempt to usurp hypothermia through shivering, patients often require paralysis to prevent shivers. All patients receiving paralytics also require concomitant sedation and mechanical ventilation. After 24 hours, paralytics and cooling devices may be discontinued with the patient being allowed to passively rewarm.

Since therapeutic hypothermia requires specialized equipment, its use is often confined to centers with experience and established institutional protocols for hypothermia. In the absence of these, clinicians should strive to maintain patient normothermia and avoid even minuscule elevation of body temperature above normal.

Patients in whom an acute coronary syndrome is posited to be the cause of cardiac arrest should undergo cardiac revascularization as soon as possible to prevent recurrent arrhythmias.

PROGNOSIS

Only approximately one in seven patients survive an in-hospital resuscitation to discharge, and of those who initially survive, only 19% are still living 6 months after IHCA. Fifty-one percent of survivors initially present in a shockable rhythm (ventricular fibrillation or ventricular tachycardia), but shockable rhythms are outnumbered in incidence to nonshockable rhythms (asystole or pulseless electrical activity) by nearly three to one in the inpatient setting.

Successful resuscitation preserves patients' neurologic function that the American Heart Association (AHA) defines using the Cerebral Performance Category score (**Table 121-4**).

Between 14 and 23% of survivors—whose pre-arrest neurological function was normal—develop moderate to severe cognitive deficits after resuscitation (Cerebral Performance Category 2–3). Fewer than 2% of survivors of IHCA will suffer prolonged coma or persistent vegetative state. While gender does not appear to predict outcomes in cardiopulmonary arrest, increased age may predict worse outcomes and lower survival probably less on the basis of age itself but rather through the accumulation of myriad comorbidities (particularly chronic kidney disease, coronary disease, and malignancy). Further multivariate data from the national registry of cardiopulmonary resuscitation (NRCPR) ultimately may help settle whether age is an independent predictor of short- and long-term survival.

TABLE 121-4 Cerebral Performance Category Score and Related Neurologic Outcome

Cerebral Performance Category	Level of functioning
CPC 1	A return to normal cerebral function and normal living
CPC 2	Cerebral disability but sufficient function for independent activities of daily living
CPC 3	Severe disability, limited cognition, inability to carry out independent existence
CPC 4	Coma
CPC 5	Brain death

PRACTICE POINT

- The focus of successful resuscitation is preservation of the patient's life and premorbid neurological function, including outcomes commensurate with a Cerebral Performance Category (CPC) of 1 (Table 121-4).

QUALITY IMPROVEMENT

Debriefing with clinicians after every resuscitation event allows input from all team members as to their feelings about the quality of the resuscitation and permits everyone to contribute their intellectual and emotional concerns. Debriefing, even just a few minutes, should occur after every resuscitation event. All resuscitations require careful post hoc analysis for team compliance with established resuscitation protocols. One very valuable source of feedback is participation in NRCPR. This international collective of nearly 15% of all U.S. hospitals, and all of the Canadian Health care System plus several other international sites, was created by the American Heart Association to collect standardized data on all inpatient cardiac arrests. Participating institutions receive quarterly reports on their resuscitations that can be compared to local, regional, national, and international norms established by all other participating institutions. These data can offer areas where improvement is needed (such as time to initial defibrillation from onset of cardiopulmonary arrest) and can serve as valuable reinforcement to team members of areas in which mastery has been accomplished. Furthermore, NRCPR data continue to help refine the cutting edge in resuscitation research and therefore meaningfully impact future patients' outcomes from cardiopulmonary arrest.

Post hoc analysis offers a stop-gap solution, but continual retraining offers the most proactive means to deliver high-quality care. Simulation labs offer an opportunity to objectively quantify team members' capabilities at performing chest compressions, BVM ventilations, and other logistics of team flow that may elude analysis during real-life resuscitations. Since studies show rapid degradation in resuscitation skills (both manual and intellectual) within days of biannual resuscitation training, clinicians require continual feedback over the intervening months to ensure an adequate skill set. Whether this feedback occurs in a formal simulation environment or one-on-one with a manikin is probably less important than ensuring that skills are adequate and reinforced over time (**Table 121-5**).

TABLE 121-5 Evidence-based Medicine Key References for Resuscitation

Study	Methods	Results	Limitations	Bottom Line
Pathophysiology				
Suzuki M, et al. *Resuscitation.* 2009;80:109–112.	Cerebral blood flow was measured in a hemorrhagic model shock in rats	Gasping increases cerebral blood flow	Animal study, but thought to closely mimic conditions in humans	Gasping causes favorable hemodynamic flow in cardiac arrest
Sillberg VAH, et al. *Resuscitation.* 2008;79:380–386.	Systematic review of the literature to assess if vasopressin and epinephrine was superior to epinephrine alone	There was no added benefit of vasopressin to epinephrine	Data could not be adequately pooled due to dissimilar constructs of many of the included studies	Epinephrine still reigns supreme as the only major drug that can impact mortality in cardiac arrest
Assessment				
Tibbals J, Russell P. *Resuscitation.* 2009;80:61–64.	Clinicians were asked to determine if children had a pulse or not while undergoing cardiopulmonary bypass	The pulse check was only 78% accurate, 86% sensitive, and 64% specific for cardiac arrest	Controlled circumstances in the absence of psychological pressure of real cardiac arrest	The pulse check remains a highly variable, though modestly sensitive and accurate test for cardiac arrest
Rapid response				
Dacey MJ, et al. *Crit Care Med.* 2007;35:2076–2082.	Prospective controlled trial investigating the impact of a rapid response team (RRT) before and after implementation of an RRT in a community hospital	RRT implementation led to reduction in hospital-wide codes from 7.6 to 3.0 cardiac arrests per 1000 discharges, reduced mortality from 2.82% to 2.35%, and reduced need for urgent ICU transfer from 45% to 29%	The RRT used physician assistants with advanced training, something that may be difficult to implement in many hospitals (which often use nurse-run RRTs)	RRTs appear to reduce key indicators of medical crises in this community hospital

(continued)

TABLE 121-5 Evidence-based Medicine Key References for Resuscitation (*continued*)

Study	Methods	Results	Limitations	Bottom Line
Rapid response				
Sharek PJ, et al. *JAMA*. 2007;298: 2267–2274.	Cohort study with historical controls to determine mortality and code rates following implementation of a physician-run RRT at a pediatric hospital	Absolute monthly mortality rate decreased by 18%, and code rates also decreased across the board	This study was conducted at quaternary referral center and would be unlikely except at rare institutions that could afford this physician-led directive	RRTs appear to reduce pediatric mortality and code rates at a teaching hospital
Sebat F, et al. *Crit Care Med*. 2007;35:2568–2575.	Prospective controlled trial investigating the impact of an RRT before and after implementation of an RRT in a referral center	Particularly in regard to patients in septic shock, an RRT resulted in significant reductions in 5 years following implementation; NNT for creation of this response team to save one life was = 3 patients	The study looked at over 7.5 years of data (2.5 before, and 5 after implementation of an RRT). Improvements in outcomes for patients in shock may have been due to overall advances in general medical care over that interval rather than the RRT itself	RRTs appear to improve outcomes in patients in shock via quicker delivery of protocolized care
Quality of life support and resuscitation				
Abella BS, et al. *JAMA*. 2005;293: 305–310.	Prospective observational study of 67 real world cardiac arrests in adult inpatients	Chest compressions were too shallow and too slow in nearly one third of cardiac arrests, ventilations were frequently more rapid than 20/min	Perhaps the most important observational study in resuscitation of humans—the study had no major limitations	Rescuers frequently fail to achieve target chest compression depth, rate, or respiratory rate goals in real-life cardiac arrests
Smith KK, et al. *Resuscitation*. 2008;78:59–65.	Evaluation of nursing retention of ACLS and BCLS following standard AHA educational guidelines	Performance of skills rapidly degrade with time for BCLS (only 58% passed at 12 months), and ACLS (only 14% passed at 12 months)	Physician skills have not been adequately assessed concomitantly to ensure code team cohesion	Rescuers feel confident about their resuscitation skills, but have little retention without ongoing education and fare worse than expected when challenged in the classroom; real-life performance degradation is just as likely
Bro-Jeppesen J, et al. *Resuscitation*. 2009;80:171–176.	Determination of neurological outcomes in patients with out-of-hospital cardiac arrest who received therapeutic hypothermia compared with historical controls	Hypothermia resulted in significantly better CPC and self-rated quality of life in survivors	This was not a randomized study, though the cohorts were remarkably similar	Therapeutic hypothermia improves quality of life in survivors of out-of-hospital cardiac arrest
Rae TD, et al. *N Engl J Med*. 2010;363:423–433.	Multicenter randomized trial of dispatcher instructions to laypeople in out-of-hospital cardiac arrest to determine if chest compressions alone with or without rescue breathing improved survival	No overall mortality difference was found, but trends were favorable for survival in patients with a primary cardiac cause of CPA and those found in shockable rhythms	This is an out-of-hospital study limited to chest compressions and rescue breathing performed by laypeople	Mounting evidence supports compression only resuscitation strategies; though this study couldn't quite clinch the issue for professionals, it does indicate the message should be compressions only for laypeople
Ehlenach WJ, et al. *N Engl J Med*. 2009;361:22–31.	Epidemiologic study of in-hospital cardiac arrest in older patients in relation to outcomes of resuscitation attempts	Blacks were almost 24% less likely to survive to hospital discharge than whites; overall survival did not change for the 13 years of the study	Study was retrospective and used Medicare billing data	Despite its limitations, black race was associated with worse outcomes in CPA; no survival benefit has occurred despite > 13 years of available data

(*continued*)

TABLE 121-5 Evidence-based Medicine Key References for Resuscitation *(continued)*

Study	Methods	Results	Limitations	Bottom Line
Quality of life support and resuscitation				
Chan PS, et al. *N Engl J Med.* 2008;358:9–17.	Using the NRCPR, the time from onset of cardiac arrest to time of defibrillation was measured and compared to outcomes	Delayed defibrillation (occurring > 2 minutes after code onset) was associated with lower survival overall but was also notably more common in patients of black race and to occur in smaller hospitals	Time keeping during cardiopulmonary arrest is a subject of considerable controversy since a code is generally quite hectic	Even with good CPR, defibrillation for patients with shockable rhythms is not only mission-critical, but time-critical as well
Kilgannon JH, et al. *JAMA.* 2010;303: 2165–2171.	Multicenter cohort study using IMPACT database to look for the effects of hyperoxia (too high a systemic arterial oxygenation level) and mortality in cardiac arrest	Patients whose arterial blood gases demonstrated a PaO_2 of > 300 mm Hg within 24 h of cardiac arrest had statistically significantly worse outcomes (18% higher relative mortality)	Large time differences between time of arrest and time of arterial blood gas determination could make some of these data difficult to differentiate	Once again proving that less is more in resuscitation: don't over-oxygenate your patients (a factor partially attributable to bag-valve-mask ventilation and hyperventilation demonstrated in resuscitation)

ACLS, advanced cardiac life support; AHA, American Heart Association; BLS, basic life support; CPA, cardiopulmonary arrest; CPC, cerebral performance category; ICU, intensive care unit; NNT, number needed to treat; NRCPR, national registry of cardiopulmonary resuscitation.

SUGGESTED READINGS

Abella BS, Alvarado JP, Myklebust H, et al. Quality of cardiopulmonary resuscitation in adult inpatients. *JAMA*. 2005;293: 305–310.

Arrich J, Holzer M, Herkner H, et al. Hypothermia for neuroprotection in adults after cardiopulmonary resuscitation. *Cochrane Database*. 2009;4:CD004128.

Bobrow BJ, Ewy GA. Ventilation during resuscitation efforts for out-of-hospital primary cardiac arrest. *Curr Op Crit Care*. 2009;15: 228–233.

Ehlenach WJ, Barnato AE, Curtis JR, et al. Epidemiologic study of in-hospital cardiopulmonary resuscitation in the elderly. *N Engl J Med*. 2009;361:22–31.

Field JM, Hazinski MF, Sayre MR, et al. Part 1: Executive Summary: 2010 American Heart Association Guidelines for Caridiopulmonary Resuscitation and Emergency Cardiovascular Care Science. *Circulation*. 2010;122:S640–S656.

Hazinski MF, Nolan JP, Billi JE, et al. Part 1: Executive summary: 2010 International Consensus on Cardiopulmonary Resuscitation and Emergency Cardiovascular Care Science with Treatment Recommendations. *Circulation*. October 2010;122(16 Suppl 2): S250–S275.

Olasveengen TM, Sunde K, Brunborg C, et al. Intravenous drug administration during out-of-hospital cardiac arrest. *JAMA*. 2009;302:2222–2229.

Zuercher M, Ewy GA. Gasping during cardiac arrest. *Curr Op Crit Care*. 2009;15:185–188.

CHAPTER 122

Intubation and Airway Support

Bisan A. Salhi, MD
Douglas S. Ander, MD

Key Clinical Questions

1. What are the indications for rapid sequence intubation?
2. What are the predictors of a difficult airway?
3. When is "awake intubation" indicated?
4. What are the alternative methods available for intubation and/or ventilation?

INTRODUCTION

Airway management can significantly affect outcomes for hospitalized critically ill patients. Failure to deliver adequate oxygen may cause irreversible brain damage or preclude successful resuscitation. Options for management may range from assisted ventilation with a bag-valve-mask (BVM) to noninvasive ventilation (NIV) support to endotracheal intubation. A successful outcome in any intubation demands proficiency in patient assessment, knowledge of the equipment (basic and advanced), requisite technical skills, appreciation of individual limitations, and an alternative plan to deal with the difficult or failed airway.

In 2006 the Society for Hospital Medicine published the Core Competencies in Hospital Medicine, which listed endotracheal intubation as one of the procedural competencies for hospitalists. However, a small survey published in 2010 noted that individual hospitalists (n = 175) performed on average only 10 endotracheal intubations in the previous year with a range of 3 to 20. This limited clinical experience with advanced airway management highlights the importance of a valuable educational program for the hospitalists as well as clinicians' understanding of their own practice and skill limitations. Depending on their clinical environment and work setting, the expectations for different hospitalists in advanced airway management will vary. However, all hospitalists should be versed in initial airway management and stabilization, including effective use of oral and nasal airway and BVM devices.

PATHOPHYSIOLOGY

AIRWAY ANATOMY

Successful intubation requires knowledge of basic airway anatomy landmarks and locations of various airway structures relative to each other to identify the glottic opening and successfully intubate. The larynx and in particular the vocal cords lie just below the epiglottis, and proper elevation of the epiglottis should allow the clinician to visualize the arytenoids and the vocal cords prior to insertion of the endotracheal tube (ETT) (**Figure 122-1**).

PREDICTORS OF A DIFFICULT AIRWAY

A *difficult airway* refers to complex or challenging BVM or endotracheal intubation. Difficult oxygenation is the inability to maintain the oxygen saturation > 90% despite using a BVM and 100% oxygen. A *failed airway* refers to the inability to either ventilate or intubate a patient after three intubation attempts by the same operator using multiple blades. Experienced operators uncommonly encounter this problem. Difficult ventilation occurs in 1 in 50 anesthesia cases. In one study of emergency department cases 2.7% were deemed failed intubation attempts due to unsuccessful first attempts requiring rescue techniques. A higher rate of poor clinical outcomes occurs when the airway is managed as an emergent (rather than elective) procedure. In addition, an increased number of airway attempts predicts poorer outcomes; thus a backup plan is necessary if initial intubation attempts are not successfully executed. Medical diagnoses that increase the likelihood of difficult airways range from congenital conditions that typically affect the airway anatomy to acquired conditions such as trauma, tumors, edema, infections, arthritis, and obesity. All affect the ability to adequately visualize the larynx during the intubation attempt (**Table 122-1**).

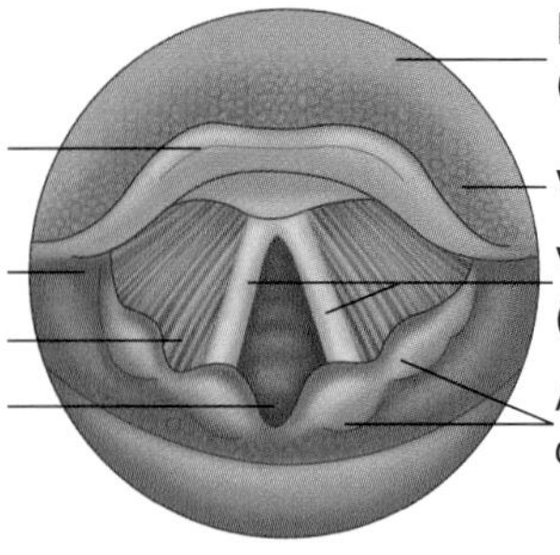

Figure 122-1 *Airway anatomy. (Reproduced, with permission, from Reichman EF, Simon RR. Emergency Medicine Procedures. New York: McGraw-Hill. Fig. 5-5.)*

Patients with large incisors, reduced distance between incisors, and reduced thyromental distance are more likely to have a poor laryngoscopic view and potentially more difficulty with intubation. Rapid assessment of these factors when one is first evaluating the patient can provide key data in development of an airway management plan. When presented with a patient that has one or more risk factors for difficult airway, additional equipment and/or personnel should be brought to the patient to assist with the airway management.

TABLE 122-1 Diagnoses Associated with a Difficult Airway

Congenital		Pierre Robin syndrome
		Down syndrome
		Anterior epiglottis
Acquired	Infectious	Ludwig angina
		Abscess
		Epiglottitis
	Arthritis	Rheumatoid arthritis
		Ankylosing spondylitis
	Tumors (benign and malignant)	Adenomas
		Goiter
		Lipoma
		Hygroma
		Carcinoma of tongue, larynx, thyroid
	Trauma	Facial injury
		Suspected or actual cervical spine injury (Cervical collar)
	Obesity	
	Acromegaly	
	Inflammation	Acute burns
		Inhalation injury
	Other	Temporomandibular joint dysfunction
		Scleroderma
		Subglottic stenosis

TABLE 122-2 Assessment for Difficult Intubation (Mnemonic: LEMON)

Look	Injury, large incisors, large tongue, beard, receding mandible, obesity, abnormal face or neck pathology or shape
Evaluate the 3-3-2 rule	Mouth opening less than 3 fingers, mandible length less than 3 fingers, or larynx to floor of the mandible less than 2 fingers
Mallampati	Class III (see base of uvula) and class IV (soft palate is not visible)
Obstruction	Any upper airway pathology that causes an obstruction (abscess, edema, masses, epiglottitis)
Neck mobility	Limited mobility of neck (trauma with cervical spine immobilization arthritis)

Many clinical assessment tools have been developed to predict a difficult airway, but insufficient evidence supports recommending any individual tool. The LEMON rule is one popular rule for assessment for difficult intubation (**Table 122-2**).

Operator and environmental factors may also contribute to challenges or failure to control the airway. Trainees and inexperienced clinicians (with low total numbers or infrequent intubations) may have greater difficulty intubating. When attempting to ventilate or intubate outside the controlled environment of the operating room, lack of proper patient positioning or inadequate equipment or medications may contribute to challenging intubations.

Many other factors have been associated with a difficult airway, but none accurately predicts, which patient will ultimately need more advanced techniques. Some patients who have several risk factors are intubated with ease while other patients who have no high-risk predictors on rare occasions have unforeseen difficulty with intubation or ventilation. In all cases the clinician should assess the potential risk for a difficult airway and always have a backup plan of action should initial attempt(s) at securing an airway prove unsuccessful.

Difficulty with BVM ventilation has been reported to occur in 5% of patients. Five independent risk factors for difficult BVM ventilation include age greater than 55 years, body mass index > 26 kg/m^2, beard, lack of teeth, and history of snoring (**Table 122-3**, MOANS assessment). BVM ventilation can effectively maintain airway patency while an alternative plan is developed and implemented. However, patients with a high risk of failing BVM ventilation may require more rapid and definitive airway evaluation and management.

TABLE 122-3 Assessment for Difficulty with Bag-valve-mask (BVM) Ventilation (Mnemonic: MOANS)

Mask seal	Inadequate mask seal (beard, blood/emesis, facial trauma, operator small hands)
Obesity	BMI > 26 kg/m^2
Age	>55 years
No teeth	No teeth (impairs BVM effectiveness)
Stiff ventilation	Asthma, COPD, ARDS, term pregnancy

ARDS, acute respiratory distress syndrome; BMI, body mass index; BVM, Bag-valve-mask; COPD, chronic obstructive pulmonary disease.

PRACTICE POINT

- Difficulty with BVM ventilation has been reported to occur in 5% of patients.

INDICATION FOR INTUBATION

All indications for endotracheal intubation can be classified as (1) failure to maintain a patent airway, (2) failure of oxygenation and/or ventilation, and (3) anticipation of a rapidly deteriorating clinical course (**Table 122-4**).

FAILURE TO MAINTAIN A PATENT AIRWAY

The ability to maintain a patent airway preserves normal oxygenation and ventilation is essential to life. Maintenance of the airway protects against aspiration of gastric contents, which can have serious short- and long-term consequences for the patient after loss of consciousness or poisoning or during major acute upper gastrointestinal bleeding.

There are several ways to effectively assess the patency of the airway. Although widely used, the presence of a gag reflex is *not* one of those methods. The gag reflex is physiologically absent in many normal adults. Additionally, stimulation of the gag reflex in an altered or obtunded patient increases the likelihood of vomiting and, consequently, aspiration of gastric contents. The ability to phonate and/or converse is a reliable indicator of a patent airway. When the patient is unable to speak, the patient's ability to handle secretions (ie, swallow) can be used as a surrogate to determine whether the airway is patent.

Noninvasive maneuvers such as a chin lift or jaw thrust or devices such as an oropharyngeal (oral) airway or a nasopharyngeal airway adjunct (nasal trumpet) may allow time to prepare for intubation by temporarily maintaining a patent airway.

PRACTICE POINT

- Presence of a gag reflex does not effectively assess airway patency. The gag reflex is physiologically absent in many normal adults. The ability to phonate and/or converse is a reliable indicator of a patent airway.

FAILURE OF OXYGENATION AND/OR VENTILATION

When a patient's inability to oxygenate does not respond to supplemental oxygen, endotracheal intubation is indicated. Rather than relying solely on the results of an arterial blood gas (ABG) value, the patient's clinical appearance, including an assessment of vital signs and mentation, guides the decision to intubate. Awaiting ABG results may delay intubation, especially if the results conflict with the clinical impression.

TABLE 122-4 Indications for Intubation

Indication	Suggestive Signs
Failure to maintain a patent airway	Inability to phonate, inability to handle secretions, high risk of aspiration
Failure to oxygenate or ventilate	Unresponsiveness to noninvasive oxygenation or ventilation methods
Anticipate deterioration in clinical condition	Patient must be unaccompanied for testing, patient unable to maintain current work of breathing, likely further studies or surgery etc.

Ventilatory failure is another indication for endotracheal intubation. Continuous pulse oximetry monitoring usually effectively determines the adequacy of oxygenation and the response to supplemental oxygen, but it does not assess ventilation. Capnography or ABG analysis can be used to determine a patient's ability to ventilate or to track the patient's response to noninvasive positive pressure ventilation. Results of these tests must also be interpreted cautiously and in conjunction with close observation of a patient's clinical course.

ANTICIPATION OF CLINICAL DETERIORATION

Despite patent airway and adequate oxygenation and ventilation, some patients may still require elective intubation to avoid emergent intubation later. Common examples include airway protection in an overdose patient or massive gastrointestinal (GI) bleeder, rest from labored breathing that cannot be sustained in a patient with severe asthma or pneumonia, or to maintain airway patency compromised from angioedema or other conditions. Anticipation of deterioration relies heavily on the physician's personal experience and judgment.

CONTRAINDICATIONS

Contraindications to endotracheal intubation can be divided into either absolute or relative but these need to be tailored to the specific clinical situation. Absolute contraindications to intubation include total airway obstruction and total loss of facial or oropharyngeal landmarks, both necessitating a surgical airway. An anticipated difficult airway as described earlier is a relative contraindication to rapid sequence intubation (RSI), and in this situation consideration of awake intubation or use of the difficult airway adjuncts should be entertained. During cardiac or respiratory arrest, ventilation with a BVM, intubation, or both should be performed despite any contraindications.

PROCEDURAL STEPS

AIRWAY PLAN

Rapid sequence intubation versus awake intubation

RSI is now the predominant and preferred method in managing the emergent airway in a patient who requires sedation (ie, not the patient requiring a crash airway). RSI is defined as the simultaneous administration of a sedative and paralytic agent to assist in endotracheal intubation, usually via direct laryngoscopy. Central to the concept of RSI is the avoidance of assisted BVM ventilation to avoid insufflation of the stomach and minimize the risk of aspiration. Outcomes evidence supports RSI as a safe and effective technique for emergency airway management that maximizes the patient and physician likelihood of timely, successful airway management.

Seven steps ("7 Ps of RSI") essential to successful rapid sequence intubation include (1) preparation, (2) preoxygenation, (3) premedication, (4) paralysis, (5) positioning, (6) placement of the ETT, and (7) postintubation care.

1. **Preparation** refers to the initial assessment of the patient's airway and the decision to intubate. The clinician assesses the patient's airway. Predictors of a difficult airway must be addressed, and backup airway devices (such as a laryngeal mask airway, gum elastic bougie, etc) prepared. Additionally, clinicians should prepare any monitors, medications, and oxygen sources. Preparation also requires appropriately trained staff to manage the airway and establishment of plans for the difficult or failed airway.
2. **Preoxygenation** involves applying 100% supplemental oxygen to induce nitrogen wash-out and maximize the amount of time available for direct laryngoscopy without oxygen desaturation. *In a normal healthy adult, adequate preoxygenation can*

permit 7–9 minutes of apnea before oxygen desaturation occurs. In patients with comorbid diseases (eg, cardiac disease, underlying lung disease, pregnancy, etc), desaturation can occur more rapidly.

3. **Premedication** involves administration of drugs *3–5 minutes before induction and paralysis* to blunt the effects of direct laryngoscopy, including bronchospasm and a strong sympathetic response. Options for pretreatment include *fentanyl (3 μg/kg)* administration in patients who are severely hypertensive, have underlying coronary disease, or intracranial hemorrhage if no contraindications exist. Additionally, lidocaine (1.5 mg/kg) may be administered in patients with asthma or elevated intracranial pressure. Premedication with lidocaine, however, may be labor intensive, adds time, and has little proven benefit. Care should be taken when considering any premedication due to the added complexity, adverse affects of the premedication agents, and limited proven benefit.
4. **Paralysis** involves administration of a paralytic agent in conjunction with a sedative agent to rapidly induce paralysis and sedation. Unless contraindicated, etomidate (for sedation) and succinylcholine (for paralysis) are the most commonly used agents in this step. Several clinical conditions preclude the use of succinylcholine (**Table 122-5**). Etomidate is relatively safe but may induce transient adrenal suppression; its use may necessitate corticosteroids supplementation in septic patients.
5. **Positioning** refers to the positioning of the patient in the "sniffing position" to improve the physician's view of the vocal cords (**Figure 122-2**).
6. **Placement of the ETT** is performed under direct visualization of the vocal cords. Methods of confirming correct ETT placement include the presence of condensation of the ETT, presence of bilateral breath sounds, absence of breath sounds over the midepigastrium, end-tidal carbon dioxide detection, and visualization on a chest X-ray. *The gold standard to confirm appropriate tube positioning is use of end-tidal carbon dioxide detection.*
7. **Postintubation care** includes the administration of sedatives, analgesics, and paralytics as needed. Patients who are medically paralyzed require sedation and pain control.

Although RSI (*by trained operators*) is the preferred method of airway management in most patients, *RSI is not advised if difficulty with BVM is predicted,* such as in patients whose airway anatomy is unknown or the ability to intubate via direct laryngoscopy is in question (eg, upper airway obstruction, stridor, angioedema, head and neck cancers). In such cases, *awake intubation or awake direct laryngoscopy* should be strongly considered as a safer option. In patients with possible upper airway or laryngeal obstruction, the administration of a topical anesthetic agent, opioid, and/or a sedative agent can allow direct visualization of the airway via direct laryngoscopy or flexible bronchoscopy. Following visualization of the airway, the patient may be intubated directly via RSI, as already described, or one of the alternative intubation methods, such as nasotracheal or fiberoptic intubation.

In general, RSI is safer and more successful than awake intubation. In select patients in which awake intubation is indicated, it should be approached with caution, and backup rescue airway methods should be readily available (**Table 122-6**).

TABLE 122-5 Contraindications to Succinylcholine Use

Condition	Time Frame
Hyperkalemia	Consider in any patient with known or suspected end-stage renal disease
Burns > 10% TBSA	5 days–6 months
Crush injury	5 days–6 months
Denervation (stroke, spinal cord injury)	5 days–6 months
Neuromuscular disease (ALS, MS)	Risk for these patients lasts indefinitely

ALS, amyotrophic lateral sclerosis; MS, multiple sclerosis; TBSA, total body surface area.

BASIC ENDOTRACHEAL INTUBATION

Bag-valve-mask ventilation

The most important skill required for inpatient clinicians in airway management is use of a BVM and airway adjuncts to ventilate and oxygenate the patient. The ability to ventilate a patient can be an effective bridge prior to intubation and is a requirement prior to use of any paralytic agents. Equipment necessary for effective ventilation includes BVM (**Figure 122-3**), an oxygen source, and airway adjuncts (oropharyngeal and nasopharyngeal airways) (**Figure 122-4**).

PRACTICE POINT

- The ability to ventilate a patient with a bag-valve-mask (BVM) can provide effective gas exchange as a bridge prior to intubation and is a requirement prior to use of any paralytic agents.

Prior to ventilating with a BVM the clinician should place an airway adjunct. *A nasopharyngeal airway is used if the patient's airway reflexes (eg, gag reflex) are still intact (see Figure 122-4). If the patient has no airway reflexes an oropharyngeal airway is placed (Figure 122-4).* These devices help maintain a patent airway and maximize ventilation during BVM ventilation. Placing the patient in a sniffing position (if no concern for cervical spine injury) optimizes the airway alignment of the oral, pharyngeal, and laryngeal axes. A rolled-up towel under the occiput of the patient can effectively align the patient in this position (see Figure 122-2). The mask is placed over the bridge of the nose and mouth. The hands are positioned to create a tight seal. The hand position is commonly described as a "C" and "E." The thumb and index finger wrap around the top of the mask and apply downward pressure to create a seal. The little finger is typically placed behind the angle of the mandible, the ring finger along the mandible, and the middle finger under the mandibular symphisis performing a chin lift and pulling the jaw forward (**Figure 122-5**). If the patient has dentures they should be left *in place* during BVM ventilation and removed just prior to insertion of the laryngoscope. If the clinician is having problems maintaining a seal or ventilating, two-hand BVM ventilation should be attempted. Pulse oximetry can be used to assess adequate oxygenation but will not provide any information about adequate ventilation.

PRACTICE POINT

- If the patient has dentures they should be left *in place* during BVM ventilation and removed just prior to insertion of the laryngoscope.

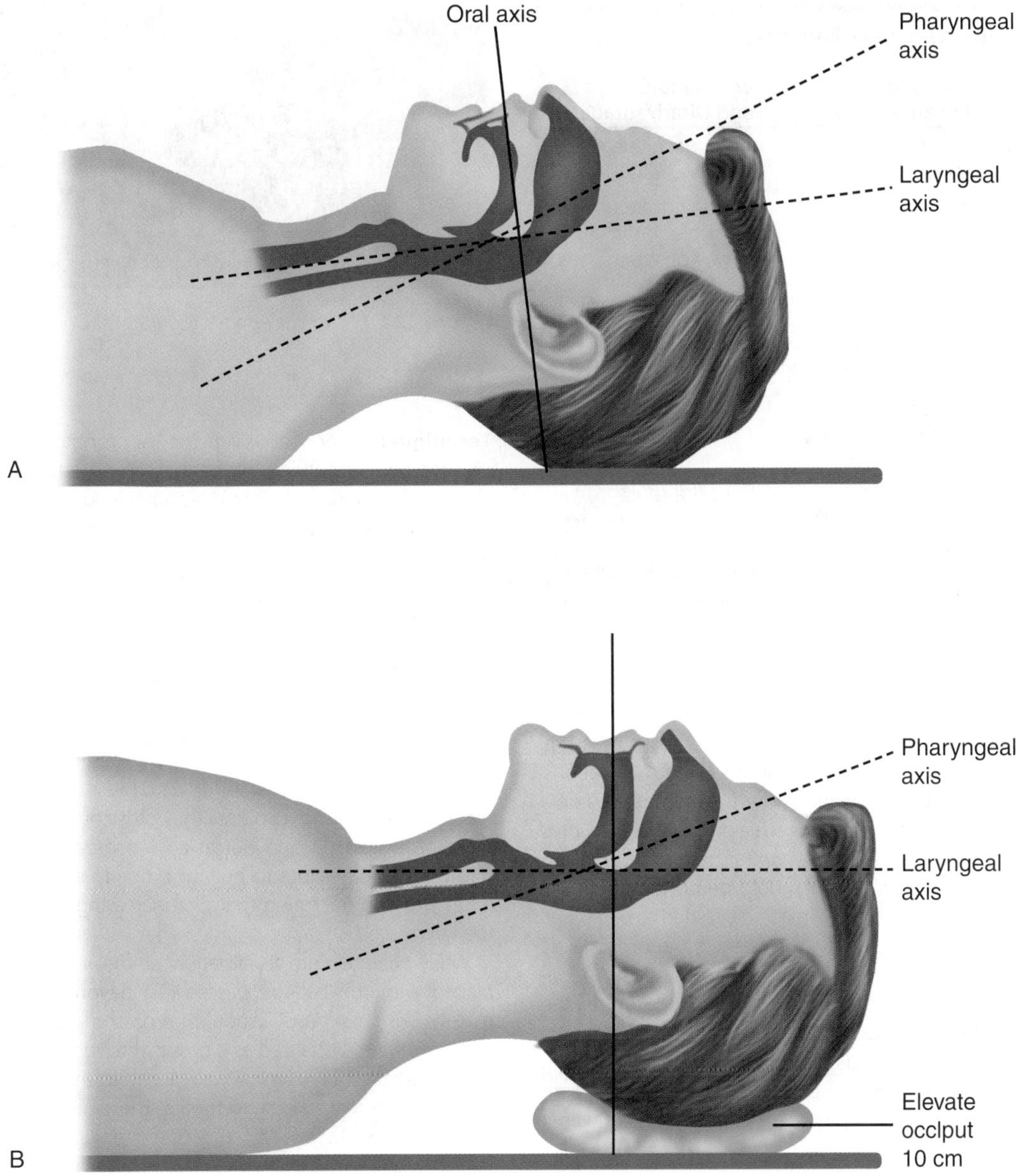

Figure 122-2 *Positioning the patient in the "sniffing" position improves alignment of the axes thereby facilitating endotracheal intubation. (Modified, with permission, from Tintinalli JE, Kelen GD, Stapczynski JS. Tintinalli's Emergency Medicine: A Comprehensive Study Guide. 6th ed. New York: McGraw-Hill, 2004. Fig. 19-1.)*

Endotracheal intubation

Airway control is typically established through direct laryngoscopy and orotracheal intubation. This technique requires several pieces of equipment, a trained operator, and a plan of action. Anyone attempting intubation, particularly if using paralytic agents, should be very comfortable with the technique, the equipment, rescue devices, and other resources available for assistance. A plan to address any contingency is advisable.

Equipment: Endotracheal intubation requires knowledge of equipment and its appropriate use. Necessary initial procedure elements include equipment availability within the facility, and organization that facilitates rapidly finding needed pieces. The equipment may be located within an airway box or crash cart. Preparation for intubation requires basic airway supplies (**Table 122-7**).

Various ETT sizes should be available (ETT sizes 7.0, 7.5, and 8.0 and more than one of the same size tube should be available in case the balloon does not function). Several blade types can be employed, curved (Macintosh) and straight (Miller). Individual preference determines which blade will be used. The tip of the curved blade is placed in the Vallecula anterior to the epiglottis and pulls the epiglottis up revealing the vocal cords. The straight blade is placed posterior to the epiglottis and pushes the epiglottis up to reveal the cords. Basic airway equipment (BVM and airway adjuncts) should always be available.

Preparation: Preparation for endotracheal intubation includes assuring all equipment is available and functions properly (eg, light on the blade works, the ETT balloon does not have an air leak). The stylet is placed within the ETT, such that the tip is *not* protruding beyond the end of the ETT. The ETT is curved either as a gentle curve or at a 45-degree angle at the distal end. The oxygen source should be available either through wall mounted oxygen or an oxygen tank. Suction should be available. Availability of several

TABLE 122-6 Adjuncts to Basic Endotracheal Intubation

Adjunct Airway Device	Uses and Advantages	Contraindications and Disadvantages
Laryngeal mask airway (LMA)	Easy to use and insert Allows selective tracheal ventilation	Not a definitive airway Contraindicated if a supraglottic airway obstruction is identified or suspected
Elastic gum bougie	Easily used when the airway is partially visualized Can pass an ETT over the device	Not useful if the airway cannot be visualized
Video laryngoscope	Allows visualization of the airway with decreased neck manipulation	Operator must be familiar with the device and intubation technique

ETT, endotracheal tube.

assistants facilitates a successful intubation. A respiratory therapist can help with ventilation, equipment, and cricoid pressure. Nurses assist with intravenous lines, monitoring, and medications. Intravenous access should be ensured and the patient placed on a cardiac monitor and pulse oximeter. *The patient should be evaluated as described earlier for a difficult airway, and if necessary expert assistance should be sought.* The patient should be positioned in the sniffing position (see Figure 122-2) by placing a folded towel, sheet, or pillow under the occiput raising the head by approximately 10 cm. The sniffing position lines up the oral, pharyngeal, and laryngeal axes optimizing the view of the cords. This maximizes the alignment of the oral, pharyngeal, and laryngeal axes to improve the visualization of the vocal cords during laryngoscopy. Neck manipulation (eg, sniffing position) is not recommended in a patient with a suspected cervical spine injury or other conditions that limit extension of the head.

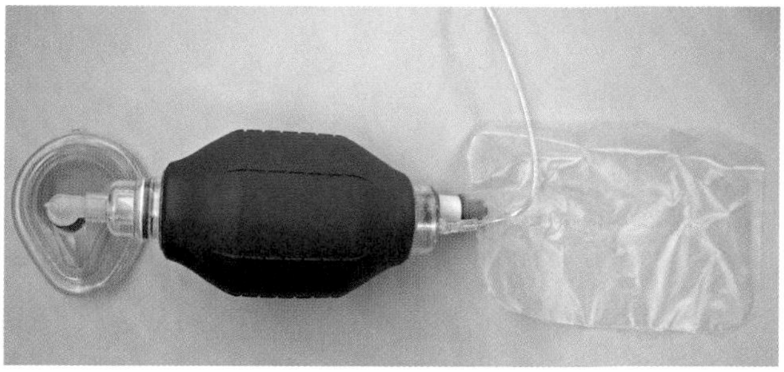

Figure 122-3 *Bag-valve-mask. (Courtesy of Douglas S. Ander, MD.)*

Technique: After choosing the appropriate equipment and positioning the patient, intubation can be attempted. *Application of the Sellick maneuver (cricoid pressure) is no longer routinely recommended during intubation.* Originally thought to decrease aspiration and improve visualization of the larynx, current evidence does not support these historical claims. The handle and blade are always held in the left hand. The mouth is opened and the blade initially placed on the right side of the mouth sweeping the tongue to the left so that the tongue does not obscure the view. The blade is advanced toward the posterior pharynx. The blade is placed into the vallecula (Miller, curved blade) or deep into the posterior pharynx (Macintosh, straight blade). If the blade is unintentionally placed into the esophagus, constant upward pressure is exerted while the blade is slowly withdrawn until the cords come into view. The blade must be pulled up and out at a 45-degree angle to the patient (**Figure 122-6**). Failure to pull up properly risks using the teeth as a fulcrum and fracturing them, or increasing the difficulty viewing the larynx.

While maintaining visualization of the vocal cords, the ETT is placed with the balloon passed just beyond the cords, approximately 2–3 cm. The ETT should be passed along the right side of the mouth and visualized as it passes through the vocal cords. In an adult male the ETT is typically advanced to the 23 cm marker at the lip and in a female 21 cm to the lip. These are approximate depths and will need to be adjusted based on auscultation and chest

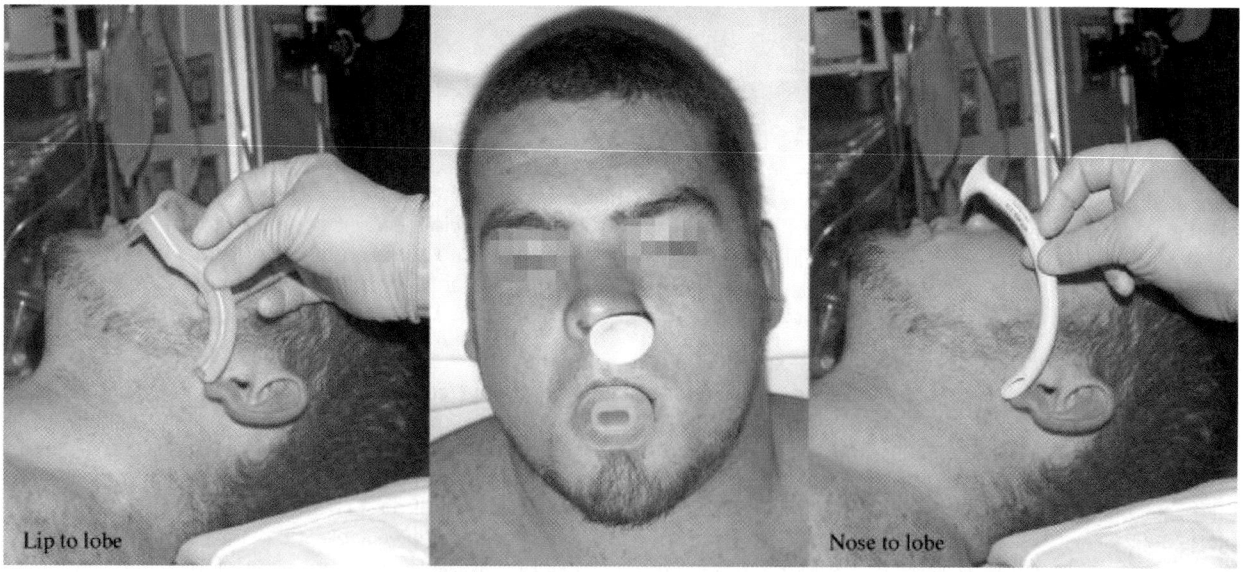

Figure 122-4 *Airway adjuncts. (Reproduced, with permission, from Knoop KJ, Stack LB, Storrow AB, et al. Atlas of Emergency Medicine. 3rd ed. New York: McGraw-Hill, 2009. Fig. 22-3. Photo contributor: Lawrence B. Stack, MD.)*

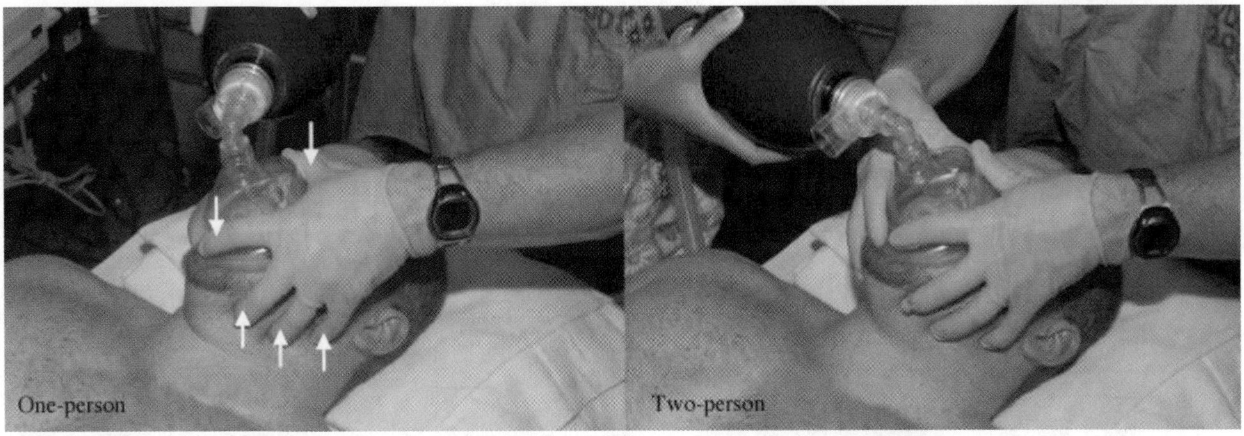

Figure 122-5 *Bag-valve-mask technique. (Reproduced, with permission, from Knoop KJ, Stack LB, Storrow AB, et al. Atlas of Emergency Medicine. 3rd ed. New York: McGraw-Hill, 2009. Fig. 22-2. Photo contributor: Lawrence B. Stack, MD.)*

radiograph. The stylet is removed, the balloon is inflated, and placement should be immediately confirmed. An assistant should monitor vital signs and pulse oximetry readings during the intubation. If oxygen saturations start to drop, the intubation should be stopped and the patient ventilated with the BVM.

PRACTICE POINT5

- In an adult male the ETT is typically advanced to the 23 cm marker at the lip and in a female 21 cm to the lip. These are approximate depths and will need to be adjusted based on auscultation and chest radiographs.

Confirmation: Confirmation that the ETT is in the trachea and properly positioned should be performed immediately after intubation. Auscultation should be performed over the bilateral chest, axilla, and epigastrium. The clinician should pay particular attention to decreased breath sounds over the left chest indicating a right mainstem intubation. An end-tidal carbon dioxide (CO_2) detection device serves as the gold standard for ETT placement confirmation. If the device does not change to the appropriate color, immediately reassess the patient since this is highly indicative of an esophageal intubation and necessitates repeat laryngoscopy after ventilation. Chest X-ray will confirm correct ETT placement (2–3 cm above the carina) and detect any other complications (eg, pneumothorax).

TABLE 122-7 Equipment for Endotracheal Intubation

Endotracheal tubes (assortment of sizes)
Oxygen (head wall or full tank)
Bag-valve-mask
Suction with Yankuer tip
Airway adjuncts (oral and nasal)
Stylets
Confirmation device (end-tidal CO_2 detector)
Stethoscope
Lubricant

Advanced skills for difficult or failed intubation: In some patients, direct laryngoscopy and endotracheal intubation present challenges to clinicians. Alternative airway devices or techniques should be considered and used when traditional airway management fails or when practitioner experience or expertise level precludes routine endotracheal intubation.

LARYNGEAL MASK AIRWAY

The laryngeal mask airway (LMA) should be considered when endotracheal intubation has failed and BVM is difficult or inadequate. The LMA is a supraglottic device that is designed to be blindly inserted into the oral cavity and, when inflated, allows selective ventilation of the trachea (**Figure 122-7**). The LMA requires minimal technical skill and has a high success rate. However, it does not provide definitive airway control and serves only as a temporizing measure while a more definitively secured airway is established. Additionally, the LMA is contraindicated in patients who have airway anomalies or upper airway deformities such as oral cancer or a supraglottic mass.

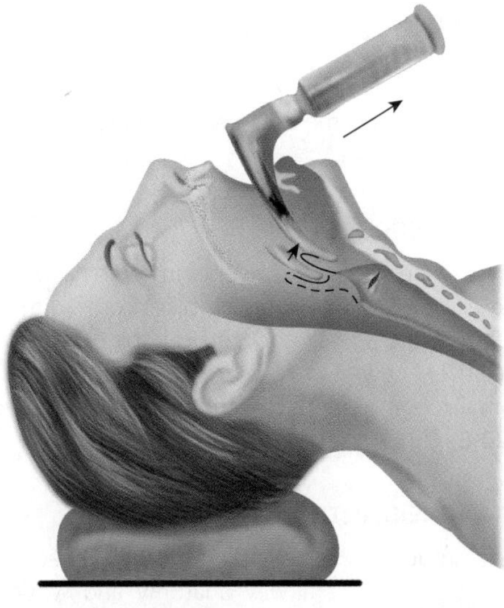

Figure 122-6 *Proper use of laryngoscope. (Reproduced, with permission, from Reichman EF, Simon RR. Emergency Medicine Procedures. New York: McGraw-Hill. Fig. 5-11.)*

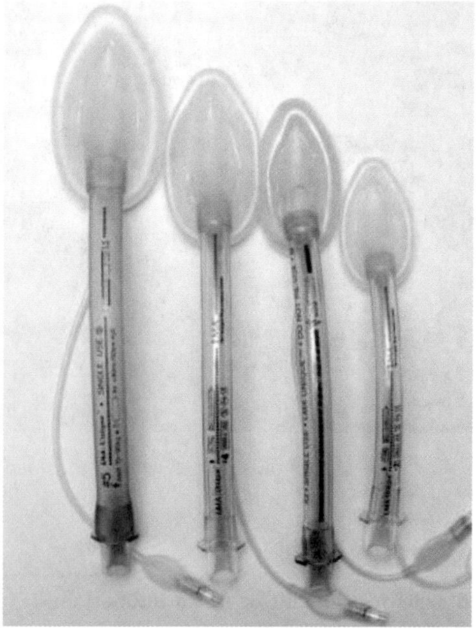

Figure 122-7 *Laryngeal mask airway. (Reproduced, with permission, from Knoop KJ, Stack LB, Storrow AB, et al. Atlas of Emergency Medicine. 3rd ed. New York: McGraw-Hill, 2009. Fig. 22-46. Photo contributor: Lawrence B. Stack, MD.)*

ELASTIC GUM BOUGIE OR TUBE CHANGER

The elastic gum bougie or tube changer can be used to assist in tube placement when the airway can be partially or fully visualized but the placement of an ETT is difficult. In this case, a flexible tube changer is placed in the airway and an ETT is advanced over the tube using the Seldinger technique, and the flexible tube is subsequently removed.

FIBEROPTIC INTUBATION

Fiberoptic intubation can be used in patients whose airway anatomy is unknown or in whom a difficult airway is anticipated. For example, patients with limited neck mobility or distorted airway anatomy may require this technique, which requires significant operator skill and experience. To perform a fiberoptic intubation, the patient must be sedated. An ETT is then placed over the fiberoptic scope. The scope is then maneuvered through the oropharynx or the nasopharynx and advanced toward the epiglottis into the trachea, and the ETT is advanced over the scope into the trachea.

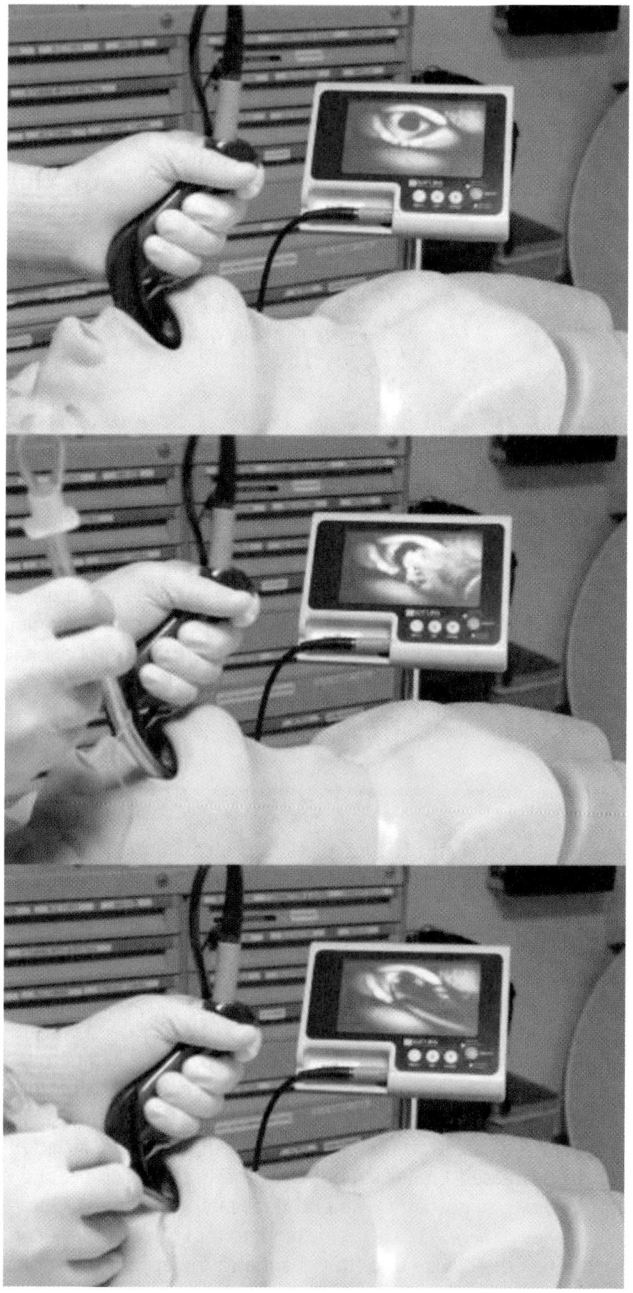

Figure 122-8 *Video laryngoscope. (Reproduced, with permission, from Knoop KJ, Stack LB, Storrow AB, et al. Atlas of Emergency Medicine. 3rd ed. New York: McGraw-Hill, 2009. Fig. 22-44. Photo contributor: Lawrence B. Stack, MD.)*

VIDEO LARYNGOSCOPE

Video laryngoscopes use laryngoscopes in combination with video imaging to allow visualization of the vocal cords with decreased manipulation of the airway and cervical spine. While this technique is relatively new, its role is quickly expanding, and it may play a central role in endotracheal intubation in the near future (**Figure 122-8**).

NASOTRACHEAL INTUBATION

Nasotracheal intubation is indicated for a spontaneously breathing patient with difficult airway anatomy and when paralysis bears high risk. Bleeding diathesis or anticipated severe epistaxis makes this procedure unadvisable. Topical anesthetic or sedative is utilized to prepare patients just prior to the procedure. In nasotracheal intubation, a blind technique, the ETT is advanced along the floor of the nare and toward the larynx. While the tube is being advanced, the operator continuously listens for breath sounds to determine proximity to the vocal cords. Additionally, auscultation is used to assess the phases in the breathing cycles and, consequently, time the advancement of the tube past the vocal cords. Nasotracheal intubation can be added with direct laryngoscopy guiding the ETT through the vocal cords with McGill forceps.

TWIN-LUMEN DEVICES (COMBITUBE)

Twin-lumen devices, such as the Combitube or the King Airway, are frequently used in prehospital airway management. The tube is inserted blindly and may enter the trachea or, more commonly, the esophagus. The tube is equipped with a proximal (high-volume) cuff and distal (low-volume) cuff. If the tube is inserted into the trachea, oxygenation and ventilation are achieved using the more distal lumen, similar to a standard ETT. If the tube is inserted into the esophagus, oxygenation and ventilation are achieved using the lumen proximal to the distal cuff (**Figure 122-9**). These devices are rarely used for definitive airway management.

CRICOTHYROTOMY

In a patient in whom the intubation cannot be achieved and BVM is inadequate in achieving adequate oxygenation and ventilation, surgical establishment of the airway (cricothyrotomy) is indicated. Although this invasive approach is rarely necessary, when emergently indicated the clinician creates a passage through the cricothyroid membrane using a tube cannula. Percutaneous cricothyrotomy technique employs a prepared kit that uses the Seldinger technique to advance an ETT over a dilator to allow oxygenation and ventilation (**Figure 122-10**).

NONINVASIVE VENTILATION

There are several clinical scenarios in which the use of NIV can decrease morbidity and mortality. NIV can be used in patients with chronic obstructive lung disease (COPD), congestive heart failure (CHF), and immunocompromised patients with respiratory distress (see Chapter 137).

NIV significantly reduces mortality, endotracheal intubation, and hospital length of stay in patients with acute exacerbation of COPD

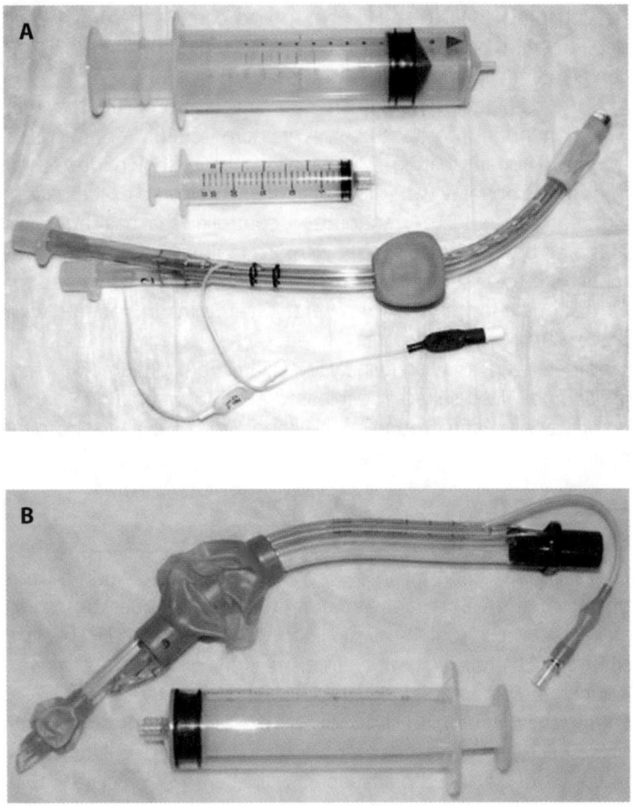

Figure 122-9 *Twin-lumen devices (A) Combitube, (B) King Airway.*

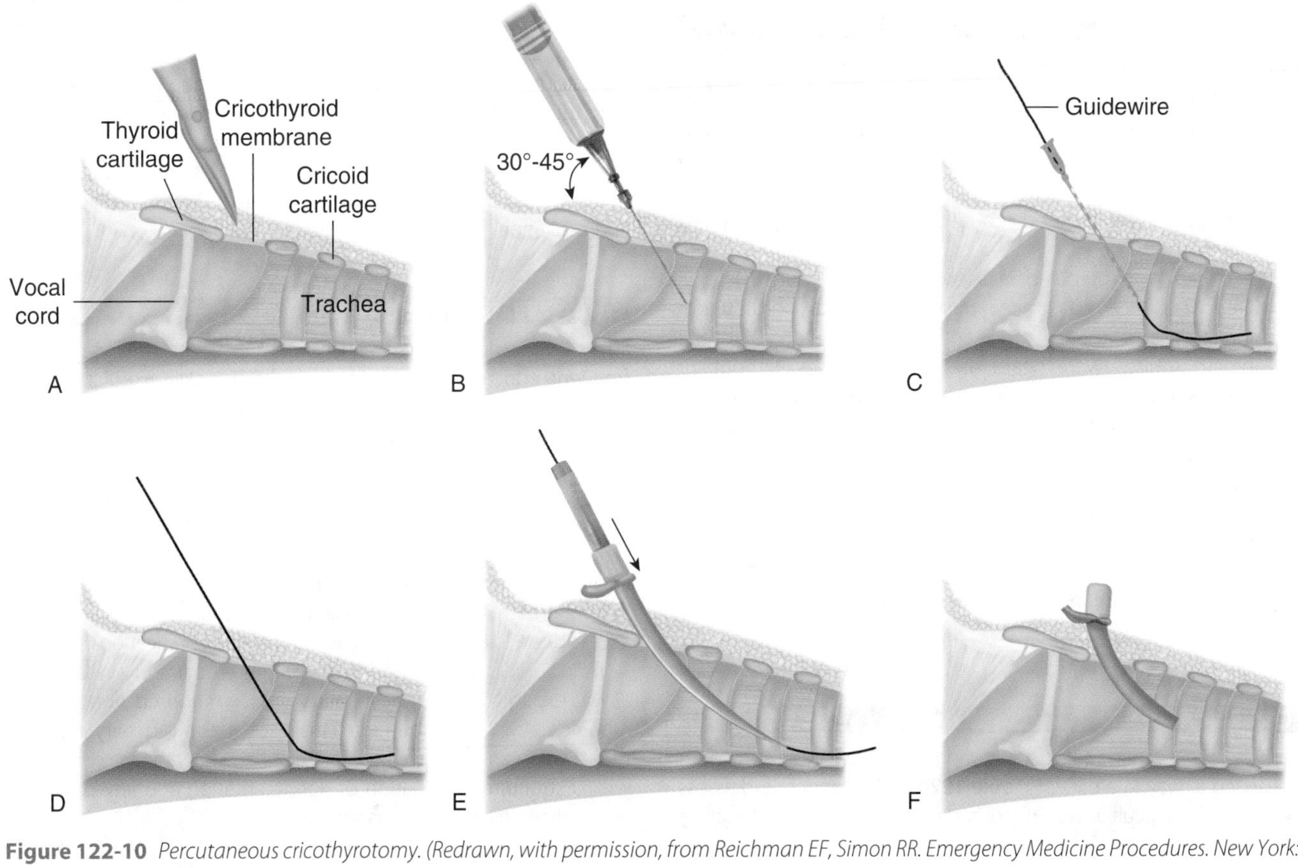

Figure 122-10 *Percutaneous cricothyrotomy. (Redrawn, with permission, from Reichman EF, Simon RR. Emergency Medicine Procedures. New York: McGraw-Hill. Fig. 14-11.)*

(see Chapter 239). NIV should be applied early in the emergency department after ABG analysis and is indicated for pH 7.25–7.35 but can be utilized cautiously with pH < 7.25.

Acute cardiogenic pulmonary edema can also be treated with NIV. Continuous positive airway pressure (CPAP) can decrease the need for intubation. Meta-analyses have shown decreased in-hospital mortality with CPAP in acute heart failure exacerbation, although a recent large, randomized, controlled trial has shown no mortality benefit but does show more rapid symptom improvement with the intervention. Overall, NIV use reduces the need for intubations and improves respiratory symptoms in patients with acute cardiogenic pulmonary edema. In selected immunocompromised patients with respiratory failure from pneumonia early initiation of NIV resulted in decreased need for intubation, serious complications, and improved likelihood of survival to hospital discharge.

CONSULTATION

The decision to consult in airway management depends on the operator's experience and comfort in the techniques described as well as the resources available to the practitioner. Hospitalists should attain proficiency and mastery of BVM skills and use of airway adjunct equipment (oral airway, nasopharyngeal airway, and LMA). Endotracheal intubation skills may be mastered by some hospitalists, especially when few other advanced practitioners intensivists to the list of advanced practitioners with such skills practice within the local facilities. Advanced practitioners with mastery in airway management—including anesthesiology, Emergency Medicine, otolaryngology, or general surgery specialists—should be consulted when a hospitalist lacks sufficient training or skill with airway techniques or when individual patient characteristics likely indicate a difficult airway.

PROCEDURE NOTE

Components of a sample procedure note for intubation are delineated as follows:

A time-out was completed verifying correct patient, procedure, site, positioning, and implant(s) or special equipment if applicable.

Patient was evaluated and required intubation for [____]. [list diagnosis]

The patient was prepared in the usual fashion, and a [____] French ET tube was placed through the vocal cords under direct visualization to [____] centimeters at the teeth. Bilateral breath sounds were heard at the lung apices without air sounds in the abdomen. Tube condensation was present. An end-tidal CO_2 monitor was used to confirm tracheal placement of the ET tube.

Sedation/Paralysis: ______________________ [list agents used]

Chest X-ray was ordered to assess for pneumothorax and ETT placement.

Patient tolerated the procedure well and there were (check one) ___no complications, or ___complications included: ________ ____.

COMPLICATIONS

Various complications can occur during the course of accessing an advanced airway in a patient (**Table 122-8**). Clinicians should assess patients for a difficult airway in an effort to prevent a failed intubation

TABLE 122-8 Endotracheal Intubation Complications

Directly Related to Laryngoscopy	Related to Endotracheal Intubation
Hemodynamic changes including hypertension, hypotension, tachycardia, and bradycardia	Tension pneumothorax
Airway trauma/perforation	Aspiration
Laryngospasm and bronchospasm	Obstruction of endotracheal tube
Trauma to teeth, lips, and tongue	Accidental extubation
Right mainstem bronchus intubation	
Raised intracranial and intraocular pressure (unclear clinical significance)	
Esophageal intubation	
Failed intubation	

attempt. Prompt recognition of an esophageal intubation will allow immediate removal of the ETT and reventilation and oxygenation with a BVM prior to reattempting intubation. Proper technique is essential to avoid any local trauma to oral anatomy and airway structures. A pneumothorax needs to be considered in a patient with hypoxia and hypotension and should be evaluated for all patients with postprocedure chest radiography. Finally accidental dislodgment of the ETT should be avoided by proper stabilization and restraint of the patient.

MAINTENANCE OF THE ENDOTRACHEAL TUBE

Proper stabilization of the ETT is critical to preventing movement of the tube or accidental dislodgment. ETTs can be taped or held in place with commercial tube holders. The site should be kept clean. Skin and mucosal assessment should occur at least every 24 hours. Placement of a nasogastric (NG) or orogastric (OG) tube following endotracheal intubation can help decompress any insufflated air that occurred during BVM use and will help reduce the risk of emesis and aspiration.

QUALITY IMPROVEMENT

Effective advanced airway management in clinical practice requires frequent education or frequent use of the skill. Simulation education can allow clinicians to practice both basic and advanced airway management techniques in a structured setting. Simulation education utilizing airway models and equipment allows mastery of psychomotor skills and practice of less common airway encounters in a safe environment. Simulation-based educational programs can be used to assess competence prior to incorporation of these skills into clinical practice (**Table 122-9**).

Furthermore, local institutional policies and protocols should be accessible and specify available equipment, medications, hospital staff (including nursing and respiratory therapy) and availability of airway experts can assist hospitalists when confronted with a patient requiring airway management. Finally, continuous quality improvement within an institution should include review of all airway cases with a structured evaluation of documentation and any complications related to airway management.

TABLE 122-9 Evidence-based Medicine Key References

Study	Methodology	Results	Limitations	Bottom Line
Epidemiology				
Thakkar R, Wright SM, Alguire P, Wigton RS, Boonyasai RT. Procedures performed by hospitalists and non-hospitalist general internists. *J Gen Intern Med.* 2010;25:448–452.	Cross-sectional survey	1059 respondents, 175 were classified as "hospitalists" and performed only 10 endotracheal intubations in the previous year with a range of 3–20.	Older survey data from 2004. Small sample size. Low overall response rate (56%).	The lack of clinical experience with airway management highlights the importance of a good educational program for the hospitalists.
Airway complications: epidemiology				
Caplan RA, Posner KL. Adverse respiratory events in anesthesia—a closed claims analysis. *Anesth.* 1990;72:828–833.	Retrospective observational study of closed claims	522 claims for adverse respiratory events. Three mechanisms accounted for three-fourths of the adverse respiratory events: inadequate ventilation (196; 38%), esophageal intubation (94; 18%), and difficult tracheal intubation (87; 17%). Most adverse outcomes (72%) were considered preventable with better monitoring.	Inability to generate risk estimates due to the lack of denominator data, absence of a control group, bias toward adverse outcome, and reliance on self-reported data.	Most adverse outcomes were considered preventable with monitoring such as pulse oximetry and capnometry.
Peterson GN, Domino KB. Management of the difficult airway—a closed claims analysis. *Anesth.* 2005;103:33–39.	Retrospective observational study of closed claims	179 claims for difficult airway. Adverse outcomes: death (71; 46%), brain damage (19; 12%), airway injury including esophageal intubation (50; 32%), pneumothorax (7; 4%), aspiration pneumonitis (3; 2%), other (7; 5%).	Inability to generate risk estimates due to the lack of denominator data, absence of a control group, bias toward adverse outcome, and reliance on self-reported data.	Despite advances in anesthesia care several significant adverse outcomes can be attributed to the difficult airway.
Bair AE, Filbin MR, Kulkarni RG. The failed intubation attempt in the emergency department: analysis of prevalence, rescue techniques, and personnel. *J Emerg Med.* 2002;23:131–140.	Prospective observational study of emergency department airway management in 30 hospitals participating in the National Emergency Airway Registry	7712 patients identified who underwent emergency intubation; 207 patients required a rescue technique for intubation after an initial unsuccessful airway. Rescue techniques: RSI (102; 49%), cricothyrotomy (43; 21%). Adjuncts were used in 22 cases and included fiberoptics, oral endotrol, LMA, and retrograde intubation.	Self-reported data from individual study sites. Bias to underreport intubation with failed initial intubations.	A total of 2.7% of emergency intubations in the emergency department required rescue.
Predicting a difficult airway				
Cattano D, Paniucci E, Paolicchi A, Forfori F, Giunta F, Hagberg C. Risk factors assessment of the difficult airway: an Italian survey of 1956 patients. *Anesth Analg.* 2004;99:1774–1779.	Prospective observational study of 1956 consecutive adult patients requiring endotracheal intubation	Mallampati score correlated with Cormack-Lehane scale but failed to reach high sensitivity (50%) or high positive predictive value (14%) for a difficult intubation.	Difficult airway was defined by the anesthesiologist.	Mallampati and other anatomical and clinical indexes had a low positive predictive value.
Langeron O, Masso E, Huraux C, et al. Prediction of difficult mask ventilation. *Anesth.* 2000;92:1229–1236.	Prospective observation study of 1502 patients requiring mask ventilation	Difficult mask ventilation was reported in 75 patients (5%; 95% CI, 3.9–6.1%). Five criteria were recognized as independent factors for difficult mask ventilation: age older than 55 years, body mass index > 26 kg/m^2, beard, lack of teeth, and history of smoking). The presence of two indicated a high likelihood of difficult mask ventilation (sensitivity, 0.72; specificity, 0.73).	Subjective determination of difficult mask ventilation. Small number of patients defined as difficult.	Difficult mask ventilation was reported in 5% of cases. Five criteria were independent risk factors and the presence of two best indicate the potential for difficulty with mask ventilation.

(continued)

TABLE 122-9 Evidence-based Medicine Key References (*continued*)

Study	Methodology	Results	Limitations	Bottom Line
RSI and airway management competency				
Sakles JC, Laurin EG, Rantapaa AA, Panacek EA. Airway management in the emergency department: a one-year study of 610 tracheal intubations. *Ann Emerg Med.* 1998;31:325–332.	Observational, consecutive series of intubations in the emergency department over a 1-year period	A total of 610 patients required airway control and 569 (93%) were intubated by Emergency Medicine residents or attendants. Rapid sequence intubation was used in 515 (84%). A total of 603 patients (98.9%) were successfully intubated. Oral tracheal intubation without paralysis was attempted in 94 patients with a success rate of 91.5% (95% CI, 84% to 96%).	Compliance rate was 88.2% requiring the authors to obtain retrospective data on 72 intubations. Self-reported data.	High success rate in the emergency department when rapid sequence intubation was used for intubation.
Reed M. Intubation training in Emergency Medicine: a review of one trainee's first 100 procedures. *Emerg Med. J* 2007;24:654–656.	Retrospective review study of the first 100 intubations by one Emergency Medicine trainee	Recorded 90 rapid sequence intubations and 10 intubations without drugs. Successful on 94 occasions with 8 complications. The complication rate improved after 30 intubations.	One trainee's experience.	Emergency Medicine residency review committee mandates 35 intubations for competency. This study supports a minimum of approximately 30 intubations to minimize complications.

LMA, laryngeal mask airway; RSI, rapid sequence intubation.

CONCLUSION

Policies regarding education, competency assessment, protocols, and quality review should be in place to maintain patient safety.

SUGGESTED READINGS

Bair AE, Filbin MR, Kulkarni RG. The failed intubation attempt in the emergency department: analysis of prevalence, rescue techniques, and personnel. *J Emerg Med.* 2002;23:131–140.

Caplan RA, Benumof JL. Practice guidelines for management of the difficult airway: an updated report by the American Society of Anesthesiologists Task Force on management of the difficult airway. *Anesth.* 2004;101:565.

Cattano D, Paniucci E, Paolicchi A, Forfori F, Giunta F, Hagberg C. Risk factors assessment of the difficult airway: an Italian survey of 1956 patients. *Anesth Analg.* 2004;99:1774–1779.

Kheterpal S, Han R, Tremper KK, et al. Incidence and predictors of difficult and impossible mask ventilation. *Anesthesiology.* 2006;105:885–891.

Masip J, Roque M, Sanchez B, Fernandez R, Subirana M, Exposito JA. Noninvasive ventilation in acute cardiogenic pulmonary edema: systematic review and meta-analysis. *JAMA.* 2005;294:3124–3130.

Pistoria M, Amin A, Dressler D, McKean S, Budnitz T. Core competencies in Hospital Medicine. *J Hosp Med.* 2006;1(S1):87.

Ram FSF, Picot J, Lightowler J, Wedzicha JA. Non-invasive positive pressure ventilation for treatment of respiratory failure due to exacerbations of chronic obstructive pulmonary disease. Cochrane Database of Systematic Reviews 2004, Issue 3. Art. No.: CD004104. DOI: 10.1002/14651858.CD004104.pub3.

Ram FSF, Wellington SR, Rowe BH, Wedzicha JA. Non-invasive positive pressure ventilation for treatment of respiratory failure due to severe acute exacerbations of asthma. Cochrane Database of Systematic Reviews 2005, Issue 3. Art. No.: CD004360. DOI: 10.1002/14651858.CD004360.pub3.

Thakkar R, Wright SM, Alguire P, Wigton RS, Boonyasai RT. Procedures performed by hospitalists and non-hospitalist. *J Gen Intern Med.* 2010;25(5):448–452.

Vital FMR, Saconato H, Ladeira MT, et al. Non-invasive positive pressure ventilation (CPAP or bilevel NPPV) for cardiogenic pulmonary edema. Cochrane Database of Systematic Reviews 2008, Issue 3. Art. No.: CD005351. DOI: 10.1002/14651858.CD005351.pub2.

CHAPTER 123

Co-management of Patients in the Emergency Department

Laurence Beer, MD, FHM
Michael A. Ross, MD, FACEP

Key Clinical Questions

1. What strategies may improve emergency department (ED) throughput and minimize ED crowding?
2. How can hospitalists and Emergency Medicine (EM) physicians collaborate to improve the care of patients boarded in the ED?
3. How can hospitalists and EM physicians improve the quality and safety of hand-offs between their departments?
4. What basic principles underlie the operation of an observation unit?

INTRODUCTION

Co-management of patients in the emergency department (ED) by Emergency Physicians and Hospital Medicine physicians has become necessary to alleviate ED crowding and optimize care of patients boarded in the ED while awaiting an inpatient bed. This chapter describes the challenge of ED crowding and how co-management strategies can improve patient flow from the ED into the hospital and improve the safety of patients who must be boarded. The chapter also examines two additional strategies for decreasing ED crowding: establishing a process for the triage of patients to appropriate services and locations within the hospital, and using ED based observation units.

EMERGENCY DEPARTMENT CROWDING

The Institute of Medicine in its 2006 report entitled *Hospital-Based Emergency Care: At the Breaking Point*[1] concluded that EDs in the United States are in crisis, with hospital crowding being the single largest contributor to long wait times and adverse clinical outcomes. Investigators have found an association between ED crowding and a higher risk of adverse cardiovascular outcomes in patients with an initial diagnosis of chest pain. Others have found that, for patients with non-ST segment elevation myocardial infarction, long ED stays are associated with decreased adherence to clinical guidelines and an increased incidence of repeat myocardial infarction. An estimated 91% of the nation's EDs are overcrowded at any given time.

The causes of ED crowding are myriad and include increased utilization, demographic changes (most significantly the aging of the population), shortages of particular types of health care providers, and changing financial trends. Most significant amongst these were increased utilization and insufficient numbers of inpatient hospital beds. From 1996 to 2006 ED visits increased 32%, from 90.3 million to 119.2 million, equating to 325,000 visits per day. During that same time the number of ED visits per 100 persons rose 18%, from 34.2 to 40.5. In 2005 approximately one-fifth of the U.S. population had visited an ED within the previous 12 months. Ironically, the increase in ED utilization has been concurrent with a decrease in the total number of EDs. From 1996 to 2006 the number of EDs in the United States declined 4.6%, from 4019 to 3833 (**Figure 123-1**).

Although increased utilization and constrained inpatient capacity are the predominant causes of ED crowding, demographic changes have also pressured ED capacity. The uninsured and the elderly, two groups of patients who tend to present with a high degree of acuity, are an increasing proportion of the patients treated in EDs. In 2006 uninsured patients accounted for 17.4% of all ED visits. In the same year patients over 75 years old were the age group with the highest per capita visit rate.

Shortages of several types of health care providers have further exacerbated the problem of ED crowding. The shortage of hospital-based nurses, estimated in July 2007 at 116,000, has left many EDs struggling to find full staffing. The well-publicized shortage of primary care physicians has left many patients with no choice but to use EDs for the initial evaluation of their medical condition, regardless of acuity. Less well publicized than nursing and primary care physician shortages is the shortage of surgeons and medical subspecialists willing to be available for calls and provide consultative or admitting services to the ED. Such physicians typically cite

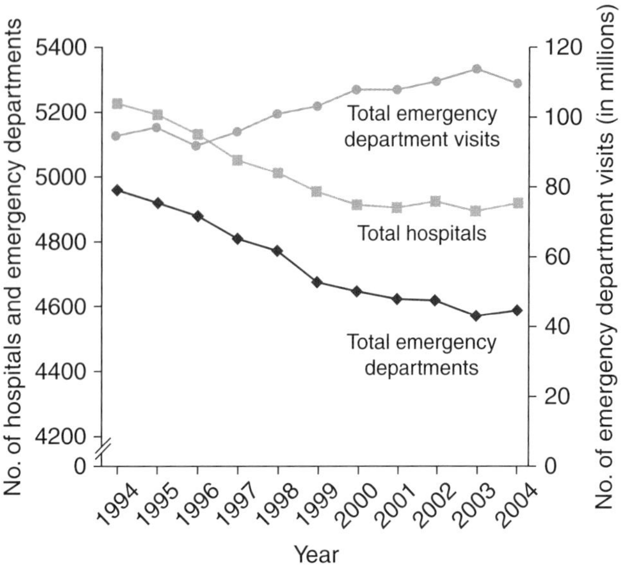

Figure 123-1 *Trends in emergency department utilization, number of hospitals, and number of emergency departments in the United States, 1994–2004. (Reproduced, with permission, from Kellermann AL. Crisis in the emergency department. N Engl J Med. 2006;355(13): 1300–1303. Copyright © 2006 Massachusetts Medical Society. All rights reserved.)*

poor compensation and the threat of increased legal liability among their reasons for avoiding covering the ED.

Staffing models have not completely accommodated the needs of EDs, now the primary portal of entry into the hospital. Most hospitals are staffed around a traditional 8 AM–5 PM, Monday through Friday model, with lower staffing during other times. Yet in 2006, 62.9% of ED visits occur outside of these hours with peak ED occupancy occurring at 7 PM. Scheduling of elective surgeries has also not evolved to accommodate ED needs. Most elective surgeries are front loaded during the week so that ancillary services such as physical and occupational therapy are available in the immediate postoperative period. This constrains operating room capacity on precisely the days that are busiest for EDs.

PRACTICE POINT

- While most hospitals are staffed around a traditional 8 AM–5 PM, Monday through Friday model, with lower staffing during other times, more than 60% of ED visits occur outside of these hours with peak ED occupancy occurring at 7 PM.

Shortages of inpatient hospital beds have paralleled those seen in EDs; high hospital census conditions limit patient flow out of the ED and hence further exacerbate ED crowding. The most frequent shortage of inpatient beds occurs in the nation's intensive care units (ICUs). One of the most frequent causes of delays in getting patients admitted from the ED is lack of ICU capacity. Across the country ICU occupancy rates at any given time are extraordinarily high, between 84% and 93% in various studies, and demand for ICU beds continues to increase. Lack of inpatient beds leads to "boarding" of admitted patients in the ED, which further restricts already constrained capacity and adversely effects clinical outcomes. The Institute of Medicine has challenged hospitals, and by extension hospitalists, to improve the flow of patients through the ED in order to eliminate ED boarding completely. Boarding and crowding have several negative consequences, including impaired flow of patients through the ED, decreased patient and provider satisfaction, poor clinical outcomes, and ambulance diversion to other less crowded EDs.

Predictably, flow of patients through the ED decreases as patient volume approaches and exceeds capacity. Under such conditions wait times for initial evaluation by a health care provider increase and the overall ED length of stay (ED LOS) increases. Although there has been significant attention to this problem over the last few years, a 2009 report by the General Accounting Office (GAO) entitled *Hospital Emergency Departments: Crowding Continues to Occur and Some Patients Wait Longer than Recommended Time Frames* illustrates that ED crowding continues as a significant issue. In 2006 patients needing *immediate care* waited an average of 28 minutes while those needing *emergent care* waited an average of 37 minutes, both exceeding time frames recommended by the National Center for Health Statistics (**Table 123-1**). In the same year the average ED LOS was 199 minutes, an increase of 12% from 178 minutes in 2001.

ED crowding also impacts overall hospital outcomes, including increased LOS and adverse events. A large, multicenter, cross-sectional study demonstrated that patients admitted to the ICU with a greater than six-hour delay in transfer from the ED had a significantly longer *hospital* length of stay and higher in-hospital mortality. In a second study increased ED LOS beyond eight hours added approximately 24 hours of total time in the hospital. Other studies have shown that patients boarded in the ED during times of crowding experience an increased number of adverse events.

EDs often resort to "diversion," the practice of alerting local emergency medical services (EMSs) that they can no longer accept patients. Several studies demonstrate that patient diversion is associated with increased mortality. Diversion also costs individual hospitals approximately $1086 per hour in lost revenue. A recent study estimates that, on average, an ambulance is diverted once every minute in the United States, roughly half a million times per year.

TABLE 123-1 Average Wait Time to See a Physician and Percentage of Visits in Which Wait Time to See a Physician Exceeded Recommended Time Frames by Acuity Level, 2006

Patient Acuity Level & Recommended Time Frame	Average Wait Time in Minutes	Percentage of Visits in which Wait Time Exceeded Recommended Time Frames
Immediate (less than 1 minute)	28	74
Emergent (1 to 14 minutes)	37	50
Urgent (15 to 60 minutes)	50	21
Semiurgent (greater than 1 to 2 hours)	68	13
Nonurgent (greater than 2 to 24 hours)	76	N/A

Data from GAO analysis of data from HHS's National Center for Health Statistics (NCHS), 2006.

PRACTICE POINT

- The Institute of Medicine has challenged hospitals, and by extension hospitalists, to improve the flow of patients through the ED in order to reduce ED crowding and eliminate ED boarding. Boarding leads to slower flow of patients through the ED, decreased patient satisfaction, and inferior outcomes. Extended delays in transfer from the ED to inpatient medical units are associated with increased length of hospital stay and increased adverse events.

REGULATORY AND PROFESSIONAL PRESSURES

Various regulatory and professional pressures on EM physicians may affect their clinical practice and also contribute to ED crowding, affecting patient flow within hospitals. Regulatory pressures include the Emergency Medical Treatment and Active Labor Act (EMTALA). EMTALA requires EDs, EM physicians, and on-call physicians covering EDs to provide a screening examination to any individual who presents to an ED and requests examination or treatment. A patient found to have an emergent condition must be treated until stabilized or transferred to another facility to receive treatment. According to EMTALA an emergency medical condition means a medical condition manifesting itself by acute symptoms of sufficient severity (including severe pain) such that the absence of immediate medical attention could reasonably be expected to result in placing the health of the individual (or, with respect to a pregnant woman, the health of the woman or her unborn child) in serious jeopardy, serious impairment to bodily functions, or serious dysfunction of any bodily organ or part.

Professional pressures affecting ED physicians include professional organization expectations, public expectations, and legal risks. The American College of Emergency Physicians (ACEP) Emergency Medicine Physician Performance Measure Set holds EM physicians accountable to consensus guidelines for a number of disease states. They address quality measures, such as aspirin on arrival for acute myocardial infarction, electrocardiogram (ECG) for syncope, and oxygen saturation (SpO_2) evaluation and empiric antibiotics for community-acquired pneumonia (CAP). The Prudent Layperson Standard (advocated by ACEP) suggests that health care coverage in EDs should be based not on diagnosis but on symptoms since the public cannot be expected to self-diagnose. High legal liability occurs in the United States compared with other English-speaking nations. Compared with the United Kingdom and Australia, the United States has 50% more medical liability claims and 350% more than Canada. Unlike Australia the United States lacks federal policies that protect physicians from litigation, even for those patients covered under EMTALA.

IMPROVING PATIENT FLOW THROUGH THE EMERGENCY DEPARTMENT

In order to identify strategies for minimizing ED crowding patient flow can be categorized into three stages: input, throughput, and output (**Table 123-2**). Hospitalists should lead collaborative efforts to improve flow through the ED and can impact various aspects of the input-throughput-output model. Since they are increasingly tasked with admitting from outpatient clinics, hospitalists can diminish ED input by selecting appropriate patients for direct admission, bypassing the ED entirely. When asked to admit from the ED, hospitalists can improve throughput by assisting EM physicians with selection of specific diagnostic tests needed to determine disposition and with triage to the most appropriate level of care. Even when they are not asked to admit, hospitalists can offer their services as consultants to assist EM physicians in developing a care plan, including initiating directed treatment or specifying optimal follow-up for patients who may not require admission. At the output stage hospitalists can standardize and streamline their admission processes and policies. They should be well versed with national as well as institution-specific admission guidelines. Hospitalist and EM leaders should partner to provide ongoing education for physicians within their departments regarding accepted guidelines and clinical care practices.

TABLE 123-2 Stages of Patient Flow Through the Emergency Department

Input	Throughput	Output
Clinic referrals Ambulance drop-offs Walk-ins Help lines	Triage Immediate assessment Stabilization Lab turnaround Radiology turnaround Reassessment Development of treatment plan Response time of consultants	Admission procedures Signout to admitting service Referals to outpatient clinics Transfer to another facility LWBS AMA Death

AMA, left against medical advice; LWBS, left without being seen.

HOSPITALIST-BASED STUDIES

Interventions directed at the ED output stage—facilitation of transfer to the appropriate inpatient level of care and proper service—have shown compelling results. In one intervention known as active bed management, a bed manager role (staffed by a hospitalist) was created to allow broad authority to assign admissions to the Department of Medicine. The bed manager conducted twice daily "prediversion rounds" in the ICU to identify bed shortages, made regular visits to the ED to assess congestion, and in consultation with EM physicians helped coordinate transfer to the appropriate hospital location. EM physicians were asked to write holding orders for patients accepted but not yet admitted. In addition, a senior hospitalist (bed director) worked to adjust hospitalist physician staffing and coordinate acceptance of patients by specialty services when the ED either began to experience excessive patient time in the department or when it went on diversion. Using these strategies, throughput for admitted patients improved on average by 98 minutes per patient, and diversion due to lack of ICU beds decreased by 27%. Institution-specific needs and current models of care and flow would affect the value of such a model at other institutions, but some organizations may benefit from a bed manager role to improve ED flow.

EMERGENCY MEDICINE–BASED STUDIES

EM-led interventions targeting the throughput stage have met with mixed results. The utilization of a triage liaison an EM physician hired to evaluate patients in the triage area, traditionally the domain of triage nurses—decreased ED LOS by an average of 36 minutes. Left-without-being-seen (LWOBS) dropped from 6.6% to 5.4% (a 20% reduction). However, time spent on ambulance diversion did not change. The duties of the triage liaison included answering incoming calls from physicians, assisting the triage nurse, assessing ambulance patients, ordering diagnostic tests, and occasionally starting directed treatment.

Another EM-led initiative entitled the Rapid Admission Policy eliminates two constraints on output: the need for patients to be seen by accepting physicians in the ED and the requirement that all diagnostic tests be completed before admission. Under this protocol once EM physicians determined that admission was necessary, a consensus inpatient location was decided upon in collaboration with the admitting physician, and the ED physician was tasked with writing brief holding orders. Once holding orders were complete, admission could not be delayed assuming a bed was available. As a result ED LOS dropped by 10.1 minutes, which, although seemingly a small improvement, actually decreased weekly minutes on diversion by 169 minutes (65%) and increased facility charges by 3.2%.

At a busy Canadian hospital a full-capacity protocol ("surge plan") was implemented to admit low-acuity patients boarded in the ED to inpatient hallways, thereby spreading the burden of boarding among different services and locations within the hospital. EM physicians coordinated with the admitting physician (usually a hospitalist) the decision about which patients to admit to floor hallway spots. Using this protocol ED LOS was reduced by five hours per patient. Inpatient hallway boarders had a *hospital LOS* one day less than their counterparts boarded in the ED; and ICU transfers and mortality were higher for patients admitted to traditional beds (hospital rooms) than for those boarded in hallway spots. However, these latter findings likely reflect selection bias rather than a clinical benefit of hallway boarding.

Based on these studies and others ACEP in 2008 identified several hospital-based solutions for ED crowding, which are likely to involve hospitalists. They have categorized these solutions into those that they consider highly effective, those that may have some efficacy, and those that have been proven ineffective (**Table 123-3**).

TABLE 123-3 "High-Impact Solutions" for Emergency Department Crowding Recommended by the American College of Emergency Physicians (ACEP) Boarding Task Force

Highly effective
Using a "full-capacity protocol" where the burden of boarding patients is shared between Emergency Medicine and Hospital Medicine departments
Coordinating discharge as early as possible in the day, preferably before noon
Possibly effective
Education programs to create institutional awareness of the dangers of ED crowding and boarding
Matching staffing to the needs of the ED, predominantly outside of traditional work hours and moving toward a 24/7 operational culture
Observation units (which may be run by EM physicians, hospitalists, or both)
Involving an EM physician or hospitalist in the ED triage process
Defining response times for both initiation and completion of consultations in the ED
Use of a whiteboard at the head of each hospitalized patient's bed that outlines what steps need to be taken before they can be discharged (as advocated by the Institute for Health care Improvement)
Have all inpatient services managed by hospitalists in order to decrease lenth of stay and eliminate time-consuming "ping-ponging" of responsibility for ED patients between different services
Hire a "Bed Czar" who has authority over all hospital bed use and is responsible for timely matching of bed needs to resources.
The use of a generic holding order admission set by EM physicians
Not effective
"Discharge lounges", specified holding areas on inpatient units for patients awaiting discharge

Data from Emergency Department Crowding: High-Impact Solutions. ACEP Boarding Task Force, July 2008.

OTHER POTENTIAL SOLUTIONS

Another valuable opportunity to improve coordination of care between the ED physicians and hospitalists arises from the Emergency Severity Index (ESI).[2] The ESI is a validated triage algorithm championed by the Agency for Health Research and Quality (AHRQ) that provides stratification of patients into five groups from 1 (most urgent) to 5 (least urgent) on the basis of acuity. It was designed specifically to improve reliability and validity of triage decision making in the ED, has high interrater reliability, and has been correlated to resource utilization and mortality. This tool has been shown to be an excellent predictor of both hospital admission and ICU admission (**Table 123-4**).

Admitting hospitalists and hospitalist bed managers can use this ESI acuity scale to anticipate floor bed and ICU bed needs. Many EDs report the ESI score on ED electronic patient boards. EM physicians can likewise alert hospitalist leadership when a large number of patients with ESI levels 1 through 3 patients are pending evaluation.

Recently, medical informatics companies have turned their attention to the issue of active bed management. Some products provide real-time assessment of bed availability and allow for more efficient patient flow and increased patient safety. Such systems typically use enterprise-wide electronic bed boards, similar to what is seen in many EDs, and simple color coding to indicate which rooms are available, occupied, or need to be cleaned. Such systems may improve overall inpatient flow of patients, and in turn ED flow.

MANAGING PATIENTS BOARDED IN THE EMERGENCY DEPARTMENT

Patients who require admission but have not left the ED due to hospital space constraints or bed availability limitations are considered "boarded" in the ED. The number of boarded patients within the ED typically increases with a higher ED census when ED staff members have to prioritize their attention to the most acute patients and to those without a care plan. Because boarded patients are physically distant from their provider of record (admitting physician), and because the "ownership" or responsibility for caring for the boarded patients is generally poorly delineated, boarded patients may receive less than optimal care. Boarders may negatively impact the care of other patients by consuming limited physical and personnel

TABLE 123-4 Emergency Severity Index (ESI) Score and Admission Risk

ESI Level	Risk of Hospital Admission	Risk of ICU Admission
1	80%	40%
2	73%	12%
3	51%	Negligible
4	Negligible	Negligible
5	Negligible	Negligible

Emergency Severity Index, Version 4. ESI Triage Research Team, 2004.

TABLE 125-5 Strategies for Improving Hand-off Communication Between Emergency Medicine and Hospital Medicine

1. Emergency Medicine (EM) and hospitalist leadership should demonstrate best practices for hand-offs
2. Leadership in both disciplines should observe physicians in their department and provide structured feedback on the quality of hand-off. Consider recording hand-offs for quality improvement (QI) review.
3. Vital signs should be rechecked at regular intervals while patients are boarded, consistent with protocol for their intended floor location.
4. Orders written in the emergency department (ED) should be readily available for hospitalists to review in the electronic medical record (EMR).
5. Formalized structured feedback should occur:

   Such feedback to EM physicians should occur expediently when adverse events occur in patients transferred to the hospitalist service. Investigators found that EM physicians were *aware of* adverse events in only 14% of the patients they admitted; yet hospitalists identified adverse events in 39% of the same patients.

   Similarly, EM physicians should provide feedback to hospitalists when patients are unexpectedly readmitted or when adverse events occur in boarded patients.
6. The Joint Commission's 2007 National Patient Safety Goals require that hospitals develop standardized hand-off tools. These tools should be service-specific to meet their needs. Content should be formalized in the form of a checklist. This helps sets expectations and provides a way to measure process. Consider including degree of certainty in diagnosis as part of the hand-off.
7. Clearly delineate the responsibility for follow-up of *pending tests results*. Results may only become available after shift change, leaving a new physician responsible. Pending test results must be part of intraservice as well as interservice hand-off. Minimize asking EM physicians to order additional tests before patient transfer to the floor as it creates ambiguity about who is responsible for the results.
8. Critical test results should be called to the clinician of record and not the ordering clinician, who may be off service. If results are called to wrong clinician, they must be redirected. This necessitates that the clinician of record is easily identified in the medical record.
9. Hospitalist changes of shift for boarded patients should be communicated to ED staff expediently.
10. Responsibilities for boarded patients should be specified at the institutional level with written policy.
11. A second hand-off should occur at the time of transfer to an inpatient unit, if the initial hand-off information was transmitted at a time distant to patient's physical movement to an inpatient bed.
12. Address hand-off problems immediately.
13. Pay particular attention to patients requiring continuing evaluation and treatment such as patients with diabetic ketoacidosis (DKA), bronchospasm, alcohol withdrawal, and hypertensive urgencies and emergencies.
14. Prioritize getting boarders out of the ED to their inpatient units.
15. Be especially cautious of hand-off difficulties that may occur when patients move from the ED first to another department (such as radiology or dialysis) prior to the inpatient unit.
16. Consider a dedicated hospitalist admitter or admission team that has no inpatient responsibilities.
17. Consider ED rotations for hospitalists and hospitalist rotations for EM physicians.

resources. Since the majority of admissions through EDs are for medical conditions, the majority of boarded patients are typically admitted to hospitalists who thus have a vested interest in addressing the problems of ED crowding and boarding.

IMPROVING COMMUNICATION

While hospitals strive to eliminate the practice of ED boarding, hospitalists can take steps to minimize boarding and improve the care of these patients. In collaboration with the ED staff, hospitalists can develop protocols that improve their care and standardize communication during a critical transition or hand-off of care from the ED to the inpatient setting. According to The Joint Commission, problematic communication is the root cause of most medical errors, adverse events, near misses, and sentinel events.

Researchers have identified several factors that can degrade the quality of the emergency physician-hospitalist hand off process:

1. Physicians from both disciplines tend to allocate inadequate time for hand-off.
2. Based on their differing needs, EM physicians and hospitalists have very different expectations for hand-off communication.
3. Hand-off occurs in a chaotic, crowded setting that is full of distractions (eg, consultant phone calls, ambulance deliveries, codes).
4. Hand-off may occur several times on a single patient when hospitalists and EM physicians change shifts or when housestaff are involved.
5. Group affiliation, which leads physicians to conform to the opinion and behavior of others within their own specialty, causes communication between specialties to require extra effort.
6. In-group and out-group biases engender mistrust.
7. Hierarchical relational issues exist between attending physicians and house staff and between senior and junior staff.

This and other research has led to several potential strategies for improving communication between hospitalist and EM providers (**Table 123-5**).

TRIAGE

The term *triage* originates from the French verb *trier*, meaning to sort. Its medical usage dates from the Napoleanic Wars when a *Hôpital de Triage* was employed as a sorting station for injured soldiers. In modern hospitals triage is the process of determining the most appropriate disposition for a patient based on the nature and severity of their illness and on hospital resources. Triage typically includes a decision about whether to admit a patient to the hospital and if so, to which clinical area and service (eg, Hospital Medicine, Surgery).

Triage complexity increases with increasing illness severity; thus patients being considered for ICU admission can present a particular challenge. Nationally accepted guidelines for ICU admission do not exist, and mortality prediction models such as the Acute Physiology and Chronic Health Evaluation IV (APACHE IV), Mortality Probability Models II (MPM II), and Simplified Acute Physiology Score (SAPS II) unfortunately have poor utility in predicting which patients should be admitted to an ICU, since all of these prognostic models were developed based on patients already in the ICU.

The most widely used framework for determining the appropriateness of ICU admission is based on the *Society of Critical Care Medicine's (SCCM) Guidelines for intensive care unit admission, discharge, and triage*, published in 1999. These guidelines implicitly acknowledge the difficulties in triaging critically ill patients by proposing three different models based on patient prioritization, diagnosis, or objective parameters. The *prioritization model* divides patients into four categories: those who need intensive monitoring and treatment (most often those requiring vasoactive drugs or mechanical ventilation), those who need intensive monitoring and *may* need immediate intervention, patients who are unstable but have a reduced likelihood of recovery, and those who are too well or too sick to benefit from intensive interventions.

Whatever model or combination thereof is used, explicit written institutional policies must exist in order to avoid confusion and to encourage consistency of practice. These policies should be made public and discussed with critically ill patients or their surrogates. Administration, nurses, support staff, and physicians should collaborate on institution-specific policies regarding ICU use. Overflow policies must also be clearly defined and readily available. The hospital should assign triage responsibilities to a single individual, with performance overseen by a multidisciplinary critical care committee. This committee should have oversight of all of the hospital's ICUs and their directors and should regularly review ICU denials and ICU rapid return or rapid readmission patients.

The Ethics Committee of SCCM in their *Consensus Statement on the Triage of Critically Ill Patients* states that providers of critical care must use some moral framework for distributing limited resources efficiently and equitably, since demand will frequently exceed supply. By necessity, in an equitable system ICU care must be restricted. Decisions should be based on the concept of medical justice, such that limited resources are allocated to those most likely to benefit from their use. Such patients should have a reasonable expectation of *substantial* recovery, as recommend by the *Consensus Statement*. Patients who are not expected to benefit should be excluded. That includes both the too-well-to-benefit and too-sick-to-benefit categories. The too-sick-to-benefit category includes not only those with end-stage chronic disease but those with irreversible conditions such as metastatic cancer unresponsive to chemotherapy, severe ischemic or anoxic brain damage, and irreversible multiorgan failure. When a patient has become critically ill with a chronic disease the desirability of ICU care should be discussed with the ICU director, the EM physician, and the patient's family at the time of initial presentation. This discussion should include specific reference to triage policies.

The role of the ICU director, often a critical care trained intensivist, should be separated from that of the triage clinician as much as possible to avoid conflicts of interest. SCCM also recommends that the ICU director have no other clinical responsibilities.

TRIAGE OF SURGICAL PATIENTS

For the sake of expediency hospitalists are sometimes asked to fill the gaps when providers in certain specialties are not immediately available or responsive to ED needs. Particularly common is the request by EM physicians to hospitalists to admit patients with surgical problems. Despite the increasing trend for such admissions, hospitalists often fear legal liability when managing patients with a primary surgical diagnosis. Hence, triage decisions for patients potentially needing surgery should follow the simple principle of placing the patient on the service where the patient will receive the most appropriate care. Oftentimes, this determination can only be made once both surgeons and hospitalists have made an in-person evaluation of the patient. In addition, the role of nursing should not be overlooked. Patients with a primary surgical diagnosis may benefit more from the care provided by surgical nurses, irrespective of who is the attending of record. Likewise, patients with a primary medical diagnosis driving admission may benefit more from the care provided by medical nurses, even if it is anticipated that they will eventually require surgery.

When the decision is made for a patient to be co-managed by surgery and Hospital Medicine, roles and responsibilities of each service must be agreed upon at the outset of care. Are the patients going to be truly co-managed where each service has the authority to write orders? or is one service or the other going to act strictly as a consultant making recommendations only? Hospital policies for the delineation of responsibilities for such patients are essential. A case-by-case approach burdens the EM physician with multiple phone calls and slows throughput. One solution that may permit more immediate evaluation and management by surgeons involves use of acute care surgeons (surgeons who spend their time caring for hospitalized patients, sometimes called surgical hospitalists or surgicalists).

CASE 123-1

A 68-year-old male with a past medical history of hypertension, type 2 diabetes, coronary artery disease, chronic obstructive pulmonary disease, and morbid obesity presented to the ED with vague abdominal pain, nausea, vomiting, cough, and a subjective fever. Vital signs included a temperature of 37.8°C, blood pressure 110/72 mm Hg, heart rate 94 beats per minuute, respiratory rate 20, and pulse oximetry 90% on room air. Physical exam revealed bilateral end-expiratory wheezing. Bowel sounds were high pitched and the abdomen was diffusely tender. Laboratory abnormalities included a blood urea nitrogen (BUN) of 32 mg/dL and a creatinine of 1.4 mg/dL, bicarbonate of mEq/L, and a white count elevated at 14,200/mm^3 with a differential of 91% neutrophils. Liver function tests and lipase are within normal limits. A chest X-ray was reportedly negative, but limited due to the patient's body habitus and an anteroposterior view. An abdominal computed tomographic (CT) scan was pending. The EM physician decided to admit the patient for hypoxia and leukocytosis, possibly pneumonia or chronic obstructive pulmonary disease (COPD) exacerbation. The admitting physician was concerned that the patient might have an acute abdomen, perhaps secondary to ischemic gut, and may need surgical intervention. He asks the ED MD to hold the patient in the ED pending the CT results. The ED MD responded that the ER was very busy and that this patient was stable enough to complete his workup on the floor.

Questions to consider:

1. If the patient is kept in the ED in order to get the CT scan, would the results change the unit the patient goes to? Would it change which service ultimately admits the patient? Would this patient remain on the medical service even with a presumptive diagnosis of ischemic gut because of his multiple comorbidities? How will a prolonged ED LOS affect this patient's care, the care of other patients in the ED, or the possibility of diversion? If the patient remained in the ED who will be responsible for following up on the results of the CT scan? Who will be responsible for consulting surgery if the patient does require it?

2. Would this patient get his CT scan as quickly on the floor as he would have in the ED?
3. Would surgeons respond to a request for consultation from a floor physician as quickly as they would to a similar request from an ED physician?
4. Is it possible that a delay in getting the CT scan done coupled with a delay in getting a surgical consultation completed would adversely affect this patient's outcome?

DISEASE-SPECIFIC CONSIDERATIONS

Disease-specific prediction models are more accurate than general guidelines in predicting need for ICU admission. Specific criteria exist only for a few medical conditions, such as gastrointestinal hemorrhage (the BLEED criteria) and pneumonia (CURB-65, Pneumonia Severity Index, SCAP score). A hospitalist should incorporate these prognostic criteria or guidelines into practice when applicable. Sepsis remains a common and life-threatening reason for presentation to the ED. Extremely common, simple sepsis is associated with low to moderate mortality risk (~16%), and may require ICU admission at presentation, but in many cases may be safely managed in the non–critical care setting. On the other hand, severe sepsis (sepsis associated with end-organ damage or hypotension) and septic shock (severe sepsis with hypotension and tissue hypoperfusion unresponsive to significant volume challenges) have an associated mortality of approximately 30% and 50%, respectively. These latter two groups of patients have unstable physiologic or hemodynamic parameters and should be admitted to the ICU, barring unusual circumstances.

OBSERVATION UNITS

The Institute of Medicine's 2007 report, *The Future of Emergency Care: Hospital Based Emergency Care at the Breaking Point*, offers several suggestions to improve the efficiency of hospital-based emergency care. The use of "Observation Units" or "Clinical Decision Units" to manage patients following their initial ED evaluation allows additional time to perform diagnostic studies or discreet time-limited management according to specific entry criteria. Such additional time can help determine the need for inpatient admission or early discharge.

PRACTICE POINT

- Observation patients are defined by the Centers for Medicare and Medicaid Services (CMS) as those patients needing further evaluation "to determine the need for inpatient admission." CMS explicitly states that most patients will require less than 24 hours to reach this goal.

Observation patients are defined by the Centers for Medicare and Medicaid Services (CMS) as those patients needing further evaluation "to determine the need for inpatient admission." CMS explicitly states that most patients will require less than 24 hours to reach this goal. Alternatively, admission review guidelines such as those published by InterQual define inpatient or observation status. By design InterQual guidelines review patient criteria for admission on a retrospective basis, whereas the CMS policy evaluates patient admission criteria prospectively. Observation patients may be best understood when considering patient lengths of stay. The Centers for Disease Control and Prevention (CDC) has reported that admitted ED patients will spend roughly five hours in the ED. Hospitals are often scrutinized for inpatient admission of one day or less, as many of those patients should have been classified as "observation" status, even though they occupy an inpatient bed.

There remains a distinct group of ED patients who clearly need more than 5 hours, but less than 24 hours, to address their clinical needs. These are the "6- to 24-hour" patients. Several prospective, randomized, controlled trials have shown that the length of stay and costs of these patients will double or triple if they are admitted to a traditional inpatient ward rather than an observation unit. Such patients will exacerbate ED overcrowding if they complete their evaluation in the ED, and they cannot be discharged without potential risks. A dedicated observation unit for appropriately selected patients can improve patient satisfaction, lower rates of missed myocardial infarction, lower diagnostic uncertainty, decrease ED and hospital overcrowding, improve diagnostic test completion rates, and maintain clinical outcomes comparable to those for patients admitted to the hospital.

PRACTICE POINT

- A dedicated observation unit for appropriately selected patients can improve patient satisfaction, lower rates of missed myocardial infarction, lower diagnostic uncertainty, decrease emergency department and hospital overcrowding, improve diagnostic test completion rates, and maintain clinical outcomes comparable to those for patients admitted to the hospital.

While observation units have been around nearly as long as EDs, it is only in the last two decades that protocol-driven units have been described. Initially units were primarily focused on patients with chest pain, subsequently giving rise to "chest pain centers." Based on clinical studies, observation units have expanded into protocols for asthma, syncope, heart failure, atrial fibrillation, and transient ischemic attacks. By design observation units are also well equipped to manage patients with dehydration, abdominal pain, renal colic, and a variety of infections. Nationally, 31% of U.S. hospitals either utilize or plan to implement an observation unit. The observation unit truly represents an interface between EM and Hospital Medicine. Fifty-three percent of observation units are geographically located within or adjacent to the ED, with the remainder either in the hospital or in both locations. Admission privileges to the unit may be "open" to any hospital physician, or "closed" and limited to only one specialty group. That group may be the EM group or Hospital Medicine group, depending on local practices. Regardless of the model, Hospital Medicine and EM need to collaborate to optimize clinical care and patient flow. Some units operate as a "hybrid" unit, caring for observation patients as well as scheduling outpatient procedure patients. This model offers the advantage of a more robust unit census, with observation patients filling the unit during the evening hours, and scheduled procedure patients filling the unit during daytime hours. This model has also been shown to improve nurse utilization for a smaller unit (3.7 vs 2.5 patients/nurse/hour).

Basic principles for the operation of an observation unit have been described by ACEP. Because the unit is designed for this specific patient population, its use should ideally be limited to patients with a well-defined reason for observation, or a working diagnosis or condition. That condition may involve a diagnostic evaluation for a potentially serious diagnosis, therapy of an acute medical condition, or management of acute psychosocial needs. Diagnostic conditions should represent a balance between the potential morbidity and mortality of the condition and the probability that the condition will be confirmed. For example, evaluation of patients with chest pain for possible acute coronary syndrome (ACS), which (if diagnosed) bears a 25% short-term adverse outcome likelihood, is often limited to patients with lower probability of disease (7% or less).

The patient's severity of illness and intensity of service requirements should be low enough to match the resources available in the observation unit. Patients actively managed in observation units have an average length of stay of 15 hours. Units are often located within or adjacent to the ED since most patients arrive from the ED. When units are remote from the ED, it becomes logistically difficult for ED physicians to participate in the care of the patient. On average, observation units are staffed with one nurse per four patients, and 20% of such units employ nurse practitioners or physician assistants. Care is best facilitated through the use of guidelines for both unit operations and the management of specific conditions developed through background research and collaboration with other relevant departments. Condition guidelines often include inclusion and exclusion criteria, interventions permitted in the observation unit, and criteria for discharge or hospital admission. From these guidelines, protocol orders may be developed. Since the observation unit functions as a limited resource within the facility and may be used as an alternative to admission, its use, processes, and outcomes require intensive and frequent review for utilization and quality. Utilization may include census, case mix, length of stay, and admission rate. Quality audits may include protocol use rates, patient satisfaction, ED or hospital return visits, hospital admission rates, ICU admission rates, and mortality. Finally the observation unit should remain cost effective and efficient for the hospital, providers, and patients.

CONCLUSION

ED crowding has become a challenging feature of the landscape of U.S. health care. The need to improve patient flow through the ED in order to alleviate crowding and minimize the practices of boarding and diversion has led EM physicians and hospitalists alike to search for solutions. This search has brought increased awareness of the need for improved communication and greater coordination of care. Several strategies to improve ED throughput include development and use of transparent and readily available guidelines for the triage of surgical and critically ill patients and the use of ED based observation units. In the event that patients do become boarded in the ED, this chapter provides suggestions for how to effectively co-manage patients until they can be placed in inpatient beds.

SUGGESTED READINGS

American College of Emergency Physicians Task Force Report on Boarding. Emergency department crowding: high-impact solutions. Irving, TX: American College of Emergency Physicians; 2008.

Full Capacity Protocol. Hospital Overcrowding website. http://hospitalovercrowding.com/policyFCPword.doc. Accessed June 19, 2010.

Guidelines for intensive care unit admission discharge and triage. Society of Critical Care Medicine Task Force of American College of Critical Care Medicine, Society of Critical Care Medicine. *Crit Care Med.* 1999;27:633–638.

Howell E, Bessman E, Kravet S, et al. Active bed management by hospitalists and emergency department throughput. *Ann Intern Med.* 2008;149:804–811.

Management of observation units. American College of Emergency Physicians. *Ann Emerg Med.* 1988;17(12):1348–1352.

Quinn JV, Mahadevan SV, Eggers G, et al. Effects of implementing a rapid admission policy in the ED. *Am J Emerg Med.* 2007;25(5): 559–563.

Ross MA, Graff LGt. Principles of observation medicine. *Emerg Med Clin North Am.* 2001;19(1):1–17.

Society of Critical Care Medicine Ethics Committee. Consensus statement on the triage of critically ill patients. *JAMA.* 1994;271: 1200–1203.

The National Report Card on the State of Emergency Medicine, American College of Emergency Physicians. (2009).

REFERENCES

1. Institute of Medicine. Committee on the Future of Emergency Care in the United States Health System. *Hospital-Based Emergency Care: At the Breaking Point.* Washington, DC: National Academies Pr; 2007.
2. Gilboy N, Tanabe P, Travers DA, et al. *Emergency Severity Index, Version 4. Implementation Handbook.*, Rockville, MD: Agency for Healthcare Research and Quality; 2005. http://www.ahrq.gov/research/esi/. Accessed July 9, 2010.

SECTION 2

Cardiovascular Medicine

CHAPTER 124

Acute Coronary Syndromes

Brian G. Hynes, MB, BCh, BAO, MRCPI
Deepak L. Bhatt, MD, MPH, FACP

Key Clinical Questions

1. What are the available tools to diagnose and risk stratify patients with suspected acute coronary syndrome (ACS)?
2. What are the American College of Cardiology and American Heart Association (ACC/AHA) class I guideline recommendations for anti-ischemia and antithrombotic therapy for unstable angina (UA) and non-ST-elevation myocardial infarction (NSTEMI)? For STEMI? Which drugs reduce mortality?
3. What are the benefits of an invasive versus a conservative strategy for managing UA/NSTEMI?
4. Which patients should undergo early invasive therapy in the setting of ACS?

INTRODUCTION

The term *acute coronary syndrome* (ACS) refers to a group of clinical symptoms consistent with acute myocardial ischemia, whether from unstable angina (UA), non-ST-segment elevation myocardial infarction (NSTEMI), or ST-segment elevation myocardial infarction (STEMI). The definition of STEMI is based on the electrocardiographic (ECG) criteria of ST-segment elevation, and this diagnosis accounts for 330,000 hospital admissions per year in the United Sstates. The definition of NSTEMI is based on the absence of ST-segment elevations on the ECG, but ST depression and T-wave inversions may be evident, and there is sufficient ischemic damage to cause biochemical evidence of myonecrosis. NSTEMI accounts for 570,000 hospital admissions per year. UA and NSTEMI have similar pathogenesis and clinical presentations, but UA is not associated with release of cardiac troponins and/or creatine kinase (CK-MB). UA accounts for 670,000 admissions per year. According to the American Heart Association (AHA), an estimated $177 billion has been spent on the treatment of coronary heart disease in 2010.

Although tremendous strides have been made in the management of cardiovascular disease, coronary heart disease currently accounts for almost 20% of deaths in the United States. The 30-day mortality associated with the diagnosis of ACS varies from 1.7% for patients with UA to 7.4% for patients with NSTEMI to 11.1% for those with STEMI.

Despite chest pain pathways to guide clinicians in risk stratification, approximately 5% of symptomatic patients with myocardial infarction are inappropriately discharged from the emergency department to the outpatient setting. In addition, nearly 50% of all myocardial infarctions (MIs) produce no symptoms.

This chapter will focus on patients diagnosed with ACS, encompassing STEMI, NSTEMI, and UA, and review the best medical evidence based on the latest pertinent clinical trials reporting diagnosis and management of ACS. Recommendations will be referenced according to the American College of Cardiology (ACC)/AHA guidelines for the management of patients with STEMI and UA/NSTEMI along with the 2007 focused update of these guidelines. This chapter will not review the rapid rule-out protocols for the more than 75% of 5 million patients who present to emergency departments in the United States annually and have no evidence of ACS. Noncardiac chest pain and chronic stable angina are covered elsewhere in this book (Specific treatments/interventions may be described in relation to ACC/AHA guideline recommendations as per the class scheme explained in **Table 124-1**).

PATHOPHYSIOLOGY

The key event in the vast majority of ACS presentations concerns the abrupt disruption of a preexisting fibrous plaque involving primarily the intima of large- and medium-sized coronary arteries. Coronary artery thrombosis may result from complete plaque rupture, superficial plaque erosion, or a calcified plaque nodule. The exact mechanisms whereby a previously stable plaque is rendered "unstable" are not fully understood, but a key role for

TABLE 124-1 Applying Classification of Recommendations and Level of Evidence

Class I	Class IIa	Class IIb	Class III
Benefit >>> Risk	*Benefit >> Risk*	*Benefit ≥ Risk*	*Risk ≥ Benefit*
	Additional studies with focused objectives needed	*Additional studies with broad objectives needed; additional registry data would be helpful*	*No additional studies needed*
Procedure/Treatment **SHOULD** be performed/ administered	**IT IS REASONABLE** to perform procedure/administer treatment	Procedure/Treatment **MAY BE CONSIDERED**	Procedure/Treatment should **NOT** be performed/administered **SINCE IT IS NOT HELPFUL AND MAY BE HARMFUL**
should is recommended is indicated is useful/effective/ beneficial	is reasonable can be useful/ effective/ beneficial is probably recommended or indicated	may/might be considered may/might be reasonable usefulness/effectiveness is unknown/unclear/uncertain or not well established	is not recommended is not indicated should not is not useful/effective/beneficial may be harmful

inflammatory cells has been advanced in the development of thin-cap fibroatheroma located predominantly in the proximal and mid sections of the three major coronary arteries and, importantly, within areas of < 50% arterial stenosis. Accurately predicting vulnerable plaques in the clinical setting is difficult because plaque composition rather than size affects both the likelihood of rupture and the exposure of prothrombotic material such as cholesterol, collagen, and fibrin to platelets, and coagulation cascade elements to the endothelium.

Transmural ischemia from occlusion of a coronary thrombus causes STEMI; whereas nonoccluding thrombus leads to UA or NSTEMI (**Figure 124-1**).

UA and NSTEMI often arise from a combination of potential mechanisms, including the following:

1. **Decreased blood delivery to the downstream myocardium**, often due to a partially occlusive thrombus overlying a disrupted atherosclerotic plaque, from microembolization of thrombus and plaque debris with resulting blockage of the distal microcirculation
2. **Fixed severe narrowing** caused by progressive atherosclerosis or in-stent restenosis resulting in sufficient collateral blood flow around the stenosis to prevent transmural infarction when a fully occlusive thrombosis occurs
3. **Dynamic obstruction** caused by intense vasospasm, often referred to as Printzmetal angina, cocaine-induced vasoconstriction, or other causes of vasoconstriction
4. **Inflammatory or infectious initiators** of arterial narrowing, plaque rupture, and/or thrombogenesis
5. **Increased myocardial oxygen demand** (fever, tachycardia, hyperthyroidism, and other hyperadrenergic states, elevations of left ventricular afterload from hypertension, severe aortic stenosis, hypertrophic cardiomyopathy) and **reduced myocardial oxygen delivery** (anemia, hypoxemia, hypotension) despite normal coronary arteries

Spontaneous coronary artery dissection is a rare cause of ACS and is often linked with hormonal imbalance in connection with pregnancy, connective tissue disorders such as Marfan and Ehlers-Danlos syndromes, or with thoracic aortic dissection.

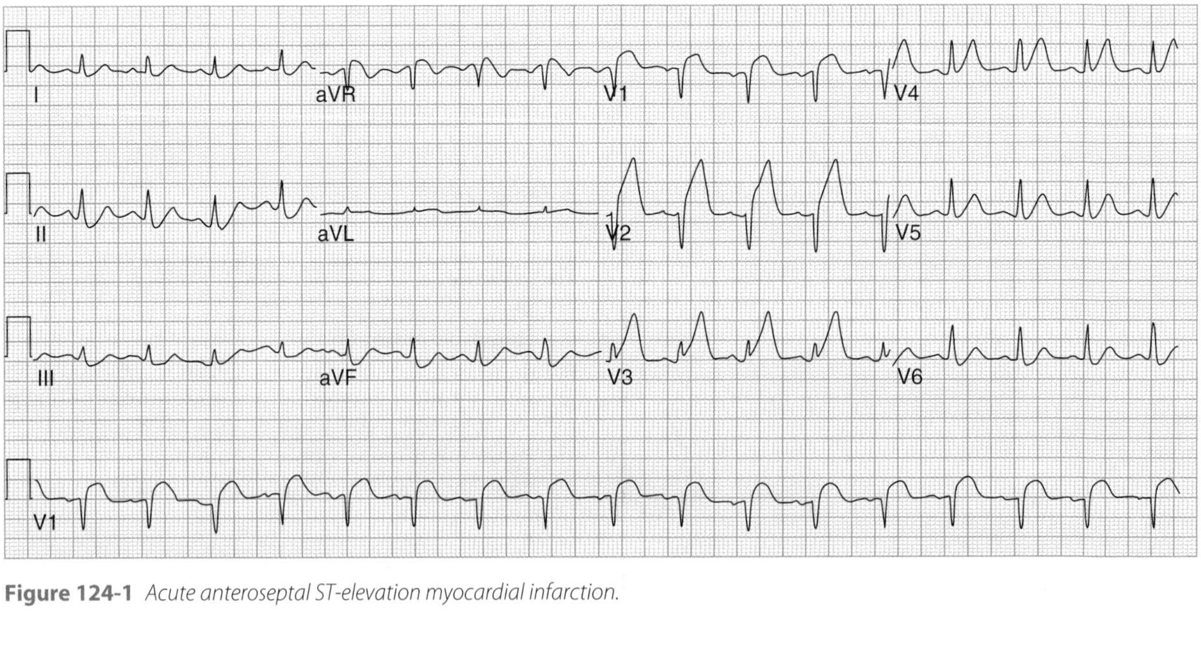

Figure 124-1 *Acute anteroseptal ST-elevation myocardial infarction.*

DIAGNOSIS

The 2007 ACC/AHA guidelines for managing UA and NSTEMI recommend that practitioners use the patient's history, physical examination, ECG interpretation, and results of cardiac biomarkers to determine the likelihood that the patient's presentation is ACS from obstructive coronary artery disease (CAD). The diagnosis for STEMI is made on the basis of ST-segment elevation in the appropriate clinical setting.

HISTORY

Classic ACS-associated symptoms include chest, upper limb extremity, and jaw or epigastric pain or discomfort at rest or associated with exertion or emotional stress. In general, diffuse, nonpositional, poorly localized chest pain or discomfort is present in three-quarters of patients presenting with acute MI. Patients may also describe upper abdominal pain or associated symptoms such as shortness of breath, diaphoresis, nausea, and presyncope or syncope. Symptoms persisting for more than 20 minutes suggest infarction rather than UA. Diabetic patients or other patients with autonomic neuropathy, women and elderly patients, and postoperative patients may not exhibit the classic symptoms of ACS. They may present with hypotension that is unexplained, pulmonary edema, delirium, or profound weakness. Vigorous physical exercise such as shovelling snow, intense emotion such as arguing with a family member, and medical or surgical stress may precipitate STEMI in as many as 50% of cases. Circadian variations may be a factor in clusters of cases within a few hours of awakening.

PRACTICE POINT

Initial evaluation

1. Patients suspected of ACS should be transported by emergency medical services rather than private transportation to an emergency room.
2. History should focus on symptoms, any past medical history of CAD, and traditional risk factors for CAD to determine the likelihood of ischemic cardiac pain and risk factors for alternative life-threatening causes.
3. Physical examination should assess possible precipitating factors (severe hypertension, hyperthyroidism, gastrointestinal bleeding), evidence of vascular disease elsewhere, and alternative life-threatening causes of symptoms.

The differential diagnosis of ACS includes acute pulmonary embolism, aortic dissection, pericardial tamponade, tension pneumothorax, esophageal rupture, and other potentially life-threatening disorders. Once the diagnosis of ACS has been made, the 2007 ACC/AHA guidelines for managing UA and NSTEMI recommend that practitioners determine

1. The likelihood that the patient's presentation is ACS from acute or subacute obstructive coronary artery disease (CAD)
2. The risk of short-term of death or nonfatal MI (risk stratification) based on the history, physical examination, ECG interpretation, and results of cardiac biomarkers

The Braunwald classification system for UA hinges on the assessment of severity of the patient's anginal symptoms (I. new-onset of severe angina or increasing angina not occurring at rest; II. angina at rest in the past month but not in the preceding 48 hours, III. rest angina within the past 48 hours), the clinical setting (A. unstable angina secondary to a non-cardiac condition that increases demand, B. primary unstable angina, and C. postinfarction angina within 14 days of acute MI), and presence or absence of accompanying transient ECG changes. **Table 124-2** lists the Canadian Classification.

TABLE 124-2 CCS Classification of Angina

- Class 0: Asymptomatic
- Class 1: Angina with strenuous exertion
- Class 2: Angina with moderate exertion
- Class 3: Angina with mild exertion
  Walking 1–2 level blocks at normal pace
  Climbing 1 flight of stairs at normal pace
- Class 4: Angina at any level of physical exertion or at rest

Data from Canadian Cardiovascular Society.

Although traditional cardiac risk factors are weak predictors of the likelihood of acute ischemia, their presence influences outcomes in patients diagnosed with ACS. For example, diabetic patients with UA/NSTEMI have a 50% greater risk of adverse cardiac outcomes than nondiabetic patients. Well-documented risk factors for obstructive CAD include age >65, hypertension, hypercholesterolemia, diabetes, and tobacco exposure, and family history of CAD especially in a sibling. The examiner should also determine risk factors for other causes of life-threatening chest pain that would alter any management strategy using antithrombotic and antiplatelet agents. (See Chapter 77 for a more detailed discussion of chest pain.) Acute aortic dissection, pulmonary embolism, esophageal rupture, tension pneumothorax and cardiac tamponade may mimic the signs and symptoms of acute MI (**Table 124-3**).

PHYSICAL EXAMINATION

Although most patients with chest pain will have an unrevealing physical examination, the examiner should first look for signs of cardiac compromise that may signify a large infarction and poor prognosis. Anterior MI may be associated with hypotension and tachycardia in approximately 25% of cases, whereas inferior MI may be associated with bradycardia and hypotension in up to 50% of cases. Low cardiac output may be suggested by the presence of low blood pressure, significantly reduced mean arterial pressure compared to the patient's baseline, and sinus tachycardia accompanied by diaphoresis, pale cool skin, confusion, and reduced urine output. Signs of elevated filling pressures include a palpable or audible S_3, audible S_4, elevated jugular venous distention, or rales. A midsystolic or late-systolic apical murmur may result from mitral valve dysfunction. Right ventricular infarction may have signs of hypotension (eg, elevated jugular venous distention) without signs of left ventricular failure. A transmural MI may produce a transient pericardial friction rub. The examiner should also look for signs of precipitating factors (eg, severe hypertension, hyperthyroidism, hemorrhage or other causes of severe anemia, and hypoxia) and for signs of vascular disease.

ECG

ECG interpretation facilitates making the diagnosis of ACS and stratifying risk. Despite limitations of the ECG in signifying ischemia of the posterior, lateral, and apical walls of the left ventricle, the admission ECG strongly predicts both early and long-term prognosis. Although a normal ECG on admission may be associated with as high as a 10% incidence of NSTEMI, and an acute MI resulting from left circumflex artery occlusion may be missed in at least 4% of cases, patients with no ECG findings have a lower risk

TABLE 124-3 Assessment of the Possibility of ACS

Feature	High Likelihood	Intermediate Likelihood	Low Likelihood
	Presence of any of characteristics below	No high-likelihood factors and presence of any of characteristics below	No high or intermediate features but may have characteristics below
History	Chest or left arm pain or discomfort as main symptom reproducing prior angina History of CAD, MI	CP or left arm pain as chief complaint Age > 70 years Male Diabetes	Probable ischemic symptoms Recent cocaine use
Exam	Transient MR, hypotension, pulmonary edema, or rales	Extracardiac vascular disease	Chest discomfort reproduced by palpation
ECG	New transient ST-segment deviation (> 1 mm) or TWI in multiple precordial leads	Fixed Q waves ST depression 0.5–1 mm or TWI > 1 mm	T-wave flattening or inversion < 1 mm in leads with dominant R waves Normal ECG
Cardiac Biomarkers	Elevated cTnI, TnT or CK-MB	Normal	Normal

ACS, acute coronary syndrome; CAD, coronary artery disease; CK-MB, creatine kinase MB fraction; CP, chest pain; cTnI, cardiac troponin I; DM, diabetes mellitus; ECG, electrocardiogram; MI, myocardial infarction; TnT, troponin T; TWI, T-wave inversion. (Adapted from Braunwald E, Mark, DB, Jones RH, et al. Unstable angina: diagnosis and management. *AHCPR Publication No. 94-0602.* 1994:1–154. Agency for Healthcare Research and Quality, US Department of Health and Human Services.)

of complications than those with new ECG abnormalities. ST deviation of only 0.5 mm (0.05 mV) increases the 30-day and 1-year risk of mortality or MI twofold.

The ACC/AHA guidelines recommend obtaining an ECG within 5 minutes of acute chest pain presentation so that it can be interpreted by an experienced physician within 10 minutes of arrival.

The patient should be placed on a cardiac monitor in immediate reach of resuscitation equipment including a cardiac defibrillator. Patients should have a bedside chest plain film that screens for alternative diagnoses and for pulmonary congestion (associated with an adverse prognosis). A bedside two-dimensional echocardiograph will detect abnormalities of wall motion in all cases of STEMI and, thus, may be indicated when there is uncertainty about the diagnosis (eg, pericardial effusion, RV infarction, ventricular aneurysm, or LV thrombus), the need for emergent reperfusion therapy, or prognosis (eg, reduced left ventricular function).

Is this patient experiencing a STEMI?

If the patient is experiencing a STEMI, a decision with regard to reperfusion strategy should be made as quickly as possible (within 10 minutes of arrival to the health care facility). ST-segment elevation of 1 mm (0.1 mV) or more in two or more contiguous leads or new left bundle-branch block (LBBB) is highly indicative of acute MI in 90% of patients. Sgarbossa's criteria refers to the ECG criteria for identifying acute MI in patients with LBBB or ventricular pacing: (1) ST-segment elevation of ≥ 5 mm in the presence of a negative QR complex, (2) ST-segment elevation of ≥ 1 mm in the presence of a positive QRS complex, and (3) ST-segment depression of ≥ 1 mm in lead V_1, V_2, or V_3. Additional ECGs encompassing right ventricular and posterior leads should be performed if inferior or posterior MI is suspected. ST-segment depression in two contiguous anterior precordial leads and/or lone ST-segment elevation in the posterior chest leads signify a true acute posterior MI. Right ventricular infarction accompanies inferior-posterior wall MI in 30% to 50% of patients. The diagnosis is made on the basis of ST-segment deviation of ≥ 1 mm (0.1 mV) in the right precordial lead V_4R. Recognition is important due to the need for volume expansion, the possibility of advanced atrioventricular nodal block, and worse prognosis relative to patients suffering from interior-posterior MI without RV infarction. ECG interpretation is needed for identification of infarct territory in acute myocardial infarction (AMI) and to differentiate common nonischemic causes of ST-segment elevation including early repolarization, acute pericarditis, pulmonary embolism, left ventricular hypertrophy, Brugada syndrome, and others. (See Chapter 102 for a detailed discussion of electrocardiographic interpretation.)

Is this Patient experiencing UA or an NSTEMI?

Patients with ST-segment depression, transient ST-segment elevation, or deep symmetrical T-wave inversion (> 2 mV) are initially diagnosed with ACS until cardiac biomarkers distinguish between UA and NSTEMI. Lesser degrees of ST-segment deviation (< 0.5 mV) and/or T-wave changes are less specific, but the more leads that have these "nonspecific" changes, the greater is the likelihood of an acute NSTEMI rather than UA.

The ACC/AHA guidelines recommend serial ECG tracings or continuous ST-segment monitoring for patients with UA and NSTEMI.

CARDIAC BIOMARKERS

Measurement of the cardiac troponins (T or I), may provide confirmatory evidence of myocardial necrosis within two to three hours in 80% of patients with acute MI. Current guidelines advocate repeated cardiac troponin (cTn) measurements at 6 and 12 hours post symptom onset to exclude MI. The biomarker of choice, cTn elevation, almost always reflects myocardial necrosis and has proved to be a powerful predictor of mortality in those with ACS. False positives may arise due to cross-reacting antibodies or as a consequence of fibrin interference. Between 15% and 53% of patients with end-sage renal disease (ESRD) may have positive cTnT measurements in the absence of myocardial necrosis compared with 10% for cTnI. However, all elevations of cTn, even in those patients without demonstrable myocardial necrosis, such as those with falsely elevated cTnT in the setting of severe renal dysfunction, are associated with increased morbidity.

PRACTICE POINT

The admission ECG

- Together with a medical history, the ECG is still the most readily available, cheapest, and simplest tool in the early diagnosis of acute MI.
- ST deviation and/or T-wave inversions in contiguous leads indicate active ischemia.
- ST-segment elevation can be correlated with the location of the MI and pathologic Q waves may suggest prior MI:
  Anteroseptal MI – Q, QS, or qrS in V_1–V_3, ST-T changes
  Anterior MI – Q, QS or qrS, in V_2–V_4, ST–T changes
  Anterolateral MI – Q, QS, qrS in V_4–V_6, ST–T changes
  Inferior MI – Q waves ST-T changes in II, III, aVF
  True Posterior MI – ECG changes in V_1–V_3, mirror image of anteroseptal MI
  Right Ventricular MI – ST elevation in right chest leads (V_4R)

Prognosis

- The admission ECG strongly predicts early and long-term prognosis for both STEMI and UA/NSTEMI.
- For STEMI, due to the larger area of myocardium at risk, anterior territory involving the left anterior descending (LAD) artery has higher rates of adverse outcomes. Right ventricular infarction (inferior MI), however, accounts for only 5% of all cases of MI-induced shock. In addition, the number of leads showing ST elevation has been correlated with mortality.
- For UA/NSTEMI, ST deviation of only 0.05 mV increases the risk of mortality or recurrent MI twofold (30 day and 1 year).
- The more leads that have "nonspecific" changes, the greater the likelihood of an acute NSTEMI. NSTEMI is 3–4 times more frequent when 3 or more ECG leads had ST-segment depression of greater than 0.2 mV (2 mm).
- Although a normal ECG on admission may be associated with as high as a 10% incidence of NSTEMI (Slater, et al, Rouan, et al.), patients with a normal ECG have a significantly lower risk of adverse cardiac endpoints.

When the initial ECG is not diagnostic

- Repeated ECGs should be obtained to evaluate for evolving changes or if chest pain recurs.
- Consider obtaining posterior leads V_{7-9} to check for posterior MI, especially if pathologic R-waves R > S in V_1–V_2 or hyperacute ST depression and large inverted T waves in V_1–V_2 (4% of acute MI patients have ST elevation in these leads alone).
- Obtain right-sided precordial leads to check for ST elevation in lead V_4R if RV infarction is suspected.

CK-MB remains part of a multi-marker test to diagnose early MI and continues to be very useful in the diagnosis of re-infarction or infarct extension or peri-procedural MI due to its shorter half-life. Commonly, CK-MB levels are relied upon to estimate infarct size despite evidence to suggest that cTn (at 72–96 hours) may reflect the extent of myocardial necrosis with greater accuracy.

PRACTICE POINT

Elevated biomarkers

- The distinction between NSTEMI and UA is made following the confirmation or absence of cardiomyocyte necrosis based on biochemical assays. Cardiac troponin levels typically increase *within three hours of the onset of ischemic chest pain* facilitating an early diagnosis of acute MI in up to 80% of cases. Levels may remain elevated for up to 15 days. Current guidelines advocate repeated cTn measurements at 6 and 12 hours post symptom onset to exclude MI. Even a slight elevation of troponin is associated with a significantly increased risk of an adverse prognosis.
- C-reactive protein and B-type natriuretic peptide (BNP) are also independent predictors of death, MI, or heart failure. The mortality risk in one study doubled as the number of elevated biomarkers rose.

Sabatine MS, Morrow DA, de Lemos JA, et al. Multimarker approach to risk stratification in non-ST elevation acute coronary syndromes: simultaneous assessment of troponin I, C-reactive protein, and B-type natriuretic peptide. *Circulation*. 2002 Apr 16;105(15):1760–1763.

TRIAGE OF PATIENTS WITH ACS

The 2007 ACC/AHA guidelines for ACS recommend early stratification for risk of short-term death or nonfatal MI to determine the site of care, specific therapy, approach (early invasive versus conservative strategy), and prognosis. Treatment of possible, probable, or definite ACS should occur in a chest pain unit (CPU), medical telemetry unit, or coronary care unit (CCU) depending on the level of suspicion or confirmation of ACS. Low-risk patients can be evaluated in a CPU or medical telemetry unit. Patients with evidence of STEMI or other significant ECG changes, as well as those with any hemodynamic instability or new arrhythmia, should be evaluated in the CCU setting.

Treatment goals depend on the underlying pathophysiology. In STEMI, the initial approach involves immediate pharmacologic or catheter-based reperfusion to obtain normal coronary blood flow in a previously totally occluded artery. Time is critical for initial perfusion therapy: the golden hour is the first 60 minutes after presentation, and total ischemic time should be less than 90 to 120 minutes. The majority of patients will receive concomitant treatments with proven efficacy. In unstable angina and NSTEMI, the goal is to identify and remedy secondary causes that may increase myocardial oxygen demand or impair myocardial oxygen delivery, provide antithrombotic therapy to prevent further thrombosis and allow endogenous fibrinolysis to dissolve the thrombus, and employ revascularization to increase blood flow and prevent reocclusion. Although reperfusion therapy improves outcomes for STEMI, fibrinolysis has no role in the management of either UA or NSTEMI ACS. A meta-analysis not only showed no benefit in this setting, but showed an increased rate of MI. Therefore, treatment hinges on distinguishing between STEMI and UA/NSTEMI and then identifying high-risk patients with UA/NSTEMI who may benefit from invasive evaluation. The goal of secondary prevention for all patients is to stabilize and halt the progression of atherosclerotic plaques.

The key question to ask is whether the patient is having a STEMI. A broad array of management strategies for STEMI requires emergent cardiology consultation and possible expedited interhospital transfer. Reperfusion therapy has the advantages of being widely available and quick to administer; percutaneous coronary

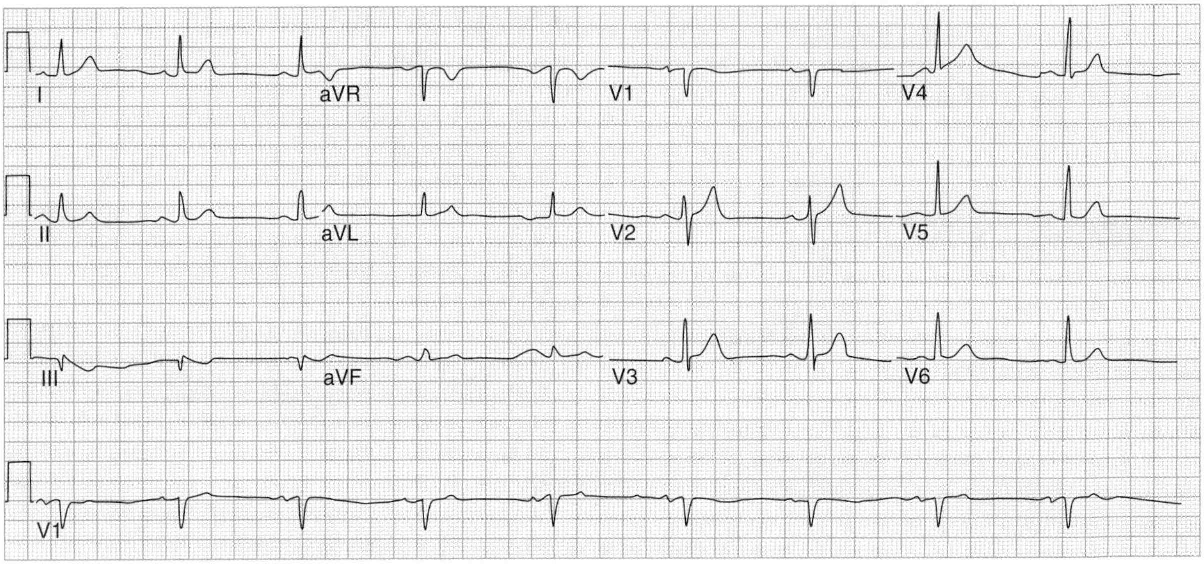

Figure 124-2 *Electrocardiogram of patient in Figure 1 one year after initial presentation.*

intervention (PCI) is more effective and has a lower bleeding risk but has limited availability and may cause treatment delays (**Figure 124-2**).

If initial testing suggests that the patient is having a NSTEMI, it is then incumbent on the practitioner to identify high-risk clinical subgroups to guide clinical decision making in order to salvage as much myocardium as possible. The clinical spectrum of non-ST-segment elevation ACS ranges from low-risk patients who would not benefit from early angiography with PCI or a selectively invasive strategy to intermediate and high-risk patients who would likely benefit due to a higher likelihood of adverse cardiac events.

TREATMENT OF STEMI

All patients with STEMI should receive dual therapy with aspirin and clopidogrel regardless of whether they undergo reperfusion with fibrinolytic therapy or do not receive reperfusion (class Ia). In patients for whom coronary artery bypass graft (CABG) surgery is planned, clopidogrel should be held at least five days, preferably seven days, unless the urgency for revascularization outweighs the risk of increased bleeding (class I). In patients less than 75 years of age, it is reasonable to administer a loading dose of clopidogrel 300 mg (class IIa); no data are available to support loading in older patients. Long-term maintenance of one year may be reasonable for patients with STEMI regardless of whether they underwent reperfusion therapy (class IIa).

Morphine for pain control remains a class I recommendation for STEMI, although it may increase adverse events in NSTEMI.

What is the optimal reperfusion strategy for this patient with STEMI?

Following recognition and diagnosis of an acute STEMI, a rapid decision with regard to reperfusion eligibility (whether fibrinolysis or PCI) and strategy must be made by the physician.

Ongoing treatment should then be carried out in the coronary care setting. The current ACC/AHA guidelines stipulate that all hospitals performing primary PCI should achieve a median door-to-balloon time of less than 90 minutes, with at least 75% of patients treated reaching this 90-minute target from first medical contact. If these time constraints cannot be met, fibrinolysis should be administered unless contraindicated.

The European Society of Cardiology (ESC) guidelines extend the 90-minute timeframe from first medical contact to PCI to 120 minutes. Furthermore, patients who present late with STEMI (> 12 hours) and who are hemodynamically stable should be transferred for PCI rather than receive thrombolysis. High-risk patients (elderly, those with anterior MI, renal impairment, or LV dysfunction) appear to sustain higher mortality rates undergoing primary PCI when a PCI-related delay is encountered.

When performed at a high-volume center (> 200 PCI procedures yearly) by experienced and skilled operators (> 75 PCI per year), primary PCI is the superior treatment modality for STEMI. Primary PCI leads to higher infarct-related artery (IRA) patency compared to fibrinolytic therapy alone. Primary PCI as opposed to thrombolysis has been shown to prevent 2 deaths per 100 patients treated (NNT = 50). Sicker STEMI patients appear to derive most benefit from PCI. Furthermore, primary PCI is associated with a lower risk of hemorrhagic stroke (0.05% versus 1.1%).

One of the major limitations to primary PCI therapy in the setting of an acute STEMI is achieving rapid transfer and access to a PCI-equipped center. It is estimated that less than one-quarter of acute care hospitals in the U.S. have PCI capabilities, though approximately 80% of the population reside within one hour of facilities with such capabilities. As the extent of myocardial necrosis and clinical outcomes are intrinsically linked to the duration of occlusion of the infarct-related artery, the point at which the delay in initiating PCI negates the advantages of prompt fibrinolysis is hotly debated. Primary PCI in a center without cardiac surgery availability is given a class IIb recommendation in 2007 ACC/AHA guidelines, although considerable data exist demonstrating excellent results compared with those facilities that have on-site cardiothoracic surgery.

Pharmacologic reperfusion is indicated in those circumstances where ECG criteria are met and symptom onset is < 12 hours (class IA) where prompt access to PCI is not possible, and no contraindications exist. Patients with a posterior STEMI presenting within 12 hours of symptom onset with no contraindications to fibrinolysis should also receive pharmacologic reperfusion (class IIA level of evidence C). Those STEMI patients who present 12 to 24 hours after symptom onset, who meet ECG criteria with recurrent ischemic symptoms also are given a class IIA recommendation for fibrinolytic therapy.

TABLE 124-4 Common Fibrinolytic Agents

Fibrinolytic	Mean Plasma Half-life (minutes)	Relative Fibrin Specificity	% Patients with TIMI-3 Flow IRA at 90 minutes	Dose
Steptokinase	23	–	32	IV infusion of 1.5 million units over 60 minutes
Alteplase	4–6	++	54	tPA 15 mg bolus, followed by 50 mg IV over first 30 minutes, followed by 35 mg over next 60 minutes
Tenecteplase	20	+++	63	Single weight-based bolus of 30 to 50 mg (depending on the exact weight) over 10 seconds

IRA, infarct related artery; IV, intravenous infusion. Adapted, with permission, from Kiernan TJ, Gersh BJ. Thrombolysis in acute myocardial infarction: current status. *Med Clin North Am.* 2007;91(4):617–637.

The U.S. Food and Drug Administration has approved tissue plasminogen activator (tPA), streptokinase, tenecteplase (TNK), and reteplase (rPA) as fibrinolytic agents, all of which promote the conversion of plasminogen to plasmin. Patients treated within one to three hours of the onset of symptoms clearly benefit the most regarding reduction of infarct size, limiting LV dysfunction, septal rupture, cardiogenic shock, ventricular arrhythmias, and death. Unlike streptokinase, newer fibrinolytic agents do not provoke an immune response and have been shown to result in greater infarct-related artery patency rates and a lower 30-day mortality benefit (**Table 124-4**).

Patients receiving fibrinolysis should be treated with dual antiplatelet therapy in addition to anticoagulation. 2007 ACC/AHA guidelines recommend that anticoagulation (unfractionated heparin [UFH], enoxaparin, or fondaparinux) should be continued for a minimum of 48 hours and up to eight days unless contraindicated. The TIMI risk score for STEMI enables the physician to rapidly assess the patient's 30-day mortality based on history and clinical exam, and ECG. Importantly, delay in treatment is associated with a higher mortality. Of 14 possible points, if the risk score is greater than 8 points, the associated mortality is 35.9% at 30 days.

The TIMI risk score for STEMI

- Age 65–74 (2 points); Age ≥ 75 (3 points) (2 or 3 points)
- Systolic blood pressure < 100 mm Hg (3 points)
- Heart rate > 100 beats per minute (2 points)
- Killip II-IV (2 points)
- Anterior ST elevation or LBBB (1 point)
- Diabetes, history of HBP, angina (1 point)
- Weight < 67 kg (1 point)
- Time to treatment > 4 hours (1 point)

When should an invasive strategy be considered post fibrinolysis for STEMI?

The timing of when to refer for PCI appears crucial in relation to maximizing potential benefits of restoring infarct-related artery (IRA) myocardial blood flow while minimizing major bleeding risks attendant with recent fibrinolysis. The process whereby a patient with acute STEMI is initially treated with a therapeutic agent with the aim of increasing the likelihood of IRA patency prior to immediate scheduled PCI is described as *facilitated PCI*. Medications used in this setting include high-dose heparin, GPIIbIIIa inhibitors, fibrinolytic therapy, or reduced-dose fibrinolysis in conjunction with a GPIIbIIIa-inhibiting drug. Possible advantages include more rapid flow restoration, thrombus burden reduction, and restoration of hemodynamic or electrical stability while awaiting PCI. Despite the conceptual appeal of such a management plan, particularly where significant delays may be unavoidable prior to PCI, the 2007 updated ACC/AHA guidelines do not recommend routine facilitated PCI, as it does not offer any evident clinical benefit. However, the guidelines do allow for a facilitated PCI strategy when a high-risk patient with a low risk of a major bleeding complication has received pretreatment with a pharmacologic regimen other than full-dose fibrinolysis (eg, for a patient with a large MI with hemodynamic or electrical instability whose transfer to the catheterization suite would involve a delay). For these patients PCI post fibrinolysis may be most beneficial if performed in the 2- to 24-hour period after administration of pharmacologic reperfusion therapy.

Approximately 5–10% of those undergoing urgent coronary angiography for STEMI are referred for urgent or deferred CABG within several days to weeks post the index event. Patients post fibrinolysis who demonstrate evidence of electrical or hemodynamic instability or recurrent ischemia should be considered for catheterization with a view to revascularization at any time after presentation.

The role of PCI within 12 hours of failed fibrinolytic therapy or rescue PCI is less clear. Guidelines recommend rescue PCI for suitable candidates less than 75 years of age who develop shock within 36 hours of MI and are suitable for revascularization that can be performed within 18 hours of the onset of hemodynamic instability (class IB), and in those with Killip class III heart failure and onset of symptoms within 12 hours (class IB).

In summary, a planned reperfusion strategy using full-dose fibrinolytic therapy followed by immediate PCI is not recommended and may be harmful (class IIIB). PCI of a significant stenosis in a patent infarct artery more than 24 hours after STEMI may be considered as part of an invasive strategy. Rescue PCI for patients who have failed fibrinolytic therapy (defined as less than 50% of ST elevation resolved after 90 minutes following reperfusion drug administration—in the lead with the greatest initial ST-segment elevation) and who have a moderate or large area of myocardium at risk (anterior MI, inferior MI with right ventricular involvement, precordial ST segment depression) is associated with a 28% risk reduction in the composite endpoints of death, re-infarction, and heart failure. PCI of totally occluded artery greater than 24 hours after STEMI is not recommended in asymptomatic patients with one- or two-vessel disease who are hemodynamically and electrically stable with no evidence of severe ischemia (class III).

Is this patient experiencing cardiogenic shock?

Cardiogenic shock due to acute MI retains a mortality rate of approximately 50%. Risk factors for cardiogenic shock include age greater 70 years, increased time from onset of symptoms of STEMI to presentation, systolic blood pressure (SBP) less than 120 mm Hg, sinus tachycardia greater than 110 beats per minute (bpm) or heart rate less than 60 bpm, and heart failure.

PROGNOSIS OF STEMI

Despite the significant advances in reperfusion therapies, the current overall STEMI 30-day mortality rate remains at 6% to 10%. Careful recognition and management of potential MI complications that may have adverse hemodynamic consequences, such as cardiogenic shock (frequently ensuing due to infarction of greater than 40% of the LV mass), RV infarction–induced hypotension or associated atrioventricular dyssynchrony, are vital.

TREATMENT OF UA/NSTEMI

What is the short-term and long-term risk of adverse cardiac events for patients experiencing NSTEMI or UA?

The TIMI, GRACE, and PURSUIT risk scores powerfully predict recurrent MI, death, or heart failure in patients with NSTEMI or UA and can be used at the bedside to tailor therapy. *Despite proven accuracy, these risk stratification tools are frequently underutilized at the bedside.*

The TIMI risk score for NSTEMI

- Age ≥65 years
- ≥3 risk factors for CAD (family history of CAD, hypertension, hypercholesterolemia, diabetes, current smoker)
- Significant coronary stenosis (stenosis ≥50%)
- ST segment deviation
- Severe anginal symptoms (≥2 anginal episodes within last 24 hrs)
- Aspirin usage within the previous 7 days
- Elevated serum cardiac biomarkers

Two phase-3 international randomized, double-blind trials totaling over 5000 patients with UA/NSTEMI validated the TIMI (Thrombolysis in Myocardial Infarction) risk score (TIMI-11B and the ESSENCE [Efficacy and Safety of Subcutaneous Enoxaparin in Unstable Angina and Non-Q-Wave MI]).

Higher TIMI scores are associated with greater risk of all-cause mortality, MI, and worsening ischemia necessitating urgent revascularization through 14 days, as follows:

- Low risk (0–2 points): 4.7 % event rates (0–1 points), 8.3% (2 points)
- Intermediate risk (3–4 points): 13.2% event rates (3 points), 19.9% (4 points)
- High risk (5–7 points): 26.2% event rates (5 points), 40.9% (6–7 points)

The TIMI III registry of over 1100 patients with ACS reinforced the validity of the TIMI scoring system. Six-week mortality increased from 1.0% to 2.9% to 5.9%, and one-year mortality increased from 3.9% to 6.5% to 21.0%, across low, intermediate, and high TIMI score groups. TACTICS TIMI-18 demonstrated that

- Early invasive strategy reduced the composite end point of death, nonfatal MI, or readmission with ACS to 15.9% versus 19.4% at six months.
- Patients in the intermediate and high-risk groups gained most from an early invasive management strategy.
- Patients classified as low risk (<3 points) derived no benefit from early angiography or PCI.

The GRACE risk score: The Global Registry of Acute Coronary Events (GRACE) risk score uses eight variables that yielded almost 90% of the prognostic information with regard to predicting the probability of *in-hospital mortality.* Risk factors include age, Killip class (a clinical classification system used in AMI based on the assessment of the patient's hemodynamic status, **Table 124-5**), SBP, ST-segment deviation, cardiac arrest upon admission, creatinine, biochemical evidence of myocardial necrosis, and heart rate. This risk model has been validated to accurately predict the risk of in-hospital mortality and the cumulative risk of death or MI in those with ACS (including STEMI) in approximately 15,000 patients derived from the GRACE multinational registry (C-statistic = 0.81 for death, C-statistic = 0.73 for death or MI). (An online risk calculator for use with this scoring system is available at www.outcomes.org/grace.)

TABLE 124-5 Clinical Findings and Associated Killip Class

Clinical Findings	Killip Class
No features of heart failure	I
Pulmonary rales, elevated jugular venous pressure or S_3	II
Pulmonary edema	III
Cardiogenic shock	IV

Data from Killip T, 3rd, Kimball JT. Treatment of myocardial infarction in a coronary care unit. A two year experience with 250 patients. *Am J Cardiol.* 1967;20(4):457–464.

PRACTICE POINT

Risk stratification NSTEMI

- Determination of site of care, selecting therapy (eg, glycoprotein IIb/IIIa inhibitors), and early invasive strategy in non-ST-segment elevation ACS hinges on risk stratification of recurrent MI, death, or heart failure.
- Older age, diabetes, vascular disease elsewhere, congestive heart failure (Killip class II or higher), and ACS despite chronic aspirin therapy (TIMI score ≥3) are clinical characteristics associated with significantly increased risk of adverse events.

According to ACC/AHA Guidelines the presence of the following predict high risk:

- Hemodynamic instability, ventricular tachycardia
- Depressed LV function, presence of congestive heart failure, worsened mitral regurgitation
- ST-segment depression
- Elevated biomarkers
- Recurrent angina at low-level exertion despite intensive therapy, angina with hypotension
- High-risk findings on stress testing
- PCI within the previous six months, prior CABG
- High-risk patients benefit from GP IIb/IIIa inhibitors (versus placebo), LMWH (versus UFH), and invasive (versus conservative) therapy

Does this patient with UA or NSTEMI require urgent coronary angiography?

Early coronary angiography allows delineation of the anatomy enabling the physician to rule out ACS in the 10% to 20% of patients with no significant coronary lesion, ensuring that they are not then inappropriately treated. Coronary angiography facilitates prognostic prediction and may appropriately direct patients with multivessel and left main disease to CABG. On the other hand, a considerable proportion of patients respond well to intensive medical therapy, and may not need to undergo an invasive procedure with its associated risks.

The ACC/AHA guidelines recommend coronary angiography leading to revascularization for patients with refractory angina or hemodynamic or electrical instability and for those patients initially managed conservatively who are judged to be at high risk unless there are concomitant severe comorbidities or specific contraindications (class IB).

Patients with higher-risk profiles should undergo catheterization within 48 hours for diagnosis and intervention.

Noninvasive testing

Contraindications to exercise testing include hemodynamic compromise, acute myocardial infarction or unstable angina, aortic dissection, acute pulmonary embolism, pericarditis or pericardial tamponade, severe anemia, critical aortic stenosis, thyrotoxicosis, pheochromocytoma, and severe uncontrolled hypertension.

> **PRACTICE POINT**
>
> **Noninvasive risk stratification in ACS**
>
> For patients who have had diagnostic angiography:
>
> 1. If the patient has undergone complete revascularization, there is usually no need for functional cardiac testing prior to discharge.
> 2. If the patient has multivessel disease and PCI of the culprit vessel, ETT with imaging is usually indicated to localize residual ischemia.
>
> For patients treated conservatively:
>
> 1. To diagnose exercise-induced ischemia and to assess extent and severity: At the time of testing patients should be free of angina at rest, the ECG should be stable for at least 24 hours prior to the test, and cardiac biomarkers should be declining.
>
> The clinical spectrum of non-ST-segment elevation ACS ranges from
>
> 1. Chronic stable angina to crescendo angina to rest pain, no ECG changes, negative biomarkers to rest pain ECG changes, negative biomarkers (UA)
> 2. Rest pain, ECG changes, positive biomarkers to transient ST elevations (NSTEMI)
>
> - Management hinges on risk stratification of individual patients with non-ST-segment elevation ACS for adverse cardiac events. Two validated, powerful risk prediction models allow for rapid bedside evaluation of individual risk. As the risk score increases, event rates significantly increase.
>
> 1. TIMI Risk Score: All-cause mortality, new or recurrent MI, severe recurrent ischemia requiring revascularization within 14 days
> 2. GRACE Risk Score: All-cause mortality from hospital discharge after any form of ACS.
>
> - Early invasive strategy (PCI) compared with medical therapy reduces the composite end point of death, nonfatal MI, or readmission with ACS to 15.9% versus 19.4% at six months in *intermediate and high-risk TIMI groups* (TIMI score 3–4 and 5–7 respectively).

The 2007 ACC/AHA guidelines recommend noninvasive testing after 12–24 hours in low- and intermediate-risk patients with either UA or NSTEMI who remain symptom free with no evidence of LV dysfunction. Limited data compare the relative prognostic value of different noninvasive testing modalities in this setting. Options include exercise or pharmacologic stress treadmill testing with or without nuclear imaging, in addition to stress echocardiography depending on the clinical circumstances of the patient (addition of imaging in presence of uninterpretable ECG) and facilities within the institution. Perfusion imaging is preferred for patients whose baseline ECG has ST-segment abnormalities, LBBB, or pacing, and for those who have a significant pretest likelihood for CAD to determine the extent of ischemia. Dobutamine or adenosine are generally reserved for those patients who cannot exercise and do not have contraindications such as severe hypertension (dobutamine) or acute bronchospasm or hypotension (adenosine).

Cardiac-computed tomography (CCT) is able to visualize nonstenotic calcified and noncalcified coronary plaques and has a very high negative predictive value (91% to 100%) of ruling out the presence of CAD. Excellent images may be obtained within five minutes, thereby facilitating rapid triage from the emergency department. Its primary use in acute chest pain should be reserved for patients with an intermediate pretest probability of CAD or for those patients at increased risk for aortic dissection and segmental pulmonary embolism that can be visualized at the same time. Patients with a low pretest probability should not be subjected to the risk of radiation; patients with a high pretest probability of CAD and suspected NSTEMI or UA would not benefit because a negative CCT would not alter the pretest probability.

Cardiac magnetic resonance (CMR) with late gadolinium enhancement may identify specific myocardial regions at risk and thereby provide additive information pertinent not only to risk stratification but also for targeting revascularization in patients with UA/NSTEMI. CMR is a rapidly evolving technology and the reported specificity, positive predictive value, and overall accuracy are likely to improve. The disadvantages of CMR include cost, long time required for scanning, the use of gadolinium in patients with reduced renal function, and contraindications (implanted pacemakers and defibrillators).

PHARMACOLOGIC THERAPY

ANTI-ISCHEMIC THERAPY (CLASS 1 RECOMMENDATIONS)

The ACC/AHA guidelines recommend bed rest for all patients and supplemental oxygen therapy to ensure adequate arterial oxygen saturation. Nonsteroidal anti-inflammatory drugs (NSAIDs), both nonselective and cyclooxygenase-2 (COX-2) selective agents, should be discontinued on admission if possible because they are associated with an increased risk of cardiovascular events in proportion to the degree of COX-2 selectivity. Regular assessment and examination of the patient including blood pressure measurement should be carried out and always prior to drug administration.

Nitroglycerin

Nitroglycerin reduces myocardial oxygen demand by venodilation (decreasing ventricular preload) and by arterial dilation of coronary arteries (improving myocardial oxygen delivery). The ACC/AHA guidelines recommend that all patients should receive nitroglycerin, sublingually or by buccal spray (0.3–0.6 mg) every five minutes for a total of three doses. If the patient's pain persists, intravenous nitroglycerin should be started at an initial rate of 5–10 µg/minute with increases of 10 μg/minute every three to five minutes until the patient is pain free or the SBP falls below 100 mm Hg or more than 30% below initial mean arterial pressure if the patient was hypertensive. Patients receiving sildenafil or other PDE-5 inhibitors should not receive nitroglycerin.

Morphine

In addition to relieving pain and anxiety, morphine may have beneficial effects in treating ACS. The use of morphine remains a class I indication for the relief of pain for patients with STEMI but may increase adverse events in UA/NSTEMI due to hypotension, respiratory depression, or confusion. For the latter, the use of morphine sulfate is a class IIa indication for the relief of ischemic pain when these symptoms do not respond to three doses of nitroglycerin or recur during treatment.

β-blocker therapy

β-blockers offer antiarrhythmic and antianginal effects and reduce myocardial contractility and heart rate, thereby decreasing myocardial oxygen demand. Beta-blockers clearly benefit patients with acute MI and are used for the same reasons in patients with ACS. The ACC/AHA guidelines recommend initiating therapy within the first 24 hours after onset of ACS for hypertensive patients unless there is a contraindication (class I recommendation). Contraindications include the presence of heart failure, low-output states, risk factors for cardiogenic shock, PR > 0.24, second- or third-degree AV block, bradycardia, hypotension, and cocaine-induced MI. Standard therapy is 5 mg metoprolol IV every five minutes times three doses, followed by 25–50 mg orally every six to eight hours if the patient is hypertensive (class IIa recommendation). Otherwise, oral therapy is prescribed to achieve a *target resting heart rate of 50–60 beats per minute.* The guidelines recommend caution in the use of IV β-blockers especially for patients at risk of cardiogenic shock (patients with hypotension, tachycardia, and evidence of CHF). Atenolol and propranolol may also be used.

Calcium channel blockers

Calcium channel blockers decrease myocardial contractility (reducing myocardial oxygen demand) and vasodilate coronary arteries (improving myocardial blood flow). The ACC/AHA guidelines recommend nondihydropyridine calcium channel blockers (eg, diltiazem, verapamil) for patients who have ischemic symptoms despite full therapeutic doses of nitroglycerin and β-blockers, for patients with Prinzmetal-variant angina, and as an alternative to β-blockers except where there is evidence of LV dysfunction or another contraindication.

Angiotensin-converting enzyme inhibitors and angiotensin II receptor blockers

The ACC/AHA guidelines recommend that angiotensin-converting enzyme (ACE) inhibitors should be given within 24 hours in those with impaired LV function (pulmonary congestion, ejection fraction (EF) < 40%) (class 1 recommendation) and should be considered for patients without impaired LV function (class IIa recommendation). These recommendations are based on a mortality benefit reported when ACE inhibitors were begun within 24 hours of MI. Patients with hypertension, renal insufficiency, diabetes, or persistent heart failure (with EF < 40%) should also receive ACE-inhibitor lifelong therapy unless contraindicated (eg, hypotension, hyperkalemia). Angiotensin receptor blockers (ARBs) are reserved for those who cannot tolerate ACE inhibitors.

ANTITHROMBOTIC THERAPY

Specific antithrombotic therapy (eg, aspirin, clopidogrel, heparin, glycoprotein IIb/IIIa inhibitors) has markedly improved clinical outcomes with ACS.

Inhibitors of platelet activation: aspirin

Aspirin (ASA) irreversibly inhibits COX-dependent platelet aggregation, decreases risk of fatal MI by 70% in the acute phase and 50% to 60% at three months to three years at a dose of 81–325 mg. Although some evidence points toward a significant role for aspirin resistance, aspirin underuse is by far a greater problem in the clinical setting. The international Reduction of Atherothrombosis for Continued Health (REACH) registry reported no antiplatelet therapy in 14% of more than 60,000 patients with CAD. In the absence of an absolute contraindication (active GI bleeding, coagulopathy, or allergy), universal, lifetime ASA should be prescribed following an ACS episode.

Inhibitors of platelet activation: clopidogrel and other diphosphate receptor blockers

Thienopyridines block adenosine-diphosphate–mediated platelet activation. In healthy volunteers 600 mg of clopidogrel inhibits about 40% of ADP-induced platelet aggregation that was detectable at two hours. After repeated daily dosing (75 mg daily) a steady state is reached where 50% to 60% inhibition occurs. Administration of 600 mg in patients about to undergo coronary angiography yields a full effect after two hours compared with lower loading doses. However, individual patients may exhibit significant differences in response to clopidogrel therapy. For patients who are allergic to aspirin, clopidogrel is an alternative first-line agent and is used as additive therapy for ACS prior to PCI (CURE trial [Clopidogrel in Unstable Angina to Prevent Recurrent Ischemic Events]). Accepted as preferred therapy for 30 days to prevent stent thrombosis in new nondrug-eluting stents (longer treatment for drug-eluting stents) and as adjunctive therapy after brachytherapy for in-stent restenosis, clopidogrel is preferred over ticlopidine for bioavailability and less agranulocytosis and thrombotic thrombocytopenic purpura (TTP). A 20% relative risk reduction and a 2% absolute reduction (NNT = 50) over one year in the primary end point of MI, stroke, or cardiovascular death occurred with the administration of clopidogrel given as a loading dose (300 mg) with a maintenance dose of 75 mg in addition to ASA compared to ASA alone (CURE trial). Patients with ACS who are intolerant of ASA should be given clopidogrel as a loading dose (usually 300 mg) followed by a maintenance dose of 75 mg daily.

ACC/AHA 2007 guidelines recommend dual antiplatelet therapy with ASA and clopidogrel in those patients undergoing coronary angiography with a view to PCI.

Recently, the thienopyridine prasugrel received FDA approval for use in patients with UA or MI who are undergoing PCI. Like clopidogrel, it binds irreversibly to the platelet ADP P2Y12 receptor but exerts a more potent antiplatelet effect with a significant reduction in the risks of recurrent MI and stent thrombosis compared with clopidogrel (TRITON–TIMI). However, an excess of major bleeding with this new agent was seen with an increased rate of fatal bleeding (approximately 3 per 1000 treated). Remaining issues such as optimal dosing in groups at high risk of bleeding need to be determined, but this antiplatelet agent may prove very useful in managing those undergoing PCI, especially those at high risk of recurrent ischemic events such as stent thrombosis.

Glycoprotein-IIB/IIIA inhibitors

Platelet aggregation may still occur despite treatment with ASA and ADP antagonists.

GPIIb/IIIa drugs block the final common pathway of platelet activation: the expression of the GPIIb/IIIa receptor. There are three agents: (1) eptifibatide (Integrilin, a peptide) and (2) tirofiban (Aggrastat, a nonpeptide) are small molecules and direct inhibitors of the GPIIb/IIIa receptor; and (3) abciximab (Reopro) is the Fab portion of the human-mouse chimeric antibody directed against the GPIIb/IIIa receptor. Many trials of each agent in UA support the use of tirofiban (PRISM, PRISM-PLUS, TACTICS-TIMI 18) and eptifibatide (PURSUIT) regardless of whether the patient will ultimately undergo cardiac angiography and abciximab (EPIC, EPISTENT, EPILOG, CAPTURE, GUSTO IV-ACS, TARGET) only if cardiac catheterization is planned within 24 hours. Tirofiban is administered as an initial dose of 0.4 μg/kg/minute for 30 minutes, followed by an infusion of 0.1 μg/kg/minute for 48 to 96 hours. Eptifibatide is given as an initial 180 μg/kg bolus, followed by an infusion of 2.0 μg/kg/minute for 72 to 96 hours. Abciximab is given as a bolus (0.25 mg/kg) followed by an infusion (0.125 μg/kg/minute (maximum of 10 μg/minute for 12–24 hours) blocks >80% of platelet receptors at two hours and requires 12 hours for bleeding times to normalize post intravenous injection. Platelet aggregation usually recovers to normal levels at 48 hours. Abciximab is currently indicated as an adjunctive antiplatelet agent in those patients with ACS/NSTEMI undergoing PCI or planned PCI within 24 hours because abciximab combined with angiography produced the best results, reducing early death by 50%.

ANTICOAGULANTS

The ACC/AHA UA/NSTEMI guidelines recommend initiation of anticoagulant therapy for all patients as soon as possible unless there are contraindications (class I recommendations).

Unfractionated heparin

Unfractionated heparin (UFH), a nonhomogeneous mixture of polysaccharide molecules with an average molecular weight of between 15,000 to 18,000 Daltons, enhances circulating antithrombin III, which in turn inactivates factor IIa, factor IXa, and factor Xa. While it does not break down existing thrombus, it prevents further thrombus formation. A meta-analysis of six randomized controlled trials from 1997 demonstrated a 33% reduction in reinfarction and recurrent ischemia when combined with ASA, although the p value was 0.06. The current recommendations include a weight-adjusted dosing regimen (60 U/kg bolus, followed by a 12 U/kg infusion), monitoring and titration according to a nomogram for target PPT 1.5–2 times the upper limits of normal (ie, approximately 50–70 seconds), aiming lower when given with GPIIb/IIIa antagonists, for at least 48 hours after presentation of UA/NSTEMI. Difficulties with UFH administration include reduced bioavailability at low doses, marked interpatient variability in anticoagulation necessitating activated partial thromboplastin–time (aPPT) measurement, and the complication of heparin-induced thrombocytopenia (HIT) may be outweighed by the ease of reversing the anticoagulant effect of UFH with protamine sulfate, and its short half-life compared with low-molecular-weight heparins (LMWHs) and the pentasaccharide fondaparinux.

Low-molecular-weight heparins

LMWHs (mean molecular weight between 4000 and 5000 Daltons) act predominantly by enhancing antithrombin, but unlike UFH they exhibit reduced thrombin-inactivating properties and have higher ratios of anti-Xa to anti-IIa. Although dalteparin, enoxaparin, and nadroparin have been compared with UFH in clinical treatment trials for UA/NSTEMI, enoxaparin appears to have a clear benefit with a 15% to 20% reduction of death, MI, and urgent revascularization at six weeks (ESSENCE, TIMI 11b). An analysis of six trials that compared enoxaparin with UFH use in almost 22,000 patients with ACS and found enoxaparin to be superior with regard to the 30-day rate of death or MI (10.1% versus 11%; OR 0.91; 95% CI, 0.83 to 0.99). Dalteparin showed an early nonsustained benefit over UFH (FRIC, FRISC, FRISCII trials). FRAXIS failed to show superiority of fraxaparine. Monitoring of anti-Xa levels is generally not advised except in certain clinical instances such as morbid obesity (>100 kg body weight), renal insufficiency, or pregnancy. Due to their renal excretion the recommended doses require reduction in patients with renal impairment (CrCl <30ml/minute, 50% of dose). Many operators still prefer UFH because the anticoagulant effect of LMWHs cannot be readily measured in the catheterization laboratory.

Factor Xa inhibitors

Despite their proven efficacy, neither UFH nor LMWH are thought to be effective attenuating existing clot-bound thrombin. This has prompted the development of more specific anticoagulants. Fondaparinux, a synthetic pentasaccharide, indirectly inhibits factor Xa and requires antithrombin for its action. The ACC/AHA guidelines recommend fondaparinux as treatment for UA/NSTEMI patients unless CABG is planned within 24 hours (class I recommendation). Though less bleeding complications have been reported with this agent compared with enoxaparin, concern remains regarding the increased propensity toward catheter thrombosis during PCI. Fondaparinux is preferred for patients receiving a conservative treatment strategy at increased risk of bleeding (class I recommendation).

Direct thrombin inhibitors

Unlike UFH, LMWH, and factor Xa inhibitors, direct thrombin inhibitors do not require a cofactor such as antithrombin in order to inhibit clot-bound thrombin. They do not interact with plasma proteins, and they are not associated with thrombocytopenia. Bivalirudin, a direct thrombin inhibitor, is a hirudin analogue that binds directly to the active site on thrombin. In patients undergoing PCI, it may be given as a bolus dose followed by a continuous infusion during the intervention. It is also used in patients diagnosed with heparin-induced thrombocytopenia who require anticoagulation. It has a short plasma half-life of only 25 minutes after administration and is only partially renally excreted. The ACC/AHA guidelines recommend bivalirudin for patients with UA/NSTEMI undergoing invasive treatment (class I recommendation). In this setting, if a thienopyridine is simultaneously administered with bivalirudin, a GP IIb/IIIa is not required (class IIa recommendation).

For patients directed toward intensive medical therapy without likely coronary intervention, the guidelines advocate enoxaparin or UFH (class IA) or fondaparinux (class IB), while patients managed conservatively, either after coronary angiography or stress testing, should receive UFH for 48 hours or enoxaparin or fondaparinux for the duration of hospitalization or up to eight days (class IA). ACC/AHA guidelines recommend that enoxaparin or fondaparinux over UFH as anticoagulant therapy for patients with UA/NSTEMI receiving conservative management unless CABG is planned within 24 hours (class IIa recommendation). The benefit of enoxaparin appears to be greater for patients at higher risk (eg, ST-segment abnormalities, elevated cardiac biomarkers, high TIMI risk scores). Enoxaparin and UFH have a class IA recommendation for patients likely undergoing PCI, while bivalirudin and fondaparinux have a class IB recommendation in this setting.

PRACTICE POINT

Discharge check list specific to non-ST-segment elevation ACS (in addition to routine discharge information):

1. Consulting cardiologist with contact information and follow-up appointment
2. Resting ECG interpretation and cardiac biomarkers
3. Results of noninvasive testing if performed (peak HR and BP, ejection fraction, imaging results)
4. Results of cardiac catheterization if performed (anatomy, ejection fraction)
5. Type of stent used if patient underwent PCI and date implanted
6. Laboratory tests (hemoglobin, TSH; baseline platelets, creatinine, lipid profile, fasting glucose, HbA1C, CRP)
7. Risk factor modification
   - Diabetes (ACE inhibitor, goal HbA1c < 7, dietary changes)
   - Obesity (goal BMI 18.5–24.9; waist circumference < 40 inches in men or < 35 inches in women)
   - Hyperlipidemia (goal LDL < 70, HDL > 40, triglycerides < 150; diet, statin)
   - Hypertension (goal BP < 130/80; beta-blocker, ACE inhibitor; home BP monitoring)
   - Congestive heart failure (ACE inhibitor, weights, heart failure program)
   - Chronic renal failure (ACE inhibitor, nephrology follow-up)
   - Smoking (smoking cessation program)
   - Depression (psychiatric consultation, treatment, follow-up)
8. New medications
   - Antiplatelet therapy (ASA, clopidogrel: dose, duration, importance of uninterrupted therapy per guidelines)
   - Medications for life: ASA, beta-blocker, ACE inhibitor, statin, nitroglycerin as needed
9. Physical activity (daily walking 30–60 minutes, cardiac rehabilitation)
   - Instructions about sexual activity, driving, working, flying.
10. Elimination of COX-2 inhibitors, NSAIDs, hormonal replacement therapy

(Data from Ali Mahajerin and Eli V Gelfand, Outpatient Visit Checklist for Patient Discharge with Diagnosis NSTECS (Table 10, p. 216) in P Toth and CP Cannon (eds.) Comprehensive Cardiovascular Medicine in Primary Care Setting. Humana Press, New York, 2010.)

Oral anticoagulation

Warfarin does not offer any additional benefit over clopidogrel plus aspirin, although combination therapy with aspirin is superior to aspirin alone. The benefit of dual antiplatelet therapy with aspirin and clopidogrel is clear for patients who undergo PCI and stenting. Therefore, warfarin is usually reserved for patients with other indications such as stroke prophylaxis (eg, atrial fibrillation, mechanical prosthetic valve, left ventricular thrombus) with a target INR of 2–2.5 in addition to dual antiplatelet therapy with 81 mg of aspirin and 75 mg of clopidogrel for various periods of time depending on patient risk.

LIPID-LOWERING THERAPY

Statins should be prescribed for all patients with UA/NSTEMI irrespective of baseline LDL cholesterol levels. The Adult Treatment Panel III guidelines and the 2007 ACC/AHA guidelines recommend dosage titration to lower the LDL cholesterol to < 70 mg/dl (class IIa recommendations). The benefit in endpoints of all-cause death, MI, UA requiring rehospitalization, or revascularization and stroke appears to be linked to statistically significant decreases in the LDL cholesterol and C-reactive protein (CRP).

A summary of the key drugs used in the initial management of ACS is provided in **Table 124-6**.

DISCHARGE PLANNING

After stabilization and treatment of ACS, continued clinical management is required for prevention of ischemia and to maximize secondary prevention. Therapy should include antiplatelet agents, beta-blockers (if intolerant, calcium channel blockers), ACE inhibitors or ARBs (class IA for LVEF < 0.4, IIA for LVEF > 0.4), and statins. Nitrates are also indicated to treat symptoms of ischemia. Patient education covering modifiable risk factors (eg, exercise, smoking, diabetic control, blood pressure) and symptom-recurrence awareness is vital. Target goals for HbA1c should be less than 7. Target goals for lipids should be LDL less than 70, HDL greater than 40, and triglycerides less than 150. Particular emphasis should be placed on compliance with dual antiplatelet agents in the post coronary artery–intervention setting. Aspirin (75–162 mg per day) should be continued indefinitely with the addition of clopidogrel 75 mg per day for one month in those managed medically (class IA). Continuation of clopidogrel for up to 1 year is given as a class IB recommendation. Patients who underwent stenting should take aspirin at a higher dose of 162–325 mg daily for the first month, and clopidogrel at 75 mg per day should be given for at least 1 month and ideally for 12 months. Those with drug-eluting stents require clopidogrel for a longer duration and a minimum of 12 months. Consideration should also be given to the need for an automated implantable cardiac defibrillator (AICD) in those with LV dysfunction. AICD placement should not be considered in the first 40 days following an acute MI (despite LV dysfunction), as trial data demonstrate no benefit to this intervention in the early post-MI period.

QUALITY IMPROVEMENT

Current guidelines advocate that primary PCI for STEMI, in a hospital with PCI capability, should be performed within 90 minutes of first contact (class IA). The practical implementation of this involves the close integration of a number of services (EMS, ED, interventional cardiology, and others). A successful model utilizes a STEMI committee to incorporate regular performance analysis and ensure target guidelines are met. Hospitalists may play a critical leadership role in improving access to primary PCI through early recognition of ACS at their community hospitals and through teamwork. In addition, hospitalists may improve provider-patient communication by taking the following steps:

1. Address disparities in health care, including facilitating access for free care for those in need.
2. Ensure patient education about the importance of therapy (eg, dual antiplatelet therapy, lifelong ASA therapy), risk-factor modification, and prescribe simple and cost-conscious drug regimens that facilitate compliance.
3. Arrange appropriate follow-up even for patients who have no evidence of CAD but have modifiable risk factors.
4. Provide availability to patients should questions arise prior to their follow-up appointments with their primary care physicians.

Hospitalists should also effectively communicate with receiving primary care physicians at the transition of care and ensure appropriate and timely follow-up.

TABLE 124-6 Summary of Core ACS Drugs

Drug	Dose	Evidence	Comments
Aspirin	325 mg (initial dose nonenteric formulation)	Nonfatal MI, nonfatal CVA, or vascular death decreased by 33%	Class IA Data from pivotal Antiplatelet Trialists' Collaboration
Clopidogrel	300–600 mg loading dose, then 75 mg per day	20% RR reduction and 2% absolute reduction in primary end point of MI, CVA, or cardiovascular death 30% reduction in CV death or MI post PCI when added to ASA	Class IA CURE trial randomized 12,000 patients with ACS
UFH	IV bolus 60–70U/kg (max 5000U bolus), followed by 12–15U/kg/hr titrate as per APTT 50–75s	Combined with ASA, reduced death or MI by 50%	Class IA
Enoxaparin	1 mg/kg twice a day SC (renal adjustment 1 mg/kg/day if CrCl< 30 cc/min)	Reduced 30-day death or MI versus UFH (10.1 versus 11%)	Class IA Meta-analysis of 22000 ACS patients
Bivalirudin	0.1 mg/kg initial IV bolus followed by 0.25 mg/kg per hour infusion	Versus UFH: Ischemic events 11.4 versus 12.2%; Bleeding 3.8 versus 9.8 (P < 0.001)	Class IB As effective as UFH at reducing in hospital ischemia with less bleeding
Fondaparinux	2.5 mg daily	Patients deemed high bleeding risk directed toward a conservative strategy Concern of increased clotting risk during PCI may necessitate addition of UFH for those needing PCI	Class IB
Nitrates	Sublingual (0.3–0.6 mg up to 1.5 mg) Or IV in first 48 hours if ongoing ischemia, heart failure, or HTN 5–200 mcg/min	Increase dose by 10 mcg every 3–5 min or as needed Aim for SBP > 110 mm Hg or < 25% drop in MAP Tolerance develops after 7–8 hours, wean off gradually (no RCT data)	Class IC Contraindicated where patient has taken phosphodiesterase inhibitor for ED (< 24 hours of sildenafil or 48 hours of tadalafil) Hypotension (SBP < 90 mm Hg) Tachycardia RV infarct
Statins		Lowered all cause mortality 3.4% versus 4.6%	Class IA Meta-analysis of > 9000 ACS patients with 23 month follow-up
Beta Blocker	Those with intrinsic sympathomimetic activity (metoprolol, propranolol, etc) given orally where no C/I exists	Controversial benefit but appear to lower 30-day mortality in those undergoing PCI for UA or MI (0.6% versus 2.0%)	Class IB Meta-analysis of patients undergoing PCI. Avoid if high risk of CS
ACE/ARB	Orally within 24 hours in those with LVEF < 0.4	Decrease mortality in those with MI and impaired LVEF	Class IA

ACE, angiotensin-converting enzyme inhibitors; ARB, angiotensin receptor blockers; CS, cardiogenic shock; C/I, contraindication; CVA, cerebrovascular accident; LVEF, left ventricular ejection fraction; MI, myocardial infarction; PCI, percutaneous coronary intervention; PO, oral; UA, unstable angina; UFH, unfractionated heparin.

CONCLUSION

Major progress has been made over the past three decades, from the establishment of coronary care units to exciting antiplatelet and antithrombotic drug developments. These have been complemented by the tremendous growth and refinement of percutaneous coronary intervention with the hope of reducing the major morbidity and mortality of cardiovascular diseases. This progress has led to a greater than 50% reduction in age-adjusted death rates for coronary heart disease in the U.S. since 1965. Despite the fact that advances in every aspect of the clinical management of patients with ACS continue unabated, opportunities to eliminate performance gaps require a coordinated team approach.

SUGGESTED READINGS

Anderson JL, Adams CD, Antman EM, et al. ACC/AHA 2007 guidelines for the management of patients with unstable angina/non-ST-Elevation myocardial infarction: a report of the American College of Cardiology/American Heart Association Task Force on Practice Guidelines (Writing Committee to Revise the 2002 Guidelines for the Management of Patients With Unstable Angina/Non-ST-Elevation Myocardial Infarction) developed in collaboration with the American College of Emergency Physicians, the Society for Cardiovascular Angiography and Interventions, and the Society of Thoracic Surgeons endorsed by the American

Association of Cardiovascular and Pulmonary Rehabilitation and the Society for Academic Emergency Medicine. *J Am Coll Cardiol.* 2007;50(7):e1–e157.

Antman EM, Anbe DT, Armstrong PW, et al. ACC/AHA guidelines for the management of patients with ST-elevation myocardial infarction; A report of the American College of Cardiology/American Heart Association Task Force on Practice Guidelines (Committee to Revise the 1999 Guidelines for the Management of patients with acute myocardial infarction). *J Am Coll Cardiol.* 2004;44(3):E1–E211.

Antman EM, Hand M, Armstrong PW, et al. 2007 Focused Update of the ACC/AHA 2004 Guidelines for the Management of Patients With ST-Elevation Myocardial Infarction: a report of the American College of Cardiology/American Heart Association Task Force on Practice Guidelines: developed in collaboration With the Canadian Cardiovascular Society endorsed by the American Academy of Family Physicians: 2007 Writing Group to Review New Evidence and Update the ACC/AHA 2004 Guidelines for the Management of Patients With ST-Elevation Myocardial Infarction, Writing on Behalf of the 2004 Writing Committee. *Circulation.* 2008;117(2):296–329.

Bavry AA, Mood GR, Kumbhani DJ, et al. Long-term benefit of statin therapy initiated during hospitalization for an acute coronary syndrome: a systematic review of randomized trials. *Am J Cardiovasc Drugs.* 2007;7(2):135–141.

Harrington RA, Becker RC, Cannon CP, et al. Antithrombotic therapy for non-ST-segment elevation acute coronary syndromes: American College of Chest Physicians Evidence-Based Clinical Practice Guidelines (8th Edition). *Chest.* 2008;133(6 Suppl): 670S–707S.

Morrow DA, Antman EM, Charlesworth A, et al. TIMI risk score for ST-elevation myocardial infarction: a convenient, bedside, clinical score for risk assessment at presentation: an Intravenous nPA for Treatment of Infarcting Myocardium Early II Trial Substudy. *Circulaiton.* 2000:102:2031–2037.

Panju AA, Hemmelgarn BR, Guyatt GH, et al. The rational clinical examination. Is this patient having a myocardial infarction? *JAMA.* 1998;280(14):1256–1263.

Rouan GW, Lee TH, Cook EF, Brand DA, Weisberg MC, Goldman L. Clinical characteristics and outcome of acute myocardial infarction in patients with initially normal or nonspecific electrocardiograms (a report from the Multicenter Chest Pain Study). *Am J Cardiol.* 1989;64(18):1087–1092.

Slater DK, Hlatky MA, Mark DB, Harrell FE, Jr., Pryor DB, Califf RM. Outcome in suspected acute myocardial infarction with normal or minimally abnormal admission electrocardiographic findings. *Am J Cardiol.* 1987;60(10):766–770.

Thygesen K, Alpert JS, White HD, et al. Universal definition of myocardial infarction. *Circulation.* 2007;116(22):2634–2653.

Van de Werf F, Bax J, Betriu A, et al. Management of acute myocardial infarction in patients presenting with persistent ST-segment elevation: the Task Force on the Management of ST-Segment Elevation Acute Myocardial Infarction of the European Society of Cardiology. *Eur Heart J.* 2008;29(23):2909–2945.

Wang K, Asinger RW, Marriott HJ. ST-segment elevation in conditions other than acute myocardial infarction. *N Engl J Med.* 2003;349(22):2128–2135.

Yusuf S, Zhao F, Mehta SR, et al. Effects of clopidogrel in addition to aspirin in patients with acute coronary syndromes without ST-segment elevation. *N Engl J Med.* 2001;345(7):494–502.

CHAPTER 125

Cardioversion

J. Ryan Jordan, MD
B. Robinson Williams III, MD

Key Clinical Questions

1. What are the indications for cardioversion?
2. What is the difference between cardioversion and defibrillation?
3. What is the difference between monophasic and biphasic cardioverter-defibrillators?
4. How much energy should be used during cardioversion?
5. What are the indications for anticoagulation prior to cardioversion?

INTRODUCTION

Cardioversion is a medical procedure whereby an abnormal heart rhythm (ie, cardiac arrhythmia) is converted back to a normal rhythm using electricity or drugs. Electrical cardioversion, also referred to as direct-current or DC cardioversion, involves the delivery of a synchronized (perfectly timed) electrical shock through the chest wall to the heart to terminate arrhythmias and restore sinus rhythm. Electrical cardioversion is an effective, rapid, and safe technique that has become a routine procedure in the management of patients with cardiac arrhythmias. Pharmacologic cardioversion, also called chemical cardioversion, uses antiarrhythmic medication instead of an electrical shock to restore the heart's normal rhythm.

Investigators at Johns Hopkins Hospital were the first to develop techniques of defibrillation by an electrical shock in the 1930s. The first human defibrillation was performed in the operating room by Claude Beck in 1947, and Paul Zoll introduced defibrillation using alternating current in 1956. Direct-current defibrillation was subsequently pioneered and introduced into clinical practice by Bernard Lown in 1962. Subsequent studies in the early 1960s demonstrated that electrical cardioversion across the closed chest could abolish other cardiac arrhythmias in addition to ventricular fibrillation (VF). Today, atrial fibrillation (AF) is the most frequent arrhythmia encountered in clinical practice and the most commonly cardioverted arrhythmia.

DISTINGUISH CARDIOVERSION AND DEFIBRILLATION

Electrical cardioversion and defibrillation procedures both use a device (eg, cardioverter-defibrillator) to deliver an electrical shock to the heart to treat abnormal heart rhythms, but they differ in the timing of the shock and energy provided. Electrical cardioversion delivers energy synchronized (ie, perfectly timed) to the QRS complex and is used to treat arrhythmias such as AF, atrial flutter (AFL), or ventricular tachycardia (VT) with a pulse. Cardioversion can be performed electively (ie, nonemergently) in stable patients or emergently in situations to correct a rapid abnormal rhythm associated with faintness, low blood pressure, chest pain, difficulty breathing, or loss of consciousness. Cardioversion is not performed in pulseless patients.

Defibrillation delivers nonsynchronized (ie, occurs at random timing) energy during the cardiac cycle and is used to treat life-threatening arrhythmias such as pulseless VT or VF. Defibrillation is the treatment of choice for the arrhythmias most commonly associated with sudden cardiac arrest. The electrical shock delivered during cardioversion or defibrillation can be delivered *externally to the heart* using electrodes (external pads or paddles) placed on the chest (most common); *directly to the heart* using internal paddles during an open chest surgery; or through the electrodes of a permanently implanted cardioverter-defibrillator (ICD).

MECHANISM OF CARDIOVERSION

Cardioversion disrupts the abnormal electrical circuit(s) in the heart and restores a normal heartbeat. The shock causes all the heart cells to depolarize simultaneously, thereby interrupting and terminating the abnormal electrical rhythm without damaging the heart. This split second interruption of the abnormal beat allows the heart's electrical system to regain control and restore a normal

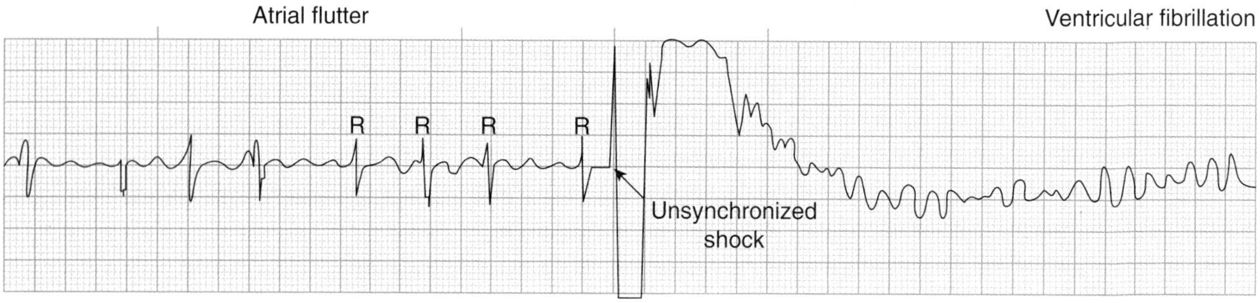

Figure 125-1 *A complication of cardioversion: induction of ventricular fibrillation. The ventricular arrhythmia occurred because the operator failed to enable the synchronizer, resulting in an inadvertent delivery of the shock on the vulnerable T wave instead of the intended delivery on the R wave. This complication is preventable by enabling the synchronizer and checking that it is properly functioning before shock delivery. (From Kerber RE. Transchest cardioversion: optimal techniques. In: Tacker WA, ed. Defibrillation of the Heart: ICDs, AEDs and Manual. St. Louis: Mosby-Year Book, 1994:164. With permission.)*

heartbeat. The delivery of energy during the shock is synchronized to the QRS complex, which represents cardiac depolarization, in order to terminate the arrhythmia safely and allow sinus rhythm to resume. The accidental delivery of an electrical shock to the T wave, which represents cardiac repolarization, is unsafe and may result in life-threatening ventricular arrhythmias (**Figure 125-1**). For this reason, synchronized cardioversion is used, rather than nonsynchronized defibrillation, for the abatement of abnormal rhythms with pulse.

PRACTICE POINT

- The accidental delivery of an electrical shock to the T wave may result in life-threatening ventricular arrhythmias. For this reason, synchronized cardioversion is used, rather than nonsynchronized defibrillation, for the abatement of abnormal rhythms with pulse.

Electrical cardioversion appears most effective in terminating arrhythmias that arise from a single reentrant circuit such as AFL, atrioventricular nodal reentrant tachycardia (AVNRT), atrioventricular reentrant tachycardia (AVRT), and monomorphic VT. The high-energy shock depolarizes the myocardium and the conduction tissue involved in the reentry circuit of the arrhythmia simultaneously. The depolarization of the myocardium is followed by a period of refractoriness that has the effect of interrupting the reentrant circuit. This interruption breaks the repeating cycle and terminates the arrhythmia. When the reentrant circuit is broken and the arrhythmia stops, the sinus node begins to fire again and a normal heart rhythm is restored. This mechanism of action does not explain how electrical cardioversion terminates AF, which arises from multiple reentrant circuits. As a result of the multiple circuits, successful cardioversion of AF often requires higher energy for termination. The exact mechanism by which electrical cardioversion terminates AF remains unknown. Other arrhythmias, such as junctional tachycardia and multifocal atrial tachycardia, originate from ectopic sites (ie, nonpacemaker) in the heart. Cardioversion is not effective for these types of arrhythmias.

TYPES OF DEFIBRILLATORS

Cardioverter-defibrillators deliver energy in a variety of waveforms, broadly characterized as monophasic or biphasic. Monophasic devices provide a unidirectional pulse of energy, meaning that electrons flow in a single direction through the heart. Monophasic energy is highly effective, and monophasic cardioverter-defibrillators remain widely used. Alternatively, biphasic devices deliver a sinusoidal biphasic waveform whereby the initial phase of energy is positive followed by a phase of opposite polarity, which means that during the shock the polarity and electron flow reverse. Biphasic cardioverter-defibrillators deliver a more consistent magnitude of current, which terminates arrhythmias more effectively and at lower energies compared to monophasic devices. As a result, biphasic cardioverter-defibrillators are increasing in use and have now become the standard for trans-chest defibrillation. Clinicians must distinguish which type of cardioverter-defibrillator is available for use, as this will dictate how much energy is required for successful cardioversion.

PRACTICE POINT

- Biphasic cardioverter-defibrillators deliver a more consistent magnitude of current, which terminates arrhythmias more effectively and at lower energies compared to monophasic devices.

INDICATIONS AND CONTRAINDICATIONS

Electrical cardioversion has become a routine procedure in the management of cardiac arrhythmias. Indications include patients in whom the rate of the arrhythmia (eg, AF) cannot be adequately controlled medically or patients who poorly tolerate the arrhythmia (eg, palpitations, angina pectoris, and heart failure). Multiple cardiac rhythms may bear indications for cardioversion or defibrillation (**Tables 125-1** and **125-2**). The most common reason for the elective cardioversion of atrial arrhythmias is to enhance cardiac performance by restoring sinus rhythm, particularly in patients with mitral stenosis, left ventricular hypertrophy (aortic stenosis, hypertrophic obstructive cardiomyopathy), and diminished myocardial reserve (heart failure, myocardial ischemia, and infarction). Urgent cardioversion may be required for patients with atrial or ventricular arrhythmias who have myocardial ischemia, acute heart failure (pulmonary edema), hypotension, mental status changes, or worsening angina pectoris.

Because electrical cardioversion is a low-risk procedure if properly performed, some authorities believe that every patient deserves one chance to achieve sinus rhythm by cardioversion, even if the short- or long-term prognosis of maintaining sinus rhythm is generally unfavorable. Other experts suggest that not all patients with newly

TABLE 125-1 Indications and Contraindications of Cardioversion

Indications	Contraindications
AF/AFL	Known atrial thrombus
1. Patient with AF/AFL > 48 hours duration and anticoagulation for > 3–4 weeks (INR 2–3)	Sinus rhythm or tachycardia
2. Acute onset AF/AFL with associated hemodynamic instability including the following:	Multifocal atrial tachycardia
Angina pectoris	Junctional tachycardia
Myocardial ischemia/infarction	Accelerated idioventricular rhythm
Hypotension/shock	Digitalis toxicity (digitalis-induced tachyarrhythmias)
Heart failure	Severe electrolyte imbalance
Pulmonary edema	Hypokalemia
Mitral stenosis	Unknown duration of AF/AFL in a stable patient not receiving therapeutic antecedent anticoagulation in the absence of a TEE
Preexcitation (WPW syndrome)	Patient that cannot be safely sedated
Left ventricular hypertrophy	
AS	
HTN	
HOCM	
3. AF/AFL of unknown duration and absence of thrombus in left atrium or atrial appendage by TEE	
4. AF/AFL < 48-hour duration	
Atrioventricular nodal reentry tachycardia	
Atrioventricular reentry tachycardia	
Ventricular tachycardia with a pulse	

AF, atrial fibrillation; AFL, atrial flutter; AS, aortic stenosis; HOCM, hypertrophic obstructive cardiomyopathy; HTN, hypertension; TEE, transesophageal echocardiogram; WPW, Wolff-Parkinson-White.

discovered AF warrant an attempt at restoring sinus rhythm since several large, randomized trials have shown that the maintenance of sinus rhythm confers no survival (or other outcome) advantage over rate control. Treatment must be determined based on clinical parameters and patient preferences.

Contraindications to electrical cardioversion include rhythms that do not respond to electrical cardioversion (eg, sinus rhythms, multifocal atrial tachycardia), digitalis toxicity, severe electrolyte imbalance (eg, hypokalemia), and known or suspected atrial thrombus. In AF or AFL, suspicion of atrial thrombus should be high if the rhythm onset is unknown or not clearly within the prior 48 hours. Transesophageal echo (TEE) evidence that the left atrium is free of thrombus may permit cardioversion for AF or AFL with unknown or > 48-hour onset.

TRIAGE/HOSPITAL ADMISSION

Cardioversion is routinely performed in most hospitals in a closely monitored setting such as an intensive care unit, an emergency department, or a specially equipped procedure room. Although patients with atrial arrhythmias are often admitted to the hospital electively for cardioversion, outpatient cardioversion is a low-risk, effective, and economical procedure. If performed on an outpatient basis, patients are observed until most of the effects of sedation have abated (1–2 hours) and require transport home safely after the procedure due to the residual effects of anesthesia. Overnight hospitalization is seldom required.

TABLE 125-2 Indications and Contraindications of Defibrillation

Indications	Contraindications
Pulseless ventricular tachycardia	Expressed wishes by patient or patient's surrogate not to be resuscitated
Ventricular fibrillation	

TREATMENT

PREPROCEDURE CHECKLIST

PRACTICE POINT

- Patients who have an abnormal airway may have increased risk for airway obstruction during sedation and may be difficult to manage if mask ventilation or intubation becomes necessary. Patients who present with any high-risk features (see Table 125-3) should be considered for anesthesiology consultation prior to cardioversion.

Prior to performing electrical cardioversion, structured measures should be integrated for all patients (**Figure 125-2**) as follows:

1. Informed consent (patient or decision maker)
2. Fasting (nothing oral) 6–8 hours prior to cardioversion (if elective)

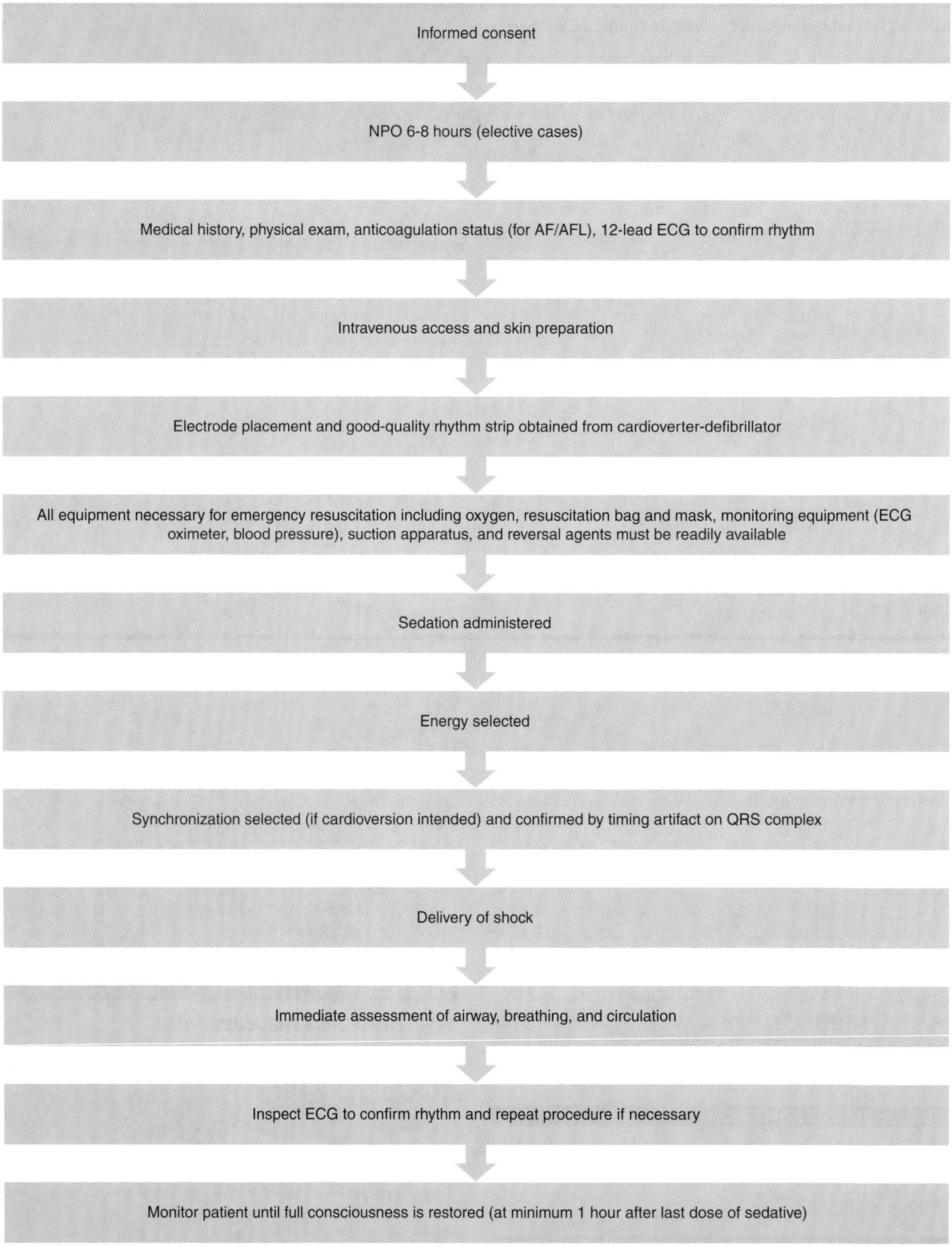

Figure 125-2 *Algorithm for external electrical cardioversion (preprocedure preparation and procedure).*

TABLE 125-3 Abnormal Physical Findings on Airway Examination

Habitus
Significant obesity (especially involving the neck and facial structures)
Head and neck
Short neck
Limited neck extension
Cervical spine trauma
Tracheal deviation
Decreased hyoid–mentum distance (<3 cm in an adult)
Mouth
Small mouth opening (<3 cm in an adult)
Edentulous
Protruding incisors
Loose or capped teeth
High-arched palate
Macroglossia
Tonsillar hypertrophy
Nonvisible uvula
Jaw
Micrognathia
Retrognathia
Trismus
Significant malocclusion

3. History and physical examination
   a. History should include current medications, allergies, previous adverse drug reactions or contraindications to sedation, diseases/disorders, prior hospitalizations, pregnancy status, nothing oral status, and anticoagulation status (if presenting arrhythmia is AF/AFL).
   b. Use history to estimate duration of AF/AFL duration and determine need for anticoagulation and/or TEE evaluation.
   c. Physical examination should include vital signs, oxygen saturation, pulmonary and cardiovascular examination, and oral cavity and airway examination. Patients who have an abnormal airway exam should be considered to be at increased risk for airway obstruction during sedation and may potentially have a difficult airway to manage if mask ventilation or intubation becomes necessary. Patients who present with any high-risk features (**Table 125-3**) should be considered for anesthesiology consultation prior to the initiation of the procedure.
4. A 12-lead electrocardiogram (ECG) is used to confirm rhythm.
5. If any electrolyte abnormality (hypokalemia, hyperkalemia) or drug toxicity (digitalis) is suspected, appropriate blood levels should be checked.
6. Peripheral venous access (for preprocedure sedation and postprocedure medications or fluids if needed) is obtained.
7. Skin preparation includes shaving of the chest hair, if present (with *electric clippers* rather than a blade) to ensure good contact of the skin and electrode pads. High-quality continuous ECG from the cardioverter-defibrillator will confirm proper contact of electrode pads to the skin.
8. Emergency resuscitation equipment available (Figure 125-2).

ANTICOAGULATION

PRACTICE POINT

- The 2008 ACCP guidelines recommend that patients undergoing urgent cardioversion be heparinized as soon as possible to prevent thrombi from forming due to atrial appendage dysfunction after cardioversion.

Cardioversion may be associated with pulmonary or systemic embolization. This complication is more likely to occur in patients with AF/AFL > 48 hours (ie, high-risk group) who have not been anticoagulated prior to cardioversion. In case-control series, the estimated risk of thromboembolism is between 1% and 5% in (nonanticoagulated patients) with AF/AFL > 48 hours undergoing cardioversion.

In patients with AF/AFL >48 hours, oral anticoagulation with warfarin (International Normalized Ratio (INR) 2.0 to 3.0) for 3–4 weeks prior to cardioversion reduces the thromboembolic risk to 0.5–0.8%. Anticoagulation before cardioversion allows time for adherence of any preexisting atrial thrombus and for prevention of new thrombus formation. Alternatively, anticoagulation with intravenous unfractionated heparin can be initiated and a TEE performed to evaluate the left atrium and left atrial appendage for evidence of thrombus. If there is no evidence of thrombus, cardioversion can safely be performed (thromboembolic risk 0.8%). The 2008 American College of Chest Physicians (ACCP) guidelines recommend that patients undergoing urgent cardioversion be heparinized as soon as possible to prevent thrombi from forming due to atrial appendage dysfunction after cardioversion. Cardioversion in patients who present with acute AF/AFL < 48 hours (ie, low-risk group) is associated with a low clinical rate of thrombembolism (0.8%).

PRACTICE POINT

- Cardioversion in patients who present with acute atrial fibrillation or atrial flutter (AF/AFL) < 48 hours (ie, low-risk group) is associated with a low clinical rate of thrombembolism (0.8%). In cardioversion of AF/AFL > 48-hour duration (not anticoagulated), the estimated risk for thromboembolism from a left atrial thrombus is 1–5%. In patients with AF/AFL > 48 hours, oral anticoagulation with warfarin (INR 2.0–3.0) for 3–4 weeks prior to cardioversion reduces the thromboembolic risk to 0.5–0.8%. Alternatively, if there is no evidence of thrombus on transesophageal echocardiogram (TEE), anticoagulation may be started, and cardioversion can be safely performed (thromboembolic risk 0.8%).

Late thromboembolic events after cardioversion are probably due to both the development of thrombus as a consequence of atrial stunning and the delayed recovery of atrial contraction after cardioversion. Pooled data from 32 studies of cardioversioon of AF/AFL suggest that 98% of clinical thromboembolic events occur within 10 days of cardioversion. Anticoagulation after the procedure prevents thrombus formation from occurring before normal atrial mechanical activity has resumed, a process that may be delayed for several weeks due to atrial stunning. The American College of Chest Physicians (ACCP) and American College of Cardiology/American Heart Association, and the European Society of Cardiology (ACC/AHA/ESC) guidelines therefore recommend continuation of warfarin therapy for at least 4 weeks after cardioversion. This recommendation only addresses

TABLE 125-4 ACC/AHA/ESC Guideline Summary: Prevention of Thromboembolism in Patients with Atrial Fibrillation Undergoing Cardioversion

Class I—There is evidence and/or general agreement that the following approaches are effective for the prevention of thromboembolism in patients with AF undergoing cardioversion

1. AF > 48 h duration, or when the duration of AF is unknown, anticoagulation (INR 2.0–3.0) recommended for at least 3 weeks prior to and 4 weeks after cardioversion, regardless of the method (electrical or pharmacologic). (*Level of evidence: B*)
2. AF > 48 h duration requiring immediate cardioversion because of hemodynamic instability; heparin should be administered concurrently (unless contraindicated) by an initial intravenous bolus injection followed by a continuous infusion in a dose adjusted to prolong the activated partial thromboplastin time to 1.5 to 2 times the reference control value. Thereafter, oral anticoagulation (INR 2.0–3.0) for at least 4 weeks, as for patients undergoing elective cardioversion. Limited data support subcutaneous administration of low-molecular-weight heparin in this indication. (*Level of evidence: C*)
3. AF < 48 h duration associated with hemodynamic instability (angina pectoris, MI, shock, or pulmonary edema), cardioversion should be performed immediately without delay for prior initiation of anticoagulation. (*Level of evidence: C*)

Class IIa—The weight of evidence or opinion is in favor of the usefulness of the following approaches for the prevention of thrombembolism in patients with AF undergoing cardioversion

1. During the first 48 hours after onset of AF, the need for anticoagulation before and after cardioversion may be based on the patient's risk of thromboembolism. (*Level of evidence: C*)
2. As an alternative to anticoagulation prior to cardioversion of AF, it is reasonable to perform TEE in search of thrombus in the LA or LAA. (*Level of evidence: B*)
   a. For patients with no identifiable thrombus, cardioversion is reasonable immediately after anticoagulation with unfractionated heparin (eg, initiate by intravenous bolus injection and an infusion continued at a dose adjusted to prolong the activated partial thromboplastin time to 1.5 to 2 times the control value until oral anticoagulation has been established with a vitamin K antagonist (eg, warfarin), as evidenced by an INR equal to or greater than 2.0.). (*Level of evidence: B*)
      i. Thereafter, oral anticoagulation (INR 2.0–3.0) is reasonable for a total anticoagulation period of at least 4 weeks, as for patients undergoing elective cardioversion. (*Level of evidence: B*).
      ii. Limited data are available to support the subcutaneous administration of a low-molecular-weight heparin in this indication. (*Level of evidence: C*)
   b. For patients in whom thrombus is identified by TEE, oral anticoagulation (INR 2.0–3.0) is reasonable for at least 3 weeks prior to and 4 weeks after restoration of sinus rhythm, and a longer period of anticoagulation may be appropriate even after apparently successful cardioversion because the risk of thromboembolism often remains elevated in such cases. (*Level of evidence: C*)
3. For patients with atrial flutter undergoing cardioversion, anticoagulation can be beneficial according to the recommendations as for patients with AF. (*Level of evidence: C*)

AF, atrial fibrillation; INR, international normalized ratio; LA, left atrium; LAA, left atrial appendage; MI, myocardial infarction; TEE, transesophageal echocardiogram.

protection from embolic events related to the cardioversion period. Patients with AF at high risk from thromboembolic events based on CHADS2 score (an acronym for Congestive heart failure, Hypertension, Age > 75, Diabetes mellitus and prior Stroke or transient ischemic attack) may require long-term anticoagulation (see Chapter 126).

Care standards require administration of anticoagulant medications when preparing patients with AF/AFL of > 48 hours for cardioversion. The ACC/AHA/ESC guidelines for the management of anticoagulation in patients with AF/AFL undergoing cardioversion recommend anticoagulation for at least 3 weeks prior and 4 weeks following cardioversion if the abnormal rhythm has been present for > 48 hours, with exceptions based on TEE evaluation (**Table 125-4**).

PROCEDURE TECHNIQUE

Following preprocedure preparation, a standardized procedure algorithm for performing electrical cardioversion should be followed (see Figure 125-2), including ECG lead and electrode pad placement, sedation, energy selection, synchronization, shock delivery, postshock patient and ECG assessment, and postprocedure monitoring.

ECG LEAD PLACEMENT

Cardioverter-defibrillators provide the option of continuously monitoring the patient's ECG using either external electrode pads or ECG leads. As a result, the ECG leads (typically three leads) are not required for cardioversion, but it is recommended that the leads be attached to the patient in nonemergent situations. Attaching the ECG leads provides additional information about the patient's heart rhythm and allows the operator to switch the lead used for monitoring and synchronization by the cardioverter-defibrillator. Using a standard three-lead (color-coded) ECG cable, the white lead is placed on the right side of the chest just below the right clavicle, the black lead is placed on the left chest just below the left clavicle, and the red lead is placed in the left midaxillary line near the apex of the heart.

ELECTRODE POSITIONING

Two electrodes (self-adhesive pads or hand-held paddles) are placed on the thorax for external cardioversion and determine the transthoracic current pathway. Electrode positioning on the chest is important to maximize current flow through the heart. The most commonly used electrodes for external cardioversion are

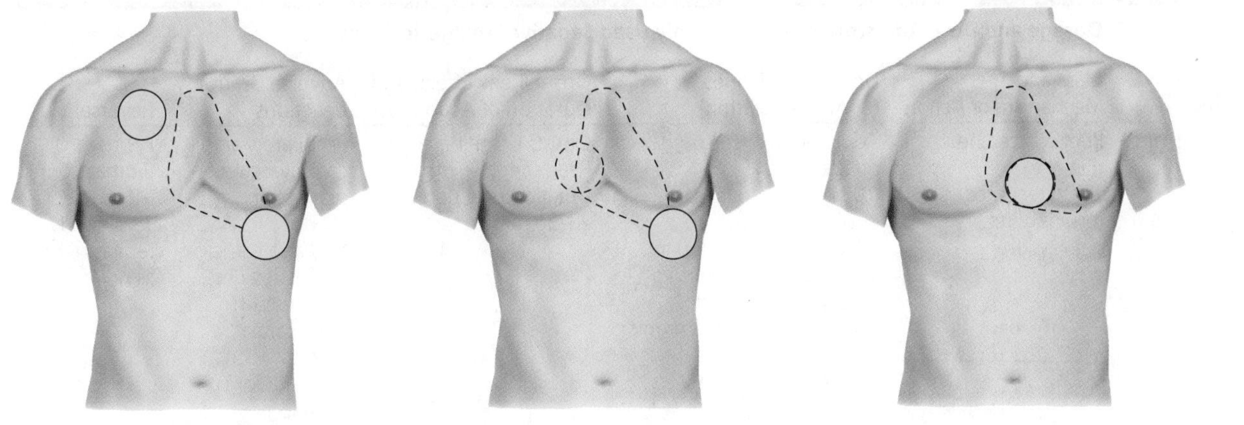

Figure 125-3 *Electrode positions commonly used for transthoracic defibrillation and cardioversion. (From Kerber RE. Transchest cardioversion: optimal techniques. In: Tacker WA, ed. Defibrillation of the Heart: ICDs, AEDs and Manual. St. Louis: Mosby-Year Book; 1994:163. With permission.)*

self-adhesive (ie, hands-free), pre-gelled, low-impedance, disposable-pad electrodes. A variety of anatomic pad placements can be used. Common electrode positions for transthoracic cardioversion/defibrillation include apex-anterior, apex-posterior, and anterior-posterior positions (**Figure 125-3**). Though all positions are effective, several studies have suggested that less energy is required, and the success rate is higher with the anterior-posterior electrode position in patients cardioverted for AF. More of the atrial mass is placed in the shock vector with anterior-posterior pads compared with apical-anterior pads. Some patients who do not respond to one method occasionally respond to another method. Therefore, if initial shocks are unsuccessful in terminating the arrhythmia, the pads should be repositioned and cardioversion repeated. Electrode pad size is an important determinant of transthoracic current flow during cardioversion, and the optimal electrode size for humans is approximately 8–12 cm in diameter.

While self-adhesive pads are convenient and safe, handheld paddles with manual pressure may be more effective than self-adhesive pads. This was illustrated in a randomized trial of patients referred for cardioversion for persistent AF, in which success rates were slightly higher for patients assigned to paddle electrodes (96% vs 88%). Improved electrode-to-skin contact and reduced transthoracic impedance with handheld electrodes may explain the benefit. Handheld paddles require the use of conducting gel to ensure good contact between the paddles and skin.

PRACTICE POINT

- Anterior-posterior electrode position requires less energy and shows higher cardioversion success rate for AF.

SEDATION

External cardioversion under conscious sedation or general anesthesia reduces pain and anxiety related to the procedure, since electrical cardioversion is an uncomfortable procedure. Prior to the initiation of sedation, the staff must determine and document the availability of a responsible adult to accompany the patient home at discharge postprocedure. Patent intravenous access must be secured in all patients. All equipment necessary for emergency resuscitation including oxygen, oxygen equipment/supplies, resuscitation bag and mask, monitoring equipment (ECG, pulse oximeter, blood pressure), functioning suction apparatus/catheters, and agents to reverse the effects of drugs administered to produce the moderate sedation (eg, naloxone, flumazenil) must be readily available. Crash cart/defibrillator and emergency airway equipment should be immediately accessible. Additionally, a physician skilled in airway management (eg, anesthesiologist) should be present or immediately available. Short-acting intravenous sedatives and short-acting analgesic agents that produce *conscious sedation* enable rapid recovery after the procedure (**Table 125-5**). As a result, overnight hospitalization is seldom required. A typical medication combination for conscious sedation would include intravenous midazolam plus fentanyl.

Conscious sedation is assessed by lack of response to tactile and verbal stimuli. The patient's ability to communicate should be preserved. Heart rate and rhythm, blood pressure, oxygen saturation, respiratory rate, and response to verbal stimuli (level of consciousness) should be continuously monitored until the patient regains consciousness and makes a full recovery. The patient usually awakens 5–10 minutes after the cardioversion. The patient should be monitored until full consciousness is restored and at least 1 hour (preferably several hours) after the last dosing of a sedative or an analgesic.

ENERGY SELECTION AND TRANSTHORACIC IMPEDANCE

PRACTICE POINT

- Obesity and severe obstructive lung disease increase thoracic impedance, which reduces the efficacy of cardioversion.

Successful cardioversion depends on the adequate delivery of energy to the heart, determined by the amount of energy provided by the cardioverter-defibrillator and the patient's transthoracic impedance. The amount of energy provided by the cardioverter-defibrillator is adjustable and selected at the time of cardioversion. The amount of energy selected for initial attempts of cardioversion-defibrillation has been controversial. More organized arrhythmias, such as AFL and VT, terminate with lower energy compared to AF and VF. In urgent settings, such as hemodynamic collapse associated with VT or VF, high-energy defibrillation (ie, 200 J max with a biphasic defibrillator; 360 J max with a monophasic defibrillator) may be used, but lower energy may be considered in this situation,

TABLE 125-5 Dosage and Dose Adjustments of Commonly Used Sedative/Analgesic Drugs

Drug	Class and Mechanism of Action	Dosing Guidelines (IV Administration)	Onset, Peak Effect, and Duration of Action	Adverse Drug Reactions	Reversal
Midazolam (Versed)	Benzodiazepine (Binds to GABA receptor resulting in CNS depression)	Adults 18–64 years of age: 0.05 mg/kg repeated every 2–3 minutes to adequate sedation up to a max dose of 0.2 mg/kg Elderly (>65) and those with COPD, CHF, or chronic debilitation: 0.02 mg/kg repeated every 2–3 minutes to adequate sedation up to a max dose of 0.2 mg/kg.	Onset: 1–3 min Peak effect: 5–7 min Duration of action: 20–30 min	Respiratory and cardiovascular depression may occur. May also cause ataxia, dizziness, hypotension, bradycardia, blurred vision, and paradoxical agitation.	Flumazenil (Romazicon): 0.2 mg over 15 seconds, may repeat at 1 min as needed
Lorazepam (Ativan)	Benzodiazepine (Binds to GABA receptor resulting in CNS depression)	Adults 18–64 years of age: 0.02–0.05 mg/kg repeated every 3–4 minutes up to a max dose of 4 mg Elderly (>65) and those with COPD, CHF, or chronic debilitation: 0.02 mg/kg repeated every 3–4 minutes up to a max of 4 mg.	Onset: 3–7 min Peak effect: 10–20 min Duration of action: 6–8 h	Respiratory and cardiovascular depression may occur. May also cause ataxia, dizziness, hypotension, bradycardia, blurred vision, and paradoxical agitation.	Flumazenil (Romazicon): 0.2 mg over 15 seconds, may repeat at 1 min as needed
Fentanyl (Sublimaze)	Opioid narcotic (Binds to opioid receptor in the CNS)	Adults 18–64 years of age: 0.5–1 μg/kg given in small incremental doses of 25–50 mcg up to a max dose of 250 μg Elderly (>65): 0.5–1 μg/kg given in small incremental doses of 25 μg up to a max dose of 100 μg. The elderly are more susceptible to CNS depression.	Onset 1–2 min Peak effect: 10–15 min Duration of action: 30–60 min	Hypotension, bradycardia, respiratory depression, nausea, vomiting, constipation, biliary spasm, and skin rash	Naloxone (Narcan): 0.4 mg initially followed by 0.1–0.2 mg every 2–3 minutes as needed Caution: Naloxone can result in a surge in sympathetic tone, hypertension, and ultimately pulmonary edema, in some cases.

CHF, congestive heart failure; CNS, central nervous system; COPD, chronic obstructive pulmonary disease; GABA, gamma-aminobutyric acid.

with monophasic defibrillators based on manufacturer recommendation (starting dose of 120 J is acceptable). There is no benefit to using greater than 360 joules. For cardioversion, lower energies effectively convert to sinus rhythm in most hemodynamically stable patients. In cardioversion, the minimum effective energy dose for shocks should be administered initially, and energy dose can be titrated up for additional shocks when the clinical situation permits (**Table 125-6**).

PRACTICE POINT

- Measures to reduce impedance and improve success during cardioversion include applying pressure to the pads, shocking during end-expiration, improving skin-electrode interface, and using conducting gels.

High transthoracic impedance, defined as the resistance of the chest to the flow of electrical current, degrades current flow through the heart. During transthoracic cardioversion, a considerably larger current must be delivered to compensate for transthoracic impedance. In animal studies, 82% of the transthoracic current was shunted to the thoracic cage, 14% to the lungs, and only 4% passed through to the heart during cardioversion. Obesity and severe obstructive lung disease increase impedance, which reduces the efficacy of cardioversion. Measures to reduce impedance should be undertaken, which include applying pressure to the pads, shocking during end-expiration, improving skin–electrode interface, and the use of conducting gels. The repeat administration of shocks also lowers impedance and improves efficacy of cardioversion. Conversely, increasing the distance between electrodes or increasing the amount of tissue or lung parenchyma between the electrodes increases impedance.

PRACTICE POINT

- In cardioversion, the minimum effective energy dose for shocks should be administered initially, and energy dose can be titrated up for additional shocks when the clinical situation permits.

TABLE 125-6 Energy Selection for Cardioversion of Commonly Encountered Arrhythmias

Arrhythmia	Energy Output (J) Monophasic	Energy Output (J) Biphasic	Synchronized	Success Rate
AF	Initial shock: 100 Subsequent shocks: 100–360 Median energy required in studies = 200 >200 may be required, particularly of AF of long duration	Initial: 50 Subsequent shocks: 50–170 Median energy required in studies = 100	Yes	75–94%
AFL	Initial shock: 50 Subsequent shocks: 50–200 Median energy required in studies = 200	Median energy required in studies = 50	Yes	90–100%
AVNRT, AVRT	Initial shock: 50 Subsequent shocks: 50–200	Not reported	Yes	Not reported
Stable VT	Initial shock: 100 Subsequent shocks: 100–200	Initial shock: 50 Subsequent shocks: 50–100	Yes	>90%

AF, atrial fibrillation; AFL, atrial flutter; AT, atrial tachycardia; AVNRT, atrioventricular nodal reciprocating tachycardia; AVRT, atrioventricular reciprocating tachycardia; VT, ventricular tachycardia.

SYNCHRONIZATION

Once the ECG leads and electrode pads are attached to the patient and the cardioverter-defibrillator is powered on, a good quality rhythm strip should be obtained to confirm the rhythm. The synchronize mode should be switched on, and confirmation of synchronization with the QRS complex should be confirmed on the monitor and on a telemetry printout. If the QRS is low amplitude or synchronization occurs with the T wave, the lead used for monitoring and synchronization on the cardioverter-defibrillator should be switched until a satisfactory QRS is seen and appropriate synchronization with each QRS complex is confirmed. *Synchronization is essential to avoid delivery of a shock during the vulnerable repolarization period, which can result in VF (see Figure 125-1).* If defibrillation is intended, the mode must be switched to asynchronous as the lack of an identifiable QRS complex will prevent the cardioverter-defibrillator from discharging in the synchronous mode.

SHOCK DELIVERY

A continuous rhythm strip should be obtained during the electroshock. Once the electrode pads are positioned and the appropriate energy and mode (synchronized or nonsynchronized) are selected, the adequacy of patient sedation should be confirmed. Next, the cardioverter-defibrillator capacitors are charged, the staff is warned to stay clear of the patient, and the shock is delivered to the patient. The patient is subsequently examined for adequacy of airway, breathing, and circulation, and the rhythm is confirmed by ECG. If the first attempt is unsuccessful, the procedure can be repeated as necessary with higher-energy shocks and/or changing the electrode pad position. This can be repeated until the arrhythmia terminates or a decision is made to abandon electrical cardioversion.

EFFICACY OF CARDIOVERSION

The overall immediate success rate of electrical cardioversion with AF is 75–94% and is inversely proportional to the duration of AF and size of the left atrium (Table 125-6). Although sinus rhythm can be restored in a substantial proportion of patients, the rate of relapse is high without concomitant antiarrhythmic drug therapy. After electrical cardioversion only 20–40% of patients maintain sinus rhythm for the first year compared to 29–53% in patients treated with antiarrhythmic drugs before electrical cardioversion and throughout follow-up. Most recurrences of AF occur within the first month after electrical cardioversion. Pretreatment with antiarrhythmic drugs (eg, amiodarone, flecanide, ibutilide, propafenone, or sotalol), recommended by the ACC/AHA/ESC, can enhance the success of electrical cardioversion and prevent recurrent AF. Pretreatment with pharmacological agents may have the greatest efficacy in patients who fail to respond to cardioversion and in those who develop acute or subacute recurrence of AF. In addition, prophylactic antiarrhythmic drug therapy may obviate the need for electrical cardioversion or reduce the energy required for the procedure by lowering the cardioversion threshold. In randomized trials of electrical cardioversion, patients pretreated with intravenous ibutilide were more often converted to sinus rhythm compared to untreated controls, and patients in whom cardioversion initially failed could more often be converted when the procedure was repeated after treatment with ibutilide.

PHARMACOLOGIC CARDIOVERSION

The development of new drugs has increased the popularity of pharmacologic cardioversion. Although pharmacologic and electrical cardioversion have not been directly compared, pharmacologic approaches appear simpler but are less effective. Unlike electrical cardioversion, pharmacologic cardioversion does not require conscious sedation or anesthesia. The major risk is related to the toxicity of antiarrhythmic drugs such as drug-induced torsades de pointes. Medications indicated for the pharmacologic cardioversion of AF less than or equal to 7 days' duration include flecanide, dofetilide, propafenone, ibutilide, or amiodarone. Pharmacologic cardioversion of AF present for more than 7 days includes dofetilide, amiodarone, or ibutilide.

Ibutilide is a class III antiarrhythmic drug (potassium-channel blocker) that prolongs the time for repolarization in atrial and ventricular myocardium. It is only available for intravenous use and is approved for the acute termination of AF/AFL of recent onset, but more effective for conversion of AFL. The 2006 practice guidelines from ACC/AHA/ESC recommend intravenous ibutilide for the pharmacologic cardioversion of AF/AFL ≤ 7 days' duration (class I recommendation) and for cardioversion of AF/AFL of more than 7 days duration (class IIA recommendation). In most patients who respond to ibutilide, arrhythmia termination is seen within 40 to 60 minutes after initiating the infusion. Ibutilide has a conversion rate of up to 75% to 80% in recent-onset atrial fibrillation and flutter; the conversion rate is higher for atrial flutter than for atrial fibrillation. Ibutilide has a 4% risk of torsades de pointes and should be avoided in patients with heart failure or prolonged QT interval.

Serum potassium and magnesium should be measured and electrolyte disturbances, especially hypokalemia or hypomagnesemia, corrected prior to use and throughout therapy with ibutilide. Ibutilide should be administered with continuous ECG monitoring at a dose of 0.01 mg/kg infused over 10 minutes for patients weighing less than 60 kg and at a dose of 1 mg over 10 minutes for patients weighing more than 60 kg. If the arrhythmia does not terminate 10 minutes after the end of the infusion, a second bolus (same dose over 10 minutes) can be given. The infusion should be stopped when the presenting arrhythmia is terminated or the patient develops sustained or nonsustained VT or marked prolongation of the QT interval. Because of the risk of QT prolongation and arrhythmias, patients treated with ibutilide should be observed with continuous ECG monitoring for at least 4 hours after the infusion or until the QT_C interval has returned to baseline. There is no evidence that the risk of thromboembolism with pharmacologic cardioversion differs from electrical cardioversion. Recommendations for anticoagulation are therefore the same for both methods.

PRACTICE POINT

- Ibutilide has a 4% risk of torsades de pointes and should be avoided in patients with depressed heart failure or prolonged QT interval.

COMPLICATIONS

Complications after electrical cardioversion are uncommon but can be serious and are mainly related to thromboembolism and arrhythmias (**Table 125-7**).

TABLE 125-7 Complications (And Incidence When Known) of Electrical Cardioversion

Electrocardiographic changes
ST segment depression (35%)
ST segment elevation (15–19%)
T wave changes
Arrhythmia and conduction abnormalities
Premature atrial contractions
Premature ventricular contractions
SVT (primarily sinus tachycardia) (30%)
Bradycardia (25%)
Left bundle branch block
Sinus arrest
High-degree atrioventricular heart block (15%)
NSVT (5%)
VT
VF (usually the result of an asynchronous shock)
Embolization (pulmonary and systemic)
1–5% nonanticoagulated patients
0.5–0.8% anticoagulated patients
Myocardial necrosis
Myocardial dysfunction
Atrial stunning
Left ventricular dysfunction
Transient hypotension
Pulmonary edema rare
Airway compromise
Painful skin burns (20–25%)
Physical trauma rare

NSVT, nonsustained ventricular tachycardia; SVT, supraventricular tachycardia; VF, ventricular fibrillation; VT, ventricular tachycardia.

THROMBOEMBOLISM

PRACTICE POINT

- Risk of thromboembolism with pharmacological cardioversion is similar to that with electrical cardioversion. Recommendations for anticoagulation are the same for both methods.

Thrombi can form within the atria (especially the left atrial appendage) due to stagnant blood flow that exists with AF/AFL. As a result, pulmonary and systemic embolization can occur after cardioversion (spontaneous, pharmacologic, or electrical) if an embolus becomes dislodged from the atria as the heart begins to contract normally. Such emboli in the systemic circulation could lead to stroke, myocardial infarction, bowel ischemia or infarction, or limb ischemia. Emboli occur less frequently in patients who have had AF/AFL < 48 hours (thromboembolic risk 0.8%). If patients with AF/AFL are appropriately anticoagulated for 3–4 weeks before cardioversion, the incidence of thromboembolism is 0.5–0.8%. The incidence is approximately 0.8% in TEE-guided cardioversion. The incidence of embolism in AF/AFL without precardioversion anticoagulation ranges from 1 to 5%. Patients with a previous embolism do not have an increased risk of embolization if anticoagulation is adequate. The risk of thromboembolism is highest in patients with rheumatic (or other) mitral stenosis, large left atrium, chronic AF, diabetes, hypertension, and prior cardiac embolic stroke.

ARRHYTHMIAS

PRACTICE POINT

- Premature atrial or ventricular beats occur commonly after cardioversion, and atrial arrhythmias—primarily sinus tachycardia—occur in up to 30% of patients. Bradycardia occurs in up to 25% of patients immediately after cardioversion. Nonsustained VT is seen in up to 5%, even without structural heart disease. Ventricular arrhythmias occur rarely, are not related to the number of shocks, and cannot be prevented by antiarrhythmic therapy.

Arrhythmias are occasionally observed after cardioversion. Premature atrial or ventricular beats are not uncommon after cardioversion, and atrial arrhythmias, primarily sinus tachycardia, are seen in up to 30% of patients. Alternatively, bradycardia is seen in up to 25% of patients immediately after cardioversion since cardioversion increases vagal tone. In one study of 75 patients undergoing cardioversion, sinus bradycardia occurred in 18 patients (24%), high-degree atrioventricular block occurred in 11 (15%), and temporary pacing was required in 10 (13%). Nonsustained VT is seen in up to 5% of patients and can occur in patients without structural heart disease. Patients receiving antiarrhythmic drugs are more prone to develop bradycardia and asystole postcardioversion. Temporary transthoracic pacing should be readily available at the time of cardioversion. Life-threatening arrhythmias are infrequent and may occur if the device is not properly synchronized. The occurrence of ventricular arrhythmias does not appear to be related to the number of shocks and cannot be prevented by antiarrhythmic therapy. Electrolyte imbalances, such as hypokalemia, and digitalis toxicity increase the risk of ventricular tachyarrhythmias.

AIRWAY COMPROMISE

Oversedation occurs most frequently in the elderly and in patients with renal and hepatic impairment and can cause respiratory depression. Dose adjustment should be considered in those populations. The patient's airway and oxygenation should be monitored carefully until complete recovery. *Reversal agents* for opiates and benzodiazepines (naloxone and flumazenil, respectively) should be readily available during the procedure. If the patient has identifiable high-risk airway features (described earlier) consultation with an anesthesiologist may be valuable.

CHEST WALL INJURY AND SKIN BURNS

PRACTICE POINT

- In order to reduce the frequency and severity of burns, proper skin–electrode interface should be confirmed, liberal conductive gel should be utilized, and the lowest effective amount of energy should be used.

First-degree skin burns of the chest wall, which can be painful, have been described with electrical cardioversion. These burns can be moderate to severe in up to 20–25% of patients undergoing cardioversion. In order to reduce the frequency and severity of burns, good skin–electrode interface should be confirmed, liberal conductive gel utilized (when using handheld paddles), and the lowest effective amount of energy should be used. Skin burns are more likely with improper technique and placement of electrodes. Though not performed routinely, the pretreatment of the skin with topical ibuprofen or steroid cream can reduce the pain and inflammation. The incidence of skin burns has been substantially reduced with the use of pre-gelled pads and biphasic defibrillators.

ELECTROCARDIOGRAPHIC CHANGES AND MYOCARDIAL INJURY

Electrocardiographic changes, including ST segment and T wave changes, can occur immediately after cardioversion. The frequency and extent of ST segment changes are lower with biphasic defibrillators. The QRS and QT intervals are not altered. Electrocardiogram findings are nonspecific, typically resolve within 5 minutes, and should not be used as the sole criteria for identifying an acute ischemic event. The pathogenesis of ST elevation is uncertain since elevations in creatine kinase MB isoenzyme or troponin are uncommon and are usually minimal when they occur. Some myocardial tissue damage or stunning may occur as a result of high-energy shocks or repeated shocks. Significant damage is uncommon, and there are generally no short- or long-term complications. Any decline in cardiac function after cardioversion is typically temporary and does not produce symptoms.

PRACTICE POINT

- ECG ST or T-wave changes following cardioversion are nonspecific, typically resolve within 5 minutes, and should not be used as the sole criteria for identifying an acute ischemic event.

INJURIES TO THE OPERATOR

Operator injuries during cardioversion occur very rarely, with an incidence of less than 1 in 1700. Cases of major electrocution have been described in extremely rare instances and have all been associated with equipment failure.

PHYSICAL TRAUMA TO THE PATIENT

Physical trauma to the patient is a rare complication and results from vigorous body movements during the delivery of the electric shock.

TROUBLESHOOTING

Failure of the monitor to work properly typically reflects a mechanical problem. The power source, lead connections, ECG leads, and electrode pads should be checked and confirmed. If the timing artifact during synchronization mode falls on the T wave, the monitoring lead should be changed until the correct position of the timing artifact is confirmed on the QRS complex. If the capacitor fails to discharge, this probably represents a failure to identify a QRS complex while in synchronized mode. The monitoring lead should be switched, synchronization on the QRS complex confirmed, and cardioversion reattempted.

CARDIOVERSION UNSUCCESSFUL

Important factors that determine the immediate and long-term success of cardioversion of atrial arrhythmias include the duration of the arrhythmia, the extent of atrial fibrosis, the size of the left atrium, and underlying structural heart disease (**Table 125-8**). If cardioversion is unsuccessful, a repeat ECG should be obtained to confirm the underlying rhythm. Next, the cardioversion telemetry strips should be carefully examined to distinguish between true failure to cardiovert and successful cardioversion that is followed by recurrence of arrhythmia. Patients with recurrence of arrhythmia might benefit from antiarrhythmic therapy before repeat attempts at cardioversion. For patients who truly fail to cardiovert, a higher level of energy, an alternate electrode pad configuration, or a biphasic device can be used on repeat attempts. In patients in whom AF recurs acutely or cardioversion fails, the combination of AV nodal blocker plus intravenous loading with amiodarone, procainamide, or ibutilide may pharmacologically restore sinus rhythm. If the AF persists, repeat cardioversion can be performed, and if successful the patient may be placed on long-term antiarrhythmic therapy.

TABLE 125-8 Factors Associated with Failed Cardioversion of Atrial Fibrillation

- Structural heart disease (eg, congestive heart failure, valvular disease)
- Underlying illness (eg, thyrotoxicosis)
- Dilated left atrium
- Extent of atrial fibrosis
- Longer duration of atrial fibrillation
- Too low energy
- Technique

Electrolyte disturbances, digitalis toxicity, and thyrotoxicosis may result in failure to cardiovert and should be corrected prior to cardioversion.

PREGNANCY

Successful cardioversion has been performed in all three trimesters of pregnancy without adverse consequences to the mother or fetus. Cardioversion does not affect the rhythm of the fetus though it is recommended that the fetal heart rhythm be monitored during the procedure.

IMPLANTABLE PACEMAKERS AND CARDIOVERTER-DEFIBRILLATORS

Several precautions are necessary when performing cardioversion in a patient with a permanent implanted device (pacemaker or ICD). Electrical cardioversion can change the settings of the device and may damage the pulse generator, the lead system, or myocardial tissue resulting in device dysfunction. To prevent this, the *electrode pads should be placed at least 12 cm from the implanted device*, preferably in the anterior-posterior position. Elective cardioversion should be initiated at low energies to reduce the risk of damage. The implantable device should be interrogated before and after cardioversion to ensure normal device function. When these precautions are employed, cardioversion with either monophasic or biphasic shocks is safe and effective in patients with implantable devices.

CONSULTATION

In 2000, an ACC/AHA task force on clinical competency published recommendations for technical and cognitive skills needed to perform external electrical cardioversion. The ACC/AHA also recommends that the minimum training necessary for competence to perform external electrical cardioversion should include competence in the interpretation of 12-lead ECGs. Previous ACC/AHA task forces recommended a minimum of eight supervised electrical cardioversions as a minimum requirement. The competence in electrical cardioversion may be achievable without formal training in cardiovascular disease. For physicians without adequate experience with electrical cardioversion, a cardiologist should be enlisted to assist with or perform the procedure. There are no published clinical competency recommendations for the use of pharmacologic cardioversion with antiarrhythmic drugs. For physicians without adequate experience with antiarrhythmic drugs, a cardiologist may be enlisted to assist with pharmacologic cardioversion as well.

QUALITY IMPROVEMENT TO ADDRESS PERFORMANCE GAPS

SECONDARY PREVENTION

Maintenance therapy with antiarrhythmic drugs is not typically recommended after electrical cardioverson in patients with a first episode of AF, particularly those at low risk for recurrence (eg, short duration and normal left atrial size) or those with a reversible cause (eg, cardiac surgery, pulmonary embolus, or hyperthyroidism). In other patients with recurrent paroxysmal or persistent AF, maintenance antiarrhythmic drug therapy may be administered to reduce the risk of recurrence *if a rhythm control strategy is chosen*. Because of the adverse effects associated with antiarrhythmic drugs and no difference in outcomes between rhythm and rate control strategies, many authorities reserve the use of long-term antiarrhythmic drug therapy to patients that remain symptomatic with rate control (**Table 125-9**).

TRANSITIONS OF CARE

After cardioversion, all patients should receive warfarin therapy for at least 4 weeks. A plan for anticoagulation and follow-up with INR monitoring with a primary physician, cardiologist, or specialized

TABLE 125-9 Evidence-based Medicine: Key References for Cardioversion

Study	Methodology	Results	Limitations	Bottom Line
Botto GL, Politi A, Bonini W, et al. External cardioversion of atrial fibrillation: role of paddle position on technical efficacy and energy requirements. *Heart*. 1999;82:726–730.	Randomized controlled trial comparing elective DCCV using AL paddle position vs AP paddle position in patients with stable AF	301 patients enrolled; higher success rate of conversion to NSR in AP group (87%) vs AL group (76%) ($p = 0.013$); arrhythmia duration was the only factor that affected the technical success of DCCV	Exclusion criteria included patients with AF duration > 2 years or of unknown duration; technical success was defined as interruption of AF for > 10 seconds; pharmacological antiarrhythmic treatment was not randomized	An AP paddle position is superior to an AL location with regard to success in DCCV of stable AF and permits lower shock energy requirements
Klein AL, Grimm RA, Murray RD, et al. Assessment of Cardioversion Using Transesophageal Echocardiography Investigators. Use of transesophageal echocardiography to guide cardioversion in patients with atrial fibrillation. *N Engl J Med*. 2001;344: 1411–1420.	Multicenter, randomized controlled trial comparing TEE-guided vs conventional treatment (warfarin for 3 weeks) in patients with AF > 48 hours undergoing elective DCCV	1222 patients enrolled; there was no significant difference between the TEE-guided group (0.8%) vs conventional treatment group (0.5%) ($p = 0.50$) in the rate of embolic events; fewer hemorrhagic events in TEE-guided group (2.9%) vs conventional treatment (5.5%) ($p = 0.03$)	Short duration of follow-up (8 weeks); there was greater use of antiarrhythmic medication in the conventional treatment group at the time of cardioversion (92.8%) vs TEE-guided group (82.2%) ($P < 0.001$)	TEE-guided cardioversion allows for early, safe cardioversion of AF and may be considered a clinically effective alternative to conventional therapy

(continued)

TABLE 125-9 Evidence-based Medicine: Key References for Cardioversion *(continued)*

Study	Methodology	Results	Limitations	Bottom line
Niebauer MJ, Brewer JE, Chung MK, et al. Comparison of the rectilinear biphasic waveform with the monophasic damped sine waveform for external cardioversion of atrial fibrillation and flutter. *Am J Cardiol.* 2004;93:1495–1499.	Retrospective trial comparing the results of DCCV using biphasic waveform to monophasic waveform in patients with AF and AFL	1361 patients in biphasic waveform group; 2025 patients in monophasic waveform group; overall success rate for AF was 99.8% in biphasic group and 92.4% in monophasic group ($P < 0.001$); successful energy for cardioversion of AF in biphasic group (median = 100 j) compared to monophasic group (median = 200 j)	Methodological limitations inherent to retrospective study design	Very high success rate for cardioversion of AF/AFL with biphasic waveform; monophasic waveform equally effective for AFL but significantly less effective in terminating AF; biphasic waveform permits lower shock energy requirements
Oral H, Souza JJ, Michaud GF, et al. Facilitating transthoracic cardioversion of atrial fibrillation with ibutilide pretreatment. *N Engl J Med.* 1999; 340:1849–1854.	Randomized controlled trial comparing DCCV with and without pretreatment with 1 mg of ibutilide in patients with AF	100 patients enrolled; conversion to NSR (100%) with ibutilide pretreatment; conversion to NSR (72%) without pretreatment ($p < 0.001$); all patients in whom DCCV alone failed, NSR was restored when cardioversion was attempted again after the administration of ibutilide	Only one technique for DCCV was used; many patients were currently being treated with antiarrhythmic drugs, and a synergistic effect with ibutilide could not be ruled out	Efficacy of DCCV for converting AF to NSR was enhanced by pretreatment with ibutilide; pretreatment with ibutilide was associated with lower shock energy requirements
Stambler BS, Wood MA, Ellenbogen KA, et al. Efficacy and safety of repeated intravenous doses of ibutilide for rapid conversion of atrial flutter or fibrillation. Ibutilide Repeat Dose Study Investigators. *Circulation.* 1996;94: 1613–1621.	Randomized controlled trial comparing intravenous ibutilide to placebo for pharmacologic cardioverson of AF or AFL	261 patients enrolled; conversion rate with ibutilide (47%) vs placebo (2%) ($P < 0.0001$); efficacy higher in AFL (63%) vs AF (31%) ($P < 0.0001$); arrhythmia termination occurred a mean of 27 minutes after start of ibutilide infusion; 8.3% patients developed polymorphic VT with ibutilide	Methodological limitations inherent to placebo-controlled design; only patients with sustained AF/AFL > 3 hours and < 45 days were enrolled	Intravenous ibutilide given in repeated doses (under monitored conditions) is effective in rapidly terminating AF and AFL and is an alternative to current cardioversion options

AF, atrial fibrillation; AFL, atrial flutter; AL, anterolateral; AP, anteroposterior; DCCV, direct current cardioversion; NSR, normal sinus rhythm; TEE, transesophageal echocardiogram; VT, ventricular tachycardia.

Coumadin clinic should be established. Patients with AF at high risk from thromboembolic events based on CHADS2 score may require long-term anticoagulation. Patients with new-onset AF should undergo thyroid function testing and receive an echocardiogram. Patients with no recurrence can follow up with their primary care physicians as outpatients and do not require any additional testing. Patients with either recurrent, symptomatic AF (despite attempts at rate control) or patients who prefer a rhythm control strategy should be referred to a cardiologist. Cardiology referral for initiation of an antiarrhythmic drug, if required, may also be indicated unless the physician is experienced with and knowledgeable of administration of these drugs. Because most antiarrhythmic agents can also be proarrhythmic, and because many have dangerous side effects to monitor, their initiation and maintenance should be performed by a clinician experienced in their use.

SUGGESTED READINGS

Botkin SB, Dhanekula LS, Olshansky B. Outpatient cardioversion of atrial arrhythmias: efficacy, safety, and costs. *Am Heart J.* 2003; 145:233–238.

Botto GL, Politi A, Bonini W, et al. External cardioversion of atrial fibrillation: role of paddle position on technical efficacy and energy requirements. *Heart.* 1999;82:726–730.

Fuster V, Rydén LE, Cannom DS, et al. ACC/AHA/ESC 2006 Guidelines for the Management of Patients with Atrial Fibrillation: a report of the American College of Cardiology/American Heart Association Task Force on Practice Guidelines and the European Society of Cardiology Committee for Practice Guidelines (Writing Committee to Revise the 2001 Guidelines for the Management of Patients with Atrial Fibrillation). *J Am Coll Cardiol.* 2006;48: e149–e246.

Kerber RE. Indications and techniques of electrical defibrillation and cardioversion. In: Fuster V, O'Rourke RA, Walsh RA, Poole-Wilson P, eds. *Hurst's the Heart.* 12th ed. New York: McGraw-Hill; 2008:1102–1108.

Klein AL, Grimm RA, Murray RD, et al. Assessment of Cardioversion Using Transesophageal Echocardiography Investigators. Use of transesophageal echocardiography to guide cardioversion in patients with atrial fibrillation. *N Engl J Med.* 2001;344:1411–1420.

Manegold JC, Israel CW, Ehrlich JR, et al. External cardioversion of atrial fibrillation in patients with implanted pacemaker or cardioverter-defibrillator systems: a randomized comparison of monophasic and biphasic shock energy application. *Eur Heart J.* 2007;28:1731–1738.

Niebauer MJ, Brewer JE, Chung MK, et al. Comparison of the rectilinear biphasic waveform with the monophasic damped sine waveform for external cardioversion of atrial fibrillation and flutter. *Am J Cardiol.* 2004;93:1495–1499.

Oral H, Souza JJ, Michaud GF, et al. Facilitating transthoracic cardioversion of atrial fibrillation with ibutilide pretreatment. *N Engl J Med*. 1999;340:1849–1854.

Stambler BS, Wood MA, Ellenbogen KA, et al. Efficacy and safety of repeated intravenous doses of ibutilide for rapid conversion of atrial flutter or fibrillation. Ibutilide Repeat Dose Study Investigators. *Circulation*. 1996;94:1613–1621.

Tracy CM, Akhtar M, DiMarco JP, et al. American College of Cardiology/American Heart Association clinical competence statement on invasive electrophysiology studies, catheter ablation, and cardioversion: a report of the American College of Cardiology/American Heart Association/American College of Physicians–American Society of Internal Medicine task force on clinical competence. *Circulation*. 2000;102:2309–2320.

CHAPTER 126

Supraventricular Tachyarrhythmias

Elbert B. Chun, MD
Gerard M. McGorisk, MD, FACC, MRCPI

Key Clinical Questions

1. What electrocardiographic findings help differentiate between the common supraventricular tachyarrhythmias (SVTs)?
2. What acute and chronic management strategies are indicated for various SVTs?
3. What comorbid conditions increase the risk of thromboembolic complications in patients with atrial fibrillation?
4. Which patients with atrial fibrillation deserve anticoagulation, and which of these patients need bridging anticoagulation until oral warfarin attains therapeutic international normalized ratio (INR)?
5. Which SVTs deserve electrophysiologic intervention over medical management?

INTRODUCTION

Supraventricular tachyarrhythmias (SVTs) comprise an array of narrow-complex arrhythmias that originate above the ventricles and include both the most commonly encountered arrhythmia, atrial fibrillation (AF), and the uncommon ones, such as Wolfe-Parkinson-White (WPW) syndrome. This chapter describes in detail the common atrial arrhythmias encountered by hospitalists, and explains the uncommon arrhythmias that hospitalists should recognize and manage with cardiologist or electrophysiologist consultation or referral. The chapter will briefly describe arrhythmia mechanisms while focusing on arrhythmia diagnosis, management options in the acute setting, and long-term management strategies—all essential for a seamless transition beyond the inpatient setting.

PRESENTATION

Common presenting symptoms of SVTs include rapid palpitations, chest discomfort, dyspnea, presyncope, and syncope. Additionally, atrial fibrillation and atrial flutter may present with new stroke symptoms. Particularly in the elderly with atrial fibrillation, palpitations and chest discomfort are often absent and excessive fatigue is the predominant symptom.

RHYTHM IDENTIFICATION

When evaluating patients with a narrow-complex arrhythmia, the QRS complex is by definition less than 120 ms. The regularity of the RR intervals then helps reduce the numerous possibilities, as indicated in the SVT recognition algorithm (**Figure 126-1**). Only four possibilities exist if the RR intervals are *irregular*: (1) atrial fibrillation, (2) atrial flutter with variable atrioventricular (AV) node blockade, (3) atrial tachycardia with variable AV node blockade, and (4) multifocal atrial tachycardia (MAT).

More challenging to diagnose is the SVT with a regular RR interval. If, however, no P wave can be identified, this indicates the most common form of *paroxysmal* SVT: atrioventricular nodal reentrant tachycardia (AVnRT). The P wave in typical AVnRT is buried within the QRS complex. If the P wave is identified, then determine if there is more than one P wave for each conducted QRS. If so, then only atrial flutter or atrial tachycardia remain as possible diagnoses.

Finally, if only a 1-to-1 relationship between the P waves and QRS complexes exists, measuring the RP interval will further narrow the likely rhythms (**Figure 126-2**). The response of the rhythm to bedside vagal maneuvers or intravenous adenosine can be used to better differentiate the regular narrow-complex arrhythmias by transiently slowing the AV conduction and revealing the P waves, converting the rhythm to sinus, or gradually slowing and reaccelerating the tachycardia (**Table 126-1**).

Proceeding through the SVT recognition algorithm (see Figure 126-1) using a sample ECG (**Figure 126-3**) the clinician first recognizes that the rate is greater than 100 beats per minute (bpm). The QRS complexes are narrow, thus leading to a generic diagnosis of SVT. Following the SVT recognition algorithm, the regularity of the RR intervals is assessed, and the absence of P waves leads to the conclusion that the SVT is attributable to typical AVnRT (see Figure 126-3).

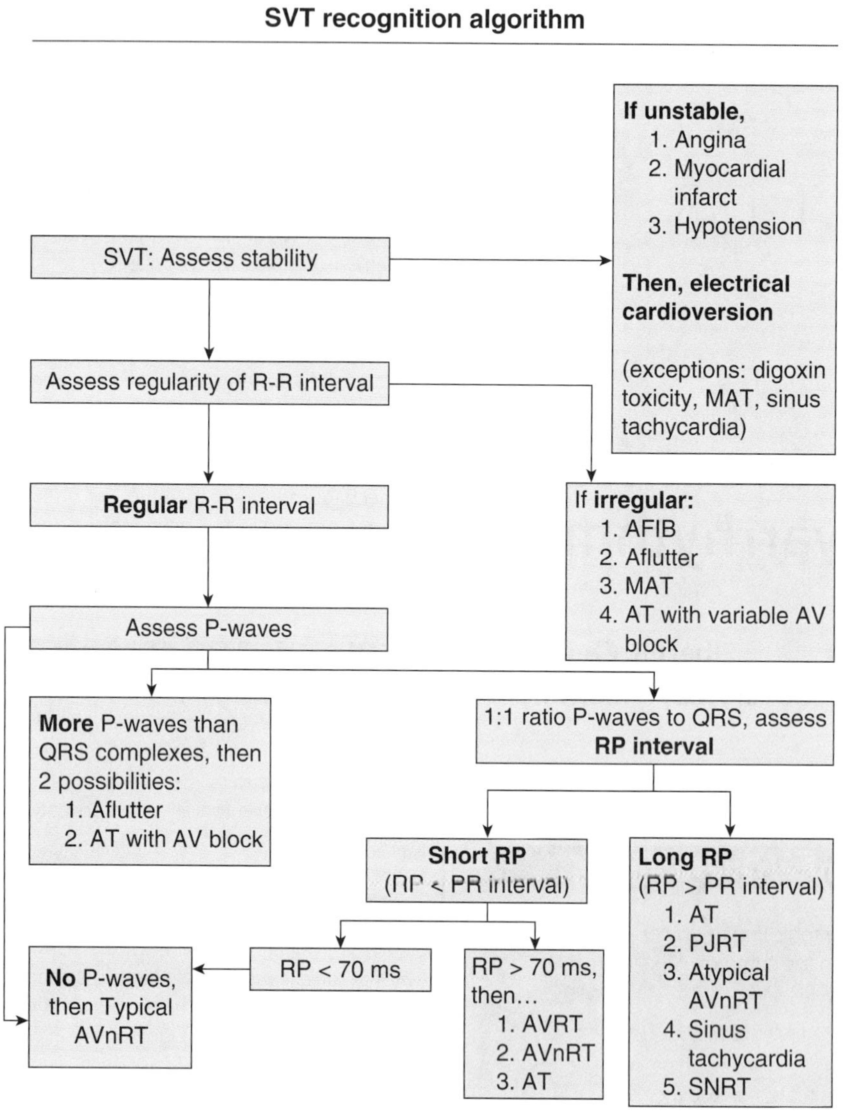

Figure 126-1 *Supraventricular tachyarrhythmia recognition algorithm. AF, atrial fibrillation; Aflutter, atrial flutter; AT, atrial tachycardia; AV block, atrioventricular block; AVnRT, atrioventricular nodal reentrant tachycardia; AVRT, atrioventricular reentry tachycardia; MAT, multifocal atrial tachycardia; PJRT, paroxysmal junctional reentrant tachycardia; SNRT, sinus node reentry tachycardia.*

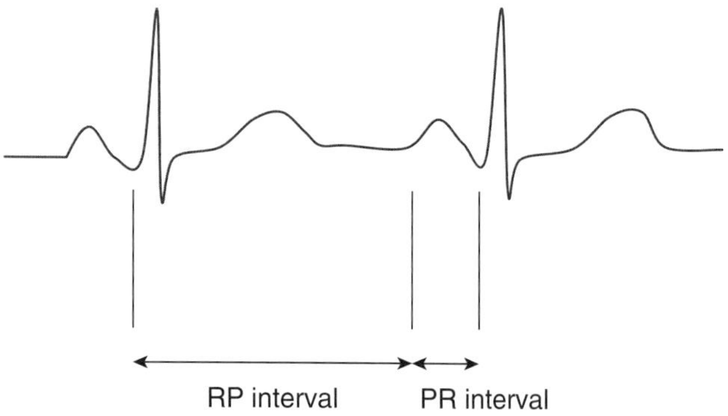

Figure 126-2 *ECG rhythm intervals demonstrating how to measure the PR and RP intervals.*

ATRIAL FIBRILLATION

EPIDEMIOLOGY

Before the age of 60, the prevalence of atrial fibrillation (AF) occurs uncommonly, in stark contrast to the prevalence estimate of 8% among those older than 80 years. As AF is the most common arrhythmia encountered by the inpatient clinician, this section will address the questions pertaining to the valvular and nonvalvular etiology of this arrhythmia, judicious utilization of cardioversion, thromboembolic and other complications, methods for estimating risk of stroke, and management strategies in the acute and chronic settings.

Patients with atrial fibrillation are classified in one of three categories: (1) paroxysmal AF, (2) persistent AF, or (3) permanent AF (**Table 126-2**).

TABLE 126-1 Effect of Transient Atrioventricular Node Blockade on Supraventricular Tachyarrhythmia Diagnosis

Rhythm	Response to Transient AV Node Blockade (vagal maneuvers or IV adenosine)
AVnRT	Sudden termination
AVRT	Sudden termination
Sinus reentry tachycardia	Sudden termination
Focal atrial tachycardia	Sudden termination, or gradual slowing and reacceleration
Ventricular tachycardia (high septal or fascicular origin)	No response
Sinus tachycardia	Gradual slowing, then reacceleration
Nonparoxysmal junctional tachycardia	Gradual slowing, then reacceleration
Atrial flutter	Persistent atrial tachycardia and transient high-grade AV blockade
Macroreentrant atrial tachycardia	Persistent atrial tachycardia and transient high-grade AV blockade

AVnRT, atrioventricular nodal reentrant tachycardia; AVRT, atrioventricular reentry tachycardia; VTACH, ventricular tachycardia.

PATHOPHYSIOLOGY

The atrium in patients with AF shows evidence of fibrosis and increased extracellular mass changes that are seen both in the myocardium of the elderly and in ischemia-induced hibernating myocardium. Within this scarred milieu, a focal-enhanced automaticity and variance in atrial tissue refractory and conduction times (known collectively as the *multiple wavelet hypothesis*) leads to this common arrhythmia. The enhanced automaticity often can be isolated to atrial tissue near the pulmonary veins. In addition to the aging process, any medical condition that leads to elevated left atrial pressure and dilated atrium—hypertension, mitral stenosis or regurgitation, and any cardiomyopathy—will predispose the patient to atrial fibrillation. Hyperadrenergic states—sepsis, alcohol ingestion or withdrawal, postoperative state, and thyrotoxicosis—also predispose to AF. *Lone atrial fibrillation* describes AF in patients younger than 60 years old in the absence of any predisposing factor.

TABLE 126-2 Atrial Fibrillation Nomenclature

Paroxysmal AF	Episodes lasting <7 days and spontaneously converting to sinus rhythm
Persistent AF	Episodes lasting >7 days unless chemical or electrically cardioverted to sinus rhythm
Permanent AF	AF resistant to multiple attempts at cardioversion
Lone AF	AF in patients younger than 60 years old in the absence of any predisposing factor

AF, atrial fibrillation.

INITIAL HOSPITAL TREATMENT

Hemodynamic compromise versus stable tachycardia

Common clinical scenarios for hospitalized patients with AF include those with stable tachycardia and those with hemodynamic compromise. For those with hypotension, a trial of *short-acting* rate-controlling agents (eg, esmolol) could be attempted to determine if slowing the tachycardia may improve the hemodynamics, keeping in mind that these very agents may exacerbate hypotension. Intravenous digoxin and amiodarone are options if hypotension prevents the use of beta-blockers and calcium channel blockers. Synchronized direct cardioversion should be performed if the hypotension does not resolve (see Chapter 125). Currently there

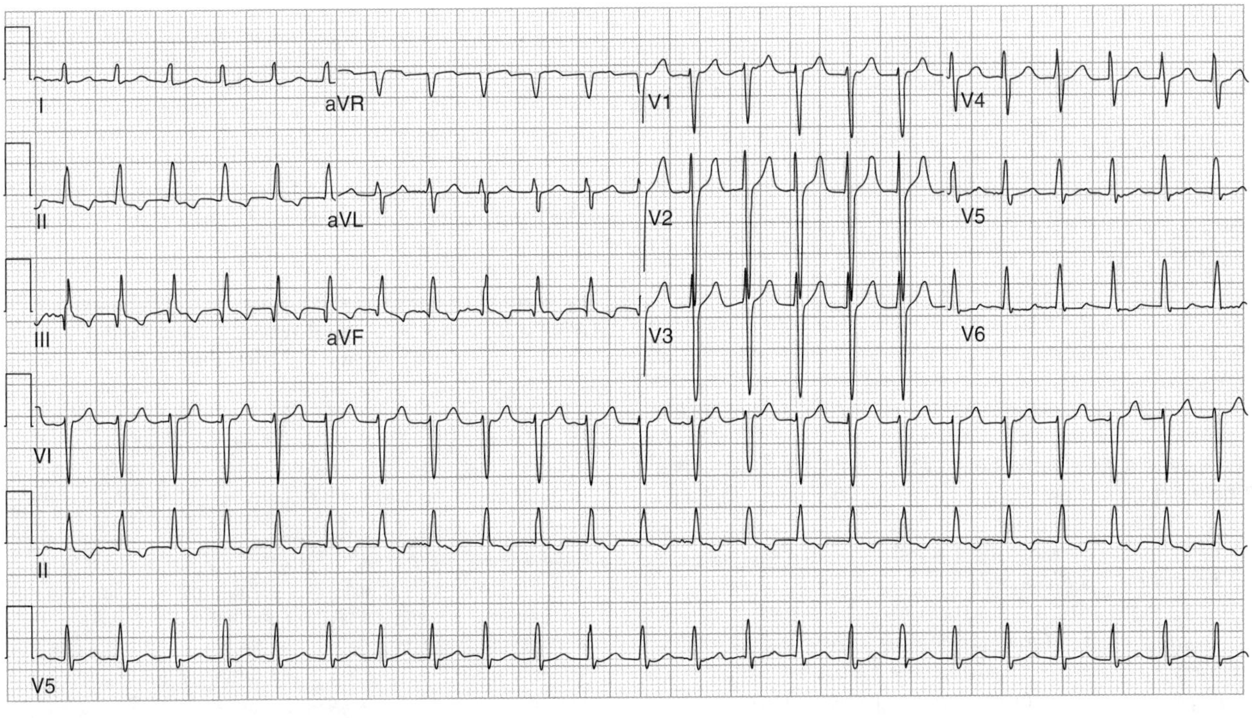

Figure 126-3 *Atrioventricular nodal tachycardia (AVnRT).*

TABLE 126-3 Intravenous Medications for Rate-Control in Atrial Fibrillation or Atrial Flutter

Medication	Loading Dose	Maintainence Dose	Side Effects
Esmolol	500 mcg/kg over 1 minute	60–200 mcg/kg/minute IV	Hypotension
Metoprolol	2.5–5 mg IV over 2 minutes Up to 3 doses	NA	Hypotension
Diltiazem	0.25 mg/kg IV over 2 minutes	5–15 mg/hour	Hypotension
Verapamil	0.075–0.15 mg/kg IV over 2 minutes	NA	Hypotension
Digoxin	0.25 mg IV every 2 hours up to total dose 1.5 mg	0.125–0.375 mg/day IV or orally	Digoxin toxicity, heart block
Amiodarone	150 mg IV over 10 minutes	0.5–1 mg/minute IV	Pulmonary toxcity, hepatitis, skin discoloration, thyroid dysfunction, corneal deposits, optic neuropathy

are two types of defibrillators: monophasic and biphasic. Biphasic defibrillators are now more common and require less energy and reduced number of shocks delivered to achieve successful cardioversion. Biphasic defibrillators also have reduced skin injury. The monophasic device should be set at a minimum of 200 joules and a maximum of 400 joules. The biphasic device demonstrates effective cardioversion at 200 joules and often times at just 100 joules for AF.

Rate control

One or multiple rate-controlling agents may be needed to provide adequate control of the ventricular response (**Table 126-3**). After 24 hours on the intravenous infusion, switching to an oral regimen can be initiated. Beta-blockers and nondihydropyridine calcium channel blockers are considered first-line agents. Intravenous digoxin and amiodarone are reasonable options, particularly in the setting of congestive heart failure. An important limitation of digoxin is that its vagally induced AV node blockade can be easily overcome in nonsedentary patients. Although very effective in rate control and even rhythm conversion, amiodarone has a long-term side-effect profile which relegates its use as a distant second option. Clinicians should target a heart rate under 110 bpm at rest but consider patient symptoms in modification of rate control.

The presence of an accessory pathway would be an absolute contraindication in the use of AV node–blocking agents. As electrical impulses are conducted nondecrementally via the accessory pathway, the ventricular response in AF will actually increase and may degenerate into ventricular fibrillation (VFIB).

Rhythm control and consultation

After assessing clinical stability and adequately controlling the rapid ventricular response, the clinician should determine if the rhythm event is new, recurrent, or an exacerbation of a permanent form of the arrhythmia. If the condition is a new event or a paroxysmal one with infrequent yet very symptomatic recurrences and has been present for *less than 48 hours*, cardioversion—chemical or electrical—followed by an attempt to maintain a sinus rhythm may offer symptom benefit and is recommended by the ACC-AHA AF guidelines from 2006 (**Table 126-4**). If the AF duration is longer than 48 hours, cardioversion remains an option after trans-esophageal echo (TEE) is negative for left atrial thrombus. Cardioverting those with new-onset AF provides the theoretical benefit of curtailing the risk of developing permanent AF.

Cardioversion can be achieved not only with electrical means, but also chemical means (**Table 126-5**). The antiarrhythmics used for cardioversion should be considered after consultation with cardiology service. A class III agent, ibutilide, can be used in select patients that have no evidence of systolic dysfunction, normal magnesium and potassium levels, and a normal corrected QT interval (QTc). Due to the risk of torsades de pointes, this should be performed in a setting equipped to handle this potential complication. Ibutilide has the advantage of increasing the efficacy of electrical cardioversion that would follow a failed chemical cardioversion. An oral class III agent, tikosyn, can be used to both convert to a sinus rhythm and also maintain a sinus rhythm. This medication should be reserved for cardiology consultants due to the need for close monitoring of the QT interval, renal dose adjustments, and limitations of use in patients with liver dysfunction. If the QT interval is greater than 500 ms, this medication should not be initiated or should be discontinued. The use of medications to maintain a sinus rhythm should remain under the care of a cardiologist due to the frequency of treatment failure and significant risk of malignant ventricular arrhythmias.

OUTPATIENT LONGITUDINAL THERAPEUTICS

Anticoagulation

The unorganized atrial contractions during AF will lead to the formation of thrombus or spontaneous echo contrast (SEC) within the left atrium or the left atrial appendage posing a substantial risk of thromboembolic phenomena to the arterial circulation, which usually manifests as stroke and, less commonly, mesenteric ischemia or an acutely ischemic limb. Although the transthoracic echocardiogram is considered the diagnostic test of choice for initial evaluation, the transesophageal echocardiogram (TEE) provides a much better resolution of the left atrium and left atrial appendage and is useful for *an early cardioversion strategy*. Thrombus or dense SEC would preclude the option for early cardioversion and necessitate the need for full anticoagulation with a vitamin K antagonist

TABLE 126-4 Indication for R-Wave Synchronized Cardioversion in Atrial Fibrillation

Rapid ventricular response not responding to pharmacologic measures in setting of ongoing angina, heart failure, myocardial ischemia, or symptomatic hypotension
Preexcitation with rapid ventricular response or hemodynamic instability
Stable hemodynamics, but poorly tolerated symptoms
Early relapse of atrial fibrillation after attempted cardioversion, proceed with administration of antiarrhythmic medications first, then repeat cardioversion
Consider patient preferences in the setting of infrequent relapses

TABLE 126-5 Medications for Pharmacologic Cardioversion of Atrial Fibrillation

Medication	Antiarrhythmic Class	Dosing	Route	Comments
Amiodarone (codarone, pacerone)	III	400 mg orally twice a day for 2 weeks (10 gm load), then 200 mg orally every day 150 mg IV over 10 minutes, then 1 mg/min for 6 hrs, then 0.5 mg/min for 18 hrs (1 gm load)	Oral	Outpatient option: oral load (gastrointestinal side effects common) Other side effects common and severe: pulmonary fibrosis, corneal deposits, thyroid dysfunction, hepatitis, skin deposition
Ibutilide (corvert)	III	If weight > 60 kg, 1 mg IV once; may repeat dose if no response in 10 mins If weight < 60 kg, then 0.01 mg/kg IV; may repeat if no response after 10 mins	IV	Inpatient only usually cardioverts within 1 hr monitor for QT prolongation Torsades 4% (more common in women) Must monitor K^+ and Mg^{+2}
Dofetilide (tikosyn)	III	500 mcg orally twice a day (restricted distribution in the U.S. to trained prescribers and facilities)	Orally	Inpatient initiation only; adjust for renal function, age, body size QT prolongation Many drug interactions (CYP3A4) Contraindicated with Bactrim, HCTZ, verapamil
Flecainide	Ic	Start 50 mg orally twice a day, may increase 100 mg/day every 4 days; max dose 300 mg every day	Orally or IV	Contraindicated in structural heart disease Adjust dose for renal dysfunction
Propafenone	Ia	Start 150 mg orally three times a day, then may increase to 225 mg orally three times a day after 4 days, then, up to 300 mg orally three times a day	Orally or IV	Contraindicated in structural heart disease including significant LVH, CHF, severe obstructive lung disease

for four weeks prior to cardioversion. In the absence of thrombus or SEC on TEE, the patient may receive early cardioversion in the setting of anticoagulation. For AF recognized greater than 48 hours after onset in patients who do not undergo TEE, full anticoagulation for four weeks is recommended followed by cardioversion, if indicated.

In either strategy, anticoagulation for a minimum of four weeks postcardioversion is necessary to reduce the risk of thromboembolic complications. The risk of embolic stroke is approximately 1% with either approach. Stroke risk postcardioversion is due to a "stunning" effect on the left atrium after any form of cardioversion (electrical, chemical, or even spontaneous). This stunning refers to a delay in the actual mechanical contraction of the left atrium, providing an environment ripe for stasis and thus thrombus formation. Benefits from an early cardioversion approach would be quicker conversion to a sinus rhythm, accelerated care for the patient, and potentially less bleeding complications associated without the preceding four weeks of anticoagulation.

PRACTICE POINT

- Transesophageal echocardiogram is a highly sensitive test to rule out thrombus within the left atrium and left atrial appendage to permit an early cardioversion strategy, if indicated.

Ablation strategies

Invasive management options for atrial fibrillation should be considered secondary options following failure of medical therapies and recurrent admissions due to symptomatic palpitations or heart failure exacerbations. The palpitations associated with atrial fibrillation can be distressing to some individuals, particularly younger patients, and have significant negative impacts on quality of life. If the use of antiarrhythmic regimens has failed, options for catheter-based interventions or even intraoperative left atrial ablation, also known as the Maze procedure can be offered. One catheter-based approach called *ablate-and-pace*, entails ablating the AV node and then pacing the ventricle. Another catheter-based approach involves isolating the focus of automaticity, usually near the pulmonary veins of the cavoatrial isthmus, ablating the foci, and initiating anticoagulation therapy thereafter. The latter approach is relatively new and long-term outcome research is still pending. The short-term safety of the procedure in centers with established experience has been proven with death rates or stroke rates under 1% and overall major complications about 6% based on international survey data. However, the mean age of the patients enrolled in these trials was 55 years old with intact systolic function and relatively nondilated atrial diameters. More long-term outcome data will be needed before catheter-based interventions can be considered a parallel option to medical treatment. A final option usually reserved for those who are undergoing open heart bypass or valve replacement is the Maze procedure, and even left atrial appendage resection, both of which may prevent the occurrence of postoperative atrial fibrillation.

COMPLICATIONS AND PROGNOSIS

Death or significant neurologic deficits occur in 71% of patients with their first episode of embolic complications associated with AF. Reducing this risk is a crucial component in the management of AF. The annual risk of strokes for AF is approximately 4.5% per year, which is reduced by two-thirds (to 1.5% per year) if patients are fully

TABLE 126-6 Antithrombotic Recommendations for Atrial Fibrillation by Etiology

AF Risk Factor	Therapy Recommendation	Level of Evidence
Thyrotoxicosis	Full anticoagulation (eg, warfarin)	Level C: Expert opinion (ACC/AHA guidelines)
Mitral stenosis	Full anticoagulation (eg, warfarin)	Level C: Expert opinion (ACC/AHA guidelines)
Mechanical valve	Full anticoagulation (eg, warfarin)	Level 1A (ACCP guidelines 2008)
$CHADS_2$ score ≥ 2	Full anticoagulation (eg, warfarin)	Level 1A (ACCP guidelines 2008)
$CHADS_2$ score = 1	Full anticoagulation (eg, warfarin) or aspirin (75–325 mg daily)	Level 1A (anticoagulation) Level 1B (asprin) (ACCP guidelines 2008)
$CHADS_2$ score = 0	Aspirin therapy (75–325 mg daily)	Level 1B (ACCP guidelines 2008)

ACC/AHA, American College of Cardiology/American Heart Association; ACCP, American College of Chest Physicians.
Level 1A (ACCP): Consistent evidence from randomized controlled trials without important limitations or exceptionally strong evidence from observational studies.
Level 1B (ACCP): Evidence from randomized controlled trials with important limitations (inconsistent results, methodologic flaws, indirect or imprecise), or very strong evidence from observational studies.
Level C (ACC/AHA): Recommendation based on expert opinion, case studies, or standards of care.

anticoagulated. However, not all patients with this condition carry the same risk of embolic events and, therefore, should be managed based on risk. Clinicians must diagnose the etiology of AF, as that will help determine risk and direct management. The vast majority of AF is *nonvalvular*, but *valvular* etiologies such as significant mitral stenosis must be considered. A severalfold increase in thromboembolic risk occurs with mitral valve stenosis–associated atrial fibrillation, and mandates full anticoagulation regardless of other stroke risk factors present. Patients with other risk factors leading to atrial fibrillation have variable levels of evidence supporting full anticoagulation, and some patients with few stroke or embolism risk factors may not attain benefit from anticoagulation that outweighs its risks (**Table 126-6**).

When considering the more common scenario of nonvalvular atrial fibrillation, multiple risk stratification strategies have been published over the decades to estimate the risk of thromboembolic complications, and to date the one most widely used and derived from large cohort data is known as the $CHADS_2$ score. **C**ongestive heart failure, **H**ypertension, **A**ge > 75, and **D**iabetes each contribute one point in this risk stratification tool whereas **S**troke contributes **2** points. The total number of points corresponds to a level of risk (incidence) of embolic stroke each year (**Table 126-7**).

TABLE 126-7 $CHADS_2$ Score and Stroke Risk

Number of Factors	Risk of Stroke (%/yr)
0 (lower risk)	1.9 (1.2–3.0)
1 (intermediate risk)	2.8 (2.0–3.8)
2 (high risk)	4.0 (3.1–5.1)
3	5.9 (4.6–7.3)
4	8.5 (6.3–11.1)
5	12.5 (8.2 –17.5)
6	18.2 (10.5–27.4)

$CHADS_2$ score is calculated by adding 1 point for each of the following: Recent **C**ongestive heart failure, **H**ypertension, **A**ge ≥ 75 years, **D**iabetes mellitus; and 2 points for prior **S**troke/transient ischemic attack.

By using this risk stratification tool clinicians can balance the benefits of therapeutic anticoagulation against the well-known complication, bleeding. With no risk factors for thromboembolic phenomena, as in the scenario of *lone atrial fibrillation,* the risk of bleeding complications with coumadin outweighs the benefit of stroke prevention. An acceptable alternative stroke risk–reduction strategy for patients who have low baseline risk ($CHADS_2$ = 0 or 1) or who have contraindications to anticoagulation is antiplatelet therapy with aspirin (81–325 mg daily).

For patients with intermediate risk ($CHADS_2$ score = 1): counsel patients with lower and intermediate thromboembolic risk that prophylaxis with warfarin is more effective than aspirin alone, but the risk of bleeding complications is higher on coumadin. The major bleeding complication risk with anticoagulation can be estimated using a risk stratification scheme with the acronym $HEMORR_2HAGES$ (**Table 126-8**). The $HEMORR_2HAGES$ risk score is calculated by adding 1 point for each of the following:

TABLE 126-8 $HEMORR_2HAGES$ Risk Score for Estimated Bleeding Risk While Receiving Anticoagulation Therapy

Risk Score	N	Number of Bleeds	Bleeds Per 100 Patient-Years of Warfarin (% Major Bleeds Per Year with Anticoagulation)
0	209	4	1.9
1	508	11	2.5
2	454	20	5.3
3	240	15	8.4
4	106	9	10.4
5	87	8	12.3

$HEMORR_2HAGES$ score is calculated by adding 1 point for each of the following:
Hepatic or renal disease, **E**thanol abuse, **M**alignancy, **O**lder age (> 75 years), **R**educed platelet countor function, **R**ebleeding risk (= previous bleeding; 2 points), **H**ypertension (uncontrolled), **A**nemia, **G**enetic factors, **E**xcessive fall risk, and **S**troke/TIA.

Hepatic or renal disease, **E**thanol abuse, **M**alignancy, **O**lder age (>75 years), **R**educed platelet count or function, **R**ebleeding risk (= previous bleeding; 2 points), **H**ypertension (uncontrolled), **A**nemia, **G**enetic factors, **E**xcessive fall risk, and **S**troke/TIA. The final score then correlates with the risk of major bleeding per 100 patients per year (ie, % major bleeds per year with anticoagulation therapy).

These risk estimation tools can be used to council patients regarding treatment choices, including benefits and risks, and help identify patients who might gain more overall benefit from antiplatelet aspirin therapy rather than anticoagulation. The $HEMORR_2HAGES$ tool might also be used to help determine which patients deserve more intensive outpatient monitoring of their anticoagulation (eg, in an anticoagulation clinic).

ATRIAL FIBRILLATION AND OLDER PEOPLE: WARFARIN CONTROVERSY

Often a difficult clinical management decision, the use of coumadin in older patients is controversial. Atrial fibrillation is the etiologic factor for 36% of strokes in individuals over the age of 80. The morbidity and mortality of a first stroke due to this disease is 71%. Meta-analysis data estimates the overall risk reduction with anticoagulation at 66% and with aspirin at 21%. Recent data has also demonstrated that patients over the age of 85 benefit more from anticoagulation than younger cohorts. Thus, the argument for anticoagulation with warfarin in this group is compelling. However, the risk of major bleeding complications is still relevant. The rate of intracranial hemorrhage (ICH) while taking warfarin is approximately 0.3% to 0.6% per year (RR ~ 2, compared to control). Aspirin also carries an increased risk of ICH (RR ~ 1.4 compared to control). Although the risk of ICH seems low, this estimate may be underestimated as older patients were underrepresented in the early randomized trials performed almost 20 years ago. More recent observational studies have estimated the risk of a major bleeding complication in individuals over the age of 80 to be 13% per year including a 2.4% per year risk of ICH.

Additional concerns for anticoagulation in older people are the increased risk for falls, likely drug interactions due to polypharmacy, complexity of coumadin regimens, need for close monitoring, and the large representation of nursing home patients. Even in research trials studying the efficacy of coumadin to prevent strokes, only two-thirds of the INRs were in the therapeutic range. Some of these concerns can be addressed with new oral thrombin inhibitors (eg, dabigatran) that eliminate the need for frequent INR monitoring and reduce the concerns for drug interactions associated with polypharmacy. The current data comparing coumadin with this direct thrombin inhibitor demonstrates better stroke prevention with the higher dose of dabigatran at 150 mg orally twice a day and even a trend toward an overall mortality benefit after a median follow-up period of two years. The downside is the increased propensity of gastrointestinal bleeding compared to warfarin. The lower dose, 110 mg orally twice a day, was found to have an equivalent reduction of stroke risk and a lower risk of major bleeding complications.

PRACTICE POINT

- New oral thrombin inhibitors (eg, dabigatran) eliminate the need for frequent INR monitoring and reduce the concerns for drug interactions associated with warfarin and polypharmacy. These medications are approved for use in atrial fibrillation for stroke prevention. However, the cost may be prohibitive.

TABLE 126-9 Risk of Postoperative Atrial Fibrillation (POAF) Based on Type of Surgery

Surgery Type	POAF/SVT %
Thoracic (noncardiac)	9–29%
Cardiothoracic	20–40%
Orthopedics	4%

Randomized trial data for the use of other antiplatelet agents (clopidogrel) in addition to aspirin for stroke prevention has been equivocal with respect to outcomes, with modest risk reduction of stroke but similar risk increase for major bleeding complications. Dual antiplatelet agents for stroke prevention are, therefore, not currently recommended.

POSTOPERATIVE ATRIAL FIBRILLATION

Postoperative atrial fibrillation (POAF) is the most common arrhythmia after surgery and observational data suggests an increased risk of short- and long-term mortality, increased length of stay, hospital costs, ICU length of stay, and stroke risk with this arrhythmia. POAF is also the most common reason for hospital readmission after open heart surgery. The risk of developing this arrhythmia varies based on the type of surgical intervention, with open heart procedures bearing the highest risk (**Table 126-9**). Some of the risk factors associated with POAF include age, atrial enlargement, procedures related to the heart such as valvular repair, and beta-blocker discontinuation.

The peak incidence of POAF occurs on the second postoperative day, and the majority occurs within five days postop. The majority of recurrent episodes of POAF occurred within several days of the first episode. The majority of POAF rhythms will spontaneously revert to sinus rhythm by the sixth postoperative week. However, if POAF is poorly tolerated due to hemodynamic compromise, anticoagulation and cardioversion would be recommended. Preoperative beta-blockade leads to significant reduction in POAF incidence, but conflicting data mires the actual effect on hospital length of stay, postoperative strokes, and mortality. The ACC/AHA 2006 guidelines for AF offer a class I recommendation of perioperative beta-blockers for prevention of POAF in patients undergoing coronary revascularization surgery (CABG).

ATRIAL FLUTTER

INTRODUCTION AND PATHOPHYSIOLOGY

Atrial flutter is the next most common form of SVT after atrial fibrillation and can manifest into the typical and atypical pattern. The typical pattern, also known as *counterclockwise flutter* due to the pattern of the macroreentry electrophysiologic mechanism, manifests as a saw-tooth pattern, typical for the P-wave negative deflections (**Figure 126-4**). The second form of atrial flutter has the opposite pattern with positive deflections in the P wave saw-tooth pattern (**Figure 126-5**). Even though the atrial rate ranges from 240 to 300 beats per minute, the AV nodal block will prevent all the atrial impulses from reaching the ventricle. The block at the AV node is frequently 2:1 but can also manifest as 3:1 and 4:1 or even variable block. The individuals that develop atrial flutter usually have a disorder that directly or indirectly involves the right atrium. Tricuspid valvular disease, various pulmonary disorders, postsurgical repair of congenital heart disease, or any process leading to the enlargement of the right atrium increase the risk for atrial flutter.

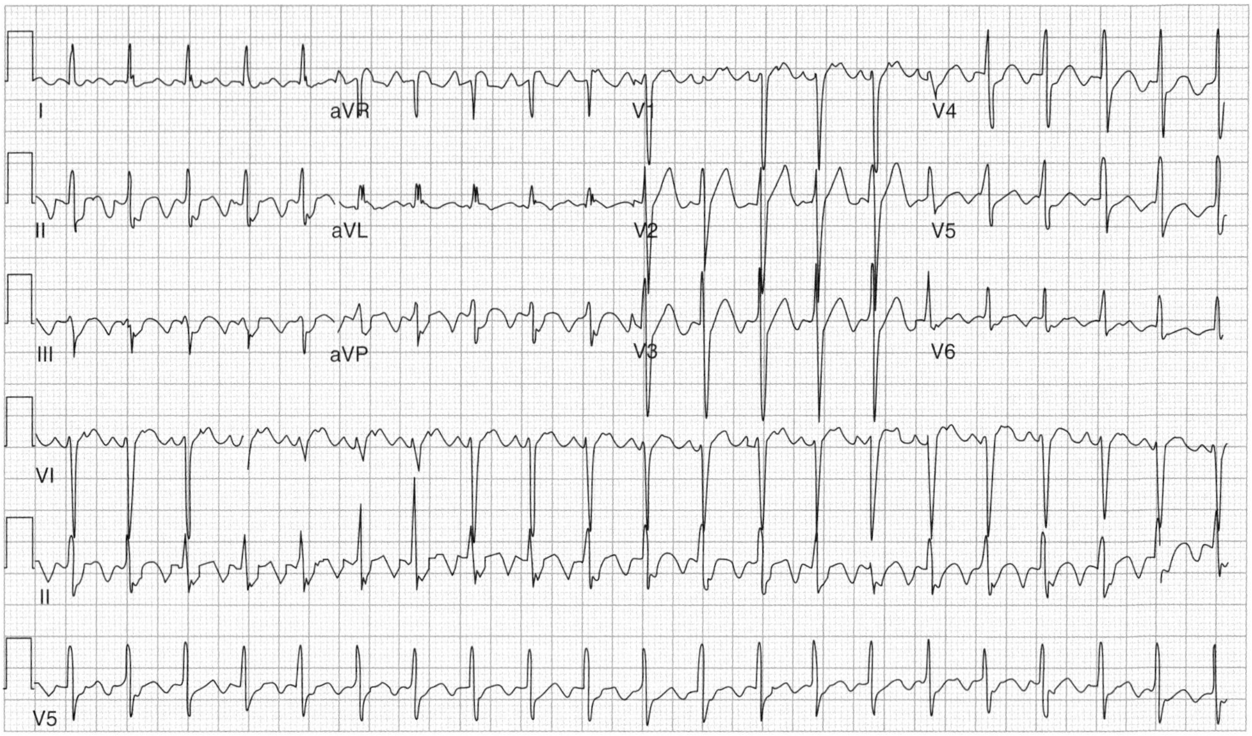

Figure 126-4 *Atrial flutter (2:1 block) with typical negative deflection P waves revealing the classic "saw-tooth" pattern.*

PRACTICE POINT

- Any disease process leading to the enlargement of the right atrium increases the risk for atrial flutter.

MANAGEMENT

The management of atrial flutter is similar to the management of atrial fibrillation. Ventricular rate control is achieved by increasing the block at the level of the AV node to reduce ventricular response to the rapid atrial rate. Certainly if the patient is hemodynamically compromised, direct cardioversion should be performed (biphasic 100 joules, monophasic 200 joules). In contrast to AF, using calcium channel blockers or beta-blockers alone are frequently insufficient in controlling the rhythm. It is often necessary to consider the addition of a class Ic antiarrhythmic, such as flecanide, to achieve satisfactory results. The class I agents are able to suppress the frequency of premature atrial beats, which trigger the development of this arrhythmia.

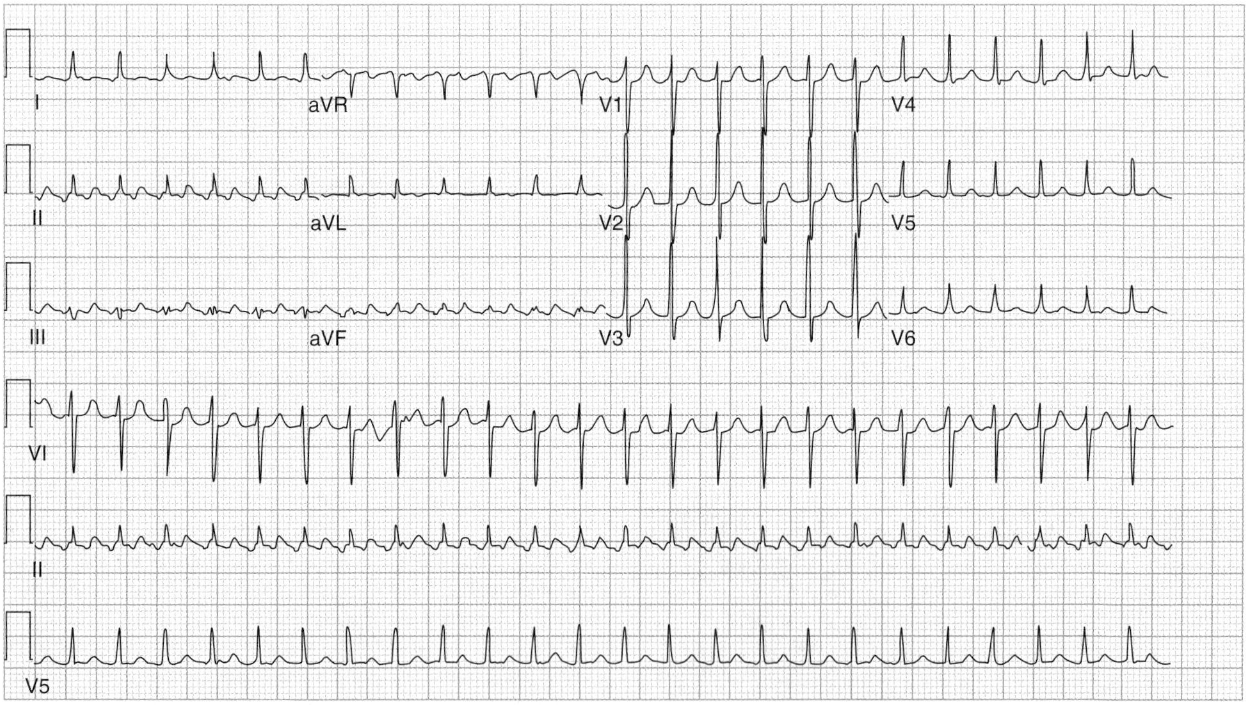

Figure 126-5 *Atrial flutter (2:1 block) with positive deflection P waves revealing an upward "saw-tooth" pattern.*

Other agents to consider would be class III agents such as ibutilide for chemical cardioversion. Sotalol and amiodarone may also be used, but side effects need to be considered in chronic management.

PRACTICE POINT

- In atrial flutter, avoid using flecainide as the sole treatment due to its ability to decrease the reentry circuit cycle length and potentially induce a fast, unstable 1:1 ventricular response and subsequent degeneration into ventricular fibrillation.

The risk of thromboembolic complications in atrial flutter is thought to be similar to that of atrial fibrillation, although there is a relative paucity of data compared with AF. For these patients, full anticoagulation should be strongly considered. In addition, approximately 75% patients with atrial flutter also develop atrial fibrillation.

In contrast to atrial fibrillation, catheter-based intervention is more strongly considered for atrial flutter due to the difficultly in achieving satisfactory rate control even with multiple medications. Success rates approaching 90% are reported with radiofrequency ablation (RFA) of the cavotricuspid isthmus, leading to a bidirectional block inhibiting the macroreentry mechanism of flutter. Due to the remaining anatomic or electrophysiologic conditions that remain after the RFA, the procedure is not considered curative. The recurrence rate is 10% to 20% over a period of two years but compares very favorably to the 60% recurrence rate of medical treatment alone. Less-frequent hospitalizations, lack of concern for medication side effects, and improved sense of quality of life are other factors weighing favorably toward a catheter-based ablative approach to atrial flutter management.

ATRIOVENTRICULAR NODAL REENTRANT TACHYCARDIA

INTRODUCTION AND EPIDEMIOLOGY

Atrioventricular nodal reentrant tachycardia (AVnRT) is the most common form of paroxysmal SVT, responsible for almost two-thirds of episodes; it is estimated that 10% of the general population has AVnRT. The palpitations characteristically start abruptly and may last for just a few minutes to as long as a few hours. They terminate as abruptly as they start. Additional symptoms include chest discomfort, dyspnea, lightheadedness, neck pulsations, and associated anxiety. These symptoms are often misdiagnosed as panic attacks if the arrhythmia is not caught while on a monitor. Signs of the arrhythmia include regular tachycardia with a heart rate between 120 and 200 bpm. Vagal maneuvers such as carotid sinus massage or the Valsalva maneuver can break the reentry circuit. This arrhythmia is usually not associated with structural heart disease and carries very little risk of death.

The mechanism of this tachyarrhythmia is a reentry circuit composed of the atrium, AV node or perinodal tissue, and the ventricle. The perinodal tissue or AV node exhibits a dual conduction physiology that reveals a slow pathway with an inherently short refractory period and a fast pathway with a relatively long refractory period.

There are three variants of AVnRT that depend on the routes of conduction. Approximately 90% of AVnRT is called typical AVnRT based on its antegrade conduction via the slow pathway and retrograde conduction via the fast pathway. With this typical conduction the surface ECG has the characteristic P waves either buried within the QRS complex or just after the QRS. As expected with fast retrograde conduction, the RP interval is shorter than the PR interval. Recognizing the relative length of the RP and PR intervals can further differentiate between the other SVTs. The ECG for the typical AVnRT often demonstrates a pseudo-R′ wave in V1 and pseudo-S′ waves in inferior limb leads. The less common variants include fast/slow and slow/slow, which will demonstrate clear P waves, inverted in the inferior limb leads with an RP interval longer than the PR interval.

MANAGEMENT

Initial hospital management

Management of AVnRT can follow a straightforward treatment sequence (**Figure 126-6**). Vagal maneuvers such as the carotid sinus massage and Valsalva maneuver can break the reentry circuit 25% of the time. If the tachycardia is refractory to these maneuvers, adenosine will convert the rhythm to sinus in approximately 90% of patients. Due to its very short half-life of less than 10 seconds, it is crucial that adenosine be given as a rapid bolus and immediately followed by 5–10 ml of saline. Adenosine is typically dosed in 6-mg increments, but patients usually respond to a 12-mg dose. The expected symptoms with the infusion are dyspnea, facial flushing, and chest discomfort that last under a minute. When using adenosine, the patient's rhythm should be monitored by telemetry via a continuously running 12-lead ECG to observe the response that occurs within 30 seconds.

PRACTICE POINT

- AVnRT can be converted to sinus rhythm with vagal maneuvers in 25% of cases and with adenosine in 90% of cases. Adenosine must be given as a rapid IV bolus and immediately followed by 5–10 ml of saline. The expected symptoms with the infusion are dyspnea, facial flushing, and chest discomfort that last under a minute. When using adenosine, the patient's rhythm should be monitored continuously with rhythm strip or 12-lead ECG to monitor the response, which occurs within 30 seconds.

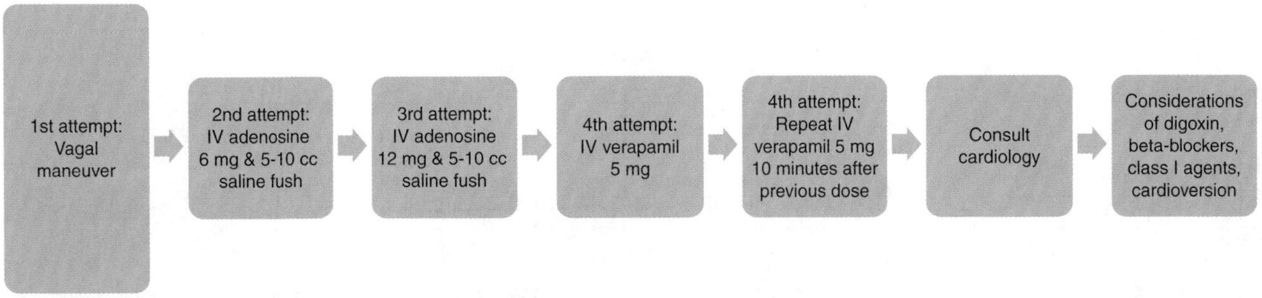

Figure 126-6 *Treatment sequence for atrioventricular nodal reentrant tachycardia (AVnRT).*

Typically, adenosine will convert the AVnRT to a sinus rhythm, but other possible rhythms include ventricular ectopy, transient sinus pause, transient bradyarrhythmias, atrial fibrillation or atrial flutter uncommonly, and, very rarely, polymorphic ventricular tachycardia. The risk of torsades de pointes is increased in patients with a baseline prolonged QTc. Factors that could decrease the efficacy of intravenous adenosine push include the use of methylxanthine products such as theophylline and caffeine, which block the A1 receptors. The use of dipyridamole (persantine, aggrenox) can augment the efficacy of adenosine by slowing its clearance. Due to the potential for exacerbating bronchospams, asthma is a relative contraindication for adenosine use. The transplanted heart is hypersensitive to adenosine, therefore a reduced dose or abandoning this approach altogether is appropriate in such patients.

Other options beside adenosine for the acute management of AVnRT include verapamil, beta-blockers, and direct cardioversion. Verapamil, a nondihydropyridine calcium channel blocker, will block both fast and slow pathways. Dosing for acute management is 5 mg IV every 10 minutes and has been reportedly 90% effective. The downside to verapamil is the potential for hypotension that could be severe and long lasting. Another option includes digoxin, although this approach is not optimal due to its delayed effect. Direct cardioversion with 10–50 joules is a final option if the previous interventions prove ineffective.

Outpatient longitudinal therapeutics

If the patient has frequent episodes that negatively impact quality of life, the use of invasive catheter ablation may be considered. The consensus approach by the ACC/AHA guidelines recommends ablation of the slow pathway due to it high efficacy (97%) and low risk of high-grade AV block (1%). The patient does need to consider the possibility of pacemaker placement if high-degree block develops as a complication. Long-term medical management is another option and includes medications such as verapamil, propanolol or class I antiarrhythmic agents such as flecanide and propafenone. The medications can be used on a daily basis to reduce the frequency of occurrences and the length of episodes. Additionally, the "pill-in-the-pocket" method obviates the daily use and could be used just during the episode. Cardiology consultation is indicated when using class I antiarrhythmics due to the risk of malignant ventricular arrhythmias.

ATRIOVENTRICULAR REENTRY TACHYCARDIA

INTRODUCTION AND PATHOPHYSIOLOGY

The next most common form of a paroxysmal SVT is atrioventricular reentry tachycardia (AVRT), which is characterized by an accessory conduction pathway between the atrium and ventricle that serves as a conduit for macroreentry. This pathway is a muscular bundle with variable properties of conduction, sometimes with bidirectional properties and in others just unidirectional capabilities. A commonly cited example of AVRT is Wolf-Parkinson-White (WPW) syndrome, a narrow-complex tachyarrhythmia that manifests symptomatically with palpitations, chest discomfort, dyspnea, presyncope or syncope, and, very rarely, sudden cardiac death.

DIAGNOSIS

A baseline ECG when in sinus rhythm may ("revealed") or may not ("concealed") demonstrate the *delta-wave* (**Figure 126-7**). The accessory pathway depolarizes the ventricular myocardium before the normal conduction system and is thus considered "preexcitation." On the ECG, this will appear as the short PR interval. Due to the relatively inefficient conduction from myocardial to myocardial cell (in contrast to the efficient His-Purkinje system), the initial portion of the QRS is slurred (delta wave) and gives the QRS a widened appearance (Figure 126-7). This accessory pathway, known as the bundle of Kent in WPW syndrome, provides the electrical wave front a conduit to move from the ventricle to the atrium, completing the macroreentry circuit.

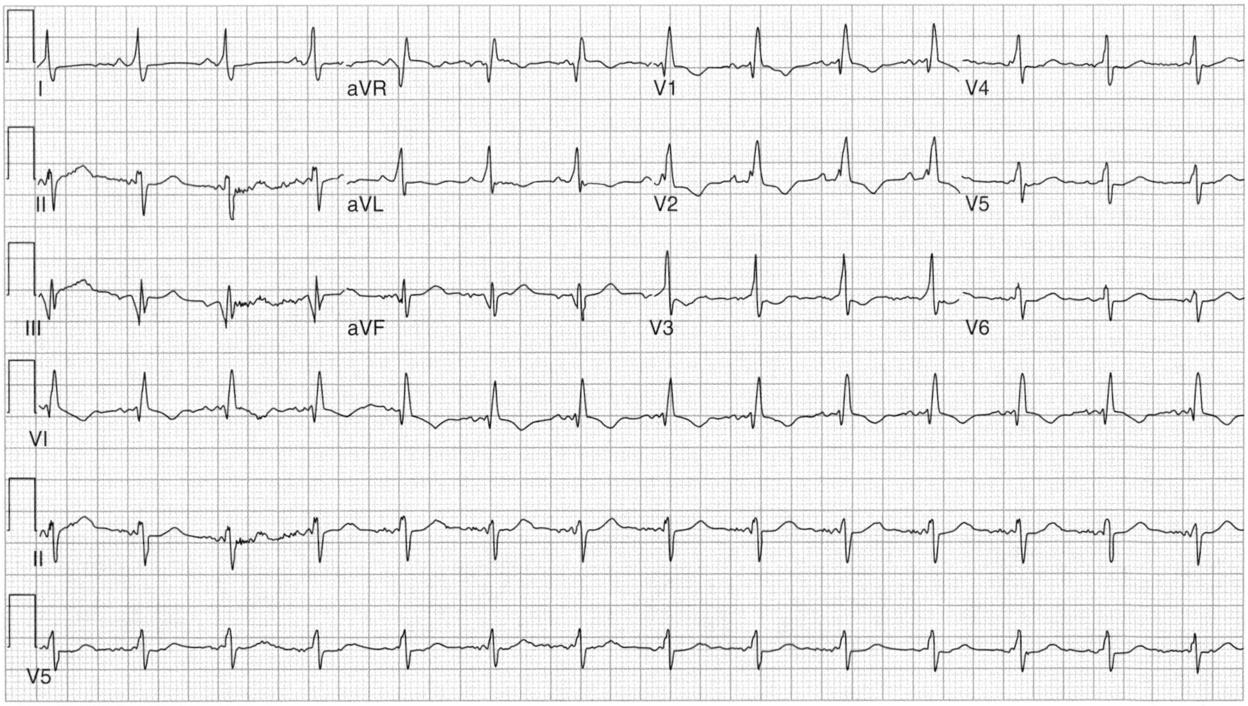

Figure 126-7 *Atrioventricular reentry tachycardia (AVRT). Wolf-Parkinson-White (WPW) syndrome with characteristic short PR interval and delta wave best seen in I, aVL, V3, and V4.*

MANAGEMENT

Initial hospital management

Management of this macroreentry arrhythmia is identical to the management for nodal reentry tachycardia with vagal maneuvers as a first option and intravenous adenosine push if unsuccessful. As discussed previously, adenosine administration usually converts the rhythm to sinus; however, less frequently atrial fibrillation or atrial flutter can develop. In very rare situations, the electrical impulse could conduct antegrade via the accessory pathway, leading to a very rapid ventricular rate, ventricular instability, and polymorphic ventricular tachycardia. This very rare complication of adenosine in AVRT requires having a crash-cart available during adenosine administration.

In some types of AVRT, the accessory pathway may not be recognizable on the ECG (considered concealed). When the accessory pathway conducts unidirectionally only from the ventricle to the atrium, the characteristic delta wave, short PR interval, and widened QRS are absent. The management remains the same as in the revealed WPW syndrome with very little concern for polymorphic ventricular tachycardia, as the accessory pathway will only conduct unidirectionally in a retrograde fashion from the ventricle to the atrium.

Outpatient longitudinal therapeutics

Beyond the acute management of AVRT, the frequency and severity of the palpitations will guide long-term treatments. Infrequent episodes that are short in duration and hemodynamically tolerable require only rest and time to resolve. A pill-in-the-pocket regimen could be considered with class Ia, Ic, or III antiarrhythmics or AV nodal–blocking agents as an option in this scenario in the absence of preexcitation. However, if the episodes are frequent and prolonged, daily use of these medications can be considered. These antiarrhythmics will prolong the refractory period for both the accessory pathway and the AV node, effectively preventing the arrhythmia or breaking the circuit during the episodes. Radiofrequency ablation of the accessory pathway provides another option (with a very high success rate and low complication rate) for permanent rhythm control that obviates the need for chronic medication in AVRT (**Figures 126-8** and **126-9**).

> **PRACTICE POINT**
>
> **Wolf-Parkinson-White with atrial fibrillation:**
>
> - Atrial fibrillation (AF) in a very young patient should lower clinicians' threshold to consider WPW syndrome. AF occurs in up to one-third of patients with WPW and is the root cause for sudden death in these patients.
> - The patient with a "revealed" WPW and atrial fibrillation will demonstrate a wide QRS complex on ECG due to the delta wave (often misinterpreted as atrial fibrillation with bundle branch block, BBB).
> - WPW with AF should *not* be rate controlled with AV node–blocking agents, as atrial impulses would be forced to the nondecrementally conducting accessory pathway. The ventricular response would become 1:1, leading to unstable ventricular tachycardia (see Figures 126-8 and 126-9).
> - Treatment: IV procainamide or IV amiodarone or electrical cardioversion

COMPLICATIONS AND PROGNOSIS

The presence of a delta wave on a resting ECG does not require a cardiology consultation. However, a delta wave with a history of palpitations, syncope, or presycope, or with a history of atrial fibrillation does require cardiology consultation. The electrophysiologist can perform invasive procedures to stratify some patients with the WPW syndrome for risk of sudden cardiac death, especially when the refractory period for the accessory pathway is short (RR interval of less than 250 ms).

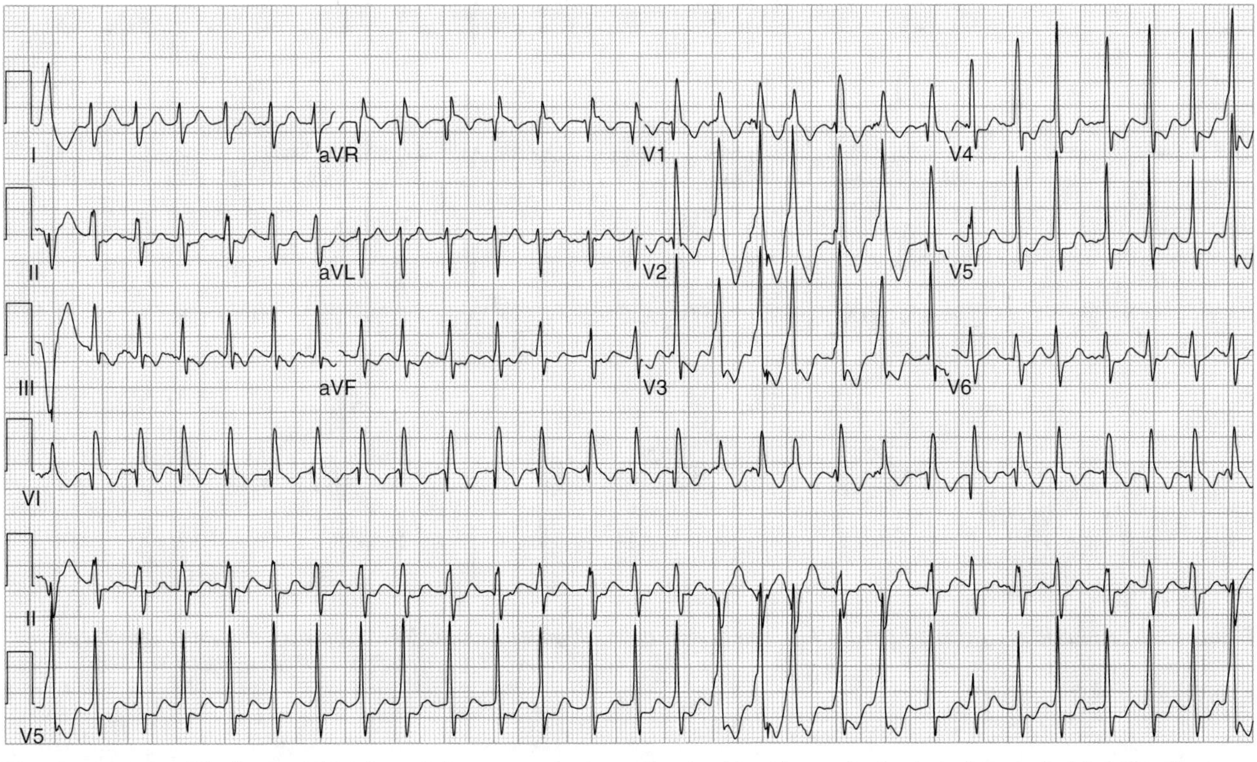

Figure 126-8 *Atrial fibrillation with brief run of aberrant conduction and noticeably wider conduction in the latter half of the ECG strip.*

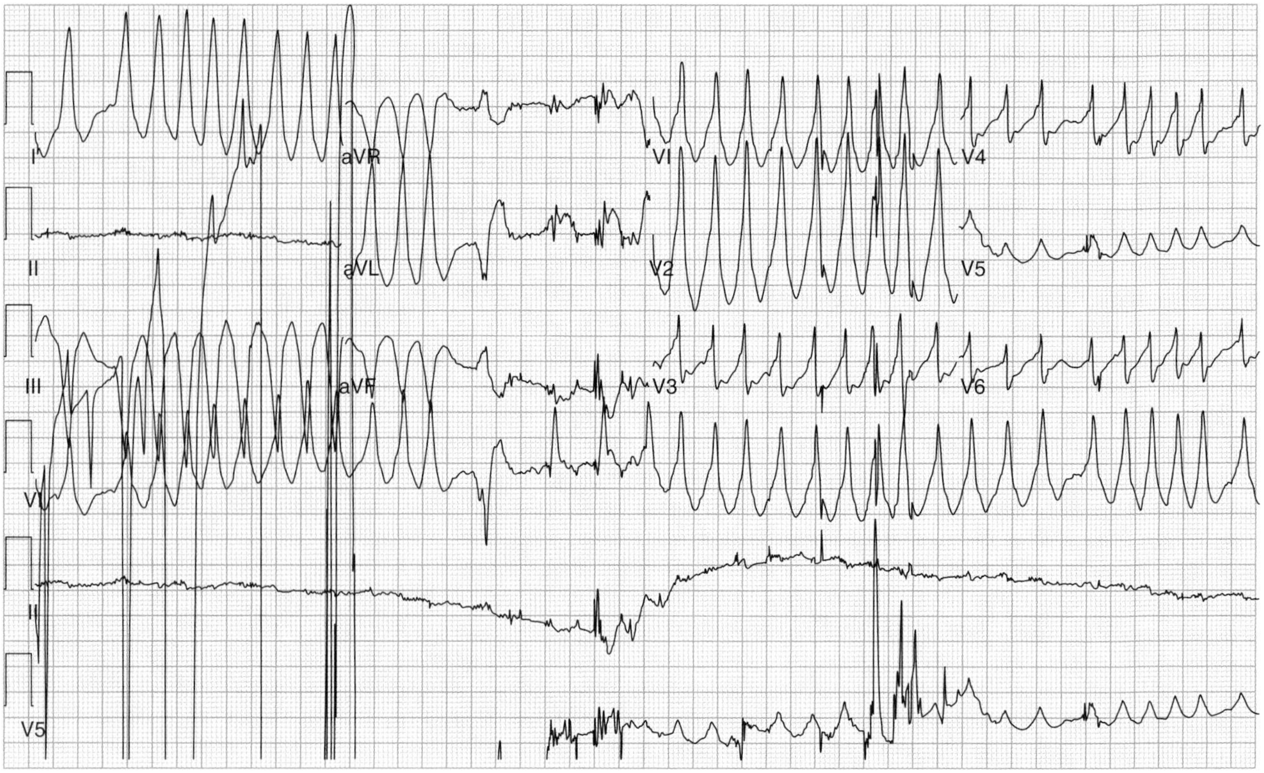

Figure 126-9 *Unstable ventricular tachycardia after patient was given IV adenosine. This AV nodal–blocking agent effectively shunted the atrial electrical impulses to the accessory pathway, which is characterized by nondecremental conduction.*

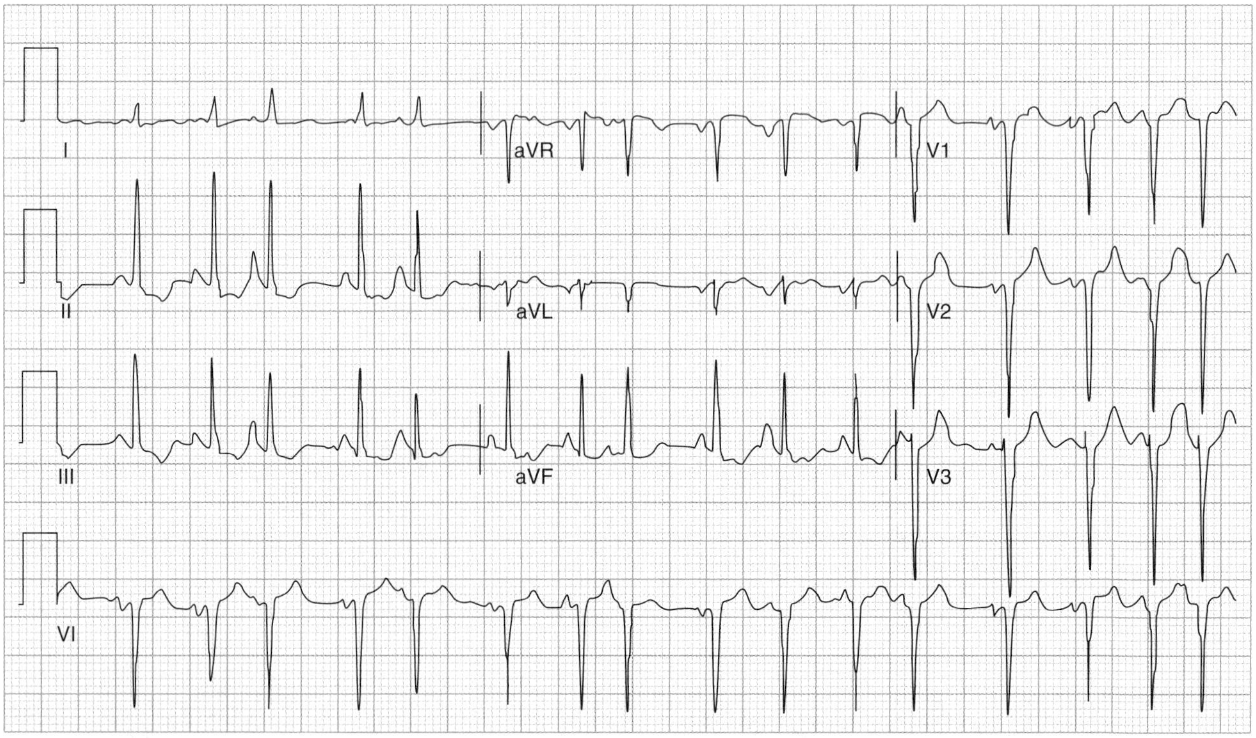

Figure 126-10 *Multifocal atrial tachycardia (MAT). Three or more distinct P-wave morphologies with an irregular rhythm. (Reproduced, with permission, from Knoop KJ, Stack LB, Storrow AB, et al. Atlas of Emergency Medicine. 3rd ed. New York: McGraw-Hill; 2009. Fig. 23-29A. Photo contributor: James V. Ritchie, MD.)*

MULTIFOCAL ATRIAL TACHYCARDIA

Multifocal atrial tachycardia (MAT) is recognized on the surface ECG by the presence of tachycardia, at least three distinct P waves, and at least three distinct PR intervals (**Figure 126-10**). Correct identification of this arrhythmia helps avoid improperly treating it as another arrhythmia. MAT usually results from another primary problem that leads to right heart strain or dysfunction (eg, severe COPD with exacerbation or pulmonary embolism). By treating the underlying condition, the arrhythmia usually resolves. However, if the tachycardia needs to be slowed based on clinical effects of the rate, beta-blockers represent the first-line treatment. A short-acting beta-blocker, IV esmolol, may be considered if concern for bronchospasm or hypotension exists. Some trials support administration of IV magnesium to slow or convert the arrhythmia; however, this has not been well studied. Finally verapamil is another therapeutic option, but may be limited by hypotension. *Electrical cardioversion is not effective and thus not recommended.* Exacerbating factors for MAT may include commonly used medications for COPD such as beta-agonists and theophylline.

JUNCTIONAL TACHYCARDIA

Junctional tachycardia originates from the AV node or the bundle of His. The paroxysmal form is considered a rare occurrence in the adult population, but the nonparoxysmal form occurs most notoriously in the setting of digoxin toxicity. Particularly with digoxin toxicity, a Wenckebach conduction block in conjunction with junctional tachycardia can manifest. Other settings in which this arrhythmia may manifest include hypokalemia, post cardiac surgery, chronic lung disease, myocardial ischemia, myocarditis, and, rarely, underlying sinus node dysfunction. Presentation of the arrhythmia under these circumstances allows the clinician to differentiate it from AVnRT, AVRT, and atrial tachycardia (AT). By addressing the underlying condition, the rhythm will correct. In the setting of digoxin toxicity, withholding the medication is the treatment of choice. Digoxin binding agents should be considered for judicious use in the setting of ventricular arrhythmias or high-grade AV block.

ATRIAL TACHYCARDIA

INTRODUCTION AND EPIDEMIOLOGY

An uncommon arrhythmia that falls under the category of SVT is atrial tachycardia. The incidence of this arrhythmia in young persons is less than 1%, however this arrhythmia is comprised of approximately 5% to 15% of patients undergoing electrophysiology studies. The arrhythmia can be seen on 24-hour Holter monitoring, but the asymptomatic patient should not be treated. If symptomatic, the patient may have typical symptoms accompanied with the SVT, including palpitations, lightheadedness, dyspnea, and perhaps syncope or presyncope.

DIAGNOSIS

The surface ECG can usually help differentiate AT from the more common rhythm sinus tachycardia by the following three features (**Figure 126-11**). The P-wave axis is usually different from the sinus P wave, which is upright in leads I and II. The onset and termination of atrial tachycardia is usually very rapid, occurring over a few beats, in contrast to the 30 seconds or minutes it takes sinus tachycardia to develop or terminate. Finally, the PR interval can be variable, which is also known as *unhooking*.

PRACTICE POINT

Atrial tachycardia features:

- P-wave axis is usually different from the sinus P wave
- Onset and termination very rapid
  - Occurring over a few beats (contrast to the 30 seconds or minutes it takes sinus tachycardia to develop or terminate)
- PR interval variable
- Potential for developing tachycardia-induced cardiomyopathy (> 70% of untreated patients) if the incessant variety
  - Reversible with correction of the tachycardia

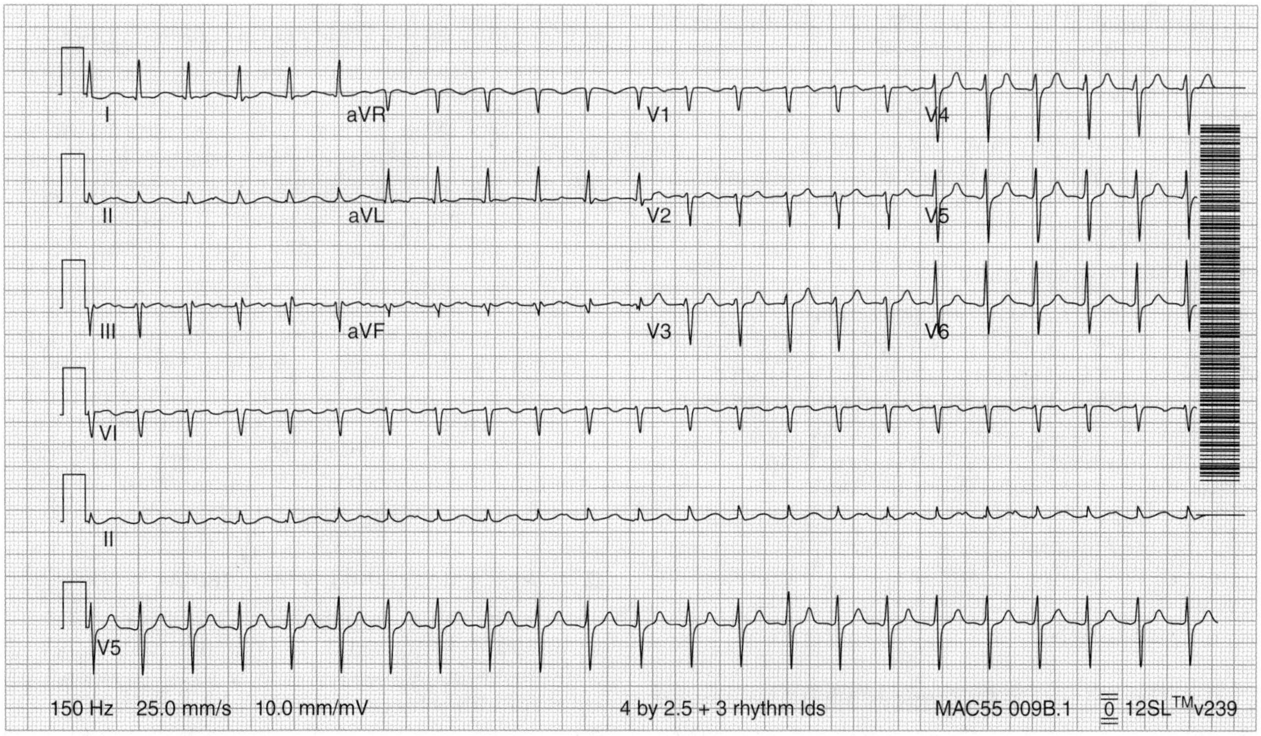

Figure 126-11 *Atrial tachycardia. Discernible P waves best seen in III and aVF. Notice the RP interval is greater than the PR interval. The tachycardia started abruptly and spontaneously and abruptly terminated after 20 minutes.*

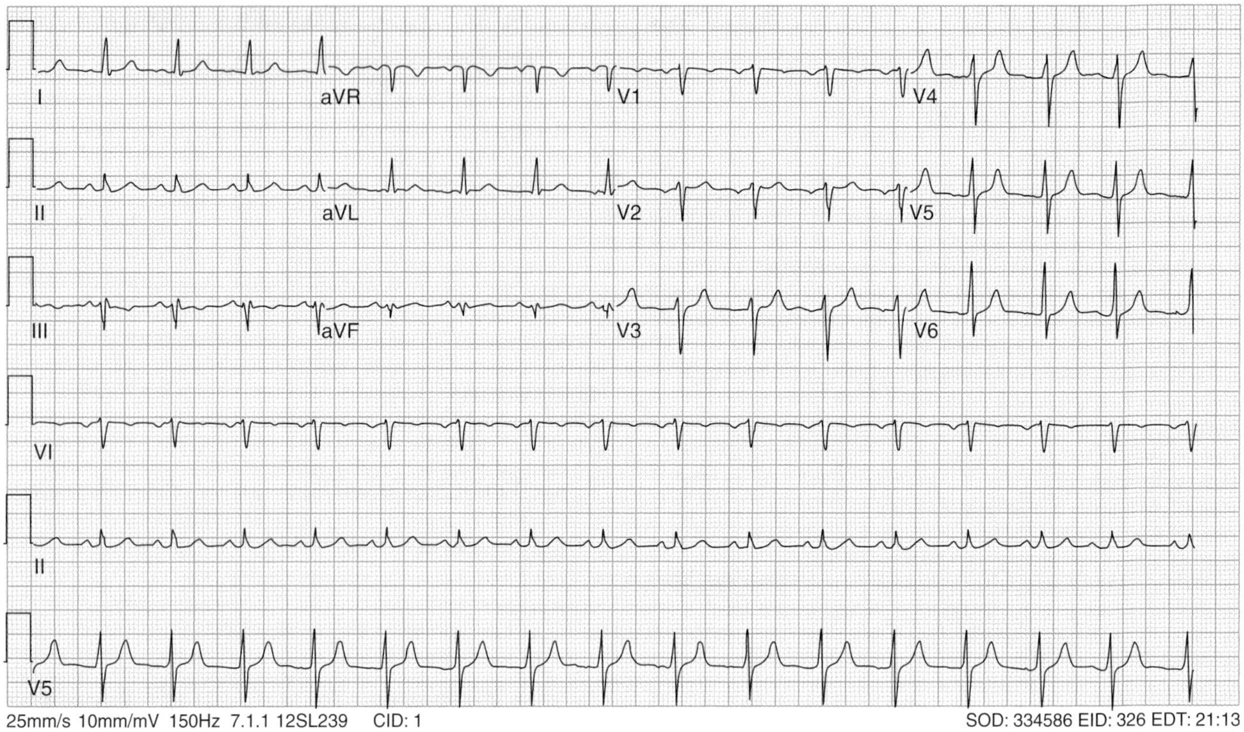

Figure 126-12 *Normal sinus rhythm of the patient in Figure 126-12 after spontaneous resolution of atrial tachycardia. Notice the distinctly different P-wave morphology between the two ECGs.*

Difficulty differentiating this rhythm from a sinus tachycardia occurs when the focus of the arrhythmia is close to the superior portion of the cristas terminalis thereby mirroring the normal P-wave axis (positive in I, II). The importance of rhythm recognition lies in the potential for developing a tachycardia-induced cardiomyopathy if left untreated. Some studies have demonstrated that with an incessant form of atrial tachycardia, over 70% patients demonstrate decreased left ventricular function. Fortunately, this complication is reversible with correction of the tachycardia. Studies have demonstrated that patients with early-onset atrial tachycardia (before the age of 25) frequently spontaneously develop a normal sinus rhythm (**Figure 126-12**). AT could also be difficult to distinguish from AVRT and AVnRT, but clues such as variable RP intervals make AT more likely. If in doubt, the electrophysiologist should be consulted.

MANAGEMENT

Initial hospital management

In the acute setting, AV node–blocking calcium channel blockers (diltiazem, verapamil) or beta-blockers can at times terminate the arrhythmia, or simply slow the ventricular rate via increased blockade at the AV node. Adenosine can also terminate the arrhythmia. The alternatives that are considered efficacious are sotalol and amiodarone; however, the side effects do need to be considered, especially if amiodarone is used for chronic management. The vagal maneuvers usually do not work, but electrical cardioversion may work, especially if the underlying reason for the AT is microreentry or triggered activity. Long-term management may include the medications discussed previously or ablation techniques via invasive electrophysiologic techniques.

SINUS TACHYCARDIAS

The sinus tachycardias represent a heterogeneous group of arrhythmias comprised of normal sinus tachycardia, inappropriate sinus tachycardia, postural orthostasis tachycardia syndrome (POTS), and sinus node reentry tachycardia (SNRT). All have the same ECG findings, which include a pulse rate >100 bpm, upright P waves in limb leads I and II (normal P-wave vector). The clinical presentation varies from the asymptomatic to regular palpitations accompanied by syncope or presycope. Normal sinus tachycardia, as one would expect, is a result of physiologic demand and requires the appropriate workup.

POSTURAL ORTHOSTASIS TACHYCARDIA SYNDROME

Postural orthostasis tachycardia syndrome (POTS) is usually found in a young population between the ages of 18 and 50 with a female predominance of 5:1. The postulated mechanisms include partial dysautonomia and the less common central beta-hypersensitivity form. POTS also has pronounced sympathetic characteristics such as tremors, anxiety, and palpitations. The evaluation of this condition includes the head-up tilt-table (HUTT) test documenting the patient's symptoms and tachycardic response greater than 30 bpm over baseline and usually greater than 120 bpm. Other diagnostic studies include 24-hour urine sodium collection, serum norepinephrine measurement (>600 pg/dl), and postganglionic antibody testing. The use of physical maneuvers to increase muscle tone in the lower extremities, compression garments, volume expanders (ie, mineralocorticoids, increased salt diet, increase fluid intake), peripheral vasoconstrictors, and centrally acting beta-blockers (ie, pindolol) are the therapeutic options.

INAPPROPRIATE SINUS TACHYCARDIA

Inappropriate sinus tachycardia (IST) characteristically has daytime tachycardia at rest or with minimal exertion and normalization of the pulse during sleep. The sinus node regulation is dysfunctional with enhanced sensitivity to sympathetic stimulus or decreased regulation by the parasympathetic system. In contrast to sinus node reentry tachycardia (SNRT), the onset and termination of this rhythm is gradual, and atrial overdrive pacing has no

TABLE 126-10 Consultation for Supraventricular Tachyarrhythmias

Rhythm	Consult Cardiology	Consider Direct Electrophysiology (EP) Consult
Atrial fibrillation	1. Refractory to multiple medications 2. Need for cardioversion (chemical, electrical, or both) 3. Desire to maintain sinus rhythm 4. Lone atrial fibrillation	1. Presence of sick sinus syndrome (SSS)—potential ablate-pace strategy 2. Refractory to medical management: potential for RFA 3. Presence of preexcitation (WPW)
Atrial flutter	1. Refractory to multiple medications 2. Need for cardioversion 3. Desire to maintain sinus rhythm	Strong consideration for RFA strategy as first-line treatment
Atrioventricular nodal reentry tachycardia	Refractory to vagal maneuvers and IV adenosine	Frequent and debilitating palpitations: potential need for RFA
Atrioventricular tachycardia	All WPW patients	1. History of syncope/ presyncope 2. Presence of atrial fibrillation or atrial flutter
Multifocal atrial tachycardia		
Atrial tachycardia		Incessant: risk of cardiomyopathy
Sinus tachycardia • Sinus reentry • Inappropriate sinus tachycardia • Postural orthostatic tachycardia syndrome (POTS)	Inability to define etiology	
Junctional tachycardia	Concern for digitalis toxicity	

RFA, radiofrequency ablation; SSS, sick sinus syndrome; WPW, Wolff-Parkinson-White syndome.

influence on the arrhythmia. Treatment of IST requires high doses of beta-blockers or calcium channel blockers. Other treatment options include antiarrhythmics or even catheter ablation in the event of medical failure.

SINUS NODE REENTRY TACHYCARDIA

Sinus node reentry tachycardia (SNRT) originates within or very close to the sinus node. It usually starts and ends abruptly. Bedside interventions such as vagal maneuvers or intravenous adenosine or verapamil can terminate this arrhythmia. Following the SVT recognition algorithm (see Figure 126-1), this rhythm is categorized within the arrhythmias with an RP interval greater than the PR interval.

CONSULTATION AND REFERRAL

A variety of instances of SVTs meet indications to consult general cardiology or electrophysiology cardiology (**Table 126-10**).

DISCHARGE PLANNING

Preventing complications of the various SVTs and readmission minimization are the mainstay of effective discharge planning. For AF and atrial flutter, strict utilization of the risk stratification tools, such as the $CHADS_2$, is crucial to better assess the need for full anticoagulation with an imperfect agent such as warfarin. On the other hand, utilizing other risk tools to estimate the risk of a major bleeding complication, such as $HEMORR_2HAGES$, can help balance the discussion with patients and aid in decision making about whether to use full anticoagulation. Prior to discharge, patient education by the physician, nutritionist, and/or the pharmacy staff about new medications and potential food or other interactions is integral. Due to known challenges in maintaining an INR in the therapeutic range, referral to an anticoagulation clinic should be strongly considered.

QUALITY IMPROVEMENT TO ADDRESS PERFORMANCE GAPS

In 2008, the ACC/AHA/Physician Consortium published guidelines to set a minimum standard for the appropriate management of AF. The conclusions from the guidelines were that two performance measures need to be tracked in the near future: the assessment of stroke risk and the frequency of full anticoagulation in high-risk patients. These conclusions were driven by consistent findings that the cause of stroke in a significant percentage of admitted patients is attributed to AF. Even when patients are known to be high risk for embolic strokes due to AF and $CHADS_2$ criteria, a large percentage of patients do not receive full anticoagulation. Other stroke studies have revealed that even when warfarin is prescribed to high-risk AF patients, the INR frequently is subtherapeutic on admission. In fact, even in the most rigorous clinical trials only 66% of the measured INR levels were therapeutic, and outside of clinical trial settings, this proportion is closer to 50%. A third performance measure, INR measurements at a monthly minimum frequency, was considered but not endorsed by the consortium.

The recent data published on the oral thrombin inhibitor, dabigatran, and the final FDA approval in 2010 provides a potentially better option for stroke prophylaxis in AF patients. Compared with warfarin, dabigatran has better stroke risk reduction and equivalent risk of major hemorrhage. Monitoring the INR or other coagulation parameters is unnecessary, and the metabolism bypasses the cytochrome P-450 enzymes, thereby decreasing the risk of drug-drug interactions. As with any new therapeutic on the market, the costs are significant. Future cost-effectiveness analysis will need to verify if the higher upfront cost of dabigatran outweighs the cost of less-effective anticoagulation with warfarin.

Some promising results are also demonstrating that oral factor Xa inhibitors (ie rivaroxaban, apixaban) are as efficacious in stroke

TABLE 126-11 Evidence-based Medicine: Key References for Supraventricular Tachyarrhythmias

Reference	Methodology	Results	Bottom Line
AFFIRM Wyse DG, et al. *N Engl J Med.* 2002;347(23):1825–1833.	Randomized trial (rate control versus rhythm control for atrial fibrillation) • $N = 4060$ • Patients age >65 or risk factors for stroke	No difference in overall mortality after 5 years of follow-up 23.8% versus 21.3% $P = 0.08$	Rhythm control not better than rate control
AF CHF Roy D, et al. *N Engl J Med.* 2008;358(25):2667–2676.	Randomized trial (rate control versus rhythm control for atrial fibrillation in systolic CHF) • $N = 1376$ • Ejection fraction ≤35%	No difference in time to death from cardiovascular causes (25% versus 27%) after 37 months	Rhythm control not better than rate control in systolic CHF
Validation of Clinical Classification Schemes for predicting stroke. Gage BF, et al. *JAMA.* 2001;285(22):2854–2870.	Comparison of $CHADS_2$ to AFI and SPAF risk classification schemes	$CHADS_2$ *c* statistic of 0.82 compared to 0.68 and 0.74 for AFI and SPAF respectively	$CHADS_2$ performs better at predicting strokes than prior classification schemes
RE-LY: Randomized evaluation of long-term anticoagulation therapy study group. Connolly SJ, et al. *New Engl J Med.* 2009;361:1139–1151.	Randomized trial in atrial fibrillation warfarin versu dabigatran • $N = 18113$ patients • Dabigatran 2 doses: 110 mg twice a day, 150 mg twice a day • primary outcome • stroke or systemic embolism • follow-up 2 years	Coumadin event rate= 1.69%/year Dabigatran 110 mg = 1.53%/year RR 0.91 P <0.001 for noninferiority Dabigatran 150 mg = 1.11%/year RR 0.66 P <0.001 for superiority	Higher-dose dabigatran prevents more strokes, but has equal major bleeding complications as coumadin

CHF, congestive heart failure.

risk reductions as warfarin with added benefits of less hemorrhagic strokes and intracranial bleeding complications and without the need for coagulation monitoring.

CONCLUSION

A systematic algorithmic approach to SVTs will aid in differentiating the common from the uncommon (see Figure 126-1). In the setting of hemodynamic instability, other concerns fall to the wayside, and direct cardioversion should be performed without delay (except with sinus tachycardia, where the underlying cause should be identified and treated) (**Table 126-11**).

SUGGESTED READINGS

Blomström-Lundqvist C, Scheinman M, Aliot E, et al. ACC/AHA/ESC guidelines for the management of patients with supraventricular arrhythmias: a report of the American College of Cardiology/American Heart Association Task Force and the European Society of Cardiology Committee for Practice Guidelines (writing committee to develop guidelines for the management of patients with supraventricular arrhythmias). *J Am Coll Cardiol.* 2003;42:1493–1531.

Fuster V, Ryden, L, Cannom M, et al. ACC/AHA/ESC 2006 guidelines for the management of patients with atrial fibrillation: a report of the American College of Cardiology/American Heart developed in collaboration with the European Heart Rhythm Association and the 2001 guidelines for the management of patients With atrial fibrillation) Cardiology Committee for Practice Guidelines (writing committee to revise association task force on practice guidelines) and the European Society of Fibrillation: a report of the American College of Cardiology/American Heart. *J Am Coll Cardiol.* 2006;48:e149–e246.

Gage B, Waterman A, Shannon W, et al. Validation of clinical classification schemes for predicting stroke: results from the National Registry of Atrial Fibrillation. *JAMA.* 2001;285:2864–2870.

Gage B, Yan Y, Milligan P, et al. Clinical classification schemes for predicting hemorrhage: Results from the National Registry ofAtrial Fibrillation (NRAF). *Am Heart J.* 2006;151:713–719.

Hylek E, Evans-Molina C, Shea C, et al. Major hemorrhage and tolerability of warfarin in the first year of therapy among elderly patients with atrial fibrillation. *Circulation.* 2007;115;2689–2696.

Kay G, Plumb V, Jayam V, et al. Atrial fibrillation, atrial flutter, and atrial tachycardia. Supraventricular tachycardia: AV node reentry and Wolff-Parkinson-White syndrome. *Hurst's The Heart*, 11th ed. New York: McGraw-Hill, 2004: pp. 825–874.

Olgin J, Zipes D, Miller J. Specific arrhythmias: diagnosis and treatment. *Braunwald's Heart Disease: A Textbook of Cardiovascular Medicine*, 8th ed. Philadelphia: *Elsevier Saunders,* 2008: pp. 863–923.

Pisters R, Oostenbrugge R, Knottberus I, et al. The likelihood of decreasing strokes in atrial fibrillation patients by strict application of guidelines. *Europace.* 12:779–784.

Singer D, Albers G, Dalen J, et al. Antithrombotic therapy in atrial fibrillation: American College of Chest Physicians evidence-based clinical practice guidelines 8th edition. *Chest.* 2008;133;546S–592S.

Wyse D, Waldo A, DiMarco J, et al. A comparison of rate-control and rhythm control in patients with atrial fibrillation. *N Eng J Med.* 2002;347:1825–1833.

CHAPTER 127

Bradyarrhythmias

Michael J. Pistoria, DO, FACP, FHM
Nainesh C. Patel, MD, FACC

Key Clinical Questions

1. Which patients with bradyarrhythmias require admission to the hospital?
2. When does the bradyarrhythmic patient require a cardiology consult?
3. Which bradyarrhythmic patients require permanent pacemaker placement?

INTRODUCTION

Bradyarrhythmia is a common finding in hospitalized patients. It can be of minimal prognostic significance or can indicate a serious cardiac condition that requires immediate attention. Broadly speaking, bradyarrhythmias are caused by depression of sinus node activity or conduction system blocks. Symptoms depend on the patient's co-morbidities, the anatomical basis for the block(s), and the location of the subsidiary pacemaker which must take over to maintain cardiac output. Clinicians must analyze historical data, and examine the patient for evidence of hypoperfusion and electrocardiographic data to determine the likelihood that the rhythm will deteriorate into a worsening bradycardia or ventricular asystole.

SINOATRIAL NODE DYSFUNCTION

EPIDEMIOLOGY

A heart rate below 60 beats per minute defines bradycardia. Resting heart rates vary among normal individuals and depends upon age and level of conditioning. One study demonstrated that resting heart rates can range from 46 to 93 beats per minute in males and 51 to 95 beats per minute in females. Additionally, heart rate varies with time of day. Heart rate during sleep may decrease between 14 and 24 beats per minute (bpm) on average, depending upon age. Due to this variability, it is difficult to fully assess the incidence and prevalence of bradycardia in the general population. Asymptomatic bradycardia portends no adverse prognostic significance in healthy individuals, including those over 40 years old.

PRACTICE POINT

- Heart rate while sleeping can decrease between 14 and 24 beats per minute on average. As a result, normotensive individuals normally experience a nocturnal dip in their blood pressure.

Sick sinus syndrome, or sinus-node dysfunction, however, does impact morbidity and mortality. The prevalence of sick sinus syndrome is estimated at 1 in 600 patients over 65 years old. Many patients with sick sinus syndrome have an elevated risk of cardiovascular events, including syncope, heart failure, and atrial fibrillation. Mortality for untreated patients with sick sinus syndrome ranges from 5 to 10% at 1 year to 25 to 30% at 5 years.

PRESENTATION

Even a significant sinus bradycardia may not produce symptoms, depending on an individual's age, physical conditioning, and co-morbidities. In these patients the bradycardia may be identified as an ECG abnormality (sinus bradycardia, sinus arrest, exit block, or alternating with a tachyarrythmia). The elderly and patients with co-existing cardiopulmonary disease are more likely to develop symptoms related to low perfusion (presyncope, fatigue, weakness, confusion) or to associated tachycardia (palpitations, angina, heart failure). See (**Table 127-1**).

PATHOPHYSIOLOGY

Vascular supply and cardiac innervations help determine etiology and pathophysiology of bradyarrhythmias (**Table 127-2**).

TABLE 127-1 Symptoms of Bradyarrhythmia

Asymptomatic Patient	Symptomatic Patient
The patient likely remains asymptomatic if he or she has the ability to increase stroke volume. Cardiac output equals stroke volume times heart rate (CO = SV × HR). Therefore, if an individual is able to compensate for a lower heart rate by increasing stroke volume, that person will remain asymptomatic. A good example of this is a well-trained athlete, whose resting heart rates may be profoundly bradycardic but who has no symptoms referable to the heart rate because of increased stroke volume.	If a patient does not have the ability to compensate for the decreased heart rate, blood pressure (SV x HR x systemic vascular resistance) will fall. The patient may therefore develop nonspecific symptoms often chronic in nature, consistent with the patient's inability to compensate for a decreased heart rate. A vagal stimulus can decrease sinus node automaticity or cause decreased impulse transmission across the atrioventricular node. In this manner, an individual can develop specific symptoms—usually manifesting as syncope.

TABLE 127-2 Causes of SA Node Bradyarrhythmias

	Etiology	Example
Intrinsic		
	Inflammatory	• Pericarditis • Myocarditis • Rheumatic heart disease
	Iatrogenic	• Postsurgical • Radiation therapy
	Aging (idiopathic conduction system fibrosis)	• Lev disease* • Lenègre-Lev syndrome* • Senile amyloidosis
	Coronary artery disease	• Acute myocardial infarction
	Infiltrative diseases	• Sarcoidosis • Amyloidosis • Hemochromatosis
	Collagen vascular diseases	• Systemic lupus erythematosus • Rheumatoid arthritis • Scleroderma • Ankylosing spondylitis
	Myotonic muscular dystrophy and Friedreich's ataxia	
	Familial and congenital heart disease	
	Infectious	• Chagas disease • Lyme disease • Rheumatic fever • Endocarditis
Extrinsic		
	Hypoxia Endotracheal suctioning (vagal maneuvers) Sleep apnea Autonomically mediated syndromes	• Neurocardiogenic syncope • Carotid-sinus hypersensitivity • Situational (cough, micturition, etc)
	Hypothyroidism	
	Hypothermia	
	Medications	• β-blockers • Calcium channel blockers • Clonidine, reserpine, methyldopa • Digoxin • Antiarrhythmics: Class IA, Class IC, Class III ▪ Adenosine ▪ Lithium carbonate ▪ Amitriptyline ▪ Phenothiazines ▪ Cimetidine ▪ Narcotics (methadone) ▪ Pentamidine
	Increased intracranial pressure	

*Acquired complete heart block due to idiopathic fibrosis and calcification of the electrical conduction system of the heart.

The sinus node, which receives flow from the sinus-node artery, spontaneously depolarizes to initiate the cardiac cycle. The sinus-node artery most often originates from the right coronary artery (RCA), but may also branch from the left circumflex (LCx) artery. Once the sinus node depolarizes, the impulse propagates through the right atrium to the atrioventricular (AV) node. The AV node, supplied by the AV nodal artery usually arises from the RCA, but as with the sinus node, may originate from the circumflex artery. Impulses then pass from the AV node to the bundle of His, which separates into the right and left bundle branches. Ischemia of the RCA or LCx can lead to SA or AV node dysfunction and subsequent bradycardia.

The innervation of the conduction system is balanced between sympathetic and parasympathetic control. Increases in parasympathetic tone decrease sinus node automaticity and slow AV nodal conduction. Therefore, a vasovagal response to external stimuli may cause a profound bradycardia due to significant parasympathetic response (Table 127-2).

PRACTICE POINT

In general, patients with bradycardias require emergent treatment if

1. there is evidence of hypoperfusion or
2. the rhythm may deteriorate further (complete heart block or ventricular asytole).

The distinction between extrinsic and intrinsic causes is important because extrinsic causes are often reversible and should be corrected before consideration of permanent pacemaker therapy.

ATRIOVENTRICULAR NODE DYSFUNCTION

EPIDEMIOLOGY

First-degree AV block, evidenced by PR interval prolongation greater than 200 msec is rare in younger patients. It occurs more frequently in patients with heart disease and the incidence of first-degree AV block may increase by nearly 10% in older patients with heart disease. Recent evidence suggests a slightly higher mortality risk in patients with first-degree AV block. Mobitz type I second-degree AV block (known as Wenckebach) is a normal variant in younger individuals, and has no known pathologic consequences. Mobitz type II second-degree AV block, however, does have increased risk of morbidity and mortality and may require aggressive

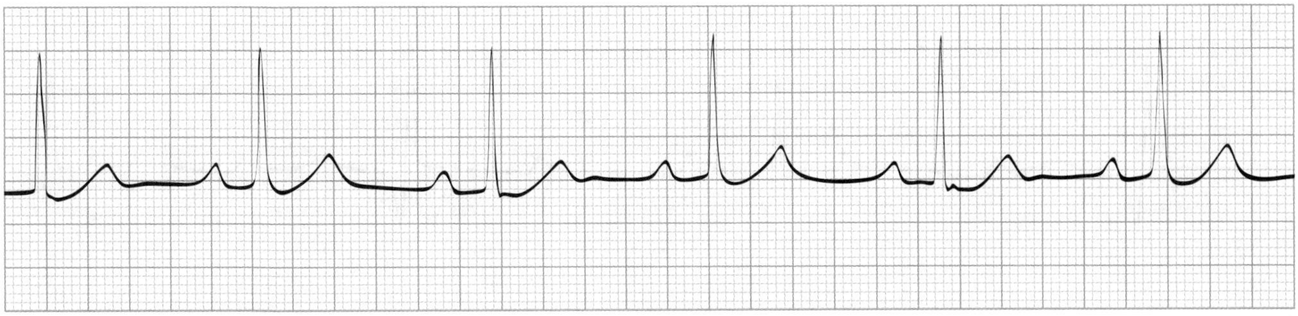

Figure 127-1 *Sinus bradycardia with first-degree atrioventricular (AV) block. First-degree AV block noted in a patient with a heart rate < 60 bpm.*

management similar to third-degree AV block. The incidence of both Mobitz type I and type II second-degree AV block increases with the presence of heart disease. In third-degree AV block, there is no AV conduction due to block at the nodal or infra nodal levels. An escape pacemaker paces the ventricles at a slower rate than the atrial rate. Acquired third-degree heart block (ie, complete heart block) is typically seen in older patients with heart disease.

PRESENTATION

First-degree and Mobitz I AV blocks are typically asymptomatic, while higher-grade AV blocks commonly present with dizziness, pre-syncope, and syncope. Patients may develop signs and symptoms consistent with heart failure.

PATHOPHYSIOLOGY

AV node dysfunction occurs when the electrical impulse moving from the atria to the ventricles is delayed or completely interrupted. This delay may be caused by an anatomic abnormality or a functional impairment and can be transient or permanent in nature. First-degree AV block occurs when conduction occurs slowly through the AV node (manifesting as a PR interval > 200 msec on ECG), while ventricular depolarization occurs without missed "beats" (**Figure 127-1**).

Classically first degree AV block is intranodal and associated with a prolonged AH (Atrial His) apical electrogram. The site of block is usually in the AV node, but may be located in the atria, AV node bundle of His, or in the His-Purkinje system. Beta-blockers, calcium channel blockers, and digitalis typically prolong the AH interval as does increased vagal tone.

In second degree AV block conduction of electrical impulses from the atrium to ventricle intermittently fail. The ECG pattern of Type I second-degree heart block—the progressive lengthening of the PR interval, shortening of the R-R interval, and a pause less than two times the immediately preceding RR interval—likely arises because of decremental conduction of electrical impulses in the AV node (**Figure 127-2**). Type II second-degree AV block commonly occurs in the distal or infra-His conduction system. It is associated with bundle branch block and is more likely to progress to higher grades of heart block than Type I. The PR interval in Mobitz II pattern is constant, and while it may be slightly prolonged, it is often normal. Eventually an atrial impulse is not conducted to the ventricles, leading to a dropped beat.

Third-degree block (or complete heart block) exhibits complete lack of impulse transmission through the AV node (**Figure 127-3**). This manifests on ECG as P waves and QRS complexes that are dissociated from one another. In complete heart block, patients often have an escape rhythm that may be narrow if originating from near the bundle of His, or wider if coming from more distal tissue.

The anatomical basis for the various degrees of AV block relates to their differing severity. In most cases, first degree AV block and Mobitz I (Wenckebach) occur within the compact AV node. The distal conduction system may be intact, and therefore intervention is often warranted only in symptomatic patients. However, Mobitz II and complete heart block occur most often within the His-Purkinje system. Because this indicates a diseased distal conduction system, intervention is often required (**Figure 127-4**).

The causes of atrioventricular block includes the intrinsic and extrinsic causes mentioned in table 127-2 for SA node disease. "Do not miss" diagnoses that require emergent treatment for the underlying cause include acute MI, acute bacterial endocarditis complicated by a valvular ring abscess, metabolic derangements (hyperkalemia and hypermagnesemia), increased intracranial pressure, and endocrine disorders (severe hypothyroidism, adrenal insufficiency). In addition to endocarditis, Lyme disease, syphilis, tuberculosis, diptheria,

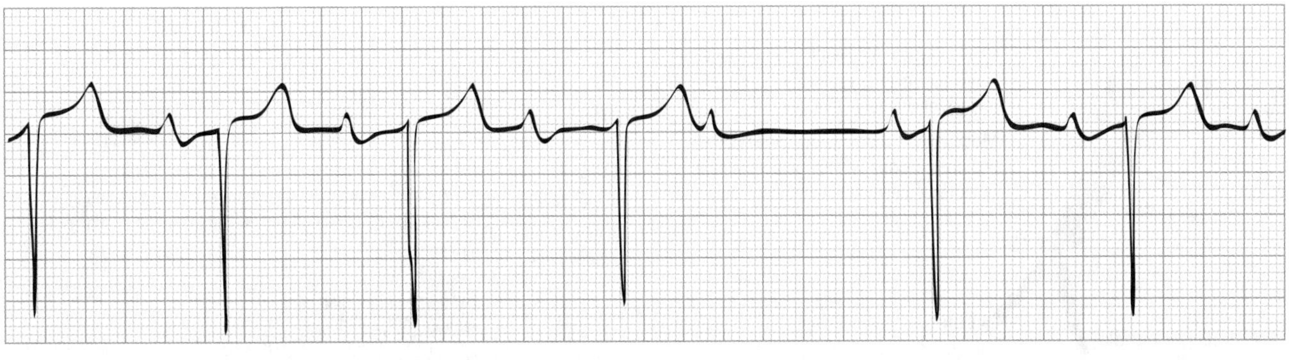

Figure 127-2 *Second-degree atrioventricular (AV) block, Mobitz type I. Second-degree AV blocks are characterized by inconsistent conduction of atrial impulses to the ventricles. In Mobitz type I second-degree AV blocks, the PR intervals vary, lengthening in duration until there is a nonconducted P wave (occurs following the fourth P wave in this rhythm strip).*

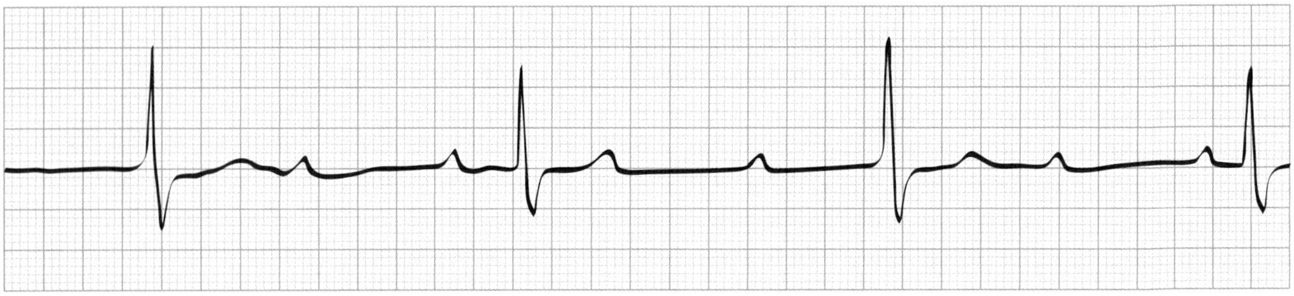

Figure 127-3 *Third-degree atrioventricular (AV) block. Third-degree AV block is often referred to as complete heart block since no atrial impulses are conducted to the ventricles. The atria and ventricular rates are completely independent on the electrocardiogram. The ventricular rate is either junctional or a ventricular escape rate. In this example, the patient has an escape rhythm near the bundle of His, as evident by the narrow QRS.*

toxoplasmosis, and Chagas disease have reportedly been associated with AV block. Iatrogenic causes include medications, catheter ablation, radiation.

Metastatic disease, specifically lymphoma, mesothelioma, and melanoma, may also affect the atrioventricular conduction system.

Other diseases (eg, Q fever, Legionella infection) may cause a relative sinus bradycardia (see **Table 127-3**).

DIAGNOSIS

All patients with bradycardia require a stepwise investigation. Clinicians should first determine if the patient has any symptoms associated with the rhythm and any signs of hypoperfusion or imminent collapse. If the rhythm is unlikely to deteriorate into an unstable rhythm such as profound bradycardia or ventricular asystole, the clinician has time to obtain a thorough history, paying particular attention to the patient's medications, including new drugs, recent dose changes, and screening for drug–drug interactions. Patients may be taking multiple AV nodal blocking agents as a result of misunderstanding or poor medication reconciliation during care transitions. A history of daytime somnolence in an obese individual may prompt an evaluation for obstructive sleep apnea. The history may also help identify precipitating events surrounding the bradycardia, possibly indicative of neurally mediated syncope, myocardial ischemia, or increased intracranial pressure.

A complete physical examination should focus on the cardiac and neurologic examinations to determine whether the patient is to identify subtle, though often nonspecific, clues that may suggest an underlying etiology for the patient's bradyarrhythmia. For example, in a patient who uses intravenous drugs, a new murmur and AV block should prompt consideration of aortic valve endocarditis with ring abscess affecting the conduction system. Clinicians should search for signs and symptoms of systemic diseases commonly associated with atrioventricular block.

All patients presenting with symptoms referable to a bradyarrhythmia or those found to be bradycardic on examination should have a 12-lead electrocardiogram to document the specific bradycardic rhythm and to look for signs of ischemia. Additional ECGs encompassing right ventricular and posterior leads should be performed if inferior or posterior MI is suspected. Other diagnostic testing is guided by symptoms and signs of systemic disease suggested by the patient's history and physical examination findings. For all patients with a potentially unstable rhythm or evidence of hypoperfusion, electrolytes, cardiac enzymes, and a complete blood count should be obtained in addition to a resting ECG.

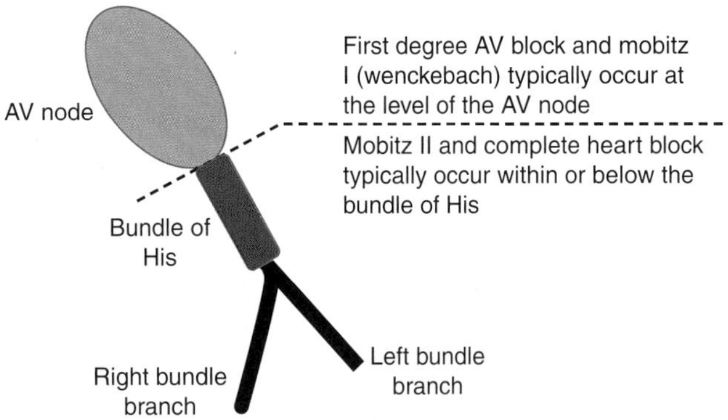

Figure 127-4 *Locations of AV-node-block. (Courtesy of Michael H. Hoskins, MD).*

TABLE 127-3 Eponyms Associated with Bradycardia

Eponym	Discussion	Significance
Faget sign (relative bradycardia in setting of fever)	Typically, when a patient is febrile, one expects an increase in pulse proportional to the elevation in temperature. The Faget sign is an inappropriately low heart rate, or *relative* bradycardia.	The Faget sign has limited diagnostic value, but it should make clinicians consider the following diagnoses in the differential: • Dengue fever • Yellow fever • *Salmonella* infection • *Brucella* infection • *Chlamydia pneumoniae* • Rickettsial infections • Q fever • *Legionella* infection • Malarial disease • Drug fever • Lymphoma
Cushing triad (bradycardia due to elevated intracranial pressure)	Elevated intracranial pressure can trigger the Cushing reflex as a means of ameliorating cerebral ischemia. The resultant changes cause hypertension, initial tachycardia followed by bradycardia, and respiratory depression.	Conditions that increase intracranial pressure: • Subarachnoid hemorrhage • Cerebral edema • Intracranial tumor • Intracranial abscess

Oxygen should be administered as necessary and continuous ECG monitoring should be provided. Derangements such as hyperkalemia or hypoxia corrected, underlying precipitants identified and treated. Persistent bradycardias unresponsive to the usual measures or clinical deterioration should prompt emergent specialty consultation.

TRIAGE/HOSPITAL ADMISSION

A patient with symptoms referable to the bradycardia should be admitted for telemetry monitoring and further evaluation.

Patients with hemodynamic compromise or life-threatening bradyarrhythmias may require admission to an intensive care unit (ICU) for intravenous (IV) drip management (pressors and/or chronotropic agents) or pacing. High-grade AV blocks (eg, third-degree AV block or Mobitz type II second-degree AV block) may require temporary external or transvenous pacing to stabilize the patient. Patients with symptomatic AV block associated with an acute MI should be admitted to a cardiac intensive care unit. Medication overdoses that present with severe bradycardia and/or high-degree AV block (with or without hemodynamic compromise) may require an ICU for administration of antidotes. Atropine may be indicated for suspected organophospate overdose, glucagon with insulin to maintain euglycemia for beta-blocker overdose, or a calcium infusion for calcium channel blocker overdose.

MANAGEMENT

INITIAL HOSPITAL TREATMENT

Initial therapy should focus on airway, breathing, and circulation. Hemodynamic compromise should be addressed immediately with active interventions following advanced cardiac life support protocol for bradycardia (**Figure 127-5**). The clinician must ensure

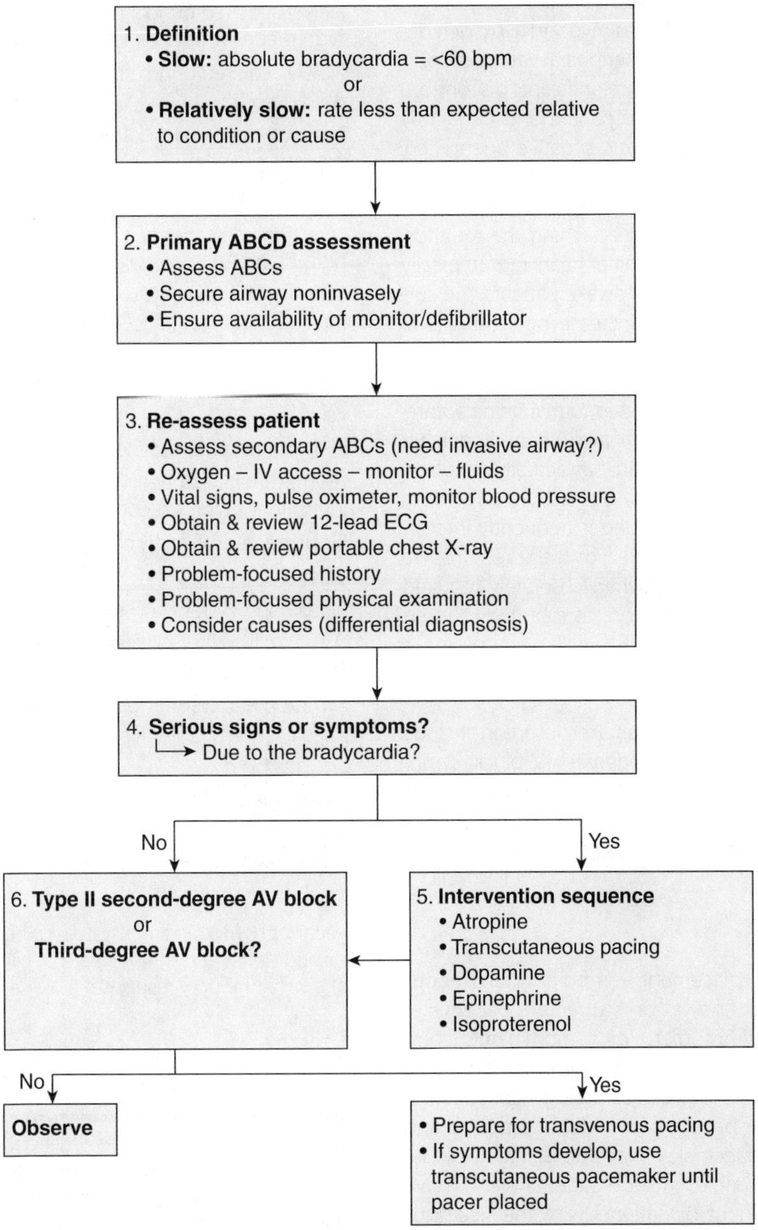

Figure 127-5 *Advanced cardiac life support algorithm for bradycardia. Medication dosing is as follows: atropine 0.5 mg IV (max 3 mg); epinephrine 2–10 μg/min IV infusion; dopamine 2–10 μg/kg/min IV infusion; isoproterenol 5–30 μg/min IV infusion (bolus IV dosing: 0.02 mg–0.06 mg initial dose with subsequent dose range of 0.01 mg–0.2 mg). (Reproduced, with permission, from Hall JB, Schmidt GA, Wood LDH. Principles of Critical Care. 3rd ed. New York: McGraw-Hill, 2005. Fig.15-3.)*

the patient has a patent airway and is able to breathe without assistance. Supplemental oxygen should be supplied when necessary, and intravenous access should be established in the event medications or resuscitative fluids are necessary.

If the patient exhibits any evidence of hypoperfusion associated with bradycardia, the clinician will need to consider intravenous medications and/or temporary pacing (see Figure 127-5). Available IV medications to treat symptomatic bradycardia include atropine, dopamine, epinephrine, and isoproterenol. The majority of sinus or AV node bradycardias respond to atropine, including some patients with infranodal blocks. IV atropine (0.5 mg) may effectively restore an adequate heart rate and abate symptoms of hypoperfusion in sinus bradycardia or in tachy-brady syndrome. Although IV atropine may be attempted in patients with high-degree AV blocks (Mobitz type II second-degree AV block or third-degree AV block) as a bridge to temporary pacing, it may be ineffective in restoring the heart rate. Atropine may be repeated to a maximum cumulative dose of 3 mg; however, doses above 2 mg are generally not effective. A second line agent, isoproterenol, may be administered as a temporizing measure but may be less effective, increases myocardial oxygen demand and ventricular ectopy, and causes peripheral vasodilation.

Transcutaneous pacing often causes significant discomfort, including pain and anxiety, for the awake patient and frequently requires opiate analgesics and/or anxiolytic sedative agents (eg, benzodiazepines) to effectively facilitate the intervention. Clinicians attempting transcutaneous pacing must have a working knowledge of the pacing equipment, including attaching the monitoring leads and pacing leads, setting the initial heart rate (typically 70–80/minute), and setting the current. In awake patients, the current should start at zero and gradually increase by 10 mA until capture is achieved. In unconscious patients, it is reasonable to begin with a high current output (200 mA) to attain rapid capture, then decrease the output to the level needed to maintain capture. Transcutaneous pacing has several inherent flaws. Often, it is difficult to determine whether capture of the heart has actually occurred. Invasive arterial waveform monitoring may be required to confirm capture. Furthermore, transcutaneous pacing is frequently ineffective and may result in intermittent capture. For these reasons, we recommend using this technique only when absolutely required during urgent or emergent clinical situations as a bridge to insertion of a temporary transvenous pacing system. External pacing is less likely to be effective if the patient has pulseless bradycardia or asystole.

Class I indications for permanent pacemaker insertion include third-degree AV block, advanced second-degree AV block, symptomatic Mobitz I or II second-degree AV block, Mobitz II with wide QRS or bifascicular block, and exercise—induced second- or third-degree AV block (without presence of myocardial ischemia) (**Table 127-4**).

CONSULTATION

New permanent pacemaker placement, temporary transvenous pacemaker placement and known or suspected pacemaker malfunction that leads to symptomatic or hemodynamic compromise with bradyarrhythmia requires prompt evaluation by a cardiologist to interrogate the device. Cardiology consultation should always occur for any patient s/p cardiac transplant and for any patient for whom pacemaker placement may facilitate optimal medical therapy. Examples include patients with known CAD who require a nodal agent or patients with the sick-sinus syndrome who are symptomatic from both the tachyarrhythmia and the bradycardia.

TABLE 127-4 Indications for Cardiac Pacing

Acquired AV block
Class I
Symptomatic permanent or intermittent AV block
Symptomatic second-degree AV block
Atrial flutter or fibrillation with advanced symptomatic AV block
Class II
Asymptomatic complete AV block with ventricular rate >40 beats/min
Asymptomatic type II second-degree AV block
After myocardial infarction
Class I
Persistent complete heart block
Persistent type II second-degree AV block
Newly acquired bundle branch block with transient high-grade AV or complete heart block
Newly acquired bundle branch block with first-degree AV block
Newly acquired bifascicular bundle branch block
Chronic bifascicular block
Class I
Symptomatic patients with fascicular block and intermittent high-grade AV or complete heart block
Symptomatic patients with bifascicular block and HV interval prolongation (>100 msec) or block distal to the His bundle at rates <100 bpm
Class II
Symptomatic patients with bifascicular block and no identifiable cause of syncope
Asymptomatic patients with bifascicular block and intermittent type II second-degree AV block.
Sinus node dysfunction
Class I
Sinus node dysfunction with symptoms of bradycardia with or without required drug therapy
Symptomatic sinus bradycardia
Symptomatic chronotropic incompetence
Class II
Sinus bradycardia <40–50 bpm or asystole >3 s and suggested symptoms not documented to be due to bradycardia
Hypersensitive carotid sinus
Class I
Recurrent syncope and asystole or heart block >3 s during carotid sinus massage or clear-cut clinical situation suggestive of a vasoinhibitory response
Class II
Recurrent syncope without clear clinical setting but abnormal response to carotid sinus massage

A, atrial; AV, atrioventricular; class I, general consensus that a pacing system is indicated; class II, consensus that a pacing system might be beneficial; H, His; V, Ventricular apical electrical recordings.

Reproduced, with permission, from Yee R, Connolly S, Noorani H: Clinical review of radiofrequency catheter ablation for cardiac arrhythmias. *Can J Cardiol.* 2003;19:1273.

TABLE 127-5 Potential Complications Associated with Pacemaker Insertion

Timing	Complication
Transvenous pacemaker insertion	• Pneumothorax • Catheter-associated bacteremia • Cardiac perforation • Cardiac tamponade
Permanent pacemaker insertion	• Bleeding • Air embolism • Pneumothorax • Cardiac perforation • Cardiac tamponade
Postoperative	• Infection (pacer pocket or other component) • Pocket hematoma • Wound dehiscence • Lead dislodgement
Long-term pacemaker	• Pacemaker syndrome • Pacemaker-mediated tachycardia

COMPLICATIONS AND PROGNOSIS

Complications may result from pacemaker insertion (**Table 127-5**). Placement of a temporary transvenous pacemaker may lead to pneumothorax, catheter-associated bacteremia, cardiac perforation and tamponade. Complications that may occur at the time of permanent pacemaker implantation include bleeding, air embolism, pneumothorax, cardiac perforation, and tamponade. Postoperative complications (occurring within approximately 30 days) include infection, pocket hematoma, wound dehiscence, or lead dislodgment.

Overall prognosis depends on the underlying etiology of the patient's bradyarrhythmia. Those with extrinsic causes of the bradyarrhythmia may have resolution of the rhythm disturbance with treatment of the underlying cause or removal of the offending drug and should suffer no long-term sequelae. When there is cardiac dysfunction, placement of a permanent pacemaker improves prognosis (**Table 127-6**).

DISCHARGE PLANNING

Any patient admitted with or found to have bradyarrhythmia must be counseled to report signs and symptoms that could be referable to the bradyarrhythmia—specifically dyspnea, lightheadedness, syncope, or palpitations.

Patients admitted for syncope or myocardial infarction with suspicion or documented evidence of bradycardia should be considered for outpatient Holter or loop monitoring. The type of monitoring depends upon the frequency of the patient's symptoms (see Chapter 99, Syncope) (**Table 127-7**).

Holter monitors should be arranged for those with daily symptoms. They continuously record the heart's electrical activity for a period of 24–48 hours. External event monitors are also worn by patients and attached to monitors worn by the patient. External event monitors are recommended for patients with less frequent symptoms (eg, symptoms at least every 1 to 3 months) and do not continuously record ECG activity. They are activated either by the patient when symptoms occur or automatically if the monitor detects an arrhythmia. Patients with very infrequent symptoms (eg, symptoms less frequent than every 3 months) can have

TABLE 127-6 Evidence-based Medicine: Key References for Bradyarrhythmias

Reference	Methodology	Results	Bottom Line
Epstein AE, DiMarco JP, Ellenbogen KA, et al. ACC/AHA/HRS 2008 guidelines for device-based therapy of cardiac rhythm abnormalities. *J Am Coll Cardiol.* 2008;51:1–62.	Expert review of the literature and consensus guidelines	Class I indications for permanent pacemaker insertion include the following: • Third-degree AV block • Advanced second-degree AV block • Symptomatic Mobitz I or II second-degree AV block • Mobitz II with wide QRS or bifascicular block • Exercise-induced second- or third-degree AV block (without presence of myocardial ischemia)	Identification of these bradyarrhythmias or AV blocks should trigger prompt cardiology consultation for evaluation and placement of a permanent pacemaker.
Cheng S, Keyes MJ, Larson MG, et al. Long-term outcomes in individuals with prolonged PR interval or first-degree atrioventricular block. *JAMA.* 2009;301(24):2571–2577.	Prospective community-based cohort study of >7500 individuals from the Framingham Heart Study	• Hazard ratio (HR) 1.44 for all-cause mortality • HR 2.06 for development of atrial fibrillation • HR 2.89 for pacemaker insertion	First-degree AV block appears to have a greater prognostic significance than previously appreciated.
Kinlay S, Leitch JW, Neil A, et al. Cardiac event recorders yield more diagnoses and are more cost-effective than 48-hour Holter monitoring in patients with palpitations. *Ann Intern Med.* 1996;124:16–20.	Randomized crossover trial, evaluating 43 patients referred for Holter monitoring	• Event monitors were twice as likely to identify a diagnostic rhythm strip than Holter monitors • A cost savings of $213 was demonstrated for each additional diagnostic rhythm strip obtained during symptoms	Patients with intermittent symptoms should be referred for an external event monitor instead of a Holter monitor.

TABLE 127-7 Ambulatory Electrocardiography

Type	Description	Indication
Holter monitor	• Worn by patient around neck or on belt for 24–48 hours • Uses several leads that are attached to patient • Records data, which are then uploaded and analyzed	• Frequent symptoms, usually occurring daily
External event monitor	• Worn continuously by the patient • Records when activated by patient when symptoms occur (records 30–60 seconds prior to activation and 2–3 minutes postactivation) • Records automatically as well, triggered by arrhythmia. Cardiologist may also program to detect specific heart rate and/or specific arrhythmias.	• Episodic symptoms, typically less frequent than every 3–4 days
Implantable loop recorder	• Small size and is inserted under the skin (similar to a pacemaker) • Programmed to record when activated by the patient (when symptoms occur) or automatically if an abnormal heart rhythm occurs	• Usually used when Holter and external event monitors are unable to identify the abnormal rhythm • Episodes are very infrequent, often less than every 2–3 months

implantable loop recorders placed for diagnosis. Generally, external event monitors are more cost-effective than Holter monitors. Implantable loop recorders are more expensive as they require implantation into the chest wall.

Follow-up with a cardiologist should always occur when a patient has a newly implanted pacemaker or is postmyocardial infarction.

QUALITY IMPROVEMENT TO ADDRESS PERFORMANCE GAPS

Changes to medications must be clearly relayed to the patient, primary care physician (PCP) and cardiologist. Reconciliation with prehospital medications is important to avoid a patient taking multiple medications from the same drug class or overmedication. Patients should notify their PCP or cardiologist if they have symptoms referable to a bradyarrhythmia, such as syncope or lightheadedness.

The American College of Cardiology/American Heart Association/Heart Rhythm Society (ACC/AHA/HRS) 2008 consensus statements on cardiac pacing do not make specific recommendations regarding follow-up. However, the Canadian Working Group on Cardiac Pacing does provide guidelines for posthospital management. Patients should have their pacemaker evaluated 72 hours postimplantation and see their cardiologist between 2 and 12 weeks following discharge. Patients should be evaluated next at 6 months and annually thereafter. This schedule will vary depending upon the patient, adherence to medical regimens, and presence of symptoms referable to rhythm abnormalities or pacemaker dysfunction. At each evaluation, the pacemaker should be interrogated and the patient screened for symptoms of lightheadedness, syncope, and heart failure.

CONCLUSION

SA node dysfunction is not associated with increased mortality but may cause distressing symptoms. Evaluation hinges upon exclusion of extrinsic causes of SA node dysfunction and correlation of the rhythm with symptoms. Temporary rate support may be required in the setting of an acute coronary syndrome, most commonly involving the right coronary artery. Regarding AV block, clinical classification was developed prior to modern understanding of the complexity of the mechanisms that impair conduction. Diagnostic testing for AV block is used to determine the level of block since the prognosis is dependent upon the location of the conduction block. Emergent intervention is required if there is evidence of hypoperfusion or the patient has a rhythm that is likely to degenerate even if asymptomatic.

SUGGESTED READINGS

Cheng S, Keyes MJ, Larson MG, et al. Long-term outcomes in individuals with prolonged PR interval or first-degree atrioventricular block. *JAMA*. 2009;301(24):2571–2577.

Epstein AE, DiMarco JP, Ellenbogen KA, et al. ACC/AHA/HRS 2008 guidelines for device-based therapy of cardiac rhythm abnormalities: executive summary: a report of the American College of Cardiology/American Heart Association Task Force on Practice Guidelines (Writing Committee to Revise the ACC/AHA/NASPE 2002 Guideline Update for Implantation of Cardiac Pacemakers and Antiarrhythmia Devices). *J Am Coll Cardiol*. 2008;51:2085–2105.

Field JM, Hazinski MF, Sayre MR, et al. 2010 International Consensus on Cardiopulmonary Resuscitation and Emergency Cardiovascular Care Science With Treatment Recommendations Part 1: executive summary: 2010 American Heart Association Guidelines for Cardiopulmonary Resuscitation and Emergency Cardiovascular Care. *Circulation*. 2010;122:S640–S656.

Fraser JD, Gillis AM, Irwin ME, et al. Guidelines for pacemaker follow-up in Canada: a consensus statement of the Canadian Working Group on Cardiac Pacing. *Can J Cardiol*. 2000;16:355–376.

Kinlay S, Leitch JW, Neil A, et al. Cardiac event recorders yield more diagnoses and are more cost-effective than 48-hour Holter monitoring in patients with palpitations. *Ann Intern Med*. 1996;124:16–20.

Mangrum JM, DiMarco JP. The evaluation and management of bradycardia. *N Engl J Med*. 2000;342:703–709.

Tresch DD, Fleg JL. Unexplained sinus bradycardia: clinical significance and long term prognosis in apparently healthy persons older than 40 years. *Am J Cardiol*. 1986;58:1009–1013.

CHAPTER 128

Ventricular Arrhythmias

Luis F. Mora, MD
Angel Rodrigo Leon, MD

Key Clinical Questions

1. What is the clinical and prognostic significance of frequent premature ventricular complexes (PVCs) and nonsustained ventricular tachycardia (NSVT), and how should they be managed?
2. In the setting of a wide complex tachycardia (WCT), what features favor a diagnosis of ventricular tachycardia (VT)?
3. What types of VT or ventricular fibrillation (VF) can occur in the absence of structural heart disease, and what types can be precipitated by exercise?
4. How should a clinician distinguish between stable VT, unstable VT, and pulseless VT diagnostically and therapeutically?
5. Which patients deserve implantable cardiodefibrillators (ICDs) for primary or secondary prevention of sudden cardiac death (SCD), and what is the role of antiarrhythmic drug therapy in primary and secondary prevention of SCD?

INTRODUCTION

Ventricular arrhythmias are a heterogeneous group of cardiac rhythm disturbances that range from benign, asymptomatic premature ventricular complexes (PVCs) to malignant and often fatal arrhythmias, such as ventricular fibrillation (VF). They can occur in both the absence and the presence of overt heart disease and have a wide spectrum of clinical significance and prognostic implications. The risk of sudden cardiac death (SCD) with some of these arrhythmias has led the medical community to identify patients susceptible to such events, and thus justify potentially dangerous and expensive treatments. Fortunately, evidence gathered from clinical trials in the last 3 decades has helped establish clear epidemiological patterns for most types of ventricular rhythm abnormalities. These patterns have proven to be vital in the development of widely accepted, evidence-based guidelines for therapy and prevention.

This chapter describes the epidemiology, pathophysiology, clinical presentation, diagnosis, treatment, and prevention of the most commonly encountered ventricular arrhythmias in current hospital practice. Care has been taken to include and cite evidence when appropriate. References to guidelines from the American College of Cardiology (ACC), American Heart Association (AHA), European Society of Cardiology (ESC), and Heart Rhythm Society (HRS) are also found throughout the text.

PREMATURE VENTRICULAR COMPLEXES

INTRODUCTION AND EPIDEMIOLOGY

PVCs, also known as ventricular premature beats (VPBs), ventricular extrasystoles (VES), or ventricular premature depolarizations (VPDs), are a frequent form of ventricular arrhythmia that occurs in both the presence and the absence of heart disease. Their prevalence depends on various demographic factors such as age, the presence or absence of heart disease, and the method used to detect them. In the Atherosclerosis Risk in the Community (ARIC) study, a review of over 15,000 healthy patients, the overall prevalence of any PVC on a 2-minute electrocardiogram (ECG) was 6% with a 34% rise for every 5-year increment in age. Conversely, published studies of healthy individuals evaluated with 24-hour ambulatory monitoring have found the prevalence of PVCs to be as high as 80%. In the background of acute myocardial infarction (AMI), the prevalence of PVCs may rise up to 93%.

Despite theoretical concerns of PVCs as a risk factor for heart disease, the occurrence of PVCs in healthy subjects has not been shown conclusively to have an impact on morbidity or mortality. A subanalysis of the Multiple Risk Factor Intervention Trial (MRFIT) found a significant threefold increase in SCD among healthy white males with any PVC on a 2-minute rhythm strip. An analysis of the Framingham Heart Study data also found significant increases in mortality when frequent or complex PVCs were identified in 1-hour ambulatory monitoring or when PVCs were identified during exercise testing. Nevertheless, several other studies do not support an association between PVCs and cardiovascular events or mortality, and no consensus exists regarding the relevance of finding them in an otherwise healthy population. Interestingly, with the exception of frequent (> 10/hour) and complex (primarily nonsustained VT) in post–myocardial infarction (MI) patients, PVCs alone do not seem to be an independent predictor of outcomes in patients with known heart disease such as left ventricular hypertrophy (LVH) and dilated or hypertrophic cardiomyopathy.

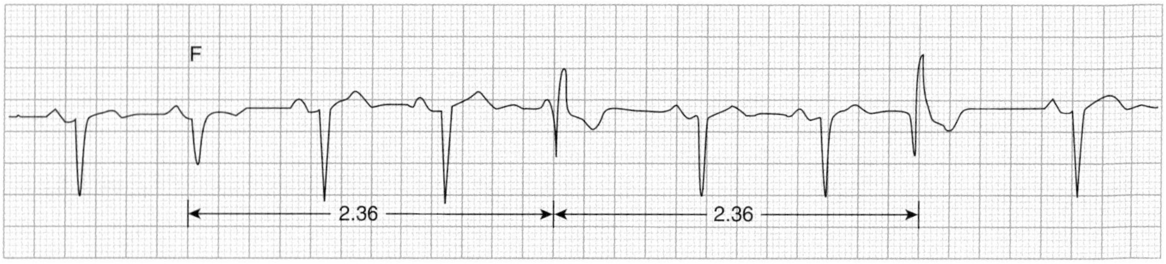

Figure 128-1 *Parasystole. The fifth and eighth ventricular complexes are premature and of similar morphology but have different coupling intervals. The second complex (F) represents a fusion beat. The interectopic interval is 2.36s.*

> **PRACTICE POINT**
>
> - In healthy patients, the occurrence of premature ventricular complexes (PVCs) does not conclusively impact morbidity or mortality. In patients with known heart disease such as left ventricular hypertrophy (LVH) or dilated or hypertrophic cardiomyopathy, PVCs alone do not independently predict adverse outcomes. However, frequent (> 10/hour) PVCs or complex PVCs—primarily nonsustained VT—in *postmyocardial infarction patients* may portend higher risk or worse outcomes.

PRESENTATION

Symptoms related to PVCs are infrequent but important to recognize. The association of specific symptoms with PVCs, along with the perceived intensity of the symptoms, has important implications for treatment. Patients may complain of palpitations, which are usually due to postextrasystolic hypercontractility, or the feeling of a "missed beat" secondary to the postextrasystolic pause. Patients may also describe neck pulsations or lightheadedness. Rarely, frequent PVCs can decrease cardiac output and cause exacerbation of underlying heart disease, particularly coronary disease and congestive heart failure (CHF). Physical exam findings vary according to the hemodynamic and electrophysiological consequences of the premature beat. Jugular venous pulsation may reveal Cannon A waves (larger than normal, sporadic, jugular venous a-waves) if there is atrial activation (normal sinus beat) simultaneous with ventricular activation by the PVC. If there is functional AV block, a variable intensity first heart sound may be heard. A PVC that has a right bundle branch block morphology (ie, originating in the left ventricle [LV]) will generate a widely split P2. Finally, murmurs vary predictably in relation with PVCs, and careful auscultation following the extrasystolic beat may provide important clues (decreased intensity in mitral valve prolapse murmur, increased dynamic obstruction in hypertrophic cardiomyopathy).

PATHOPHYSIOLOGY

The mechanisms responsible for the generation of PVCs are similar to those causing most tachyarrhythmias. Although increased automaticity, reentry, and triggered activity can all be causes of PVCs, each mechanism may have some distinguishing features on the surface ECG. PVCs often occur with a predictable and constant relationship to the preceding sinus beat (ie, fixed coupling). When this is the case, the mechanism of PVC generation is usually reentry. Examples of this type of PVC include bigeminy (a PVC after every sinus beat), trigeminy (a PVC after every two sinus beats), and quadrigeminy (a PVC after every three sinus beats). When fixed coupling is not present, the mechanism responsible for the generation of the PVC is generally increased automaticity or triggered activity from one or more ectopic ventricular foci. A specific example of this type of PVC, *parasystole*, refers to a protected automatic ventricular focus that is not reset or altered by surrounding ventricular activation (ie, entrance block). Because the focus is independent of sinus activity and ventricular activation, there will be no fixed coupling but the interectopic intervals (interval between successive PVCs) will have a common denominator (**Figure 128-1**).

DIAGNOSIS

A PVC is characterized on the surface ECG by a wide (> 120 msec) and bizarre QRS that is premature and is commonly followed by a fully compensatory pause (**Figure 128-2**). The T wave that follows a PVC will usually have a vector that is directed opposite that of the mean PVC-QRS vector. These characteristics have notable exceptions. The fully compensatory pause that follows PVCs depends on the PVC not influencing atrial depolarization or AV conduction. In most cases, PVCs will not conduct retrograde to the atria and thus will have no effect on sinus impulse formation. When these PVCs occur, the sinus impulse that happens during the PVC will not be able to conduct antegradely to the ventricles because the ventricle is refractory. However, because the sinus node is not reset by the PVC, the sinus beat following the PVC will come at a predictable time that is usually equal to twice the basic R–R interval (Figure 128-2), and usually described as a fully compensatory pause.

Occasionally, PVCs will have no influence on the subsequent sinus impulse and propagation. These premature beats are termed interpolated PVCs **(Figure 128-3)**. Although PVCs with fully compensatory pauses are most common, sometimes PVCs are conducted retrograde and may result in atrial activation. This will manifest on the ECG as inverted P waves in the inferior leads after the PVC. If the sinus node is reset by this retrograde atrial activation, the pause that follows the PVC will be less than compensatory. In other cases, the PVC may not conduct to the atria but may be blocked retrograde in the AV node, rendering the node refractory. This can result in prolongation of the PR interval for the sinus beat following the PVC or even block of the next sinus P wave. The consequence of both these situations is a more than compensatory pause. Finally, with regard to the T wave vector, the usual relationship between the PVC-QRS and its subsequent T wave may be altered if there is a preexisting repolarization abnormality in the myocardium where the PVC is being originated.

MANAGEMENT

Currently no data support suppressive treatment of PVCs in asymptomatic healthy individuals. The evidence describing long-term mortality risk in healthy patients with PVCs is conflicting. These patients should be reassured and offered standard cardiac risk factor

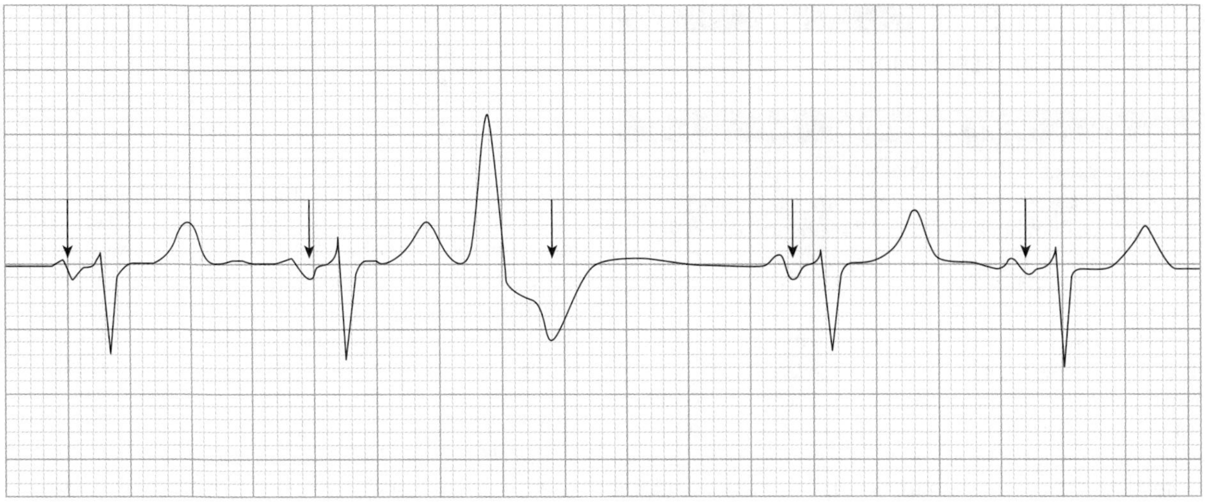

Figure 128-2 *A typical premature ventricular complex (PVC) (third QRS from left to right). Sinus activity (arrows) is usually not disrupted by the PVC. The beat following the PVC will come at a predictable moment that is equal to twice the basic R–R interval (fully compensatory pause). (Reproduced, with permission, from Tintinalli JE, Stapczynski JS, Cline DM, et al. Tintinalli's Emergency Medicine: A Comprehensive Study Guide. 7th ed. New York: McGraw-Hill; 2011. Fig. 22-23B.)*

evaluation and modification. The clinician should also thoroughly investigate possible exacerbating factors such as current medications (eg, stimulants), possible comorbidities (eg, hyperthyroidism), and electrolyte abnormalities.

When PVCs are clearly *symptomatic*, intervention should also be aimed at reducing anxiety and identifying precipitating factors, but consideration can be given to suppression of the PVCs with antiarrhythmic agents. The decision to treat with antiarrhythmics, however, must be carefully balanced. While most antiarrhythmic agents are effective at decreasing PVCs, many of these agents have known proarrhythmic properties that may render the net outcome as harm rather than benefit. As an example, in the Cardiac Arrhythmia Suppression Trials (CAST I and II), patients with a prior myocardial infarction and frequent PVCs were randomized to receive placebo versus one of three antiarrhythmic agents (flecainide, encainide, or moricizine). Although antiarrhythmic therapy proved efficacious in suppressing PVCs, the study was discontinued after 2 years' follow-up because of an increase in overall mortality in the group that was randomized to antiarrhythmic agents. Similarly, more recent trials using amiodarone for suppression of PVCs in the setting of post-MI patients and heart failure patients have shown antiarrhythmic therapy to be effective at reducing ventricular ectopy and arrhythmic mortality but have failed to demonstrate an effect on overall mortality. Based on the available evidence, even if PVCs may have some prognostic value in the setting of certain specific cardiac conditions, there is no indication to treat PVCs in the presence or absence of heart disease to reduce mortality risk. Nonetheless, the presence of structural heart disease may warrant therapy with PVC-suppressing agents, such as beta-blockers, even when the primary aim is not to treat the PVCs (ie, beta-blockers in heart failure and post-MI).

PRACTICE POINT

- There is no indication to treat premature ventricular complexes (PVCs) in the presence or absence of heart disease to reduce mortality risk. If PVCs do warrant therapy based on clinically significant symptoms, beta-blockers are first-line therapy.

If PVCs do warrant therapy based on clinically significant symptoms, beta-blockers are first-line therapy. This class of drug is particularly useful for daytime PVCs or PVCs that are related to stress, thyrotoxicosis, and mitral valve prolapse. The lowest possible dose that alleviates symptoms should be used. Other pharmacological alternatives include amiodarone and sotalol, but referral to a cardiologist is generally warranted before initiation of these latter medications. The 2006 ACC/AHA/ESC guidelines for management of patients with ventricular arrhythmias recommend radiofrequency ablation for PVCs (class IIa indication) if PVCs are frequent, symptomatic, and have proven refractory to medical therapy and if the patient is otherwise at low risk for sudden cardiac death (ie, does not meet criteria for device therapy).

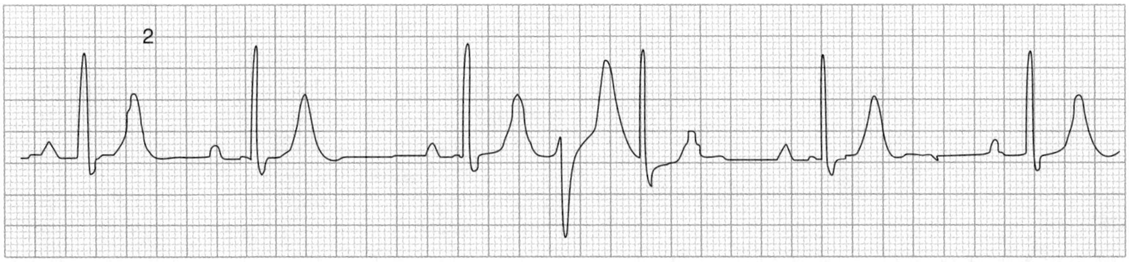

Figure 128-3 *An interpolated premature ventricular complex (fourth QRS from left to right). (Reproduced, with permission, from Fauci AS, Braunwald E, Kasper DL, et al. Harrison's Principles of Internal Medicine. 17th ed. New York: McGraw-Hill; 2008, Fig. 226-3C.)*

VENTRICULAR TACHYCARDIA

INTRODUCTION AND EPIDEMIOLOGY

PRACTICE POINT

- Sudden cardiac death (SCD), commonly defined as death from an arrhythmic cause occurring within 1 hour of the onset of symptoms, accounts for up to 460,000 deaths annually in the United States.

VT is another common form of ventricular arrhythmia that has a variety of different presentations. In the most severe of cases, VT may precipitate cardiac collapse and cause SCD. SCD, commonly defined as death from an arrhythmic cause occurring within 1 hour of the onset of symptoms, accounts for up to 460,000 deaths annually in the United States. VT and VF lead to more than 80% of monitored cases of SCD. Although VT may occur in the setting of structurally and genetically normal hearts, most patients with potentially malignant ventricular arrhythmias will have some form of underlying heart disease. As an example, approximately 70% of patients with SCD will have severe coronary disease. Furthermore, over 50% of patients treated for recurrent VT will have ischemic heart disease, and most others will have some form of cardiomyopathy. The prognosis of VT largely depends on the presence of underlying heart disease. VT in the presence of structural heart disease usually confers a high risk of SCD, whereas VT in the absence of structural heart disease or inherited sudden cardiac death syndromes generally has a good prognosis.

PRACTICE POINT

- Ventricular tachycardia (VT) in the presence of structural heart disease usually confers a high risk of sudden cardiac death, whereas VT in the absence of structural heart disease or inherited sudden cardiac death syndromes generally has a good prognosis.

PRESENTATION

In VT, symptoms are nonspecific and depend largely on the degree of hemodynamic compromise that occurs—*determined by the duration of the arrhythmia, the ventricular rate, and the presence of underlying heart disease.* Palpitations, heart failure, symptomatic hypotension or hemodynamic collapse, and SCD may all be presenting features of VT. VT may occur with minimal hemodynamic consequences, and the absence of symptoms and hemodynamic instability does not necessarily favor the diagnosis of another type of arrhythmia (ie, supraventricular tachycardia with aberrancy). Specific physical exam findings, as occurs with PVCs, include cannon A waves (secondary to AV dissociation), first heart sound variability, and split-second heart sounds.

PATHOPHYSIOLOGY

The mechanisms responsible for the generation of VT are identical to those discussed for tachyarrhythmias and PVCs (ie, reentry, increased automaticity, or triggered activity) and vary according to the clinical context in which they are encountered (ie, normal heart, long QT interval, ischemic heart disease).

DIAGNOSIS

VT is defined as the occurrence of three or more consecutive ventricular beats at a rate of more than 100 beats per minute (bpm). Although ventricular beats typically originate in ventricular muscle, they can also be initiated anywhere in the specialized conduction tissue distal to the bifurcation of the His bundle. *Because of its ventricular origin, the QRS in VT is usually wide (> 120 msec), bizarre, and has a T-wave vector opposite the main QRS deflection* (**Figure 128-4**). Rarely, however, ventricular beats originating in the basal septum or high in the fascicular system may produce a narrow complex QRS (less than 5% of all VTs). VT is usually regular but slight R–R variability may exist. The rate varies anywhere from 60 to 250 bpm depending on the specific type of VT.

To classify VT, the morphology of consecutive beats and the duration of the VT episode are considered. The morphology of consecutive ventricular beats may be close to identical (ie, monomorphic VT) or may vary from beat to beat (polymorphic VT). Occasionally, the QRS axis will alternate predictably from beat to beat, a VT that is known as bidirectional VT (**Figure 128-5**), usually seen in the setting of digitalis toxicity, cardiomyopathy, or catecholaminergic polymorphic VT. The duration of VT also helps classify the tachycardia as nonsustained (arbitrarily defined as lasting less than 30 seconds), or sustained (lasting more than 30 seconds or requiring termination due to hemodynamic collapse).

PRACTICE POINT

- Ventricular tachycardia (VT) is defined as the occurrence of three or more consecutive ventricular beats at a rate of more than 100 beats per minute (bpm). The rate varies anywhere from 60 to 250 bpm depending on the specific type of VT. Nonsustained ventricular tachycardia (NSVT) is arbitrarily defined as lasting less than 30 seconds. Sustained VT lasts more than 30 seconds or requires termination due to hemodynamic collapse.

DIFFERENTIAL DIAGNOSIS

The differential diagnosis of wide complex tachycardias (WCT) includes three major categories: VT, supraventricular tachycardia (SVT) with aberrant conduction, and SVT with antegrade conduction through an accessory pathway (ie, preexcitation). Though a clear distinction is often difficult to make, several clues support a diagnosis of VT in the setting of a WCT (**Table 128-1**). The most important clinical predictor of VT is the presence of structural heart disease. As such, a patient with a reduced ejection fraction or previous MI and a wide complex tachycardia should always be presumed to have VT (over SVT with aberrancy or preexcitation) unless there is very compelling evidence otherwise.

In addition, careful observation of the ECG tracing for evidence of fusion beats, capture beats, or atrioventricular (AV) dissociation will provide important clues for the diagnosis. Fusion and capture beats (**Figures 128-6** and **128-7**) imply activation of the ventricle from two different electrical sites during the tachycardia. Because both fusion and capture beats result in a QRS that is narrower than the QRS seen during the rest of the tachycardia, they imply intermittent partial (fusion) or complete (capture) conduction to the ventricles from a supraventricular focus and thus rule out a supraventricular origin for the tachycardia. Although evidence of AV dissociation during a WCT has long been considered a forceful argument in favor of VT, retrograde activation of the atria (ie, ventricular to atrial conduction) is seen in up to 25% of VT. Thus identification of independent atrial activity and AV dissociation during a WCT is helpful in identifying VT, but these conditions are not always present (see Figures 128-4 and 128-7), and if present they may represent retrograde conduction. If the patient is stable and there is any doubt that the rhythm is VT versus SVT, immediate expert consultation should be sought.

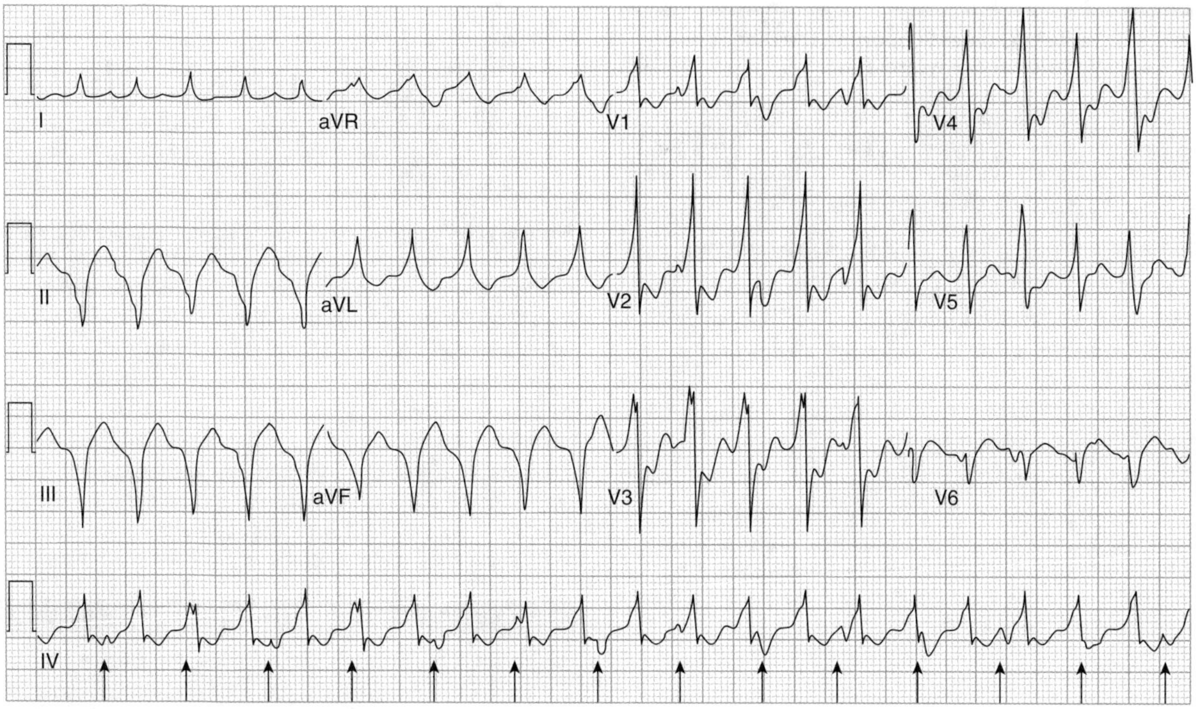

Figure 128-4 *Ventricular tachycardia. Electrocardiogram showing a wide complex tachycardia with independent atrial activity (arrows). Atrioventricular dissociation (seen here), although not always present, is very specific for a tachycardia of ventricular origin. (Reproduced, with permission, from Fauci AS, Braunwald E, Kasper DL, et al. Harrison's Principles of Internal Medicine. 17th ed. New York: McGraw-Hill; 2008, Fig. 226-10.)*

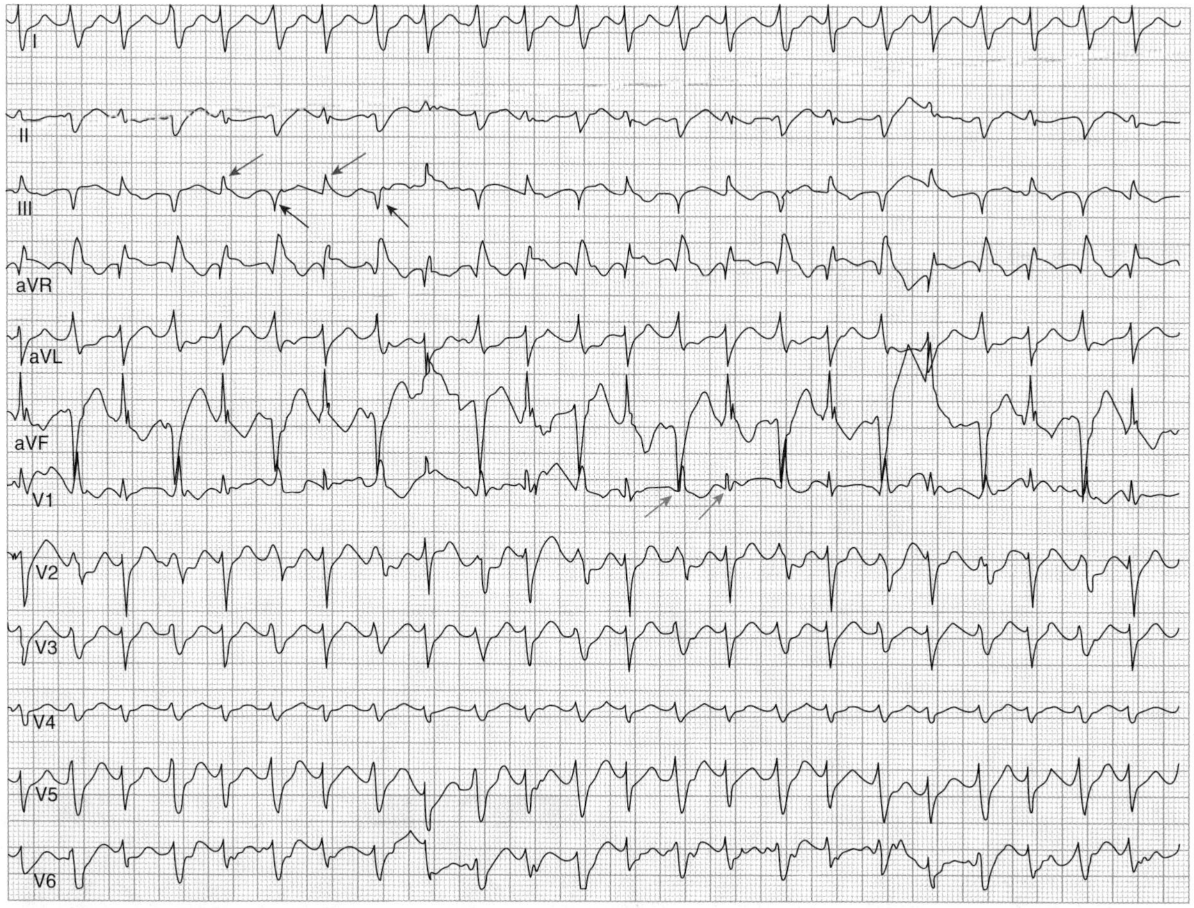

Figure 128-5 *Bidirectional ventricular tachycardia. Wide QRS tachycardia with relatively narrow QRS complex with right bundle branch block (RBBB) (green arrows) morphology and alternating inferior (red arrows) and superior (blue arrows) axes. (Reproduced, with permission, from Knoop KJ, Stack LB, Storrow AB, et al. Atlas of Emergency Medicine. 3rd ed. New York: McGraw-Hill; 2009. Fig. 23-32C. Photo contributor: Marc Mickiewicz, MD.)*

TABLE 128-1 Table ECG Clues Supporting the Diagnosis of Ventricular Tachycardia

AV dissociation (atrial capture, fusion beats)
QRS duration > 140 ms for RBBB type V1 morphology; V1 > 160 ms for LBBB type V1 morphology
Frontal plane axis –90° to 180°
Delayed activation during initial phase of the QRS complex
LBBB pattern—R wave in V1, V2 > 40 ms
RBBB pattern—onset of R wave to nadir of S > 100 ms
Bizarre QRS pattern that does not mimic typical RBBB or LBBB QRS complex
Concordance of QRS complex in all precordial leads
RS or dominant S in V6 for RBBB VT
Q wave in V6 with LBBB QRS pattern
Monophasic R or biphasic qR or R/S in V1 with RBBB pattern

Note: AV, atrioventricular; RBBB/LBBB, right/left bundle branch block. Reproduced, with permission, from Fauci AS, Braunwald E, Kasper DL, et al. *Harrison's Principles of Internal Medicine.* 17th ed. New York: McGraw-Hill; 2008:1437.

PRACTICE POINT

- A patient with a reduced ejection fraction or previous myocardial infarction and a wide complex tachycardia should always be presumed to have VT (over SVT with aberrancy or preexcitation).

MANAGEMENT

Initial hospital treatment

Stable and unstable VT with a pulse The initial management of suspected ventricular rhythm disturbances requires careful assessment of stability. Stable patients bear no significant hemodynamic consequences related to the arrhythmia. Treatment of significant hemodynamic consequences (eg, extreme hypotension) or other symptoms related to hypoperfusion (ie, angina, heart failure, altered mental status) in the setting of a suspected ventricular arrhythmia should occur emergently (ie, within seconds to minutes), precluding any further diagnostic maneuvers. The diagnostic exercise of distinguishing VT from SVT with aberrancy or preexcitation by using historical, clinical, and ECG data should only be undertaken in stable patients. Synchronized cardioversion (CV) with 100–200 J (monophasic) or 50–100 J (biphasic) is the treatment of choice in patients who are unstable as a result of VT. Required knowledge and practice of both basic life support (BLS) process and algorithms and advanced cardiac life support (ACLS) process and algorithms aid successful resuscitative measures in unstable ventricular arrhythmias.

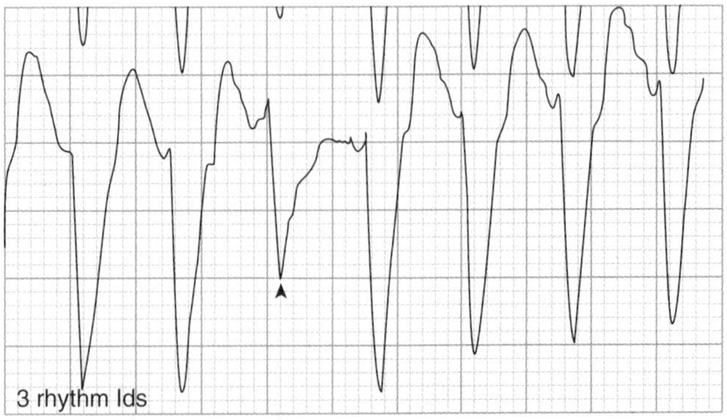

Figure 128-6 *Fusion beat. The QRS that is highlighted by the arrowhead represents fusion of a QRS originated from both a supraventricular focus and the ventricles. (Electrocardiogram contributor: Marc Mickiewicz, MD.) (Reproduced, with permission, from Knoop KJ, Stack LB, Storrow AB, et al. Atlas of Emergency Medicine. 3rd ed. New York: McGraw-Hill, 2009. Fig. 23-32B. Photo contributor: Marc Mickiewicz, MD.)*

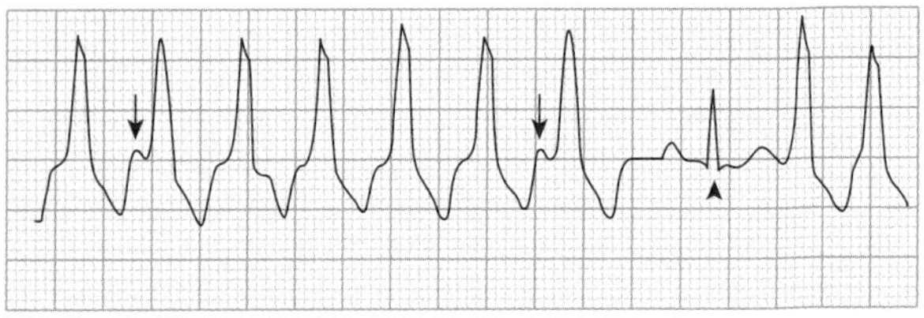

Figure 128-7 *Capture beat. Ventricular tachycardia (VT) with atrioventricular dissociation (arrows show P waves). A capture beat occurs following a lapse in the VT (arrowhead). (Reproduced, with permission, from Knoop KJ, Stack LB, Storrow AB, et al. Atlas of Emergency Medicine. 3rd ed. New York: McGraw-Hill, 2009. Fig. 23-33B.)*

PRACTICE POINT

- Treatment of significant hemodynamic instability in the setting of a suspected ventricular arrhythmia should occur emergently, within seconds to minutes. The diagnostic exercise of distinguishing ventricular tachycardia from supraventricular tachycardia with aberrancy or preexcitation by using historical, clinical, and electrocardiographic data should only be undertaken in stable patients.

Clinically stable VT allows more time to identify the diagnosis and plan specific therapy. The yearly incidence of SCD in patients who present with stable VT is only 2%. Nonetheless, patients should be hospitalized and a judicious search for underlying, reversible conditions (ischemia, heart failure, and electrolyte abnormalities) should be performed, as correction of an underlying disorder may decrease or abolish the arrhythmic phenomena without any other antiarrhythmic therapy. If the diagnosis of VT is certain, nonemergent synchronized CV, starting at monophasic doses of 100–200 J, remains a first-line option for treatment. If antiarrhythmic agents are used, amiodarone, procainamide, and lidocaine are all options. The medication choice depends on patient-specific information (eg, avoidance of procainamide in heart failure or renal failure). Amiodarone is most often used in current hospital practice. Other therapeutic strategies are effective in specific circumstances. Magnesium sulfate, for example, has a specific role in torsade de pointes. Adenosine and verapamil can be used in certain types of idiopathic VT (yet to be discussed). Digitalis-induced VT must be treated with digoxin-specific Fab fragments (Digibind). In selected cases (eg, VT associated with a scar from a previous MI), the tachycardia can be acutely suppressed by overdrive pacing or terminated by anti-tachycardia pacing (ATP). In the absence of a previously implanted device (ie, ICD), overdrive pacing and ATP both require the placement of a pacemaker lead in the right ventricle (RV), a procedure that is usually reserved for specialized cardiology or electrophysiology (EP) teams.

PRACTICE POINT

- Synchronized cardioversion serves as the treatment of choice in unstable (but not pulseless) ventricular tachycardia (VT) and in stable VT, when the diagnosis of VT is certain, Cardioversion energy dosing is 50–100 J (biphasic) or 100–200 J (monophasic). Narcotic sedative and/or analgesic agents should be administered intravenously prior to cardioversion when possible.

Pulseless VT with no discernible pulse is defined as pulseless arrest and not unstable VT. This has important implications for treatment. Pulseless VT and VF are both nonperfusing rhythms that require immediate defibrillation to restore effective circulation. Early identification of the rhythm with earliest possible defibrillation is the most critical aspect of care. In VF, survival decreases by approximately 7–10% with every minute of VF that goes unattended. The selection of energy for defibrillation depends on the mechanism of delivery. With a monophasic defibrillator, a 360 J voltage single dose is applied once before resuming cardiopulmonary resuscitation (CPR) (no "stacking" of shocks as previously recommended prior to 2005). With biphasic defibrillators, manufacturer recommendations should be followed. When recommendations are unknown, biphasic devices should be used at voltage of 200 J.

PRACTICE POINT

- Pulseless ventricular tachycardia and ventricular fibrillation are both nonperfusing rhythms that require immediate defibrillation (starting dose 120 J biphasic, 360 J monophasic) to restore effective circulation.

PRACTICE POINT

- Antiarrhythmic medications (eg, amiodarone or lidocaine) that successfully aborted the arrest should be continued as an intravenous drip after successful resuscitation. Nearly all patients should be treated with a beta-blocker agent following arrest due to a ventricular arrhythmia if the patient's blood pressure and heart rate will tolerate it.

Though defibrillation is essential in pulseless VT or VF, adequate chest compressions also affect outcomes. Pulse checks are no longer recommended after defibrillation, and other interruptions in chest compressions, including time to place an advanced airway, should be kept to a minimum. The importance of these changes is highlighted by a recent study that showed significantly improved mortality in patients with witnessed VF cardiac arrest after implementation of the 2005 AHA CPR guidelines (see Chapter 121).

Following initial stabilization from any serious ventricular arrhythmia, efforts should continue in identifying and correcting the underlying cause. Most patients will need monitoring in an intensive care unit (ICU) setting for further stabilization and quick recognition of recurrences and complications. Antiarrhythmic medications (eg, amiodarone or lidocaine) that successfully aborted the arrest should be continued as an IV drip after successful resuscitation. Nearly all patients should be treated with a beta-blocker agent following arrest due to a ventricular arrhythmia if the patient's blood pressure and heart rate will tolerate it. Induced hypothermia to mitigate postarrest anoxic brain injury should be employed in postresuscitative care. The 2010 AHA CPR guidelines recommend cooling to 32–34°C for 12–24 hours in survivors of VF arrest (class I recommendation). Induced hypothermia also may be considered for comatose adult patients after cardiac arrest of any initial rhythm other than VF (class IIb recommendation).

PRACTICE POINT

- Induced hypothermia to mitigate postarrest anoxic brain injury should be employed in postresuscitative care. The 2010 American Heart Association guidelines recommend cooling to 32°–34°C for 12–24 hours in survivors of ventricular fibrillation arrest.

Longitudinal/outpatient therapeutics: primary and secondary prevention

Long-term therapy for secondary prevention of ventricular arrhythmias is aimed at preventing symptomatic recurrences and SCD. Consequently, not all patients with VT or VF will require long-term treatment. For example, episodes of asymptomatic NSVT in patients without structural heart disease will usually not be treated with chronic antiarrhythmic therapy or device implantation. Primary prevention may be indicated in selected patient populations based on their risk factor profile.

Primary prevention Considerable evidence supports primary prevention for patients at high risk of SCD. Reduced left ventricular ejection fraction (LVEF) has consistently proven to be an independent risk factor for SCD. The Candesartan in Heart Failure Assessment of Reduction in Mortality and Morbidity (CHARM) study showed a 39% relative risk increase for every 10% reduction in ejection fraction (EF) below 45%. Though antiarrhythmic drugs still may have a role in some patients for symptom control, the ICD provides the most significant impact on primary prevention strategies.

The European and Canadian Myocardial Infarct Amiodarone Trials (EMIAT and CAMIAT) demonstrated reduced arrhythmic mortality with pharmacological therapy (amiodarone) but failed to show an impact on total mortality. Other large antiarrhythmic trials such as CAST and SWORD (Survival With d-Oral Sotalol) actually reported increased mortality in the treatment arms. These and other trials have provided a strong foundation for endorsing avoidance of antiarrhythmic drugs for purposes of primary prevention of SCD. The experience with ICD therapy has been quite the opposite. Initial trials like the Multicenter Automatic Defibrillator Implantation Trial (MADIT) and the Multicenter Unsustained Tachycardia Trial (MUSTT) focused on patients with known coronary disease and low EF who had inducible VT; mortality was significantly reduced in both these trials. MADIT-II later showed improved mortality in the ICD arm with patients selected based only on EF and not presence/absence of inducible VT. Subsequent trials that included patients with both nonischemic and ischemic cardiomyopathy (CM) and low EF also demonstrated improved mortality in the ICD treatment arms. Based on these results, the AHA/ACC/ESC/HRS have provided clear recommendations for the use of ICDs in their 2006 guidelines for ICD implantation (**Table 128-2**) and 2008 Guidelines for Device-Based Therapy of Cardiac Rhythm Abnormalities. Patients post-MI with low EF have a class I recommendation for ICD implantation only *after 40 days following the initial event.* One trial that specifically examined early implantation (5–32 days post-MI) of an ICD in patients with low EF following MI failed to show a significant effect on overall mortality.

PRACTICE POINT

- Antiarrhythmic drugs are ineffective for primary prevention of sudden cardiac death (SCD), even in patients with high risk (eg, systolic heart failure). Implantable cardiac defibrillators (ICDs) effectively prevent SCD in patients with low ejection fraction (EF < 30–35%).

Secondary prevention Patients who have survived an episode of SCD are at very high risk for recurrent, life-threatening arrhythmic events. Secondary prevention trials have shown significant mortality benefit associated with ICD implantation. The Cardiac Arrest Study Hamburg (CASH), Antiarrhythmics versus Implantable Defibrillators (AVID), and Canadian Implantable Defibrillator Study (CIDS) trials all demonstrated reduced mortality in cardiac arrest survivors randomized to ICD. Although drugs like amiodarone have also been

TABLE 128-2 ACC/AHA/ESC 2006 Guidelines for Internal Cardioverter-Defibrillator Implantation

Class I

1. ICD therapy is recommended for secondary prevention of SCD in patients who survived VF or hemodynamically unstable VT, or VT with syncope and who have an LVEF 40%, are receiving chronic optimal medical therapy, and have a reasonable expectation of survival with a good functional status for > 1 year (Level of Evidence: A).
2. The ICD is effective therapy to reduce mortality by a reduction in SCD in patients with LV dysfunction caused by prior MI who present with hemodynamically unstable sustained VT, are receiving chronic optimal medical therapy, and have reasonable expectation of survival with a good functional status for > 1 year (Level of Evidence: A).
3. An ICD should be implanted in patients with nonischemic DCM and significant LV dysfunction who have sustained VT or VF, are receiving chronic optimal medical therapy, and have reasonable expectation of survival with a good functional status for > 1 year (Level of Evidence: A).
4. ICD therapy is recommended for primary prevention to reduce total mortality by a reduction in SCD in patients with LV dysfunction caused by prior MI who are at least 40 days post-MI, have an LVEF 30% to 40%, are NYHA functional class II or III, are receiving chronic optimal medical therapy, and have reasonable expectation of survival with a good functional status for > 1 year (Level of Evidence: A).
5. ICD therapy is recommended for primary prevention to reduce total mortality by a reduction in SCD in patients with nonischemic heart disease who have an LVEF 30% to 35%, are NYHA functional class II or III receiving chronic optimal medical therapy, and have reasonable expectation of survival with a good functional status for > 1 year (Level of Evidence: B).

Class IIa

1. ICD implantation is reasonable for treatment of recurrent sustained VT in patients post-MI with normal or near normal ventricular function who are receiving chronic optimal medical therapy and have reasonable expectation of survival with a good functional status for > 1 year (Level of Evidence: C).
2. Implantation of an ICD is reasonable in patients with LV dysfunction caused by prior MI who are at least 40 days post-MI, have an LVEF 30% to 35%, are NYHA functional class I on chronic optimal medical therapy, and have reasonable expectation of survival with a good functional status for > 1 year (Level of Evidence: B).
3. ICD implantation can be beneficial for patients with unexplained syncope, significant LV dysfunction, and nonischemic DCM who are receiving optimal medical therapy and who have a reasonable expectation of survival with a good functional status for > 1 year (Level of Evidence: C).
4. ICD therapy is reasonable in patients who have recurrent stable VT, a normal or near normal LVEF, and optimally treated HF and who have a reasonable expectation of survival with a good functional status for > 1 year (Level of Evidence: C).
5. ICD therapy combined with biventricular pacing can be effective for primary prevention to reduce total mortality by a reduction in SCD in patients with NYHA functional class III or IV receiving optimal medical therapy, in sinus rhythm with a QRS complex of at least 120 msec and who have reasonable expectation of survival with a good functional status for > 1 year (Level of Evidence: B).
6. ICD therapy is reasonable for primary prevention to reduce total mortality by a reduction in SCD in patients with LV dysfunction caused by prior MI who are at least 40 days post-MI, have an LVEF 30% to 35%, are NYHA functional class I, are receiving chronic optimal medical therapy, and have reasonable expectation of survival with a good functional status for > 1 year (Level of Evidence: B).

Class IIb

1. ICD therapy may be considered for primary prevention to reduce total mortality by a reduction in SCD in patients with nonischemic heart disease who have an LVEF 30% to 35%, are NYHA functional class I receiving chronic optimal medical therapy, and have a reasonable expectation of survival with a good functional status for > 1 year (Level of Evidence: B).

DCM, dilated cardiomyopathy; ICD, internal cardioverter-defibrillator; LV, left ventricular; LVEF, left ventricular ejection fraction; MI, myocardial infarction; NYHA, New York Heart Association; SCD, sudden cardiac death; VF, ventricular fibrillation; VT, ventricular tachycardia.

Reproduced, with permission, from Fuster V, O'Rourke RA, Walsh RA, et al. *Hurst's the Heart.* 12th ed. New York: McGraw-Hill; 2008:1007.

shown to be superior to placebo, comparisons favor ICD therapy. A meta-analysis of secondary prevention ICD trials showed a mortality benefit in the ICD population when compared to amiodarone. The benefit, however, was restricted to patients with EF lower than 35%. AHA/ACC/HRS guidelines provide class I recommendation for ICD implantation in patients who present with SCD from VF or sustained VT, irrespective of EF. Additionally, patients who have near-normal hearts and sustained VT that does not result in cardiac arrest have a class IIa recommendation for ICD implantation.

The role of antiarrhythmic therapy is relegated to patients who refuse, or are poor candidates for, ICD therapy and for patients who have recurrent arrhythmias and ICD shocks. Poor candidates include patients who do not have a reasonable expectation of survival (> 1 year) with an acceptable functional status, patients with incessant VT/VF or VT/VF that is amenable to catheter ablation, and patients with no structural heart disease and ventricular dysrhythmias due to a completely reversible disorder (eg, electrolyte imbalance, drugs, or trauma). Amiodarone effectively reduces the frequency of ventricular arrhythmias that result in symptoms or shocks and may also reduce the ventricular rate enough to allow for pace-termination of the arrhythmia. When amiodarone fails, other drugs such as sotalol, procainamide, or flecainide may be used. Radiofrequency ablation (RFA) may also be effective in selected patients (ie, VT/VF precipitated by preexcitation, RV or LV outflow tract VT, idiopathic VT, or fascicular VT in the absence of structural heart disease).

VENTRICULAR FLUTTER AND FIBRILLATION

INTRODUCTION AND EPIDEMIOLOGY

Ventricular flutter (VFl) and fibrillation (VF) are extreme derangements of the electrical activity in the heart that usually terminate fatally within minutes if no intervention is made. As with VT, the incidence of VF can be inferred from the epidemiology of SCD; *VF is the implicated arrhythmia in approximately 70% of reported cases of monitored SCD (including those preceded by VT).* VF likely is responsible for the majority of unmonitored, out-of-hospital cardiac

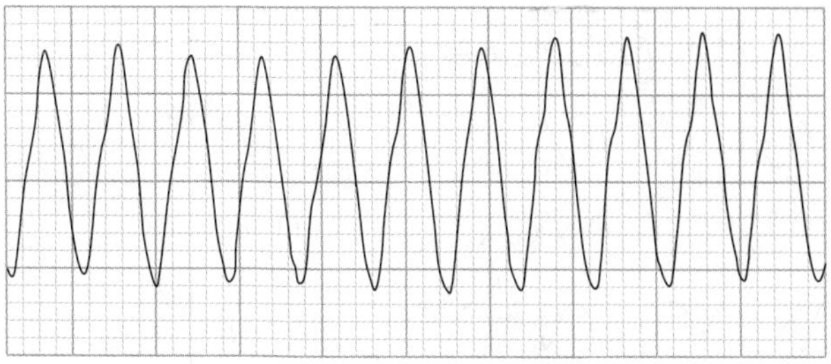

Figure 128-8 *Ventricular flutter. Very rapid, regular, wide-complex tachycardia with sine-wave appearance. The rate in this example is 330 bpm. Differential diagnosis includes Wolff-Parkinson-White with atrial flutter. (Reproduced, with permission, from Knoop KJ, Stack LB, Storrow AB, et al. Atlas of Emergency Medicine. 3rd ed. New York: McGraw-Hill, 2009. Fig. 23-33B.)*

arrests. Though most cases of VF happen in the setting of underlying ischemic heart disease, VF may also be a manifestation of myocardial viral infection, valvular disease, hypertrophic cardiomyopathy, long and short QT syndromes, dilated cardiomyopathy, drugs (eg, class I and III antiarrhythmics, digoxin, tricyclic antidepressants, cocaine), hypoxia, ion channel disorders, and electrolyte and acid–base disorders. VF can also happen in the setting of atrial fibrillation (AF) with rapid antegrade conduction over an accessory pathway (eg, AF in Wolff-Parkinson-White syndrome).

PRESENTATION

Patients with VF always present in complete hemodynamic collapse. Blood pressure is unobtainable, heart sounds are absent, and agonal breathing or apnea is typical. Asystole and death are the inevitable result if prompt resuscitation efforts are not initiated.

PATHOPHYSIOLOGY

VF happens as a consequence of multiple localized areas of microreentry, usually seen in structurally or genetically abnormal hearts that harbor an environment of heterogeneous ventricular depolarization and dispersion of ventricular repolarization. Electrical impulses traveling through myocardium with these derangements get fragmented, and multiple areas of functional reentry are produced. This results in multiple, dynamic, reentry spiral waves of myocardial activation that manifest on the surface ECG as VF.

DIAGNOSIS

VFl is a very fast (usually 150–300/min), sine wave appearing rhythm that is almost invariably associated with hemodynamic collapse (**Figure 128-8**). Under normal circumstances it cannot be differentiated from rapid VT or atrial flutter with underlying preexcitation. VF is characterized by a very rapid, irregular, and polymorphic ventricular rhythm with no clearly defined QRS or T wave (**Figure 128-9**). The absence of organized electrical activity precludes the generation of normal myocardial contraction, and cardiac output becomes negligible leading to hemodynamic collapse. Most cases of VF are preceded by an increase in ventricular ectopy (ie, PVCs) and repetitive nonsustained arrhythmias that include both monomorphic and polymorphic VT.

> **PRACTICE POINT**
>
> - Most cases of ventricular fibrillation are preceded by an increase in ventricular ectopy (ie, premature ventricular complexes) and repetitive nonsustained arrhythmias that include both monomorphic and polymorphic ventricular tachycardia.

MANAGEMENT

VFl and VF are medical emergencies. Acute treatment has already been detailed in the management section of pulseless VT within this chapter. Long-term primary and secondary prevention of malignant ventricular arrhythmias has also been discussed previously.

SPECIFIC SUBTYPES OF VENTRICULAR TACHYCARDIA AND VENTRICULAR FIBRILLATION

VT and VF occur most commonly in the setting of identifiable heart disease. One autopsy report found that 95% of patients who presented with SCD had evidence of structural abnormalities. Moreover, many patients with SCD and seemingly normal hearts have nonstructural cardiac pathology in the form of conduction disease, inherited ion channel abnormalities, or structural protein derangements. Nonetheless, a small subset of patients with VT/VF will have no detectable cardiac abnormality.

The fact that VT and VF can occur in either the absence or the presence of structural heart disease leads to considerable heterogeneity in clinical features and implications. Specific examples are detailed in the following sections.

VT/VF IN THE ABSENCE OF STRUCTURAL HEART DISEASE

Idiopathic VT

Idiopathic monomorphic VT (10% of all VT referrals) occurs in structurally normal hearts and has a relatively benign prognosis. These tachycardias represent the nonmalignant end of the spectrum for VT and are considered specific syndromes rather than compensated forms of malignant VT. Although terminology varies, there are at least three well established forms of idiopathic VT:

1. Repetitive monomorphic VT (RMVT, also known as right ventricular outflow tract [RVOT] tachycardia)
2. Paroxysmal sustained VT
3. Idiopathic left ventricular tachycardia (ILVT).

RMVT is a type of idiopathic VT that usually originates in the septal or anterior aspect of the RVOT. Surface ECG reveals a left bundle branch morphology and inferior axis (**Figure 128-10**) because of the origination site. RMVT originates in the LV outflow tract in about 10–15% of cases. RMVT has a variety of synonymous descriptions in the literature, most relevant of which are catecholamine-sensitive VT, verapamil-sensitive VT, and exercise-induced VT. Typically, RMVT presents as nonsustained VT in young

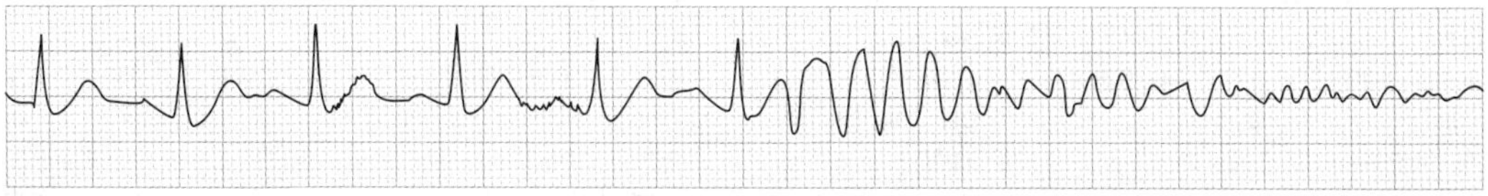

Figure 128-9 *Ventricular fibrillation. After six beats, sinus rhythm degenerates into ventricular fibrillation. (Reproduced, with permission, from Stone KC, Humphries RL. Current Diagnosis & Treatment: Emergency Medicine 6th ed. New York: McGraw-Hill, 2008. Fig. 33-19.)*

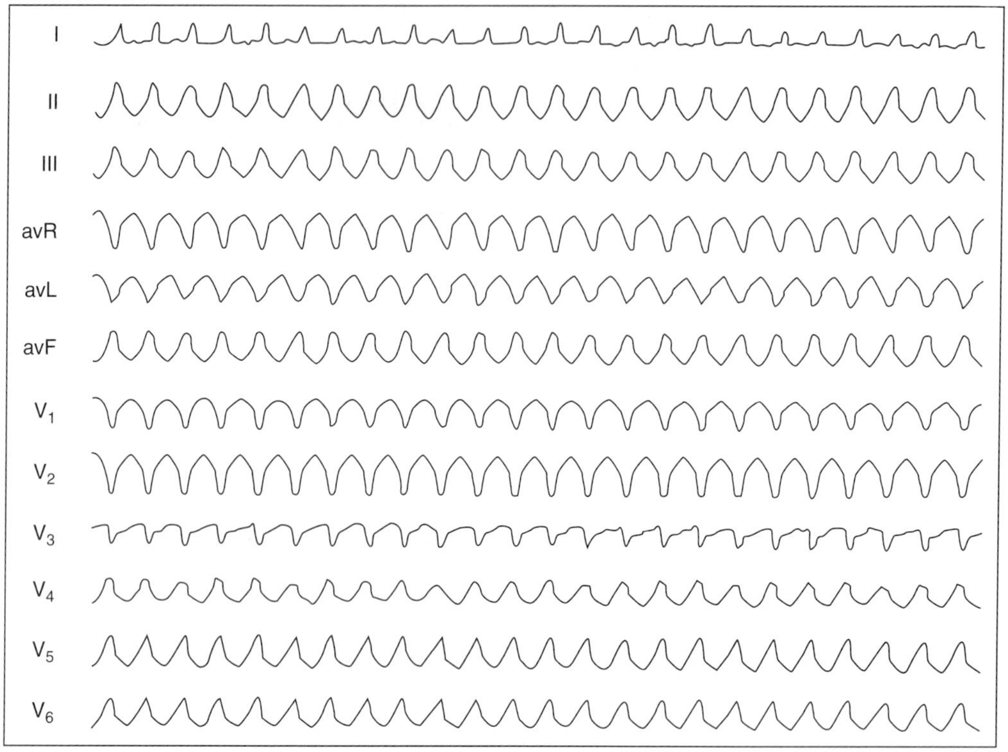

Figure 128-10 *Repetitive monomorphic ventricular tachycardia (VT). Twelve-lead electrocardiogram that is typical of VT in the absence of structural heart disease, originating in the right ventricular outflow tract. There is left bundle branch block morphology with late transition (V_4) in the precordial leads and an inferior axis in the limb leads. Negative QRS complex in lead avL suggest a septal origin. (Reproduced, with permission, from Badhwar N, et al. Idiopathic ventricular tachycardia: diagnosis and management. Curr Probl Cardiol. 2007;32:7.)*

to middle-aged patients during periods of high levels of circulating catecholamines (such as stress or exercise). The pathophysiology of the arrhythmia involves abnormalities in cardiac sympathetic function and triggered activity. Prognosis for patients with RMVT is usually good, but malignant variants have been described. These are, however, the exception, and most cases of RMVT will not be treated as malignant unless certain high risk features such as syncope, fast VT (> 230 bpm), or frequent ectopy is present. The treatment of RMVT is relatively unique because the arrhythmia is sensitive to adenosine, verapamil, and beta-blockers. Any of these drugs may be used to terminate the acute episode, and verapamil and beta-blockers are usually prescribed for prevention of recurrence. Class III antiarrhythmics such as amiodarone and sotalol can also be used. RFA is an alternative for refractory symptomatic patients that is being used with increased frequency and that has a success rate that ranges from 80 to 100% (for typical RVOT RMVT).

Paroxysmal sustained VT is another type of RV idiopathic VT that also typically arises from the RVOT and that may respond to drugs like adenosine. Because of its obvious similarities with RMVT, it is considered by some not to be a distinct syndrome. Treatment for paroxysmal sustained VT is similar to that for RMVT.

ILVT usually originates in the inferoapical or midseptal region of the LV. Because of its location, the QRS on the surface ECG will usually be relatively narrow (0.12–0.14 s) with a right bundle branch block (RBBB) morphology and a left superior axis. It typically presents as palpitations in young adults, and is usually not precipitated by exercise; SCD is rare. Reentry has been proposed as the underlying electrophysiological mechanism. ILVT is especially sensitive to verapamil in the acute setting, and it is often used for long-term treatment. As with RMVT, RFA is an option for patients who are drug refractory or drug intolerant.

Catecholaminergic polymorphic VT

Polymorphic VT is less common than monomorphic VT in the absence of structural heart disease and inherited ion channel disorders. When clearly associated with a family history of SCD or stress-induced syncope, it is known as catecholaminergic polymorphic VT (CPVT). There is also a sporadic version in which no family history is identified. The disorder typically presents in childhood or adolescence as life-threatening VT (that is often bidirectional VT) or VF that is precipitated by physical or emotional stress. The arrhythmia is easily inducible during EP testing. Many patients with CPVT will have mutations in the cardiac ryanodine receptor, a receptor that mediates calcium release from the sarcoplasmic reticulum. Long-term beta-blockade has variable reported efficacy but is accepted as first-line treatment. Most patients with life-threatening VT or symptomatic VT despite beta-blockers should be offered an ICD in accordance with the 2008 ACC/AHA/HRS guidelines for device-based therapy.

Long QT syndrome (congenital, acquired) and torsade de pointes

The QT interval on a surface ECG represents the time it takes for myocardial cells to depolarize and repolarize. Although the normal value for a corrected QT (QTc, adjusted for heart rate) is usually quoted as < 440 msec, normal QT length also depends on other variables such as age and gender. Measurements are usually made in the lead with the longest clearly identifiable QT. Though expert opinion varies, U waves, when present, should probably be included as part of the QT only when they are clearly merged with the T wave. The long QT syndromes (LQTS) are a heterogeneous group of disorders that are due to defects in the ion currents that

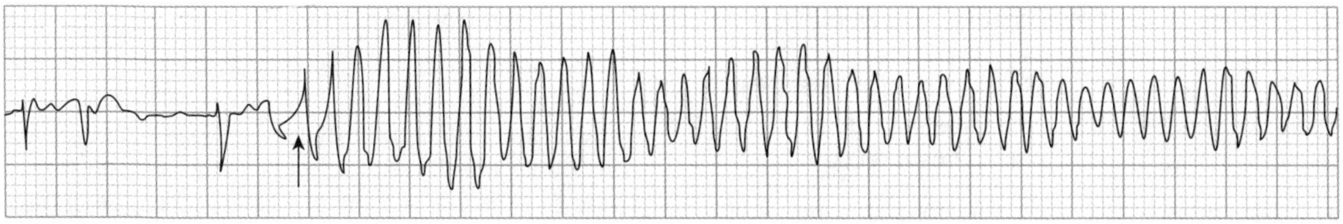

Figure 128-11 *Torsade de pointes. A polymorphic, "twisting," tachycardia is preceded by a short R–R interval followed by a long R–R interval with a premature ventricular complex falling during repolarization; the R on T phenomenon (arrow). (Reproduced, with permission, from Fuster V, O'Rourke RA, Walsh RA, et al. Hurst's the Heart. 12th ed. New York: McGraw-Hill, 2008. Fig. 94-4.)*

are responsible for repolarization. These defects may be acquired or congenital and are especially important because they can lead to a very serious form of polymorphic VT that is termed torsade de pointes (TdP). TdP is a polymorphic VT that is characterized by QRS complexes that vary in amplitude and cycle length in a pattern that seems to "twist" around the baseline (**Figure 128-11**). It is by definition associated with a long QT, usually in excess of 600 msec. The pathophysiology, clinical presentation, and management of the acquired and congenital forms of LQTS have several distinctive features.

PRACTICE POINT

- U waves, when present, should probably be included as part of the QT only when they are clearly merged with the T wave.

PRACTICE POINT

- Torsade de pointes (TdP) is a polymorphic ventricular tachycardia that is characterized by QRS complexes that vary in amplitude and cycle length in a pattern that seems to "twist" around the baseline (see Figure 128-11). It is by definition associated with a long QT, usually in excess of 600 msec.

Acquired Acquired LQTS is by far more common than congenital LQTS and is usually secondary to medications or electrolyte imbalances such as hypomagnesemia, hypokalemia, and hypocalcemia. The TdP that is seen in acquired LQTS tends to start after a PVC with a compensatory pause or during bradycardia. Although not clearly a cause in itself, bradycardia aggravates the potential of certain drugs to prolong the QT interval and precipitate TdP.

PRACTICE POINT

- Many drugs have been implicated in acquired long QT syndrome (LQTS) (see Table 128-3). A more detailed list, that is updated frequently, is available on the internet (www.torsades.org or www.qtdrugs.org).

Many drugs have been implicated in acquired LQTS (**Table 128-3**). A more detailed list, which is updated frequently, is available on the Internet (www.torsades.org or www.qtdrugs.org). The medications most frequently responsible for QT prolongation and TdP are antiarrhythmics, macrolides, certain antipsychotics, and antihistamines. The overall incidence of drug-induced LQTS varies according to the drug and population studied. Two commonly cited drugs, sotalol and cisapride, have reported TdP incidences of 2–4% and 5.7%, respectively. Though drug-related LQTS is thought to be an idiosyncratic event, most patients who develop the syndrome will have one or more risk factors. These risk factors include female sex, concomitant electrolyte disturbances or bradycardia, baseline QT prolongation or silent congenital LQTS mutations, underlying heart disease, high drug concentrations, and concurrent use of medications that prolong the QT interval (eg, erythromycin and cimetidine).

Hypomagnesemia, hypokalemia, and hypocalcemia can also cause acquired LQTS and predispose to TdP. The QT-prolonging effects of these electrolyte imbalances are likely a consequence of decreased activity in normal outward repolarizing currents and enhanced drug-related blockade of these currents. Other causes of

TABLE 128-3 Selected Medications Associated with Prolonged QT Interval

Antiarrhythmic drugs
Quinidine
Procainamide hydrochloride
Disopyramide phosphate
Sotalol hydrochloride
Amiodarone
Ibutilide fumarate
Dofetilide
Propafenone
Anesthetics/antiasthmatics
Droperidol
Adrenaline
Antibiotics
Clarithromycin
Erythromycin
Pentamidine
Trimethoprim-sulfamethoxazole
Ketoconazole
Fluconazole
Antihistamines
Terfenadine
Diphenhydramine
Antihyperlipidemic
Probucol
Central nervous system active drugs
Droperidol
Haloperidol
Pimozide
Risperidone
Gastrointestinal stimulants
Cisapride

Reproduced, with permission, from Fuster V, O'Rourke RA, Walsh RA, et al. *Hurst's the Heart.* 12th ed. New York: McGraw-Hill; 2008:1838.

acquired LQTS include stroke (both ischemic and hemorrhagic) and nutritional disorders.

Treatment for acquired LQTS is focused on rapid identification and correction of reversible causes and acute management of TdP when present (as detailed in the VT management section).

Congenital The incidence of the congenital long QT syndromes in the general population is estimated to be 1 in 2500 to 1 in 10,000 and accounts for approximately 3000 to 4000 cases of SCD in the U.S. annually. Two clinical phenotypes have been described. They are differentiated based on their inheritance pattern and presence of sensorineural hearing loss. The Romano Ward *syndrome* is the autosomal dominant variant of the LQTS and is not associated with hearing loss. *The Jervell and Lange-Nielsen syndrome* is the autosomal recessive variant of the LQTS that is associated with sensorineural hearing loss. In addition to the clinical phenotypes, the LQTS may be classified based on their underlying genetic mutation. Over 10 different types of genetic mutations (LQT1-LQT10) have been described. However, mutations within LQT1, LQT2, and LQT3 represent over 90% of cases.

Symptoms related to congenital LQTS are nonspecific and are mostly a consequence of the development of arrhythmias. In the international QT registry, an ongoing study of patients with LQTS and their families started in 1979, 76% of proband patients (ie, index subjects with LQTS) had a cardiac event defined as cardiac arrest, SCD, or syncope.

The pathophysiology of LQTS is incompletely understood, but congenital LQTS is generally accepted as a disease of ion channels. The common denominator of all these mutations is abnormal repolarization and prolongation of the QT interval. In the setting of a long QT, triggered activity (ie, early after depolarizations [EADs] that reach threshold potential) are thought to be the most common initiating factor for VT. The development of EADs and malignant arrhythmias is facilitated by bradycardia, electrolyte disturbances, and increased sympathetic activity.

The diagnosis of congenital LQTS is clinical and based on historical data (eg, family history, syncope), ECG findings (long QT interval, especially QTc > 480 msec), and exercise testing (abnormal shortening of the QT interval is insensitive but may help in the diagnosis). Genetic testing is not used routinely for diagnosis but may be useful to identify family members of patients with a known diagnosis of congenital LQTS, to confirm the diagnosis in cases where clinical criteria are not conclusive, and to identify patients with LQT1, where strenuous exercise is particularly dangerous and beta-blockers are especially useful.

The treatment of congenital LQTS is focused on the prevention of malignant arrhythmias and SCD. Avoidance of drugs that prolong the QT and close monitoring of electrolyte abnormalities is paramount. Restriction of activity to low-intensity exercise is also recommended, especially in confirmed LQT1 cases. Beta-blockers should be prescribed in all patients with congenital LQTS, as they reduce cardiac events and overall mortality in this population. Mexiletine may be used as add-on therapy in patients with LQT3. Based on ACC/AHA/HRS guidelines for cardiac device therapy, primary prevention of SCD with ICD implantation is recommended (class IIa) only for patients with LQTS who have VT or syncope while on beta-blocker therapy. Other therapeutic strategies considered by electrophysiologists may include left cardiac sympathetic denervation, cardiac pacing, and RFA.

PRACTICE POINT

- Beta-blockers should be prescribed in all patients with congenital long-QT syndrome, as they reduce cardiac events and overall mortality in this population.

Brugada syndrome

The Brugada syndrome (BS) is a distinct form of inherited ion-channel disorder that can lead to VF and SCD in hearts with no evident structural abnormalities. The prevalence of ECG findings compatible with BS ranges from 0.4% in a report from the United States to 1.0% in a report from Japan. BS has an autosomal dominant genetic pattern of inheritance and occurs more commonly in men. Up to one-third of families with BS have mutations in the SCN5A gene that encodes the alpha subunit of the cardiac sodium channel. Collectively, mutations in the SCN5A gene may lead to a wide range of different phenotypes, including sudden unexpected nocturnal death syndrome (SUNDS), atrial standstill, LQT3, and isolated progressive cardiac conduction defect. The mutations seen in BS are "loss of function" mutations that result in defective sodium channels with impaired activation or accelerated inactivation. These alterations ultimately reduce the duration of normal cardiac action potentials.

The characteristic ECG changes in the BS are thought to arise from differential expression of these defective channels within the layers of the RV. It has been proposed that epicardial cells in the RV, which are preferentially affected, lose their action potential dome and thus promote a current directed toward them from the unaffected RV endocardial cells. This results in the typical ST segment changes seen in the three types of BS. The heterogeneity of electrophysiological properties within the RV also provides the substrate for reentry arrhythmias (phase 2 reentry). The typical ECG in BS has a pseudo-RBBB pattern with permanent ST segment elevation in the anterior precordial leads. Specific alterations in the appearance of the ST segment differentiate the syndrome into three "types" (**Figure 128-12**).

Diagnosis of BS, as with LQTS, is based on a combination of electrocardiographic, historical, and clinical findings. Genetic testing, while available, is not routinely recommended due to its lack of sensitivity and specificity. EP testing is also not routinely performed but may have a role in risk stratifying asymptomatic patients with characteristic ECG findings.

The ACC/AHA/ESC currently recommends ICD therapy for patients with BS and previous cardiac arrest (class Ia), BS and previous VT without arrest (class IIa), and BS and syncope (class IIa). Some groups also advocate ICD use in asymptomatic patients with inducible VT or VF during EP testing. Antiarrhythmic therapy is reserved for patients with frequent, recurrent episodes of VT and VF to reduce the amount of ICD discharges.

VENTRICULAR TACHYCARDIA AND FIBRILLATION IN THE PRESENCE OF STRUCTURAL HEART DISEASE VT/VF AND ISCHEMIC HEART DISEASE

The incidence of VT/VF in ischemic heart disease depends on the underlying pathology. In the GUSTO-1 trial, which included over 40,000 patients with ST-elevation MI (STEMI) treated with thrombolysis, the incidence of VT and VF was 3.5% and 4.1%, respectively. In a pooled analysis of over 25,000 patients with non-STEMI or unstable angina (UA), the incidence of VT and VF was only 0.8% and 1%, respectively.

Patients with ischemic heart disease are at risk for developing ventricular arrhythmias from a variety of different mechanisms. As an example, acute ischemia leading to VT or VF is likely a consequence of local electrophysiological alterations in ischemic myocardium. Other rhythm disturbances, such as accelerated idioventricular rhythm (AIVR), are usually seen in the setting of reperfusion. VT in the patient with a remote history of an MI is usually due to reentry circuits around/in scarred myocardial tissue.

The pathogenesis of abnormal ventricular rhythms in ischemic heart disease varies according to the timing of the ischemic insult.

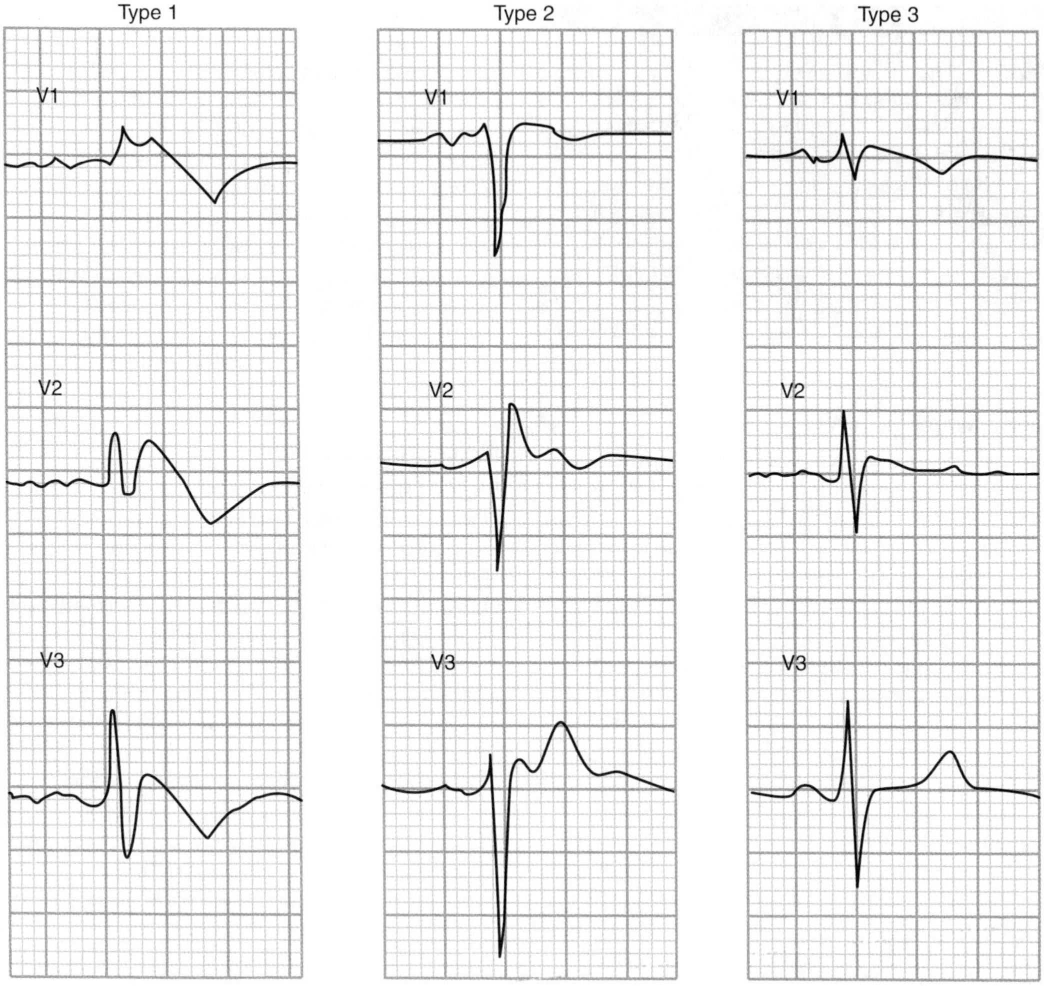

Figure 128-12 *Electrocardiographic patterns in Brugada syndrome (BS). Only type 1 ST-segment elevation is considered diagnostic for BS when associated with clinical features such as syncope and spontaneous/inducible ventricular arrhythmias. Types 2 and 3 may indicate the presence of BS but drug challenge is required for diagnosis. The electrocardiograms in the right and left panels are from the same patient before (right panel, type III) and after (left panel, type I) intravenous administration of 1 mg/kg of ajmaline in 10 minutes. (Reproduced, with permission, from Fuster V, O'Rourke RA, Walsh RA, et al. Hurst's the Heart. 12th ed. New York: McGraw-Hill, 2008. Fig. 33-7.)*

The various time-dependent changes in ischemic myocardial cells provide a substrate for all the possible electrophysiological mechanisms of arrhythmia induction (ie, reentry, triggered activity, increased automaticity). Specifically, acute ischemia causes resting cardiomyocyte membrane potential to become less negative. In addition, acute ischemia significantly reduces the duration, amplitude, and velocity of the cardiac myocyte action potential. These alterations in resting membrane potential and conduction may lead to reentry, triggered activity, and increased automaticity. Chronic consequences (ie, scar) of an acute ischemic insult incite reentry as the predominant mechanism for ventricular arrhythmia. Although some ventricular rhythms may occur in the setting of reperfusion ("reperfusion arrhythmias"), these appear not to be life threatening and do not seem to carry any prognostic significance. Moreover, while the appearance of a typical reperfusion rhythm (AIVR) has long been considered a marker of relieved coronary occlusion, it is neither sensitive nor specific for successful reperfusion. AIVR, also known as slow VT, is identified on the ECG as a wide-complex ventricular rhythm with a rate of 40–100 bpm (usually 60–100 bpm).

VT/VF in hypertrophic cardiomyopathy

Patients with hypertrophic cardiomyopathy (HCM) are at increased risk for malignant ventricular arrhythmias and SCD. In one community-based study of patients with HCM, the incidence of SCD was 1.1% at 5.5 years follow-up. Despite this, the use of routine electrophysiological testing as a screening tool is controversial. Instead, major society guidelines have advocated prevention and treatment decisions based on clinical data. High-risk clinical features for the development of VT include family history of SCD, syncope (especially exercise induced or repetitive), NSVT, failure to increase BP during exercise testing, and massive (≥ 30 mm) LV hypertrophy.

Current evidence for treatment of HCM is limited. As randomized, controlled trial data are lacking, the ACC/AHA/HRS guidelines recommend ICD implantation, based on observational data, for patients with HCM who (1) are survivors of an episode of sustained VT or SCD, (2) have one of the five high-risk features (see sidebar), or (3) have end-stage HCM with LV dysfunction and dilation.

PRACTICE POINT

- Major society guidelines do not recommend routine electrophysiological (EP) testing in hypertrophic cardiomyopathy (HCM). Rather, they recommend evaluation when high risk clinical features for the development of ventricular tachycardia exist, including family history of sudden cardiac death, syncope (especially exercise induced or repetitive), nonsustained ventricular tachycardia, failure to increase blood pressure during exercise testing, and massive (≥ 30 mm) left ventricular hypertrophy.

VT/VF in arrhythmogenic right ventricular cardiomyopathy (ARVC)

Arrhythmogenic right ventricular dysplasia (ARVC), a specific type of cardiomyopathy that is characterized by fibrofatty replacement of ventricular myocardium, initially affects the RV producing typical wall motion abnormalities and RV dysfunction. Though predominantly described as a disease of the RV, the LV is eventually involved in up to 60% of cases. *The mean age at diagnosis is 30, and exercise is often a precipitating factor.*

Approximately 50% of patients with ARVC present with symptomatic ventricular arrhythmias. The patchy nature of the fibrofatty infiltration presumably provides a substrate for reentry. Monomorphic VT is the most common form of arrhythmia in this population and is characterized by an LBBB pattern with an inferior axis, similar to RV outflow VT. Though rare, polymorphic VT associated with sympathetic stimulation may also be present in some forms of ARVC. *The resting ECG in sinus rhythm is normal in up to 50% of cases.* When abnormal, ECG findings include incomplete or complete RBBB, inverted T waves in the right precordial leads, and increased QT dispersion (variability in the QT between leads). A terminal notch following the QRS, commonly known as an *epsilon wave*, is seen only in 30% of patients (**Figure 128-13**).

The diagnosis of ARVC is based on clinical criteria that include the presence of ventricular arrhythmias, ECG findings, and echocardiographic and historical information. Myocardial biopsy is insensitive owing to the segmental nature of the disease.

Treatment, as with HCM, focuses on the prevention of SCD. Patients with ARVC are instructed to avoid high-demand physical activities, including competitive sports. ICDs are recommended as secondary prevention for patients with sustained VT or VF and as primary prevention in patients with high-risk features (eg, extensive RV involvement, LV involvement, family with SCD, unexplained syncope). Antiarrhythmics are used in cases where ICDs are contraindicated or when ventricular arrhythmias and ICD discharges are frequent. RFA is an option for patients who have failed antiarrhythmic therapy.

ELECTRICAL STORM

Electrical storm (ES) is commonly used to describe the occurrence of multiple episodes of unstable VT or VF in a short amount of time. Definitions vary but most authors agree that at least more than two episodes in a 24-hour period constitute ES. ES is a relatively rare phenomenon in the absence of a known predisposition to ventricular arrhythmias, but prevalence as high as 23% per year has been reported in secondary prevention ICD trials. Secondary prevention trials have also found ES to be an independent predictor for mortality, including cardiac nonsudden death. The most common identifiable precipitating factor for ES is ischemia.

The cornerstone of ES management is identifying and correcting any possible reversible cause. Ischemia, decompensated heart failure, and electrolyte disturbances must all be considered and treated accordingly. Patients who present with ES and have not had an ICD implanted previously should be resuscitated according to current ACLS guidelines. Reperfusion, beta-blockade, and IV antiarrhythmics are essential in ES secondary to ischemia. Once stabilized, most patients who survive an episode of ES should undergo implantation of an ICD. Although antiarrhythmics may be used, ICD therapy has

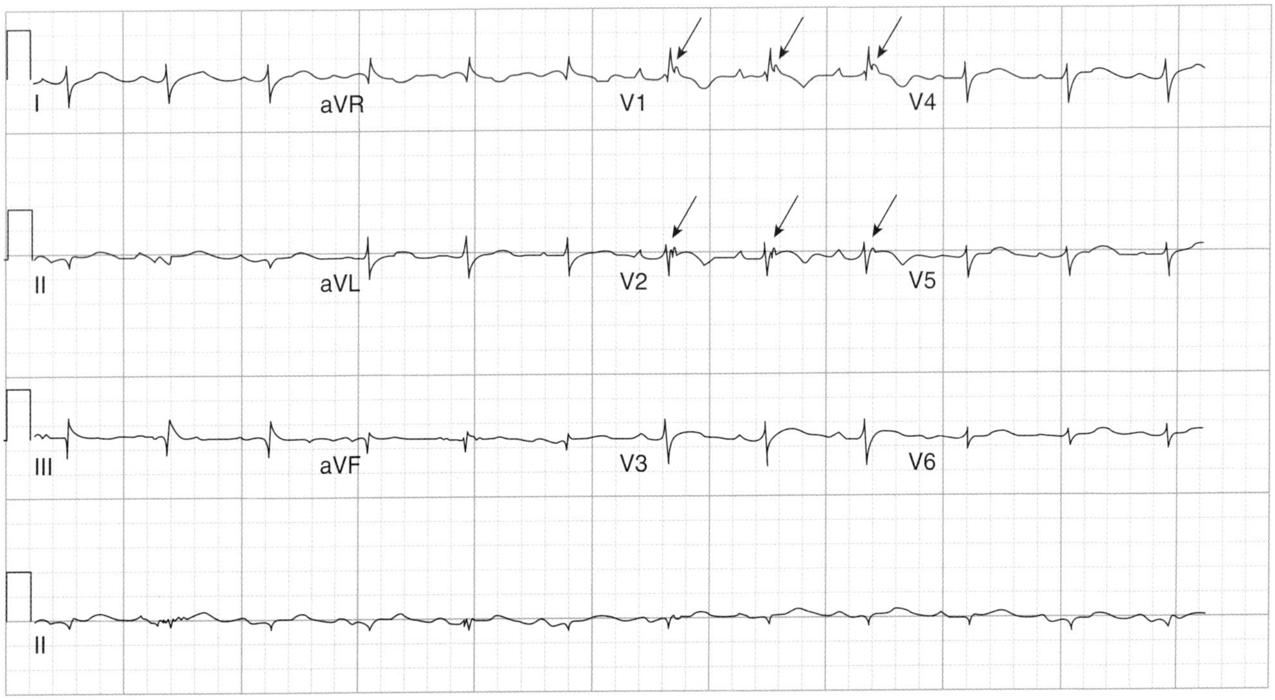

Figure 128-13 *Epsilon waves (arrows) in a patient with arrhythmogenic right ventricular cardiomyopathy. This is an important diagnostic feature for this condition. (Reproduced, with permission, from Fuster V, O'Rourke RA, Walsh RA, et al. Hurst's the Heart. 12th ed. New York: McGraw-Hill, 2008. Fig. 39-3.)*

TABLE 128-4 Evidence-based Medicine: Key References for Ventricular Arrhythmias

Reference	Methodology	Results	Bottom Line
CAST Echt DS, et al. *N Engl J Med.* 1991;21;324(12): 781–788	Randomized trial (flecainide, encainide vs placebo) • $n = 1498$ • Post-MI • EF ≤ 40% • ≥6 PVC/h	Significantly increased arrhythmic mortality in treatment arms (3.9 vs 1.0%). Nonarrhythmic cardiac mortality also increased in treatment arms.	Arrhythmic and cardiac death increased with all treatment arms, PVCs post-MI should not be suppressed with antiarrhythmic medication.
MADIT II Moss AJ, et al. *N Engl J Med.* 2002;1;346(12): 877–883	Randomized trial (ICD vs conventional medical therapy) • $n = 1232$ • Post-MI (> 30 d) • EF ≤ 30% • > 10 PVC/h or couplets	Significantly reduced mortality in ICD arm (14.2 vs 19.8%) at 20 months HR = 0.65	Improved survival in ICD arm for patients with preexisting MI
COMPANION Bristow MR, et al. *N Engl J Med.* 2004;20;350(21): 2140–2150	Randomized trial (ICD-CRT vs CRT alone vs optimal medical therapy • $n = 1520$ • Ischemic or NICM • EF ≤ 35%	Significant reduction in the all-cause mortality and all-cause hospitalization for both CRT arms (56 vs 68%). Only the ICD-CRT groups had significant reduction in only all-cause mortality.	Improved survival in ICD-CRT group > CRT group > medical therapy group in both ischemic and NICM
SCD-HeFT Bardy GH, et al. *N Engl J Med.* 2005;20;352(3): 225–237	Randomized trial (ICD vs amiodarone vs medical therapy • $n = 2521$ • Ischemic and NICM (NYHA II–III) • EF ≤ 35%	Significantly reduced overall mortality in ICD arm (29 vs 36% with placebo) HR = 0.77	Improved survival in ICD group for both ischemic and NICM patients. No benefit from amiodarone compared to placebo

CRT, cardiac resynchronization therapy; EF, ejection fraction; HR, heart rate; ICD, implantable cardiodefibrillator; MI, myocardial infarction; NICM, nonischmic cardiomyopathy; NYHA, New York Heart Association; PVC, premature ventricular complex.

proven to significantly improve mortality for survivors of cardiac arrest from ventricular arrhythmias when compared to drugs alone. For patients who already have an ICD, antiarrhythmics, especially amiodarone, are often used for suppression of frequent symptomatic arrhythmic episodes and ICD discharges. Overdrive pacing, RFA, and spinal cord modulation are also alternatives in selected cases.

QUALITY IMPROVEMENT TO ADDRESS PERFORMANCE GAPS

COSTS AND UTILIZATION

Most estimates have projected costs of ICD per year of life saved to be approximately $50,000 to $100,000, within the accepted range for developed countries. A cost-effectiveness study that used data from six extensively cited ICD *primary prevention* trials found that ICD implantation had a cost-effectiveness of $34,000 to $70,200 per quality-adjusted life-years (QALYs) gained. However, other analyses have yielded results as high as $235,000 dollars per year of life saved in one primary prevention trial and $213,543 in one secondary prevention trial. Because of this disparate information, ICD implantation for primary and secondary prevention of SCD remains an intervention requiring longer-term cost effectiveness evaluation.

DISPARITIES IN CARE

Gender and racial disparities have been reported in both primary and secondary prevention populations eligible for ICD therapy. An analysis of ICD utilization in a sample Medicare population found ICDs were significantly less used in women than men for both primary and secondary prevention. In another analysis of over 13,000 eligible ICD candidates for primary prevention, women were also less likely to receive the intervention than men, and black patients were less likely to receive an ICD when compared to white men. Finally, a recently published meta-analysis that was designed specifically to assess the benefits of ICD therapy in women for primary prevention found no significant reduction in all-cause mortality for women treated with ICDs. The reason for such disparities is likely multifactorial and requires sensitive evaluations by part of the medical community at large. The potential lack of benefit of ICD therapy in women must be further explored with specific prospective trials targeted to this population. **Table 128-4** lists evidence-based medicine key resources for ventricular arrhythmias.

SUGGESTED READINGS

Antzelevitch C, Brugada P, Borggrefe M, et al. Brugada syndrome: report of the second consensus conference: endorsed by the Heart Rhythm Society and the European Heart Rhythm Association. *Circulation.* 2005;111:659.

Connolly SJ, Hallstrom AP, Cappato R, et al. Meta-analysis of the implantable cardioverter defibrillator secondary prevention trials. *Eur Heart J.* 2000:21:2071–2078.

Epstein AE, DiMarco JP, Ellenbogen KA, et al. ACC/AHA/HRS 2008 Guidelines for Device-Based Therapy of Cardiac Rhythm Abnormalities: a report of the American College of Cardiology/American Heart Association Task Force on Practice Guidelines (Writing Committee to Revise the ACC/AHA/NASPE 2002 Guideline Update for Implantation of Cardiac Pacemakers and Antiarrhythmia Devices): developed in collaboration with the American Association for Thoracic Surgery and Society of Thoracic Surgeons. *Circulation.* 2008;117:e350.

Field JM, Hazinski MF, Sayre MR, et al. 2010 American Heart Association Guidelines for Cardiopulmonary Resuscitation and Emergency Cardiovascular Care. Part 1: Executive summary. *Circulation*. 2010 Nov 2;122(18 Suppl 3):S640–S656.

Hohnloser SH, Al-Khalidi HR, Pratt CM, et al. Electrical storm in patients with an implantable defibrillator: incidence, features, and preventive therapy: insights from a randomized trial. *Eur Heart J*. 2006;27:3027.

Huikuri HV, Castellanos A, Myerburg RJ. Sudden death due to cardiac arrhythmias. *N Engl J Med*. 2001;345(20):1473–1482.

Josephson ME, Zimethbaum P. The tachyarrythmias. In: Kasper DL, Braunwald E, Fauci AS, Hauser SL, Longo DL, Jameson JL, eds. *Harrison's Principles of Internal Medicine*. 16th ed. New York: *McGraw-Hill*; 2004:1343.

Rho RW, Page RL. Ventricular arrhythmias. In: Fuster V, O'Rourke RA, Walsh RA, et al., eds. Hurst's the Heart. 12th ed. http://accessmedicine.com/resourceTOC.aspx?resourceID=664/October 21, 2011

Sanders GD, Hlatky MA, Owens DK. Cost-effectiveness of implantable cardioverter-defibrillators. *N Engl J Med*. 2005;353:1471.

Zipes DP, Camm AJ, Borggrefe M, et al. ACC/AHA/ESC 2006 Guidelines for Management of Patients With Ventricular Arrhythmias and the Prevention of Sudden Cardiac Death—Executive Summary: a report of the American College of Cardiology/American Heart Association Task Force and the European Society of Cardiology Committee for Practice Guidelines (Writing Committee to Develop Guidelines for Management of Patients with Ventricular Arrhythmias and the Prevention of Sudden Cardiac Death). *J Am Coll Cardiol*. 2006;48:1064.

CHAPTER 129

Pacemakers, Defibrillators, and Cardiac Resynchronization Devices in Hospital Medicine

Michael H. Hoskins, MD
David B. De Lurgio, MD, FACP

Key Clinical Questions

1. What are the components of an implantable pacing or defibrillation system?
2. How do pacemakers interact with the heart's natural rhythm to know when to and when not to pace?
3. What do the common pacing codes (ie, VVI, DDD) mean, and how do they affect the electrocardiogram (ECG)?
4. When should patients be referred for cardiac resynchronization therapy (CRT)?
5. How should clinicians evaluate the patient who has received an implantable cardiac defibrillator (ICD) shock?
6. When should a pacemaker or ICD be interrogated in the inpatient setting?

INTRODUCTION

Advances in technology and the expansion of indications have greatly increased the number of patients receiving pacemakers and implantable cardiac defibrillators (ICDs). Approximately 200,000 pacemakers and 100,000 defibrillators are implanted annually for the management of cardiac arrhythmias, treatment of congestive heart failure, and the prevention of sudden cardiac death. These devices have progressed from relatively simple components with basic pacing and defibrillation features, to more advanced systems with a significant impact on patient morbidity and mortality. The increasing number and complexity of devices encountered in hospitalized patients frequently presents a clinical management challenge. The purpose of this chapter is to introduce basic concepts of pacing and defibrillation, review standard indications for cardiac rhythm devices, and highlight pertinent clinical considerations for hospitalist care of patients with these devices.

EQUIPMENT AND HARDWARE

Cardiac pacing and defibrillating systems consist of pulse generators and leads. The pulse generator is the "device" that contains the battery, circuitry, and capacitors. It is typically encased in a titanium housing that ranges in size and shape depending on the manufacturer. Defibrillator pulse generators are about two to three times larger than pacemakers (**Figure 129-1**).

The leads are connected to the pulse generator at the time of implant and are attached distally to the myocardium. They are secured to the myocardium either "actively" by means of a small screw, or "passively" by means of small tines near the lead tip. Pacemaker leads consist of conducting wires, a silicone or polyurethane insulation coating, and platinum electrodes used for pacing. Defibrillation leads have one or two additional wire coils capable of delivering high-voltage impulses for defibrillation (**Figure 129-2**).

Technologic advancements in the field of cardiac rhythm devices have resulted in smaller batteries with increased life spans. Most batteries used in modern devices are lithium-based and are nonrechargeable with a finite life span. Typically, a pacemaker battery will last approximately 10 years, while an ICD battery will last approximately five years. Once exhausted, these batteries must be exchanged.

PRACTICE POINT

- Pacemaker batteries will last approximately 10 years, while an ICD battery will last approximately five years. Once exhausted, these batteries must be exchanged.

Battery longevity depends on several factors, the most important of which include pacing output, the relative amount of time pacing is required, and the number of programmable features that are activated on the device. Furthermore, frequent ICD therapies represent a common cause for battery drain. The cardiologist managing the patient will tailor device programming to maximize battery life without sacrificing the clinical function of the device.

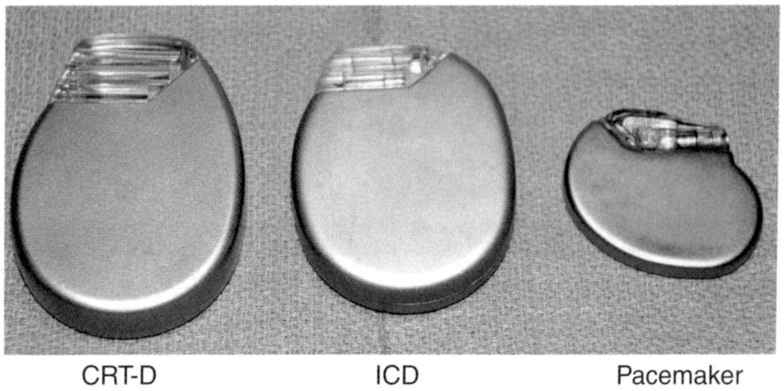

Figure 129-1 *Examples of cardiac resynchronization therapy with defibrillator (CRT-D), implantable cardiac defibrillator (ICD), and pacemaker devices. Note the size difference between the defibrillator and pacemaker devices.*

The remaining life of a battery is displayed each time the device is interrogated. As battery life declines, the device will enter a period called *elective replacement interval* (ERI). This alerts the physician that there are approximately two to three months of remaining battery life and the patient should be scheduled for elective replacement of the device. Further depletion of the battery will lead to the *end-of-life* (EOL) period, an indication that the battery should be replaced as soon as possible. Importantly, as batteries enter the ERI and EOL periods, certain features of the device will automatically turn off to preserve as much battery life as possible. This may result in a reduction in the clinical benefit a patient receives from the device.

BASIC PACING CONCEPTS

SENSING AND PACING

The two primary functions of pacemakers are *sensing* and *pacing*. Sensing refers to the ability of the device to detect native impulses originating from the heart. These sensed events are used to time subsequent events based on programmable settings. The ability of the device to sense a native impulse depends on the amplitude of the electrical signal generated by the heart, as seen by the device. *Undersensing* occurs when the amplitude of the signal is insufficient for detection by the pacemaker and results in inappropriate pacing by the device (**Figure 129-3**). *Oversensing* occurs when the device inappropriately interprets signals as native impulses. Oversensing leads to inappropriate inhibition of pacing, and may occur as a result of internal or external "noise" detected by the device (**Figure 129-4**). When oversensing occurs in an ICD, the device can misinterpret the signals as a ventricular arrhythmia and inappropriately shock the patient.

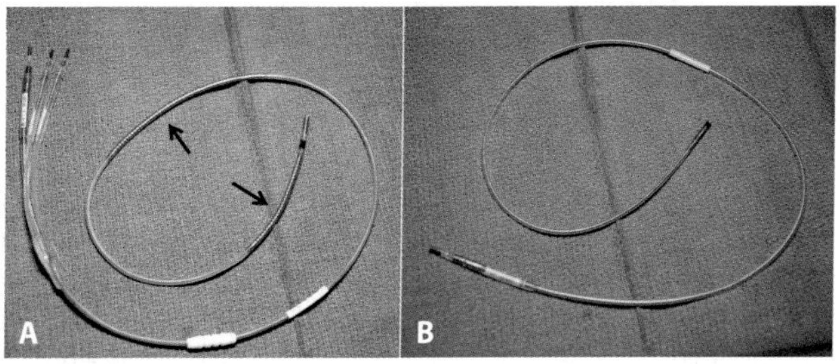

Figure 129-2 *Examples of (A) an implantable cardiac defibrillator (ICD) lead and (B) a pacemaker lead. Note the high-voltage defibrillation coils on the ICD lead (indicated by arrows).*

PRACTICE POINT

- *Undersensing* occurs when the amplitude of the signal is insufficient for detection by the pacemaker and results in inappropriate pacing by the device (Figure 129-3). *Oversensing* occurs when the device inappropriately interprets signals as native impulses. Oversensing leads to inappropriate inhibition of pacing, and may occur as a result of internal or external "noise" detected by the device (Figure 129-4).

Pacing output is the electrical stimulation that results in myocardial depolarization and contraction of the heart. The minimal amount of electrical energy required to cause depolarization is termed the *capture threshold,* and it is a function of the electrode-tissue interface. Pacing output is programmed sufficiently above the capture threshold to provide an adequate safety margin. This output is seen on surface electrocardiograms as a discrete "spike" called a pacing stimulus artifact. Importantly, modern devices with bipolar pacing and low energy outputs can generate a relatively small stimulus artifact that may be difficult to see on surface tracings. Careful attention to the tracing will usually reveal these small artifacts.

When insufficient energy is delivered by the device, the electrical stimulus may fail to depolarize the myocardium. This is called *failure to capture.* It is recognized when a pacing stimulus artifact is not followed by a P wave or QRS complex (depending on which chamber is being paced), and occurs as a result of either inappropriately low output or poor electrode-tissue interface from lead dislodgement. Failure to capture is relatively uncommon in chronic devices with stable leads. When failure to capture occurs in patients who are pacemaker dependent, dangerously low heart rates may result (**Figure 129-5**).

PRACTICE POINT

- Failure to capture occurs when a pacing stimulus artifact is not followed by a P wave or QRS complex (depending on which chamber is being paced), and occurs as a result of either inappropriately low output or poor electrode-tissue interface from lead dislodgement.

TIMING INTERVALS

There are multiple programmable intervals pacemakers use to determine when to deliver pacing output. The most important of these include *lower rate limit, AV interval,* and *upper rate limit* (**Figure 129-6**). The *lower rate limit* is the slowest rate that a pacemaker will allow the heart to reach. When the heart rate drops below this rate, the pacemaker will begin pacing. However, as long as the heart rate exceeds this rate, pacing will not occur. Therefore, lack of pacing on a surface ECG in this instance does not indicate device malfunction.

PRACTICE POINT

- Pacemaker *lower rate limit* is the slowest rate that a pacemaker will allow the heart to reach. When the heart rate drops below this rate, the pacemaker will begin pacing. However, as long as the heart rate exceeds this rate, pacing will not occur.

The *AV* (atrioventricular) *interval* is the time allowed after an atrial event before ventricular pacing will occur. This is analogous

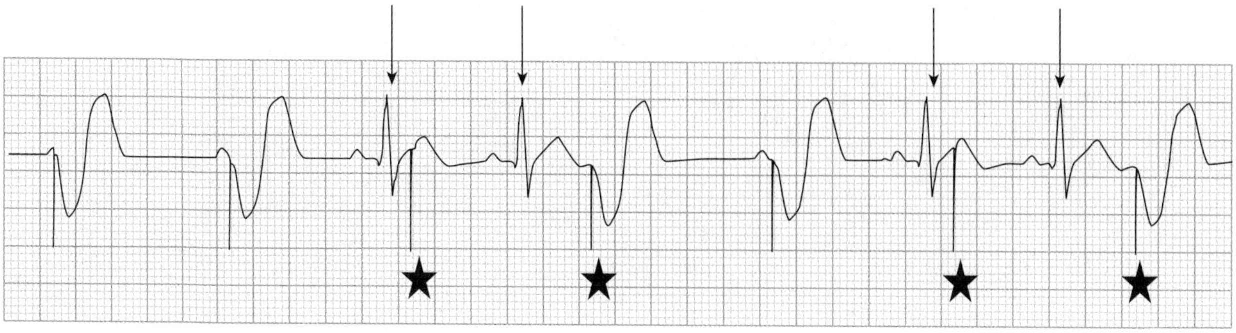

Figure 129-3 *Ventricular undersensing. The QRS complexes marked with arrows are not sensed by the pacemaker. As a result, the device continues to deliver pacing stimuli inappropriately (stars).*

to the PR interval. As long as native AV conduction occurs within this interval, ventricular pacing will be inhibited. However, if the AV interval expires before native AV conduction occurs, then ventricular pacing will occur.

The AV interval is typically programmed sufficiently long to promote native conduction, as chronic right ventricular pacing increases morbidity in certain patient populations. The most important exception to this is in the case of cardiac resynchronization in patients with biventricular pacemakers. In this situation, the AV interval is programmed relatively short, to provide the physiologic benefits of biventricular resynchronization.

The *upper rate limit* is a programmed rate above which the pacemaker will not pace. In patients with sinus or atrial tachycardia that exceeds the upper rate limit, the pacemaker will pace the ventricle only as fast as the upper rate limit. This may result in atrial events that are not followed by ventricular pacing, and may lead to misinterpreting pacemaker function from the surface electrogram.

Most surface electrograms in patients with pacemakers can be explained by these basic pacing functions. However, there are an increasing number of programmable features in modern devices designed to enhance overall pacing function. These features may mimic device malfunction in the form of oversensing, undersensing, or other strange phenomena, and may require the assistance of a cardiologist to interpret. While true device malfunction does occur, it is relatively uncommon. Apparent malfunction based on surface electrograms can usually be explained by normal device function.

NOMENCLATURE (NASPE CODES)

One common source of confusion is interpretation of the nomenclature used to describe pacemaker function. The current system in use was revised in 2002 by the North American Society of Pacing and Electrophysiology (NASPE) and uses a letter system to describe pacemaker function (**Table 129-1**). The first and second letters are used to identify the chamber(s) in which there is pacing and sensing, respectively. The third letter indicates the effect of sensing on subsequent pacing stimuli. Sensed events can induce (trigger) pacing, inhibit pacing, or both.

Modern pacemakers also have mechanisms to detect patient activity and increase the pacing rate accordingly to compensate for increased physiologic demands. This is particularly useful in patients with chronotropic incompetence who cannot increase their heart rate on their own. Depending on the manufacturer, patient activity may be sensed either by physical motion or changes in minute ventilation. When this feature is activated, a fourth letter, R (for *R*ate response), is used in the pacing code.

Most modern devices have the ability to pace in all modes, as long as they are connected to both the atrium and ventricle. The most commonly used modes are described below.

AAI/VVI

AAI and VVI modes function to pace and sense only in the atrium or ventricle respectively. The "I" in the third letter position

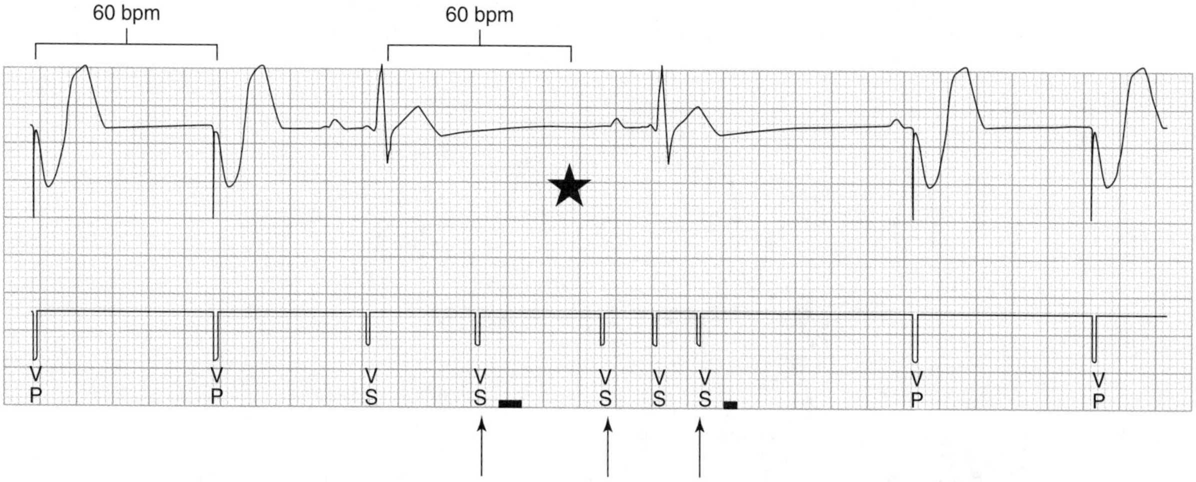

Figure 129-4 *Ventricular oversensing. This device is programmed VVI with a lower rate limit of 60 bpm. The markers noted by arrows show where ventricular oversensing occurs (VS). This causes an inhibition of pacing. Had oversensing not occurred, pacing would have occurred at the point marked by the star.*

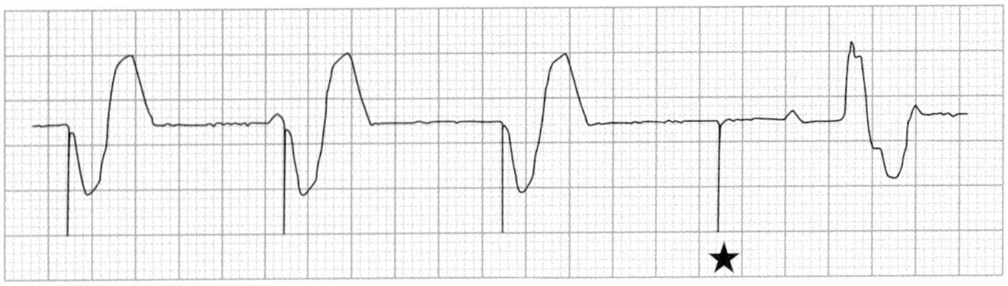

Figure 129-5 *Failure to capture. Ventricular pacing spikes precede the first three QRS complexes. The fourth pacing spike (star) fails to capture the ventricle, and is not followed by a QRS complex.*

refers to the fact that sensed events in a given chamber will inhibit pacing in that chamber. For instance, in AAI mode, if the atrial lead senses a native atrial depolarization, the pacemaker will inhibit pacing until the lower rate limit is exceeded. If a subsequent atrial event has not been sensed within that time, pacing will occur.

AAI mode is typically used for patients with isolated sinus node dysfunction to prevent sinus bradycardia or sinus pauses. The device will pace the atrium at a programmed lower rate unless the sinus node rate exceeds the lower rate limit. This mode has the benefit of limiting ventricular pacing but requires intact AV conduction. Similarly, VVI mode is used to pace and sense only in the ventricle. This mode is usually used as a "back-up" mode to prevent the heart rate from dropping below a programmed lower rate. It is commonly used in patients with permanent atrial fibrillation and high-grade or complete AV block.

DDD

Pacemakers in DDD mode offer the ability to pace and sense in both chambers. This mode provides the benefit of maintaining AV synchrony. DDD mode is programmed with lower and upper rate limits. A native atrial (sinus) impulse that occurs before the lower rate limit has "timed-out" is sensed by the device. If a native impulse does not occur in this time, an atrial pacing stimulus is delivered. The device then waits for native AV conduction, with a subsequent ventricular sensed event, to occur within a programmed AV interval. If a ventricular sensed event does not occur within this period, a ventricular pacing stimulus is delivered. **Figure 129-7** illustrates the various ways DDD pacing can manifest on the ECG.

VOO

VOO mode is often referred to as "asynchronous" pacing. This mode will pace the ventricle at a programmed rate, whether or not a native ventricular impulse occurs. Sensing (and thus inhibition) does not occur. This mode is typically used to prevent inappropriate inhibition (ie, from electromagnetic interference) in the pacemaker-dependent patient. It is commonly used during surgery in pacemaker dependent patients to avoid inhibition of pacing caused by noise from electro-cautery devices.

DEVICE INDICATIONS

PACEMAKERS

Multiple common cardiac conditions serve as indications for permanent pacemaker implantation for patients with sinus and/or AV node dysfunction (**Table 129-2**).

The indications for permanent pacemaker implantation relate primarily to bradycardia caused by sinus and/or AV node dysfunction. In general, permanent pacemakers should be considered in patients with sinus node dysfunction only when the patient is symptomatic as a result of bradycardia. Sinus node dysfunction that manifests as symptomatic sinus bradycardia, sinus pauses, or chronotropic incompetence (inability of the sinus node to adequately accelerate in response to physical activity) are class I indications for pacing. Additionally, when drugs (ie, beta-blockers) that may result in symptomatic sinus bradycardia are required for other indications, pacing should be considered.

The indications for cardiac pacing in patients with AV node disease are more varied. Similar to sinus node dysfunction, pacing is generally used in symptomatic patients. However, in the case of AV node disease, permanent pacemakers are required in certain conditions even in asymptomatic patients. For instance, patients with third-degree AV block or type 2 second-degree AV block (Mobitz 2) should be considered for pacing regardless of symptoms. Even in patients with type 1 second-degree AV block (Mobitz 1 or Wenkebach) pacing should be used if the patient is symptomatic. Occasionally, evaluation of the AV conduction system during electrophysiologic study is required to identify patients with advanced

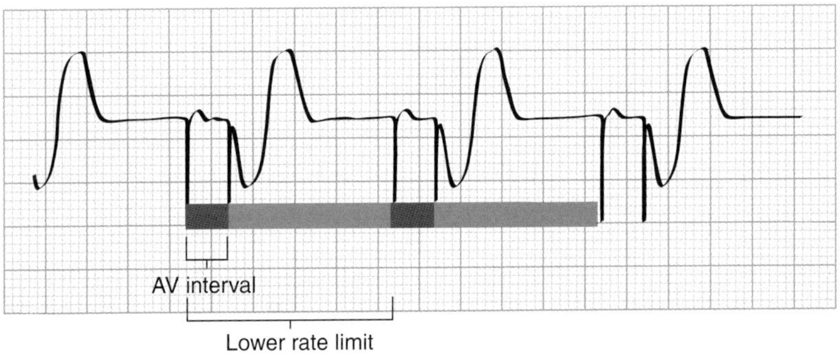

Figure 129-6 *Schematic demonstrating the concepts of lower rate limit and AV interval. This device is programmed DDD. An atrial event is not sensed before the lower rate limit expires, so atrial pacing occurs at the programmed rate. Native AV conduction does not occur within the programmed AV interval, so ventricular pacing occurs. See text for details.*

TABLE 129-1 Coding System for Pacemakers

I	II	III	IV	V
Chambers paced	Chambers sensed	Response to sensing	Rate modulation	Multisite pacing
O = None	O = None	O = None	O = None	O = None
A = Atrium	A = Atrium	T = Triggered	R = Rate modulation	A = Atrium
V = Ventricle	V = Ventricle	I = Inhibited		V = Ventricle
D = Dual (A + V)	D = Dual (A + V)	D = Dual (T = I)		D = Dual (A + V)

AV node disease. In this situation, certain criteria exist to suggest the need for pacing.

Slow AV conduction during atrial fibrillation is a common indication for permanent pacing. This may occur as a result of native AV nodal disease, medications that slow AV conduction but are required for other indications, or iatrogenic ablation of the AV node for rapid ventricular rates. With the exception of patients who have undergone AV nodal ablation, pacing should be used only in patients who have symptoms from slow ventricular rates. However, in patients with atrial fibrillation and pauses of five seconds or longer, pacing is indicated even in the absence of symptoms.

DEFIBRILLATORS

Multiple cardiac conditions serve as common indications for ICD implantation (**Table 129-3**). ICDs were initially designed for patients who survived cardiac arrest from sustained ventricular tachycardia (VT) or ventricular fibrillation (VF). However, in the

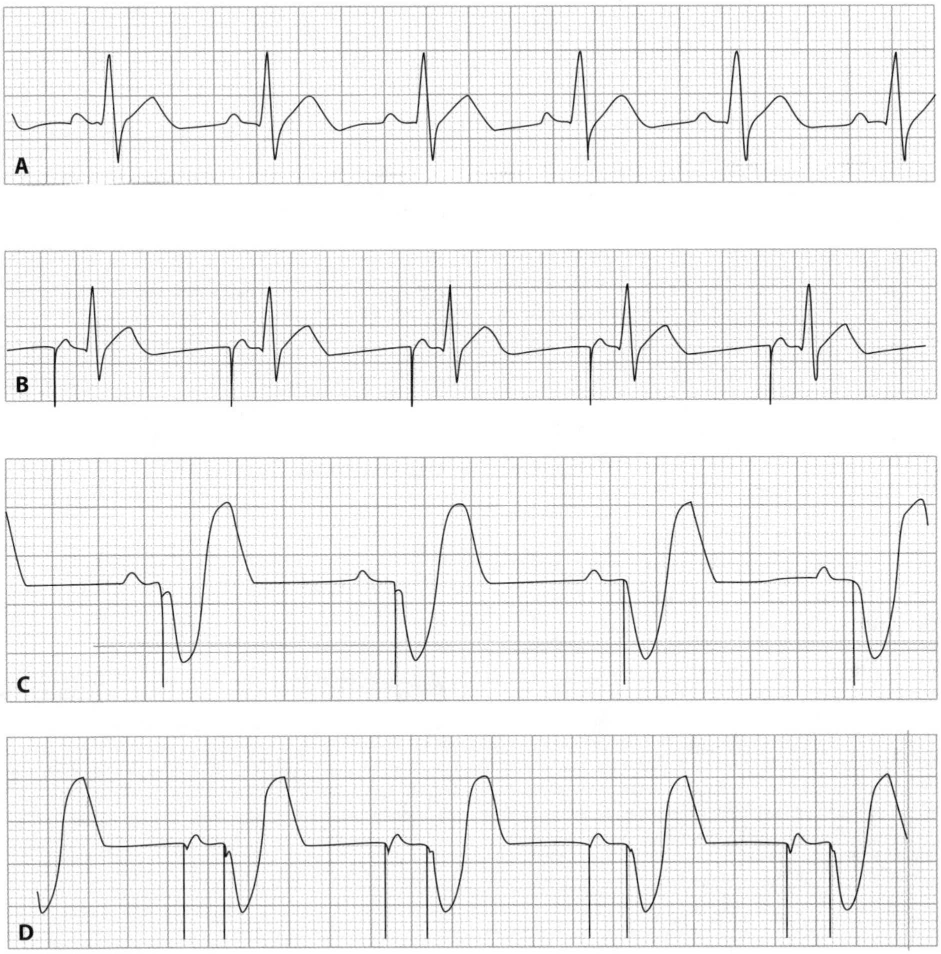

Figure 129-7 *Four appearances of DDD pacing. In each panel, the device is programmed DDD with a lower rate of 60 bpm and an AV interval of 200 msec. (A) The underlying sinus rate exceeds the lower rate limit, so atrial pacing does not occur. Native AV conduction is faster than 200 msec, so ventricular pacing does not occur. (B) The atrial rate has slowed to a rate below the lower rate limit, so atrial pacing occurs at 60 bpm. However, native AV conduction is still faster than 200 msec, so ventricular pacing does not occur. (C) The atrial rate exceeds the lower rate limit, so atrial pacing does not occur. However, native AV conduction is slower than the AV interval. Therefore, ventricular pacing occurs 200 msec after the atrial event is sensed. (D) Both the atrial rate and AV conduction are slower than the programmed intervals. Therefore, atrial pacing occurs at a rate of 60 bpm and ventricular pacing occurs 200 msec later.*

TABLE 129-2 Common Indications for Permanent Cardiac Pacemakers

Sinus node dysfunction • Symptomatic sinus bradycardia • Symptomatic sinus pauses • Symptomatic chronotropic incompetence • Required use of a medication that causes symptomatic sinus node dysfunction
Atrioventricular nodal dysfunction • Symptomatic type I second-degree AV block (Mobitz I or Wenkebach) • Type II second-degree AV block (Mobitz II) • High-grade or complete AV block • Atrial fibrillation with symptomatic slow ventricular response • AV block caused by ablation of the AV node • Required use of a medication that causes symptomatic AV nodal dysfunction

past two decades, indications for ICDs have expanded significantly. Multiple trials have established their superior mortality benefit when compared to antiarrhythmic medications for primary prevention of sudden cardiac arrest. Their current use can be divided into primary prevention of sudden cardiac arrest or secondary prevention for patients who have survived cardiac arrest from VT or VF.

The use of ICDs for primary prevention of sudden death is indicated in patients with ischemic or nonischemic cardiomyopathy, ejection fraction less than or equal to 35%, and New York Heart Association (NYHA) class II-III heart failure symptoms. Patients with ejection fraction less than or equal to 30% and class I symptoms may also be candidates for ICD implantation. When properly selected, these patients experience a 25–30% relative reduction in mortality when implanted with an ICD. Primary prevention is the largest indication for ICDs and remains an important way for hospitalists to intervene on long-term patient outcome. When hospitalists encounter these patients, inpatient cardiology or electrophysiology consult can help determine if an ICD is appropriate.

TABLE 129-3 Common Indications for Implantable Cardiac Defibrillators

Primary prevention of sudden cardiac arrest • Ischemic cardiomyopathy, EF < 35%, NYHA class II-III, at least 40 days after myocardial infarction • Ischemic cardiomyopathy, EF < 30%, NYHA class I • Nonischemic cardiomyopathy, EF < 35%, NYHA class II-III
Secondary prevention of sudden cardiac arrest • Survivors of sudden cardiac arrest from VF or sustained VT without reversible causes • Structural heart disease and sustained VT • Syncope with inducible hemodynamically significant VT of VF during EP study
Special patient populations • Long QT syndrome with VT or syncope • Brugada syndrome with VT or syncope • Hypertrophic cardiomyopathy with risk factors for sudden cardiac arrest* • Arrhythmogenic right ventricular dysplasia with risk factors for sudden cardiac arrest

*Risk factors include nonsustained VT, syncope, severe LVH, and hypotension with exercise.

Patients who have survived cardiac arrest from VT or VF should undergo ICD implantation regardless of the presence or absence of structural heart disease, unless a clearly reversible cause of the arrest can be identified and corrected. In patients with moderately reduced ejection fraction (less than or equal to 40%), nonsustained VT, and inducible VT or VF during electrophysiologic study, ICD implantation is appropriate.

There are several considerations when timing ICD implantation. For patients with newly diagnosed nonischemic cardiomyopathy, the exact timing of ICD implantation varies. An ICD is indicated when the cardiomyopathy is nonreversible and patients are receiving appropriate heart failure medications. In patients with ischemic cardiomyopathy from myocardial infarction, ICDs should not be implanted within the first 40 days after the infarct. This recommendation is based on data that suggests no overall mortality benefit from ICDs implanted within this peri-infarct period.

Other patient populations who may benefit from ICD therapy in certain situations include those with hypertrophic cardiomyopathy, long QT syndrome, Brugada syndrome, and cardiac sarcoid.

CARDIAC RESYNCHRONIZATION THERAPY

Patients with advanced heart failure and a severely reduced ejection fraction often have intraventricular conduction disturbances that result in mechanical "dyssynchrony" of the left ventricle. This dyssynchrony leads to inefficient ventricular contraction and increased maladaptive ventricular remodeling. Prolongation of the QRS duration (in particular, left bundle-branch block) is often used as an electrical surrogate for mechanical dyssynchrony. Many of these patients benefit from biventricular pacing (otherwise known as *cardiac resynchronization therapy* or CRT). Cardiac resynchronization is obtained by positioning a lead in the coronary sinus to pace the lateral wall of the left ventricle, in addition to the standard right ventricular lead. A CRT device can be programmed to pace the right and left ventricles at specific times to maximize cardiac output.

The ideal candidates for cardiac resynchronization include patients in sinus rhythm with ejection fractions < 35%, NYHA class III symptoms, and left bundle-branch block with a QRS > 120 msec. When patients are properly selected for this therapy, they experience an approximate 30% reduction in heart failure hospitalizations and mortality. Roughly two-thirds of patients who undergo CRT implantation will receive clinical benefit from this therapy.

PRACTICE POINT

- Candidates for cardiac resynchronization therapy (CRT) include patients in sinus rhythm with ejection fractions < 35%, NYHA class III symptoms, *and* left bundle-branch block with a QRS > 120 msec. When patients are properly selected for this therapy, they experience approximately a 30% reduction in heart failure hospitalizations and mortality.

Chronic right ventricular apical pacing may worsen heart failure symptoms and ejection fraction. Thus, another patient population that may benefit from CRT is patients with decreased ejection fraction and a need for chronic ventricular pacing. Cardiac resynchronization in these patients may reduce maladaptive left ventricular remodeling and preserve ejection fraction. One common example of CRT used in this setting is a patient with decreased ejection fraction and atrial arrhythmias who undergoes ablation of the AV node for control of rapid ventricular rates.

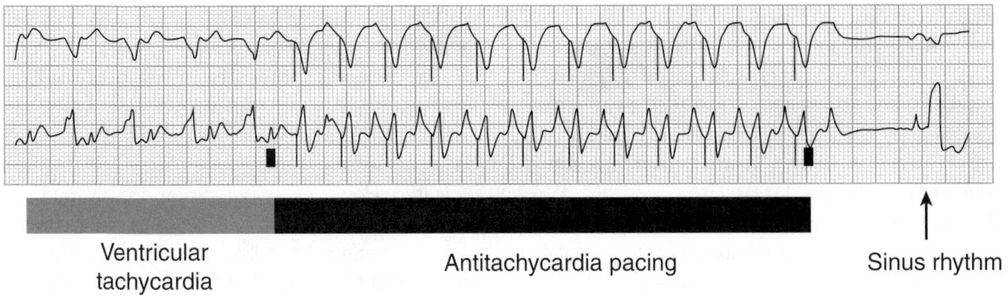

Figure 129-8 *Telemetry strip showing antitachycardia pacing (ATP) for ventricular tachycardia (VT). The patient is initially in a slow VT (approximately 130 bpm). A 12-beat burst of ATP is administered by the implantable cardiac defibrillator (ICD), which terminates the VT. A sinus beat is seen at the end of the strip.*

IMPLANTABLE CARDIAC DEFIBRILLATOR (ICD) THERAPY

ICDs are used to treat ventricular tachyarrhythmias. To do this, the device must recognize the arrhythmia, and then treat it appropriately. Ventricular arrhythmias are initially recognized by the device when the ventricular rate exceeds a programmed rate cutoff. If this ventricular rate is maintained for a given number of beats, the device will recognize the fast rhythm as VT or VF and begin to treat the arrhythmia. Nonsustained VT typically does not last long enough to meet criteria for the device.

Because the initial detection of the arrhythmia is based entirely on rate, it may be difficult for the device to discern whether a fast rhythm is ventricular or supraventricular in origin. Therefore, once VT or VF has been identified by the rate cutoff, ICDs use a series of programmable algorithms to discriminate true ventricular arrhythmias from other tachyarrhythmias such as sinus tachycardia, supraventricular tachycardia, or atrial fibrillation with rapid ventricular rates. These algorithms are designed to limit ICD therapy to only true VT or VF. These algorithms are very effective but not perfect. When optimally programmed, inappropriate shocks due to nonventricular rhythms can be minimized. Nonetheless, inappropriate ICD shocks remain one of the most common adverse events associated with ICD use.

The goal of ICD therapy is to terminate potentially life-threatening ventricular arrhythmias. Modern devices perform this function with a combination of high-voltage defibrillation shocks and less painful bursts of rapid pacing. Typical programming includes several initial attempts to pace the ventricle at a rate slightly faster than the ventricular tachycardia (termed "antitachycardia pacing"). In some patients, this will terminate the arrhythmia, and a shock can be avoided. However, if antitachycardia pacing is not successful, then the device will deliver a series of high-voltage shocks until the arrhythmia terminates (**Figures 129-8** and **129-9**).

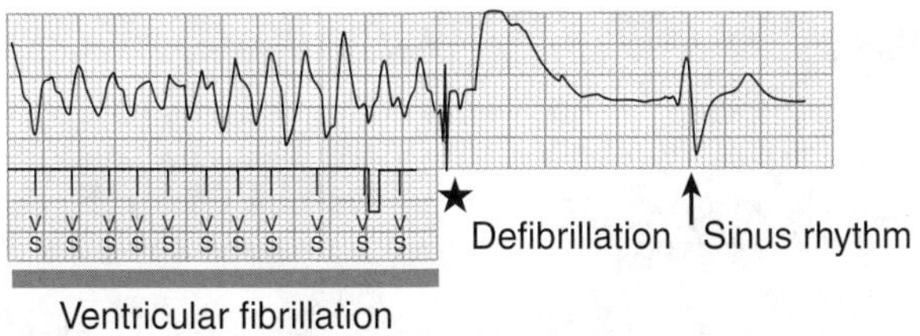

Figure 129-9 *Intracardiac electrograms during an implantable cardiac defibrillator (ICD) interrogation shows ventricular fibrillation that is successfully treated with a shock, indicated by the star. The resultant rhythm is sinus.*

PRACTICE POINT

- The goal of ICD therapy is to terminate potentially life-threatening ventricular arrhythmias. Often, initial attempts to overpace the ventricle at a rate slightly faster than the ventricular tachycardia (termed "antitachycardia pacing") will terminate the arrhythmia, and a shock can be avoided.

EVALUATING THE PATIENT WITH ICD SHOCKS

Approximately 15–30% of patients will experience an appropriate ICD shock within three years of implant. When a patient receives an ICD shock, the goal of the physician is to determine whether the therapy was appropriate. An important consideration is the number of shocks a patient receives. Most often, a single shock represents appropriate therapy for VT or VF. If the patient is otherwise stable, hospitalization is usually not warranted. A common practice is to have the patient call his or her physician's office to arrange follow-up within 24 hours. In this situation, if it is determined that the ICD shock was appropriate, the focus should be on addressing any exacerbating factors, most often congestive heart failure.

When a patient receives more than two shocks within 24 hours he or she should be evaluated immediately, as this may indicate inappropriate shocks, failed device therapy, or recurrent ventricular arrhythmias. Whereas shocks preceded by syncope or presyncope are usually appropriate, shocks without such a prodrome may be inappropriate. Inappropriate shocks may result from sinus tachycardia, SVT, or atrial fibrillation with rapid ventricular response, external electromagnetic interference (electrical "noise"), or true device or lead malfunction. The precise management of inappropriate ICD shocks will depend on the underlying cause.

PRACTICE POINT

- When a patient receives a single ICD shock, it often represents appropriate therapy for VT or VF. If the patient is otherwise stable, hospitalization is usually not warranted. When a patient receives two or more shocks within 24 hours he or she should be evaluated immediately, as this may indicate inappropriate shocks, failed device therapy, or recurrent ventricular arrhythmias.
- Inappropriate shocks may result from sinus tachycardia, SVT or atrial fibrillation with rapid ventricular response, external electromagnetic interference (electrical "noise"), or true device or lead malfunction.

The term *electrical storm* describes multiple appropriate shocks within 24 hours, and indicates recurrent VT or VF. This is a potentially life-threatening condition, and these patients should be hospitalized with a focus on correcting any underlying causes such as ischemia, electrolyte abnormalities, or worsening heart failure. Often, these patients will require short- or long-term antiarrhythmic medications to suppress recurrent ventricular arrhythmias.

Even single ICD shocks can result in considerable distress and anxiety for the patient and can reduce their quality of life. Attention should be paid to the patient's psychological status after any ICD shock, and when needed, anxiolytic medications should be offered. Less commonly, professional psychological treatment may be required.

IMPLANTATION AND PERIOPERATIVE CONSIDERATIONS

Implantation of pacemakers and defibrillators should be performed by experienced physicians with appropriate training, and in a sterile environment with trained ancillary staff. Usually this is done in an electrophysiology (EP) laboratory or in an operating room with fluoroscopic capabilities. Most often, conscious sedation is used in combination with local anesthesia. An incision is made in the upper anterior chest or in the delto-pectoral groove. A pocket is then made in the subcutaneous or subpectoral space to house the pulse generator. Venous access is obtained either by needle puncture of the subclavian or axillary vein, or by direct cut-down of the cephalic vein. The leads are then advanced transvenously into the heart and positioned in their appropriate locations (**Figure 129-10**). The proximal ends of the leads are connected to the pulse generator, which is then inserted into the pocket. The incision is sutured closed and dressed with a sterile dressing.

While implantation of cardiac rhythm devices is a relatively safe procedure, complications may develop. Complications that occur at the time of implant may include bleeding, air embolism, pneumothorax, cardiac perforation, and tamponade. Postoperative complications (occurring within approximately 30 days) include infection, pocket hematoma, wound dehiscence, or lead dislodgement.

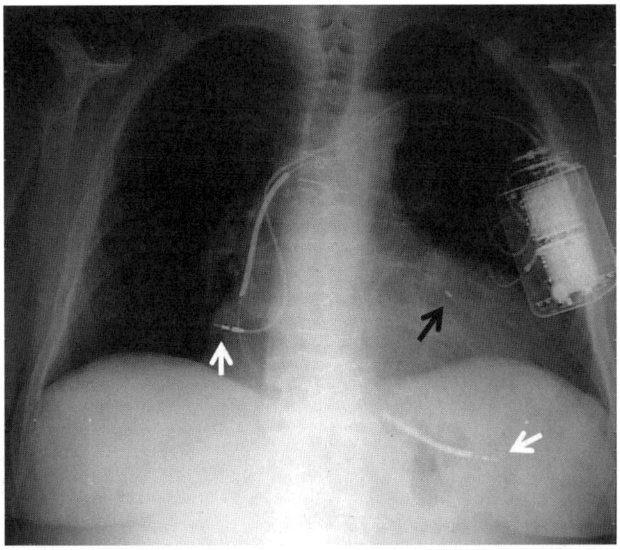

Figure 129-10 *Chest X-ray showing proper placement of a cardiac resynchronization therapy with defibrillator (CRT-D) device. Note the positions of the right atrial and right ventricular leads (white arrows). The left ventricular lead is positioned in the coronary sinus (black arrow).*

Patients receiving cardiac rhythm devices often concomitantly receive anticoagulation therapy with aspirin, clopidogrel, warfarin, and/or heparin products for other medical conditions. Each of these agents increases the risk of postoperative bleeding complications, albeit to varying degrees. In general, anticoagulation should be continued around the time of device implantation as medically indicated. However, as heparin and enoxaparin place the patient at particularly high risk of developing a hematoma, avoiding these agents whenever possible for 12 hours prior to the procedure and one to two days after the procedure may reduce the risk of hematoma formation. When withholding anticoagulation is not possible (ie, mechanical heart valves), the timing of the procedure is considered on a case by case basis. Therapeutic treatment with warfarin usually does not cause significant bleeding complications if the INR is kept below 2.5.

Guidelines for antibiotic therapy in the perioperative period for cardiac rhythm devices are not well defined. While the risk of infection is relatively low (< 1%), patient morbidity and associated health care costs can be high. Therefore, intravenous antibiotics to cover gram-positive skin flora should be given at the time of implantation.

DISCHARGE PLANNIG: OUTPATIENT DEVICE FOLLOW-UP

When patients are discharged from the hospital after device implantation, they should have explicit follow-up instructions. They should be seen by a physician or nurse approximately one week after implantation to have their wound examined and any stitches removed. Thereafter, regular follow-up with a cardiologist or a specialized device clinic should be arranged every three to six months. Newer devices have accompanying home monitoring systems that are capable of transmitting device data telephonically. These systems allow the physician to monitor the status of the device and communicate with the patient by phone, thereby reducing the frequency of office visits for the patient.

INDICATIONS FOR DEVICE INTERROGATION AND CONSULTATION

Interrogation of cardiac rhythm devices should be scheduled as an outpatient on a regular basis (every six months). Routine inpatient interrogation of a device is usually not warranted unless there is specific concern for a device-related issue. Examples of such issues include recent ICD shocks, failure of proper capture or sensing, decompensated heart failure, and specific patient complaints such as palpitations or syncope.

Occasionally patients will describe a vibration or beeping that originates from the device. These are programmed alerts designed to notify patients to have their device interrogated. The majority of the times, these alerts are used to indicate battery depletion or lead malfunction.

PRACTICE POINT

- Routine *inpatient* interrogation of a device is usually not warranted unless there is specific concern for a device-related problem. Examples include recent ICD shocks, failure of proper capture or sensing, decompensated heart failure, syncope or palpitations.
- Occasionally patients will describe a vibration or beeping that originates from the device. These programmed alerts notify patients to have their device interrogated (often they indicate battery depletion or lead malfunction).

TABLE 129-4 Evidence-based Medicine Key References for Pacemakers, Defibrillators, and Cardiac Resynchronization Devices

Study	Methodology	Results	Limitations	Bottom Line
AVID Investigators. *New Engl J Med.* 1997;337:1576.	Multicenter, randomized trial comparing antiarrhythmics vs. ICDs in patients with decreased EF (< 40%) and surviving sustained ventricular arrhythmias	1016 patients enrolled; patients receiving ICDs had 31% RRR in mortality at three-year follow-up.	No control group; amiodarone dosing was empiric and not determined by electrophysiologic testing.	For secondary prevention, ICDs reduce mortality in survivors of life-threatening ventricular arrhythmias with reduced EF.
Moss, et al. *New Engl J Med.* 2002;346:877.	Multicenter, randomized trial comparing ICDs vs. standard medical therapy in patients with prior myocardial infarction and reduced EF (< 30%).	1232 patients randomized; patients receiving ICDs had HR for risk of death of 0.69 at four-year follow-up.	No control group; patients receiving ICDs had higher rates of heart failure exacerbations.	For primary prevention, ICDs reduce mortality in patients with coronary disease and reduced EF.
Abraham, et al. *New Engl J Med.* 2002;346:1845.	Multicenter, randomized trial comparing cardiac resynchronization vs. standard medical therapy in patients with moderate to severe CHF, EF ≤ 35%, and QRS ≥ 130 milliseconds.	453 patients enrolled; patients receiving CRT had improvement in quality of life, six-minute walk distance, and functional class. CRT patients had a 7% ARR in CHF hospitalizations.	Investigators only blinded for initial six months after randomization.	In patients with moderate to severe CHF, reduced EF, and interventricular conduction delay, CRT improves clinical parameters and reduces CHF hospitalizations.

Cardiac rhythm devices are typically interrogated by a trained nurse or device company representative. The information collected is then routinely reviewed by an electrophysiologist or cardiologist. If abnormal device function is identified, simple programming changes can often correct the problem. However, an electrophysiologist should be consulted if a hospitalist has any concerns about device function that cannot be managed with programming changes. The most common examples of such concerns include frequent ICD shocks, lead malfunction/fracture, or device infection.

While most device evaluations can be done with the help of surface tracings (ECGs), when necessary consultation with a cardiologist or electrophysiologist can assist with diagnostic and management strategies (**Table 129-4**).

QUALITY IMPROVEMENT TO ADDRESS PERFORMANCE GAPS

COST UTILIZATION

Implantable defibrillators are associated with increased cost to the health care system. The estimated cost per life-year added is between $30,000 and $50,000, which compares with the standard benchmark of $50,000 for renal dialysis. The exact cost effectiveness depends on a patient's individual risk for sudden death and his or her other comorbidities. Proper patient selection is necessary for this therapy to remain cost effective. However, when restricted to appropriate patients, the cost effectiveness of ICD implantation is comparable to other long-term cardiovascular therapies.

DISPARITIES IN CARE

Gender and ethnic disparities persist in patients who receive cardiac rhythm devices. Female gender and nonwhite race are both associated with decreased rates of device implantation (odds ratio of 0.86 [95% CI 0.79–0.93] and 0.70 [95% CI 0.66–0.76], respectively), even after accounting for multiple clinical and demographic variables. The causes behind these disparities are likely multifactorial, but may include differences in access to health care and physician-patient relationships among patients of varying race and gender.

SUGGESTED READINGS

Abraham WT, Fisher WG, Smith AL, et al. Cardiac resynchronization in chronic heart failure. *New Engl J Med.* 2002;346:1845.

Bardy GH, Lee KL, Mark DB, et al. Amiodarone or and implantable cardioverter-defibrillator for congestive heart failure. *New Engl J Med.* 2005;352:225.

Bernstein AD, Daubert J-C, Fletcher RD, et al. The revised NASPE/BPEG generic code for antibradycardia, adaptive-rate, and multisite pacing. *Pacing Clin Electrophysiol.* 2000;25:260.

Buxton AE, Lee KL, Fisher JD, et al. A randomized study of the prevention of sudden death in patients with coronary artery disease. *New Engl J Med.* 1999;341:1882.

El-Chami MF, Hanna IR, Bush H, et al. Impact of race and gender on cardiac device implantations. *Heart Rhythm.* 1007;4:1420.

Epstein AE, DiMarco JP, Ellenbogan KA, et al. ACC/AHA/HRS 2008 Guidelines for Device-Based Therapy of Cardiac Rhythm Abnormalities: A Report of the American College of Cardiology/American Heart Association Task Force on Practice Guidelines (Writing Committee to Revise the ACC/AHA/NASPE 2002 Guideline Update for Implantation of Cardiac Pacemakers and Antiarrhythmia Devices) Developed in Collaboration With the American Association for Thoracic Surgery and Society of Thoracic Surgeons. *J Am Coll Cardiol.* 2008;51:e1.

Germano JJ, Reynolds M, Essebag V, et al. Frequency and causes of implantable cardiovertor-defibrillator therapies: Is device therapy proarrhythmic? *Am J Cardiol.* 2006;97:1255.

Hohnloser SH, Kuck KH, Dorian P, et al. Prophylactic use of an implantable cardioverter-defibrillator after acute myocardial infarction. *New Engl J Med.* 2004;351:2481.

Moss AJ, Zareba W, Hall WJ, et al. Prophylactic implantation of a defibrillator in patients with myocardial infarction and reduced ejection fraction. *New Engl J Med.* 2002;346:877.

The Antiarrhytmic Versus Implantable Defibrillators (AVID) Investigators. A comparison of antiarrhythmic-drug therapy with implantable defibrillators in patients resuscitated from near-fatal ventricular arrhythmias. *New Engl J Med.* 1997;337:1576.

CHAPTER 130

Heart Failure

Julio A. Barcena, MD
James C. Fang, MD, FACC

Key Clinical Questions

Reduced Ejection Fraction

1. What is the definition and classification of heart failure?
2. What is the mortality and morbidity of heart failure?
3. What is the recommended testing for a patient with newly diagnosed heart failure?
4. What are the standard therapies for heart failure?
5. How can we remove congestion in heart failure?

Preserved Ejection Fraction

1. How do you diagnose heart failure (HF)?
2. What are the predisposing risk factors for HF with preserved ejection fraction?
3. What is the recommended evaluation for patients newly diagnosed with HF?
4. How do you treat HF?

REDUCED EJECTION FRACTION

CASE 130-1

A 66-year-old man presents with progressive history of breathlessness, decrease in activity tolerance, orthopnea and paroxysmal nocturnal dyspnea. His past medical history includes diabetes and a myocardial infarction 5 years ago.

On physical examination the patient appears dyspneic with a blood pressure of 145/90 mm Hg and a heart rate of 100 beats per minute (bpm). The jugular venous pressure is 14 cm H_2O, the point of maximum impulse is displaced laterally, and the heart sounds are distant with an S_3 gallop. There are rales in the lung bases with abdominal right upper quadrant fullness; the lower extremities are cold with significant pitting edema.

EPIDEMIOLOGY/OVERVIEW

Heart failure (HF) is a condition that affects millions in the United States, and over half a million people are newly diagnosed each year. The incidence of HF increases with age, affecting 6% to 10% of people age older than 65. It is the leading cause of hospital admissions in the United States and is responsible for 6.5 million hospital-days each year and up to 15 million office visits. Over the past decade, the rate of hospitalizations for HF has increased by 159%, and 45% of patients hospitalized with acute heart failure will be rehospitalized at least once (and 15% at least twice) within 12 months.

Approximately 260,000 patients die of HF in the United States each year. The number of HF deaths has increased steadily despite advances in treatment, in part because of aging of the population and improved survival after acute myocardial infarction (MI). The estimated direct and indirect cost of HF is $27.9 billion per year, and approximately $2.9 billion annually is spent on drugs for the treatment of HF.

Heart failure has been identified by The Joint Commission on Accreditation of Health care Organizations (JCAHO) as a priority focus for hospital core measure development. The four HF core measures are

HF-1—Discharge instructions
HF-2—Evaluation of left ventricular systolic function
HF-3—Angiotensin-converting enzyme (ACE) inhibitor or angiotensin receptor blocker (ARB) for left ventricular systolic dysfunction
HF-4—Adult smoking cessation advice/counseling.

PATHOPHYSIOLOGY

Heart failure is a complex clinical syndrome that can result from any structural or functional cardiac disorder that impairs the ability of the ventricle to fill or eject blood and maintain metabolic demands of the body. It is characterized by specific signs and symptoms, such as dyspnea, fatigue which may limit exercise tolerance, and fluid retention which leads to pulmonary and peripheral edema.

Heart failure may result from disorders of the pericardium, heart valves, myocardium, or coronary circulation as well as rhythm disturbances. The majority of patients have symptoms due to an impairment of left ventricular (LV) myocardial function, with or without a reduced ejection fraction. The etiologies for LV

TABLE 130-1 Etiologies of Left Ventricular Systolic Dysfunction

Coronary artery disease
Idiopathic dilated cardiomyopathy
Familial cardiomyopathy
Neuromuscular disorders (eg, muscular dystrophies)
Chagas cardiomyopathy
Toxins (eg, alcohol, cocaine)
Medications (eg, adriamycin)
Diabetes mellitus
Myocarditis (lymphocytic, hypersensitivity, giant cell)
Infiltrative (amyloidosis, sarcoidosis, hemochromatosis)
Metabolic disorders (hypothyroidism)
Peripartum
Untreated valvular heart disease (aortic stenosis or regurgitation, mitral regurgitation)
Tachyarrhythmias (atrial and/or ventricular arrhythmias)
Autoimmune disorders (lupus, rheumatoid arthritis)
Hypertension

dysfunction are broad, coronary artery disease being the leading cause in developed countries (**Table 130-1**).

Heart failure is generally a progressive disorder that results after an insult or stress to the myocardium resulting in cardiac remodeling (eg, ventricular enlargement and hypertrophy) with myocyte hypertrophy and apoptosis, myocardial fibrosis, and changes in calcium cycling. These processes increase hemodynamic wall stress causing a further decline in myocardial mechanical performance; ventricular enlargement leads to incompetence of the mitral valve and regurgitation. Mitral regurgitation leads to decreased forward stroke volume, elevated pulmonary venous pressure, increased wall stress and ultimately more remodeling. In response to progressive cardiac dysfunction, neurohormonal systems (in particular the renin-angiotensin-aldosterone and adrenergic systems) become activated to provide acute hemodynamic stabilization. Patients with HF have elevated circulating or tissue levels of norepinephrine, angiotensin II, aldosterone, endothelin, vasopressin, and cytokines. However, when chronically stimulated, these systems act to adversely affect the structure and function of the heart. Neurohormonal activation increases the hemodynamic stresses on the ventricle by causing sodium retention and peripheral vasoconstriction that subsequently lead to further remodeling and more neurohormonal stimulation. The remodeling process precedes the development of symptoms, and in conjunction with the activation of the neurohormonal cascade, continues after the appearance of symptoms and contributes to worsening of symptoms, development of arrhythmias, and ultimate mortality despite optimal therapy.

The 2005 ACC/AHA task force developed a new classification scheme outlining four stages in the evolution of the HF syndrome (**Figure 130-1**), recognizing established risk factors, structural prerequisites, asymptomatic and symptomatic phases, and appropriate therapeutic interventions at each stage to reduce morbidity and mortality.

There are two states of heart failure, compensated and acute decompensated heart failure (formerly "congestive heart failure"). Heart failure is predominantly characterized by an elevation in left atrial and subsequently pulmonary venous and arterial pressures. The net result may be transudation of excess fluid into the alveolar spaces, leading to decreased diffusing capacity, hypoxia, and shortness of breath. Inadequate cardiac output may also complicate the hemodynamic and clinical picture and generally represents a poor prognostic feature.

DIAGNOSIS

Clinical manifestations vary among individuals. The chronicity, severity and degree of hemodynamic decompensation as well as patient specific factors such as age, gender, and other comorbidities influence symptoms. Clinical signs and symptoms of HF lack sensitivity and specificity. Exercise intolerance, usually a predominant symptom, but does not correlate with the degree of LV dysfunction as assessed by ejection fraction. The New York Heart Association (NYHA) functional classification is used to assess exercise tolerance and should be determined in the ambulatory and compensated state.

I = No symptoms
II = Symptoms with moderate or marked levels of activity
III = Symptoms with mild activity
IV = Symptoms at rest

Elevated left atrial and pulmonary capillary wedge pressures are responsible for "congestive" symptoms such as shortness of breath, cough, orthopnea, paroxysmal nocturnal dyspnea, and peripheral edema. Early satiety, right upper quadrant tenderness, and anorexia may be subtle signs of volume overload. A reduced cardiac output may be manifest as easy fatigability, mental status changes and/or a decrease in exercise tolerance. Angina may be present in both ischemic and nonischemic cardiomyopathies.

A careful physical examination is the cornerstone of the evaluation of patients with heart failure. The examination helps to determine the status and severity of the hemodynamic profile which then guides a therapeutic plan. The examination should focus on determining the hemodynamic picture along two axes: degree of volume overload ("wet" or "dry") and adequacy of perfusion ("warm" or "cold"). Findings consistent with elevated cardiac filling pressures and fluid overload include elevated jugular venous pressure, hepatojugular reflux, gallops (S_3 and S_4), murmurs of tricuspid or mitral regurgitation, pulmonary rales, hepatomegaly, ascites, and edema. Narrow pulse pressure, cool extremities, altered mentation, Cheyne-Stokes respiration, and a resting tachycardia suggest a marked reduction in cardiac output. Hypotension may indicate severe ventricular dysfunction and impending cardiogenic shock. The presence of peripheral edema and pulmonary rales, although relatively specific, are not sensitive and may be absent. The etiology of cardiac dysfunction may also be apparent at the time of examination although the differential diagnosis is broad (**Table 130-2**). A comprehensive evaluation should be performed.

TABLE 130-2 Mimickers of Heart Failure

Myocardial ischemia
Pulmonary disease (pneumonia, asthma, chronic obstructive pulmonary disease, pulmonary embolus, pulmonary arterial hypertension)
Sleep disordered breathing
Obesity
Malnutrition
Hepatic failure
Renal failure
Hypoalbuminemia
Venous insufficiency
Depression and deconditioning
Pericardial disease

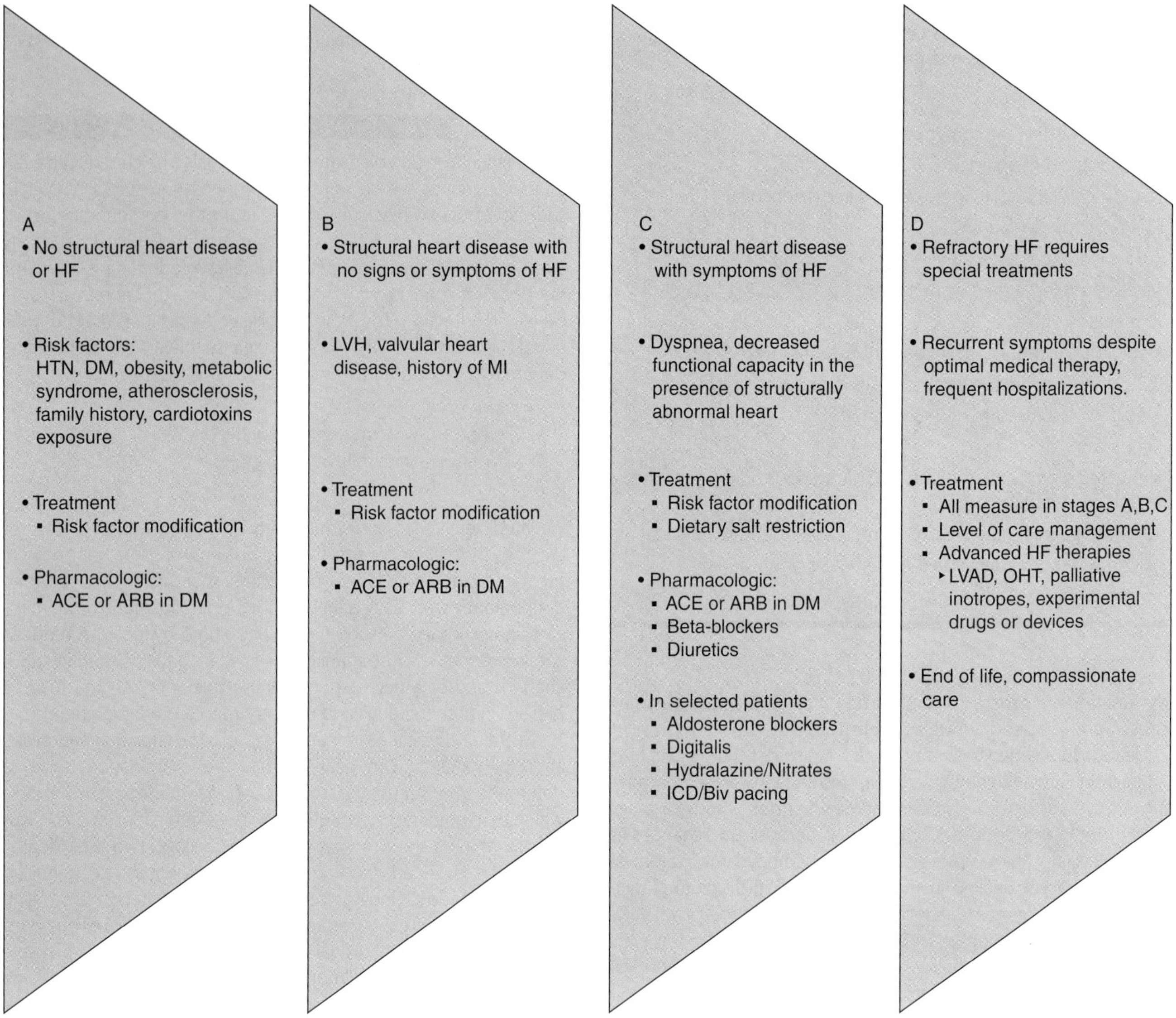

Figure 130-1 *Stages in the development of heart failure/recommended therapy by stage. ACEI, angiotensin-converting enzyme inhibitor; ARB, angiotensin II receptor blocker; EF, ejection fraction; FHx CM, family history of cardiomyopathy; HF, heart failure; LV, left ventricular; LVH, left ventricular hypertrophy; and MI, myocardial infarction.*

Echocardiography is critical to the determination of etiology, particularly distinguishing those patients with predominantly systolic heart failure from those with valvular heart disease or preserved ejection fraction (eg, >50%). Electrocardiogram, full laboratory assessment, and a chest x-ray should be performed in all patients presenting for the first time with heart failure. Additional testing (eg, right heart catheterization, brain natriuretic peptide [BNP] or N-terminal proBNP) should be considered but individualized.

TRIAGE AND INITIAL MANAGEMENT

The goal of the initial triage is to establish a cause for decompensation (**Table 130-3**) as well as defining the hemodynamic picture using the physical examination and history. As noted above, the hemodynamic picture can be described as one of four states on the basis of two axes: volume status (overload ["wet"] or euvolemic ["dry"]) and perfusion or cardiac output (well perfused ["warm"] or low output ["cold"]) in order to place the patient in one of four categories (**Figure 130-2**).

Acute decompensated heart failure, whether in the context of new onset or chronic, requires urgent treatment and should focus on hemodynamic stabilization, oxygenation and organ perfusion, and restoring filling pressure to optimal levels.

Initial laboratory evaluation of patients with HF should include complete blood count, urinalysis, serum electrolytes (including

TABLE 130-3 Precipitating Factors in Acute Decompensated Heart Failure

Acute coronary syndrome
Uncontrolled hypertension
Acute arrhythmia (ventricular or supraventricular)
Valvular heart disease
Acute severe myocarditis
Medical or dietary noncompliance
Infections
Perioperative volume resuscitation
Drug or alcohol abuse

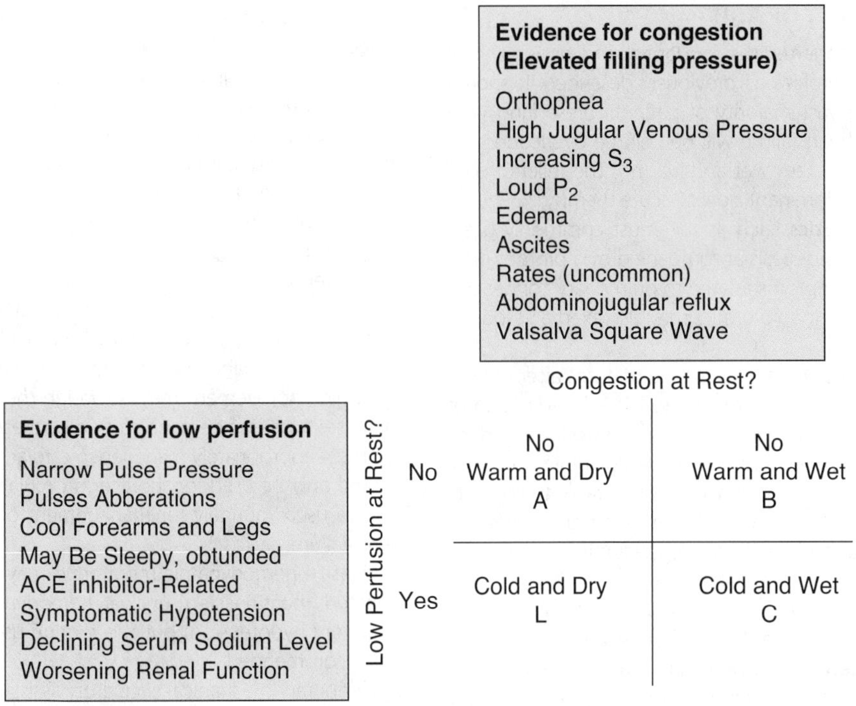

Diagram indicating 2 x 2 table of hemodynamic profiles for patients presenting with heart failure. Most patients can be classified in a 2-minute bedside assessment according to the signs and symptoms shown although in practice some patients may be on the border between the warm-and-wet and cold-and-wet profiles. This classification helps guide initial therapy and prognosis for patients presenting with advanced heart failure. Although most patients presenting with hypoperfusion also have elevated filling pressure (cold and wet profile), many patients present with elevated filling pressures without major reduction in perfusion (warm and wet profile). Patients presenting with symptoms of heart failure at rest or minimal exertion without clinical evidence of elevated filling pressures or hypoperfusion (warm and dry profile) should be carefully evaluated to determine whether their symptoms result from heart failure.

Figure 130-2 *Hemodynamic profiles in Heart failure. (Reprinted, with permission, Nohria A, Lewis E, Stevenson W L. Medical Management of Advanced Heart Failure. JAMA. 2002;287(5):628–640. Copyright 2002 American Medical Association. All rights reserved.)*

calcium and magnesium), blood urea nitrogen, serum creatinine, fasting blood glucose, liver function tests, lipid profile, thyroid function tests, and cardiac biomarkers. Screening for sleep-disordered breathing, HIV, rheumatologic disorders, and pheochromocytoma are reasonable in selected situations.

Twelve-lead electrocardiogram should be obtained to assess for rhythm, conduction system abnormalities and rule out acute coronary syndromes. Chest x-ray is useful in identifying cardiomegaly, pulmonary congestion, and concomitant pulmonary disorders such as pneumonia or chronic obstructive pulmonary disease.

Echocardiography is critical in the initial evaluation of patients with new onset HF to obtain information on left ventricular wall thickness, end diastolic and end systolic dimensions, right ventricular function, ejection fraction, valvular and pericardial disease. Serial assessments may be useful after optimizing medical and device therapy or a change in clinical status. Coronary angiography should be performed in patients presenting with HF who have angina or significant ischemia unless they are not candidates for revascularization. Endomyocardial biopsy is reserved for patients in whom a specific diagnosis is suspected (eg, hemochromatosis, amyloidosis, sarcoidosis) if it would change management. Brain natriuretic peptide or *N*-terminal pro-BNP (secreted by the cardiac ventricles in response to wall stress) can be useful in the urgent care setting when the diagnosis in patients presenting with dyspnea is uncertain. Both markers have good negative predictive values to exclude HF and can provide prognostic information if HF is confirmed. Their use to guide therapy has not yet been established.

A risk stratification tool developed from the Acute Decompensated Heart Failure National Registry (ADHERE) identified the following variables as predicting higher risk for in-hospital mortality:

- Blood urea nitrogen >43 mg/dL
- Admission systolic blood pressure <115 mm Hg
- Serum creatinine >2.75 mg/dL

Other parameters that have been correlated with clinical outcomes in patients hospitalized with HF include age, heart failure etiology (ischemic cardiomyopathy has poorer prognosis), anemia, hyponatremia, B-type natriuretic peptide levels, and left ventricular ejection fraction (LVEF).

TREATMENT AND COMPLICATIONS

The management of acute decompensated heart failure (ADHF) can be divided into two aspects. The acute management is directed toward hemodynamic recovery to improve symptoms and identification of complicating comorbidities; chronic treatment is directed at preserving functional capacity, preventing rehospitalizations, and improving long-term survival.

ACUTE MANAGEMENT OF ADHF

The initial phase of management is to identify and target one of the four hemodynamic profiles as previously described. It should be recognized that the vast majority of patients presenting with acute decompensated heart failure will be volume overloaded yet adequately perfused (so-called "wet and warm"). The relief of congestion is therefore a predominant goal of acute therapy.

Intravenous **loop diuretics** such as the most commonly used, furosemide, will produce a diuresis accompanied by a prompt drop in preload and relief of symptoms related to pulmonary congestion (**Table 130-4**). Intravenous loop diuretics may also exert a vasodilating effect.

The peak diuretic effect typically occurs 30 minutes after administration and should be titrated to response. The administration of a thiazide diuretic, such as metolazone, 30 minutes prior to a dose of furosemide can potentiate its effect. Continuous infusions may be considered although they appear to be comparable to properly dosed bolus treatment. Overly rapid diuresis with an excessively rapid reduction in intravascular volume may result in symptomatic hypotension and/or worsening renal function.

Morphine may be useful because it induces venodilation and mild arterial dilatation and relieves breathlessness and anxiety.

Supplemental oxygen should be initiated and pulse oximetry monitored. Noninvasive positive pressure ventilation, if necessary for acute respiratory failure, is associated with a significant reduction in the need for tracheal intubation and mechanical ventilation.

Vasodilator therapy should be initiated in the absence of symptomatic hypotension. Short-acting ACE inhibitors, ARBs, or hydralazine are the drugs of choice in most situations. Intravenous vasodilator therapy may be considered if rapid improvement of congestive symptoms is needed but requires close hemodynamic monitoring, ideally in an ICU setting.

Nitrates decrease systemic and pulmonary vascular pressures and are also coronary vasodilators.

TABLE 130-4 Suggested Diuretic Dosing in Heart Failure

Drug	Initial Dose	Maximum Daily Doses
Loop diuretics		
Bumetanide	1 mg	5–10 mg
Torsemide	20 mg	100–200 mg
Furosemide	40 mg	160–320 mg
Thiazide diuretics (given 30 min before loop diuretic to augment diuresis)		
Hydrochlorothiazide	25 mg	100 mg
Chlorothiazide	250–500 mg IV once or twice daily plus loop diuretic	
Metolazone	2.5–10 mg orally once or twice daily with loop diuretic	
IV continuous infusion		
Bumetanide	1 mg IV load then 0.5–1 mg/h	
Torsemide	20 mg IV load then 5–10 mg/h	
Furosemide	20–80 mg IV load then 5–20 mg/h	

Nitroprusside is indicated when there is a need for acute combined afterload and preload reduction (hypertensive emergency, acute aortic regurgitation, acute mitral regurgitation).

Nesiritide has venous, arterial, and modest coronary vasodilatory properties that reduce preload and afterload and has no direct inotropic effects. It is currently only approved for the acute relief of dyspnea in the patient with decompensated heart failure. Because of its hypotensive effects, it should be used only at recommended doses and with caution.

Intravenous inotropic agents (dobutamine, milrinone, dopamine) are indicated in the presence of peripheral hypoperfusion (hypotension, decreased renal function) with or without pulmonary edema refractory to the above treatment modalities. The benefit of hemodynamic improvement may outweigh the risk of arrhythmias and increase in oxygen demand caused by these agents. These patients are most appropriately managed in cardiac care units. These agents should only be used for short-term circulatory support and should not be used routinely for management of acute decompensated heart failure.

Invasive hemodynamic monitoring may be required in carefully selected situations (eg, unclear hemodynamic picture, medically refractory hypotension) but the routine use of such monitoring is not recommended.

Temporary mechanical circulatory assistance (intra-aortic balloon counter-pulsation pump or ventricular assist device) may be indicated in patients not responding to pharmacologic therapy when there is reasonable potential for myocardial recovery with specific interventions (eg, bypass surgery). They can also be considered to help "bridge" appropriate patients to mechanical circulatory support or cardiac transplantation.

Ultrafiltration may benefit patients with acute decompensated HF accompanied by renal insufficiency or diuretic resistance. Advantages include adjustable fluid removal volumes and rates, no effect on serum electrolytes, and decreased neurohormonal activity.

Emergent coronary angiography is indicated if an acute coronary syndrome is the cause of acute HF.

Continuous electrocardiographic monitoring is necessary during the acute decompensation phase. Arrhythmias may be a cause or complicating factor of HF.

SUPRAVENTRICULAR ARRHYTHMIAS (SVTs)

SVTs often complicate the course of patients with heart failure, in particular atrial fibrillation and flutter, which affect 10% to 30% of patients with chronic HF. It may occur as a primary myocardial process affecting the atria or as a result of atrial remodeling secondary to volume or pressure overload of the right and left ventricles. Atrial arrhythmias are associated with a decrease in exercise capacity and worse long-term prognosis. SVTs are poorly tolerated in heart failure for four reasons:

1. The loss of atrial "kick" decreases cardiac output
2. Rapid ventricular rates increase myocardial oxygen demand and decrease coronary perfusion
3. Rapid ventricular rates impair relaxation
4. Blood stasis in fibrillating atria predisposes to systemic and pulmonary embolism.

The primary management strategy for atrial arrhythmias complicating ADHF is to control the ventricular rate and to provide anticoagulation to reduce thromboembolic complications. A target resting heart rate of < 80 bpm and < 110 bpm during exercise are reasonable goals. Rate control with beta-blockers and digoxin should be considered but overly aggressive beta-blocker therapy may be poorly tolerated. Improvements in volume status alone may decrease the ventricular response. Early involvement of a cardiovascular medicine specialist should be considered since restoration of sinus rhythm with advanced therapies (eg, cardioversion, antiarrythmics, catheter ablation) may be of benefit in carefully selected patients.

RENAL INSUFFICIENCY

Renal insufficiency complicating heart failure management is known as the cardiorenal syndrome. Patients with HF often have baseline impaired renal function as a result of decreased renal perfusion, intrinsic renal disease, elevated central and renal vein pressure, neurohormonal activation, and/or drugs used to treat HF. Renal function may also acutely decline during treatment with diuretics and ACE inhibitors. Although these changes may be short-lived, asymptomatic and reversible, such declines in renal function often result in a prolonged hospitalization and portend a poor prognosis. As HF worsens, an accompanying decline in renal perfusion limits the ability of the kidneys to respond to diuretic therapy. In this situation, higher doses of diuretics and/or the addition of other diuretics with synergistic effects (eg, sequential nephron blockade) are needed. Current studies suggest no significant benefit to the use of continuous intravenous diuretic regimens over intravenous bolus dosing. If diuretic management is ineffective or complicated by progressive renal insufficiency, mechanical fluid removal (ultrafiltration) can be considered in well-selected patients, although anticoagulation and special intravenous access is required. Cardiovascular and renal consultation should be sought when cardiorenal syndrome is present.

PRACTICE POINT

- Current studies suggest no significant benefit to the use of continuous intravenous diuretic regimens over intravenous bolus dosing. If diuretic management is ineffective or complicated by progressive renal insufficiency, mechanical fluid removal (ultrafiltration) may be considered in well-selected patients, although anticoagulation and special intravenous access is required. Cardiovascular and renal consultation should be sought when cardiorenal syndrome is present.

CHRONIC MANAGEMENT

A crucial goal in the management of decompensated HF is optimizing the pharmacologic regimen in the chronic ambulatory state when the patient stabilizes. Goals shift to enhancing survival, minimizing symptoms and disability, improving functional capacity, and delaying disease progression. All patients should receive dietary instructions, including a daily low sodium restriction <2 gram Na^+. Fluid restriction (<2 L/d) is recommended in patients with moderate hyponatremia (serum sodium <135 mEq/L) and should be considered in all patients with fluid overload. Patients should record their weight on a daily basis. See Figure 130-1 and below for recommended pharmacologic therapy by HF stage.

THERAPIES FOR HEART FAILURE WITH LEFT VENTRICULAR SYSTOLIC DYSFUNCTION

Diuretics treat the sodium and fluid retention of HF. Once a decompensated HF patient achieves a compensated volume status, an oral regimen using the lowest diuretic doses to maintain euvolemia should be determined. Possible and frequent complications of poorly monitored diuretic management include hypotension and worsening renal function.

Angiotensin-converting enzyme inhibitors are vasodilators and potent neurohormonal antagonists that have been shown to alleviate symptoms, improve clinical status, and reduce the risk of death and hospitalization and should be prescribed to *all patients with HF with reduced LVEF* unless contraindicated (angioedema, pregnancy, significant renal artery stenosis, or hyperkalemia) (**Table 130-5**). Renal insufficiency and cough are relative contraindications. Treatment with an ACE inhibitor should be initiated at low doses followed by gradual increments in dose as tolerated to the target doses used in clinical trials (eg, captopril 50 mg three times a day, enalapril 10 mg twice a day, lisinopril 20–40 mg daily). When excessive hypotension is a concern, short-acting ACE inhibitors should be considered with a transition to long acting agents titrated to appropriate target study doses. Adverse effects of ACE inhibitors include hypotension, worsening renal function, hyperkalemia, cough, rash, leukopenia, dysgeusia, and angioedema. In patients who are hemodynamically or clinically unstable, it is recommended to interrupt treatment with the ACE inhibitors temporarily until the patient stabilizes. ***Angiotensin II receptor blockers*** should be used in patients who are ACE inhibitor intolerant.

Beta-blockers decrease the symptoms of HF as well as reduce the risk of death and hospitalization. Beta-blockers antagonize the sympathetic nervous system and thereby block the adverse consequences of adrenergic stimulation in HF. Three beta-blockers have been shown to be effective in reducing the risk of death in patients with chronic HF: bisoprolol, sustained-release metoprolol succinate, and carvedilol. Beta-blockers should be prescribed to all patients with stable compensated HF due to reduced LVEF unless they have a contraindication to their use. See (**Table 130-6**). Acceptable patients for beta-blocker therapy should have no or minimal evidence of fluid overload or volume depletion and should not have required recent treatment with an intravenous positive inotropic agent.

TABLE 130-5 Selected Angiotensin-converting Enzyme Inhibitor Trials in Heart Failure

Clinical Trial	No. Patients	Inclusion	Study Drug	Initial Dosing	Target Dose	Relative Risk, Mortality
Save	2231	3 days post MI survivors with LVEF < 40% without HF	Captopril	6.25 mg three times a day	50 mg three times a day	0.81 (0.68–0.97); $P = 0.019$
Consensus	253	NYHA IV Symptoms with heart size > 600 mL/m^2	Enalapril maleate	2.5 mg twice a day	10 mg twice a day	0.60; $P = 0.002$; power 90%
Solvd	2569	Congestive heart failure with LVEF < 35%	Enalapril maleate	2.5 mg twice a day	10 mg twice a day	0.82 (0.74–0.95); $P < 0.0036$

TABLE 130-6 Beta-blocker Use in Heart Failure

Clinical Trial	No. Patients	Inclusion	Study Drug	Initial Dose	Target Dose	Relative Risk, Mortality
CIBIS II	2647	NYHA III–IV Symptomatic HF with EF < 35%	Bisoprolol	1.25 mg daily	10 mg daily	RR 0.66 (0.54–0.81); $P < 0.0001$
Copernicus	2289	NYHA III–IV HF with EF < 25%	Carvedilol	3.125 mg twice a day	25–50 mg twice a day	RR 0.65 (0.52–0.81); $P = 0.000013$
Comet	3029	NYHA II–IV Symptomatic EF < 35%	Carvedilol	3.125 mg twice a day	25–50 mg twice a day	RR 0.83 (0.74–0.93); $P = 0.002$
US Carvedilol HF study	1094	NYHA II–III Mostly ischemic etiology	Carvedilol	3.125 mg twice a day	25–50 mg twice a day	RR 0.35 (0.20–0.61); $P < 0.001$
Merit HF	3991	NYHA II–IV Symptomatic HF with LEF < 40%	Metoprolol succinate	12.5–25 mg/d	200 mg daily	RR 0.6 (0.53–0.81); $P < 0.001$

Treatment with a beta-blocker should be initiated at very low doses followed by gradual increments to target doses used in the clinical trials (eg, carvedilol 25–50 mg twice a day, metoprolol succinate 200 mg daily, bisoprolol 10 mg daily). Initiation of beta-blockers can cause fluid retention, fatigue, bradycardia and heart block, and hypotension, and therefore, requires very close monitoring and follow-up. If patients develop fluid retention with or without symptoms on beta-blockers, the beta-blocker can be continued while the dose of diuretic is increased. If a patient deteriorates significantly demonstrating hypoperfusion or requires intravenous inotropic drugs, it is recommended to stop or reduce treatment with beta-blockers temporarily until the patient stabilizes (**Table 130-7**).

Aldosterone antagonists (spironolactone and eplerenone) have been shown to reduce mortality and hospitalizations and improve functional class in patients with advanced heart failure (spironolactone) as well as patients with HF after an acute MI (eplerenone). Addition of an aldosterone antagonist is recommended in patients with NYHA class 3 or 4 symptoms of HF and reduced LVEF who can comply with laboratory monitoring to assess renal function and potassium concentration. Creatinine should be less than or equal to 2.5 mg/dL in men or less than or equal to 2.0 mg/dL in women (to reduce the risk of hyperkalemia) and potassium should be less than 5.0 mEq/L (**Table 130-8**).

Digitalis can improve symptoms, quality of life, exercise tolerance, and reduce hospitalization rates in patients with mild to moderate HF, but has no effect on mortality. Because of its narrow therapeutic window, it is currently considered second-line therapy for chronic heart failure (eg, class II recommendation in ACC/AHA guidelines).

The chronic HF guidelines suggest that the addition of ***hydralazine***, an arterial vasodilator, and ***nitrates*** is reasonable in patients with reduced LVEF who have persistent symptoms yet are already taking target doses of ACE inhibitors and beta-blockers for symptomatic HF. The combination can also be considered in symptomatic patients who cannot be given an ACE inhibitor or ARB. A prospective, double-blind randomized trial conducted in African American patients with NYHA class III/IV HF demonstrated a mortality/morbidity benefit of isosorbide dinitrate plus hydralazine when added to a standard HF regimen. Time to first hospitalization and quality of life were also improved. The target doses used in this trial was hydralazine 75 mg three times a day and isosorbide dinitrate 40 mg three times a day.

TABLE 130-7 Selected Angiotensin-receptor Blocker Heart Failure Trials

Clinical Trial	No. Patients	Inclusion	Study Drug	Initial Dose	Target Dose	Relative Risk, Mortality
Val-Heft	5010	NYHA II–IV LVEF < 40% EDD 2.9 cm.m[2]	Valsartan	40 mg twice a day	160 mg twice a day	1.02 (0.88–1.18); $P = 0.8$
CHARM-Added	2548	NYHA II–IV LVEF < 40%	Candesartan	4–8 mg daily	32 mg daily	0.85 (0.75–0.96); $P = 0.011$
VALIANT	14703	0.5–10 days post MI with clinical or radiologic signs of HF and LVEF < 35% by echo or < 40 by LV gram	Valsartan	40 mg twice a day	160 mg twice a day	1.00 (0.90–1.11); $P = 0.98$

TABLE 130-8 Other Drugs Used in Heart Failure

Clinical Trial	No. Patients	Inclusion	Study Drug	Initial Dose	Target Dose	Relative Risk, Mortality
Rales	1663	NYHA III-IV LVEF <35%	Spironolactone	25 mg daily	25 mg daily	0.7 (0.60–0.82); $P < 0.0001$
Ephesus	6642	3–14 d post MI with LVEF <40% and HF symptoms	Eplerenone	25 mg daily	50 mg daily	0.85 (0.75–0.96); $P = 0.008$
V-Heft	642	Chronic CHF with LVEF <45% peak O_2 consumption <25 mL/kg/min	Hydralazine Isosorbide dinitrate	25 mg four times a day 10 mg four times a day	75 mg four times a day 40 mg four times a day	0.66 (0.46–0.96); $P < 0.082$
A-Heft	1050	NYHA III-IV LVEF <35% or <45% with EDD >6.5 cm by echo self ID Black	Hydralazine Isosorbide dinitrate	37.5 mg three times a day 20 mg three times a day	75 mg three times a day 40 mg three times a day	0.57 (−0.1–1.9); $P = 0.01$
DIG	6800	HF and LVEF <45% and sinus rhythm	Digoxin	0.125 mg daily	0.25 mg daily	1.01

Anticoagulation with ***warfarin*** is indicated in patients with HF who have experienced a previous thromboembolic event or who have paroxysmal or persistent atrial fibrillation. Anticoagulation should also be considered in patients with underlying disorders that may be associated with an increased thromboembolic risk (eg, amyloidosis, myocarditis). The evidence for benefit of chronic warfarin anticoagulation in patients with systolic heart failure in the absence of these previous indications is limited and is considered a class II indication.

Certain drugs should be avoided or used with caution in HF patients. Nonsteroidal anti-inflammatory drugs can cause sodium retention, peripheral vasoconstriction, and precipitate renal insufficiency and should be avoided. If analgesia is required, acetaminophen and judicious use of narcotics should be considered. Thiazolidinediones have been associated with increased peripheral edema and symptomatic HF and should be avoided, particularly in those with NYHA III/IV symptoms. Most calcium channel blockers should generally be avoided because of their cardiodepressant effects. Routine combined use of an ACE inhibitor, ARB, and aldosterone antagonist is not recommended given the risk for hyperkalemia, particularly in diabetic patients.

DEVICE THERAPY: INTRACARDIAC DEFIBRILLATORS (ICD) AND CARDIAC RESYNCHRONIZATION THERAPY (CRT)

Patients with systolic HF are at risk for sudden cardiac death due to ventricular arrhythmias. ICDs have been shown to decrease sudden death and all-cause mortality in several randomized prospective clinical trials of patients with left ventricular systolic dysfunction. The impact of ICD therapy is limited to a reduction in death from lethal arrhythmias; they do not improve quality of life or symptoms due to heart failure. The use of ICD therapy in primary prevention of sudden death must always be weighed against other factors that may affect long-term survival and individualized quality of life. Current guideline recommendations for ICD therapy include the following:

1. Secondary prevention to prolong survival in patients with current or prior symptoms of HF and reduced LVEF who have a history of cardiac arrest, ventricular fibrillation, or hemodynamically destabilizing ventricular tachycardia (ACC/AHA class I recommendation)
2. Primary prevention to reduce total mortality by a reduction in sudden cardiac death in patients with either ischemic heart disease (at least 40 days post-MI) or nonischemic cardiomyopathy (at least 9 months) who have an LVEF less than or equal to 30%, with NYHA functional class II or III symptoms while undergoing chronic optimal medical therapy, and have reasonable expectation of survival with a good functional status for more than 1 year (class I)

ICDs are not warranted in patients with refractory symptoms of HF (stage D) or in patients with concomitant diseases that would shorten their life expectancy independent of HF.

Electromechanical dyssynchrony (as evidenced by a prolonged QRS duration) has been associated with increased myocardial oxygen consumption, mitral regurgitation, ventricular remodeling, and neurohormonal activation. In patients with systolic heart failure, these changes are associated with heart failure symptoms and increased mortality. Dyssynchronous contraction can be alleviated by electrically activating the right and left ventricles in a synchronized manner with a biventricular pacemaker device (known as cardiac resynchronization therapy). CRT improves symptoms and quality of life as well as improving ventricular size and function and decreasing mitral regurgitation. These benefits result in improved survival and decreased hospitalizations in patients with persistently symptomatic HF despite optimal medical therapy who have prolonged QRS duration. The ACC/AHA/HRS class I recommendation for cardiac resynchronization therapy is for patients with LVEF less than or equal to 35%, sinus rhythm, and NYHA functional class III or ambulatory class IV symptoms despite recommended, optimal medical therapy and who have cardiac dyssynchrony, which is currently defined as a QRS duration greater than 120 milliseconds.

REVASCULARIZATION

The 2009 ACC/AHA guidelines on HF suggest coronary angiography in the following situations unless the patient is not eligible for revascularization of any kind:

1. HF patients who have angina or significant ischemia (class I). In patients with both HF and angina, coronary revascularization can relieve symptoms of myocardial ischemia; coronary artery

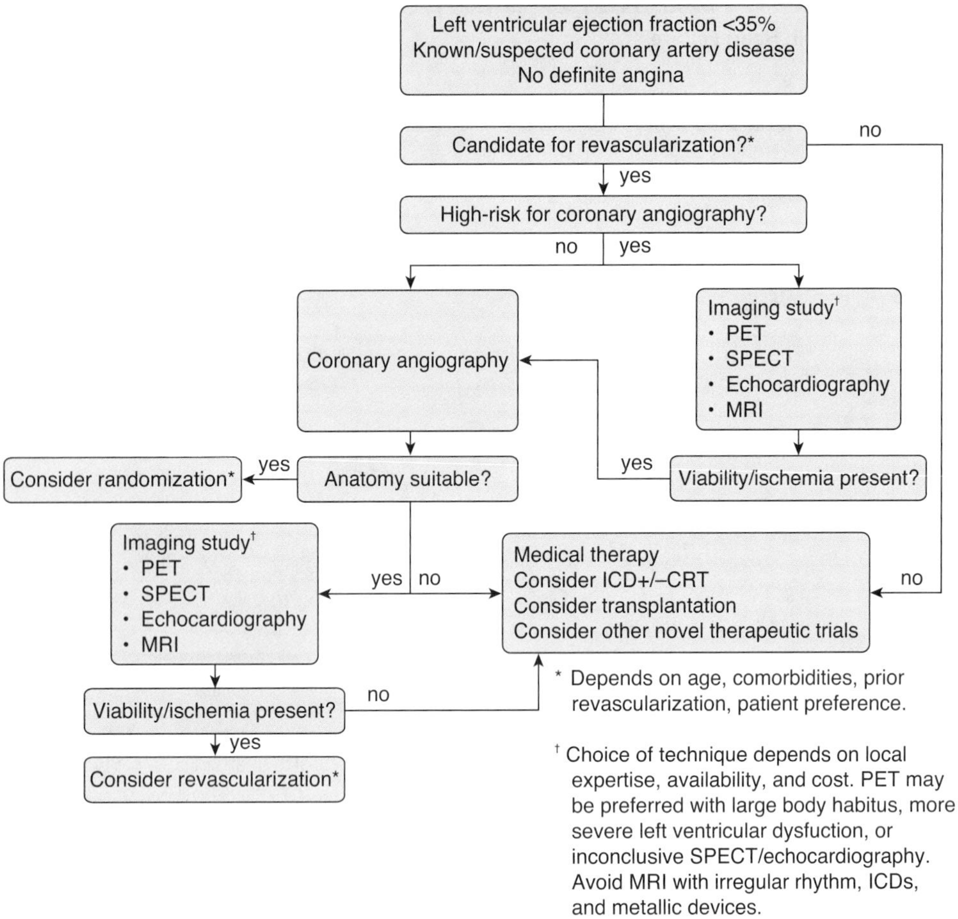

Figure 130-3 *When to revascuarize. (Reprinted, with permission, from Chareonthaitawee P, Gersh BJ, Araoz PA, et al. Revascularization in severe left ventricular dysfunction—the role of viability testing. J Am Coll Cardiol. 2005;46(4);567–574.)*

bypass surgery has been shown to lessen angina and reduce the risk of death in patients who have multivessel disease, reduced LVEF, and stable angina.
2. HF patients with chest pain that may or may not be of cardiac origin who have not had evaluation of their coronary anatomy (class IIa)
3. HF patients who have known or suspected coronary artery disease but who do *not* have angina (class IIa)

Less well supported by evidence, noninvasive imaging may be considered to define the likelihood of coronary artery disease in patients with HF and LV dysfunction (class IIb).

Observational data suggests that patients who have ischemic cardiomyopathy, HF, and no symptoms of angina, but have viable myocardium (by noninvasive imaging) demonstrate improved LV function and survival with revascularization compared with medical therapy (**Figure 130-3**). Alternatively, patients without viable myocardium should not be revascularized.

Noninvasive imaging to detect myocardial ischemia and viability is reasonable in patients who have *known* coronary artery disease and *no* angina unless the patient is not eligible for revascularization (class IIa).

CARE TRANSITIONS (DISCHARGE CONSIDERATIONS)

Rehospitalization occurs in 30% to 50% of patients within 3 to 6 months after heart failure hospitalization. Failure to meet criteria for discharge may increase the likelihood for readmission. Criteria for discharge should include

1. Achieving optimal volume status, resolution of heart failure symptoms, and use of appropriate medications that are tolerated without hypotension or renal insufficiency.
2. An understanding of the discharge instructions by patients and their families regarding medications, diet, activity, daily weights, identification of symptoms, and scheduled follow-up.

Follow-up with a primary care physician or cardiologist within a week of discharge is mandatory to assess the patient's clinical status, tolerance of medications, and to assess the need for laboratory evaluation. Closer follow-up after discharge may be necessary by telephone to assure stable weights or continuing weight loss if needed and to adjust diuretic dosing. Direct communication with the outpatient provider or disease management team should be standard practice. Hospital or practice-based disease management programs are of great benefit if available and have been shown to improve patient quality of life and reduce heart failure hospitalizations. Cardiology consultation should be strongly considered during inpatient care and is critical for follow-up to address the multiple issues relevant to the management of chronic systolic heart failure. This consideration is particularly relevant since heart failure admissions are markers for subsequent mortality.

Patients with stage D HF, or refractory HF, have marked symptoms at rest despite maximal medical therapy are best cared for by heart failure specialists. They may be eligible for specialized advanced treatments, such as mechanical circulatory support, procedures to facilitate fluid removal (ultrafiltration or dialysis), invasive hemodynamic guided therapy, or cardiac transplantation. End-of-life and palliative care can also be reviewed and offered when appropriate.

DISEASE MANAGEMENT STRATEGIES AND QUALITY IMPROVEMENT

Hospital admission for HF can be prevented by multidisciplinary disease management programs. Such programs can also improve functional status and quality of life for these patients. Appropriate patients (including those with a history of multiple readmissions, moderate to severe heart failure, or multiple comorbidities, and/or those at high risk due to cognitive impairment or persistent nonadherence) should be referred to heart failure management programs where available. A multidisciplinary team made up of physicians, HF nurses, dietitians, and pharmacists can provide

- Individualized education and counseling to the patient, family members, and caregivers that emphasize self-care
- Assistance with medication and dietary compliance
- Optimization of drug therapy
- Medicine reconciliation
- Low-cost scales to measure daily weights
- Increased access to health care
- Early attention to signs and symptoms of fluid overload
- Close telephone follow-up after hospital discharge to assess symptoms and daily weights and to adjust diuretic dosing

Hospitalists are in a key role to lead quality improvement initiatives to facilitate patient education and discharge planning, ensure adherence to evidence-based guidelines to improve patient outcomes, and to implement national quality measures. Initiatives include the use of HF clinical pathways and preprinted HF discharge instructions and educational material. Discharge planning most importantly should include a visiting nurse or telephone follow-up soon after discharge and a clinic visit within 1 week of discharge.

Educating patients with HF and their families is critical and should start early in the hospitalization. This can be achieved through discussions, videotapes, and reading materials at the appropriate educational level in the patient's native language. The aim of education should be to empower patients and their families to embrace the patient's self-care so they may recognize symptoms, implement therapy, and self-evaluate the effect of treatments.

Patient noncompliance with medications and diet is a common cause of clinical deterioration and readmission. *Discharge instructions* must address the following:

- Medications (prescribed and what to avoid)
- Dietary restrictions (low-salt diet and fluid restriction)
- Activity recommendations
- Signs and symptoms of heart failure and what to do
- Close follow-up
- Weight monitoring (and what to do with weight gain)
- National guidelines strongly recommend *smoking cessation counseling* for smokers with cardiovascular disease, including heart failure
- Exercise training (aerobic) improves exercise capacity and quality of life in patients with mild to moderate heart failure in the short term. Optimal exercise protocols are not defined, but excessively strenuous physical exertion should be discouraged
- Immunization with influenza and pneumococcal vaccines is recommended
- Nutritional supplements and hormonal therapies should be avoided according to current guidelines

PRESERVED EJECTION FRACTION

CASE 130-2

A 70-year-old woman with a past medical history of atrial fibrillation and long-standing hypertension experiences dyspnea on exertion, some orthopnea, and peripheral edema. On physical examination her blood pressure is 160/80 mm Hg and heart rate is irregular at 90 beats per minute. Jugular venous pressure is elevated, estimated at 14 cm H_2O, point of maximal impulse sustained, and heart sounds are irregular without murmurs, rubs, or gallops. Lung examination reveals diffuse rales in both lung fields. Extremities are warm with 2 + pitting edema.

EPIDEMIOLOGY/OVERVIEW

Heart failure (HF) with preserved left ventricular ejection fraction (LVEF), commonly known as diastolic heart failure, has surpassed systolic dysfunction as a cause for heart failure admissions. It is estimated that as many as 20% to 60% of patients with HF have a relatively normal LVEF. The prevalence of this patient population is increasing due to the aging population, the increasing incidence of hypertension and diabetes mellitus, and a growing awareness and ability to make the diagnosis. The rate of hospitalizations for HF is similar in patients with preserved and reduced LVEF. Patients with HF with preserved EF have similar rates of survival to those with HF and depressed ejection fraction.

Patients with HF with preserved LVEF are more likely to be older, female, and have a history of hypertension and atrial fibrillation when compared with patients with reduced EF. Obesity, anemia, and diabetes are also commonly present. In contrast to HF with low LVEF, few clinical trials have been done in HF patients with preserved LVEF. No therapy has been shown to improve survival in this type of HF.

PATHOPHYSIOLOGY

Heart failure with preserved LVEF or diastolic heart failure is poorly understood, heterogeneous disorder. Heart failure with preserved ejection fraction (HFPEF) is the preferred designation, since it remains unclear if the primary abnormality in this syndrome is diastolic dysfunction. The definition of "preserved" LVEF is variable in both clinical trials and in practice and can range from >40% to 60%. Heart failure with preserved LVEF has traditionally been attributed to reduced ventricular compliance and abnormal relaxation during diastole. Abnormal renal sodium and water handling, reduced vascular compliance, and anemia also appear to play roles in HFPEF. Diastolic function is often abnormal in patients with HF and reduced LVEF as well as those with preserved LVEF. The nature and extent of diastolic dysfunction is variable in HFPEF. Cardiac output, especially during exercise, may be limited by abnormal filling characteristics of the left ventricle as well as chronotropic incompetence and lack of vasodilator reserve. In restrictive cardiomyopathies, the "purest" form of HFPEF, ventricular chamber dimensions are reduced, intraventricular pressures are elevated, and cardiac output is essentially heart rate dependent.

Chronic hypertension with resultant left ventricular hypertrophy is a major cause of HFPEF. Elevations in systemic blood pressure increase left ventricular wall stress and systolic load, which can impair myocardial relaxation in patients with diastolic HF.

Several myocardial disorders that may present as HFPEF should be considered in the differential diagnosis, including restrictive cardiomyopathy, hypertrophic cardiomyopathy, and infiltrative cardiomyopathies. Patients with diastolic heart failure may have difficulty tolerating atrial fibrillation since the loss of atrioventricular synchrony can greatly reduce left atrial emptying, left ventricular (LV) filling, and LV stroke volume. Patients with diastolic HF may not tolerate tachycardia since increases in heart rate shorten the duration of diastole and truncate the late phase of diastolic filling. Paradoxically, tachycardia may be important to preserve exercise tolerance when stroke volume is limited. Ischemia can worsen diastolic dysfunction and symptoms of heart failure. Ischemia can result from coronary heart disease and/or LV hypertrophy with subendocardial ischemia.

CLINICAL PRESENTATION AND MAKING THE DIAGNOSIS

Diastolic dysfunction alone is insufficient to make the diagnosis of HFPEF. Signs and symptoms of heart failure must be present. The signs and symptoms of HFPEF are similar to those in HF with low LVEF and cannot be used to distinguish between the two. Echocardiography remains the cornerstone of making the distinction between systolic and diastolic HF. See **Table 130-9** for differential diagnosis in a patient with HF and normal LVEF.

Heart failure, whatever the etiology, is a clinical diagnosis. The diagnosis is generally based on the presence of typical signs or symptoms of HF in a patient who has preserved systolic function, typically defined by the LVEF. There may or may not be evidence of abnormal left ventricular relaxation, filling, or stiffness. Evidence for diastolic dysfunction is often made by Doppler echocardiography but is load dependent. Echocardiographic signs of diastolic dysfunction include abnormalities in mitral inflow, tissue Doppler, and pulmonary venous inflow. Plasma concentrations of brain natriuretic peptide (BNP) and N-terminal proBNP may be increased in patients with diastolic HF and can improve diagnostic accuracy, particularly in the presence of signs and symptoms of heart failure. A documented increase in left ventricular end-diastolic or pulmonary capillary wedge pressure is also diagnostic of HFPEF if the ejection fraction is preserved.

TRIAGE AND INITIAL MANAGEMENT

Regardless of the cause of acute heart failure (eg, HFPEF or systolic HF), initial treatment should focus on hemodynamic stabilization, oxygenation, and restoring filling pressure to optimal levels while searching for precipitating causes. No proven therapy for heart failure with preserved EF currently exists. Treatment should be directed toward symptoms, comorbid conditions, and physiologic factors known to contribute to impaired ventricular relaxation such as control of systolic and diastolic hypertension, control ventricular rate in patients with atrial fibrillation, control of pulmonary congestion and peripheral edema with diuretics, and coronary revascularization in patients with coronary heart disease. See **Table 130-10** for a summary of treatment recommendations.

Occult coronary heart disease is a potentially reversible cause of diastolic heart failure and should be excluded. Obesity, anemia, and sleep disordered breathing should be treated. One randomized clinical trial (candesartan in heart failure assessment of reduction in mortality and morbidity [CHARM] study) showed a reduction in hospital admissions for HF in patients with New York Heart Association (NYHA) functional class II–IV and LVEF higher than 40% taking candesartan compared with placebo but there was no difference in cardiovascular mortality. Three other trials have failed to demonstrate a significant benefit for other ARBs or beta-blockers. See **Table 130-11** for a summary of randomized clinical trials in HFPEF.

TABLE 130-9 Diagnostic Considerations in Heart Failure with Preserved Ejection Fraction Syndrome

- Valvular pathologies
- Infiltrative heart disease
  - Amyloidosis
  - Sarcoidosis
  - Hemochromatosis
- Constrictive pericarditis
- Systemic hypertension
- Ischemic heart disease
- High output states
  - Anemia
  - Thyrotoxicosis
  - AV communications
- Obesity
- Pulmonary hypertension associated with pulmonary vascular disorders
- Right-sided heart failure resulting from chronic lung disease

TABLE 130-10 Therapeutic Recommendations for Heart Failure with Preserved Ejection Fraction Syndrome

Class I A
Systemic blood pressure control
Class I C
Diuretic use to control pulmonary congestion and peripheral edema
Rate control in patients with atrial fibrillation
Class IIa C
Coronary revascularization is reasonable in patients with coronary artery disease in whom symptomatic or demonstrable myocardial ischemia is judged to be having an adverse effect on cardiac function.
Class IIb C
Restoration and maintenance of sinus rhythm in patients with atrial fibrillation might be useful to improve symptoms
The use of beta-adrenergic blocking agents, angiotensin-converting enzyme inhibitors, angiotensin II receptor blockers, or calcium antagonists in patients with controlled hypertension might be effective to minimize symptoms of heart failure.

DISEASE MANAGEMENT STRATEGIES

Studies suggest that hospital admission for HF can be prevented with multidisciplinary disease management programs. Functional status and quality of life can also be improved for HF patients. Appropriate patients (multiple readmissions, high risk due to cognitive impairment or multiple comorbidities, persistent nonadherence) should be referred to HF management programs if available. A multidisciplinary team made up of physicians, HF nurses, dietitians, and pharmacists can provide individualized education and counseling to the patient, family members, and caregivers that emphasize self-care, optimization of drug therapy, increased access to health care, early attention to signs and symptoms of fluid overload, and close telephone follow-up after hospital discharge to assess symptoms and daily weights, adjust diuretic dosing, and answer questions regarding diet and medications. As with patients with systolic HF, patient and family education about diastolic HF is critical and

TABLE 130-11 Outcomes of Randomized Clinical Trials in Heart Failure with Preserved Ejection Fraction

	CHARM-Preserved	I-Preserve	PEP-CHF	Seniors (s)
Therapy	Candesartan	Irbesartan	Perindopril	Nebivolol
Age (yr)	> 18 (67)	≥ 60 (72)	≥ 70 (75)	≥ 70 (76)
EF (%)	≥ 40 (mean 54)	≥ 45 (mean 60)	≥ 40 (mean 65)	≥ 35 (mean 49)
Patients (N)	3023	4128	850	752
Female (%)	40%	60%	55%	38%
Primary endpoint	CV death or HF hospitalization	Death or CV hospitalization	Death or HF hospitalization	Death or CV hospitalization
Relative risk	0.89 (0.77–1.03); $P = 0.051$	0.95 (0.86–1.05); $P = 0.35$	0.92 (0.70–1.21); $P = 0.545$	0.88 (0.73–1.05); $P = 0.21$

should start early in the hospitalization. Patient noncompliance with medications and diet is a common cause of clinical deterioration and readmission. *Discharge instructions* must address the following:

- Medications (prescribed and what to avoid)
- Dietary restrictions (low-salt diet and possibly fluid restriction)
- Activity recommendations
- Signs and symptoms of worsening condition and what to do
- Close follow-up
- Weight monitoring (and what to do with weight gain)

National guidelines strongly recommend *smoking cessation counseling* for smokers with cardiovascular disease, including heart failure. Immunization with influenza and pneumococcal vaccines is recommended.

CARE TRANSITIONS

Clinically, HF patients can be discharged once optimal volume status is obtained, symptoms have resolved, and appropriate medications have controlled heart rate and blood pressure without hypotension or renal insufficiency. Patient and family should demonstrate an understanding of the discharge instructions regarding medications, diet, activity, daily weights, worsening symptoms, and follow-up. Close follow-up with a primary care physician or cardiologist within a week is mandatory to assess the patient's clinical status and tolerance of medications and to check for electrolyte abnormalities. Closer follow-up by telephone may be necessary to monitor weights and symptoms. Direct communication with the outpatient provider should be standard practice.

SUGGESTED READINGS

Bhatia RS, Tu JV, Lee DS, et al. Outcome of heart failure with preserved ejection fraction in a population-based study. *N Engl J Med.* 2006;355:260–269.

Chareonthaitawee P, Gersh BJ, Araoz PA, et al. Revascularization in severe left ventricular dysfunction. *J Am Coll Cardiol.* 2005;46:567–574.

Cleland JGF, Daubert JC, Erdmann E, et al. The effect of cardiac resynchronization on morbidity and mortality in heart failure. *N Engl J Med.* 2005;352:1539–1549.

Fonarow GC, Adams KF, Abraham WT, et al. Risk stratification for in-hospital mortality in acutely decompensated heart failure. *JAMA.* 2005;293:572–580.

Forrester JS, Diamond GA, Swan HJ. Correlative classification of clinical and hemodynamic function after acute myocardial infarction. *Am J Cardiol.* 1977;39:137–145.

Heart Failure Society of America. Executive summary: HFSA 2006 comprehensive heart failure practice guideline. *J Card Fail.* 2006;12:10–38.

Hunt SA, Abraham WT, Marshall CH, et al. ACC/AHA 2009 guideline update for the diagnosis and management of chronic heart failure in the adult: a report of the American College of Cardiology/American Heart Association task force on practice guidelines (Writing Committee to Update the 2005 Guidelines for the Evaluation and Management of Heart Failure): developed in collaboration with the American College of Chest Physicians and the International Society for Heart and Lung Transplantation: endorsed by the Heart Rhythm Society. Jessup M, Brozena S. Heart failure. *Circulation.* 2009;119:e391–e479.

Jessup M, Brozena S. Heart failure. *N Engl J Med.* 2003;348:2007–2018.

Leite-Moreira AF. Current perspectives in diastolic dysfunction and diastolic heart failure. *Heart.* 2006;92:712–718.

Mueller C, Scholer A, Laule-Kilian K, et al. Use of B-type natriuretic peptide in the evaluation and management of acute dyspnea. *N Engl J Med.* 2004;350:647–654.

Nieminen MS, Bohm M, Cowie MR, et al. Guidelines on the diagnosis and treatment of acute heart failure. The task force on acute heart failure of the European society of Cardiology. *Eur Heart J.* 2005:1–36.

Nohria A, Lewis E, Stevenson W L. Medical management of advanced heart failure. *JAMA.* 2002;287(5):628–640.

Owan TE, Hodge DO, Herges RM, et al. Trends in prevalence and outcome of heart failure with preserved ejection fraction. *N Engl J Med.* 2006;355:251–259.

Pitt B, Zannad F, Remme WJ, et al. The e ffect of spironolactone on morbidity and mortality in patients with severe heart failure. *N Engl J Med.* 1999;341:709–717.

Rees K, Taylor RS, Sing S, et al. Exercise-based rehabilitation for heart failure. Cochrane Database of Systematic Reviews. 2004, Issue 3. CD003331. DOI: 10.1002/14651858.CD003331.pub2.

Taylor AL, Ziesche S, Yancy C, et al. Combination of isosorbide dinitrate and hydralazine in blacks with heart failure. *N Engl J Med.* 2004;351:2049–2057.

Yusuf S, Pfeffer MA, Swedberg K, et al. Effects of candesartan in patients with chronic heart failure and preserved left-ventricular ejection fraction: the CHARM-preserved trial. *Lancet.* 2003;362:777–781.

Zipes DP, Libby P, Bonow RO, et al. Braunwald's Heart Disease. A Textbook of Cardiovascular Medicine. 7th ed. Philadelphia, PA: Elsevier Saunders; 2005:509–624.

CHAPTER 131

Valvular Heart Disease

Patrick Willis, MD
Zahid Junagadhwalla, MD
Vasilis C. Babaliaros, MD

Key Clinical Questions

1. What are the key factors that determine when to proceed to aortic valve repair, implantation, or replacement for patients with aortic stenosis? What guides decision-making relating to aortic surgery for acute aortic regurgitation?
2. When should patients with chronic aortic regurgitation undergo surgery?
3. What are the indications for surgery in patients with mitral stenosis? What are the goals of medical therapy for mitral regurgitation and when should patients be considered for mitral valve repair or replacement?
4. What are the objectives of treatment of pulmonic stenosis? When should a patient with pulmonic regurgitation be referred for surgery?
5. What are the factors that determine medical versus surgical treatment of tricuspid stenosis or tricuspid regurgitation?

INTRODUCTION

Valvular heart disease is a common disorder seen by hospitalists. Often a cardiologist and/or cardiac surgeon is consulted to comanage these patients; however, a comprehensive understanding and appropriate screening by an internist is important for both an inpatient and outpatient practice. This chapter provides practical information regarding the pathophysiology, diagnosis, and therapy of the valvular abnormalities that commonly affect each of the four valves.

AORTIC VALVE DISORDERS

AORTIC STENOSIS

Pathophysiology

Aortic stenosis (AS) is a disease of the aortic valve that causes obstruction to the ejection of blood from the left ventricle into the aorta. It is caused by three distinct abnormalities: congenital, rheumatic, and degenerative. Degenerative stenosis (also known as calcific or senile AS) is the leading cause of valvular cardiac surgery in adults. The prevalence is estimated from 2–7% in populations over the age of 65.

Calcific aortic disease represents a spectrum ranging from aortic sclerosis, defined as leaflet thickening without significant obstruction, to severe AS (defined below). Several risk factors have been associated with aortic sclerosis including smoking, hypertension, diabetes, LDL-cholesterol, and C-reactive protein (CRP). Though calcification can occur during the degeneration of all aortic valves, it tends to be more pronounced in patients with congenital abnormalities of the valve (ie, bicuspid valves) than the calcification of the trileaflet valve (the most common anatomy of AS).

Rheumatic heart disease has historically been an important cause of AS, but due to improvements in therapy and diagnosis it is uncommon in industrialized countries. Rheumatic disease remains an important cause of AS in developing nations, and should be considered in immigrant populations. Other uncommon causes of AS include connective tissue diseases, radiation therapy, and hyperlipoproteinemia syndromes. Chronic renal disease is associated with abnormal calcium homeostasis, and has been shown to hasten the progression of AS.

More recent data supports the hypothesis that aortic valve calcification is an active process that may not completely reflect patient age (and "over-use") of the valve. Abnormalities of blood flow across the valve can lead to damage of the valvular endothelium. Endothelial injury initiates an inflammatory process similar to atherosclerosis and ultimately leads to deposition of calcium on the valve and eventual stenosis. Patients with congenitally bicuspid valves are exposed to more profound abnormalities in blood flow and develop AS earlier than trileaflet valves, usually in their fifth to sixth decade, but it can occur as early as their fourth decade. In rheumatic disease, an autoimmune inflammatory reaction is triggered by prior *Streptococcus* infection that targets the valvular endothelium leading to inflammation and eventual calcification.

Stenosis of the aortic valve occurs slowly and is subclinical until the disease is fairly advanced. Progressive calcium deposition and inflammation limit aortic leaflet mobility. The stenosis imposes a pressure burden on the left ventricle, which concentrically hypertrophies in response to maintain normal wall stress (afterload). With advanced disease, the adaptive mechanism fails and left ventricular wall stress increases. Systolic ventricular function declines as wall stress increases, and heart failure is inevitable in untreated disease.

PRACTICE POINT

- In aortic stenosis, hypertrophied heart muscle requires more blood flow than normal heart muscle during exercise and may exhibit areas of relatively ischemic heart muscle—potential sources of arrhythmia, including ventricular tachycardia and sudden cardiac death.

Many of the symptoms of AS can be attributed to left ventricular hypertrophy (LVH). The consequence of concentric LVH is a smaller, less compliant chamber. Thus, left ventricular end-diastolic pressure is often increased to maintain stroke volume, especially during periods of increased cardiac output (eg, exercise), leading to the sensation of dyspnea. Furthermore, hypertrophied heart muscle requires more blood flow than normal heart muscle during exercise (supply-demand mismatch) and is subject to ischemia manifesting as chest pain even in the absence of coronary atherosclerotic disease. Areas of relatively ischemic heart muscle are potential sources of arrhythmia that can result in ventricular tachycardia and sudden cardiac death.

Diagnosis: does the patient have AS?

Aortic stenosis may exhibit a variety of possible clinical presentations and symptoms (**Table 131-1**). An ECG is indicated in the initial workup of all patients with valvular disease and is abnormal in more than 90% of patients with AS (**Figure 131-1**). The most common abnormality seen on the ECG is LVH due to pressure overload. Evidence of LVH and absent Q waves helps distinguish AS from other conditions such as aortic sclerosis with ischemic heart disease. Patients with AS often have conduction disease manifesting as AV block, hemiblock, or bundle branch block.

Transthoracic echocardiography is the test of choice in the evaluation of suspected AS and for the evaluation of all pathologic murmurs detected on physical exam (**Figure 131-2**). Echocardiography

TABLE 131-1 Symptoms and Physical Exam Findings in Aortic Stenosis

Aortic Stenosis Symptoms	Aortic Stenosis Physical Exam Findings
Decreased exercise tolerance, shortness of breath on exertion, chest pain, syncope/near syncope, heart failure	Late peaking systolic ejection murmur best auscultated at the right second intercostal space, which can obscure S_2 when severe
	Gallavardin phenomena (often heard loudest at the right upper sterna border but can also be heard along the left upper sterna border and apex of the heart)
	Murmurs can radiate to the carotid arteries; carotid upstroke is delayed and diminished (parvus et tardus)
	Jugular venous pressure (may be present in patients with pulmonary hypertension secondary to AS)

can accurately detect the presence of a pressure gradient across the aortic valve. It can also assess left ventricular function and the presence of LVH. Anatomical details of the valve stenosis can be seen and used to determine the etiology of AS. An aortic valve area of > 1.5 cm^2 is mild stenosis; aortic valve area of 1.0–1.5 cm^2 is moderate stenosis; aortic valve area < 1.0 cm^2 is severe stenosis.

PRACTICE POINT

- An aortic valve area of < 1.0 cm^2 is severe stenosis. The onset of symptoms in AS portends a poor prognosis, with an average survival of only two to three years unless replacement is performed. Symptomatic patients are at risk of sudden death (8–34%). Patients with failing left ventricular function or severe AS should be referred for treatment regardless of symptoms.

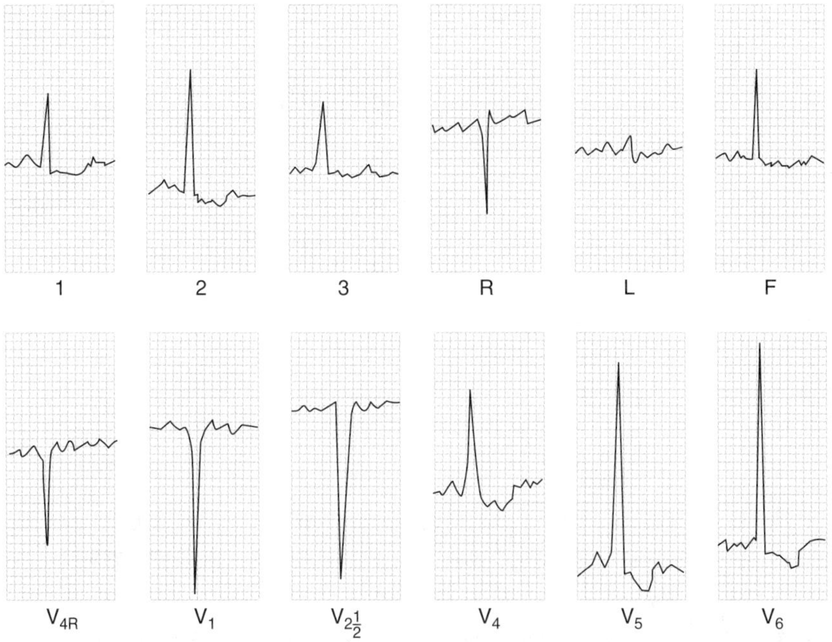

Figure 131-1 *ECG of a patient with aortic stenosis is consistent with severe left ventricular hypertrophy. (Reproduced, with permission, from Fuster V, O'Rourke RA, Walsh RA, et al. Hurst's the Heart. 12th ed. New York: McGraw-Hill, 2008. Fig. 82-23.)*

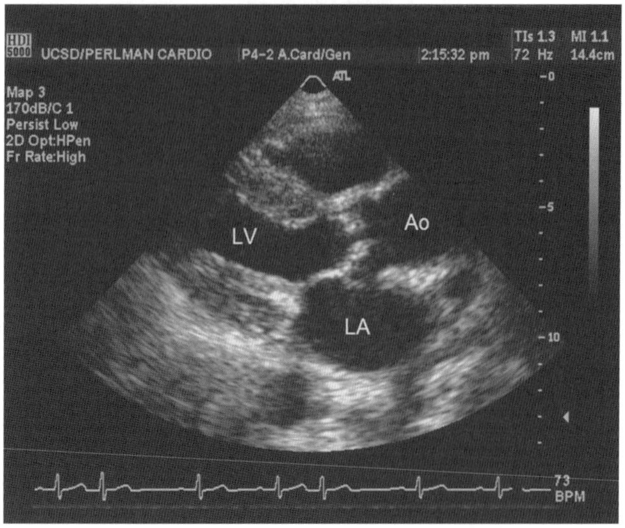

Figure 131-2 *Cardiac echocardiography in the parasternal long axis view shows thickened, stenotic aortic valve and left ventricular hypertrophy. Ao, aorta; LA, left atrium; LV, left ventricle. (Reproduced, with permission, from Fuster V, O'Rourke RA, Walsh RA, et al. Hurst's the Heart. 12th ed. New York: McGraw-Hill, 2008. Fig. 16-59.)*

Cardiac catheterization is no longer the test of choice for the diagnosis of AS. Catheterization is used only when echo-Doppler exam is inconclusive or there is a discrepancy between noninvasive findings and the physical exam. Catheterization remains essential, however, prior to aortic valve replacement for the evaluation of coronary artery disease.

Treatment

The key factors to proceed to aortic valve repair, implantation, or replacement are the onset of symptoms and left ventricular function. The onset of symptoms portends a poor prognosis with an average survival of only two to three years unless replacement is performed. Additionally, symptomatic patients are at risk of sudden death (8–34%), and thus, a strategy of "watchful waiting" should never take the place of prompt referral. Patients with failing left ventricular function and severe AS should be referred for treatment regardless of symptoms.

Surgical aortic valve replacement Surgical aortic valve replacement is the only therapy with proven survival benefit (**Figure 131-3**). A thorough discussion between the surgeon and patient exploring the risks and benefits of valve replacement should take place before proceeding with surgery. Physicians should also discuss the merits and drawbacks of the different types of valves (bioprosthetic versus mechanical) before the operation. Current bioprosthetic valves are made of porcine or bovine pericardial tissue and require reoperation 10 to 20 years after implantation; these valves do not require long-term anticoagulation. Mechanical valves are not prone to degeneration but patients are exposed to the risks of lifelong anticoagulation. Therefore the patient's bleeding risks are very important when selecting the type of valve to implant.

Balloon aortic valvuloplasty For patients who are highly symptomatic yet too high-risk to undergo an operation because of risk factors such as severe lung disease or porcelain aorta, balloon valvuloplasty is a reasonable option. This is a percutaneous procedure done in the cardiac catheterization lab in which a balloon is used to dilate the aortic valve and relieve stenosis and almost all patients do have symptomatic relief. Unfortunately, all patients

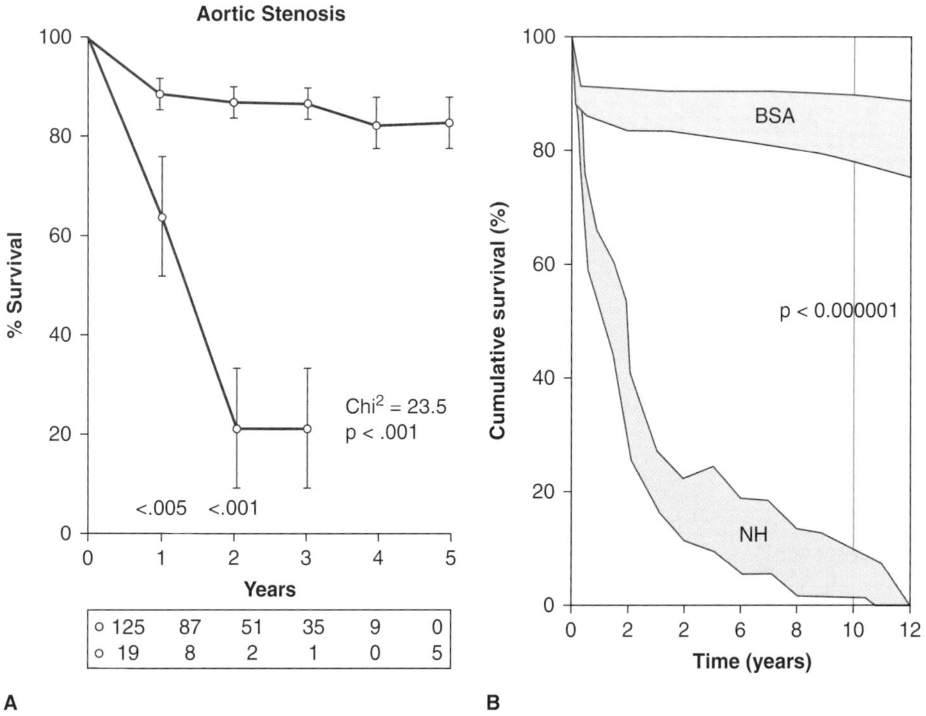

Figure 131-3 *Plot of survival versus time in patients with severe, symptomatic aortic stenosis that underwent surgical valve replacement (blue lines, BSA) versus best medical therapy (red lines, NH, natural history of aortic stenosis). (Reproduced, with permission, from Fuster V, O'Rourke RA, Walsh RA, et al. Hurst's the Heart. 12th ed. New York: McGraw-Hill, 2008. Fig. 75-6.)*

restenose eventually at 6–12 months, some earlier and some later, and there is no improvement in mortality. Currently this technique is used for palliation in patients with no further options, or as a bridge to surgical or transcatheter aortic valve implantation.

Transcatheter aortic valve implantation Transcatheter aortic valve implantation (TAVI), placement of a stent-mounted bioprosthetic aortic valve using a catheter delivery system) is quickly becoming the treatment of choice in high risk or nonoperable patients. This approach avoids the morbidity of sternotomy and may be safer for elderly patients with serious and multiple comorbidities. Early experience in Europe and Canada has demonstrated the feasibility of the procedure, and follow-up, though relatively short, has been encouraging. Currently in the United States this therapy is only available through randomized trials that are currently underway to further evaluate the safety and efficacy of TAVI.

AORTIC REGURGITATION

Pathophysiology

Aortic regurgitation (AR) is the diastolic reversal of blood flow from the aorta back into the left ventricle. It occurs as result of inadequate coaptation of valve leaflets due to either valve abnormalities or dilation of the aortic root. AR is a serious cardiac abnormality and may occur as part of systemic or congenital disease. In developing countries, rheumatic heart disease is the most common cause, but bicuspid aortic valve and aortic root dilatation account for most of the cases in developed countries. Causes of aortic root dilatation include (1) Marfan syndrome and other related connective tissue diseases, and (2) aortitis secondary to syphilis, Behcet, Takayasu, Reiter syndrome, and ankylosing spondylitis. Endocarditis can lead to the rupture of leaflets, and vegetations on the valvular cusps can cause inadequate closure of leaflets. Aortic root dissection is a cause of *acute* AR.

The prevalence of at least mild AR is approximately 13% in men and 8.5% in women, and increases with age. Of asymptomatic people over the age of 55, 29% have AR of which a minority (13% of the patients with AR) have moderate to severe AR. In younger patients (23 to 35 years), the prevalence of AR is 1.3%.

AR can be classified as acute or chronic. Acute AR is secondary to acute aortic dissection, endocarditis, and deceleration injury (motor vehicle accident). With acute *severe* AR, the end-diastolic pressure in the left ventricle rises dramatically and the heart tries to compensate by increasing the heart rate and contractility (Starling law) to keep up with the preload. Often the compensatory mechanisms are insufficient to maintain the normal stroke volume and heart failure ensues. Chronic *severe* AR presents differently, as the patients remain asymptomatic for months to years while the heart compensates for gradual increased preload. The heart wall undergoes eccentric hypertrophy to decrease wall stress. Eventually, left ventricle systolic dysfunction supervenes and left ventricle end-diastolic pressure rises, resulting in symptomatic congestive heart failure. Timing aortic valve repair/replacement before irreversible myocardial dysfunction develops is of critical importance.

Diagnosis: does the patient have aortic regurgitation?

The signs and symptoms of AR depend on the acuity of disease. In *acute* AR, the patient can present with sudden onset of pulmonary edema and hypotension or cardiogenic shock. Patients may present with signs and symptoms of myocardial ischemia or aortic root dissection. The left ventricular size is normal on exam, and the diastolic murmur may be short and/or soft due to equalization of diastolic pressure between aorta and ventricle.

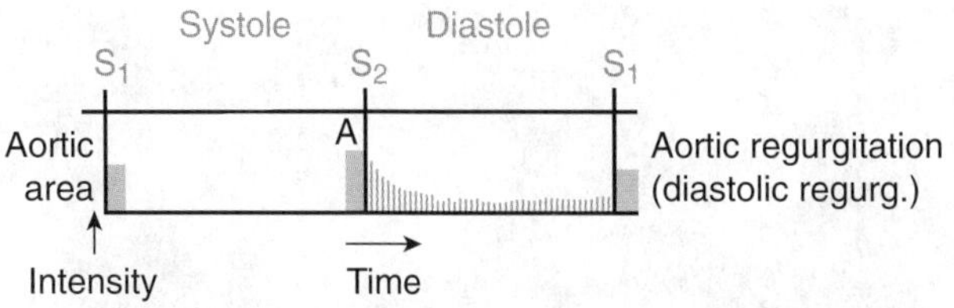

Figure 131-4 *Diagram representation of the heart murmur of aortic regurgitation. The murmur is a decrescendo murmur in early diastole that can also continue into late diastole when listening at the apex (Austin Flint murmur). (Reproduced, with permission, from LeBlond RF, DeGowin RL, Brown DD. DeGowin's Diagnostic Examination, 9th ed. New York: McGraw-Hill, 2009. Fig. 8-39.)*

An apical diastolic rumble may be present (Austin Flint murmur, see below) (**Figure 131-4**). Pulse pressure may not be increased due to reduced systolic pressure. The transthoracic echocardiogram confirms the presence, severity, and etiology of AR. Transesophageal echocardiogram is one of the best tests that can be performed if aortic root dissection is suspected in the setting of acute AR.

History and physical exam findings may be suggestive of AR (**Table 131-2**). Because physical signs are often not specific enough to judge the severity of the AR, transthoracic echocardiography is performed to better delineate disease severity (**Figure 131-5**). Echocardiography evaluates the valvular anatomy, aortic root, and impact of AR on ventricular size and function. Several echo indexes are used to assess severity. Color Doppler provides visualization of the origin of regurgitant jet and its width (color jet width > 65% of left ventricular outflow tract is severe AR). Continuous wave Doppler can estimate the degree of AR, assuming the left ventricular end diastolic pressure is not very elevated (pressure half time < 250 msec is severe AR). Diastolic reversal of flow in the descending aorta can also be seen by echo and is indicative of severe AR.

TABLE 131-2 Symptoms and Physical Exam Findings in Aortic Regurgitation

Aortic Regurgitation Symptoms	Physical Exam Findings
Decreased exercise tolerance, shortness of breath on exertion, chest pain, syncope/near syncope, heart failure	Arterial pulse shows rapid rise and a quick collapse (Corrigan pulse or water hammer pulse) resulting in widened pulse pressure greater than 50 mm Hg
	High-pitched early-peaking diastolic, decrescendo blowing murmur, which is heard best with the diaphragm of the stethoscope just after A_2
	The murmur is usually soft and can be accentuated with the patient sitting up, leaning forward, and breath holding at the end of expiration
	Maneuvers that increase arterial pressure such as squatting, accentuate the murmur; inhalation of amyl nitrate or Valsalva maneuver, which lower arterial pressure, decrease the intensity of the murmur

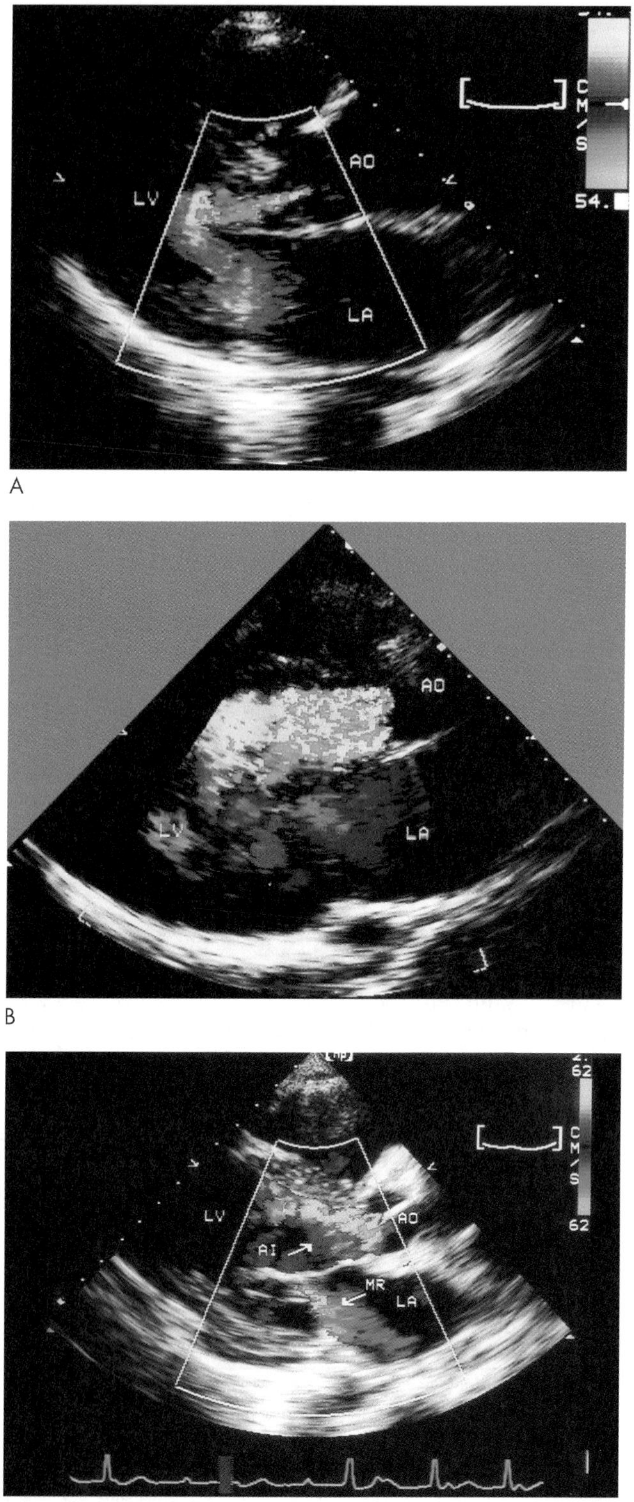

Figure 131-5 *Cardiac echocardiography in the parasternal long axis view shows mild (A) and severe (B and C) aortic regurgitation by color doppler (seen as turbulent color flow originating from aortic valve). Ao, aorta; AI, aortic insufficiency; LV, left ventricle; LA, left atrium; MR, mitral regurgitation. (Reproduced, with permission, from Fuster V, O'Rourke RA, Walsh RA, et al. Hurst's the Heart. 12th ed. New York: McGraw-Hill, 2008. Fig. 16-64.)*

PRACTICE POINT

- In aortic regurgitation, timing aortic valve repair/replacement before irreversible myocardial dysfunction develops can lead to reversal of left ventricular dilatation and improvement in ejection fraction (EF). Valve replacement surgery should be performed before the EF is ≤ 50% and/or before the left ventricular end systolic dimension is ≥ 55 mm to preserve the left ventricle even in asymptomatic patients.
- Medical therapy with vasodilators (hydralazine, nifedipine, and angiotensin converting enzyme inhibitors) does not improve mortality.

If the results of echocardiogram (transthoracic and transesophageal) are of insufficient quality or if the impact of the AR on the patient is unclear, other tests can be ordered. In chronic severe AR, treadmill exercise testing is helpful to assess the functional status and symptomatic response in sedentary patients. Multigated Acquisition Scan (MUGA) or magnetic resonance imaging (MRI) can be used to assess left ventricular function. Fluoroscopic angiography evaluates AR and concomitant coronary disease preoperatively, which is particularly useful in patients undergoing valvular surgery that have risk factors for coronary disease (men > 35 years, premenopausal women > 35 years, and postmenopausal women).

Treatment

Acute severe AR is often a surgical emergency. Surgery should be performed as soon as possible in patients with hemodynamic instability or congestive heart failure, particularly if medical therapy is ineffective. Recommended initial management for patients with acute AR includes airway management (intubation), positive inotropic agents (dobutamine), and a vasodilator therapy (nitroprusside).

Chronic AR has a protracted course and patients may remain asymptomatic for decades. Many patients with mild or moderate AR remain stable and may never require corrective surgery. Treatment of chronic AR depends on five factors: (1) severity, (2) symptoms, (3) left ventricular function, (4) left ventricular dilatation, and (5) operability. Medical therapy with vasodilators (hydralazine, nifedipine, and angiotensin converting enzyme inhibitors) does not improve mortality. Aortic valve replacement is performed in the majority of patients requiring surgery, though aortic valve repair may be possible in selected patients at specialized centers. The majority of the patients show reversal of left ventricular dilatation and improvement in ejection fraction (EF). Preoperative left ventricular function is the best predictor of long-term prognosis in patients undergoing surgery. Patients with normal preoperative EF or a brief duration of left ventricular dysfunction (less than 14 months) have greater improvement in left ventricular dimensions and early and late postoperative improvement in left ventricular function. Patients with impaired preoperative ventricular function have a greater risk of developing congestive heart failure postoperatively. In general, surgery should be performed before the EF is ≤ 50% and/or before the left ventricular end systolic dimension is ≥ 55 mm to preserve the left ventricle even in asymptomatic patients.

MITRAL VALVE DISORDERS

MITRAL STENOSIS

Pathophysiology

Mitral stenosis (MS) impedes the flow of blood from the left atrium into the left ventricle. In the United States, more than 95% of MS

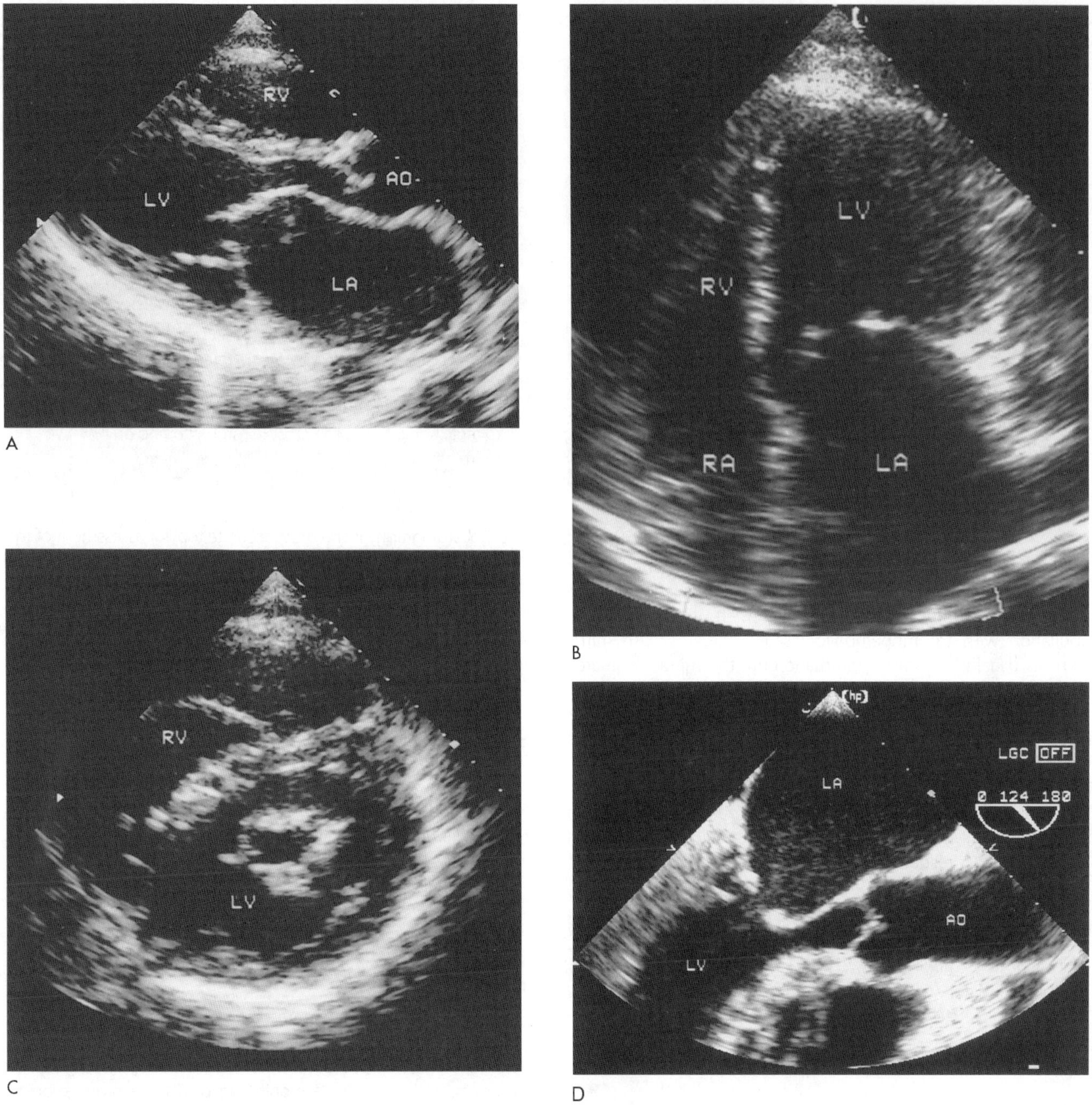

Figure 131-6 *Cardiac echocardiography in the parasternal long axis view (A), apical 4 chamber view (B), short axis view (C) and 3 chamber TEE (transesophageal) view (D) shows thickened and stenotic mitral valve. Ao, aorta; LA, left atrium; LV, left ventricle; RV, right ventricle. (Reproduced, with permission, from Fuster V, O'Rourke RA, Walsh RA, et al. Hurst's the Heart. 12th ed. New York: McGraw-Hill, 2008. Fig. 16-73.)*

results from a prior episode of rheumatic fever (RF) with secondary changes of the valve leading to rheumatic heart disease. RF affects the mitral valve in isolation approximately 25% of the time, and has 35% prevalence for multivalve involvement (aortic and mitral) with the tricuspid or pulmonic valves rarely involved. The clinical course between initial RF episode and valvular obstruction or regurgitation is variable. The prevalence of RF is 1 case per 150,000 in the United States and as high as 50 per 100,000 with frequent recurrence in undeveloped or underdeveloped countries. Symptomatic MS often presents at an older age in developed countries and as early as the teenage years in undeveloped ones. The prevalence of MS is decreasing in the United States because of the decreased prevalence of streptococcal strains that cause RF and the earlier detection and treatment of streptococcal pharyngitis.

Rheumatic MS results from an autoimmune process between the streptococcal protein and the valvular tissue causing inflammation and edema of the leaflets during bouts of RF, causing thickening of leaflet edges, commissural fusion, chordal shortening, and calcification of the mitral apparatus. These changes culminate in valve stenosis and/or regurgitation. Aschoff bodies (another pathological finding) are more consistently found in the myocardium and rarely seen on the valvular tissue at autopsy (**Figure 131-6**). The valvular pathological changes of RF mainly affect the anterior leaflet and result in a "doming" motion during ventricular diastole and the characteristic "fish-mouth" appearance seen by transthoracic echocardiogram (**Figure 131-7**).

As RF progresses, the normal mitral valve opening area (> 4 cm^2) can be restricted to a mild (1.5–2.0 cm^2), moderate (1.0–1.5 cm^2),

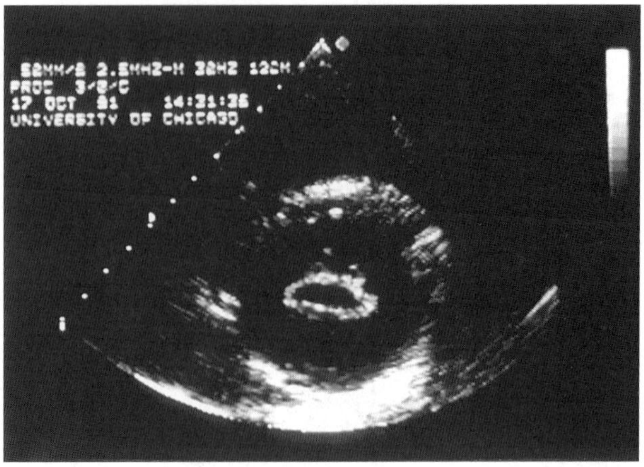

Figure 131-7 *Characteristic "fish-mouth" appearance of mitral stenosis seen by transthoracic echocardiogram. (Reproduced, with permission, from Hall JB, Schmidt GA, Wood LDH. Principles of Critical Care. 3rd ed. New York: McGraw-Hill, 2005. Fig. 29-7.)*

or severe (< 1.0 cm²) degree. The reduction in valve orifice leads to an elevated transmitral gradient, elevation in left atrial and pulmonary pressures, enlargement of the left atrium, and atrial fibrillation with thromboembolic disease. Patients with mitral stenosis usually are not symptomatic until the mitral valve area is < 1.0 cm² or the valve stenosis is moderate with associated tachycardia. Tachycardia for any reason decreases the time for diastolic emptying of the left atrium, and therefore increases left atrial and pulmonic pressures, elevates transmitral gradient, and reduces cardiac output (under-filling of the left ventricle). Dyspnea and acute pulmonary edema can occur suddenly in an asymptomatic MS patient that develops atrial fibrillation with rapid ventricular response.

PRACTICE POINT

- Patients with mitral stenosis usually are not symptomatic until the mitral valve area is < 1.0 cm² or the valve stenosis is moderate with associated tachycardia.

Diagnosis: Does the patient have mitral stenosis?

In developed countries, MS is a slowly progressive disease and thus patients can remain asymptomatic simply by adjusting their lifestyles to a more sedentary level. Dyspnea is the most common presenting complaint along with fatigue during minimal exertion; other signs and symptoms of more advanced disease are orthopnea, paroxysmal nocturnal dyspnea, and pulmonary edema. Symptoms in MS can be precipitated by changes in heart rate or volume status such as atrial fibrillation, emotional stress, pregnancy, fever, or exercise. Other symptoms include hemoptysis (due to rupture of bronchial vessels in patients with pulmonary hypertension), chest pain, palpitations, and hoarseness because of compression of the left recurrent laryngeal nerve from the dilated left atrium and pulmonary artery (Ortner syndrome).

An irregular pulse is the most common finding on physical examination (atrial fibrillation). Increased jugular venous pressure is common when the patient has developed pulmonary hypertension. *The ausculatory findings are more evident when examining the patient in the left lateral decubitus position and listening at the apex.* If right heart dilatation second to pulmonary hypertension is present, the left ventricular apex is displaced more posteriorly. Classically, there is an accentuated first heart sound and an opening snap (snapping open of the domed leaflets into the left ventricle) though calcification and valvular thickening can reduce leaflet excursion and both sounds may be absent with severe MS. The *diastolic murmur is low pitched and best heard with the bell of the stethoscope*; the intensity of the murmur does not correlate with the severity of the MS as it can be altered by numerous factors, especially exercise. Repeat auscultation after exercise (eg, sit-ups) makes the murmur of MS more audible.

PRACTICE POINT

- Symptoms in MS include hemoptysis, chest pain, palpitations, and hoarseness and can be precipitated by changes in heart rate or volume status such as atrial fibrillation, emotional stress, pregnancy, fever, or exercise. An irregular pulse due to atrial fibrillation is the most common finding on physical examination.

Echocardiography is the most accurate tool for assessment of the valve anatomy, valve area, transvalvular gradient, and the presence of multivalvular disease. If transthoracic images are suboptimal, transesophageal images can aid in delineating the valvular apparatus and in evaluation for clot in the left atrium or left atrial appendage. The echocardiographer should be able to categorize the MS as mild, moderate, or severe (< 1.0 cm² valve area), and determine the etiology of disease. Electrocardiography (ECG) is relatively nonspecific for the diagnosis of MS, though left atrial and right atrial abnormalities with right axis deviation of the QRS complex should alert the clinician of the possibility of MS (**Figure 131-8**). Chest X-ray may show left atrial enlargement (splaying of the main stem bronchi), left atrial appendage enlargement (straightening of the left cardiac silhouette), enlargement of the pulmonary arteries and pulmonary edema. Diagnostic catheterization can be helpful for quantifying transvalvular gradient and area if the echocardiographic data is inconsistent with clinical findings.

Treatment

Patients with mild to moderate MS can remain asymptomatic for years; therefore, the medical management of MS is focused on preventing further complications/recurrences of RF, optimizing hemodynamics, and appropriate monitoring of disease progression to allow referral for surgical or nonsurgical intervention (**Table 131-3**).

Asymptomatic patients with moderate MS can be evaluated yearly with a physical examination and echocardiogram. Symptomatic patients with severe MS, however, should be referred for percutaneous or surgical therapy as the five-year survival rate without intervention is approximately 40%. The therapy recommended for the patient is usually made after consultation with a cardiologist or cardiothoracic surgeon who has experience in percutaneous balloon mitral valvuloplasty (BMV) or surgical mitral repair or replacement. BMV, if feasible, is the first-line therapy recommended for patients with symptomatic moderate to severe MS, asymptomatic severe MS with significant pulmonary hypertension, and patients with severe MS and new onset atrial fibrillation.

PRACTICE POINT

- Symptomatic patients with severe MS should be referred for percutaneous or surgical therapy as the five-year survival rate without intervention is approximately 40%.

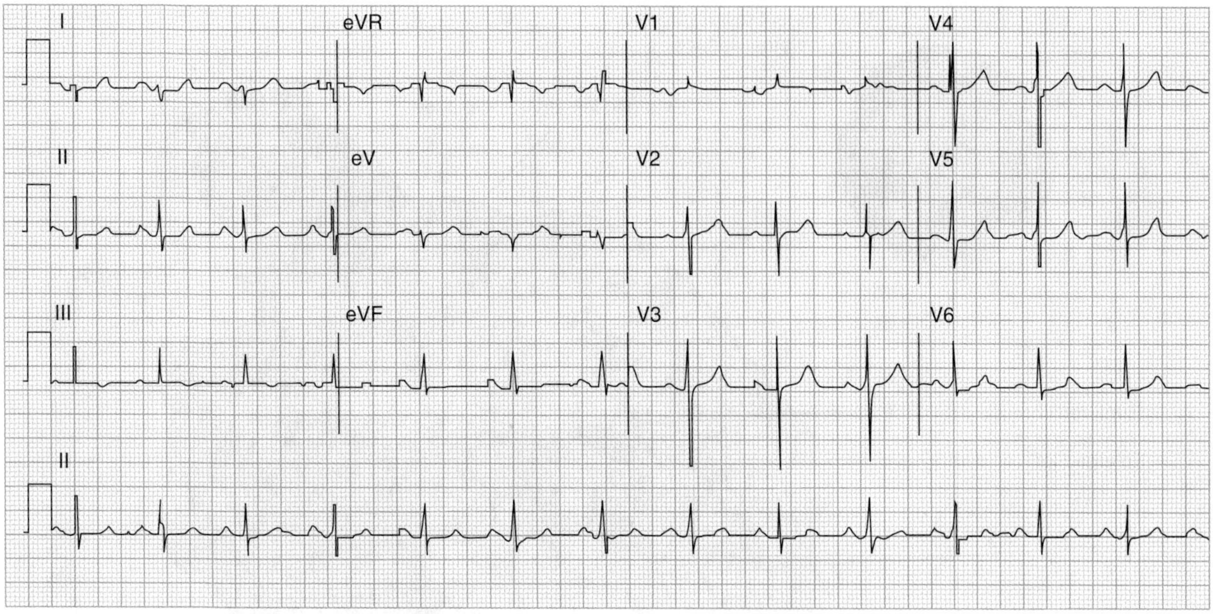

Figure 131-8 *ECG of a patient with mitral stenosis shows left and right atrial abnormality and right axis deviation of the QRS. (Reproduced, with permission, from Fauci AS, Braunwald E, Kasper DL, et al. Harrison's Principles of Internal Medicine. 17th ed. New York: McGraw-Hill, 2008. Figure 19-15. http://www.accessmedicine.com.)*

Complications associated with BMV are uncommon and include embolism with stroke, severe mitral regurgitation, pulmonary edema, and complications from the transseptal puncture (perforation of the left atrium or the aorta requiring surgical repair). Patients who are not favorable candidates for BMV, usually because of extensive leaflet calcification or significant mitral regurgitation, are considered for surgical valve repair or replacement with either a mechanical or bioprosthetic valve, depending on variables such as patient age and ability to take anticoagulation.

MITRAL REGURGITATION

Pathophysiology

Mitral regurgitation (MR) occurs when the coaptation between the mitral leaflets is inadequate to prevent blood from returning back to the left atrium from the left ventricle during systole. A thorough understanding of MR requires knowledge of the mitral valve anatomy and function (**Figure 131-9**). The mitral valve apparatus consists of the anterior and posterior leaflets, which are attached at their base to the fibrous skeleton of the heart at the anterior annulus and to the left ventricle at the posterior annulus respectively. The leaflet tips are connected by the chordae tendinae to the papillary muscles, which originate from the left ventricle. During systole, contraction of the left ventricle and papillary muscles constricts the mitral annulus and steadies the position of the leaflets via the chordate tendinae, allowing adequate coaptation of the anterior and posterior leaflets. The pathophysiology of MR can involve derangements in one or all components of the mitral apparatus (**Table 131-4**).

Acutely, MR enhances left ventricular emptying because a portion of the stroke volume regurgitates into the low pressure left atrium. This regurgitant volume subsequently increases the preload. The decrease in afterload and increase in preload results in a supra-normal left ventricular ejection fraction (eg, EF 75% or 85%). As regurgitation becomes more chronic progressing to severe, the left ventricle hypertrophies and dilates maintaining cardiac output. Over time, the left ventricle will be unable to maintain the cardiac output, the ejection fraction will decrease, the left atrium will dilate and the pulmonary pressure will increase. At that point, the patient will be symptomatic. If the MR is secondary to ventricular dilation (also known as functional MR), the progression of MR occurs after, not before, ventricular failure.

TABLE 131-3 Treatment of Mitral Stenosis

Maintain sinus rhythm if patients develop atrial fibrillation/flutter with antiarrhythmics such as class III and 1C agents and cardioversion.
Rate controlling agents such as beta-blockers, calcium antagonists, and digoxin will help with rate control and moderate transvalvular gradients.
Maintain a low sodium intake and patients often benefit from scheduled diuretics to optimize fluid status.
Anticoagulation in MS patients is recommended for atrial fibrillation (paroxysmal or permanent) regardless of CHADS2 score, as this is a high risk population even in sinus rhythm.

Diagnosis: Does the patient have mitral regurgitation?

The disease progression of MR is variable and depends on the etiology, initial severity of MR, and baseline heart function. Patients with mild, primary MR usually remain asymptomatic for several years unless an acute event occurs such as atrial fibrillation, ruptured chordae, or flail leaflet. Symptoms tend to be a function of the progression of left atrial pressure and pulmonary hypertension rather than left ventricular function. Therefore, *fatigue and exhaustion* can be subtle clues to significant MR with progressively decreasing cardiac output and elevating pulmonary pressure with preserved ejection fraction. At times, significant and sometimes irreversible ventricular dysfunction has occurred by the time symptoms develop. Patients with mild secondary MR have ventricular dysfunction of a varying degree. Progression of MR reflects

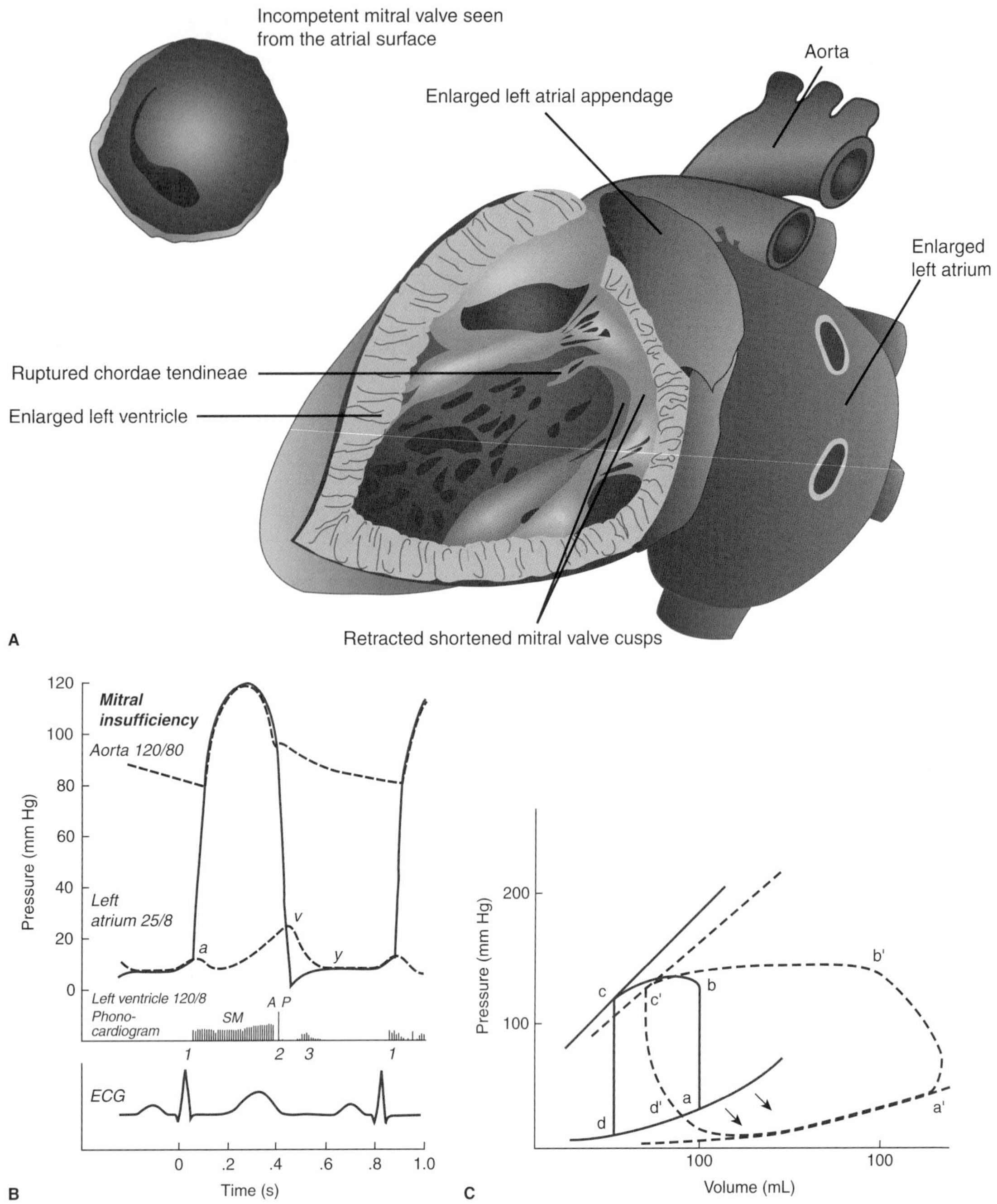

Figure 131-9 *Anatomical drawing (A), pressure tracings (B), and pressure-volume flow loop (C) in a patient with mitral regurgitation. (Reproduced, with permission, from McPhee SJ, Hammer GD. Pathophysiology of Disease: An Introduction to Clinical Medicine. 6th ed. New York: McGraw-Hill; 2010. Fig. 10-26.)*

progression of LV disease with remodeling. Symptoms of heart failure reflect a combination of the severity of MR and the amount of LV dysfunction. Physical exam findings include holosystolic murmur and diastolic rumble (**Table 131-5**).

Evaluation and management of MR requires echocardiography to evaluate for complications and candidacy for medical or surgical interventions. Echocardiography aids the diagnosis, quantification, etiology, and potential repair of MR. Transthoracic echocardiography can assess left atrial size, pulmonary pressures, and LV dimensions, which can be followed serially for subtle progression of disease prior to symptom onset. Transesophageal echocardiography better visualizes the mitral valve for assessing etiology and repair options. MR severity is often qualified by the size of the color regurgitant jet and whether it reaches the posterior wall of the left atrium. Other methods of quantitating MR severity include reversal of the pulmonary vein flow during systole, an effective regurgitant orifice of >0.40 cm^2 and a regurgitant volume $>50\%$. Electrocardiography (ECG) typically shows left atrial abnormality and/or atrial fibrillation and may show signs of right ventricular enlargement if pulmonary hypertension is significant (**Figure 131-10**). On chest radiography, LV enlargement, left atrial enlargement, and pulmonary edema may be seen (**Figure 131-11**). Calcification on the lateral projection in the position of the annulus may be present, especially prominent

TABLE 131-4 Mitral Regurgitation (MR) Causes

Primary Causes Disease of the leaflets	Secondary Causes Disease of the ventricle with normal leaflets
Redundancy, retraction, deformity, or perforations of the leaflets: • Myxomatous degeneration (ie, mitral valve prolapse or fibroelastic deficiency) • Rheumatic fever (RF) • Endocarditis **Abnormalities of the chordae** • Shortening (inflammation secondary to RF or endocarditis) • Lengthening (mitral valve prolapse) **Papillary muscle dysfunction** • Coronary ischemia/infarct • Can cause severe MR because of leaflet tethering or flail leaflet	**Dilatation of the mitral annulus** • Left ventricular dilation • Mitral annular calcification **Ischemia causing regional myocardial dysfunction at the papillary muscle insertion** • May result in papillary dysfunction with resultant MR

TABLE 131-5 Mitral Regurgitation Physical Examination Findings

Severe MR Physical Exam
Diminished S_1 due to defective leaflet closure and loud P_2 component of S_2 heralding significant pulmonary hypertension
Audible diastolic rumble and an S_3 due to the increased volume across the valve into the ventricle
Holosystolic murmur, high pitched, at the apex, sternum or back depending on the direction of the regurgitant jet
When the murmur is not holosystolic it is likely not severe and one should consider mitral valve prolapse, which exhibits a late peaking murmur and is preceded by a midsystolic click

PRACTICE POINT

- Symptoms in mitral regurgitation (MR) correlate with progression of left atrial pressure and pulmonary hypertension rather than left ventricular function. Therefore, *fatigue and exhaustion* can be subtle clues to significant MR.
- Echocardiographic findings of left atrial size, pulmonary pressures, and LV dimensions can be followed serially for progression of disease prior to symptom onset.

in end stage renal disease and elderly patients. Cardiac magnetic resonance imaging can quantitate regurgitant volume and assess details of the valve apparatus, particularly when the echocardiogram is difficult to interpret. Regurgitant severity can also be assessed in the catheterization lab with left ventricular angiography.

Treatment

Medical therapy is targeted at decreasing the amount of MR and treating underlying left ventricular dysfunction. The amount of MR depends on the size of the regurgitant orifice and the pressure

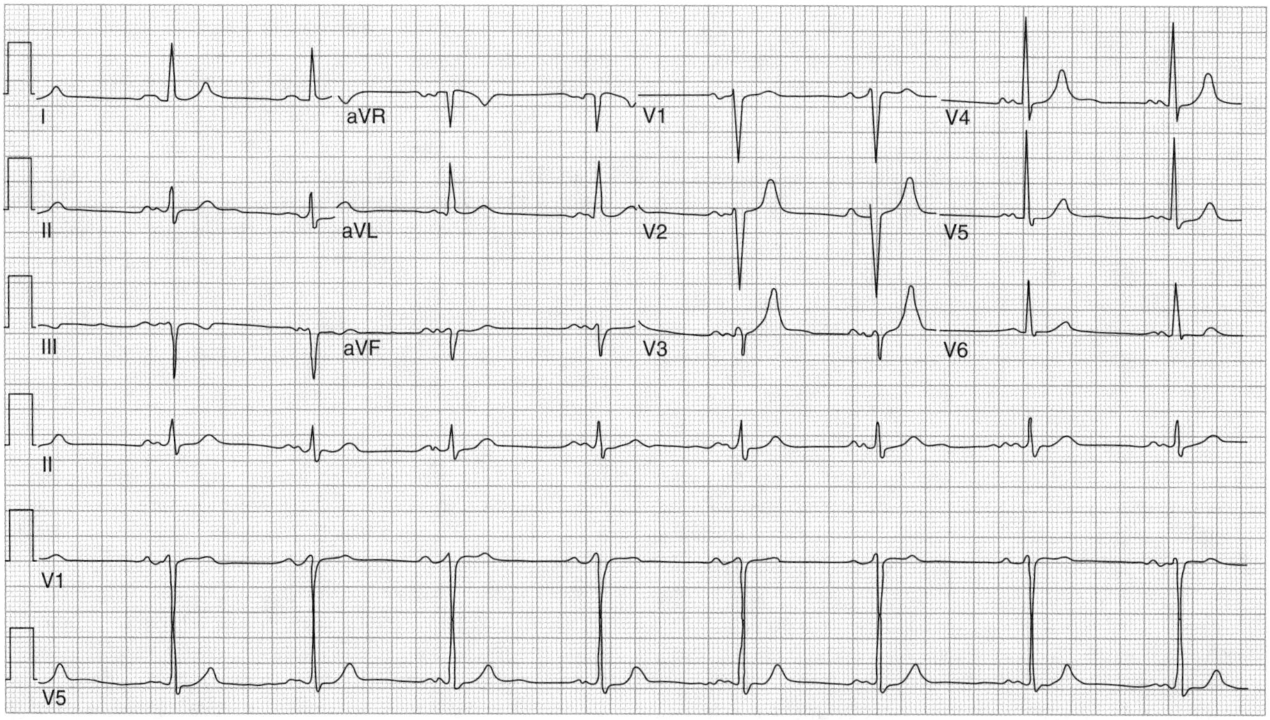

Figure 131-10 *ECG in a patient with mitral regurgitation demonstrating left atrial abnormality, based on p-wave with a "double-hump" in leads II, V4, V5, and V6. (Reproduced, with permission, from Fuster V, O'Rourke RA, Walsh RA, et al. Hurst's the Heart. 12th ed. New York: McGraw-Hill, 2008. Fig. 76-9.)*

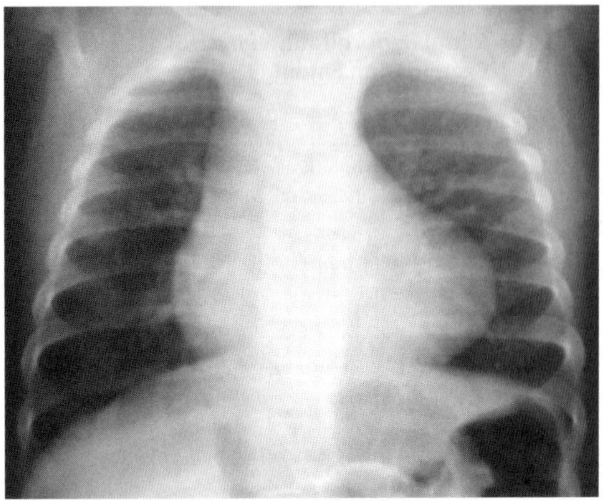

Figure 131-11 *Chest radiograph from a patient with mitral regurgitation shows enlarged left atrium, left ventricle and mild pulmonary edema. (Reproduced, with permission, from Chen MYM, Pope TL, Ott TJ. Basic Radiology. New York: McGraw-Hill. Fig. 3-36.)*

difference between the left ventricle and left atrium. Decreasing left ventricular preload and afterload will decrease the pressure (and size) of the ventricle and thus, medical therapy consists of preload reducing agents (eg, diuretics) and afterload reducing agents (eg, angiotensin converting enzyme [ACE] inhibitors). These therapies are effective for acute MR. In chronic MR however, the systemic vascular resistance is usually decreased and debate regarding benefit of afterload reduction in affecting forward volumes and preserving systolic function leads to some practice variation.

In patients with primary LV dysfunction and secondary MR, medical therapy consists of beta blockade and possibly ACE-inhibitors. Endocarditis prophylaxis is not recommended and any patients exhibiting atrial fibrillation should have chronotropic control and anticoagulation if appropriate. Ultimately, surgical intervention should be considered for patients with significant symptoms and/or mild to no symptoms, but with signs of deteriorating ventricular function. Outcomes of surgical valve repair or replacement are significantly improved if the ejection fraction is >60% and/or left ventricular end systolic dimensions are <40 mm at time of surgery for primary MR. Asymptomatic patients with significant MR and normal ejection fraction and dimensions should be followed with serial transthoracic echocardiograms every 6–12 months along with regular physical examinations. Indications for surgical repair of secondary MR are more controversial, particularly for ischemic MR, and should be discussed in detail with a cardiac surgeon and cardiologist who have extensive experience in valvular heart disease.

Surgical treatment consists of mitral repair or replacement. Mitral valve repair is the preferred therapy if possible. Repair consists of leaflet reconstruction and an annuloplasty ring with excellent results based on appropriate patient selection. Repair also offers greater chance for preservation of the subvalvular apparatus and a lower risk of thromboembolism, structural deterioration, or endocarditis compared with valve replacement. Patients with deformed leaflets secondary to rheumatic heart disease, rigid calcified leaflets second to end stage renal disease, or older patients may have better outcomes with valve replacement. Regardless of whether repair or replacement is selected, preservation of the chordae and papillary muscles helps preserve left ventricular function.

Mitral valve repair or replacement has the potential to significantly improve ventricular function when the valve has primary dysfunction, whereas functional or secondary MR has less potential for ventricular recovery as the primary problem is the cardiomyopathy. Catheter-based therapies for valve replacement and repair are under investigation and may become an effective therapy for MR in the future.

PULMONARY VALVE DISORDERS

PULMONIC STENOSIS

Pathophysiology

Pulmonic stenosis is a valvular abnormality that obstructs blood flow between the right ventricle and the pulmonary arteries. Pulmonic valve stenosis is normally uncommon and when present is usually secondary to congenital pulmonic stenosis (PS), prevalent in 8–10% of pediatric and up to 15% of adult congenital cases. A congenitally malformed valve can range from a trileaflet valve with fusion at the commissures, a thickened dysplastic valve, an imperforate membrane, or atresia. PS can occur in isolation or as part of a multiorgan congenital disease such as Noonan syndrome. Acquired etiologies such as rheumatic heart disease are rare and rheumatic disease usually involves other valves if present on the pulmonic valve. Malignant carcinoid can involve the pulmonic valve in addition to the tricuspid valve (see below). Obstruction of the valve can also be extrinsic to the valve as a consequence of cardiac tumors or sinus of valsalva aneurysm. The right ventricle usually tolerates mild to moderate obstruction well, with minimal dilatation or reduction in function.

Diagnosis: Does the patient have pulmonic stenosis?

Adults with mild to moderate obstruction usually remain asymptomatic and infrequently progress to significant PS. In 15–20% of the patients, the obstruction can worsen with outflow tract obstruction leading to symptoms of fatigue, dyspnea, and chest pain.

On physical exam, the murmur of PS depends on the pliability of the valve. The murmur is best auscultated in the left upper sternal border (LUSB) and may be associated with an ejection click. Often, a singular second heart sound without an ejection click is heard if the valve motion is significantly restricted. The ECG may be normal in mild to moderate cases. As severity progresses, right ventricular hypertrophy and strain can manifest on the ECG as a tall R wave or an rSR′ in lead V_1 with predominant S waves in the lateral leads (**Figure 131-12**). Chest radiography reveals normal heart borders and vasculature in mild to moderate disease but with severe obstruction there can be right atrial and ventricular enlargement. Echocardiography is the definitive tool to assess for severity, cause, and characterization of the valve to determine appropriate therapy. A peak gradient >50 mm Hg across the pulmonic valve is considered significant.

Treatment

The options for therapy for PS focus on relief of the obstruction but depend on the status of the valve and cause of obstruction. A membrane or atresia usually requires creation of a tract and dilatation surgically. If stenosis is secondary to a valve with commissural fusion, balloon valvuloplasty can be performed with excellent long-term results. Even in the setting of a dysplastic valve, the results with valvuloplasty are usually favorable, though not as long lasting as with commissural fusion. For patients who are not candidates for valvuloplasty, surgical replacement of the valve is indicated usually in conjunction with patch repair of any supravalvular obstruction. Regardless of the therapy, the prognosis

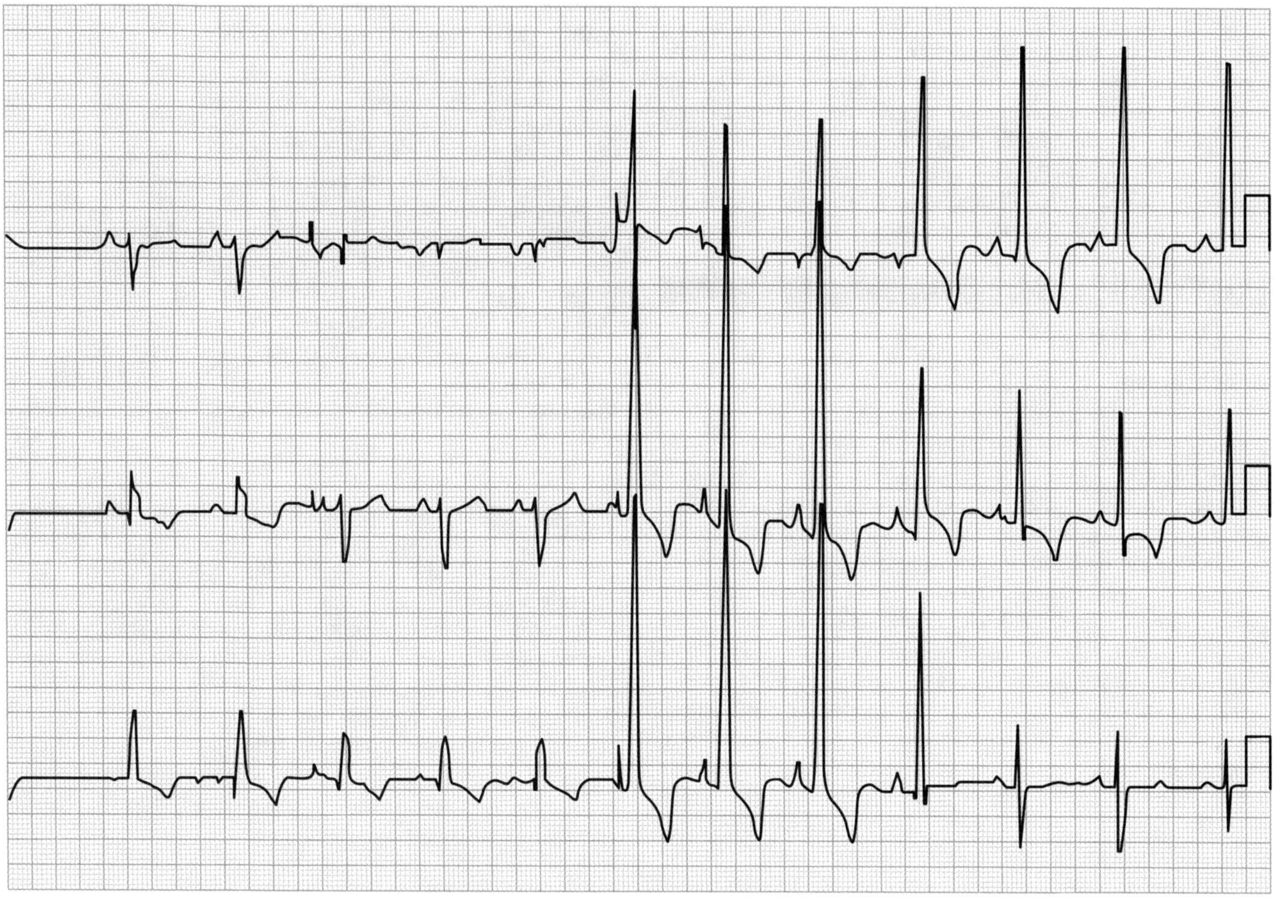

Figure 131-12 *Electrocardiograph in congenital pulmonic stenosis with sereve right ventricular hypertrophy and marked right-axis deviation. (Reproduced, with permission, from Crawford MH. Current Diagnosis & Treatment: Cardiology. 3rd ed. New York: McGraw-Hill, 2009. Fig. 28-3.)*

of PS is excellent if there is adequate relief of the obstruction and preserved right ventricular function and size.

PULMONIC REGURGITATION

Pathophysiology

The most common etiology of pulmonic regurgitation (PR) is dilatation of the annular ring secondary to pulmonary hypertension (eg, pulmonary hypertension with MS), or connective tissue disorder (eg, dilation of the pulmonary artery with Marfan syndrome). Less commonly, diseases that cause deformation in the architecture of the leaflets can lead to regurgitation. These include rheumatic heart disease, endocarditis, malignant carcinoid, and congenital malformation of the valve (also associated with other cardiac anomalies such as Tetralogy of Fallot and pulmonic stenosis). Direct trauma from right heart catheterization or surgical misadventure has been documented.

Diagnosis: Does the patient have pulmonic regurgitation?

PR can lead to right ventricular volume overload and is usually tolerated well over years without symptoms unless right ventricular failure or pulmonary hypertension ensues. Patients with PR from endocarditis can have septic pulmonary emboli, which can lead to pulmonary hypertension. If pulmonary hypertension develops, PR can progress and worsen right-sided failure. Most patients complain of dyspnea and fatigue. In addition to classic cardiac exam findings (**Table 131-6**), physical examination findings can include peripheral edema and ascites with liver dysfunction with severe right heart failure.

The electrocardiogram often is normal in mild to moderate cases but will begin to reflect right ventricular overload and hypertrophy as failure worsens and pulmonary hypertension ensues. The chest radiograph is usually nonspecific but may show pulmonary artery and right ventricular enlargement at the borders. Cardiac magnetic resonance is especially usefully in quantifying the regurgitant volume and assessing the valve structure, geometry, and function of the right ventricle. Echocardiography remains the gold standard for assessing regurgitant severity, valve anatomy, and pulmonary hypertension. Criteria for severity of PR by echocardiography are similar to that of AR.

TABLE 131-6 Pulmonic Regurgitation Physical Examination Findings

Diastolic murmur best auscultated at the left parasternal third to fourth intercostal spaces, usually low pitched, occurring immediately after P_2
The murmur can be high pitched in the presence of significant pulmonary hypertension (Graham Steell murmur)
P_2 accentuated in the presence of pulmonary hypertension
Palpable tap in the second intercostal space, reflecting pulmonic valve closure at elevated pressures

Treatment

PR usually remains clinically unimportant and rarely requires intervention. Often therapy directed at the causal event (eg, MS) will relieve PR by decreasing pulmonary hypertension. Surgical therapy for primary PR is indicated for progressive right heart failure and volume overload. As a rule, a pulmonic allograft or porcine bioprosthesis are typically chosen. Catheter-based valve implantation is currently available for high risk surgical patients with PR and/or PS.

TRICUSPID VALVE DISORDERS

TRICUSPID STENOSIS

Pathophyisology

Triscuspid stenosis (TS) is an uncommon condition that obstructs the flow of blood from the right atrium to the right ventricle during diastole. Distortion of the tricuspid valve apparatus with commissural fusion, shortened chordae, and decrease in valve orifice are the findings of TS regardless of etiology. Because the pressures in the right side of the heart are normally low, a pressure gradient ≥5 mm Hg across the tricuspid valve can result in elevated right atrial pressures. Chronically elevated right atrial pressures lead to signs and symptoms of systemic venous congestion, including prominent jugular venous pulsations with an exaggerated a-wave, lower extremity edema, ascites, and liver congestion/dysfunction. In more severe forms of TS, pulmonary blood flow is significantly decreased and cardiac output can become limited, especially with exercise. Right atrial enlargement and hypertrophy can contribute to the development of atrial fibrillation, which significantly exaggerates the symptoms of venous congestion. The most common etiologies include rheumatic heart disease (RHD), carcinoid disease, congenital heart disease, and infective endocarditis.

RHD is the most common cause of TS in the U.S. and throughout the world. Isolated tricuspid valve involvement is rare, and clinical TS is usually discovered concomitantly with mitral and aortic valve disease. The overall incidence of TS in patients with RHD has been estimated at 9% to 15%, with clinically significant and more severe forms occurring in only 5%.

Carcinoid heart disease occurs in patients who have primary intestinal tumors with metastasis to the liver. The incidence of carcinoid heart disease is approximately 1 in 300,000 of the population. The metastatic carcinoid tumors produce paraneoplastic substances (serotonin), which lead to the characteristic endocardial fibrous white plaque formation within the valve leaflets and tricuspid valve chordal apparatus. These fibrous depositions lead to valve distortion with foreshortened leaflets that are unable to open or close (frozen valve), resulting in TS and often tricuspid valve regurgitation.

Infective endocarditis affecting the tricuspid valve can also lead to TS and is most common among those who are intravenous illicit drug users or those who have anatomically abnormal tricuspid valves at baseline. Congenital TS is extremely rare with an incidence occurring in less than 0.1% of the population.

Diagnosis: Does the patient have tricuspid stenosis?

Although the age range can vary, patients usually present in their third or fourth decades (age 40 to 60 years). Most patients with symptomatic TS will present with fatigue, extremity swelling, abdominal discomfort, or dyspnea that is slowly progressive over a period of months to years. Antecedent history of rheumatic fever (RF) or heart murmur should be elicited on history. Many adult patients may not have been informed of their actual diagnosis during childhood or the disease may never have been discovered. These patients may only remember an illness with a prolonged fever, rash, or severe joint pain requiring prolonged bed rest and absence from school. A history of persistent heart murmur beginning in late childhood that has been passed off as benign or innocent may also be the only historical clue to antecedent episode of RF.

TABLE 131-7 Signs of Tricuspid Stenosis

Physical Exam
Jugular venous pulsations elevated and a prominent presystolic a-wave during atrial contraction
Hepatomegaly, ascites, and peripheral edema with moderate-to-severe TS
Low frequency presystolic murmur *usually* auscultated at the lower left sternal border in the fourth intercostal space, intensified with maneuvers that increase blood flow across the valve (eg, inspiration, squatting, and isotonic exercise)
An opening snap sometimes heard, but diminishes as severity worsens

Features of flushing, diarrhea, and bronchospasm should raise the possibility of carcinoid syndrome, and these patients have a 50% chance of cardiac involvement. The vast majority of patients with cardiac involvement present with signs of right heart failure secondary to severe dysfunction of the tricuspid and pulmonary valves. TS patients may also present with symptoms and signs of endocarditis, including unremitting or recurrent fever with generalized malaise and other physical stigmata. The patient may have an antecedent history of tricuspid valve replacement or intravenous drug use.

Cardiac findings on physical examination can be subtle or misinterpreted (**Table 131-7**). The presystolic murmur of TS is often missed or attributed to mitral valve stenosis. Although characteristics of the two murmurs can help differentiate one from the other, a high index of suspicion must be maintained for tricuspid valve involvement in a patient with multivalvular rheumatic heart disease. Patients with endocarditis-associated TS may present with the physical stigmata of bacterial endocarditis (eg, splinter hemorrhages, Osler nodes, and Janeway lesions).

A comprehensive metabolic profile helps evaluate for significant hepatic congestion associated with systemic venous hypertension and serves as a surrogate for end-organ dysfunction (eg, renal insufficiency). Twenty-four hour urinary excretion of 5-hydroxyindole acetic acid (5-HIAA) may be used to determine whether carcinoid heart disease is present. Blood cultures can help evaluate the possibility of bacterial endocarditis.

Ancillary tests should include CXR, ECG, echocardiogram, and possibly cardiac catheterization. Although there are no clearly defined criteria for tricuspid stenosis severity, severe tricuspid stenosis (TS) is often defined by the onset of overt symptoms accompanied by a mean gradient by echocardiogram or cardiac catheterization of >3 mm Hg, though a gradient >8–10 mm Hg is often observed. Mild to moderate TS is usually asymptomatic, and has no clearly-defined gradient range beyond the definition of TS diagnosed with a gradient of ≤3 mm Hg.

Treatment

The main goal of treatment is to relieve the symptoms that result from restricted diastolic filling of the right ventricle and diminished pulmonary blood flow. Medical care consists of (1) assessment and treatment of the underlying etiology for the valvular pathology (eg, antibiotics for bacterial endocarditis or somatostatin analogs for carcinoid syndrome); (2) fluid and sodium restriction; (3) medications to treat cardiac arrhythmias secondary to right atrial distension (usually

TABLE 131-8 Causes of Tricuspid Regurgitation

Functional causes
Dilatation of the right ventricle/tricuspid annulus from any cause
Secondary causes
Primary leaflet such as Ebstein anomaly, infective endocarditis, trauma, RF, carcinoid syndrome, papillary muscle dysfunction or rupture, marantic endocarditis, and myxomatous degeneration
Tricuspid valve injury from permanent pacemakers, implantable cardioverter-defibrillators, and endomyocardial biopsies
Anorectic drug (eg, fenfluramine and phentermine, "Fen-Phen")
Carcinoid syndrome

atrial fibrillation and/or flutter); and (4) pharmacotherapy with diuretics to reduce morbidity associated with systemic venous congestion.

Surgical valve replacement or commissurotomy is indicated if right heart failure persists or if low cardiac output develops. Successful percutaneous balloon valvotomy has been performed when the subvalvar structures are normal.

TRICUSPID REGURGITATION

Pathophyisology

Tricuspid regurgitation (TR) occurs commonly. Often it is asymptomatic and discovered initially by echocardiography. TR is characterized by backflow of blood into the right atrium from the right ventricle during systole. Since the right atrium is compliant, no major hemodynamic consequences manifest in mild or moderate TR. With severe TR, right atrial and venous pressures rise and patients present with signs and symptoms of right-sided heart failure (**Table 131-8**).

In the past, an association between TR and the combined use of the anorectic drugs fenfluramine and phentermine ("Fen-Phen"), has been described. The dopamine agonist pergolide may induce TR by a mechanism similar to that of anorectic drugs and carcinoid syndrome.

Does the patient have triscupid regurgitation?

The findings of mild to moderate TR are not striking other than an audible murmur. With *severe TR*, patients may exhibit right-sided congestive heart failure including painful hepatosplenomegaly, ascites, and peripheral edema as well as a sensation of pulsation in the neck (from distended and pulsatile jugular veins). In some patients however, no symptoms manifest for many years despite severe regurgitation.

PRACTICE POINT

- In severe tricuspid regurgitation, symptoms of right-sided congestive heart failure (painful hepatosplenomegaly, ascites, and peripheral edema) and a sensation of pulsation in the neck (from distended and pulsatile jugular veins) may occur. Jugular venous distension may be more prominent with inspiration. However, patients may have no symptoms for many years despite severe regurgitation.

Physical examination findings can suggest the presence of TR even in the absence of significant symptoms (**Table 131-9**). The jugular veins of patients with severe TR are distended and prominent, which reflects elevation in right atrial pressure. A prominent

TABLE 131-9 Signs of Tricuspid Regurgitation

Physical Exam
Holosystolic murmur best heard at right or left mid-sternal border or at the subxiphoid area
Physical maneuvers that result in an increase in venous return (leg raising, exercise, hepatic compression) intensify the murmur of TR
Deep inspiration increases venous return to the right ventricle and the murmur of TR becomes louder and longer (Rivero-Carvallo sign)
Right ventricular heave on precordial palpation of the chest due to a dilated right ventricle
Abdominal exam with an enlarged, tender, and pulsatile liver; ascites, peripheral edema, and/or anascara
Unilateral or bilateral pleural effusions when pulmonary hypertension is present

"c-v" wave due to systolic regurgitation into the right atrium is seen. Jugular venous distension may be more prominent with inspiration; this finding may not be obvious with marked venous distension. A systolic thrill may be palpated over the jugular vein in patients with severe TR.

The abdominal exam may reveal an enlarged, tender, and pulsatile liver. The murmur associated with severe TR can be auscultated over the liver coupled with a palpable thrill. The abdominal exam can also reveal ascites, peripheral edema, and in very severe cases anascara. Unilateral or bilateral pleural effusions may occur in the presence of pulmonary hypertension or left-sided cardiac disease.

The ECG often reveals no characteristic changes unless other concomitant disorders are present such as right ventricular infarction, pulmonary hypertension, pulmonary embolus. Chest radiographs of patients with TR reveal cardiomegaly due to right ventricular enlargement. A prominent cardiac silhouette is observed on the right in the PA view, and the enlarged right ventricle fills the retrosternal space in the lateral view. Additional findings may include right atrial enlargement, a prominent azygos vein, pleural effusion, and upward displacement of the diaphragm due to ascites. When the etiology of the TR is pulmonary hypertension secondary to a left-sided cardiac abnormality, other radiographic findings may be seen, particularly prominent right and left pulmonary artery hilar segments.

Echocardiography is the mainstay of testing in the evaluation of the TR. Tricuspid valve motion may be normal or abnormal. Characteristic primary valvular abnormalities that can be seen by echocardiography include Ebstein anomaly, carcinoid heart disease, RF, prolapse, flail leaflet, and endocarditis. The right ventricle and right atrium are usually dilated in the presence of moderate to severe TR, unless the TR is acute. Doppler color flow establishes the severity of TR. The major Doppler criteria for severe TR are a color jet (vena contracta) width > 0.7 cm and systolic flow reversal in the hepatic veins. Systolic flow reversal may not be accurate when atrial fibrillation is present. Other findings include a dilated tricuspid annulus and paradoxical, interventricular septal motion, which reflect increased volume within the right ventricle (diastolic overload).

Cardiac catheterization and contrast right ventriculography are often not helpful for the diagnosis or evaluation of TR. However, in some patients, invasive evaluation may be performed to determine pulmonary vascular resistance or to evaluate the left heart pressures for causes of functional TR.

Treatment

The treatment of TR depends on the etiology. In functional TR, correction of high pulmonary artery pressures can result in improvement in TR. This has been demonstrated in patients with reversible causes of pulmonary hypertension such as mitral stenosis and chronic thromboembolic pulmonary hypertension. Among patients who undergo surgery for correction of left-sided heart disease, concurrent tricuspid valve annuloplasty is often performed (eg, mitral valve repair with concurrent tricuspid valve repair). Tricuspid annuloplasty for functional TR is rarely ever performed as an isolated procedure as the recurrence rate is high. Treatment of primary TR (often replacement with a tissue or mechanical valve) should be done by a cardiac surgeon that has experience in congenital heart or valvular heart disease.

CONCLUSION

Valvular heart disease is rapidly emerging as a separate subspecialty within cardiology and cardiac surgery. It encompasses multiple pathophysiologic processes due to a myriad of systemic and congenital diseases. Therapies for valvular heart disease continue to evolve as minimally-invasive surgical and catheter-based approaches gain experience. The internist and hospitalist remain the gatekeepers of these patients and should maintain a working understanding of diagnoses and therapies to optimize patient care. Collaboration with a cardiologist or cardiac surgeon that has expertise in this area is essential.

SUGGESTED READINGS

Babaliaros V, Block P. State of the art percutaneous intervention for the treatment of valvular heart disease: a review of the current technologies and ongoing research in the field of percutaneous valve replacement and repair. *Cardiology*. 2007;107:87–96.

Baumgartner H, Hung J, Bermejo J, et al. Echocardiographic assessment of valve stenosis: EAE/ASE recommendations for clinical practice. *J Am Soc Echocardiogr*. 2009;22:1–23; quiz 101–102.

Bonow RO, Carabello BA, Chatterjee K, et al. 2008 focused update incorporated into the ACC/AHA 2006 guidelines for the management of patients with valvular heart disease: a report of the American College of Cardiology/American Heart Association Task Force on Practice Guidelines (Writing Committee to revise the 1998 guidelines for the management of patients with valvular heart disease). Endorsed by the Society of Cardiovascular Anesthesiologists, Society for Cardiovascular Angiography and Interventions, and Society of Thoracic Surgeons. *J Am Coll Cardiol*. 2008;52:e1–e142.

Bonow RO, Carabello BA, Chatterjee K, et al. ACC/AHA 2006 guidelines for the management of patients with valvular heart disease: a report of the American College of Cardiology/American Heart Association Task Force on Practice Guidelines (Writing Committee to Revise the 1998 guidelines for the management of patients with valvular heart disease) developed in collaboration with the Society of Cardiovascular Anesthesiologists endorsed by the Society for Cardiovascular Angiography and Interventions and the Society of Thoracic Surgeons. *J Am Coll Cardiol*. 2006;48:e1–e148.

Carabello BA, Crawford FA Jr., Valvular heart disease. *N Engl J Med*. 1997;337:32–41.

Carabello BA. Is it ever too late to operate on the patient with valvular heart disease? *J Am Coll Cardiol*. 2004;44:376–383.

Feldman T, Leon MB. Prospects for percutaneous valve therapies. *Circulation*. 2007;116:2866–2877.

Zoghbi WA, Enriquez-Sarano M, Foster E, et al. Recommendations for evaluation of the severity of native valvular regurgitation with two-dimensional and Doppler echocardiography. *J Am Soc Echocardiogr*. 2003;16:777–802.

CHAPTER 132

Myocarditis, Pericardial Disease, and Cardiac Tamponade

Benjamin D. Mackie, MD
Matthew E. Certain, MD
Stephen D. Clements Jr., MD

Key Clinical Questions

1. What are the most common etiologies of pericarditis and myocarditis?
2. How are pericarditis and myocarditis diagnosed?
3. Which imaging modality is most accurate in diagnosing myocarditis?
4. What are the evidence-based physical examination, radiographic, electrocardiographic, and imaging findings used in the diagnosis of cardiac tamponade, and how is it managed?
5. What are the differences in physical examination, testing results, and treatment of constrictive pericarditis versus cardiac tamponade?

MYOCARDITIS

INTRODUCTION

Acute myocarditis is an inflammatory infiltration of the myocardium. The clinical sequelae of this disease include subclinical disease to fulminant cardiogenic shock.

Acute myocarditis can present a challenging diagnostic dilemma. Traditionally, the diagnosis of myocarditis is made by endomyocardial biopsy. In acute myocarditis, biopsy shows areas of necrosis with a lymphocytic infiltration. However, endomyocardial biopsy is subject to procedural risks, sampling bias, and poor sensitivity. Noninvasive cardiac magnetic resonance imaging (MRI) has become an alternative mechanism for diagnosing myocarditis.

PATHOPHYSIOLOGY

The most common cause of myocarditis is a viral pathogen. However, other infectious, autoimmune, and toxic causes occur as well. Initial studies in the latter half of the 20th century indicated Coxsackie B virus as the frequent causative agent in endomyocardial biopsies. However, since the 1990s adenovirus has emerged as the more frequent viral agent. Since that time, parvovirus and other viruses have been seen in the biopsy results of patients with myocarditis. Other viral causes of acute myocarditis have been reported in patients with hepatitis C virus (HCV), Epstein-Barr virus, and cytomegalovirus (CMV).

Infectious etiologies other than viruses have been implicated as a cause of myocarditis, including mycoplasma and *Borrelia burgdorferi* (Lyme disease). In developing countries, *Trypanosoma cruzi* has been known to infect the myocardium causing Chagas disease.

PRESENTATION

The clinical presentation of patients with myocarditis can range from mild dyspnea and chest discomfort to fulminant cardiogenic shock. Patients may report a viral prodrome in the weeks preceding presentation, including fevers, respiratory, or GI symptoms. According to the European Study of Epidemiology and Treatment of Inflammatory Heart Disease, patients with myocarditis present with dyspnea (72%), chest pain (32%), and arrhythmias (18%). Patients may also present with symptoms related to congestive heart failure, including fatigue, orthopnea, paroxysmal nocturnal dyspnea, palpitations, and syncope.

As an infiltrative process, the amount of affected myocardium can be highly variable in myocarditis. Some patients may present with ventricular arrhythmias if the conducting system is involved while other patients may present with a dilated cardiomyopathy.

The physical examination of patients with acute myocarditis may correlate with the patients' symptoms. In patients with mild symptoms, the physical examination may be relatively normal. However, patients with severe myocarditis may appear in cardiogenic shock. Diaphoresis, rales, jugular venous distention, hypotension, and peripheral edema can all be seen in patients with myocarditis.

DIAGNOSIS

The electrocardiogram (ECG) in myocarditis may show sinus tachycardia and nonspecific ST-segment changes and T-wave inversion. ST-segment elevation and Q-waves that suggest acute myocardial ischemia can occur in myocarditis. Patients may also present with bundle-branch blocks, atrioventricular block, or ventricular tachyarrhythmias. An associated pericarditis may be present in patients with myocarditis, so called myopericarditis, which can also cause diffuse ST-segment elevation in addition to PR-segment depression.

PRACTICE POINT

ECG findings in acute pericarditis include:

- Diffuse ST-segment elevation
  - Hexaxial and precordial leads with the exception of AVR and V_1 which may have ST-segment depression
  - Concave shape and no accompanied by reciprocal changes
  - No T-wave inversion and no associated Q-waves
- PR depression, all leads except AVR and V_1 which may show PR elevation
- ECG changes last up to two weeks

Patients with myocarditis can have elevated biomarkers, such as troponin-I, CK-MB, and CPK. Troponin-I levels are more commonly elevated than other cardiac biomarkers. However, troponin-I elevation has a low sensitivity (34%) for myocarditis.

The white blood cell count may range from completely normal to a mild leukocytosis in patients with myocarditis. Viral myocarditis may cause a nonspecific lymphocytic predominance. Eosinophilia may be associated with drug-induced myocarditis or an infiltrative disease like Churg-Strauss. Thrombocytopenia may be present due to the acute viral illness, or from splenic sequestration due to splenomegaly, which may accompany congestive heart failure.

The serum chemistry in patients with suspected myocarditis varies according to the disease burden of the myocardium. Severely affected individuals may have chemistries that correlate with congestive heart failure, including hyponatremia due to sodium dysregulation and reduced kidney function due to poor cardiac output. Elevated liver transaminases (AST and ALT) along with markers of synthetic function (PT/INR, PTT) may be elevated due to hepatic congestion.

Chest radiography may reveal pulmonary vascular congestion and cardiomegaly due to a dilated cardiomyopathy or pneumonia if the myocarditis is caused by mycoplasma.

The role of echocardiography in the diagnosis of myocarditis is nonspecific. Even in severe cases of myocarditis, echocardiography may only identify a dilated cardiomyopathy or, less commonly, hypertrophic or restrictive cardiomyopathies. Regional wall motion abnormalities may mimic changes commonly seen with ischemia.

Although echocardiography has been the traditional imaging modality of choice, it can be normal in less severe cases of myocarditis. Therefore, computed tomography or magnetic resonance imaging may be considered in the diagnosis of myocarditis when echocardiography is nondiagnostic. MRI identifies myocarditis in 30% of patients with chest pain, elevated troponins, and normal coronary arteries. In cases where edema, capillary leak and necrosis can be assessed, cardiac MRI has a sensitivity of 67%, a specificity of 91%, and a diagnostic accuracy of 78%.

PRACTICE POINT

- Computed tomography or magnetic resonance imaging can assist in the diagnosis of myocarditis when echocardiography is nondiagnostic. MRI identifies myocarditis in 30% of patients with chest pain, elevated troponins, and normal coronary arteries. Cardiac MRI has a sensitivity of 67%, a specificity of 91%, and a diagnostic accuracy of 78%.

Endomyocardial biopsy is the gold standard for diagnosing myocarditis. However, the biopsy procedure has obvious risks, can vary by interpreter, lacks prognostic value, and has a low sensitivity due to sampling error. For these reasons, endomyocardial biopsy should be reserved for cases when other infiltrative disorders are in the differential diagnosis, such as cardiac sarcoidosis or giant cell myocarditis. Histologically, an inflammatory cellular infiltrate may be seen with or without myocyte necrosis.

PRACTICE POINT

- Endomyocardial biopsy should be reserved for cases when other infiltrative disorders are in the differential diagnosis, such as cardiac sarcoidosis or giant cell myocarditis.

MANAGEMENT

The low incidence of myocarditis precludes performing randomized controlled trials with sufficient power to assess therapeutic regimens. The basis of therapy for patients with myocarditis remains largely supportive. The majority of patients with myocarditis will recover fully. For the patients with a stable clinical course, the basis of therapy resides in angiotensin-converting enzme (ACE) inhibitors, beta-blockers, and diuretic therapy. Patients with severe left ventricular (LV) dysfunction can rapidly progress to cardiogenic shock. These patients may require a left ventricular assist device (LVAD) or extracorporeal membrane oxygenation (ECMO) as a bridge to cardiac transplantation.

Patients with myocarditis may have an increased risk of arrhythmias, requiring temporary pacemakers for bradycardia or complete heart block, or antiarrhythmic agents such as amiodarone for ventricular tachyarrhythmias. For patients who present with or have ventricular arrhythmias after the diagnosis of myocarditis, implantable cardiac defibrillators (ICD) may be considered once the acute phase of the illness has resolved. In addition to patients with ventricular tachycardia or fibrillation, those patients with an ejection fraction less than 35% following resolution of the acute phase of myocarditis, should be considered for ICD implantation. It should be noted that patients under consideration for ICD placement should have a life expectancy longer than one year on optimal medical therapy.

While myocarditis is a lymphocytic infiltrative disease, immunosuppressive agents show only marginal beneficial effects. One small trial suggests that patients with human leukocyte antigen expression on biopsy have modest benefit (ejection fraction improvement and New York Heart Association [NYHA] class) from prednisone and azathioprine.

PERICARDITIS

INTRODUCTION

Acute pericarditis is defined as signs and/or symptoms consistent with pericardial inflammation of less than three weeks' duration. The true incidence of pericarditis is difficult to quantify since many cases go undiagnosed. Pericarditis may account for up to 1% of cases of ST elevations on ECG, and account for 5% of emergency room visits. Eighty percent to 90% of cases of pericarditis are idiopathic.

PATHOPHYSIOLOGY

Pericarditis can be an acute, subacute, or chronic process. The etiology of acute pericarditis is often idiopathic or viral, though the pericardium can be affected by numerous other disease processes including infectious, neoplastic, autoimmune, and traumatic causes (**Table 132-1**).

TABLE 132-1 Causes of Pericardial Heart Disease

Idiopathic
Infectious
Bacterial (*Pneumococcus, Streptococcus, Staphylococcus, Haemophilus influenzae*, gram-negative rods, *Brucella melitensis, Francisella tularensis, Legionella pneumophila, Neisseria gonorrhoeae, Neisseria meningitidis, Borrelia burgdorferi* [Lyme disease], *Mycoplasma*)
Viral (Coxsackievirus, echovirus, adenovirus, varicella, influenza, cytomegalovirus, HIV, hepatitis B, mumps, infectious mononucleosis)
Mycobacterial (*Mycobacterium tuberculosis, Mycobacterium avium-intracellulare*)
Fungal (*Histoplasma, Coccidioidomycosis, Blastomyces, Candida albicans, Nocardia, Actinomyces*)
Protozoal (*Toxoplasma, Echinococcus*, amebae)
AIDS associated
Neoplastic
Primary (mesothelioma, fibrosarcoma)
Secondary (breast, lung, melanoma, lymphoma, leukemia)
Immune/Inflammatory
Connective tissue diseases (rheumatoid arthritis, systemic lupus erythematosus, scleroderma, acute rheumatic fever, dermatomyositis, mixed connective tissue disease, Wegener granulomatosis)
Arteritis (temporal arteritis, polyarteritis nodosa, Takayasu's arteritis)
Acute myocardial infarction and post myocardial infarction (Dressler syndrome)
Postcardiotomy, posttraumatic
Metabolic
Nephrogenic, myxedema, amyloidosis, aortic dissection
Drugs
Hydralazine, procainamide, daunorubicin, isoniazid, anticoagulants, cyclosporine, methysergide, phenytoin, dantrolene, mesalazine
Traumatic
Blunt trauma, surgical trauma, penetrating trauma, instrument/device trauma (implantable defibrillators, pacemakers, catheters)
Congenital
Pericardial cysts, congenital absence of pericardium, Mulibrey nanism

Although the pericardium is not required to maintain life, it serves many functions within the thorax. The pericardium is composed of two layers. An inner layer, the visceral pericardium, adheres to the epicardial surface of the heart and consists of a layer of mesothelial cells. The outer layer is an avascular, fibrous parietal layer and consists of elastin fibers embedded within compact layers of collagen. The visceral pericardium reflects back near the great vessels and forms the inner layer of the parietal pericardium. The pericardial space is formed from these two layers and normally contains up to 50 mL of an ultrafiltrate of plasma. In the pericardium, villi and cilia enhance the resorption of fluid. The capacity of the pericardium to accept increased fluid volume depends on the rate of accumulation. A rapid addition of 50 to 200 mL will dramatically increase pressure and affect cardiac function, whereas a very slow accumulation of large amounts of fluid as in myxedema will have little effect on pressure or hemodynamics.

The collagen matrix of the parietal pericardium gives the pericardium its unique mechanical properties. Functionally, the pericardium facilitates contraction and relaxation of the ventricles and atria, allowing pressure changes on one side of the heart to be transmitted to the other side. Additionally, the pericardium's mechanical properties may determine cardiac output during exercise via the pericardium's direct limitation of the cardiac filling volumes.

PRESENTATION

Acute pericarditis presents with chest pain of abrupt onset as the most common complaint. The pain can be quite severe, sharp in character, and nearly always pleuritic in nature. The sharp pain of acute pericarditis differs from the pressure-like discomfort of myocardial ischemia. The pain may be located substernally or located in the anterior chest, and radiation to the neck, arms and shoulders can also occur (**Figure 132-1**).

The phrenic nerve, which innervates the trapezius muscles, traverses the pericardium; therefore, radiation to the either trapezius ridge of the left shoulder is very specific for pericardial pain. Classically, the pain associated with pericarditis will improve with sitting up and leaning forward and is exacerbated by lying flat or with slight changes in position. Associated symptoms include dyspnea from splinting due to pain, cough, myalgia, arthralgias, and occasionally hiccoughs.

Vital signs in patients with pericarditis may be normal or show low-grade fever and tachycardia. High fever may indicate a bacterial cause, and these patients should undergo echocardiographic evaluation. There may be associated tachypnea from the dyspnea or pain. The most specific, and pathognomonic, finding associated with pericarditis is the pericardial friction rub. This scratchy, superficial sound likely results from inflamed visceral and parietal pericardium rubbing against each other. Classically, there are three components correlating with ventricular systole, ventricular diastole, and atrial systole. All components, two components, one component, or none may be present, as the finding is not sensitive. Two components would be expected in atrial fibrillation due to loss of the atrial component; rapid heart rates may only produce two components due to summation of the early diastolic rub and presystolic rub. The rub may be composed solely of the ventricular component, which is the last to leave over the course of illness. These rubs, described as triphasic, biphasic, or monophasic, may be confused with other cardiac abnormalities, especially in patients with a monophasic rub, which may be mistaken for a murmur.

The pericardial friction rub is best heard at the left sternal border, often in a well-localized spot but may be heard only at the apex. Therefore, the examiner needs to take a systematic approach to auscultation; position the patient forward or even on his hands and knees with the chest down or lying on his abdomen propped up on his elbows; use the diaphragm of the stethoscope against the chest wall with forced expiration; and listen over the entire left precordium. Frequent examinations may be required to hear the friction rub given its fleeting nature. The sound has been described as the sound produced when walking through snow, or pulling apart two pieces of Velcro. The rub of pericarditis may sound very similar to the harsh sound of Hamman crunch (heard in some patients with pneumomediastinum); care should be taken to differentiate these two auscultatory findings. In uncomplicated pericarditis, the jugular venous waveforms remain unchanged.

DIAGNOSIS

The initial approach to the patient with suspected pericarditis is based on a thorough history, physical examination and testing—ECG, cardiac enzymes, basic chemistry, complete blood count, erythrocyte sedimentation rate (ESR) or C-reactive protein (CRP),

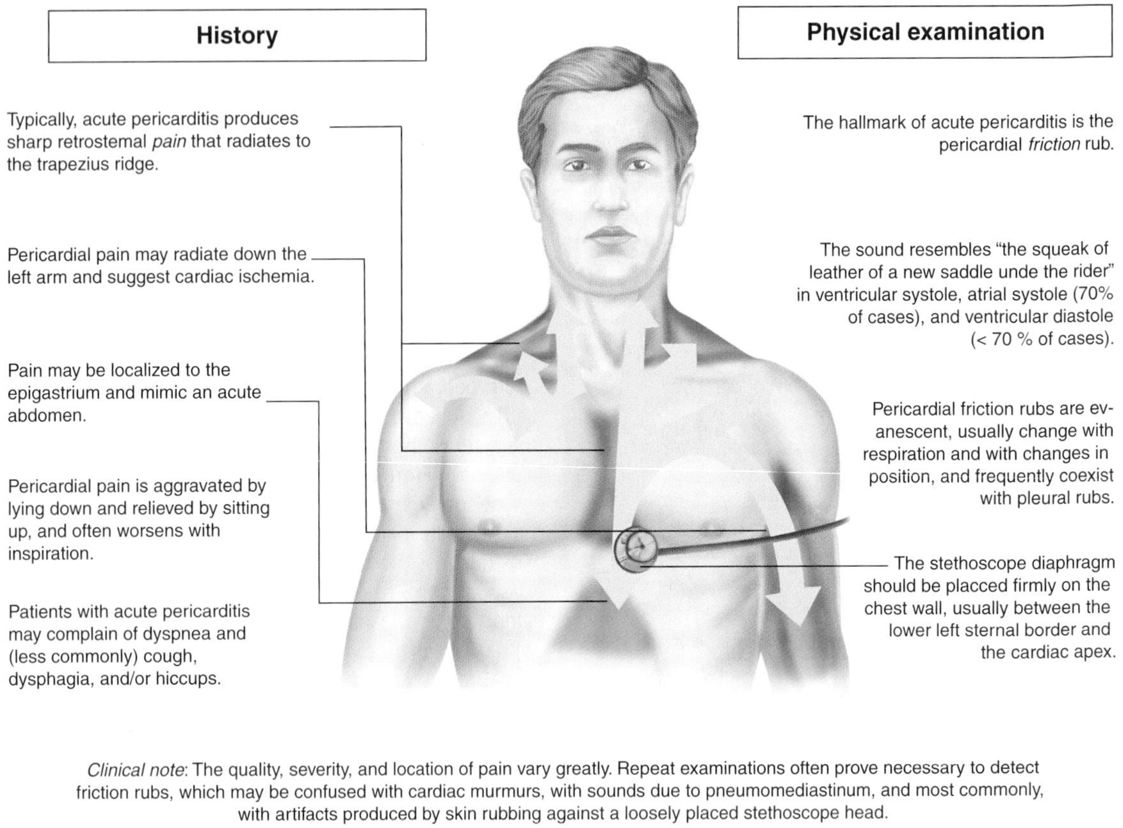

Figure 132-1 *Clinical features of acute pericarditis. A prodrome of fever, malaise, and myalgia may herald the chief complaint of chest pain. (Modified, with permission, from Fuster V, O'Rourke RA, Walsh RA, et al. Hurst's the Heart. 12th ed. New York: McGraw-Hill; 2008. Fig. 84-3.)*

and chest radiograph. ECG demonstrates valuable findings for the diagnosis of acute pericarditis (**Figure 132-2**). Abnormalities are found in approximately 90% of the cases. The most sensitive ECG change of acute pericarditis is ST-segment elevation due to abnormal repolarization secondary to pericardial inflammation. Classically, the ECG of acute pericarditis shows ST elevation in the hexaxial and precordial leads with the exception of AVR and V_1 which may have ST-segment depression. The ST elevations have concave shape and are not accompanied by reciprocal changes. In ischemia, on the other hand, the slope of ST elevation is more often convex in

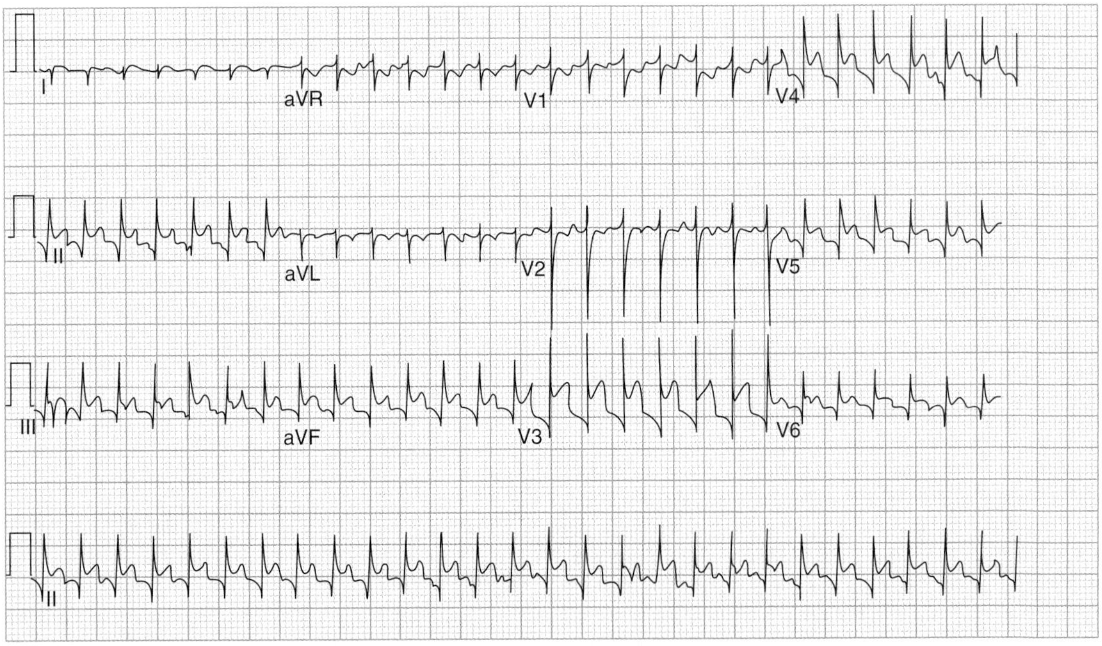

Figure 132-2 *Twelve-lead electrocardiogram of patient with acute pericarditis. (Modified, with permission, from Fuster V, O'Rourke RA, Walsh RA, et al. Hurst's the Heart. 12th ed. New York: McGraw-Hill; 2008. Fig. 84-4.)*

shape and accompanied by reciprocal changes on the ECG. These two differences help to distinguish the ST elevation of pericarditis from that of ischemia. In addition, ST-segment elevation, which typically occurs during the first few days of pericardial inflammation, may last up to two weeks. T-wave inversion does not occur at the time of ST-segment elevation nor are there associated Q-waves. PR depression is very specific of acute pericarditis and is attributed to subepicardial atrial injury. In fact, PR depression found in all leads except AVR and V_1, which may show PR elevation. This finding may be very useful when the patient has no friction rub and equivocal ST elevation. Electrical alternans, the presence of alternating QRS amplitudes may suggest the presence of a significant pericardial effusion. Serial ECGs at presentation are especially useful because of how the changes evolve in contrast to acute myocardial ischemia or J-point elevation.

PRACTICE POINT

- Pericarditis account for up to 1% of cases of ST elevations on ECG, and account for 5% of emergency room visits. Eighty percent to 90% of cases of pericarditis are idiopathic.

Creatinine kinase MB fraction and/or troponin I values may be elevated in 8% to 22% of patients presenting with acute pericarditis. Evidence of elevated troponin or CK-MB laboratory values correlate with ST elevation on the electrocardiogram. The elevation of cardiac enzymes may represent silent myocarditis in addition to pericarditis, or the epicardial inflammation that can accompany acute pericarditis. Acute pericarditis may accompany endocardial ischemia, such that coronary disease may need to be ruled out in patients presenting with pericarditis who have concomitant significant elevations in cardiac biomarkers.

Acute pericarditis may be associated with mild elevations in the total white blood cell count, usually with a lymphocytic predominance. The differential of the white blood cell count may reflect the underlying etiology; viral or idiopathic pericarditis may present with a lymphocytic predominance, whereas bacterial pericarditis may have a neutrophilic predominance.

The erythrocyte sedimentation rate may have mild elevation, but significant elevations in the ESR may suggest an autoimmune etiology, uremia, bacterial processes, or tuberculosis. Patients presenting with uremia may have a pericardial friction rub on exam.

The chest radiograph may be completely normal in viral or idiopathic acute pericarditis. Pericardial effusion should be suspected in the setting of an abnormal cardiac silhouette. An accumulation of more than 200 mL of pericardial effusion will enlarge the cardiac silhouette, indistinguishable from other causes of cardiomegaly. As more fluid accumulates, however, a "water bottle" configuration may develop. In the absence of pulmonary venous congestion, considerable cardiomegaly may be a clue that a pericardial effusion is present. Fluid between the two pericardial layers may show separation of the epicardial fat pad from the outer border of the cardiac silhouette. An abnormal chest radiograph may suggest the etiology for the pericarditis, or a different diagnosis. An infiltrate on chest X-ray may suggest bacterial pericarditis as the etiology. An upper lobe infiltrate, or a completely normal chest X-ray may accompany tuberculosis pericarditis. Pulmonary congestion may suggest ischemia or myocarditis.

Echocardiography is the imaging modality of choice in acute pericarditis because of its availability, lack of radiation exposure, and ability to rule out potentially fatal complications such as tamponade. An echocardiogram is recommended for most patients with pericarditis, especially patients with fever, currently on anticoagulation therapy, in an immunocompromised state, a recent history of trauma, or if there is suspected myocardial involvement. Echocardiography in patients with uncomplicated acute pericarditis may be completely normal. A small effusion may be present which does not necessitate intervention. Large pericardial effusions are uncommon in acute pericarditis and should trigger the clinician to pursue other diagnoses. Focal wall motion abnormalities may suggest that myocarditis may be present.

CT and MRI are emerging as valuable methods for detecting complicated pericarditis. The inflamed pericardium in both acute and chronic pericarditis can be visualized by MRI. The ability to assess fluid attenuation on both CT and MRI allows a noninvasive assessment of the etiology. The thickened pericardial layers and any pericardial effusion can be effectively visualized on cardiac MRI. Furthermore, MRI may be the noninvasive imaging modality of choice for the diagnosis of myocarditis, which can accompany pericarditis.

MANAGEMENT

Patients with a history, physical examination, and testing consistent with pericarditis should receive nonsteroidal anti-inflammatory drugs (NSAIDs) as the initial treatment. Aspirin is preferred over NSAIDs if acute myocardial infarction is the cause of acute pericarditis, as NSAIDs may promote ventricular rupture. Therapeutic options include: aspirin (2–4 g daily), ibuprofen (1600–3200 mg daily), or other NSAIDs at high therapeutic dosing for 2 to 4 weeks' duration. If there is no large effusion and cardiac enzymes are normal, the patient can be discharged and followed up within two to four weeks to ensure resolution. If the pain has resolved, therapy can be discontinued at that time.

Patients that do not have an adequate response to NSAIDs may require narcotic analgesics for pain control. Colchicine in combination with aspirin is an alternative regimen in the treatment of acute pericarditis, and reduces recurrences of pericarditis in comparison to aspirin alone. Colchicine alone is an alternative agent when aspirin or an NSAID is contraindicated. Colchicine should be initiated at a 2 mg loading dose, then 1 mg daily for 2 weeks, but may require maintenance therapy for up to 3 months.

Alternately, a prednisone taper over the course of a week, starting at 60 mg orally can be used. However, patients receiving steroid therapy for acute pericarditis have a higher relapse rate than with other medications. Corticosteroids are indicated in acute pericarditis due to systemic inflammatory diseases or uremia. Corticosteroids also should be considered in patients who are refractory to or have contraindications to aspirin, NSAIDs, and colchicine. However, *corticosteroids may promote the development of recurrent pericarditis* and should not be used in patients with acute pericarditis due to bacterial infection or tuberculosis. They should also be avoided in patients with postinfarction pericarditis due to the risk of ventricular aneurysm formation.

The most common complication of acute pericarditis is recurrent pericarditis, occurring in 15% to 30% of patients presenting with acute pericarditis. Colchicine is the treatment of choice for recurrent acute pericarditis and can prevent recurrences. In patients with a first episode of pericarditis, patients treated with colchicine therapy (1.0–2.0 mg/d for the first day, then 0.5–1.0 mg/d for 6 months) decreases recurrence (24% vs 51%) over standard therapy plus aspirin.

PERICARDIAL EFFUSIONS AND CARDIAC TAMPONADE

INTRODUCTION

Many inflammatory and noninflammatory conditions lead to excess fluid in the pericardial space, thereby, overwhelming the villi and cilia that physiologically reabsorb fluid and optimize the movement of the pericardial layers over one another (Table 132-1). Often, pericardial effusions accompany episodes of pericarditis and share the same etiology. Sometimes, pericardial effusions are incidentally noted during imaging for other indications. Therefore, clinicians need to quickly determine if a pericardial effusion is a factor in the patient's clinical syndrome, identify any hemodynamic consequences of the effusion, and then appropriately manage with the help of consultants.

PATHOPHYSIOLOGY

Effusion formation is most often part of an inflammatory process involving the pericardium. Less commonly, accumulation of lymphatic drainage or blood can occur. The latter is termed hemopericardium and is most commonly associated with ascending aortic dissection, perforation of the atrial or ventricular walls, or direct injury to the pericardium itself. Patients with anasarca, uremia, or myxedema may also develop a significant pericardial effusion. Cardiac tamponade can develop irrespective of the pathophysiology responsible for the development of the effusion. Whether cardiac tamponade is present depends upon many factors, most importantly is the acuity with which the effusion has accumulated. The pericardium is a compliant collagen-based structure with the intrinsic ability to stretch and accommodate a large amount of fluid without causing hemodynamic consequences when effusions accumulate subacutely or chronically. The hemodynamic consequences of a pericardial effusion are determined by the amount of increased pressure within the pericardial sac and the heart's ability to compensate or accommodate this increased pressure. Rapid accumulation of pericardial fluid can lead to very high intrapericardial pressures within a very short amount of time causing hemodynamic collapse despite a small volume effusion. However, even large chronic effusions will eventually reach a critical volume at which intrapericardial pressures will lead to hemodynamic collapse.

PRACTICE POINT

- Rapid accumulation of pericardial fluid can cause hemodynamic collapse despite a small volume effusion. Even large chronic effusions will eventually reach a critical volume at which intrapericardial pressures will lead to hemodynamic collapse.

Right atrial and ventricular diastolic pressures rise as intrapericardial pressure increases. Eventually, these pressures equalize at which time the hemodynamic consequences of cardiac tamponade become clinically evident. These hemodynamic effects are best appreciated as loss of the *y* descent in the RA venous waveform (**Figure 132-3**) and the presence of a paradoxical arterial pulse. In cardiac tamponade total heart volume is fixed while the inspiratory augmentation of venous return to right sided circulation is retained. In contrast to the hemodynamics of constrictive physiology, intrathoracic pressure changes are transmitted through the pericardium in cardiac tamponade.

The *y* descent represents the decrease in RA pressure during passive filling of the right ventricle (RV) immediately after the tricuspid valve opens signifying the beginning of ventricular diastole. In cardiac tamponade the normal pressure gradient between the right atrium and right ventricle is lost since diastolic pressures in all four cardiac chambers are equalized causing an abbreviated and minimized decrease in RA pressure represented by a "blunted" *y* descent (**Figure 132-4**).

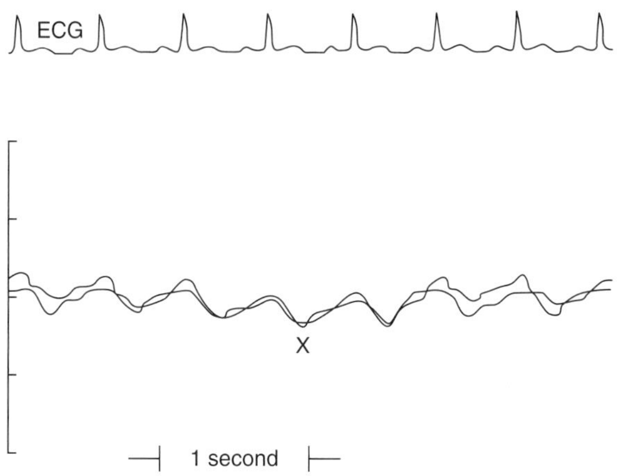

Figure 132-3 *Simultaneous right atrial and pericardial pressures from a patient with severe cardiac tamponade. The pressures are elevated and equal to one another, and only the x descent on the right atrial tracing is present; the y descent is absent. The pressures fall normally during inspiration. (Reproduced, with permission, from Fuster V, O'Rourke RA, Walsh RA, et al. Hurst's the Heart. 12th ed. New York: McGraw-Hill; 2008. Fig. 84-10.)*

The paradoxical pulse or "pulsus paradoxus" is defined as a >10 mm Hg decrease in systolic blood pressure during inspiration. The decreased intrathoracic pressure accompanying inspiration leads to increased filling of the right heart. Since total cardiac vol-

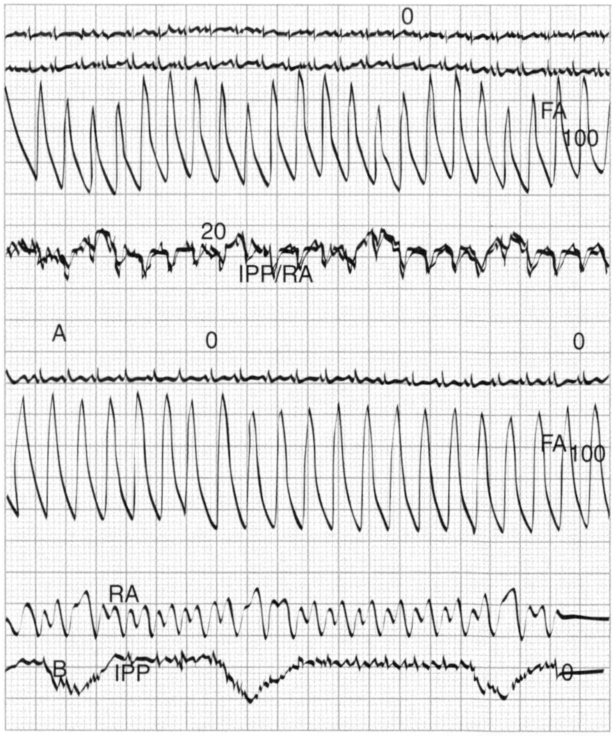

Figure 132-4 *Hemodynamic record from a patient with cardiac tamponade before (A) and after (B) pericardiocentesis. (A) Pulsus paradoxus is evident from the femoral artery (FA) pressure tracing. Note the absent y descent on the right atrial (RA) tracing and the equal and elevated RA and pericardial (IPP) pressures. (B) After removal of pericardial fluid, pericardial and right atrial pressures decrease and the pulsus paradoxus disappears. (Modified, with permission, from Fuster V, O'Rourke RA, Walsh RA, et al. Hurst's the Heart. 12th ed. New York: McGraw-Hill; 2008. Fig. 84-15.)*

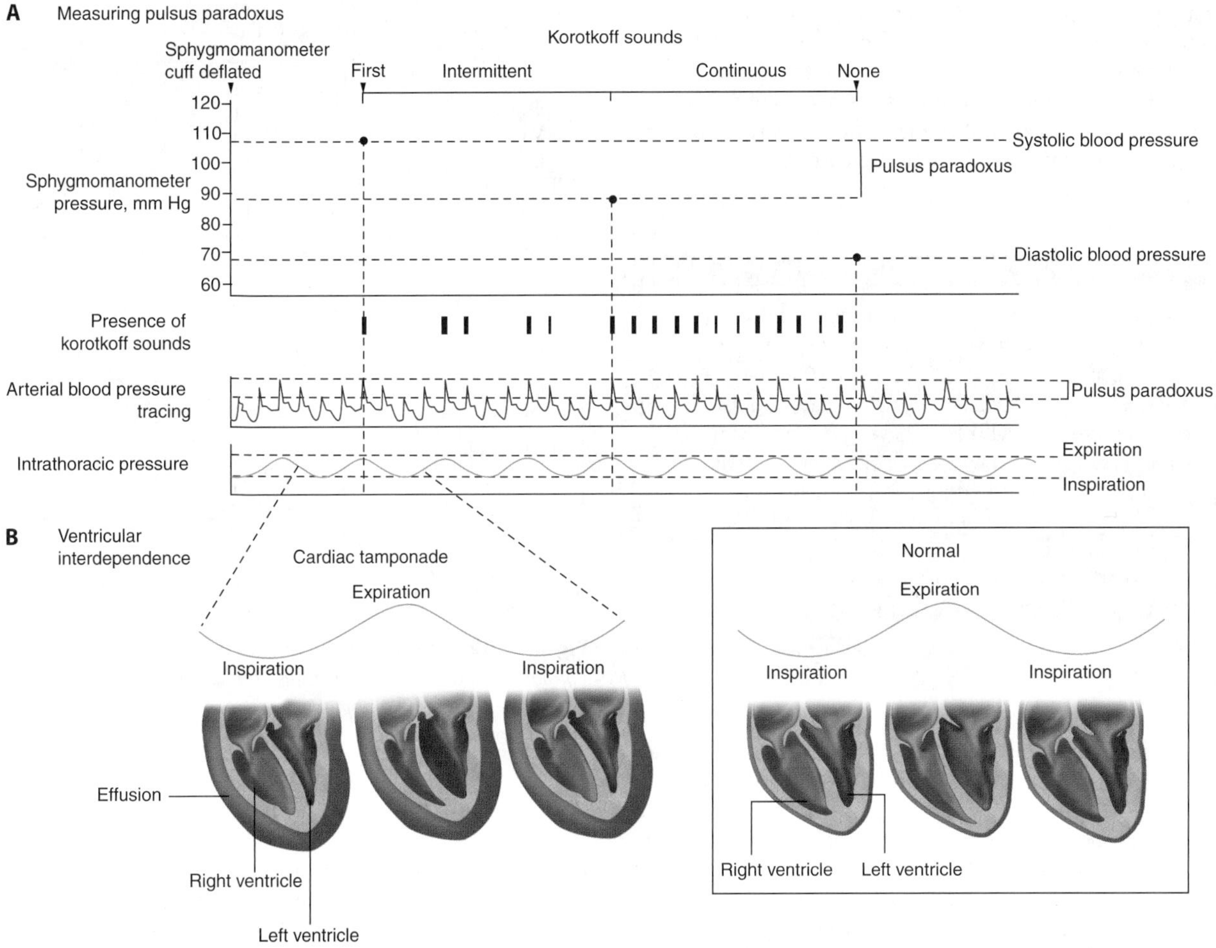

Figure 132-5 *Pathophysiology and measurement of pulsus paradoxus. (A) The examiner inflates the sphygmomanometer cuff fully, listens for Korotkoff sounds as the cuff is slowly deflated, and then notes the pressure at which Korotkoff sounds are initially audible only during expiration. As the cuff is further deflated, the examiner notes the pressure at which Korotkoff sounds become audible during expiration and inspiration. The difference between these 2 pressure is the pulses paradoxus. In cardiac tamponade, the pulsus paradoxus measure greater than 10 mm Hg. Inspiratory dimunition in the pulse wave amplitude seen on this arterial tracing demonstrate pulsus paradoxus. A similar phenomenon may be observed on a pulse oximeter waveform. (B) During inspiration in the normal heart, negative intrapleural pressures increase venous returns to the right ventricle and decrease pulmonary venous return to the left ventricle by increasing pulmonary reservoir for blood. As a result of increased right ventricular distention, the interventricular septum bows slightly to the left, and the distensibility, filling, and stroke volume of the left ventricle are mildly reduced. In expiration, these changes are reciprocal, resulting in the septum bowling to the right and a mild reduction in right ventricular filling. In the presence of cardiac tamponade, the reciprocal changes seen in the normal heart are exaggerated when the pericardial sac is filled with fluid, thus limiting distensibility of the entire heart. This results in a more dramatic reduction in filling of the left ventricle during inspiration, exacerbating the normal inspiratory decrease in stroke volume and blood pressure. (Reproduced, with permission, from Roy CL, Minor MA, Brookhart A, et al. Does this patient with pericardial effusion have cardiac tamponade? JAMA. 2007;297:1810–1818.)*

ume is fixed, this increase in right sided filling comes at the expense of decreased left heart volumes mediated through interventricular dependence or exaggerated leftward shift of the interventricular septum. Consequently, there is decreased LV filling and therefore stroke volume. The increased right sided filling does lead to increased RV stroke volume. However, several cardiac cycles are required before this causes increased LV filling. As intrapericardial pressure increases, total intracardiac volume is further diminished, and the above hemodynamic effects are accentuated, potentially leading to hemodynamic collapse (**Figure 132-5**).

PRESENTATION

Pericardial effusions do not usually cause symptoms beyond those associated with any concomitant pericardial inflammation. However, cardiac tamponade commonly causes chest pain, dyspnea, or chest fullness. Additionally, symptoms of hepatic and visceral congestion, fever, fatigue, and lethargy have been reported. Importantly, these symptoms may be absent or unobtainable in patients with acute cardiac tamponade if they are in shock or critically ill. Of these symptoms dyspnea has the highest sensitivity reported in observational studies of 87% to 88%.

Physical exam findings can be helpful in the assessment of a patient with suspected cardiac tamponade. Beck's triad (hypotension, tachycardia, and distant heart sounds) was originally described in 1935 by Dr. Claude Schaeffer Beck, a thoracic surgeon. Notably, hypotension and distant heart sounds are insensitive physical findings in the assessment of cardiac tamponade. While these findings can be useful, more recent evidence based analysis of clinical, electrocardiographic, and radiographic findings are available. The presence of a paradoxical pulse, defined as a > 12 mm Hg decrease in systolic blood pressure upon inspiration has a sensitivity of 98% and a specificity of 83% with a positive likelihood ratio of 5.9. When the paradoxical pulse was < 10 to 12 mm Hg the negative LR was 0.03. In pooled analyses, elevated jugular venous pressure and tachycardia were shown to be reasonably sensitive markers (sensitivity of 76% and 77%,respectively) that, when absent, decreases the likelihood of cardiac tamponade.

PRACTICE POINT

- A paradoxical pulse is the most helpful clinical test for cardiac tamponade, with sensitivity of 98%, specificity of 83%, a positive likelihood ratio (LR+) of 5.9, and a negative likelihood ratio (LR–) of 0.03. Elevated jugular venous pressure and tachycardia have good sensitivity (76% and 77%, respectively) that, when absent, decreases the likelihood of cardiac tamponade. Hypotension and distant heart sounds are insensitive physical findings in the assessment of cardiac tamponade. (Roy CL, Minor MA, Brookhart MA, Choudhry NK. Does this patient with cardiac pericardial effusion have cardiac tamponade? *JAMA.* 2007;297(16):1810–1818.)

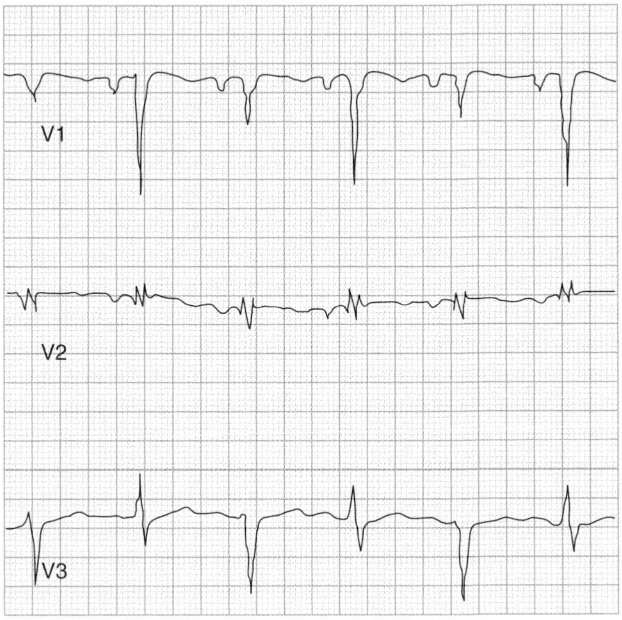

Figure 132-6 *Electrocardiogram (leads V_1–V_3) of a patient with cardiac tamponade demonstrates marked electrical alternans, with varying or alternating amplitude of the QRS complex with each cardiac contraction.*

The bedside evaluation of pulsus paradoxus may be initially appreciated by the disappearance of the radial pulse on inspiration. Smaller degrees of pulsus paradoxus may be noted while gradually reducing finger pressure on the radial or femoral artery similar to the gradual lowering of blood pressure from the point of obliterating the pulse to the point when only expiratory pulses are felt to the point of feeling all pulses. The accurate measurement of the paradoxical pulse is quantified using cuff sphygmomanometry, and is represented by the differences in recorded pressures between that recorded when the first Korotkoff sound is auscultated and that at which Korotkoff sounds are heard with every heart beat (Figure 132-5). Importantly, a paradoxical pulse may be absent when preexisting conditions exist that elevate LV diastolic pressures such as aortic regurgitation, LV hypertrophy, or LV failure, and conditions that limit right heart filling such as pulmonary hypertension. When cardiogenic shock develops, pulsus paradoxus may be difficult to detect. Additionally, a paradoxical pulse can be present in the absence of tamponade in patients with a multitude of disorders including COPD, asthma, pulmonary embolism, or shock.

DIAGNOSIS

Electrocardiographic findings of low voltage, electrical alternans, and PR depression have specificities ranging from 89% to 100%, but are very insensitive findings for the diagnosis of pericardial effusions. Electrical alternans is caused by "swing" of the heart within the fluid-filled pericardium (**Figure 132-6**). Similarly the finding of an enlarged cardiac silhouette on chest radiography has a high sensitivity (~89%) and low specificity (~50%) for pericardial effusions. The cardiac silhouette may appear flask-like with "tenting" that often obscures the left heart border at the level of the left atrial appendage (**Figure 132-7**).

The primary diagnostic imaging modality for cardiac tamponade is transthoracic Doppler echocardiography, a noninvasive study that provides accurate information regarding the hemodynamic effects of a pericardial effusion. Echocardiography can accurately detect and quantify effusions of any size and serve as a useful tool to evaluate effusions on a serial basis. Right atrial and right ventricular collapse during early ventricular diastole signify that an effusion is severe enough to cause some degree of hemodynamic compromise. On echocardiogram, RA collapse is the most sensitive finding, while RV collapse is the most specific finding for cardiac tamponade (**Figure 132-8**). Importantly, large pleural effusions can also cause these findings to be present. Exaggerated respiratory variation of right and left sided venous and valvular flow patterns are highly specific for tamponade as well.

Both CT and MRI are useful adjuncts to echocardiography, providing accurate quantification of pericardial effusions and real-time imaging to quantify septal shift and chamber collapse with accuracy similar to that of echocardiography. Detailed assessment of the

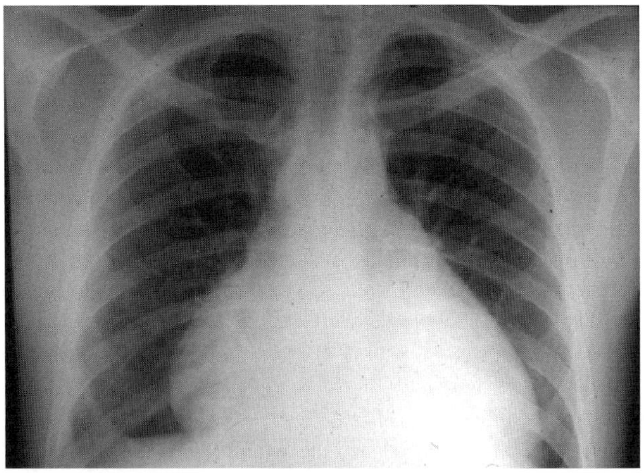

Figure 132-7 *Chest X-ray (anterior) of a patient with rapidly increasing pericardial effusion and hemodynamic evidence of cardiac tamponade. Note how the cardiac silhouette is rounded in its lower portion and tapers at the base of the heart, resembling a plastic bag filled with water sitting on a table ("water-bottle" heart).*

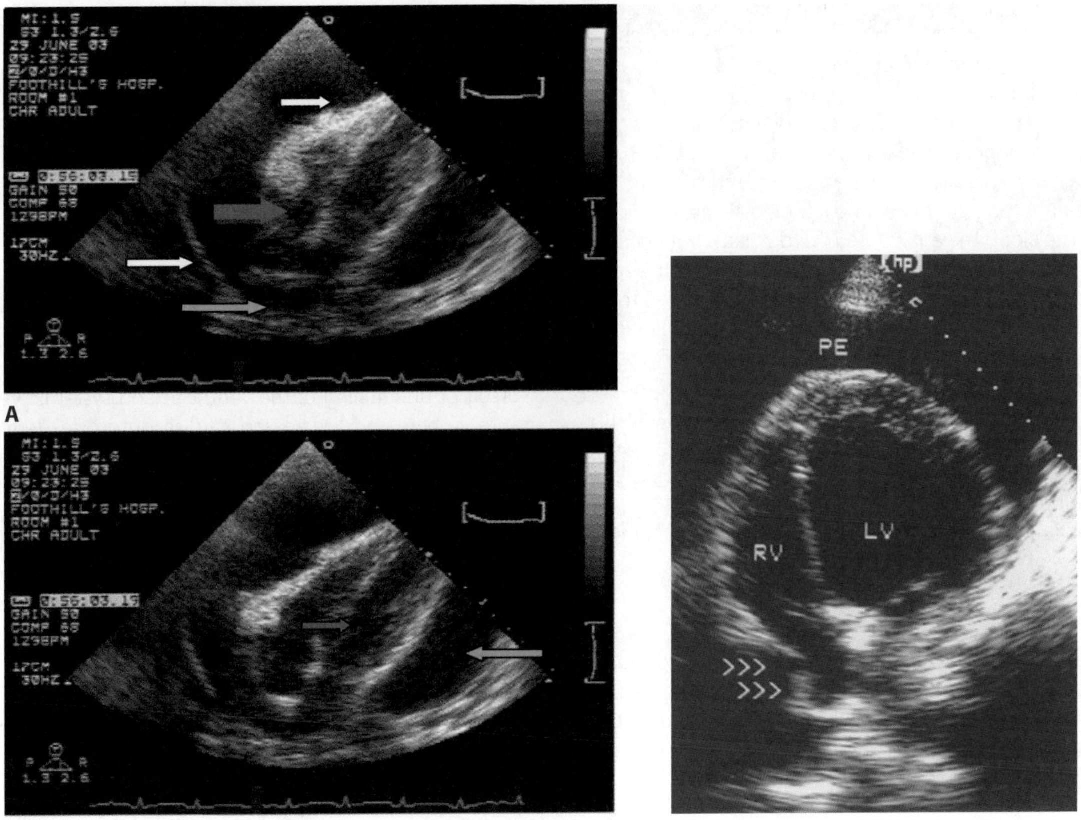

B C

Figure 132-8 *(A) An early diastolic frame of a two-dimensional echocardiogram in a patient with cardiac tamponade. There is a very large pericardial effusion (white arrows) and right atrial (blue arrow) and right ventricular (red arrow) collapse. (B) A late diastolic frame from the same cardiac cycle; both ventricles are underfilled. Right and left ventricles labeled with red and blue arrows, respectively. (Reproduced, with permission, from Hall JB, Schmidt GA, Wood LDH. Principles of Critical Care. 3rd ed. New York: McGraw-Hill; 2005. Fig. 28-7.) (C) Two-dimensional echocardiogram in the apical four-chamber view. During late diastole, there is inversion of the lateral wall of the right atrium. (Reproduced, with permission, from Fuster V, O'Rourke RA, Walsh RA, et al. Hurst's the Heart. 12th ed. New York: McGraw-Hill; 2008. Fig. 16-138.)*

pericardium and the pericardial fluid, and other pathology occurring within the chest are advantages over echocardiography.

MANAGEMENT

Management of pericardial effusions is first determined by the presence or absence of tamponade physiology. If tamponade physiology is present the threshold for urgent pericardiocentesis should be low. The presence of cardiac tamponade should be considered a medical emergency, warranting admission to an intensive care unit with prompt consultation of a cardiovascular diseases specialist. In patients whom the decision to perform pericardiocentesis has been deferred, invasive hemodynamic monitoring with pulmonary artery catheter can be useful. Volume resuscitation is beneficial in patients with hypovolemia; however, it can be detrimental in the euvolemic or hypervolemic patient. In the absence of hypovolemia, excessive fluid resuscitation can cause increased intracardiac and pericardial pressures thus decreasing the transmural myocardial pressures and cardiac filling eventually leading to circulatory collapse. If the patient's volume status is difficult to determine, then it is reasonable to give a fluid challenge and monitor closely for clinical improvement or deterioration. The use of inotropes, specifically dobutamine, has some temporizing benefit in animal studies; however, in most patients with tamponade physiology compensatory mechanisms are already maximized.

PRACTICE POINT

- The presence of cardiac tamponade should be considered a medical emergency, warranting admission to an intensive care unit with prompt consultation of a cardiovascular diseases specialist to perform an urgent pericardiocentesis. If the patient becomes pulseless, pericardiocentesis should be performed immediately, even by inexperienced practitioners.
- Volume resuscitation is beneficial in patients with hypovolemia, but can be detrimental in the euvolemic or hypervolemic patient.

Removal of the pericardial fluid with pericardiocentesis is the definitive treatment for cardiac tamponade. When available, pericardiocentesis is performed in the cardiac catheterization laboratory using echocardiographic guidance. In the emergent situation this may be performed blindly at the bedside. If the procedure is performed by a cardiovascular disease specialist, a pigtail catheter can be placed over a wire to facilitate further drainage of the effusion; however, this may not be possible in the emergent setting. Repeated echocardiography should be performed immediately postprocedurally to evaluate for hemodynamic improvement. The pericardiocentesis procedure is delineated in the Practice Point.

PRACTICE POINT

- Pericardiocentesis procedure: Patient is positioned at a 30° head-up angle to allow pericardial fluid to pool at the apex. A long 16- or 18-gauge pericardiocentesis needle attached to a stopcock and a large syringe filled with 10 to 15 cc of 1% lidocaine is inserted in the subxiphoid area one fingerbreadth below the left medial costal margin. Anesthetize along the anticipated needle path. The needle is slowly advanced at a 15° to 30° angle directed at the left shoulder with the injection of lidocaine as needed to minimize discomfort to the patient. Intermittent aspiration should occur during advancement of the needle. Once fluid is aspirated, the operator should immediately turn the stopcock to pressure to verify the location of the needle. In cardiac tamponade the pressure waveform will resemble that of the right atrium. A RV waveform is abnormal and the needle should be promptly withdrawn. Usually only 50 to 100 cc of fluid needs to be removed before hemodynamic improvement is observed.

Pericardial fluid should be sent to the laboratory for analysis, including cell count with differential, hematocrit, total protein, LDH, Gram and acid fast bacilli (AFB) stains, as well as bacterial, fungal, and AFB cultures when appropriate. Additionally, cytology can be helpful if there is a suspicion of a malignant etiology. Lights criteria, commonly used to evaluate pleural effusions can be applied to determine if pericardial fluid is exudative or transudative. In the setting of pericarditis a pericardial biopsy is often required to make a diagnosis.

Long-term management involves treating the underlying pathology causing the effusion and serial echocardiography to monitor for recurrence of effusion. We recommend a repeat transthoracic echocardiogram 48 to 72 hours following initial drainage of a pericardial effusion. If there is no evidence of recurrence then further transthoracic echocardiography should be performed as clinically indicated. If there is evidence of recurrence within the first 72 hours then repeat pericardiocentesis, or more definitively, a pericardial window may be indicated, with consultative assistance from a cardiovascular disease specialist. Transudative pericardial effusions are more likely to recur and to require a pericardial window procedure performed by a cardiothoracic or thoracic surgeon. All patients diagnosed with a pericardial effusion warrant short and long term follow up with a cardiovascular disease specialist. Follow-up for two weeks following hospital discharge is indicated.

CONSTRICTIVE PERICARDITIS

INTRODUCTION

Constrictive pericarditis is the late stage manifestation of any inflammatory process resulting in constriction and loss of elasticity of the pericardium. Any process leading to acute pericarditis can also result in constrictive pericarditis. In the developed world the three most common etiologies are postviral (idiopathic), postsurgical, and radiation induced. In less developed parts of the world tuberculosis is still a major infectious etiology of constrictive pericarditis.

PATHOPHYSIOLOGY

Once scarring of the pericardium takes place, its intrinsic elasticity is lost. An inelastic pericardium results in restricted filling of both atria and ventricles. The stiffened pericardium effectively limits total cardiac volume causing equilibration of filling pressures in all four chambers of the heart. A consequence of this is accentuated ventricular filling during early diastole driven by elevated atrial pressures. This rapid early filling continues until mid-diastole when the ventricles reach their filling limit set by the stiffened pericardium. At this point, ventricular filling ceases and filling pressures equalize throughout the heart. The rapid early ventricular filling is represented by an accentuated *y* decent in both right and left atrial pressure tracings. This presents as a dominant negative wave in the already distended neck veins. The equalization of ventricular filling pressures is represented by the "square root" sign seen on diastolic ventricular pressure tracings (**Figure 132-9**), both of which are distinguishing features of constrictive physiology. Overall, cardiac output is decreased as a result of underfilling of the ventricles and systemic venous pressure is increased. Decreased cardiac output leads to increased sympathetic activity and upregulation of the renin-angiotensin, aldosterone-system, enhancing sodium and water retention leading to volume overload. Systemic venous pressures can be significantly increased leading to congestive hepatopathy and cachexia in advanced stages of disease. Ventricular contraction is usually preserved; however, it may be slightly diminished because of a decreased preload effect.

The decrease in intrathoracic pressure seen with inspiration is not transmitted to any of the intracardiac chambers, but is transmitted to the pulmonary vasculature. This results in a diminished filling gradient between the pulmonary veins and the left atrium causing a decrease in mitral inflow velocities and decreased filling of the left ventricle during inspiration. Consequently, RV filling is enhanced via right to left septal shift. These events are reversed during expiration. This is an important difference from the hemodynamics seen in restrictive cardiomyopathy and cardiac tamponade physiology that is useful in delineating the underlying cardiac physiology when measuring hemodynamic parameters invasively.

Effusive-constrictive pericarditis occurs when tamponade physiology occurs from a pericardial effusion in the setting of a fibrotic pericardium. Once the pericardial fluid is removed, constrictive physiology remains. The most common etiologies are malignancy, radiation therapy, connective tissue disease, and idiopathic pericarditis.

PRESENTATION

Patients with constrictive physiology usually present with complaints of volume overload, dyspnea on exertion, and fatigue. Additionally symptoms of hepatic congestion may also be prominent, sometimes leading to the misdiagnosis of chronic hepatic disease. Important physical exam findings include the presence of Kussmal sign (lack of decline in jugular venous pressure with inspiration), which is seen only in 20% of cases. Kussmal sign can also be present in cases of severe right-sided heart failure and tricuspid valve disease. A paradoxical pulse is appreciated in 20% of cases as well. Additionally, a pericardial friction rub and pericardial knock can be present; however both are uncommon.

DIAGNOSIS

There are no specific features on electrocardiogram to aid in the diagnosis of constrictive pericarditis. Atrial fibrillation, low voltage, and nonspecific ST-T wave changes can be seen in up to 33% of cases, however these findings are nonspecific. Chest radiography may reveal ringed calcification of the cardiac silhouette, especially on the lateral view (**Figure 132-10**).

Transthoracic Doppler echocardiography, a class I recommendation by the American College of Cardiology, remains a useful imaging modality to obtain valuable hemodynamic and anatomic

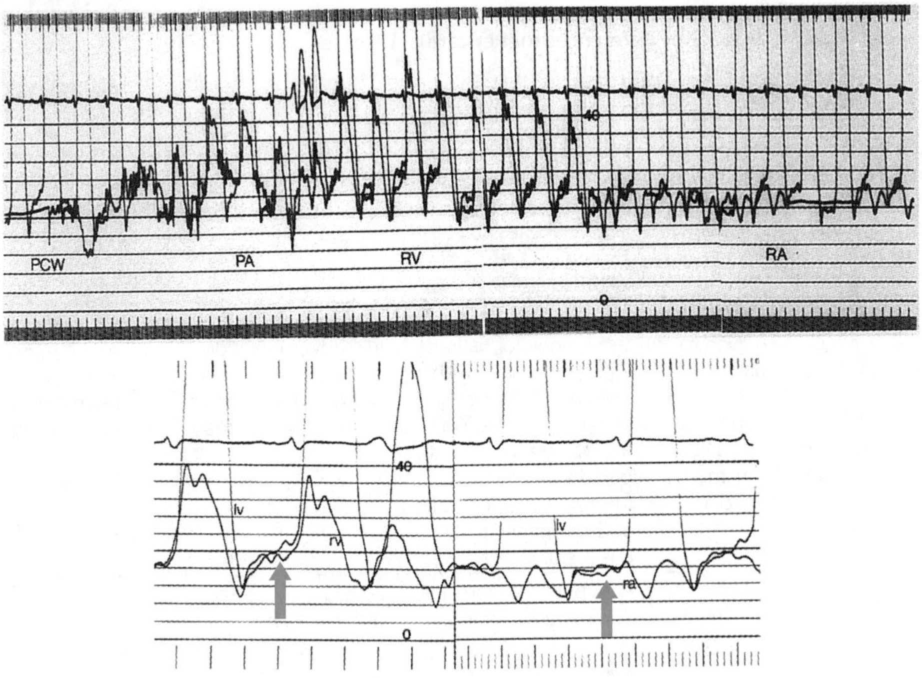

Figure 132-9 *Hemodynamic record of a patient with surgically proven constrictive pericarditis. (Top) Slow-paper-speed recording of high-gain left ventricular (LV) pressure and simultaneous right heart pullback from pulmonary capillary wedge (PCW) to pulmonary artery (PA), right ventricle (RV), and right atrium (RA). (Bottom) Fast-paper-speed recording of LV and simultaneous RV and RA pressure tracings. Note the increased and equal atrial and diastolic pressures (blue arrows), the prominent x and y descents on the RA tracing, and the dip and plateau on the RV and LV tracings during longer diastoles. (Reproduced, with permission, from Fuster V, O'Rourke RA, Walsh RA, et al. Hurst's the Heart. 12th ed. New York: McGraw-Hill; 2008. Fig. 84-22.)*

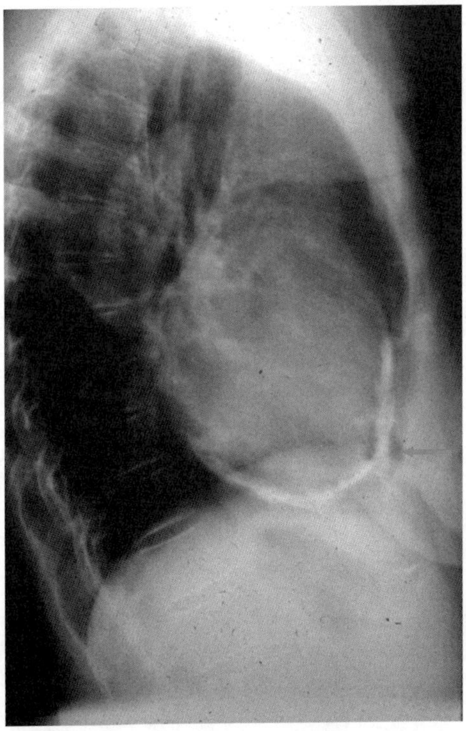

Figure 132-10 *Standard lateral view of a chest X-ray of a patient with constrictive pericarditis. Note the calcification appreciated in the apical region denoted by the blue arrow.*

information in the to evaluation of constrictive pericarditis. If further information is needed, evaluation with cardiac MRI can be pursued. Both cardiac CT and MRI provide direct visualization of the pericardium and allow for precise measurement of pericardial thickness. Cardiac MRI can also provide useful information regarding hemodynamics, and is considered by some to be the imaging modality of choice for pericardial diseases. In some cases the diagnosis of constrictive pericarditis cannot be made based solely on noninvasive imaging modalities. In these cases, a right and left heart catheterization is required to determine the diagnosis.

MANAGEMENT

Pericardiectomy is the treatment of choice for chronic symptomatic constrictive pericarditis (**Table 132-2**). Complete pericardiectomy (which has been likened to peeling an orange) is preferred to partial resection as recurrence rates decrease with complete resection. Additionally, patients surgically treated with complete pericardiectomy achieve more rapid normalization of hemodynamics and have lower long-term mortality rates when compared with those treated with partial pericardial resection, 83.8% versus 73.9%, respectively. Patients with very early or very advanced disease are not optimal surgical candidates because a small percentage of patients with acute pericarditis will also have some constrictive symptoms that will spontaneously resolve. The mortality associated with pericardiectomy can reach 30% to 40% in patients with advanced disease and NYHA class IV symptoms.

TABLE 132-2 Evidence-based Medicine: Key References for Pericardial Diseases

Reference	Methodology	Results	Limitations	Bottom Line
Imazio M, et al. Colchicine as first-line therapy for recurrent pericarditis. *Arch Intern Med.* 2005;165: 1987–1989.	A prospective, randomized, open-label design comparing the addition of colchicine to standard therapy with aspirin versus standard therapy alone.	Treatment with colchicine significantly decreased the recurrence rate (actuarial rates at 18 months were 24.0% vs 50.6%; P = .02).	Open-label trial design	Colchicine therapy led to a clinically important and statistically significant benefit over conventional treatment, decreasing the recurrence rate in patients with a first episode of recurrent pericarditis.
Roy CL, et al. Does this patient with a pericardial effusion have cardiac tamponade? *JAMA.* 2007;297(16): 1810–1818.	Meta-analysis of 787 sources from 1966 to 2006. Systematically reviews the accuracy of the history, physical examination, and basic diagnostic tests for the diagnosis of cardiac tamponade.	Five features occur in the majority of patients with tamponade with statistically significant sensitivities: dyspnea, tachycardia, pulsus paradoxus, elevated jugular venous pressure, and cardiomegaly on chest radiograph.	Significant heterogeneity in study population, design, and reference standard for the diagnosis of cardiac tamponade	A pulsus paradoxus >10 mm Hg among patients with a pericardial effusion helps distinguish those with cardiac tamponade from those without. Diagnostic certainty of presence of tamponade requires additional testing.
Bertog SC, et al. Constrictive pericarditis: etiology and cause-specific survival after pericardiectomy. *J Am Coll Cardiol.* 2004;43:1445–1452.	A retrospective case review of 163 patients who underwent pericardiectomy for CP over a 24-year period at a single surgical center.	Perioperative mortality was 6%. Idiopathic CP had the best prognosis followed by postsurgical and postradiation CP	Retrospective review with results from a single surgery center, significant heterogeneity of patient population, present cardiac physiology, and severity of disease at time of surgery	Long-term survival after pericardiectomy for CP is related to underlying etiology, LV systolic function, renal function, serum sodium, and PAP.

CP, constrictive pericarditis; LV, left ventricular; PAP, pulmonary artery systolic pressure.

Medical therapy with diuretics and digoxin can provide some minor clinical improvement as well. In selected patients, cardiac transplantation may be an option. In patients with tuberculous involvement, rapid treatment with appropriate antimicrobial therapy should be initiated.

SUGGESTED READINGS

Cooper LT Jr. Myocarditis. *N Engl J Med.* 2009;360:1526–1538.

Curtiss E, Reddy, Uretsky B, Cecchetti A. Pulsus paradoxus: definition and relation to the severity of cardiac tamponade. *Am Heart J.* 1988;115:391–398.

Lange RA, Hillis LD. Clinical practice. Acute pericarditis. *N Engl J Med.* 2004;351:2195–2202.

Little WC, Freeman GL. Pericardial disease. *Circulation.* 2006;113: 1622–1632.

Imazio M, Bobbio M, Cecchi E, et al. Colchicine as first-choice therapy for recurrent pericarditis. *Arch Intern Med.* 2005;165:1987–1991.

Reddy P, Curtiss E, O'Toole J, Shaver J. Cardiac tamponade: hemodynamic observations in man. *Circulation.* 1978;58:265–272.

Roy CL, Minor MA, Brookhart MA, Choudhry NK. Does this patient with cardiac pericardial effusion have cardiac tamponade? *JAMA.* 2007;297(16):1810–1818.

Spodick DH. Acute pericarditis. *JAMA.* 2003;289:1150–1153.

Spodick D. Acute cardiac tamponade. *N Engl J Med.* 2003;349: 684–690.

Troughton RW, Asher CR, Klein AL. Pericarditis. *Lancet.* 2004;363: 717–727.

SECTION 3

Critical Care

CHAPTER 133

The Role of the Hospitalist in Critical Care

Kristin R. Wise, MD
Michael Heisler, MD, MPH

Key Clinical Questions

1. How did intensive care units (ICUs) and critical care medicine develop in the United States?
2. Who currently provides critical care in the United States?
3. What is an intensivist?
4. What are the evidence-based recommendations for ICU staffing?
5. What are some of the challenges of nationwide ICU staffing?
6. What is the role of hospitalists in future critical care provision?

INTRODUCTION

Current estimates indicate that approximately 6000 adult intensive care units (ICUs) provide complex care for 55,000 to 70,000 patients per day in the United States. The number of ICUs continues to rise despite a nationwide decrease in hospitals. ICU beds account for over 10% of all US hospital beds with over 4.4 million patient admissions annually. Costs associated with ICUs account for 1% of the US annual gross national product and approximately 20% of individual hospital expenditures. These national trends are the likely results of medical advances compounded by the surge of baby boomers reaching more advanced age and the growing obesity epidemic.

The United States faces current and future ICU critical care physician staffing shortages. The most recent estimates suggest that only one-third of critically ill patients receive medical care from a physician with specialized critical care training, commonly referred to as an "intensivist." The intensivist shortage coupled with the explosive growth of hospitalists over the past decade has led to more than 75% of hospitalists providing critical care as part of their clinical practice. A brief historical review of ICU development and of relevant medical literature will provide insight into current US physician staffing practices. While their role is not yet clearly defined, hospitalists will certainly continue to play a major role in future critical care provision.

HISTORICAL BACKGROUND

The first American ICU is attributed to Dr. W. E. Dandy, a surgeon who created a three-bed unit in 1926 dedicated to the post-operative care of neurosurgical patients at The Johns Hopkins Hospital in Baltimore. In response to the nursing shortages after World War II, patients requiring intensive postoperative care or mechanical ventilation were located together within hospitals to improve medical care efficiency. The polio epidemic in the late 1940s and subsequent advances in mechanical ventilation in the early 1950s fostered the expansion of ICUs. An anesthesiologist and pioneer of cardiopulmonary resuscitation, Dr. Peter Safar, started the first 24-hour, physician-staffed ICU in 1958 at Baltimore City Hospital. Since the 1960s, most hospitals have maintained at least one ICU. There are presently more than 65,000 adult ICU beds and 20,000 pediatric ICU beds distributed unevenly among hospitals in the United States.

In 1970, a group of subspecialists with shared interests established the Society of Critical Care Medicine (SCCM) and defined critical care medicine as "the multidisciplinary health care specialty that cares for patients with acute, life-threatening illness or injury." SCCM remains the largest multispecialty medical group in the United States today with 14,000 current members. In 1979, the American Board of Medical Specialties (ABMS) proposed to make critical care a multidisciplinary subspecialty of four existing primary boards—anesthesia, internal medicine, pediatrics, and surgery. These boards failed to reach consensus on training requirements; therefore, in 1986 the ABMS approved separate critical care board certification in concurrence with fellowship program development in these fields. Each discipline has its own board-eligibility requirements and subspecialty exams in critical care which remain separate today. Fellowship programs span from 1 to 2 years for anesthesia or surgery and 2 to 3 years for critical care medicine, combined pulmonary-critical care medicine or pediatric critical care. There are less than 1000 critical care fellowship positions offered each year between the four disciplines of anesthesia, internal medicine, pediatrics, and surgery. Almost 80% of adult intensivists initially train in internal medicine while less than 10% train in anesthesia and surgery. The most current estimates report there are almost 11,000 intensivists who provide care in the ICU setting as part, or all, of their patient responsibilities and approximately half maintain their critical care board certification.

A few critical care medicine fellowship programs have accepted Emergency Medicine residency graduates but have not granted them critical care board eligibility upon fellowship completion. Instead, many of these graduates have completed the European Society of Intensive Care Medicine examination to document competency. In 2009, the ABMS and the boards of Emergency Medicine and internal medicine agreed to accept Emergency Medicine residency graduates in all 2-year critical care medicine fellowships and to grant critical care board eligibility upon completion.

MEDICAL LITERATURE REVIEW

The medical literature on ICU physician staffing is scant and relies heavily on small, observational trials that often use historical controls. One of the first published studies was led by Li, et al in 1984 and examined mortality outcomes with the use of onsite physicians. Specifically, two internists were hired to provide care exclusively for hospitalized patients at one institution, replacing two physicians who had concurrent inpatient and outpatient responsibilities. This study showed decreased ICU and hospital mortality correlating with the use of onsite physician staffing. The greatest limitation of this study was its small size, but its design is characteristic of subsequent larger studies by other investigators. Despite its limitations, this published article was well received by the medical community. Li's study is often inaccurately referred to as the first one to examine intensivists; under closer inspection, the two physicians studied are actually hospitalists by today's definition.

PRACTICE POINT

- Most studies regarding ICU staffing do not compare hospitalists to intensivists despite the fact that 75% of hospitalists care for critically ill patients.

Later studies using critical care trained physicians in lieu of hospitalists consistently suggest improved patient outcomes when intensivists provide care to ICU patients. A meta-analysis by Pronovost, et al (2002) of 19 studies, including the original one by Li, et al, reported decreases in both hospital and ICU mortality and length of stay with the use of intensivists. All studies compared intensivists to traditional control models—physicians with both hospital and clinic responsibilities—and not to hospitalists. Other limitations of this meta-analysis include the retrospective or observational designs of the included studies, single-center studies, small sample sizes, and an inappropriate outcome adjustment based on proposed study quality in the analysis. Despite these study limitations, the specialized training of intensivists likely improves critical care provision and patient outcomes.

Aside from the study by Li, et al, no published trials compare adult hospitalists' ICU care to intensivists' (or other clinicians) ICU care since the "hospitalist movement" began in the 1990s and critical care board certification began in 1986. A recent study from Emory University School of Medicine suggests favorable outcomes when ICUs are staffed by hospitalists utilizing selective intensivist consultation (unpublished data, awaiting peer review). To date, one published trial evaluated pediatric patient outcomes with the use of pediatric hospitalists at a single institution. Tenner, et al reported decreased mortality and length of stay when pediatric hospitalists provided after-hour care rather than pediatric residents.

A study by Levy, et al in 2008 examined the impact of intensivists by utilizing a large, multicenter database. The study produced controversial findings that suggested intensivist-staffed ICUs may have higher mortality rates. Although this retrospective study had a sample size of more than 100,000 patients from multiple medical centers, the authors concluded that confounding factors contributed to their findings. The database relied on the accuracy of diagnosis coding and self-identified specialty by physicians. Hospitalists were included among the nonintensivist physicians but were not evaluated separately, nor compared directly, with the intensivists. This paper received critical editorial review by some intensivist peers but most agreed that further well-designed studies are needed to more accurately define the impact of intensivists and hospitalists.

ICU PHYSICIAN STAFFING

Based on available medical literature and expert opinions, an advocacy group made a recommendation in 2000 to staff *urban* ICUs with intensivists. This advocacy organization—the Leapfrog Group—is a nonmedical business consortium that strives to improve the quality of American medical care by using employer health care purchasing power as a compelling influence. One of its initial "three leaps" to improve patient safety focused on the use of intensivist-led ICU Physician Staffing (IPS) and had four principle components: (1) physicians with board certification in critical care manage or co-manage all ICU patients; (2) physician clinical responsibilities are exclusively to the ICU; (3) physicians are present in the ICU during daytime hours (8 hours per day); and (4) physicians are accessible at all other times with an assistant who can reach the ICU in less than 5 minutes. When the Leapfrog Group proposed IPS, estimates suggested that 10% of American ICUs already used this staffing model. A follow-up study in 2006 by Angus, et al estimated that merely 4% of ICUs met these stringent IPS standards. Nearly 25% of ICUs attained "high intensity" staffing, defined as intensivist management or co-management of at least 80% of ICU patients. Several barriers to IPS implementation include the perceived loss of control or potential income by primary physicians and other subspecialists. Interestingly, hospitalists have faced and overcome similar concerns over the past two decades regarding their role in inpatient care. Other barriers to IPS include the significant costs to hospitals for recruitment and retention of intensivists and the limited availability of intensivists for hire. The latter reason has received the most attention.

In 2000, the Committee for Manpower for Pulmonary and Critical Care Societies (COMPACCS) published the first large-scale assessment of the American intensivist workforce. With representation from key professional groups, including the American College of Chest Physicians, the American Thoracic Society, and the Society of Critical Care Medicine (SCCM), this committee carefully examined the current and future supply and demand for adult intensivists. It discovered that most intensivists spend considerable time on activities outside the ICU and on average allocate only 26% of their clinical time to the ICU itself. COMPACCS demonstrated a projected widening disparity between intensivist supply and demand, with a predicted shortfall of intensivist hours that will equal 22% by 2020 and 35% by 2035 (**Figure 133-1**). This study's findings suggest the future growth of critical care needs in the United States will outpace the ability to train and retain intensivists.

Subsequent workforce evaluations have reached similar conclusions to COMPACCS when performed by critical care professional societies in 2004 and 2007 and the governmental department of Health Resources and Services Administration in 2006. All analyses

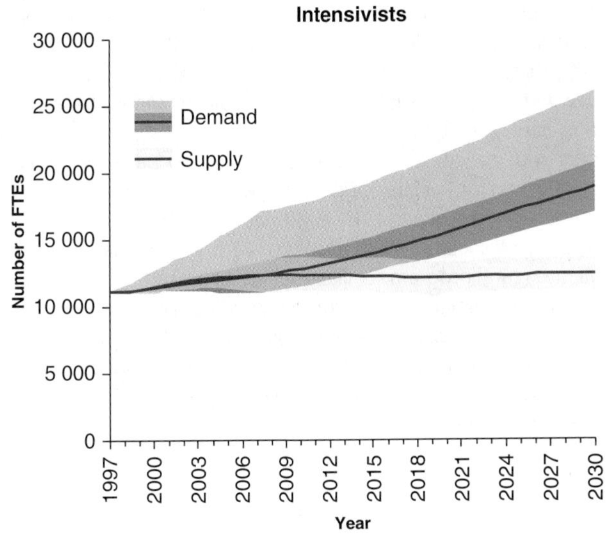

Figure 133-1 *Forecast of supply and demand for intensivists. FTEs, full-time equivalents. (Reproduced, with permission, from Angus DC, Kelley MA, Schmitz RJ, et al. Current and projected workforce requirements for the care of The critically ill and patients with pulmonary disease: can we meet the requirements of an aging population? JAMA. 2000;284(21):2766. Copyright © 2000 American Medical Association. All rights reserved.)*

distinguish between the "physician supply" and the "effective supply." The intensivist physician supply reflects the total number of active intensivists and nears 11,000. The intensivist effective supply reflects the total amount of pooled ICU services provided by all intensivists and is merely equivalent to 2000 to 2500 full-time physicians. This underscores the severity of the staffing shortage and raises concerns that implementing the Leapfrog Group's intensivist-led IPS nationwide is not feasible.

One answer to the intensivist shortage has been hospitalist practice in the ICU, either alongside or in place of critical care specialists. Hospital Medicine remains the fastest growing specialty in the United States (**Figure 133-2**). The Society of Hospital Medicine (SHM) 2007/2008 National Survey revealed that 75% of Hospital Medicine physician respondents care for critically ill patients. However, critical care encompasses only a small portion of their overall activities. In academic centers where intensivists are more prevalent, a remarkable 45% of hospitalists reported that they provide critical care.

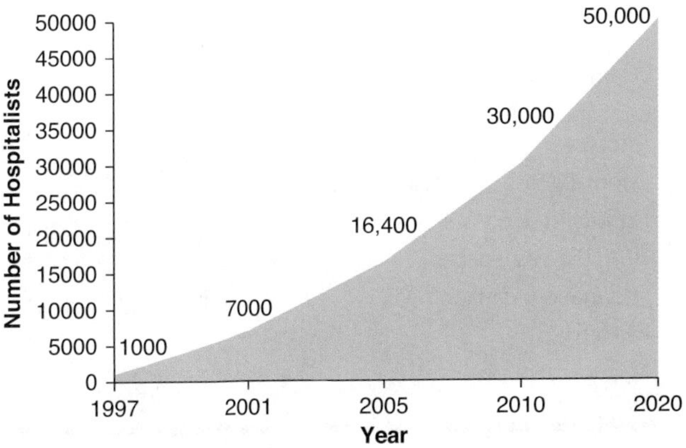

Figure 133-2 *Actual and projected growth of Hospital Medicine in the United States.*

Surveys conducted by other Hospital Medicine groups demonstrate comparable findings. Hospital Medicine's prevalence in the ICU has become so significant that a few editorials refer to hospitalists as the 'new intensivists' while others describe this staffing solution as merely a "stop-gap." Anecdotal evidence suggests facilities that currently utilize co-management for ICU patients benefit from an arrangement that capitalizes on hospitalists' onsite availability and intensivists' critical care proficiency. Proponents of hospitalists in the ICU argue that patient outcomes are more important than strict adherence to the Leapfrog Group's standards.

The expanding future needs for critical care provision stem from several trends. First, the acuity of hospitalized patients is rising as a result of medical advances and the increasing shift of lower acuity medical care to outpatient settings or other health care facilities. Second, the predictions account for the anticipated health care needs of the aging American population, specifically the baby boomer generation. Data from the US Census Bureau predicts that the population over the age of 65 will grow in size by 50% between 2000 and 2020 as compared to a 10% growth in the population under the age of 65. Patients over 65 years consume the greatest amount of health care services and account for more than half of all ICU patients. Health care expenditures 2 years before death are greater than any other period of life. Almost 500,000 people die in the ICU every year. For patients older than 65 years, the primary inpatient providers are hospitalists who are expected to continue providing care for the majority of older hospitalized patients.

ICU ORGANIZATION

ICUs are often divided broadly into two formats, "open" and "closed," according to admitting physicians. In open systems, primary care physicians retain the responsibilities of patient care and may choose to involve specialists, if available, with critical care expertise. In closed systems, the patient care is directed by critical care specialists either through the transfer of all care responsibilities or mandatory consultation upon arrival to the ICU. Hospitalists commonly practice in open formats and in facilities without intensivists. Critical care specialists are more prevalent in academic institutions where closed formats predominate. The closed format minimizes the number of physicians and thus reduces provider practice variability which can contribute to medical errors. In open formats, however, hospitalists also tend to narrow the range of admitting physicians. The Leapfrog Group's IPS model commonly is interpreted to favor closed formats though this is not a requirement to meet its four principles. Instead, the Leapfrog Group aims to increase critically ill patients' exposure to intensivist knowledge and skills. Comanagement with hospitalists meets this goal, and both the SHM and SCCM express support of such collaborative efforts.

While many published studies compare patient outcomes between open and closed formats, additional studies have demonstrated that it takes more than an intensivist to provide high-quality critical care. A growing body of ICU literature focuses broadly on the organizational components associated with successful systems. One crucial component of a "systems approach" is the consistent use of ICU protocols and checklists which can outperform treatments by individual providers. Frequently updated protocols ensure evidence-based practice, reduce provider practice variability, and likely result in improved patient outcomes as well as more efficient consumption of resources. Additionally, ICUs benefit from the leadership of a director who can maximize material and personnel resources, standardize practices, oversee unit data collection for quality and system improvement, and ensure effective communication and teamwork among the disciplines of physicians, nonphysician providers, nursing staff, respiratory therapists, and critical care pharmacists. A study by Kim, et al in 2010 showed that daily rounds by multidisciplinary teams in the ICU may reduce mortality. The

SCCM has endorsed an intensivist-led multidisciplinary team model as the optimal approach to critical care provision for many decades. In centers without intensivists, hospitalists are ideal candidates to serve as ICU directors with their skill sets in quality improvement, protocol development, health care resource management, and hospital leadership.

FUTURE DIRECTIONS

The limited intensivist workforce combined with expanding critical care needs mandates more efficient utilization and effective dissemination of critical care resources. Two special task forces convened to address the critical care "crisis" and raise awareness before Congress. Those task forces included FOCCUS (Framing Options for Critical Care in the United States) in 2004 and PrOMIS (Prioritizing the Organization and Management of Intensive Care Services in the Unites States) in 2007. Each published conference reports with recommendations to optimize, redistribute and expand the critical care workforce.

OPTIMIZING THE CRITICAL CARE WORKFORCE

Both FOCCUS and PrOMIS emphasize the importance of standardized critical care practices since significant regional and institutional variations exist. To date, the disciplines which provide critical care board certifications—anesthesia, internal medicine, pediatrics, and surgery—do not have well-defined homogeneous core competencies or a common competency examination. FOCCUS recommends identification and endorsement of core competencies similar to those reached by the international, transdisciplinary consensus from the European Society of Intensive Care Medicine. PrOMIS encourages these four disciplines to reach agreement on a common competency-based examination. Uniform standards for accreditation of critical care capacity need development as well. On an institutional level, the designation of an ICU director, either an intensivist or hospitalist, and consistent use of uniform ICU protocols are recommended immediately. Future investment in health services research is needed to enhance unit organization and to define the optimal roles of hospitalists and intensivists in the ICU.

While most recommendations concentrate on provider supply, FOCCUS and PrOMIS do also address critical care demand. The development and enforcement of clear admission and discharge criteria on institutional, regional, and national levels could minimize less effective or less efficient ICU use. Since hospitalists care for patients before, often during, and after the ICU stay, Hospital Medicine must actively participate in the development of ICU transfer criteria. Public education could confront the sometimes unrealistic expectations often held by patients and their families of critical care effectiveness. An emphasis on end of life discussions, preferably in the outpatient setting, combined with widespread use of advance directives could help ensure critical care provision to appropriate populations.

PRACTICE POINT

- In 2008, the ABMS formally recognized Hospice and Palliative Medicine as a subspecialty with its own board certification. More than 50 fellowships programs train physicians in this specialty.

In the inpatient setting, hospital palliative care programs offer an excellent means to address end of life issues. Such programs decrease ICU admission and length of stay during the last 6 months of life, while increasing patient and family satisfaction with medical care. In 2008, the ABMS formally recognized Hospice and Palliative Medicine as a subspecialty with its own board certification, and more than 50 fellowships programs train physicians within this specialty. Hospital Medicine incorporates palliative care into its core competencies and shares overlapping tenets with palliative medicine—availability to patients, families and referring physicians; ability to work in teams; and interest in inpatient care quality. The presence of a hospitalist program is strongly associated with hospitals starting and maintaining a palliative care program, a likely result of hospitalists' constant exposure to patients with chronic medical problems and life threatening illnesses. Currently more than half of the hospitals with greater than 50 beds have palliative care programs, a rate that has doubled during the past 5 years and is expected to continue its rapid growth.

TABLE 133-1 Core Competencies in Hospital Medicine

Core competencies	
Acute coronary syndrome	Diabetes mellitus
Acute renal failure	Gastrointestinal bleed
Alcohol and drug withdrawal	Hospital-acquired pneumonia
Asthma	Pain management
Cardiac arrhythmia	Perioperative medicine
Cellulitis	Sepsis syndrome
Chronic obstructive pulmonary disease	Stroke
Community-acquired pneumonia	Urinary tract infection
Congestive heart failure	Venous thromboembolism
Delirium and dementia	
Procedures	
Arthrocentesis	Lumbar puncture
Emergency procedures:	Paracentesis
Advanced cardiac life support	Thoracentesis
Endotrachael intubation	Vascular access
Ventilator management	
Health care systems	
Care of the elderly patient	Nutrition in the hospitalized patient
Care of vulnerable populations	Palliative care
Communication	Patient education
Diagnostic decision making	Patient handoff
Drug safety, pharmacoeconomics	Patient safety
Equitable allocation of resources	Practice-based learning
Evidence-based medicine	Prevention of health care infections
Hospitalist as consultant	Prevention of antimicrobial Resistance
Hospitalist as teacher	Professionalism and medical ethics
Information management	Quality improvement
Leadership	
Management practices	

Data from Pistoria MJ, Amin AN, Dressler DD, et al. The core competencies in Hospital Medicine: A framework for curriculum development. *J Hosp Med.* 2006;1(S1):2–67.

TABLE 133-2 Evidence-based Medicine: Key References for ICU Physician Staffing

Study	Methodology	Results	Limitations	Bottom Line
Landmark trial				
Li TC, et al. *JAMA.* 1984;252: 2023–2027.	Prospective, observational	• 517 patients enrolled in 1 year; 480 patients from previous year as historical controls; 4 physicians • Lower hospital mortality (OR, 0.62), fewer ICU readmissions	• Small size • Single center • Historical controls	• Onsite physicians associated with improved mortality outcomes
Historical review				
Fuchs RJ, et al. *Best Pract Res Clin Anaesthesiol.* 2005;19:125–135.	Review article of published evidence supporting intensivists	• Summarizes 13 articles from 1984 to 2004	• Review article	• Intensivist-led staffing models are cost-effective and improve mortality and LOS
Epidemiology				
Angus DC, et al. *JAMA.* 2000;284: 2762–2770.	Prospective, national surveys; estimates current and future US physician requirements for adult critical care	• 393 ICU directors, 421 specialists surveyed • Intensivists care for 36.8% of ICU patients • Predicts shortfall of intensivist hours equal to 22% of demand by 2020 and 35% by 2030	• Future projections may be imprecise • Potential inaccuracies in administrative reports of patient-level data	• US critical care needs will outpace future supply of intensivists
Recent trials				
Pronovost PJ, et al. *JAMA.* 2002;288: 2151–2162.	Systematic literature review; compares patient outcomes between intensivists and nonintensivists	• Reviewed 19 studies of intensivists • 16 report lower hospital mortality; 14 report lower ICU mortality • 10 report shorter hospital LOS; 14 report shorter ICU LOS	• Many small, observational studies; no RCT • Methodology may bias results in favor of intensivists	• Need more rigorous study of intensivists • Mandatory ICU intensivist staffing may improve patient outcomes
Levy MM, et al. *Ann Intern Med.* 2008;148: 801–809.	Retrospective analysis of prospectively collected national database of ICU patients; compares intensivists to nonintensivists	• Database of 101,832 patients in 100 US hospitals with 123 ICUs from 2000 to 2004 • Adjusted OR 1.42 for mortality with intensivists	• Database relies on accurate physician documentation • Referral and patient selection biases • Unrecognized confounders of illness severity may affect results	• Contradicts prior published findings • Need more research to explain findings and further evaluate intensivists

ICU, intensive care unit; LOS, length of stay; RCT, randomized control trials.

REDISTRIBUTING CRITICAL CARE RESOURCES

An important proposal by FOCCUS and PrOMIS is to regionalize critical care as a means to best distribute limited ICU resources. Trauma care in the US is a successful example of this approach and could be replicated by creating tiered critical care centers. Regionalization takes advantage of the higher intensivist prevalence in tertiary centers. Secondary care centers could utilize hospitalists or other providers with critical care competency. Barriers to regionalization include the existing institutional and regional practice variation and the absence of a general consensus approach to critical care.

To encourage appropriate resource distribution, the Leapfrog Group's IPS could be liberalized to the 'high-intensity' models described by critical care experts. This staffing model requires only 80% of ICU patients, rather than 100%, have intensivist management or comanagement. Such a model could realign intensivists to care for the ICU populations that benefit most from their involvement—those with the most severe critical illnesses.

Telemedicine extends critical care expertise to remote facilities without relocating intensivists to low demand areas. Forty electronic ICU (e-ICU) programs provide remote critical care services in the US, and that number continues to grow. Fostering research to enhance the role of medical informatics, including decision support systems, may further help the delivery of care to remote areas and the development of a regional tiered system. Little information describes hospitalists' current participation or future role in telemedicine. Unique opportunities for Hospital Medicine may exist in this area.

EXPANDING CRITICAL CARE SERVICES

Most importantly, the FOCCUS and PrOMIS task forces sought ways to expand the critical care workforce. When intensivists serve as *consultants*, rather than admitting physicians, they are able to see more patients. Likewise, an *intensivist-led* team with non-physician providers allows a greater reach of intensivist expertise to a broader patient population than a single critical care provider could offer alone. The numbers of acute care nurse practitioners and physician assistants available for hire unfortunately limits this option. Additional recommendations include increasing intensivist fellowship training positions and creating incentives to attract and retain health care professionals to critical care careers.

PRACTICE POINT

- The PrOMIS Report describes the potential impact of hospitalists to address the critical care staffing crisis. The role of hospitalists in critical care is anticipated to expand, although it needs better definition and consensus agreement.

The provider shortage that precludes intensivists from caring for *all* critically ill patients has precipitated an interest in certifying others who provide critical care additionally. The PrOMIS Report described the potential impact of hospitalists to address the staffing crisis and called for "cross-training of hospital-based providers to provide intensive care services in lower 'tier' hospitals." Many illnesses managed in the ICU are merely more complicated or more critically ill versions of the common medical conditions found in the Hospital Medicine Core Competencies, and hospitalists may be able to offer significant critical care provision. Similarly, procedures necessary to practice in the ICU setting are also contained within the Hospital Medicine Core Competencies (**Table 133-1**). Furthermore, the growth curve for the Hospital Medicine workforce continues to rise sharply and currently exceeds 30,000, already outnumbering intensivists. Graduates of Emergency Medicine residency programs, another hospital-based specialty, could participate in training and credentialing options as well.

The format, length of training, and type of certification for critical care competency remains controversial and proposals vary widely. Some recommendations include identifying hospitalists with specific ICU interest and skills who could be required to dedicate at least 50% of their clinical time to the ICU and complete annual critical care continuing medical education. More aggressive suggestions include a rigorous, comprehensive education and skills training process accomplished with a combination of onsite training and distance learning. Critical care certification would distinguish recipients as possessing capabilities beyond those obtained in residency, but it would *not* be equivalent to critical care board certification. Several institutions are moving forward with training designs.

Another strategy to augment the critical care workforce could be the establishment of basic competency criteria by appropriate governing bodies such as SCCM and SHM. Individual institutions could implement customized programs appropriate for their institution and their patient populations that meet this established competency criteria. One means to develop clear consensus and guidelines for such criteria would be to convene the proposed PrOMIS II working group to further the efforts of the original PrOMIS Task Force.

CONCLUSION

The growing US critical care needs coupled with the predicted intensivist workforce shortage require innovative solutions to provide health care to the critically ill without compromising the quality of patient care (**Table 133-2**). The organizational framework of ICUs needs revision to facilitate judicious utilization of costly and limited ICU material and personnel resources. Based on current training models, the number of intensivists is unlikely to change significantly over the next 25 years. Therefore, our health care system must adapt with solutions to provide care for our critically ill patient population. The role of hospitalists in critical care is anticipated to expand, although it needs better definition and consensus agreement. The question is no longer *if* hospitalists should be involved in ICU care, but rather *how* to assure clinician competency, care quality, and improved clinical outcomes through enhanced collaboration between Hospital Medicine and critical care medicine.

SUGGESTED READINGS

Angus DC, Kelley MA, Schmitz RT, et al. Current and projected workforce requirements for care of the critically ill and patients with pulmonary disease: can we meet the requirements of an aging population? *JAMA*. 2000;284:2762–2770.

Angus DC, Shorr AF, White A, et al. Critical care delivery in the United States: Distribution of services and compliance with Leapfrog recommendations. *Crit Care Med*. 2006;34(4):1016–1024.

Barnato AE, Kahn JM, Rubenfield GD, et al. Prioritizing the organization and management of intensive care services in the United States: The PrOMIS conference. *Crit Care Med*. 2007;35(4):1003–1011.

Ewart, GW, Marcus L, Gaba MM, et al. The critical care medicine crisis: A call for federal action. *Chest*. 2004;125(4):1518–1521.

Fuchs RJ, Berenholtz SM, Dorman T. Do intensivists in the ICU improve outcome? *Best Pract Res Clin Anaesthesiol*. 2005;19:125–135.

Kim M, Barnato AE, Angus DC, et al. The effect of multidisciplinary care teams on intensive care unit mortality. *Arch Intern Med*. 2010;170(4):369–376.

Levy MM, Rapoport J, Lemeshow S, et al. Association between critical care physician management and patient mortality in the intensive care unit. *Ann Intern Med*. 2008;148(11):801–809.

Li TC, Malcolm CP, Shaw L, et al. On-site physician staffing in a community hospital intensive care unit. *JAMA*. 1984;252:2023–2027.

Pronovost PJ, Angus DC, Dorman T, et al. Physician staffing patterns and clinical outcomes in critically ill patients. *JAMA*. 2002;288:2151–2162.

Tenner PA, Dibrell H, Taylor RP. Improved survival with hospitalists in a pediatric intensive care unit. *Crit Care Med*. 2003;31:847–852.

CHAPTER 134

Acute Respiratory Distress Syndrome

Corey D. Kershaw, MD
Greg S. Martin, MD, MSc

Key Clinical Questions

1. What are the predisposing diseases/conditions that lead to acute respiratory distress syndrome (ARDS)?
2. How can ARDS be differentiated from other causes of hypoxemic respiratory failure?
3. What is the correct strategy in the management of mechanical ventilation in ARDS?
4. What adjunctive therapies may be beneficial in ARDS management?
5. What is the expected morbidity for patients who survive ARDS to hospital discharge?

INTRODUCTION

The acute respiratory distress syndrome (ARDS) describes a common disorder encountered in the critical care unit that remains a significant cause of morbidity and mortality since its initial description in 1967. Standardization of ventilator strategies and overall improvement in critical care management, however, has resulted in significant improvements in outcomes in the last decade. Early recognition is essential in order to admit and/or transfer the patient to a higher level of care, when indicated.

EPIDEMIOLOGY

Since the publication of the American-European Consensus Conference (AECC) (see Diagnosis) definitions for acute lung injury (ALI) and ARDS, the incidence has been identified in several studies. Without differentiating between ALI and ARDS, the incidence may range from 20 to 50 cases per 100,000 person-years. When rigorous screening for ALI and ARDS was applied in King County, Washington in 2000, investigators reported an incidence of 78.9 cases/100,000 person-years and 58.7 cases/100,000 person-years, respectively. Methodological differences may explain the disparity in incidence, as some reports retrospectively review prior ARDS studies while others prospectively identify patients admitted to an intensive care unit (ICU) or among those requiring mechanical ventilation. Inaccuracies in true incidence are magnified by a nonspecific case definition—the AECC ARDS criteria—and the relative lack of validation studies for said criteria (see Diagnosis).

PRESENTATION

Patients presenting with acute lung injury or impending ARDS may be difficult to differentiate initially from other causes of hypoxemic respiratory failure. A predisposing cause of ALI/ARDS should be present, with pulmonary and non-pulmonary sepsis most common (**Table 134-1**). Knowledge of the common etiologies of ARDS is important as early vigilance in regards to moving the patient to a higher level of care (eg, transferring to the ICU) and initiation of appropriate ICU interventions can minimize morbidity and mortality. Furthermore, identification of an underlying cause or inciting event is important in differentiating ARDS from other lung diseases or syndromes that may be misidentified as ARDS. Early and efficient identification of predisposing syndromes may prevent progression to ALI or ARDS. The evolution from inciting cause to ARDS typically occurs within 3 to 5 days, giving the clinician a window of suspicion for ARDS to develop.

PRACTICE POINT

- The evolution from inciting cause to ARDS typically occurs within 3 to 5 days, giving the clinician a window of suspicion for ARDS to develop.

The presenting complaint may be nonspecific and herald a more serious problem which accompanies the predisposing condition. Shortness of breath, dyspnea, and cough are likely present. Fever and sputum production may indicate a pulmonary infection, while hypoxemia requiring high fractions of inspired supplemental oxygen suggests evolving acute lung injury with worsening ventilation-perfusion (V/Q) mismatching and worsening shunt

TABLE 134-1 Common Predisposing Causes of ARDS

Direct Lung Injury	Indirect Lung Injury
Pneumonia	Nonpulmonary sepsis
Gastric aspiration	Acute pancreatitis
Chest trauma/lung contusion	Nonchest trauma
Inhalation injury	Massive transfusions
Near-drowning	Surface burns

physiology. The evaluating clinician may describe declining level of consciousness secondary to severe hypoxemia or concomitant hypercapnia. Concerning findings such as altered mentation and hypercapnia usually warrant immediate endotracheal intubation. Tachypnea and auscultation of rales on physical examination is typical of ALI/ARDS but may also present in other causes of acute respiratory failure such as congestive heart failure, pneumonia, or occult interstitial lung disease. Laboratory studies are not specific for ARDS. Severe hypoxemia is part of the diagnostic criteria of ALI and ARDS. Concomitant hypercapnia may indicate failure of compensatory ventilatory mechanisms. Failure to compensate for a respiratory acidosis or inadequate clearance of carbon dioxide in the face of tachypnea is especially worrisome and warrants immediate attention. Leukocytosis, also nonspecific, may belie the predisposing cause as in severe pneumonia or sepsis.

Chest radiography reveals bilateral, diffuse airspace infiltrates. Patchy infiltrates may become more confluent as the syndrome evolves (**Figure 134-1**). Cardiomegaly suggests preexisting cardiac disease and thus left ventricular dysfunction as an etiology for the patient's hypoxemia and chest radiograph abnormality. In cases where there is concern about coexistent or predominant heart failure, additional testing (echocardiogram or pulmonary artery catheter, for example) may be required to confirm the diagnosis of ARDS or rule out other conditions.

PATHOPHYSIOLOGY

Integrity of the alveolar-capillary membrane is required to maintain a dry alveolar space and to ensure adequate gas exchange between the alveolar epithelium across the interstitial space to the pulmonary capillaries. The predisposing injury leading to ARDS results in several pathophysiological changes at every level of the alveolar-capillary compartment (**Figure 134-2**).

The alveolar epithelium is composed primarily of two types of cells. Type I pneumocytes function primarily in architectural support as well as fluid and solute transport through its aquaporin-5 surface proteins. The larger, but fewer, type II pneumocytes are capable of differentiating into type I cells. These cells primarily produce and recycle surfactant. The type I cell is more susceptible to injury, and during the early phases of ARDS (the *acute, exudative phase*) barrier integrity is disrupted as type I cells are damaged. Dilution of edema fluid in the alveolus and decreased production following type II cell damage impairs surfactant function. This contributes to atelectasis and worsening pulmonary compliance.

Similar injury occurs on the capillary endothelial side of the compartment. In ALI/ARDS, the alveolar-capillary barrier loses its ability to limit egress of fluids, proteins, and debris from the vascular space. The combination of vascular hydrostatic and protein osmotic pressures, together with vascular integrity, sets the stage for accumulation of proteinaceous pulmonary edema according to Starling's equation, first described in 1896:

$$J_v = K_{f,c}[(P_c - P_i) - \sigma(\pi_{pp} - \pi_{ip})]$$

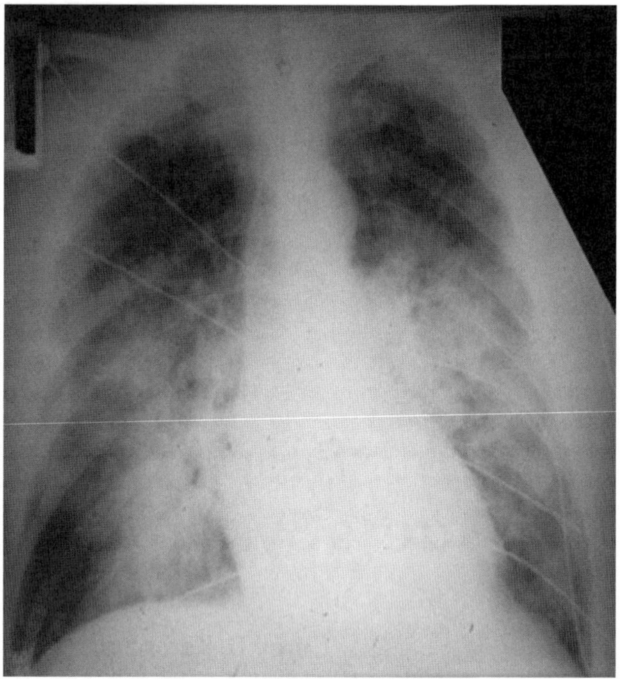

A

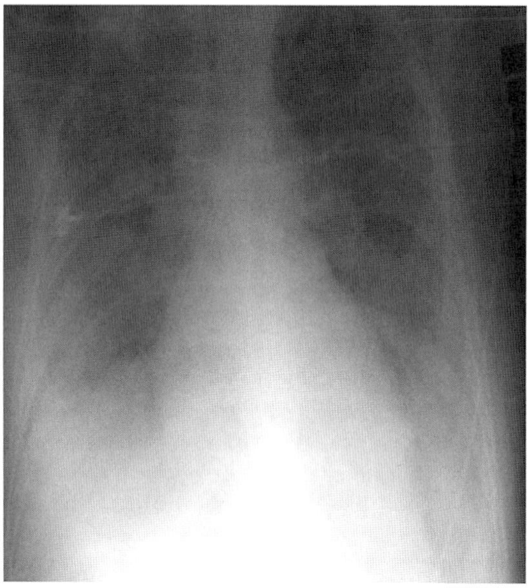

B

Figure 134-1 *Chest radiographs depicting ARDS with a patchy airspace pattern (A). ARDS can progress to a more confluent airspace pattern over time (B).*

The Starling equation states that movement of fluid across a capillary barrier into an interstitial space is governed by balances in the hydrostatic pressure in the capillary and interstitium (P_c and P_i, respectively) and the plasma and interstitial oncotic pressures (π_{pp} and π_{ip}, respectively). Increases in capillary hydrostatic pressure or decreases capillary oncotic pressure will result in net movement of fluid out of the plasma space and in to the interstitial subcompartment. The capillary reflection coefficient (σ) and the bulk transfer coefficient (K_f) describe the integrity of the capillary barrier: as σ approaches zero the barrier loses its ability to segregate oncotically active substances, while increases in K_f linearly increase movement of fluid across the membrane. The injury seen early in acute lung

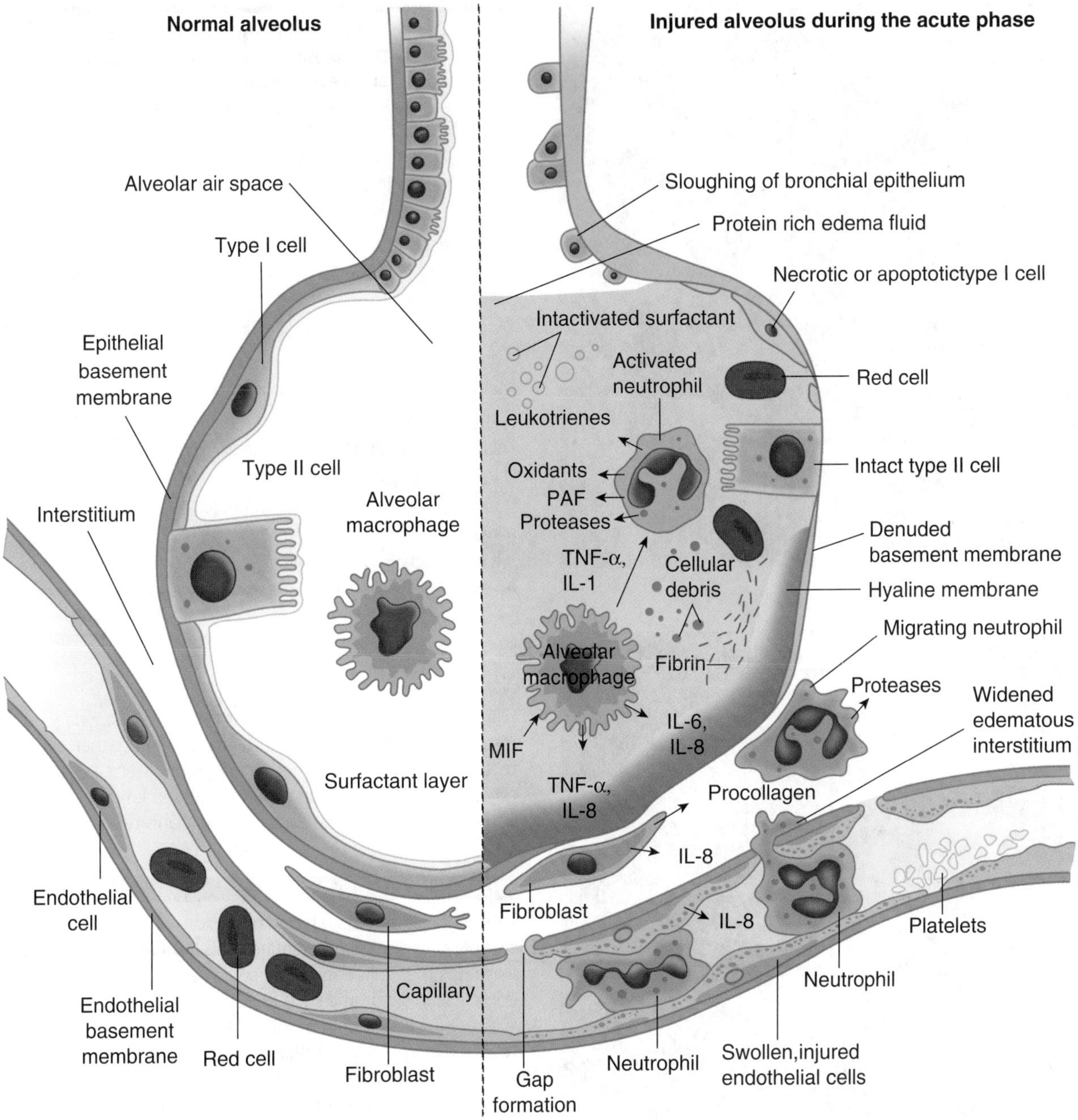

Figure 134-2 *Normal alveolus on the left (a) and injured alveolus during the acute phase of the acute respiratory distress syndrome on the right (b). (Reproduced, with permission, from Ware LB, Matthay MA. The acute respiratory distress syndrome. N Engl J Med. 2000;342:1334).*

injury facilitates movement of fluid out of the capillary compartment by a combination of these changes.

In this early stage of ARDS, shunting and hypoxemia dominate the clinical picture. The flooding of the alveolar unit with *proteinaceous Edema* leads to worsening V/Q mismatching and physiologic shunt that is increasingly refractory to oxygen supplementation. The *atelectasis* caused by surfactant defects requires higher pressures to maintain alveolar patency for ventilation. *Increases in pulmonary artery pressures* secondary to hypoxemic pulmonary vasoconstriction, decreases in pulmonary circulation due to *microthrombi* and direct damage to the vascular endothelium lead to worsening dead space ventilation. Together, each of these contributes to increased work of breathing. The histological change seen in the exudative phase is known as *diffuse alveolar damage* (**Figure 134-3A**). Nonspecific for ARDS, diffuse alveolar damage is not considered diagnostic and a lung biopsy is not necessary unless other alternative diagnoses are seriously considered.

PRACTICE POINT

- Diffuse alveolar damage is nonspecific for ARDS and not considered diagnostic. Lung biopsy is not necessary unless other alternative diagnoses are seriously considered.

These changes in the exudative phase of ARDS are heterogeneous and of variable duration, typically lasting 7 to 10 days. Following the exudative phase, the lungs progress to the second stage of disease known as the *proliferative phase* (**Figure 134-3B**). Type II pneumocytes begin to regenerate in order to reconstitute the surfactant layer, and type I cells rebuild the damaged alveolar epithelium. Depending on the effectiveness of this reparative process, recovery from ARDS in days 7 through 21 may be rapid. Some patients, however, have a prolonged course as procollagen III is deposited in the interstitial space with subsequent fibrosis.

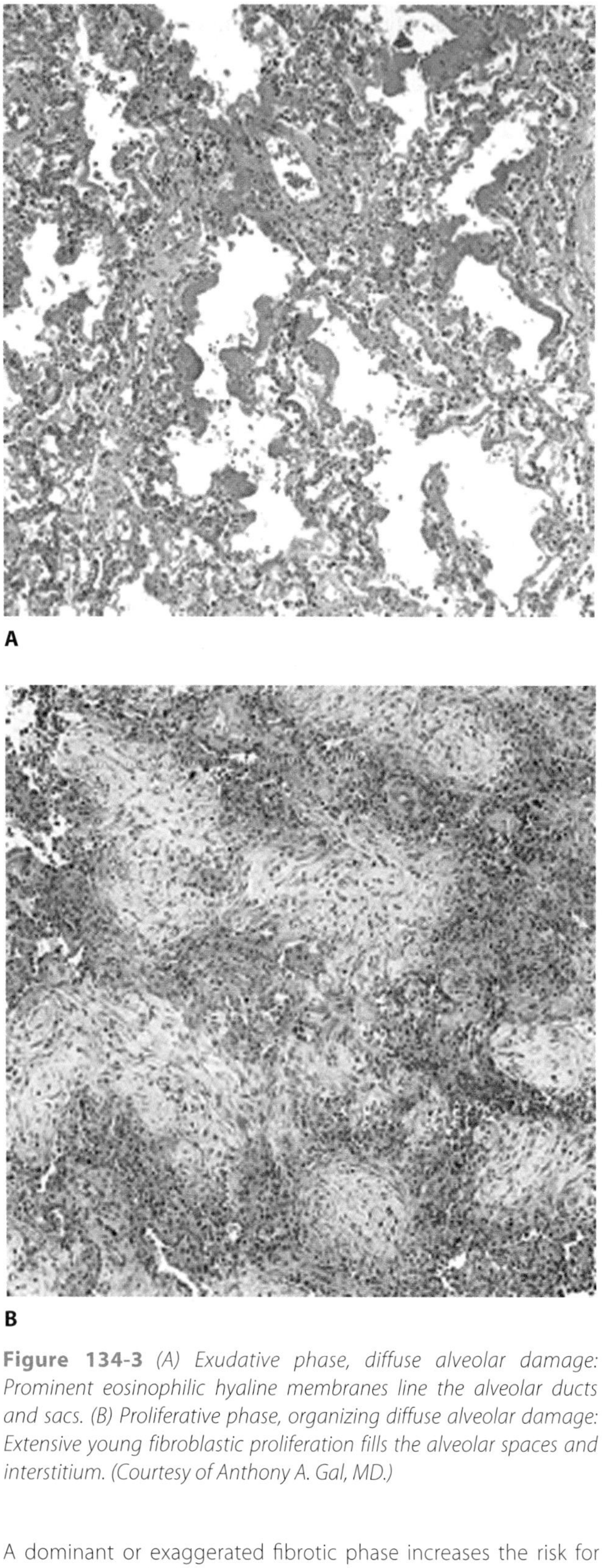

Figure 134-3 *(A) Exudative phase, diffuse alveolar damage: Prominent eosinophilic hyaline membranes line the alveolar ducts and sacs. (B) Proliferative phase, organizing diffuse alveolar damage: Extensive young fibroblastic proliferation fills the alveolar spaces and interstitium. (Courtesy of Anthony A. Gal, MD.)*

A dominant or exaggerated fibrotic phase increases the risk for prolonged morbidity or mortality and may require prolonged mechanical ventilation. As the vascular changes that occur in the exudative phase become more irreversible, pulmonary hypertension may result.

PRACTICE POINT

- Depending on the effectiveness of the reparative process, recovery from ARDS in days 7 through 21 may be rapid.

TABLE 134-2 Differential Diagnosis of Diseases Causing Diffuse Airspace Pattern on Chest Radiography and Severe Hypoxemia

Infectious
Pneumocystis jiroveci pneumonia
Viral pneumonitis
Severe community-acquired pneumonia
Noninfectious
Hydrostatic pulmonary edema: heart failure or other volume overload state
Acute interstitial pneumonia (Hamman-Rich syndrome)
Diffuse alveolar hemorrhage
Acute eosinophilic pneumonia
Lymphangitic spread of cancer or leukemic infiltration
Acute onset of cryptogenic organizing pneumonia
Drug toxicity (eg, amiodarone, methotrexate, bleomycin)
Immunologic (eg, lupus pneumonitis, Goodpasture disease, Wegener disease)
Hypersensitivity pneumonitis

In summary, the acute respiratory failure secondary to ARDS results from both permeability damage—from either direct injury to the alveolar-capillary membrane or an overzealous inflammatory response to the injury—and decreased lung compliance that deranges the normal gas exchange mechanisms.

DIFFERENTIAL DIAGNOSIS

The diagnosis of ARDS is based on clinical criteria and requires exclusion of other diseases presenting in a similar manner. This challenge illustrates the limitation of using clinical parameters to diagnose a complicated syndrome such as ARDS.

Acute infectious pneumonias that cause either an interstitial pattern or diffuse airspace disease can be indistinguishable on clinical grounds from ARDS. *Pneumocystis jiroveci* pneumonia (previously PCP), pneumonitis secondary to viral infection (varicella zoster, for example), or a severe bacterial community-acquired pneumonia may present with a chest x-ray and refractory hypoxemia without the same cellular toxicity seen in ARDS. Further, these pulmonary infections may lead to the development of ARDS and complicate the diagnosis more.

There are also multiple noninfectious diseases that can mimic the refractory hypoxemia and chest x-ray pattern in ARDS (**Table 134-2**).

DIAGNOSIS

In 1994, the American-European Consensus Conference on ARDS published the clinical definition of acute lung injury and acute respiratory distress syndrome. Since that time, ALI has been defined by the following three criteria: (1) PaO_2:FiO_2 ≤ 300, (2) bilateral infiltrates on chest x-ray (see Figures 134-1A, B), and (3) the absence of left atrial hypertension or a pulmonary artery occlusion pressure ≤ 18 mm Hg. The third criterion excludes pulmonary edema of hydrostatic or cardiogenic origin. ARDS is defined by the same criteria but with worse oxygenation (PaO_2:FiO_2 ≤ 200), representing the subset of ALI patients with more severe hypoxemia.

PRACTICE POINT

- **Acute lung injury** definition (three criteria): (1) $PaO_2:FiO_2 \leq 300$, (2) bilateral infiltrates on chest x-ray (Figures 134-1A, B), and (3) absence of left atrial hypertension or a pulmonary artery occlusion pressure ≤ 18 mm Hg.
- **Acute respiratory distress syndrome** definition: same criteria but with worse oxygenation—$PaO_2:FiO_2 \leq 200$—representing the subset of ALI patients with more severe hypoxemia.

While this definition allows for standardization in clinical trials enrollment, limitations arise when attempting to exclude other causes of refractory hypoxemia and bilateral airspace opacifications on chest x-ray. While many diseases can mimic this pattern and present in a similar fashion, the mechanisms by which these abnormalities develop differ from mechanisms that generate ARDS. The absence of a means to identify the known cellular toxicity changes that cause increases in vascular permeability may lead to an erroneous diagnosis and delay appropriate therapies.

Using confirmatory scientific methods in concert with less specific clinical criteria to define ALI and ARDS would allow clinicians to apply the most appropriate therapy earlier in the disease course and further advance the clinical research studies of this patient population.

Gallium scanning to quantify radioactive-labeled tracer movement out of the vascular space (changes in alveolar-capillary membrane permeability) has been studied but failed to differentiate ALI-induced edema from noncardiogenic pulmonary edema. Measurements of extravascular lung water using indicator dilution techniques may identify patients with ALI as opposed to edema from increased hydrostatic pressure. Studies are currently under way to assess the accuracy of these methods in comparison to the clinical criteria for ARDS. Until more sophisticated methods gain study evidence support to differentiate increased vascular permeability in the lung, the clinical definition of ARDS will be the method for diagnosis. Because of the definition's limitations, alternative causes of hypoxemia and bilateral infiltrates on chest x-ray should always be considered.

TRIAGE AND HOSPITAL ADMISSION

A patient presenting with new-onset or worsening hypoxemia must be admitted to the hospital; admission to the ICU should be pursued for patients with respiratory distress or hypoxemia refractory to supplemental oxygen. Initiation of mechanical ventilation qualifies for ICU admission, and some facilities require that patients placed on noninvasive ventilation also be admitted to a higher level of monitored care. Clinically unstable patients who require closer monitoring or higher levels of nursing care than can be provided on a typical medical/surgical floor setting should also be admitted or transferred to a progressive or intensive care unit.

MANAGEMENT

As a consequence of the underlying precipitant and resultant lung injury, ARDS leads to mechanical abnormalities in the lung parenchyma. This requires increased work of breathing in order to meet ventilatory demands. While noninvasive methods of oxygen delivery may temporarily eliminate hypoxemia, definitive management often requires invasive mechanical ventilation to correct the underlying gas exchange abnormalities (ie, hypoxemia) without the expense of causing further lung damage. **Table 134-3** provides a detailed summary of the management strategies that have been studied in ARDS.

MECHANICAL VENTILATION STRATEGIES

Application of mechanical ventilation allows decreased work of breathing by off-loading respiratory muscles and improving effective minute ventilation. As the work of breathing decreases, CO_2 production is decreased and overall acid-base status is improved. The poor lung compliance and heterogeneity of ARDS, however, places the lung in a position of vulnerability from the positive pressure generated by the ventilator. Atelectatic segments, especially those in an area of transition near normal lung, are especially susceptible to overstretching during the inspiratory phase of respiration. Further, the abnormalities in surfactant physiology characterizing ARDS lead to excessive closure of some alveoli during expiration. Repeated closure and overdistention leads to additional alveolar damage, a phenomenon known as ventilator-induced lung injury.

Strides in improving overall survival from ARDS were realized with the publication of a successful trial using low-tidal volume ventilation in a lung-protective strategy. The ARDS Network, a consortium of academic centers in the United States and funded by the National Institutes of Health (NIH), reported in 2000 an 8.8% absolute reduction in mortality when using 6 cc/kg target tidal volume compared with the common standard of 12 cc/kg. The investigation also employed aggressive management of acid-base derangements and used a standardized protocol for the application of positive end-expiratory pressure (PEEP) for a given FiO_2. The use of low-tidal volume ventilation was confirmed in a follow-up study published in 2004 that examined a higher PEEP/FiO_2 strategy in comparison to the one used in the ARDS Network study of 2000. While there was no mortality difference between the two treatment arms, the mortality was similar to the earlier trial.

Subsequent clinical trials have explored alternative methods of ventilation in ARDS. These include studies of various recruitment maneuvers and prone ventilation. While prone ventilation and recruitment maneuvers increase oxygenation in the majority of patients, this strategy has no improvement in mortality. This may serve to underscore the cause of death in patients with ARDS is typically not hypoxemia but rather multisystem organ failure.

High-frequency oscillatory ventilation (HFOV), a more advanced ventilator mode that employs very high respiratory rates and very small tidal volumes, is occasionally used in severely ill patients with respiratory failure. Very small tidal volumes at high rates are delivered at rather stable end-expiratory distending pressures. The technology allows for maximal alveolar recruitment but with a lower risk of overdistention because of the smaller tidal volumes delivered. Because of the high frequency, gas exchange is adequate despite the small volumes. A mortality benefit has not been demonstrated in two randomized-controlled trials to date, but earlier application may be valuable based on some study data. Other advanced modes of ventilation, such as adaptive support ventilation (ASV) or airway pressure-release ventilation (APRV), are becoming more prominent as ventilator technology advances. In ASV, a target percentage minute ventilation is set. Using a close loop algorithm, the ventilator determines and delivers an appropriate frequency and tidal volume combination based on its determination of the lung's mechanics. Spontaneous breaths are delivered with either pressure support or in a pressure-controlled manner, the amount of which is determined by the ventilator. APRV, like HFOV, employs a stable distending pressure, but with a periodic decrease in pressure—the "release"—for CO_2 removal. The patient can breathe spontaneously above the distended pressure. Neither of the modes have been extensively studied in well-designed clinical trials of ARDS at this point.

NONVENTILATORY STRATEGIES

The management of ARDS entails more than attention to proper ventilatory support, particularly as it relates to fluid status. In

TABLE 134-3 Summary of Management Strategies for Acute Respiratory Distress Syndrome

Management Strategy	Effect	Reference
Low-tidal volume ventilation	Reduced mortality, shortened duration of mechanical ventilation	Brower RG, et al; and The Acute Respiratory Distress Syndrome Network. Ventilation with lower tidal volumes as compared with traditional tidal volumes for acute lung injury and the acute respiratory distress syndrome. *N Engl J Med.* 2000;342:1301–1308.
Fluid restriction and/or diuretics	Reduced duration of mechanical ventilation	Wiedemann HP, et al; and the Acute Respiratory Distress Syndrome Network. Comparison of two fluid-management strategies in acute lung injury. *N Engl J Med.* 2006;354:2564–2575.
Corticosteroids	Reduced duration of mechanical ventilation and shock, improved oxygenation and respiratory-system compliance. Higher rates of neuromuscular weakness and increased mortality at 60 and 180 days if treated > 14 days after ARDS onset of ARDS	Steinberg KP, et al; and the Acute Respiratory Distress Syndrome Network. Comparison of two fluid-management strategies in acute lung injury. *N Engl J Med.* 2006;354:1671–1684.
Inhaled nitric oxide	Improved oxygenation; no impact on the duration of mechanical ventilation or survival	Taylor RW, et al. Low-dose inhaled nitric oxide in patients with acute lung injury: a randomized controlled trial. *JAMA.* 2004;291(13):1603–1609. Griffiths MJ, Evans TW. Inhaled nitric oxide therapy in adults. *N Engl J Med.* 2005;353:2683–2695.
Albumin and diuretics	Improved oxygenation and hemodynamics; no impact on the duration of mechanical ventilation or survival	Martin GS, et al. Albumin and furosemide therapy in hypoproteinemic patients with acute lung injury. *Crit Care Med* 2002;30:2175–2182. Martin GS, et al. A randomized, controlled trial of furosemide with or without albumin in hypoproteinemic patients with acute lung injury. *Crit Care Med.* 2005;33:1681–1687.
Surfactant	No impact on duration of mechanical ventilation or survival	Spragg RG, et al. Effect of recombinant surfactant protein C-based surfactant on the acute respiratory distress syndrome. *N Engl J Med.* 2004;351:884–892.
Beta-agonists	Potential reduction in lung water; no impact on duration of mechanical ventilation or survival	NHLBI ARDS Network. http://www.ardsnet.org/studies/alta Perkins GD, et al. The beta-agonist lung injury trial (BALTI): a randomized placebo-controlled clinical trial. *Am J Respir Crit Care Med.* 2006;173:281–287.
Prone positioning	Potential improvement in oxygenation, no certain impact on duration of mechanical ventilation or survival (severe ARDS may have survival benefit)	Taccone P, et al. Prone positioning in patients with moderate and severe acute respiratory distress syndrome: A randomized controlled trial. *JAMA.* 2009;302:1977–1984.
Recruitment maneuvers	Potential improvements in oxgyenation; possibly reduced duration of mechanical ventilation and other organ dysfunction	Meade MO, et al. Ventilation strategy using low tidal volumes, recruitment maneuvers, and high positive endexpiratory pressure for acute lung injury and acute respiratory distress syndrome: A randomized controlled trial. *JAMA.* 2008;299:637–645. Mercat A, et al. Positive end-expiratory pressure setting in adults with acute lung injury and acute respiratory distress syndrome: A randomized controlled trial. *JAMA.* 2008;299:646–655.
High frequency oscillatory ventilation	No clear impact on the duration of mechanical ventilation or survival	Fessler HE, et al. A protocol for high-frequency oscillatory ventilation in adults: results from a roundtable discussion. *Crit Care Med.* 2007;35:1649–1654.
Extracorporeal membrane oxygenation	No clear impact on the duration of mechanical ventilation or survival	Peek GJ, et al. Efficacy and economic assessment of conventional ventilator support versus extracorporeal membrane oxygenation for severe adult respiratory failure (CESAR): A multicentre randomised controlled trial. *Lancet.* 2009;374:1351–1363.

a trial published by the ARDS Network investigators in 2006, a conservative fluid management strategy reduced the number of days of ventilator support and ICU stay without causing nonpulmonary organ dysfunction. The same study found that use of a pulmonary artery catheter to direct fluid management was not superior to central venous catheter use, and indeed resulted in more arrhythmias.

Based on the pathophysiological mechanisms in ARDS, multiple targets for pharmacotherapy have been identified. Despite numerous trials of various therapies, no definitive agent has shown a benefit in clinically important outcomes. These include surfactant therapy, inhaled nitric oxide, phosphodiesterase inhibitors, and activated protein C, among others.

The role of corticosteroids in ARDS deserves special mention as the inflammatory response that produces diffuse alveolar damage suggests that corticosteroids may be beneficial. Corticosteroids have been studied extensively in differing doses and timing, yet no trial has yet defined a clear benefit in these patients. The best trial to date reported improvements in lung and cardiovascular physiology and a shortened duration of mechanical ventilation, but without an improvement in mortality and at the expense of steroid-induced neuromyopathy.

Future therapies may lie in the realm of genomics and cell-based therapy, as preliminary studies of mesenchymal stem cells and GM-CSF hold promise. As of 2010, these trials are in the early stages, and their benefit awaits definitive investigation.

The underlying source of the patient's ARDS must always be addressed. Patients with ARDS in the ICU are at risk for ICU-related complications pertaining to their stay. Thus, preventive measures should be employed. This includes appropriate prophylaxis against stress ulcers bleeding and deep venous thrombosis, raising the head of the bed at least 30° to guard against ventilator-associated pneumonia, and daily screening for readiness-to-liberate from the ventilator in conjunction with daily interruption of all sedative and analgesic infusions. Clinicians should minimize procedures to those deemed absolutely necessary.

CONSULTATIONS

Involvement of a clinician with special expertise in critical care medicine and/or management of mechanical ventilation is appropriate, if available. Early consultation to physical and occupational therapy specialists to initiate the rehabilitation of the patient and counter any strength deconditioning is an emerging area of interest in the ICU.

PROGNOSIS AND COMPLICATIONS

PREDICTORS

As the majority of patients with ARDS die not of worsening respiratory failure but rather nonpulmonary conditions such as multisystem organ failure or nosocomial infection, oxygenation carries uncertain weight in determining ARDS prognosis. The presence of refractory hypoxemia has little bearing on overall prognosis at the time of presentation, unless the hypoxemia is especially severe ($PaO_2/FiO_2 < 50$). A more important poor prognostic predictor, in considering oxygenation, is the time to recovery. Patients not demonstrating recovery in terms of lower oxygen requirements by day 7 of presentation have a more protracted ICU course, are at increased risk for long-term ventilator dependency, and face a longer recovery to regain strength and conditioning should they survive to hospital discharge. Additional factors, such as increasing age, length-of-stay net positive volume status, and sepsis as the predisposition to ARDS are also predictors of higher morbidity and mortality.

PRACTICE POINT

Management strategies:

- Low tidal volumes: 8.8% absolute reduction in mortality (NNT = 11) when using 6 cc/kg target tidal volume in ARDS compared with the common standard of 12 cc/kg.
- Prone ventilation: While prone ventilation and recruitment maneuvers increase oxygenation, no mortality improvement is gained.
- Fluid management: Conservative fluid management strategy, compared to aggressive fluid resuscitation, reduces ventilator days and ICU length of stay.
- Pulmonary artery catheters: PA catheter-directed fluid management does not improve outcomes compared to central venous catheter directed management, and results in more arrhythmias.
- Corticosteroids: After extensive study, no trial data has delineated a clear benefit of steroids in ARDS patients.

SURVIVAL

Studies differ in regard to the current trend in ARDS mortality. Disparity exists in trends between academic and community medical centers, as mortality has improved in the last 10 to 15 years in the former but perhaps not the latter. Analyzing pooled mortality over time in retrospective literature reviews demonstrates a *mortality rate of 35% to 50%*. Consensus is lacking on whether this number is truly static or decreasing on an annual basis, and it further depends on the patient population investigated and the site in which said investigation occurred. As an example, there has been an improvement in mortality from 35% to 26% in the last 15 years in patients enrolled in studies as part of the ARDS Network. Based on other discrepant studies, this trend may not be widely generalizable.

Any improvement in mortality may be due to not only the administration of low-tidal volume ventilation, but also overall improvement in ICU care over time. In the ARDS Network mortality analysis, the mortality improvement trend persisted after adjusting the statistical model for low-tidal volume ventilation and other clinical covariates. An improvement in the general management of ICU patients, such as sepsis, has occurred over time. Simple interventions such as daily ventilator liberation screening, proper oral care, venous thromboembolic disease prophylaxis, and other routine applications have likely made a significant impact on ARDS survival.

COMPLICATIONS

Patients who survive ARDS have surprisingly few respiratory system sequelae at 1 and 2 years after hospital discharge. A review of 1-year ARDS survivors found that none of the patients were requiring oxygen supplementation and their lung function testing, with the exception of low diffusion capacity, had returned to normal. Most frequently patients experienced functional limitation caused primarily by muscle weakness and fatigue. Corticosteroid administration and prolonged duration of respiratory failure are associated with more functional sequelae in these ARDS survivors.

Inability to perform functionally at pre-morbid levels adversely impacts patients' overall sense of well-being after going home. Their health-related quality of life is self-rated as lower than normal, a finding that is still present at two years from discharge. Half of survivors at 2 years report significant anxiety and depression not present prior to their critical illness. They also perform poorly on standardized neurocognitive tests, especially those assessing memory, attentiveness, and executive function (such as planning or abstract thinking).

TABLE 134-4 Evidence-based Medicine: Key References for Acute Respiratory Distress Syndrome

Study	Methodology	Results	Limitations	Bottom Line
The Acute Respiratory Distress Syndrome Network. *N Engl J Med.* 2000;342:1301–1308.	Randomized, double-blind trial of 6 cc/kg vs 12 cc/kg tidal volume per ideal body weight for ventilating ARDS	861 patients enrolled; 8.8% absolute reduction in mortality in low-tidal volume ventilation group	Control group tidal volume goals perhaps harmful	Low-tidal volume ventilation with increased PEEP at higher inspired oxygen levels and aggressive pH management improves mortality
Rubenfeld GD, et al. *N Engl J Med.* 2005; 353:1685–1693.	Prospective, population-based, cohort study to identify incidence and outcomes of acute lung injury	Incidence of ALI was 79.8 per 100,000 person-years, with a mortality of 38.5%, estimated US deaths 74,500 per year	Single-region cohort (Pacific Northwest); demographics may differ in other regions; relied on medical and public health records for data—some cases may have been misclassified	Incidence of ALI in the US may be higher than expected and carries a substantial burden on public health
Herridge MS, et al. *N Engl J Med.* 2003; 348:683–693.	Longitudinal, prospective cohort study; 109 survivors of ARDS followed to assess pulmonary and nonpulmonary function at 1 year after ICU discharge	Except DLCO, lung function normal at 6 months; no oxygen requirements; patients reported functional limitation, primarily due to muscle weakness and fatigue	Small number of patients followed; no control group (non-ARDS ICU survivors)	ARDS survivors have persistent functional disability, more due to weakness than pulmonary dysfunction 1 year after ICU discharge
Wiedemann HP, et al. *N Engl J Med.* 2006;354: 2564–2575.	Prospective, randomized study of conservative vs liberal fluid management in acute lung injury	1000 patients; no difference in 60-day mortality; conservative-strategy cohort had more ventilator-free days and lower ICU length of stay; organ failures not increased	Strategy to guide fluid/diuresis management may be challenging to apply in clinical practice	In hemodynamically stable patients with acute lung injury, targeting a central venous pressure of <4 mm Hg improves time off the ventilator and in the ICU without an increase in organ failure

DISCHARGE PLANNING

Patients who survive to ICU and hospital discharge have functionally limiting deficits. Thus, early planning for referral to a physical rehabilitation facility is often indicated. Most recently, studies of physical and occupational therapy suggest that starting these therapies in the ICU, even in patients still requiring mechanical ventilatory support, leads to quicker and better functional recovery months after discharge (**Table 134-4**). Therefore, engaging physical and occupational therapy early in the ARDS course is warranted and likely offers benefit to patient outcomes.

PRACTICE POINT

- Refractory hypoxemia at presentation has little bearing on overall prognosis, except when hypoxemia is especially severe ($PaO_2/FiO_2 < 50$).
- Physical and occupational therapy initiation in the ICU—even in patients still requiring mechanical ventilatory support—leads to quicker and better functional recovery months after discharge.

For patients who do not recover quickly from ARDS or who require prolonged mechanical ventilation, the rehabilitation phase will likely involve some time in a long-term acute care (LTAC) facility. LTACs—health care facilities that provide lower intensity acute inpatient care—permit a smoother transition to physical rehabilitation while still providing a higher level of care in patients who are near ventilator liberation or have a tracheostomy in place. The ultimate goal of complete liberation from the ventilator and decannulation of the tracheostomy tube may be accomplished in parallel with physical, occupational and speech/swallowing therapies. The transfer to a long-term acute care facility can be difficult on families as they adjust to a less intensive level of care as their loved ones recover. Hospitals make use of liaisons between the two facilities to make this transition easier.

SUGGESTED READINGS

Briel M, Meade M, Mercat A, et al. Higher vs lower positive end-expiratory pressure in patients with acute lung injury and acute respiratory distress syndrome: systematic review and meta-analysis. *JAMA.* 2010;303:865–873.

Cribbs SK, Martin GS. Fluid balance and colloid osmotic pressure in acute respiratory failure: optimizing therapy. Expert Rev Respir Med. 2009;3:651–662.

Erickson SE, Martin GS, Davis JL, et al. Recent trends in acute lung injury mortality: 1996–2005. *Crit Care Med.* 2009;37:1574–1579.

Herridge MS, Cheung AM, Tansey CM, et al. One-year outcomes in survivors of the acute respiratory distress syndrome. *N Engl J Med.* 2003;348:683–693.

NHLBI ARDS Clinical Trials Network. Comparison of two fluid-management strategies in acute lung injury. *N Engl J Med.* 2006;354:2564–2575.

NHLBI ARDS Clinical Trials Network. Efficacy and safety of corticosteroids for persistent acute respiratory distress syndrome. *N Engl J Med.* 2006;354:1671–1684.

Piantadosi CA, Schwartz DA. The acute respiratory distress syndrome. *Ann Intern Med.* 2004;141:460–470.

Putensen C, Theuerkauf N, Zinserling J, et al. Meta-analysis: ventilation strategies and outcomes of the acute respiratory distress syndrome and acute lung injury. *Ann Intern Med.* 2009;151: 566–576.

Rubenfeld GD, Caldwell E, Peabody E, et al. Incidence and outcomes of acute lung injury. *N Engl J Med.* 2005;353:1685–1693.

Ware LB, Matthay MA. The acute respiratory distress syndrome. *N Engl Med J.* 2000;342:1334–1349.

CHAPTER 135

Analgesia, Paralytics, and Sedation

Gary Margolias, MD
Robert S. Harris, MD

Key Clinical Questions

1. What are the clinical and pharmacologic effects of single agent versus multiple agent sedative and analgesic administration?
2. What is the best way to dose sedative, analgesic, and paralytic agents in the intensive care unit (ICU)?
3. How do the pharmacokinetics and dosing of sedative, analgesic, and paralytic agents change with duration of infusion?
4. What is the proper sequence to initiate sedatives, analgesics, and/or paralytics, and how does dosing refinement affect time to weaning and other predictors of favorable outcome?
5. How should a hospitalist select individual sedative, analgesic, or paralytic agents in critically ill patients?
6. When should a hospitalist decide to paralyze a ventilated patient?

INTRODUCTION

The appropriate delivery of critical care to patients in the intensive care unit (ICU) requires a judicious use of sedative and analgesic regimens for many patients as well as the occasional need for neuromuscular blockade. Providers utilize various sedative-analgesic strategies to accomplish this goal, and pharmacologically induced paralysis may be undertaken in upwards of 10% of specific ICU populations. While management of the discomfort of mechanical ventilation serves as the primary indication for most sedative and analgesic regimens in the ICU, the increased myocardial oxygen consumption as well as immunosuppression resulting from catechol upregulation also represent important untoward outcomes to aggressively manage by treating pain and anxiety with analgesic and sedative medications.

Critically ill patients are subject to adverse stimuli that arise not only from endotracheal support apparatus, but also from indwelling monitoring lines and catheters and from surgical and other wounds. Sleep deprivation and encroachments on personal modesty also provoke further intolerance of the ICU environment. The significant discomforts of the ICU setting may be palliated with the use of sedative and analgesic therapy.

DOSING PRINCIPLES

Sedative, analgesic, and paralytic therapies are administered by intravenous (IV) *bolus* or by IV *infusion*, as intramuscular and enteral titration are unreliable.

Principles of dose initiation and maintenence

Bolus dosing has the advantage of a rapid onset of action, but has the associated risk of either over- or undershooting the therapeutic goal. As such, nursing vigilance with frequent assessment and bolus titration to defined therapeutic outcomes is necessary. On the other hand, infusion drug dosing reflects a more gradual and refined titration to clinical effect, but does carry a greater risk of drug accumulation with protracted infusion. As such, an unwanted prolongation of time to awakening may occur when clinical circumstances allow for drug discontinuation. For this reason, infusions should only be undertaken in the ICU when bolus dosing has failed to produce the desired sedative effect.

Clinicians should follow a structured algorithm for ICU sedation, pain control, and paralysis (**Figure 135-1**). While sedative and analgesic agents help to maintain mechanical ventilation their prolonged use can become an obstacle to liberation from life support. Because planning for weaning should occur as soon as ventilatory support is begun, the sedative and analgesic goals should be defined and dosing plan structured for each individual agent such that their sum individual dosing requirements are minimized.

Analgesic goals should be addressed first. Once adequate analgesia is achieved, sedation can be targeted to the patient's clinical need. For instance, a patient with acute respiratory distress syndrome (ARDS) ventilated with a high-frequency oscillator may require deep sedation and analgesia (and possibly neuromuscular blockade), whereas a patient requiring minimal volume ventilation or pressure support may need only mild analgesia and sedation. An initial targeted focus on the patient's analgesic need will help curtail sedative requirements, as adequate pain control decreases anxiety and sedative need.

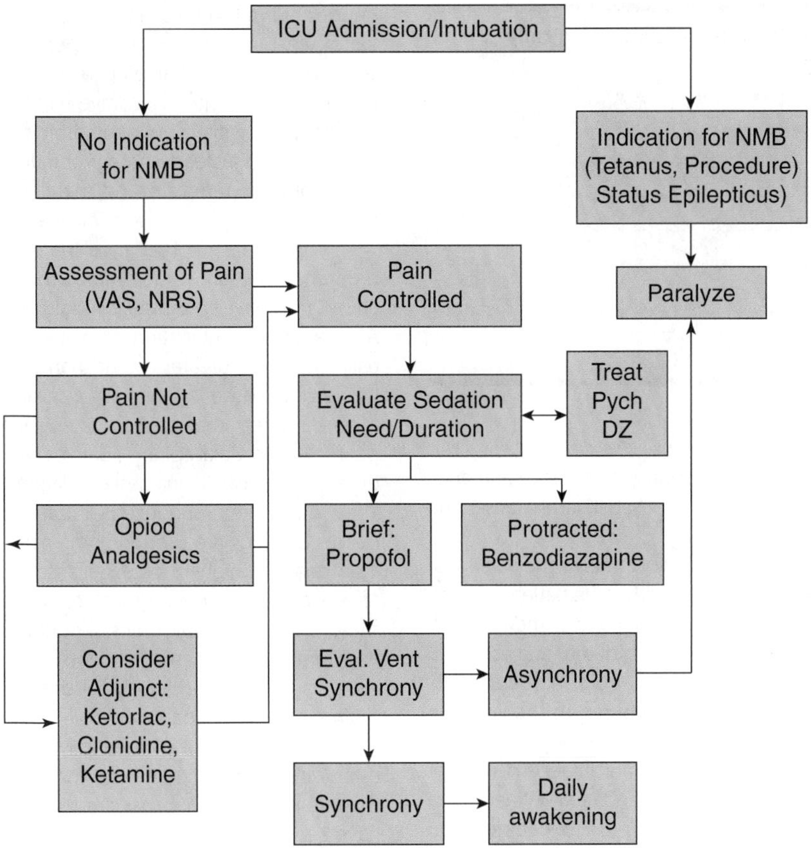

Figure 135-1 *Algorithm for ICU sedation, pain control, and paralysis.*

Recent clinical evidence supports that sedation need not be applied as a routine aspect of ICU care even in the most severely ill intubated patients provided that adequate bolus analgesia (morphine) is carefully administered. Patients treated in this manner demonstrated shorter ICU stays and fewer ventilator days without suffering any untoward clinical outcomes. It may be reasonable to consider analgesia only in some patients and utilize sedation only for "rescue" purposes for patients intolerant of a purely analgesic regimen.

During the initiation phase of sedation and analgesia, the patient's chronic comorbid conditions must be considered in guiding analgesic requirement. For instance, the patient may have a source of chronic pain such as musculoskeletal pain or neuropathy. This could be an overlooked source of discomfort if not factored in the appraisal of a patient's analgesic need. Once pain and anxiety are controlled, sedation can also be reduced as tolerated. Similarly, preexisting psychiatric disorders such as psychosis should be taken into account in targeting sedation and anxiolysis.

Dose or infusion maintenance: Analgesic and sedative titration and active management should continue throughout the ICU stay. If the patient's dyssynchrony with the ventilator is primarily a manifestation of untreated pain, continued escalation in dosing with sedative medications (eg, propofol) could lead to unnecessary hemodynamic compromise and drug accumulation. Alternately, adding a medication or switching to a medication with intrinsic analgesic properties may better benefit some patients.

Dose or infusion weaning and discontinuation: Withdrawal of sedative and analgesic medications may result in the development of delirium that may impede liberation from mechanical ventilation and unnecessary diagnostic workup. This type of delirium is common, having been reported in upwards of one-third of patients who have been sedated in the ICU for greater than a week.

A sensitivity to the signs of withdrawal from opioids (diaphoresis, tachycardia, papillary dilatation, lacrimation, piloerection, hypertension, vomiting, abdominal cramping, restlessness, anxiety, fever, yawning) and bezodiazapines (tremor, diaphoresis, anxiety, tachycardia, nausea) should be maintained. Some advocate a 10% decrement in narcotic use every day, but a tailored approach may be appropriate for some patients.

PHARMACOKINETIC PRINCIPLES

Caring for critically ill patients represents an extremely dynamic practice in which drug regimens with rapid clinical effects and short durations of action are frequently best suited. In general, drugs without active metabolites and with few pharmacologic interactions offer the greatest efficacy with the fewest side effects. Furthermore, medications with smaller volumes of distribution are more easily titrated. Drugs that do not manifest significant tachyphylaxis also lend themselves to titration in ICU practice. Sedatives and analgesics with increased risk of hemodynamic side effects are avoided when possible, as are medications with higher risk of withdrawal symptoms upon their discontinuation.

Table 135-1 contains a list of the pharmacologic characteristics of the ideal drug. While no single drug possesses every one of these ideal properties, sedative and analgesic medications are selected based on these parameters and the individual patient's clinical condition. ICU patients can have depressed or changing hepatic and renal clearance profiles, as well as dynamic hepatic synthetic function and nutritional flux. Drug concentrations and protein binding can change as well. Similarly, alterations in gut absorption affect serum levels of enterally administered agents. Each patient's

TABLE 135-1 Characteristics of the Pharmacologically Ideal Drug

Clinical onset	Rapid
Clinical effect	Short
Active metabolites	None
Pharmacologic interactions	None
Volume of distribution	Small
Tachyphylaxis	None
Hemodynamic side effects	None
Withdrawal symptoms	None

prevailing physiology as well as the response to sedative and analgesic therapy should impact the titration of sedative, analgesic, and paralytic medications in the ICU.

Drugs do not attain an immediate steady state, as they are influenced by the volume of distribution (Vd) within the patient and the variable redistribution into different anatomic compartments. Upon administration, drugs are preferentially distributed to vessel-rich organ systems. Drugs with lipophilic biochemical properties (eg, fentanyl, midazolam) are more rapidly distributed to the lipid-rich regions of the body, which includes the central nervous system (CNS) (**Figure 135-2**). Hydrophilic drugs (eg, morphine) on the other hand penetrate fatty tissue relatively poorly and are confined more to the lower Vd that is the plasma, with slower CNS penetration and clinical effect.

An administered drug will undergo renal and hepatic metabolism, but certain highly lipophilic drugs with relatively long elimination half-times by kidney and liver distribute rapidly at first into the vessel-rich group (including CNS), and then redistribute into a second "compartment" (plasma), thereby rapidly terminating their clinical (sedative) effect. With time and ongoing infusion, this termination of clinical effect by redistribution becomes attenuated as a new steady state is established between compartments (**Figure 135-3**). Broadly, these phenomena of variable pharmacokinetics contribute to the context-sensitive half-time of an agent. This principle represents a clinically useful way to understand how greater length of infusion prolongs clinical effect. Classical ways of thinking about drug elimination half-lives after bolus dosing by renal and hepatic metabolism have little clinical utility with ongoing infusion and changing distribution between compartments. The concept of *context-sensitive half-time* describes changing time to elimination of half of the current plasma concentration with discontinuation of a drug at that point in time. These dynamic pharmacokinetics have important implications in the ICU setting. Suitable arousal for ventilator weaning is very much dependant on CNS concentration of sedative agents at that particular point in time, which in turn is reliant on the context-sensitive half-time of the drug. With passing time, and with continued administration, lipophilic drugs that have come to a steady state within lipid rich compartments may redistribute systemically and manifest a declining dose requirement and a longer time to clinical awakening.

Concomitant use of sedative and analgesic agents will affect the properties of each of the drugs. Drugs of different pharmacologic classes may have synergistic or additive sedative or analgesic effects. A synergistic combination magnifies the relative clinical effect of each drug to a greater extent than would be predicted based on its individual dose potency, whereas an additive combination finds a clinical effect that approximates each drug's individual relative potency. Benzodiazepine sedatives and opiate analgesic agents display synergism in analgesia, sedation, and respiratory depression. Therefore, more pronounced clinical effects occur when these two classes of drugs are used in combination than when each is used individually at higher doses. Because of this, unpredictable clinical effects can occur when drugs are coadministered, and combining these classes of medications should be done with caution in the nonventilated or weaning patient.

Similarly, changing individual doses of drugs in a combination regimen should be done with the same care as the administration of a new drug because an entirely new pharmacodynamic state is established with differing combination drug concentrations. Drugs that are not primarily considered sedative agents, but nonetheless have sedating properties (eg, anticholinergic agents or neuroleptics), should also be used with cognizance of their potential additive or synergistic sedative capability. Finally, unlike the benzodiazepines, many commonly used sedative medications, such as propofol, have no individual analgesic properties or potentiation when used in combination with opioids.

SEDATION IN THE ICU

SEDATIVE MEDICATION SELECTION AND PRECAUTIONS

The benzodiazepines and propofol represent the most commonly used agents for sedation and anxiolysis in critically ill patients. Both classes of drugs potentiate GABA inhibition within the CNS with anxiolytic, sedative, and hypnotic effects. Both have similar amnestic potential, which may be desirable within the ICU setting, and both have similar respiratory depressant effects due to shifting of the carbon dioxide (CO_2) response curve rightward (decreased respiratory drive at physiologic CO_2 levels) and blunting of hypoxic drive.

The individual drugs in both classes are lipid soluble. However, propofol is carried in a lipid emulsion that renders it much more lipophilic, which in turn accounts for the very rapid uptake into

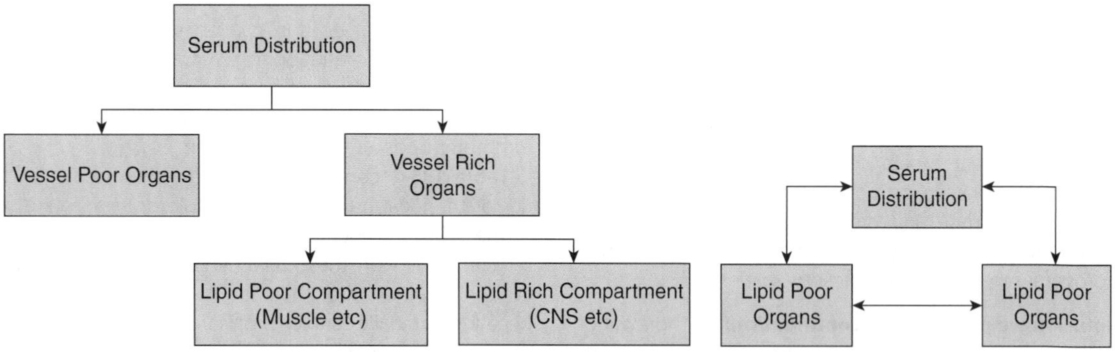

Figure 135-2 *(A) Distribution of lipophilic drug with initial bolus dosing. (B) Redistribution of lipophilic drug over time.*

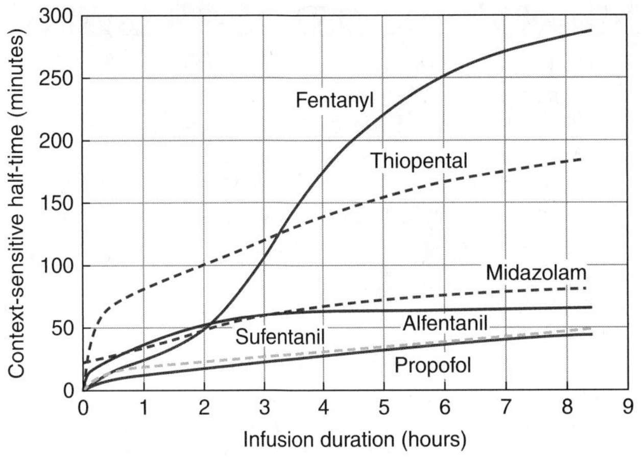

Figure 135-3 *Context-sensitive half-time of various sedative and analgesic drugs. (Reproduced, with permission, from Longnecker DE, Brown DL, Newman MF, et al. Anesthesiology. New York: McGraw-Hill, 2008. Fig. 68-5.)*

the lipid-rich and highly vascular CNS with subsequent quick redistribution out of the CNS after bolus dosing or brief infusions. This redistribution terminates propofol's clinical sedative effect. Like all lipophilic agents, propofol and benzodiazepines will demonstrate a prolongation of clinical effect once they have been discontinued if their protracted use has resulted in saturation of the body's "lipid compartment."

The choice of whether to use a benzodiazepine or propofol depends on pharmocokinetic considerations and the matching of the time needed for sedation in a particular clinical circumstance to the pharmacokinetic properties of the drug. Propofol is more often the agent of choice for sedation for brief procedural interventions or short-term mechanical ventilation (less than one to three days), whereas the benzodiazapines might serve as a more cost-effective choice for sedation that is expected to last more than a few days. Based on the pharmacologic properties and important clinical considerations of the commonly used sedatives, benzodiazepines also often serve as the preferred agents for sedation when refractory hypotension is a concern, as they do not have the same degree of direct vasodilation that can occur with propofol.

Benzodiazepines

Pharmacologic properties of commonly used benzodiazepine agents vary (**Table 135-2**) as do dosing regimens and costs of both benzodiazepine and opioid drugs (**Table 135-3**). The pharmacokinetic properties and dosing of sedative and analgesic agents were derived from studies of healthy volunteers who have received single bolus drug doses. These data may not accurately reflect dynamic context-sensitive half-times with continuous infusion, especially in critically ill patients with shifting volumes of distribution, serum drug-protein binding, severely compromised hepatic perfusion, and metabolism changes.

Midazolam and lorazepam are the most commonly used benzodiazepines in the ICU. Although midazolam is thought of as a rapid-onset, short-acting agent, when used in the short term its high lipid solubility results in accumulation with prolonged infusion. This characteristic, along with the fact that its primary metabolite (1-hydroxymidazolam glucuronide) is clinically active for up to 36 hours after drug cessation, makes lorazepam a preferred sedative especially in the obese and in patients requiring greater than 48 hours of sedation.

PRACTICE POINT

- Midazolam has high lipid solubility and an active metabolite clinically active for up to 36 hours after drug cessation. Both of these properties result in accumulation with prolonged infusion of the drug. Therefore, lorazepam may be a preferred sedative for infusions, especially in obese patients and in patients requiring more than 48–72 hours of sedation.

Benzodiazepine precautions

Benzodiazepine withdrawal can occur with weaning from these drugs. Longer-acting agents such as diazepam or lorazepam may be used as a bridge to complete discontinuation of sedation.

Patients receiving greater than 50 mg total dose or greater than 1 mg/kg of IV lorazepam per day are at risk for toxicity from *propylene glycol*, a solvent in which the drug is dissolved. Propylene glycol toxicity can cause renal injury and acute tubular necrosis (ATN), tissue necrosis, and significant anion-gap acidosis. Patients receiving greater than the recommended daily dose of this drug should be monitored for toxicity with daily osmolar gap measurements.

PRACTICE POINT

- Lorazepam at high doses of infusion or high total dose can cause propylene glycol toxicity—potentially leading to acute tubular necrosis, tissue necrosis, and significant anion-gap acidosis—due to the solvent in which the drug is dissolved. Daily osmolar gap measurements are necessary in patients receiving > 50 mg total dose or > 1 mg/kg of IV lorazepam daily.

TABLE 135-2 Pharmacologic Properties of Commonly Used Intravenous Opioids

Opioid Medications	Equianalgesic IV Dose	Intermittent Dosing	Infusion Dose	Onset (minutes)	Half-Life (hours)	Lipophilicity	Active Metabolites
Fentanyl	100–200 mcg	0.35–0.5 mcg/kg every 0.5–1 hour	0.7–10.0 mcg/kg/hour	Immediate	1.5–6	+++	Yes
Morphine	10 mg	0.01–0.15 mg/kg every 1–2 hours	0.07–0.5 mg/kg/hour	<5	3–7	+	Yes
Hydromorphone	1.5 mg	10–30 mcg/kg every 1–2 hours	7–15 mcg/kg/hour	<5	2–3	++	No
Meperidine	70–100 mg	Not recommended	Not recommended	<5	3–4	+++	Yes
Methadone	10 mg	10 mg every 6 hours	Not recommended	10–20	15–30	+++	No

TABLE 135-3 Equianalgesic Comparison of Commonly Utilized Opioids

Opioid Agent	Equianalgesic Potency (mg)
Morphine	1
Fentanyl	75–125 (mcg)
Hydromorphone	0.15
Meperidine	0.1

Propofol

Propofol, a hydrophobic drug, demonstrates rapid onset and offset due to its ability to rapidly penetrate the CNS with initiation and then redistribute to other tissues with discontinuation. The drug is metabolized to inactive products by the liver and then excreted by the kidneys. *Hepatic and renal diseases do not alter clinical effect in any appreciable manner.* Prolonged infusion times and deeper depths of sedation result in drug accumulation and sedation. Propofol use is associated with fewer ventilator days compared to patients treated with bolus dosing of lorazepam.

Propofol precautions

The lipid emulsion of the drug has a significant caloric load (1.1 Kcal/cc) that should be factored as part of the daily intake. Propofol is also associated with the development of hypotriglyceridemia, especially in those predisposed to this condition or in those receiving concurrent total parenteral nutrition (TPN).

In patients receiving high-dose propofol infusions (>83 mcg/kg/min for >48 hours), a rare (39 published cases) but serious condition—propofol related infusion syndrome (PRIS)—associated with rhabdomyolysis, myocardial failure, acute renal failure, severe metabolic acidosis, bradyarrhythmias, cardiac arrest, and hypotension has been described. PRIS occurs more often in patients receiving vasopressors or glucocorticoids or those with mitochondrial metabolic deficiencies.

PRACTICE POINT

- Propofol has no individual analgesic properties or potentiation when used in combination with opioids.

Other sedative drugs

Other drugs used less frequently as alternatives for sedation in the ICU include neuroleptic drugs (eg, haloperidol), alpha-agonist drugs, ketamine, and inhalational agents. Neuroleptic drugs (eg, haloperidol 2 mg IV/IM doubled as needed every 15 minutes) are helpful as single agents or in combination with benzodiazepine sedatives, but their use should be undertaken with cognizance of possible associated prolongation of the QTc interval (monitored with intermittent ECG) and torsades de pointes. Other medications that might prolong the QT interval (azole antifungal drugs, amiodarone, macrolides, etc) should be used with caution in combination with these medications and electrolyte balance (especially magnesium) should be maintained. Cumulative haloperidol dose (>35 mg) has been shown to increase the risk of torsades as has higher-dose IV administration (>20 mg) and prior cardiac disease. Extrapyramidal symptoms and neuroleptic malignant syndrome are other clinical entities associated with neuroleptic medication use.

PRACTICE POINT

- Cumulative haloperidol dose > 35 mg, higher-dose IV administration (> 20 mg), and history of cardiac disease have been shown to increase the risk of torsades de pointes. Haloperidol should be used with caution for sedation and only after a screening ECG that confirms a normal QTc interval. Electrolyte levels including magnesium and potassium should be monitored and maintained while prescribing haloperidol for sedation.

A more recently available drug used for sedation is the alpha-agonist drug *dexmetatomidine*. It is especially useful for short-term sedation, has very little respiratory depressant effect, and has some analgesic properties. These characteristics frequently permit—unlike the other sedative agents—ventilator weaning without full discontinuation of the drug, a property advantageous in patients whose weaning is hindered by primarily nonpulmonary considerations such as pain and agitation.

Ketamine offers similar pharmacologic advantages to dexmetatomidine, but its use is limited by undesirable, dose-dependant, psychotropic effects. Inhalational anesthetics remain rarely utilized "niche drugs" in ICU practice and are unlikely to make their way into routine ICU practice due to difficultly in monitoring and scavenging of exhaled drug into the ambient environment.

MONITORING AND MANAGEMENT OF SEDATION

Daily awakening

Evidence well supports scheduled daily awakening of intubated patients; this practice should be a routine aspect of ICU care. Daily awakening permits reassessment of sedative and analgesic requirements on a routine basis, and once the patient has demonstrated lucidity and is examined by the provider, sedative protocols can be reinitiated at half their previous dose, which allows a step-wise decrement in sedative requirements. Daily awakening protocols reduce ICU length of stay (LOS), decrease the number of tracheostomy procedures, decrease the number of diagnostic studies ordered to diagnose altered mental status, and decrease the amount of overall sedating drugs required by intubated patients.

PRACTICE POINT

- Daily awakening of intubated patients is an evidence-based practice part of routine ICU care. Daily awakening protocols reduce ICU length of stay and decrease tracheostomy procedures, diagnostic studies ordered, and the amount of sedating drugs required. Daily awakening also reduces PTSD incidence during recovery from critical illness. Following daily awakening, sedative protocols can be reinitiated at a lower dose to allow a step-wise decrement in sedative requirements. Daily awakening should be avoided in patients requiring ongoing paralytic use.

During these sedation-free windows, ICU staff can facilitate ventilator weaning. Initial concerns that these hiatuses in sedation would be psychologically traumatic for patients have not been observed. In fact, daily awakening leads to lower incidence of post-traumatic stress disorder (PTSD) when compared to patients not participating in daily awakening protocols. Concerns over an increased risk of myocardial ischemic episodes secondary to the anxiety incumbent in arousal have not been observed. Daily awakening should be undertaken with more care in those with hypertensive emergencies or status asthmaticus and should clearly be avoided in those whose care requires ongoing paralytic use.

Sedation assessment

Several instruments have been developed to assess the level of sedation and aid in the titration of sedating medications. The therapeutic goal of sedative-analgesic medications in intubated patients is to achieve comfort that includes a calm and cooperative disposition and ability to follow commands. However, for patients with a need for higher levels of mechanical ventilator support, deeper sedation goals may be necessary.

Clinical instruments can help define sedation goals for individual patients and guide therapy to achieve these goals. While several clinical instruments have been developed to assess sedation goals, none has been validated as a tool for rapidly titrating sedative drug dosing in a dynamic minute-by-minute or hour-by-hour fashion. Nevertheless, clinical use of some of these assessment tools occurs in many ICU settings. Instrument scales utilized in the ICU setting include: the Riker Sedation-Agitation Scale (SAS), the Motor Activity Assessment Scale (MAAS), the Ramsay Scale, the Adaptation to the Intensive Care Environment (ATICE) instrument, the Minnesota Sedation Assessment Tool (MSAT), the Vancouver Interaction and Calmness Scale (VICS), and the Richmond Agitation-Sedation Scale (RASS). Some of these scales utilize descriptors of behavior (eg, SAS), whereas others use descriptors of motor activity (eg, MAAS) or of observed levels of sleep states (eg, Ramsay). The individual choice of a particular scale may represent institutional preference; however, the Ramsay scale does have the benefit of a relatively broad body of reference within the literature comparing sedation protocols, and the RASS is becoming more widely accepted for assessing changes in sedation over days in the ICU.

Sedation reversal

Flumazenil is a benzodiazepine derivative with high affinity for the benzodiazepine receptor and acts as a competitive inhibitor for benzodiazepine drugs. Although this intrinsic effective inhibition has found indications for use in clinical practice, especially for reversal of benzodiazepine anesthetic use, the drug has little benefit in the ICU setting. Use of flumazenil after prolonged benzodiazepine use in the ICU might provoke withdrawal symptoms or seizures. The drug has no indication in those with any clinical predisposition toward seizure (eg, epilepsy, intracranial pathology, electrolyte disturbances, benzodiazepine, or alcohol dependence) or in the setting of cyclic antidepressant overdose. Use of the drug is also complicated by the relatively short elimination half-life (one hour) that might result in benzodiazepine resedation after flumazenil metabolism. A better approach for a patient thought to be suffering respiratory compromise due to benzodiazepine overdose might be supportive.

ANALGESIA IN THE ICU

Analgesia is indicated in mechanically ventilated patients and other ICU patients with pain or other unpleasant symptoms (eg, shortness of breath) related to their medical conditions or for prophylactic use prior to surgical or procedural interventions. Individual self-report of pain represents the most reliable assessment of patient discomfort. However, impediments to communication—physical, such as endotracheal intubation, or physiologic, such as delirium—make appropriate titration of analgesic medications difficult.

ANALGESIA ASSESSMENT

Instruments that standardize patient self-report of discomfort include the Visual Analogue Scale (VAS), which uses linear descriptors of pain that patients can designate by pointing to their level of discomfort; the Numeric Rating Scale (NRS), which uses a similar principle to assign patient assessment of pain on a scale of 1 to 10, with 10 being the most severe; and the Faces Pain Scale (**Figure 135-4**), which graphically demonstrates pain by facial expression. This simplified approach of assigning a single number to pain is preferred in the ICU environment where verbal communication is limited. These scales have been validated largely outside of the ICU setting, but serve a practical clinical use in ICU care. More objective tools for the assessment of patient discomfort by medical personnel or family members have also been developed. These instruments could conceivably circumvent the problems inherent to patient self-report in the ICU; however, currently the NRS remains the preferred means of pain assessment by the Association for Critical Care Nurses (ACCN) and the Society of Critical Care Medicine (SCCM).

ANALGESIC MEDICATION SELECTION AND PRECAUTIONS

Nonopioid analgesics, such as acetaminophen and nonsteroidal anti-inflammatory medications, maintain a minor, adjunctive role in analgesic treatment in the ICU. Ketamine and alpha-agonist drugs (eg, dexmedetomidine) also have analgesic properties, but they are utilized primarily for their sedative properties rather than primary analgesic therapy. Opioids serve as the primary pharmacologic class to treat pain in the ICU setting.

Opioid pharmacology

Opioid analgesics provide the clinically desirable effects of pain control and a blunting of the sensation of dyspnea. Various opioid agents exhibit slightly different time to onset and varying durations of effect (see Table 135-3). Dosing and cost of different agents also vary widely. The analgesic action of these drugs occurs primarily due to interaction with the mu (μ) receptors in both the CNS and periphery. More lipid-soluble drugs (eg, fentanyl) have more rapid onset of action, as they are quickly distributed to the lipid-rich CNS tissue. Conversely, these same agents will have a protracted redistribution phase after they have been discontinued, as they will continue a slow release into circulation from these same lipid-rich compartments.

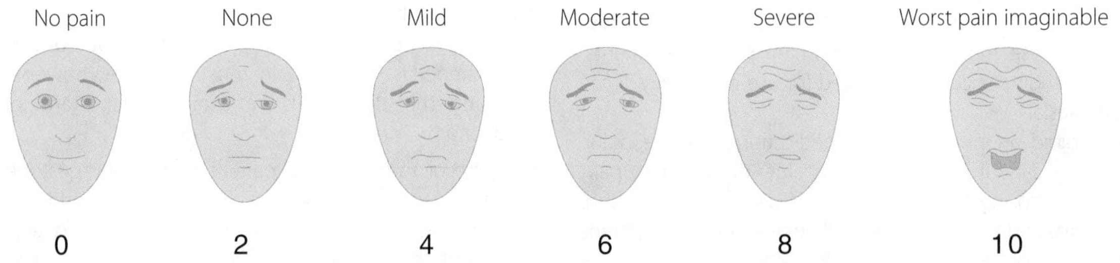

Figure 135-4 *The Faces pain scale (The Faces Pain Scale—Revised. From Pain 2001;93:173–183. Used with permission from IASP.)*

TABLE 135-4 Conditions Associated with Possible Hyperkalemia after Succinylcholine Use

Neurologic	Metabolic	Anatomic
CVA	Metabolic acidosis	Third-degree burn
CNS/PNS tumor	Renal failure*	Severe intraabdominal infection
Closed head injury		Crush injury
Prolonged neuromuscular block with nondepolarizing agent		
Prolonged Immobilization		

*Normal rise in serum potassium is superimposed on preexisting hyperkalemia
CVA, cerebrovascular accident (stroke); CNS, central nervous system; PNS, peripheral nervous system.

Drugs with greater hepatic or renal metabolism may have extended activity in patients in whom comorbid disease or age impacts the function of these organ systems. Agents that are metabolized to active compounds usually have longer clinical effect, and the pharmacologic properties of metabolites may be clinically important.

Equianalgesic assessment is made using morphine as the standard-bearer to which other agents are compared (**Table 135-4**). These comparisons are extrapolated from studies with intramuscular dosing in healthy volunteers, and entirely different pharmacokinetics might exist with infusion dosing, opioid switching, and especially in critically ill patients with attendant renal and hepatic compromise as well as altered volume of distribution (Vd) and protein-drug binding.

Opioid selection

Morphine, fentanyl, and hydromorphone are the agents most often used in the ICU. Intravenous fentanyl, a commonly used, highly lipophilic agent with no active metabolites, attains almost immediate CNS effect, but may accumulate after prolonged infusion and in patients with renal dysfunction. Fentanyl patches are avoided in the ICU due to delayed and unpredictable onset and offset.

Morphine, on the other hand, has an active metabolite (morphine-6-gluconoride) that can also accumulate in patients with renal dysfunction and may result in prolonged respiratory depression. This agent also has more antihistamine effects than other opioid agents. Compared to morphine, hydromorphone induces less histamine release and has fewer accumulating metabolites in renal failure patients.

Methadone has N-Methyl-D-aspartic acid (NMDA)-receptor antagonism properties that may be exploited for the treatment of neuropathic pain. Its long duration of action also makes it useful for weaning from shorter-acting agents.

Meperidine has a neurotoxic metabolite (normeperidine) that may accumulate, especially in patients with renal dysfunction, leading to cerebral excitation, seizures, and even death. The drug has interactions with other drug classes (eg, MAOIs, SSRIs), which may further make its use more complicated than with other agents. Therefore, meperidine should be avoided for use in critically ill patients for analgesia.

Once an opioid agent is selected, medications may be bolus dosed—utilizing careful assessment of analgesic effect (eg, pain scales)—as bolus dosing is less likely to result in drug accumulation, and steady states and analgesic effect will be more rapidly apparent than with titration of narcotic infusions. Narcotic dosing should be guided by clinical effect and not by defined "upper dose limits," as determined in pharmacologic manuals. When dose escalation fails to demonstrate analgesia, a different opioid medication should be tried because opioid receptor affinity may change with continued exposure to a single agent.

PRACTICE POINT

- When opioid dose escalation fails to demonstrate analgesia, a different opioid medication should be tried because opioid receptor affinity may change with continued exposure to a single agent.

Opioid precautions

Histamine release can occur on rare occasions with opioid use (especially with morphine). This is associated with hypotension, bronchospasm, flushing, and urticaria. For those with compromised hemodynamics or reactive airways disease, the concern for histamine release may factor into the choice of analgesic agent.

Clinically undesirable effects of opioids include the ablation of the hypoxic respiratory drive and the displacement of the carbon dioxide response curve rightward. These effects increase the likelihood of respiratory acidosis and respiratory failure. Worsening hypotension may also occur in hemodynamically compromised patients due either to an indirect blunting of intrinsic catecholamine-mediated vasomotor tone during a stress response, or, rarely, from the direct vasodilating effect of histamine release with bolus doses of certain opioids (eg, morphine, meperidine). Opioid analgesics may also cause or potentiate reduced gut transit or ileus as well as urinary retention in critically ill patients.

Rapid tapering of opioids may lead to withdrawal in patients exposed to high doses of narcotics for more than one week. Opioid infusions should not be decreased more than 25% per day.

PRACTICE POINT

The significant side effects and precautions of opiods include:

- **Histamine release:** May lead to hypotension, bronchospasm, flushing, and urticaria (especially with morphine; use with caution in patients with compromised hemodynamics or reactive airways disease)
- **Respiratory acidosis and respiratory failure** due to blunting of hypoxic respiratory drive
- **Worsening hypotension** in hemodynamically compromised patients
- **Reduced gut transit or ileus**
- **Urinary retention**
- **Opioid withdrawal:** For patients exposed to high-dose narcotics for more than one week, opioid infusions should be decreased no more than 25% per day to avoid withdrawal symptoms

Analgesia reversal

Naloxone is the most widely used competitive inhibitor of opioid medications. It is primarily used in the ICU setting to reverse the acute respiratory depressant effects of narcotic drugs. Its use in this manner is likely safe in most instances; however, nuances to using this drug that are clinically important include the following:

- Use of the drug in a patient in the early postoperative setting can result in acute analgesic reversal and an associated hyperadrenergic surge that can be devastating (eg, ventricular arrhythmias, acute congestive heart failure, hypertension), and incremental naloxone dosing is usually curtailed tenfold in these patients.

- Administration of the drug to those chronically dependent on opioids (eg, cancer patients, opioid abusers) might precipitate severe withdrawal.

If naloxone is used, it can be administered intravenously, subcutaneously, or intramuscularly. Intravenous dosing (in patients who are not postoperative) is 0.4 mg intravenously, repeated as needed. Intravenous infusion (eg, 0.4 mg/hour) might be necessary to prevent recurrent narcotic sedation, as the drug half-life is fairly short (one to four hours).

PARALYSIS IN THE ICU

Neuromuscular blocking (NMB) agents should be used sparingly and only for narrow indications. Outside of planned surgical procedures in the operating room, rare occasions in the ICU (or for patients heading to the ICU) necessitate paralysis of critically ill patients. Indications for paralysis in the ICU include the following:

- Eliminate spontaneous breathing and promote mechanical ventilation (eg, eliminate the patient's urge to fight the ventilator).
- Cause a pharmacologic restraint to prevent patient self-harm or to facilitate a necessary procedure or diagnostic study.
- Decrease oxygen consumption.

Induced paralysis may be indicated in selected ICU patients, but NMB agents should be prescribed only by clinicians experienced with using these agents. At times, when lung injury is especially severe and associated with severely limited pulmonary compliance, change in mechanics—including increased chest wall compliance—is needed to facilitate safe airway pressures. Rising airway pressures may not be remedied in this circumstance with changes in ventilation modes and other ventilatory parameters, and paralysis may represent the sole therapeutic option available to diminish the risk of barotrauma. Similarly, if conventional ventilatory strategies have not successfully addressed restricted compliance and increasing airway pressures, then an oscillating ventilator may be employed to greatly restrict tidal breathing and lung expansion. This nonphysiologic approach to ventilation requires pharmacologic paralysis and sedation for its implementation.

Rare nonpulmonary indications exist for the use of NMB drugs. Mechanically ventilated patients may, in rare situations, need NMB agents to facilitate an invasive procedure in the ICU or a critical diagnostic test (eg, magnetic resonance imaging [MRI]) where motion must be minimized. NMB agents can decrease the muscle rigidity of status epilepticus, tetany, and neuroleptic malignant syndrome. While previous data have suggested benefit with the use of NMB to diminish intracranial pressures during suctioning in patients with head trauma, studies have failed to provide evidence of improved outcome with this practice.

PARALYTIC MEDICATION SELECTION AND PRECAUTIONS

Neuromuscular blocking agents are broadly divided between the depolarizing agent succinylcholine and the myriad of other nondepolarizing agents (eg, vecuronium, rocuronium, atracurium). Succinylcholine results in depolarization of the motor endplate with the onset of paralysis, whereas the nondepolarizing agents do not. Succinylcholine is used primarily for intubation, whereas nondepolarizing NMBs are used for intubation and for the maintenance of paralysis.

In critically ill patients, density of the nicotinic acetylcholine (Ach) receptor (nAChR) at the nerve terminal increases over time. The result of this increase in receptor density in clinical practice is tachyphylaxis to the nondepolarizing NMB agents with time, as a greater concentration of NMB is needed to achieve sufficient receptor saturation and paralysis. Another important consideration occurs with the use of succinylcholine in disease states where chronically denervated muscle groups exist (eg, stroke, metabolic acidosis, renal failure, burns). In these cases, an upregulation of Ach receptors at the motor endplate has occurred, and the use of the depolarizing NMB agent succinylcholine for intubation could result in massive exaggerated muscle depolarization with attendant dangerous hyperkalemia (**Table 135-5**).

PRACTICE POINT

- Tachyphylaxis is defined as rapid decrease in the response to a drug due to previous (long-term) exposure to that drug. Increasing the dose of the drug will not increase the pharmacologic response. Tachyphylaxis may develop with an initial dose. This can sometimes be caused by depletion or marked reduction of the amount of neurotransmitter responsible for creating the drug's effect.

Neuromuscular blocking agents

Multiple NMB agents are available for use in the ICU setting. Pharmacology and dosing varies based on the agent selected (**Table 135-6**). Vecuronium, the most commonly used paralytic in the ICU setting, serves as a cost-effective option and is only impacted to a minor degree by moderate renal and hepatic disease. Cisatacurium has the benefit of *Hoffman degradation*, a pH-dependent serum elimination that is not influenced at all by kidney or liver function. Therefore, cisatacurium is used in patients with severe renal or hepatic impairment. Bolus or continuous infusion is appropriate dosing for paralysis. Switching or combining NMB agents might result in unanticipated synergistic potentiation and prolonged neuromuscular blockade.

TABLE 135-5 Pharmacologic Properties of Commonly Used Intravenous Sedatives

Drug	IV Dose	Intermittent Dosing	Infusion Dosing	Time to Onset	Half-Life	Lipophilicity	Active Metabolites
Midazolam	0.5–4.0 mg	0.02–0.08 mg/kg every 0.5–2 hours	0.04–0.2 mg/kg/hour	2–5 min	3–12 hours	+++	Yes
Lorazepam	0.04 mg/kg	0.02–0.06 mg/kg every 2–6 hours	0.01–0.1 mg/kg/hour	5–20 min	10–20 hours	++	No
Diazepam	2–10 mg	0.03–0.1 mg/kg every 0.5–6 hours	NA	2–5 min	20–50 hours	+++	Yes
Propofol	Infusion dosing	NA	5–80 mcg/kg/min	1–2 min	1.5–12.4 hours	+++	No

TABLE 135-6 Pharmacology of Commonly Used Neuromuscular Blocking Agents

Drug	Intubating Dose (mg/kg)	Infusion Rate (μg/kg/min)	Onset to Intubating Conditions (seconds)	Duration of Action	Clinical Niche
Rocuronium	0.9–1.2	9–12	60–90	Intermediate	Rapid-onset nondepolarizing NMB
Vecuronium	0.08–0.12	1–2	90–150	Intermediate	Cost effective
Atacurium	0.5	3–12	90–150	Intermediate	ESRD/cirrhotic patients (nonrenal/hepatic metabolism)
Cisatacurium	0.15–0.2	1–3	90–120	Intermediate	Similar to atracurium but without risk of histamine release
Succinylcholine	1.5	NA	30–90	Very short	Emergent airway (most rapid onset)

PRACTICE POINT

- Cisatracurium elimination is not influenced by kidney or liver function and can be used in patients with severe renal or hepatic impairment.

Various medical conditions, medications, and clinical circumstances affect the duration of action and degree of neuromuscular weakness (**Table 135-7**). If sedation and analgesia fail to allow adequate ventilatory support and neuromuscular agents are thought to be clinically indicated, they should be utilized in patients who are normothermic, free of electrolyte or acid-base disturbances, lack concomitant neuromuscular disease, and are not receiving steroids or specific antibiotics that are known to potentiate neuromuscular blockade.

TABLE 135-7 Clinical Effect of Drug and Metabolic States on Neuromuscular Blockers

Agent or Clinical Condition	Effect on Neuromuscular Blockers
Phenytoin Carbemazepine Ranitidine Azathioprine	Decrease sensitivity
Aminoglycosides Polymyxin Tetracycline Clindamycin Lidocaine Quinidine	Potentiate action
Hypermagnesemia	Enhance weakness
Hyperthermia Respiratory alkalosis Hypercalcemia	Decrease sensitivity
Hypokalemia Hyponatremia Hypocalcemia Respiratory acidosis Metabolic alkalosis Hypophosphotemia	Increased sensitivity
Hypothermia	Prolonged action

Paralysis assessment

The paralytic effect of NMB agents is usually evaluated with neuromuscular monitors (with train-of-four [TOF] appraisal) rather than by clinical assessment of neuromuscular strength. Whenever a paralytic agent is used, the TOF test measures the degree of neuromuscular blockade using a peripheral nerve stimulator. A baseline measurement is performed prior to starting the paralytic agent to determine the current necessary to obtain twitch. The clinician should complete the TOF test and document until a TOF ratio of 2/4 is achieved. TOF assessments should occur every four hours while a patient is receiving an NMB agent (intermittent bolus or infusion) for continued paralysis.

PRACTICE POINT

Instructions for train-of-four (TOF) assessment prior to and during paralysis

1. Attach two electrodes along the course of the ulnar nerve (temporal nerve may be used).
2. Connect the lead to the peripheral nerve stimulator by inserting the jacks into the proximal (red) and distal (black) output jacks. Connect the other end to the patient electrodes.
3. Turn the stimulator on. Select the current necessary (usually 20 mA) for that patient to twitch when the stimuli are applied.
4. Press the TOF once. It will deliver a train of four pulses where each is 0.5 seconds apart. Do not use the other buttons on the stimulator.
5. Count the number of twitches the patient had out of four (0/4, 1/4, 2/4, 3/4, 4/4.) Adjust the medication as ordered. The goal ratio is between 1/4 to 2/4 twitches.

Paralytic precautions

The complications of protracted NMB agent use include significantly compromised ability to detect patient distress or potentially lethal medical conditions such as stroke, peritonitis, myocardial infarction, or hypoglycemia. A paralyzed patient shows no obvious outward signs of distress, and inadvertent ventilator disconnection could be lethal. Inadequate sedation in an otherwise paralyzed patients can occur and may result in significant psychological trauma. Additionally, with ongoing NMB use, up to 10% of patients may develop neuropathies or critical care myopathy, especially with concomitant steroid use. Secondary nerve or soft tissue injury may also arise (eg, decubitus ulcer) from the pressure of limbs and dependent body segments against hard surfaces in pharmacologically immobilized patients. For all of these reasons, paralytic use should be punctuated by "drug holidays" during which a clinical appraisal of ongoing need and a survey for occult complications is undertaken.

TABLE 135-8 Evidence-based Key References for Sedation, Analgesia, and Paralysis in the Intensive Care Unit

Study	Methodology	Results	Limitations	Bottom Line
Kress, et al. *N Engl J Med.* 2000;342: 1471–1477.	RCT of standard care versus daily interruption of sedation (and analgesia) until awareness/agitation are manifest then restarting at half the prior dose.	Lower combined use of midazolam/morphine (not propofol); shorter ICU length of stay; decreased ICU-related complications.	Power to detect all adverse effects of removing sedation (eg, self-extubation) limited. Effect on PTSD, myocardial infarction risk not addressed until later study by same authors.	Protocol-based approaches that allow for interruption of sedation allow for recognized windows for weaning and fewer days of mechanical ventilation.
Kress, et al. *Am J Respir Crit Care Med.* 2003;168: 1457–1461.	Psychological screening interview applied to individuals previously in ICU (minimum 6 months prior) who underwent DIS compared with contemporaneous controls.	Daily interruption of sedation results in less PTSD and improved psychological adjustment.	Retrospective study. Controls assigned from same institution from same period of time (potential for bias).	Concerns for psychological trauma with lightened sedation are unwarranted. Shorter durations of sedation and DIS are associated with improved psychological outcomes.
Strom, et al. *Lancet.* 2010; 375:475–438.	Single institution RCT of critically ill patients receiving morphine prn analgesia versus analgesia with sedative protocol (propofol changing to midazolam) with DIS.	Patients not assigned to receive sedation had fewer ventilator-dependent days and shorter ICU stays.	Single-center, unblinded. 140/428 eligible patients included in study due to need for sedation for medical condition (status epilipticus, etc); 18% of pts without sedation were intolerant of protocol.	Treatment of pain in the ICU should be primary focus with sedation a secondary concern. Withholding sedation may improve outcome in pts expected to require intermediate to long-term mechanical ventilation.

DIS, daily interruption of sedation; ICU, intensive care unit; PTSD, post-traumatic stress disorder; RCT, randomized controlled trial.

CONSULTATION

Accessing critical care, anesthesia, or other specialty consultation to assist with the use of sedative, analgesic, or paralytic medications in the ICU should be left to the individual clinician's experience and comfort level in utilizing these agents. As part of a planned and measured approach for use of these agents (see Figure 135-3), a hospitalist may solicit assistance early in the ICU course with management of comorbid psychiatric, rheumatalgic, or other chronic uncontrolled painful disease or for management of long-standing opioid or drug dependence.

If lung mechanics require nonconventional modes of ventilation (eg, oscillating ventilation) or paralysis to allow patient synchrony with the ventilator, follow the critical care consultation protocol for neuromuscular blockade.

Anesthesia consultation in particular should be considered in patients when a complex or very difficult intubation is anticipated, when preexisting neurologic or metabolic disease preclude the use of succinylcholine, or when hemodynamic compromise may complicate anesthetic induction at the time of intubation.

Prolonged ICU stays that require longer-term use of sedative, analgesic, or paralytic agents may benefit from consultation with various ancillary services. Clinical pharmacists can help to guide dosing as pharmacokinetics shift with the clinical picture and the length of drug utilization. Nutritionists can guide assessment of caloric need in the setting of ongoing propofol infusion. Wound care specialists can help prevent and treat soft tissue breakdown when prolonged sedation or neuromuscular blockade is used.

Upon weaning off sedative, analgesic, and paralytic agents, consultation consideration from psychiatry or a pain specialist may be indicated if a patient suffers delirium or drug withdrawal symptoms that preclude successful liberation from the ventilator. Such consultation should be done on a case-by-case basis.

QUALITY IMPROVEMENT

While the use of sedative, hypnotic, and neuromuscular blocking regimens represent an integral part of ICU care, allowing for tolerance of and synchronization with the ventilator, they should be carefully monitored and adjusted to specific patient needs. Nursing and physician staff should work in concert to assess and implement an appropriate level of sedation that allows for ongoing ventilatory needs without representing an impediment to efficient weaning, as increased ventilator-dependent days are associated with greater risk of pneumonia and other significant ICU morbidity.

Daily awakening should be an integral part of ICU care in intubated nonparalyzed patients to allow opportunities for successful weaning and refinement of the goal for sedation and analgesia.

Neuromuscular blocking agents should be instituted with well-defined goals in mind, usually related to severely compromised lung compliance and the use of unconventional ventilatory strategies. Patients should be weaned off these drugs as soon as feasible (**Table 135-8**).

SUGGESTED READINGS

Devlin J, Roberts R. Pharmacology of commonly used analgesics and sedatives in the ICU: benzodiazepines, propofol, and opioids. *Crit Care Clin.* 2009;25:431–449.

Kress JP, Pohlman AS, O'Connor MF, et al. Daily interruption of sedative infusions in critically ill patients undergoing mechanical ventilation. *N Engl J Med.* 2000;343:814–815.

Kress JP, Gehlbach B, Lacy M, et al. The long-term psychological effects of daily sedative interruption on critically ill patients. *Am J Respir Crit Care Med.* 2003;168:1457–1461.

Gehlbach BK, Kress JP. Sedation in the intensive care unit. *Curr Opinion Critic Care.* 2002;8(4):290–298.

Jacobi J, Fraser GL, Coursin DB, et al. Clinical practice guidelines for the sustained use of sedatives and analgesics in the critically ill adult. *Crit Care Med.* 2002;30:119–139.

Murphy G, Vender J. Neuromuscular-blocking drugs. *Crit Care Clin.* 2001;17:925–942

Ostermann ME, Keenan SP, Seiferling RA, et al. Sedation in the intensive care unit: a systematic review. *JAMA.* 2000;283:1451–1459.

Sessler C, Varney K. Patient-focused sedation and analgesia in the ICU. *Chest.* 2008;133:552–556.

Strom T, Martinussen T, Toft P. A protocol of no sedation for critically ill patients receiving mechanical ventilation: a randomised trial. *Lancet.* 2010;375:475–480.

CHAPTER 136

Prevention in the Intensive Care Unit Setting

Laura Evans, MD, MSc
Nishay Chitkara, MD

Key Clinical Questions

1. What are the common preventable complications of intensive care unit (ICU) care?
2. What components are included within the care bundles to reduce catheter-related blood stream infections and ventilator-associated pneumonia?
3. What pharmacologic and nonpharmacologic interventions may be used for prevention of venous thromboembolism in the ICU?
4. Which ICU patients are high risk for stress ulcer bleeding and require pharmacologic prophylaxis? When should prophylaxis be discontinued?
5. What are the essential elements of interdisciplinary care in the ICU?

INTRODUCTION

Critical illness places patients at high risk for various complications during hospitalization. Invasive monitoring devices, mechanical ventilatory support, immobility, and debility due to illness all contribute to susceptibility to these complications. Previously considered unavoidable consequences of critical illness, many ICU-related complications can be prevented.

In recent years, the Institute for health care Improvement (IHI) and other national organizations have advocated the adoption of a series of "bundles" with the goal of reducing the rate of complications in the ICU. Bundles aggregate evidence-based practices relevant to a diagnosis or procedure into a single intervention. The rationale for the use of bundles is that, when their elements are reliably applied together, they allow more uniform application of best practices and, thus, improve patient outcomes. Bundles represent one of many tools needed to prevent ICU-related complications (**Table 136-1**).

PRACTICE POINT

- Care bundles allow for more uniform application of all elements of evidence based practice and, thus, result in improved patient outcomes.

For each preventable ICU complication, this chapter will address epidemiology and strategies for prevention. Finally, daily goals of care will be addressed. Critical care practitioners can ensure the essential elements of preventive care in the ICU are implemented by incorporating a worksheet for daily goals of care.

COMMON COMPLICATIONS IN THE ICU

CATHETER-RELATED BLOOD STREAM INFECTIONS

Catheter-related blood stream infections (CR-BSIs) cause significant morbidity and mortality in the ICU, and increased length of stay as well as cost. Primary blood stream infections are most often related to infected intravascular devices, mostly central venous catheters. At least 80,000 new cases of CR-BSIs occur each year in the United States. Extra costs due to bloodstream infections among survivors averaged greater than $40,000 per patient.

Hospital-acquired infection rates now serve as a publicly reported quality indicator. Many states in the U.S. currently require mandatory reporting of CR-BSIs to the Centers for Disease Control and Prevention (CDC), and some states have made hospital-specific data publicly available. These publicly reported infection rates are based on the National health care Safety Network (NHSN) surveillance definition (**Table 136-2**). As of October 1, 2008, the Centers for Medicare and Medicaid Services (CMS) no longer reimburses hospitals for costs associated with some hospital-acquired conditions, including CR-BSIs.

The organisms most commonly causing BSIs include coagulase-negative staphylococci (31%), *Staphylococcus aureus* (20%), *Enterococcus* species (9%), *Candida* species (9%), and *Escherichia coli* (6%) (**Table 136-3**). The emergence of coagulase-negative staphylococcal infections and Candida species as virulent organisms can be attributed to increased use of intravascular catheters and the selection pressure created by broad spectrum antibiotic use.

TABLE 136-1 Components of the Institute for health care Improvement Central Line and Ventilator Bundles

IHI Central Line Bundle*	IHI Ventilator Bundle†
1. Hand hygiene	1. Elevation of the head of bed (to between 30 and 45 degrees)
2. Maximal barrier precautions	2. Daily interruption of sedation and assessment of readiness to extubate
3. Chlorhexidine skin antisepsis	3. Prophylaxis for peptic ulcer disease
4. Optimal catheter site selection, with avoidance of the femoral vein for central venous access in adult patients	4. Prophylaxis for deep venous thrombosis
5. Daily review of line necessity, with prompt removal of unnecessary lines	5. Daily oral care with chlorhexidine

*5 Million Lives Campaign. *Getting Started Kit: Prevent Central Line Infections How-to Guide*. Cambridge, MA: Institute for Healthcare Improvement; 2008. (Available at www.ihi.org).

†5 Million Lives Campaign. *Getting Started Kit: Prevent Ventilator-Associated Pneumonia* How-to Guide. Cambridge, MA: Institute for Healthcare Improvement; 2010. (Available at http://www.ihi.org).

TABLE 136-2 National Health Care Safety Network Surveillance Definition of Central Line–Associated Bloodstream Infection

Laboratory-confirmed bloodstream infection requires one of the following criteria:

1. A recognized pathogen cultured from one or more blood cultures; the organism is not related to an infection at another site
2. The patient has at least one of the following signs or symptoms: fever (> 38°C), chills, or hypotension *and* signs and symptoms and positive laboratory results are not related to infection at another site
3. Organisms considered to be usual skin contaminants require that the patient have fever, chills, or hypotension, as well as one of the following: (1) the common skin contaminant is isolated from two blood cultures drawn on separate occasions, and the organism is not related to infection at another site, or (2) the common skin contaminant is isolated from a single blood culture in a patient with an intravascular access device and appropriate antibiotic therapy is instituted.
4. A patient less than 12 months of age has one of the following: fever (> 38°C), hypothermia (< 37°C), apnea, bradycardia, as well as one of the above organism criteria

Clinical sepsis is defined by either of the following criteria:

1. One of the following clinical signs or symptoms with no other recognized cause: fever (> 38°C), hypotension (systolic pressure < 90 mm Hg), oliguria (< 20 mL/h). ALSO, blood culture is not done or no organism or antigen is detected in blood, and there is no apparent infection at another site.
2. The patient is less than 12 months of age with one of the following signs or symptoms and no other recognized cause: fever (> 38°C); hypothermia (< 37°C); apnea; bradycardia AND the following conditions all apply: blood culture is not done or no organism or antigen is detected in blood; there is no apparent infection at another site.

TABLE 136-3 Most Common Pathogens Isolated From Nosocomial Bloodstream Infections.

	Percentage of BSIs	
Pathogen	Total	ICU
Coagulase-negative staphylococci	31.3	35.9
Staphyloccocus aureus	20.2	16.8
Enterococcus species	9.4	9.8
Candida species	9.0	10.1
Escherichia coli	5.6	3.7
Klebsiella species	4.8	4.0
Enterobacter species	4.3	4.7
Pseudomonas aeruginosa	3.9	4.7
Acinetobacter baumanii	1.7	2.1
Serratia species	1.3	1.6

Susceptibility to CR-BSIs is increased by a number of intrinsic host factors including malnutrition, burns, loss of skin integrity, neutropenia, extremes of age, severity of underlying illness, and immunosuppression. The single most important extrinsic factor related to development of primary BSIs is the catheter itself. Peripheral intravenous catheters have the lowest associated rate of infection (0.5 per 1000 catheter days), while pulmonary artery catheters have the highest rates of CR-BSIs (3.7 per 1000 catheter days), followed by central venous catheters (2.7 per 1000 catheter days for nonmedicated, nontunneled central venous catheters).

PRACTICE POINT

Measures indicated for the prevention of catheter-related blood stream infections:

- Maximal sterile-barrier precautions
- Chlorhexidine skin antisepsis (rather than iodine-based antiseptic solutions)
- Preferred site to lower risk of CR-BSI: subclavian venous site (or if not available, internal jugular site)
- Avoiding antibiotic ointment at the catheter site
- Removing central venous catheters as soon as no longer needed. Peripheral intravenous lines are preferred
- Antimicrobial-impregnated catheters

A number of measures can be employed for the prevention of CR-BSIs. Some of the most effective efforts to reduce CR-BSIs include (1) appropriate site selection for the catheter, (2) use of proper skin antiseptic agents, (3) use of maximal sterile barrier precautions during the procedure (Table 136-4), (4) early central catheter removal when no longer needed, and (5) use of antimicrobial-impregnated catheters. Table 136-1 summarizes the elements of the IHI's central line bundle for reduction of CR-BSIs. The insertion of catheters into the subclavian vein has been associated with a significantly lower rate of infection compared to the femoral vein in a randomized controlled trial. Observational data suggest that the subclavian site is also associated with a lower risk of infection than the internal jugular site. However, no single randomized controlled trial has compared the infection risk for all three insertion sites. Since the subclavian site may be associated with higher rates of mechanical complications such as bleeding and pneumothorax, decisions regarding site selection for CVC insertion should take into account the clinical circumstances of the individual patient.

TABLE 136-4 Maximal Sterile Barrier Precautions During Central Venous Catheter Insertion

1. Persons placing the central venous catheter should wear a cap, mask, sterile gown, and sterile gloves
2. A large sterile drape should cover the patient from head to toe, with an opening at the site of insertion
3. A sterile sleeve should be used to protect pulmonary artery catheters during insertion.

Skin antisepsis at the catheter insertion site should be performed with 2% aqueous *chlorhexidine* gluconate. Tincture of iodine, an iodophor, or 70% alcohol may be used as alternatives if chlorhexidine is contraindicated, but is less effective than chlorhexidine in infection prevention. Maximal sterile-barrier precautions should always be used during catheter insertion (**Table 136-4**).

The use of antimicrobial-impregnated catheters significantly reduced the rate of CR-BSIs and reduced overall medical costs in randomized clinical trials. Three such types of catheters are currently available: chlorhexidine and silver sulfadiazine impregnated, platinum and silver impregnated, and minocycline and rifampin impregnated. CDC guidelines recommend the following; (1) use of an antimicrobial- or antiseptic-impregnated central venous catheter (CVC) in adults whose catheter is expected to remain in place more than five days if an institution's rate of CR-BSI remains high, or above the institutional goal, despite education of staff who insert and maintain catheters; (2) use of maximal sterile barrier precautions; (3) and use of 2% chlorhexidine preparation for skin antisepsis during CVC insertion.

CVCs should be removed promptly when they are no longer needed or when a peripheral IV can be reasonably inserted and serve the same function as the CVC. Maintaining a CVC when it is not absolutely necessary increases the risk of bacterial colonization and subsequent CR-BSIs over time. Routine catheter changes do not reduce the risk of CR-BSIs, and routine guidewire catheter exchanges may actually increase the rate of infections. Therefore, routine or scheduled CVC changes should not be performed. Rather, catheters should be changed only when concern arises for infection or catheter malfunction. If a catheter infection is suspected and a CVC is still needed, a new catheter should be placed at a different insertion site. *Antibiotic ointments promote emergence of antibiotic-resistant bacteria when applied to catheter-insertion sites and therefore should be avoided.*

Clinical manifestations of CR-BSIs are often limited to fever, but more specifically can include inflammation or purulence at the site of catheter insertion and bacteremia with no apparent source. The diagnosis of CR-BSIs requires microbiological data to fulfill the CDC criteria for a laboratory-confirmed bloodstream infection (LCBI).

When a CR-BSI is suspected in a patient with fever and a CVC in place, the possibility of bacteremia should be evaluated with *two cultures of blood from peripheral sites*. A positive blood culture from the central venous catheter does not differentiate catheter colonization or hub contamination from a true CR-BSI. A negative blood culture from the catheter makes a CR-BSI unlikely. When diagnosis of a CR-BSI is highly suspected or confirmed—either clinically or microbiologically—the catheter should be removed immediately and antibiotics should be rapidly initiated. When the organism is identified antibiotics should be tailored to the sensitivity of the organisms grown in culture (**Figure 136-1**).

VENTILATOR-ASSOCIATED PNEUMONIA

Ventilator-associated pneumonia (VAP) is commonly considered a subtype of hospital-acquired pneumonia, which develops in mechanically ventilated patients more than 48–72 hours after endotracheal intubation. Incidence estimates range from 9% to 27% of mechanically ventilated patients, and the development of VAP is associated with increased mortality, increased ICU and hospital length of stay, and increased cost. Common pathogens

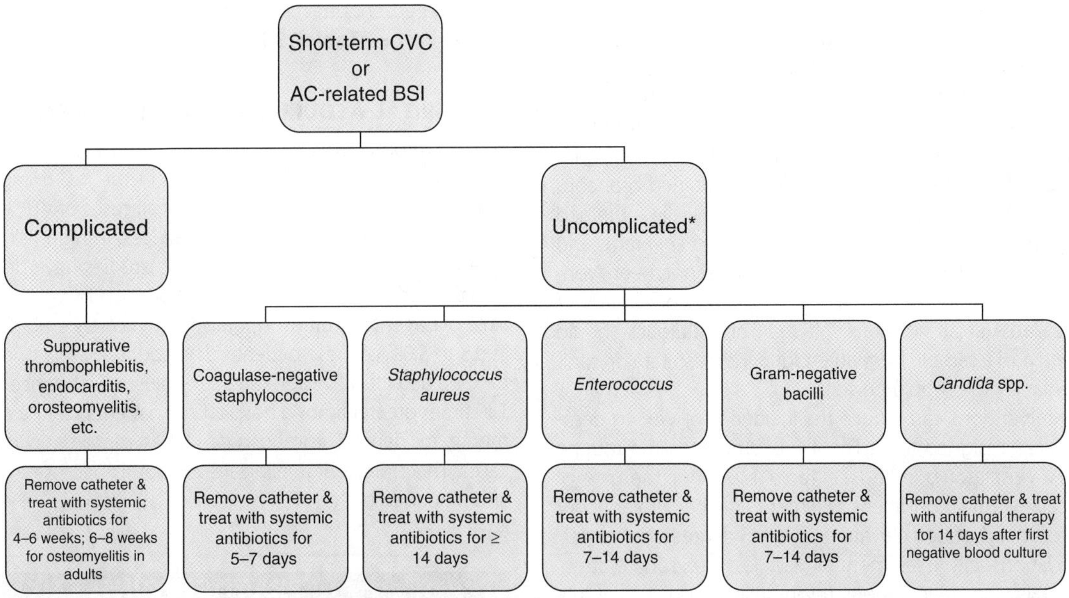

Figure 136-1 *Algorithm for management of patients with short-term CVC–related or arterial catheter–related blood stream infection. AC, arterial catheter; BSI, blood stream infection; CVC, central venous catheter. *Uncomplicated BSI = resolution of BSI within 72 hours; no intravascular hardware; no evidence of endocarditis, suppurative thrombophlebitis, or S aureus infection; no active malignancy; and no immunosuppression.*

TABLE 136-5 Strategies for the Prevention of Ventilator-Associated Pneumonia

Head-of-bed elevation	Elevation of the head of the bed to at least 30–45 degrees decreases the risk of aspiration of gastric contents compared to the supine position. A single RCT demonstrated a decrease in VAP incidence in patients managed in the semirecumbent position.
Subglottic suction	Continuous aspiration of subglottic secretions may decrease aspiration and risk of VAP. Studies have suggested that endotracheal tubes designed to permit continuous subglotttic suction are most effective in patients who are intubated for greater than 72 hours.
Silver-coated endotracheal tubes	Silver-coated endotracheal tubes may reduce bacterial colonization and biofilm formation. A large RCT published in 2008 demonstrated a absolute risk reduction of 2.7% (NNT = 37) and a relative risk reduction of VAP of 35.9% for patients intubated longer than 24 hours. There was also a delayed time to occurrence of VAP with silver-coated endotracheal tubes.
Oral care	Decontamination of the oropharynx may decrease the burden of microbes that are aspirated. Use of chlorhexidine for oral decontamination has been demonstrated to decrease the risk of VAP in patients after cardiac surgery and in patients intubated greater than 24 hours, but does not impact mortality. A single large RCT using a combination of tobramycin, colistin and amphotericin B for oral decontamination found a decrease in the risk of VAP and a reduction in the odds ratio of death (0.86 (95% CI 0.74–0.99), NNT = 35).
Selective digestive tract decontamination	Selective digestive tract decontamination typically refers to topical (oropharyngeal or through a nasogastric tube) administration of a combination of nonabsorbable antibiotics and antifungals, sometimes in combination with intravenous therapy to reduce oropharyngeal and gastric colonization. A large RCT of SDD (topical application of tobramycin, colistin, and amphotericin B in the oropharynx and stomach every six hours until ICU discharge, and intravenous cefotaxime for four days) demonstrated a modest decrease in mortality without any short-term increase in bacterial resistance. Some clinicians remain concerned about longer-term effects on bacterial resistance patterns.
Stress ulcer prophylaxis	Modification of gastric pH may decrease the risk of stress ulcer bleeding, but may increase the risk of VAP. One RCT demonstrated a lower incidence of VAP with less change in gastric pH in patients receiving sulcralfate for stress ulcer prophylaxis compared to antacids or H2 receptor blockers. More recent data has suggested that use of PPI increases the risk of hospital-acquired pneumonia. H2 blockers and PPIs may be more effective at reducing the risk of stress ulcer bleeding than sucralfate, but may confer an increased risk of VAP. Selection of stress ulcer prophylaxis should include all these factors as well as local cost.
Ventilator circuit changes	Currently the Center for Disease Control recommends changing ventilator circuits no more frequently than every 48 hours while the American Association of Respiratory Care recommends against routine changes. More frequent changes are associated with increased risk of VAP.

H2, Histamine-2; NNT, number needed to treat; PPI, proton pump inhibitors; RCT, randomized controlled trial; SDD, Selective digestive tract decontamination; VAP, ventilator-associated pneumonia.

include *Staphylococcus aureus, Klebsiella pneumoniae, Pseudomonas aeruginosa, Escherichia coli, Enterobacter species,* and *Acinetobacter* species. The diagnosis of VAP should be considered in mechanically ventilated patients with fever, change in respiratory secretions, leukocytosis, or change in oxygen requirements; and with a new or persistent infiltrate on chest radiography. A lower respiratory tract sample should be obtained for culture when VAP is suspected, prior to the initiation of antibiotics. Samples may be obtained bronchoscopically or nonbronchoscopically. Bronchoscopically obtained cultures may lead to narrower-spectrum antibiotic coverage and more frequent deescalation of therapy, but have not been convincingly shown to decrease mortality. As bronchoscopy may not always be available at all hospitals, initiation of antibiotics should not be delayed and a sample from an endotracheal aspirate or mini-bronchoalveolar lavage should be sent.

Multiple interventions can reduce the incidence of VAP, as demonstrated in well-designed trials. The IHI recommends the routine use of the IHI ventilator bundle (see Table 136-1) for the care of all mechanically ventilated patients. Elements of the IHI ventilator bundle include: head-of-bed elevation of 30–45 degrees, daily interruption of sedation, daily assessment of readiness to extubate, stress ulcer prophylaxis, and deep venous thrombosis prophylaxis. While the ventilator bundle does not specifically address VAP prevention and observational studies have reported mixed results as to the bundle's effect on VAP prevention, use of the ventilator bundle is recommended in the care of all mechanically ventilated patients. Strategies for the prevention of VAP may include subglottic suction, silver-coated endotracheal tubes, oral care, and limiting ventilator circuit changes (**Table 136-5**).

HOSPITAL-ACQUIRED VENOUS THROMBOEMBOLISM

Venous thromboembolism (VTE) is a significant cause of morbidity, preventable illness, and mortality in the ICU. Hospitalization is associated with approximately 25% of all cases of VTE, with a majority of cases occurring on medical services. In high-risk patients not receiving any prophylaxis, prospective studies have detected deep vein thrombosis in 10.5% to 14.9% of patients by venography, and in 5.0% of patients by ultrasonography. Pulmonary embolism occurred in 0.3 to 5.0% of these patients. One county-based study from 1980 to 1990 detected the age- and sex-adjusted incidence of VTE to be 130 times greater among hospitalized patients compared with community residents. Thrombosis can be asymptomatic in over 70% of cases. Therefore, a high clinical suspicion is necessary for detection and management of VTE.

PRACTICE POINT

- Thrombosis can be asymptomatic in over 70% of cases. A high clinical suspicion is necessary for detection and management of VTE.

TABLE 136-6 Risk Factors for Venous Thromboembolism in Hospitalized Patients

Admitting Conditions	Clinical Characteristics
Acute infectious disease	Previous venous thromboembolism
Congestive heart failure (New York Heart Association Class III or IV disease)	Advanced age (particularly >75 years)
Acute myocardial infarction	Recent surgery (especially orthopedic) or trauma
Acute respiratory disease	Immobility or paresis
Stroke	Obesity (body mass index >30)
Rheumatic disease (ie, acute arthritis)	Central venous catheterization
Inflammatory bowel disease	Inherited or acquired thrombophilic states
Malignancy	Varicose veins
Spinal cord injury	Estrogen therapy
Pregnancy/peripartum	Mechanical ventilation
Nephrotic syndrome	
Sepsis or septic shock	

TABLE 136-7 Prophylaxis for Venous Thromboembolism

Drug	Route of Administration	Dose
Pharmacologic options		
Unfractionated heparin	Subcutaneous	5000 U every 8 hours
Low-molecular-weight heparins		
Dalteparin	Subcutaneous	5000 units once daily
Enoxaparin	Subcutaneous	40 mg once daily
Fondiparinux	Subcutaneous	2.5 mg once daily
Nonpharmacologic options*		
Ambulation		
Exercises involving foot extension		
Graduated compression stockings		
Pneumatic compression devices		

*Nonpharmacologic prophylaxis is recommended for patients at high risk for bleeding, including those with recent or active gastrointestinal bleeding, patients with hemorrhagic stroke, and patients with severe thrombocytopenia or other coagulopathic conditions.

Admitting medical conditions associated with a high rate of VTE include acute infectious diseases, congestive heart failure, acute myocardial infarction, acute respiratory disease, stroke, acute renal failure, malignancy, and rheumatic disease—many of which lead to immobilization. Sepsis and the systemic inflammatory response syndrome, conditions managed frequently in critically ill patients, are also hypercoagulable states. Clinical characteristics or past history increasing the risk for VTE include previous VTE, older age, recent surgery or trauma, immobility or paresis, obesity (body mass index [BMI] >30), central venous catheterization, inherited thrombophilic states, varicose veins, estrogen therapy (oral contraceptives and hormone replacement), pregnancy, and active tobacco use (**Table 136-6**).

Safe and effective VTE prophylaxis begins with identification of patients at risk. While systems for VTE risk estimation based on the number and type of risk factors have been proposed, no formal, prospectively validated risk assessment models exist for determining the need for pharmacologic prophylaxis for medical patients. However, patients who will benefit from pharmacologic prophylaxis for VTE include those over 40 years of age, those having limited mobility for three days or more, and those possessing at least one thrombotic risk factor (see Table 136-6). Presence of multiple risk factors increases the risk.

Prophylactic treatments against VTE (**Table 136-7**) target the two major factors behind its pathogenesis: venous stasis by improving venous blood flow and hypercoagulabilty by reducing blood coagulability.

Pharmacologic prophylaxis, as provided with unfractionated heparins (UFH), low-molecular-weight heparins (LMWHs), or fondaparinux, is the preferred preventive therapy for VTE. Clinical trials involving surgical patients provided the initial documentation of the efficacy of this type of treatment, with one trial showing a significant reduction in the incidence of fatal pulmonary embolism following general surgery. A subsequent meta-analysis confirmed the ability of low-dose UFH (5000 units subcutaneously, given every 8–12 hours) to significantly reduce the rates of postoperative VTE (risk reduction 67%), total pulmonary embolism (PE) (risk reduction 47%), and fatal PE (risk reduction 64%). Studies in medical patients have shown pharmacologic prophylaxis to significantly reduce the relative risks of PE and nonfatal PE, with a nonsignificant reduction in the relative risk of DVT. In various studies of hospitalized patients at high risk for VTE, LMWHs, low-dose unfractionated heparin, and fondaparinux have each significantly reduced the rate of VTE. No mortality benefit has been shown, and data on rates of major bleeding with pharmacologic prophylaxis are inconsistent.

Nonpharmacologic therapies for prevention of VTE include ambulation, foot extension exercises to improve venous flow, and graduated compression stockings. Currently, no data on the use of graduated compression stockings are available from large studies of hospitalized medical patients, but a Cochrane Systematic Review has shown them to be effective in reducing VTE in postoperative hospitalized patients by 50%. Intermittent pneumatic compression devices offer another option for nonpharmacolgic prophylaxis, preventing venous stasis by enhancing blood flow in the deep veins and reducing plasminogen activator inhibitor-1 (thus increasing endogenous fibrinolytic activity). Pneumatic compression devices should not be used in the setting of peripheral vascular disease. A Cochrane Systematic Review has shown them to be effective in reducing the incidence of VTE, and even more so when used in combination with pharmacologic prophylaxis. Nonpharmacologic prophylaxis should be implemented in patients with contraindications to pharmacologic prophylaxis, including those at high risk for bleeding, such as patients with active or recent gastrointestinal bleeding, those with hemorrhagic stroke, or those with defects of hemostasis (ie, severe thrombocytopenia).

Protocols that promote increased use of pharmacologic VTE prophylaxis in hospitalized patients, and particularly in ICU patients, can improve prophylaxis rates and reduce VTE events and complications. Educational programs, computer prompts reminding physicians to consider VTE prophylaxis, and computer programs identifying high-risk patients have all increased the use of prophylaxis by clinicians. Recently, a protocol for VTE risk assessment and prevention was validated in a prospective observation study. Its implementation improved VTE prophylaxis and substantially reduced the incidence of hospital-acquired VTE.

STRESS ULCER BLEEDING

Stress ulcer bleeding can lead to significant morbidity in at-risk hospitalized patients. In one large North American study, 1.5% of ICU patients developed clinically relevant overt bleeding due to stress ulceration. Postulated mechanisms include excessive acid secretion, mucosal ischemia, and impaired mucus production. Risk factors identified in the large Canadian cohort study included respiratory failure (mechanical ventilation >48 hours) and coagulopathy (INR > 1.5, PTT > 2 times the upper limit of normal, or platelet count < 50,000/μL). Patients with one or both of these risk factors had a 3.7% rate of clinically important bleeding, compared to 0.1% in patients without either risk factor. Other likely risk factors for stress ulcer bleeding include

- Burns, major trauma, head injury
- Sepsis, hypotension
- Mechanical ventilation, coagulopathy, acute renal failure

Pharmacologic agents can reduce the risk of stress ulcer bleeding. The most commonly studied agents are H2 blockers and proton pump inhibitors (PPI) (**Table 136-8**). Both classes are effective at reducing the risk of overt gastrointestinal bleeding. No convincing evidence supports superiority of one class over another. Both H2 blockers and PPIs increase gastric pH, and some data suggests that this may increase the risk of hospital- or ventilator-associated pneumonia, particularly with PPIs. Sucralfate does not alter gastric pH and evidence suggests that the rate of nosocomial pneumonia is lower with sucralfate compared to antacids and H2 blockers. However, sucralfate does not appear to be as effective as H2 blockers in the prevention of stress ulcer–related bleeding. A trial of 1200 mechanically ventilated patients compared the H2 blocker ranitidine with sucralfate and found a significant reduction in clinically important GI bleeding with ranitidine (1.7% of patients) compared to sucralfate (3.8% of patients). A meta-analysis has shown stress ulcer prophylaxis with a PPI to confer a 4% absolute risk reduction in GI bleeding compared with prophylaxis with an H2 blocker (NNT = 25). Enteral nutrition may also reduce risk of stress ulcer bleeding.

TABLE 136-8 Pharmacologic Therapies for Stress Ulcer Prophylaxis*

Sucralfate suspension, 1 gram via nasogastric tube every 6 hours
H2-receptor blockade†
Cimetidine, continuous infusion (up to 50 mg/hr IV) or bolus dose (up to 300 mg IV every 6 hours)
Ranitidine, bolus dose (50 mg IV every 8 hours)
Famotidine, bolus dose (20 mg IV twice daily)
Proton pump inhibitors†
Omeprazole, bolus dose (40 mg orally or via nasogastric tube daily)
Pantoprazole, bolus dose (40 mg orally, via nasogastric tube, or IV daily)
Esomeprazole, bolus dose (40 mg orally, via nasogastric tube, or IV daily)
Lansoprazole, bolus dose (30 mg orally or via nasogastric tube daily)
Rabeprazole, bolus dose (20 mg orally daily)

*This table includes the most commonly used medications for stress ulcer prophylaxis. Due to numerous side effects, antacids are rarely used to prevent stress ulcers. Prostaglandin analogs (such as misoprostol) are not effective in preventing stress ulcer formation.

†IV preparations are unnecessary and costly unless patient is unable to tolerate enteral-route medication.

Guidelines from the American Society of Health System Pharmacists suggest that stress ulcer prophylaxis should be limited to patients at high risk of overt gastrointestinal bleeding, including patients with respiratory failure or coagulopathy (INR > 1.5 or platelet count < 50,000/μL), or two or more of the following risk factors: sepsis, ICU admission lasting more than one week, occult GI bleeding lasting six or more days, and glucocorticoid therapy (more than 250 mg of hydrocortisone or the equivalent daily). Selection of either an H2 blocker or PPI should consider local cost.

Stress ulcer pharmacologic prophylaxis should be discontinued when risk factors resolve or when patients transfer out of the ICU to the medical floor.

PRESSURE ULCER RISKS AND PREVENTION

When critically ill patients are sedated, ventilated, and confined to bed for long periods, they are invariably at risk for the development of skin breakdown. Multiple factors contribute to the progression of pressure ulcers, and it is a testament to preventive measures that such injury does not occur more frequently.

The European Pressure Ulcer Advisory Panel (EPUAP) defines a pressure ulcer as "an area of localized damage to the skin and underlying tissue caused by pressure, shear, friction, or a combination of these." Pressure ulcers occur when the balance of compressive or shearing forces overwhelms the tissue tolerance for pressure or the tissue tolerance for changes in oxygen concentration. Additionally, external pressure exceeding capillary pressure results in occlusion and thrombosis of the capillary, leading to tissue anoxia, release of toxic metabolites, cell death, and formation of ulcers.

PRACTICE POINT

Classification of pressure ulcers:

- Grade I: Nonblanchable erythema of intact skin; indicators may also include discoloration, warmth, edema, induration
- Grade II: Partial thickness skin loss involving epidermis, dermis or both; a superficial ulcer
- Grade III: Full-thickness skin loss, with damage or necrosis of subcutaneous tissue
- Grade IV: Destruction, tissue necrosis, or damage to muscle, bone, or supporting structures; full-thickness skin may or may not be present

The International Pressure Ulcer Prevalence Survey (IPUP) documented overall prevalence and facility-acquired pressure ulcer rates of 13.5% and 6% in 2008 (N = 90,938) and 12.3% and 5% in 2009 (N = 92,408), respectively. Highest rates of facility-acquired pressure ulcer rates occurred in adult ICUs: 9.2% in the general cardiac care unit (2008), 12.1% in the medical ICU (2008), 10.3% in the surgical ICU (2009). The prevalence rates of both overall and facility-acquired pressure ulcers were lower in 2008 and 2009 compared with 2006 and 2007.

A number of risk assessment scales have been identified to determine patients at high risk for developing pressure ulcers. These scales should ideally identify those patients who would most benefit from preventive measures. However, none have been validated for ICU patients or developed especially for this population. The four most significant external factors for development of pressure ulcers are: pressure (in excess of arteriolar pressure), shearing forces, friction (which can cause abrasion), and moisture. Host risk factors include immobility, incontinence, nutritional compromise, tissue perfusion (which may be compromised by hypotension, dehydration, vasoconstriction in shock states, and heart failure), and neurologic diseases (leading to immobility).

Prevention of pressure ulcers requires relief of high degrees and extended durations of pressure. Frequent patient repositioning forms the cornerstone of prevention and should be employed every two to three hours. Regular turning reduces interface pressure and maintains microcirculatory perfusion. Pressure-reducing support surfaces for bedbound patients come in numerous types. Nonpowered support surfaces are made of gel, foam or water, and distribute local pressure over a wider body surface area. Powered (dynamic) surfaces use electricity to alternate air currents in order to redistribute pressure on the body.

Supportive interventions are equally important for reducing the rate of pressure ulcers. Immobility can be prevented through physical therapy and the interruption of sedative medications. Incontinence should be managed since excess moisture contributes to skin breakdown. However, urinary catheters should not be used to prevent stress ulcers, but may be considered for patients to prevent the progression of otherwise severe or evolving pressure ulceration. Adequate nutrition prevents ulcer formation, and promotes healing of ulcers. Therefore, nutritional assessment should ensure adequate intake of protein and calories. Finally, skin assessment should recognize changes in integrity, color, turgor, and moisture status. The skin should be kept clean and dry, with the use of mild cleansing agents that minimize irritation.

Regulatory organizations, such as the Joint Commission, now consider significant pressure ulcers that develop during a hospital stay as a "never event" and a marker of poorer-quality care. Additionally, the Centers for Medicare and Medicaid Services (CMS) may no longer reimburse facilities for pressure ulcers that develop during a hospital stay. Therefore, health care organizations should work to systematically implement interventions that help ensure prevention of pressure ulcers in hospitalized patients who are at risk for developing this condition.

ESSENTIAL ELEMENTS OF CARE IN THE ICU

Other essential elements of high-quality and efficient ICU care include hand hygiene, interdisciplinary communication, patient and family communication, sedation interruption and daily awakening in intubated patients, and assessment of delirium.

1. **Hand hygiene and infection control:** Scrupulous adherence to hand hygiene has been demonstrated to help terminate infectious outbreaks in health care facilities, reduce transmission of multidrug-resistant organisms, and reduce overall hospital-acquired infection rates. The CDC has issued comprehensive recommendations for hand hygiene in health care settings. These guidelines highlight the importance of handwashing with soap and water when hands are visibly soiled or contaminated, and before and after direct patient contact. Alcohol-based solutions may be used when hands are not visibly soiled. In the presence of *Clostridium difficile* infection, handwashing with soap and water is essential to preventing the transmission of infectious spores. In this era of increasing microbial resistance to antibiotics, adherence to hand hygiene and appropriate infection control precautions is a central tenet in safe ICU (and hospital) care.
2. **Interdisciplinary communication:** The ICU is an extremely complex environment and patient safety research has shown poor communication among intensive ICU nurses and doctors to be a common causal factor underlying critical incidents in the ICU. All members of the interdisciplinary ICU team must be committed to promoting teamwork and open communication across disciplines. Use of daily goals checklists in the ICU has been shown to improve interdisciplinary communication, improve team members' understanding of patient care plans in the ICU, and decrease ICU length of stay (**Table 136-9**). A more detailed description of interdisciplinary communication is described in other parts of the text (see Chapters 7 and 9).

TABLE 136-9 Sample Daily Goals Checklist for ICU Care

Date					
Problems to be addressed today					
What is the patient's greatest safety risk?					
Discharge plan or needs					
Pain management/sedation					
Cardiac/volume status					
Pulmonary/ventilation					
Mobilization (Risk for falls?)					
Medication changes (Can any be discontinued?)					
Diet/nutrition					
Consultations today					
Tests/procedures					
Nursing bedside treatments					
Can catheters or invasive devices be removed?					
Is this patient receiving venous thromboembolic and stress ulcer bleeding prophylaxis?					
Patient/family safety concerns; patient/family education and communication					
Print name/title Signature					
Print name/title Signature					

TABLE 136-10 Evidence-based Medicine Key References: Prevention in the ICU

Study	Methodology	Results	Limitations	Bottom Line
Catheter-related blood stream infections				
Pronovost P, Needham D, Berenholtz S, et al. An intervention to decrease catheter-related infections in the ICU. *N Eng J Med.* 2006;355(26):2725–2732.	Prospective, observational	• 103 intensive care units in Michigan instituted a central line bundle consisting of (1) handwashing, (2) using full barrier precautions, (3) skin prep with chlorhexidine, (4) avoiding the femoral site, and (5) discontinuing unnecessary catheters. • Median infection rates decreased from 2.7 per 1000 catheter days to 0 per 1000 catheter days after 3 months.	Before and after study design	Catheter-related blood stream infections are largely preventable with use of a central line bundle.
Ventilator-associated pneumonia				
Drakulovic MB, Torres A, Bauer TT, et al. Supine body position as a risk factorfornosocomialpneumonia in mechanically ventilated patients: a randomised trial. *Lancet.* 1999;354:1851–1858.	Randomized trial of the effect of supine versus semi-recumbent positioning of mechanically ventilated patients on incidence of ventilator associated pneumonia	• 90 patients randomized, 86 patients included for analysis • Frequency of clinically suspected VAP was lower in the semirecumbent group versus the supine group—8% versus 34%; ($p = 0.003$). • Frequency of microbiologically confirmed pneumonia was lower in the semirecumbent group versus supine group—5% versus 23%; ($p = 0.018$).	• Single center • Analysis not intention to treat	Semirecumbent body position may decrease the incidence of VAP.
Kollef MH, Afessa B, Anzueto A, et al. Silver-coated endotracheal tubes and incidence of ventilator-associated pneumonia: the NASCENT randomized trial. *JAMA.* 2008;300(7):805–813.	Mullticenter randomized, controlled, single-blind trial of silver-coated versus standard low-pressure, high-volume endotracheal tubes and incidence of VAP	• Among patients intubated for ≥24 hours, rates of microbiologically confirmed VAP were 4.8% (95% CI, 3.4–6.6%) in the group receiving the silver-coated tube and 7.5% (95% CI, 5.7–9.7%) (p =.03) in the group receiving the uncoated tube; (NNT = 37).	• Single-blind study • VAP rates low in both groups	Patients receiving a silver-coated endotracheal tube had a statistically significant reduction in the incidence of VAP.
Hospital-acquired venous thromboembolism				
Geerts WH, Bergqvist D, Pineo GF, et al. Prevention of venous thromboembolism: American College of Chest Physicians evidence-based clinical practice guideline (8th edition). *Chest.* 2008;133:381S–453S.	Evidence-based clinical practice guideline for prevention of venous thromboembolism	• Evidence-based recommendations for prevention pf venous thromboembolism in various patient populations	Clinical practice guideline	Synthesis of many clinical trials with evidence-based recommendations
Stress ulcer bleeding				
Cook DJ, Fuller HD, Guyatt GH, et al. Risk factors for gastrointestinal bleeding in critically ill patients. *N Eng J Med.* 1994; 330(6):377–381.	Prospective observational study of intensive care unit patients	• 4.4% of patients had overt bleeding and 1.5% of patients had clinically important bleeding. • Respiratory failure (odds ratio 15.6) and coagulopathy (ods ratio 4.3) were strong independent risk factors for clinically important bleeding	Observational study	Respiratory failure (mechanical ventilation for >48 hours) and coagulopathy are risk factors fro clinically important stress ulcer bleeding in ICU patients
Pressure ulcers				
Reddy M, Gill SS, Rochon PA. Preventing pressure ulcers: a systematic review. *JAMA.* 2006;296(8):974–984.	Systematic review of randomized controlled trials of pressure ulcer prevention	• Use of support surfaces, repositioning the patient, optimizing nutritional status, and moisturizing sacral skin are appropriate strategies to prevent pressure ulcers.	Systematic review	Multiple strategies may help prevent pressure ulcers.

CI, confidence interval; NNT, number needed to treat; VAP, ventilator-associated pneumonia.

3. **Communication with patients and families:** In evaluations of family satisfaction with ICU care, communication with physicians consistently receives low marks. One study found that half of the families of ICU patients surveyed failed to comprehend the patient's diagnoses, prognosis, or treatment plan. Among patients that died in the hospital, one in four had concerns about communication with their physician and half wanted more contact with their physicians. In addition, family members of critically ill patients have a high prevalence of symptoms of anxiety, depression, and posttraumatic stress disorder (PTSD) associated with having a loved one in the ICU. In 2007, an important study from France showed that implementing a program of a proactive ICU family conference in combination with a bereavement pamphlet decreased anxiety, depression, and PTSD among family members three months after a death in the ICU. In a separate study, family meetings within the first three ICU days for patients at highest risk for poor outcomes achieved significant reductions in ICU length of stay and conflict over the goals of care. Good quality, early communication with patients and families in the ICU should be a priority for all members of the interdisciplinary ICU team. See Chapter 140 for additional information on patient and family communication.
4. **Daily interruption of sedation and daily assessment of readiness to extubate:** Achieving the appropriate balance of sedation and analgesia in mechanically ventilated patients is challenging. Both excessive and insufficient sedation may increase the risk of iatrogenic complications and potentially impede recovery. Kress and colleagues randomized 128 adult patients on mechanical ventilation to daily interruption of sedation or interruption at the clinician's discretion. Daily interruption of sedation resulted in a significant reduction duration of mechanical ventilation from 7.3 days to 4.9 days ($p = 0.004$). Paired spontaneous awakening trials (daily interruption of sedation) and spontaneous breathing trials were assessed in the Awakening and Breathing Controlled (ABC) Trial. This protocolized approach to interruption of sedation and spontaneous breathing resulted in an increased number of days free from mechanical ventilation, decreased ICU and hospital length of stay, and decreased one-year mortality. A recent single-center study demonstrating the feasibility and safety of mechanical ventilation without sedation will likely prompt further research.
5. **Assessment of delirium:** Delirium, a fluctuating disturbance of consciousness with reduced ability to focus, sustain, or shift attention, develops rapidly in the ICU setting. Delirium is a significant contributor to ICU and hospital length of stay, morbidity, and mortality in the ICU, and patients with delirium have lower six-month survival rates. ICU patients, therefore, require frequent monitoring to assess for delirium. The Confusion Assessment Method in the ICU (CAM-ICU) allows physicians, nurses, and other clinicians to rapidly perform a bedside delirium assessment. This tool (available at http://www.icudelirium.org/docs/CAM_ICU.pdf) permits evaluation of changes in mental status, attention level, thought organization, and level of consciousness. The assessment of ICU delirium should be performed every shift. Patients' delirium risk may be reduced by modification of some factors, including sedative and analgesic medications. Strategies for prevention and treatment are currently being investigated in multiple studies (**Table 136-10**).

SUGGESTED READINGS

American Society of Health-System Pharmacists therapeutic guidelines on stress ulcer prophylaxis. *Am J Health Syst Pharm.* 1999; 56(8):729.

Cook DJ, Fuller HD, Guyatt GH, et al. Risk factors for gastrointestinal bleeding in critically ill patients. Canadian Critical Care Trials Group. *N Engl J Med.* 1994;330(6):377.

Geerts WH, Bergqvist D, Pineo GF, et al. Prevention of venous thromboembolism: American College of Chest Physicians evidence-based clinical practice duidelines (8th edition). *Chest.* 2008;133:381S–453S.

Girard TD, Kress JP, Fuchs BD, et al. Efficacy and safety of a paired sedation and ventilator weaning protocol for mechanically ventilated patients in intensive care (Awakening and Breathing Controlled trial): a randomised controlled trial. *Lancet* 2008; 371(9607):126–134.

Guidelines for prevention of intravascular catheter-related infections, 2002. Center for Disease Control and Prevention. Available at http://www.cdc.gov/ncidod/dhqp/gl_intrvascular.html.

Lautrette A, Darmon M, Megarbane B, et al. A communication strategy and brochure for relatives of patients dying in the ICU. *N Engl J Med.* 2007;356(5):469.

Niederman MS, Craven, DE. Guidelines for the management of adults with hospital-acquired, ventilator-associated, and healthcare-associated pneumonia. *Am J Respir Crit Care Med.* 2005;171:388.

Pronovost P, Needham D, Berenholtz S, et al. An intervention to decrease catheter-related infections in the ICU. *N Eng J Med.* 2006; 355(26):2725.

CHAPTER 137

Respiratory Failure

Eric M. Siegal, MD, SFHM

Key Clinical Questions

1. How should a clinician rapidly assess the severity and stability of a patient with acute respiratory distress?
2. How can principles of respiratory physiology be effectively applied to guide diagnosis and therapy?
3. What are the indications and contraindications for noninvasive positive pressure ventilation (NPPV), and what outcomes does this intervention affect?
4. When does a patient require advanced airway management?

CASE 137-1

A 53-year-old with COPD was hospitalized with acute pancreatitis. He had received substantial fluid resuscitation and parenteral morphine for severe epigastric pain. He became increasingly confused and somnolent, and his oxygen saturation acutely decreased to 82 percent on 2 liters per nasal cannula. On a nonrebreather face mask, his SpO_2 increased to 98 percent. He appeared uncomfortable, was tachycardic, tachypneic, and moderately confused. His expiratory phase was prolonged, and breath sounds were nearly absent at the lung bases. He had moderate peripheral edema, and his epigastrium was moderately tender.

INTRODUCTION

Acute respiratory failure, a common inpatient medical emergency, mandates rapid assessment of the patient and initiation of appropriate and potentially life-saving therapy. Treatment decisions often must be made with limited information and well before a definitive diagnosis can be established. In this time-pressured, high-risk environment, clinicians must develop a diagnostic and therapeutic schema that facilitates a rapid and comprehensive approach to the patient with acute respiratory failure. The four key steps to approaching the patient with acute respiratory failure are

1. Rapid assessment of the severity of the presentation and of the patient's stability
2. Determination of the likely cause or causes
3. Initiation of treatment
4. Assessment of the efficacy of treatment

PATHOPHYSIOLOGY AND DIFFERENTIAL DIAGNOSIS

Understanding the pathophysiologic underpinnings of acute respiratory failure simplifies and increases the accuracy of the diagnostic approach and the likelihood of choosing a successful therapeutic intervention. The five main etiologies of acute respiratory failure are

- Shunt
- Ventilation/perfusion (V/Q) mismatch
- Impaired diffusion
- Decreased mixed venous oxygen saturation
- Alveolar hypoventilation

SHUNT

Shunt occurs when a portion of pulmonary blood flow does not participate in gas exchange. *Physiologic shunt*, the most common cause of acute hypoxemia in the hospitalized patient, develops when pulmonary perfusion is inappropriately maintained to injured, atelectatic or collapsed alveolar units. A relatively small area of infiltrate or atelectasis may cause profound hypoxemia if there is significant shunt to that area. *Anatomic shunts* describe physical conduits that divert deoxygenated blood into the systemic circulation, as occurs with right to left intracardiac shunt or intrapulmonary shunt. In both anatomic and physiologic shunts, deoxygenated blood enters the systemic circulation. As the degree of shunt (shunt fraction) increases, the partial pressure of arterial oxygen (PaO_2) becomes increasingly independent of the fraction of inspired oxygen (FiO_2), and once the shunt fraction exceeds 50%, increasing FiO_2 does not increase PaO_2. In conditions characterized by high shunt fractions, the FiO_2 can often be lowered without compromising the PaO_2.

VENTILATION/PERFUSION MISMATCH

V/Q mismatch describes lung ventilation in excess of perfusion. Any process that increases dead space ventilation, such as alveolar overdistension (auto-PEEP), lung parenchymal destruction (emphysema), hypoperfusion (hypovolemia, acute RV failure), or obstruction of the pulmonary arterial circulation (pulmonary embolus) will generate V/Q mismatch. V/Q mismatch is characterized primarily by hypercapnia rather than hypoxemia. As a case in point, although tachypnea and respiratory distress are common clinical manifestations of acute pulmonary embolism (PE), marked hypoxemia is uncommon. Patients who become markedly hypoxemic after an acute PE generally have a secondary lung process or may have developed right-to-left intracardiac shunting due to acute right ventricular pressure overload.

PRACTICE POINT

- In most circumstances, PE does not cause marked hypoxemia. Patients who become markedly hypoxemic should be evaluated for another pulmonary process or acute right-to-left intracardiac shunt.

IMPAIRED DIFFUSION

Processes that damage or thicken the alveolar-capillary membrane, such as pulmonary edema, inflammation, fibrosis, or hemorrhage, increase the time required for gas to move between the alveolus and the pulmonary capillary. Under normal circumstances, gas exchange occurs very early as blood transits the pulmonary microcirculation. However, as cardiac output increases to meet metabolic demand (eg, during sepsis or exercise), blood spends proportionately less time in the pulmonary microcirculation. Impaired diffusion capacity will become clinically evident when the time required for gas exchange exceeds the amount of time that blood spends in the pulmonary capillary bed. This phenomenon explains why measuring exercise capacity remains the most sensitive and predictive indicator of disease progression in disorders characterized by progressive loss of diffusing capacity, such as pulmonary fibrosis.

DECREASED MIXED VENOUS OXYGEN SATURATION

Mixed venous oxygen saturation (MvO_2) reflects tissue oxygen extraction (VO_2), or whether oxygen delivery is meeting metabolic demands. Oxygen delivery (DO_2) is dependent upon cardiac output, hemoglobin level, and oxygen saturation. Decreases in any of these variables may significantly compromise oxygen delivery. When impaired oxygen delivery is coupled with increased metabolic demand (eg, septic shock), oxygen consumption will exceed oxygen delivery, at which point the MvO_2 will decrease; normal MvO_2 is 70%. If highly deoxygenated blood is returned to the right heart and gas exchange is impaired, blood may not fully oxygenate in the pulmonary circuit. Consequently, as gas exchange worsens, the MvO_2 plays an increasingly important role in dictating the PaO_2. Theoretically, the MvO_2 can be increased by manipulating oxygen delivery with red blood cell transfusion or treatment with inotropic agents. Studies in which DO_2 has been manipulated have demonstrated conflicting outcomes, and this practice remains controversial.

ALVEOLAR HYPOVENTILATION

Finally, alveolar hypoventilation may also cause acute respiratory failure if minute ventilation decreases below a patient's minimum metabolic requirements.

DIAGNOSIS

The etiology of acute respiratory failure is often multifactorial, and physiologic derangements can be synergistic. A patient with a simple opiate overdose may initially present with hypoventilatory respiratory failure, but subsequent atelectasis or aspiration may cause physiologic shunting and impaired gas exchange.

V/Q mismatch, shunt, and diffusion abnormalities all reflect derangements in pulmonary gas exchange, while hypoventilation reflects abnormalities with the mechanics or control of ventilation. The arterial blood gas and calculation of the alveolar-arterial (A-a) gradient effectively differentiate impaired gas exchange from impaired ventilatory control. The A-a gradient is widened by processes that impair gas exchange, but remains normal in pure hypoventilatory respiratory failure.

$$\text{A-a gradient} = FiO_2 \times (P_{barometric} - P_{H_2O}) - PaO_2 + PaCO_2/0.8$$

At sea level breathing room air:

$$\text{A-a gradient} = 0.21 \times (760 - 50) - PaO_2 - (PaCO_2 \times 1.25)$$

Simplified:

At sea level: $\text{A-a gradient} = 150 - PaO_2 - (PaCO_2 \times 1.25)$
Normal $\text{A-a gradient} = (\text{Age}/4) + 4$

The A-a gradient increases by approximately 6 mm Hg for every 10% increase in FiO_2, presumably due to blunting of physiologic pulmonary hypoxic vasoconstriction. Thus, a healthy patient with a baseline A-a gradient of 10 mm Hg on room air will develop an A-a gradient of 60 mm Hg when breathing 100% oxygen. As a result, the A-a gradient becomes progressively more difficult to interpret as the FiO_2 increases. In patients with high FiO_2 requirements, the ratio of oxygenation to supplementation (PaO_2/FiO_2 ratio) is a better and more reliable gauge of gas-exchange impairment.

PRACTICE POINT

- The A-a gradient increases by approximately 6 mm Hg for every 10 percent increase in the FiO_2 in a normal individual. Therefore, the A-a gradient becomes progressively more difficult to interpret as the FiO_2 increases. In patients with high FiO_2 requirements, the PaO_2/FiO_2 ratio is a more sensitive and reliable gauge of impairment than the A-a gradient.

Despite its limitations in severely hypoxemic states, the A-a gradient is a useful first step to a physiologic approach to acute respiratory failure (**Figure 137-1**). While it is helpful to approach respiratory failure based on physiologic principles, it is equally instructive to assess the primary anatomic systems required for effective respiration—specifically, the control of respiration, the airway, chest mechanics, the lung parenchyma, and vascular perfusion (**Table 137-1**). These complimentary physiologic and anatomic approaches to acute respiratory failure facilitate a rapid and comprehensive approach to diagnosis and treatment. Once a provisional diagnosis has been established, clinicians must initiate therapy that is specifically targeted to reversing the pathophysiology. A full discussion of these interventions is beyond the scope of this chapter, but rapid initiation of effective adjunctive therapy may prevent progression to acute intubation and ventilation.

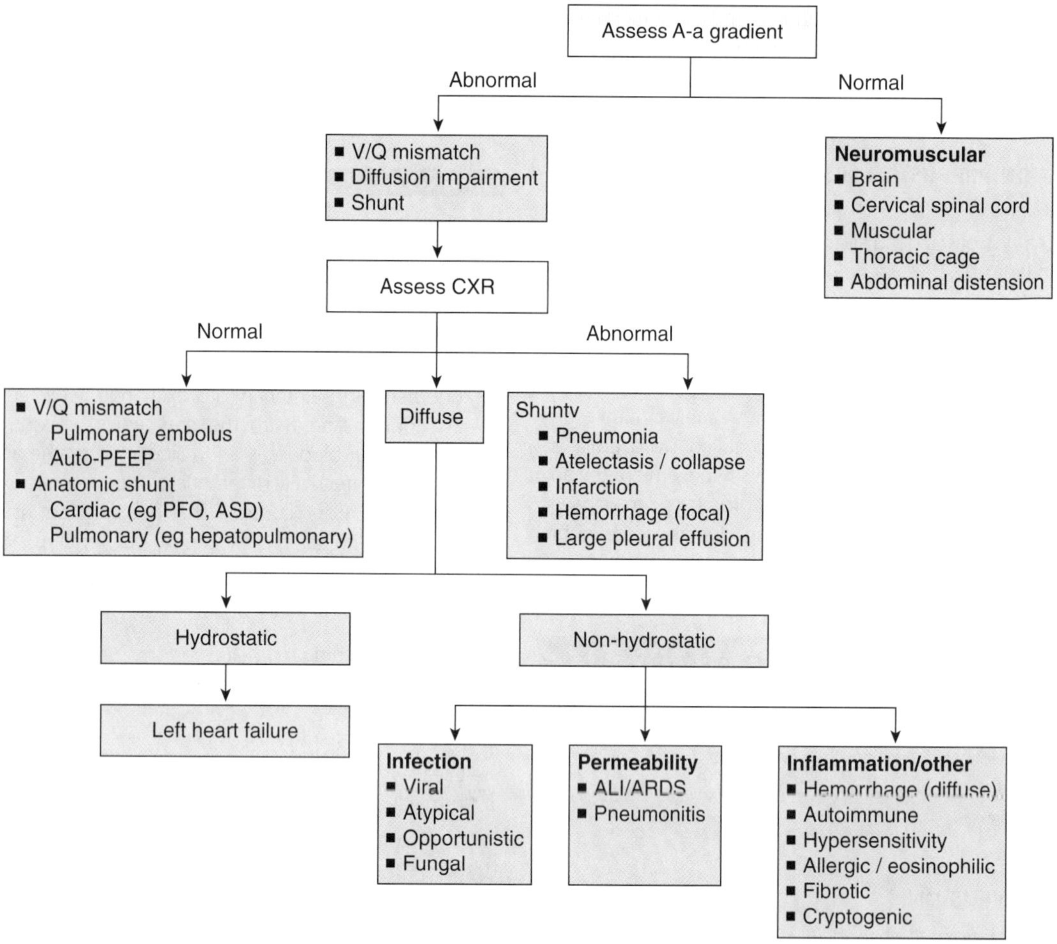

Figure 137-1 *A physiology-based algorithm for acute hypoxemic respiratory failure. ALI, acute lung injury; ARDS, acute respiratory distress syndrome ASD; atrial septal defect; CXR, chest X-ray; PFO, patent foramen ovale. (Adapted, with permission, from Dr. Kenneth E. Wood.)*

TRIAGE

RAPID ASSESSMENT OF SEVERITY AND STABILITY

Assessing the severity and stability of acute respiratory failure at the extremes of illness is generally straightforward. The patient who is awake, can speak in full sentences, and appears relatively comfortable is unlikely to acutely decompensate or require emergent interventions. On the other hand, the patient who is obtunded, hemodynamically unstable, or who appears exhausted due to respiratory effort should almost always be intubated and mechanically ventilated without delay. The challenge lies in assessing presentations that fall between these two extremes. The initial survey must occur quickly and systematically to determine the degree of respiratory distress, the patient's stability, and the likelihood of further deterioration. This assessment can be distilled to four key questions:

1. **How severe is the patient's respiratory distress?**
   The degree of respiratory distress can be quickly and accurately assessed with a focused physical examination. Altered mental status, the use of accessory muscles of respiration (sternocleidomastoid, scalene, intercostals, and abdominal musculature), tachypnea, and signs of adrenergic stimulation (tachycardia, diaphoresis, hypertension and agitation) indicate a high degree of respiratory distress or effort. The presence of one or more of these findings should serve as a red flag that the patient may have impending respiratory failure. A patient's age, comorbid diseases, and estimated physiologic reserve should also be factored into the severity assessment. Intuitively, a fit 25-year-old will tolerate a greater degree of respiratory distress than a chronically ill 75-year-old.
2. **Is the patient protecting his or her airway?**
   The airway assessment includes an evaluation of the patient's mental status, ability to manage secretions, risk for aspiration, and the patency of the airway itself. This assessment can often be performed in seconds. A patient who is awake, responsive, managing secretions, and phonating audibly is protecting the airway. Contrary to popular teaching, the gag reflex does not reliably indicate whether the patient is protecting his airway. Healthy adults may have a diminished or absent gag reflex, while comatose patients may not. Coma, defined as a Glasgow Coma Scale (GCS) score of eight or less, is a better predictor of actual or impending airway compromise (**Table 137-2**). As a general rule, any patient who is comatose and unlikely to awaken very rapidly should be immediately intubated for airway protection.

PRACTICE POINT

- A patient who is awake, responsive, managing secretions, and phonating audibly is protecting his airway. The gag reflex does not reliably indicate whether the patient is protecting the airway.

TABLE 137-1 Systems-based Approach to Acute Respiratory Failure

Cause	Potential Intervention
Neurologic	
Decreased level of consciousness (drugs, toxins, infection, metabolic derangements, stroke, hypercarbia)	Reversal agents (naloxone, flumazenil)
Impaired central control (obesity-hypoventilation, central apnea)	Acute bag-mask ventilation, BPAP
Spinal cord injury	BPAP
Neuromuscular disease (myasthenia, Guillain-Barre', motor neuron disease, critical illness polyneuropathy)	Pyridostigmine, BPAP
Airway	
Upper airway obstruction (tumor, trauma, foreign body, infection/abscess, edema, dynamic obstruction)	Foreign body removal, head positioning, oral airway, heliox, inhaled racemic epinephrine, corticosteroids
Lower airway obstruction (foreign body, mucus plug, tumor, bronchospasm)	Bronchodilators, corticosteroids, heliox, catheter suctioning, bronchoscopic suctioning
Chest Mechanics	
Chest wall trauma	Analgesia
Extrathoracic restriction (kyphosis, obesity)	BPAP
Pneumothorax, hemothorax	Tube thoracostomy ("chest tube")
Pleural effusion	Thoracentesis
Pain/splinting (rib fracture, upper abdominal surgery)	Analgesia (oral, parenteral, epidural, intercostal block)
Abdominal distension	Nasogastric decompression, paracentesis, release of abdominal binder
Lung Parenchyma	
Edema (hydrostatic or nonhydrostatic)	Diuresis, vasodilators (nitroglycerin, nesiritide, morphine)
Atelectasis	Cough, incentive spirometry, intermittent positive pressure ventilation, chest percussion
Infiltrate	Position patient with "good" side in dependent position (except in pulmonary hemorrhage)
Vascular	
Pulmonary embolus	Anticoagulation, thrombolysis
Right ventricular failure	Inotropes, inhaled nitric oxide
Decreased MvO_2	Inotropes, red blood cell transfusion

BPAP, bilevel positive airway pressure.

TABLE 137-2 The Glasgow Coma Scale

		Score
Best eye opening	Spontaneous	4
	To voice	3
	To pain	2
	None	1
Best verbal response	Oriented	5
	Confused	4
	Inappropriate words	3
	Incomprehensible	2
	None	1
Best motor response	Obeys commands	6
	Localizes to pain	5
	Withdraws from pain	4
	Flexion to pain	3
	Extension to pain	2
	None	1
Total		15

Secretion management depends upon the competency of the swallow mechanism and the volume of secretions such as saliva, sputum, blood, or gastric contents. As respiratory effort and confusion worsen, patients become increasingly unable to manage secretions, and this too should be factored into the assessment.

As the stability of an airway often evolves over time, airway assessment should include an estimation of the clinical course as a key component. A patient with acute hypercarbia and a GCS of seven may awaken within minutes of initiation of bag-mask ventilation, while a patient with mild airway compromise due to acute epiglottitis may rapidly progress to complete airway obstruction. Whatever the etiology, early intubation of a potentially threatened airway should always be entertained unless rapid and sustained improvement is expected. Extreme caution should be taken if airway compromise is due to anatomic compression or obstruction. In such circumstances, it is often safer to delay intubation until a clinician with expertise in difficult airway management is available.

3. **Is gas exchange adequate?**

Clinical signs of hypoxemia or hypercarbia may include headache, altered mental status, cyanosis, or acute end-organ failure, but these findings are neither sensitive nor specific. Pulse oximetry is generally the first measurement available at the bedside, and it provides rapid, real-time quantification of peripheral oxygenation.

The presence of carboxyhemoglobinemia or methemoglobinemia may falsely elevate the SpO_2, while motion artifact and hypoperfusion due to occlusive arterial disease, hypotension, or vasoconstriction may degrade signal quality and artificially depress the SpO_2 (**Table 137-3**).

Due to the sigmoidal shape of the oxyhemoglobin dissociation curve, the accuracy of pulse oximetry rapidly deteriorates once the SpO_2 falls below 80%. Most importantly, pulse oximetry provides no information about ventilation or acid-base status. The arterial blood gas, while mildly invasive and more difficult to obtain than pulse oximetry, therefore remains the gold standard in the assessment of acute respiratory failure.

TABLE 137-3 Factors Affecting the Accuracy of Pulse Oximetry

Falsely lowered SpO_2
• Probe malposition
• Impaired perfusion (peripheral vasoconstriction, peripheral arterial disease)
• Dark skin pigmentation
• Nail polish
• Methylene blue
• Motion artifact
Falsely elevated SpO_2
• Carboxyhemoglobin
• Methemoglobin
• Hypothermia

4. **What is the likely progression of the acute presentation?** Predicting the natural history of an acute presentation of respiratory distress is as important as assessing its severity. A patient with severe acute respiratory distress due to cardiogenic pulmonary edema may respond quickly and dramatically to adjunctive therapies, while a patient with tachypnea and metabolic acidosis due to septic shock will likely deteriorate before getting better. Patients who are expected to significantly worsen before they improve should almost always be intubated.

With these four screening questions, a clinician can rapidly and efficiently obtain a snapshot of the severity of the presentation, how much "reserve" the patient has, and the likely natural course of the condition. Any patient who "fails" one or more of these screening questions should either be intubated immediately or placed under close observation.

MANAGEMENT

OXYGEN SUPPLEMENTATION AND OXYGEN FLOW DEVICES

Supplemental oxygen therapy improves arterial oxygenation by increasing the oxygen diffusion gradient across the alveolar-capillary membrane. Each liter per minute of supplemental oxygen increases the FiO_2 by approximately 3%. Basic oxygen delivery devices such as the nasal cannula and simple face mask deliver *low-flow* oxygen to supplement inspired room air. They are widely available, comfortable and generally well tolerated, but they cannot be titrated to deliver a precise FiO_2. However, with each breath, room air is admixed with supplemental oxygen, which limits the maximum effective FiO_2 to approximately 40%. Consequently, *low-flow devices* contribute little benefit to increasing oxygen flow rates beyond six liters per minute. As respiratory distress worsens and minute ventilation increases, low-flow devices lose efficacy because patients entrain an increasing proportion of room air relative to supplemental oxygen.

High-flow oxygen devices utilize the venturi effect to deliver supplemental oxygen. A jet of high-flow oxygen entrains room air through a side port in the device, mixing supplemental oxygen with room air. As in low-flow systems, the effective FiO_2 is limited to about 50%. Venturi devices offer two main advantages over low-flow devices: (1) they can be set to deliver a precise FiO_2, and (2) their high flows may better match the respiratory demands of patients with high minute ventilation.

Closed systems such as the nonrebreather or reservoir face mask deliver oxygen into a reservoir bag from which the patient breathes. Entrainment of room air and rebreathing of exhaled gas are minimized by a tight face seal and a one-way exhalation valve on the side of the mask. Although a well-fitted reservoir face mask can theoretically deliver nearly 100% FiO_2, under most circumstances the FiO_2 ranges from 60% to 90%. Closed systems such as the reservoir mask should be used cautiously in patients with acute hypercarbic respiratory failure, as they may exacerbate hypercarbia.

VENTILATORY SUPPORT

The physiology of positive pressure ventilation

The effects of positive pressure ventilation (PPV) on cardiopulmonary performance are complex and vary depending upon intravascular filling pressures, autonomic tone, lung compliance, and ventricular performance.

PPV decreases the work needed for breathing in patients with acute respiratory distress by reducing the metabolic load imposed upon respiratory muscles. At rest, respiration consumes roughly 3% of the cardiac output, but this may increase to up 40% during acute respiratory distress. Positive end-expiratory pressure (PEEP) [essentially synonymous with continuous positive airway pressure [CPAP]) increases mean airway pressure, which recruits collapsed alveoli and prevents end-expiratory collapse of damaged lung units; both of these functions decrease physiologic shunting.

However, PPV can also be deleterious. In acute lung injury, the distribution of injury is often heterogeneous, with areas of injured and noncompliant lung often juxtaposed with uninjured areas with normal compliance. Positive pressure will preferentially distend compliant lung, which, if not monitored, may lead to overdistension of healthy lung segments. This overdistention may increase dead space ventilation, impair perfusion to healthy lung segments, increase work of breathing, and provoke barotrauma.

PEEP also has important hemodynamic effects, including reducing right ventricular (RV) preload and stroke volume as well as left ventricular afterload. The net effect is to unload the left ventricle (LV) by decreasing both LV preload and afterload. Thus, PEEP is a physiologically attractive treatment for acute cardiogenic pulmonary edema. High levels of PEEP (generally greater than 10 cm H_2O) may impair venous return to the RV, leading to hypotension in patients who are hypovolemic or who have impaired RV function due to pericardial disease, tamponade, infarction, or severe pulmonary hypertension.

Noninvasive positive pressure ventilation (NPPV)

In appropriately selected patients, NPPV offers the benefits of mechanical ventilation without the morbidity and discomfort of an endotracheal tube (**Figure 137-2**). The two most commonly used NPPV modalities are continuous positive airway pressure (CPAP) and bilevel positive airway pressure (BPAP). (Note: Bi-PAP is a registered trademark). BPAP is CPAP with cyclic inspiratory positive pressure added to augment ventilation.

The three main BPAP settings are the inspiratory positive airway pressure (IPAP), the expiratory positive airway pressure (EPAP, synonymous with CPAP), and the FiO_2. Generally, the initial EPAP is set between 5 and 10 cm H_2O, and the IPAP is set between 5 and 15 cm H_2O *above* the EPAP. It is important to recognize that the IPAP and EPAP are additive; thus a setting of EPAP 5 and IPAP 10 means that the patient is receiving 15 cm H_2O of inspiratory positive pressure. Higher EPAP settings may be required to compensate

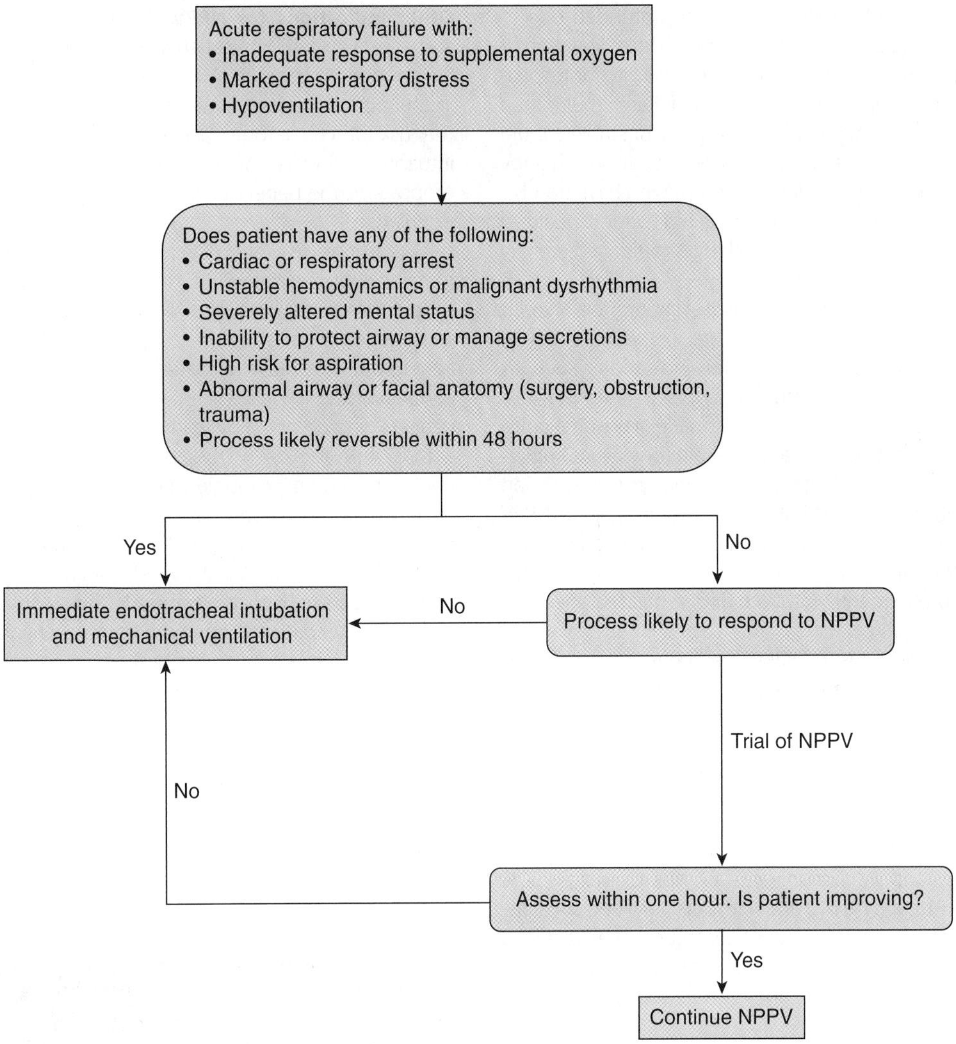

Figure 137-2 *Algorithm for invasive ventilation versus noninvasive ventilation decision making in patients with acute respiratory failure.*

for extrathoracic pressure exerted by obesity, kyphoscoliosis, or abdominal distension. Increased IPAP may be necessary to meet the high inspiratory flow needs of patients who are young and fit or who have diseases characterized by inspiratory air hunger, such as COPD or asthma.

NPPV may be delivered through a face mask, nasal mask, or nasal prongs. As patients in respiratory distress almost invariably mouth-breathe, the face mask is the preferred initial choice for treatment of acute respiratory failure. The face mask is generally less comfortable than nasal masks and restricts access for suctioning secretions or administering oral medications. Face masks should be used with extreme caution when there is potential for vomiting or aspiration. NPPV rarely induces barotrauma or adversely impacts hemodynamics. The primary side effects of NPPV include discomfort or claustrophobia due to dyssynchrony with positive pressure breaths, sinus pressure or discomfort, mild gastric distension, and pressure injury to the bridge of the nose or face after extended use.

Patient selection for NPPV: Patient selection is by far the most important predictor of successful response to NPPV. NPPV is most effective in patients who are young, have low APACHE II scores, and who can cooperate with nurses and respiratory therapists. As a good face-mask seal is extremely important to maintain positive pressure ventilation, NPPV may be less effective in patients who have abnormal facial anatomy, are edentulous, or who have copious facial hair. NPPV should be limited to patients who are expected to improve within 48 to 72 hours of initiation of therapy for acute respiratory failure. The best predictors of NPPV efficacy are decreased respiratory effort and decreased respiratory acidosis. Patients who fail to respond to NPPV within one to two hours of therapy initiation are unlikely to improve and should be promptly intubated and mechanically ventilated.

PRACTICE POINT

- The best predictors of NPPV efficacy include decreased work of breathing and decreased respiratory acidosis. Patients who fail to respond to NPPV within one to two hours of initiation of therapy are unlikely to improve and should be promptly intubated and mechanically ventilated.

An unprotected airway and high risk for aspiration are near-absolute contraindications to NPPV (see Figure 137-2). Cautious exceptions may be made for patients who are obtunded due to hypercarbia and who are likely to rapidly improve after initiation of NPPV. Patients who have a status of post acute cardiac or respiratory arrest, have nonrespiratory acute organ failure, multiorgan failure, or who are significantly hemodynamically unstable should be intubated. NPPV has been successfully used as salvage therapy for patients who should ideally be intubated but who have do-not-resuscitate status. Treatment in this setting is highly individualized and the potential risks and benefits of NPPV should be carefully considered.

NPPV used for chronic respiratory failure should be treated very differently than NPPV used for acute respiratory failure. Patients who chronically require NPPV for indications such as obesity-hypoventilation or neuromuscular disease are generally stable and can be safely managed in most inpatient hospital units. In contrast, NPPV as a treatment for acute respiratory failure implies patient instability and high risk for rapid decline and progression to endotracheal intubation. Hospital units that allow acute NPPV should provide close patient monitoring, have staff trained to manage acute respiratory failure, maintain on-site respiratory therapy, and be prepared to emergently intubate and ventilate patients in the event of treatment failure.

The two primary indications for NPPV in acute respiratory failure are hypercarbic COPD exacerbations and acute cardiogenic pulmonary edema.

COPD exacerbation: NPPV is the treatment of choice for patients with moderate to severe acute hypercarbic COPD exacerbation (pH 7.10–7.35). A meta-analysis of 14 randomized trials comparing NPPV with conventional therapy demonstrated that NPPV decreased *mortality* and *intubation* rates by approximately 50% (number-needed-to-treat [NNT] 10 and 4 respectively) and substantially reduced hospital lengths of stay. NPPV offers no advantages over supplemental oxygen therapy for patients with nonhypercarbic COPD exacerbations (pH > 7.35) and is often poorly tolerated in this population.

PRACTICE POINT

- In COPD exacerbations, NPPV decreases *mortality* and *intubation* rates by approximately 50 percent (number-needed-to-treat [NNT] 10 and 4 respectively) and substantially reduces hospital lengths of stay.

Acute cardiogenic pulmonary edema: Due to its salutary effects on left ventricular function, NPPV is an attractive nonpharmacologic therapy for acute cardiogenic pulmonary edema (ACPE). The physiologic benefit of NPPV in decompensated heart failure primarily derives from CPAP or PEEP, which recruits or maintains inflation of alveoli. The use of inspiratory positive pressure (IPAP) in the absence of acute hypercarbia appears to offer no additional benefit and may increase patient discomfort. The role of NPPV in ACPE remains somewhat controversial. Many early studies demonstrated reductions in intubation rates, ICU admissions, and mortality. However, a recent large randomized multicenter trial failed to show a meaningful benefit for NPPV for ACPE. A subsequent meta-analysis that included this trial demonstrated a net reduction in mortality and intubation rates, especially for patients with acute myocardial ischemia. NPPV use in ACPE should be limited to CPAP in the absence of respiratory acidosis or hypercarbia.

Other indications for NPPV: NPPV may reduce complications and mortality rates in patients with acute hypoxemic respiratory failure due to pneumonia. This benefit is most prominent in immunocompromised patients, primarily due to elimination of the risk of ventilator-associated pneumonia (VAP) by avoiding intuabtion. However, as overall VAP rates have declined with better prophylaxis, the benefit of NPPV may become less apparent in this population.

The routine use of NPPV for treatment of status asthmaticus remains controversial. While NPPV is frequently used for this indication, there remains only a single randomized trial (performed in an emergency department) to support this indication. It is reasonable to attempt NPPV for patients with status asthmaticus and no contraindications while maintaining a low threshold for intubating patients who do not show early improvement.

NPPV has also been studied for preintubation and postextubation management. A single trial demonstrated that NPPV is more effective than bag-valve-mask (BVM) ventilation for preoxygenation prior to emergent intubation. Patients who received preintubation BPAP rather than standard BVM ventilation had fewer desaturations and fewer severe hypoxemic episodes during intubation. NPPV may also expedite patient liberation from mechanical ventilation by providing a "step-down" mode between mechanical ventilation and supplemental oxygen therapy. Postextubation NPPV is beneficial *only* if it is initiated immediately after extubation, before a patient develops signs of respiratory failure. A well-designed randomized trial demonstrated that NPPV used to treat postextubation respiratory failure delayed reintubation and markedly increased mortality. Thus, most patients who develop postextubation respiratory failure should be promptly reintubated rather than attempting treatment with NPPV.

PRACTICE POINT

- Patients who develop postextubation respiratory failure should be promptly reintubated rather than attempting treatment with NPPV.

Finally, NPPV may be a lifesaving temporizing intervention for patients with airway compromise from anatomic obstruction or compression. Difficult airways should be managed by clinicians with advanced airway management skills and equipment, neither of which may be emergently available. NPPV can be used to physiologically stent open a compromised airway, buying time to marshal the resources necessary to facilitate a safe intubation or surgical airway.

The decision to intubate: The decision to intubate rests upon the four key questions posed at the beginning of this chapter (see Figure 137-2):

1. How severe is the patient's respiratory distress?
2. Is the patient protecting his or her airway?
3. Is gas exchange adequate?
4. What is the likely progression of this acute presentation?

Finally, the ultimate question a clinician must answer in any individual patient management situation is whether the preponderance of evidence supports safe management without an endotracheal tube (**Table 137-4**). It is always appropriate to approach acute respiratory failure with the expectation that the patient will require intubation unless she or he "proves" otherwise (see Figure 137-2).

TABLE 137-4 Evidence-based Medicine: Key References for Acute Respiratory Failure

Study	Methodology	Results	Limitations	Bottom Line
Ram, et al. *Cochrane DB Syst Rev.* 2004(3): CD004104.	Meta-analysis of 14 randomized controlled trials (RCT) comparing NPPV with conventional care for acute hypercarbic COPD exacerbation.	NPPV was superior to conventional care for multiple outcomes, with marked reductions mortality (RR: 0.52), intubation (RR: 0.41), and treatment failure (RR: 0.48). Hospital length of stay was reduced by 3.24 days.	Meta-analyses are subject to bias, and should be interpreted with caution. However, the magnitude of the benefit of NPPV demonstrated across multiple important outcomes is very persuasive.	NPPV should be first-line therapy for patients with moderate-to-severe acute hypercarbic COPD exacerbations who have no contraindications to treatment.
Gray, et al. *NEJM.* 2008;359 (2):142–151.	1069 patients enrolled in multicenter RCT comparing CPAP, Bi-level PAP and O_2 therapy for acute cardiogenic pulmonary edema (ACPE)	For primary endpoints of 7d mortality and intubation rates, NPPV was equivalent to conventional O_2 therapy. Patients receiving NPPV had faster symptom relief and improvement in tachypnea and acidosis.	Intervention was, by necessity, not blinded. Very high O_2 flow rates in conventional arm may have confounded results.	The role of NPPV for treatment of ACPE remains controversial. Although a well-designed, large, multicenter RCT failed to show a benefit for NPPV, the preponderance of data supports NPPV treatment for ACPE. The benefit may be more pronounced in patients with ACPE and concomitant ACS. At absolute minimum, NPPV speeds symptom relief and does not appear to be harmful.
Weng, et al. *Ann Intern Med.* 2010;52(9): 590–600.	Recent meta-analysis of RCTs comparing NPPV versus conventional therapy for ADHF. Includes results of Gray trial (above).	CPAP reduced mortality (RR: 0.64) and need for intubation (RR: 0.44). Benefits were more prominent in trials with high proportion of patients with acute coronary syndromes (ACS).	Patient characteristics, clinical settings, as well as definitions, cause, and severity of ACPE differed among the trials.	
Baillard, et al. *Am J Respir Crit Care Med.* 2006;174(2): 171–177.	Small ICU-based RCT comparing three minutes of preoxygenation prior to intubation using bag-valve mask ventilation versus bi-level PAP.	Preoxygenation SpO_2 was higher in the NPPV group as compared with the control group. There were fewer desaturations during intubation, and fewer severe desaturations (< 80%) (45% versus 7%).	Very small trial (53 patients) performed in two ICUs. Results may not generalize to all ICU populations. The study was not powered to analyze complications that might affect outcomes.	For patients undergoing urgent/emergent rapid sequence intubation, consider preoxygenation with NPPV rather than bag-valve mask ventilation. The common practice of removing NPPV to "bag" a patient prior to intubation may be counterproductive.
Esteban, et al. *NEJM.* 2004; 350(24): 2452–2460.	Multicenter, RCT to evaluate the effect of NPPV on mortality for postextubation respiratory failure developing after > 48 hours of mechanical ventilation. 221 patients enrolled.	NPPV did not reduce rate of reintubation (48% in both groups). Median time to reintubation was longer in the NPPV group (12 hours versus 2.5 hours). ICU mortality was higher in the NPPV group (25% versus 14%)	Posthoc analysis suggested that NPPV might reduce intubation rates for the subset of patients with COPD and hypercarbic respiratory failure. Benefit was not statistically significant.	While NPPV may be an effective bridge to speed liberation from the ventilator, patients who develop overt respiratory postextubation should be immediately reintubated. This may not apply to patients with COPD and postextubation hypercarbic respiratory failure.
Moulton, et al. *BMJ.* 1991; 303:1240.	Observational study of relationship between gag reflex and GCS in 111 sequential patients evaluated in an emergency dept.	Poor correlation between the GCS and presence or absence of a gag reflex. Attenuated gag reflex was seen in patients with normal GCS (15), and normal gag reflex was seen in patients meeting criteria for coma (GCS < 8)	Small study with highly observer-dependent finding.	The gag reflex is an unreliable indicator of ability to protect an airway. Assessment should include other measurements such as the GCS.

SUGGESTED READINGS

Esteban A, Frutos-Vivar F, Ferguson ND, et al. Noninvasive positive-pressure ventilation for respiratory failure after extubation. *N Engl J Med*. 2004;350:2452–2460.

International consensus conferences in intensive care medicine: Noninvasive positive pressure ventilation in acute respiratory failure. *Am J Res Crit Care Med*. 2001;163:283.

Keenan SP, Sinuff T, Cook DJ, Hill NS. Which patients with acute exacerbation of chronic obstructive pulmonary disease benefit from noninvasive positive-pressure ventilation? A systematic review of the literature. *Ann Intern Med*. 2003;138(11):861–870.

Masip J, Roque M, Sanchez B, et al. Noninvasive ventilation in acute cardiogenic pulmonary edema: systematic review and meta-analysis. *JAMA*. 2005;294(24):3124–3130.

Moulton C, Pennycook A, Makower R. Relation between Glasgow coma scale and the gag reflex. *BMJ*. 1991;303:1240.

Ram FS, Picot J, Lightowler J, Wedzicha JA. Non-invasive positive pressure ventilation for treatment of respiratory failure due to exacerbations of chronic obstructive pulmonary disease. *Cochrane Database Syst Rev*. 2004;(3):CD004104.

Raoof S, Khan FA. Mechanical ventilation manual. 1998; *American College of Physicians Publishing*.

Theodore AC, Parsons PE, Wilson KC. Oxygenation and mechanisms of hypoxemia. Up To Date; Version 18.2, May, 2010.

West, JB. Respiratory Physiology: The Essentials. Philadelpha: Wolters Kluwer Health/Lipincott Williams & Wilkins; 2008.

Winck JC, Azevedo LF, Costa-Pereira A, Antonelli M, Wyatt JC. Efficacy and safety of non-invasive ventilation in the treatment of acute cardiogenic pulmonary edema—a systematic review and meta-analysis. *Crit Care*. 2006;10(2):R69.

CHAPTER 138

Sepsis

Kevin Felner, MD
Robert L. Smith, MD

Key Clinical Questions

1. What is the definition of systemic inflammatory response syndrome (SIRS) and how do you differentiate SIRS from sepsis, severe sepsis, and septic shock?
2. Which patients presenting with sepsis need admission to the intensive care unit (ICU)?
3. Which septic patients need invasive monitoring (arterial catheter, central venous catheter)?
4. What interventions in the treatment of sepsis improve mortality?
5. Which septic patients deserve empiric steroids as part of the therapeutic regimen?

INTRODUCTION

Sepsis is a clinical syndrome that complicates severe infection and is characterized by systemic inflammation and widespread tissue injury. The incidence and number of sepsis-related deaths has increased from 1979 to 2000, and sepsis remains the tenth most common cause of death in the United States. Despite the rising number of cases, earlier identification of sepsis and improved intensive medical care has been shown to reduce the overall mortality rate to approximately 17.9%. Severity is correlated with mortality; up to 40% of patients with severe sepsis and 60% of patients with septic shock die due to sepsis-related complications (**Table 138-1**).

Successful shock resuscitation may be associated with considerable morbidity and mortality. Multiple organ dysfunction syndrome (MODS) refers to severe acquired dysfunction of at least two organ systems lasting at least 24 to 48 hours in the setting of sepsis, trauma, burns, or severe inflammatory conditions so that homeostasis cannot be maintained without intervention. Mortality is directly correlated with the number of dysfunctional organs and the duration of dysfunction (**Table 138-2**). An uncontrolled hyperinflammatory response is believed to be the cause of multiple organ dysfunction.

The American College of Chest Physicians (ACCP) and the Society of Critical Care Medicine (SCCM) defined in 2001 at the International Sepsis Definitions Conference the following terms to describe the spectrum of systemic inflammation and sepsis. *Systemic inflammatory response syndrome* (SIRS) is defined as a clinical syndrome that results from activation of the immune system whether due to infection, trauma, burns, or a noninfectious inflammatory process. It includes at least two of the following: (1) temperature >38 degrees Celsius or <36 degrees Celsius; (2) heart rate >90 beats/minute; (3) respiratory rate >20 breaths/minute or $paCO_2$ <32 mm Hg; a (4) white blood cell count >12,000 cells/mm^3, or <4000 cells/mm^3, or >10% immature (band) forms.

Sepsis is defined as a clinical syndrome that results from activation of the immune system with a documented infection. The definition of sepsis includes the above SIRS criteria plus a culture-proven infection or presumed presence of an infection. The severity of sepsis is graded according to the associated organ dysfunction and hemodynamic compromise. *Severe sepsis* is defined as the presence of sepsis and one or more organ dysfunctions. *Organ dysfunction* can be defined as acute lung injury including acute respiratory distress syndrome (ARDS), disseminated intravascular coagulation, thrombocytopenia, altered mental status, mottled skin, capillary refill greater than three seconds, renal dysfunction, hepatic dysfunction, cardiac dysfunction based on echocardiography or measurement of cardiac index, or lactic acidosis indicating hypoperfusion. *Septic shock* is defined as the presence of sepsis and refractory hypotension with mean systemic blood pressure lower than 65 mm Hg *unresponsive to crystalloid fluid challenge of 20 to 40 cc/kg* leading to acute circulatory collapse.

PATHOPHYSIOLOGY

Sepsis is as an uncontrolled inflammatory response to an infection in which a dysregulated host immune response leads to multiorgan involvement not limited to the source infected organ. Microbial antigens such as lipopolysaccharides (LPS) from Gram-negative bacteria bind to Toll-like receptors on inflammatory cells, thereby causing a complex immune reaction involving T-cells,

TABLE 138-1 Sepsis Syndromes, Definitions, and Mortality Risk

Syndrome	Definition	Approximate Mortality
Systemic inflammatory response syndrome (SIRS)	At least two of the following four clinical features: 1. Temperature > 38 degrees Celsius or < 36 degrees Celsius 2. Heart rate > 90 beats/minute 3. Respiratory rate > 20 breaths/minute **or** $PaCO_2$ < 32 mm Hg 4. White blood cell (WBC) count > 12,000 cells/mm^3, **or** < 4000 cells/mm^3, **or** > 10% immature (band) forms	10%
Sepsis	SIRS criteria plus a culture-proven infection *or presumed presence of an infection*	20%
Severe sepsis	Sepsis plus presence of one or more organ dysfunctions including: • Pulmonary dysfunction (eg, acute respiratory distress syndrome) • Cardiac dysfunction • Renal dysfunction • Hepatic dysfunction • Neurologic dysfunction (altered sensorium) • Hematologic dysfunction (eg, disseminated intravascular coagulation [DIC], thrombocytopenia) • Lactic acidosis (indicating end-organ hypoperfusion)	20–40%
Septic shock	Sepsis and refractory hypotension with mean systemic blood pressure lower than 65 mm Hg unresponsive to crystalloid fluid challenge of 20–40 cc/kg	40–60%

macrophages, neutrophil, endothelial cells, and dendritic cells. Cytokines (such as IL-1, IL-6, IL-8), growth factors (such as TNFa), high-mobility group box-1 (HMGB-1), arachidonic acid metabolites, and nitric oxide and host genetics likely determine the nature of the response. The complement cascade, coagulation cascades, platelets, and leukocytes interact at the vascular endothelium level resulting in microvascular injury, thrombosis, and loss of endothelial integrity, which altogether results in tissue ischemia. This diffuse endothelial disruption is responsible for the various organ dysfunctions and global tissue hypoxia that accompany severe sepsis and septic shock. Global tissue hypoxia can occur from multiple mechanisms including decreased preload, vasoregulatory dysfunction, myocardial depression, and impaired tissue extraction due to microcirculatory dysfunction or mitochondrial dysfunction (cytopathic hypoxia). Some noninfectious processes (eg, pancreatitis) can also lead to a dysregulated host immune response and multiorgan dysfunction, and these conditions are categorized using the term SIRS. These patients appear septic without a clear infectious source.

DIFFERENTIAL DIAGNOSIS

The differential diagnosis for sepsis is broad, including conditions that present with high-output states and those with low-output shock. While many patients present with common conditions that meet SIRS criteria—nonmassive pulmonary embolus, alcohol withdrawal, even COPD exacerbations—other conditions can mimic sepsis with high cardiac output state and wide pulse pressure without shock including thyrotoxicosis, aortic regurgitation, arteriosclerosis, and cirrhosis. While all patients with sepsis do not present in shock, the differential diagnosis for shock should always be considered. In addition to septic shock, conditions that belong to the category of vasodilatory, or high cardiac output, shock include anaphylaxis, adrenal insufficiency, and neurogenic shock.

The other causes of shock should always remain in the differential for patients with sepsis as the presentation may combine two or more processes or may simply mimic two processes. For example, a patient with underlying poor cardiac function who becomes septic may not be able to generate the high cardiac outputs expected in sepsis and may not have the typical findings on physical examination of a septic patient. Moreover, the phenomenon of sepsis-induced myocardial dysfunction occurs when patients have normal cardiac function prior to their infection and the sepsis induces a global cardiac dysfunction, seen on echocardiography as global hypokinesis, which may impair the expected high cardiac output usually associated with a vasodilated circulation. The other causes of shock all fall into a category of low-output states, including cardiogenic shock, hypovolemic shock, and obstructive shock (**Table 138-3**).

TABLE 138-2 Correlation Between Organ Failure and Mortality in Sepsis

Organ Failure	Mortality
One lasting more than one day	20%
Two lasting more than one day	40%
Three lasting more than three days	80%

PRACTICE POINT

- Sepsis-induced myocardial dysfunction occurs when sepsis induces a global cardiac dysfunction, seen on echocardiography as global hypokinesis, which may impair the expected high cardiac output usually associated with a vasodilated circulation.

DIAGNOSIS

A high index of suspicion for the clinical sepsis syndrome facilitates early identification of the inciting stimulus, and intervention may limit the ongoing immune response. Septic patients present with

TABLE 138-3 Differential Diagnosis of Shock

Vasodilatory shock	Sepsis
	Anaphylaxis
	Adrenal insufficiency
	Neurogenic
Low-output shock states	Cardiogenic (eg, massive myocardial infarction, myocarditis, valvular disease)
	Hypovolemic (eg, hemorrhagic, gastrointestinal losses, burns, pancreatitis)
	Obstructive (eg, massive PE, tension pneumothorax, auto-PEEP, tamponade, abdominal compartment syndrome)

PE, pulmonary embolus; PEEP, positive end expiratory pressure.

signs and symptoms ranging from fever and chills to delirium to shock. Presentation often varies according to infection source, patient age, underlying comorbidities (including immune system function and cardiac status), and timing of presentation relative to onset of sepsis. Early manifestations of sepsis—tachycardia, oliguria, and hyperglycemia—may be subtle and easily overlooked in the hospitalized patient. Signs of established sepsis include altered mental status, metabolic acidosis and respiratory alkalosis, hypotension with decreased systemic vascular resistance (SVR) and elevated cardiac output, and coagulopathy. Late manifestations include acute lung injury (ALI), ARDS, acute renal failure, hepatic dysfunction, and refractory shock. Sepsis can occur related to a systemic inflammatory response to any infectious source, but less than 50% of septic patients will have positive blood cultures. Therefore, aggressive clinical evaluation should occur inquiring about symptoms including fever, rigors, mental status changes, cough, shortness of breath, vomiting, diarrhea, dysuria, hematuria, and many other symptoms that might suggest the source of infection. Patients may also present with obvious or subtle physical examination findings. In an analogous manner to the thorough history, a complete physical examination can assess for potential infection sources from any organ system. Sometimes inconspicuous and missed infection sources may include the skin and soft tissue, central nervous system, gastrointestinal tract, and indwelling devices.

PRACTICE POINT

- Less than 50% of septic patients will have positive blood cultures, and 20% to 30% of patients will have no microbial cause identified from any source. Aggressive clinical evaluation includes a detailed history and review of systems. A complete physical examination can assess for sometimes inconspicuous and missed infection sources, including skin and soft tissue, central nervous system, gastrointestinal tract, and indwelling devices.

In addition to stabilizing the patient, it is critical to identify the cause of the ongoing immunologic response. Obtaining cultures for blood, urine, and other fluids early, prior to administration of antibiotics, helps preserve the integrity of results and should be an extremely high priority, but not at the expense of administering antibiotics expediently. Identification of the underlying source remains paramount, and lack of source identification and control may render choice of antibiotics meaningless. The most common sites of infection in sepsis are the urinary and respiratory tracts, but any organ system may be involved. Urinary sources include cystitis, pyelonephritis, and perinephric abscess. Patients with kidney stones may develop Gram-negative septicemia. Sinusitis, mastoiditis, pneumonia, lung abscess, and empyema may be associated with sepsis. Gastrointestinal sources of sepsis may include esophageal rupture or perforation following a procedure or after vomiting, cholangitis, cholecystitis, intestinal infarction or perforation, acute pancreatitis, *Clostridium difficile* colitis, diverticulitis, and intraabdominal abscess. Postoperative mediastinitis and acute bacterial endocarditis may lead to sepsis. It is also critical to consider skin and soft tissue sources of sepsis because of the possibility of an infected decubitus ulcer, postoperative wound, soft tissue abscess, or necrotizing fasciitis. Vascular causes include catheter infections (central and peripheral lines, arterial catheters, dialysis catheters, ventriculoperitoneal shunts) and septic thrombophlebitis. Infected articular prosthetic devices have also been associated with sepsis. Meningitis and intracranial abscess, sometimes associated with neurosurgery, are also considerations.

Relevant diagnostic studies based on symptoms, signs, and clinical suspicion in patients may include chest or abdominal radiography and culture of blood, urine, sputum, or other relevant body fluids that may be infected—cerebrospinal fluid (CSF) analysis, paracentesis in patients with ascites, or thoracentesis in patients with pleural effusion. Bacteremia is found in only approximately 50% of cases of severe sepsis and septic shock, while 20% to 30% of patients will have no microbial cause identified from any source. When relatively basic diagnostic evaluations—including plain films, blood cultures, and fluid cultures—do not yield a likely infectious culprit, advanced imaging including chest and abdominal computed tomography can assess for pulmonary infiltrates, intraabdominal abscesses, and obstructing renal stones. Biliary pathology may be better imaged with ultrasound, magnetic resonance imaging (MRI), or endoscopic retrograde pancreatography (ERCP) if necessary. Echocardiography to assess for endocarditis may be necessary based on physical examination findings, blood culture results, and the clinical picture.

TRIAGE AND HOSPITAL ADMISSION

All patients with a presentation of *severe sepsis* or *septic shock* should be admitted to or transferred to a monitored setting that is capable of continuous vital sign monitoring with the ability to measure central venous pressure (CVP) and central venous oxygen saturations ($ScvO_2$). Those patients with SIRS and sepsis should be monitored closely if not placed in an intensive care unit setting so that they can be treated promptly if they start to show signs of deterioration. Vital signs should be monitored frequently and a low threshold to utilize other monitoring (telemetry and continuous pulse oximetry) should be considered. Patient response to initial resuscitation in the emergency department or on a medical floor should guide the clinician with respect to intensive care unit (ICU) admission with the capability of intraarterial blood pressure measurement and the delivery of vasoactive medications. Intermediate care units (sometimes called *step-down units* or *transitional care units*) vary from facility to facility in their capabilities for invasive monitoring and use of vasoactive agents. The protocols and policies at individual institutions will help determine placement of these patients, based on monitoring requirements. Due to the emphasis placed on early aggressive resuscitation, early antibiotics, and early source identification and control, septic patients require careful evaluation to determine admission location, and patients with marginally stable clinical parameters should be admitted to an ICU setting to expeditiously meet early care goals to improve outcomes.

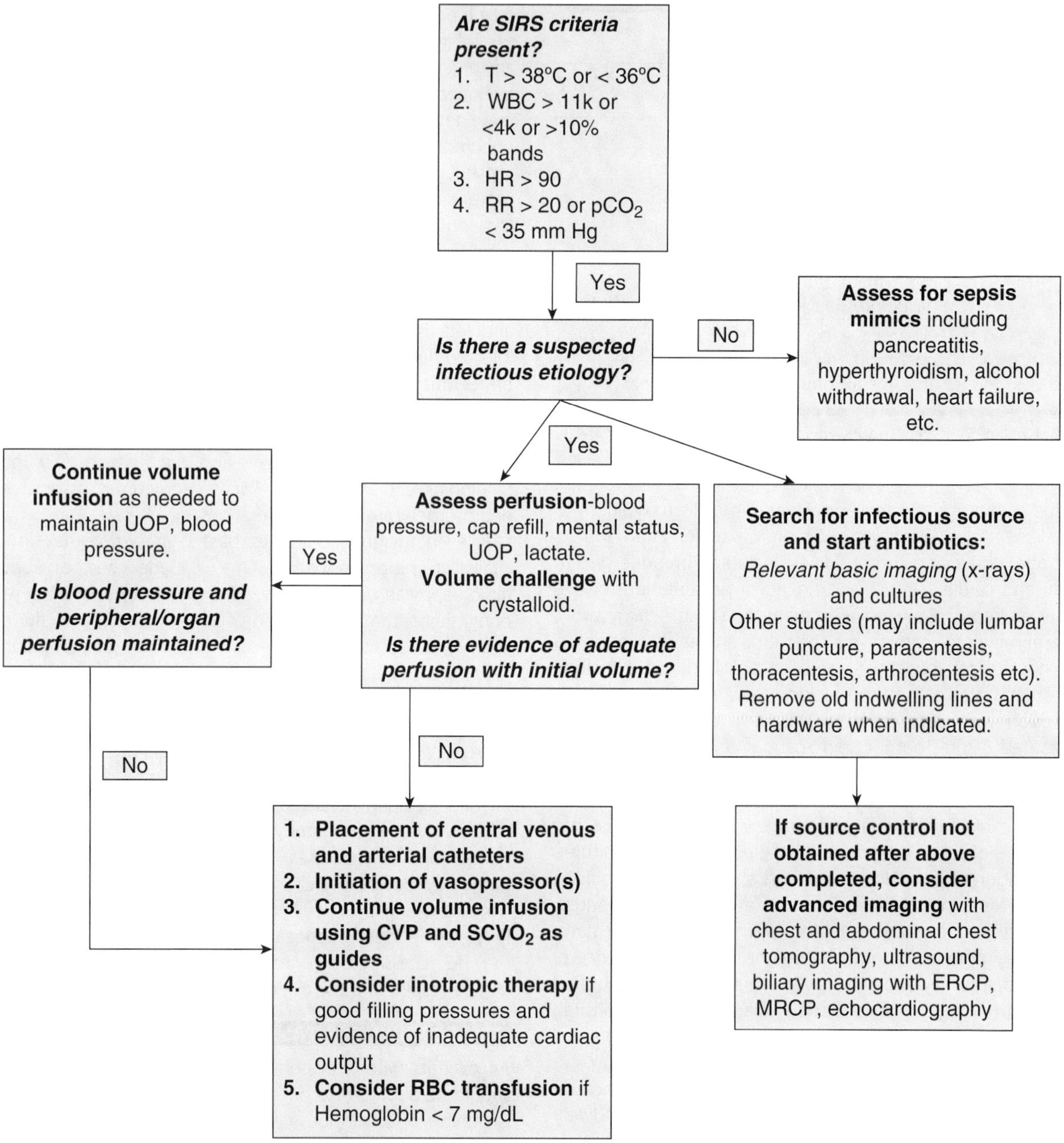

SIRS, Systemic Inflammatory Response Syndrome; T, temperature; WBC, white blood cells; HR, heart rate; RR, respiratory rate; UOP, urine output; CVP, central venous pressure; $SCVO_2$, central venous oxygenation saturation.

Figure 138-1 *Sepsis algorithm.*

PRACTICE POINT

- Early aggressive resuscitation, early antibiotics, and early source identification and control improve outcomes in patients with severe sepsis and septic shock. These patients require careful evaluation to determine admission location, and patients with marginally stable clinical parameters should be admitted to an intensive care unit setting to expeditiously meet early care goals to improve outcomes.

MANAGEMENT

Management of severe sepsis and septic shock requires a structured approach that assures proper diagnostic evaluation and implementation of evidence-based interventions in an expedient manner to improve outcomes (**Figure 138-1**). This approach requires (1) empiric antibiotic coverage of an infectious source while cultures are pending, (2) optimal fluid resuscitation, (3) pressor and/or inotrope therapy for selected patients, and (4) consideration of additional therapies such as drainage of abscesses, removal of lines, moderate (but not intensive) control of hyperglycemia, and (5) consideration of steroids in selected patient subsets when indicated.

ANTIBIOTIC THERAPY

Initial emergency department management of patients with sepsis begins with a high awareness of the condition by assessing all patients for the presence of SIRS criteria. Numerous studies have shown that early and appropriate antibiotics are associated with markedly improved outcomes. Antibiotics should be directed against the likely organisms based upon the presumptive infection source. In many situations, especially when the presumptive source of infection is not obvious, multiple antibiotic agents should be initiated to offer broad antimicrobial coverage. Such broad coverage should then be reevaluated daily to optimize dosing and minimize drug interactions and the development of resistance. Choice of antibiotic depends upon penetration into the suspected infection site, local resistance patterns, efficacy against the most likely organisms, and risks of side effects. Therapeutic drainage of an infected space is critical to diagnose the source of infection, guide the choice of antibiotic therapy, and facilitate recovery. In patients with devices, clinicians may need to evaluate and consider early and rapid removal of potentially or known infected invasive devices including central venous catheters (CVCs), peripherally inserted central venous catheters (PICCs), foley catheters, and other implanted hardware.

Recent evidence suggests that mortality increases with delay of antibiotics more than one hour after identification and management of severe sepsis or septic shock. In selected patients, including abdominal surgery patients and patients receiving total parenteral nutrition (TPN) or long-standing steroids, the suspicion for fungal infections should be raised and may require adding empiric antifungal agents to the antimicrobial regimen.

PRACTICE POINT

- Antibiotic therapy must be initiated early in patients with sepsis, as mortality increases with delay of antibiotics more than one hour after identification of patients with severe sepsis or septic shock.

INTRAVENOUS FLUIDS

Volume resuscitation should begin simultaneously with empiric antibiotic therapy in patients suspected of having sepsis. In the vasodilatory state low blood pressures with decreased venous return lead to an underfilled, but hyperdynamic heart. Rivers and colleagues showed that early goal-directed therapy (EGDT), initiated in the emergency department, improved mortality in patients with severe sepsis and septic shock. That early goal-directed therapy includes early aggressive volume resuscitation in the first six hours of care, and other measures over the first hours and days of care (see Figure 138-1). As part of EGDT, a central venous catheter placed in the internal jugular or subclavian vein allows close monitoring of central venous pressure (CVP). If the patient remains hypotensive (mean arterial pressure [MAP] < 65 mm Hg) after a reasonable fluid challenge with crystalloid (approximately 20–40 cc/kg) to optimize filling pressures, CVP and $ScvO_2$ monitoring allows adjustment of or addition of interventions based on the parameters measured within the individual patient to achieve the goal of $ScvO_2$ at 70%. Studies evaluating resuscitation with crystalloid intravenous (IV) fluids versus colloid fluid (eg, albumin) support no added benefit of colloid fluid over crystalloid. The Saline Versus Albumin Fluid Evaluation (SAFE) study evaluated nearly 7000 critically ill patients, 18% of whom had severe sepsis. Patients were randomly assigned to receive 4% albumin versus normal saline, and investigators reported no differences in mortality at 28 days. Additionally, there were no significant differences seen in the sepsis subgroup. Despite a theoretic benefit to using albumin in highly selected patients with significant volume overload, no studies support this approach. For routine use in sepsis, crystalloid fluid (normal saline) should be used first due to evidence of benefit, markedly lower expense, and demonstrated safety (lacking the inherent risks of blood product administration with albumin).

The EGDT algorithm uses a CVP goal of 8–12 cm H_2O, which is a reasonable estimate goal. However, that goal should not be applied blindly to all patients without knowledge of coexisting conditions including pulmonary arterial hypertension, dilated cardiomyopathy, and old right ventricular infarction. Clinicians should follow the trend of the CVP and correlate it with the $ScvO_2$, patient hemodynamics, and evidence of organ perfusion including mental status and urine output. Ample data suggests that the CVP serves as a poor predictor of volume responsiveness, and multiple factors are necessary to determine the need for continued volume resuscitation. The $SCVO_2$ carries valuable information and weight, offering the clinician an assessment of cardiac function and oxygen delivery balanced against oxygen consumption.

PRACTICE POINT

- *Central venous saturation* ($ScvO_2$) is a measure of oxygen saturation taken from the distal tip of a central venous line inserted just proximal to the right atrium. The $ScvO_2$ measures the balance between oxygen delivery and oxygen consumption, with normal $ScvO_2$ ranging between 65% and 75%. Lower values reflect a high oxygen extraction state, usually seen in states of shock with low cardiac output (cardiogenic, hypovolemic, obstructive).
- In sepsis, as in other vasodilatory or high cardiac output states, low oxygen extraction—possibly due to mitochondrial dysfunction—leads to higher values of $ScvO_2$. Often, these higher values of $ScvO_2$ are not apparent until the patient has been adequately resuscitated with intravascular volume expansion. The mean $ScvO_2$ in the Rivers study was 55%, which is lower than values seen in other sepsis trials.
- Early goal-directed therapy (EGDT) studies suggest that clinicians should augment therapeutic interventions when $ScvO_2$ is less than 70% in patients with severe sepsis or septic shock.
- The order of therapy augmentation includes: volume expansion (to achieve CVP 8–12 mm Hg) → pressor agents (to achieve MAP ≥ 65 mm Hg) → transfusion of packed RBCs (to achieve an $ScvO_2 \geq 70\%$) → inotropic agents (to achieve an $ScvO_2 \geq 70\%$).

BLOOD TRANSFUSION

Patients with severe sepsis or septic shock who have been resuscitated adequately will usually demonstrate the physiology of a low oxygen extraction state with high $ScvO_2$ values, but importantly, preresuscitation values may make patients appear as high oxygen extractors, with low $ScvO_2$ values more consistent with a low cardiac output state. EGDT protocol includes transfusing red blood cells if the hematocrit is less than 30% and the $ScvO_2$ remains less than 70% after meeting CVP and blood pressure goals. While a subgroup analysis favored transfusions to improve outcomes, potential deleterious effects from red blood cell transfusions, including questionable efficacy of older stored blood, the immunomodulating effects of red blood cell transfusions, and the risk of transfusion reactions, make this part of the EGDT protocol more difficult to recommend broadly for every patient meeting EGDT criteria. Routine transfusion of red blood cells should likely be avoided unless patients exhibit evidence of active bleeding, active ischemia, or hemologlobin is below 7 gm/dL. Expert opinion is conflicting with regard to blood transfusion threshold in sepsis management because other evidence-based literature supports no improvement in ICU patients who are transfused to a goal hemoglobin of 10 gm/dL rather than 7 gm/dL.

VASOACTIVE MEDICATIONS

An important aspect of sepsis management includes vasoactive medications. Pressors are often needed to maintain mean arterial blood pressures (MAP) and the choice of agent depends on the physiologic need (**Table 138-4**). The EGDT protocol recommends

TABLE 138-4 Vasoactive Medications in Sepsis

Medication (Dose)	Inotropy	Chronotropy	Arterial Vasoconstriction	Practical Uses
Norepinephrine 0.01–3.00 mcg/kg/minute; 8–30 mcg/minute typical dosing	Yes	Yes	Yes	• First line for many patients with severe sepsis or septic shock • Significant vasoconstriction with inotropy which is helpful for patients with poor left ventricular reserve or sepsis-related cardiomyopathy
Dopamine 1–5 mcg/kg/minute, increased renal blood flow; 5–10 minute mcg/kg, increased chronotropy/inotropy; > 10 mcg/kg/minute, predominant vasoconstriction, increased blood pressure	Yes	Yes	Yes	• Also first line for sepsis • Randomized comparison to norepinephrine showed no significant differences in mortality, but *increased arrhythmias with dopamine* • More tachycardia than with norepinephrine • More potent inotrope than norepinephrine • Differing effects at escalating doses with vasoconstriction at highest dose • Available in premixed or preprepared bags and therefore can be initiated quickly during emergent need
Phenylephrine 0.4–9.1 mcg/kg/minute	No	No	Yes	• Pure vasoconstrictor • Used primarily in sepsis in patients with excessive tachycardia or arrhythmias to avoid medications with chronotropic effect • Used in severe aortic stenosis with hypotension to raise mean arterial pressure and preserve coronary perfusion • Decrease outflow tract gradient in patients with hypertrophic cardiomyophathy
Epinephrine 2–10 mcg/minute	Yes	Yes	Yes	• More recent data supporting its role in septic patients • Increased production of lactate, especially gastrointestinal, as well as significant tachycardia has kept this a second-line medication
Vasopressin 0.01–0.04 units/minute	No	No	Yes	• Used due to relative depletion of vasopressin in sepsis • Nonadrenergic vasoconstrictor • Data not clear on role and effect, but does spare adrenergic receptors • Concern over decrease in splanchnic perfusion • *Should not be used as the sole vasopressor agent in sepsis, and should not be titrated for effect*
Dobutamine 2.5–20.0 mcg/kg/minute	Yes	Yes	Vasodilator	• Used for patients exhibiting evidence of low-output state with sepsis due to underlying poor cardiac reserve or sepsis-induced cardiomyopathy • Can lead to hypotension, and should be used with a vasoconstrictor initially if hypotension occurs due to vasodilatory effects
Milrinone 0.375–0.75 mcg/kg/minute	Yes	Yes	Vasodilator	• Similar to dobutamine, though works through nonadrenergic receptors. May be useful in patients on long-acting beta blockers who need inotropy/chronotropy • Dose adjustment needed in renal failure

vasopressor agents to maintain MAP ≥ 65 mm Hg. There is no firm evidence favoring one pressor agent over another, but norepinephrine likely has the greatest vasoconstrictor potency along with some inotropic effect. Dopamine can be used if a more inotropic and chronotropic effect is desired and should be avoided if cardiogenic shock is suspected due to demonstrated increased mortality and arrhythmias in that patient population. Low-dose dopamine does *not* provide renal protection, and should not be used solely for that purpose. Phenylephrine may be the preferred agent for blood pressure elevation in patients with prohibitive tachycardia or arrhythmias. Vasopressin, a pure vasoconstrictor, has been used to lessen the doses of adrenergic pressor agents; however, current available data does not support its routine use in sepsis.

PRACTICE POINT

- Dopamine should be avoided if cardiogenic shock is suspected, due to demonstrated increased mortality and arrhythmias in that patient population. Similarly, vasopressin should not be used routinely or as the sole vasopressor agent in septic shock.

The reversible global myocardial dysfunction that often occurs during sepsis may manifest as poor organ perfusion or as persistently low $ScvO_2$ values despite seemingly adequate filling pressures. Echocardiography or a pulmonary artery (PA) catheter may aid in this diagnosis; however, a PA catheter is rarely necessary in the management of septic shock. The addition of an inotropic agent such as dobutamine or milrinone may be temporarily required until the myocardial dysfunction improves. The EGDT protocol recommends inotropic agents to meet a goal $ScvO_2$ of 70% —after achieving CVP, MAP, and hematocrit goals—in order to improve tissue oxygen delivery.

NUTRITION

Septic patients typically have increased catabolic physiology (breakdown of protein in order to generate amino acids for gluconeogenesis) due to inflammatory response. Supplying calories early in the clinical course of sepsis can limit catabolic activity; gut integrity and immune function may be better maintained, leading to decreased infections in critically ill patients. In general, gastrointestinal (GI) tract (enteral) feeding should begin when patients are unable to feed themselves or meet nutritional goals on their own. Several studies have shown a decrease in infectious complications and stress ulcer complications in patients who are started on early (<48 hours) enteral nutrition. Multiple factors, including existing nutritional status as well as the potential for harm from temporarily withholding enteral nutrition or starting parenteral nutrition, play into the decision of initiating enteral nutrition. Patients who are hemodynamically unstable or on high-dose vasopressors may bear risk of bowel ischemia if fed enterally. Total parenteral nutrition (TPN) should be reserved for a minority of patients, typically patients post gastrointestinal surgery. TPN leads to more infectious complications (including fungemia) than enteral feeding, though there is no data showing that enteral feeding improves mortality versus TPN.

GLYCEMIC CONTROL

Guidelines recommend moderate glycemic control (blood glucose [BG] 140–180 mg /dL) in medical ICU patients, including septic patients. Tight glycemic control (keeping BG 80–110 mg/dL) in critically ill medical patients leads to worse mortality outcomes. No significant mortality benefit is achieved with tight glycemic control in critically ill patients except for those undergoing cardiothoracic surgery. Since tight glycemic control (80–110 mg/dL) is associated with significant morbidity due to hypoglycemia, endocrine and critical care authorities recommend more moderate glycemic control (140–180 mg /dL) protocols in medical ICUs and for septic patients.

TABLE 138-5 Recommendations for Use of Steroids in Septic Shock

- Intravenous hydrocortisone (300 mg/day, split into every-6-hour or every-8-hour dosing) for adult patients in septic shock when hypotension responds poorly to fluid resuscitation and vasopressors. Avoid steroids in absence of shock (unless patient's underlying endocrine history requires it).
- ACTH (Corsyntropin) stimulation test is not recommended.
- Hydrocortisone is preferred to dexamethasone.
- Steroid therapy may be weaned once vasopressors are no longer required.

ACTH, adrenocrticotropic hormone.

STEROIDS

Relative or functional adrenal insufficiency refers to suboptimal adrenal response to severe sepsis. While some debate has focused around when to prescribe corticosteroids to septic patients and how to make that decision, recent guidelines offer some assistance to clinicians making this decision (**Table 138-5**). In patients with septic shock, defined by systolic blood pressure less than 90 mm Hg despite volume resuscitation and vasopressor medications, corticosteroids offer benefit. The duration of the corticosteroids should be less than seven days and they should not be given with mineralocorticoid. Since the most recent guidelines by the Society of Critical Care Medicine (SCCM) in 2008, a 2009 meta-analysis summary of randomized controlled trial data suggests that low-dose (< 300 mg hydrocortisone per day) short-course (< 5 days) therapy offers significant mortality benefit (relative risk reduction 16%, number needed to treat 14) and length-of-stay reduction (average reduction 4.5 days) to patients with severe sepsis or septic shock.

PRACTICE POINT

- In patients with septic shock, corticosteroids may offer mortality benefit. The duration of the corticosteroids should be less than seven days and not be given with a mineralocorticoid. A 2009 meta-analysis summary of randomized controlled trial data suggests that low-dose (< 300 mg hydrocortisone per day) short-course (< 5 days) therapy offers significant mortality benefit (relative risk reduction 16%, number needed to treat 14) and length-of-stay reduction (average reduction 4.5 days) to patients with severe sepsis or septic shock.

ACTIVATED PROTEIN C

Sepsis induces a procoagulant response and this leads to the development of recombinant human activated protein C (APC), a protein that promotes fibrinolysis and inhibits thrombolysis. The original PROWESS study (see Table 138-6) demonstrated that APC improved mortality in patients with severe sepsis or septic shock who have the highest baseline risk (defined as an APACHE II score >25 or multiple organ dysfunction); patients with lower risk (APACHE II score <25 or single organ dysfunction) receive no mortality benefit. In addition, there was concern that APC would lead

TABLE 138-6 Evidence-based Medicine: Key References for Sepsis

Reference	Methodology	Results	Limitations	Bottom Line
Rivers, et al. *NEJM.* 2001;345(19): 1368–1377.	Randomized controlled trial of 263 patients with sepsis or severe sepsis assigned to receive six hours of early goal-directed therapy (EGDT) versus standard of care in the emergency room prior to admission to the intensive care unit. In-hospital mortality was the primary outcome.	Hospital mortality was 30.5% for the EGDT group versus 46.5% for the control group ($p = 0.009$).	Single-center study and bundled elements included transfusion of red blood cells in a way that has been proven to be unnecessary and possibly harmful. The utility of the central venous pressure to guide fluid responsiveness has been proven unreliable.	The importance of early and aggressive volume resuscitation in septic patients is emphasized. The difference in the two groups is essentially related to the amount of volume they each received in the first six hours. It is not clear that using the CVP and the hematocrit are ideal ways to manage sepsis resuscitation as there is strong independent evidence against both of them.
Ibrahim, et al. *CHEST.* 2000;118:146–155.	Prospective cohort study of 142 patients with blood stream infections admitted to intensive care units comparing hospital survival and adequacy of antimicrobial therapy.	Hospital mortality rate of patients on inadequate antimicrobial treatment (61.9%) was greater than the hospital mortality (28.4%; CI 1.77–2.69; $p < 0.0001$) of the patients on adequate antimicrobial treatment.	Single-center study. Mixed group of medical and surgical patients may not be applicable to other types of intensive care unit patients. Antibiotic decisions based on physician judgment, which may differ from places where guidelines/protocols are in place and mandatory.	Appropriate antibiotics are crucial in caring for patients with bloodstream infections. Suggests using broad coverage initially and allowing culture data to narrow later to limit inappropriate use, which can breed resistance and not be cost effective.
Gaieski, et al. *Crit Care Med.* 2010;38: 1045–1053.	Prospective cohort study of 261 patients with severe sepsis or septic shock undergoing EGDT to study the association between time to antibiotic administration and survival.	Mortality was markedly better for patients who received appropriate antibiotics both less than one hour from triage (mortality 19.5% versus 33.2%) and less than one hour from qualification for EGDT to appropriate antibiotics (25.0% versus 38.5%).	Single-center study. May not be applicable to other institutions not using an ER-initiated EGDT algorithm.	Early appropriate antibiotics are essential for patients with severe sepsis or septic shock. This cohort was treated with EGDT, which controls for volume resuscitation, and the vasoactive medication aspects of sepsis. The results support this important intervention.
The NICE-SUGAR Study Investigators. *N Engl J Med.* 2009;360: 1283–1297.	Multicenter randomized controlled trial of 6104 medical and surgical intensive care unit (ICU) patients expected to require ICU care for three or more consecutive days. Patients were assigned to intensive glucose control with target of 81–108 mg/dL or a conventional-control target of < 180 mg. Primary outcome was death at 90 days.	Significant mortality day 90 seen in patients in the intensive-control group versus the conventional-control group (27.5% versus 24.9%, $p = 0.02$). Severe hypoglycemia found in 6.8% of the intensive-control group versus 0.5% in the conventional-control group ($p < 0.0001$).	Open-label design, imbalance between the study groups with respect to number of patients on glucocorticoid therapy.	No additional benefit in lowering blood glucose levels below the range of approximately 140–180 mg/dL in critically ill patients.

Sprung, et al. *N Engl J Med.* 2008;358:111–124.	Multicenter, randomized, double-blind, placebo-controlled trial of 499 patients with septic shock with study patients assigned to 50 mg intravenous hydrocortisone every six hours for five days and tapered over six days versus placebo. Primary outcome was death at 28 days.	At 28 days there was no significant difference in mortality between the two groups with mortality 34.3% in the steroid group versus 31.5% in the placebo group ($p = 0.51$). There was no significant difference in mortality between the patients in the two study groups who did not have a response to cosintropin or between those who had a response to cosintropin.	The use of etomidate in 26% of the patients, which can inhibit corticosteroid production. Study lacked power due to early stop in patient enrollment due to slow recruitment, termination of funding, and time expiration of the study drug.	Based on this study, general use of corticosteroids for septic shock is not recommended. As well, corticotropin testing cannot be recommended to determine which patients should receive corticosteroid therapy. Steroids did lead to more rapid reversal of shock, but no change in mortality. Subgroup with refractory septic shock showed a mortality benefit from steroids, similar to Annane study. Patients on hydrocortisone also had more cases of superinfection and hyperglycemia.
Annane, et al. *JAMA.* 2002;288:862–871.	Multicenter, randomized, double-blind, placebo-controlled trial of 300 patients with septic shock with study patients receiving hydrocortisone 50 mg every six hours intravenously and once daily administration of 50 mcg of fludocortisone via nasogastric tube versus indiscernible placebos for total seven days. Primary outcome was 28-day survival in nonresponders to the short corticotropin test.	There were 229 nonresponders to the corticotropin test and 70 responders to the corticotropin test with equal numbers of study and placebo in each group. In nonresponders, there was a significant ($p = .02$) decrease in death in the corticosteroid group and withdrawal of vasopressor therapy within 28 days in the corticosteroid group ($p = .001$) compared to placebo. No significant differences seen between responders.	The patients studied were in refractory shock, defined as systolic blood pressure < 90 mm Hg after one hour despite fluid resuscitation and vasopressor therapy. Significant number of patients received etomidate (24%) prior to enrollment, which is known to cause transient adrenal insufficiency.	Significant reduction in risk of death in patients with refractory septic shock given seven-day treatment with low-dose hydrocortisone and fludrocortisone with relative adrenal insufficiency (nonresponders to corticotropin stimulation).
Bernard, et al. (PROWESS study group).* *N Eng J Med.* 2001;344:699–709.	Multicenter randomized, double-blind, placebo-controlled trial of 1690 patients with severe sepsis assigned to received intravenous infusion of activated protein C (drotrecogin alfa activated) for a total of 96 hours versus placebo. Primary end point was mortality at 28 days after initiation of the infusion.	The mortality was 30.8% in the placebo group versus 24.7% in the treatment group. Absolute risk reduction of death was 6.1% ($p = 0.005$). Serious bleeding was high in the group treated with activated protein C (3.5% versus 2.0%, $p = 0.06$).	Patients with high risk of bleeding (eg, chronic liver disease, chronic kidney failure on dialysis, thrombocytopenia) were excluded and these are commonly encountered in patients with severe sepsis. Majority improvement seen in sickest patients, those with APACHE II (Acute Physiology and Chronic Health Evaluation) scores > 25.	Activated protein C should be administered to patients with severe sepsis who meet the inclusion criteria. Recommendation cannot be made for patients with less-severe sepsis.
Abraham, et al. (ADDRESS Study Group).* *N Engl J Med.* 2005;353:1332–1341.	Multicenter randomized, double-blind, placebo-controlled trial of 2640 patients with severe sepsis and low risk of death (defined by APACHE II score < 25 or single organ failure) assigned to receive intravenous infusion of activated protein C (drotrecogin alfa activated) versus placebo. Primary end point was death at 28 days after initiation of infusion.	No statistically significant reduction in the 28-day mortality rate with the use of activated protein C (17% in the placebo group versus 18.5% in the treated group, $p = 0.34$). Rate of serious bleeding was greater in the activated protein C group than in the placebo group (2.4% versus 1.2%, $p = 0.02$) during the infusion.	Enrollment was discontinued due to the low likelihood of meeting defined objective.	Activated protein C should not be given to patients without severe sepsis, APACHE II scores < 25. Subsequent studies have shown some economic validation of the more ill patients in PROWESS, but have also demonstrated increased bleeding in patients receiving it as well. Treatment must be individualized, due to both side effects and cost effectiveness.

*Please refer to Activated Protein C section of chapter text in reference updated information related to this Activated Protein C that was recently pulled from the US market by the manufacturer.

to an increase in bleeding and extreme caution was recommended in the following patients: (1) severely thrombocytopenic (platelet count <30,000/mm^3); (2) conditions that increase risk of bleeding (eg, recent surgery requiring general or spinal anesthesia within 12 hours of infusion, intracranial surgery, recent stroke, cerebral aneurysm, recent gastrointestinal bleed); (3) recent anticoagulant therapy including unfractionated heparin, low-molecular-weight heparin, Coumadin, thrombolytics, glycoprotein IIb/IIIa antagonists; (4) portal hypertension. These patients were all excluded from the original study on APC. The decision to prescribe APC should be individualized (though limited to patients with severe sepsis or septic shock with high mortality risk) with respect to the patient's goals, values, and coexisting medical conditions including terminal illnesses. Because this medication bears high cost and risk of fatal or devastating bleeding, the decision to prescribe it should be carefully considered in consultation with critical care specialists when available.

After much debate about its efficacy and questionable FDA approval, activated protein C (trade name Xigris) was recently pulled from the market. Because of the lack of conclusive benefit demonstrated in subsequent studies after the original PROWESS study, the European Medicines Agency felt the risk-benefit ratio of activated protein C needed to be clarified and the maker of Xigris, Eli Lilly, was asked to conduct a new placebo-controlled trial for patients with septic shock. The study was named PROWESS-SHOCK and its results were recently revealed, failing to meet the primary endpoint of statistically significant reduction in 28-day all-cause mortality in patients treated with activated protein C (Xigris). The risk of severe bleeding events was similar in both arms, suggesting no harm. These results call into question the overall risk-benefit balance of activate protein C for the severe sepsis and septic shock patient population, and Eli Lilly has thus decided to withdraw the product from the market worldwide.

CONSULTATION

The multidisciplinary environment of the ICU often requires inclusion of many different consultants to aid in the care of critically ill patients, as in the setting of sepsis, severe sepsis, and septic shock. A team that includes critical care nursing, intensivists, infectious disease specialists, nephrologists, endocrinologists, surgeons, palliative care experts, nutritionists, social workers, and many others may be necessary to optimize the care of patients with sepsis.

Many patients with sepsis will not require the care of an intensivist; however, consultation should be considered for persistent hemodynamic instability, incipient progression to multiorgan failure, and when uncertainty exists regarding diagnosis or management. Septic patients with multiorgan failure or those requiring advanced airway and/or ventilator management likely deserve intensivist involvement in their care. Consultation with an intensivist should also be considered if invasive monitoring is needed including placement of central venous and arterial catheters, and especially if placement of pulmonary artery catheters is contemplated. In addition, intensivist consultation may assist with decision making to prescribe recombinant APC or corticosteroids in the setting of septic shock.

Not uncommonly, consultation with a nephrologist is required for patients with acute kidney injury who may need renal replacement therapy while critically ill.

The multidisciplinary approach required in the care of complex critically ill patients often requires collaboration and consultation of other clinical specialists, including critical care nursing; respiratory care; physical, occupational, and speech therapy; wound care nursing; social services; pastoral care; palliative care; and others. Clinicians caring for patients in the critical care setting should have a low threshold to involve necessary services in the care of their critically ill patients to optimize care quality and efficiency.

COMPLICATIONS AND PROGNOSIS

Uncomplicated sepsis that is treated appropriately and aggressively will often have very few untoward outcomes and patients may return to baseline within a very short time frame. Sepsis that progresses to severe sepsis or septic shock more frequently leads to a complicated course for the patient (see Table 138-1). Patients will often require invasive procedures including central venous catheter and arterial catheter placement, as well as possible endotracheal intubation and mechanical ventilation to manage airway, refractory hypoxemia, and/or increased work of breathing. Patients with acute lung injury, also known as noncardiogenic pulmonary edema or acute respiratory distress syndrome (ARDS), may require a prolonged course of mechanical ventilation; their lung function typically improves over time, though not back to baseline. Other patients may suffer kidney injury requiring dialysis therapy. The typically reversible acute tubular necrosis may take days, weeks, or months to resolve, and some patients may require chronic hemodialysis permanently. A relatively common neurologic disorder encountered in sepsis is the development of critical illness polyneuropathy, which will typically manifest in difficulty liberating a patient from mechanical ventilation due to profound weakness. This condition usually resolves, but often can take several months. Psychological stress, often described as posttraumatic stress disorder, is related to the common complication of ICU delirium. Daily awakening in the ICU may minimize delirium.

DISCHARGE PLANNING

Patients may transition from a closely monitored setting—either intensive care unit or intermediate care unit—to a medical floor when they are hemodynamically stable (ie, off vasoactive medications) and not in need of frequent CVP and $ScvO_2$ measurement. Any septic patient requiring mechanical ventilation, or even noninvasive mechanical ventilation intermittently, should remain in an ICU setting until their gas exchange or work of breathing problems have resolved and they no longer require supportive devices. Discharge from the hospital may occur quickly if a patient has mild sepsis that is treated and resolves quickly. For a more prolonged hospitalization including mechanical ventilation, a patient may require significant physical rehabilitation within an acute or subacute rehabilitation facility before returning to the home environment.

QUALITY IMPROVEMENT TO ADDRESS PERFORMANCE GAPS

Institutional sepsis protocols likely will standardize and improve overall care for septic patients admitted to hospitals and ICUs. Since outcomes in severe sepsis and septic shock highly depend on expedient administration of evidence-based interventions, institutions and individual clinicians should consider measuring process outcomes (eg, time to antibiotics in sepsis, use of $ScvO_2$ monitoring) as well as patient outcomes to help best delineate areas of heterogeneous care and help drive consistent evidence-based or guideline-based practice to improve overall outcomes.

Sepsis prevention requires early recognition of disease and prompt treatment to prevent progression to severe sepsis and septic shock. A lower threshold for sepsis evaluation and aggressive therapy needs to be applied to immunosuppressed patients, including patients with HIV, asplenia, neutropenia, and patients receiving immunosuppressive agents. Early removal of urinary catheters, central venous catheters, and liberation from mechanical ventilation to prevent ventilator-associated pneumonia will lower the incidence of sepsis. The cost of caring for septic patients exceeds $22,000 per hospitalization, and much opportunity exists to improve outcomes and reduce hospital lengths of stay and costs for a medical condition that bears high morbidity and mortality (**Table 138-6**).

SUGGESTED READINGS

Annane D, Bellissant E, Bollaert PE, et al. Corticosteroids in the treatment of severe sepsis and septic shock in adults: a systematic review. *JAMA*. 2009;301(22):2362–2375.

Dellinger RP, Levy MM, Carlet JM, et al. Surviving sepsis campaign: international guidelines for management of severe sepsis and septic shock: 2008. *Crit Care Med*. 2008;36(1):296–327.

Finfer S, Chittock DR, Su SY, et al. Intensive versus conventional glucose control in critically ill patients. *N Engl J Med*. 2009;360(13): 1283–1297.

Garnacho-Montero J, Garcia-Garmendia JL, Barrero-Almodovar A. Impact of adequate empirical antibiotic therapy on the outcome of patients admitted to the intensive care unit with sepsis. *Crit Care Med*. 2003;(12):2742–2751.

Heffner AC, Horton JM, Marchick MR, et al. Etiology of illness in patients with severe sepsis admitted to the hospital form the emergency department. *Clin Infec Dis*. 2010;50(6):814–820.

Hollenberg SM, Ahrens TS, Annane D, et al. Practice parameters for hemodynamic support of sepsis in adult patients: 2004 update. *Crit Care Med*. 2004;(9):1928–1948.

Kumar A, Ellis P, Arabi Y, et al. Initiation of inappropriate antimicrobial therapy results in a fivefold reduction of survival in human septic shock. *Chest*. 2009;136(5):1237–1248.

Kumar A, Roberts D, Wood KE, et al. Duration of hypotension before initiation of effective antimicrobial therapy is the critical determinant of survival in human septic shock. *Crit Care Med*. 2006;34(6):1589–1596.

Rivers E, Nguyen B, Havstad S. Early goal-directed therapy in the treatment of severe sepsis and septic shock. *N Engl J Med*. 2001; 345(19):1368–1377.

Van den Berghe G, Wilmer A, Hermans G, et al. Intensive insulin therapy in the medical ICU. *N Engl J Med*. 2006;354(5):449–461.

Vincent JL, Bernard GR, Beale R, et al. Drotrecogin alfa (activated) treatment in severe sepsis from the global open-label trial ENHANCE: further evidence for survival and safety and implications for early treatment. *Crit Care Med*. 2005;33(10):2266–2277.

CHAPTER 139

Surgical Critical Care

Zara Cooper, MD, MSc
Selwyn O. Rogers Jr., MD, MPH

Key Clinical Questions

1. Which surgical patients require admission to the intensive care unit?
2. How should postoperative bleeding be best managed?
3. What contributes to postoperative pulmonary insufficiency, and how should it be managed?
4. What is damage control surgery?
5. What are the indications for open abdomen and delayed abdominal closure?

INTRODUCTION

INVASIVE MONITORING

Several measurements can be obtained in the intensive care unit (ICU) to guide management. Central venous monitoring is used to measure central venous pressure, a marker of volume status and right atrial pressure. The central oxygen venous saturation, obtained from the distal port of a multilumen catheter, can be measured as a surrogate for mixed venous oxygen saturation instead of using a pulmonary artery catheter (PAC). The central venous oxygen saturation is usually 10% lower than the mixed venous oxygen saturation from the PAC, but this measure can vary due to multiple factors such as anemia or sepsis. Arterial vascular access monitors blood pressure and measures arterial blood gases (ABG). The base deficit in the ABG is a particularly useful aggregated index for determining tissue perfusion. The arterial base deficit is the amount of additional base that must be added to raise one litre of whole blood pH as predicted by the arterial partial pressure of carbon dioxide ($PaCO_2$). Base deficit, which is used as a surrogate marker of metabolic acidosis, is a calculated value; can be classified as mild (2–5 mmol/L), moderate (6–14 mmol/L), and severe (>15 mmol/L); and is used as a surrogate marker of metabolic acidosis. Serial measurements are useful in guiding resuscitation and have been shown to predict hospital mortality, length of stay, severity of sepsis, and organ failure in both medical and surgical ICU patients. The PAC can be used to monitor ventricular filling pressures, cardiac output and index, vascular resistance, and venous oxygen saturation. The routine use of PACs in postoperative patients is controversial. A large meta-analysis and randomized trials in medical and surgical patients have not demonstrated any benefit in PAC use. However, a recent study using 53,000 trauma patients showed a survival benefit with the use of PACs in severely injured, elderly patients with high base deficits. The results of invasive monitoring should not be used as isolated values. Rather, they should be trended and used in the broader context of the clinical exam.

TRIAGE

CRITERIA FOR ADMISSION TO THE ICU

Patients may be admitted to the ICU preoperatively, immediately postoperatively, or postoperatively after initial admission to the ward. Preoperative admission may be required for resuscitation in the event of preoperative respiratory failure, cardiogenic shock, or sepsis. ICU admission may also be required for patients who need invasive monitoring for blood pressure management in the setting of severe cardiovascular disease, such as a stroke or acute myocardial infarction.

Postoperatively, patients may be admitted to the ICU for respiratory failure, hemodynamic instability, or close monitoring for complications such as bleeding or physiologic alterations. Patients may also require admission to the ICU due to exacerbation of underlying comorbidities or after procedures with significant blood loss or massive fluid shifts seen in peritonitis or bowel obstruction. Some patients need prolonged mechanical ventilation due to the prolonged effects of general anesthesia, airway edema, or volume overload. Patients with preoperative renal, hepatic, or pulmonary insufficiency may also benefit from elective postoperative ICU admission, as they may be more susceptible to the adverse effects of narcotics and less likely to tolerate hemodynamic perturbations.

MANAGEMENT

NUTRITIONAL MANAGEMENT

Malnutrition in surgical patients is associated with poor wound healing, increased rates of infection, longer hospital stay, and higher mortality. Volume shifts, increased hemodynamic changes, and tissue injury all contribute to an acute phase reaction, which increases metabolic demands. Catecholamines and cortisol increase protein turnover and muscle breakdown as fat and protein are shuttled to essential organs. Weakened respiratory muscles contribute to atelectasis, pneumonia, and prolonged respiratory failure. Immunity is impaired as cell growth and cell turnover are decreased.

From the VA Cooperative study comparing outcomes of patients with mild, moderate, and severe malnutrition, preoperative nutritional supplementation is indicated for severely malnourished patients awaiting major surgery but who cannot tolerate oral intake for five days prior to intervention. Such high-risk patients include cancer patients who have lost more than 10% of their body weight, or other patients who have lost 15% of their body weight in the preceding six months.

Enteral nutrition reduces complications and improves outcomes over parenteral nutrition. Enteral feeding prevents atrophy associated with disuse and helps the gastrointestinal tract provide a barrier to infection. Trials comparing enteral and parental nutrition have consistently found that enteral nutrition has fewer complications and improved survival compared with parenteral nutrition. Patients with head and neck malignancies and other anatomic barriers to oral intake may benefit from placement of a gastrostomy or jejenostomy tube. Postpyloric feeding is indicated in cases of gastric outlet obstruction or early satiety.

Nasogastric and orogastric routes are indicated for short-term feeding because they are relatively minor interventions and are associated with fewer complications. However, caution must be taken when placing nasogastric or orogastric tubes in obtunded patients who are at increased risk for aspiration and inadvertent placement in the respiratory tract. Postplacement radiographs of styleted tubes confirming placement are indicated for all patients.

PRACTICE POINT

- For nasogastric (NG) and orogastric (OG) tubes, postplacement radiographs of styleted tubes to confirm placement are indicated for all patients to reduce risk for aspiration and inadvertent placement in the respiratory tract.

Enteral nutrition is not safe for patients with bowel obstruction. Patients with an ileus should not be fed enterally until the ileus resolves; feeding in some instances puts the patient at risk for vomiting and possible aspiration. Most patients with escalating vasopressor requirements should not be enterally fed because the gut mucosal integrity may be impaired; these patients also have an increased risk for intestinal ischemia. Some clinicians advocate for restricting all forms of enteral nutrition for patients who are hypotensive or receiving pressor agents due to the resultant ileus and relative bowel ischemia that may ensue. Enteral nutrition may be used cautiously in patients receiving low-dose vasopressor support, while monitoring for gut ischemia and ileus.

Most nutritional formulas provide all essential elements and minerals and contain 1–2 kcal/ml. Specific tube feeding formulas have been developed for patients with renal disease, respiratory failure, hepatic insufficiency, and diabetes. Elemental formulas are provided to patients with malabsorptive disorders. Patients taking enteral formulas should be monitored for feeding intolerance, hypernatremia, and diarrhea. Patients fed through their stomach should have gastric residuals checked every six hours, and feeds should not be held if residuals are less than 300 ml. Patients fed through the small bowel do not have to have residuals checked. When diarrhea occurs in a tube-fed patient, infectious causes should be ruled out. Whenever there is any doubt about how best to meet a patient's nutritional needs, consultation with a nutritional support service or the surgeon should be initiated.

PRACTICE POINT

- Patients receiving gastric tube feeding should have gastric residuals checked every six hours, and feeds should be held only when residuals are greater than 300 ml. Patients fed through the small bowel do not require residuals to be checked.

In cases where enteral nutrition is not possible, total parenteral nutrition (TPN) may be used but is accompanied by an increased risk of central line–associated blood stream infections (CLABSI) and hyperglycemia. Most patients should receive 150% of their total nonprotein calorie needs to optimize their nutrition. Patients should receive at least 1.5 gm/kg of protein as well. For those who are severely malnourished, caloric provision should be reintroduced in a graduated fashion to avoid refeeding syndrome. Refeeding syndrome may occur when nutritional support is given to severely malnourished patients, and metabolism suddenly shifts from a catabolic to an anabolic state. Carbohydrate intake triggers insulin release, with subsequent cellular uptake of potassium, phosphate, and magnesium. When the serum concentrations of these electrolytes are reduced, arrhythmias and severe muscle weakness can occur.

Improvements in nutritional status should be monitored through weekly prealbumin and C-reactive protein (CRP) levels. Traditionally, protein status was monitored by albumin levels. However, albumin has a half-life of 20 days and is not an appropriate measure of short-term nutritional improvement. Its levels are also affected by fluid balance, and so patients with volume overload will have low relative levels.

The half-life of prealbumin is 48 hours, making it a more reliable marker of response to feeding. Unfortunately, during inflammation hepatic synthesis of transport proteins is suppressed, with resultant low levels of prealbumin due to inflammation alone. C-reactive protein (CRP) is an acute phase reactant that peaks 48 hours after the inflammatory insult, and levels of CRP are routinely used to monitor the degree of inflammation and assist in the interpretation of prealbumin levels.

Guidelines from the American Society of Parenteral and Enteral Nutrition (ASPEN) do not recommend nutritional support in well-nourished patients who will resume oral feeding within 7–10 days post surgery. However, patients following emergency surgery, burns, head injury, and orthopedic trauma have particularly high metabolic demands and may need up to 2 gm/kg of protein per day to maintain nitrogen balance. If the need for prolonged enteral support is determined intraoperatively, placement of a gastrostomy or jejenostomy tube during the initial operation should be considered. In this case, feeds can usually be started within a day or two following surgery.

Patients receiving tube feeds may remain malnourished if they never obtain their daily requirements due to frequent interruptions secondary to medication administration or radiologic tests or other procedures. Commonly, tube feeds are held in surgical ICU patients because of high gastric residuals and impending procedures or planned extubation. Clinicians should maintain vigilance in assessing patients' nutritional needs, monitoring patients' actual nutritional intake, and adjusting nutritional provision actively and frequently to support postoperative needs. Consultation with nutrition specialists may be necessary to optimize support.

Candidates for TPN include patients who have undergone massive intestinal resection or who cannot tolerate enteral feeds. Central venous access is required to administer the high levels of dextrose in TPN. Either a subclavian or internal jugular approach is most appropriate for short-term access as femoral catheters have higher risks of thrombosis, infection, and hematomas. TPN poses an increased risk for line sepsis and bacteremia. A peripherally inserted central venous catheter (PICC) or a subclavian tunneled line is preferred for patients requiring long-term parenteral nutrition (more than six to eight days).

■ BLOOD TRANSFUSIONS

In the surgical settings, some surgeons liberally transfuse blood and use triggers of a hematocrit less than 30 or a hemoglobin level less than 10 mg/dL. Liberal use of blood transfusion has been associated with higher mortality. Transfusion has been associated with immunosuppression and increased infectious complications. Despite the risks, clear indications for transfusion remain. Platelet transfusion is indicated in the setting of microvascular bleeding and normothermia. Hypothermia should be corrected before transfusion because cold body temperature can increase platelet dysfunction.

Cryoprecipitate, which contains fibrinogen, factor VIII, von Willebrand factor (VWF), and fibronectin, treats fibrinogen deficiency in consumptive coagulopathy, Von Willebrand deficiency, and hemophilia. Fresh frozen plasma (FFP) contains all of the clotting factors as well as fibrinogen. It is used for emergent transfusion in warfarin-induced coagulopathy, liver disease, and disseminated intravascular coagulation (DIC) prior to procedures or in the event of spontaneous bleeding. In patients without cardiovascular disease, transfusion of packed red blood cells is indicated when the hemoglobin level is 7 mg/dL or less.

Recombinant factor VIIa

Recombinant factor VIIa (rFVIIa) is a synthetic form of factor VII, which activates factors X and IX when it interacts with factor II (thrombin) on the subendothelium. Due to its cost, use of factor rFVIIa has been limited to treatment of coagulopathy from hemorrhagic shock and reversal of warfarin-induced coagulopathy in head injured patients. Recombinant FVIIa has been shown to increase the risk of thrombosis.

Massive transfusion

Massive transfusion is defined as the transfusion of more than 10 units of packed red blood cells (pRBCs). Transfusion of pRBCs and crystalloid can cause a dilutional coagulopathy. Recent investigations from the wars in Iraq and Afghanistan have demonstrated improved outcomes with a 1:1:1 ratio of platelets, FFP, and packed red cells. Many trauma centers have resorted to this strategy for massive transfusions. Institutional guidelines vary, and clinicians should work within the guidelines of their local practice environment.

■ SPECIAL CASES

Damage control surgery and the open abdomen

Damage control surgery is the term most often applied to (1) trauma patients in extremis, and (2) patients with major intraabdominal injury needing immediate control of hemorrhage and contamination but too unstable for definitive immediate repair. After surgical hemorrhage is controlled in the operating room (OR), patients are usually taken to the ICU for resuscitation and stabilization before definitive surgical repair, which is delayed to manage hypothermia, metabolic acidosis, and coagulopathy in the ICU. Typically, patients will have an open abdomen with a temporary closure device. Once stabilized, further evaluation and definitive repairs can be completed.

The SICU as an operating room

Transporting critically ill and unstable patients can pose serious risks to the patient and require considerable resources to transfer monitoring devices and ensure that drugs are readily available. A dedicated nurse and a respiratory therapist must travel with an intubated patient, and, if emergent surgery is required, an operating room (OR) must be immediately available. Increasingly, the ICU is used as an alternative to the OR. Unfortunately, ideal operating conditions cannot usually be replicated. The OR provides access to inhalational agents, sterility, room lights, and temperature control that cannot be moved to other locations. However, there are times when scarce OR availability and the patient's condition make bedside procedures preferable. Bedside laparotomy, open and percutaneous tracheostomy, feeding tube placement, and fasciotomies are examples of procedures that can be done at the bedside in emergent or elective circumstances. Emergent laparotomy for abdominal compartment syndrome is sometimes performed at the bedside.

Patients should be prepared as they would be for the OR. Informed consent should be obtained, coagulopathy corrected, and preoperative antibiotics given, if appropriate. If general anesthesia is necessary, an anesthesiologist should be present to manage anesthetics and the airway. At a minimum, one nurse should be present for patient recovery. Blood pressure monitoring, pulse oximetry, and cardiac telemetry should be used during the procedure to monitor vital signs.

Bedside procedures should be handled similarly to those in the OR. All personnel should understand their role. It may be helpful to have OR staff come to the bedside if ICU staff are unfamiliar with OR procedures. Sterile procedures and technique must be used, and all personnel in the room should have caps and masks on. It may be useful to bring sterile drapes from the OR, as they will be large enough to provide ample coverage. Surgeons and instrument technicians should scrub as they would for the OR. Foot traffic in the space should be kept to a minimum.

COMPLICATIONS

■ POSTOPERATIVE BLEEDING

Hypotension and tachycardia in the postoperative setting presumptively indicates hemorrhage, until proven otherwise (**Figure 139-1**). Hemorrhagic shock is a potentially lethal postoperative complication. Bleeding should be ruled out before other types of shock are considered. Bleeding in the postoperative period may be due to surgical site bleeding or diffuse coagulopathy. Clues to surgical bleeding include hemorrhage from surgical wounds, tubes, and drains. Any appreciable output (eg, >100 mL) should prompt surgical consultation. Surgical compartments, such as the abdomen, retroperitoneum, and thighs, can harbor multiple units of blood depending on the patient's body habitus. These can be assessed on physical exam looking for ecchymosis, swelling, or tense soft tissue. Computed tomography (CT) with intravenous (IV) contrast can reveal active bleeding or old hematoma. Nonsurgical bleeding is multifactorial and may be associated with hypothermia, acidosis, or impaired coagulation. Hypothermia and acidosis from shock cause a complex coagulopathy due to ineffective clotting. Hypothermia may also occur with systemic inflammatory response syndrome and sepsis, where decreased oxygen consumption impedes maintenance of core body temperature. Hypothermia slows enzymatic proteolysis and causes defective platelet adhesion and aggregation and decreased thromboxane production, which contributes to overall platelet dysfunction and impaired hemostasis. Treatment includes rewarming with warmed intravenous fluids, warming blankets, and increasing the room temperature. Surgical bleeding exacerbates coagulopathy which, in turn, exacerbates bleeding; therefore, significant hemorrhage needs to be addressed expediently. Acidosis also contributes to coagulopathy

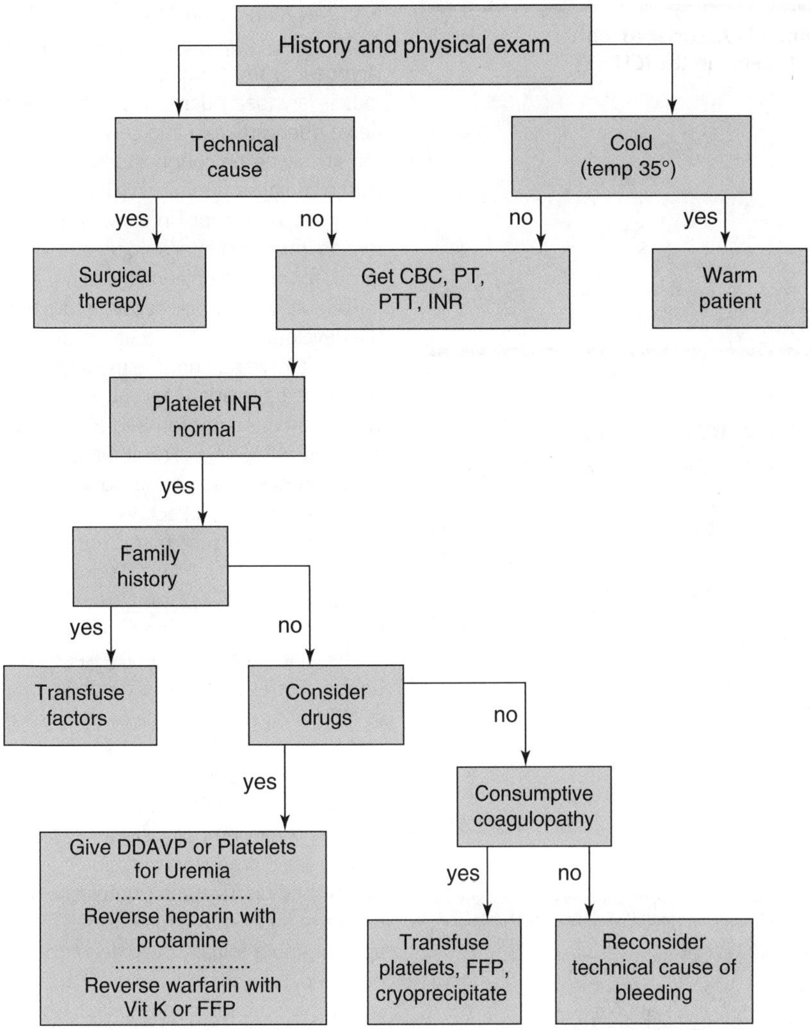

Figure 139-1 *Management of postoperative bleeding. CBC, complete blood count; ddAVP, desmopressin; FFP, fresh frozen plasma; INR, international normalized ratio; PT, prothrombin time; PTT, partial thromboplastin time; Temp, temperature (oC); Vit K, vitamin K.*

by decreasing thrombin generation. Treatment includes volume administration to increase tissue perfusion and correction of the underlying etiology.

PRACTICE POINT

- Surgical compartments, such as the abdomen, retroperitoneum, and thighs, can harbor multiple units of blood depending on the patient's body habitus.

Coagulopathy may be associated with congenital bleeding deficiencies, such as Von Willebrand disease (VWD) or hemophilia A or B, or more commonly, acquired bleeding disorders. Postoperative sepsis can cause coagulopathy through inflammatory mediators, platelet sequestration, and consumption. Tissue factor inhibits fibrinolysis and increases fibrin deposition with subsequent tissue thrombosis. Thrombin generation also consumes factors in the clotting cascade, contributing to a consumptive coagulopathy. Sepsis can also cause DIC, which is a consumptive coagulopathy characterized by microvascular thrombosis and platelet aggregation. DIC can also occur during other inflammatory states, including pancreatitis, malignancy, and transfusion reactions. Laboratory markers include thrombocytopenia, prolonged prothombin time (PT) and partial thromboplastin time (PTT), elevated fibrin split products, and schistocytes on peripheral smear. DIC should be suspected in the setting of coagulopathy and microvascular bleeding. Treatment is directed at eradicating the inflammatory source.

Platelet transfusions can correct thrombocytopenia and may be necessary even in the face of normal platelet levels in uremic patients with evidence of ongoing bleeding. Fresh frozen plasma (FFP) can be used to correct an elevated INR and associated coagulation deficiencies. Cryoprecipitate may be used to replace fibrinogen in settings with a low fibrinogen such as cirrhosis, thrombosis, and hemmorhage.

Thrombocytopenia can be caused by decreased platelet production, as seen in malignancy or with chemotherapy, platelet sequestration and consumption found in sepsis or DIC, and immune mechanisms associated with certain drugs such as heparin, H2-histamine blockers, and sulfa drugs (**Table 139-1**). Transfusion and fluid resuscitation can also contribute to a dilutional thrombocytopenia, but the volume of the transfusion is not proportional to the drop in platelets. Dilution may contribute to thrombocytopenia, but it should not be attributed as the only cause. Platelet dysfunction can also be seen in renal and hepatic insufficiency. In the event of active bleeding, platelet transfusion is indicated at platelet levels less than 50,000/dL. In the absence of active bleeding, many patients can tolerate lower platelet counts as low as 20,000/dL.

TABLE 139-1 Drugs Commonly Associated with Thrombocytopenia in the ICU

Heparin
Sulfonamides
Furosimide
Penicillins
Ranitidine
Digoxin
Quinidine

POSTOPERATIVE PULMONARY INSUFFICIENCY

Postoperative pulmonary failure is defined as postoperative intubation for more than 48 hours or intubation within 48 hours postoperatively. Decreased vital capacity (VC), functional residual capacity (FRC), and pulmonary edema may all contribute to a decrease in pulmonary function exhibited following surgery and general anesthesia. Decreases in VC and FRC and increases in pulmonary edema will continue into the immediate postoperative period and return to normal function after one to two weeks. In many patients, the VC drops to 40% of preoperative levels within the first 12 hours after surgery. Decreased FRC is caused by shallow breathing without maximal inspiration at regular intervals. Normally, maximal inspiration a few times each hour prevents atelectasis. However, without these maximal breaths, the FRC decreases to 70% of the preoperative value within 24 hours.

PRACTICE POINT

- Maximal inspiration a few times each hour prevents atelectasis. However, without these maximal breaths, the FRC decreases to 70% of the preoperative value within 24 hours. Therefore, chest physiotherapy, early mobilization, incentive spirometry (and/or deep breathing exercises), and adequate pain control serve to prevent postoperative pulmonary complications and pulmonary failure.

Pain limits diaphragmatic excursion and contributes to shallow breathing. Adequate pain control and increased maximal inspiration with pulmonary toilet, including chest physiotherapy, early mobilization, and incentive spirometry (and/or deep breathing exercises) are the main cornerstones of postoperative pulmonary care. Patients who smoke and those with preexisting lung disease are at increased risk for postoperative respiratory failure. Patients greater than age 65 are also at significant risk for postoperative pulmonary impairment because of relatively compromised pulmonary function compared to younger patients. Other risk factors for postoperative pulmonary complications include American Society of Anesthesiologists (ASA) Class II or higher, heart failure, and functional dependence.

Pulmonary edema is most often seen in patients with left ventricular failure, volume overload, or capillary permeability as seen in sepsis. Edema increases the risk of pneumonia and atelectasis. Pulmonary toilet, judicious management of fluids, and infection prevention all minimize the risk of postoperative pulmonary edema.

Patients with pulmonary comorbidities may benefit from noninvasive strategies, such as noninvasive ventilation. Causes of respiratory failure in the immediate postoperative period include volume overload, sepsis, and mechanical failure. Upper airway edema from volume overload, prolonged prone positioning, or trauma after intubation may also cause prolonged ventilator dependence. The airway edema usually resolves in a few days and can be treated with elevation of the head of the bed and judicious fluid management. In cases where airway edema is suspected or confirmed by laryngeal exam, steroids may be prescribed prior to extubation to reduce laryngeal edema and stridor. Injury to the recurrent laryngeal nerve during thyroid and cervical esophageal or other neck dissections can weaken cough and increase the risk of aspiration. Patients with bilateral recurrent nerve injury are candidates for tracheostomy for airway protection. In some thoracic surgical cases, patients will remain intubated after surgery to increase lung expansion in an attempt to minimize pleural bleeding.

Patients with shock, sepsis, and trauma are at increased risk for the development of the acute respiratory distress syndrome (ARDS). Inflammatory and immune mediators cause microvasculature leaks, plasma extravasation, and alveolar edema. Both oxygenation and ventilation are compromised as gas exchange across the alveoli is impaired. ARDS is a clinical diagnosis manifested by bilateral infiltrates on chest radiograph (due to diffuse inflammatory infiltrate and capillary leak), a PaO_2 to FiO_2 ratio less than 200, and a pulmonary wedge pressure consistent with noncardiogenic pulmonary edema (< 18) or no clinical signs of heart failure. Lung-protective ventilation strategies, using low tidal volumes of 6 ml/kg ideal body weight, have been shown to reduce mortality.

The fat embolism syndrome, seen in patients with traumatic long bone fractures and after orthopedic surgery, presents very similarly to ARDS. Diagnosis is made by the Sudan blue stain test in the blood and eosinophilia. The two syndromes are treated in the same manner with supportive care.

Pulmonary contusions from trauma, postoperative pneumonia, and pulmonary embolus can all lead to acute postoperative respiratory failure. Pulmonary contusion is associated with blunt chest wall trauma and rib fractures. Contusions can blossom days after the initial injury, and hypoxia may worsen before it improves. Patients who appear stable initially may decompensate and should be closely observed. Pain control and mechanical ventilation are often necessary to give the lung time to heal. Surgical patients, in general, and especially those with malignancy, obesity, or hypercoagulable states have increased risk of pulmonary embolus. Pulmonary embolus can present with severe hypoxia or isolated tachycardia. Therefore, a high degree of clinical suspicion is necessary. Patients may complain of dyspnea, chest pain, or be totally asymptomatic. Arterial blood gas measurement will show an elevated arterial-alveolar gradient. The diagnosis is confirmed with a high-resolution chest and lower extremity CT with IV contrast. If patients are too ill to tolerate a CT or cannot tolerate IV contrast, empiric treatment with therapeutic anticoagulation is warranted if the clinical suspicion of pulmonary embolus is high. Decisions about anticoagulation should be made in concert with the surgical team.

Surgical patients have increased risk of aspiration for a number of reasons. First, they are often immobile and may even be supine for long periods of time. Second, they may have impaired consciousness from postoperative delirium, narcotic use, or prolonged effects of anesthesia. Third, disruption of the oropharyngeal sphincters by nasogastric or endotracheal tubes may precipitate aspiration. Not all aspiration events cause pneumonia or pneumonitis, and empiric antibiotics are not indicated in the absence of fever, sputum production, and/or infiltrates on chest X-ray. However, if aspiration pneumonia is suspected, antimicrobial coverage should be initiated.

POSTOPERATIVE RENAL FAILURE

Postoperative renal failure presents with oliguria (< 500 mL/day) with rising blood urea nitrogen and creatinine. The patients at greatest risk for postoperative renal failure have baseline renal impairment. The most likely causes of postoperative renal failure are hypovolemia and acute tubular necrosis caused by transient hypotension or nephrotoxic agents. Transient hypotension may be seen in the operating room during or after anesthesia induction, after considerable blood loss, following premature use of diuretics, and after aortic cross clamping during abdominal aneurysm repair. Clinicians evaluating postoperative renal failure should closely review the intraoperative anesthesia report to evaluate for transient hypotension as an etiology. Nephrotoxic agents include contrast dye, nonsteroidal anti-inflammatory drugs (NSAIDS), sulfa-based drugs, and certain antibiotics. Treatment for renal failure is entirely supportive and includes restoration of intravascular volume in hypovolemic patients and cessation or avoidance of nephrotoxic agents. For those with progressive renal failure with hyperkalemia, intractable acidosis, or volume overload, temporary renal replacement therapy with continuous or intermittent dialysis may be required, depending on the condition of the patient. ICU admission with arterial monitoring and measurement of central venous pressures or wedge pressures may be necessary to manage volume status.

POSTOPERATIVE DELIRIUM

Postoperative delirium, an acute decline in cognitive function with confusion, agitation, and disorientation, complicates 11% to 25% of operative cases. Comorbid conditions increasing the likelihood of postoperative delirium include older age, alcohol abuse, malnutrition, baseline dementia, and a history of prior postoperative delirium. Postoperative factors contributing to delirium include pain, excessive sedatives and analgesics, and immobility. Decreased mobility contributes to atelectasis, leading to hypoxemia, a risk factor for delirium.

Delirium leads to prolonged ICU and hospital length of stay. Patients with delirium have increased risk for aspiration and falls and may pull at indwelling catheters and surgical drains. Patients who pose a risk to themselves or others require monitoring in the ICU.

Evaluation for delirium should include a search for infectious sources, electrolyte imbalances, and hypoxemia. Head CT is indicated in patients who cannot cooperate with a neurologic examination, who have focal neurologic deficits, and who have risk factors for stroke. Close communication with family members can assist with a valuable history of the patient's preoperative mental status.

Once the diagnosis of delirium is established, inciting factors should be addressed. Alcohol withdrawal can lead to postoperative delirium but is also associated with a sympathetic response, which can lead to hemodynamic instability and even death. An alcohol history should be solicited from all preoperative surgical patients and readdressed postoperatively if there is concern regarding the etiology of delirium. Even small doses of daily alcohol intake can lead to physiologic dependence that needs to be addressed pre- and postoperatively. Surgical and nosocomial infections, especially in the presence of high fever, can cause delirium. Hypoxemia secondary to a pneumonia, atelectasis, or pulmonary embolus can present as delirium. Similarly, anemia and profound dehydration may manifest as delirium. Sedating medications should be minimized. Antipsychotics, such as haloperidol or quetiapine, better manage agitation than narcotic anxiolytic agents (eg, benzodiazepines), except in the setting of alcohol withdrawal, where benzodiazepines may be more effective. Patients may require one-to-one observation, which is preferable to restraints, as the latter will exacerbate delirium. Clinicians should promote normal sleep-wake cycles for patients with delirium. Familiar environmental cues help to reorient patients. Support from family members, hearing aids, glasses, and dentures can help the patient regain a sense of self. Early identification and management of delirium offers best care for this challenging postoperative complication.

SURGICAL SITE INFECTIONS

Surgical site infections (SSIs) are the most common postoperative complication, and include superficial and deep space infections. Closed space infections spread along tissue planes and may cause severe tissue destruction requiring debridement for source control. Wound infections are most common in diabetic and obese patients and after surgery in a contaminated space.

Most superficial wound infections can be managed by opening the wound at the bedside to allow drainage. Antibiotics may be added if systemic signs and symptoms exist. The development of necrotic tissue in the wound warrants debridement, possibly in the operating room. The classic "salmon-colored drainage" is typical of an abdominal wound dehiscence (eg, fascial separation) and does not necessarily signify infection. In some cases, a small dehiscence can be managed without surgery. Large dehiscences require urgent surgical treatment. Evisceration or protrusion of the bowel contents from the abdominal cavity is a surgical emergency. The individual approach will be left to surgical judgment, and the surgical team should be notified if there is any concern about wound disruption.

Closed space infections and abscesses must be drained either percutaneously (eg, by interventional radiology) if deep, or with incision and drainage if superficial. Superficial wounds should be left open to heal by secondary intention until they close. Dressing changes one to three times per day is typical depending on the amount of debridement required. Most commonly, dressings are initially changed three times per day until the wound bed starts to show granulation. At that time, the frequency of dressing changes can be progressively decreased. Alternatively, once the wound is adequately debrided, a vacuum-assisted closure device—where negative pressure is exerted to the wound—can be applied.

Anastomotic leaks typically occur between postoperative days five and seven and are accompanied by abdominal pain, fever, and elevated white count. This constellation of symptoms after an enteric anastomosis should warrant an abdominal/pelvic CT scan with oral contrast. Most often these leaks can be managed with percutaneous drainage. Inability to control the infection or sepsis warrants operative intervention. Surgical consultation is warranted.

PRACTICE POINT

- Anastomotic leaks typically occur between postoperative days five and seven and are accompanied by abdominal pain, fever, and elevated white count. *Abdominal/pelvic CT scan with oral contrast is indicated for diagnosis.*

Necrotizing soft tissue infections (NSTI) are potentially lethal surgical infections and most often seen in previous surgical and traumatic wounds. Risk factors for NSTI include obesity, diabetes, and immunosuppression. The necrosis tends to spread along tissue planes with poor blood supply and relative hypoxemia. Toxins spread rapidly causing thrombosis along these planes and worsening necrosis. Eighty percent of infections are polymicrobial. The hallmarks of necrotizing fasciitis are erythema, pain out of proportion to exam or anesthesia, vesicles and bullae, and dusky skin changes or frank gangrene.

PRACTICE POINT

- The hallmarks of necrotizing fasciitis are erythema, pain out of proportion to exam or anesthesia, vesicles and bullae, and dusky skin changes or frank gangrene.

Suspicion of NSTI warrants emergent surgical consultation and biopsy, which can be done at the bedside or, preferably, in the operating room. *Imaging studies should not delay operative treatment.* Pathologic diagnosis is confirmed on frozen section by finding polynuclear cells and bacteria in the fascia. Cultures should be sent from the operating room. Treatment includes wide debridement, supportive care, resuscitation, and delayed reconstruction, if indicated. The patients are usually systemically quite ill with severely elevated white blood cell counts, high fevers, and organ dysfunction and/or failure. Empiric antimicrobials indicated for treatment include vancomycin to cover methicillin-resistant *Staphylococcus aureus* (MRSA), a quinolone or third-generation cephalosporin to cover gram-negatives, and clindamycin for anaerobic coverage and toxin elimination. Infectious disease consultation for these challenging cases is highly recommended. Antibiotics can be narrowed after culture results return.

ABDOMINAL COMPARTMENT SYNDROME

Abdominal compartment syndrome (ACS) is most often the result of massive fluid resuscitation to treat hemorrhagic or septic shock. It can occur from fluid resuscitation in the ICU or OR. If attempts to close the fascia at the end of surgery cause increased airway pressures (measured on the ventilator), the patient has intraabdominal hypertension (IAH). In those cases, the fascia should be left open until the IAH remits. ACS is marked by multiorgan dysfunction that may progress to failure secondary to the anatomic effects of increased abdominal compartment pressure. Abdominal pressures can be estimated by measuring transmitted bladder pressures by connecting a pressure transducer to a clamped Foley catheter. In the nonobese patient, intraabdominal pressures higher than 30 mm Hg warrant surgical exploration and decompression. Obese patients may have elevated abdominal pressures at baseline, thus body habitus should be considered when evaluating the patient for ACS. Patients in extremis may be too unstable for transport and may need bedside exploration. Exploration mandates a midline abdominal incision large enough to release the compartment pressure.

PRACTICE POINT

- To assess for ACS, abdominal pressures can be estimated by measuring transmitted bladder pressures by connecting a pressure transducer to a clamped Foley catheter. In the nonobese patient, intraabdominal pressures higher than 30 mm Hg warrant surgical exploration and decompression. Obese patients may have elevated intraabdominal pressures at baseline.

When the abdominal fascia can not be closed safely because of concerns for the development of ACS, the patient is left with an open abdomen. The term open abdomen indicates that the fascia is not closed after surgery, and that the abdominal viscera are no longer covered by soft tissue. The abdomen is left open to avoid the development of ACS. Sometimes the patient is in extremis in the OR, and it is best to delay closure. At other times, reexploration is planned within a few days to remove packing left in the abdomen to achieve hemostasis or a "second-look" laparotomy is indicated to inspect ischemic bowel. The abdomen is usually contained with a Bogota bag or similar device. The *Bogota bag*, a term coined during the gun violence of the 1980s drug wars in Bogota, Colombia, consists of a nonadhesive plastic dressing covering the abdominal viscera, covered with some absorbent material such as a vacuum sponge, burn dressings, or gauze, followed by a plastic dressing that is attached to the skin by suture or adhesive. The entire dressing is placed to suction and drains excess abdominal fluid. Patients with an open abdomen can lose liters of insensible fluid through their abdomen each day, which should be accounted for in their volume management. Patients with an open abdomen are almost always intubated and sedated to minimize agitation and the risk of evisceration. Feeding with an open abdomen is controversial, but there are no clear contraindications to feeding the hemodynamically stable patient with bowel continuity. There is no indication for prophylactic antibiotics in this setting, but sterile management of the wound is imperative. Treatment of the open abdomen includes multiple trips to the operating room for washouts to prevent tertiary peritonitis and eventual abdominal wall reconstruction and delayed hernia repair.

Once the patient is stabilized, edema is improved, and no further laparotomies are anticipated, the abdomen can be closed. Primary closure is ideal but often impossible because the fascia retracts when left open for too many days. Closure may employ a variety of techniques tailored to the individual patient. Management of the wounds may be a multidisciplinary effort between general and plastic surgeons and wound care nurses. Damage control surgery is reserved for severely critically ill patients at high risk for ACS, rebleeding, or ongoing intestinal ischemia. Meticulous management of these patients impacts their surgical course and requires close communication between the surgeon and other physicians caring for these challenging patients.

QUALITY IMPROVEMENT

CHECKLISTS IN THE SICU

Checklists are being used with increasing frequency in complex health care settings to reduce medical errors and improve compliance with best practices. Checklists have been used with particular success in the ICU to reduce rates of bloodstream infections, achieve compliance with guidelines for thromboembolism prophylaxis, and clarify the daily goals of patient care. In one early use of checklists in the ICU, Pronovost and colleagues demonstrated that a comprehensive checklist of daily goals increased understanding of the care plan by nurses and house staff from 10% to 95% and cut the average length of stay in half. In a similar intervention that used a checklist during the insertion of central lines, catheter-related blood stream infections (CRBSI) were reduced from 11.3/1000 catheter days to 0/1000 catheter days. The improvement was sustained for a year after the intervention. It was estimated that the intervention prevented eight deaths. These checklists have been adopted in hospitals nationwide. In 2008 the Surgical Safety Checklist was launched by the World Health Organization. This program, which includes a safety check at three key stages of surgical procedures and has now been adopted worldwide, has been shown to drop hospital death rates and surgical infections. Checklists have been used to effectively address a number of complex health care problems and will play an increasingly prominent role in quality delivery and risk reduction.

PHYSICIAN STAFFING IN THE SICU

Traditionally, the surgical ICU has been an "open unit" where operating surgeons manage their patients while they are in the ICU. Increasingly, a "closed" or "hybrid" model, where the operating surgeon comanages their patients with an intensivist while the patient is in the ICU, has been promulgated as an effective model. The intensivist may be another surgeon, anesthesiologist, pulmonologist, internist, or Emergency Medicine physician. In this setting, the surgeon manages the wound, postoperative drains, and other factors that most directly affect surgical recovery, while

TABLE 139-2 Evidence-based Medicine Key References

Study	Methodology	Results	Limitations	Bottom Line
Epidemiology				
Friese, et al. *Care Med.* 2006;34(6):1597.	Retrospective database analysis	• Logistic regression analysis demonstrated decreased mortality when a pulmonary artery catheter (PAC) was used in the management of patients with the following severe injury characteristics: Injury Severity Score of 25–75, base deficit of less than −11, or age of 61–90 years.		Trauma patients managed with a PAC are more severely injured and have a higher mortality.
Sandham. *NEJM.* 2003;348:5–14.	Randomized trial	• A total of 77 of 997 patients who underwent surgery without the use of a PAC (7.7%) died in the hospital, as compared with 78 of 997 patients in whom PAC was used (7.8%). • There was a higher rate of pulmonary embolism in the catheter group than in the standard-care group. • The survival rates at 6 months among patients in the standard-care and catheter groups were 88.1% and 87.4%, respectively. At 12 months, the rates were 83.9% and 83.0%, respectively.	Only patients 60 years or older.	No benefit to therapy directed by PAC over standard care in elderly, high-risk surgical patients requiring intensive care.
Nuttall, et al. *Anesthesiology.* 2006;105: 198–208.	Practice guidelines	• Practice Guidelines for Perioperative Blood Transfusion and Adjuvant Therapies.	Practice guidelines are not intended as standards or absolute requirements. The use of practice guidelines cannot guarantee any specific outcome.	These guidelines focus on the perioperative management of patients undergoing surgery or other invasive procedures in which significant blood loss occurs or is expected.
Hébert, et al. *N Engl J Med.* 1999;340(6): 409–417.	Randomized controlled clinical trial.	• 838 patients were enrolled in the study. • 30-day mortality was similar in the restrictive-strategy group and the liberal-strategy group. • The rates were significantly lower with restrictive transfusion strategy among patients who were less acutely ill.	• Only 1 tertiary-level and 3 community intensive care units in Canada were included. • Study exluded age of less than 16 years; inability to receive blood products; active blood loss at the time of enrollment; chronic anemia; pregnancy; brain death or imminent death (within 24 hours).	A restrictive strategy of red-cell transfusion is at least as effective as, and possibly superior to, a liberal transfusion strategy in critically ill patients, with the possible exception of patients with acute myocardial infarction and unstable angina.
Holcomb, et al. *Ann Surg.* 2008;248(3): 447–458.	Retrospective cohort.	• Among 466 massive transfusion (MT) patients, survival varied by center from 41% to 74%. • Mean injury severity score varied by center from 22 to 40. • Thirty-day survival was increased in patients with high plasma: RBC ratio relative to those with low plasma: RBC ratio. • 30-day survival was increased in patients with high platelet: RBC ratio relative to those with low platelet: RBC ratio.	• Only plasma and platelets levels were recorded	Massive transfusion practice guidelines should aim for a 1:1:1 ratio of plasma: platelets: RBCs.
Jaber, et al. *Crit Care.* 2009;13(2):R49.	Meta-analysis of randomized controlled trials.	• Seven prospective, randomized, double-blinded trials, including 1846 patients, (949 of which received steroids) were selected. • Steroids significantly decreased the risk of reintubation. • The effect of steroids on reintubation and stridor was more pronounced for selected high-risk patients, as determined by a reduced cuff-leak volume.	• Only adults included. • Evaluation based on reintubation mainly.	The benefit of steroids remains unclear when patients at high risk are not selected.

(continued)

TABLE 139-2 Evidence-based Medicine Key References (*continued*)

Study	Methodology	Results	Limitations	Bottom Line
Epidemiology				
Ely, et al. *JAMA.* 2004;291(14): 1753–1762.	Prospective cohort study.	• Of 275 patients, 51 (18.5%) had persistent coma and died in the hospital. • Patients who developed delirium had higher 6-month mortality rates (34% versus 15%, $p = .03$) and spent 10 days longer in the hospital than those who never developed delirium.	Small study *N*.	Delirium was an independent predictor of higher 6-month mortality and longer hospital stay even after adjusting for relevant covariates including coma, sedatives, and analgesics in patients receiving mechanical ventilation.
McClave, et al. ASPEN. *Guidelines in Adult Critically Ill JPEN.* 2009;33:277.	Guidelines	• Guidelines for the Provision and Assessment of Nutrition Support Therapy in the Adult Critically Ill Patient.		Practice guidelines are not intended as absolute requirements. The use of these practice guidelines does not in any way project or guarantees any specific benefit in outcome or survival.
Beltrame, et al. *Minerva Anestesiol.* 2008;74(10): 529–535.	A cohort study.	• 528 mechanically ventilated patients underwent tracheostomy at the bedside. • Percutaneous dilational tracheostomy (PDT) was performed more rapidly than surgical tracheostomy (ST). • The overall ICU stay and mean duration of mechanical ventilation were lower in the PDT than in the ST group. • There were no statistically significant differences in ICU and hospital outcome between the two techniques.	Only two ICUs included.	PDT is associated with a shorter duration of mechanical ventilation and a reduced ICU length of stay.

the intensivist manages the ventilator, vascular access, nutritional status, and infectious issues. Obviously, significant overlap in care domains occurs, and aggressive communication from all care providers is paramount to an optimal patient outcome. The operating surgeon, who will usually be the attending of record, should be notified of any changes in the patient's condition and any plans for interventions. Alternately, the surgical team should notify the critical care service with any significant changes in plans or clinical expectations. With the aging population and increasing complexity and specialization of surgery, critical care management is increasingly a team approach with intensivists comanaging these complex and critically ill patients with the surgeons. Excellent and frequent communication optimizes patient care (**Table 139-2**).

CONCLUSION

Patients in the surgical intensive care unit require monitoring to either prevent postoperative morbidity and mortality or treat complications that have already occurred. Like all intensive care unit patients, SICU patients benefit from multi-disciplinary, evidence-based, quality-driven care. Hospitalists should recognize that as compared to medical patients, strategies for volume resuscitation, blood product transfusion, and nutritional supplementation may differ in surgical patients due to their unique physiology. To provide the best care for the patient, treating physicians need to understand the patient's surgical procedure, indications for that procedure, and the expected postoperative course. Communication among all treating physicians and caregivers helps achieve the best possible outcomes.

SUGGESTED READINGS

Lawrence VA, Cornell JE, Smetana GW. American College of Physicians. Strategies to reduce postoperative pulmonary complications after noncardiothoracic surgery: systematic review for the American College of Physicians. *Ann Intern Med.* 2006;144(8):596–608.

Osland E, Yunus R, Khan S, Memon MA. Early enteral nutrition within 24 h of intestinal surgery versus later commencement of feeding: a systematic review and meta-analysis. *J Gastrointest Surg.* 2009;13(3):569–575.

Rapoport J, Teres D, Steingrub J, Higgins T, McGee W, Lemeshow S. Patient characteristics and ICU organizational factors that influence frequency of pulmonary artery catheterization. *JAMA.* 2000;283(19):2559–2567.

Sagraves SG, Toschlog EA, Rotondo MF. Damage control surgery—the intensivist's role. *J Intensive Care Med.* 2006;21(1):5–16.

Spinella PC, Holcomb JB. Resuscitation and transfusion principles for traumatic hemorrhagic shock. *Blood Rev.* 2009;23(6):231–240.

CHAPTER 140

The Family Meeting in the ICU

Allison S. Friedenberg, MD
Mitchell M. Levy, MD, FCCM, FCCP
J. Randall Curtis, MD, MPH

Key Clinical Questions

1. When should the ICU clinicians meet with the family of a critically ill patient and how should these meetings be conducted?
2. Who should be included in an ICU family meeting?
3. What are the elements of shared decision making?
4. How should ICU clinicians discuss prognosis with ICU patients and their families, and specifically, how should the clinicians break the bad news?

INTRODUCTION

In the United States, approximately 20% of all deaths occur in the intensive care unit (ICU) each year. Critically ill patients frequently lack decisional capacity and the ability to express their preferences for treatment, and thus decisions regarding goals of care often involve family members. In these circumstances the concept of surrogate decision making is enacted, which generally involves a person, often a family member, who knows the values and preferences of the incapacitated patient and who is willing to serve as a surrogate decision maker. However, prior studies have reported poor communication and conflicting goals of care between ICU clinicians and patients' families. Communicating effectively and compassionately with families will help improve medical decision making for the patient and improve family outcomes after the critical illness of a loved one. The ICU family conference is a central component of this communication. This chapter provides a framework of how to plan, structure, and lead an effective meeting with families of critically ill patients.

IMPACT OF A FAMILY MEETING

MEDICAL DECISION MAKING

Relatives, partners, and friends often provide support and care for a patient, which for some will include the responsibility of surrogate decision making. Surrogate decision makers bear an enormous amount of emotional stress, and decision making during these circumstances can be difficult. In addition, one study revealed that despite discussions with ICU physicians, only half of families of critically ill patients adequately understood their relatives' diagnoses, prognoses, or treatments. Despite this, clinicians and health systems often neglect the care of the family as part of the overall care of a patient.

PRACTICE POINT

- Families and physicians function interdependently, and their partnership must be established in order to make good medical decisions and provide optimal care for the patient.

The American Medical Association endorses an interdependence of families and physicians, and their partnership must be established in order to make good medical decisions and provide optimal care for the patient. High quality ICU care depends on effective clinician-family communication to improve the family members' level of understanding and their ability to provide surrogate decision making that accurately reflects the wishes of the patient.

FAMILY OUTCOMES: ANXIETY, DEPRESSION, POSTTRAUMATIC STRESS DISORDER

Up to 25% of families report dissatisfaction with their communication with ICU caregivers. Furthermore, the approach to communication may cause anxiety, depression, and posttraumatic stress disorder among family members. Many physicians who work in critical care units conduct family meetings only after ICU patients are actively dying. However, critical care teams should meet with all families of ICU patients early during the ICU stay. In fact, family members of patients who survive the ICU also have a high burden of anxiety and depression and are more dissatisfied with communication in the ICU than family members of patients who die. Interventions have been developed and evaluated that can reduce the symptom burden of families in the ICU. One randomized trial demonstrated that a structured family meeting in conjunction with an informational brochure about the dying process results in a significant reduction in anxiety, depression, and posttraumatic stress reaction among family members.

INTERDISCIPLINARY TEAM COLLABORATION

While the methods of physician communication with families can have a significant impact on satisfaction, interdisciplinary communication also has a significant impact on important patient and family outcomes. Observational studies show increased survival, shorter ICU lengths of stay, and improved patient satisfaction when nurses and physicians communicate effectively. In addition, patients and families have reported that interdisciplinary communication plays an important role in end-of-life care, and existing studies demonstrate that most interventions that improve end-of-life care include an interdisciplinary team in the intervention.

COMPOSITION OF FAMILY MEETINGS

In the initial steps in planning a family meeting clinicians should define who should be involved in the process. They must identify who the "family members" are for the patient and who among them should be involved in this process. To answer this question, the clinician must identify any assigned health care proxy or durable power of attorney for health care. If there has been no designation, or if the designation is unknown, then the legal next of kin should be located. Definitions of legal decision makers vary state by state and hospitalists should refer to local and state statutes or risk management departments to help determine legal next of kin. When approaching either the proxy or the legal next of kin to schedule a family meeting, the clinician should determine who that person believes is important to attend the meeting. Sometimes, others involved in the patient's life can contribute information about who should be involved in decision making. When patients have large families, an effective meeting with all family members present may prove challenging. Nonetheless, all family members who desire to participate should be involved, and, in these circumstances it may be beneficial to seek the assistance of other, skilled members of the interdisciplinary team, such as a social worker, clinical psychologist, or ethicist.

The large interdisciplinary team—including consulting physicians, nurses, social workers, and spiritual care providers—that provides care for ICU patients frequently know the patient and family from different perspectives, and holding a meeting without attempting to have all relevant members present may result in miscommunication and missed opportunities to provide families with the best possible resources.

Holding an initial family meeting within 72 hours of ICU admission reduces the number of ICU days (by one day on average) and improves ratings of quality of dying by family members of ICU patients. Therefore, meeting with the family within 72 hours, and ideally within the initial 24 hours of admission can maintain high quality ICU care.

The location of the family meeting can augment the family experience. The chaotic ICU environment, with constant noise from alarms and frequent disruptions due to patient care interventions, can overwhelm families who may not retain the information or have difficulty discussing their concerns and emotions at the bedside. If no dedicated family conference room is available, the physician should find a private, quiet place away from the patient room, and large enough to accommodate the family and the members of the interdisciplinary team.

PRACTICE POINT

- The ideal location for a family meeting in the ICU is a dedicated family conference room or a private, quiet place away from the patient room. Meeting with the family at the bedside should be discouraged except when the patient is able to participate.

DECISION MAKING ABOUT LIFE-SUSTAINING TREATMENTS

The approach to decision making about life-sustaining treatments in the ICU can vary from "patient autonomy"—or more commonly surrogate autonomy—on one end of the spectrum to "parentalism" on the other end of the spectrum. Although many patients desire autonomy, when it comes to decisions about life-sustaining therapy in the ICU, often the decisions fall to the surrogate. In the extreme, the autonomy model may make family members feel like they are being abandoned and may place unnecessary stress on the family. On the other hand, the extreme parentalism model takes all decisions away from the patient and family, limiting the input of their values and perspectives in decision making. The model of shared decision making encourages clinicians and patients or surrogates to communicate and exchange information and come to a decision jointly. In 2005, five European and North American critical care societies issued a joint statement supporting the model of shared decision making when caring for ICU patients.

PRACTICE POINT

- The model of shared decision making encourages clinicians and patients or surrogates to communicate and exchange information and come to a decision jointly.

Multiple components in the shared decision model are essential to have an adequate exchange of information and to make joint decisions with the family (**Table 140-1**). Although the shared decision making model is the preferred model, clinicians may need to adjust it based on unique patient and family situations. As circumstances and prognosis change, the role the family wishes to play may change. Therefore, the initial meeting should model shared decision making, beginning with the exchange of information regarding the status of the patient and the patient's treatment preferences, followed by an assessment of the role the family wishes to play in the decision making process.

The decision making model should adjust dynamically and may change several times throughout the course of an ICU stay. As patients become more critically ill and fail to reach certain milestones, such as extubation, the physician should be willing to respond to the needs of the family and, when family members are struggling with responsibility for such decisions, be willing to actively relieve them of the burden of the decision making process.

PRACTICE POINT

- As patients become more critically ill and the prognosis is more certain, the physician should be willing to take on a more active role in the decision making process in order to relieve the family of the burden of decision making in these circumstances.

TABLE 140-1 Dimensions of Shared Decision Making

	Example Physician Behaviors and Questions
Providing medical information and eliciting patient values and preferences	Discuss nature of decision *What are the essential clinical issues we are addressing?* Describe alternatives and pros/cons *What are the clinically reasonable choices and the pros and cons of each treatment choice?* Discuss prognosis and uncertainty *What is the likelihood of success of treatment and how confident are we in this estimate?* Assess understanding *Is the family now an "informed participant," with a working understanding of the decision?* Explore patient's values/preferences *What is known about the patient's medical preferences or values? What is important to the patient?*
Exploring the family's preferred role in decision making	Discuss family's role *What role should the family play in making the decision?* Assess desire for others' input *Is there anyone else the family would like to consult?*
Deliberation and decision-making	Explore "context" *How will the decision impact the patient's life?* If the family is to participate in decision making, elicit family opinion about best treatment choice *What does the family think is the most appropriate decision for the patient?*

KEY STRATEGIES FOR FAMILY MEETINGS

A simplified outline of the elements used to plan and execute a family meeting should be utilized (**Figure 140-1**).

Prior to meeting with the family, a brief preconference meeting involving all members of the interdisciplinary team provides an opportunity to share information about the patient and family and will assure that all members of the health care team have a shared understanding of the diagnosis, prognosis, prognostic uncertainty, and indicated treatments. A frequent cause of families' dissatisfaction with ICU care is receiving inconsistent information from different members of the health care team. Although a preconference requires some additional time, this preplanning may actually save time by allowing the actual meeting to be more efficient and effective. This preconference is also a time during which conflicts or controversial issues surrounding the patient's care can be discussed and resolved prior to meeting with the family.

FACILITATE COMMUNICATION

After the preconference is held, a time and place should be scheduled to meet with the interdisciplinary team and the appropriate members of the family. In the beginning of any family meeting, all members present should be introduced by name and their role or relation to the patient described.

PRACTICE POINT

- In the beginning of any family meeting, all members present should be introduced by name and their role or relation to the patient described.

After introductions, clinicians leading the meeting should express empathy for the family and patient. Empathic statements by physicians have been associated with increased family satisfaction and encourage openness and trust at the beginning of the meeting. The three most common types of empathic statements that may be appropriate in this setting (depending on what has been discussed with the family) include those that explicitly acknowledge the difficulty of being a surrogate decision maker, the difficulty of having a critically ill loved one, and the sorrow of contemplating a loved one's death.

PRACTICE POINT

Examples of empathic statements:

1. "It is extremely difficult to be in a position to have to put your own wishes aside in order to think about what your Dad would want if he could tell us."
2. "I can imagine how painful this must be for you to watch someone you care so much about be so sick."
3. "I know it must be really sad to think about losing your Mom, but I can promise you that she will not suffer. We will be here right here with her, and with you."
4. "I understand that it feels really unfair when bad things are happening to someone you care about so much. It's a very helpless feeling."

LISTEN AND BREAK BAD NEWS

Exchange of medical information usually occurs early in a family meeting. Clinicians should start the meeting by *allowing the family to describe what they understand about the status of their loved one* and, when the family has a story to tell, allow the family to speak without interruptions. Family members are more satisfied with communication when clinicians spend less time talking and more time listening. Allowing the family to express their concerns and provide information about their loved one helps the team identify the needs of the family and the goals of care for the patient.

PRACTICE POINT

- Clinicians should start the family meeting by allowing the family to describe what they understand about the status of their loved one and allow the family to speak without interruptions.

Allowing the family to talk uninterrupted may cause physicians and other members of the team to experience the emotions of the family and often requires the caregivers to think about death in a way that makes many uncomfortable. The ability to listen closely to the family takes discipline and patience. The skills needed to deal with death and the uncertainty about death require self-reflection about the process of dying, and ultimately, consideration of the possibility of one's own death.

Studies suggest that physicians often do not discuss prognosis with patients or family in part because of uncertainty. Even in the context of uncertainty, treating physicians have the obligation to provide prognostic information to patients and their families.

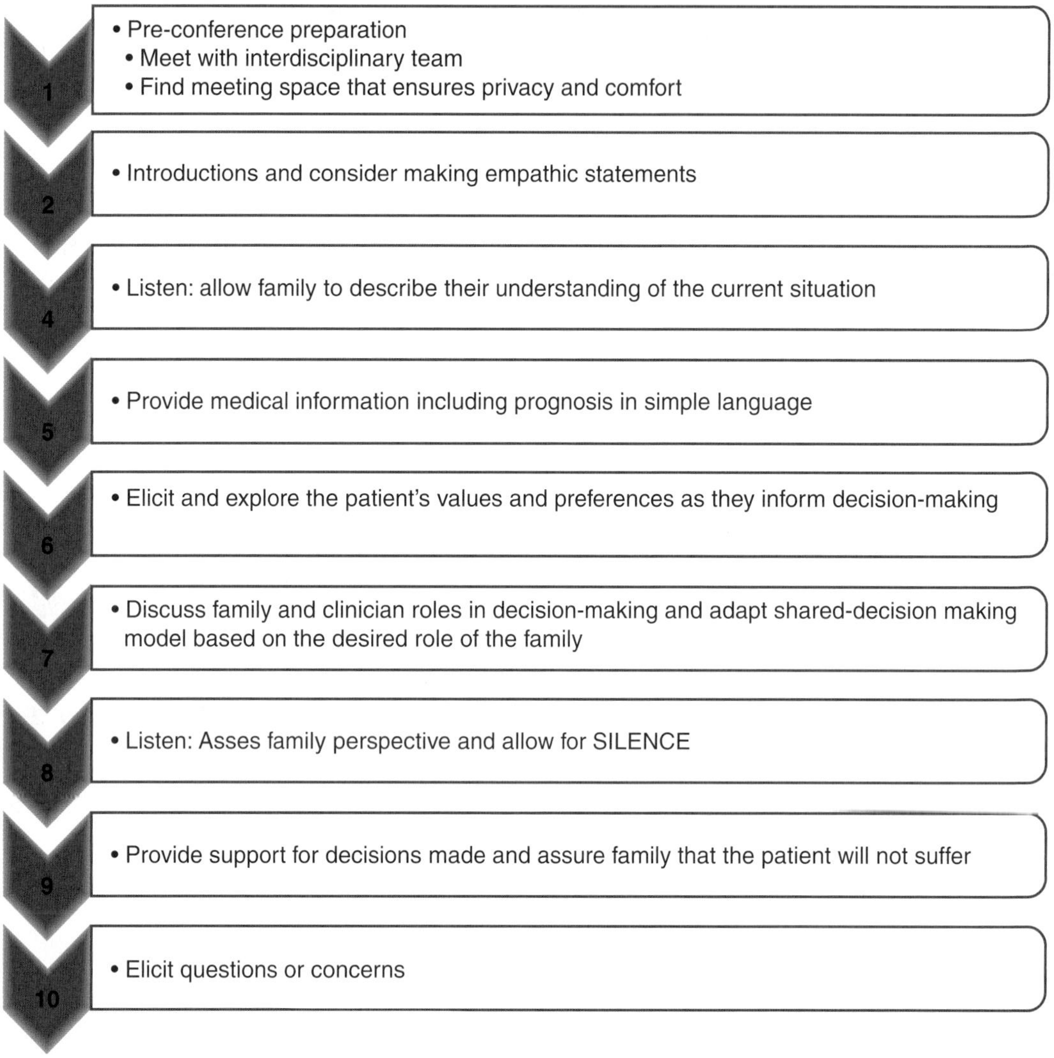

Figure 140-1 *Organizational process for an ICU family meeting.*

> **PRACTICE POINT**
>
> - When conducting prognostic discussions, clinicians should utilize numeric expressions of risk—which lead to better understanding of prognosis—rather than vague qualitative expressions.
>
>   Recommended: "Your Dad has a number of organs that are not working, and 80% of people as sick as your Dad do not survive."
>
>   Not recommended: "Your Dad is very sick and overall his chance of survival is poor."

Many physicians avoid using the word "death" for fear of causing hopelessness or provoking more suffering; however, families have greater difficulty accepting death if they never heard it or understood it to be a possibility. Even if it seems obvious to the physicians that death is a possibility, it is important for the term "death" to be explicitly stated to the family. Using expressions like "pass away" may be misunderstood by families. Simple language and information when talking with families also facilitate better understanding, and clinicians should describe which organ systems are not working. For example, stating: "Your father's lungs aren't working, which is why he is on the breathing machine, sometimes called a respirator or ventilator, and his kidneys are failing. When patients are as sick as your father, 90% of them will die." Families may ask more specific medical questions, but it is generally important to start by using the most simple language and information.

When clinicians allow for silence and serve as patient listeners during the information exchange, the family meeting allows families to process information and time to develop and ask questions. Rushing through a family meeting by filling the silence will only undermine the goal of the meeting, as families will leave feeling unheard and with unanswered questions. This may result in flawed surrogate decision making due to miscommunication, and treatments provided may not reflect the values of the patient.

After this process of exchanging medical information is complete, clinicians need to assess the family's understanding of the information. Families often do not understand the diagnoses or prognoses despite meeting with physicians. Therefore, any misunderstandings can be discovered by asking family members to repeat back the diagnoses and prognoses as they understand them, and then be resolved prior to proceeding to medical decision making.

PRACTICE POINT

- Rushing through a family meeting by filling the silence will only undermine the goal of the meeting, as families will leave feeling unheard and with unanswered questions. When clinicians allow for silence and serve as patient listeners during the information exchange, the family meeting is often more effective.

After the assessment of understanding, clinicians may transition to discuss the patient's values and preferences, so that the care team can understand the patient's preferences if the patient is unable to participate in the discussion. In this context, the family attempts to provide substituted judgment based on previously stated preferences and values of the patient. Surrogate decision makers should be encouraged to recall information about what the patient would want, rather than use their own wishes for the patient as the basis for decision-making. Clinicians should specifically ask the surrogate(s) if they ever had conversations with the patient about what they would want regarding life sustaining treatments, or if they ever made reference to others who had to make similar decisions. When surrogates are unsure about what the patient would want, clinicians can explore what was important for the patient's quality of life prior to coming to the hospital. This process of "evoking" the patient's values from surrogates can often serve to alleviate anxiety around surrogate decision making.

PRACTICE POINT

- Surrogate decision makers should be encouraged to recall information about what the patient would want, rather than use their own wishes for the patient as the basis for decision making.

After discussing the patient's values and goals for treatment, the clinician should next assess the role the family wishes to play in terms of medical decision making. Families can simply be asked how involved they want to be in making the medical decisions for their loved one, although families may feel uncomfortable saying they do not want to be involved. Clinicians may offer this option more directly if the family gives indications that they would prefer not to be directly involved in decisions. The decision making role can change over time and can be revisited as frequently as necessary, especially when there is a change in the patient's status.

Finally, clinicians should forge an agreement with family members about the plans for treatment that reflect the patient's preferences. When there is uncertainty about the desire for or effectiveness of aggressive life-sustaining therapies, clinicians should consider introducing a "time-limited trial of therapy" that may alleviate concerns about prolonged, ineffective care. For example, the physician may recommend a trial of life-sustaining therapy for 48 hours, but if at that time the patient is not improving or is getting worse, the team and family will meet again and the focus may shift toward comfort measures.

Physicians and other clinicians should reassure the family that no matter what decisions are made, the patient will not be allowed to suffer and will not be abandoned. In addition, the family should understand that the plan can change depending on the outcomes of the interventions. Prior to concluding the family meeting, the meeting leader should ask the family if anyone has any other questions or needs that can be addressed.

PRACTICE POINT

- During the final decision making process physicians and other clinicians should reassure the family that no matter what decisions are made, the patient will not be allowed to suffer and will not be abandoned.

DISCUSSING WITHDRAWAL OF LIFE-SUSTAINING TREATMENT

If the decision is made to withdraw life-sustaining therapy, clinicians should emphasize several important points to family members:

1. Life-sustaining therapy was not able to reverse the underlying disease.
2. The surrogate decision makers and the ICU team did "everything they could" for their loved one.
3. The removal of life-sustaining therapy is allowing the disease to take its natural course.
4. Aggressive therapy in the form of palliative care will be provided to ensure the patient's comfort.

PRACTICE POINT

- Clinicians should appreciate that "life-sustaining therapies," not "care" is being withdrawn. Therefore, the phrase "withdrawal of care" should not be used.

When clinicians and families decide to withdraw life-sustaining therapy, physicians should provide education to families about the likely time from withdrawal of life support to death and the variability and uncertainty in determining this time frame, as well as treatments available to prevent or treat pain, dyspnea, and suffering during the withdrawal of life-sustaining therapy. (See Chapter 219 Care of the Imminently Dying Patient.)

QUALITY IMPROVEMENT

Many interventions that have demonstrated benefit to improve care for ICU patients are incorporated as a standard procedure or protocol within the ICU. Utilization of a protocol for family conferences will encourage consistency across the ICU and help prevent oversights and miscommunication. Obviously, communication with families cannot be performed in a manner in which the team appears rigid or uncaring. Each individual patient and family functions differently and must be treated individually. Nevertheless, key components of the family conference should be systematically applied in an individualized way. A simple mnemonic features five key elements to help guide clinicians in communicating with families: VALUE (**Figure 140-2**). As demonstrated in clinical studies, the use and implementation of the facets and principles of this mnemonic reduces anxiety, depression, and posttraumatic stress reaction in families (**Table 140-2**).

CONCLUSION

In the ICU, patients receive some of the most advanced medical care available. Experts from all specialties and disciplines collaborate to make medical decisions, perform procedures, and apply life-sustaining treatments. Equally important to patients and their loved ones is effective and frequent communication and interaction with members of the interdisciplinary ICU team to determine the goals of care. ICU clinicians can meet the diverse needs of patients and their families in the ICU by using empathy, effective listening skills, and an adaptable model of shared decision making. Focusing on

VALUE - 5-step approach to Improving Communication with Families in the ICU	
V	Value family statements
A	Acknowledge family emotions
L	Listen to the family
U	Understand the patient as a person
E	Elicit family questions

Figure 140-2 *VALUE: A five-step approach to improving communication with families in the ICU.*

TABLE 140-2 Evidence-based Medicine: Key References for ICU Family Meetings

Reference	Methodology	Results	Limitations	Bottom Line
Lautrette A, et al. A communication Strategy and brochure for relatives of patients dying in the ICU. *NEJM.* 2007;356:469–478.	Randomized trial of structured family meeting and bereavement brochure vs. customary end of life conference in 126 families of ICU patients.	The intervention group had lower PTSD-related symptoms (45% vs. 69%), anxiety (45% vs. 67%), and depression (29% vs. 56%). Withdrawal of life-sustaining therapies was more common in intervention group than control (mechanical ventilator withdrawal 27% vs. 14%)	The study was performed in France, where the physician-patient relationship is perceived as more parentalistic than in other countries. Unknown how many families actually read the brochure and what that impact may be. PTSD, anxiety, and depression scores were not evaluated before the intervention.	Utilizing a structured approach for meetings with families of ICU patients predicted to die and the use of a bereavement brochure reduces PTSD-related symptoms, anxiety, and depression in family members of ICU patients. This approach also reduces the use of nonbeneficial life-sustaining therapies.
White D, et al. Toward Shared Decision Making at the End of Life in Intensive Care Units: Opportunities for Improvement. *Arch Intern Med.* 2007;167:461–467.	Observational study evaluating 51 family-physician conferences to assess for shared decision making and to measure the association of shared decision making with family satisfaction.	Only 2% of all decisions met all criteria for shared decision making. The least frequently addressed elements were the family's role in decision making (31%), and the family's understanding of the decision (25%). Lower family educational level was associated with less shared decision making. Higher levels of shared decision making were significantly associated with greater family satisfaction.	Only 46% of families who were eligible to have their physician conference audio-taped agreed to enroll. Knowledge of being audio-taped may alter the behavior and communication of physicians and families.	Physicians rarely incorporate all of the elements of shared decision making. Physicians often do not assess what role the family prefers to have in the decision making process. Shared decision making results in higher levels of family satisfaction.
Azoulay E, et al. Meeting the Needs of Intensive Care Unit Patient Families. A Multicenter Study. *Am J Respir Crit Care Med.* 2001;163:135–139.	Prospective study evaluating family satisfaction in 920 family members of 637 ICU patients.	There were seven predictors of family satisfaction: family members of French descent, knowledge by family members of the specific role of each caregiver in the ICU, patient to nurse ratio ≤ 3, information provided by a junior physician, no perceived contradictions in information given by caregivers, adequate time spent by caregivers providing information, and help from the primary doctor.	The study was performed in France, where the decision making model is often perceived as more parentalistic and therefore the results may not pertain to families in other countries. Survey bias may exist based on those who did not complete the surveys.	Six of the seven predictors of improved family members' satisfaction are related to the ICU clinician. Explaining the roles of each ICU clinician and spending more time providing consistent information about the patient's condition results in improved family satisfaction.

effective and timely communication and utilizing a communication protocol (Figure 140-2) to help facilitate family meetings allow for consistency and efficiency in medical decision making that best reflects the wishes of patients and facilitates provision of the highest quality of critical care.

SUGGESTED READINGS

Curtis JR, Rubenfeld GD. *Managing Death in the Intensive Care Unit: The Transition from Cure to Comfort.* New York, NY: *Oxford University Press Inc.*; 2001.

Curtis JR, Rubenfeld GD. Improving palliative care for patients in the intensive care unit. *J Palliat Med.* 2005;8:840–854.

Curtis JR and White DB. Practical Guidance for Evidence-Based ICU Family Conferences. *Chest.* 2008;134:835–843.

Davidson JE, Powers K, Hedayat KM, et al. Clinical practice guidelines for support of the family in the patient-centered intensive care unit: American College of Critical Care Medicine Task Force 2004–2005. *Crit Care Med.* 2007;35:605–622.

Lautrette A, Darmon M, Megarbane B, et al. A communication strategy and brochure for relatives of patients dying in the ICU. *N Engl J Med.* 2007;356:469–478.

Stapleton RD, Engelber RA, Wenrich MD, et al. Clinician statements and family satisfaction with family conferences in the intensive care unit. *Crit Care Med.* 2006;43:1679–1685.

Truog RD, Campbell ML, Curtis JR, et al. Recommendations for end-of-life care in the intensive care unit: A consensus statement by the American Academy of Critical Care Medicine. *Crit Care Med.* 2008;36:953–963.

Vincent, JL. Communication in the ICU. *Intensive Care Med.* 1997;23: 1093–1098.

SECTION 4

Dermatology

CHAPTER 141

Flushing and Urticaria

Lisa M. Grandinetti, MD
Timothy J. Patton, DO
Joseph C. English III, MD

Key Clinical Questions

1. What mechanisms cause cutaneous flushing?
2. How does one differentiate benign and malignant etiologies of flushing?
3. What tests and studies are useful to evaluate each potential diagnosis?
4. What treatments are available for each etiology?
5. What is the difference between acute and chronic urticaria?
6. What are the common causes of acute urticaria and chronic urticaria?
7. What is the appropriate workup for patients with acute or chronic urticaria?
8. In what clinical scenario is a skin biopsy indicated?
9. What is the appropriate workup when vasculitis is present on skin histology?
10. What therapies are available for acute and chronic urticaria?

FLUSHING: CLINICAL MANIFESTATIONS AND CAUSES

Flushing results from vasodilation in the skin, produced by release of vasoactive mediators or activity of the vasomotor nerves. It is characterized by sudden warmth and visible erythema, affecting the head (**Figure 141-1**), neck, and upper chest, regions of abundant superficial cutaneous vasculature. Flushing may be episodic or constant. When persistent, it may produce fixed facial erythema with a cyanotic tinge, secondary to the development of telangiectasias and large cutaneous blood vessels, containing slow-moving, deoxygenated blood (**Figure 141-2**).

The overwhelming majority of patients with flushing have common and relatively innocuous causes, with only a small proportion of cases being associated with tumors and other significant underlying medical problems (**Table 141-1**).

BENIGN CUTANEOUS FLUSHING

Flushing is most often physiologic (benign cutaneous flushing). It is more common in women than men. Common precipitants include fever, exercise, warm temperatures, spicy foods, and alcohol. In fair-skinned persons, flushing (or blushing) often occurs in response to strong emotion, which perhaps evolved as a nonverbal means to express arousal or display vigor. Although blushing historically was thought attractive, it may produce anxiety and distress in some contemporary patients.

ROSACEA

Rosacea is characterized by acneiform inflammation of the central face, with erythema, flushing episodes, telangiectasias, and often papules and pustules. Eye lesions, such as blepharitis, conjunctivitis, episcleritis, and keratitis with corneal ulcers also occur. It is common in fair-skinned patients of middle age; the prevalence among Caucasian women in the United States is approximately 16%. The etiology is unknown. There seems to be a genetic predisposition. *Helicobacter pylori* and the face mite *Demodex folliculorum* have been invoked as possible causes, with equivocal data. Antimicrobial peptides (AMPs) have also been suggested to play a role. These peptides, such as cathelicidins and beta-defensins, are components of the innate immune system, with broad antimicrobial activity. They are released with any injury to the skin. LL-37 canthelicidin is expressed in abnormally high amounts in the skin of rosacea patients, compared to controls. When LL-37 has been injected into the skin of mice, the mice demonstrate a phenotype similar to rosacea patients, with erythema, inflammation and telangiectasias. Rosacea must be distinguished from systemic lupus erythematosus and photosensitivity eruptions. Rosacea is confined to the face; extrafacial lesions suggest another etiology.

CLIMACTERIC FLUSHING

Climacteric flushing occurs in 50% to 85% of menopausal women not taking estrogen replacement. It may be experienced as a wave of heat radiating outward from the upper body, and typically lasting 3 to 4 minutes. Skin temperature is elevated about 1°C during hot flashes, and heart rate also rises. The physiology is poorly understood, but may relate to changes in hypothalamic thermoregulation associated with fluctuations in estrogen levels. Episodes are often associated with the same

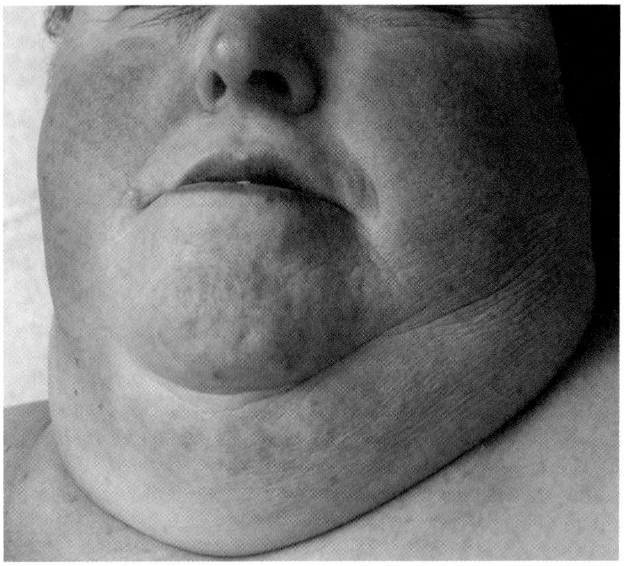

Figure 141-1 *Acute flushing.*

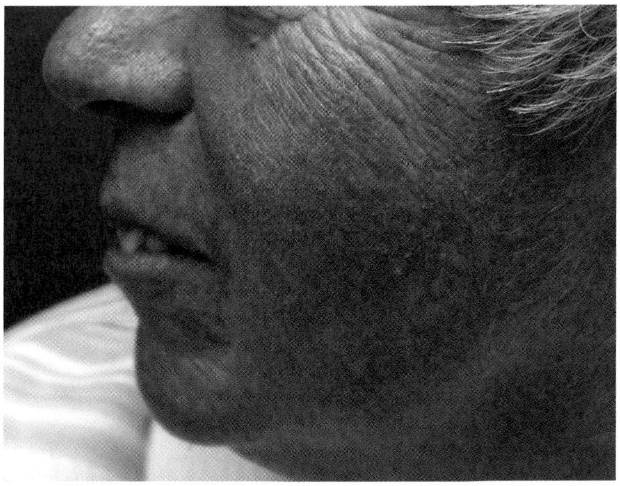

Figure 141-2 *Chronic persistent flushing.*

precipitants as benign physiologic flushing, but they may also be unprovoked. If frequent, concentration and sleep may be disturbed, and depression and fatigue may result. Lifestyle measures, including keeping the body cool and avoiding triggers, may be helpful. Estrogen replacement is the most effective drug therapy, but should only be prescribed after a detailed discussion of risks and benefits.

TABLE 141-1 Differential Diagnosis of Flushing

Common benign flushing
Benign cutaneous flushing
Emotion, fever, hyperthermia, psychiatric or anxiety disorders, ingestion of food and alcoholic beverage, idiopathic
Rosacea
Climacterium
Iatrogenic (medications related)
Niacin, calcium channel blockers, beta-blockers, nitroglycerin, sildenafil citrate, ACE inhibitors, vancomycin, NSAIDs, chemotherapeutic agents, morphine and other opioids (partial list)
Uncommon to rare potentially life-threatening flushing
Carcinoid syndrome
Pheochromocytoma
Systemic mastocytosis
Anaphylaxis
Medullary thyroid carcinoma
Pancreatic islet cell tumor (VIPoma)
Renal cell carcinoma
Histamine fish poisoning
Ciguatera fish poisoning
Neurologic disorders
Parkinson disease, dysautonomia and orthostatic hypotension, migraines, multiple sclerosis, brain tumors, epilepsy, autonomic hyperreflexia, Horner syndrome, Frey syndrome

DRUGS, ALCOHOL, AND FOODS

All vasodilator drugs, such as nitroglycerine, sildenafil, and calcium channel blockers, may lead to flushing. Niacin-induced flushing is due to the subcutaneous release of prostaglandin D2, along with the formation of vasodilatory prostanoids. Morphine and other opiates may trigger histamine release from mast cells, leading to flushing. Sulfonylurea drugs interfere with the metabolism of alcohol, leading to acetaldehyde-related flushing when these patients imbibe alcohol.

Alcohol and its metabolite acetaldehyde are both vasodilators and may lead to flushing. Wines may contain several substances which provoke flushing, including tyramine, histamine, and sulfites. Asian populations have a prevalence rate of alcohol-related facial flushing of up to 36%, often related to an inherited deficiency of aldehyde dehydrogenase 2, which leads to a buildup of acetaldehyde. Spicy foods and foods containing tyramine (aged cheeses and meats, soy products), sulfites (wines, dried fruits), or nitrites (cured meats) may lead to flushing. Flushing from scombroid poisoning (histamine fish poisoning) results from eating fish which has been left at room temperature too long, leading to conversion of histidine to histamine by surface bacteria. It is not a true allergy.

NEOPLASMS

An uncommon cause of flushing, **carcinoid tumors** are, in general, quite rare and occur in approximately 2 per 100,000 people. Carcinoid syndrome occurs in about 10% of patients with carcinoid tumors. Carcinoid syndrome (CS) occurs in approximately 10% of all patients with carcinoid tumors. Flushing is the most frequent clinical sign, appearing in up to 95% of patients at some point during the course of their disease. The likelihood of flushing in carcinoid syndrome is dependent on the production of tumor-derived mediators such as 5-hydroxytryptamine and substance P and on the anatomic location of the carcinoid tumor. The flushing associated with CS is distinctive, occurring as well-defined, intensely pruritic reddish-brown wheals all over the body, including the palms and soles.

The annual incidence of **pheochromocytoma** in the United States is estimated to be approximately 500 to 1100 cases per year. Medullary carcinoma of the thyroid gland, another uncommon malignancy associated with flushing, is a tumor of the parafollicular, or C cells, of the thyroid gland and accounts for approximately 5% to 8% of all thyroid tumors. Pancreatic VIPoma, a neuroendocrine tumor of the pancreatic islet cells, is associated with watery diarrhea, abdominal pain, and flushing. VIPoma occurs at a rate of approximately 0.05 to 0.2 new cases per million adults.

Systemic mastocytosis is a condition that presents with increased mast cells in the skin and visceral organs. When the mast cells degranulate, they release many mediators including histamine, which as discussed above, is believed to cause flushing through its vasodilatory effect on vascular smooth muscle.

Malignant causes, such as pheochromocytoma produce flushing by the elevated production of endogenous catecholamines. These substances are well-described mediators of flushing when administered exogenously.

Medullary carcinoma of the thyroid gland produces calcitonin and carcinoembryonic antigen (CEA). The flushing associated with this entity is believed to be due to the overproduction of these products, especially calcitonin. Flushing, and diarrhea, can sometimes be the presenting symptoms of medullary thyroid cancer.

Pancreatic islet cell tumors are neuroendocrine tumors of the gut and include insulinoma, gastrinoma, glucagonoma, somatostatinoma and VIPoma. VIPoma, a tumor of the delta cells of the pancreas, specifically produces increased amounts of vasoactive intestinal peptide (VIP). VIP relaxes vascular smooth muscle which produces the cutaneous flush associated with this tumor.

ANAPHYLAXIS

An uncommon but potentially life-threatening cause of flushing is anaphylaxis. Acute anaphylaxis is mediated by the massive release of histamine and prostaglandin D2, as well as tryptase, to a lesser degree. It is felt that both histamine and prostaglandin D2, through its vasodilatory activity on vascular smooth muscle produces the cutaneous manifestation of flushing.

NEUROLOGIC DISEASE

Neurologic disorders that may affect the autonomic nervous system, such as Parkinson disease, multiple sclerosis, and migraine, may occasionally lead to flushing. Cluster headache and paroxysmal hemicrania may cause ipsilateral facial pain and autonomic disturbances, including flushing. Patients with Horner syndrome may have ipsilateral ptosis, miosis, anhidrosis, and loss of flushing. Flushing is preserved on the contralateral side, leading to asymmetric physiologic flushing ("harlequin syndrome"). The patient may erroneously perceive the contralateral flushing as the abnormality. Causes of Horner syndrome include Pancoast tumors of the lung, carotid aneurysm, brainstem stroke, and multiple sclerosis. Aberrant nerve regeneration after parotid gland injury or surgery may result in ipsilateral flushing and sweating with eating and salivation (Frey syndrome).

DIAGNOSIS

Once you have identified the patient's complaint as consistent with flushing, it is necessary to evaluate for the underlying etiology. While episodic flushing can be a normal physiologic response to external factors such as heat or alcohol, persistent flushing is uncommon and should raise a red flag to the clinician that further investigation is warranted. Consideration of associated signs and symptoms may help to guide your decision making (**Figures 141-3** and **141-4**).

If the patient's flushing is triggered by spicy foods, hot drinks, alcohol, caffeine, and extremes in temperature, you should consider the diagnosis of rosacea. The diagnosis is made on clinical findings, as there is no specific confirmatory laboratory testing. Rosacea can be a condition that not only involves the skin, but can also have ocular symptoms; therefore, the patient should preferably be evaluated by a dermatologist and an ophthalmologist.

Establishing the diagnosis of climacteric-related flushing is often based on a constellation of clinical symptoms and can be supported by laboratory testing of the patient's hormone levels including follicle-stimulating hormone (FSH) and estradiol.

Flushing may be a prominent sign in intoxicated patients. Alcohol combined with other medications, such as disulfiram, sulfonylureas, and oral antifungal agents may cause severe reactions, including flushing, and should be also considered.

Medication reactions are a very common cause of flushing in the hospitalized patient. The list of provocative medications is

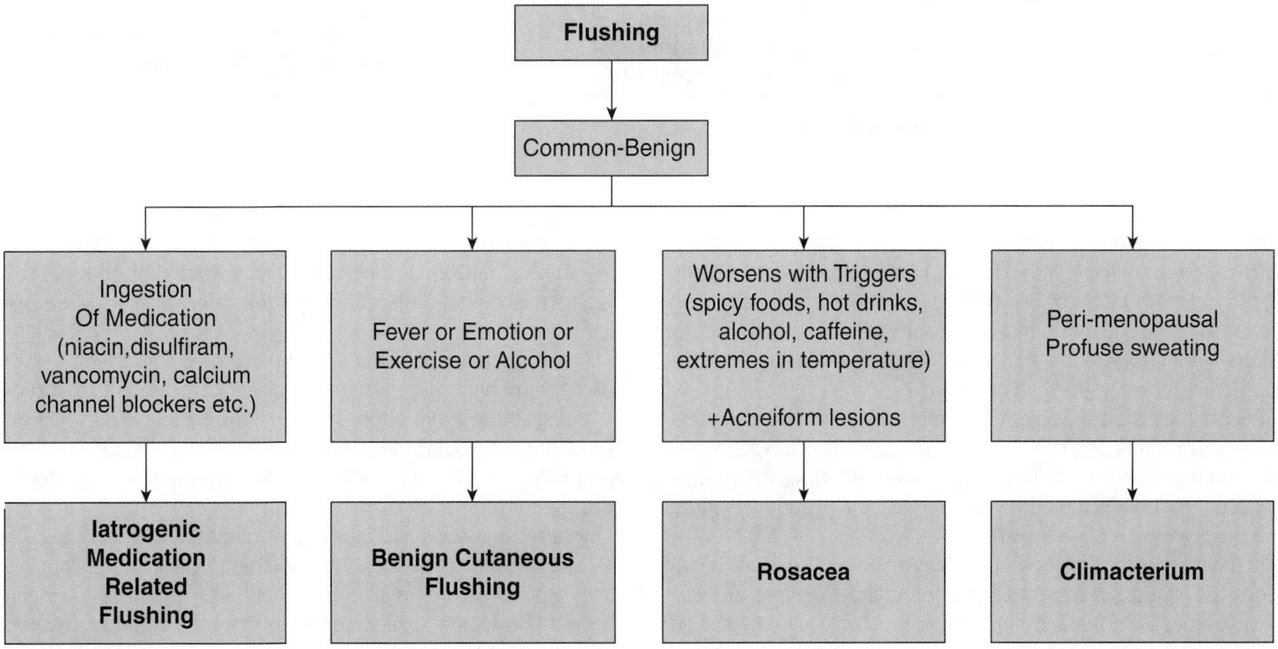

Figure 141-3 *Diagnostic approach to common, benign causes of flushing.*

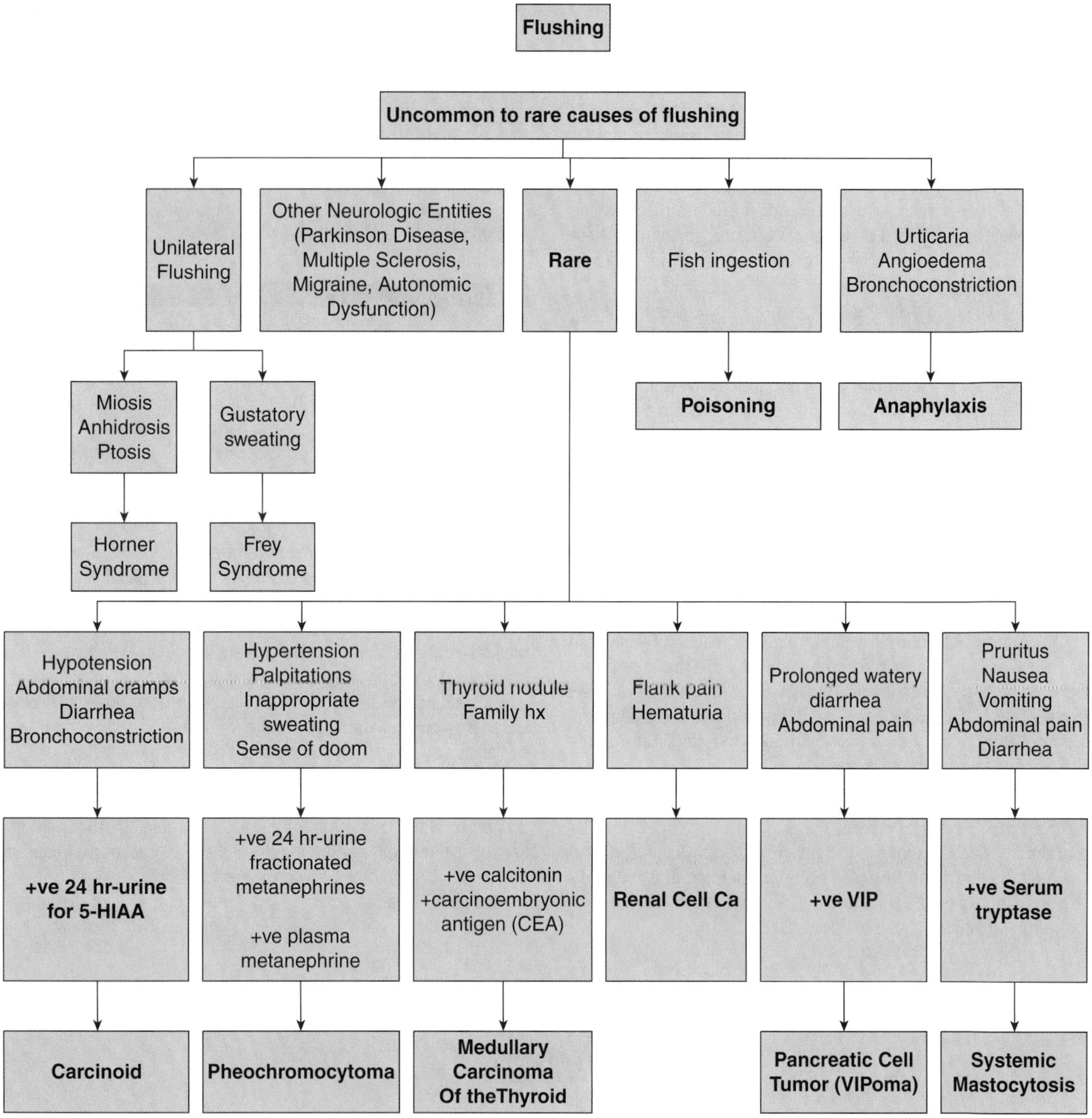

Figure 141-4 *Diagnosis of less common causes of flushing.*

extensive and listed, in part, in Table 141-1. Consideration of the patient's medication regimen, including over-the-counter supplements including niacin or nicotinic acid is integral to determining the cause of the patient's symptom. Niacin-related flushing typically occurs within 20 minutes to 1 hour after niacin dosing, and the duration is generally less than one hour.

Anaphylaxis is a severe type I hypersensitivity response. Clinical symptoms include angioedema, urticaria and bronchospasm and require urgent treatment. There are numerous causes for an anaphylactic reaction including foods, such as peanuts and tree nuts, and medications, such as aspirin.

If the patient has associated paroxysmal hypertension, headaches, palpitations, tachycardia, inappropriate sweating, anxiety, tremulousness, nausea and vomiting, pheochromocytoma should be considered. As these are some of the cardinal manifestations of pheochromocytoma, laboratory testing including urinary normetanephrine and platelet norepinephrine are warranted. ^{123}I-metaiodobenzoguanidine scintigraphy is another option if the diagnosis is clinically suspected and the catecholamine measurements are normal.

If the patient presents with symptoms of gastrointestinal hypermotility and flushing, evaluation for carcinoid tumor including 24-hour urine levels of 5-hydroxyindoleoacetic acid (5-HIAA) should be performed. Levels greater than 25 mg per 24 hours are usually indicative of the diagnosis. Imaging studies may also be considered.

Systemic mastocytosis rarely may manifest with flushing, in association with pruritus, nausea, vomiting, abdominal pain, diarrhea, headache and vascular instability. Serum tryptase has been shown to be an adequate screening test for this condition. Elevated serum tryptase levels should warrant a consultation by hematology/oncology and possible bone marrow biopsy.

When evaluating for medullary carcinoma of the thyroid gland, fine needle aspiration of the thyroid in addition to blood testing for calcitonin and CEA can be performed. This malignancy is also seen in multiple endocrine neoplasia Types II-A and II-B and further evaluation of these patients to rule out additional malignancy is warranted.

Pancreatic islet cell tumors, specifically VIPoma, may present with watery diarrhea, hypokalemia and achlorhydria. Diagnosis requires obtaining blood VIP levels from patients when they are symptomatic and appropriate imaging studies, including MRI.

Neurologic disease associated with flushing is important to recognize, especially in the acute setting, such as Horner syndrome secondary to trauma, internal carotid or aortic artery dissection, or in autonomic hyperreflexia that is seen in spinal cord lesions. In other settings, the patient may already have the underlying diagnosis of multiple sclerosis, migraines or Parkinson disease, for which flushing has been reported to occur in.

TRIAGE/HOSPITAL ADMISSION

Common and benign flushing is most frequently addressed in the outpatient setting. Flushing is seldom the primary indication for hospital admission. However, the hospitalist should be familiar with the causes of flushing, both benign and potentially life threatening, as they are sometimes seen in the hospitalized patient admitted for other reasons. Flushing can be seen in febrile inpatients, patients who are having an adverse medication reaction, and intoxicated patients requiring urgent care. Flushing associated with systemic or neurologic symptoms, as discussed above, may require admission for further investigation and workup of the etiology, for stabilization of blood pressure, as seen in the associated malignant hypertension of pheochromocytoma and carcinoid syndrome, for fluid resuscitation as required for pancreatic VIPoma, and for observation and treatment of an anaphylactic episode.

TREATMENT OPTIONS

Treatment options are again based on the underlying etiology responsible for the flushing response. In the case of benign entities, such as rosacea, the use of targeted laser therapy, such as pulsed dye laser, to the facial telangiectasias often results in a significant decrease in facial flushing. Oral antibiotics such as tetracycline and doxycycline are frequently used in the treatment of rosacea for their antimicrobial and anti-inflammatory properties. Emotional (or idiopathic) flushing has been treated anecdotally with nonselective beta-blockers, such as nadolol, with mixed results.

Niacin, or nicotinic acid, is frequently utilized for its lipid-lowering capacity. The side effect profile of this medication often makes compliance with therapy difficult. Coadministration of aspirin 650 mg with extended release niacin resulted in significantly reduced flushing incidence. Reduction in flushing was also seen at the 325 mg dose of aspirin.

Estrogen replacement therapy provides symptomatic relief for many women suffering from climacteric flushing. The use of this treatment is fraught with controversy and should be judged on a case by case basis.

The diagnosis of anaphylaxis is based on the patient's clinical symptoms, including angioedema, urticaria, and bronchospasm. Treatment often requires the use of subcutaneous epinephrine, antihistamines, or beta-adrenergic agents such as albuterol and intravenous corticosteroids.

Treatment of mastocytosis varies with the subtype. Cutaneous mastocytosis without evidence of visceral involvement usually has a very favorable prognosis and treatment is aimed at symptomatic relief. Antihistamines, cromolyn, avoidance of triggers and phototherapy have been described as viable options. Systemic mastocytosis may require medications such as imatinib mesylate or even bone marrow transplant.

Flushing related to carcinoid syndrome can be treated with somatostatin, octreotide, or lantreotide, which decrease the secretion of vasoactive mediators. Successful treatment of pheochromocytoma requires surgical consultation and the use of alpha-receptor blockers.

Once the diagnosis of medullary thyroid carcinoma is confirmed, patients frequently require total thyroidectomy and surrounding lymph node dissection. Surgical treatment is also the standard of care for VIPomas. After correcting dehydration and slowing the patient's diarrhea with medications like octreotide, surgery to remove the tumor provides the best chance for a cure.

If the patient has known underlying neurologic disease, such as Parkinson disease or multiple sclerosis, consultation with the patient's neurologist regarding symptom alleviation should be performed. If the flushing occurs in the acute setting, in the absence of known neurologic disease, further investigation including appropriate imaging studies should be performed.

DISCHARGE PLANNING

In addition to a thorough inpatient workup, patients should be referred to the appropriate consulting physician, as deemed necessary, based on the underlying etiology of the patient's flushing.

QUALITY IMPROVEMENT

While the majority of patients with cutaneous flushing will be diagnosed as having a benign entity such as emotionally induced flushing or rosacea, these patients must be appropriately evaluated as to not miss a rare, but more life threatening condition such as pheochromocytoma or carcinoid syndrome. Clinical history will help to guide your decision regarding the need for an extensive workup. Evidence-based medicine is, unfortunately, lacking with respect to providing clear direction in the most accurate and cost-effective means of evaluating the flushing patient.

Improving patient satisfaction is a good marker of quality improvement. Addressing common causes of flushing such as rosacea, medication-related flushing, and emotional flushing can provide patients with significant satisfaction. These entities, while not life-threatening, are often very aggravating and cosmetically unappealing. A means to address this performance gap is to provide patients with options for treatment, or suggest a referral to another physician who has expertise in the cosmetic management of these conditions.

URTICARIA: INTRODUCTION/EPIDEMIOLOGY

Urticaria is a cutaneous disorder characterized by the presence of transient, pruritic, erythematous, slightly edematous plaques. Urticaria, or hives, is not a specific disease but is a reactive process of the skin with enumerable etiologies. The lesions of urticaria tend to be pruritic, can last from a few minutes to several hours, and are irregularly shaped with an adjacent zone of pallor (**Figure 141-5**). Individual lesions commonly last less than 24 hours, with crops of lesions recurring over a period of less than 6 weeks in acute urticaria, or over a period lasting more than 6 weeks in chronic urticaria. Urticaria can occasionally be accompanied by edema of deeper tissues known as angioedema. In highly sensitive individuals, the inflammatory processes that lead to urticaria and angioedema can progress to include symptoms of airway compromise and hypotension, a condition defined as anaphylaxis.

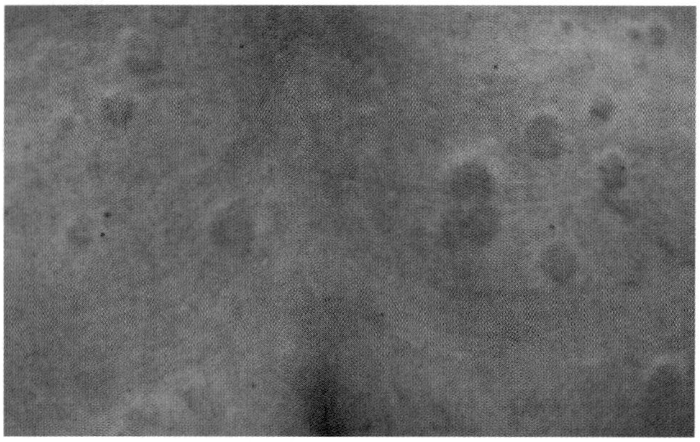

Figure 141-5 *Urticarial wheals with circumferential pallor.*

The cumulative incidence of acute urticaria was recently determined to be 18.7% among individuals 18 and older, which is in agreement with previous studies that measured the lifetime incidence of acute urticaria. The prevalence of chronic urticaria in the same population was estimated as 0.6%.

PATHOPHYSIOLOGY

The primary effector cell involved in the pathogenesis of urticaria, both acute and chronic, is the mast cell. In response to various stimuli, the mast cell is capable of releasing multiple mediators of the urticarial response. These mediators include histamine, interleukins and other cytokines, and products derived from the metabolism of arachidonic acid such as prostaglandins and leukotrienes. The precise stimuli involved in causing the release of these mediators depend on the clinical scenario in which hives are encountered and can be nonimmunologic and immunologic in nature. Some medications, such as opioids, directly stimulate mast cell degranulation. Neuropeptides and components of the complement pathway can also act directly on the mast cell. Many of the immunologic causes of mast cell degranulation work through the high-affinity IgE receptor (FcεRI) that is present on the surface of the mast cell. The allergen-IgE-FcεRI complex that forms on mast cells can cause mediator release. Antibodies directed against the FcεRI receptor or the IgE molecule itself can also stimulate mast cell degranulation.

DIFFERENTIAL DIAGNOSIS

COMMON CONDITIONS

Some cases of contact dermatitis can present with pruritic urticarial lesions. Often, in the setting of acute contact dermatitis, bullae and vesicles may be present, which are not a feature of urticaria. Contact dermatitis often occurs on a limited area of the skin (ie, eyelids, hands, feet), whereas the lesions of urticaria tend to be more widespread in nature. Latex and some foods as a cause of contact urticaria has also been well described and could hopefully be identified by patient history. Erythema multiforme (EM) occurs most often as the result of a hypersensitivity reaction to the herpes simplex virus (HSV). Lesions of EM can be urticarial in nature, but classically appear as target lesions. Evidence of HSV infection can sometimes be demonstrated in patients that have been diagnosed with EM. The terms urticarial dermatitis and dermal hypersensitivity reaction (DHR) can be encountered in the pathologic descriptions of a number of different clinical conditions. Some patients with the pathologic diagnosis of DHR may actually have urticaria or one of its differential diagnoses. Other patients with urticarial dermatitis/DHR are not able to be classified into a specific clinical condition and can have urticarial lesions that persist for longer than 24 hours. The etiology of the hypersensitivity reaction in these patients is often unknown and is similar to hives in that enumerable etiologies can be the trigger.

The cutaneous lesions of Lyme disease, known as erythema chronicum migrans, are urticarial in nature. Only one lesion is present in early localized infection of Lyme disease, which would be unusual for urticaria. The lesions of early disseminated Lyme disease can be multiple in nature, but these lesions tend to be more macular then edematous, are not pruritic, and do not typically have the zone of pallor that is present in urticaria.

POTENTIALLY LIFE-THREATENING CONDITIONS

Acute neutrophilic dermatosis, or Sweet syndrome, can begin as urticarial lesions. These lesions tend to become a much darker red with much greater edema than what is commonly seen in urticaria. Patients with Sweet syndrome also have systemic symptoms of fevers and joint pain which are not commonly present in urticaria. Sweet syndrome is a reactive process that occurs as a response to a number of different stimuli including, in about 20% of cases, a hematologic malignancy such as acute myelogenous leukemia or myelodysplastic syndrome. While the classic lesions of vasculitis are described as palpable purpura, some lesions of vasculitis are urticarial in nature. The lesions of urticarial vasculitis typically last longer than 24 hours in contrast to acute and chronic urticaria and tend to elicit symptoms of burning as opposed to pruritus. Lesions often resolve with purpuric or ecchymotic changes. When urticarial vasculitis occurs in the setting of low complement levels, it can be associated with systemic lupus erythematosus. In the setting of normal complement, urticarial vasculitis can be associated with a number of autoimmune or infectious etiologies, including Sjogren, hepatitis C, or cryoglobulinemia.

Bullous pemphigoid (BP) is an autoimmune blistering disease of the skin. In about one-third of cases, patients may have widespread urticarial lesions without any evidence of bullae or vesicles. These patients tend to be older than the typical urticarial patient and are readily diagnosed with direct immunofluorescence testing of the skin. If early diagnosis of BP does not occur, lesions can evolve into bullae and erosions which, if widespread, can lead to sepsis.

DIAGNOSIS

The diagnosis of urticaria is made by history and physical examination in the majority of instances. Details regarding foods, medications, and recent signs of infection are all important aspects of the patient's history. Physical provocation tests are performed if the history suggests that there is a specific cause for the urticaria (ie, ice cube application to the skin if cold urticaria is suspected, an ultraviolet or visible light source if solar urticaria is suspected). In general, the lesions of urticaria appear the same no matter what the etiology may be. One exception to this rule is cholinergic urticaria, where the lesions appear as small urticarial papules on an erythematous background (**Figure 141-6A, B**). These lesions can be duplicated in the clinic by having the patient run in place in the examination room. Dermatographism, a form of urticaria whereby lesions occur on the skin from nonspecific physical stimuli, can be elicited by scratching the skin and seeing if a wheal and flare response occurs (**Figure 141-7**). In the vast majority of instances, a biopsy is not routinely performed in order to diagnose urticaria and is only done if there is a high suspicion that one of the other differential diagnoses may be present.

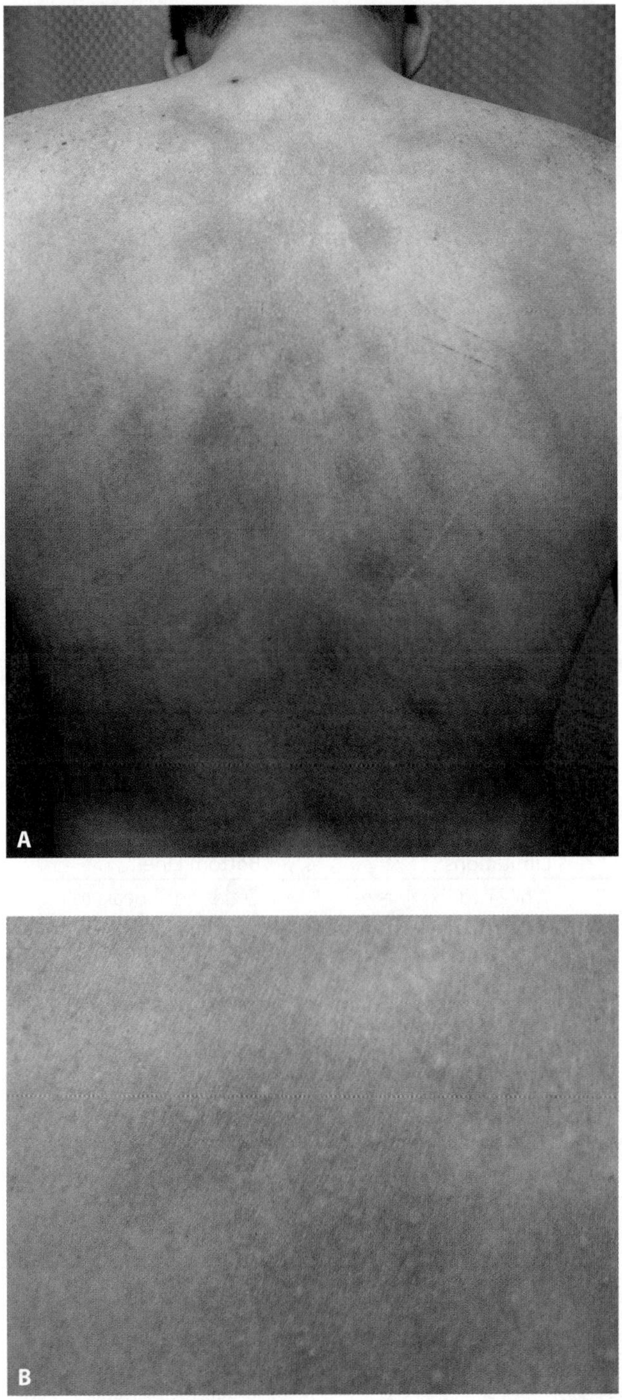

Figure 141-6 *Cholinergic urticaria. (A) Multiple erythematous flares, typically provoked by sweating and changes in body temperature. (B) Close-up view reveals pruritic papules on a red base.*

TRIAGE/HOSPITAL ADMISSION

The hospitalist will most likely encounter urticaria in the setting of a patient that has already been admitted. This will occur in the form of an urticarial, angiodema or anaphylactic response to medications or from procedures requiring IV contrast dye. The hospitalist may admit a patient for observation after being treated for extensive urticaria with angiodema or anaphylaxis in the emergency department with IV steroids, IV/IM Benadryl and subcutaneous epinephrine. An algorithmic approach is outlined in **Figure 141-8**.

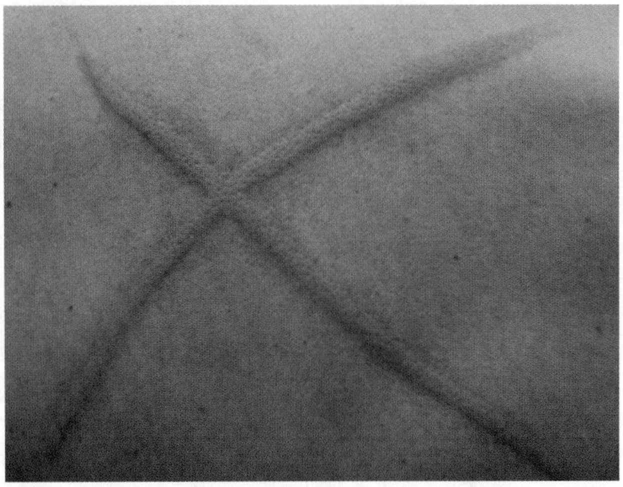

Figure 141-7 *Dermatographism.*

In acute urticaria (urticaria lasting less than 6 weeks), if no triggers can be identified, the next step is to proceed with therapy to control symptoms until the disease runs its course. In chronic urticaria, the next step is to consider if additional workup needs to be done for these patients. Many triggers have been implicated as being a cause of chronic urticaria, including chronic infections, autoimmune diseases, and parasitic infestations, among others. Performing an exhaustive workup to rule out other conditions is not likely to be of benefit in the vast majority of patients that present with chronic urticaria. An autologous serum skin test, while frequently mentioned as a tool to diagnose chronic autoimmune urticaria, is rarely performed. More recently, commercial laboratories have made the urticaria index available, which can detect the presence of antibodies to FcεRI. While this may serve to elucidate the cause of urticaria in some instances, the treatment plan is not significantly altered by the presence of these antibodies. Some also advocate testing for thyroid autoantibodies, but without overt thyroid disease, it is not always clear what the presence of these antibodies indicates in terms of the management of the patient. Skin prick testing or intradermal testing can be performed when a specific allergen is suspected as the cause of urticaria.

TREATMENT

In the cases where the cause of urticaria is clearly identified, either avoidance or treatment of the triggering stimulus is obviously indicated. In the instances where a clear etiology cannot be found, patients are most commonly prescribed antihistamines (**Table 141-2**), which act as antagonists with histamine at the H1 receptor, as first-line therapy. Some patients are prescribed a combination of a first generation antihistamine in the evening (due to a potential side effect of drowsiness) and a second generation antihistamine in during the day. Others advocate the use of maximum doses of the first generation antihistamines (25–100 mg of diphenhydramine every 6 hours) before considering the second generation options. While some articles suggest the addition of a H2-receptor antagonist may be helpful, this is not routinely prescribed.

Systemic corticosteroids consistently demonstrate effectiveness, but if used for long periods are associated with a number of adverse side effects. In cases of chronic urticaria that do not respond to conventional therapies, steroid-sparing immunosuppressive therapies are sometimes added. These can include cyclosporine, azathioprine, and mycophenolate mofetil. The risks versus benefits

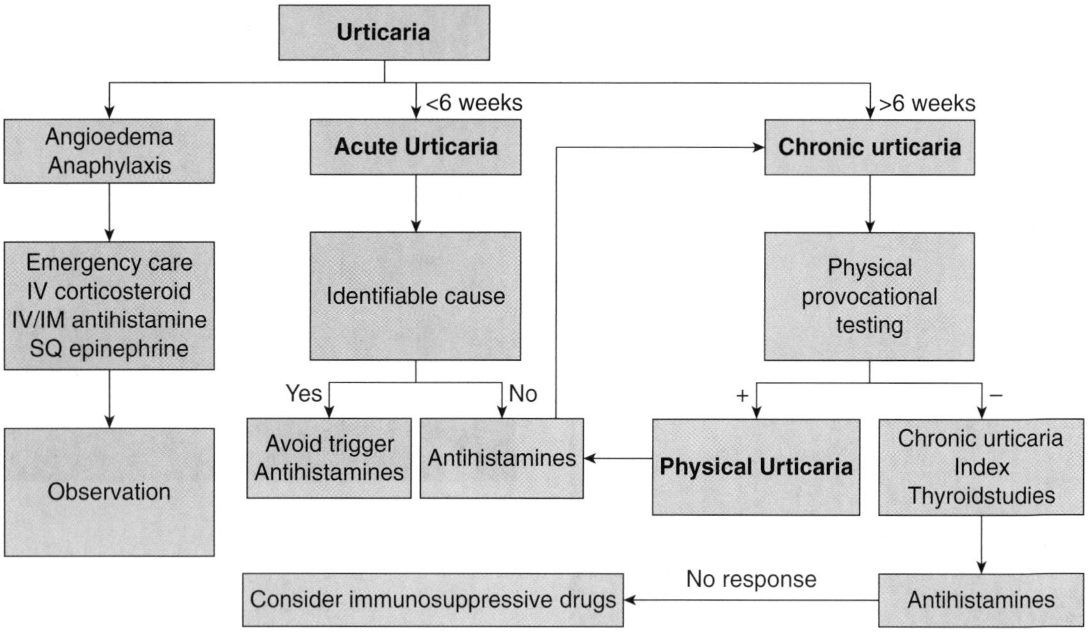

Figure 141-8 *Diagnosis of urticaria.*

TABLE 141-2 Evidence-based Medicine: Key References for Urticaria

Study	Methodology	Results	Limitations	Bottom Line
Kalivas J, et al. *J Allergy Clin Immunol.* 1990;86: 1014–1018.	Multicenter, double-blind, placebo-controlled safety and efficacy study comparing cetirizine (5–20 mg/d) to hydroxyzine (25–75 mg/d) to placebo for treatment of chronic idiopathic urticaria	Cetirizine was as effective as hydroxyzine with significantly lower incidence of somnolence	While hydroxyzine was significantly more sedating than placebo, difference in sedation between hydroxyzine and cetirizine did not reach statistical significance	Cetirizine appears to be as effective as first-generation antihistamines, and is not more sedating than placebo
Monroe EW. *Clin Ther.* 1992; 14:17–21.	Double-blind, placebo-controlled study comparing loratidine (10 mg/d) to hydroxyzine (25 mg three times a day) to placebo in the treatment of urticaria or atopic dermatitis	Loratadine was as effective of hydroxyzine, with lower incidence of side effects	Of the 59 patients studied, only 18 patients had urticaria (rest of patients studied had atopic dermatitis)	Loratadine as a single daily dose may be as effective as hydroxyzine, with lower risks of sedation and somnolence
Nelson HS, et al. *Ann Allergy Asthma Immunol.* 2000;84:517–522.	Double-blind, randomized, placebo-controlled study comparing twice daily placebo with four different doses of fexofenadine (20, 60, 120, or 240 mg twice a day)	All four doses of fexofenadine were significantly better at controlling pruritus and number of wheals when compared to placebo	Study compared fexofenadine to placebo, rather than another antihistamine	Compared to placebo, fexofenadine reduces pruritus and wheals in patients with chronic idiopathic urticaria
Grattan CE, et al. *Br J Dermatol.* 2000;143: 365–372.	Randomized, double-blind, placebo-controlled study comparing cyclosporine (Sandimmun 4 mg/kg/d) to placebo in the control of urticaria activity score of wheal numbers and itch	Overall response to cyclosporine was 65% (19/29 patients)	Study only included patients with positive autologous serum skin test (ASST); only 8 of 20 patients in cyclosporine group responded during blinded portion of trial; rest of responders were during unblinded portion of the study	As ASST is not routinely performed in evaluation of urticaria patients, results of study may not be applicable to urticaria patients who are seen in everyday clinic, but cyclosporine is well tolerated and is probably worth considering for 4–8 week course in patients not responding to antihistamine therapy

of these medications need to be completely understood by the patient before proceeding. Patients also need to be reassured that in most instances, even in idiopathic cases where no cause of the urticaria can be identified, the urticaria will spontaneously remit. It may take several years for this to occur, but remission is the rule.

COMPLICATIONS

When urticaria is accompanied by significant angioedema of the oral mucosa, airway integrity may be compromised. In these instances, administration of dilute epinephrine may be required, followed by admission to a hospital with close observation.

DISCHARGE PLANNING

If the patient develops an urticarial eruption in the hospital appropriate referral for outpatient follow up is indicated. Acute or chronic urticaria is not a cause for hospital admission and most patients are sent home from outpatient clinic with follow-up planned for about 6 weeks in order to determine the effectiveness of therapy.

CONCLUSION

Patients with urticaria may be profoundly uncomfortable, and it is tempting to prescribe systemic corticosteroids in these patients to alleviate symptoms. If patients continually seek this therapy for short-term relief, it can make appropriate management with antihistamines or other nonsteroid medications difficult. Performing many tests in order to elucidate the cause of the urticaria should also be discouraged when it is not directed by patient history and physical examination. The results of these tests are seldom helpful in the management of the patient.

SUGGESTED READINGS

Flushing

El Tal AK, Tannous Z. Cutaneous vascular disorders associated with internal malignancy. *Dermatol Clin*. 2008;26:45–57.

Heymann WR. Flushing, pheochromocytoma, and the dermatologist. *J Am Acad Dermatol*. 2006;55:1075–1077.

Huang AJ, Sawaya GF, Vittinghoff E, et al. Hot flushes, coronary heart disease, and hormone therapy in postmenopausal women. *Menopause*. 2009;16(4):639–643.

Izikson L, English JC, Zirwas MJ. The flushing patient: differential diagnosis, workup and treatment. *J Am Acad Dermatol*. 2006;55: 193–208.

Ray D, Williams G. Pathophysiological causes and clinical significance of flushing. *Br J Hosp Med*. 1993;50:594–598.

Urticaria

Brown NA, Carter JD. Urticarial vasculitis. *Curr Rheumatol Rep*. 2007;9(4):312–319.

Kaplan AP, Greaves M. Pathogenesis of chronic urticaria. *Clin Exp Allergy*. 2009;39(6):777–787.

Khan DA. Chronic urticaria: diagnosis and management. *Allergy Asthma Proc*. 2008;29(5):439–446.

Lee EE, Maibach HI. Treatment of urticaria. An evidence-based evaluation of antihistamines. *Am J Clin Dermatol*. 2001;2(1):27–32.

Poonawalla T, Kelly B. Urticaria: a review. *Am J Clin Dermatol*. 2009;10(1):9–21.

CHAPTER 142

Adverse Cutaneous Drug Reactions

Nicole F. Velez, MD
Arturo P. Saavedra, MD, PhD

Key Clinical Questions

1. What are the red flags that should alert the hospitalist to an adverse cutaneous reaction?
2. When must the offending drug be discontinued?
3. How do you treat through a cutaneous reaction?
4. What is the recommended treatment for Stevens-Johnson syndrome/toxic epidermal necrolysis?
5. When should you call a dermatology consult?
6. How do you counsel the patient at time of discharge?

INTRODUCTION

Complications of drug therapy are the most common adverse events associated with inpatient admissions and hospital discharge. In the United States, adverse drug events account for up to 140,000 deaths and $136 billion in costs annually. Skin involvement occurs frequently in drug reactions, and may be a presenting manifestation. While most cutaneous reactions are benign and self-limiting, serious adverse cutaneous reactions affect 2% to 3% of inpatients, and lead to 0.1% to 0.3% of hospital fatalities. However, early recognition of clinical findings (**Table 142-1**) is critical to ensure prompt drug discontinuation and prevent further complications. Risk factors include female gender, age, immunosupression, and greater number of medications. Common culprits are penicillins, sulfonamides, and nonsteroidal anti-inflammatory agents (NSAIDs).

PATHOPHYSIOLOGY

Cutaneous drug reactions occur by both immunologic and nonimmunologic mechanisms. Genetic predisposition, host characteristics, and probably other poorly understood factors also play important roles.

Nonimmunologic mechanisms are predictable drug reactions, related to overdose, cumulative toxicity, and delayed toxicity. Immunologic mechanisms are often unpredictable. They are classified into four categories. Type I reactions are IgE-mediated responses that activate mast cells, and produce urticaria, angioedema, and hemodynamic instability. Type II reactions involve cytotoxic IgG responses, and often cause blood cell dyscrasias, such as hemolytic anemia, thrombocytopenia, and leukopenia. In type III reactions, immune complex deposition and complement activation produce a vasculitis or serum sickness-like presentation. Finally, type IV reactions are T-cell mediated, and account for most drug exanthems. The character of the skin rash may depend on the type of T-cell response elicited. For example, T-helper 2 responses produce interleukin-4 and -5 secretion and the classic exanthem or morbilliform rash with both erythematous macules and papules (**Figure 142-1**). A predominantly cytotoxic T-cell response may lead to keratinocyte necrosis and vesicular and pustular eruptions. The T-cell response elicited is determined by the antigenic epitopes of the drug, which depend upon the drug's chemical reactivity, prior metabolism, and protein binding. In Stevens-Johnson syndrome (SJS) and toxic epidermal necrolysis (TEN), keratinocyte death is also influenced by activation of fatty acid synthetase (Fas) receptors, leading to caspase activation and keratinocyte apoptosis.

Host characteristics that influence drug reactions include alterations in drug metabolism pathways, concurrent medications, immunosuppression, and underlying disease. Patients who have low levels of the enzyme epoxide hydrolase and are taking aromatic anticonvulsants, such as phenytoin, carbamazepine, and phenobarbital, accumulate toxic metabolites (arene oxides). This predisposes to the development of drug reaction with eosinophilia and systemic symptoms (DRESS). Reactivation of latent viral infections, such as human herpesvirus 6 and 7, also predispose patients to more severe cutaneous drug reactions.

TABLE 142-1 The "Red Flags" of Adverse Cutaneous Drug Reactions

Cutaneous signs	
	Blisters
	Palpable purpura
	Confluent erythema
	Epidermal necrosis
	Ulcers
	Mucosal involvement
	Facial edema
Systemic signs	
	Fever (> 40°C)
	Skin tenderness
	Lymphadenopathy
	Arthralgias
	Shortness of breath, wheezing
	Hypotension
Laboratory findings	
	Liver function tests > 3x normal
	Eosinophilia (> 1500/mm^3)
	Neutropenia

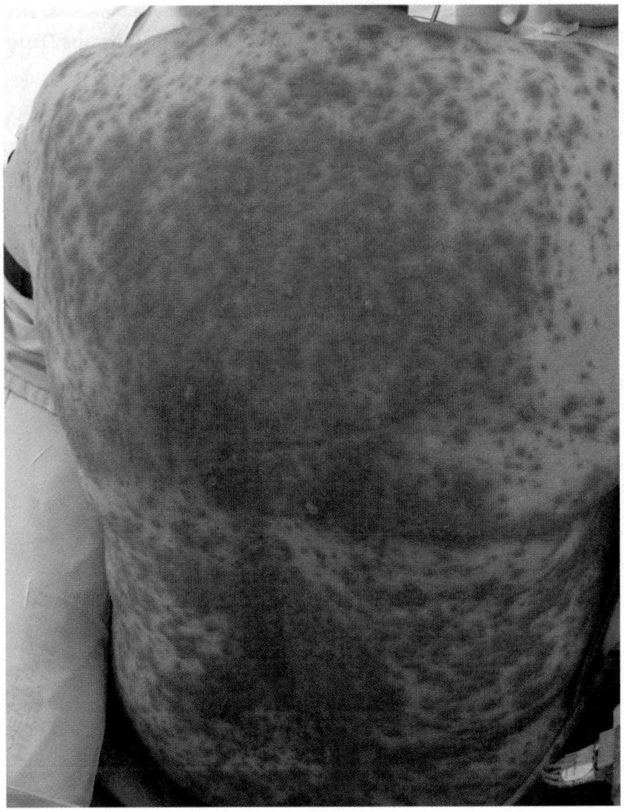

Figure 142-1 *Morbilliform drug rash. Erythematous macules and papules coalescing in dependent areas.*

DOES THIS PATIENT HAVE AN ADVERSE CUTANEOUS DRUG REACTION?

THE FEBRILE PATIENT WITH MUCOSAL SYMPTOMS

Stevens-Johnson syndrome and toxic epidermal necrolysis

Mucosal symptoms should always prompt the clinician to consider an early cutaneous drug reaction. Although the incidence of SJS and TEN are low (1.2–6 per million and 0.4–1.2 per million, respectively), they are associated with a combined mortality of 20% to 25%. SJS and TEN represent a clinical spectrum of disease which should not be confused with erythema multiforme. Whereas erythema multiforme is typically a postinfectious process with limited skin findings (**Figure 142-2**) and low morbidity, SJS/TEN represents a drug-induced systemic spectrum of disease characterized by epidermal necrosis, mucosal membrane involvement, rapid course, and poor prognosis (**Table 142-2**).

Diagnosis should be suspected in the patient with fever, mucosal symptoms, and progressive skin findings. There may be a prodrome of fever, malaise, and upper respiratory tract symptoms. Conjunctival lesions are seen in 85% of cases, and range from asymptomatic hyperemia to keratitis, corneal erosions and pseudomembrane formation. Erosions of the trachea, bronchi, gastrointestinal tract and urethra may also occur, leading to respiratory compromise, impaired alimentation, and painful micturition. Ill-defined erythematous and violaceous macules with two zones of color (atypical target lesions) begin on the upper trunk, and spreads to the extremities over 1 to 4 days. Keratinocyte necrosis produces flaccid blisters that spread with pressure (positive Nikolsky sign) and lead to epidermal sloughing (**Figure 142-3**). Although controversial, the distinction between SJS and TEN is based on the percentage of body surface area (BSA) with epidermal detachment (< 10% SJS, > 30% TEN, 10–30% overlap SJS/TEN). This is important for prognosis and treatment. Laboratory findings may include anemia and lymphopenia. Neutropenia is rare, and associated with worse prognosis.

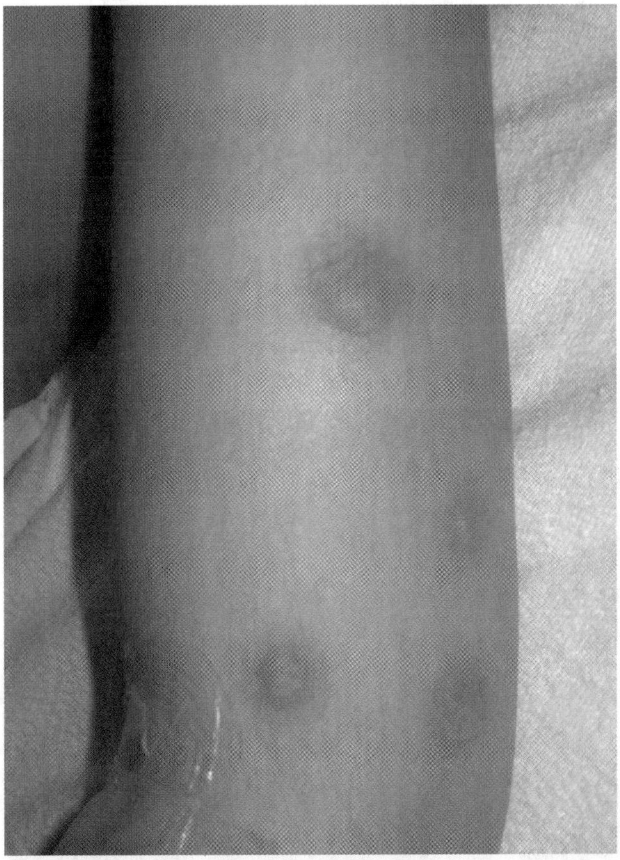

Figure 142-2 *Erythema multiforme. Typical target lesions with three zones of color (dusky and bullous center surrounded by an erythematous ring and an outer, light pink halo) with limited skin involvement.*

TABLE 142-2 Characteristics of Major Severe Cutaneous Drug Reactions

Drug Reaction	Cutaneous Findings	Mucosal Involvement	Percentage that are Drug Induced (%)	Time Interval from Start of Drug and Onset of Reaction	Mortality (%)	Selected Responsible Drugs
Stevens-Johnson syndrome	Dusky, atypical target lesions, < 10% of BSA	Yes	50	1–3 wk	5	Sulfonamides Anticonvulsants NSAIDs Allopurinol
Toxic epidermal necrolysis	Confluent erythema, large sheets of necrotic epidermis, > 30% BSA	Yes	> 80	1–3 wk	30	
DRESS	Facial edema, edematous plaques with perifollicular accentuation	No	70–90	2–6 wk	5–10	Anticonvulsants Sulfonamides Allopurinol Minocycline Lamotrigine
AGEP	Widespread erythema with nonfollicular sterile pustules	Rare (20%)	70–90	< 4 days	1–2	Beta-lactam antibiotics Macrolides Calcium channel blockers

AGEP, acute generalized exanthematous pustulosis; BSA, body surface area; DRESS, drug reaction with eosinophilia and systemic symptoms.

Diagnosis is clinical, but skin biopsy and immunoflourescence studies may be of value in excluding other nondrug-related bullous and mucosal disorders, such as staphylococcal scalded skin syndrome, bullous pemphigoid, pemphigus vulgaris, and paraneoplastic pemphigus. The hospitalist should also ask about risk factors for other blistering disorders, such as thermal burns, phototoxic burns, and pressure blisters.

THE PATIENT WITH CUTANEOUS FINDINGS AND SIGNS OF END ORGAN DAMAGE

Drug reaction with eosinophilia and systemic symptoms

Previously associated with the aromatic anticonvulsant agents, DRESS is now known to be associated with other medications, including sulfonamides, calcium channel blockers, and allopurinol.

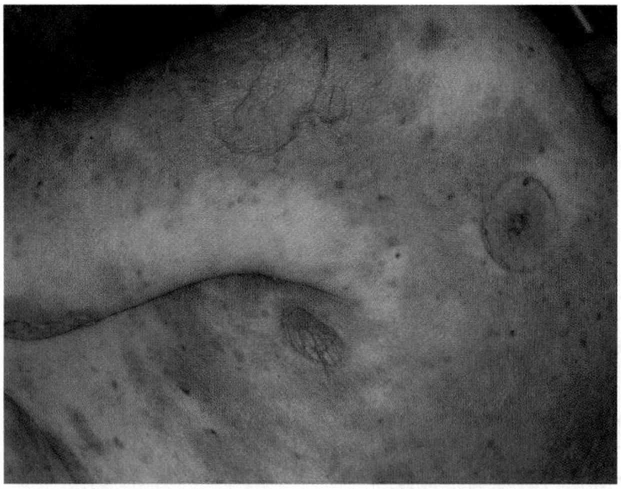

Figure 142-3 *Toxic epidermal necrolysis. Large dusky patches with flaccid blisters and areas of desquamation.*

Symptoms usually begin 2 to 6 weeks after drug initiation (Table 142-2). Diagnosis should be suspected in the febrile patient with an evolving morbilliform rash (**Figure 142-4**), lymphadenopathy, eosinophilia (> 1500/mm^3), atypical lymphocytes, and transaminitis. Macules and papules evolve to form edematous and confluent plaques with perifollicular accentuation. Facial edema is often prominent. The cutaneous findings may resemble SJS if vesicles form secondary to dermal edema. Rarely, small pustules are observed, and the diagnosis may be confused with acute generalized exanthematous pustulosis. Dermatotologic consult and a skin biopsy can help to distinguish these entities (**Table 142-3**). Evidence of visceral involvement may also be a distinguishing feature of DRESS. Up to 50% of patients develop a potentially life-threatening hepatitis (as compared with 10% of patients with SJS/TEN). Other visceral complications include arthralgias, pericarditis, pulmonary infiltrates, and interstitial nephritis. Reactivation of human herpesvirus 6 (HHV-6) is frequently found in these patients, and may predispose them to immunosuppression and subsequent bacterial infections. No prognostic factors have been identified. Mortality is 10%.

Drug-induced pseudolymphoma (**Table 142-4**) may also present with infiltrated plaques, lymphadenopathy, and similar histologic findings on lymph node biopsy. However, unlike DRESS, pseudolymphoma presents insidiously, lacks systemic involvement, and has a much better prognosis.

Urticaria, angioedema, and anaphylaxis

In a patient with urticaria, facial edema, or stridor and wheezing, drug-induced angioedema and anaphylaxis must be considered. IgE-mediated hypersensitivity reactions can occur within minutes to hours of drug exposure. The presence of urticaria, defined as itchy, edematous papules and plaques of varying size with central pallor, may signal an IgE-mediated reaction. Pale, pink swellings of the face and mucosal surfaces that are painful rather than itchy, often persisting for > 24 hours, are suggestive of angioedema and must be evaluated more closely. Anaphylaxis, or cardiopulmonary compromise in the setting of systemic vasodilatation, is rare

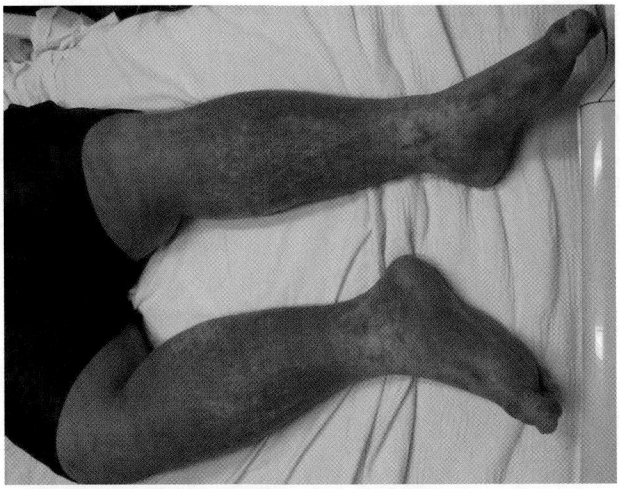

A

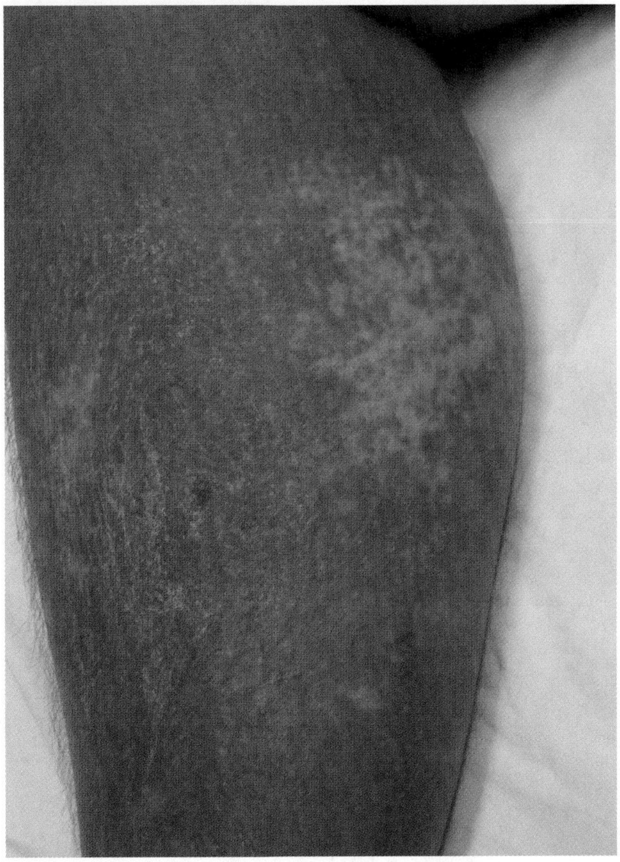

B

Figure 142-4 *(A) Drug reaction with eosinophilia and systemic symptoms. Erythematous macules and papules coalescing into patches on the back of a patient with early drug reaction with eosinophilia and systemic symptoms. (B) Lesions progress to form edematous plaques with perifollicular accentuation.*

(80–100 cases/million/year). Drug allergies account for 18% of cases of anaphylaxis. The most common drug culprits are penicillins, anesthetic agents, and radiocontrast.

Non-IgE–mediated mechanisms also produce angioedema. Angiotensin-converting enzyme inhibitors (ACEi)–induced angioedema affects up to 0.1 to 0.7% of patients taking this class of medications. It presents as acute-onset nonpitting edema that may occur weeks to years after the medication was started. African Americans, hemodialysis patients, and those with a history of idiopathic angioedema are at higher risk. While swelling of the lips and anterior tongue are the most common presentations and often the most visibly concerning, clinicians should carefully evaluate the palate and oropharynx, as swelling of these sites is more predictive of need for intubation.

Other causes of urticaria and angioedema that must be considered include infections and exposures, such as insect bites and food. Urticaria without angioedema can also be seen in common drug rashes, vasculitis, neutrophilic dermatoses, and early bullous pemphigoid. When angioedema occurs without urticaria and drug reactions have been excluded, the clinician should consider C1 esterase deficiency.

TABLE 142-3 Indications for Considering Dermatologic Consultation in Adverse Cutaneous Drug Reaction

Uncertainty regarding indication for skin biopsy
Uncertainty regarding indication for systemic steroids or intravenous immunoglobulin in patient with Stevens-Johnson syndrome and toxic epidermal necrolysis
Clinicopathologic correlation

Drug-induced vasculitis

Adverse drug reactions account for approximately 10% of cases of leukocytoclastic vasculitis, or cutaneous small vessel vasculitis. Blood vessel inflammation and even necrosis may occur from drug-induced immune complex deposition, complement activation, and granulocyte recruitment. Common medication culprits are NSAIDs, penicillins, cephalosporins, sulfonamides, allopurinol, and propylthiouracil. Signs and symptoms begin within 1 to 2 weeks of first exposure and less than 3 days after re-exposure. Palpable purpura on the lower extremities is the classic cutaneous finding, but hemorrhagic blisters, ulcers, nodules and urticaria may also be observed. While systemic involvement is rare, blood vessel inflammation can become widespread and affect the kidney, liver, gastrointestinal tract, or nervous system. Patients should be screened for systemic symptoms including fever, headache, abdominal pain, hematuria, and peripheral neuropathy. Urinary sediment and fecal occult blood should be checked in addition to a complete blood count and basic metabolic panel. Histopathology shows fibrinoid necrosis and direct immunofluorescence may reveal IgM and C3 deposits in the capillary wall. Patients who develop drug-induced vasculitis to propylthiouracil, hydralazine or minocycline may have a positive antimyeloperoxidase antibody.

In the evaluation of a suspected drug-induced vasculitis, the possibility of an underlying infection must be excluded first. Other diagnoses which can be differentiated by skin biopsy include Henoch-Schönlein purpura, polyarteritis nodosa, and Wegener granulomatosus. Symptoms should resolve with drug discontinuation. Systemic steroids are only indicated if there is visceral involvement.

THE PATIENT WITH CONFLUENT ERYTHEMA

Acute generalized exanthematous pustulosis

Acute generalized exanthematous pustulosis (AGEP) is a rare drug reaction associated with low mortality that may present with widespread erythema and resemble other more life-threatening entities. AGEP presents within the first few days of drug exposure. Initial signs include high fevers (38°C), and widespread erythema that begins on the face and spreads centrifugally, favoring the intertriginous areas. Numerous, small, nonfollicular, sterile pustules appear on top of the

TABLE 142-4 Drug Reactions that Mimic Systemic Disease

Presentation	Clinical Findings	Time Between Start of Drug and Onset of Symptoms	Resolution with Drug Discontinuation	Common Drug Culprits
Erythema nodosum	Bilateral, tender, erythematous nodules (mainly on shins)	Weeks	Yes	Oral contraceptive pills Estrogens Sulfonamides Penicillin Bromides Iodides Azathioprine
Subacute cutaneous lupus-like reaction	Psoriasiform or annular lesions on trunk, arms, and extensor surfaces	At least 1 year	Sometimes	Hydrochlorothiazide Calcium channel blockers Terbinafine NSAIDs Griseofulvin Docetaxel PUVA Interferon
Systemic lupus-like reaction	Fever, weight loss, serositis; cutaneous findings are uncommon	Variable	Yes	Procainamide Hydralazine Chlorpromazine Isonlazid Methyldopa Propylthiouracil Quinidine Practolol D-penicillamine PUVA Minocycline
Neutrophilic eccrine hidradenitis	Erythematous papules and plaques surrounding eccrine glands	7–14 days	Yes	Cytarabine Mitoxantrone Bleomycin Anthracyclines Methotrexate Cyclophosphamide Acetaminophen
Sweet syndrome (acute febrile neutrophilic dermatoses)	Painful, erythematous plaques (mainly on face and upper extremities)	Days	Yes	G-CSF All-*trans*-retinoic acid
Pseudoporphyria	Skin fragility, erosions, blisters, and scarring (mainly on dorsal hands, face and extensor surfaces of legs)	Variable	Yes	NSAIDs Furosemide Tetracycline Retinoids UVA exposure (including tanning beds) Hemodialysis
Pseudolymphoma	Solitary or widespread erythematous to violaceous papules, plaques, and nodules; lymphadenopathy and erythroderma may occur	Months to years	Yes	Phenobarbital Carbamazepine Chlorpromazine Promethazine Imatinib mesylate Angiotensin-2–receptor antagonists

(continued)

TABLE 142-4 Drug Reactions that Mimic Systemic Disease (*continued*)

Presentation	Clinical Findings	Time Between Start of Drug and Onset of Symptoms	Resolution with Drug Discontinuation	Common Drug Culprits
Pemphigus	Flaccid blisters, erosions of skin, and mucous membranes	Weeks to months	Sometimes	Penicillamine ACE inhibitors Gold sodium thiomalate Pyritinol
Linear-IgA bullous dermatosis	Tense vesicles in an annular configuration	1–15 days	Yes	Vancomycin Beta-lactam antibiotics Captopril NSAIDs
Granulomas	Firm, mobile cutaneous nodules; may be tender and ulcerate	Years	No	Injection of talc or starch products
Skin necrosis	Painful plaques and hemorrhagic blisters evolve into necrotic ulcers and ischemic infarcts; most common sites: breasts, thighs, and buttocks	2– 5 days	No	Warfarin Heparin

ACE, angiotensin-converting enzyme; G-CSF, granulocyte colony-stimulating factor; NSAID, nonsteroidal anti-inflammatory drug; PUVA, psoralen ultraviolet-A radiation.

erythema (**Figure 142-5**). Pustules may persist for up to 10 days. A characteristic pinpoint pattern of desquamation follows. Edema of the hands and face may be observed. Patients frequently report skin pain and burning. Mucosal involvement occurs in only 20% of patients, and usually presents as a localized oral erosion. Leukocytosis (> 10,000/mL) and a mild eosinophilia may be present in a third of patients. Systemic involvement is rare. Estimated incidence is 1 to 5 cases/million. The most common culprits are beta-lactam antibiotics, macrolides, calcium channel blockers, and antimalarials.

Distinguishing AGEP from pustular psoriasis and Sneddon-Wilkinson disease (a recurrent, superficial pustular dermatosis with a polycyclic pattern and flexural accentuation) may be challenging. Features that distinguish AGEP include its short course, association with new drug exposure and histopathologic characteristics (namely superficial dermal edema, leukocytoclastic vasculitis, eosinophils, and focal keratinocyte necrosis). If the pustules are not appreciated

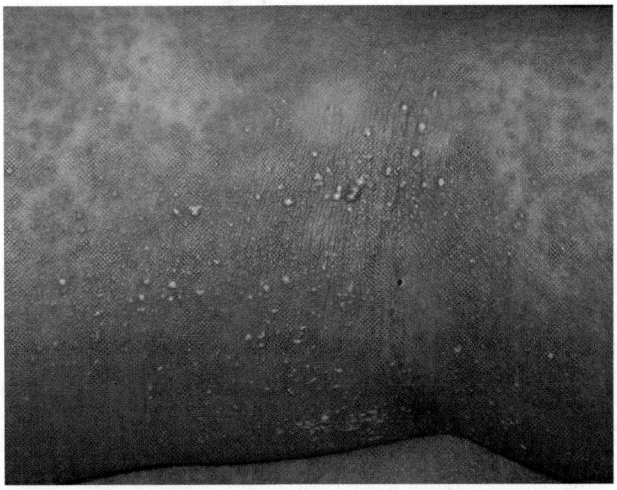

Figure 142-5 *Acute generalized exanthematous pustulosis. Widespread erythema with numerous, pinpoint, nonfollicular, sterile pustules.*

on exam, the disease may resemble drug-induced erythroderma, toxic epidermal necrolysis or staphylococcal scalded skin syndrome. Skin biopsy and dermatologic consultation may be of value if the diagnosis is unclear (Table 142-3).

Erythroderma

Erythroderma, or exfoliative dermatitis, is defined as a generalized erythema and scaling that involves more than 90% of the skin surface. Common associated signs and symptoms include fever, lymphadenopathy, edema, and pruritus. Medications are the second most common cause of erythroderma (20%). Other causes include generalization of an underlying dermatosis (50%), neoplasms (10%), and infections (**Table 142-5**). No etiology is identified in up to 25% of cases. Drug-induced erythroderma is characterized by its acute onset, initial morbilliform appearance, and relatively short course, resolving within 2 to 6 weeks of drug discontinuation. Increased peripheral blood flow can produce facial edema, hepatomegaly, and systemic complications including tachycardia, high output heart failure, and thermoregulatory disturbances. A higher prevalence of erythroderma has been reported among patients with human immunodeficiency virus (HIV), and an HIV test should be checked in all patients with risk factors. Of the many medications implicated, the most common culprits include allopurinol, beta-lactam antibiotics and aromatic anticonvulsants. Histopathology is often helpful in ruling out other potential causes, and multiple skin biopsies may be required if the initial pathology is inconclusive.

SPECIAL CONSIDERATIONS IN THE IMMUNOCOMPROMISED POPULATION

Studies of adverse cutaneous drug reactions consistently demonstrate that patients with underlying immunosuppression, including malignancy, connective tissue disease, liver failure, renal failure and HIV, are at increased risk for drug rashes. Diagnosis is more challenging in these populations because they are also at risk for developing other clinical syndromes with skin findings that may mimic a drug eruption.

TABLE 142-5 Differential Diagnosis of Erythroderma

1. Primary dermatoses
   - Atopic dermatitis
   - Seborrheic dermatitis
   - Psoriasis
   - Pityriasis rubra pilaris
   - Pemphigus foliaceous
2. Infections
   - Human immunodeficiency virus
   - Staphylococcal scalded skin syndrome
   - Hepatitis
3. Neoplasm
   - Cutaneous T-cell lymphoma
   - Sezary syndrome
   - Malignant histiocytosis
   - Acute and chronic leukemias
   - Solid tumors (colon, lung, prostate, thyroid, fallopian tubes, larynx, and esophagus)
   - Reticular cell sarcoma
4. Medications (common examples)
   - Allopurinol
   - Beta-lactam antibiotics
   - Aromatic anticonvulsants
   - Sulfonamides
5. Idiopathic

Among HIV-positive patients, drug-related eruptions are one hundred times more common than in the general population. Contributing factors to this risk include multiple chronic medications, altered pathways of drug metabolism, increased oxidative stress, and immune hyperactivation. Higher risk of rash is associated with decreasing CD4+ cell count, age, underlying skin disease, and viral reactivation. If the medication is necessary and the reaction is limited to the skin, the medication may be continued. However, the clinician should be aware that HIV patients are more liable to progress to SJS/TEN. Other serious conditions that may masquerade as a morbilliform exanthem in the HIV patient include Kawasaki disease, recalcitrant erythematous desquamating disorder (a chronic staphylococcal infection), and exacerbation of an underlying dermatoses.

Morbilliform rash in the transplant population is most often due to an antibiotic or chemotherapeutic agent. As these patients are frequently thrombocytopenic, the eruption may appear more purpuric. Other diagnoses that must be considered include eruption of lymphocyte recovery, acute cutaneous graft-versus-host disease (GVHD), engraftment syndrome, and viral infection. Acute GVHD may be difficult to distinguish from a drug reaction, and skin biopsy may not be diagnostic. Features that suggest acute GVHD include a rash that favors the scalp, ears, hands and feet, associated diarrhea, and elevated liver function tests. Once acute GVHD is suspected, systemic steroids should be initiated.

Some immunocompromised patients develop cutaneous drug reactions as expected side effects of their potent medications. An example is the papulopustular eruption associated with epidermal growth factor receptor inhibitors. This reaction is rarely life-threatening, and most patients are able to continue the medication with symptomatic treatment for the rash.

A PATIENT WITH SIGNS OF NEW SYSTEMIC DISEASE

Medications may provoke a wide spectrum of systemic diseases, including lupus, erythema nodosum, and neutrophilic dermatoses. In a patient on multiple medications who presents with signs or symptoms of a new systemic disease, a drug reaction should always be excluded prior to initiating treatment. Drug-induced syndromes usually resolve once the medication is discontinued. Table 142-4 provides a brief overview of the major classes of systemic disease which may be drug-induced, the most common culprits, and the effect of medication discontinuation.

DIFFERENTIAL DIAGNOSIS

EXANTHEMATOUS DRUG REACTION (THE "COMMON DRUG RASH")

Exanthematous or morbilliform eruptions account for more than 90% of drug reactions. Skin lesions may appear within 4 to 14 days of drug initiation, and typically consist of pink to red macules and papules that begin symmetrically on the trunk and upper extremities. The eruption is polymorphic, spreads distally, and often becomes confluent on the thorax. Pruritus is a common complaint. The benign drug rash lacks mucosal involvement, skin tenderness, and signs of end organ damage. Symptomatic management consists of both sedating (eg, diphenhydramine or hydroxyzine 25 mg po every 6 hours) and non-sedating (eg, cetirizine 5–10 mg PO daily or fexofenadine 180 mg PO daily) antihistamines. Potent (class I) topical steroids, such as clobetasol 0.05% ointment, can be applied daily to the trunk and extremities. Sensitive areas, including the face, axilla, inframammary skin and genitals, should be treated with a mild (class 4) topical steroid, such as hydrocortisone 2.5% cream. Topical steroid use should be limited to two week intervals to avoid side effects such as skin atrophy, striae, pigmentary change, contact dermatitis, and infection. Hypothalamus-pituitary-adrenal axis suppression is rare, unless the steroid is applied to large areas of denuded skin or mucosal surfaces where absorption levels are higher.

FIXED-DRUG ERUPTION/GENERALIZED BULLOUS FIXED-DRUG ERUPTION (GBFDE)

Fixed-drug eruptions are characterized by well-demarcated pink to violaceous plaques, with or without blisters. Lesions favor the face, extremities and genitalia, and typically occur at the same sites upon re-exposure. Affected areas resolve with postinflammatory hyperpigmentation. Onset is usually within 1 to 2 weeks of first exposure to the culprit medication, and then within 24 hours of subsequent exposures. In the generalized form, there are multiple cutaneous lesions, often with central blisters and areas of detached epidermis. Histopathology may reveal necrotic keratinocytes and resemble SJS/TEN. However, unlike more severe drug reactions, GBFDE has limited mucosal involvement, mild systemic symptoms, no visceral involvement, and good prognosis. The history of similar lesions at the same sites upon prior medication exposure is most helpful in distinguishing this entity. These patients usually do not require transfer to a burn unit.

BACTERIAL INFECTIONS

Bacterial infections should always be excluded before diagnosing an adverse cutaneous drug reaction, in order to avoid delay of a necessary antibiotic. Staphylococcal scalded skin syndrome (SSSS) presents with fever, skin tenderness and a confluent erythema with overlying superficial blisters, which may initially resemble TEN. Although almost exclusively a disease of infants, SSSS can occur in adults with a history of renal failure, immunosuppression, malignancy, chronic alcohol abuse, or HIV. The disease is mediated by an exfoliative toxin of *Staphylococcal aureus* that targets desmoglein I, causing interdesmosmal splitting and blistering in a superficial layer of the epidermis. Features that distinguish SSSS from TEN include the superficial nature of the blister and its fragility (TEN forms subepidermal blisters), a negative Nikolsky sign, although this test is imperfect, and the absence of significant mucosal findings. Cultures of bullae are negative, but *S aureus* may be isolated from the nasopharynx or blood. Early diagnosis is critical, as mortality among adults can be greater than 50%.

Staphylococcal and streptococcal toxic shock syndromes are characterized by fever, macular erythema, and multiorgan system failure and may also resemble SJS/TEN. Recent surgery, upper respiratory tract infection, or tampon use are classically associated with staphylococcal toxic shock syndrome, whereas a history of recent trauma or soft tissue infection may be more suggestive of streptococcal toxic shock. In patients with this constellation of signs and no recent medication exposure, these diagnoses should be strongly considered. Blood cultures are positive in 15% of staphylococcal toxic shock cases and 50% of streptococcal toxic shock cases.

VIRAL INFECTIONS

Many viral infections present with prodromal symptoms, a morbilliform eruption, and systemic findings that may mimic an adverse cutaneous drug eruption. Measles and rubella are still reported among communities with poor vaccination rates, and are rarely complicated by secondary bacterial infections, encephalitis, or thrombocytopenic purpura. In adults, parvovirus B19 presents with a diffuse, web-like (reticulate) rash, fever, and arthralgias. Epstein-Barr virus (EBV) usually follows a self-limited course with fever, pharyngitis, and lymphadenopathy. A macular rash is seen in 10% of patients, but the incidence rises to 90% if the patient has received ampicillin. Severe complications of EBV include hepatitis and airway compromise. In bone marrow transplant patients, the most common viral infection is cytomegalovirus, which typically presents 30 to 100 days after transplant, and may lead to a fatal pneumonitis. Patients may develop a morbilliform eruption and perianal erosions. Some centers perform weekly antigen tests in post-transplant patients. Finally, primary HIV infection must always be considered. A nonpruritic, photodistributed, macular rash is seen in 40% to 50% of patients during acute HIV infection (2–6 weeks postexposure).

ANGIOIMMUNOBLASTIC T-CELL LYMPHOMA

Angioimmunoblastic T-cell lymphoma (AITL), the second most common peripheral T-cell lymphoma, may present acutely with a diffuse, pruritic morbilliform rash, fever, and lymphadenopathy. The constellation of symptoms and the frequent accompanying eosinophilia may closely resemble drug reaction with eosinophilia and systemic symptoms. Distinguishing features of AITL include a polyclonal hypergammaglobulinemia (seen in 80% of patients), hemolytic anemia, and specific findings on lymph node biopsy. Treatment involves corticosteroids or cytotoxic agents. Prognosis is poor, with mortality of 50% to 72%, and a median survival of 11 to 30 months.

PRIMARY DERMATOLOGIC DISEASE

Exacerbation of an underlying dermatologic disease may have an acute and impressive presentation. Patients with psoriasis who are treated with systemic steroids for another condition may experience a severe generalized pustular version of psoriasis when the steroids are discontinued. A review of the patient's past dermatologic history should be performed when evaluating a potential drug reaction.

TRIAGE/HOSPITAL ADMISSION

Hospital admission is not required for reliable patients with classic morbilliform eruptions to a known culprit, in the absence of mucosal or systemic involvement. These patients may be observed in the outpatient setting and managed symptomatically, as long as they are aware of possible complications (the "red flags" of Table 142-1) and have access to an emergency department. In these patients, the culprit drug should be discontinued. In extraordinary circumstances where the culprit drug is required, no alternative exists, and the cutaneous eruption is benign, the drug may be continued with frequent monitoring for systemic involvement. Symptomatic treatment of associated pruritus includes oral antihistamines and topical steroids.

Hospital admission is indicated for any patient with a progressive cutaneous eruption of unclear etiology or the patient with a known cutaneous drug reaction who has mucosal involvement, immunocompromise, blisters, or signs of a systemic inflammatory response, including two or more of the following: fever, tachycardia, tachypnea, and leukocytosis or leukopenia.

COMPLICATIONS

MUCOSAL DAMAGE

Ocular sequelae may affect up to 35% of patients who survive SJS/TEN. The most common complication is a dry eye syndrome. More serious sequelae include corneal scarring and ocular vascularization, which may lead to permanent visual loss. Ocular sequelae cannot be predicted by percentage of body surface area involved, currently used SJS/TEN severity scores, or ocular symptoms during the acute stage. No preventive treatment regimens have been identified, but early studies suggest that amniotic membrane transplantation may be of use in some cases as an anti-inflammatory mediator. All patients with SJS/TEN should be evaluated routinely by ophthalmology during hospitalization and after discharge.

HEPATITIS

Fulminant hepatitis is the most common cause of death associated with DRESS. Liver biopsies show an eosinophilic infiltrate, granulomas and hepatocyte necrosis. Early recognition of DRESS and discontinuation of the culprit drug are critical to prevent hepatic damage. Of note, hepatitis may persist for several weeks after drug withdrawal and patients should be monitored closely.

SEPSIS

In patients with toxic epidermal necrolysis, sepsis is the most common cause of death. Early transfer to an intensive care unit, daily wound care, and periodic blood cultures can help prevent the morbidity and mortality associated with sepsis.

TREATMENT

SJS/TEN

Early discontinuation of the culprit drug reduces mortality and should be the primary intervention. All medications, especially those introduced within one month of the reaction, should be considered as a possible culprit, and discontinued. If widespread skin involvement is present (>30% BSA), the patient should be transferred to an intensive care unit or burn unit. A severity scoring system has been developed to predict prognosis (**Table 142-6**). Important complications to consider are fluid loss (approximately 3–4 liters daily in adults with 50% BSA involved), renal insufficiency, diffuse interstitial pneumonitis, and sepsis. Supportive measures including daily wound care, eye lubrication, pain control, nutritional support, and fluid replacement are the mainstays of treatment. All patients should have a routine ophthalmologic evaluation, and gynecologic evaluation should be considered when appropriate. Patients may require mechanical ventilation.

TABLE 142-6 SCORTEN: Severity-of-illness Score for Toxic Epidermal Necrolysis

Variables	Points
Age (≥ 40 y)	1
Heart rate (≥ 120/min)	1
BSA involved at day 1 > 10%	1
Serum urea level (> 10 mmol/L)	1
Serum bicarbonate level (> 14 mmol/L)	1
Score	**Mortality**
0–1	3
2	12
3	35
4	58
≥ 5	90

BSA, body surface area.
Data from Bastuji-Garin S, et al. *J Invest Dermatol.* 2000;115:149–153.

No clear consensus has emerged on systemic treatment modalities. As SJS/TEN are rare entities, designing randomized placebo controlled trials is challenging. Thalidomide, cyclosporine, and cyclophosphamide have been studied to date and show mixed results. Several studies support the use of systemic corticosteroids in SJS, advocating that if administered within the first two days, mortality may be decreased. An ongoing controversy exists on the role of human intravenous immunoglobulin (IVIg). A proposed mechanism argues that IVIg may provide Fas-blocking antibodies which interfere with Fas ligand-induced keratinocyte apoptosis. Of the eight clinical studies of IVIg use in adults with SJS/TEN to date (with > 10 patients), five showed reduction in mortality associated with a total dose of > 2 g/kg of IVIg over 3 to 4 days (**Table 142-7**). Effect of IVIG likely depends on timing of treatment in disease course, variability in the IVIG batch, dosing, and the patient's comorbidities (particularly renal insufficiency).

DRESS

In addition to withdrawal of the offending medication, systemic corticosteroids are often advocated for treatment of DRESS, especially when there is associated inflammation of the heart and lungs. The typical starting dose is prednisone 1 mg/kg/day. Steroid dose should be tapered slowly over several weeks to avoid the risk of relapse.

ANGIOEDEMA

All patients with progressive angioedema or a concern for anaphylaxis should be hospitalized and closely monitored. Severe angioedema must be treated with epinephrine. Otolaryngology should be consulted for airway management. Oral antihistamines, systemic steroids, or both, along with discontinuation of the culprit drug, are the treatment of choice in other cases.

AGEP

Treatment of AGEP consists of withdrawal of the culprit medication, topical corticosteroids, and antipyretics. Once the culprit medication is discontinued, resolution of symptoms occurs in a few days.

TABLE 142-7 Evidence-based Medicine: Key References for Use of IVIg in SJS/TEN

Study	Methodology	Number of Patients	Total IVIg Dose (g/kg)	Results	Adverse Effects	Authors' Conclusion
Prins C, et al. *Arch Dematol.* 2003;139:26–32.	Retrospective, noncontrolled study	38	2.7	90% had resolution of TEN within 15 days. 88% survival	None	Effective
Brown KM, et al. *J Burn Care Rehabil.* 2004;25:81–88.	Retrospective, controlled	24 (vs 21 placebo)	1.6	No difference in mortality or days until wound closure	More complications in TEN group	Ineffective
Bachot N, et al. *Arch Dermatol.* 2003;139:33–36.	Prospective, observed vs expected deaths	20	1.9	11 deaths, 8 expected	Overall decrease in renal function	Ineffective
Campione E, et al. *Acta Derm Venereol.* 2003;83:430–432.	Prospective	20	2	Stopped progression of disease within 2 days	Headache, nausea, GI distress	Effective
Shortt R, et al. *J Burn Care Rehabil.* 2004;25(3):246–255.	Retrospective, controlled	16 (vs 16 control patients)	2.8	No significant differences in progression of TEN	None	Ineffective
Al-Mutairi N, et al. *Int J Dermatol.* 2004;43:847–851.	Prospective, noncontrolled	12	3.2	Stopped progression of disease within average of 2 days. 100% survival	None	Effective
Trent JT, et al. *Arch Dermatol.* 2003;139:39–43.	Prospective, observed vs predicted death	10	3.9	1 patient died vs 5.8 predicted	None	Effective
Viard I, et al. *Science.* 1998;282:490–493.	Prospective, noncontrolled	10	2.5	Stopped progression of disease, rapid skin healing	None	Effective

GI, gastrointestinal; TEN, toxic epidermal necrolysis.
Data from Mittman N, et al. *Am J Clin Dermatol.* 2006;7:359–368.

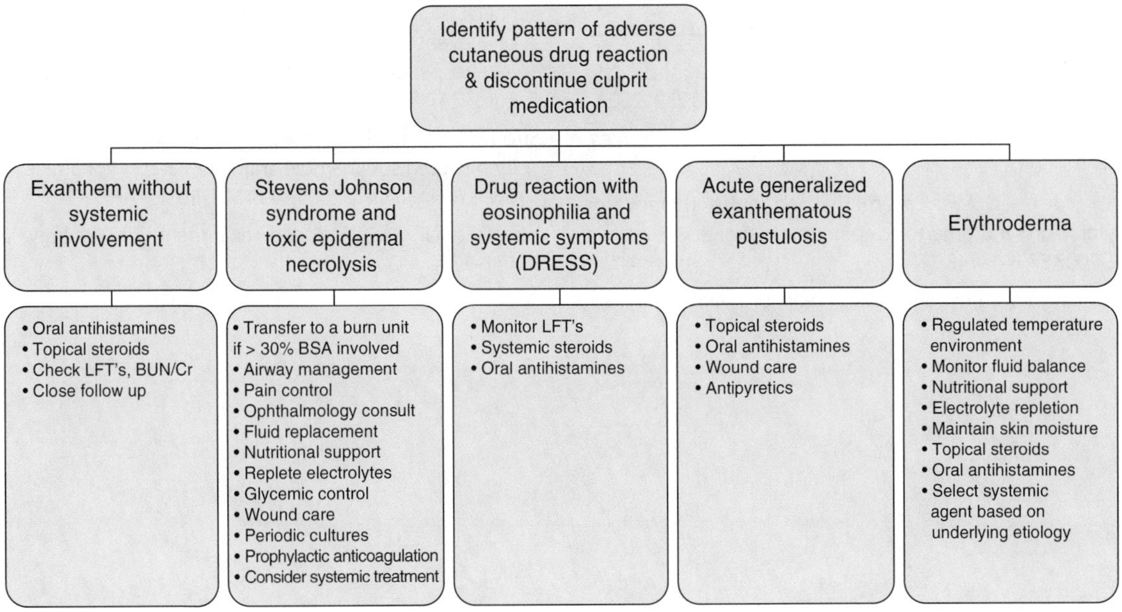

Figure 142-6 *Summary of treatment approaches for adverse cutaneous drug reactions.*

ERYTHRODERMA

Patients with erythroderma and signs of systemic inflammatory response or a history of immunosupression should be hospitalized to avoid complications related to high output heart failure, thermoregulatory disturbances, and the hypercatabolic state. Selection of systemic therapies must be carefully guided by the underlying cause of the erythroderma. While steroids may be beneficial in drug-induced erythroderma, they exacerbate psoriasis, and are contraindicated in staphylococcal scalded skin syndrome (**Figure 142-6**).

DISCHARGE CONSIDERATIONS

Several important considerations must be addressed prior to discharge. The adverse cutaneous drug reaction should be carefully recorded in the patient's medical record. Information should include the date the culprit drug was initiated and discontinued, the time of onset of the reaction, associated symptoms, systemic complications (if any), and the treatment provided. Patients who develop symptoms that are known side effects of a medication (eg, nausea while on doxycycline) should not be listed as allergic to the medication.

Patients must be clearly educated on what classes of medications to avoid. Patients with a history of DRESS associated to an aromatic anticonvulsant should avoid all other aromatic anticonvulsants (phenytoin, phenobarbital, and carbemazepine), as cross-reactivity approaches 70% to 80%. However, patients with adverse cutaneous drug reactions to sulfonamide antibiotics may not need to avoid other nonantibiotic sulfonamide agents. Research shows that while these patients are at a higher risk of future adverse drug reactions, there may not be cross-reactivity between the antibiotic and nonantibiotic sulfonamide agents. When the culprit medication is not clearly identified, patch tests have been shown to be helpful to avoid future recurrences of AGEP, but their sensitivity and specificity are low. Patients should be aware of signs and symptoms that require emergency department evaluation, and should also understand that certain reactions may rebound with steroid taper.

QUALITY IMPROVEMENT

Improvements in online medical records, communication, and a team-oriented systems approach may help avoid adverse cutaneous drug reactions. Online medical records must accurately record previous drug reactions. Already, many order entry systems can be programmed to prompt warnings and alarms when a similar drug class is ordered on readmission. Physicians and pharmacists should review these reactions and medication interactions routinely to ensure they are up to date.

National standards should exist for documentation of care when patients are transferred from one hospital system to another. If the receiving physician does not have access to information on the timing and dosing of medications received prior to arrival, recognition of an adverse cutaneous drug reaction and identification of the culprit medication may be delayed. The receiving physician should then communicate back to the transferring hospital so that they can update their patient record system as well. In the future, national drug databases should be easily accessible to all clinicians.

PRACTICE POINT

- Benign morbilliform drug reactions can be impressive in appearance. They will frequently generalize and develop a violaceous hue in the dependent areas. Outpatient management of a cutaneous drug reaction is appropriate if the patient is reliable, immunocompetent, and well appearing without mucosal membrane involvement or systemic symptoms, and if the culprit medication is identified. Patients who are not hospitalized should understand what signs/symptoms require further evaluation. Patients should also be aware that their skin findings and the associated pruritus may persist for up to 2 weeks after drug discontinuation.

SUGGESTED READINGS

Frigas E, Park MA. Acute urticaria and angioedema: diagnostic and treatment considerations. *Am J Clin Dermatol.* 2009;10:239–250.

Gruchalla RS, Pirmohamed M. Antibiotic allergy. *N Engl J Med.* 2006;354:601–609.

Kardaun SH, Jonkman MF. Dexamethasone pulse therapy for Stevens-Johnson syndrome/toxic epidermal necrolysis. *Acta Derm Venereol.* 2007;87:144–148.

Pichler WJ. Delayed drug hypersensitivity reactions. *Ann Intern Med.* 2003;139:683–693.

Schneck J, Fagot JP, Sekula P. Effects of treatments on the mortality of Stevens Johnson syndrome and toxic epidermal necrolysis: a retrospective study on patients included in the prospective EuroSCAR Study. *J Am Acad Dermatol.* 2008;58:33–40.

Strom BL, Shinnar R, Apter AJ, Margolis DJ. Absence of cross-reactivity between sulfonamide antibiotics and sulfonamide nonantibiotics. *N Engl J Med.* 2003;349:1628–1635.

Yawalkar N. Drug-induced exanthems. Toxicology 2005;209:131–134.

CHAPTER 143

Papulosquamous Disorders

Anne E. Allan, MD
Timothy R. Quinn, MD, CH

Key Clinical Questions

1. When should a patient with an erythematous scaly eruption be evaluated for an underlying infectious process?
2. How should the patient with diffuse erythroderma be evaluated?
3. What are the best topical treatments for psoriasis?
4. Are oral steroids useful in the treatment of psoriasis?
5. Are there physical findings that help differentiate between contact and irritant dermatitis?

INTRODUCTION

Papulosquamous disorders are a group of unrelated dermatologic conditions in which patients present with red, raised lesions with scale. While psoriasis is the prototypical papulosquamous disorder, similar skin lesions are seen in infections, lymphomas, and allergic conditions. The conditions described in this chapter are ubiquitous, and primarily inflammatory in nature. From a clinical point of view, the history, the distribution of the lesions, and careful evaluation of the primary lesion are most helpful in helping establish the diagnosis. Ancillary tests include a KOH preparation, a skin biopsy and, if necessary, dermatologic consultation. It should be remembered that treating a condition without a definitive diagnosis can lead to unnecessary patient aggravation and added expense.

PSORIASIS

Psoriasis, a chronic relapsing condition with genetic and environmental triggers, can be readily diagnosed on skin examination. It is very common. Approximately 2% of the population is affected by psoriasis. In the United States, the prevalence may be as high as 4.6%.

PATHOGENESIS

Psoriasis was formerly likened to "wound healing gone wrong." It was blamed on abnormally rapid keratinocyte growth and maturation, with a reduction of the epidermal turnover time from the normal 4 weeks to only 3 to 4 days. However, psoriasis is now recognized to be a T-cell–mediated disease. Several Th-1 helper lymphocyte-associated cytokines drive epidermal proliferation, such as interferon-α, tumor necrosis factor, and certain interleukins. Circulating levels of IL-22 are especially correlated with disease activity. Biopsy reveals epidermal hyperplasia with tortuous papillary dermal blood vessels, and a loss of the granular layer with abundant parakeratotic scale. In pustular lesions, neutrophils form collections in the epidermis.

CLINICAL FEATURES

The lesions are well demarcated and associated with a characteristic silvery white, plate-like adherent scale (**Figure 143-1**).

When the thick scale is forcibly removed, small punctate bleeding points develop (the Auspitz sign) (**Figure 143-2**).

Psoriasis may affect the entire body surface, including the nails. As injury can trigger psoriasis, lesions are typically seen on the elbows, knees, and buttocks (**Figure 143-3**).

While some patients are only troubled by pruritus, most are ashamed of their appearance and the unsightly scaling. Variants include the chronic plaque type, guttate psoriasis, and pustular psoriasis, all of which can evolve into the erythrodermic variant.

In plaque-type psoriasis, the most common presentation, patients develop well-demarcated erythematous scaly plaques distributed symmetrically over the extremities, often involving both elbows and knees. Psoriasis of the gluteal cleft is also common (**Figure 143-4**).

The lesions are chronic and persistent. In the guttate variant, which usually involves a younger age group, the lesions develop acutely, are smaller, have less scale, and are distributed widely over the trunk and buttocks (**Figure 143-5**).

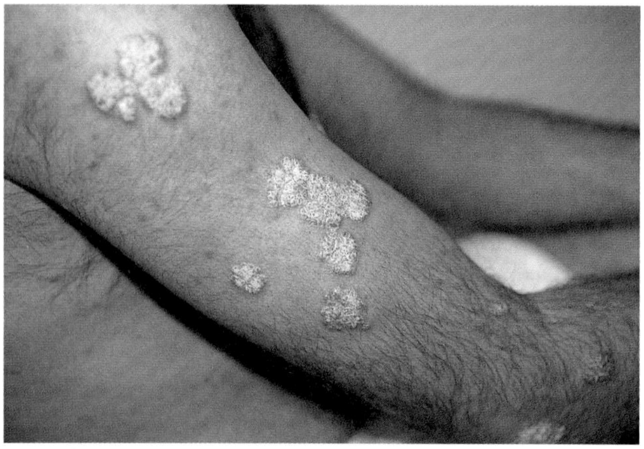

Figure 143-1 *Chronic plaque psoriasis with classic scale.*

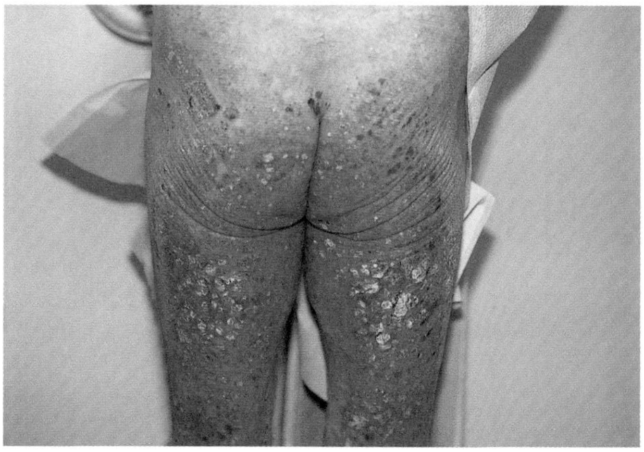

Figure 143-3 *Jockey with worsening psoriasis in areas of trauma.*

This variant is often triggered by an antecedent upper respiratory infection. In the rarer pustular variant, numerous pustules can be seen in a limited distribution involving acral sites (pustulosis of the palms and soles) or in a more generalized distribution associated with diffuse erythema (von Zumbusch variant). Common nail changes in psoriasis include nail pitting (**Figure 143-6**), onycholysis (separation of the nail plate from the nail bed), and subungual hyperkeratosis.

Occasionally a yellow shiny lesion, or "oil spot," develops in the nail bed. About 10% of patients have concomitant arthritis, which may be severe.

DIFFERENTIAL DIAGNOSIS

In a patient with a few isolated, red, raised lesions, tinea corporis, atopic dermatitis, contact and irritant dermatitis, seborrheic dermatitis, and cutaneous T-cell lymphoma should be considered. In tinea corporis the lesions are more annular with central clearing and have a raised border, often with only fine peripheral scale. A KOH preparation of the scale demonstrating fungal hyphae is diagnostic. In atopic, contact, and irritant dermatitides, the lesions are not so well demarcated and the distribution is different. Cutaneous T-cell lymphoma often presents on the buttocks and posterior thighs, but the plaques are thin and somewhat less red. A skin biopsy revealing atypical T lymphocytes within the epidermis is helpful in confirming this diagnosis. The differential diagnosis of the guttate variant includes drug eruption, viral exanthem, secondary syphilis, and pityriasis rosea. In the pustular variant involving the palms and soles, infections and impetiginized dyshidrotic eczema are in the differential diagnosis. In the more generalized pustular variant of psoriasis, pustular drug eruption and acute generalized exanthematous pustulosis (AGEP) should be excluded.

TREATMENT

In the hospitalized patient with chronic plaque-type psoriasis, it is reasonable to continue the patient's outpatient regimen. Topical steroid creams and ointments containing the vitamin D derivative calcipotriol or the retinoid tazarotene are mainstays of treatment. Both modify epidermal proliferation. Anthralins and tars are also effective, but not as widely used. Patients with a few lesions of the guttate variant may be treated with topical steroids alone. However, underlying streptococcal pharyngitis should be excluded, and treated if present. Systemic high-dose corticosteroids should be used with great caution in patients with psoriasis, as a severe flare of psoriasis with total body erythroderma may occur as glucocorticoids are tapered.

In patients with more generalized lesions of the chronic type and the guttate variant, which often involve 20% of the body or more, therapeutic options include ultraviolet (UV) therapy with narrow or broadband UVB, or psolaren UVA therapy, combining oral methoxy-psoralen with UVA radiation. The guttate variant usually resolves spontaneously over three months, but phototherapy hastens resolution. Additional therapies for diffuse recalcitrant psoriasis include acitretin, cyclosporine and methotrexate. Newer biologic agents, targeting either specific cytokines or specific T-cells, should be used in consultation with a dermatologist.

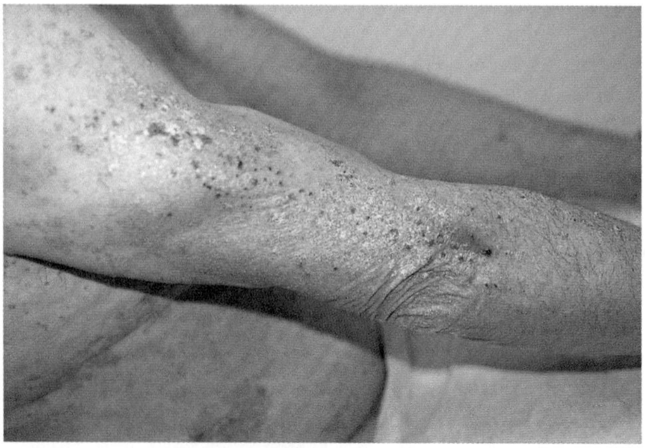

Figure 143-2 *Chronic plaque psoriasis with Auspitz sign.*

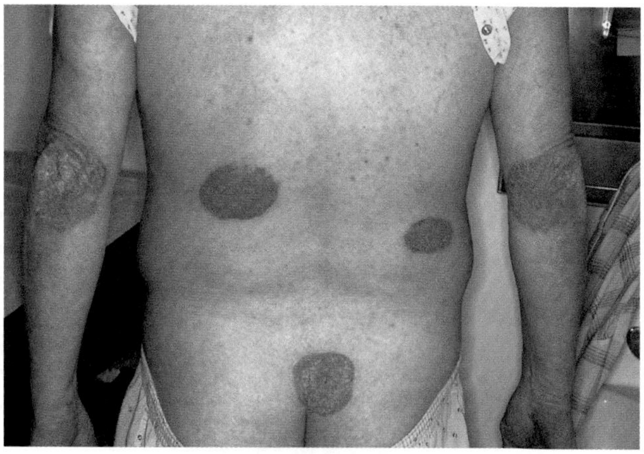

Figure 143-4 *Symmetrical involvement of psoriasis.*

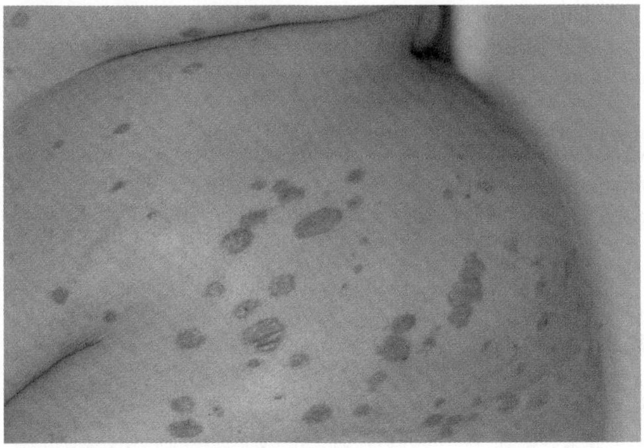

Figure 143-5 *Guttate psoriasis in the typical distribution.*

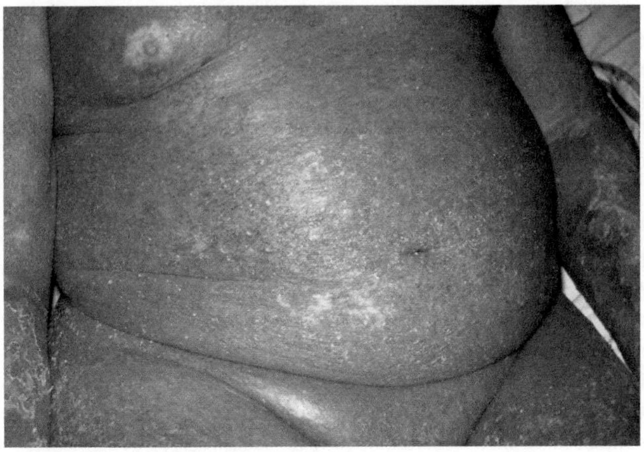

Figure 143-7 *Erythroderma.*

ERYTHRODERMA

Erythroderma, or exfoliative dermatitis, refers to extensive body redness often associated with scale. Diffuse erythroderma may be produced by several different underlying skin conditions. In 25% of cases, no clear cause is found. Erythroderma is rare, with a reported incidence of 1 to 2 per 100,000 of the population. Men are more often affected. The mean age of onset is 60 years.

PATHOPHYSIOLOGY

In erythroderma, inflammation leads to diffuse cutaneous vasodilation, with thermoregulation problems due to rapid heat loss through the skin. Patients may become hypothermic. Shunting of blood to the periphery may increase cardiac output and aggravate underlying heart disease. High-output cardiac failure has been reported. Inflammation also leads to epidermal hyperplasia and shortened transit time of keratinocytes through the epidermis. The new stratum corneum is poorly formed, compromising the normal barrier function of the epidermis, and leading to increased transepidermal water and protein loss. The risk of skin infection is also increased. As careful fluid, electrolyte, and cardiac monitoring are needed, patients with erythroderma are best managed in the hospital setting with dermatology consultation.

CLINICAL FEATURES

Over 90% of the patient's body surface area is diffusely erythematous (**Figure 143-7**).

There is minimal scale early on, with more developing a week after the onset of the erythema. The skin is warm. The patient complains of pruritus, and feels cold. On physical examination, 50% of patients have diffuse lymphadenopathy. When the exfoliative dermatitis is chronic, there may be associated hair loss and nail thickening. Hyperkeratosis of palms and soles also develops over time. Chronic periorbital edema and scale may lead to bilateral ectropion.

DIFFERENTIAL DIAGNOSIS

In evaluating the patient with diffuse erythema, it is important to seek a history of a prior skin condition (**Table 143-1**).

In more than 50% of patients, erythroderma results when a preexisting skin condition such as atopic dermatitis, psoriasis, or cutaneous T-cell lymphoma becomes generalized. A complete drug history should also be obtained; over 60 different drugs have been implicated in erythroderma. Skin biopsy determines the cause of erythroderma in over 60% cases, revealing subtle changes of the underlying chronic condition on microscopy. Patients with apparently idiopathic erythroderma ("red person syndrome") must be monitored and reevaluated over time.

Erythroderma usually develops gradually in those with a preexisting dermatosis, but may evolve rapidly and explosively when caused by lymphoma or a drug hypersensitivity reaction. Over 90% of patients present with pruritus. This is particularly severe in those with Sezary syndrome, the erythrodermic and leukemic variant of cutaneous T-cell lymphoma. Generalized lymphadenopathy is

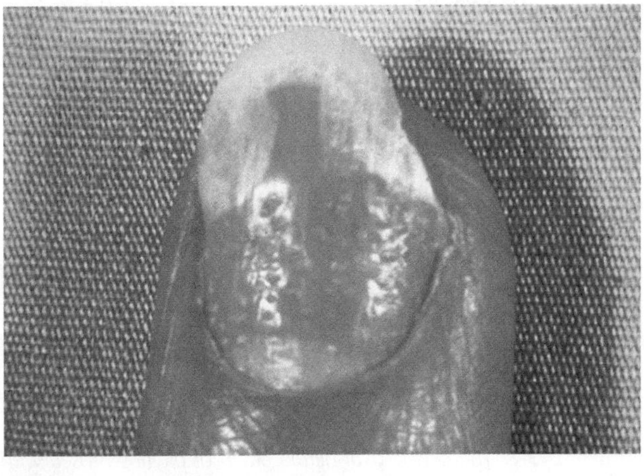

Figure 143-6 *Nail pitting in psoriasis.*

TABLE 143-1 Underlying Causes of Erythroderma

Preexisting conditions: psoriasis, atopic dermatitis, seborrheic dermatitis, contact dermatitis, pityriasis rubra pilaris, ichthyoses, cutaneous T-cell lymphoma, stasis dermatitis, scabies, sarcoid, bullous pemphigoid, pemphigus foliaceus, lichen planus, graft-vs-host disease, reactive arthritis, connective tissue disease, human immunodeficiency virus
Drugs: allopurinol, amiodarone, antimalarials, aspirin, anticonvulsants, angiotensin-converting enzyme inhibitors, cimetidine, ranitidine, furosemide, thiazides, isoniazid, lithium, nonsteroidal anti-inflammatory drugs, quinidine, sulfonamides
Lymphoma: cutaneous T-cell lymphoma, Sezary syndrome, extracutaneous lymphoma
Idiopathic: unclear cause at time of presentation, follow-up over time required; some will be reclassified into the lymphoma group at a later date

seen in half of those affected; it is usually dermatopathic in nature, driven by T cell expansion in response to antigen presentation by dendritic cells in the setting of skin inflammation. However, if lymphadenopathy is prominent, a Sezary count on peripheral blood and biopsies of skin or lymph node may be needed to rule out lymphoma.

TREATMENT

Definitive therapy of erythroderma depends on the underlying condition. Emollients and topical mild to mid-potency corticosteroid ointments under occlusion (to enhance absorption of the steroids) are helpful in most cases. Antihistamines can be given for pruritus. Cessation of all unnecessary drugs, including over-the-counter supplements, is advisable while the patient is being evaluated. Oral corticosteroids may be used in erythroderma due to drugs, but they are generally avoided in erythroderma secondary to underlying psoriasis. General care includes attention to the underlying metabolic and hemodynamic changes, and correction of fluid and electrolyte abnormalities.

SEBORRHEIC DERMATITIS

Seborrheic dermatitis is an erythematous, scaly eruption that develops in skin that is rich in sebaceous glands. Affected locations vary depending on the patient's age. In babies, the scalp and diaper regions are the major areas affected. In adults, the face, scalp, and chest are commonly involved. The prevalence is approximately 3% to 5%.

PATHOPHYSIOLOGY

The pathogenesis of seborrheic dermatitis has not been clearly established. Factors which may play a role include infection with the lipophilic yeast *Malassezia globosa,* increased sebaceous secretions, and genetic susceptibility. Patients with alcoholism and neurologic disorders such as Parkinson disease have an increased incidence of this condition, perhaps because of a reduced ability to perform skin care and hygiene. It is also common in HIV, presumably because of immune perturbations.

CLINICAL FEATURES

In adults, flaky, erythematous, thin, poorly demarcated patches and plaques are identified over the scalp, eyebrows, nasolabial folds, and ears. The chest can also be involved. The scale is yellower and greasier than that seen in psoriasis.

DIFFERENTIAL DIAGNOSIS

The presence of yellow scale and the absence of well-demarcated lesions help to distinguish seborrheic dermatitis from psoriasis. Actinic keratoses occur on sun-damaged areas, especially in fair-skinned persons; the scale is drier and crustier than that of seborrheic dermatitis. Additional entities that may be confused with seborrheic dermatitis include both contact and irritant dermatitis.

TREATMENT

Seborrheic dermatitis is generally a chronic relapsing condition. Topical therapies include a mild to mid-potency topical steroid cream combined with an antifungal cream, usually ketoconazole (2% cream applied daily). Attention to scalp involvement is also important, with frequent shampooing with 2% ketoconazole and antidandruff (zinc pyrithione) shampoos. In hospitalized patients with new onset or worsening seborrheic dermatitis, HIV testing should be considered. Seborrheic dermatitis is one of the most common cutaneous manifestations of AIDS, affecting between 20% to 80% of patients. Rarely, underlying zinc deficiency in those receiving parenteral nutrition has been also associated with this condition.

PITYRIASIS ROSEA

Pityriasis rosea is a self-limited skin eruption with a striking appearance, usually lasting 6 weeks, and most common in those between the ages of 10 and 35 years. The prevalence is 0.13% in women and 0.14% in men.

PATHOPHYSIOLOGY

A viral etiology for pityriasis rosea has long been suspected, as it is more prevalent in cooler months in the temperate zones, and outbreaks occur in confined populations. In addition, many patients report low-grade fever and upper respiratory symptoms prior to the eruption. Recent studies have implicated human herpesvirus 6 and 7 (HHV-6 and -7), but these are not conclusive.

CLINICAL FEATURES

The typical patient develops a single red scaly lesion, 2 to 10 cm in diameter, usually on the trunk or extremity (**Figure 143-8**).

This lesion, termed the herald patch, is usually slightly raised and salmon-red. This plaque or patch is ringed by a fine, wrinkled scale that forms a collar (collarette scale). After a few days to 2 weeks, additional smaller oval lesions with the same collarette scale develop over the trunk, distributed over the back along skin tension lines, a pattern likened to the drooping limbs of a Christmas tree. Most patients report some pruritus. The palms and soles are spared.

DIFFERENTIAL DIAGNOSIS

Classic pityriasis rosea is unlikely to be mistaken for other conditions by experienced clinicians. Unfortunately, atypical presentations occur. Patients may lack a typical herald patch. When only a few lesions are present, tinea corporis should be excluded, and a KOH examination performed. In those with more diffuse involvement, a drug eruption, a viral exanthem, guttate psoriasis, and secondary syphilis should be considered. Serologic testing for syphilis should be performed if the clinical diagnosis of pityriasis rosea is not definitive. Rarely, drugs such as captopril, hydrochlorothiazide, and imatinib have been reported to cause pityriasis rosea-like drug eruptions.

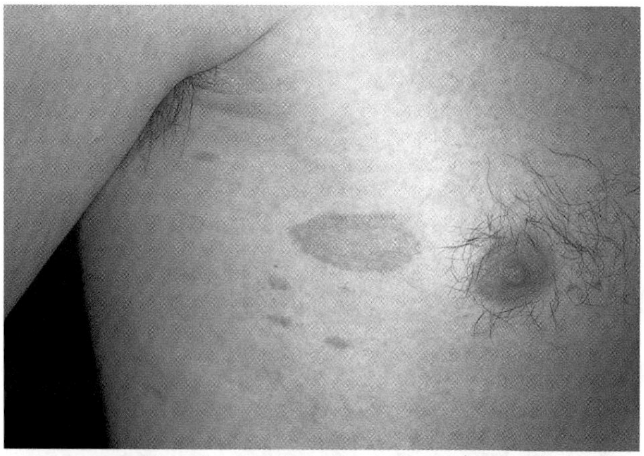

Figure 143-8 *The classic oval herald patch of pityriasis rosea with associated smaller lesions.*

■ TREATMENT

Most patients only require reassurance that the eruption will dissipate and does not cause additional problems. Patients must be informed that the eruption can last for as long as 12 to 14 weeks. Oral antihistamines and topical steroids may mollify the pruritus. Broadband UVB with daily erythemogenic dosages of UVB may also relieve pruritus and hasten the resolution of the eruption. All therapies work best when begun within two weeks of the onset.

ATOPIC (ECZEMATOUS) DERMATITIS

Atopic dermatitis (AD) is the prototype of the group of eczematous dermatidites. It is a chronic pruritic eruption commonly found in individuals with a personal or family history of an atopic diathesis (atopic dermatitis, asthma, allergic rhinitis). The prevalence in children in northern Europe, America, and Australia ranges from 10% to 20%, with a slight female preponderance. While it usually arises before the age of 5 years, the disorder may persist into childhood and adulthood. Clinical findings include an erythematous exudative papulovesicular rash involving the flexural and extensor surfaces of the upper and lower extremity. Over time, scaly lichenified patches and plaques appear, and tend to localize to the flexural regions. AD is associated with xerosis, and an increased susceptibility to exogenous irritants.

■ PATHOGENESIS

Immunologic factors contributing to atopic dermatitis include respiratory and food allergies, and possibly autoallergy. The impaired barrier function of the skin in AD makes it susceptible to environmental factors such as microbial pathogens, irritants, and allergens which exacerbate the inflammatory process. Genetic factors also play a role in AD. Up to 73% of patients have a family history of atopy. Chromosomal regions 3q21 and 5q31 have been linked to elevated serum IgE levels and AD. Genes mapping to loci that are involved in T-cell activation, Th-2 cytokines, the high affinity IgE receptor, and mast cell chymase have also been linked to AD.

■ CLINICAL FEATURES

While acute dermatitis predominates in childhood, and chronic changes are characteristic of adulthood, lesions may show acute, subacute, or chronic epidermal patterns at any age. Acute lesions are characterized by erythematous and edematous papules and plaques. In severe cases, these progress to vesicles with extensive crust. Superimposed excoriations are frequently present. Subacute and chronic lesions are characterized by increased epidermal thickening and hyperkeratosis with lichenification. Papular eczema with perifollicular accentuation is a variant commonly observed in patients with Asian and African heritage. In adults, AD is localized predominantly in a flexural distribution involving the antecubital and popliteal fossae and posterior neck. Wrists, hands, and feet are also commonly involved. Characteristic secondary findings include pruritus, xerosis, keratosis pilaris, ichthyosis vulgaris, and if lichenification is severe, prurigo nodularis. Erythroderma may develop at any stage of AD.

■ DIFFERENTIAL DIAGNOSIS

In adults, diagnostic considerations include allergic or irritant contact dermatitis, cutaneous T-cell lymphoma (CTCL), psoriasis, asteatotic eczema, lichen simplex chronicus, scabies, fungal infection, and drug reactions. The history and pattern of distribution should allow separation of AD from contact dermatitis and drug eruption. Biopsy will distinguish AD from most cases of psoriasis, CTCL, infection, and lichen simplex chronicus.

■ TREATMENT

Prevention and supportive care includes reducing triggers such as soaps and chemicals. Liberal use of emollients to avoid xerosis helps maintain the barrier function of the skin. Drug therapy includes topical corticosteroids and topical calcineurin inhibitors, such as tacrolimus and pimecrolimus. Adjunctive therapies include antihistamines for pruritus and antimicrobials for superinfection. Phototherapy, systemic steroids, and immunosuppressant therapies such as cyclosporine, methotrexate, and azathioprine are used in patients with severe and recalcitrant disease.

ALLERGIC CONTACT DERMATITIS

Allergic contact dermatitis (ACD) is a delayed-type hypersensitivity reaction from exposure to an allergen to which an individual has been previously sensitized. Common triggers include nickel-containing jewelry, cosmetics, topical medications, plants, and chemicals at home and in workplace. ACD is common, representing approximately 4% to 7% of all dermatologic consultations. No specific age, race or sex difference can be observed when controlled for exposure patterns.

■ PATHOGENESIS

Re-exposure to an allergen after sensitization results in antigen presentation to primed T-cells, ultimately producing an eczematous epidermal reaction pattern. On biopsy, ACD is characterized by spongiotic microvesicles in the epidermis, imparting a "Swiss cheese" appearance. Subacute and chronic lesions are indistinguishable from other forms of chronic eczematous dermatitis.

■ CLINICAL FEATURES

ACD presents as a pruritic papulovesicular eruption, often exhibiting discrete or bizarre-appearing patterns, depending on the extent of contact with the allergen. Classic examples include linear streaks on the legs after contact with poison ivy, and lesions under earrings, necklaces, or watches in individuals with nickel allergy.

■ DIFFERENTIAL DIAGNOSIS

The differential diagnosis includes other forms of eczematous dermatitis, such as irritant contact dermatitis, atopic dermatitis, stasis dermatitis, and seborrheic dermatitis. Hand and foot contact dermatitis should be distinguished from psoriasis and tinea. The history and the pattern of distribution are generally most helpful in making a diagnosis. Patch testing and biopsy evaluation may be useful when the history and physical exam is not diagnostic.

■ TREATMENT

If the allergen is identified, removal of the offending agent and patient education are paramount for avoiding future contact reactions. Topical and systemic corticosteroids in the case of severe reactions are useful to reduce inflammation. Generous use of emollients will allow the reestablishment of the barrier function of the skin.

IRRITANT CONTACT DERMATITIS

Irritant contact dermatitis (ICD) is a localized nonimmune-mediated reaction secondary to the direct cytotoxic effect of an irritant compound. Offending agents include soaps, detergents, feces, urine, solvents, and wool. ICD is a leading cause of occupational morbidity in the hospital setting.

■ EPIDEMIOLOGY

ICD represents approximately 80% of all cases of contact dermatitis. High at-risk occupations with frequent irritant exposure include hospital workers; kitchen and catering staff; hair stylists; chemical, metal, and textile workers; and dry cleaner workers. Epidermal barrier function has a direct bearing on susceptibility to ICD, with infants and the elderly being more often affected. Any substance that reduces the barrier function of the skin, such as water or detergents, commonly increases the incidence of ICD.

PATHOGENESIS

Offending agents commonly associated with ICD may either act acutely, by provoking cytotoxic damage to keratinocytes, or chronically, gradual damaging cell membranes by disrupting the barrier function of keratinocytes and surface lipids. After keratinocyte injury, T-cells are activated, with cytokine production resulting in epidermal proliferation and an eczematous irritant epidermal reaction. On biopsy, epidermal necrosis with mild spongiosis is characteristic.

CLINICAL FEATURES

Skin findings include erythema, eczematous changes, vesiculobullous lesions, and frank epidermal necrosis. The lesions have sharply demarcated borders, and are limited to the area of irritant exposure.

DIFFERENTIAL DIAGNOSIS

In most cases, ICD is a diagnosis of exclusion, with ACD being the most important differential consideration. Clinically, patients frequently report a sensation of burning or stinging, rather than the pruritus of ACD.

TREATMENT

Avoidance of and protection from causative agents is the principal treatment for ICD. Preventive measures include protective equipment, barrier ointments, and emollients. Topical steroids and immune modulators are generally not helpful in the treatment of ICD.

SUGGESTED READINGS

Chang C, Keen CL, Gershwin ME. Treatment of eczema. *Clin Rev Allergy Immunol.* 2007;33:204–225.

Drago F, Broccolo F, Rebora A. Pityriasis rosea: an update with a critical appraisal of its possible herpesviral etiology. *J Am Acad Dermatol.* 2009;61:303–318.

Levine D, Gottlieb A. Evaluation and management of psoriasis: an internist's guide. *Med Clin North Am.* 2009;93:1291–1303.

Naldi L, Rebora A. Clinical practice: seborrheic dermatitis. *N Engl J Med.* 2009;360:387–396.

Nosbaum A, Vocanson M, Rozieres A, Hennino A, Nicolas JF. Allergic and irritant contact dermatitis. *Eur J Dermatol.* 2009;19:325–332.

CHAPTER 144

Pressure Ulcers

Courtney H. Lyder, MD, GNP, FAAN

Key Clinical Questions

1. What is a pressure ulcer and how do you stage severity?
2. How do you assess individual risk for the development of pressure ulcers?
3. What measures are effective in pressure ulcer prevention?
4. How should pressure ulcers be cleansed, debrided, and dressed?
5. What role do adjunctive therapies have in pressure ulcer treatment?

INTRODUCTION

Pressure ulcers, or "bedsores," are a key clinical indicator of quality of care in hospitals. Their occurrence is widely seen as a marker for substandard care, triggering anger and sometimes litigation on the part of patients and families. However, they remain common in hospitalized patients. In 1993, pressure ulcers were diagnosed during 280,000 hospital stays in the United States, a number that rose to 455,000 in 2004. Up to 15% of elderly patients develop pressure ulcers within the first week of hospitalization. Mortality may be as high as 60% for older persons with pressure ulcers in the year after hospital discharge.

Pressure ulcers are also expensive, with an average charge per stay of $43,180. In 2007, the Centers for Medicare and Medicaid Services (CMS) made payouts of more than $11 billion for beneficiaries admitted to hospitals who developed stage III and stage IV pressure ulcers. The Centers for Medicare and Medicaid Services subsequently stopped reimbursement for hospital-acquired stage III and stage IV pressure ulcers in October 2008.

PATHOPHYSIOLOGY

Pressure ulcers are focal injuries of skin and subcutaneous tissue resulting from pressure, shear forces, friction, or some combination of these. They most often overlie bony prominences of the pelvis and lower extremities, such as the sacrum, greater trochanter of the hip, and heels, but they may appear in other locations, depending on patient positioning (**Figure 144-1**).

Tissue ischemia occurs when external pressures exceed perfusion pressures. Normal blood pressure within capillaries ranges from 20 to 40 mm Hg; 32 mm Hg is considered average. An external pressure less than 32 mm Hg usually suffices to prevent pressure ulcers. However, capillary blood pressure may be less than 32 mm Hg in critically ill patients due to hemodynamic instability and comorbid conditions.

Frictional forces, like those generated between the heels and bedsheets, can lead to blisters and skin breakdown, favoring the development of pressure ulcers. Bedbound patients are also prone to shear forces, which occur when bone and soft tissue move relative to the skin, which is held in place by friction.

Older patients are more susceptible to shear forces, as their soft tissues are atrophied and contain less elastin. Moisture, as in urine, stool, and sweat, acts synergistically with pressure, friction, and shear forces to facilitate skin breakdown.

PREVENTION

Pressure ulcer prevention requires a team effort, involving physicians, nurses (including wound, ostomy, and continence nurses), dietitians, and physical therapists. Studies have demonstrated that comprehensive pressure ulcer prevention programs can decrease incidence rates, although not to zero. For optimal effectiveness, pressure ulcer prevention must begin as soon as patients enter the hospital. There are five basic components to comprehensive pressure ulcer prevention: risk assessment, skin care, mechanical loading, support surfaces, and nutritional support.

RISK ASSESSMENT

The identification of patients at greatest risk of pressure ulcers involves the use of a risk assessment tool, skin assessment, and

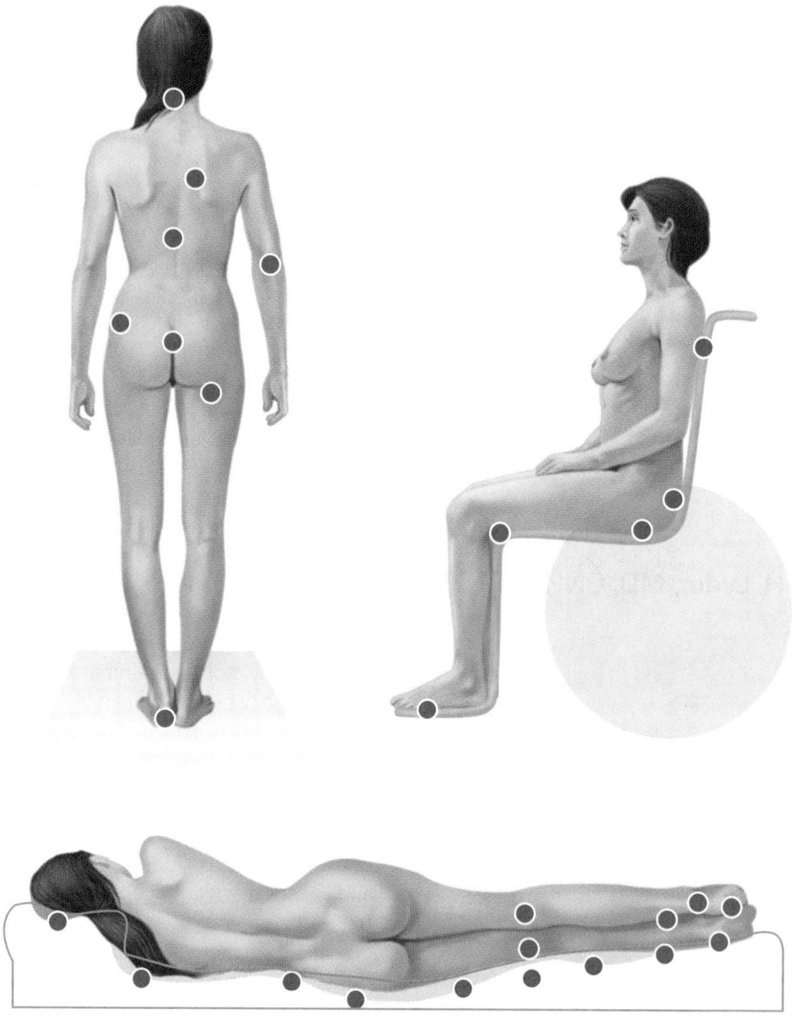

Figure 144-1 *Pressure ulcer locations. The most common sites of pressure ulceration are the sacrum and coccyx, heels, and greater trochanters of the hip. (From Preventing Pressure Ulcers: A Patient's Guide. Washington, DC: U.S. Department of Health and Human Services; USGPO 617-025/68298,1992).*

clinical judgment. More than 20 pressure ulcer prediction tools are used throughout the world, with the most popular being the Braden, Norton, and Waterlow scales. The Braden Scale for Predicting Pressure Sore Risk is the most widely used in U.S. hospitals. (The copyrighted tool is available at http://www.bradenscale.com/images/bradenscale.pdf.) The Braden Scale is designed for use with adults, and consists of six subscales: sensory perception, moisture, activity, mobility, nutrition, and friction and shear. Total scores on the Braden Scale range from 6 (high risk) to 23 (low risk); a score of 18 is the cut-off score for onset of pressure ulcer risk.

There is general consensus from most pressure ulcer clinical guidelines to do a risk assessment on admission, at discharge, and whenever the patient's clinical condition changes. Skin assessment should also be correlated with risk assessment. Close attention should be paid to greater trochanters, heels, sacrum, and coccyx, as more than 60% of all pressure ulcers occur at these locations.

SKIN CARE

The skin of patients at risk of pressure ulceration should be inspected regularly for erythema. This includes pressure points, as well as areas of contact with medical devices, such as catheters, oxygen tubing, ventilator tubing, and semi-rigid cervical collars, as these may also cause ulceration. Pain over an erythematous area may herald skin breakdown. It is not always possible to see redness on darkly pigmented skin. However, depending on the degree of pigmentation, erythema may appear blue or purple, compared to adjacent skin. Erythema should be categorized as blanching or nonblanching. Localized heat, edema, and induration over the pressure points are additional warning signs for pressure ulcer development. The frequency of inspection may need to be increased in response to any deterioration in overall patient condition.

Protecting skin from excessive moisture with barrier paste or other products is essential, as the mechanical properties of the stratum corneum may be changed by moisture and warmth. Massaging areas of reddened skin should be avoided, as these may contain damaged blood vessels or fragile skin. Skin emollients to hydrate dry skin should be considered.

MECHANICAL LOADING

One of the most important preventive measures is decreasing mechanical load and pressure exposure. High pressures over bony prominences for short periods of time and low pressures over bony prominences for long periods of time are equally damaging. Repositioning frequency should be determined by the patient's skin condition and tissue tolerance, level of activity and mobility, general medical condition, overall treatment objectives, and support surfaces applied to the bed or chair. Turning and repositioning hospitalized patients every two hours while in bed, and every one hour while seated, is reasonable for most hospitalized patients. Those who are critically ill may require hourly repositioning, while stabilized patients on specialty beds, such as low air loss or air fluidized, may only need repositioning every four hours.

The patient should be repositioned to relieve or redistribute pressure. Transfer aids, such as the Hoyer lift or trapeze, that reduce friction and shear forces should be used. Avoid positioning the patient directly on a bony prominence or directly onto medical devices, such as tubes or drains. The 30-degree-tilt position and the standard 90-degree side-lying position seem to be equivalent in protection against the development of pressure ulcers.

SUPPORT SURFACES

Pressure should be distributed as evenly as possible across the patient's body to reduce the incidence of pressure ulcers. The use of support surfaces may assist in pressure redistribution. The Centers for Medicare and Medicaid Services have divided support surfaces into three categories for reimbursement purposes. Group 1 devices are static and do not require electricity. Static devices include air, foam (convoluted and solid), gel, and water overlays or mattresses. These devices are ideal when a patient is at low risk for pressure ulcer development. The devices have some drawbacks: foam may degrade and lose its stiffness over time, and gel mattresses can increase skin heat and moisture. Group 2 devices are dynamic and powered by electricity or pump action. These devices include alternating and low-air-loss mattresses. These mattresses are better for patients at moderate to high risk for pressure ulcers, or who have full-thickness pressure ulcers (stage III and stage IV). Critically ill patients are excellent candidates for this group of support surfaces.

Group 3 devices, also dynamic, comprise only air-fluidized beds. These are electric, and contain silicone-coated beads that liquefy when air is pumped through the bed. These beds are used for patients at very high risk for pressure ulcers, patients with nonhealing full-thickness pressure ulcers, and patients with numerous truncal full-thickness pressure ulcers. The National Pressure Ulcer Advisory Panel has suggested new definitions for support surfaces that move away from these categories and divide support surfaces into simply powered or nonpowered. Whether these new definitions will be embraced by the Centers for Medicare and Medicaid Services is yet to be determined.

Approximately 20% of all pressure ulcers are found on the heels. Heel-protection devices should be considered for hospitalized patients at risk for pressure ulcers. The heels should be elevated and offloaded to distribute the weight of the leg along the calf without putting pressure on the Achilles tendon. The knee should also be in slight flexion to avoid hyperextension of the knee, which could lead to obstruction of the popliteal vein and deep vein thrombosis. Some hospitals may alternatively use a pillow to "float" the heels. If the use of a pillow is preferred, then the pillow should be placed under the calves to elevate the heels from the mattress.

NUTRITION

While nutritional status in patients with pressure ulcers is often poor, the evidence for a relationship between nutrition intake and pressure ulcer prevention is not always supported by randomized controlled trials. There is also a lack of empirical evidence to link the use of vitamin and mineral supplementation to the prevention of pressure ulcers. Therefore, while nutritional status should be optimized in patients at risk for pressure ulcers, overtreatment should also be avoided.

TREATMENT

When a pressure ulcer develops, the hospitalist must provide local care of the ulcer, but also assess the patient's overall physical health, nutritional status, pain level, and psychosocial health, considering the whole patient, not merely the hole on the patient. In addition to mechanical loading and support surfaces, as discussed above, pressure ulcer management includes the following.

ULCER ASSESSMENT

The ulcer bed should first be cleansed with a nontoxic solution. Cleaning removes necrotic debris and bacteria that may delay healing. Normal saline (0.9% sodium chloride) or water solutions are best, as neither is toxic to healthy tissue. Although the active ingredients in newer wound cleansers may be nontoxic surfactants, the inert carrier may be toxic to healthy granulation tissue.

The pressure ulcer should be assessed for location, stage, size (length, width and depth), sinus tracts, undermining, tunneling, exudate (quality and quantity), necrotic tissue, and the presence or absence of granulation tissue and epithelialization. This comprehensive assessment establishes the baseline for measuring ulcer healing or deterioration. Ulcer assessment should be done at least weekly.

STAGING

Upon completing the pressure ulcer assessment, the ulcer should be staged. The most commonly used pressure ulcer staging system was developed by the National Pressure Ulcer Advisory Panel. Their system classifies skin changes into five levels of skin ulceration (**Table 144-1** and **Figure 144-2**).

This system rates the pressure ulcer from superficial tissue damage (stage I) to full-thickness skin loss involving muscle or bone (stage IV) and deep tissue injury. If the pressure ulcer is covered with necrotic tissue (eschar), it is noted as unstageable.

WOUND BED PREPARATION

A recent concept in the healing of chronic ulcers is wound bed preparation. The goal of wound bed preparation is to provide the ulcer with an optimal environment for healing: a wound bed that is highly vascularized, with minimal exudate. The three main principles are debridement, bacterial balance, and exudate control.

There is no optimal debridement method. The preferred method is determined by the goals of the patient, the presence or absence of infection, the amount of dead tissue present, and cost considerations. There are five common types of debridement: mechanical, autolytic, enzymatic, sharp, and biosurgery. *Mechanical debridement* uses wet-to-dry gauze to adhere to the necrotic tissue, which is then removed. Upon removal of the gauze dressing, necrotic tissue and wound debris are removed. The challenge with mechanical debridement is the possibility that healthy granulation tissue may also be removed along with the devitalized tissue, thereby delaying wound healing. *Autolytic debridement* involves semi-occlusive, transparent film dressings, and occlusive dressings, such as hydrocolloids and hydrogels, which create a favorable environment for the body's enzymes to break down the necrotic tissue. *Enzymatic debridement* employs proteolytic enzymes, such as papain-urea, collagenase, and trypsin, to remove necrotic tissue. While enzymatic debridement is effective, it is slower than other types and often costly. *Sharp debridement* with scalpel or laser is probably the most rapid and effective type of debridement, and should be strongly considered when the patient is suspected of having cellulitis or sepsis. Finally, *biosurgery* (maggot therapy) is another effective and relatively quick method of debridement. Maggot therapy is very specific for devitalized tissue, although patient and provider unease have limited its acceptance.

TABLE 144-1 National Pressure Ulcer Staging System

Pressure Ulcer Stage	Previous NPUAP Staging Definitions	2007 NPUAP Definitions	2007 NPUAP Descriptions to Accompany Revised Definitions
Deep tissue injury	A pressure-related injury to subcutaneous tissues under intact skin. Initially, these lesions have the appearance of a deep bruise, and they may herald the subsequent development of a Stage III–IV pressure ulcer, even with optimal treatment.	Purple or maroon localized area of discolored intact skin or blood-filled blister due to damage of underlying soft tissue from pressure and/or shear.	• The area may be preceded by tissue that is painful, firm, mushy, boggy, warmer, or cooler, as compared to adjacent tissue. • Deep tissue injury may be difficult to detect in individuals with dark skin tones. • The area may rapidly evolve to expose additional layers of tissue, even with optimal treatment.
Stage I	An observable pressure-related alteration of intact skin whose indicators as compared to an adjacent or opposite area on the body may include changes in one or more of these parameters: skin temperature (warmth or coolness), tissue consistency (firm or boggy feel), sensation (pain, itching), and/or a defined area of persistent redness in lightly pigmented skin; in darker skin tones, the ulcer may appear with persistent red, blue, or purple hues.	Intact skin with nonblanchable redness of a localized area, usually over a bony prominence.	• The area may be painful, firm, soft, warmer, or cooler, as compared to adjacent tissue. • Stage I may be difficult to detect in individuals with dark skin tones. • May indicate at-risk persons (a heralding sign of risk).
Stage II	Partial thickness skin loss involving the epidermis and/or dermis. The ulcer is superficial and presents clinically as an abrasion, blister, or shallow crater.	Partial thickness loss of dermis presenting as a shallow open ulcer with a red, pink wound bed without slough. May also present as an intact or open/ruptured serum-filled blister.	Presents as a shiny or dry shallow ulcer without slough or bruising. This stage should not be used to describe skin tears, tape burns, perineal dermatitis, maceration, or excoriation.
Stage III	Full thickness skin loss involving damage or necrosis of subcutaneous tissue that may extend down to, but not through, underlying fascia. The ulcer presents clinically as a deep crater with or without undermining of adjacent tissue.	Full thickness tissue loss. Subcutaneous fat may be visible, but bone, tendon, or muscle are *not* exposed. Slough may be present but does not obscure the depth of tissue loss. *May* include undermining and tunneling.	• The depth of a Stage III pressure ulcer varies by anatomical location. The bridge of the nose, ear, occiput, and malleolus do not have subcutaneous tissue, and Stage III ulcers can be shallow. In contrast, areas of significant adiposity can develop in extremely deep Stage III pressure ulcers. • Bone/tendon is not visible or directly palpable.
Stage IV	Full thickness skin loss with extensive destruction; tissue necrosis; or damage to muscle, bone, or supporting structure (such as tendon, or joint capsule).	Full thickness tissue loss with exposed bone, tendon, or muscle. Slough or eschar may be present on some parts of the wound bed. *Often* includes undermining and tunneling.	• The depth of a Stage IV pressure ulcer varies by anatomical location. The bridge of the nose, ear, occiput, and malleolus do not have subcutaneous tissue, and these ulcers can be shallow. • Stage IV ulcers can extend into muscle and/or supporting structures (eg, fascia, tendon, or joint capsule), making osteomyelitis likely to occur. • Exposed bone/tendon is visible or directly palpable.
Unstageable		Full thickness tissue loss in which *actual* depth of the ulcer is *completely* obscured by slough (yellow, tan, gray, green, or brown) and/or eschar (tan, brown, or black) in the wound bed.	Until enough slough and/or eschar is removed to expose the base of the wound, the true depth, and therefore stage, cannot be determined. Stable (dry, or adherent, intact without erythema or fluctuance) eschar on the heels serves as the "the body's natural (biological) cover" and should not be removed.

Reproduced, with permission, from National Pressure Ulcer Advisory Panel.

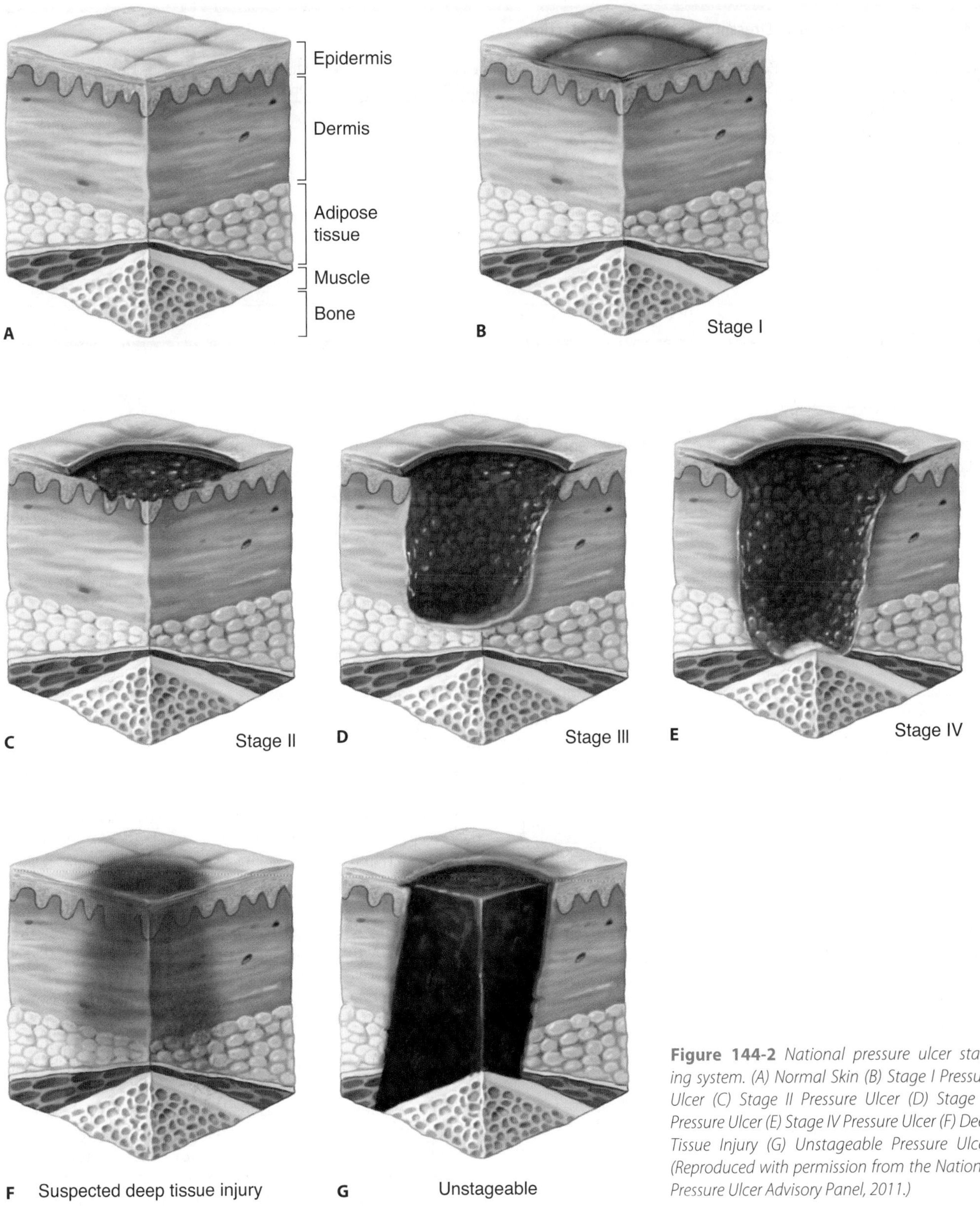

Figure 144-2 *National pressure ulcer staging system. (A) Normal Skin (B) Stage I Pressure Ulcer (C) Stage II Pressure Ulcer (D) Stage III Pressure Ulcer (E) Stage IV Pressure Ulcer (F) Deep Tissue Injury (G) Unstageable Pressure Ulcer. (Reproduced with permission from the National Pressure Ulcer Advisory Panel, 2011.)*

Managing bacterial burden is an important consideration in wound bed preparation. All pressure ulcers contain a variety of bacteria. Bacteria are more likely to impede wound healing when their concentration reaches 105 or 106 organisms per gram in the ulcer. Certain strains of bacteria may impair ulcer healing at lower concentrations. Clinical signs of ulcer infection include odor, purulent exudate, excessive draining, bleeding, and pain. If these are present, wound cultures should be obtained, and treatment with oral or intravenous antibiotics should be considered based on antimicrobial sensitivity testing. Other strategies to reduce bacterial bioburden include the use of silver impregnated dressings and topical sulfa silverdiazine.

Exudate management is the last component of wound bed preparation. Excessive exudate decreases ulcer healing, and may damage healthy surrounding tissue. Exudates are managed by selecting an appropriate dressing. Dressings can be classified as

TABLE 144-2 Pressure Ulcer Dressing Classification Selection

Dressing Classification	Partial Thickness (Stages I and II)	Full Thickness (Stages III and IV)	Moderate Drainage	Heavy Drainage
Transparent films	X			
Hydrocolloids	X	X (As a secondary dressing)	X	X
Alginates	X (Stage II only)	X		X
Foams	X (Stage II only)	X	X	X
Composites	X (Stage II only)	X	X	X
Hydrogels	X (Stage II with dry wound bed only)	X (Dry wound beds only)		
Hydrofibers		X		X
Antirecalcitrant dressings		X	X	X

gauze, petroleum-based nonadherent gauze, transparent films, hydrocolloids, foam islands, alginates, hydrogels, composites, and combinations (**Table 144-2**).

No matter what dressing is selected, the goal should be to keep the pressure ulcer moist, which optimizes healing. Since no studies exist that demonstrate that one dressing heals all pressure ulcers within an ulcer classification, a careful assessment of the pressure ulcer, needs of the patient, and environmental factors (frequency of dressing changes to increase adherence) must be considered.

Since wet-to-dry gauze dressings are a form of debridement, they should only be used in necrotic wounds. Once healthy granulation tissue is observed, wet-to-dry dressing should be stopped, and other dressings should be used. Negative pressure therapy, or vacuum-assisted closure (VAC) therapy, should also be considered for exudating ulcers. Negative pressure therapy removes excess exudate, increases local blood flow, and promotes granulation tissue. Negative pressure therapy should not be used in pressure ulcers with suspected osteomyelitis, eschar, or exposed blood vessels or viscera.

NUTRITION

Many patients with pressure ulcers are malnourished. High protein diets in poorly nourished patients with pressure wounds are reasonable, although there is a paucity of evidence to support their use.

PAIN MANAGEMENT

Pressure ulcers are often painful, especially stage IV ulcers. Strategies to reduce pain include the use of dressings that may mitigate pain, such as those containing soft-silicone, and administering analgesic prior to dressing changes.

MONITORING HEALING

There is considerable debate regarding the use of reverse staging of pressure ulcers to monitor healing. Staging of pressure ulcers is only appropriate for defining the maximum anatomic depth of tissue damage. Since pressure ulcers heal to progressively more shallow depth, they do not replace lost muscle, subcutaneous fat, or dermis before they reepithelialize. Instead, pressure ulcers are filled with granulation (scar) tissue composed primarily of endothelial cells, fibroblasts, collagen, and extra cellular matrix. Thus, a stage IV pressure ulcer cannot become a stage III, stage II, or subsequently stage I. When a stage IV pressure ulcer has healed, it should be classified as a healed stage IV pressure ulcer, not a Stage 0. Therefore, reverse staging does not accurately characterize what is physiologically occurring in the pressure ulcer.

The Pressure Ulcer Scale for Healing (PUSH) and the Bates-Jensen Wound Assessment Tool (BWAT) are both valid and reliable for measuring pressure ulcer healing. The PUSH tool requires less time, having only three items, compared to the 13 items of the BWAT tool. For both tools, a lower score indicates a greater degree of healing. Both tools are usually used weekly.

ADJUNCTIVE THERAPY

When the pressure ulcer is not showing signs of healing within two to four weeks, adjunctive therapies should be considered. The most commonly adjunctive therapies include electrical stimulation, hyperbaric oxygen, growth factors, and autologous skin. Electrical stimulation is the use of electrical current to stimulate cellular processes important to pressure ulcer healing. These processes include increasing fibroblasts, neutrophils, and macrophages, collagen and DNA synthesis, and increasing the number of receptor sites for specific growth factors. Electrical stimulation is most effective in healing stage III and IV pressure ulcers.

Hyperbaric oxygen is believed to promote wound healing by stimulating fibroblast, collagen synthesis, epithelialization, and control of infection. However, there remains a dearth of studies investigating the association of hyperbaric oxygen and healing pressure ulcers. The use of growth factors and skin equivalents in healing of pressure ulcers is relatively new. The use of cytokine growth factors, such as recombinant platelet-derived growth factor-BB (rhPDGF-BB) and fibroblast growth factors (bFGF), and skin equivalents are currently being studied. Much research is needed to identify the appropriate ulcer environment for growth factors to be optimally effective.

QUALITY IMPROVEMENT

Quality improvement measures to prevent pressure ulcers include risk assessment at admission, discharge, and when the patient's clinical condition changes; staff education; better documentation; increased use of mechanical loading and support surfaces to reduce pressure, friction, and shear forces; and the creation of a dedicated wound care team to improve care practices.

PRACTICE POINT

- All wounds may be painful, and they may become more sensitive over time. Light touch or even air movement across a pressure ulcer may be exquisitely painful for some patients. Control of background pain and incident pain (that occurring at dressing changes) may require basal pain medication as well as premedication for dressing changes. Nonpharmacologic measures that may reduce patient discomfort during dressing changes include measures that make the environment less stressful, such as noise reduction, engaging family members and ancillary personnel in hand holding when appropriate, frequent explanation and verbal engagement with the patient, and limiting wound manipulation and exposure to the minimum necessary.

CONCLUSION

The effective prevention and management of pressure ulcers remains a challenge for physicians. However, careful interventions coupled with continuous vigilance by all members of the health care team usually result in positive outcomes. However, despite aggressive prevention and treatment strategies, not all pressure ulcers can be prevented or healed, making documentation of quality of care important.

SUGGESTED READINGS

Ayello EA, Braden B. How and why to do pressure ulcer risk assessment. *Adv Skin Wound Care.* 2002;15:125–132.

Bolton LL, van Rijswijk L, Shaffer FA. Quality wound care equals cost-effective wound care: a clinical model. *Adv Skin Wound Care.* 1997;10(4):33–38.

Centers for Medicare & Medicaid Services. Department of Health and Human Services; 2004. CMS Manual System, Pub. 100–107: State operations, provider certification.

European Pressure Ulcer Advisory Panel and National Pressure Ulcer Advisory Panel. Treatment of pressure ulcers: Quick Reference Guide. Washington DC: National Pressure Ulcer Advisory Panel; 2009. Available at: http://www.npuap.org/Final_Quick_Treatment_for_web_2010.pdf. Accessed August 6, 2011.

Lyder CH, Preston J, Grady J, et al. Quality of care for hospitalized Medicare patients at risk for pressure ulcers. *Arch Intern Med.* 2001;161:1549–1554.

Lyder C, Grady J, Mathur D, et al. Preventing pressure ulcers in Connecticut hospitals using the plan-do-study-act model for quality improvement. *Jt Comm J Qual Patient Saf.* 2004;30:205–214.

Panel on the Prediction and Prevention of Pressure Ulcers in Adults. Pressure ulcers in adults: prediction and prevention Clinical Practice Guideline No 3. Rockville, MD: Agency for Health Care Policy and Research; 1992. AHCPR Publication No. 92-0047.

Reddy M, Gill SS, Rochon PA. Preventing pressure ulcers: a systematic review. *JAMA.* 2006;296:974–984.

CHAPTER 145

Diabetic Foot Infections

John M. Embil, MD, FRCPC
Elly Trepman, MD

Key Clinical Questions

1. What clinical screening methods may detect the risk of potential foot problems in a diabetic patient?
2. If a foot ulcer occurs, what treatment options are available?
3. How are skin and soft tissue infections of the lower extremities classified and treated in diabetic patients?
4. How is osteomyelitis diagnosed and treated in diabetic patients?
5. How is the Charcot foot diagnosed and managed?
6. What preventive measures may be taken to protect the diabetic foot?

INTRODUCTION

During the past decade, the number of patients in the United States with diabetes mellitus has increased by 50%, from 15.7 million people to 23.6 million people. This rising prevalence is associated with the soaring numbers of the overweight and elderly in the population. Patients with diabetes mellitus are susceptible to peripheral neuropathy, peripheral vascular disease, and foot and ankle ulcers. Approximately 15% of diabetics develop a foot ulcer during their lifetime. Ulcers may heal or may be complicated by cellulitis, abscess formation, osteomyelitis, gangrene, and amputation. The financial burden of a foot ulcer is approximately $28,000 within two years of diagnosis, and the lifetime cost of an amputation is approximately $50,000. Nonhealing ulcers precede amputation in 84% of lower extremity amputations in diabetic patients. The mortality rate of diabetic patients after lower extremity amputation ranges from 11–41% within one year and 39–68% by five years.

PATHOPHYSIOLOGY

Diabetic foot infections usually are caused by direct bacterial invasion from a skin ulcer or a break in the skin barrier, such as from tinea pedis. Other contributing factors include oxidative stress, poor nutritional condition, immunocompromised status, impaired neutrophil function associated with hyperglycemia, and tissue ischemia from vascular insufficiency and inflammation. These factors may contribute to polymicrobial infection commonly noted in the diabetic foot.

Peripheral neuropathy in diabetic patients may cause sensory, motor, and autonomic disturbances that may contribute to the development of foot ulcers. In individuals with normal sensation in their feet, minor injuries cause pain, leading to rest and treatment that promote healing. However, diabetic sensory neuropathy may cause loss of protective sensation. Injuries, including repetitive minor trauma or persistent pressure from poorly fitting footwear, may go unnoticed and evolve to a necrotic lesion. Motor neuropathy causes contracture of intrinsic muscles and secondary claw toe deformities, with increased pressure points on the toes or metatarsal heads. Autonomic neuropathy may cause skin dryness and cracking, allowing bacteria to invade and destroy the subcutaneous tissues.

Charcot neuroarthropathy is another complication of diabetic neuropathy that may contribute to ulcer development. Charcot neuroarthropathy arises from repetitive microtrauma in the absence of protective sensation, leading to macroscopic fracture and joint injury. Furthermore, arteriovenous shunting associated with autonomic neuropathy may contribute to abnormal bone vascularity and associated osteopenia, resulting in increased susceptibility to fracture and joint injury. Damage to the bones and joints may cause collapse of the longitudinal arch of the foot or other foot deformity, resulting in bony prominence, points of pressure, and instability that may result in ulcer.

When an ulcer occurs, there may be initial bacterial colonization of the wound base. Subsequently, bacterial invasion of tissue may occur with development of overt infection, such as cellulitis, osteomyelitis, septic tenosynovitis, septic arthritis, or abscess. Rapid spread of infection along tissue planes may be facilitated by impaired immune function and poor vascularity. Therefore, a minor abrasion on a deformed toe that was caused by a poorly fitting shoe may rapidly evolve to a limb-threatening septic tenosynovitis, sometimes within one or two days.

EVALUATION AND DIAGNOSIS

Evaluation of the diabetic patient, with or without a foot lesion, includes the history and physical examination, with attention to the foot and ankle (**Table 145-1**). Guidelines for recommended frequency of screening evaluations and use of protective footwear are based on presence of neuropathy, history of ulcer, and foot deformity (**Table 145-2**).

HISTORY

History includes diabetes control and relevant diabetic complications such as neuropathy and vascular disease. Prior foot ulcers are associated with a high risk of a new foot ulcer or infection. Traumatic injury, even if minor, may cause tissue necrosis leading to an ulcer or initiate Charcot neuroarthropathy. The earliest indication of a diabetic foot infection may be a worsening of blood glucose control, which may precede fever, rigors, and local signs of sepsis.

PHYSICAL EXAMINATION

Physical examination includes inspection for ulcer, skin cracks, drainage, erythema, nail problems, and deformities (**Table 145-3**). Sensory neuropathy is confirmed by the absence of sensation upon contact with a 10 gram (Semmes-Weinstein) monofilament. Inspection between the toes may reveal maceration, ulcer, or purulent drainage, especially between the fourth and fifth toes. Erythema, swelling, and increased warmth may be early signs of Charcot neuroarthropathy, but presence of these signs with an ulcer or previous history of an ulcer will increase suspicion for presence of an associated infection. Erythema associated with infection persists during foot elevation, but erythema associated with Charcot neuroarthropathy may decrease when the foot is elevated. Palpable pulses do not exclude the presence of major microvascular disease.

When an ulcer is present (**Figure 145-1**), documentation includes size (diameter), depth, anatomic location, associated deformity, odor, drainage, and presence of visible bone, joint, or tendon tissue. The ulcer base may consist of moist red granulation tissue or dry grey necrotic debris. Drainage may be serous, serosanguinous, or purulent. When the ulcer base is probed with a sterile metal probe, palpation of exposed bone suggests the presence of osteomyelitis unless proven otherwise. Ulcers are classified based on depth and associated presence of exposed deep structures, infection, and status of distal perfusion (gangrene). Although several classification systems have been described, the Wagner classification system remains the most commonly used (**Table 145-4**).

VASCULAR ASSESSMENT

Vascular assessment may include determination of toe blood pressures, oxygenation, and Doppler arterial waveforms. Ankle-brachial index (ratio of arm to ankle blood pressure) of 0.8 to 1.0 is considered normal, and ratios of less than 0.8 may be associated with delayed wound healing. A ratio of less than 0.5 indicates inadequate arterial inflow associated with a very poor chance of wound healing. It is important to note that normal ABI results may occur in the presence of major vascular disease because of calcified blood vessels that may result in spuriously elevated occlusion pressure at the ankle. Toe pressures less than 40 mm Hg may indicate inadequate arterial inflow for promotion of healing, and vascular surgical consultation frequently is considered. Radiographs may reveal calcified small blood vessels in the forefoot or toes, bony changes consistent with osteomyelitis, or fractures and dislocations indicative of Charcot neuroarthropathy. Osteomyelitis may be present concurrent with Charcot neuroarthopathy, especially when ulcers are present.

SPECIALIZED IMAGING STUDIES

Specialized imaging studies may be sensitive, but not necessarily specific for infection. Technetium bone scintigraphy may be abnormal in the presence of osteomyelitis, fracture, or Charcot neuroarthropathy, but a false negative result may occur in the presence

TABLE 145-1 Evaluation of the Diabetic Foot

History
Duration of diabetes
Previous foot ulcer
Previous Charcot neuroarthropathy
Trauma, injury
Erythema
Swelling
Increased warmth
Dependent rubor
Pain or paresthesias
Exertional pain
Nail problems
Shoes
Changes in blood sugar control
Fever, rigors, chills
Physical examination
Inspection: erythema, swelling, increased warmth, dryness, dependent rubor
Joint stiffness
Tendon contractures
Ulcers: probe to bone
Deformity
Corns, calluses
Neuropathy: Semmes-Weinstein monofilament (10 gram)
Vascular: pulses, capillary refill
Laboratory investigations
Blood sugar, especially changes in glucose control
Hemoglobin A_{1c}
Complete blood count and differential
Erythrocyte sedimentation rate
C-reactive protein
Albumin
Blood cultures
Wound cultures
Biopsy and culture of infected tissue
Vascular studies
Ankle brachial index (ABI)
Doppler waveforms
Toe pressures
Imaging studies
AP, lateral, and oblique foot radiographs
AP, lateral, and mortise ankle radiographs
Nuclear medicine (technetium bone scan, indium-labelled white blood cell scan, gallium scan)
Ultrasonography
Computed tomography
Magnetic resonance imaging (with or without gadolinium enhancement)

TABLE 145-2 Risk Categories and Preventive Management of Diabetic Patients with Peripheral Neuropathy*

Risk Category†	Classification†	Preventive Management
0	Protective sensation intact Foot morphology normal	Patient education and daily self-examination Foot examination at each visit or at least four times per year Appropriately fitted footwear
1	Protective sensation absent Foot morphology normal No history of ulcers	Patient education and daily self-examination Foot examination at each visit or at least four times per year Appropriately fitted footwear with soft insoles
2	Protective sensation absent Foot deformity present No history of ulcers	Patient education and daily self-examination Foot examination at each visit or at least four times per year Appropriately fitted footwear with a suitable insole
3	Protective sensation absent Foot deformity History of plantar ulcer or amputation	Patient education and daily self-examination Foot examination at each visit or at least four times per year Appropriately fitted footwear with a suitable insole (may need custom-made footwear)

*Modified from Foot screening: care of the foot in diabetes. The Carville approach. Department of Health and Human Services, USA. US Government Printing Office, 1994.

†The Semmes-Weinstein 10 gram monofilament assessment for the presence of peripheral neuropathy is used in conjunction with a history of ulcers to establish the risk category. Higher risk category is associated with a greater risk of ulceration.

TABLE 145-3 Common Foot Complications in Diabetic Patients

Clinical Manifestations	Explanation	Treatment Suggestions
Nonblanching erythema over pressure points	Indicates unrelieved pressure; skin can break down, leading to ulcer; appropriate footwear and orthoses may reduce pressure	Custom-made, pressure-relieving insole If deformity present, custom-made orthopedic footwear and/or corrective surgery
Calluses and corns	Ongoing unrelieved mechanical pressure or friction causing the keratin layer of skin to thicken May act as abnormal points of high plantar foot pressure and lead to skin ulcers and undermining of the underlying soft tissues Subkeratotic hematoma or hemorrhage in or under the callus is a sign of unrelieved pressure and underlying soft tissue injury A corn is a callus with a hard central core	Paring (debridement) to relieve pressure Care to avoid trauma to underlying intact skin Patient, family member, or care giver may use a pumice stone to minimize buildup If visual impairment is present or the area to be treated with the pumice stone cannot be adequately visualized, then a care provider must be designated to perform this foot care Callus around the rim of a neuropathic ulcer is debrided to visualize ulcer and promote healing Appropriate footwear to minimize formation
Tinea pedis	Fungal infection, often related to increased moisture in the web spaces between toes Complications include fissuring of skin, which may act as a portal of entry for bacteria	The web spaces in between the toes must be kept dry; foot powder, lamb's wool, and footwear with a wide toe box may be helpful Topical antifungal therapy
Onychomycosis	Fungal infection of the toenails White/yellow discoloration of the nail, with nail hypertrophy and irregularity Most frequently due to *Trichophytin rubrum* and *T mentagrophytes* Yeasts such as *Candida albicans* and other nondermatophyte molds have been associated with onychomycosis Topical creams and ointments are ineffective because microorganisms have invaded the nail bed and plate With conventional oral therapy, disease-free nail can be achieved in approximately 25–50% of patients	Nail clippings may be submitted to the microbiology laboratory for culture and identification of the dermatophyte Systemic therapy may be necessary to eradicate the infection in the nail bed and plate Oral therapy may include itraconazole, terbinafine, or fluconazole, but the risks and benefits of these agents must be carefully considered before embarking upon lengthy treatment courses For most people, treatment of onychomycosis is not necessary, as the clinical and cosmetic effects are minor Treatment may be indicated for recurring paronychia or psychological complications

(continued)

TABLE 145-3 Common Foot Complications in Diabetic Patients *(continued)*

Clinical Manifestations	Explanation	Treatment Suggestions
Onychogryphosis	Hypertrophic nails that are thickened and horn-like These nails may disintegrate, get caught in socks, traumatize adjacent toes, or get torn off inside footwear	Regular nail care every 3–6 weeks may minimize complications Nails are cut straight across and the edges smoothed down Nail care provided by caregiver knowledgeable about diabetic foot complications, with avoidance of injury to surrounding tissues
Onychocryptosis	Ingrown toenail Results from altered fit of the nail plate in the lateral nail groove as a result of improper footwear and poor nail-trimming technique Classification: Stage I—mild complications with local inflammation and slight infection Stage II—worsening of the process with infection and marked discomfort Stage III—most advanced process with lateral wall hypertrophy and infection; infection may be severe and lead to amputation	Regular nail care and properly fitted footwear may minimize occurrence Stage I disease may be managed by proper nail trimming and elevation of the nail edges Stage II disease may require systemic antimicrobial therapy and more aggressive surgical debridement of the nail Stage III disease may require partial nail avulsion and destruction of the nail matrix
Paronychia	Infection of the lateral nail fold May be a consequence of an ingrown toenail	Best managed by partial nail excision, twice-daily saline solution soaks, antimicrobial therapy, and adequate nail care Systemic antibiotics and local surgical debridement may be indicated Assess appropriateness of footwear

of vascular disease or abscess. Indium-labeled white blood cell scans and gallium scintigraphy may be positive in the presence of infection and Charcot neuroarthropathy, and may not distinguish between these two conditions. Magnetic resonance imaging may be sensitive but not specific for infection, and specificity of gadolinium enhancement for infection is unproven.

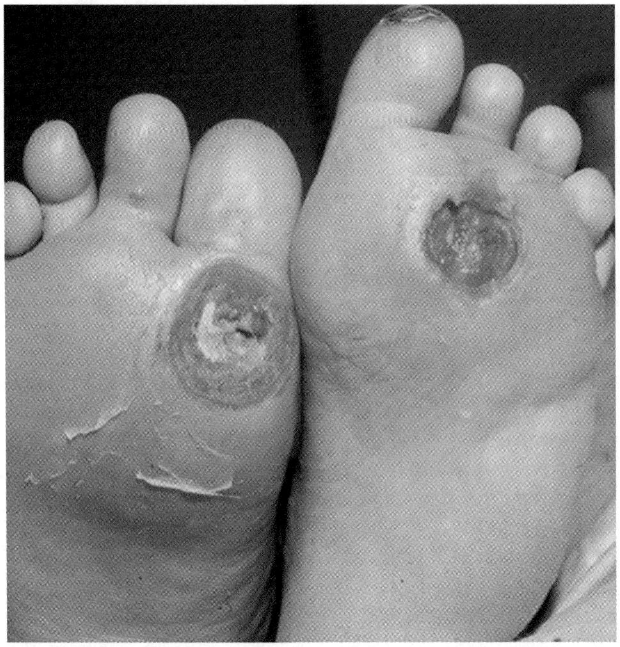

Figure 145-1 *This patient has an ulcer under the right first metatarsal head and sesamoids with central eschar and necrosis, and a clean granulating ulcer under the left second metatarsal head. Neuropathic deformities are also present. (Reproduced, with permission, from Wolff K, Johnson RA, Suurmond D. Fitzpatrick's Color Atlas & Synopsis of Clinical Dermatology. 5th ed. New York, NY: McGraw-Hill; 2005. Fig. 15-3.)*

WOUND CULTURES

Wound cultures by means of a swab from the ulcer base may be misleading, because the results frequently do not correlate with those of a deep wound or bone culture. Diabetic foot infection is a condition that may spread and destroy tissue, potentially leading to amputation, systemic sepsis, or death. Thus, superficial wound specimen cultures may document surface contamination rather than the true pathogens responsible for the infection. Specimens for culture are best obtained from infected tissue that does not communicate with the skin surface. The ideal specimen for culture assessment of infection is a curettage specimen from the base of the ulcer or bone biopsy specimens if osteomyelitis is suspected. If such specimens are not available, cultures of purulent exudate from within the ulcer base or sinuses may be an acceptable alternative. However, in the absence of a current or previous foot ulcer, a swollen, warm, erythematous foot may indicate presence of early Charcot neuroarthropathy, and open biopsy has the risk of potentially causing a deep, limb-threatening infection.

TREATMENT

Treatment of diabetic foot infection requires management of patient factors, antimicrobial treatment, wound care, and management of associated complications (**Table 145-5**).

Some early localized diabetic foot infections may be managed on an outpatient basis. However, many foot infections present with associated systemic sepsis and may be both limb- and life-threatening. If the patient has signs of systemic sepsis or a foot-at-risk because of abscess or septic tenosynovitis, then hospital admission, surgical and infectious diseases consultation, extensive operative debridement, and parenteral antimicrobial therapy usually are required.

TABLE 145-4 Diabetic Foot Ulcers: Wagner Classification and Management Options

Grade	Wagner Classification (Wagner, 1981)	Management Options
Grade 0	Skin intact, no open lesions Callus may be present at sites of localized pressure Nonblanching erythema may be present at sites of unrelieved pressure	Pare calluses Footwear and orthoses fitted for weight displacement
Grade 1	Superficial skin ulcer, often at high pressure areas (metatarsal heads, toes)	Pare calluses to expose ulcer base Deep swabs or curettage specimen from ulcer base for bacterial culture if clinical evidence of infection present Radiographs to exclude unsuspected bone infection (if this is detected, the ulcer is classified as a Grade 3 lesion) Moist dressings such as moist-to-dry saline gauze or hydroactive gel Infected ulcers (cellulitis) treated with systemic antimicrobials Pressure relief with appropriate footwear, crutches, wheelchairs, and casting (casts are applied by an experienced individual and monitored on a regular basis) Surgical debridement may be indicated
Grade 2	Deeper ulcer that may involve ligament, tendon, joint, bone, or fascia, usually associated with infection such as cellulitis	Management similar to Grade 1 lesions
Grade 3	The ulcer extends to deeper tissue layers such as bone If bone can be probed at the base of an ulcer, osteomyelitis is present, unless proven otherwise Tendinitis, tenosynovitis, and deep space abscesses may also be present	Noninvasive assessment of the adequacy of peripheral circulation (ankle-brachial index) Radiographs to screen for foreign bodies, gas, and magnitude of bony involvement Aggressive surgical debridement of infected bone, especially if abscess or systemic sepsis is present Appropriate antimicrobial therapy. Antimicrobials may be administered orally in most patients, but parenteral therapy may be of benefit depending upon the extent of involvement Vascular surgical opinion may be necessary if vascular insufficiency is present
Grade 4	Localized gangrene (toes, forefoot, heel) Gangrene may be dry or wet Infection may or may not be present	Management as for a Grade 3 lesion Urgent noninvasive assessment of peripheral circulation and vascular surgical opinion, possibly including angiography Angioplasty or bypass surgery may be indicated if a suitable stenotic lesion is demonstrated on angiography Local surgery to remove gangrenous tissue may be attempted, but single ischemic toes may be kept dry and allowed to mummify and auto-amputate Painting gangrenous digits with povidone-iodine may prevent or minimize the risk of progression to wet gangrene
Grade 5	Gangrene of entire foot	Urgent assessment as outlined for Grade 4 lesions Control of diabetes and infection Amputation guided by the level and adequacy of circulation

Timing of surgical debridement is based on clinical judgment and patient factors. In some instances, delay of surgical debridement may be prudent to allow reduction of swelling and abscess localization with parenteral antimicrobial therapy and bedrest, and to improve hemodynamic stability of the septic patient prior to anesthesia. However, in other cases, emergency debridement may be limb-saving or life-saving. Radical debridement includes excision of all purulent and necrotic tissue, including bone, joint, and tendon, and may include amputation of gangrenous portions of the foot. Emergency amputation is uncommon, but may be indicated for life-threatening, rapidly spreading infection such as gas gangrene or necrotizing fasciitis.

Antimicrobial treatment for diabetic foot infection may include parenteral, oral, and combination (parenteral and oral) antimicrobial therapy. Many diabetic foot infections are polymicrobial, and initial treatment may include empiric broad spectrum antimicrobials for coverage of gram-positive cocci, gram-negative rods, and anaerobic organisms. Subsequently, after culture results are available and early clinical improvement is noted, culture-directed antimicrobial agents are selected. Suggested empiric regimens for the management of infection in the diabetic foot are listed in Table 145-5.

The duration of therapy and route of administration of antimicrobial agents may vary depending on clinical response to therapy, severity of infection, availability of outpatient intravenous therapy, cost of treatment, and patient compliance issues. Diabetic foot infections confined to the skin and soft tissue infections are usually managed with either a brief course of parenteral followed by oral antimicrobial therapy, or oral therapy alone. Osteomyelitis may require surgical debridement and either a prolonged course of parenteral or oral antimicrobial therapy. Recommendations about route and duration of antimicrobial therapy frequently are

TABLE 145-5 Empiric Therapy for Infection in the Diabetic Foot*

Infection Severity	Antimicrobial Agent†
Mild infections Neither limb- nor life-threatening Usually associated with cellulitis surrounding an ulcer Purulent debris may be present at the base of the ulcer Usual organisms: aerobic gram positive cocci Frequently treated with outpatient oral antimicrobial therapy	• Cephalexin • Cloxacillin • Trimethoprim-sulfamethoxazole (TMP-SMX) • Clindamycin • Amoxicillin-clavulanic acid • Linezolid • Doxycycline
Moderate infections Include more extensive cellulitis, plantar abscess Initial antimicrobial therapy against staphylococci, streptococci, anaerobes, and common *Enterobacteriaceae* species Patients who are not toxic may be treated with debridement and oral antimicrobial therapy Patients who are ill or toxic despite moderate local signs are treated as having a severe infection [see below]	• TMP-SMX and metronidazole • TMP-SMX and clindamycin • Ciprofloxacin (or levofloxacin) and clindamycin • Ciprofloxacin, linezolid, and metronidazole • Amoxicillin-clavulanic acid • Moxifloxacin • Linezolid
Severe infections Limb- or life-threatening Patients may be critically ill or toxic and usually are treated with initial parenteral therapy until stable, then oral therapy Frequently polymicrobial Immediate hospitalization, early surgical debridement, and parenteral antimicrobial therapy If MRSA is present or suspected, addition of vancomycin, linezolid, or ceftobiprole may be considered	• Cefoxitin • Third (ceftriaxone or cefotaxime) generation cephalosporin and metronidazole • Combination of β-lactam antibiotic and β-lactamase inhibitor (eg, piperacillin and tazobactam) • Clindamycin and third generation cephalosporin (ie, cefotaxime, ceftriaxone, or ceftazidime) • Carbapenem (ie, imipenem/cilastatin, meropenem, or ertapenem) • Tigecycline
Osteomyelitis Treated with intravenous therapy or long-term oral antimicrobial therapy with agents that are well absorbed from the gastrointestinal tract and have good distribution to bone and tissue Surgical debridement indicated to removed necrotic debris, abscess, or sequestrum If MRSA is present or suspected, addition of vancomycin, linezolid, or ceftobiprole may be considered	Parenteral options • Combination of β-lactam antibiotic and β-lactamase inhibitor (eg, piperacillin and tazobactam) • Clindamycin and third generation cephalosporin (ie, cefotaxime, ceftriaxone, or ceftazidime) • Carbapenem (ie, imipenem/cilastatin, meropenem, or ertapenem) Oral options (when supported by culture data) • Cloxacillin • Cephalexin • TMP-SMX • Clindamycin • Amoxicillin-clavulanic acid • Linezolid • Doxycycline • TMP-SMX and metronidazole or clindamycin • Levofloxacin or ciprofloxacin and metronidazole or clindamycin

*Antibacterial therapy should always be guided by available culture results. If in doubt about the most appropriate antimicrobial regimen, discussion with an infectious diseases consultant may be prudent.

†Dosage may depend on renal function and drug levels. Prior to initiating antimicrobial therapy, verify creatinine clearance and modify dose and interval accordingly.

The agents suggested in this section are for empiric therapy prior to the availability of final culture and susceptibility results. Knowledge of local epidemiology must also guide therapeutic choices, and some agents (β-lactams) are ineffective against methicillin-resistant *Staphylococcus aureus* (MRSA).

Many of the agents identified in this table do not have a specific Food and Drug Administration (FDA) indication for the management of diabetic foot infections including osteomyelitis, but may have an indication for the management of skin and soft tissue infections or may have antimicrobial activity effective against the typical pathogens encountered in osteomyelitis of the diabetic foot. Therapy must be refined based upon the final culture and susceptibility profiles for the pathogens recovered.

Duration of therapy is based on clinical response. However, typical treatment courses for skin and soft tissue infections range from 7 (mild) to 21 (severe) days, and the treatment of osteomyelitis may require 4 to 6 weeks of parenteral or several months of oral antimicrobial therapy. When possible, it is desirable to switch to oral antimicrobial therapy to avoid complications from parenteral administration.

not evidence-based; therefore, clinical course and response to therapy are the best guides to the treatment approach. Foot infections restricted to soft tissue are commonly treated for one to four weeks, depending on severity. When bone is infected and complete debridement of nonviable bone and tissue has been performed, treatment duration is typically four to six weeks. When diabetic foot infections involve bone, and debridement has not been performed or residual dead bone remains after debridement, failure rates of antibiotic treatment are high. Some clinicians opt to treat for three months or longer in this scenario.

Response to antimicrobial therapy is monitored with frequent clinical examination and periodic tests including white blood cell count, differential, and C-reactive protein. The erythrocyte sedimentation rate may remain elevated, despite adequate initial control of infection. Radiographs or CT scanning may demonstrate bony consolidation and maturation of healed bone, or may reveal regions of ongoing bone destruction or sequestrum that may require further surgical debridement. The role of routine follow-up cultures is controversial and is considered on a case-by-case basis; repeating specimens for cultures may be indicated if clinical response to therapy is incomplete or if recurrent infection is suspected.

Wound care may include offloading, wound dressings, and surgical reconstruction. Offloading—removal of mechanical factors that may prevent wound healing—may include crutches and nonweightbearing gait, removable walker boots, bivalved or other casts, wheelchairs, and periods of bedrest. The risks of immobilization, including thromboembolic disease and cardiac deconditioning, must be weighed against the risks of ambulation resulting in spread of infection and delayed wound healing.

Advances in wound dressings are beyond the scope of this review. Despite the development of diverse (and sometimes costly) wound dressings, effective and cost-efficient basic wound care is based on maintaining a moist wound environment to expedite healing. The mainstay of wound treatment consists of basic gauze dressings moistened with saline and allowed to dry. This helps the debridement process and provides a moist environment for granulation tissue. Excessive moisture in the applied gauze is avoided because of potential maceration of the wound margins (hence, the term "moist-to-dry" instead of "wet-to-dry" dressing). After necrotic debris has been removed from the wound base, gauze dressings may be continued until the wound is healed. Other commercially available (and more costly) dressing products, such as hydroactive gels or paraffin impregnated gauzes, may be used to maintain a moist environment. Topical antimicrobial dressings are not recommended. There are limited data to support any added benefit to their use, and complications may include hypersensitivity reactions and the development of antimicrobial-resistant pathogens. The development of so called "negative pressure" suction sponge wound systems, such as the Vacuum Assisted Closure™ device, that decrease localized edema and wound size to facilitate wound healing after surgical debridement, have shown some benefit in the management of acute surgical wounds in the diabetic foot.

Management of associated complications, such as peripheral vascular disease or Charcot deformity, may be indicated for effective infection control and prevention of recurrence. If an infection does not respond to antimicrobial and wound treatment because of ischemia, peripheral vascular reconstruction may be indicated if the patient has an occlusion amenable to angioplasty or surgical correction. Charcot deformity may cause ongoing or recurrent pressure and wound breakdown, and surgical reconstruction of the Charcot foot may be indicated to remove areas of local bony pressure or to control instability. The healed foot is frequently managed with custom-molded orthoses and orthopedic footwear to decrease potential risk of recurrent ulcer and associated infection.

TABLE 145-6 Prevention of Diabetic Foot Ulcer and Infection

Patient education (classes, handouts)
Self-examination
Footwear and orthoses
Lotion and lamb's wool
Nutrition and glycemic control
Foot screening examinations
Aggressive early evaluation and treatment of foot lesions
Multidisciplinary clinic setting
Antimicrobial prophylaxis for elective surgery

DISCHARGE CONSIDERATIONS

Hospital discharge may be considered when systemic symptoms have subsided and control of infection has been established. Patients being discharged on intravenous antibiotics will need early planning for long-term vascular access and arrangements for home antimicrobial administration. Outpatient providers should be informed about diagnosis, therapeutic decisions and duration, and required monitoring. Patients with osteomyelitis benefit from infectious diseases follow-up. Prior to discharge, the patient's diabetic regimen should be assessed and modified if glycemic control is inadequate. Patients may benefit from outpatient teaching regarding diabetes management and foot care, and involvement of foot care specialists, as below.

PREVENTION

Preventive programs have the potential to reduce the enormous personal morbidity and societal costs of diabetic foot ulcers (**Table 145-6**). Patient education, including group classes, individual teaching, and information sheets, may improve patient awareness of the importance of daily self-examination of the foot and shoes, and early evaluation of seemingly minor symptoms. For the patient with established neuropathy, specialized footwear and orthoses may protect the limb from external pressure and shear stresses that may result in ulcers or abrasions. Lotions may prevent cracking of dry exposed skin, and lamb's wool may prevent maceration and skin breakdown between the toes. Nutritional management with a low-glycemic program may reverse the early signs of metabolic syndrome and type 2 diabetes mellitus.

Physician and staff education may result in more frequent foot screening examinations and prompter evaluation of patient complaints. Aggressive early evaluation and treatment of foot injuries or wounds may decrease the risk of uncontrolled, limb-threatening infection. In regional centers, prompt evaluation and treatment may be facilitated in a multidisciplinary diabetic foot program with specialized physicians, nurses, pedorthists (specialists in medical footwear), orthotists (clinicians who fit and fabricate orthotic insoles), physiotherapists, and support staff. Office staff may be trained to arrange urgent evaluation of early problem signs in the diabetic neuropathic patient.

PRACTICE POINT

- Poor footwear may lead to foot injury in diabetics. The shoes of diabetics should be evaluated to ensure that they fit properly, provide support, and are in good repair. Inspection of the shoes may reveal blood stains, foul odor, rough seams, or an embedded foreign body, such as a thumb tack or nail. Diabetics should wear shoes with a wide, high toe box to prevent chafing and injury of the toes and metatarsal heads, and removable insoles to accommodate molded orthotics, if necessary.

SUGGESTED READINGS

Apelqvist J, Bakker K, van Houtum WH, Schaper NC. International Working Group on the Diabetic Foot (IWGDF) Editorial Board. Practical guidelines on the management and prevention of the diabetic foot: based upon the International Consensus on the Diabetic Foot (2007) Prepared by the International Working Group on the Diabetic Foot. *Diabetes Metab Res Rev*. 2008;24(Suppl 1): S181–S187.

Embil JM, Rose G, Trepman E, et al. Oral antimicrobial therapy for diabetic foot osteomyelitis. *Foot Ankle Int*. 2006;27:771–779.

Embil JM, Trepman E. Microbiological evaluation of diabetic foot osteomyelitis. *Clin Infect Dis*. 2006:42:63–65.

Lipsky BA, Berendt AR, Derry HG, et al. Infectious Diseases Society of America Guideline: diagnosing and treating diabetic foot infections. *Clin Infect Dis*. 2004;39:885–910.

Pinzur MS, Slovenkai MP, Trepman E, Shields NN. Guidelines for diabetic foot care: recommendations endorsed by the Diabetes Committee of the American Orthopaedic Foot and Ankle Society. *Foot Ankle Int*. 2005;26:113–119.

Sella EJ. Diagnostic imaging of the diabetic foot. *Foot Ankle Int*. 2009;30:568–576.

Trepman E, Bracilovic A, Lamborn KK, et al. Diabetic foot care: multilingual translation of a patient education leaflet. *Foot Ankle Int*. 2005;26:64–107.

Trepman E, Nihal A, Pinzur MS. Current concepts review: Charcot neuroarthropathy of the foot and ankle. *Foot Ankle Int*. 2005;26:46–63.

CHAPTER 146

Venous Ulcers

Katherine L. Brown, MD, MPH
Tania Phillips, MD, FACPC

Key Clinical Questions

1. Does this patient have a venous ulcer?
2. What is the diagnostic approach to a patient with a suspected venous ulcer?
3. What are appropriate treatments for venous ulcers?
4. How might patients prevent venous ulcers?

INTRODUCTION/EPIDEMIOLOGY

Up to 80% of all leg ulcers are venous ulcers. Approximately 1–2% of the U.S. adult population has a history of a venous ulcer. Several risk factors (**Table 146-1**) are associated with venous ulcers. Coexisting diseases are not uncommon; 5–12% of venous ulcer patients have diabetes mellitus, and 10–15% have rheumatologic disease.

Because of their unpredictable and often chronic course, venous ulcers impose a significant economic burden, accounting for 1–3% of the total health care budgets in developed countries, and approximately $3 billion per year in the United States. Venous ulcers also result in substantial indirect costs, including an estimated loss of 2 million working days per year in the United States, as well as decreased work productivity, premature disability, and other impacts on quality of life.

PATHOPHYSIOLOGY

The lower extremity venous system is made up of superficial veins, communicating (perforating) veins, and deep veins. These veins have one-way valves that, under normal conditions, prevent reflux and promote cephalad blood flow with leg muscle contraction.

Venous ulcers typically occur in the setting of chronic venous insufficiency, due to reflux through incompetent valves, venous outflow obstruction, as in venous thrombosis, or failure of the calf-muscle pump. Valvular incompetence may occur in the superficial (45%) or deep (12%) venous systems, or both (43%). Obesity, leg immobility, inflammatory conditions of muscles or joints, fibrosis, and neuropathies can result in calf-muscle pump failure.

Several mechanisms may contribute to the development of venous ulcers. Elevated venous pressures may lead to capillary distention and leakage of fibrin, resulting in fibrin cuff formation around dermal capillaries and decreased oxygen diffusion to tissues. Abnormalities in fibrinolysis may contribute to this process. Fibrinogen and other macromolecules that have leaked into tissues may trap growth factors, making them unavailable for tissue maintenance and repair. Trapping of white cells may cause enzyme release and inflammation that further increases vessel permeability and damages tissues.

DOES THE PATIENT HAVE A VENOUS ULCER?

HISTORY

Patients should be assessed for risk factors (Table 146-1), symptoms, prior treatments, and ulcer course. Patients with venous ulcers have variable symptoms that tend to be worse at the end of the day, and improve with leg elevation. These include aching, cramping, swelling, heaviness, tingling, itching, burning, copious, sometimes malodorous drainage, and restless legs. Symptoms are greater in individuals with higher CEAP (clinical, etiologic, anatomical, and pathophysiological) classifications (**Table 146-2**). It is not unusual for venous ulcers to persist for years. Venous ulcers often recur at the same site.

Although venous ulcers are often less painful than other ulcer types, up to 75% of venous ulcer patients complain of pain. Deep ulcers around the ankles and ulcers with surrounding *atrophie blanche* (stellate white scars) can be particularly painful. Patients with venous ulcers may also have problems with physical function, mobility, depression, and social isolation that significantly impact their quality of life.

TABLE 146-1 Risk Factors

Heredity
Age (peak prevalence between 60–80 years)
Female sex (1.6 female: 1 male)
Obesity
History of
Leg injury
Varicose vein surgery
Phlebitis
Deep vein thrombosis
Congenital absence of valves
Venous valve or wall degeneration
Arteriovenous shunts
Pregnancy
Prolonged standing
Taller height
Inadequate treatment of chronic venous Insufficiency or edema

CLINICAL PRESENTATION

Clinical signs of venous disease are listed in **Table 146-3**. Up to 76% of venous ulcers may be diagnosed by clinical evaluation. Venous ulcers are typically ill-defined with irregular borders, a shallow wound bed, and may have a yellowish fibrinous exudate or pink granulation tissue. Around the ulcer, there can be skin dyspigmentation (darkening or lightening), purpura, and thickening of the skin. Venous ulcers tend to be located over the medial malleolus or within the "gaiter area" (the distal third of the leg, from the mid-calf to the ankle). Ulcers outside this area should raise the possibility of another cause.

DIFFERENTIAL DIAGNOSIS

When pain is particularly severe, the ulcer is of long duration, or fails to improve with treatment, one should consider the possibility of concomitant infection, allergic contact dermatitis (to topical wound treatments), malignancy, or other ulcer etiologies.

Infection

All nonhealing ulcers should be evaluated with *tissue* cultures (not surface cultures) for bacterial, fungal, viral, mycobacterial, and atypical mycobacterial infection.

TABLE 146-2 CEAP (Clinical, Etiologic, Anatomical, and Pathophysiological) Classification of Chronic Venous Disease

Class	Definition
C_0	No visible or palpable signs of venous disease
C_1	Telangiectases (dilated venules, < 1 mm diameter), reticular veins (dilated, nonpalpable, veins, ≤ 3 mm diameter), malleolar venous flare (arrays of small veins about the ankles)
C_2	Varicose veins (dilated, palpable veins, > 3 mm diameter)
C_3	Edema without skin changes
C_4	Skin changes*
C_5	Skin changes* with healed ulceration
C_6	Skin changes* with active ulceration

*As described in Table 146-3.

TABLE 146-3 Clinical Signs of Chronic Venous Disease

Sign	Description
Pitting edema	Swelling of lower legs that retain an indentation after applying firm pressure
Venous eczema/ stasis dermatitis	Redness, scaling, itch, +/– exudates
Dyspigmentation	Reddish-brown discoloration, especially around the ankle
Purpura	Nonblanching red to purple spots
Hemosiderosis	Cayenne pepper-appearing specks on shins
Varicosities	
Malleolar venous flares	Arrays of small veins around the ankles
Varicose veins	Large tortuous superficial veins
Atrophie blanche	Stellate white scars
Induration/ dermatosclerosis	Hardening of the skin
Lipodermatosclerosis	
Early changes	Acute noninfectious cellulitis with redness and swelling
Late changes	Sharply demarcated hardening associated with skin discoloration of the distal third of the lower leg, giving the lower leg the silhouette of an inverted champagne bottle

Malignancy

Patients with chronic nonhealing ulcers should have a skin biopsy to evaluate for malignancy.

Arterial ulcers

Arterial ulcers can present with claudication or rest pain, and are often exquisitely painful. They present as sharply demarcated, punched-out ulcers with a fibrinous yellow base or black necrotic eschar, sometimes with exposure of deep tissues, such as tendons. They often occur distally, especially on the foot, or over bony prominences. Associated clinical findings include absent dorsalis pedis pulse, prolonged capillary refill time (>4–5 seconds), pallor with limb elevation and reactive hyperemia on dependency (dependent rubor), loss of hair, shiny skin, cool feet, abnormal toenails, and a low ankle/brachial pressure index (ABI) ≤ 0.5.

Neuropathic ulcers

Neuropathic ulcers are common in diabetic patients. They are often associated with numbness, burning, and tingling, but can also be asymptomatic. They tend to occur over pressure-bearing areas, such as the soles of the feet. These ulcers are often deep, and associated infections of soft tissue and bone are common.

Inflammatory conditions

Inflammatory conditions commonly associated with ulceration include pyoderma gangrenosum and vasculitis. Pyoderma gangrenosum often begins as a small pustule that rapidly enlarges. It develops violaceous, undermined borders with a cribriform (perforated, sieve-like) base and tends to worsen with trauma, including debridement. Two-thirds are associated with inflammatory bowel disease, rheumatoid arthritis, or hematologic malignancies.

Vasculitis can be associated with palpable purpura (nonblanching red to blue papules), livedo reticularis (netlike, red-purple erythema, especially on the legs), and necrosis. Rheumatoid arthritis, systemic lupus erythematosus, scleroderma, and other connective tissue diseases may also be associated with lower extremity ulcers in the absence of overt vasculitis.

Procoagulant disorders

Sickle cell anemia, anticardiolipin antibodies, and other procoagulant disorders can result in chronic wounds similar to venous ulcers.

WHAT IS THE APPROACH TO A PATIENT WITH A SUSPECTED VENOUS ULCER?

Table 146-4 outlines key components of ulcer evaluation. A thorough history may support the diagnosis of venous stasis or suggest alternative diagnoses. Patients should be questioned about risk factors for venous ulcers (Table 146-1), associated symptoms and modifying factors, and response to prior treatments. Patients with venous leg ulcers often experience worsening symptoms in the dependent position and symptom relief with elevation. Claudication (calf pain or cramping with ambulation) is more consistent with arterial disease. Decreased or altered sensation in distal extremities suggests a neuropathic ulcer. Patients with pyoderma gangrenosum ulcers may note ulcer enlargement after trauma, such as mechanical debridement. Ulcers can be multifactorial and may have secondary complications, such as infection.

Ulcer location and surrounding skin changes are crucial elements of the physical examination. Venous ulcers usually occur in the gaiter area (between the mid-calf and ankle), and typically are shallow with irregular shapes and ragged borders. Associated skin changes include dyspigmentation, purpura, and thickening of the skin (Table 146-3). While the edema of cardiac, renal, and hepatic disease is typically soft and painless, venous disease is associated with hard, indurated edema. Other ulcer etiologies should be excluded by palpating distal pulses and testing skin sensation with a 10-g Semmes-Weinstein monofilament. An ankle-brachial index (ABI) < 0.8 supports an arterial component to the ulcer.

The duplex ultrasound scan is preferred for evaluating venous anatomy and diagnosing venous insufficiency, due to its accuracy, noninvasiveness, and reproducibility. When ordering duplex ultrasonography, ask for evaluation of venous insufficiency (reflux). Failure to do so may result in testing for only the presence or absence of deep vein thromboses (DVT). Other less common studies include continuous-wave Doppler studies for superficial vein anatomic information and air plethysmography or photoplethysmography for evaluating calf-muscle pump function. Invasive phlebography is reserved for evaluation before vascular surgery.

State-of-the-art ulcer care will fail unless underlying related diseases are first addressed. Laboratory testing may be performed to exclude concurrent inflammatory, infectious, and coagulopathic diseases (Table 146-4). Any nonhealing ulcer should be biopsied for histological examination and tissue cultures. This can be

TABLE 146-4 Diagnostic Workup

History	Screen for risk factors (Table 146-1) Are symptoms worse in the dependent position and alleviated with elevation? Does the patient have other systemic diseases? Does the patient experience calf pain or cramping with walking (claudication)? Does he or she complain of numbness or altered sensation? Does the ulcer historically worsen with invasive procedures (eg, following debridement)?
Physical examination	Ulcer location Surrounding skin changes (Table 146-3) Palpate pulses Measure ankle-brachial index (ABI) Test sensation with 10g Semmes-Weinstein monofilament
Studies	Duplex ultrasonography (gold standard) for confirming venous reflux, and excluding thromboses Segmental arterial pulse waveform analysis, magnetic resonance angiography, arteriography if arterial disease suspected. If osteomyelitis is suspected, consider bone scans, magnetic resonance imaging (MRI), computed tomographic scans (CT), and bone biopsy
Laboratory testing for possible underlying systemic disease	Antinuclear antibody (ANA) Glucose, HbA1c Anticardiolipin antibody Lupus anticoagulant antibody ANCA Protein C, protein S, antithrombin III Cryoglobulins Cryofibrinogens Rheumatoid factor (RF) Factor V Leiden, prothrombin gene mutation
Biopsy (for any nonhealing ulcer)	For histopathologic examination For tissue cultures (bacterial, viral, fungal, mycobacterial, atypical mycobacterial)

accomplished with either two small punch biopsies, or one large wedge biopsy that is bisected with a scalpel, providing a sample for each study. Tissue should be cultured for bacteria, fungi, viruses, and mycobacteria, including atypical mycobacteria.

WHAT ARE APPROPRIATE TREATMENTS FOR VENOUS ULCERS?

COMPRESSION

By raising local hydrostatic pressure and lowering superficial venous pressure, compression (typically 35–40 mm Hg at the ankle) reduces edema and vascular leakage, increases cutaneous blood flow and lymph transport, approximates valve leaflets, and increases ulcer healing rates compared to controls. Contraindications to compression therapy include arterial insufficiency and decompensated congestive heart failure. Walking and exercise involving the calf-muscle pump enhance compression therapy effectiveness. Unfortunately, patients with severe lipodermatosclerosis (**Figure 146-1**) may have difficulties with the ankle dorsiflexion required in these exercises.

Compression choices include the Unna boot, multilayer compression wraps, graduated compression elastic stockings, orthotic compression devices, and compression pumps. The Unna boot is a zinc-impregnated, semirigid paste bandage applied in the clinic at least weekly with the foot at a 90° angle. One clear benefit is patient adherence, due to its cast-like properties and mandated close clinical follow-up. Disadvantages include the need to keep dry when bathing, unpleasant odor from wound exudates, inability to accommodate large leg volume fluctuations, need for frequent clinic visits, and potential for contact dermatitis. The Unna boot does not provide effective compression for immobile patients. Because of its low resting pressure, it is unsuitable for patients with venous ulcers who also have borderline arterial disease.

Alternatively, there are a number of elastic compression therapies. Compression bandages are applied spirally, with a 50% overlap from right above the toes to just below the knees. Compression bandages are adjustable for changes in leg volume, provide increased rest and working pressures, conform to the leg better than more rigid bandages, and allow for more frequent dressing changes. Disadvantages include complications related to improper application, unraveling, and patient compliance. The three classes of single-layer compression bandages range from light compression (class I) to moderate-high pressure (class III) bandages (eg, Tensopress, Setopress, and Surepress) for severe edema, postthrombotic venous insufficiency, and severe varicosities. Multilayer bandage systems, like Dynaflex and Profore, provide 40–45 mm Hg of support, can adapt to changing leg sizes, and are more cost effective despite higher up-front costs. They are effective in immobile patients, but have high resting pressures and should not be used for patients with concomitant arterial disease. In clinical trials, multicomponent bandages work better than single-component bandages, and multicomponent systems including an elastic bandage appear more effective than those composed mainly of inelastic components.

Orthotic compression devices consist of multiple Velcro straps. They are adjustable for changes in leg circumference and easily removed for frequent dressing changes. Intermittent pneumatic compression (IPC) devices, originally designed for deep venous thrombosis prophylaxis, work by inflating and deflating an airtight bag around the leg. They require immobility for several hours per day. Studies of IPC have demonstrated increased healing relative to no compression, but it is unclear whether IPC is equivalent to other forms of compression, or whether it may be used as an adjunct to other compression therapies (**Figures 146-2** and **146-3**).

DEBRIDEMENT

Frequent venous ulcer debridement may facilitate healing by removing impediments to wound bed granulation and epithelialization. There are four types of wound debridement. **Autolytic** debridement uses occlusive dressings to maintain contact between the wound and enzyme-rich bodily fluids to selectively liquefy necrotic tissue. **Enzymatic** debridement employs commercially available topical agents, like collagenase (Santyl) and trypsin (Granulex). **Mechanical** debridement includes wet-to-dry dressings, hydrotherapy, and irrigation for nonselectively removing viable and necrotic wound tissue. As this may be painful, many clinicians apply topical anesthetic agents, such as lidocaine/prilocaine combinations (marketed as Eutectic Mixture of Local Anesthetics, or EMLA) during mechanical debridement. **Surgical** debridement is typically performed under anesthesia for wounds with a large amount of necrotic tissue.

WOUND PREPARATION AND TOPICAL TREATMENTS

Venous stasis ulcers should be kept moist and cleansed with physiologic saline. Hydrogen peroxide, povidone iodine, acetic acid, and sodium hypochlorite, which are toxic to healthy granulation tissue as well as bacteria, should be avoided. Silver sulfadiazine (Silvadene), a topical medication commonly used for inhibiting bacterial and fungal growth in burn wounds, has variable efficacy in the treatment of venous ulcers. Uncomplicated stasis dermatitis without ulceration

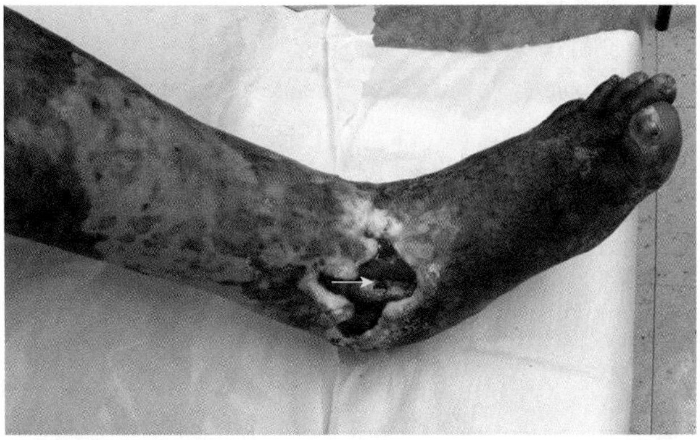

Figure 146-1 *Venous ulcer overlying the medial malleolus. Note the irregular shape of the ulcer, the fibrinous yellow exudate in the wound bed (yellow arrow) and the skin changes involving the gaiter region (the area between the mid-calf and ankle). In addition, this patient has significant pitting edema, skin hardening, and decreased ankle range of motion.*

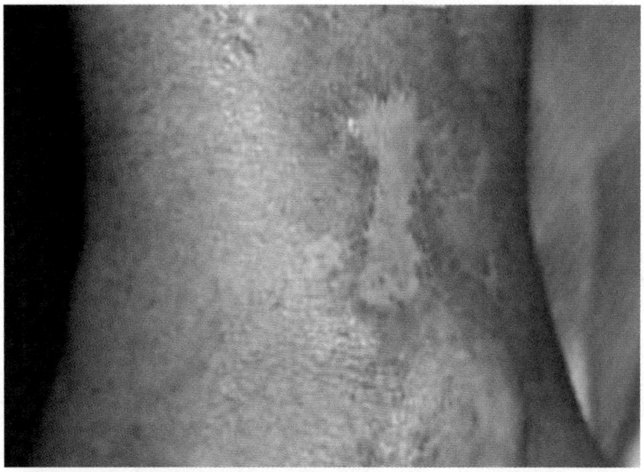

Figure 146-2 *Atrophe blanche, appearing as a whitish scar with stellate borders near the medial malleolus.*

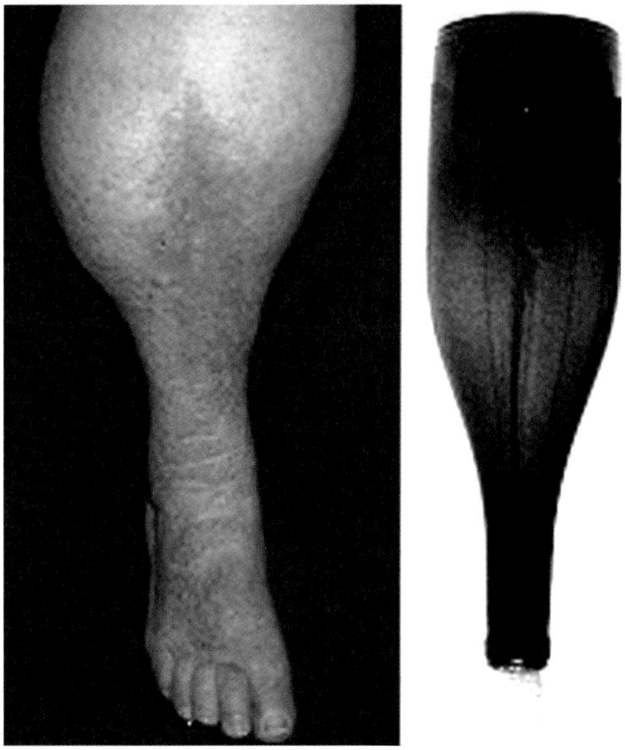

Figure 146-3 *Lipodermatosclerosis presents as redness, swelling, and skin hardening that gives the lower leg the silhouette of an inverted champagne bottle.*

that is wet and oozing usually improves with topical corticosteroid creams; ointments may be used for stasis dermatitis that is dry, thickened, and pruritic.

DRESSINGS

Dressings differ in many characteristics, including absorptiveness (**Table 146-5**). The wound should be covered with a moisture-retentive dressing, such as hydrocolloid or hydrogel, to promote autolysis of necrotic material and soothe pain. Highly absorptive dressings, such as foams and alginates, should be reserved for profusely exudative wounds. Dressings should be applied with adequate margins around the wound, and the frequency of dressing changes should be adjusted to avoid leakage. Compressive therapy should be applied over dressings.

SKIN GRAFTING AND VENOUS SURGERY

Skin grafts may be considered for refractory venous ulcers. Grafts may be harvested or grown from the patient's own intact skin (autografts), or bioengineered from donor cells (allografts). Compared to compression alone, treatment with skin grafts plus compression results in more healed ulcers at six months and a shorter time to wound closure, as well as better healing of large ulcers, deep ulcers, and ulcers of >6 months duration. Two-layer tissue-engineered skin grafts have also been shown to increase ulcer healing.

Adjunctive surgical therapies aim to reduce ulcer recurrence by stopping flow through incompetent superficial veins, thus decreasing venous reflux and hypertension. Surgical therapies include venous stripping, superficial vein ligation, and deep perforator vein ligation. Sclerotherapy is a nonsurgical means of accomplishing

TABLE 146-5 Dressings

Type	Indications	Pros	Cons
Simple, nonadherent Telfa, Vaseline Adaptic	Minimal to mild exudate Superficial wound	Less expensive	Require second dressing
Films Tegaderm, Omiderm, Opsite, Biooclusive, Blisterfilm, Transeal	Minimal exudate	Clear Adhesive Bacterial barrier	Wound adherence Fluid collection
Hydrocolloids Duoderm, NuDerm, Comfeel, Cutinova, Replicare, Granulex, Tegasorb, Biofilm	Mild to moderate exudate Deep wounds	Autolytic debridement Absorbent Bacterial barrier	Opaque Odor
Hydrogels Vigilon, Tegagel, Curagel, Clearsite, Curafil, Elasto-Gel, Solosite wound gel, 2nd Skin	Painful wounds Dry or mild exudate Crusted exudate	Semitransparent Soothing Hydrating No wound adherence	Require second dressing Frequent dressing changes
Foams Allevyn, Flexzan, Hydrasorb, Lyofoam, Vigifoam	Moderate to heavy exudate Pressure relief Protection of bony prominences	Absorbent Conforms to contours	Opaque Require second dressing
Alginates Algiderm, Algisite, Algisorb, Kaltostat, Curasorb, Polymen, SeaSorb, Sorbsan, Cutinova	Heavy exudate Deep wounds	Highly absorbent Hemostatic No wound adherence Fewer dressing changes	Require second dressing

the same goal by injection of incompetent veins with an irritant solution. The ESCHAR study, a randomized controlled trial of 500 patients, showed that venous ulcer surgery with compression did not significantly improve ulcer healing compared to compression alone, but surgery did significantly reduce rates of ulcer recurrence at three years (56% recurrence with compression alone, vs. 31% recurrence with compression and surgery).

Minimally invasive venous surgical techniques include subfascial endoscopic perforator vein ligation (SEPS) for patients with chronic or recurrent venous ulceration associated with incompetent perforator veins, and investigational percutaneous techniques (eg, endovenous laser therapy and radiofrequency ablation) for ablating the great saphenous vein. Surgery is contraindicated in patients with increased risk for infection, deep venous thrombosis, or anesthetic complications.

ADJUCTIVE THERAPIES

Adjunctive therapies may be considered in patients whose wounds fail to heal despite appropriate dressings and compression therapy. These include systemic medications, growth factors, alternative medicine, and hyperbaric oxygen therapy. Evidence in support of these therapies is limited.

Diuretics have a limited role in chronic venous insufficiency. They may help reduce edema that is difficult to mobilize, but may also lead to volume depletion. Though most venous ulcers are heavily colonized with bacteria, routine administration of topical or systemic **antibiotics** does not improve healing rates, and may be complicated by emergence of resistant organisms and contact dermatitis. Antibiotics should be reserved for ulcers with signs of infection, such as increasing erythema, pain, and ulcer size. Tissue cultures should be obtained prior to starting antibiotics. Empiric treatment should cover both Gram-positive and Gram-negative bacteria, including *Pseudomonas*, and should be tailored according to culture results.

Although one small trial found a benefit of **aspirin** in speeding healing of venous ulcers, there is currently insufficient evidence to recommend it as routine therapy. No **growth factors** are currently approved by the FDA for venous ulcer treatment. **Pentoxifylline** is an oral medication with antiplatelet and anti-inflammatory effects, and it also reduces blood viscosity. It appears effective as an adjunct to compression bandaging, and is possibly effective in the absence of compression for enhancing venous ulcer healing.

Herbal remedies for chronic venous insufficiency include horse chestnut extract, rutoside extracts, and pycnogenol (French maritime pine bark extract). A Cochrane Review concluded that these extracts reduced such pain, edema, and pruritus, with no significant differences between these substances, except that pycnogenol appeared somewhat more efficacious than horse chestnut extract for edema. It is unclear whether these substances provide additional benefit to patients on standard therapy, as most patients in these studies were not treated with compression therapy.

In **hyperbaric oxygen therapy** (HBOT), very high arterial oxygen tensions are achieved by placing patients in an airtight chamber filled with pure oxygen at pressures greater than one atmosphere. It may improve short-term wound healing, but no improvement in long-term outcomes has been shown.

PRACTICE POINT

- Caregivers should encourage patients with venous disease to elevate their legs above the level of the heart whenever possible. Lesser degrees of elevation, such as placing the feet on a footstool or ottoman while seated in an armchair, are ineffective in increasing venous return.

TABLE 146-6 Prognostic Indicators of Venous Ulcer Healing

Favorable	Unfavorable
Baseline ulcer surface area < 5 cm^2	Baseline ulcer surface area > 5 cm^2
Ulcer duration < 1 year	Previous operations (eg, knee or hip surgery)
Ankle-brachial index (ABI) greater than 0.8	ABI less than 0.8
Reduction in calf circumference ≥ 3 cm during the first 50 days of treatment	History of venous ligation or venous stripping
Emergence of new skin islets on > 10% of wound in 50 days	Body mass index (BMI) > 33 kg/m^2
	Daily walking distance < 200 meters
	History of surgical wound debridement
	> 50% of wound covered with fibrin
	Wound depth > 2 cm
	Fixed ankle joint
	Reduced ankle range of motion
	Calf:ankle circumference ratio < 1.3

PROGNOSIS

The strongest predictors of failure of venous ulcers to heal are ulcer size and duration (**Table 146-6**). Healing occurs in 64% of venous ulcers present for less than 1 year, 48% of ulcers present for 1–3 years, and 24% of ulcers present more than 3 years. With regard to size, 72% of venous ulcers with baseline areas < 5 cm^2 heal, while only 40% of ulcers with a baseline area > 5 cm^2 heal.

PREVENTION

Compression stockings are effective in improving venous hemodynamics and edema and preventing primary and recurrent ulcers in patients with venous disease. Since recurrence rates are as high as 72%, patients with healed venous ulcers should wear lifelong compressive elastic stockings. This does not include patients with severe concurrent arterial disease, in whom compression stockings are contraindicated. There are four classes of compression stockings: class I (20–30 mm Hg, for varicose veins and mild edema), class II (30–40 mm Hg, for moderate venous insufficiency, moderate edema, and severe varicosities), class III (40–50 mm Hg, for severe edema), and class IV (≥ 60 mm Hg, for elephantiasis and severe venous insufficiency with postthrombotic edema).

Elderly patients and those with arthritis find it difficult to put on compression stockings. Helpful tips include washing new compression stockings prior to wear to reduce stiffness and applying stockings early in the morning when edema is least. Some stockings have modifications like silk liners or zippers for easier application and removal. There are also various aids (eg, Stocking Donner, Easy Slide, and Circaid) to assist with application of traditional compression stockings (**Table 146-7**).

CONCLUSION

Clinical diagnosis of venous disease should be confirmed by duplex ultrasound scan. Once arterial disease has been excluded, compression is the cornerstone of therapy.

Treatment of superfical venous incompetence and consistent use of compression stocking can reduce the risk of recurrence.

TABLE 146-7 Evidence-based Medicine: Venous Ulcers

Paper	Methodology	Results	Limitations	Bottom Line
O'Meara S, Cullum NA, Nelson EA. Cochrane Database of Syst Rev. 2009;1:CD000265	Systematic review of randomized trials of compression bandages or stockings in the treatment of venous ulcers	Venous ulcers healed more quickly with compression than without, with a number needed to treat of two to demonstrate benefit; multicomponent systems are more effective than single-component compression	Data on ulcer recurrence were inadequate to draw conclusions; significant heterogeneity in study designs	Venous ulcers heal more quickly with compression than without
Gohel MS, Barwell JR, Taylor M, et al. *BMJ.* 2007;335(7610):83 (Effect of Surgery and Compression on Healing and Recurrence, or ESCHAR trial)	Randomized controlled trial of superficial venous surgery, guided by duplex scanning and compression vs. compression only in 500 patients with open or recently healed venous ulcers	Overall ulcer healing rates at three years were not significantly different (89% in the compression group and 93% in the compression plus surgery group); recurrence rates at four years were lower in the compression plus surgery group compared with the compression group (31% vs. 56%; $P < 0.001$)	Patients were given written and verbal advice to wear compression stockings after ulcer healing to prevent relapse, but compliance with stocking use was not formally assessed	Superficial vein surgery does not increase the likelihood of healing in venous ulcers, but it does reduce the risk of relapse
Williams D, Enoch S, Miller D, et al. *Wound Repair Regen.* 2005;13:131–137	Concurrently controlled prospective cohort study, comparing the effect of a single sharp debridement in 28 venous ulcers with slough, nonviable tissue, and no granulation tissue, compared to 27 control venous ulcers without slough and with slight granulation tissue; both groups received compression therapy	At four weeks post-debridement, the study ulcers showed a 6 cm^2 reduction in mean surface area vs. a 1 cm^2 reduction in controls ($P = 0.02$). By week 20 post-debridement, the study ulcers achieved a 7.4 cm^2 reduction in the MSA vs. an increase of 1.3 cm^2 in controls ($P = 0.008$)	Over the relatively short follow-up time of 20 weeks, there was no difference between groups in the number of patients with ulcer resolution	A single sharp debridement in venous ulcers with necrotic tissue may speed early healing when used in conjunction with compression therapy

SUGGESTED READINGS

Briggs M, Nelson EA. Topical agents or dressings for pain in venous leg ulcers. *Cochrane Database Syst Rev*. 2010;4:CD001177.

Fonder MA, Lazarus GS, Cowan DA, et al. Treating the chronic wound: a practical approach to the care of nonhealing wounds and wound care dressings. *J Am Acad Dermatol*. 2008;58:185–206.

Jones JE, Nelson EA. Skin grafting for venous leg ulcers. *Cochrane Database Syst Rev*. 2007;2:CD001737.

Jull AB, Arroll B, Parag V, Waters J. Pentoxifylline for treating venous leg ulcers. *Cochrane Database Syst Rev*. 2007;3:CD001733.

Kranke P, Bennett MH, Debus SE, Roeckl-Wiedmann I, Schnabel A. Hyperbaric oxygen therapy for chronic wounds. *Cochrane Database Syst Rev*. 2004;1:CD004123.

Milic DJ, Zivic SS, Bogdanovic DC, Karanovic ND, Golubovic ZV. Risk factors related to the failure of venous leg ulcers to heal with compression treatment. *J Vasc Surg*. 2009;49:1242–1247.

Miller OF, Phillips TJ. Leg ulcers. *J Am Acad Dermatol*. 2000;43:91–95.

Nelson EA, Mani R, Vowden K. Intermittent pneumatic compression for treating venous leg ulcers. *Cochrane Database Syst Rev*. 2008;2:CD001899.

Phillips TJ, Machado R, Trout R, et al. Prognostic indicators in venous ulcers. *J Am Acad Dermatol*. 2000;43:627–630.

CHAPTER 147

Dermatologic Findings in Systemic Disease

Jennifer K. Tan, MD
Ruth Ann Vleugels, MD

Key Clinical Questions

1. What are the most common cutaneous manifestations of gastrointestinal, renal, rheumatologic, and endocrinologic disease? What are rare but important cutaneous findings which should not be missed?
2. How does systemic amyloidosis manifest in the skin?
3. What key features are necessary to recognize nutritional deficiencies?
4. What is the systemic approach to purpura?
5. When should an inpatient dermatology consultation be obtained?

INTRODUCTION

This chapter will focus on the integument and its unique ability to exhibit disease that lies beneath. Though an all encompassing review of this subject is beyond the scope of this chapter, we will discuss the cutaneous manifestations of systemic disease that are commonly encountered during the daily practice of hospitalist medicine. A helpful approach to this subject is to consider whether a cutaneous lesion represents *skin involvement* by an internal condition, such as amyloidosis or cutaneous metastases, or a *reactive process* to underlying disease, such as neutrophilic dermatoses related to inflammatory bowel disease, or cutaneous vasculitis due to a drug hypersensitivity reaction. Additionally, cutaneous lesions can be characterized as *specific* to an underlying systemic process, or as a *nonspecific* manifestation that may occur in the setting of multiple disorders. Cutaneous findings may represent the sole clinical manifestation of a systemic disorder. Thus, a basic knowledge of these dermatologic conditions is essential not only for recognizing an underlying association, but also for determining when an inpatient dermatology consult may be useful in the diagnosis and management of an otherwise puzzling patient.

CUTANEOUS MANIFESTATIONS OF GASTROINTESTINAL DISEASE

GASTROINTESTINAL HEMORRHAGE

Disorders in which vascular lesions are found in both the skin and viscera may occasionally manifest with gastrointestinal (GI) hemorrhage. Though rare, this group of disorders should be considered when approaching a patient with a gastrointestinal bleed, particularly in the context of recurrent hemorrhage, familial history of hemorrhage, or multiple vascular lesions noted on the skin.

Telangiectasia in the setting of GI or pulmonary vascular lesions raises suspicion for ***hereditary hemorrhagic telangiectasia*** (HHT, also known as Osler-Weber-Rendu syndrome). This is a familial autosomal dominant or spontaneous disorder, characterized by cutaneous telangiectasias and visceral arteriovenous anomalies. Epistaxis in childhood is often the presenting sign, followed by the development of well defined 2–3 mm macular or papular telangiectasias on the face, lips, tongue, ears, and chest during late childhood to young adulthood (**Figure 147-1**). Telangiectasias represent dilations of the superficial capillary network, which typically blanch upon pressure. GI bleeding from mucosal telangiectasias occurs in about 20–40% of cases, with onset typically after the fourth decade. The stomach and duodenum are often sources of this potentially life-threatening bleeding. Additional visceral manifestations of HHT include hepatic or pulmonary arteriovenous fistulae, which may lead to shunting, dyspnea, hemoptysis, or systemic embolism and infection, and cerebral arteriovenous malformations, which may lead to intracranial hemorrhage.

Blue rubber bleb nevus syndrome (BRBNS) is a spontaneous or autosomal dominantly inherited disorder characterized by multiple venous malformations of the skin, GI tract, and other viscera. Cutaneous findings include multiple dark blue to violaceous compressible, rubbery skin lesions known as blebs, most commonly located on the trunk and upper extremities. Initially characterized in the literature as "hemangiomas," the lesions associated with BRBNS are actually venous malformations that may appear macular, papular, or nodular. The classic "blue rubber nipple" demonstrates delicate

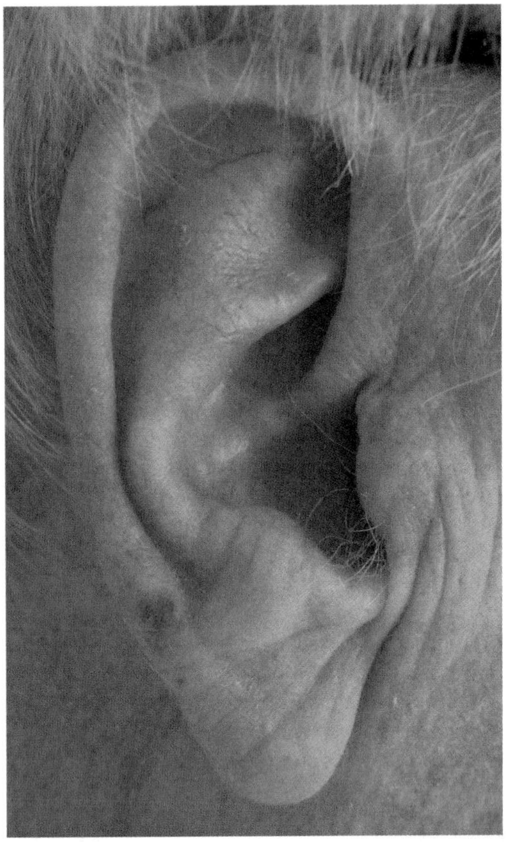

Figure 147-1 *Telangiectasia on the ear of a patient with hereditary hemorrhagic telangiectasia.*

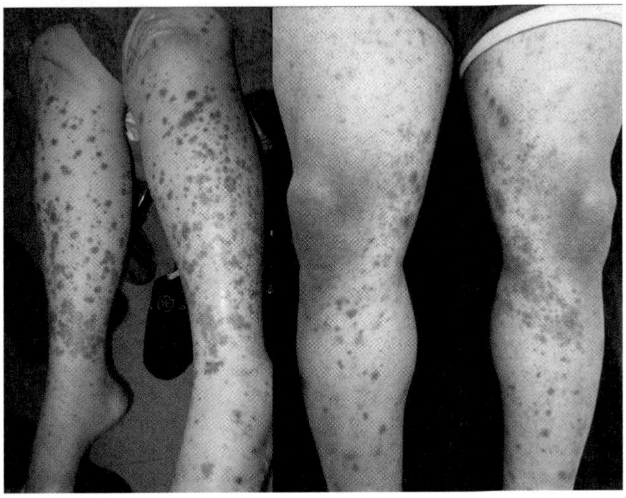

Figure 147-2 *Palpable purpura on the legs of two patients with Henoch-Schönlein purpura. This small vessel vasculitis results in non-blanchable papules that appear red to violaceous, depending on skin type and lesion duration.*

crumpling when compressed with slow refill upon release. Notably, cutaneous lesions tend not to bleed but are characteristically tender due to the high content of vascular smooth muscle. Most blebs are present at birth or by 2 years of age, but may enlarge and become more prominent with age. It is important for hospitalists to be familiar with BRBNS, as potentially life-threatening GI bleeding is generally the most serious complication of BRBNS. Patients thought to have BRBNS should be screened with colonoscopy to evaluate for potential GI involvement.

Henoch-Schönlein purpura (HSP) is a systemic vasculitis characterized by involvement of the skin, gastrointestinal tract, kidneys, and joints. Often considered a disease of childhood, HSP also occurs in adults. The major cutaneous manifestation of HSP is palpable purpura, the hallmark of small vessel vasculitis, presenting as 2–5 mm erythematous to violaceous papules that do not blanch with pressure (**Figure 147-2**). These lesions typically appear on the buttocks and lower extremities in HSP; lesions above the waist are anecdotally associated with an increased risk of renal involvement. Periumbilical purpura has also been noted to occur. Gastrointestinal signs and symptoms include abdominal pain, bleeding, and intussusception; these symptoms may precede the cutaneous findings. GI bleeding is often occult, and is suspected to occur in 40–60% of cases. If findings are limited solely to the skin, no treatment is necessary. If renal or GI involvement is present, more aggressive systemic immunosuppressive therapy may be necessary. Other systemic vasculitides, such as microscopic polyangiitis and polyarteritis nodosa, can also result in GI hemorrhage.

Kaposi sarcoma (KS) may occasionally present with gastrointestinal bleeding, though KS in general is much less common since the advent of highly active antiretroviral therapy for HIV. Cutaneous KS is a vascular neoplasm associated with human herpesvirus-8. The epidemic form of KS, which occurs in association with HIV, presents with violaceous patches, plaques, or nodules, most commonly on the chest, face, and oral cavity (**Figure 147-3**). Among patients with epidemic KS, involvement of the gastrointestinal tract is observed in 50–80% of patients with cutaneous disease, and more than 90% of patients with oral disease.

Pseudoxanthoma elasticum (PXE), a rare genetic disorder resulting in degeneration of elastic tissue, may affect the elastic media of blood vessels producing hemorrhage. Upper GI bleeding is more common than lower GI bleeding, and often presents in the third to fourth decade. Unlike the other disorders discussed in this section, the dermatologic manifestations of PXE do not typically include cutaneous vascular lesions. Instead, PXE manifests as yellow, cobblestoned papules that resemble "chicken skin" on the neck, axillae, antecubital fossae, and groin. Similar lesions or diffuse superficial erosions may be observed on mucosal surfaces during endoscopy. Ophthalmic signs of PXE include retinal neovascularization, producing angioid streaks. Other systemic manifestations include hypertension, premature vascular disease, cardiac disease, and cerebral hemorrhage. GI hemorrhage can be devastating in patients with PXE, and this hemorrhage may precede the classic dermatologic and ophthalmologic signs.

MALABSORPTION SYNDROMES

Malabsorption syndromes often produce nutritional deficiencies due to vitamin and mineral loss. An associated cutaneous eruption may suggest the correct diagnosis. Zinc deficiency may result from genetic, autosomal recessive abnormalities in zinc absorption, or be acquired from poor diet, geophagia (clay eating), chronic diarrhea, cystic fibrosis, total parenteral nutrition, renal disease, liver disease, alcoholism, or medications such as diuretics and sodium valproate. Zinc deficiency leads to a characteristic skin eruption known as ***acrodermatitis enteropathica***. Eczematous, vesicular, or pustular skin lesions typically appear in an acral, perirectal, or perioral distribution. The diaper area is frequently involved. Alopecia, glossitis, and nail dystrophy may also be observed. Diagnosis is made via plasma zinc level, though alkaline phosphatase, a zinc-dependent enzyme, is also often low in this deficiency.

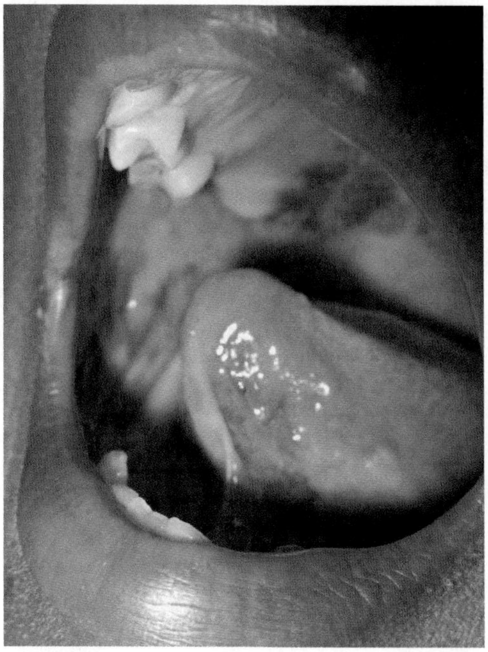

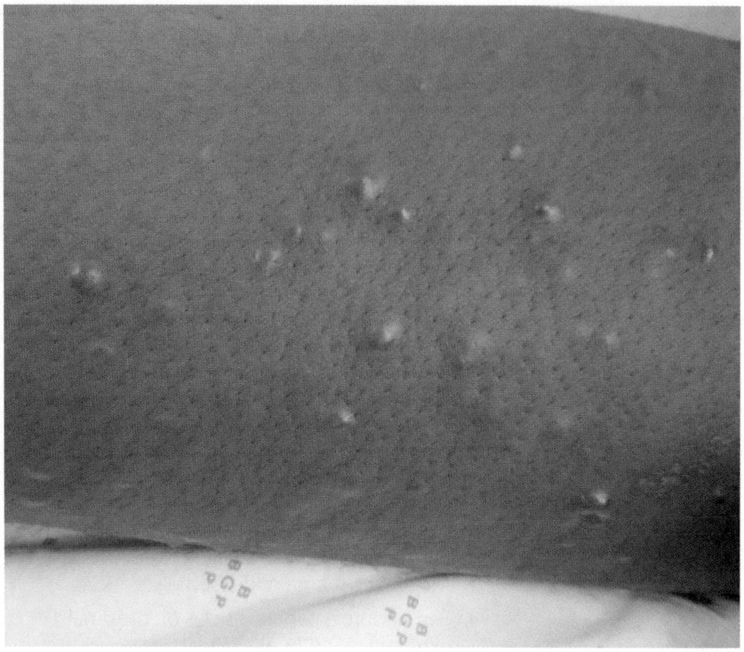

Figure 147-3 *Kaposi sarcoma of the oral cavity (left) and thigh (right) in patients with AIDS. Lesions may appear as brown to violaceous patches, plaques, nodules, or tumors.*

Dermatitis herpetiformis (DH) is characterized by a pruritic papulovesicular eruption on the extensor surfaces of the limbs, especially the forearms, elbows, and knees (**Figure 147-4**). The buttocks and posterior scalp are also often affected. As DH is intensely pruritic, patients often present only with excoriations, rather than well-defined vesicles, in the classic areas of involvement. DH is a cutaneous manifestation of gluten-sensitive enteropathy (celiac disease). Though more than 85% of DH patients demonstrate small bowel inflammation on biopsy, less than 10% have severe malabsorption. Patients may demonstrate an associated autoimmune disease or endocrinopathy, including thyroid disease, diabetes mellitus, or Addison disease. Treatment of DH includes gluten avoidance and antineutrophilic agents such as dapsone.

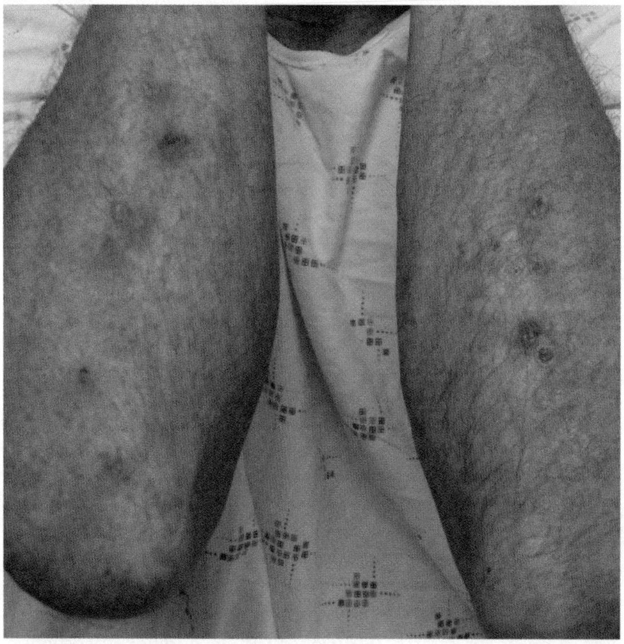

Figure 147-4 *Grouped erosions and bullae on the elbows and forearms in a patient with dermatitis herpetiformis. Small crusted papules and vesicles may also occur.*

INFLAMMATORY BOWEL DISEASE

Ulcerative colitis (UC) and Crohn disease (CD) produce skin findings in as many as one-third of affected patients. Clinical manifestations range from specific lesions, such as fistulae formation and metastatic disease, to nonspecific reactive conditions. Many of these skin lesions may be manifestations of either UC or CD, though some findings are more often associated with a specific entity. Erythema nodosum and pyoderma gangrenosum will be discussed in detail. Other cutaneous manifestations of inflammatory bowel disease are listed in **Table 147-1**.

Erythema nodosum is the most common panniculitis or inflammatory disorder of fat. It presents with erythematous, tender nodules, characteristically on the shins (**Figure 147-5**). It is not specific for IBD. Erythema nodosum is often a hypersensitivity reaction to systemic disease or an antigenic trigger, although 30–50% of cases are idiopathic. Fever, malaise, and arthralgias may occur, and females are affected more commonly than males. It is typically self-limited and resolves within several weeks, with lesions appearing bruise-like later in the disease course. Ulceration usually does not occur. Erythema nodosum may precede the diagnosis of IBD or occur concomitantly with a disease flare. It occurs in 1–10% of patients with UC and in less than 2% of patients with CD. Common associations, evaluation, and treatment are provided in **Table 147-2**. The differential diagnosis includes other forms of panniculitis, such as connective tissue panniculitis, infectious panniculitis, pancreatic panniculitis, and erythema induratum or nodular vasculitis, which is often associated with tuberculosis.

In 1930, Brunsting and colleagues characterized painful ulcers in several patients with underlying bowel disease. These skin lesions, which they called ***pyoderma gangrenosum*** (PG), were pustules that evolved into undermined ulcers with overhanging, gray borders and peripheral erythema (**Figure 147-6**). Although they were correct in identifying an association with bowel disease, the condition is not

TABLE 147-1 Cutaneous Manifestations of Inflammatory Bowel Disease

Disease	Cutaneous Exam Findings	Association	Treatment
	Nonspecific associations		
Urticaria	Transient, edematous, pruritic wheals	UC, Crohn	Antihistamines
Aphthous ulcers	Painful oral erosions	UC, Crohn	Topical steroids
Small vessel vasculitis	Multiple, small (~3–5 mm), nonblanchable red to purple macules and papules, known as "palpable purpura"	UC, Crohn	Systemic steroids if there is systemic involvement, otherwise supportive care
Erythema nodosum	Tender erythematous nodules on anterior shins, representing inflammation of the fat (panniculitis)	UC > Crohn	NSAIDs, bedrest, potassium iodide, systemic steroids, dapsone, colchicine
Neutrophilic dermatoses 1. Pyoderma gangrenosum 2. Sweet syndrome 3. Behçet disease 4. Bowel bypass syndrome	1. Pustules and boggy ulcerations with gray borders, typically on legs; can be peristomal 2. Very edematous, tender red to purple plaques and nodules, typically on face/neck/upper extremities and trunk 3. Recurrent oral and genital ulcerations, acne-like and erythema noduosum-like lesions 4. Red or purple papulovesicles on proximal extremities and trunk	UC >> Crohn	Treat underlying IBD (if present), systemic steroids, dapsone, colchicine, cyclosporine, mycophenolate mofetil, infliximab *AVOID debriding these lesions; the cutaneous eruption may worsen due to pathergy*
Cutaneous polyarteritis nodosa	Purple lacelike eruption on legs (livedo), with nodules or ulcerations.	Crohn	Systemic steroids, cytotoxic agents such as cyclophosphamide if systemic involvement
	Specific associations		
Fissures and fistula	Painful erosions and draining sinus tracts, most commonly in the perineum	Crohn > UC	Treat underlying Crohn; sinus tracts may require surgery
Cutaneous or metastatic Crohn	Cutaneous granulomas manifesting as erythematous plaques, nodules, and linear ulcerations, typically in inguinal crease	Crohn	Treat underlying Crohn
Mucosal Crohn	Cobblestoning and ulceration of oral mucosa appearing identical to bowel lesions	Crohn	Treat underlying Crohn
	Rare associations		
Erythema multiforme	Target lesions on extremities and trunk +/– ocular inflammation, hemorrhagic crusting on lips, oral/genital mucosal erosions	UC and Crohn (as well as infections and medications)	Supportive care, possible systemic steroids
Vitiligo	Depigmented macules on extremities, face, trunk	UC and Crohn (also thyroid disease)	Topical steroids, phototherapy
Epidermolysis bullosa acquisita (EBA)	Bullae and ulcerations with scarring over elbows and knees; may be peristomal (with differential diagnosis often including PG)	UC and Crohn	Treat underlying IBD, supportive care to bullae

due to bacterial infection, as they had originally postulated. PG is now recognized as an inflammatory disorder sometimes associated with systemic diseases, including IBD, paraprotenemia, malignancy, and rheumatoid arthritis, although many cases are idiopathic. Though IBD is the single most common cause of PG, only 1–5% of patients with inflammatory bowel disease develop PG. In the setting of IBD, PG is usually associated with active colitis and may be an indication for surgery. PG typically presents on the leg, but lesions can present anywhere. Peristomal PG is also common in IBD patients. Disease associations and treatment for PG are summarized in **Table 147-3**.

PG is a neutrophilic dermatosis, with diffuse skin infiltration by mature neutrophils. Other neutrophilic dermatoses include Behçet disease, neutrophilic eccrine hidradenitis, bowel bypass syndrome, rheumatoid neutrophilic dermatitis, and Sweet syndrome (acute febrile neutrophilic dermatosis). An important characteristic of each of these entities is the phenomenon of ***pathergy***, meaning that pustular, neutrophil-rich skin lesions develop or worsen following intradermal trauma. The pathergy test used in the diagnosis of Behçet disease is based on this phenomenon. Evidence of pathergy may be found within sites of vaccinations, venipuncture, indwelling catheters, or recently performed procedures (**Figure 147-7**).

It is useful to differentiate pathergy from another term commonly used in dermatology known as the ***Koebner phenomenon*** (also called the isomorphic effect). First described in patients with psoriasis by Heinrich Koebner in the late nineteenth century, the Koebner phenomenon more generally refers to the development of lesions after minor traumatic insult. It occurs in up to 25% of patients with psoriasis, often resulting from mild trauma such as a sunburn or scratch (**Figure 147-8**). In addition to psoriasis, skin conditions that may demonstrate the Koebner phenomenon include lichen planus, vitiligo, and leukocytoclastic vasculitis. Unlike pathergy, koebnerization involves the development of lesions

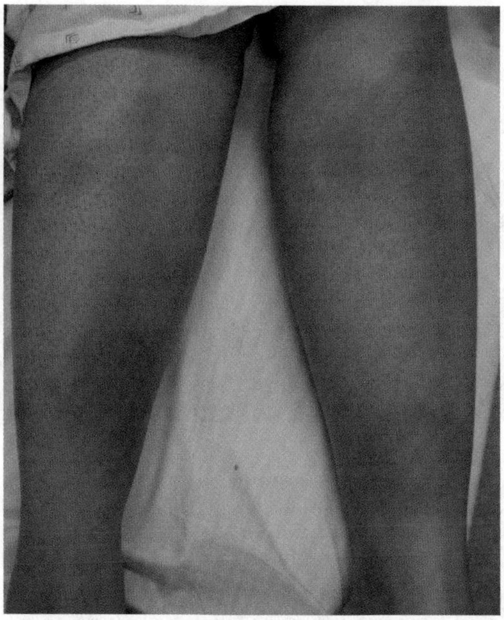

Figure 147-5 *Erythema nodosum: typical erythematous, tender nodules involving the pretibial region.*

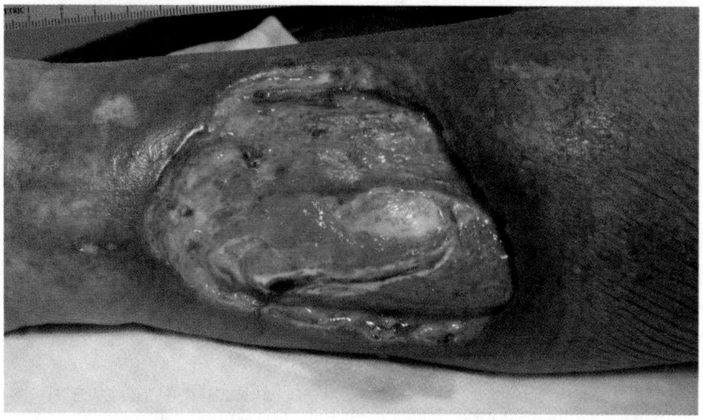

Figure 147-6 *Pyoderma gangrenosum in a patient with ulcerative colitis. Note the large, deep ulceration with overhanging, gray-colored borders.*

characteristic to an underlying disorder, and it is not a phenomenon limited to the neutrophilic dermatoses.

LIVER DISEASE

Cholestasis and cirrhosis have several cutaneous findings that are not specific to any particular etiology of liver disease. Diffuse ***pruritus*** and ***xerosis*** of the skin are common. ***Jaundice*** results from the binding of bilirubin to elastin, and may be observed initially in the conjunctivae, lingual frenulum, and on the soft palate, where elastic fibers are highly concentrated. ***Spider angiomata***, with punctate central arterioles and branches towards the periphery (**Figure 147-9A**), are common in chronic liver disease, but may also be seen with oral contraceptive use, increasing age, alcohol use, and in chronic inflammatory conditions. ***Palmar erythema***, affecting the thenar and hypothenar eminences, is another clinical sign of liver disease (**Figure 147-9B**). It is also seen in pregnancy, rheumatoid arthritis, lupus, thyrotoxicosis, diabetes, neoplasms, where it is thought to result from systemic release of angiogenic factors, and as an idiopathic condition. In liver disease, the pathogenesis of spider angiomata and palmar erythema is thought to involve increased levels of circulating estrogens.

Dupuytren contracture, a thickening of the palmar aponeurosis that may lead to fixed flexion of the fourth and fifth digit, is seen in some cirrhotic patients. It has also been associated with diabetes, anticonvulsant use, a positive family history, and possibly repetitive trauma. The nails are also commonly affected in liver disease. ***Terry nails***, the classic nail finding in liver failure, demonstrate whitening of the majority of the nail plate, with retention of only a small band of pink nail plate along the distal portion of the nail (**Figure 147-9C**). Terry nails are also seen in renal disease and malnutrition. Chronic infection with ***hepatitis B virus*** (HBV) or ***hepatitis C virus*** (HCV) may be associated with these nonspecific findings of liver disease. Several skin disorders are also specifically associated with either HBV or HCV (**Table 147-4**).

CUTANEOUS MANIFESTATIONS OF CHRONIC RENAL DISEASE

COMMON AND BENIGN CUTANEOUS DISEASE

The most common cutaneous complication of chronic renal failure is ***pruritus***, which occurs in more than 50% of hemodialysis (HD) patients. Renal pruritus may be generalized, localized, sporadic, or continuous, and is exacerbated by HD. Though the precise etiology is unknown, it is suspected to involve an interplay between xerosis,

TABLE 147-2 Causes, Diagnostic Considerations, and Treatment for Erythema Nodosum

Select Causes	Diagnostic Considerations	Treatment
Idiopathic (30–50%)	*(as appropriate)*	**General**
Infections	CBC	Identify and treat underlying cause
Bacterial: streptococcal (most common), GI (*Yersinia, Salmonella, Campylobacter*)	HCG	Bed rest and leg elevation
	ESR or C-reactive protein	**Recommended based on large case series**
Viral: respiratory, HBV	CXR	Potassium iodide
Fungal: coccidioidomycosis, histoplasmosis	Antistreptolysin O or anti-DNAse B titers	**Recommended based on small series or case reports**
Mycobacterial: tuberculosis	Throat swab (for streptococcal infection)	
Medications: OCPs, estrogens, sulfonamides, penicillin, others	Tuberculin test	Nonsteroidal anti-inflammatory drugs
	Stool ova and parasite	Systemic corticosteroids
Sarcoidosis	Hemetest stool	Dapsone
Inflammatory bowel disease	Biopsy	Colchicine
Pregnancy		Mycophenolate mofetil
Neutrophilic dermatoses: Behçet disease, Sweet syndrome		

TABLE 147-3 Systemic Associations and Treatment Options for Pyoderma Gangrenosum

Select Systemic Associations	Treatment
Gastrointestinal	**General**
Inflammatory bowel disease	Rule out infection (biopsy, tissue culture for bacteria, mycobacteria, fungi)
Diverticulosis	Avoid trauma/debridement/excision (given pathergy response)
Primary biliary cirrhosis	Careful local wound care in conjunction with specialist
Chronic hepatitis	**Recommended based on prospective controlled trial**
Rheumatologic	Infliximab
Rheumatoid arthritis	**Recommended based on retrospective trial or large case series**
Ankylosing spondylitis	Prednisone
Polychondritis	Intralesional corticosteroids
Systemic lupus erythematosus	Cyclosporine
Wegener granulomatosis	Thalidomide
Hematologic	Oral antibiotics (eg, minocycline)
Leukemia	Clofazamine
Myeloproliferative disease	Dapsone
Myelodysplasia	Topical tacrolimus
Monoclonal gammopathy	**Recommended based on small series or case reports**
Myeloma	High-potency topical corticosteroids
Solid organ malignancy	Colchicine
Colon	Tacrolimus
Breast	Methotrexate
Prostate	Mycophenolate mofetil
Lung	Azathioprine
Endocrinologic	Cyclophosphamide
Diabetes mellitus	Intravenous immunoglobulin
Thyroid disease	Potassium iodide
Idiopathic	Topical cromolyn sodium
	Hyperbaric oxygen
	Etanercept

neuropathy, mast cells, and possibly the HD membrane. Treatment strategies include emollients, narrowband phototherapy (to be used with caution in transplant patients or possible future transplant recipients due to an increased risk of nonmelanoma skin cancer, particularly squamous cell carcinoma), antihistamines, gabapentin, serotonin reuptake inhibitors, and opiate receptor antagonists.

Chronic renal failure is also associated with nail changes. Approximately 10% of patients with chronic renal failure demonstrate ***Lindsay nails***, also known as half-and-half nails, in which the proximal portion of the nail appears white, while the distal half appears normal. In nephrotic syndrome, multiple white bands may appear parallel to the lunula of the nail; these bands are known as ***Muehrcke lines***, and may also be seen with hypoalbuminemia due to liver disease or malnutrition.

Acquired perforating dermatosis is an uncommon, nonspecific manifestation of chronic renal disease (**Figure 147-10A**). These lesions, characterized by relatively small, dome-shaped papules with

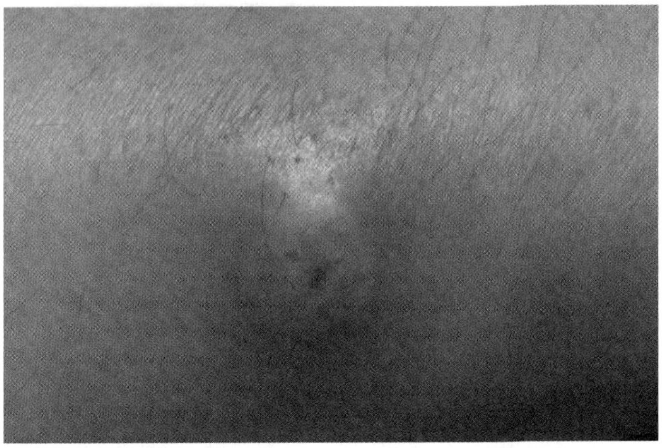

A

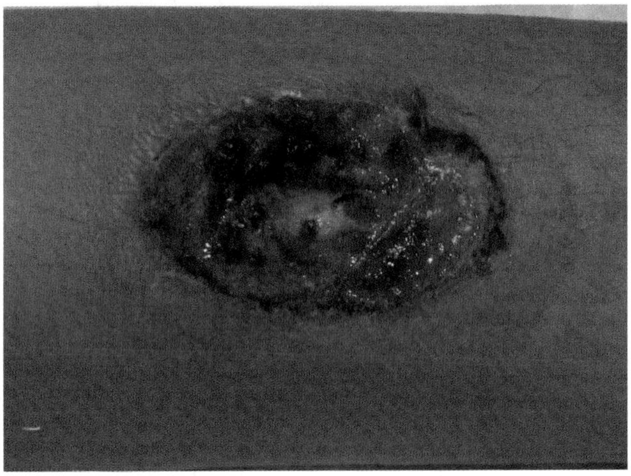

B

Figure 147-7 *Demonstration of pathergy in a patient with pyoderma gangrenosum. A large pustule developed in this patient with ulcerative colitis (A), which was initially suspected to represent an infectious process; all cultures were negative. Following debridement of the lesion, an ulcer characteristic of pyoderma gangrenosum developed (B). This patient's condition improved with systemic corticosteroids.*

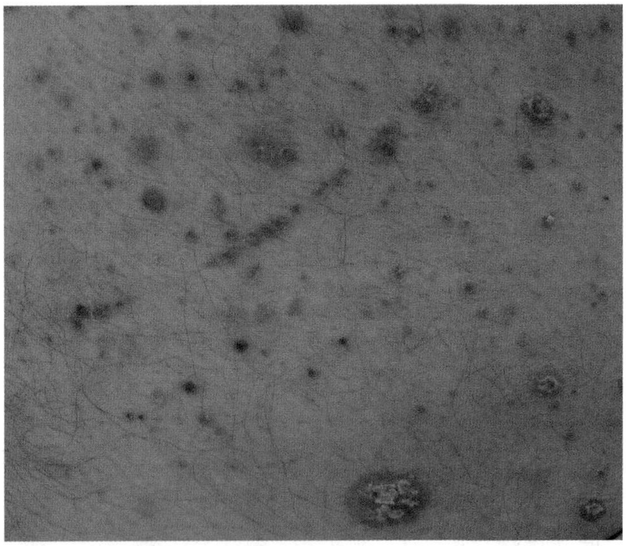

Figure 147-8 *Koebner phenomenon in a patient with psoriasis. Erythematous, scaly papules developed in a linear array after scratching. Typical psoriasiform papules and plaques are also seen in this patient.*

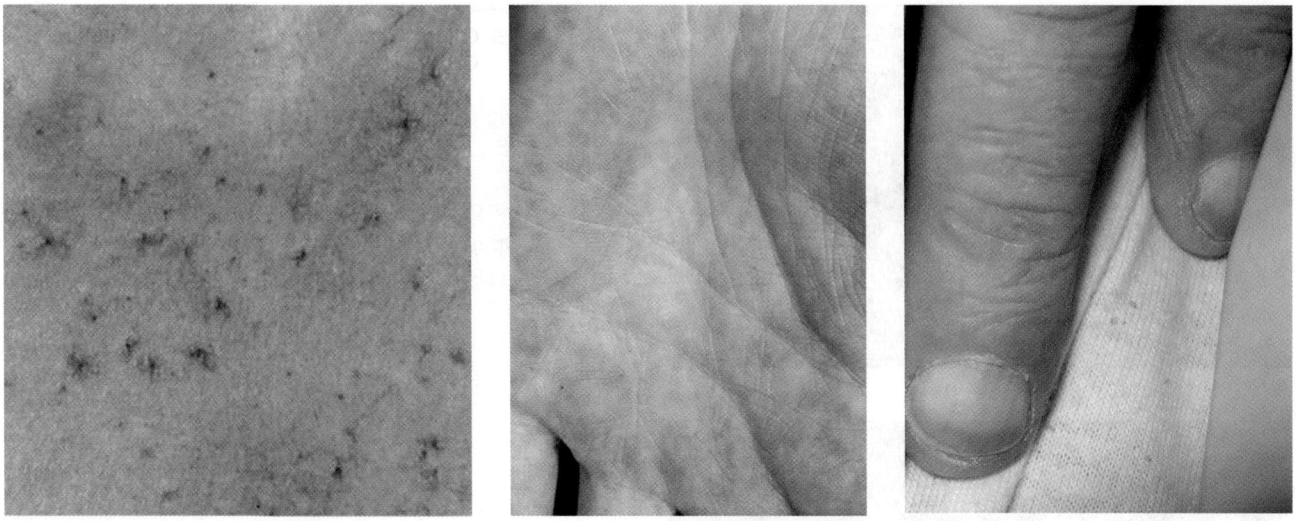

A B C

Figure 147-9 *Cutaneous manifestations of liver disease. (A) Multiple spider angiomata. (Reproduced, with permission, from Wolff K, Johnson RA, Suurmond D. Fitzpatrick's Color Atlas & Synopsis of Clinical Dermatology. 5th ed. New York: McGraw-Hill; 2005. Fig. 151-9.) (B) Palmar erythema. (Reproduced, with permission, from Wolff K, Johnson RA, Suurmond D. Fitzpatrick's Color Atlas & Synopsis of Clinical Dermatology. 5th ed. New York: McGraw-Hill; 2005. Fig. 151-8). (C) Terry nails (Courtesy of Dr. Adam Lipworth).*

a hyperkeratotic central core or plug, occur in up to 10% of dialysis patients. Most patients have end-stage renal disease due to diabetic nephropathy and are undergoing HD. However, lesions may develop prior to dialysis, as well as in patients without renal disease who have diabetes, liver disease, or malignancy. The arms and trunk are predominantly affected, particularly on the extensor aspects. No intervention is necessary for these benign lesions, however, associated pruritus may be challenging to manage.

RARE AND SERIOUS DISEASE

Nephrogenic systemic fibrosis (NSF), previously known as nephrogenic fibrosing dermopathy, is a progressive, fibrotic thickening

TABLE 147-4 Cutaneous Manifestations of HBV and HCV

Hepatitis	Disease	Cutaneous Manifestations	Systemic Manifestations
HBV	Serum sickness reaction	Urticarial or morbilliform eruption	Proteinuria, hematuria, arthritis, hypocomplementemia
	Polyarteritis nodosa	Purple lacelike eruption on legs (livedo), with nodules or ulcerations	Fever, abdominal pain, arthralgias, myalgias, mononeuritis multiplex, congestive heart failure, renal hypertension
	Papular acrodermatitis of childhood (Gianotti-Crosti Syndrome)	Skin-colored to red raised papules on extremities, buttocks and face, with sparing of the trunk	None
HCV	Urticaria/urticarial vasculitis	Edematous wheals	Arthralgias, abdominal pain, nausea, vomiting, diarrhea, proteinuria, hematuria
	Cryoglobulinemia	Red to violaceous raised papules on legs known as "palpable purpura," purple lacelike eruption on legs (livedo), ulceration of skin	Arthralgias, neuropathy, membranoproliferative glomerulonephritis; rheumatoid factor (RF) positive in cases associated with HCV
	Lichen planus	Violaceous, pruritic, polygonal papules, often on extremities. Can demonstrate Koebner phenomenon. Oral involvement is most closely associated with HCV.	None
	Porphyria cutanea tarda (PCT)	Vesicles and bullae, predominantly on dorsal hands. Hyperpigmentation and fragility of skin, milia formation, hypertrichosis.	Porphyrins are typically detectable in the urine. Bright coral red fluorescence of patient's urine with a Wood's lamp allows for bedside diagnosis.
	Necrolytic acral erythema	Papulosquamous or vesicobullous eruption on hands and feet	May be associated with zinc deficiency
	Sarcoidosis (associated with interferon and ribavirin therapy for HCV)	Red to brown papules, plaques, rarely subcutaneous nodules	Hilar lymphadenopathy, respiratory or cardiac involvement, hepatomegaly, arthralgias/arthritis, nervous system involvement, ocular involvement (including lacrimal gland enlargement, uveitis)

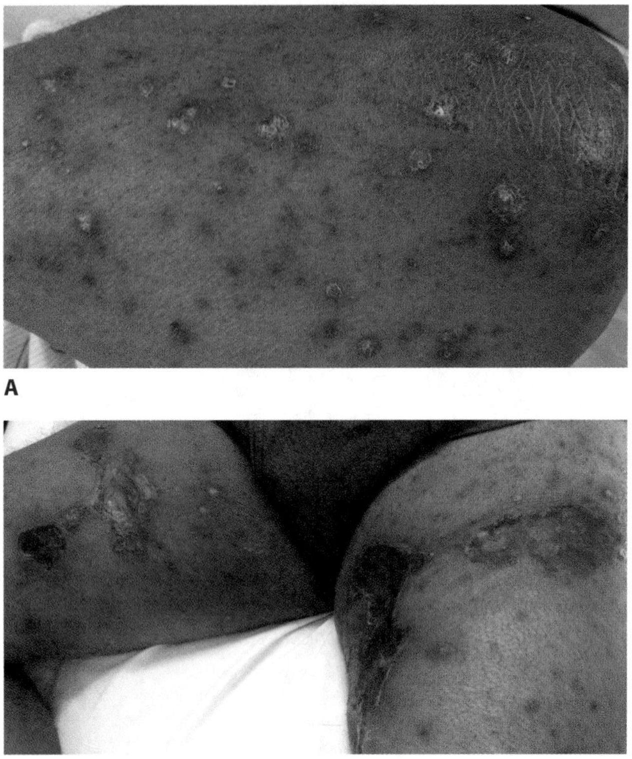

Figure 147-10 *Cutaneous manifestations of renal disease. (A) Acquired perforating dermatosis: dome-shaped papules with hyperkeratotic central cores. Lesions are often pruritic. (B) Calciphylaxis: painful necrotic ulcers on the thighs.*

of the skin, beginning on the lower extremities. As the disease progresses, joint contractures may occur, limiting mobility and ultimately disabling the patient. The pathogenesis of NSF seems to relate to oxidative tissue damage from free gadolinium ions in patients, typically those with renal failure, who undergo MRI contrast imaging studies; the risk is increased with progressive degrees of renal insufficiency, which lead to a longer tissue half-life of gadolinium, and is higher in patients who receive less-stable gadolinium chelates. Unfortunately, treatment options for NSF are limited. Patients should undergo physical therapy to limit loss of movement and avoid additional exposure to gadolinium. Pharmacologic therapy with immunosuppressives, thalidomide, and phototherapy has only a modest effect. Treatment with imatinib has shown some promising results in case series, though large randomized controlled trials have not been conducted.

Calciphylaxis is a serious, potentially lethal condition that affects 1–4% of patients with end-stage renal disease (ESRD) on dialysis. Calciphylaxis can also occur in other settings, including coumadin use and primary hyperparathyroidism. It is a cutaneous vasculopathy characterized by arterial wall calcification and proliferation with subsequent fibrosis and thrombosis. The overlying skin develops progressive ischemia, with resultant severe pain and necrosis (**Figure 147-10B**). The pathophysiology is likely multifactorial, but may be related to prolonged hyperphosphatemia from secondary or tertiary hyperparathyroidism.

Clinically, calciphylaxis manifests as red to violaceous plaques that progress to nodules and deep, necrotic ulcers. Lesions may have an overlying eschar and appear stellate, or star-shaped, outlining the area of vascular compromise. There may be associated livedo racemosa or retiform purpura, a patchy, net-like pattern of violaceous erythema on the skin. There is a predilection for the thighs,

TABLE 147-5 Calciphylaxis: Diagnostic and Therapeutic Considerations

Clinical Associations	Suggested Workup	Treatment Options
ESRD	BUN/Creatinine	Sodium thiosulfate
Alcoholic liver disease	Calcium	Parathyroidectomy
Coumadin use	Phosphorus	Cinacalcet
Protein C and S deficiency	Serum PTH	Etidronate
		Thrombolytics
Primary Hyperparathyroidism		Surgical debridement (controversial)
Malignancy		
Diabetes		Pain management
Crohn disease		Meticulous wound care

abdomen, breasts, and other areas with a thick layer of adipose tissue. Women who are obese or who have type 2 diabetes are at increased risk.

Calciphylaxis can be rapidly progressive and potentially fatal, requiring prompt recognition and treatment. A skin biopsy should be performed for confirmation of diagnosis. Treatment options are limited (**Table 147-5**). Therapies aim to mitigate hyperparathyroidism and the attendant hypercalcemia and hyperphosphatemia. The severe pain associated with tissue ischemia must be addressed. Complications are common, including infection and poor wound healing due to chronic ischemia. Overall, the prognosis is poor, with a mortality rate of up to 85% following diagnosis. Proximal lesions have a higher mortality. The major cause of mortality in patients with calciphylaxis is sepsis from wound infections, indicating a crucial need for meticulous wound care.

RENAL-CUTANEOUS SYNDROMES

There are several rare but important syndromes associated with cutaneous lesions and renal disease, including renal cell carcinoma. In many of these syndromes, the cutaneous findings may precede the development of malignancy. Thus, recognition of these syndromes may lead to earlier diagnosis of renal cancer. The cutaneous manifestations, gene defects, and renal manifestations of these rare entities are listed in **Table 147-6**.

RHEUMATOLOGIC DISEASE AND THE SKIN

LUPUS ERYTHEMATOUS

Lupus erythematosus is a complex polygenic autoimmune disease linked to several HLA subtypes and genes involved in immune signaling, as well as to environmental factors. These factors seem to lead to autoantibody production by B cells, abetted by derangements in T cell regulatory function. Lupus may either be systemic (systemic lupus erythematosus, SLE) or localized to the skin (cutaneous lupus erythematosus). Cutaneous lupus has many different variants, each with characteristic findings, prognosis, and treatment options.

Cutaneous lupus erythematosus has three main subtypes: acute, subacute (SCLE), and chronic (CCLE), as summarized in **Table 147-7**. Localized acute cutaneous lupus erythematosus (ACLE) manifests as the characteristic malar or butterfly rash (**Figure 147-11**). Subacute cutaneous disease commonly presents as scaly, red psoriasiform plaques or as annular lesions (**Figure 147-12**). Chronic cutaneous lupus is further subdivided into discoid lupus, tumid lupus, and lupus panniculitis. These cutaneous lupus variants have different

TABLE 147-6 Renal-cutaneous Syndromes

Disease	Gene Defect, Inheritance Pattern	Cutaneous Findings	Renal Manifestations
Birt-Hogg-Dube	Folliculin, AD	Achrochordon, fibrofolliculomas, trichodiscomas (may be a variant of fibrofolliculoma)	Renal cell carcinoma, especially the chromophobe and oncocytic types
Fabry disease	Alpha-galactosidase A, X-linked recessive	Angiokeratoma corporis diffusum	Glomerulonephritis and "Maltese crosses" in the urine
Familial leiomyomatosis (Reed syndrome)	Fumarate hydratase, AD	Multiple skin colored leiomyomas (patients may also have uterine leiomyomas)	Renal cell carcinoma, papillary type
POEMS Syndrome (Polyneuropathy, organomegaly, endocrinopathy, monoclonal gammopathy, and skin changes)	No known genetic defect, cases are sporadic	Scleroderma like thickening of the skin, hyperpigmentation, glomeruloid hemangiomas (of the skin), hypertrichosis	Proteinuria, hematuria, and renal failure
Tuberous sclerosis	Hamartin, AD	Ash-leaf macules, facial angiofibromas, connective tissue nevi (shagreen patch), periungual fibromas	Angiomyolipomas, multicystic kidneys

TABLE 147-7 Overview of Cutaneous Lupus, and Strength of Association with Systemic Lupus

Lupus Type	Cutaneous Findings	Systemic Findings	Autoantibody Profile	Treatment Options
Acute cutaneous lupus (ACLE)	Bilateral malar erythema (butterfly rash) Erythematous eruption on dorsal fingers, with sparing over the joints Periungal erythema Photosensitivity	*Strongest association with SLE* Oral ulcers Arthritis Renal involvement CNS involvement Pleuritis/pericarditis Blood abnormalities (leukopenia, anemia, thrombocytopenia)	ANA+ Anti-ds DNA+ (correlates with renal involvement) Anti-Ro, La, Sm+ Anti-phospholipid antibodies	Sun protection Topical corticosteroids Antimalarials (hydroxychloroquine) Oral steroids Steroid-sparing immunosuppressants (including methotrexate, azathioprine, mycophenolate mofetil)
Subacute cutaneous lupus (SCLE)	Lesions are often strikingly photodistributed (V of chest, back, arms) with sparing of mid-face. Types: 1. Annular (ring shaped) or polycyclic, erythematous plaques with clear center 2. Erythematous, psoriasiform scaly plaques	50% of patients meet criteria for SLE; however, a much lower percentage have renal or CNS involvement 40–50% with arthritis/arthralgias 20% with leukopenia	80% with ANA+ Anti-Ro+ (correlates with photosensitivity)	Sun protection Topical corticosteroids Antimalarials (hydroxychloroquine) Immunosuppressants for refractory cases
Chronic cutaneous lupus (CCLE)				
Discoid lupus (DLE)	Hyperpigmented plaques with central atrophy and scarring; lesions favor the scalp, nose, malar areas, and ears	5–10% of patients develop systemic involvement (increased if lesions on body in addition to face/scalp)	20% ANA+	Sun protection Topical corticosteroids Antimalarials (hydroxychloroquine) Immunosuppressants for refractory cases
Tumid lupus	Erythematous, edematous plaques on mid-chest, back, and face	5–10% of patients develop systemic involvement	40% ANA+	Sun protection Topical corticosteroids Antimalarials (hydroxychloroquine)

(*continued*)

TABLE 147-7 Overview of Cutaneous Lupus, and Strength of Association with Systemic Lupus ***(continued)***

Lupus Type	Cutaneous Findings	Systemic Findings	Autoantibody Profile	Treatment Options
Lupus panniculitis	Firm, tender subcutaneous nodules with normal overlying skin or with discoid lupus changes on overlying skin; typically on proximal upper extremities, thighs, buttocks, or face. Chronic lesions become depressed plaques	5–10% of patients develop systemic involvement	30% ANA+	Antimalarials (hydroxychloroquine) Immunosuppressants
Neonatal lupus	Annular (ring-shaped), polycyclic, or scaly erythematous plaques with clear center, similar to SCLE. Typical involvement on face, particularly around eyes. Mother often has anti-Ro+ SCLE, and must be evaluated	50% of children will have permanent third degree heart block (must therefore check ECG); hepatobiliary disease; thrombocytopenia	Anti-Ro, La, or U1RNP antibodies passively acquired from mother	If no heart block or systemic disease, supportive care only, as once the antibodies are degraded by the child, cutaneous eruption resolves. If there is heart block, must involve cardiology. Mother should be evaluated and treated for SCLE / autoimmune disease.

risks of systemic involvement, autoantibody profiles, and cutaneous findings, depending on the location and depth of the inflammatory infiltrate. Acute cutaneous lupus has the strongest association with systemic disease, and is always considered a manifestation of active SLE, followed by subacute and chronic cutaneous lupus, which may or may not be associated with SLE.

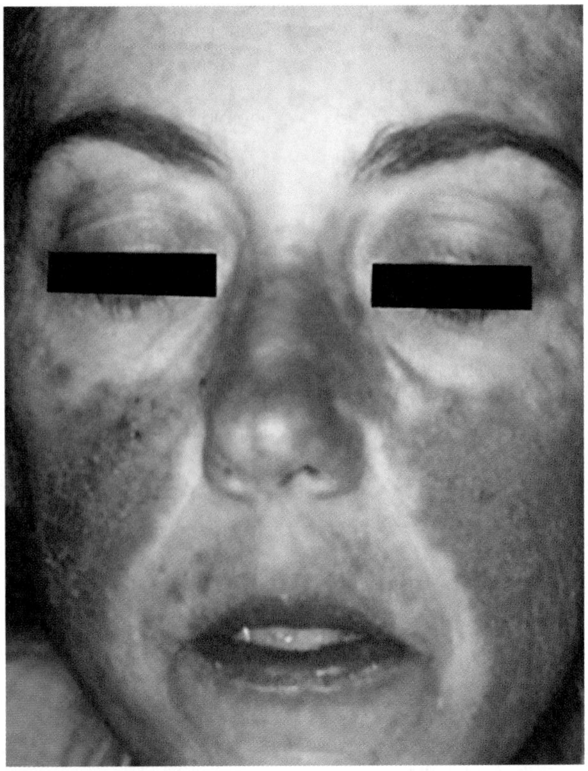

Figure 147-11 *Acute cutaneous lupus erythematosus (ACLE) typically manifests as the characteristic malar "butterfly" rash. (Reproduced, with permission, from Wolff K, Johnson RA, Suurmond D. Fitzpatrick's Color Atlas & Synopsis of Clinical Dermatology. 5th ed. New York: McGraw-Hill; 2005. Fig. 156-3.)*

Drug-induced SLE presents with arthralgias, serositis, and other systemic findings, with less frequent cutaneous involvement, whereas drug-induced SCLE presents with cutaneous findings similar to SCLE, without systemic findings. Drug-induced SLE has been associated with hydralazine, isoniazid, procainamide, quinidine, propylthiouracil, minocycline, statins, and tumor necrosis factor-alpha inhibitors, among others, while medications such as hydrochlorothiazide, calcium channel blockers, angiotensin converting-enzyme inhibitors, interferons, griseofulvin, and terbinafine are associated with drug-induced SCLE. Minocycline, a commonly prescribed tetracycline antibiotic, has been associated with more than 75 cases of drug-induced SLE and is sometimes C-ANCA positive.

In addition to aggressive photoprotection and topical corticosteroids, antimalarial therapy, typically hydroxychloroquine, is a mainstay of therapy for cutaneous lupus. If systemic disease is present or if cutaneous disease is refractory to antimalarial therapy, more aggressive immunosuppression with oral steroids or steroid-sparing immunosuppressive agents is necessary. A comprehensive discussion of therapeutic options is reviewed elsewhere in this text.

SYSTEMIC SCLEROSIS/CREST

Systemic sclerosis is an autoimmune connective tissue disease characterized by fibrosis of skin and internal organs and extensive damage to the microvasculature. Cutaneous fibrosis without internal organ involvement can occur, and is known as localized scleroderma or morphea. This discussion will focus only on systemic sclerosis.

Systemic sclerosis can be divided into localized and diffuse systemic sclerosis, depending on the extent of cutaneous involvement. In both localized and diffuse cases, Raynaud phenomenon is often the first manifestation of disease. Severe Raynaud may lead to pitted scars and ulcerations of the fingertips, and gangrenous digital lesions and fingertip amputation may ensue. Patients often go through a phase of hand swelling and edema, followed by progressive sclerosis. Both localized and diffuse systemic sclerosis initially demonstrate symmetric induration and fibrosis of the skin on the hands (**Figure 147-13A**), fingers, and face. Diffuse disease may then progress to involve the proximal extremities, trunk, and pelvis. Facial involvement characteristically affects the mouth, leading to decreased oral aperture, and occasionally the

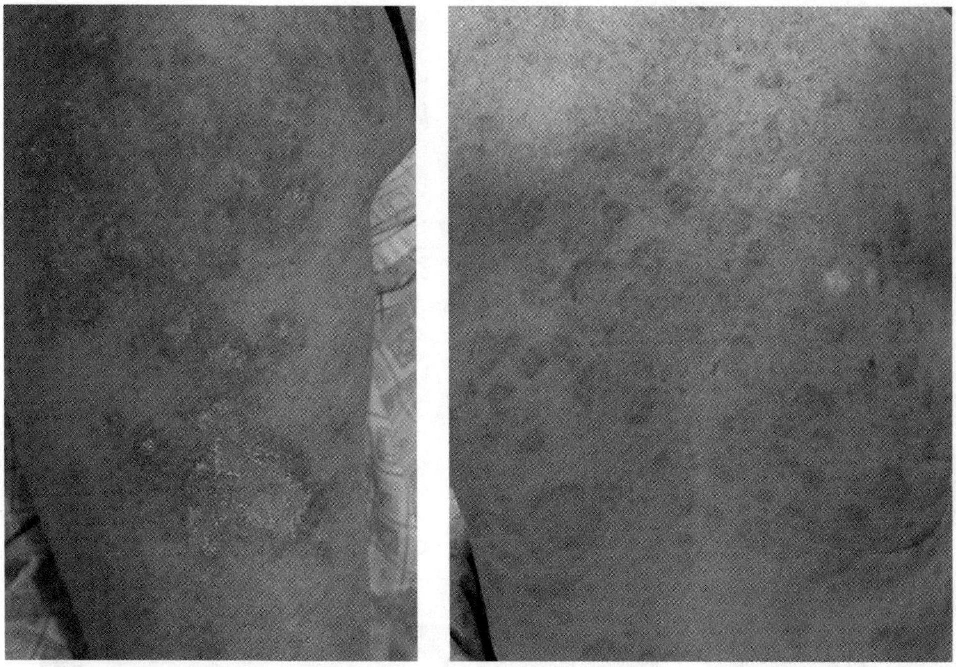

A B

Figure 147-12 *Subacute cutaneous lupus (SCLE). There are two main clinical variants: psoriasiform, scaly erythematous plaques (A) and erythematous, annular plaques (B).*

nose, giving it a beaked appearance. Patients may initially note a loss of wrinkles, and they may appear younger than their stated age. Ultimately, loss of facial movement and microstomia develop as the disease progresses. Diffuse hyperpigmentation of the skin, or patchy follicular hypopigmentation along with hyperpigmentation ("salt-and-pepper" appearance), may also be observed (**Figure 147-13B**).

CREST syndrome refers to a subset of patients with localized systemic sclerosis, characterized by calcinosis cutis, Raynaud phenomenon, esophageal dysmotility, sclerodactyly, and telangiectasias (**Figure 147-13C**). Not all patients with localized systemic sclerosis have all of the diagnostic criteria for CREST, and some patients with diffuse disease have multiple features of CREST. Patients with limited disease and exaggerated CREST features have a higher frequency of anticentromere autoantibodies, and a higher incidence of pulmonary hypertension and gastrointestinal complications.

Organ involvement may develop before or after the characteristic cutaneous eruption in both localized and diffuse systemic sclerosis. Common extracutaneous manifestations include interstitial lung disease and pulmonary hypertension, esophageal dysmotility and reflux, right- or left-sided heart failure, and renal hypertension. Pulmonary hypertension is the most common cause of death (scleroderma renal crisis was formerly the leading cause of death, but outcomes have improved with aggressive ACE inhibitor treatment). Patients with diffuse systemic sclerosis and antitopoisomerase I autoantibodies generally have a worse prognosis, and are more likely to develop early, severe internal organ involvement. Localized systemic sclerosis has a better prognosis, with patients tending to develop internal organ involvement years later in the course of their disease.

The pathogenesis of fibrosis in systemic sclerosis is unknown, though autoimmunity is thought to be involved. Most patients have a positive ANA. Patients with localized systemic sclerosis also may have anticentromere antibodies, while patients with diffuse systemic sclerosis may have anti-Scl-70 (antitopoisomerase) antibodies. However, the sensitivity of each of these autoantibodies

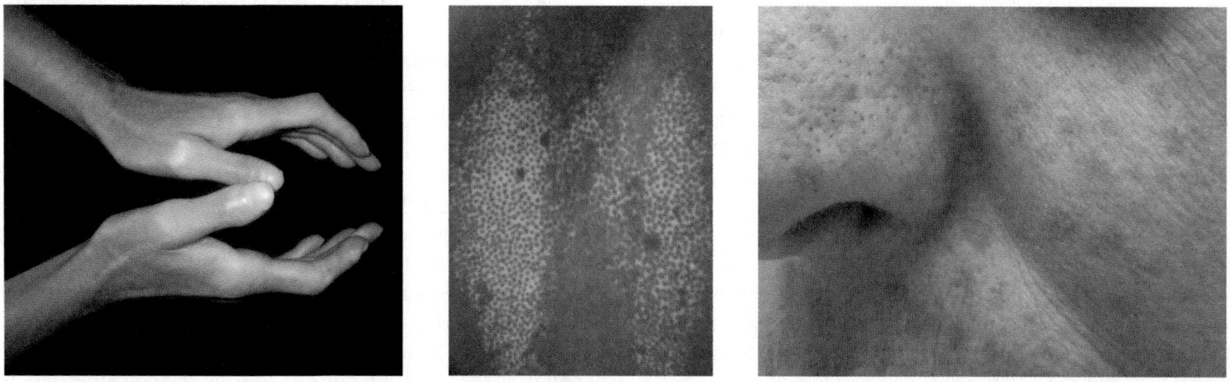

A B C

Figure 147-13 *Cutaneous findings in systemic sclerosis. (A) Sclerodactyly, or thickening of the skin of the digits of the hands and feet. Digital ulceration, calcinosis, and joint contractures may also develop. (B) "Salt-and-pepper" appearance of the skin, produced by a combination of patchy hyperpigmentation and follicular hypopigmentation. (C) In the CREST variant of systemic sclerosis, mat telangiectasias are common on the face, upper trunk, and extremities.*

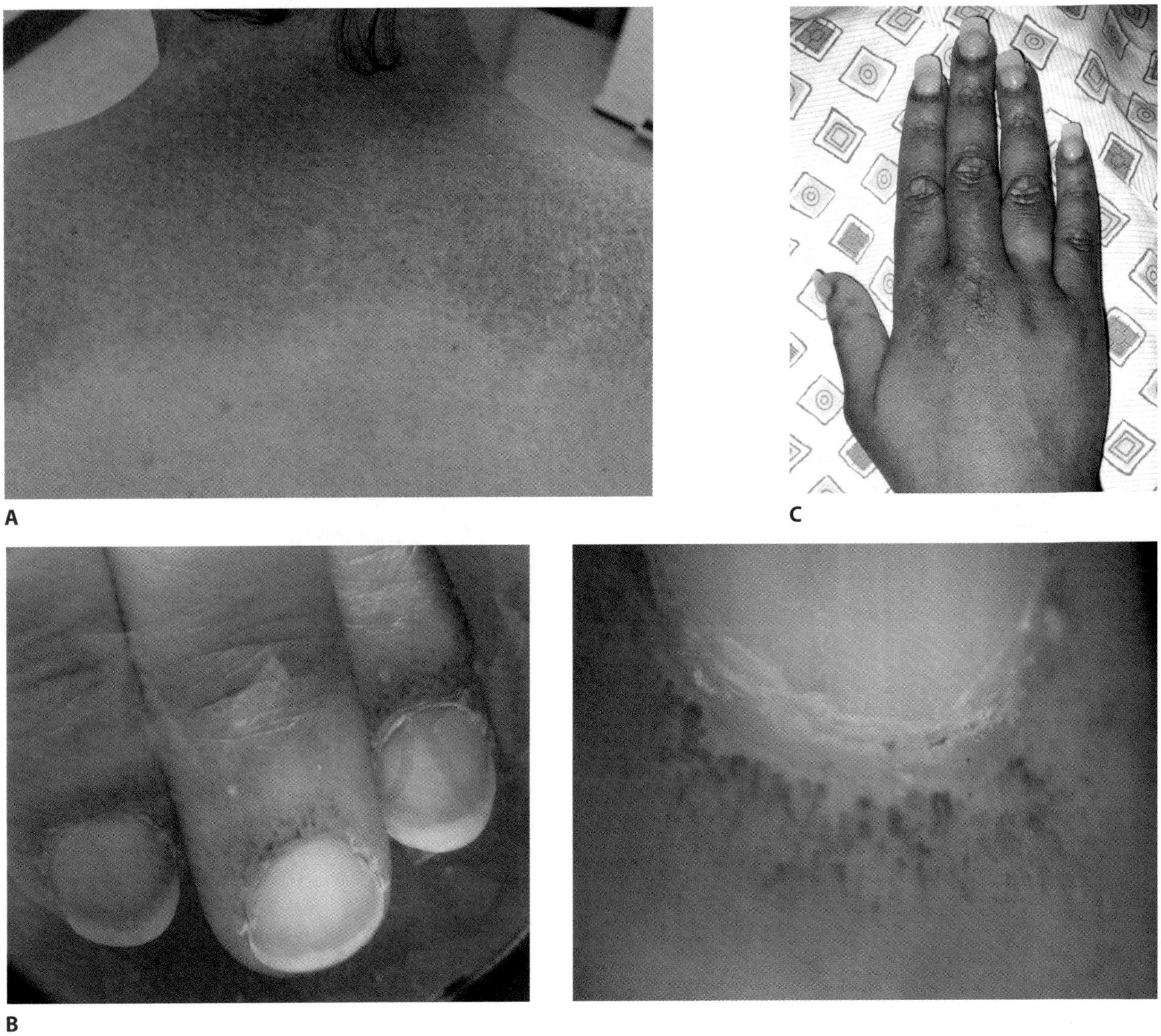

Figure 147-14 *Cutaneous findings in dermatomyositis. (A) Typical shawl sign demonstrating poikiloderma (atrophy, telangiectasia, hyperpigmentation, and hypopigmentation). (B) Dilated capillary loops within the nailfold, along with hypertrophic cuticles. (C) Gottron papules: violaceous papules overlying the joints. (Courtesy of Dr. Peter Lio).*

is relatively low. Cytokines and growth factors, particularly TGF-β and connective tissue growth factor (CTGF), may contribute to the pathogenesis by increasing collagen synthesis. Current treatment is directed toward the manifestations of systemic sclerosis, rather than the underlying pathogenesis. Raynaud phenomenon responds well to calcium channel blockers. Phosphodiesterase inhibitors such as sildenafil citrate and endothelial receptor antagonists such as bosentan have been used for both refractory Raynaud phenomenon with ulcerations and pulmonary hypertension. ACE inhibitors have substantially reduced the mortality associated with renal hypertension, and immunosuppressive therapies have been shown to be an effective treatment for pulmonary fibrosis. Cutaneous disease has been treated with agents including D-penicillamine, methotrexate, mycophenolate mofetil, imatinib mesylate, and cyclophosphamide, amongst others, although prospective studies are essentially lacking. Most recently, antibodies to TGF-β and CTGF have been studied in clinical trials, but the results have been limited.

■ DERMATOMYOSITIS

Dermatomyositis (DM) is an autoimmune connective tissue disease involving skin and proximal muscles. However, the characteristic rash may occur without notable muscle involvement, as in amyopathic or hypomyopathic dermatomyositis. Muscle involvement without a cutaneous eruption (polymyositis) is now thought to occur through a different pathogenetic mechanism.

The cutaneous eruption of dermatomyositis typically begins on the face, with noticeable eyelid edema and violaceous-colored erythema (heliotrope rash). Erythema and poikiloderma (atrophy, telangiectasia, hyperpigmentation, and hypopigmentation) may develop on the mid-face or on the upper back and shoulders, called the shawl sign (**Figure 147-14A**). Dilated blood vessels or telangiectasias at the nailfold, with overgrowth of the cuticle, may be present (**Figure 147-14B**). Nail bed telangiectasias may also be seen in other connective tissue diseases. Pruritus, particularly of the scalp, can be a frustrating symptom for patients. Erythematous to violaceous papules and plaques, with or without associated scale, may develop on the dorsal hands with involvement most prominent over the joints, known as Gottron's papules (**Figure 147-14C**). By contrast, patients with lupus can have an erythematous eruption, which typically involves the interphalangeal components of the dorsal fingers, with joint sparing.

Symmetric proximal muscle weakness is common in dermatomyositis, with particular involvement of the shoulders and hips. Myopathy can be diagnosed by measuring creatine kinase and

TABLE 147-8 Autoantibodies Associated with Dermatomyositis, Systemic Sclerosis, and Mixed Connective Tissue Disease

Autoantibody	Cutaneous Findings	Systemic Findings
Anti-Mi2	"Classic" cutaneous dermatomyositis, particularly shawl sign and cuticular overgrowth	Better prognosis, better response to treatment, less risk of pulmonary fibrosis
Anti-tRNA synthetases (including Jo-1)	Erythema and nonpruritic, scaly patches on the hands, particularly lateral and volar fingers, so-called "mechanic's hands" Raynaud phenomenon	Increased risk of interstitial lung disease; fever, arthritis, myositis, Raynaud (so-called anti-synthetase syndrome)
Anti-PM-Scl	Sclerodermoid skin changes (thickening and induration of the skin) Sclerodactyly	Increased risk of systemic sclerosis
Anti-U1RNP	Mixed connective tissue disease, with overlapping cutaneous features of lupus, systemic sclerosis, and dermatomyositis	Myositis, arthritis, increased risk of pulmonary fibrosis, decreased risk of nephritis compared to lupus

aldolase levels or by obtaining an electromyogram. Muscle biopsies and magnetic resonance imaging (MRI) studies are also used. In addition, patients may develop arthritis and arthralgias, as well as pulmonary fibrosis or even cardiac involvement. Esophageal involvement can present as either reflux or dysphagia. Baseline esophageal studies, pulmonary function tests with diffusion studies, and electrocardiogram are recommended. Similar to other autoimmune connective tissue diseases, specific autoantibodies can be associated with systemic involvement in DM (**Table 147-8**).

Between 10–50% of cases of DM in adults are associated with underlying cancer. The diagnosis of malignancy may precede or follow the diagnosis of DM. Underlying malignancies include adenocarcinoma of the ovary, lung, pancreas, colon, and stomach, as well as lymphoma. In female patients, there is a strong association with ovarian cancer, and in Southeast Asian patients, there is an association with nasopharyngeal carcinoma. Routine malignancy screening is not considered sufficient to detect potentially associated malignancies, and more advanced laboratory and imaging studies, such as computed tomography (CT) of chest, abdomen, and pelvis, along with a transvaginal pelvic ultrasound in women, are warranted. Screening tests should be performed at the time of diagnosis and on an annual basis for the next 3–5 years to detect possible malignancies (**Table 147-9**). Juvenile dermatomyositis is usually not associated with underlying malignancy, but may instead be associated with an increased risk of calcinosis cutis and vasculitis, particularly of the GI tract.

Oral steroids remain the initial treatment of choice for myositis. Steroid-sparing agents, such as methotrexate, azathioprine, or mycophenolate mofetil, may also be beneficial. For patients who have failed these treatments, intravenous immunoglobulin (IVIG) or rituximab may help. Cutaneous disease is treated with strict photoprotection, topical corticosteroids, antimalarials including hydroxychloroquine, and immunosuppressive medications in more refractory cases.

TABLE 147-9 Malignancies Associated with Dermatomyositis and Suggested Evaluation

Malignancies associated with dermatomyositis (reported frequency 10–50%)	Suggested malignancy workup (consider annually for 3–5 years following diagnosis)
Genitourinary, especially ovarian cancer	Full physical examination
Colon	CBC, complete metabolic panel, TSH
Breast	Stool occult blood testing
Lung	Breast and gynecologic in women; Pap smear and mammography
Gastric	CT of the chest, abdomen, and pelvis
Pancreatic	Transvaginal pelvic ultrasound in women
Lymphoma	CA-125
Nasopharyngeal carcinoma (overrepresented in Southeast Asians)	Gastrointestinal endoscopy (age-appropriate)

CUTANEOUS MANIFESTATIONS OF ENDOCRINE DISORDERS

THYROID DISEASE

Similar to its role elsewhere in the body, thyroid hormone is instrumental in regulating the development and homeostasis of the skin and hair. Specifically, thyroid hormone regulates skin thickness, protein synthesis, cell division, and temperature. As a result, hypo- and hyperthyroidism result in characteristic cutaneous findings, in addition to systemic manifestations.

Hypothyroidism results in a decreased metabolic state with reduced core temperature, vasoconstriction, and xerosis (dry skin). As a result, acquired ichthyosis or keratoderma may develop, in addition to brittle nails. The skin may be slightly yellow from carotenemia, as hypothyroidism diminishes the transformation of carotene to vitamin A. The patient may have myxedema, swollen, pale, and waxy skin with diffuse deposits of mucopolysaccharides. There is often associated swelling of the eyelids, lips, and tongue. Finally, loss of the lateral aspects of the eyebrows (madarosis) and scalp hair can also occur in hypothyroidism.

Hyperthyroidism can also produce diffuse alopecia. However, in contrast to hypothyroidism, hyperthyroidism results in cutaneous thinning and warm, moist skin. Hyperhidrosis may also occur due to increased vasodilation. Finally, hyperpigmentation similar to that observed in Addison disease may be associated with hyperthyroidism.

The most common cause of hyperthyroidism is ***Graves disease***, caused by autoantibodies to the TSH receptor. Up to 25% of patients with Graves disease develop ophthalmopathy (or orbitopathy), with exophthalmos and proptosis caused by orbital fat accumulation and edema of the ocular muscles. Hyperthyroid patients may have lid retraction and widening of the palpebral fissures without necessarily having Graves' ophthalmopathy.

About 4% of patients with Graves disease have ***pretibial myxedema*** or dermopathy, manifesting as symmetric, indurated, firm plaques and nodules with a peau d'orange texture on the anterior shins. Rarely, patients with Graves disease have ***thyroid acropachy***, consisting of the triad of digital clubbing, soft tissue swelling of the hands and feet, and periosteal bone formation.

DIABETES MELLITUS

Type I and type 2 diabetes mellitus are complicated by a variety of cutaneous manifestations (**Figure 147-15**). Contributing factors include vascular insufficiency, microangiopathy, metabolic derangement, neutrophil dysfunction from hyperglycemia, poor wound healing, and neuropathic complications.

Skin infections occur in 20–50% of diabetic patients. These include candidal intertrigo, tinea, diabetic foot infections, malignant otitis externa due to Pseudomonas, and mucormycosis in the setting of ketoacidosis. It is particularly important to recognize and treat tinea pedis in this population, as minute regions of skin breakdown from tinea often serves as a portal of entry for diabetic foot infections.

Irregular, red-brown papules or plaques on the pretibial areas should raise suspicion for ***diabetic dermopathy***. Once the inflammatory stage has subsided, these lesions heal over months to years, leaving atrophic, hyperpigmented scars. Diabetic dermopathy may precede the onset of abnormal glucose metabolism, and has been associated with a greater susceptibility for microvascular complications such as retinitis, nephropathy, and neuropathy. There is no specific therapy. Glycemic control should be optimized. Insulin resistance is associated with the development of ***acrochordons*** (skin tags), fleshy, soft papules on the eyelids, neck, axillae, and inguinal folds, and ***acanthosis nigricans***, velvety, hyperpigmented, asymptomatic plaques in the neck, axilla, and groin.

Patients with diabetes often develop ***nail changes***. In type 2 disease, 40–50% of patients demonstrate yellow nails, often most prominent along the distal portion. This may be confused with onychomycosis. In addition to yellow nails, patients may develop periungual telangiectasia, with ragged cuticles and nailfold erythema.

Necrobiosis lipoidica (NL) manifests as yellow to red-brown plaques with atrophy and telangiectasia on the lower legs. Central atrophy may develop, sometimes with painful ulceration. Though NL is seen in less than 2% of patients with diabetes, a third of patients with NL have frank diabetes, and another third have impaired glucose tolerance. Topical or intralesional corticosteroids may arrest the progression of plaques. Ulceration usually responds to topical wound care. ***Diabetic bullae*** (bullous diabeticorum) also occur on the lower legs. They are generally noninflamed, asymptomatic blisters on the dorsal and lateral legs, which heal with supportive care in 2–6 weeks. Wound care is necessary to prevent bacterial secondary infection.

Patients with both types of diabetes may demonstrate skin thickening, ranging from nonspecific thickening of the dorsal hands (observed in 20–30% of diabetics), to marked thickening of the upper back, known as ***scleredema diabeticorum*** (2.5–14% of diabetics). Diabetes is responsible for only about a third of scleredema cases; scleredema may also be seen in paraproteinemia, hyperparathyroidism, and as a postinfectious streptococcal complication.

Similar to patients with chronic renal failure, diabetes has been associated with ***acquired perforating dermatoses*** and ***calciphylaxis***, though less frequently. It is unknown whether these conditions tend to affect patients with diabetes alone, or patients who have concomitant diabetes and renal failure. ***Vitiligo***, which presents with depigmented patches of skin, is observed in 1–7% of patients with type 1 diabetes. The coexistence of these two conditions suggests the polyglandular autoimmune syndrome.

Disseminated granuloma annulare is weakly associated with type 2 diabetes. This condition consists of hundreds of small, oval to ring-shaped thin pink papules that appear over the trunk and limbs. It tends to resolve spontaneously over time. Treatment options include topical or intralesional corticosteroids, amongst other anti-inflammatory therapeutic regimens.

AMYLOIDOSIS

Amyloid is a homogenous, eosinophilic, waxy material that can be deposited in any of the body's organ systems. Amyloidosis may be either acquired or hereditary, and may be further subdivided into systemic and localized forms. Acquired amyloidosis may be primary, due to deposition of monoclonal immunoglobulin light chains, or secondary, due to accumulation of serum amyloid A in patients with longstanding systemic inflammatory conditions, as in untreated tuberculosis or rheumatoid arthritis.

The clinical presentation depends on the organ of deposition. Cutaneous lesions range from hyperpigmented patches, seen in macular amyloid, to macroglossia and pinch purpura, seen in primary systemic disease. **Table 147-10** summarizes the different subtypes of amyloidosis, as well as their cutaneous manifestations and treatment options.

Primary systemic amyloid is a clonal disorder of plasma cells. While myeloma is sometimes complicated by amyloidosis, most patients with primary systemic amyloid do not meet diagnostic criteria for myeloma. Organ involvement in primary amyloidosis includes the skin, gastrointestinal tract, kidneys, and especially the cardiovascular system; the most common causes of death are refractory heart failure and ventricular arrhythmia. Cutaneous involvement is observed in 40% of patients with primary systemic amyloidosis. Skin findings include macroglossia, often manifesting with indentations on the side of the tongue from the teeth, waxy or shiny nodules, and purpuric papules and nodules, particularly around the eyes, oral cavity, and extremities. In contrast, visceral disease predominates in secondary systemic amyloid from inflammatory states or infection, and skin lesions are usually absent. Despite the ostensible lack of skin involvement in secondary systemic amyloidosis, biopsy of clinically normal skin may demonstrate perivascular amyloid deposition in 50% of cases; sensitivity may be increased by use of rectal biopsies, rather than abdominal fat pad biopsies.

Treatment is directed at the underlying causative disease. Primary systemic amyloid requires hematology-oncology consultation for evaluation and treatment of a potentially associated plasma cell dyscrasia. Secondary systemic amyloidosis, on the other hand, requires evaluation to determine the chronic inflammatory or infectious etiology.

NUTRITIONAL DEFICIENCIES

In developing countries, nutritional deficiencies arise from malnutrition or starvation, particularly in infants and young children. In contrast, nutritional deficiencies in developed countries are often manifestations of alcoholism, total parenteral nutrition (TPN), restricted diets, and malabsorption syndromes.

As many essential nutrients are involved in interrelated steps in metabolic pathways of fatty acids, vitamin deficiencies may have similar cutaneous eruptions (**Table 147-11**). These include: acral or intertriginous desquamative eruptions, which may initially be confused with atopic dermatitis or fungal infections; seborrheic eruptions, consisting of scaly erythematous plaques on the mid-chest, back, perioral areas, and central face; glossitis; diffuse alopecia; and peripheral edema. Unfortunately, these lesions are nonspecific and may be subtle. The histopathologic findings of the different nutritional deficiencies are also nonspecific, consisting of pallor of the epidermis with edema and bulla (blister) formation.

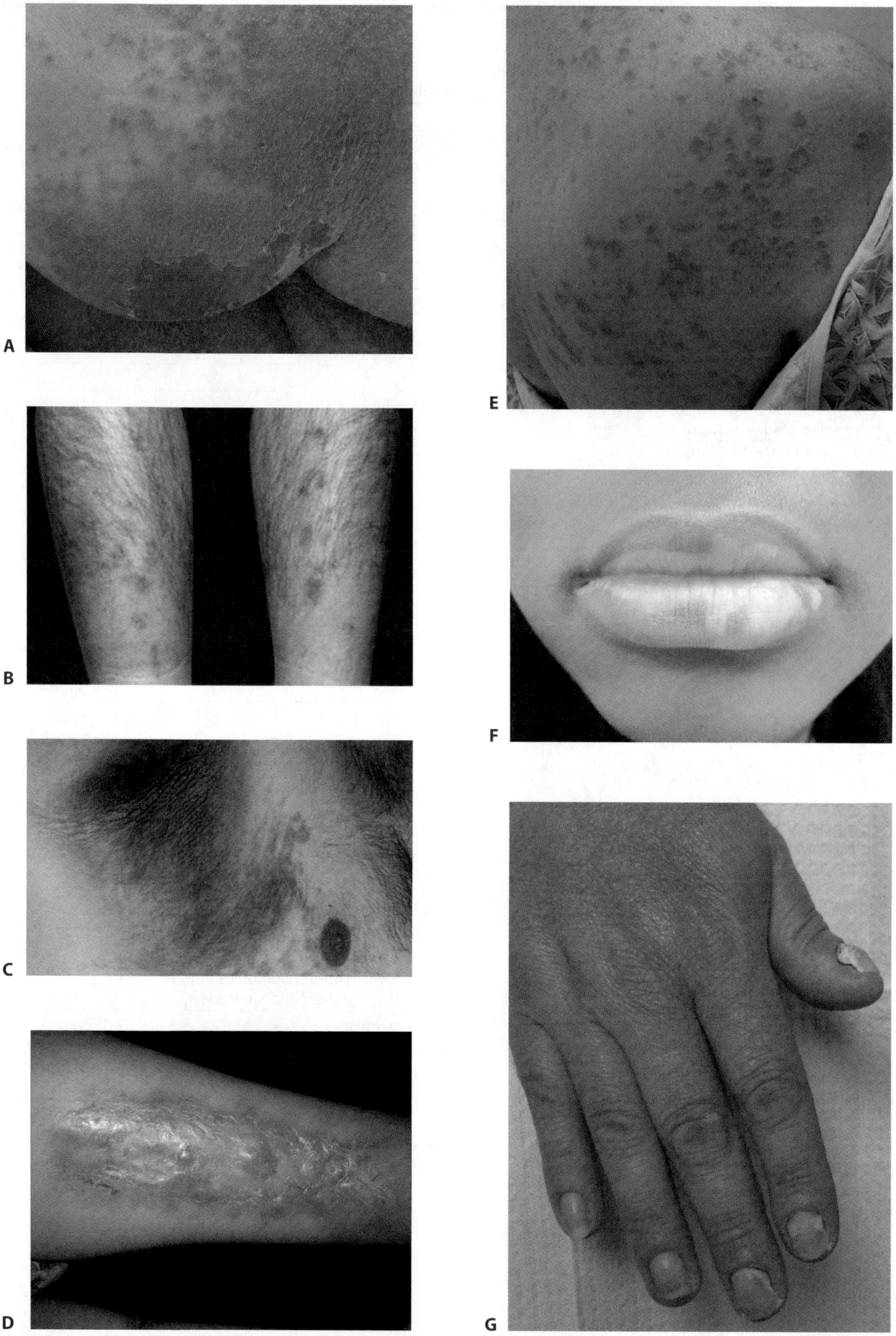

Figure 147-15 *Cutaneous manifestations of diabetes. (A) Eroded plaques with satellite papules and pustules, characteristic of cutaneous candidiasis. (B) Diabetic dermopathy: brown papules and plaques on the pretibial region. (Reproduced, with permission, from Wolff K, Johnson RA, Suurmond D. Fitzpatrick's Color Atlas & Synopsis of Clinical Dermatology. 5th ed. New York: McGraw-Hill; 2005. Fig. 152-8.) (C) Acanthosis nigricans: typical hyperpigmented, velvety, verrucous axillary plaques. (Reproduced, with permission, from Wolff K, Johnson RA, Suurmond D. Fitzpatrick's Color Atlas & Synopsis of Clinical Dermatology. 6th ed. New York: McGraw-Hill; 2005. Fig. 5-1.) (D) Yellow to red-brown plaques of necrobiosis lipoidica, with atrophy of the overlying epidermis and telangiectasias. (E) Disseminated granuloma annulare, many small, oval to ring-shaped pink papules over the trunk and limbs. (F) Depigmented patches on the lips in vitiligo. (G) Yellow nail changes.*

TABLE 147-10 Summary of Amyloidosis

Disease	Underlying Disease	Type of Amyloid Deposited	Clinical Manifestations	Treatment
Systemic amyloidosis: involvement of multiple organ systems				
Primary systemic amyloid	Multiple myeloma or other plasma cell dyscrasias	AL amyloid	Cutaneous: macroglossia, pinch purpura (petechial and purpuric papules/nodules around eyelids, neck, axilla), and waxy or purpuric papules/plaques on body Systemic: Carpal tunnel syndrome, arthritis, CHF, hepatomegaly, neuropathy	Treat underlying myeloma/plasma cell dyscrasia, typically with chemotherapy
Secondary systemic amyloid	Chronic inflammatory conditions (such as RA) or chronic infections (such as TB)	AA amyloid	Cutaneous: usually none Systemic: amyloid deposited around parenchymal organs (kidneys, liver, spleen)	Treat underlying causative inflammatory or infectious condition
Localized amyloidosis: involvement of a single organ system				
Primary cutaneous amyloid	Deposition of amyloid likely due to chronic rubbing and irritation of the skin	Keratin-derived amyloid	Cutaneous lesions: 1. Macular amyloid: rippled, hyperpigmented patches, typically located on upper back between scapula 2. Lichen amyloid: Hyperpigmented, scaly, pruritic papules, typically located on anterior shins or extensor surfaces Systemic: none	Avoid scratching and rubbing the area, as this worsens the hyperpigmentation Topical steroids Phototherapy
Primary cutaneous amyloid (AL-derived)	Cause unknown, but amyloid likely from localized plasma cells	AL amyloid	Nodular amyloid: single or multiple nodules on trunk, extremities or face	No treatment necessary Surgical excision or destruction may be useful
Secondary cutaneous amyloid	Amyloid deposited in preexisting skin tumors, such as basal cell carcinomas, dermatofibromas, seborrheic keratoses	Keratin-derived amyloid	Cutaneous lesions: amyloid not appreciated clinically, but seen only on microscopic examination. Systemic: none	No treatment necessary for the amyloid
Cerebral amyloidosis	Alzheimer disease		Cutaneous lesions: none Systemic: CNS amyloid deposits	No effective treatment
Hereditary amyloid syndromes: may involve multiple organ systems				
Familial Mediterranean fever (FMF)	Mutations in pyrin gene, leading to increased secretion of interleukin-1β	AA amyloid	Cutaneous: erysipelas-like eruption on lower extremities Systemic: fever, pleuritis, peritonitis, synovitis, amyloid deposition in kidneys	Colchicine (anti-neutrophil agent)
Muckle-Wells syndrome	Proinflammatory mutation in cryopyrin gene	AA amyloid	Cutaneous: urticaria Systemic: fever, limb pains, deafness, amyloid deposition around kidneys	Anakinra (IL-1 receptor antagonist)

TABLE 147-11 Cutaneous and Other Manifestations of Vitamin Deficiencies

Vitamin/Nutrient Deficiency	Clinical Manifestations
Vitamin A	Night blindness; some patients demonstrate a follicular hyperkeratotic eruption that resembles "toad skin" (phrynoderma)
Vitamin B (and subtypes)	Cutaneous manifestations vary based on subtype. Pellagra (B3 deficiency) consists of photodistributed (forearms, face, neck, and V of chest) eczematous eruption. Other Vitamin B deficiencies consist of seborrheic dermatitis-like eruption, glossitis, and cheilitis
Vitamin C (scurvy)	Easy bruising, bleeding gums, corkscrew hairs with perifollicular hemorrhage
Zinc (acrodermatitis enteropathica)	Eczematous dermatitis, with crusting, in seborrheic distribution (perioral, inguinal regions) as well as acral sites (hands/feet)
Marasmus (caloric deficiency)	Shrunken, wasted appearance with height and weight > 2 standard deviations below normal
Kwashiorkor (protein deficiency)	Edema, ascites, xerosis (dry skin)

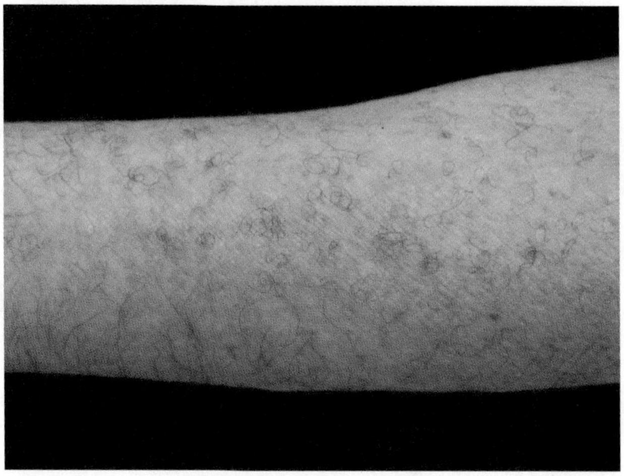

A

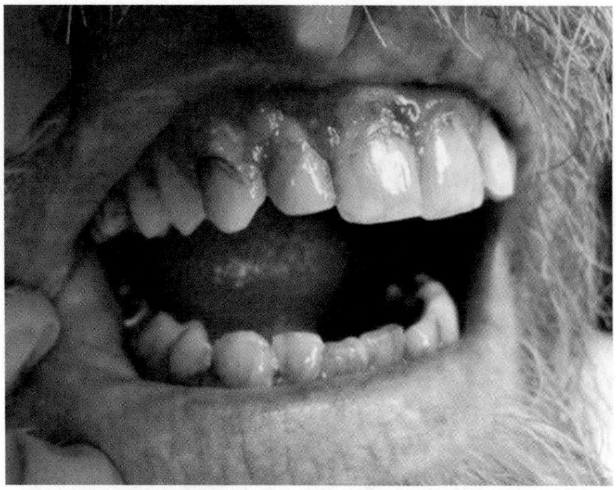

B

Figure 147-16 *Clinical features of vitamin C deficiency (scurvy): corkscrew hairs (A) and gingival friability and bleeding (B).*

Patients with nutritional and vitamin deficiencies are often initially misdiagnosed. Frequently, children are diagnosed with atopic dermatitis, but do not respond to traditional eczema treatments. Adults are often misdiagnosed as having seborrheic dermatitis or psoriasis, but similarly fail to improve.

Diagnosing a possible nutritional deficiency requires a detailed dietary history, including total food intake, use of dietary supplements or suppressants, and a prior history of GI disease, including inflammatory bowel disease and previous gastrointestinal surgery. Physicians should consider coexisting psychiatric issues, such as alcoholism, substance abuse, anorexia, or bulimia. Laboratory values can be beneficial, including complete blood count, zinc levels, alkaline phosphatase levels (a zinc-dependent enzyme), vitamin A, vitamin B and subtypes, vitamin C, and vitamin D. In infants, metabolic nutritional panels can be checked for possible inborn errors of metabolism causing dietary deficiency. Once the deficiency is determined, appropriate supplementation can be initiated (**Figure 147-16**).

CUTANEOUS SARCOIDOSIS

Sarcodoisis is a disease of unknown etiology that most commonly affects the lungs, eyes, lymphoid organs, liver, and skin. Approximately 70% of patients presenting with cutaneous involvement actually have systemic sarcoidosis. Diagnosis is made on clinical exam and confirmed by the presence of noncaseating granulomas on histology. Nonspecific cutaneous conditions are also associated with sarcoid, including erythema nodosum, pruritus, erythema multiforme, and erythroderma.

Sarcoidosis mimics many types of cutaneous disease. The most common presentation is ***papular sarcoid***, presenting as small, 3–5 mm red-brown to violaceous papules typically on the face (**Figure 147-17A**). Papules may coalesce into larger, annular plaques that appear serpiginious (**Figure 147-17B**). Lesions may be hypopigmented on darker skin. When the scalp is involved, there may be scarring alopecia. Sarcoidosis sometimes produces red, indurated plaques with telangiectasias on the central face or neck, a condition known as ***lupus pernio***; involvement of the nasal rim indicates increased risk for upper airway involvement. Sarcoidosis may develop within scars (**Figure 147-17C**) or areas previously affected by infection, trauma, or radiation. Less common manifestations of cutaneous sarcoidosis include ichthyosis-like lesions, pustular lesions, verrucous lesions, and subcutaneous sarcoid.

MALIGNANCY AND THE SKIN

Malignancy may manifest in the skin as direct metastatic spread, or by inducing an inflammatory dermatosis or other paraneoplastic skin changes. These paraneoplastic phenomena may resolve following treatment of the underlying malignancy.

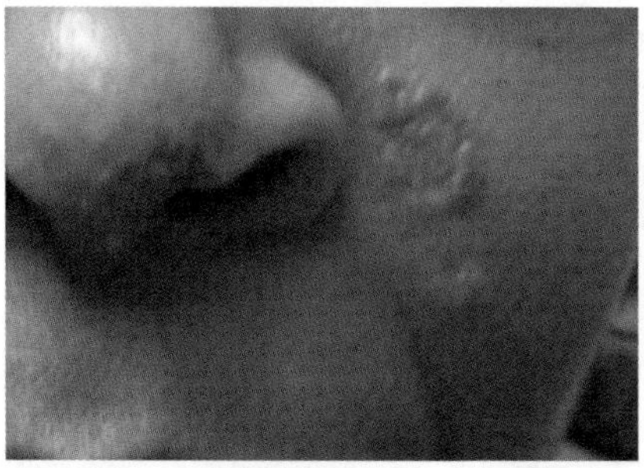

A

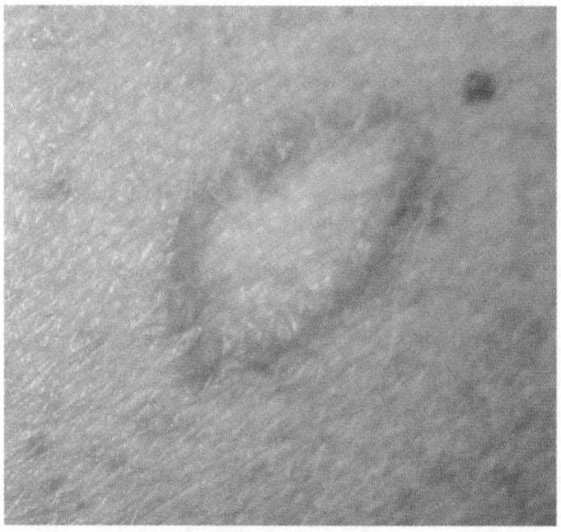

B

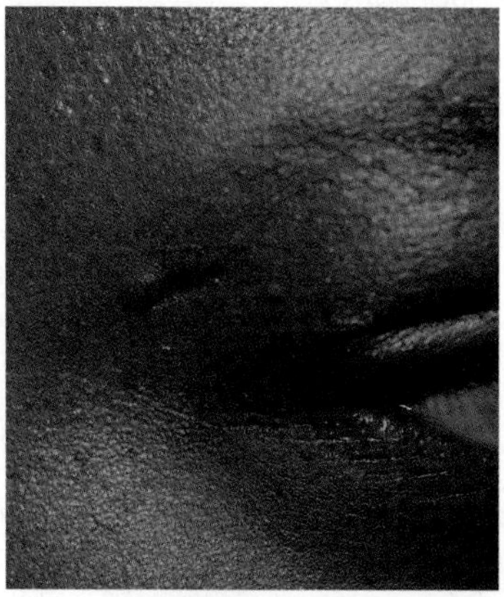

C

Figure 147-17 *The variable presentations of sarcoidosis: (A) papular sarcoid on the face; (B) orange-brown, annular plaque on the trunk; (C) in a scar (Courtesy of Dr. Richard A. Johnson).*

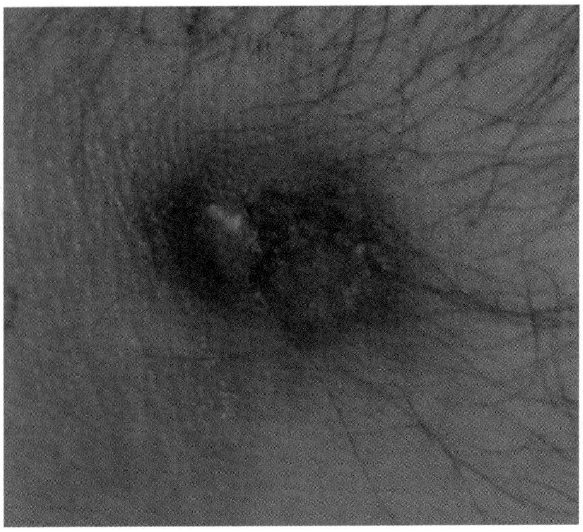

Figure 147-18 *Acute febrile neutrophilic dermatosis (Sweet syndrome). Edematous, violaceous, vesiculated plaques and papulonodules.*

PARANEOPLASTIC CUTANEOUS SIGNS

Sweet syndrome, or acute febrile neutrophilic dermatosis, presents with fever, neutrophilia, and painful red-purple papules, nodules, and plaques that often appear indurated or vesiculated (**Figure 147-18**). It has three main types: classical, malignancy-associated, and drug-induced (**Table 147-12**). Malignancy-associated Sweet syndrome may precede, appear concurrently with, or arise after the patient's cancer diagnosis; it is often associated with hematologic malignancies, especially acute myelogenous leukemia. Sweet syndrome occurs relatively frequently, in comparison with other paraneoplastic phenomenon. Not surprisingly, it is often confused with an infectious process due to the presence of fever, leukocytosis, and tender skin lesions. Pustular lesions may develop in sites of trauma (pathergy). Systemic complications include pulmonary infiltrates, oral ulcers, hepatosplenomegaly, aortitis, glomerulonephritis, sterile osteomyelitis, blepharitis, and conjunctivitis.

Seborrheic keratoses are waxy, wart-like lesions with a stuck-on appearance, sometimes confused for melanoma when they are dark colored. ***The sign of Leser-Trélat***, or the sudden appearance or growth of extensive seborrheic keratoses, has been associated with underlying adenocarcinoma, including colon, breast, stomach, lung, kidney, liver, and pancreas. High levels of epidermal growth factor and other cytokines have been suggested as a possible mechanism. The presence of many such lesions is extremely common in the adult population, and is most often a normal variant. The validity of this association has also been questioned in recent years.

Acanthosis nigricans, focal, symmetric, thickened, velvety plaques in the intertriginous folds of the axillae, groin, posterior neck, and oral mucosa, may occur in conjunction with underlying malignancy. It is most frequently associated with adenocarcinoma of the GI or GU tract, particularly with gastric cancer, though associations with ovarian, endometrial, and lung cancers have also been reported. However, most cases of acanthosis nigricans are not associated with malignancy. Acanthosis nigricans is also associated with obesity and insulin resistance, and may also be seen in patients taking nicotinic acid, corticosteroids, growth hormone, and oral contraceptives. Familial forms also exist.

Tripe palms, a thickened, moss-like covering of the palms resembling the coarse folds of gastric ruggae, are often a paraneoplastic phenomenon. When tripe palms and acanthosis nigricans are observed together, they are associated with gastric cancer; tripe palms occurring in isolation is most often related to underlying lung cancer.

Thickening of pressure-point areas on the soles can be seen in ***Howel-Evans syndrome***. This autosomal-dominant condition results in an acquired, focal keratoderma (thickening of the skin on the palms and soles) and is associated with esophageal cancer. Diffuse thickening of the skin on the palms and soles (acquired palmoplantar keratoderma) has also been observed with lung, breast, renal, and colon carcinoma.

Bazex syndrome, also known as acrokeratosis paraneoplastica, is an acquired keratoderma associated with malignancy, most commonly squamous cell cancer of the head and neck, as well as lung and esophageal cancer. Bazex syndrome has three progressive phases that parallel the course of the tumor. The initial eruption consists of violaceous, ill-defined, thin, slightly scaly papules on acral regions, including the fingers, toes, ears, and nose. Palmoplantar

TABLE 147-12 Sweet Syndrome: Associations, Diagnostic Criteria, and Treatment

Associations	Diagnostic Criteria*	Treatment
Classical • Infection (URI, GI) • Inflammatory bowel disease • Pregnancy • Idiopathic Malignancy-associated • AML and other hematologic malignancies • GU, GI, breast Drug-induced • G-CSF or GM-CSF • All-trans retinoic acid • Antibiotics: trimethoprim-sulfamethoxazole, tetracyclines • OCPs	Major criteria • Abrupt onset of typical skin lesions • Pathology consistent with Sweet syndrome Minor criteria • Preceded by associated infection, vaccination; accompanied by associated malignancy, disorder, or drug • Fever, constitutional signs, and symptoms • Leukocytosis • Response to corticosteroids	Prednisone (1 mg/kg/day, tapered over wks-mos) Potassium iodine (900 mg/day) Colchicine (0.6 mg three times in a day) Dapsone (100–200 mg/day) Indomethacin (150 mg/day × 1 wk, then 100 mg/day) Cyclosporine (2–3 mg/kg/day, tapered over weeks)

*Proposed by Su and Liu in 1986. Diagnosis requires two major and two minor criteria.

keratoderma appears in the second stage, along with spread of the initial lesions. In the third stage, the eruption generalizes, though the acral predominance, violaceous color, and thickened palms and soles predominate.

Paraneoplastic pemphigus (PNP) is characterized by severe mucosal erosions and ulcers as well as variable skin lesions, ranging from lichenoid papules to erythema multiforme-like target lesions and frank blisters. In fact, PNP is often mistaken for severe erythema multiforme Stevens-Johnson syndrome. Common associated malignancies include lymphoma, thymoma, and other lymphoproliferative disorders, such as Castleman disease. Patients with PNP must be followed carefully for involvement of the respiratory tract epithelium, manifesting as a rapidly progressive and potentially fatal form of brochiolitis obliterans with organizing pneumonia.

Generalized redness, swelling, and scaling of the skin is known as ***erythroderma*** (**Figure 147-19**). Though most cases are caused by an underlying skin disease such as psoriasis, seborrheic dermatitis, or ichthyosis, amongst others, 10–15% of cases may be paraneoplastic. Leukemia and lymphoma are common associations, including cutaneous T cell lymphomas. Viral infections such as HIV can also result in erythroderma. Erythema in a serpiginous, figurate pattern may represent a rare entity called ***erythema gyratum repens***. Lesions demonstrate a polycyclic appearance resembling wood-grain. This condition is nearly always associated with a malignancy, particularly underlying lung carcinoma.

Recurrent and migratory thrombophlebitis is known as ***Trosseau syndrome***. Veins on the neck, chest, abdomen, and legs are typically involved, possibly by an underlying coagulopathy. This syndrome is associated with adenocarcinomas with abundant mucin production, such as pancreatic or prostate cancer.

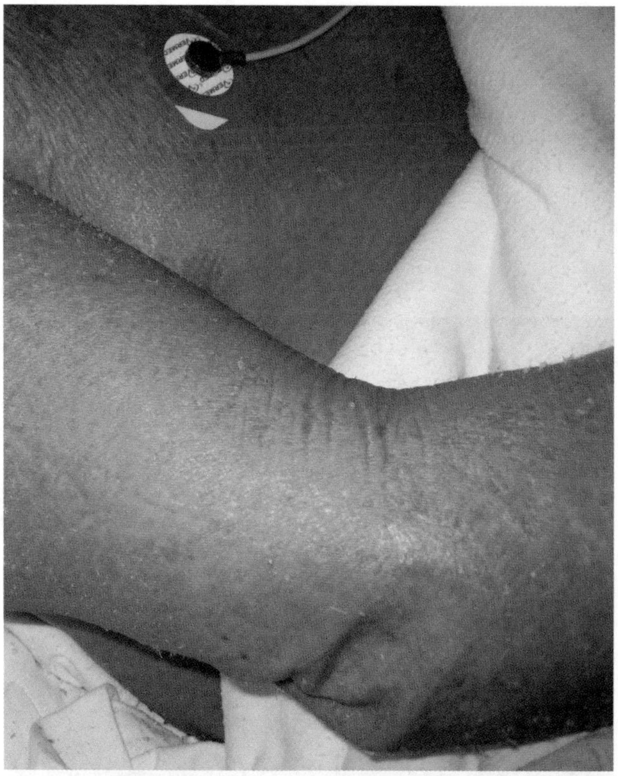

Figure 147-19 *Subacute erythroderma, presenting as full-body redness and scaling. Psoriasis, seborrheic dermatitis, ichthyosis, and other underlying skin diseases, along with medications, HIV, and malignancy can all result in erythroderma.*

TABLE 147-13 Most Common Malignancies Producing Cutaneous Metastases

Women	Men
• Breast	• Lung
• Colon	• Colon
• Melanoma	• Melanoma

METASTATIC DISEASE

Though uncommon, metastases to the skin can be the first sign of malignancy, affording a relatively straightforward opportunity for diagnosis. It may be difficult to discern the origin of a metastatic tumor on physical examination alone. Patient gender may be helpful in suggesting likely sources (**Table 147-13**). Skin lesions are often firm papules, plaques, or nodules. There may be secondary ulceration. Lesions are often violaceous in color, and individual lesions tend to vary in size and shape (**Figure 147-20**). The distribution is usually irregular, but lesions are sometimes found close to the primary tumor. Biopsy and histologic analysis are required for definitive diagnosis.

CUTANEOUS FINDINGS IN LEUKEMIA AND LYMPHOMA

The skin lesions associated with leukemia and lymphoma may also be reactive, or less often, the result of direct skin infiltration with malignant cells. Reactive skin conditions in hematopoietic malignancies include acquired ichthyosis, pruritus, erythroderma, and purpuric lesions. Direct infiltration of the skin with leukemic or lymphomatous cells often presents with skin colored to red or violaceous papules, plaques, nodules, or ulcers (**Figure 147-21A**). Size and distribution is variable, and the lesions often demonstrate a firm or rubbery texture. Rarely, patients may present with friable gingiva, exuberant responses to insect bites, or leukemic cells within cutaneous sites of inflammation such as a recent outbreak of herpes zoster (**Figure 147-21B**). The pathophysiology underlying these clinical presentations is poorly understood.

In acute myelomonocytic or monocytic leukemia, lesions may actually present several months before systemic disease is apparent. This phenomenon, known as aleukemic leukemia cutis, occurs when atypical blast cells appear in the skin prior to evidence of disease within the blood and bone marrow.

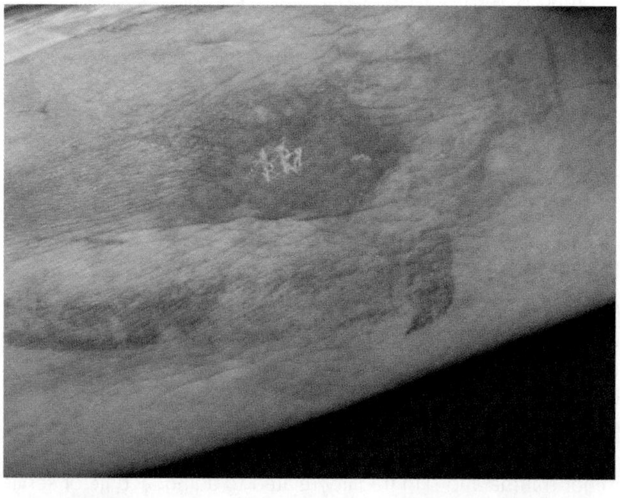

Figure 147-20 *Metastatic breast cancer to the skin. A firm, indurated, violaceous to erythematous plaque on the chest wall. The lesion was asymptomatic.*

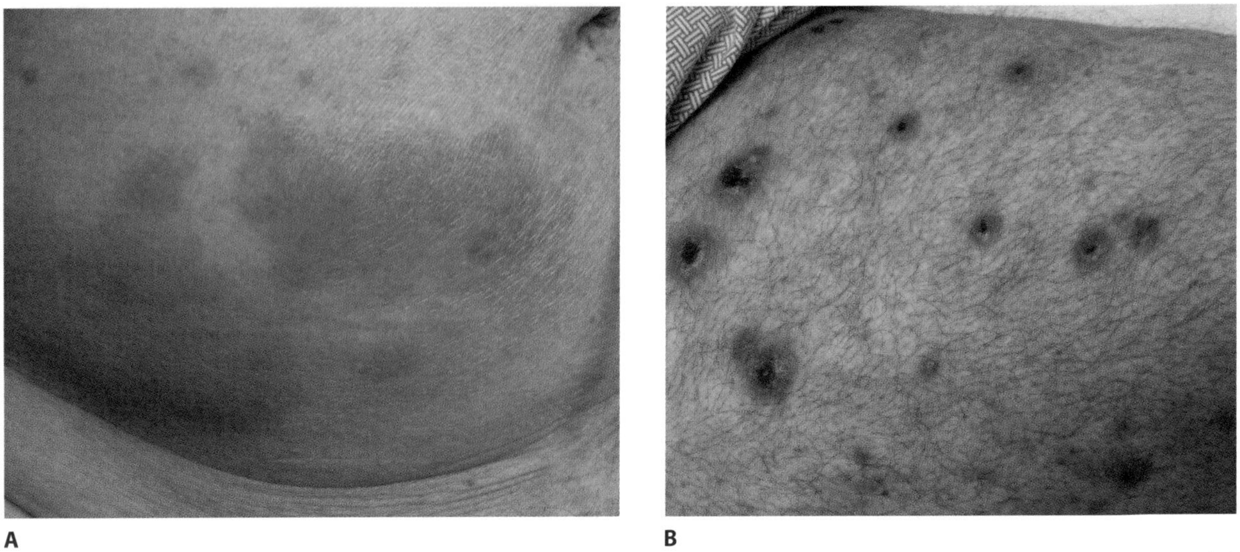

Figure 147-21 *Cutaneous findings in leukemia and lymphoma. (A) Several infiltrated, erythematous papules and plaques in a patient with lymphoma. Skin biopsy confirmed cutaneous involvement of lymphoma and lesions resolved with chemotherapy. (B) Seeding of recently active lesions of herpes zoster (shingles) with leukemic cells in a patient with CLL, producing chronic, violaceous nodules.*

PURPURA

Purpura results from the extravasation of blood into the skin. Clinical manifestations range from nonpalpable purple macules to red-purple papules to large net-like plaques with hemorrhage and blister formation. Older lesions may have a greenish-yellow tinge from hemoglobin breakdown. Purely purpuric lesions are nonblanching, although some purpura may partly blanch due to an associated inflammatory component.

Purpura may arise from intravascular, vascular, or extravascular pathology. Intravascular etiologies include platelet or coagulation hemostatic abnormalities. Vascular causes include inflammatory disorders, such as vasculitis, and noninflammatory conditions such as microvascular occlusion syndromes and thrombosis. Scurvy, corticosteroids, tissue swelling, and trauma are examples of extravascular causes of purpura.

Purpura commonly develops in hospitalized patients, especially with the use of anticoagulation for prevention of deep vein thrombosis. Although purpura may result from incidental trauma, it can also represent the sole manifestation of overwhelming sepsis and thrombosis. The history should ascertain purpura duration, how the lesions began and progressed, distribution, and associated systemic symptoms. The patient's reason for hospital admission, comorbidities, and recent medication history should be reviewed. Physical examination should include a complete cutaneous examination, as well as cardiovascular, pulmonary, abdominal, and neurologic examinations, to determine whether the patient has a systemic illness or disease limited to the skin.

MACULAR PURPURA

Macular purpura is the most common type of purpura, (**Figure 147-22**) presenting as flat, red-purple lesions. Petechiae are the smallest type, presenting as 2–3 mm round purpuric macules. Larger lesions are known as ecchymoses (bruises). The largest and deepest of these lesions are known as hematomas.

Macular purpura in the community is frequently caused by minor trauma and skin fragility related to aging (actinic or senile purpura). Macular purpura in the hospital setting is often related to a bleeding diasthesis, as from therapeutic anticoagulation with heparin or warfarin, disseminated intravascular coagulation, platelet dysfunction from uremia, or drug-induced thrombocytopenia.

Small macular purpuric lesions are not concerning. However, as the macular purpuric lesions become larger or more confluent, the level of concern should increase. ***Purpura fulminans*** is the most aggressive and dangerous form of macular purpuric lesions. Purpura fulminans may begin as small petechial lesions, but rapidly progresses to large ecchymoses, particularly over the extremities and pressure points. The eruption subsequently generalizes with hemorrhagic skin necrosis on the hands, feet, and other acral areas. When this occurs, patients are typically hypotensive, septic, and unstable. Infectious causes of purpura fulminans include meningococcal meningitis, streptococcal or pneumococcal sepsis, or bacteremia of any organism. Noninfectious causes include antiphospholipid antibody syndrome, deficiencies of protein C or protein S, or Factor V Leiden.

Figure 147-22 *Macular purpura: petechiae in a patient on anticoagulant therapy.*

Purpura fulminans can be rapidly fatal. Patients who do survive may require amputation of several digits. Thus, it is imperative to recognize these patients and begin treatment as soon as possible. As soon as the diagnosis is suspected, blood cultures should be performed, and patients should be started on broad spectrum antibiotics and receive aggressive supportive care, including intubation, hemodynamic support, and replacement blood products, if necessary.

PALPABLE PURPURA

These lesions are typically small 0.5–1 cm purpuric papules and plaques that are slightly elevated and firm to the touch (**Figure 147-23**). There is often mild surrounding inflammation. Palpable purpura most commonly results from inflammation of the small vessels of the skin, known as leukocytoclastic vasculitis. In the hospitalized patient, palpable purpura are most often due to a drug hypersensitivity reaction. Common offenders include antibiotics, NSAIDs, thiazides, and allopurinol. Infections are another common cause of palpable purpura, typically bacterial infections or hepatitis B and C. Less common causes of palpable purpura and leukocytoclastic vasculitis include Churg-Strauss syndrome, microscopic polyangiitis, Henoch-Schönlein purpura, and cryoglobulinemia.

Palpable purpura alone requires only symptomatic treatment with topical corticosteroids. However, as palpable purpura implies cutaneous vasculitis, it is important to evaluate for potential systemic vasculitis. Systemic small vessel vasculitis may affect the cardiovascular, renal, gastrointestinal, pulmonary, neurologic, and musculoskeletal systems. Typical systemic manifestations include fever, arthralgias, weakness, shortness of breath, chest pain, abdominal pain, hemoptysis, hematuria, and hematochezia. Patients with systemic vasculitis may require more aggressive treatment with systemic corticosteroids or steroid sparing immunosuppressive agents. Thus, all patients with palpable purpura should be evaluated closely for signs of systemic vasculitis; a careful review of systems, blood pressure evaluation, blood urea nitrogen, creatinine, urinalysis and urine microscopy, and testing for fecal occult blood are warranted.

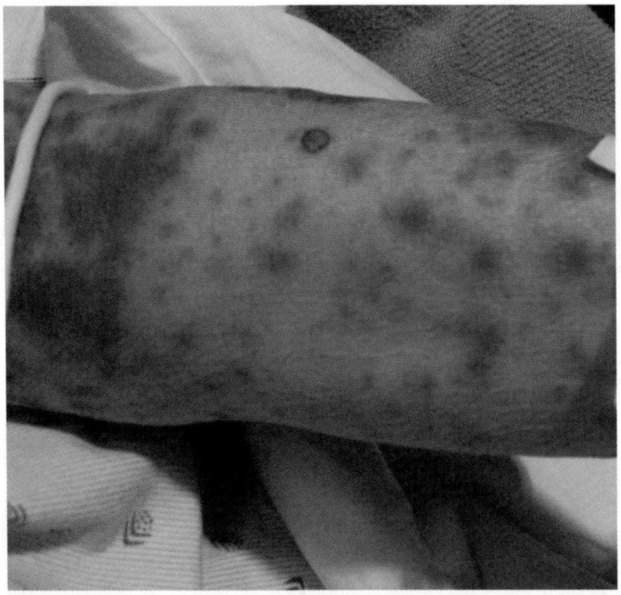

Figure 147-23 *Palpable purpura in a patient with small vessel vasculitis.*

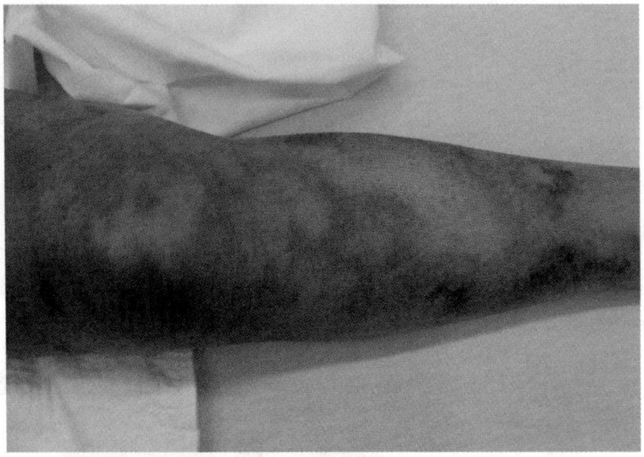

Figure 147-24 *Retiform purpura manifesting as net-like, nonblanchable erythema with minimal surrounding inflammation. This patient presented with Gram-negative sepsis with superficial cutaneous thrombosis.*

RETIFORM PURPURA

Retiform purpura form a net-like pattern of interconnecting blue or purple lines (**Figure 147-24**). Livedo reticularis, a physiologic manifestation of cool skin, appears clinically similar, but is nonpurpuric; the pattern is blanching, and resolves with warming of the skin. Retiform purpura are due to slow blood flow or occlusion of the cutaneous vessels, resulting in localized areas of decreased blood supply to the skin. Frank necrosis of the skin, manifested as a dusky violaceous to gray color, may also be present. Ulcerations often develop in extensive cases, with acral hemorrhage or gangrene being a relatively common clinical manifestation.

Potential pathophysiologic causes include microvascular platelet plugs, such in thrombocytosis or thrombotic thrombocytopenic purpura, cold-related agglutination, as with cryoglobulins, angioinvasive organisms, such as mucormycosis or *Aspergillus*, altered coagulation, as in heparin-induced thrombocytopenia sepsis and coumadin skin necrosis, crystal deposition, such as cholesterol emboli or calciphylaxis, red blood cell occlusion, as in sickle cell anemia, and inflammatory vasculitis, particularly medium vessel vasculitides, such as rheumatoid vasculitis or polyarteritis nodosa, which can also present with nodules and ulcers.

Patients with retiform purpura should be considered extremely ill. Since retiform purpura is a cutaneous manifestation of vascular occlusion, vascular occlusion of internal organs may also be present. These patients may rapidly decompensate and require aggressive supportive measures, including intubation and hemodynamic support. The underlying cause should be identified as quickly as possible to initiate specific therapy (**Figure 147-25**).

WHEN SHOULD AN INPATIENT DERMATOLOGY CONSULTATION BE OBTAINED?

As a general rule, if a patient is admitted for a complex skin condition, such as a diffuse blistering disorder, generalized erythroderma, or a severe cutaneous drug reaction, a dermatology consult should be obtained to facilitate diagnosis and management. Consultation should also be considered in cases that appear to be atypical presentations of an otherwise routine skin condition, such as a refractory or exuberant cellulitis or drug hypersensitivity reaction. Finally, consultation should be obtained early in the course of patients with dermatologic emergencies, such as Stevens-Johnson

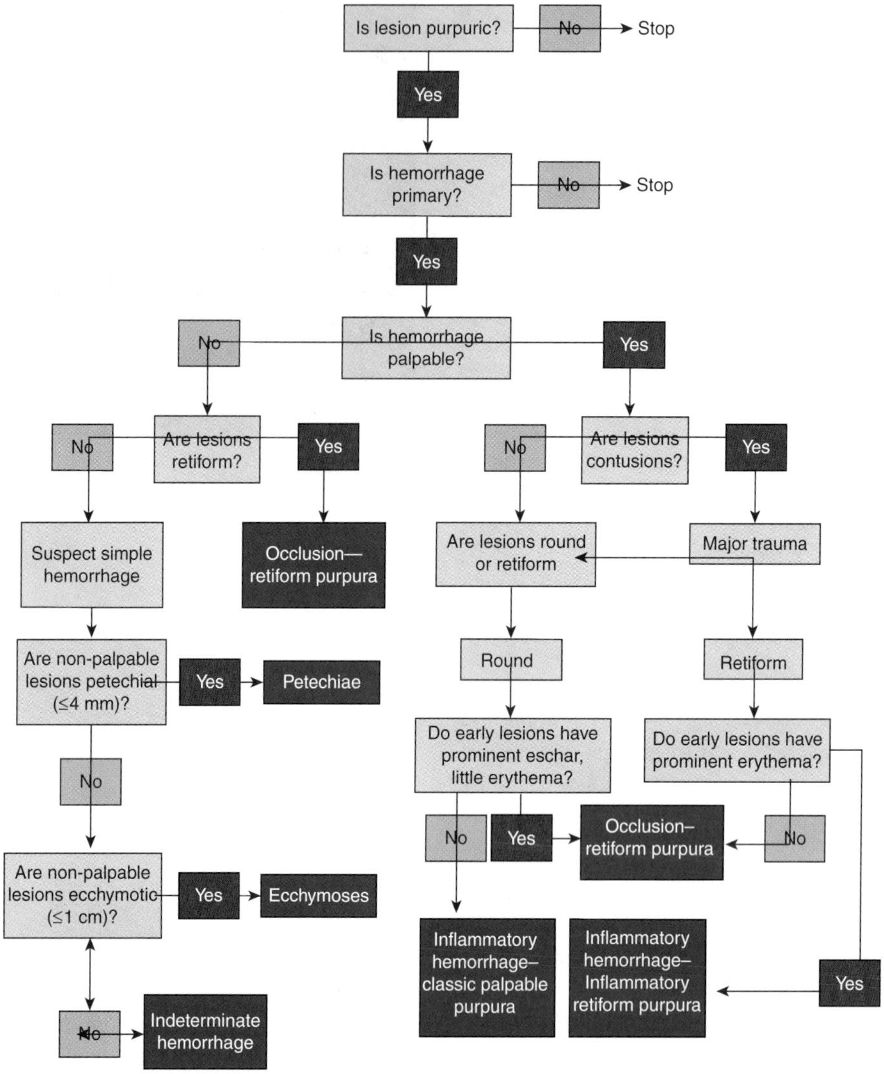

Figure 147-25 *Diagnostic algorithm for purpura. (Reproduced, with permission, from Fauci AS, Braunwald E, Kasper DL, et al. Harrison's Principles of Internal Medicine. 17th ed. New York: McGraw-Hill; 2008. Figure 145-1.)*

syndrome/toxic epidermal necrolysis, bullous graft-versus-host disease, staphylococcal scalded skin syndrome, meningococcemia, and retiform purpura.

Dermatology involvement may help to determine an accurate diagnosis early in a patient's hospital stay and decrease the patient's length of stay. Dermatologists may also maximize the patient's topical and systemic therapy, helping the patient to improve more rapidly. Although inpatient dermatology consults are not readily available at all hospitals, there has been a move to increase access to prompt, high-quality dermatologic care through the establishment of dermatology hospitalist programs at some institutions. Indications for dermatology consultation are summarized in **Table 147-14**.

TABLE 147-14 When Should an Inpatient Dermatology Consult Be Obtained?

- Patient is admitted for a skin disorder.
- Atypical presentation of common condition.
- Common condition not responding to appropriate therapy.
- Diagnostic challenge with cutaneous manifestation.
- Dermatologic emergencies (including Stevens Johnson Syndrome/Toxic Epidermal Necrolysis, bullous graft versus host disease, staphylococcal scalded skin syndrome, meningococcemia, and retiform purpura)
- Prompt diagnosis may result in early discharge.

CONCLUSION

Many common and rare systemic diseases present with cutaneous manifestations. The hospitalist's ability to recognize these skin conditions often provides helpful diagnostic and/or therapeutic clues in approaching the patient's overall care.

SUGGESTED READINGS

Callen JP, Jorizzo JL, Bolognia JL, Piette W, Zone JJ, eds. *Dermatological Signs of Internal Disease.* 4th ed. London, England: Elsevier; 2009.

Chen KR, Carlson JA. Clinical approach to cutaneous vasculitis. *Am J Clin Dermatol.* 2008;9:71–92.

Cohen PR, Kurzrock R. Sweet syndrome revisited: a review of disease concepts. *Int J Dermatol.* 2003;42:761–778.

Costner MI, Grau RH. Update on connective tissue diseases in dermatology. *Semin Cutan Med Surg.* 2006;25:207–220.

Doherty CB, Rosen T. Evidence-based therapy for cutaneous sarcoidosis. *Drugs.* 2008;68:1361–1383.

Dyachenko P, Shustak A, Rozenman D. Hemodialysis-related pruritus and associated cutaneous manifestations. *Int J Dermatol.* 2006;45:664–667.

Robinson-Bostom L, DiGiovanna JJ. Cutaneous manifestations of end-stage renal disease. *J Am Acad Dermatol.* 2000;43:975–986.

Ruocco E, Sangiuliano S, Gravina AG, Miranda A, Nicoletti G. Pyoderma gangrenosum: an updated review. *J Eur Acad Dermatol Venereol.* 2009;23:1008–1017.

Sontheimer RD. Skin manifestations of systemic autoimmune connective tissue disease: diagnostics and therapeutics. *Best Pract Res Clin Rheumatol.* 2004;18:429–462.

Van Hattem S, Bootsma AH, Thio HB. Skin manifestations of diabetes. *Cleve Clin J Med.* 2008;75:772, 774, 776–777.

SECTION 5
Endocrinology

CHAPTER 148

Glycemic Emergencies

Margo S. Hudson, MD
Graham T. McMahon, MD, MMSc

Key Clinical Questions

1. How are diabetic ketoacidosis and hyperosmolar hyperglycemic syndrome diagnosed and treated?
2. How is hypoglycemia treated?
3. What are the causes of hypoglycemia in nondiabetic patients?
4. How is hypoglycemia avoided in the hospital?

INTRODUCTION

Admissions with diabetic ketoacidosis (DKA) as the primary diagnosis have increased over the past 30 years, with 120,000 recorded in the United States in 2005. However, mortality has been reduced to less than 5%. Hyperosmolar hyperglycemic syndrome (HHS) is less common, but it is associated with a mortality of up to 11% because of the greater age and comorbid conditions of the at-risk patient population.

DIABETIC KETOACIDOSIS

PATHOPHYSIOLOGY

DKA arises in patients with absolute or severe insulin deficiency. The resulting hyperglycemia combined with an increase in counter-regulatory hormones, including glucagon, catecholamines, cortisol, and growth hormone, precipitate proteolysis and lipolysis. Lipolysis causes the accumulation of acidic ketones, and hyperglycemia leads to osmotic diuresis and electrolyte loss, precipitating the characteristic metabolic acidosis and severe dehydration.

SYMPTOMS AND SIGNS

Symptoms of DKA generally develop over a short period of time and include polyuria, polydipsia, and weight loss. Abdominal pain and vomiting are common with acidosis, and must be distinguished from an acute abdomen. Decreased mentation and deep, labored Kussmaul respirations are advanced findings. Symptoms and signs of intercurrent illness should be sought. Leukocytosis and hyperamylasemia are often detectable at presentation and normalize with treatment.

DIAGNOSIS

A recent consensus statement has clarified diagnostic criteria for DKA (**Table 148-1**). Five laboratory conditions are typically present: plasma glucose greater than 250 mg/dl (13.9 mmol/L), anion gap of greater than 10 mEq/L, the presence of ketonuria or ketonemia, serum bicarbonate below 18 mEq/L, and arterial pH less than 7.30. DKA is graded as mild, moderate, or severe, with increasing severity associated with lower pH and deterioration in mental status. Arterial blood gas measurement should be obtained at the outset; measurements of venous blood pH can be used to track the resolution of the acidosis thereafter.

As 3-beta-hydroxybutyrate is the most abundant ketone in the early stages of DKA, but is not measured in the nitroprusside assay for ketones, assessment should also include direct measurement of 3-beta-hydroxybutyrate when available; a level over 3 mmol/liter is considered clinically significant. Although a glucose of at least 250 mg/dl is included among the diagnostic criteria, patients who are pregnant or who have a high glomerular filtration rate can be in DKA at glucose levels under this threshold.

PRECIPITANTS

Precipitating factors fall into two categories: lack of insulin or development of another illness. Approximately one-quarter of DKA admissions occur at the onset of diabetes. Although type 1 diabetes accounts for the majority of these initial presentations, as many as half of adult African Americans and Hispanics with new-onset diabetes presenting in DKA may actually have

TABLE 148-1 Diagnostic Criteria for DKA and HHS

Diagnostic Criteria and Classification	DKA			
	Mild	Moderate	Severe	HHS
Plasma glucose (mg/dl)	> 250	> 250	> 250	> 600
Arterial pH	7.25–7.30	7.00 to < 7.25	< 7.00	> 7.3
Serum bicarbonate (mEq/l)	15–18	10 to < 15	< 10	> 15
Urine ketone	Positive	Positive	Positive	Small
Serum ketone*	Positive	Positive	Positive	Small
Effective serum osmolality (mOsm/l)	Variable	Variable	Variable	> 320
Anion gap (mEq/l)	> 10	> 12	> 12	< 12
Mental status	Alert	Alert/ drowsy	Stupor/ Coma	Variable

Adapted, with permission, from Kitabchi AE, Umpierrez GE, Murphy MB, et al. Hyperglycemic crises in adult patients with diabetes: a consensus statement from the American Diabetes Association. *Diabetes Care.* 2009; 32:1335–1343.

Anion gap = $Na - (C1 + HCO_3)$.

*β hydroxy-butyrate is preferred with value > 3 mmol/liter significant.

type 2 diabetes, and ultimately may be able to discontinue insulin therapy. In the patient with a prior history of diabetes, poor adherence to insulin is the most common precipitating factor, particularly in adolescence. Technical problems with pumps, improper storage of insulin, or psychological or cognitive disorders should also be considered.

Among intercurrent illnesses, infection is a particularly common precipitating factor and must be assiduously excluded. Other causes include myocardial infarction, stroke, pancreatitis, and medications such as glucocorticoids and antipsychotic medicines.

DIFFERENTIAL DIAGNOSIS

DKA is not the only cause of an anion gap acidosis. Differential diagnoses include alcoholic ketoacidosis, starvation ketosis, severe chronic renal failure, lactic acidosis, and toxic ingestions such as salicylate, methanol, ethylene glycol, and paraldehyde.

TREATMENT

Treatment of diabetic ketoacidosis should simultaneously address each of the components that contribute to the syndrome: dehydration, hyperglycemia, electrolyte loss, and acidosis. A stepwise approach can facilitate management of these patients (**Figure 148-1**). Most patients with DKA are managed initially in critical care units, but local experience may facilitate management in a monitored general unit.

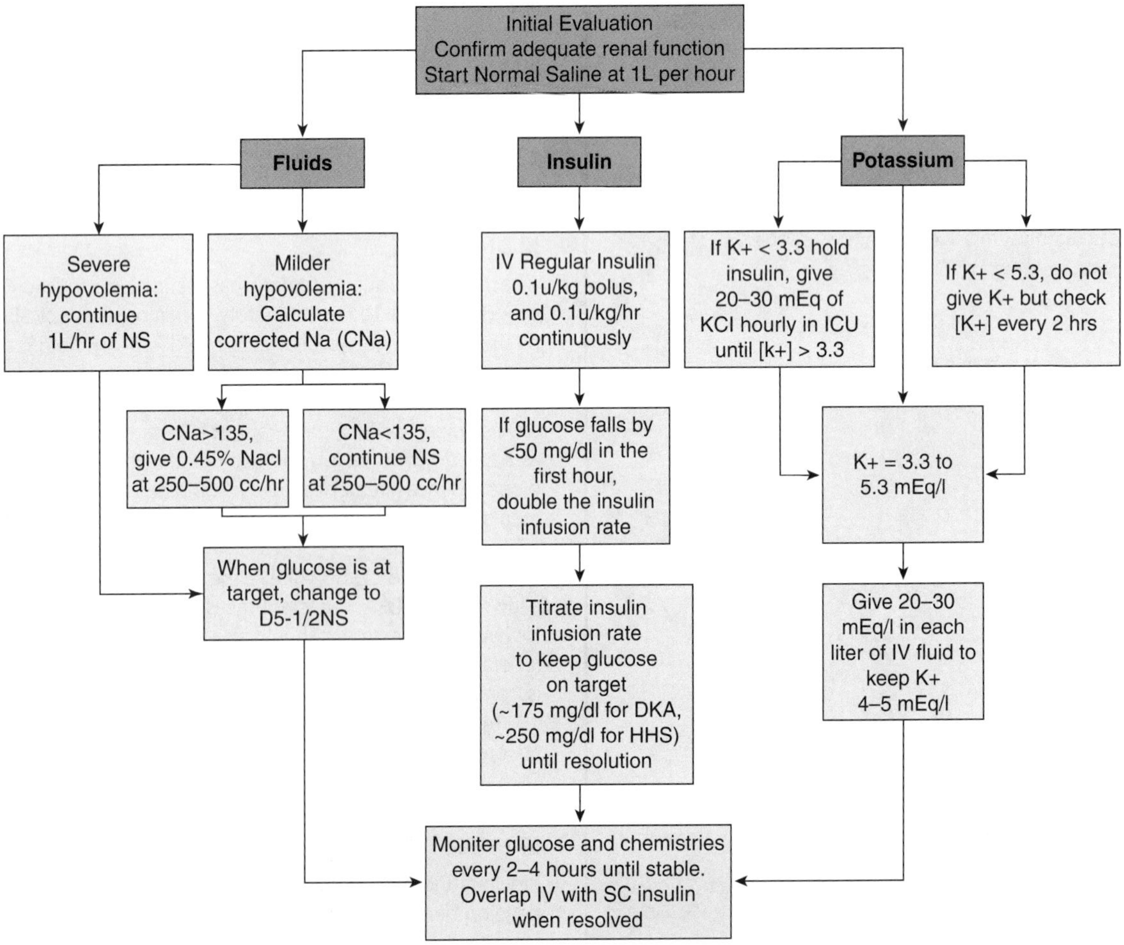

Figure 148-1 *Flowchart for the management of DKA and HHS. (Adapted, with permission, from Kitabchi AE, Umpierrez GE, Murphy MB, et al. Hyperglycemic crises in adult patients with diabetes: a consensus statement from the American Diabetes Association. Diabetes Care. 2009;32:1335–1343.)*

TABLE 148-2 Estimating Water and Electrolyte Deficits in DKA and HHS

Calculation	Equation	Normal Range
Corrected Na (CNa)	Na (in mEq/L) + .016 (glucose [in mg/dl] - 100)	135–145 mEq/L
Effective osmolarity	$2\ Na(mEq/L) + \frac{glucose\ (mg/dl)}{18}$	280–290 mOsm/L
Water deficit	0.6 (wt in kg) ([CNa-140]/140)	<0.5 L

Fluid replacement

Patients with diabetic ketoacidosis are invariably dehydrated. Initial fluid resuscitation in the average adult without cardiac dysfunction should be 1 liter of 0.9% sodium chloride, infused over one hour. Subsequent fluid replacement will depend on the degree of dehydration and corrected sodium level. Equations that are helpful in guiding therapy are presented in **Table 148-2**.

After the first liter of normal saline is infused, hypotonic fluids are appropriate if either corrected sodium level or serum osmolarity are elevated. Typical total body water deficit in DKA in adults is 6 liters, which should be replaced in the first 24 to 36 hours. Once serum glucose falls to between 200 and 250 mg/dl (11.1–13.9 mmol/L), dextrose should be added to the intravenous fluids to maintain glucose between 150 and 200 mg/dl (8.3–11.1 mmol/L).

Insulin

Intravenous insulin therapy is the standard of care for the management of hyperglycemia in DKA, although subcutaneous insulin algorithms have been used successfully in some patients with mild and uncomplicated DKA. The goal of intravenous insulin therapy is to lower serum glucose by approximately 50 to 70 mg/dl (2.8–4.2 mmol/L) per hour. This is usually accomplished with a 0.1 U/kg intravenous bolus of regular insulin, followed by a 0.1 U /kg/hr insulin infusion, with the drip rate adjusted as needed to achieve the desired decrease in glucose. A bolus dose of insulin may not be necessary with an infusion rate of 0.14 U/kg/hr.

Intravenous insulin should be continued until ketoacidosis has resolved. The current American Diabetes Association consensus criteria suggest that the patient can be transitioned to subcutaneous insulin when the glucose is below 200 mg/dl (11.1 mmol/L), the serum bicarbonate is greater than 18 mEq/L, and the venous pH is greater than 7.30. In addition, intravenous insulin should not be stopped prior to normalization of the anion gap. Urinary ketosis may remain detectable after clearance of serum ketones, and therefore is an unreliable indicator for resolution of the acidosis.

Once DKA has resolved, intravenous insulin should be continued for two to four hours after the first subcutaneous dose of basal and rapid-acting insulin; premature discontinuation of the insulin infusion is the most common reason for recurrence of DKA in the hospitalized patient. Subcutaneous insulin must be dosed to ensure that both basal needs and prandial needs are met when the patient resumes eating. A well-established outpatient insulin dose can be used to determine the insulin replacement strategy in patients with known diabetes. Patients new to insulin can be started on a weight-based dose of 0.5–0.6 U/kg/day, divided into 0.25 U/kg/day of long-acting insulin for basal requirements and 0.1 U/kg of a rapid-acting insulin before meals.

Potassium

Acidosis tends to raise serum potassium, even when total body potassium stores are depleted. Intravenous insulin, fluid replacement, and correction of acidosis lower serum potassium and can precipitate serious hypokalemia. In the absence of hyperkalemia, between 20 and 30 mEq of potassium should be added to each liter of intravenous fluids during treatment of DKA. Intravenous insulin treatment in a patient who is hypokalemic can be dangerous, so if it is less than 3.3 mEq/L at the initial evaluation, potassium should be administered through a central line and the patient should be monitored in the intensive care unit Adequate renal function should be established prior to starting potassium replacement.

Bicarbonate

Bicarbonate is not recommended for the management of acidosis in patients with DKA as long as the initial pH is greater than 7.0, as it may provoke hypokalemia in adults and cerebral edema in children. Judicious use of bicarbonate may be helpful for patients whose pH is less than 7.0.

Phosphate

Serum phosphate may be normal or high at the time of presentation of DKA, despite total body phosphate deficits. Serum phosphate falls rapidly with treatment. Aggressive phosphate replacement in DKA is generally not recommended, because of concerns of precipitating hypocalcemia and an absence of proven efficacy. If phosphate is below 1 mg/dL, it can be replaced in intravenous fluids as potassium or sodium phosphate at a dose of 20–30 meq infused over 6–12 hours. When the patient is eating and drinking again, milk is an excellent source of phosphate.

COMPLICATIONS

Cerebral edema is the most feared complication of DKA treatment. It is extremely rare in adults, but occurs in up to 1% of episodes in children and is associated with a high mortality in this group. A high rate of initial fluid resuscitation or bicarbonate therapy has been associated with cerebral edema, but its etiology has not been clearly determined. Treatment with intravenous mannitol is recommended if cerebral edema develops, but outcomes are often poor.

PREVENTION

Patients should be educated about the dangers of insulin omission and guidelines for insulin adjustment during illness. In the hospitalized patient, diabetic ketoacidosis is preventable with adequate monitoring and should never occur *de novo*. DKA can develop in hospitalized patients with diabetes if glucose levels are not monitored, or when only correctional (sliding scale) insulin is prescribed, omitting basal insulin from the patient's regimen.

HYPEROSMOLAR HYPERGLYCEMIC STATE

PATHOPHYSIOLOGY

Though DKA and hyperosmolar hyperglycemia (HHS) exist on a hyperglycemic continuum, HHS is associated with more severe hyperosmolarity and is not associated with acidosis or ketosis. Diagnostic criteria are listed in Table 148-1. HHS tends to occur in older patients and is not seen in patients with type 1 diabetes. This may be because patients who develop HHS retain some insulin production and can suppress ketogenesis, and are therefore less prone to become acidotic.

CLINICAL PRESENTATION

Most patients present with a several days to weeks of increasing polyuria and polydipsia, with the gradual onset of mental status changes. Patients often have additional factors that contribute to the inability to maintain hydration, such as diuretic therapy or poor functional status. Patients with severe metabolic changes can present with obtundation, seizures, and hemiparesis or other focal neurological findings. On presentation, patients are severely dehydrated, frequently hypotensive, and may have hyperthermia or hypothermia.

PRECIPITANTS

Intercurrent illness, especially infection, is the most common precipitating event of HHS. Other causes can include myocardial ischemia, stroke, pancreatitis, corticosteroid use, and initiation of diuretics.

TREATMENT

A stepwise approach to the treatment of HHS is outlined in Figure 148-1. Rehydration is the mainstay of management.

Fluids

Fluid resuscitation is the most important and urgent treatment modality, but must be managed carefully. The effective osmolarity and the total body water deficit should be calculated using the corrected sodium (Table 148-2). In the absence of cardiac decompensation, the initial therapy will generally be one liter of normal sodium chloride over one hour. Normal saline is used since it is hypotonic to the patient's serum when profound dehydration is present. The remaining calculated fluid deficit should be replaced over 24 to 36 hours. Typical fluid deficits are as high as nine liters. The serum osmolarity should be corrected gradually, as rapid correction has been associated with slower neurologic recovery.

Insulin

Subcutaneous insulin is not appropriate for patients with HHS because poor tissue perfusion limits the absorption of insulin from the skin. Intravenous insulin is recommended, using a similar protocol to that used in DKA. Once the serum glucose falls to below 300 mg/dl (16.7 mmol/L), dextrose infusion should be initiated, with a target glucose of between 250 and 300 mg/dl (13.9–16.7 mmol/L), until mental status and serum osmolarity have normalized.

Potassium

Potassium should be replaced carefully in HHS, since these patients have more significant renal insufficiency than in DKA, and potassium may accumulate.

HYPOGLYCEMIA IN HOSPITALIZED PATIENTS

Hypoglycemia is relatively common among hospitalized patients, and is almost always a complication of the treatment of diabetes mellitus. However, hypoglycemia can also be the presenting feature of an underlying disease. True spontaneous hypoglycemia is likely only when Whipple triad is present. This triad is comprised of: (1) typical hypoglycemic symptoms, (2) low measured plasma glucose, and (3) reversal of symptoms with restoration of normal glucose levels. A plasma value for glucose lower than 55 mg/dl (3.1 mmol/L) is generally needed for diagnosis. However, because some people normally have glucose levels below this cut-off and laboratory errors are possible, it is important that the other components of Whipple triad be present before initiating an evaluation.

Hypoglycemia symptoms are due to either autonomic activation or neuroglycopenia. Autonomic symptoms due to sympathetic and parasympathetic activation, including palpitations, tremors, sweating and hunger, appear as the plasma glucose falls below 65 mg/dl (3.6 mmol/L). Neuroglycopenic symptoms such as behavioral changes, obtundation, focal neurologic deficits, seizures, and ultimately coma emerge as the glucose falls below 40 mg/dl (2.2 mmol/L). Patients with frequent hypoglycemia, with or without underlying diabetes, may develop hypoglycemia unawareness, and have attenuated or absent autonomic symptoms, leaving them more vulnerable to develop severe neuroglycopenia. Many hospitalized patients have significant baseline neurologic or autonomic impairment, and may be unable to manifest the typical symptoms other than seizure or coma. Consequently, caregivers must be vigilant to recognize hypoglycemia in the hospitalized patient, particularly if consciousness is blunted. Diabetic patients with longstanding poor glycemic control may also develop symptoms of hypoglycemia at higher glucose levels than normal persons, because of alterations in cerebral glucose transport.

Glucose values are usually measured in the hospital using point-of-care testing devices that are not as precise as laboratory measures. Although 95% of values obtained on a glucometer are within 20% of the laboratory measured value, only 69% are within 10% at values below 70 mg/dl. Therefore, when unexpected hypoglycemia is noted at the bedside, the findings should be confirmed in the laboratory. When accurate measurement is critical, the blood glucose should be sent to the laboratory in a tube with an inhibitor of glycolysis, and the plasma separated from formed blood elements as quickly as possible.

EVALUATION AND TREATMENT OF HYPOGLYCEMIA IN PATIENTS WITHOUT DIABETES

CLINICAL PRESENTATION

Hypoglycemia should be evaluated in patients who fulfill Whipple triad. If hypoglycemia is recurrent, expeditious evaluation is imperative. To avoid misinterpretation, diagnostic testing must be performed during a hypoglycemic episode, which may need to be provoked by fasting. Precipitants of hypoglycemia, timing of the hypoglycemia in relation to fasting or food intake, and the patient's overall condition can be helpful clues to establishing the diagnosis, as discussed below.

CAUSES OF HYPOGLYCEMIA

The causes of hypoglycemia can be divided into two categories: those associated with high insulin levels and those associated with suppressed insulin levels (**Table 148-3**). An excess of endogenous insulin can cause hypoglycemia even in the presence of a robust counter-regulatory hormone response. Insulinomas are rare, with an incidence of 4 cases per 1 million patient-years. These islet cell tumors usually occur sporadically but can be associated with multiple endocrine neoplasia syndromes. Fasting hypoglycemia is the most common presentation, but some patients present exclusively with postprandial hypoglycemia. Postprandial hypoglycemia is the most common presentation of two recently described conditions featuring diffuse islet cell hypertrophy, noninsulinoma pancreatogenous hypoglycemia, and postgastric bypass hypoglycemia.

Glyburide, glipizide, and other sulfonylurea medications, as well as meglitinides, boost endogenous insulin secretion. Repaglinide appears to be the only available member of the meglitinide class that causes significant hypoglycemia. Surreptitious use of any of these drugs can present with typical manifestations of insulinoma. Some genetic defects can cause hyperinsulinemic hypoglycemia, but these are rare and usually present early in life. Rarely, antibodies to insulin or the insulin receptor may lead to fluctuations in serum insulin levels and hypoglycemia in nondiabetic patients who typically have other autoimmune diseases. Surreptitious insulin injection

TABLE 148-3 Causes of Hypoglycemia

I. Insulinmediated
   A. Insulinoma
   B. Noninsulinoma pancreatogenous hypoglycemia
   C. Postgastric bypass hypoglycemia
   D. Oral diabetes secretagogue medications
      1. Glyburide
      2. Glipizide
      3. Gimepiride
      4. Gliclazide
      5. Repaglinide
   E. Genetic mutations
   F. Antibody-mediated
   G. Exogenous insulin (factitious or malicious)
II. Noninsulin mediated
   A. Critical illness
      1. Hepatic, renal, cardiac failure
      2. Sepsis
      3. Inanition/malnutrition
   B. Adrenal insufficiency
   C. Nonislet cell tumor
   D. Toxins
      1. Alcohol
      2. Salicylate excess
      3. Hypoglycin

must always be considered as a cause of cryptic hypoglycemia with elevated insulin levels.

Noninsulin-mediated hypoglycemia may develop during critical or chronic illness. Severe protein and calorie malnutrition in the hospital setting impairs the ability to maintain normal glycogen stores, increasing susceptibility to hypoglycemia. Hepatic and renal insufficiency decrease gluconeogenesis and glycogenolysis. Patients with sepsis are particularly prone to hypoglycemia, and its presence in infection is associated with increased mortality. Hypoglycemia in heart failure is usually related to secondary hepatic dysfunction. Adrenal insufficiency, either primary or secondary to hypopituitarism, is only rarely a cause of hypoglycemia, but it should be considered in the appropriate clinical context.

Nonislet tumors producing insulin-like growth factor 2 (IGF-2) may cause hypoglycemia. Although IGF-2 has its own receptor, it can bind to the insulin receptor and have insulin-like effects. Tumors producing IGF-2 tend to be bulky and intraabdominal or retroperitoneal, and include sarcomas, hepatomas, lymphomas, and teratomas. They produce a precursor form of IGF-2 ("big" IGF-2). This form is not measured by conventional assays but is implied by suppressed levels of insulin, growth hormone, and IGF-1. IGF-1 secreting tumors leading to hypoglycemia have also been described.

Toxins should be considered in the evaluation of the hypoglycemic patient. Ethanol inhibits hepatic gluconeogenesis and suppresses the release of counter-regulatory hormones. Hypoglycemia is especially common in poorly nourished alcoholics. Salicylates in high doses also suppress hepatic glucose output. Excess consumption of Jamaican ackee fruit can cause hypoglycemia; the fruit contains the compound hypoglycin, which interferes with hepatic gluconeogenesis. A variety of medications (**Table 148-4**) have been

TABLE 148-4 Drugs Associated with Hypoglycemia with Moderate Confidence

Cibenzoline
Glucagon
Fluoroquinolones
IGF-1
Indomethacin
Lithium
Octreotide
Pentamidine
Propoxyphene/dextropropoxyphene
Quinine
Sulfonamides

Data from Murad MH, Coto-Yglesias F, Wang AT, et al. Drug-induced hypoglycemia: a systematic review. *J Clin Endocrinol Metab.* 2009;94:741–745.

reported to cause hypoglycemia, with variable reliability of evidence. Pentamidine, quinine, fluoroquinolones, glucagon, and rarely sulfonamides may lead to hypoglycemia by enhancing endogenous insulin release. Mechanisms of hypoglycemia for other listed drugs are diverse, if known, or uncertain.

DIAGNOSTIC TESTING

Initial investigation of the patient with confirmed hypoglycemia should include tests of hepatic and renal function and a complete blood count. Biochemical testing comprising levels of insulin, C-peptide level, beta-hydroxy-butyrate, and cortisol should be obtained when the patient is symptomatic and the serum glucose is less than 55 mg/dl (3.1 mmol/L). Screening for sulfonylureas, meglitinides, alcohol, and salicylates should be considered. While "big" IGF-2 cannot be measured, growth hormone, IGF-1, and native IGF-2 can be obtained if a nonislet cell malignancy is suspected. Insulin antibodies can be measured if an autoimmune disease is suspected and the patient has not been previously treated with insulin.

Beta-hydroxybutyrate levels are generally low (less than 2.7 mmol/L) when the cause of the hypoglycemia is insulin-mediated, as insulin suppresses lipolysis. This test is rapidly available, and can incriminate insulin as the etiology before other laboratory results return. Because high levels of insulin generally suppress glycogenolysis, an increase in the glucose level of more than 25 mg/dl (1.4 mmol/L) after administration of 1 mg of glucagon intravenously while hypoglycemic can also be used as an indicator of hyperinsulinemia. If hypoglycemia does not occur spontaneously, either a monitored fast of up to 72 hours until hypoglycemia develops or a mixed meal challenge can be used to induce hypoglycemia and obtain necessary samples. **Table 148-5** outlines expected results in various hypoglycemic disorders.

TREATMENT

Normoglycemia should be maintained until definitive treatment for the underlying diagnosis can be initiated. Normoglycemia can usually be accomplished with an initial dose of 25 grams of glucose given intravenously, followed by a constant infusion of 5% or 10% dextrose in water. Symptoms generally resolve within 15–20 minutes after the glucose level normalizes. The time to recovery can be prolonged if the patient has had a recent seizure or is comatose. If endogenous insulin is felt to be the cause of hypoglycemia and

TABLE 148-5 Differential Diagnosis of Hypoglycemic Disorders

	Insulinoma	Sulfonylurea (SU)	Exogenous Insulin	NIPH/Gastric Bypass	IGF-2	Insulin Ab or Insulin-receptor Ab	Cortisol Deficiency
Insulin (high when > 3 μU/ml)	↑	↑	↑	↑	↓	↑	↓
C-peptide (high when > 0.2 nmol/l)	↑	↑	↓	↑	↓	*	↓
Beta-hydroxy-butyrate (high when > 2.7 mmol/l)	↓	↓	↓	↓	↓	↓	↑
Cortisol (suggestive if < 15 μg/dl when hypoglycemic)	↑	↑	↑	↑	↑	↑	↓
Sulfonulylurea/meglitinide screen	–	++	–	–	–	–	–
IGF-2 associated findings†	–	–	–	–	++	–	–
Insulin antibody	–	–	+/–	–	–	++	–

*Free-C-peptide reported to be low.
†See text.
Data from Cryer PE, Axelrod L, Grossman AB, et al. Evaluation and management of adult hypoglycemic disorders: an Endocrine Society Clinical Practice Guideline. *J Clin Endocrinol Metab.* 2009;94:709–728.

intravenous dextrose is not sufficient for maintaining normoglycemia, octreotide or diazoxide therapy can be initiated.

HYPOGLYCEMIA IN DIABETIC PATIENTS IN THE AMBULATORY SETTING

EPIDEMIOLOGY

Improved glucose control has been associated with reductions in diabetes-related morbidity and mortality. However, tight glucose control is generally associated with an increased incidence of hypoglycemia, which can sometimes be severe and dangerous. Severe hypoglycemia is variably defined, but any episode requiring assistance of another person generally qualifies. The rate of severe hypoglycemic episodes is approximately 115 and 35 events per 1000 outpatients per year with type 1 and type 2 diabetes, respectively. Among inpatients, hypoglycemia is generally defined as any glucose level below 70 mg/dl (3.9 mmol/L) and severe hypoglycemia as any confirmed glucose level below 40 mg/dl (2.2 mmol/L). Patients with either type 1 or type 2 diabetes, particularly those with autonomic insufficiency, can develop hypoglycemia unawareness and may be especially susceptible to severe hypoglycemia.

CONSEQUENCES

Acute effects of hypoglycemia are primarily neurologic and have been previously discussed. However, acute hypoglycemia may also predispose to a prolonged QTc interval and precipitate major cardiovascular events. Long-term effects on cognitive function of recurrent hypoglycemia are unclear at this time, with some studies showing no significant effects and others demonstrating neurologic sequelae.

SIGNS AND SYMPTOMS

When hypoglycemic symptoms and signs are typical, the diagnosis is generally straightforward, given the wide availability of point-of-care testing. Nevertheless, diabetic patients with any change in neurologic status should have their glucose measurement checked, given the broad spectrum of neuroglycopenic symptoms.

CAUSES

Hypoglycemia develops in diabetic patients because of a mismatch between insulin (either injected or endogenously produced with the aid of a secretagogue) and carbohydrate availability. Accidental or intentional overdose of medications, deterioration in renal function, exercise, and a missed or delayed meal are common precipitants of hypoglycemia in the community. Alcohol ingestion suppresses hepatic glucose output such that oral hypoglycemic drugs in conjunction with alcohol can cause severe and prolonged hypoglycemia. This is particularly the case with metformin, which usually will not cause hypoglycemia independently.

TREATMENT

Initial treatment is 15–20 grams of carbohydrate orally, such as 4 oz (120 mL) of juice or full-calorie soda, or 8 oz (240 mL) of nonfat milk. If the patient cannot take oral glucose, it should be given as an intravenous bolus of 25 g of dextrose 50% in water. In the absence of a functioning intravenous line, 1 mg of glucagon can be administered intramuscularly, although this may induce emesis. Glucose should be rechecked in 15–20 minutes and the treatment repeated if necessary.

PRACTICE POINT

- Factitious, or self-induced, hypoglycemia should be considered in all patients with unexplained hypoglycemia. Patients are more likely to be female, have a health care background, and have psychiatric comorbidities. In patients without diabetes, clinicians should attempt to determine if the patient has access to hypoglycemic drugs through work, friends, or family members. Patients with factitious hypoglycemia due to insulin injection will have a suppressed C-peptide, indicative of the exogenous origin of circulating insulin, sometimes with very high serum insulin levels, in contrast to the slightly high or inappropriately normal insulin levels typical of patients with hypoglycemia from insulinoma. Patients should be screened for sulfonylurea and meglitinide use as well. It should be born in mind that medication-induced hypoglycemia may be accidental, as in the older patient who mistakenly uses a spouse's pill bottle that resembles his or her own. Outbreaks of hypoglycemia due to the use of counterfeit medications have also occurred, such as sexual enhancement products contaminated with sulfonylureas.

Medication-induced hypoglycemia can result in prolonged and recurrent hypoglycemic episodes. The duration of action of the responsible medication can be used to determine the required duration of monitoring. Many sulfonylureas have a duration of action close to 24 hours. The duration of action of insulin varies by formulation, but is prolonged with higher doses, intentional overdose, and renal failure. Since many types of insulin are transparent, patients may not correctly recall which insulin was administered in error, so clinicians should be cautious in prematurely discharging patients with insulin-induced hypoglycemia.

Prevention of future episodes necessitates an understanding of the underlying cause of the precipitating episode. Medication adjustment, adequate glucose monitoring, and patient education are all important. A glucagon emergency kit should be prescribed to patients at risk for recurrence.

HYPOGLYCEMIA IN THE HOSPITALIZED PATIENT WITH DIABETES

HYPOGLYCEMIA IN THE INTENSIVE CARE UNIT

The association of hyperglycemia with poor inpatient outcomes has prompted more aggressive management of glucose in patients with known diabetes and those with new-onset hyperglycemia. Maintaining glucose in the normal range during critical illness has been associated with reductions in morbidity and mortality in some studies, and has resulted in widespread use of intravenous insulin administered using titration protocols. However, tighter control of glucose in critically ill patients results in an increased incidence of hypoglycemia, with 6–17% of patients experiencing at least one glucose value below 40 mg/dl (2.2 mmol/L). Concerns about the effect of hypoglycemia on patient outcomes have led to recommendations to change the glucose range for critically ill patients to between 140–180 mg/dl (7.8–10 mmol/L). Increasing the familiarity of staff with the chosen intravenous insulin protocol and frequent monitoring appear to offer protection from hypoglycemia.

HYPOGLYCEMIA IN THE NON-ICU PATIENT

Oral agents are cumbersome to adjust and potentially dangerous in the hospital setting and generally should be stopped on admission. Subcutaneously administered insulin is the preferred medication for management of hyperglycemia in the non–critically ill hospitalized patient. Insulin is among the top 10 drugs causing preventable adverse drug events during hospitalization; some 69% of inpatient hypoglycemia events are preventable. Many situations that lead to insulin-induced hypoglycemia can be anticipated. Careful attention to glucose testing, timing of insulin delivery, and synchrony with meals can play an important role in the prevention of hypoglycemia. Hypoglycemia in non-ICU patients with diabetes has recently been associated with higher inpatient mortality, as well as mortality at one year post discharge, highlighting the need for prevention.

TREATMENT OF HYPOGLYCEMIA IN THE HOSPITAL

Both ambulatory and inpatient areas of the hospital should have protocols in place to deal with hypoglycemia. Caregivers must be able to act quickly and independently to restore normoglycemia. Initial response is as outlined above. To avoid repeat episodes, patients should be assessed regarding the need for an intravenous glucose infusion after initial stabilization.

PREVENTION OF HYPOGLYCEMIA IN HOSPITALIZED PATIENTS

To avoid unnecessary hypoglycemia, insulin is optimally dosed in three components, including basal insulin, prandial insulin (for the patient taking meals), and correctional (often called sliding scale) insulin. A combination of these three elements can achieve more stable glucose levels during hospitalization than sliding scale insulin alone. Initial dosing of insulin in the hospitalized patient can be difficult because of many changing factors that contribute both to hyperglycemia, such as infection and corticosteroids, and hypoglycemia, such as poor oral intake. In the well-controlled patient on established insulin as an outpatient, a 20% decrease from the usual outpatient dose is recommended.

QUALITY IMPROVEMENT

Several measures may improve the hospital management of glycemic crises. These include the adoption and promotion of standard protocols for the management of patients with hyperosmolar hyperglycemic syndrome and diabetic ketoacidosis, and monitoring for protocol adherence in the care of patients admitted with these diagnoses. The quality of inpatient diabetes care may be improved with standard insulin order sets, based on the principles of physiologic insulin control and adjustment for oral intake or lack thereof. Hospitals should have ongoing metrics to assess the quality of diabetes care and the incidence of inpatient hypoglycemia and hyperglycemia. Electronic monitoring may be a useful adjunct to these efforts, for example, to track the utilization of 50% dextrose or the unwarranted use of oral hypoglycemic agents in the inpatient setting. Physician, nurse, and patient education should be part of any quality improvement initiative.

SUGGESTED READINGS

Braithwaite SS, Buie MM, Thompson CL, et al. Hospital hypoglycemia: not only treatment but also prevention. *Endocr Pract.* 2004;10(suppl 2):89–99.

Cryer PE, Axelrod L, Grossman AB, et al. Evaluation and management of adult hypoglycemic disorders: an Endocrine Society Clinical Practice Guideline. *J Clin Endocrinol Metab.* 2009;94:709–728.

Kitabchi AE, Umpierrez GE, Murphy MB, et al. Hyperglycemic crises in adult patients with diabetes: a consensus statement from the American Diabetes Association. *Diabetes Care.* 2009;32:1335–1343.

Moghissi ES, Korytkowski MT, DiNardo M, et al. American Association of Clinical Endocrinologists and American Diabetes Association consensus statement on inpatient glycemic control. *Diabetes Care.* 2009;32:1119–1131.

Murad MH, Coto-Yglesias F, Wang AT, et al. Clinical review: Drug-induced hypoglycemia: a systematic review. *J Clin Endocrinol Metab.* 2009;94:741–745.

Smith WD, Winterstein AG, Johns T, et al. Causes of hyperglycemia and hypoglycemia in adult inpatients. *Am J Health Syst Pharm.* 2005;62:714–719.

Turchin A, Matheny ME, Shubina M, et al. Hypoglycemia and clinical outcomes in patients with diabetes hospitalized in the general ward. *Diabetes Care.* 2009;32:1153–1157.

CHAPTER 149

Inpatient Management of Diabetes and Hyperglycemia

Jeffrey L. Schnipper, MD, MPH, FHM

Key Clinical Questions

1. Why control diabetes and hyperglycemia in the hospital?
2. What are the goals of glycemic management in critical care and noncritical care settings?
3. When should patients be treated with oral agents, with subcutaneous insulin, and with continuous insulin infusions?
4. Is it safe to prescribe subcutaneous insulin for the first time in a hospitalized patient?
5. How should insulin orders be adjusted in response to poor inpatient glucose control?
6. What should be considered when discharging a patient with diabetes or inpatient hyperglycemia?
7. How may the quality of glucose management be improved in hospital settings?

INTRODUCTION

Diabetes mellitus is common in hospitalized patients. In 2007, diabetes was listed as a diagnosis in approximately 19% of all hospital discharges in the United States. Because discharge diagnoses may not capture undiagnosed diabetes or hospital-related hyperglycemia, the true prevalence of diabetes or hyperglycemia in hospitalized patients is likely much higher. For example, in one study of 1886 general medicine and surgery admissions, hyperglycemia (defined as a fasting plasma glucose of ≥ 126 mg/dL or a random plasma glucose of ≥ 200 mg/dL) was found in 38% of patients. Of these, 68% had known diabetes, but the other 32% had no previous diagnosis and consisted of patients with undiagnosed diabetes, "prediabetes" unmasked by the stress of illness, and pure "stress hyperglycemia."

Hyperglycemia is associated with worse outcomes among hospitalized patients, including infections, increased length of stay, decreased independent living after discharge, and increased mortality. Hyperglycemia among known diabetics in the hospital carries a 2.7 relative risk of in-hospital death; even more dramatic is the 18-fold increased risk of death associated with hyperglycemia among those without a previous diagnosis of diabetes. Similar results have been seen in patients with pneumonia, myocardial infarction, chronic obstructive pulmonary disease, stroke, and those receiving total parenteral nutrition. Some of this excess mortality reflects the role of hyperglycemia as a marker for physiologic stress and severity of underlying disease. However, even when rigorous adjustment for severity of illness is conducted, excess mortality remains.

RATIONALE FOR INPATIENT GLUCOSE CONTROL

Does correcting inpatient hyperglycemia improve outcomes? In the noncritical care setting, this question has remained unanswered until recently.

RABBIT Surgery was a dual-site randomized controlled trial of 211 patients with type 2 DM admitted to general surgery services. The intervention group received a basal-bolus regimen with glargine once daily and glulisine before meals with a goal pre-meal glucose of 100–140 mg/dL. The control group received sliding scale regular insulin 4 times daily for glucose > 140 mg/dL. Mean glucose for the hospitalization was 157 vs. 176 mg/dL in favor of the intervention. Proportion of patients with any glucose < 40 mg/dL was 3.8% in the intervention group and 0% in the control group. Most importantly, the primary outcome, a composite of hospital complications including postoperative wound infection, pneumonia, respiratory failure, acute renal failure, and bacteremia, occurred in 24% in the control group and only 9% in the intervention group ($p = .003$; number needed to treat of 7 to prevent one complication). In the critical care setting, several studies of tight glycemic control have been performed, with mixed results. Early studies, such as the Leuven study conducted by van den Berghe, et al, in surgical intensive care unit (ICU) patients, were clearly positive. In Leuven I, patients were randomized to an insulin infusion protocol triggered when the blood glucose was > 100 mg/dL or a protocol that was triggered when glucose was > 215 mg/dL. The mean achieved glucose was 103 mg/dL vs. 153 mg/dL. Outcomes in the intervention arm included a 46% reduction in sepsis, 41% reduction in the need for dialysis, 50% reduction in blood transfusions, 44% reduction in polyneuropathy, and a 34% reduction in inpatient mortality. However, subsequent studies have not been so favorable. A follow-up study conducted by the same group on medical ICU patients was equivocal: mortality did not improve except in a post hoc analysis of patients with an ICU length of stay of three days or more, although morbidity was lessened (faster weaning from mechanical ventilation, discharge from the ICU, and discharge from the hospital). Of note, separation of glucose control was less pronounced than in the SICU study (mean glucose 153 mg/dL vs. 111 mg/dL), and rates of severe hypoglycemia were much higher (19% vs. 3% of patients with at least one glucose < 40 mg/dL). More recently, the NICE-SUGAR study was even less favorable to tight glucose control. In this open-label study of 6104 critically ill patients (medical and surgical), the intervention arm had a slightly increased 90-day mortality rate (27.5% vs. 24.9%), and a much higher rate of severe hypoglycemia (6.8% vs. 0.5%).

Some providers have interpreted NICE-SUGAR as justifying lax glucose control in critically ill patients. There are many reasons to avoid this approach:

1. In the NICE-SUGAR study, "control patients" actually had reasonably good glucose control: 69% were on an insulin infusion, and the median glucose was 141 mg/dL.
2. The high rates of hypoglycemia observed may be a specific problem with the Leuven insulin infusion protocol. Lower rates of hypoglycemia are seen with the use of other insulin infusion protocols, such as Yale and Glucommander, which are easier to administer and take better account of trends in glucose control over time (**Table 149-1**).
3. Septic patients may be particularly prone to hypoglycemia (medical ICU patients in these studies always have higher rates of hypoglycemia than surgical ICU patients; Table 149-1). The rational clinical response should be higher glucose targets in these patients, not lack of any target at all.
4. Insulin is one of the highest risk medications used in the hospital, and yet its inpatient use has been historically haphazard and irrational. A standardized approach to insulin use can prevent both severe hyperglycemia and hypoglycemia, both known to be hazardous to patients.
5. Several quality improvement studies, including several conducted by hospitalists, have shown the ability to institute processes that reduce hyperglycemia, while maintaining or even reducing the rate of hypoglycemia.

In response to recent studies, the American Association of Clinical Endocrinologists (AACE) and the American Diabetes Association (ADA) have updated their guidelines. In critically ill patients, extrapolating from NICE-SUGAR's control group, they recommend starting insulin infusions at a threshold no higher than 180 mg/dL, and aiming for a target range of 140–180 mg/dL. Recommendations for noncritically ill patients remain essentially unchanged: goals of premeal glucose readings < 140 mg/dL and random glucose readings < 180 mg/dL, with more or less stringent goals depending on previously achieved control and medical comorbidities (note that these goals might change in response to RABBIT Surgery, published after the release of these guidelines).

We agree with the approach of the National Quality Forum, whose Recommended Safe Practice advocates taking "actions to improve glycemic control by implementing evidence-based intervention practices that prevent hypoglycemia and optimize the care of patients with hyperglycemia and diabetes." Future studies will hopefully provide further guidance on which goals apply to which patient populations and which protocols are most safe and effective.

PATHOPHYSIOLOGY

Even short-term hyperglycemia may be hazardous in the context of medical illness. Hyperglycemia is associated with immune dysfunction, specifically neutrophil impairment. The secondary metabolic perturbations associated with hyperglycemia, such as overproduction of free fatty acids, reactive oxygen species, ketones, and lactic acid, may lead to cellular injury, inflammation, and defective wound repair. These adverse effects are likely to be most evident in patients with infections (eg, pneumonia), wounds (eg, sternotomy), and

TABLE 149-1 Rates of Hyperglycemia in Trials Using Different Insulin Infusion Protocols

Study	Patient Population	Hypoglycemia Rate*
Leuven Protocol		
Leuven 1 (*N Engl J Med.* 2001;345:1359–1367)	Surgical	5.1%
Leuven 2 (*N Engl J Med.* 2006;354:449–461)	Medical	19%
Glucontrol (*Intensive Care Med.* 2009;35:738–748)	Medical /Surgical	8.6%
VISEP (*N Engl J Med.* 2008;358:125–139)	Medical	17%
NICE-SUGAR (*N Engl J Med.* 2009;360:1283–1297)	Medical /Surgical	6.8%
Yale Protocol		
Yale 1 (*J Cardiothorac Vasc Anesth.* 2004;18:690–697)	Surgical	0%
Yale 2 (*Diabetes Care.* 2004;27:461–467)	Medical	4.3%
Glucommander Protocol		
Glucommander 1 (*Diabetes Care.* 2005;28:2418–2423)	Surgical	2.6%

*Proportion of patients with any glucose < 40 mg/dL.

infarction or ischemia (eg, myocardial infarction, stroke), exactly the populations in which observational data linking hyperglycemia to increased mortality are the strongest. Hyperglycemia may also lead to fluid and electrolyte imbalances once thresholds for glucosuria are reached (generally around 200 mg/dL). These can be potentially catastrophic in patients already suffering from acute renal failure, hypernatremia, and lactic acidosis. In addition preventing to these short-term problems, good inpatient glucose management may lead to better glucose control after discharge, for example, triggering a change to insulin use in a patient poorly controlled on maximal doses of oral agents. Measures to improve outpatient glucose control can have sustained effects on long-term diabetic complications such as neuropathy, nephropathy, retinopathy, and cardiovascular disease.

DIAGNOSIS

Hyperglcyemia is not usually the primary reason for hospitalization in diabetic patients. When it is, it is usually clinically obvious, as in diabetic ketoacidosis (DKA) in patients with type 1 diabetes, and hyperglycemic hyperosmolar state (HHS, formerly known as hyperosmolar nonketotic coma) in patients with type 2 diabetes. Diagnostic errors that may occur in the management of patients with diabetes and hyperglycemia include the following.

1. Failure to recognize hyperglycemia in a patient without a previous diagnosis of diabetes (eg, failure to notice a routine laboratory glucose of 200 mg/dL as abnormal). Any routine glucose reading over 180 mg/dL should trigger further evaluation and monitoring, including at least 24 hours of point-of-care (POC) glucose testing before meals and a hemoglobin A1c test. The hemoglobin A1c may be useful in the diagnosis of type 2 diabetes and helps assess the prior 90 days of glucose control, enabling the provider to distinguish diabetes from stress hyperglycemia. It is also extremely useful for discharge planning.
2. Failure to recognize type 1 diabetes, as opposed to type 2 diabetes. While the diagnosis may be obvious in a young, thin patient who presents for the first time in DKA, it should also be considered in the patient with chronic pancreatitis and pancreatic insufficiency, the patient who has had complete or partial pancreatectomy for malignancy, and other situations in which beta cell failure may be the predominant problem. These patients must receive insulin at all times, are more insulin sensitive, and typically have more labile glucose control due to the lack of pancreatic reserve. Many of these patients would benefit from endocrinology input for both diagnosis and management.

Glucose monitoring should be obtained in any patient with a history of diabetes, inpatient hyperglycemia, or receiving treatment that might cause hyperglycemia (such as systemic corticosteroids). In the setting of corticosteorids, monitoring can be stopped after 24 hours if hyperglycemia is not observed and increases in glucocorticoid doses are not planned. Patients eating discrete meals should generally be tested before each meal and before bedtime, while patients who are receiving nothing by mouth (NPO), receiving continuous enteral nutrition (tube feeds), or total parenteral nutrition (TPN) should be tested every six hours. Additional testing is optional depending on the circumstance. For example, testing at 3 AM can be used to rule out nocturnal hypoglycemia, while testing one to two hours after meals can be used to test the adequacy of nutritional insulin dosing (see Treatment, below).

TRIAGE

Patients admitted with DKA may be best admitted to an ICU. Insulin infusions are usually required for these patients, as well as frequent (every one to two hours) monitoring and repletion of fluids and electrolytes. These considerations alone may mandate ICU-level care. However, some hospitals may be able to safely manage these patients in intermediate care areas. Beyond DKA, if the clinical situation otherwise requires IV insulin infusions (see below), and such infusions can only be delivered in an ICU, then that would also mandate triage to an ICU.

TREATMENT

The management of inpatients with diabetes or hyperglycemia is inherently unstable. Patients suffer from nutritional and clinical instability, from acute illness and stress-related hyperglycemia that is dynamic and difficult to measure and predict, and from the use of diagnostic and therapeutic interventions that impact glycemic control and the actions of antihyperglycemic therapies. Most patients will require changes from their home regimen to an inpatient regimen that takes these factors into account.

USE OF ORAL ANTIDIABETIC AGENTS

Broadly speaking, there are three options for controlling inpatient hyperglycemia: oral agents, intravenous (IV) insulin infusions, and subcutaneous insulin injections. Most experts recommend against the routine use of oral agents in the hospital for a variety of reasons.

1. They are slow-acting and difficult to titrate.
2. Insulin secretatogogues such as glipizide, glyburide, and repaglinide inhibit pancreatic auto-regulation and can easily cause hypoglycemia, especially in the setting of reduced oral intake. Many are also long-acting.
3. Metformin can cause nausea, vomiting, and diarrhea, and is contraindicated in conditions that can predispose to lactic acidosis, including renal failure, use of intravenous iodinated contrast, heart failure, and liver failure.
4. Thiazolidinediones such as pioglitazone and rosiglitazone are very slow-acting and can cause fluid retention and pulmonary and peripheral edema.

Oral agents should only be continued in patients with good glucose control before and at the time of admission, who are not very ill, have a short projected length of stay, will not be NPO for any procedure, and will not be undergoing studies that use IV contrast. Oral agents should also be avoided in hospitalized patients who either have or are at risk for developing renal failure, heart failure, liver failure, or peripheral edema during the hospitalization. In the small population of patients who are eligible to continue oral agents, glycemia should be closely monitored. If glucose control is poor, oral agents should be stopped and insulin begun.

USE OF INTRAVENOUS INSULIN INFUSIONS

IV insulin infusions are rapidly effective and generally safe with frequent glucose monitoring. The benefit of IV insulin infusion is most proven in the settings of critical illness, before major surgical procedures, after organ transplantation, acute myocardial infarction, DKA, prolonged fasting in a patient with type 1 diabetes, and labor and delivery. Insulin infusions should be used in critically ill patients with hyperglycemia in accordance with updated AACE/ADA guidelines. Insulin infusions are generally under-utilized in noncritically ill patients, especially in patients with infections, wounds, or organ damage with several days of poor glucose control on subcutaneous regimens. In these patients, an insulin infusion can usually restore good glucose control within hours, although this may create safety issues. Policies can usually be adopted to protect patients and staff from unsafe situations, such as restricting their use in noncritical areas to daytime hours and only for one day, and guaranteeing availability of clinical personnel to adjust the drip rate every hour.

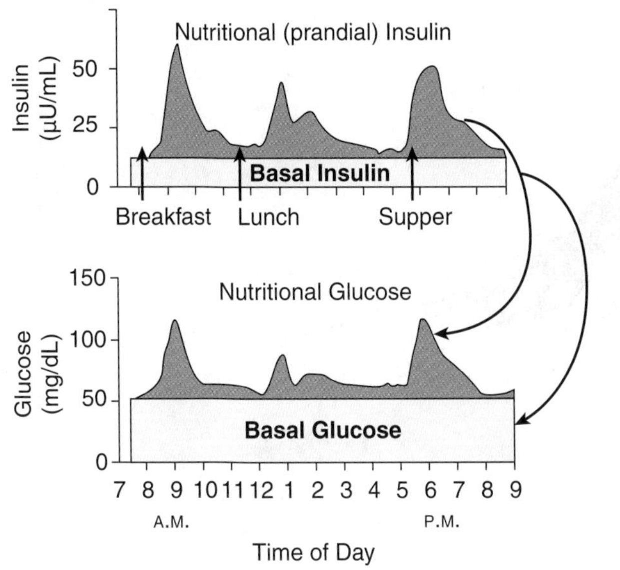

Figure 149-1 *Physiologic relationship between basal and nutritional glucose levels and basal and nutritional insulin levels in nondiabetic individuals.*

SUBCUTANEOUS INSULIN

The best treatment for most inpatients with diabetes and hyperglycemia is subcutaneous insulin injections, prescribed in an anticipatory and physiologic fashion. Three types of insulin orders should be provided: basal, nutritional ("bolus"), and correctional. Basal insulin is required in all patients with type 1 diabetes, and most patients with type 2 diabetes, to maintain euglycemia by preventing gluconeogenesis. It mimics the continuous, low-level endogenous insulin produced by the body at all times (**Figure 149-1**). Long-acting insulins such as glargine, detemir, and NPH are most appropriate for use as basal insulin (**Figure 149-2**). Nutritional insulin provides for the spike in blood glucose with meals, mimicking the rapid rise in blood insulin levels in response to eating (Figure 149-1). It should not be given to patients who are NPO. In patients eating discrete meals, rapid-acting insulins such as insulin lispro, aspart, and glulisine are most appropriate (Figure 149-2). For patients on continuous tube feeds, a short- to intermediate-acting insulin, such as regular insulin every 6 hours, is appropriate. In nondiabetics, the amount of basal insulin produced is approximately equal to the amount of nutritional insulin produced. This 50/50 ratio of basal-to-nutritional insulin is generally recommended for the treatment of inpatient hyperglycemia.

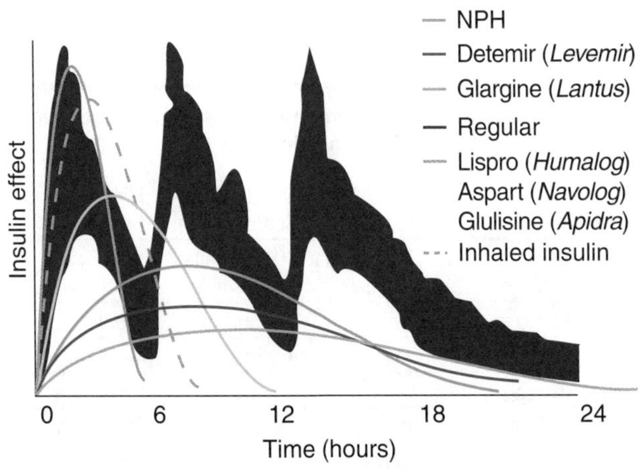

Figure 149-2 *Pharmacokinetics of various types of insulin.*

Correctional insulin is extra insulin given to correct hyperglycemia that occurs despite basal and nutritional insulin. The term "correctional insulin" is now preferred to the term "sliding scale," in order to emphasize that correctional insulin should not be used alone and is ineffective in maintaining euglycemia without basal and nutritional insulin. It is often written in a "stepped" format, so that more severe hyperglycemia is treated with higher doses. The steps should be customized to the patient, based on the patient's estimated insulin sensitivity (so that a patient receiving 100 units of scheduled insulin a day is not receiving a 1–5 unit scale). Correctional insulin that is required consistently (eg, two or more times a day) suggests a need to modify the basal or nutritional insulin doses.

Physiologic subcutaneous insulin regimens should be used in

- All patients with type 1 diabetes, unless they require an insulin infusion
- Patients with type 2 diabetes that are already insulin-requiring, are poorly controlled despite oral agents, or known to require high doses of oral agents that will be held in the hospital
- Any patient with blood glucose levels during hospitalization consistently above the target range (eg, >180 mg/dL in noncritical care patients)

HOW TO ORDER PHYSIOLOGIC SUBCUTANEOUS INSULIN IN THE HOSPITAL

Most experts recommend a step-wise approach to physiologic insulin dosing in the hospital:

1. Decide if a patient is appropriate for subcutaneous insulin, and discontinue all oral antidiabetic agents.
2. Calculate the estimated total daily dose (TDD) of insulin.
3. Determine the distribution of the TDD, based on the patient's nutritional regimen.
4. Reevaluate and adjust the TDD daily, based on the glycemic control of the previous 24 hours.

CALCULATING THE TOTAL DAILY DOSE

The TDD can be estimated in several ways. For patients well-controlled on a preadmission insulin regimen, we recommend adding up all the scheduled insulin doses to derive the TDD. For patients not on insulin prior to admission, a weight-based calculation is most appropriate. A typical starting dose is 0.4 to 0.6 units/kg/day. Patients with renal failure, recent hypoglycemia, who are older, thin, or insulin-sensitive (eg, type 1), should start at the lower end of this range (or even 0.3 units/kg/day if multiple risk factors for hypoglycemia apply). Patients who are obese, on corticosteroids, or have a history of hyperglycemia should start at the higher end of this range, and may in fact eventually need much higher doses. For patients transferred out of an ICU whose glucose level has been well-controlled on an insulin drip at a stable dose for at least six hours, the TDD can be estimated by multiplying the hourly drip rate by 20. This is likely to slightly underestimate the TDD, but is done to avoid hypoglycemia. This also assumes the patient was receiving nutrition in the ICU (eg, tube feeds); if the patient was not being fed, the above calculation estimates the basal insulin requirement only, and the TDD would be double this amount.

DIVIDING THE TOTAL DAILY DOSE INTO BASAL AND NUTRITIONAL COMPONENTS

Once the TDD has been estimated, the daily basal dose can be calculated as approximately half the TDD, while the daily nutritional dose can be estimated as the other half of the TDD. Basal insulin can be given as one daily dose (eg, insulin glargine at night), or split (eg, NPH at morning and at night). The type, dose, and frequency

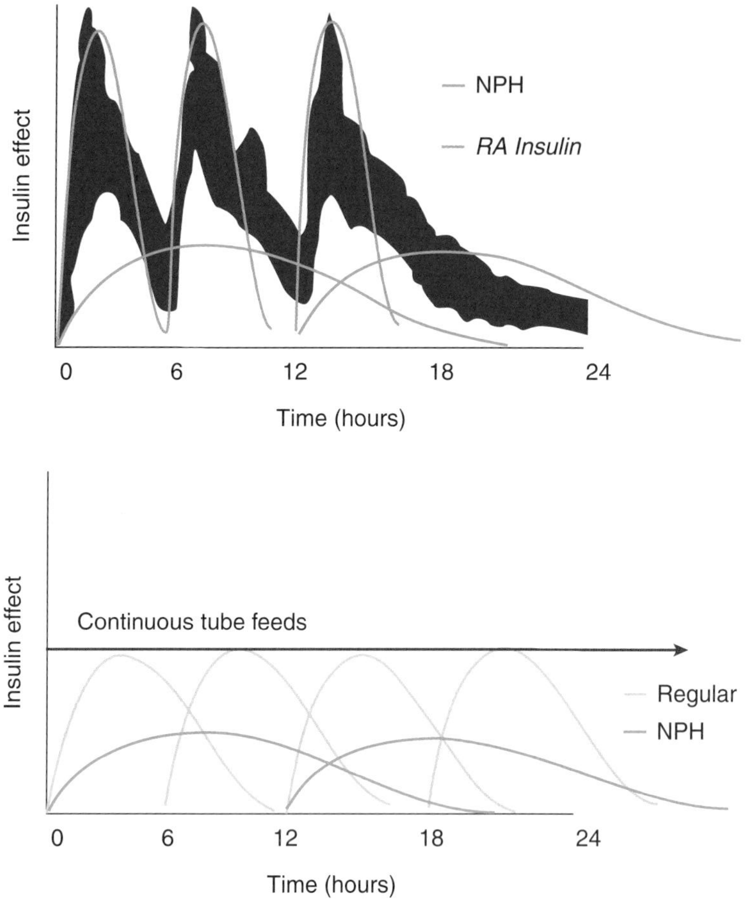

Figure 149-3 *Examples of insulin regimens for patients with diferent kinds of nutritional intake. 3A: Patients eating discrete meals. 3B: Patients receiving continuous enteral nutrition (tube feeds).*

of nutritional insulin will depend on the patient's nutritional status (**Figure 149-3**). For example, for patients receiving discrete meals, it can be written as rapid-acting insulin before meals (ie, split in three doses; Figure 149-3A). For a patient receiving continuous tube feeds or TPN, it can be written as regular insulin every six hours (ie, split in four doses; Figure 149-3B). Even in patients on continuous tube feeds, this approach is recommended over giving the entire TDD as insulin glargine, for example, in case tube feeds have to be discontinued (eg, for testing, or because of gastric tube malfunction or GI transit issues). In this case, the basal dose can remain unchanged, nutritional insulin can be discontinued, and the risk of hypoglycemia should persist for no more than six hours, rather than 24 hours. Nutritional insulin is not ordered in patients who are NPO.

In patients with unpredictable oral intake, it may be appropriate to wait until the meal has been eaten before giving nutritional insulin. If a patient eats all the food provided to him/her, the entire dose of rapid-acting insulin can be given immediately after the meal. If half the food is eaten, the dose can be halved, and so on. Assuming a patient has been written for a consistent carbohydrate meal (which is recommended), this approach resembles "carb-counting" (multiplying the carbohydrate intake by a factor to determine the insulin dose), but is easier to implement.

ORDERING CORRECTIONAL INSULIN

Correctional insulin is usually given in the same form as the patient's nutritional insulin. It may be given at the same time as nutritional insulin (eg, 6 units "standing" nutritional insulin, plus 4 units for a glucose of 260 mg/dL, for a total of 10 units rapid-acting insulin given before the meal). In patients who are NPO, it can be written as regular insulin every six hours or rapid-acting insulin every four hours. As noted above, stepped dosing orders should take insulin sensitivity into account. One way to do this is to have three different strengths of sliding scales using the TDD as the estimate of insulin sensitivity (see **Table 149-2** as an example).

DANGERS OF SLIDING SCALE INSULIN USED ALONE

In patients well-controlled on oral agents at home, or in nondiabetics started on corticosteroids, it may be appropriate to write for routine POC glucose testing and a correctional insulin protocol alone. But if this approach results in hyperglycemia, it should be

TABLE 149-2 Examples of Correctional Insulin Scales Based on Total Daily Insulin Dose

	Low Scale	Medium Scale	High Scale
Pre-meal Blood glucose	<40 Units Insulin/day	40–80 Units Insulin/day	>80 Units Insulin/day
150–199 mg/dL	1 unit	1 units	2 units
200–249 mg/dL	2 units	3 units	4 units
250–299 mg/dL	3 units	5 units	7 units
300–349 mg/dL	4 units	7 units	10 units
>349 mg/dL	5 units	8 units	12 units

abandoned in favor of the approach described above. Correctional insulin by itself does not work: by definition, it is reactive and predictably causes hyperglycemia, it leads to a roller-coaster pattern of glycemia (which in itself may be dangerous), it increases the risk for stacking of insulin doses and hypoglycemia, and it promotes an illusion of control and clinical inertia. Several studies have shown that sliding scale insulin alone leads to higher rates of hyperglycemia, compared with any other approach to glucose management. Moreover, even in the patients described above, starting physiological insulin on the first hospital day is completely safe. In anyone with a functioning pancreas (ie, anyone except patients with type 1 diabetes), endogenous insulin production will automatically adjust as exogenous insulin is given. Patients will not become hypoglycemic, as long as the TDD given is less than or equal to the patient's true insulin requirements, the dosing principles above are followed, and the patient is not receiving an insulin secretagogue. In our experience, patients with mild or no diabetes do well on physiologic insulin regimens because of the degree of pancreatic reserve.

INSULIN ADJUSTMENT

As a rule, insulin orders require daily adjustment in response to changes in patient status and glucose control. Unfortunately, there is currently no consensus on the best method of daily insulin adjustment. Some experts recommend adjusting the basal dose separately from the nutritional dose (eg, using the morning fasting glucose to guide basal dose adjustment, and glucose levels later in the day to guide nutritional dose adjustment). Others recommend using global glucose control to guide adjustments to the TDD and then distributing it into basal and nutritional components. At our institution, we use the following approach:

1. Add up the total insulin administered the previous day (scheduled plus correctional).
2. Make adjustments to the TDD (10–30% up or down) based on the degree of hypoglycemia or hyperglycemia, as well as changes in renal function, corticosteroid dose, nutritional intake, and physiologic stress caused by illness.
3. Distribute the new TDD into basal and nutritional components, keeping nutritional intake in mind, and the fact that the morning fasting glucose best reflects the adequacy of the basal insulin dose.
4. Change the correctional insulin scale as needed based on the new TDD.

COMPLICATIONS

Common inpatient complications include hypoglycemia and iatrogenic DKA. Hypoglycemia often occurs because of unexpected reductions in nutritional intake, such as vomiting or tube feeds that have to be held. This can be prevented with the following measures.

1. Proactively identifying patients at risk for hypoglycemia, including patients with type 1 diabetes, patients who are older, who have renal dysfunction, or unpredictable nutritional intake, and lower insulin doses and monitor glucose levels more frequently in these patients.
2. Writing balanced basal and nutritional insulin doses. Many patients have preadmission regimens that are predominantly basal insulin because they are easier to administer. But when these patients have reduced orally intake in the hospital, hypoglycemia may result. This is why we recommend splitting the patient's home TDD in half as the basal insulin dose, even if this results in a basal dose lower than that prescribed at home. The nutritional insulin can then be written based on the patient's degree of nutritional intake.
3. Giving nutritional insulin after meals in patients with unpredictable oral intake, as described above.
4. Being aware of patients with inpatient insulin requirements that are much higher than preadmission requirements because of physiologic stress, and that these high requirements may resolve quickly as a patient's illness improves.

Iatrogenic DKA is best prevented by ensuring that all patients with type 1 diabetes (including patients with pancreatic disease) are receiving basal insulin at all times.

DISCHARGE CONSIDERATIONS

Several factors must be considered in discharge planning for patients with diabetes or inpatient hyperglycemia. First is the adequacy of their preadmission medication regimen. This is best determined by obtaining a hemoglobin A1c at admission, if one is not available from the previous month. The hemoglobin A1c may be misleading if patients have recently undergone rapid red cell turnover, as in bleeding, transfusion, and hemolytic anemia. If the hemoglobin A1c is close to 7, then most patients can be discharged on their preadmission regimen, with the possible exception of patients being discharged on a long course of high-dose corticosteroids. If the A1c is significantly greater than 7, then the home regimen probably needs to be adjusted. This might include higher doses of preadmission oral agents, or minor (10–20%) increases in preadmission insulin doses. Regimens that worked well in the hospital may not be best for patients after discharge. In particular, inpatient regimens may be more complex than some patients can manage. Patients on maximum doses of two oral agents prior to admission with an elevated hemoglobin A1c pose a particular challenge. If possible, these patients should be discharged on insulin, using the simplest regimen possible (eg, insulin glargine once a day, perhaps with a rapid-acting insulin to cover their biggest meal of the day). They should have inpatient insulin teaching, monitoring by a visiting nurse in the week after discharge, and follow-up with a diabetes educator and endocrinologist within a week of discharge.

Hospitalization should be viewed as a unique opportunity for patient education. It should be determined as early as possible if the patient will require home fingerstick glucose monitoring and insulin, and if so, what type of insulin and what means of injection (needle and syringe or insulin pen). Once these decisions are made, education can be tailored accordingly for patients or their caregivers. Education should focus first on necessary survival skills, such as recognizing symptoms of hypoglycemia and how to manage it, and when and who to call for problems. Hospitals should develop, adapt, or borrow standard sets of educational materials to facilitate this process. Regardless of the quality of inpatient education, it needs to continue once patients leave the hospital.

QUALITY IMPROVEMENT

True gains in the quality of care among patients with diabetes and hyperglycemia can only come with hospital-wide, multidisciplinary efforts. In fact, inpatient diabetes management lends itself rather well to quality improvement (QI) efforts. A full discussion of this topic is beyond the scope of this chapter, but the Society of Hospital Medicine (SHM) is an invaluable resource in this area. Its website includes an implementation guide that takes the hospitalist leader step-by-step through process improvement at his or her institution. SHM also sponsors a Glycemic Control Mentored Implementation program, in which experts help hospitals around the country develop their programs over the course of a year.

As with most QI efforts, necessary steps include obtaining institutional commitment, forming an interdisciplinary team with expert knowledge and the ability to influence change, process-mapping of present practice, and understanding gaps between current and ideal processes. Actions should be prioritized based on potential costs and benefits. Goals should be set that are specific, measurable, aggressive, achievable, relevant, and time-bound. Rapid-cycle continuous quality improvement methods (ie, plan-do-study-act) should be used to develop, test, refine, and spread interventions to improve care. In the case of inpatient diabetes, likely interventions consist of protocols to specify care processes for various clinical situations, education of physicians, nurses, and pharmacists, patient educational materials, and order sets that specify and provide decision support for all aspects of inpatient care.

Once interventions have been refined, steps should be taken to ensure that they are implemented with high reliability. These may include electronic reminders, real-time actionable reports of patients with poor glycemic control, and use of personnel such as nurses or pharmacists to help clinicians identify and act on patients with suboptimal control. Other steps may include building proper care into the workflow, such as disallowing insulin orders except via an approved order set and automatically triggering 24 hours of POC glucose testing in response to hyperglycemia found on routine laboratory testing. Several studies have shown that such broad-based QI efforts can successfully improve glycemic control, while maintaining or even reducing rates of hypoglycemia.

CONCLUSION

Inpatient hyperglycemia is associated with adverse patient outcomes. Although more research is needed to clarify the optimal glucose targets in various patient populations and how best to achieve them, a strong argument can be made for a standardized, rational approach to the inpatient management of diabetes and hyperglycemia, based on existing evidence. For most noncritical care patients, guidelines recommend physiologic use of subcutaneous insulin divided into three components: basal, nutritional, and correctional, with daily adjustment of orders as necessary to prevent hypo- and hyperglycemia. Discharge orders should be based on the patient's preadmission regimen and hemoglobin A1c. Patient education is crucial for improving outcomes after discharge. Broad-based, multidisciplinary efforts are required for hospitals to improve their management of these patients. Hospitalists should be involved in these efforts whenever possible.

SUGGESTED READINGS

Davidson PC, Steed RD, Bode BW. Glucommander: a computer-directed intravenous insulin system shown to be safe, simple, and effective in 120,618 h of operation. *Diabetes Care.* 2005;28:2418–2423.

Finfer S, Chittock DR, Su SY, et al. Intensive versus conventional glucose control in critically ill patients. *N Engl J Med.* 2009;360:1283–1297.

Moghissi ES, Korytkowski MT, DiNardo M, et al. American Association of Clinical Endocrinologists and American Diabetes Association consensus statement on inpatient glycemic control. *Endocr Pract.* 2009;15:353–369.

Preiser JC, Devos P, Ruiz-Santana S, et al. A prospective randomised multi-centre controlled trial on tight glucose control by intensive insulin therapy in adult intensive care units: the Glucontrol study. *Intensive Care Med.* 2009;35:1738–1748.

Schnipper JL, Liang CL, Ndumele CD, et al. Effects of a computerized order set on the inpatient management of hyperglycemia: a cluster-randomized controlled trial. *Endocr Pract.* 2010;16:209–218.

Society of Hospital Medicine. Glycemic Control Implementation Guide. 2008; http://www.hospitalmedicine.org/ResourceRoomRedesign/html/GC_Imp_Guide.cfm#. Accessed April 18, 2010.

Umpierrez GE, Isaacs SD, Bazargan N, You X, Thaler LM, Kitabchi AE. Hyperglycemia: an independent marker of in-hospital mortality in patients with undiagnosed diabetes. *J Clin Endocrinol Metab.* 2002;87:978–982.

Umpierrez GE, Smiley D, Jacobs S, et al. Randomized study of basal-bolus insulin therapy in the inpatient management of patients with type 2 diabetes undergoing general surgery (RABBIT 2 Surgery). *Diabetes Care.* Feb 2011;34(2):256–261.

Van den Berghe G, Wilmer A, Hermans G, et al. Intensive insulin therapy in the medical ICU. *N Engl J Med.* 2006;354:449–461.

Van den Berghe G, Wouters P, Weekers F, et al. Intensive insulin therapy in the critically ill patients. *N Engl J Med.* 2001;345:1359–1367.

CHAPTER 150

Thyroid Emergencies

Jill M. Paulson, MD
Anthony N. Hollenberg, MD

Key Clinical Questions

1. How does one interpret thyroid function tests in the inpatient setting?
2. How can one distinguish nonthyroidal illness from other thyroid conditions?
3. How does myxedema coma differ from a normal hypothyroid state and how is it treated?
4. What characterizes thyroid storm and how is it distinct from thyrotoxicosis?
5. How is thyroid storm treated?

INTRODUCTION

Thyroid disease is important to hospitalists for two reasons. Rarely, patients are admitted to the hospital with myxedema coma or thyrotoxicosis, conditions that must be recognized early as prompt diagnosis and treatment reduce patient morbidity and mortality. More often, patients have thyroid function tests performed in the hospital because of nonspecific symptoms such as fatigue, weight loss, and palpitations, and the hospitalist has to distinguish between true thyroid disease and nonthyroidal illness syndrome (euthyroid sick syndrome). To understand the diagnosis and treatment of thyroid disease, it is necessary to review the normal physiology of thyroid hormone.

THYROID HORMONE PHYSIOLOGY AND TESTING

Thyroid hormone usually refers to both thyroxine (T_4) and triiodothyronine (T_3). The thyroid synthesizes primarily T_4, but can also synthesize T_3. T_3 is felt to be the biologically active form of the hormone; T_4, which has a longer half-life, functions as a prohormone. Eighty percent of T_3 is produced by deiodination of the tyrosine rings of T_4 by a family of deiodinases, which are expressed in a variety of tissues. Both the type 1 and 2 deiodinases convert T_4 to T_3. In contrast, the type 3 deiodinase converts T_4 to inactive reverse T_3 (rT_3) and also inactivates T_3.

Both T_4 and T_3 likely gain access to cells by a variety of transporters that are still being elucidated. T_3 acts mainly in the nucleus, binding to thyroid hormone receptors (TRs) to regulate gene expression. This genomic action accounts for many of T_3's physiologic effects including thermogenesis, decreased systemic vascular resistance, and increased cardiac chronotropy and inotropy. T_3 and the TR may also act directly in the cytoplasm on other cell signaling pathways that influence physiologic function.

T_3 feeds back at the level of the hypothalamus and pituitary to regulate thyrotropin-releasing hormone (TRH) and thyroid stimulating hormone (TSH) synthesis and secretion respectively. TSH governs the amount of thyroid hormone synthesized by the thyroid gland. TSH is a heterodimeric glycoprotein hormone that can be measured by rapid, sensitive, and reliable immunoassays in the laboratory. A suppressed TSH demonstrates excessive thyroid hormone and hyperthyroidism, while an elevated TSH indicates inadequate thyroid hormone and hypothyroidism (**Figure 150-1**).

In certain clinical situations, including patients with central hypothyroidism (secondary hypothyroidism) due to hypothalamic-pituitary dysfunction, those treated with medications such as dopamine and glucocorticoids, and critically ill patients, the TSH is not able to reliably determine thyroid status and should not be used as a screening test (**Table 150-1**).

Thyroid status can also be assessed by measuring circulating T_4 and T_3 levels. Because thyroid hormones are protein bound, the most common test used to measure peripheral thyroid hormone is an analogue free T_4 (fT_4) assay. While this assay is usually reliable, the indirect methodology used may make it difficult to interpret in severe illness or pregnancy. In these circumstances, measurement of total T_4 (TT_4) and total T_3 (TT_3), together with an index of protein binding such as thyroxine binding globulin (TBG) or resin uptake, is the preferred method. Also available, but rarely used due to limited availability and cost, is direct measurement of fT_4 by equilibrium dialysis. Free T_3 levels can also be measured, but have limited clinical utility. In the hospital or outpatient setting,

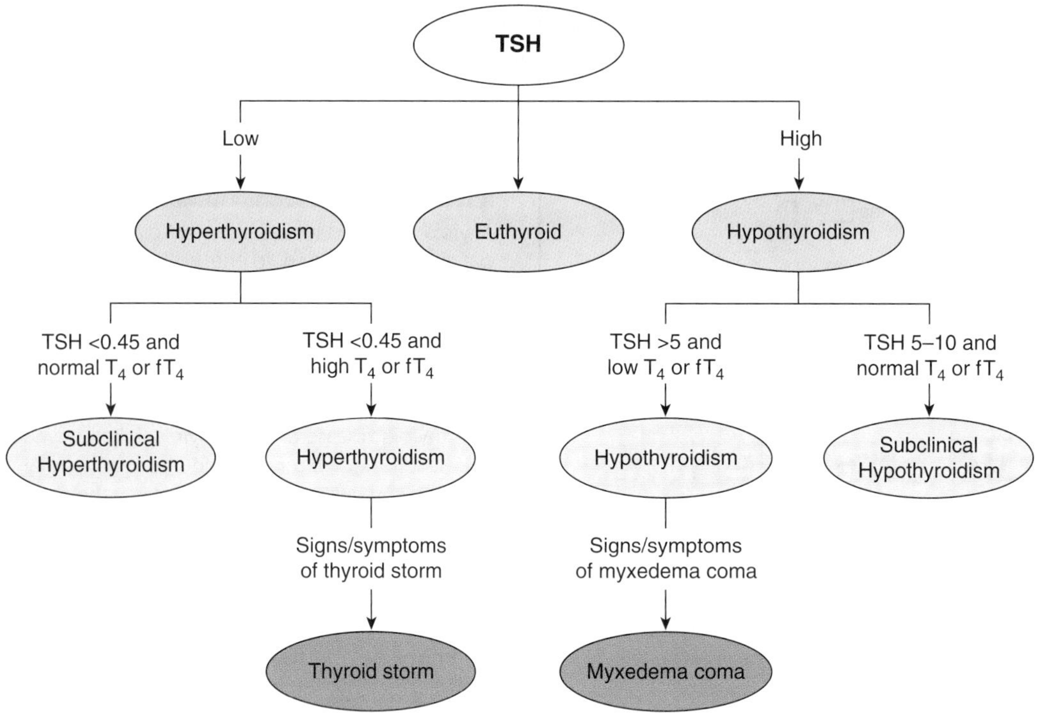

Figure 150-1 *Algorithm for thyroid function tests. This algorithm does not apply in patients with hypothalamic-pituitary disease, serious illness, or those who are taking certain medications such as amiodarone, glucocorticoids, and dopamine.*

once thyroid disease is clinically suspected, it is usual to screen with a TSH and if abnormal proceed to determine circulating thyroid hormone levels by measuring fT_4 and potentially TT_3. However, in the critically ill patient suspected of having thyroid dysfunction, it is reasonable to obtain a full panel of thyroid tests, including TSH, fT_4, TT_4, and TT_3.

NONTHYROIDAL ILLNESS SYNDROME (EUTHYROID SICK SYNDROME)

ALTERATED THYROID FUNCTION IN NONTHYROIDAL ILLNESS SYNDROME

Ideally, routine laboratory testing of thyroid function is best done outside the hospital. In severe illness, changes in thyroid function make it difficult to determine whether thyroid disease is present. Studies show abnormalities in thyroid function testing in 40–70% of intensive care unit (ICU) patients. Nonthyroidal illness syndrome, known as the "euthyroid sick syndrome" or "low T_3 syndrome," is characterized by low serum T_3, high rT_3, normal-low T_4, and normal-low TSH. As these changes somewhat resemble central hypothyroidism, the clinical scenario must be taken into consideration when interpreting thyroid testing. The nonthyroidal illness syndrome is due to a complex interplay of changes in the hypothalamic-pituitary-thyroid axis and in the peripheral metabolism of thyroid hormone. There is controversy over whether these changes are maladaptive or are adaptive, but it is likely that they are an effort to decrease energy utilization during extreme stress and illness.

TABLE 150-1 Commonly Used Medications that Affect Thyroid Function Tests

Drug	Affect on Thyroid Function Tests
Amiodarone	Acute effects (up to three months after initiation): Transient increase in TSH (< 10 μU/mL) Increase in T_4 and fT_4 Decrease T_3 Long-term can lead to hypo- or hyperthyroidism
Dopamine	Decreases TSH (not undetectable)
Glucocorticoids	Decreases TSH (not undetectable)
Interferon-alpha	Hypothyroidism and hyperthyroidism can occur (transient in many cases)

LOW T_3 AND HIGH rT_3 IN NONTHYROIDAL ILLNESS

Nonthyroidal illness syndrome is sometimes termed "low T_3 syndrome," as this is the earliest and most persistent abnormality. Uniformly, T_3 is low and rT_3 is high, with the T_3 level bearing an inverse relationship to the severity of disease. In acute illness, these changes may occur within hours. Alterations in deiodinase activity appear to be responsible. Type 1 deiodinase is inhibited, leading to diminished conversion of T_4 to T_3. Action of type 3 deiodinase is increased, which metabolizes T_4 to inactive rT_3, and also lowers T_3 by increasing its degradation. Thus, T_3 levels are rapidly lowered and rT_3 levels are elevated.

T_4 AND TSH IN NONTHYROIDAL ILLNESS

TSH and T_4 levels may be normal in nonthyroidal illness. However, a normal TSH in nonthyroidal illness may be inappropriate in the face of an already low T_3 level. In a healthy individual with an intact hypothalamic-pituitary-thyroid axis, this would lead to an increase in TSH. As the patient's underlying illness worsens, changes in hypothalamic and pituitary action also occur, leading to low TSH levels. TSH is usually detectable in this setting (> 0.05 μU/mL), whereas in clinical thyrotoxicosis it is completely suppressed. Once TSH falls, serum T_4 usually follows suit. However, severe illness can also cause decreased binding of T_4 to its serum binding proteins. As a result, fT_4 concentrations can be low, normal, or high in nonthyroidal illness depending on the assay used. When TSH is low, the possibility of secondary hypothyroidism should also be considered. Production of other pituitary hormones is usually also affected, and it is important to remember that both gonadotropins and growth hormone can be suppressed in acute illness.

In recovery from nonthyroidal illness, the axis tends to reset from the top down. TSH rises, sometimes above the normal range in the initial period of the recovery, though typically not above 20 μU/mL, in order to allow for the recovery of T_4. However, T_3 may still remain low in this setting. The TSH eventually returns to its physiologic normal level as the recovery continues. If TSH concentrations rise above 20 μU/mL in presumed nonthyroidal illness, primary hypothyroidism should be considered. Outpatient thyroid function tests prior to hospitalization may be very helpful, as this may establish a previous baseline.

When interpreting thyroid testing in hospitalized patients, it should be borne in mind that dopamine, glucocorticoids, amiodarone, and other medications often administered to the critically ill, may affect the results of thyroid function testing (Table 150-1).

SHOULD NONTHYROIDAL ILLNESS SYNDROME BE TREATED?

In patients with a persistently low T_3 from nonthyroidal illness, the T_3 level is an independent predictor of morbidity and mortality. Does replacement of thyroid hormone to normal levels in such patients lead to lower morbidity and mortality? Treatment of nonthyroidal illness with T_4 therapy has not shown to be of clinical benefit. In one study of ICU patients with nonthyroidal illness, those treated with T_4 to normalize serum T_4 values did not have a significant rise in their T_3 levels. Furthermore, the T_4-treated group had the same mortality rate as the untreated control group.

Thyroid hormone replacement with T_3 has been tried in patients with low T_3 in a variety of clinical settings, including renal failure, congestive heart failure, and coronary artery bypass graft (CABG). T_3 replacement has not been found to be beneficial in the majority of studies. Although T_3 supplementation appears to temporarily improve hemodynamics in critically ill patients with cardiac disease, there is no evidence of a mortality benefit. Because of the potential for morbidity and harm with both T_4 and T_3 replacement, we do not believe that there is adequate evidence to treat patients who have nonthyroidal illness with thyroid hormone.

MYXEDEMA COMA

CASE 150-1

MYXEDEMA COMA

A 69-year-old woman is brought to the hospital after she is found unresponsive in her apartment. A neighbor told emergency medical personnel that the patient had lately seemed withdrawn and apathetic.

Her primary care physician was contacted. She noted that the patient had a history of severe depression and hypothyroidism, and had missed several recent office appointments.

On examination, the patient was barely rousable, with a temperature of 34.4°C (94°F), pulse 48 beats per minute, and respirations 12 breaths per minute. Her skin was dry and doughy, and her hair was coarse and sparse. Macroglossia was present, and the thyroid appeared diffusely enlarged. There were crackles at both lung bases. Delayed relaxation of the deep tendon reflexes was noted.

Laboratory tests were notable for TSH 162 μU/mL (normal range, 0.27–4.62 μU/mL); free thyroxine (fT_4), which was undetectable (normal range, 0.7 to 2.2 ng/dL); and serum sodium 126 mmol/L. A chest radiograph showed bibasilar infiltrates. Her respiratory status deteriorated, and she developed hypotension. She started Bilevel Positive Airway Pressure (BiPAP) for hypoxemic and hypercarbic respiratory failure, and was transferred to the intensive care unit, where she was mechanically ventilated and passively rewarmed.

She received a loading dose of 250 μg of intravenous levothyroxine, followed by a daily dose of 75 μg of levothyroxine thereafter, as well as stress dose hydrocortisone and ampicillin-sulbactam. She was eventually discharged to a skilled nursing facility, and resumed drug therapy for depression and thyroid replacement.

Myxedema coma is a rare and life-threatening manifestation of decompensated or previously undiagnosed hypothyroidism. Hallmarks include hypothermia, altered mental status, and a precipitating cause, such as concomitant severe illness, cold exposure, or drug effect from lithium or sedatives. As mortality rates are greater than 50% in many case series, clinical suspicion must be high as survival depends on early recognition, treatment of the underlying illness, and thyroid hormone replacement.

CAUSES OF MYXEDEMA COMA

Approximately 90–95% of cases are due to primary hypothyroidism, and 5–10% are due to secondary hypothyroidism. Precipitating factors are almost always present in myxedema coma. Underlying infection must be assumed to be present until ruled out, and should be treated empirically and promptly. Leukocytosis and fever will often be absent in infection in the setting of myxedema. Cold exposure increases susceptibility to myxedema coma, although the exact mechanism for this is not fully understood. Many drugs may predispose to myxedema coma, including lithium, narcotics, benzodiazepines, barbiturates, and amiodarone. Surgery, trauma, burns, hypoxia, hypercapnia, acidosis, gastrointestinal bleed, and infections are also commonly implicated.

CLINICAL MANIFESTATIONS OF MYXEDEMA COMA

Most cases of myxedema coma occur in older women, as hypothyroidism is five to eight times more common in women. About 80–90% of cases of myxedema coma occur in winter. The patient interview should assess for symptoms of hypothyroidism, such as cold intolerance, decreased appetite, and fatigue. The patient should be asked about a history of thyroid disease, adherence to thyroid medications, a history of head and neck irradiation, and radioactive iodine treatment.

On examination, defective thermoregulation is always present, usually with marked hypothermia resulting in rectal temperatures less than 35.6° C (96.0° F). In patients with an underlying infection, body temperature may be close to normal, when fever would usually be expected. Other signs of severe hypothyroidism are common, but not all classic findings are present in all patients. The skin may be dry, with a thickened and doughy feel. The face may be swollen, with periorbital edema and macroglossia. The hair may be coarse, dry, and brittle, with the eyebrows missing the outer one-third of the hair (**Figure 150-2**). Deep tendon reflexes will have a delayed relaxation phase. Goiter or a thyroidectomy scar may be found.

Neurological manifestations are invariably present. The patient may display somnolence, lethargy, depression, and rarely coma (myxedema coma is a misnomer, as coma is not necessary for diagnosis). Seizures are present in up to 25% of cases. Sensory

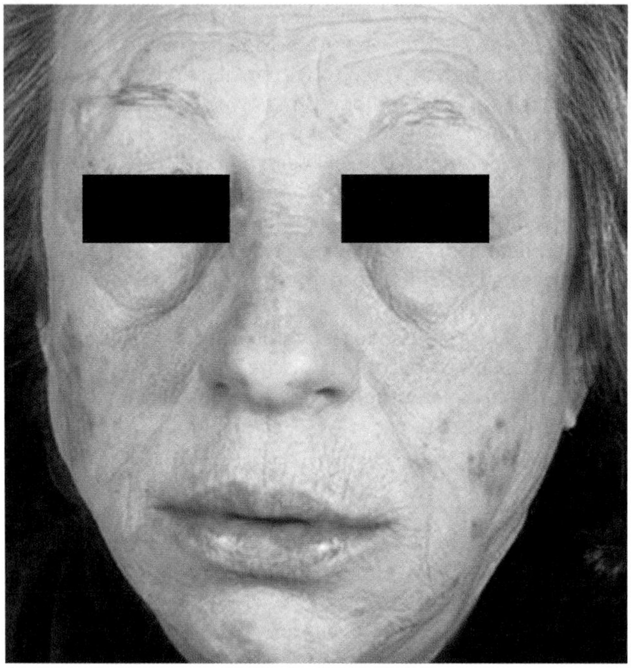

Figure 150-2 *Typical features of severe hypothyroidism, including dry doughy skin, coarse hair, periorbital puffiness, lateral thinning of the eyebrows, and a dull and apathetic facial expression. (Reproduced with permission from Wolff K, Goldsmith LA, Katz SI, et al. Fitzpatrick's Dermatology in General Medicine. 7th ed. New York, NY: McGraw-Hill; 2008. Fig. 152-12.)*

and motor peripheral neuropathies may be present. Neurogenic dysphagia may lead to aspiration events.

Cardiovascular involvement includes bradycardia, dilated cardiomyopathy, pericardial effusion, and QT prolongation. In long-standing compensated hypothyroidism, the pulse pressure may be narrowed, with an elevated diastolic blood pressure from increased systemic vascular resistance. However, in myxedema coma, cardiac contractility, stroke volume, and cardiac output may all be reduced, and hypotension and shock may occur. Hypotension in myxedema cannot be reversed without thyroid hormone therapy.

Other organ systems are also involved in myxedema. Pneumonia may be a complication of myxedema or a precipitant of it. Decreased respiratory drive, diaphragmatic weakness, pleural effusions, and airway obstruction from macroglossia may all lead to hypercapnic respiratory failure. Constipation is frequent in hypothyroidism. In myxedema coma, this may progress to paralytic ileus and megacolon. Ascites may also be found. The glomerular filtration rate is often reduced from decreased cardiac output and vasoconstriction, and most patients have hyponatremia from decreased free water excretion. Features of myxedema coma are summarized in **Table 150-2**.

LABORATORY FINDINGS IN MYXEDEMA COMA

Individuals with myxedema coma have profoundly elevated TSH, with low T_4 and T_3, in addition to neurological aberrations, hypothermia, and usually another precipitating illness. In myxedema due to secondary hypothyroidism, TSH may be low or normal, and there may be other evidence of pituitary dysfunction. Routine blood testing may reveal hyponatremia and renal insufficiency. Hypoglycemia may result from hypothyroidism, concurrent adrenal insufficiency in secondary hypothyroidism, or impaired gluconeogenesis in critical illness and starvation. Hypercarbia and hypoxia may be present.

TABLE 150-2 Potential Clinical Manifestations and Exam Findings in Myxedema Coma

Defective thermoregulation (can be normal temperature)
Thyroid
Goiter
Neurological
Somnolence, lethargy, depression, coma
Seizures in 25%
Sensory and peripheral neuropathies
Reflexes with delayed relaxation phase
Skin
Dry, coarse, myxedematous skin
Periorbital edema
Macroglossia
Cardiovascular
Bradycardia
Dilated cardiomyopathy
ECG abnormalities (prolonged QT)
Pericardial effusion
Elevated diastolic blood pressure
Hypotension and shock
Respiratory
Pneumonia
Aspiration events
Pleural effusions
Diaphragmatic weakness
Hypoventilation and hypoxemia
Tongue and pharynx can be edematous
Gastrointestinal
Paralytic ileus
Megacolon
Ascites

There may be a mild normocytic anemia. Creatinine kinase and serum total cholesterol are often elevated.

THYROID REPLACEMENT IN MYXEDEMA COMA

Thyroid hormone replacement in myxedema must be adequate to reverse symptoms, but not be excessive, as atrial arrhythmias and cardiac ischemia may result. Unfortunately, there are no randomized prospective trials of treatment. Various treatment protocols with thyroid replacement have been proposed, including T_3 alone, T_3 and T_4 together, and T_4 alone.

It is also not clear if such patients should be treated with intravenous or oral T_4 replacement. We favor using intravenous thyroid replacement initially, as patients may be prone to aspiration because of altered mental status, and ileus may compromise absorption. Many experts prefer to use T_3 in myxedema coma due to its rapid onset, shorter half-life, and the decreased conversion to T_4 to T_3 in myxedema. Our preference is to use T_4 alone, particularly if the diagnosis is questionable and the patient appears stable. For patients in true myxedema coma, administration of both T_4 and T_3 is reasonable to restore thyroid levels quickly. Dosing of T_4 depends on the patient's age, comorbidities, cardiovascular function, and severity of illness. It is estimated that the total body pool of T_4 is 500 μg; many give high doses of T_4, up to 500 μg as a loading dose. We often give 200–250 μg of IV T_4 as an initial loading dose; in older patients and those with comorbid medical conditions, we withhold a loading dose. If a loading dose was given, we start replacement therapy with T_4 24 hours later based on body weight. We change to oral T_4 replacement when the patient is swallowing safely, and adequate absorption can be ensured. In selected patients, therapy with T_3, at a dose of 5–10 μg every 8–12 hours, may be given until clinical improvement is observed, usually for 1–3 days.

GENERAL CARE IN MYXEDEMA COMA

Thyroid hormone replacement alone will not reverse myxedema coma. Patients need vigorous supportive care and treatment of precipitating conditions. All patients should be considered for treatment in the ICU. An infectious workup should be performed, including chest radiograph, blood cultures, urinalysis, and urine culture. Vasopressor support and hydration may be required for hypotension and shock. Due to the potential for arrhythmia and heart failure, cardiovascular status should be closely watched. Hypothermia should be treated. Active rewarming methods and direct heat should be avoided, as this may lead to peripheral vasodilatation and worsen hypotension and shock. Passive rewarming with blankets and other methods is preferred. Noninvasive ventilation or mechanical ventilation may be necessary for patients with hypercapnia and hypoxia. Parenteral nutrition may be required until swallowing is assessed and found to be safe.

Though most cases of myxedema coma are due to primary hypothyroidism (90–95%), missing a case of secondary hypothyroidism will greatly increase the risk of death. Most cases of secondary hypothyroidism are due to pituitary dysfunction, and thyroid and adrenal dysfunction may both be present. If adrenal insufficiency cannot be excluded, glucocorticoids should be administered intravenously at stress dose levels. If possible, a random cortisol should be checked prior to administration, as there may not be time to perform a cosyntropin stimulation test. These patients usually will require formal testing of the adrenal axis at a later date, after glucocorticoids doses are tapered.

DISCHARGE MANAGEMENT

The patient should be discharged on oral levothyroxine. If patients were previously stable on a known levothyroxine dose with which they were not adherent, they should return to that dosage, adjusted if necessary based on new data. In elderly patients, replacement doses of levothyroxine are generally lower than in younger patients. Additional tests may be undertaken on an outpatient basis to identify the etiology of hypothyroidism, if unknown. Thyroid function tests should be repeated six weeks after discharge. Interventions to improve medication adherence should be considered, such as the use of pill boxes and engaging the support from visiting nurses and family members.

THYROID STORM

CASE 150-2

THYROID STORM

A 33-year-old man was brought in from a homeless shelter with a fever of 39°C (102.2F). He had worked in retail sales until losing his job some months ago. On interview, he had pressured speech and loosening of associations, and was anxious to leave the hospital. Workers at the shelter noted that he had been acting erratic recently, and losing weight in spite of a ravenous appetite. The patient was ill during a recent influenza outbreak, and had been taking high doses of aspirin for fever.

On examination, he was thin and diaphoretic, with a regular pulse of 130 beats per minute. The thyroid gland was diffusely enlarged. Hyperreflexia and a fine tremor were present.

Laboratory testing was notable for calcium 11.1 mg/dL (2.78 mmol/liter), TSH <0.02 μU/mL (normal range 0.27–4.62), total T_4 51.1 μg/dL (normal range 4.6–12.0), and total T_3 534 ng/dL (normal range 80–200).

He was admitted to the intensive care unit and treated with methimazole, hydrocortisone, propranolol, saturated solution of potassium iodide, and intravenous fluids. His mental and cardiovascular status normalized over several days, and he was discharged in good condition. He was subsequently treated successfully with radioactive iodine for Graves disease.

Thyroid storm, also called thyrotoxic crisis, decompensated thyrotoxicosis, and accelerated thyrotoxicosis, is a life-threatening form of severe hyperthyroidism. The distinction of thyroid storm from compensated thyrotoxicosis is clinical, as thyroid function test abnormalities are similar in the two conditions. In addition to typical features of hyperthyroidism, such as tachycardia and tremulousness, thyroid storm is accompanied by other features, such as fever, mental status changes, diarrhea, vomiting, hepatitis, arrhythmia, myocardial ischemia, and congestive heart failure. Mortality may be as high as 20–30%.

CAUSES OF THYROID STORM

Graves disease is the most common cause of hyperthyroidism and thyroid storm. It is caused by autoantibodies to the TSH receptor, leading to enhanced production and release of thyroid hormone. Toxic adenoma (hot nodule) and toxic multinodular goiter may also cause hyperthyroidism and thyroid storm. Subacute thyroiditis is a common cause of thyrotoxicosis but rarely leads to thyroid storm. Other rare causes of thyrotoxicosis include TSH-producing pituitary adenomas, trophoblastic tumors that produce HCG, which are able to bind to the TSH receptor, and struma ovarii, a rare ovarian tumor that ectopically produces thyroid hormone.

As with myxedema coma, infection is the most common precipitant of thyroid storm in patients with underlying thyrotoxicosis. Other precipitants include trauma, myocardial infarction, diabetic ketoacidosis, pulmonary embolism, surgery, pregnancy, stroke, emotional distress, poor adherence to antithyroid medications, sympathomimetic drugs such as pseudoephredine, and salicylates, which displace thyroid hormone from binding proteins. Iodine loads from radiocontrast agents or amiodarone also predispose to thyroid storm. In the past, hyperthyroid patients undergoing thyroidectomy were at risk of thyroid storm due to release of thyroid hormones after thyroidal manipulation, in addition to the acute stress of surgery. This is currently rare because of pretreatment with antithyroidal medications. Uncommonly, patients go into thyroid storm after receiving radioactive iodine to treat underlying hyperthyroidism, probably from excessive thyroid hormone release from radiation thyroiditis.

CLINICAL MANIFESTATIONS OF THYROID STORM

Features of thyroid storm are summarized in **Table 150-3**. Patients should be questioned about common symptoms of thyrotoxicosis, including weight loss despite ample appetite, poor energy, difficulty sleeping, heat intolerance, hyperdefecation, palpitations, chest pain, anxiety, emotional labilitiy, and diplopia (from ophthalmopathy). Additionally, a history of past thyrotoxicosis, recent radioactive iodine treatment, and recent surgery should be sought.

TABLE 150-3 Potential Clinical Manifestations and Exam Findings in Thyroid Storm

Fever (can have hyperpyrexia, temperatures > 105°F)
Thyroid
Nodule
Diffuse enlargement
Ophthalmologic
Ophthalmopathy
Neurological
Anxiety, psychosis, or coma
Seizure
Hyperreflexia
Skin
Moist
Pretibial myxedema
Cardiovascular
Sinus tachycardia
Hyperdynamic precordium
Atrial fibrillation
Other arrhythmias
Congestive heart failure
Gastrointestinal
Nausea/vomiting
Diarrhea
Severe abdominal pain
Jaundice
Hepatosplenomegaly/vascular congestion

TABLE 150-4 Diagnostic Criteria for Thyroid Storm

Thermoregulatory dysfunction		**Cardiovascular dysfunction**	
Temperature		Tachycardia	
99–99.9	5	90–109	5
100–100.9	10	101–119	10
101–101.9	15	120–129	15
102–102.9	20	130–139	20
103–103.9	25	≥ 140	25
≥ 104	30		
Central nervous system effects		**Congestive heart failure**	
Absent	0	Absent	0
Mild	10	Mild	5
Agitation		Pedal edema	
Moderate	20	Moderate	10
Delirium		Bibasilar rales	
Psychosis		Severe	15
Extreme lethargy		Pulmonary edema	
Severe	30		
Seizure			
Coma			
Gastroentestinal-hepatic dysfunction		**Atrial fibrillation**	
Absent	0	Absent	0
Moderate	10	Present	10
Diarrhea		**Precipitating event**	
Nausea/vomiting		Absent	0
Abdominal pain		Present	10
Severe	20		
Unexplained jaundice			

A score of 45 or greater is highly suggestive of thyroid storm; a score of 25–44 is suggestive of impending storm, and a score below 25 is unlikely to represent thyroid storm. (Adapted, with permission, from Burch HB and Wartofsky L. *Endocrinol Metab Clin North Am.* 1993;22:263–277.)

On physical examination, a goiter with possible bruit, ophthalmopathy, and rarely pretibial myxedema will help make the clinical diagnosis of Graves disease. Thyroid exam may reveal nodules or diffuse enlargement. Skin may be moist. On cardiovascular exam, the patient may have sinus tachycardia and a hyperdynamic precordium. Atrial fibrillation is present in 10–35% of thyrotoxic individuals. Congestive heart failure, persistent arrhythmias, and cardiovascular collapse may be present. The patient may have neurologic and psychiatric pathology, including anxiety, mania, psychosis, seizure, or coma. Muscles may be weak and wasted, and reflexes are brisk. In thyroid storm, there is also fever, often with hyperpyrexia in excess of 40.5°C (105°F). Severe nausea, vomiting, and abdominal pain may be present. Jaundice, hepatosplenomegaly from vascular congestion, and hepatic necrosis are seen in severe cases.

Elderly patients with thyroid storm may have a clinical picture dominated by apathetic thyrotoxicosis where typical hyperadrenergic symptoms are blunted. The major clinical features are apathy, depression, somnolence, and coma, in addition to more typical symptoms of hyperthyroidism such as weight loss, weakness, and arrhythmias. Apathetic thyrotoxicosis and thyroid storm should be in the differential diagnosis of altered mental status and coma of unclear cause.

Due to the difficulty in diagnosis of thyroid storm, Burch and Wartofksy developed a point system to help distinguish severe thyrotoxicosis from thyroid storm (**Table 150-4**). Diagnostic criteria include fever, central nervous system effects, gastrointestinal and hepatic dysfunction, tachycardia and atrial fibrillation, the presence and degree of congestive heart failure, and the presence of a precipitating factor. A score of 45 or greater is highly suggestive of thyroid storm. However, the Burch-Wartofsky score has not been validated prospectively.

LABORATORY FINDINGS IN THYROID STORM

As above, thyroid function tests are similar in the patient with compensated thyrotoxicosis and the patient with thyroid storm; only the clinical manifestations distinguish the two. TSH is suppressed, except in the extremely rare case of a thyrotropin-secreting pituitary adenoma. Both T_4 and T_3 are markedly elevated. The T_3 may be lower than expected due to concurrent nonthyroidal illness syndrome. Because TBG may be low in the patient with thyroid storm, and other inhibitors of protein binding may be present, the response to therapy is best followed by checking total T_4 with either TBG or resin uptake, yielding a free thyroxine index. The TSH may remain suppressed for months, so this is not followed acutely. Other laboratory findings may include hyperglycemia, due to increased glycogenolysis and catecholamine-mediated inhibition of insulin release. Mild hypercalcemia and elevated alkaline phosphatase occur, perhaps due to bone resorption provoked by thyroid hormone. Elevation of liver transaminases and total bilirubin occurs. There may be a slight

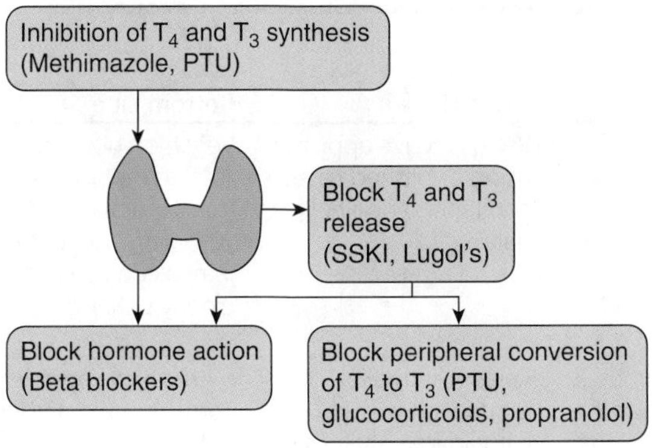

Figure 150-3 *Treatment of thyroid storm.*

leukocytosis with left shift, even in the absence of infection. While hepatic metabolism of cortisol is accelerated, and conversion of biologically inactive cortisone to active cortisol is decreased, there is also increased synthesis of cortisol, and adrenal function is usually normal. In long standing thyrotoxicosis, adrenal cortical reserve is impaired. Diagnostic nuclear scanning of the thyroid should be delayed until the patient is stable.

TREATMENT OF HYPERTHYROIDISM IN THYROID STORM

In thyroid storm, one must treat the underlying precipitant, use supportive care to treat the multiorgan and systemic complications, and decrease circulating thyroid hormone levels. Patients need intensive monitoring and likely should be in the ICU.

Treatment of hyperthyroidism in thyroid storm or accelerated thyrotoxicosis involves four steps (**Figure 150-3**): suppression of thyroid hormone synthesis; preventing T_4 and T_3 release from the thyroid; inhibition of peripheral conversion of T_4 to T_3; and blocking the action of thyroid hormone on target organs.

Thionamides, such as propylthiouricil (PTU) and methimazole, inhibit thyroid hormone synthesis, and they may also have immunomodulatory effects. Because PTU inhibits peripheral conversion of T_4 to T_3 and methimazole does not, PTU has been favored for treatment of thyroid storm in the past. However, due to the longer half-life of methimazole and the use of other agents in thyroid storm that prevent peripheral conversion of T_4 to T_3, many clinicians now prefer methimazole, especially as PTU has more side effects, especially hepatic. Our practice is to use either high doses of methimazole, typically 20–30 mg every 6 hours, or PTU 200–400 mg every 4–6 hours orally or through the nasogastric tube, until the patient's thyroid function and clinical condition is improving. We then decrease the antithyroidal medication dosage accordingly. Patients who cannot take oral medications, or who do not have a nasogastric tube, may be treated with intravenous methimazole or PTU in enema or suppository form, as described in case reports. Major side effects of the thionamides include rash or urticarial reactions in 5%, agranulocytosis in 0.2–0.4%, and liver function abnormalities in approximately 0.2%.

Iodine is given to prevent stored T_4 and T_3 release from the thyroid. In high doses, iodine inhibits iodine organification in the thyroid (Wolff-Chaikoff effect). Iodine may be given as a saturated solution of potassium iodide (SSKI), up to 5 drops every 6 hours, or Lugol's solution, up to 8 drops every 8 hours. Radiocontrast iodine agents can also be used orally but because of the paucity of data we prefer SSKI or Lugol's. Iodine should be given only *after* antithyroidal medication has been started, waiting at least one hour, because of the potential for patient deterioration from increased iodination of thyroid hormone. In patients allergic to iodine, lithium may be given at a dose of 300 mg every 8 hours. This is rarely done, as lithium levels require close monitoring, and alternative agents are usually available. In patients who require an antiarrhythmic, the use of amiodarone may be desirable. Amiodarone is 37.3% iodine by weight, and inhibits thyroid hormone release and also blocks conversion of T_4 to T_3.

Peripheral conversion of T_4 to T_3 should also be inhibited in thyroid storm. This may be accomplished with PTU, as noted above. Glucocorticoids are also effective. We prefer hydrocortisone 100 mg every 8 hours, with dexamethasone 4 mg every 12 hours as an alternative. As steroid breakdown is accelerated in thyrotoxicosis, high doses of hydrocortisone may need to be given for several days prior to tapering. This has the added benefit of treating the relative adrenal insufficiency that may be present. Iopanoic acid, which is no longer available in the United States, is another potent inhibitor of peripheral conversion of T_4 to T_3.

Beta-blockade is useful to antagonize the effects of T_3 on the heart and sympathetic nervous system. Propranolol is most often used, as it also inhibits T_4 to T_3 conversion. An intravenous loading dose up to 1 mg can be given, followed by oral doses of 60–80 mg every 4–6 hours, with appropriate titration. Some authorities prefer intravenous esmolol, due to its short half-life and ability to be rapidly titrated. Cardioselective beta-blockers can also be used, such as atenolol and metoprolol.

Rarely used therapies include potassium perchlorate, which is a competitive inhibitor of iodine transport. It has fallen out of favor because of its side effect profile, which includes aplastic anemia and nephrotic syndrome. Cholestyramine reduces enterohepatic thyroid hormone absorption, but may also interfere with absorption of a number of other medications. Treatments of last resort include plasmapheresis or emergency thyroidectomy, which is avoided if at all possible because of substantial perioperative mortality.

TREATMENT OF SYSTEMIC DECOMPENSATION

Besides lowering thyroid hormone levels, the multiorgan and systemic complications need to be treated. Hyperpyrexia and fever should be treated with acetaminophen, as aspirin at high dosages can displace thyroid hormone from TBG, increasing fT_4. Cooling blankets, alcohol sponging, and ice packs may also be needed. Fluids should be aggressively repleted, as sensible and insensible losses can be extensive. Intravenous fluids with dextrose help to replenish glycogen stores. Cardiac arrhythmias and congestive heart failure may be present and need aggressive treatment. If arrhythmias are present, amiodarone may be a preferred therapy, as its high iodine content and ability to block thyroid hormone release and peripheral conversion are beneficial side effects. Underlying precipitants should be identified and treated, and infection should be excluded by performing a chest radiograph, urinalysis, and blood and urine cultures.

DISCHARGE MANAGEMENT

Priorities at discharge for patients with thyroid storm include simplifying therapy to optimize adherence, and arranging for definitive diagnosis and therapy on an outpatient basis. The patient should be switched to methimazole if not already on it, due to its lower frequency of dosing, higher compliance rate, and better side effect profile. If the cause of hyperthyroidism is unclear, a radioactive iodine uptake scan should be done as an outpatient, if not already performed. The patient should be discharged on a daily dose of methimazole and beta-blockers as indicated, and outpatient follow-up with endocrinology should be coordinated. Patients hospitalized for complicated thyrotoxicosis are more likely to be of lower socioeconomic class, uninsured, or covered by Medicaid. Barriers to

TABLE 150-5 Evidence-based Medicine: Thyroid Emergencies

Paper	Methodology	Results	Limitations	Bottom Line
Yamamoto T, Fukuyama J, Fujiyoshi A. *Thyroid.* 1999;9:1167–1174.	Retrospective study of factors associated with mortality in myxedema coma, with 8 original cases and 82 cases reported in the literature	Older age, cardiac complications, and high-dose thyroid hormone replacement ($T_4 \geq 500$ µg/d or $T_3 \geq 75$ µg/d) were significantly associated with death within one month of treatment	Retrospective approach using published cases and limited original data	Very high doses of thyroid replacement may be associated with worse outcomes in myxedema coma in elderly patients
Dutta P, Bhansali A, Masoodi SR, et al. *Crit Care.* 2008;12(1):R1.	Study of predictors of outcome in 23 patients with myxedema coma from a tertiary referral institution in India	87% of patients were women, 65% presented in winter, and 74% had infection (usually pneumonia); mortality was 52%; predictors of mortality included hypotension, bradycardia, need for mechanical ventilation, unresponsive hypothermia, sepsis, low Glasgow coma score, and high APACHE II score; outcome did not differ according to route of levothyroxine replacement (oral vs. intravenous)	Relatively small, retrospective study with limited abilities to detect differences in outcome	Mortality of myxedema coma is high; method of thyroid hormone replacement did not appear to affect outcome
Arlot S, Debussche X, Lalau JD, et al. *Intensive Care Med.* 1991;17:16–18.	Retrospective study of clinical and laboratory response of seven patients with myxedema coma, all older women, to either intravenous or oral thyroid hormone replacement	All patients received high loading doses of T_4, either intravenously or orally, followed by daily maintenance doses; laboratory improvement in patients receiving oral therapy lagged behind the clinical response, which occurred within 24–72 hours. In one patient with myxedema ileus, absorption of oral T_4 was minimally affected	Small, retrospective study	The oral route of replacement of T_4 seems to be effective in many patients with myxedema coma, and is associated with a more gradual rise in serum T_3, which might be beneficial in elderly patients
Sherman SI, Simonson L, Ladenson PW. *Am J Med.* 1996;101: 192–198.	Case control study of 59 patients admitted to an urban teaching hospital with complicated thyrotoxicosis, compared to 118 hyperthyroid outpatients	Compared to uncomplicated controls, patients with complicated thyrotoxicosis were more likely to be uninsured or covered by Medicaid, to be < 30 or > 50 years old, and to have serum T_4 concentrations greater than twice the upper limit of normal	Retrospective study design; findings may not apply to other patient populations	Difficulties with access to medical care may be an important factor in the development of thyrotoxicosis

care, whether social, economic, logistical, or psychiatric, should be identified in the discharge process, and steps taken to ameliorate them (**Table 150-5**).

SUGGESTED READINGS

Adler SM, Wartofsky L. The nonthyroidal illness syndrome. *Endocrinol Metab Clin North Am.* 2007;36:657–672.

De Groot, LJ. Dangerous dogmas in medicine: the nonthyroidal illness syndrome. *J Clin Endocrinol Metab.* 1999;84:151–164.

Hodak SP, Huang C, Clarke D, Burman KD, Jonklaas J, Janicic-Kharic N. Intravenous methimazole in the treatment of refractory hyperthyroidism. *Thyroid.* 2006;16:691–695.

Nayak B, Burman K. Thyrotoxicosis and thyroid storm. *Endocrinol Metab Clin North Am.* 2006;35:663–686.

Pingitore A, Galli E, Barison A, et al. Acute effects of triiodothyronine (T_3) replacement therapy in patients with chronic heart failure and low-T_3 syndrome: a randomized, placebo-controlled study. *J Clin Endocrinol Metab.* 2008;93:1351–1358.

Tsatsoulis A, Johnson EO, Kalogera CH, Seferiadis K, Tsolas O. The effect of thyrotoxicosis on adrenocortical reserve. *Eur J Endocrinol.* 2000;142:231–235.

Walter RM, Jr., Bartle WR. Rectal administration of propylthiouracil in the treatment of Graves disease. *Am J Med.* 1990;88:69–70.

Wartofsky L. Myxedema coma. *Endocrinol Metab Clin North Am.* 2006;35:687–698.

CHAPTER 151

Adrenal Insufficiency

Elaine C. Lin Liew, MD, FRCA
Ann S. Sheehy, MD, MS
Kenneth E. Wood, DO, FCCP
Douglas B. Coursin, MD, FCCP

Key Clinical Questions

1. What are normal and stress production of endogenous corticocosteroids?
2. What are the types of adrenal insufficiency?
3. Which patients are at high risk of adrenal insufficiency or critical illness-related corticosteroid insufficiency and therefore may benefit from physiologic or pharmacologic steroid treatment of their illnesses?
4. For those patients who need corticosteroid supplementation, which agents should be used, and for how long?

INTRODUCTION

Adrenal insufficiency (AI) was described by Thomas Addison in 1855 as a fatal disease caused by tuberculous adrenalitis and adrenal gland failure. In 1949, the synthesis of cortisone resulted in life-saving therapy for Addison disease. However, this was shortly followed by reports of patient deaths from presumed adrenal crisis due to abrupt cortisone withdrawal in the perioperative period. These reports resulted in a new standard of administration of high doses of supplemental corticosteroids during periods of physical stress, although this practice may not be universally warranted.

Primary AI (Addison disease) refers to primary adrenal gland dysfunction. It has a prevalence of 40–110 cases per million people and an incidence of six cases per million people per year. Secondary AI denotes pituitary disease with adrenocorticotropic hormone (ACTH) hormone deficiency. The prevalence of secondary AI is approximately 150–280 per million. Hypothalamic dysfunction is responsible for tertiary AI. It usually arises after abrupt withdrawal or reduction in corticocosteroid dose, in the setting of chronic exogenous corticosteroids, and is reasonably common in the hospital setting, although the exact prevalence is unknown (**Table 151-1**).

PRACTICE POINT

- Common scenarios for AI in the hospital include patients on long-term glucocorticoid therapy not receiving adequate replacement or supplemental glucocorticoids during major illness, and critically ill patients with sepsis. Other patients at risk include those with a history of brain injury or intracranial aneurysm.

PATHOPHYSIOLOGY

The adrenal gland consists of a cortex that produces steroid hormones and a medulla that produces catecholamines. The adrenal cortex is divided into three layers. The outermost layer, the zona glomerulosa, produces mineralocorticoids, primarily aldosterone. The middle layer, the zona fasciculata, produces glucocorticoids, primarily cortisol and to a lesser extent, cortisone. The zona reticularis, the innermost layer, produces adrenal androgens.

The release of glucocorticoids is controlled by the hypothalamic-pituitary-adrenal (HPA) axis. The hypothalamus secretes corticotropin-releasing hormone (CRH), which acts on the pituitary to produce adrenocorticotropic hormone (ACTH). ACTH stimulates the adrenal glands to produce cortisol, which inhibits further production of CRH. Cortisol secretion is diurnal, with the highest levels in the morning and lowest around midnight. Daily endogenous secretion of glucocorticoid is equivalent to 5–7 mg/day of oral prednisone or 20–30 mg/day of hydrocortisone (Table 151-5). During stress, cortisol synthesis can increase tenfold.

All cells in the human body have glucocorticoid receptors, reflecting the integral role of glucocorticoids in physiologic homeostasis. Glucocorticoids regulate carbohydrate, lipid and amino acid metabolism, facilitate catecholamine production and action, and maintain cardiovascular integrity, with additional effects on wound healing, the immune system and the nervous system.

TABLE 151-1 Primary, Secondary, and Tertiary Adrenal Insufficiency

Type	Incidence	Features	Etiologies
Primary	Prevalence: 40–110 cases/million Incidence: 6 cases/million/year	ACTH-independent > 90% of destruction of adrenal cortex Loss of mineralocorticoid and glucocorticoid production Patients may be hyperpigmented Requires lifetime therapy	Autoimmune ~80% of cases in United States Isolated autoimmune adrenalitis APS 1 – associated with hypoparathyroidism, chronic mucocutaneous candidiasis APS 2 – associated with thyroid disease, type 1 diabetes mellitus Infection Tuberculous AIDS: CMV, MAC, Kaposi sarcoma 30% of patients with AIDS develop AI Fungal infections (histoplasmosis, coccidiomycosis, blastomycosis) Inflammation Cancer Metastases from breast, lung, and melanoma may infiltrate and replace normal adrenal tissue Acute Addisonian crisis Infectious – meningococcemia with purpura fulminans (Waterhouse-Friederichsen syndrome); sepsis with other bacteria Stress Hemorrhage Shock Drug-induced adrenal insufficiency Mitotane, ketoconazole, suramin, etomidate, aminoglutethimide
Secondary	Prevalence: 150–280 per million	Pituitary disease that interferes with ACTH secretion Clinical features due to loss of glucocorticoid function Intact mineralocorticoid function Rarely hypovolemic, more commonly hypoglycemic	Panhypopituitarism Pituitary tumors, craniopharyngomas Infection Infiltrative diseases Head trauma Intracranial artery aneurysms Sheehan syndrome Isolated ACTH deficiency Rare, likely autoimmune process
Tertiary	Most common form	Processes that interfere with hypothalamic CRH secretion	Abrupt cessation of glucocorticoid therapy Correction of Cushing syndrome

APS, autoimmune polyglandular syndrome 1 (APS-1); MAC, mycobacterium avium complex.

CAUSES OF ADRENAL INSUFFICIENCY

PRIMARY ADRENAL INSUFFICIENCY

Primary AI arises when greater than 90% of adrenal tissue is destroyed, resulting in loss of glucocorticoid and mineralocorticoid function. Absence of glucocorticoids result in an increase in ACTH and melanocyte-stimulating hormone levels, while the absence of aldosterone results in increased renin levels.

Autoimmune adrenalitis

In developed nations, 80% of primary AI is due to autoimmune disease, which may occur in isolation or as a manifestation of a polyglandular autoimmune syndrome. Autoimmune polyendocrine syndrome type I (APS-I) underlies up to 15% of autoimmune adrenalitis. It usually presents with hypoparathyroidism or chronic mucocutaneous candidiasis during childhood, with adrenal insufficiency developing by 10 to 15 years of age. It is also frequently associated with primary hypogonadism, childhood alopecia, and malabsorption. It is caused by mutations in the autoimmune regulator (*AIRE*) gene, inherited in an autosomal recessive fashion. Mutations in *AIRE* interfere with the normal culling of autoreactive T cells, leading to the eventual autoimmune destruction of endocrine glands.

Autoimmune polyglandular syndrome type II (APS-II) is more prevalent than APS-I, and has autosomal dominant transmission with incomplete penetrance. In half the cases, AI is the first manifestation, often associated with the later development of autoimmune thyroid disease and type 1 diabetes mellitus. The clinical spectrum may also include hypogonadism, vitiligo (seen in up to 15% of primary AI), myasthenia gravis, rheumatoid arthritis, antiphosholipid antibody syndrome, and celiac disease.

Infectious adrenalitis

Tuberculosis is the most common cause of primary AI worldwide, and was the cause of adrenal failure in most of Addison's original patients. Adrenal involvement in tuberculosis is not common except in disseminated disease, in which it is found in up to 50% of cases. Although recovery of adrenal function is possible after appropriate antituberculous treatment, it often does not occur. AIDS is currently the principal infectious cause of AI in the United States. Causes of AI in AIDS patients include cytomegalovirus, *Mycobacterium avium-intracellulare*, cryptococcosis, and metastatic Kaposi sarcoma. Other factors may contribute to AI in HIV patients, such as peripheral resistance to glucocorticoid action from chronic inflammation, or use of the appetite stimulant megestrol acetate, which has intrinsic glucocorticoid activity and suppresses the hypothalamic-pituitary-adrenal (HPA) axis. The endemic mycoses, such as histoplasmosis, coccidoidomycosis, and blastomycosis, may rarely cause granulomatous disease of the adrenals severe enough to cause AI.

The adrenal glands may be infiltrated by metastatic disease, most commonly from lung, breast, stomach, or colon cancer, melanoma, or lymphoma. However, metastases rarely destroy enough adrenal tissue for AI to manifest.

Hemorrhagic infarction

The adrenal gland is vascular and somewhat prone to hemorrhage. Bilateral adrenal hemorrhage may cause AI. It may result from meningococcal septic shock with disseminated intravascular coagulation (Waterhouse-Friderichsen syndrome), as well as overwhelming sepsis with other organisms, including Staphylococcus aureus, *Streptococcus pyogenes, Streptococcus pneumoniae, Pseudomonas aeruginosa*, and *Escherichia coli*. Other risk factors for adrenal hemorrhage include anticoagulants, coagulopathy, trauma, carcinoma, adrenal vein thrombosis, pregnancy, and any acute medical or surgical illness. Patients often present with back pain and hypotension; CT imaging reveals enlarged adrenal glands with high attenuation.

Drugs

Drugs cause AI by various mechanisms. Etomidate, ketoconazole, metyrapone, and suramin inhibit cortisol synthesis. However, AI only becomes evident in patients with limited pituitary or adrenal reserve, and those previously on glucocorticoid therapy. Phenytoin, rifampin, and barbiturates accelerate the metabolism of cortisol, as well as the metabolism of synthetic steroids, such as dexamethasone and fludrocortisone.

Miscellaneous

Rare causes of primary AI include adrenoleukodystrophy, congenital adrenal hypoplasia, glucocorticoid insensitivity, and defective cholesterol metabolism.

SECONDARY ADRENAL INSUFFICIENCY

Any process that interferes with pituitary ACTH secretion may lead to secondary AI. Unlike primary AI, mineralocorticoid secretion is preserved because it is under the control of the renin-angiotensin system. Another distinguishing characteristic of secondary AI is decreased or absent plasma ACTH levels, compared to normal or elevated ACTH levels in primary AI. The most frequent cause of secondary AI is panhypopituitarism, and less commonly isolated ACTH deficiency.

Panhypopituitarism

Panhypopituitarism may result from pituitary tumors, traumatic brain injury, intracranial aneurysm, and pituitary surgery or radiotherapy. Up to 30% of patients with head trauma experience pituitary dysfunction months or years after the initial insult. Less often, panhypopituitarism can be caused by infection (tuberculosis, histoplasmosis), infiltrative diseases, and autoimmune lymphocytic hypophysitis. Although pituitary metastases are frequently found in patients with disseminated cancer, these metastases rarely impede hormone secretion. Sheehan syndrome is massive peripartum blood loss precipitating hypovolemic shock and anterior pituitary infarction. Pituitary apoplexy from hemorrhage into an enlarging pituitary adenoma may also lead to panhypopituitarism during or after pregnancy.

Isolated ACTH deficiency

Isolated ACTH deficiency is a rare cause of secondary AI and may have an autoimmune origin. It is frequently associated with autoantibodies to pituitary cells and with other autoimmune endocrine disorders, most commonly thyroid disease.

TERTIARY ADRENAL INSUFFICIENCY

Tertiary AI occurs due to any process that involves the hypothalamus and interferes with the secretion of CRH and subsequent ACTH release. The most common cause of tertiary AI is abrupt cessation of glucocorticoid therapy.

Chronic glucocorticoid therapy

Prolonged corticosteroid therapy in excess of 5 mg/day of prednisone or its equivalent suppresses CRH and ACTH secretion, resulting in adrenal atrophy. Tertiary iatrogenic AI may then become apparent with abrupt cessation of exogenous glucocorticoid therapy, or when inadequate supplementation is provided in times of physiologic stress. There is inconsistent data to accurately predict the degree of adrenal suppression that occurs with exogenous glucocorticoid therapy. However, a reduced response to exogenous ACTH has been reported after discontinuation of oral prednisone 25 mg twice a day for as brief a period as five days. Patients who receive 5 mg/day or less of prednisone appear to have an intact HPA axis. It may require more than a year for the HPA axis to recover after cessation of exogenous glucocorticoids.

CLINICAL PRESENTATION

The diagnosis of AI may be delayed because signs and symptoms are nonspecific, and frequently misleading (**Table 151-2**). Most patients encounter several physicians prior to diagnosis, and many are only diagnosed after presenting with adrenal crisis. Recognition of patients at risk facilitates diagnosis. Common scenarios for AI in the hospital include patients on long-term glucocorticoid therapy not receiving adequate replacement or supplemental glucocorticoids during major illness, and critically ill patients with sepsis. Other patients at risk include those with a history of brain injury or intracranial aneurysm.

Clinical features of AI include weakness, fatigue, anorexia, nausea, diarrhea, abdominal pain, weight loss, and hypotension. Hypotension occurs as a result of depressed myocardial contractility, reduced responsiveness to catecholamines, and hypovolemia with hyponatremia. Along with the above signs and symptoms, patients with Addison disease or primary adrenal failure exhibit salt craving and a characteristic diffuse hyperpigmentation with accentuation in

TABLE 151-2 Clinical Features of Adrenal Insufficiency

Glucocorticoid Deficiency	Mineralocortocoid Deficiency	Adrenal Androgen Deficiency
Fatigue	Salt craving (primary AI)	Dry and itchy skin
Anorexia, weight loss	Dizziness	Loss of libido
Abdominal pain	Hypotension, orthostatic symptoms	Loss of pubic hair
Nausea, vomiting	Hyponatremia	
Myalgia	Hyperkalemia (primary AI)	
Hypotension		
Anemia, lymphocytosis, eosinophilia		
Hypercalcemia		
Hypoglycemia		
Increased TSH (primary AI)		

the palmar folds, scars, and oral mucosa (**Figures 151-1** and **151-2**). Vitiligo may be present in up to 15% of patients, particularly in those with autoimmune-related adrenal failure. Low sodium and increased potassium are associated with mineralocorticoid deficiency. Adrenal crisis is life-threatening, and typically presents with severe, refractory hypotension. In addition to other signs of AI, hypoglycemia, fever, confusion, or coma may also be present.

DIAGNOSIS

PRIMARY AI

CASE 151-1

A 33-year-old previously healthy female presented to the emergency room with several days of diarrhea, general malaise, and weakness. Family history was significant for thyroid disease in her mother and sister. Her initial blood pressure was 78/47 mm Hg, with a low-grade fever of 100.5°F. Physical examination revealed a slightly hypovolemic female in mild distress, with no other obvious findings. Laboratory studies demonstrated leukocytosis of 15,3000/mm^3, with mild eosinophilia, creatinine 1.6 mg/dL, potassium 5.8 mmol/L, and sodium 124 mmol/L. Blood, urine, and stool cultures were obtained. She received 3 liters of normal saline, with a blood pressure of 82/50 mm Hg after rehydration. Empiric antibiotics were started, and she was admitted to the hospital. A cortisol level drawn at 7:00 AM the following morning was 6 μg/dL. Cosyntropin stimulation test with 250 μg was performed, and cortisol rose to 8 μg/dL 60 minutes following injection of cosyntropin. ACTH was 138 pg/mL (normal 7–69 pg/mL), confirming primary adrenal insufficiency. Intravenous hydrocortisone was initiated, with dramatic improvement in the patient's blood pressure and sense of well-being.

While gastroenteritis with dehydration would be the most common diagnosis in an otherwise healthy young woman with this history, her electrolyte abnormalities, leukocytosis, eosinophilia, mild fever, and refractory hypotension suggest adrenal failure. Hospitalized patients with suspected AI should have a morning cortisol drawn between 7:00 and 9:00 AM. Cortisol values less than 3 μg/dL or greater than 18–19 μg/dL essentially rule in or out the disease, respectively. Patients with cortisol between 3 and 18 μg/dL should receive a 250 μg cosyntropin (ACTH) stimulation test. A cortisol level drawn 30–60 minutes following injection of cosyntropin should be greater than 18 μg/dL, with lower values indicating adrenal insufficiency. (Of note, the cortisol rise of less than 9 μg/dl sometimes used to diagnose AI in the critical care literature is not used in noncritically ill patients.)

ACTH levels should be drawn to differentiate primary AI from secondary and tertiary AI, with high values suggesting primary AI. Abdominal CT may be performed in patients with primary AI of unclear etiology; adrenal glands affected by autoimmune disease are usually small and atrophic. Brain MRI may be considered for those with suspected secondary AI.

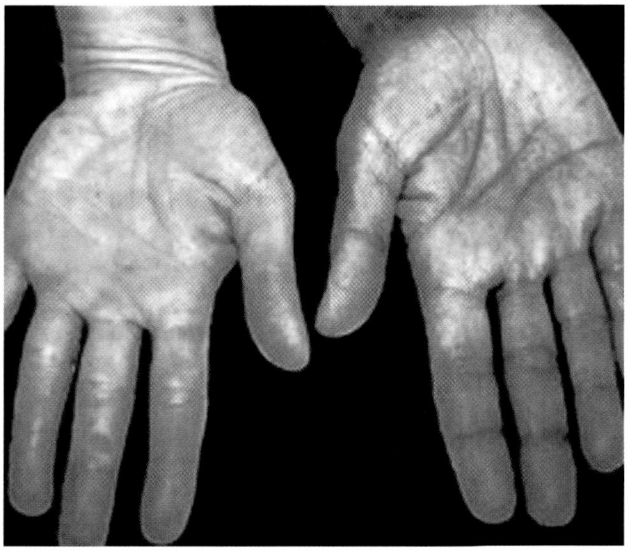

Figure 151-1 *Hyperpigmentation of the palmar creases in primary adrenal insufficiency is seen in the hand at the right, with the hand of an unaffected individual at left. Hyperpigmentation and freckling in primary adrenal insufficiency is more marked in sun-exposed areas, gums, buccal mucosae, axillae, pressure points, genitals, nail beds, nipples, areolae, and recent scars. (Reproduced, with permission, from Wolff K, Goldsmith LA, Katz SI, et al. Fitzpatrick's Dermatology in General Medicine. 7th ed. New York: McGraw-Hill, 2008. Fig. 152-16.)*

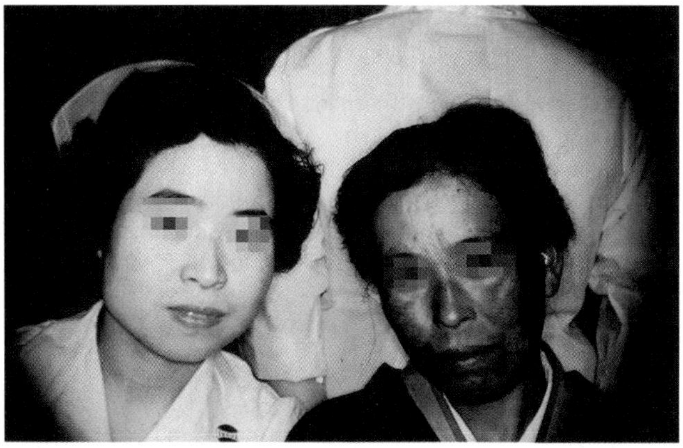

Figure 151-2 *Addison disease. Japanese patient in whom tuberculosis was the etiology of the adrenal insufficiency. Note the striking contrast in the skin color of a normal Japanese female nurse compared to the diffuse brown hyperpigmentation in the patient with Addison disease. (Reproduced, with permission, from Fitzpatrick TB, Johnson RA, Polano MK, et al. Fitzpatrick's Color Atlas and Synopsis of Clinical Dermatology: Common and Serious Diseases. 2nd ed. New York: McGraw-Hill, 1992. Fig. 647.)*

Patients with confirmed or suspected acute adrenal crisis who are hypotensive and symptomatic should be given 100 mg of hydrocortisone intravenously immediately, with 100–300 mg of hydrocortisone given in divided doses daily until symptoms and signs normalize. In patients with suspected adrenal crisis, treatment should not be delayed until confirmatory test results are available. However, caution should be used in interpreting morning cortisol values in patients already started on exogenous corticosteroids, as ACTH and cortisol production will be appropriately blunted in patients without adrenal dysfunction. As well, replacement corticosteroids may be metabolized to plasma cortisol, resulting in a false normal or elevated value. Replacement therapy with dexamethasone should be considered until ACTH stimulation testing is performed. Although dexamethasone depresses basal cortisol levels, it is less likely to inhibit the cortisol response to an ACTH challenge.

PRACTICE POINT

- Adrenal crisis is more likely in patients with primary adrenal insufficiency than secondary or tertiary adrenal insufficiency. Patients with primary adrenal insufficiency are both glucocorticoid and mineralocorticoid deficient. By contrast, most patients with secondary or tertiary adrenal insufficiency have intact aldosterone synthesis, and usually require only glucocorticoid replacement.

SECONDARY AND TERTIARY AI

In secondary (pituitary origin) or tertiary (hypothalamic origin) adrenal insufficiency, serum cortisol and ACTH are both low when these are measured simultaneously in the absence of exogenous glucocorticoids. This may be confirmed with the 48-hour ACTH stimulation test. Patients with secondary or tertiary adrenal insufficiency should boost cortisol production with prolonged ACTH dosing, whereas no effect on cortisol production will be seen in those with primary AI. Secondary and tertiary adrenal insufficiency can be distinguished by the CRH test. Administration of CRH to patients with tertiary AI will result in a surge in ACTH levels, but will not boost ACTH levels in patients with secondary AI. (This distinction usually does not affect patient management.)

TERTIARY AI FROM CHRONIC EXOGENOUS CORTICOSTEROIDS

CASE 151-2

A 67-year-old man with a medical history of hypertension and oxygen-dependent chronic obstructive pulmonary disease (COPD) presented to his primary care physician for evaluation of increasing dyspnea, fever, and productive cough, as well as generalized weakness and lack of energy. He has had approximately four clinic visits a year for COPD exacerbations necessitating oral steroids, with use of an inhaled corticosteroid between exacerbations. Examination revealed a temperature of 101.2°F, blood pressure 92/50 mm Hg, heart rate 110 beats/minute, and an oxygen saturation of 84% on his usual home oxygen of 2 liters. On chest auscultation, breath sounds were distant, but without audible wheezing. Crackles and egophony were heard at the left lung base. A chest radiograph revealed hyperinflation, with left lower lobe consolidation. He was admitted to the hospital, and antibiotics were begun. After 48 hours, his oxygen requirement was reduced, but he continued to complain of fatigue, and his blood pressure remained low, despite holding his oral antihypertensive agents. Morning cortisol was 2.5 μg/dL, indicating adrenal insufficiency. Intravenous steroids were initiated, with marked improvement in symptoms and signs.

This patient developed tertiary AI from sequential courses of oral corticosteroids, in combination with his daily corticosteroid inhaler. Symptoms became manifest in the setting of pneumonia. While patients on daily oral glucocorticoids are most likely to develop tertiary AI, patients on intermittent corticosteroids are also at risk for tertiary AI, as are patients on chronic inhaled corticosteroids, potent topical corticosteroids, and those receiving frequent musculoskeletal corticosteroid injections. The diagnosis of tertiary AI is supported by the finding of a low morning cortisol or abnormal ACTH stimulation test.

MANAGEMENT

ACUTE ADRENAL INSUFFICIENCY

Acute AI should be treated immediately. Diagnostic testing must not delay treatment of the patient in adrenal crisis. Management should proceed as follows:

1. Draw blood for serum cortisol, renin, ACTH, and chemistries.
2. Fluid resuscitation: 1–3 liters 0.9% saline (or 5% dextrose in 0.9% saline if hypoglycemic), titrated to volume status and urine output. Avoid hypotonic saline, which will worsen hyponatremia.
3. 100 mg IV hydrocortisone or 4 mg IV dexamethasone (if performing a cosyntropin stimulation).
4. 250 μg cosyntropin stimulation test, with 30 minute cortisol level if dexamethasone administered.
5. IV hydrocortisone 200 mg continuous infusion over 24 hours, or 50 mg every six hours. In uncomplicated cases, an oral maintenance dose should commence after taper of IV therapy over 1–3 days.
6. Diagnostic evaluation to determine the cause of AI.

CHRONIC ADRENAL INSUFFICIENCY

In chronic AI, glucocorticoid replacement is usually given in morning and evening doses to mimic diurnal cortisol secretion. Oral administration of a total daily dose of 15–25 mg hydrocortisone is equivalent to the daily cortisol production of 5–10 mg/m^2. The optimal dose is that which avoids signs and symptoms of glucocorticoid excess, while relieving symptoms of glucocorticoid deficiency.

The short half-life of hydrocortisone enables dosing to mimic the normal physiologic diurnal variation. The morning dose (about one-half to two-thirds of total) should be given as soon as possible after waking, with the evening dose administered about 6–8 hours later. Long-acting glucocorticoids, such as prednisolone and dexamethasone, may be preferred for patients with afternoon fatigue or who are poorly adherent. Monitoring of the adequacy of glucocorticoid replacement is clinical, because reliable, objective measurements are lacking. Under treatment with glucocorticoid manifests as an impaired sense of well-being, while over treatment causes osteoporosis, excessive weight gain, and features of Cushing syndrome.

Patients with primary AI require replacement with both glucocorticoids and mineralocorticoids. Fludrocortisone, a potent synthetic mineralocorticoid, is typically started at 0.1 mg/day, with a dose range of 0.05–0.2 mg/day. Signs of excess mineralocorticoid replacement include hypertension, edema, and hypokalemia. Monitoring of mineralocorticoid replacement includes measurement of orthostatic blood pressure, serum sodium, potassium, and plasma renin. If hypertension develops, the dose of fludrocortisone should be reduced, with close monitoring of serum sodium and potassium. As the sodium-retaining effects of fludrocortisone require several days to develop, sodium deficits in acute AI should be replaced with intravenous normal saline. Mineralocorticoid doses do not need to be increased during stress or minor illness, as stress doses of hydrocortisone have mineralcorticoid properties. However, mineralcorticoid dosing may need to be increased during periods of increased salt loss, such as hot weather, and liberal salt intake should be encouraged in these circumstances.

Dehydroepiandrosterone (DHEA) levels, which are diminished in patients with primary AI, may be initially replaced with a 25–50 mg daily dose, with subsequent doses titrated to clinical response. DHEA replacement may have modest effects on sense of well-being and quality of life, although evidence to support claims of improved sexual function and satisfaction in women is not robust.

DISCHARGE CONSIDERATIONS

Patients and their families should be educated about the importance of taking corticosteroid replacement therapy as directed, and the potentially fatal consequences of failing to do so. They should also be instructed about stress-related glucocorticoid dose adjustment, with advice to double their hydrocortisone dose during infections requiring antibiotics or associated with fevers. All patients should carry a steroid emergency card or medical alert bracelet or necklace. An emergency hydrocortisone kit with prefilled syringes should be given to patients, particularly those who live in remote areas with limited access to medical care. Patients should have outpatient follow-up with an endocrinologist, as well as their primary care physician.

USE OF CORTICOSTEROIDS IN PATIENTS WITH CRITICAL ILLNESS

CRITICAL ILLNESS-RELATED CORTICOSTEROID INSUFFICIENCY (CIRCI)

The stress response in critical illness is a well-recognized physiologic phenomenon that parallels the adaptive "fight-or-flight" response seen in animals. This phenomenon involves activation of the HPA axis and the sympathetic nervous system, with resultant increases in cortisol, epinephrine, norepinephrine, and cytokines and other inflammatory mediators. However, in some critically ill patients, there may be inadequate production of corticosteroids and decreased peripheral responsiveness to corticosteroids, resulting in what has been called critical illness-related corticosteroid insufficiency (CIRCI). The prevalence of CIRCI may be as high as 60% in septic shock patients.

The definition and treatment of CIRCI remain controversial. Universal use of glucocorticoids in septic shock patients has not been shown to be beneficial. Two criteria that have been used for diagnosis are a random cortisol of less than 10 μg/dl in the presence of critical illness and a cortisol rise of less than 9 μg/dl on ACTH stimulation testing. However, ACTH stimulation testing does not identify patients who benefit from glucocorticoids. At present, the American College of Critical Care Medicine recommends consideration of corticosteroids in patients remaining in shock despite adequate fluid resuscitation and vasopressor administration. If steroids are administered, intravenous hydrocortisone 50 mg every 6 hours for 7 days should be used, and subsequently tapered off. Fludrocortisone use merits further study, but is considered optional per the recent Society of Critical Care Medicine consensus statement.

As the current literature has mostly focused on intensive care unit patients with septic shock, these recommendations cannot be applied to other critically ill patients without sepsis, or to non-critically ill patient populations. Additionally, side effects of steroid use in the critically ill are substantial, and include hypertension, electrolyte abnormalities, volume overload, immunosuppression, delayed wound healing, neuromuscular weakness, and hyperglycemia. These side effects, the narrow scope of existing literature, and the lack of robust proven benefit make glucocorticoids a treatment modality that should be used in critically ill septic patients on a case-by-case basis only.

TABLE 151-3 Guidelines for Adrenal Supplementation Therapy for Patients on Chronic Corticosteroids*

Severity of Stress	Corticosteroid Dose	Frequency and Duration of Therapy
Mild Mild febrile illness Endoscopy	25 mg intravenous hydrocortisone	Day of procedure only
Moderate Routine abdominal surgery Significant febrile illness	50–75 mg intravenous hydrocortisone	Day of procedure, with 1–2 day taper back to usual dose
Severe Major surgery (cardiac) Severe pancreatitis	100–150 mg intravenous hydrocortisone	Day of procedure, with 1–2 day taper back to usual dose

*Patients using less than 5 mg/prednisone equivalent a day typically do not require supplementation in the setting of medical or surgical stress.

PREEXISTING ADRENAL INSUFFICIENCY AND NEED FOR CORTICOSTEROID AUGMENTATION

Patients with primary and secondary adrenal insufficiency, as well as the many patients on oral glucocorticoid therapy at risk of tertiary AI, may require supplemental steroids in the setting of acute illness. Patients on potent topical corticosteroids may also be at slight risk for tertiary AI. While dose augmentation in the setting of surgical procedures or severe illness should be considered for patients receiving more than 5 mg/day of prednisone or its equivalent, there is debate over optimal duration and dose recommended. Suggested glucocorticoid dosing is found in **Table 151-3**, based on existing evidence and expert opinion. Mineralocorticoid use is a topic of ongoing investigation. Currently, supplementation is not routinely recommended except in patients with primary AI and selected patients with refractory septic shock.

GLUCOCORTICOID USE IN SELECT POPULATIONS

There are many other hospitalized patients for whom corticosteroid use should be considered. However, aside from studies in septic shock patients, large randomized controlled trials are lacking for most other patient populations. Several recent trials in patients with the acute respiratory distress syndrome (ARDS) have shown improved outcomes with glucocorticoid use, reflected by decreased mechanical ventilation time and reduced mortality. In patients with severe or critical, relatively early ARDS (less than two weeks),

TABLE 151-4 Recommended Uses of Supplemental Corticosteroids

Clinical Condition*	Recommended Dose†	Notes
Critical illness-related corticosteroid insufficiency (CIRCI)	50 mg IV hydrocortisone every 6 hours for 7 days	Recommended for patients with shock refractory to volume and vasopressor administration, ACTH stimulation should not be used to determine who may benefit
Acute respiratory distress syndrome (ARDS)	1 mg/kg/day IV methylprednisolone for 14 days	Start within 14 days, taper slowly over one month
Pneumocystis pneumonia (PCP)	40 mg oral prednisone twice daily for 5 days, then 40 mg daily for 5 days, then 20 mg daily for 11 days	Steroids indicated only for hypoxic patients (partial pressure of oxygen < 70 mm Hg or alveolar-arterial gradient > 35); doses recommended are for HIV patients, non-HIV patients with PCP pneumonia may require higher doses than listed)
Chronic obstructive pulmonary disease (COPD) exacerbation	30–60 mg of oral prednisone for 7–10 days	
Asthma exacerbation	40–80 mg of oral prednisone in divided doses daily for 10–14 days	
Solid organ transplant	Doses vary	
Bacterial meningitis	Dexamethasone 10 mg IV every 6 hours for 4 days	First does given before or with first dose antibiotics
Alcoholic hepatitis	40 mg oral prednisolone for 4 weeks followed by taper	When discriminant function is > 32 and/or evidence of hepatic encephalopathy
Acute spinal cord injury	30 mg/kg IV methylprednisolone bolus followed by 5.4 mg/kg/hour for 23 hours	Practice guidelines suggest this as optional therapy
Others (cardiac surgery, end-stage liver disease, hepato-adrenal syndrome, severe pancreatitis, community-acquired pneumonia)	Variable	Consensus is lacking, data is limited

ACTH, adrenocorticotropic hormone; IV, intravenous; kg, kilogram; mg, milligram.

*Side effects of steroids, including hyperglycemia, poor wound healing, hypertension electrolyte abnormalities, volume overload, neuromuscular weakness are numerous and should be considered in a risk-benefit fashion for every decision to use corticosteroids.

†Doses, duration of therapy, and choice of particular corticosteroid are largely empiric or based on expert opinion.

methylprednisolone doses of 1 mg/kg/day continuous infusion is currently recommended for at least 14 days, followed by slow taper over one month.

Despite more limited data, such as small randomized trials, observational data, and expert opinion, recommendations supporting routine corticosteroid use can still be made for several other patient populations. These guidelines can be found in **Table 151-4**, and with comparative data on different corticosteroid medications in **Table 151-5**. Because data is limited for many patient groups, suggested doses, duration of therapy, and the choice of a particular corticosteroid are largely empiric, or based upon expert opinion. Risks need to be considered in any decision about corticosteroid use, particularly in situations in which benefits are not well defined (**Table 151-6**).

PRACTICE POINT

- If adrenal crisis is suspected and a cosyntropin (ACTH) stimulation test has not yet been performed, dexamethasone 4 mg IV every 6 hours is preferred to hydrocortisone, as it is less likely to interfere with test interpretation.

TABLE 151-5 Characteristics of Commonly Used Steroids

	Glucocorticoid Activity	Mineralocorticoid Activity	Half-life (Hours)	Approximate Equivalent Dose (mg)
Hydrocortisone	1	1	6–8	20
Prednisone	4	0.1–0.2	18–36	5
Methylprednisolone	5	0.1–0.2	18–36	4
Dexamethasone	30	< 0.1	36–54	0.75
Fludrocortisone	0	20	18–36	0.05–2

TABLE 151-6 Evidence-based Medicine: Adrenal Insufficiency

Paper	Methodology	Results	Limitations	Bottom Line
Sprung CL, Annane D, Keh D, et al. *N Engl J Med.* 2008;358:111–124	499 patients with septic shock randomized to receive 50 mg of hydrocortisone every 6 hours or placebo; 233 of these patients were found to have an abnormal ACTH (cosyntropin) stimulation test, defined as an increase in the cortisol level of less than 9 µg/dL	Mortality at 28 days was similar in both treatment and control groups, including the subset of patients with an abnormal cosyntropin stimulation test; patients who received hydrocortisone had more rapid reversal of septic shock, but were also more likely to develop new infections	Most patients were admitted to surgical, rather than medical, intensive care units; the study did not reach targeted enrollment, and it was somewhat underpowered	There is no evidence to support the routine administration of corticosteroids to patients with septic shock, even if the cosyntropin stimulation test is abnormal
Yong SL, Marik P, Esposito M, Coulthard P. *Cochrane Database Syst Rev.* 2009;(4):CD005367	Systematic review and meta-analysis of supplemental perioperative steroids for surgical patients with adrenal insufficiency	Only 2 randomized, controlled trials involving 37 patients with known adrenal insufficiency randomized to placebo vs. extra perioperative corticosteroids have been published in the last 61 years; no difference in outcomes was observed	This represents an insufficient amount of high-quality literature to address the question of efficacy	Current evidence is inadequate to determine whether patients with adrenal insufficiency on stable replacement doses routinely require additional corticosteroids perioperatively
Alkatib AA, Cosma M, Elamin MB, et al. *J Clin Endocrinol Metab.* 2009;94:3676–3681	Meta-analysis of randomized placebo-controlled trials of dehydroepiandrosterone (DHEA) treatment effects on quality of life in women with adrenal insufficiency	10 eligible trials were identified; DHEA showed small but significant effects on depression and quality of life; effects on anxiety and libido did not attain significance; side effects were minor and well tolerated	Trials were small, yielded inconsistent results, and used different measures of health-related quality of life	DHEA confers modest benefits on health-related quality of life and mood in women with adrenal insufficiency, without significant effects on anxiety or sexual function

SUGGESTED READINGS

Arlt W, Allolio B. Adrenal insufficiency. *Lancet.* 2003;361:1881–1893.

Bornstein SR. Current concepts: predisposing factors for adrenal insufficiency. *N Engl J Med.* 2009;360:2328–2339.

Coursin DB, Wood KE. Corticosteroid supplementation for adrenal insufficiency. *JAMA.* 2002;287:236–240.

Marik PE. Critical illness-related corticosteroid insufficiency. *Chest.* 2009;135;181–193.

Marik PE, Pastores SM, Annane D, et al. Recommendations for the diagnosis and management of corticosteroid insufficiency in critically ill adult patients: consensus statements from an international task force by the American College of Critical Care Medicine. *Crit Care Med.* 2008;36:1937–1949.

Meduri GU, Marik PE, Annanne D. Prolonged glucocorticoid treatment in acute respiratory distress syndrome: evidence supporting effectiveness and safety. *Crit Care Med.* 2009;37:1800–1803.

CHAPTER 152

Pituitary Disease

Shilpa H. Jain, MD
Laurence Katznelson, MD

Key Clinical Questions

1. How and when do you evaluate pituitary hormonal function?
2. How do you treat patients with excess or deficient pituitary hormonal function?
3. How do you classify pituitary tumors?
4. Which patients with pituitary disease require hospital admission?
5. What are the indications for consultation with endocrinology and/or neurosurgery?
6. What are the complications associated with neurosurgical resection of pituitary tumors?

INTRODUCTION

Pituitary disorders are characterized by tumors that lead to excessive hormone secretion or by inadequate hormone production from a multitude of causes. Pituitary disease is more common than popularly supposed. In unselected autopsies, the prevalence of pituitary adenomas averages about 14%. However, the prevalence of clinically significant pituitary adenomas is much lower, about 94 per 100,000 people. At least 30% of survivors of traumatic brain injury and subarachnoid hemorrhage have chronic anterior hypopituitarism at 24–36 months; therefore, clinicians must consider this diagnosis in populations at risk, such as wounded combat veterans. Hypopituitarism is also frequent after cranial irradiation, and may complicate pituitary disease of any cause. This chapter discusses the basic function of the pituitary gland, the evaluation of hypopituitarism, and the approach to patients with pituitary tumors.

PITUITARY GLAND ANATOMY AND PHYSIOLOGY

The pituitary gland is located at the base of the brain within the sella turcica, which is the bony roof of the sphenoid sinus. It lies outside the dura mater. The pituitary stalk, containing neurovascular bundles, extends from the hypothalamus through a dural opening to the pituitary gland. This anatomical arrangement renders the pituitary stalk vulnerable to traumatic injury. The optic chiasm is located above the pituitary gland and anterior to the pituitary stalk. The pituitary gland is bordered on the sides by the cavernous sinuses, which consist of vascular lakes containing cranial nerves III, IV, V, and VI and a portion of the carotid artery. The pituitary gland consists of two lobes, anterior and posterior (**Figure 152-1**).

The anterior lobe, or adenohypophysis, is composed of secretory cells that manufacture at least six hormones: corticotropin (ACTH), thyroid stimulating hormone (TSH), growth hormone (GH), follicle stimulating hormone (FSH), luteinizing hormone (LH), and prolactin (PRL). Secretion of the first five hormones is triggered by hypothalamic releasing factors that travel down the pituitary stalk through a portal venous system. In contrast, anterior pituitary secretion of prolactin, which promotes lactation, is tonically inhibited by hypothalamic secretion of dopamine. Any disorder that compresses or interferes with the pituitary stalk can cause prolactin elevation.

In contrast, the posterior lobe, or neurohypophysis, is comprised of axons of cell bodies arising in the hypothalamus. These axons store and secrete vasopressin (antidiuretic hormone, or ADH) and oxytocin. Vasopressin has a key role in fluid and electrolyte balance by promoting retention of water by the kidney. Oxytocin stimulates uterine contractions at parturition.

HYPOPITUITARISM

CAUSES

The most common cause of hypopituitarism is a **pituitary adenoma**. Other causes include **nonpituitary sellar masses**, such as craniopharyngiomas and meningiomas, damage to normal pituitary tissue during **neurosurgery** for pituitary adenoma, and sudden hemorrhage into a pituitary adenoma (**pituitary apoplexy**). **Sheehan syndrome** is pituitary necrosis related to postpartum hemorrhage and hypotension; presumably the pituitary is at greater risk of ischemic injury in this setting because of its normal increase in volume during pregnancy. Patients usually

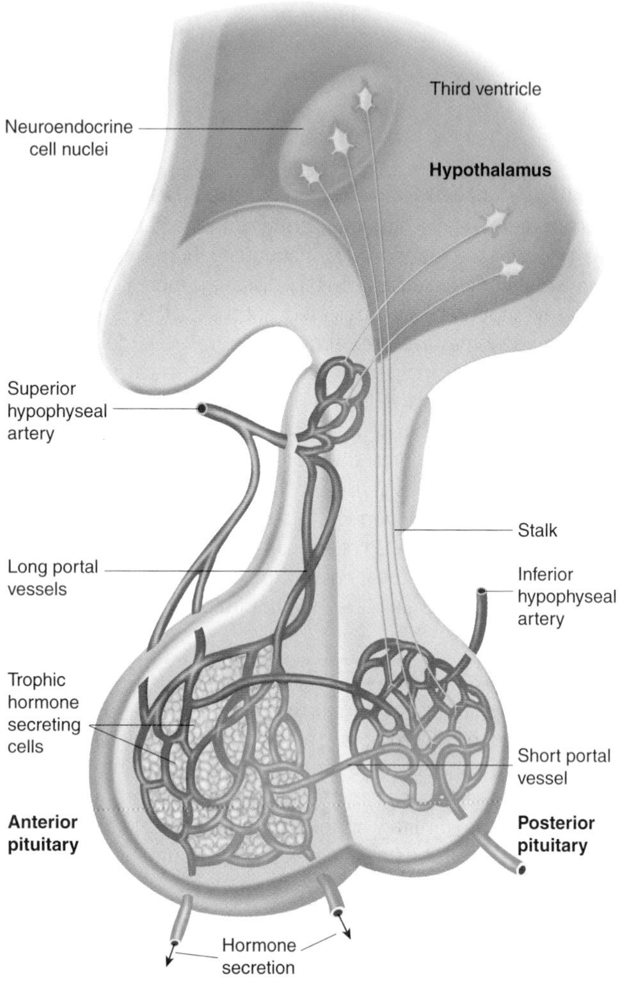

Figure 152-1 *The hypothalamic-pituitary axis. Hypothalamic nuclei secrete hormones in a pulsatile fashion into a portal venous system, which perfuses anterior pituitary secretory cells and regulates its activity. Posterior pituitary hormones are derived from direct neural extensions from the hypothalamus. (Reproduced, with permission, from Fauci AS, Braunwald E, Kasper DL, et al. Harrison's Principles of Internal Medicine. 17th ed. New York, NY: McGraw-Hill, 2008. Figure 333-2.)*

present with failure of lactation, followed by slowly progressive symptoms and signs of hypopituitarism. **Cranial irradiation** causes hypopituitarism in approximately 40% of patients over a 10-year period, with the precise risk depending on the total radiation dose and length of time after exposure. The prevalence of hypopituitarism after **traumatic brain injury** (TBI) and **subarachnoid hemorrhage** (SAH) has been reported to be approximately 30% and 50%, respectively. Growth hormone deficiency is the most common endocrine abnormality following both TBI and SAH. **Developmental and genetic causes** of hypopituitarism are rare, and include pituitary aplasia or hypoplasia, hypothalamic defects, mutations in transcription factors, and genetic conditions, such as Kallman syndrome and Prader-Willi syndrome. Other rare causes include metastatic disease from breast, lung, or skin cancer, histiocytosis X, and sarcoidosis.

PRESENTATION AND DIAGNOSIS

Specific tests are used to assess each hormonal axis (**Table 152-1**).

Central or secondary adrenal insufficiency, caused by decreased pituitary ACTH release, is associated with anorexia, orthostasis, arthralgias, fatigue, vomiting, and hyponatremia. Hyperpigmentation is absent and serum potassium is normal, unlike Addison disease (primary adrenal insufficiency). The evaluation of central adrenal insufficiency is somewhat controversial, as the criteria for diagnosis depend on the severity of the patient's condition. In a stable, noncritically ill patient, a fasting serum cortisol > 15 μg/dl is considered normal. Central adrenal insufficiency is clearly present when the morning serum cortisol is < 3 μg/dl and ACTH is low or inappropriately normal. If the serum cortisol is between 3 and 15 μg/dl, then further testing is appropriate. Such testing may include a standard 250 μg ACTH (cosyntropin) stimulation test, in which serum cortisol is measured at baseline and 30 and 60 minutes after intravenous cosyntropin administration. Alternatively, serum cortisol may be measured 45–60 minutes after an intramuscular injection of cosyntropin. A peak serum cortisol of > 18 μg/dl is considered normal in this test. An important limitation of the use of cosyntropin stimulation testing in central adrenal insufficiency is that it may be normal in the acute setting of pituitary disease (such as following pituitary surgery) because the adrenal gland can respond normally to cosyntropin in the first few weeks following a pituitary insult. Over time, ACTH deficiency leads to adrenal atrophy, and at that point the response to cosyntropin stimulation is blunted. It is also possible that the pharmacologic dose of cosyntropin may overshadow mild central adrenal insufficiency, and a normal result may give a false sense of security that adrenal function is intact. Other measures of ACTH reserve, such as metyrapone stimulation or insulin-induced hypoglycemia testing, may be more reliable as they measure integrity of the entire axis, but they are also less practical and rarely used in clinical practice. The diagnosis of central adrenal insufficiency in the presence of physiologic stress is less clear, as a "normal" cortisol value may be inappropriately low for the setting. Change in serum cortisol following cosyntropin has been used as a marker for adrenal function in the intensive care unit, but there is controversy as to the interpretation of such tests.

The symptoms of **central hypothyroidism** are similar to those of primary hypothyroidism, and include cold intolerance, fatigue, mild weight gain, dry skin, alopecia, and constipation. Findings include delayed tendon reflexes, facial puffiness and coarsening, bradycardia, slowed mentation, nonpitting edema, pleural effusions, and carpal tunnel syndrome. Diagnosis is based on the presence of a low serum free T4 with low or normal TSH, in contrast to the elevated TSH seen in primary hypothyroidism. However, low free T4 can be the first thyroid abnormality associated with nonthyroidal illnesses (sick euthyroid), common in the inpatient setting. Therefore, the definitive diagnosis of central hypothyroidism may sometimes be delayed until the subject recovers from acute illness.

Hypogonadism (testosterone and estrogen deficiency) cannot be reliably diagnosed in the inpatient setting, as levels of both hormones decline markedly during acute illness. In men, secondary hypogonadism is associated with decreases in sexual function, libido, and muscle mass. In women, secondary hypogonadism is associated with secondary amenorrhea and symptoms of estrogen deficiency, such as hot flashes, vaginal dryness, or decreased libido. In the outpatient setting, secondary male hypogonadism is diagnosed based on low levels of testosterone and low or normal FSH and LH. In women, secondary hypogonadism is suggested by irregular or absent menses and low or normal FSH and LH.

Growth hormone (GH) deficiency in children is characterized by short stature, and in adults by increased body fat, reduced muscle mass and bone density, and diminished quality of life. GH is secreted in pulsatile fashion, and most secretion is nocturnal.

TABLE 152-1 Hormonal Profile in Excessive and Insufficient Anterior Pituitary Function

Pituitary Hormone	End Organ and its Hormone	Criteria for Hormonal Excess	Criteria for Hormonal Deficiency
ACTH	Adrenal glands: Cortisol	⇑ Cortisol • 24 hr urine cortisol > 3 times upper limit of normal × 2 collections • Overnight 1 mg dexamethasone suppression test with serum cortisol > 1.8 μg/dl Normal/⇑ ACTH	⇓ Cortisol • 8 AM serum cortisol < 3 μg/dl Normal/⇓ ACTH
TSH	Thyroid gland: T4, T3	⇑ T4, T3 Normal/⇑ TSH	⇓ T4 Normal/⇓ TSH
Growth hormone (GH)	Liver: IGF-1	⇑ IGF-1 • Serum IGF-1 > age and gender specific upper limit of normal ⇑ GH • Oral glucose tolerance test with nadir GH > 1 μg/l	⇓ IGF-1 • Serum IGF-1 < age and gender specific upper limit of normal ⇓ GH • Insulin-induced hypoglycemia, with peak GH < 5.1 μg/l • Glucagon stimulation with peak GH < 3 μg/l
FSH, LH	Testes: testosterone	⇑ Testosterone Normal/⇑ FSH, LH	⇓ Testosterone Normal/⇓ FSH, LH
	Ovaries: estradiol, progesterone	Abnormal/absent menses Normal/⇑ FSH, LH	Abnormal/absent menses Normal/⇓ FSH, LH
Prolactin	Mammary glands	⇑ Prolactin	⇓ Prolactin (rare)

During the day, GH levels in normal subjects may be low or undetectable. Therefore, random daytime GH levels are of little clinical utility. As GH stimulates production of insulin-like growth factor-1 (IGF-1) by the liver, IGF-1 is a surrogate marker of recent GH levels. A low serum IGF-1 level supports the diagnosis of GH deficiency, especially in the setting of other pituitary disease. Further evidence of GH deficiency may be provided by an insufficient GH response to insulin-induced hypoglycemia or to growth hormone-releasing hormone (GHRH).

Central diabetes insipidus (DI) due to ADH deficiency presents with polyuria and polydipsia. The physical examination is normal unless dehydration has developed. If hypernatremia is present, the patient may be obtunded, but most patients are able to maintain eunatremia with a high fluid intake. The diagnosis is confirmed with a carefully supervised fluid deprivation test, demonstrating the inability to appropriately concentrate urine osmolality despite rising plasma sodium and osmolality. Patients with central DI will subsequently increase their urine osmolality more than 50% with desmopressin administration, whereas patients with nephrogenic DI will not.

PITUITARY TUMORS

Pituitary tumors are classified based on hormonal secretion and size. Tumors that secrete excessive amounts of pituitary hormones are referred to as functional or secretory tumors, and tumors that do not produce biologically active hormone are known as nonfunctioning or nonsecretory tumors. Pituitary tumors are classified as microadenomas if the diameter is less than 10 mm, and macroadenomas if the diameter is greater than 10 mm.

PRESENTATION

Patients with functioning pituitary adenomas present with classic manifestations specific to each hormone (**Table 152-2**). These benign tumors usually secrete in order of decreasing incidence excessive quantities of prolactin, growth hormone, ACTH, and rarely thyrotropin, or gonadotropin.

TABLE 152-2 Clinical Presentations of Pituitary Tumors

1. Functioning tumors
   a. Prolactinoma
   b. Acromegaly
   c. Cushing disease
   d. Hyperthyroidism
2. Mass effects
   a. Hypopituitarism
      i. Adrenal insufficiency
      ii. Hypothyroidism
      iii. Hypogonadism
      iv. Growth hormone deficiency
   b. Headaches
   c. Neurological deficits
      i. Visual changes: decreased visual acuity, visual field deficits, ophthalmoplegia
      ii. Ptosis
      iii. Facial sensory syndromes
   d. Cerebrospinal fluid leakage +/– meningitis
   e. Nasopharyngeal obstruction
3. Pituitary apoplexy
4. Asymptomatic
   a. Nonfunctioning tumors

In addition, pituitary macroadenomas that extend beyond the sella may compress local structures, leading to temporal visual loss and hypopituitarism. The overwhelming majority of pituitary tumors are benign pathologically. Rarely, however, adenocarcinoma may arise in the pituitary.

Prolactinomas account for approximately 30–40% of all pituitary tumors. Symptoms in women include amenorrhea or oligomenorrhea, infertility, and galactorrhea. Postmenopausal women with prolactinomas are unlikely to develop galactorrhea, as their estrogen levels are usually very low. Men with prolactinomas may present with decreased libido, erectile dysfunction, and infertility.

The second most common functional pituitary tumor is a growth hormone-secreting adenoma (approximately 10%), which results in **acromegaly**. Clinical manifestations of acromegaly include enlargement of soft tissues, cartilage and bones in face, hands, and feet and enlarged viscera (heart, liver, thyroid). Cutaneous symptoms include excessive sweating, oily skin, and skin tags. Patients may also note changes in ring, hat, and shoe size over many years. Patients may have arthralgias, arthritis, carpal tunnel syndrome, hyperglycemia, obstructive sleep apnea, and congestive heart failure. On physical examination they have signs of hypertension, enlarged hands and feet with characteristically enlarged finger pulps and heel pads, jaw prognathism, gaps between teeth, frontal bone bossing, macroglossia, and coarse, soft, doughy skin. Acromegaly is associated with an increased risk of early mortality, primarily from cardiovascular disease.

Cushing disease, or hypercortisolemia due to an ACTH-secreting pituitary tumor, can present with truncal obesity, violaceous striae, moon facies, facial plethora, dorsocervical and supraclavicular fat deposition, bruising, proximal muscle weakness and wasting, edema, hirsutism, acne, mood disorders, hyperglycemia, hypokalemia, hypertension, increased susceptibility to infections, thromboembolism, and fractures related to osteoporosis. **TSH-secreting adenomas**, characterized by TSH induced hyperthyroidism, are very rare, accounting for approximately 1–2% of pituitary tumors.

Nonfunctioning pituitary tumors, the most common type of pituitary adenoma accounting for up to 40% of all tumors, commonly stem from pituitary cells that produce the gonadotropins LH and FSH. They may be diagnosed during evaluation of headache, visual loss, or hypopituitarism. They may also be detected incidentally. Approximately 10% of the normal adult population has a clinically unsuspected microadenoma on brain magnetic resonance imaging (MRI). While these patients may not have symptoms, subtle hormonal or neurological abnormalities may be present, and they should be evaluated for hormonal excess and deficiency, and carefully examined for visual field defects and other neurologic abnormalities.

COMPLICATIONS

MASS EFFECTS

Compression of the native pituitary gland may lead to hypopituitarism. The presence of a sellar mass and diabetes insipidus points to a nonpituitary lesion, as pituitary tumors rarely present with diabetes insipidus. Extension into the adjacent cavernous sinus can lead to diplopia, ophthalmoplegia, ptosis, and facial sensory syndromes due to cranial nerve involvement. Superior tumor extension may impinge upon the optic chiasm, leading to visual field deficits, classically bitemporal hemianopsia (**Figure 152-2**).

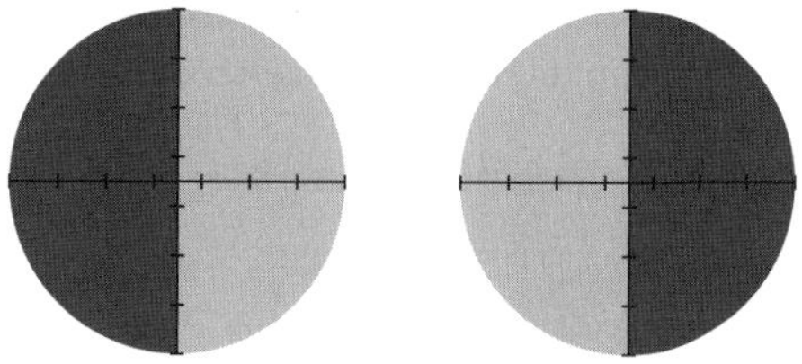
Bitemporal Hemianopia

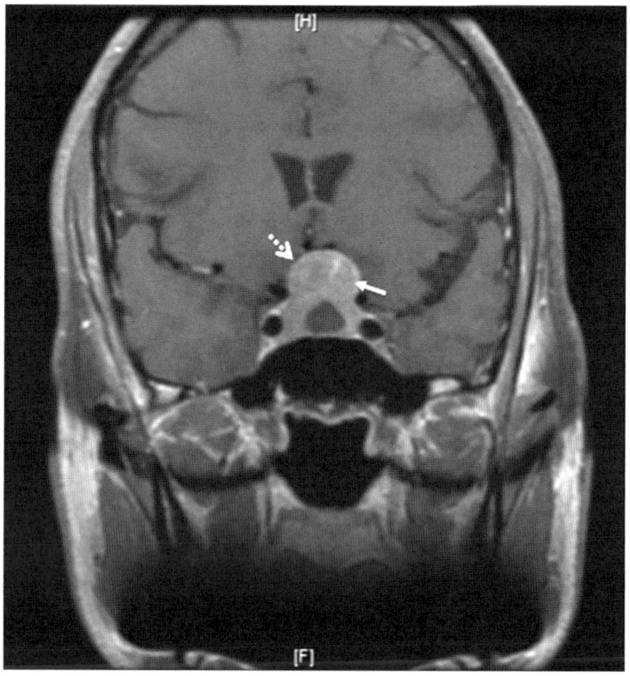

Figure 152-2 *Magnetic resonance imaging scan, coronal view, of a pituitary macroadenoma (solid arrow) with superior extension and compression of the optic chiasm (dashed arrow).*

PRACTICE POINT

- Checking visual fields may suggest that a lesion exists near the optic chiasm, which is closely associated with the pituitary fossa. Involvement of the upper quadrants first, a sign of compression of the optic chiasma from below, suggests pituitary adenoma, nasopharyngeal carcinoma, or sphenoid sinus mucocele. Involvement of the lower quadrants first, signaling compression of the optic chiasma from above, suggests a craniopharyngioma or third ventricular tumor.
- Some pituitary tumors may expand laterally, compressing nerves lying within the walls of the cavernous sinus, especially cranial nerve III. Rarely, vertical expansion obstructs the foramen of Munro, leading to hydrocephalus and/or hypothalamic compression.

PITUITARY APOPLEXY

Rarely, patients may present with pituitary apoplexy, or acute hemorrhagic infarction of a pituitary adenoma. This is an endocrine emergency because of frequent associated acute adrenal insufficiency. Patients with apoplexy may present with severe headaches, visual field deficits, opthalmoplegia, and altered consciousness. Immediate management includes glucocorticoid coverage, intravenous fluids, and neurosurgical consultation. Predisposing factors include hemodynamic instability and anticoagulation.

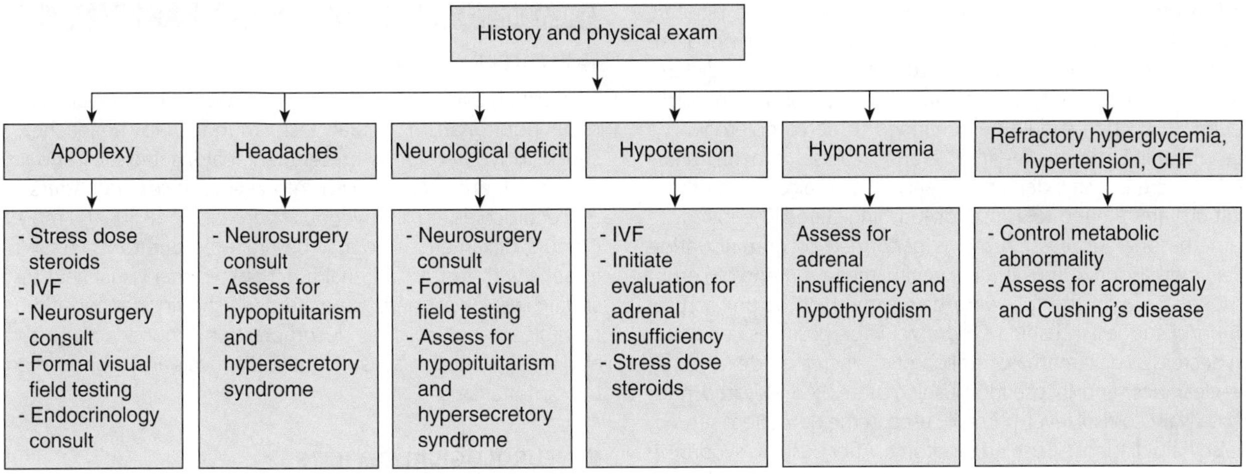

Figure 152-3 *Approach to the patient with a pituitary tumor.*

EVALUATION

The approach to a patient with a pituitary tumor is outlined in **Figure 152-3**.

Patients with suspected pituitary tumors should be asked about headaches, visual changes, and symptoms of hormonal excess and deficiency. Patients with suspected acromegaly should be asked about surreptitious GH use for athletic purposes or purported antiaging effects. Signs of special interest on physical examination include abnormalities of blood pressure readings with orthostatics, heart rate, cranial nerves with visual field testing, and signs of hormone excess and deficiency.

The initial endocrine laboratory evaluation for patients with suspected hypersecretory syndromes includes measurements of serum prolactin, IGF-1, free T4, and TSH. Either 24-hour urinary free cortisol or overnight 1 mg dexamethasone suppression test should be performed to exclude Cushing disease. Patients with suspected hypopituitarism should have measurements of serum 8 AM cortisol, ACTH, free T4, TSH, FSH, LH, testosterone (in men), IGF-1, and a cosyntropin stimulation test.

All patients should have a brain MRI, with thin sections through the pituitary gland, with and without contrast enhancement. Neuro-opthalmological examination with formal visual field testing should be performed, especially in the presence of visual symptoms or compression of optic chiasm.

CONSULTATION

Endocrinology consultation is indicated for patients with suspected hypersecretory syndromes, hypopituitarism, sellar masses, pituitary apoplexy, and postoperative diabetes insipidus or syndrome of inappropriate ADH secretion. Neurosurgery consultation is indicated for patients with pituitary apoplexy, neurological deficits from pituitary disease, acromegaly, Cushing disease, TSH-secreting adenoma, cerebrospinal fluid leak, nasopharyngeal obstruction, and resistance or intolerance of medical therapy for prolactinoma

DIAGNOSIS

Prolactinomas are diagnosed on the basis of an elevated serum prolactin, exclusion of other causes of hyperprolactinemia, and pituitary imaging confirming the presence of a pituitary adenoma. Macroprolactinomas (tumors > 10 mm in greatest diameter) usually produce prolactin levels > 150 ng/mL. When the serum prolactin is only mildly elevated (ie, up to 40 ng/mL), it should be repeated, as transient factors such as food, exercise, stress, and chest wall stimulation may cause modest hyperprolactinemia. Modest hyperprolactinemia is also seen in pregnancy, primary hypothyroidism, renal failure, cirrhosis, and with medications such as metoclopramide, calcium channel blockers, phenothiazines, selective serotonin reuptake inhibitors, and risperidone. Lastly, any sellar mass may compress the pituitary stalk, reduce dopamine delivery to the pituitary, and lead to elevations in prolactin levels of up to approximately 150 ng/mL. For this reason, imaging studies should be performed in any patient with unexplained, modest hyperprolactinemia.

PRACTICE POINT

- Macroprolactinemia is a laboratory pitfall in the diagnosis of prolactinoma. In some patients, serum prolactin levels may be high because of circulating aggregates of a biologically inert, glycosylated form of prolactin (macroprolactin). Macroprolactinemia appears to be a benign variant, and is not associated with pituitary adenomas or typical symptoms of prolactinoma. It may be distinguished from true hyperprolactinemia by gel filtration or polyethylene glycol precipitation.

Acromegaly is a chronic, debilitating disease characterized by episodic hypersecretion of GH and continuously elevated levels of IGF-1. The best screening test for acromegaly is measurement of a random IGF-1 level, which shows less normal variability than serum GH. If IGF-1 is elevated after adjustment for age and gender, then a 75 g oral glucose tolerance test should confirm the diagnosis, with measurement of GH levels at baseline and one and two hours after glucose ingestion. The diagnostic value for acromegaly is a nadir GH level > 1 µg/L. Most tumors are macroadenomas at diagnosis.

PRACTICE POINT

- Because of mitogenic and antiapoptotic effects of GH and IGF-1, acromegaly is associated with an increased risk of colon carcinoma, thyroid cancer, and possibly other malignancies. All acromegalic patients should have a colonoscopy and careful physical examination for thyroid nodules.

In **Cushing disease**, an ACTH-secreting tumor of the pituitary gland leads to overproduction of cortisol. Demonstration of an elevated 24-hour urinary free cortisol or an abnormal dexamethasone suppression test is diagnostic of Cushing syndrome. The urine collection should be confirmed to be complete with a urine creatinine measurement. The urine cortisol can be mildly high in severe obesity, depression, anxiety, and alcoholism; these conditions are referred to as pseudo-Cushing states. The low-dose dexamethasone suppression test is performed by administration of dexamethasone 1 mg at 11 PM, with measurement of serum cortisol at 8 AM on the following day. A morning serum cortisol >1.8 μg/dl suggests Cushing syndrome. False positives can result from decreased dexamethasone absorption, increased dexamethasone clearance, and in pseudo-Cushing states. An elevated midnight salivary cortisol level, primarily used in the outpatient setting, can also help diagnose Cushing syndrome. After Cushing syndrome has been diagnosed, serum ACTH should be measured. A normal or increased ACTH level confirms ACTH-dependent Cushing syndrome. If a sellar mass >6 mm is present, a tentative diagnosis of Cushing disease (pituitary tumor) is made. If the source of the ACTH-dependent hypercortisolism is unclear, additional tests such as high-dose dexamethasone suppression testing, corticotropin-releasing hormone stimulation, or inferior petrosal sinus sampling may be necessary to determine whether ACTH secretion is pituitary or ectopic in origin.

As both nonfunctional and functional pituitary adenomas may compress the normal pituitary gland leading to hypopituitarism, adrenal insufficiency and hypothyroidism should be excluded in these patients.

DIFFERENTIAL DIAGNOSIS

The differential diagnosis of a pituitary adenoma includes several other sellar lesions. Meningiomas in or near the sella may affect pituitary function and compress the optic chiasm. Remnants of Rathke pouch, the embryological origin of the anterior pituitary lobe, may form a nonneoplastic cyst (Rathke cleft cyst) or low-grade tumor (craniopharyngioma). Rathke cleft cysts are typically asymptomatic, but can present with hypopituituitarism and headaches. They may be differentiated from pituitary adenomas based on imaging features. Craniopharyngiomas most often present during childhood and adolescence with diabetes insipidus, which is rare in pituitary adenoma, as well as headaches and anterior pituitary deficiencies. Lymphocytic hypophysitis, or autoimmune inflammation and destruction of the pituitary gland, is most common in young women, and may present in pregnancy. Up to 25% of patients also have autoimmune thyroid disease. Infiltrative diseases such as sarcoidosis and hemochromatosis may involve the pituitary. Rarely, lymphoma involves the pituitary stalk and hypothalamus. Metastases, especially from breast, lung, and gastrointestinal tract, can spread to the pituitary, particularly to the posterior lobe. Any sellar mass may have compressive effects, including hypopituitiarism. The presence of diabetes insipidus and a sellar mass usually points away from a diagnosis of a pituitary tumor.

HOSPITAL ADMISSION

Most patients with pituitary tumors do not require inpatient evaluation and management. Indications for admission include pituitary apoplexy; major neurological deficits, especially sudden and progressive loss of vision or diplopia; major complications of hypopituitarism, such as hypotension, severe hyponatremia, and hypernatremia; and major complications of acromegaly and other hyperfunctioning syndromes, such as refractory hyperglycemia, refractory hypertension, and congestive heart failure.

TREATMENT

PITUITARY APOPLEXY

Hemorrhagic infarction of the pituitary gland may lead to acute panhypopituitarism, visual loss, thunderclap headache, and shock. If hypotension is present, adrenal insufficiency should be presumed, and treated with intravenous fluids and stress dose glucocorticoids (eg, intravenous hydrocortisone 50–100 mg every 8 hours; dexamethasone may be preferred due to its lesser interference with tests of adrenal function). Formal visual field testing should be performed. Neurosurgery should be consulted for possible urgent surgical decompression. Endocrinology should also be consulted to assist with the diagnosis and management of hypopituitarism.

NEUROLOGICAL DEFICITS

Visual difficulties, such as visual field cuts and diplopia, are the most common neurological symptom of pituitary neoplasms. Transsphenoidal tumor resection may decompress cranial nerves and improve vision or restore it to normal. If surgery is not feasible, medical therapies or radiation may help shrink the tumor and alleviate the neurological deficit.

HYPOTENSION

Hypotension in the presence of a pituitary adenoma strongly suggests central adrenal insufficiency. Ideally, serum should be collected for diagnostic workup of adrenal insufficiency prior to initiation of treatment. However, if the patient is hemodynamically unstable, stress dose steroids should be started prior to confirmation of adrenal insufficiency. As hydrocortisone and prednisone are detected in the serum cortisol assay, the serum cortisol value is not informative while the patient is taking these medications. As dexamethasone is not detected by this assay, it may be used while evaluation of the hypothalamic-pituitary-adrenal axis is ongoing. After recovery from the acute illness, the glucocorticoid dose can be tapered to hydrocortisone 20–30 mg per day or prednisone 5–7.5 mg per day. Some patients may require repeat testing on an outpatient basis to confirm the diagnosis of adrenal insufficiency.

HYPONATREMIA

Hyponatremia in patients with sellar masses may reflect either central adrenal insufficiency or central hypothyroidism. Therapy of central adrenal insufficiency is discussed above. Central hypothyroidism is treated with levothyroxine, with typical oral starting doses of 25–50 μg, depending on the patient's age and cardiovascular status. Over time, levothyroxine can be increased to full replacement dose, which is usually 1.6 μg/kg. The levothyroxine dose should be titrated until the free T4 is within the normal range. Serum TSH should not be used for dose titration, as the TSH concentration is not an appropriate marker of thyroid function in patients with hypothalamic or pituitary disease. If the patient cannot take oral medications, then levothyroxine can be administered as a daily intravenous dose of 50–66% of the oral dose. In central hypothyroidism, glucocorticoids should be administered when thyroid hormone replacement is initiated, as levothyroxine increases the metabolism of cortisol, and can precipitate an adrenal crisis if borderline adrenal function is present.

PITUITARY ADENOMA

Indications for treatment of prolactinoma include macroadenoma or enlarging microadenoma, headache, amenorrhea, infertility, acne, hirsutism, undesired galactorrhea in women, and gynecomastia and testosterone deficiency in men. Dopamine agonists are the primary mode of therapy for prolactinoma. These agents rapidly reduce prolactin secretion and adenoma size in most subjects. The dopamine agonists indicated for prolactinoma treatment in the United States are bromocriptine and cabergoline. Bromocriptine is less expensive, but is more often associated with nausea than cabergoline. It is typically started at a dose of 1.25 mg at bedtime, and then slowly titrated to a maximum dose of 2.5 mg twice daily. Cabergoline, a longer-acting dopamine agonist, may be more effective and better tolerated than bromocriptine, but it is more expensive. Cabergoline is started at a dose of 0.25 mg once weekly, and increased up to a maximum of 1 mg twice a week. High doses of cabergoline used in Parkinson disease are associated with an increased risk of cardiac valvular regurgitation, possibly due to stimulation of 5-HT_{2B} receptors on myofibroblasts. There is currently no definite evidence that this occurs with the lower doses of cabergoline used in the treatment of prolactinoma.

Serum prolactin levels should be monitored to determine the dose and efficacy of dopamine agonist. Patients with macroadenomas should be intermittently followed with pituitary MRI. Transsphenoidal surgery is offered for prolactinoma when medical therapy fails or is poorly tolerated, or when there is a significant cystic component that does not respond fully to dopamine agonist therapy. Radiotherapy is an option in patients who fail pharmacological and surgical therapy. Because prolactinomas may enlarge with gestation, serial visual field testing should be performed during pregnancy.

Aggressive treatment of **acromegaly** is essential, as it is associated with increased mortality and multiple morbidities. Transsphenoidal surgery is preferred for most patients, because it leads to the most rapid fall in serum GH levels, it is necessary for tumor debulking if there are local mass effects, and it is more often associated with biochemical cure than medical therapy. Approximately 70–80% of patients with microadenomas and < 50% of patients with macroadenomas attain biochemical normalization after surgery. Medical therapy is largely used as adjuvant therapy in patients who have failed surgery. Somatostatin analogs (octreotide and lanreotide) are available in monthly depot preparations, and control GH and normalize serum IGF-1 levels in approximately 50–70% of cases. Dopamine agonists, including cabergoline and bromocriptine, are less effective than somatostatin analogs. The GH receptor antagonist pegvisomant is highly effective in reducing serum IGF-1 levels, and is often utilized as a secondary agent for subjects with incomplete or lack of response to somatostatin analogs. Radiation therapy is an adjuvant option for patients who have failed surgery and are unresponsive to or intolerant of medical therapy.

The primary therapy for **Cushing disease** is transsphenoidal resection. Remission rates in patients with a microadenoma undergoing selective adenomectomy by an expert pituitary surgeon are in the range of 65–90%. However, recurrence rates approach 20% at 10 years, and may reflect dura mater invasion. In patients with persistent disease despite surgery, further options include radiation therapy, medical adrenalectomy, and surgical adrenalectomy. Medical therapy uses inhibitors of adrenal cortisol synthesis, such as ketoconazole, metyrapone, aminoglutethamide, and mitotane. It is largely utilized as a temporizing option during radiotherapy or while further surgery is being planned. Bilateral surgical adrenalectomy is a definitive treatment that provides immediate control of hypercortisolism, though the resultant adrenal insufficieny will require lifelong glucocorticoid and mineralocorticoid replacement therapy. After bilateral adrenalectomy, up to 25% of patients develop Nelson syndrome, characterized by high serum ACTH levels, hyperpigmentation, and progressive pituitary enlargement with aggressive, often invasive tumor behavior. Surgical resection may be difficult. Directed radiotherapy may be indicated.

The primary therapy for **nonfunctioning adenomas** is surgery. However, because these tumors are often detected incidentally and there is a delay in diagnosis, these adenomas are often macroadenomas with extrasellar extension at diagnosis, and surgery is utilized for decompression of adjacent structures and is usually subtotal in extent. Medical therapies, including somatostatin analogs, are of limited use for these tumors. Radiation therapy is utilized in an adjuvant role for residual tumors following surgery, particularly in adenomas involving the cavernous sinus.

PITUITARY SURGERY AND ITS COMPLICATIONS

Transsphenoidal, endonasal surgery is used to remove the majority of pituitary tumors. Rarely, craniotomy is required for a large pituitary tumor with significant suprasellar and extrasellar extension. Outcome depends on surgical expertise, tumor size, degree of invasiveness, preoperative hormone levels, and prior pituitary surgery. There is a robust relationship between transsphenoidal surgery complication rates and experience, with operators who have performed < 200 procedures having complication rates two or three times higher than operators who have performed > 500 procedures. The most common complications are anterior pituitary insufficiency (7–21% of procedures) and diabetes insipidus (8–19%). The endonasal approach may lead to sinusitis and nasal septum perforation. CSF leak occurs in 1.5–4% of transsphenoidal surgeries, and is typically corrected via reconstruction of the sellar floor with subcutaneous fat harvested from the abdomen or thigh. A temporary lumbar drain may be required if the CSF leak is persistent. Other complications, including carotid artery injury, intracranial hemorrhage, epistaxis, visual deficits, meningitis, and other central nervous system (CNS) injuries occur in < 1% of cases when surgery is performed by a highly experienced neurosurgeon. Mortality rates range from 0.2–1.2%.

As acute adrenal insufficiency is a common complication, patients are either treated with stress dose glucocorticoids perioperatively or closely monitored for steroid sufficiency. The glucocorticoid dose is tapered based on the patient's hemodynamic status after surgery. If steroids can be successfully weaned to physiologic doses (prednisone 5 mg or hydrocortisone 20–30 mg daily), then a morning serum cortisol should be obtained prior to discharge to determine optimal dosing. Steroids can be stopped if the serum cortisol is > 10 μg/dl. However, if the morning serum cortisol is < 10 μg/dl, then glucocorticoids should be continued and a morning serum cortisol repeated one week postoperatively.

Within 24–48 hours of surgery, reduction in ADH secretion may lead to diabetes insipidus. Approximately 7–12 days postoperatively, this may be followed by the syndrome of inappropriate ADH secretion (SIADH), presumably because of release of preformed ADH from the posterior pituitary. If damage to the hypothalamus or pituitary stalk is permanent, then posterior pituitary stores of ADH are not replenished and diabetes insipidus may relapse. This postsurgical response has been called the triple phase response: diabetes insipidus, SIADH, and diabetes insipidus again. Close monitoring of electrolytes is therefore imperative following surgery. Patients with acromegaly often have significant polyuria following surgery, reflecting appropriate diuresis of the associated volume overload. However, if polyuria and hypernatremia develops in acromegaly patients postoperatively, this suggests diabetes insipidus, not physiologic diuresis.

Diabetes insipidus is characterized by polyuria (> 3 L/day) and polydipsia. It is diagnosed based on a low urine osmolality (< 250 mosmol/kg) in the setting of a high serum osmolality (> 290 mosmol/kg) in the absence of hyperglycemia. When fluids are withheld or the thirst mechanism is impaired, then hypernatremia can also occur. Treatment consists of intravenous fluid replacement and administration of desmopressin (DDAVP) to control polyuria.

TABLE 152-3 Evidence-based Medicine: Key References for Pituitary Disease

Study	Methods	Results	Limitations	Bottom Line
Webster J, et al. *N Engl J Med.* 1994; 331:904–909.	Randomized trial of 24 weeks of cabergoline vs. bromocriptine in 459 women with amenorrhea and high serum prolactin	Cabergoline was more effective at achieving normal prolactin levels (83% vs. 59%, $p < 0.001$) and ovulatory cycles or pregnancy (72% vs. 52%, $p < 0.001$) and better tolerated than bromocriptine	Double blind study for only first eight weeks	Cabergoline is superior to bromocriptine in women with amenorrhea associated with high serum prolactin levels
Freda PU, et al. *J Clin Endocrinol Metab.* 2005;90: 4465–4473.	Meta-analysis of 44 prospective trials on efficacy of long-acting somatostatin analog therapy for acromegaly	GH and IGF-1 normalization occurred in up to 67% of subjects receiving somatostatin analogs	Heterogeneity of studies including variability in inclusion criteria, GH and IGF-1 assays, drug dosing, and reporting of drop outs could have affected efficacy estimates	Long-acting somatostatin analogs are effective agents for lowering GH levels
Elamin MB, et al. *J Clin Endocrinol Metab.* 2008;93: 1553–1562.	Meta-analysis and review of 27 studies on the accuracy of diagnostic tests for Cushing syndrome	Positive 24-hour urinary free cortisol had likelihood ratio LR+ 10.6 and LR- 0.16; 1 mg overnight dexamethasone suppression test had LR+ 16.4 and LR- 0.06	Study population enriched with high prevalence of Cushing syndrome; heterogeneous studies	Common diagnostic tests for Cushing syndrome are accurate in a referral population
Ayuk J, et al. *Clin Endocrinol (Oxf).* 2004;61:747–752.	Retrospective study of patients with pituitary apoplexy who underwent surgery ($n = 15$) if worsening visual deficits vs. conservative management ($n = 18$) if no progressive visual deficits	Visual deficits resolved in 60% of surgical group and 100% of conservatively managed group; both groups had similar prevalence of hypopituitarism	Nonrandomized small retrospective study	Surgery can resolve progressive visual deficits caused by pituitary apoplexy, but may not prevent or correct hypopituitarism

Urine output, urine osmolality, and serum sodium should be closely monitored to help adjust fluids and DDAVP dosing. As diabetes insipidus may be a transient postoperative phenomenon, the need for continued DDAVP should be reassessed on an ongoing basis.

In SIADH, hyponatremia is associated with a low plasma osmolality and an inappropriately normal to high urine osmolality (at least >100 mosmol/kg). Other causes of hyponatremia in the postoperative setting include central adrenal insufficiency, central hypothyroidism, over-replacement with hypotonic fluids, and possibly cerebral salt wasting. SIADH is treated by restriction of free water. If the patient has symptomatic or severe hyponatremia, hypertonic fluids may rarely be required (**Table 152-3**).

DISCHARGE CONSIDERATIONS

Patients with pituitary adenomas can be discharged after resolution of acute complications and appropriate follow-up has been arranged. For hypersecretory syndromes and hypopituitarism, patients should have endocrinology follow-up. After neurosurgery, patients should have both endocrinology and neurosurgery follow-up. Patients who were diagnosed with adrenal insufficiency should be given medical alert identification and extra glucocorticoid tablets. During a febrile syndrome or other illness, patients should be instructed to take double to triple their glucocorticoid dose and call their endocrinologist or primary care physician. If they cannot maintain oral intake, they should go to their local emergency room for parenteral fluids and glucocorticoids.

QUALITY IMPROVEMENT

Effective communication between the hospitalist, endocrinology, and neurosurgery teams can significantly improve the quality of care for patients with pituitary tumors. The consult services should be contacted immediately when indicated, but the primary medical team can provide life-saving care with early recognition of acute complications and initiating important temporizing measures.

CONCLUSION

Clinical manifestations of pituitary disease range from consequences of hormonal excess and hypopituitarism to direct local mass effects of tumors. Evaluation of pituitary disease includes testing of each hypothalamic-pituitary-end organ axis, MRI of the pituitary gland, and visual field testing. Endocrinology and neurosurgical consultation are indicated for treatment of hormonal abnormalities and control of tumor activity and mass effects. Coordination of care between the hospitalist and specialist teams results in optimal care of patients with pituitary disease.

SUGGESTED READINGS

Agha A, Sherlock M, Brennan S, et al. Hypothalamic-pituitary dysfunction after irradiation of nonpituitary brain tumors in adults. *J Clin Endocrinol Metab.* 2005;90:6355–6360.

Ciric I, Ragin A, Baumgartner C, Pierce D. Complications of transsphenoidal surgery: results of a national survey and review of the literature, and personal experience. *Neurosurgery*. 1997;40:225–236.

Dumont AS, Nemergut EC 2nd, Jane JA Jr, Laws ER Jr. Postoperative care following pituitary surgery. *J Intensive Care Med*. 2005;20:127–240.

Freda PU, Beckers AM, Katznelson L, et al. Pituitary incidentaloma: an endocrine society clinical practice guideline. *J Clin Endocrinol Metab*. 2011;96:894–904.

Grinspoon SK, Biller BM. Laboratory assessment of adrenal insufficiency. *J Clin Endocrinol Metab*. 1994;79:923–931.

Melmed S, Casanueva FF, Hoffman AR, et al. Diagnosis and treatment of hyperprolactinemia: an endocrine society clinical practice guideline. *J Clin Endocrinol Metab*. 2011;96:273–288.

Melmed S, Colao A, Barkan A, et al. Acromegaly Consensus Group. Guidelines for acromegaly management: an update. *J Clin Endocrinol Metab*. 2009;94:1509–1517.

Nieman LK, Biller BM, Finding JW, et al. The diagnosis of Cushing's syndrome: an Endocrine Society clinical practice guidelines. *J Clin Endocrinol Metab*. 2008;93:1526–1540.

Schneider HJ, Kreitschmann-Andermahr H, Ghigo E, Stalla GK, Agha A. Hypothalmopituitary dysfunction following traumatic brain injury and aneurysmal subarachnoid hemorrhage: a systematic review. *JAMA*. 2007;298:1429–1438.

SECTION 6

Gastroenterology

CHAPTER 153

Dysphagia, Aspiration and Swallowing Dysfunction

Anupama Ravi, MD
Jennifer Christie, MD

Key Clinical Questions

1. What symptoms are consistent with oropharyngeal versus esophageal dysphagia?
2. What etiologies and mechanisms lead to dysphagia?
3. What tests and studies are useful to evaluate dysphagia, based on symptoms and signs?
4. What treatments are available for each etiology of dysphagia?
5. What is the long-term prognosis and follow-up for dysphagia, based on the diagnosis?

INTRODUCTION

Dysphagia is caused either by lack of coordination of the muscles required to transfer food material from the mouth to the stomach or by a fixed obstruction between the mouth and the stomach.

EPIDEMIOLOGY

Dysphagia is a common complaint, especially in the elderly. Fifteen percent of people older than 60 years who live independently complain of dysphagia, whereas 30–60% of residents in institutional settings experience dysphagia. Incidence and prevalence also varies according to underlying neurological problems. Various neurological disorders have increased risk of dysphagia (**Table 153-1**). Furthermore, dysphagia is associated with high mortality and morbidity. Patients with stroke who have dysphagia are twice as likely to die as patients without dysphagia. Several studies have also demonstrated that patients with dysphagia have higher incidence of aspiration pneumonia, longer length of hospital stay, as well as more severe levels of disability years after their stroke.

PATHOPHYSIOLOGY

Swallowing is divided into three phases: the oral preparatory phase, the pharyngeal phase, and the esophageal phase. Oral preparatory phase starts with the food bolus being placed in the mouth and being chewed with the help of the muscles of mastication. From the oropharynx, the food bolus is propelled by the back of the tongue and other muscles into the pharynx, with voluntary elevation of the soft palate in order to prevent food from entering the nose. The cranial nerves involved in this stage of swallowing include the trigeminal, facial, and hypoglossal nerves.

The pharyngeal phase starts as the bolus reaches the pharynx. Special sensory receptors activate this involuntary phase of swallowing. The reflex, which is mediated by the swallowing center in the medulla, causes the food to be further pushed back into the pharynx and esophagus by rhythmic, involuntary contractions of several muscles in the back of the mouth, pharynx, and esophagus.

The esophageal phase begins with the opening of the upper esophageal sphincter. The lower esophageal sphincter relaxes and food passes into the stomach. The passage of food through the esophagus during this phase requires the coordinated action of the vagus nerve, the glossopharyngeal nerve, and nerve fibers from the sympathetic nervous system.

Dysphagia can occur when there is an abnormality in any of these phases. Based on the presenting symptoms and signs, the specific pathophysiology can be determined (**Table 153-2**).

DIAGNOSIS

WHAT IS CAUSING THE DYSPHAGIA?

Evaluation of patients with dysphagia involves distinguishing oropharyngeal dysphagia from esophageal dysphagia during a thorough history and physical examination (**Figure 153-1**). In patients with oropharyngeal dysphagia, swallow initiation may be delayed or absent. Symptom onset often occurs immediately after swallowing rather than later. The patient may also express a need to reposition the body to facilitate transfer. Aspiration may manifest as cough after swallowing. Nasopharyngeal regurgitation or change in tone of speech may be reported. A sensation of fullness in neck

TABLE 153-1 Incidence/Prevalence of Dysphagia in Different Neurological Conditions

Neurological Disorder	Incidence/Prevalence of Dysphagia
Acute cerebral infarct	5–60% develop dysphagia acutely, but 86% of them recover after acute phase
Bulbar poliomyelitis	60% have persistent long-term dysphagia
Parkinson disease	15–20% have clinical symptoms of dysphagia, but 95% have silent aspiration
Myotonic dystrophy	50%, have clinical symptoms of dysphagia, but 95% have silent aspiration
Myasthenia gravis	30–40% have prominent dysphagia

or chest is most likely reported by patients with oropharyngeal dysphagia, but it can also be experienced in patients with GERD or esophageal dysphagia. Additionally, weight loss, nutritional deficiency, and recurrent aspiration pneumonia are common presenting problems.

The differential diagnosis for a patient presenting with dysphagia is extensive (**Table 153-3**). The examiner should perform a thorough physical exam, including a complete head and neck exam as well as neurological exam, to delineate between various causes of dysphagia. The presence of cervical lymphadenopathy should raise the possibility of a malignant etiology of the patient's symptoms or upper extremity weakness and/or myopia a myopathic etiology such as myastenia gravis. Oropharyngeal etiologies of dysphagia may include iatrogenic, infectious, inflammatory, metabolic, myopathic, neurologic, and structural causes. Esophageal etiologies include reflux, infiltrative diseases, connective tissue disorders, motility disorders, and structural disorders (Table 153-3).

The patient's presenting history and other clinical information should direct testing towards the most likely possibilities. Diagnostic modalities employed in the workup of dysphagia include barium swallow (modified or nonmodified), fiberoptic endoscopic evaluation of swallowing (FEES), manometry, and scintigraphy (**Table 153-4** and **Figure 153-2**).

TRIAGE AND HOSPITAL ADMISSION

The acuity of onset of dysphagia as well as other underlying medical problems dictates the need for hospital admission. A patient with gradually progressive dysphagia can be evaluated as an outpatient. However, a patient with acute onset of dysphagia needs more urgent attention in the hospital. Patients with acute esophageal dysphagia, namely in cases of a food impaction, can be treated in the emergency room with emergent endoscopy and dislodgement of the food bolus. Patients who have life-threatening conditions—including head trauma, stroke, infections, or other acutely presenting dysphagia—require emergent evaluation in the hospital (Table 153-3). The prognosis of the patient with dysphagia largely depends on the etiology. Nonetheless, early diagnosis and appropriate management help prevent complications and improve outcomes.

DYSPHAGIA SCREENING

Screening for dysphagia should be considered for any critically ill patient in the hospital, especially in patients with neurological problems. Dysphagia screening is one of the core measures for Joint Commission primary stroke center certification. Specialized hospital stroke centers stabilize and treat patients who have sustained a stroke, and initiate the evaluation and management of stroke patients with dysphagia.

Patients with prolonged intubation represent another population with particularly high risk for dysphagia. Several studies have shown that the duration of endotracheal intubation is a strong predictor of subsequent dysphagia that both prolongs the return to normal oral feeding and delays subsequent hospital discharge. Thus, routine dysphagia screening in patients who require prolonged intubation may help to reduce the risk of complications such as aspiration pneumonia.

TABLE 153-2 Clinical Vignettes Illustrating the Pathophysiology of Dysphagia

Case Presentation	Analysis	Differential Diagnosis	Pathophysiology
A 60-year-old man with past medical history of hypertension, hyperlipidemia, and diabetes mellitus presents to the ED with sudden onset of inability to use right arm and leg. He also has slurring of speech with difficulty swallowing.	Sudden onset of symptoms suggest a central nervous system acute event.	Cerebrovascular accident involving either MCA territory or extracranial ICA territory, multiple sclerosis, Guillain-Barre syndrome and polio	Oral preparatory and pharyngeal phases involved
A 45-year-old woman presents with gradual onset of difficulty swallowing. The symptoms occur a few minutes after swallowing. It is accompanied by nasal regurgitation and change in tone of her voice. She also coughs every time she tries to eat. Symptoms are preceded by difficulty climbing stairs and combing her hair.	Gradual onset of dysphagia with symptoms of muscle weakness is suggestive of an underlying myopathic cause of dysphagia.	Connective tissue disorders like dermatomyositis and polymyositis, sarcoidosis, paraneoplastic syndromes, and myasthenia gravis	Oral preparatory, pharyngeal and esophageal phases involved
A 30-year-old man presents with difficulty swallowing for both solids and liquids over several months. He has complaints of significant weight loss and regurgitation of undigested food several hours after eating the meal. He also has history of recurrent pneumonias.	Gradual onset of dysphagia for solids and liquids in a young individual is suggestive of esophageal dysmotility.	Diffuse esophageal spasm, ineffective esophageal motility, scleroderma, lupus, mixed connective tissue disorders, and achalasia	Esophageal phase involved

ED, emergency department; ICA, inferior cerebral artery; MCA, middle cerebral artery.

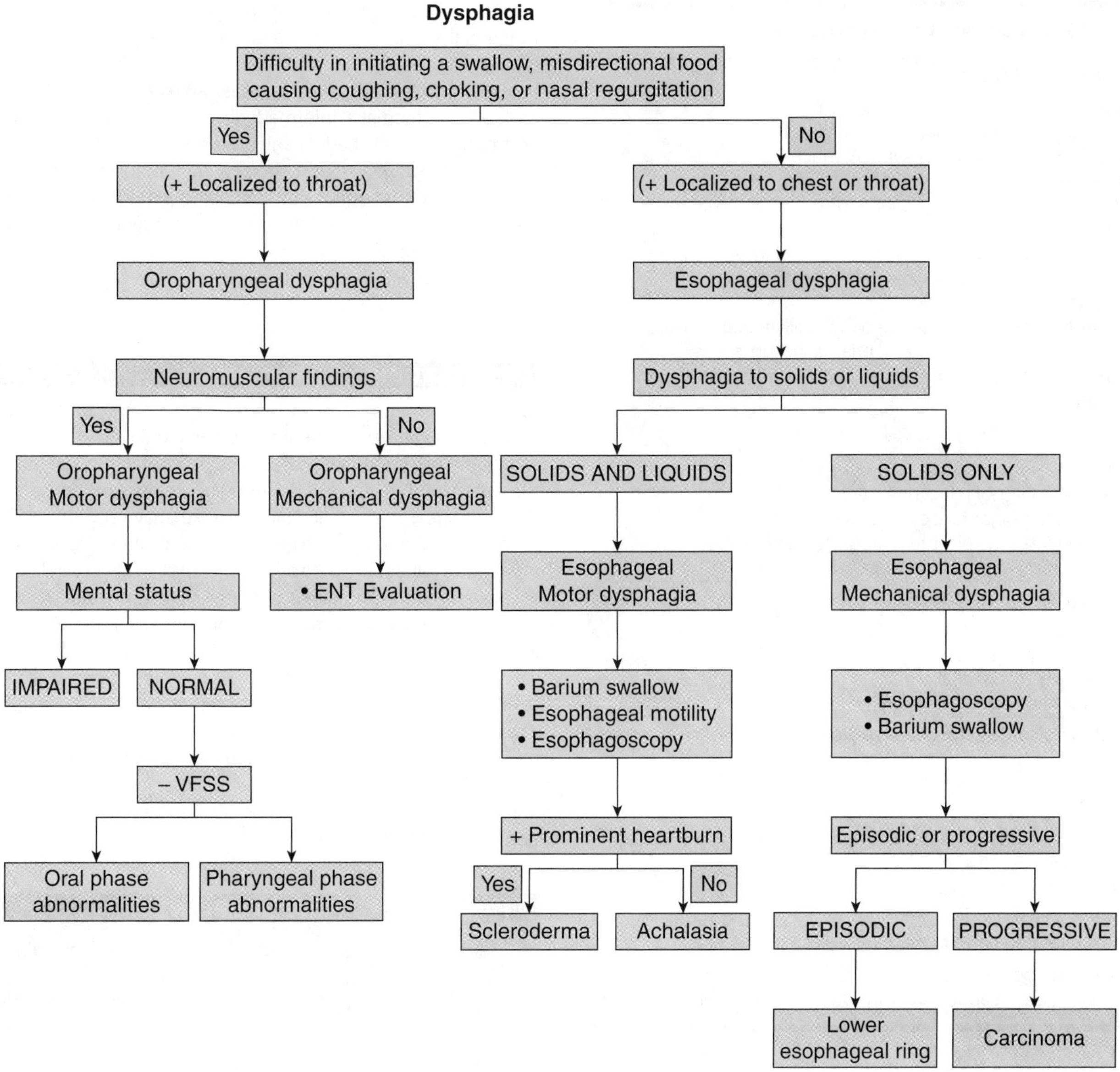

Figure 153-1 *Approach to Patient with Dysphagia. ENT, Otolaryngology; VFSS, Videofluoroscopic Swallowing Study. (Reproduced, with permission, from Fauci AS, Braunwald E, Kasper DL, et al. Harrison's Principles of Internal Medicine. 17th ed. New York: McGraw-Hill; 2008. Figure 38-1.)*

MANAGEMENT

INITIAL HOSPITAL TREATMENT

Dysphagia treatment goals include improving food transfer and preventing aspiration. The treatment should focus on the underlying etiology as treatment modalities vary based on the etiology of dysphagia (**Table 153-5**). In general, patients need to be kept NPO to prevent aspiration. All essential medications need to be given intravenously.

CONSULTATIONS

The common specialties involved in the care of patients with dysphagia include neurology, general surgery, gastroenterology, otolaryngology, speech therapy, and nutrition services. Early consultations with speech therapy and nutrition services can help facilitate diagnosis and improve patient education and management. Speech therapists can perform a bedside swallowing evaluation that provides information about the locus of the patient's dysphagia (oropharyngeal or esophageal), patient's readiness for a radiographic study, laryngeal function, best food consistency and coughing status. Treatment of common causes of dysphagia based on etiology often requires appropriate specialty consultation (Table 153-5).

> **PRACTICE POINT**
>
> - Early consultations with speech therapy and nutrition services can help facilitate diagnosis and improve patient education as well as management in patients with dysphagia or aspiration.

LONGITUDINAL/OUTPATIENT THERAPEUTICS

Regardless of the etiology, safe swallowing methods are the cornerstone of management in patients with oropharyngeal dysphagia (**Table 153-6**). Modalities to improve swallowing include standard speech and swallow rehabilitation. Based on the functional abnormality, the speech and swallowing therapist can devise a rehabilitation plan that includes some of the safe swallowing techniques

TABLE 153-3 Common Causes of Dysphagia

Oropharyngeal causes
• **Iatrogenic:** medication side-effects, radiation, postsurgical, postintubation
• **Infectious:** Lyme disease, syphilis, mucositis
• **Inflammatory:** caustic ingestion, radiation
• **Metabolic:** amyloidosis, Cushing disease, thyrotoxicosis, Wilson disease
• **Myopathic:** connective tissue disorders, dermatomyositis, polymyositis, sarcoidosis, paraneoplastic syndromes, myasthenia gravis
• **Neurological:** stroke, cerebral palsy, Guillian-Barre syndrome, multiple sclerosis, polio, dementia, Parkinson disease
• **Structural:** cricopharyngeal bar, Zenker diverticulum, webs, oropharyngeal tumors
Esophageal causes
General
• Gastroesophageal reflux disease
• Infiltrative: eosinophilic esophagitis
• Connective tissue disorders: lupus, scleroderma, mixed connective tissue disorders, etc
Esophageal motility disorders
• Achalasia
• Diffuse esophageal spasm
• Ineffective esophageal motility
• Nonspecific esophageal motility disorder
Structural disorders: Mechanical disorders
• Peptic stricture
• Schatzki ring
• Diverticula
• Carcinoma and benign tumors
• Foreign bodies (Acute)
• Vascular compression
• Mediastinal masses
Life-threatening conditions
• Infectious: botulism, diphtheria
• Neurological: head trauma, brainstem tumors, stroke

(Table 153-6). Additionally, neuromuscular electrical stimulation (NMES), and thermal tactile stimulation (TTS) may be implemented for stroke patients or patients with a neuromuscular etiology of their dysphagia. NMES involves direct stimulation of muscles to recruit motor units and increase muscle strength and has demonstrated benefit in some small studies. TTS involves increasing "oral awareness" by touching the anterior facial pillars with a cold probe prior to having the patient swallow. This is thought to alert the brain cortex and facilitate the pharyngeal stage of a swallow more quickly. The utility of the sensory modalities is currently under debate.

If the dysphagia persists for a prolonged period of time (more than three days), other enteral feeding methods may be considered, such as nasogastric tubes (NGTs), percutaneous gastrostomy (PEG), or jejunostomy (PEJ) tubes. PEG tubes are indicated in patients with prolonged dysphagia for more than 4–6 weeks. The timing and indications of PEG tube placement vary based on individual patient characteristics. Robust data supports the use of PEGs in patients with head and neck cancers to improve the patients' nutritional status as well as overall outcomes. On the other hand, PEG tubes in patients with advanced dementia and other progressive neurological disorders do not improve mortality or morbidity. In fact, studies have shown that PEG tubes are not effective in preventing aspiration pneumonia, improving nutritional or functional status, or in extending life. In these instances, patients and/or families should work with a multidisciplinary care team (including physicians, nurses, social workers, speech therapists, and others) to make informed decisions regarding swallowing and nutrition. Each patient must be assessed on a case-by-case basis to determine the best short- as well as long-term approach to nutrition. Other options for managing patients with dysphagia and resultant aspiration include surgical procedures that divert or close off the upper airway from the esophagus. However, these are often reserved for patients who maintain a high aspiration risk despite tracheaostomy alone.

COMPLICATIONS AND PROGNOSIS

Aspiration pneumonia is the most common cause of death from dysphagia due to neurological etiologies. It occurs due to aspiration of oropharyngeal secretions containing bacteria into the larynx and lower respiratory tracts. Temporary depression of the immune system following a stroke may facilitate development of pneumonia. Aspiration risk is best assessed through inpatient evaluation by a speech therapist, with possible further assessment with a modified barium swallow. A modified barium swallow is usually performed in the presence of a speech/swallowing therapist. The patient is instructed to swallow substances of varying consistencies under fluoroscopy. A technician will acquire lateral and anteroposterior views of the oral as well as pharyngeal phases of swallowing. The therapist is able to obtain information regarding the level and mechanism of swallowing dysfunction as well as risk of aspiration. Additionally, therapies and techniques to improve swallowing can often be devised based on the information obtained from this study.

PRACTICE POINT

- Aspiration pneumonia is the most common cause of death from dysphagia due to neurological etiologies.

In patients with documented aspiration, safe swallowing methods should be employed (Table 153-6). In the absence of improvement with these techniques, feeding through nasogastric tubes (NGTs) or gastrostomy tubes (PEG) may be considered. However, the risk of aspiration is not diminished with gastrostomy tubes as compared to NGTs. Furthermore, NGT are not without risk. Often, patients will pull on the tube causing it to coil or migrate proximally into the oropharynx. This can subsequently increase the risk of aspiration pneumonia. Epistaxis is a potential complication of NGTs in patients with bleeding disorders, coagulopathy, or receiving anticoagulants. Furthermore, large bore tubes can obstruct breathing in a small percentage of adult patients and cause irritation of the nasal mucosa resulting in sinusitis. With persistent aspiration risk despite extended therapy for 4–6 weeks, a PEG tube may be considered. Despite preventive measures, if a patient develops clinical and laboratory signs and symptoms of aspiration pneumonia, antibiotics should be prescribed (Refer to Community-Acquired Pneumonia chapter 189 for therapy).

PRACTICE POINT

- In patients with dysphagia, the risk of aspiration is not diminished with gastrostomy (PEG) tubes as compared to nasogastric tubes (NGTs).

TABLE 153-4 Diagnostic Modalities for Evaluation of Dysphagia

Diagnostic Test	Clinician Involved	Presentation Where Test Indicated	Invasiveness	Technique	Information Obtained
Modified barium swallow	Speech pathologist, fluoroscopic radiologist	Nasal regurgitation, change in tone of voice, cough with eating, recurrent pneumonia	No	Lateral and anteroposterior views of oral and pharyngeal phases of swallow are assessed by speech pathologist	• Mechanism and severity of oropharyngeal dysfunction • Qualitative aspiration
Barium swallow	Fluoroscopic radiolologist	Gradual/sudden dysphagia for solids progressing to liquids	No	Series of radiographs that look at esophageal phase of swallowing during passage of contrast liquid/pill	• Anatomy of esophagus • Peristaltic activity • Presence or absence of reflux
Fiberoptic endoscopic evaluation of swallowing	Otolaryngologist	Nasal regurgitation, change in tone of voice, cough with eating, recurrent pneumonia	Yes	Direct visualization of all mucosal surfaces of oral cavity, nasopharynx, pharynx, and larynx by nasal endoscope	• Pharyngeal phase of swallowing
Manometry	Gastroenterologist	Gradual dysphagia for solids/liquids, regurgitation of undigested material hours after eating	Yes	Intraesophageal pressures within esophagus are measured by transnasal transducer	• Peristaltic activity • Degree of pharyngeal and esophageal contraction • Upper and lower esophageal sphincter relaxation
Scintigraphy	Nuclear radiologist	Nasal regurgitation, change in tone of voice, cough with eating, Recurrent pneumonia	No	Neck and chest images of passage of technetium-99m labeled oral secretions	• Quantitative aspiration • Esophageal clearance

TABLE 153-5 Treatment of Common Causes of Dysphagia Based on Etiology

Etiology of Dysphagia	Interventions to Consider	Success Rate	Consultation
Neoplasm	Radiation/chemotherapy/surgical resection	Early disease 5-y survival rate 15–59%	Medical/surgical oncology/nutrition/ gastroenterology
Esophageal rings/webs	Upper endoscopy with dilation	50%	Gastroenterology
Achalasia	Surgical incision of LES (Heller myotomy) in appropriate patients.* If not an option, endoscopic rupture of LES (pneumatic balloon dilation) or botulinum injection	62–100% depending on type and mode of toxin	Gastroenterology, general or thoracic surgery. If not surgical candidate, consult gastroenterology. Nutrition
Stroke	Anticoagulation if appropriate, blood pressure control, rehabilitation- physical therapy/ occupational therapy	Varies based on severity of dysphagia	Neurology/speech/ nutrition/ gastroenterology/ physical and occupational therapy
Degenerative neurological disorders	Appropriate medications, rehabilitation (physical therapy/ occupational therapy)	Varies based on severity of dysphagia and underlying disease	Neurology/speech/nutrition, physical and occupation therapy
Zenker diverticulum (Figure 153-2)	Cricopharyngeal myotomy along with possible diverticulum suspension	80–100%	ENT/thoracic surgery/gastroenterology

ENT, otolaryngology; LES, lower esophageal sphincter.
*Procedure of choice.

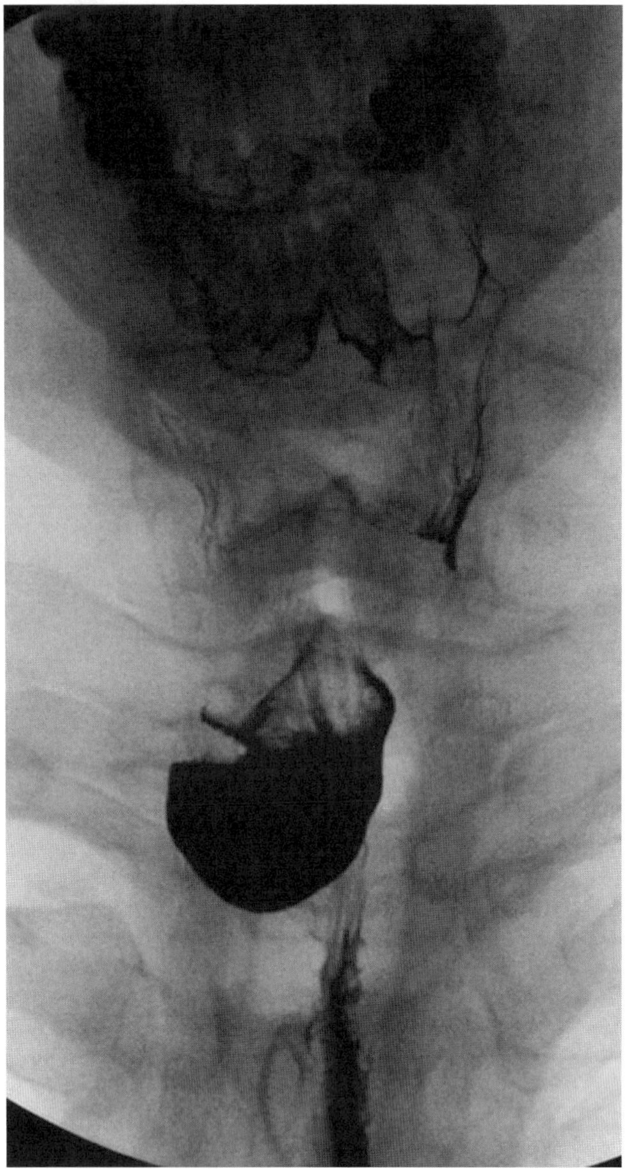

Figure 153-2 *Anteriolateral view of a patient with dysphagia due to a Zenker diverticulum. (Courtesy of Deborah Baumgarten, MD, MPH; Department of Radiology, Emory School of Medicine.)*

Dehydration is a common complication of dysphagia and may be a risk factor for aspiration pneumonia due to decreased salivary secretion and possible lethargy or confusion. Dehydration can also lead to immune status depression. Clinicians should maintain a low threshold to suspect and evaluate patients for dehydration. Adequate fluid intake can be achieved through simple interventions, such as systematically offering patients preferred liquids or foods with high fluid content. In patients who cannot eat or swallow, maintaining hydration through NGT, PEG fluid supplementation, or with intravenous fluids may be necessary.

Malnutrition occurs commonly following stroke. Up to 50% of stroke patients and 65% of dysphagia patients admitted for rehabilitation after a cerebrovascular event will develop malnutrition. Malnutrition increases the risk of aspiration and decreases immunity. It also contributes to overall functional decline, muscle breakdown, osteoporosis, osteopenia, iron-deficiency anemia, skin breakdown, and poor wound healing. These poor outcomes can be avoided by careful nutritional assessment by a nutritionist early during the disease course and by providing adequate oral or enteral supplementation. Early collaboration and consultation with an inpatient nutrition service will help mitigate malnutrition and some of its associated complications.

TABLE 153-6 Safe Swallowing Methods

- **Thickening liquids** by adding thickeners to modify the texture.
- **Oral motor exercises** reinforce the lip and tongue and control drooling while assisting bolus formation and propulsion.
- **Intentional multiple swallows** help clear pooling in the pharynx.
- **Bending the neck forward** can offset delayed pharyngeal contraction by assisting laryngeal elevation and closure.
- **Placing the food bolus posteriorly after tilting the head back** may facilitate swallowing.
- In ***unilateral pharyngeal dysfunction,*** **turning the head to the weaker side while tilting it to the stronger side** can help propel food forward.
- **Effortful swallow** can offset impaired tongue base retraction and decreased pharyngeal control.

DISCHARGE PLANNING

Discharge planning requires a multidisciplinary approach including follow-up with a variety of different specialties. Importantly, the care team must confirm that the patient can safely swallow recommended consistency, ingest calories, as well as medications required as an outpatient.

PEG tubes are indicated for patients who are unable to consume sufficient nutrition over a period of more than four to six weeks, despite a functioning gastrointestinal tract. Though clinical data suggests that patients can be safely fed through NGTs until that time period, many patients may receive a PEG tube earlier to allow a more consistent and reliable enteral feeding source and for patients' comfort. Therefore, if appropriate or required prior to discharge, a decision regarding the need for a PEG tube should be made and the PEG should be placed several days before discharge.

REHABILITATION

Rehabilitative therapy, especially in patients with neurological disorders, should begin in the hospital after the patient's medical condition has been stabilized, usually within 24 to 48 hours after an acute neurologic event. After the initial therapy (physical therapy, occupational therapy, and/or speech therapy, as indicated) in the hospital, there are several different types of continued rehabilitation that can be pursued following the acute care hospital stay. The different rehabilitation approaches are determined by the patient's ability to perform physical activity, medical necessity, amount of neurological impairment, and the amount of support available at home. While a patient with minimal medical necessity and good physical capacity may benefit from acute inpatient or outpatient rehabilitation, a patient with limited physical capacity and multitude of medical problems may benefit more from subacute rehabilitation or long-term acute care setting. Additionally, home-based rehabilitation (home health) may be enough for certain patients, if they do not require intensive inpatient rehabilitation or they lack transportation to get to an outpatient rehabilitation center. Home health rehabilitation requires adequate support systems at home. Yet, home rehabilitation therapy can also assure a safer home environment for the patient. Occupational therapists can help with this transition.

FOLLOW-UP

Discharge planning should also include outpatient follow-up with the primary care physician and any other relevant specialists. Prior to discharge, the hospital care provider should speak with a representative from all of the services that helped to manage the patient to determine if additional tests or swallowing therapies are recommended as an outpatient. For instance, patients diagnosed with peptic strictures of the esophagus may need outpatient follow-up with a gastroenterologist to have serial dilations of their strictures until the dysphagia resolves. While stroke or dysphagia centers may provide this service to all patients, many hospitals do not have a multidisciplinary care team in place. Therefore, the hospitalist in conjunction with the primary care physician must play a key role in coordinating the appropriate outpatient care for their patients.

Follow-up with a primary care physician should occur within one to four weeks following hospital discharge.

QUALITY IMPROVEMENT TO ADDRESS PERFORMANCE

EARLY RECOGNITION OF SWALLOWING IMPAIRMENT

Several steps can be taken to improve the quality of care given to patients in the hospital and help transition their care smoothly. One tool that can be employed for early recognition of dysphagia in stroke patients is the Modified Mann Assessment of Swallowing Ability (MMASA), a bedside screening test that can be employed by physicians or other clinicians to screen for dysphagia (**Figure 153-3**). It scores different facets of the physical exam including alertness, cooperation, respiration, expressive dysphasia, dysarthria, tongue movement, and strength. The tool may facilitate earlier identification of dysphagia prompting more rapid comprehensive evaluation and intervention.

DISPARITIES IN HEALTH CARE

One prospective cohort study from Ontario, Canada shows that patients older than 80 years old have almost 15% 30-day risk adjusted fatality rate after an acute stroke. Older patients require longer hospitalization and have higher pneumonia risk and higher disability at discharge. Other data has shown that Asians have a higher incidence of dysphagia compared to blacks or whites (OR-1.64; CI, 1.50–1.79), but it is unclear why these disparities exist.

COSTS AND RESOURCE UTILIZATION

When aspiration pneumonia is highly suspected or diagnosed, clinicians should specify that the pneumonia may be due to aspiration. Such patients often bear a worse prognosis as well as a longer length of hospital stay. Thus, care providers can implement strategies to effectively treat the pneumonia and to reduce recurrent aspiration pneumonia. Aspiration in the setting of pneumonia is taken into account and contributes significantly to the case mix index for hospitals (**Table 153-7**).

Modified Mann Assessment of Swallowing Ability (MMASA)
INSTRUCTIONS:
Circle the most appropriate clinical findings for each indicator.
Calculate the total score by adding the points for each indicator.
Patient Name____________________
Date____________________

1. Alertness
Task: Observe and evaluate the patient's response to speech, limb movement, or painful stimulation

Grade:
10 = Alert
8 = Drowsy-fluctuating awareness/alert level
5 = Difficult to arouse by speech or movement
2 = Coma or nonresponsive

2. Cooperation
Task: Gain patient's attention and attempt to initiate communication or activity

Grade:
10 = Cooperative-engages in some form of verbal or nonverbal exchange
8 = Fluctuating co-operation
5 = Reluctant co-operation
2 = No co-operation/response

3. Respiration
Task: Assess status of patient's Task: Assess status of patient's

Grade:
10 = Chest clear, no clinical or radiographic evidence of abnormality
8 = Sputum in the upper airway or other respiratory condition (eg, asthma/bronchopasm, chronic obstructive pulmonary disease)
6 = Fine basal crepitations/self-clearing
4 = Coarse basal crepitations
2 = Suspected infection/frequent suctioning/respirator dependent

4. Expressive Dysphasia
Task: Assess for disturbances expression

Grade:
5 = No abnormality
4 = Mild difficulty finding words/expressing ideas
3 = Expresses self in a limited manner/short phrases or words
2 = No functional speech sounds or undecipherable single words
1 = Unable to assess

Figure 153-3 *Modified Mann Assessment of Swallowing Ability (MMASA), a bedside screening test that can be employed by physicians to screen for dysphagia. (Reproduced, with permission, from Giselle Denya Mann, MPH, PhD.)*

5. Auditory Comprehension
Task: Ability to understand basic verbal communication

Grade:
10 = No abnormality
8 = Follows ordinary conversation with little difficulty
6 = Follows simple conversation/instructions with repetition
4 = Occasional response if cued
1 = No response

6. Dysarthria
Task: Assess articulation

Grade:
5 = No abnormality
4 = Slow with occasional hesitation and sluring
3 = Speech intelligible but obviously defective rate/range/strength/coordination
2 = Speech unintelligible
1 = Unable to assess

7. Saliva
Task: Observe patient's control of of saliva; note any escape of secretions from the side of the mouth

Grade:
5 = No abnormality
4 = Forthy/expectorated into cup
3 = Drooling at times, during speech, while side lying or fatigued
2 = Some drool consistently
1 = Gross drooling, unable to control drooling

8. Tongue Movement
Task: Assess tongue movement
Protrusion: Have patient extend tongue as forward as possible, and then retract
Lateralization: Have patient touch each corner of the mouth, then repeat altering lateral movements
Elevation: With mouth wide open, have patient raise tongue upto palate;alternate elevation and depression in this way

Grade:
10 = Full range of movements/no abnormality detected
8 = Mild impairment in range
6 = Incomplete movement
4 = Minimal movement
2 = No movement or unable to perform

9. Tongue Strength
Task: Assess bilateral tongue strength
Have patient push laterally and anteriorly against tongue blade

Grade:
10 = No abnormality
8 = Minimal weakness
5 = Obvious unilateral weakness
2 = Gross weakness or unable to perform

10. Gag
Task: Contact posterior pharyngeal wall on either side separately

Grade:
5 = No abnormality
4 = Diminished bilaterally
3 = Diminished unilaterally
2 = Absent unilaterally
1 = No gag response

11. Cough Reflex
Task: Ask patient to cough as strong as possible
Observe strength and clarity of cough

Grade:
10 = No abnormality
8 = Cough attempted, but hoarse in quality
5 = Attempt inadequate
2 = No attempt or unable to perform

12. Palate
Task: Ask patient to produce a strong as "AH" several times and sustain each one for several seconds
Observe for hypernasality and note action of palate elevation

Grade:
10 = No abnormality
8 = Slight asymmetry noted; mobile palate
6 = Unilaterally weak and inconsistently maintained
4 = Minimal movement, nasal regurgitation, nasal air escape
2 = No elevation of palate or unable to perform

MMASA SORE = ___________

Interpretation
Score ≥ 95: Start oral diet and progress as tolerated. Monitor first oral intake and consult SPEECHPATHOLOGY if patient has difficulty eating or drinking.
Score ≤ 94: Nothing by mouth and consult SPEECHPATHOLOGY for a formal swallow evaluation.

Figure 153-3 *(continued)*

TABLE 153-7 Evidence-based Medicine: Key References for Management of Dysphagia

Reference	Methodology	Results	Limitations	Bottom Line
Hinchey JA, et al. *Stroke.* 2005;36(9): 1972–1976.	Prospective chart review to compare rate of aspiration pneumonia in sites with formal dysphagia screen as compared to sites with no formal screen	The pneumonia rate at sites with formal dysphagia screen was 2.4% vs 5.4% ($P = 0.0016$) at sites with no formal screen	Was not a randomized, double-blinded study. Levels of dysphagia varied among patients	Formal dysphagia screen is associated with higher adherence rate to dysphagia screens and significantly decreased risk of pneumonia
Barker J, et al. *Can J Surg.* 2009;52(2): 119–124.	Retrospective chart review. Multivariate regression analysis and parametric modeling were used to identify patient-specific characteristics associated with postextubation dysphagia and subsequent resumption of normal oral feeding after cardiac surgery	Incremental factors associated with increased risk for postextubation dysphagia included duration of endotracheal intubation ($P < 0.001$); occurrence of perioperative cerebrovascular event ($P = 0.014$); and presence of perioperative sepsis ($P = 0.016$)	Retrospective study with small sample size in one particular population of patients with prolonged intubation	Duration of postoperative endotracheal intubation is strong predictor of subsequent dysphagia that both prolongs return to normal oral feeding and delays subsequent hospital discharge. Swallowing surveillance should be undertaken with prolonged post-extubation
Fay DE, et al. *Am J Gastroenterol.* 1991;86(11): 1604–1609.	Retrospective chart review to compare long-term clinical outcomes in patients receiving nutrition via nasogastric tubes vs gastrostomy tubes	Cumulative rates of minor and major complications (including aspiration pneumonia) were similar in both groups during follow-up. Mortality was similar	Retrospective study with small sample size	In patients with dysphagia, risk of aspiration is not diminished with gastrostomy tubes as compared to nasogastric tubes

SUGGESTED READINGS

Antonios N, Carnaby-Mann G, Crary M, et al. Analysis of a physician tool for evaluating dysphagia on an inpatient stroke unit: MMASA. *Journal of Stroke and Cerebrovascular Diseases.* 2010;19:49–57.

Cook IJ, Kahrilas PJ. AGA technical review on management of oropharyngeal dysphagia. *Gastroenterology.* 1999;116:455.

Cook. Oropharyngeal Dysphagia. *Gastroenterol Clin N Am.* 2009;38: 411–431.

Ha L, Hauge T. Percutaneous endoscopic gastrostomy (PEG) for enteral nutrition in patients with stroke. *Scand J Gastroenterol.* 2003;38(9):962–966.

Langmore S, Grillone G, Ekackattu A, et al. Disorders of Swallowing: Palliative care. *Otolaryngol Clin N Am.* 42:87–105.

Lim, KB, Lee HJ, Lim SS, et al. Neuromuscular electrical and thermal-tactile stimulation for dysphagia caused by stroke: A randomized controlled trial. *J Rehabil Med.* 2009;41:174–178.

Metheny N, Meert K, and Clouse R. Complications related to feeding tube placement. *Curr Opin Gastro.* 2007;23:178–182.

Walter G. Bradley, Robert B. Daroff, Gerald Fenichel, Joseph Jankovic. Neurology in Clinical Practice, 5th ed. Butterworth-Heinemann.

White GN, O'Rourke F, Ong BS, et al. Dysphagia; Causes, assessment, treatment, and management. *Geriatrics.* 2008;63(5):15–20.

CHAPTER 154

Gastroesophageal Reflux Disease and Esophagitis

Walter W. Chan, MD, MPH
Robert Burakoff, MD, MPH

Key Clinical Questions

1. What is the approach to patients presenting with reflux, heartburn, or noncardiac chest pain?
2. How should patients with esophagitis and gastroesophageal reflux disease (GERD) be managed in the inpatient setting?
3. What are the possible complications resulting from esophagitis and GERD?

INTRODUCTION

Gastroesophageal reflux disease (GERD) and other esophageal disorders account for a significant number of physician office visits, hospital admissions, and endoscopic procedures each year. Annual management costs for GERD alone have been estimated to exceed $9 billion and continue to escalate. GERD results from the backflowing of gastroduodenal contents into the esophagus, leading to a variety of symptoms including heartburn, chest discomfort, regurgitation, and dysphagia. Compromise in the physiological barrier of reflux at the gastroesophageal junction is believed to be the primary mechanism of reflux. Esophagitis is defined as the presence of signs of inflammation of the esophageal mucosal surfaces, both macroscopically and microscopically. GERD is the most common cause of esophagitis, followed closely by medication-induced and infection-induced inflammation. Symptoms of esophagitis may range from mild chest discomfort to significant dysphagia and odynophagia.

EPIDEMIOLOGY

The prevalence of GERD and esophagitis in the U.S. has been increasing in recent years. Epidemiological studies have shown that approximately 25% of the Western population report having symptoms of heartburn at least once a month, with up to 5% noting daily symptoms. While the prevalence of heartburn symptoms appears to be similar in both genders, female patients less likely possess objective findings of reflux on physiological studies. Moreover, numerous clinical studies have shown a lower response rate to antireflux treatment for female patients. No definite relationship between age and GERD has been concluded. At least one study has suggested less reflux symptoms in older individuals. However, the elderly also seem to possess more severe esophagitis, suggesting a higher prevalence of asymptomatic reflux. Strongly positive association has been demonstrated between obesity and reflux symptoms in clinical studies. An increase in body mass index (BMI) both causes reflux and exacerbates existing symptoms.

PRESENTATION

GERD most typically presents as heartburn, regurgitation, and dysphagia. Patients often describe heartburn as a retrosternal, "burning" discomfort in the lower chest or epigastric region that often travels up toward the neck region. Symptoms often worsen after meals or when patients are in a supine position. As a result, patients frequently complain of symptoms or exacerbation of symptoms at night that may wake them up from sleep. Physiological studies suggest that gastric distention caused by meals and sleep can each induce transient relaxation of the lower esophageal sphincter (LES). Dysphagia is a common symptom of GERD, and it is often a result of esophageal mucosal inflammation. However, it is also one of the "alarming" signs of GERD that indicate the need for further evaluation to exclude possible underlying malignancy. Other "alarming" signs of GERD include odynophagia, weight loss, signs of gastrointestinal (GI) bleeding, advanced age, and a family history of upper GI tract malignancy. When one or more of the "alarming" signs is present, further evaluation with endoscopy or other radiographic imaging should be considered.

> **PRACTICE POINT**
>
> - "Alarming" signs of GERD include dysphagia, odynophagia, weight loss, signs of GI bleeding, advanced age, and a family history of upper GI tract malignancy. When any is present, further evaluation with endoscopy or other radiographic imaging is indicated.

In addition to the typical esophageal presentation, GERD may also cause a variety of atypical, extra-esophageal manifestations. Coexisting pulmonary disease with GERD occurs commonly, with the diagnosis established in 40% to 80% of asthmatics. Although airway irritation resulting from microaspiration of refluxed contents has been implicated as a possible trigger for asthma, certain medications used for asthma, such as bronchodilators, may also cause transient LES relaxation. However, consistent treatment benefit for asthma has not been demonstrated using acid suppression medications or anti-reflux surgery. Nevertheless, GERD likely plays a role in the pathogenesis of pulmonary disorders such as asthma, chronic bronchitis, bronchiectasis, aspiration pneumonia, and pulmonary fibrosis, as well as upper airway manifestations such as pharyngitis, laryngitis, or postnasal drip. Oral problems such as dental erosions, halitosis, and aphthous ulcers have also been linked to GERD.

Patients with GERD or esophagitis may also present with noncardiac chest pain, often described by patients as nonspecific retrosternal discomfort. Such chest discomfort may be a result of mucosal inflammation or esophageal spasm or dysmotility, and it may mimic other causes of chest pain such as acute coronary syndrome or pulmonary disorders. Noncardiac chest pain resulting from esophageal disorders is a common presentation leading to emergency room visits and hospital admission for further workup.

PATHOPHYSIOLOGY

GERD

The lower esophageal sphincter, a tonic smooth muscle located in the lower esophagus around the gastro-esophageal junction, serves as the major barrier to reflux of gastric content into the esophagus. Disruption in the tonic contractile pressure of the LES may result in the backflowing of gastric content into the esophagus. Such a disruption may present in the form of a general decrease in the tonic pressure of the LES (hypotensive LES) or inappropriate relaxation of the LES not during swallowing (pathologic transient LES relaxation). Many factors have been associated with disruption of the tonic contraction of the LES. For example, a hiatal hernia leads to anatomic disruption of the gastroesophageal junction and is associated with an increased risk of transient LES relaxation. Certain medications such as sedatives, food items such as caffeine and chocolate, and lifestyle behavior including alcohol and tobacco use can also lead to LES relaxation, resulting in GERD symptoms. In addition to LES relaxation, the barrier between the stomach and esophagus may also be pathologically overcome if the intragastric pressure exceeds the tonic contractile pressure of the LES. Most commonly, this situation results from obesity, delayed gastric emptying, or certain postoperative states.

While GERD symptoms are often thought to be a result of the presence of acidic gastric content in the esophagus, leading to burning sensation and inflammation, the backflow of nonacidic contents such as bile can also generate similar symptoms. Since certain diagnostic modalities including pH study and the use of acid-suppression medications for treatment of GERD targets the presence of acid in the esophagus, the identification of nonacid reflux patients would help identify patients who may not respond to common medical therapy for GERD symptoms.

ESOPHAGITIS

Esophagitis presents with inflammatory changes in the esophageal mucosa, with or without signs of erosion. The inflammatory reactions in the esophagus can be elicited by direct caustic injury, most commonly by acid, trauma, infection, or autoimmune processes. In the case of reflux-induced esophagitis, the diffusion of hydrogen ions into the esophageal mucosa leads to cellular acidification and necrosis. As a result, erosion and inflammatory cells infiltration ensue. Caustic injuries may also be caused by direct erosion or chemical reactions between the substance and the esophageal mucosa.

DIFFERENTIAL DIAGNOSIS

GERD

A variety of risk factors have been linked to GERD. Certain medications can cause a decrease in LES pressure, including beta adrenergic agonists, alpha adrenergic antagonists, anticholinergics, benzodiazepines, calcium channel blockers, narcotics, progesterone, estrogens, and tricyclic antidepressants. Lifestyle behaviors such as smoking, alcohol ingestions, and food ingestion prior to incumbency have been linked to GERD symptoms. Some food items and beverages can also cause heartburn symptoms by reducing LES pressure. Examples include fatty food, chocolate, citrus fruits, tomato-based products, peppermint, vinegar, carbonated drinks, and caffeinated beverages.

In addition to lifestyle behavior and ingestions, other known risk factors for GERD include obesity, gastroparesis, and hiatal hernia. Obesity may lead to an increase in intra-abdominal pressure that can cause LES relaxation. Gastroparesis causes intragastric distention, which may in turn activate stretch receptors of the stomach, resulting in decrease in LES pressure.

> **PRACTICE POINT**
>
> - Sedative medications, caffeine, chocolate, alcohol or tobacco each can lead to LES relaxation, resulting in GERD symptoms. Medications that can cause a decrease in LES pressure include beta adrenergic agonists, alpha adrenergic antagonists, anticholinergics, benzodiazepines, calcium channel blockers, narcotics, progesterone, estrogens, and tricyclic antidepressants.

ESOPHAGITIS

Inflammation of the esophagus is most commonly related to GERD. Other risk factors for the development of esophagitis include medication, infection, radiation, or less common causes such as autoimmune disorders. Medication-induced esophagitis ("pill esophagitis") causes direct injury to the esophageal mucosa. Common examples include alendronate, aspirin, nonsteroidal anti-inflammatory drugs, iron salts, potassium chloride tablets, quinidine, and tetracycline. However, any medication or foreign object can lead to direct injury and erosion into the esophageal mucosa if its transit through the esophagus is prolonged.

Infectious esophagitis usually occur in immunocompromised hosts such as patients with acquired immune deficiency syndrome (AIDS), posttransplantation, or undergoing chemotherapy. The most common etiologies for infectious esophagitis are fungal and viral infections. Esophageal candidiasis is one of the most common opportunistic infections in immunocompromised patients (**Figure 154-1**). Often it represents the initial presentation leading to the diagnosis of HIV infection, and candida esophagitis (unlike simple thrush alone) is an AIDS-defining illness. Patients

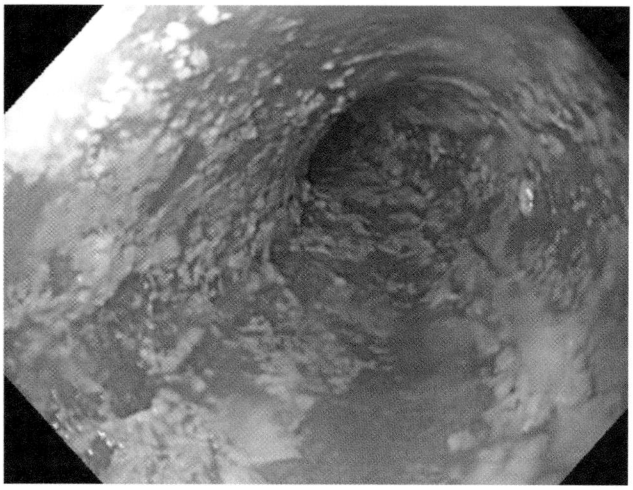

Figure 154-1 *Endoscopy revealing Candida esophagitis.*

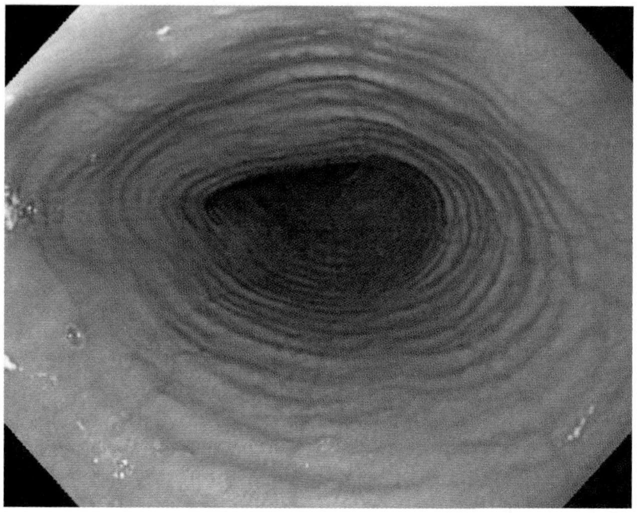

Figure 154-2 *Eosinophilic esophagitis. Findings of longitudinal markings and concentric rings in the middle third of the esophagus ("feline esophagus") consistent with eosinophilic esophagitis. Biopsies obtained revealed infiltration of > 40 eosinophils/hpf.*

with esophageal candidiasis often complain of dysphagia and occasionally odynophagia. Esophageal candidiasis appears as whitish plaques on the esophageal mucosa that are easily scraped off, and oropharyngeal disease (thrush) often coexists. Therefore, in immunosuppressed patients who present with dysphagia, a careful oral examination can often provide clues to possible esophageal candidiasis. Empiric treatment with antifungals can often be considered in these high-risk patients. The most common agents causing viral esophagitis are human herpes simplex virus (HSV) and cytomegalovirus (CMV). Similar to fungal candidiasis, HSV and CMV esophagitis often present with dysphagia and odynophagia, although odynophagia presents more commonly in these cases. Concomitant oropharyngeal disease often occurs. Diagnosis requires endoscopic visualization of the typical HSV or CMV ulcers.

Cancer patients with prior chest radiation therapy may also develop radiation-induced esophagitis. Symptom onset can be immediate (within 3 weeks) or delayed (usually 3 or more months), with significant variation in the severity often unrelated to the dosage of radiation received. Symptoms can range from mild dysphagia to severe odynophagia or structuring requiring enteral tube feeding. As these patients are often also immunocompromised from chemotherapy, infectious esophagitis may coexist and must first be ruled out or treated.

Patients with a history of hematologic malignancy who have undergone bone marrow transplantation may develop graft-versus-host disease (GVHD), which can involve any part of the gastrointestinal tract. GVHD of the esophagus often leads to significant inflammation and ulceration, resulting in symptoms of significant dysphagia, odynophagia, or bleeding. Therefore, this diagnosis must be considered in bone marrow transplant patients presenting with upper gastrointestinal bleeding or new-onset dysphagia symptoms, and mucosal biopsies can establish the diagnosis. Similar to other cancer patients, infectious esophagitis is also very prevalent in this population and may coexist with GVHD due to chronic immunosuppression.

Autoimmune disorders remain an uncommon cause of esophagitis. Inflammatory diseases such as Crohn disease or Behçet disease may involve the esophagus, leading to inflammation and often ulcerations. Another one of such disorders, eosinophilic esophagitis, appears to be increasing in incidence in recent years. Eosinophilic esophagitis is defined by the infiltration of large number of eosinophils in the esophageal mucosa. Etiology of eosinophilic esophagitis remains unclear; however, it is often linked to other allergic disorders such as asthma or dermatitis. Patients with eosinophilic esophagitis are often young and they often first present with an episode of food impaction. While eosinophilic esophagitis can be associated with characteristic endoscopic appearances, its diagnosis requires histopathologic confirmation of eosinophilic infiltration (**Figure 154-2**).

DIAGNOSIS

ACID SUPPRESSION AS A DIAGNOSTIC TOOL

GERD diagnosis is most frequently achieved thorough history of classic symptoms combined with response to empiric antacid medical therapy, most commonly a proton pump inhibitor (PPI). A meta-analysis of studies on the diagnostic value of PPI response in GERD revealed a pooled sensitivity of 78% and specificity of 54% (positive likelihood ratio 1.70). In most cases, no further diagnostic testing is needed in patients with typical GERD symptoms who have no alarming signs that resolve with a trial of PPI. However, patients who fail to respond to a trial of PPI or report alarm signs should undergo further diagnostic workup, including endoscopy, radiographic imaging, or physiologic testing such as manometry, impedance, and pH studies.

UPPER ENDOSCOPY

Upper endoscopy or esophageal gastroduodenoscopy (EGD) serves as an appropriate initial evaluation of GERD as it allows direct visualization of the esophageal mucosa to exclude the presence of other diseases such as tumors and evaluate for signs and severity of GERD-induced esophagitis. The Los Angeles classification is the most commonly used system in the endoscopic grading of severity of reflux esophagitis. It measures the length and circumferential involvement of mucosal breaks and assigns the findings into four different grades (A–D). In addition to evaluation of esophagitis, endoscopy also allows the diagnosis of complications from GERD, including strictures or the presence of Barrett esophagus. If reflux-induced strictures were discovered, endoscopic dilation can be performed for treatment. Overall, endoscopy has been shown to exhibit high specificity (> 90%) for the diagnosis of GERD but only a moderate sensitivity (~50%). The lack of endoscopic signs of GERD does not exclude its diagnosis. Previous studies have shown that many symptomatic patients with negative initial studies develop mucosal lesions during follow-up endoscopic examinations. Therefore, *symptomatic patients with negative endoscopies should undergo further diagnostic workup.*

RADIOGRAPHIC STUDIES

Radiographic studies such as barium swallow or upper GI series can also be used to detect esophagitis, hiatal hernias, esophageal strictures, or tumors. The primary goal of these studies is to rule out other significant diseases in patients with low clinical suspicion for them. Although they have the advantage of being noninvasive, inexpensive, and widely available, they are less sensitive and specific and should only be used over upper endoscopy if no endoscopist is available or if the patient cannot tolerate an endoscopic procedure.

MOTILITY STUDIES

Several kinds of motility studies have been used for the workup of reflux disease.

Ambulatory esophageal pH monitoring records the distal esophageal pH continuously using a transnasal probe or a pill-sized capsule (Bravo capsule) placed 5 cm above the LES. A battery-powered device carried by the patient records data from the probe, as well as the time of meals and symptom onset. This allows correlation between patient-reported symptoms and objective signs of acid exposure in the distal esophagus, described as symptom association probability (SAP) or symptom index (SI). SAP > 95% or SI > 50% indicates significant association between symptoms and acid exposure. A pH < 4 measured by the probe is defined as acid exposure. In normal individuals, the total amount of time with esophageal pH < 4 (total acid exposure time) over a day should be less than 4%. Although esophageal pH monitoring provides the most sensitive test for identifying presence of acid in the esophagus, its use should be reserved for selected patients: those with symptoms refractory to therapy, atypical symptoms unresponsive to acid suppression, or history of antireflux surgery.

Esophageal manometry measures the strength, duration, and sequential nature of esophageal smooth muscle contraction. An array of pressure sensors along a small catheter passed through the nose into the esophagus and stomach measures the esophageal body contraction, as well as the resting pressure and relaxation of the LES. With each swallow, different pattern of muscle contraction along the probe allows identification of the presence of any motility abnormalities, LES hypotension, or transient relaxation. This test is particularly important as a part of the preoperative evaluation for anti-reflux surgery. In addition to obtaining valuable information regarding LES pressure, manometry also identifies patients with underlying esophageal disorders such as achalasia or diffuse esophageal spasm that would be a contraindication to fundoplication.

Impedance monitoring is a technique in measuring bolus transit through the esophagus. Similar to manometry, it contains a small, flexible catheter placed through the nose into the esophagus. In GERD patients, impedance can identify fluid bolus refluxing into the esophagus and measure the extent of reflux. The combined impedance-pH monitoring device can further classify the refluxed fluid bolus as acidic, weakly acidic, or nonacidic.

TRIAGE AND HOSPITAL ADMISSION

Although GERD and esophagitis can cause significant morbidity for patients, they are still generally managed in the outpatient setting. In rare instances, patients who cannot tolerate oral diet due to significant dysphagia or odynophagia caused by severe esophagitis may require hospitalization for nutritional support. These patients may demonstrate clinical signs of significant dehydration, including hypotension and tachycardia. In the setting of prolonged poor nutritional status, clinical signs related to deficiency of other nutritional elements such as folate and certain vitamins may also be present. In these cases, intravenous hydration needs to be initiated, and other forms of nutritional support such as tube-feeding or TPN may need to be considered.

Another important reason for hospital admission in patients presenting with GERD or esophagitis-related symptoms is to rule out other significant illnesses. Certain GERD and esophagitis symptoms may mimic more significant cardiovascular diseases such as acute coronary syndrome. Patients presenting with chest discomfort should undergo careful cardiac evaluation, and the diagnosis of GERD and esophagitis should not be assumed until cardiac causes can be ruled out.

MANAGEMENT

SYMPTOMATIC MANAGEMENT

Treatment of patients with GERD or esophagitis should aim at the control of symptoms as well as healing of esophageal inflammation. In the case of GERD and reflux esophagitis, management focuses on eliminating acid exposure to the esophagus using both pharmacological and surgical means. Medical treatment for GERD centers around the use of antacid and antisecretory agents. Over-the-counter antacids neutralize refluxed gastric acid, are inexpensive and convenient, and can be used as short-term treatment for patients with occasional symptoms.

Antisecretory agents include histamine-2 (H2) receptor antagonists and PPI. H2 blockers inhibit gastric acid secretion by competitively binding the H2 receptors on gastric parietal cells. They prevent heartburn symptoms when taken before meals and relieve post-prandial heartburn if taken after meals. In patients with frequent GERD symptoms, twice daily H2 blockers may be required for maximal effects. Previous studies have demonstrated that H2 blockers offer a 10% to 24% therapeutic gain over placebo in healing mild to moderate esophagitis, but not effective in healing moderate to severe esophagitis. No differences in efficacy among the different H2 blockers have been found. If a patient remains symptomatic after 6 weeks of standard dose, twice daily H2 blocker therapy, increasing dose or prolonged therapy do not appear to provide additional relief. H2 blockers are appropriate for treating patients with mild to moderate GERD.

Proton pump inhibitors directly block the hydrogen-potassium ATPase on the apical surface of the parietal cells and act on a more downstream pathway than H2 blockers to decrease acid secretion. Compared to H2 blockers, PPIs have greater effectiveness in treating esophagitis after 4 to 8 weeks of therapy. All first-generation PPIs (all except esomeprazole) have similar effects on healing of esophagitis and gastric acidity. Esomeprazole has been shown to have a statistically significant advantage in average gastric pH and percentage of time with nonacidic pH when compared to other PPIs after 5 days of therapy. However, no objective evidence has demonstrated any significant benefit of esomeprazole over other PPIs in symptoms control or esophagitis healing. The timing of PPI use is important as its efficacy depends on the presence of proton pumps on the parietal cells. Therefore, PPIs should be taken during fasting state approximately 30 minutes before meals to allow for maximal effects.

PRACTICE POINT

- PPIs should be taken during fasting state approximately 30 minutes before meals to allow for maximal effects.

While short-term side effects associated with PPI use is rare and relatively mild, increasing evidence has emerged over the past few years suggesting that prolonged use of PPI may have long-term, systemic consequences. Malabsorption, including vitamin B12 and vitamin D, osteoporosis, Clostridium difficile colitis, community-acquired pneumonia, and symptomatic small intestinal bacterial overgrowth have all been linked to chronic PPI use. Recently, concerns regarding absorption and treatment effects of certain medications have been raised in patients with concurrent PPI use. In particular, the concomitant use of PPI and clopidogrel has been under intense scrutiny given the large number of cardiac patients taking clopidogrel who also require PPI therapy. Several in vitro studies have demonstrated evidence of a decrease in efficacy of clopidogrel with PPI using serum markers for platelet response, leading the FDA to issue a warning advising the avoidance of PPI and clopidogrel co-administration. A large number of nonrandomized, observational clinical studies have been published, with the results ranging from no clinical effect to a mild to moderate increase in clinical events such as recurrent MI or hospitalization. The only large, randomized trial studying the effect of PPI (omeprazole) vs placebo on clinical outcome in patients taking clopidogrel (COGENT) demonstrated no difference in cardiovascular events (HR, 1.02; 95% CI, 0.70–1.51), but a significant decrease in GI events (HR, 0.55; 95% CI, 0.36–0.85). Furthermore, a meta-analysis published in April, 2010 showed no significant association between concomitant PPI-clopidogrel use and overall mortality (RR, 1.09; 95% CI, 0.94–1.26). Given the short half-life of both PPI and clopidogrel, some experts have suggested that separating their intake by 12 to 20 hours (eg, one taken before breakfast and the other before bedtime) should, in theory, minimize any potential clinical interaction. Recent AGA practice guidelines found no current evidence to suggest that concurrent PPI and clopidogrel use result in an increase in cardiovascular events. Regardless, use of PPI should be judicious in light of evidence of potential long-term side effects, and dose reduction or discontinuation should be considered after symptom-control or mucosal healing has been achieved.

Newer pharmacological agents developed for the management of GERD, especially in those with nonacidic or weakly acidic reflux include arbaclofen placarbil, a prodrug of the active R-isomer baclofen, currently under investigation for the treatment GERD. Previous studies have shown baclofen to be effective in inhibiting transient lower esophageal sphincter relaxation, thereby decreasing acid reflux. However, the use of baclofen has been limited by its short half-life and poor patient tolerability. Arbaclofen is absorbed throughout the small intestine with longer half-life and better tolerated by patients. Several recent clinical trials have shown that arbaclofen decreases reflux, particularly post-prandial reflux, in patients with GERD. It is currently undergoing further clinical trials and represents a promising option for pharmacological treatment of GERD.

While most patients achieve adequate treatment response with pharmacotherapy, some may experience symptoms refractory to acid suppression or wish to discontinue medication use. In these cases, barrier enhancing antireflux therapy either surgically or endoscopically can be attempted. Antireflux surgeries have been safely performed since the 1950s, and the advance of laparoscopic approach further decreases the complication rate and postoperative hospital stay. *Nissen fundoplication*, either open or laparoscopic, involves enhancing the pressure at the LES region by wrapping and attaching part of the gastric fundus around the distal esophagus. Studies have shown a symptom response of 80% to 90% postoperatively. However, long-term studies demonstrated that the majority of patients experience recurrent symptoms and require acid-suppression medications again within 10 years. Complication rate of fundoplication range from 5% to 20%, most commonly due to dysphagia, chest pain, gas-bloat syndrome, flatulence, and vagal nerve injuries. Dysphagia remains the most commonly encountered complication from fundoplication. It may occur early in 0% to 20% of patients, or late in up to 6% of patients at 2 years. Preoperative physiologic studies including manometry and pH testing can help identify patients with higher likelihood of positive or negative outcomes. Increased LES relaxation and positive pH testing results are positive predictors of fundoplication outcome, while patients with normal pH testing or normal LES pressure are less likely to respond to fundoplication. In addition, patients with advanced spastic esophageal disorders or signs of achalasia on manometry are contraindicated for surgery given the high risk of postoperative dysphagia.

NUTRITIONAL SUPPORT

In rare cases of patients with significant esophagitis causing severe dysphagia or odynophagia, nutritional support may be needed due to their inability to tolerate adequate oral diet or hydration. Enteral feeding and hydration through a gastrostomy or jejeunostomy tube may be required. Intravenous hydration or parenteral nutrition may be needed in certain patients with severe malnutrition or other concurrent gastrointestinal disorder. Clinicians should pay particular attention to any signs of deficiency of specific elements such as vitamin B12, vitamin D, and calcium and the need for replacement.

LONGITUDINAL/OUTPATIENT THERAPEUTICS

Outpatient care of patients with GERD or esophagitis focuses on medical treatment of underlying disorders as well as lifestyle modification. Acid suppression medications, such as PPI or H2 receptor antagonists, are the mainstay of therapy as described above. Once symptoms resolve or esophagitis heals, dosages of acid suppression medications may be slowly tapered as tolerated. Lifestyle modifications remain a cornerstone of GERD treatment. Avoiding foods and acid-containing beverages that exacerbate their symptoms should be advocated. Patients should be educated about not lying down after eating for at least 3 hours to avoid refluxing of ingested food. Similarly, eating smaller and frequent meals can help decrease GERD symptoms. For patients with significant nocturnal reflux, elevation of the head of the bed to 30° to 45° angle can help reduce nocturnal symptoms. Such elevation may be achieved by placing blocks underneath the front feet of the bed or triangular wedge underneath the mattress. In addition, avoidance of alcohol or tobacco use may reduce GERD symptoms or esophagitis. Weight loss in overweight or obese patients is also a significant part of GERD management.

INFECTIOUS ESOPHAGITIS

Treatment strategy for infectious etiologies of esophagitis can be broadly divided into acute eradication and prevention of recurrence. In patients with acute, symptomatic infectious esophagitis, antimicrobial therapy should be initiated and targeted toward the organism responsible. Determination of the duration of therapy, mode of administration (oral vs parenteral), and choice of antimicrobial agent should depend on a combination of factors including the patients' symptoms, other medical comorbidities, and underlying immune function. Intravenous administration may be needed in those with significant odynophagia or patients who are acutely ill or severely immunosuppressed. Increased treatment duration and more potent agents should also be considered in these patients.

Patients with suspected or diagnosed esophageal candidiasis can be first treated with a 14-day course of fluconazole (400 mg loading dose on first day followed by 200 mg daily on subsequent days), administered orally or intravenously. Fungal esophagitis unresponsive to fluconazole may require more potent antifungals such as amphotericin and should be managed with input from infectious diseases specialists. First-line therapy for HSV esophagitis in immunosuppressed patients involves a course of acyclovir (5 mg/kg IV every 8 hours for 7–14 days or 400 mg orally 5 times daily for 7–10 days), while CMV esophagitis requires the use of ganciclovir (5 mg/kg IV every 12 hours or 900 mg daily twice daily) for 3 to 6 weeks. Again, more potent antivirals such as foscarnet may be necessary in cases unresponsive to first-line agents and infectious diseases specialists should be involved in management of these cases. HSV or CMV esophagitis in immunocompetent hosts usually resolve without treatment after 1 to 2 weeks. Experience with orogenital HSV suggests that antiviral treatments may hasten symptom recovery. Therefore, some clinicians suggest treating immunocompetent patients with a shorter course of therapy.

COMPLICATIONS AND PROGNOSIS

Complications from chronic GERD can be divided by the sites of manifestations: esophageal vs extra-esophageal. Esophageal complications include ulcers, erosions, strictures, Barrett esophagus, and malignancy. Extra-esophageal complications mainly involve pulmonary manifestations of aspirated gastric contents.

Esophageal ulcers may result from esophagitis caused by chronic GERD or impacted foreign bodies. They may account for up to 2% of all upper GI bleeding. However, the vast majority heal completely with acid-suppressive medications. Chronic GERD and esophagitis may also lead to peptic esophageal strictures, which have been described in up to 10% of patients seeking medical attention for reflux symptoms. Patients with strictures usually present with dysphagia to solid food but can tolerate fluid without difficulties. Weight loss is uncommon and malignancy needs to be ruled out when present. Treatment for peptic strictures involves a combination of acid-suppression therapy and endoscopic dilation. Food and foreign body impaction is another common complication for patients with esophageal strictures or significant esophagitis. In addition to reflux esophagitis, another form commonly associated with food impaction is eosinophilic esophagitis. Treatment strategies for eosinophilic esophagitis include the use of antihistamine, leukotrienne inhibitors, or steroids.

Chronic GERD may also predispose patients to the development of Barrett esophagus and esophageal adenocarcinoma. Barrett esophagus is the metaplastic change of the esophageal lining due to chronic reflux injury and esophagitis. It involves the replacement of the normal squamous epithelium of the distal esophagus with specialized intestinal metaplasia. Such metaplastic change may protect the esophagus against further injury by gastric acid, but it also increases the risk for esophageal adenocarcinoma. The prevalence of Barrett esophagus in GERD patients is approximately 5% to 10%, which is considerably higher than the estimated 1.6% to 1.7% reported in the general population. The prevalence in those with esophageal strictures is even higher at about 30%. Caucasians, male, and middle-aged patients are more commonly affected. Other risk factors for Barrett esophagus include tobacco and alcohol use. The exact risk of esophageal adenocarcinoma in patients with Barrett esophagus remains debated, but is believed to be around 0.5% to 1%. The use of EGD to screen for Barrett in patients with a history GERD symptoms remains controversial, as there is no direct clinical data to support the utility of screening. In the most recent medical position statement published by the AGA in 2008, no specific recommendation was made regarding the screening of GERD patients for Barrett with EGD due to the lack of sufficient evidence. Surveillance for signs of dysplastic changes should be performed periodically, however, if a diagnosis of Barrett has been confirmed on biopsy. Conservative treatment with continued surveillance remains the mainstay of therapy for Barrett without dysplasia. For those with high-grade dysplasia present on biopsies, treatment strategy includes endoscopic ablative therapy or surgical resection. Treatment strategy for low-grade dysplasia remains controversial but involves ablative therapy or conservative surveillance. Acid control should be continued as part of medical therapy for Barrett's esophagus.

Extra-esophageal complications of GERD may manifest in many forms, mainly resulting in pulmonary or upper airway abnormalities. GERD is believed to play a role in the pathogenesis of pulmonary disorders such as asthma, chronic bronchitis, bronchiectasis, aspiration pneumonia, and pulmonary fibrosis. Studies have also linked GERD to upper airway manifestations such as pharyngitis, laryngitis, or postnasal drip. Oral problems such as dental erosions, halitosis, and aphthous ulcers have also been associated with GERD. However, despite evidence of increased prevalence of these disorders in patients with GERD, treatment with acid suppression medications has not consistently demonstrated clinical improvement in patients with these manifestations. Despite the lack of clear evidence, current clinical practice usually involves a workup for GERD in patients presenting with these disorders of unclear etiology or refractory to standard treatment.

The main goal of GERD and esophagitis treatment is to keep patients symptom free with the least amount of acid-suppression medications that abates symptoms. Therefore, in patients who have responded to medical therapy or lifestyle changes, a trial of tapering and withdrawing medications should be attempted. In general, symptoms relief should be sustained for at least 2 to 3 weeks prior to the start of dosage tapering. Tapering should involve the sequential decrease in dosage or frequency for PPI, which may ultimately be switched to H2 receptor antagonists. Abrupt withdrawal of PPI should be avoided as "rebound hypersecretion" may ensue when parietal cells secrete an elevated amount of acid after prolonged blockade. Adhering to lifestyle or dietary choices that decrease symptoms usually allows most motivated GERD patients to wean off medications. However, in patients with erosive esophagitis, relapse of symptoms and mucosal damage occurs in more than 80% of patients when therapy is stopped.

Patients with infectious esophagitis often respond well to first-line antimicrobial therapy. Those at highest risks of nonresponse are usually patients with profound immunosuppression. Clinical studies have demonstrated a decrease in candida-, CMV-, or HSV-related diseases in immunosuppressed patients receiving respective prophylactic therapy. However, given the high acute treatment response rate, ease and low cost of therapy, and risk for development of drug resistance and sensitivity, long-term maintenance or secondary prophylaxis is not routinely recommended for infectious esophagitis, even in immunosuppressed patients. Some experts suggest consideration for maintenance therapy only in immunosuppressed patients with severe or frequent relapses of their infectious esophagitis.

DISCHARGE PLANNING

In the rare instances where patients were admitted for complications from their GERD or esophagitis, discharge planning mainly involves ensuring proper follow-up with a gastroenterology specialist, continuation of medical therapy, and patient education for secondary prevention. For patients with significant nutritional deficits requiring feeding tube placement, discharge planning should also include education on the proper use of the feeding tube, home nursing care or transfer to skilled nursing facilities, adequate equipment for continuation with tube-feeding after discharge, and instructions regarding caloric count. Follow-up for these patients should also include visits with a nutritionist for continued management of tube-feeding regimen. Educational materials regarding the prevention of recurrent GERD and esophagitis such as lifestyle modification strategies should be given, targeting their underlying etiologies.

TABLE 154-1 Evidence-based Medicine Key References for GERD and Esophagitis

Study	Methodology	Results	Limitations	Bottom Line
Khan M, et al. *Cochrane Database Syst Rev.* 2007;2:CD003244.	Cochrane review	• 137 treatment trials (36,978 patients) included • PPI superior to placebo (83% vs 18% at 8 wk, NNT = 1.7) and H2RA (84% vs 52%, RR = 0.51) for esophagitis healing • PPI superior to placebo (56% vs 8% at 4 wk, NNT = 2–3) and H2RA (77% vs 48% at 4–12 wk) for heartburn resolution	Pooled data with significant heterogeneity	PPI is superior to H2RA in the treatment of reflux esophagitis and heartburn symptoms.
Locke GR, et al. *Gastroenterology.* 1997;112:1448–1456.	Population-based, observational, cohort	• 2200 Olmsted county residents aged 25–74 • 19.8% experienced at least weekly heartburn or acid regurgitation • Heartburn and acid regurgitation significantly associated with noncardiac chest pain (OR = 4.2), dysphagia (OR = 4.7), dyspepsia (OR = 3.1), and globus (OR = 1.9)	Single-county patient population, questionnaire based	GERD is an important cause of noncardiac chest pain symptoms. Dysphagia, dyspepsia, and globus sensation are other manifestations of reflux.
Bhatt DL, et al. *N Engl J Med.* 2010;363(20): 1909–1917.	Randomized, placebo-controlled trial	• 3873 patients with indication for dual antiplatelet therapy • Randomized to clopidogrel with omeprazole or placebo • Omeprazole decreased GI bleeding rate compared to placebo (1.1% vs 2.9%, HR 0.18–0.63) • No difference in rate of cardiovascular event (4.9% vs 5.7%, HR 0.68–1.44)	Trial prematurely terminated due to loss of financing (planned enrollment = 5000 patients)	When used with clopidogrel, omeprazole decreased GI bleeding rate but showed no difference in cardiovascular event compared to placebo.
av-Citrin O, et al. *Aliment Pharmacol Ther.* 2005;21: 269–275.	Prospective, controlled, observational trial	• 345 pregnant PPI users and 787 pregnant controls • No difference in rate of major congenital abnormalities: omeprazole (3.6%), lansoprazole (3.9%), and pantoprazole (2.1%) vs controls (3.8%)	Different doses of PPI	PPI does not represent a major teratogenic risk in humans.
American Lung Association Asthma Clinical Research Centers. *N Engl J Med.* 2009;360(15): 1487–1499.	Randomized, placebo-controlled trial	• 412 patients with minimal to no reflux symptoms and inadequately controlled asthma randomly assigned to receive esomeprazole 40 mg twice a day or placebo for 24 wk • No difference in episodes of poor asthma control, pulmonary function, airway reactivity, symptoms score, nocturnal awakening, and quality of life		PPI does not improve outcome of inadequately controlled asthma in patients with minimal to no reflux symptoms.
Vakil N, Fennerty MB. *Aliment Pharmacol Ther.* 2003;18(6): 559–568.	Systematic review	• 32 trials comparing efficacy of different doses and formulations of PPI in the treatment of GERD and peptic ulcer disease • For GERD symptoms, all five PPI demonstrated similar efficacy after 1–2 wk of treatment, but lansoprazole and esomaprazole demonstrated faster symptom relief • Esomeprazole is superior in esophagitis healing	Pooled data with significant heterogeneity, inclusion of low-quality trials	All five PPI are equally efficacious in treatment of GERD symptoms. Esomeprazole demonstrated slight superiority in healing esophagitis. Overall, there is insufficient evidence to establish the superiority of one agent over the others across all GERD-related complications.

QUALITY IMPROVEMENT

SECONDARY PREVENTION

Secondary prevention plays a big role in the outpatient management of patients with GERD and esophagitis. It also represents an area where greater improvements can be made in decreasing the morbidity of the diseases. Lifestyle modifications such as dietary and sleeping habits as described above have been shown to be effective in decreasing symptoms in patients with GERD. Education, encouragement and assistance may sometimes be needed in aiding patients to adhere to lifestyle changes. In addition to providing educational materials, assistance from nutritionists and social workers may help patients achieve their lifestyle modification goals. In addition to lifestyle changes, continued use of medications such as acid suppression drugs can help prevent recurrent symptoms or development of complications. However, patients who adhere to lifestyle changes and achieve symptom relief should attempt a trial of medication weaning to allow maintenance on the lowest dose of medications possible. In patients with esophagitis, endoscopic surveillance to evaluate for mucosal healing can aide in adjustment of medical therapy and in the evaluation of treatment efficacy, especially in other forms of esophagitis.

TRANSITION OF CARE

Follow-up after initial diagnosis of GERD or esophagitis remains important. Patients should continue care with a gastroenterology specialist for management of their diseases until symptoms resolve or condition stabilizes. Continued consultation with nutrition specialists may be needed for selected patients with ongoing GERD symptoms or difficulties adhering to lifestyle modifications. Certain underlying causes of esophagitis may require further care by other specialists, for example, patients found to have infectious esophagitis such as candidiasis or HSV may require further workup for underlying immunosuppression. Patients diagnosed with eosinophilic esophagitis should undergo allergen testing by an allergy/immunology specialist to identify any particular immunological trigger of disease.

OUTCOMES TO MONITOR

Symptoms resolution remains the main outcomes for monitoring in patients with GERD and esophagitis. Esophageal mucosal healing in patients with esophagitis, or endoscopic and pathologic evidence of resolution of underlying disease in patients with eosinophilic esophagitis or Barrett esophagus serve as other outcomes for monitoring and surveillance.

COSTS AND RESOURCE UTILIZATION

As the most common gastrointestinal disease, GERD also represents the most costly digestive disorder. The annual management cost of GERD has been estimated to exceed $9 billion. Much of the costs may be related to overuse of acid suppression medications or unnecessary endoscopic or other diagnostic procedures. In both the primary care and inpatient settings, there have been signs of PPI overuse in treatment of nonspecific gastrointestinal complaints. In addition, inappropriate use of high-dose PPI and lack of tapering or withdrawal strategies result in many patients being kept on more acid suppressive medications than they require. As stated above, empiric PPI should be used only in patients with signs and symptoms suggestive of GERD or esophagitis. Atypical symptoms or complaints should be thoroughly evaluated before PPI therapy is started. PPI tapering and withdrawal should be attempted in all patients with controlled symptoms. Lifestyle modification should be better promoted as its success often complements the tapering of medications. Endoscopic and other diagnostic procedures should be reserved for patients with atypical or alarming symptoms, or those who failed empiric PPI therapy (**Table 154-1**). Adherence to this strategy allows the delivery of the most cost-effective care for one of the most common and costly disorders today.

SUGGESTED READINGS

Bhatt DL, Cryer BL, Contant CF, et al. Clopidogrel with or without omeprazole in coronary artery disease. *N Engl J Med.* 2010;363(20):1909–1917.

DeVault KR, Castell DO. American College of Gastroenterology. Updated guidelines for the diagnosis and treatment of gastroesophageal reflux disease. *Am J Gastroenterol.* 2005;100:190.

Gerson LB, Huff FJ, Hila A, et al. Arbaclofen placarbil decreases postprandial reflux in patients with gastroesophageal reflux disease. *Am J Gastroenterol.* 2010;105(6):1266–1275.

Inadomi JM, Jamal R, Murata GH, et al. Step-down management of gastroesophageal reflux disease. Gastroenterology 2001;121:1095–1100.

Kahrilas PJ. GERD pathogenesis, pathophysiology and clinical manigestations. *Cleve Clin J Med.* 2003;70(Suppl 5):S4–S19.

Kahrilas PJ, Shaheen NJ, Vaezi M. American Gastroenterological Association Medical Position Statement on the Management of Gastroesophageal Reflux Disease. Gastroenterology. 2008; 135:1383.

Klok RM, Postma MJ, van Hout BA, et al. Meta-analysis: comparing the efficacy of proton pump inhibitors in short-term use. Aliment Pharmacol Therapeut 2003;(10):1237–1245.

Numans ME, Lau J, de Wit NJ, et al. Short-term treatments with proton pump inhibitors as a test for gastroesophageal reflux disease: a meta-analysis of diagnostic test characteristics. *Ann Intern Med.* 2004;140:518–527.

Richter JE. Diagnostic tests for gastroesophageal reflux disease. *Am J Med Sci.* 2003;326:300–308.

Spechler SJ, Lee E, Ahnen D, et al. Long-term outcome of medical and surgical therapies for gastroesophageal reflux disease: follow-up of a randomized controlled trial. *JAMA.* 2001;285:2331–2338.

CHAPTER 155

Upper Gastrointestinal Bleeding

Brian H. Hyett, MD
John R. Saltzman, MD

Key Clinical Questions

1. What is the timing and treatment of peptic ulcer disease?
2. What are the factors in diagnosis and treatment of aortoenteric fistula?
3. What treatments are available for each etiology of upper GI bleeding?
4. What is the appropriate management and follow-up of variceal bleeding?
5. How do you estimate the severity of bleeding so that you can triage appropriate patients to the ICU, medical floor, or observation unit?
6. Which patients are more likely to rebleed and hence require continued observation in the hospital after their bleeding has apparently stopped, and for how long?

INTRODUCTION

Upper gastrointestinal (GI) bleeding is responsible for over 300,000 hospitalizations per year in the United States. An additional 100,000 to 150,000 patients develop upper GI bleeding during hospitalizations. The annual cost of treating nonvariceal acute upper GI bleeding in the United States exceeds $2.5 billion. In 2004, for patients *with* and *without* complications of non-variceal upper GI bleeding in the United States, mean lengths of stay were 4.4 and 2.7 days, respectively, and hospitalization costs were $5632 and $3402, respectively.

Upper GI bleeding is defined as a bleeding source in the GI tract proximal to the ligament of Treitz. The presentation varies depending on the nature and severity of bleeding and includes hematemesis, melena, hematochezia (in rapid upper GI bleeding), and anemia with heme-positive stools. Bleeding can be associated with changes in vital signs, including tachycardia and hypotension. Given the range of presentations, pinpointing the nature and severity of GI bleeding can be a challenging task.

The natural history of nonvariceal upper GI bleeding is that 80% of patients will stop bleeding spontaneously and no further urgent intervention will be needed. However if a patient rebleeds, there is a 10-fold increased mortality rate. In contrast, only 50% of patients with a variceal hemorrhage stop bleeding spontaneously. Following cessation of active variceal bleeding, there is a high risk of recurrent bleeding within six weeks.

The mortality rate for nonvariceal upper GI bleeding is 5% to 14%. This mortality rate is essentially unchanged since 1945, despite the development of new medications, endoscopy (both diagnostic and therapeutic), intensive care units, and advances in surgical management. The mortality remains high since patients with GI bleeding now are older, have more comorbidities, and are taking more medications including nonsteroidal anti-inflammatory drugs (NSAIDs), anticoagulants, and antiplatelet agents. For variceal bleeding, mortality is between 15% to 50% for each bleeding episode, and 70% to 80% in those with continuous bleeding. Variceal hemorrhage is responsible for one-third of all deaths due to cirrhosis.

PRACTICE POINT

- In nonvariceal upper GI bleeding, 80% of patients will stop bleeding spontaneously and no further urgent intervention will be needed. However, if a patient rebleeds, there is a 10-fold increased mortality rate. In contrast, only 50% of patients with a variceal hemorrhage stop bleeding spontaneously. The period of greatest risk of variceal rebleeding is within the first 48 to 72 hours, and over 50% of all subsequent rebleeding episodes occur within the first 10 days. For variceal bleeding, mortality is between 15% to 50% for each bleeding episode, and 70% to 80% in those with continuous bleeding.

DIFFERENTIAL DIAGNOSIS

NONVARICEAL BLEEDING

Peptic ulcer disease

Diagnosis Peptic ulcer disease is a common condition stemming from an imbalance of protective and disruptive factors of the GI mucosa. Ulcers most commonly are found in the stomach and proximal

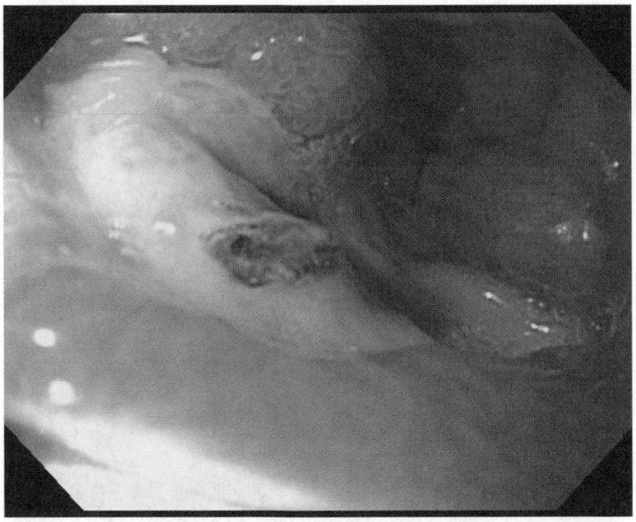

Figure 155-1 *Duodenal ulcer.*

duodenum (**Figures 155-1** and **155-2**). Peptic ulcer disease is the most common cause of upper GI bleeding and accounts for up to 50% of total cases and over 100,000 hospital admissions per year in the United States. The annual incidence of peptic ulcer disease in patients infected with *Helicobacter pylori* is about 1% per year, which is 6 to 10 times higher than patients who are uninfected. Diagnosis is made by endoscopy performed when symptoms prompt endoscopic investigation. An initial step in management is to identify *H pylori* infection and users of NSAIDs. These two risk factors account for the vast majority of ulcers in the upper GI tract.

Disruptive factors that can damage the mucosa of the GI tract include acid, pepsin, bile salts, ischemia, and *H pylori*. Exogenous causes are predominately medications (NSAIDs and aspirin). Stress-induced ulcers are a common cause of bleeding in patients hospitalized for other severe illnesses. Risk factors for stress-induced ulcers include respiratory failure (especially intubated patients) coagulopathy (INR > 1.5 or platelets < 50,000/microliter), trauma, sepsis, renal failure, burns, ICU admission, and surgery.

Pathophysiology The defensive forces of the esophagus include esophageal motility with clearance of refluxed materials, the lower esophageal sphincter to prevent reflux, and salivary secretions that contain bicarbonate. Gastric protective factors include the mucous layer as well as tissue mediators. *H pylori* is a flagellated bacterium with several unique attributes which aid in its ability to break down gastric mucosa. These factors include its production of urease which neutralizes the acidic gastric environment. NSAIDs inhibit cyclooxygenase, thus decreasing mucosal protective prostaglandin levels in the stomach. They also increase gastric vascular endothelial adhesion molecules, thus leading to neutrophil adherence and mucosal injury.

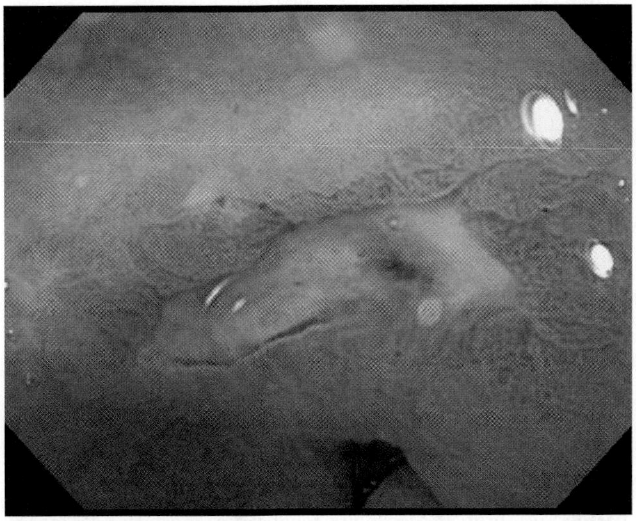

Figure 155-2 *Gastric ulcer.*

Clinical findings Peptic ulcer disease presents in a variety of ways. Patients can experience epigastric pain, melena, hematochezia, dyspepsia, bloating, or can be asymptomatic with or without anemia. On examination pain may be epigastric and reproducible, but many patients are have right sided pain or no pain at all.

CASE 155-1

A 57-year-old woman developed epigastric pain and black stools. Blood tests revealed antibodies to *H pylori* and anemia. She was found to be guaiac positive on examination. Based on the symptoms of anemia, black stool and her age, an upper endoscopy was performed which revealed a proximal duodenal ulcer with no visible vessel. She was treated with triple therapy (antibiotics and a PPI) and her symptoms quickly improved and her anemia resolved in 3 months.

Prognosis Response to treatment and outcomes vary for peptic ulcer disease. Treatment is with proton pump inhibitor (PPI) therapy until asymptomatic and/or mucosal healing is demonstrated via and esophagogastroduodenoscopy (EGD) and/or antibiotics where indicated and removal of offending agents (eg, NSAIDs) leads to mucosal healing (**Table 155-1**). Chronic, nonhealing ulcers should prompt consideration of underlying illness or an alternative diagnosis, such as malignancy.

Mallory-Weiss tears

Diagnosis Mallory-Weiss tears occur at the gastroesophageal junction in the distal esophagus or proximal stomach (**Figure 155-3**). Typically, these tears form after repeated and severe vomiting or retching. The tears may extend into the underlying blood vessels. Acute upper GI bleeding is the major clinical finding, which may be associated with epigastric pain which may radiate to the back. Endoscopy is used to document the presence of a gastroesophageal tear and allows the possibility of therapeutic intervention.

TABLE 155-1 Recommended Treatment Regimens for *H Pylori* Infection

Three-drug regimens
Proton pump inhibitor (PPI) orally twice daily + clarithromycin 500 mg orally twice daily + amoxicillin 1 gm orally twice daily. Eradication 85–90%. Duration 10–14 days.
Proton pump inhibitor orally twice daily + clarithromycin 500 mg orally twice daily + metronidazole 500 mg orally twice daily. Eradication 75–85%. Duration 10–14 days. This regimen is generally used for PCN allergic patients.
Four-drug regimen
Proton pump inhibitor orally twice daily + bismuth subsalicylate 525 mg 4 times daily + Tetracycline 500 mg 4 times daily + metronidazole 500 mg orally 3–4 times daily. Eradication 75–90%. Duration 2 weeks.

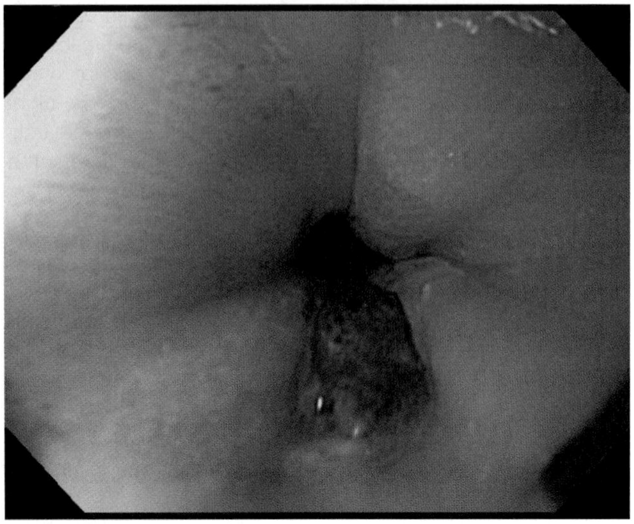

Figure 155-3 *Mallory-Weiss tear.*

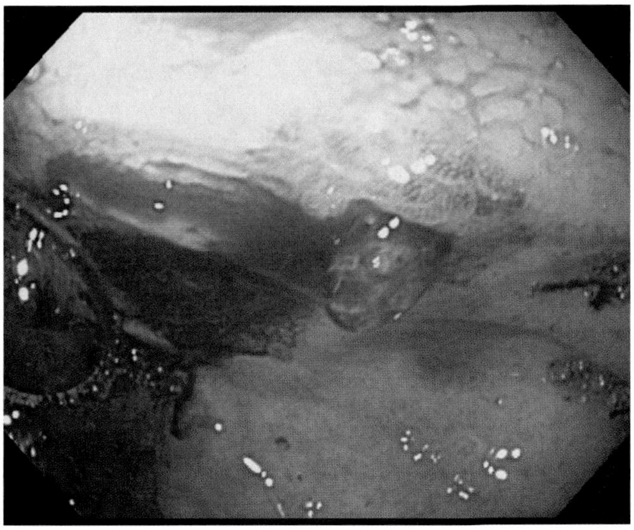

Figure 155-4 *Dielafoy lesion.*

PRACTICE POINT

- Although 40% to 70% of patients with bleeding Mallory-Weiss tears require blood transfusions, most tears heal spontaneously within 24 to 48 hours of presentation.

Bleeding occurs when the tear involves the underlying esophageal venous or arterial plexus. Patients often have a history of nonbloody vomiting or retching before the onset of hematemesis. The tears are located at the esophagogastric junction, and can be within a hiatal hernia. Tears can extend downward into the cardia or, less commonly, upward into the esophagus.

Pathophysiology Mallory-Weiss syndrome is characterized by longitudinal mucosal lacerations in the distal esophagus and proximal stomach, which are usually associated with forceful retching.

Prognosis Although 40% to 70% of patients with bleeding Mallory-Weiss tears require blood transfusions, most tears heal spontaneously within 24 to 48 hours of presentation. Risk factors for rebleeding include portal hypertension and coagulopathy. Patients with active or ongoing bleeding can be treated with endoscopic hemostatic methods. For the rare patient with ongoing bleeding unresponsive to endoscopic control, intravenous infusions of octreotide, arterial embolization via angiography and esophageal balloon tamponade have been used. In refractory bleeding, surgery with over-sewing of the bleeding vessel may be required.

Dieulafoy lesions

Essentials of diagnosis A Dieulafoy lesion is a dilated, aberrant submucosal vessel which erodes through normal surrounding epithelium and is not associated with an ulcer (**Figure 155-4**). Dieulafoy lesions are typically located just below the gastroesophageal junction on the lesser curvature of the stomach but can be found in areas throughout the GI tract, including the esophagus, duodenum, and colon. When a Dieulafoy lesion bleeds, massive arterial bleeding can occur. In the absence of active bleeding, the lesion is difficult to see, as it may appear as a small and subtle raised area, such as a nipple or visible vessel without an associated ulcer. In patients with massive bleeding and no obvious cause, the lesser curvature of the stomach within 6 centimeters of the gastroesophageal junction should be carefully inspected endoscopically for evidence of a Dieulafoy lesion.

The typical patient with a Dieulafoy lesion is a man, with multiple comorbidities, already hospitalized for other problems. Diagnosis is confirmed with finding a visible vessel or active arterial pumping, without an associated ulcer or mass. The diagnosis can be difficult, as bleeding may be massive such that the area may be covered with blood and the source may not be visualized. It is especially challenging to diagnose Dieulafoy lesions that are not bleeding as the absence of an associated ulcer makes detection of the vessel difficult.

Pathophysiology The cause of a Dieulafoy lesion is unknown. The arteries are 1 to 3 mm in size, which is approximately 10 times the caliber of mucosal capillaries. The typical location is in the upper stomach along the high lesser curvature, within 6 cm of the gastroesophageal junction.

Clinical findings A Dieulafoy lesion often presents with a massive acute upper GI bleed, although the bleeding may be self-limited in nature. The diagnosis is confirmed with finding a visible vessel or with active arterial pumping without an associated ulcer or mass.

Prognosis Endoscopic treatment is the mainstay for bleeding control of a Dieulafoy lesion via cautery, clips or the combination of epinephrine injection and one of these two treatment modalities. The risk of recurrent bleeding following endoscopic treatment is relatively high due to the size of the underlying artery. In patients with recurrent bleeding, repeat endoscopic therapy is often the next step, however, surgical therapy may be necessary and consultation by a surgeon early on is recommended. Surgical treatment of a Dieulafoy lesion is typically a wedge resection, as simple oversewing has a high rebleeding rate.

VASCULAR MALFORMATIONS

Angiodysplasia

Diagnosis Angiodysplasias may occur throughout the GI tract, may be multiple in one gastrointestinal region, or coexist in several different gastrointestinal locations. Although angiodysplasias are a relatively common source of small bowel bleeding, they are a rare source of massive bleeding from the stomach. Bleeding from an upper GI vascular malformation is typically intermittent and low grade in nature, although it can be acute and overt.

Pathophysiology It is unknown what causes most vascular malformations. Vascular malformations can be present at birth although they do not appear to be hereditary. They occur equally in both sexes and in different races. Vascular malformations may be caused by a rupture or clotting of a blood vessel during fetal development, although not associated with other problems at birth.

Clinical findings Bleeding from upper GI vascular malformations is typically intermittent and low grade in nature, although it can be acute and overt. The endoscopic appearance can be variable, but includes a superficial collection or tuft of blood vessels.

Prognosis Endoscopic therapy with thermal coagulation is the treatment of choice with cautery applied first to the periphery and then to the center of the lesion. Argon plasma coagulation has been applied to the treatment of vascular malformations and is an effective therapy. Certain medications have been utilized in an attempt to treat vascular malformations in the upper gastrointestinal tract. Combination estrogen/progesterone therapy has been widely used, but overall has yielded inconsistent results. Angiography or surgery can be offered for failures of endoscopic and medical therapy, but is rarely necessary.

Gastric antral vascular ectasia

Diagnosis Gastric antral vascular ectasia (GAVE), also known as "watermelon stomach," is an idiopathic condition often associated with portal hypertension. GAVE is a relatively unusual cause of upper GI bleeding. The bleeding that occurs is typically chronic and low grade, often associated with iron deficiency anemia and occult bleeding. It is unusual to have acute or massive upper GI bleeding from GAVE.

Pathophysiology The etiology of watermelon stomach is not known; however, it has been theorized to be due to gastroduodenal prolapse and occurs in patients with cirrhosis, portal hypertension, and systemic sclerosis. Patients with concomitant portal hypertension have bleeding that is more difficult to control, requiring treatment of the underlying portal hypertension.

Clinical findings Vascular malformations occur in rows of reddish stripes that radiate outward from the pylorus, in a pattern which resembles the stripes on a watermelon; hence this entity has been referred to as "watermelon stomach." These stripes represent rows of vascular malformations and the entity is easy to recognize in the classic form. However, GAVE may have a less organized appearance making it more difficult to diagnose. Although the diagnosis is by endoscopy, it can be confirmed by histology from endoscopic biopsy. Biopsies of GAVE show areas of vascular ectasia associated with spindle cell proliferation and fibrohyalinosis.

Prognosis Most patients will respond to endoscopic therapy most commonly with argon plasma coagulation. However, surgery with an antrectomy may be required for patients who have persistent bleeding despite endoscopic management.

Aortoenteric fistula

Diagnosis Aortoenteric fistulas occur when there is a direct communication between the aorta and the gastrointestinal tract and can lead to massive bleeding. Patients may have a "herald" bleed with initial hematemesis or hematochezia, which may spontaneously remit. This may then be followed by torrential bleeding, including exsanguination, making it important to quickly diagnose this condition. Intermittent bleeding can occur if a blood clot overlies a fistulous connection. There may be abdominal or back pain (which occurs in about half of patients), or signs of fever and infection. On physical examination, a bruit may be heard and a pulsatile mass may be palpable at any point along the midabdomen representing the course of the abdominal aorta.

A high index of suspicion is needed to promptly diagnose a patient with an aortoenteric fistula for successful management. In a patient who has a known risk factor such as previous aortic grafting this diagnosis should be considered early in the course. In fact, it should always be suspected in patients with massive bleeding from the second to third portion of the duodenum. The diagnosis can be confirmed by computed tomography with angiography or with traditional angiography. Diagnostic tests need to be done in an expeditious manner along with cardiothoracic surgical evaluation as the management of an aortoenteric fistula is surgical. The mortality rate of an unrecognized fistula is 100%, whereas the mortality for a recognized fistula is 30%.

Hemobilia

Diagnosis Hemobilia is a rare cause of acute upper GI bleeding that occurs from the hepatobiliary tract in less than 1% of patients who undergo a procedure to the biliary tree (ERCP or surgery) and almost never spontaneously with the rare exception of invasive tumors. **The classic triad of hemobilia is biliary colic, obstructive jaundice, and gastrointestinal bleeding.** The diagnosis of hemobilia can be difficult by upper endoscopy which may not clearly visualize the ampulla. A side-viewing duodenoscope is often utilized to access the ampulla directly or to perform endoscopic retrograde cholangiopancreatography (ERCP).

Hemobilia should be considered in patients who have had a recent history of hepatic or biliary tract injury. This includes trauma to the area, percutaneous (or transjugular) liver biopsies, and percutaneous transhepatic cholangiograms, ablations of liver tumors or biopsies. Hemobilia can also occur secondary to gallstones, cholecystitis, hepatobiliary tumors, hepatic abscesses, and aneurysms. Obstructive jaundice may be associated with biliary sepsis. Patients with these findings should be considered as potentially having hemobilia. Treatment is directed at the primary cause of bleeding although ERCP may also be needed to remove clot from the bile duct causing obstruction. While treatment can occasionally be performed endoscopically, it may need to be done angiographically (such as by arterial embolization) or surgically.

Hemosuccus pancreaticus

Diagnosis Hemosuccus pancreaticus is another rare cause of upper GI bleeding which occurs due to bleeding from the pancreatic duct. This can be secondary to chronic pancreatitis, pancreatic pseudocysts, and pancreatic tumors. This can also occur after a therapeutic endoscopy of the pancreas, including pancreatic sphincterotomy or stone removal. Hemosuccus pancreaticus can be difficult to detect by routine endoscopy, thus a side-viewing duodenoscope and ERCP may be needed to reveal the source of the bleeding. The diagnosis can be confirmed by abdominal CT scan, angiography, or intraabdominal exploration.

Bleeding occurs when there is erosion into a vessel, forming a direct communication with the pancreatic duct. Mesenteric angiography is important for diagnosis and treatment, often with coil embolization to control the acute bleeding. For persistent or massive bleeding, surgery with resection of the bleeding area or ligation of bleeding vessel may be required.

Cameron lesion

Diagnosis Cameron lesions are erosions or ulcers that occur in the distal aspect of a hiatal hernia. Although this may be an incidental finding on upper endoscopy, these lesions can be responsible for iron deficiency anemia or acute or chronic upper GI bleeding.

The mechanism of formation of a Cameron lesion is not well understood. Potential etiologies include gastroesophageal reflux and mechanical trauma of the area. Management of a Cameron lesion depends on the clinical situation. Patients with acute bleeding can be treated by endoscopic methods. Patients who do not have acute bleeding, but have chronic blood loss may be treated with medical therapy, such as a proton pump inhibitor and iron repletion. Surgical repair of the hiatal hernia is curative, but rarely necessary.

Upper gastrointestinal tumors

Diagnosis Neoplasms of the upper GI tract are a rare cause of upper GI bleeding. These tumors may be esophageal squamous carcinomas, malignant lymphomas or adenocarcinomas (primary or metastatic), or benign such as leiomyeiomas or gastrointestinal stromal tumors. The symptoms that suggest bleeding may be from a gastrointestinal tumor include symptoms that may be attributable to the primary tumor such as dysphagia from esophageal cancer, but symptoms may be nonspecific including cachexia, weight loss, and early satiety. If the diagnosis of a tumor is not previously known, it may be detected at the time of endoscopy and confirmed by brushings or biopsies. Endoscopic ultrasound may be needed to evaluate submucosal masses.

Bleeding from an upper gastrointestinal tumor can be from mucosal erosions or ulcerations, or from invasion of the tumor into an underlying vessel. Typically endoscopic treatments are a temporizing measure prior to more definitive measures such as surgery, because rebleeding will frequently occur after endoscopy. Medical therapy is often ineffective in this setting, although palliative measures may be provided including chemotherapy and radiation of the primary tumor. Patients who have bleeding due to an upper GI malignancy have a very poor prognosis. The majority of patients (>60%) will die within 3 months. However, patients who have a benign upper gastrointestinal tumor that bleeds will be cured by surgical resection.

VARICEAL BLEEDING

Gastroesophageal varices

Diagnosis Varices are dilated venous collaterals that have a tendency to rupture and can bleed massively. Esophageal and gastric varices develop as a result of portal hypertension usually due to advanced liver disease and cirrhosis (**Figures 155-5** and **155-6**). Varices may be isolated to the stomach if they are due to splenic vein thrombosis, acute pancreatitis, or a pancreatic tumor. Esophageal and gastric varices may occur without any clinical symptoms.

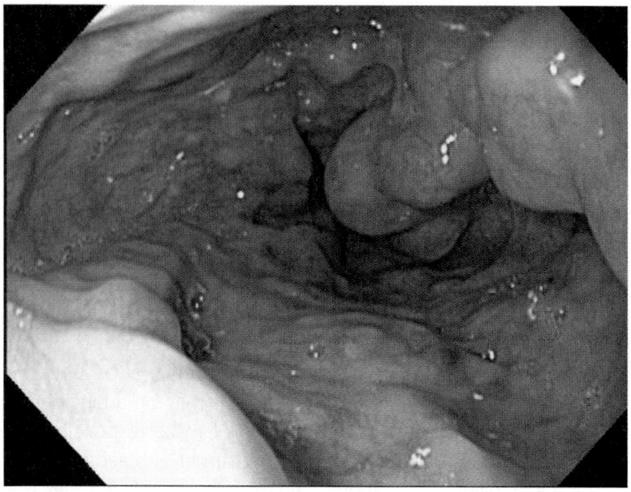

Figure 155-5 *Esophageal varices.*

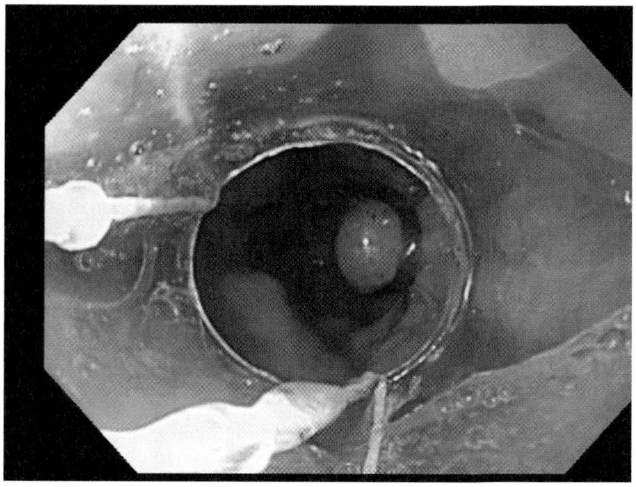

Figure 155-6 *Banded esophageal varix.*

Acute variceal bleeding is different from nonvariceal bleeding in many respects. Upper endoscopy is the primary diagnostic modality and allows for direct visualization of columns of esophageal varices. If varices are suspected as the source of upper GI bleeding, endoscopy should be performed quickly (within 24 hours) for potential intervention. Abdominal CT and ultrasound may show the presence of collateral veins. Portal vein angiography may also demonstrate the presence of collaterals or recanalization of the umbilical vein.

Variceal hemorrhage is responsible for one-third of all deaths due to cirrhosis. Mortality is between 15% to 50% for each bleeding episode, and 70% to 80% in those with continuous bleeding. Following cessation of active variceal bleeding, there is a high risk of recurrent bleeding within 6 weeks (>50%). The time of greatest risk is within the first 48 to 72 hours (90% of rebleeds will occur in this time period), and over half of all subsequent rebleeding episodes occur within the first 10 days. Recurrent variceal bleeding may occur in up to 70% of patients within six weeks of the index bleed if preventive measures are not performed.

Survival during the 6 weeks following the index bleed is directly related to rebleeding. Risk factors include age greater than 60 years, large varices, severe initial bleed (hemoglobin < 8 g/dL on admission) and renal failure. Patients with acute variceal bleeding are typically treated with multiple modalities simultaneously, including medical therapies and endoscopic management. Over resuscitation should be avoided as over vigorous volume repletion has been associated with precipitation of further bleeding. While early intervention in the form of transfusions (for low hemoglobin) and intravenous fluids may be warranted in the setting of hypotension, patients who are suspected to have significant bleeding should undergo endoscopy early in the course of resuscitation. In addition radiologic and surgical treatments may be needed. Endoscopic variceal band ligation is a commonly applied therapy. This is a method of placing elastic bands over varices, similar to the technique of banding hemorrhoids. Varices are suctioned into a banding device and the bands are released around the base of the varices. It is typically performed in the distal 5 cm of the esophagus. **Esophageal variceal band ligation controls acute bleeding in 90% of patients, but has a rebleeding rate up to 30%.**

Pathophysiology Normal pressure in the portal vein is 5 to10 mm Hg. An elevated portal venous pressure of greater than 10 mm Hg (due to obstruction) increases capillary pressure. The connection between the portal and systemic circulation may enlarge to allow blood to bypass the obstruction and pass directly into the systemic circulation. One of the known sites of such anastomosis is the distal esophagus. Studies have demonstrated the role of endothelin-1 and nitric oxide in the pathogenesis of portal hypertension and esophageal varices. Endothelin-1 is a powerful vasoconstrictor synthesized by sinusoidal endothelial cells that has been implicated in the increased hepatic vascular resistance of cirrhosis and in the development of liver fibrosis. Nitric oxide is a vasodilator substance that is synthesized by sinusoidal endothelial cells. In the cirrhotic liver, the production of nitric oxide is decreased, and endothelial nitric oxide synthase activity and nitrite production by sinusoidal endothelial cells are reduced.

Clinical findings The symptoms of variceal bleeding are nonspecific and include hematemesis, melena, and hematochezia. Patients may feel light-headed and dizzy; and those with severe liver disease may have hepatic encephalopathy, which may be the sole presenting feature in a cirrhotic patient who is bleeding from the upper GI tract. Other associated signs and symptoms are the clinical manifestations of cirrhosis including the laboratory abnormalities associated with cirrhosis (see Chapter 159). The objective of upper endoscopy is to find and define the source of bleeding and to treat it. Varices are evaluated for signs of either active bleeding or markers of recent bleeding. These markers include large tortuous varices with red wale marks (longitudinal red streaks on varices that resemble red, corduroy wales), cherry red spots (discrete cherry red spots that are flat on a varix) and hemocystic spots (raised discrete red spots that overlie varices that appear as "blood blisters"). Platelet or fibrin plugs are white nipple-like projections that project from a varix indicative of a site with recent bleeding and with a very high risk of bleeding.

Prognosis Variceal bleeding is a significant cause of rebleeding and mortality. Variceal bleeding will stop in approximately 50% of patients, but those who have continued bleeding have a mortality that approaches 80%. Patients have a high risk of rebleeding (up to 70%) until the gastroesophageal varices are obliterated. If a patient survives the initial bleeding episode, repeated courses of band ligation are performed approximately every 2 weeks until the varices are obliterated. This is combined with medical therapy using nonselective beta-blockade to reduce portal pressures. Current data supports the use of nonselective beta-blockers for grades III and IV varices prophylactically and for any grade of varix found to bleed. The prognosis for patients with bleeding gastroesophageal varices is poor even with control of bleeding varices as this is indicative of progressive liver disease. Patients die from hepatic decompensation, rebleeding, infections, renal failure, and other complications. Bacterial infections occur in up to 20% of cirrhotics with GI bleeding and subsequently develop in an additional 50% of patients during hospitalization for variceal bleeds. These include spontaneous bacterial peritonitis, pneumonia, sepsis (urosepsis, etc) and skin infections. The use of prophylactic antibiotics in patients with acute variceal bleeding has been shown to decrease the rates of subsequent infection, spontaneous bacterial peritonitis, bacteremia, and death. Data for the use of fluoroquinolones as the prophylactic antibiotic of choice is supported by frequent clinical use but a growing resistance of organisms to this class must be considered in choosing an antibiotic and alternatives include third-generation cephalosporins.

PRACTICE POINT

- Variceal bleeding will stop in approximately 50% of patients, but those who have continued bleeding have a mortality that approaches 80%. Nonselective beta-blockers are indicated for grades III and IV varices prophylactically and for any grade of varix found to bleed. Prophylactic antibiotics are indicated in patients with acute variceal bleeding to decrease the rates of subsequent infection, spontaneous bacterial peritonitis, bacteremia, and death.

Portal hypertensive gastropathy

Diagnosis In patients with cirrhosis and portal hypertension, gastric mucosal blood flow is increased, leading to congestion and hyperemia of the stomach. Portal hypertensive gastropathy occurs when edema and capillary venous dilatation in the stomach causes friability. This can subsequently result in bleeding with rupture of ectatic vessels. The endoscopic appearance is a mosaic-like pattern of pink mucosa, with a characteristic "snakeskin" appearance. Overall this is a rare cause of acute upper GI bleeding, although it may be a source of chronic blood loss in cirrhotics.

Portal hypertensive gastropathy may develop after treatment of esophageal varices. A proposed mechanism is that following treatment of varices there is increased backpressure into the stomach vasculature, leading to the development of gastric congestion. Thus the goal of treatment of portal hypertensive gastropathy is to decrease portal pressures and therefore stop bleeding. The affected area is diffuse and pharmacologic agents which decrease blood flow, such as octreotide, can be used acutely. Nonselective beta-blockers (nadolol and propranolol) are often given, with the dose then increased and adjusted if side effects occur. Endoscopic treatments are ineffective in this disorder. Patients with uncontrolled bleeding may need transjugular intrahepatic portal systemic shunt therapy or a surgical shunt. In patients with decompensated liver disease, liver transplantation is indicated.

DIAGNOSIS

All upper GI bleeding can be life-threatening. Factors that portend a favorable or a poor prognosis in patients with nonvariceal upper GI bleeding can be used to appropriately triage and manage patients. The role of nasogastric (NG) tube aspiration is controversial, but may provide useful information. NG tube aspirates, however, can be falsely negative; false-negatives most commonly occur in patients with bleeding from duodenal ulcers due to spasm of the pylorus, and can occur in other conditions, including gastric ulcers and rarely esophageal varices (if the tube is positioned in a nondependent area of the stomach).

PRACTICE POINT

- Patients with a clear NG tube aspirate have a 6% mortality, whereas those with red blood from hematemesis or NG tube aspirate have an 18% mortality, and patients with red blood from above as well as hematochezia have a 30% mortality rate.

HISTORY TO AID DIAGNOSIS

Similar to utilizing laboratory values to aid in diagnosis, a thorough history can help to predict a source of bleeding and prognosticate outcomes. For instance, an alcoholic with cirrhosis who has not recently undergone variceal screening endoscopy and presents with a large volume upper GI bleed should be managed as a variceal bleed until proven otherwise and should be started on octreotide and undergo urgent endoscopy. Conversely, a patient with no history of liver disease or physical stigmata of cirrhosis probably has a nonvariceal source of bleeding. A patient with an extensive NSAID use history most likely has peptic ulcer disease.

CASE 155-2

A 79-year-old man with a history of retching in the setting of nausea and vomiting presented with a day of melena. Vital signs revealed a normal BP but tachycardia with a pulse of 104. He was feeling well until he ate undercooked fish and vomited for

12 hours the day before admission. He reported some epigastric pain. Laboratory values indicated an elevated BUN and a rectal exam revealed black, guaiac positive tarry stool. Cardiac enzymes and ECG were unremarkable. His subsequent labs revealed a hematocrit of 33% (baseline 45%). He underwent urgent upper endoscopy and a small Mallory Weiss tear was identified in the posterior gastroesophageal junction with no active bleeding. He was initially treated with an IV PPI and transitioned to an oral PPI and discharged home the following day.

LABORATORY TESTING TO ESTABLISH GI BLEEDING SOURCE

While it is difficult to predict a source of bleeding without direct visualization, the laboratory values can present valuable clues which may aid in steps towards diagnosis. For instance, *the BUN will be elevated out of proportion to the creatinine due to digestion of blood in most patients with upper GI bleeding.* In variceal bleeding, abnormalities of the liver enzymes (ALT, AST) are seen in patients with active hepatocellular damage. Patients may have hyperbilirubinemia and poor synthetic function, with hypoalbuminemia and an elevated INR. Patients with bone marrow suppression from alcohol may have pancytopenia or those with hypersplenism may have low platelet counts. In patients with liver failure, hypoglycemia may be detected. Low albumin states may predict worse outcomes from bleeding. Although laboratory values cannot predict a source of bleed, they help define the clinical status of the bleeding patient.

TRIAGE/HOSPITAL ADMISSION

RISK ASSESSMENT: CLINICAL PREDICTORS AND GUIDELINES

Clinical guidelines have been developed to help optimize the management of patients with nonvariceal upper GI bleeding. The aim of guidelines is to identify low-risk patients who can be discharged either directly from the emergency room or at an early stage of hospitalization, and to identify high-risk patients who will need more resources. Several such guidelines include both clinical data and information obtained at the time of endoscopy. Newer guidelines focus on clinical data to determine which patients bear increased mortality risk and therefore merit urgent endoscopy and/or ICU level care.

Two main prognostic scores for upper GI bleeding have been used clinically. The Rockall score (**Table 155-2**) is a scoring system used to predict rebleeding and mortality in patients with nonvariceal upper GI bleeding. In this scoring system, scores of zero to 3 are assigned to the factors of age, the presence of shock, comorbidity, diagnosis, and endoscopic stigmata. A low-risk patient has a score of two or less and about 30% of patients will belong to this category. In this low-risk group, there was a 4.3% risk of rebleeding and 0.1% mortality. Patients with Rockall scores of three to five have intermediate rates of rebleeding and mortality (2.0–7.9%) whereas patients with a score of 6 or greater have a high rebleeding and mortality rate (15.1–39.1%). Limitations of this scoring system include that it was derived from a relatively small number of patients and the full score requires both clinical and endoscopic information to calculate.

A scoring system that only uses clinical information (and not endoscopic data) obtained at the time of presentation, developed by Blatchford and colleagues (**Table 155-3**), helps determine urgency of endoscopy and intervention need. The clinical information incorporated in this scoring system includes hemoglobin, BUN, pulse, systolic blood pressure, the presence of syncope, melena, liver disease, and heart failure. A new scoring system that also only uses information available at the time of initial presentation is the AIMS65 score. This score includes five factors: albumin < 3.0 g/dL, INR > 1.5, altered mental status, systolic blood pressure < 90 mm Hg, and age > 65 years. In this score, each factor is assigned a score of 1 and high-risk patients have an AIMS score > 1.

MANAGEMENT

INITIAL HOSPITAL TREATMENT

While the early goals of treatment for GI bleeding include identification of the bleeding source and facilitation of bleeding cessation, the *primary task is stabilization of the patient.* Patients need to have at least two large bore peripheral intravenous (IV) access catheters (18 gauge or larger) or central venous access. Supplemental oxygen should be administered routinely. Crystalloid fluids should be initially administered to maintain an adequate blood pressure. Patients who are not able to adequately protect their airways (including patients with ongoing, severe hematemesis) or at risk for aspiration should be considered for elective endotracheal intubation.

Patients who are high risk, such as the elderly or those with coronary artery disease, should be transfused to maintain a hematocrit above 30%. Young and healthy patients should be transfused to maintain a hematocrit of above 20%. In patients with a coagulopathy, this should be corrected if possible with transfu-

TABLE 155-2 The Components and Score Assignments of the Rockall Risk Assessment Score for Upper GI Bleeding

	Score			
Variable	0	1	2	3
Age (yr)	< 60	60–79	> 79	
Shock	BP > 100 mg Hg Pulse < 100 bpm	BP > 100 mg Hg Pulse > 100 bpm	BP < 100 mg Hg Pulse > 100 bpm	
Comorbidity	None		Cardiac disease, any other major comorbidity not listed in next column	Renal failure, liver failure Disseminated malignancy
Endoscopic diagnosis	Mallory-Weiss tear, no lesion	All other diagnoses	Upper GI tract malignancy	
Major stigmata of recent hemorrhage	None, or dark spots only		Blood in upper GI tract, adherent clot or spurting vessels	

BP, blood pressure; GI, gastrointestinal; bmp, beats/min. Max score = 11; low risk = < 2; high risk = > 5 (although this varies in the literature).

TABLE 155-3 The Components and Interpretation of the Blatchford Scoring System

Variables	Points
Systolic blood pressure (mm Hg)	
100–109	1
90–99	2
< 90	3
Blood urea nitrogen (mmol/L)	
6.5–7.9	2
8.0–9.9	3
10.0–24.9	4
> 25	6
Hemoglobin: Men (g/dL)	
12.0–12.9	1
10.0–11.9	3
< 10	6
Hemoglobin: Women (g/dL)	
10.0–11.9	1
< 10	2
Other variables	
Pulse > 100	1
Presentation with melena	1
Hepatic disease	2
Cardiac failure	2
Total	—

A score of > 1 is considered "high risk" while ≤ 1 is "low risk" in terms of predicting need for intervention.

sion of fresh frozen plasma (starting with 1 unit and then more may be required based on subsequent INR) or administration of vitamin K (10 mg orally if at all possible but equivalent SC or IV dosage is effective as well). In patients with a low platelet count (< 50,000/mL), transfuse platelets with an initial 1 to 2 units and subsequent recheck prior to procedure with a goal platelet count of > 50,000.

Medications

Medications useful for management of acute upper GI bleeding include proton pump inhibitors and octreotide. Other medications including H2 blockers have not been demonstrated to favorably influence the natural history of acute GI bleeding.

Proton pump inhibitor therapy

Proton pump inhibitors in patients with significant nonvariceal GI bleeding prevents rebleeding and assists in the initial cessation of bleeding. Endoscopic therapy is considered the standard of care for patients with active bleeding and nonbleeding visible vessels. Patients with peptic ulcer and successful endoscopic therapy have less rebleeding with the addition of intravenous PPI therapy. In patients initially treated in the emergency room with a bolus infusion of omeprazole followed by a continuous infusion, active bleeding lesions found at endoscopy decreased and clean-based ulcers at endoscopy increased. Recommended dosing for PPIs includes an initial intravenous (IV) bolus followed by an IV infusion for 72 hours after endoscopic therapy (**Table 155-4**). Patients who remain stable may then transition to standard dose oral PPIs.

TABLE 155-4 Commonly Used Oral Proton Pump Inhibitors (PPIs) and Their Recommended Dose Regimen for Acute Upper Gastrointestinal (GI) Bleeding

PPI Name	Initial Bolus Dose	Continuous IV Infusion Dose	Duration
Lansoprazole (Prevacid)	60 mg	6 mg/h	Up to 72 h
Pantoprazole (Protonix)	80 mg	8 mg/h	Up to 72 h
Esomeprazole (Nexium)	80 mg	8 mg/h	Up to 72 h

Octreotide

The somatostatin analogue octreotide can be used to treat patients with both variceal and non-variceal upper GI bleeding. This medication is indicated in patients with variceal bleeding or acute upper GI bleeding thought secondary to varices, using a loading dose of 25 to 50 mcg followed by an intravenous infusion of 25 to 50 mcg per hour. Octreotide may also be helpful in patients with nonvariceal bleeding. While a useful adjunctive treatment in patients with nonvariceal upper GI bleeding, octreotide should not be prescribed routinely to patients with nonvariceal upper GI bleeding. For all suspected etiologies of upper GI bleeding, the use of octreotide should be considered in patients who have persistent bleeding on optimal medical management, including PPIs, who are poor surgical risks (such as those with multiple comorbidities already in the hospital).

Endoscopic treatments

Endoscopic therapy for upper GI bleeding has been demonstrated to yield significant improvement in hemostasis, number of units of blood transfused, number of emergency interventions, hospital length of stay, and hospital costs. Endoscopic therapy is the standard of care for patients with the high-risk stigmata of recent hemorrhage of active bleeding or a nonbleeding visible vessel. The management of adherent clots has been controversial in the literature and guidelines with recent data suggesting a possible role for endoscopic therapy.

For many conditions including active bleeding, visible vessels, and esophageal varices, endoscopic techniques are the mainstay of treatment. The timing and occasion for endoscopic treatment often depends on the clinical presentation and/or findings at time of endoscopy. An upper endoscopy examination is indicated within 24 hours of presentation for patients with suspected upper GI bleeding. Conditions which warrant rapid triage and planned endoscopy include bleeding in the setting of known varices, persistent hypotension requiring pressors, and increasing transfusion requirement. However, hemodynamic stability, protection of the airway (if necessary), and platelets or vitamin K administration when applicable may be necessary steps prior to endoscopic evaluation regardless of the urgency. In addition, data supports endoscopic evaluation within 24 hours and does not support a need for more urgent endoscopy in most patients.

PRACTICE POINT

- Upper endoscopy is indicated within 24 hours of presentation for patients with suspected upper GI bleeding but most patients do not require more urgent endoscopy. Hemodynamic stability and correction of thrombocytopenia and coagulopathy are necessary prior to endoscopy.

Optimization of visualization

One of the challenges of managing patients with GI bleeding is visualization due to blood within the gastrointestinal tract. This problem may be overcome by the use of a variety of techniques or a combination of endoscopic techniques including the use of double-channel or large channel endoscopes and vigorous irrigation.

In addition to endoscopic techniques, intravenous erythromycin (250 mg IV bolus or 3 mg/kg over 30 minutes) can be used for its prokinetic properties to increase gastric emptying and clear the stomach of blood. The erythromycin is given intravenously 30 to 120 minutes prior to endoscopy as a useful adjunctive treatment in patients with large gastrointestinal bleeds. It can be used either initially or after an endoscopy shows large amounts of blood remaining in the stomach with withdrawal of the endoscope and the use of erythromycin before proceeding again with endoscopy. Metoclopramide may also be used similarly, although there is less available data about its effectiveness in patients with upper GI bleeding.

Methods to control bleeding

The current endoscopic modalities to treat non-variceal GI bleeding include the use of injection therapies (primarily with dilute epinephrine), contact thermal therapies including heater and bipolar probes, noncontact thermal methods (predominantly argon plasma coagulation), mechanical treatments including a variety of hemoclips and band ligation techniques, and a combination of the above treatment modalities (typically injection therapies combined with one of the other modalities) (**Table 155-5**). For nonvariceal upper GI bleeding, combination therapy and use of hemoclips improve outcomes and decrease recurrent bleeding. For esophageal variceal bleeding, banding with small rubber bands placed endoscopically to tamponade blood flow offers the effective treatment and outcomes. Success with injection of glues in the treatment of gastric varices has been demonstrated. Decompression of portal pressures when possible is the optimal therapy.

While endoscopic injection sclerotherapy and banding ligation in conjunction with pharmacologic treatment are the primary methods for controlling acute variceal bleeding, tamponade with a Sengstaken-Blakemore tube may be indicated when these methods fail or before endoscopy if a rapid bleed occurs. The use of these tubes is indicated for acute bleeding from esophageal or gastric varices unresponsive to medical therapy, tears at the gastroesophageal junction, Mallory-Weiss tears unresponsive to medical therapy or esophageal exclusion to manage distal esophageal perforation. The Sengstaken-Blakemore tube is absolutely contraindicated for patients in whom bleeding has stopped and in those with recent surgery of the gastro-esophageal junction or known esophageal stricture.

TABLE 155-5 Available Modalities for Endoscopic Therapy

Injection therapy
a. Epinephrine
b. Hypertonic saline
c. Sclerosant (absolute alcohol, polidoconol)
d. Tissue adhesives: cyanoacyralate, thrombin/fibrin glue
Thermal therapy
a. Contact: HP, bipolar (gold probe, BICAP)
b. Non-contact: APC, Nd: YAG laser
Mechanical therapy
a. Endoclips
b. Endoscopic band ligation
Dual therapy (combination of above modalities)

APC, argon plasma cautery; BICAP, bipolar probe; HP, heater probe.

CASE 155-3

A 62-year-old man with a history of NSAID use and tobacco abuse sought medical attention for intermittent hematemesis for 1 day. His vital signs revealed a heart rate of 114 bpm and a low-normal BP (100/60 mm Hg). NG tube lavage revealed bright red blood which continued to be suctioned. Laboratory studies reported anemia with a hematocrit of 21% (baseline 45%). His physicians administered erythromycin intravenously and initiated a PPI infusion. After stabilization with two large bore IVs, and initiation of blood transfusions, a gastroenterologist performed an upper endoscopy which identified a visible bleeding vessel in a deep duodenal ulcer. The ulcer was injected with dilute epinephrine, and clips were placed to achieve hemostasis. The patient was monitored in an intensive care unit and had an uneventful post-procedure course.

■ CONSULTATION

Hospitalists should involve a gastroenterologist early in the course of upper GI bleeding. Emergent consultation is appropriate with rapid bleeds in the setting of hypotension, a very low hematocrit, known varices or other instances when urgent endoscopy might be required. In most cases, however, patient stabilization is a crucial first step before gastroenterology intervention can be considered (**Figure 155-7**). A gastroenterology consultant can provide

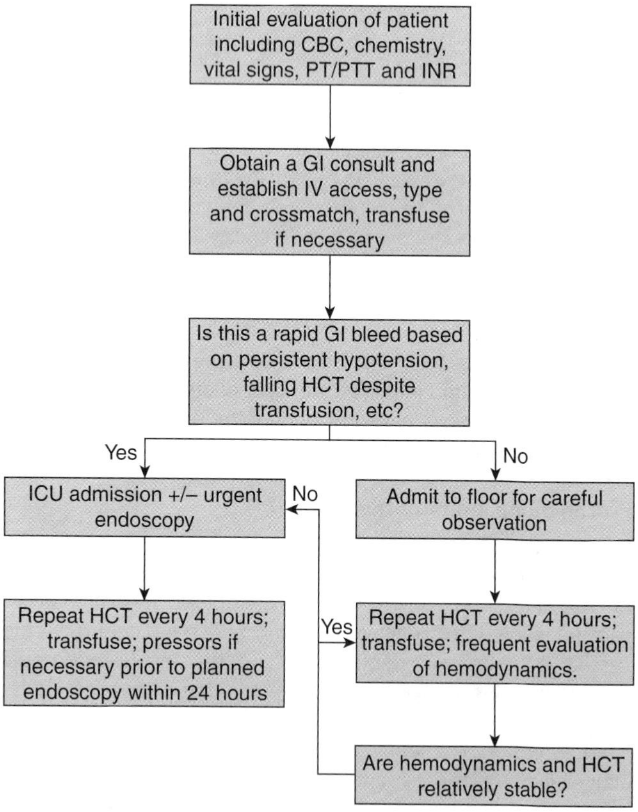

Figure 155-7 *Initial diagnostic algorithm for upper GI bleeding. (CBC, complete blood count; HCT, hematocrit; ICU, intensive care unit; INR, international normalized ratio; IV, intravenous; PT, prothrombin time; PTT, partial thromboplastin time.)*

diagnostic and therapeutic advice early in the course of treatment and may be called as soon as a suspected upper GI bleeding patient is identified. In addition, surgery consultation is indicated in certain circumstances including patients requiring the ICU, those who require multiple blood transfusions or those who undergo endoscopy without identification of a source of bleed or ability to stop the bleeding. Likewise, interventional radiology should be consulted if a bleeding source distal to the ligament of Treitz is suspected either prior to or after EGD. In these "mid" (small bowel) or lower GI bleeding patients, the patient may benefit from a tagged red blood cell scan and subsequent angiography. **The key to consultation is to involve the consultant early and to report any significant clinical changes.**

COMPLICATIONS AND PROGNOSIS

COMPLICATIONS OF GI BLEEDING

The reported mortality of upper GI bleeding generally ranges from 5% to 14%. Complications of GI bleeding include hypotension and subsequent shock which can lead to organ failure and death if not addressed in a timely manner. Aspiration of blood contents and subsequent hypoxemia and respiratory failure represents another adverse outcome. Tachycardia in the setting of preexisting coronary heart disease can lead to ischemia. Anemia can also further lead to under-perfusion of vital organs and some patients die of complications subsequent to inadequate resuscitation with blood and fluids as discussed above.

COMPLICATIONS OF TREATMENT

The majority of the complications associated with treatment of upper GI bleeding stem from endoscopic treatments. Major complications include myocardial infarction, perforation, aspiration, hemorrhage, and death. Minor complications of endoscopy include mucosal tears, medication reactions and hypoxemia. In addition, a small risk exists of infection or bleeding from the endoscopic intervention itself. If sedatives are utilized for the procedure, the individual risks of each medication are added to the overall risk of the procedure. Many of the complications of GI endoscopy are cardiopulmonary in origin.

The initial evaluation of patients with upper GI bleeding should include risk assessment to triage patients to appropriate levels of care and perform resuscitation measures. Elective endotracheal intubation should be considered in patients at high risk of aspiration, such as those with massive upper GI bleeding. Attention must be given to provide the proper level of sedation required to perform the procedure.

Epinephrine is a vasoconstrictor which can lead to local ischemia and can also cause tachycardia. Large doses of injected epinephrine during endoscopic therapy especially in the region of the esophagus and upper stomach are associated with significant elevations of systolic blood pressure and tachycardia. The use of cautery can lead to direct tissue injury, which may further damage the GI tract. The use of cautery may lead to perforation, especially if excessive pressure is exerted on the site of therapy. The depth of penetration of tissue injury may be lessened by the use of injection therapy that lifts the tissue and provides a safety barrier.

PROGNOSIS

In patients presenting with upper GI bleeding, a number of clinical prognostic factors have been shown to be helpful in predicting a poor outcome. These include older age (age >60 years), the presence of shock, hematemesis and/or hematochezia, onset of bleeding in a patient hospitalized for other reasons, bleeding from malignancies of the upper GI tract or varices, increasing comorbid diseases, and patients with severe coagulopathies.

DISCHARGE PLANNING

RESTARTING ANTICOAGULATION IN UPPER GI BLEEDING

Patients who require anticoagulants (eg, warfarin) or platelet function inhibitors (eg, clopidogrel, aspirin) may develop signs of upper GI bleeding. Most GI bleeding episodes on antiplatelet agents or anticoagulants occur within the first year of therapy. Once a source of bleeding is identified, the timing of restarting anticoagulants represents a difficult decision. Part of the decision-making process is evaluating the benefit of the anticoagulant or platelet inhibitor compared to the risk of bleeding. A patient with high-risk thromboembolic disease should have careful consideration of reversal of anticoagulation in consultation with the prescribing cardiologist or neurologist before endoscopy. A patient with low-risk thromboembolic disease can have complete reversal of anticoagulation followed by endoscopy. When to resume anticoagulation depends on the source and severity of bleeding as well as the underlying condition being treated. After hemostasis is achieved, patients who need to be restarted on anticoagulants have to be monitored carefully.

OUTPATIENT SYMPTOM MONITORING

Patients discharged after upper GI bleeding require education about signs and symptoms to help identify any early bleeding. Patients should look for the return of black stool as a sign of a developing bleed. However, for the first 24 to 48 hours following an endoscopy which yielded a bleeding source, patients can expect to see subsequent passage of blood which may be maroon or black. Resting pulse with evaluation for tachycardia can be measured by patients. In addition, patients require education about over-the-counter medications to avoid which may affect GI bleeding, including drugs that contain NSAIDs or aspirin. Bismuth subsalicylate (eg, Pepto-Bismol) should also be avoided as it causes the stool to appear dark and the stool color can be confused with melena.

OUTPATIENT LAB MONITORING

Patients who had bleeding related to supra-therapeutic levels of warfarin need careful monitoring of the INR if the medication is subsequently resumed. Clinics which specialize in anticoagulation can reduce bleeding outcomes. In addition, anemic patients should have hemoglobin levels checked in the outpatient setting 1 to 2 weeks following discharge, as asymptomatic recurrent bleeding can present with worsening anemia. For upper GI bleeding, an elevated BUN can be a useful marker of recurrent bleeding. Patients with *H Pylori*–related bleeding should have an *H pylori* breath test or stool antigen performed if upper endoscopy is not scheduled to confirm that *H pylori* has been successfully eradicated.

QUALITY IMPROVEMENT TO ADDRESS PERFORMANCE GAPS

PREVENTION

Primary and secondary prevention of upper GI bleeding requires careful evaluation of a patient's underlying medical problems and current medications. NSAID use should be minimized whenever possible and, if necessary, one should monitor frequently for symptoms and signs of GI bleeding which may indicate peptic ulcer disease, esophagitis, gastritis or duodenitis which can follow NSAID use. Beta-blocker therapy with propranolol or nadolol should be used in patients with cirrhosis and a prior history of esophageal variceal bleeding (secondary prophylaxis) regardless of grade, or grades III and IV esophageal varices without previous hemorrhage (primary prophylaxis). The comparison of nonselective beta-blockers and placebo in several randomized controlled trials demonstrates a greater than 20% absolute risk reduction in subsequent bleeding from esophageal varices. Prevention of GI bleeding in admitted patients requires careful monitoring of medications (eg, anticoagulants and antiplatelet agents) and comorbidities. Patients at high risk for stress ulcer bleeding (eg, mechanical ventilation) benefit from prophylactic PPI dosing.

TRANSITIONS OF CARE

As patients transition from in hospital care to outpatient management several factors must be considered. Medications must be adjusted from the inpatient setting to appropriate outpatient regimens. For example, although patients with upper GI bleeding are often managed with high dose proton pump inhibitors in the hospital, at discharge most patients can be managed on a once daily standard dose oral proton pump inhibitor.

Findings at endoscopy may require changes in the medical regimen or subsequent endoscopies. In patients with peptic ulcer disease, biopsy results positive for *H pylori* infection indicate a necessary outpatient antibiotic regimen. Most patients with significant gastric ulcers will require repeat endoscopy examinations in 8 to 12 weeks to confirm healing of the ulcer and to exclude malignancy.

Communication of inhospital care givers with outpatient physicians is critical to the successful management of patients with significant upper GI bleeding. Follow-up with a primary physician should take place for repeat blood draws and physical examination within 7 to 14 days of hospital discharge, and follow-up with a gastroenterologist either for a planned repeat endoscopy or office visit should take place within 2 to 4 weeks depending on the source of bleeding. For example, variceal bleeding may require a 2-week follow-up endoscopy for further banding and assessment of healing. Outpatient planning for follow up with gastroenterology, general surgery, and primary care should take place prior to discharge with the consulting specialists and the outpatient primary care provider.

DISPARITIES IN HEALTH CARE

While scarce literature identifies disparities in health care in gastroenterology, one recent study showed significant proportion of visits to US emergency departments for acute GI illnesses are associated with a delay in initial clinical assessment. Of the patient visits analyzed, there were an estimated 1.6 million emergency department visits for acute pancreatitis, 2.2 million visits for appendicitis, 1.2 million visits for cholecystitis, and 3.9 million visits for upper GI bleeding. The study showed that Hispanic patients waited longer and had a higher frequency of delays compared with other racial and ethnic groups. Future investigations into racial, ethnic, gender and other disparities in health delivery and performance in upper GI bleeding are needed.

SUGGESTED READINGS

Banares R, Albillos A, Rincon D, et al. Endoscopic treatment versus endoscopic plus pharmacologic treatment for acute variceal bleeding: a meta-analysis. *Hepatology.* 2002;35:609–615.

Barkun AN, Bardou M, Kuipers EJ, et al. International Consensus Upper Gastrointestinal Bleeding Conference Group. International consensus recommendations on the management of patients with nonvariceal upper gastrointestinal bleeding. *Ann Intern Med.* 2010;152(2):101–113.

Bjorkman DJ, Zaman A, Fennerty MB, et al. Urgent vs. elective endoscopy for acute non-variceal upper-GI bleeding: an effectiveness study. *Gastrointest Endosc.* 2004;60:1–8.

Blatchford O, Murray WR, Blatchford M. A risk score to predict need for treatment for upper-gastrointestinal hemorrhage. *Lancet.* 2000;356:1318–1321.

Gralnek IM, Barkun AN, Bardou M. Management of acute bleeding from a peptic ulcer. *N Engl J Med.* 2008;359(9):928–937.

Hay JA, Maldonado L, Weingarten SR, et al. Prospective evaluation of a clinical guideline recommending hospital length of stay in upper gastrointestinal tract hemorrhage. *JAMA.* 1997;278:2151–2156.

Pfau PR, Cooper GS, Carlson MD, et al. Success and shortcomings of a clinical care pathway in the management of acute nonvariceal upper gastrointestinal bleeding. *Am J Gastroenterol.* 2004;99:425–431.

Rockall TA, Logan RFA, Devlin HB, et al. Steering Committee of the National Audit of Acute Upper Gastrointestinal Haemorrhage. Risk assessment after acute upper gastrointestinal hemorrhage. *Gut.* 1996;38:316–321.

Rockall TA, Logan RFA, Devlin HB, Northfield TC. National audit of acute upper gastrointestinal haemorrhage. Selection of patients for early discharge or outpatient care after acute upper gastrointestinal hemorrhage. *Lancet.* 1996;347:1138–1140.

Wolf AT, Wasan SK, Saltzman JR. Impact of anticoagulation on rebleeding following endoscopic therapy for non-variceal upper gastrointestinal hemorrhage. *Am J Gastroenterol.* 2007;102(2):290–296.

CHAPTER 156

Acute Pancreatitis

Bechien U. Wu, MD, MPH
Darwin L. Conwell, MD, MS

Key Clinical Questions

1. What are the criteria for the diagnosis of acute pancreatitis?
2. What efforts should be made to determine etiology during hospitalization, and what is the optimal timing of diagnostic and/or intervention studies in acute pancreatitis?
3. What are the key components of early management?
4. What is the management of late complications?
5. When should consultation with gastroenterology, surgery, or interventional radiology be considered?
6. When are specific interventions such as ERCP, fine-needle aspiration, or prophylactic antibiotics indicated?

INTRODUCTION

Acute pancreatitis is a common cause for hospitalization in the United States. Recent data from the National Center for Health Statistics has indicated a rising frequency of admissions for acute pancreatitis attributed to the increase in gallstone-related disease. Annually, more than 300,000 hospital admissions for acute pancreatitis present in the United States at a direct cost of more than $2 billion. Although acute pancreatitis is typically a mild, self-limited disease, a wide range of severity exists. Fifteen to 20% of patients experience a more severe form of disease with overall inhospital mortality estimated to range between 3–5% of cases.

Risk factors for acute pancreatitis include both genetic susceptibility and environmental exposures. Genes involving mutation in the cystic fibrosis transmembrane conductance regulator (CFTR), cationic trypsinogen gene (PRSS1), and secretory trypsin inhibitor (SPINK1) have been identified in patients with recurrent acute pancreatitis. Other patient-related factors such as obesity have also been demonstrated to be associated with increased severity of disease.

ETIOLOGIES

The most common etiology for acute pancreatitis is now gallstone-related disease, followed by alcohol and post-ERCP (endoscopic retrograde cholangiopancreatography) pancreatitis (**Table 156-1**). Additional etiologies include metabolic derangements (hypercalcemia, hypertriglyceridemia) and medications (**Table 156-2**). Less common etiologies include autoimmune and hereditary forms of pancreatitis. Whether pancreas divisum itself is a cause for acute pancreatitis remains controversial.

Obstructive causes for pancreatitis secondary to pancreatic mass or cystic lesions, such as intraductal papillary mucinous neoplasm (IPMNs), are increasingly recognized due to improvements in imaging techniques.

CLINICAL PRESENTATION

Patients with acute pancreatitis usually complain of sudden onset unrelenting epigastric pain that is sharp in nature. This pain often radiates to the back. Nausea and vomiting are common as is anorexia. Patients may present with signs of volume depletion in the setting of decreased oral intake as well as potential third-space losses. Signs of systemic inflammation are common at the time of presentation including fever, tachycardia, and leukocytosis. Rarely, physical exam findings may include evidence of hemorrhagic pancreatitis such as flank (Grey-Turner sign) or periumbilical (Cullen sign) ecchymosis.

PATHOPHYSIOLOGY

Acute pancreatitis results from local tissue injury to the pancreas. Ordinarily, digestive enzymes are sequestered in an inactivated form within vesicles (zymogen granules) of the acinar cell. However, in acute pancreatitis, an insult (alcohol, gallstones, medications, oxidative stress) leads to premature zymogen activation as well as retention of activated enzymes within the acinar cell. This leads to a process of auto-digestion that is associated with increased activation of the transcription factor NF-kb that in turn leads to increased release of proinflammatory cytokines (interleukins 1, 2, 6, 8 and TNF-alpha). This local inflammatory response leads to increased recruitment of neutrophils and macrophages. If left unchecked, this local

TABLE 156-1 Etiologies of Acute Pancreatitis

Etiology	Notes
Gallstone	Most common cause. Combined use of abdominal ultrasound and liver tests enhances diagnosis.
Alcohol	Usually in setting of long-standing alcohol history.
Post-ERCP	Placement of prophylactic pancreatic duct stent associated with reduced incidence.
Medication	Recent classification system based on level of evidence for potentially offending medications.
Hypercalcemia	Should prompt evaluation for underlying cause.
Hypertriglyceridemia	Triglyceride levels can be falsely elevated during an acute episode; levels > 1000 mg/dL are fairly specific.
Autoimmune	US and Asian criteria differ. Usually associated with classic radiologic findings. IgG4 is specific but has only ~50% sensitivity.
Pancreas divisum	Controversial. Anatomic anomaly of pancreatic ducts. Should only be considered if alternative etiologies have been excluded.
Hereditary	Most commonly associated with mutation in cationic trypsinogen (PRSS1) gene.
Idiopathic	Despite thorough evaluation, a cause for pancreatitis is unable to be identified in 15–20% of cases.

TABLE 156-2 Drug-induced Pancreatitis

Class I Medications (Implicated in > 20 reported cases of acute pancreatitis with at least one documented case following reexposure)	Class II Medications (Implicated in more than 10 cases of acute pancreatitis)
Didanosine	Rifampin
Asparaginase	Lamivudine
Azathioprine	Octreotide
Valproic acid	Carbamazepine
Pentamidine	Acetaminophen
Mercaptopurine	Phenformin
Mesalamine	Interferon alfa-2b
Estrogens	Enalapril
Opiates	Hydrochlorothiazide
Tetracycline	Cisplatin
Cytarabine	Erythromycin
Steroids	Cyclopenthiazide
Trimethoprim/sulfamethoxazole	
Sulfasalazine	
Furosemide	
Sulindac	

inflammation can lead to systemic inflammation and subsequent multiorgan dysfunction syndrome (MODS). In patients with CFTR mutations, the decreased ductal secretion of chloride is believed to cause plugging in the secondary pancreatic ducts leading to acute pancreatic inflammation. In hereditary pancreatitis, an imbalance between acinar cell protective mechanisms results in the inability to inactivate a defective "supertrypsin" (PRSS1 mutation) or the presence of a defective trypsin inhibitor (SPINK1).

DIFFERENTIAL DIAGNOSIS

The presence of epigastric pain with an elevation in amylase/lipase ≥ 3 times normal is highly accurate for the diagnosis of acute pancreatitis. Additional considerations should include acute cholecystitis or ascending cholangitis (both of which may be concurrent with an attack of biliary pancreatitis). Less common considerations include a penetrating duodenal ulcer, renal colic or diabetic ketoacidosis. Further potentially life-threatening conditions include a perforated viscus, bowel obstruction or myocardial infarction. Serum amylase may also be elevated in salivary disorders, ectopic pregnancy or macroamylasemia.

DIAGNOSIS

The diagnosis of acute pancreatitis requires at least two of the following: (1) typical epigastric abdominal pain, (2) amylase/lipase evaluation ≥ 3 times upper limit of normal, and/or (3) confirmatory findings on cross-sectional imaging. Findings on abdominal ultrasound in conjunction with liver function tests have very high sensitivity for the detection of gallstone-related illness. Specifically, an elevated ALT level > 2 to 3 times normal has been found to have a 95% positive predictive value for gallstone-related illness. More recently, magnetic resonance cholangiopancreatography (MRCP) has emerged as a highly accurate, noninvasive means to evaluate for the presence of biliary pancreatitis (**Figure 156-1**).

PRACTICE POINT

- The diagnosis of acute pancreatitis requires at least two of the following: (1) typical epigastric abdominal pain, (2) amylase/lipase evaluation ≥ 3 times upper limit of normal, and/or (3) confirmatory findings on cross-sectional imaging.

The finding of hypercalcemia in the setting of acute pancreatitis should prompt a thorough evaluation for the potential underlying etiology such as hyperparathyroidism or occult malignancy.

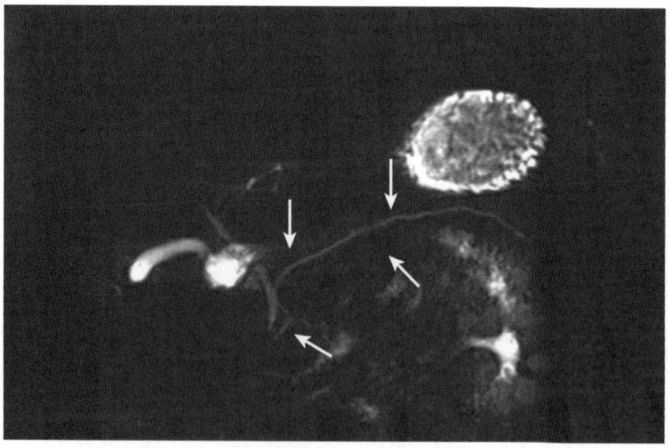

Figure 156-1 *Secretin-enhanced MRCP image demonstrating normal pancreatic duct anatomy (arrow).*

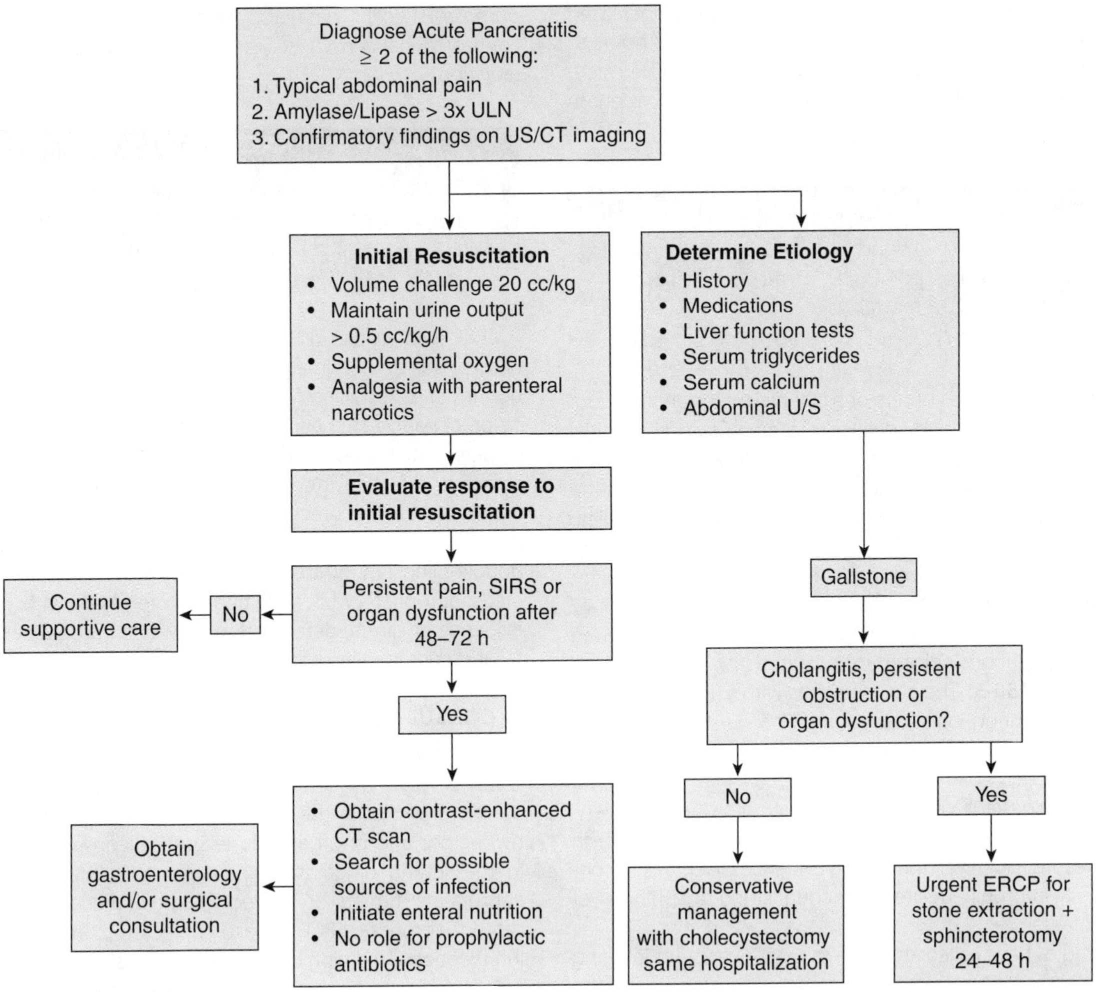

Figure 156-2 *Suggested initial management algorithm for acute pancreatitis. (CT, computed tomography; ERCP, endoscopic retrograde cholangiopancreatography; ULN, upper limits of normal; US or U/S, ultrasound; SIRS, systemic inflammatory response syndrome).*

Autoimmune pancreatitis is a rare cause of acute pancreatitis that has recently gained increasing attention in the medical literature. An otherwise unexplained episode of acute pancreatitis in a patient with CT scan findings of an enhancing "rim" or diffusely enlarged pancreas or retrograde pancreatogram features of an irregularly narrowed pancreatic duct are suggestive of autoimmune pancreatitis on imaging. A serum IgG4 level is relatively specific in this patient population though lacks sensitivity for the diagnosis.

TRIAGE/HOSPITAL ADMISSION

CRITERIA FOR ADMISSION

All patients with confirmed acute pancreatitis should be managed as inpatients because they need vigorous intravenous fluid resuscitation and intravenous analgesia. The potential role for management in an observation unit with less intensive monitoring for mild cases of acute pancreatitis is currently under study.

CRITERIA FOR ICU ADMISSION

Persistent or worsening organ dysfunction after initial fluid resuscitation or patients with significant comorbid or concurrent illness (eg, congestive heart failure and/or chronic kidney disease) should be considered for hemodynamic monitoring in an intensive care setting. Also, patients with a rise in either hematocrit or BUN after initial resuscitation efforts should strongly be considered for hemodynamic monitoring to guide further resuscitation efforts.

Multiorgan dysfunction and infection are two major complications that can develop in the patient hospitalized for acute pancreatitis. Patients with organ dysfunction are best managed in an intensive care setting. In addition to extra-pancreatic infection, infected necrosis continues to be associated with a high morbidity and mortality. Infected necrosis is best managed in a multidisciplinary setting involving gastroenterology, surgery, and interventional radiology services.

MANAGEMENT

INITIAL HOSPITAL TREATMENT

Initial management of acute pancreatitis should include determination of etiology, assessment of severity, fluid challenge, and analgesia (**Figure 156-2**). Etiology may guide subsequent management, as in the case of gallstone pancreatitis. Nearly all clinical practice guidelines recommend abdominal ultrasound (in preference to abdominal computed tomography) in the early assessment of patients with acute pancreatitis. Further assessment should include routine laboratory tests (liver profile, calcium, complete blood count). A recent simplified prognostic scoring system allows rapid assessment of a patient's risk for mortality during the initial phase (first 24 hours) of illness. This bedside index of severity in acute pancreatitis (BISAP) assigns points for each of the following: BUN > 25, impaired mental status, systemic inflammatory response syndrome (SIRS), age >60, and pleural effusion. The presence of three or more of these findings signals a substantially increased risk of mortality. Unlike the Ranson score that requires 48 hours to complete, the BISAP has the advantage of being able to be calculated within the first 24 hours of hospitalization—a critical phase for early intervention.

PRACTICE POINT

- A BISAP score in the first 24 hours of 0–1 point = < 1% mortality, 2 points = 2% mortality, 3 points = 5–8% mortality, 4 points = 13–19%, 5 points = > 20% mortality.

Fluid resuscitation is the cornerstone of initial treatment for acute pancreatitis. Clinical practice guidelines recommend vigorous initial fluid resuscitation with the thought of potentially preventing complications such as necrosis. Although aggressive fluid resuscitation has not been demonstrated to directly prevent specific complications, a rise in hematocrit or BUN in the setting of intravenous hydration has been associated with necrosis and inhospital mortality, respectively. Specifically, an elevated BUN at admission > 25 mg/dL and/or a rise in BUN during the initial 24 hours in the setting of volume resuscitation indicate an increased risk for in-hospital mortality (**Figure 156-3**). Therefore, patients with a rise in either hematocrit or BUN during initial resuscitation efforts should strongly be considered for hemodynanmic monitoring to guide further resuscitation efforts.

Adequate analgesia is central to patient comfort and recovery. Limited data is available regarding treatment options for pain in acute pancreatitis. However, there is no evidence to suggest a contraindication to morphine-related compounds due to sphincter of oddi spasm.

Recent studies have called attention to extensive use of imaging associated with acute pancreatitis. In an attempt to standardize use of imaging services, the American College of Radiology has issued appropriateness criteria for imaging tests in acute pancreatitis. Current recommendations are for the use of abdominal ultrasound early in the disease course to evaluate for biliary-related complications. Computed tomography is generally reserved for patients with evidence of systemic inflammation (SIRS) after 48 hours of illness or signs of clinical deterioration. If suspicion for biliary disease is high then magnetic resonance cholangiopancreatography (MRCP) may be considered as a noninvasive alternative to ERCP for diagnostic purposes. Recent data also recommends the judicious use of contrast enhanced CT scans due to reduce patient exposure to radiation.

PRACTICE POINT

- Clinical practice guidelines recommend abdominal ultrasound (in preference to abdominal computed tomography) in the early assessment of patients with acute pancreatitis.

ERCP is indicated in the setting of persistent biliary obstruction (stone visualized on imaging with persistent elevation in liver function tests) or suspicion for ascending cholangitis. Fine-needle aspiration of pancreatic necrosis is indicated in a patient with evidence of persistent systemic inflammation in the absence of alternative source of infection (generally after 7 days of illness). Prophylactic antibiotics for the prevention of infected pancreatic necrosis are currently not recommended based on results from several recent double-blind randomized controlled trials. Antibiotics are considered appropriate while awaiting culture results in a patient with evidence of clinical deterioration. However, most experts advocate tailoring or removing antibiotics once culture results are known.

CONSULTATION

Gastroenterology should be consulted when gallstone pancreatitis is suspected, in the setting of a patient with persistent (>48 hours duration) SIRS or in the setting of acute pancreatitis complicated by necrosis and/or organ failure. Surgical consultation is indicated in the setting of gallstone pancreatitis in order to arrange for appropriate timing of cholecystectomy. Recent data has indicated that routine ERCP prior to cholecystectomy is not indicated. Interventional radiological services can assist in the identification of infected necrosis through CT-guided fine-needle aspiration and gram stain of necrosis in a patient with ongoing fever or systemic inflammation. A multidisciplinary team approach is indicated for the management of infected necrosis as care may need to be individualized (surgical debridement vs. temporizing maneuvers such as percutaneous drainage until the patient is stabilized). In general, a multidisciplinary care can help optimize use of procedures, antibiotics and imaging studies.

Nutritional support services may be required for initiation of enteral or parenteral nutrition in a patient that is not anticipated

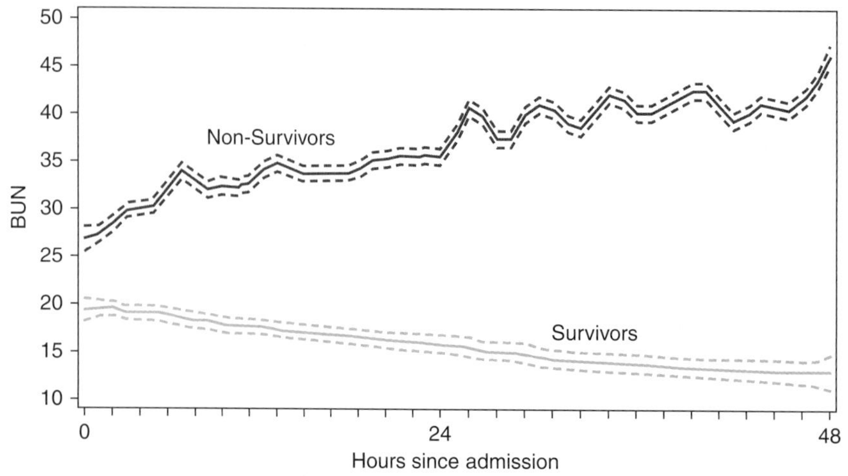

Figure 156-3 *Plot of early BUN changes among survivors vs nonsurvivors of acute pancreatitis. Data from 5819 cases of acute pancreatitis from 69 US hospitals. Solid lines represent mean BUN values, and dashed lines indicate 95% confidence limits.*

to begin oral feeding within 7 days of hospitalization. In addition, both consultation with gastroenterology and interventional radiology may assist in placement of a nasojejunal catheter for purposes of enteral nutrition in a patient that is not anticipated to begin oral feeding within 7 days.

LONGITUDINAL OUTPATIENT THERAPEUTICS OR REGIMEN AUGMENTATION

During the convalescent or recovery phase from acute pancreatitis, attention should focus on prevention of future recurrence and management of long-term complications. Recent data from a randomized-controlled trial has indicated that repeated alcohol counseling can reduce the recurrence of alcohol-associated pancreatitis when compared to a single, one-time intervention. In addition, cases of "idiopathic" pancreatitis should be further evaluated with either repeat abdominal ultrasound (which may detect abnormalities such as biliary sludge often missed in the context of acute illness) or secretin enhanced MRCP to evaluate for anatomical anomalies including IPMN and pancreas divisum. More invasive interventions such as endoscopic ultrasound or ERCP are generally reserved for patients with recurrent episodes of idiopathic acute pancreatitis.

COMPLICATIONS

Long-term sequelae that may arise in the setting of acute pancreatitis include both local and systemic complications. *Local complications* include development of fluid collections that may either comprise a pseudocyst (homogeneous fluid-filled collection) or a postnecrotic collection (heterogeneous cavity filled with fluid and necrotic debris) (**Figure 156-4**). The distinction can be important given that it may influence approach to treatment. In general, intervention in fluid collections that arise in the setting of acute pancreatitis is only indicated in the setting of symptoms or infection. A symptomatic or infected fluid collection following an episode of acute pancreatitis is an indication for consultation with gastroenterology and surgical services. Although far less common, an additional potentially serious local complication is development of a pseudoaneurysm. Hemorrhage from a pseudoaneurysm can be life-threatening and is best managed by angiography with surgical treatment reserved for failure to achieve hemostasis by alternative measures.

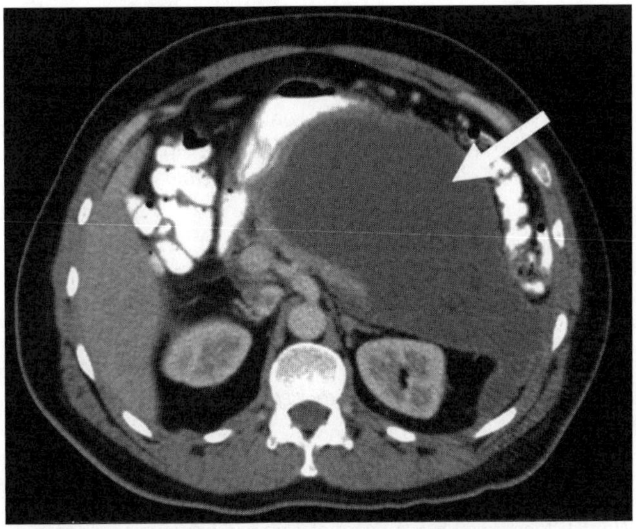

Figure 156-4 *Contrast-enhanced abdominal computed tomography demonstrating large heterogeneous post-necrotic collection (arrow) arising in a patient with necrotizing pancreatitis (8 weeks after initial episode).*

PRACTICE POINT

- A rise in hematocrit or BUN in the setting of intravenous hydration has been associated with necrosis and inhospital mortality, respectively. Specifically, an elevated BUN at admission > 25 mg/dL and/or a rise in BUN during the initial 24 hours in the setting of volume resuscitation indicate an increased risk for inhospital mortality.

PRACTICE POINT

- For pancreatic pseudocysts (homogeneous fluid filled collections) or a postnecrotic collections (heterogeneous cavity filled with fluid and necrotic debris), intervention is only indicated in the setting of symptoms or infection. A symptomatic or infected fluid collection following an episode of acute pancreatitis is an indication for consultation with gastroenterology and surgical services.

Additional long-term *systemic complications* that can result from acute pancreatitis include both exocrine and endocrine insufficiency of the pancreas. Patients with symptoms of steatorrhea or signs of fat-soluble vitamin deficiency should be evaluated with a fecal elastase to screen for pancreatic exocrine insufficiency. If the diagnosis is unclear, referral to a pancreas center for formal pancreatic function testing may confirm the diagnosis. Treatment with pancreatic enzyme supplementation is then indicated (generally at least 30,000 IU lipase with each meal). Patients suffering necrotizing pancreatitis and especially those who have undergone pancreatic debridement are at increased risk of worsening or new-onset diabetes. Fasting glucose or hemoglobin A1C can be useful to screen for development of diabetes in this high-risk category of patients. Patients may develop brittle diabetes in the setting of extensive necrosis in which case referral to endocrinology may be useful in order to optimize glycemic control.

DISCHARGE PLANNING

Goals of discharge planning for acute pancreatitis include (1) arrangement for adequate follow-up, (2) prevention of disease recurrence, and (3) initiation of appropriate secondary evaluation. Although follow-up interval should be based on an individual patient's needs, a 2-week interval has been routinely utilized. Patients with severe disease complicated by necrosis or fluid collections should be referred for outpatient follow-up with gastroenterology services. The two most important interventions for secondary prevention are cholecystectomy for gallstone-related acute pancreatitis and alcohol counseling for patients with alcohol-associated disease. In the case of gallstone pancreatitis, cholecystectomy is strongly recommended during the same hospitalization to reduce the likelihood of recurrent episode of biliary complications while awaiting surgery. Prior studies have also shown this to be a cost-effective strategy for the prevention of gallstone pancreatitis. In the case of alcohol associated disease, longitudinal alcohol cessation therapy is recommended.

QUALITY IMPROVEMENT TO ADDRESS PERFORMANCE GAPS

There are several active areas of research to address quality improvement in acute pancreatitis (**Table 156-3**), including the following:

1. Optimization of fluid resuscitation: a multicenter randomized controlled trial is currently ongoing to evaluate the efficacy of a standardized, goal-oriented resuscitation protocol for use in patients with acute pancreatitis (TIGER study NCT00853515).

TABLE 156-3 Evidence-based Medicine Key References for Acute Pancreatitis

Study	Methodology	Results	Limitations	Bottom Line
Dellinger EP, et al. *Ann Surg.* 2007;245(5):674–683.	Double-blind randomized controlled trial; N = 100 patients with severe necrotizing pancreatitis: meropenem 1 g iv every 8 hours vs placebo	No reduction in either infected necrosis or mortality	Study did not address impact of reduction in extra-pancreatic infection	Prophylactic antibiotics no longer recommended for necrotizing pancreatitis
Nordback I, et al. *Gastroenterology.* 2009;136(3):848–855.	Open-label, randomized controlled trial; N = 120 patients with initial episode of alcohol-induced pancreatitis: single alcohol counseling session vs repeated 6 month intervention	Reduction in recurrence of acute pancreatitis (9 vs 20; $P = 0.02$) among intervention arm	Significant loss to follow-up in both arms (25% control arm, 35% treatment arm)	Repeated alcohol counseling likely has more impact on prevention than single intervention
van Santvoort HC, et al. *N Engl J Med.* 2010;362(16): 1491–1502.	Randomized-controlled trial; N = 88 patients with necrosis and suspected infection: open necrosectomy vs step-up approach with initial percutaneous drainage ± minimally invasive surgery	Reduction in composite clinical outcome of major complications in step-up approach (40% vs 69%; $P = 0.006$)	One-third of patients in step-up approach responded to catheter alone	Open necrosectomy should be reserved for patients who do not respond to minimally invasive techniques for management of suspected or confirmed infected necrosis
Marik PE, Zaloga GP. *BMJ.* 2004;328(7453):1407.	Meta-analysis of trials evaluating enteral vs parenteral nutrition	Pooled analysis determined that enteral nutrition was associated with reduced infectious complications compared to parenteral route	Unable to address optimal timing of nutrition or route of enteral nutrition	Enteral nutrition is preferred over parenteral route for management of patients with severe pancreatitis

2. Optimization of pain management: more data is needed to help determine an optimal approach to analgesia in patients with acute pancreatitis.
3. Prevention of hospital-acquired infection: recent data has identified a high rate of extra-pancreatic infections that substantially impact patient outcomes. Strategies to prevent development hospital-acquired infection should be a major target for future research.
4. Cost-effective management and resource utilization: recent efforts have been directed at enhancing risk-assessment strategies in acute pancreatitis in order to better direct resources. The question of whether some patients may benefit from a brief stay in an observation unit setting rather than hospitalization is currently being investigated.
5. Transitions of care: we are studying the impact of a streamlined process of care for inpatients hospitalized for acute pancreatitis to ensure early follow-up in our Center for Pancreatic Disease at Brigham and Women's Hospital.
6. Quality metrics still need to be evaluated. Candidate measures include rates of inhospital mortality, nosocomial infection, as well as implementation of appropriate timing of cholecystectomy.

SUGGESTED READINGS

Badalov N, Baradarian R, Iswara K, et al. Drug-induced acute pancreatitis: an evidence-based review. *Clin Gastroenterol Hepatol.* 2007;5(6):648–661; quiz 4.

Banks PA, Freeman ML. Practice guidelines in acute pancreatitis. *Am J Gastroenterol.* 2006;101(10):2379–2400.

Dellinger EP, Tellado JM, Soto NE, et al. Early antibiotic treatment for severe acute necrotizing pancreatitis: a randomized, double-blind, placebo-controlled study. *Ann Surg.* 2007;245(5): 674–683.

Forsmark CE, Baillie J. AGA Institute technical review on acute pancreatitis. *Gastroenterology.* 2007;132(5):2022–2044.

Gaisano HY, Gorelick FS. New insights into the mechanisms of pancreatitis. *Gastroenterology.* 2009;136(7):2040–2044.

Nordback I, Pelli H, Lappalainen-Lehto R, et al. The recurrence of acute alcohol-associated pancreatitis can be reduced: a randomized controlled trial. *Gastroenterology.* 2009;136(3): 848–855.

van Santvoort HC, Besselink MG, Bakker OJ, et al. Dutch Pancreatitis Study Group. A step up approach or open necrosectomy for necrotizing pancreatitis. *N Engl J Med.* 2010;362(16): 1491–1502.

Wu BU, Conwell DL. Acute pancreatitis part I: approach to early management. *Clin Gastroenterol Hepatol.* 2010;8(5):410–416, quiz e56–e58.

Wu BU, Conwell DL. Acute pancreatitis part II: approach to follow-up. *Clin Gastroenterol Hepatol.* 2010;8(5):417–422.

Wu BU, Johannes RS, Sun X, et al. The early prediction of mortality in acute pancreatitis: a large population-based study. *Gut.* 2008;57(12):1698–1703.

CHAPTER 157

Biliary Disease: Jaundice, Obstruction, and Acute Cholangitis

John Baillie, MB, ChB, FRCP(Glasg.), FACG, FASGE

Key Clinical Questions

1. What causes jaundice?
2. How are biliary obstruction and cholangitis diagnosed?
3. What are the best imaging modalities?
4. What treatment strategies should be employed in patients with biliary obstruction or cholangitis?
5. When should procedure or surgical intervention be considered in patients with cholangitis?

INTRODUCTION: JAUNDICE

This chapter describes clinical conditions manifested as a result of acute or subacute biliary disease. Particular focus is on conditions that frequently present to the inpatient setting, including jaundice, which is frequently a symptom of biliary or liver disease, as well as acute obstruction or infection within the biliary tract.

Jaundice is a yellowish discoloration of the skin, the conjunctivae, and other mucous membranes caused by hyperbilirubinemia (**Figure 157-1**). Generally, the serum bilirubin level needs to exceed 2.5 to 3 times the upper limit of normal (0.5–1.0 mg/dL) before jaundice is apparent. Jaundice is typically recognized earliest under the tongue, followed by within the sclera (sclera icterus), prior to it manifesting in the skin. Jaundice usually results from a pathologic process that interferes with the normal metabolism and excretion of bilirubin (Figure 157-1). Physiologically, bilirubin is the product of the breakdown of the hemoglobin in senescent red blood cells. Splitting of the four pyrrole ring of heme produces biliverdin, which is then reduced to bilirubin. Water-insoluble bilirubin is transported from the spleen to the liver, where it is rendered more water soluble by conjugation to glucuronic acid. Conjugated bilirubin is excreted into bile and subsequently into the gut, where it is broken down by bacteria into urobilinogen, some of which is converted into stercobilinogen and excreted in the stool, and some of which is transported to the kidneys and excreted in the urine. The stools of patients with obstructive jaundice, who cannot excrete bilirubin into the gut, have pale stools and dark urine, the latter due to greater-than-normal urinary excretion of urobilinogen.

TYPES OF JAUNDICE

Prehepatic

Prehepatic jaundice results from any process that causes an increased rate of hemoglobin breakdown (hemolysis) (**Figure 157-2**). Congenital and acquired conditions cause hemolysis. Congenital conditions that lead to hemolysis include sickle cell syndrome, thalassemia, and spherocytosis; these conditions lead to increased breakdown of red blood cells and hemolysis. Infectious etiologies may lead to massive lysis of red cells, including the malaria parasite (*Plasmodium falciparum* causes blackwater fever). Iatrogenic causes of hemolysis due to various drugs can occur, and autoimmune hemolytic syndromes can also lead to prehepatic jaundice. More than 900 drugs, toxins, and herbs are known to cause liver injury, and more than 2000 deaths per year are attributed to this cause in the United States. The mechanisms of—and predispositions to—drug-related liver injury are complex. However, many of these reactions result in cholestasis, which is often reversible when the drug is withdrawn. Drugs frequently associated with cholestasis include anabolic steroids, oral contraceptives, chlorpromazine, ciprofloxacin, cimetedine, phenytoin, captopril, erythromycin, amoxicillin/clavulanic acid, and others.

Fractionation of the unconjugated and conjugated bilirubin in the serum of patients with hemolysis and other causes of prehepatic jaundice will typically show a predominance of unconjugated (indirect, or water-insoluble) bilirubin. Laboratory findings in hemolysis include a decreased serum haptoglobin level and an elevated peripheral blood reticulocyte count.

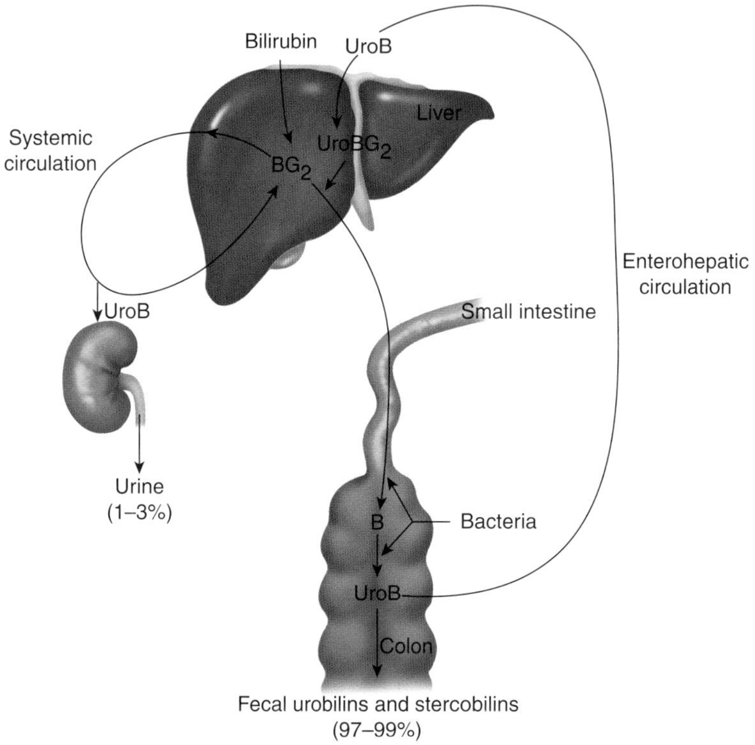

Figure 157-1 *Cycling of bilirubin and its products through the liver, intestines, portal and systemic circulations, and kidneys. (B, bilirubin; G, glucuronide; UroB, urobilinogen).*

Hepatic

Intrahepatic mechanisms of jaundice include liver cell (hepatocyte) swelling or death (necrosis), and may be caused by viral hepatitis, alcoholic hepatitis, drug or chemical toxicities, or autoimmune disease. Congenital abnormalities of bilirubin metabolism, such as unconjugated (indirect) hyperbilirubinemia seen in Gilbert disease, can occasionally cause sufficient elevation of serum bilirubin for an individual to develop clinical jaundice. Replacement of normal liver parenchyma by malignancy (primary or metastatic) can cause jaundice by compressing normal adjacent tissue and compressing bile canaliculi.

Prehepatic:
- **Any cause of increase hemoglobin breakdown** (congenital and acquired forms of hemolysis)

Hepatic:
- **Congenital abnormalities of hemoglobin** metabolism (eg, Gilbert disease), conditions causing liver cell (hepatocyte) swelling or death (eg, chemical (toxic), viral, autoimmune), replacement of normal tissue by tumor/space-occupying lesions

Posthepatic:
- **Mechanical obstruction to bile flow,** including biliary stones and strictures (benign and malignant), biliary parasites, biliary varices, chronic pancreatitis (incl autoimmune), inflammatory pseudotumor

Figure 157-2 *Causes of jaundice.*

Posthepatic

Mechanical obstruction to bile flow will cause jaundice. Common causes are bile duct stones (choledocholithiasis) and cancers involving the head of the pancreas. Rare causes include benign biliary strictures (eg, postsurgical, those associated with chronic pancreatitis, primary sclerosing cholangitis), pancreatic pseudocysts, bile duct parasites, biliary varices, and inflammatory pseudotumor.

INTRODUCTION: BILIARY OBSTRUCTION AND ACUTE CHOLANGITIS

Acute cholangitis describes infection of the bile, typically by gram-negative bacteria (eg, *Escherichia coli*, *Enterococcus*, *Serratia*, *Pseudomonas*). The presenting symptoms of pain, jaundice and fever constitute Charcot triad, and are indicative of acute bile infection. When the biliovenous pressure exceeds about 40 mm Hg, bacteria can migrate into the bloodsteam. The addition of hypotension and confusion to Charcot triad suggests sepsis, and the combination of five symptoms makes up the Pentad of Reynolds. Unrelieved, acute cholangitis carries close to 100% mortality. Even when the biliary tree is decompressed, acute cholangitis carries a mortality of around 5%.

DIFFERENTIAL DIAGNOSIS

In developed countries, the common causes of acute cholangitis include bile duct stones, benign biliary strictures (eg, postsurgical, chronic pancreatitis, primary sclerosing cholangitis and obstructed biliary stents and drains (catheters) (**Figure 157-3**). Malignant biliary strictures rarely present with acute cholangitis, but unrelieved, the chronic biliary obstruction of biliary and pancreatic cancers can lead to biliary sepsis and liver abscesses. In tropical climates, biliary parasites (eg, *Clonorchis sinesis*, *Fasciola hepatica*) can cause biliary obstruction and cholangitis.

Benign biliary obstruction:

- Choledocholithiasis (bile duct stones)
- Mirizzi syndrome
- Strictures (postsurgical, those associated with chronic pancreatitis, primary sclerosing cholangitis
- Biliary parasites (eg, Clonorchis senensis, Fasciola hepatica)
- Occluded biliary stent or drain

Malignant biliary obstruction:

- Pancreatic, bile duct (cholangiocarcinoma)
- Gallbladder, hepatoma, metastatic, lymphoma

Figure 157-3 *Causes of acute cholangitis.*

PRESENTATION AND DIAGNOSIS

Physical findings

Fever, diaphoresis, and tachycardia commonly occur in acute cholangitis, but may be absent in elderly patients. Patients with acute cholangitis typically complain of abdominal pain, which may be localized to the right upper abdomen or more diffuse. Surgical signs, such as abdominal rigidity and rebound tenderness, are absent, unless there is concurrent acute cholecystitis. Jaundice is almost always present, most obvious in the sclerae of the eyes or sublingually. Patients should not exhibit stigmata of chronic liver disease—spider nevi, palmar erythema, finger clubbing, parotid enlargement—unless the patient also has chronic liver disease. The liver and spleen should not be enlarged, and no mass should be present, unless the gallbladder is acutely distended in mechanical obstruction (rare in benign disease, but is the cause of *Courvoiser sign* in malignant obstructive jaundice). With cholangitis and sepsis, patients may become confused.

Laboratory findings

Appropriate blood tests on presentation include a complete blood count, a comprehensive metabolic panel (including a liver panel), basic coagulation studies, and arterial blood gas estimation. Aerobic and anaerobic blood cultures should be drawn before the institution of antibiotics, and treatment modified as necessary when results are available. Most cases of acute cholangitis are caused by gram-negative bacteria. The bile is normally sterile. In the presence of gallbladder or common duct stones, however, the incidence of bactibilia increases. The most common organisms isolated in bile are *E coli* (27%), *Klebsiella* species (16%), *Enterococcus* species (15%), *Streptococcus* species (8%), *Enterobacter* species (7%), and *Pseudomonas aeruginosa* (7%). Organisms isolated from blood cultures are similar to those found in bile. The most common pathogens isolated in blood cultures are *E coli* (59%), *Klebsiella* species (16%), *Pseudomonas aeruginosa* (5%), and *Enterococcus* species (4%). In addition, polymicrobial infection is commonly found in bile cultures (30–87%) and less frequent in blood cultures (6–16%).

Imaging

Abdominal ultrasound may show dilatation of the biliary tree (normal diameter ≤ 8 mm), with or without the presence of stones in patients with choledocholithiasis. Abdominal ultrasound also provides useful information about the gallbladder (stones, acute cholecystitis) Similar information is available from cross-sectional imaging (computed tomography [CT], magnetic resonance imaging [MRI]). Endoscopic ultrasound (EUS) may now serve as the gold standard for diagnosing gallbladder and bile duct stones. MRI focusing on the biliary tree and pancreas is called magnetic resonance cholangiopancreatography (MRCP), and provides outstanding views of fluid-containing organs and ducts. Cholangiography performed during endoscopic retrograde cholangiopancreatography (ERCP) will confirm the presence of biliary obstruction from choledocholithiasis and benign and malignant strictures. Percutaneous transhepatic cholangiography is also diagnostic and therapeutic in biliary obstruction.

MANAGEMENT

Initial hospital treatment

Acute cholangitis requires rapid relief of biliary obstruction by endoscopic, radiologic, or surgical intervention. Patients who present with signs and symptoms of acute cholangitis should have liver and biliary ultrasound and basic blood work (complete blood count, comprehensive metabolic panel, blood cultures) performed without delay to support the diagnosis. If the patient is clinically stable, it is acceptable to wait 6 to 12 hours to observe the effect of intravenous fluids and broad spectrum antibiotics. If the patient's clinical condition suggests severe sepsis, and especially if it cannot be stabilized with the above interventions, urgent ERCP for biliary decompression is indicated. If possible the patient should be managed in an intensive care setting. General anesthesia may be necessary during ERCP to ensure that vital functions, such as oxygenation and maintenance of blood pressure, can be continuously monitored and corrected where necessary. Acute cholangitis should be regarded as a medical emergency and treated aggressively.

ERCP can access the biliary tree in the least invasive manner. Biliary stones can be removed after endoscopic sphincterotomy, with or without balloon dilation (**Figure 157-4**). When large stones cannot be removed, a plastic biliary endoprosthesis (stent) or nasobiliary drain should be placed across the obstruction to ensure bile flow. Placing a nasobiliary drain is more demanding than stenting, but allows monitoring of the output, flushing of the tube, and a way

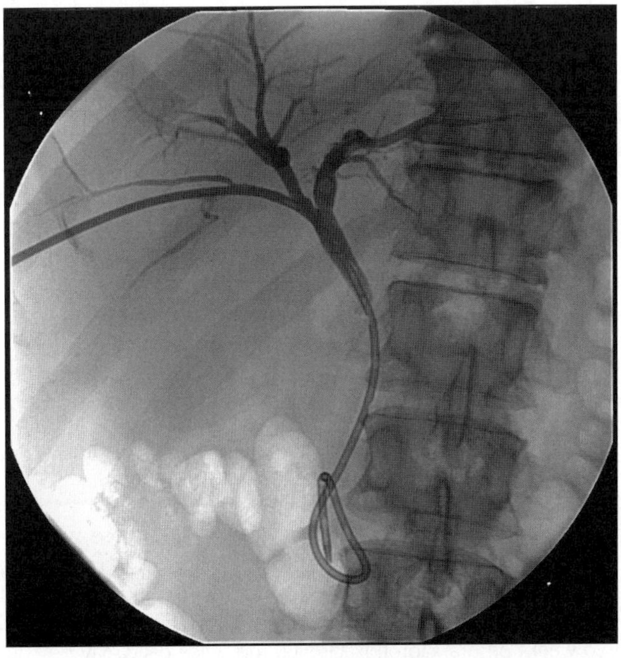

Figure 157-4 *Internal-external percutaneous biliary drain for managing a biliary stricture.*

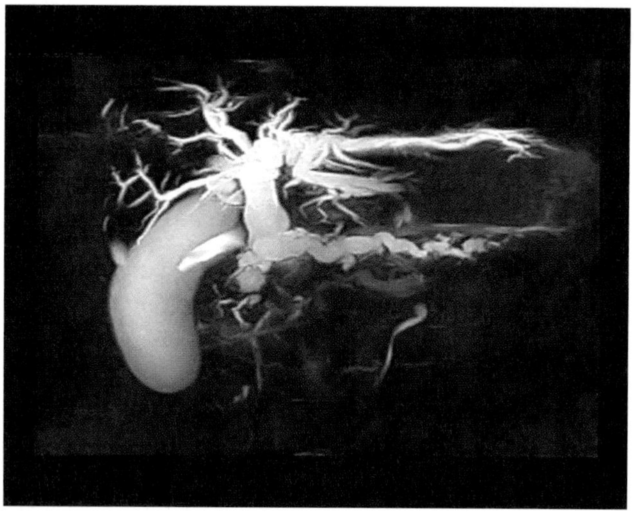

Figure 157-5 *Dilated gallbladder, bile ducts, and pancreatic duct in pancreatic head cancer.*

to obtain a subsequent cholangiogram. If ERCP fails or is inadequate to reestablish bile drainage, percutaneous transhepatic cholangiography, a more invasive procedure, can allow external access. Once access to the biliary tree has been obtained, a percutaneous drain can be inserted for decompression. If the obstruction can be traversed, an internal-external drain is placed, with the distal end left in the duodenum (though the duodenal papilla) (**Figure 157-5**). The drain is usually held in position at the skin access site by a suture. Initially, the bile is allowed to drain externally into a bag. After the sepsis has resolved, the drain is internalized (capped off at skin level), so that the bile has to track into duodenum through the catheter. To maintain patency, the internalized drain is typically flushed with sterile water two or three times a day. It is unusual for surgery to be performed to manage cholangitis alone. In the setting of acute cholecystitis with acute cholangitis, open cholecystectomy with common bile duct exploration may be performed, with the placement of a T-tube for biliary drainage. However, most surgeons prefer to have preoperative biliary decompression by ERCP when obstruction and sepsis is present. If acute cholecystitis is identified complicating acute cholangitis, the placement of a cholecystostomy tube under radiologic guidance is a useful temporizing maneuver until resolution of the infectious cholangitis. Elective cholecystectomy may then be considered.

Medical management in acute cholangitis includes fluid resuscitation, correction of electrolyte abnormalities, correction of infection-related complications (eg, disseminated intravascular coagulation), and administration of broad-spectrum antibiotics (see below). Patients with severe sepsis or shock should be managed in an intensive care setting, with aggressive diagnostic and therapeutic measures—central venous catheterization, urine output strict measurement, volume resuscitation, and pressor agents when needed—applied similar to any patient who presents with critical illness due to infection.

Longitudinal and outpatient therapeutics

Patients with recurrent cholangitis—for example those with primary sclerosing cholangitis or recurrent choledocholithiasis—may benefit from cycling oral antibiotics. No standard guidelines exist for antibiotic regimens to maintain bile sterility. One week on and two weeks off oral ciprofloxacin 500 mg twice daily may be considered. Metronidazole may be added for anerobic coverage, although many patients find this drug causes nausea and metallic taste in mouth; and patients taking metronidazole must abstain from alcohol during treatment. Length of cyclical therapy does not have supporting studies to guide practice. A trial of three to six months may be reasonable before a trial off of cycling antibiotics, and clinicians should monitor and record episodes of recurrence while on and off preventive antimicrobial therapy. Episodes of cholangitis while on oral antibiotic therapy suggests unrelieved biliary obstruction or antibiotic resistance, or both. Antibiotics should be changed if concern for resistance or recurrence while on prophylactic therapy.

COMPLICATIONS AND PROGNOSIS

Unrelieved acute cholangitis is associated with mortality approaching 100%. Since the introduction of antibiotics effective against gram-negative bacteria and nonsurgical means of decompressing the biliary tree (ERCP and percutaneous drainage), the mortality has decreased dramatically to approximately 5%. Severely ill patients with cholangitis who have major comorbidities may not survive, even if effective biliary drainage can be reestablished. Biliary sepsis should be regarded as a medical emergency and managed with appropriate urgency. Unrelieved chronic biliary obstruction is often associated with a low-grade cholangitis, typically seen in the setting of chronic strictures of the biliary tree. Eventually, the part of the liver affected by the obstruction may undergo atrophy or develop secondary biliary cirrhosis. Chronic obstruction may also lead to the development of multiple abscesses within the liver.

Cholangitis due to an unusual organism (eg, *Serratia*, *Pseudomonas*) seen after ERCP may indicate iatrogenic infection introduced by the endoscopic procedure. If many patients within one center develop the same type of post-ERCP biliary or pancreatic infection, iatrogenic etiology should be considered and sought. Modern disinfection regimens for endoscopes, which employ automated washing machines, have largely eliminated endoscope-transmitted infection, but sporadic cases still occur. Such outbreaks of endoscope-associated infection should be aggressively investigated with assistance from the hospital epidemiologist and suspect endoscopes and washing machines taken out of service.

DISCHARGE PLANNING

Discharging clinicians should assure adequate biliary drainage for patients leaving the hospital. Patients who have undrained or inadequately drained bile ducts are likely to return to hospital with recurrent cholangitis, even if taking appropriate antibiotics. Sometimes the most effective form of biliary drainage is external; elderly patients with complex malignant hilar strictures may need an internal-external biliary drainage to manage their jaundice and itching. Biliary drains need to be flushed with sterile water several times a day. Discharging physicians should arrange for home health nursing to assist with drains and train patients in their management until outpatient follow-up.

When nonsurgical interventions have failed, surgical intervention may ameliorate recurrent cholangitis. For example, when patients with postsurgical strictures fail endoscopic or percutaneous stenting, as evidenced by progressive liver damage and/or recurrent attacks of acute cholangitis, surgical bypass (eg, choledocho-jejunostomy) can alleviate recurrent episodes and worsening organ dysfunction. In a small subset of patients with primary sclerosing cholangitis, liver transplantation may be necessary to manage progressive deterioration due to recurrent cholangitis, culminating in liver failure. Patients who have chronic biliary sepsis are generally considered unsuitable for liver transplantation; therefore, aggressive management of acute cholangitis episodes is paramount.

QUALITY IMPROVEMENT TO ADDRESS PERFORMANCE GAPS

TRANSITIONS OF CARE

Patients with recurrent cholangitis should be referred to and followed by a physician who understands the natural history of the disorder—a gastroenterologist or a surgeon with interest and expertise in the management of hepatobiliary disorders. Patients who may need surgery in the future should be jointly managed by a gastroenterologist and a surgeon. Patients with chronic liver disease related to biliary obstruction and cholangitis should also be followed by a transplant hepatologist who can coordinate evaluation and listing for liver transplantation when indicated. Physicians managing patients on cyclical antibiotics often should consult infectious disease colleagues who can advise on the choice of antibacterial agents and their rotation, if needed. Patients at risk for recurrent cholangitis who do not receive long-term antibiotics (cyclical or otherwise) should be provided with a standing prescriptions for antibiotics, which they can start at the first sign of infection.

DISPARITIES IN HEALTH CARE

Patients who lack medical insurance frequently delay seeking care for their cholangitis, potentially with fatal results. Indigent patients with comorbidities, such as chronic viral hepatitis or human immunodeficiency virus have particular risk for overwhelming sepsis when they develop cholangitis. The underinsured and uninsured typically lack outpatient health care providers in the community, and rely on emergency department care when they become seriously ill. Such patients should be identified when they present to health care facilities, so that social services and related resources can be applied to find longitudinal care by appropriate physicians and other care providers. Health care reform may benefit these patients such that they may receive timely and necessary experienced care in the outpatient setting, thus preventing recurrent episodes and hospitalization.

OUTCOMES TO MONITOR

Patients with acute cholangitis do not always present with the classical Charcot triad of pain, jaundice, and fever. Their symptoms may be quite subtle, such as vague abdominal pain with or without shaking chills or a flu-like illness. This is especially true for patients whose cholangitis is chronic, and modified by intermittent courses of antibacterial agents. In some patients, the only symptom signaling biliary obstruction or cholangitis may be pruritus. Patients at risk for recurrent attacks of cholangitis should be educated to recognize the early clinical signs, and encouraged to seek medical care. Cholangitis may be asymptomatic, and lead insidiously to chronic liver disease, including secondary biliary cirrhosis. One clue to asymptomatic cholangitis includes progressive worsening liver alkaline phosphatase. When liver disease is established, decompensation accompanying biliary sepsis may present as confusion due to hepatic encephalopathy. Other complications of cirrhosis, especially bleeding from esophageal varices, may supervene. Regular clinic review and monitoring liver tests can identify those patients who have inadequate biliary drainage predisposing to recurrent cholangitis and risk of chronic liver disease.

COSTS AND RESOURCE UTILIZATION

Early, aggressive management of acute cholangitis will help avoid costly complications, and reduce overall mortality. Tertiary care center referral for acute cholangitis is indicated if a community hospital is not equipped to perform ERCP or other necessary testing and interventions. Late transfer of a very ill patient to a specialist or referral center likely worsens morbidity and mortality. Timely recognition and referral to a specialist center should be considered in a community setting that is not equipped to care for this condition.

CONCLUSION

The management of jaundice requires integration of bilirubin metabolism physiology with the pathologic processes that may interfere with this complex metabolic process (prehepatic, hepatic and post-hepatic mechanisms). Mechanical biliary obstruction may be benign (eg. bile duct stones) or malignant. Unrelieved biliary obstruction often leads to infection (acute cholangitis), which is potentially fatal. Early recognition of acute cholangitis and the prompt re-establishment of free biliary flow, usually by therapeutic endoscopic retrograde cholangiopancreatography (ERCP), is the key to successful management. As elderly and immunosuppressed patients often fail to exhibit the classic signs and symptoms of acute cholangitis (ie. Charcot's Triad), a high index of suspicion is necessary to make the diagnosis.

SUGGESTED READINGS

Abdallah AA, Krige JE, Bornman PC. Biliary tract obstruction in chronic pancreatitis. *HPB (Oxf)*. 2007;9(6):421–428.

Attasaranya S, Fogel EL, Lehman GA. Choledocholithiasis, ascending cholangitis, and gallstone pancreatitis. *Med Clin North Am*. 2008;92(4):925–960.

Catalano OA, Sahani DV, Forcione DG, et al. Biliary infections: spectrum of imaging findings and management. *Radiographics*. 2000;29(7):2059–2080.

Lee JG. Diagnosis and management of acute cholangitis. *Nat Rev Gastroenterol Hepatol*. 2009;6(9):533–541.

Leung JW, Yu AS. Hepatolithiasis and biliary parasites. *Baillieres Clin Gastroenterol*. 1997;11(4):681–706.

Rösch T, Meining A, Frühmorgen S, et al. A prospective comparison of the diagnostic accuracy of ERCP, MRCP, CT, and EUS in biliary strictures. *Gastrointest Endosc*. 2002;55(7):870–876.

Rosing DK, De Virgilio C, Nguyen AT, et al. Cholangitis: analysis of admission prognostic indicators and outcomes. *Am Surg*. 2007;73(10):949–954.

Scheiman JM, Carlos RC, Barnett JL, et al. Can endoscopic ultrasound or magnetic resonance cholangiopancreatography replace ERCP in patients with suspected biliary disease? A prospective trial and cost analysis. *Am J Gastroenterol*. 2001;96:2900–2904.

Sharma BC, Kumar R, Agarwal N, Sarin SK. Endoscopic biliary drainage by nasobiliary drain or by stent placement in patients with acute cholangitis. *Endoscopy*. 2005;37(5):439–443.

van Erpecum K. Gallstone disease. Complications of bile-duct stones: Acute cholangitis and pancreatitis. *Best Pract Res Clin Gastroenterol*. 2006;20(6):1139–1152.

CHAPTER 158

Acute Liver Disease

Ryan M. Ford, MD
Ram M. Subramanian, MD
James R. Spivey, MD

Key Clinical Questions

1. How is acute liver failure (ALF) defined and diagnosed, and how does it differ from acutely decompensated cirrhosis?
2. Which causes of decompensated chronic liver failure can also be classified as "acute" failure with respect to transplant candidacy?
3. How should clinicians acutely evaluate, triage, and manage ALF patients, including initial diagnostic testing follow-up testing?
4. What clinical and laboratory parameters should be frequently monitored?
5. What complications of ALF lead to high mortality, and how are they managed?
6. How is intracranial hypertension and cerebral edema managed medically?
7. What prognostic measures best identify ALF patients who will require liver transplant in order to survive?
8. What evidence-based interventions improve outcomes in patients with acute liver failure? Are they etiology specific?

INTRODUCTION

DEFINITION

Acute liver failure (ALF) is a rare clinical syndrome that is defined by coagulopathy and encephalopathy that occurs over a span of less than 6 months in a patient without preexisting liver disease. Based on the time to encephalopathy from the onset of jaundice, three types of ALF have been described: hyperacute (0–7 days), acute (8–28 days), and subacute (29 days–12 weeks).

Patients with subacute liver failure often pose a clinical challenge, as they may show signs suggesting chronic liver disease, such as ascites or prolonged encephalopathy. Also, patients with subacute liver failure (eg, drug induced) may follow a variable and unpredictable course, often leading to heightened anxiety for the patient, family, and medical providers.

As an exception to the definition of ALF, patients with Wilson disease, reactivation/superinfection of chronic hepatitis B, or autoimmune hepatitis may be considered to have ALF despite the presence of underlying chronic liver disease.

EPIDEMIOLOGY

Approximately 2000 cases of ALF occur each year in the United States. ALF can affect people of all ages and is associated with high morbidity and mortality. Multiorgan failure (MOF) is the most common cause of death (>50% of cases), with infection and intracranial hypertension responsible for most of the remaining deaths. With recent improvements in care, spontaneous recovery and overall survival now exceed 40% and 65%, respectively. Over the past 25 years in the United States, overall mortality from ALF has decreased from more than 80% to 33%.

PATHOPHYSIOLOGY

ALF involves massive hepatocellular necrosis and liver dysfunction. A resulting cytokine storm leads to oxidative stress and a systemic inflammatory response syndrome. HIV medications, Wilson disease, and acute fatty liver of pregnancy may uniquely cause severe mitochondrial dysfunction with resulting lactic acidosis. Ultimately, multiorgan dysfunction occurs.

Intracranial hypertension (ICH) and cerebral edema may result from both elevated ammonia levels, which causes direct astrocyte toxicity, and loss of cerebral blood flow autoregulation. Loss of cerebral autoregulation in ALF leads to ICH, and intracranial contents are rapidly damaged by both hydrostatic and osmolar shifts. Noncardiogenic pulmonary edema (acute respiratory distress syndrome, ARDS) and renal failure may result from cytokine-induced damage and hemodynamic derangements. Cardiovascular collapse can be seen with a severe depression of systemic vascular resistance, another process that is driven by cytokines and derangements in vasoactive substances. Loss of the normal synthetic function of the liver also leads to both a coagulopathy and prothrombotic state. Metabolism of medications and other physiologic mechanisms, such as biliary excretion, are also disrupted in the setting of ALF.

Acute liver failure *differs* from acute on chronic liver failure. Although there are some examples of overlap (eg, Wilson disease, autoimmune hepatitis, acute on chronic hepatitis B), the pathophysiology of the two clinical syndromes differ with respect to physiologic adaptation. For instance, patients with ALF are at risk for elevated intracranial pressure (ICP) because neuronal adaptation does not have time to occur as the ammonia levels rapidly rise.

DIFFERENTIAL DIAGNOSIS

In the setting of possible ALF, clinicians must exclude chronic liver disease. Only a few chronic hepatic conditions may present with true ALF: (1) Wilson disease, (2) autoimmune hepatitis, and (3) acute on chronic viral hepatitis B.

A nodular appearing liver on imaging studies can be misleading, as an irregular contour may represent regenerative nodules interspersed with areas of acute injury and necrosis. Similar to acute alcoholic hepatitis, acute portal hypertension and ascites may also be seen with ALF. Finally, sepsis with disseminated intravascular coagulation in a patient who has cirrhosis can also mimic ALF, as such a patient can present with altered mental status, coagulopathy, and jaundice.

CAUSES OF ALF

In the United States, acetaminophen toxicity is the number one cause of ALF (39%). Approximately 20% to 25% of these patients undergo orthotopic liver transplantation. Whereas most cases of acetaminophen-induced ALF involve ingestions exceeding 10 g/day, severe liver injury can occur with doses as low as 3to 4 g/day, as is seen with therapeutic misadventure. Therapeutic misadventure, referring to therapeutic doses of acetaminophen in the setting of alcohol, malnutrition, or cytochrome p450-inducing medications, occurs in nearly half of acetaminophen toxicity cases (**Table 158-1**).

In addition to acetaminophen, multiple other causes can lead to ALF, and in the United States approximately 20% of ALF cases have no discernible cause (**Table 158-2**). Non-acetaminophen drug or toxin-induced liver injury accounts for 13% of cases (**Table 158-3**). Toxins may include *Amanita phalloides* (mushrooms), sea anemone sting, or carbon tetrachloride. Acute hepatitis A and B account for 4% and 7% of ALF cases, respectively. The remainder of cases may be due to other viruses (herpes simplex virus [HSV], Epstein-Barr virus [EBV], cytomegalovirus [CMV]), Wilson disease, Budd-Chiari syndrome, sinusoidal obstruction syndrome, acute fatty liver of pregnancy, autoimmune hepatitis, malignant infiltration, or ischemia.

DIAGNOSIS

PRESENTATION

A patient can present at any point along the disease severity spectrum. Multiorgan failure may rapidly ensue and manifest with abrupt clinical decompensation. Some patients, such as those who recently ingested an acetaminophen overdose, or those with subacute liver failure, may initially present asymptomatically, despite having markedly abnormal blood work. Nonspecific symptoms may include nausea, vomiting, abdominal pain, fever, malaise, fatigue, arthralgias, itching, bleeding, headache, and diarrhea. Nonspecific clinical signs may include abdominal pain, altered mental status, jaundice, or ascites.

HISTORY

A detailed history, including a careful review of possible exposure to viruses, drugs, or toxins, may help uncover a possible cause of liver failure. Clinicians must question about over the counter medications, alternative therapies, herbs, and supplements (Table 158-3). If the patient is encephalopathic, a collateral history from friends or family is important, as identifying a cause can be paramount in the management of ALF.

Acetaminophen toxicity may involve intentional overdose or may involve high doses over an extended period of time. For example, a patient who takes over the counter acetaminophen in addition to prescribed acetaminophen-containing pain medications may exceed a critical daily dose that leads to severe liver injury. Alcoholics and malnourished patients are at greater risk for acetaminophen-induced liver injury.

TABLE 158-1 Cytochrome P450–inducing Medications

Cytochrome P450 Inducers
Ethanol
Isoniazid
Rifampin or rifabutin
Phenobarbital
Glucocorticoids
Phenytoin
Pioglitazone
Omeprazole
Insulin
Carbamazepine
Nafcillin
HIV antiretrovirals (efavirenz, nevirapine)
St John's wort

TABLE 158-2 Causes of Acute Liver Failure

Category	Examples
Drug induced	See Table 158-3
Acute viral	Hepatitis A
	Hepatitis B
	Hepatitis D (superimposed on Hepatitis B)
	Hepatitis E
	Hepatitis C
	Herpes simplex virus
	Varicella zoster virus
	Cytomegalovirus
	Epstein-Barr virus
Indeterminate	
Toxin exposure	*Amanita phalloides* (mushrooms)
	Organic solvents
	Herbal medicines
	Bacterial toxins (eg, *Bacillus cereus*)
	Sea anemone sting
	Carbon tetrachloride
Wilson disease	
Pregnancy related	Acute fatty liver of pregnancy
	HELLP syndrome
Autoimmune hepatitis	
Malignancy	Lymphoma
	Diffuse metastatic disease
Hepatic ischemia	Shock
	Acute arterial thrombosis/injury
Vascular	Acute Budd-Chiari syndrome (hepatic vein thrombosis)
Heat stroke	
Postextensive hepatic resection	

HELLP, hemolytic anemia, elevated liver enzymes, and low platelet counts.

TABLE 158-3 Drug-induced Hepatotoxicity

Category	Drug Name
Prescription medications	
Antimicrobials	Ampicillin-clavulanate
	Trimethoprim-sulfamethoxazole
	Fluoroquinolones
	Macrolides
	Nitrofurantoin
	Tetracycline
	"-azole" antifungals (eg, fluconazole, voriconizole, etc)
	Isoniazid
	HIV antiretroviral drugs
Anticonvulsants	Valproic acid
	Phenytoin
	Carbamazepine
Lipid-lowering drugs	Statins
	Niacin
Anti-hypertensive drugs	Antiotensin-converting enzyme inhibitors
	Methyldopa
	Metformin
Diabetic drugs	Thioglitazones (eg, pioglitozone, rosiglitazone)
	Tricyclic antidepressants
Antidepressants	Tamoxifen
Hormonal therapy	
Chemotherapy agents	Propylthiouracil
Other	Amiodarone
	Allopurinol
Over-the-counter medications	
	Acetaminophen
	Nonsteroidal anti-inflammatory drugs
	Niacin
Recreational drugs	
	Cocaine
	MDMA (ecstasy)
	Methamphetamines

Most idiosyncratic drug-induced liver injuries are not dose-related and tend to occur within the first 6 months of drug initiation (Table 158-3).

PRACTICE POINT

- Most idiosyncratic **drug-induced liver injuries** are not dose related and tend to occur within the first 6 months of drug initiation.
- Mechanisms of injury include hepatocellular necrosis, cholestasis, a mixed pattern, steatosis, autoimmune, hypersensitivity, phospholipidosis, mitochondrial toxicity, and sinusoidal obstruction syndrome.
- If suspected, immediate withdrawal of the offending agent is paramount.
- If autoimmune or hypersensitivity is suspected, steroids may be beneficial.

A history of IV drug abuse may indicate risk for infections such as acute hepatitis B and D. Travel to endemic regions (eg, Russia, Pakistan, India, Mexico) may place a patient at risk for acute hepatitis E infection. Immunosuppressed patients and women in their 3rd trimester of pregnancy are at increased risk for herpes simplex infection. A history of preeclampsia in a pregnant woman increases the risk of acute fatty liver of pregnancy, which also occurs in the 3rd trimester. Previous or coexisting autoimmune diseases (thyroiditis, insulin dependent diabetes, lupus, vitiligo, etc) may indicate an increased risk for autoimmune hepatitis. Cardiac disease (congestive heart failure, myocardial infarction, arrhythmia) or hemodynamic instability may lead to "shock liver" from hypoperfusion. Documented hypotension is not always found with ischemic liver injury. A history of malignancy or hypercoagulable state may raise concern for malignant infiltration or Budd-Chiari syndrome (hepatic vein thrombosis), which often presents with acute abdominal pain, ascites, and striking hepatomegaly. Finally, a history of chemotherapy may place a patient at risk for sinusoidal obstruction syndrome, formerly known as veno-occlusive disease, which can present in a similar manner as Budd-Chiari syndrome (**Table 158-4**).

PHYSICAL EXAMINATION

With ALF, the most important step in the physical examination is assessing mental status and performing frequent neurological examinations. Clinicians must also examine closely for any signs of chronic liver disease including spider angiomata, telangiectasias, Terry nails (fingernails and/or toenail appear white with a characteristic "ground glass" appearance, with no lunula), palmar erythema, asterixis, splenomegaly, caput medusa, collateral venous patterns, and gynecomastia. Whereas ascites and varices are classically seen with chronic liver disease, these signs of portal hypertension can be seen with acute liver disease as well (eg, alcoholic hepatitis, venous thrombosis, pre-sinusoidal portal hypertension).

In patients suspected of Wilson disease, a slit lamp examination of the eye should be performed to assess for the presence of Kayser-Fleischer rings. In patients with ICH from cerebral edema, Cushing triad—hypertension, bradycardia, irregular respirations—may or may not be present. Pupillary dilation or signs of decerebrate posturing typically occur late in the course of ALF and indicate a grave prognosis.

LABORATORY

When ordering laboratory testing for patients admitted with ALF, a standard protocol can facilitate a thorough evaluation, since the initial lab survey is often extensive. Even if a diagnosis seems clear, evaluating for concomitant diseases such as viral hepatitis or human immunodeficiency virus is important in a patient who may require a liver transplant. Frequent hepatic function testing often necessitates indwelling vascular access (central venous catheter or arterial catheter) for serial blood draws and other clinical management (**Table 158-5**). No consensus guidelines recommend specific laboratory testing in the setting of probable ALF; however, laboratory testing is necessary in anticipation of possible liver transplantation (Table 158-5).

Upon presentation, very high transaminase levels (AST and ALT levels > 1000 U/L) may limit the differential to a few possible etiologies: acute viral infection, acetaminophen-induced injury, shock liver, or autoimmune hepatitis. AST and ALT levels exceeding 3500 U/L are highly correlated with acetaminophen poisoning. Whereas transaminase levels may be helpful initially, they do not add much information once the diagnosis of ALF is established. Transaminase levels that appear to be normalizing may indicate an obliterated liver, especially if associated with hypoglycemia and an unabated rise in the international normalized ratio (INR). Alternatively,

TABLE 158-4 Historical Clues to ALF Etiology

Historical Clue	Potential Etiology
Witnessed or confessed overdose	Acetaminophen or other drug-induced liver injury
History of polysubstance abuse, including intravenous drug use	Drug-induced, toxin (eg, mushrooms), hepatitis B, hepatitis D, hepatitis C
Travel to Russia, Pakistan, India, Mexico, or other endemic regions	Hepatitis E
Immunosuppressed state	Herpes simplex virus, varicella zoster virus, cytomegalovirus
Third trimester of pregnancy	Acute fatty liver of pregnancy, HELLP syndrome, herpes simplex virus, or any other cause of ALF
History of autoimmune disease (eg, Hashimoto thyroiditis, type 1 diabetes mellitus, Addison disease, lupus, vitiligo)	Autoimmune hepatitis
Hemodynamic instability (heart failure, arrhythmia, myocardial infarction)	Shock liver
History of hypercoagulable state	Budd-Chiari syndrome, shock liver from arterial thrombosis, malignant infiltration
History of chemotherapy	Sinusoidal obstruction syndrome
History of chronic Hepatitis B	Acute hepatitis B flare, superinfection with hepatitis D
Northwestern United States	*Amanita phalloides* (mushroom toxicity)
History of malignancy	Diffuse hepatic metastases
Hemolytic anemia, renal failure, low-normal alkaline phosphatase, or low uric acid	Wilson disease

HELLP, hemolytic anemia, elevated liver enzymes, and low platelet counts.

normalizing liver enzymes may also indicate improving hepatic injury facilitated by removal of a toxic exposure, natural history of a virus, or a treatment response (eg, autoimmune hepatitis, herpes simplex, hepatitis B). A bilirubin level on presentation carries prognostic significance, especially with drug-induced liver injury (*Hy's law*, a prognostic indicator that suggests that drug-induced liver injury leading to jaundice, without hepatic transplantation, has a case fatality rate of 10–50%). Initial INR and creatinine also provide prognostic information.

IMAGING

Ordering a multitude of imaging tests that require patient transport and movement may present unnecessary risk for a critically ill patient with ALF. Nevertheless, imaging—when safe to perform—can provide diagnostic information to direct management. All patients with ALF should undergo an abdominal ultrasound with Doppler to assess for signs of chronic liver disease, and to assess the hepatic vasculature (hepatic veins, portal vein, hepatic artery). Computed tomography (CT) scan of the abdomen without contrast is preferred if the patient's body habitus (eg, obesity, ascites, bowel distension) precludes an adequate ultrasound examination. Avoidance of IV contrast is important since many patients with ALF are at risk for developing acute kidney injury. MRI of the abdomen with IV gadolinium is an alternative imaging modality that is center specific and depends on radiologic expertise.

PRACTICE POINT

- Clinicians should avoid use of iodinated IV contrast in patients presenting with ALF as many of these patients bear high risk for developing acute kidney injury.

In a patient with worsening mental status, a noncontrast brain CT will help evaluate for intracranial hemorrhage or cerebral edema. Cerebral edema, while prognostically ominous if seen on CT, may indicate the need for placement of an ICP monitor. In a patient with suspected brain damage, transcranial Doppler ultrasounds or continuous electroencephalograms (EEGs) may provide prognostic information. To assess heart function and valves, a transthoracic echocardiogram may be necessary, especially if a patient is a possible liver transplant candidate. Plain films, such as chest x-rays and abdominal radiographs, may also be ordered as clinically indicated but are generally performed at the patient bedside (portable machine) to avoid unnecessary patient transport.

LIVER BIOPSY

When specific diseases such as autoimmune hepatitis, Wilson disease, HSV hepatitis, or lymphoma are suspected, a liver biopsy may be useful in assisting with diagnosis. A liver biopsy may also help determine the extent of necrosis and regeneration in cases of subacute liver failure. *For the majority of ALF cases, a liver biopsy is not necessary and may even lead to complications such as hemorrhage or infection.* In cases of severe ALF, a biopsy will most likely show extensive necrosis and "ghosts" of hepatocytes.

TRIAGE AND HOSPITAL ADMISSION

Any patient with suspected ALF should be admitted to the hospital for a thorough evaluation and consideration for liver transplant. If a patient is being admitted to a hospital that is not a transplant center, early transfer to a transplant center should be considered, especially if both encephalopathy and coagulopathy are present. Rapid deterioration in clinical and biochemical status following an initial stable presentation can occur. Some centers may use prognostic models to determine who should be transferred. At the present time, there are no validated criteria that dictate when to transfer a patient. Prior to transfer, a detailed communication between the receiving and transferring facility should address the existing neurologic, cardiopulmonary, hepatic, hematologic, and renal status. Prior to transfer, it may be necessary to electively intubate a patient for airway protection, as advancing encephalopathy can occur unexpectedly during transit.

TABLE 158-5 Initial Comprehensive and Serial Laboratory Tests to Order for Patients with Acute Liver Failure*

Initial (Comprehensive)	Laboratory Tests to Consider Ordering Initially	Laboratory Tests to Monitor Serially
Complete blood count with differential	24-h urine copper level	Complete blood count with differential every 6–8 hours
Comprehensive metabolic profile	Coombs test	Comprehensive metabolic profile every 6–8 hours
Coagulation studies (INR/PT/PTT)	Peritoneal fluid analysis (if ascites is present)	Coagulation studies (INR/PT/PTT) every 6–8 hours
Arterial blood gas	Lactate dehydrogenase	Arterial blood gas every 6–8 hours
Arterial lactate	Haptoglobin	Coagulation factor levels (factor V, VII) once or twice a day
Acetaminophen level	Uric acid	Fibrinogen daily
Coagulation factor levels (factors V, VII, VIII)	Serum ferritin	Serum osmolarity every 6 hours (if patient is receiving IV mannitol therapy)
Urinalysis with microscopy	Arterial ammonia	
Urine drug screen for cocaine, amphetamines, opiates, barbiturates, benzodiazepines, and marijuana	Quantitative serum immunoglobulins	
Fibrinogen	EBV quantitative PCR	
Hepatitis B quantitative DNA	HIV viral load	
Hepatitis C quantitative RNA	D-dimers	
Hepatitis A IgM antibody	Blood cultures	
Hepatitis B surface antigen	Urine culture	
Hepatitis B core antibody (IgM and IgG)		
Hepatitis B surface antibody		
CMV IgG antibody		
CMV quantitative PCR		
EBV serologic panel		
HSV quantitative PCR		
HIV antibody		
Rapid plasma regain (RPR)		
Ceruloplasmin		
Alpha-1-antitrypsin level and phenotype		
Antinuclear antibody		
Antismooth muscle antibody		
Antimitochondrial antibody		
Serum osmolarity		

*Based on expert opinion of the authors; not based on any consensus guidelines.

PRACTICE POINT

- ALF patients admitted to a nontransplant center should be considered for early transfer to a transplant center, especially in patients with both encephalopathy and coagulopathy. Prior to transfer, it may be necessary to electively intubate a patient for airway protection, as advancing encephalopathy can occur unexpectedly in transit.

Patients that develop grade II, III, or IV encephalopathy should be managed in an ICU (**Table 158-6**). Patients with grade III or IV encephalopathy may require both intubation for airway protection and possible ICP monitoring. Even though a patient may appear stable, rapid changes in clinical status may occur and should be dealt with in an urgent manner. Frequent neurologic evaluation, serial laboratory testing, and 24-hour monitoring in an ICU

TABLE158-6 Grades of Encephalopathy

Grade	Clinical Picture
I	Mood instability
	Shortened attention span
	Insomnia
	Mild confusion
II	Lethargy
	Personality changes
	Moderate confusion/disorientation
III	Marked confusion
	Somnolence
	Incoherent
IV	Coma (unresponsive to verbal or noxious stimuli)

together provide the best opportunity to detect clinically significant changes in status.

MANAGEMENT

INITIAL MANAGEMENT (OVERVIEW)

A directed history and physical examination, extensive laboratory panel, and relevant imaging should be performed as quickly and safely as possible. A careful history and physical examination needs to focus on the potential causes of liver injury, and any evidence of chronic liver disease that would preclude a diagnosis of ALF. Any barriers to potential liver transplant (comorbidities, lack of social support, active neoplastic or infectious processes, etc) should be assessed.

In known or suspected cases of acetaminophen toxicity, acetaminophen nomograms are unreliable if the time from ingestion is not known, or if a single large ingestion was not taken. Activated charcoal may be given to patients within the first 4 hours of intentional acetaminophen overdose. Serial measurements of liver enzymes, coagulation parameters (INR and factor V levels), arterial pH, and arterial lactate will help to prognosticate the extent of liver damage. Serial assessments of mental status help determine stage of encephalopathy and direct further intervention (eg, head CT, ICP monitor) (**Table 158-7**).

ROLE OF N-ACETYL-CYSTEINE (NAC)

The administration of NAC can provide protection from hepatotoxicity, especially if given within 12 hours of nonstaggered ingestion of acetaminophen. The main effects of NAC are to increase hepatic glutathione production and act as an antioxidant. The first dose of NAC may still be beneficial up to 48 to 72 hours following acetaminophen ingestion.

NAC may also offer benefit in non-acetaminophen causes of liver failure, as it seems to improve overall hemodynamic status and oxygen delivery to peripheral tissues. A recent trial randomized patients with non-acetaminophen ALF to intravenous NAC or placebo. Transplant-free survival improved in patients who received NAC. NAC also improved one-year overall survival in the subset of patients with mild (grade 1–2) encephalopathy.

Based on available evidence, all patients with ALF, regardless of etiology, should receive NAC. In the absence of significant upper GI symptoms, NAC may be given orally or by NG tube as follows: 140 mg/kg (5% dextrose solution) loading dose followed by 70 mg/kg every 4 hours for 17 doses. Oral NAC has several potential side effects that include nausea, vomiting, rare urticaria, and bronchospasm. NAC may also be administered intravenously as follows: 150 mg/kg (5% dextrose solution) loading dose over 15 minutes, followed by 50 mg/kg given over 4 hours, followed by 100 mg/kg given over 16 hours. Intravenous NAC may lead to rare anaphylaxis, ECG abnormalities, bronchospasm, and false improvements in INR. The US Food and Drug Administration (FDA) has not yet approved the intravenous use of NAC for ALF. NAC therapy can be stopped when the patient proceeds to liver transplantation, or when there is evidence that hepatic dysfunction is resolving, defined by improved encephalopathy and coagulopathy (INR < 1.5).

PRACTICE POINT

- All patients with ALF, regardless of etiology, should receive N-acetyl cysteine (NAC) therapy to improve transplant-free survival.

TABLE 158-7 Overview of Management in Patients with Acute Liver Failure

Rapid assessment and stabilization	Mental status? Adequate IV access? Need for intubation?
Directed history and physical exam	Cause of acute liver failure? Grade of encephalopathy? Medical comorbidities?
Activated charcoal within 4 h of known acetaminophen overdose	
Initiation of N-acetylcysteine	Intravenous or enteral, depending on patient stability
Full panel of lab tests	See Table 158-5 Assess coagulopathy
Abdominal imaging study	Is there evidence of chronic liver disease?
Head imaging study (based on mental status)	Any evidence of cerebral edema?
Multiple consultations	Transplant hepatology Transplant surgery Pulmonary/critical care Nephrology Hematology Infectious disease Social services Psychiatry Anesthesiology Ethics?
Admission to ICU	
Organ-specific management of complications	See Table 158-8
Assessment of transplant candidacy (may include collateral history from family and friends)	Usually a multidisciplinary assessment based on consultations
Estimate prognosis of survival without transplant	King's College criteria (See Table 158-9) MELD score APACHE score

CONSULTATION

Depending on the severity and extent of multiorgan involvement, patients with ALF often require multiple consultations (Table 158-7). A multidisciplinary approach is also very important for patients who may be candidates for liver transplantation. Consultations may include providers from critical care medicine, transplant hepatology (surgical and medical), anesthesiology, cardiology, nephrology, infectious diseases, pulmonary, psychiatry, social services, and possibly the ethics committee.

COMPLICATIONS AND PROGNOSIS

Since patients with advanced ALF present with multiorgan system failure, management should follow a systems-based, goal-directed approach. Management of ALF in an organ system based manner requires multiple disciplines and coordinated care (**Table 158-8**).

TABLE 158-8 Organ-specific Management of Acute Liver Failure

Organ System	Complication(s)	Management
Neurologic	Cerebral edema and intracranial hypertension	1. Consider placing an intracranial monitor 2. Maintain a cerebral perfusion pressure of 60–80 mm Hg 3. Maintain an ICP < 25 mm Hg 4. Maintain head of bed somewhat elevated (45°) 5. Medical management of elevated ICP (see Figure 158-1) 6. Avoid stimulation of patient 7. Serial neurologic examinations 8. Consider EEG
Pulmonary	Mechanical ventilation for either airway protection from altered mental status or due to respiratory failure from ALI/ARDS	1. Lidocaine IV or endotracheal during intubation 2. Propofol for sedation 3. Consider cis-atracurium paralysis 4. Either volume or pressure controlled ventilation 5. Low tidal volumes of 6 mL/kg of ideal body weight 6. Maintain maximal plateau pressure < 30 cm H_2O 7. Avoid bronchoscopy
Cardiovascular	Hypotension (hemodynamic collapse)	1. Arterial catheter for direct measurement 2. Fluid resuscitation (often less volume than is required with sepsis) 3. Vasopressor support with norepinephrine as first choice 4. Avoid alpha-adrenergic agents 5. Consider a pulmonary artery catheter 6. Monitor mixed or central venous oxygen saturation
Renal	Acute kidney injury, volume overload, and metabolic disturbances	1. Early initiation of renal replacement therapy with CRRT preferred over HD 2. Nephrology consultation 3. Bicarbonate buffered hemofiltration 4. Renal ultrasound
Hematology	Thrombocytopenia and coagulation abnormalities involving both a bleeding and thrombosis risk	1. Vitamin K 10 mg SQ x 3 days 2. Avoid FFP unless there is bleeding, and monitor serial INR/PT/PTT 3. Transfuse platelets based on Practice Point recommendations (page 1293) 4. Subcutaneous heparin for DVT prophylaxis 5. Consider recombinant factor VII if placing an intracranial pressure monitor
Infectious Disease	Bacterial and fungal infections; acute viral causes of ALF	1. Maintain a low clinical threshold to culture and start empiric antimicrobials 2. Follow hospital protocols to reduce iatrogenic infections from central lines and catheters 3. Early antiviral therapy for acute hepatitis B, HSV, CMV, or VZV
Endocrine	Relative adrenal insufficiency	1. Maintain a low clinical suspicion if hypotension seems refractory 2. Consider stress dose steroid therapy
Electrolytes	Hypoglycemia, hypophosphatemia, hyponatremia, hypo- or hyperkalemia, low magnesium levels, metabolic acidosis	1. Frequent serum glucose checks; dextrose-containing fluids 2. Bicarbonate buffered solutions with CRRT 3. Replete phosphorous, potassium, and magnesium 4. Treat hyperkalemia 5. Early CRRT
GI/Nutrition	Stress ulcerations, severe catabolic state	1. Early enteral feedings should be considered 2. TPN if enteral feeds not possible (ileus, etc) 3. H2-blocker or PPI therapy

ALI/ARDS, acute lung injury/acute respiratory distress syndrome; CMV, cytomegalovirus; CRRT, continuous renal replacement therapy; DVT, deep vein thrombosis; EEG, electroencephalogram; HD, hemodialysis; HSV, herpes simplex virus; ICP, intracranial pressure; PPI, proton pump inhibitor; TPN, total parenteral nutrition; VZV, varicella zoster virus.

CEREBRAL EDEMA AND INTRACRANIAL HYPERTENSION

Intracranial hypertension and cerebral edema remain serious complications of ALF, often leading to fatal herniation. ICH develops in approximately 20% to 30% of patients with ALF. Cerebral edema occurs more often in patients with a short time interval (28 days or less) between the development of jaundice and the onset of encephalopathy. Younger patients, with less cerebral atrophy than older patients, may not tolerate rapid shifts in ICP. Young age and high arterial ammonia correlate with increased risk of death from herniation. Cerebral edema is rarely seen in patients with mild (grades I–II) encephalopathy. Risk factors for progression to encephalopathy and cerebral edema include the presence of systemic inflammatory response syndrome, the need for vasopressors, the need for continuous renal replacement therapy (CRRT), or the presence of infection.

The exact mechanisms underlying elevated ICP in patients with ALF are not fully understood and are likely multifactorial. Both retrospective and prospective studies have shown that higher arterial ammonia levels portend a higher risk of cerebral herniation and death. An arterial ammonia >124 micromoles/L predicts mortality with a 77.5% diagnostic accuracy (sensitivity 78.6%, specificity 76.3%). Elevated ammonia levels lead to osmotic shifts that negatively affect astrocytes. When ammonia levels rise in subacute or chronic liver disease, there is time for adaptation. In ALF, the rapidity of the rise in serum ammonia is thought to limit the time for adaptation.

ICP MONITORING

No randomized controlled trials demonstrate an overall survival benefit in ALF with the use of ICP monitoring. The utility of ICP monitors is extrapolated from the neurointensive care literature regarding management of traumatic brain injury. Clinical signs of elevated ICP are not always present, and pupillary dilation, decerebrate posturing, or changes on brain CT scans are often discovered late in the course. Therefore, a more accurate and potentially objective measure of ICP using a monitoring device can enable determination of ICH and guide decisions of therapy, prognosis, and candidacy for liver transplantation.

Significant ICH is defined as a sustained (>10 min) elevation of ICP >25 mm Hg. In addition to the ICP, the cerebral perfusion pressure (CPP)—defined as the difference between the mean arterial pressure (MAP) and ICP (ie, CPP = MAP − ICP) with optimal CPP 60 to 80 mm Hg—guides patient management. Augmentation of MAP with vasoactive agents in order to maintain adequate CPP in the setting of an elevated ICP may be necessary.

Refractory ICH or decreased CPP are considered contraindications to liver transplantation in many centers. One study showed that prolonged high ICP (>25 mm Hg) and low CPP (<40 mm Hg) for greater than 2 hours portended poor neurologic recovery and should preclude liver transplantation. However, absolute pressure thresholds predicting irreversible neurologic damage or precluding transplantation should be used with caution, since such pressure thresholds have been challenged by reports of complete neurologic recovery after prolonged (>24 h) ICH (ICP > 35 mm Hg) with low CPP (<50 mm Hg). For patients with ALF who are listed for transplantation, ICP monitoring may help with ICU management of cerebral edema and ICH prior to transplantation. Furthermore, since elevated ICP can persist perioperatively, ICP monitors can also be useful both during and after the liver transplant surgery. Given the absence of large randomized controlled trials, the use of ICP monitors currently remains center dependent.

The major risks involved with placing an intracranial device include infection and bleeding, with mortality from bleeding reported to be 1% to 3%. Intraventricular catheters bear greater risk than intraparenchymal or subdural catheters, which in turn bear greater risk than epidural devices. The intraparenchymal location appears to offer the optimal balance between accuracy and safety. Aggressive correction of coagulation parameters, along with the use of recombinant activated factor VII, may reduce bleeding risk and allow wider use of ICP monitoring devices.

MEDICAL MANAGEMENT OF ELEVATED ICP

Patients with ALF can progress rapidly from grade 1 to 4 encephalopathy. Frequent and detailed neurological examinations are vital, as subtle changes of increasing ICP can be missed. Once a head CT has ruled out any other process, patients with suspected ICH should have as little stimulation as possible. Visitors, lights, and noises should be reduced. The head of the bed should be elevated to 30°. CPP should be maintained at 60 to 80 mm Hg, and this may require cautious titration of MAP to compensate for increasing ICP. Clinicians should avoid the placement of bilateral internal jugular lines for access, as this may collectively compromise intracranial venous drainage.

Lactulose may be used with early encephalopathy, but it lacks long-term benefit. Lactulose may also lead to gaseous distension of the bowel, which can complicate subsequent transplant surgery. The role of nonabsorbable antibiotics, such as rifaximin, has not been demonstrated.

Patients with grade III or IV encephalopathy should be intubated for airway protection. Endotracheal or intravenous lidocaine prior to intubation may be helpful in reducing spikes of ICP. For intubation, small doses of propofol may be used with caution, as the half-life of propofol is prolonged in hepatic failure. Propofol may also cause a decrease in MAP, thus compromising CPP.

Seizure activity should be treated with phenytoin or fosphenytoin; however, prophylactic antiepileptic therapy is not indicated.

With ALF, the ICP should be maintained below 25 mm Hg in order to improve CPP. Treatment of elevated ICP is usually instituted when there is either a sustained rise in ICP (>10 min) or if clinical signs suggest ischemia or herniation. Increased sedation with propofol may be used for transient spikes of ICP due to agitation. Once ICH is established, an algorithmic treatment approach can be followed (**Figure 158-1**).

Osmotic diuresis with IV mannitol effectively reduces cerebral edema and improves survival, based on a prospective, controlled study performed at King's College in London. A bolus dose of 0.5-1 g/kg may be repeated once or twice as needed, as long as the serum osmolarity does not exceed 320 mOsm/L. Since mannitol is cleared by the kidneys, there is risk of intravascular hypervolemia and high pressure pulmonary edema in the setting of renal failure. As mannitol is removed by dialysis, it may be used in patients on CRRT. Serum osmolarity and sodium level should be monitored every 6 to 8 hours when mannitol is used. In the absence of ICH, prophylactic mannitol is not indicated.

In the past, patients were mechanically hyperventilated in order to reduce the serum partial pressure of carbon dioxide (pCO_2) and cause cerebral vasoconstriction, thus reducing both cerebral blood flow and ICP. This effect is very transient, perhaps only lasting several minutes. Out of concern for cerebral hypoxia with reduced cerebral blood flow, hyperventilation is no longer a mainstay of therapy. Short-term hyperventilation has not been shown to improve outcome in ALF, but it does prolong survival in the ICU; therefore, it may occasionally be used as bridge therapy in selected patients who await a liver transplant.

In the setting of ICH refractory to mannitol therapy, induction and maintenance of hypernatremia may be used to prevent rising ICP. The efficacy of hypertonic saline in the prevention and treatment of ICH has been demonstrated in the neurologic

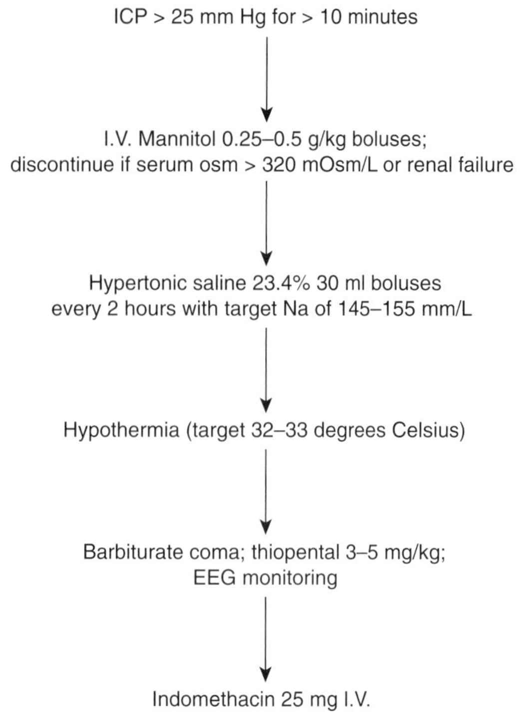

Figure 158-1 *Algorithm for management of elevated intracranial pressure in acute liver failure. (EEG, electroencephalogram).*

intensive care literature. The goal of therapeutic hypernatremia is a serum sodium of 145 to 155 mmol/L, which can be obtained using 30% hypertonic saline in boluses of 20 mL. In contrast to mannitol, boluses of hypertonic saline have less tachyphylaxis to multiple doses. In the presence of CRRT, achieving the desired level of therapeutic hypernatremia may be a challenge, since a relatively hyponatremic replacement fluid is often used in the CRRT circuit.

Moderate hypothermia, with a goal core temperature of 32° to 34°C, may also prevent or control elevated ICP. Patients may be iatrogenically hypothermic from transfusions or a CRRT circuit. Cooling blankets can be added to further reduce core temperature. Hypothermia can also prevent ICP spikes during liver transplant surgery.

In cases of elevated ICP refractory to osmotherapy (ie, mannitol and hypernatremia) and hypothermia, induction of a barbiturate coma using thiopental or pentobarbital can be considered. Significant myocardial depression and systemic hypotension may limit the use of a barbiturate coma. Some ICUs choose paralytic therapy over barbiturate coma. A continuous EEG can monitor burst suppression, the primary goal of either coma induction or paralysis with sedation.

Finally, intravenous indomethacin induces cerebral vasoconstriction and may temporarily reduce ICP; however, this medication is not easily prepared and it may be quite expensive for only a transient benefit.

AIRWAY AND VENTILATION

Patients with ALF who reach grades III to IV encephalopathy require intubation and mechanical ventilation. When intubating, a clinician skilled in the procedure should maintain adequate pre-oxygenation, prevention of hypercapnea, and avoidance of hypotension. Propofol sedation and lidocaine (endotracheal or intravenous) may help to minimize spikes in ICP. Pre-intubation, clinicians may utilize neuromuscular blockade. When indicated, cis-atracurium—a nondepolarizing agent, metabolized independently of liver or renal function—is the paralytic of choice and permits neurologic assessment 40 to 60 minutes after the bolus. No consensus drives practice regarding the specific mode of mechanical ventilation; therefore, either volume or pressure controlled mode can be utilized. Initial ventilator settings should include a low tidal volume strategy of 6 mL/kg of ideal body weight and a maximum plateau pressure of 30 cm H_2O, in order to minimize the effects of mechanical ventilation-induced barotrauma. If a low tidal volume strategy increases pCO_2, this may lead to cerebrovascular dilation and increase in ICP. Therefore, clinicians should strictly manage pCO_2 through minute ventilation and adjust respiratory rate accordingly.

Optimal patient-ventilator synchrony with adequate sedation and analgesia helps prevent spikes in ICP. Critical care physicians should employ paralysis if patient-ventilator asynchrony occurs despite aggressive sedation and analgesia. While mechanical hyperventilation does not improve outcomes, spontaneous hyperventilation should not be inhibited, as it does result in mild hypocapnia and cerebrovascular constriction, thus reducing ICP. Whenever possible, to avoid any spikes in ICP, bronchoscopy should be avoided in patients with ALF.

CIRCULATION

Circulatory changes associated with ALF can resemble changes seen with endotoxinemia-induced septic shock. The pattern observed depends on the etiology and rapidity of ALF. In hyperacute liver failure due to acetaminophen overdose, patients can develop fulminant peripheral cardiovascular collapse that can lead to early death. Early hemodynamic changes in ALF include increased portal pressures, splanchnic sequestration of blood, and decreased central venous return. Fluid resuscitation and vasopressor support may be necessary, but fluid requirements in ALF may be less than in patients with septic shock. Some experts recommend placement of a pulmonary artery catheter to aid in assessing volume status. NAC benefits hemodynamic stabilization and improves oxygen consumption in patients with ALF.

In order to maintain an adequate CPP, systemic vasopressor support may be necessary, especially if the patient is hypotensive from ALF-induced vasodilation. Clinicians should maintain close monitoring and titration of oxygen delivery while using vasoconstrictors. A mixed, or central, venous oxygen saturation can guide the institution and titration of vasoactive agents.

Careful pressor selection facilitates adequate blood flow to the liver and brain. Norepinephrine serves as the vasopressor of choice in cases of ALF. It increases hepatic blood flow in parallel with cardiac output, and has less tachycardia than dopamine. Norepinephrine also leads to less lactate production than epinephrine. Alpha-adrenergic agents (epinephrine, high dose vasopressin, terlipressin) can worsen peripheral oxygen delivery and lead to splanchnic ischemia. Terlipressin increases both cerebral blood flow and ICP, due to breakdown of autoregulation.

Relative adrenal insufficiency can occur with ALF, and stress dose steroids (hydrocortisone up to 200–300 mg daily) have been shown to reduce norepinephrine requirements. Intravenous steroids should be given to patient with ALF who develop persistent hypotension despite adequate IV fluids and vasopressor support.

Hemodynamics and intracranial hypertension frequently improve after removal of the native liver during liver transplant surgery. Therefore, ALF patients who are listed for transplantation but who have persistent circulatory dysfunction despite maximal medical measures, should be considered for a bridging, last-resort hepatectomy.

RENAL FAILURE

Acute renal failure occurs frequently in the setting of ALF, with an incidence up to 70%, and portends a poor prognosis. Causes of renal failure may include a pre-renal insult (systemic vasodilation, hypovolemia, sepsis), direct renal injury (acute tubular necrosis from hypoperfusion, acetaminophen, or other toxins), or post-renal obstruction. The nephrotoxic effects of acetaminophen usually reverse spontaneously, but whether NAC contributes has not been proven.

Based on randomized trials, early initiation of CRRT improves outcomes over intermittent hemodialysis in order to reduce dramatic fluid shifts and avoid spikes in ICP. High-volume hemofiltration improves laboratory (lactate, base deficit) abnormalities and reduces vasopressor requirements, but may not affect survival in ALF. Because patients with ALF do not tolerate a lactate load, bicarbonate buffered hemofiltration is recommended.

BLEEDING AND CLOTTING

Coagulation abnormalities, due to both decreased synthesis and increased consumption, occur frequently in patients with ALF. Thrombocytopenia occurs in 50% to 70% of patients, but only 5% of patients with ALF experience significant bleeding. Variceal bleeding almost never occurs, as chronic portal hypertension is absent. Spontaneous intracranial bleeding (in the absence of an ICP monitor) is rare as well. Practice-based recommendations for platelet transfusion in ALF include (1) all patients with platelet count $< 10{,}000/mm^3$, (2) patients with sepsis and platelet count $< 20{,}000/mm^3$, or (3) patients with a planned invasive procedure or active bleeding and a platelet count $< 50{,}000/mm^3$. Patients with ALF also bear increased thrombosis risk due to reduced protein C and protein S production; therefore, venous thromboembolism prophylaxis with subcutaneous heparin may be instituted.

PRACTICE POINT

Platelets and coagulation factors

- Platelet transfusion recommendations in ALF:
  1. All patients with platelet count $< 10{,}000/mm^3$
  2. Sepsis with platelet count $< 20{,}000/mm^3$, or
  3. Planned invasive procedure or active bleeding with platelet count $< 50{,}000/mm^3$
- Hepatically synthesized factors (factor V, factor VII) and INR provide the most sensitive biochemical indicators of hepatic synthetic function and recovery
- Administration of fresh frozen plasma—which can obscure the picture of endogenous coagulation factor production—should be avoided in the absence of active bleeding
- Vitamin K (5–10 mg subcutaneously daily for 3 days) can help eliminate any component of malnutrition as a source for coagulopathy

Hepatically synthesized factors (factor V, factor VII) and INR provide the most sensitive biochemical indicators of hepatic synthetic function and recovery. Therefore, administration of fresh frozen plasma (FFP)—which can obscure the picture of endogenous coagulation factor production—should be avoided in the absence of active bleeding. Vitamin K (5–10 mg subcutaneously daily for 3 days) can help eliminate any component of malnutrition as a source for coagulopathy. FFP transfusion and plasmapheresis carry additional risks of volume overload and transfusion-related acute lung injury. If an invasive procedure, such as an ICP monitor, is planned, activated recombinant factor VII can temporarily correct the INR. A minimum dose of 40 mcg/kg is recommended in order to achieve a transient (therapeutic window of 60–90 min) reversal of coagulopathy. Repeat dosing can be administered as necessary. Factor VIIa has been associated with rare cases of thromboembolism and cerebrovascular accident. Bleeding rarely poses a major problem with transplant surgery itself, and the preoperative degree of coagulopathy does not predict posttransplant outcome.

INFECTION

Patients with ALF have altered immune function and, in the setting of multiple intravenous lines, catheters, and devices, have moderate to high risk for bacterial and fungal sepsis. Up to 80% of ALF patients develop bacterial infections, and 30% of patients develop fungal infections. Most infections are diagnosed within 72 hours of hospital admission and are commonly localized to the respiratory tract, urinary tract, or bloodstream. Gram-positive infections with *Staphylococcus* or *Streptococcus* species occur more commonly than gram negative or *Candida* infections.

Clinicians should maintain a low threshold to evaluate for infection since the usual signs of infection may be absent in nearly one-third of individuals with ALF. Because active infection may preclude liver transplantation, some centers advocate starting empiric antimicrobial therapy upon hospital admission. While antibiotic prophylaxis reduces the incidence of infection and may reduce the risk of ICH and cerebral edema, such prophylaxis has not shown an overall survival benefit. Empiric antibacterial and antifungal therapy should be administered in the setting of shock, and may be considered in advanced encephalopathy or in patients listed for transplantation.

METABOLIC ABNORMALITIES AND NUTRITION

Metabolic derangements are common in patients with ALF. Alkalosis and acidosis may both occur and are best managed by identifying and treating the underlying disorder. Hypoglycemia should be managed with continuous glucose infusions and frequent serum glucose checks. Sodium, potassium, and magnesium levels are often low and should be supplemented. Hypophosphatemia is common and, while necessitating supplementation, may be a good prognostic sign, as it may reflect the consumption of ATP in a regenerating liver. High or normal phosphate levels may indicate a lack of hepatic regeneration and renal impairment. ALF patients frequently have increased energy expenditure and a catabolic state. Therefore, in order to reduce infectious complications, early enteral feedings should be initiated, including 60 g of protein per day. Enteral feedings may also reduce the risk of GI bleeding due to stress ulcerations in critically ill patients.

LIVER SUPPORT SYSTEMS AND AUXILIARY GRAFTS

Several liver replacement devices have been tested in patients with liver failure, but there have been few controlled trials. A recent meta-analysis that considered all available bioartificial devices failed to prove efficacy in the treatment of ALF. Currently, liver support systems are not recommended outside of clinical trials. Strategies to reduce serum ammonia levels by continuous venous hemofiltration or by plasma exchange can be considered. High volume (>8 L) plasma exchange may reduce serum ammonia and improve hemodynamics in patients with ALF. For patients in whom a liver graft donor has been identified, total hepatectomy may be considered, as it removes the major source of pro-inflammatory cytokines that contribute to cerebral vasodilation.

The use of auxiliary liver transplants (reduced size graft from living or deceased donor) to provide temporary hepatic function while awaiting recovery of the native liver has gained interest in Europe. The best outcome has been seen in patients younger than 40 years of age with either acute viral hepatitis or acetaminophen toxicity.

PROGNOSIS

Regardless of the acuity, the etiology of ALF best predicts the likelihood of spontaneous recovery without transplantation. Patients with ALF due to acetaminophen, hepatitis A, shock liver, or pregnancy-related disease have >50% transplant-free survival, whereas patients with other etiologies have a <25% transplant-free survival. Patients with autoimmune hepatitis, acute hepatitis B, or acute HSV may improve with specific therapy and not require a liver transplant.

Clinicians should use accepted prognostic models to evaluate patients with ALF. The King's College prognostic criteria separate patients with acetaminophen-induced ALF from those with non-acetaminophen-induced ALF (**Table 158-9**).

The King's College model has high specificity (92%) in determining who will need a liver transplant, but low sensitivity (69%). If a patient fulfills the King's College criteria, the likelihood ratio positive for a poor prognosis without transplant is 8.63. On the other hand, the likelihood ratio negative for a patient with unfulfilled King's College criteria is 0.34. Therefore, the King's College criteria may misclassify a substantial number of patients who will die without a liver transplant. A recent meta-analysis found that the King's College criteria and a pH <7.30 were both fairly specific in predicting a poor outcome.

One small study showed that an APACHE II score >15 on admission for patients with acetaminophen-induced ALF shows a specificity of 92% and a sensitivity of 81% (likelihood ratio positive 10.1, likelihood ratio negative 0.21) for predicting need of liver transplant. The Model for End Stage Liver Disease (MELD) score may eventually prove to be superior to the King's College criteria in cases of non-acetaminophen induced ALF. A single study in Argentina showed a MELD score of greater than 30 to be superior to the King's College criteria in predicting poor prognosis without transplant in patients with non-acetaminophen induced ALF. The positive predictive value and negative predictive value of a MELD >30 was found to be 91% and 100%, respectively (diagnostic accuracy 95%). Further studies are needed for validation.

Finally, multiple clinical predictors correlate with poor outcome in the absence of transplant. Encephalopathy at the time of admission predicts a worse prognosis. Patients presenting with grade III or IV encephalopathy die or require transplant in 60% to 90% of cases. Age, renal failure, and severity of coagulopathy are also independent predictors of mortality without transplant. Even the King's College criteria lack the sensitivity to replace an experienced transplant physician's clinical judgment.

TABLE 158-9 King's College Criteria—Prognostic Model for Determining Poor Outcome without Liver Transplantation in Acute Liver Failure (ALF)

For acetaminophen-Induced ALF	For non-acetaminophen–Induced ALF
Arterial pH <7.3	INR >6.5
OR	*OR*
All 3 of the following:	3 out of 5 of the following criteria:
INR >6.5	Age <11 or >40
Serum creatinine >3.4 mg/dL	Serum bilirubin >18 mg/dL
Grade III or IV encephalopathy	Time from jaundice to coma >7 days
	INR >3.5
	Etiology non-A or non-B viral hepatitis *OR* drug-induced liver injury

DISCHARGE PLANNING

If a patient recovers from ALF with or without transplant, he or she should receive education about the disease and ways to prevent future injury. Depending on the etiology of ALF, ongoing treatment and follow-up may be necessary. For example, a patient with autoimmune hepatitis will need close hepatology follow-up and treatment with immunosuppressant medications. Also, a patient with acute on chronic hepatitis B will require hepatology follow-up, not only for antiviral treatment but also for hepatocellular carcinoma screening. The need for rehabilitation depends on overall performance and details of the hospitalization.

If a patient undergoes a liver transplant, a strong social network is vital, and close follow-up in the transplant center must be arranged. Rehabilitation or a skilled nursing facility may be necessary for some patients, especially if social support becomes a limitation. In contrast to patients transplanted for chronic liver disease, social support breakdown occurs more commonly when a patient undergoes liver transplantation for ALF, likely due to less time for education and a comprehensive assessment.

QUALITY IMPROVEMENT

Since fatal outcome occurs frequently in ALF without liver transplant, and because liver transplant is not always an option (eg, organ availability, poor candidate), public health measures should focus on prevention of ALF. Controlling distribution of acetaminophen could reduce overdoses. Some countries limit acetaminophen access by regulating the number of blister packs that can be purchased. Education about unintentional acetaminophen overdose, and education about drug and alcohol interactions, may help reduce acetaminophen-related ALF in the United States. Finally, early recognition of drug-induced hepatoxicity, along with cessation of offending agents, may prevent some cases from progressing to liver failure.

In some cases, patients with ALF who are good candidates for liver transplant die before a donor liver becomes available. Increasing organ donation will lead to more lives saved, and additional education and outreach programs to increase liver donation are needed. Also, other creative ways to increase the donor pool (eg, extended criteria donors, paired exchanges, and partial-liver living donors) may augment the pool of available transplant organs.

Due to the low incidence of ALF, there are few controlled trials that can help guide management (**Table 158-10**). Standards of intensive care in this patient population have not been well established and are mostly guided by expert opinion. Management may differ from center to center. Multicenter collaborations and prospective trials may improve future management of patients with ALF.

TABLE 158-10 Evidence-based Medicine Key References for Acute Liver Failure (ALF)

Reference	Methodology	Results	Limitations	Bottom Line
Epidemiology and Diagnosis				
Ostapowicz G, et al. *Ann Intern Med.* 2002;137:947–954.	Multicenter prospective cohort from 17 tertiary centers (United States Acute Liver Failure Study Group)	308 consecutive patients over 41 mo; 73% women, median age 38; acetaminophen-induced ALF most common etiology and with best prognosis; 29% of all patients underwent transplant, 43% of patients survived without transplant	Liver transplant not always available	Important multicenter study to define etiology, clinical features, and short-term outcomes in patients with ALF
N-acetylcysteine (NAC)				
Prescott L, et al. *BMJ.* 1979;2:1097–1100.	Outcome data of 102 patients with acetaminophen overdose who were treated with IV NAC as compared to a retrospective control group (n = 57) without NAC	IV NAC within 8 h of acetaminophen ingestion offers complete protection; within 10 h, only 1 of 62 patients developed severe hepatotoxicity	Not a randomized controlled trial	Give IV NAC asap with acetaminophen overdose
Smilkstein MJ, et al. *N Eng J Med.* 1988;319:1557–1562.	Analysis of a national multicenter study (1976–1985); outcome data from 2,540 patients treated with investigational oral NAC for acetaminophen overdose	If given within 8 h of ingestion, oral NAC confers complete protection from severe hepatotoxicity (regardless of acetaminophen level); 72 h oral NAC protocol is as effective as 20 h IV regimen	Not a randomized controlled trial; no control group	Oral NAC is equivalent to 20 h IV NAC if a patient can take oral dosing
Smilkstein MJ, et al. *Ann Emerg Med.* 1991;20:1058–1063.	Nonrandomized multicenter study of 179 patients with acetaminophen overdose and IV NAC over 48 h	If given within 10 h of ingestion, 10% risk of severe hepatotoxicity; 14% of patients developed mild urticaria or rash during loading dose	Not a randomized controlled trial	48 h IV NAC protocol is safe and effective, especially if given within 10 h of acetaminophen ingestion
Keays R, et al. *BMJ.* 1991;303:1026–1029.	Prospective randomized controlled trial of 50 patients with acetaminophen-induced ALF; 25 patients received IV NAC until recovery or death; 25 patients received 5% dextrose (England)	IV NAC group had 48% survival vs 20% survival in control group ($P = 0.037$); IV NAC group had a lower incidence of cerebral edema and less hypotension requiring pressor support	Single center; 25 patients in each arm	IV NAC has survival benefit in patients with acetaminophen-induced ALF; give IV NAC regardless of time from acetaminophen ingestion
Prognosis and complications				
Clemmesen JO, et al. *Hepatology.* 1999;29:648–653.	Retrospective study of 44 patients with ALF (Denmark)	Patients with cerebral herniation (n = 14) had higher arterial ammonia levels than patients who did not herniate ($P < 0.001$)	Retrospective study	Higher arterial ammonia levels in patients with ALF portend a higher risk of cerebral herniation/death
Bhatia V, et al. *Gut.* 2006;55:98–104.	Prospective study of 80 patients admitted with ALF over 2 yr (New Delhi)	42 patients died (median arterial ammonia level of 175); median ammonia level was 105 in survivors	Single center in India	Arterial ammonia > 124 predicted mortality with a sensitivity of 79% and specificity of 76%
Bailey B, et al. *Crit Care Med.* 2003;31:299–305.	Meta-analysis of prognostic criteria determining need for transplant in acetaminophen-induced ALF	King's College criteria (9 studies); sensitivity 69%, specificity 92%; APACHE II score > 15 had LR+ of 16.4 and a LR– of 0.19 (1 study)	Only one study evaluated APACHE II score	KCH criteria and possibly APACHE II scores are useful but not perfect in predicting need for transplant in patients with acetaminophen-induced ALF
Yantorno SE, et al. *Liver Transpl.* 2007;13: 822–828.	Retrospective cohort of 120 patients with non-acetaminophen causes of ALF (Argentina)	MELD > 30 predicted need for transplant with diagnostic accuracy of 95%, PPV 91%, NPV 100%	Single center; did not include acetaminophen-induced cases of ALF	MELD score > 30 may better predict need for transplant in non-acetaminophen induced cases of ALF when compared to King's College

(continued)

TABLE 158-10 Evidence-based Medicine Key References for Acute Liver Failure (ALF) (*continued*)

Reference	Methodology	Results	Limitations	Bottom Line
Katoonizadeh A, et al. *Liver Int.* 2007;27: 329–334.	Retrospective analysis of prospective cohort; 99 patients with non-acetaminophen induced ALF	King's College criteria and MELD > 30 had similar NPV (91–92%) and low PPV (52–56%); MELD > 35 had sensitivity 86%, specificty 75%	Excluded acetaminophen-induced cases of ALF	Both King's College criteria and MELD score may have similar prognostic value in cases of non-acetaminophen ALF
Management				
Lidofsky SD, et al. *Hepatology.* 1992; 16:1–7.	Retrospective cohort study of 20 adults and 3 children with ALF who had intracranial pressure monitors placed (UCSF)	10 patients required medical therapy for sustained elevation of ICP, 6 had refractory ICH and died	Not a randomized controlled trial	ICP monitors may have a role in diagnosis and treatment of ICH in patients with ALF
Blei AT, et al. *Lancet.* 1993;341:157–158.	Survey of US centers; 262 patients with ALF who received an ICP monitor	Epidural most common and lowest risk (1% fatal bleed) compared to other types (4–5% fatal bleed)	Survey data	If using an ICP monitor, an epidural device is most common and preferred for safety
Vaquero J, et al. *Liver Transpl.* 2005;11: 1581–1589.	Retrospective data from US ALF Study Group centers (24 sites)—332 patients	28% of patients underwent ICP monitor placement (center dependent); 30-d survival post liver transplant was equal with or without ICP monitor; pts with ICP monitor required more medical therapy and vasopressor support	Variation among centers	ICP monitors may be useful in patients who are potential transplant candidates, but this remains controversial
Shami VM, et al. *Liver Transpl.* 2003;9: 138–143.	Comparative trial assessing FFP (8 patients) vs FFP/recombinant activated factor VII (7 patients) in 15 patients with poor prognosis based on King's College criteria	100% of patients who received FFP and recombinant activated factor VII could undergo placement of ICP monitor (vs 38% in FFP alone group)	Not a prospective, randomized controlled trial	Recombinant activated factor VII facilitates placement of an ICP monitor by reducing risk of bleeding
Canalese J, et al. *Gut.* 1982;23:625–629.	Controlled trial comparing mannitol (17 patients) to no mannitol (17 patients) for treating cerebral edema in 34 patients with ALF	IV mannitol group had a 47% survival compared to 6% in the control group ($P = 0.008$)	Single center (all patients had an ICP monitor and were given IV dexamethasone)	IV mannitol treats ICH/cerebral edema and confers a survival benefit
Murphy N, et al. *Hepatology.* 2004;39:464–470.	Randomized controlled trial of 30 patients with ALF and severe (grade III–IV) encephalopathy; 15 patients with hypertonic saline; 15 patients with standard care	30% saline with a goal serum sodium of 145–155 mmol/L reduces the incidence and severity of ICH	Single center; all patients had an ICP monitor (Camino subdural)	Hypertonic saline is indicated in cases of ALF and advanced encephalopathy
Jalan R, et al. *Lancet.* 1999;354:1164–1168.	Retrospective analysis of moderate hypothermia in 7 consecutive patients with elevated ICP not responding to mannitol or ultrafiltration	4 patients who underwent transplant had good outcomes	Not a randomized controlled trial	Moderate hypothermia should be used in cases of ALF with elevated ICP that does not respond to mannitol
Rolando N, et al. *Hepatology.* 1990;11:49–53.	Retrospective study of a prospective cohort of 50 consecutive patients with ALF and grade II encephalopathy	53 bacterial infections in 40 patients (47% respiratory, 23% urinary, 4% CVC related); 70% gram-positive; 32% of patients developed fungal infections (15 *Candida*, 1 *Aspergillus*, and all had concominant bacterial infections; all deaths after 7 d were from infection; fever and leukocytosis absent in 30% of infections	Single center data	Maintain a high suspicion for bacterial and fungal infections in patients who present with ALF
Kjaergard LL, et al. *JAMA.* 2003;289: 217–222.	Meta-analysis for artificial and bioartificial support systems in acute (2 studies) and acute-on-chronic (10 studies) liver failure	No effect on mortality	Only 2 studies looking at acute liver failure	No role for artificial support systems at the present time, more studies needed

SUGGESTED READINGS

Chenard-Neu MP, Boudjema K, Bernuau J, et al. Auxiliary liver transplantation: regeneration of the native liver and outcome in 30 patients with fulminant hepatic failure–a multicenter European study. *Hepatology.* 1996;23:1119–1127.

Farmer DG, Anselmo DM, Ghobrial RM, et al. Liver transplantation for fulminant hepatic failure: experience with more than 200 patients over a 17-year period. *Ann Surg.* 2003;237:666–675; discussion 675–676.

Hoofnagle JH, Carithers RL Jr, Shapiro C, Ascher N. Fulminant hepatic failure: summary of a workshop. *Hepatology.* 1995;21:240–252.

O'Grady JG, Alexander GJ, Hayllar KM, Williams R. Early indicators of prognosis in fulminant hepatic failure. *Gastroenterology.* 1989;97:439–445.

Ostapowicz G, Fontana RJ, Schiodt FV, et al. Results of a prospective study of acute liver failure at 17 tertiary care centers in the United States. *Ann Intern Med.* 2002;137:947–954.

Polson J, Lee WM. AASLD position paper: the management of acute liver failure. *Hepatology.* 2005;41:1179–1197.

Ringe B, Lubbe N, Kuse E, et al. Total hepatectomy and liver transplantation as two-stage procedure. *Ann Surg.* 1993;218:3–9.

Shakil AO, Kramer D, Mazariegos GV, et al. Acute liver failure: clinical features, outcome analysis, and applicability of prognostic criteria. Liver Transpl 2000;6:163–169.

Stravitz RT, Kramer DJ. Management of acute liver failure. *Nat Rev Gastroenterol Hepatol.* 2009;6:542–553.

van Hoek B, de Boer J, Boudjema K, et al. Auxiliary versus orthotopic liver transplantation for acute liver failure. EURALT Study Group. European Auxiliary Liver Transplant Registry. *J Hepatol.* 1999;30:699–705.

CHAPTER 159

Cirrhosis and its Complications

Patricia Wong, MD, MSCE
Jennifer C. Price, MD
H. Franklin Herlong, MD

Key Clinical Questions

1. What findings are commonly seen on physical examination, laboratory studies, and imaging studies in patients with cirrhosis?
2. How is the etiology of ascites determined and by sending what studies of ascitic fluid?
3. What are common causes of renal failure in patients with cirrhosis?
4. How is hepatorenal syndrome diagnosed and treated?
5. How can hepatic encephalopathy present clinically, and what are the treatment options?

INTRODUCTION

Cirrhosis describes the end stage of chronic liver disease from any etiology. Histologically, injured and regenerating hepatocytes are surrounded by extracellular matrix or fibrosis, creating a nodular appearance to the liver parenchyma. A presumptive diagnosis of cirrhosis without histologic confirmation can often be made on clinical grounds alone. A palpable, enlarged left liver lobe with a small right lobe is highly suggestive of cirrhosis. Splenomegaly implies the presence of portal hypertension and cirrhosis. Cutaneous changes, such as spider angiomata and palmar erythema (**Figure 159-1**) and complications of end-stage liver disease, such as ascites and hepatic encephalopathy, are also strongly associated with underlying cirrhosis. While these physical findings have a high specificity for cirrhosis, their sensitivity is low.

Laboratory tests that assess hepatic synthetic capacity such as prothrombin time (PT) or international normalized ratio (INR) and albumin concentration may be helpful in making the diagnosis of cirrhosis but can be confounded by variables such as nutritional status and comorbid conditions. Thrombocytopenia in a patient with chronic liver disease is the most sensitive and specific laboratory abnormality for cirrhosis. In patients with chronic hepatitis C infection, a ratio of AST to ALT that is greater than one has a high correlation with cirrhotic changes seen on liver biopsy. Cross-sectional imaging studies of the liver, including computed tomography, ultrasonography, and magnetic resonance imaging, are not sensitive for diagnosing cirrhosis, particularly in its early stages. However, they are reasonably accurate for detecting changes associated with late stages of cirrhosis, such as a small, nodular-appearing liver, splenomegaly, prominent collateral vessels in the portal circulation, and ascites.

PRACTICE POINT

- Thrombocytopenia in a patient with chronic liver disease is the most sensitive and specific laboratory abnormality for cirrhosis. Cross-sectional imaging studies of the liver, including computed tomography (CT), ultrasonography (US), and magnetic resonance imaging (MRI), are not sensitive for diagnosing cirrhosis, particularly in its early stages.

Patients with cirrhosis may be asymptomatic (compensated) or have symptoms resulting from complications of end-stage liver disease (decompensated). Patients with compensated liver disease have no increase in mortality compared to healthy patients. However, over a 10-year period, approximately 50% of these patients will develop decompensated liver disease. The most common complications of cirrhosis include ascites, variceal bleeding, and encephalopathy. Decompensation dramatically affects survival. The median survival of patients with decompensated cirrhosis is two years.

This chapter focuses on the pathophysiology, diagnosis, and management of four types of cirrhotic decompensation: ascites, spontaneous bacterial peritonitis, hepatorenal syndrome, and hepatic encephalopathy. Management of variceal bleeding is discussed in Chapter 155 on Upper Gastrointestinal Bleeding.

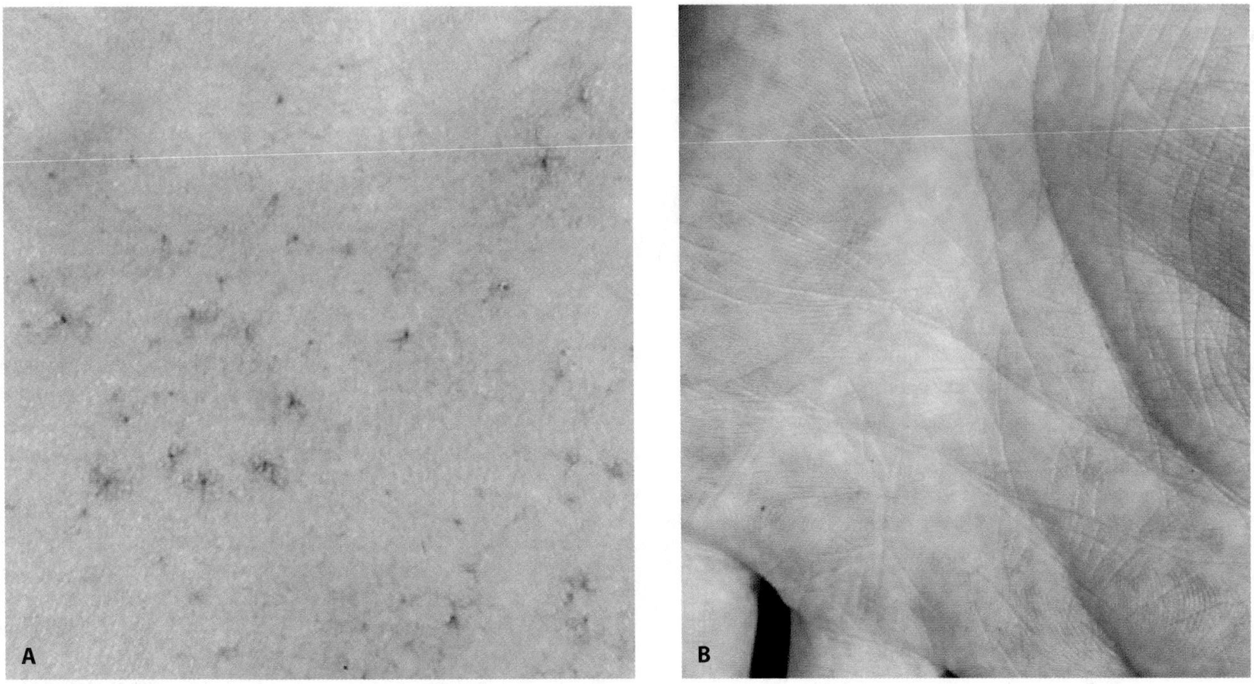

Figure 159-1 *(A) Spider angiomata. (Reproduced, with permission, from Wolff K, Goldsmith LA, Katz SI, et al. Fitzpatrick's Dermatology in General Medicine. 7th ed. New York: McGraw-Hill; 2008. Fig. 151-9.) (B) Palmar erythema (Reproduced, with permission, from Wolff K, Goldsmith LA, Katz SI, et al. Fitzpatrick's Dermatology in General Medicine. 7th ed. New York: McGraw-Hill; 2008. Fig. 151-8.)*

ASCITES

Ascites is an accumulation of fluid within the peritoneal cavity. Many diseases can lead to the formation of ascitic fluid (**Table 159-1**). Ascites usually results from either portal hypertension or peritoneal disease. By far the most common cause of ascites is cirrhosis, accounting for 85% of cases. The remaining 15% is caused by peritoneal malignancy, followed by congestive heart failure. Tuberculous peritonitis is a common cause of ascites in endemic regions (developing countries) of the world, but is rarely seen in the U.S.

Ascites is the most common complication of cirrhosis and the most frequent reason for hospitalization in cirrhotic patients. The development of ascites represents an important transition point in the natural history of cirrhosis, as approximately 15% of patients with cirrhosis die within one year of forming ascites, and 50% die within five years. Many practitioners consider new-onset ascites an indication for liver transplantation evaluation.

PATHOPHYSIOLOGY OF ASCITES

The pathogenesis of ascites in cirrhosis involves two key factors: high pressure in the hepatic sinusoids (portal hypertension) and increased renal retention of sodium (**Figure 159-2**). Distortion of normal hepatic vascular architecture from formation of regenerating nodules and fibrous tissue results in increased resistance to blood flow and an increase in sinusoidal pressure. Splanchnic arterial vasodilation, mediated by increased production of nitric oxide, increases flow in the vessels entering the liver and exacerbates portal hypertension. Cirrhotic patients with ascites have significantly higher portal pressures than cirrhotic patients without ascites. Ascites develops when the hepatic venous pressure gradient, which estimates intrahepatic vascular resistance, exceeds 12 mm Hg.

Dilation of the splanchnic circulation decreases the "effective" circulating arterial blood volume and activates the sympathetic nervous system. Activation of the renin-angiotensin-aldosterone (RAA) system promotes renal arterial vasoconstriction, increased sodium and water absorption, and plasma volume expansion. Increased plasma volume increases lymph formation through splanchnic capillaries and hepatic sinusoids. Lymph formation is further augmented by hypoalbuminemia, which decreases intravascular oncotic pressure.

Early in cirrhosis, the lymphatic system efficiently returns excess lymph produced in the hepatic and splanchnic compartments to the systemic circulation. Increased lymph resorption is evidenced by dilation of hepatic lymphatics and the thoracic duct in some patients with cirrhosis. However, as cirrhosis progresses, the expanded plasma volume and lymph production eventually exceeds return, and continuous formation of ascites occurs within the peritoneal cavity.

DIAGNOSIS OF ASCITES

Accurate detection of ascites is difficult based on the physical exam alone. Shifting dullness is the most reliable sign of ascites but is only 77% sensitive and 72% specific for diagnosing ascites. Fluid wave is the most specific sign for ascites (90% specificity), but lacks sensitivity (62%). Dullness in the flanks is only observed when there is at least 1500 ml of ascitic fluid in the abdomen. Because ascites may result from congestive heart failure or constrictive pericarditis, the jugular veins should be carefully examined for evidence of increased right atrial pressure in all patients with ascites. Diagnosing ascites on the physical exam is particularly challenging in patients who are obese or when the volume of ascites is small and usually requires ultrasonographic confirmation. Ultrasonography can also determine a site where a diagnostic paracentesis can be performed safely and provide information about the liver parenchyma and surrounding vasculature.

A diagnostic paracentesis should be performed in the initial evaluation of all patients with new-onset of ascites. It is the most effective and efficient method of determining the etiology of ascites.

TABLE 159-1 Causes of Ascites

Portal hypertension	Cirrhosis Alcoholic hepatitis Fulminant hepatitis Hepatic veno-occlusive disease Massive liver metastasis Congestive heart failure Constrictive pericarditis Budd-Chiari syndrome (Hepatic vein thrombosis)
Hypoalbuminemia	Nephrotic syndrome Protein-losing enteropathy Malnutrition
Peritoneal disease	Malignant ascites Peritoneal mesothelioma, peritoneal carcinomatosis Tuberculosis Chlamydia trachomatis Fungal peritonitis Candida albicans, Histoplasma capsulatum, Coccidioides immitis, Cryptococcus neoformans Parasitic peritonitis Schistosoma mansoni, Strongyloides stercoralis, Entamoeba histolytica Sarcoidosis Barium peritonitis Vasculitis Systemic lupus erythematosus Henoch-Schonnlein purpura Eosinophilic gastroenteritis Whipple disease
Miscellaneous	Myxedema Ovarian disease Carcinoma, benign tumors, ovarian hyperstimulation syndrome Pancreatic ascites Biliary ascites Chylous ascites Nephrogenic ascites Acquired immune deficiency syndrome (AIDS)

It should also be performed in all cirrhotic patients with signs of decompensation such as encephalopathy, fever, or renal insufficiency. Infected ascitic fluid can cause or exacerbate all of these complications of cirrhosis. The optimal site for needle insertion is in the left lower quadrant, 3 cm cephalad and 3 cm medial to the anterior superior iliac spine (See Chapter 116, Paracentesis procedure chapter, for more detailed description of Paracentesis procedure). The abdominal wall is thinner and fluid tends to pool at this location. A diagnostic paracentesis is a safe procedure, with serious complications occurring in less than 1/1000 procedures. In a study of more than 1000 paracenteses, no significant bleeding complications occurred, even in the setting of significant thrombocytopenia and prolongation of the prothrombin time. Bleeding complications occur almost exclusively in patients with underlying renal failure, presumably from platelet dysfunction.

Routine analysis of ascitic fluid (**Table 159-2**) should include total protein and albumin concentrations and a cell count with differential. Simultaneous serum albumin concentration should be determined in order to calculate the serum-to-ascites albumin gradient (SAAG). The SAAG is the most helpful test in determining the etiology of ascites (**Figure 159-3**). In patients with cirrhosis and ascites, the SAAG correlates with the degree of sinusoidal hypertension (sinusoidal pressure of 11 mg Hg = SAAG of 1.1 g/dl). If the SAAG is greater than 1.1 g/dl, it is assumed that the sinusoidal pressure is at or exceeds 12 mm Hg and that the ascites is secondary to portal hypertension (presinusoidal, sinusoidal, or postsinusoidal). If the SAAG is less than 1.1 g/dl, the cause of ascites is not related to portal hypertension. Total protein is usually low in cirrhosis (< 1g/dl) and high (> 2.5 g/dl) in most other disease states. Low ascitic protein and albumin in cirrhotic ascites is believed to be secondary to "capillarization" of hepatic sinusoids in cirrhotic livers, where fibrosis occurs within the endothelial lining, obliterating fenestrae and preventing macromolecules such as proteins and complement from entering into the subendothelial space. Spontaneous bacterial peritonitis (SBP) can be diagnosed by a total polymorphonuclear (PMN) cell concentration that exceeds 250/mm^3.

Based on the results of these initial screening tests, additional tests can be ordered when appropriate. If there is a reasonable index of suspicion for bacterial peritonitis, 10–20 ml of ascitic fluid should be inoculated into blood culture bottles at the bedside (see SBP section). Milky (chylous) ascites should be tested for elevated triglyceride levels, which may suggest lymphatic obstruction, or, rarely, cirrhosis. If the SAAG is low and there are reasons to suspect tuberculosis, it is appropriate to check an adenosine deaminase level and AFB culture. In the setting of peritoneal carcinomatosis, ascitic cytology is positive in more than 95% of cases. Patients with chronic pancreatitis or pancreatic duct leak may form pancreatic ascites when ascitic fluid amylase concentration exceeds serum amylase concentrations. Clinicians should exclude malignancy and tuberculosis as causes of ascites if risk factors and clinical suspicion support these diagnoses, as these diseases are associated with high mortality and require specialized treatments.

MANAGEMENT OF ASCITES

Management of ascites (Figure 159-2) in the hospitalized patient depends on the etiology of the ascites. Hospitalized patients with *tense ascites* due to portal hypertension may benefit symptomatically from large-volume paracentesis. Large volume paracentesis should not be performed in patients with SBP, as it may precipitate renal dysfunction.

To prevent reaccumulation of fluid, the mainstay of therapy for ascites is sodium restriction and diuretic therapy. Mobilization of ascites requires a negative sodium balance, which is determined by dietary intake and renal sodium excretion. The degree of sodium restriction depends on renal sodium retention. Patients who excrete relatively higher amounts of sodium (24-hour urine sodium ≥ 25 mEq) can be placed on a 2g/day sodium restriction. Patient who are sodium avid (24-hour urine sodium < 25 mEq) require 1g/day restriction. Because fluid retention in ascites results from inappropriate renal retention of sodium, *free water restriction* generally is not necessary unless the patient is hyponatremic, with a serum sodium of less than 125 mEq/L.

Spironolactone and furosemide are the most commonly used diuretics in the management of ascites. They promote natruesis through different mechanisms. Spironolactone acts as a competitive inhibitor of aldosterone in the distal nephron. Furosemide inhibits

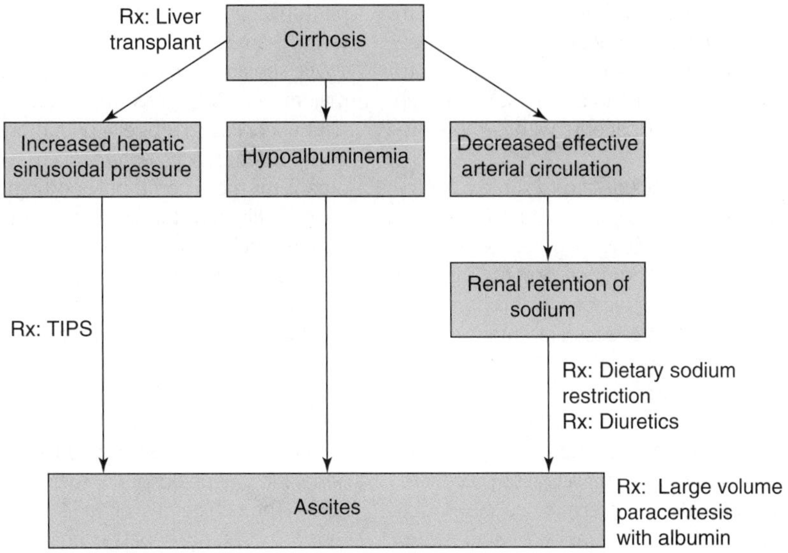

Figure 159-2 *Pathophysiology and available treatment (Rx) of ascites in cirrhosis. TIPS, transjugular intrahepatic porto-systemic shunt.*

the Na^+-$2Cl^-$-K^+ transport system in the ascending limb of the loop of Henle. Simultaneous administration increases the natriuretic effect of both drugs and reduces the incidence of potassium imbalance that can occur when given alone. Diuretics should be initiated with a diuresis goal of approximately 1 liter per day. If the patient does not have signs of peripheral edema, a smaller diuresis goal of 500 cc per day is appropriate, as more rapid removal can lead to plasma volume depletion.

Oral spironolactone is initiated first at 100 mg daily, followed by oral furosemide at 40 mg daily. These medications can be slowly increased at the same ratio if the patient's renal function tolerates it, to a maximum dose of spironolactone 400 mg daily and furosemide 160 mg daily. A spot urine sodium to potassium concentration ratio that exceeds 1 indicates that a patient has effective aldosterone blockade and should respond to sodium restriction. In contrast to hospitalized patients with ascites due to congestive heart failure, patients with cirrhotic ascites should *not* be treated with aggressive *intravenous diuresis*, as this often leads to azotemia.

PRACTICE POINT

- Diuretics should be initiated with a diuresis goal of approximately 1 liter per day (or 500 cc per day if no peripheral edema is present). Oral spironolactone is initiated first at 100 mg daily, followed by oral furosemide at 40 mg daily. These medications can be slowly increased at the same ratio if the patient's renal function tolerates it, to a maximum dose of spironolactone 400 mg daily and furosemide 160 mg daily. Intravenous diuretics should be avoided in patients with ascites due to cirrhosis.

Patients with continued fluid accumulation despite sodium restriction and diuretic therapy have refractory ascites. There are two subtypes of refractory ascites. Diuretic-resistant ascites cannot

TABLE 159-2 Analysis of Ascitic Fluid

Routine analysis: performed in all patients with new onset ascites or cirrhotic patient with encephalopathy, fever, or renal insufficiency
Total protein
Albumin
Cell count and differential
Culture
Additional tests: performed as appropriate based on suspicion of underlying disease
Triglyceride (chylous ascites)
Cytology (malignant ascites)
Amylase (pancreatic ascites)
Adenosine deaminase (Tuberculous peritonitis)
AFB culture (Tuberculous peritonitis)

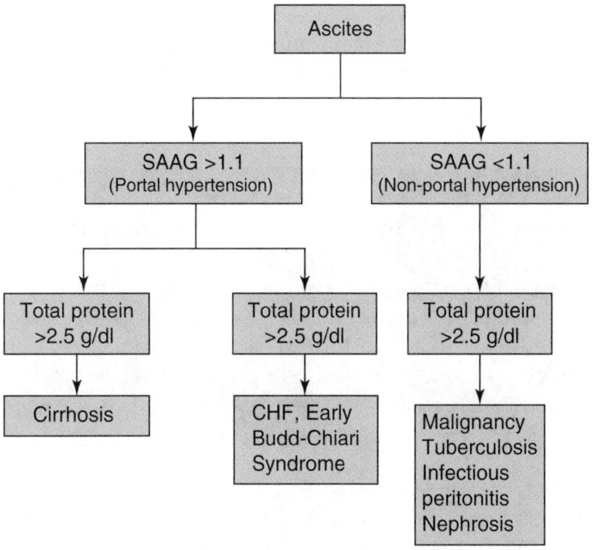

Figure 159-3 *Differential diagnosis of ascites. CHF, Congestive Heart Failure; SAAG, Serum to Ascites Albumin Gradient.*

be mobilized or recurs quickly despite maximal dietary sodium restriction and diuretic doses. Diuretic-intractable ascites is persistent ascites due to limitations in diuretic usage secondary to diuretic-induced complications, such as rise in creatinine or hepatic encephalopathy. Approximately 10% of patients with cirrhotic ascites develop refractory ascites.

Treatment options for these patients include large volume paracentesis (LVP), transjugular intrahepatic portosystemic shunt (TIPS), and liver transplantation. Serial paracenteses, usually 4–6 liters per session, can be effective at symptomatically treating these patients. Albumin replacement during LVP (10 grams per liter removed) remains controversial. Its administration is for prevention of postparacentesis circulatory dysfunction caused by further activation of the sympathetic nervous system and RAA system due to fluid shifts that result in decreased systemic blood volume. Colloid replacement with 25% intravenous albumin appears to be most appropriate when more than 5 liters are removed, and should be initiated during the paracentesis procedure. Placement of TIPS is usually performed by an interventional radiologist. It has been demonstrated to be very effective at decreasing ascites recurrence but it is associated with increased risk of encephalopathy and is poorly tolerated in patients with advanced liver disease.

Nonsteroidal anti-inflammatory drugs (NSAIDS) should be avoided in patients with cirrhosis and ascites because they can lead to sodium retention and renal insufficiency through inhibition of cyclooxygenase and prostaglandin synthesis. This is particularly critical in cirrhotic patients who maintain high renin levels and rely on prostaglandin synthesis to ensure sufficient renal blood flow and adequate GFR.

COMPLICATION OF ASCITES

Spontaneous bacterial peritonitis

Spontaneous bacterial peritonitis (SBP) is a bacterial infection of ascitic fluid without an apparent intra-abdominal source of infection, and thought to be due to translocation of bacteria across the bowel wall. Pathogenesis of SBP may involve disruption of intestinal permeability barrier and increased susceptibility of cirrhotic ascites to infection due to low complement concentration. The classic clinical manifestations of SBP include ascites, abdominal pain, fever, and altered mental status. However, patients with SBP may be asymptomatic or present with much more subtle symptoms, such as mild confusion. Because of this and the importance of early treatment to prevent adverse outcomes, all patients hospitalized with ascites should undergo diagnostic paracentesis at the time of admission to evaluate for SBP. Patients should have a repeat diagnostic paracentesis during their hospitalization if they develop clinical symptoms or laboratory abnormalities concerning for infection.

PRACTICE POINT

- The classic clinical manifestations of spontaneous bacterial peritonitis (SBP) include ascites, abdominal pain, fever, and altered mental status. However, patients with SBP may be asymptomatic or present with much more subtle symptoms, such as mild confusion. Therefore, all patients hospitalized with ascites should undergo diagnostic paracentesis at the time of admission to evaluate for SBP.

The diagnosis of SBP is made through analysis of ascitic fluid (**Table 159-3**). A neutrophil absolute cell count ≥250 cells/mm^3 or a positive ascitic culture without evidence of an intra-abdominal source of infection is diagnostic of SBP. The exception is tuberculous peritonitis, in which ascitic WBC may exceed 500 cells/mm^3 but fewer than 50% are PMNs. *In evaluating grossly bloody ascitic fluid, 1 WBC should be subtracted for every 750 red blood cells in the fluid.* The majority of pathogens implicated in SBP are Gram-negative rods (Escherichia coli, Klebsiella pneumoniae) followed by Gram-positive cocci (Streptococci, enterococcus, pneumococcus). Gram-positive organisms more commonly occur in patients on selective intestinal decontamination for SBP prophylaxis. Culture negative, neutrophil positive ascites occurs commonly (15–50%), and a positive ascitic fluid culture is not necessary for the diagnosis of SBP. Findings of polymicrobial infection, anaerobes, high protein concentration (>1g/dl), high PMN counts (≥250 cells/mm^3), low glucose (<50 mg/dl) or high LDH (>serum upper limit of normal), should raise suspicion for secondary peritonitis, such as perforated viscus, diverticulitis, or intra-abdominal abscess.

Uncomplicated SBP should be treated for five days with a third generation cephalosporin such as cefotaxime 2g IV every eight hours. The choice of antibiotic can be adjusted based on results of sensitivity testing. Renal failure is a common and serious complication of SBP. To reduce this risk and improve survival, IV albumin, which acts as a plasma expander, is indicated in addition to antibiotics. Albumin is dosed at 1.5 g/kg body weight on day one of SBP diagnosis and 1 g/kg on day three. Patients with secondary bacterial peritonitis should undergo abdominal computed tomography (CT) scanning and surgery as indicated. They should also receive approximately two weeks of a third generation cephalosporin plus metronidazole for anaerobic coverage.

PRACTICE POINT

- Uncomplicated SBP should be treated with antibiotics for five days. Intravenous albumin reduces the risk of renal failure and improves survival in patients with SBP. Albumin is dosed at 1.5 g/kg body weight on day one of SBP diagnosis and 1 g/kg on day three.

Repeating the paracentesis after 48 hours of treatment is not routinely necessary in patients with SBP but should be performed if the patient is not responding clinically to treatment or in cases of secondary peritonitis. Following an episode of SBP,

TABLE 159-3 Evaluation and Management of Spontaneous Bacterial Peritonitis (SBP)

Criteria for the diagnosis of SBP (only 1 necessary)
Ascitic fluid neutrophil count ≥250 cell/mm^3
Ascitic culture grows typical organism(s)
Antibiotic use
Treatment: all patients who meet criteria for SBP
Third generation cephalosporin (IV) for five days (based on sensitivity of organism)
Albumin 1.5 g/kg body weight (day one) and 1.0 g/kg body weight (day three)
Prophylaxis: all patients with a history of SBP
Oral fluoroquinolone (norfloxacin 400 mg) once daily or double strength trimethoprim-sulfamethoxazole once daily
Prophylaxis: all patients with cirrhosis and acute gastrointestinal bleeding
Third generation cephalosporin (IV) and/or oral fluoroquinolone for seven days total

antibiotic prophylaxis with either an oral flouroquinolone, such as norfloxacin 400 mg daily, or trimethoprim-sulfamethoxazole one double strength tablet daily reduces recurrence of SBP. Patients with a history of SBP should be prescribed prophylactic antibiotics at hospital discharge. Prophylaxis may also be indicated for inpatients without a history of SBP but at higher risk of SBP due to a low-protein ascites (ascitic fluid total protein < 1 g/dl). However, the benefit of long-term prophylaxis is controversial in these patients, and current guidelines recommend prophylaxis during inpatient admission only. Finally, a seven-day course of SBP prophylaxis is also warranted in patients with cirrhosis and upper gastrointestinal bleeding, independent of the presence of ascites. Antibiotic choice should target Gram-negative bacteria. Third generation cephalosporins have efficacy in this situation. The antibiotic can be changed to oral norfloxacin 400 mg daily if the patient is discharged prior to completion of the seven-day course.

HEPATORENAL SYNDROME

The hepatorenal syndrome (HRS) is a functional renal impairment associated with abnormalities of the arterial circulation and endogenous vasoactive systems. Other causes of acute renal failure, including intrinsic renal disease, prerenal azotemia, acute tubular necrosis, and toxic insult to the kidneys must be excluded to make the diagnosis. HRS is considered functional because the kidneys themselves are morphologically intact, and renal function can be restored in these patients following liver transplantation.

The incidence of HRS in patients with cirrhosis who are hospitalized for ascites is approximately 10%. The incidence of HRS in patients with cirrhosis and ascites without azotemia, was 18% within one year and 39% within five years, according to one study. Patients with HRS typically present with oliguria, a rising serum creatinine, and marked sodium retention (urine sodium < 10 mEq/L). Renal function does not improve with 1.5 liter of a plasma volume expander. There are two different types of HRS (**Table 159-4**) that share the same pathogenic mechanism but vary in clinical presentation of the renal failure. Type I HRS is the more aggressive form and is defined by a rapid doubling of serum creatinine to > 2.5 mg/dl or a 50% reduction in creatinine clearance to < 20 ml/min in less than two weeks. Type I HRS is associated with a very poor prognosis and high mortality. Without treatment, the median survival of patients with type 1 HRS is less than two weeks and most patients die within 8–10 weeks after the onset of renal failure. Type II HRS is characterized by impaired renal function in which serum creatinine > 1.5 mg/dl, but criteria for Type 1 HRS are not met. These patients have a better prognosis than patients with Type 1 HRS.

TABLE 159-4 Definitions of Two Types of Hepatorenal Syndrome (HRS)

HRS Type 1
Rapidly progressing renal failure (< 2 weeks)
≥ 2-fold increase of serum creatinine to > 2.5 mg/dL (221 umol/L) or
50% decrease of creatinine clearance to < 20 mL/min
HRS Type 2
Serum creatinine > 1.5 mg/dL (132.6 umol/L) or
Creatinine clearance < 40 mL/min
Criteria for HRS type 1 not met

PATHOPHYSIOLOGY OF HEPATORENAL SYNDROME

HRS is primarily mediated by renal arterial vasoconstriction. The pathogenesis of renal vasoconstriction in HRS is not completely understood, but it is related to changes in systemic hemodynamics, similar to those described in the pathogenesis of ascites. Vasodilation of the splanchnic circulation leads to a drop in effective circulating systemic blood volume, which activates the sympathetic nervous system. Vasoconstrictor mechanisms are triggered including release of ADH and activation of the renin-angiotensin-aldosterone system (RAA). Activation of the RAA system promotes renal arterial vasoconstriction, increased sodium and water absorption, and plasma volume expansion. Local renal vasodilators cannot overcome the systemic vasoconstrictor systems and renal function becomes progressively compromised.

HRS can develop spontaneously or can be triggered by a precipitating factor. The most common precipitating trigger for type 1 HRS is SBP. Other triggers include systemic bacterial infection and large volume paracentesis without adequate plasma expansion.

PRACTICE POINT

- The most common precipitating trigger for type 1 hepatorenal syndrome (HRS) is spontaneous bacterial peritonitis (SBP). Other triggers include systemic bacterial infection and large volume paracentesis without adequate plasma expansion.

DIAGNOSIS OF HEPATORENAL SYNDROME

Criteria for the diagnosis of HRS proposed by the International Ascites Club include five major and five minor criteria (**Table 159-5**). All major criteria must be present to make the diagnosis of HRS.

TABLE 159-5 Criteria for the Diagnosis of Hepatorenal Syndrome (HRS) According to the Consensus of the International Ascites Club*

Major Criteria
Chronic or acute liver disease with advanced hepatic failure and portal hypertension
Low glomerular filtration rate, as indicated by serum creatinine of > 1.5 mg/d or 24 h creatinine clearance < 40 mL/min
Absence of shock, ongoing bacterial infection, and current or recent treatment with nephrotoxic drugs. Absence of gastrointestinal fluid losses or renal fluid losses
No sustained improvement in renal function (decrease in serum creatinine to 1.5 mg/dL or less or increase in creatinine clearance to 40 mL/min or more) following diuretic withdrawal and expansion of plasma volume with 1.5L of isotonic saline
Proteinuria < 500 mg/dL and no ultrasonographic evidence of obstructive uropathy or parenchymal renal disease
Minor Criteria
Urine volume < 500 mL/d
Urine sodium < 10 mEq/L
Urine osmolality greater than plasma osmolality
Urine red blood cells < 50 per high power field
Serum sodium concentration < 130 mEq/L

*All major criteria must be present for the diagnosis. Minor criteria support the diagnosis but are not necessary.

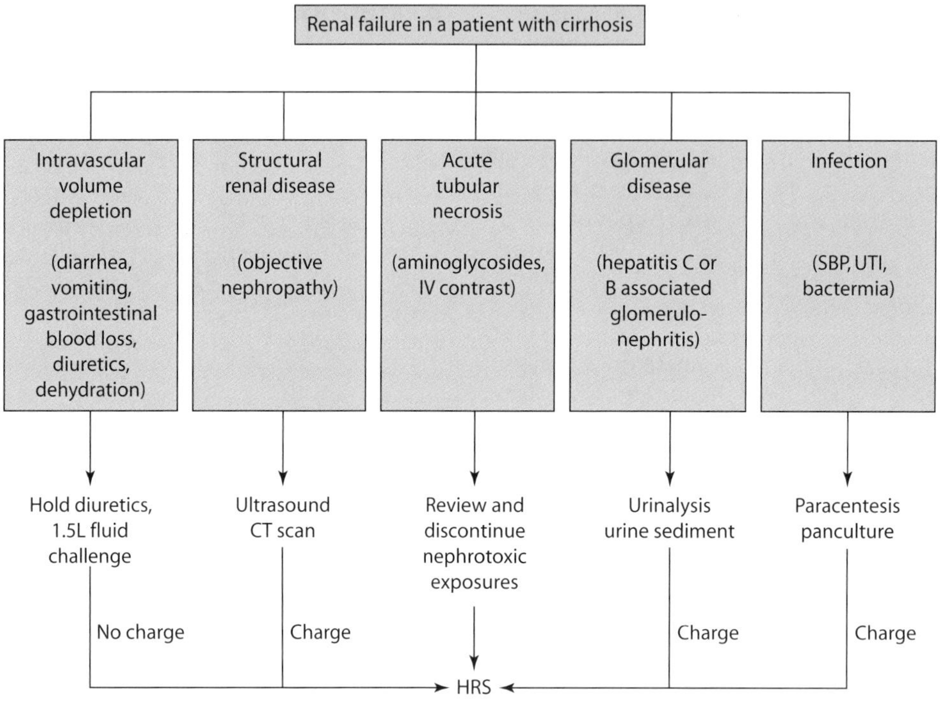

Figure 159-4 *Evaluation of renal failure in cirrhosis. CT, computed tomography; HRS, hepatorenal syndrome; IV, intravenous; SBP, spontaneous bacterial peritonitis; UTI, urinary tract infection.*

Minor criteria are not required but provide additional evidence supporting the diagnosis.

The diagnosis of HRS requires a thorough evaluation for and exclusion of alternative causes of renal failure (**Figure 159-4**). Patients with cirrhosis have increased risk for multiple causes of renal failure, including hypovolemia (secondary to large-volume paracentesis, over-diuresis, poor fluid intake, diarrhea, GI bleeding), acute tubular necrosis (secondary to shock, infection, GI bleeding), nephrotoxic medications (including NSAIDS and aminoglycosides), contrast nephropathy, allergic interstitial nephritis, and intrinsic renal disease. Although it can be difficult to distinguish HRS from acute tubular necrosis or prerenal azotemia, this is an important distinction to make given the poorer prognosis associated with HRS. One way to differentiate HRS and prerenal azotemia is to assess the patient's renal response to a 1.5 liter fluid challenge; a lack of improvement in renal function is required for the diagnosis of HRS.

MANAGEMENT OF HEPATORENAL SYNDROME

Several pharmacologic agents have been investigated for the treatment of HRS, including systemic vasoconstrictors, renal vasodilators, endothelin blockers, and N-acetylcysteine. Of these, the combination of vasoconstrictors and plasma expanders has shown the most promise in terms of efficacy and safety. Intravenous albumin (1 g/kg on day 1, then 20–40 g/day), combined with the alpha-1 adrenergic agonist midodrine (7.5 mg to 12.5 mg orally three times daily) and the somatostatin analogue octreotide (100 μg to 200 μg subcutaneously three times daily) improved renal function and decreased mortality in small studies of patients with HRS. Medications should be titrated to achieve at least a 15 mm Hg increase in mean arterial pressure.

The vasopressin analogs ornipressin and terlipressin cause splanchnic vasoconstriction, thereby counteracting the splanchnic vasodilation that is central to the pathophysiology of HRS. Though effective at improving renal function in HRS, ornipressin is associated with ischemic side effects, thus precluding its use in treating HRS. Terlipressin has been shown to improve renal function in randomized controlled trials among patients with HRS. However, it has not been shown to improve survival and is associated with more cardiovascular complications than placebo. Currently, terlipressin is not available for use in the United States.

PRACTICE POINT

- Intravenous albumin (25%, 1 g/kg on day 1, then 20–40 g/day), combined with midodrine (7.5 mg to 12.5 mg orally three times daily) and octreotide (100 μg to 200 μg subcutaneously three times daily) improved renal function and decreased mortality in hepatorenal syndrome (HRS). Medications should be titrated to achieve at least a 15 mm Hg increase in mean arterial pressure.

Though TIPS may be useful in treating HRS by decreasing portal hypertension, there are limited data supporting its use for the management of HRS. Many patients who meet the diagnostic criteria for HRS are not TIPS candidates due to the severity of their liver disease. In those stable enough to undergo TIPS, the procedure may improve renal function in the short term but there is no evidence for improved survival.

Renal replacement therapy (RRT) in HRS is generally used as a bridge to liver transplantation, although there have been no controlled studies evaluating the effectiveness of dialysis in HRS or the survival benefits of dialysis pretransplant. The likelihood of recovery of renal function in HRS depends on the improvement of liver function, and survival on dialysis correlates with severity of liver disease. For this reason, patients with potentially reversible liver disease, as in acute fulminant hepatitis, may benefit from RRT. However, dialysis is not recommended for patients with irreversible liver

TABLE 159-6 Stages of Hepatic Encephalopathy

Stage	Consciousness	Intellect	Neuromotor Abnormalities
Subclinical	Normal	Normal	Present on testing
1	Lack of awareness	Forgetful	Uncoordination
2	Lethargic, drowsy	Disorientation	Asterixis
3	Somnolent, arousable	Incommunicative	Abnormal reflexes
4	Coma	Absent	Decerebrate

damage who are not liver transplantation candidates. Patients with decompensated cirrhosis and HRS often tolerate intermittent hemodialysis poorly and require continuous veno-venous hemodialysis.

Liver transplantation is the best treatment for HRS because it offers a potential cure for both the liver disease and renal dysfunction. Liver transplantation reverses the primary pathophysiologic circulatory abnormalities that underlie HRS. Most patients recover renal function after transplantation. However, the longer a patient has had HRS prior to transplantation, the less likely he or she is to recover normal renal function post-transplant. HRS is also associated with increased morbidity and early mortality after transplantation.

HEPATIC ENCEPHALOPATHY

Hepatic encephalopathy (HE) is a complex syndrome that results in neuropsychiatric disturbances in patients with cirrhosis or acute liver failure. Symptoms can range from subtle abnormalities, detectable only through specialized neuropsychological testing, to overt coma. The various stages of encephalopathy are based on level of consciousness, cognitive function, behavioral disturbances, and neuromuscular features (**Table 159-6**). Mild symptoms such as sleep pattern reversal, confusion, irritability, or altered personality may be apparent only to close contacts. For this reason, it is often helpful to evaluate a cirrhotic patient in the presence of family members.

A classification system for HE was established by the World Congress of Gastroenterology in 1998 (**Table 159-7**). This system is based on the nature of the underlying liver disease and the persistence and severity of symptoms. HE can be associated with acute liver failure, porto-systemic shunting without intrinsic liver disease, and cirrhosis. HE encephalopathy associated with cirrhosis can be further characterized as episodic, persistent, or minimal. Episodic HE develops over a short period of time and fluctuates in severity.

TABLE 159-7 World Congress of Gastroenterology Classification System for Hepatic Encephalopathy (HE)

Type A: encephalopathy associated with *acute* liver failure
Type B: encephalopathy caused by portal-systemic bypass without intrinsic hepatocellular disease
Type C: encephalopathy associated with cirrhosis and portal hypertension or porto-systemic shunt
Episodic—delirium that develops over a short period of time and fluctuates in severity
Persistent—continuous overt neurologic or behavioral abnormalities
Minimal—no clinically overt cognitive dysfunction, but cognitive impairment seen on neuropsychological studies

Patients with persistent HE exhibit continuous overt neurologic or behavioral abnormalities. Minimal hepatic encephalopathy (MHE) is a milder form of HE in which impairment in cognitive function is only detectable through neuropsychological testing. The etiology and management of each of these forms of HE varies.

PATHOPHYSIOLOGY OF HEPATIC ENCEPHALOPATHY

Multiple factors contribute to the development of hepatic encephalopathy, but the exact pathogenesis remains unclear. Most theories postulate that the brain is exposed to toxic substances that are produced by bacterial flora. These substances are generated through processing of nitrogenous dietary compounds and are incompletely cleared from the blood by the compromised liver. Ammonia was the first neurotoxic substance identified and has been extensively studied. The majority of patients with overt HE have elevated plasma levels of ammonia. However, *the level of hyperammonemia does not necessarily correlate with degree of hepatic encephalopathy.*

There are several mechanisms by which ammonia affects central nervous system (CNS) function. Patients with HE have increased ammonia diffusion across the blood-brain barrier. Ammonia enters CNS astrocytes and combines with the neurotransmitter glutamate to form glutamine. Glutamine is converted back to ammonia and glutamate within astrocyte mitochondria. Mitochondrial ammonia stimulates production of reactive oxygen species and aquaporin 4, which results in astrocyte swelling and histologic changes known as Alzheimer type II astrocytosis. Ammonia also has deleterious effects on cerebral perfusion and glucose metabolism, which contribute to CNS impairment.

Gamma-aminobutyric acid (GABA), the primary inhibitory neurotransmitter in the CNS, may also play an important role in the pathogenesis of HE. Increased GABA levels have been associated with liver injury and hyperammonemia. The proposed mechanism of increased GABA activity is through increased production of endogenous benzodiazepine ligands by gut bacteria that bind the benzodiazepine site of GABA receptors and upregulates GABA-ergic transmission. The best supporting evidence for this theory is the observation of improvement in mental status in some patients with HE after administration of the benzodiazepine antagonist flumazenil even in the absence of exposure to exogenous benzodiazepines.

Other substances, such as mercaptans, neurosteroids, and manganese may also contribute to HE through neuronal and astrocytic injury. Most likely, all of these factors have varying influences in individual patients with HE depending on the etiology, acuity, and severity of the underlying liver disease.

DIAGNOSIS OF HEPATIC ENCEPHALOPATHY

The diagnosis of HE remains largely clinical. There are no specific signs, symptoms, or laboratory tests that are diagnostic of the disorder. Patients with HE may exhibit a range of altered levels of consciousness and cognitive-behavioral changes. Symptoms commonly associated with HE, however, are nonspecific and can be associated with other conditions such as hypoglycemia, intracranial pathology, uremia, or intoxication. Other causes of altered mental status therefore must be excluded before making the diagnosis of HE. Asterixis, a flapping tremor of the outstretched hands, is a common feature of HE but may also be seen in other metabolic encephalopathies, such as uremia. Focal neurologic deficits such as hemiplegia or hemiparesis, and seizures are rarely observed in patients with HE and should prompt further CNS evaluation, including imaging, to exclude structural lesions. Laboratory abnormalities such as elevated plasma levels of ammonia are commonly seen in HE but are not universal. Routine ordering of plasma ammonia levels in cirrhotic patients with delirium is not recommended to evaluate for or follow the course of HE. Ordering of ammonia levels should be reserved for patients in whom *another etiology* for encephalopathy is reasonably likely to help evaluate the likelihood of HE. Patients with levels above 150 μmol/L are more likely to have hepatic encephalopathy, but elevated levels below that threshold may or may not have hepatic encephalopathy. EEG testing is always abnormal in overt HE, but observed changes, such as triphasic waves, are not specific.

PRACTICE POINT

- The diagnosis of hepatic encephalopathy (HE) remains largely clinical, based on history and physical examination, while ruling out other potential etiologies of encephalopathy. There are no specific signs, symptoms, or laboratory tests that are diagnostic of the disorder. Ammonia levels should not be ordered routinely to evaluate for or follow the course of hepatic encephalopathy.

MANAGEMENT OF HEPATIC ENCEPHALOPATHY

Management of patients with HE associated with acute and chronic liver disease is detailed below. Encephalopathy associated with portal-systemic shunting without intrinsic liver disease will not be discussed.

Hepatic encephalopathy associated with cirrhosis: episodic

In most patients with episodic HE associated with cirrhosis, a precipitating factor can be identified (**Table 159-8**). In general, precipitants alter CNS function by increasing toxin generation, by impairing liver function and enhancing portosystemic shunting of toxins to the brain, by decreasing clearance of toxins, or by enhancing the effects of toxins on the CNS. Common precipitants include gastrointestinal bleeding, infection, hypokalemia, azotemia, acute hepatitis, and drug side effects. A thorough evaluation for precipitating factors is indicated for all hospitalized patients with HE. Identified precipitants must be treated.

TABLE 159-8 Common Precipitants of Episodic Hepatic Encephalopathy Associated with Cirrhosis

Gastrointestinal bleeding
Infection
Hypokalemia
Azotemia
Drug side effects
Excessive protein ingestion
Constipation

Gastrointestinal bleeding is the most common precipitant of episodic HE in patients with cirrhosis. This occurs through a combination of impaired hepatic function from decreased hepatic perfusion and increased production of nitrogenous byproducts from digestion of blood proteins. Evaluation of gastrointestinal blood loss and control of active bleeding must be performed in all patients with episodic HE.

PRACTICE POINT

- Gastrointestinal bleeding is the most common precipitant of episodic hepatic encephalopathy (HE) in patients with cirrhosis. Evaluation of gastrointestinal blood loss and control of active bleeding must be performed in all patients with episodic HE. All patients with HE and ascites should undergo a diagnostic paracentesis to exclude SBP, the most common bacterial infection in hospitalized patients with cirrhosis.

A high prevalence of infection occurs in patients with HE, and a careful assessment for occult infection is indicated in all patients with HE. All patients with HE and ascites should undergo a diagnostic paracentesis to exclude SBP, the most common bacterial infection in hospitalized patients with cirrhosis. If there is a high index of suspicion for infection, empiric antibiotic therapy should be started after cultures have been drawn and before results are known. Cirrhotic patients frequently have baseline neutropenia from hypersplenism and may not exhibit leukocytosis in response to bacterial infections. Patients with advanced liver disease are also often hypothermic and do not mount a fever in response to infection. The mechanism by which infection causes HE in patients with cirrhosis is believed to be cytokine-mediated. Activation of cytokines exacerbates astrocyte swelling, and bacterial cell wall compounds augment the effects of ammonia on cerebral blood flow.

Azotemia and electrolyte disturbances can also cause HE in patients with cirrhosis. Cirrhotic patients, particularly those with ascites, are often exposed to potent diuretics. Intravascular volume depletion from vigorous diuresis can reduce renal perfusion and result in azotemia and increased ammonia production. A hypoklalemic alkalosis can enhance both renal ammonia production and ammonia transport across the blood brain barrier by favoring ammonia over ammonium ion. In these patients, reestablishing intravascular volume and correcting electrolyte imbalances can often reverse encephalopathy without any other specific therapy.

A careful review of medications and diet is also important when evaluating patients with cirrhosis and HE. Exposure to sedatives and analgesics, especially benzodiazepines, can potentiate the effects of putative neurotoxins in HE and should be avoided. In a minority of patients, increased dietary protein intake can precipitate an episode of encephalopathy by increasing the nitrogen load in the gastrointestinal tract. This can often be reversed with simple dietary modifications; however, protein restrictions should not be applied routinely for all patients with cirrhosis or hepatic encephalopathy.

Hepatic encephalopathy associated with cirrhosis: persistent

In patients with cirrhosis and persistent encephalopathy, or those with episodic encephalopathy whose symptoms continue after treatment of underlying precipitating factors, specific therapy directed toward encephalopathy is indicated. All proposed therapies reduce gut bacterial production of toxins derived from intraluminal nitrogenous substances. Although commonly used, the efficacy of most of these therapies remains equivocal based on data from clinical trials and meta-analyses.

Cathartics The nonabsorbable disaccharides (lactulose and lactitol) have remained the mainstay of therapy for HE. Theoretically, lactulose increases ammonia clearance through its cathartic action and decreases intestinal ammonia absorption by "trapping" it in the acidic colonic lumen that results from the accumulation of short-chain fatty acids. Patients often show improvement in symptoms of HE within hours of lactulose administration. However, a Cochrane review concluded that "there is insufficient evidence to determine whether non-absorbable disaccharides are of benefit in patients with HE" and "nonabsorbable dissacharides should not be used as the comparator in randomized trials of HE."

Despite the absence of compelling evidence to support its use, lactulose remains the most commonly used agent for the treatment of HE. It may have the greatest efficacy in patients with HE precipitated by gastrointestinal bleeding, since its cathartic action rapidly evacuates the colon of blood, thereby reducing bacterial protein load. Lactulose is titrated to a goal of producing 3–5 soft bowel movements per day. In most patients, 30 cc administered twice a day is sufficient. Higher or more frequent dosing may cause bloating and excessive diarrhea. For patients who are not able to take oral medications, lactulose can be administered per rectum (300 cc lactulose with 700 cc water). There are few adverse side effects from lactulose other than occasional hypernatremia.

Diet High dietary protein intake may be associated with hepatic encephalopathy. In theory, dietary protein intake stimulates nitrogenous toxin production in the gut. While dietary protein restriction may improve HE in certain individuals, this benefit has been difficult to establish in controlled trials. Many studies of severe acute alcoholic hepatitis even observed that administration of high protein/high calorie diets improved, rather than exacerbated, encephalopathy. Furthermore, protein restriction to less than 40 g per day can accelerate catabolism and contribute to malnutrition. During episodes of severe encephalopathy, dietary protein intake is negligible during the first few days in the hospital. After this initial period, it is reasonable to modestly restrict dietary protein to 1.0 g/kg/day and to observe the patient for clinical improvements. Protein from vegetable sources may be better tolerated than animal-derived protein.

Antibiotics Orally administered poorly absorbed antibiotics may improve HE by decreasing toxin production by gut flora. Several clinical trials have assessed the efficacy of various antibiotics in patients with different classes of HE. Studies of oral metronidazole and oral vancomycin have yielded equivocal results. Rifaximin, a derivative of rifamycin, has broad spectrum activity against Gram-negative rods and Gram-positive cocci. Several studies suggest that rifaximin is superior to disaccharides in patients with both overt and minimal encephalopathy. One recent study showed no increased risk for bacterial overgrowth or fungal colonization with rifaximin therapy for prolonged periods. The recommended dose of rifaximin is 400 mg three times daily. Its use may be limited by cost ($1200–$2000 per month), and FDA approval is still pending. Neomycin, an aminoglycoside, is contraindicated in patients with HE due to the risk of ototoxicity and renal failure.

Other therapies Therapies that enhance ammonia clearance include sodium benzoate, zinc, and L-ornithine L-asparate (LOLA). Sodium benzoate combines with ammonia to produce hippurate, which is renally excreted. It has been used extensively in children with urea cycle deficits and compares favorably with lactulose in patients with HE in limited trials. LOLA increases hepatic conversion of ammonia and performs better than placebo at lowering plasma ammonia and improving encephalopathy grade. Zinc lowers plasma ammonia by increasing ornithine transcarbamylase activity, but its benefits in HE have been inconsistent. Flumazenil, a benzodiazepine receptor antagonist, has been shown to improve HE grade but is not currently FDA-approved for treatment of HE. Branched chain amino acids in several different formulations improve symptoms but not survival and are relatively expensive. Probiotics reduce substrate for other gut bacteria; early trials suggest a possible benefit in minimal encephalopathy.

Hepatic encephalopathy associated with cirrhosis: minimal

Minimal hepatic encephalopathy (MHE) is a milder form of HE in which impairment in cognitive function is only detectable through neuropsychological testing such as the number connection test and block design test. The deficits in MHE are primarily related to visual-spacial orientation, attention deficits, and impaired short-term memory. Oral and written skills are grossly intact. Neuroimaging studies have shown changes in cerebral blood flow and abnormalities on neuropsychological testing. While patients with MHE have no overt symptoms of encephalopathy, they may have a diminished capacity to work or drive. One study comparing physical requirements of employment with concurrent psychomotor and motor deficits concluded that more than half of "blue-collar" workers and one quarter of "white collar" workers with MHE were unfit to work. Studies assessing the effect of MHE on driving through simulator and on-road testing have yielded inconsistent results. Some studies observe no impairment in ability to drive. Other studies have shown that patients with MHE have more collisions and have difficulty following traffic rules and road signs. At present, there is no consensus on driving restrictions for patients with MHE. Several recent controlled trials have suggested that both lactulose and rifaximin improve neuropsychological testing and quality of life in patients with MHE.

Hepatic encephalopathy associated with acute liver failure

The clinical presentation and management of HE associated with acute liver failure differs from HE in cirrhosis and portal hypertension. Cerebral edema and intracranial hypertension is common in HE associated with acute liver failure but rare in chronic liver disease. The risk of cerebral edema correlates with encephalopathic grade. The risk is very low in grades 1 and 2 but progresses to 35% in grade 3 and 75% in grade 4. The reason for the association between cerebral edema and acute liver failure is not known. HE associated with both acute and chronic liver disease can present with marked hyperammonemia and consequences of ammonia on cerebral function should be similar in both types of liver disease. It is possible that markers of systemic inflammation commonly seen in acute liver failure, but not chronic liver disease, may be a contributing factor. Excess free water with hyponatremia may exacerbate ammonia-induced cerebral edema.

PRACTICE POINT

- Cerebral edema and intracranial hypertension is common in hepatic encephalopathy (HE) associated with acute liver failure but rare in chronic liver disease. The risk of cerebral edema correlates with encephalopathic grade, low risk in HE grades 1 and 2 but progresses to 35% in HE grade 3 and 75% in HE grade 4. Patients with acute liver failure who develop grade 2 HE should be admitted to an intensive care unit with integrated monitoring and multiorgan support. Patients with grade 3 HE should be ventilated for airway protection and the head should be elevated to 30 degrees.

TABLE 159-9 Evidence-based Medicine: Key References for Complications of Cirrhosis

Reference	Methodology	Results	Limitations	Bottom Line
Runyon B. *Hepatology.* 2009;49:2087–2107.	Review article	Discusses diagnosis and management of ascites, SBP, and HRS.	Review	AASLD Practice guidelines for management of adult patients with ascites from cirrhosis
Runyon BA, et al. *Ann Intern Med.* 1992;117:215–220.	Prospective observational	SAAG is superior to exudates/transudate concept in establishing cause of ascites	Heterogeneous patient population	The study provides guidelines for the use of the SAAG from ascitic fluid analysis to determine whether ascites is due to cirrhosis
Stanley MM, et al. *N Engl J Med.* 1989;321:1632–1638.	Randomized controlled trial	Used a combination of sodium restriction, spironolactone, and furosemide to treat ascites	Multicenter trial comparing diuretic therapy with peritoneovenous shunt	Ascites can be controlled with medical therapy in 90% of patients
Gines P, et al. *Gastroentrology.* 1987;93:234–241.	Randomized controlled trial	Compared paracentesis with diuretics in the treatment of ascites	Evaluated tense ascites	Large volume paracentesis can be safely performed for control of tense ascites in cirrhosis
Haynes GR, et al. *Eur J Anaesth.* 2003; 20:771–793.	Meta-analysis	79 randomized trials in multiple settings showed albumin infusion reduces rises in creatinine, but no effect on mortality	Included only 10 trials in patients with ascites	No consensus statement as to value of albumin after paracentesis
Salerno F, et al. *Gastroenterology.* 2007;133:825–834.	Meta-analysis	Evaluated TIPS for refractory ascites; included individual patient data; significant improvement in survival ($p = 0.035$) with TIPS and similar likelihood of encephalopathy	Systematic review	Shows improved survival with TIPS compared to medical therapy in patients with refractory ascites
Hoefs JC, et al. *Hepatology.* 1982; 2:399–407.	Observational study	Establishes criteria for diagnosis of SBP as positive culture with PMN count > 250 cells/mm^3	Small study N, limited follow-up time	Established criteria for empiric therapy for SBP
Felisart J, et al. *Hepatology.* 1985;5:457–462.	Randomized controlled trial	Cefotaxime covers 95% of SBP flora	Treatment effectiveness compared to ampicillin-tobramycin only	Suggests Cefotaxime as preferred therapy for suspected SBP
Salerno F. *Gut.* 2007;56: 1310–1318.	Review	Established criteria for diagnosis of 2 types of hepatorenal syndrome	Review	Report of a consensus group on criteria for the diagnosis of hepatorenal syndrome
Esrailian E, et al. *Dig Dis Sci.* 2007;52:742–748.	Retrospective nonrandomized controls	Midodrine/octreotide reduced mortality 43% versus 71% compared to albumin treated controls	Retrospective nonrandomized control	Suggests potential benefit of midodrine/octreotide in type 1 HRS
Ferenci P, et al. *Hepatology;* 2002;35:719.	Review article	Discusses definition and criteria for diagnosis of hepatic encephalopathy	Review article	Defines the three types of encephalopathy
Sundaram V, et al. *Med Clin North Am.* 2009;93:819–836.	Review article	Discussion of pathophysiology, clinical features, and treatment of encephalopathy	Review article	Comprehensive review of the management of hepatic encephalopathy
Als-Nielsen B, et al. *BMJ.* 2004;328:1046.	Meta analysis	Disaccharides compared to placebo or no intervention showed modest but statistically significant benefit	Review article	Nonabsorbable disaccharides improve symptoms in about 75% of patients with overt encephalopathy
Bass N, et al. *N Engl J Med.* 2010;362:1071–1081.	Randomized placebo controlled trial	Rifaximin 550 mg twice a day maintained remission from hepatic encephalopathy more effectively than placebo and reduced risk of hospitalization	6 month study 90% received concomitant lactulose	Over a short interval rifaximin reduced episodes of overt encephalopathy compared to placebo in patients also receiving lactulose

(continued)

TABLE 159-9 Evidence-based Medicine: Key References for Complications of Cirrhosis (*continued*)

Reference	Methodology	Results	Limitations	Bottom Line
Prasad S, et al. *Hepatology*. 2007;45:549–549.	Randomized trial	Lactulose improved cognitive function and quality of life in patients with minimal hepatic encephalopathy	Short duration	Lactulose was beneficial in patients with minimal encephalopathy
Stravitz RT, et al. *Crit Care Med.* 2007 Nov;35(11): 2498–2508.	Guideline	ICP monitoring recommended in advanced hepatic encephalopathy awaiting liver transplantation. For high ICP, use osmotic therapy with IV mannitol to maintain mildly hyperosmotic state and high normal serum sodium to minimize cerebral edema.	Divergent practices exist for some areas of management, and some recommendations supported by limited evidence or expert opinion.	Concensus guidleines direct ICU management of acute liver failure and may direct future studies.

Accurately assessing intracranial pressure (ICP) on clinical grounds is difficult. Physical findings such as papillary changes, abnormalities in the oculovestibular reflex, and decerebrate posturing are indicators of intracranial hypertension but often become apparent at an irreversible stage of HE. Some medical centers advocate the use of invasive monitoring devices to accurately measure ICP. However, one retrospective report from the U.S. Acute Liver Failure Study reported a 10% complication rate associated with invasive ICP monitoring, of which 5% could have contributed to death. There was also no significant improvement in outcomes in patients with invasive monitoring. Therefore, while ICP monitoring generally provides important information, particularly in patients with high grade HE, risks and benefits of its usage are largely dependent on local expertise on placement and interpretation of the devices.

Patients with acute liver failure who develop grade 2 HE should be admitted to an intensive care unit with integrated monitoring and multiorgan support. Patients with grade 3 HE should be ventilated for airway protection, and the head should be elevated to 30 degrees. Intravenous hypotonic solutions should be avoided because of the risk of hyponatremia-induced cerebral edema. Bolus infusions of mannitol (0.5 to 1.0 g/kg) or hypertonic saline should be given to patients with objective evidence of increased ICP. Temporary hyperventilation with a goal $PaCO_2$ of 25 mm Hg may be helpful if the ICP cannot be adequately lowered with mannitol. Most patients require renal replacement therapy (RRT) to lower ammonia levels since lactulose is ineffective in acute liver failure. Intracranial hypertension refractory to medical management should prompt consideration for liver transplantation. More detailed instructions for the management of patients with acute liver failure can be found in recommendations published by the U.S. Acute Liver Failure Study Group (**Table 159-9**).

CONCLUSION

Ascites, spontaneous bacterial peritonitis, hepatorenal syndrome, and hepatic encephalopathy are common complications of cirrhosis, and each requires detailed evaluation and specific management in patients presenting to the hospital.

Multidisciplinary care involving hepatologists, nutritionists, and hospitalists and when appropriate palliative care specialists should promote optimal medical care by ensuring patient safety, preventing complications from end stage disease, and respecting the patients' wishes.

SUGGESTED READINGS

Arroyo V, Guevara M, Gines P. Hepatorenal syndrome in cirrhosis: pathogenesis and treatment. *Gastroenterology*. 2002;122:1658.

Ferenci P, Lockwood A, Mullen K, et al. Hepatic encephalopathy—definition, nomenclature, diagnosis, and quantification: final report of the working party at the 11th World Congresses of Gastroenterology, Vienna, 1998. *Hepatology*. 2002;35:716–721.

Gines P, Schrier RW. Renal failure in cirrhosis. *N Engl J Med.* 2009; 361:1279.

Hou W, Sanyal A. Ascites: diagnosis and management. *Med Clin N Am*. 2009;93:801–817.

Mackelaite L, Alsauskas ZC, Ranganna, K. Renal failure in patients with cirrhosis. *Med Clin North Am*. 2009;93:855–869.

Munoz S. Hepatic encephalopathy. *Med Clin North Am*. 2008;92: 795–812.

Runyon B. Management of adult patients with ascites due to cirrhosis: an update. *Hepatology*. 2009;49:2087–2107.

Salerno A, Gerbes, Gines P, et al. Diagnosis, prevention and treatment of hepatorenal syndrome in cirrhosis. *Gut*. 2007;56:1310–1318.

Sundaram V, Shaikh O. Hepatic Encephalopathy: pathophysiology and emerging therapies. *Med Clin North Am*. 2009;93:819–836.

Williams JW, Simel DL. Does this Patient Have Ascites? How to Divine Fluid in the Abdomen. *JAMA*. 2002;267(19):2645–2648.

CHAPTER 160

Acute Lower Gastrointestinal Bleeding

Linda S. Lee, MD

Key Clinical Questions

1. What risk factors increase the severity of lower gastrointestinal (GI) bleeding?
2. What are the categories and individual causal factors for colonic ischemia?
3. What are the indications for tagged red blood cell scan and angiography in the setting of lower GI bleeding?
4. What are the indications for surgery in patients with diverticular bleeding and ischemic colitis?

INTRODUCTION

Lower gastrointestinal (GI) bleeding is defined as bleeding that occurs from a source distal to the ligament of Treitz. This chapter will discuss only colonic sources of bleeding, as other chapters explore both upper gastrointestinal and small intestinal bleeding.

Lower GI bleeding accounts for about 20% of major gastrointestinal bleeding and is less common and generally less severe than upper GI bleeding. There are 20 to 27 hospitalizations per 100,000 adults in the United States due to lower GI bleeding. It generally occurs in the older population with a mean age between 63 and 77 years old. Nearly 80% of lower GI bleeding stops spontaneously, similar to upper GI bleeding. The overall mortality rate of lower GI bleeding is 2% to 4%. Similar to upper GI bleeding, patients who begin lower GI bleeding as an outpatient have a significantly lower mortality rate (3.6%) than inpatients who develop lower GI bleeding (23%).

PRACTICE POINT

- Nearly 80% of lower GI bleeding stops spontaneously, and the mortality rate of lower GI bleeding is 2% to 4%. Patients who begin lower GI bleeding as an outpatient have a significantly lower mortality rate (3.6%) than inpatients who develop lower GI bleeding (23%).

PRESENTATION

Definitions of bleeding

Hematochezia is defined as bright red blood per rectum and usually implies a left colonic source, although it can be caused by a more brisk, proximal source of bleeding. Maroon stools are maroon-colored blood mixed with stool that is often associated with a right colonic source of bleeding; however, it can also result from a more brisk, proximal source of bleeding. Melena refers to black, tarry, foul smelling stool that results from the bacterial degradation of hemoglobin over a period of at least 14 hours. It usually implies an upper GI source of bleeding, although it may be associated with right colonic bleeding in cases of slow motility. Ingestion of iron, bismuth, charcoal, and licorice should be excluded as they all can turn stool black. Occult blood refers to the presence of small quantities of blood in the stool that does not change its color and can only be detected by performing a stool guaiac card test. Blood loss of at least 5–10 mL per day can be detected by stool guaiac card tests. The gastrointestinal tract normally loses about 0.5–1.5 mL of blood per day, which is not usually detected by guaiac tests.

PRACTICE POINT

- Ingestion of iron, bismuth, charcoal, and licorice should be excluded as they all can turn stool black.

SIGNS AND SYMPTOMS

History in these patients should focus on factors associated with potential etiologies (**Table 160-1**). Differential diagnosis should be

TABLE 160-1 History Features Based on Bleeding Etiology

Etiology of Lower GI Bleeding	Historical Features
Hemorrhoidal bleeding	Blood coating the stool
	Pain with defecation
Proximal large bowel bleeding	Blood mixed in the stool
IBD	Bloody diarrhea
	Tenesmus
	Abdominal pain
Infectious colitis	Bloody diarrhea
	Fever
	Abdominal pain
	Recent travel history
Anal fissure	Pain with defecation
Colon cancer	Change in stool caliber
	Weight loss
Ischemic colitis	Abdominal pain
	Pain out of proportion to exam
Diverticulosis	Painless bleeding
	NSAID use
AVM	Painless bleeding
Radiation proctitis	Painless bleeding
Colon ulcer	NSAID use
Postpolypectomy bleed	Recent colonoscopy

developed based on presenting complaints and physical examination. Patients should be asked about symptoms that might indicate hemodynamic compromise including dyspnea, chest pain, lightheadedness, and fatigue.

The physical examination and initial testing should focus on

1. **Vital signs.** Orthostatic hypotension with decrease of 20 mm Hg in the systolic blood pressure implies at least a 20% loss of blood volume.
2. **Abdominal examination** for tenderness, masses, liver span, and splenomegaly.
3. **Rectal examination** including inspection of the anus, characterization of the stool color, and stool guaiac card test.

TRIAGE/HOSPITAL ADMISSION

APPROACH TO PATIENTS WITH ACUTE LOWER GASTROINTESTINAL BLEEDING

When patients initially present with acute lower GI bleeding, they should be triaged and managed based on the severity of the hemorrhage (**Figure 160-1**).

INITIAL CLINICAL ASSESSMENT AND MANAGEMENT

During the initial clinical evaluation of patients with suspected acute lower GI bleeding, resuscitation should proceed simultaneously with the placement of two large-bore (18-gauge or larger) peripheral catheters or a large bore central line (eg, cordis) followed by administration of intravenous fluids including normal saline and/or packed red blood cells. **Blood tests** should be performed including complete blood count, prothrombin time, partial thromboplastin time, electrolytes, and typing and cross-matching for

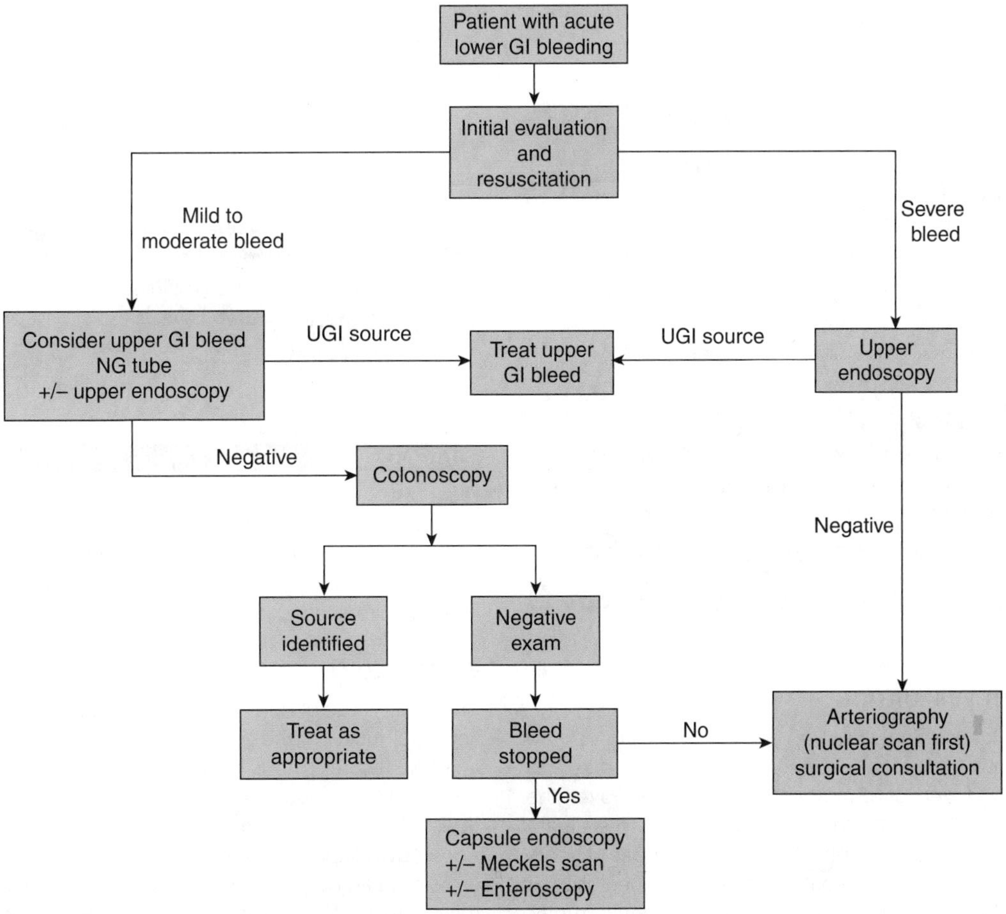

Figure 160-1 *Algorithm for management of patients with suspected lower GI bleeding.*

blood products. Coagulopathy and thrombocytopenia should be immediately corrected if possible. Platelets should be maintained above 50,000/mL and coagulopathy should be corrected with vitamin K or fresh frozen plasma. Vitamin K should be taken orally unless the patient has cirrhosis or biliary obstruction, in which case it should be administered subcutaneously. It takes 12 to 24 hours for the full effect of vitamin K to occur, unlike fresh frozen plasma, which rapidly reverses coagulopathy. The effects of fresh frozen plasma last about three to five hours and large volumes (over 2–3 liters) may be required to completely reverse coagulopathy depending on the initial INR. Recombinant activated factor VII has been approved for use in patients with hemophilia A and B with factor 8 and 9 inhibitors. Evidence of possible benefit in patients with cirrhosis and gastrointestinal bleeding has been demonstrated, although the optimal dose is unclear and recombinant activated factor VII is very expensive with a single 90 mcg/kg dose costing at least $4500.

PREDICTION OF MORBIDITY AND MORTALITY

Multiple validated scoring systems help predict the probability of rebleeding, surgery, and mortality in *upper* GI bleeding. These scoring systems enable appropriate triage and aggressive management of high risk patients and potentially early discharge of low risk patients. Few studies stratify patients by severity in *lower* GI bleeding. The strongest predictors of mortality include age over 70, ischemic colitis, and presence of at least two comorbidities.

Risk factors identified for increased *severity* of lower GI bleeding are heart rate greater than 100 beats per minute, systolic blood pressure less than 115 mm Hg, syncope, nontender abdomen, rectal bleeding within four hours of presentation, aspirin use, and more than two comorbidities. Patients with none of these risk factors have a low risk (6%) of severe bleeding; those with one to three of these have a moderate risk (43%); and those with more than three risk factors have a high risk (79%) of severe bleeding.

PRACTICE POINT

Increased severity of lower GI bleeding is associated with the following risk factors (RF):

- heart rate greater than 100 beats per minute
- systolic blood pressure less than 115 mm Hg
- syncope
- nontender abdomen
- rectal bleeding within four hours of presentation
- aspirin use
- more than two comorbidities

Zero RFs equates to a low incidence (6%) of severe bleeding.

One to three RFs equates to a moderate incidence (43%) of severe bleeding.

More than three risk factors equates to a high risk (79%) of severe bleeding.

OUTPATIENT EVALUATION

Patients who have *minor bleeding with scant hematochezia* represent 75% to 90% of all patients with lower GI bleeding and may be evaluated as outpatients. For patients over the age of 50 years, colonoscopy should be performed to evaluate the source and to screen for colon cancer. In younger patients with rectal bleeding, there is debate regarding the necessity of a colonoscopy versus flexible sigmoidoscopy. Several studies demonstrate that 10% to 30% of patients with rectal bleeding had proximal lesions, which would have been missed by a flexible sigmoidoscopy. Other studies found that no cancers and only a very few polyps would have been missed by flexible sigmoidoscopy in patients with "outlet-type bleeding," defined as blood seen during or after defecation on the toilet paper or in the toilet bowl without symptoms or special risk factors for colorectal neoplasia. Physicians are unable to reliably predict based on history alone which patients with rectal bleeding will have significant pathology. As patients grow older, it becomes cost-effective to perform a full colonoscopy. Patients in their mid-30s or older should likely be evaluated with a colonoscopy while patients in their 20s with "outlet-type bleeding" may have a flexible sigmoidoscopy. If no lesion is discovered to explain the hematochezia, those patients should then undergo a full colonoscopy.

Another category of patients presents with *chronic, intermittent bleeding*, which manifests as guaiac positive stool and/or iron deficiency anemia. Evaluation of these patients can usually occur in the outpatient setting; however, if the patients are severely anemic with cardiopulmonary symptoms and/or disease, inpatient admission should be considered for further monitoring, evaluation, and management. All of these patients must be evaluated with colonoscopy. About 25% to 41% of these patients will have abnormalities on upper endoscopy. Therefore, if no source is identified on colonoscopy or if the patient has upper gastrointestinal symptoms, an upper endoscopy should be performed. Asymptomatic patients may also harbor upper gastrointestinal abnormalities, and those with iron deficiency anemia should undergo an upper endoscopy.

Other patients with lower GI bleeding include those with episodic, severe bleeding and continuous active bleeding who must be evaluated in the hospital. Approximately 10% to 15% of initially suspected lower GI bleeding cases ultimately have an upper gastrointestinal source. Clues to the possible upper gastrointestinal source include hematochezia with hemodynamic instability, melena, and a history of upper GI bleeding. Placement of a nasogastric tube or obtaining a prompt upper endoscopy examination may be helpful to rule out an upper GI source in patients with severe bleeding.

PRACTICE POINT

- Approximately 10% to 15% of initially suspected lower GI bleeding cases ultimately have an upper gastrointestinal source.

DIAGNOSIS

Diagnostic evaluation must be performed after patients have been adequately resuscitated. If an upper GI source is suspected, an upper endoscopy should be performed first. Lower GI evaluation can be performed with anoscopy, flexible sigmoidoscopy, colonoscopy, rarely barium enema, and various radiologic studies.

ANOSCOPY

Anoscopy is useful only for diagnosing bleeding sources from the anorectal junction and anal canal including internal hemorrhoids and anal fissures. This is performed using an anoscope, which is a tube about the width of an average to large bowel movement and three to four inches long through which a light can be shone. Anoscopy is superior to flexible sigmoidoscopy for detecting hemorrhoids in an outpatient setting, and can be performed quickly in the office or at the bedside as an adjunct to flexible sigmoidoscopy and colonoscopy.

FLEXIBLE SIGMOIDOSCOPY

Flexible sigmoidoscopy uses a 65 cm long sigmoidoscope that visualizes the left colon. It can be performed without sedation and only minimal preparation with enemas. However, the diagnostic yield of flexible sigmoidoscopy in acute lower GI bleeding is only 9%. The role of anoscopy and flexible sigmoidoscopy in inpatients with acute lower GI bleeding is limited as most patients should undergo colonoscopy.

COLONOSCOPY

Colonoscopy is the test of choice in the majority of patients with acute lower GI bleeding as it can be both diagnostic and therapeutic. The diagnostic accuracy of colonoscopy in lower GI bleeding ranges from 48% to 90% and urgent colonoscopy appears to increase diagnostic yield. This wide range in yield is partially explained by different criteria for diagnosis, as often if no active bleeding, nonbleeding visible vessel, or adherent clot is found, bleeding is attributed to a lesion if blood is present in the area. The presence of fresh blood in the terminal ileum is presumed to indicate a noncolonic source of bleeding.

The overall complication rate of colonoscopy in acute lower GI bleeding is 1.3% with 0.3% risk of perforation. Bowel preparation is safe and well-tolerated in most patients. The complication rate of colonoscopy in an unprepped colon may be higher. About 2% to 6% of colonoscopy preparations in acute lower GI bleeding are poor. Between 4 to 8 liters (1–2 gallons) of Golytely should be administered orally or via nasogastric tube until the effluence is clear. Antiemetics and prokinetics such as metoclopramide 10 mg should be given as needed during the preparation. In patients at risk of aspiration or fluid overload the preparation should be cautiously administered although complication rates are low with PEG-based preparations. Colonoscopy can be performed within one to two hours after the stool clears. There is no role for enemas in colonoscopy preparation.

It is not clear that aggressive treatment with urgent colonoscopy improves the outcome in patients with severe lower GI bleeding. There are two prospective randomized trials to date of patients with significant lower GI bleeding who were randomized to standard care or urgent colonoscopy. Patients in the standard care arm underwent elective colonoscopy within four days of admission while patients undergoing urgent colonoscopy were administered 4–6 L of a balanced electrolyte-polyethylene glycol (PEG) prep solution orally or via a nasogastric tube over three to four hours and underwent colonoscopy within 8 to 12 hours of hospitalization or diagnosis of hematochezia. More sources of bleeding were identified in the urgent colonoscopy group in one study, but there was no difference in early or late rebleeding, length of hospital stay, surgery, mortality, or complications in either study. Therefore, it is unclear whether urgent colonoscopy influences patient outcome despite the increased identification and treatment of a source of bleeding, and further larger studies are needed.

BARIUM ENEMA

There is no role for barium enema in acute lower GI bleeding. It may impede the performance of a colonoscopy or subsequent angiography due to the presence of barium in the colon. In young patients with minor hematochezia who have a negative flexible sigmoidoscopy, barium enema can be an alternative to colonoscopy.

TAGGED RED BLOOD CELL SCAN

Tagged red blood cell scan and angiography may be the tests of choice in patients with massive lower GI bleeding that prevents colonoscopy, in those with ongoing bleeding and a negative colonoscopy, or in patients who have not yet been prepared for a colonoscopy. Although tagged RBC scan is solely a diagnostic exam, angiography, like colonoscopy, can be both diagnostic and therapeutic.

A bleeding rate of at least 0.1 to 0.5 mL/min is required to be detected by tagged RBC scan. An injected radiotracer circulates in the blood and extravasation of blood into the gastrointestinal lumen can be identified on a series of static images captured after injection or on multiple sequential dynamic images obtained at 15- or 30-second intervals (**Figures 160-2A, B**). Two radiotracers have been used for tagged RBC scan: technetium (Tc) 99 m sulfur colloid and technetium 99m-labelled RBC, which involves labeling the patient's red blood cells *in vitro* and then reinjecting them into the patient. Sulfur colloid is rapidly cleared by the reticuloendothelial system and, therefore, leaves the blood pool within minutes, which provides an approximate 10-minute window to detect extravasation. RBC labeling is superior because the red blood cells persist for at least 24 hours in the circulation. This allows for longer imaging and repeated imaging if the patient rebleeds during this time window. Typically a 90-minute imaging period is used as the diagnostic yield plateaus at this time.

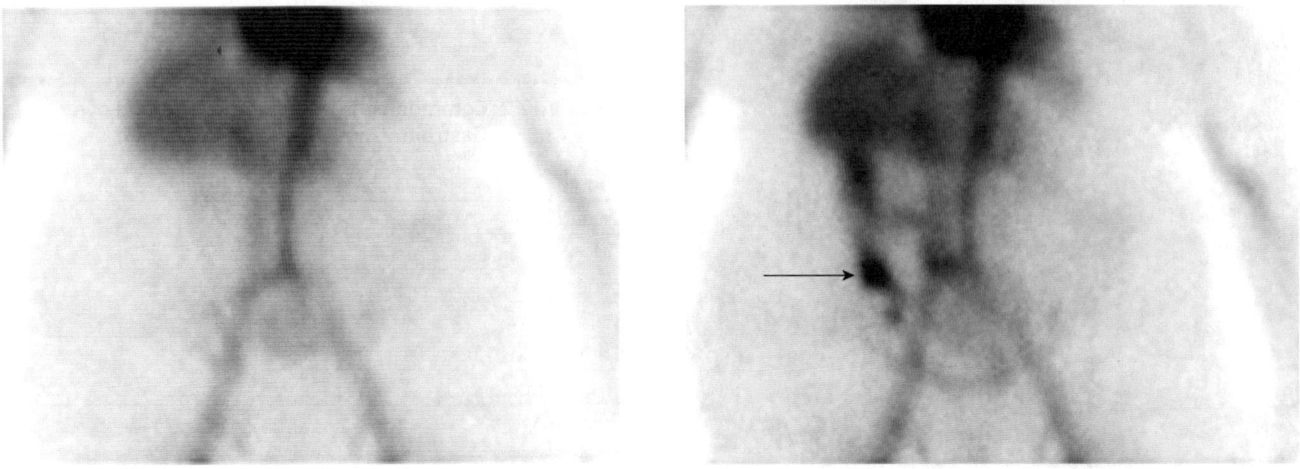

A B

Figure 160-2 *(A) Baseline tagged RBC scan. (B) Tagged RBC scan with active bleeding from right colon (arrow).*

About 45% of tagged RBC scans for lower GI bleeding are positive. Accuracy of localization of the bleeding site ranges from 24% to 91%. Scans that are positive within two hours were 95% to 100% accurate in localizing the bleeding site compared to 57% to 67% accurate for scans positive after two hours. Because of the relatively high rate of false localization, confirmatory studies are required before proceeding to surgery.

The tagged RBC scan can be useful before angiography because it selects patients who are bleeding sufficiently for an angiogram and it may allow more targeted angiography with decreased contrast load. A positive tagged RBC scan increases the diagnostic yield of angiography 2.4 times by selecting outpatients who are not actively bleeding at the time of tagged RBC scan. Following a positive tagged RBC scan, urgent angiography should be performed within one hour if feasible. Delaying angiography may lead to increased negative results, as lower GI bleeding is often episodic and intermittent.

PRACTICE POINT

- Tagged RBC scan selects patients who are bleeding sufficiently for evaluation with angiogram, and it may allow more targeted angiography with decreased contrast load.
- Following a positive tagged RBC scan, urgent angiography should be performed within one hour. Delaying angiography may lead to increased negative results, as lower GI bleeding is often episodic and intermittent.

ANGIOGRAPHY

A more rapid rate of bleeding compared to tagged RBC scan of at least 0.5 to 1.5 mL/min is necessary to be detected during angiography (**Figure 160-3**). Patients who are massively bleeding and hemodynamically unstable should be resuscitated and proceed directly to angiography without tagged RBC scan. The diagnostic yield of angiography ranges from 27% to 77% with a mean of 47%; sensitivity and specificity are 47% and 100%, respectively. Complications of angiography occur in 10% to 20% and include renal failure, hematoma, ischemia, and infarction. Provocative testing using anticoagulants (eg, intravenous heparin and intra-arterial tPA) and vasodilators (intra-arterial tolazoline) can increase diagnostic yield although concern for significant complications exist. This approach may be undertaken in very select situations after extensive discussion with the patient, gastroenterologist, surgeon, and radiologist. Further studies are necessary to optimize the efficacy and prove the safety of this approach.

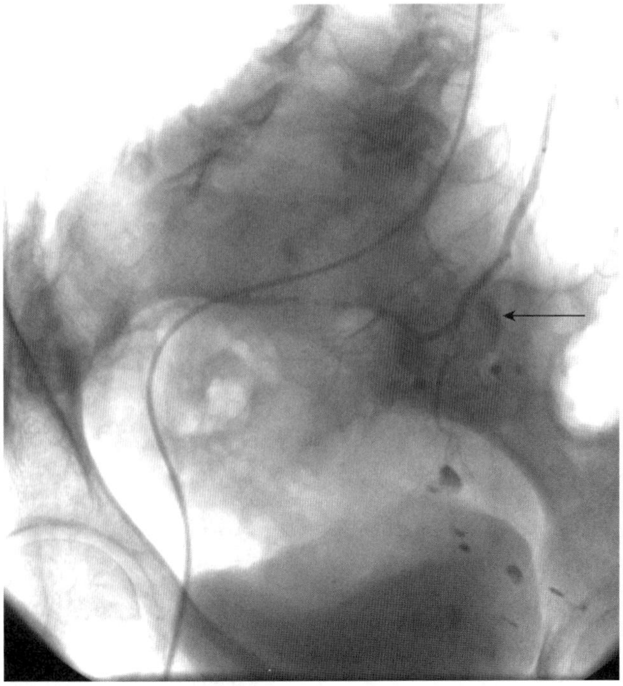

Figure 160-3 *Angiography with active bleeding from right colon (arrow).*

MULTIDETECTOR ROW COMPUTED TOMOGRAPHY

Recent advances in CT technology may lead to a future role for CT scan in lower GI bleeding. Multidetector row computed tomography (MDCT) incorporates several improvements that allow enhanced delineation of mesenteric vessels: faster scanning time, more accurate acquisition of images in arterial and venous phases, and improved 3D display. Patients do not ingest any water or contrast material orally and after an initial unenhanced CT scan, images are obtained during the arterial phase to identify extravasation of contrast into the bowel lumen. Preliminary studies using angiography as the gold standard demonstrate sensitivity and specificity of 83–91% and 99%, respectively, for detecting acute GI bleeding with MDCT and 100% accuracy in localization of bleeding site. Single-detector CT scan can detect bleeding rates of 0.3 mL/min and MDCT may approach the detection ability of tagged RBC scans.

MAGNETIC RESONANCE ANGIOGRAM

Magnetic resonance (MR) angiogram is not typically used in acute lower GI bleeding because it lacks the resolution to detect hemorrhage from small blood vessels. A new blood pool MR contrast agent may help localize the bleeding to a bowel segment. This contrast agent remains in the intravascular space for many hours and subsequent imaging could identify extravascular contrast.

DIFFERENTIAL DIAGNOSIS

The differential diagnosis for lower GI bleeding is broad although the vast majority is due to diverticulosis, ischemic colitis, arteriovenous malformations (AVM), neoplasia and hemorrhoids (**Table 160-2**) Following initial evaluation, the cause of lower GI bleeding remains uncertain in about 12% of cases.

TABLE 160-2 Common Sources and Prevalence of Lower Gastrointestinal Bleeding*

Source	Prevalence (%)
Diverticulosis	17–44
Colonic Angiodysplasia	2–30
Ischemia	9–21
Malignancy	4–14
Hemorrhoids/Anorectal	4–11
Postpolypectomy	6
Unknown	8–12

*Data from Longstreth GF. *Am J Gastroenterol.* 1997;92:419; Strate L. *Arch Int Med.* 2003;163:838; Zuccaro G. *Am J Gastroenterol.* 1998;93:1202; Barnert J. *Nat Rev Gastroenterol Hepatol.* 2009;6:637–646.

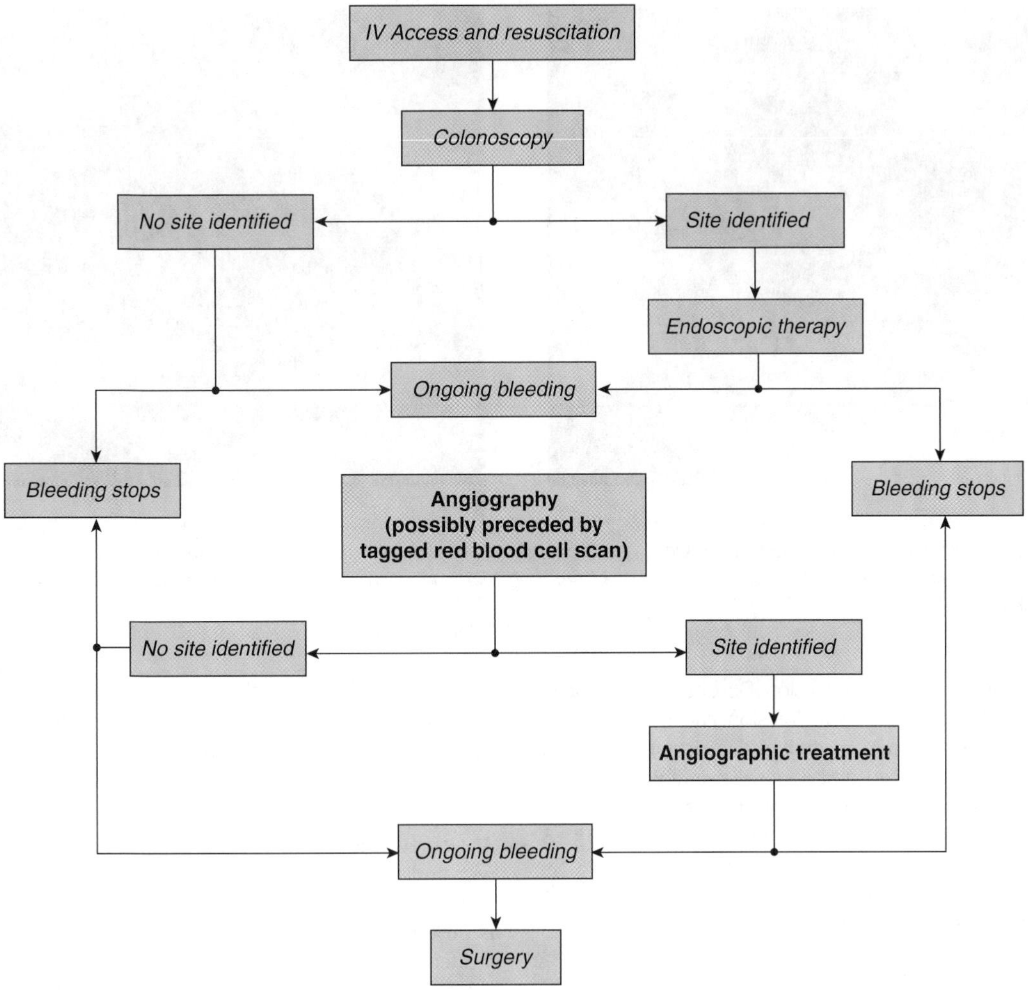

Figure 160-4 *Algorithm for management of diverticular bleeding.*

DIVERTICULOSIS

Diverticulosis is the most common etiology of lower GI bleeding. It is more prevalent in developed countries and older patients. While 5% to 10% of people under the age of 40 have diverticulosis, nearly two-thirds of people older than 80 years are affected.

Presentation and pathophysiology

About 75% to 80% of people with diverticulosis are asymptomatic; however, 3% to 20% experience diverticular bleeding. Massive bleeding can occur in 3% to 5% of patients. Risk factors for diverticular bleeding include the use of NSAIDs, advanced age, and right colon location. Bleeding occurs at the site of penetration of the vasa recta, with the vasa recta stretched over the dome of the diverticula resulting in segmental wall weakness and predisposing to rupture. Abrupt painless bleeding characterizes diverticular bleeding; mild lower abdominal cramping may occur before passage of bright red or maroon blood due to the cathartic nature of blood in the intestines. Melena is unusual for arterial bleeding from diverticulosis. Guaiac positive stool alone and iron deficiency anemia are not consistent with diverticular bleeding.

Diagnosis

More than 75% of diverticulosis are located in the left colon, although about 60% of bleeding diverticula detected during angiography occur in the right colon compared to 60% found bleeding during colonoscopy are located in the left colon. The vast majority of diverticular bleeding stops spontaneously. Colonoscopy is often the initial diagnostic procedure performed to rule out other lesions and determine the bleeding site, which is found in less than 22% of cases. Urgent colonoscopy increases the chance of detecting a bleeding site. If bleeding without a clear source persists or recurs, tagged RBC scan can be performed followed by immediate angiography if positive. If tagged RBC scan is negative, repeat colonoscopy can be considered. An algorithm delineating a recommended approach to diverticular bleeding can assist clinicians with management (**Figure 160-4**).

Management

Endoscopic options There are multiple endoscopic options if a bleeding diverticulum is identified, including epinephrine injection, bipolar coagulation, combination therapy, or mechanical therapy. Epinephrine injection in four quadrants can control bleeding or close the mouth of the diverticulum by tamponade. The majority of bleeding vessels or nonbleeding visible vessels identified during endoscopy are located on the neck of the diverticulum. Thermal therapy should be avoided at the dome of the diverticulum. A small study suggested that endoscopic treatment is successful long-term with no recurrent bleeding over a median of 30 months, while 53% of patients treated conservatively rebled. Mechanical therapy with endoclips or endoscopic band ligation may also be used to treat bleeding diverticula (**Figure 160-5**).

Interventional radiology options Angiography offers another treatment option. Continuous, selective intra-arterial vasopressin infusion stops bleeding in about 90% of cases with up to 50%

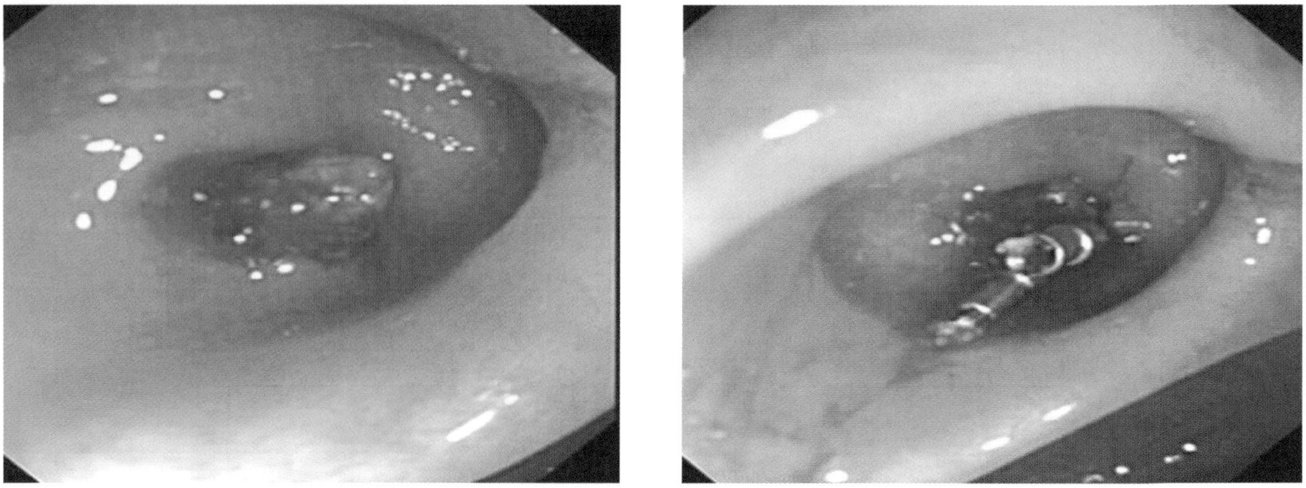

A B

Figure 160-5 *(A) Diverticulum with large, oozing visible vessel. (B) Posttreatment of diverticulum with two hemoclips. (Reproduced, with permission, from Greenberger N, Blumberg R, Burakoff R. Current Diagnosis & Treatment: Gastroenterology, Hepatology, and Endoscopy. New York: McGraw-Hill, 2008. Plates 64–65.)*

rebleeding after discontinuing the infusion. Despite this temporary effect in many patients, vasopressin infusion can be helpful to allow bowel preparation before a semielective definitive surgical procedure. However, it can cause abdominal pain and should be avoided in patients with known coronary artery disease.

Superselective embolization with microcatheters uses 2.5 to 3 French microcatheters, which are advanced through conventional 5 French catheters to access smaller, more distal vessels. Various embolic agents are used, including gel foam, polyvinyl alcohol, and microcoils. Recurrent bleeding one month after embolization occurs in less than 15% of diverticular hemorrhage compared to more than 40% of nondiverticular causes such as arteriovenous malformation. Major ischemic complications requiring surgery appear to occur in less than 6% of patients.

Surgical options Persistent massive hemorrhage, transfusion requirement over 4 units in 24 hours, and recurrent diverticular bleeding meet potential indications for surgery, necessary in up to 25% of people requiring transfusions. Mortality rate is still relatively high at 10% even with directed segmental resection with a rebleeding rate of 14% at one-year follow-up. Blind segmental resection should be avoided due to rebleeding rates as high as 33% with mortality rates ranging from up to 50% or more. Blind total colectomy yields rebleeding rates as low as 0% but mortality rates range from 0% to 33%. Therefore, aggressive efforts should be made to localize a bleeding site preoperatively.

Repeat diverticular bleeding occurs in 25% to 35%, while 50% of these people experience a third episode of diverticular hemorrhage. NSAID use is a potential risk factor; however, whether avoiding NSAIDs reduces the chance of rebleeding is unclear.

ARTERIOVENOUS MALFORMATION

Arteriovenous malformations (AVMs) are the reported source of lower GI bleeding in 3% to 40% of patients, which are usually congenital and occur in 1% to 2% of colon autopsy specimens.

Presentation and pathophysiology

AVMs are ectatic mucosal and submucosal blood vessels with a direct communication between the arteries and veins without intervening capillaries. Over half are located in the right colon and 47% of patients experience *painless hematochezia* similar to diverticular hemorrhage. Bleeding AVMs can present with chronic, intermittent bleeding. Risk factors for bleeding include advanced age (greater than age 60 years), right-sided location, and possibly certain conditions (aortic stenosis and chronic renal failure).

Diagnosis

Angiography is considered the gold standard in diagnosing AVMs with findings including ectatic slowly emptying veins, vascular tufts, or early filling veins. The **diagnostic sensitivity of colonoscopy is 80% to 90%** with the characteristic finding of a 2 to 10 mm, red fern-like flat lesion with ectatic vessels radiating from a central vessel. Poor bowel preparation and use of meperidine, which transiently decreases mucosal blood flow, could potentially hinder the identification of AVMs. Use of naloxone may enhance colonic vasculature and AVM identification.

Management

Bleeding AVMs discovered during colonoscopy can be treated with a variety of thermal therapies. Contact electrocautery can begin with the outer feeder vessels and progress toward the central vessel (**Figure 160-6**). Argon plasma coagulation (APC) has become a popular noncontact method with approximately 80% success rate. Nonbleeding AVMs without evidence of GI bleeding should not be treated. However, if there is a history of guaiac positive stool or iron deficiency anemia, AVMs should be treated even if not actively bleeding.

There is a potential role for medical treatment of AVMs. Only case series and reports have suggested the benefit of octreotide administered subcutaneously in doses ranging from 100 mcg to 500 mcg two times a day by decreasing the need for transfusions. Long-term estrogen-progesterone treatment for one year did not decrease rebleeding from AVMs in a randomized trial. Another study that suggested benefit from hormone therapy had a study population containing 50% of patients with Osler-Weber Rendu disease. Therefore, this subset of patients may experience decreased bleeding from AVMs with hormone therapy.

ISCHEMIC COLITIS

Colonic ischemia, which most commonly occurs in the elderly with multiple comorbidities, is caused by a reduction in colonic blood flow due to vasospasm, occlusion, and/or hypoperfusion. Eighty-five percent of patients with colonic ischemia have a benign

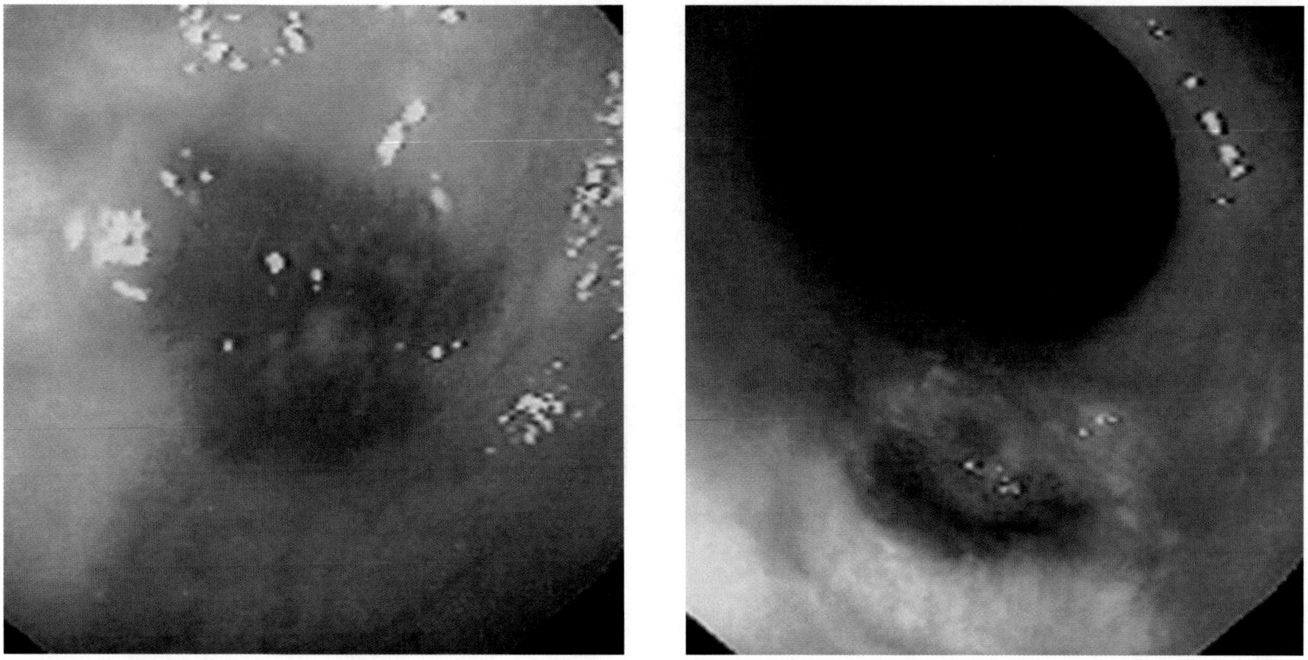

A **B**

Figure 160-6 *(A) AVM in patient with lower GI bleeding. (B) Posttreatment of AVM with bipolar cautery. (Reproduced, with permission, from Greenberger N, Blumberg R, Burakoff R. Current Diagnosis & Treatment: Gastroenterology, Hepatology, and Endoscopy. New York: McGraw-Hill, 2008. Plates 66–67.)*

course called nongangrenous ischemia with transient ischemia that resolves without sequelae. However, life-threatening complications occur in 15% of patients who develop gangrenous colonic ischemia.

PRACTICE POINT

- The majority of patients with colonic ischemia have no identifiable cause.

Presentation and pathophysiology

The potential causes of colonic ischemia are varied (**Table 160-3**). However, the majority of patients with colonic ischemia have no identifiable cause. The colonic circulation is supplied by three arterial sources: the superior mesenteric artery (SMA) branches into the ileocolic (supplies terminal ileum, appendix, cecum, and proximal ascending colon), right colic (supplies distal ascending colon and hepatic flexure) and middle colic arteries (supplies proximal transverse colon); the inferior mesenteric artery (IMA) branches into the left colic (supplies distal transverse and splenic flexure), sigmoid (supplies descending and sigmoid colon) and superior rectal arteries (supplies majority of rectum); and the internal iliac artery branches into the internal pudendal and middle rectal arteries (supplies remainder of rectum). Colonic blood supply helps determine the areas of weak blood supply due to narrow terminal branches. This occurs with the SMA in the area of the splenic flexure and with the IMA in the area of the rectosigmoid junction. These are called the watershed areas, which are most vulnerable to systemic hypotension.

PRACTICE POINT

- Watershed areas of the large colon occur at the splenic flexure and at the rectosigmoid junction and are most vulnerable to systemic hypotension leading to colonic ischemia.

TABLE 160-3 Causes of Colonic Ischemia

Vascular occlusion	**Iatrogenic**
Mesenteric artery thrombosis	Cardiopulmonary bypass
Aortic reconstruction	Aortoiliac reconstruction
Aortic dissection	Colonoscopy
Cholesterol emboli	Renal transplant
Venous thrombosis	**Drugs**
Hypercoagulable state	Alosetron
Portal hypertension	Carboplatin
Pancreatitis	Cocaine
Sickle cell disease	Digitalis
Shock	Diuretics
Cardiac failure	Danazol
Anaphylaxis	Estrogens
Pancreatitis	NSAIDs
Mechanical	Paclitaxel
Adhesion	Simvastatin
Strangulated hernia	Sumatriptan
Colon cancer	Tegaserod
Rectal prolapse	**Miscellaneous**
Small vessel disease	Hemodialysis
Diabetes	Long distance running
Amyloidosis	Airplane flight
Rheumatoid arthritis	Neurogenic
Takayasu arteritis	Spontaneous (young adults)
Wegener arteritis	
Systemic lupus erythematosus	
Buerger disease	
Polyarteritis nodosa	
Vasculitis	

Colonic ischemia usually is due to a sudden reduction in colonic blood flow due to local or systemic compromises of the circulation. Most patients have nonocclusive ischemia and evaluation with angiography would not detect any specific occluding lesion. Nonocclusive ischemia commonly affects the watershed areas of the colon, with the left colon involved in about 75% of cases including 25% at the splenic flexure. A common cause of colonic ischemia is aortoiliac surgery with an incidence of colonic ischemia of 1% to 7%. The most commonly affected area is the distal left colon and risk factors for developing this complication postsurgery include older age, prior colectomy, surgeon experience, renal disease, cross-clamping time, and ligation of both iliac arteries.

The clinical manifestations of colonic ischemia vary depending on the cause of the ischemia and the clinical setting. The onset of symptoms is typically rapid with pain over the affected area of bowel, often on the left side. Within 24 hours, patients may develop rectal bleeding and bloody diarrhea. There are three progressive clinical stages. The hyperactive phase occurs soon after injury with abdominal pain and frequent bloody diarrhea. As most patients have injury confined to the mucosal and submucosal layers, symptoms will respond to conservative therapy in more than 80% of patients with resolution of symptoms and no long-term sequelae. The paralytic phase is characterized by less severe but more generalized abdominal pain along with a distended bowel and decreased bowel sounds. The last phase, found in *10% to 20% of patients*, is called the shock phase associated with *gangrenous bowel* and the clinical manifestations of shock. Patients who develop metabolic acidosis and white blood cell counts greater than 20,000 μL may require rapid progression to surgery.

PRACTICE POINT

- Ten percent to 20% of ischemic colitis patients will develop gangrenous bowel and the clinical manifestations of shock.

Diagnosis

The diagnosis of colonic ischemia is established by a combination of clinical setting, physical diagnosis, and diagnostic studies. The differential diagnosis includes infectious colitis, inflammatory bowel disease, diverticulitis, radiation enteritis, and colon cancer. In hospitalized patients *C difficile* infection must be excluded. Although there are no specific blood tests for colonic ischemia, elevations may be noted in the white blood cell count, amylase, CPK, and serum lactate. Most plain x-rays in colonic ischemia have nonspecific findings, although thumb printing due to submucosal edema and pneumatosis may be seen typically in patients with more advanced disease.

Diagnostic testing with CT scans may reveal segmental thickening of the involved colon. Endoscopic evaluation with sigmoidoscopy or colonoscopy may be used to confirm the diagnosis in patients whose diagnosis is unclear and who do not have signs of peritonitis or perforation. Care must be taken to avoid overdistension with air during the examination to prevent worsening of ischemic damage. Endoscopic findings typically occur in a segmental distribution and vary depending on the degree of damage, ranging from pale mucosa with petechial bleeding to cyanotic, necrotic bowel. **Figure 160-7** demonstrates a focal area of erythema with superficial ulceration in a patient with mild ischemic colitis. Angiography is usually not indicated in colonic ischemia as the blood flow to the colon returns to normal by the time of clinical presentation.

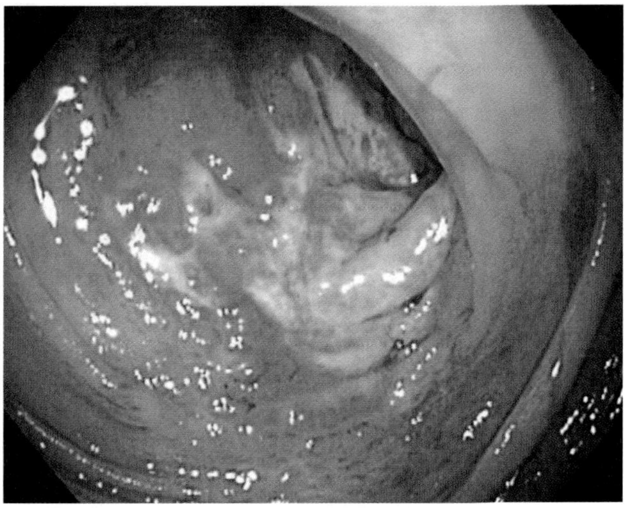

Figure 160-7 *Area of colonic ischemia.*

PRACTICE POINT

- Angiography is usually not indicated in colonic ischemia as the blood flow to the colon returns to normal by the time of clinical presentation.

Management

Treatment of colonic ischemia is supportive in the absence of signs of colonic gangrene or perforation. Patients are placed on bowel rest and supported with intravenous fluids. Antibiotics are recommended only for patients with moderate to severe disease. In patients with clinical deterioration—manifested by high leukocytosis, persistent fever, peritoneal signs, and ongoing GI bleeding—despite supportive measures, surgery with segmental resection is indicated. Patients with evidence of mesenteric venous thrombosis or hypercoagulability should be treated with anticoagulants.

Prognosis

The natural history of patients with ischemic colitis is that *most patients with nonocclusive colonic ischemia will improve in one to two days with complete resolution within two weeks.* Patients with more severe disease may develop segmental colitis or strictures. Most patients will not experience a recurrence, especially if potentially predisposing factors are identified and corrected.

NEOPLASM

Neoplasms of the colon may present with GI bleeding. In patients over the age of 50, rectal bleeding is due to a neoplasm in about 10% of cases; however, neoplasms are an uncommon source of rectal bleeding in persons younger than age 50.

Presentation and pathophysiology

Although most bleeding from colonic neoplasms tends to be low grade and occult, bleeding may be brisk and overt at times. Bleeding occurs due to erosion or ulceration of the lesion. Distal lesions (left side and rectum) are more likely to present with bright red blood per rectum, whereas more proximal lesions tend to present with maroon stool, melena, or occult blood.

Diagnosis

The diagnosis of a neoplasm as the source of lower GI bleeding is typically done by colonoscopy with biopsies performed to confirm the diagnosis. Larger neoplasms may be detected on CT scans.

Management

The therapeutic options for those patients with bleeding neoplasms are limited. Standard endoscopic therapies have marginal effectiveness. The use of fibrin glue has been reported to be effective anecdotally and in small studies (**Figure 160-8**). The treatment for most patients with bleeding colonic neoplasms is surgical resection.

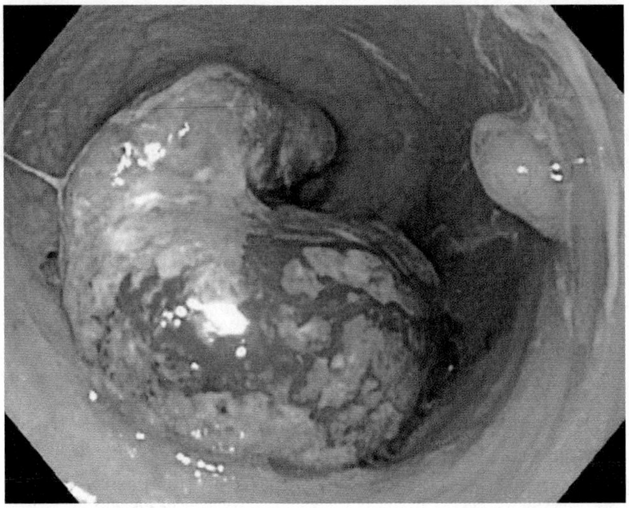

A

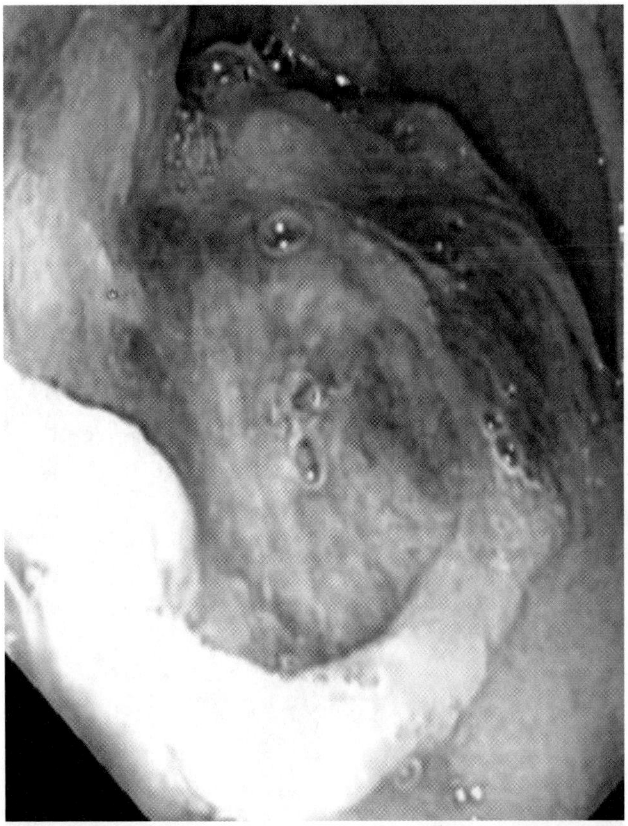

B

Figure 160-8 *(A) Colon cancer. (B) Posttreatment with Tisseel fibrin glue. (Reproduced, with permission, from Greenberger N, Blumberg R, Burakoff R. Current Diagnosis & Treatment: Gastroenterology, Hepatology, and Endoscopy. New York: McGraw-Hill, 2008. Plates 68–69.)*

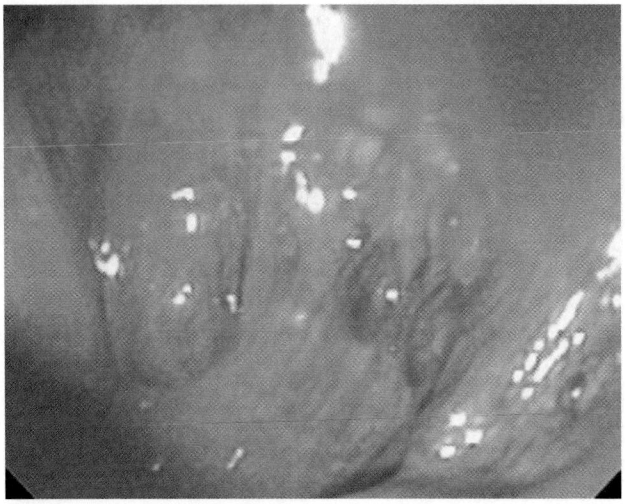

Figure 160-9 *Multiple internal hemorrhoids. (Reproduced, with permission, from Greenberger N, Blumberg R, Burakoff R. Current Diagnosis & Treatment: Gastroenterology, Hepatology, and Endoscopy. New York: McGraw-Hill, 2008. Plate 70.)*

HEMORRHOIDS

Hemorrhoids and other anorectal disorders (solitary rectal ulcers and anal fissures) are an important source of lower GI bleeding.

Presentation and pathophysiology

Hemorrhoids are dilated submucosal vessels in the anus, which are considered internal if above the dentate line (**Figure 160-9**) and external if below. Hemorrhoids are extremely common and usually asymptomatic, but can present with pruritus, thrombosis, or hematochezia. Bleeding from hemorrhoids occurs when there is rupture of a blood vessel.

The clinical manifestations of bleeding hemorrhoids include painless hematochezia with the stool being coated with bright red blood. Further bleeding may occur with blood dripping into the toilet bowl or staining underwear. Although bleeding from hemorrhoids is usually low-grade, high volume or massive bleeding may occur rarely. Severe bleeding from hemorrhoids may occur in patients with a coagulopathy.

Management

Acute treatment for most patients with bleeding hemorrhoids is not needed as most episodes are mild and resolve spontaneously. Topical medical treatments, such as hydrocortisone cream or hydrocortisone acetate/pramoxine cream, help decrease inflammation, and surgery is rarely needed for those with persistent or massive bleeding.

POSTPOLYPECTOMY

Postpolypectomy bleeding occurs after 1% to 6% of polypectomies and is the leading major complication following colonoscopy with polypectomy. Acute hemorrhage occurring at the time of polypectomy accounts for less than 50% of cases. Although bleeding usually occurs within seven days, delayed bleeding can occur within 20 days following polypectomy when the eschar falls off the site.

Risk factors for postpolypectomy bleeding include removal of large polyps (greater than 1 cm in diameter), age over 65 years, cardiovascular or chronic renal disease, platelet dysfunction, and

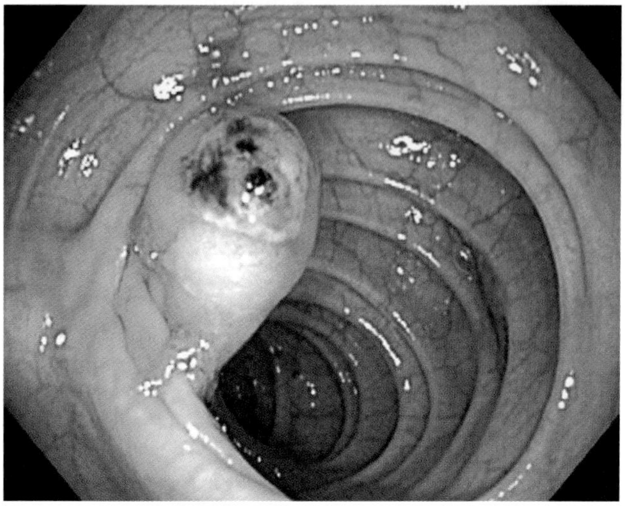

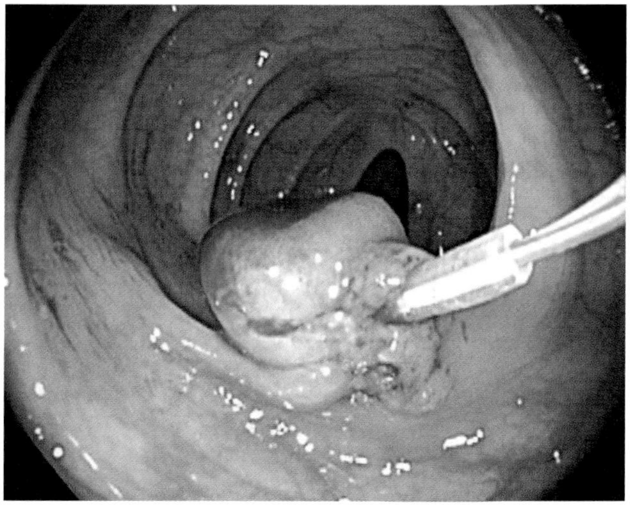

A B

Figure 160-10 *(A) Visible vessels at polypectomy site. (B) Bleeding controlled with placement of endoloop. (Reproduced, with permission, from Greenberger N, Blumberg R, Burakoff R. Current Diagnosis & Treatment: Gastroenterology, Hepatology, and Endoscopy. New York: McGraw-Hill, 2008. Plates 71–72.)*

coagulopathy. Multiple studies have tried to identify techniques to reduce the risk of postpolypectomy bleeding. Only submucosal injection of saline has proven useful in large polyps, while it is unclear whether the type of electrical current (blended versus cutting), placement of prophylactic endoclips, or use of an endoloop decreases the risk of bleeding.

Management

Polypectomy bleeding is usually self-limited with more than 70% resolving with supportive care. Therapeutic options for persistent bleeding include resnaring the stalk of the polypectomy site to apply pressure, injection therapy with epinephrine, contact or noncontact thermal treatment with bipolar coagulation or APC, and endoclip application (**Figure 160-10**).

NSAID-INDUCED BLEEDING

While most appreciate that NSAIDs commonly cause peptic ulcer disease and upper GI bleeding, fewer clinicians appreciate that NSAIDs can damage the large intestine and cause lower GI bleeding. Characteristic endoscopic findings include single or multiple well-defined ulcers with normal intervening mucosa that are classically found in the terminal ileum and proximal colon and a single or multiple diaphragm-like strictures with normal intervening mucosa. Only 21% of patients with colonic ulcers have simultaneous gastric ulcers. Clinical presentation is variable and includes guaiac positive stool, iron deficiency anemia, hematochezia, crampy abdominal pain, weight loss, and change in bowel habits. NSAID-induced colonic ulcers may also be an incidental finding in asymptomatic patients.

Because pathology from NSAID-induced colonic ulcers is nonspecific, diagnosis is made after excluding other potential causes of colonic ulcers including infectious, ischemic, and inflammatory. Symptomatic patients usually respond within a few days after cessation of NSAIDs. If NSAIDs cannot be discontinued, concomitant therapy with misoprostol, sulfasalazine, or metronidazole may protect the mucosa from damage and help heal ulcers.

RADIATION PROCTITIS

Pelvic radiation can cause both acute and chronic radiation proctitis.

Presentation

Acute damage presents within three months of radiation therapy with diarrhea, tenesmus and rarely, bleeding. Chronic radiation proctitis typically occurs 9 to 14 months following radiation in up to 20% of patients, but can occur years later (**Figure 160-11**). Bleeding is a prominent symptom due to mucosal atrophy and fibrosis leading to chronic mucosal ischemia.

Management

There are no standardized recommendations for treatment of bleeding from radiation proctitis. Endoscopic therapy appears superior to medical treatment in reducing severe bleeding with nearly 75% success following endoscopic treatment compared to 33% undergoing medical therapy. Multiple oral and topical

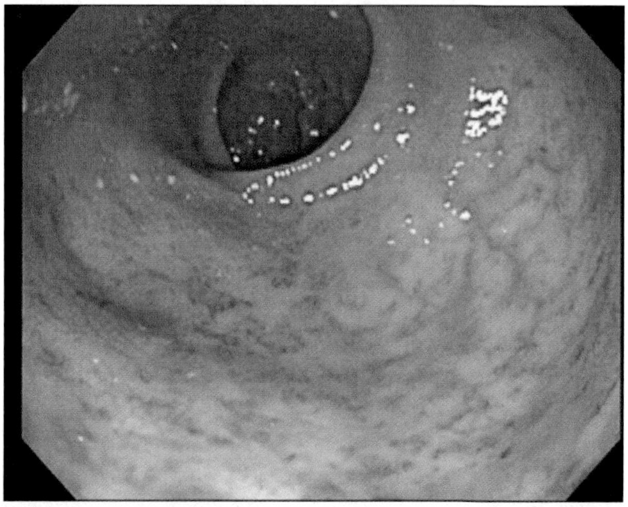

Figure 160-11 *Chronic radiation proctitis. (Reproduced, with permission, from Greenberger N, Blumberg R, Burakoff R. Current Diagnosis & Treatment: Gastroenterology, Hepatology, and Endoscopy. New York: McGraw-Hill, 2008. Plate 73.)*

therapies have been investigated (mainly in small clinical trials or case series), and a few may be effective including sucralfate enema, short-chain fatty acid enema, and topical formalin therapy.

Endoscopic management with heater probe and bipolar coagulation effectively controls bleeding during a mean of four treatment sessions performed every four to six weeks. Argon plasma coagulation has received more attention recently with 85% to 100% success in reducing or stopping bleeding over a mean of two to three treatments every one to two months. All visible telangiectasias are obliterated at each session while rectal ulcers resulting from previous treatments are avoided. Short-term complications occur in 7% including rectal pain or fever. Rare major complications include rectovaginal fistula, anal/rectal stricture, and perforation, presumed secondary to accumulation of combustible gas. A full bowel preparation is safest as there are rare reports of explosions of gas during APC when an enema preparation was used. During long-term follow-up over one to five years, recurrent bleeding occurred in 0% to 8% of patients.

Hyperbaric oxygen may represent another therapeutic option, and is believed to promote angiogenesis and collagen formation leading to reepithelialization. The few recent case series selected patients who had failed previous medical and/or endoscopic therapy for hyperbaric oxygen treatment, and report a 75% to 100% decrease or cessation of bleeding. A recent randomized trial confirms complete or partial healing of radiation proctitis in 89% treated with hyperbaric oxygen compared with 63% in the control group. The treatment regimen is rigorous with patients in a hyperbaric chamber at a pressure of 2.4 atmospheres with 100% oxygen for 90 minutes five days per week for 30–40 sessions. Hyperbaric oxygen therapy may be considered in patients refractory to standard medical and endoscopic treatment before proceeding to surgery.

SUGGESTED READINGS

Barnert J, Messmann H. Diagnosis and management of lower gastrointestinal bleeding. *Nat Rev Gastroenterol Hepatol.* 2009;6:637–646.

Czymek R, Kempf A, Roblick UJ, et al. Surgical treatment concepts for acute lower gastrointestinal bleeding. *J Gastrointest Surg.* 2008;12:2212–2220.

Davila RE, Rajan E, Adler DG, et al. ASGE Guideline: the role of endoscopy in the patient with lower-GI bleeding. *Gastrointestinal Endoscopy.* 2005;62(5):656–660.

Green BT, Rockey DC, Portwood G, et al. Urgent colonoscopy for evaluation and management of acute lower gastrointestinal hemorrhage: a randomized controlled trial. *American Journal of Gastroenterology.* 2005;100(11):2395–2402.

Laine L, Shah A. Randomized trial of urgent vs. elective colonoscopy in patients hospitalized with lower GI bleeding. *Am J Gastroenterol.* 2010;105:2636–2641.

Song LWK, Baron TH. Endoscopic management of acute lower gastrointestinal bleeding. *American Journal of Gastroenterology.* 2008;103:1881–1887.

Strate LL, Ayanian JZ, Kotler G, Syngal S. Risk factors for mortality in lower intestinal bleeding. *Clinical Gastroenterology and Hepatology.* 2008;6;1004–1010.

Strate LL, Naumann CR. The role of colonoscopy and radiological procedures in the management of acute lower intestinal bleeding. *Clin Gastroenterol Hepatol.* 2010;8:333–343.

Strate LL, Saltzman JR, Ookubo R, Mutinga ML, Syngal S. Validation of a clinical prediction rule for severe acute lower intestinal bleeding. *American Journal of Gastroenterology.* 2005;100(8):1821–1827.

Theodoropoulou A and Koutroubakis IE. Ischemic colitis: clinical practice in diagnosis and treatment. *World J Gastroenterology.* 2008;14:7302–7308.

CHAPTER 161

Small Bowel Disorders

Anne C. Travis, MD, MSc
John R. Saltzman, MD

Key Clinical Questions

Malabsorption and Celiac Disease

1. Does this patient have malabsorption?
2. Is the malabsorption due to celiac disease?
3. What other diseases need to be considered?
4. What are the consequences of malabsorption?
5. How is malabsorption managed?

Small Bowel Obstruction

1. What are common causes of small bowel obstruction?
2. How do patients present with small bowel obstruction?
3. When do patients with small bowel obstruction need to go to surgery and when can they be managed medically?
4. Can small bowel obstruction be prevented?

Small Bowel Ileus

1. What conditions predispose to small bowel ileus?
2. Can small bowel ileus be prevented?
3. How is small bowel ileus treated?
4. When can a patient resume oral intake?

Acute Mesenteric Ischemia

1. Does this patient have acute mesenteric ischemia?
2. What conditions predispose to mesenteric ischemia?
3. How does mesenteric ischemia differ from colonic ischemia?
4. Is emergent surgery necessary?

MALABSORPTION AND CELIAC DISEASE

INTRODUCTION AND EPIDIEMIOLOGY

Numerous causes lead to malabsorption and maldigestion, ranging from the common to the obscure. Lactose intolerance, for example, is present in 7% to 20% of Caucasian adults, 50% of Hispanics, 65% to 75% of African Americans, and 90% in some East Asian populations. Celiac disease is most commonly seen in whites of northern European ancestry. In a large screening study from the United States, the prevalence of celiac disease in average risk individuals was 1:133. The prevalence was highest in first-degree relatives of a patient with celiac disease (1:22). Other disorders, such as primary intestinal lymphangiectasias, occur so rarely that it is difficult to estimate their true prevalence.

PRESENTATION

Patients with malabsorption often report weight loss, diarrhea, anorexia, flatulence, borborygmi, and/or greasy, foul smelling, voluminous pale stools. Patients may also have symptoms related to specific micronutrient deficiencies (**Table 161-1**). Some patients, however, are asymptomatic.

PATHOPHYSIOLOGY

Malabsorption refers to impaired nutrient absorption, whereas maldigestion refers to impaired digestion of nutrients within the gut lumen or at the brush border. The term malabsorption, however, is often used to encompass both processes since digestion is a required step for absorption. Three steps comprise nutrient absorption. The first is luminal processing, in which ingested nutrients are broken down into absorbable subunits. The second is absorption of nutrients into the intestinal mucosa. The third is the transport of the nutrients into the circulation. Malabsorption can occur if any of these steps are disrupted.

Malabsorption can be either global or partial. *Global malabsorption* occurs when there is diffuse mucosal involvement or reduced absorptive surface, seen in disorders such as short gut syndrome or celiac disease. *Partial malabsorption* refers to the malabsorption of specific nutrients, such as vitamin B_{12} malabsorption in pernicious anemia or Crohn disease with involvement of the terminal ileum (the site of vitamin B_{12} absorption).

FAT DIGESTION

Fat digestion and absorption depend upon fat hydrolysis, primarily by pancreatic enzymes (lipase, colipase). The fatty acids then combine with bile salts, lipids, and fat soluble vitamins to form micelles and liposomes, which subsequently cross the microvillus membrane. Once within the enterocytes, the fatty acids are transported to the endoplasmic reticulum where chylomicrons form and are transported into the lymphatics. Diseases such as chronic pancreatitis interfere with fat digestion and absorption, resulting in fat malabsorption (**Table 161-2**).

CARBOHYDRATE DIGESTION

Carbohydrate digestion involves the breakdown of complex carbohydrates (starches) and disaccharides into monosaccharides, which

TABLE 161-1 Symptoms and Laboratory Abnormalities Associated with Nutrient Deficiencies

Nutrient	Symptoms of Malabsorption	Laboratory Abnormalities
Fat	Pale, voluminous stool	Steatorrhea
	Diarrhea without flatulence	Stool fat >6 gm/day on diet of 100 gm of fat/day
Carbohydrates	Watery diarrhea	Acidic stool
	Flatulence	Increased stool osmotic gap
	Dairy intolerance	
Protein	Edema	Hypoalbuminemia
	Muscle atrophy	Hypoproteinemia
	Amenorrhea	
Vitamin B_{12}	Fatigue	Macrocytic anemia
	Dyspnea on exertion	Low serum B_{12} level
	Pallor	Elevated homocysteine and methylmalonic acid
	Ataxia	
	Paresthesias	
	Loss of vibration and position sense	
Folate	Fatigue	Macrocytic anemia
	Dyspnea on exertion	Decreased serum and red blood cell folate
	Pallor	Elevated homocysteine
Iron	Fatigue	Microcytic anemia
	Dyspnea on exertion	Low serum iron and ferritin
	Pallor	Increased total iron binding capacity
	Glossitis	
	Pagophagia (ice consumption)	
Calcium and vitamin D	Paresthesias	Hypocalcemia
	Tetany	Increased alkaline phosphatase
	Pathologic fractures	Low vitamin D
	Positive Chvostec and Trousseau signs	Low bone density
Vitamin A	Follicular hyperkeratosis	Decreased serum carotene
	Night blindness	
B vitamins	Chelosis	Decreased serum levels
	Painless glossitis	
	Acrodermatitis	
	Angular stomatitis	
Vitamin K	Hematomas	Prolonged prothrombin time
	Bleeding disorders	Decreased vitamin K dependent clotting factors (II, VII, IX, X)

are then absorbed by active and passive transport into enterocytes. Starch digestion requires amylase (salivary and pancreatic) to break the complex sugars into oligo- and disaccharides, which are then broken down into monosaccharides by brush border enzymes (primarily disaccharidases). Ingested disaccharides, such as lactose and sucrose, are also broken down by brush border disaccharidases. Disorders leading to carbohydrate malabsorption (Table 161-2) result in the maldigested and malabsorbed carbohydrates passing into the colon, where they are degraded by bacteria through fermentation, resulting in the production of short chain fatty acids, hydrogen, carbon dioxide, and methane.

PROTEIN DIGESTION

The goal of protein digestion is to break proteins down into components that are capable of being absorbed. As with fat and carbohydrate digestion, disorders that impair protein digestion or absorption result in protein malabsorption (Table 161-2). Protein digestion starts with gastric pepsins. Then proteases secreted by the pancreas into the duodenum act on the partially digested proteins, resulting in the production of amino acids, dipeptides, and tripeptides. Selective transporters move neutral, basic, and acidic amino acids, as well as dipeptides and tripeptides, from the gut into the bloodstream.

VITAMINS, MINERALS, AND TRACE ELEMENTS

Vitamins, minerals, and trace elements have many different transport mechanisms including passive diffusion, carrier-mediated passive transport, and active transport. Most are absorbed in the proximal half of the small intestine. Two notable exceptions are vitamin B_{12} and magnesium, which are absorbed distally. Some examples of disorders associated with vitamin, mineral, and trace element deficiencies are shown in Table 161-2.

TABLE 161-2 Disorders Associated with Malabsorption

Disorder	Affected Nutrient(s)	Mechanism(s)
Chronic pancreatitis	Fat	Lipase and colipase deficiencies
	Carbohydrate	Pancreatic amylase deficiency
	Protein	Protease deficiencies
Cystic fibrosis	Protein	Impaired protease excretion
Zollinger-Ellison syndrome	Fat, protein	Digestive enzyme inactivation
Cirrhosis	Fat, fat soluble vitamins	Decreased bile salt production
Chronic cholestasis	Fat, fat soluble vitamins	Impaired bile salt secretion
Bacterial overgrowth	Fat, fat soluble vitamins	Bile salt deconjugation
	Carbohydrate	Damage to brush border enzymes
	Protein, carbohydrate, vitamin B_{12}	Consumption of nutrients by bacteria
Lactose intolerance	Lactose	Lactase deficiency
Celiac disease, tropical sprue, common variable immunodeficiency	Carbohydrate	Decreased brush border enzyme activity due to villous damage
	Carbohydrate, protein, fat	Decreased absorptive surface area
Short bowel syndrome	Fat, carbohydrate, protein, vitamin B_{12}	Decreased absorptive surface area
Pernicious anemia	Vitamin B_{12}	Impaired production of intrinsic factor
Ileal disease (eg, Crohn, lymphoma, amyloid)	Vitamin B_{12}	Decreased absorptive surface
Intestinal lymphangiectasia	Fat, fat soluble vitamins	Impaired transport into lymphatics

CELIAC DISEASE

Celiac disease occurs as a result of immune mediated damage to the small bowel mucosa. Certain gliadin peptides can initiate an innate immune response in macrophages, monocytes, dendridic cells, and intestinal epithelial cells. Intraepithelial lymphocytes and autoantibodies to tissue transglutaminase may also play a role in the pathogenesis of celiac disease. The end result is damage to the small intestinal villi, which results in malabsorption due to decreased surface area and damage to brush border enzymes.

DIFFERENTIAL DIAGNOSIS

Numerous conditions cause malabsorption, including celiac disease, small bowel bacterial overgrowth, Crohn disease with small bowel involvement, chronic pancreatitis, short bowel syndrome, protein losing enteropathy, intestinal lymphangiectasias, amyloid, small bowel lymphoma, eosinophilic gastroenteritis, common variable immunodeficiency, lactose intolerance and other disaccharidase deficiencies, and Zollinger-Ellison syndrome (Table 161-2).

Disorders that may mimic malabsorption include irritable bowel syndrome with diarrhea and/or bloating, microscopic colitis, and laxative abuse. In the case of irritable bowel syndrome and microscopic colitis, patients should not have nutrient deficiencies or lose weight.

DIAGNOSIS

HISTORY

Taking a careful history is the first step in diagnosing malabsorption. In addition to eliciting symptoms that are suggestive of malabsorption, the history can also help identify possible causes of malabsorption (eg, short bowel syndrome in a patient who has undergone a partial small bowel resection), as well as guide further testing. Conditions associated with celiac disease include dermatitis herpetiformis, diabetes mellitus, selective IgA deficiency, Down syndrome, liver disease, and thyroid disease.

PHYSICAL EXAM

The physical exam can give clues about underlying conditions that predispose to malabsorption, such as an abdominal scar in the case of a patient who has had a small bowel resection. The exam may also show evidence of nutritional deficiencies, such as pallor in the setting of anemia and neurologic abnormalities in the setting of vitamin B_{12} deficiency (Table 161-1).

LABORATORY EVALUATION

Various routine laboratory tests may suggest malabsorption (**Table 161-3**). To test for fat malabsorption, the initial test often obtained is a Sudan stain of the stool. This test will identify more than 90% of patients with clinically significant steatorrhea. However, its overall sensitivity and reliability are limited by variability in the performance and interpretation of the test. If fat malabsorption is suspected, a 72-hour fecal fat determination serves as the gold standard. Normal individuals will absorb 94% of the fat that is ingested. The stool should be collected and refrigerated for 72 hours with the patient on a 100 gm of fat per day diet. Excretion of more than 6 gm of fat is abnormal, though values up to 14 gm per day have been seen in volunteers in whom diarrhea was induced and in patients with a stool weight of greater than 1000 gm per day (normal is < 200 gm per day). Patients with true steatorrhea typically have fecal fat excretion of more than 20 gm of fat per day. While testing for protein malabsorption is not generally performed, enteral protein loss can be demonstrated by measuring alpha-1 antitrypsin clearance. In this test, stool is collected for 24 hours, along with a serum measurement of alpha-1 antitrypsin. Clearance is calculated by dividing the product of the fecal alpha-1 antitrypsin and the stool volume by the serum concentration of alpha-1 antitrypsin. In protein losing enteropathy, the value is typically greater than 100 mg/mL.

Laboratory testing can be particularly useful in the evaluation of celiac disease. In addition to nonspecific findings, such as iron deficiency, specific tests for celiac disease include antibodies to tissue transglutaminase (anti-TTG), which are highly sensitive and

TABLE 161-3 Laboratory Abnormalities in Malabsorption

Decreased	Increased
Hemoglobin, iron, ferritin, total iron binding capacity	Urine oxalate
Folate (serum or red blood cell)	Prothrombin time
Vitamin B_{12}	Stool fat
Calcium	
Magnesium	
Cholesterol	
Carotene	
Albumin	

specific (95% and 94%, respectively). Tests can detect both IgA and IgG individually, which is important, since celiac is associated with selective IgA deficiency.

If celiac disease is suspected, serologic testing should be obtained for antitissue transglutaminase and antiendomysial antibodies (with testing to confirm normal IgA levels). If IgA levels are low, IgG-based testing for antitissue transglutaminase or antigliadin antibodies should be obtained. An IgA endomysial assay is highly specific, but only moderately sensitive for detecting celiac disease in untreated patients, and will frequently be falsely negative in patients with celiac disease who are on a gluten free diet. Antigliadin antibody testing has only moderate sensitivity and specificity and the positive predictive value in a general population is poor.

PRACTICE POINT

- In the diagnosis of celiac disease, antibodies to tissue transglutaminase (anti-TTG) are highly sensitive and specific (95% and 94%, respectively). Celiac disease is associated with selective anti-TTG IgA deficiency. Antigliaden antibodies have poor sensitivity and specificity for celiac disease.

ENDOSCOPIC EVALUATION

Upper endoscopy

Some causes of malabsorption will be apparent on upper endoscopy. In the case of celiac disease, the duodenal mucosa may appear scalloped with a mosaic pattern and decreased duodenal folds (**Figure 161-1**). In Crohn disease the mucosa may have a cobblestone appearance. (See Chapter 163 Inflammatory Bowel Disease.) Biopsies should always be obtained, as the findings may be subtle and not discernable to the endoscopist. Biopsies in celiac disease will demonstrate villous blunting with crypt elongation and an increase in intraepithelial lymphocytes. However, not all villous blunting is due to celiac disease. Other conditions that may result in villous blunting include bacterial overgrowth, common variable immunodeficiency, autoimmune enteropathy, Crohn disease, eosinophilic gastroenteritis, giardiasis, lymphoma, peptic duodenitis, gastroenteritis, tropical sprue, Zollinger-Ellison syndrome, and other immunodeficiency states.

Colonoscopy

Colonoscopy with intubation and biopsy of the terminal ileum may aid in making a diagnosis of Crohn disease. Additionally, random biopsies obtained from the colon may help to exclude alternative diagnoses, such as microscopic colitis.

Wireless capsule endoscopy

An advantage of wireless capsule endoscopy over standard endoscopy is that it allows for visualization of the entire small bowel. While generally not required to make a diagnosis of celiac disease (which typically involves the proximal small bowel), the procedure can be helpful in diagnosing other small bowel disorders with mucosal involvement, such as Crohn disease and lymphoma. It is also useful in patients with known celiac disease who are not responding to a gluten free diet. In these patients, considerations include inadvertent gluten ingestion, enteropathy associated T-cell lymphoma, ulcerative jejunitis and refractory celiac disease (ie, celiac disease that does not respond to strict gluten restriction). A disadvantage of wireless capsule endoscopy is that it does not allow for biopsies

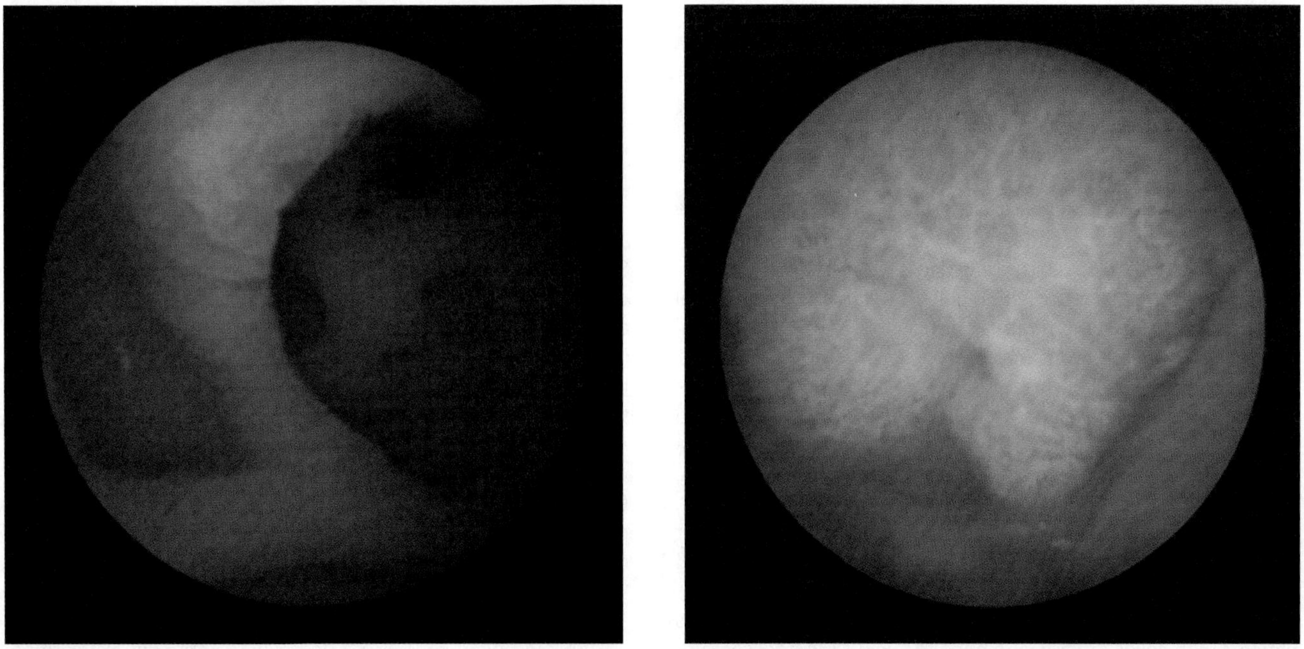

A **B**

Figure 161-1 *Celiac disease. (A) Scalloping of the mucosa. (B) Mosaic mucosal pattern.*

to be obtained. Additionally, it is contraindicated in patients with suspected small bowel obstructions.

Endoscopic retrograde cholangiopancreatography (ERCP) and endoscopic ultrasound (EUS)

ERCP and EUS are sometimes employed to help make a diagnosis of chronic pancreatitis. Findings on ERCP include a dilated, irregular pancreatic duct and stones within the pancreatic duct. However, a normal ERCP does not exclude the diagnosis of chronic pancreatitis. Findings on EUS include both parenchymal and ductal abnormalities. The parenchymal abnormalities of chronic pancreatitis seen on EUS include hyperechoic (white) foci and strands, lobularity, atrophy, cysts, and calcifications. The ductal changes include ductal dilation, irregularity, visible side branches, hyperechoic walls, and pancreatic duct stones. However, the most sensitive finding for chronic pancreatitis is pancreatic function testing, with a reported sensitivity of 80% to 90%. At the time of endoscopy, samples of pancreatic juice are obtained from the duodenum following secretin stimulation. In the setting of chronic pancreatitis, the bicarbonate concentration will be low.

Radiologic evaluation

Radiologic testing has only limited value in the evaluation of malabsorption. Small bowel barium studies may show small bowel diverticula that can be associated with small bowel bacterial overgrowth, or mucosal disease that is not easily reached endoscopically (though capsule endoscopy is superior to small-bowel follow-through for detecting mucosal disease). Computed tomography and magnetic resonance cholangiopancreatography (MRCP) may aid in the diagnosis of chronic pancreatitis.

Breath testing

Bacterial fermentation of undigested carbohydrates is the basis for breath testing. The fermentation results in increases in breath hydrogen, or in the elaboration of radio-labeled carbon dioxide. The tests commonly help diagnose bacterial overgrowth (in which case bacteria digest the carbohydrates within the small bowel) and lactose intolerance. Tests also exist for fructose, sucrose, and isomaltose malabsorption.

TRIAGE/HOSPITAL ADMISSION

While generally managed as outpatients, patients with severe malnutrition or dehydration may need admission for nutritional support, volume repletion, and to correct electrolyte abnormalities.

MANAGEMENT

Treatment of malabsorption aims at correcting nutritional deficiencies and, when possible, correcting the underlying disorder resulting in malabsorption (eg, antibiotic treatment for bacterial overgrowth). Consultation with a dietician is frequently helpful in managing patients with malabsorption. In complicated cases, however, a physician who specializes in nutrition support should be consulted. Significant weight loss (> 10 percent) is associated with increased morbidity and mortality and should be treated aggressively. In some cases, patients may need total parenteral nutrition. Vitamin and mineral deficiencies should be corrected if present. Typically, oral supplementation is sufficient. Patients with significant steatorrhea may need supplementation with fat-soluble vitamins (A, D, E, and K).

Some patients benefit from nutritional restriction, such as patients with celiac disease who need to avoid all gluten-containing foods. Patients should receive counseling from a nutritionist to help them understand what is involved with being gluten free.

TABLE 161-4 Sources of Gluten

Grains/Flours Containing Gluten	Foods Easier to Identify as Containing Gluten	Foods and Products That May Contain Hidden Gluten
Barley	Biscuits	Baked beans
Bulgur	Bread and rolls	Blue cheese
Farina	Cakes	Bran
Graham flour	Cereal	Chutney
Kamut	Communion wafers	Curry powder
Matzo	Cookies	Dry mustard powder
Oats*	Couscous	Farina
Rye	Malted beverages	Gravy powders
Seitan	Muffins	Hydrolyzed vegetable protein
Semolina	Pancakes	Imitation bacon
Spelt	Pasta	Imitation crab meat
Triticale	Pastries and pie crust	Inexpensive chocolate
Wheat	Pizza	Instant coffee
Wheat germ	Pretzels	Licorice
Wheat grass	Scones	Lipstick
	Stuffing	Luncheon meat
	Yorkshire pudding	Malt vinegar
		Marinades
		Meat and fish pastes
		Meat loaf
		Monosodium glutamate
		Pickles
		Potato chips
		Salad dressing
		Sausages
		Self basting turkeys
		Soups/broths
		Soy sauce
		Stock cubes
		Supplements and pills
		Toothpaste
		White pepper

*May be contaminated with gluten.

Some patients believe they are following a gluten free diet because they are avoiding bread products, not realizing that gluten is present in numerous other foods and products (eg, soy sauce, soups, lunch meats, some toothpastes) (**Table 161-4**). For patients with isolated carbohydrate malabsorption (such as lactose intolerance), foods containing the offending carbohydrate should be avoided. Additionally, patients with celiac disease or bacterial overgrowth will often have lactose intolerance until their villi return to normal, and therefore should minimize intake of lactose-containing food products until adequately treated. Patients with steatorrhea should restrict their intake of long chain fatty acids to below 40 gm/day. Some patients may require supplementation with medium-chain triglycerides to maintain adequate caloric intake.

Managing diarrhea is also a necessary component in treatment of malabsorption conditions. Agents that may be helpful in controlling diarrhea include loperamide, diphenoxylate with atropine, deodorized tincture of opium, and bile acid binding agents such as cholestyramine. (See Chapter 80 Diarrhea.)

In the case of chronic pancreatitis, patients should follow a low fat diet and receive pancreatic enzyme supplements with meals. A typical dose is 30,000 IU of encapsulated pancreatic lipase. The efficacy of pancreatic enzymes may be increased by giving H_2-receptor antagonists or proton pump inhibitors to decrease inactivation of the enzymes by gastric secretions.

SMALL BOWEL OBSTRUCTION

INTRODUCTION

Small bowel obstructions (SBOs) account for 15% of emergency admissions for abdominal pain (more than 300,000 hospitalizations per year in the United States). Mortality rates are significant, with an estimated 30,000 deaths per year.

ETIOLOGY

SBOs can be due to mechanical causes (eg, adhesions) or may be functional (pseudoobstruction). In the case of mechanical obstructions, clinicians must differentiate between complete obstructions and partial obstructions, as the former generally require urgent surgical treatment, whereas the latter may be managed medically.

ADHESIONS

In adults, adhesions are responsible for 75% of SBOs, and the incidence of SBO from adhesions has increased over the past 30 years due to an increasing number of laparotomies and laparoscopies. Approximately 5% of abdominopelvic surgeries are complicated by SBOs, with rates of up to 10% for colorectal surgery. The risk of SBO from adhesions is highest in the first few years following surgery, but can occur decades later.

PRACTICE POINT

- Approximately 5% of abdominopelvic surgeries are complicated by SBOs, with rates of up to 10% for colorectal surgery. The risk of SBO from adhesions is highest in the first few years following surgery, but can occur decades later.

HERNIAS

Hernias also commonly cause SBOs, though the frequency of SBOs due to hernias has decreased due to an increase in the rate of prophylactic herniorraphy. The incidence has decreased from 30% to 15% over the last 30 years. Hernias can either be external (femoral, inguinal, midventral, periumbilical, and incisional hernias) or internal. Internal hernias can be subdivided further into congenital (obturator, paraduodenal, transmesenteric, and transomental hernias) or acquired (due to surgery).

TUMORS

Tumors account for 5% to 10% of SBOs. The most common mechanism is extrinsic small bowel compression by gastrointestinal or gynecologic malignancies (especially colon and ovarian cancer). Small bowel cancer is a much less common cause.

OTHER CAUSES

Other causes of SBOs occur much less frequently and include strictures (due to small bowel Crohn disease, medications such as nonsteroidal anti-inflammatory drugs, radiation enteritis, or ischemia), gallstone ileus, phytobezoars, foreign bodies, intussusception, and infection (peritoneal tuberculosis, actinomycosis, and enteric parasites). In children, common causes of SBOs include intussusception, intestinal atresia, and meconium ileus.

PATHOPHYSIOLOGY

SIMPLE OBSTRUCTION

Simple obstruction occurs when the bowel is occluded at one point. When this occurs, fluid accumulates proximal to the obstruction. This results in volume depletion due to impaired intestinal water and electrolyte absorption and increased intestinal secretion. Because of stasis within the small bowel, bacterial overgrowth also develops, with a marked increase in the number of anaerobic bacteria. Fermentation by the bacteria then leads to gas production. The resultant bowel dilation with fluid and gas induces inflammation in the involved small bowel, which leads to an increase in enteric propulsive activity as the bowel attempts to overcome the obstruction. As the muscle fatigues, bowel motility decreases. Vascular perfusion is also compromised because of increasing intraluminal pressure and intramural tension. Because of its high metabolic activity, the small bowel mucosa is very sensitive to ischemia.

CLOSED-LOOP OBSTRUCTION

A closed-loop obstruction occurs when the small bowel is occluded at two points. This can be seen in the setting of an incarcerated hernia, with the hernia sack compressing the small bowel, or with a volvulus, in which the small bowel twists around itself. Because the accumulated gas and fluid cannot escape the loop either proximally or distally, dilation occurs rapidly with resultant mucosal ischemia. In addition, the mesenteric vessels supplying the small bowel may be strangulated as they enter the hernia sack or at the point of occlusion from a volvulus, which exacerbates the ischemia. This ischemia then rapidly results in necrosis and perforation of the small bowel.

DIFFERENTIAL DIAGNOSIS

Nonobstructive intestinal motility disorders (eg, paralytic ileus, intestinal pseudoobstruction) should be considered in patients suspected of having an SBO (see section on small bowel ileus, below). Paralytic ileus is present to some degree in most patients who have undergone open abdominal surgery and may be exacerbated by electrolyte disorders.

DIAGNOSIS

CLINICAL PRESENTATION

Patients with SBOs will often complain of colicky abdominal pain, nausea and vomiting, abdominal distension, and progressive obstipation. However, patients with partial obstructions may not have typical presentations. The pain is frequently sharp with a sudden onset. As the bowel fatigues, the pain may diminish. In addition, vomiting may temporarily relieve the pain by decompressing the distended bowel. Once ischemia or perforation develops, the pain becomes more severe and constant. Since closed-loop obstructions may be associated with mesenteric ischemia, the pain in these cases may be out of proportion to the examination (see section on mesenteric ischemia, below).

Patients with proximal obstructions typically complain of epigastric pain that occurs every three to four minutes. They also frequently have associated bilious emesis. In contrast, distal obstructions typically result in periumbilical pain that occurs every 15 to 20 minutes. Feculent emesis may also occur with distal obstructions, though it is infrequent.

HISTORY

In addition to determining if patients have a prior history of SBO, clinicians should inquire about conditions that predispose to SBO, such as a history of abdominal surgery, abdominal or pelvic radiation, abdominal cancer, symptoms of hernias, inflammatory bowel disease, or pelvic inflammatory disease. Clinicians should inquire of female patients about the timing of their last menstrual period.

Failure to pass flatus is suggestive of a complete small bowel obstruction, whereas rigors, high fever, or systemic toxicity suggest possible intestinal necrosis or peroration.

PHYSICAL EXAMINATION

While findings will vary based on the degree of obstruction, in severe cases patients appear acutely ill, restless, and are febrile. Signs suggestive of intravascular volume depletion may be present, including tachycardia, orthostatic hypotension, dry mucous membranes, and poor skin turgor. The abdomen is moderately distended in the case of proximal obstruction, whereas it may be severely distended with distal obstruction. Bowel sounds are high-pitched and hyperactive initially, with audible rushes or borborygmi that coincide with episodes of abdominal pain. As time progresses, the bowel sounds become progressively hypoactive and softer, eventually disappearing as a result of bowel fatigue. On percussion tympani may be present. Peritoneal signs (eg, rebound tenderness, guarding) are generally absent, unless necrosis or perforation have occurred.

Signs that may point to a possible etiology for the obstruction include jaundice in the case of obstruction due to a pancreatobiliary malignancy or gallstone ileus. Other signs of malignancy include a palpable abdominal mass, hepatomegaly, splenomegaly, and lymphadenopathy. Abdominal scars suggest possible adhesions, whereas external hernias should be examined for signs of incarceration. A rectal examination should be performed to rule out fecal impaction or a rectal malignancy.

LABORATORY TESTING

Laboratory testing is generally nonspecific. Third-spacing of fluids may lead to electrolyte imbalances, azotemia, and hemoconcentration. Intestinal ischemia may result in lactic acidosis. Other signs of possible ischemia include a marked leukocytosis with a left-shift and hyperamylasemia. However, laboratory findings of ischemia may develop late, so their absence should not be seen as an indication of adequate perfusion. Because surgery may be indicated, a coagulation profile as well as platelet count should be obtained. Women of childbearing potential should have a serum pregnancy test.

RADIOGRAPHIC EVALUATION

Radiologic examination significantly aids the diagnosis of SBO since the physical examination and laboratory findings are nonspecific. A plain upright and supine abdominal x-ray is diagnostic in 50% to 70% of cases. The x-ray reveals a dilated, gas-filled proximal small bowel, with collapsed, gasless small bowel distal to the obstruction (**Figure 161-2**). The finding of a transition zone is highly specific for an SBO, but has poor sensitivity. Gas may not be present in cases of a closed-loop obstruction, resulting in a normal x-ray. The accuracy of plain films is highly dependent upon the experience of the radiologist interpreting the study.

> **PRACTICE POINT**
>
> - A plain upright and supine abdominal X-ray is diagnostic in 50% to 70% percent of SBO cases. The X-ray reveals a dilated, gas-filled proximal small bowel, with collapsed, gasless small bowel distal to the obstruction. The finding of a transition zone is highly specific for an SBO, but has poor sensitivity.

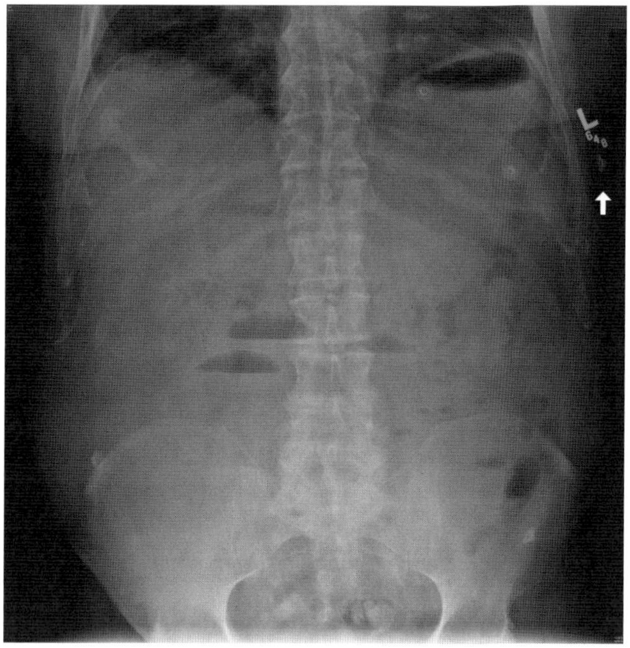

Figure 161-2 *Upright abdominal radiograph of small bowel obstruction (SBO). Eighty-seven-year-old man with early SBO from adhesions due to prior surgery.*

In cases where an x-ray is inconclusive, additional imaging is required. Options include abdominal ultrasound, small bowel follow-through (SBFT), abdominal computed tomography (CT), or abdominal magnetic resonance imaging (MRI). While abdominal ultrasound is as sensitive as an x-ray, with higher specificity, it is infrequently used for suspected SBO due to the availability of more accurate tests.

In patients with suspected *partial SBOs* a small bowel follow-through may provide prognostic information, changing the diagnosis in about half of cases. Water-soluble contrast is given and followed through the small bowel with serial x-rays. The presence of contrast within the colon is highly sensitive (97%) and specific (96%) for predicting resolution without surgery. The disadvantages of SBFT include the time required for completion of the test and the lack of mucosal detail due to dilution of the contrast in the fluid-filled small bowel.

Abdominal computed tomography (CT) allows for rapid and accurate diagnosis (**Figure 161-3**). Like SBFT, the presence of contrast in the colon suggests a partial SBO, with a sensitivity of 92% and a specificity of 93% for diagnosing a complete SBO. When intravenous contrast is used, CT can help identify the cause of the SBO, diagnose strangulation, and identify other pathology that may mimic an SBO (eg, superior mesenteric artery or vein thrombosis causing an ileus). CT is 60% sensitive for identifying a closed-loop obstruction. Where available, CT enteroclysis or multidetector row CT improves the accuracy in identifying the cause of SBO.

MRI with T2-weighted images is more accurate than contrast-enhanced helical CT for identifying the point of obstruction (96% vs. 93%) and in identifying the cause (88% vs. 57%). MRI enterography is another alternative for diagnosing SBO.

Wireless capsule endoscopy is contraindicated in patients with suspected SBO (partial or complete) because of a very high risk of capsule retention at the site of obstruction.

TRIAGE/HOSPITAL ADMISSION

All patients with suspected SBO should be admitted to the hospital. Patients with confirmed or highly suspected complete obstruction should be admitted to a surgical team, while patients

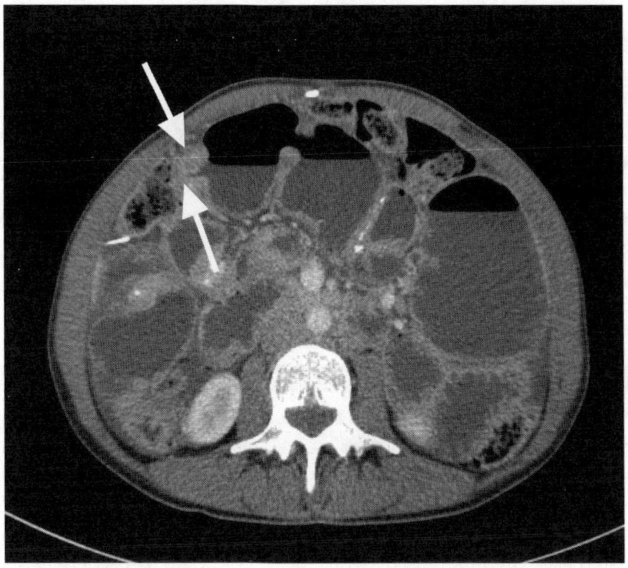

Figure 161-3 *Computed tomography (CT) image of small bowel obstruction (SBO). CT shows the transition point (arrows) of an SBO in a 49-year-old woman with metastatic ovarian cancer.*

with a partial obstruction that has a reasonable likelihood of resolving with medical management alone, may be admitted to a Hospital Medicine or internal medicine team with surgical consultation.

MANAGEMENT

Initial treatment in all cases of SBO includes aggressive intravenous volume repletion and bowel rest. Liberal use of antiemetics can provide symptomatic relief to patients with nausea and vomiting.

Nasogastric tube (NGT) decompression is used to clear gastric contents, decompress the proximal small bowel, and prevent aspiration. This may be done with a soft, lubricated 14 Fr tube and placed with the patient in an upright position. Ideally, the tip of the tube should be in the most dependent portion of the stomach. Once the tube is in proper position it should be taped to the nose, taking care to avoid pressure on the nares. The tube should then be placed on intermittent low wall suction and its output recorded. If the gastric aspirate is feculent it is suggestive of a distal small bowel obstruction. When the obstruction resolves, the tube can be removed and the patient's diet can be advanced, starting first with liquids. The rate at which the diet is advanced will depend upon the patient's tolerance of oral intake. If obstruction resolution is uncertain, the NGT can be clamped for four hours at a time. If the patient does not report nausea and the gastric residuals are less than 100 mL, the tube can be removed and the patient's diet advanced.

Conservative therapy will lead to resolution of a partial SBO in about 90% of cases. Any patients being managed conservatively require serial examinations to look for evidence of worsening obstruction. Surgery is required emergently if there is evidence of complete obstruction, peritonitis, pneumotosis intestinalis, or strangulation. In addition, surgery is indicated in patients with partial SBOs who have not shown signs of improvement after 24 to 72 hours. Patients requiring surgery should receive preoperative antibiotic therapy to cover anaerobic and Gram-negative bacteria.

PRACTICE POINT

- Conservative therapy will lead to resolution of a *partial* SBO in about 90% of cases. Medically managed patients require serial abdominal examinations to look for evidence of worsening obstruction. Surgery is required emergently if there is evidence of complete obstruction, peritonitis, pneumotosis intestinalis, or strangulation. In addition, surgery is indicated in patients with partial SBOs who have not shown signs of clinical improvement after 24 to 48 hours.

During surgery, ischemic, necrotic, or poorly viable small bowel is resected. It is important that only viable small bowel be left to decrease the risk of an anastomotic leak, intra-abdominal abscess, or chronic structuring. Viable bowel should not be removed due to the risk of increased operative mortality and short bowel syndrome. Bowel viability can be assessed at the time of surgery by inspection, palpation, and the use of vital dyes and/or Doppler flowmetry. In some cases, a second-look laparotomy is performed 24 hours after the initial surgery to ensure that no ischemic bowel was left in place.

While most patients who require surgery undergo open laparotomy, less invasive approaches may occasionally be appropriate (eg, for an incarcerated inguinal hernia).

COMPLICATIONS AND PROGNOSIS

SBOs are complicated by strangulation in 30% of cases and necrosis in 15%. Patients with strangulation are at much higher risk for mortality (up to 31%) compared with patients who have a simple mechanical obstruction. Postoperative morbidity is 23% and mortality is 5%. Old age, comorbidities, nonviable strangulated bowel, and a delay in surgery are risk factors for mortality.

PREVENTING RECURRENCE

For patients with SBO who undergo surgery for adhesions, 15% will have a recurrent SBO within five years, and up to 50% will have a recurrence by ten years. After a second episode, the incidence of recurrence increases to 85%. Risk factors for recurrence include conservative management of the SBO, younger age, and dense/multiple adhesions.

Surgical techniques to prevent bowel adhesions include gentle handling of abdominal tissues, avoidance of irritating materials, careful hemostasis, avoidance of bowel ischemia or tissue desiccation, and early surgery (prior to the onset of sepsis). The use of barriers such as sodium hyaluronate- or cellulose-based bioresorbable membranes decreases the frequency of adhesions and may reduce the rate of SBO. Laparoscopic surgery also appears to decrease the risk of adhesions and SBO compared with open laparotomy.

SMALL BOWEL ILEUS

EPIDEMIOLOGY

Postoperative ileus (POI) occurs commonly following both abdominal and nonabdominal surgery. It occurs almost universally after abdominal surgery, but also develops following major nonabdominal surgery, such as knee or hip arthroplasty (2.1%) and infrarenal endovascular aneurysm repair (3.9%). Normal gut function typically returns following surgery within 0 to 24 hours for the stomach, 24 to 48 hours for the small intestine, and 48 to 72 hours for the

TABLE 161-5 Factors that Predispose to Prolonged Postoperative Ileus

Abdominal surgery
Mechanical ventilation
Increased intracranial pressure
Burns
Infections/sepsis
Abdominal compartment syndrome
Volume overload
Hypotension
Use of vasoactive drugs
Electrolyte disorders
Hypokalemia
Hyponatremia
Hypomagnesemia
Hypermagnesemia
Hypocalcemia
Hypercalcemia
Use of opioids
Uremia
Diabetic ketoacidosis
Hypoparathyroidism

colon. More recent data suggest that the recovery of normal gut function may be shorter, with gastric and small intestinal activity returning to normal within hours of surgery, and the colon in one to two days. In some cases, however, POI is prolonged (three to five days), resulting in increased pain, decreased mobility, and prolonged hospitalization.

PRACTICE POINT

- Normal gut function typically returns following surgery within 0 to 24 hours for the stomach, 24 to 48 hours for the small intestine, and 48 to 72 hours for the colon. In some cases, postoperative ileus is prolonged (three to five days), resulting in increased pain, decreased mobility, and prolonged hospitalization.

Direct annual health care costs for POI in the United States exceed $1 billion. Multiple factors predispose to prolonged POI (**Table 161-5**).

PRESENTATION

Patients with POI often present with nausea and/or vomiting; abdominal distension and bloating; diffuse, persistent abdominal pain; inability to pass flatus; and inability to tolerate oral intake.

PATHOPHYSIOLOGY

Gastrointestinal motility is mediated by various neural networks as well as neurohormonal peptides. The enteric nervous system is composed of neurons located within the gut wall. These intrinsic neurons synapse with the extrinsic neural network, which is composed of the visceral sensory afferents in the vagus, splanchnic, and pelvic nerves, along with the motor efferents of the autonomic nervous system.

Gastrointestinal motility can be disrupted in many ways, leading to POI. Inflammation as a result of intestinal manipulation and trauma can result in muscle dysfunction, which may extend to involve the entire GI tract, not just the manipulated segment. Noxious spinal afferent signals increase inhibitory sympathetic activity in the GI tract, and neurohormonal peptides such as nitric oxide, vasoactive intestinal polypeptide, and possibly substance P, act as inhibitory neurotransmitters. Opioids exert their effects primarily at the level of the enteric nervous system, where they increase resting tone, decrease gastric emptying, increase small intestinal periodic spasms, and decrease colonic propulsion.

DIFFERENTIAL DIAGNOSIS

The primary entity that needs to be considered in a patient who is suspected of having POI is small bowel obstruction (SBO; see section on small bowel obstruction, above). Many of the diagnostic tests employed in the evaluation of POI are aimed at ruling out small bowel obstruction. The signs and symptoms can be similar, which can make differentiation difficult. SBO occurs in up to 1% of patients within 30 days of abdominal surgery. Acute colonic pseudoobstruction (Ogilvie syndrome) should also be considered, and like POI, it is often seen following surgery.

DIAGNOSIS

CLINICAL PRESENTATION

The patient's history is an important factor in the evaluation of SBO. The history should be reviewed to look for medical illnesses, medications, and prior surgeries that could predispose to POI or SBO. Patients with POI typically have abdominal distension along with mild, poorly localized abdominal pain. Patients may report the lack of passage of flatus or stool, intolerance of oral intake, or nausea and vomiting. Because many patients with POI are critically ill, they may be unable to communicate their symptoms.

The examination may reveal abdominal distension and tympani, hypoactive or absent bowel sounds, and mild, diffuse abdominal tenderness. Signs of volume depletion (tachycardia, orthostatic hypotension, dry mucous membranes) may also manifest.

Patients with POI typically develop symptoms immediately after surgery, whereas patients with SBO develop symptoms at variable times after surgery. Additionally, patients with SBO tend to have more severe symptoms, progress more rapidly, and appear more ill overall.

LABORATORY EVALUATION

Laboratory testing helps determine the cause of POI and identify evidence of alternative diagnoses (mainly SBO). Electrolyte disturbances contribute to POI, and patients should have their serum electrolytes (sodium, potassium, magnesium, calcium) checked to look for abnormalities. SBO can result in a metabolic acidosis, so patients should have their serum chloride and bicarbonate levels checked as well. An elevated white blood cell count should raise suspicion for a possible perforation, whereas evidence of hemoconcentration (elevated hematocrit, elevated BUN, elevated creatinine) suggests volume depletion.

RADIOGRAPHIC EVALUATION

Plain abdominal radiographs often demonstrate dilated loops of small bowel. While air-fluid levels are typically thought of as signs of SBO, they can also be seen in patients with POI. If the diagnosis remains in question after obtaining the history, performing a physical examination, and obtaining plain abdominal radiographs and abdominal computed tomographic (CT) can distinguish POI from a complete SBO, with sensitivity and specificity of 90–100%. Unfortunately, CT is less reliable in distinguishing POI from a *partial* SBO. Upper GI contrast studies with water-soluble radio-opaque contrast (eg, Gastrografin) can further elucidate the diagnosis if it is still uncertain after CT.

MANAGEMENT

Initial management of POI is conservative and largely supportive. Patients should receive intravenous fluids and correction of any electrolyte abnormalities. Underlying conditions that may be contributing should be sought and treated (eg, antibiotics for sepsis), and drugs that promote GI dysmotility should be discontinued.

Traditionally, oral intake was restricted until patients started passing flatus or stool. More recent studies, however, suggest that early enteral feeding not only is safe, but it also decreases the duration of POI and hospital stay. In cases of severe or protracted vomiting, a nasogastric tube may be required.

PRACTICE POINT

- In postoperative ileus, *early enteral feeding* should be employed as it decreases the duration of POI and hospital length of stay.

Peripheral opiate antagonists (eg, methylnaltrexone; available orally, subcutaneously, or intravenously) for the treatment of postoperative ileus block the peripheral antimotility effects of opioids without interfering with their analgesic effects. They act on the mu-opioid receptor and have limited to no ability to cross the blood-brain barrier.

Additional strategies for treating prolonged POI with little or no supporting evidence for benefit include bran/fiber, metoclopramide, erythromycin, neostigmine, early ambulation (though it has other benefits in the postoperative patient), and gum chewing.

COMPLICATIONS AND PROGNOSIS

When POI is prolonged, patients may have compromised nutrition, leading to increased catabolism, poor wound healing, increased rates of infection, and the need for parenteral nutrition. Patients often will also have decreased mobility as a result of pain. Each of these factors may result in prolonged hospitalization. Additionally, patients with POI have increased risk of pulmonary complications and nosocomial infections.

PREVENTING POSTOPERATIVE ILEUS

Prevention of POI is important given the paucity of effective strategies for managing it. The use of midthoracic epidural anesthesia with local anesthetics both intraoperatively and postoperatively for pain control has been associated with more rapid return of postoperative function compared with using systemic or epidural opioids. This approach blocks both the nociceptive spinal sensory afferents and the inhibitory sympathetic efferents.

Minimally invasive surgery also can reduce POI in animal models and in randomized controlled trials in GI and gynecology laparoscopy rather than open approaches. These findings may have been confounded, however, by decreased opioid use and earlier postoperative feeding after laparoscopic surgery. For patients in whom minimally-invasive surgery is not an option, gentle handling of the intestines is recommended.

Minimizing opioid use postoperatively may aid in the prevention of POI. Increased use of nonsteroidal anti-inflammatory drugs (NSAIDs) may reduce reliance upon opioid analgesics and may decrease inflammation, another component in the development of POI. Ongoing studies may help determine if methylnaltrexone, a peripheral mu-opioid receptor antagonist that is used in the treatment of POI, could also be used to prevent the development of POI.

ACUTE MESENTERIC ISCHEMIA

EPIDEMIOLOGY

Acute mesenteric ischemia is an uncommon, but frequently catastrophic, vascular emergency. In the United States, it occurs in 1 in 1000 patients admitted to acute care hospitals, but its incidence is increasing as the population ages. Even with surgical intervention, it has a high mortality rate, ranging from 60–70%. Recognizing acute mesenteric ischemia quickly is critical, as delays in diagnosis and intervention portend a poor outcome.

PATHOPHYSIOLOGY

Acute mesenteric ischemia occurs when prolonged reduction in the splanchnic blood flow occurs. There are four types of acute mesenteric ischemia, categorized based on their cause: arterial embolism, arterial thrombosis, nonocclusive, and venous thrombosis. The most common cause is *arterial embolism*, which accounts for 50% of cases, a third of whom will have a history of a prior embolic event. The emboli most commonly originate from a cardiac source. Risk factors for developing the mural thrombi that embolize to the mesenteric arteries include myocardial ischemia/infarction, atrial arrhythmias (specifically atrial fibrillation and atrial flutter), valvular disorders, cardiomyopathies, endocarditis, and ventricular aneurysms. A mesenteric artery embolus can also occur following coronary or cerebral angiography. Most emboli lodge in the superior mesenteric artery (SMA) because of the angle from which it takes off from the aorta.

Arterial thrombosis accounts for 15–25% of acute mesenteric ischemia cases. Like arterial emboli, arterial thrombosis most commonly involves the SMA. Almost all cases occur in the setting of severe atherosclerotic disease. Patients with arterial thromboses often have developed collateral blood flow due to the slow progression of atherosclerosis. These patients therefore frequently tolerate obstruction of a major visceral artery. Ischemia or infarction occurs when there is occlusion of the last remaining major visceral artery or of an essential collateral artery. Because of this, the extent of ischemia or infarction is much more extensive (duodenum to transverse colon).

Nonocclusive mesenteric ischemia is seen in 20–30% of cases and is poorly understood. It often occurs in the setting of decreased cardiac output with diffuse mesenteric vasoconstriction. Splanchnic vasoconstriction occurs in response to decreased cardiac output, hypotension, hypovolemia, and vasopressors. Intestinal hypoxia results from the low flow state. While not all patients will have clear risk factors for nonocclusive mesenteric ischemia, some predisposing factors include age greater than 50 years, myocardial infarction, aortic insufficiency, congestive heart failure, cardiopulmonary bypass, renal disease, liver disease, and major cardiovascular or abdominal surgery.

Mesenteric venous thrombosis is the cause of acute mesenteric ischemia in 5% of cases. The majority are due to primary clotting disorders, though in 10% no cause is found. The thrombi typically originate in the venous arcades and propagate to the arcuate channels. Occlusion of the intramural vessels results in hemorrhagic infractions. The superior mesenteric vein is the most commonly involved vessel, whereas involvement of the inferior mesenteric

TABLE 161-6 Differential Diagnosis of Acute Mesenteric Ischemia

Gastrointestinal	Gynecologic	Cardiovascular
Cholangitis	Ectopic pregnancy	Abdominal angina
Cholecystitis	Ovarian torsion	Abdominal aortic aneurysm
Choledocholithiasis	**Pulmonary**	Aortic dissection
Cholelithiasis	Pneumonia	Myocardial infarction
Colonic obstruction	Pneumothorax	**Other**
Diverticulitis		Boerhaave syndrome
Gastric volvulus		Intra-abdominal abscess
Ileus		Porphyria
Intestinal perforation		Pyelonephritis
Intestinal pseudoobstruction		Sepsis
Pancreatitis		Testicular torsion
Small bowel obstruction		

vein is uncommon. Predisposing conditions include primary clotting disorders (up to 75% of cases) and a history of deep vein thrombosis, inflammatory bowel disease, right-sided heart failure, pancreatitis, malignancy, hepatosplenomegaly, hepatitis, recent abdominal surgery or infection, estrogen use, sickle cell disease, and polycythemia.

DIFFERENTIAL DIAGNOSIS

The differential diagnosis for acute mesenteric ischemia is broad and includes gastrointestinal, gynecologic, pulmonary, and cardiovascular considerations (**Table 161-6**).

DIAGNOSIS

CLINICAL PRESENTATION

The presentation of acute mesenteric ischemia is variable, depending on the underlying cause. The classic description includes rapid onset of severe abdominal pain, often out of proportion to findings on physical examination. Some patients will also report forceful bowel evacuation coinciding with the onset of pain. However, in patients with mesenteric venous thrombosis, the onset of symptoms may be insidious, occurring over weeks to months. These patients may complain of nausea, vomiting, and nonspecific abdominal pain.

Delays in the diagnosis of acute mesenteric ischemia may occur due to the nonspecific clinical presentation. Patients frequently complain of severe abdominal pain, but have few objective clinical findings. Mental status changes occur commonly (~one-third of cases) in elderly patients with mesenteric ischemia.

In cases of arterial embolism, symptoms typically have a sudden onset, with patients often complaining of severe periumbilical abdominal pain associated with nausea, vomiting, and diarrhea, which may turn bloody. The sudden onset of symptoms occurs because these patients often lack developed collateral circulation. These patients classically have "pain out of proportion to exam." As ischemia and infarction progress, these patients can become dehydrated, with massive third-spacing of fluids. These patients may present with mental confusion, tachycardia, and ultimately circulatory collapse.

PRACTICE POINT

- Acute mesenteric ischemia due to arterial embolism presents with sudden onset severe periumbilical abdominal pain *("pain out of proportion to exam")*, associated with nausea, vomiting, and diarrhea (sometimes bloody). As ischemia and infarction progress, patients may have massive third-spacing of fluids, mental confusion, tachycardia, and ultimately circulatory collapse.

The presentation of patients with arterial thrombosis is frequently subacute. In the case of patients with SMA thromboses, prodromal symptoms include postprandial pain, nausea, and weight loss. Once acute ischemia has occurred, however, these patients develop symptoms like those seen with arterial embolism.

The presentation of nonocclusive mesenteric ischemia can be particularly difficult to recognize, as many of these patients are elderly and critically ill prior to the onset of the ischemia, which may overshadow the signs of mesenteric ischemia. In patients who are intubated and sedated, the indication that mesenteric ischemia is present may be an unexplained worsening of their clinical status or a failure to improve as anticipated.

Mesenteric venous thrombosis, unlike arterial causes of acute mesenteric ischemia, typically presents late. One to two weeks after the onset, patients will complain of diffuse, nonspecific abdominal pain, anorexia, and diarrhea. Signs on exam include fever, abdominal distension, and hemoccult positive stool. These patients have fewer prodromal symptoms compared with those with arterial thrombosis. Additional findings include bloody ascites and third-spacing of fluid with dehydration and hypotension.

Regardless of the cause, once infarction has occurred, patients develop peritoneal signs, hemodynamic instability, sepsis, and multiorgan failure.

LABORATORY EVALUATION

Laboratory findings do not generally aid in diagnosis, as the findings are nonspecific; patients with acute mesenteric ischemia can have normal laboratory values. Abnormalities may include leukocytosis with a left shift, hemoconcentration, and metabolic acidosis. Other laboratory abnormalities include elevated serum lactate, elevated serum amylase, elevated aspartate aminotransferase (AST), elevated phosphate, elevated potassium, elevated creatinine kinase-BB isoenzyme (but not total creatinine kinase), and elevated lactate dehydrogenase. Unfortunately, many of these laboratory abnormalities occur late, once infarction has occurred.

RADIOGRAPHIC EVALUATION

Plain abdominal radiographs may be normal in 25% of patients with early acute mesenteric ischemia. If abnormal, the findings, while nonspecific, may include thumbprinting, thickening of the bowel loops (<40 percent) or ileus. Pneumatosis intestinalis and air in the portal vein are late findings and associated with a poor prognosis. The primary role for plain radiographs is to exclude other causes that explain the patient's symptoms.

Barium enemas are contraindicated as they can interfere with angiography, offer little information, and can increase intraluminal pressure, further decreasing perfusion of the bowel wall, possibly leading to perforation.

Traditional abdominal computed tomography (CT) is frequently employed in the evaluation of patients with abdominal pain. Unfortunately, in the case of acute mesenteric ischemia, CT has poor sensitivity and specificity for making the diagnosis. Sensitivity may improve to 64% and specificity to 92% if dynamic contrast enhanced CT is used. Findings on CT include focal or segmental bowel wall thickening, intestinal pneumatosis with portal vein gas, lack of enhancement of the arterial vasculature (due to arterial occlusion), and liver or splenic infarcts. CT scanning, however, is the test of choice for diagnosing mesenteric venous thrombosis, with a sensitivity of 90%.

Newer radiographic imaging methods include magnetic resonance angiography and multidetector row CT, which provide more detailed information. These modalities, however, need to be compared to angiography.

The gold standard for diagnosing acute mesenteric ischemia is angiography, though it is less sensitive than CT for detecting mesenteric venous thrombosis. Angiography in both anteroposterior and lateral views are needed to obtain adequate visualization. In cases of arterial emboli or thrombosis, findings include lack of visualization distal to the obstruction. In nonocclusive mesenteric ischemia, areas of narrowing and irregularity in the major arteries may be seen, with decreased or absent flow in the smaller vessels. In the case of mesenteric venous thrombosis, venous filling defects or absent flow may be seen during the venous phase of the exam.

PRACTICE POINT

- The gold standard for diagnosing acute mesenteric ischemia is angiography, though it is less sensitive than computed tomography (CT) for detecting mesenteric venous thrombosis. Standard contrast-enhanced CT has poor sensitivity and specificity for making the diagnosis, but sensitivity improves to 64% and specificity to 92% if dynamic contrast enhanced CT is used. Findings on CT include focal or segmental bowel wall thickening, intestinal pneumatosis with portal vein gas, lack of enhancement of the arterial vasculature, and liver or splenic infarcts. CT scanning is the test of choice for diagnosing mesenteric venous thrombosis, with a sensitivity of 90%.

TRIAGE/HOSPITAL ADMISSION

Diagnosis of acute mesenteric ischemia requires a high clinical suspicion, especially in patients with risk factors. Due to its high mortality, any patient with suspected mesenteric ischemia should be admitted to the hospital for prompt evaluation and treatment.

MANAGEMENT

Once the diagnosis is made, treatment should be initiated immediately. The goals of treatment are to resuscitate the patient, treat the underlying condition if possible, reduce vasospasm, prevent propagation of intravascular clotting, prevent infection, and minimize reperfusion injury.

INITIAL MANAGEMENT

Management starts with administration of intravenous fluids and blood products. Crystalloid intravenous fluid volume replacement up to 100 mL/kg will support these patients who may have significant third-spacing of fluid. A nasogastric tube should be placed for gastric decompression. Patients should receive broad spectrum antibiotics immediately. In the absence of contraindications, intravenous heparin is indicated, with a goal partial thromboplastin time (PTT) of twice the upper limit of normal. Data are lacking regarding the use of low-molecular-weight heparin in this setting. Long-term anticoagulation may be indicated, based on the etiology of the ischemia, other interventions performed, and whether the patient continues to have risk factors for recurrent mesenteric ischemia.

REDUCING MESENTERIC VASOSPASM

Once the patient's hemodynamic condition has been optimized and anticoagulation initiated, the next step is to decrease mesenteric vasospasm. If angiography was used in making the diagnosis, the angiographic catheter is left in the SMA for infusions of papaverine (a phosphodiesterase inhibitor that increases mesenteric blood flow) or other vasodilators. If the diagnosis was made without angiography, glucagon may be infused to help reduce vasospasm (starting at 1 mcg/kg, titrated up to 10 mcg/kg, as tolerated).

Vasoconstrictors and digitalis should be avoided since they can worsen mesenteric ischemia. If patients require pressor agents or inotropes in their management, low-dose dopamine, dobutamine or milrinone affect mesenteric profusion less than the other agents, and may be considered.

ANGIOGRAPHIC THERAPIES

Patients undergoing angiography, both for diagnosis and for treatment, must be hemodynamically stabilized prior to the procedure, since mesenteric vasoconstriction is a normal response to hypotension or hypovolemia, potentially leading to a false-positive result in a patient who has not been adequately resuscitated. Angiography allows for the administration of intra-arterial vasodilators or thrombolytic agents, angioplasty, stent placement, and embolectomy. Papaverine is used to prevent vasoconstriction in both occlusive and nonocclusive acute mesenteric ischemia. The specific treatments employed will depend on the underlying cause of the ischemia. Consideration of angiographic therapies should be done in consultation with vascular surgery colleagues, if available.

SURGERY

If intestinal infarction or perforation is suspected (based on clinical, laboratory, or radiographic findings) emergency laparotomy is required. Even in patients without infarction, surgery is usually required. The exception is in patients with nonocclusive acute mesenteric ischemia, where patients are managed medically in the absence of infarction (treatment of underlying condition if possible, infusion of papaverine). The goal of surgery is to reestablish blood flow via revascularization (embolectomy, thrombectomy, endarterectomy, or bypass). Once revascularization has been performed, infarcted bowel is resected. Determining intestinal viability at the time of surgery can be difficult, and some patients will require a "second-look" laparotomy to ensure that all infarcted bowel was removed.

COMPLICATIONS AND PROGNOSIS

Survival in acute mesenteric ischemia depends on expediency of diagnosis. Diagnosis within 24 hours of symptom onset portends a 50% survival, while further delays can lead to less than 30% survival. Additionally, recurrence is not uncommon and carries with it a poor prognosis. Patients who undergo significant small bowel resections are at risk of developing short gut syndrome and could require long-term total parenteral nutrition or small bowel transplantation.

PREVENTION OF RECURRENCE

The approach to preventing recurrences of acute mesenteric ischemia depends upon the cause of the ischemia. For patients with mesenteric arterial emboli, treatment is typically aimed at preventing future emboli using an anticoagulant (eg, warfarin). An anticoagulant may also be used for patients with mesenteric venous thrombosis. In patients with mesenteric venous thrombosis it is typically continued for six months, but long-term treatment may be warranted in patients with coagulation disorders. Antiplatelet agents such as aspirin may help prevent recurrent acute mesenteric ischemia that is due to mesenteric arterial thrombosis or nonocclusive mesenteric ischemia, though data are limited.

SUGGESTED READINGS

American Gastroenterological Association medial position statement: guidelines for the evaluation and management of chronic diarrhea. *Gastroenterology*. 1999;116:1461.

Batke M, Cappell MS. Adynamic ileus and acute colonic pseudo-obstruction. *Med Clin N Am*. 2008;92:649–670.

Brandt LJ, Boley SJ. AGA technical review on intestinal ischemia. *Gastroenterol*. 2000;118:954–968.

Cappell MS, Batke M. Mechanical obstruction of the small bowel and colon. *Med Clin N Am*. 2008;92:575–597.

Eltarawy IG, Etman YM, Zenati M, et al. Acute mesenteric ischemia: the importance of early surgical consultation. *Am Surg*. 2009;75:212–219.

Hadithi M, von Blomberg BM, Crusius JB, et al. Accuracy of serologic tests and HLA-DQ typing for diagnosing celiac disease. *Ann Intern Med*. 2007;147:294.

Kehlet H, Holte K. Review of postoperative ileus. *Am J Surg*. 2001;182:3S–10S.

Kumar S, Saar MG, Kamat PS. Mesenteric venous thrombosis. *N Engl J Med*. 2001;345:1683–1688.

Oldenburg WA, Lau LL, Rodenberg TJ, et al. Acute mesenteric ischemia: a clinical review. *Arch Intern Med*. 2004;164:1054–1062.

Zeinali F, Stulberg JJ, Delaney CP. Pharmacological management of postoperative ileus. *Can J Surg*. 2009;52:153–157.

CHAPTER 162

Large Bowel Disorders

Shachi Tyagi, MD
Mitchell S. Cappell, MD, PhD

Key Clinical Questions

1. When should ischemic colitis be suspected?
2. What are the key diagnostic tests for ischemic colitis, diverticulitis, acute appendicitis, colonic obstruction, and colonic pseudoobstruction?
3. How is diverticulitis medically managed? What are the indications for surgery in patients with diverticulitis?
4. What are the therapeutic options for colonic obstruction? for colonic pseudoobstruction?

INTRODUCTION

Large bowel disorders (LBD) impose a substantial burden on Americans, accounting for more than 1% of all inpatient admissions, contributing as comorbidities to other hospitalizations, and resulting in expenditures of more than $20 billion annually, which is likely to increase as the population ages. This chapter describes disorders of ischemic colitis, diverticulitis, acute appendicitis, colonic obstruction, and colonic pseudoobstruction. Other disorders, including lower gastrointestinal bleeding, inflammatory bowel diseases, tumors and cancer of the colon, and diarrhea are described in chapters dedicated to those disorders. **Table 162-1** describes key diagnostic tests and therapeutic options for important large bowel disorders, while **Table 162-2** describes the colonoscopic findings.

COLONIC ANATOMY

The colon is a tubular structure approximately 30 to 40 cm in length at birth, but grows to nearly 150 cm in adulthood. It has a much larger diameter than that of the small bowel. The colon extends from the small bowel at the ileocecal valve to terminate at the anal verge. The longitudinal muscle fibers coalesce around the colonic circumference to form three discrete bands called *teniae.* The colon is divided into cecum, ascending colon, hepatic flexure, transverse colon, splenic flexure, descending colon, sigmoid colon, and rectum. The first portion of the ascending colon, called the *cecum*, is a sacculated structure 6 to 8 cm in length and breadth that generally lies in the right iliac fossa and projects downward as a blind pouch below the entrance of the ileum. The large diameter of the cecum makes it particularly vulnerable to rupture from distal colonic obstruction. Its large diameter also provides ample space for cecal tumors to grow before producing obstruction. The mobility of the cecum is normally restricted by a small mesocecum, but 10% to 20% of people lack this mesocecum and are thereby predisposed to cecal volvulus. The *vermiform appendix* is a blind, digitiform outpouching of the cecum that begins inferior to the ileocecal valve. The *ascending colon* extends about 20 cm along the right side of the peritoneal cavity from the cecum to the hepatic flexure. The colon turns medially and anteriorly at the hepatic flexure to emerge as the *transverse colon*, which drapes itself across the anterior abdomen for 40 to 50 cm between the hepatic and splenic flexures. This is the most mobile colonic segment. This segment may dip down into the pelvis in the upright posture. The temporary festooned arrangement of transverse colon can become entrenched by adhesions, such as adhesions after hysterectomy. Such adhesions can result in a technically difficult colonoscopy. The *descending colon*, about 30 cm in length, continues as the S-shaped *sigmoid colon* in the retroperitoneum. The colonic diameter is narrowest (2.5 cm) in the sigmoid colon. The sigmoid colon does not provide ample space to accommodate local tumors or strictures and therefore sigmoid colon tumors or strictures result in early obstruction. The shape, tortuosity, mobility, and spasticity of the sigmoid colon create challenges for the colonoscopist, as well as render it susceptible to volvulus.

Despite individual anatomic variations, the colon generally has a specific vascular arrangement. The *superior mesenteric artery* (SMA) in addition to supplying nearly the entire small intestine, supplies the entire right colon, including the cecum, ascending colon, hepatic flexure, and most of the transverse colon. The *inferior mesenteric artery* (IMA) supplies most of the left colon including the descending colon, sigmoid colon, and part of the rectum. The rectum is

TABLE 162-1 Key Diagnostic Tests and Therapies for Important Large Bowel Diseases in Hospitalized Patients

Disease or Disorder	Key Diagnostic Tests	Major Therapeutic Options
Lower gastrointestinal bleeding	Colonoscopy – localizes site and determines etiology. Nuclear scintigraphy using radio-labelled erythrocytes – locates approximate site. Mesenteric angiography – can determine site and cause if lesion is actively bleeding. CT enterography or capsule endoscopy – second line tests if other tests are unrevealing.	Colonoscopy – injection, ablation, or mechanical therapy to stop the bleeding. Angiography – intra-arterial vasopressin infusion or gelfoam or coil embolization. Surgery – for ongoing bleeding refractory to colonoscopic or angiographic therapy.
Ischemic colitis	Colonoscopy – highly sensitive and specific. Mesenteric angiography – can be diagnostic and therapeutic, test mandatory for involvement of major branches of superior mesenteric artery. Abdominal computed tomography – important to exclude other conditions and often helps suggest the diagnosis.	Medical therapy – usually supportive, including bowel rest, intravenous fluids, antibiotic therapy, and reversal of precipitating factors. Surgery – required for frankly infarcted bowel, impending peritonitis, and sepsis refractory to antibiotic therapy.
Inflammatory bowel disease (IBD)	Blood tests – complete blood count, ESR or C reactive protein. Stool tests – for bacterial culture, fecal leukocytes, ova and parasites, *C difficile* toxin. Abdominal computed tomography – helpful to suggest IBD and to diagnose alternative conditions. Colonoscopy – highly diagnostic in combination with colonic biopsies; examination of terminal ileum recommended for Crohn disease.	General therapy – bowel rest, intravenous hydration, correct electrolyte disorders. Medications – typically first corticosteroids, consider biologic anti-TNF alpha therapy, antibiotics for abscesses or fistulas. Surgery – for large or refractory abscesses, refractory toxic megacolon, severe disease refractory to medical therapy.
Diverticulitis	Abdominal computed tomography – radiologic test of choice for diagnosis and evaluating complications. Colonoscopy – avoided in the setting of acute diverticulitis.	Medical therapy – bowel rest, intravenous antibiotics, intravenous hydration. Percutaneous drainage – for large, walled-off abscess. Surgery – multiple recurrent attacks, advanced Hinchey stage III or IV disease, severe abscesses, refractoriness to medical therapy, colonic perforation.
Acute appendicitis	Abdominal computed tomography – inflamed, distended appendix that fails to fill with contrast or air, appendicolith, mural thickening, pericecal fluid collection, periappendiceal fat stranding. Abdominal ultrasound – valuable only in certain circumstances such as pediatric patients, pregnant women, and thin adults.	Preoperative resuscitation – intravenous hydration, antibiotics, replete electrolytes. Surgery – either open or laparoscopic appendectomy.
Acute diarrhea	Stool studies – for bacterial culture and sensitivity, for ova and parasites, for *C difficile* toxin, stool for fecal leukocytes, stool for fecal occult blood. Abdominal CT – helpful to exclude other diseases and can help define extent of colitis. Colonoscopy – generally only indicated if stool studies do not reveal a cause and if patient is still having diarrhea despite medical therapy.	Supportive therapy – bowel rest, intravenous fluids, replete missing electrolytes. Antibiotic therapy – indicated for certain specific infections or for systemic toxicity.
C difficile colitis	Stool assay for *C difficile* toxin or PCR of stool specimen for *C difficile* gene encoding for toxin B. Colonoscopy – sometimes required to detect characteristic pseudomembranes.	Established therapy – discontinue offending antibiotic, treat with flagyl or vancomycin. Novel or experimental therapies – immunglobulin, rifaxmin, cholestramine, nitazoxanide or fecal transplant.
Colonic obstruction	Radiologic tests – obstructive series, abdominal computerized tomography, occasionally barium enema or CT colonography. Small bowel series or small bowel enterography – for suspected small bowel obstruction.	Supportive therapy – complete bowel rest, antibiotics, intravenous hydration, replete lost electrolytes. Treatment – depends upon etiology. Malignant obstruction or any complete obstruction refractory to medical therapy requires surgery. Sigmoid volvulus often initially responds to sigmoidoscopy or colonoscopy.

(continued)

TABLE 162-1 Key Diagnostic Tests and Therapies for Important Large Bowel Diseases in Hospitalized Patients *(continued)*

Disease or Disorder	Key Diagnostic Tests	Major Therapeutic Options
Colonic pseudoobstruction	Daily abdominal flat plates – to monitor cecal and transverse colon diameters. Colonoscopy – mostly for therapeutic decompression, but helpful diagnostically to exclude other disorders such as mechanical obstruction (eg, volvulus), and detect severity of colonic involvement (especially secondary colonic ischemia).	General measures – bowel rest, correct underlying reversible etiologic factors, discontinue narcotics, nasogastric tube suction, rectal tube, antibiotics in selected circumstances. Neostigmine – must be administered in an ICU. Colonoscopic decompression – usually done on an unprepared colon, emphasis on aspirating air. Surgery – for pseudoobstruction refractory to general measures, neostigmine therapy, and colonoscopic decompression.

also supplied by the inferior and middle rectal (hemorrhoidal) arteries derived from the internal pudendal and internal iliac arteries. Ischemia of the rectum is rare because it is supplied by both the IMA and the systemic circulation via the internal pudendal and internal iliac arteries. Contrariwise, the splenic flexure is vulnerable to ischemia because it lies at a watershed area that is supplied by end arteries of the SMA and the IMA, which have a low perfusion pressure. The splenic flexure can become ischemic when the systemic blood pressure declines in shock.

Extensive anastomotic and collateral circulations exist individually within the SMA and within the IMA and between these two arteries. A series of arcades interconnect neighboring branches of the SMA, while a similar series of arcades interconnect neighboring branches of the IMA. These collateral pathways protect against intestinal ischemia because they open up immediately when one branch of a major vessel is occluded.

The venous system generally parallels the arterial system. The superior mesenteric vein (SMV) drains the cecum, ascending colon, hepatic flexure, and transverse colon, whereas the inferior mesenteric vein (IMV) drains the descending colon, sigmoid colon, and proximal rectum. The IMV drains into the splenic vein, which then joins the SMV to form the portal vein.

ISCHEMIC COLITIS

Ischemic colitis (IC) is defined as inflammation of the colon secondary to diminished blood perfusion that leads to bowel wall ischemia. The colon is the most common site of gastrointestinal ischemic injury. Ischemic colitis encompasses numerous clinical entities that produce insufficient blood perfusion to a segment or the entire colon, and result in variably severe ischemic necrosis ranging from superficial mucosal involvement to full-thickness transmural

TABLE 162-2 Colonoscopic Findings with Large Bowel Disorders in Hospitalized Patients

Disease or Disorder	Colonoscopic Findings
Colonic diverticular bleeding	Stigmata of recent hemorrhage: active bleeding, feeding vessel, adherent clot. Blood pooling in area around diverticulum. No other significant lesion seen at colonoscopy.
Internal hemorrhoids	Purplish lesions just proximal to dentate line bulging into the lumen detected by anoscopy or by rectal retroflexion during colonoscopy.
Angiodysplasia	Macular, intensely erythematous, reticular lesions with an internal structure (eg, starburst pattern or fern tree). Must distinguish lesion from colonoscopic trauma.
Colon cancer	Irregular, exophytic mass with induration and superficial Ulceration, or irregular or asymmetric stricture.
Dieulafoy lesion	Raised, pigmented (visible) vessel without surrounding ulceration. Most common in proximal stomach but can occur in colon or rectum.
Radiation colitis	Acute – sloughed off mucosa, mucosal exudate, edema. Chronic – irregular telangiectasias, mucosal friability, active bleeding, mucosal pallor, fibrotic strictures.
Ischemic colitis	Mottled, grey, or dusky bowel, mucosal friability, mucosal edema, mucosal erythema, superficial ulcers, abrupt transition from normal colon to colitis, rectal sparing, hemorrhagic nodules, de novo colitis, colonoscopic changes rapidly disappear.
Ulcerative colitis	Mucosal granularity, erythema, blunting of normal vascular pattern, mucosal friability or bleeding, mucopus, superficial ulcers, pseudopolyps, rectum involved, continuous involvement without skip lesions.
Crohn disease	Deep linear ulcers, cobblestoning, fistulas, fibrotic strictures, rectal sparing, terminal ileal involvement, skip lesions.
Diverticulitis	Colonoscopy not recommended in the setting of acute diverticulitis due to increased risk of colonic perforation because of colonic spasm and tortuosity. Colonoscopy generally recommended about six weeks after acute diverticulitis to exclude colon cancer in the elderly.
Pseudomembranous colitis	Characteristic raised, yellow-to-green, densely adherent, plaques that are 2–8 mm wide and are randomly scattered over colonic mucosa with relatively normal intervening mucosa.
Colonic pseudoobstruction	Highly dilated, air-filled, compliant colon with poor or no muscular activity and no mechanical obstruction or stricture. At colonoscopy evaluate colon for mucosal ischemia. Abort colonoscopy if dusky or frankly necrotic bowel encountered during the procedure.

necrosis. The term *ischemic colitis* describes the phenomenon of colonic ischemic injury, especially as observed on colonoscopy, but lacks specificity because it fails to specify the obstructed vessel, mechanism, and etiology. The physician should not accept ischemic colitis as a final diagnosis but should assiduously analyze the cause to determine the *site* of occlusion, including colonic branches of the SMA, SMV, IMA, and IMV; the *mechanism* of occlusion, including embolus, thrombus, or vasospasm; and the *cause* of occlusion, including atherosclerosis, vasculitis, low flow states, and hypercoagulable states.

ETIOLOGY

IC is caused by diminished colonic perfusion due to a decrease in systemic perfusion or an anatomic occlusion that is so severe that colonic metabolic demands are not met. Anatomic factors predisposing to colonic ischemia include the narrow caliber of the IMA and occasional vascular variations that lack significant collaterals between the SMA and IMA. Predisposing physiologic factors include the low perfusion pressure at the splenic flexure, a watershed area, a decrease in perfusion associated with colonic motility, and sustained mesenteric vasospasm associated with systemic hypotension or other severe physiologic stress produced by sympathetic activity. **Table 162-3** lists various conditions associated with ischemic colitis.

Ischemic colitis most often occurs in the elderly; the average age is 70 years. Age-related tortuosity of colonic arteries as well as cumulative atherosclerotic disease increases vascular resistance and contributes to colonic ischemia in elderly patients. Mesenteric arterial emboli, thrombosis, or trauma may lead to occlusive vascular disease and impaired colonic perfusion. Colonic hypoperfusion due to congestive heart failure, transient perioperative hypotension, strenuous physical activity, or shock due to various causes, such as hypovolemia or sepsis, can result in IC. About 10% to 15% of patients with ischemic colitis have colonic obstruction from colon cancer, benign colonic stricture, or colonic diverticulitis.

A hypercoagulable state is often a significant factor in the pathogenesis of IC in young patients. Vasculitidies can cause thrombosis and occlusion of small vessels perfusing the colon, resulting in IC (Table 162-3). Various medications predispose to colonic ischemia (**Table 162-4**). Rare causes of ischemic colitis include aortic dissection, intra-abdominal inflammatory disease, and colonic infections such as schistosomiasis or cytomegalovirus. Severe constipation is a risk factor for ischemic colitis. Constipation, however, is an exceedingly common complaint so that patients with mild to moderate constipation without other risk factors rarely develop ischemic colitis.

Infectious colitis and ischemic colitis may present similarly with acute abdominal pain. Various clinical characteristics can help differentiate ischemic colitis from infectious colitis (**Table 162-5**).

TABLE 162-3 Etiologies of Ischemic Colitis

Primary circulatory abnormalities
Atherosclerosis with thrombosis of the IMA or SMA
Systemic hypotension with a low-flow state (nonocclusive mesenteric ischemia, NOMI)
Shock
Hypovolemia or dehydration
Long distance running
Emboli of SMA or IMA
Aortic injury
Aortic surgery (intraoperative injury to IMA)
Aortic dissection
Extrinsic disease compressing the vasculature
Cancer infiltrating the mesentery
Retroperitoneal fibrosis
Vasculitis
Behcet disease
Buerger disease (thromboangiitis obliterans)
Polyarteritis nodosa
Rheumatoid arthritis with vasculitis
Systemic lupus erythematosus with vasculitis
Takayasu disease
Wegener granulomatosis
Hypercoagulopathy/blood dyscrasia
Anticardiolipin antibodies
Antithrombin III deficiency
Factor V Leiden mutation
Protein C deficiency
Protein S deficiency
Sickle cell disease
Extrinsic compression of bowel vasculature associated with intestinal obstruction
Incarcerated hernia
Sigmoid volvulus
Cecal volvulus
Intussusception
Bowel adhesions
Colonic obstruction with colonic distention
Colon cancer with stricture
Benign colonic stricture
Colonic diverticular stricture
Toxic megacolon
Colonic pseudoobstruction
Drug induced injury (see Table 162-4)
Other
Amyloidosis

CLINICAL PRESENTATION

The clinical presentation varies with the underlying cause, extent of vascular obstruction, rapidity of ischemic insult, degree of collateral circulation, presence of comorbidities, and time of presentation. Patients typically present with a sudden onset of crampy abdominal pain, diarrhea, and an urge to defecate. The pain is commonly localized to the left lower quadrant because the left colon is most commonly affected, but localized ischemia to other areas of the colon will often lead to pain localized within the corresponding area of the abdomen. Gastrointestinal bleeding, manifesting as bright red or maroon blood mixed with stool, frequently occurs. The bleeding is generally mild and does not cause hemodynamic instability or require blood transfusion. Other symptoms include anorexia and nausea and vomiting from an associated ileus.

Signs include mild to moderate tenderness over the involved intestinal segment, abdominal distention, low-grade pyrexia, tachycardia, and fecal occult blood. In 10% to 20% of cases, marked tenderness with peritoneal signs may be present on physical examination accompanied by metabolic acidosis and septic shock due to severe ischemia, especially with transmural infarction.

TABLE 162-4 Drugs Associated with Colonic Ischemia

Well-established associations – proposed mechanisms
Cocaine – vasoconstriction due to noradrenergic stimulation
Ergotamine – vasospasm
Estrogen (with progesterone) contraceptives – thrombosis due to hypercoagulability
Pseudoephedrine – alpha-adrenergic vasoconstrictor
Sodium polystyrene (kayexalate) – electrolyte shifts due to medication
Vasopressin – vasospasm
Probable associations – proposed mechanisms
Amphetamines – sympathetic vasoconstriction
Digitalis – mesenteric vasoconstrictor at toxic levels
Dopamine – potent vasoconstrictor
Epinephrine or norepinephrine – potent vasoconstrictors
Methysergide – mesenteric vascular compression from retroperitoneal fibrosis
Nonsteroidal anti-inflammatory drugs – decreased synthesis of local prostaglandins that promote intestinal vasodilation
Possible associations – proposed mechanisms
Alosetron – unknown mechanism related to 5-HT(3) antagonism, induced constipation may play a role
Alpha-interferon – unknown mechanism
Danazol – ischemia from constipation and bowel dilatation
Diuretics – cause volume depletion and decreased colonic perfusion
Tegaserod – serotonin 5HT(4) antagonist that may cause severe diarrhea and ischemic colitis.
Tricyclic antidepressants – may decrease colonic perfusion

Data from Cappell MS. Colonic toxicity of administered drugs and chemicals. *Am J Gastroenterol.* 2004;99(6):1175–1190 and Cappell MS. Intestinal (mesenteric) vasculopathy: II. Ischemic colitis and chronic mesenteric ischemia. *Gastroenterol Clin North Am.* 1998;27(4):827–860.

TABLE 162-5 Distinguishing Ischemic Colitis from Infectious Colitis

Clinical Characteristic	Ischemic Colitis	Infectious Colitis
Symptoms		
Acuity of symptoms	Often sudden	Often gradual
Abdominal pain	Predominant symptom, may be severe	Secondary symptom
Diarrhea	May occur early as minor symptom	Predominant symptom
Gastrointestinal bleeding	Frequent, mild blood per rectum	Sometimes bloody diarrhea
Risk factors		
Risk factors for atherosclerosis	Frequent	Sometimes
Prior manifestations of vascular disease	Frequent	Occasionally
Risk factors for ischemic colitis (Table 162-3)	Frequent	Occasionally
Physical examination		
Physical findings of dehydration (eg, dry mucous membranes)	Occasional	Frequent with severe diarrhea
Bowel sounds	Early hyperactive, then hypoactive	Hyperactive bowel sounds
Lab tests		
Serum bicarbonate level	Often low	Often normal
Serum lactate	Often elevated	Usually normal
Fecal leukocytes	Often present	Often present
Stool culture	Nondiagnostic	May be diagnostic
Plain abdominal roentgenogram		
Thumbprinting	Characteristic later finding	Uncommon
Thickened colonic wall	Common	Common
Colonoscopy		
Grey or dusky bowel	Characteristic of colonic infarction	Rare
Rectal involvement	Rectum spared due to dual blood supply	Rectum often involved
Splenic flexure involvement	Frequent due to "watershed effect"	Sometimes involved
Segmental involvement	Characteristic	Frequently widespread colitis
Skip lesions	Uncharacteristic	Occasionally occurs
Abrupt transition from normal to abnormal colon	Characteristic	Uncommon
Hemorrhagic nodules	Fairly characteristic finding	Rare

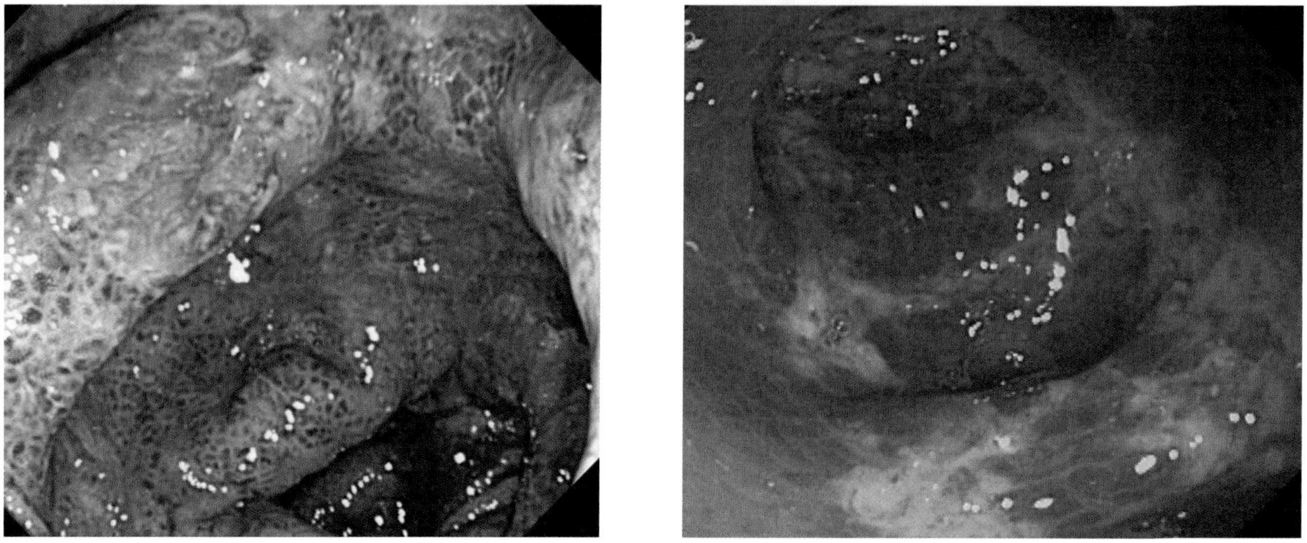

A B

Figure 162-1 *(A) Colonoscopic video-photograph showing submucosal edema and hemorrhage (hemorrhagic nodules) in a patient with colonic ischemia. The patient presented with acute lower abdominal pain and rectal bleeding. (B) Colonoscopic video-photograph showing segmental erythema and ulcerations that develop in ischemic colitis several days after clinical presentation, as the hemorrhagic nodules disappear.*

DIAGNOSIS

Because mild to moderate IC is nonspecific and variable, the diagnosis largely depends on a high index of clinical suspicion, often based on predisposing conditions, as those presented in Table 162-3.

PRACTICE POINT

- In ischemic colitis, the degree of laboratory abnormalities parallels the severity of ischemia. Severe ischemia manifests with leukocytosis, neutrophilia, and a shift to immature leukocyte forms on the leukocyte differential. Necrosis can cause metabolic acidosis, as well as elevations of the serum lactate. Patients with a clinical suspicion of IC should have stool cultures for *Salmonella, Shigella, Campylobacter,* and *Escherichia coli* O157:H7. Infection with parasites or viruses such as cytomegalovirus should also be excluded.

Plain abdominal roentgenogram shows nonspecific findings in about 20% of cases such as dilated and air-filled (exhausted) bowel loops, colonic aperistalsis, and mural thickening, but it is often valuable to exclude other abdominal disorders. Barium enema may suggest colonic ischemia, with thumbprinting, from submucosal hemorrhage and edema. Computed tomography (CT), often the initial diagnostic test to assess patients with nonspecific abdominal pain, can reveal mural thickening, thumbprinting, and pericolonic stranding, with or without peritoneal fluid. Mural thickening with IC is typically concentric, symmetric, and smooth.

Colonoscopy is the best diagnostic test in IC because of high sensitivity, the ability to obtain mucosal biopsy specimens to exclude other pathologic entities, and the ability to perform subsequent angiography, which is indicated for suspected superior mesenteric arteriopathy. Flexible sigmoidoscopy is adequate to evaluate colonic ischemia after aortic surgery or aortic aneurysm rupture because in these situations the ischemia almost always involves the distal colon and colonoscopy is inadvisable in such critically ill patients. Colonoscopy may reveal hemorrhagic nodules, which represent submucosal edema and hemorrhage that correspond to the thumbprints present at barium enema (**Figure 162-1A**).

Hemorrhagic nodules localized to the ascending colon suggest SMA occlusion and a need for angiography. Colonoscopy should be performed early because the hemorrhagic nodules usually disappear within several days. Segmental erythema, with or without ulcerations and bleeding, may be subsequently observed (**Figure 162-1B**). With transmural bowel infarction from severe ischemia, the mucosa may appear dusky, gray, or black. The colonoscopist should discontinue colonoscopic intubation when encountering frankly necrotic bowel because of a high risk of colonic perforation. Colonoscopic evidence favoring the diagnosis of ischemic colitis rather than inflammatory bowel disease includes a segmental distribution of injury, abrupt transition between injured and uninjured mucosa, rectal sparing, de novo colitis, occurrence in the elderly, and rapid mucosal healing on repeat colonoscopy.

TREATMENT

Treatment of IC depends on etiology, disease severity, timing of presentation, and presence of comorbidities. Most cases of IC are transient and treated expectantly with medical therapy. Patients should be placed on bowel rest and given intravenous fluids to replete intravascular volume and reduce intestinal oxygen requirements. Patients with malnourishment, profuse diarrhea, or a prolonged clinical course should receive parenteral hyperalimentation. Empiric broad-spectrum intravenous antibiotics, such as piperacillin/tazobactam, ceftriaxone plus metronidazole, ciprofloxacin plus metronidazole, or imipenem, are recommended to minimize bacterial translocation and sepsis due to the loss of mucosal integrity. A nasogastric tube should be placed if ileus is present. A rectal tube may help decompress a distended colon. Antiplatelet agents have not been evaluated in the treatment of IC and are generally not administered. Signs and symptoms often disappear within 24 to 48 hours, and colonoscopic and roentgenographic abnormalities often completely resolve within several weeks. Colonoscopy should be repeated several weeks after the initial presentation to verify disease recovery and thereby confirm the diagnosis.

About 20% of patients with acute IC require surgery because of signs or laboratory findings of peritonitis. The intraoperative appearance of the serosal surface of infarcted colon ranges from that of wet tissue paper to mottled or dusky bowel. It is important at surgery to resect all devitalized bowel to ensure normal surgical margins. Primary anastomosis is usually not performed because of the increased risk of anastomotic dehiscence. The proximal colonic loop is exteriorized to form a colostomy, and the distal loop is either exteriorized to form a mucous fistula or closed to form a Hartmann pouch.

PRACTICE POINT

- In ischemic colitis, vasopressors should be discontinued or avoided whenever possible. Narcotic analgesics should be withheld early in treatment because these agents blunt the signs of peritonitis and promote abdominal distention. Cathartics are relatively contraindicated because they can precipitate colonic perforation.

DIVERTICULITIS

Diverticula are small mucosal herniations that protrude through the smooth muscle layers of the intestines via the openings of vasa recta or nutrient vessels. Although diverticula can occur throughout the gastrointestinal tract, they most commonly occur in the colon, especially the sigmoid colon, which experiences much higher intraluminal pressures than the rest of the gastrointestinal tract. Diverticula are common, frequently asymptomatic, and are associated with a low-fiber diet, obesity, and constipation. Diverticulosis denotes the presence of uninflamed diverticula. Its incidence increases with age, from less than 5% before age 40 years to greater than 65% by age 85 years.

About 10–15% of patients with diverticulosis develop diverticulitis, defined as inflammation of one or more diverticula (**Figure 162-2**). While generally a disease of the elderly, 20% of cases occur in patients less than 50 years old. The pathogenesis is unclear. Fecal material or undigested food particles may collect in a diverticulum, cause obstruction, and result in distension of a diverticulum, which leads to vascular compromise and colonic microperforation causing inflammation in the colonic wall and paracolonic tissues. Alternatively, inspissated food particles or fecaliths can abrade the mucosal wall of diverticula, resulting in focal inflammation, necrosis, and microperforation. Typically microperforations are walled off by pericolonic fat and mesentery, and the inflammation remains contained and mild. However, macroperforations from extensive disease lead to abscess formation and, rarely, intestinal rupture or peritonitis. Fistulae or abscesses are complications of diverticulitis. Frank bacterial peritonitis is a rare, life-threatening complication. Multiple episodes of diverticulitis can lead to scarring, clinically manifesting as a colonic stricture.

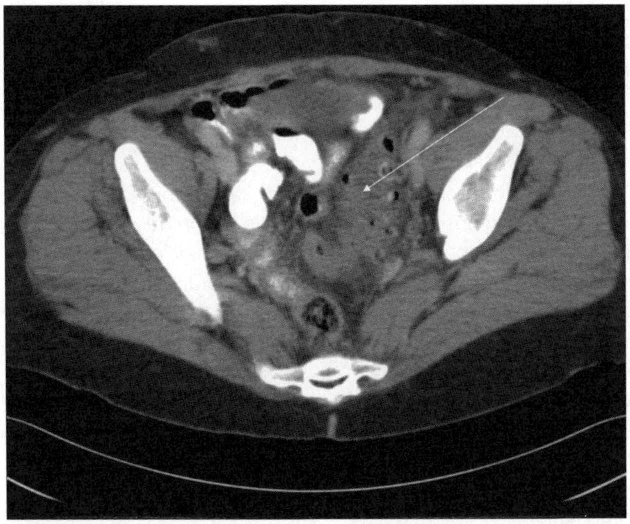

Figure 162-2 *CT of abdomen in a 60-year-old female presenting with left lower quadrant abdominal pain showing sigmoid colon mural thickening, several colonic diverticula, and associated mesocolic fat infiltration, findings consistent with acute diverticulitis.*

CLINICAL PRESENTATION

Patients typically present with crampy, left lower quadrant abdominal pain and low-grade pyrexia. The pain may be intermittent or constant, and may be associated with a change in bowel habits, either diarrhea or constipation. Other symptoms include anorexia, nausea, and vomiting. Patients may complain of urinary symptoms, such as dysuria, urgency, and frequency due to bladder irritation from the inflamed adjacent sigmoid colon.

Signs reflect the severity of inflammation and the presence of complications. Common signs with uncomplicated diverticulitis are pyrexia and localized abdominal tenderness. The tenderness is usually located in the left lower quadrant where the sigmoid colon is located. Right lower quadrant tenderness, mimicking acute appendicitis, can occur with right-sided diverticulitis. Guarding, localized rebound tenderness, and a tender, palpable mass can occur with diverticulitis complicated by abscess formation. The abdomen may be distended and tympanitic. Bowel sounds are typically hypoactive, but may be normoactive in mild cases or hyperactive if obstruction occurs. If a fistula forms, the findings vary depending on the type of fistula. Colovesicular fistulas may present with suprapubic, flank, or costovertebral angle tenderness. Female patients with colovaginal fistulas may present with purulent vaginal discharge. Complicated diverticulitis is classified according to Hinchey's classification based on clinical findings, imaging studies, and presence of complications (**Table 162-6**).

LABORATORY EVALUATION

Laboratory studies are often nonspecific. A hemogram may reveal leukocytosis, neutrophilia, and a shift to immature neutrophil forms, indicating acute infection. An absence of leukocytosis does not, however, exclude diverticulitis. Serum chemistries help assess electrolyte abnormalities in patients with vomiting or diarrhea. Blood cultures should be obtained prior to empiric administration of parenteral antimicrobial therapy in patients who are febrile, severely ill, or have complicated disease.

Further studies are needed if the diagnosis is unclear or if complications are suspected. Upright and supine abdominal films are recommended in patients with significant abdominal pain. An upright chest radiograph should be obtained to exclude pneumoperitoneum or lower-lobe pneumonia. Abdominal radiographs are abnormal in 30% to 50% of patients with acute diverticulitis, with findings of bowel dilation, from obstruction or ileus, or findings of a soft tissue density suggesting an abscess.

Abdominal computed tomography (CT) is the radiologic test of choice. It is superior to intraluminal examinations, such as barium enema. CT can image mural and extramural disease. Sensitivity and specificity, especially with helical CT and colonic contrast, are as high as 97%. CT findings include colonic diverticulosis, pericolonic fat infiltration or "stranding," mural thickening, phlegmon, and abscess. Ultrasonography (US) is a low cost, convenient, noninvasive, alternative diagnostic modality for acute diverticulitis, but it has limitations. Supportive findings include diverticulosis, mural thickening, mural

TABLE 162-6 **Classification and Treatment of Complicated Diverticulitis According to Hinchey Classification**

Stage	Description	Treatment
	Uncomplicated diverticulitis	Treatment as outlined under stage I.
I	Small or confined pericolic or mesenteric abscess	An immunocompetent and reliable patient who can tolerate a diet, has no systemic symptoms, and no diffuse peritoneal signs can be managed as an outpatient with a clear liquid diet and oral antibiotics. Contraindications for outpatient management include immunocompromised state, corticosteroid therapy, severe comorbidities, and patient age >85 years old. Patients failing outpatient management should be hospitalized for bowel rest, intravenous antibiotics, and surgical consultation.
II	Large abscess, often confined to the pelvis	Hospitalization for intravenous antibiotics, bowel rest, CT-guided percutaneous drainage, and surgical consultation.
III	Generalized peritonitis due to rupture of a pericolic or pelvic abscess (noncommunicating with the colonic lumen because of obliteration of the diverticular neck by inflammation)	Urgent surgical intervention after patient resuscitation in an ICU.
IV	Feculent peritonitis due to free perforation of a diverticulum (communicating with colonic lumen)	Urgent surgical intervention after patient resuscitation in an ICU.

hyperechogenicity, and abscesses. It is a second-line diagnostic tool because it is highly operator-dependent.

Colonoscopy or sigmoidoscopy is generally avoided in the initial evaluation of suspected acute diverticulitis because of the risk of colonic perforation from the instrument or from air insufflation alone due to colonic spasticity, tortuosity, and inflammation. If the diagnosis is ambiguous, a limited flexible sigmoidoscopy with minimal air insufflation can help exclude alternative diagnoses, such as inflammatory bowel disease or ischemic colitis. A colonoscopy should be electively performed about six weeks after initiating therapy, after the acute disease has resolved, to evaluate the extent of diverticulosis and to exclude colonic neoplasia.

TREATMENT

Patients with acute diverticulitis typically present with signs and symptoms sufficient to justify the clinical diagnosis and the institution of empiric therapy. **Figure 162-3** shows an algorithm for the management of acute diverticulitis. Acute diverticulitis is treated according to Hinchey stage (Table 162-6).

Medical management

Patients hospitalized for acute diverticulitis should have complete bowel rest (NPO) and receive intravenous hydration and intravenous broad-spectrum antibiotics, with coverage for common anaerobic microorganisms such as *Bacteroides fragilis*, *Peptostreptococcus* and *Clostridium*, as well as aerobic microorganisms such as *Escherichia coli*, *Klebsiella*, *Proteus*, *Streptococcus*, and *Enterobacter*. Recommended antibiotic regimens include anaerobic antibiotic coverage with metronidazole, and Gram-negative antibiotic coverage with an aminoglycoside, monobactam, or third-generation cephalosporin. Single-agent coverage, with second-generation cephalosporins or combined beta-lactamase inhibitors such as ampicillin/sulbactam or ticarcillin/clavulanate, is a reasonable alternative. Pain management is important. Morphine is preferred over meperidine for pain control because of less toxicity. Nonsteroidal anti-inflammatory drugs (NSAIDs) and corticosteroids should be avoided due to an increased risk of colonic perforation.

Once the diagnosis is established and the patient has been stabilized, patients hospitalized with moderate disease should undergo daily abdominal examinations to monitor the illness. With appropriate treatment, symptomatic improvement should occur within two to three days, at which time the diet may be advanced. If improvement continues, the patient may be discharged with instructions to complete a 7 to 10 day course of oral antibiotics. If pyrexia and leukocytosis do not resolve after two to three days of therapy or serial examinations reveal worsening signs or new peritoneal findings, repeat abdominal CT is recommended to exclude complications.

Percutaneous drainage

CT-guided percutaneous drainage is indicated for a peridiverticular abscess that is *more than 4 cm in diameter* (Hinchey stage II disease, Table 162-6). The abdominal pain, pyrexia, and leukocytosis usually promptly decrease after drainage. Percutaneous drainage has eliminated the need for a multistage procedure with initial colostomy, and instead permits temporary palliative drainage with subsequent single-stage resection. The timing of surgery following drain placement depends upon resolution of the local inflammatory response. Follow-up CT scan is recommended six to eight weeks after percutaneous drainage to plan elective surgical intervention. Colonoscopy to exclude other colonic pathology can be safely performed at this time, as long as the inflammation has resolved. Rarely, the percutaneous drains inadequately control the local infection and urgent surgical intervention is required.

Elective surgery

The American Society of Colon and Rectal Surgeons currently recommends consideration of elective colon resection on an individual basis for recurrent, uncomplicated diverticulitis to prevent further recurrences. Considerations regarding elective surgery include patient age, comorbidities, severity and frequency of the attacks, residual symptoms after resolution of the acute attack, and immunocompromised state. Single-stage resection with primary anastomosis is the standard elective surgery for uncomplicated diverticulitis. After excluding colonic perforation, bowel preparation is essential before single-stage surgery, using either a one-day polyethylene glycol electrolyte lavage or two- to three-day mechanical preparation.

Emergency surgery

Urgent surgical intervention is required for patients who present with Hinchey stages III or IV, uncontrolled perforation, or failure of

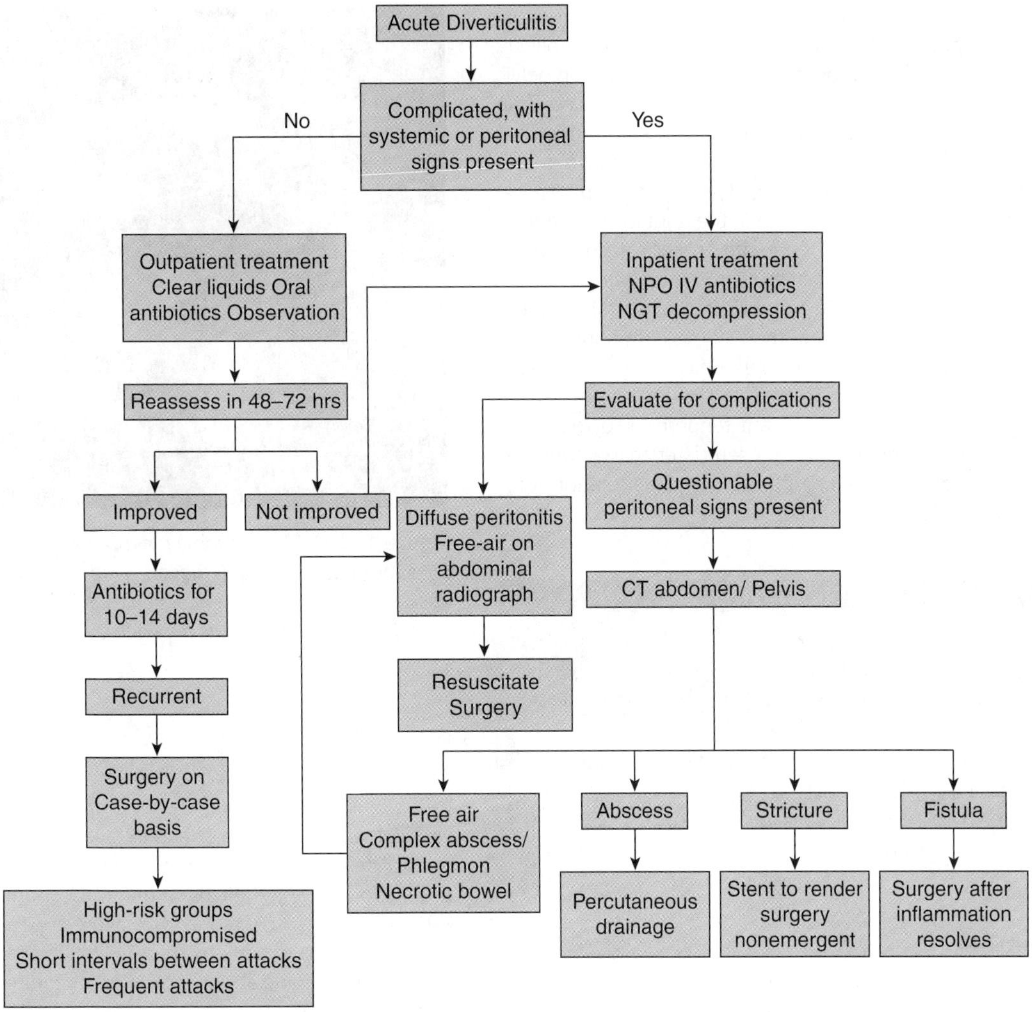

Figure 162-3 *An algorithm for the management of acute diverticulitis, depending on severity and presence of complications. (IV, intravenous; NGT, nasogastric tube; NPO, nothing per os.)*

medical therapy (Table 162-6). Early identification of peritonitis is critical. A CT scan can confirm the diagnosis in ambiguous cases, but an abdominal series showing pneumoperitoneum together with a high clinical suspicion is sufficient to justify laparotomy. The surgical approach in an emergent setting is a two-stage procedure: primary resection of diseased bowel with proximal end colostomy and oversewing of the distal stump (Hartmann pouch), followed by takedown of the colostomy and reanastomosis after the inflammation has resolved, usually three to six months later. When concerned about potential peritoneal contamination from bowel perforation, bowel lavage can be performed on the operating table during urgent or emergent surgery to permit a single stage, primary anastomosis.

ACUTE APPENDICITIS

Appendicitis is the most common abdominal surgical emergency in the United States, with more than 250,000 appendectomies per annum. The peak incidence occurs in the second and third decades of life; it is relatively rare at the extremes of age. However, perforation is more common in infancy and in old age. Mortality is highest among the elderly. Males and females are affected equally. Appendicitis may result from apendiceal luminal obstruction due to fecaliths, lymphoid hyperplasia, parasites, or tumors. Venous engorgement, with consequently impaired arterial flow, leads to ischemia and necrosis of mucosa and then muscularis propria. Mucosal necrosis, erosions, and ulcers permit bacterial invasion that produces a local inflammatory response.

CLINICAL PRESENTATION

Acute appendicitis presents initially with vague, mild to moderate epigastric or periumbilical discomfort. The periumbilical abdominal pain is visceral, resulting from distention of the appendiceal lumen. This pain sensation is transmitted by slow-conducting C nerve fibers and is usually poorly localized in the periumbilical or epigastric region, and is generally mild and crampy, visceral pain. After the inflammation spreads to parietal peritoneum, the pain migrates to the right lower quadrant, and becomes somatic, steady, more severe, and aggravated by motion or cough. Parietal afferent nerves are A delta fibers, which are fast-conducting and unilateral. These nerve fibers localize the pain to the right lower quadrant. This classic sequence occurs in two-thirds of patients.

Physical findings vary according to time after onset and location of the appendix, which may be situated deep in the pelvic cul-de-sac, in the right lower quadrant, or occasionally in the right upper quadrant (especially during pregnancy). Localized right lower quadrant tenderness is an important finding when present, but its absence does not exclude appendicitis. Tenderness is sometimes absent early in the visceral stage of appendicitis, but ultimately always develops at locations that correspond to the appendiceal location. Point tenderness typically occurs at McBurney point, anatomically located on a line one-third of the distance between the anterior superior iliac spine (ASIS) and the umbilicus. Abdominal tenderness may be absent if a retrocecal or pelvic appendix is present, in which case the tenderness may occur in the flank or on rectal or pelvic examination. Rebound tenderness often manifests late in appendicitis. Flexion of the right hip and guarded movement by the patient are due to parietal peritoneal involvement. Cutaneous hyperesthesia of the right lower quadrant and the psoas or obturator signs are late findings. Tachycardia is uncommon with simple appendicitis, but common with complications. Most patients with simple appendicitis have a temperature less than 38°C; temperature greater than 38°C is commonly associated with perforated or gangrenous appendicitis. The diagnosis is challenging in elderly patients. They often lack the classic pattern of pain migration, right lower quadrant tenderness, pyrexia, and leukocytosis. Elderly patients often present later than young patients. For these reasons, the complication and perforation rates can be as high as 50% in the elderly.

PRACTICE POINT

- Psoas sign – Passive right hip flexion elicits right lower quadrant pain and may cause the patient to draw up the right knee. This sign indicates an inflamed (retrocecal) appendix lying against the psoas muscle.
- Obturator sign – Passive flexion of the right hip and knee, followed by internal rotation of the right hip, elicits right lower quadrant pain. This sign indicates an inflamed (pelvic) appendix that lies against the right obturator internus muscle.

EVALUATION

All patients with potential appendicitis should have urgent surgical consultation. Laboratory abnormalities include markers of acute inflammation, such as leukocytosis and a shift to immature neutrophil forms. Leukocytosis of >20,000 cells/μL suggests appendiceal perforation. Abdominal radiographs are rarely helpful. Only 5% have an opaque fecalith in the right lower quadrant. Consequently, abdominal radiographs are obtained only if other conditions, such as intestinal obstruction or ureteral calculus, are in the differential diagnosis. Contrast-enhanced or nonenhanced CT is superior to abdominal ultrasound and abdominal radiographs. CT findings include an inflamed, distended (>6 mm wide) appendix that fails to fill with contrast or air (**Figure 162-4**); findings of an appendicolith; appendiceal mural thickening; periappendiceal inflammation; cecal apical thickening; and pericecal fluid collections. Pneumoperitoneum is uncommon, even in perforated appendicitis. CT visualization of a normal appendix, nonvisualization of the appendix altogether, or demonstration of alternative intra-abdominal pathology constitutes a negative study. The positive predictive value of CT is 95% to 97%, and accuracy is 90% to 98%.

The diagnostic role of abdominal ultrasound is controversial. A shadowing appendicolith, pericecal inflammation, or localized pericecal fluid collection suggest appendicitis. Appendicitis is excluded by ultrasonographic visualization of a normal appendix, but a study in which the appendix is nonvisualized does not exclude acute appendicitis. Unfortunately, a normal appendix is demonstrated by ultrasonography less than 50% of the time when there is no appendicitis. Ultrasound is more sensitive and specific in children (>90% sensitivity and specificity in children) than in adults. Abdominal ultrasound is an alternative first imaging study for appendicitis, especially for institutions with experienced ultrasonographers, in pregnant women, thin adult patients, and pediatric patients.

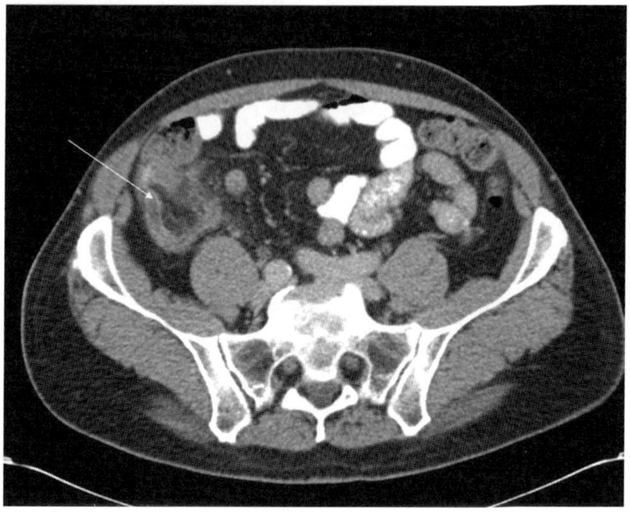

Figure 162-4 *CT of abdomen in a 24-year-old male presenting with an acute abdomen reveals massive dilation of the appendix with mural thickening and severe periappendiceal inflammatory changes (see arrow) consistent with acute appendicitis.*

TREATMENT

Patients are administered preoperatively intravenous antibiotics to prevent bacterial invasion, intravenous fluids to correct intravascular volume depletion, and intravenous electrolytes to correct electrolyte imbalances. Appendectomy is uniformly recommended, even though appendicitis sometimes spontaneously resolves. Patients highly suspected to have acute appendicitis by an expert clinician can go directly to surgery after emergency resuscitation without undergoing abdominal CT or other radiologic studies. Both open and laparoscopic appendectomies are safe and effective for nonperforated appendicitis. Laparoscopic appendectomy may be superior to open appendectomy for uncomplicated appendicitis but this has not been definitively proven. Laparoscopic appendectomy takes more operative time and is more expensive, but after laparoscopic appendectomy, patients require less pain medication, have a shorter hospitalization, and have a lower rate of wound infection than after open appendectomy. Yet, patients experience an increased rate of intra-abdominal abscesses after laparoscopic appendectomy. Laparoscopic appendectomy is preferable for patients who need to rapidly return to work or who have an uncertain preoperative diagnosis.

Patients with perforation and a palpable right lower quadrant mass usually have extensive periappendiceal inflammation or an abscess. In patients without diffuse peritonitis or systemic toxicity, initial management can be operative or nonoperative. With initial nonoperative management, patients are placed at bowel rest and administered intravenous fluids and antibiotics. A CT scan of the abdomen is obtained. If a single abscess greater than 3 cm is discovered, percutaneous drainage of the abscess under CT guidance is performed. If multiple abscesses are found or if the patient does not improve within 24 to 48 hours of conservative therapy, operative drainage of the abscess(es) is/are performed. Success rates of 90% to 95% have been reported with initial nonoperative management. Following complete resolution of the acute illness, colonoscopy or barium enema should be performed in elderly patients to exclude cecal cancer. Interval appendectomy after 6 to 12 weeks when the acute inflammation has resolved is recommended, but the role of interval appendectomy remains controversial because the rate of recurrent appendicitis is less than 20% at one year.

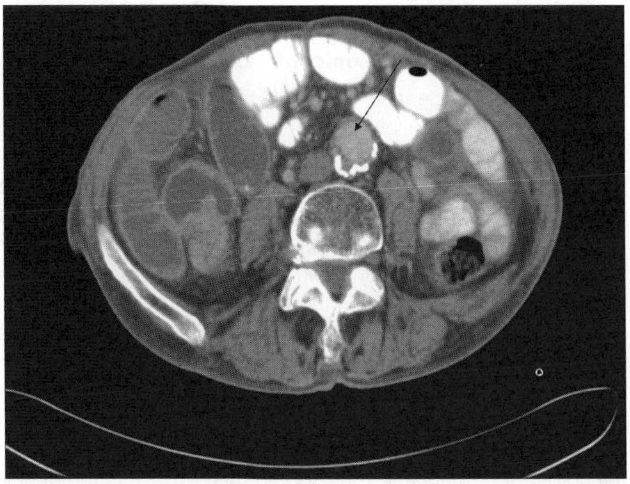

Figure 162-5 *CT of abdomen in an 89-year-old male with an intraluminal mass lesion (see arrow) in ascending colon. The mass almost totally obstructs the lumen, with only a thin margin of contrast medium seen circumferentially. Contrast is present in bowel proximal to the mass. The colon is decompressed distally via a patent rectum. Note the shift of the ascending colon from its normal position in the left lower quadrant to the central pelvis due to the dilated bowel proximal to the obstructing lesion.*

COLONIC OBSTRUCTION

Colonic obstruction can occur as the primary problem requiring hospitalization or as a secondary complication during hospitalization. Common causes of colonic obstruction include malignancy, volvulus, and diverticular stricture. Infrequent causes include Crohn disease, endometriosis, intussusception, extrinsic tumors, and fecal impaction. Colonic obstruction is more common in the elderly because the incidence of neoplasms and other causative diseases is higher in this population.

ADENOCARCINOMA

Malignant neoplasms, nearly always adenocarcinomas, cause more than 50% of all cases of colonic obstruction (**Figure 162-5**). About 20% of patients with colorectal cancer present with obstructive symptoms, and half of these require emergency operative decompression. Three-fourths of obstructing adenocarcinomas occur distal to the splenic flexure, many within reach of a flexible sigmoidoscope. Carcinomas of the left colon can manifest as a scirrhous tumor causing progressive stenosis of the lumen, whereas cancers of the right colon typically grow as a polypoid or fungating mass (**Figure 162-6**) that obstructs the colon only upon reaching a large size that occludes the lumen, or rarely, by acting as a lead point for a colonic intussusception.

VOLVULUS

Colonic volvulus is an axial twist of the colon on its vascular pedicle. It causes 10% to 15% of colonic obstructions. Anatomic factors promoting volvulus include a redundant, highly mobile, colonic segment that has two closely adjacent points of fixation to peritoneal structures. In sigmoid volvulus, the redundant sigmoid colon is fixed across a narrow base by the lateral peritoneal attachments proximally and the rectum distally. Failure of fusion of parietal peritoneum to the cecum and ascending colon permits formation of cecal volvulus in which the distal ileum, cecum, and ascending colon rotate and twist or fold. In the variant of a *cecal bascule,* the cecum folds upward. Volvulus typically produces a closed-loop obstruction with ischemia from occluding the vascular pedicle and from increased wall tension due to rapid distention. The ischemia rapidly leads to gangrene and perforation. Volvulus of the transverse colon is uncommon and is related to a congenital or surgical absence of supporting ligaments and tissues.

BENIGN COLONIC STRICTURES

Benign colonic strictures occur most commonly from diverticulitis and less commonly at the site of a surgical anastomosis. Benign colonic strictures account for less than 10% of cases of colonic obstruction.

EVALUATION

Mechanical obstruction must be differentiated from acute colonic pseudoobstruction, which is characterized by clinical and radiological findings resembling that of large bowel obstruction in the absence of a mechanical blockage. Colonic pseudoobstruction may

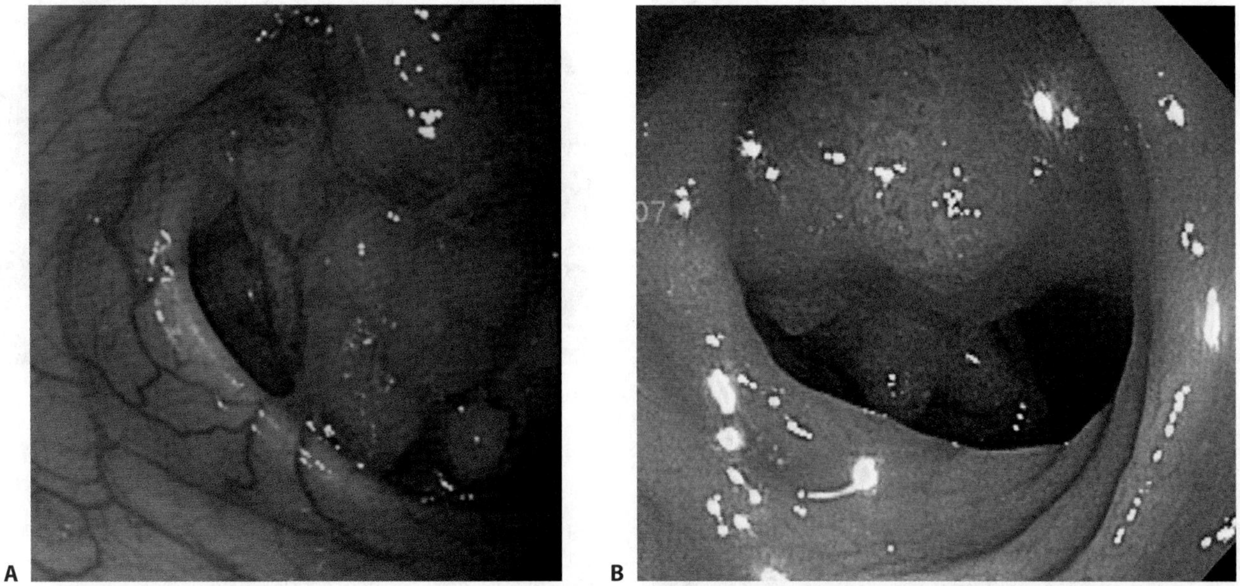

Figure 162-6 *Colonoscopic video-photographs of a multinodular mucosal mass mostly obstructing the lumen of the colon illustrated in two different patients (A and B) presenting with symptoms of colonic obstruction. In both cases, the mass was due to colon cancer.*

result from impaired function of gastrointestinal muscle, innervating neurons, or pacemaker cells. This condition usually affects elderly people with underlying comorbidities, and early recognition and appropriate management are essential to prevent life-threatening complications.

> **PRACTICE POINT**
>
> - Upright chest and abdominal radiographs and supine abdominal radiographs constitute the standard "obstruction series" that should be obtained in every patient with suspected bowel obstruction.

With colonic obstruction, flat and upright abdominal radiographs demonstrate dilation of the small and/or large bowel and air-fluid levels. An upright chest radiograph helps exclude pneumoperitoneum, a radiologic sign of gastrointestinal perforation. An abrupt cutoff in colonic air suggests the anatomic location of an obstruction. *A dilated, air-filled colon without air in the rectum is more consistent with obstruction than pseudoobstruction.* The presence of air in the rectum is consistent with obstipation, pseudoobstruction, or partial obstruction. This finding can, however, be misleading, particularly if the patient has undergone rectal examinations or enemas.

The classic radiologic feature of sigmoid volvulus is a distended and ahaustral sigmoid loop ("bent inner-tube" appearance), the apex of which is often directed toward the patient's right shoulder (**Figure 162-7**). The classic radiologic features of cecal volvulus include (1) a massively dilated cecum located in the epigastrium or left upper quadrant; (2) a coffee-bean appearance of distended cecum; (3) distended loops of small bowel suggesting small bowel obstruction (SBO); and (4) a single, long air-fluid level present on upright or decubitus radiographs. CT or magnetic resonance imaging is not routinely necessary.

TREATMENT

Benign and malignant colonic strictures

Resuscitation of patients with colonic obstruction includes restoration of intravascular volume, correction of electrolyte disorders, and nasogastric aspiration for intestinal decompression. The need and urgency for surgical decompression depends upon the degree of obstruction (partial versus complete) and the presence versus absence of strangulation. The goals of surgery include (1) prompt decompression of the obstructed colon; (2) definitively treating the obstructing lesion; and (3) reestablishing intestinal continuity. All these goals may not be achieved with one operation. Patients with partially obstructing benign or malignant strictures and no evidence of peritonitis may undergo semielective resection of the stricture after resuscitation and nasogastric aspiration. Conversion of an emergent to a semielective operation permits preparation of the colon for primary anastomosis and thereby lowers the operative risk. Complete, unremitting, colonic obstruction necessitates emergency operative decompression.

Obstruction proximal to the splenic flexure is most frequently due to adenocarcinoma and can usually be treated with right hemicolectomy and primary ileocolonic anastomosis. Acute colonic obstruction from advanced colonic malignancy is a surgical emergency. Obstructed patients who are medically unable to withstand resection should undergo tube cecostomy, colostomy, or loop ileostomy. Obstruction at or distal to the splenic flexure may be from either adenocarcinoma or diverticular stricture, differentiation of which may be difficult during laparotomy. Patients who are medically fit with relatively small tumors or inflammatory masses of the left colon or sigmoid may undergo left hemicolectomy or sigmoid colectomy with an end colostomy and closure of the distal bowel or the creation of a distal mucous fistula. Recently, self-expanding metallic stents have been successfully deployed at colonoscopy to relieve malignant colonic obstruction prior to definitive resection

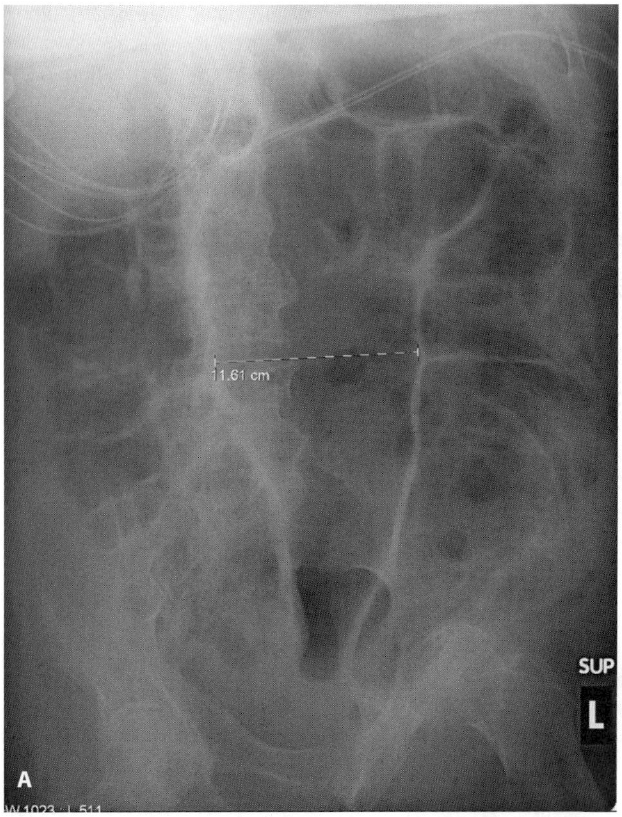

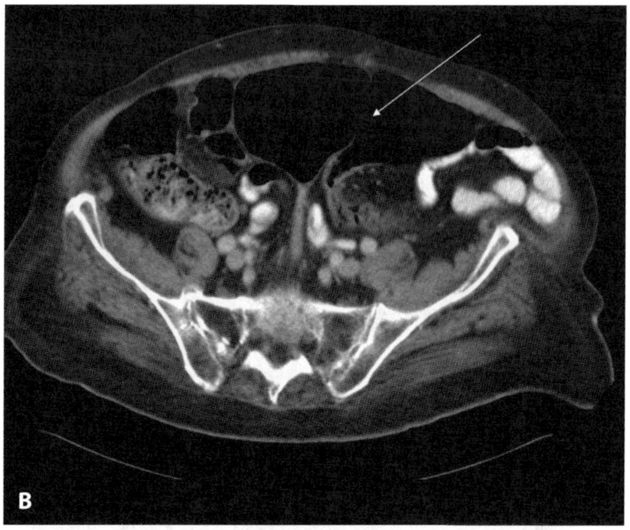

Figure 162-7 *(A) Upright abdominal radiograph of an 80-year-old male showing massively dilated loops of sigmoid colon measuring 11.6 cm maximally, findings consistent with sigmoid volvulus. (B) CT of abdomen in the same patient showing a massively dilated segment of sigmoid colon filled with air from sigmoid volvulus (see arrow).*

or to palliate obstructive symptoms in patients with advanced, unresectable cancer. This approach permits subsequent mechanical bowel preparation and primary colo-colonic anastomosis, after treatment of significant concomitant medical illnesses.

Colonic volvulus

The initial management of sigmoid volvulus without peritonitis is sigmoidoscopic or colonoscopic decompression and placement of a rectal tube beyond the point of obstruction. The procedure may, indeed, detort the volvulus. Colonoscopy must, however, be performed carefully with minimal insufflation of air (or preferably with insufflation of carbon dioxide) to minimize the risk of perforation of the distended, thin-walled, and inflamed bowel. Endoscopic reduction of sigmoid volvulus is associated with a 25% to 50% recurrence rate, so elective sigmoid resection and coloproctostomy, or in medically compromised patients, end colostomy, is recommended after endoscopic decompression and bowel preparation. This approach reduces recurrence rates to 3% to 6%. Patients requiring emergency laparotomy for strangulated sigmoid volvulus require sigmoid resection with end colostomy and a Hartmann pouch.

The role of initial nonsurgical management of patients with cecal volvulus is poorly defined. Although colonoscopy has been successfully employed to reduce cecal volvulus, the risk of perforation of the thinned, often ischemic cecum is substantial, as is the danger of missing a short segment of necrotic bowel at colonoscopy with delay in definitive resection. Surgical options for cecal volvulus include cecopexy, cecostomy, and resection. Detorsion alone, or when combined with appendectomy, is associated with a high recurrence rate.

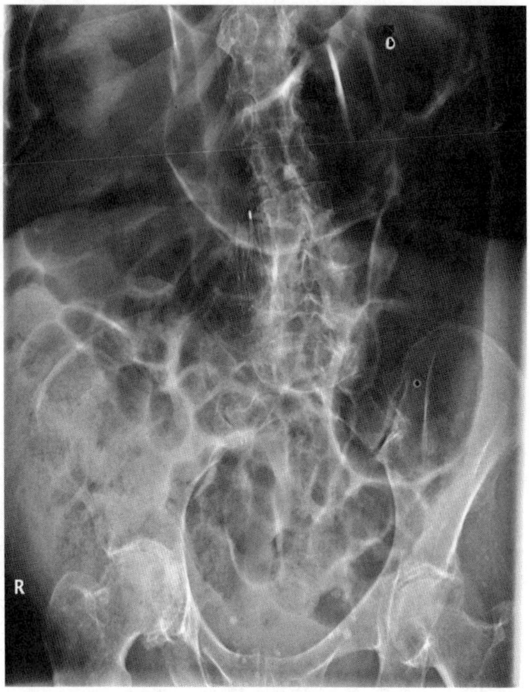

Figure 162-8 *Upright abdominal radiograph of a 90-year-old female showing dilation of both small and large bowel loops, including the rectum. This pattern of dilation throughout the bowel without a transition point to nondilated bowel is characteristic of colonic pseudoobstruction.*

COLONIC PSEUDOOBSTRUCTION

Acute colonic pseudoobstruction, or Ogilvie syndrome, is a clinical disorder with the symptoms, signs, and radiographic appearance resembling those of acute large bowel obstruction but without mechanical obstruction (**Figure 162-8**). Colonic pseudoobstruction typically occurs in a setting of a recent serious medical illness or surgical procedure. Narcotic administration for postoperative pain may aggravate the usual postoperative ileus and precipitate acute intestinal pseudoobstruction. Patients with colonic pseudoobstruction typically present with severe abdominal distention, without passage of stool or gas. Some patients with intestinal pseudoobstruction, however, still pass some gas or even have bowel movements. Nausea and vomiting can be present.

EVALUATION

Evaluation of these patients is similar to that discussed for colonic obstruction.

TREATMENT

PRACTICE POINT

- The mainstay of treatment of colonic pseudoobstruction is correction of underlying reversible etiologic factors, such as infection, hypotension, hypoxemia, and electrolyte imbalances, especially of potassium and calcium. Antikinetic agents such as narcotics or anticholinergics should be promptly discontinued.

Patients should receive nothing per os (NPO). Nasogastric suction may be helpful but does not produce major intestinal decompression because the functional obstruction is primarily colonic. Rectal tube decompression can be effective for sigmoid colon involvement. Morbidity and mortality from this condition is reduced by careful daily monitoring of abdominal radiographs, leukocyte counts, and serum electrolytes. Increasing abdominal pain and tenderness associated with leukocytosis warrants urgent surgical consultation to exclude bowel perforation.

If after 72 hrs of conservative measures the cecal diameter is still >9 cm, neostigmine (1–2 mg) can be rapidly infused intravenously. Contraindications to neostigmine include bradycardia, hypertension, severe renal insufficiency, signs of bowel perforation, and active bronchospasm. If neostigmine is ineffective or contraindicated, colonoscopic decompression is strongly considered. The main risk of colonoscopic decompression is cecal perforation.

Patients occasionally require surgery. Tube cecostomy may be performed for colonic venting. Percutaneous cecostomy may also be performed under CT guidance, but this procedure entails significant morbidity. Surgical decompression by cecostomy, colostomy, or resection, is associated with a poor outcome, possibly because it is performed in patients with more severe disease in whom less invasive measures have failed. Surgery is essential for suspected perforation or peritonitis.

CONCLUSION

Large bowel diseases constitute an important cause of hospitalization, encompassing more than 1% of all hospitalizations and contributing as comorbid conditions to other hospitalizations. This chapter reviews many important in-hospital large bowel diseases, including ischemic colitis, diverticulitis, acute appendicitis, colonic obstruction, and colonic pseudoobstruction. This chapter emphasizes the inpatient evaluation and treatment of these diseases and deemphasizes the outpatient management of these diseases. This work also excludes or deemphasizes many important colonic disorders primarily diagnosed and medically treated in the outpatient setting, such as colon cancer, chronic diarrhea, and irritable bowel syndrome. **Table 162-7** summarizes data from key recent studies on the discussed colonic disorders using an evidence-based approach.

TABLE 162-7 Evidence-based Medicine: Key References for Colonic Disorders

Study	Methodology	Results	Limitations	Bottom Line
Ischemic colitis				
Midian-Singh R, et al. *South Med J.* 2004;97:120–123.	Case series of prospective evaluation for hypercoagulopathy in 18 of 28 patients who presented with "idiopathic" ischemic colitis during a two-year period. Hypercoagulopathy panel included 11 blood tests.	Five of 18 patients with "idiopathic" ischemic colitis had significant hypercoagulopathies, including factor V and protein C resistance, protein S deficiency, prothrombin mutation, and anticardiolipin antibody.	Small study. Potential selection bias because 10 of the 28 patients did not undergo hypercoagulopathy testing. Case series approach with no control group.	Hypercoagulopathy syndromes can frequently underlie otherwise "idiopathic" ischemic colitis. Tests for hypercoagulopathy should be performed in patients with "idiopathic" ischemic colitis who lack other risk factors.
Mosele M, et al. *Scand J Gastroenterol.* 2010;45:428–433.	Retrospective chart review at one hospital during a six-year period of 46 elderly patients diagnosed with ischemic colitis based on computerized identification of discharge diagnoses vs. elderly controls (without vascular gastrointestinal insufficiency or gastrointestinal inflammatory or infectious diseases).	Independent risk factors for ischemic colitis: constipation (odds ratio = 4.8, 95%-CI: 1.1–20.1), vasculopathy (odds ratio = 4.9, 95%-CI: 1.4–16.6), hepatitis C virus infection (OR = 9.9, 95%-CI: 1.1–92.90), and cancer (odds ratio = 7.5, 95%-CI: 1.6–56.5).	Retrospective study, only moderate size of study and control populations. Potential selection bias when patients selected according to discharge diagnoses.	Constipation, vasculopathy, hepatitis C virus infection, and cancer appear to be strong risk factors for ischemic colitis in the elderly.
Won Chung J, et al. *Dis Colon Rectum.* 2010;53:1287–1294.	Retrospective analysis of 153 of 173 patients who were diagnosed with ischemic colitis. Univariate and multivariate analysis to identify clinical, laboratory, and endoscopic parameters associated with a poor prognosis.	The following were independent predictors of severe ischemic colitis: tachycardia (OR = 4.6, 95% CI: 1.4–14.7), early shock (OR = 6.5, 95%-CI: 2.0–21.2), and endoscopic evidence of colonic ulceration (OR = 9.9, 95%-CI: 2.0–48.8).	Small size of subgroup with severe ischemic colitis (20 patients), retrospective analysis, potential selection bias due to loss of 20 patients unavailable for analysis.	Tachycardia, early shock, or endoscopic evidence of colonic ulceration may be early predictors of a severe or complicated clinical course. Patients with these findings may require intensive care monitoring, aggressive diagnostic testing, and aggressive therapy.
Diverticulitis				
Andeweg C, et al. *World J Surg.* 2008;32:1501–1506.	Retrospective, observational study of 183 patients studied over 18-yr period. Patients identified by a computerized pathology database.	Recurrence rate of diverticulitis after limited colon resection for diverticulitis was 8.7% over a mean of 7.2 years of follow-up. Only identified risk factors for postoperative recurrence of diverticulitis: younger age (mean age with recurrence = 54 yr, mean age no recurrence = 64 yr, $p < 0.02$), persistent postoperative abdominal symptoms (recurrence rate = 22.2% with symptoms vs. 5.4% without symptoms, $p < 0.01$).	Retrospective, observational study. Computerized identification of study patients from a pathology database may not have captured all treated patients.	Younger age and persistent postoperative abdominal complaints may identify subgroups at high risk of recurrent diverticulitis after surgery.
Morris CR, et al. *Br J Surg.* 2008;95: 876–881.	Retrospective observational study of incidence, mortality, and risk factors for mortality of perforated diverticulitis at five hospitals over a five-year period. Patients identified by computerized search of discharge diagnostic codes.	Incidence of diverticular perforation for adults was 3.9 per 100,000 per annum. Mortality was 24.3%. Risk factors for mortality included: age >65 yrs (odds ratio =10.3, 95%-CI: 3.0–35.4, $p < 0.001$), renal disease (odds ratio = 13.6, 95%-CI: 1.5–124, $p = 0.02$), prior NSAID use (odds ratio = 2.8, 95% CI: 1.4–5.7, $p = 0.004$), and ASA score>II (odds ratio = 8.9, 95%-CI: 3.8–20.7, $p = <0.001$).	Retrospective, observational study. Computerized identification of patients may have biased study towards more severe episodes of diverticulitis.	High mortality of diverticulitis associated with colonic perforation. Yet, most patients recover with early, aggressive surgical therapy, even in presence of high risk factors.

Appendicitis				
Ingraham AM, et al. *Surgery*. 2010; 148:625–635.	Retrospective observational study of patient outcomes after laparoscopic vs. open appendectomy using a large multicenter database maintained by the American College of Surgeons that includes more than 200 hospitals.	Of 32,683 analyzed patients, 76.4% underwent laparoscopic appendectomy and 23.6% underwent open appendectomy. Patients undergoing laparoscopic appendectomy had less overall morbidity (4.5% vs. 8.8%, odds ratio = 0.60, 95%-CI: 0.54–0.68), had less frequent site specific infections (3.3% vs. 6.7%, odds ratio = 0.57, 95%-CI: 0.50–0.65), and had less frequent serious morbidity or mortality (2.6% vs. 4.3%, odds ratio = 0.87, 95%-CI: 0.74–1.01).	Retrospective study. Clinical parameters not collected in database were unstudied. Study results may not apply to community hospitals that do not participate in this database.	Laparoscopic appendectomy is a relatively low risk procedure for acute appendicitis and may be generally associated with superior outcomes compared to open appendectomy.
Lugo JZ, et al. *J Surg Res*. 2010;164:91–94.	Retrospective observational study of 46 patients undergoing interval laparoscopic appendectomy after nonoperative management of complication of right lower quadrant abscess or phlegmon from acute appendicitis during a six-year period.	84% of operated patients had persistent or chronic appendicitis, complicated inflammatory bowel disease, or neoplasm and therefore likely benefited from surgical exploration.	Retrospective, observational study. Limited study size. Method to identify study patients not described, but apparently based on computerized review of computed tomographic reports. Analysis may not have captured all treated patients. No comparison to unoperated control group.	Interval appendectomy following conservative management for complicated acute appendicitis is justified due to the high rate of problems requiring surgical therapy.
Colonic obstruction				
Vemulapalli R, et al. *Dig Dis Sci*. 2010;55:1732–1737.	Retrospective, observational study comparing 53 patients undergoing self-expanding stent placement vs. 70 patients undergoing palliative surgery for obstructing, incurable colon cancer. Patients identified by a computerized pathology database.	Success rate at relieving obstruction: 94% for stent vs. 100% for surgery. Median hospital stay: two days for stent vs. eight days for surgery. Complication rate: 8% for stent vs. 30% for surgery. In hospital mortality 0% for stent vs. 8.5% for surgery.	Retrospective study, nonrandomized treatments, single center study. Computerized analysis of pathology database may not have captured all treated patients.	Self-expanding metal stents may be a highly effective and safe therapy when compared to surgery for palliation of incurable, obstructing colon cancer.
Larkin JO, et al. *Ann R Coll Surg Engl*. 2009;91:205–209.	Retrospective study comparing nonoperative vs. operative management of acute sigmoid volvulus. Patients identified by operating room registry and admissions office records.	27 patients treated for sigmoid volvulus during 11 years at one hospital, including 11 patients managed with colonoscopic decompression alone vs. 15 requiring surgery. Of 11 patients undergoing only colonoscopy, four died and five were readmitted with recurrent volvulus, whereas only 1 of 15 patients initially undergoing surgery died. There was no mortality in eight patients with ASA scores of IV undergoing surgery.	Retrospective study, nonrandomized treatments, small study size. Nonrandomized treatment may have led to bias of nonsurgical treatment for sickest patients, who then had a higher mortality.	Given the high risk of recurrence of sigmoid volvulus treated colonoscopically and the relatively low surgical mortality, all patients should be strongly considered for definitive surgery after successful colonoscopic decompression of sigmoid volvulus.

(continued)

TABLE 162-7 Evidence-based Medicine: Key References for Colonic Disorders (*continued*)

Study	Methodology	Results	Limitations	Bottom Line
Colonic pseudoobstruction				
Loftus CG, et al. *Am J Gastroenterol.* 2002;97:3118–3122.	Retrospective, observational study of 18 patients receiving neostigmine for acute colonic pseudoobstruction that did not respond to conservative therapy. Patients identified using computerized database of patients classified according to diagnosis.	Only 18 of 151 patients presenting with colonic pseudoobstruction received neostigmine. Among the 18 patients receiving neostigmine, 11 (61%) had a sustained therapeutic response. The remaining 7 (39%) required colonoscopic decompression or surgery for persistent colonic dilatation. Neostigmine responders were more likely to be older (mean age: 76 vs. 54 yr, $p = 0.03$), and had faster resolution of colonic pseudoobstruction than patients treated conservatively (without neostigmine or colonoscopy) (mean resolution 2 vs. 4 days, $p = 0.038$).	Retrospective study, nonrandomized treatments, limited number of patients treated with neostigmine. Computerized analysis may not have captured all treated patients.	Neostigmine was effective in resolving acute colonic pseudoobstruction in the majority of cases. This therapy is likely underutilized.
Mehta R, et al. *J Gastroenterol Hepatol.* 2006;21:459–461.	Prospective study of factors predicting successful outcome in 19 patients treated with neostigmine for colonic pseudoobstruction.	Of 19 treated patients, 16 (84%) had an initial response with neostigmine and 10 (63%) had a sustained response. Of nine patients retreated with neostigmine, five had a sustained response. Neostigmine responders were more likely to be postoperative patients (73% vs. 25%, $p = 0.07$), less likely to have electrolyte disturbances (20% vs. 100%, $p = 0.01$), and less likely to be on antimotility agents (13% vs. 100%, $p = 0.003$).	Small study size. Lack of control group to compare outcome in patients not receiving neostigmine.	Neostigmine leads to about a 65% sustained response in patients with acute colonic pseudoobstruction. For neostigmine to be effective electrolyte imbalances should be corrected and antimotility agents (eg, opiates) should be discontinued.

SUGGESTED READINGS

Antolovic D, Reissfelder C, Koch M, et al. Surgical treatment of sigmoid diverticulitis–analysis of predictive risk factors for postoperative infections, surgical complications, and mortality. *Int J Colorectal Dis.* 2009;24:577–584.

Byrnes MC, Mazuski JE. Antimicrobial therapy for acute colonic diverticulitis. *Surg Infect (Larchmt).* 2009;10:143–154.

Cappell MS. Colonic toxicity of administered drugs and chemicals. *Am J Gastroenterol.* 2004;99:1175–1190.

Cappell MS. Intestinal (mesenteric) vasculopathy. II. Ischemic colitis and chronic mesenteric ischemia. *Gastroenterol Clin North Am.* 1998;27:827–860.

Cappell MS, Friedel D. The role of sigmoidoscopy and colonoscopy in the diagnosis and management of lower gastrointestinal disorders: technique, indications, and contraindications. *Med Clin North Am.* 2002;86:1217–1252.

Martel J, Raskin JB. History, incidence, and epidemiology of diverticulosis. *J Clin Gastroenterol.* 2008;42:1125–1127.

Moriwaki Y, Sugiyama M, Toyoda H, et al. Lethal obstructive colitis: how and when patients with colonic obstruction should be prevented from falling into a lethal condition. *Hepatogastroenterology.* 2009;56:659–662.

Pappagallo M. Incidence, prevalence, and management of opioid bowel dysfunction. *Am J Surg.* 2001;182:11S–18S.

Xu M, Zhong Y, Yao L, et al. Endoscopic decompression using a transanal drainage tube for acute obstruction of the rectum and left colon as a bridge to curative surgery. *Colorectal Dis.* 2009;11:405–409.

Vanek VW, Al-Salti M. Acute pseudo-obstruction of the colon (Ogilvie's syndrome). An analysis of 400 cases. *Dis Colon Rectum.* 1986;29:203–210.

CHAPTER 163

Inflammatory Bowel Disease

Jan-Michael A. Klapproth, MD
Mohammad Wehbi, MD

Key Clinical Questions

1. What factors predispose to the development of IBD?
2. Which patients with IBD require hospital admission?
3. How can clinicians induce and maintain remission quickly and safely to prevent progression of disease and surgical intervention in hospitalized patients with inflammatory bowel disease (IBD)?
4. How can clinicians minimize adverse events related to IBD, its medications, and related surgery?

INTRODUCTION

Significant heterogeneity in the geographic distribution of inflammatory bowel disease (IBD) exists, but a north-south gradient has been confirmed in multiple studies. Both conditions, ulcerative colitis (UC) and Crohn disease (CD), are more common in commercially insured and individuals of the upper middle class than those covered by Medicaid. A total of approximately 1.5 million Americans are affected by UC and CD. In adults, the prevalence of UC and CD was 238 and 201 per 100,000 people, respectively. The incidences for UC and CD range from 7.6–8.8 and 6.9–7.9 per 100,000 people, respectively. In developed countries, incidence rates have been increasing for CD, but are stable for UC. Further, in comparison to the general population, patients with IBD are more likely to visit the emergency room, be admitted for medical management of their disease, and be admitted for surgery during the first five years following diagnosis.

PRESENTATION

UC and CD are chronically remitting inflammatory conditions. Both diseases are extremely variable in their presentation and course, and both have bimodal age distributions (average age of presentation 28 years with a second peak at age 50 years). The clinical presentation is more variable in CD due to the transmural nature of the condition, variability in the extent of inflammation, and extraintestinal manifestations of the disease.

SYMPTOMS COMMON IN UC AND CD

Presentation of IBD varies considerably and can be subtle. The most common presentation for both diseases includes increase in stool frequency and decrease in consistency. The second most common presenting symptom is abdominal pain. In UC, this pain is cramping, located in the left lower quadrant, and improves with bowel movement, whereas in CD pain is felt in the right lower quadrant and worsens with food intake. The third most common symptom is weight loss, which is more prevalent in CD than UC, and the presenting symptom in 87% of patients with CD. Both CD and UC may exhibit extraintestinal manifestations as well (**Table 163-1**).

Up to one-third of patients with IBD suffer from extraintestinal manifestations that can be divided into three groups. Patients with either UC or CD involving the colon frequently suffer from inflammatory conditions in the form of peripheral and axial arthropathy, erythema nodosum and pyoderma gangrenosum, episcleritis and uveitis. Inflammatory conditions involving joints, skin, and eyes usually run a course parallel to the intestinal IBD activity. Independent of the inflammatory activity in the gut are manifestations like ankylosing spondylitis, primary sclerosing cholangitis, uveitis, and sacroileitis. For these extraintestinal manifestations specific associations with human leukocyte antigens have been established. The third group of extraintestinal manifestations is due to metabolic derangements and include kidney stones, amyloidosis, and bone loss. They are parallel to intestinal activity.

SYMPTOMS MORE COMMON IN UC

Symptoms more frequently encountered with UC are left lower quadrant pain, urgency, frequency, bleeding, and mucoid discharge. **Table 163-2** summarizes clinical symptoms and findings related to the extent of intestinal involvement.

TABLE 163-1 Summary of Extraintestinal Manifestations of IBD

Parallel Course	Peripheral arthritis	5–20%
	Erythema nodosum	10–20%
	Episcleritis	1.6–6.3%
	Aphthous stomatitis	25%
	Pyoderma gangrenosum	1–10%
	Uveitis	0.5–9%
Independent course	Ankylosing spondylitis	5–10%
	Sacroileitits	3–5%
	Uveitits	1.6–6.3%
	Primary sclerosing cholangitis	2.4–7.5%
Metabolic manifestations	Nephrolithiasis	7–10%
	Osteopenia, osteoporosis	23–59%
	Amyloidosis	0.07–0.9%

SYMPTOMS MORE COMMON IN CD

As opposed to UC with its continuous inflammation limited to the colon and occasionally the terminal ileum, CD may affect any portion of the gastrointestinal tract, from the mouth to the anus, in a discontinuous fashion, termed *skip lesions*. Involvement of the esophagus and stomach is uncommon, occurring in only 5% of all patients with CD. Usually, CD presents with right lower quadrant pain, nocturnal diarrhea, obstructive symptoms (nausea, vomiting, abdominal distention), fever, and weight loss (**Table 163-3**).

CLASSIFICATION OF UC AND CD ACCORDING TO ANATOMIC LOCATION

With inflammation limited to the mucosal layer of the colon, UC is clinically classified according to anatomical involvement into

- Proctitis (mainly rectal involvement), affecting the distal 10 cm to 15 cm
- Left-sided disease with inflammation extending to the descending colon
- Pancolitis, defined as disease activity extending proximally beyond the splenic flexure

In CD, transmural inflammation can affect any part of the gastrointestinal system with involvement of

- The small bowel in 80% of patients
- The ileocolon (both the ileum and the colon) in 50% of patients
- The colon in 20% of patients

CD is further defined by the inflammatory process as inflammatory, fibrostenotic, or fistulizing.

TABLE 163-2 Symptoms of UC According to Extent of Colonic Inflammation

Site Involved in UC	Symptoms
Rectum	Tenesmus, rectal prolapse, bloody and mucoid discharge, constipation
Left-sided disease	Pain improves with bowel movement, blood mixed with stool
Pancolitis	Diffuse abdominal pain, abdominal distention, absent bowel sounds

TABLE 163-3 Symptoms of CD in Correlation to Anatomic Site

Site Involved in CD	Symptoms
Gastroduodenum	Dyspepsia, vomiting, epigastric pain
Small bowel	Diarrhea, obstruction, periumbilical pain
Ileo-colon	Right lower quadrant pain, bleeding uncommon, obstruction
Colon	Tenesmus, rectal prolapse, fistula, skin maceration

PATHOPHYSIOLOGY

GENETICS

IBD manifests due to an inappropriate immune response that occurs in genetically susceptible individuals as the result of a complex interaction among environmental and microbial factors and the intestinal immune system. Incidence and prevalence of IBD are two- to four-fold and two- to nine-fold higher in Ashkenazi Jews than the nonJewish populations, respectively. A positive family history can be established in 10–20% of CD cases, which is higher in comparison to UC.

Thus far, more than 30 novel genetic IBD-susceptible gene loci have been identified and the number is growing rapidly. However, while several promising associations between IBD and gene variants have been identified and replicated effectively, *genotyping is not currently standard diagnostic procedure.*

ENVIRONMENT

Smoking has a dose-dependent beneficial effect on disease activity in UC, but not CD. More exsmokers develop UC as compared with current smokers. This is in stark contrast to CD, as smoking has a detrimental effect on disease activity. Smoking is associated with clinical recurrence of CD, and a shorter time to clinical recurrence. Both a positive family history of IBD and smoking at the time of the initial ileocolic resection are associated with an increased risk of a second ileocolic resection. Following surgically-induced remission, the time to clinical relapse for smokers was shorter (130 weeks versus 234 weeks in nonsmokers, $P < 0.001$). In comparison to nonsmoking patients with CD, smokers have a 2.5- and 2-fold increased risk of surgical and clinical recurrence, respectively. Therefore, aggressive strategies for smoking cessation are warranted.

DIFFERENTIAL DIAGNOSIS

POTENTIALLY LIFE-THREATENING CONDITIONS

Multiple conditions may mimic an IBD flare (**Table 163-4**). In-hospital acquisition of *Clostridium difficile* is a major concern in all patients, but especially patients with IBD. *C difficile* colitis is associated with a significant health care burden in hospitalized IBD patients, carries a higher mortality risk (28%), and is associated with higher resource utilization. Infection with *C difficile* can occur at any point in the IBD patient's hospital admission, and the prevalence is highest among patients with UC (37.5 per 1,000 patients), followed by CD (10.9 per 1,000 patients), and lowest among patients admitted for nongastrointestinal etiologies (4.5 per 1,000 patients). Clinical deterioration in an IBD patient who has required multiple days of hospitalization should raise the suspicion for *C difficile*. The diagnosis is established by, preferably, three stool samples tested for toxin A and B produced by *C difficile* (Table 163-4).

TABLE 163-4 IBD Differential Diagnosis and Characteristics

Disease	Diagnostic Clues
Irritable bowel syndrome	No red flags, like weight loss, bloody diarrhea, obstruction
Colonic ischemia	Presence of vascular diseases
Cytomegalovirus	Colonic IBD not improving despite therapy
Clostridium difficile colitis	Colonic IBD not improving despite therapy
Behçet disease	Mediterranean descent, skin ulcerations
Intestinal tuberculosis	Immigrant to the U.S.
Yersinia enterocolitica	Exposure to cattle, deer, and pigs

PRACTICE POINT

- Despite an overall normal life expectancy for patients with ulcerative colitis, patients older than 50 years of age and with extensive colitis at diagnosis have an increased mortality within the first two years after diagnosis.

Cytomegalovirus (CMV) infection of the colon is another potentially life-threatening condition that may mimic an IBD flare. Severe, therapy-refractory UC and CD should raise a high level of suspicion for this infection. High risk groups include female IBD patients presenting with fever, lymphadenopathy, splenomegaly, leukopenia, and mild hepatitis. The diagnosis is established by immunohistochemistry for viral early antigen performed on a biopsy specimen, which is significantly more sensitive than serological tests.

DIAGNOSIS

IBD diagnosis is based on clinical history and physical examination with particular emphasis on family history and perianal examination. Currently, no single test is pathognomonic for CD or UC, and the diagnosis is supplemented by laboratory investigations, including complete blood count, liver function tests, and C-reactive protein measurement. Due to their acceptable specificity but low sensitivity, serologies for perinuclear anti-Neutrophil Cytoplasmic Antibodies (pANCA) and anti-*Saccharomyces cerevisiae* Antibodies (ASCA) should be used with caution in patients with a low pretest probability of IBD to prevent a delay in the correct diagnosis and consequently inappropriate treatment. Patients with CD have a positive ASCA in 50–70% of cases with a specificity of 92% if negative for pANCA. In contrast, individuals with UC are positive for pANCA in 40–80% of cases and with a specificity of 98% when found negative for ASCA. However, serologies for pANCA and ASCA might be useful for the diagnosis of indeterminate colitis.

Endoscopy serves as the mainstay for IBD diagnosis, and in particular ileo-colonoscopy, with biopsies for histological examination (**Table 163-5**, **Figures 163-1** and **163-2**). Even though colonoscopy is a simple and safe procedure in patients with mild to moderate disease, it should be limited during hospitalization for a severe IBD flare to prevent perforation. Exceptions include cases of therapy-refractory disease in which limited colonoscopic intervention by an experienced operator should be considered to rule out infectious complications like *C difficile* colitis or CMV colitis. Ileocolonoscopy can be supplemented by wireless capsule endoscopy (WCE) for small bowel examination, but WCE should not be used during severe disease. WCE has a higher diagnostic yield than enteroclysis in the detection of CD of the small bowel, both in patients with known and newly suspected CD. Enteroclysis is a rarely performed procedure, but very helpful examination by which barium is administered through a nasogastric tube directly into the small bowel, excluding the upper gastrointestinal tract.

TABLE 163-5 Endoscopic Features of UC and CD

UC	CD
Rectum inflamed	Rectum spared
Continuous inflammation	Skip lesions
Loss of vascularity	Aphthous ulcerations
Mucosal granularity	Linear and serpiginous ulcerations
Normal ileo-cecal valve	Fistulae
	Ulcerated terminal ileum

As an alternative to endoscopy, severity of inflammation can be analyzed by radiographic studies (**Figures 163-3** and **163-4**). Magnetic resonance (MR) enterography can reliably assess small bowel disease severity in the evaluation of ileocolonic Crohn disease. Dynamic contrast-enhanced MR imaging can help determine disease activity in perianal CD and might be helpful in selecting a subpopulation of patients who should be monitored more closely for development of more extensive disease. Alternatively, MR and CT enterography have similar sensitivities for detecting active small-bowel inflammation, and CT may have superior image quality based on study cohorts. CT was found to provide higher sensitivity in detecting enterovesical, enterocutaneous, and perianal fistulae, as well as extraluminal disease and complications, including abscesses, most commonly identified in the ischiorectal fossa, psoas muscle, and neighboring solid organs. However, CT studies raise the concern of cumulative radiation exposure, and therefore may not be a valuable option to monitor disease (**Table 163-6**).

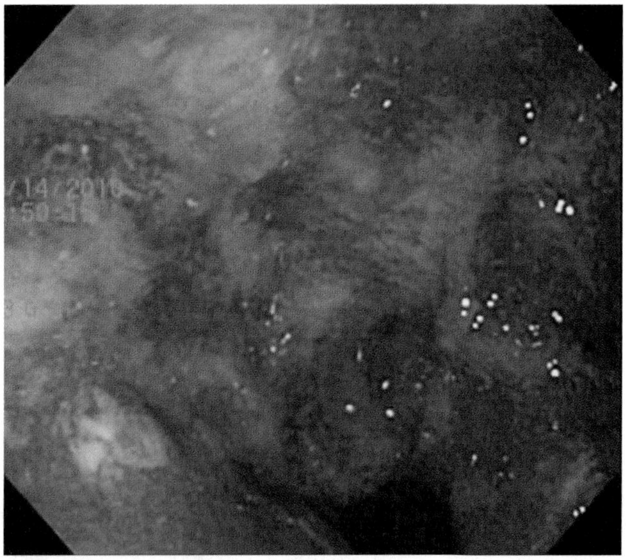

Figure 163-1 *Endoscopic image of inflamed colon in a patient with UC. Macroscopic features supporting a diagnosis of UC are loss of vascularity and granularity.*

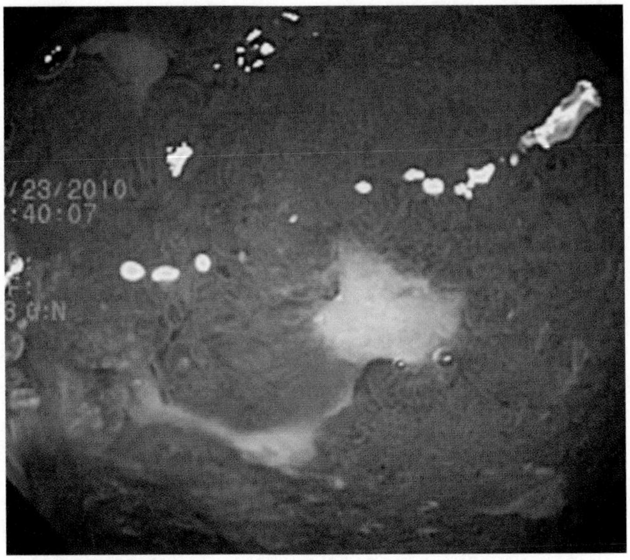

Figure 163-2 *Endoscopic findings during colonoscopy of a patient with CD. Large serpiginous ulceration on the ileocecal valve in a patient with CD.*

CLINICAL COURSE

Initially, approximately 10% of patients with UC will present with severe disease, and 15% will develop a severe flare during the course of their lifetime (**Table 163-7**). Relapses of UC are unpredictable, except that disease activity in the foregoing years indicates with 70–80% probability that the disease will continue the following year. Activity of UC during the first two years after diagnosis correlates significantly with disease activity during the ensuing five consecutive years. During years three to seven after diagnosis, 25% of patients will be in remission, 18% have flares annually, and 57% will have intermittent relapses.

About half of patients with UC will be in remission at any given time, although 90% will have an intermittent course. Despite an overall normal life expectancy for patients with ulcerative colitis, patients older than 50 years of age and with extensive colitis at diagnosis have an increased mortality within the first two years after diagnosis, most likely due to colitis-associated postoperative complications and comorbidities.

As opposed to UC, the majority of patients with CD experience a chronic intermittent disease course, while 13% have an unremitting disease course, and 10% experience prolonged remission (**Table 163-8**). For the majority of affected patients, the location remains stable over the course of the disease, and only 16% of patients experience a change in location over ten years. However, 46% of patients will have a change in disease behavior. The most prominent change is from nonstricturing, nonpenetrating disease to either stricturing (27%) or penetrating (29%) disease. Ileal CD is predominantly stricturing, whereas colonic or ileocolonic CD is more often penetrating, which is evident at time of diagnosis and more prominent during the ensuing ten years. When examined over 15 years, 15% of affected individuals will become incapable of

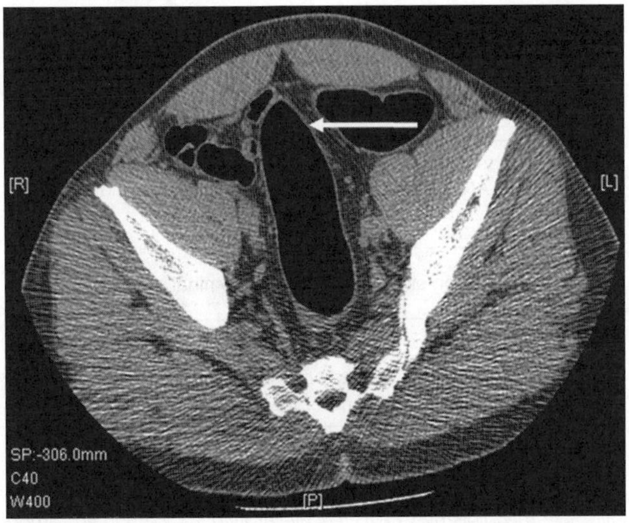

Figure 163-3 *CT findings in a patient with pancolitis due to moderately active UC. Image from a virtual colonoscopy in a patient with long-standing, difficult to control, UC. The characteristic findings are wall thickening and a loss of haustrations (arrow).*

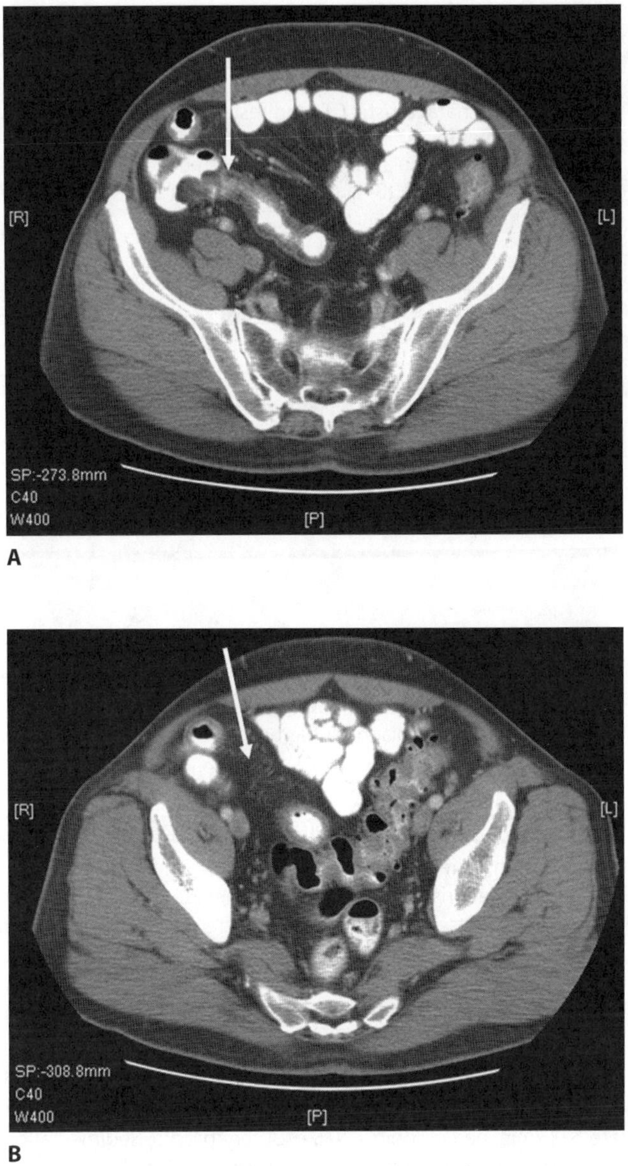

Figure 163-4 *Characteristic CT manifestations of CD involving the terminal ileum. (A) Inflamed terminal ileum and ileocecal valve resulting in irregular contrast enhancement and bowel wall thickening (arrow). (B) Encasement of terminal ileum by fat tissue, termed "creeping fat."*

TABLE 163-6 Summary of Radiographic CT Scan Findings Differentiating UC and CD

Figure 163-4: Characteristic CT manifestations of CD involving the terminal ileum. (A) Inflamed terminal ileum and ileocecal valve resulting in irregular contrast enhancement and bowel wall thickening (arrow). **(B)** Encasement of terminal ileum by fat tissue, termed "creeping fat."

UC	CD
Colon mural wall thickening, 8 mm	Large and small bowel wall thickening 11–13 mm
Colon mural fat deposition	Perienteric stranding
Rectal narrowing, widening of presacral space	Mesenteric fat attenuation, adenopathy, creeping fat
Inhomogeneous enhancement with mural stratification (target sign)	Mesenteric hypervascularity (comb sign)

regular work and obtain disability, while 75% of the patients remain fully capable of work. Within a time period of ten years, 50% of the patients will not have experienced any year with impaired capacity for work. Age at time of diagnosis has no influence on either location or behavior of disease.

TRIAGE AND HOSPITAL ADMISSION

Hospitals with more than 145 admissions per year for IBD and associated complications confer a mortality benefit for patients with CD. Therefore, patients with severe disease or requiring intensive unit care may require transfer to a tertiary care hospital (**Figure 163-5**).

CRITERIA FOR GENERAL ADMISSION

In addition to failure of medical therapy, criteria for admission established by Truelove and Witts in 1955 have not changed and consist of six and more stools per day, temperature >37.8°C, heart rate >90/min, hemoglobin <10.5 g/dL, erythrocyte sedimentation rate >30 mm/hour with evidence of systemic toxicity. In addition to intravenous hydration and bowel rest, these patients require hospitalization to facilitate monitoring of response to therapy, including frequent abdominal examinations by auscultation, palpation, and flat plate abdominal X-ray and adjustment of their medications.

TABLE 163-7 Truelove and Witts Classification of Ulcerative Colitis Disease Activity

Classification of Disease Activity in UC	Characteristics
Mild	<4 stools/day Mild anemia ESR <30 mm/hr
Moderate	Intermediate of mild and severe activity
Severe	>6 stools /day Temperature >37.5°C Heart Rate >90/minute Hemoglobin <75% of baseline ESR >30 mm/hr

ESR, erythrocyte sedimentation rate.

TABLE 163-8 Classification of Disease Activity in CD

Classification of Disease Activity in CD	Characteristics
Mild to moderate	Ambulatory patient, normal diet, no evidence of toxicity, weight loss <10%
Moderate to severe	Therapy failure, weight loss, abdominal pain, anemia, nausea, vomiting
Severe to fulminant	Unresponsive to steroids, fever, vomiting, obstruction, rebound tenderness, cachexia, abscess formation

CRITERIA FOR ICU ADMISSION

Multiorgan failure and hemodynamic instability predicts poor outcomes and is associated with high mortality rates of more than 70% in UC patients. Early signs of multiorgan failure include disproportionate tachycardia, tachypnea, oliguria, jaundice, hypoxemia, and mental confusion. These symptoms and signs should prompt an aggressive therapeutic approach including transfer to the ICU and consideration of early colectomy.

MANAGEMENT

VTE PROPHYLAXIS

Systemic thromboembolic events are recognized clinically in 1–7.7% of patients admitted for management of IBD. However, the incidence is significantly higher in postmortem studies, reaching 39–41%, translating into a greater than threefold increased risk of thromboembolic complications in comparison to control populations. For patients with active colitis, this risk is increased 15-fold. The most common sites involved are the deep veins of the extremities and/or pulmonary vasculature.

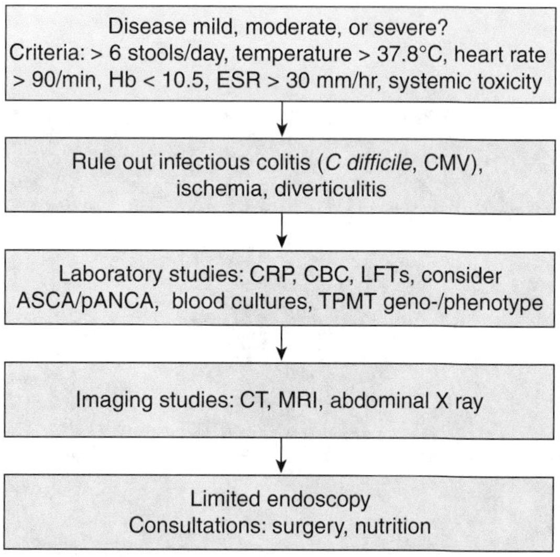

Figure 163-5 *Initial assessment of severe IBD exacerbation. ASCA, anti-Saccharomyces cerviciae antibody; CBC, complete blood count; CMV, cytomegalovirus; CRP, C-reactive protein; CT, computed tomography; ESR, erythrocyte sedimentation rate; Hb, hemoglobin; IBD, inflammatory bowel disease; LFTs, liver function tests; MRI, magnetic resonance imaging; pANCA, perinuclear anti-neutrophil cytoplasmic antibody; TPMT, thiopurine methyltrasnferase.*

TABLE 163-9 Medications for the Management of Severe IBD Exacerbation

Medication	Indication	Mechanism	Contraindication	Side Effect	Outcome
Hydrocortisone methylprednisolone	Initial treatment for severe UC, CD	Inhibition of proinflammatory cytokines (interleukins, arachidonic acid metabolites), leucocyte function, and migration	Tubercular, syphilitic, bacterial, and fungal infections	Hypertension, diabetes, psychotic behavior, sleep disturbances, impaired wound healing, bone loss	CD remission rate 50–75%, UC remission rate 84%
Cyclosporine	Steroid failure treatment for severe UC	Calcineurin mediated T cell suppression	Uncontrolled infections and hypertension	Hypertension headache, renal dysfunction, opportunistic infections	UC response rate 82%
Infliximab	Alternative steroid failure treatment for severe UC, CD	Neutralization of TNF-α	Untreated chronic infection (TB), moderate to severe heart failure, hypersensitivity to murine products	Upper respiratory tract and urinary tract infections, cough, rash, back pain, nausea, vomiting, abdominal pain, headache, fever	CD response rate 80%; UC remission 60–70%, colectomy 21% at 8 weeks

Therefore, primary prophylaxis is indicated for any patient admitted to the hospital for management of an IBD flare. Mechanical measures include ambulation, compression stockings, or pneumatic boots, all improving peripheral circulation. Alternative or additional interventions may include physical therapy. In addition to mechanical measures, acutely ill patients unable to ambulate should receive primary pharmacologic prophylaxis. This decision requires balancing the risk of gastrointestinal hemorrhage versus the very high risk of VTE. This appears to be true in particular for patients with UC, but not CD. At this point, no firm recommendation regarding the length of prophylactic treatment can be made.

Treatment of thromboembolic complications fundamentally does not differ from other patients, but bleeding from active disease has to be taken into consideration. If the risk of bleeding is high, consideration should be given to catheter-directed thrombolysis performed by interventional radiology. For patients unable to tolerate anticoagulation or who develop recurrent thrombosis, placement of an inferior vena cava filter is recommended (**Table 163-9**).

INDUCTION OF REMISSION IN PATIENTS WITH UC

The mainstay for the management of moderate to severe UC remains systemic steroids, either hydrocortisone at 300 mg daily (divided doses) or methlyprednisolone 60 mg daily (**Figure 163-6**). Continuous dosing bears no benefit compared to bolus dosing. However, 30% of patients become steroid refractory after five to seven days of IV steroids. Therefore, clinicians should monitor basic clinical and laboratory parameters predicting who will require surgical intervention. After three days of IV steroid therapy, patients with more than eight bowel movements per day (or more than three bowel movements per day plus a CRP greater than 45 mg/dl) have an 85% likelihood of requiring colectomy.

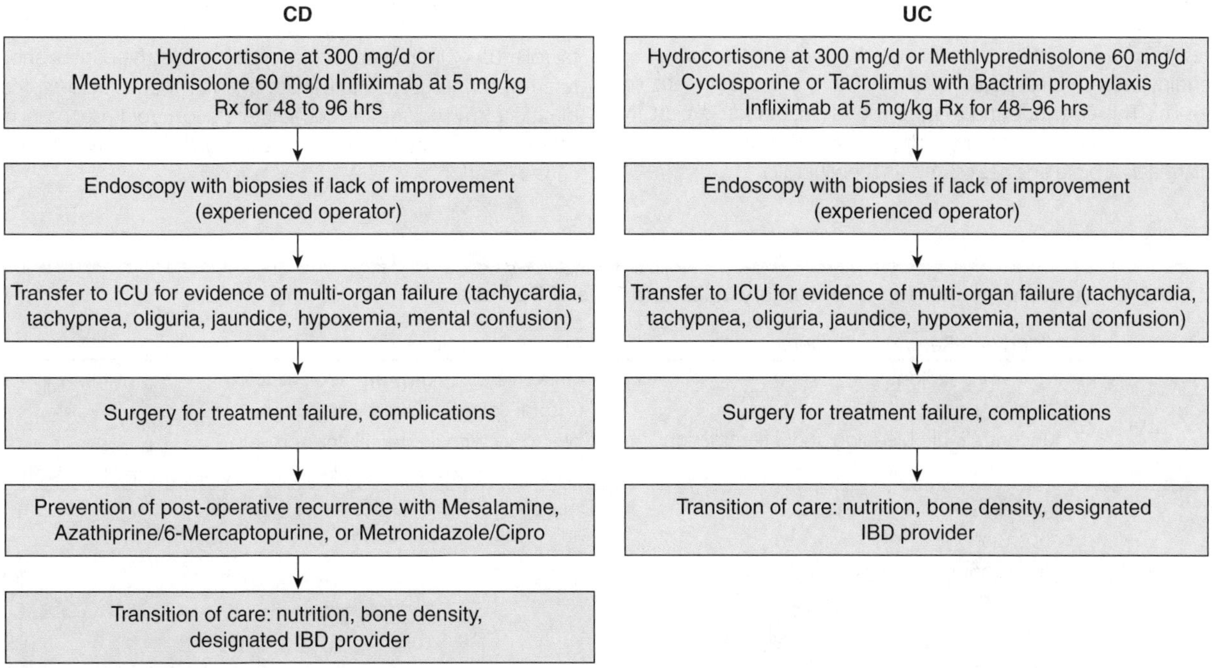

Figure 163-6 *Outline for inpatient IBD therapy.*

PRACTICE POINT

- Thirty percent of patients with UC flare become steroid refractory after five to seven days of IV steroids. After three days of IV steroid therapy, patients with more than eight bowel movements per day (or more than three bowel movements per day plus a CRP greater than 45 mg/dl) have an 85% likelihood of requiring colectomy.

Patients with severe ulcerative colitis who are refractory to corticosteroid should be referred for surgery. When a patient is not agreeable to surgery or if the clinical picture does not permit surgery, evidence supports the use of intravenous cyclosporine, or alternatively tacrolimus or infliximab, a chimeric antibody directed against TNF-α. The adverse effects associated with cyclosporine, including nephrotoxicity, are dose dependent. Hence, therapy should be initiated with the lower 2 mg/kg/day dose. Subsequent doses should be adjusted based on cyclosporine blood concentrations of 150–250 ng/ml. In addition, cyclosporine can be used in patients with contraindications for steroid therapy (avascular necrosis, psychosis). Cyclosporine should be used only to induce remission and serve as a "bridge" for the maintenance of remission with immunomodulators azathioprine or 6-mercaptopurine. This approach prevents colectomy at five years in up to 80% of cyclosporine responders. Cyclosporine should not be used as a long-term monotherapy to avoid surgery or the maintenance of remission. When this medication is used, it is pertinent to provide prophylaxis with bactrim to prevent *Pneumocystis (carinii) jiroveci* pneumonia. Serum concentrations of magnesium and cholesterol should be monitored, as a low level for both increases the likelihood of seizures with the use of cyclosporine. Cyclosporine does not increase the rate of perioperative complications.

Infliximab reduces the need for colectomy in moderate-to-severe disease. The decision to utilize cyclosporine or infliximab is based on provider preference, as studies comparing infliximab and cyclosporine have not been conducted. However, infliximab might be the preferred drug for patients already on azathioprine or 6-mercaptopurine as those medications combined with cyclosporine show a poor short- and long-term response. *The sequential administration of infliximab and cyclosporine should not be prescribed given that it is associated with significant morbidity.*

Certain interventions have no benefit in the management of severe UC. These include the routine use of antibiotics (except in impeding perforation), nutritional support with TPN, and the use of antidiarrheals, opioid analgesics, and anticholinergics.

PRACTICE POINT

- Interventions with no benefit in the management of severe UC include the routine use of antibiotics (except in impeding perforation), nutritional support with TPN, and the use of antidiarrheals, opioid analgesics, and anticholinergics.

INDUCTION OF REMISSION IN PATIENTS WITH CD

The mainstay for the management of moderate to severe CD is the use of intravenous steroids or infliximab. Steroid therapy includes hydrocortisone at 300 mg daily (divided doses) or methlyprednisolone 60 mg daily. Alternatively, clinical response to infusion with infliximab at 5 mg/kg, occurs rapidly when given at zero, two, and six weeks. However, clinical response is often short lived, generally only three to four months. A follow-up trial showed that the duration of effect could be sustained in 46% of patients with maintenance doses of infliximab when given at eight-week intervals. As opposed to therapy for UC, a recent review demonstrated that low dose oral cyclosporine is *not* effective for treatment of active CD. Higher oral doses and injections of cyclosporine have not been sufficiently evaluated.

CONSULTATIONS

Cases of severe CD or UC should be managed by a team of physicians, consisting of the hospitalist, a gastroenterologist, and a surgeon experienced in IBD surgery. In addition, nutritional support and wound care (stoma) specialists add valuable input in management early during hospital stay, especially in cases in which colectomy is entertained.

INDICATIONS FOR SURGERY

UC

Eighty percent of severe UC patients will not require surgical intervention (**Table 163-10**). However, the critical window of opportunity should not be missed to identify patients that would benefit from a surgical intervention. Most studies now define 48 to 96 hours as an adequate trial of medical therapy in which significant clinical improvement should occur. Depending on the individual patient, an alternative regimen might be offered, like cyclosporine, tacrolimus, or infliximab. If this is not feasible, the patient should be referred for surgery. Multivariate analysis found factors predictive of colectomy include concomitant corticosteroid use, baseline CRP serum concentrations of at least 2 mg/dl, and a North American center location.

TABLE 163-10 Summary of Indications for Surgery in IBD and Type of Operation

Disease	Condition Requiring Surgery	Surgical Procedure
UC	Toxic megacolon	Transverse colostomy and loop ileostomy
	Toxic colitis, perforation, medically uncontrollable bleeding and inflammation	Subtotal colectomy with ileostomy
		Colectomy with ileorectal anastomosis
		Proctocolectomy with Brooke ileostomy or continent ileostomy
CD	Medically refractory disease	Depending on anatomical site, segmental resection, colectomy with ileostomy, stricturoplasty
	Obstruction	
	Fulminant colitis, toxic megacolon	
	Perforation with acute abdomen	
	Perianal and intra-abdominal abscesses	
	Fistula (enteroenteric, enterovesicular)	

PRACTICE POINT

- In ulcerative colitis acute flare, patients who do not respond to an adequate trial of medical therapy within 48 to 96 hours with significant clinical improvement should be referred for surgical intervention.

CD

Surgical intervention in CD is common, as 70–90% of patients will need a surgical intervention at some point during their lifetime. Failure of medical therapy, defined by symptoms that cannot be controlled or progress with maximum medical therapy, intractable side effects, inability of a patient to maintain compliance with a medical regimen, and complications of the disease process are indications to proceed with surgical intervention. Indications for surgery include worsening signs and symptoms of colitis, numerous bloody stools per day, fever, elevated heart rate, anemia, elevated sedimentation rate, radiographic evidence of colonic distension, and abdominal distension with tenderness on physical examination.

Failure to improve within a few days following an initial stabilization period, or worsening colitis should trigger consideration for operative intervention. Patients with severe colitis or those with findings of eight bowel movements or more per day (or three to eight bowel movements per day with a CRP level greater 45 mg/mL) despite three days of therapy require a colectomy in 85% of cases. Other indications for emergent surgery include the development of toxic megacolon, particularly in the context of perforation, progressive colonic dilatation, massive hemorrhage or hemodynamic instability. For these cases, total abdominal colectomy and end ileostomy is the procedure of choice. Postoperative complication rates range from 23–33% with a low mortality rate (0–4%) in the absence of a perforation, and laparoscopic resection of ileocolonic CD is associated with less blood loss, fewer respiratory complications, faster return of bowel function, and shorter hospital stay.

PREVENTION OF POSTOPERATIVE RECURRENCE IN CD

Postoperative recurrence defined as radiographic, endoscopic, and pathologic evidence of CD can develop within weeks of resection and is related to luminal factors. Endoscopic recurrence rates range from 58–93% one year out from surgery and are highest for ileocolonic anastomosis. It is therefore pertinent to initiate therapy as soon as the patient is able to tolerate, preferably oral, medications. Recurrence of CD has been shown to be related to patient's age, smoking history, duration and course of disease prior to surgery, severity, extension, and stricturing and penetrating phenotype.

Mesalamine has minimal benefit when compared to placebo. In contrast, metronidazole 20 mg/kg/day—when started within seven days postoperatively and continued for three months—results in significant reduction of severe endoscopic recurrence. However, metronidazole use is frequently limited by its side effect profile consisting of peripheral neuropathy, metallic taste, and disulfiram-like effect. Azathioprine and 6-mercaptopurine are more efficient in comparison to mesalamine in decreasing postoperative recurrence of CD, and allow for a switch from metronidazole with its unfavorable side effect profile. Prior to the initiation of azathioprine and 6-mercaptopurine, a determination of thiopurine methyltransferase (TPMT) geno- or phenotype is indicated. Testing predicts adverse events and reduces the chance of clinical response when TPMT activity is greater than 35 pmol/h/mg/Hb. The goal is to attain serum thioguanine concentrations above 100 pmol/8 × 10^8 RBC, which correlates with a clinical response. In addition to mesalamine, antibiotics, and immunomodulators, infliximab has been shown to reduce postoperative endoscopic recurrence when given at zero, two, and six weeks postoperatively (9% vs. 85% placebo). This study also showed that recurrence was more severe in the placebo group in comparison to patients treated with infliximab. Therefore, infusion of infliximab should be considered for patients with severe recurrence discovered on follow-up endoscopy at 6–12 months postoperatively.

Budesonide given at 6 mg per day for up to one year prevented endoscopic postoperative recurrence in patients with inflammatory, but not fibrostenotic CD.

OUTPATIENT MEDICATIONS FOR CD AND UC

After disease severity has decreased to mild to moderate in activity, patients may be switched to oral medications (with the exception of infliximab, which remains by infusion), and advanced to a regular diet, both prerequisites for discharge (**Table 163-11**). If IV steroids were part of the medical regimen, prednisone should be given at 60 mg/d and tapered over the ensuing weeks. It is also appropriate to consider testing for TPMT geno- or phenotype prior to initiation of immunomodulatory therapy with 6-mercaptopurine or azathioprine. Infliximab should be continued at intervals of every eight weeks. Oral antibiotics are an option in postoperative, right-sided colonic and perianal CD. Sulfasalazine at 4g/day in divided dosages improves outcomes in patients with UC, but has limited utility in CD.

COMPLICATIONS AND PROGNOSIS

UC ADVERSE OUTCOMES

Toxic megacolon, defined by a transverse colon diameter exceeding 6 centimeters, has been reported in 7–17% of patients requiring hospitalization and is thought to have a lifetime incidence of 0.5–2.5%. However, the mortality rate from toxic megacolon is only 0.2%. Other complications include a change in diagnosis. A recent study showed that in patients with ulcerative colitis, 13% had their diagnosis altered postoperatively to either CD or indeterminate colitis. Long-term evaluations of emergency surgery for toxic megacolon and creation of an ileostomy indicate that 38% of patients elected not to reverse the ileostomy, choosing either completion of colonic resection with proctectomy or no further surgery at all.

CD ADVERSE OUTCOMES

Intestinal obstruction represents a frequent complication of small bowel CD. Colonic strictures in CD are less frequent, but still present in 17% of patients with colitis. Chronic obstruction due to a fixed fibrostenotic lesion will require surgical management. Fistulas with associated abscess are another common complication of small bowel CD that requires surgical intervention. *Intra-abdominal abscesses recur more frequently in CD when drained percutaneously in comparison to surgically drained abscesses, 56% vs. 12%, respectively.* Almost half of patients with fistulizing CD initially managed nonoperatively will eventually require surgery during the ensuing year, frequently secondary to medical intractability. Surgical management of fistulizing disease usually involves resection of the primary site with active disease and simple debridement and primary closure of the secondary site that is usually normal. Complicated enteral fistulas to the vagina and urinary bladder require surgery with primary site resection and repair of the secondary site. Free perforation is associated with a high mortality if not treated, and surgical management will involve resection, rather than repair, of the diseased segment. Surgery is

TABLE 163-11 Medications for Induction and Maintenance of Remission Following Hospitalization

Medication	Indication	Mechanism	Contraindication	Side Effect	Outcome
Azathioprine/6-MP	Steroid sparing, prevention of postoperative recurrence of CD	Inhibition of DNA synthesis in lymphocytes	Low/absent TPMT activity	Bone marrow suppression, hepatitis, pancreatitis, rash	Better prevention of postoperative recurrence in comparison to mesalamine in CD
Methotrexate	Alternate immunomodulator for the management of CD	Inhibition of dihydrofolate reductase, resulting in decreased nucleic acid production	Pregnancy, bone marrow suppression, liver disease	Anemia, bruisability, neutropenia, stomatitis, nausea	Induction and maintenance of endoscopic and clinical CD remission
Mesalamine	Prevention of postoperative recurrence CD, treatment for induction of remission of mild to moderate UC and CD	Control of peroxisome proliferator-activated receptor-γ resulting in modification of inflammatory and cytokine response	Hypersensitivity to mesalamine or aminosalicylates	Diarrhea, nausea, abdominal cramping, rarely interstitial nephritis	Marginal decreases in clinical and endoscopic CD recurrence rate at anastomosis at two years
Metronidazole	Prevention of postoperative recurrence, treatment of fistulizing and colonic CD	Bactericidal for anaerobic bacteria	Hypersensitivity to imidazole derivatives	Nausea, antabuse effect, metallic taste, peripheral neuropathy	Prevents endoscopic recurrence of CD at three months and clinical recurrence at one year
Ciprofloxacin	Fistulizing CD, prevention of postoperative recurrence	Bacteriostatic against Gram-positive and negative bacteria	Hypersensitivity to quinolones, panic disorders and depression	Peripheral neuropathy, toxic epidermal necrolysis, pancreatitis, hemolytic anemia, spontaneous tendon rupture	Use as alternative single agent or in combination with metronidazole for rectal and fistulizing CD
Budesonide	Prevention of postoperative recurrence, mild to moderately active ileocecal CD	Broad inhibition of immune activation	Hypersensitivity	Risk of perforation, headache, nausea	Prevented postoperative recurrence in inflammatory CD
Infliximab	Prevention of postoperative recurrence	Neutralization of TNF-α	Untreated chronic infection (TB), moderate to severe heart failure, hypersensitivity to murine products	Upper respiratory tract and urinary tract infections, cough, rash, back pain, nausea, vomiting, abdominal pain, headache, fever	Most dramatic effect in preventing endoscopic recurrence of postoperative CD

also indicated for a proven malignancy, high-grade dysplasia, or dysplasia-associated lesion of mass discovered during endoscopy in colonic CD, whereas diagnosis and management of low-grade dysplasia is still controversial.

DISCHARGE PLANNING

Hospitalization rates for UC and CD are highest among patients in their third decade (20 to 29 years old). The average length of stay for patients with either disease fell from about two weeks in 1983/84 to 9 or 10 days in 2000/01. However, more than a quarter of patients hospitalized for CD and more than 20% of those with UC were readmitted within the same year. Optimal management of patients with IBD requires a multidisciplinary approach involving gastroenterologists, surgeons, pathologists, and radiologists, with the support of dermatologists and rheumatologists. In particular for CD, nutritional support serves an essential role in the patient care. Continuity of care and expertise by a designated IBD provider provides clinical expertise and establishment of patient-provider trust.

QUALITY IMPROVEMENT TO ADDRESS PERFORMANCE GAPS

SECONDARY PREVENTION

Early optimization and maintenance of nutrition and body weight, particularly toward lean tissue mass, helps prevent IBD-related bone disease. In CD, the reported prevalence of osteopenia and osteoporosis is 22–55% and 3–57.6%, respectively, for the lumbar spine and femoral neck, and in UC the reported prevalence of osteopenia and osteoporosis is 32–67% and 4–50%. More importantly, this results in an increased risk of fracture—symptomatic or asymptomatic—that may be up to 40–60% higher than in the control population. As for diagnosis, Dexa scans are the best way to predict fractures. Therapy with vitamin D and calcium (660–800 mg/day premenopausal, 800–1200 mg/day postmenopausal) is indicated, as intake of both is decreased in patients with IBD. Outcomes for bisphosphonates use in IBD have been controversial, except in steroid-induced loss of bone mineral density (BMD), low impact fractures, and T score less than 2.5. However, patients should be warned of relevant side effects, especially esophagitis, and these medications should be monitored carefully in pregnant women.

TRANSITION OF CARE

Frequently, patients with IBD do not receive optimal medical therapy, particularly with dosing of 5-ASA and immunomodulatory medications, the prolonged use of corticosteroids, failure to use steroid-sparing agents, inadequate measures to prevent metabolic bone disease, and inadequate screening for colorectal cancer. Transition to outpatient care with an expert IBD provider will permit high quality continued care.

DISPARITIES IN HEALTH CARE

Comparing African American and whites, both races' populations were similar with respect to age of CD onset, lag in time to diagnosis, and number of gastrointestinal-related hospitalizations and surgeries. Medication usage patterns were also similar in both groups.

After adjusting for age, sex, health insurance, comorbidities, median neighborhood income, and hospital characteristics, the relative rate ratio of undergoing bowel resection for African Americans, Hispanics, and Asians compared to whites was 0.68 [95% confidence interval (CI): (0.61–0.76), 0.70 (95% CI: 0.60–0.83), and 0.31 (95% CI: 0.16–0.59], respectively. Compared to those with private insurance, the relative risk of surgery for those with Medicare, those with Medicaid, and those who were "self-pay" was 0.48 (95% CI: 0.44–0.54), 0.52 (95% CI: 0.46–0.59), and 0.67 (95% CI: 0.58–0.77), respectively. Women were less likely than men to undergo bowel resection (incidence rate ratio [IRR] = 0.80; 95% CI: 0.76–0.85). The in-hospital mortality of individuals who resided in neighborhoods whose median income was above the national median was lower (IRR = 0.71; 95% CI: 0.50–0.99).

TABLE 163-12 Evidence-based Medicine KEY REFERENCES in Inflammatory Bowel Disease

Reference	Methodology	Results	Limitations	Bottom Line
Carter, et al. Guidelines for the management of inflammatory bowel disease in adults. *Gut.* 2004;53(suppl 5):V1–V16	Review article	Extensive review for the management of IBD on an in- and outpatient base in bullet format	Review article, published in 2004	Reference publication for quick access to clinically highly relevant information, including drug actions and side effects, and summary of recommendations
Doherty GA, et al. Meta-analysis: pre-operative infliximab treatment and short-term post-operative complications in patients with ulcerative colitis. *Expert Rev Gastroenterol Hepatol.* 2009;3:395–405	Review article about the management of severe UC	Up-to-date summary of UC management	Review article	Helpful treatment algorithms for the management of severe UC exacerbation, extensive discussion of infliximab utilization
El-Hachem S, et al. Postoperative Crohn's disease: prevention and treatment. *Expert Rev Gastroenterol Hepatol.* 2009;3:249–256	Review article weighing medical options and diagnostic interventions to prevent postoperative recurrence of CD	Up-to-date summary of postoperative management of CD	Review article	Detailed discussion of advantages and disadvantages of medications used postoperatively, helpful tables to grade endoscopic recurrent disease and efficacy of medications
Hwang JM, et al. State-of-the-art of irritable bowel syndrome and inflammatory bowel disease research in 2008. *World J Gastroenterol.* 2008;14:2678–2690	Review article		Review article	Overview of most common elective and emergent indications and operations for IBD with anticipated outcome and complications
Nielsen OH, et al. Diagnosis and management of fistulizing Crohn's disease. *Nat Clin Pract Gastroenterol Hepatol.* 2009;6:92–106	Review article	Extensive review article about the management of this most complicated form of CD	Review article	Clinically relevant summary for the management of complicated fistulizing CD
Sandborn WJ, et al. Colectomy rate comparison after treatment of ulcerative colitis with placebo or infliximab. *Gastroenterology.* 2009;137:1250–1260	Randomized, double-blind, placebo-controlled studies evaluating the role of infliximab in preventing colectomy	Infliimab significantly reduces colectomy rate at 54 weeks	Higher likelihood in the treatment group to develop infections (tuberculosis, histoplasmosis, listeriosis), and malignancy	Infliximab might become medication of choice after steroid failure in the management of severe UC

Approximately 25% of all IBD-related hospitalizations are for patients older than 65 years of age. This population was less likely to be hospitalized with fistulizing (4.0% versus 8.8%, $P < 0.001$) or stricturing (4.0% versus 5.8%, $P = 0.001$) disease. Even after adjusting for comorbidities, patients over the age of 65 years had higher in-hospital mortality (odds ratio [OR] 3.91, 95% confidence interval [CI] 2.50–6.11). In addition, older patients with fistulizing disease are more likely to undergo surgery (OR 1.55, 95% CI 1.00–2.40) and had a longer postoperative stay.

OUTCOME MONITORING

It is pertinent to establish activity of CD six months after surgically-induced remission to devise commencement of prophylactic therapy, even in patients that are asymptomatic. This is usually achieved with ileocolonoscopy, which is superior to WCE. Particularly patients with severe disease in the neoterminal ileum are at higher risk of early symptomatic recurrence compared to patients with either no or mild lesions.

COSTS AND RESOURCE UTILIZATION

Mean annual costs for CD and UC are $8265 and $5066, respectively. As for CD, 31% of costs are attributable to hospitalization, 33% to outpatient care, and 35% to pharmaceutical claims. The corresponding distribution for UC was 38%, 35%, and 27%, respectively. Medical expenses are significantly higher for children younger than 20 years of age in comparison to adults, regardless of gender or geographic region, demonstrating a significant economic burden of IBD. Independent of disease duration, outpatient utilization was more than twice as likely among IBD cases compared with controls whether or not the contact was made for IBD-specific reasons. Inpatient stays for IBD-specific reasons are dependent on disease duration. For non-IBD-specific reasons, IBD cases were 1.5 times as likely to have inpatient stays, regardless of disease duration. Within the first two years from disease diagnosis the most costly resources are employed (**Table 163-12**).

SUGGESTED READINGS

Carter MJ, Lobo AJ, Travis SP. Guidelines for the management of inflammatory bowel disease in adults. *Gut*. 2004;(53)(suppl 5): V1–V16.

Doherty GA, Cheifetz AS. Management of acute severe ulcerative colitis. *Expert Rev Gastroenterol Hepatol*. 2009;3:395–405.

El-Hachem S, Regueiro M. Postoperative Crohn's disease: prevention and treatment. *Expert Rev Gastroenterol Hepatol*. 2009;3: 249–256.

Hwang JM, Varma MG. Surgery for inflammatory bowel disease. *World J Gastroenterol*. 2008;14:2678–2690.

Nielsen OH, Rogler G, Hahnloser D, Thomsen OO. Diagnosis and management of fistulizing Crohn's disease. *Nat Clin Pract Gastroenterol Hepatol*. 2009;6:92–106.

Sandborn WJ, Rutgeerts P, Feagan BG, et al. Colectomy rate comparison after treatment of ulcerative colitis with placebo or infliximab. *Gastroenterology*. 2009;137:1250–1260; quiz 520.

SECTION 7

Geriatrics

CHAPTER 164

Principles of Geriatric Care

William L. Lyons, MD

Key Clinical Questions

1. How do elderly patients differ from younger patients?
2. What are the risk factors for functional decline in the hospital?
3. What are the risk factors for the development of geriatric syndromes as a complication of hospitalization?
4. What items in the history and physical exam require customization for the geriatric patient?
5. What are the factors that predict higher mortality post-discharge of elderly patients?

INTRODUCTION

Elderly patients differ from younger ones in many ways, including some that influence their care in the hospital. Optimal geriatric hospital care takes these special characteristics into account, and entails the use of a particular systematic approach, no matter what patients' admitting diagnoses may be. This chapter begins with a description of differences between older and younger hospital patients; describes the importance of self-care function among the elderly; summarizes key features of well-studied acute geriatric interventions; provides tips for care of the older patient on admission day, daily work rounds, and discharge; and finishes with information about prognosis in this population.

HOW OLDER PATIENTS DIFFER

One characteristic difference between older and younger patients is in how they present with common diseases. Younger patients generally present with complaints and findings that anatomically point to the diseased organ: they have productive cough and dyspnea with pneumococcal pneumonia, or chest pain with myocardial infarction. Older patients may demonstrate the same signs and symptoms, but often they present with one of two often-overlapping pictures. The first is acute functional loss—the sudden loss of self-care capability, such as independence in bathing or dressing. The other is the geriatric syndrome, which is a clinical syndrome (such as acute confusion, fall, dizziness or syncope, new-onset urinary incontinence) reflecting the presence of diminished physiological reserve. A frail elder with pneumonia may have no complaints directed at the thorax, but instead may be brought in by family because of confusion, falls, and new difficulties in the shower.

A variety of physiological changes occur as a result of normal aging in humans; **Table 164-1** summarizes some of the most prominent.

It is apparent that, in every physiologic system, aging results in a loss of physiological resilience, a reduced ability of the older body to maintain normal functioning when confronted with an external stressor. (Common stressors include pharmacologic adverse effects as well as acute illnesses.) Chronic diseases like heart failure, Alzheimer disease, or emphysema detract still further from the older patient's physiological reserve. Geriatricians have long noted the "weakest link principle" among their patients—an elder's illness presentation will reflect failure of that physiological system with the least reserve, rather than the system that is the locus of the new acute ailment. Hence, the elder whose circulatory system is weak comes to attention for syncope when struck down by a viral infection.

Two corollaries result from older patients' atypical presentations and chronic multimorbidity. First, the wise diagnostician casts a wide net when confronted with sick older patients. Whether the frail elder's complaint is new confusion or a fall, the admitting physician should consider a wide variety of incipient illnesses, and conduct a correspondingly comprehensive evaluation. Second, Occam's razor, which motivates us to uncover a unifying diagnosis for multiple findings, more often fails in treating older patients.

Another crucial difference between older and younger patients is that the former show greater fragility in the hospital. Elderly

TABLE 164-1 Selected Physiological Changes that Occur with Normal Aging

System	Changes
Nervous	Brain perfusion shows impaired autoregulation
	Slowed reaction time
	Impaired balance from reduced vestibular responsiveness
Circulatory	Decreased maximal HR and CO
	Impaired diastolic filling, greater dependence on atrial systole
	Reduced pacemaker cells in SA node
	Reduced response to beta-adrenergic stimulation
	Reduced elasticity of large arteries (increased systolic BP)
Respiratory	Reduced FEV1 and FVC
	Impaired ciliary clearance
	Reduced PaO_2 from V/Q mismatch
	Lungs less elastic
	Chest wall stiffer
Musculoskeletal	Reduced muscle mass with age
	Reduced bone mass
Renal/Urinary	Steady drop in GFR with age
	Reduced sodium conservation and excretion
	Reduced ability to concentrate or dilute urine
	Reduced ability to excrete acid load
	Renal perfusion more dependent on local prostaglandins
	Impaired bladder emptying
Sensory	Reduced contrast sensitivity (vision)
	Impaired dark adaptation (vision)
	Loss of high-frequency tones (hearing)
Immune	Diminished cell-mediated immunity
	Antibodies have lower affinity
Hematologic	Reduced erythropoietic response to EPO

BP, blood pressure; CO, cardiac output; EPO, erythropoietin; FEV1, forced expiratory volume in 1 second; FVC, forced vital capacity; GFR, glomerular filtration rate; HR, heart rate; PaO_2, arterial partial pressure of oxygen; SA, sinoatrial; V/Q, ventilation-perfusion ratio.

hospitalized patients have been shown to suffer almost twice the incidence of preventable adverse events related to medical procedures, drug effects, and falls than do younger patients. Older age is also a well-established risk factor for activities-of-daily-living decline in the hospital.

Finally, older patients, by virtue of the fact that they are closer to the end of their lives than the beginning, often evince different health care goals than younger patients. The typical younger patient seeks rescue or life prolongation as a consequence of hospital care. Many older patients, of course, have the same desires, but a substantial number emphasize instead maintenance of independence or achieving symptomatic relief. This greater diversity in health care goals among older patients compels hospital providers to address the issue head on, a matter taken up later.

THE IMPORTANCE OF FUNCTION

Function refers to the set of behaviors needed to remain independent in daily life. Functional domains include the following:

- Basic activities of daily living (ADLs): bathing, dressing, toileting, transfers, continence, and feeding.
- Instrumental activities of daily living (IADLs): using the telephone, shopping, food preparation, housekeeping, laundry, transportation, managing medications, and managing money.
- Mobility: including the ability to ambulate in the home or community, negotiate stairs, etc.

The trajectories of physiological and functional measures often differ greatly during elders' hospitalizations. Whereas physiological markers (vital signs, laboratory assessments) typically improve by discharge, functional measures commonly show worse status. Studies have shown, for example, that 20% to more than 30% of older patients admitted to hospital general medical wards lose independence in one or more ADLs by the time of discharge. One study of almost 2300 elders on the general medical service of two hospitals found that 35% were discharged with worse-than-baseline function. This 35% was composed of the following subgroups: 12% showed decline in the hospital only, 18% had prehospital decline from baseline but failed to recover, and 5% demonstrated both prehospital and in-hospital decline.

Scholars of geriatric patients' function have enunciated certain principles of ADLs and IADLs: (1) ADLs reflect more than simply physical function, but reflect the match between a patient's physical abilities and her environment (including social support). (2) As people age, ADLs are typically lost in an orderly fashion: the ability to bathe independently is lost first, the ability to feed oneself last. (3) ADL loss progresses through predictable stages: first, one can do the ADL without difficulty; later, one can do it, but with difficulty; still later, one can't do it alone, but can do it with assistance; and finally, one can't do it, as there is insufficient help. (4) IADLs reflect higher-order cognitive skills needed for individuals to live independently, and with most conditions (especially dementing disorders). IADLs are lost before ADLs.

Patients' mobility often follows a different trajectory than their ADL or IADL function. Cognitively impaired patients, in particular, commonly maintain their mobility while suffering ADL and IADL losses. An older patient's mobility may be assessed by asking: *Do you have difficulty walking up or down stairs? Do you have difficulty walking several blocks? Do you have difficulty walking across a room?*

Although physicians appear in some studies to be unaware of their patients' functional abilities or at least commonly neglect to document them, functional capacity is a potent predictor of outcomes in older patients. Function reveals the extent to which a patient is impacted by her various diagnoses. Poor function has been shown to predict mortality, institutional placement, caregiver burden, quality of life, length of stay, and cost of care.

Functional loss in the hospital probably reflects complex interactions between diseases, age, and hospital care itself.

Table 164-2 lists factors that have been found in various studies to increase the risk of in-hospital functional decline. Predictors include preexisting functional impairment, brain disease (dementia, delirium, depression), malnutrition, mobility difficulties (including bed rest), and older age. Regarding age, one research group found that older hospitalized patients are less likely to recover ADL function that they lost from their baseline preceding admission, and are more likely to develop new functional impairments during their hospital stay. Others have reported that cognitive impairment present at hospital admission predicts failure of functional recovery at three months following hospital discharge.

TABLE 164-2 Risk Factors for In-Hospital Functional Decline in Older Patients

Age over 75
Presence of preadmission ADL disability
Presence of preadmission IADL disability
Cognitive impairment at admission
Delirium, including subsyndromal delirium
Pressure sores
Depression symptoms
Low body mass index
Longer hospital length of stay
Mobility impairment (use of assistive device) or bed rest
Institutional residence
Lower social activity level
Certain diagnostic categories (ICD-9 codes)

Risk factors for the development of geriatric syndromes in the hospital have been established as well. One group found the following predictors of four specific geriatric syndromes (pressure sores, urinary incontinence, fecal incontinence, and falls): cognitive impairment, advanced age, prolonged hospital length of stay, and severe ADL disability. Not surprisingly, these resilience-sapping properties predict ADL decline as well (Table 164-2).

ENGINEERING IMPROVED GERIATRIC HOSPITAL CARE

A number of approaches have been designed to improve the hospital care processes for geriatric inpatients. Rubenstein and coworkers demonstrated the benefits of an inpatient "GEM" (for geriatric evaluation and management) unit to which older adults are admitted after stabilization in another acute ward. In a later multicenter, randomized trial conducted at 11 Veterans Affairs medical centers, GEM units were demonstrated to improve ADL function and physical performance relative to usual hospital care.

The Acute Care for Elders ("ACE") system, in contrast to GEM units, allows for direct admission of acutely ill patients to the special inpatient ward without prior stabilization. ACE employs a proactive, "prehabilitative" approach, designed to help hospitalized elders maintain or achieve functional independence. Key elements of the ACE program are summarized in **Table 164-3**. ACE was shown, in a randomized controlled trial set in an academic medical center, to result in greater ADL independence at the time of hospital discharge, and in less frequent need for nursing home placement. A follow-up study performed at a community hospital showed a more modest difference in function between ACE and control patients. The performance of ACE (and other special geriatric acute care systems) is probably sensitive to factors that depend on interdisciplinary team function.

TABLE 164-3 Key Components of Acute Care for Elders ("Ace") Units

Component	Description
Prepared environment for mobility and orientation	Carpeting, abundant grab bars, raised toilet seats, low beds, clocks, and calendars
Nursing-initiated protocols for patient-centered care	Targeted at independence in self care, nutrition, sleep hygiene, skin care, mood, cognition
Planning for home	Early involvement of social services
Medical care review	Geriatrician advises about optimal medication prescribing, risk assessment of procedures, and so on.

A recent systematic review and meta-analysis examined seven studies in which older hospital patients were randomized to either usual care or inpatient geriatric assessment and management. (This analysis included two studies of ACE units, as well as studies of Veterans Affairs GEM units, and a number of European programs.) The meta-analysis found that specialized geriatric inpatient programs showed statistically significant improvements in both functional status at discharge and need for institutionalization at one year. Nonsignificant trends toward improvement were found in readmission risk, institutionalization within one year, and mortality.

The Hospital Elder Life Program ("HELP") differs from the programs described above because enrolled patients are admitted to wherever open beds exist, rather than to specialized inpatient wards. This multicomponent intervention was designed to prevent incident delirium in hospitalized elders. The program makes extensive use of well-trained and committed volunteers. At admission, older patients are assessed for the presence of six risk factors for delirium (cognitive impairment, sleep deprivation, immobility, vision impairment, hearing impairment, and dehydration), and protocols are triggered to manage identified risks. In a randomized, controlled study, delirium incidence in the intervention patients was 9.9%, significantly less than 15% in the control group. Both severity and duration of delirium appeared to be unaffected by the intervention.

Targeting of patients appropriate for the above-described interventions is probably crucial to assure cost-effective care. Leaders of such programs typically establish admission criteria in order to exclude older patients who are too vigorous, too functionally dependent, profoundly demented, or terminally ill.

TIPS FOR ADMISSION DAY

A comprehensive and systematic geriatric evaluation, employing the assessment features of GEM or ACE units or HELP, complements the traditional medical approach learned in most physicians' training. The section that follows highlights special geriatric issues to consider within the traditional categories learned in medical school. The traditional admission mantra—history of present illness, past medical history, medications, family history, and do on—still works well with the geriatric patient, but the constituent items need customization for the older patient.

History of present illness

Older patients with chronic cognitive impairment or delirium should have their illness stories corroborated by family, friends, or nursing facility staff as appropriate. Also, patients (or informants) should be questioned not only about signs and symptoms but about new functional problems that have arisen as a result of the illness—trouble walking, transferring, bathing, shopping, managing medications, and so on.

Past medical history

A well-documented past medical history for many elders will include not only the usual medical problems like diabetes mellitus and hypertension, but functional diagnoses like gait impairment or dysphagia. Sophisticated clinicians recognize these functional diagnoses as multifactorial and attributable to sundry medical conditions, and will document them accordingly: *"Gait impairment and frequent falls, secondary to Parkinson disease and knee osteoarthritis," or "Dysphagia secondary to a cerebrovascular accident in 2002."*

Medications

A patient's as-taken medication regimen often deviates substantially from the theoretical one listed in the outpatient medical record. (This discrepancy may become apparent when, for example, a hypertensive patient's blood pressure plummets in the hospital when admitting orders are written that parrot the outpatient drug list.) Although the following advice applies of course to the care of all patients, it is especially helpful when admitting the elderly: determine not only the complete outpatient drug regimen, but ask about the patient's method for remembering to take doses and for an estimate of how often doses are missed. The complete outpatient regimen of many patients often includes a blend of pills ordered by multiple prescribers and bought at multiple pharmacies, as well as over-the-counter agents and herbal or nontraditional remedies.

Family history

It is very unusual for an older patient's family history to provide the clue needed to make a difficult diagnosis. Uncovering genetic predispositions to various diseases is probably less important than simply asking about the health of people in a patient's family. A very ill spouse may be unlikely to serve as your patient's future caregiver; rather, your patient may be the one serving in the care-giving role. The family history also may provide glimmers of insight into a patient's views on preferred intensity of health care, and attentive listening to an older person's narrative of a family member's grave illness can pay dividends in that domain.

Social history

The older patient's social history includes a number of items not always collected from a younger individual:

a. What is the extent of social support? Who lives in the patient's home, and how much of the time? Who is in the expanded social network and would be able and willing to help in the event of prolonged illness or functional dependence?
b. In the event of lost decisional capacity, who is the patient's surrogate?
c. Does the patient have difficulty with or need assistance with ADLs and IADLs? Who provides the assistance, and what do they do? Does the patient receive Meals on Wheels?
d. Is there any reason to suspect elder mistreatment? Consider asking, *"Do you feel safe returning to where you live?"*
e. In addition to wishes regarding attempts at resuscitation, inquire about the patient's global health care goals. The author broaches the subject along the following lines: *"You know, Mrs. Green, I have a lot of patients about your age and with similar medical problems, and they tell me, 'Doctor, I want you to do anything you can to help me live as long as possible. Use any treatment or surgery or put me on a ventilator, but staying alive is very important to me.' And I have other patients who have said, 'Doctor, at this point in my life it's more important to me that I am comfortable and in my own home. That's more important than being kept alive.' Do you have any thoughts along these lines, Mrs. Green?"* Another way to begin a goals-of-care discussion is to ask, *"Can you imagine any way of living that would be worse than death?"*

Review of systems

In addition to the usual review conducted on younger patients, it is important to inquire about the following:

a. Weight loss and poor appetite. Malnutrition in older hospitalized patients has been shown to predict increased risk for mortality, dependence in ADLs, and institutionalization, even after correction for comorbid and acute illnesses. Some 15% of elders have severe protein-calorie malnutrition at admission, and 25% of older patients suffer nutritional decline during the course of their hospital stay. Patients with weight loss should be assessed for reversible causes (oral cavity disease, dysphagia, medication adverse effects, etc.) and considered for oral nutritional supplementation.
b. Mobility problems and falls. Recent hospitalization is an independent risk factor for hip fracture among older patients. Restricted activity or bed rest predicts the development of disability in this population as well. Older patients admitted to the hospital should be encouraged to ambulate (with assistance if necessary) several times a day, or at least spend time out of bed in a chair if they cannot ambulate. "Bed rest" activity orders are generally appropriate only for patients whose care goals are palliative. Patients with falls and mobility difficulties may benefit from involvement of physical therapy.
c. Impaired vision, impaired hearing. Impairment in these two vital sensory modalities predicts the development of delirium in the hospital, and efforts to identify and manage these impairments have been demonstrated to reduce this risk. Elders admitted to the hospital should be asked about these sensory problems, and hospital staff should ask that assistive devices such as glasses or hearing aids be brought in from home by family.
d. Depression. Depression among hospitalized elders is common and often undiagnosed. The presence of depression in this population is associated with increased risk of death, ADL dependence, and need for institutional placement. Older hospitalized patients can be screened for depression with use of questions directed at the two cardinal symptoms of the disorder: depressed mood (*"Have you been feeling sad, depressed, or hopeless?"*) and anhedonia (*"Have you lost your usual interest or pleasure in doing things?"*). Possibly depressed patients identified on screening should be evaluated more thoroughly, and those diagnosed with depression can be treated or flagged for additional care in the discharge summary.

Physical examination

The following components of the physical examination deserve particular attention during the admission of an elderly patient:

a. General appearance. Does the patient exhibit vitality or frailty when moving in bed to facilitate the examination? Is there an odor of incontinence or poor hygiene?
b. Nutritional status. Malnutrition is apparent from low body mass index, loss of subcutaneous fat, and diminished muscle bulk (look for concave temporal fossae, squared-off shoulders reflecting thinning of deltoids, and diminished intrinsic hand muscles).
c. Mental status. Dementia is a risk factor for the development of delirium, as well as for difficulty adhering with therapy, and patients in early stages commonly go undetected. Some form of mental status assessment should be incorporated into the admission evaluation, such as the Folstein Mini-Mental State Examination. Delirium should be suspected in the inattentive patient with acute onset and fluctuating course, and is more likely in a patient having difficulty with a task such as reciting the months of the year in reverse.

d. Oral cavity. Assess the health of older patients' teeth and gums. Poor dentition and periodontal disease may explain an elder's poor nutritional status.
e. Mobility. Observe patients' ability to arise from a seated position without use of the arms; inability to do so typically reflects quadriceps weakness. Gait (speed, symmetry, stride length, truncal posture, arm swing) reflects neurological and musculoskeletal health.
f. Vision and hearing. Use a pocket Snellen chart to evaluate vision in older patients. Hearing can be assessed using an audioscope or by checking the patient's ability to hear a whispered word in each ear.
g. Frail elders admitted to the hospital should be checked for the presence of pressure ulcers. The earliest stage of such ulcers is nonblanching erythema. Common locations for ulcers are skin over the following bony prominences: occiput, scapulae, sacrum, ischial tuberosities, greater trochanter, and posterior calcaneus.

TIPS FOR DAILY WORK ROUNDS

Perhaps the most advantageous practice to adopt in caring for hospitalized elders is to maintain a focus on certain "low-tech" considerations critical to good outcomes, in spite of the presence of disease-specific and technological distractions. Choosing the proper imaging modality is essential, but should not cause the physician to ignore that a patient has not eaten or walked in two days. A suggested checklist of items to review daily when seeing older patients on hospital rounds is provided in **Table 164-4**. The items in this table reflect lessons learned from specialized inpatient geriatric programs (such as ACE units), in which patients are frequently assessed for ADL status and mobility, nutrient intake and bowel function, mental status, presence of risky devices (such as bladder catheters or restraints), skin health, polypharmacy, and determination of a discharge plan.

DISCHARGE OF THE OLDER PATIENT

The older hospitalized patient should generally be discharged to the least restrictive environment that will support her functional, rehabilitative, and clinical needs. In order to recommend a venue, the hospital team should assess the patient's ADL and mobility function; inquire about the capabilities and willingness of family caregivers, as well as the patient's physical home environment; clarify the needed rehabilitative disciplines (physical therapy, occupational therapy, speech therapy) and the intensity of their anticipated programs; and specify the technical components of the patient's treatment plan (intravenous therapy, wound and ostomy care, etc.). Based on findings of studies on ACE units and similar programs, patients' length of stay is probably reduced when hospitals' interdisciplinary teams commence discharge planning from the day of admission.

TABLE 164-4 Tips for Daily Work Rounds

1. ADL status and trajectory: Is the patient approaching baseline function?
2. Oral intake: How much of each meal is being eaten? Consider between-meal supplements.
3. Bowel function: When was the last bowel movement? Consider a laxative.
4. Mobility: Has the patient been out of bed? Encourage ambulation, consider physical therapy.
5. Physical examination: Document attachments (central lines, bladder catheters, etc) and discontinue them when possible.
6. Physical examination: Check mental status daily to identify incident delirium.
7. Physical examination: In the mobility-impaired patient, check high risk sites for pressure ulcers.
8. Pharmacotherapy: Practice good drug list hygiene by reviewing the medication list and discontinuing nonessential agents.
9. Discharge planning: Discharge destination identified? Family and Social Services recruited to help with arrangements?

Home health care agencies help to provide care for complex, clinically stable discharged elders. Medicare provides funding for care deemed reasonable and necessary, provided that it is difficult for the patient to leave the home. There also must be a "skilled need," meaning a need for a registered nurse, physical therapist, or speech pathologist. After a patient has been admitted to an agency's service under the care of one of these three disciplines, other disciplines (occupational therapy, medical social work) may be involved as needed. Hospitalists discharging frail, complex, or precarious patients to a home environment should consider involving visiting nursing for vital signs measurements and assessments of clinical stability.

Potential "red flags," findings or symptoms that suggest that a clinical condition is worsening, should be routinely communicated to the patient and caregiver before discharge. Further, it is important to clarify *who* (the hospitalist? or primary care provider?) should be called in the event that a problem arises.

Older hospital patients typically have longer medication lists than younger ones. These lists must be meticulously reconciled at the time of hospital discharge for the benefit of the patient and any new set of providers. The end result of the medication reconciliation process is a document that lists the following: (a) What medications (including doses, frequencies, any tapering or stop schedules, and indications) are to be taken after hospital discharge? (b) Which of these medications is new, when compared with the regimen taken before hospital admission? (c) Which drugs from the preadmission regimen are to be stopped?

In most instances a well-constructed and timely discharge summary provides adequate communication between hospital-based and post-acute clinicians. At times, however, a telephone call from the hospitalist to the receiving provider is appropriate. An example of such a time would be to warn the next provider of the need to watch for a critical, but still awaited, laboratory result. Other examples include the provision of delicate, psychosocial context that a discharge summary could not properly cover, or the relating of ongoing discussions with the patient about shifting global health goals.

PROGNOSIS

Older hospitalized patients are at greater risk of readmission than younger ones. Other factors predicting rehospitalization are the presence of certain medical diagnoses (cardiovascular disease, diabetes, and cancer), psychosocial considerations (depression, inadequate social support, Medicaid eligibility), previous hospital use, worse self-rating of health, and failure of the hospital team to provide discharge-related counseling prior to dismissal.

For many elderly patients, hospitalization is a milestone marking a terminal decline. Inouye, et al demonstrated that, after adjustment for disease burden and severity, three risk factors independently predict mortality for older patients following hospitalization: impairment in IADLs, cognitive impairment, and depression. Walter and coworkers created and validated a prognostic index for post-discharge mortality. Factors in this index predicting greater mortality were male sex, ADL dependence, congestive heart failure, cancer, elevated creatinine, and low albumin.

CONCLUSION

Elderly patients often present with atypical presentations of common diseases, necessitating wide-ranging diagnostic workups. They are at greater risk of injury and functional decline in the hospital, and optimal outcomes result from adopting a systematic approach to their care, regardless of admitting diagnosis. Approaches that have demonstrated improved outcomes employ comprehensive geriatric assessment of patients at admission, and those patients found to have predetermined risk factors for functional decline or geriatric syndromes reliably undergo targeted treatments designed to reduce those risks. The challenge for the hospitalist caring for older patients is to attend to the technical, disease-focused issues that prompt admission in the first place without neglecting the "prehabilitative" orientation that can prevent discharge to a nursing home.

SUGGESTED READINGS

Cohen HJ, Feussner JR, Weinberger M, et al. A controlled trial of inpatient and outpatient geriatric evaluation and management. *N Engl J Med*. 2002;346:905–912.

Covinsky KE, Justice AC, Rosenthal GE, et al. Measuring prognosis and case mix in hospitalized elders. The importance of functional status. *J Gen Intern Med*. 1997;12(4):254–255.

Covinsky KE, Palmer RM, Fortinsky RH, et al. Loss of independence in activities of daily living in older adults hospitalized with medical illnesses: Increased vulnerability with age. *J Am Geriatr Soc*. 2003;51:451–458.

Inouye SK, Bogardus ST, Carpentier PA, et al. A multicomponent intervention to prevent delirium in hospitalized older patients. *N Engl J Med*. 1999;340:669–676.

Inouye SK, Peduzzi PN, Robinson JT, et al. Importance of functional measures in predicting mortality among older hospitalized patients. *JAMA*. 1998;279:1187–1193.

Landefeld CS, Palmer RM, Kresevic D, et al. A randomized trial of care in a hospital medical unit especially designed to improve the functional outcomes of acutely ill older patients. *N Engl J Med*. 1995;332:1338–1344.

Mecocci P, von Strauss E, Cherubini A, et al. Cognitive impairment is the major risk factor for development of geriatric syndromes during hospitalization: Results from the GIFA study. *Dement Geriatr Cogn Disord*. 2005;20:262–269.

Sands LP, Yaffe K, Covinsky KE, et al. Cognitive screening predicts magnitude of functional recovery from admission to 3 months after discharge in hospitalized elders. *J Gerontol A Biol Sci Med Sci*. 2003;58A:37–45.

Van Craen K, Braes T, Wellens N, et al. The effectiveness of inpatient geriatric evaluation and management units: A systematic review and meta-analysis. *J Am Geriatr Soc*. 2010;58:83–92.

Walter LC, Brand RJ, Counsell SR, et al. Development and validation of a prognostic index for 1-year mortality in older adults after hospitalization. *JAMA*. 2001;285(23):2987–2994.

CHAPTER 165

The Geriatric History and Physical Examination

Arline D. Bohannon, MD
Peter A. Boling, MD

Key Clinical Questions

1. What are the essential aspects of geriatric assessment that should occur routinely in the hospital?
2. How should the geriatric assessment differ from admission assessments of younger patients?
3. What should the assessment of the physical function domain include? The psychological domain? The social domain?

INTRODUCTION

The U.S. population of adults age 65 years and older will double within 20 years. In 2005, an estimated 35 million nonfederal hospital discharges occurred in the U.S. excluding newborns, and while older adults (65+) comprise 12% of the population, they accounted for 35% of hospital stays. Increasingly often, geriatric patients enter the hospital through the emergency room. For example, for patients 80 and older, 64% came through the emergency room in 2002, compared with 55% in 1997.

Risk of ICU admission and utilization also rise with age, peaking in the very old: in those age 85 years or more there were 58.2 admissions per 1,000 residents and 195.8 days per 1,000 residents, compared with 3.8 admissions per 1,000 residents and 11.5 days per 1,000 residents in those 18 to 44 years old. Residents 85 years old and older were 3.75 times more likely to be admitted to the ICU than those age 18–44 after controlling for comorbid illness. Risk of ICU admission increased with admission to surgical units, and presence of multiple comorbid illnesses especially cardiovascular and renal disease.

In addition to high personal costs, the impact on health care costs is also high. As one example, the occurrence of delirium more than doubles the impact on health care costs. Annual estimated costs in the U.S. attributable to delirium range from 38 billion to 152 billon dollars due to increased mortality and morbidity, prolonged hospital stay, functional decline, and institutionalization. With 42% of the U.S. national health care budget spent on inpatient care, and readmissions accounting for one-quarter of Medicare inpatient expenditures, reduction in readmissions is becoming a focal point in health care policy, and hospitals may lose reimbursement when preventable readmissions occur.

HAZARDS OF HOSPITALIZATION

Normal aging reduces physiologic reserve and the ability to maintain homeostasis under physiologic stress even in the best of circumstances. Chronic disease, the stress of acute illness precipitating admission, and polypharmacy then add to vulnerability in this heterogeneous population. Furthermore, the hospital experience disrupts normal life rhythms in a foreign environment away from familiar cues and supports. Hospital procedures and policies promote dependency and immobility that is often related to physical restraints and expose the patient to multiple unfamiliar people, further exacerbated by unit transfers. Hospitals disrupt sleep and nutrition due to lighting, unit noise, and interruptions such as frequent blood drawing and performance of vital signs and tests. Use of sedatives or medications with anticholinergic side effects—though sometimes unavoidable during anesthesia—and inadequate pain management further exacerbate the risk of hospital acquired complications, including delirium, depression, infection, malnutrition, deconditioning, falls, and pressure ulcers. Adverse outcomes include in death, a prolonged hospital stay, nursing home placement, and increased long-term dependency.

Incident delirium, which is one of the most troublesome complications during hospitalization, ranges from 11% to 42% of admissions and functional deficits related to delirium may persist long after hospital discharge. While the classic association of delirium with urinary tract infection is common and well recognized, many cases of hospital-acquired delirium result from an underlying predisposition complicated by medication side effects, undertreated pain, restraints, constipation, and disrupted routines, producing a cascade of adverse effects. (Refer to section on Infectious Diseases for hospital-acquired infections and delirium).

Studies have also shown that 30% to 60% of older people develop new dependencies in activities of daily living (ADL) during their hospital stay, with a dramatic loss of muscle strength for each day at bed rest. And pressure ulcers, considered a preventable complication of hospitalization, are associated with increased length of stay and health care cost, to the point that they are being called "never" events for which Medicare will refuse to pay. The median incidence of pressure ulcers in hospitalized elderly persons varies from 5% to 16% and has not decreased in recent years. Some pressure ulcers develop early during hospitalization, after only a few hours of immobility induced pressure. One large study found that 6% of patients developed one or more hospital-acquired pressure ulcers within two days of hospital admission. Risk factors for new pressure ulcers include increased age, male gender, African-American ethnicity, immobility (requiring assistance with turning in bed), transfer from nursing home, nutritional compromise, BMI < 18.5, the presence of another pressure ulcer, and urinary and fecal incontinence. (See Chapter 144 Pressure Ulcers and Chapter 164 Principles of Geriatric Care for a discussion of evidence-based models of care to prevent inpatient complications.)

The elderly patient admitted to the hospital should be considered a "high-risk senior," defined as those at risk for developing health-related crises, simply by virtue of being hospitalized. The admission of any elderly patient to the hospital offers a window of opportunity for identifying those at risk for further functional disability and clarifying targets for timely intervention to prevent or delay further decline and a cascade of readmissions. Patients with five or more chronic illnesses and deficits in activities of daily living or ADLs are at dramatically higher risk of preventable readmission. The hospitalist should provide an actionable assessment that will lead to a multidisciplinary approach utilizing case management, appropriate consultation, disease management programs in patients with lower degrees of comorbidity, and coordinated posthospital care. Optimal practice involves targeting posthospital services to be cost-effective and efficient: the right care, in the right place, at the right time, based on need. And there is a need for an effective handoff, which is too often overlooked.

THE GERIATRIC HISTORY AND PHYSICAL EXAMINATION

The admission history and physical examination is the starting point. This is a multistep process of acquiring data that in aggregate leads to a provisional diagnosis. Physicians are taught to seek one diagnosis that will explain all or most aspects of a patient's signs and symptoms at presentation. However, elderly patients commonly have multiple comorbid conditions of varying severity that may affect the initial presentation of a new illness. Unlike younger patients, whose signs and symptoms refer to the diseased organ, ill elderly patients commonly develop nonspecific symptoms such as lethargy, confusion, falls, and incontinence and decreased ability to perform ADLs. Painless myocardial infarction, pneumonia without cough or fever, apathetic hyperthyroidism, and depression masquerading as dementia are examples of common yet atypical presentations. A change in mental status, gradual debilitation, and nonspecific symptoms are also characteristic of tuberculosis in the elderly; yet this patient population has weakened delayed hypersensitivity reactions so that only 5–10% of 90-year-olds will have a positive initial PPD despite prior exposure. In addition, there may not be one unifying diagnosis to explain all symptoms, some of which may be from drug side effects. Therefore, clinicians need to maintain a high index of suspicion, incorporate risk factors into clinical decision making, carefully review all medications and treatment, obtain information from multiple sources, and perform a comprehensive examination.

To guide the care process, geriatric medicine focuses on functional domains—physical, cognitive, psychological, and social—that can be used to assess quality of life and goals of care. In addition to treating the cause for admission, a multifaceted approach may improve outcomes by identifying disability, taking steps to improve functional performance, instituting preventive measures to limit iatrogenic complications and disability, and by promoting wellness and independence. This chapter will describe the essential history and physical exam components that should routinely be performed for hospitalized elderly patients in addition to the admission history and physical examination ordinarily performed for younger patients, and explains how to factor this information into discharge planning.

In order to obtain a complete patient history, clinicians should communicate with family members and caregivers for information about baseline functioning, and if possible, contact the primary care physician or geriatrician on the day of admission. Providers need this information to achieve goals of hospitalization, which include avoidance of complications that might exacerbate preexisting conditions that make the patient even more vulnerable to prolonged hospital stay and the need for permanent placement upon discharge. The team should encourage liberal visiting by family and friends, especially during meals and evening hours, inform the family of the risks of hospitalization, and engage them in preventive measures such as orienting the patient, explaining the hospital routine, and assisting with ambulation. The family should bring in the patient's hearing aid, glasses, and assistive devices that will facilitate optimal function. Care must then be taken not to lose these sometimes expensive items during the hospital care process.

Effective communication during the patient interview always begins with speaking in the patient's native language and at the level appropriate for the patient's educational background and cognitive function. The clinician should

- Address the patient by his or her last name.
- Try to minimize extraneous noise and interruptions.
- Sit opposite the patient at eye level, smiling, speaking slowly with a low-pitched voice.
- Inquire about hearing deficits, confirming that the patient can hear the conversation, and ask him or her to repeat back what has been heard.
- Raise the volume of his or her voice, if necessary, but not shout; shouting may be misinterpreted as anger.
- Write questions down in a large print, if the patient does not have his or her hearing aid or still cannot hear.
- Allow plenty of time for the patient to respond to questions.
- Try to reassure the patient that he or she is in a safe environment.
- Engage the patient to speak about his or her interests.
- Use visual aids in the room to identify care providers and be available when family members visit.

THE COGNITIVE DOMAIN

The prevalence of cognitive impairment doubles every five years after the age of 65. By age 90, 40% to 50% of patients have some dementia. Family members and friends often notice the changes seen in dementia but may deny the symptoms or neglect to mention the symptoms to busy medical practitioners, especially in the early stages of the condition. Many patients do not complain or volunteer information about memory loss and this problem will be overlooked unless they are specifically questioned or tested to detect the early signs. In general, physicians often fail to identify or document early or mild cognitive impairment. The interviewer should ask the patient and any family caregivers whether the patient suffers from memory loss sufficient to interfere with social functioning in the months or years preceding the acute illness. Dementia is a potent risk factor for hospital-acquired complications including delirium, and recognizing it will help with preventive measures. The sometimes subtle symptoms and signs of dementia are noticeable to the people who live with the older adult and these also may precipitate a hospital admission for "placement," again requiring a proactive approach from day one. Consider the following example, as it might normally occur and as it might be improved.

CASE 165-1

AN ELDERLY PATIENT, TWO VIEWS

View One

A 79-year-old female with hypertensive heart disease and mild chronic obstructive lung disease is admitted to the hospitalist service from the ED late at night after calling an ambulance for chest pain. Her symptoms are vague. There have been three visits for chest pain to area hospitals in the past year.

She is hypertensive in the ED (210/80) and has "mild interstitial edema" on chest X-ray, negative cardiac enzymes, and a normal acute phase myocardial imaging study. She is given medications for ACS, has a Foley catheter inserted, which she pulls throughout the night and first two hospital days. She receives a dose of haldol (2 mg IV) and is diuresed 2 liters with resulting rise in BUN and creatinine from 32 and 1.2 to 46 and 1.5 respectively. A stress test and echocardiogram show no new conditions.

At discharge on hospital day four, her carvedilol dose, which was 12.5 mg twice a day on a prior admission, is increased to 25 mg twice a day and her furosemide dose is increased from 20 to 40 mg daily. She is given a new patient appointment with a cardiologist affiliated with the hospital and told to see her primary care physician in one week. A referral is made to home health care and the dictated summary is sent as a "cc" to the PCP.

A week later she is readmitted through the ER, this time with altered mental status, worsened renal function, hypotension, and urosepsis with a resistant hospital-acquired organism. After a 10-day inpatient stay she is transferred to a skilled nursing facility for rehab as a result of deconditioning and persistent confusion to the point that she is incapable of self care.

View Two

A 79-year-old female with hypertensive heart disease and mild chronic obstructive lung disease is admitted to the hospitalist service from the ED late at night after calling an ambulance for chest pain. Her symptoms are vague and she says she keeps going to the hospital for this but "they don't tell me anything."

She is hypertensive in the ED (210/80) and has "mild interstitial edema" on chest X-ray, negative cardiac enzymes, and a normal acute phase myocardial imaging study. She is given initial medications for ACS.

On exam, the hospitalist screens for dementia and delirium, and finds that while she is verbal and sociable and does not meet any criteria for delirium by the confusion assessment method (CAM) (0/4 points), she has significantly impaired memory. There is no listed family and the patient lives alone. Needing third party information, the hospitalist asks the care coordinator to help connect the dots, which leads to a call to a neighbor, an e-mail to her primary care physician (PCP), and a look at her external medication history in the e-prescribing database.

The PCP agrees with discharging her home with no additional intervention. In particular, past attempts at increasing diuretics caused worrisome volume contraction. She had missed several appointments, had made countless calls to the police to say that burglars were at her door, and kept going to the ED. She had undergone noninvasive cardiac testing multiple times and often ran out of medications both because of cost and dementia for which she had also been tested. There were a variety of cardiovascular medications ordered in the past six months by several different physicians. Her son lived nearby but was often away. Attempts to manage this problem with home health agency care were unsuccessful since she was afraid of strangers and refused to let them in.

The primary care physician, who is a geriatrician, had been considering house calls and said this would be the next step, thanking the hospitalist for the courtesy of reaching out. The hospital social worker places a call to Adult Protective Services.

On admission, clinicians should interview caregivers about baseline and recent changes in mental status. While delirium can develop in the hospital, it is often present on admission as well. Delirium is an acute decline in attention and cognitive function that is characterized by waxing and waning mental status that likely started in the last few days or weeks. Delirium should not be confused with dementia, which has an insidious onset and is chronically present for years by the time of diagnosis. Changes in alertness, confusion, agitation, change in daily routines (sleeping more or less than normal, eating poorly) are common signs of delirium. Delirium is much more common in patients with existing dementia, but in the face of a potent stressor it can occur in patients with no prior cognitive deficits. The examiner should inquire about all risk factors for developing delirium, poor baseline cognitive status, frailty, polypharmacy, and number of medical comorbidities, particularly cerebrovascular and cardiovascular diseases, chronic liver or kidney disease, and visual or hearing impairment. See Chapter 79 Delirium and Chapter 166 Agitation in Older Adults.

PHYSICAL FUNCTION

The ability to perform daily activities depends on many body systems including special senses (vision and hearing), and it impacts nutrition and medication compliance. Functional status should be assessed by determining the elder's ability to perform basic and instrumental activities of daily living (ADL). Basic ADLs, essential to independent living, include seven items in a standardized, widely accepted scale: bathing, dressing, eating, toileting, transferring, ambulating, and maintaining continence. ADL difficulties are the most common cause for needing help at home. Bathing is the basic ADL with the highest prevalence of disability. As the patient perceives difficulty with bathing, he or she may change to sponge baths or neglect bathing altogether. Similarly, changes occur in dressing routines, and clothes may become soiled. Deficits in transferring or eating convey a higher degree of dependency. Lack of bathing or signs of incontinence may suggest the need for more detailed questions about physical or cognitive abilities or social supports. In patients with intact cognition, self-report of daily function is reliable; in those with impaired cognition a third party interview should confirm this information. Mobility may be assessed by asking if the patient has difficulty walking outside, from room to room, or climbing a flight of stairs. Presence of new ADL deficits, sometimes acquired during hospitalization, is the strongest predictor of mortality and institutionalization.

Memory loss, medical illness, depression, inability to shop, and financial issues may impact nutritional status. Dysfunction and diseases of the oral cavity may affect overall health, social interactions, and increase risk of malnutrition. Oral hygiene and nutrition may be compromised due to alterations in vision, manual dexterity, upper extremity function, poorly fitting dentures, or alterations in salivary flow. The examiner should specifically inquire whether the patient has regular dental care. Dysphagia, either inability to swallow successfully or a sensation that materials do not pass easily from the mouth to the stomach, odynophagia, and severe vascular disease of the celiac axis that causes intestinal angina all may cause fear of eating and result in malnutrition. Weakness of the soft palate or pharyngeal constrictors can cause dysarthria and nasal regurgitation of food. One other neglected factor related to poor eating is constipation. In addition to observing nutritional status, when there is a potential deficit, the interviewer should inquire about meals, whether the patient prepares them or has assistance, and whether the patient can get food when he or she wants it. An unintentional weight loss of 10 pounds in the preceding 6 months or 5% of body weight in the past month is a red flag. Time should be taken to inquire about these issues rather than simply prescribing medication in response to poor oral intake, such as megestrol acetate (Megace) or metoclopramide (Reglan) which have significant side effects.

The interview should also address the IADLs (instrumental activities of daily living): use of the telephone, shopping and cooking meals, managing finances, doing housework and laundry, and managing transportation. In particular among the IADLs, the examiner should inquire about how the patient obtains, organizes, and takes all medications. Make sure to include over-the-counter medications such as antihistamines (Tylenol PM contains 25 mg of diphenhydramine), which can exacerbate cognitive impairment and may affect appetite, bowel, and bladder function. Anticholinergic medicines, antihistamines, and certain antihypertensives can worsen dental hygiene by decreasing salivary flow. See Chapter 171 Polypharmacy in the Hospitalized Elderly.

Vision and hearing impairment increases the risk of falling and may be associated with depression, social isolation, and further decline. For hospitalized patients, vision and hearing impairment, combined with unfamiliar settings and routines, contribute to sensory deprivation. Sensory deficits interfere with communication and increase the risk for delirium, and hence, morbidity. Visually impaired patients may have no idea who is examining them. The physician should inquire whether the patient is still driving, has difficulty seeing the television, reading, or identifying people in the room. If a patient is visually impaired, there should be a sign in the room to alert people to identify themselves upon entering. Many elderly patients are also unaware of hearing deficits due to the slowly progressive nature of sensorineural loss or deny the problem due to the stigma of wearing a hearing aid. Family members should be asked whether the patient hears them or plays the radio or television too loud. Clinicians too often misinterpret hearing loss for cognitive impairment.

PSYCHOLOGICAL DOMAIN

Depression has an adverse impact on quality of life, risk of physical disability, and recovery from an acute illness, and it is associated with increased medical care costs even after adjusting for the severity of chronic medical diseases. Depression may be confused with dementia and may be chronic. These conditions also may coexist. Suspect depression when the patient is oriented, alert, and relatively coherent but apathetic and failing to progress in his or her recovery. Depression is also typically of recent onset, rather than insidious and chronic like dementia. In older patients, depression tends to have a stronger cognitive and biobehavioral presentation, while less prominent are reports of disturbed mood. The depressed patient may be disengaged and make little effort to perform a task, which is sometimes confused with dementia by the provider. For example, a depressed patient may simply refuse to work with physical therapy. Clinicians should ask the patient whether he or she often feels depressed, sad, downhearted or "blue," treat underlying depression, and try to address anxiety and worries that inevitably develop during hospitalization. Some patients need help with the bereavement process if they have recently lost friends or family. Bear in mind that antidepressant drug therapy, if used, will take two to three weeks to become effective and also be aware of the side effect profiles of some antidepressants, which include nausea and anxiety. In certain selected older patients with impaired cognition, a rapid-acting option is methylphenidate, which should be ordered by clinicians experienced in its use.

SOCIAL HISTORY

In addition to lifestyle habits such as tobacco and alcohol use that are commonly asked, social history in geriatric patients should explore the current living situation and any economic issues that interfere with patient well-being plus support systems for ADLs and IADLs. Specifically, it is important to know if the patients live alone or with others, whether they have to go up and down stairs, what kinds of help are already provided in the home, how reliable the caregivers are, and whether patients have trouble affording or obtaining their medications. The clinician should also note symptoms that may suggest elder mistreatment. See Chapter 167 Elder Mistreatment. The physician can then combine an awareness of functional limitations that is gained during the medical history with knowledge of social supports to enhance the posthospital care plan. The patient's caregiver support rather than the patient's primary diagnosis or functional disability often determines whether the patient can be discharged to his or her home. The admission assessment should identify patient's primary support, health care proxy, and any potential barriers for return to the community.

The examiner should search for and document preexisting conditions at the time of admission that predispose elderly patients to complications during hospitalization such as malnutrition, frailty, and dementia and take steps to avoid further deterioration. The baseline neurologic examination should assess cognitive function (documenting the presence of possible dementia, delirium, or depression), functional status (including evidence of deconditioning), the presence of pressure ulcers, and hearing and vision deficits.

VITAL SIGNS

The first step is to review vital signs not only in the context of the complaint precipitating admission but also to assess prognosis. Ideally, the examiner should personally take the patient's blood pressure in both arms. The pulse pressure (PP) and the systolic blood pressure (SBP) typically increase with age, whereas the diastolic blood pressure (DBP) declines. According to Framingham data, with age there is a gradual shift in predictors of coronary artery disease from the DBP in people less than 50 years of age to DBP, to SBP and PP as approximately equal predictors in people aged 50–59, and then SBP and PP as the strongest predictors in people over age 60. According to the Multiple Risk Factor Intervention Trial, isolated systolic hypertension (SBP > 140 mm Hg and DBP < 90 mm Hg) triples the risk of coronary heart disease and all-cause mortality in men over the age of 50. A higher PP (>60 mg) is an additional independent risk factor for myocardial infarction, carotid artery stenosis, end-stage renal disease, renovascular hypertension, left ventricular hypertrophy, cardiovascular events, and mortality. (Refer to Chapter 89 Hypertension). A wide PP greater than 50% of the SBP is also seen in aortic regurgitation and may be a clue to high flow states such as hyperthyroidism, fever, symptomatic anemia, Paget disease, and severe exfoliative dermatitis.

A narrow pulse pressure PP less than 25% of the systolic blood pressure (SBP) coupled with cool extremities, altered mentation, Cheyne-Stokes respiration, and a resting tachycardia may portend severe ventricular dysfunction and impending cardiogenic shock.

A narrow pulse pressure may also be seen in aortic stenosis, pericardial tamponade, constrictive pericarditis, and tachycardia.

And, while momentary blood pressures recorded in the hospital are important, these values are often affected by acute illness, pain, changes in medications, or medication compliance around the acute episode. Care should be taken to avoid overinterpretation and overtreatment. In particular, if the patient or family have reported dizziness, syncope, or falling, or if antihypertensive medications are increased in the hospital, the blood pressure and pulse should be recorded while the patient is supine and again after standing for one to two minutes to detect orthostatic changes. Postural hypotension is defined as a drop in mean blood pressure (MBP), namely, one-third of the SBP and two-thirds of the DBP, of 20% or more. Alterations of the conduction system by disease or medications such as beta-blockers may prevent a corresponding rise in pulse. In an era of evidence-based guidelines developed in younger and healthier populations, care must be taken when applying algorithms to the care of frail elders.

The examiner should personally observe the patient's breathing and respiratory rate (often recorded incorrectly on the vital sign sheet). If tachypnea is noted at rest, the patient may have functional limitations due to respiratory insufficiency with hypoxia during exercise that may not be apparent at rest or have incipient heart failure or sepsis for which increased work of breathing may be the only clue. An elderly patient with increased intracranial pressure following stroke or a patient with severe heart failure may have Cheyne-Stokes breathing, as may any patient with prior stroke and superimposed metabolic derangement. Kussmaul breathing suggests metabolic acidosis in older patients, just as it does in the young. Biot breathing with irregular periods of apnea often seen in the setting of multiple strokes carries a poor prognosis. During quiet breathing the examiner may check for pulsus paradoxicus, an exaggeration of the normal decrease in SBP with inspiration. Normally during inspiration the SBP may drop 0–10 mm Hg. Many conditions may cause an exaggerated pulsus paradoxicus such as constrictive pericarditis, tamponade, pulmonary embolism, right ventricular failure, and asthma, and its presence is correlated with physiologic severity of illness.

The patient should be weighed on admission and periodically during the hospitalization. A body mass index (BMI) of 18.5 kg/m^3 or less is a practical measure of undernourishment. Another common complication of inpatient care in older patients who enter the hospital seriously ill is excess fluid gain related to acute volume resuscitation; weight may be the best clue as edema may initially settle in areas not easy to see.

OBSERVATION

Nothing tells the story like first-hand observation. If the patient is asleep, observe breathing before waking up the patient. Does the patient open his or her eyes when you enter the room? Does the patient fall asleep during your conversation? Does the patient appear malnourished? Does the patient have tethers that can be removed such as oxygen, Foley catheters, IV lines, or monitoring devices? Is the patient wearing a diaper? Can the patient sit up without assistance during the examination? The examiner should refrain from assisting the patient until the determination is made that the patient cannot do this on his or her own. If the patient can sit up without assistance, can the patient stand or walk without risk of falling? Simply watching the hospitalized patient get out of bed and take a few steps or use the telephone provides valuable insight into the patient's ability to perform ADLs. There are formally validated measures such as timed walk or timed "Get Up and Go" which provide numeric data: 20 seconds on the Up and Go defines high risk of institutional care. See Chapter 168 Functional Decline. A physician who does not attempt to get the patient out of bed or pay attention to his or her ability to participate in self care will often miss the mark when it comes to making proactive plans for continuing care, resulting in last minute scrambling for alternative options and dissatisfaction.

PRESSURE ULCERS AND THE SKIN EXAM

Alongside clinical importance, there are both medical-legal and regulatory reasons for a thorough, documented skin assessment upon admission and at regular intervals during hospitalization, with special attention to high-risk areas. Much of this work can and should be done by nurses, but the physician should lead this initiative, confirm nurses' findings when problems are found, and perform independent assessments based on clinical judgment and patient risk factors. In addition to the sacrum, ischial areas, and trochanters, physicians should pay attention to the heels, an area often overlooked, and be alert to erythema of intact skin in high pressure areas that does not resolve when pressure is removed (thus consistent with a Stage 1 pressure ulcer). Physicians should recognize immobility as a major risk factor for skin damage and when making rounds, ask the nurses about the skin, and examine the skin of immobilized patients. See Chapter 144 Pressure Ulcers. Reducing the incidence of pressure ulcers requires a multidisciplinary team approach, identifying patients at risk and intervening early. Preventive strategies shown to be effective include risk assessment on admission and 48 hours later.

Pressure ulcers observed early in the hospital stay may fall into two major groups: (1) superficial ulcers induced by friction or transient pressure and that usually resolve quickly; and (2) deep ulcers reflecting a sustained, pressure-related ischemic injury to deep layers of the skin and subcutaneous tissues, occurring days earlier, sometimes before hospitalization, but delayed in clinical presentation and appearing days later. These wounds may take months to heal.

COGNITIVE DOMAIN

Although busy inpatient physicians cannot be expected to do an in-depth mental status examination on every patient, the usual "alert and oriented" questions are inadequate to detect clinically significant dementia and delirium. A more complete assessment is needed for every older inpatient. The diagnosis of "dementia" is too often added to the patient's record when the real diagnosis is delirium or depression, and may become virtually indelible in this era of electronic documentation. Memory loss is the cardinal feature of dementia. Dementia should be considered only when there is a history of chronic impairment dating back several months and sufficiently severe to affect social functioning. If the patient cannot pay attention due to delirium, then screening for dementia will not reveal valid results. Several brief screening tools for delirium are available and should be familiar to inpatient care providers. The CAM is the most studied. A positive CAM score requires evidence of an acute onset and fluctuating course plus a deficit in attention (the hallmark features), and at least one of two other features, which are disorganized thinking and change in level of alertness. The CAM-ICU version helps when patients cannot communicate verbally. The Delirium Rating Scale can be used to rate symptom severity.

Validated measures to screen for dementia are available, such as the Mini Mental State Exam (MMSE); these require three to five minutes and some MMSE components may be physically difficult for acutely ill patients to complete. One strategy is to use the most reliable single component within the MMSE as an initial screen. That component is a three-item recall (learning a list of three words and repeating them after a brief distraction), which tests short-term memory, the common ground of all dementias. Three-item recall is a useful clue but is not sufficient by itself. Combining recall with clock drawing is the Mini-Cog and in testing for dementia, the Mini-Cog has comparable sensitivity and specificity to the full MMSE. However, clock drawing may also be difficult in the inpatient setting.

Whatever cognitive evaluation strategy is used by the hospital physician, it should go beyond simply testing orientation to person, place, and time, and mental status testing should be a routine feature of all inpatient geriatric history of physical exams. And, when present, impaired cognition found in the hospital should be placed in context with the history.

DISCHARGE PLANNING

Despite recent advances in electronic records, patient pathways, and technology-assisted decision support, the following factors identified nearly 20 years ago still cause delayed or ineffective discharge from the hospital: inadequate assessment of the patient by health care professionals resulting in poor knowledge of the patient's social circumstances; poor organization, for example late booking of transport preventing timely discharge from the hospital; and poor communication between the hospital and providers of clinical services in the community after discharge, which remains pervasive and a serious quality problem for providers in the inpatient care setting.

When preparing for discharge, incorporating a solid understanding of the geriatric patient's functional status, clinical condition and social support needs, and ensuring adequate provision of continuing care following discharge may reduce return to hospital with preventable problems such as falls. Discharge planning begun at the time of admission can have impressive results. One classic 1995 study found 50% fewer readmissions after applying focused care processes designed for selected older patients with recurrent admissions for heart failure related to uncontrolled hypertension or ischemia. Geriatric cardiologist medication review, intensive patient education, and specific home nursing follow-up were the main interventions.

The literature on discharge planning is extensive and offers both success stories and failures. The most successful studies select and concentrate on patients who are inherently vulnerable to poor transitions from hospital to home, and provide a focused intervention. At Virginia Commonwealth University over the past 10 years, the transitional care program has been associated with more than 60% reduction in hospital costs for the enrolled patients during the 6 months post-discharge as compared to the prior 6 months. The transitional care model employs nurse practitioners making home visits and has helped extremely complex patients remain in the community.

Many discharge planning programs have reported increased quality of life and patient satisfaction. Neither optimal care nor health care utilization benefits occur when team members work in isolation. Multidisciplinary intervention—a combination that includes discharge planning, geriatric assessment with functional and cognitive evaluation, and medication review—is far more likely to be effective. In-person intervention after discharge (rather than telephonic care management) is found in the most successful models, and the experience and expertise of discharge planners also make a difference. Of note, there are varied control group costs in the formal studies of transitional care interventions, and combined with the differences in magnitude of impact, one must conclude that each institution should consider targeted populations, usual care settings, and local resources when designing its strategies.

An important element is direct communication with post-hospital care providers. Expert panel recommendations developed in 2005 by the Society for Hospital Medicine and hosted on the website provide a specific list of items, still too often overlooked to this day.

AREAS FOR FUTURE RESEARCH

Care of the hospitalized elder is challenging, and requires a multidisciplinary approach to prevent and manage complications like delirium and decline in functional status. Geriatric focused history and physical exams are the starting point to identify patients at increased risk. One method to improve documentation of risk factors is use of templates, consultation notes, or inpatient notes adapted to an electronic medical record. Templates provide cues to document physical function, mental status, social supports, and complete skin assessments. The electronic medical record can then trigger use of care sets or treatment protocols that restrict use of medications known to precipitate delirium, encourage early mobilization, and promote pressure relief. There remains a paucity of high quality published research on preventing complications in hospitalized elders, examining mortality, quality of life, caregiver issues, health care utilization and cost. As the aging population is growing exponentially, it is imperative that interventions are developed, tested, and proven to be reproducible in order to systematically improve the care of hospitalized elders nationwide.

Initiatives are now being pursued actively by many providers and organizations to improve inpatient geriatric care and post-hospital care, with a focus on both care processes and transitions. Among these is Project Boost, supported by the Society for Hospital Medicine and tested at several medical centers nationwide.

CONCLUSION

Limited physiologic reserves, high comorbidity, and complex social issues make the needs of elderly inpatients relatively unique among adults. Circumstances vary across settings and studies, including such issues as financial assets, extent of managed care penetration in communities, availability of community assets, and strength of the local primary care workforce. Solid evidence shows that improved care processes and careful assessment can materially reduce the incidence and consequences of delirium, pressure ulcers, institutional care, hospital readmission, and avoidable health care costs. We have described the importance of the geriatric focused history and physical that can provide valuable information to target interventions to improve outcomes. Beyond what is known there is much research work yet to be done in further refining our clinical care of older patients.

SUGGESTED READINGS

Bowles KH, Ratcliffe SJ, Holmes JH, Liberatore M, Nydick R, Naylor MD. Post-acute referral decisions made by multidisciplinary experts compared to hospital clinicians and the patients' 12-week outcomes. *Med Care.* 2008;46(2):158–166.

Boyd CM, Landefeld CS, Counsell SR, et al. Recovery of Activities of Daily Living in older adults after hospitalization for acute medical illness. *J Am Geriatr Soc.* 2008;56:2171–2179.

Covinsky KE, Palmer RM, Fortinsky RH, et al. Loss of independence in activities of daily living in older adults hospitalized with medical illnesses: Increased vulnerability with age. *J Am Geriatr Soc J.* 2003;51:451–458.

Kortebein P, Symons TB, Ferrando A, et al. Functional impact of 10 days of bed rest in healthy older adults. *J Gerontol A Biol Sci Med Sci.* 2008;63(10):1076–1081.

Luetz A, Heymann A, Radtke FM, et al. Different assessment tools for intensive care unit delirium: Which score to use? *Crit Care Med.* 2010;38(2):409–418.

Sochalski J, Jaarsma T, Krumholz HM, et al. What works in chronic care management: the case of heart failure. *Health Affairs.* 2009;28(1):179–189.

CHAPTER 166

Agitation in Older Adults

Caroline N. Harada, MD
Heather L. Herrington, MD

Key Clinical Questions

1. When is agitation due to delirium versus dementia?
2. What are the most common causes of agitation in hospitalized older patients?
3. What are the best non-pharmacologic techniques to manage agitation in older patients?
4. Which medications are best for treating agitation in older patients?
5. What are the potential complications of agitation?
6. How can agitation due to delirium or dementia be prevented?

INTRODUCTION

It is horrible to see an agitated patient in the hospital, even worse to try to care for one, and probably worst of all to be an agitated patient. There is often significant internal and external pressure on hospital staff to "control the patient" and this can lead to thoughtless action. But the best (and often the only) way to address the agitation is to think carefully about the problem before acting. This chapter will attempt to present a thoughtful approach to agitation in hospitalized older adults.

Agitation in an older patient can take multiple forms: aggression, psychomotor agitation, and psychosis. Aggression refers to verbal or physical aggression often involving resistance to care. Psychomotor agitation includes restless motor activity such as pacing, rocking, or other purposeless movement, as well as sleep disturbances, repetitive vocalizations, and restlessness. Psychosis includes delusions, hallucinations, and misidentifications. Patients can experience any combination of these symptoms.

EPIDEMIOLOGY OF AGITATION IN OLDER HOSPITALIZED PATIENTS

Agitation is a common symptom in older hospitalized adults; it may be present on admission or develop during the hospital stay. Reports of the incidence of agitation in this population vary widely, but may be as high as 52% in older ICU patients. The risk of behavioral disturbance is highest for patients who have cognitive impairment on hospital admission.

IMPACT OF AGITATION IN HOSPITALIZED PATIENTS

Agitation causes significant distress for patients, caregivers, and hospital staff. Hallucinations and delusions have been associated with the highest levels of distress for patients, but agitation and aggression were most distressing for hospital staff.

In addition to psychological distress, agitation in hospitalized patients is associated with increased length of hospital stay and increased health care costs. It increases the risk of injury to patients and staff, as well as the risk of complications such as falls, restraint-related injuries, and unintended removal of indwelling catheters and tubes.

DIFFERENTIAL DIAGNOSIS

Agitation can have multiple causes in an older hospitalized patient. The most common causes are delirium, dementia, and psychiatric disorders.

DELIRIUM

Delirium is present in 14–24% of patients admitted to the hospital, and arises in 6–56% of patients during hospitalization. The prevalence of delirium increases with age. Among older adults, it can be the sole presenting symptom for medical illness such as infection or cardiac ischemia. The diagnosis of delirium is made from bedside observation, and although the diagnostic criteria are still evolving, most agree that it consists of an acute change in cognition that results in inattention, altered level of consciousness, and disorganized thinking, usually with a fluctuating course. There is significant heterogeneity in the clinical presentation of delirium: many patients develop the hypoactive form of delirium, which does not involve agitation and is often overlooked. Other patients have agitation, which can include delusions or hallucinations in 30% of delirious patients.

Delirium tends to occur in people with predisposing factors, such as advanced age, dementia, functional impairment, and multiple coexisting medical conditions. It usually is triggered by one or multiple precipitating factors, including medications, medical illness, neurologic disease, surgery, or environmental stressors.

DEMENTIA

Dementia affects approximately 13.9% of the U.S. population over age 70. Prevalence increases with age, and in the population of adults age 90 and older prevalence approaches 40%. It is estimated that by 2050, over 9 million people in the U.S. will have dementia. Sixty percent to ninety-eight percent of patients with dementia may have agitation at some point during the course of their disease. It typically occurs in the moderate and severe stages of the disease, and symptoms are often transient. When these patients are admitted to the hospital with acute medical illness, it is common for these symptoms to persist or worsen.

PRACTICE POINT

- In patients with dementia, it can be difficult to distinguish between delirium superimposed on dementia and agitation due to the dementia itself. Agitation that is a symptom of dementia is commonly called "behavioral and psychiatric symptoms of dementia" (BPSD). How do you distinguish between the two? The key differences are that delirium has an acute onset and usually results in inattention. In BPSD, on the other hand, agitated behaviors are often long-standing and are usually not associated with a change in the level of attentiveness.

Alzheimer disease is the most common type of dementia, followed by cerebrovascular dementia, and then dementia with Lewy bodies (DLB). Other forms of dementia such as frontotemporal dementia, Creutzfeldt-Jakob disease, and Parkinson dementia are significantly less common. Agitation can accompany any type of dementia. Patients with DLB commonly suffer from visual hallucinations, and those with frontotemporal dementia often exhibit impulsiveness, lack of judgment, and personality changes that can result in agitated behaviors.

The diagnosis of dementia is best made when patients are medically stable in the outpatient setting. Unfortunately, dementia is commonly overlooked by primary care providers, who fail to document cognitive problems in up to two-thirds of cases. If dementia is suspected, it is prudent to defer the full diagnostic workup until the patient is truly at his or her medical and cognitive baseline, since even mild delirium will interfere with accurate diagnosis and staging. It is appropriate, however, to perform a thorough neurologic examination and to check for reversible causes of cognitive impairment such as thyroid disease, vitamin B12 deficiency, and normal pressure hydrocephalus. Laboratory tests such as TSH, vitamin B12 levels, and possibly brain imaging can be done while the patient is hospitalized to facilitate the outpatient workup. A complete discussion of the evaluation of a person with cognitive impairment is outside the scope of this chapter.

PSYCHIATRIC DISORDERS

Although psychiatric disorders such as depression with psychotic features, acute mania, and schizophrenia are significantly less common than delirium or dementia, they can cause agitation in older, hospitalized adults. In patients with a history of psychiatric disease, this should be entertained in the differential diagnosis of agitation. In patients without such history, new onset bipolar disorder with mania could be considered, as it does occur in older patients, although it is quite rare. Depression is common in older adults, so depression with psychotic features should also be considered.

PATHOPHYSIOLOGY

The pathophysiology of agitation in hospitalized older adults varies based on the underlying cause of the agitation, and it is poorly understood for most dementias and delirium. In both cases, cholinergic deficiency plays a key role. For this reason, drugs with anticholinergic properties often cause increased confusion and agitation in patients with dementia and delirium. Multiple other neurotransmitters have also been implicated in the pathophysiology of delirium, including dopamine, glutamate, serotonin, and melatonin. Mediators of inflammation such as interleukins, tumor necrosis factor alpha, interferon, cytokines, and cortisol also tend to be elevated in delirium and in many types of dementia, and these may also play a role in agitation.

DIAGNOSIS: WHAT IS THE CAUSE OF THIS PATIENT'S AGITATION?

As discussed above, it is not always easy to distinguish between delirium and dementia. Many agitated patients suffer from both simultaneously. Yet no matter what the diagnosis, the key is the same: to identify and address the underlying trigger for the agitation. Because there is often no test to definitively determine if a particular factor is causing the patient's agitation, the diagnosis is sometimes achieved by correcting as many factors as possible and observing for improvement in symptoms (**Table 166-1**).

TRIAGE/HOSPITAL ADMISSION

Older patients with new onset agitation require hospitalization, usually on a general medicine ward, since medical illness is a common cause of agitation and one that must be identified and addressed in a timely manner. In addition, hospitalization is often required to control the agitated behaviors and keep the patient from harming him- or herself and others.

Admission to a geriatric psychiatry unit is preferable in patients with known dementia and a long history of dementia-related agitation that has recently escalated. Evaluation for new medical illness is still required, but it is less likely to reveal a cause. For patients of this type, a geriatric psychiatry unit is ideal because the staff is experienced in both pharmacologic and nonpharmacologic management of agitation. During the hospitalization, staff and family can determine the best living arrangement for the patient in the future. Many of these patients will require nursing home placement.

Patients who develop symptoms of agitation while hospitalized for another reason can often stay on the ward to which they were originally admitted. If the patient is complex, consultation with geriatrics, geriatric psychiatry, or neurology can also be considered.

Some hospitals have created specialized medical care units for older patients. These units are designed to minimize stressful hospital stimuli and offer structured activities and therapy during the day, open access to family caregivers, and nurses who are specially trained to deal with behavioral disturbances. These units are associated with lower rates of agitation and delirium among patients.

TREATMENT OPTIONS

NONPHARMACOLOGIC MANAGEMENT OF AGITATION

Management of agitation should begin with nonpharmacologic treatments. Recognizing the cause of the patient's agitation and removing it is often the only treatment necessary. Recognize

TABLE 166-1 Causes of Agitation in Older Patients

Acute medical illness	
	Infection
	Acute coronary syndrome
	Hypoxia
	Shock
	Fever or hypothermia
	Dehydration
	Metabolic derangements
	Stroke
	Intracranial bleeding
	Other intracranial lesions (eg, brain tumors, NPH)
	Surgery
Drugs	
	Sedative hypnotics
	Narcotics
	Anticholinergic drugs
	Alcohol or drug withdrawal
	Illicit drugs
Basic needs	
	Hunger or thirst
	Pain
	Boredom or immobilization
	Fatigue or sleep deprivation
	Wet or soiled
	Unable to hear or see
	Constipation or urinary retention
Environmental triggers*	
	Unfamiliar environment
	Intensive care unit
	Physical restraints
	Bladder catheter
	Multiple procedures
	Change in daily routine
	Too cold/hot
Interpersonal issues*	
	Strain in relationship with caregiver
	Grief/bereavement

*Cause agitation primarily in people with dementia—less likely to cause agitation in those who are cognitively intact.

agitation for what it is: a response to an unpleasant condition. A patient who is constantly throwing off his hospital gown and bed sheets may simply be attempting to "cool off" in an overly-warm room. Nursing staff education is essential to the effective treatment of agitation, and there are many Web-based resources for nurse education related to this topic; please refer to the Suggested Reading section for a list. **Table 166-2** summarizes the most helpful nonpharmacologic strategies to manage a patient with agitation.

Family members can be extremely helpful in calming and reorienting an agitated patient, but they often require education about the patient's symptoms and their role in the treatment plan. Using the term "delirium," when applicable, and explaining that in many cases the only predictable feature of delirium is that it is unpredictable, may help family members and others better understand this condition.

Also, untreated pain may cause or exacerbate agitation, and it is essential to evaluate for, recognize, and treat pain. Patients who are agitated and confused may not be able to adequately or appropriately communicate their experience of pain, but various nonverbal assessments of pain can help identify pain in these patients. Standard pain protocols and training to help doctors, nurses, and other staff recognize nonverbal indicators of pain (such as grimacing or moaning) may help reduce agitation. Also, it is important to recognize that the older patient with agitation may not be able to reliably ask for pain medication, so it may be necessary to order scheduled analgesic medications for these patients.

TABLE 166-2 Nonpharmacologic Management of Agitation*

Review medication list carefully and discontinue or taper possible contributors		
	Ask about nonprescription medications (over-the-counter medications, herbal medications, alcohol, and illicit drug use)	
Address basic needs		
	Maintain hydration and nutrition	
	Encourage use of hearing aids, glasses, and dentures to avoid sensory deprivation and improve orientation	
	Avoid unnecessary nighttime interruptions to promote normal sleep-wake cycles (vital sign checks, blood draws, bathing, and turning)	
	Physical therapy or nursing to mobilize patient as soon as it is safely possible	
Keep the environment calm		
	Avoid physical restraints	
		Use sitters, bed alarms, low beds, move the patient to a room closer to the nurses' station for closer monitoring
		Consider removing other irritants/barriers to mobility such as urinary catheters, supplemental oxygen, telemetry monitors, continuous intravenous infusions
	Encourage family members to stay at the bedside as much as possible	
	Educate family members so they can help calm and reorient the patient	
	Encourage family members to place familiar items (photos, blankets, etc) at the bedside	
	Keep clocks and calendars visible to assist with orientation	
	Minimize staff and room changes	
	Minimize excess noise, especially at night	
	Ensure adequate lighting during the day (but avoid overly bright light in patients with cataracts)	
	Ensure relative darkness at night	
	Complementary therapy: music, art, pet, and massage therapy†	
	Create a dayroom for activities (this will help motivate patients to stay awake and mobile during the day)	
	Enlist hospital volunteers to provide companionship, activities, frequent reorientation	
Promote helpful interpersonal interactions		
	Frequent reorientation: "Mrs. Smith, today is Thursday and you are in the hospital with pneumonia."	
	Reassuring statements: "Mrs. Smith, you are in the hospital and we are here to help you."	

*These strategies should be employed for ALL older patients, not just those with agitation, as many have been shown to prevent delirium.

†Complementary therapies can worsen agitation in some patients, so use should be individualized.

Agitation and delirium are often accompanied by use of physical restraints. Though restraints are presumed to prevent falls and other safety problems, there is little evidence to support this notion, and quite a bit to refute it. Restraints, including bed side rails, are barriers to mobility, which lead to deconditioning and a higher risk for falls. They are also associated with entrapment and asphyxiation.

In addition, restraints often worsen agitation. Nurses may also be distressed by the use of restraints, even though (and perhaps because) they requested that restraints be placed. Again, staff education is essential. Recognize the person's strengths. Can you redirect the agitated person who is pulling at the bed sheets by giving her laundry to fold? A patient with dementia who can still play the piano may soothe herself and others by doing just that. Consider asking a family member or sitter to stay with the patient to help redirect the patient toward safer activities. Employ all available resources to avoid the use of physical restraints.

In addition, discontinue urinary catheters, supplemental oxygen, telemetry monitors, continuous intravenous infusions, and other barriers to mobility as soon as these treatments are no longer necessary, as these tethers act both as barriers to mobility and irritants that add to the stress of hospitalization. Using protocols to continually reassess the need for these interventions can help minimize their use.

Finally, review all medications, paying particular attention to medications that are known to be high risk for causing agitation in older adults. Potentially inappropriate medications to avoid in the older adult include antihistamines such as diphenhydramine, anticholinergics such as promethazine, muscle relaxants such as cyclobenzaprine, and benzodiazepines. Review the patient's home medication list, review the actual medications and bottles if they are available, and inquire specifically about the use of anxiolytic medications, over-the-counter medications, and alcohol. Institutional protocols, such as automatic electronic prompts or reminders for potentially inappropriate medication use in older patients, may help avoid these contributors to agitation

PHARMACOLOGIC MANAGEMENT OF AGITATION

Patients who are at acute risk of harming themselves or others may require immediate pharmacologic treatment of agitation. Patients who are not at risk of harming themselves or others, but whose symptoms seem to cause significant distress, may also benefit from pharmacologic treatment. There is no FDA-approved drug for the treatment of agitation in patients with dementia, so all drugs discussed here are used "off-label."

Antipsychotic medications are often considered first-line therapy for psychotic and aggressive forms of agitation. They are less effective for psychomotor forms of agitation. There is, unfortunately, variable evidence to support the efficacy of these medications. Antipsychotic medications may cause adverse side effects including sedation, tardive dyskinesia, and extrapyramidal symptoms. In addition, antipsychotics have been associated with increased mortality in patients with dementia. (See **Table 166-3**, Evidence-based Medicine.) Increased risk of mortality with the use of antipsychotics has not been found for hospitalized older patients with delirium without dementia.

TABLE 166-3 Evidence-based Medicine: Antipsychotics for Patients with Dementia

Study	Methodology	Results	Limitations	Bottom Line
Schneider LS, et al. Risk of death with atypical antipsychotic drug treatment for dementia. *JAMA.* 2005; 294:1934–1943	Meta-analysis of 15 randomized, placebo-controlled trials of atypical antipsychotics in patients with dementia, lasting 10–12 weeks	Death occurred more often among patients on antipsychotics than among patients on placebo. OR 1.54; 95% CI 1.06–2.23	Secondary data analysis. Study not designed to detect differences between drugs, effects of long-term use, or cause of death.	Atypical antipsychotics may be associated with a small increase in risk of death in patients with dementia.
Wang PS, et al. Risk of death in elderly users of conventional vs. atypical antipsychotic medications. *N Engl J Med.* 2005;353:2335–2341	Retrospective cohort study of 22,890 patients over age 65 on antipsychotics for any reason (not just dementia)	Adjusted risk of death 37% higher with conventional compared to atypical antipsychotics. Adjusted HR 1.37 (95% CI 1.27–1.49).	Observational study, so subject to possible confounders. Cause of death not included in study.	Conventional antipsychotics like haloperidol are, like atypical antipsychotics, associated with a small increase in risk of death in older patients.
Schneider LS, et al. Effectiveness of atypical antipsychotic drugs in patients with Alzheimer's disease. *N Engl J Med.* 2006;355:1525–1538	Randomized placebo-controlled trial of olanzapine, quetiapine, or risperidone for psychosis or agitation in 421 outpatients with Alzheimer disease (the CATIE-AD study). Primary outcome: time to drug discontinuation for any reason.	Time to discontinuation due to lack of efficacy for olanzapine and risperidone was longer than placebo, but this was offset by discontinuations due to adverse effects. Sixty-three percent discontinued antipsychotics at 12 weeks.	Because relied on study physicians to titrate or discontinue medications to maximize efficacy and minimize side effects, results reflect physician behavior as well as pharmacologic efficacy.	Atypical antipsychotic medications have modest efficacy and significant side effects when used for treatment of psychosis, aggression, or agitation in patients with Alzheimer disease.
Sultzer DL, et al. Clinical Symptom Responses to Atypical Antipsychotic Medications in Alzheimer's Disease: Phase 1 Outcomes from the CATIE-AD Effectiveness Trial. *Am J Psychiatry. 2008*;165:844–854	Randomized placebo-controlled trial of olanzapine, quetiapine, or risperidone for psychosis or agitation in 421 outpatients with Alzheimer disease (the CATIE-AD study).	Risperidone and olanzapine (but not quetiapine) resulted in modest improvement in Neuropsychiatric Inventory scores, as well as on scales measuring hostile suspiciousness and psychosis but not quality of life or functioning.	Same as above. In addition, because many patients were treated only briefly with study drugs, full drug effects may not have been captured (medial duration of treatment 7.1 weeks).	Olanzapine and risperidone had modest efficacy for agitation, but not quality of life, in patients with Alzheimer disease.

CATIE-AD, Clinical Antipsychotic Trials of Intervention Effectiveness—Alzheimer disease; CI, confidence interval; OR, odds ratio.

PRACTICE POINT

Antipsychotics

- Antipsychotics now come with a "black box" warning from the FDA advising that these drugs should not be used for patients with dementia due to the risk of increased mortality. It is essential to discuss the risks and benefits of treatment with health care surrogates prior to administration of these medications. Surrogates will often agree that the slightly increased risk of death is outweighed by the potential benefit of relief from distressing psychiatric symptoms.

If these medications are prescribed, it is essential to identify the target symptoms and use the lowest possible dose for the shortest possible time. For example, starting doses of haloperidol should be 0.25 mg to 0.5 mg intravenous or by mouth. For quetiapine, 12.5 mg to 25 mg by mouth every twelve hours is appropriate. Monitor the patient carefully for the target symptoms, and as they resolve, taper and discontinue these medications.

Other medications have been implicated in the treatment of agitation. Though the evidence base is scant, studies suggest that cholinesterase inhibitors and memantine may have some efficacy for behavioral disturbances in patients with dementia. There is insufficient evidence to support using these drugs as primary pharmacologic treatments for agitation, but they should certainly be continued in patients who are already taking them at the time they develop agitation.

Antidepressants such as citalopram may be modestly efficacious in the treatment of agitation, and one study found no difference in the efficacy of citalopram and risperidone when treating agitation in patients with dementia. Mood stabilizers and anticonvulsants such as valproate preparations and carbamazepine are also used as second-line therapies, but evidence to support their efficacy is still lacking.

PRACTICE POINT

Avoid benzodiazepines

- Benzodiazepines are rarely indicated for agitation in older patients as they may cause unintended side effects, particularly paradoxical agitation. However, in patients with alcoholism or chronic benzodiazepine use, benzodiazepines are often essential therapy to prevent withdrawal syndromes. Benzodiazepines may also be used in the treatment of dying patients, when delirium is terminal and nonreversible.

COMPLICATIONS

The agitated patient is at high risk for complications; preventing these is of utmost importance. Please refer to **Table 166-4** for a list of possible complications and recommended preventive strategies.

DISCHARGE PLANNING

A substantial number of patients are discharged from the acute care setting with persistent, mild agitation. This may be distressing to family or other caregivers, but agitation and delirium may continue to improve after discharge, especially once the patient is back in a more familiar or calmer environment.

Continued agitation will often determine the setting of the patient's care after discharge. Such patients are sometimes discharged back to their home with the addition of 24-hour supervision. Some patients with agitation may be discharged for skilled rehabilitation. During this rehabilitation period, they will be reevaluated regarding the need for long-term nursing home care versus a more independent setting. Behavioral symptoms are one of the most common reasons for nursing home placement among patients with dementia.

TABLE 166-4 Preventing Complications of Agitation

Complication	Preventive Strategy
Adverse drug reactions	Avoid drugs that can cause confusion or oversedation, especially benzodiazepines[1]
Aspiration	Protect the patient's airway
Deconditioning	Encourage mobilization (even if just "out of bed to chair")
Deep vein thrombosis or pulmonary embolus	Encourage mobilization, avoid restraints
Dehydration or malnutrition	Monitor for signs of each and intervene early, offer water often, ensure patient can access water when thirsty, food when hungry
Injuries	Avoid restraints, avoid falls
	Promote nighttime sleep
	Enlist a sitter or encourage family to stay with patient
Pain	Careful observation for signs of pain, empiric treatment may be necessary
Pressure ulcers	Avoid restraints, encourage early mobilization or frequent repositioning if patient is bedbound

PRACTICE POINT

Antipsychotics Part II

- Due to the risk of increased morbidity and mortality with antipsychotics, if these drugs are initiated to treat agitation in hospitalized older adults they should be discontinued or tapered at discharge if possible. A plan regarding taper of any continued psychoactive medications should be clearly communicated to both the patient's family and the clinician who will be assuming care at the time of discharge.

QUALITY IMPROVEMENT

There are many areas for improvement. Studies have shown that rates of delirium can be lowered by adhering to the nonpharmacologic strategies discussed above. Hospital protocols to prevent delirium should be put into place. These can include automatic electronic reminders regarding the risks of delirium that appear when a physician tries to order a potentially inappropriate medication. Similar reminders can also appear when physical restraints or bladder catheters are ordered. More comprehensive programs such as the "Hospital Elder Life Program," which institutionalizes many of the nonpharmacologic strategies listed in Table 166-2, can prevent or minimize delirium in the hospitalized older adult.

Care transitions are the optimal time to prevent or minimize complications related to agitation. At the time of the patient's admission to the hospital, it is imperative to get a good history from the patient's caregivers. Speak with either the nursing home staff or the patient's family or caregivers regarding both the events that precipitated hospitalization and the patient's baseline behaviors. For example, did the patient previously participate in all social activities and then suddenly become agitated, or does the patient have a history of behavioral disturbances due to dementia and now has suddenly become more agitated? This will help in understanding the agitation syndrome and in planning strategies to address it.

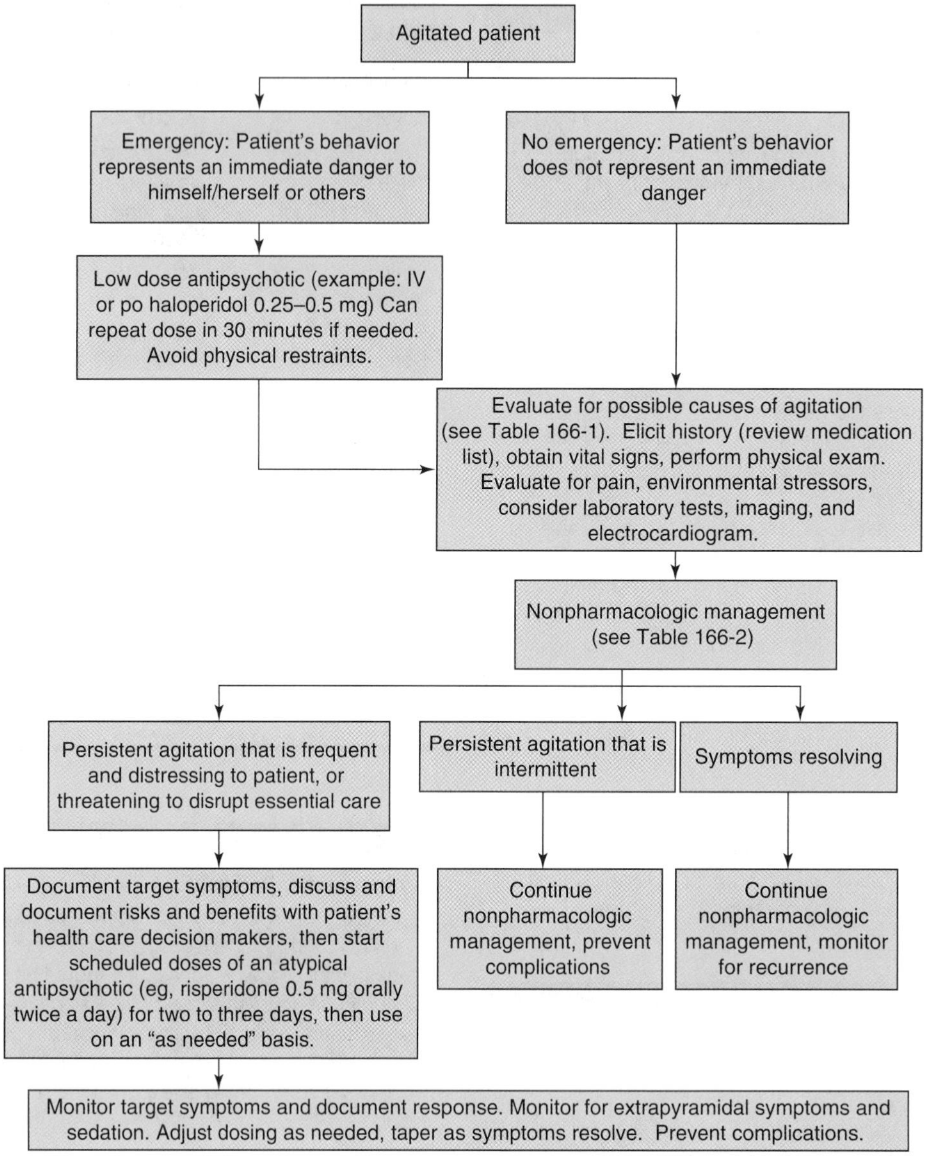

Figure 166-1 *Approach to agitation in older adults.*

Once the patient is medically stable and ready for discharge from the acute hospital setting, it is important, as noted above, to communicate with the receiving team regarding the plan for tapering antipsychotic or other psychoactive medications as an outpatient (**Figure 166-1**).

SUGGESTED READINGS

Ballard CG, Gauthier S, Cummings JL, et al. Management of agitation and aggression associated with Alzheimer disease. *Nat Rev Neurol*. 2009;5(5):245–255.

Blass DM, Rabins PV. In the clinic: Dementia. *Ann Intern Med*. 2008;148(7):ITC4-1-ITC4–16.

Inouye SK. Delirium in older persons. *N Engl J Med*. 2006;354(11): 1157–1165.

Inouye SK, Bogardus ST Jr, Baker DI, Leo-Summers L, Cooney LM Jr. The Hospital Elder Life Program: a model of care to prevent cognitive and functional decline in older hospitalized patients. Hospital Elder Life Program. *J Am Geriatr Soc*. 2000;48(12): 1697–1706.

Salzman C, Jeste DV, Meyer RE, et al. Elderly patients with dementia-related symptoms of severe agitation and aggression: consensus statement on treatment options, clinical trials methodology, and policy. *J Clin Psychiatry*. 2008;69(6):889–898.

REFERENCE

1. Fick DM, Cooper JW, Wade WE, Waller JL, Maclean JR, Beers MH. Updating the Beers criteria for potentially inappropriate medication use in older adults: results of a US consensus panel of experts. *Arch Intern Med*. 2003;163(22):2716–2724.

Helpful websites for nurse education:

http://consultgerirn.org/

http://www.nicheprogram.org/

http://elderlife.med.yale.edu/public/public-main.php

CHAPTER 167

Elder Mistreatment

Karin Ouchida, MD
Mark S. Lachs, MD, MPH

Key Clinical Questions

1. When should you suspect elder mistreatment? What are the signs or red flags?
2. How do you assess for elder mistreatment?
3. What should you document in your assessment?
4. When does a patient require hospital admission?
5. If you suspect elder mistreatment, when must you report it and who should you contact?
6. Which experts are available for consultation?
7. How do you create a safe discharge plan to ensure a smooth transition to the next setting?

INTRODUCTION

Multiple definitions of elder abuse and neglect exist. For practitioners of hospitalist medicine, a useful definition comes from the American Medical Association (AMA), which classifies elder abuse and neglect as "acts of commission or omission that result in harm or threatened harm to the health or welfare of an older adult."[1] This broad description reminds the clinician to look beyond the image of the bruised and battered victim for the often subtle signs of neglect and other types of abuse. Both the World Health Organization and the U.S. National Academy of Sciences definitions add that the "perpetrators" of abuse and neglect are typically persons whom the older adult holds in a position of trust.[2,3] These responsible individuals may either cause the mistreatment or fail to prevent it. The AMA emphasizes, however, that mistreatment may be intentional or unintentional. Unintentional mistreatment is often due to a caregiver's ignorance, inexperience, or inability, often stemming from his or her own medical or mental health problems.

Despite the varying definitions of abuse and neglect, agreement exists for the following six types of mistreatment (listed in order of frequency substantiated by Adult Protective Services in the 1998 National Elder Abuse Incidence Study).[4]

1. **Neglect:** The refusal or failure of a designated caregiver to meet needs necessary for an older adult's physical and mental well-being. Neglect includes, but is not limited to, the failure to provide basic necessities like food, water, clothing, shelter, and medicine. It also encompasses the failure to ensure an older adult's comfort, safety, and personal hygiene.
2. **Self-neglect:** The refusal or failure of an older adult to meet his or her own physical and mental needs resulting in threats to personal health or safety. Self-neglect includes, but is not limited to, an elder's failure to take medications, adhere to medical treatment or maintain adequate nutrition, personal hygiene, and shelter. In its most extreme form, self-neglect is manifest by domestic squalor, social withdrawal, hoarding behaviors, lack of shame, and refusal to accept help. While self-neglect is a fundamentally different phenomenon than elder abuse by another actor, hospitalists may confront it even more frequently than elder abuse when neglected health problems cause or contribute to the reasons for hospital admission. Additionally, the same community resources (ie, adult protective services) are often called upon to address self-neglect.
3. **Psychological abuse:** Verbal or nonverbal acts intended to cause anguish, pain, or distress. Psychological abuse includes, but is not limited to verbal assaults, insults, threats (including threat of abandonment or institutionalization), intimidation, humiliation, and harassment. Additional examples include the infantilization or the social isolation of an older adult.
4. **Financial or material exploitation:** The illegal or improper use of an elder's funds, property, or assets. Financial abuse includes, but is not limited to, cashing an older adult's checks without permission, forging an older adult's signature, stealing money or possessions, coercing or deceiving an older adult into signing documents (eg, contracts, wills, or property deeds), and improper use of conservatorship, guardianship, or power of attorney status.
5. **Physical abuse:** Acts intended to cause impairment, physical pain, or bodily injury. Physical abuse includes, but is not limited to, acts of violence such as striking (with or without an object),

pushing, shoving, shaking, kicking, pinching, and burning. Additional examples include the inappropriate use of drugs or physical restraints, force feeding, and physical punishment of any kind.
6. **Sexual abuse:** Any type of nonconsensual sexual contact including situations in which an older adult is unable to consent. Sexual abuse includes, but is not limited to unwanted, sexually explicit photographing, and all types of sexual assault and battery such as rape, sodomy, and coerced nudity.

Many quoted statistics on elder mistreatment are outdated and reported frequencies depend on the definition employed and the setting(s) examined. The commonly cited 1998 National Elder Abuse Incidence Study (NEAIS) utilized Adult Protective Services records from 15 states and reports from "sentinels" at community agencies who frequently work with elderly clients. The NEAIS found more than 550,000 adults age 60 and older reported experiencing abuse, neglect, or self-neglect in domestic settings. This figure is considered a gross underestimate, as nearly 80% of incidents were not reported to Adult Protective Services, the major agency tasked with receiving and investigating reports of abuse and neglect.

Two recent studies have shed more light on the prevalence of abuse and neglect in community-dwelling older Americans. In 2008, Laumann, et al surveyed 3005 adults ages 57 to 85 years about physical, verbal, and financial abuse experienced in the last year by adding three questions about mistreatment to the National Social Life, Health, and Aging Project.[5] Verbal abuse was most frequently reported (9%), followed by financial (3.5%) and physical abuse (0.2%). Female sex and physical vulnerability appeared to be associated with a higher risk of verbal mistreatment and African-Americans were more likely to report financial abuse. In February 2010, Acierno and colleagues published the results of a national survey of 5770 cognitively intact, community-dwelling adults age 60 and older. They found 11.4% experienced some form of neglect or abuse within the last year. The study specifically assessed reports of "potential neglect" defined as an identified but unmet need for assistance, financial mistreatment perpetrated by family, and physical, sexual, and emotional abuse. The majority of the respondents self-identified as white (88%), 60% were female, and the average age was 71.5 years. The prevalence of mistreatment by type was 5.2% for financial abuse by a family member, 5.1% for potential neglect, 4.6% for emotional abuse, 1.6% for physical abuse, and 0.6% for sexual abuse. Factors associated with increased risk of mistreatment included a history of trauma, low social support, and dependence in activities of daily living.

Elder mistreatment occurs among men and women of all racial, ethnic, and socioeconomic groups. Risk factors associated with the older victim of mistreatment include a shared living situation, social isolation, and conditions that increase his or her dependence on others (eg, cognitive impairment, functional decline, and mental illness). In cases of financial abuse, however, the older adult more often lives alone. Characteristics that appear more frequently amongst perpetrators of elder mistreatment include mental illness, substance abuse, and emotional or financial dependency on the older adult, and a history of violence or antisocial behavior. Other commonly cited perpetrator risk factors include external stressors (medical illness, financial stress), inexperience, and caregiver burnout.

In clinical practice, risk factors that create an imbalance between the older adult's needs and the ability of the caregiver/support system to meet those needs led to increased vulnerability. Three key risk factors leading to this critical imbalance include cognitive impairment, physical frailty, and social isolation.

Clinicians should also be aware that elder mistreatment is an independent risk factor for death. Lachs and colleagues conducted a prospective cohort study of 2800 community-dwelling adults age 65 and older. The mortality rate was three times higher in the elder mistreatment group and 1.7 times greater in the self-neglect group. In the group with any elder mistreatment, the survival rate was 9% versus 40%.

Despite being ideally suited to detect, manage, and prevent elder mistreatment, a 2004 study conducted by the National Center on Elder Abuse found that physicians are one of the least likely groups of individuals to report abuse and neglect. Explanations for physician underreporting include insufficient knowledge of assessment protocols and mandatory reporting guidelines, concerns about a negative effect on relationships with patients and caregivers, reluctance to get involved with the legal system, and time constraints. While the intent of this chapter is to equip hospitalists with the knowledge and skills to assess and intervene on elder mistreatment, time constraints are a valid concern. An assessment for elder abuse and neglect is rarely a quick and simple endeavor. It often requires taking a detailed history from the patient and other caregivers and a thorough physical exam that includes a cognitive evaluation. A comprehensive evaluation may conflict with pressures to manage length of stay by focusing on the diagnosis and treatment of only the acute medical issues. We will discuss how to utilize an interdisciplinary team as well as expert consultants to lessen the burden on any one provider. Hospitalists can also make use of time-based billing in order to maximize reimbursement for managing these complex cases. Elder mistreatment cases often unfold over time, for example, over the course of a single lengthy admission or multiple admissions, and hospitalists commonly "hand off" these complex patients to their colleagues in subacute, home care, or ambulatory settings. Because we understand the limitations of what can be reasonably accomplished in an acute care setting, we have devoted portions of this chapter to "handoffs" and how to ensure safe transitions between care providers.

UNIQUE CHALLENGES AND OPPORTUNITIES FOR HOSPITALISTS

Most importantly, the busy practicing clinician may encounter at least one victim of elder abuse for every 20 to 40 older adults seen. Hospitalists are caring for an increasing proportion of older adults in acute care settings. A 2009 study of Medicare patients by Yong-Fan, et al in the *New England Journal of Medicine* revealed that the odds of a hospitalized older adult being cared for by a hospitalist increased nearly 30% every year from 1997 to 2006.[6] This underscores the imperative for hospital-based clinicians to know which older adults are at greatest risk for elder mistreatment and how to properly assess them.

POTENTIAL FOR POSITIVE INTERVENTION

While we acknowledge the challenges of performing assessments for elder mistreatment in an acute care setting, the critical opportunity inpatient providers to positively impact on the lives elder mistreatment victims and their caregivers must be emphasized. The acute care admission may signal a crisis coming to a head or the first sign that an older adult is being abused or neglected. Both represent chances to intervene to ensure safety and prevent further harm. For example, the elderly woman with dementia admitted with a fall in the setting of hypoglycemia is being cared for by her increasingly frail husband who left her alone while he went to his doctor's office. She didn't feel well and assuming it was her "sugar" took an extra dose of her oral diabetes medications. The husband's decision to leave his wife alone at home is most likely unintentional neglect but the resulting hospitalization provides an opportunity to educate and to intervene. Perhaps the patient's medication regimen can be simplified and short-term home care services ordered for nursing and physical therapy visits. While she is receiving home health care, a social worker can also visit the home to explore entitlements since the husband and wife will require additional help and supervision once the short-term services end.

Hospital-based providers may be the only individuals outside of family allowed access to an abused or neglected older adult and are uniquely qualified to order the proper workup to document the presence or absence of mistreatment, to recommend admission or transfer to another setting, and to order services such as home health care. For known cases of ongoing abuse in the community, hospitalization is often a sentinel juncture that provides new opportunities such as (1) the ability to assess clients free from the influence of abusers or their environments, (2) to counsel victims in a different setting about the range of possible options, and (3) an opportunity to bring new resources to bear on the problem that would prove difficult in other settings (including psychiatric consultation, physical therapy, and social services).

POTENTIAL FOR HARM WITH INACTION

Conversely, when the hospital-based clinician fails to recognize the signs of abuse or neglect and misses an opportunity for intervention, significant harm can come to the patient and his/her caregivers. For example, the frail bed-bound elderly female with multiple sclerosis admitted with several worsening pressure ulcers may confide in the physician that she fears her son because he frequently yells and shakes his fist at her. Recently he broke the hospital bed and air mattress she had at home and would not allow her aides to turn and reposition her. If the patient's report was dismissed and she was not asked, in private, whether she wanted to return home or go to a subacute facility for wound care, she could suffer increasing morbidity or mortality if violence at home escalates. Furthermore, if the inpatient provider "fumbles the handoff" and fails to properly document the assessment and planned intervention, the patient and the health care system could pay the consequences. If the example patient was discharged to a subacute facility that was unaware of the patient's fears of her son, the receiving clinicians might inadvertently discharge the patient home several weeks later. Or, should the patient be readmitted to the acute care setting under a different hospitalist, that physician might also unknowingly involve the patient's son in discharge planning.

CASE 167-1

THE "SOCIAL ADMIT"

An 86-year-old woman with a history of diabetes mellitus, hypertension, atrial fibrillation, and venous insufficiency presents to the emergency department after a fall at home. The patient was admitted two weeks ago after a similar fall at home and was discharged with home care services. The patient reports she was walking to the bathroom and tripped over a throw rug falling forward onto her hands and knees. She did not lose consciousness or bump her head. The patient lives with her adult son who helps with chores, shopping, and medication, including insulin administration.

Triage vital signs:
Temperature 98.0°F BP 180/90 mm Hg HR 110 irregularly irregular O_2 sat 99% Finger stick blood sugar: 300

Laboratory data:

Na^+ 148 mmol/L, K^+ 5.0 mmol/L, Cl^- 100 mmol/L, HCO_3^- 30 mmol/L, BUN 40 mg/dL, Cr 1.3 mg/mL, glucose 280 mg/dL
CBC: WBC 6.0 × 10^9/L, Hgb 14.0 g/dL platelets 320,000/μL
PT/INR: 1.0
LFTs normal except for albumin 2.8
UA: positive for glucose, negative for nitrites, leukocyte esterase; 0–3 WBC, Specific gravity 1.030
Head CT report: negative for acute stroke or bleed.
Plain films of her pelvis, hips, and knees report: no fractures.

The social worker is concerned about the patient's safety at home and is unable to reach the patient's son who is at work. The patient reports the home care services ended and she no longer has a home health aide. The patient is admitted to the hospitalist service as a "social admission."

A closer look at the "Social Admit"

In this case, multiple red flags suggest that she is the victim of elder neglect. Concerning details from her history include the recent admission, her repeated falls, the discontinuation of home care services, and the inability to reach her primary caregiver. She has signs of poorly controlled chronic illness such as an elevated blood pressure and blood glucose level, tachycardia, and glucosuria. The subtherapeutic PT/INR level suggests an inadequate amount of warfarin or missed doses. Finally, the low albumin level and elevations in her serum BUN and creatinine and urine specific gravity imply possible malnutrition and dehydration. Any one of these "medical diagnoses" like rapid atrial fibrillation, poorly controlled diabetes, and volume depletion could be used to "medically justify" an acute care admission and further evaluation for neglect.

Recommendations

In this case, much could be gained by speaking separately with the patient and with her son. The hospitalist's role consists of evaluating her understanding of her medical problems, explaining her current health status, and assessing her functional status.

- Does she understand that she has atrial fibrillation and diabetes?
- Does she have a neuropathy that is contributing to her falls?
- What is her current health status? A hemoglobin A1C would give a sense of her glucose control over the past eight weeks.
- Does she have regular follow-up with an outpatient physician?
- Does she have sufficient medications at home and is she getting them every day as directed?
- Does she need assistance with toileting and transfers. Who is present to help her with these activities of daily living while her son is at work?
- Why were her home care services discontinued?

Similar questions could be directed toward her son. As caregiver neglect may be due to ignorance, inexperience or inability, perhaps the son does not understand the importance of adhering to a diabetic diet or is unaware of what foods she should or should not eat. He may not be comfortable administering her insulin or believes she does not require it every day. He may not understand the impact of her poorly controlled illnesses on her functional status.

CASE 167-2

THE "FREQUENT FLIER"

An 86-year-old woman with a history of coronary artery disease, chronic systolic congestive heart failure with an ejection fraction of 35%, hypothyroidism, and atrial fibrillation presents to the emergency room with progressive dyspnea on exertion and chest pain. She always comes in with the same diagnosis, responds quickly to diuretics, she is "in and out in 3 days."

Triage vital signs:
Temperature 96.7°F, BP 110/60 mm Hg, heart rate 130 irregularly irregular, room air O_2 saturation 90%.

Her examination is notable for signs of congestive heart failure; she has decreased breath sounds at the lung bases, rales in the mid and upper lung fields, and 3+ lower extremity edema.

Laboratory data:
Na^+ 142 mmol/L, K^+ 4.6 mmol/L, Cl^- 100 mmol/L, HCO_3^- 30 mmol/L, BUN 40 mg/dL, Cr 1.5 mg/mL, glucose 140 mg/dL
CBC: WBC 6.0 x 10^9/L Hgb 12.0 g/dL platelets 320,000 μL
BNP: 10,000
PT/INR: 1.2
Digoxin level 0.0
Chemistry profile normal except for albumin 2.4
UA: negative

She is admitted to the hospitalist service for acute systolic congestive heart failure and rapid atrial fibrillation.

A closer look at Case 167-2

Several red flags indicate possible elder neglect, including frequent admissions for decompensated congestive heart failure and a quick positive response to medications provided in the hospital. On exam, she has the expected signs of heart failure but her laboratory values suggest an inadequate amount of both warfarin and digoxin. While the indication for acute hospital admission is not disputed in this situation, the hospitalist should take the extra time to investigate the reasons behind the failed hospital-to-home transition.

Recommendations

The evaluation and documentation of decision-making capacity in a potential elder mistreatment victim are critical. The description "alert and oriented times three" is insufficient documentation of a patient's decision-making capacity. To demonstrate capacity, the individual must be able to understand the relevant information or choices being presented, articulate a choice, and provide a reasonable explanation for that choice. Cognitive impairment does not automatically indicate a lack of capacity. The assessment of capacity must be decision-specific (eg, does this patient have capacity to participate in discharge planning?).

These two cases may on the surface appear as routine admissions that hospitalists see every week on their services. However, subtle red flags in each case should raise the possibility of elder mistreatment. This chapter will help hospitalists recognize the signs of elder abuse and neglect and provide them with the skills to perform an assessment and devise appropriate multidisciplinary interventions. These examples underscore the need for hospital-based providers to be aware of the signs and symptoms of elder mistreatment and the appropriate forms of intervention. We now detail the components of assessment, intervention, and follow-up.

HOW TO CONDUCT AN ASSESSMENT FOR ELDER MISTREATMENT

WHEN TO ASSESS

Hospitalists should adopt the practice of "universal precautions" for elder mistreatment. This entails maintaining a high index of suspicion, especially when a patient's caregiver and support system is clearly inadequate to meet his or her needs. The risk factors for elder abuse and neglect that most often lead to an imbalance between needs and supports are cognitive impairment, physical frailty, and social isolation. If one type of abuse or neglect is suspected, the hospitalist should screen for all other forms. The American Medical Association considers certain signs "red flags" indicating potential elder neglect or abuse (**Table 167-1**).

Often medical providers must act like detectives, putting together the smallest of details to form a larger picture. The presence of any one or a combination of these indicators should trigger an assessment for elder mistreatment (**Figure 167-1**).

TABLE 167-1 Red Flags or Indicators of Possible Elder Neglect and Abuse

Neglect and self-neglect
• Inappropriate dress for season
• Poor hygiene
• Dehydration
• Malnutrition
• Hypothermia or hyperthermia
• Pressure ulcers
• Lack of assistive devices
• Nonadherence with medications
• Nonadherence with recommendations for services (eg, refusal of home care services)
• Abandonment
Emotional or psychological abuse
• Depression
• Anxiety
• Agitation
• Passivity
• Evasiveness
• Fear
• Confusion
Financial or material exploitation
• Nonadherence with medications
• Nonadherence with recommendations for services (eg, refusal of home care services)
• Frequent emergency department visits
• Frequent hospital admissions
• Unpaid bills or rent; impending eviction
• Abrupt changes in an older adult's will or financial documents
• Unexplained or frequent withdrawals from bank accounts
• Disappearance of funds or possessions
• Unauthorized credit card charges
Physical abuse
• History inconsistent with injuries
• Delay in presentation
• Repeated emergency department or office visits
• Frequent hospital admissions
• Suspicious pattern or bruising or burns (eg, circumferential abrasions consistent with wrist restraints)
• Changes in demeanor or activity level
• Caregiver refusal to leave older adult alone
• Drug levels consistent with overdosing or underdosing of medications (eg, warfarin, antiepileptic drugs)
Sexual abuse
• Difficulty walking or sitting
• Vaginal or urinary symptoms
• Bruising around the breasts, genital area, and/or inner thighs
• Torn or stained undergarments
• Unexplained sexually-transmitted diseases
• Behavioral changes including withdrawal, depression, insomnia, aggressive behavior, sexual behavior

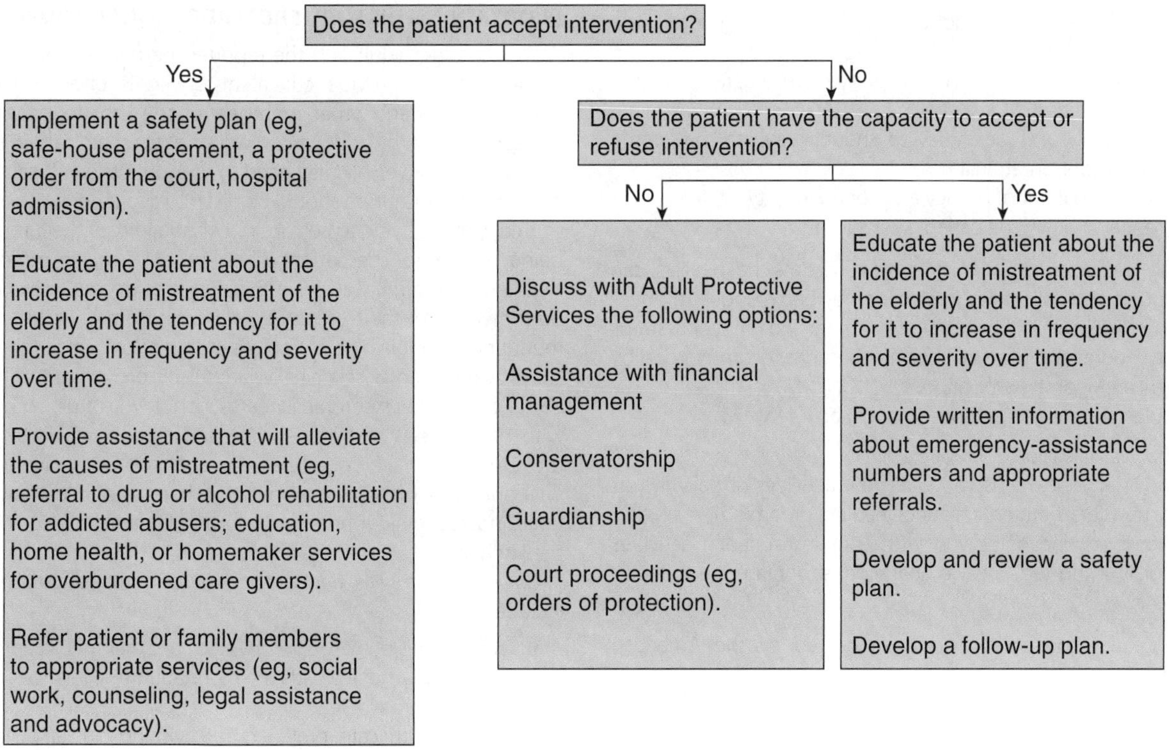

Figure 167-1 *Approach to patient. (Reproduced, with permission, from Abuse and neglect of elderly persons. Lachs MS, Pillemer K. N Engl J Med. 1995(332):437–443. Copyright Massachusetts Medical Society. All rights reserved.)*

WHAT TO ASSESS

The presence of any one of the red flags in Table 167-1 in a patient with an insufficient support system should prompt a full assessment for elder mistreatment. A comprehensive assessment similar to any admission or consultation includes a thorough history and physical exam.

In obtaining the history, the hospitalist should address and document the following:

- History from the older adult
- History from the suspected abuser/neglector
- History from any collateral sources (eg, caregivers, outpatient physicians, home care personnel)
- Assessment of functional status
- Assessment of social and financial resources

In performing a full physical exam the hospitalist should note and document the following:

- General appearance (hygiene, cleanliness, and appropriateness of attire)
- Vital signs (orthostatic blood pressure and pulse measurements) and weight
- Head and neck exam (fit of dentures, dental hygiene, venereal lesions, deviated septum)
- Full skin exam (ecchymoses, burns, lacerations, abrasions, pressure ulcers)
- Musculoskeletal exam (fractures or signs of previous fractures)
- Genitorectal exam (bruising, venereal lesions, inguinal rash, fecal impaction) including rape kit if indicated
- Mood and affect
- Assessment of cognitive function and decision-making capacity
- Gait

HOW TO ASSESS

When assessing for elder mistreatment, it is imperative to interview the older adult and suspected perpetrator separately. The older adult's willingness to accept help will ultimately determine the intervention strategies employed (Figure 167-1). The hospitalist can matter-of-factly inform the caregiver or family member that the hospital's policy requires the physician interview each patient privately and provide assurance that time will be allotted for the caregiver's questions/concerns to be addressed as well. For time efficiency, another member of the interdisciplinary team (eg, the social worker, a resident, or fellow) can elicit the history from the caregiver or family member while the hospitalist completes the patient interview and physical exam. If the caregiver or suspected abuser/neglector refuses to allow the older adult to be interviewed alone, it should raise the examiner's suspicions and should be documented in the medical record. Special attention should be paid to how the older adult acts in the caregiver's presence. Note any comments or glances the person gives to the older adult conveying a message to "keep your mouth shut or else." Subtle changes in the older adult's demeanor when being interviewed alone can also signal abuse or neglect. The older adult may appear withdrawn or depressed, speak in low tones or make poor eye contact.

Older adults with cognitive impairment and/or sensory impairments can pose an additional challenge during the assessment. Providers, in a rush to obtain the history may ignore the older adult completely and allow the caregiver to provide all of the details. Remember, however, that the elderly who suffer from cognitive deficits may be more vulnerable to mistreatment. Do not assume that these individuals cannot adequately describe the mistreatment. When interviewing older adults with cognitive impairment, helpful tips for the hospitalist include the following:

- Allot extra time for the interview or break the interview up over several encounters.
- Ensure that the patient has his/her assistive devices (eg, eyeglasses, hearing aid, dentures).

- Minimize background noise when possible (eg, draw the curtain, close the door).
- Position yourself so that you are at eye level (eg, raise head of the patient's bed, sit in a chair).
- Speak slowly and clearly; avoid shouting, which may come across as confrontational.
- Assure the patient of privacy and confidentiality.
- Repeat and clarify the patient's responses.

For all suspected elder mistreatment victims, hospitalists can build rapport and collect key information by beginning with open-ended questions about the living environment and functional status and then progressing to more specific questions recommended by the American Medical Association.

Examples of general questions to begin an interview:

- Who lives with you?
- Who, if anyone, helps you with your activities of daily living? (eg, transfers, bathing, toileting, feeding, grooming)
- Who, if anyone helps you with your instrumental activities of daily living (eg, meal preparation, shopping, medications, bills)?

Examples of specific questions suggested by the American Medical Association:

- Do you feel safe in your home?
- Does anyone ever threaten you or verbally assault you?
- Has anyone ever touched you without your consent?
- Has anyone ever asked you to sign documents you don't understand?
- Has anyone ever taken your things without your permission?
- Are you afraid of anyone in your home?
- Are you alone a lot?
- Has anyone ever failed to help you when you were unable to help yourself?

When interviewing caregivers or suspected perpetrators, the health care provider should remain nonjudgmental and avoid confrontation. One should also try to provide empathy for the burden of caregiving. Pay attention to inconsistencies in the explanations provided or frequently changing stories.

Helpful questions for caregivers or suspected perpetrators include the following:

- How long have you been caring for (the patient)?
- What are your primary caregiving responsibilities?
- Do you feel you have adequate support? Why or why not?
- How are you coping with your responsibilities?
- What is your understanding of the patient's medical conditions and needs?
- Can you tell me in your words what happened? (if physical signs of injury or history of injury)

If elder mistreatment is disclosed, be prepared to validate the patient's experience and listen supportively as you might be the first person the victim has confided in. It may take several conversations with a provider or providers before the victim reveals information about elder mistreatment.

Some victims choose not to disclose or refuse assistance. There are many reasons why a victim might refuse help, including a fear of escalating abuse or neglect if the nature of the relationship is altered or exposed. An abuser may not demonstrate aggression in front of the medical providers, often because he or she does not want any outsider to detect a problem. A caregiver who is neglecting an older adult may attribute signs of neglect like malnutrition, dehydration, uncontrolled chronic diseases, or mood disorders to the patient (eg, "She refuses to eat or take her medications") or to the aging process (eg, "Wouldn't anyone be depressed in this situation?").

OBTAINING HISTORY FROM ADDITIONAL SOURCES

While the older adult and the reported perpetrator of the abuse or neglect can provide critical history, it is often insufficient. The hospitalist and other members of the inpatient team may be approached by individuals wanting to share "their side of the story" or conversely may need to seek out other critical sources of information. Caution should be taken to avoid believing any one source without trying to corroborate the validity of the information being presented. The patient who reports her niece came in the middle of the night and stole thousands of dollars from her may be the victim of theft or may be suffering from cognitive impairment and paranoia. The patient's outpatient or community medical providers can be especially helpful by providing information about the patient's chronic illnesses, cognitive status, compliance with medications and office visits, and caregivers. Home health providers who have visited patients at home can provide critical environmental history for example, is there evidence of clutter or hoarding, is the neighborhood safe, and is there sufficient food in the kitchen?

Collateral history is frequently required and potential sources include

- The patient's primary care physician or other medical providers
- Individuals who live with the older adult (eg, relatives, friends, personal care workers)
- Home health care providers (eg, visiting nurse, physical or occupational therapist, social worker, home health aide)
- Neighbors, friends, additional family members
- Apartment superintendent or landlord
- Bank or financial institution officials

The responsibility to gather collateral information should be shared amongst members of the inpatient team. The hospitalist must interview and examine the patient but can and should engage physician assistants, medical trainees (residents and medical students), social work, physical and occupational therapy, nutrition, and others to help assess the patient's functional and psychosocial status and to elucidate any reports of abuse or neglect.

INDICATIONS FOR HOSPITAL ADMISSION

Most indications for admission of a suspected victim of elder mistreatment are the same as for all geriatric patients and include

- Hemodynamic instability
- New diagnoses requiring acute hospital care such as acute myocardial infarction or cerebrovascular accident
- Exacerbations of chronic illnesses requiring acute hospital care such as uncontrolled diabetes with hyperosmolarity or worsening of chronic obstructive pulmonary disease
- Change in mental status
- Trauma with major fracture, inability to ambulate, or uncontrolled pain

APPROACH TO THE "SOCIAL ADMIT"

Less clear are those situations in which the hospitalist is called by the emergency department to admit a patient who is unsafe to return to the previous care setting. If coming from home, these patients may have been referred by a home care agency, a concerned neighbor, or a family member. Patients may also be transferred out of institutional settings such as rehabilitation facilities or nursing homes by caregivers dissatisfied with the care being provided. While there is a tendency for hospital-based physicians to dread these "social admits," any reports of abuse or neglect must be carefully and systematically addressed.

It may be easier to conceptualize a set of conditions or parameters for safe discharge from the emergency department rather than to list criteria for hospital admission. Patients sent from post-acute settings such as rehabilitation facilities or nursing homes with any allegation of abuse or neglect will require admission and workup before transfer back to a post-acute setting. Patients coming to the emergency department from home settings (private homes, assisted livings, etc) can be safely transitioned back if their functional status is accurately assessed and measures to ensure their safety can be put into place.

Consider an elderly man with a history of dementia brought in by his daughter for a fall at home and worsening confusion. The patient has a mild forehead laceration and abrasions on his knees but a negative CT scan of the brain. The emergency department staff describes him as "belligerent and agitated." He is given a benzodiazepine in the emergency department, he has a bladder catheter placed to obtain a urinalysis, and he is placed in wrist restraints. The daughter appears overwhelmed by his care and the emergency department feels he is "unsafe to return home."

The hospitalist must consider neglect in the differential and be prepared to investigate whether the patient was inappropriately left alone for an extended period of time, whether there is evidence of uncontrolled chronic illness, malnourishment or dehydration, and whether the patient reports any abuse or neglect. However, the hospitalist may also recognize delirium and simultaneously explore etiologies and remove exacerbating factors such as the urinary catheter and restraints. Perhaps the patient has a urinary tract infection and dehydration with a sodium level of 148. Once the benzodiazepine wears off and with some intravenous free water, it's possible that his mental status will improve and he will be able to demonstrate an ability to eat and drink on his own. The hospitalist must confirm that the patient has appropriate access to food and medications, follow-up medical care, and supervision. He could qualify for short-term home health care with a visiting nurse and physical therapist plus a few hours of a home health aide. Depending on the amount of supervision needed and how involved his daughter and other caregivers are, he could be discharged home. A safe transition home will require interdisciplinary coordination with social work, the home health agency, and the patient's outpatient provider.

DIFFERENTIAL DIAGNOSIS

DIFFERENTIATING SIGNS OF ABUSE AND NEGLECT FROM "NORMAL" AGING

Some signs of abuse and neglect can be indistinguishable from "normal" changes associated with aging. Other signs of mistreatment may mimic the symptoms or consequences of medical conditions common to the older adult population. For example, bruising or skin tears may be due to thinning skin or use of blood-thinning medications. Multiple fractures may be a consequence of falls, osteoporosis, or underlying malignancy. Pressure ulcers may occur in the absence of neglect in a patient with end-stage dementia, malnutrition, and immobility. Changes in mood and behavior can reflect depression or anxiety independent of elder mistreatment.

A 2005 study by Mosqueda, et al in the *Journal of the American Geriatrics Society* examined the life cycle of bruises in older adults and found that 90% of accidental bruises occurred on the extremities and no accidental bruises occurred on the neck, ears, genital area, or soles of the feet.[7] However, location of bruising alone is insufficient to prove abuse has occurred. Unlike child abuse, there are no pathognomonic signs of elder mistreatment. Therefore, obtaining a comprehensive history from the older adult, involved caregivers, and other collateral sources remains paramount. When documenting signs of skin breakdown or injury on physical exam, it is critical to describe the location, color, shape, and size of what is visualized as opposed to an overall impression or judgment. For example, bruises can be marked on a standard body diagram with notations for the color, shape, and exact size instead of being interpreted and documented in the medical record as "old," "fading," or "resolving." Mosqueda's study looking at the life-cycle of bruises in the elderly found that the color of the bruise did not predict its age (ie, some bruises were predominantly yellow during the first 24 hours after onset).

TREATMENT AND INTERVENTION STRATEGIES

CLEAR DOCUMENTATION

When conducting an elder mistreatment assessment, the hospital-based provider should adopt a "forensic approach" to documentation. This entails being mindful of the potential legal implications of one's findings.

The following should be clearly detailed in the medical record:

- Names of individuals present during the interview and exam and relationship to the patient
- The patient's demeanor and any observed reactions to caregivers
- Verbatim descriptions of events from the patient and caregivers
- Timeline of events
- Functional status
- Hygiene and dress
- Physical exam
- Cognitive evaluation
- Referrals made (eg, social work, home care, adult protective services)
- Education provided to the patient and/or caregivers
- Safety plan discussed

PHOTOGRAPHS AND PHYSICAL EVIDENCE

If possible, use photographs (with victim's consent) or body diagrams to document injuries. Photographs should be taken before any medical treatment is given (without jeopardizing health of patient). Photographs should be labeled with the victim's name, the location of the injury, the date and time, and the name of the photographer. Take photographs from several angles and use a coin or ruler to provide a sense of scale. Preserve all physical evidence (eg, torn or stained clothing, broken eyeglasses, or damaged assistive devices) as this might be used in court.

ENLIST THE HELP OF AN INTERDISCIPLINARY TEAM

Cases of suspected elder mistreatment can be both complex and time-consuming. Hospitalists should involve their interdisciplinary colleagues as soon as possible to benefit from their expertise in safety planning and development of interventions and to share responsibility for various components of the assessment.

SOCIAL WORK

In the acute care setting, hospitalists will most often collaborate with social workers to assess and treat victims of abuse and neglect. Inpatient social workers can be instrumental by obtaining collateral information from the patient's caregivers and/or family members, clarifying the patient's current level of social support, and investigating financial resources. Without sound knowledge of the patient's insurance coverage and potential entitlements, a safe discharge plan cannot be developed. For example, the hospitalist may want to discharge a patient with 24-hour supervision at home to ensure his safety but most insurances, including Medicare and state Medicaid plans, will not cover this level of personal care and the patient may not have the financial resources to pay for a private home attendant. Hospitalists should also be aware the home health care agencies often employ social workers who can relay critical information about the suspected victim's psychosocial functioning, resources, and entitlements prior to hospitalization.

PHYSICAL AND OCCUPATIONAL THERAPY

Physical and occupational therapists can assist the hospitalist in assessing the suspected victim's functional status. Knowing the patient's current level of function and the extent of decline is essential for setting goals for medical therapy and determining the appropriate discharge destination. It can also be helpful when trying to substantiate history provided by a caregiver or the patient. For example, if the caregiver reports the patient sustained a head laceration and periorbital bruising by falling out of bed, the physical therapist's assessment of the patient's ability to transfer in and out of bed and to ambulate will be critical. Similarly, if a patient is admitted with profound dehydration and reports she is able to perform her own shopping and feed herself, the occupational therapist's evaluation of the patient's ability to perform activities of daily living will become significant.

CONSULT EXPERTS

The hospitalist who suspects elder mistreatment may also benefit from specialty consultations from geriatrics, psychiatry, geriatric psychiatry if available, and ethics. While a geriatrician may have experience in performing a complete assessment for elder abuse and/or neglect, the hospitalist should be prepared with a specific question or questions when calling the consultant. Geriatricians can assess functional status and assist with clarifying goals of care. Psychiatrists and geriatric psychiatrists can be especially particularly helpful in assessing a patient's decision-making capacity or determining whether cognitive impairment or a mood disorder is impacting the patient's care. Elder mistreatment cases often involve ethical dilemmas, so if the hospital utilizes an ethicist or ethics committee, a formal consultation can prove invaluable. For example, when treating the self-neglecting patient who puts himself at risk by refusing home services or not using assistive devices, the hospitalist must weigh the patient's autonomy against the duty to avoid harm (nonmaleficence). In extreme cases of self-neglect that are associated with hoarding, patients may put other roommates, neighbors, or even pets at risk as well. In these situations, physicians must also consider the impact of the patient's choices and behaviors on the safety of the surrounding community.

INVOLVE RISK MANAGEMENT AND LEGAL DEPARTMENTS

Risk management and the hospital's legal department represent other interdisciplinary team members to whom the hospitalist can access for assistance. The primary role of risk management is to minimize potential liability through continuous monitoring and evaluation of the processes and outcomes of patient care. Risk management teams are often composed of a combination of clinicians (nurses, physicians) and quality management experts. Elder mistreatment cases may reveal gaps in quality of care and/or inefficient processes. The hospitalist should involve risk management in cases in which the discharge plan may be disputed by the patient or caregivers, when the discharge plan is complicated by a patient who lacks decision-making capacity and no surrogate or proxy exists, and when the hospitalist suspects an ongoing or imminent threat to patient safety. Risk management will often guide the hospitalist as to whether the legal department's assistance is required. The legal department is frequently consulted in cases in which the patient lacks decision-making capacity due to cognitive impairment or psychiatric illness and a court-appointed guardian is needed to establish a safe discharge plan.

As with all members of the interdisciplinary team, hospitalists should contact risk management and legal as early as possible.

ACCESS COMMUNITY RESOURCES

In addition to the interdisciplinary and expert services available to the hospitalist in the acute care setting, extensive community resources should be utilized to create safe discharge plans for elder mistreatment victims. These organizations can also be valuable sources of collateral information if already involved with the victim prior to hospitalization.

HOME HEALTH CARE

The term home health care may refer to an extensive range of services provided in patients' homes from certified home health agencies providing short-term skilled care from nurses and physical therapists to privately hired personal care workers providing assistance with activities of daily living. Multiple types of home care services are often utilized as a critical intervention in elder mistreatment situations because it increases the number of "eyes and ears" on the patient and his/her caregivers. Especially in cases in which mistreatment is suspected but not confirmed, added supervision and monitoring can help clarify what is actually occurring in the patient's home. Here we will focus primarily on Medicare-certified home health care programs. Following a hospitalization for acute illness, elder mistreatment victims often meet the criteria for skilled services, that is, they need a visiting nurse or physical therapist. The hospitalist must also certify that the patient is homebound (ie, leaving home requires a considerable and taxing effort), requires short-term intermittent care, and has an outpatient physician to supervise home care services in order for the patient to quality for home health care post-discharge.

While the home health nurse's primary role may be to monitor a wound and instruct a caregiver to perform dressing changes, he or she can also report back to the outpatient physician on the caregiver's ability and willingness to provide appropriate care, the sanitary conditions in the home, and the patient's overall medical status. The physical therapist's orders may be to perform gait training and muscle strengthening exercises, but he or she can also alert the outpatient physician to red flags for mistreatment such as the patient/caregiver refusing visits, the patient's prescriptions going unfilled, and signs of uncontrolled medical illness.

While home health agencies can and do play a vital role in increasing the short-term supervision and monitoring of elder mistreatment victims, the hospitalist should know that agencies must also maintain the safety of their employees and will not accept patients whose home environments are compromised by extreme disrepair, bug or vermin infestation, or the presence of occupants who are suspected of engaging in criminal activity.

ADULT PROTECTIVE SERVICES

In most states, Adult Protective Services (APS) represents the first responders to reports of abuse, neglect, and exploitation of vulnerable adults. Established in 1975 under Title XX of the Social Security Act, APS exists in all 50 states. Because little or no federal funding was allotted, each state has developed its own program based on the state's individual laws and regulations. States may differ in their definitions of mistreatment, types of abuse and neglect addressed by state law, eligibility criteria, and settings covered. For example, California APS agencies investigate reports of abuse in private homes as well as in hospitals, whereas in New York, APS serves physically and/or mentally impaired adults at risk for harm in the community.

Similarities exist across state APS agencies in terms of the services provided, for example, receipt and investigation into reports of mistreatment, evaluation of client risk and capacity to consent to services, development and implementation of a case plan, client counseling, assistance with services and benefits, and monitoring of ongoing service delivery. According to the National Adult Protective Services Association, APS encompasses "those services provided to older people and people with disabilities in danger of being mistreated or neglected, are unable to protect themselves, and have no one to assist them." Most states implemented a social casework model of service delivery designed to enable vulnerable elderly to continue living independently in the community.

Despite state differences, certain basic principles shape APS practice. These include the client's right to self-determination, the use of the least restrictive alternative, the maintenance of the family unit when possible, and the use of community-based services instead of institutions. Knowing these fundamental tenets may assist hospitalists in understanding the limitations of Adult Protective Services. For example, in New York State, APS cannot evaluate clients in an acute care setting. A referral to APS can be a key component of ensuring a safe discharge plan but if the patient has decision-making capacity and refuses to allow APS representatives to perform an evaluation of the home or investigate potential entitlements, they cannot force the client to accept their services.

LAW ENFORCEMENT/DISTRICT ATTORNEY'S OFFICE

In cases of elder mistreatment in which the hospitalist suspects a crime has been committed and the victim wishes to press charges against the responsible party (eg, physical, financial, and/or sexual abuse), the hospitalist should file a report with law enforcement by contacting 911. The hospital's risk management and legal teams should also be immediately consulted. In accordance with the hospital's policies, they will provide further direction about involving law enforcement and involving the appropriate district attorney's office. In situations in which the hospitalist is unsure whether a crime has been committed, it can be helpful to contact the district attorney's office directly. Each office may have an attorney specifically assigned to an elder mistreatment unit and/or a community liaison who can offer guidance to the hospitalist. For example, the elderly gentleman who discloses to the nursing staff that he cannot afford his medications because he loaned his much younger girlfriend $25,000 for her dress business and she has failed to pay him back may be ambivalent about whether to press charges so the hospitalist can contact the district attorney's office to obtain advice for the patient should he decide he wants legal assistance.

MANDATORY REPORTING GUIDELINES

The majority of states have mandated reporting laws for elder mistreatment and except for Puerto Rico and South Dakota, "good faith reporting" provisions protect physicians from liability for having informed Adult Protective Services or other investigative agencies of their suspicions even if the reports are not substantiated. The five states that at the time of this writing have no mandatory reporting laws include Colorado, New Jersey, New York, North Dakota, and South Dakota. Social service employees such as Adult Protective Services workers are mandated reporters even in states like New York where physicians are not. Even in the absence of legal mandates, health and mental health professionals have an ethical and moral obligation to report elder mistreatment. Hospitalists need only have a reasonable suspicion of mistreatment to report. In cases in which abuse or neglect occurs in the community, APS is typically the agency tasked with investigation. For patients who reside in a nursing home or long-term care setting, the hospitalist and/or social worker may be required to alert the state Department of Health, APS, and/or the ombudsman.

TESTIFYING IN COURT

Concerns about being called to testify in court can pose a barrier to screening and assessment for elder mistreatment. In many cases, thorough documentation in the medical record can avert the need for in-court testimony by the physician. In other cases, the hospitalist's testimony may be required either as an expert witness or as a layperson to present general observations of behavior or statements made. When called as an expert witness, the physician may be asked to render opinions about the signs of neglect, the patient's decision-making capacity, and whether an explanation given is consistent with the victim's injuries.

The American Medical Association advises physicians providing testimony to

- Meet with the attorney presenting you as a witness before the trial to practice
- Suggest questions for the attorney to ask you if acting as an expert witness
- Propose questions for the opposing expert if acting as an expert witness
- Make sure you understand both the legal and factual issues and how they relate to your testimony
- Determine what evidence (ie, photographs) should be part of your testimony
- Answer only the questions asked; do not volunteer additional information
- Ask for questions to be repeated if necessary
- Explain when a one-word answer is insufficient
- Calmly correct an attorney who incorrectly reports prior testimony

PREVENTION

Just as an acute care stay can provide hospitalists with the chance to stop the cycle of abuse and neglect, it can also represent a critical window to intervene on an at-risk patient and prevent mistreatment from occurring in the first place. Prevention begins with knowing the risk factors for abuse and neglect so that hospitalists can identify the most vulnerable patients and gather an interdisciplinary team to devise a safety plan. Remember that the "vulnerable" patient is not always the one who is admitted with bruising or trauma but also the patients who are admitted monthly for uncontrolled chronic illness and have been nonadherent with their medications, the patients who come with worsening wounds or signs of poor nutrition, and the patients whose caregivers appear overwhelmed by their responsibilities. The same interventions for active abuse and neglect cases detailed above eg, the early and intense involvement of an interdisciplianry team during the hospitalization and establishment of links to post-discharge community resources, can prevent situations from escalating into mistreatment.

SYSTEMS ISSUES

The hospitalist model has been associated with reduced length of stay, lower inpatient costs, and improved patient care in multiple complex conditions. However, the use of hospitalists also complicates the care coordination process by increasing the number of handoffs amongst providers and muddying lines of accountability to ensure safe transitions. In a 2007 study published in the *Archives of Internal Medicine*, Southern, et al found a stronger association between lower length of stay and hospitalist care amongst patients requiring discharge with home care services or transfer to a skilled nursing facility.[8] They hypothesized that the greater reduction in length of stay associated with such "complex discharge planning" reflects the hospitalists' experience and skills in working with interdisciplinary team members such as social workers and discharge planners.

Elderly patients at risk for abuse and neglect or victims of frank mistreatment represent a highly complex group of patients, and hospitalists may truly dread the potential for these patients to increase their workload and their average length of stay. We argue, however, that medical, financial, and ethical incentives exist for providing extra attention to the care transitions of suspected or confirmed elder mistreatment victims. Even in states without mandated reporting laws for elder abuse, physicians have an ethical obligation to protect victims of elder abuse and neglect. Ethical dilemmas that arise when attempting to establish a safety plan for elder mistreatment victims typically involve weighing the need to protect patient autonomy against the physician's duty to promote beneficence and nonmaleficence.

Medically, the hospitalist who recognizes that ongoing abuse or neglect underlies the uncontrolled diabetes, congestive heart failure, or major depression will not only treat the victim's acute exacerbations but will introduce the supports and supervision necessary to give the patient an improved chance of success in controlling his or her illness. This strategy of addressing both the acute medical issue and the psychosocial factors contributing to it also makes financial sense if the inpatient team's interventions prevent unnecessary health care utilization, especially hospital readmissions. As Medicare begins to limit reimbursements to hospitals for readmissions for the same diagnosis, hospitals will also have an incentive to end the revolving door phenomenon. Contrary to the belief that bringing elder mistreatment victims into the medical system will result in a dramatic, downstream increase in health care utilization, in their 2008 study in the *Journal of the American Geriatrics Society*, Franzini and Dyer found that self-neglectors were no more expensive to the system than matched controls.[9] Self-neglectors by definition are nonadherent to medical interventions and typically refuse services they are entitled to, putting themselves at risk for serious mental and physical decline. Yet after undergoing a comprehensive geriatric assessment and when given access to longitudinal primary care, these patients were not hospitalized more or for a significantly greater length of stay.

The essential components of transitional care for all hospitalized patients include physician-to-physician communication across care sites, medication reconciliation, patient education to encourage self-efficacy, and assurance of appropriate social supports. Ensuring a safe transition for hospitalized elder mistreatment victims starts with an accurate assessment of baseline and current functional status to determine the appropriate discharge destination and requires communication between the sending (hospitalist and inpatient team) and receiving providers (primary care physician, home health agency, APS). The transfer of information between the inpatient and outpatient providers is especially imperative in elder mistreatment cases because often there is a suspicion of abuse or neglect but no confirmation. In these situations, patients will often be discharged to short-term rehabilitation facilities or to their homes with referrals for home health care and an APS referral. Hospitalists should communicate directly with the patient's primary care provider or the nursing home to alert the receiving physician about abuse and/or neglect concerns. When home health care is part of the intervention for a victim, the agency should be made aware of the concerns about mistreatment and should know how to contact the outpatient physician if one of its employees witnesses abuse and/or neglect.

CONCLUSION

Identifying and treating victims of elder abuse and neglect can be a daunting challenge but each inpatient admission should be viewed by the hospitalist as an opportunity to have a potentially life-saving impact of the life of the elder mistreatment victim. The hospitalist may be the first individual to notice the medical consequences of abuse or neglect or may be viewed as a trusted individual in whom the patient confides. In either case, the hospitalist possesses the capacity to guide the inpatient workup and management, document his or her assessment, and enlist the help of an interdisciplinary team to devise a safety plan.

SUGGESTED READINGS

Ahmad M, Lachs MS. Elder abuse and neglect: What physicians can and should do. *Cleve Clin J Med*. 2002;69:801–808.

Kleinschmidt KC. Elder abuse: a review. *Ann Emerg Med*. 1997:309: 463–472.

Kripalani S, Jackson AT, Schnipper JL, et al. Promoting effective transitions of care at hospital discharge: a review of key issues for hospitalists. *J Hosp Med*. 2007;(2):314–323.

Lachs MS, Pillemer K. Abuse and neglect of elderly persons. *N Engl J Med*. 1995;333:437.

Lachs MS, Pillemer K. Elder abuse. *The Lancet*. 2004;364:1263–1272.

Liao S, Mosqueda L. Physical abuse of the elderly: The medical director's response. *J Am Med Dir Assoc*. 2007 Mar;8(3 Suppl 2): e61–e64.

Lindenauer PK, Rothberg MB, Pekow PS, et al. Outcomes of care by hospitalists, general internists and family physicians. *NEJM*. 2007;357(25):2589–2600.

Pham HH, Grossman JM, Cohen G, et al. Hospitalists and care transitions: the divorce of inpatient and outpatient care. *Health Affairs*. 2008;27(5):1315–1327.

Texas Elder Abuse and Mistreatment Institute Medical Management of Elder Abuse: A practical approach. http://www.dfps.state.tx.us/everyonesbusiness/PDFs/English-APSinserts.pdf. Accessed on November 11, 2011.

REFERENCES

1. American Medical Association Diagnostic and Treatment Guidelines on Elder abuse and Neglect. Chicago, IL: American Medical Association; 1992.
2. National Academies of Sciences. Bonnie R, Wallace R, eds. *Elder abuse: abuse, neglect, and exploitation in an aging America*. Washington, D.C.: National Academy Press;2002.
3. WHO. The Toronto declaration on the global prevention of elder abuse. Geneva, Switzerland: WHO; 2002.
4. Acierno R, Hernandez MS, Amstadter AB, et al. Prevalence and correlates of emotional, physical, sexual, and financial abuse and potential neglect in the United States: The National Elder Mistreatment Study. *Am J Public Health*. 2010;100:292–297.
5. Laumann EO, Leitsch SA, Waite LJ. Elder mistreatment in the United States: prevalence estimates from a nationally representative study. *J Gerontol B Psychol Sci Soc Sci*. 2008;63(4):S248–S254.
6. Yong-Fang K, Gulshan S, Freeman JL, et al. Growth in the Care of Older Patients by Hospitalists in the United States. *N Engl J Med*. 2009;360:1102–1012.
7. Mosqueda L, Burnight K, Liao S. The life cycle of bruises in older adults. *J Am Geriatr Soc*. 2005;53:1339–1343.

8. Southern WN, Berger MA, Bellin EY, et al. Hospitalist care and length of stay in patients requiring complex discharge planning and close clinical monitoring. *Arch Int Med*. 2007;167(17): 1869–1874.
9. Franzini L and Dyer CB. Healthcare costs and utilization of vulnerable elderly people reported to adult protective services for self-neglect. *J Am Geriatr Soc*. 2008(56):667–676.

WEB-BASED RESOURCES

Centers for Medicare and Medicaid Services. Medicare and Home Health Care [Online] http://www.medicare.gov/Publications/Pubs/pdf/10969.pdf. Accessed March 20, 2010.

Liao S, Smith S. Reporting elder mistreatment. ACP Pier. [Online] October 30, 2006. http://pier.acponline.orgphysicians/ethical_legal/el056.html. Accessed on September 29, 2008.

Otto, JM. National Adult Protective Services Association. History of NAPSA: The role of Adult Protective Services in Addressing Abuse. [Online] http://www.apsnetwork.org/About/history.htm. Accessed March 20, 2010.

The American Bar Association Commission on Law and Aging. Laws Related to Elder Abuse. [Online] http://new.abanet.org/aging/Pages/elderabuse.aspx. Accessed February 9, 2010.

The National Center on Elder Abuse at the American Public Human Services Association in Collaboration with Westat, Inc. The National Elder Abuse Incidence Study, 1998. http://www.aoa.gov/AoARoot/AoA_Programs/Elder_Rights/Elder_Abuse/docs/ABuseReport_Full.pdf. Accessed on September 24, 2009.

The National Center on Elder Abuse. The 2004 Survey of State Adult Protective Services: Abuse of Adults 60 Years of Age and Older [Online]; http://www.ncea.aoa.gov/NCEAroot/Main_Site/pdf/2-14-06%20FINAL%2060+REPORT.pdf. Accessed on September 24, 2009.

CHAPTER 168

Functional Decline

Melissa Mattison, MD, SFHM, FACP

Key Clinical Questions

1. How is functional ability assessed?
2. What is functional decline?
3. What are the risk factors for developing functional decline?
4. How does hospitalization contribute to functional decline?
5. How can functional decline be prevented?

INTRODUCTION

Approximately 30% of people living in the community that are older than 65 fall each year and more than half of these people will fall again. The yearly costs for acute hospital care for fall-related fractures are estimated in the billions in the United States; and lifetime costs associated with fall injuries for this age group is rising as the U.S. population ages. Falls are the 6th leading cause of death and a common reason for loss of independent living. Some of these falls occur within 30 days of admission to the hospital, and may be the result of deconditioning that occurred during the index hospitalization.

Many hospital environments are not designed for maintaining or improving patient function. Hospitalization is often associated with bed rest, decreased mobility, sleep deprivation, and poor nutritional intake. These factors can cause a cascade of events that reduce functional ability in a patient of any age including a decrease in cardiovascular conditioning. Older patients, in particular, tend to be more vulnerable to functional disability and are particularly susceptible to loss of functional independence during hospitalization. This frequently results in placement upon discharge in nursing facilities, sometimes for short-term rehabilitation, but often for long-term residence.

Today, approximately half of all hospitalized adults are over the age of 65 and this proportion will likely increase as the overall number of elderly increases. Mitigating the factors that contribute to functional decline during hospitalization will improve the quality of care provided to patients, reduce readmissions, and decrease the disability and cost that extends well beyond hospitalization.

FUNCTIONAL ASSESSMENT

Inpatient physicians should perform a functional assessment on all patients. Oftentimes, it is inferred—a middle-aged mother of three admitted for gallstones is assumed to be independent. A 60-year-old employed carpenter with angina is assumed to be fully independent. These assumptions are usually right. However, as patients age, assumptions are often incorrect. Clinicians may care for a 72-year-old fully dependent nursing home resident and at the same time care for a 94-year-old fully independent resident living at home alone.

There is no all-purpose test to determine a patient's functional abilities. Rather, clinicians must rely upon yes/no questions around specific tasks as well as bedside assessment tools.

Several assessment tools have been developed to aid clinicians in determining a patient's functional status (**Table 168-1**). The Activities of Daily Living (ADLs) have been used for the past 30 years to assess a patient's ability to feed and clean themselves, dress, transfer from bed to chair, maintain continence, and toilet independently. The Instrumental Activities of Daily Living (IADLs) include the ability to use the telephone, take transportation, manage finances, shop, cook, clean, do laundry, and take medications.

While ADLs and IADLs can give a clinician a good sense of how a patient functions with life tasks, clinicians should also assess gait, hearing, vision, and nutritional status. The Get Up and Go Test is useful to determine how well a patient can walk. Ask the patient to stand from a seated position without using her arms, walk 10 feet, turn around, and return to the chair and sit down. The inability to get up without using one's arms, trouble with

TABLE 168-1 Assessment of Function

Assessment	Components	Specifics	Notes
ADLs	Toileting, bathing, dressing, feeding, transferring, continence	Can you dress yourself? Do you need help going to the bathroom?	ADL disability is strongly correlated with nursing home placement
IADLs	Shopping, cooking, using transportation, managing finances, using the telephone, laundry, taking medications	Who pays your bills? Do you do your own cooking and cleaning? How do you get to your doctor's appointments?	
Get Up and Go Test	Gait	Rise from chair without using arms, walk 10 feet, turn around and return to chair. *If unable, ask about history of falls*	Inability to rise without use of arms, showing poor balance, judgment or taking more than 15 seconds to complete this task is associated with increased risk of falling
Whisper Test	Hearing	After exhaling, whisper, into each ear individually while occluding opposite ear	
Snellen Chart	Vision	Stand 20 feet away, or use handheld chart 14 inches from eyes	
Nutrition	Assess for weight loss, calculate BMI, measure intake	Risk factors for malnutrition include dementia, social isolation, inability to prepare meals, alcohol abuse, poverty, dental problems	More than half of all patients ≥65 years admitted to hospital may be malnourished

ADLs, Activities of Daily Living; IADLs, Instrumental Activities of Daily Living; BMI, body mass index.

balance or turning, using adaptive devices, or taking longer than 15 seconds are markers for increased risk of falling. Also note whether these tests are associated with an abnormal cardiac response: systolic blood pressure drops or heart rate increases abnormally. Orthostatic changes from the sitting to standing position are likely to have a negative impact on the patient's mobility. Likewise, for a patient with lung disease, significant hypoxia during walking should be noted and corrected.

Gross testing of auditory and visual acuity can be easily performed at the bedside. Test vision at the bedside with the Snellen chart. Assess hearing with the Whisper Test.

While physical function is important, a cognitive evaluation should also be performed. A patient's cognitive function is critical to understanding whether the patient will be able to adhere to recommended therapies, participate in informed consent, and take prescribed medications correctly. Clinicians should not make assumptions about a patient's cognitive ability since there can be wide variations that are not predicted by age or other factors. Chapter 165 addresses formal assessment of cognition.

A patient's nutritional status impacts physical and cognitive function. For instance, poor nutritional status negatively impacts immune function. All patients should be screened for malnutrition by calculating their body mass index (BMI) and should be questioned about weight loss and access to food. See Chapter 54.

HOSPITALIZATION AND DISABILITY

Hospitalization is associated with a decline in function for many patients. Losing function is a marker for increased morbidity and mortality. It both increases the risk of nursing home placement, and the risk of death. While younger patients tend to have enough "reserve" to absorb a small decline without affecting independence, this is often not true for older patients whose functional reserve decreases with advancing age. Many older people are marginally able to function independently at baseline. Then, an illness strikes. The physiologic stress of battling the illness combined with hospitalization often leaves elderly patients dependent upon others to complete their ADLs or IADLs. Losing the ability to transfer from bed to chair or to prepare one's meals can necessitate placement in a nursing home at the time of discharge. Regaining this function can be difficult.

Homeostenosis is a term coined by physiologists used to explain this vulnerability in older patients due to each organ system having diminished reserve with advancing age. Without any stress or insult, the whole body continues to function without difficulty. However, when illness strikes and one organ system fails, homeostasis is disrupted and other organ systems lack the reserve necessary to compensate. This lack of reserve is manifested by decreased resilience. It is postulated that older people often must dip into their functional reserves just to maintain homeostasis, leaving them vulnerable to multiple system breakdowns during a time of illness or stress. For example, a patient with mild cognitive impairment who normally can function independently commonly develops delirium with marked confusion in the setting of concurrent infection.

In addition to the physiologic effects of illness, hospitalization itself places elderly patients at risk for further functional decline. Immobility is a major factor leading to disability. Older patients are more prone to suffer from cognitive impairment, decreased muscle strength, hearing and visual impairment, as well as difficulty with balance, orthostasis, and arthritis (**Table 168-2**). All of these factors can contribute to immobility. Bed rest orders and fall

TABLE 168-2 Risk Factors for Immobility

Cognitive impairment
Hearing and visual impairment
Balance/gait difficulty
Orthostasis
Arthritis
Use of indwelling catheters, continuous IV infusions, telemetry leads ("tethers")

TABLE 168-3 Risk Factor Modification

Risk Factor	Intervention
Immobility	Encourage ambulation, limit bed rest, involve physical therapy early during hospitalization, address limits to mobilization (eg, remove catheters, IVs, etc as soon as they are longer medically necessary)
Malnutrition	Daily multivitamin supplementation, nutrition/dietary consultation, mealtime assistance with feeding, increase access to food, limit "nothing by mouth" orders
Dehydration	Offer fluids by mouth if able to tolerate, IVF if necessary
Falls	Avoid medications associated with falls, assess for orthostasis, provide supervision with ambulation and safe, lighted environment, address risks for immobility (see above)

precautions forbidding patients to leave bed unattended, though well intentioned, add to inactivity and further loss of cardiovascular reserve and muscle strength. Foley catheters, continuous intravenous lines, and telemetry leads ("tethers") make it difficult to safely move from bed to chair or to the bathroom.

By the second hospital day, a decline in functional status can be detected in many patients. Identifying patients who are most vulnerable—those in whom any further loss will throw them over the brink to dependency—is important for all clinicians at the time of hospital admission.

PREVENTING FUNCTIONAL DECLINE

Preventing disability from developing during hospitalization is a challenge. Hospitalization itself is cited as a major cause of functional decline. It is not clear if this is due to the underlying illness necessitating the hospital stay or intrinsic factors of hospitalization. It is likely a combination of both. Given the heterogeneity and complexity involved, few studies address this issue.

Based on studies of outpatients who develop disability and expert opinion, some recommendations can be made. The functional status of all patients should be determined on admission and interventions should be targeted accordingly. Clinicians should encourage mobility in all hospitalized patients. Bed rest orders should be minimized to situations of absolute medical necessity because of the association with loss of muscle mass, impaired balance, functional incontinence, decreased ventilation, pressure sores, and bone loss.

There are a few populations that merit special mention. Patients who fall or are at risk for falling are particularly vulnerable for growing physical dependence during hospitalization. These patients are commonly placed in bed with alarms activated to prevent unsupervised mobility. This may be warranted to prevent a cognitively impaired patient from rising without needed assistance. However, this can contribute to immobility. Specific recommendations to limit immobility in this population and reduce the risk of falling are:

- Consult physical therapy early during the hospitalization and have someone walk with the patient in hallway twice daily.
- Encourage taking meals out of bed.
- Avoid the use of medications associated with falling such as benzodiazepines, narcotics, antidepressants (serotonin-reuptake inhibitors and tricyclics), and certain antiarrhythmics.
- Look for evidence of orthostatic hypotension and treat accordingly.
- Provide proper lighting and supervision with ambulation.
- Remove indwelling catheters, telemetry leads, and IV lines as soon as they are no longer medically required.

Using the list above, consider creating a daily checklist and incorporate the maneuvers outlined above into everyday practice of clinical staff.

Patients who appear malnourished on admission or who have limited access to nutrition during hospitalization also require special attention. Protein intake is often not sufficient during an acute illness and protein intake may be insufficient in patients who otherwise appear overweight. Lack of sufficient nutrition is seen in more than half of elders admitted to the hospital. Poor nutrition contributes to decreased muscle strength, diminished respiratory function, development of pressure ulcers, longer hospital stays, and increased mortality. Optimizing nutritional status during hospitalization, avoiding extended periods of time when the patient is NPO, and involving nutrition experts early can be helpful. Some experts recommend a supplemental multivitamin for all older patients admitted to the hospital because of evidence that this may reduce length of stay.

Older patients are particularly prone to becoming dehydrated in the hospital. The sense of thirst is commonly impaired with advanced age. Renal function also diminishes with age and this may result in decreased sensitivity to antidiuretic hormone. Additionally, patient access to fluids in the hospital can be limited, especially in patients unable to feed themselves or being kept "nothing by mouth" for treatment purposes. Dehydration can frequently result and cause electrolyte imbalance, orthostatic hypotension, and increased risk of falling. Ensuring adequate fluid intake by mouth (preferred) or by intravenous access is an important component to minimizing these risks (**Table 168-3**).

INTERVENTIONS AT DISCHARGE/TRANSITION OF CARE

With the rise of the Hospital Medicine specialty, the discharging physician will usually stop providing care for the patient and turn patient care over to an outpatient provider. Many patients with functional decline at the time of discharge will be discharged to a skilled nursing facility or to home with supportive care. This transition of care can be a vulnerable time for the patient. Physicians completing the discharge paperwork can use this as an opportunity to communicate with outpatient providers and should include important information outlined below:

- Patient's baseline level of physical and cognitive functioning at the time of *admission* and *discharge*
- Mobility goals
- Preferred intensity of care
- Unique needs or diagnoses that bear special consideration (eg, orthostatic hypotension or malnourished requiring nutritional supplements)

CONCLUSION

Hospitalization can result in significant physical functional decline. The innate aspects of a hospital environment combined with the stress of the physical illness necessitating the hospitalization can lead patients to lose muscle mass, strength, and balance. This is particularly difficult for patients who at baseline have little physical

TABLE 168-4 The Bedside Mobility Evaluation

History
Falls: Have you fallen within the last year? Why? What were you doing? Did you hurt yourself? How many times have you fallen?
• Look for a pattern to the falls: environment, medical, medication related?
Function: How do you get around? Do you use a cane, a walker, a wheelchair? Have you had any education in how to use it? If you need help, who helps you?
Medical conditions: Do you suffer from arthritis, Parkinson disease, incontinence, or lightheadness? Have you ever had a stroke? Do you have problems with your memory? Do you have trouble rising from a chair?
• Orthostasis, cognitive impairment, limited mobility due to significant arthritis or neuromuscular disease can hinder function. Assess for reduced lower extremity strength, reduced grip strength, hip or knee pain.
Sensory impairments: Do you have trouble seeing or hearing? Can you see well enough to read? Can you taste your food?
Physical exam
Observe: Can the patient sit up in bed without assistance? Can the patient get out of bed without help? If yes, can the patient perform the Get Up and Go Test? Can the patient perform the functional reach test while maintaining balance?
Gait, balance, and physical performance: Assess for gait abnormalities, reduced walking speed, postural sway, impaired balance, difficulty rising from a chair, difficulty transferring.
Cognitive and psychological deficits: Assess mental status, cognitive function and for the presence of depression.
Medications: Review medications for presence of sedatives, hypnotics, anxiolytics, and antidepressants.
Intervene
1. Educate patients and family about fall prevention
2. Evaluate medical disorders for remedial causes
3. Review medications for psychoactive drugs, antihypertensives
4. Order: Physical therapy evaluation for problems with balance and gait, therapy for muscle weakness, transfer training, deconditioning, need for walking aids; home safety evaluation; and arrange for evaluation and treatment of vision problems, incontinence
5. Consider: Alerting system if patient lives alone and continues to have risk factors for falling

reserve and prior to admission were living on the brink of dependency. Inpatient physicians must assess patient function at the time of admission. They must then customize therapy for the most vulnerable patients by addressing nutritional and physical needs, including limiting bed rest orders, encouraging early mobilization, and avoiding medications that contribute to falls and delirium. Finally, at discharge, inpatient physicians must communicate with providers assuming post-hospital care so that the unique needs of each patient are met (**Table 168-4**).

SUGGESTED READINGS

Creditor MC. The hazards of hospitalization in the elderly. *Ann Intern Med.* 1993;118:219–223.

Gill TM, Allore HG, Holford TR, Guo Z. Hospitalization, restricted activity, and the development of disability among older persons. *JAMA.* 2004;292:2115–2124.

Gill TM, Baker DI, Gottschalk M, Peduzzi PN, Allore H, Byers A. A program to prevent functional decline in physically frail, elderly persons who live at home. *N Engl J Med.* 2002;347:1068–1074.

Gill TM, Williams CS, Tinetti ME. The combined effects of baseline vulnerability and acute hospital events on the development of functional dependence among community-living older persons. *J Gerontol A Biol Sci Med Sci.* 1999;54:M377–M383.

Katz S, Ford AB, Moskowitz RW, Jackson BA, Jaffe MW. Studies of illness in the aged. The Index of ADL: A Standardized Measure of Biological and Psychosocial Function. *JAMA.* 1963;185:914–919.

Thomas DR. Focus on functional decline in hospitalized older adults. *J Gerontol A Biol Sci Med Sci.* 2002;57:M567– M568.

Tinetti ME. Clinical practice. Preventing falls in elderly persons. *N Engl J Med.* 2003;348:42–49.

Tinetti ME, Williams CS. Falls, injuries due to falls, and the risk of admission to a nursing home. *N Engl J Med.* 1997;337:1279–1284.

Wells JL, Dumbrell AC. Nutrition and aging: assessment and treatment of compromised nutritional status in frail elderly patients. *Clin Interv Aging.* 2006;1:67–79.

Williams ME, Owens JE, Parker BE Jr, Granata KP. A new approach to assessing function in elderly people. *Trans Am Clin Climatol Assoc.* 2003;114:203–216; discussion 16–17.

CHAPTER 169

The Frail Hospitalized Patient

Elizabeth Lindenberger, MD
Kenneth Boockvar, MD, MS

Key Clinical Questions

1. How do you identify frail, hospitalized older patients?
2. What adverse outcomes are common among this population?
3. How can an interdisciplinary team prevent adverse outcomes for frail older patients?
4. What are the opportunities to improve long-term health outcomes?
5. What are the steps for establishing a safe and thorough discharge plan?

INTRODUCTION

Older patients disproportionately face many complications during hospitalization, including deconditioning from immobility, nosocomial infections, pressure ulcers, falls, and delirium. Hospital-associated deconditioning may lead to rapid functional decline. One in three older hospitalized patients loses the ability to perform at least one activity of daily living (ADL) by the time of discharge. Losing the ability to bathe or toilet independently may result in discharge to a nursing home for a patient who has previously lived independently. One in five hospitalized older patients is discharged to a nursing home due to a new loss of function. The frailest patients are at highest risk for hospital-associated functional decline and institutionalization.

If asked what a frail older patient looks like, many physicians would say, "I know it when I see it." The thin older person who slowly ambulates with a walker is easily identified as frail. Nevertheless, recognizing frailty in clinical practice may not always be so straightforward. Frailty does not fit into classic organ-specific models of disease, and it may not be evident to clinicians, patients, or family members that there has been a decline in health. Declines in strength, mobility, cognitive function, and nutrition may be gradual. Patients or clinicians may attribute these changes to old age and not appreciate that a response is indicated to reverse the process.

Frailty may be particularly difficult to identify in the hospital setting. A physically robust older patient may be indistinguishable from a frail older patient at first glance if they are both acutely ill, dressed in hospital gowns, and lying in hospital beds. Without asking the right questions and assessing important factors such as mobility, cognitive function, and nutritional status, the health care team may fail to identify the frail patient and take appropriate steps to reduce the hazards of hospitalization.

PATHOPHYSIOLOGY

Frailty manifests with a variety of clinical features including loss of strength, weight loss, low levels of activity, and slowed performance. The biological basis of frailty involves a combination of age- and disease-related physiological changes including skeletal muscle loss, changes in endocrine function, and chronic inflammation. Endocrine changes include decreases in estrogen, testosterone, growth hormone, and insulin-like growth factor, each of which has been implicated in muscle loss. Frail older patients have been shown to have increased levels of proinflammatory cytokines, such as interleukin-6 and C-reactive protein. Although these laboratory findings contribute to our understanding of the physiologic basis of frailty, they are not useful for diagnostic purposes, especially in hospitalized patients who have changes in inflammatory markers and endocrine function stemming from acute illness. Frailty remains a clinical diagnosis based on history, physical examination, and functional assessment. Frailty is perhaps best assessed in the absence of acute illness, thus making the diagnosis in the hospital particularly challenging.

While frailty is a clinical syndrome associated with physiologic changes, the most clinically useful way to conceptualize frailty among hospitalized patients is by asking the question, "Is my patient fragile?" Frailty may be broadly defined as a diminished capacity to withstand stress that, in turn, places individuals at risk for adverse health outcomes. Hospitalization is one of the greatest stressors an older patient may face. Therefore, in the context of the hospitalized older patient, frailty may best be defined as the patient characteristics most highly associated with adverse outcomes. Frail hospitalized patients are, therefore, those who are the most "fragile."

THE FRAGILE PATIENT: A 4-STEP APPROACH

Caring for a fragile patient in the hospital has much in common with caring for any fragile entity. We propose a 4-step approach for managing the fragile older patient and demonstrate how each step compares to caring for a fragile vase. In step 1, we recognize that our patient is fragile and at risk for adverse events. This is analogous to receiving an heirloom vase from a relative and recognizing that its ceramic characteristics increase the likelihood of breaking. In step 2, we outline a plan for protecting the patient from adverse events in the hospital, similar to how we plan to keep our vase from breaking. In step 3, we identify the ways that we can promote positive health outcomes analogous to polishing the vase, optimizing its beauty and well-being. In step 4, we prepare a safe discharge plan, just as we decide how we will safely transfer our vase to another home.

CASE 169-1

Is this patient frail?

An 88-year-old man presents to the hospital with confusion and decreased appetite over 3 days. Past medical history is significant only for hypertension and benign prostatic hypertrophy, and his medications include tamsulosin, amlodipine, and diphenhydramine for insomnia. He wears glasses but did not bring them to the hospital. He lives with his wife of 60 years. She prepares his meals and he has not lost any weight over the past 6 months. This couple has three daughters who live locally and shop for them.

On examination, he appears thin and well groomed. His body mass index is 22. He is mildly tachypneic and has crackles at the left base on lung exam. His attention is poor, and he frequently drifts off to sleep during the interview. His speech is disorganized. He knows his name but is not oriented to time or place. He is unable to recall three words in 5 minutes, and is unable to draw a clock.

His laboratory tests are notable for an elevated white blood cell count, a blood urea nitrogen level of 42, and a creatinine of 1.5. His chest x-ray reveals an infiltrate consistent with a left lower lobe pneumonia.

History from patient's wife

Although the patient was apparently walking without difficulty up until 3 days ago, he now requires assistance to walk due to an unsteady gait. He had an abrupt decline in his thinking and appetite 3 days ago, but prior to that he was "fine." He was independent in all of his basic activities of daily living and walks regularly with his wife in the neighborhood. He has no history of a dementia diagnosis.

On detailed questioning, his wife admits that her husband has had a mild decline in his memory over the past several years and that he is no longer able to manage the couple's finances. He has difficulty with short-term memory and frequently repeats questions. She has to remind her husband to take his medications each morning. She has begun to feel nervous letting her husband go outside by himself for fear that he might get lost. She is with her husband all the time and takes care of the cooking, cleaning, and laundry.

Assessment of frailty

In addition to his *advanced age*, he has multiple characteristics of frailty:

- *Delirium*, as demonstrated by his poor attention, acute worsening of cognition, and disorganized speech; risk factors include dementia, dehydration, pneumonia.
- *Likely underlying dementia*
- *Functional impairment*, as evidenced by his dependence in an IADL, ie, needing assistance with medication management and his unsteady gait, a departure from his baseline
- *Dehydration* on clinical exam and laboratory tests

Due to his acute delirium, it is not possible to pursue a vision or depression screening at this time. He does wear glasses and should be encouraged to use them during his hospitalization.

Prevention of adverse outcomes

Key interventions to limit the course of his delirium and also reduce the risk of falls and fall-related injury

- Promote hydration
- Provide glasses
- Mobilize early on during hospitalization
- Avoid psychoactive medications, indwelling urinary catheter, physical restraints

Nursing team

- Provides him with a low bed
- Initiates a toileting schedule, every 2 hours during the day

Physicians

- Determine that the patient lacks decision-making capacity
- Identify his wife as next of kin and surrogate decision maker
- Address goals of care

Family

- Clarifies his wishes that he "loves life" and continues to take great pleasure in his daily life with family. Although his wife knows he would not desire prolonged artificial life support if his prognosis were poor, she does not desire limitations on his health care at this time.

Promotion of this patient's long-term health and well-being with a safe and effective discharge plan

- Assess effectiveness of appropriate treatment—resolution of pneumonia and delirium with hydration and 3 days of appropriate antibiotics.
- Assess cognitive function—he is oriented to place, month, and year and knows that he is in the hospital. He has a general but not detailed understanding of his medical conditions. His wife confirms that this is his baseline level of cognition.
- Assess functional status—despite working closely with physical therapy, his ambulation has remained unsteady. He can ambulate independently and safely over 100 feet with a rolling walker. He needs assistance with bathing but is otherwise independent in basic ADL.
- Review medication regimen—stop diphenhydramine, as this is likely to increase fall risk and confusion. Add only a short-course of oral antibiotics to his discharge medications.
- Provide written instructions to his wife regarding both these changes.
- Refer to a home care agency that can provide him with home physical therapy under his Medicare benefit. The agency will also provide short-term home health aide support for the duration of his home physical therapy benefit that will give his wife some respite from caregiving.

- Educate family about community services such as community adult day health programs that can provide the socialization for the patient and respite for his wife.

DIAGNOSIS

STEP 1: IDENTIFY FRAIL PATIENTS

Recognition is the first step in caring for the frail hospitalized patient. Although there are many potential adverse outcomes of hospitalization for frail older patients, outcomes commonly studied include functional decline, delirium, and institutionalization. These outcomes not only greatly impact on patients' quality of life, but they incur high costs to society.

Despite the absence of a simple diagnostic test for frailty, this clinical syndrome manifests signs and symptoms that can be identified at the time of hospital admission. **Table 169-1** lists 10 "frailty characteristics" and methods to assess each one. Each of these characteristics is associated with at least one major adverse outcome, including hospital-associated delirium and/or functional decline. Assessing for these ten frailty characteristics at admission facilitates identification of potentially treatable conditions and implementation of preventative measures.

TABLE 169-1 Step 1: Is My Patient Frail/Fragile? Assess at Hospital Admission

Frailty Characteristics*	Evidence	Assessment
Advanced age	Covinsky KE, et al. *J Am Geriatr Soc.* 2003;51(4):451–458.	Age ≥ 85
Dementia	Inouye SK, et al. *J Am Geriatr Soc.* 2007;51(4):451–458. Sands LP, et al. *J Gerontol A Biol Sci Med Sci.* 2003;58(1):37–45.	MiniCog (name 3 objects/re-ask in 5 minutes; draw 8-inch circle and ask patient to draw a clock with a specified time) *Or* MMSE *And* History from caregiver/family regarding progressive decline in cognitive function and ADL/IADL
Delirium	McAvay GJ, et al. *J Am Geriatr Soc.* 2006;54(8):1245–1250. Givens JL, et al. *J Am Geriatr Soc.* 2009;57(8):1347–1353.	Recognize key features: acute onset of confusion, fluctuating course, inattention, and either disorganized thinking or altered consciousness
Functional impairment (ADL, IADL)	Inouye SK, et al. *J Am Geriatr Soc.* 2007;51(4):451–458. Covinsky KE, et al. *J Am Geriatr Soc.* 2003;51(4):451–458.	Basic—ADLs *"2 weeks ago, did you need any help with bathing? Dressing? Moving from bed to a chair? Using the toilet? Did you have any difficulty with these things?"* Higher Level—IADLs *"2 weeks ago, did you need any help with paying bills? Handling your medications? Did you have any difficulty with these things?"*
Impaired or unsteady walking	Boyd CM, et al. *Am J Med.* 2005;118(11): 1225–1231. Lindenberger EC, et al. *J Am Geriatr Soc.* 2003;51(5);621–626.	*"2 weeks ago, were you able to walk without help? Did you use a cane? Walker? Wheelchair? Are you unsteady with walking?"*
Hospitalized for fall	Gill TM, et al. *JAMA.* 2004;292(17):2115–2124.	Obtain history
Vision impairment	Inouye SK, et al. *J Am Geriatr Soc.* 2007;51(4):451–458. Inouye SK. *Ann Med.* 2000;32(4):257–263.	*"Do you have problems with your vision?"* Or Snellen eye chart or Jaeger Card each eye (with glasses) abnormal (< 20/70 visual acuity)
Dehydration	Inouye SK. *Ann Med.* 2000;32(4):257–263.	BUN/creatinine ratio ≥ 18
Malnutrition	Boyd CM, et al. *Am J Med.* 2005;118(11): 1225–1231. Fried LP, et al. *J Gerontol A Biol Sci Med Sci.* 2001;56A(3):M146– M156.	*"Have you lost weight in the past 6 months? How much?"* Or Body mass index < 21
Depressive symptoms	Givens JL, et al. *J Am Geriatr Soc.* 2009;57(8):1347–1353. McAvay GJ, et al. *J Am Geriatr Soc.* 2006;54(8):1245–1250.	*"Over the past month, have you often been bothered by (a) feeling sad, depressed, or hopeless? (b) little interest or pleasure in doing things?"* Or Geriatric Depression Scale
Social Isolation	Jones DM, et al. *J Am Geriatr Soc.* 2004;52(11):1929–1933.	*"Where do you live? Who lives at home with you? Who are the people that help you the most day to day?"*

ADLs, Activities of Daily Living; IADLs, Instrumental Activities of Daily Living.
*Older patients with one or more of these characteristics should be considered fragile and at risk for adverse outcomes. Risk factors for adverse outcomes such as functional decline, delirium, and institutionalization.

Some frailty characteristics may be identified immediately without a detailed, time-consuming assessment. Simple questions about function and social supports can be incorporated into the social history component of the patient interview for patients aged 85 and older, for cognitively impaired elders, and those hospitalized for a fall or fall-related injury. Social workers and physical and occupational therapists working with the medical team can complete more detailed assessments of function and social supports for these high-risk patients. Inpatient geriatric consultation may address challenging cases of delirium, dementia, or concerns regarding inadequate home supports.

Assessments of key frailty characteristics—delirium and dementia—should be made at the time of hospital admission to identify patients having one or both of these diagnoses. Many fragile patients will present with delirium, and others will develop delirium during their hospitalization. Delirium is associated with a variety of adverse outcomes including functional decline, institutionalization and death. Delirium may be distinguished from dementia by its abrupt onset and characteristics of impaired attention, fluctuating consciousness, and incoherent or disorganized speech. Approximately 30% of patients with delirium have underlying dementia. See Chapter 166: Agitation in Older Adults.

Another frailty characteristic, impaired functional status ie, activities of daily living, and impaired or unsteady walking can be assessed quickly and easily at the time of hospital admission, and treatment of impaired physical function may prevent post discharge falls. Table 169-1 describes simple interview questions to assess function. Many frail older patients will already have lost physical abilities in the days immediately preceding hospital admission due to acute illness. It is therefore critical to ask patients not only about baseline function, ie, 2 weeks prior to admission, but also to assess their function at admission and during the hospital course.

Vision impairment and dehydration are frailty characteristics highly associated with the development of delirium. Randomized controlled trials have shown that multifactorial interventions including maximizing vision, eg, making certain patients have their glasses in the hospital, and treating dehydration may decrease the incidence of hospital-associated delirium.

Malnutrition, common among frail older adults both in and out of the hospital, is associated with hospital-associated functional decline. Evidence of weight loss and low body mass may be red flags for fragility among the hospitalized older patient. Depressive symptoms and social isolation are additional frailty characteristics associated with adverse outcomes in older adults. Table 169-1 lists questions and simple screening tools to assess for each of these conditions. See case example.

TREATMENT

■ STEP 2: PREVENT ADVERSE OUTCOMES

Table 169-2 lists five key strategies for avoiding hospital-associated adverse events in frail patients that include baseline and daily clinical assessments. Each of these strategies requires an interdisciplinary team approach, ie, collaborative assessments and plans by the physician, nursing staff, social workers, and pharmacists. Table 169-2 describes the core physician roles for each strategy in addition to roles for other non-physician team members.

Assess mental status daily, if not more frequently, to recognize symptoms of delirium, which can wax and wane. Assess physical function, including walking ability, not only on admission but also throughout the hospital stay to avoid the common and often avoidable complication of functional decline. For those patients with impaired mobility, frequently assess skin integrity in order to identify and prevent progression of early pressure ulcers.

Avoid potentially harmful orders for bed rest and routine orders for medical devices that restrict mobility, including unnecessary intravenous lines, cardiac monitors, oxygen cannulas, and indwelling urinary catheters. Urinary catheters, in particular, are rarely necessary except in cases of urinary retention. Avoid physical restraints at all times as they promote deconditioning, exacerbate delirium, and increase the risk of fall-related injury. Mobilize the frail patient early during the hospital stay and engage in physical therapy as soon as possible. See Chapter 258: Physical Therapy and Rehabilitation.

Review medications daily and avoid

- Inappropriate medications, especially benzodiazepines and anticholinergic, which increase risk for both falls and delirium
- Standing medication orders for anxiety, sleep, and agitation.

For many frail patients with serious illness, procedures intended to diagnose occult conditions or prolong life may be more burdensome than beneficial. Studies suggest that the highest priorities of patients with serious endstage conditions, such as cancer, endstage kidney disease, or ADL disability, are to have their quality of life optimized, to avoid being a burden to their family, and to maintain a sense of control. Elicit frail patients' goals and values regarding medical care and desired health care proxies. For patients lacking decision-making capacity, these discussions take place with the patients' surrogates. Advance care planning discussions, paired with appropriate transfer of this information at discharge, may reduce the risk for medical error and should promote patient centered care during hospitalization and beyond. Advance care planning first requires determination of decision-making capacity for the discussion. Patients with mild dementia may have limited capacity, eg, the patient may have the capacity to appoint a health care proxy but lack capacity to make complex medical decisions. The second step of advance care planning involves assigning a health care proxy by encouraging patients with decision-making capacity to complete an advance directive.

When discussing goals of care, physicians often focus heavily on particular procedures such as resuscitation or artificial ventilation. It is difficult, however, for patients to make decisions regarding particular interventions or procedures out of the context of particular health circumstances and without addressing expected outcomes. Conversations with patients should instead focus on eliciting general goals and values that can be translated into particular decisions. Open-ended questions may include the following: "How do you think about balancing quality of life with length of life?," "What are the things that give your life meaning day-to-day?," "Would there be any circumstances under which you would find life not worth living?," and "What do you consider your quality of life to be like now?"

In the hospital setting, it is frequently necessary to assist patients and surrogates in translating their goals and values into treatment decisions. Decisions regarding CPR, invasive mechanical ventilation, and feeding tubes are frequently important in the hospital setting. Once the physician has assessed the patient's or surrogate's goals and values, he or she may then present specific treatment options. The physician may assist patients and surrogates in the decision-making process by explaining the treatment options at hand, describing likely outcomes based on the patient's condition, and exploring how acceptable these treatments and outcomes may be based on the patient's expressed goals and values. See case example.

■ STEP 3: IDENTIFY OPPORTUNITIES TO IMPROVE LONG-TERM HEALTH OUTCOMES

The Boy Scout motto "try and leave this world a little better than you found it" translates well to the physician's role in caring for a frail hospitalized patient. Although most physicians are aware of the

TABLE 169-2 Step 2: Strategies to Prevent Adverse Outcomes for the Fragile Patient

Strategy	Physician Interventions	Interventions by Other Disciplines	Potential Quality Improvement Targets
Prevent delirium	Assess and monitor mental status daily Assess for malnutrition and dehydration Avoid immobilizing devices (eg, indwelling urinary catheters, intravenous lines, cardiac monitors) Avoid drugs that may trigger delirium	Make adaptations for vision and hearing impairment (nursing, audiology) Maintain nutrition and hydration, including hand feeding when necessary (dietician, nursing)	Reduction of urinary catheter use
Maintain mobility and avoid fall-related injury	Assess baseline function (ADL/IADL) and reassess mobility/function daily Avoid immobilizing devices (eg, indwelling urinary catheters, intravenous lines, cardiac monitors) Order OT/PT Avoid standing medication orders for sleep, anxiety, agitation Avoid drugs that are inappropriate for the elderly	Mobilize early (nursing, OT/PT) Provide appropriate assistive devices (OT/PT) Have patient walk to toilet every 2 hours during the day (nursing) Lower mattress height to height of mattress at home (nursing)	Physical and occupational therapy within first 24 hours Reduction of physical restraint use
Minimize psychoactive medications	Avoid standing prescriptions for sleep, anxiety, agitation Avoid drugs that are inappropriate for the elderly Review and reduce medications regularly	Use nonpharmacologic approaches for sleep, anxiety, agitation (nursing) Review medications for potential errors or interactions (pharmacist)	Reduction of benzodiazepine use
Prevent pressure ulcers	Examine skin and order appropriate wound care Avoid immobilizing devices	Monitor skin (nursing) Provide pressure-relief, including appropriate mattresses (nursing) Maximize nutrition (dietician, nursing) Mobilize early (nursing, OT/PT)	Reduction of hospital-associated pressure ulcers
Address advance care planning	Assess capacity for discussion of advance care planning Establish goals of care with patient or surrogate; readdress upon changes in health condition; initiate family meetings when needed Identify proxy	Complete or update advance directives when necessary (social work) Participate in interdisciplinary family meetings to establish goals of care (social work, nursing)	Increased documentation of advance care planning discussions Increased incidence of advance directives

ADLs, Activities of Daily Living; IADLs, Instrumental Activities of Daily Living; OT, occupational therapy; PT, physical therapy.

potential for hospital-associated harm, the potential opportunities for promoting long-term health in the hospital setting may be less obvious. **Table 169-3** lists five areas of health promotion for fragile hospitalized patients. With just a small amount of extra attention, physicians may be able to discharge patients home with safer medication regimens, greater home supports, and better symptom control compared to pre-hospitalization.

Many of the health promotion strategies listed in Table 169-3 aim to improve longer-term function outcomes and quality of life. Hospital physicians may, for example, identify and treat potentially reversible frailty conditions such as depression, weight loss, and falls; and they may initiate treatment for chronic symptoms such as pain or dyspnea. Physicians may also employ strategies to help patients maintain their health at home and reduce the risk of medical error. In addition to avoiding the prescribing of new potentially harmful medications, hospital physicians should review patients' chronic medication list for potentially harmful medications.

Hospitalization provides a key opportunity to identify older patients who will benefit from increased home supports. Initiating appropriate referrals for home health aides, adult day health, or home-delivered meals, for example, may provide the additional support a fragile older patient needs to remain independent and avoid hospital readmission and institutionalization.

DISCHARGE PLANNING

STEP 4: IMPLEMENT A SAFE AND THOROUGH DISCHARGE PLAN

The fragile patient requires special planning and precautions upon discharge. **Table 169-4** outlines the major tasks for promoting a safe and effective discharge plan.

The first two steps of discharge planning involve reassessment of clinical stability and patient function. Once the patient is clinically stable and functional status has been reassessed, the physician will determine the patient's need for any skilled nursing or rehabilitation services. A patient hospitalized for hip fracture, for example, will require physical and occupational therapy. Rehabilitation services may be provided in a rehabilitation hospital, a community nursing home or at home, depending on the patient's condition, living

TABLE 169-3 Step 3: Opportunities to Improve Long-term Health Outcomes

Treat conditions that contribute to frailty
1. Depression: listen to concerns, inform about support groups and centers, and consider selective serotonin-reuptake inhibitors and/or psychotherapy
2. Weight loss: liberalize diet, recommend small frequent feedings, consider nutritional drinks, address oral care and denture problems, and inquire about food access
3. Falls: eliminate psychotropic or other implicated medication, treat underlying conditions such as vision impairment or pain, counsel on home safety or refer for home safety inspection, consider referral for physical therapy, treat osteoporosis
Treat symptoms
Assess for pain, dyspnea, and other bothersome symptoms
Offer pharmacologic treatment, eg, acetaminophen or opioids
Offer nonpharmacologic treatments, eg, energy conservation techniques for dyspnea
Reduce medications
Eliminate potentially harmful classes of medications, eg, benzodiazepines and anticholinergic medications
Examples of specific potentially harmful medications: • Avoid meperidine; replace with alternative opioid • Avoid amitriptyline and imipramine; replace with nortriptyline or desipramine (less anticholinergic) • Identify medications causing side effects
Maximize home supports
Offer community services such as home health aides, adult day health, case management
Identify patients meeting hospice criteria and offer home hospice service
Address advance care planning
Identify surrogate decision maker
Establish goals of care
Provide legal forms (living will, durable power of attorney for health care, or do-not-resuscitate)

situation, and insurance. Medicare provides payment for short-term rehabilitation services in hospital, nursing home, and home settings. Similarly, if a patient has skilled nursing needs such as short-term antibiotics or dressing changes for a wound, these services can be provided in the home or nursing home settings and paid for under the Medicare benefit.

Patients with active delirium are generally considered stable for discharge only after clinical triggers have been identified and treated and once there is evidence of improvement. The physician, with help from physical and occupational therapy, must reassess functional status when planning for discharge. Functional assessment should focus on ability to ambulate, transfer, and bathe independently. When planning a home discharge plan, physicians must consider home characteristics such as whether the patient will need to negotiate stairs. Occupational therapists can help determine whether a frail patient returning home will benefit from home safety equipment such as a bedside commode or bathroom grab bars.

Transitions of care, particularly those between hospital discharge and home or long-term care setting, are frequently associated with medical error due to poor communication. For patients returning home, physicians should provide detailed

TABLE 169-4 Step 4: Discharge Planning

Task	Physician's Role
Assess clinical stability	Assess for fever, uncontrolled hypertension or hypotension, and delirium
Reassess functional status	Reassess patient's Activities of Daily Living, with particular emphasis on ability to walk, bathe, and transfer independently
Identify needs for skilled services	Work with social worker to make appropriate referrals, eg, home care agency for rehabilitation services or skilled nursing, hospice care
Identify place of discharge	Elicit goals and preferences from patient (or surrogate) Recommend appropriate level of care, eg, skilled nursing facility versus home options, based on available home supports, needs for rehabilitation services, and patient preferences
Provide discharge instructions	Communicate clearly with patient and/or caregivers regarding discharge medications, follow-up appointments, and how/whom to contact for health-related concerns

information to patients and caregivers regarding medication changes. Patients and caregivers should be provided detailed information about follow-up appointments and when and whom to call for health concerns.

QUALITY IMPROVEMENT TO ADDRESS PERFORMANCE GAPS

There are numerous opportunities for quality improvement interventions in the care of frail hospitalized patients. Quality improvement initiatives are most effective when they are led by invested individuals, when there is "buy-in" from the involved team members, and when they target meaningful outcomes that are measurable.

Table 169-2 describes five important strategies for avoiding adverse outcomes in frail older patients. The third column outlines one to two quality improvement opportunities for each of these strategies. All of the targets listed are measurable and may serve as markers of quality care processes. For example, measuring and reducing the prevalence of physical restraint and urinary catheter reflect safe care practices.

Early mobilization of frail older patients may be measured in a variety of ways, including by the presence of a physical or occupational therapy assessment within the first 24 hours of admission. Quality improvement interventions targeting a decreased rate of hospital-associated pressure ulcers and decreased prescribing of potentially inappropriate medications, eg, benzodiazepines, may also lead to improved patient safety.

Lastly, quality improvement efforts to improve advance care planning in the hospital may lead to improved patient outcomes, specifically increasing the chance that patients' goals and wishes will be known and honored at the end of life. An increase in documented advance care planning discussions and incidence of completed advance directives are potential quality improvement targets for frail older patients.

CONCLUSION

The health care team should recognize important factors associated with frailty and intervene to reduce the hazards of hospitalization for this vulnerable population. This assessment begins with asking the right questions on hospital admission for each patient at risk: Is this patient frail? What key strategies can be implemented to prevent adverse outcomes? Are there any opportunities to improve long-term health outcomes? What steps should be taken to implement a safe and thorough discharge plan? Hospitalists should also try to improve hospital care for all frail elders by engaging in quality improvement initiatives that establish process measures, measure outcomes, and develop performance targets.

SUGGESTED READINGS

Boockvar KS, Meier DE. Palliative care for frail older adults. *JAMA*. 2006;296(18):2245–2253.

Caring for the Hospitalized Elderly: Current Best Practice and New Horizons. *A Special Supplement to The Hospitalist*. 2004. http://www.hospitalmedicine.org/AM/Template.cfm?Section=The_Hospitalist&Template=/CM/ContentDisplay.cfm&ContentFileID=1447

Inouye SK, Brown CJ, Tinetti ME. Medicare Nonpayment, hospital falls, and unintended consequences. *N Engl J Med*. 2009;360(23): 2390–2393.

Inouye SK. A multicomponent intervention to prevent delirium in hospitalized older patients. *N Engl J Med*. 1999;340(9): 669–676.

Inouye SK. A practical program for preventing delirium in hospitalized elderly patients. *Cleve Clin J Med*. 2004;71(11): 890–896.

Landefeld CS. Improving health care for older persons. *Ann Intern Med*. 2003;139(5):421–424.

Messinger-Rapport BJ, Baum EE, Smith ML, et al. Advance care planning: beyond the living will. *Cleve Clin J Med*. 2009;76(5): 276–285.

CHAPTER 170

Incontinence

Alayne D. Markland, DO, MSc
Catherine E. DuBeau, MD

Key Clinical Questions

1. What are the prevalence and impact of urinary and fecal incontinence in the inpatient setting?
2. What are the causes and mechanisms of urinary and fecal incontinence in hospitalized adults?
3. Which serious underlying diseases or conditions can present with urinary or fecal incontinence?
4. What are the common causes of urinary retention in hospitalized patients?
5. Which tests and studies are most useful in the evaluation of urinary and fecal incontinence in the hospital setting?
6. What treatments are available for urinary and fecal incontinence?
7. What are the treatments for urinary retention in hospitalized patients?
8. What are the guidelines for urinary catheter use and management in hospitalized patients?
9. What are the important elements of incontinence management in transitions of care?

INTRODUCTION AND EPIDEMIOLOGY

Urinary incontinence (UI) is a common condition that increases with age and affects up to one-third of community-dwelling persons. Although fecal incontinence (FI) is less prevalent, two-thirds of patients with FI also have urinary UI (dual incontinence); only about 20% of patients with UI have dual incontinence. In the hospital setting both UI and FI may coexist with urinary retention (UR). Relatively few studies have addressed the prevalence of both types of incontinence in acute care settings. It has been estimated that 22% to 35% of patients on general medical wards have UI and the prevalence of FI is 10% in acute care settings.

Although incontinence care is often delegated to nursing staff, failure to recognize, evaluate, and treat incontinence and UR as significant "hazards of hospitalization," especially in older patients, can increase morbidity and functional impairment and increase length of stay. Incontinence can cause skin breakdown, pressure ulcers, increased use of indwelling catheters, and falls. Catheter-associated urinary tract infection (CAUTI) is a "never event" that impacts reimbursement as well as quality of care. Poor quality incontinence management also increases costs from absorbent and containment products, increased use of already limited resources (eg, nursing and aide time), and can lead to increased caregiver burden after discharge.

PATHOPHYSIOLOGY OF INCONTINENCE AND URINARY RETENTION

Normal micturition and defecation involve similar neural control and muscular coordination. Efferent nerves arising from the sacral micturition center at S2–S4 mediate bladder muscle (detrusor) contraction via muscarinic receptors. Contraction of smooth muscle in the proximal urethral and internal anal sphincters is medicated by sympathetic, adrenergic nerves arising from T11-L2. The distal urethral sphincter and the external anal sphincter are voluntarily controlled via somatic cholinergic nicotinic nerves arising from the sacral micturition center. Urethral and anal closure are also maintained through contraction and support from striated muscle and fascial elements in the pelvic floor. Coordination of bladder filling and emptying is controlled by a micturition center in the pons linked to subcortical and frontal pathways that inhibit voiding. Less is known about neurological control of defecation, although similar mechanisms have been proposed that coordinate relaxation of the external anal sphincter with the change of the ano-rectal angle with valsalva. Normal defecation also depends on stool consistency (affected by diet and colonic transit time), rectal compliance and sensation (ability to retain stool in the rectum and delay defecation until socially appropriate), and integrity of the internal and external anal sphincters and the puborectalis muscles.

Especially relevant in the hospital setting, urinary and fecal incontinence also can result or be exacerbated by impaired functional (mobility, manual dexterity) and cognitive status, and the presence of comorbid conditions (**Table 170-1**) and medications (**Table 170-2**) that can directly or indirectly affect neural and muscular control of micturition and defecation. Recognition and management of these potentially remediable factors are essential for effective incontinence treatment. Procedures and monitoring in the acute care setting can also impact continence status (**Table 170-3**). Imposed bed rest makes toileting impossible, and predisposes to impaired bladder emptying and constipation that can lead to dual incontinence.

TABLE 170-1 Comorbid Conditions Causing or Exacerbating Urinary and/or Fecal Incontinence

Comorbidity	Effect on Continence
Cardiovascular disease	
Acute coronary syndrome	Altered mental status
Congestive heart failure	Nocturnal polyuria; treatment with loop diuretics
Metabolic disease	
Diabetes mellitus	Osmotic diuresis from hyperglycemia, altered mental status from hyper- or hypoglycemia, urinary retention from constipation, gastroparesis, neuropathy
Hypercalemia	Diuresis, altered mental status
Vitamin B12 deficiency	Impaired bladder sensation, peripheral neuropathy
Thyroid disease	Changes in cecal transit time from hypo- or hyperthyroidism
Neurologic disease	
Cerebrovascular disease, stroke	Upper motor neuron disease with impaired bladder sensation, acutely impaired physical function and cognition
Seizures	Acute loss of motor control/sphincter impairment
Delirium	Impaired cognitive function
Dementia	Impaired cognitive function
Parkinson disease	Impaired CNS control, impaired physical function, constipation
Spinal cord injury or impairment	Dependent on level: suprasacral—uninhibited contractions and dyssynergia between bladder and sphincter contraction; sacral—impaired detrusor contractility, sphincter incompetence
Psychiatric disease	
Affective disorders, psychosis	Decreased motivation; cognitive impairment
Alcoholism	Functional and cognitive impairments; acute intoxication: diuresis, diarrhea, urinary retention
Gastrointestinal disease	
Constipation	Urinary retention, impaired urgency sensation, impaction
Diarrhea (infectious causes)	Increase in rectal volume, impaired ability to voluntarily contract external anal sphincter
Malabsorptive syndromes	Loose stool, increased bowel frequency
Inflammatory bowel disease	Stool consistency changes, altered recto-anal anatomy, reduced rectal storage capacity
Others	
Musculoskeletal disease	Functional impairment, detrusor overactivity from cervical myelopathy in rheumatoid arthritis and osteoarthritis
Peripheral venous insufficiency	Nocturnal polyuria
Pulmonary disease	Exacerbation of stress incontinence and fecal leakage with chronic cough

Adapted, with permission, from DuBeau CE. Incontinence. In: Pompei P, Murphy JB, eds. *Geriatric Review Syllabus*. 7th ed. American Geriatric Society.

TABLE 170-2 Medications Associated with Urinary and Fecal Incontinence

Medication	Effect on Continence
Alcohol	Frequency, urgency, sedation, delirium, immobility, change in stool consistency
Alpha-adrenergic agonists	Outlet obstruction (men)
Alpha-adrenergic blockers	Stress leakage (women)
Angiotensin-converting enzyme inhibitors	Associated cough worsens stress and urge leakage in persons with impaired sphincter function
Antibiotics/antifungals	Increased gastrointestinal side effects, including diarrhea
Anticholinergics	Impaired emptying, retention, delirium, sedation, constipation, fecal impaction
Anticholinesterase inhibitors	Increased gastrointestinal side effects, including diarrhea
Antipsychotics	Anticholinergic effects, rigidity, and immobility
Calcium channel blockers	Impaired detrusor contractility and retention, constipation, dihydropyridine agents increase pedal edema and may lead to nocturnal polyuria
Cholinesterase inhibitors	Urge incontinence
Colchicine	Increase in bowel frequency, diarrhea
GAGAnergic agents (gabapentin, pregablin)	Pedal edema leading to nocturia
Loop diuretics	Polyuria, frequency, urgency
Narcotic analgesics	Urinary retention, fecal impaction, sedation, delirium
Nonsteroidal anti-inflammatory drugs	Pedal edema leading to nocturnal polyuria, constipation
Nonsulfonurea glucose-lowering drugs (metformin)	Alterations in stool consistency
Osmotic laxatives (lactulose, polyethylene glycol)	Diarrhea
Sedative hypnotics	Sedation, delirium, immobility
Thiazolidinediones	Pedal edema leading to nocturnal polyuria

Adapted, with permission, from DuBeau CE. Incontinence. In: Pompei P, Murphy JB, eds. *Geriatric Review Syllabus*. 7th ed. American Geriatric Society.

UI is typically classified into four main symptom types: urge, stress, mixed, and impaired bladder emptying (formerly called "overflow") (**Table 170-4**). Hospitalized patients are at risk for uncommon causes of UI, particularly extra-urethral urine leakage from vesico-vaginal or vesico-rectal fistulas.

The main types of fecal leakage are urge (associated with urgent need to pass stool), passive (without sensation), or seepage (low volume staining in underwear). Iatrogenic changes in stool consistency are major causes of hospital incontinence. Constipation and impaction can cause UI by impairing bladder emptying by mechanical obstruction and/or a reflex sympathetic stimulation. They also cause FI when watery stool "leaks" around impacted stool. Impaction in the rectal canal also can impair afferent sensations of bladder and rectal

TABLE 170-3 Other Hospital-Acquired Causes of Urinary and Fecal Incontinence

Causes	Impact on Continence
Prolonged use of transurethral catheters	Stress UI from urethral damage; urge UI from bladder irritation
Prolonged use of rectal tubes	Fecal incontinence (urge and passive types) due to weakness in anal sphincters
Epidural or spinal anesthesia	Urinary retention, UI and FI from interruption of efferent and afferent pathways
Decreased mobility from physical or chemical restraints, Foley catheters, IV lines, casts, etc	Limit toilet access leading to UI and FI

UI, urinary incontinence; FI, fecal incontinence.

TABLE 170-5 Common Causes of Urinary Retention in Hospitalized Patients

Mechanical	Neurogenic	Medications
Stool impaction Catheter obstruction (eg, blood clot, twisted catheter)	Acute cauda equina syndrome Sacral/subsacral spinal cord injury Bed rest Sacral herpes zoster Urinary tract infection Bladder overdistention from rapid diuresis	Anesthesia Opiates Anticholinergics (eg, phenergan, metoclopramide, antispasmodics)

fullness, leading to leakage without sensory awareness. Anal fissures, hemorrhoids, fistulas, and abscesses in close approximation to the anal sphincters can all lead to FI by impairing anal sphincter function. Large volume, watery diarrhea may cause FI by overwhelming the rectal capacity and voluntary anal sphincter contraction.

Urinary retention can be acute or chronic, and partial (patient may still void or leak urine) or complete (inability to void). Acute UR presents with a relatively sudden difficulty or inability to pass urine with suprapubic pain; bladder distention may not be evident by either palpation or percussion. Pain may be absent if sensory afferents are impaired (eg, with cauda equina syndrome). Chronic retention may be asymptomatic except for associated UI.

TABLE 170-4 Types of Urinary Incontinence

Type	Symptoms	Common Pathophysiology
Urge	Leakage associated with urgency, the relatively sudden and compelling need to void. Often coexists with urinary frequency and nocturia	Uninhibited bladder contractions due to • Increased afferent signaling from the detrusor and urothelium • Impairment in CNS inhibitory control • Interruption/damage to suprasacral spinal pathways • Idiopathic
Stress	Leakage with increased abdominal pressure (coughing, laughing, change in position, straining)	• Impaired urethral support • Impaired urethral closure
Mixed	Combination urge and stress symptoms	Combination urge and stress causes
Incomplete emptying	Elevated postvoiding residual Other symptoms nonspecific; may include dribbling, urgency, stress, stranguria	• Urethral obstruction • Weak or absent detrusor contractility • Combination of both

The causes of UR fall into three general categories: increased outflow resistance (mechanical or dynamic); interruption of detrusor sensory afferents or motor efferents; and decreased detrusor contractility (neurogenic, myogenic, or iatrogenic [medications]) (**Table 170-5**). UR is common after spinal or epidural anesthesia. Although prostate enlargement is common in older men and if advanced can cause outlet obstruction and chronic UR, acute UR is usually precipitated by other factors. Outlet obstruction in women is uncommon; when present, it is usually due with prior anti-incontinence surgery or marked pelvic organ prolapse.

EVALUATION

The basic evaluation for UI should include a focused history, physical examination, laboratory evaluation, and, less frequently, radiology tests (Table 170-5). Postvoiding residual (PVR) volume should be done in all hospitalized patients with acute UI or suspected retention. Risk factors for elevated PVR, in addition to medications (Table 170-2), include previous history of UR, new stroke, untreated UTI, hip fracture, fecal impaction, male gender, bedrest, and benign prostatic enlargement. There are no evidence-based criteria for "abnormal" PVR; in general, PVR >150 to 200 mL is considered clinically significant in men. Women may tolerate PVRs in this range without symptoms or morbidity; thus, PVR interpretation should be individualized. While it is reasonable to screen men with acute UR for hydronephrosis, the prior probability of hydronephrosis due to elevated PVR in women is very low, and upper-tract imaging is not necessary in the absence of new renal impairment.

Urinalysis should be interpreted with caution to avoid overtreatment of asymptomatic bacteriuria (see chapter on urinary tract infections), which is found in at least 20% of older women. Diagnosis of urinary tract infection requires relevant symptoms and/or positive urinary nitrite in addition to pyuria, bacteriuria, and leukocyte esterase. In catheterized patients, urine samples should be taken only from a newly placed catheter.

The basic FI evaluation is similar to that for UI, with particular focus on the perineal and anorectal exam. Further workup may include anoscopy, flexible sigmoidoscopy, or colonoscopy to rule out mucosal disease or for the evaluation of rectal bleeding.

The evaluation of urinary retention also is similar to that of UI and FI (Table 170-5). The gold standard for the diagnosis of outlet obstruction is urodynamic pressure-flow study; cystoscopy alone is nonspecific and insensitive. In hospitalized men, prostate specific antigen (PSA) testing is even less specific for prostate cancer, as PSA can be elevated by acute UR and urethral instrumentation/catheterization.

TREATMENT

Treatment of UI and FI in hospitalized patients begins with addressing contributing comorbidity, iatrogenic complications, and medications. General measures include removal of impediments that limit access to toilets or commode, regular nursing assistance to reach the toilet if needed, bedside urinals, condom catheters, and handheld urinals.

Urge UI can be treated with antimuscarinic agents (oxybutynin, darifenacin, tolterodine, solifenacin, trospium, fesoterodine). Adverse effects include dry mouth, constipation, and dyspepsia. Shorter-acting immediate-release formulations (available for oxybutynin and tolterodine) may be preferable in patients with preexisting constipation or at risk for impaired bladder emptying. Most patients with stress UI can be referred for appropriate gynecology or urology follow-up after discharge; however, inhospital neurology consultation should be considered if neurgogenic sphincter dysfunction is suspected. Treatment of UI with indwelling catheters should be reserved for only specific indications (**Table 170-6**). Clean intermittent catheterization has little role in the acute care setting.

TABLE 170-6 Evaluation of Incontinence in Acute Care

Focused history	• Acute vs chronic • Onset, duration, frequency, previous evaluation/treatment • Review of comorbid conditions, medications, mobility, access to toilet/commode • Review nursing assessment for bladder and bowel function • Fluid status—intravenous and oral
Physical examination	• General • Volume status • Abdomen (masses, suprapubic tenderness) • Neurological (motor strength, sensation) • Cognition (eg, MiniCog, Confusion Assessment Method; see Chapter 79: Delirium) • Bedside pelvic (check for significant pelvic organ prolapse, pain on bimanual exam) • Rectal (in all patients, check for impaction and masses; in patients with retention, check sacral nerve innervation by perineal sensation, sphincter tone, and anal wink* and/or bulbocavernosus reflex) • Perineal skin (dermatitis, cellulitis, pressure ulcers)
Laboratory	• Urinalysis • If diarrhea, consider stool studies appropriate to patient's condition (eg, *Clostridium difficile* antigen, ova and parasites, culture, fecal leukocytes, fecal fat) • Other: if chronic UR, consider vitamin B12 level; with chronic diarrhea or constipation, thyroid studies
Radiology	• Post-void residual volume (by bladder ultrasound, if available) • Abdominal KUB if constipation • Neurological and/or pelvic imaging if indicated by known or suspected comorbidity (eg, pelvic mass, new neurological deficits) • Indigo carmine or methylene blue testing if urinary tract fistula suspected

*To do anal wink, lightly scratch perineal skin lateral to anus and visually check for anal contraction; for bulbocavernosus reflex, lightly squeeze either the clitoris or glans and check for anal contraction (either visually or with finger inserted in rectum).

TABLE 170-7 Indications for Indwelling Urethral Catheters

Indication	Management
Acute urinary retention or obstruction	• Remove catheter as soon as possible (eg, after reversible causes identified and removed) • Arrange appropriate outpatient care following hospitalization
Accurate measurement of urinary output in critically ill patients	• Minimize time with catheter inserted • Remove catheter when alternative means of urinary collection are available
Perioperative use	• Urologic surgery or other surgery on contiguous structures in the genitourinary tract • Anticipated long duration surgery (with catheter removal in postanesthesia care unit) • Need for intraoperative urinary output measurement • Large volume fluids or diuretics during surgery
Stage 2 or greater open sacral or perineal wounds in incontinent patients	• To improve healing and reduce exposure to moisture
Comfort care at the end of life	• When goal is to improve quality of life for patient and caregivers

Adapted from the Centers for Disease Control and Prevention: Guidelines for Prevention of Catheter-Associated Urinary Tract Infections 2009. http://www.cdc.gov/ncidod/dhqp/dpac_uti_pc.html. Accessed April 1, 2010.

For acute retention, all patients should have bladder decompression with an indwelling catheter for several days while being treated for potentially remediable causes such as medications and impaction (**Table 170-7**). Catheters coated with silver alloys reduce asymptomatic bacteriuria in hospitalized patients requiring short-term urethral catheterization. A voiding trial without catheter should follow decompression. With the patient adequately hydrated, the catheter is removed (never clamped), and a PVR checked after the first void (or bladder volume checked if there is no void after about 6 hours). If the PVR is <100 to 150 mL, the catheter can stay out but the patient should have close follow-up—both in the hospital and after discharge—to ensure that retention does not recur. If the PVR remains high, the catheter should be reinserted while further evaluation and treatment of the inability to void continues. Patients who must leave the hospital with catheter in place should have a follow-up appointment within one week and another voiding trial attempted at that time.

Medications may expedite catheter removal in selected patients. Alpha-adrenergic antagonists (eg, terazosin, doxazosin, tamsulosin, alfuzosin) can be used for UR due to prostatic obstruction. 5-alpha reductase inhibitors (finasteride and dutasteride) are not useful in the acute care setting because of the delayed onset of treatment effect (up to 6 months). Methylnaltrexone (0.15 mg/kg of body weight) may be used for opioid-induced and possibly postoperative urinary retention. Bethanecol chloride is ineffective.

Management of FI with diarrhea may include medications (bulking agents and antidiarrheals); containment by absorbent products or external fecal collectors, bowel management systems, or diversion by rectal tube. Data on the efficacy and utility of most of these options in the acute care setting are limited. Diphenoxylate should be avoided because of potential drug interactions and cognitive changes. External fecal collectors are preferable to rectal tubes, which can damage anal sphincters continence and rectal mucosa, and block fecal passage as diarrhea resolves. They are contraindicated in patients with recent rectal or prostate surgery, recent myocardial infarction, rectal mucosal disease, clotting disorders, and impaired immune status. FI due to impaction is treated with laxatives and enemas; methylnaltrexone is effective for opiod-induced impaction.

Select patients may need further evaluation by a specialist in urology, gynecology, gastroenterology, colorectal surgery, or neurology depending on the type of incontinence and potential etiologies. Nurses specializing in wound, ostomy, and continence care are also a valuable resource in the acute care setting.

IMPLICATIONS FOR TRANSITIONS OF CARE

Incontinence management and treatment has implications for transitions of care to either home, skilled nursing facility, or acute rehabilitation. Medication reconciliation should consider possible drug interactions between previous or new bladder antimuscarinics and other medications at discharge. These drugs (with the exception of trospium and fesoterodine) are metabolized by CY34A and 2D6, with potential interactions with antifungals and macrolide antibiotics. Hospital-acquired deconditioning can greatly impact continence; discussion with the patient, family, and other care providers must anticipate and help with new home needs such raised toilet seats, bedside commodes or urinals, protective garments, adsorbent products, and skin care. If long-term catheter use is indicated, specific instructions for management and follow-up are needed for subacute care settings; nursing care should be arranged for patients returning home.

QUALITY IMPROVEMENT CONSIDERATIONS

Daily order renewal and review of indwelling catheter need have been implemented at hospitals for the reduction of catheter-associated urinary tract infection. Screening and recognition of a prior UI, FI, and UR history upon hospital admission is needed to identify hospitalized patients at risk for these conditions. Development of pharmacy reminders for medications that are associated with incontinence and UR among hospitalized patients may also help improve outcomes. Lastly, improvements in bowel regimens, especially for hospitalized patients on narcotics and at risk for constipation, are needed.

CONCLUSION

Impaired functional status and immobility, cognitive impairment, co-morbid conditions, and medications are potential remedial factors that can lead to incontinence in the hospital setting. Hospitalists are in a position to prevent, recognize, evaluate, and treat these "hazards of hospitalization" which can otherwise lead to increased morbidity, functional impairment, and cost of care, especially for elderly patients. Hospitalists should also try to improve hospital care for all vulnerable patients by developing hospital wide quality improvement initiatives that reduce iatrogenic complications such as incontinence.

SUGGESTED READINGS

Centers for Disease Control and Prevention. Guidelines for Prevention of Catheter-Associated Urinary Tract Infections 2009. http://www.cdc.gov/ncidod/dhqp/dpac_uti_pc.html. Accessed April 1, 2010.

Johnson JR, Kuskowski MA, Wilt TJ. Systematic review: antimicrobial urinary catheters to prevent catheter-associated urinary tract infection in hospitalized patients. *Ann Intern Med.* 2006:144(2):116–126.

McCormick KA, Scheve AA, Leahy E. Nursing management of urinary incontinence in geriatric inpatients. *Nurs Clin North Am.* 1988;23(1):231–264.

Ostaszkiewicz J, O'Connell B, Millar L. Incontinence: managed or mismanaged in hospital settings? *Int J Nurs Pract.* 2008;14(6):495–502.

Petrilli CO, Traughber B, Schnelle JF. Behavioral management in the inpatient geriatric population. *Nurs Clin North Am.* 1988;23(1):265–277.

Pfisterer MH, Johnson TM 2nd, Jenetzky E, et al. Geriatric patients' preferences for treatment of urinary incontinence: a study of hospitalized, cognitively competent adults aged 80 and older. *J Am Geriatr Soc.* 2007;55(12):2016–2022.

Saint S, Kowalski CP, Kaufman SR, et al. Preventing hospital-acquired urinary tract infection in the United States: a national study. *Clin Infect Dis.* 2008;46(2):243–250.

Schumm K, Lam TB. Types of urethral catheters for management of short-term voiding problems in hospitalised adults. *Cochrane Database Syst Rev.* 2004;(1):CD004013; PMID:14974052.

Sier H, Ouslander J, Orzeck S. Urinary incontinence among geriatric patients in an acute-care hospital. *J Am Med Assoc.* 1987;257(13):1767–1771.

CHAPTER 171

Polypharmacy in the Hospitalized Elderly

Emily R. Hajjar, PharmD, BCPS, CGP
Gina DeSevo, PharmD
Joseph T. Hanlon, PharmD, MS

Key Clinical Questions

1. What really defines polypharmacy?
2. What are the consequences of polypharmacy?
3. Who is at risk for polypharmacy?
4. How can clinicians reduce polypharmacy?

INTRODUCTION

Polypharmacy is most often defined in one of two ways: the use of multiple medications categorized by medication count or the use of unnecessary medications. Medication counts ranging from two to nine medications have been used to classify a patient as having polypharmacy. Lacking consensus about the specific medication count threshold, studies describing the occurrence of polypharmacy have chosen various numbers to operationalize their definition. As most elderly patients have multiple comorbidities requiring multiple medications based on established medical guidelines, this controversial definition fails to consider medication appropriateness. In fact, polypharmacy, measured by medication count only, may be appropriate to treat a patient with a number of medical conditions. The second definition of polypharmacy requires a review of medication appropriateness. Drugs deemed unnecessary include those that lack an indication or efficacy for a condition or therapeutically duplicate another medication, such as a prescription of a proton pump inhibitor for a patient with no history of peptic ulcer disease or a need for stress-ulcer prophylaxis. Few studies have evaluated this definition of polypharmacy despite its clinical relevance.

PREVALENCE OF MEDICATION USE

An in-home survey of 3005 participants of whom 58% ≥65 years of age reported that overall 94% of older adults took one or more medications and the average number of prescription medications was 3.6 per person. Over a third of men and women aged 75 to 84 years took ≥5 prescription (Rx) drugs. Moreover, nearly half of men and women ≥65 years of age reported the use of over-the-counter (OTC) drugs.

Table 171-1 lists the most common prescription and OTC drugs reported by gender. It is also important to note that 54% of older men and women reported use of dietary supplements.

Table 171-2 lists the most common dietary supplements reported by gender.

Hospitalized older adults have even higher medication use. Surprisingly, no national US data provide information about the epidemiology of drug use in hospitalized elders. One study of 834 older frail inpatients from 11 VA hospitals found that the average number of prescription drugs was 7.6 whereas the number of nonprescription drugs used was 2.6. This contrasts with a study from Ireland where the average number of medications was 5 per elderly hospitalized patient.

Table 171-3 lists the most common medications taken by older adults in a single US hospital. As a reflection of indications of hospitalization, hospitalized compared to community dwelling elders more commonly take opioid analgesics and antibiotics.

UNNECESSARY DRUGS

Few studies have measured the prevalence of unnecessary drug use in the elderly population and only one study has evaluated the prevalence of unnecessary drug use specifically in the inpatient setting. That study reported in a population of 384 frail hospitalized veterans aged 65 and older, 44% of patients had at least one unnecessary drug at time of discharge from the hospital. The reasons for a medication to be classified as unnecessary included lack of indication (33%), lack of efficacy (19%), and therapeutic duplication (8%). This study also noted that approximately 75% of those receiving an

TABLE 171-1 Most Common Rx and OTC Drugs Used by Community-dwelling Elders

Men	Women
Aspirin	Aspirin
Lisinopril	Levothyroxine
Hydrochlorothiazide	Hydrochlorothiazide
Atorvastatin	Atorvastatin
Simvastatin	Metoprolol
Metoprolol	Lisinopril
Atenolol	Acetaminophen
Amlodipine	Atenolol
Furosemide	Alendronate
Levothyroxine	Simvastatin
Metformin	Amlodipine
Warfarin	Furosemide
Acetaminophen	Metformin
Ezemibe	Conjugated estrogen

Data from Qato DM, Alexander GC, Conti RM, et al. Use of prescription and over-the-counter medications and dietary supplements among older adults in the United States. *JAMA*. 2008;300:2867–2878.

TABLE 171-2 Most Common Dietary Supplements Used by Community-dwelling Elders

Men	Women
MVI/min	MVI/min
Vitamin E	Calcium
Vitamin B	Vitamin C
Vitamin C	Vitamin E
Calcium	Chondroitin/glucosamine
K+ supplements	K+ supplements
Folic acid	Vitamin B
Chondroitin/glucosamine	Vitamin D
Omega-3 fatty acids	Folic acid
Saw palmetto	Omega-3 fatty acids

Data from Qato DM, Alexander GC, Conti RM, et al. Use of prescription and over-the-counter medications and dietary supplements among older adults in the United States. *JAMA*. 2008;300:2867–2878.

unnecessary drug were prescribed that medication prior to admission while the remaining 25% had an unnecessary drug started during hospitalization.

RISK FACTORS FOR POLYPHARMACY

Older adults are particularly at high risk for polypharmacy and for the adverse effects associated with polypharmacy. Factors associated with polypharmacy include multiple chronic medical conditions, use of multiple providers and multiple pharmacies, especially with lack of communication amongst these parties, frequent hospitalizations, lack of information on the effects of new drugs in the elderly and clear endpoints of therapy, and continued use of drugs without re-evaluation. One study of 523 elderly patients, ≥ 75 years of age in Finland, found that poor self-reported health, obstructive pulmonary disease, diabetes, depression, heart disease, and pain were significantly associated with polypharmacy (defined as six to nine drugs). Additionally, age 85 years and older, female gender, and moderately poor self-reported health were significantly associated with excessive polypharmacy (defined as 10 or more drugs). Several potential predictors of unnecessary drug use have also been identified. Although the associations were not statistically significant, in a study of 128 veterans age 60 years and older prescribed at least five medications per day, factors found to be associated with unnecessary drug use included white race, income less than $30,000 per year, number of prescription medications, and lack of belief in a "powerful other" for their health locus

TABLE 171-3 Most Common Medications Used by Hospitalized Elders

1. Warfarin	18. Atenolol	35. Metronidazole
2. Potassium	19. Levofloxacin	36. Allopurinol
3. Pantoprazole	20. Oxycodone	37. Captopril
4. Metoprolol	21. Acetaminophen/hydrocodone	38. Donepezil
5. Furosemide	22. Acetaminophen/propoxyphene napsylate	39. Temazepam
6. Digoxin	23. Lorazepam	40. Rofecoxib
7. Acetaminophen/oxycodone	24. Tamsulosin	41. Trimethoprim/sulfamethoxazole
8. Levothyroxine	25. Quinapril	42. Paroxetine
9. Nizatidine	26. Nitroglycerin	43. Azithromycin
10. Lisinopril	27. Alprazolam	44. Carvedilol
11. Clopidogrel	28. Gabapentin	45. Glyburide
12. Amlodipine	29. Zolpidem	46. Phenytoin
13. Prednisone	30. Hydrochlorothiazide	47. Spironolactone
14. Simvastatin	31. Losartan	48. Metformin
15. Atorvastatin	32. Citalopram	49. Mirtazapine
16. Isosorbide	33. Amiodarone	50. Sertraline
17. Diltiazem	34. Enalapril	

Data from Steinmetz KL, Coley KC, Pollock BG. Assessment of Geriatric Information on the Drug Label for Commonly Prescribed Drugs in Older People. *J Am Geriatr Soc*. 2005;53:891–894.

of control. In another study of 384 frail veterans aged 65 and older, nine or more medications and multiple prescribers significantly predicted unnecessary drug use.

CONSEQUENCES OF POLYPHARMACY

Polypharmacy is the most consistent risk factor for adverse drug reactions. Up to 16% of hospitalizations in older adults are due to adverse drug reactions (ADR). Moreover, between 10% to 20% of older hospitalized patients experience an ADR. Polypharmacy also increases the risk of functional status decline, and geriatric syndromes such as cognitive impairment, delirium, and falls.

Polypharmacy increases the risk of medication adherence problems, medication errors due to suboptimal prescribing due to inappropriate choice and drug interactions, and cost. A recent study reported that 49% of hospitalized older adults received one or more potentially inappropriate drugs (defined as those whose risk outweighs potential benefit). The use of one inappropriate medication of particular concern, diphenhydramine, can increase the risk of well-documented complications of hospitalization (delirium and falls) due to anticholinergic side effects. Clearly, the risk exceeds any potential benefit, because diphenhydramine has been shown to be ineffective sedative/hypnotic for older hospitalized adults and safer alternatives exist such as zolpidem which has a moderate half-life. The use of another inappropriate drug of concern for older hospitalized adults, propoxyphene, also frequently results in adverse effects, and an FDA advisory committee has recommended that this agent be removed from the market. Clearly, the risk exceeds any potential benefit, because a meta-analysis published over a decade ago showed that propoxyphene relieves pain no more effectively than acetaminophen alone and safer alternatives exist such as tramadol, a well-studied analgesic agent that is not a schedule II drug.

INTERVENTIONS TO REDUCE POLYPHARMACY

There have been few specific randomized controlled trials restricted to older hospitalized adults conducted to reduce polypharmacy. One study conducted by Schmader, et al, found that geriatric evaluation and management in older hospitalized veteran patients reduced the number of unnecessary medications compared to control patients. Owens, et al, found that adding a clinical pharmacist to a geriatric team resulted in fewer medications being added to intervention patients when compared to control patients. Another strategy of providing computerized decision support is effective in improving prescribing in general and may be most instrumental to improve the prescribing and monitoring of primarily renally cleared medications in older hospitalized patients. Finally, it cannot be stressed enough the importance of performing medication reconciliation and discontinuing medications started in hospital before discharge that do not address ongoing clinical problems that threaten quality of life/functional status of older adults.

QUALITY IMPROVEMENT

The first step to prevent or detect polypharmacy is to complete a thorough medication history upon hospital admission, including all prescription and non-prescription medications, vitamins, herbal products, and alternative therapies. Some OTC products such as ibuprofen or diphenhydramine may in fact contribute to the patient's hospital admission. Direct questions should include asking pointed questions about OTC drugs to prompt each patient to report the use of various products purchased on his own initiative. If a patient is unable to communicate which medications he is taking, the information should be obtained from the person who provides medications for the patient on a daily basis as well as from the patient's pharmacy.

The medication history should also evaluate medication adherence. When all medications are administered by the hospital staff, noncompliant patients may suffer adverse drug reactions due to an abrupt increase in dosage.

The second step evaluates whether each medication is truly necessary for the patient in the appropriate dosage.

- *Is each medication indicated for either an acute or chronic medical indication?* If yes, determine effectiveness, optimal dosage given the patient's current circumstances or whether an alternative new drug therapy is preferable. Some medical conditions in the elderly may no longer require medication therapy or the risks associated with drug therapy outweigh the potential benefits. If medication therapy is determined to be necessary, consider the drug's pharmacokinetic and side effect profile, the patient's renal and hepatic function as well as patient preference and formulary constraints for proper selection and dosing. Frequently, starting doses in the elderly are reduced and medications are administered in extended dosing intervals compared to younger patient's medication regimens in order to prevent toxicity from occurring. Health care providers must also consider concomitant medical conditions with medication regimens to avoid drug-disease or drug-drug interactions. Dosage adjustments may also be required as new drugs are added to the drug regimen.
- *If the drug does not have an indication for either an acute or chronic condition, was it prescribed to treat an adverse effect of another medication?* For many patients adding a second medication to manage the side effect of another medication unnecessarily complicates the patient's medication regimen. An example of this would be the use of a proton-pump inhibitor to control dyspepsia associated with bisphosphonate therapy. To avoid a prescribing cascade, determine the cause of any new symptoms which may result from previous drug therapy or from a medical condition.
- *Is the patient near the end of life?* Continuing drug therapy such as a statin in a dying patient is inappropriate as the patient's remaining life expectancy will not be changed by this medication class. Always consider time until onset of benefit, treatment goals, and life expectancy when starting or continuing medications as a patient nears the end of his or her life.
- *If you plan to discontinue a medication, does the drug require tapering rather than abrupt discontinuation?* Medications such as opioids and benzodiazepines require tapering to avoid withdrawal symptoms; antidepressants and corticosteroids to minimize a resurgence of the underlying condition, or in the case of corticosteroids to avoid creating a new problem, adrenal insufficiency. A hospital admission may be the ideal time to discontinue medications because it affords a setting where close monitoring can be conducted.
- *Are all underlying medical problems optimally treated with drug therapy according to established guidelines?* Medical conditions that have no associated medication should also be evaluated to see if additional therapy is needed to properly treat the patient.

The process of medication reconciliation helps to prevent polypharmacy. Reconciliation should be done whenever a patient is transferred between levels of care during a hospital admission, at hospital discharge, on nursing home admission, or transfer to independent living. Constant reevaluation of a patient's medication regimen at each transfer of care and communication with the patient's primary care physician can prevent the continuation of any unnecessary medications as well as those that may be omitted. For instance, stress-ulcer prophylaxis agents should be discontinued once a patient is no longer determined to be in an environment where a stress-ulcer may form. Formulary changes can also be addressed when the medication reconciliation process occurs to avoid duplication of medications upon return home. For example, a drug class such as an ACE inhibitor is likely continued during hospitalization but the specific drug may change due to reimbursement such as ramipril in one setting and lisinopril or captopril in the other. Discharge medications should be reconciled with admission medications so that the patient continues only one ACE inhibitor. A system should be in place to educate all patients not only about new medications but all medications—dosages, frequency, when to stop, and what medications should be discarded upon return home.

PRACTICE POINT

On admission, throughout hospitalization, and with any transition of care

- Determine whether drug side effects are responsible any new symptoms or exacerbating underlying medical conditions
- Establish clear and practical therapeutic goals and monitoring plans
- Review periodically medications and perform drug reconciliation with each transition, including screen for adverse drug reactions, therapeutic failures, and adverse drug withdrawal events
- Taper or discontinue ineffective or redundant or possibly harmful medications
- Minimize adverse effects by screening for drug–drug and drug–disease interactions before prescribing a medication to a patient
- Develop expertise in prescribing a few select drugs—the medication's dosing, therapeutic and adverse effects—to manage common problems in the elderly
- When in doubt, consult with a pharmacist

CONCLUSION

Polypharmacy commonly occurs in hospitalized older persons. While guideline adherence may necessitate the use of multiple medications, the use of unnecessary medications must be avoided to prevent negative patient health outcomes. Health care providers must be aware of inappropriate medications when managing the medication regimens of older patients and should adhere to the principles of geriatric pharmacotherapy when prescribing.

SUGGESTED READINGS

Hajjar ER, Cafiero AC, Hanlon JT. Polypharmacy in elderly patients. *Am J Geriatr Pharmacother.* 2007;5:345–351.

Holmes HM, Hayley DC, Alexander GC, Sachs GA. Reconsidering medication appropriateness for patients late in life. *Arch Intern Med.* 2006;166:605–609.

Montamat SC, Cusack B. Overcoming problems with polypharmacy and drug misuse in the elderly. *Clin Geriatr Med.* 1992;8:142–158.

Rochon PA, Gurwitz JH. Optimising drug treatment for the elderly: the prescribing cascade. *BMJ.* 1997;315:1096–1099.

Spinewine A, Schmader KE, Barber N, et al. Appropriate prescribing in elderly people: How can it be measured and optimized? *Lancet.* 2007;370:173–184.

Stewart RB. Polypharmacy in the elderly: A fait accompli? *DICP.* 1990;24:321–323.

CHAPTER 172

Hospital Discharge to the Nursing Home

Miguel A. Paniagua, MD, FACP
Christine Bradway, PhD, CRNP
Manuel A. Eskildsen, MD, CMD

Key Clinical Questions

1. What are the levels of care provided in skilled nursing facilities?
2. What types of interdisciplinary care services are provided at skilled nursing facilities?
3. What are the roles and responsibilities of hospital and facility providers in ensuring adequate transitions to and from the hospital?
4. What is the future of skilled care after hospital discharge?

INTRODUCTION

With the assistance of hospital interdisciplinary professionals, hospitalists plays an integral role in ensuring timely and efficient discharge planning for a spectrum of patients, including those who require skilled nursing or nursing home care. Having knowledge of both the level of care provided as well as the challenges in care transitions to these settings is imperative.

SKILLED NURSING FACILITIES: STRUCTURE AND TYPES OF CARE PROVIDED

Skilled nursing facility (SNF) or "subacute" care is provided mostly after an acute hospitalization, and consists of nursing or rehabilitative services that may not be practical on an outpatient basis, like intravenous injections and frequent physical therapy. These facilities are a common site for hospital discharge: 12% of all discharges in 2006 were to "long-term care and other facilities." Knowing about the types of services provided at SNFs is important for hospital-based physicians, as the scope and intensity of the care their patients will get after they are discharged to these facilities will differ significantly from that which they will have received in the hospital up to that point.

LONG-TERM VS SUBACUTE CARE

There are two major categories of patients in nursing homes: those who reside in the facilities and receive long-term care, and those who are admitted for SNF care, most often following hospitalization. These two groups differ in terms of their clinical features, as well as in the financing sources for their nursing facility stays.

Long-term care is the more traditional service provided in a nursing facility. These "residents," as they are called, when they stay in a nursing facility for the long term, receive custodial care and help with their Activities of Daily Living (ADLs), and have their medications administered to them by a nurse. Of note, elder caregivers' most common reasons for seeking placement are difficult-to-manage, dementia-related behaviors, as well as increased functional needs. Long-term care is not reimbursed by Medicare, so as a result, residents have to pay for their stays out-of-pocket, until the cost of their care exceeds their income ("spend down") to qualify for Medicaid, which does cover long-term nursing facility stays.

Skilled nursing facility care may be provided in freestanding nursing facilities or hospital-based units, though the trend has been toward freestanding community-based facilities. Hospital-based facilities made up only 7% of all SNFs in 2008, compared to 12% in 2000. These units provide services for posthospital stays, mainly for the purpose of rehabilitation, wound care, or other postacute care. Skilled nursing facility care is reimbursed by Medicare and many other private insurance programs, at a higher rate than Medicaid, which may explain the growth in this sector as a percentage of overall services provided at skilled nursing facilities.

Medicare provides coverage of up to 100 days after a medically necessary hospital stay of at least 3 consecutive days. The most common reason for SNF admission in 2006 was rehabilitation after orthopedic surgery, such as total hip replacement. The next most common diagnoses were congestive heart failure and pneumonia.

TABLE 172-1 Comparison Between Acute Hospital Services and Skilled Nursing Facility Care

Services Provided	Skilled Nursing Facility	Hospital
Physician Services	Physicians have a requirement to see patients at least monthly	Physicians see patients daily
Advanced practice nurses (APNs) and physician assistants	More present in the nursing facility	Physicians are less likely to rely on APNs
Nursing	Primarily licensed practical nurses (LPNs) with RN oversight, as well as nonlicensed (CNA) caregivers	Typically registered nurses (RNs)
Ancillary services (eg, blood drawing, laboratory testing, x-rays, ECG)	Rarely present on-site, and thus services are provided via contract arrangement	Usually on-site
Rehabilitation	Frequently emphasized more than medical care	Often only gets initiated after patient becomes medically stabilized

Data from Ouslander JG, Osterweil D, Morley J. Medical Care in the Nursing Home. 2nd ed. New York: McGraw-Hill; 1997.

Generally, the main purpose of a SNF stay is rehabilitation or other skilled nursing service (eg, wound care) to ensure the highest possible level of function in order to return to the previous living arrangement in the community. Skilled nursing facility care also differs from that which is provided in the hospital, as detailed in **Table 172-1**.

SKILLED SERVICES

The complexity of SNF care varies greatly throughout the country, from the provision of short-term rehabilitative services to returning long-stay residents to a facility, to more specialized facility programs, such as ventilator weaning. However, there are a core set of skilled services which generally merit reimbursement from Medicare or other payers.

These are

- Rehabilitation: The three main therapy disciplines which perform rehabilitative services at SNFs are physical, occupational, and speech therapy. Generally, therapists work with patients 5 to 7 days per week.
  - Physical therapy: Therapists work with patients on gait, balance, and lower extremity strength and mobility.
  - Occupational therapy: Activities include training on performing ADLs, as well as upper-extremity strength training.
  - Speech therapy: Diagnoses treated include dysphagia, as well as aphasia, especially in the context of acute or subacute neurologic disease (eg stroke).
- Wound care performed by nurses at least daily.
- Intravenous (IV) therapy: This may include simple IV fluids, as well as medications such as antibiotics.
- Provision of feedings in the context of a new percutaneous gastrostomy tube.
- Supervision of clinical conditions by nurses or physicians: Examples of this would include frequent laboratory monitoring, skilled nursing observation of congestive heart failure, and renal hemodialysis.

ROLES AND RESPONSIBILITIES

HOSPITAL TEAM

Understanding predischarge resources available can better ensure the hospitalist can facilitate a successful transition to the nursing home setting. Most hospital settings have a relatively large team of professionals from different disciplines who work together to provide acute care for complex, hospitalized older patients. An understanding of the importance of the team approach as well as an appreciation for other team members' roles is critical to good geriatric care. Team members that physicians regularly collaborate with include the following:

Therapist

Physical and occupational therapists and speech language pathologists are involved as indicated throughout the hospitalization in order to help determine what level of care and rehabilitation patients will need upon discharge. Indications for consultation of physical therapy include

- Change in functional status such as new loss of range of motion, sensory changes or focal weakness
- Altered weight-bearing status
- Falling or gait unsteadiness
- Need for walkers, canes, or crutches for ambulation or fabricated back braces
- Assessment of home discharge plan that may require physical therapy versus transfer to SNF

Indications for occupational therapy consultation include

- New upper-extremity weakness or sensory impairments
- Splinting or recommendations for adaptive equipment
- Management of edema
- Cognitive or safety issues
- New visual or perceptual impairments
- Impairment of ADLs
- Evaluation of home safety

Indications for speech and swallow consultation include assessment of aspiration risk due to

- Recurrent pneumonia
- Vocal cord paralysis
- Impaired speech or language
- Weight loss associated with eating more slowly
- Coughing during or soon after eating or drinking, or choking
- Wet sounding voice during or after eating and drinking

Social work

Social workers are usually involved from the time of hospital admission to provide support for patients and their families, and to work with other team members on an appropriate discharge plan. Indications for consultation with social workers include concerns about

- Elder abuse
- Ability to pay for medications
- Ethical issues

- Financial issues stemming from illness such as unemployment, lack of insurance, need for assistance to fill out forms for Medicaid, social security, or other government programs
- Access to community services

These team members have extensive training and knowledge of the continuum of home and community-based health services for older adults, health care systems, available resources, Medicare, Medicaid, and insurance reimbursement, and how patients' individual financial situations affect care needs. Social workers may also assess the patient's psychosocial and emotional needs and work with other team members to provide necessary hospital or postdischarge evaluation and treatment.

Nursing

Nursing staff play a key role in the care of hospitalized older adults. Nursing staff include licensed (registered nurses [RNs], licensed practical nurses [LPNs]), and unlicensed (certified nursing assistants [CNAs]) personnel who provide bedside care on a 24-hour basis for hospitalized patients. This includes complete or partial assistance with ADLs such as bathing, toileting, and eating; medication monitoring and administration; assessment and management of acute conditions in collaboration with physicians; and education of staff, patients, and family members. Nurses also work very closely with other team members to assure that individualized care, specific goals, and plans for discharge are met. This should involve including family caregivers (or in the case of patients admitted from a long-term care setting, the facility staff) early in care plan discussions and decision-making. In many hospitals, a nurse, social worker, or nurse/social worker team act as discharge planner or care manager and work with staff and families regarding posthospital care needs. Hospitalized older adults with a diagnosis of preexisting dementia are particularly at risk of developing serious comorbid disease and often have complex discharge planning needs requiring special attention.

TRANSITIONAL ISSUES IN DISCHARGES TO THE SKILLED NUR.SING FACILITY

Patients who are discharged from the hospital to a SNF incur many risks as their care shifts from one set of providers to another, frequently in the context of multiple chronic medical problems. These "care transitions," as they are known, increase the risks for adverse outcomes in these patients, partly due to the difficulties inherent in handing off the care of frail, ill patients from one care setting to the next when communication of all the details of patient care between sites is poor. Research into care transitions has shown that these communication problems frequently result in medication errors, as well as nonelective hospital readmissions.

When patients are transferred from hospital to SNF, physicians and nurses in the receiving facility require timely and accurate information in order to resume their care as seamlessly as possible (**Table 172-2**). Legible and accurate medication lists, as well as pertinent written or formal dictated discharge summaries of patients' clinical experiences in the hospital enable smooth care transitions. However, medication errors and medication gaps are frequent, sometimes leading to adverse outcomes.

TABLE 172-2 Roles of the Hospitalist in Discharge to Long-term Care

Assist with identification of a physician or provider who will care for the patient following hospital discharge. Do so as soon as discharge appears imminent
Consult with the nursing home physician or provider to assist in discharge/transfer planning if he or she is on the hospital staff
Call a physician or provider (if not on hospital staff) prior to transfer of the patient to discuss reason for hospitalization, hospital course, and established goals of care
Review and sign all transfer orders, and provide a contact number if questions arise concerning the transfer
Dictate a discharge/transfer summary at the time of discharge and request stat transcription so the summary may accompany the patient to the receiving facility

Data from Brechtelsbauer D. My patients arrive with poor documentation: how to handle tricky transition issues. *Caring for the Ages*. April 2005:26–27. http://www.amda.com/managementtools/bibliography/CFA4_05.pdf.

COMMUNICATION

Care transitions between the hospital and any other setting are fraught with communication problems, not just between providers and patients, but between different providers as well. Qualitative studies of interviews with patients and family members have revealed that family members are frequently not prepared to handle their role as caregivers in managing patients' medical problems, and do not feel like they have enough access to their health care providers in order to obtain appropriate support or information. Older adults who are ethnic minorities and recent immigrants are extremely vulnerable during transitions from one health care setting to another and communication may be adversely affected by the older adult's reliance on family and friends (rather than health care providers) for postdischarge information as well as linguistically inappropriate reading materials and services. As for SNF discharges, surveys have also shown that patients and caregivers feel that hospital providers do not adequately prepare them for what's involved in the transition, and that they do not transfer information appropriately across settings. These communication gaps make adverse outcomes from care transitions more likely.

Communication between providers is also important. The hospital discharge summary is a crucial element in the handoff between the sending and accepting provider which should contain the most relevant elements of the patient's hospital stay, and outline the plan of care from that point forward (**Figure 172-1**).

Unfortunately, the information sent to nursing facilities is frequently inadequate. A study of 300 consecutive transfers from hospitals to nursing homes in New York City found that discharge summaries were available 72% of the time, with clinical data often missing, and contact information for referring physicians present in less than half of cases. A systematic review of studies on hospital discharges found that discharge summaries frequently did not identify the responsible hospital physician, discharge medications, or the intended follow-up plan for the patient.

MEDICATION ERRORS

When patients are discharged from the hospital to skilled nursing facilities, gaps in communication and transcription can occur, resulting in threats to patient safety, including medication errors. One study of elder patients followed in the month after hospital discharge found that 20% reported adverse drug reactions. Another study of elder patients discharged home from the hospital found that 14% had at least one medication discrepancy.

The issues described previously with the potential loss of information in the transition from the hospital to the nursing home are not limited to communication lapses. In one pilot study, patients

Universal Transfer Form

AMDA has developed and recommends the use of the Universal Transfer Form (UTF) to facilitate the transfer of necessary patient information from one care setting to another. Patient transfers are fraught with the potential for errors stemming from the inaccurate or incomplete transfer of patient information. Use of the UTF can help to minimize the occurrence of such errors by ensuring that patient information is transmitted fully and in a timely fashion.

Patient's name: ____________ Patient Identifier #: ____________
Setting Discharged from: ____________ Patient's date of birth: ____________
Setting Discharged to: ____________ Patient's gender Male: ______Female: ____________
Attending physician in setting discharged from: ____________
Admission date: / / Discharge date: / /

A. Admitting diagnosis: ____________

B. Other diagnoses from this admission:
1.________ 4. ________
2. ________ 5. ________
3. ________ 6. ________

C. Current diagnoses prior to admission:
1.________ 4. ________
2. ________ 5. ________
3. ________ 6. ________

D. Surgical procedures and endoscopies during admission (include name of physician who performed the procedure) None __ Physician name: ____________
1.________ Date/results ________ (may attach)
2. ________ Date/results ________ (may attach)
3. ________ Date/results ________ (may attach)

E. Laboratory values (please record most recent results, with date)

WBC	/ /	_____	BUN	/ /	_____
Hgb	/ /	_____	Creatinine	/ /	_____
Na+	/ /	_____	CL	/ /	_____
K+	/ /	_____	CO_2	/ /	_____
Fasting glucose	/ /	_____	Other	/ /	_____

F. Results and dates of pertinent studies (radiology, CT, MRI, nuclear scans, etc.) (may attach)
1. ____________
2. ____________
3. ____________
Chest X-ray: Date performed:_______ Results: No active disease:______
Or description if abnormal:____________

G. Allergies:
Medication: ____________ Reaction:____________
Medication: ____________ Reaction:____________
Foods: ____________ Reaction:____________
Other: ____________ Reaction:____________

H. Admission weight_______ Discharge weight:________

I. Advance directives:

	Yes	No
CPR	__	__
Artificial Nutrition	__	__
Further hospitalization	__	__

Other: ____________
(Attach copies)

Figure 172-1 *Universal Transfer Form (UTF). (Reprinted with permission. Table 6. American Medical Directors Association. Transitions of Care in the Long-Term Care Continuum Clinical Practice Guideline. Columbia, MD: AMDA; 2010. Copyright © 2010 American Medical Directors Association, All rights reserved.)*

J. Has patient had a recent fall? Yes __ No__ Did the patient wander unsafe while hospitalized? Yes __ No__

K. Comments on inpatient course: (may attach narrative)

L. Is the patient aware of his/her diagnosis(es)? Yes __ No __
If No, why not? ______

M. Patient's cognitive status for decision-making:
___ Independent ____Modified independence (some difficulty in new situations)
___ Moderately impaired (decisions poor) ___Severely impaired (never/rarely makes decisions)

N. Is the patient a candidate for rehabilitation therapy? Yes __ No __
If yes, state goals for rehabilitation:

O. Discharge medication orders:
1.______ Rationale: ______
Dose ______ Route ______ Frequency ______

2. ______ Rationale: ______
Dose ______ Route ______ Frequency ______

3. ______ Rationale: ______
Dose ______ Route ______ Frequency ______

4.______ Rationale: ______
Dose ______ Route ______ Frequency ______

5. ______ Rationale: ______
Dose ______ Route ______ Frequency ______

6. ______ Rationale: ______
Dose ______ Route ______ Frequency ______

7.______ Rationale: ______
Dose ______ Route ______ Frequency ______

8. ______ Rationale: ______
Dose ______ Route ______ Frequency ______

9. ______ Rationale: ______
Dose ______ Route ______ Frequency ______

10. ______ Rationale: ______
Dose ______ Route ______ Frequency ______

11. ______ Rationale: ______
Dose ______ Route ______ Frequency ______

Figure 172-1 *(continued)*

P. Diet: ____

Q. Immunizations: Influenza: ___ Date: _____ Pneumococcal: ___ Date: _____
Tetanus -Diphtheria: ___ Date: ____
Tests: PPD: __ Results: __+/- __ Date: ____

R. Additional orders: ____

____

____

____

____

S. Follow-up on consults/tests/procedures recommended: ____________________

____

____

____

____

T. Is patient the primary decision maker? Yes __ No: __
If no, name of the substitute or surrogate:

____

Name of physician /designee completing form:____________________________
Contact phone number: ( ) _____-____________ Extension or beeper: ____________________
Date form completed: / /

Name of Primary Care Physician
Contact phone number: ( ) _____-____________ Extension or beeper: ____________________

Figure 172-1 *(continued)*

making the transition from hospital to nursing home (NH) experienced a greater than 12-hour delay in medication administration, and the mean number of missed doses of medications was three or more.

HOSPITAL READMISSIONS

Unsuccessful care transitions may also result in nonelective readmissions to the hospital after discharge. Hospital readmissions can set back the patient's goal of recovery and functional independence, and are also more costly for the health care system in general. They are also increasingly seen as a measure of the quality of care provided in the hospital setting. Even though most readmissions to the hospital are thought to be due to progression of patients' chronic illnesses, up to 48% of them are thought to be preventable. Readmissions to the hospital are common. One study of Medicare beneficiaries found that 19.6% of all patients admitted to the hospital were rehospitalized within 30 days, and that 67.1% of patients who had been discharged with medical conditions were rehospitalized or died within a year.

STRATEGIES FOR SUCCESSFUL HOSPITAL-SNF TRANSITION

Patient transfers from the hospital to the SNF are laden with the potential for errors stemming from the inaccurate or incomplete transfer of patient information. The timely transfer of information to receiving providers is also important. Transitional care has been defined as "care and services that promote the safe and timely transfer of patients from one level of care to another (eg, acute to sub-acute) or from one type of setting to another (eg, hospital to home)."

DISCHARGE SUMMARY

The key components of an effective summary for a SNF include the standard requirements of a typical hospital discharge. In addition, the inclusion of changes in diet, functional status as indicated by rehabilitation discipline assessments, and advance directives should also be included. More important is to ensure timely communication with SNF providers on the discharge diagnoses and plans (see Table 172-2).

DISCHARGE MEDICATIONS AND ORDERS

Any newly prescribed medications and concurrent medications changes from the prior medication list should be clearly documented prior to discharge or readmission to the SNF. This should include any skilled nursing needs there were not present prior to the hospitalization, such as wound care, intravenous fluids or medications, and specialized enteral feedings.

A "HAND-OFF" SUMMARY SHEET

A hand-off summary sheet is useful, particularly if the hospital discharge summary is to be delayed (due to dictation or transcription delays) that includes discharge diagnoses, brief hospital course, list of previous and new or changed medications. The American Medical Directors Association, the professional association of long-term care medicine practitioners and advocates, has developed a Universal Transfer Form (UTF) to facilitate the transfer of necessary patient information from one care setting to another (see Figure 172-1). Use of the UTF can help to minimize the occurrence of such errors by ensuring that patient information is transmitted fully and in a timely fashion.

THE FUTURE OF SNF CARE AFTER DISCHARGE

ADVANCED PRACTICE NURSES FOR TRANSITIONS

Successful models of interdisciplinary care where advanced practice nurses (APNs, nurse practitioners (nurse practitioners [NPs], and clinical nurse specialists [CNSs]) play key roles have been demonstrated for many years in nursing homes. Four workforce models that have been identified include the following:

- Model 1: APNs Employed by or contracted with primary care physicians or physician groups

- Model 2: APNs Employed by managed care organizations
- Model 3: APNs Employed directly by or contracted with a facility part-time or shared
- Model 4: Independent APN provider

In most cases, APNs supplement, rather than replace care given by the NH resident's primary care physician. In addition, the APN role often differs from the physician role as the APN may participate or take leadership in staff development, committee work, quality initiatives, and other aspects of the day-to-day work that occurs in the NH. Studies suggest that APNs in NHs act as collaborators, educators, counselors, communicators, clinicians, and care managers. Moreover, APN care has been found to be cost-effective, can prevent unnecessary emergency department visits and hospital admissions, and improves NH staff confidence.

For older adults and lay caregivers, transitions from one setting to another are filled with physical, emotional, environmental, and system factors that can result in unmet needs, dissatisfaction with care, and high rehospitalization rates. Since the early 1980s, models of care utilizing APNs have demonstrated numerous positive outcomes in easing transitions between hospital and home settings for vulnerable individuals, including frail patients. Within these models, APNs use a holistic approach to care that includes an in-depth understanding of health care systems, the ability to work with a wide variety of health professionals, and a focus on individualizing care, empowering patients and caregivers, anticipating outcomes, crossing barriers, and creating solutions.

Frail elders, including those admitted to the hospital from a NH or who require a SNF stay postdischarge, are particularly vulnerable during the transition from one setting to another. Although not yet formally tested, it seems likely that using highly skilled APNs in a future model targeting the transition to a SNF following hospital discharge may include similar elements of previous models and hopefully, result in similar positive outcomes. For example, a future model focused on the SNF environment might include the following:

1. An APN (with expertise in geriatrics and the long-term care environment) meets with the patient early on in the hospital stay and communicates regularly with hospital caregivers, SNF personnel, and family members to coordinate individualized hospital care and discharge plans.
2. Ideally, the same APN follows the patient after discharge and works with the SNF resident's primary care physician and other providers to assure that hospital discharge instructions are communicated, understood, and followed in a timely fashion.
3. The APN continues to provide SNF follow-up on a regular basis (early on, this might include numerous in-person visits to the SNF), is involved in resident assessment and management as necessary, educates SNF staff and family members on the resident's condition and plan of care as needed, and participates in SNF resident care conferences.
4. The APN uses his/her judgment to determine further resident, family, and SNF staff needs, is available by telephone 7 days a week to answer questions or help staff with decision making, and follows the resident until the resident is stable and risk of readmission is minimal.

Thus, proven strategies that have made the APN transitional care model work in other settings may also be congruent with the needs of patients and SNF staff, such as the focus on individualized care, an understanding of multiple health care settings, excellent clinical skills, and the ability to foster positive communication among a wide variety of professional caregivers, families, and patients. That said, it is also important to be aware of the differences between SNF and home settings and consider plans that incorporate additional, or in some cases, different skill sets and strategies as the model is tested and if the model is to be successful.

CONCLUSION

The hospitalist physician's role in ensuring successful patient discharge planning, including those who require skilled nursing or nursing home care is a crucial role on the care continuum. This includes ensuring the transfer of necessary patient information from one care site to another in addition to having knowledge of both the level of care and services provided in the diverse assortment of nursing home settings.

SUGGESTED READINGS

Coleman EA, Berenson RA. Lost in transition: challenges and opportunities for improving the quality of transitional care. *Ann Intern Med*. 2004;140:533–536.

Coleman EA. Falling through the cracks: challenges and opportunities for improving transitional care for persons with continuous complex care needs. *J Amer Geriatr Soc*. 2003;51:549–555.

Jencks SF, Williams MV, Coleman EA. Rehospitalizations among patients in the Medicare fee-for-service program. *N Engl J Med*. 2009 Apr 2;360(14):1418–1428.

Naylor M, Brooten D, Jones R, et al. Comprehensive discharge planning for the hospitalized elder: A randomized clinical trial. *Ann Intern Med*. 1994;120:999–1006.

SECTION 8

Hematology

CHAPTER 173

Abnormalities in Red Blood Cells

Madeleine Verhovsek, MD, BSc
Andrew McFarlane, MLT, ART

Key Clinical Questions

Anemia

1. How does peripheral blood smear aid in the diagnosis of anemia?
2. How do I interpret iron studies?
3. What are the best tests to diagnose hemolytic anemia?
4. How do I determine the cause of hemolytic anemia?
5. When should I investigate for hemoglobinopathy?
6. What factors suggest the need for bone marrow examination?
7. What is the most effective way to administer oral iron?
8. When and how should I use erythropoietin (EPO) in anemia of renal dysfunction or anemia of chronic disease? (How is it dosed and when should I expect a response?)

Polycythemia and Secondary Erythrocytosis

1. How do I distinguish primary and secondary erythrocytosis in a patient who smokes or has chronic lung disease?
2. When should I be concerned about carbon monoxide poisoning?
3. How do I manage secondary erythrocytosis?
4. What tests should I do to rule out a myeloproliferative disorder?
5. What complications can occur in patients with myeloproliferative disorders?
6. When is phlebotomy indicated?

(continued)

ANEMIA

INTRODUCTION

Anemia is one of the most common blood disorders worldwide and, in developed countries, commonly affects older adults. The primary function of a red blood cell is to deliver oxygen to the tissues. Red blood cells are made in the bone marrow and must contain adequate amounts of hemoglobin to perform this function. Normal production is dependent on the availability of the required "ingredients" (ie, iron, folic acid, vitamin B_{12}), a normal functioning bone marrow, and erythropoietin for stimulation of red cell production. Anemia can result from defects affecting hemoglobin production, dozens of disease states, including renal impairment and chronic inflammatory conditions, and may also be caused by other external or internal factors influencing the circulatory survival of red blood cells through premature destruction or blood loss. This chapter will provide a framework for investigation in order to navigate the many diagnostic tests and treatment options.

Anemia is defined as a reduction in the number of circulating red cells that results in a hemoglobin level lower than an age- and sex-matched population (**Table 173-1**).

In addition to the RBC count, hemoglobin, and hematocrit, which make the diagnosis of anemia possible, the complete blood count (CBC) provides essential information that helps tailor the investigation. One of the RBC indices, the mean corpuscular volume (MCV), permits classification of hypoproliferative anemias into hypochromic microcytic anemia (MCV < 80fl), normocytic anemia (MCV 80 to 100 fl), or macrocytic anemia (MCV > 100 fl). An increase in the reticulocyte count by 1% will increase the MCV by approximately 2 fl. The red cell distribution width (RDW) reflects the variation in RBC size or anisocytosis. Useful in distinguishing between certain hypoproliferative anemias, it is normally 11.5% to 14.5%. Normally between 0.5% and 2.5%, the reticulocyte count is calculated as a percentage of the total RBC; therefore, it must be corrected in the presence of anemia. The reticulocyte production index (RPI) is one method frequently used. The RPI = % reticulocytes × (patient Hct/45)/maturation time. With increasingly severe anemia, more reticulocytes are released from the marrow. The maturation time equals 1 if the patient's Hct is 45. Each 10-point drop in the patient's Hct increases the maturation time by 1.5 days. A low reticulocyte count suggests an underlying defect in RBC production; an elevated reticulocyte count suggests an underlying problem in RBC survival. Likewise, a RPI less than 2.5 suggests that the anemia stems from a hypoproliferative process; a RPI greater than 2.5 suggests that the anemia is due to bleeding or hemolysis. Examination of the peripheral smear may reveal morphologic abnormalities of the RBC that permit an accurate and timely diagnosis (**Table 173-2**).

PATHOPHYSIOLOGY

Although there are many causes of anemia, clinicians most commonly encounter iron deficiency anemia, thalassemia trait, and anemia of chronic disease.

Acute anemia results from bleeding or hemolysis. In someone who has been injured or who has suffered complications of surgery, the source of acute bleeding is normally clear. Hemolysis-related anemia due to increased destruction of red blood cells occurs by various mechanisms and can be broadly categorized as intrinsic red cell defects or extrinsic processes (**Figure 173-1**).

Key Clinical Questions

7. How frequently should phlebotomy be performed and what are the monitoring parameters?
8. Is there a role for antiplatelet agents and anticoagulants in patients with a myeloproliferative disorder?

Thalassemia and Hemoglobinopathies

1. Which hemoglobinopathies are considered to be clinically significant?
2. How is thalassemia differentiated from iron deficiency anemia?
3. When should one investigate for hemoglobinopathies?
4. When should transfusion therapy be considered?
5. What are the common complications in patients with thalassemia?

Sickle Cell Disease

1. What are triggers for admission in a patient with sickle cell disease?
2. What is appropriate hydration for acute chest syndrome or painful crisis?
3. What clinical presentations benefit from red blood cell transfusion or red cell exchange?
4. What is an appropriate transfusion threshold?
5. How is pain optimally managed?
6. What are special considerations in management of sickle cell disease in pregnancy or in labor?
7. What are special considerations perioperatively?
8. When should hydroxyurea be used?

Internally, problems of the red cell membrane (hereditary spherocytosis), the hemoglobin (eg, sickle cell anemia) or the deficiency of glycolytic pathway enzymes [glucose-6 phosphate dehydrogenase (G6PD) and pyruvate kinase (PK)] result in shorter life span. External mechanisms can be further classified as immune mediated or nonimmune resulting from infection, drugs, or mechanical injury. Hemolysis can occur intravascularly or extravascularly (ie, via the reticuloendothelial system), although many times it may be difficult to determine the site of cell destruction due to overlap in overwhelming acute cases.

The differential diagnosis of chronic anemia, whether microcytic, normocytic, or macrocytic, is broad. One of the most common causes of chronic blood loss is occult blood loss, particularly from the GI tract, or in younger women through menses, leading to iron deficiency anemia. Once the bone marrow receives the signal from erythropoietin, it requires building blocks from which to assemble the components of the red blood cell. Iron deficiency is one of the most common causes of anemia, often due to dietary deficiency or occult blood loss.

Underproduction of RBC results from a number of chronic diseases. The bone marrow, which produces the majority of red cells, relies on erythropoietin secreted by the kidneys to signal the need for new red blood cell production. In renal impairment, a decreased erythropoietin level leads to chronic anemia. In bone marrow failure states, underproduction may be caused by a decrease of precursor cells (eg, aplastic anemia, pure red cell aplasia), crowding out of normal RBC precursors by malignant cells (eg, leukemia, metastatic cancer) or abnormal maturation (eg, myelodysplastic syndrome, vitamin B_{12}, or folate deficiency). Inflammatory conditions can also cause chronic anemia by a combination of mechanisms due to proinflammatory cytokines that produce a "functional" iron deficiency in which iron is trapped in storage (eg, inside macrophages) instead of being available for hemoglobin production, abnormal proliferation of RBC progenitors in the bone marrow, insufficient erythropoietin, and reduced RBC life span.

TABLE 173-1 World Health Organization's Hemoglobin Threshold used to Define Anemia

Age or Gender Group	Hb Threshold (g/dl)
Children (0.5–5.0 yrs)	11.0
Children (5–12 yrs)	11.5
Children (12–15 yrs)	12.0
Women, nonpregnant (> 15yrs)	12.0
Women, pregnant	11.0
Men (> 15yrs)	13.0

DIAGNOSIS: HOW DO I DETERMINE THE CAUSE OF ANEMIA?

A complete blood count (CBC) is the backbone for the evaluation of anemia. The World Health Organization (WHO) defines anemia in an adult as a hemoglobin < 13g/dL for men and < 12 g/dL for women. A patient with chronic, mild, stable anemia can comfortably be evaluated in an outpatient setting. However, any patient with acute and/or severe anemia will benefit from the intensive investigations, monitoring, and treatment offered in the hospital. Anyone who is hemodynamically unstable due to blood loss should receive care in a monitored setting. After the diagnosis of anemia is confirmed, the next step is to determine why so that appropriate treatment can be administered (Figure 173-1).

Since the potential causes of anemia are numerous, a thorough and broad history should include query about:

- Any associated symptoms, in particular, bleeding (gastrointestinal, including melena, menses, hematuria) and constitutional B symptoms
- Past medical history, in particular, autoimmune/inflammatory disorder, chronic infection, liver disease, renal impairment, thyroid dysfunction, previous diagnosis, and treatment of anemia
- Medication history
- Social history, in particular, dietary intake, alcohol use, risk of sexually transmitted infections
- Family history of anemia
- Full review of systems, which may uncover symptoms of previously undiagnosed inflammatory disorders or organ dysfunction

Most prominent symptoms in severe anemia include fatigue, dizziness, palpitations, or breathlessness on physical exertion. Information about the onset of symptoms may help to determine whether the anemia is acute or chronic. The patient should also be questioned as to whether he or she has had a recent complete blood count.

PRACTICE POINT

- The average red blood cell survives for 120 days after it is released into circulation. If anemia is due to underproduction alone, the hemoglobin should decrease by less than 25% in a 30-day period (roughly 0.1g/dL per day).

TABLE 173-2 The Peripheral Smear

RBC Size and Hemoglobin Content		Etiology
Hypochromic microcytic anemia with 1. RDW > 15% 2. RBC < 4.6 x 10^{12} 3. Smear—anisocytosis, poikilocytosis	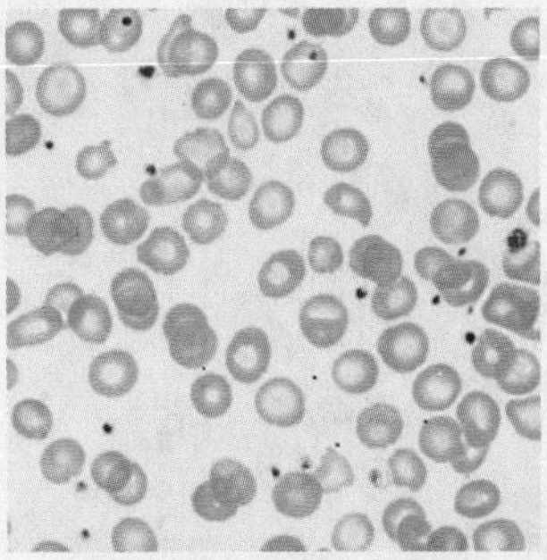	**Iron deficiency anemia** (low serum ferritin < 12µg/L; low iron, high TIBC, < 9% TS, high RDW) **Anemia of chronic disease** (normal/high ferritin, low serum iron, low TIBC, > 9% TS, normal RDW) **Sideroblastic anemia** (dimorphic population of hypochromic and normochromic cells, normal/high ferritin, high serum iron, normal TIBC, normal RDW)
Hypochromic microcytic anemia with 1. RDW < 15% 2. RBC > 4.6 x 10^{12} 3. Smear—uniform RBCs with basophilic stippling and target cells	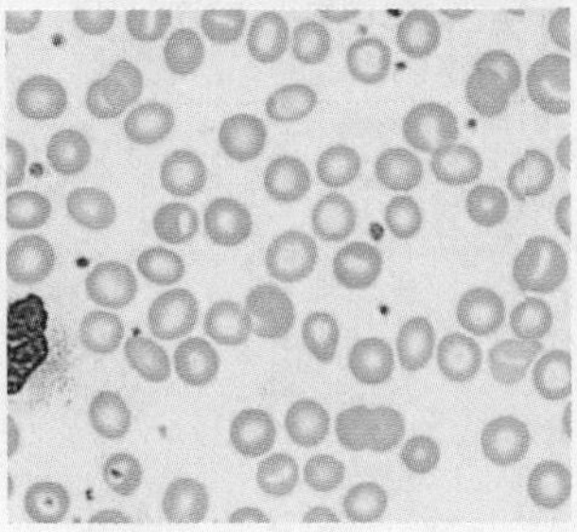	**Thalassemia** (normal/high ferritin, normal/high serum iron, normal TIBC, normal/high RDW—check Hb electrophoresis and Hb A_2 quantitation) **Anemia of chronic disease** (normal pattern, increased iron stores, < 15% ringed sideroblasts RS) **Aplastic anemia, myelofibrosis, anemia from metastatic cancer** (normal to increased iron stores, < 15% RS) **Refractory anemia with RS, lead poisoning** (> 15% RS)
Normochromic normocytic anemia with 1. Immature myeloid cells 2. Nucleated RBCs 3. Teardrop cells and/or 4. Elliptocytes	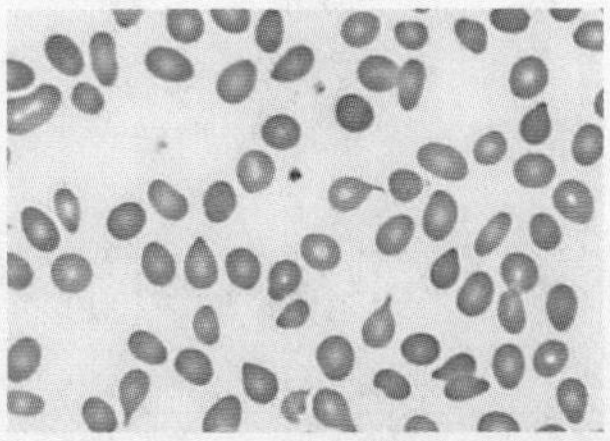	**Early iron deficiency** **Secondary BM failure; due to liver disease, hypothyrodism, immflamation or renal impairment**
Normochromic normocytic anemia without abnormal cells on smear	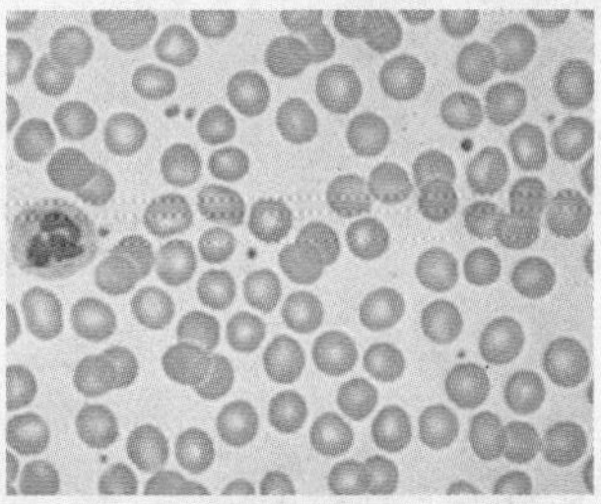	**Early iron deficiency** **Secondary BM failure from liver disease, hypothyroidism, inflammation, uremia**
Macrocytic anemia with hypersegmented neutrophils (one six-lobed nucleus or five-lobed nucleus in > 5% of neutrophils)	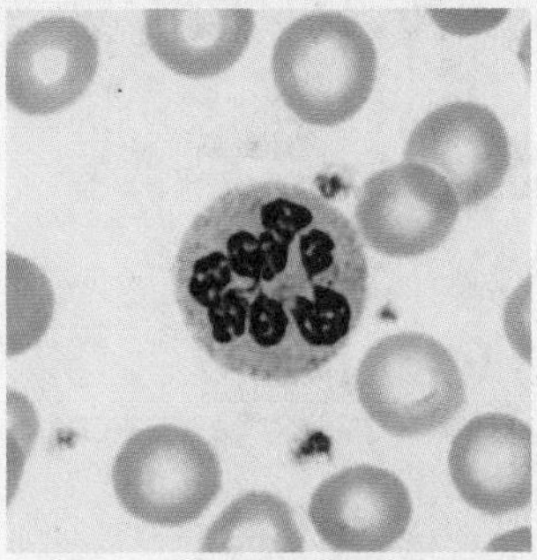	**Megaloblastic anemia** (check serum B_{12}, serum folate, RBC folate; if all normal, BM for myedysplastic syndrome and myeloproliferative disorder)
Macrocytic anemia without macroovalocytes and hypersegmented neutrophils	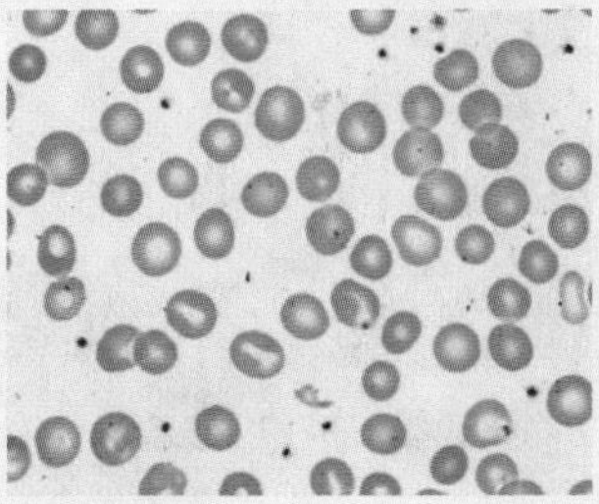	**Reticulocytosis** **Liver disease** **Thyroid disease** **Cold agglutinin disease** **Drugs**

(continued)

TABLE 173-2 The Peripheral Smear *(continued)*

Abnormal cell type		
Basophilic stippling	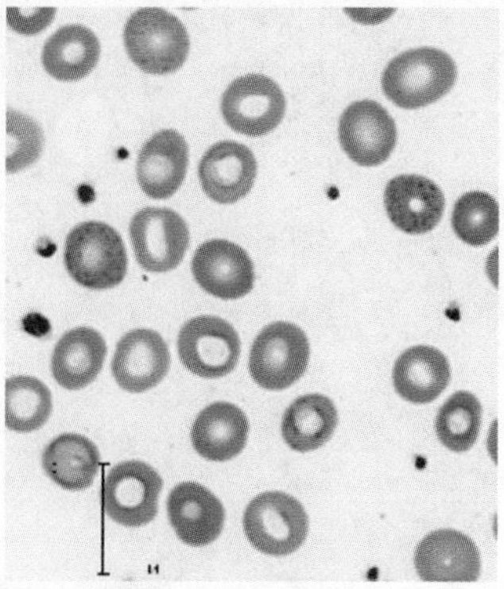	Hemolytic anemias, thalassemias, lead poisoning
Bite cells (Heinz bodies removed by splenic macrophages)	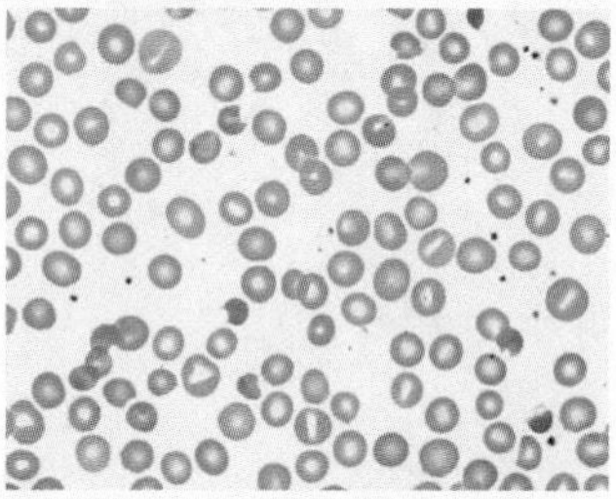	G6PD deficiency, oxidative drugs or unstable hemoglobin
Burr cells, spur cells (acanthocytes)	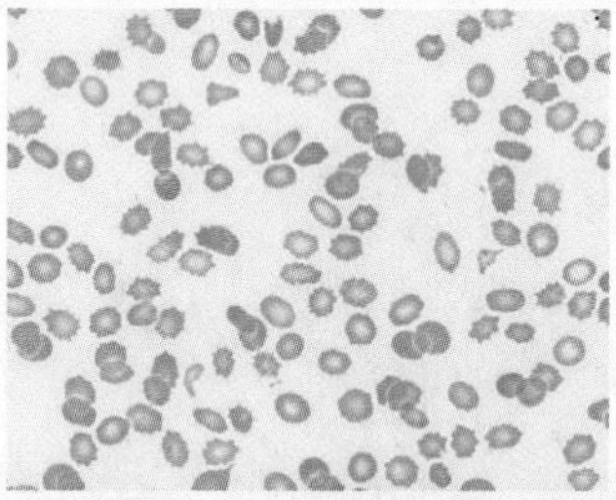	Liver disease, uremia, hypersplenism
Elliptocytes	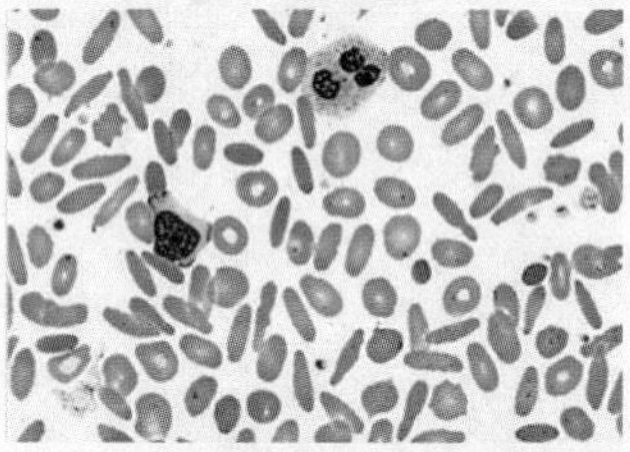	Iron deficiency anemia Hereditary elliptocytosis
Hemolysis of RBC	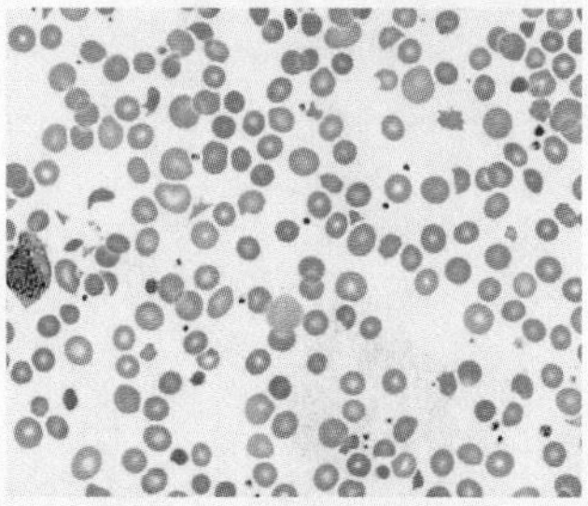	Hemolytic anemia
Howell-Jolly bodies	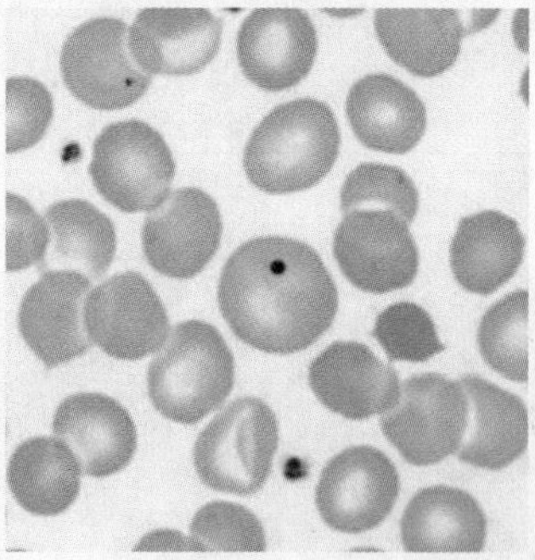	Postsplenectomy or functional asplenia

(continued)

TABLE 173-2 The Peripheral Smear (*continued*)

Abnormal cell type		
Nucleated RBC Schistocytes (fragmented RBCs)	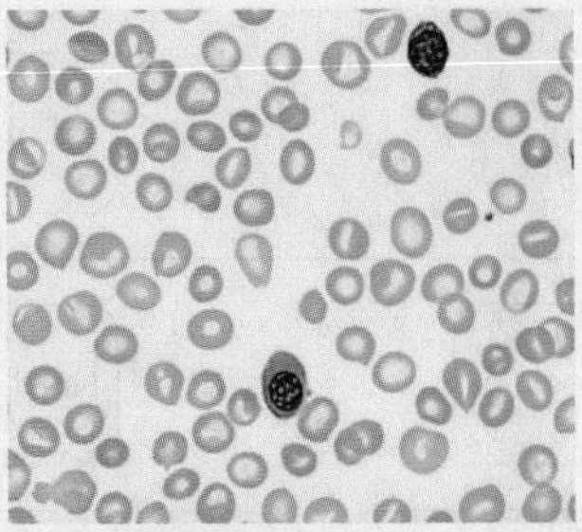	Microangiopathic or macroangiopathic hemolysis eg, DIC, TTP
Sickled forms	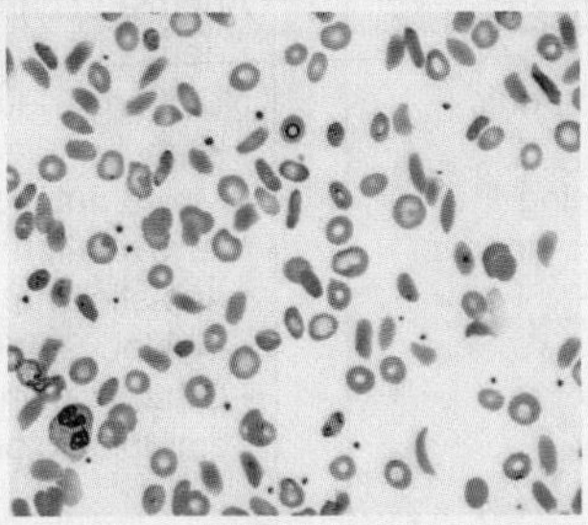	Sickle cell disease
Spherocytes (RBCs lack central pallor)	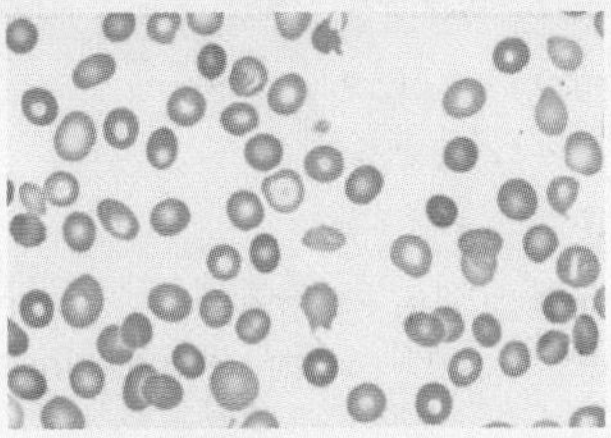	Immune-mediated hemolysis, hereditary spherocytosis, hypersplenism
Target cells	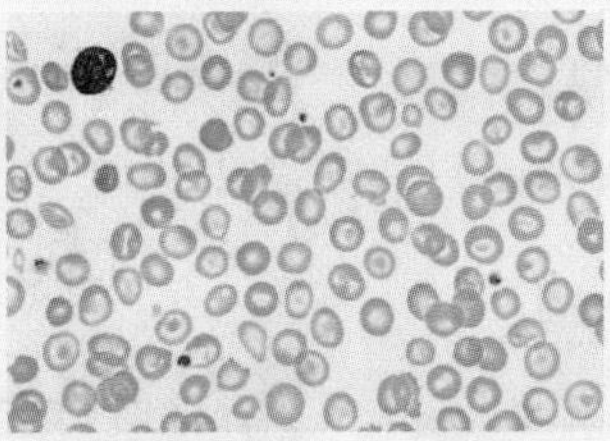	Thalassemias, hemoglobin C, hemoglobin E, hemoglobin S, liver disease, postsplenectomy
Teardrop cells	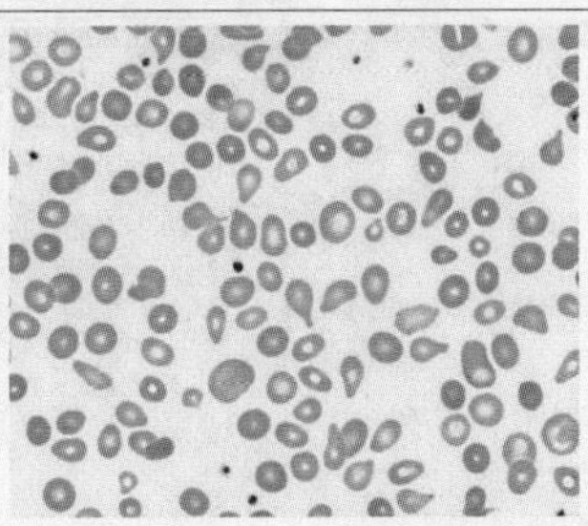	Myelopthisis, hypersplenism

BM, bone marrow; CML, chronic myelogenous leukemia; DIC, disseminated intravascular coagulation; G6PD, glucose-6-phosphate dehydrogenase; RBC, red blood cell; RDW, red cell distribution width; RS, ringed sideroblasts; TIBC, total iron binding capacity; TS, transferrin saturation; TTP, thrombotic thrombocytopenic purpura.

The physical examination may reveal evidence of decompensation as in acute blood loss (eg, unstable vital signs) or chronic extreme anemia (eg, congestive heart failure), signs of severe anemia (eg, pallor of the skin, conjunctivae, tongue, nail beds, and palmar creases, or tachycardia and the presence of a flow murmur), or help to identify previously unknown systemic disease (eg, signs of chronic liver disease).

Recent blood tests showing a previously normal hemoglobin level may confirm that the anemia is acute. Elevated reticulocyte count or reticulocyte percent is suggestive of acute or ongoing blood loss or hemolysis. If the anemia is not acute, workup can be guided by the peripheral blood smear and the mean corpuscular volume (MCV) of the red blood cells—small (microcytic), large (macrocytic), or normal size (normocytic). It is also important to note the white blood cell and platelet counts. Pancytopenia can be seen in aplastic anemia, vitamin B_{12} deficiency, myelodysplastic syndrome, primary bone marrow malignancies, or in liver disease with portal hypertension and splenomegaly. A normal white blood cell and platelet count with isolated anemia is unlikely to be due to marrow failure, with the exception of pure red cell aplasia. The reticulocyte count may also be useful to distinguish conditions associated with hyporegenerative anemia having low values of $< 50 \times 10^9$/L (aplastic anemia, pure red cell aplasia, or marrow infiltration) from a regenerative anemia seen with hemolysis or hemorrhage.

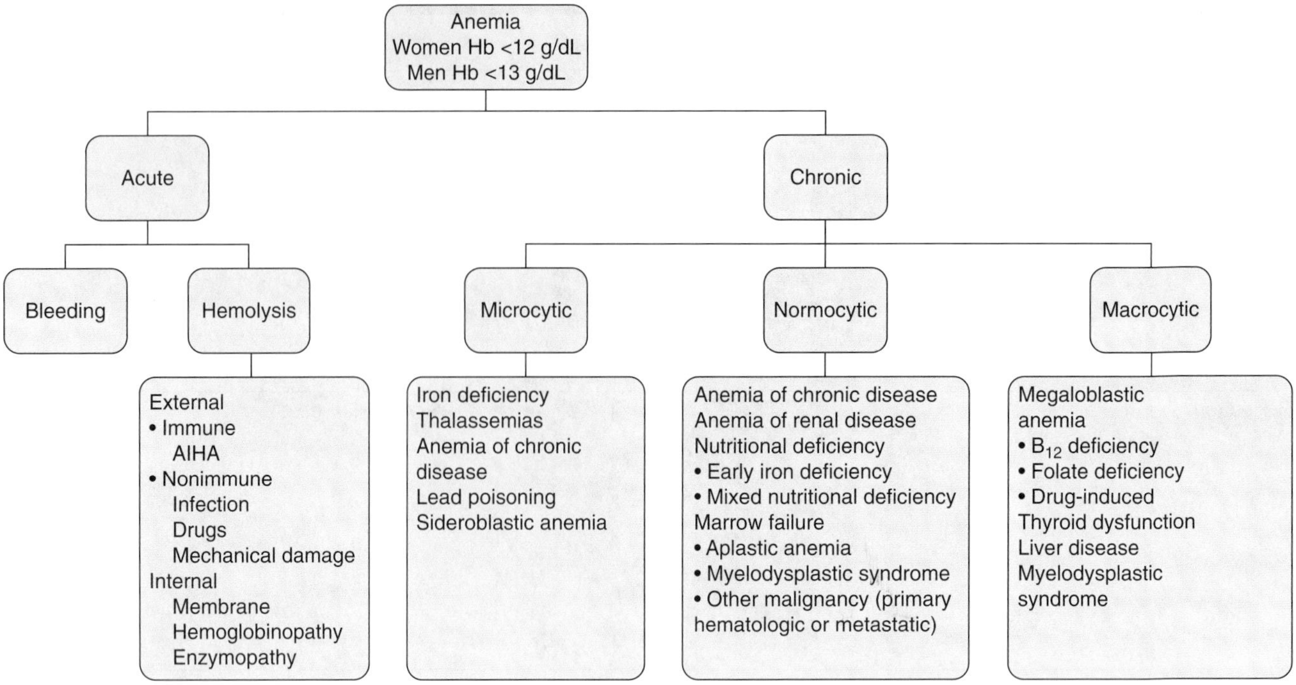

Figure 173-1 *Differential diagnosis of anemia. AIHA, autoimmune hemolytic anemia.*

The appearance of the red cells in a peripheral blood film can be associated with the different causes of anemia, and offers suggestions for relevant subsequent investigations (Table 173-2).

PRACTICE POINT

- The first question to ask in the evaluation of anemia is whether the anemia is due to acute or chronic blood loss, decreased production of red blood cells, or increased destruction. The first step is a complete history and physical examination, followed by a review of the complete blood count (CBC), the reticulocyte count, and the peripheral blood smear. The objective is to make the correct diagnosis without subjecting the patient to unnecessary laboratory tests and invasive procedures.

MICROCYTIC ANEMIA

Peripheral blood smear in iron deficiency anemia (IDA) shows small ("microcytic" or low MCV) red blood cells that are very pale ("hypochromic") containing less hemoglobin as indicated by a reduced mean corpuscular hemoglobin (MCH). Other changes of note may include anisocytosis (variable size of red blood cells) and poikilocytosis (variable shape of RBCs, for example target cells and pencil cells). Based on the blood smear alone it is difficult to discern IDA from a thalassemia trait. Therefore, further laboratory testing to investigate iron status and for exclusion of a possible hemoglobinopathy may be required.

Serum ferritin is considered a good measure of iron stores; levels below 30 mg/L in otherwise healthy patients are reflective of iron deficiency. However, ferritin is an acute phase reactant and may be higher in iron deficient patients with other medical problems. For this reason, the ferritin threshold may need to be increased. If the diagnosis is unclear, bone marrow examination, which is considered the "gold standard" test to confirm iron deficiency anemia, should be considered. Other tests that may be useful for the confirmation of a diagnosis in microcytic anemia include serum iron, total iron-binding capacity (TIBC), serum transferrin receptor, and measurement of zinc protoporphyrin (ZPP) and free erythrocyte protoporphyrins (FEP) (**Table 173-3**).

PRACTICE POINT

- Stages of iron deficiency are
  1. Storage iron depletion (decrease in serum ferritin levels, a reflection of total iron body stores).
  2. Iron-deficient erythropoiesis (a transferrin saturation < 9%, an indicator of impaired iron supply for the developing RBC).
  3. Microcytic hypochromic RBCs (RDW > 15% and variation in RBC shape, poikilocytosis, unlike Thalassemia).
- The bottom line: The MCV, serum iron, total iron-binding capacity, and percentage of transferrin saturation can predict the presence or absence of bone marrow iron in most patients without requiring a bone marrow exam.

TABLE 173-3 Typical Patterns of Iron Investigations in Iron Deficiency Anemia and Anemia of Chronic Disease

Biochemical Marker	Iron Deficiency Anemia	Anemia of Chronic Disease/Inflammation
Serum ferritin	Decreased	Normal or increased
Serum iron	Decreased	Deceased or normal
Total iron-binding capacity	Normal to increased	Decreased or normal
Transferrin saturation	Decreased	Decreased or normal
Serum transferrin receptor	Increased	Normal
ZPP or FEP	Increased	Increased

FEP, free erythrocyte protoporphyrin; ZPP, zinc protoporphyrin.

A hemoglobinopathy should be considered if the patient is healthy, not iron deficient, has a family history of microcytic anemia or thalassemia, or if the patient's ethnic group is known to commonly have thalassemia or variant hemoglobins associated with microcytosis (Hb E). Initial hemoglobinopathy investigations will quantify normal and abnormal hemoglobins to identify beta-thalassemia trait, homozygous beta-thalassemia, and Hb E. However, further DNA analysis may be required for diagnosis of alpha-thalassemia or may be useful to confirm the presence of other globin gene deletions or mutations. Pregnant women with microcytosis should always be considered for hemoglobinopathy testing regardless of iron status due to the risk of genetic transmission of a severe form of hemoglobinopathy or thalassemia to the fetus.

NORMOCYTIC ANEMIA

Normocytic anemia is the most frequently encountered category of anemia, and is often the most difficult to work up because it can result from many disparate disorders; it can be due to decreased RBC production, either primary (eg, aplastic anemia, acute leukemia) or secondary (eg, renal failure, anemia of chronic disease). Hemolytic anemia, both immune and nonimmune, and acute bleeding can also present as normocytic anemia.

Hemolytic anemia: increased red cell destruction

Hemolytic anemia may present in many ways; it can be acute and uncompensated or chronic and well compensated, or anything in between. Therefore most patients presenting with anemia of unclear etiology should be screened for hemolysis. The red cells in hemolytic anemia often vary in appearance depending on the underlying process. Examination of the peripheral smear is a useful tool for the differential diagnosis. Spherocytes can be present in autoimmune hemolytic anemia (AIHA) or in hereditary spherocytosis when the patient has a negative Coombs test. Sickle cell anemia manifests with characteristic sickle-shaped cells. Schistocytes are a hallmark of red cell destruction and can be correlated with platelet numbers for differentiating a microangiopathic hemolytic anemia from macroangiopathic hemolytic conditions 9 eg, caused by heart valves. Decreased platelets are seen in disseminated intravascular coagulation (DIC), thrombotic thrombocytopenic purpura (TTP), and hemolytic uremic syndrome (HUS). Platelets are normal in macroangiopathic hemolytic conditions caused by heart valves.

Screening tests that suggest the possibility of hemolysis include elevated lactate dehydrogenase, elevated unconjugated bilirubin, and elevated reticulocyte count. The level of haptoglobin, a protein that binds free hemoglobin in the circulation, may be a useful indicator for hemolysis. A low level or absence of haptoglobin, along with the presence of free hemoglobin in circulation, is suggestive of hemolysis. However, low haptoglobin can also be seen in liver disease. Haptoglobins are an acute phase reactant and therefore may be falsely elevated during any inflammatory process.

Often further specialized testing is required to confirm and identify the cause of hemolytic anemia. This can include direct antiglobulin test (DAT or Coombs test), hemoglobinopathy testing, and/or enzymopathy testing, as indicated. The DAT identifies IgG and/or complement on the RBC surface and can be positive in AIHA, drug-induced anemia, or a hemolytic transfusion reaction. A hemoglobinopathy investigation separates and quantifies the expected hemoglobins (Hb A, A2, and F) but will also identify many variant hemoglobins (eg, HbS, C, or E) or other rarer unstable hemoglobin variants (eg, Hb Köln, Hb Hasharon) known to cause hemolysis. To assess for enzyme deficiencies, quantitative testing of red cell pyruvate kinase and G6PD is performed. More recently, flow cytometry has been used to identify paroxysmal nocturnal hemoglobinuria (PNH) using the GPI-anchored antigens CD55 and CD59 on red cells or neutrophils. The osmotic fragility (OF) test is useful for confirmation of hereditary spherocytosis. However, the eosin-5-maleimide (EMA) dye binding test by flow cytometry has shown to have higher specificity and sensitivity than OF for red cell cytoskeleton disorders causing hemolysis.

Decreased red blood cell production

If anemia is due to decreased RBC production, the reticulocyte count will be low or "inappropriately normal." Serum erythropoietin level can be helpful but it is nondiagnostic; if it is high, it may indicate a primary bone marrow problem, which could be confirmed with a bone marrow aspirate and/or biopsy. Serum erythropoietin level will be low or inappropriately normal in any of the secondary causes of normocytic anemia, particularly in renal dysfunction. Moderate renal impairment can present with anemia, therefore renal function testing is essential, regardless of serum EPO level.

Anemia of chronic disease (ACD) is a difficult diagnosis to pin down. Essentially it is a clinical diagnosis in a patient who has had a sufficient and negative workup for other causes of anemia, and who has an underlying inflammatory condition. Measurement of iron indices or inflammatory markers (eg, erythrocyte sedimentation rate or C-reactive protein) may be a useful adjunct in testing. Bone marrow exam should reveal normal or increased amounts of stored iron and decreased iron staining in erythroid precursors, reflecting impaired iron utilization.

MACROCYTIC ANEMIA

B_{12} deficiency

Vitamin B_{12} (also known as cobalamin) is obtained by intake of animal products, including red meat, poultry, fish, dairy, and eggs. The total body store of vitamin B_{12} is 2–5 mg, primarily stored in the liver. Approximately 2–5 mcg of B_{12} is lost daily, most of which is excreted in the bile.

Although a typical Western diet contains 5–20 mcg/day of vitamin B_{12}, which is more than sufficient to replace daily losses, B_{12} deficiency can occur in individuals following a strict vegan diet.

In patients with gastritis, gastric atrophy, or history of gastrectomy, absence of gastric acid and pepsin prevents release of cobalamin from the protein to which it is bound. Furthermore, production of gastric intrinsic factor (IF), a molecule that binds free cobalamin in the gastrointestinal tract and facilitates cobalamin absorption in the terminal ileum, may be impaired. Malabsorption can also occur if there is inadequate absorption at the terminal ileum, due to prior resection or Crohn disease.

One of the most common causes of B_{12} deficiency is pernicious anemia, in which there is a deficiency of IF due to presumed autoimmune destruction of gastric parietal cells or the IF itself.

Vitamin B_{12} deficiency presents most commonly with hematologic abnormalities and/or neuropsychiatric signs and symptoms. Macrocytic anemia, with macro-ovalocytes on peripheral blood smear, is the classic hematologic abnormality. Neutrophils have hypersegmented nuclei. There may also be leukopenia and/or thrombocytopenia. Bone marrow examination reveals megaloblastosis.

The classic neurological manifestation is subacute combined degeneration of the spinal cord, resulting in sensory and motor disturbances that cause ataxia. Peripheral and cranial neuropathies may also be seen. In severe cases, patients may present with stroke or dementia-like syndromes. Physical exam may reveal classic findings such as glossitis and jaundice.

A serum B_{12} level < 200ng/L (148pmol/L) is very sensitive (97%) for the diagnosis of B_{12} deficiency. Because some patients with normal or low-normal serum B_{12} levels may be truly deficient and benefit from vitamin replacement, elevated methylmalonic acid (MMA) and homocysteine can help to clarify the diagnosis. Elevated MMA and hemocysteine are both sensitive early markers of B_{12} deficiency. Elevated levels should, however, be interpreted in the context of individual patients: homocysteine is also elevated in folate deficiency and hereditary homocyteinemia. MMA may be elevated in renal insufficiency and methylmalonic aciduria, and in some patients with folate deficiency. Serum MMA may be lowered in B_{12}-deficient patients receiving antibiotic treatment. A Schilling test, involving oral administration of radiolabeled cocyanocobalamin, has historically been used to assess vitamin B_{12} absorption. Unfortunately, the Schilling test is not widely available. Anti-intrinsic factor antibodies are highly specific for pernicious anemia (specificity >95%) and therefore, if positive, help to confirm the diagnosis; however sensitivity is poor (50–70%).

Folate deficiency

Folate is found in animal products and leafy green vegetables. As such, the most common cause of folate deficiency is inadequate nutritional intake. With universal folate supplementation, folate deficiency has become increasingly rare. However, patients with alcohol abuse remain at risk due to folate malabsorption and impaired folate metabolism in the liver. Individuals with increased folate requirements are also at increased risk. This includes pregnant women (for whom folate deficiency is associated with an increased risk of fetal spina bifida) and patients with chronic hemolytic anemia. The widespread use of routine, prophylactic folic acid supplementation in these groups can prevent deficiency. Use of some drugs has been linked to folate deficiency, including trimethoprim, pyrimethamin, methotrexate, and phenytoin.

Similar to vitamin B_{12} deficiency, folate deficiency can result in megaloblastic anemia. However, folate deficiency has no neurologic sequelae.

Diagnosis is made when the serum or red blood cell folate is below the normal range. Serum folate concentration may be normal in approximately 5% of individuals with folate deficiency; therefore if there is still a high index of suspicion, red blood cell folate should be tested.

Drug-induced anemia

A number of drugs can cause macrocytosis or macrocytic anemia. These include the following:

- Pyrimidine and purine analogs that inhibit DNA synthesis (eg, 5-FU, azathioprine)
- Antifolates (eg, methotrexate)
- Hydroxyurea
- Zidovudine

Other causes of macrocytic anemia

Occasionally, an exceptionally brisk reticulocytosis in response to anemia results in the average red blood cell being larger, thus increasing the MCV measurement. Other causes of macrocytosis that should be considered include liver disease, hypothyroidism, alcohol abuse, and myelodysplastic syndrome.

PRACTICE POINT

- Many anemias in their early stages have a normal MCV and then become either microcytic or macrocytic.
- The peripheral smear may provide important clues such as a myelopthisis (elliptocytes, teardrop cells, immature myeloid forms, nucleated RBCs), sickle cell disease (sickled RBCs), infectious disease (malaria).

TREATMENT

IRON DEFICIENCY ANEMIA

The goal of treatment for IDA is to improve the hemoglobin level and replenish iron stores. This typically requires 150–200 mg elemental iron per day for four to six months, or until serum ferritin has increased to approximately 50 mg/L. Iron is given orally unless the patient has severe gastrointestinal intolerance, malabsorption, or uncontrolled blood loss. The relative amounts of elemental iron in different preparations are listed below:

Ferrous gluconate:	300 mg	35 mg elemental iron
Ferrous sulfate:	300 mg	60 mg elemental iron
Ferrous fumarate:	300 mg	100 mg elemental iron
Polysaccharide iron complex:	150 mg	150 mg elemental iron

In the absence of ongoing blood loss, hemoglobin should increase by 1–2 g/dL within three weeks of starting adequate oral replacement, and iron stores should be replete in three months. Failure to respond may be due to nonadherence, poor iron absorption, or an incorrect diagnosis. If instead the patient has thalassemia, iron supplementation could be harmful, in that it will increase iron overload.

To improve iron absorption, the iron tablets should be taken on an empty stomach or with orange juice or a tablet of ascorbic acid. Concurrent administration of antacids should be avoided. Many patients complain of nausea or dyspepsia 30–60 minutes following a dose. This often subsides with ongoing treatment but, if it is an ongoing issue, night time dosing or administration of higher doses with food may improve symptoms and maintain adequate absorption.

Intravenous iron is an option for patients who are intolerant of or who do not respond to oral iron. These must be administered in a medically supervised area because of risks of hypotension, allergic, or anaphylactic reactions. Several iron preparations are available for intravenous administration, of which iron dextran has the highest risk of adverse reactions.

B_{12} DEFICIENCY

Vitamin B_{12} replacement can be divided into initial management (designed to quickly build up the tissue stores) and long-term maintenance treatment. A common initial regimen consists of intramuscular cyanocobalamin 1000 mcg/day for one or two weeks, followed by 1000 mcg/week for one month. Hematologic response should be evident one week after the first dose. In particular, there should be a noticeable increase in the reticulocyte count. If reticulocytosis is mild or absent, the original diagnosis should be questioned. By the eighth week, the MCV should have returned to the normal range.

Maintenance treatment can be given parenterally or orally. Parenteral cyanocobalamin may be given at a dose of 1000 mcg/month until the cause of deficiency is corrected, or lifelong in pernicious anemia. Oral therapy for pernicious anemia is 1000 mcg/day. Lower doses (eg, 125–500 mcg/day) can be given for other causes of deficiency; however the cost and risk of a higher dose are negligible and a standard dose of 1000 mcg/day is commonly prescribed.

FOLATE DEFICIENCY

Treatment is with oral folic acid (1–5 mg/day) until complete hematologic recovery. Patients with an ongoing cause of folate deficiency (eg, chronic hemolytic anemia or pregnancy) should continue on long-term supplementation. Because treatment with folic acid can partially reverse the hematologic abnormalities seen in vitamin B_{12} deficiency, but do not attenuate the progression of neurologic sequelae, serum vitamin B_{12} levels should be measured prior to therapy.

ANEMIA OF CHRONIC RENAL DISEASE

As the glomerular filtration rates decline, anemia becomes increasingly common in patients with chronic renal disease. Erythropoiesis-stimulating agents (ESAs) are widely used in treatment. Other options include red blood cell transfusions or androgens.

ESAs may be started if the hemoglobin level is ≤10 g/dL for predialysis and peritoneal dialysis patients, and if the hemoglobin is ≤11 g/dL in dialysis patients. Adequate iron stores should be confirmed, and other causes of anemia should be ruled out. Epoetin alpha or darbepoeitin may be used, with a target hemoglobin of 10–12 g/dL. Levels above 13 g/dL have been associated with increased risk of thrombotic events. Epoetin alpha can be started at a dose of 10,000 units subcutaneously once weekly or 20,000 units subcutaneously every other week. Lower starting doses may be appropriate for smaller patients or those with higher pretreatment hemoglobin. For dialysis patients, EPO can be administered intravenously during hemodialysis sessions. Throughout ESA therapy, iron supplementation should be used to maintain a transferrin saturation of 20–50% and a serum ferritin level of 100–500 ng/mL. Ongoing clinical trials are evaluating the precise determinants of cardiovascular risk and the optimal hemoglobin target. Updated clinical practice guidelines should be consulted.

HEMOLYTIC ANEMIA

Any hemolysis caused by an underlying disorder (eg, AIHA due to a lymphoproliferative disorder) is treated in the long term by bringing the disease under control. A short-term treatment may include high-dose oral corticosteroids. Hemolytic anemia caused by cold agglutinins typically improves with avoidance of cold exposure.

MYELODYSPLASTIC SYNDROMES

The anemia of myelodysplatsic syndromes (MDS) is typically treated with chronic transfusions or erythropoiesis-stimulating agents (ESAs). Patients with MDS-related anemia with serum EPO level <100–200 mU/mL and lower-risk disease are most likely to respond to ESAs. Relatively high doses of epoetin-alpha or darbepoetin are usually required. Patients who do not qualify for or respond to ESAs are likely to require chronic red blood cell transfusions. Unfortunately, transfusion-dependent MDS patients have decreased overall survival, especially those in lower-risk categories. Decreased overall survival in these individuals is linked to elevated ferritin levels, indicating that transfusional iron overload is at least partially responsible for worsened outcomes. Serum ferritin and transferrin iron saturation should be monitored in transfusion-dependent MDS patients. T2-weighted magnetic resonance imaging (MRI) may be used to evaluate for cardiac and liver iron deposition. Chelation therapy should be considered in patients with evidence of iron overload.

COMPLICATIONS

Bone marrow examination may aid diagnosis if anemia is apparently due to underproduction, or if anemia is associated with leukopenia, thrombocytopenia, and/or other morphologic abnormalities suggesting bone marrow disease. Rarely, bone marrow examination is necessary to help quantify iron stores in a patient with normal serum ferritin but microcytic anemia is felt to be due to iron deficiency.

Consultation with a hematologist should be considered in complex cases and for patients with thalassemia, sickle cell disease, other variant hemoglobins, bone marrow failure syndromes, or autoimmune hemolytic anemia. Patients with anemia due to end-stage renal disease may be best managed by a renal specialist.

RARE CAUSES FOR CONSIDERATION

Thrombotic thrombocytopenic purpura (TTP) is caused by impaired cleavage of ultra large multimers of von Willebrand factor, causing increased platelet aggregation in small vessels. TTP presents with hemolytic anemia and thrombocytopenia. Other features can include fever, neurologic symptoms (headache, seizures, or coma), and acute renal impairment. Blood film shows red blood cell fragments (schistocytes) that result from damage to red cells in the microvasculature.

When a cause of microcytic or normocytic anemia is not found, remember to test for paroxysmal nocturnal hemoglobinuria (PNH), which typically presents with episodes of intravascular hemolysis and red urine. As a result of chronic and recurrent hemoglobinuria, patients can become iron deficient. PNH is a clonal disorder that can result in aplastic anemia or acute leukemia. Patients with PNH are at increased risk of thromboembolism. The diagnosis of PNH is made when flow cytometry shows a clone of WBCs (PB or BM) lacking cell markers CD55 or CD59.

There are several rare congential bone marrow failure syndromes that result in lifelong anemia. These include Diamond-Blackfan anemia, Fanconi anemia, Schwachman-Diamond syndrome, and congential dyserythropoietic anemia. These disorders will typically present in early childhood and require ongoing follow-up. First diagnosis in adulthood is rare but does occur.

QUALITY IMPROVEMENT

Anemia is a common finding in hospitalized patients. Typically, low hemoglobin is caused by one or more of the numerous underlying problems describe above. However, daily in-hospital blood testing can exacerbate anemia. As a result, in all hospital patients, in particular those with preexisting anemia, blood sampling should be minimized by careful use of laboratory investigations. In any patient diagnosed with anemia, discharge planning should include a plan for routine monitoring of hemoglobin. The frequency and duration of follow-up will be tailored to the cause and severity of anemia.

POLYCYTHEMIA AND SECONDARY ERYTHROCYTOSIS

INTRODUCTION

Erythrocytosis is the term used to describe unusually high hematocrit, hemoglobin, and/or red blood cell count. An increased red blood cell count is a medical concern for two reasons: (1) It can be the "red flag" for some underlying medical problem that needs attention and (2) erythrocytosis itself can cause problems with sluggish blood flow and subsequent ischemic phenomena, particularly neurologic signs and symptoms. Investigations to determine the cause of erythrocytosis enable proper classification (ie, primary or secondary process), which guides the therapeutic strategy.

PATHOPHYSIOLOGY

True erythrocytosis (as opposed to spurious erythrocytosis, see below) is defined as having both an increased hematocrit and an increased red cell mass that can be classified as either primary or secondary. Primary erythrocytosis is due to a group of clonal bone marrow disorders known as myeloproliferative disorders (MPD) that include polycythemia rubra vera resulting in autonomous production of too many red blood cells, essential thrombocythemia in which the platelet counts are elevated, and primary myelofibrosis. The MPDs are discussed in Chapter 179 Hematologic Malignancies.

Secondary erythrocytosis can occur by three mechanisms, all involving increased erythropoietin (EPO) signalling in the bone marrow.

1. **"Appropriate" increase in EPO production:** In healthy homeostasis, the kidneys make and secrete EPO based on the oxygen tension (PO_2) in the renal blood vessels. If oxygen delivered

TABLE 173-4 Classification of Absolute Erythrocytosis

Primary erythrocytosis
Polycythemia vera (and other myeloproliferative neoplasms)
Secondary erythrocytosis
Congenital
Chuvash polycythemia (*VHL* mutation)
Other defects in oxygen sensing pathway (eg, *PHD2* or *HIF*-2α mutations)
EPO receptor mutation
High oxygen-affinity hemoglobin
2,3-Biphosphoglycerate mutase deficiency
Acquired
EPO Mediated
Central hypoxia
High altitude
Right-to-left cardiopulmonary vascular shunts
Chronic lung disease
Obstructive sleep apnea
Carbon monoxide poisoning
Smoking
Local renal hypoxia
Renal artery stenosis
Renal cysts
Post-renal transplant erythrocytosis
Pathologic EPO production
Renal cell carcinoma
Hepatocellular carcinoma
Cerebellar hemangioma
Meningioma
Uterine fibroids (leiomyomas)
Pheochromocytoma
Drugs
Testosterone administration
EPO agonist administration
Idiopathic erythrocytosis

EPO, erythropoeitin.
Data from McMullen MF, et al. Guidelines for the diagnosis, investigation and management of polycythaemia/erythrocytosis. *British Journal of Haematology*. 2005;130:174–195.

to the kidneys decreases, the kidneys release more EPO as a signal to the bone marrow that the blood needs increased oxygen-carrying capacity in the form of hemoglobin. Oxygen delivery to the body tissues may be decreased as a result of hypoxemia or anemia. Hypoxemia may be due to reasons listed in **Table 173-4**. Relative renal hypoxia due to renal artery stenosis will cause increased EPO by the same mechanism.

2. **Autonomously produced erythropoietin:** Several types of neoplasm are known to produce excess EPO, including renal cell carcinoma, uterine fibroids, hemangioblastoma, and hepatocellular carcinoma. EPO production can also be increased following renal transplant, although this dysregulated EPO production effect is not completely understood. Inherited causes of up-regulated EPO production due to defects in the oxygen-sensing pathway have been described with genetic mutations in the von Hippel-Lindau (VHL) gene including the Chuvash polycythemia (VHL 598C > T) mutation.
3. **Exogenous EPO:** Patients with anemia of renal disease or anemia that is associated with cancer may be on erythropoietin-stimulating agents. If the prescribed dose is too high or the patient takes the medication incorrectly, it can result in erythrocytosis.

EPO production is also increased with elevated testosterone levels. Elevated testosterone levels stimulate EPO release, and also increase bone marrow activity and iron incorporation into RBCs. This is why the hemoglobin reference range for men is higher than that for women. Exogenous androgen administration (eg, "blood doping" by some body builders and athletes) or increased endogenous testosterone (eg, germ cell tumors) can result in increased hemoglobin.

SPURIOUS ERYTHROCYTOSIS

Spurious erythrocytosis occurs when either the patient or the patient's blood sample has reduced plasma volume, giving a false increase in hemoglobin concentration. Common causes of dehydration should be excluded (eg, illness, diuretic medications, caffeine-containing beverages, smoking).

DIAGNOSIS: WHY DOES THIS PATIENT HAVE POLYCYTHEMIA?

The detection of erythrocytosis is largely based on laboratory findings of increased hemoglobin, hematocrit, and red cell counts; however, some findings on history and physical exam can suggest a primary polycythemia. As well, a good clinical evaluation of the patient may direct the clinician to the underlying cause of erythrocytosis.

History should include:

- History of prior polycythemia
- Date and results of most recent CBC
- Questions about possible causes of secondary polycythemia
- Symptoms and complications resulting from polycythemia, which can include:
  - Thromboembolic—transient ischemic attack (TIA) or stroke, myocardial infarction, venous thromboembolism
  - Hyperviscosity—headache, dizziness, tinnitus, dyspnea, chest pain
  - Erythromelalgia (painful paresthesias in the hands and feet)
  - Aquagenic pruritis (itch after skin exposure to water [eg, after a bath])
  - Gout

Physical examination should be performed, with particular attention to vital signs, cardiac, and respiratory exams. Low oxygen saturation on pulse oximetry may suggest hypoxemia as the cause of polycythemia. Polycythemia can lead to chronic hypertension. True polycythemia will commonly be accompanied by "plethora," a ruddy appearance of the skin, particularly apparent on the face. If cyanosis is present, it may be due to polycythemia alone (increased red blood cell mass and relatively increased deoxygenated hemoglobin) or may reflect an underlying hypoxemic condition. Presence of splenomegaly suggests a myeloproliferative disorder.

BLOOD TESTS

As per WHO guidelines, polycythemia is suspected when complete blood count results show a hemoglobin of >16.5 in women or >18.5 g/dL in men or other evidence of increased red cell volume (eg, hematocrit > 99th percentile of method-specific reference range for age, sex, and altitude of residence). A patient with polycythemia may also have an elevated red blood cell count. However, this may not be reliable as it also occurs in patients with thalassemia minor or having high O_2 affinity hemoglobin variants.

When polycythemia is suspected, spurious polycythemia should be ruled out. Repeat CBC may be done to rule out transient clinical dehydration or laboratory error.

To classify absolute polycythemia as primary or secondary (Table 173-1), a serum erythropoietin level is essential. Evidence of chronic respiratory disease or hypoxemia on physical exam should be followed up with arterial blood gas to confirm low arterial oxygen saturation. Co-oximetry of arterial blood can also quantify carboxyhemoglobin, which will be elevated in polycythemia caused by chronic carbon monoxide exposure. Other laboratory investigations should be guided by clinical assessment of the most likely underlying cause of polycythemia, but may include screening tests for renal and liver function, serum ferritin level, hemoglobin electrophoresis, hemoglobin oxygen-affinity (p50) testing, and *JAK2* mutation analysis (see MPD in Chapter 179 Hematologic Malignancies).

IMAGING

Chest X-ray and/or computed tomography (CT) scan may be used to confirm findings on clinical evaluation or to exclude occult disease. Ultrasound can evaluate for splenomegaly (associated with MPDs), local renal vascular disease, or neoplastic processes causing increased EPO or testosterone production.

OTHER INVESTIGATIONS

A formal sleep study is indicated if the patient has clear signs and symptoms of obstructive sleep apnea. Bone marrow exam is rarely useful in the workup of polycythemia.

TRIAGE AND HOSPITAL ADMISSION

Many of the conditions causing secondary polycythemia can present with acute illness and these cases should be triaged accordingly. Polycythemia in and of itself is not an indication for hospital admission, but it can be associated with severe symptoms and complications (see Diagnosis earlier in this chapter), which may necessitate acute medical attention.

TREATMENT

Goals of treatment in primary polycythemia include decreasing chronic symptoms due to hyperviscosity and increased RBC turnover, and reducing the long-term risk of thrombotic complications. Reduction of hemoglobin concentration may be achieved by a program of repeated phlebotomies and/or cytoreductive agents, such as hydroxyurea. Acetylsalicylic acid has been shown to reduce the risk of thrombotic events in polycythemia vera, with minimal increase in risk of bleeding. Traditional risk factors for vascular disease should be managed as appropriate.

For patients with secondary erythrocytosis, the main principle of management is treatment of the underlying disorder.

COMPLICATIONS

Complications of primary polycythemia can include venous or arterial thrombotic events. Over time, a small percentage of patients develop myelofibrosis or, more rarely, acute myeloid leukemia. Bone marrow exam should be performed if progression of marrow disease is suspected.

RARE CAUSES FOR CONSIDERATION

In rare instances, primary or secondary polycythemia can be congenital. Congenital mutation of the EPO receptor can result in the EPO receptor being chronically "switched on." Congenital low 2,3-bisphosphoglycerate is associated with less off-loading of oxygen by hemoglobin at the peripheral tissues, and a compensatory increase in endogenous EPO.

DISCHARGE CONSIDERATIONS

In any patient diagnosed with polycythemia, discharge planning should include a plan for routine monitoring of hemoglobin. The frequency and duration of follow-up will be tailored to the cause and severity of polycythemia.

THALASSEMIA AND HEMOGLOBINOPATHIES

INTRODUCTION

The hemoglobinopathies are genetic disorders affecting the production, structure, or function of the globin chains that form hemoglobin contained within red cells. These are one of most common genetic diseases known, with worldwide estimates of 270 million carriers, and more than 300,000 infants born each year with clinically severe abnormalities. The hemoglobin tetramer is made from two pairs of globin chains, each attached to a heme group. Normally three types are of hemoglobin can be detected by electrophoretic techniques: Hb A ($\alpha_2\beta_2$), the predominant adult form; Hb F ($\alpha_2\gamma_2$), found at high levels in newborns; and a minor amount of HbA_2 ($\alpha_2\delta_2$). The genes responsible for producing these globin proteins are found on two gene clusters; chromosome 16p13.3 is the location for two alpha (α) globin genes, and on chromosome 11p15.5 are the beta (β), delta (δ), and gamma (γ) globin genes. Currently more than 1,000 mutations have been described in the α, β, δ, and γ globin genes, which are categorized and listed on the World Wide Web (http://globin.cse.psu.edu) with novel mutations continually being discovered. Heterozygous carriers of globin gene mutations are typically asymptomatic but can present with microcytosis, hemolysis, anemia, cyanosis, or erythrocytosis, depending on the underlying defect. Individuals who are homozygous or compound heterozygous for specific types of globin gene mutations can present with serious disease states ranging from thalassemia major, a condition that requires lifelong transfusion therapy, to severe sickling syndromes presenting with chronic hemolysis and periodic painful sickle cell crises. The detection and diagnosis of the hemoglobinopathies largely relies on a good clinical history and the correlation of physical findings, such as splenomegaly, with results of diagnostic laboratory tests. The most common hemoglobin disorders—sickle cell disease and thalassemia—can be diagnosed easily in most clinical laboratories; however, complex unusual cases may require further more sophisticated investigations including DNA-based procedures. Sickle cell disease is covered in more detail in this chapter.

PATHOPHYSIOLOGY

The hemoglobin (Hb) tetramer contains four subunits, each containing a globin attached to a molecule of heme, a protein structure that transports oxygen efficiently. The major hemoglobin found in individuals older than six months is Hb A, or adult hemoglobin, consisting of two α- and two β-globin subunits. The hemoglobin disorders are genetic mutations in these globin chains that can be divided into two broad categories: the "variants," in which qualitative changes in the globin chain structure may result in an abnormal function or electrophoretic properties, and the "thalassemias," in which reduced production of globin chains leads to a decrease in hemoglobin, resulting in a microcytic, hypochromic anemia. Hemoglobin disorders are most commonly found in people from malaria-endemic regions, where high gene prevalence has been attributed to a survival advantage for carriers. However, due to global population migration, these disorders are now found in all regions, including North America and northern Europe. Thus, consideration for an individual's ethnicity may be useful, but should not be the sole criterion to determine if a search for a hemoglobin disorder is indicated.

HEMOGLOBIN VARIANTS

Most hemoglobin variants are due to single nucleotide point mutations in the globin genes that change the amino acid sequence. A variant hemoglobin can also result from deletions or gene rearrangements that lead to fusion of two globin genes, changes in the stop codon of the globin gene resulting in extending globin chains, or multiple nucleic acid substitutions at two different positions in the globin gene. Although most mutations are rare and of no clinical consequence, some can cause severe or lifelong conditions. Examples are Hb S (β codon 6 GAG > GTG Glu > Val) causing sickle cell disease or Hb C (β codon 6 GAG > AAG Glu > Lys), which, when combined with Hb S, also causes a significant sickling disorder; and Hb E (β codon 26 GAG > AAG or Glu > Lys), which can contribute to severe β-thalassemia syndromes. Other common variants are Hb D, Hb Lepore, Hb O, and Hb Constant Spring.

THALASSEMIA

The most important thalassemia syndromes are those that affect either the α- or β-globin chains. Thalassemias can be caused by point mutations that reduce or eliminate the globin gene production. Thalassemia may also be the result of insertions or deletions in the gene itself that down-regulate gene expression, or from a total deletion of the globin gene. Abnormalities affecting α-globin chain production are termed α-thalassemia and those affecting β-globin production are called β-thalassemia. Some mutations that affect globin gene expression may also produce detectable hemoglobin variants. The most common variants that present with a thalassemia phenotype are Hb E (β codon 26 GAG > AAG or Glu → Lys), Hb Lepore (caused by a δ-β fusion globin chain), or Hb Constant Spring (α2 codon 142 TAA > CAA or Ter → Gln).

CLINICALLY SIGNIFICANT HEMOGLOBINOPATHIES

The most common clinically significant hemoglobinopathies can be divided into three distinct syndromes: the sickle cell syndromes, the α-thalassemia syndromes, and the β-thalassemia syndromes. They are normally inherited as autosomal recessive abnormalities (ie, heterozygous individuals are asymptomatic), whereas homozygous or compound heterozygous individuals are severely affected. Other rare globin gene mutations may be inherited as autosomal dominant expression. These include the unstable hemoglobins (implicated in Heinz body-induced hemolysis), the high oxygen affinity hemoglobins (presenting with secondary compensated erythrocytosis), the low oxygen affinity hemoglobins, and Hb M variants.

Therefore reasons to correctly diagnose the hemoglobinoapthies are:

1. Diagnosis of serious or life-threatening hemoglobin abnormalities to plan for appropriate preventative management (eg, penicillin prophylaxis and pneumococcal vaccination in infants with sickle cell disease) and medical treatment (eg, chronic transfusion program and chelation therapy in β-thalassemia major).
2. Investigation of microcytic anemia to identify individuals with thalassemia trait so that unnecessary investigations (eg, endoscopy) and treatment for presumed iron deficiency can be avoided.
3. Identification of individuals of reproductive age who are carriers of clinically significant hemoglobin mutations to initiate proper genetic counselling and guide future reproductive decisions.

α-THALASSEMIA SYNDROMES

Normally, individuals have four α globin genes—two on each chromosome 16. Carriers of α thalassemia have deletions of one (-α/αα) or two (--/αα or -α/-α) of the α globin genes. Deletion of three α globin genes results in hemoglobin H disease (HbH: --/-α). Deletion of all four α globin genes typically results in hydrops fetalis, which is not compatible with life unless antenatal diagnosis is followed by in utero transfusion. Rarely, α-thalassemia syndromes are caused by nondeletional mutations, such as Hb Constant Spring, which have the same effect as a single α gene deletion. Deletion of one α globin gene (referred to as α^{+}-thalassemia) is often seen in individuals of African, Mediterranean, and Southeast Asian ethnic backgrounds, while deletion of two α globin genes in *cis* (--αα; referred to as α^{0}-thalassemia) is most often seen in the Southeast Asian population. The most commonly reported α-thalassemia genotypes are presented with the clinical presentation and reproductive significance in **Table 173-5**.

β-THALASSEMIA SYNDROMES

Normally, individuals inherit two β-globin genes, one on each chromosome 11. β-thalassemia syndromes are most often a result of point mutations, or small deletions or insertions in the β-globin gene. These mutations either reduce the β-globin chain production (β^{+}-thalassemia mutations) or completely eliminate β-globin production from the affected gene (β^{0}-thalassemia mutations). Also

TABLE 173-5 The Clinical Presentation, Genotypes, and Reproductive Significance of the Various α–Thalassemia Syndromes

Hemoglobinopathy	Clinical Presentation	Genotypes	Reproductive Significance
α^{+}-Thalassemia heterozygous	Normal to mild microcytosis	*–α/αα* or $\alpha^{T}\alpha/\alpha\alpha$	Carrier for Hb H disease
Hb Constant Spring	Normal to mild microcytosis	$\alpha^{CS}\alpha/\alpha\alpha$	Carrier for Hb H/Hb Constant Spring Disease
Homozygous α^{+}-thalassemia	Microcytosis, normal Hb or mild anemia	*–α/–α*	Carrier for Hb H disease
α^{0}-Thalassemia trait	Microcytosis, normal Hb or mild anemia	*– –/–αα*	Carrier for Hb Bart Hydrops fetalis, and Hb H disease
Hb H disease, Hb H/Hb Constant Spring disease	Mild to moderate microcytosis with hemolytic anemia	*– –/–α* or $\alpha^{T}\alpha$/– – or $\alpha^{CS}\alpha$/– –	Carrier for Hb Bart hydrops fetalis and Hb H disease
Hb Bart hydrops fetalis	High-risk pregnancy with fetal death without *in utero* transfusion interventions	– –/– –	Carrier for Hb Bart hydrops fetalis and Hb H disease

–α/αα, α thalassemia caused by a single-gene deletion; $\alpha^{T}\alpha/\alpha\alpha$, *α* thalassemia caused by a point mutation; *– –/αα, αα* thalassemia caused by a two-gene deletion in *cis*; α^{CS}, Constant Spring mutation of alpha gene.

Adapted, with permission, from Lafferty JD, Waye JS, Chui DH, et al. Good practice guidelines for laboratory investigation of hemoglobinopathies. *Lab Hematol.* 2003;9(4):237–245.

TABLE 173-6 The Clinical Presentation and Reproductive Significance of the Various β-Thalassemia Syndromes

Hemoglobinopathy	Clinical Presentation	Genotypes	Reproductive Significance
β-Thalassemia trait	Microcytosis with normal Hb or mild anemia, elevated Hb A2	β^A/β^0, β^A/β^+	Carrier for β thalassemia major or β thalassemia intermedia or HbS/β thalassemia
δ-β-Thalassemia trait	Microcytosis with normal Hb or mild anemia, normal Hb A2 and elevated Hb F	β^A /δβ Thal	Carrier for β thalassemia intermedia
Hb E trait or homozygous Hb E	Normal to microcytosis, normal Hb or mild anemia	β^A/δ^E or β^E/β^E	Carrier for β thalassemia intermedia or major
Hb Lepore trait	Microcytosis with normal Hb or mild anemia	β^A/β^{Lepore}	Carrier for β thalassemia intermedia or major
β-Thalassemia intermedia	Moderate microcytosis with anemia sometimes requiring intermittent transfusion	β^+/β^E or β^+/β^+ or β^+/β^0 or β^+/β^{Lepore} or β^0/δβ, or β^+/δβ or δβ/δβ or β Thal with excess α globin genes	Carrier for β thalassemia intermedia or major or HbS/β^+ or Hb S/β^0 thalassemia
β-Thalassemia major	Transfusion-dependent microcytic anemia	β^0/β^0 or β^0/β^E or β^0/β^{Lepore} or $\beta^{Lepore}/\beta^{Lepore}$	Carrier for β thalassemia intermedia or major

β^A, normal β-globin gene; β^0, beta-zero mutation (no β-globin gene produced); β^+, beta-zero mutation (reduced β-globin gene production); δ-β, delta-beta thalassemia deletion; β^E, Hb E; β^{Lepore}, Hb Lepore.

Adapted, with permission, from Lafferty JD, Waye JS, Chui DH, et al. Good practice guidelines for laboratory investigation of hemoglobinopathies. *Lab Hematol*. 2003;9(4):237–245.

some β-chain variants can present as thalassemia phenotypes that are clinically severe when inherited as compound heterozygous (eg, Hb E/β thalassemia and Hb Lepore/β thalassemia). There is a high prevalence of β-thalassemia in the African, Mediterranean, Middle Eastern, Indian, and Southeast Asian ethnic populations. Hemoglobin E is most commonly found in Southeast Asian populations, while Hb Lepore is found in Mediterranean, African, and Southeast Asian populations. These most commonly detected β-thalassemia genotypes are presented with the clinical presentation and reproductive significance in Table 173-5. "β-thalassemia major" is used to describe patients who are transfusion dependent from infancy or early childhood (usually due to homozygosity or compound heterozygosity for β^0-thalassemia), whereas "β-thalassemia intermedia" refers to patients with anemia that is more severe than that of someone with β-thalassemia trait, but less severe than typical β-thalassemia major (**Table 173-6**).

DIAGNOSIS: DOES THIS PATIENT HAVE A CLINICALLY SIGNIFICANT HEMOGLOBINOPATHY?

A patient who has an ethnic background with a high prevalence of hemoglobinopathies and a positive family history of anemia, chronic transfusions, painful sickle cell crises, or hydrops fetalis should alert the physician to the possibility of congenital hemoglobin disorders. However, heterozygous carriers of most hemoglobinopathies are asymptomatic and clinically well. A good clinical history is important, including demographic information.

The laboratory diagnosis of hemoglobinoapthies begins with a CBC and peripheral blood smear, specifically looking at the appearance of the RBCs, the hemoglobin level, and erythrocyte indices (**Figure 173-2**).

A low mean corpuscular volume (MCV) and mean corpuscular hemoglobin (MCH) are associated with microcytosis and hypochromasia. These values may be indicative of thalassemia but need to be differentiated from iron deficiency anemia (IDA) or anemia of chronic disease (ACD), which may also present with microcytic, hypochromic anemia (see the Anemia section earlier in this chapter). Individuals with uncomplicated α- or β-thalassemia trait will usually have normal iron studies. However, a diagnosis of IDA or ACD does not rule out coexisting thalassemia trait.

HEMOGLOBIN SEPARATION

Separation of the hemoglobin fractions are used to detect variant hemoglobins. In a normal adult, HbA, HbA_2, and HbF should all be present. Traditionally, hemoglobin separation has been done using alkaline and acid electrophoresis. Although these methods are still used in some laboratories as initial screening for variant hemoglobin identification, automated methods are available that not only separate the hemoglobin fractions but also provide accurate quantification of the hemoglobin fractions.

1. **High performance liquid chromatography (HPLC):** One of the automated systems commonly used for hemoglobinopathy screening is a cation-exchange HPLC, a method based on elution of hemoglobin fractions on a chromatography column. The HPLC system quantifies the hemoglobin fractions, provides accurate levels of Hb A, Hb A_2, and Hb F, and has good resolving power to detect many of the variant hemoglobins.
2. **Capillary electrophoresis (CE):** Capillary electrophoresis is a relatively new automated system available for hemoglobin separation and quantification. A hemoglobin solution migrates through a buffer solution contained in fine capillary tubes when an electrical current is applied. These automated systems have excellent resolving power, providing a rapid and sensitive method of hemoglobin separation and quantification.

Functional investigations:

1. **P_{50} analysis:** Hemoglobins that have changed oxygen affinity can be identified by performing a P_{50} analysis or oxygen dissociation curve. Some variant hemoglobins will have a high O_2 affinity resulting in erythrocytosis or low oxygen affinity causing anemia or cyanosis. Several of these hemoglobin variants will show no differences in electrophoretic mobility from Hb A.
2. **Stability testing:** Hemoglobin instability can be demonstrated by exposing hemoglobin to excessive heat or incubating it with a buffered isopropyl alcohol. These unstable hemoglobin variants may also be identified by increased Heinz body detection and the presence of bite cells and dense fragments in the peripheral red cell morphology.

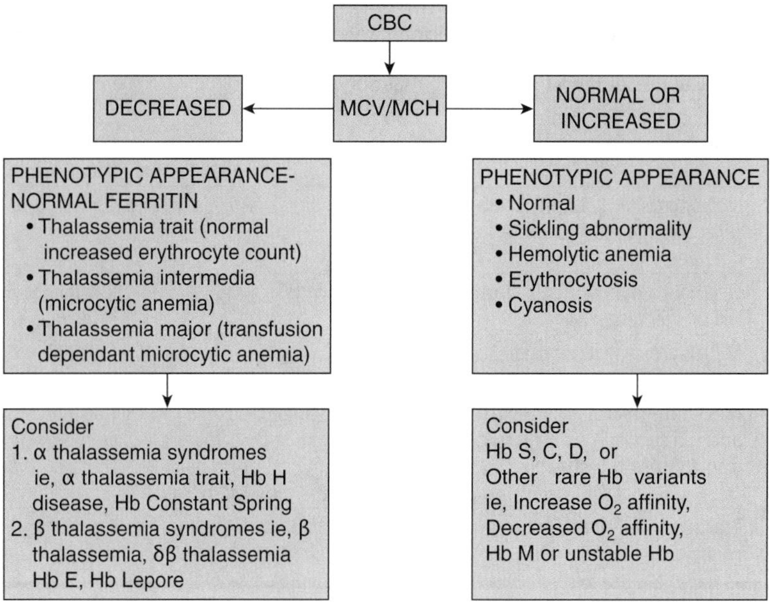

Figure 173-2 *Preliminary hemoglobinopathy considerations based on the MCV/MCH. (A normal RDW is not a reliable indicator of the thalassemia trait as it can be normal in some genotypes of thalassemia and abnormal in others.) MCV, mean corpuscular volume; MCH, mean corpuscular hemoglobin. (Adapted, with permission, from Lafferty JD, Waye JS, Chui DH, et al. Good practice guidelines for laboratory investigation of hemoglobinopathies. Lab Hematol. 2003;9(4):237–245.)*

3. **Hb M testing:** Some variants will produce a methemoglobinemia that can be identified through performing a unique absorption spectral scan. These are a specific group of variant hemoglobins that produce methemoglobin called the Hb Ms.

Molecular diagnostics: Molecular diagnosis and DNA analysis are used for positive characterization of variant hemoglobins or confirmation of thalassemia. These are performed on DNA and include PCR, direct nucleotide sequencing, and southern hybridization techniques.

INTERPRETATION OF LABORATORY INVESTIGATIONS

In the setting of a suspected hemoglobin disorder, one must correlate laboratory findings with the patient's age, gender, ethnicity, and reproductive status. Standard investigations cannot definitively diagnose all clinically important variant hemoglobins. Interpretation of hemoglobinopathy investigations can be challenging. Therefore guidance from a knowledgeable laboratory professional can be helpful in determining if a clinically significant hemoglobin disorder is present.

Alpha-thalassemia syndromes are associated with microcytosis (see Table 173-5). Silent carriers (-α/αα) may have microcytosis without significant anemia, whereas individuals with two α genes deleted (- -/αα or –α/–α) generally have a mild microcytic anemia. Hb H disease (- -/-α) is associated with moderate microcytic anemia that becomes more severe during pregnancy or acute illness. Unfortunately, hemoglobin separation methods do not always add additional information when α thalassemia syndromes are suspected; it is most common to find normal proportions of HbA, HbF, and HbA_2. If HbH (β^4) is detected, it can aid in diagnosis. However, this hemoglobin is fast moving on gel electrophoresis, and may run off the gel prior to completion of the test. Furthermore, HbH is not always present in sufficient quantities for detection by standard methods. In practice, DNA analysis is often required to confirm α thalassemia syndromes. After sufficient investigations have ruled out other common causes of microcytic anemia (eg, IDA, ACD), DNA analysis for α-thalassemia may be required to confirm most α-thalassemia syndromes. DNA testing for α thalassemia is advised in all pregnant women with unexplained microcytic anemia.

β-thalassemia trait is also associated with a microcytic anemia (see Table 173-6). Furthermore, HbA_2 is characteristically elevated (> 3.5%) (**Table 173-7**). In cases in which there is δβ-thalassemia trait or β-thalassemia trait with a coexisting δ-globin mutation, HbA_2 level may be normal. In β-thalassemia major, the patient, by definition, is making very little or no HbA. In practice, because these patients require routine transfusion of donor blood, hemoglobin separation methods will show normal proportions of HbA, HbF, and HbA_2 expected from donor RBCs. Thalassemias can also be diagnosed in patients that have an elevated HbF quantity in the

TABLE 173-7 Typical Adult Hemoglobin Patterns*

	Hb A	Hb A2	Other Hemoglobins
Normal	95–98%	< 3.5%	—
α-Thalassemia—all types	95–98%	< 3.5%	—
β-Thalassemia Trait	95%	> 3.5%	—
δ-β-Thalassemia Trait	80–90%	< 3.5%	Will have elevated HbF (5–15%)
Hb E Trait	~ 70%	< 5%	Hb E = 25–30%
Hb E Homozygous	—	< 5%	Hb E = 85–95%

*Hb F will also be present in small quantities with all of the above genotypes. Proportion varies, based on several genetic modifiers but typically represents < 2%.

presence of a low MCV and MCH. Alternately, elevated HbF can be seen in individuals with hereditary persistence of fetal hemoglobin (HPFH) who are clinically well, with a normal MCV and MCH.

Hb E is another cause of microcytic anemia. Heterozygous Hb E is asymptomatic and is not associated with anemia, but RBCs can be slightly microcytic (MCV 80 +/- 5 fL). Homozygous Hb E is also asymptomatic, with most individuals having a mild anemia (11.4 +/- 1.8) and microcytosis (MCV 70 +/- 4 fL). Target cells represent 20–80% of RBCs. Typical adult hemoglobin patterns are presented in Table 173-7.

Homozygosity for the HbS mutation (HbSS), or compound heterozygosity for HbS and other beta globin mutations (eg, beta-thalassemia, HbC, HbO, HbD) are associated with important clinical complications (see Sickle Cell Disease section of this chapter). Most other variant hemoglobins are not clinically significant and do not cause disease. An individual who is heterozygous for a β-globin gene mutation will present with one variant hemoglobin in a quantity slightly less in amount than Hb A (eg, Hb E in Table 173-7). When a patient is heterozygous for an α-globin gene mutations, he or she will usually have one variant hemoglobin in a quantity of approximately 10–25%, and the majority of the remaining hemoglobin will be normal Hb A.

TRIAGE AND HOSPITAL ADMISSION

The thalassemias and hemoglobinopathies can present in diverse ways. Heterozygosity for globin gene deletions and mutations is usually asymptomatic or may be associated with mild anemia. These patients can be investigated as an outpatient.

Individuals with clinically significant disorders of hemoglobin, including β-thalassemia major, are usually diagnosed in early childhood and require close medical care and follow-up. Illness requiring inpatient treatment may develop due to acute worsening of anemia or transfusion related complications, including organ dysfunction due to chronic iron overload (see Complications below).

TREATMENT

Patients with β-thalassemia major require routine, chronic transfusion of RBCs (eg, every three to four weeks). For most patients, a target pretransfusion hemoglobin of 9–11 g/dL is appropriate. Higher levels (11–12 g/dL) may be necessary for patients with cardiorespiratory disease. Post-transfusion hemoglobin should not exceed 14–15g/dL.

As a result of the frequency and volume of RBC transfusions, most patients develop significant iron overload early in childhood and require lifelong chelation therapy. Care of these patients is optimally provided by a specialized, multidisciplinary, comprehensive care clinic.

COMPLICATIONS

Complications of thalassemia can be divided into complications of the disease itself, and complications of transfusion therapy. Historically, patients who have received inadequate chronic transfusion develop diffuse bone marrow expansion. Expansion of marrow production in atypical sites (eg, skull and maxillary bones) leads to the characteristic "thalassemic facies," with frontal bossing and prominent maxillae. Expansion of bone marrow in the pelvis and long bones leads to thinning of the boney cortex, high risk of fractures, and delayed growth.

With modern practices of regular RBC transfusion, many of these historical complications are now avoided. However, RBC transfusion is associated with risks that may include hemolytic transfusion reactions, alloimmunization, febrile nonhemolytic transfusion reaction, or transfusion-transmitted infection. All patients who are on a program of chronic transfusion should be vaccinated for hepatitis B virus.

Iron overload is an expected complication in all chronically transfused patients, since each milliliter of RBC transfusion contains 1 mg of iron—at least 200 mg of iron per unit of RBCs transfused. Since the human body has no mechanism for excreting excess iron, once body iron stores are replete, unnecessary free iron is deposited in the tissues, leading to organ dysfunction. Serum ferritin and transferrin saturation are easy tests to screen for iron overload. Although there is no widely accepted target for serum ferritin, it is well understood that increasing serum ferritin concentrations are associated with increased risk of iron deposition in the liver. Over time, significant iron overload of the heart, pancreas, and pituitary will follow if chelation is not initiated. Current practice in patients with β-thalassemia major is to start chelation after the first 20 transfusion or when the serum ferritin level rises above 1000. Chelation treatment usually commences at two to three years of age and continues throughout life. The most common chelating agents in North America are deferoxamine (parenteral) and deferasirox (oral). Deferiprone is another oral chelator that is used widely in Europe and Asia (**Table 173-8**).

RARE CAUSES FOR CONSIDERATION: DETECTION AND DIAGNOSIS OF RARE HEMOGLOBIN VARIANTS

To date more than 1,000 globin chain mutations have been described. The majority are not clinically significant and can be detected by routine testing. Variants found in patients who are clinically well and hematologically normal are unlikely to be clinically significant. However, some rare variants that are clinically significant are difficult to detect through conventional hemoglobin separation techniques and may require further specialized analysis as outlined

TABLE 173-8 Dosing, Administration, and Possible Adverse Effects with Iron Chelating Agents

	Common Starting Dose and Administration	Maximum Daily Dose	Possible Adverse Effects
Deferoxamine	20 mg/kg administered by subcutaneous infusion over 8–12 hours, 5–7 nights per week (up to a maximum of	60 mg/kg	Infusion site reactions; vision or hearing abnormalities; skeletal and growth abnormalities; zinc deficiency; Yersinia enterocolitica infection
Deferasirox	20–40 mg/kg administered by mouth daily (suspended in water)	40 mg/kg	Rash, GI symptoms; mild elevation in transaminases; hearing impairment; nonprogressive elevation in serum creatinine
Deferiprone	75 mg/kg/d in three divided doses	100 mg/kg	Agranulocytosis; arthalgias, zinc deficiency; mild GI symptoms and mild aminotransferase elevations

TABLE 173-9 Detection and Diagnosis of Clinically Significant Rare Hemoglobinopathy Syndromes

Rare Syndrome	Presentation	Detection	Hb Variant Identification
Unstable Hemoglobins	Chronic or sporadic hemolytic anemia.	• Abnormal erythrocyte morphology • Elevated Heinz body counts • Abnormal Hb instability testing (heat or isopropanol) • Suspicious Hb H inclusion bodies	DNA sequencing
High oxygen affinity	Erythrocytosis	Hb oxygen affinity analysis -(p50)	DNA sequencing
Low oxygen affinity	Anemia, cyanosis	Hb oxygen affinity analysis -(p50)	DNA sequencing
Hemoglobin M	Cyanosis	Methemoglobin absorption spectrum	DNA sequencing

Adapted, with permission, from Lafferty JD, Waye JS, Chui DH, et al. Good practice guidelines for laboratory investigation of hemoglobinopathies. *Lab Hematol.* 2003;9(4):237–245.

in **Table 173-9**. DNA investigation may be the only analysis that can definitively identify these hemoglobins and should be considered in patients who have pertinent symptoms.

The unstable hemoglobins

Rare hemoglobin variants may denature readily, causing chronic hemolysis and anemia. The denatured globin precipitates in the RBC, producing Heinz bodies that are removed from the red cells by the spleen. Peripheral blood smear shows bite cells, irregularly contracted erythrocytes, or dense fragments. Other laboratory findings provide supporting evidence for active hemolysis (eg, elevated reticulocyte count, reduced haptoglobin). Unstable hemoglobins can fall into two categories: spontaneously unstable variants that result in congenital Heinz body hemolysis (eg, Hb Köln) or milder forms that present with hemolysis after ingestion of oxidative drugs. The unstable hemoglobins can be difficult to detect using conventional hemoglobin variant detection techniques and the diagnosis may rely on the erythrocyte morphology, Heinz body count, specialized tests to demonstrate in vitro instability, and DNA investigations.

High oxygen affinity hemoglobin variants

Hemoglobin variants that hold on to oxygen more avidly than Hb A are called "high oxygen affinity" hemoglobins. Increased oxygen affinity results in tissue hypoxia that stimulates the production of erythropoietin leading to an erythrocytosis. These patients tend to be asymptomatic but can present with symptoms of increased blood viscosity. Since many of these variants do not separate by routine hemoglobin separation techniques, specialized analysis to measure oxygen equilibration curve and the partial pressure of oxygen at 50% saturation (called the P_{50} value) can be used in diagnosis. Alternately the P_{50} can be calculated by venous blood gas values. DNA analysis can confirm and characterize high oxygen affinity variants.

Low oxygen affinity hemoglobin variants

Some hemoglobin variants have a lower affinity for oxygen and therefore release oxygen more readily than Hb A. This can suppress the production of erythropoietin, leading to a lower hemoglobin level. Like the unstable and high oxygen affinity variants, many hemoglobins with a low oxygen affinity will not separate from Hb A using conventional Hb separation techniques. The detection of an abnormal low oxygen affinity often relies on the clinical presentation correlated with the P_{50} value and a DNA investigation.

The M hemoglobins

Patients presenting with cyanosis can also have an Hb M. These hemoglobin variants have an accumulation of methemoglobin in the circulating red cells that causes a pseudocyanosis or brownish/slate pigmentation of the skin. The M hemoglobins also can be difficult to detect using conventional Hb variant detection techniques. Detection relies on demonstration of abnormal absorption spectra followed by DNA investigation.

DISCHARGE CONSIDERATIONS

Close follow-up should be arranged for patients with complications of hemoglobinopathy. For patients with clinically symptomatic thalassemia syndromes, follow-up with a comprehensive care clinic is suggested.

SICKLE CELL DISEASE

INTRODUCTION

Sickle cell disease (SCD) is characterised by atypical red cells that assume a sickle shape when deoxygenated. The inheritance of a single sickle cell gene (heterozygous Hb S, or sickle cell trait) offers a survival advantage against malaria, which has contributed to the high gene prevalence of Hb S in many regions of Sub-Saharan Africa, the Middle East, India, and the Mediterranean. In part due to global immigration patterns, sickle cell disease has become one of the most common hemoglobinopathies seen worldwide. Patients with sickle cell disease are homozygous for the sickle gene (Hb SS) or compound heterozygous for the Hb S gene mutation and another beta globin gene mutation. Individuals with SCD have a decreased life expectancy and may present with severe clinical complications that can lead to death if not properly treated. Screening for this disorder has been the focus for many newborn screening programs across most of North America and Europe to ensure early prophylaxis is given for reduced mortality and morbidity.

PATHOPHYSIOLOGY

Hemoglobin S is the result of a substitution of valine for glutamic acid at the sixth amino acid of the β-globin chain that decreases the solubility of the hemoglobin molecule in the deoxygenated state causing hemoglobin polymerization and sickle cell formation. The homozygous expression of Hb S and the corresponding absence of Hb A cause a severe sickling disorder, in which hemoglobin polymerization initiates an elaborate pathophysiological cascade involving RBC injury, release of free hemoglobin into the blood, and adhesive interactions among sickle RBCs, endothelial cells, and other blood cells. Damaged RBCs initiate vessel occlusion and ischemia. Furthermore, the ongoing premature destruction of these sickle cells leads to chronic anemia.

The compound heterozygous inheritance of Hb S with other β-globin chain variants (Hb C, Hb D, Hb O^{Arab}, or β-thalassemia trait) may also result in an absence of Hb A and a severe sickling

TABLE 173-10 The Genotypes, Clinical Presentation, and Reproductive Significance of the Sickle Cell Syndromes

Hemoglobinopathy	Clinical Presentation	Genotypes	Reproductive Significance
Hb S trait	None	β^A/β^S	Carrier for all sickling disorders
Hb C trait	None	β^A/β^C	Carrier for Hb SC disease and Hb C disease
Hb C disease	Occasional mild hemolytic anemia	β^C/β^C	Carrier for Hb SC disease and Hb C disease
Hb D trait	None	β^A/β^D	Carrier for Hb SD disease
Hb O^{Arab} trait	None	β^A/β^{OArab}	Carrier for Hb SO disease
β-Thalassemia trait	Microcytosis with normal Hb or mild anemia	β^A/β^0 or β^A/β^+	Carrier for Hb S/β-thalassemia
Sickle cell disease	Severe sickling abnormality	β^S/β^S	Carrier for all sickling disorders
Hb Sβ^0-thalassemia,	Microcytosis, severe sickling abnormality	β^S/β^0	Carrier for all sickling disorders or Hb Sβ^0-thalassemia or thalassemia intermedia or major
Hb SD disease	Severe sickling abnormality	β^S/β^D	Carrier for Hb SD or all sickling disorders
Hb Sβ^+ thalassemia	Microcytosis, mild to moderate sickling abnormality	β^S/β^+	Carrier for all sickling disorders or Hb Sβ^+-thalassemia or β-thalassemia intermedia
Hb SC disease, Hb SO disease	Mild to moderate sickling abnormality	β^S/β^C or β^S/β^{OArab}	Carrier for all sickling disorders

β^A, normal β globin gene; β^S, Hb S gene; β^C, Hb C gene; β^D, Hb D gene; $\beta^{O\text{-}Arab}$, Hb O-Arab gene; β^0, beta-zero mutation (no β globin gene produced); β^+, beta-zero mutation (reduced β globin gene production).

Adapted, with permission, from Lafferty JD, Waye JS, Chui DH, et al. Good practice guidelines for laboratory investigation of hemoglobinopathies. *Lab Hematol.* 2003;9(4):237–245.

syndrome. These genotypes are detailed in **Table 173-10**. Sickle cell disease is associated with an increased risk of death from sepsis, acute chest syndrome or stroke, and chronic complications that accumulate with age.

DIAGNOSIS: DOES THIS PATIENT HAVE ACUTE COMPLICATIONS OF SICKLE CELL DISEASE?

Evaluation of a patient with sickle cell disease will begin with a thorough history and physical. History should include details of clinical symptoms (eg, boney pain, chest pain, or shortness of breath) and a history of previous complications and medical care. In patients with pain, it is critical to determine whether the pain is due to a vaso-occlusive crisis (pain related to sickling of RBCs) or whether another process may be responsible (eg, abdominal pain due to acute cholecytitis). As the patient is likely to have had numerous sickle painful episodes in his or her lifetime, asking the patient, "Is this your typical sickle cell pain?" can help guide whether further investigations are required.

Vital signs should be measured, including pulse oximetry. Hypoxemia can suggest an underlying acute chest syndrome, pneumonia or pulmonary embolism. Hypoxemia is also a risk factor for worsened RBC sickling.

Adult patients are usually aware of their diagnosis of sickle cell disease. However, if the diagnosis or the genotype is in question, further testing may be performed. A CBC will show variable degrees of anemia. Peripheral blood smear should show sickled RBCs. Target cells and Howell-Jolly bodies suggest functional asplenia, associated with splenic autoinfarction—a common complication of sickle cell disease in childhood. Reticulocytes are elevated due to hemolysis of sickle cells. White blood cell count may be elevated if infection is present.

THE SICKLE SOLUBILITY TEST

The Hb S solubility test is a simple screening test able to detect Hb S. When reduced with sodium dithionite, Hb S is insoluble and precipitates in high molarity phosphate buffer at neutral pH. A Hb S solubility test is useful as a screening test for Hb S in adult patients and as a confirmatory test when Hb S is detected by either electrophoresis or HPLC, helping to distinguish Hb S from other variants with similar migrating mobility as Hb S. The sickle solubility test cannot distinguish between sickle cell trait, sickle cell disease, or Hb S/β-thalassemia. The test is negative when the concentration of Hb S is less than 15%, and thus it is not used to test blood samples from infants or patients who have received RBC transfusion. Importantly, the test cannot detect hemoglobin variants such as Hbs C, D Punjab, and O Arab, which can cause a sickling disorder in combination with Hb S. Thus, Hb S solubility tests should not be used for assessment of potential reproductive risk, for genetic counseling, or as a primary diagnostic test.

HEMOGLOBIN SEPARATION AND MOLECULAR DIAGNOSTICS

Methods such as gel electrophoresis, HPLC, and CE are effective for identifying the presence of Hb S and/or other variant hemoglobins involved in compound heterozygous sickle cell disease. For more details on these methods, see Hemoglobin Separation in Thalassemia and Hemoglobinopathies section of this chapter. Molecular diagnostics and DNA analysis are used for positive characterization of the variant hemoglobin(s). Methods used include PCR, direct nucleotide sequencing, and southern hybridization.

TRIAGE AND HOSPITAL ADMISSION

Painful episodes are the most frequent complication in sickle cell disease. Patients who have had recurrent episodes may be treated at home with oral analgesics (acetaminophen, NSAIDs, or opiates). If the episode is more severe, they may require higher-dose therapy in a hospital-based setting. Severe pain requiring repeated doses of IV analgesia is best treated as an in-patient. Other supportive care should include judicious administration of intravenous fluid. Supplemental oxygen is indicated if the SpO_2 or SaO_2 are low. Painful episodes may take several days to a week or more to resolve.

Other indications for admission include acute chest syndrome, sepsis, stroke, and hyperhemolysis. These complications are best managed in an intensive care setting.

TREATMENT

Outpatient treatment of sickle cell disease can be divided into preventative care and symptom management. Preventative care includes penicillin prophylaxis in children, immunizations (especially against encapsulated organisms such as *Streptococcus pneumoniae*, *Hemophilus influenzae*, and *Neisseria meningitides*) and patient education to avoid extremes of heat, remain hydrated, and seek rapid medical attention in case of symptoms. In pediatric populations, there is evidence that chronic RBC transfusion is effective at preventing stroke in certain high-risk groups.

Hydroxyurea is increasingly used to prevent vaso-occlusive crises and hemolysis. There is good evidence in patients with Hb SS that hydroxyurea leads to significantly fewer painful episodes, fewer episodes of chest syndrome, and reduced need for transfusion and hospitalization, with few side effects. Long-term follow-up data suggest that there is also a decrease in mortality proportional to the number of years on hydroxyurea therapy. The exact mechanism of improved clinical outcomes with hydroxyurea in SCD is unknown, although it is known that hemoglobin level and Hb F percentage improve while on the medication, both of which are associated with less severe sickle cell disease phenotype. Hydroxyurea also results in reduced leukocyte count, which may have an anti-inflammatory effect.

The goal of hydroxyurea is to titrate to the maximal tolerated dose for each patient, based on maintaining safe blood counts. Laboratory testing of CBC, reticulocyte count, Hb F levels, renal, and liver function tests should be performed prior to initiating hydroxyurea and should be repeated at regular intervals thereafter. Although the expected decrease in WBC and platelets and increase in HbF can be seen within weeks to months, a clinical response may not be seen until after three to six months of treatment. In addition to laboratory monitoring and dose adjustment, follow-up appointments should be used to assess symptoms and to encourage continued adherence. Because of increased rates of leukemia and skin cancers in patients who have taken hydroxyurea for myeloproliferative disorders, there has been concern about the risk of malignancy after long-term use of hydroxyurea in SCD. However, rates of cancer do not seem to be elevated in adults or children who have taken hydroxyurea for SCD. Although unsubstantiated in human studies, concern remains about possible teratogenesis and impaired spermatogenesis based on animal studies. As a result, contraception is advised for both men and women taking hydroxyurea, and hydroxyurea is contraindicated during pregnancy or breast-feeding.

Other preventative care in SCD disease involves monitoring for end-organ complications, including proliferative sickle retinopathy, pulmonary hypertension, renal impairment, avascular necrosis, and iron overload.

Inpatient treatment may be required for management of acute complications, the diagnosis and treatment of which are discussed in the proceeding section.

COMPLICATIONS

ANEMIA

Patients with SCD will be anemic at baseline, even during periods of good physical health. The anemia in sickle cell disease is caused by red cell destruction or hemolysis. Red cell survival is only 10–20 days, compared with 120 days in individuals without SCD. The bone marrow increases RBC production dramatically, but it is unable to keep pace with the destruction. Red cell production increases by five- to ten-fold in most patients with sickle cell disease.

However, anemia in SCD may become more severe acutely, due to acute-on-chronic hemolysis, sepsis, hyperhemolysis, or aplastic crisis (eg, pure red cell aplasia due to parvovirus B19), or patients may become more symptomatic due to hypoxemia or increased oxygen demand. Red cell transfusions increase the oxygen-carrying capacity of blood, decrease the percentage of sickle RBCs, and improve microvascular perfusion. Simple transfusion is used when the patient has symptoms of anemia and the therapeutic goal is an increase in hemoglobin level. Transfusion is not advised in uncomplicated painful episodes.

Exchange transfusion involves removing the patient's RBCs and replacing them with Hb S-negative donor RBCs. The main advantage of exchange transfusions over simple transfusions is avoidance of hyperviscosity and volume overload, while reducing the percentage of sickle hemoglobin. Acute chest syndrome and stroke are two indications for exchange transfusion. Exchange transfusion requires the availability of skilled staff to perform the procedure as well as adequate vascular access in the patient. For automated exchange transfusion (erythrocytapheresis), specialized equipment is also required. Any patient who is expected to need RBC transfusion should be vaccinated for hepatitis B virus.

PAINFUL EPISODES

Painful episodes (sometimes referred to as "painful crises" or "vaso-occlusive crises") are the most frequent complication in sickle cell disease, and are presumed to be due to vaso-occlusive ischemia in bones and other tissues. Triggers may include hypoxia, dehydration, cold, or fever. The frequency and duration of the vaso-occlusive crisis may vary considerably between patients but it is the most common cause of morbidity and mortality in sickle cell disease. Patients who have had recurrent episodes should have a supply of appropriate oral analgesics (acetaminophen, NSAIDs, or opiates) at home so that pain can be treated quickly and effectively. If the episode is more severe, patients may require higher-dose therapy in a hospital-based setting. Often parenteral therapy (eg, NSAIDs or opiates) is most effective. Patients should be taken at their word about the severity of their pain. There is no objective measure of severity of a vaso-occlusive episode, and undertreatment or delays in analgesic administration lead to unnecessary suffering and weakening of the patient-provider relationship.

ACUTE CHEST SYNDROME

Acute chest syndrome (ACS) is an acute complication of SCD that may be defined as fever and respiratory symptoms in the presence of a new pulmonary infiltrate on chest X-ray. ACS is a leading cause of hospitalization in patients with SCD and a significant risk factor for early mortality. The incidence of ACS is highest in patients with Hb SS genotype. Causes of ACS include pulmonary infections (eg, influenza, bacterial, or viral pneumonia), pulmonary infarction, or fat embolism from necrotic bone marrow. SCD patients who have undergone abdominal surgery are at risk of developing ACS in the immediate postoperative period. SCD patients with asthma are twice as likely to develop ACS as SCD patients who do not have asthma. The most frequent symptoms at diagnosis of ACS include fever, cough, chest pain, shortness of breath, and tachypnea. Acute chest syndrome requires admission to the hospital. If signs and symptoms are severe, patients should be treated in an intensive care setting. Supplemental oxygen should be administered to maintain oxygen saturation of ≥95%. Adequate analgesia is required for pain. CBC, CXR, arterial blood gases, blood cultures (if febrile), sputum cultures, RBC blood grouping, and crossmatch should be done rapidly. Regardless of the etiology, management of ACS includes intravenous broad-spectrum antibiotics, bronchodilators, incentive spirometry, and careful hydration. Patients who are hypoxemic (SaO_2 < 80 mm Hb) should receive supplemental oxygen. Transfusion can be an important adjunct, especially if the patient is hypoxemic. There have been no randomized trials comparing simple and exchange transfusions in this setting. It is generally accepted that in severe acute chest syndrome, the goal of transfusion is to maintain a hemoglobin concentration >10g/dL and a Hb S level of <30%.

■ STROKE

Individuals with SCD are at higher risk of stroke than the general population. Patients with the homozygous form of SCD, HbSS, have the highest risk, with an 11% chance of developing a first stroke by the age of 20 years, compared with a 2% risk for patients with Hb SC disease. Those age 2 to 5 years have the highest incidence of first stroke followed by those between 6 and 9 years of age. Most strokes in children with SCD are ischemic. Clinical features of ischemic stroke include focal weakness (usually hemiparesis); seizures; altered consciousness and mentation; confusion; and visual, speech, and sensory disturbances. In children, symptoms may be transient.

Known risk factors include low hemoglobin levels, high white cell count, hypertension, and a recent history of acute chest syndrome. Genetic factors and nocturnal hypoxemia may also contribute to stroke risk. Transcranial Doppler ultrasonography (TCD) is used as a screening tool for stroke prevention in children with SCD. Children with abnormal TCD receive prophylactic blood transfusion, based on the results of a randomized trial showing a 92% reduction in stroke risk with a chronic RBC transfusion strategy versus observation.

No large studies of stroke prevention have been done in adults with SCD. Early detection is important. Although treatment of acute stroke in children focuses on hydration and exchange transfusion, there is less consensus on SCD-specific interventions for adults with stroke. Practice guidelines from the National Institutes of Health (NIH) and the National Heart, Lung, and Blood Institute (NHLBI) are based on current recommendations for prevention and management of stroke in adults without SCD.

■ SEPSIS

Patients with sickle cell disease are at increased risk of infection and bacteremia. Increased incidence of infection is partially explained by functional asplenia—immunization against encapsulated organisms should help to decrease the risk. SCD patients with fever should receive an appropriate septic workup, with consideration of their immunization status and past history of sickle cell complications. Acute chest syndrome, osteomyelitis, and skin and soft tissue infections should be ruled out, as appropriate.

■ PRIAPISM

Priapism occurs in 30–45% of male patients with SCD and it is defined as a prolonged, unwanted, and uncomfortable or painful erection. Priapism occurs when sickle veno-occlusion causes a pathologic decrease in venous outflow from the penile vascular chambers. Minor episodes can be uncomfortable but tolerable and self-limited, lasting up to several hours. Major episodes can last a few hours to several days and are often extremely painful. Prolonged priapism (>4 hours) can lead to ischemia and fibrosis and is considered a medical emergency. Prolonged or recurrent priapism can result in impotence.

Initial self-treatment by patients has some reported benefit, including analgesia, oral hydration, and exercise. However, for some patients the duration of the episode seems unresponsive to conservative measures. If a patient presents for medical attention, he should be treated rapidly and in a sensitive manner. First-line intervention includes supportive care measures such as intravenous hydration and narcotic analgesia. If the episode persists for more than two hours, additional measures must be considered. Use of exchange transfusion in this setting is controversial because of conflicting evidence for efficacy and reports of ASPEN syndrome (association of sickle cell disease, priapism, exchange transfusion, and neurologic events). If the episode does not resolve rapidly, a urology specialist should become involved.

■ BONE AND SOFT TISSUE COMPLICATIONS

In SCD patients presenting with bone pain, clinicians must distinguish between common causes, including acute vaso-occlusive crisis, osteomyelitis (OM), and avascular necrosis, while also considering more rare complications such as abscesses or septic arthritis. It is useful to know that bone pain in sickle cell disease is much more likely to be due to vaso-occlusion than to OM; in one pediatric series, VOC was at least 50 times more likely.

A thorough evaluation begins with assessing historical features of the pain. If the onset of symptoms was acute, it may be suggestive of vaso-occlusion or OM versus the chronic pain and disability caused by AVN. Concurrent infectious symptoms (eg, fever, rigors) may be present in OM. Any prior history of boney complications can also guide further investigations.

Physical examination should include a musculoskeletal examination, targeting the joint or other location of symptoms. Elevated temperature may be suggestive of OM or other infectious etiology, while other abnormalities in vital signs (eg, tachycardia, hypotension) would be late signs and potentially indicative of progression to sepsis.

Leukocytosis and increased erythrocyte sedimentation rate (ESR) are nonspecific findings that may be present in both infectious and noninfectious processes. If infection is suspected, blood cultures should be drawn. Cultures of the suspected site of infection also aid in diagnosis (eg, joint aspiration, abscess drainage, bone aspirate, or bone biopsy), as indicated by clinical suspicion and results of imaging.

Plain radiography, radioisotope bone scanning, and radiolabelled leukocyte scanning are not always useful in the routine diagnostic evaluation of bone pain in SCD as these modalities can detect acute infarction but changes are often difficult to distinguish from those seen in OM. Ultrasonography is a rapid, simple, and noninvasive modality that is moderately sensitive for detecting acute osteomyelitis. The main ultrasonographic finding in OM is subperiosteal fluid. MRI can be useful in the diagnosis of OM. As with other imaging modalities, there is overlap between the changes seen in infection and infarction. Although still not 100% specific for differentiating OM from VOC, gadolinium enhancement improves the accuracy of MRI.

Management of bone pain may include oral, intravenous, or subcutaneous opiates, depending on severity of pain. More specific management should be tailored to the underlying process.

■ PERIOPERATIVE COMPLICATIONS

Surgical procedures such as splenectomy, cholecystectomy, or orthopedic surgery are commonly required in patients due to complications of their SCD. In addition, patients with SCD may require surgeries due to unrelated medical problems during their lifetimes. Patients with SCD have a higher risk of perioperative complications than the general population for several reasons. First, patients with SCD are already anemic and any procedural bleeding will further drop hemoglobin levels, leading to more severe anemia and decreased oxygen carrying capacity. Second, intraoperative hypoxia, postoperative atelectasis, and decreased oral intake can trigger sickling of red blood cells. Sickling of red blood cells can lead to painful crisis or acute chest syndrome, among other SCD-related complications. All patients should undergo consultation with an anesthesiologist prior to surgery. Patients undergoing medium- and high-risk surgery should receive prophylactic red blood cell transfusions to target a hemoglobin of 100 mg/L. Red cell exchange transfusion can be considered in very high risk procedures (eg, orthopedic surgery requiring tourniquet, vascular surgery requiring arterial clamping) or in patients with a history of postoperative complications. Cross-matched units of red blood cells should be on hold in the blood bank. Importantly, all patients should receive adequate hydration prior to surgery. If the patient is required to remain in NPO status prior to surgery, he or she should be admitted for intravenous hydration with isotonic solution during the NPO period. Postoperatively, isotonic intravenous fluids should be administered until the patient is drinking and eating well. Supplemental oxygen should be used as needed. Deep breathing exercises and/or incentive spirometry may be used to reduce the risk of postoperative atelectasis.

An in-depth discussion of chronic complications of SCD is beyond the scope of this chapter. An excellent resource for further information is the NIH/NHLBI Guidelines (2002) ("The Management of Sickle Cell Disease"). Close follow-up should be arranged for patients with complications of SCD.

CONCLUSION

Discharge considerations: Patients admitted for complications od sickle cell disease require close monitoring of symptoms and laboratory parameters during their hospital stay. If they are being treated for a painful episode, doses of pain medication should be carefully titrated downward as pain symptoms improve. Intravenuos opiates should be switched over equianalgesic doses of oral medication prior to discharge. Eligibility for discharge will depend on stable clinical status and ability of the patient to manage symptoms effectively at home. Follow-up with a comprehensive care clinic is suggested.

SUGGESTED READINGS

Brawley OW, Cornelius LJ, Edwards LR, et al. National Institutes of Health Consensus Development Conference statement: hydroxyurea treatment for sickle cell disease. *Ann Intern Med.* 2008;148(12):932–938.

Capellini M, Cohen A, Eleftheriou A, et al. Guidelines for the Clinical Management of Thalassemia. Second ed. Thalassemia International Federation, November 2008. Online at: www.thalassaemia.org.cy/pdf/Guidelines_2nd_revised_edition_EN.pdf

Chui DHK, Fucharoen S, Chan V. Hemoglobin H disease: not necessarily a benign disorder. *Blood.* 2003;101:791–800.

Clement FM, Klarenbach S, Tonelli M, Johnson JA, Manns BJ. The impact of selecting a high hemoglobin target level on health-related quality of life for patients with chronic kidney disease: a systematic review and meta-analysis. *Arch Intern Med.* 2009;169(12):1104–1112.

Dhaliwal G, Cornett PA, Tierney LM, Jr. Hemolytic anemia. *Am Fam Physician.* 2004;69(11):2599–2606.

Lanzkron S, Strouse JJ, Wilson R, et al. Systematic review: hydroxyurea for the treatment of adults with sickle cell disease. *Ann Intern Med.* 2008;148(12):939–955.

McMullin MF, Bareford D, Campbell P, et al. Guidelines for the diagnosis, investigation and management of polycythaemia/erythrocytosis. *Br J Haematol.* 2005;130(2):174–195.

NIH/NHLBI Guidelines. Management of adults with sickle cell disease, 2002. Available at http://www.nhlbi.nih.gov/health/prof/blood/sickle/sc_mngt.pdf.

Platt OS, Brambilla DJ, Rosse WF, et al. Mortality in sickle cell disease. Life expectancy and risk factors for early death. *N Engl J Med.* 1994;330(23):1639–1644.

Zempsky WT. Treatment of sickle cell pain: fostering trust and justice. *JAMA.* 2009;302(22):2479–2480.

CHAPTER 174

Disorders of the White Cell

Blair J. N. Leonard, MD, PhD, FRCP
Brian Leber, MD, FRCP(C)

Key Clinical Questions

1. What are the most common causes of leukocytosis in the hospital inpatient setting?
2. Which medications can cause neutropenia and agranulocytosis?
3. What are the most common causes of eosinophilia?
4. What key white blood cell (WBC) findings indicate an impending medical emergency and warrant immediate action?
5. What are the indications for a bone marrow biopsy and aspirate?
6. What is the role of molecular testing in the diagnostic work up of common WBC disorders?
7. What is the role for granulocyte colony-stimulating factors (GCSF) in nonmalignant hematologic disorders?

INTRODUCTION

Deviation from the normal range in the leukocyte count is one of the most common laboratory abnormalities in the inpatient setting and frequently indicates the onset of clinical conditions that significantly impact hospitalized patients. Individual laboratory values may vary from day to day depending on fluid status and other factors,. Hence, a "normal" white blood cell (WBC) or differential count has a typical distribution of values (**Table 174-1**).

A natural response to the physiologic fluctuations of the host's hormonal and cytokine milieu, WBC counts also vary with the time of day and the season of the year. Typically, the hormonal variation associated with pregnancy will also increase the absolute WBC count due to an increase in circulating neutrophils.

There is also a significant genetic component to the ranges expressed on a WBC count, as neutrophil counts have been shown to vary considerably among ethnic groups. People of African descent, Yemenite and Ethiopian Jews, and people of Middle Eastern decent all have been shown to possess WBC counts with medians well below those established in predominantly Caucasian populations. Typically, these values do not fall below the threshold of mild neutropenia ($< 1.5 \times 10^9$) for any significant period of time, and thus are not usually associated with significant infection risk. In fact, these physiologic deviations are not known to result in any clinically measurable increase in morbidity or mortality, and do not require any specific intervention once underlying pathology has been ruled out.

Recognizing abnormalities of the complete blood count (CBC) and, more specifically, the composition of the differential count are critical for formulating a differential diagnosis of disorders involving the WBC lineages. Valuable time and resources can be saved and best directed if careful attention is paid to these simple tests in the context of a good history and physical examination performed when abnormalities are first detected. As a general rule of thumb, malignant causes should always be considered in the differential diagnosis when red blood cell (RBC) or platelet lineages are also abnormal, or if there is a history of unexplained weight loss, anorexia, lymphadenopathy, or other systemic symptoms. This chapter will review each WBC lineage and the common nonmalignant conditions associated with their abnormalities. Hematologic malignancies will be addressed in Chapter 179.

EPIDEMIOLOGY OF WHITE BLOOD CELL ABNORMALITIES

In one recent large retrospective study of over 45,000 hospitalized patients, leukocytosis had a prevalence of 31.2%, and leucopenia was prevalent in 6.1%. Underlying bacterial infection is the most common reason for both leukocytosis and leukopenia in the inpatient setting, and thus the overwhelming majority of these variations in WBC counts are due to disorders involving neutrophils. Therefore, practically speaking, the terms *leukocytosis* and *neutrophilia* are commonly interchanged in the medical literature. While disorders involving other components of the WBC differential are far less common, they can represent vastly different pathological processes, and thus require different diagnostic investigation. Not all leukocytoses are neutrophilias, and thus the timely identification of the cell lineage involved in a WBC abnormality can have a significant impact on clinical outcome.

TABLE 174-1 The Normal White Blood Cell Count

White Blood Cell Type	Typical Range of Values
Neutrophils	4–11 × 10^9/L
Lymphocytes	1.5–3.5 × 10^9/L
Monocytes	0.2–0.8 × 10^9/L
Eosinophils	0.05–0.4 × 10^9/L
Basophils	0.01–0.1 × 10^9/L

PROGNOSIS

The WBC count can be thought of as equilibrium, with deviations above or below the normal distribution correlating with adverse outcomes in patients. Large, retrospective, population-based analysis of abnormalities in WBC magnitude have indicated that absolute WBC count correlates with all-cause mortality in an otherwise healthy population. As might be expected, this association is J-shaped, with both increasing leukopenia and increasing leukocytosis correlating with increased mortality. In hospitalized patients the presence of either abnormality has been shown to correlate with an increase in 30-day overall mortality. WBC deviations correlate with morbidity and mortality not only across patient settings, such as the intensive care unit and emergency department, but also across disease states.

Leukocystosis is a robust prognostic indicator of overall mortality in the hospitalized patient with underlying infection, such as profound sepsis, with several studies confirming that the absolute magnitude of the leukocytosis directly correlates with the overall mortality rate. Leukocytosis is also prognostic in cardiac conditions, including coronary artery disease (CAD) and acute coronary syndrome (ACS). Though it is unclear if WBC abnormalities have an active or passive role in mortality of these pathologies, it is clear that abnormalities in WBC count herald a poorer outcome in such patients.

PRACTICE POINT

- An abnormal WBC count is a clear indicator of failing health in a broad spectrum of patient settings and, thus, is an important laboratory result that requires further investigation to ascertain etiology.

The bulk of experience with morbidity and mortality in leukopenic patients comes from patient populations with malignancies, where there is a direct correlation between depth of neutropenia and infection and mortality rates. However, patients without malignancy or primary bone marrow pathology can also develop significant leukopenia. In this setting leukopenia may represent a myriad of pathologic mechanisms, such as direct cytokine suppression of marrow precursors or bone marrow infiltration, and is an ominous sign of profound immunocompromisation of the patient. Such patients typically require specialized clinical care as well as intensive support and monitoring. Despite the widespread availability of WBC growth factors, these medications have not shown significant efficacy in septic patients who are otherwise not immunocompromised and are not routinely recommended for septic hospitalized patients.

DISORDERS OF THE NEUTROPHIL

NEUTROPHILLIA

Infection and physiologic stress cause the overwhelming proportion of neutrophillia and, thus, leukocytosis (**Table 174-2**).

TABLE 174-2 Differential Diagnosis of Leukocytosis in the Hospitalized Patient

Diagnosis	Incidence
Infection	52%
Physiologic stress	38%
Medications or drugs	11%
Hematologic condition	6%
Necrosis/inflammation	6%
Unknown	4%

Data from Wanahita A, Goldsmith EA, Musher DM. Conditions associated with leukocytosis in a tertiary care hospital, with particular attention to the role of infection caused by clostridium difficile. *Clinical Infectious Diseases.* 2002;34:1585–1592.

Common sources of infection include the pulmonary, urinary, and gastrointestinal tracts, as well as soft tissue infections. A burgeoning infective etiology in hospitalized patients in the era of widespread antibiotic use is *Clostridium difficile* colitis, and this diagnosis should be considered in the workup of an unexplained leukocytosis in a hospitalized patient, especially if there is a history of recent exposure to systemic antibiotic therapy.

PRACTICE POINT

- Given the importance of timely intervention with goal-directed therapy in septic patients, this paradigm underscores the need for initial consideration of infection in all hospitalized patients with an unexplained leukocytosis.

Both pathologic and physiologic stressors can cause glucocorticoid hormone release, and the elevated circulating cortisol will liberate neutrophils from the endothelium where they are normally marginalized. Thus, any state causing stress can potentially cause an elevated neutrophil count in hospitalized patients. Common causes of the neutrophilia that is associated with stress include the presence of a hyperdynamic cardiac output state from cardiorespiratory exertion, or a prolonged state of extreme anxiety. Though initially differentiating infection from physiologic stress as a cause of neutrophilia can be challenging, a few key elements may be more suggestive of the likely cause. Stress-related neutrophilia is typically characterized by an antecedent initiating event, followed by a transient process, such as seizure, rigors, hyperthermia, or hyperemesis, that commonly reverses within hours after the initiating stimulus. In addition, stress hormone–mediated neutrophil demarginalization does not typically cause the characteristic morphologic findings of the activated neutrophil, such as toxic granulation of the cytoplasm or the presence of Dohle bodies. A history, physical examination, and review of the peripheral smear often identifies an obvious etiology and saves time and resources in the diagnostic workup.

Although less common than infection or stress, some medications frequently cause neutrophilia in the hospitalized patient. These medications include systemic corticosteroids, anesthetic agents, beta-agonists, and epinephrine. As there is often no easy way to confirm a medication-induced neutrophilia, it is a diagnosis of exclusion and should only be considered when infection has been essentially ruled out. Much like stress-induced neutrophilia, a drug-induced cause is less likely to show toxic changes to neutrophils on morphologic examination, and the presence of such changes or other concerning symptoms should lead the hospitalist to further investigate the possibility of infection as a cause.

NEUTROPENIA

Neutropenia is often classified into mild (< 1.5×10^9/L neutrophils), moderate (< 1.0×10^9/L), or severe (< 0.5×10^9/L), with infection risk and mortality highest in the severely neutropenic patient. Such patients are at high risk of death, and specialty care and consultation with a hematologist should be sought. In contrast to the outpatient setting where primary hematologic and "unknown" causes predominate, the most common causes of acquired neutropenia in the hospitalized setting include infection (both bacterial and viral), medication, and autoimmune and systemic inflammation. From a causal standpoint, neutropenia is relatively nonspecific for bacterial infections, and is more likely a reflection of the depth of immunocompromisation rather than a reflection of any specific organism. Acute viral infections, such as with parvovirus B19, may give rise to a transient isolated neutropenia, typically associated with nonspecific viral infection symptoms and reticulocytopenia. Some chronic viral infections are also classically associated with an isolated neutropenia, including HIV and hepatitis C infection, and should be considered in the differential diagnosis of a persisting neutropenia if the history or physical examination is suggestive.

After infection, other benign causes of neutropenia are less common. A hypersplenic state can sequester neutrophils much like RBCs, causing a mild chronic neutropenia. Dietary insufficiency can cause megaloblastosis, which may initially manifest as neutropenia with classic megaloblastic changes of hypersegmented neutrophils indicating nuclear-cytoplasmic maturation dyssynchrony. Serum B12 and RBC folate levels are important to investigate if this abnormality is observed, as deficiencies in these nutrients are a common reversible cause of megaloblastosis. These findings may appear before a macrocytic anemia is present. Prevalence of B12 deficiency has been noted in the 10% to 15% range in older patients in the community, however, and perhaps as high as 30% to 40% in hospitalized patients. Metformin-related B12 deficiency is an underappreciated cause, and positively correlates with both the dose and duration of metformin therapy. In addition, common medications interfering with cellular metabolism, such as methotrexate or hydroxyurea, may also give rise to neutropenia with a megaloblastic picture, though without B12 or folate deficiency.

Acquired autoimmune neutropenia may occasionally be seen in hospitalized patients, and is associated with autoantibodies generated toward antigens on the neutrophil's surface. In elderly hospitalized patients these antibodies are typically secondary to systemic inflammatory conditions such as systemic lupus erythematosus or rheumatoid arthritis, though they may also be associated with a recent transfusion or the presence of a thymoma. Diagnosis is largely based on supportive history, physical, and diagnostic testing for the underlying systemic diseases, as the antineutrophil antibodies are often nonspecific and haven't been validated for diagnosis. The course may be complicated with other autoimmune phenomena such as hemolytic anemia, antiphospholipid antibody syndrome, or Felty syndrome. Patients are at risk of overwhelming infection when profoundly neutropenic and need to be closely monitored for infection, with rapid initiation of therapy should infection arise. Treatment is largely supportive and aimed at treating the underlying condition, though occasionally granulocyte colony-stimulating factor (GCSF) may be used in selected patients. It is advisable to avoid fresh unwashed fruits and vegetables or flowers during the neutropenic period due to the potential increased risk of infection associated with such exposures.

A large population-based cohort study identified several drugs that have been associated with medication-induced agranulocytosis—a failure of bone marrow to produce neutrophils. Many of these medications are commonly used in hospitalized patients (**Table 174-3**).

TABLE 174-3 List of Drugs Causing Agranulocytosis in Hospitalized Patients

Medication	Attributable Risk
Metamizole sodium	16.29
Beta-Lactam antibiotics	12.01
Ticlopidine	11.19
Antithyroid drugs	7.21
Sulfonamides	5.44
Calcium dobesilate	5.02
Diclonfinac	4.19
Spironolactone	3.22
Carbamazapine	2.57

Data from Ibáñez L, Vidal X, Ballarín E, Laporte JR. Population-based drug-induced agranulocytosis. *Arch Intern Med.* 2005;165(8):869–874.

Cyclic neutropenia, chronic benign neutropenia, and congenital bone marrow failure syndrome such as Kostmann disease can also occasionally present with asymptomatic neutropenia in a hospitalized patient. These patients typically will have a history of such a condition and given the rarity of these diagnoses, should be considered only when the more common etiologies have been ruled out.

ACQUIRED NEUTROPHIL DYSFUNCTION

Outside of absolute number, neutrophils can also be functionally impaired by conditions such as poorly controlled diabetes, chronic iron overload states, and chronic renal insufficiency. Typically these patients are more susceptible to bacterial infections secondary to neutrophil dysfunction, often with uncommon organisms such as *Vibrio Vulnificus* or *Yersenia Enterocolitica* as in the case of chronically iron-overloaded patients. Neutrophil dysfunction can occur as a result of the underlying condition as well as from instituted therapies, such as hemodialysis in renal failure patients. Treatment paradigms involve appropriate antimicrobial and supportive therapies, as well as control or resolution of the underlying condition if possible.

DISORDERS OF LYMPHOCYTES

Lymphocytes are generated in the bone marrow from a common precursor. They can differentiate in the bone marrow (B-cells) and become involved in antibody, or humoral, immunity, or they can differentiate in the thymus (T-cells) and become involved in cell-mediated immunity. Abnormalities of the lymphocyte are the next most common nonmalignant WBC abnormality encountered in the hospital after those involving the neutrophil. These can be broadly categorized as inherited or related to acquired lymphocyte abnormalities; the acquired variety will predominate in the hospitalist setting.

INHERITED LYMPHOCYTE DISORDERS

Inherited lymphocyte abnormalities are relatively infrequent, and typically the care of such patients would lie beyond the scope of the practicing hospitalist with few exceptions. However, selective IgA deficiency is a relatively common abnormality seen in the Caucasian population (~ 1 in 600) and, thus, will likely be encountered in the course of practice. Awareness for selective IgA deficiency should be raised when patients report recurrent pyogenic infections, typically involving skin and/or lungs. Appropriately focused antibiotic therapy is the treatment of choice in these patients, and there is no role for intravenous immunoglobulin (IVIG) supplementation, as IVIG does not contain IgA. Importantly, adverse reactions can occur upon transfusion of IgA-deficient patients with blood products, including life-threatening anaphylactic reactions. This is due to the presence of preformed IgA antibodies in IgA-deficient patients that react to contaminating IgA in the administered blood products. Autoimmune conditions such as systemic lupus erythematosus (SLE) or rheumatoid arthritis (RA) are also commonly associated with IgA deficiency, and a further workup for these conditions in newly diagnosed patients would be prudent.

ACQUIRED LYMPHOCYTE DISORDERS: LYMPHOCYTOSIS

Acquired nonmalignant lymphocytosis is a relatively common finding in the hospitalized population, and typically represents a reactive process secondary to infection, most commonly of a viral nature. Mononucleosis syndromes, typically associated with characteristic morphologic changes to lymphocytes on the peripheral blood film (atypical lymphocytes), suggests viral etiologies such as acute cytomegalovirus or Epstein-Barr virus. Potential bacterial etiologies for lymphocytosis would be a less common finding, but would include such bacterium as *Bordetella pertussis* and *Toxoplasmosis gondii*.

Less common causes of an acquired lymphocytosis include a reactive process secondary to administration of a drug or medication such as a corticosteroid. Reactive lymphocytosis can also occur secondary to a variety of underlying systemic conditions such as Graves disease, Hodgkin lymphoma, or SLE. These less common etiologies should be considered if the lymphocytosis persists once infectious etiologies have been ruled out.

Monoclonal B-cell lymphocytosis (MBL) is an increasingly appreciated cause of chronic, persisting lymphocytosis in the elderly hospitalized patient with no obvious underlying etiology. MBL is similar to the monoclonal gammopathy of unknown significance (MGUS) in that a clonal population of cells is apparent with increasing age, with an unknown clinical significance. While MBL in and of itself does not require specific treatment, these patients are more likely to develop chronic lymphocytic leukemia (CLL) and, thus, would benefit from closer monitoring for the development of features of CLL. A lymphocytosis less than 5000/mm^3 but greater than the normal range without clinical features of CLL would suggest MBL, whereas persistent lymphocyte counts of greater than 5000/mm^3 would suggest a diagnosis of CLL. A diagnosis of MBL can be made on flow cytometry; does would not require a bone marrow aspirate or biopsy unless associated cytopenias are involved and the diagnosis of symptomatic CLL with bone marrow involvement is being considered.

ACQUIRED LYMPHOCYTE DISORDERS: LYMPHOCYTOPENIA

In the general population, the acquired immune deficiency syndrome (AIDS) is the most common cause of an acquired nonmalignant lymphocytopenia, typically skewing the CD4:CD8 ratio by selectively depleting the CD4 T-cell subpopulation. A persistent unexplained lymphocytopenia warrants further investigation, as occult chronic HIV infection would be high on the differential diagnosis and requires prompt recognition and treatment.

Other less common causes include hypersplenism, a reactive response to active inflammatory conditions, or concomitant corticosteroid use. Similar to chronic alcohol consumption, malnutrition may present with other findings, such as a transient lymphocytopenia, Serum immunoglobulins should be quantified in persistently lymphocytopenic patients, as IgG-deficient patients will be more susceptible to bacterial infections, such as pneumonia or sinusitis, and may respond well to IVIG supplementation. The reverse is not always true, however, and IgG-deficient patients may not be lymphocytopenic at all, with the diagnosis of IgG deficiency only suspected with a history of repeated unexplained infections in an otherwise healthy patient.

TABLE 174-4 Differential Diagnosis of Secondary Causes of Monocytosis

Infection
CMV Infection, bacterial endocarditis
Tuberculosis, syphilis
Malignancy
Hodgkin disease, multiple myeloma
Systemic inflammatory conditions
Ulcererative colitis, connective tissue diseases
Sarcoidosis
Alcoholic hepatitis

DISORDERS OF MONOCYTES AND MACROPHAGES

Monocytes are typically released into circulation once generated in the marrow and are sequestered in the red pulp of the spleen then released into the bloodstream to differentiate into functional macrophages at their destination. These WBCs are involved in phagocytosis, cytokine release, and appropriate antigen presentation at sites of infection. Benign abnormalities include monocytosis and monocytopenia, the dysregulation of function associated with the hemophagocytic syndromes, and the rare heterogeneous histiocytic diseases, which are beyond the scope of this review.

MONOCYTOSIS

The benign causes of a monocytosis are reactive processes and are numerous (**Table 174-4**), including infection, malignancy, and autoimmune processes.

MONOCYTOPENIA

Monocytopenia is less common and is associated with neoplastic processes such as hairy cell leukemia or autoimmune processes like SLE. Systemic corticosteroid use can cause a transient monocytosis, as can an associated thermal insult.

HEMOPHAGOCYTIC SYNDROMES

Hemophagocytic syndromes are characterized by a highly dysregulated immune response toward an underlying stimulus and may be associated with infection, products of host tissue damage, or underlying autoimmune or malignant conditions. They can be acquired or familial, and the presence of activated macrophages that consume host RBCs (hemophagocytosis) is the cardinal feature of these rare, but potentially fatal syndromes. The timely identification of a hemophagocytic syndrome is important, as death can occur rapidly due to the associated hyperinflammatory state. Clinical suspicion should be raised for this condition in any patient with cytopenias, splenomegaly, and a recurring or prolonged fever without any organism isolated and that is unresponsive to empirical antimicrobial therapy. No specific blood tests confirm hemophagocytic syndrome, though an elevated ferritin and fasting triglyceride with decreased fibrinogen levels accompanying the clinical findings are highly suggestive and are part of the diagnostic criteria. The hemophagocytic syndrome associated with fulminant Epstein-Barr virus (EBV) infection is particularly concerning due to the high mortality associated with it, and urgent hematologic consultation should always be sought when the diagnosis is considered.

TABLE 174-5 Differential Diagnosis of Secondary Causes of Eosinophilia

Allergic disorders
Helmenthitic parasitic infections
Drug hypersensitivity reactions
Pulmonary syndromes (eg, Loeffler syndrome)
Tuberculosis
Primary causes (eg, chronic eosinophilic leukemia)
Neoplastic process (eg, Hodgkin disease)
Hypereosinophilic syndrome
Myeloproliferative disorders (eg, chronic myelomonocytic leukemia)

DISORDERS OF EOSINOPHILS

Eosinophils are highly granular cells capable of producing a multitude of destructive enzymes, reactive oxygen species, and cytokines to combat parasitic and viral infections. Benign abnormalities of eosinophils, typically manifested as an eosinophilia, are a relatively rare abnormality of WBC. However, its timely identification in the hospitalized patient can help to appropriately direct the inquisition for an underlying etiology. Common causes of peripheral blood eosinophilia are listed in (**Table 174-5**).

Classically, the diagnostic pathway of eosinophilia branches with the initial identification of a primary or clonal process versus a reactive or secondary process. For example, eosinophilia defined as an absolute eosinophil count of greater than 500/mm^3 (or range 400–600/mm^3) can be associated with HIV infection, syphilis, tuberculosis, parasitic infections, new medications, allergic bronchopulmonary aspergillosis (ABPA), adrenal insufficiency, and hematologic malignancies such as Hodgkin disease. If an appropriate history and physical examination do not reveal an obvious reactive cause such as an acute inflammatory state, infection, or malignancy, further investigations should include a bone marrow biopsy with testing for eosinophilic clonality. Tests for clonality include conventional G-banding cytogenetics and molecular testing for cloncal markers such as the X-linked HUMARA gene in females, the mutated c-Kit gene, or the FIP1L1-PDGF fusion protein. This latter molecular target is important to look for, as its presence portends a high likelihood of response to oral tyrosine kinase therapy, such as imatinib. If established as a clonal disorder, primary eosinophilic processes include the myelodysplastic/myeloproliferative disorders and acute or chronic eosinophilic leukemia. The idiopathic hypereosinophilic syndrome (HES) is a diagnosis of exclusion and should only be made in the absence of identification of either a primary clonal or secondary reactive process.

Drug reactions should also be considered in the differential diagnosis of a reactive eosinophilia, with common candidates including antibiotics such as the penicillins and cephalosporins, ACE inhibitors, and anticonvulsants such as phenytoin.

The immediate danger of eosinophilia is that eosinophils are highly granular cells, possessing a variety of toxic proteins, such as peroxidase, and major basic protein; an excess can lead to indiscriminate and widespread tissue infiltration and damage. Regardless of etiology, eosinophils are exquisitely sensitive to large doses of corticosteroids. Other potential treatments include interferon alpha and selected tyrosine kinase inhibitors. Specialized consultation should be sought and treatment should be initiated promptly in cases of a severe eosinophilia to minimize the extensive tissue damage that can accompany this condition.

DISORDERS OF BASOPHILS AND MAST CELLS

Basophils and mast cells are related cells, sharing functional properties (such as histamine release) that help protect the host from parasitic infection. They also play a role in the innate immune system of the host against bacterial infection and are involved in the IgE-mediated hypersensitivity reaction. Benign abnormalities involving basophils or mast cells are very uncommon; typically, abnormalities of absolute number, as functional disorders of basophils, are rare.

BASOPHILIA

Primary basophilia is highly suggestive of chronic myelogenous leukemia (CML), and investigations should be initiated to rule out this condition when basophilia is found. Secondary basophilia can be seen in allergic reactions such as those accompanying drug or food hypersensitivity. In addition, it can accompany underlying infections such as varicella and/or autoimmune conditions, the classic being ulcerative colitis. Endocrine dysfunction such as that observed in hypothyroidism can also cause basophilia. In children and, less frequently, in adults, cutaneous mastocytosis typically presenting as urticarium pigmentosum may be seen, with characteristic lesions that become intensely pruritic when stroked. Though clonal in nature, in children this condition is not considered malignant and often resolves spontaneously. In adults the malignant counterpart, systemic mastocytosis, is more frequently found.

BASOPHILOPENIA

Basophilopenia is a relatively nonspecific finding associated with increased levels of stress and glucocorticoid levels, such as may be seen in sepsis, systemic inflammation conditions, and acute hemorrhage. Endocrine fluctuations such as those occurring in hyperthyroidism or ovulation can also be associated with a transient basophilopenia.

LEUKEMOID REACTIONS

Leukemoid reactions are elevated WBC counts (typically $>50.0 \times 10^9$/L) characterized by the presence of immature cell types, such as promyelocytes and metamyelocytes, in the peripheral blood—the so-called "left shift" along the flow of leukocyte differentiation (**Figure 174-1**).

These represent the pool of stored polymorphonuclear neutrophils (PMNs) typically harbored in the bone marrow. Unlike the similar presentation of CML, the leukemoid reaction is reactive and not of clonal origin. Historically, the elevated leukocyte alkaline phosphatase (LAP) score was more suggestive of the functional leukocytes of a leukemoid reaction than the suppressed LAP observed in CML. With the higher sensitivity and specificity of polymerase chain reaction (PCR) testing of peripheral blood samples for the breakpoint cluster region (BCR)–Abelson leukemia (ABL) virus transcript of CML, the LAP is largely of historical note only.

The leukemoid reaction can be seen in hospitalized patients secondary to several acute medical conditions, all of which appear to essentially "shock" the bone marrow into mobilizing its cellular components via cytokine- and growth factor–mediated processes. Such conditions include the massive hemorrhage that can accompany trauma or a gastrointestinal bleed or the profound immunosuppression of severe sepsis. Infrequently, leukamoid reactions can be related to the administration of certain medications such as corticosteroids. Leukemoid reactions typically occur suddenly and can result in startling and impressive acute increases in the WBC count. Though reflective of the severity of the pathologic stress, leukemoid

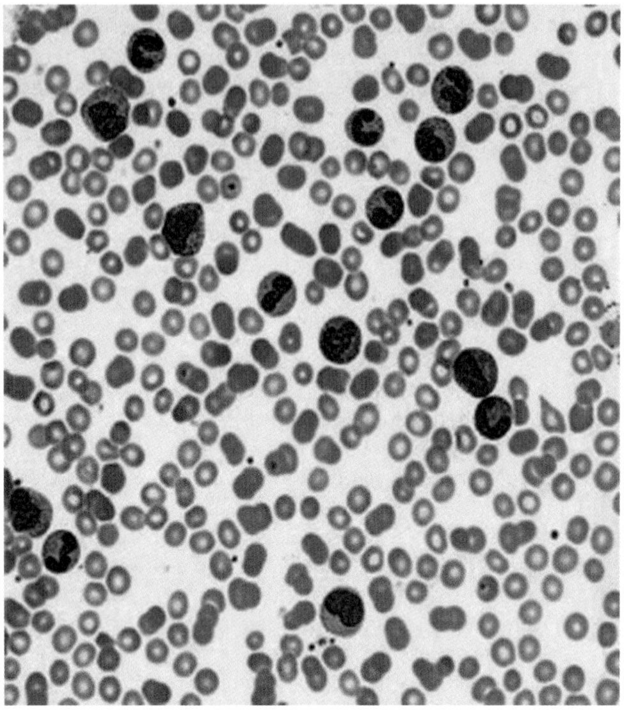

Figure 174-1 *Left-shifted peripheral blood film.*

reactions are not known to be dangerous to the patient and will typically resolve with appropriate treatment and resolution of the underlying cause.

LEUKOERYTHROBLASTIC REACTION

The leukoerythroblastic reaction has a similar presentation to that of the leukemoid reaction. However, the presence of circulating RBC precursors, or nucleated red cells (NERCS), as well as teardrop shaped RBCs will also be noted. The presence of the leukoerythroblastic reaction is indicative of an infiltrative process involving the bone marrow, with displacement of bone marrow contents by extramedullary cells such as those of a malignant tumor or of granulomatous disease. Infiltration of the bone marrow with fibroblastic tissue can also present in this fashion (eg, the marrow fibrosis that accompanies myeloproliferative disorders such as primary myelofibrosis). However, the line between the leukemoid reaction and the leukoerythroblastic reaction is not a rigid one from an etiologic standpoint, and many of the acute clinical scenarios that cause the former can also precipitate the latter if the challenge to the bone marrow itself is severe enough.

When associated with metastatic malignancies such as breast, lung, or prostate cancer, the presence of the leukoerythroblastic reaction indicates advanced and disseminated metastatic disease. Thus, prognostically the leukoerythroblastic reaction is associated with a less favorable outcome. Much like the leukemoid reaction, the leukoerythroblastic response requires no specific treatment other than that aimed at addressing the underlying cause.

LIFE-THREATENING EMERGENCIES INVOLVING NONMALIGNANT ABNORMALITIES IN WHITE BLOOD CELLS

LEUKOSTASIS

Leukostasis is a hematologic condition that demands emergent action to prevent the severe life-threatening pulmonary and cerebral sequelae that will ultimately result if this condition progresses untreated. Though more commonly associated with a malignant condition such as acute leukemia, leukostasis can also occur as a sequela of a nonmalignant WBC condition, such as might accompany a profound reactive eosinophilia. Absolute WBC values at which leukostasis can occur are not rigid and differ among the cell type of origin, thus guidelines for cutoff values cannot be reliably applied. Suspicion should be raised when otherwise unexplained ischemic symptoms occur in a patient in the context of a grossly elevated WBC count.

Typical ischemic symptoms, such as dyspnea and chest pain, or both focal and general neurologic findings, such as a decreased level of consciousness, are often present. Fluid hydration and acute leukocytoreduction with leukapheresis are the mainstays of treatment, with the later shown in retrospective studies to have a significant impact on mortality at presentation for these patients. Hydroxyurea as a form of cytochemical reduction can be used initially if timely access to leukapheresis is an issue. Maintaining a high index of suspicion and recognizing the signs and symptoms are of the utmost importance in making the diagnosis quickly to allow for timely intervention.

PATHOBIOLOGY OF NONMALIGNANT WHITE CELL DISORDERS

EXAMINATION OF THE PERIPHERAL BLOOD SMEAR

Microscopic examination of the peripheral blood smear is a simple, expedient, and widely available analytical method that can be of tremendous diagnostic significance for the hospitalist in unexplained cases of WBC abnormalities. A preliminary examination of the peripheral smear can identify several obvious pathologic findings, such as the previously mentioned leukemoid reaction or the hypersegmented neutrophils of megaloblastosis (**Figure 174-2**).

In addition, several subtle but classic features of the peripheral blood smear can be readily identified and can aid the hospitalist in directing further investigations.

The presence of *toxic granulation*, seen as dark and dense azurophilic granules on Wright staining, can also be observed in the cytoplasm of activated neutrophils (**Figure 174-3**). These granules contain a variety of antimicrobial enzymes and mediators, and their presence is strongly suggestive of underlying

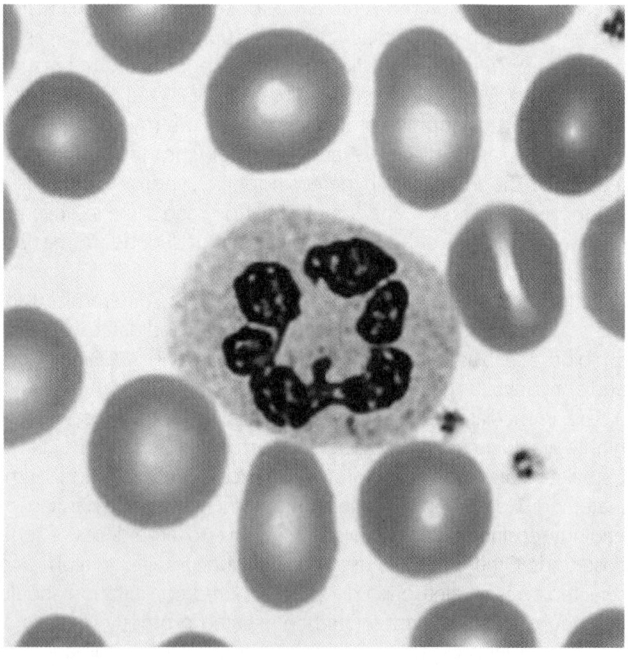

Figure 174-2 *Hypersegmented neutrophil of megaloblastosis.*

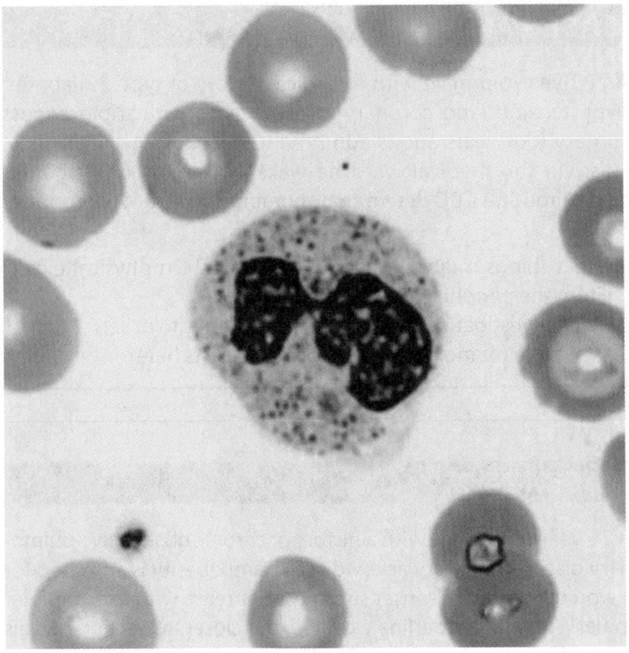

Figure 174-3 *Activated neutrophil with toxic granulation and Dohle bodies.*

infection. They can also be seen upon administration of colony-stimulating factors such as GCSF. When due to infection, the magnitude of the level of toxic granulation observed in leukocytes can be informative, as it has been shown to roughly correlate with sensitive serum markers of inflammation such as serum levels of C-reactive protein.

Dohle bodies, light blue-gray ovular inclusions seen typically on the periphery of activated neutrophils (see Figure 174-3), are thought to be caused by clumping of ribosomes and endoplasmic reticulum. These accumulate when the neutrophil is metabolically active, such as when fighting active infection. Cytoplasmic vacuolization of the neutrophil is another microscopically visible sign of an activated neutrophil and, thus, the presence of underlying infection. Vacuolization correlates with the extent of lysosomal function and autophagy and is considered strongly suggestive for the presence of more severe sepsis and systemic bacteremia.

Leukoagglutination, another morphologic finding, is a possible cause of spurious leucopenia and the characteristic clumping of WBCs are easily diagnosed on examination of the peripheral blood smear. Leukoagglutination is a nonspecific finding and may be associated with malignancy, hepatic disorders, and infections; the associated infections are typically gram-negative septicemia. However, leukoagglutination may be associated with the ethylenediaminetetraacetic acid (EDTA) anticoagulation used on blood sample collection similar to that seen with platelets, and recollection of the sample in alternate anticoagulants such as citrated or heparinized container may be enough to unmask the etiology.

Occasionally the presence of *reactive* or *atypical* lymphocytes, large lymphocytes with abundant basophilic cytoplasm and polymorphic nucleoli, can be noted in the peripheral blood. These are thought to represent antigenically-stimulated lymphocytes responding to underlying active infection. Classically associated with viral infections such as CMV and EBV, the atypical lymphocyte is somewhat nonspecific and can also be associated with bacterial infections, drug reactions, and endocrinopathies such as Addison disease. These cells may be mistaken for the blasts of acute leukemia, especially in the context of a severe acute infection with marrow suppression. Thus, if there is any ambiguity on history and physical examination, more aggressive investigation, such as flow cytometry on a peripheral blood sample, should be performed to help elucidate the etiology.

PRACTICE POINT

- Microscopic examination of the peripheral blood smear is a simple, expedient, and widely available analytical method that can be of tremendous diagnostic significance in unexplained cases of WBC abnormalities.

FLOW CYTOMETRY ANALYSIS

Flow cytometry is an extremely useful investigational tool that allows simultaneous multiparametric analysis of the physical characteristics defining WBC types using the principles of light scattering, excitation, and fluorochrome emission. As such, it can allow for the rapid identification and quantification of populations of WBC in any given patient sample based on the characteristic immunophenotype of the population subset. This is an important characteristic, as conventional cell counters used in the CBC identify cell types based on size alone and can easily misidentify atypical cell types.

Flow cytometry can be a vital investigational tool for the hospitalist; for example, it can be used in the initial workup of a new leukocytosis to identify a malignant versus a benign reactive cause. Flow cytometry also has direct uses in nonmalignant hematologic conditions, such as in the determination of CD4/CD8 count ratios in HIV-associated lymphocytopenia or in the diagnosis of rarer conditions such as paroxysmal nocturnal hemoglobinuria and Langerhans cell histiocytosis. Unfortunately, flow cytometry cannot reliably determine clonality, and further molecular techniques, such as T-cell receptor or B-cell light chain sequencing, would be required to confirm clonality.

EXAMINATION OF THE BONE MARROW ASPIRATE AND BIOPSY

Bone marrow aspiration and biopsy can be exceedingly helpful in the diagnosis and management of hematologic malignancies as well as in ascertaining overall bone marrow function when investigating the etiology of unexplained cytopenias. It is important in the diagnosis and management of the myelodysplastic syndromes and acute leukemia. It also has a role in the investigation of certain infections, such as tuberculosis, and is central in the diagnostic workup of a fever of unknown origin. It is the gold standard for determining body iron stores and helpful for the diagnosis of cellular storage disorders such as Gaucher disease and infiltrative conditions such as sarcoidosis or amyloidosis.

Samples of bone marrow are typically taken under local anesthetic from the posterior superior iliac crest, as it is the easiest accessible site. The anterior superior crest and the sternum are alternative accessible sites when the posterior crest cannot be accessed; the sternum is an option only for aspiration because biopsy is contraindicated at this site. A bone marrow aspirate is typically sent for flow cytometry, morphologic, conventional G-banded cytogenetic, and specialized molecular studies, as the diagnostic question requires. Molecular testing with PCR-based assays or fluorescent in situ hybridization (FISH) can only be performed if the molecular targets being looked for are previously known. A trephine biopsy of the trabecula should also be taken to appropriately assess bone marrow cellularity and morphologic cellular associations; the morphologic cellular associations may be characteristic of the underlying condition and, thus, of significant aid in establishing the diagnosis.

ROLE OF SUPPORTIVE MOLECULAR TESTING

After a complete history and physical exam and examination of the peripheral blood smear and bone marrow biopsy and aspirate, there are a few specific molecular tests that can be helpful in the workup of a WBC abnormality. These tests are of utility in the initial workup to differentiate between a malignant and a benign cause of a hematologic abnormality, thus facilitating the timely and appropriate request for a hematologic consultation.

Examples of molecular tests widely available on peripheral blood samples include PCR analysis for the presence of the BCR-ABL fusion transcript in granulocytes in the diagnostic workup of an unexplained left shift. Other common tyrosine kinase mutations such as those found in the Janus kinase 2 (Jak2) or myeloproliferative leukemia virus (MPL) can be tested for, as a persisting leukocytosis can accompany myeloproliferative disorders such as essential thrombocythemia. Platelet-derived growth factor (PDGF) fusion proteins on FISH of peripheral blood or marrow aspirate samples in eosinophilia can both identify clonality and establish the role of tyrosine kinase inhibitor therapy, as can *c-kit* mutations in mastocytosis. PCR-based sequencing of the T-cell receptor on T lymphocytes and the kappa and lamda light chain genes in B lymphocytes can also be done to confirm a clonal population of lymphocytic cells such as that in MBL or CLL.

Molecular testing will become more widespread and will gain prominence for identifying clonal disorders that may respond to targeted therapy in the future, so a working knowledge of the basics of molecular testing can be of great benefit to the hospitalist in the workup of hospitalized patients. Currently, however, the majority of molecular tests are specific for malignant conditions and, thus, of limited utility for benign abnormalities.

CLINICAL USE OF COLONY-STIMULATING FACTORS IN BENIGN HEMATOLOGIC CONDITIONS

The cornerstone of treatment for benign causes of WBC disorders is identification and removal of the underlying etiology whenever possible. However, the clinical development of colony-stimulating factors (CSF) has enabled the practitioner to augment transient periods of neutropenia when elimination of the underlying cause in a timely fashion is not feasible.

The two clinically available CSFs are granulocyte macrophage colony-stimulating factor (GM-CSF), which stimulates production of neutrophils, monocytes, and eosinophils, and granulocyte colony-stimulating factor (GCSF), which stimulates production only of neutrophils. Administration of these CSFs not only augments the magnitude of the total WBC pool, but also appears to improve mature neutrophil function as well. Currently, only GCSF (Filgrastim) has approval for use in benign WBC conditions, specifically for reducing both the incidence and the duration of complications in patients with congenital, cyclic, and idiopathic neutropenia.

Despite the limited licensed indication, several off-label uses for GCSF in benign leukopenic conditions have also been reported in the literature. These include minimizing the sequelae of neutropenia associated with HIV disease or HIV drug–associated neutropenia, as well as supporting neutropenia in benign conditions that require myelosuppresive drugs such as methotrexate. Case reports have also described usage for treating prolonged neutropenia related to autoimmune neutropenia as well as drug-induced agranulocytosis. Although efficacious and promising, the overall safety profile of these medications in such settings has not been completely determined, and, thus, their use remains largely investigational and should only be employed in conjunction with specialty consultation.

CASE 174-1

An 82-year-old male with a medical history of type 2 diabetes, hypertension, and coronary artery disease with triple bypass surgery four years ago is admitted to hospital for a workup of falls. On the medical ward he wakes with new-onset confusion. A routine CBC drawn that morning shows a WBC count of 38,000.

1. What things might be helpful on history? On physical exam? From the peripheral blood film?
2. What investigations would be the next ones to order?
3. What role for molecular testing, if any, exists here?

CASE 174-2

A 74-year-old female with a history of chronic obstructive pulmonary disease, coronary artery disease, and obesity is admitted for a workup of gradual-onset shortness of breath with exertion. Her initial WBC was borderline elevated, but closer inspection reveals a lymphocyte count of 4.2×10^9/L.

1. What potential nonmalignant diagnosis should be considered?
2. What investigations would be helpful to determine the diagnosis?
3. Is a bone marrow biopsy and aspirate helpful or required in this case?

CASE 174-3

A 78-year-old female with a history of recurring bladder infections over the past year is admitted to the hospital with recent-onset confusion and weakness and is subsequently found to have pyelonephritis. Her most recent CBC shows a WBC count of 1.8.

1. What aspect of the CBC would be directly related to her mortality risk?
2. Does she require a bone marrow biopsy and aspirate? What features of the peripheral smear may make you want to perform this test?
3. Is there a role for granulocyte colony-stimulating factor (GCSF) in the care of this patient?

CONCLUSION

Recognizing the composition of the differential white blood cell count and associated abnormalities is critical for formulating a differential diagnosis of disorders involving the WBC lineages and for initiating potentially life-saving treatment. Although benign causes should resolve with treatment of the underlying cause, the severity of the deviation of the WBC provides important prognostic information that may influence triage decisions and management. The WBC count may also provide important clues to previously undiagnosed underlying congenital and acquired disorders such as HIV or immunoglobin deficiency so that directed therapy can be initiated during hospitalization. Valuable time and resources can be saved and best directed if careful attention is paid to these simple tests in the clinical context of the acutely ill patient.

SUGGESTED READINGS

Hoffbrand AV, Moss PAH, Pettit JE. Essential Haematology. Fifth Edition. Oxford, UK: Blackwell Publishing.

Ibáñez L, Vidal X, Ballarín E, Laporte JR. Population-based drug-induced agranulocytosis. *Arch Intern Med.* 2005;165(8): 869–874.

Kho AN, Hui S, Kesterson JG, McDonald CJ. Which observations from the complete blood cell count predict mortality for hospitalized patients? *J Hosp Med.* 2007;2(1):5–12.

Wanahita A, Goldsmith EA, Musher DM. Conditions associated with leukocytosis in a tertiary care hospital, with particular attention to the role of infection caused by clostridium difficile. *Clinical Infectious Diseases.* 2002;34:1585–1592.

CHAPTER 175

Quantitative Abnormalities of Platelets: Thrombocytopenia and Thrombocytosis

Theodore E. Warkentin, MD

Key Clinical Questions

Thrombocytopenia

1. Does the patient have true thrombocytopenia or pseudothrombocytopenia?
2. What is the timing of onset, progression, and severity of the thrombocytopenia?
3. Is the thrombocytopenia isolated, or is there concomitant anemia, leukopenia, or both?
4. What are the findings of the peripheral blood film?
5. What tests and studies are useful to evaluate each etiology?
6. What is the frequency of specific causes of thrombocytopenia in defined clinical circumstances?
7. Is the thrombocytopenia a marker of bleeding risk, thrombosis risk, or adverse prognosis?
8. What treatments are available for each etiology?

Thrombocytosis

1. Is the thrombocytosis newly acquired during the hospitalization?
2. Is there concomitant splenomegaly and/or abnormalities in hemoglobin or white blood cell levels?
3. Does the thrombocytosis predate the hospitalization?
4. Is the red cell size (mean corpuscular volume) increased or decreased?

THROMBOCYTOPENIA

INTRODUCTION

The normal platelet count range is approximately 150 to 400 × 10^9/L (150,000 to 400,000 per mm^3). An individual's platelet count usually remains relatively constant during life. The platelet count decreases normally during pregnancy (gestational thrombocytopenia). The platelet count increases to above the usual value following an acute self-limited thrombocytopenia (eg, postsurgery thrombocytosis).

PRACTICE POINT

- Evaluation of thrombocytopenia should include review of the peripheral smear. The timing of onset of thrombocytopenia is a valuable clue regarding its possible etiologies. Identification of the cause of the thrombocytopenia determines next steps, including identification of those patients with low platelet counts who are likely to benefit from platelet transfusions in select circumstances.

Many clinicians equate thrombocytopenia with increased bleeding risk. Indeed, severe immune-mediated thrombocytopenia does pose increased bleeding risk. But certain other thrombocytopenic disorders are associated with greatly increased risk of thrombosis (eg, heparin-induced thrombocytopenia [HIT], antiphospholipid syndrome, cancer-associated hypercoagulability), or increased mortality (thrombocytopenia complicating septicemia or multi-organ system dysfunction).

The various explanations for thrombocytopenia differ depending on the clinical setting. For patients who present to the emergency room with acute, severe thrombocytopenia, certain life-threatening disorders must be considered, such as thrombotic thrombocytopenia purpura (TTP), drug-induced immune thrombocytopenic purpura (D-ITP), and acute leukemia. In postoperative patients, the timing of onset of thrombocytopenia is important since early thrombocytopenia is usually due to postoperative hemodilution, whereas later-onset thrombocytopenia suggests heparin-induced thrombocytopenia, septicemia, or other postoperative complications. Thrombocytopenia in the intensive care unit is often due to poorly defined platelet consumption complicating multiorgan system dysfunction.

The hospitalist may be the first physician called upon to evaluate a thrombocytopenic patient, especially when the platelet count decline begins during hospitalization. The hospitalist needs to appreciate the circumstances when referral to a hematologist is appropriate.

PHYSICAL EXAMINATION

The physical examination should focus on the presence of signs of bleeding (petechiae, purpura), fever, or chills (infection, anaphylactoid reaction secondary to acute HIT), the presence of invasive catheters and the integrity of the surrounding skin (source of infection), ventilator status (risk for pneumonia, indicator of multiorgan system failure), hemodynamic status (shock with risk of multiorgan failure–associated thrombocytopenia and disseminated intravascular coagulation [DIC]), pulses and distal limb ischemia (HIT-associated arterial or venous thrombosis), lymphadenopathy (lymphoproliferative disorders), hepatosplenomegaly (hypersplenism), and miscellaneous skin lesions (necrotizing skin lesions at heparin injection sites). Note that acral (distal extremity) tissue ischemic necrosis—despite palpable or Doppler-identifiable pulses—is a hallmark of disturbed procoagulant-anticoagulant balance that underlies several hematologic disorders such as overt (decompensated) DIC and HIT-associated venous limb gangrene (usually caused by warfarin).

The hallmark of severe thrombocytopenia is mucocutaneous bleeding, particularly pinpoint intradermal hemorrhages known as *petechiae*. These are nonpalpable, nonblanching, and indicate bleeding from capillaries. Petechiae are most evident in dependent areas (eg, the legs and feet in outpatients and the back and posterior thighs in bedridden patients) because of the effects of hydrostatic pressure. Generalized "oozing" from mucosal sites (eg, nose and genitourinary and gastrointestinal tracts) can be seen in severe thrombocytopenia. A classic finding is "blood blisters" (hemorrhagic vesicles of the oral mucosa or tongue) when the platelet count is less than $10 \times 10^9/L$ in the setting of autoimmune, alloimmune, or drug-induced immune thrombocytopenia. *Ecchymosis* denotes intradermal hemorrhage greater than 2 mm (ie, larger than petechiae); however, ecchymoses are less specific than petechiae for thrombocytopenic bleeding.

PATHOPHYSIOLOGY

Table 175-1 lists the five general mechanisms of thrombocytopenia, plus a sixth category of spurious thrombocytopenia ("pseudothrombocytopenia").

Pseudothrombocytopenia

A key question when evaluating a patient for thrombocytopenia is, Does the patient have true thrombocytopenia or pseudothrombocytopenia? Platelet clumping that occurs ex vivo (ie, only after the blood has been drawn into an anticoagulant) can be caused by naturally occurring antibodies that bind to platelets, resulting in platelet agglutination, but only in the presence of anticoagulant. This is most often seen when blood is collected into the purple tube (containing ethylenediaminetetraacetic acid [EDTA]) for determination of the complete blood count (CBC) (ie, EDTA-induced pseudothrombocytopenia). The thrombocytopenia is spurious because the electronic particle counter fails to detect the clumped platelets. Examination of the blood film reveals platelet clumping. Usually, platelet clumping does not occur, or is less marked, when blood is collected into another anticoagulant (eg, citrate, heparin). Pseudothrombocytopenia is clinically insignificant except when inappropriate treatment results from a wrong diagnosis of thrombocytopenia.

Hemodilution

A decline of 20% to 70% occurs universally in patients following major surgery, a phenomenon that is most dramatic in post–cardiac surgery patients. The platelet count nadir usually occurs between postoperative days 1 and 4 (median, day 2), with a subsequent rise in the platelet count that peaks at approximately day 14, at levels that are usually two to three times the patient's preoperative baseline (postthrombocytopenia thrombocytosis). The platelet count decline is roughly proportional to the amount of crystalloid, colloid, or blood products administered, plus some component of platelet consumption. Dilutional coagulopathy generally accompanies the thrombocytopenia, accounting for the minor increases in prothrombin time (PT) and activated partial thromboplastin time (APTT) that are commonly seen immediately after surgery. Hemodilution occurs universally after major surgery and represents the most common explanation for thrombocytopenia in the early postoperative period.

The diagnosis of dilutional thrombocytopenia is a good example of considering the key question, What is the timing of onset, progression, and severity of the thrombocytopenia? Here, the timing is abrupt in onset (directly follows surgery), the thrombocytopenia progresses to its usual nadir at approximately day 2 (range, days 1 to 4), and is mild to moderate in severity depending on the nature of the surgery and the amount of fluids and blood products administered. In the case of cardiac surgery utilizing extracorporeal circulation (cardiopulmonary bypass), the maximum decline in platelet count averages 50%, but can be as high as 70%. Furthermore, the natural history of dilutional thrombocytopenia is for the platelet count—after attaining its nadir—to progressively increase to peak levels at approximately day 14 that are considerably greater than the preoperative baseline.

TABLE 175-1 Six General Explanations for Thrombocytopenia

Explanation	Comment	Examples
Pseudothrombocytopenia	Antibody-mediated platelet clumping that occurs ex vivo (spurious thrombocytopenia)	EDTA-induced pseudothrombocytopenia
Hemodilution	Abrupt platelet count fall due to administration of fluids or blood products	Early postoperative thrombocytopenia
Hypersplenism	Splenomegaly may require imaging studies to detect; concomitant leukopenia and (to lesser extent) anemia are usually present	Cirrhosis-associated portal hypertension
Decreased platelet production	Usually there is concomitant leukopenia and anemia (a notable exception is certain types of hereditary thrombocytopenia)	Myelodysplasia; aplastic anemia; marrow infiltration by metastatic cancer; MYH9-associated thrombocytopenia
Platelet consumption	Accelerated platelet clearance due to pathologically increased thrombin generation or other poorly defined mechanisms of increased platelet clearance	Disseminated intravascular coagulation; septicemia; multiorgan system failure
Platelet destruction	Accelerated platelet clearance due to pathologic mechanisms that target platelets, especially due to autoantibodies	Autoimmune thrombocytopenic purpura; HIT; drug-induced immune thrombocytopenia; TTP/HUS

EDTA, ethylenediaminetetraacetic acid; HIT, heparin-induced thrombocytopenia; HUS, hemolytic uremic syndrome; MYH9, myosin heavy chain 9 (nonmuscle); TTP, thrombotic thrombocytopenic purpura.

TABLE 175-2 The Blood Film in The Evaluation of Thrombocytopenia

Feature	Suggested Diagnosis	Comment
Platelet clumping; platelet rosetting around neutrophils and/or monocytes (rare)	Pseudothrombocytopenia	Clinically insignificant (other than potential for false diagnosis of thrombocytopenia)
Neutrophilia; "toxic" white cells (increased granules, vacuoles)	Septicemia or other marked proinflammatory conditions	Blood cultures should be ordered, as bacteremia/fungemia is common cause of thrombocytopenia
Giant platelets; neutrophil inclusions	MYH9-associated macrothrombocytopenia	Inclusions may be difficult to discern without special stains
Red cell macrocytosis, "target" red cells, acanthocytes (spur cells), pancytopenia	Liver disease with portal hypertension and hypersplenism	Thrombocytopenia and neutropenia usually parallel one another in severity
Hypogranular leukocytes, left shift, Pelger-Huët anomaly (*pince-nez* appearance)	Myelodysplasia, myeloid leukemia	*Pince-nez* (French: "eyeglasses clipped to the bridge of the nose") appearance of leukocyte nuclei
Red cell fragments (schistocytes, eg, "helmet" cells); polychromasia	Microangiopathic hemolysis (TTP, HUS), DIC	Red cell fragments more prominent in TTP and HUS than in DIC
Red cell microbial inclusions	Malaria, babesia, *Cryptococcus* (rarely seen in red cells)	Type of malaria can be determined, eg, "ring forms" of *Plasmodium falciparum*

DIC, disseminated intravascular coagulation; HUS, hemolytic uremic syndrome; MYH9, myosin heavy chain 9; TTP, thrombotic thrombocytopenic purpura.

Hypersplenism

When approaching the diagnosis of hypersplenism, consider the following question: Is the thrombocytopenia isolated, or is there concomitant anemia and/or leukopenia? Whereas isolated thrombocytopenia usually indicates consumption or destruction of platelets (eg, DIC or immune thrombocytopenia) or hereditary thrombocytopenia (eg, MYH9-associated thrombocytopenia), thrombocytopenia associated with anemia and leukopenia can indicate hemodilution (discussed previously), hypersplenism, or marrow failure (eg, leukemia, marrow infiltration by metastatic cancer), or the combination of anemia and thrombocytopenia (eg, a disorder such as TTP).

Normally, about one-third of the circulating platelets are exchangeably sequestered within the spleen. Increased spleen size leads to greater splenic pooling (as high as 70–90%) and, thus, thrombocytopenia ("hypersplenism"). Two factors determine the extent of splenic pooling: splenic blood flow and splenic transit time. The most important determinant of splenic blood flow is spleen size, and the most important determinant of splenic transit time is splenic perfusion (spleen blood flow/spleen volume). However, since disorders that alter splenic transit time (eg, congestive heart failure, rheumatologic disorders) usually have counterbalancing effects on splenic blood flow, in practical terms, spleen size itself correlates well with the degree of splenic platelet pooling. Hence, radiologic imaging of spleen size can assess whether thrombocytopenia is caused by hypersplenism. A more recent concept is that reduced hepatic production of thrombopoietin (TPO) also contributes to thrombocytopenia of hypersplenism, in the setting of severe liver disease.

Decreased platelet production

Decreased platelet production can be caused by congenital or acquired bone marrow disorders, often manifesting as pancytopenia. However, isolated thrombocytopenia is seen in the MYH9-associated thrombocytopenias. Suspicion of decreased marrow production is often based on the answer to the question, What are the findings of the peripheral blood film? The blood film often points to a diagnosis of a primary bone marrow disorder, eg, primitive cells such as leukoblasts (acute leukemia) or abnormal lymphoid cells (neoplastic lymphoproliferative disorders), dysplastic white cells (myelodysplasia), tear drop red cells (infiltrative marrow disorders such as carcinoma metastatic to the bone marrow, myeloproliferative neoplasms with increased marrow fibrosis), and large red and white cells (megaloblastic anemia of vitamin B12 deficiency). The presence of very large platelets, together with neutrophil inclusions, is suggestive of MYH9-associated thrombocytopenia. **Table 175-2** lists some of the findings of the peripheral blood film in patients with decreased platelet production, as well as some other disorders.

Demographics trends, particularly increasing numbers of elderly patients, suggest that clonal marrow disorders such as myelodysplasia ("preleukemia") and chronic lymphoid leukemia will become more common. These are often "incidental" findings when patients are admitted for nonhematologic problems, and a routine CBC can lead to detection of thrombocytopenia.

Platelet consumption

Pathological activation of the coagulation system, often termed *disseminated intravascular coagulation* (DIC) or *consumptive coagulopathy*, is usually accompanied by thrombocytopenia. Underlying problems can include shock, trauma/burns, septicemia, multiorgan system failure, malignancy, envenomations, severe hemolysis, certain complications of pregnancy (eg, placental abruption, retained products), and so forth. Sometimes, thrombocytopenia due to increased platelet consumption occurs even when the global coagulation assays (PT, PTT) are not markedly elevated; this can be seen in some infections or in multiorgan system failure, and might reflect nonthrombin-mediated mechanisms of accelerated physiologic platelet clearance.

A key question is, What tests and studies are useful in evaluating each etiology? Testing for DIC should include the global coagulation assays (PT, APTT) in addition to fibrinogen and one or more markers of fibrin formation, such as the fibrin d-dimer, fibrin(ogen) degradation products (FDPs), fibrin monomer, and the protamine sulfate paracoagulation test (the last test is infrequently performed nowadays). Blood cultures should be done because bacteremia is a common explanation for consumptive thrombocytopenia (with or without laboratory evidence for DIC) in hospitalized patients; when a consumptive thrombocytopenia occurs in a patient who has received antibiotics for a prolonged period, fungemia becomes

TABLE 175-3 Laboratory Tests Used to Investigate a Patient with Thrombocytopenia

Test	Comment
Complete blood count (CBC)	Electronic particle counters; detects thrombocytopenia
Review of blood film	See Table 175–2
Blood cultures	Bacteremia, fungemia
Antinuclear antibody test	Systemic lupus erythematosus (associated with immune thrombocytopenia)
Direct antiglobulin test (if anemic)	Combined immune hemolysis and immune thrombocytopenia (Evan syndrome)
Coagulation tests: PT/INR, APTT, TCT	Screen for deficiency of coagulation factor (or factors), or detect presence of inhibitor (anticoagulant or antibody inhibitor)
Coagulation tests: fibrinogen; fibrin d-dimer, FDPs, fibrin monomer, protamine sulfate paracoagulation assay	Low fibrinogen and presence of other markers can indicate DIC or hyperfibrinolysis (caveat: fibrinogen levels can be normal in DIC)
Coagulation assays: "nonspecific inhibitor"; anticardiolipin; anti-β2-glycoprotein I	APS suggested by positive tests for antiphospholipid antibodies detected either by functional (coagulation) or immunologic assays
Serum protein electrophoresis; quantitative immunoglobulin levels	Plasma cell or lymphoproliferative disorders (usually monoclonal) or chronic hepatitis/hypersplenism (polyclonal hypergammaglobulinemia)
HIV serology	HIV-associated thrombocytopenia
Bone marrow aspirate and biopsy	Assess megakaryocyte numbers and morphology; evaluate for primary or secondary (eg, metastatic neoplasm) bone marrow disorder

APS, antiphospholipid syndrome; APTT, activated partial thromboplastin time; DIC, disseminated intravascular coagulation; FDPs, fibrin degradation products; HIV, human immunodeficiency virus; PT/INR (prothrombin time/international normalized ratio); TCT, thrombin clotting time.

Note: This table excludes certain specialized tests, such as those for antibodies that cause heparin-induced thrombocytopenia, flow cytometry-based immunophenotyping, and cytogenetic studies of peripheral blood or marrow blood cells.

an increasingly plausible explanation for a consumptive thrombocytopenia. **Table 175-3** lists some of the laboratory tests that can be helpful in evaluating thrombocytopenia.

Platelet destruction

The term *platelet destruction* (or *destructive thrombocytopenia*) refers to disorders in which pathologic factors destroy platelets in a nonphysiologic manner, most often as a direct or indirect result of antibodies. **Table 175-4** lists different antibody-mediated

TABLE 175-4 Antibody-Mediated Thrombocytopenia

Disorder	Comment
Platelet count often $<20 \times 10^9$/L	
(Auto) immune thrombocytopenic purpura	Primary (idiopathic) or secondary (eg, associated with systemic lupus erythematosus, lymphoproliferative disorders, viral hepatitis, HIV infection)
Posttransfusion purpura	Severe thrombocytopenia 5–10 days after blood transfusion
Drug-induced immune thrombocytopenia	See Table 175–5
Thrombotic thrombocytopenic purpura-hemolytic uremic syndrome	Idiopathic thrombotic thrombocytopenic purpura in many cases is caused by autoantibodies that bind to the von Willebrand factor–cleaving metalloprotease, ADAMTS13
Platelet count often $>20 \times 10^9$/L	
Heparin-induced thrombocytopenia	Prothrombotic adverse drug reaction characterized by high risk of venous and arterial thrombosis; risk factor for warfarin-associated microthrombosis

thrombocytopenic disorders. Heparin-induced thrombocytopenia (HIT) overlaps the differing concepts of destructive and consumptive thrombocytopenia: it arises from pathologic platelet-activating antibodies (destructive thrombocytopenia) and, in its severe form, can also feature overt DIC (consumptive thrombocytopenia).

A key question is, What is the frequency of specific causes of thrombocytopenia in defined clinical circumstances? For example, when a patient has very severe thrombocytopenia (platelet count $<20 \times 10^9$/L), destructive thrombocytopenia is the likely problem (eg, ITP [autoimmune], D-ITP [drug-induced], TTP, and occasionally, very severe HIT or DIC) as it is unusual for consumptive thrombocytopenia or hypersplenism to produce such severe thrombocytopenia. Severe thrombocytopenia due to primary bone marrow disorders is usually clinically obvious (eg, pancytopenia with circulated myeloblasts). The next section deals with some of the possible explanations for thrombocytopenia when it occurs following the patient's admission to hospital, particularly in the postsurgery context.

ONSET OF THROMBOCYTOPENIA AFTER HOSPITALIZATION

In hospitalized patients, the timing of onset of thrombocytopenia is a valuable clue regarding its possible etiologies. **Figure 175-1** shows the typical evolution of platelet counts after surgery: after an early postoperative decline, the platelet count increases steadily, reaching levels that are usually two to three times the preoperative baseline, peaking at postoperative day 14, before gradually declining over the third week. The figure also shows the usual timing of onset of several common (and rare) explanations for thrombocytopenia.

Diagnostic considerations

Hemodynamic compromise and circulatory or septic shock: Thrombocytopenia with or without overt DIC is a common finding in patients with early postsurgery circulatory shock,

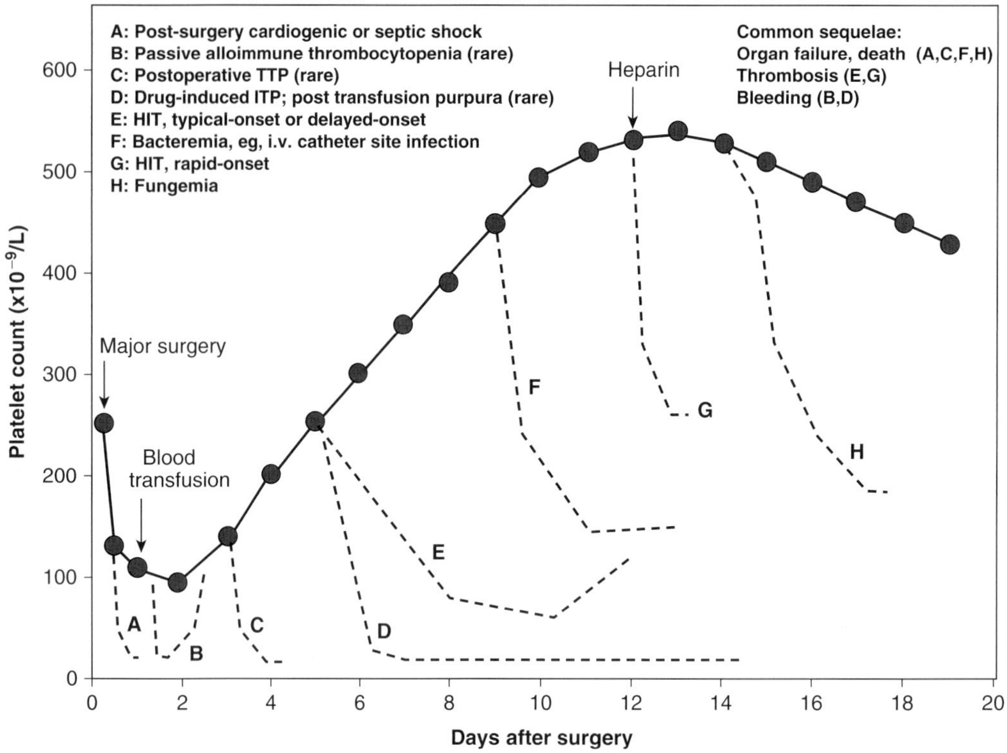

Figure 175-1 *Timing of onset of thrombocytopenia in a postoperative patient: diagnostic implications. The circles connected by a solid line indicate the typical evolution of postoperative thrombocytopenia (usual nadir, day 2) to postoperative thrombocytosis (usual peak, day 14). The dashed lines indicate various temporal profiles of unexpected postoperative thrombocytopenia and associated diagnostic considerations. In profile D, it is assumed that the responsible drug or blood product was started (or given) in the intra- or perioperative period. Note: For profile G, thrombosis is the usual reason why heparin is given, leading to rapid-onset HIT.*

such as resulting from cardiac failure or sepsis (see profile A in Figure 175-1). Hypotension and vasopressor use can contribute to acral limb ischemia, but there is usually also a prominent role of microvascular thrombosis that is related to failure of natural anticoagulants (protein C pathway, antithrombin III) to control pathologic thrombin generation.

Passive alloimmune thrombocytopenia: Rarely, blood products contain cell-specific alloantibodies that cause life-threatening sequelae. Best known is transfusion-associated acute lung injury (TRALI), where transfusion of blood product—usually from a multiparous female donor—containing antigranulocyte alloantibodies causes life-threatening pulmonary edema. The platelet analogue of TRALI is passive alloimmune thrombocytopenia (PAT), which is characterized by severe thrombocytopenia that begins abruptly after administering a blood product (eg, fresh frozen plasma [FFP], red cell concentrates) containing platelet-reactive alloantibodies (see profile B in Figure 175-1).

Postoperative TTP: Rarely, patients develop TTP in the early postoperative period, probably because postoperative proinflammatory factors trigger someone already predisposed to TTP to develop overt disease (see profile C in Figure 175-1). TTP itself is a rare disease, and postoperative TTP constitutes only about 1% of all TTP presentations. The clinical picture is that of severe postoperative thrombocytopenia (often $<20 \times 10^9$/L) and microangiopathic hemolysis (anemia, red cell fragments, greatly elevated lactate dehydrogenase, negative direct Coombs test). Treatment is managed by a hematologist (plasma exchange, high-dose corticosteroids).

Drug-induced immune thrombocytopenic purpura and posttransfusion purpura: The onset of severe thrombocytopenia (platelet count $<20 \times 10^9$/L) beginning approximately one week after the institution of a new drug or the receipt of blood products, suggests the diagnosis of drug-induced immune thrombocytopenic purpura (D-ITP) or posttransfusion purpura (PTP), respectively (see profile D in Figure 175-1). **Table 175-5** lists some of the drugs most frequently implicated in classic (typical) D-ITP, as well as other atypical drug-induced thrombocytopenic syndromes. Petechiae and purpura are common in D-ITP and PTP, and when such signs of bleeding are encountered, platelet transfusions with or without high-dose intravenous immunoglobulin G (IVIgG) may be appropriate.

Heparin-induced thrombocytopenia: This immune-mediated drug reaction involving platelets is more common than all of the causes of D-ITP combined. The frequency is highly variable, but in patients who have all of the risk factors—unfractionated heparin use for more than one week, postoperative thromboprophylaxis, female sex—the frequency is 1–5%. The typical picture (~65% of patients; see profile E in Figure 175-1) is an otherwise unexpected platelet count fall that begins 5 to 10 days after receiving heparin, most often in the setting of postsurgical thromboprophylaxis. The frequency of HIT is approximately tenfold less with low-molecular-weight heparin (LMWH), and even less common (although reported) with the pentasaccharide anticoagulant, fondaparinux.

Approximately 25% to 30% of patients (see profile G in Figure 175-1) present with rapid-onset HIT, in which the platelet count falls abruptly after resuming heparin in a patient who has circulating HIT antibodies that resulted from a recent preceding

TABLE 175-5 Drug-Induced Immune Thrombocytopenic Purpura: Implicated Drugs (Selected List)

Typical D-ITP
Quinine, quinidine
Antibiotics (ceftriaxone, levofloxacin, nafcillin, piperacillin, rifampin, sulfamethoxazole, trimethoprim, vancomycin)
Antiinflammatory (acetaminophen*, ibuprofen*, naproxen)
Antineoplastic (oxaliplatin)
Cardiac (amiodarone, furosemide)
Neurologic (carbamazepine, phenytoin)
Atypical
GPIIb/IIIa antagonist–induced thrombocytopenia (abciximab, eptifibatide, tirofiban)†
HIT (see also Table 175-6)
TTP/HUS (quinine, ticlopidine, clopidogrel, cyclosporine, gemcitabine, mitomycin C)

D-ITP, drug-induced immune thrombocytopenic purpura; HIT, heparin-induced thrombocytopenia; HUS, hemolytic-uremic syndrome; TTP, thrombotic thrombocytopenic purpura.

Note: This is a partial list only. Readers should consult published lists (see Suggested Reading) or a Web site (www.ouhsc.edu/platelets/DITP.html) for additional drugs.

*Drug metabolites implicated.

†An atypical feature of D-ITP caused by GPIIb/IIIa antagonists is that ~ 1% of patients who receive one of these agents for the first time develop abrupt-onset D-ITP because of naturally occurring antibodies.

heparin exposure. HIT antibodies are transient (median time of detectability, 50–80 days, depending upon the assay performed), which explains why recent—rather than remote—preceding exposure to heparin is a crucial factor in accounting for rapid-onset HIT. About one-quarter of patients who develop rapid-onset HIT following a heparin bolus evince an anaphylactoid reaction. It is increasingly recognized that patients can present with HIT several days after their last exposure to heparin (delayed-onset HIT); here, the patient can present to the emergency room with thrombosis and thrombocytopenia one or two weeks following a preceding exposure to heparin, which can be quite brief (eg, administered only during cardiac or vascular surgery).

HIT is a "clinicopathologic disorder," and its diagnosis rests on two criteria: (1) the presence of one or more clinically evident events (most often, thrombocytopenia with or without thrombosis) bearing a temporal relationship to a preceding immunizing heparin exposure; and (2) detectability of heparin-dependent platelet-activating antibodies against PF4/heparin complexes. **Table 175-6** lists the various sequelae of HIT.

Two types of laboratory assays—platelet activation assays (eg, serotonin-release assay [SRA]) and PF4-dependent enzyme-immunoassays (EIAs)—are very sensitive for HIT, and, thus, a negative assay generally rules out the diagnosis. Platelet activation assays have superior sensitivity-specificity tradeoffs compared with EIAs, and a positive SRA is more diagnostically specific for HIT than the EIA. The "strength" of an EIA (measured in optical density units) corresponds strongly to the presence of platelet-activating antibodies and, hence, risk of HIT. Therefore, one should be skeptical about the diagnosis of HIT if the EIA is only weakly positive (eg, 0.4–1.0 units; usual cutoff, 0.4 U).

When HIT is strongly suspected or serologically confirmed, the heparin is stopped, and an alternative anticoagulant is given, usually in therapeutic doses (options include danaparoid [outside the U.S.], fondaparinux, lepirudin, argatroban, bivalirudin [note: dosing guidelines for these anticoagulants is outside the scope of this chapter]). *It is important not to give warfarin during the acute thrombocytopenic phase of HIT* for three reasons: (1) warfarin does not inhibit HIT-associated hypercoagulability; (2) warfarin causes depletion of protein C (vitamin K–dependent natural anticoagulant), a finding characteristic of devastating microthrombosis syndromes in HIT, such as venous limb gangrene (limb necrosis despite palpable pulses in the setting of deep-vein thrombosis); and (3) warfarin use leads to systematic underdosing of alternative anticoagulants that are usually monitored by the APTT (lepirudin, argatroban, bivalirudin). Indeed, if warfarin has already been given when HIT is diagnosed, the warfarin

TABLE 175-6 Heparin-Induced Thrombocytopenia: Clinical-Pathologic Criteria for Diagnosis

Clinical	Pathologic
At least one of the following: • **Thrombocytopenia*** • **Thrombosis** (eg, *venous*: deep-vein thrombosis, pulmonary embolism, venous limb gangrene, adrenal hemorrhage,† cerebral vein thrombosis, splanchnic vein thrombosis; *arterial*: limb artery thrombosis, stroke, myocardial infarction, mesenteric artery thrombosis, miscellaneous artery; *microvascular*) • Necrotizing skin lesions at heparin injection sites‡ • Acute anaphylactoid reactions§	Heparin-dependent, platelet-activating IgG** • Positive platelet activation assay (eg, serotonin-release assay) • Positive anti-PF4/polyanion-IgG EIA (infers possibility of platelet-activating IgG††)
Timing: Above event (or events) demonstrates temporal relation to a preceding immunizing heparin exposure¶	
Absence of another more compelling explanation	

*Greater than 50% platelet count fall is seen in ~ 90% of patients; in 5–10%, the platelet fall is 30–50%.

†Adrenal hemorrhagic necrosis is a consequence of adrenal vein thrombosis.

‡Nonnecrotizing lesions (erythematous plaques) are less specific for heparin-induced thrombocytopenia (HIT).

§Usually occur 5–30 minutes after intravenous heparin bolus and, rarely, after subcutaneous heparin.

¶Typical onset is 5–10 days after immunizing heparin exposure (usually, given intra- or perioperatively); rapid-onset HIT can occur if heparin is given to a patient who already has circulating HIT-Abs, usually due to heparin given in the last 5–100 days.

**Acute serum or plasma should be used for testing, as HIT-Abs are transient.

††In the appropriate context, a strong-positive EIA (IgG-specific or polyspecific assay that detects IgG/A/M antibodies) can be used to infer presence of platelet-activating HIT-Abs.

Reprinted, with permission, from Warkentin TE. Agents for the treatment of heparin-induced thrombocytopenia. *Hematol/Oncol Clin N Am.* 2010;24(4):755.

should be reversed with intravenous vitamin K. Other tenets of HIT management include avoiding, if possible, prophylactic platelet transfusions (as petechiae and other platelet-mediated bleeding are not features of HIT) and imaging for lower-limb deep vein thrombosis (DVT, the most common complication of HIT).

For a patient with a previous history of HIT, repeat exposure to heparin can be considered in special circumstances, most often for cardiac or vascular surgery, provided that platelet-activating antibodies are no longer detectable.

The relative high frequency of HIT raises important issues regarding hospital quality control through platelet count monitoring for HIT. Recently, the American College of Chest Physicians (ACCP) evidence-based clinical practice guidelines (8th edition) opined that intensity of platelet count monitoring should reflect the risk of HIT in any given situation. Thus, for patients at highest risk (> 1%), such as postoperative patients receiving antithrombotic prophylaxis with unfractionated heparin (UFH), platelet count monitoring should occur at least every other day between postoperative days 4 and 14 (or until UFH is stopped, whichever occurs first). For patients at intermediate risk (0.1–1%) (eg, postoperative patients receiving LMWH or medical patients receiving UFH), monitoring should occurs "at least every 2 or 3 days from day 4 to day 14 (or until heparin is stopped, whichever occurs first), when practical" (Warkentin, et al, 2008). However, when HIT risk is rare (< 0.1%), such as with use of LMWH for medical or obstetric patients, or fondaparinux for any indication, routine platelet count monitoring for purposes of early detection of HIT is not advised. Of course, routine platelet count monitoring itself can be problematic if it leads to overdiagnosis of HIT and inappropriate cessation of heparin.

Bacteremia and fungemia: Infection is a relatively common explanation for thrombocytopenia in hospitalized patients, and usually indicates microbial invasion of the blood (hence, the importance of performing blood cultures in patients with unexplained thrombocytopenia). Supporting blood film abnormalities include leukocyte "left-shift" (bands, metamyelocytes) and "toxic" features (eg, cytoplasmic vacuolation, toxic granules). Coagulation assays for DIC should be performed, although in many cases there is elevation in fibrin D-dimer levels with normal INR, APTT, and fibrinogen levels. In patients with overt DIC (elevated INR, reduced fibrinogen), there is risk for microvascular thrombosis (eg, acral ischemia) and special treatment approaches (eg, use of recombinant activated protein C or heparin) may be appropriate. The pathogenesis of thrombocytopenia is multifactorial (thrombin-mediated, increased macrophage clearance of platelets, decreased marrow platelet production, effects of microbial toxins). Persistence of thrombocytopenia in sepsis is a poor prognostic factor. As a general rule, fungemia occurs later in the course of hospitalization than does bacteremia (compare profile H with profiles A and F in Figure 175-1).

CHRONIC THROMBOCYTOPENIA

Thrombocytopenia in a hospitalized patient can indicate the presence of a preexisting disorder of platelet number, such as hypersplenism, chronic (auto)immune thrombocytopenic purpura (ITP), or a primary bone marrow disorder, either congenital (eg, hereditary thrombocytopenia) or acquired (eg, myelodysplasia). Sometimes, there is an exacerbation of the chronic thrombocytopenia, such as a relapse of ITP or infection-associated worsening of thrombocytopenia in a patient with myelodysplasia.

Diagnostic considerations

Hypersplenism: Table 175-7 lists various explanations for splenomegaly. In North America, the most common cause is cirrhosis, and, thus, concomitant coagulopathy due to liver dysfunction is

TABLE 175-7 Differential Diagnosis of Splenomegaly and Hypersplenism

Congestive splenomegaly
Intrahepatic
Cirrhosis*
Extrahepatic
Portal vein obstruction
Splenic vein obstruction
Hepatic vein occlusion (Budd-Chiari syndrome)
Chronic passive congestion
Heart failure
Infections
Acute
Viral (viral hepatitis, infectious mononucleosis, cytomegalovirus infection)
Bacterial (septicemia, salmonellosis, brucellosis, splenic abscess)
Parasite (toxoplasmosis)
Subacute and chronic
Subacute bacterial endocarditis
Tuberculosis
Malaria
Kala-azar
Fungal disease
Inflammation
Felty syndrome
Systemic lupus erythematosus
Serum sickness
Rheumatic fever
Sarcoidosis
Hematologic disorders
Red cell disorders: hemolytic anemias, thalassemia, sickle cell disorders
Neoplasia
Malignant
Myeloproliferative disorders
Myeloid metaplasia
Polycythemia rubra vera
Essential thrombocythemia
Chronic leukemia
Chronic myeloid leukemia
Chronic lymphocytic leukemia
Hairy cell leukemia
Lymphoma
Acute leukemia
Malignant histiocytosis
Benign
Hamartoma
Hemangioma
Lymphangioma
Fibroma
Storage diseases
Gaucher disease
Niemann-Pick disease
Miscellaneous
Amyloidosis
Cysts

*The most common cause of hypersplenism in North America.

common. Often, incidentally detected mild or moderate thrombocytopenia is the first clue that a patient has cirrhosis due to alcohol abuse or chronic viral hepatitis.

Chronic autoimmune thrombocytopenia: Immune thrombocytopenic purpura, also known as autoimmune or idiopathic thrombocytopenic purpura, is an acquired, antibody-mediated disorder of adults and children characterized by persistent decrease of the platelet count ($< 100 \times 10^9$/L) and, depending upon its severity, increased bleeding risk. Unlike children, most adults with acute ITP exhibit persistence of thrombocytopenia, ie, *chronic* ITP. When there is an associated illness (eg, systemic lupus erythematosus, HIV infection, monoclonal lymphoproliferative disorder), the ITP is called *secondary*; in their absence, the patient is said to have *primary* ITP. Although the role of autoantibodies in ITP is not disputed, there is no clear role for laboratory testing in the diagnosis of ITP.

Most patients are benefited at least transiently with therapies such as oral corticosteroids, intravenous IVIgG, or Rh immune globulin, although the latter is only potentially effective if the patient is Rh(D) positive. Unfortunately, the thrombocytopenia often relapses during corticosteroid tapering, or one to three weeks following administration of IVIgG or Rh immune globulin. Thus, many patients will eventually undergo splenectomy, since durable remissions are observed in 60% to 70% of patients. The large number of third-line treatment approaches (immunosuppressives, danazol, rituximab, thrombopoietin analogues) speaks to the challenge in managing chronic ITP that is refractory to the first- and second-line treatment approach of corticosteroids followed by splenectomy. Two thrombopoietin receptor agonists, eltrombopag (oral agent) and romiplostim (administered by subcutaneous injection), are approved in the U.S. for treatment of chronic ITP, but their high cost and requirement for ongoing use are drawbacks. Platelet transfusions are usually indicated only to manage life-threatening bleeding.

Hereditary thrombocytopenia: Hereditary (or congenital) thrombocytopenia (eg, MYH9-associated macrothrombocytopenia) is more common than generally recognized. Although there are different syndromes, most common is MYH9-associated macrothrombocytopenia, so named because the defect is in the nonmuscle myosin heavy chain, and affected patients have very large platelets. Often, the platelet count is greater than that reported by the electronic particle counter, as it fails to count the largest-sized platelets. Inheritance is autosomal dominant. Depending on the exact location of the mutation, patients can have one or more of the following features: leukocyte inclusions, sensorineural hearing loss, presenile cataracts, and renal disease. Most patients have no or minimal bleeding symptoms and signs. Many patients are misdiagnosed as having chronic ITP.

Myelodysplasia and other primary marrow disorders: Numerous primary marrow disorders can cause thrombocytopenia, usually with leukopenia and anemia (pancytopenia). If there are increased numbers of circulating neoplastic cells, leukocytosis can be seen (eg, acute or chronic myeloid or lymphoid leukemia). *Myelodysplasia* (preleukemia) refers to clonal disorders of myeloid cells in which the marrow "blast" count is less than 30%; diagnostic clues include anemia with elevated red cell size (macrocytosis), leukopenia/leukocytosis with dysplastic white cells changes (eg, Pelger-Huet appearance, hypogranular leukocytes), and thrombocytopenia; characteristic chromosomal abnormalities of affected blood and bone marrow cells are common. Sometimes, isolated thrombocytopenia is the presenting feature of myelodysplasia.

Myelophthysis and other secondary marrow disorders: *Myelophthysis* refers to marrow replacement by tumor or fibrosis, yielding a characteristic peripheral blood picture known as *leukoerythroblastosis* (leukocyte left shift, circulating nucleated red blood cells) together with tear-drop red cells. When the cause of marrow infiltration is metastatic adenocarcinoma, there may also be red cell fragments and coagulopathy indicating overt DIC. In that setting, thrombocytopenia reflects both decreased marrow production and increased consumption.

ACUTE THROMBOCYTOPENIA PRECIPITATING ADMISSION TO HOSPITAL

Sometimes, acute thrombocytopenia is *the* major feature of the patient's presentation, and the emergency room and early hospitalization period are aimed at establishing diagnosis and treatment. Many of these disorders are life threatening.

Diagnostic considerations

Drug-induced immune thrombocytopenic purpura: Certain drugs newly started in outpatients, such as sulfa antibiotics and carbamazepine, can cause severe immune thrombocytopenia (see Table 175-5). Always ask about possible exposure to quinine, as this component of "tonic water" is a relatively common cause of severe thrombocytopenia in patients presenting to the emergency room. Treatment includes stopping any suspected drugs, and administering one or more of the following: corticosteroids, high-dose IVIgG, or platelet transfusions. The presence of oropharyngeal blood blisters indicates a higher risk of life-threatening bleeding (intracranial, pericardial) than cutaneous purpura (petechiae, ecchymoses) alone.

Acute immune thrombocytopenic purpura: Most adults have chronic ITP, but the initial presentation of this disorder by definition is *acute*, as the natural history of persisting chronic thrombocytopenia is not yet known. Treatment with corticosteroids and/or IVIgG is usually given only if there are bleeding symptoms or signs, and platelet transfusions are reserved for life-threatening bleeding, as their therapeutic benefit is transient and sensitization to platelet antigens could develop.

Thrombotic thrombocytopenic purpura and hemolytic-uremic syndrome: Thrombocytopenia and microangiopathic (or schistocytic) hemolysis constitute the TTP duad. Affected patients can exhibit organ dysfunction due to platelet–von Willebrand factor (vWF) thrombi in small arteries and arterioles, most commonly involving the central nervous system (confusion, dysarthria, coma), kidneys (oliguric renal failure), and muscles (elevated creatine kinase, cardiac dysrrhythmias including sudden death). A useful diagnostic clue is measurement of lactate dehydrogenase: levels are typically markedly elevated in patients with TTP. TTP has female predominance, and increased risk in African Americans. Most often, the disorder is idiopathic, although autoantibodies against the shear-dependent vWF-cleaving protease, known as ADAMTS13 (a disintegrin and metalloproteinase with thrombospondin motifs, member 13), have been identified in a high proportion of affected patients. TTP can also occur in association with autoimmune disorders (eg, systemic lupus erythematosus), with certain drugs (eg, quinine, ticlopidine, clopidogrel, cyclosporine, gemcitabine, mitomycin C), or soon after surgery or acute pancreatitis.

Untreated, the mortality of TTP approaches 100%. Even when successfully treated with corticosteroids and pheresis, there is a relatively high risk (at least one-third) of subsequent relapse, although this might occur months or years in the future. Rituximab appears to be an effective treatment for patients with refractory or relapsing TTP.

A related syndrome known as hemolytic uremic syndrome (HUS) has prominent renal dysfunction and often occurs with a diarrheal prodrome, as a common precipitant is preceding infection with verotoxin-producing *E coli*. Rarely, quinine can cause a syndrome that strongly resembles HUS.

Delayed-onset heparin-induced thrombocytopenia with thrombosis: Thrombocytopenia accompanying venous or arterial thrombosis, or adrenal hemorrhagic infarction (itself an indicator of adrenal vein thrombosis) in a recently hospitalized patient should prompt consideration of *delayed-onset HIT*. Patients have strong-positive tests for HIT antibodies and often concomitant DIC. Interestingly, some patients have not had any preceding exposure to heparin (eg, they received warfarin for postsurgery thromboprophylaxis). Thus, it has been proposed that surgery itself can rarely precipitate the anti-PF4/heparin immune response that underlies HIT. Ideally, heparin should be avoided in patients with delayed-onset HIT, but if given, a further abrupt decline in platelet count—with or without an anaphylactoid reaction—is characteristic.

THROMBOCYTOSIS

INTRODUCTION

Thrombocytosis (platelet count > 450 × 10^9/L) is often an unexpected abnormality detected by routine CBC. Usually, thrombocytosis arises *during* hospitalization as a physiologic response to preceding acute thrombocytopenia. When thrombocytosis is already apparent at the time of admission, it most often represents a *secondary* (or reactive) thrombocytosis, and usually does not pose thrombotic or other risks. In contrast, *primary* thrombocytosis indicates that the increase in platelets is caused by alterations targeting hematopoietic cells and can indicate risk of thrombosis and/or bleeding. **Table 175-8** classifies various explanations for thrombocytosis.

PRACTICE POINT

- Similar to thrombocytopenia, evaluation of thrombocytosis should include review of the peripheral smear and determination of whether other cell lines are abnormal. The timing of the onset of thrombocytosis is also an important clue to the cause. Thrombocytosis that arises *during* hospitalization is usually a physiologic response to preceding acute thrombocytopenia. Thrombocytosis already apparent at the time of admission most often represents a secondary (or "reactive") thrombocytosis, but sometimes a primary thrombocytosis (eg, myeloproliferative neoplasm).

PHYSIOLOGIC THROMBOCYTOSIS

Platelet count regulation through constitutive production of thrombopoietin (TPO) infers that any acute self-limited thrombocytopenia will naturally be followed by transient, self-limited thrombocytosis. Another physiologic tenet is that absence of a spleen (and associated splenic pooling) will yield approximately a 30% increase in the platelet count on a chronic basis.

Diagnostic considerations

Postthrombocytopenia thrombocytosis: Consider the key question, Is the thrombocytosis newly acquired during the hospitalization? If so, it is likely that there was a transient drop in the platelet count approximately one to two weeks earlier, as exemplified in Figure 175-1. Typically, the platelet count peaks approximately two weeks following any acute drop in platelet count and represents a physiologic response to increased TPO levels that occur as a direct result of the preceding platelet count decline (**Figure 175-2**). In this author's opinion, the finding of thrombocytosis in this clinical setting does not require any additional antithrombotic measures over what would already be prudent in the same clinical situation, had thrombocytosis not been evident.

TABLE 175-8 Causes of Thrombocytosis

Physiologic
Post-thrombocytopenia thrombocytosis (2nd and 3rd week post-any acute platelet count decline)
Post-splenectomy or congenital/acquired asplenia
Secondary or "reactive"
Inflammatory/infectious, eg, polymyalgia rheumatica (giant cell arteritis), rheumatoid arthritis, polyarteritis nodosa, inflammatory bowel disease, tuberculosis, other chronic infections), solid tumors, especially metastatic carcinoma
Iron deficiency
Hemolytic anemia
Pseudothrombocytosis (eg, burns)
Primary
Hereditary or familial thrombocytosis
Neoplastic (myeloproliferative disorders, eg, polycythemia rubra vera, chronic myeloid leukemia, essential thrombocythemia, myeloid metaplasia, myelodysplasia [eg, 5q- syndrome, refractory anemia with ringed sideroblasts])

Postsplenectomy thrombocytosis: Greatly elevated platelet counts can occur following splenectomy. This is because physiologic thrombocytosis that follows acute surgery–associated thrombocytopenia is exacerbated by the lack of splenic sequestration of platelets. Thus, peak platelet counts as high as 1500 to 2000 × 10^9/L can be seen approximately two weeks post splenectomy, before returning to a "baseline" that is approximately one-third higher than the patient's usual presplenectomy platelet count.

SECONDARY (REACTIVE) THROMBOCYTOSIS

It is important to identify the underlying explanation for secondary thrombocytosis, as the causes can be life threatening (eg, giant cell arteritis, occult abscess, lung carcinoma, iron deficiency anemia secondary to colon cancer). Further, management of the thrombocytosis necessarily focuses on treatment of the underlying disease.

Diagnostic considerations

Inflammatory/infectious thrombocytosis: Answering yes to the key question, "Does the thrombocytosis predate the hospitalization?" suggests that the patient may have a subacute or chronic inflammatory/infectious cause of thrombocytosis (see Table 175-8 for representative disorders). Unlike neoplastic disorders, increased risk of thrombosis is not usually a feature of reactive thrombocytosis that represents a response to inflammatory cytokines, although exceptions to this general rule exist. For example, the author once encountered a patient who presented with cerebral venous (dural sinus) thrombosis who had an incidental finding of thrombocytosis; this proved to be one of the clues (along with mild diarrhea) that the patient had undiagnosed inflammatory bowel disease.

Iron deficiency anemia or hemolytic anemia: Anemia with microcytosis suggests iron deficiency anemia as the cause of thrombocytosis, whereas anemia with elevated mean corpuscular volume (MCV) suggests that acute or chronic hemolytic anemia should be ruled out (young red cells known as reticulocytes have MCV values of ~160 fL, and thus the MCV is usually elevated in patients with hemolysis). The key question should be, Is the MCV increased or decreased? Of course, elevated MCV is also a feature of many primary hematologic disorders, such as myelodysplasia, considered earlier.

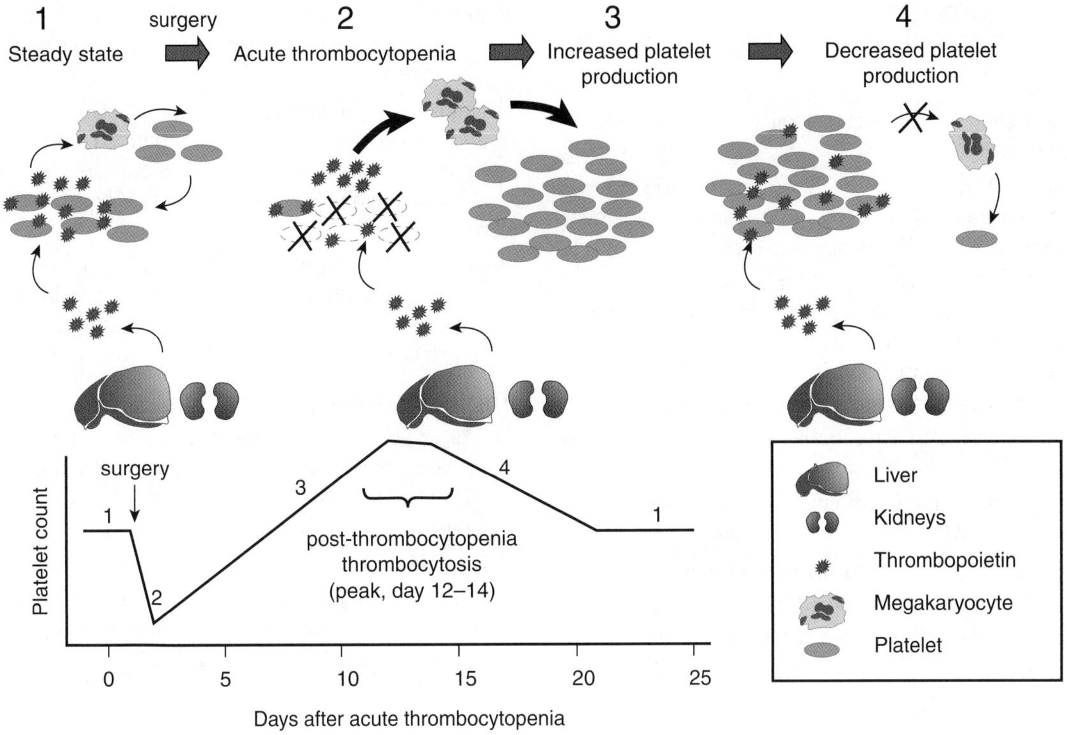

Figure 175-2 *Pathophysiology of postthrombocytopenia thrombocytosis. Thrombopoietin (TPO) binds to platelets and megakaryocytes via a specific receptor (c-Mpl, not shown). The receptor-bound TPO is removed from circulation and degraded. The level of circulating TPO is, thus, inversely related to the mass of platelets and megakaryocytes. In thrombocytopenia, fewer binding sites are available, and, consequently, free TPO levels are high, stimulating megakaryocyte proliferation and differentiation and leading to increased platelet production. In thrombocytosis, the high platelet mass acts as a "sink" for removing TPO, with decreased stimulus for platelet production. Thus, following acute thrombocytopenia, TPO levels rise about twofold, leading to increased platelet production that begins on days 2 to 4, with resulting thrombocytosis that generally peaks about days 12 to 14 (postthrombocytopenia thrombocytosis), and returns to baseline by approximately day 21. (Reprinted, with permission, from Arnold DM, Warkentin TE. Thrombocytopenia and thrombocytosis. In: Wilson WC, Grande CM, Hoyt DB, eds. Trauma: Critical Care (vol. 2). New York: Informa Healthcare USA; 2007:983–1005).*

PRIMARY THROMBOCYTOSIS

Primary thrombocytosis disorders are important to recognize as patients can be at increased bleeding or thrombotic risk, and sometimes both. Moreover, specialized care by a hematologic oncologist is standard.

Diagnostic considerations

Hereditary or familial thrombocytosis: The pathophysiologic explanation for hereditary thrombocytosis is usually unknown. However, in 10% to 20% of patients, an underlying genetic abnormality in thrombopoiesis has been identified (eg, mutations in thrombopoietin or its receptor).

Primary neoplastic disorders: The key question, "Is there concomitant splenomegaly and/or abnormalities in hemoglobin or WBC levels?", aims to address the possibility of a primary hematologic neoplasm. Any of the classic myeloproliferative neoplasms (MPN)—polycythemia vera (PV), chronic myeloid leukemia (CML), essential thrombocythemia (ET), or primary myelofibrosis (PMF)—can feature thrombocytosis, generally without significant dysmyelopoiesis. In contrast, myelodysplastic syndrome (MDS) is characterized by dysplastic bone marrow hyperplasia (sometimes, hypoplasia), with variable degrees of peripheral blood cytopenias. However, sometimes MDS features prominent elevations in blood count: the "5q-syndrome" is a specific type of MDS that features severe anemia, thrombocytosis with dysmegakaryopoiesis, and a more benign clinical course.

The presence of thrombocytosis does not necessarily indicate increased thrombotic risk: for example, platelet counts $> 1500 \times 10^9$/L can be associated with bleeding (due to acquired vWF syndrome from accelerated vWF clearance); further, platelet dysfunction is common in bone marrow neoplasia. Also, thrombotic risk factors besides elevated platelet count values per se are also important, such as elevated hematocrit in polycythemia rubra vera (PRV) and possibly elevated WBC levels.

SPURIOUS THROMBOCYTOSIS

Pseudothrombocytosis

Sometimes, spurious thrombocytosis results when the electronic particle counter misclassifies tiny red cell fragments, which can result in burn victims, as platelets.

CONCLUSION

Quantitative platelet disorders, thrombocytopenia and thrombocytosis, have diverse causes. Clinicians should focus on determining the probable cause of the patient's abnormal platelet count, as this will direct the management approach and prognosis.

SUGGESTED READINGS

Thrombocytopenia

Althaus K, Greinacher A. MYH9-related platelet disorders. *Semin Thromb Haemost.* 2009;35:189–203.

Aster RH, Curtis BR, McFarland JG, Bougie DW. Drug-induced thrombocytopenia: pathogenesis, diagnosis, and management. *J Thromb Haemost.* 2009;7:911–918.

Rodeghiero F, Stasi R, Gernsheimer T, et al. Standardization of terminology, definitions and outcome criteria in immune thrombocytopenic purpura of adults and children: report from an international working group. *Blood.* 2009;113:2386–2393.

Warkentin TE. Drug-induced immune-mediated thrombocytopenia—from purpura to thrombosis. *N Engl J Med.* 2007;356: 891–893.

Warkentin TE. Agents for the treatment of heparin-induced thrombocytopenia. *Hematol/Oncol Clin N Am.* 2010;24:755–775.

Warkentin TE, Kelton JG. Temporal aspects of heparin-induced thrombocytopenia. *N Engl J Med.* 2001;344:1286–1292.

Warkentin TE, Kelton JG. Delayed-onset heparin-induced thrombocytopenia and thrombosis. *Ann Intern Med.* 2001;135:502–506.

Warkentin TE, Elavathil LJ, Hayward CPM, et al. The pathogenesis of venous limb gangrene associated with heparin-induced thrombocytopenia. *Ann Intern Med.* 1997;127:804–812.

Warkentin TE, Greinacher A, Koster A, Lincoff AM. Treatment and prevention of heparin-induced thrombocytopenia. American College of Chest Physicians evidence-based clinical practice guidelines (8th edition). *Chest.* 2008;133(6 Suppl.): 340S–380S.

Warkentin TE, Sheppard JI, Moore JC, Sigouin CS, Kelton JG. Quantitative interpretation of optical density measurements using PF4-dependent enzyme-immunoassays. *J Thromb Haemost.* 2008;6:1304–1312.

Thrombocytosis

Kelaidi C, Eclache V, Fenaux P. The role of lenalidomide in the management of myelodysplasia with del 5q. *Br J Haematol.* 2008;140:267–278.

Skoda R. Thrombocytosis. *Hematology Am Soc Hematol Educ Program.* 2009:159–167.

Tefferi A, Thiele J, Vardiman JW. The 2008 World Health Organization classification system for myeloproliferative neoplasms: order out of chaos. *Cancer.* 2009;115:3842–3847.

CHAPTER 176

Approach to Patients with Bleeding Disorders

Kathryn Webert, MD, MSc, FRCPC
Catherine P.M. Hayward, MD, PhD

Key Clinical Questions

1. When should a bleeding disorder be suspected?
2. How should patients suspected of bleeding disorders be evaluated?
3. How does one interpret the results of hemostasis testing?
4. What is the general approach to management of an individual with a bleeding disorder?

INTRODUCTION

In general, severe bleeding disorders are uncommon, unlike mild bleeding problems, which can be more challenging to diagnose. Most episodes of clinically significant bleeding requiring medical attention result from local causes (eg, a duodenal ulcer), surgery, or trauma. However, it is important to recognize when bleeding problems are more serious due to an underlying hemostatic abnormality.

Abnormal bleeding represents an important health care problem. For example, in the United States, it has been estimated that at least 5% to 10% of women of childbearing age seek medical care for menorrhagia and have bleeding severe enough to require medical intervention. Among the many defects that can cause abnormal bleeding, inherited and acquired von Willebrand disease (vWD) and platelet function disorders are much more common than defects in coagulation and fibrinolytic proteins.

PATHOPHYSIOLOGY

REVIEW OF NORMAL HEMOSTASIS

Hemostasis consists of the following steps: (1) initiation and formation of the platelet plug, also known as primary hemostasis; (2) propagation and amplification of the clotting "cascade" or secondary hemostasis, which involves activation of a series of coagulation factors resulting in the generation of thrombin that cleaves fibrinogen to fibrin; (3) cross-linking of fibrin; (3) termination of procoagulant response by antithrombotic control mechanisms; (4) removal of the clot by fibrinolysis; and (5) tissue repair and regeneration.

When a vessel is injured, platelets adhere to exposed collagen and other components of the subendothelium as the first defense against bleeding. This initial adhesion is dependent on von Willebrand factor (vWF) as well as specific platelet receptors (eg, glycoprotein [GP] IbIXV) for vWF and collagen. This adhesion leads to platelet activation and shape change as well as platelet aggregation, which promotes recruitment of additional platelets.

Coagulation is initiated *in vivo* when endothelial or vascular cells are damaged. This results in exposure of blood to tissue factor (TF), which binds to factor VII (FVII) and its activated form, factor VII (FVIIa). TF-FVIIa complexes (extrinisic tenase) then activates factors IX and X directly. Activated factor IX can also form a complex with factor VIIIa as well as phospholipids and calcium, called the *intrinsic tenase complex*, that promotes further conversion of factor X to factor Xa. The generated factor Xa associates with activated factor V, phospholipids, and calcium to form the prothrombinase complex that activates prothrombin to thrombin. Intrinsic and extrinsic tenase are needed to generate enough thrombin for normal hemostasis. Once thrombin is generated, it cleaves fibrinogen to fibrin, which leads to formation of a fibrin clot and promotes platelet activation and the generation of activated factors V and VIII. Thrombin also results in the formation of activated XIII, an enzyme that crosslinks fibrin to make the clot more resistant to fibrinolysis (the cleavage of the fibrin clot).

When coagulation is activated, fibrinolysis is activated, leading to slow dissolution of the clot as part of wound healing. The process of fibrinolysis requires activation of plasminogen to plasmin, which is a serine protease that cleaves crosslinked fibrin. Fibrinolysis results in the formation of fibrinogen degradation products, including D-dimers. The generation of plasmin is controlled by both activators (ie, tissue-type and urinary-type plasmin activators) and inhibitors (ie, plasminogen activator inhibitor 1 and α2 plasmin inhibitor).

GENERAL CLASSIFICATION OF BLEEDING DISORDERS ACCORDING TO PATHOPHYSIOLOGY

Bleeding disorders may be classified according to whether they are inherited or acquired, and by their underlying pathophysiology. The latter classification is often divided into the following broad categories: vascular disorders (eg, hemorrhagic telangiectasia and diseases of the connective tissue in the vessel wall, which are often challenging to diagnose); disorders of primary hemostasis (eg, platelet and vWF deficiencies and defects); disorders of secondary hemostasis (eg, clotting factor defects and deficiencies); and disorders of fibrinolysis (see **Table 176-1**). Some disorders (eg, severe vWD) impair hemostasis by impairing both platelet adhesion and fibrin formation, due to the associated factor VIII deficiency. Drugs that inhibit platelet function (eg, aspirin, nonsteroidal anti-inflammatory drugs, serotonin reuptake inhibitors) and those that inhibit coagulation (eg, heparin, warfarin) are important causes to consider when evaluating and managing an individual with bleeding.

TABLE 176-1 Questions to Consider when Evaluating a Patient for a Possible Bleeding Disorder

What are the patient's bleeding symptoms?
- Is there a personal or family history of bleeding with trauma or procedures?
- What are the site(s) of bleeding?
- For women: Is there a history of prolonged, heavy periods or bleeding with childbirth?
- What is the severity of bleeding?
- What is the duration of bleeding events?
- Has the patient required any treatments for bleeding?

Does the history suggest a congenital or acquired problem?
- Note: For congenital bleeding disorders, the bleeding symptoms may date back to childhood and may affect other family members; acquired bleeding disorders should be considered when the bleeding problems are more recent, and a drug-induced defect should be excluded.

What is the timing of the bleeding?
- Is the bleeding immediate or delayed (onset one or more days after challenges)?

Is the bleeding systemic or local?
- Note: Local bleeding is suggestive of a local cause, although acquired or inherited bleeding disorders can make it worse.

Are there any aggravating or contributing factors?
- Note: The drug history (prescription, nonprescription, and other supplements) should be carefully reviewed.

What is the patient's general medical history?
- Does the patient have a history of liver, kidney, or thyroid diseases? The patient should also be questioned about relevant symptoms of these disorders.
- Does the patient have a history of pregnancy loss (may be associated with disorders of fibrinogen).
- Does the patient have a history of poor wound healing (can occur in a variety of bleeding disorders).

How many times has the patient experienced a significant hemostatic challenge, and how many of these were associated with abnormal bleeding?
- Note: A history of bleeding with only some challenges suggests a mild or acquired bleeding problem.

DOES THIS PATIENT HAVE A BLEEDING DISORDER?

WHEN TO SUSPECT A BLEEDING DISORDER

In general, a bleeding disorder should be suspected when bleeding occurs with minimal or no provocation, when it is more severe than expected for a given challenge, and when bleeding episodes occur repeatedly with challenges. Care should be taken to avoid asking very subjective questions about bleeding. For example, it is preferable to ask women about menstrual periods lasting longer than seven days, with more than two to three days of heavy flow, and/or periods that interfere with their lifestyle than to ask if they experience "heavy" periods. Similarly, asking about bruises as big as or larger than oranges and/or bruises appearing without provocation is better than asking about "easy bruising."

While individuals with severe bleeding problems may report spontaneous bleeding and serious bleeding with major and minor hemostatic challenges, individuals with milder defects can report abnormal bleeding with some but not all significant hemostatic challenges. The clinical assessment should be directed toward identifying the type and severity of bleeding problems experienced by an individual, in order to plan appropriate laboratory testing and therapy.

KEY COMPONENTS OF THE HISTORY

What are the patient's bleeding symptoms?

The patient should be questioned about his or her current bleeding symptoms and past bleeding symptoms and a family history of bleeding problems (**Table 176-2**). The following characteristics of the bleeding should be determined: association with trauma or procedures and if it occurred with some or all minor and major procedures; site(s) (including joint bleeds); severity (eg, bleeding resulting in additional interventions such as blood transfusions, intensive care unit admission, and/or prolongation of hospitalization stay); duration of bleeding; and any treatments that were given to control bleeding (types of drugs or blood products). It may be helpful to determine if the patient received anticoagulants or drugs that inhibit platelet function. Female patients should be asked questions about menstrual periods and abnormal bleeding with childbirth and pregnancy losses. Mucocutaneous bleeding (ie, abnormal bruising, gum bleeding, and epistaxis) is more suggestive of a defect in primary hemostasis. Some bleeding symptoms, such as deep tissue bleeding, joint hemorrhages, and spontaneous unexplained hematuria are uncommon but can occur in severe inherited coagulation protein deficiencies. Some bleeding problems, such as epistaxis, can be experienced by individuals without bleeding disorders. Bleeding after trauma should be considered but can be difficult to evaluate because it is not specific to individuals with bleeding disorders.

PRACTICE POINT

- The timing of the bleeding relative to the surgical or dental procedure may be an important clue to the etiology of the bleeding disorder. Patients with disorders of primary hemostasis will often describe abnormal bleeding during or within a few hours whereas disorders of secondary hemostasis typically manifest as delayed-onset bleeding evident days following trauma or surgery.

What is the timing of bleeding?

The bleeding history is often used to assess when abnormal bleeding occurred (eg, same day or days later) relative to invasive

TABLE 176-2 General Classification of Bleeding Disorders According to Pathophysiology

Vascular disorders
- Congenital (eg, hereditary hemorrhagic telangiectasis, Ehlers-Danlos syndrome)
- Acquired (eg, secondary to steroid use, vitamin C deficiency)

Disorders of platelets and their function
- Thrombocytopenia
  - Acquired (eg, drug-induced, immune-mediated)
  - Congenital (eg, inherited platelet or bone marrow disorders)
- Disorders of platelet function
  - Congenital (secretion defects are the most common)
  - Acquired (eg, drug-induced, renal failure)
- Von Willebrand disease
  - Congenital
  - Acquired

Disorders of coagulation
- Coagulation factor deficiencies
  - Congenital (ie, hemophilia A [factor VIII deficiency], hemophilia B [factor IX deficiency], deficiencies or defects of factors II, V, VII, X, XI, fibrinogen, or XIII)
  - Acquired (vitamin K deficiency, liver disease, anticoagulant therapy, massive blood loss [hemodilution], acquired coagulation factor inhibitors)

Disorders of fibrinolysis
- Congenital (ie, alpha-2 antiplasmin deficiency, plasminogen activator inhibitor-1 deficiency, Quebec platelet disorder)
- Acquired (ie, hyperfibrinolytic syndrome, disseminated intravascular coagulation)

Other
- Acquired bleeding secondary to other disorders such as renal failure, thyroid disease, or Cushing syndrome

surgical or dental procedures. Bleeding during, immediately after, or on the same day as the challenge is suggestive of a disorder of primary hemostasis (see Disorders of Primary Hemostasis later in this chapter), whereas bleeding that becomes problematic one or more days after a challenge is more typical of a factor deficiency or a fibrinolytic defect.

Is the bleeding disorder congenital or acquired, and are there aggravating or contributing factors?

Inherited problems tend to present earlier in life than acquired problems unless they are mild. Inherited problems are often associated with a positive family history, which may be negative if the condition is recessive or X-linked. A thorough bleeding history should include questions about potential aggravating or contributing factors such as new medications (eg, aspirin or antidepressant therapy).

Individuals with acquired bleeding disorders often describe bleeding that is more recent in onset. Causes of an acquired bleeding disorder are listed in Table 176-2 and include liver disease, vitamin K deficiency, autoimmune-mediated conditions (eg, immune thrombocytopenic purpura), hypothyroidism, acquired factor VIII deficiency or acquired vWD, and other conditions such as Cushing syndrome

It is important to emphasize that the patient's entire bleeding history must be assessed in order to determine if the problem is mild or severe and if it is likely congenital or acquired.

Has the patient experienced any hemostatic challenges?

Patients should be questioned about how many operative and invasive dental procedures they have undergone, and how many of these were associated with abnormal bleeding. It may be helpful to ask if the patient has experienced any unusually large ecchymosis around incisions when evaluating the surgical bleeding history. It is important to note that individuals who have undergone a number of common surgical and dental procedures (eg, tonsillectomy, wisdom tooth extraction) without experiencing abnormal bleeding might still have a mild bleeding problem (particularly if other aspects of their bleeding history are abnormal); however, they are unlikely to have a severe bleeding disorder. Alternately, it is important to recognize that sometimes abnormal bleeding occurs in healthy individuals undergoing a major procedure due to technical complications.

What is the patient's general medical history? Is there a systemic disease that is causing or contributing to the patient's bleeding symptoms?

An evaluation of a patient's general medical history for new or worsening bleeding, and other changes in health, is important for assessing undiagnosed liver, kidney, or endocrine disorders such as thyroid disease or Cushing syndrome. The manifestations of some bleeding disorders, such as severe fibrinogen deficiency, can include recurrent pregnancy losses (due to hemorrhagic abruptions) and poor wound healing. Intracranial hemorrhage is seen more frequently in severe bleeding disorders (such as severe congenital factor XIII deficiency, severe coagulation factor, or fibrinolytic protein deficiencies and/or defects). Anemia can make bleeding worse and a history of iron deficiency (with or without anemia) can suggest chronically increased blood loss (eg, due to menorrhagia). Sometimes the history can suggest a rare inherited syndrome such as a platelet disorder associated with albinism, hearing loss, renal insufficiency, or skeletal malformations.

Has the patient ingested any medications that may have caused or worsened bleeding?

It is helpful to obtain a list of all medications (including prescription, nonprescription, and herbal) that the patient was taking in order to determine what might have caused or worsened their bleeding. Drugs can cause or worsen bleeding by a variety of mechanisms inducing: thrombocytopenia (eg, quinine, penicillin); impaired platelet function (eg, due to nonsteroidal anti-inflammatory drugs such as aspirin, clopidogrel, serotonin reuptake inhibitors, or fish oil supplements); or defective coagulation (eg, due to heparin or warfarin).

PHYSICAL EXAMINATION

The physical examination is often not very informative in individuals with a bleeding disorder. An initial assessment of acute bleeding should determine the patient's hemodynamic status and if there are signs of anemia. Blood blisters in the mouth, hemorrhages on the bite margins in the mouth, and petechiae (tiny red-colored skin lesions that reflect small hemorrhages into the skin, particularly on dependent parts of the body and at sites of trauma) may suggest significant thrombocytopenia. Large bruises or purpura may suggest a defect in primary hemostasis or acquired hemophilia. Sometimes the purpuric skin lesions of severe anticoagulant protein deficiencies (eg, purpura fulminans due to severe congenital protein C deficiency) are mistaken for skin bleeding. Abnormalities in joints, lymph nodes, spleen, and liver should raise concern for the possibility of a secondary bleeding disorder.

DIFFERENTIAL DIAGNOSIS BASED ON CLINICAL ASSESSMENT

Table 176-3 outlines the differences between disorders of primary and secondary hemostasis.

Disorders of primary hemostasis

Patients with disorders of primary hemostasis will often describe experiencing abnormal bleeding during or within a few hours of a surgical or dental procedure. These problems, with or without mucocutaneous bleeding symptoms, should raise questions about vWF and platelet abnormalities (both qualitative and quantitative) or, less commonly, blood vessel abnormalities. Defects in primary hemostasis can also present as troublesome epistaxis and/or gingival bleeding, petechiae, superficial bruising or ecchymosis, and menorrhagia. Petechiae are very suggestive of a platelet or vascular disorder.

Disorders of secondary hemostasis

Disorders of secondary hemostasis typically manifest as delayed-onset bleeding that becomes evident in the days following trauma or surgical procedure. When there is a severe factor deficiency, there can be spontaneous bleeding into joint spaces (hemarthroses) and into deep, soft tissues (eg, muscle hematomas). The most common inherited disorders of secondary hemostasis include hemophilia A (factor VIII deficiency) and hemophilia B (factor IX deficiency). Acquired hemophilia, due to an antibody directed against factor VIII, accounts for about 10% of all hemophilia. Factor XIII deficiency and fibrinolytic disorders can also present with delayed bleeding, but these conditions are less common.

TABLE 176-3 Distinction between Disorders of Primary and Secondary Hemostasis

	Disorders of Primary Hemostasis	Disorders of Secondary Hemostasis
Timing of bleeding	Immediate	Delayed (starts one or more days after trauma or surgery)
Petechiae	Common (especially with thrombocytopenia)	Not seen
Ecchymoses	Common	May occur (usually large)
Deep hematomas	Not common	Common in severe factor deficiencies
Joint bleeding (hemarthoses)	Not common	Common in severe factor deficiencies
Mucous membrane bleeding	Common	Uncommon
Epistaxis	Common, particularly in childhood	Uncommon
Menorrhagia	Common	May occur
Inheritance (if congenital)	Dominant or recessive	Most common cause (hemophilia) is X-linked

HOW SHOULD THIS PATIENT WITH A SUSPECTED BLEEDING DISORDER BE INVESTIGATED?

Investigations for bleeding problems need to consider the etiologies of mild and severe and common and rare disorders. **Figure 176-1** summarizes a stepwise approach to investigation, some of which may be performed at the time of a specialist evaluation. Often, a broad range of tests is needed to assess an individual with a suspected bleeding disorder (see Figure 176-1). A complete blood count is helpful to evaluate for thrombocytopenia and to determine if there are other hematologic abnormalities such as anemia (which may reflect acute or chronic bleeding), or white blood cell abnormalities that may suggest an underlying bone marrow disorder. An assessment for iron deficiency (which may be present without anemia) should be considered. A blood group and antibody screen should be done before surgery in individuals with a history of abnormal bleeding and can be helpful when interpreting vWD testing results.

When selecting tests of hemostasis to investigate a bleeding problem, it is helpful to consider that coagulation defects are generally much rarer than defects in platelets and vWF. Like the bleeding time, closure times measured by the platelet function analyzer (PFA)-100 are optional and cannot be used to exclude vWD or platelet disorders. While it is common practice to order a prothrombin time (PT, sometimes reported as an international normalized ratio [INR]) and an activated partial thromboplastin time (APTT) in individuals with bleeding problems, the results are often normal. A fibrinogen level and a thrombin time should be considered because the PT and APTT are insensitive to fibrinogen problems. **Table 176-4** lists the different causes of abnormal coagulation tests.

To assess for vWD, a vWF antigen, vWF ristocetin cofactor activity, and factor VIII level should be ordered. The vWF level can be mildly low in blood group O individuals.

Platelet disorders are typically evaluated by specialized tests of platelet aggregation and secretion assays, which may require referral to a bleeding disorder specialist.

Additional tests can be helpful to evaluate if there is a history of acquired bleeding, which could reflect liver or renal disease or an endocrine disorder such as hypothyroidism or Cushing syndrome. As fibrinolytic defects are uncommon, testing is rarely done except by specialists.

PRACTICE POINT

- In general, the patient's symptoms, not the laboratory values, should be treated. Local factors can be significant contributors to bleeding and should be considered in the plans for investigation and treatment, even in patients with documented coagulopathies. Always consider risks and benefits (including those of treating or not treating) when deciding on appropriate therapies as the risks of certain therapies include increased prothrombotic risks. Patients with congenital bleeding disorders are best managed in a multidisciplinary care setting to plan treatment and prevention of acute bleeding episodes and to deal with complications (eg, hemophilic arthropathy). Information on the patient's bleeding problem and the treatment plans must be communicated to both the patient and their health care providers.

HOW SHOULD THIS PATIENT WITH A BLEEDING DISORDER BE TREATED?

The management of each patient with a bleeding disorder depends on the cause and severity of their bleeding disorder.

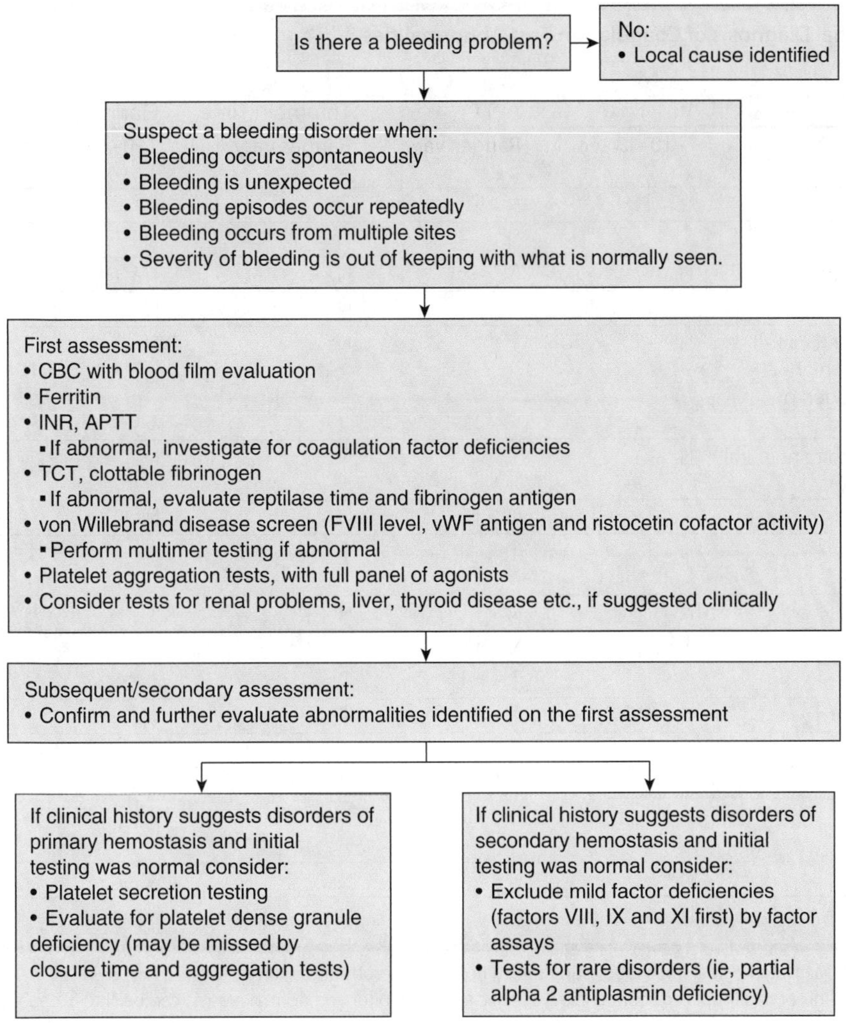

Figure 176-1 *A staged assessment to the diagnostic testing of bleeding disorders. (APTT, activated partial thromboplastin time; CBC, complete blood count; INR, international normalized ratio; TCT, thrombin clot time; vWF, von Willebrand factor.)*

GENERAL CONSIDERATIONS

- The patient's symptoms, not the laboratory values, should be treated. In general, treatment should be considered when the patient is bleeding or when the risk of bleeding is high (for example, if the patient is undergoing an invasive procedure).
- Local factors can be significant contributors to bleeding and should be considered in the plans for investigation and treatment, even in patients with documented coagulopathies.
- It is necessary to consider risks and benefits (including those of treating or not treating) when deciding on appropriate therapies, as the risks of certain therapies include increased prothrombotic risks. Other risks of hemostatic therapies (for treatment or propylaxis) include risks for viral transmission (ie, with blood products; recombinant products are generally preferred over blood-derived products to minimize these risks), and hyponatremia (with desmopressin acetate, if fluid restriction is not imposed for 12 hours post therapy). In addition, treatment plans need to consider whether standard treatments (eg, use of intramuscular injections, postoperative anticoagulants, anti-inflammatory drugs that inhibit platelet function) should be modified because of the patient's bleeding problems.
- Information on the patient's bleeding problem and the treatment plans must be communicated to both the patient and his health care providers. Patients with congenital bleeding disorders must be "taught" that prophylactic treatment is required prior to invasive procedures.
- Patients with congenital bleeding disorders are best managed in a multidisciplinary care setting to plan treatment and prevention of acute bleeding episodes and to deal with complications (eg, hemophilic arthropathy).

OTHER ISSUES TO CONSIDER FOR TREATMENT OF CONGENITAL BLEEDING DISORDERS

Treatments for factor deficiencies

Individuals with moderate-to-severe clinically significant factor deficiencies often require factor concentrates (recombinant products generally preferred over plasma-derived products), although some conditions and circumstances (eg, mild hemophilia due to factor VIII deficiency with mild bleeding) may be managed with desmopressin. Fibrinolytic inhibitor drugs (aminocaproic acid and tranexamic acid) are often used as an adjunctive therapy for some procedures, such as dental and oral-nasal surgeries.

Von Willebrand disease

The treatment of vWD depends on the type and severity of the disease. With mild vWD, which is more common, treatment with

TABLE 176-4 Differential Diagnosis of Coagulation Test Abnormalities

	PT	APTT	Thrombin Time	Fibrinogen	Platelet Count
Reference intervals	~ 10–13 sec	Ranges vary	Ranges vary	150–400 mg/dL 1.5–4.0 g/L	150–400 × 106/mL
Fibrinogen deficiency	N – ↑	N – ↑	↑	↑	N
Factor VII deficiency	↑	N	N	N	N
Factor VIII, IX, or XI deficiency	N	↑	N	N	N
Factor II, V, X deficiency	↑	↑	N	N	N
Factor deficiencies not associated with bleeding (factor XII, high-molecular-weight kininogen or prekallikrein deficiency)	N	↑	N	N	N
Acquired hemophilia and congenital hemophilia with inhibitors	N	↑*	N	N	N
Lupus anticoagulant	N – ↑	N – ↑†	N – ↑	N	N
Heparin therapy or sample contamination	N – ↑	↑	↑↑	N	N
Liver disease	N – ↑	N – ↑	N – ↑	↓ – N – ↑	↓ – N
Vitamin K deficiency	↑	N – ↑	N	N	N
Fibrinolytic therapy	↑	↑	↑	↓	N
Consumptive coagulopathy	N – ↑	↑	↑	↓	↓
Dilutional coagulopathy	N – ↑	N – ↑	N – ↑	↓ – N	↓
Von Willebrand disease	N	N – ↑	N	N	N ↓ in type 2B and platelet type
Thrombocytopenia	N	N	N	N	↓
Platelet function disorders	N	N	N	N	↓ – N

↑, elevated; ↓, reduced; APTT, activated partial thromboplastin time; N, normal; PT, prothrombin time.

*An APTT of a 1:1 immediate mix of patient plasma containing a specific factor inhibitor and normal plasma can be N to ↑ depending on the features of their inhibitor. If a specific factor inhibitor is suspected, factor assays and tests for specific factor inhibitors should be performed.

†APTT reagents have different sensitivities to lupus anticoagulants. A lupus anticoagulant usually prolongs the APTT with a 1:1 mix of patient and normal plasma.

desmopressin acetate may be sufficient for many situations. In general, the treatment goal is to raise the levels of vWF (by giving the medication desmopressin acetate or vWF concentrates) to normal.

Platelet function disorders

Most platelet function disorders are mild bleeding disorders that respond to treatment with desmopressin acetate. Other options for therapy include fibrinolytic inhibitors (eg, for menorrhagia, oral-nasal surgery, or dental extractions), platelet transfusions (reserved for rare, severe disorders, such as Glanzmann thrombasthenia and Bernard Soulier syndrome and also given when bleeding is serious and not adequately controlled by desmopressin), and sometimes activated factor VII concentrate (generally reserved for situations where there is a wish to avoid platelet transfusions and other drug therapies, such as desmopressin, are not adequate).

GENERAL MANAGEMENT OF COMMON ACQUIRED BLEEDING DISORDERS

Liver disease

The coagulopathy related to liver disease is multifactorial, as the liver is the major source of all hemostatic proteins in plasma except for vWF and tissue plasminogen activator. Individuals with liver disease often have deficiencies of multiple coagulation factors, and in mild liver disease, there can be low levels of factors VII and, at times, factors XI and XII. Fibrinogen deficiency is typically only seen with severe liver disease. In fact, fibrinogen levels are often elevated in mild liver disease. Sometimes patients with liver disease have additional hemostatic defects such as vitamin K deficiency, thrombocytopenia, dysfibrinogenemia, platelet function abnormalities, and disseminated intravascular coagulation (DIC). If an individual with coagulopathy from liver disease requires treatment (ie, before a procedure associated with a significantly increased risk of bleeding), one or more of the following treatment options should be considered: vitamin K replacement, plasma infusion (typically requires four or more units to have measurable effects), and/or platelet transfusion.

Anticoagulant medications

Treatment of serious bleeding due to anticoagulants may require reversal of the anticoagulant. Patients on an oral vitamin K antagonist, who require reversal to treat bleeding, should receive vitamin K, and when more rapid reversal is required (eg, to treat life-threatening gastrointestinal bleeding), prothrombin complex concentrate (if available) or plasma infusion should be considered. Protamine sulfate can be considered when there is a need to rapidly reverse unfractionated heparin or low-molecular-weight heparin because of bleeding. However, this treatment reverses only about 60% of the anti–factor Xa activity of low-molecular-weight heparin. Unfortunately, agents are not available to rapidly reverse some of the newer, novel anticoagulants that are direct inhibitors of thrombin or factor Xa. It is unclear whether bleeding from these newer agents is improved by treatment with desmopressin acetate, fibrinolytic inhibitor drugs, or other treatments, such as prothrombin complex concentrates and factor VIIa.

Vitamin K deficiency

Acquired bleeding due to vitamin K deficiency results from decreased gamma-carboxylation of the vitamin K–dependent factors II, VII, IX, and X and can be treated by administration of vitamin K.

CONCLUSION

Abnormal bleeding in an important health care problem that should be suspected when bleeding occurs spontaneously, is more severe than expected or occurs on repeated occasions.

SUGGESTED READINGS

Hayward CP. Diagnostic approach to platelet function disorders. *Transfus Apher Sci.* 2008;38:65–76.

James AH. Guidelines for bleeding disorders in women. *Thromb Res.* 2009;123(Suppl 2):S124–S128.

Keeling D, Tait C, Makris M. Guideline on the selection and use of therapeutic products to treat haemophilia and other hereditary bleeding disorders. A United Kingdom Haemophilia Center Doctors' Organisation (UKHCDO) guideline approved by the British Committee for Standards in Haematology. *Haemophilia.* 2008;14:671–684.

Mannuci PM, Duga S, Peyvandi F. Recessively inherited coagulation disorders. *Blood.* 2004;104:1243–1252.

Nichols WL, Hultin MB, James AH, et al. von Willebrand disease (VWD): evidence-based diagnosis and management guidelines, the National Heart, Lung, and Blood Institute (NHLBI) Expert Panel report (USA). *Haemophilia.* 2008;14:171–232.

Verhovsek M, Moffat KA, Hayward CP. Laboratory testing for fibrinogen abnormalities. *Am J Hematol.* 2008;83:928–931.

CHAPTER 177

Transfusion of Blood Components, Derivatives and Their Adverse Effects

Elianna Saidenberg, MD, FRCP(C)
Morris A. Blajchman, MD, FRCP

Key Clinical Questions

1. What are the indications for transfusion of blood products?
2. What are the common complications of transfusion?
3. What interventions minimize the need for transfusion?

INTRODUCTION

The transfusion of blood products is a regular, daily occurrence in hospital practice. In 2006, in the United States, approximately 22.3 million transfusions of various blood products were carried out. Depending on the size of the hospital and the range of services offered, only a few patients a month or many patients each day may be transfused. Similarly, blood banks may carry as few as one or two to more than a dozen different types of blood products. **Table 177-1** shows a list of most of the blood products provided to Canadian hospitals for patient use by Canadian Blood Services.

It is not necessary for physicians outside the field of transfusion medicine to have detailed information about each of these many products. However, clinicians should be able to explain the indications for transfusion of the most commonly used blood products and recognize transfusion reactions. Each of the five cases demonstrates how certain blood products might be used and the adverse outcomes that are potentially associated with their use.

CASE INFORMATION

1. A 73-year-old male with a lower GI bleed.
2. A 31-year-old woman undergoing therapy for AML with bruising, petechiae, and uncontrolled epistaxis.
3. A 67-year-old man on oral anticoagulant therapy with a profusely bleeding scalp laceration.
4. A 28-year-old female s/p recent pregnancy termination, now acutely unwell with a purpuric rash and heavy vaginal bleeding.
5. A victim of a hit and run motor vehicle accident who has sustained multiple injuries, including a fractured pelvis.

Each of these patients would likely benefit from the transfusion of different products and at least one of them would probably benefit from the transfusion of multiple blood products.

RED BLOOD CELL TRANSFUSIONS

CASE 177-1

RECTAL BLEEDING AND THE TRANSFUSION DECISION (RBCs)

A 73-year-old male with a history of hypertension and angina presented to the emergency department with rectal bleeding. Colonoscopy revealed the source of the bleeding to be a tumor in the colon. Surgeons plan to remove the affected portion of the colon. Prior to surgery, the patient's hemoglobin was found to be 8.5 g/dL (85 g/L). He reported chest discomfort on ambulating from his hospital bed to the bathroom. The chest discomfort was relieved by sublingual nitroglycerine spray. His physical examination was notable for his vital signs—heart rate of 110 beats per minute (bpm) and BP of 130/75 mm Hg.

Since Mr. A was likely having symptoms from his anemia he was transfused one unit of packed red blood cells (RBCs). His hemoglobin rose to 9.3 g/dL (93 g/L) and he no longer experienced symptoms of breathlessness or chest pain with

ambulation. The surgeon anticipated that there will be additional surgical blood loss and requested that an additional transfusion be given prior to surgery. The attending hospitalist argued that there was no clear evidence indicating a benefit to additional RBC transfusions and, there was a risk of volume overload associated with additional RBC transfusions. The decision was made to hold off on further RBC transfusions but to alert the blood bank of the possible need for intraoperative or postoperative transfusion. The transfusion laboratory crossmatched two additional RBC units for the patient, to be on hand on the day of the surgery.

The treatment of anemia, with the consequent improvement in tissue oxygen delivery, is the key indication for the transfusion of red blood cells (RBCs). One unit of RBCs has a volume of about 250 mL and should contain a hematocrit of less than 0.80 L/L. Transfusion of one RBC unit will increase the hemoglobin by about 1.0 g/dL (10 g/L) and can often relieve the symptoms in patients with anemia. Treating anemia may also be associated with improved outcomes in certain patient groups. However, there is no hemoglobin level at which a transfusion is indicated for all patients. The preexisting physical condition of an individual, the rate at which the hemoglobin has dropped, as well as the degree of anemia all impact on how well the patient will compensate for the low hemoglobin. The decision to transfuse should be individualized for each patient based on clinical condition. Additionally, the decision should be made with a clear understanding of the risks, as well as the benefits of RBC transfusions.

TABLE 177-1 Products Supplied in Canada by Canadian Blood Services

- Packed red blood cells (RBCs)*
- Platelets*
  - Single donor apheresis
  - Pooled from multiple donors
- Fresh frozen plasma (FFP)
- Cryoprecipitate units
- Prothrombin complex concentrates (PCCs)
- Albumin
- Antithrombin concentrates
- C-1 esterase inhibitor concentrates
- Recombinant human factor VIIa (rhFVIIa)
- Factor VII concentrates
- von Willebrand factor/factor VIII concentrates
- Intravenous immune globulin (IVIg)
- Recombinant factor VIII concentrates
- Recombinant factor IX concentrates
- Factor XI concentrates
- Factor XIII concentrates
- Fibrinogen concentrates
- Immune globulins (Ig) preparations:
  - Anti-D Ig
  - Anti-CMV Ig
  - Anti-hepatitis B Ig
  - Anti-varicella Ig
- Starch volume expanders
- Protein C concentrates
- Factor eight inhibitor bypassing activity agent (FEIBA)

*In Canada, cellular products are universally leukoreduced before storage. These products may also be provided irradiated, provided as CMV negative, concentrates, or as washed cells. Additionally, RBCs of rare blood types may be stored frozen for up to 10 years, and processed just prior to transfusion in the liquid state.

It is generally accepted that patients with acute blood loss due to active bleeding will need RBC transfusions to maintain the hemoglobin above 7.0 g/dL (70 g/L). Transfusion therapy in such cases should always be considered only one part of a resuscitative measure. Attention should be focused on treating the source of blood loss. In patients with chronic anemia, compensatory mechanisms often have the opportunity to come into play and consequently, patients with chronic anemia may tolerate much lower hemoglobin levels than those with acute blood loss. Indeed, young patients with uncompromised cardiac or pulmonary function may tolerate very low hemoglobin levels. RBC transfusions are usually recommended in older patients or those with poor cardiopulmonary reserve whose hemoglobin levels are less than 7.0 g/dL (70 g/L). Transfusion to higher levels may be necessary in symptomatic patients but transfusion is not usually appropriate if the hemoglobin level is greater than 10 g/dL (100 g/L).

Though the above recommendations are generally accepted, the literature regarding when to transfuse anemic patients presents some conflicting data and can be difficult to interpret. One of the key areas of conflict is the prophylactic transfusion of patients with moderate degrees of anemia (hemoglobin 7.0–10.0 g/dL or 70–100 g/L), especially in patients who are perioperative or critically ill. The best available data regarding the transfusion of critically ill patients come from the Transfusion Requirements in Critical Care (TRICC) trial in which critically ill patients were randomized to either a restrictive or a liberal transfusion protocol and followed prospectively to assess for difference in mortality. Those in the restrictive transfusion group were transfused to maintain their hemoglobin between 7.0–9.0 g/dL (70–90 g/L) and those in the liberal arm were transfused to maintain their hemoglobin between 10.0–12.0 g/dL (100–120 g/L). Mortality at 30 days was similar in the two groups and there was some indication that the restrictive strategy might be superior in younger patients who were less critically ill. This was not the case in the subgroup of patients who experienced myocardial ischemia. These data are usually interpreted to indicate that critically ill patients may safely tolerate a drop in hemoglobin level below 90 g/L before RBC transfusions are indicated, but higher levels may be required in the more severely ill or those with active coronary artery disease.

A large retrospective study examined the effect of perioperative transfusion on mortality at 30 days and 90 days after surgery. No correlation between transfusion and mortality could be found and the results suggested that patients whose hemoglobin levels were as low as 8.0 g/dL (80 g/L) did not suffer increased mortality. However, these conclusions are limited by the fact that nearly all patients in the study with a hemoglobin less than 8.0 g/dL (80 g/L) received transfusions. Despite the large numbers of patients evaluated in the above-noted trials and other studies, there can be no consensus on a threshold hemoglobin value at which all patients should be transfused. It merits frequent repetition that clinical signs and symptoms, not a hemoglobin number, should inform the decision to transfuse RBCS. Most importantly, the potential risks of transfusions should always be weighed against the anticipated benefits.

There are certain special groups of patients whose transfusion requirements differ from that of the general population. For example, patients with sickle cell anemia suffer chronic anemia caused by ongoing hemolysis and often tolerate low levels of hemoglobin. However, when complications arise, transfusion therapy is an important part of their therapy. Two types of RBC transfusions may be indicated in these situations. One is a simple transfusion, the other is an exchange transfusion in which the patient's RBCs are removed at the same time that donor RBCs are transfused. Simple RBC transfusions are indicated for the relief of the complications of sickle cell disease including, but not limited to, acute anemia due to blood loss, aplastic crisis, acute

TABLE 177-2 Donor ABO Blood Group Compatibility for RBC Transfusions

Recipient Type	Donor RBC Types which can be Used
A	A, O
B	B, O
AB	AB, A, B, O
O	O

splenic or hepatic sequestration crisis, and acute chest syndrome. Additionally, there is evidence that such patients may require preoperative transfusion to reach a goal of a hemoglobin level of 10.0 g/dL (100 g/L) if the patient will be undergoing a general anesthetic or if the surgery is ophthalmologic.

When it seems likely that a patient will require an RBC transfusion certain tests should be done in the transfusion medicine laboratory to ensure that a safe product is chosen for the patient. These tests are commonly referred to as the group, screen, and crossmatch. Grouping consists of determining the patient's ABO and Rh(D) blood groups. It is mandatory that all patients be transfused with RBC units that are ABO compatible (see **Table 177-2**). It is preferable to transfuse Rh(D) matched units to all patients, but it is especially important to do so in young girls and women of child-bearing age who are Rh(D) negative and therefore at risk of having hemolytic disease of the newborn if they become alloimmunized with anti-Rh(D) antibodies. When blood is needed urgently and grouping cannot be performed, group O Rh(D) negative units, the universal blood donor type, should be used.

Screening of a recipient's blood sample refers to assessing a patient's serum for presence of antibodies against RBC antigens. Crossmatching is the final step to ensure compatibility between donor and the recipient. These tests fall into one of two general categories: those tests that involve mixing donor and recipient serum, and those which can be done electronically, known as computer crossmatches. If an actual laboratory test is done, the RBCs of the donor and serum of the recipient are mixed and donor RBCs are evaluated for the presence of agglutination. If no RBC agglutination occurs, then the donor RBCs are compatible for transfusion to the recipient and no further testing is required. If RBC agglutination is seen, further testing on both the donor blood and the recipient's sample is needed. In an electronic crossmatch, the computer will select an appropriate unit from the blood bank's supply. The donor unit must have been tested twice to confirm the ABO group and the recipient should have two recent ABO groups and one antibody screen recorded in the hospital's laboratory information system. The recipient must not have had any transfusions subsequent to these tests being done.

PLATELET TRANSFUSIONS

CASE 177-2

THROMBOCYTOPENIA AND THE TRANSFUSION DECISION (PLATELETS)

A 31-year-old woman underwent consolidation chemotherapy for the treatment of acute myeloid leukemia (AML). The treatment has, predictably, caused a significant thrombocytopenia and her platelet count on this day was 4×10^9/L. She has noticed petechiae and purpura on her trunk and extremities and has also experienced spontaneous epistaxis that has been difficult to control with local measures.

This patient was transfused with one unit of apheresis platelets. Shortly after the transfusion her epistaxis stops. Later that evening she became febrile and the epistaxis resumed. She was again transfused with platelets. During the remainder of her hospital stay she was transfused one dose of platelets when her platelet count is less than 10×10^9.

In general, patients with low platelet counts or documented platelet function abnormalities who are bleeding are likely to benefit from platelet transfusions. However, while all causes of anemia may be treated with transfusion, not all causes of thrombocytopenia may be safely treated with the transfusion of platelet products. Thrombocytopenia caused by bone marrow failure, chemotherapy, bone marrow transplantation, or mechanical peripheral destruction (as occurs with use of cardiopulmonary bypass pumps) may be safely treated with platelet transfusions, whereas conditions associated with immune destruction of platelets (ex ITP or HIT) or microangiopathic hemolysis (ex TTP) can be dangerously aggravated by platelet transfusions.

PRACTICE POINT

- Just as symptomatic anemia is the key indication for RBC transfusions, so is symptomatic thrombocytopenia the main indication for platelet transfusions. However, there are notable exceptions. Conditions associated with immune destruction of platelets (ex ITP or HIT) or microangiopathic hemolysis (ex TTP) can be dangerously aggravated by platelet transfusions.

While decisions to transfuse platelets should always be made on an individual case-by-case basis, the transfusion threshold for platelet transfusions is generally well accepted. The majority of platelet transfusions currently are for the prophylactic treatment of chronic hypoprolifative thrombocytopenia. There is evidence from prospective randomized trials that withholding platelet transfusion until platelet counts drop below 10×10^9/L is a safe practice that enables a rational use of a very limited resource. A higher threshold of 20×10^9/L should be used in patients with additional bleeding risks such as sepsis. Patients requiring surgery or other invasive procedures who are also thrombocytopenic should be treated with prophylactic platelet transfusion. The final decision about what platelet count might be appropriate should be made in conjunction with the physician performing the procedures. Some general recommendations can be made, despite the lack of good evidence-based studies providing guidelines in such circumstances. A platelet count of greater than 100×10^9/L should probably be maintained for neurosurgical procedures and in patients who have suffered head trauma. For other types of procedures associated with an estimated blood loss of greater than 500 mL and those being performed under epidural anesthesia, platelets should be transfused to keep the count above 50×10^9/L. For those procedures associated with lower blood losses, a platelet count between $20–50 \times 10^9$/L should usually be sufficient.

The above recommendations are not the subject of much debate; however, questions remain about the dose of platelets that should be given, especially for those patients receiving prophylactic transfusions. A typical dose of platelets contains about 300×10^9 platelets. Studies looking at the safety and efficacy of lower doses versus these standard doses of platelet concentrates for transfusion have provided conflicting results. A recent large clinical study (PLADO) has provided evidence that a platelet dose as low as 110×10^9 is not different from a dose of 440×10^9 in bleeding risk. Until additional high level evidence becomes available, platelet transfusion doses such as those listed above should continue to be prescribed.

Multiple methods exist for the production of platelet products for transfusion. Two general preparation methods are the platelet rich plasma (PRP) method and the buffy coat method. In the PRP method, platelets are separated from a unit of whole blood and suspended in plasma from the same donor. One such platelet unit typically contains 55 × 10^9 platelets; and five units usually represent an average adult dose. The five units must be pooled in the blood bank just prior to being released for transfusion. In the buffy coat method, platelets from four donors are pooled by the blood collection agency and suspended in plasma from one of these donors. This prepooled unit constitutes one dose and usually contains at least 240 × 10^9 platelets. The buffy coat method is considered advantageous in that it decreases the number of donors to which the recipient is exposed, more plasma is made available for other uses, and since the units are pooled during production, there is no need to pool them in the hospital, thereby, they are available to leave the blood bank quicker.

Platelet concentrates are also prepared by an apheresis procedure that removes only platelets from the donor's circulation. Such a unit usually contains approximately 250 × 10^9 platelets and one unit constitutes one adult dose. While platelets prepared from any of these methods are safe for transfusion, there are some situations in which apheresis platelets may be particularly beneficial. In patients who are likely to be transfused multiple times, apheresis platelets may help reduce the risk of alloimmunization to platelet and WBC antigens by limiting the number of donors to which the recipient is exposed.

THE TRANSFUSION OF PLASMA PRODUCTS AND PLASMA DERIVATIVES

CASE 177-3

BLEEDING AND THE TRANSFUSION DECISION (PLASMA PRODUCTS)

A 67-year-old male with a history of atrial fibrillation had an INR of 5.4 due to coumadin prescribed for stroke prophylaxis. He had fallen and sustained some bruises and a scalp laceration that was bleeding profusely, but had no other serious injuries. The ER physician did not feel that he could stitch the laceration until the bleeding stopped. His CBC did not show evidence of anemia caused from his bleeding.

A dose of a prothrombin complex concentrate was given. One hour after its administration Mr. C's INR was found to be 1.4. Reversal of the anticoagulation in combination with local measures succeeded in decreasing the bleeding risk. The emergency physician successfully sutured the laceration and the patient was discharged home. Mr. C was advised to resume his anticoagulant medication the following day and attend a local laboratory for further monitoring of his INR.

The correction of coagulation abnormalities of differing etiologies may be accomplished through the use of plasma and plasma derivatives such as cryoprecipitate and prothrombin complex concentrates. However, not all patients with coagulation abnormalities require transfusion therapy. The 2008 American College of Chest Physicians clinical practice guidelines on the management of anticoagulation recommend using blood products to reverse the anticoagulant effect of oral vitamin K antagonists only if there is evidence of serious bleeding or when urgent surgery is needed. In such situations the use of fresh frozen plasma (FFP) or

TABLE 177-3 ABO Blood Group Compatibility for Plasma Transfusion

Recipient ABO Group	Safe Plasma Donor ABO Group
A	A, AB
B	B, AB
AB	AB
O	O, A, B, AB

prothrombin complex concentrates (PCCs) in combination with oral or intravenous vitamin K is suggested. Indeed, whatever the etiology of the coagulation abnormality, only if there is evidence of bleeding or the need for invasive procedures should plasma component or derivative therapy be used.

Immediately following collection, an average unit of FFP contains approximately one clotting factor unit/mL of all the coagulation factors. However, concentrations of the labile factors, V and VIII, decrease rapidly in unfrozen plasma. Consequently, plasma intended for transfusion must be frozen shortly after collection and maintained in a frozen state to ensure that there will be adequate levels of these clotting factors at the time of transfusion. To achieve a level of at least 30% of these clotting factors, a dose of 10–15 ml/kg of FFP is usually needed. The units selected for transfusion must be ABO compatible (see **Table 177-3**). While group O RBCs are safe for transfusion to patients of all ABO types, this is not the case for plasma. The universal plasma donor is group AB and this ABO type of plasma should be used for emergency transfusions when the recipient ABO group is not known.

Prothrombin complex concentrates (PCCs) contain the vitamin K dependent clotting factors II, VII, IX, and X at a concentration about 25 times that found in frozen plasma. Their main clinical indication is for patients requiring the reversal of the anticoagulant effect of coumadin. PCCs have several advantages over frozen plasma that make them well suited for this clinical indication. Up to two liters of plasma may be needed to bring the INR into the reference range in a patient who is excessively anticoagulated with coumadin. The usual therapeutic dose of a PCC is contained in one-quarter of that volume. This is especially relevant for patients who have poor left ventricular function or those who are receiving large volumes of other products. Additionally, this smaller volume can be infused much more quickly, allowing the desired outcome to be achieved faster, which is of key relevance in treating life-threatening bleeding. Another important advantage is that PCC products have all been treated with viral inactivation procedures during manufacturing. These processes, which include heat pasteurization and nanofiltration, cannot be performed on blood intended for transfusion as plasma. As a result of the viral inactivation procedures, the risk of viral transmission from these products is extremely low, though not nil. The use of pathogen-inactivated plasma is available in some European countries.

THE TRANSFUSION OF MULTIPLE BLOOD PRODUCTS

CASE 177-4

TRANSFUSION OF MULTIPLE BLOOD PRODUCTS

A 28-year-old female presented two days after a pregnancy termination with vaginal bleeding and a new purpuric rash. Her blood pressure was 80/60 mm Hg and her heart rate was 98 bpm. Blood work showed hemoglobin 11.0 g/dL (110 g/L), platelets

156 × 10^9/L, WBC 8.5 × 10^9/L, elevated INR and a PTT, and decreased plasma fibrinogen. Pelvic ultrasound showed retained products of conception and a diagnosis of disseminated intravascular coagulation was made.

This patient received volume resuscitation with normal saline and transfusion of one dose of cryoprecipitate. She appeared clinically unwell and repeat blood work showed that her hemoglobin has now fallen to 7.7 g/dL (77 g/L) and her platelets to 80 × 10^9/L. En route to the OR for evacuation of retained products of conception she was transfused one unit of RBCs and one dose of platelets. The procedure was successful and shortly thereafter the bleeding stopped. Blood work the following morning showed correction of the INR and aPTT; the hemoglobin level was 8.0 g/dL (80 g/L) and the platelet count was up to 150 × 10^9/L. She was discharged home with a prescription for oral iron supplementation and a follow-up appointment with her gynecologist.

Cryoprecipitate is made when FFP is thawed at between 1–6°C, centrifuged, and refrozen. Each unit of cryoprecipitate typically contains 80–100 clotting units of factor VIII, 150–250 mg of fibrinogen, as well as von Willebrand factor and factor XIII. The usual dose of one unit per 10 kg of body weight will increase the fibrinogen level by about 0.5 g/L. The major reason cryoprecipitate is transfused is to increase the fibrinogen concentration in bleeding patients with a fibrinogen concentration of less than 1 g/L. Though congenital causes of hypofibrinogenemia do exist, the etiology most frequently seen in hospitals will be acquired hypofibrinogenemia due to DIC or fibrinolysis. Though cryoprecipitate may be given empirically in cases of massive transfusion or uncontrolled bleeding it is recommended that the fibrinogen level be documented before administering this product. The goal of therapy with cryoprecipitate transfusion should be to increase the fibrinogen level to greater than 1 g/L. It is important to recognize that transfusion of cryoprecipitate will only temporarily increase the fibrinogen level if the causative pathologic process is ongoing. Efforts thus should be directed to correcting the underlying condition.

■ MULTIPLE PRODUCTS (MASSIVE TRANSFUSIONS)

CASE 177-5

SEVERE TRAUMA AND THE MASSIVE TRANSFUSION PROTOCOL (MTP)

An unidentified male, age approximately 25 years, who has been hit by a car. Upon arrival to the emergency department he was unconscious and hypotensive. Initial assessment revealed multiple injuries including an open book fracture of the pelvis. Urgent resuscitative efforts began with administration of fluids and RBCs.

Further evaluation of the patient revealed a great deal of internal bleeding whose source cannot be determined. Plans were made to take the patient to OR for a laparotomy to investigate, and hopefully treat, the source of bleeding. As per the hospital massive transfusion protocol (MTP), once six units of RBCs have been transfused FFP and platelets should be given. Cryoprecipitate was also administered when a low fibrinogen was reported. Additional blood products continued to be transfused as per the MTP. In the OR, the trauma surgeon reported ongoing excessive bleeding and that he cannot visualize the source. He requested recombinant activated human factor VII (rhFVIIa) from the blood bank.

Traumatic injury is an important cause of death in adults in developed countries. Early trauma-related mortality is most frequently due to head injury or hemorrhage; later mortality is usually due to multiorgan failure. Severe hemorrhage in traumatic injuries, as well as in other settings such as operative misadventure, variceal bleeding, and obstetrical complications, requires urgent transfusion therapy, often with multiple doses of different blood products. Transfusion of more than 10 units of RBCs within a 24-hour period is referred to as massive transfusion. Such situations of large volume transfusions present a challenge to the blood bank as well as to the health care workers performing the resuscitation.

Acutely injured patients often require transfusion faster than grouping and screening can be performed. In such settings it is recommended that uncrossmatched, group O RBCs (UORBC) be given. Though such cells may be safely given to patients of any ABO blood type, there remain risks for complications related to the mismatching of other blood groups. A 2005 study assessed blood bank and trauma registries for an entire year to assess the incidence of complications related to the transfusion of UORBC. The authors found that this approach enabled rapid resuscitation and was not associated with increased risk of serological transfusion complications. Specifically, the study found that the rate of development of Rh(D) alloantibodies was lower than would be predicted for the general population. This may be due to the relatively immune suppressed status of critically ill patients.

While transfusion can be a life-saving therapy in hemorrhaging patients, the need for massive transfusion portends a high rate of mortality and is associated with multiple complications. Additionally, it has been identified as an independent risk for later development of multiorgan failure. Coagulopathy is an important complication of massive transfusion, which develops in more than half of the patients who are massively transfused. Both elevations in INR and aPTT as well as thrombocytopenia can develop. This occurs as a result of both dilution and the consumption of some of the coagulation factors. Hypothermia and acidosis are also important contributing factors. In some massive transfusion cases DIC may also be present, which renders the patient even more coagulopathic. The hypothermia that contributes to coagulopathy may be caused by infusion of cold fluids and blood products during volume resuscitation. Use of a blood warmer is a critical step in preventing this complication. Hypothermia can also lead to cardiac arrhythmias and hypotension.

Citrate is used as an anticoagulant in the blood products used for transfusion. Normally it is a completely safe additive because it is rapidly metabolized by the liver. In the event of a massive transfusion, the liver's ability to metabolize citrate can be exceeded and citrate toxicity will develop. Presence of excessive amounts of citrate can lead to hypocalcemia, hypomagnesemia, and metabolic alkalosis with all of their attendant signs and symptoms. The hypocalcemia should be promptly treated with intravenous calcium. Hyperkalemia is another important metabolic complication of massive transfusion. RBCs release potassium during storage and transfusion of large amounts of stored RBCs can introduce significant amounts of potassium into the circulation. This will be exacerbated if there is presence of acidosis or renal failure and should be treated as for hyperkalemia due to any other cause (**Table 177-4**).

When massive transfusion occurs it is always in the setting of a complicated clinical case and the very time-sensitive resuscitative effort. It is easy to imagine how errors can occur in such settings, especially when multiple departments of the hospital, such as the patient care area, the hematology laboratory, and the blood bank, need to work together under stressful circumstances. MTP are algorithms often created by a hospital's transfusion committee that aim to enable this type of coordinated effort. Such protocols typically have several components—a procedure for initial resuscitation with

TABLE 177-4 Complications of Massive Transfusion

Complication	Signs and Symptoms	Prevention and Management
Hypothermia caused by transfusion	• Reduced platelet and coagulation factor function • Decreased citrate metabolism • Increased stored RBC hemoglobin oxygen affinity and consequent decreased oxygen delivery to tissues • Decreased myocardial function	• Use of blood warming devices • Use of other measures to warm patient
Coagulaopathy	• Greater than expected blood loss • ↑ INR and aPTT • Thrombocytopenia	• Transfusion of platelets, FFP, and cryoprecipitate
Hypocalcemia due to citrate toxicity	• Tetany • Cardiac arrhythmias	• Monitoring of serum calcium • IV calcium therapy
Hyperkalemia due to potassium leakage from stored RBCs	• Cardiac arrhythmias	• Monitor serum potassium • Treat hyperkalemia as needed

crystalloids and RBCs, a procedure for the transfusion of appropriate products while hemorrhage is ongoing, and a procedure for laboratory monitoring.

While the goals and general structure of MTPs are similar, there is no consensus on optimal laboratory monitoring or the best schedule for blood product administration. Additionally, there is more than one type of approach that can be dictated by the MTP. Some protocols begin with a RBC and crystalloid resuscitation phase, which is followed by additional components such as platelets and FFP depending on the patient's laboratory values. Such an approach allows the rational use of blood products and may minimize wastage. However, to be successful it requires timely availability of laboratory values to guide therapy. This approach has been criticized as some physicians feel that conventional laboratory tests are not necessarily reflective of in vivo coagulation. An alternative approach is to administer predetermined blood product packages that are delivered consecutively until resuscitation is complete or the patient expires. It is thought that such an approach might help to prevent the coagulopathy of massive transfusion by providing plasma products earlier in the resuscitation. Additionally, such transfusion packages may prevent the delays associated with the ordering, preparing, and the issuing of blood products (**Table 177-5**).

OTHER CLOTTING FACTOR CONCENTRATES AND RHFVIIA

In the cascade model of coagulation, when tissue factor (TF) is exposed at the site of vessel injury, activated factor VII binds to the exposed TF. This TF-VIIa complex triggers the extrinsic pathway leading to the generation of thrombin and subsequent platelet activation and formation of a fibrin clot. When given in pharmacologic doses that far exceed the amount of circulating activated factor VII in vivo, rhFVIIa will also bind to activated platelets and directly activate factor X. The rhFVIIa was initially developed for the treatment of patients with hemophilia and inhibitors to factor VIII or IX. In that clinical setting there is abundant evidence of rhFVIIa's efficacy and safety and the treatment of hemophilia with inhibitors and acquired antibodies to FVIII remain the sole licensed indications for its use in Canada, the U.S., and many other countries. Given its potential as procoagulant therapy for serious bleeding in various settings, there have been many investigations of its use for indications not approved by regulatory authorities, or "off-label" uses.

Some of the settings in which the use of rhFVIIa has been assessed include variceal bleeding in cirrhotic patients, traumatic injury, intracranial hemorrhage, and cardiac surgery. These studies have failed to show a clinically relevant difference in outcome for patients treated with rhFVIIa compared to the placebo-treated

TABLE 177-5 Features of Massive Transfusion Protocols

Component of MTP	To be Included	Desired Outcome
Multidisciplinary communication	• Early notification of transfusion service • Concise and effective communication between clinical area and blood bank	• Enables rapid issue of blood products • Allows blood bank to assess inventory and order additional products if needed
Laboratory	• Adequate laboratory support to ensure rapid, repeated, evaluation of hemoglobin, platelet count, INR, aPTT, fibrinogen, calcium, pH, electrolytes, and renal function	• Ability to monitor outcomes of resuscitative efforts and direct rational use of additional blood products
Quality improvement	• Quality indicators to be assessed at predetermined intervals • Examples: Blood product turnaround time, laboratory value turnaround time, blood product wastage, adverse events related to transfusion, mortality	• Enable ongoing quality improvement to ensure MTP is meeting goals of improving patient outcomes in massive transfusion

groups. However, these studies have revealed that use of rhFVIIa may be associated with serious adverse outcomes related to thrombosis. A review of the American Food and Drug Agency's Adverse Event Reporting System (AERS) from March 1999 to December 2004 identified 185 thromboembolic complications related to use of rhFVIIa; 151 of these occurred in patients in whom the drug was used for unlabeled indication; 54.1% of the events were arterial thromboses; 40.4% were venous; and 5.5% were cases of device occlusions. Fifty of the adverse events were fatal and the deaths were deemed to be due to thromboembolic causes in 36 (72%) of the cases.

Given the lack of evidence for efficacy of rhFVIIa and the abundant evidence of harm, at this time the use of rhFVIIa in patients who do not have hemophilia should be considered experimental and should only be used in the context of a properly designed clinical trial.

COMPLICATIONS OF TRANSFUSION

Transfusion therapy can be life-saving in some circumstances. However, it is not a benign intervention. There are many known adverse events associated with blood product transfusions, which can range from mild to life-threatening. These adverse events can occur immediately during a transfusion or may not be recognized for days, weeks, months, or years. Adverse outcomes of transfusion related to viral diseases have been the subject of much media attention in recent decades and are often the cause of great concern for clinicians and patients. However, today, these are among the least frequently encountered complications of transfusion. Certainly, hospital-based practitioners must be aware of the risk of transmission of viral infections through blood transfusion in order to give the patients all the information needed to gain informed consent. However, it is the nonviral adverse events associated with transfusions that currently represent the more common serious risks of transfusion. It is incumbent upon the hospitalist physician to know how to recognize and manage such reactions.

PRACTICE POINT

- Informed consent requires that clinicians inform patients of infectious and other potential complications of transfusion. It is the nonviral adverse events associated with transfusions that currently represent the more common serious risks of transfusion.

It cannot be sufficiently stressed that the best way to prevent transfusion-associated adverse events is to avoid transfusions as much as possible. Though transfusion safety has increased in recent decades, transfusion is not a benign therapy. Each order for transfusion should be carefully considered to ensure that the anticipated benefits of treatment are likely to outweigh potential adverse events.

FEVER

CASE 177-2 (continued)

The patient is admitted for another cycle of chemotherapy. Again she became thrombocytopenic and required further platelet transfusions. During such a transfusion her temperature rose from 36.8°C to 38.3°C.

Approximately 1 in 300 transfusions will be complicated by fever. Febrile transfusion reactions are defined as a greater than 1°C rise in temperature or a temperature of greater than 38°C during, or within four hours after the end of a transfusion. Such reactions may have several etiologies but the initial management of all febrile reactions is similar. Once fever is detected the transfusion should be stopped while IV access is maintained with normal saline. The other vital signs must be checked and recorded. Identification of the patient should be rechecked against the identification of the blood product to ensure that there has not been erroneous transfusion of the wrong blood to the patient. Additional measures may be necessary, depending on the presence of additional symptoms and the suspected etiology of the fever. It is important to remember that in sick, hospitalized patients etiologies outside of those related to transfusion should be considered when trying to determine the cause of the fever.

One possible cause of a febrile transfusion reaction is bacterial sepsis due to bacterial contamination of the blood product. Since platelet components are stored at room temperature they provide favorable conditions for bacterial growth and are the blood product most frequently involved in transfusion-associated sepsis. However, all types of blood products have been implicated. Most regulatory agencies now require blood collection agencies to perform bacterial testing on all platelet units and there is evidence that this practice significantly decreases the rate of transfusion associated sepsis, but this risk remains a concern associated particularly with platelet transfusions.

Contamination of the blood product from skin bacteria on the donor may occur at the time of donation. Such contamination is minimized by the careful cleansing of the venipuncture site and also diverting the first aliquot of blood collected. Bacteremia in the donor can also result in bacterial contamination. Predonation screening is the most important step in reducing this risk. Contamination rarely also occurs during the processing and handling of blood products.

The range of symptoms reported to accompany fever in transfusion-associated sepsis is quite variable and depends on the patient's underlying medical condition, the type of bacteria, and the bacterial load present in the unit. Most patients only experience fever and chills with no other symptoms or clinical sequelae. However, more severe symptoms and serious outcomes, including death, have been reported. In both the U.S. and the U.K., transfusion-associated sepsis is reported to be the third leading cause of transfusion-associated mortality. The most severe tend to occur with Gram-negative bacteria because of endotoxin production. Some implicated Gram-negative bacteria include *Klebsiella pneumonia*, *Serratia marcenscens*, and *Yersinia enterocolitica*. *Yersinia* infections may complicate RBC transfusions as the bacteria are capable of growing at the cold temperatures at which RBCs are stored. When contamination is with Gram-positive bacteria, the bacteria are usually *Staphylococcus* species from the donor's skin.

Transfusion-associated bacterial sepsis should be suspected if the fever is accompanied by tachycardia, hypotension, dyspnea, nausea, or vomiting or clinical symptoms of DIC. If this diagnosis is suspected the transfusion should not be restarted. The remainder of the offending unit and the tubing should be returned to the blood bank for additional testing including culture. Additional blood samples should be drawn from the patient for culture, CBC, and routine chemistry. These should come from a venipuncture site distant from the transfusion infusion site. Antimicrobial therapy should be started immediately with a broad spectrum antibiotic and the patient should be monitored in the appropriate clinical setting, such as an intensive care unit.

Acute hemolytic transfusion reactions (AHTRs) are another important cause of fever and serious symptoms during transfusion.

AHTRs occur due to the presence, in the recipient's circulation, of preformed antibody directed against an antigen present on the donor's RBCs. The antibody reacts with the antigen on the transfused RBCs, which leads to complement activation and intravascular hemolysis. The massive hemolysis can lead to a cytokine storm that can activate the coagulation system and result in DIC. The additional signs and symptoms of AHTR include hemoglobinuria, hypotension and possible shock, flank pain, pain at the site of the infusion, chest tightness, vomiting, diarrhea, and symptoms of DIC such as oozing at IV sites. The combination of the circulatory changes that can lead to decreased renal blood flow and the nephrotoxic properties of the products of RBC hemolysis can result in acute renal failure, which is not always reversible. AHTRs can also lead to a fatal outcome. The severity of the symptoms and outcomes usually correlates with the amount of incompatible blood transfused. Most fatal AHTRs have occurred after transfusions of more than 200 mL of incompatible blood.

If an AHTR is suspected the transfusion should be stopped and not restarted. However, it is imperative to ensure that IV access is maintained and sufficient fluids infused to ensure good urine output. This may require high infusion rates in excess of 500 mL per hour. The patient identification should be rechecked against the product identity and the remaining product should be returned to the blood bank. A patient sample should also be sent to the blood bank for ABO group retesting. Additional samples should be drawn to check CBC, INR, aPTT, fibrinogen, electrolytes, BUN, creatinine, bilirubin, LDH, and haptoglobin. Additional supportive care may be necessary and patient transfer to a monitored setting, such as the ICU, is usually warranted.

The antigens most frequently implicated in AHTRs are those of the ABO blood group. ABO incompatible transfusions usually occur as the result of human error leading to incorrect blood component transfusion. How to improve systems for checking patient and blood product identity is the subject of ongoing research and new technologies are becoming more readily available. Surveillance of processes surrounding blood issuing and transfusion should be part of quality assurance initiatives of every hospital's transfusion medicine service.

The third potential etiology of fever during transfusion is what is called a febrile nonhemolytic transfusion reaction (FNHTR). Such reactions are mainly caused by cytokines that have accumulated in the transfused product. The incidence of these reactions is highest with platelet transfusions, but can occur with the transfusion of any cellular blood component. The symptoms of FNHTRs are usually limited to only fever and chills. These reactions may be treated with antipyretic medication such as acetaminophen. If severe rigors are present, meperidine at a dose of 25–50 mg IV may be effective. If the cause of fever during transfusion is deemed to be FNHTR and the symptoms are not too severe, the transfusion may be restarted.

CASE 177-2 (continued)

The patient's transfusion was stopped and normal saline infused to keep the IV line open. The blood product identification was checked against the patient's wristband. There was no evidence that she received the incorrect blood product. Her blood pressure, heart rate, respiratory rate, and oxygen saturation were found to be normal. She admitted to some chills but no other symptoms. The attending physician felt that the fever likely represented a febrile nonhemolytic transfusion reaction, ordered acetaminophen for the patient, and administered the rest of the unit of platelets. The remainder of the transfusion was uneventful.

SHORTNESS OF BREATH

CASE 177-1 (continued)

Postoperatively this patient's hemoglobin was 8.1 g/dL (81 g/L) and he developed symptoms associated with his anemia: chest pain and shortness of breath. A transfusion of RBCs was ordered. After the infusion of the RBC unit Mr. B complained of increasing shortness of breath.

The sensation of shortness of breath is a common complaint among hospitalized patients and there are many possible etiologies that could be related to the patient's underlying disease, complications of hospitalization such as hospital-acquired-pneumonia, pulmonary embolus, or complications of therapy. When dyspnea is reported during or shortly after a transfusion a complication of the transfusion therapy should always be considered as a possible cause. The adverse events that should be considered include transfusion-related acute lung injury (TRALI), transfusion-associated circulatory overload (TACO), and anaphylaxis.

When a patient complains of shortness of breath around the time of a transfusion the infusion should be stopped and IV access maintained. The patient's vital signs should be evaluated and monitored and a cardiac and respiratory exam should be performed. Concurrently, the identification of the blood product and the patient should be rechecked. The remainder of the unit and attached tubing should be returned to the blood bank for investigation. There are no circumstances in which the transfusion may safely be restarted. A stat chest X-ray should be ordered. Appropriate therapies such as supplemental oxygen or diuresis should be provided and the patient should be moved to a monitored setting if clinically necessary. Additional investigations or therapies may be warranted based on the diagnosis suspected.

Transfusion related acute lung injury (TRALI) is an important, serious adverse event of blood transfusion whose diagnosis can often be complicated. Acute lung injury (ALI) is an entity defined by the acute onset of hypoxemia with presence of bilateral lung infiltrates on CXR and no evidence of circulatory overload. Risk factors for ALI include direct and indirect lung injuries. Direct injuries include aspiration, toxic inhalation, pneumonia, and drowning. Causes of indirect lung injury include sepsis, shock, trauma, burns, pancreatitis, cardio-pulmonary bypass, and drug overdose. TRALI should be suspected when new ALI symptoms occur during or within six hours after completion of a transfusion and no other risk factors for ALI are present. TRALI may still be possible if other risk factors for ALI are present and it should be included in the differential diagnosis (**Table 177-6**).

Two mechanisms for the etiology of TRALI have been proposed. The first theory proposes that donor antibodies against HLA or neutrophils present in the blood product bind to neutrophils in the recipient's pulmonary endothelium, which leads to release of toxic biologic response modifiers that result in pulmonary capillary leak. The second proposed mechanism is that biologically active lipids in the transfused blood cause the pulmonary complications. TRALI has been reported following the transfusion of all types of blood products, but the majority of reported cases have been associated with transfusion of plasma-containing products collected from multiparous women who have developed antineutrophil antibodies during pregnancy. When TRALI is suspected the hospital blood bank should be notified so that additional studies can be ordered to look for such antibodies in the donor. If the antibodies are found, the donor should be permanently deferred from donating blood in an effort to prevent similar adverse events in other recipients. As part of this effort to reduce the incidence of TRALI, some blood collection

TABLE 177-6 TRALI Diagnosis Checklist

Is ALI present?

All four criteria must be met:

- Acute onset of signs and symptoms
- Hypoxemia present
  - $PaO_2/FiOs < 300$ mm Hg or $SaO_2 < 90\%$ on room air
- Bilateral lung infiltrates seen on chest X-ray
- No evidence of circulatory overload

Is TRALI definitely present?

All three criteria must be met:

- No ALI present prior to transfusion
- Evidence of ALI apparent during, or within six hours of completion of transfusion
- No other risk factors for ALI present

Is TRALI possibly present?

- New ALI is present and has occurred during or within six hours of transfusion
- Other risk factors for ALI are present

agencies have stopped using blood from female donors for the manufacture of plasma-containing products.

All patients with TRALI require treatment with supplemental oxygen and more than half will also need mechanical ventilation. Such supportive measures are usually the only therapy that is indicated as the syndrome usually resolves within a few days of the transfusion. However, TRALI can be a fatal complication of transfusion with a fatality rate reported to be between 5–10%.

TRALI should always be differentiated from transfusion-associated circulatory overload (TACO), which is a frequent complication of transfusion. Patients with a compromised cardiopulmonary system and those with renal failure are at highest risk for TACO. Symptoms other than dyspnea include cough, tachycardia, elevated blood pressure, and widened pulse pressure. Elevations in the jugular venous pressure may also be seen. The chest X-ray findings are as for pulmonary overload from any other cause. Diuretic drugs represent the cornerstone of therapy and subsequent transfusions should be given at reduced infusion rates if possible. Although TACO can readily be recognized and treated, fatalities have been reported. Accurate diagnosis and rapid treatment are the keys to preventing such outcomes.

The final cause of transfusion-induced shortness of breath is anaphylaxis, which is a rare complication of transfusion but an extremely serious one. Symptoms of anaphylactic transfusion reactions include dyspnea, hypotension, bronchospasm, and stridor as well as gastrointestinal symptoms. The transfusion must not be restarted if anaphylaxis is suspected. Treatment with epinephrine, corticosteroids, and supportive care including intubation if needed, should be administered immediately. Any clinical area in which transfusions are given should have the necessary drugs and instruments to perform such resuscitation.

The most important risk factor for the development of transfusion-related anaphylaxis is IgA deficiency with anti-IgA antibodies. Patients who experience anaphylaxis during transfusion should be tested for the presence of these conditions. If a patient is found to have anti-IgA antibodies he or she should be made aware of this fact and informed to alert his or her physician should he or she require transfusion in the future. The patient may consider wearing a medic-alert bracelet as well. The local blood bank should ensure that the condition is noted in the patient's file and that only washed RBCs or plasma products from IgA deficient donors be used in future transfusions.

CASE 177-1 *(continued)*

This patient's vital signs revealed him to be tachycardic and hypoxic. Supplemental oxygen was started. The attending physician's differential diagnosis was TRALI or TACO. The chest X-ray showed bilateral pulmonary infiltrates, which could be consistent with either diagnosis. However, careful physical exam showed signs of congestive heart failure with an elevated JVP and a widened pulse pressure. A dose of furosemide achieved a good diuresis with prompt resolution of symptoms and radiologic findings.

URTICARIA

CASE 177-5 *(continued)*

The young victim of a hit-and-run accident survived his surgery and was transferred to the intensive care unit in critical condition. His INR and aPTT were somewhat elevated because of DIC, and a dose of FFP was ordered to correct the coagulopathy before inserting an additional central line. During the infusion of FFP he develops urticaria on his face and trunk.

Mild allergic reactions are relatively common complications of transfusion, occurring in approximately 1 in 100 transfusions of plasma-containing products. Such reactions may be very mild with only a handful of urticarial lesions and range to more severe reactions with most of the body surface covered in urticaria. Associated symptoms can include pruritus, nausea, vomiting, diarrhea as well as some wheezing and coughing. The exact etiology is not known but urticarial reactions are thought to be caused by soluble antigens in the donor blood to which the recipient has previously been sensitized.

When an allergic reaction occurs during a transfusion the infusion should be stopped immediately. The patient's vital signs should be checked and the patient should be examined to determine the extent of the urticarial rash. The patient should be questioned about the presence of any accompanying symptoms. If the rash is on less than two-thirds of the body surface and there are no other symptoms present the reaction would be classified as a minor allergic reaction. Diphenhydramine can be given orally or by IV to relieve symptoms and the transfusion may be restarted while the patient is carefully observed. If additional symptoms develop or the urticaria worsens, the transfusion should be permanently discontinued.

When a more severe allergic reaction is present the transfusion should not be restarted. Such a patient should be carefully monitored to assess for the presence or development of anaphylactic symptoms. Anaphylaxis should be treated with epinephrine and steroids as well as supportive care including possible intubation. Other severe allergic reactions may not require epinephrine treatment but may need treatment with corticosteroids and diphenhydramine. Patients having these types of reactions should be monitored carefully and not discharged or moved to an unmonitored setting until symptoms have resolved.

The blood bank should be notified of the reaction and investigations of the patient for possible IgA deficiency should be undertaken.

Some patients experience recurrent urticarial reactions with transfusion. Such patients often benefit from premedication with diphenhydramine or steroids for subsequent transfusions. An alternative measure to help prevent recurrent reactions is to provide plasma depleted or washed platelet and RBC units. The precise efficacy of these measures is not known. Routine premedication

TABLE 177-7 Transfusion Triggers and Risks of Transfusion

RBC criteria for transfusion	**RBC risks per unit (all blood products)**
Indication: to improve oxygen delivery Shelf life: 42 days from donor collection Each RBC unit: 250–300 ml containing 55–80% RBC Transfuse an otherwise young healthy person with Hg 6 g/dl and no transfusion is required for any patient with Hg > 10 g/dL (100 g/L) (American Society of Anesthesiologists) Preoperative patients with expected blood loss, pregnant patients, and oncology/BMT patients may require an individualized approach to maintain a Hg between 8 g/dL (80 g/L) and 9 g/dL (90 g/L). In patients with myocardial ischemia the liberal trigger may be preferred Restrictive trigger for transfusion (Hg > 7 g/dL – 70 g/L) versus liberal trigger (10 g/dL – 100 g/L) showed better outcomes in the restrictive group (Canadian Critical Care Trials Group)	Infections directly traceable to donor have been dramatically reduced due to donor restrictions and increased surveillance: HIV (1:2,000,000), hepatitis C (1:2,000,000), hepatitis B (1:200,000), West Nile Virus (approaching 0) Infectious agents not yet screened for: Bacteria, viruses, parasites Yersinia enterocolitica (1 in 65,000) variant Creutzfeld-Jakob disease Clerical error (1 in 12,000) Close temporal relation to transfusion: hemolytic reactions due to ABO blood type incompatibility, febrile nonhemolytic and allergic reactions (1:100), acute lung injury (1 in 5000), volume overload (1:400), metabolic derangements Immunologic alloimmunization, graft versus host
Platelets criteria for transfusion	**Platelet risks**
Indication: to prevent or reduce bleeding due to thrombocytopenia or platelet dysfunction Shelf life: limited to five to seven days Except for oncology patients undergoing chemotherapy that suppresses the bone marrow, there are no consensus guidelines so the following statements reflect common practice: Nonbleeding patients without risk factors (sepsis, fever, DIC): withhold transfusion until platelet count falls to 5–10 x 10^3/mm^3 (5–10 x 10^9/L) Nonbleeding patients with risk factors: withhold transfusion until platelet count falls to 20 × 10^3/ mm^3 Uncomplicated surgery: 50 × 10^3/ mm^3 (50 × 10^9/L) There is insufficient data to guide recommendations for patients with platelet counts between 50 100 × 10^3/mm^3 (50–100 × 10^9/L) or at risk for bleeding.	Risks of RBC and plasma products Bacterial contamination (1 unit in every 2000–3000 units) Febrile reactions Venous thromboembolism Alloimmunization
Fresh frozen plasma (FFP) criteria	**FFP risks**
Replacement of single clotting factor when individual factors unavailable Reversal of warfarin (active bleeding or prior to invasive procedure, target INR 1.5) Thrombotic thrombocytopenic purpura (TTP), DIC Hemorrhagic disease of the newborn	With the exception of bacterial contamination, similar to platelet transfusions
Cryoprecipitate criteria (limited data)	**Cryoprecipitate risks**
Each unit: plasma enriched with Factor VIII, vWF, Factor XIII, fibronectin, and fibrinogen Normal but dysfunctional fibrinogen levels or fibrinogen levels < 100 mg/dL (1g/L) Bleeding due to congenital Factor XIII deficiency von Willebrand disease who require vWF replacement	Viral transmission multiple FFP (due to collection from multiple units of FFP)
Prothrombin complex concentrates	**Prothrombin complex concentrates risks**
Each unit: Pooled plasma from multiple donors, major component Factor IX Possibly a better option than FFP and Vitamin K to reverse warfarin-related bleeding, including intracerebral hemorrhage Avoid in patients with liver disease	Infection Allergic reactions Hemolysis Fluid overload Thrombosis
Albumin	**Albumin risks**
Use for volume expansion controversial	Similar to pooled plasma

Data from Shander A, Goodnough LT. Update on Transfusion Medicine. *Pharmacotherapy*. 2007;27:57S–68S.

for all patients to help prevent allergic transfusion reactions is not a practice supported by available evidence and exposes patients to undue risks of the medications. Hence, this practice should be discouraged.

CASE 177-5 (continued)

The transfusion was stopped and 25 mg IV diphenhydramine was given. Since the patient was intubated and in a monitored setting and the procedure was deemed important, the decision was made to continue with the transfusion. The urticaria resolved and no further complications were seen.

HYPOTENSION

CASE 177-3 (continued)

Several weeks after this patient's scalp laceration was sutured, he was again seen in the ED with injuries related to a fall. He has multiple bruises and a large hematoma on his knee. His INR was 2.0 and a CBC showed his hemoglobin to be 79 g/L. The emergency physician decided to transfuse one unit of RBCs. Shortly after the transfusion was given, his blood pressure dropped to 80/60 mm Hg.

Hypotensive transfusion reactions are defined as a more than 30 mm Hg drop in systolic or diastolic blood pressure during a transfusion. A drop in blood pressure can be seen in association with multiple transfusion reactions such as sepsis, acute hemolytic transfusion reactions, TRALI, and serious allergic reactions. When hypotensive transfusion reactions occur separate from these other syndromes they are usually mediated by bradykinins present in the transfused product. Angiotensin-converting enzyme (ACE) is the key mediator of bradykinin degradation in vivo, and the most frequent etiology of bradykinin-mediated hypotensive transfusion reactions is therapy with ACE-inhibitor drugs that prevent their breakdown. Other rare individuals have a genetic polymorphism that results in decreased bradykinin degradation.

When a hypotensive transfusion reaction occurs, the transfusion should be discontinued and not restarted. Supportive care, including fluids and vassopressor medications may be warranted. A careful examination and investigation for other transfusion reactions associated with hypotension should be undertaken. This should include the monitoring of other vital signs, blood bank investigations to rule out hemolytic transfusion reaction, and possibly CXR to rule out TRALI. If it is determined that ACE-inhibitor therapy is implicated in the reaction the patient should be placed on an alternative medications prior to future transfusions if possible.

CASE 177-3 (continued)

This patient's transfusion was stopped and he was placed in the reverse Trendelenberg position and an infusion of IV normal saline started. Within the hour his blood pressure stabilized and no other symptoms were observed. A careful drug history revealed that he takes an ACE-inhibitor for treatment of his hypertension. Review of the patient's medical history noted that he suffers from chronic anemia believed to be the anemia of chronic disease. His hemoglobin level is normally in the range of 8 g/dL (80 g/L) and he tolerates this reasonably well. Had this been determined earlier, this RBC transfusion and the transfusion reaction may have been avoided.

CONCLUSION

Transfusion of allogeneic blood products is an important part of modern medical care. There are well-recognized indications for transfusion of a variety of cellular blood components as well as plasma and its derivatives. It is incumbent upon the physician to be aware of these indications in order to ensure that patients who would benefit from transfusion receive this therapy that can be life-saving. However, it is of equal importance that physicians recognize the risks of transfusion and carefully weigh these risks against perceived possible benefits of every single transfusion ordered. Additionally, physicians must be aware of how to manage any untoward outcomes of transfusion from those that are mild irritants to those that are life-threatening. Utilization of interventions to minimize the need for transfusion is another important way medical staff can ensure rational use of a scarce resource and reduce patients' exposures to the risks of transfusion therapy (**Table 177-7**).

SUGGESTED READINGS

Key trials and editorials in transfusion medicine:

Birchall J, Stanworth SJ, Duffy MR, et al. Evidence for the use of recombinant Factor VIIa in the prevention and treatment of bleeding in patients without hemophilia. *Transf Med Rev. 2008*;22: 177–187.

Blajchman MA, Vamvakas EC. The continuing risk of Transfusion-Transmitted Infections. *N Engl J Med.* 2006;355:1303–1305.

CRASH-2 trial collaborators. Effects of tranexamic acid on death, vascular occlusive events, and blood transfusion in trauma patients with significant haemorrhage (CRASH-2): a randomized, placebo-controlled trial. *Lancet.* 2010;376:23–32.

Fergusson DA, Hebert PC, Mazer D, et al. A comparison of aprotinin and lysine analogues in high-risk cardiac surgery. *N Eng J Med.* 2008;358:2319–2331.

Goldman M, Webert KE, Arnold DM, et al. Proceedings of a consensus conference: towards an understanding of TRALI. *Transf Med Rev.* 2005;19:2–31.

Hebert PC, Wells G, Blajchman MA, et al. A multicentre, randomized, controlled clinical trial of transfusion requirements in critical care. *N Eng J Med.* 1999;340:409–417.

Levi M, Levy JH, Anderson HF, Truloff D. Safety of recombinant activated Factor VII in randomized clinical trials. *N Eng J Med.* 2010;363:1791–1800.

O'Connell KA, Wood JJ, Wise RP, et al. Thromboembolic adverse events after use of recombinant human coagulation Factor VIIa. *JAMA.* 2006;295:293–298.

Slichter SJ, Kaufman RM, Assmann SF, et al. Dose of prophylactic platelet transfusions and prevention of hemorrhage. *N Eng J Med.* 2010;362:600–613.

Vamvakas EC, Blajchman MA. Transfusion-related mortality: the ongoing risks of allogeneic blood transfusion and the available strategies for their prevention. *Blood.* 2009;113:3406–3417.

Useful review articles:

Key NS, Negrier C. Coagulation factor concentrates: past, present and future. *Lancet.* 2007;370:439–448.

Klein HG, Spahn DR, Carson JL. Red blood cell transfusion in clinical practice. *Lancet.* 2007;370:415–426.

Stroncek DF, Rebulla P. Platelet transfusions. *Lancet.* 2007;370: 427–438.

CHAPTER 178

Hypercoagulable States

Sam Schulman, MD, PhD
Karina Meijer, MD, PhD

Key Clinical Questions

1. Which hospitalized patients are at risk for venous thromboembolism?
2. Who is at increased risk for complications from thromboprophylaxis?
3. How do you make sure that thromboprophylaxis is prescribed to all patients who should get it?

INTRODUCTION

Many patients have an increased baseline propensity for thrombosis due to underlying hypercoagulable states, the majority of which are acquired. An acute insult may then result in hospitalization, which usually further increases the risk due to immobilization, procedures including central venous catheter placement or pacemaker, and/or administration of certain drugs. The main question in most patient groups detailed below is whether they can expect a net benefit from pharmacologic thromboprophylaxis, mainly low-molecular-weight heparins (LMWHs). Ideally, one has to balance the risk and consequences of venous thromboembolism (VTE) with the risk of bleeding and other complications of anticoagulants in every patient, while also taking the values and preferences of that patient into consideration. To facilitate this balancing process, institutions and national and international organizations have developed guidelines for the use of thromboprophylaxis. The use of these guidelines and local protocols has greatly improved patient outcomes, mainly by increasing the use of pharmacologic thromboprophylaxis in patients at risk for VTE. The authors strongly advise the development and implementation of a local protocol.

THROMBOPHILIA AND VENOUS THROMBOEMBOLISM

DEFICIENCIES OF NATURAL INHIBITORS OF COAGULATION

Less than 1% of the general population has a congenital deficiency of one of the natural inhibitors of coagulation: antithrombin, protein C, and protein S. These deficiencies are associated with a high lifetime risk of VTE (60–70% in a recent study) and with a high risk of recurrence after a first event (50% after 10 years). A limitation to these data is that they are derived from highly selected families, which might have led to an overestimation of risk. No population-based data are available.

Acquired protein C deficiency may be seen with disseminated intravascular coagulation (DIC), extensive deep vein thrombosis (DVT), severe liver disease, infection, malignancy, acute respiratory distress syndrome (ARDS), the hemolytic uremic syndrome, thrombotic thrombocytopenic purpura (TTP), and following L-asparaginase therapy. Although levels of protein C may decrease postoperatively, the significance is unknown. Acquired protein S deficiency may be seen with DIC and severe liver disease. Total and free protein S decrease steadily during pregnancy, with the lowest levels at term. Acquired antithrombin deficiency may be seen due to decreased synthesis (liver disease, following L-asparaginase therapy), malnutrition, or consumptive states (acute thrombosis, DIC, malignancy, preeclampsia). Most patients, however, will have normal antithrombin levels within 24 hours of initiation of heparin therapy. A clue to antithrombin deficiency may be inadequate or failure of activated partial thromboplastin time (PTT) to prolong during intravenous heparin therapy. Because protein C and protein S are vitamin K–dependent factors, warfarin-induced skin necrosis may occur with these deficiencies.

Patients with a known deficiency, primarily of antithrombin but to some extent also protein C and protein S, have a strong indication for pharmacologic thromboprophylaxis in any situation that increases the risk of thrombosis, including lower-limb immobilization, pregnancy, and bed rest as a medical patient. Given the high risk of recurrence, long-term anticoagulation should be considered in these patients after the first episode of VTE, especially if it was unprovoked (ie, not associated with a transient major risk factor for VTE, such as major surgery or trauma).

The utility of testing for a deficiency of a natural inhibitor is strongly debated, mainly because of its low prevalence. Testing in the context of thromboprophylaxis is not indicated. Even in patients who present with DVT, the prevalence of these deficiencies is so low that testing is rarely cost effective. Most centers limit thrombophilia testing to those patients who are young, who have recurrent VTE, or who have a strong family history.

COMMON THROMBOPHILIC MUTATIONS

Heterozygous factor V Leiden (causing resistance to degradation by activated protein C) and prothrombin mutation occur in 5% and 2% to 3%, respectively, of the Caucasian population and rarely in other races. The lifetime risk of VTE associated with these mutations is 5% to 10% in unselected populations. While the risk of a first VTE is increased, these mutations hardly increase the risk of recurrence after a first event. Testing for factor V Leiden and prothrombin mutation is not recommended in routine clinical practice, as their (heterozygous) presence does not influence the indication for, or intensity of, thromboprophylaxis or the duration of treatment for VTE.

ELEVATED LEVELS OF FACTOR VIII

Increased levels of coagulation factor VIII are a mild risk factor for VTE. As with heterozygous factor V Leiden and prothrombin mutation, routine testing for high factor VIII in patients who present with VTE is not useful. A previously documented high level of factor VIII does not influence the indication or intensity of thromboprophylaxis.

However, evidence is accumulating that high levels of factor VIII and D-dimers in patients one month after discontinuation of anticoagulation for VTE might predict a high risk of recurrence of VTE. It is not yet common clinical practice to tailor duration of anticoagulation according to these tests, but trials are ongoing.

HOMOCYSTEINEMIA AND HOMOCYSTINURIA

Deficiency of folic acid or vitamin B12 accounts for approximately two-thirds of patients with elevated plasma homocysteine levels. This condition becomes more prevalent with increasing age, end-stage renal disease, and in pregnancy, and has been associated with occlusive arterial disease and with VTE, often at unusual sites (thrombosis in the central, cerebral, or splanchnic veins). Certain mutations that result in a high homocysteine level have only been weakly associated with VTE, and lowering of the level with vitamin supplementation has not been shown to be effective in reducing the risk of thromboembolism.

Homocystinuria, an autosomal recessive disease resulting from cystathionine beta-synthase deficiency, is associated with a tenfold or greater increase in homocysteine levels and has a prevalence of four per million. Approximately 20% of affected patients suffer from arterial and venous thromboembolism.

ANTIPHOSPHOLIPID SYNDROME

The antiphospholipid syndrome (APS) is defined as a combination of laboratory evidence (ie, presence of lupus anticoagulant or antibodies against cardiolipin or β2-glycoprotein I) and clinical manifestations (ie, at least one thrombotic event or obstetric complications). Thromboembolic events are more often venous than arterial and often involve unusual locations. The strongest laboratory association with thromboembolism is for lupus anticoagulant, followed by β2-glycoprotein I antibodies, and then cardiolipin antibodies; combined serologic abnormalities result in even stronger associations. When the APS is secondary to systemic lupus erythematosus, the presence of lupus anticoagulant or antibodies against cardiolipin increases the risk of VTE sixfold and twofold, respectively.

Primary prophylaxis with anticoagulation in APS should be provided for high-risk situations (surgery, trauma, puerperium), whereas aspirin is suggested for prophylaxis during pregnancy.

After a VTE event, secondary prophylaxis should be with the same intensity (warfarin with a target international normalized ratio (INR) of 2.0–3.0) as for other VTE. The duration of anticoagulation needs to be assessed after three to six months, taking into account whether the event was unprovoked, the presence of multiple serologic abnormalities, the serologic titer, compliance, and patient preferences. The risk of recurrence, including fatal events, is increased and some patients may experience recurrence in spite of anticoagulant therapy. This may be due to falsely prolonged coagulation times, and a switch from warfarin to long-term LMWH, or to monitoring warfarin with a coagulation factor X method, is then helpful. Patients with APS and arterial events should receive aspirin since there is no evidence that warfarin is more effective. Pregnancy loss in APS is most typical in patients with systemic lupus or with previous pregnancy complications. For these patients, heparin (unfractionated or LMWH) in combination with aspirin provides the highest success rate regarding live births.

The catastrophic APS (cAPS, Asherson syndrome) is characterized by microthrombi, anemia with schistocytes, and thrombocytopenia and is often triggered by an infection. The clinical course is rapid with multiorgan failure (usually pulmonary, cardiac and renal) and about 50% mortality, but this occurs only in 1% of patients with APS. Treatment with a combination of intravenous heparin, high-dose corticosteroids, and plasma exchange results in the highest rate of recovery (78%). The addition of intravenous immunoglobulin does not seem to improve the prognosis. The survivors may sometimes develop additional APS manifestations, but relapse of cAPS is very unusual.

MEDICALLY ILL PATIENTS AND VTE

Medically ill patients have a moderately increased risk of VTE, depending on their conditions, age, and treatments. In addition to potentially preventable mortality due to pulmonary embolism, VTE in medically ill patients prolongs hospitalization and increases costs. A growing body of evidence shows that thromboprophylaxis is underused in this patient group.

Pharmacologic prophylaxis is recommended for all patients admitted with congestive heart failure, severe respiratory disease, and those in intensive care unless there is an increased risk of bleeding. Hospitalized patients who have no contraindications should be prescribed pharmacologic prophylaxis if they have additional risk factors for VTE, including previous VTE, known thrombophilic states pregnancy (discussed later), inflammatory diseases, or malignancy. In case of recent, current, or high risk of bleeding, compression therapy of the legs should be used.

The elderly have a higher risk of VTE but also a higher risk of bleeding. Clinicians tend to overestimate the risk of bleeding and to underestimate the risk (and consequences) of VTE, thus withholding thromboprophylaxis from patients who are likely to benefit. However, older patients are more likely than younger patients to have renal dysfunction, which increases the bleeding risk with any anticoagulant. In patients with a creatinine clearance less than 30 ml/min, unfractionated heparin or vitamin K antagonists might be preferred over LMWH.

Sickle cell disease is associated with hypercoagulability through activation of both plasma coagulation and platelets. Ischemic stroke, pulmonary hypertension, avascular joint necrosis, and leg ulcers are viewed as thrombotic complications. The hypothesis that antiplatelet agents, warfarin, and heparin can prevent vasoocclusive events and subsequent complications has been tested, but studies were small and results not conclusive. Therefore, maintenance antithrombotic therapy is not routinely given. Patients who are hospitalized with a sickle cell crisis should be given thromboprophylaxis to prevent VTE.

Patients with the nephrotic syndrome have an increased risk of renal vein thrombosis, deep vein thrombosis, and pulmonary embolism. This is probably mediated by imbalances between pro- and antithrombotic factors. Estimates of the absolute risk vary from 2% to 40% of patients during their course of disease, with higher incidences in older studies. Randomized studies to guide prophylactic anticoagulant treatment in these patients have not been performed. Clinical practice is to consider vitamin K antagonists in patients with serum albumin below 2.0 to 2.5 g/dL (20 to 25 g/L) who do not have an increased risk of bleeding, especially when other risk factors including previous VTE, positive family history, and high body mass index are present.

POSTOPERATIVE PATIENTS AND VTE

The risk of VTE and need for adequate thromboprophylaxis in postoperative patients is well established. Early ambulation is sufficient in low-risk patients who undergo minor or laparoscopic or arthroscopic procedures, and mechanical prophylaxis can be used in patients with increased risk of bleeding, but all others should receive pharmacologic prophylaxis. This includes patients who undergo major general, orthopedic, gynecologic, urologic, and thoracic surgery. A prophylactic dose of LMWH is adequate for most patients, with fondaparinux as an alternative, and subcutaneous unfractionated heparin for patients with renal dysfunction. In most patients, thromboprophylaxis is given until discharge. For very high-risk patients (for example, major surgery for malignancy in a patient with previous VTE), thromboprophylaxis should be continued for about a month after surgery.

Patients after hip fracture surgery or hip or knee arthroplasty are at very high risk of VTE. This is illustrated by the fact that the first phase 3 studies with new anticoagulants are almost always performed in these patient groups. They should receive pharmacologic prophylaxis for at least 10 but preferably 35 days after surgery. The preferred agents are fondaparinux and LMWH, with vitamin K antagonists recommended for patients with renal dysfunction.

The main challenge in postoperative patients, as in the medically ill patients, is to ensure that thromboprophylaxis is prescribed for all patients who do not have contraindication. Every hospital should use a protocol or guideline, and adherence should be monitored.

PREGNANCY AND HYPERCOAGULOPATHY

During pregnancy and the postpartum period, women have a four to five times increased risk of VTE. One to two per 1000 pregnancies are complicated by VTE, which is the cause of 20% to 30% of all maternal deaths in the developed world. The risk of VTE is equal in the three trimesters of pregnancy, but does increase postpartum. About one-third of all pregnancy-associated deep vein thrombosis and about half of all pregnancy-related pulmonary embolism occur during the six weeks postpartum, as compared to the nine months antepartum. The increased risk of VTE during and after pregnancy is caused by both altered hemostatic balance and compromised venous flow. The risk of VTE is higher in obese and older women and after caesarian section as compared with vaginal delivery. Black women seem to be at higher risk than Caucasian women, while the risk is probably lower in Asian women.

Thromboprophylaxis is not indicated in healthy women during uncomplicated pregnancy or after uncomplicated vaginal delivery. There are no high-quality studies on routine thromboprophylaxis after caesarean section. The American College of Chest Physicians guidelines advise against it, while it is commonly used in European practice. Thromboprophylaxis should be used after caesarean section in patients with additional risk factors, such as emergency indication, delayed immobilization, and obesity (**Table 178-1**).

Antepartum thromboprophylaxis is indicated in women with a markedly increased risk of VTE (see Table 178-1). This includes women with a history of spontaneous or recurrent VTE and those with high-risk thrombophilia (deficiency of antithrombin, antiphospholid syndrome, and homozygous/compound heterozygous factor V Leiden or prothrombin mutation). Thromboprophylaxis should also be considered in hospitalized pregnant patients if they are ill or bedridden. Thromboprophylaxis for six weeks postpartum is given at a lower threshold of risk than prophylaxis antepartum, as the daily risk of VTE is much higher. In addition to women with an antepartum indication, this includes women with any history of VTE and lower-risk thrombophilia (deficiencies of protein C or protein S). For asymptomatic patients with low-risk thrombophilia (heterozygous factor V Leiden or prothrombin mutation), throm-

TABLE 178-1 Prophylaxis Against Venous Thromboembolism During and After Pregnancy

Condition	Pregnancy	Antepartum	In Hospital After	Puerperium Delivery
VTE during pregnancy or previous VTE with indefinite duration of VKA	LMWH/UFH	LMWH/UFH	LMWH/UFH	LMWH/VKA
Previous unprovoked VTE	(LMWH/UFH)	LMWH/UFH	LMWH/UFH	LMWH/VKA
No VTE but antithrombin deficiency; *or* previous VTE *with* antithrombin deficiency, APLA, homozygosity or compound heterozygosity for FVL and prothrombin mutation *and* not on VKA		LMWH/UFH	LMWH/UFH	LMWH/VKA
Previous VTE in pregnancy or on estrogen *or* previous VTE with low—risk thrombophilia		(LMWH/UFH)	LMWH/VKA	LMWH/VKA
Previous VTE and transient risk factor			LMWH/VKA	LMWH/VKA
Cesarian section and at least one additional risk factor			LMWH/UFH	
APLA and recurrent pregnancy loss		LMWH/UFH		

APLA, anti-phospholipid antibodies; LMWH, low-molecular-weight heparin; UFH, unfractionated heparin; VTE, venous thromboembolism.

boprophylaxis is not usually prescribed. In many cases of increased risk of VTE, the decision to give or withhold thromboprophylaxis is not clear-cut, and the pros and cons should be discussed with the patient.

In the setting of thromboprophylaxis in pregnant women, LMWHs are preferentially used. They do not pass the placenta and do not have the potential for teratogenicity or fetal bleeding. However, they are associated with hypersensitivity skin reactions. If these appear, patients can be switched to another brand of LMWH, although the skin reactions tend to recur after a number of weeks. Fondaparinux or danaparoid can then be used as an alternative. Unfractionated heparin has the disadvantages of increased risk of osteoporosis when used for long (greater than one month) periods of time, heparin-induced thrombocytopenia, and inferior efficacy when used in nonpregnant populations. Warfarin is associated with teratogenicity when used between 6 and 12 weeks of gestation and with risk of fetal bleeding. If long-term use of LMWH is not feasible, warfarin might be an acceptable alternative between 12 and 36 weeks of gestation. For postpartum prophylaxis, both LMWH and warfarin are good options. Warfarin can be safely used in breastfeeding women.

CANCER AND HYPERCOAGULABILITY

One fifth of patients with a first event of VTE have undiagnosed cancer. The neoplasm causes hypercoagulability via production and secretion of procoagulant substances, by endothelial injury, platelet and monocyte activation, and by vascular occlusion. Solid tumors with the greatest risk of associated venous thromboembolism include glioma and adenocarcinoma of the pancreas, stomach, biliary tree, breast, and lung. Many chemotherapeutic agents and growth factors increase the risk of thrombosis further, and the risk also increases with the extent of the disease. In myeloproliferative disease, presence of the JAK2 mutation has been associated with increased risk for thrombosis. Strategies for screening for cancer in patients with VTE are shown in **Table 178-2**.

All hospitalized patients with active cancer should receive primary prophylaxis. If unfractionated heparin is used, the dose should be 5000 units three times a day. Prophylaxis should be given for at least a week after surgery and extension to one month is suggested. When a patient with cancer has developed VTE, anticoagulant treatment is more challenging than in other patients. The risk of recurrence despite adequate treatment is paralleled with an increased risk of bleeding complications. LMWH is a better choice than warfarin for secondary prophylaxis and should be given at full therapeutic dose for at least one month and may then be reduced to three-quarters of that dose. Anticoagulation should continue as long as there is active cancer but may be switched to warfarin (INR, 2 to 3) after three to six months.

TABLE 178-2 Screening for Malignancy in Patients with Venous Thromboembolism

When to be Alert for Underlying Malignancy	How to Screen
All unprovoked VTE Recurrence on therapeutic anticoagulation Multiple-site VTE simultaneously Recurrent unprovoked superficial thrombosis (Trousseau sign)	All patients with VTE: history and physical examination and age appropriate routine malignancy screening Low degree of suspicion: Further testing without clues is not useful Moderate degree of suspicion: CT of abdomen and pelvis High degree of suspicion: Routine chemistry, CBC, CT of chest, abdomen, and pelvis; mammography and gynecology consultation in females, PSA in males

CBC, complete blood count; CT, computed tomography, PSA, prostate-specific antigen; VTE, venous thromboembolism.

DISSEMINATED INTRAVASCULAR COAGULATION

Disseminated intravascular coagulation (DIC) is an acquired syndrome, caused typically by sepsis, trauma, organ destruction, cancer, obstetric complications, vascular malformations, severe liver failure, or severe toxic or immunologic reactions. Any of these may trigger excessive activation of the blood coagulation, with or without concomitant inflammation. The result is widespread fibrin formation in the microvasculature, rather than the normal concentration of a clot to an injured locus. In severe, uncompensated DIC organ dysfunction will ensue. In the early phase microthrombi will cause organ hypoxia, but if the DIC is not controlled and the hemostatic components are consumed faster than they can be replaced the patient will develop bleeding tendency, which eventually becomes generalized. The International Society on Thrombosis and Hemostasis has proposed an algorithm for diagnosis of overt DIC (**Table 178-3**).

The underlying cause has to be identified and treated or removed. The hypercoagulability may be controlled with active protein C concentrate in severe sepsis. Other treatment modalities include replacement fresh frozen plasma or more specific components (fibrinogen or cryoprecipitate, prothrombin complex concentrate, antithrombin). Unfractionated or low-molecular-weight heparin in subtherapeutic doses is sometimes used but should not be combined with antithrombin.

TABLE 178-3 Diagnosis: Disseminated Intravascular Coagulation

1. **Risk Assessment:** Does the patient have an underlying disorder known to be associated with disseminated intravascular coagulation (DIC)? *If yes, proceed. If no, do not use this algorithm.*
2. **Order global coagulation tests (DIC screen):** Platelet count, prothrombin time (PT), fibrinogen, soluble fibrin monomers, or fibrin degradation products.
3. **Score these coagulation test results:**
   a. Platelet count *(> 100 = 0; < 100 = 1; < 50 = 2)* ☐
   b. Elevated fibrin-related marker *(soluble fibrin monomers or fibrin degradation products)* ☐ *(No increase = 0; moderate increase = 2; strong increase = 3)* ☐
   c. Prolonged prothrombin time *(< 3 s = 0; 3–5 s = 1; > 5 s = 2)* ☐
   d. Fibrinogen level *(< 1.0 g/L = 0; ≥ 1 g/L = 1)* ☐
4. Score ≥ 5 is compatible with overt DIC; repeat score daily: Score < 5 is suggestive (not affirmative) of nonovert DIC; repeat next 1–2 days.

Reproduced, with permission, from Taylor FB, Toh CH, Hoots WK, et al. Towards definition, clinical and laboratory criteria, and a scoring system for disseminated intravascular coagulation. *Thromb Haemost.* 2001;86;1327–1330.

THROMBOTIC THROMBOCYTOPENIC PURPURA

Thrombotic thrombocytopenic purpura (TTP) is a disease defined by microangiopathic hemolytic anemia (**Figure 178-1**) and thrombocytopenia, without an alternative explanation (for example, DIC, malignancy, or obstetric disorders).

Patients often present with fever and renal and neurologic abnormalities, but these are not required for the diagnosis. The annual incidence is low at about four per million. Primary TTP is caused by a deficiency or inhibition of ADAMTS13. This protein cleaves and inactivates the large, very active von Willebrand multimers that interact with platelets at the site of vascular injury. The absence of ADAMTS13 leads to unchecked accumulation of platelets and growth of thrombi, particularly microvascular thrombosis. ADAMTS13 levels can be measured, but turnaround times are commonly too long to help in making the diagnosis. A test result can be helpful to confirm the diagnosis though, especially when the response to therapy is not optimal. The natural course of TTP is fatal in over 90% of patients. Observations in the 1960s and 1970 led to the conclusion that normal plasma contained a factor that could reverse TTP (ie, what is now known to be ADAMTS13). A subsequent randomized trial showed that plasma exchange has even better results than plasma infusion: 78% versus 63% survival at six months. The current standard of care is that plasma exchange should be started the same day a clinical diagnosis of TTP is made. When plasma exchange is not immediately available, plasma infusion should be started first. A useful strategy is to continue daily exchanges of the patient's plasma volume until the neurologic status, platelet count, and lactate dehydrogenase (LDH) level have normalized. After this, plasma exchange on alternate days is continued for about a week. Some centers start low-dose aspirin (80 mg) as soon as the platelet count rises above 50×10^9/L. Although most patients will respond to this therapy, relapse is expected in about 30%. Nonresponding or relapsing patients are treated with immunosuppression, either steroids or rituximab.

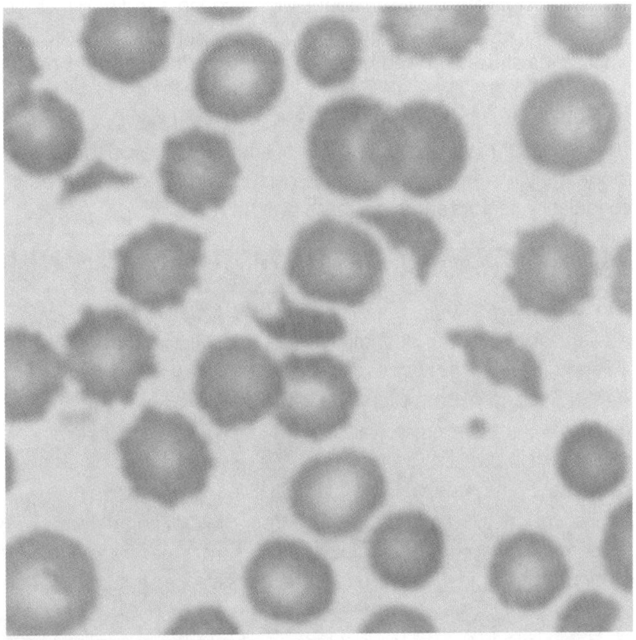

Figure 178-1 *Schistocytes and decreased platelets in microangiopathic hemolytic anemia, one of a pentad of findings seen with thrombotic thrombocytopenic purpura. (Reproduced, with permission, from Fauci AS, Braunwald E, Kasper DL, et al. Harrison's Principles of Internal Medicine 17th ed. New York: McGraw-Hill; 2008: Fig. 109-1D.)*

THE VASCULITIDES

The vasculitides have inflammation and fibroid necrosis in vessel walls as common denominators, but they differ regarding the size and type of blood vessels affected, cellular reactions, and serologic manifestations. In systemic lupus erythematosus both arterial disease with accelerated atherosclerosis, typically affecting the heart and the kidneys, and venous thrombosis are seen. Behçet disease (oral ulcers, genital ulcers, uveitis, retinitis, cutaneous vasculitis, synovitis, meningoencephalitis) is also associated with arterial and venous thrombosis in up to 40% of the patients, but pulmonary embolism is rare due to adherence to the vessel wall. Thromboembolic events may be the initial presentation of disease. In Buerger disease small arteries and veins distally in the extremities manifest occlusions. Conversely, in Kawasaki disease the systemic vasculitis has a predilection for the coronary arteries. In patients with antineutrophil cytoplasmic antibody–associated vasculitis the incidence of venous thrombosis is high. The interaction between the inflammatory process and the hemostatic mechanisms appears in both directions, and, therefore, the risk of thrombotic complications relates to the activity of the vasculitis.

Treatment with antiplatelet agents is recommended in giant cell arteritis and in Kawasaki disease, and for the latter, anticoagulation and thrombolytic therapy are indicated in certain phases. Long-term anticoagulation is also required in association with the antiphospholipid syndrome (discussed earlier). In general, there is a lack of evidence-based guidelines on antithrombotic prevention and therapy in the vasculitides.

DRUG-INDUCED HYPERCOAGULABILITY

Drug-induced hypercoagulapathy is associated with a number of drugs (**Table 178-4**).

HEPARIN-INDUCED THROMBOCYTOPENIA

Because millions of people are exposed to heparin each year, a high index of suspicion is required to prevent the sequelae of HIT which is associated with a increased thrombosis risk greater than 30 times that of a control population. HIT risk factors depend on:

- duration of heparin exposure (11–14 days > 5–10 days > 1–4 days)
- type of heparin (UFH (2.6%) > LMWH (0.2%)
- type of patient (surgery>medical>pregnancy)

TABLE 178-4 Therapeutic Agents that Increase the Risk of Thromboembolism

Estrogens (oral administration; dose dependent)
Tamoxifen
Aromatase inhibitors (less so than tamoxifen)
Chemotherapy in general
L-asparaginase (decreased antithrombin levels)
Mitomycin (TTP)
Corticosteroids
Growth factors
Protease inhibitors (against HIV)
Paradoxical effects
Heparin (via HIT), both venous and arterial
Warfarin during initiation (inbalance between pro-and anticoagulant factors)

HIT, heparin-induced thrombocytopenia; HIV, human immunodeficiency virus; TTP, thrombotic thrombocytopenic purpura.

TABLE 178-5 Determination of Pretest Probability of HIT Using the 4T Model

4T's	2 Points	1 Point	0 Point
Thrombocytopenia	Platelet count fall > 50% and platelet nadir ≥ 20 × 10^9/L	Platelet count fall 30–50% or platelet nadir 10–19 × 10^9/L	Platelet count fall < 30% or platelet nadir < 10 × 10^9/L
Timing* of platelet count fall	Clear onset between days 5–10 or platelet fall ≤ 1 day (prior heparin exposure within 30 days)	Consistent with fall days 5–10, but not clear (eg, missing platelet counts); onset after day 10, or fall ≤ 1 day (prior heparin exposure 30–100 days ago)	Platelet count fall <4 days without recent exposure
Thrombosis or other sequelae	New thrombosis (confirmed); skin necrosis; acute systemic reaction postintravenous unfractionated heparin bolus	Progressive or recurrent thrombosis; non-necrotizing (erythematous) skin lesions; suspected thrombosis (not proven)	None
Other causes for thrombocytopenia	None apparent	Possible	Definite

*Timing refers to 1st dose of immunizing heparin exposure
Pretest Probability Score
Score 6–8 = high
Score 4–5 = intermediate
Score 0–3 = low
If the pretest probability of HIT is low, it is not recommended to screen for HIT because most patients with positive PF4 antibodies will not have HIT.
Lo GK, Juhl D, Warkentin TE, et al. Evaluation of pretest clinical score (4 T's) for the diagnosis of heparin-induced thrombocytopenia in two clinical settings. *J Thromb Haemost*. 2006;4:759–765. Reprinted with permission.

Patients receiving unfractionated heparin for more than five days after surgery constitute a typical risk group for heparin-induced thrombocytopenia (HIT, see Chapter 175), which is an antibody reaction with new epitopes exposed on platelet factor 4 when it is bound to heparin. HIT may, however, also occur in medical patients and occasionally with LMWH. Only a small proportion of patients with this antibody reaction develop symptoms of venous or arterial thromboembolism, but in those few patients the hypercoagulability is pronounced and can result in loss of limb or life. Other symptoms indicative of HIT are necrotic skin reactions at the site of heparin injection, adrenal necrosis, and in the case of intravenous injection of heparin, anaphylactoid reactions. Patients at risk for HIT should be monitored with platelet count every two to three days for the first two weeks while on unfractionated heparin. Diagnosis using the 4T model is described in **Table 178-5**. When the platelet count falls by at least 50% or if a thrombotic event is observed within two weeks from starting treatment with heparin, even if already discontinued, screening for HIT antibodies should be done, heparin should immediately be replaced by a nonheparin parenteral anticoagulant, and warfarin should be reversed with vitamin K and should only be resumed when the platelet count has normalized or HIT is excluded. Alternative anticoagulants are lepirudin, argatroban, danaparoid, bivalirudin, and fondaparinux. Reexposure to heparin within 100 days from HIT is likely to cause recurrent symptoms without any delay and must be avoided.

WARFARIN (COUMADIN) INDUCED SKIN NECROSIS

Vitamin K antagonists may cause skin necrosis in approximately 1 in 5000 patients with 85% of the affected cases being women. The mechanism is an imbalance between the rapidly occurring profound depression of the natural anticoagulants protein C and protein S, and on the other hand a slower and mild reduction of the procoagulant vitamin K–dependent coagulation factors. Therefore, preexisting deficiency of protein C, protein S, or antithrombin is also a risk factor. Fibrin is then deposited in subcutaneous small veins and venules, typically in the breasts, thighs, or buttocks. The syndrome starts with localized pain and a maculopapular rash 3–10 days after initiation of warfarin therapy, and then progresses within 24–48 hour to hemorrhagic lesions, hemorrhagic bullae, and finally necrosis. This develops into an eschar with slow healing but often requiring plastic surgery or mastectomy. Immediately upon recognition of the syndrome, vitamin K should be given, warfarin should be stopped, the natural anticoagulants should be replaced with plasma or a specific concentrate (protein C or antithrombin), and anticoagulation with heparin should be continued. After healing of the lesions, the vitamin K antagonist may be resumed extremely carefully (start dose 1–2 mg/day) or more appropriately use of an alternative agent.

OTHER ASSOCIATIONS

PAROXYSMAL NOCTURNAL HEMATURIA

Venous thrombosis occurs in about 40% of patients and may include unusual sites (eg, intraabdominal veins, cerebral veins and sinuses, small veins of the skin, and hepatic vein (Budd-Chiari) thrombosis).

INFLAMMATORY BOWEL DISEASE

The risk of thromboembolism in inflammatory bowel disease is moderately increased. It is often associated with increased levels of coagulation factors and a decrease in antithrombin.

PRACTICE POINT

Do not miss:

- Catastrophic antiphospholipid syndrome: Microthrombi, anemia with schistocytes, thrombocytopenia. High-dose steroids and plasma exchange usually result in recovery.
- Disseminated intravascular coagulation: *Early*: microthrombi, organ hypoxia; *late*: consumption coagulopathy with bleeding. Removal of causative factors is crucial. APC in sepsis.
- Thrombotic thrombocytopenic purpura: Microangiopathic hemolytic anemia, thrombocytopenia, sometimes fever, and neurologic signs. Plasma exchange can save life and until then give FFP.
- Heparin-induced thrombocytopenia: Thrombocytopenia or dropping platelet count, timely after start of heparin, sometimes arterial or venous thrombosis. Stop heparin and vitamin K antagonists, start alternative anticoagulant, monitor effect to save life and limb.

CONCLUSION

Most hospitalized patients have multiple risk factors for VTE due to underlying hypercoagulability that they have acquired during their lives. The key questions to ask is whether the patient is at low risk of developing VTE (only a small minority of patients), is there a contraindication to pharmacologic prophylaxis (due to bleeding or allergy), and whether the patient is undergoing a procedure that makes pharmacologic prophylaxis problematic. All other patients should receive pharmacologic prophylaxis. The risk of VTE also extends beyond hospitalization and clinicians should include information about what the patient received and recommendations about prophylaxis when they transition patients to another care setting. Patients' first lifetime VTE may present in the community but have been acquired during a recent hospitalization.

SUGGESTED READINGS

Bates SM, Greer IA, Pabinger I, Sofaer S, Hirsh J. Venous thromboembolism, thrombophilia, antithrombotic therapy, and pregnancy. American College of Chest Physicians evidence-based clinical practice guidelines (8th edition). *Chest.* 2008;133:844S–886S.

Cohen AT, Tapson VF, Bergmann J-F, et al. Venous thromboembolism risk and prophylaxis in the acute hospital care setting (ENDORSE) study: a multinational cross-sectional study. *Lancet.* 2008;371:387–394.

Crowther MA, Kelton JG. Congenital thrombophilic states associated with venous thrombosis: a qualitative overview and proposed classification system. *Ann Intern Med.* 2003;138:128–134.

Geerts WH, Bergqvist D, Pineo GF, et al. Prevention of venous thromboembolism: American College of Chest Physicians evidence-based clinical practice guidelines (8th edition). *Chest.* 2008;133:381S–453S.

Lim W, Crowther MA, Eikelboom JW, et al. Management of antiphospholipid antibody syndrome: a systematic review. *JAMA.* 2006;295:1050–1057.

Rock GA, Shumak KH, Buskard NA, et al. Comparison of plasma exchange with plasma infusion in the treatment of thrombotic thrombocytopenic purpura. Canadian Apheresis Study Group. *N Engl J Med.* 1991;325:393–397.

Taylor FB, Toh CH, Hoots WK, et al. Towards definition, clinical and laboratory criteria, and a scoring system for disseminated intravascular coagulation. *Thromb Haemost.* 2001;86:1327–30.

Warkentin TE, Greinacher A, Koster A, et al. Treatment and prevention of heparin-induced thrombocytopenia. *Chest.* 2008; 133(Suppl):340S–380S.

CHAPTER 179

Hematologic Malignancies

Elizabeth F. Krakow, MD,CM, FRCPC
Graeme Fraser, MD, MSc (HRM), FRCPC

Key Clinical Questions

1. What are the "classic" clinical and basic laboratory features of each of the common hematologic malignancies? ("How do I prove the diagnosis?")
2. What is the natural history of each disease entity without therapy?
3. What is the goal of treatment for each disease entity (cure, prolongation of survival, or purely palliation)?
4. Which modalities may be employed for each disease entity (chemotherapy, immunotherapy, radiation, stem cell transplant)?
5. What is the prognosis with therapy? How can the prognosis estimate be refined?
6. What needs to be done to prepare the patient for therapy (to communicate risks and benefits and to reduce toxicity)?
7. How do we assess the response?
8. How do we monitor the patient after completion of therapy, both early on (for relapse) and later (for delayed toxicities of therapy)?

SECTION 1: THE CONCEPT OF MALIGNANCY

INTRODUCTION

Practitioners need to be familiar with the broad classes of hematologic malignancy (acute and chronic leukemias, aggressive and indolent lymphomas, myeloma, myeloproliferative neoplasms, and myelodysplastic syndromes). They should also be familiar with the side effects of therapy, for example, acute and chronic cardiotoxicity from anthracyclines, long-lasting immunosuppression from purine analogs, and the expected timing of neutropenia (**Table 179-1**). He or she should also be comfortable managing a number of hematologic emergencies, which are described in the following chapter. The specifics of diagnosis and treatment can be both subtle and complex. Subspecialty consultation with a hematologist or oncologist is essential in caring for a patient who is suspected or known to suffer these conditions.

PATHOPHYSIOLOGY

In general, each nucleated somatic cell belonging to a given person contains an identical DNA sequence. The exception occurs in normal lymphocyte development, in which the actual DNA sequences encoding immunoglobulin genes (in the case of B cells) or the T cell receptor (in the case of T cells) are altered. Because different cell types do not derive their unique features from differences in the DNA sequence, the **regulation of gene expression** is crucial to ensure that growth, proliferation, cell-specific functions, and cell death occur at the appropriate times in the life of the cell.

Clonal proliferation is the *sine qua non* of malignancy. Clonal proliferation refers to the concept that an entire population of malignant cells arises from a single ancestral cell that, due to one or more genetic or epigenetic changes, develops the ability to proliferate autonomously, independent of physiologic growth stimuli. The cancer-initiating cell is often conceptualized as a "cancer stem cell," but whether the inciting genetic mutations actually occur in a normal stem cell or in a more mature cell that then reactivates primitive or "embryonic" gene expression programs, and so regresses in differentiation, is a matter of active investigation. The hallmark of a stem cell is its ability to "self-renew" an unlimited number of times. Self-renewal may be accomplished through symmetric cell division in which the stem cell gives rise to two identical daughter stem cells, or through asymmetric cell division in which the stem cell divides in a way that yields one copy of itself and one daughter cell that will launch a differentiation program.

Two basic mechanisms of genetic alteration contribute to **neoplastic transformation:** mutations in the DNA sequence, and chromosomal aberrations. Genomic instability is an important consequence of DNA mutations and chromosomal aberrations. Fusions may corrupt transcription factors that would otherwise activate genes needed for DNA mismatch repair and for repair of double strand breaks. The p53 protein normally pauses the cell cycle long enough for DNA repair to occur or if the damage is extensive, directs the cell toward apoptotic cell death. In hematologic malignancies, as in solid tumors, p53 function is often sabotaged. This allows accumulation of additional defects in tumor suppressor and oncogenic pathways, which leads to continued evolution of the malignant clone and favors the emergence of more aggressive subclones.

Although clonal proliferation is necessary for malignancy, it is not sufficient. Secondary clonal events due to genomic instability must

TABLE 179-1 Common Antineoplastic Agents and their Side Effects

Drug	Mechanism	Uses	Side Effects	Comments
Chemotherapy and targeted therapy				
All-trans retinoic acid (ATRA) and arsenic trioxide (ATO)	Differentiating agents	Acute promyelocytic leukemia	Life-threatening hyperleukocytosis and the differentiation syndrome, marked by weight gain and edema, progressing to dyspnea, interstitial pulmonary infiltrates, pleural and/or pericardial effusions, unexplained fevers, and acute renal insufficiency. Other toxicities unique to differentiating agents include pseudotumor cerebri with ATRA and dangerously prolonged QT intervals and hyperglycemia with ATO. If a patient on ATO presents with syncope or palpitations and the absolute QT interval is > 500 msec, ATO should be withheld, electrolytes repleted, and QT-prolonging drugs stopped.	Dexamethasone 10 mg IV twice a day should be started at the earliest sign of differentiation syndrome, even if other etiologies like sepsis or primary CHF are possible. In patients with acute renal failure or requiring ICU admission for respiratory distress, ATRA or ATO should be temporarily held.
Anagrelide	A prostaglandin synthetase inhibitor, specifically inhibits platelet production but occasionally causes mild anemia	Myeloproliferative neoplasms	Palpitations, CHF, noncardiac edema, diarrhea, abdominal pain, headache, bleeding, anemia	In the MRC PT-1 trial, aspirin + hydroxyurea were compared to aspirin + anagrelide treatment for ET. There were more arterial events and fewer venous thromboses in the anagrelide arm. Anagrelide increased progression to marrow fibrosis and conferred a higher risk of serious hemorrhage. More patients withdrew from the anagrelide arm due to adverse effects. A starting dose of 0.5 mg twice a day is appropriate.
Anthracyclines (daunorubicin, doxorubicin, idarubicin, epirubicin)	Inhibit DNA synthesis by intercalating between DNA base pairs, causing single-strand and double-strand breaks; Generate free radicals that cause oxidative damage to DNA and cellular proteins.	Acute leukemias (eg, daunorubicin in "3 + 7"), lymphomas (eg, doxorubicin is the H in "CHOP").	Myelosuppression. Early cardiotoxicity may manifest as transient asymptomatic sinus tachycardia or ECG abnormalities and does not predict late cardiotoxicty. Late cardiotoxicity is dose-dependent. Extravasation may cause tissue necrosis days to weeks later. Radiation recall, high emetogenicity, reversible alopecia, and secondary leukemia are other considerations.	Baseline assessment of ejection fraction is advised. Anthracyclines are contraindicated if the EF is < 45%, if the patient suffered an MI in the past three months, or in the presence of severe arrhythmias. Cumulative lifetime doses are limited to 450–550 mg/m^2 doxorubicin, 800 mg/m^2 daunorubicin, 150 mg/m^2 idarubicin.
5-Azacitidine and decitabine	At low doses, they act as demethylating agents (inhibit DNA methyltransferase)	Myelodysplastic syndromes	Both drugs cause nausea, diarrhea, constipation, and cytopenias. SC injection site reactions. neuropathy, hepatotoxicity, rash, hypokalemia, and renal failure have occurred with 5-aza.	Profound cytopenias may herald an eventual response to treatment rather than progressive disease.

(continued)

TABLE 179-1 Common Antineoplastic Agents and their Side Effects (*continued*)

Drug	Mechanism	Uses	Side Effects	Comments
Bleomycin	A glycopeptide antibiotic, it causes scission of single- and double-stranded DNA and interferes with DNA repair	Hodgkin lymphoma, uncommonly used today in NHL	Fever and chills occur in half of patients within hours of treatment. Anaphylactoid reactions may occur. Interstitial pneumonitis and pulmonary fibrosis may be life threatening. The presentation may be subtle: nonproductive cough, dyspnea, unexplained fever. CXR usually shows bilateral reticular or nodual opacities without pleural effusions, but may be normal, and reduced D_LCO is the first PFT abnormality. Flagellate erythema is a rare but distinctive rash that may appear from one day to several months following bleomycin administration. Bleomycin enhances radiation injury. Alopecia.	Bleomycin should be withheld if the D_LCO falls to 30–35% of the initial value, if the FVC falls significantly, or if there are clinical or radiographic features suggesting pulmonary toxicity. Prednisone 1 mg/kg should be employed in patients with pneumonitis. Since oxygen may synergize with bleomycin to produce fibrosis, supplemental oxygen administered during operative procedures and critical illnesses should be minimized.
Bortezomib	A proteosome inhibitor	Multiple myeloma. Investigational and salvage use in certain lymphomas.	Peripheral neuropathy that is sometimes painful, orthostatic hypotension, gastrointestinal upset, constipation, ileus, thrombocytopenia, herpes zoster, tumor lysis syndrome.	Zoster prophylaxis is advisable in VZV+ patients. The neuropathy may require dose reductions and usually improves or resolves within two years of discontinuing treatment.
Busulfan	An alkylating agent, it forms DNA intrastrand and interstrand crosslinks.	Conditioning for allogeneic stem cell transplant. At lower doses, it may be used for palliation in myeloproliferative neoplasms and CML.	Myelosuppression may be prolonged. An Addisonian-like syndrome with skin hyperpigmentation and weakness but normal adrenal function may occur. Alveolar and interstitial pneumonitis are well described. Seizures may occur in the setting of transplant conditioning and busulfan may potentiate cyclophosphamide in causing sinusoidal obstruction syndrome.	In the transplant conditioning setting, drug level monitoring with dose adjustment to achieve 800–1000 ng/mL reduces serious toxicity and phenytoin or, less commonly, lorazepam seizure prophylaxis is employed. Pulmonary toxicity is treated with steroids (eg, prednisone 50–100 mg/day) and minimizing inspired oxygen.
Chorambucil	An alkylating agent	CLL, low-grade lymphoma	Generally well-tolerated. Myelosuppression is the usual dose-limiting toxicity. Pulmonary toxicity, rash, and toxic epidermal necrolysis are rare occurrences.	CBCs should be monitored closely, especially with continuous administration.
Cyclophosphamide	An alkylating agent, it interferes with DNA replication and transcription of RNA	Lymphoma, transplant conditioning	Myelosuppresion is the major dose-limiting toxicity. Hemorrhagic cystitis is common (10%, up to 40% with high doses). Tumor lysis syndrome may occur. Nasal stuffiness and facial discomfort are common complaints with rapid infusions. Pulmonary toxicity occasionally occurs and has a high fatality rate. SIADH is seen. In the transplant setting, Cy is the main drug responsible for sinusoidal obstruction syndrome and cardiac necrosis can occur at high doses. Alopecia, radiation recall, and secondary leukemia and other cancers are other considerations.	Patients should be well hydrated and prophylactic mesna is used to minimize the occurrence of hemorrhagic cystitis. When this complication does supervene, treatment includes aggressive hydration (to ensure a diuresis of 3 L/24 h) and maintaining platelets $> 50 \times 10^9$/L. If the urine does not clear, pain is severe, or renal insufficiency develops, then obtain a renal ultrasound and start continuous bladder irrigation adding 300 mg of hydrocortisone to each 3 L bag of irrigation fluid. Additional measures include cystoscopic evacuation of clots and fulguration, and intravesical carboprost.

Cytarabine	An analogue of cytidine, AraC inhibits DNA polymerase, thus stopping DNA elongation. It is also incorporated into DNA leading to errors in replication and transcription.	AML induction and consolidation, MDS, high-grade lymphomas	Myelosuppression. Cytarabine sometimes provokes a generalized rash, fever, and myalgia 6–12 hours after administration of high doses. Palmar–plantar erythrodysesthesia manifests as painful paresthesias and edematous erythema of the palms and soles, followed weeks later by desquamation. Rash is due to build up of the drug in areas that lack sweat glands, not an allergic reaction, and further treatment with this agent is permissible. Chemical conjunctivitis is common with high doses and prophylactic steroid eye drops are required. Cerebellar degeneration can occur and may be irreversible. Hepatotoxicity and pulmonary toxicity may occur.	Test for cerebellar dysfunction (include handwriting) before each high dose infusion used in consolidation therapy. Cerebellar toxicity mandates cessation of this therapy. Steroids may be used to treat pulmonary toxicity, which may present as a capillary leak syndrome 2–21 days after the first dose.
Fludarabine	A purine analogue, it inhibits DNA and RNA polymerase, DNA primase, DNA ligase and ribonucleotide reductase	CLL, lymphomas, salvage regimens for AML, conditioning regimens in nonmyeloablative stem cell transplantation	Myelosuppression may persist for many months. Profoundly reduces B and T lymphocytes; this degree of immunosuppression can lead to opportunistic infection with intracellular pathogens (PCP, *Listeria*) and transfusion-related graft-versus-host disease. Interstitial pneumonitis and dose-dependent irreversible neurotoxicity (including confusion, cortical blindness, and necrotizing leukoencephalopathy) rarely occur in current protocols. Autoimmune haemolytic anemia is common when used in DAT+ CLL patients.	Blood banks and patients themselves should be aware of the need to irradiate cellular blood products. PCP prophylaxis is required.
Hydroxyurea	Considered an antimetabolite, it inhibits ribonucleotide reductase, which leads to depletion of the deoxynucleoside triphosphate pool.	Myeloproliferative neoplasms, CML, temporary control of AML	Dose-related neutropenia, macrocytic anemia, thrombocytopenia. Vasculitic ulcerations in patients with MPNs. Mouth ulcers. Enhances the toxicity of radiation and may cause radiation recall.	Hydroxyurea will ameliorate splenomegaly and hypercatabolic symptoms. Women on chronic hydroxyurea therapy who are contemplating pregnancy should be switched to interferon-alpha.
Imatinib (first generation), nilotinib, dasatinib (second generation)	Tyrosine kinase inhibitors with varying specificity for *BCR-ABL* and other kinases	CML, Ph+ ALL, and subsets of CMML, chronic eosinophilic leukemia, and systemic mastocytosis	Imatinib: Nausea, diarrhea, muscle cramps, fluid retention, periorbital edema, hepatotoxicty, rashes. Nilotinib: Indirect hyperbilirubinemia, asymptomatic lipase elevations, hyperglycemia, rashes. Dasatinib: Pleural and pericardial effusions, pulmonary edema. Both nilotinib and dasatinib may prolong the QT interval. All TKIs cause neutropenia and thrombocytopenia (often before resumption of nonclonal hematopoiesis).	The three currently available TKIs have very different drug-drug interactions and side effect profiles. Toxicity from one agent does not preclude switching to another TKI.
Glucocorticoids (eg, prednisone, dexamethasone, methylprednisolone)	Upregulate or downregulate gene transcription, and cause apoptosis of lymphocytes.	ALL, CLL, NHL, Hodgkin lymphoma, myeloma	Short-term: Euphoria, psychosis, insomnia, hyperglycemia, appetite stimulation, myopathy, fluid retention, hypertension, hypokalemia. Chronic use: Cushingoid appearance, peptic ulcers, osteoporosis, avascular necrosis, cataracts, impaired cellular immunity.	Side effects should be actively managed. Fungal and PCP prophylaxis may be indicated, depending on dose, duration of use, and prior history of candidal or mold infections. In patients in whom a prolonged (≥ 3 month) course of glucocorticoids is envisioned, primary osteoporosis prevention with a bisphosphonate in addition to calcium and vitamin D should be considered, especially if the baseline T-score is ≤ −1.

(*continued*)

TABLE 179-1 Common Antineoplastic Agents and their Side Effects *(continued)*

Drug	Mechanism	Uses	Side Effects	Comments
L-asparaginase	By hydrolyzing asparagine, it deprives lymphoid cells of this required amino acid, impairing protein synthesis.	ALL	Hypersensitivity reactions, acute pancreatitis, hyperglycemia, hepatotoxicity. Thrombosis is frequent but hemorrhage may also occur, as asparagine depletion interferes with liver synthesis of both anticoagulant and procoagulant proteins. Lethargy, confusion, and personality changes resolve within days of drug discontinuation.	For allergic patients, *Erwinia*-derived asparaginase should be substituted for standard *E Coli*-derived asparaginase. Asparaginase is poorly tolerated in adults, particularly because of thrombotic complications. Serum amylase should be obtained prior to each cycle, and significant elevations or symptomatic pancreatitis preclude further therapy with this drug.
Lenalidomide and thalidomide	Immunomodulators with antiangiogenic activity	Myeloma (both). 5q- syndrome/ MDS (lenalidomide). Investigational use in many other hematologic cancers.	Thalidomide: Somnolence, constipation, peripheral neuropathy. Lenalidomide: myelosuppression, especially thrombocytopenia, rare pneumonitis. Both agents are associated with thrombosis. Rashes and rare cases of toxic epidermal necrolysis have been reported. Both agents are teratogenic.	The risk of thrombosis is augmented by concurrent glucocorticoids or erythropoietin. The optimal VTE prophylaxis is debated.
Melphalan	An alkylating agent	Low dose: elderly or unfit patients with myeloma; High-dose: conditioning for autologous stem cell transplant in myeloma, NHL, and HL	Mucositis is the limiting effect of high dose treatment. Pneumonitis and pulmonary fibrosis rarely occur. Tissue necrosis occurs with extravasation.	Prolonged alkylator exposure precludes subsequent autologous stem cell collection, which is why melphalan is avoided as initial therapy in transplant-eligible patients.
6-Mercaptopurine	A purine analogue	Maintenance therapy in ALL and APL	Myelosuppression, especially in patients with thiopurine methyltransferase deficiency; hepatotoxicity, immunosuppression, radiation recall.	Allopurinol significantly increases plasma concentrations of 6-MP. When administered together, the 6-MP dose should be reduced by 25–33%. 6-MP should be stopped promptly at the first indication of myelosuppression, since the nadir may be delayed.
Methotrexate	As an antifolate, it prevents *de novo* purine and pyrimidine biosynthesis.	High-grade NHL, ALL, prevention of graft-versus-host disease in the transplant setting	Myelosuppression, stomatitis, mucositis, tumor lysis syndrome, hepatotoxicity, acute renal insufficiency, idiosyncratic pulmonary toxicity, radiation recall, chemical meningitis with intrathecal administration.	Many drugs can reduce renal clearance of MTX or displace MTX from albumin, increasing bioavailability. For example, penicillins should not be administered with high-dose MTX. MTX also accumulates in effusions and edema fluid, which can lead to substantial toxicity. Effusions should be evacuated before MTX is given. Leucovorin rescue, hydration, and urinary alkalinization are the mainstays of treating MTX toxicity. High flux hemodialysis may be tried, and glucaripidase may be available on a compassionate basis.

Vinca alkaloids (vincristine and vinblastine)	Antimicrotubule agents	ALL, NHL, Hodgkin lymphoma, myeloma	Vincristine's dose-limiting effect is neurotoxicity. Commonly, this includes peripheral sensory impairment, paresthesias, and loss of deep tendon reflexes. Painful dysesthesia, motor impairment that includes foot drop and difficulty with fine finger movements, ataxia, cranial nerve palsies manifesting as hoarseness, ptosis, facial nerve palsies, or jaw pain, and in extreme cases paralysis can occur. Autonomic toxicity includes constipation and ileus. Vinblastine is less neurotoxic. Both drugs are vesicants.	With vincristine, aggressive bowel regimens are needed to prevent obstipation and ileus. Extravasation may be treated by infiltrating the area with 1–2 mL of hyaluronidase, 150 U/mL, then applying warm compresses for 72 hours.
Immunotherapy				
Alemtuzumab	A monoclonal anti-CD52 antibody	CLL, T-cell lymphomas	Infusion reactions, as described for rituximab below, are common during the first week of therapy. Profound cytopenias are very common. Opportunistic infections due to profound lymphopenia are frequent.	Prophylaxis against PCP and herpetic infections, and prophylactic or preemptive therapy for CMV is mandatory. Blood products administered prior to recovery from lymphopenia should be irradiated to avoid transfusion-related graft-versus-host disease.
Rituximab	A monoclonal anti-CD20 antibody	CLL, B-cell NHL	Infusion reactions including fevers, rigors, urticaria, bronchospasm and hypotension are common. The incidence of infusion reactions is highest with the first dose (77%) and diminishes with subsequent doses. Anaphylaxis may occur, usually at the second or subsequent infusion. Pulmonary reactions that manifest with dyspnea, bronchospasm, hypoxia, and lung infiltrates may occur acutely (one to two hours after initiation of the first infusion) or be delayed (one to four weeks after infusion). Tumor lysis syndrome is well-recognized (particularly in CLL). Due to immunosuppression, hepatitis reactivation and extremely rarely progressive multifocal leukoencephalopathy may occur; the risk of PML is likely augmented when rituximab is combined with chemotherapy.	Most infusion reactions are mild-to-moderate and can be managed by interrupting or slowing the infusion and supportive care (saline, antihistamines, methylprednisolone, acetaminophen, bronchodilators, ± epinephrine if severe).

lead to loss of cell cycle control, increased self-renewal, and escape from apoptosis. Dissemination of malignant cells is facilitated by down-regulation of adhesion molecules that anchor cells to their stromal niches, up-regulation of surface molecules that promote interaction with the endothelium, and expression of particular cytokines to promote extravasation. The neoplastic cells must also evolve mechanisms to escape immune surveillance.

Cell of origin: myeloid versus lymphoid

Lymphoid neoplasms Lymphoid neoplasms appear to recapitulate stages of normal B cell or T cell differentiation, so they are largely classified according to the normal counterpart of the neoplastic cell. For example, B cell neoplasms can be related to one of four stages: (1) precursor B cells, (2) pregerminal center B cells, (3) germinal center B cells (centroblasts and centrocytes), and (4) post-germinal center B cells (memory B cells and plasma cells).

Classification of lymphoid neoplasms is not based on any single parameter. Morphology and various surface markers in combination (as detected by immunohistochemistry or flow cytometry) usually suffice to render a diagnosis. The subtleties in refining the diagnosis are complex; morphology can be atypical and no surface marker is 100% sensitive and specific for any particular lymphoid neoplasm. Chromosome translocations, overexpression of particular gene products (like the ALK enzyme or bcl2), rearrangement of the immunoglobulin genes or TCR, and detection of viral components (eg, Epstein-Barr virus, human T cell leukemia/lymphoma virus) are considered when they are appropriate to the pathologic differential diagnosis.

Myeloid neoplasms The acute and chronic myeloid leukemias likewise can be classified according to the normal counterpart that most closely resembles them in morphology and immunophenotype. The analogy is not ideal, as most myeloid leukemias likely arise from a primitive hematopoietic stem cell or progenitor cell, even if the ultimate differentiation block produces a more mature-appearing neoplasm. By contrast, the lymphoid neoplasms might have actually arisen from the presumed normal counterpart. The French-American-British classification first produced in 1976 and updated through 1989 distinguished eight subtypes of acute myeloid leukemia based on morphology and simple immunohistochemical stains. These include M0 (minimally differentiated), M1 (without maturation), M2 (with granulocytic maturation), M3 (promyelocytic), M4 (myelomonocytic), M5a (monoblastic) and M5b (monocytic), M6a (erytholeukemia) and M6b (pure erythroid leukemia, which is extremely rare), and M7 (megakaryocytic). The FAB also identified subtypes of myelodysplastic syndrome (eg, refractory anemia) and myeloproliferative disorders (eg, polycythemia vera). FAB terms are still widely used in common speech, but the current standard classification was issued by the World Health Organization and most recently updated in 2008. The WHO classification of myeloid neoplasms relies upon surface markers, genetic aberrations, clinical presentation and prognosis, and any relation to known inciting factors.

The terms "lymphoma" and "leukemia" are often confusing. In general, "leukemia" means there are cancerous cells of hematopoietic origin in the bone marrow and usually also circulating in the peripheral blood. These cells may be of myeloid or of lymphoid origin. "Lymphoma" means that there are tumors of lymphoid origin causing enlargement of lymph nodes or spleen, or causing masses in organs like the liver or gut.

More precisely, the exact definition of leukemia versus lymphoma depends on the clinical and pathologic features of specific disease entities. For example, in acute lymphoblastic diseases, some treatment protocols use the term "leukemia" if malignant blasts comprise more than 25% of nucleated cells in the bone marrow and the term "lymphoma" if there are fewer than 25% marrow blasts, regardless of whether the patient bears other masses, such as enlarged lymph nodes or tumors in the anterior mediastinum. This 25% cut-off is arbitrary. The current WHO classification advises using the term "lymphoblastic leukemia" when marrow and blood involvement is extensive. In acute myeloid leukemias, the WHO considers 20% marrow involvement to represent the lowest threshold at which to diagnose "leukemia" as opposed to "myelodysplasia" (barring certain genetic aberrations that flip the diagnosis to "leukemia" even at lower proportions of blasts). By contrast, in the WHO classification, there is no "lower threshold" for bone marrow involvement in the diagnosis of acute lymphoblastic leukemia.

As another example, for CLL/SLL, we use the term "chronic lymphocytic leukemia" if there are more than 5×10^9/L circulating malignant B cells with or without lymph node, spleen, or liver enlargement, but we use the term "small lymphocytic lymphoma" if there is lymphadenopathy (or spleen or liver enlargement) with fewer than 5×10^9/L circulating malignant lymphocytes and no cytopenias attributable to marrow infiltration. Finally, if the blood shows fewer than 5×10^9 cells/L malignant lymphocytes and nodal and organ enlargements are absent, we diagnose "monoclonal B lymphocytosis of unknown significance" (MBUS). MBUS can be found in 3–4% of healthy adults over age 40 and occasionally evolves to CLL.

On the other hand, lymphadenopathy and "masses" are not unique to neoplasms of lymphoid origin. Myeloid leukemias do occasionally form masses and do occasionally cause lymph node enlargement. Masses of myeloid blasts infiltrating organs (other than bone marrow) and effacing normal tissue architecture are called "myeloid sarcomas." (Old terms include "granulocytic sarcoma" and "chloroma.") Simple enlargement of the spleen due to infiltrating AML or simple infiltration of the skin or gingival without effacement of the normal tissue architecture would not be considered a myeloid sarcoma.

MOLECULAR DIAGNOSTICS

In the course of establishing a diagnosis, hematologists increasingly rely on advanced molecular laboratory methods to detect DNA mutations, chromosomal aberrations, and chimeric proteins. For example, polymerase chain reaction (PCR) can be used to detect jak2 harboring the V617F mutation that characterizes most cases of polycythemia vera. Standard G-banded karyotypes often reveal chromosomal aberrations of diagnostic importance. Fluorescence *in situ* hybridization (FISH) can be used to detect fusion genes such as *BCR-ABL* in CML or *PDGFRβ-FLIPI* in chronic myelomonocytic leukemia. Several techniques are available to study the immunoglobulin genes and the T cell receptor in order to prove clonality of suspected lymphoid malignancies. PCR or immunohistochemistry can also be used to detect certain viruses (like Epstein-Barr virus or human T cell leukemia/lymphoma virus) that are associated with particular lymphoid cancers.

The results of such investigations often influence treatment decisions based upon their prognostic properties. For example, certain chromosomal aberrations, such as t(8;21) and inversion of chromosome 16, confer a good prognosis in AML. Consequently, hematologists would not recommend frontline allogeneic stem cell transplants to these patients. If acute promyelocytic leukemia is associated with t(15;17)(q22;q12) fusing *PML* to *RARα*, the patient is likely to respond well to *all-trans retinoic acid* (ATRA). Other chromosomal aberrations, such as loss of part of chromosome 5 or 7, or inversion of chromosome 3, confer a dismal prognosis in AML. Hematologists would routinely offer allogeneic stem cell transplant to young, fit patients with these karyotypes. DNA sequence mutations can also inform prognosis. For example, a particular type of mutation in the Flt3 tyrosine kinase (internal tandem duplication in the DNA sequence encoding the juxtamembrane domain of the molecule) confers a poor prognosis in AML.

Bone marrow aspiration

When a clinician performs a bone marrow aspiration in a patient suspected of harboring an undiagnosed hematologic malignancy, three draws should normally be performed: one for histopathology smears (prepared at the bedside or drawn into EDTA for immediate preparation in the lab), one for flow cytometry (sodium heparin or EDTA tube, per institutional guidelines), and one for cytogenetics/molecular testing (sodium heparin tube). For the smears and flow cytometry samples, only 0.5–1 mL should be withdrawn with each pull to avoid diluting the sample with blood. The bone marrow biopsy is useful to assess cellularity, infiltration with carcinoma, and fibrosis. Although not all hospital laboratories can perform the more specialized tests, the samples can normally be sent to reference centers.

EPIDEMIOLOGY

Acute leukemias

Acute myeloid leukemia (AML) occurs in 3.5 persons per 100,000 per year. It comprises 80–90% of adult acute leukemias. Acute lymphoblastic leukemia (ALL) occurs in 1 person per 100,000 per year. It comprises only 10–20% of adult acute leukemias but accounts for the majority of childhood leukemia.

Chronic leukemias

Chronic myeloid leukemia (CML) accounts for 15% of all adult leukemias. Its global incidence is 1.6 per 100,000 persons per year. The median age at diagnosis is 53 years and the incidence increases with age, although CML can even occur in childhood. While ionizing radiation is associated with CML and its incidence is increased among survivors of the Hiroshima nuclear bomb, most cases have no known cause. The incidence of chronic lymphocytic leukemia (CLL) in Western countries is 2–6 per 100,000 persons per year. The incidence rises sharply with increasing age; above 75 years, the incidence is 35 to 40/100,000 persons per year. The median age at diagnosis is 72 years. There is a 2:1 male to female predominance. CLL is not associated with radiation exposure.

Myelodysplasia

The median age at diagnosis is around 70 years. While the crude incidence is around 2 per 100,000 persons annually, the age-adjusted incidence is around 20 per 100,000 persons over age 70. Ten percent to 15% of cases are estimated to be related to prior chemotherapy or radiation.

Myeloproliferative neoplasms

The incidence of each of the major non-CML myeloproliferative neoplasms (MPNs) ranges from 0.2 to 3 cases per 100,000 persons per year. They can occur at any age but are more common in older adults. Essential thrombocythemia (ET) shows a second peak in younger women in the third to fifth decade, and these women usually suffer few complications. Familial predisposition to adult-onset MPNs is also described. Radiation exposure has been linked to polycythemia vera (PV).

Non-Hodgkin lymphoma

NHL is the fifth most common cancer in adults, with a crude incidence of around 20 per 100,000 persons per year. Its incidence rises with age. For unknown reasons, its incidence in the Western hemisphere and Australia has been rising at a rate of 2–3% per year for the past three decades.

HODGKIN LYMPHOMA

HL is uncommon with an annual incidence of 2.5 per 100,000 persons. The peak incidence is around age 30, but there is a second, smaller peak in adults older than 65 years.

MONOCLONAL GAMMOPATHY OF UNDETERMINED SIGNIFICANCE (MGUS) AND MYELOMA

Monoclonal gammopathy, detected as an abnormal spike on serum protein electrophoresis, is common. In the absence of cytopenias (anemia), renal insufficiency, hypercalcemia, lytic lesions attributable to plasma cell expansion, or conditions such as cryoglobulinemia or cold agglutinin disease, the presence of an asymptomatic monoclonal component is termed "monoclonal gammopathy of undetermined significance" (MGUS). MGUS was detected in 3% of persons 50 years of age or older, 5% percent of persons 70 years of age or older, and 7.5% of those above age 85 in a predominantly Caucasian cohort. The prevalence is about three-fold higher among African Americans. MGUS evolves to myeloma, related plasma cell dyscrasias, or less frequently to lymphoma at a rate of approximately 1% per year, but the risk can be more precisely quantified for the individual patient by taking into account the immunoglobulin isotype (IgG vs. non-IgG), the size of the monoclonal peak (risk increasing above 15 g/L), and the serum free light chain ratio. It is thought that most myeloma evolves from antecedent MGUS.

The incidence of myeloma is 5.4 per 100,000 persons per year, but it is twice as high among African Americans, who have higher physiologic immunoglobulin levels and a higher prevalence of MGUS. Like MGUS, the incidence of myeloma increases with age.

SECTION 2: THE ACUTE LEUKEMIAS

This section will discuss acute myeloid leukemia (AML) and acute lymphoblastic leukemia (ALL) together, comparing and contrasting them at times, because the salient clinical features are similar in adults. The acute leukemias are very aggressive hematologic cancers, are usually fatal within weeks if not properly treated, and require urgent inpatient management. The goal of care in young, fit patients is to cure the disease with chemotherapy and possibly stem cell transplantation. In elderly patients (above age 60), outcomes are poor, with less than 10% survival in those with unfavorable cytogenetics, even with the most aggressive therapy. In this population, palliation with periodic "gentle" chemotherapy or investigational agents, treatment of infections, and supportive red cell and platelet transfusions may be more appropriate.

PATHOGENESIS

AML and ALL are due primarily to increased proliferation and failure of differentiation. Most leukemias arise *de novo*. AML may also result from evolution of myelodysplastic syndromes or progression of myeloproliferative neoplasms. Either AML or ALL may evolve from CML. Prior chemotherapy can initiate DNA damage that, if not repaired, leads to AML. If alkylating agents or radiation is implicated, the usual latency is 5–10 years and loss of chromosomes 5 or 7 is frequent. If topoisomerase II inhibitors are implicated, the usual latency is one to five years and translocations involving 11q23 are frequent. Prior chemotherapy may also lead to ALL, but rarely. Certain chemical exposures, such as benzene, are also leukemogenic. Down syndrome is characteristically associated with acute megakaryocytic leukemia, other AML subtypes, or ALL, as well as a transient myeloproliferative disorder in newborns. Familial predisposition to AML is described. Examples include kindreds with germline *RUNX1* (*AML1*) gene mutations that are sometimes associated with thrombocytopenia and platelet function defects and kindreds with germline *CEBPA* mutations that are sometimes associated with increased eosinophils. Sporadic aplastic anemia and certain inherited bone marrow failure syndromes predispose to AML. Other syndromes that predispose to development of various solid tumors, such as Li Fraumeni syndrome and Bloom syndrome, also increase the risk of leukemia. In short, a family history of hematologic cancer, bone marrow failure, bleeding diathesis, and solid tumors should be sought.

DIAGNOSIS

The WHO classification, revised in 2008, is widely accepted but the old French-American-British (FAB) classification is still used in common parlance. The FAB classification relies upon microscopy and simple immunohistochemistry, while the WHO classification also incorporates immunophenotyping and molecular investigations.

Per the WHO, the diagnosis generally requires that very immature cells, called "blasts," comprise at least 20% of circulating peripheral blood white cells or of nucleated bone marrow cells. There are three exceptions to this rule: (1) cases with particular recurrent, balanced translocations or inversions are considered AML even at lesser blast counts; (2) certain AML subtypes when abnormal promyelocytes, promonocytes, monocytes, or proerythroblasts count as "blast equivalents"; and (3) myeloid sarcomas, which may be unaccompanied by circulating leukemia or increased bone marrow blasts, but for all intents and purposes are a form of AML. Normal bone marrow comprises < 5% blasts and normal blood contains none.

It is often impossible to distinguish the lineage of poorly differentiated leukemia under the light microscope. Auer rods are pathognomonic of AML (**Figure 179-1**). In AML, immunophenotyping by flow cytometry will show typical combinations of myeloid markers (eg, CD33, CD13, CD15, HLA-DR), monocytic markers (eg, CD4, CD14, CD11b, CD11c, CD64, CD36, CD68, CD163, lysozyme), and rarely megakaryocytic or erythroid markers. In ALL, lymphoid markers are expressed (eg, TdT and CD10, as well as B cell markers CD19, cytoplasmic CD79a, cytoplasmic or surface CD22, or T cell markers CD2, CD3, CD5, CD7). Either leukemia may express markers of primitive blasts (eg, CD34, CD117). Biphenotypic and bilineage leukemias are encountered occasionally.

Immunohistochemistry is still useful; myeloperoxidase stains myeloblasts, nonspecific esterase stains monoblasts, and periodic acid Schiff (PAS) stains lymphoblasts. Cytogenetics or molecular analyses (FISH or PCR) may show characteristic translocations, deletions, or fusion genes. These are routine investigations. Sequencing for point mutations and internal tandem duplications of Flt3 and other genes is increasingly performed for risk stratification, and the results may steer some patients toward trials of Flt3 inhibitors or to transplant.

PRESENTATION

Blasts overtake the marrow, preventing normal hematopoiesis. Patients may come to clinical attention because of classic symptoms related to anemia, infection (due to neutropenia), bruising, or abnormal bleeding (usually with platelets $< 20 \times 10^9/L$). Some patients are leukopenic, even when the marrow is "packed" with blasts, but most have normal to extremely elevated white counts. Blasts are ineffective at fighting infections. Although fever may be disease related, cultures of blood and urine should be done in all cases, and sputum and stool cultures when localizing symptoms are present. Gram-negative sepsis due to translocation of gut organisms is common when the neutrophil count is $< 0.5 \times 10^9/L$. In the setting of neutropenic fever or suspected infection, broad spectrum antibiotics that cover *Pseudomonas aeruginosa* and other gut pathogens should be initiated promptly (eg, piperacillin/tazobactam 4.5 gram IV every 6 to 8 hours, ceftazidime 2 gram IV every 8 hours). Bone pain may occur as a result of rapid bone marrow expansion from proliferating blasts. In such cases, narcotic analgesia may be appropriate; nonsteroidal anti-inflammatory drugs and acetaminophen are usually avoided owing to increased bleeding risks (in the setting of thrombocytopenia) and masking of fevers respectively. Despite narcotics, pain relief may be suboptimal until chemotherapy takes effect, often just a few days into the treatment course.

Tissue infiltration is typical of certain AML subtypes, especially monoblastic and monocytic forms (FAB subtype M4/5) and M2 with t(8;21). Rarely, AML cells can form a solid tumor, called a myeloid sarcoma. These may be located anywhere in the body including skin, lymph nodes, gastrointestinal tract, bone, soft tissue, testes, and mediastinum. Lymphadenopathy is rarely seen with AML but is more common with ALL. Splenomegaly may occur with either. Large anterior mediastinal tumors are typical of T cell ALL. When associated with airway obstruction or the superior vena cava syndrome they are medical emergencies that should be handled with the involvement of anesthesia and intensive care teams. Prompt institution of steroids is required and chemotherapy should follow as soon as the diagnosis is confirmed. Mediastinal radiation is indicated only if the patient's condition deteriorates and the mass grows despite these measures. Leukostasis is much more likely to occur in AML with white counts exceeding $200 \times 10^9/L$ and is rare in ALL. Hyperfibrinolysis and disseminated intravascular coagulation are classically described with acute promyelocytic leukemia (M3) but can occur in other subtypes and should be routinely evaluated in all newly diagnosed patients. Markers of tumor lysis need to be checked in all patients; abnormalities detected prior to initiating chemotherapy (spontaneous tumor lysis) must be promptly treated. Patients with normal tumor lysis markers prior to chemotherapy also require treatment to prevent the development of tumor lysis syndrome, which commonly complicates the management of aggressive hematologic malignancies once chemotherapy is started (see chapter 180 for more details). Hypokalemia sometimes complicates FAB M4 or M5 AML subtypes because monocytic forms release lysozyme that damages renal tubules, causing potassium wasting. It should not be over-vigorously corrected because hyperkalemia may supervene once chemotherapy is initiated.

Central nervous system involvement is more frequent with ALL. Neurologic symptoms are usually due to leptomeningeal disease.

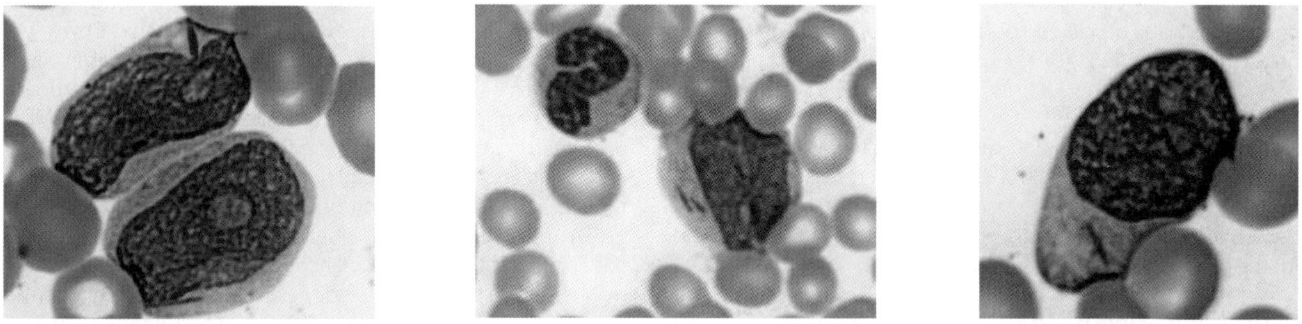

A B C

Figure 179-1 *AML with Auer rods (A-C). Auer rods are needle-like inclusions in the cytoplasm of myeloblasts (and are not seen in monoblasts or lymphoblasts). (Courtesy Wendy Patterson, McMaster University and Hamilton Health Sciences.)*

Early CNS involvement is very rare in AML. ALL protocols all mandate a diagnostic lumbar puncture at presentation, even in the absence of neurologic symptoms. Patients with CNS disease are treated with intensified intrathecal chemotherapy and, depending on the extent of CNS involvement and the protocol, cranial irradiation. ALL patients without CNS involvement have a sufficiently high risk of future CNS disease that intrathecal chemotherapy, high dose systemic chemotherapy that crosses the blood-brain barrier, and cranial irradiation on a prophylactic schedule are routinely included in treatment protocols.

TREATMENT PRINCIPLES AND SUPPORTIVE CARE

Induction therapy requires admission to the hospital. Central venous access is essential for multiagent intravenous chemotherapy. Supportive care includes prevention and management of tumor lysis syndrome (see chapter 180), treatment of neutropenic fever and infections, and administration of blood products.

CHEMOTHERAPY

Acute myeloid leukemia

For AML and ALL, the first day of chemotherapy is considered "Day 1." A typical AML induction regimen is "3 + 7", that is, three daily infusions of an anthracycline overlapping with seven days of continuous-infusion cytarabine, although other acceptable regimens exist. Marrow aplasia generally lasts four to six weeks. Some institutions examine the bone marrow around the fourteenth day of induction. If the bone marrow is hypoplastic and contains < 5% blasts, the patient is considered to have responded to chemotherapy. If the marrow is > 20% cellular with > 5% blasts, the response is inadequate and a second round of induction (usually with alternative drugs) may be administered. Intermediate results such as a hypoplastic marrow with > 5% blasts might prompt reexamination of the marrow in a few days' time. Other institutions only examine the marrow once reconstitution of blood counts has occurred. The bone marrow is then examined to confirm histologic remission (ie, a normocellular marrow with < 5% blasts), although cytogenetic and molecular testing may still detect the malignant clone at this point. Patients are generally discharged after peripheral blood counts recover.

Consolidation therapy generally consists of three to four monthly cycles. Again, several acceptable regimens exist. One common regimen employs high-dose cytarabine administered every 12 hours on days 1, 3, and 5. Patients may be hospitalized for the few days of chemotherapy infusion but are usually discharged immediately thereafter. Supportive transfusions are routinely provided through the outpatient hematology-oncology clinics, but it is common for patients to be readmitted to hospital for fever/infection.

For acute promyelocytic leukemia (FAB M3), the differentiating agents ATRA and arsenic are added to induction and consolidation therapy. APL is currently the only type of AML for which maintenance therapy is employed.

Acute lymphoblastic leukemia

Regimens for ALL are generally more complicated. They entail four phases: remission induction, intensification (also called consolidation in some protocols), continuation (also called maintenance), and CNS therapy. In adults, four anchor drugs are included in induction: glucocorticoids, vincristine, L-asparaginase, and an anthracycline. Some regimens incorporate other drugs too. The intensification phase lasts many weeks. Intensification employs multiagent chemotherapy. Continuation relies on oral daily 6-mercaptopurine and weekly oral or IV methotrexate with pulses of vincristine and steroids for one to two years or even longer in some protocols. CNS-directed treatment is given throughout all phases with intrathecal methotrexate and/or cytarabine, but an aggressive schedule of CNS prophylaxis with intrathecal drugs and/or cranial irradiation is intercalated into many protocols between segments of intensification therapy. Residual mediastinal masses are generally irradiated. Patients may be offered allogeneic stem cell transplantation in lieu of intensification or continuation therapy depending on their risk stratification. Recent studies suggest that allogeneic transplant offers a substantial survival advantage compared to chemotherapy alone in certain patient subgroups, but also that transplant-related mortality may be considerable in patients older than 35 years.

A coagulopathy related to depletion of specific proteins involved in maintenance of normal hemostasis, particularly fibrinogen and antithrombin III, can develop in patients treated with L-asparaginase. Usually this is subclinical, but bleeding and thrombotic complications occasionally develop. Patients at increased risk for bleeding complications who develop abnormalities in coagulation testing (eg, severe hypofibrinoginemia) should be considered for prophylactic factor replacement. Adults presenting with venous thrombosis should be treated with unfractionated heparin (UFH) or low molecular weight heparin (LMWH). Our general practice is to use a full-dose UFH or LMWH at platelet counts above 50×10^9/L and to consider reduced doses of UFH or LMWH at platelet counts lower than 50×10^9/L. Patients sometimes receive platelet transfusions to permit adequate anticoagulation, but this approach is not feasible for many because of eventual platelet refractoriness. For those who cannot be safely anticoagulated because of more profound thrombocytopenia or recent bleeding, a temporary inferior vena cava filter is placed. Other reasons to suspend anticoagulation are intramuscular injection of L-asparaginase and planned lumbar punctures.

The Philadelphia chromosome (*BCR-ABL* p190 variant) occurs in about 30% of adult ALL cases and portends a particularly poor prognosis. Appropriate candidates are offered up-front allogeneic stem cell transplant for Ph+ ALL as soon as they enter complete remission.

CNS prophylaxis

CNS prophylaxis is established in ALL but is not routinely required in AML. Patients with AML who should be considered for a screening LP include those with monocytic or myelomonocytic subtypes, those with t(8;21), biphenotypic leukemia, or a presenting WBC $> 100 \times 10^9$/L. Some guidelines also recommend CNS surveillance in APL patients who develop hyperleukocytosis during therapy. If CSF cytology is positive, intrathecal chemotherapy is given twice a week until blasts clear, then weekly for four to six weeks.

SUPPORTIVE CARE

Because several weeks of aplasia are anticipated following induction, and to a lesser extent consolidation chemotherapy, excellent supportive care is integral to patients' survival.

Infections

Neutropenia is the central immune defect induced by antileukemic chemotherapy. Enteric Gram-negative bacteria, due to mucositis, and catheter-related Gram-positive bacteria are the most frequent causes of neutropenic sepsis. With prolonged neutropenia, opportunistic fungal infections become important. These include invasive candidal infections and pulmonary Aspergillosis. In patients with AML, viral infections and *Pneumocystis jiroveci* are less frequently encountered, as cell-mediated immunity is relatively preserved.

Antibiotics The use of broad-spectrum antibiotics for febrile neutropenia, even in the absence of an isolated pathogen, is imperative. Health care providers must be familiar with guidelines for the management of neutropenic fever and consultation with the infectious disease service is recommended if available/appropriate.

The use of prophylactic antibiotics is controversial. The National Comprehensive Cancer Network (NCCN) and the Infectious Disease Society of America (ISDA) state that prophylactic fluoroquinolone antibiotics may be offered to leukemia patients who are anticipated to be neutropenic (ANC $< 1 \times 10^9$/L) for longer than seven days. There is evidence from placebo-controlled, randomized trials in leukemia and lymphoma and from large meta-analyses that such antibiotics dramatically decrease the frequency of fever and of documented Gram-negative infections and may decrease overall mortality. Levofloxacin may be superior to other quinolones because of its additional Gram-positive coverage. Prophylactic antibiotics are likely cost effective in high risk patients, but they may increase the frequency of *Clostridium difficile* infection and of Gram-positive infections like *Streptococcus viridans*. PCP prophylaxis is recommended for patients with ALL, but is not used in all protocols.

The use of prophylactic antifungals during induction is widely accepted. Fluconazole covers most but not all *Candida* species while the other antifungals mentioned below cover molds as well as yeast. In a randomized trial, prophylactic posaconazole led to fewer invasive fungal infections and reduced overall mortality compared to fluconazole or itraconazole in neutropenic AML patients receiving induction chemotherapy and the NCCN recommends its use in this setting. Many institutions continue to use fluconazole, which is less expensive and available intravenously. Also, ALL patients should receive fluconazole prophylaxis despite its narrower spectrum of activity because posaconazole, itraconazole, and voriconazole reduce clearance of vinca alkaloids, which might cause neurotoxicity. Patients with chronic severe neutropenia due to aplastic anemia or MDS should also receive prophylactic antifungal therapy. There is insufficient data to advise primary antifungal prophylaxis in consolidation therapy of leukemia.

Prophylactic growth factor support Granulocyte colony stimulating factor (G-CSF, filgrastim) is widely used in neutropenic patients with ALL. Prophylactic G-CSF enables ALL protocols in adults to be intensified, approximating the more successful pediatric protocols. However, the American Society of Clinical Oncology (ASCO) does advise caution in prescribing G-CSF to children with ALL because there is some suggestion that growth factors increase the risk of secondary MDS/AML.

Institutional practice varies with regard to the use of G-CSF in AML. G-CSF shortens the duration of neutropenia following AML induction by two to six days and decreases the incidence of infections. However, most studies do not show a survival benefit for G-CSF in AML. Current ASCO recommendations are to refrain from using G-CSF before or concurrent with chemotherapy because "priming" with G-CSF does not improve survival. The ASCO guidelines note that it is reasonable to use prophylactic G-CSF after induction to decrease the duration of hospitalization and the incidence of severe infections, but study results have been modest and variable. Post-induction growth factor support does not improve complete remission (CR) rates, CR duration, or overall survival (OS). The rare elderly patients who receive aggressive induction therapy might benefit most. ASCO does recommend the use of prophylactic G-CSF after consolidation treatments to avoid hospitalization for infection, despite the lack of impact on CR duration or OS. The long-acting pegylated filgrastim is not recommended for AML patients pending further trials.

Therapeutic growth factor support G-CSF is not routinely given as adjunctive therapy to febrile neutropenic patients. However, it may be considered in patients at high risk of complications. These include those aged >65 years, those expected to be profoundly neutropenic with ANC $< 1 \times 10^9$/L for longer than 10 days, those with pneumonia, hypotension, multiorgan dysfunction, invasive fungal infection, uncontrolled primary disease, or who were hospitalized at the time the fever developed.

Transfusion support

Platelet transfusion Cytopenias result both from the disease and from chemotherapy. Platelet transfusions are generally administered prophylactically at platelet counts below 10,000 to 20,000/uL (10 to 20×10^9/L). One randomized trial showed no difference in the proportion of major bleeding events in patients allocated to a transfusion threshold of 10,000/ul compared with those allocated to a threshold of 20,000/uL despite receiving 21.5% fewer platelet transfusions. Because modern randomized studies have not tested a transfusion threshold below 10,000/uL, and because current ASCO evidence-based guidelines advise the use of the 10,000 to 20,000/uL threshold to trigger prophylactic transfusion, this is the "community standard" and most physicians are reluctant to deviate from it. Higher triggers are necessary in the presence of fever, DIC, splenomegaly, leukostasis, active bleeding, neurologic symptoms, recent ingestion of antiplatelet drugs, or planned invasive procedures.

Fever, splenomegaly, and large body habitus increase platelet transfusion requirements. In the absence of these factors, two consecutive one-hour post-transfusion increments below 15,000/uL (15×10^9/L) should provoke suspicion for platelet refractoriness and may warrant consultation with the Transfusion Medicine service.

Red cell transfusion Packed red cells are generally transfused when the hemoglobin falls below 80 g/L, not only to ameliorate symptoms of anemia, but also to preserve the rheologic properties of the blood so that the platelets flow along the periphery of the vessels, maximizing their hemostatic efficacy. Patients whose marrow is infiltrated with leukemia or whose marrow was recently ablated by chemotherapy do not respond to erythropoietin, so red cell transfusion is the mainstay of anemia management.

Coagulopathy Clinically significant DIC should be investigated and corrected with cryoprecipitate, fresh frozen plasma, and platelets as required, and monitored closely until resolution.

Other considerations Cellular blood products (including platelets) should be from CMV negative donors in patients who may be future allogeneic stem cell transplant candidates. CMV status should be determined serologically in such patients. The use of CMV negative blood products needs only to continue in transplant candidates who are CMV negative. Beware that recent IVIG administration frequently leads to falsely positive CMV serology.

Transplant recipients and patients treated with purine analogue chemotherapy (eg, fludarabine) should receive irradiated blood products to prevent transfusion-associated graft-versus-host disease. Irradiation is not necessary for cryoprecipitate or fresh frozen plasma. Local institutions vary in their policies as to which other groups of patients receive irradiated blood products.

Fertility and contraception Oral contraceptive pills or other hormonal therapy may prevent or ameliorate severe menstrual bleeding during the period of thrombocytopenia. Sperm banking and oocyte collection should be considered, particularly for young ALL patients, because chemotherapy increases the risk of infertility. Unfortunately, the urgency to institute therapy often does not allow for clomiphene stimulation and oocyte harvesting. Cryopreservation of unfertilized oocytes is suboptimal, so treatment is usually reserved for women in stable relationships that allow fertilized eggs to be cryopreserved. Regardless, all patients should be counselled about the fertility risks associated with treatment and offered referral to an appropriate clinic to review options for fertility preservations prior to initiating therapy if possible. Due to teratogenicity of treatment, all patients should be counseled to use appropriate contraception.

Avoiding cardiotoxicity Both AML and ALL induction regimens (in adults) contain anthracyclines. Acute cardiotoxicity is rare, appears unrelated to total dose, manifests as sinus tachycardia, flat T waves, ST segment depression, pericarditis/myocarditis, or left ventricular failure, and usually reverses within months. Early onset progressive and late onset cardiotoxicity often present as resting tachycardia in an asymptomatic patient. Patients may have a nonproductive cough or jugular venous distention and progress to frank congestive heart failure.

The occurrence of late cardiotoxicity is dose dependent. Although there is no cumulative dose that is "definitely safe," current protocols limit cumulative lifetime doses to 450–550 mg/m^2 doxorubicin, 800 mg/m^2 daunorubicin, 150 mg/m^2 idarubicin, 900 mg/m^2 epirubicin, or 160 mg/m^2 mitoxantrone. Echocardiography or rest radionucleotide scanning to assess the ejection fraction should be performed prior to anthracycline administration. Anthracyclines are contraindicated when the ejection fraction is below 45%, if the patient suffered an MI in the past three months, and in the presence of severe arrhythmia. Anthracycline-induced congestive heart failure is managed with the same drugs and devices used for nonischemic dilated cardiomyopathy with left ventricular dysfunction from other causes.

PROGNOSIS

Median five-year overall survival for AML and ALL is about 30% in adults. This figure varies widely according to age (with fewer than 15% of adults > age 60 surviving) and the presence or absence of specific cytogenetic and molecular abnormalities.

Cytogenetic abnormalities are the most powerful prognostic factors in AML and ALL. The poor outcomes among older adults are in part due to over-representation of unfavorable cytogenetics in this cohort, in addition to a higher likelihood of therapy-related disease and antecedent hematologic disorders, and to comorbidities that increase treatment-related morbidity. Higher blast counts, delayed time to clearance of blasts from the blood and marrow, expression of multidrug resistance proteins, and mutations in various genes that control cell cycling, proliferation, and propensity to apoptosis are other important prognostic factors.

SECTION 3: CHRONIC MYELOID LEUKEMIA

MOLECULAR PATHOGENESIS

Peter Nowel and David Hungerford's discovery of a small stump on routine G-banded karyotypes in Philadelphia in 1960 proved for the first time that cancer is attributable to abnormal DNA. In 1973, Janet Rowley recognized that the Philadelphia chromosome (Ph) is due to a reciprocal translocation between chromosomes 9 and 22. In 1982, scientists identified the translocation partners as *ABL* (chromosome 9q34) and *BCR* (chromosome 22q11) genes. Later, scientists showed how the BCR-ABL fusion protein can transform cells.

Highly sensitive methods can detect the *BCR-ABL* fusion gene in about 30% of people. However, these mutations likely arise in and are restricted to the myeloid progenitor cells or their progeny. Their limited self-renewal capacity is thought to explain why frank CML does not develop; the mutation-bearing cells eventually die off. Thus, a final important discovery was that the disease-causing *BCR-ABL* fusion gene arises in a multipotent hematopoietic stem cell (HSC, **Figure 179-2**).

Additional mutations eventually accumulate in myeloid progenitors, causing them to acquire unlimited self-renewal (ie, stem cell-like) capacity and paving the way for transformation to myeloid blast crisis. Alternatively, the HSC or lymphoid progenitor compartments may accumulate additional mutations that lead to lymphoid blast crisis.

CLINICAL PRESENTATION

Roughly 20–40% of cases are discovered by routine blood counts, when patients are still asymptomatic. Other patients may present with fatigue, weight loss, night sweats, or symptomatic anemia. Splenomegaly is common and may cause symptoms such as early satiety, left upper quadrant pain, or pain referred to the shoulder. Hepatomegaly is less frequent and usually asymptomatic, and liver function is almost invariably normal. Rare patients present with leukostasis and require urgent leukapheresis (see Chapter 180, Management of Emergencies in Patients with Hematologic Malignancies). The majority (~85%) of patients are diagnosed during the chronic phase.

LABORATORY FEATURES

The median white count at diagnosis is ~100–170/mm^3 and it will be left-shifted. Myelocytes and metamyelocytes may be seen, but blasts are rare. Absolute basophilia occurs in almost all patients, and eosinophilia occurs in some. Monocytes should not comprise more than 3% of the white cells, even though the absolute monocyte count may be increased. (The exception here is rare cases with the p190 BCR-ABL isoform, which may exhibit sufficient monocytosis to be confused with chronic myelomonocytic leukemia. This emphasizes the need to test for *BCR-ABL* in any disorder that presents similarly.) Occasional patients present with significant thrombocytosis, and rarely patients may have a marked isolated thrombocytosis. It is important to exclude CML when evaluating a patient with suspected essential thrombocythemia that lacks the *jak2* V617F mutation.

DIFFERENTIAL DIAGNOSIS

The differential diagnosis of a marked granulocytic, left-shifted leukocytosis (WBC > 50/mm^3) includes a leukemoid reaction, as might be seen with infections like *Clostridium difficile* colitis. In the hospital context, a recently normal neutrophil count essentially excludes CML and the rarer disorder, chronic neutrophilic leukemia (CNL). Unlike CML, a leukemoid reaction will not exhibit basophilia. An outmoded test, the leukocyte alkaline phosphatase (LAP) score, will be high in leukemoid reactions and CNL and low in CML. If serious doubt exists, the peripheral blood should be tested for *BCR-ABL* by FISH or PCR to exclude CML, and clonality assays could be performed to exclude CNL. A high, markedly left-shifted white count along with evidence of stressed erythropoiesis, such as nucleated red cells and erythroblasts, as well as bizarre red cell shapes including teardrop forms, should raise suspicion for a leukoerythroblastic process (**Figure 179-3**). In adults, a leukoerythroblastic blood film suggests either bone marrow fibrosis or neoplastic infiltration. In that situation, a bone marrow biopsy should be stained for reticulin, collagen, and epithelial cells (to detect occult carcinoma).

NATURAL HISTORY

Classically, CML exhibits three phases. **The chronic phase** is characterized by a prolonged period of stable or gradually rising white count and a hypercellular marrow with less than 5% blasts. Untreated, the median duration of the chronic phase is two to three years. The WHO denotes **the accelerated phase (AP)** by any of the following: increasing WBC, increasing splenomegaly, persistent thrombocytosis (> 1000/mm^3) unresponsive to therapy, thrombocytopenia (< 100/mm^3) unrelated to therapy, or clonal cytogenetic evolution occurring after the initial diagnostic karyotype. The delineation between phases is not always clear cut. Basophilia exceeding 20% of peripheral blood white cells and an increase in bone marrow or blood myeloblasts to 10–19% may indicate progression from the chronic to accelerated phase, but are more likely to signify imminent progression to blast crisis. Untreated,

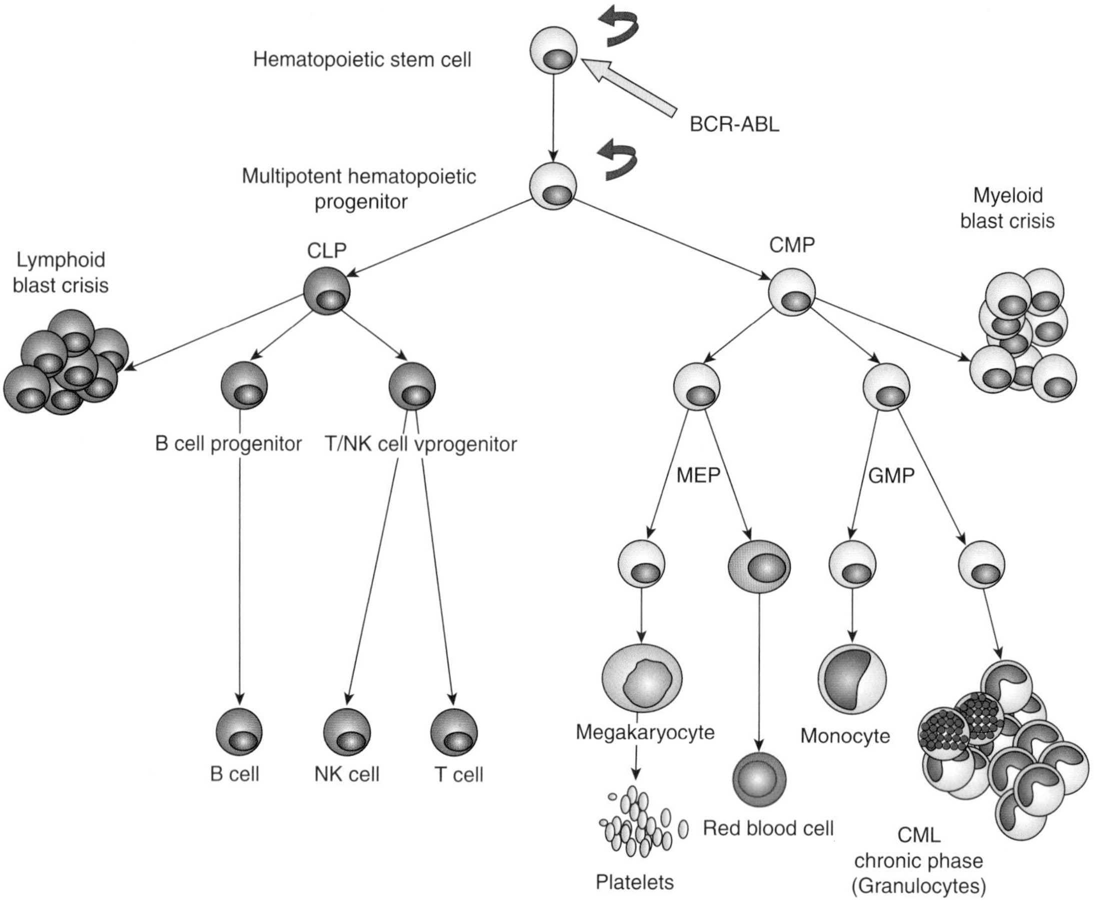

Figure 179-2 *The pathogenesis of chronic myeloid leukemia (CML). The hematopoietic stem cell (HSC) is generally quiescent but its self-renewal capacity persists for the life of the organism. HSCs can differentiate into common myeloid progenitors (CMPs), which then differentiate into granulocyte/macrophage progenitors (GMPs) and megakaryocyte/erythrocyte progenitors (MEP). CML is initiated by the expression of the BCR-ABL fusion gene in HSCs. Initially, the result is chronic expansion of the myeloid progenitor cell pool, which still maintains its ability to differentiate along the usual granulocytic lineages. Although the primitive HSC bearing the Philadelphia chromosome gives rise to common lymphoid progenitors (CLP) too, B cells derived from the malignant clone are detectable only at low levels and T cells bearing the BCR-ABL fusion gene are rare. These findings imply that BCR-ABL impairs lymphocyte development in the chronic phase. Eventually, additional genetic aberrations accumulate, leading to transformation to myeloid or lymphoid blast crisis.*

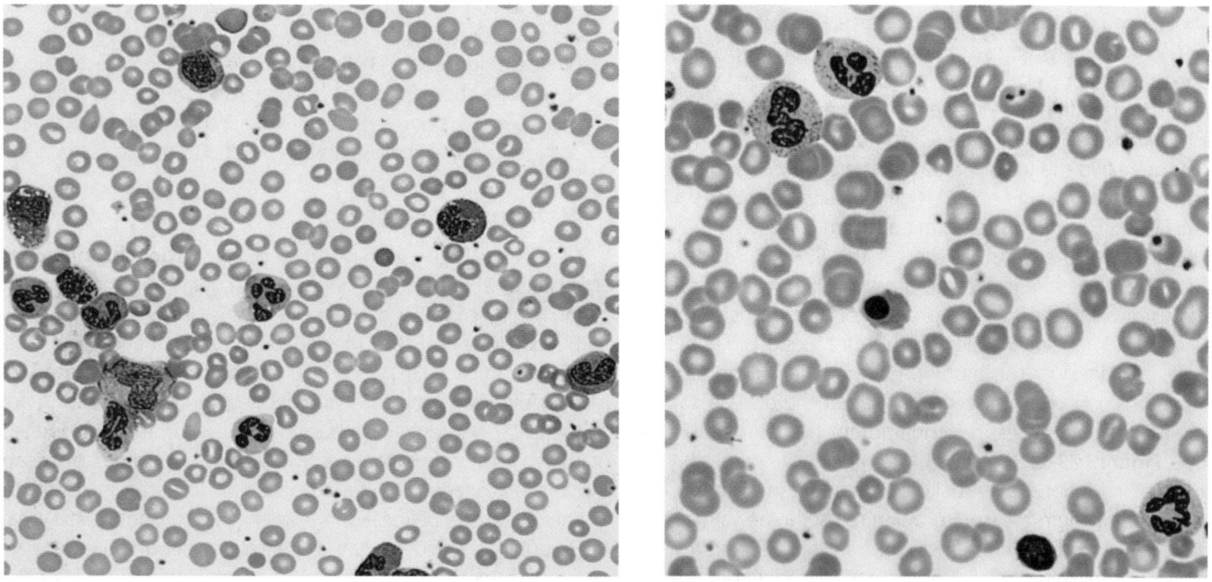

Figure 179-3 *CML (left). Leukoerythroblastic blood film (right). (Courtesy Wendy Patterson, McMaster University and Hamilton Health Sciences.)*

the median duration of the accelerated phase is less than one year. Finally, the definition of **blast crisis (BC)** rests on the presence of ≥ 20% blasts in the blood or bone marrow, or extramedullary blast proliferation, which is generally in the skin, lymph nodes, spleen, bone, or central nervous system. In two-thirds of cases, the blast crisis is myeloid. In the other third, it is lymphoid. Normal white cells and platelets are markedly decreased. Blast crisis is difficult to treat and usually fatal. The median survival in myeloid blast crisis is three to six months and in lymphoid blast crisis, nine months.

TREATMENT

The goal of therapy is to slow excessive granulocytic (and sometimes megakaryocytic) proliferation and to slow or stop disease progression. At present, short of allogeneic stem cell transplantation, the disease is not considered curable, although research programs aimed at devising curative approaches are active.

Treatment of chronic phase

The IRIS trial established imatinib, a *BCR-ABL* tyrosine kinase inhibitor, as the new standard for chronic phase disease. There are no head-to-head trials comparing up-front allogeneic stem cell transplant to imatinib therapy. Historically, transplant in the first chronic phase was associated with 26% mortality at two years. Although surviving transplant patients are generally cured of disease, this compares poorly to the imatinib six-year survival data. First-line transplant may still be considered for young patients (< age 40) with high Sokal risk scores (see below) and matched sibling donors. However, transplant as a first-line strategy has generally fallen out of favor.

Monitoring response

The main goal of therapy is to achieve a complete cytogenetic response (CCyR), which is the most important predictor of long-term freedom from progression. Even when a patient achieves a complete molecular response (undetectable *BCR-ABL*), current recommendations are to continue tyrosine kinase inhibitor (TKI) therapy lifelong. TKIs should not be discontinued outside of ongoing clinical studies aimed at characterizing the rates and risk factors for relapse.

Neutropenia and thrombocytopenia are common with all TKIs because in untreated CML, the majority of myelopoiesis is from the malignant clone. Once growth of the CML clone is inhibited, peripheral blood count recovery lags until normal myelopoiesis is replenished.

Treatment of accelerated phase and blast crisis

Dasatinib and nilotinib are second generation TKIs that improve peripheral blood counts in about half of patients in AP for whom imatinib was ineffective or intolerable, and some AP patients even achieve cytogenetic and molecular responses. Nonetheless, responses may be transient, so appropriate transplant candidates should be HLA typed and potential donors should be identified. The final decision on whether to proceed to transplant may depend on the individual patient's response to the alternative TKI therapy, the presence of other cytogenetic abnormalities, and the patient's preference.

On the other hand, patients in BC fair uniformly poorly. Myeloid BC should be treated with induction chemotherapy as for AML. Lymphoid BC should be treated with induction protocols for ALL. TKI therapy may be added to chemotherapy, at the risk of added toxicity.

Survival of patients transplanted while in AP or BC is poor (47% and 16% at two years, per the European Blood and Marrow Transplant registry). Therefore, a concerted effort should be made to achieve a second chronic phase with chemotherapy and TKIs prior to proceeding with transplant. Nontransplant candidates who do not respond to TKI therapy may be palliated with drugs like busulfan and hydroxyurea.

PROGNOSIS

A number of prognostic scores take into account such factors as age, spleen size, platelet count, and percentages of blasts, eosinophils, and basophils in the blood. The most popular is the Sokal Score (published in 1984). It has been validated in the imatinib era. In the IRIS trial, the overall survival at six years was 76.3%, 86.9%, and 93.9% in the high, intermediate, and low Sokal risk groups, respectively.

Clonal evolution, as evidenced by the acquisition of additional cytogenetic abnormalities in Ph+ cells on G-banded bone marrow karyotypes, is prognostically important. Certain aberrations, such as trisomy 8, duplication of the Ph chromosome (implying amplification of *BCR-ABL*), isochromosome 17q, and del(der)9, stereotypically herald progression through accelerated phase and into blast crisis. Failure to meet the NCCN milestones for hematologic, cytogenetic, and molecular responses within the specified time frames and loss of a previous cytogenetic or molecular response also signify the likelihood of progression.

SECTION 4: CHRONIC LYMPHOCYTIC LEUKEMIA

PATHOGENESIS

Chronic lymphocytic leukemia (CLL) is due to the accumulation of monoclonal small lymphocytes that have low proliferative capacity. The etiology of CLL is unknown. The existence of structurally similar B cell receptors across CLL cases suggests that the malignant B cells might recognize similar epitopes. Familial CLL has been described but most cases are sporadic. However, there may be an increased incidence of other hematologic malignancies in first-degree relatives of CLL patients. Also, the rarity of CLL in the Far East persists in emigrant populations, implying that genetic background predisposes to this leukemia.

CLINICAL PRESENTATION

Most patients are diagnosed while asymptomatic because a blood count is performed for other indications. Others present with fatigue, B symptoms (fever, weight loss, night sweats), lymphadenopathy, or hepatosplenomegaly. Immune dysfunction accounts for infectious, autoimmune cytopenias, and other malignant complications.

Leukostasis is extremely unusual, even at white counts well in excess of 500×10^9/L. The physical examination should identify which nodal areas are involved and detect liver or spleen enlargement.

Infections

Secondary T cell, NK cell, neutrophil, and macrophage impairments are well described. Hypogammaglobulinemia results from the CD95 ligand/CD95 interaction between plasma cells and malignant B cells that inhibits plasma cells from secreting immunoglobulin and induces their apoptosis, and from T cell dysfunction. Zoster and respiratory tract infections due to viruses, *Streptococcus pneumoniae* or *Haemophilus influenzae* are frequently encountered as the disease progresses. Two randomized studies and one cross-over study in CLL show that low-dose intravenous immune globulin (IVIG) infusions reduce the incidence of infections, especially at IgG levels below 3 g/L, but there was no improvement in quality of life or survival. This finding was confirmed in a meta-analysis that also included studies in myeloma patients. In addition, IVIG prophylaxis is expensive and generally not considered cost effective. As a result, IVIG (0.4 mg/kg every 3–4 weeks) is usually reserved for selected patients with recurrent serious infections requiring hospitalization.

All patients with CLL should be vaccinated against viral influenza and pneumococcus. Haemophilus influenzae type b and meningococcal vaccines are advised pre-splenectomy and might be given to all patients too. Live vaccines are generally contraindicated.

Autoimmunity

Autoimmune phenomena are generally directed against red cells or platelets. Between 10% and 25% of patients develop autoimmune hemolytic anemia (AIHA) at some point during the course of disease. The direct antiglobulin test (DAT) should be checked at diagnosis and periodically thereafter, even in the absence of ancillary evidence of hemolysis such as elevated bilirubin, LDH, or reduced haptoglobin. ITP occurs in 2–3% of patients, while pure red cell aplasia and autoimmune neutropenia complicate the course of CLL even less frequently (the latter are more commonly associated with T cell large granular leukemia).

By themselves, AIHA and ITP are not indications for chemotherapy, but if more conservative measures such as a course of corticosteroids are ineffective, then treating the underlying CLL may be required. The majority of patients respond to steroids (eg, prednisone 1 mg/kg/day) within one to two weeks. The successful dose should be maintained for two to six weeks and tapered slowly over three months. If there is no response to steroids, then rituximab-containing combination chemotherapy, splenectomy, or other ITP-appropriate immunosuppressive drugs are considered. In urgent situations, high-dose IV methylprednisolone and full-dose IVIG (eg, 1 gram/kg/day for two days) may work rapidly.

Secondary malignancy

Immune dysregulation is implicated in the increased incidence of solid tumors among patients with CLL. These include an excess of colorectal, lung, and squamous cell skin cancers. Age-appropriate cancer screening, sun protection, and annual dermatologic examination are advised.

LABORATORY FEATURES

The National Cancer Institute (NCI)-sponsored International Working Group definition of CLL, endorsed by the WHO, requires the presence of $\geq 5 \times 10^9$/L monoclonal B cells with typical CLL immunophenotype circulating in the peripheral blood (kappa or lambda restriction, dim surface IgM or IgD, CD5 positive, CD23 positive, dim CD20) sustained over three months. The blood film will show small, fairly normal-appearing lymphocytes as well as smudge cells, but these are not pathognomonic for CLL. Fewer than 55% of lymphocytes should be prolymphocytes (medium-sized cells with moderately more open chromatin and a single, prominent nucleolus); otherwise, the diagnosis is prolymphocytic leukemia, an entity that behaves quite differently from CLL. When arising *de novo,* prolymphocytic leukemia is usually CD5 and CD23 negative. Small lymphocytic lymphoma is the nonleukemic counterpart of CLL with identical tissue morphology and immunophenotype, circulating monoclonal B-lymphocytes $< 5.0 \times 10^9$/L, and no cytopenias related to bone marrow infiltration. Monoclonal B lymphocytosis is a recently described entity in which the relevant circulating cells fall below the concentration threshold for diagnosing CLL (see Natural History, below).

A bone marrow is not necessary at diagnosis but might be useful before aggressive therapy to assess "marrow reserve" or to elucidate the etiology of reticulocytopenic anemia (eg, heavy marrow infiltration with CLL vs. pure red cell aplasia) or thrombocytopenia (eg, ample megakaryocytes imply ITP).

Other investigations should include standard chemistries, quantitative serum immunoglobulins, serum and urine protein electrophoresis (a small monoclonal component is common), LDH, uric acid, and a direct antiglobulin test. Spherocytes may be noticed on the blood film if there is significant extravascular hemolysis. Baseline HIV and hepatitis B and C serological studies should be ordered at diagnosis; this applies to all the diseases discussed in this chapter.

Outside of a clinical trial, no imaging is required. However, a baseline chest X-ray is recommended to aid assessment when suspected pulmonary infections develop and many clinicians do order a computed tomography (CT) of the chest, abdomen, and pelvis before initiating treatment.

NATURAL HISTORY

In general terms, CLL is considered an indolent, albeit incurable, lymphoproliferative disease with progression in most cases over months to years. It is managed primarily in the outpatient setting, especially in the early, asymptomatic phase. The natural history and prognosis are extremely heterogeneous with median survivals ranging from 2 to 20 years within specific subgroups of patients. A number of novel prognostic markers have recently been discovered that provide powerful prognostic information in addition to clinical stage and help to explain some of the observed heterogeneity. These tests are often obtained at diagnosis and/or prior to initiating chemotherapy by sending peripheral blood or bone marrow samples to an appropriate molecular diagnostics laboratory. Examples include assessment of CD38 and ZAP-70 expression on leukemic B-cells as measured by flow cytometry (negativity conferring a favorable prognosis), mutational status of the immunoglobulin heavy chain gene (unmutated IgV_H associated with poorer prognosis), interphase FISH cytogenetic evaluation (high risk markers include deletions of 17p and 11q), and beta-2 microglobulin. Testing for ZAP-70 and IgV_H sequencing are not available at most centers.

The most frequent cause of death is infection. Death from secondary malignancies and from non-CLL related causes follows in frequency. Richter transformation to an aggressive, treatment-refractory large B cell lymphoma occurs in 1% to 10% of patients. Transformation to prolymphocytic leukemia occurs in up to 10% of patients. Rare patients develop other lymphomas, including Hodgkin disease.

The factors determining whether monoclonal B lymphocytosis evolves into CLL are under active investigation. A recent study found that the rate of progression to symptomatic CLL needing treatment is only 4% per year in the first seven years, and negligible thereafter. Currently, asymptomatic patients with low level CLL-phenotype clones should be considered to have "monoclonal B lymphocytosis of unknown significance (MBUS)," analogous to patients with monoclonal gammopathy of undetermined significance (MGUS), and followed clinically at approximately 6–12 month intervals to monitor for disease progression.

TREATMENT

Asymptomatic patients do not require chemotherapy and should be placed on clinical observation, often referred to as "watchful waiting." Data from more than 2000 patients with early-stage disease enrolled in randomized clinical trials of immediate versus delayed alkylator-based chemotherapy have been synthesized in a meta-analysis. These studies showed no survival benefit to immediate therapy. According to the National Cancer Institute, indications for initiating therapy include B-symptoms (fever, drenching night sweats, weight loss), severe fatigue, massive lymphadenopathy (>10 cm), massive splenomegaly (>6 cm below the costal margin), anemia, or thrombocytopenia (Rai Stage 3 or 4) that is due to marrow infiltration or autoimmune mediated and not responsive to steroids; or a lymphocyte doubling time <6 months. Patients with cytopenias due to marrow infiltration usually do not respond to growth factors (G-CSF or erythropoietin);

chemotherapy is required. However, growth factors may be useful to support patients through periods of chemotherapy-induced cytopenias.

Symptomatic patients generally require treatment with chemotherapy. There are a number of first-line treatment options, depending on the clinical circumstance. Fit, younger patients are candidates for combination chemo-immunotherapy incorporating a purine analogue and monoclonal antibody. In a recent landmark randomized trial, the addition of rituximab (an anti-CD 20 monoclonal antibody) to fludarabine plus cyclophosphamide (FCR) increased overall survival compared with fludarabine and cyclophosphamide alone without a substantial increase in toxicity. This trial is the only randomized controlled trial to demonstrate a survival benefit for a first-line treatment regimen and FCR is now recommended for this indication. Toxicities associated with FCR include myelosuppression, neutropenic fever, and infections, including the potential for opportunistic infections such as *Pneumocystis jiroveci* (formerly: *Pneumocystis carinii*) and reactivation of herpes simplex and varicella zoster viruses; appropriate prophylaxis is required during and after therapy (eg, Septra, acyclovir). If preventative measures are implemented (allopurinol, oral hydration), clinically important tumor lysis syndrome is relatively uncommon.

Very elderly or frail patients with significant comorbidity may not be suitable candidates for aggressive treatment and may fair best with conservative therapy, such as single-agent oral chlorambucil. To date, the results of prognostic marker testing have had little impact on treatment decision making because their predictive properties remain unclear in most cases. Detection of del17p (approximately 5–7% of patients) or del11q (approximately 15–20% of patients) are notable exceptions that may impact initial choice of chemotherapy regimen in selected cases.

Transformation to a large B cell lymphoma is generally refractory to treatment. An attempt is often made to control disease with regimens for aggressive lymphomas that include anthracyclines.

MONITORING RESPONSE

In general practice, response is monitored by history, physical exam, CBC, and differential white counts. Follow-up CT scans are increasingly being performed, particularly in clinical trials. Immunophenotyping of blood or marrow lymphocytes is used to confirm suspected complete remission. A marrow aspirate need only be done to investigate cytopenias of unclear cause. For clinical trials, more stringent disease assessment is performed.

SECTION 5: MYELODYSPLASIA

Myelodysplasia is a condition in which ineffective hematopoiesis in one or more lineages is accompanied by increased cell turnover in the bone marrow and morphologic dysplasia. Clinically, it manifests as peripheral blood cytopenias affecting one or more lineages, while the bone marrow is classically hypercellular. Patients might die of infections, bleeding, transfusion-related iron overload, or progression to acute leukemia.

PATHOGENESIS

The myelodysplastic syndromes (MDS) are clonal disorders. The transforming event probably occurs in a myeloid stem cell. Clonal hematopoiesis encompasses the myeloid, erythroid, and megakaryocytic compartments. Immature cells tend to die prematurely by programmed cell death, and those cells that reach terminal differentiation states are defective. For example, mature neutrophils may lack myeloperoxidase and mature platelets might be unable to aggregate effectively. A number of genetic lesions have been described, but the driving defects remain elusive.

Sideroblastic anemia generally exhibits reticulocytopenia and erythroid marrow hyperplasia with iron-laden mitochondria ringing the nucleus, as demonstrated by a Prussian blue stain. Congenital forms present with microcytic anemia, whereas the acquired form is generally normocytic or macrocytic. Reversible acquired sideroblastic anemia may be due to alcohol, drugs (isoniazid, chloramphenicol), copper deficiency/zinc toxicity, or hypothermia; in these instances, the marrow is often hypocellular and other cytopenias may also occur.

DIAGNOSIS

The possibility of MDS is raised when a patient presents with one or more refractory cytopenias. The WHO classification mandates that minimally 10% of bone marrow cells in at least one lineage (erythroid, myeloid, or megakaryocytic) are morphologically dysplastic. In the absence of definitive morphologic dysplasia, the presence of specified unbalanced or balanced chromosomal abnormalities is considered presumptive evidence of MDS. Further subcategorization is based on the number of cytopenias and dysplastic lineages (eg, refractory anemia with unilineage dysplasia vs. refractory anemia with multilineage dysplasia), the presence of ≥ 15% ringed sideroblasts, and the percentage of blasts in the blood and marrow. MDS with isolated del(5q) occupies a unique category. Nutritional deficiencies (including B12 and folate deficiency), medications, toxins (eg, arsenic, alcohol), growth factor therapy, regenerative stress erythropoeisis (eg, following an episode of hemolytic anemia), and systemic infection (eg, tuberculosis) should be excluded before a diagnosis of primary MDS is rendered.

CLINICAL PRESENTATION

Patients usually present with gradually progressive macrocytic (and sometimes normocytic) anemia. Neutropenia and thrombocytopenia are much less frequent initial manifestations but develop as the condition progresses. Organomegaly is quite uncommon. Rarely, autoimmune complications like vasculitis, monoarticular arthritis, or a syndrome of fever, edema, and pulmonary infiltrates occur.

LABORATORY INVESTIGATIONS

Initial investigations should include a CBC, reticulocyte count (which will be inappropriately low), erythropoietin level, and iron studies. Attention should be paid to the blood monocyte count, which should be below 1×10^9/L, otherwise the diagnosis of chronic myelomonocytic leukemia is more likely. Bone marrow aspiration and biopsy with iron stain, cytogenetics, flow cytometry (to assess the blast count), and reticulin stain are crucial. In most instances, the marrow is hypercellular. Hypoplastic MDS may be difficult to distinguish from aplastic anemia. A minimal amount of dysplasia may accompany the latter entity too. Hypocellular MDS is more likely to show a normal or high percentage of CD34+ cells in the marrow (mean 3.5%, range 1–7%). In aplastic anemia, CD34+ stem cells are under immune attack and are often extremely low by flow cytometry or immunohistochemistry (mean 0.13%, range 0.02–0.36%). Apart from those chromosomal abnormalities listed by the WHO, many other cytogenetic aberrations are frequently seen but not specific for MDS and may occur in aplastic anemia too. Therefore, cytogenetic findings cannot always be used to distinguish the two entities. HLA-DR15 is associated with both aplastic anemia and MDS in younger patients and > 40% of these MDS patients may respond to immunosuppressive therapy, but responses drop sharply as age increases. HLA typing is also warranted in younger patients for whom allogeneic transplant may be warranted.

NATURAL HISTORY

Most patients die of progressive marrow failure, either due to infections in the setting of neutropenia or to cardiac failure from transfusion-associated iron overload. Others progress to overt AML. Certain WHO subtypes, including MDS with isolated del(5q) and refractory anemia with ringed sideroblasts confer a better prognosis and rarely transform to AML.

Two prognostic scores, the International Prognostic Scoring System (IPSS) and the WHO-classification based scoring system (WPSS) are commonly used to predict the risk of leukemic evolution and overall survival. Among patients older than 60, survival is shortened further. The WPSS has the advantage of applicability at any time during the disease course.

TREATMENT

Specific therapies such as hypomethylating agents (azacitidine, decitabine), lenalidomide, growth factor support, and possibly chelation therapy in those with transfusion-associated iron overload are generally administered on an outpatient basis and will not be discussed here. MDS is usually a chronic illness, often not directly related to the reason for hospitalization. Physicians should be sensitized to the cardiac complications resulting from iron overload. When cytopenias are severe or when MDS progresses to AML, the same supportive care as discussed above applies (ie, transfusion of blood products to support hemoglobin and platelets, and prompt management of infection-related complications, especially in neutropenic patients). Younger patients with poor risk disease may be offered allogeneic stem cell transplant.

SECTION 6: MYELOPROLIFERATIVE NEOPLASMS

The classic myeloproliferative neoplasms (MPNs) include CML (already discussed), polycythemia vera (PV), essential thrombocythemia (ET), and primary myelofibrosis (PMF). There are also a number of less common (eg, chronic eosinophilic leukemia, systemic mastocytosis) and extremely rare (eg, chronic basophilic leukemia) MPNs. By definition, MPNs feature <20% blasts in blood and marrow. The goal of treatment is to relieve symptoms and to prevent complications such as thrombosis. MPNs are not curable with available pharmacologic therapies.

PATHOGENESIS

MPNs likely result from increased sensitivity to growth-promoting cytokines due to activating somatic mutations. Whether the different disease phenotypes are due to different cell types in which the same culprit mutation originates, to other interacting genetic factors, to the "dosage" of heterozygously or homozygously *jak-2* mutated cells, or to genetic lesions that precede *jak-2* mutation is not clear; evidence exists to support each of these hypotheses.

DIAGNOSIS

The diagnosis of MPNs rests on demonstrating clonal proliferation leading to accumulation of mature circulating blood cells. Clonal proliferation may not be demonstrable in all cases and some instances of essential thrombocythemia are probably truly polyclonal. In such cases, reactive thrombocytosis (eg, due to iron deficiency, infection, or metastatic cancer) should be carefully excluded. Similarly, when considering a diagnosis of PV, it is important to rule out physiologic and nonphysiologic causes of erythrocytosis, such as (1) hypoxia from chronic pulmonary disease, sleep apnea, and right-to-left cardiac shunts; (2) elevated carboxyhemoglobin from smoking or occupational exposure to hydrocarbon fumes; (3) inappropriate renal, hepatic, or paraneoplastic erythropoietin production; and (4) relative polycythemia due to decreased plasma volume (as in dehydration, diuretic use, or alcoholism). An algorithm for evaluating erythrocytosis is presented in Chapter 173 Abnormalities in Red Blood Cells. Myelofibrosis might be secondary to a separate hematologic neoplasm, including antecedent PV or ET, to carcinoma metastatic to the marrow, or to other inflammatory conditions. The WHO classification should be consulted for the specific diagnostic criteria for each entity.

CLINICAL PRESENTATION

In addition to elevated blood counts, the classic MPNs share many clinical features, including frequent hepatosplenomegaly, hyperuricemia that can lead to gout, a risk of arterial and venous thrombosis, and hypercatabolism leading to fatigue. Symptoms due to hyperviscosity, histamine release, and microvascular vasomotor instability include aquagenic pruritus and erythromelalgia. Facial plethora is often described in patients with PV. Hyperviscosity may lead to epistaxis or gastrointestinal bleeding (often occult), particularly in PV. One-fifth of PV patients and 10–25% of ET patients present with thrombotic complications, including transient ischemic attacks, ischemic stroke, myocardial infarction, deep venous thrombosis, hepatic vein thrombosis (Budd-Chiari syndrome), or splanchnic vein thrombosis. Extreme thrombocytosis, as may occur with ET or PV (platelets $>1000 \times 10^9$/L), may paradoxically lead to hemorrhage, including hemorrhagic stroke, because of qualitative platelet dysfunction such as acquired type 2 von Willebrand disorder as the platelet surface binds and cleaves large vWF multimers. About 10% of patients with ET present with a hemorrhagic event. Pulmonary hypertension is a serious complication, which portends poor survival. Extramedullary hematopoeisis is unique to primary and secondary myelofibrosis. It results from neoplastic hematopoietic cells migrating to the spleen and liver, not resumption of fetal hematopoiesis.

LABORATORY FEATURES AND INVESTIGATIONS

PV is considered when the hemoglobin is above 185 g/L in men or 165 g/L in women, when the hematocrit is above the ninety-ninth percentile for age, sex, and altitude, or when there is other evidence of elizabeth increased red cell mass. The patient is usually overtly iron deficient, but iron supplementation should not be prescribed because it can precipitate a rapid, dangerous rise in the red cell count. The white count and platelet count are frequently elevated too. The oxygen saturation should be normal and if carboxyhemoglobinemia is possible, then an arterial blood gas should be obtained. Nocturnal monitoring to exclude sleep apnea may be needed. If the erythropoietin level is inappropriately normal or elevated, abdominal imaging should be performed to rule out renal and liver tumors, and rarely uterine, ovarian, and adrenal tumors. Cerebellar hemangiomas, parotid neoplasms, and lymphomas are occasionally implicated in ectopic erythropoietin production.

ET is considered when the platelet count is persistently above 450×10^9/L in the absence of underlying reactive etiologies and once alternative myeloproliferative neoplasms have been excluded. Myelofibrosis often comes to attention because of a leukoerythroblastic peripheral blood smear featuring teardrop red cell forms, nucleated red blood cells, and left-shifted granulocyte series.

Bone marrow aspiration and biopsy are not mandatory in straightforward instances of PV or ET, in which *jak2* or *c-mpl* mutations in the peripheral blood granulocytes are detected in the setting of a classic clinical picture, but this procedure might still be useful to prove clonality with karyotypes in *jak-2* negative cases and to evaluate the degree of fibrosis.

NATURAL HISTORY

Untreated, 40–50% of PV patients will suffer thrombosis, 20–40% will die of thrombosis, 15% will develop significant bleeding, and

5–10% will die of bleeding. In PV, two-thirds of thrombotic events in the ECLAP study were arterial and one-third venous. In ET, arterial thrombosis is about three times as frequent as venous thrombosis and the incidence of bleeding is lower than in PV. PV and ET may evolve from a proliferative phase to a "spent" phase with progressive marrow fibrosis and poor median survival of < 3 years. The risk of developing myelofibrosis increases with duration of PV or ET. Because of overlapping features, some of the ET patients who are "early" progressors might actually have had primary myelofibrosis (PMF) all along. PMF characteristically also evolves from a proliferative, prefibrotic phase to a fibrotic stage. All three conditions can transform to AML. PV transforms to AML at a rate of 0.3–1% per year and although it has been difficult to demonstrate, this risk probably increases with duration of disease. In ET, transformation to AML is rare in the first decade after diagnosis and increases thereafter. The risk of transformation is increased by alkylating agents (eg, chlorambucil, busulfan) and radioactive phosphate (P^{32}). Whether or not hydroxyurea is associated with increased risk of leukemic transformation remains controversial based upon currently available data; however, definitive evidence to support claims of increased risk is lacking in our opinion. Nonetheless, the risks and benefits need to be carefully considered prior to recommending lifelong cytoreductive treatment.

TREATMENT

Traditional cardiovascular risk factors, including smoking, diabetes, age > 60–65 years, and a history of prior venous or arterial thrombosis are associated with increased risk of thrombotic events in PV and ET. Based on the ECLAP study, low-dose aspirin is recommended for all PV patients and extrapolated to ET patients as well. Weekly or twice weekly phlebotomy to achieve a target hematocrit below 45% in men, 42% in women, and 37% in pregnant women is advised for all patients with PV. Once iron-limited hematopoiesis develops, the frequency of phlebotomy can usually be decreased to two to four times per year to maintain the target hematocrit. PV and ET patients who have suffered a prior thrombotic event should be treated with cytoreductive therapy to reduce their risk of recurrent, potentially fatal thrombosis. Patients older than age 60 and those with extreme thrombocytosis (> 1500–2000 × 10^9/L) in the absence of prior thrombosis have an intermediate risk of thrombotic complications and bleeding, and should also be considered for hydroxyurea therapy, although the evidence for pharmacologic cytoreduction in these populations derives largely from observational data and expert opinion. Hydroxyurea is titrated to achieve a normal platelet count (150–400 × 10^9/L) while maintaining adequate counts in other cell lines. All modifiable cardiac risk factors should be aggressively managed according to current guidelines. *Jak-2* inhibitors are now entering clinical trials with early promising results.

Finally, it is crucial to delay elective surgery in the face of uncontrolled blood counts. Up to 80% of uncontrolled PV patients will suffer postoperative thrombotic or hemorrhagic events, but only 5–10% will develop such complications if hemoglobin and platelet counts are normalized for several weeks preoperatively. Perioperative DVT prophylaxis should be prescribed.

Erythromelalgia responds to aspirin. Refractory vasomotor symptoms may respond to hydroxyurea or anagrelide. Pruritus may respond to antihistamines, SSRIs, cholestyramine, or psoralen/ultraviolet light (PUVA). Allopurinol should be used prophylactically until cell counts and hyperuricemia are controlled. Symptomatic splenomegaly refractory to cytoreductive drugs may be treated with splenectomy or splenic irradiation. Splenectomy carries risks of portal vein thrombosis propagating from the ligated splenic vein, operative mortality around 10%, post-splenectomy thrombocytosis, and late massive hepatomegaly. Splenic irradiation carries the risk of prolonged, profound cytopenias. Radiation is also used to treat extramedullary hematopoietic tumors that threaten the spinal cord. Growth factors (including erythropoietin) or androgens may be helpful in patients with advanced fibrosis. Extreme thrombocytosis should be treated with pharmacologic cytoreduction but in the setting of severe or life-threatening bleeding, plateletpheresis is recommended together with the initiation of cytoreductive therapy. Iron chelation may be appropriate for transfusion-dependent patients with PMF, ferritin > 1000 ug/L, and good life expectancy. Transformation to AML is associated with a very poor prognosis (median survival < six months). Management may include induction chemotherapy followed by allogeneic stem cell transplantation if the patient is young and fit; otherwise, experimental or palliative therapy is more appropriate.

Acute thrombotic events are managed with the same methods applied to non-MPN patients, including cardiac catheterization, thrombolysis, heparinization, and warfarin. These treatments need to be instituted judiciously as the risk of bleeding might be high, particularly with extreme thrombocytosis or hyperviscosity. The hemoglobin should be controlled with phlebotomy. Whether the platelet count should be controlled with plateletpheresis or with cytoreductive agents in the setting of acute thrombosis and the optimal target platelet count are controversial. Concurrent with introducing hydroxyurea in all such cases, we generally recommend plateletpheresis in instances of life-threatening thrombosis (or bleeding) with platelets above 1500 × 10^9/L, to achieve a target platelet count below 600 × 10^9/L. DDAVP, Humate P (vWF/FVIII concentrate), or cryoprecipitate may be helpful to control hemorrhage in patients with acquired type 2 vWD. Antiplatelet and anticoagulant drugs should be discontinued in the face of bleeding.

PROGNOSIS

Older patients with PV can expect a normal life expectancy if they adhere to treatment. Young adults can expect long-term survival, but their life expectancy is still reduced compared to age-matched healthy populations. The survival with ET is likewise long, but reduced after the first decade of disease. The prognosis with PMF is generally poorer and may be estimated using the International Working Group for Myelofibrosis Research and Treatment score, or for adults < 56 years old, the Cervantes scoring system; they take into account factors such as anemia, constitutional symptoms, low or high white count, and blast percentage in the blood. Cytogenetic aberrations do not predict progression to AML, progression to fibrosis, or survival in PV and ET, but they are predictive in PMF.

SECTION 7: NON-HODGKIN LYMPHOMA

Non-Hodgkin lymphomas are clinically and pathologically heterogeneous and their presenting signs and symptoms protean. Some are indolent diseases which, untreated, progress over years. Others are aggressive neoplasms that can take the patient's life in a matter of weeks. The propensity for extranodal and secondary CNS dissemination depends on the histologic subtype and the patient's underlying immune status (eg, concurrent HIV infection, post transplant immunosuppression, congenital immunodeficiency syndromes). The importance of obtaining appropriate biopsy material to facilitate a timely and accurate histologic diagnosis cannot be overstated.

PATHOGENESIS

For most patients diagnosed with non-Hodgkin lymphoma, known risk factors are absent and the underlying etiology remains elusive. Well-established risk factors for the development of non-Hodgkin lymphomas include prior exposure to ionizing radiation, congenital and acquired immunodeficiency states (eg, post-transplant lymphoproliferative disorders [PTLD], HIV-associated lymphoma), and a variety of infectious agents. Examples of the latter include the association of (1) Epstein-Barr virus (EBV) with nasal T/NK cell lymphoma, endemic Burkitt lymphoma, HIV-associated lymphoma, and PTLD among others; (2) hepatitis C with splenic marginal zone lymphoma; (3) human herpes virus 8 (HHV-8) with Castleman disease and primary effusion lymphoma; (4) human T cell lymphotropic virus 1 (HTLV-1) with adult T cell leukemia/lymphoma; and (5) bacterial infections such as *Helicobacter pylori*, *Chlamydia*, and *Borrelia burgdorferi* with marginal zone lymphomas in the gastrointestinal tract, eye, and skin respectively. Pesticide and herbicide exposure has been linked to the higher incidence of NHL in agricultural workers and rural populations.

Many lymphomas are marked by characteristic and even diagnostic chromosome translocations. Typically, the promoters belonging to the immunoglobulin heavy chain gene (IgH) on chromosome 14q32, the kappa light chain gene on 2p12, or the lambda light chain gene on 22p11 are translocated to a partner chromosome where they upregulate transcription of a known or putative oncogene. Common examples include follicular lymphoma t(14;18), mantle cell lymphoma t(11;14), and Burkitt lymphoma t(8;14) that involve the genes for bcl-2, bcl-1, and c-myc respectively.

CLASSIFICATION AND STAGING

Non-Hodgkin lymphomas (NHL) are classified according to the 2008 WHO Classification of Tumours of Haematopoietic and Lymphoid Tissues. NHL is broadly classified into B cell neoplasms that comprise approximately 85–90% of cases, and T cell/NK cell neoplasms that account for the remaining 10–15%. More than 50 different lymphoma subtypes are now recognized, exclusive of Hodgkin lymphoma and plasma cell neoplasms; however more than 60% of cases are due to the two most common varieties: diffuse large B cell lymphoma (an aggressive subtype) and follicular lymphoma (an indolent B cell neoplasm). It is essential that sufficient tissue be obtained from an adequate biopsy to allow accurate diagnosis of the specific lymphoma subtype; not infrequently, more than one attempt at biopsy is needed. Once an accurate histologic diagnosis of NHL is made, staging investigations, including at a minimum CT scanning of the chest, abdomen, and pelvis and unilateral bone marrow aspirate and biopsy, are generally performed. NHL is staged according to the Cotswolds Modification of the Ann Arbor System (**Figure 179-4**).

CLINICAL PROGNOSTIC SCORES

Relapse-free and overall survival for patients diagnosed with NHL can be estimated using one of several clinical prognostic scores. In general, these prognostic models are developed and validated by retrospectively analyzing large patient data sets to determine pretreatment clinical factors that correlate with clinical outcomes. The original International Prognostic Index (IPI) evaluated patients with aggressive histology lymphoma treated with anthracycline-containing chemotherapy. Ultimately, five equally weighted factors were independently associated with poor patient outcomes and included in the IPI score. One point is assigned for each of the following: age greater than 60, ECOG performance status 2 or greater, LDH above the upper limit of normal, stage III or IV disease, and two or more extranodal sites. Patients are assigned to one of four risk groups based upon the number of factors present at diagnosis as follows: low (zero or one factor present), low-intermediate (two factors), high-intermediate (three factors), and high risk (four or five factors). The IPI provides substantially more prognostic information than disease stage alone and has subsequently been applied to other patient and histologic subgroups. Examples that illustrate the application of the IPI are shown in **Table 179-2**.

Recently, a number of disease-specific prognostic scores have been developed that have improved prognostic discrimination compared with the IPI. The most commonly used in clinical practice is the follicular lymphoma IPI (FLIPI), which assigns 1 point for the number of involved nodal areas (≤4 vs. ≥5), elevated LDH, age ≥60 years, stage III or IV disease, and hemoglobin < 120 g/L.

For aggressive diseases, progression free survival and overall survival times are similar because second and third-line "salvage" treatment is often unsuccessful. By contrast, for indolent diseases, overall survival far exceeds progression free survival because although incurable, the lymphoma can usually be controlled with subsequent lines of treatment and patients might experience long survivals despite persistent disease.

ESSENTIAL INVESTIGATIONS

The evaluation of a patient with suspected or confirmed lymphoma begins with a thorough history, focused on presenting and associated symptoms (eg, B symptoms), risk factors, and performance status, and a complete physical exam with attention to node-bearing areas (including Waldeyer ring), liver, and spleen size, CNS, and testicular exam. Routine laboratory tests should include CBC with differential white count and examination of a peripheral blood smear, chemistry including electrolytes, renal function and liver profile, LDH, calcium, albumin, phosphate, uric acid, serum protein electrophoresis, beta-2 microglobulin, hepatitis B, hepatitis C, and HIV testing, and exclusion of pregnancy in women of child-bearing age. An echocardiogram or resting radionucleotide scan should confirm an adequate ejection fraction prior to instituting anthracycline chemotherapy. CT of the chest, abdomen, and pelvis with contrast is appropriate for most types of lymphoma. Imaging of the head and neck with CT or MRI are appropriate in selected cases as dictated by the clinical presentation. Diagnostic lumbar puncture is recommended for symptoms referable to the CNS (following CT head to exclude increased intracranial pressure), and for patients with specific histologic subtypes or presenting features associated with increased risk for CNS involvement (eg, Burkitt lymphoma, lymphoblastic lymphoma, aggressive histology lymphomas with paranasal/sinus, testicular, or diffuse marrow involvement). Endoscopic evaluation of the GI tract should be considered for patients with mantle cell lymphomas and for patients with involvement of Waldeyer ring because of a high incidence of simultaneous involvement at distant gastrointestinal sites.

An abnormal lymph node should be excised or involved tissue (liver, lung) should be biopsied. Although fine needle aspiration biopsy (FNAB) may be able to distinguish lymphoma from carcinoma if there is suspicion of the latter, it has no role in the investigation of suspected lymphoma because the material obtained through this approach is invariably insufficient to provide accurate histologic classification. We recommend proceeding directly to excision of a palpably enlarged lymph node when suspicion of lymphoma exceeds that of metastatic carcinoma or other neoplasm. In cases in which palpable nodes are absent and a more invasive surgical procedure would be required to obtain an excisional biopsy (eg, laparotomy/mediastinoscopy), image-guided percutaneous large bore core biopsies are often attempted first. However, because the histologic pattern of disease relative to the architecture of a normal lymph node is often crucial for accurate diagnosis and because sampling errors may occur, core biopsy is more likely to lead to nondiagnostic sampling compared with an excisional node biopsy. To allow for determination of immunophenotype by flow cytometry, a portion

Stage I	Involvement of a single lymph node region (I) or single extralymphatic site (IE)
Stage II	Involvement of two or more lymph node regions on the same side of the diaphragm, with (IIE) or without (II) limited contiguous extension into an extralymphatic organ or structure.
Stage III	Involvement of lymph node regions on both sides of the diaphragm which may include spleen (IIIS) or limited contiguous extension into an extralymphatic organ or structure (IIIE).
Stage IV	Diffuse or disseminated involvement of one or more extralymphatic tissues with or without lymphatic involvement
• *All cases are subclassified to indicate the absence (A) or presence (B) of systemic symptoms during the 6 months prior to diagnosis (unexplained fever, night sweats, or weight loss > 10% of body weight)* • *The subscript 'X' is used if bulky disease is present (nodal mass > 10 cm in maximal dimension or a mediastinal mass ≥ one-third of the internal transverse diameter of the thorax at the T5/6 level on imaging).*	

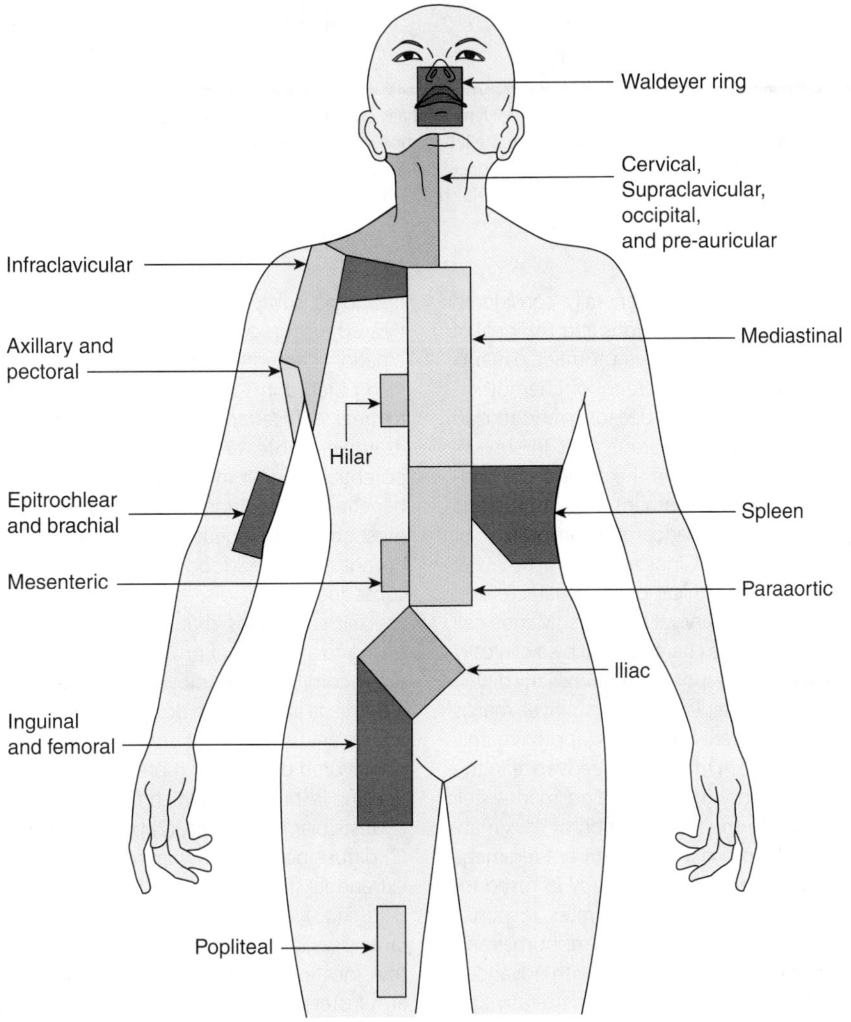

Figure 179-4 *Nodal areas for staging Non-Hodgkin and Hodgkin Lymphoma (figure) and the Ann Arbor staging system with Cotswolds modifications (table). (Modified from http://en.wikipedia.org/wiki/File:Lymph_node_regions.svg. Accessed July 24, 2011.)*

of the biopsy sample should be sent directly to the pathology lab without being placed in formaldehyde.

TREATMENT

Indolent lymphomas

The treatment of indolent NHL is dictated primarily by histologic subtype, disease stage, and patient factors such as presence or absence of symptoms and comorbid illnesses. This group of diseases includes follicular lymphoma, mantle cell lymphoma, marginal zone lymphomas, small lymphocytic lymphoma, lymphoplasmacytic lymphoma/Waldenstrom macroglobulinemia, and hairy cell leukemia, among others. A detailed discussion of specific treatment approaches and chemotherapy regimens for each subtype is beyond the scope of this chapter; however it is useful to review guiding principles in the management of such patients. Patients with localized disease (ie, stage I or II) are generally offered involved field radiation therapy with the potential for long-term disease-free survival and possibly

TABLE 179-2 Utility of the International Prognostic Index

Peripheral T Cell Lymphoma: Outcome According to the IPI

Risk group	Number of factors	Portion of patients	Five-year failure-free survival	Five-year overall survival
Low	0, 1	28%	35%	52%
Low-intermediate	2	35%	16%	33%
High-intermediate	3	22%	13%	16%
High	4, 5	15%	8%	13%

Diffuse Large B Cell Lymphoma Treated with R-CHOP: Outcome According to the Revised IPI

Risk group	Number of factors	Portion of patients	Four-year progression-free survival	Four-year overall survival
Very good	0	10%	94%	94%
Good	1, 2	45%	80%	79%
Poor	3, 4, 5	45%	53%	55%

Data from Savage KJ, Harris NL, Vose JM, et al. ALK⁻ anaplastic large-cell lymphoma is clinically and immunophenotypically different from both ALK⁺ ALCL and peripheral T-cell lymphoma, not otherwise specified: report from the International Peripheral T-Cell Lymphoma Project. *Blood.* 2008;111(12):5496–5504 and Sehn LH, Berry B, Chhanabhai M, et al. The revised International Prognostic Index (R-IPI) is a better predictor of outcome than the standard IPI for patients with diffuse large B-cell lymphoma treated with R-CHOP. *Blood.* 2007;109(5):1857–1861.

cure. Advanced stage disease (stage III/IV) is generally considered incurable with available chemotherapeutic options and the goal of treatment is primarily to alleviate symptoms. Asymptomatic patients are managed with clinical observation and deferral of chemotherapy until symptomatic disease progression because randomized controlled trials have not demonstrated improvement in survival or quality of life with immediate treatment. In the setting of symptomatic disease, (for example, the development of symptomatic lymph node or spleen enlargement, presence of B symptoms), or progressive cytopenias, chemotherapy is indicated. In most cases, response rates are excellent and the clinical course characterized by prolonged disease-free and overall survival (ie, years). Mantle cell lymphoma is a notable exception that is characterized by a clinically aggressive course with relatively brief response duration, early development of chemo-resistance, and median overall survival that is significantly shorter than related indolent histologies (approximately 3–4 years vs. 8–10 years respectively). A major recent advance in the management of indolent B-cell lymphomas including mantle cell lymphoma has been achieved with the incorporation of rituximab, a monoclonal anti-CD20 antibody, into first-line treatment regimens (chemo-immunotherapy) and as maintenance therapy in responding patients. This approach has improved response rates, response duration, and survival across the spectrum of B-cell lymphomas and is now considered standard. Unfortunately, patients with advanced stage indolent lymphoma invariably relapse following therapy and require sequential chemo-immunotherapeutic protocols associated with successively shorter treatment-free intervals before the development of chemo-resistance or large cell transformation. The role of autologous stem cell transplantation in selected patients as part of first-line treatment (mantle cell lymphoma) or as treatment for relapsed disease (follicular lymphoma) is evolving rapidly. Allogeneic stem cell transplant is associated with a strong "graft-versus-lymphoma" effect in indolent subtypes; however, it is associated with substantial toxicity related to infections and graft-versus-host disease and is therefore reserved for a highly selected population of younger, fit patients with relapsed/refractory disease.

Aggressive lymphomas

Treatment decisions for aggressive lymphomas are based on whether the disease is limited or advanced, in addition to the histologic subtype. Patients with adequate cardiac function are treated using cyclically administered anthracycline-based combination chemotherapy with curative intent. Radiation therapy is incorporated in specific instances. NCCN-endorsed strategies used to treat diffuse large B cell lymphoma (DLBCL) serve as a useful example (**Table 179-3**). Patients diagnosed with DLBCL have the potential to recur in the CNS. Patients at particularly high risk may benefit from additional therapy directed toward the CNS because most chemotherapeutic drugs commonly used to treat lymphoma do not cross the blood brain barrier sufficiently to protect against subsequent CNS disease. The optimal treatment regimens and specific subgroups that warrant prophylaxis remain controversial owing to a paucity of prospective and randomized clinical trials. The most commonly employed strategies include repeated doses of intrathecal and/or high dose systemic methotrexate; however, other agents are used and schedules vary widely. Whole brain radiation is not favored because of more frequent and long-term neurotoxicity. Specific instances in which CNS prophylaxis is considered include (1) testicular lymphoma, (2) paranasal, sinus, or orbital involvement, (3) diffuse bone marrow involvement, and (4) high IPI and multiple extranodal sites.

Burkitt lymphoma is a highly aggressive subtype that warrants special consideration. Classically associated with a t(8;14) translocation involving the c-myc gene, Burkitt lymphoma proliferates faster than any other mature B-cell neoplasm. The importance of CNS prophylaxis is universally accepted in the case of Burkitt lymphoma when the risk of CNS involvement or recurrence is so high that treatment directed to the CNS is routinely included in regimens used to treat this particular subtype. Patients with limited, low risk disease may receive an abbreviated course of intensive chemotherapy (eg, CODOX-M), and approximately 80% of younger such patients will be cured. By contrast, those with high risk disease receive a longer course of intensive treatment (eg, CODOX-M/IVAC) with long-term remission and cure achieved in approximately 60% of those younger than 60 years. Patients with Burkitt lymphoma have a particularly high risk of severe tumor lysis syndrome and require careful management to prevent this complication; rasburicase is useful in this instance.

Unique approaches and treatment protocols also apply to the management of cutaneous lymphomas and primary CNS lymphoma

TABLE 179-3 NCCN Version 3.2011 Strategies to Treat Diffuse Large B-Cell Lymphoma

Stage and Presentation	Strategy (and Level of Evidence)
Limited (stage I or II) without bulky* adenopathy, B symptoms† or elevated LDH	Three cycles of R-CHOP followed by RT, (30–36 Gy if CR, 40–50 Gy if residual disease; category 2A) or six cycles of R-CHOP with or without RT (category 2B for RT after six chemotherapy cycles)
Limited disease with poor risk factors (elevated LDH, stage II disease, age >60, ECOG performance status ≥2)	As above (all category 2A)
Bulky* stage I or II disease	Six cycles of R-CHOP followed by RT (category 1)
Progressive disease during first-line chemotherapy	Switch to salvage chemotherapy followed by an autologous stem cell transplant with or without RT to previously involved sites (category 1 for autologous transplant if CR or PR is achieved after salvage chemotherapy), or enter a clinical trial (category 2A). If not a transplant candidate, choices include single-agent rituximab or lenalidomide (for patients with non-germinal center DLBCL), certain multiagent regimens, or clinical trials (category 2A).
Advanced disease (Stage III or IV, B symptoms†)	Six to eight cycles of R-CHOP (category 1), possibly followed by radiation to sites of prior bulk (category 2B for radiation)

*Bulk is defined as a mass ≥10 cm, but chest masses ≥ one-third the thoracic diameter may be considered for radiation too.
†Patients with B symptoms are generally considered to have advanced disease, even if apparently limited stage, although this is not explicitly stated in the NCCN guideline. Consult the NCCN guidelines at http://www.nccn.org/professionals/physician_gls/f_guidelines.asp.
Gy, Gray; R-CHOP; rituximab, cyclophosphamide, doxorubicin, vincristine ("Oncovin"), prednisone administered every three weeks, RT; Radiation treatment.

among others. The specifics are beyond the scope of this chapter. Aggressive histology T cell lymphomas are managed with similar principles as their B-cell counterparts. However, in many instances they are associated with an inferior prognosis.

The management of relapsed or refractory aggressive histology lymphoma remains challenging. Younger, fit patients who respond to second-line chemotherapy are treated with high dose chemotherapy followed by autologous stem cell transplant; approximately 40–50% will achieve long-term remission and cure. Patients not eligible for transplant and those not responsive to second-line chemotherapy have a poor prognosis and are generally treated with palliative measures emphasizing gentler chemotherapeutic regimens and radiation therapy. Allogeneic transplants for relapsed transformed or aggressive lymphoma are still considered experimental and outcomes have been poor.

RESPONSE ASSESSMENT

The reader is referred to internationally agreed-upon criteria for response assessment (Cheson, *Journal of Clinical Oncology*, 2007;25:579–586). Response is usually assessed with imaging studies midway through a planned course of therapy (eg, after three cycles of R-CHOP for DLBCL) and sometimes after only a single cycle of therapy (eg, for Burkitt lymphoma) to guide the decision of whether to continue with the planned treatment (in the case of a good response), to extend the planned treatment (eg, from six to eight cycles, in the case of a slow or partial response), or to switch to a salvage regimen (in the case of progressive or chemo-refractory disease).

Often, residual masses are visible on CT at the end of therapy. These masses may signify fibrosis or persistent lymphoma. While tissue biopsy remains the gold standard, positron emission tomography (CT/PET) scanning is increasingly popular for end-of-treatment evaluation of DLBCL and Hodgkin lymphoma (HL). Pretreatment PET is recommended for these two entities to serve as a basis for comparison. For now, interim PET scanning should be limited to clinical trials. To be designated in complete remission, complete disappearance of lymphoma-related symptoms, biochemical abnormalities (eg, increased LDH), and clinically and radiographically detectable disease is required. (In certain situations, PET-negative residual masses are compatible with CR.)

POST-TREATMENT MONITORING

Each type of NHL has a characteristic interval in which relapses tend to occur. For example, most DLBCL relapses occur within two to three years of achieving remission. Burkitt lymphoma tends to relapse within two years. The median time to progressive or relapsed follicular lymphoma after modern rituximab-containing therapy is approximately four to five years. Patients are generally monitored with a clinical exam and routine laboratory investigations every three months for two years, then every six months for three years. Outside a clinical trial, there is no role for routine surveillance CT or PET scanning. Beyond five years the risk of recurrence is likely sufficiently low that patients are deemed cured and follow-up may revert to the primary care physician for ongoing monitoring of treatment-related late effects. Regular, lifelong monitoring of the CBC is required to detect early myelodysplasic syndrome. The risk of secondary MDS/AML varies, depending on the specific treatment regimen. Patients who received radiation therapy as part of their treatment are at increased risk of early atherosclerotic vascular disease and second malignancies within exposed tissues. As a result, aggressive management of cardiovascular risk factors and strict adherence to cancer screening guidelines are essential.

SECTION 8: CLASSIC HODGKIN LYMPHOMA

Hodgkin lymphoma is characterized by contiguous disease progression from one lymph node region to adjacent regions. This distinguishes it from NHL, which frequently involves distant, noncontiguous sites. Pathologic and epidemiologic features also distinguish the two major groups. While therapeutic approaches are similar, different drug combinations are required.

PATHOGENESIS

Hodgkin lymphoma (HL) is distinguished from NHL by the Reed-Sternberg cell, a large binucleated or multinucleated germinal-center derived B cell with a characteristic immunophenotype (CD15 and CD30 positive). Reed-Sternberg cells are clonal and neoplastic. However, they tend to be scantily distributed in the abnormal lymph node. The surrounding inflammatory reaction is the more prominent feature. The WHO classifies classic HL into four subtypes according to the inflammatory response. The evidence for a microbiologic trigger includes expression of EBV proteins in 30–50% of Western HL patients and virtually all HIV-associated HL, an association with antecedent infectious mononucleosis, and a high incidence among HIV positive patients that is unaffected by HAART. Nodular lymphocyte-predominant Hodgkin lymphoma (NLPHL) differs from classic HL in important clinical and phenotypic ways. NLPHL will not be addressed here.

CLINICAL PRESENTATION

Typical presentations include an asymptomatic neck or supraclavicular mass, B symptoms, or alcohol-induced pruritis or pain. A mediastinal mass should raise suspicion for HL, but the pathologist must be careful to differentiate it from primary mediastinal large B-cell lymphoma, T-cell lymphomas, and overlap lymphomas.

DIAGNOSTIC WORKUP

An adequate lymph node or tissue biopsy is essential. Pretreatment CT and gallium or PET scans are required for accurate staging and to evaluate response. A bone marrow aspiration and biopsy is routinely performed for staging purposes, although marrow involvement is rare in the absence of advanced stage, B symptoms, cytopenias, or HIV positivity. Bone scans are indicated if the patient endorses bone pain. Lumbar puncture is not required. The erythrocyte sedimentation rate (ESR) should be measured as part of risk assessment; an elevated ESR is a poor prognostic marker. In anticipation of anthracycline and bleomycin-containing chemotherapy, baseline evaluation of left ventricular function and pulmonary function studies are recommended. The remaining investigations are as outlined for NHL. Staging is performed according to the Ann Arbor system with Cotswolds modifications (Figure 179-4).

NATURAL HISTORY

At diagnosis, HL is usually a slow-growing malignancy. It is not uncommon for a lymph node involved by HL to wax and wane in size over time. However, the disease eventually spreads through contiguous nodal regions. This is in contradistinction to NHL, which can seemingly "skip" to distant nodal or extranodal sites. Modern treatment regimens are associated with high cure rates and aim to minimize late morbidity and mortality due to the late effects of treatment, particularly cardiovascular disease and second cancers associated with radiation therapy. Relapsed disease often behaves aggressively and is frequently difficult to treat, thus disease control remains a priority in initial treatment decisions.

TREATMENT

Accurate staging is key to selecting the optimal therapeutic approach. Criteria for "limited stage" include stage I or II disease without any bulky disease or B symptoms. Bulky stage I/II, stage III or IV, or B symptoms assign patients to the "advanced disease" group. European criteria for "favorable early stage" disease include stage I or II disease, age < 50 years, absence of B symptoms, absence of bulky mediastinal disease, normal ESR, and fewer than four involved sites. The remaining patients with stage I or II disease are considered to have "unfavorable early stage disease."

Current management of limited stage and advanced disease has evolved through a series of well-conducted trials. Patients with limited stage disease are usually treated with combined modality therapy consisting of three to four cycles of adriamycin, bleomycin, vinblastine, and dacarbazine (ABVD) plus involved field radiation. Ongoing studies aim at defining algorithms for risk-adapted therapy (based on CT/PET evaluation after two cycles of ABVD) and at testing reduced radiation doses, narrower radiation fields, and the potential to eliminate radiation entirely in selected favorable risk subgroups. Treatment of advanced disease usually consists of six to eight cycles of ABVD chemotherapy. More aggressive chemotherapeutic regimens may improve disease-free survival at the expense of increased toxicity, including secondary acute leukemia.

Younger (eg, < age 65), fit patients with chemo-sensitive systemic relapse are candidates for potentially curative high dose chemotherapy and autologous stem cell transplant. For transplant ineligible patients, options included radiation, palliative chemotherapy, and/or clinical trials. Experience with allogeneic stem cell transplant is limited and outcomes have been poor.

Bleomycin toxicity

The potential for patients to develop life-threatening pulmonary toxicity is a major limitation of bleomycin therapy. Bleomycin is inactivated in vivo by bleomycin hydrolase, an enzyme that is poorly expressed in lung and skin tissues and a fact that may be responsible for the organ specific drug toxicity. The clinical presentation varies, depending on the type of lung injury; bleomycin-induced interstitial lung disease typically presents subacutely one to six months post therapy, while hypersensitivity pneumonitis may develop and progress more rapidly. Patients presenting with dyspnea, nonproductive cough, chest discomfort, unexplained fever or a large A-a gradient should be evaluated with a chest X-ray and PFTs if they have received bleomycin. Bilateral reticular or nodular opacification without pleural effusions is the most frequent CXR finding, but alveolar infiltrates or a normal CXR do not exclude the diagnosis. The first PFT abnormality is reduced D_LCO, which may progress to a restrictive pattern. Prednisone 1 mg/kg or IV equivalent should be instituted immediately. Hypersensitivity pneumonitis is more responsive to steroids than interstitial pulmonary fibrosis. In cases of suspected toxicity, further bleomycin is contraindicated.

Prognosis

For early stage disease, long-term progression or event-free survival is achieved in 81% to 97% of patients across studies and overall survival exceeds 90%. In advanced stage disease, anticipated survival varies widely and is best predicted using the Hasenclever score. Between 10% and 30% of patients relapse, depending on initial disease stage, bulk, and therapy.

Monitoring post therapy

After completing treatment, patients are clinically monitored for relapse every two to four months for one year, then every three to six months for three to five years. Importantly, the risk of death from other causes surpasses the risk of death from HL at 15 years. Secondary breast and thyroid carcinomas are common after radiation to the mediastinum and neck respectively. Hypothyroidism occurs in half of patients treated with neck radiation. They should be given sufficient doses of thyroxine to suppress the TSH to low-normal to minimize the risk of stimulating thyroid cancer. Breast self-exam and serial MRI or mammography are indicated within 8 to 10 years of radiation therapy or when a woman turns 40 (whichever comes first). In patients who were younger than 30 at the time of radiation, the incidence of breast cancer exceeds 30% by age 40. Lung cancer may be detected by surveillance CXRs. Smoking should be avoided. The lifelong incidence of other solid tumors is likewise increased. Coronary artery disease, pericardial disease, and myocardial damage are late manifestations of radiation and/or anthracycline chemotherapy. Secondary AML is less common with ABVD than with previous alkylator-based regimens. Radiation also contributes to the risk of AML. Dental follow-up is required for patients who received high neck radiation. Vaccinations against encapsulated bacteria in those who received splenic irradiation and annual influenza vaccination, especially in patients who received bleomycin, is important. Finally, patients with HL have a higher incidence of subsequent NHL. Any suspected recurrence of HL should be confirmed with a tissue diagnosis.

SECTION 9: PLASMA CELL DYSCRASIAS

Plasma cell dyscrasias include monoclonal gammopathies of undetermined significance (MGUS), multiple myeloma, extramedullary plasmacytoma, solitary plasmacytoma of bone, primary amyloidosis and the heavy and light chain deposition diseases, as well as very rare conditions like heavy chain diseases and POEMS (peripheral neuropathy, organomegaly, endocrinopathy, monoclonal gammopathy, skin changes) syndrome. This section focuses on multiple myeloma.

PATHOGENESIS

Exposure to fertilizers, pesticides, asbestos, aromatic hydrocarbons, other occupational toxins, and ionizing radiation has been linked to development of both MGUS and myeloma. Like other B-cell malignancies so far discussed, myeloma exhibits recurrent translocations involving the immunoglobulin heavy chain locus fused to one of several potential partner genes. Beyond the aberrations detected in the neoplastic plasma cell clones, the development of myeloma is promoted by the bone marrow microenvironment, including IL-6-secreting stromal cells and neoangiogenic endothelial cells. Finally, myeloma cells secrete RANK ligand (RANKL) and induce stromal cells to do the same. RANKL binds RANK (Receptor Activator for Nuclear Factor κ B) on osteoclast precursors and osteoclasts, triggering osteoclast differentiation and activation. Myeloma cells also produce Dickkopf homolog 1 (DKK1) that inhibits osteoblasts. Osteopenia, osteoporosis, and osteolytic bone lesions result.

CLINICAL PRESENTATION

Clinical features are related to skeletal destruction (bone pain, fractures, hypercalcemia), marrow infiltration (anemia), extramedullary plasmacytomas (mass effects, airway compromise), and abnormally low levels of uninvolved immunoglobulins (recurrent infections). Rarely, symptomatic hyperviscosity occurs. This complication is more often seen with IgA myeloma and high IgM levels in Waldenstöm macroglobulinemia (an indolent B-cell lymphoproliferative disease associated with a lymphoplasmacytic marrow infiltrate and a monoclonal IgM paraprotein).

Renal insufficiency most frequently results from light chain casts damaging renal *tubules*. This condition is called "myeloma kidney" and is detected by finding mainly light chain proteinuria in the urine collection. "Light chain deposition disease" can occur with or without concurrent multiple myeloma. LCDD is due to light chain deposits damaging the *glomeruli*. It is detected by finding mainly albumin in the urine collection, sometimes in the nephrotic range. Light chain (AL) amyloidosis can be considered a form of LCDD in which the light chains form insoluble beta-pleated sheets that aggregate into fibrils and stain with Congo red histologically to produce apple green birefringence under polarized light. LCDD generally predominates in the kidneys, although heart and liver may be affected. AL amyloidosis may present with nephrotic syndrome (with or without renal insufficiency), restrictive cardiomyopathy with characteristic interventricular septal thickening, gastrointestinal infiltration with recurrent hematochezia, hepatomegaly and transaminitis, macroglossia, or purpura. Periorbital purpura ("raccoon eyes") precipitated by a valsalva maneuver are rare but characteristic of AL amyloidosis. About 10% of patients with AL amyloidosis have coexisting myeloma, while even fewer have Waldenström macroglobulinemia. Hypercalcemia, dehydration, hyperuricemia, and nonsteroidal anti-inflammatory drugs used for bone pain also contribute to renal dysfunction. Rarely, patients acquire type 2 renal tubular acidosis, a normal anion gap acidosis with bicarbonate wasting above the reabsorptive threshold such that plasma HCO^{3-} usually stabilizes between 12 and 20 mmol/L, sometimes associated with hypophosphatemia, hypouricemia, and glucosuria due to proximal tubule wasting.

DIAGNOSIS

Multiple myeloma will usually yield abnormally elevated IgG (55%) or IgA (25%) in association with kappa or lambda light chains. Light chain-only myeloma occurs in about 15% of patients. IgM myeloma is extremely rare; elevated IgM is more likely due to lymphoplasmacytic lymphoma (called "Waldenström macroglobulinemia" if the level exceeds 30 g/L) or other NHL. Monoclonality must be confirmed with serum or urine protein electropheresis and the heavy and light chain isotype must be confirmed with immunofixation. Approximately 15% of patients will manifest light chain proteinuria without concurrent abnormalities on serum protein electrophoresis, so it is important to order urine free light chains when considering the diagnosis. Polyclonal immunoglobulin elevations may be due to underlying infection, connective tissue disease, or cirrhosis. Serum free light chains (kappa or lambda chains not associated with a heavy chain) are a new, very sensitive test for plasma cell dyscrasias. Approximately 70% of previously-designated nonsecretory myeloma actually does secrete excess monoclonal kappa or lambda light chain and can be detected by this assay. True nonsecretory myeloma is rare. Similarly, if the serum protein electrophoresis indicates a monoclonal peak in the gamma region but the standard immunofixation is negative for heavy chains, the immunology laboratory should perform immunofixation with antibodies to IgD and IgE heavy chains to exclude the unusual instance of IgD or IgE secreting myeloma (< 1%). Biclonal gammopathies (eg, monoclonal IgG-kappa and IgG-lambda or IgG and IgA) occur in approximately 1% of patients. The monoclonal component should be quantitated at diagnosis and a 24-hour urine collection should measure light chain excretion, realizing that it may be less reliable than the serum free light chain level in patients with significant renal impairment. Nonetheless, the two tests are complementary.

Evaluation should minimally include a CBC, assessment of renal function (including a measured creatinine clearance if the serum creatinine is elevated), determination of the presence and extent of proteinuria (light chains are not detected by urine dip stick, but the presence of albumin and other filtered proteins may point to light chain deposition disease or amyloidosis), a skeletal survey (plain radiographs of the skull, ribs, spine, pelvis, bilateral humeri, and femurs), and a bone marrow aspirate and biopsy. MRI of the head, spine, and pelvis is advisable in patients suspected of harboring a solitary plasmacytoma, to exclude multiple plasmacytomas.

If these tests are normal, the diagnosis of MGUS is more likely but semiannual or annual follow-up should be arranged. A bone marrow examination does not necessarily need to be performed in cases in which MGUS is very likely, but if the monoclonal component exceeds 10 to 15 g/L or the serum kappa or lambda free light chain is markedly elevated, it is recommended. Cytogenetic abnormalities are common in MGUS and cannot distinguish MGUS from myeloma. When myeloma is diagnosed, the albumin and beta-2 microglobulin levels are important for estimating prognosis.

The WHO defines symptomatic plasma cell myeloma as the presence of monoclonal immunoglobulin in the serum and/or urine (generally > 30 g/L for IgG and > 25 g/L for IgA, but no lower limit is specified), clonal plasma cell expansion in the marrow (generally representing > 10% of nucleated cells) or a plasmacytoma, and related organ damage (hypercalcemia, renal insufficiency attributed to myeloma, anemia, lytic bone lesions or osteoporosis with compression fractures, symptomatic hyperviscosity, amyloidosis or recurrent bacterial infections). Asymptomatic (also called smoldering) myeloma is defined by the serum monoclonal protein exceeding 30 g/L or bone marrow clonal plasma cells exceeding 10% in the absence of related organ damage.

STAGING AND PROGNOSIS

The International Staging System (ISS) is simple and robust. Based on a β2-microglobulin cut-off below 3.5 mg/L or above 5.5 mg/L and serum albumin above or below 3.5 g/dL, patients are stratified into three stages. Median survival is 62, 44, and 29 months for stage I, II, and III disease, respectively.

Patients with IgA myeloma generally experience a more rapid and deeper response to induction therapy, but are also more likely to relapse early and their overall survival is inferior to that of patients with IgG myeloma.

Patients with renal impairment fare worse than those with normal renal function. Plasmablastic morphology confers a worse prognosis compared to finding mature-appearing plasma cell expansion in the marrow. A plasma cell labeling index ≥3% indicates a high proliferation rate and more aggressive disease. Elderly patients are more likely to have indolent disease, while younger patients more frequently exhibit high-risk cytogenetics. Patients with plasma cell leukemia ($\geq 2 \times 10^9$/L circulating plasma cells or ≥20% of the white cell differential) face a dismal prognosis; survival is only a few months. Plasma cell leukemia may present *de novo* or evolve from late stage, longstanding myeloma.

TREATMENT

Prevention of renal and musculoskeletal complications

Aminoglycosides and intravenous radiographic contrast dye should be avoided even in myeloma patients with normal renal function. Renal function in myeloma patients is often exquisitely sensitive to even low doses of NSAIDs, which should be avoided.

Bisphosphonates infused intravenously each month sharply reduce skeletal events in patients with lytic bone lesions. Osteonecrosis of the jaw is an infrequent complication of bisphosphonate therapy. The risk should be minimized by performing any required dental work prior to initiating therapy and by discontinuing infusions after approximately two years. Patients should also be monitored for reversible albuminuria and for the rare occurrence of irreversible renal impairment.

Common medical complications

Patients presenting in renal failure should be aggressively hydrated. They should receive hemodialysis for the usual indications. Plasmapheresis is no longer considered standard care for myeloma-attributed renal failure. Ultrasound of the kidneys, ureters, and bladder is recommended to exclude obstructive uropathy, which may rarely be due to an extramedullary plasmacytoma. NSAIDs and other nephrotoxins should be discontinued. Pyelonephritis should be excluded with urinalysis and culture. Antimyeloma treatment with agents that are safe in renal failure (eg, dexamethasone) should be instituted as expeditiously as possible. Uric acid levels should be monitored and allopurinol, in doses adjusted for the renal impairment, is appropriate, particularly in patients not requiring dialysis.

Patients with multiple myeloma commonly experience acute bone pain, which may respond to steroids and radiation in addition to liberal use of narcotic analgesia. Drugs like pregabalin, carbamazepine, and amitriptyline may ameliorate neuropathic pain but local nerve blocks and epidural anesthesia are sometimes required. Two invasive options are available to patients with vertebral compression fractures. Percutaneous vertebroplasty may be used for vertebral stabilization or for pain relief. The procedure, usually performed by an interventional radiologist, involves injection of polymethylmethyl acrylate (PMMA, a component of bone cement) into the vertebral body. Kyphoplasty is a variation of vertebroplasty in which inflatable bone tamps are placed in the vertebral body. Bone cement is then injected into the bone tamp. The goal is to reexpand the collapsed vertebral body to its original height. No randomized controlled trials of vertebroplasty or kyphoplasty in the myeloma population exist, although large case series are encouraging, so it is not possible to know whether the pain relief and increased mobility often observed within one to two days after injection is due to a placebo effect, local anesthetic injected for the procedure, or the bone cement itself. Although leakage of PMMA is common and usually asymptomatic, serious complications occasionally result, including mobility restriction, pain or radiculopathy, and rarely spinal cord compression.

Anemia may be due to marrow infiltration and to renal impairment. It usually improves with therapy directed at the underlying myeloma, but some patients require recombinant erythropoietin or red cell transfusions. The risks of recombinant erythropoietin in cancer patients are discussed in the chapter on red cell disorders.

Reduced levels of normal immunoglobulins predispose to infection. Periodic IVIG infusions are usually reserved for the occasional patient with severe recurrent infections, as reviewed above for CLL.

Treatment of the myeloma itself

Multiple myeloma is currently considered incurable. The goal of treatment is to prevent complications such as fractures and renal impairment, improve cytopenias, eliminate symptoms like bone pain, and prolong life. Median survival has improved recently due to the development of effective novel agents that have been successfully incorporated into treatment algorithms and include immunomodulatory drugs (thalidomide and lenalidomide), and proteasome inhibitors (bortezomib, tradename Velcade).

Patients are divided into those who are candidates for autologous stem cell transplantation and those who, due to advanced age or comorbidities, are not. Transplant eligible patients are first treated with four to six cycles of induction therapy that ideally includes one or more novel agents often in combination with dexamethasone. Treatment with stem cell toxic medications (eg, melphalan) must be avoided. Responding patients undergo stem cell mobilization into the peripheral blood using drugs such as cyclophosphamide and G-CSF with or without plerixafor (a CXCR4 inhibitor). Stem cells are subsequently harvested by apheresis and cryopreserved for later use. After induction and harvesting are complete, myeloablative "conditioning" chemotherapy (typically melphalan 200 mg/m^2) is administered followed by rescue with autologous stem cell infusion. Patients who achieve only partial remission or stable disease post transplant may be offered a second ("tandem") transplant, while those who achieve a complete or very good partial response (VGPR, defined as ≥ 90% reduction in serum monoclonal protein and < 100 mg/24 hr monoclonal protein in the urine) are unlikely to benefit from a planned tandem transplant. Several trials have evaluated the role of maintenance therapy post transplant and have demonstrated improved progression free survival compared with observation. Options include thalidomide, lenalidomide, prednisone, other novel agents or combinations, and interferon alpha. Despite improved PFS, steroid and thalidomide-based regimens have not been proven to improve overall survival and drug-induced toxicity can significantly impair quality of life. Better-tolerated novel agents such as lenalidomide and bortezomib are currently being evaluated as maintenance regimens. Patients who achieve less than a VGPR post transplant are most likely to benefit from maintenance therapy. Allogeneic transplant is still experimental; studies have yielded conflicting results.

Historically, transplant ineligible patients were treated with melphalan and prednisone (MP), a well tolerated oral regimen associated with median overall survival of approximately three years. The incorporation of novel agents to MP has led to improved overall survival in recent randomized controlled trials and is now considered standard. Examples include MP plus thalidomide (MPT) and MP plus Velcade (MPV); alternative, perhaps more effective combination therapy is rapidly evolving through sequential and parallel clinical trials.

Immunomodulatory drugs carry an increased risk of deep vein thrombosis. Optimal prophylaxis (aspirin, warfarin, or low-molecular-weight heparin) has not been definitively established. However, patients at lower risk for thrombosis are generally candidates for aspirin while higher risk individuals (eg, prior history of venous thrombosis) are usually prophylaxed with anticoagulation (ie, low-molecular-weight heparin [LMWH] or vitamin K antagonists such as warfarin). Thalidomide causes fatigue, sedation, and constipation. Thalidomide and bortezomib both cause peripheral neuropathy that may be painful. The neuropathy is more likely to be irreversible when caused by thalidomide. Toxic epidermal necrolysis is a rare but recognized potentially fatal complication of thalidomide. Lenalidomide can cause significant myelosuppression. Because it is renally excreted, the dose must be reduced for patients with renal impairment and is generally contraindicated in those with renal failure. Bortezomib is also associated with suppressed myelopoiesis, particularly predictable/reversible thrombocytopenia, and may cause acute or delayed gastrointestinal upset.

Judging the survival impact of any therapy is difficult because life may be prolonged by any of various available salvage treatments. Strategies to treat relapsed myeloma are beyond the scope of this text.

A WORD ABOUT SPECIAL PATIENT POPULATIONS

A detailed discussion of special populations will not be embarked upon here. However, the clinician should always bear in mind the uniqueness of individual patients. Populations that merit specific thought include pregnant women, the elderly, those with congenital or acquired immunodeficiency (HIV/AIDS), those with chromosomal fragility syndromes, and those with chronic infections such as hepatitis B that can reactivate during chemotherapy.

CONCLUSION

A hospitalist may be the first physician to investigate an abnormal CBC, a severe metabolic abnormality, an enlarged lymph node, an acute fracture, or a mediastinal mass, and hence to diagnose a hematologic malignancy. Hospitalists are increasingly called upon to manage complications that develop during treatment. This chapter aims to provide a basic knowledge of the different disease entities, drugs employed, and expected disease course, but consultation with a hematologist or oncologist is always advisable, especially if chemotherapy or radiation is to be prescribed.

PRACTICE POINT

- Consultation with a hematologist or oncologist is always advisable for any patient hospitalized for known or suspected malignancies of hematopoietic cell lines. The patient's primary hematologist should also receive complete discharge information, including any complications of treatment discovered during the patient's hospitalization.

SUGGESTED READINGS

Cheson BD, Pfistner B, Juweid ME, et al. Revised response criteria for malignant lymphoma. *J Clin Oncol*. 2007;25:579–586.

Coiffier B, Lepage E, Briere J, et al. CHOP chemotherapy plus rituximab compared with CHOP alone in elderly patients with diffuse large-B-cell lymphoma. *N Engl J Med*. 2002;346:235–242.

Friedman DL and Constine LS. Late effects of treatment for Hodgkin lymphoma. *J Natl Compr Canc Netw*. 2006;4:249–257.

Gafter-Gvili A, Fraser A, Paul M, Leibovici L. Meta-analysis: antibiotic prophylaxis reduces mortality in neutropenic patients. *Ann Intern Med*. 2005;142:979–995.

Grimwade D, Hills RK, Moorman AV, et al. Refinement of cytogenetic classification in acute myeloid leukemia: determination of prognostic significance of rare recurring chromosomal abmormalities among 5876 younger adult patients treated in the United Kingdom Medical Research Council Trials. *Blood*. 2010;116:354–365.

Hallek M, Cheson BD, Catovsky D, et al. Guidelines for the diagnosis and treatment of chronic lymphocytic leukemia: a report from the International Workshop on Chronic Lymphocytic Leukemia updating the National Cancer Institute-Working Group 1996 guidelines. *Blood*. 2008;111:5446–5456.

Hallek M, Fischer K, Fingerle-Rowson G, et al. Addition of rituximab to fludarabine and cyclophosphamide in patients with chronic lymphocytic leukaemia: a randomized, open-label, phase 3 trial. *Lancet*. 2010;376:1122–1124.

Hochhaus A, O'Brien SG, Guilhot F, et al. Six-year follow-up of patients receiving imatinib for the first-line treatment of chronic myeloid leukemia. *Leukemia*. 2009;23:1054–1061.

Kyle RA, Therneau TM, Rajkumar SV, et al. Prevalence of monoclonal gammopathy of undetermined significance. *N Engl J Med*. 2006;354:1362–1369.

Landolfi R, Marchioli R, Kutti J, et al. Efficacy and safety of low-dose aspirin in polycythemia vera. *N Engl J Med*. 2004;350:114–124.

National Comprehensive Cancer Network. Clinical Practice Guidelines in Oncology. Prevention and Treatment of Cancer-Related Infections. v.2.2011, at nccn.org/professionals/physician_gls/pdf/infections.pdf. Accessed July 24, 2011.

Sanz MA, Grimwade D, Tallman MS, et al. Management of acute promyelocytic leukemia: recommendations from an expert panel on behalf of the European LeukemiaNet. *Blood*. 2009;113:1875–1891.

Slichter SJ, Kaufman RM, Assmann SF, et al. Dose of prophylactic platelet transfusions and prevention of hemorrhage. *N Engl J Med*. 2010;362:600–613.

CHAPTER 180

Management of Emergencies in Patients with Hematologic Malignancies

Elizabeth F. Krakow, MD,CM, FRCPC
Graeme Fraser, MD, MSc (HRM), FRCPC

Key Clinical Questions

1. What emergencies might arise at presentation of a hematologic malignancy, and how should they be treated?
2. What emergencies might arise in the course of treatment, and how should they be handled?

INTRODUCTION

This chapter will review common emergencies uniquely associated with hematologic malignancies and their treatment.

TUMOR LYSIS SYNDROME

CASE 180-1

A 30-year-old Caucasian man developed lethargy and nausea. He recently started chemotherapy for Burkitt lymphoma. He was mildly tachycardic, afebrile, and had a large, easily palpable abdominal mass. In addition to anemia and thrombocytopenia, the blood work was notable for potassium of 5.8 mmol/L and creatinine of 3.9 mg/dL (350 umol/L). The nurse reported that he had produced only 200 mL of urine in the previous 8 hours. What other blood tests should be ordered? What measures can be taken to prevent permanent renal failure?

The serum uric acid was 15.6 mg/dL (925 mmol/L), the phosphate is 7.9 mg/dL (2.57 mmol/L), and the calcium was 7.88 mg/dL (1.97 mmol/L). Urinalysis showed marked uric acid crystals. The electrocardiogram was essentially normal. Glucose, insulin and Kayexalate for the hyperkalemia, normal saline 200 mL/h, aluminum hydroxide 60 mL four time a day, and rasburicase 0.2 mg/kg intravenously was administered. A Foley catheter was inserted and the patient was monitored closely for signs of fluid overload. Serum electrolytes and renal function were checked every four hours overnight, and the covering physician alerted the nephrologist and the patient's treating hematologist to the situation.

CASE 180-2

A 56-year-old woman presented to the emergency room for five days of progressive shortness of breath and headache, for which she took aspirin. Her oxygen saturation was 87% on room air, and she was tachycardic, mildly hypotensive, and febrile. Her examiners noted a palpable spleen 4 cm below the costal margin, lower extremities covered in petechia, and engored retinal veins. They did not identify focal neurologic deficits.

Her white count was 135×10^9/L with large, monocytic-appearing blasts on the peripheral blood film, hematocrit 22%, and platelet count 18×10^9/L. Her chemistry profile revealed hyperkalemia, a creatinine double her baseline, a uric acid level of 17 mg/dL, and an INR of 1.5. Her chest X-ray showed diffuse bilateral infiltrates.

Physician orders includec hydroxyurea 3 g orally stat, then 2 g every 8 hours, a platelet transfusion, normal saline at 125 mL/hour (2 L/m^2/day), continuously monitoring O_2 saturation, treatment of the hyperkalemia, and ceftazidime and rasburicase. Unfortunately, while her physicians were arranging transfer to a tertiary care hospital, the patient's level of consciousness deteriorated. A stat brain CT showed a large parietal hemorrhage with midline shift and herniation. The patient was immediately intubated, but the neurosurgeon concluded that

surgical intervention would be futile. Two days later, her family elected to withdraw ventilator support and she passed away in the intensive care unit.

PATHOPHYSIOLOGY

Tumor lysis syndrome (TLS) may occur spontaneously or upon initiation of treatment for hematologic malignancies with high proliferation rates or large tumor burden (as reflected in high lactate dehydrogenase [LDH]), or exquisite sensitivity to chemotherapy, radiation, glucocorticoids, or cytotoxic antibodies. TLS usually occurs within 12 to 72 hours of initiating cytotoxic treatment. Burkitt lymphoma and acute lymphoblastic leukemia (ALL) account for the majority of cases, but TLS is observed frequently with acute myeloid leukemia (AML), aggressive lymphomas like diffuse large B-cell lymphoma (DLBCL) or extensive mantle cell lymphoma, and some newer regimens for chronic lymphocytic leukemia (CLL). Massive tumor lysis releases potassium, phosphate, and nucleic acids in the circulation. Purines are catabolized to uric acid, which may precipitate in renal tubules and lead to acute renal failure.

PREVENTION

It is better to institute preventive measures rather than wait for overt TLS to develop. In patients with spontaneous TLS, it is preferable to defer cytotoxic therapy for a couple days, if possible, until the patient is prehydrated and metabolic derangements are controlled.

Either allopurinol or rasburicase may prevent hyperuricemia. Allopurinol inhibits urate production by blocking xanthine oxidase. Uric acid and, to a lesser degree, xanthine solubility is higher in alkaline urine, so urine alkalinization was traditionally attempted when employing allopurinol to reduce precipitation of uric acid and xanthine crystals in the renal tubules, but is no longer recommended (discussed in more detail later in this chapter). Allopurinol does not decrease already-formed uric acid and takes several days to meaningfully decrease hyperuricemia. Rasburicase is a recombinant urate oxidase enzyme that catalyses the conversion of uric acid to allantoin, an inactive metabolite of purine metabolism; allantoin is 5 to 10 times more soluble than uric acid, so its renal excretion is more effective. Rasburicase is effective within four hours of administration and is the treatment of choice in patients with marked hyperuricemia (>450 umol/L or >7.5 mg/dL) or in patients deemed at high risk for TLS. Note that rasburicase continues to degrade uric acid while the blood sample is sitting at room temperature, so it is important to keep the sample on ice to avoid spuriously low values in patients who have received this drug. Rare instances of hemolytic anemia, methemoglobinemia, and hypersensitivity are reported. The drug is contraindicated in those with glucose-6-phosphate dehydrogenase (G6PD) deficiency.

The best choice of intravenous (IV) fluids is controversial. Urinary alkalinization to a minimum pH of 6.5–7.0 using IV sodium bicarbonate (eg, 3 ampules = 150 mEq $NaHCO_3$ added to each liter of 5% dextrose in water solution [D5W]) or acetazolamide was previously recommended in patients treated with allopurinol. However, an animal study suggests that high tubular flow, whether induced by water or solute diuresis, is critically important to preventing urate nephropathy while urinary alkalinization plays at most a minor protective role. Current guidelines advise against routine alkalinization because of the lack of evidence of efficacy and the risk of promoting precipitation of calcium-phosphate crystals, but the advisability of alkalinization in patients receiving allopurinol is unclear. Alkalinization is not required in patients receiving rasburicase. In adults, the total fluid intake should be approximately one to two times greater than a standard maintenance IV rate (2–3L/m^2/day) with a goal urine output of 80–100 ml/hr. Diuretics may be used to enhance tubular flow but caution must be exercised to avoid intravascular volume depletion.

TREATMENT

Electrolytes, uric acid, and renal function should be monitored at least one to two times daily until evidence of TLS has resolved. Hyperkalemia should be treated by the usual algorithms. In patients with hyperleukocytosis, blood potassium levels should be measured in the plasma, since serum results may be factitiously high due to potassium release from leukemic blasts during clotting. Alkalinization may be useful in patients with metabolic acidosis; consultation with a nephrologist is advised. Dialysis may be required for any of these metabolic complications.

Patients with asymptomatic hypocalcemia should be closely monitored with serial electrocardiographs (ECGs) and telemetry. Intravenous calcium gluconate or calcium carbonate can worsen nephrocalcinosis, but symptomatic hypocalcemia should be treated. Hypocalcemia can also cause cardiac arrhythmias and tetany. A phosphate binder such as aluminum hydroxide (30–60 mL three to four times a day with meals) prevents and treats hyperphosphatemia. Phosphate precipitates with calcium, resulting in nephrocalcinosis, currently the leading cause of TLS-induced renal failure.

HYPERLEUKOCYTOSIS WITH LEUKOSTASIS

PATHOPHYSIOLOGY

Hyperleukocytosis (white blood cell count $>100 \times 10^9$/L) may present with symptomatic leukostasis. *Leukostasis* refers to impaired microcirculation by leukemic cells resulting in tissue hypoxia. The elaboration of cytokines and toxic metabolic products also contributes to endothelial damage and resulting hemorrhage. Leukostasis is most often seen in myelomonocytic or monocytic AML (FAB M4 or M5) because tissue infiltration by blasts contributes to the pathology. Usually, the circulating AML blast count is above $50–100 \times 10^9$/L. Patients with chronic myeloid leukemia (CML), even in chronic phase, may develop symptomatic leukostasis at white counts above 250×10^9/L. Leukostasis is rare in patients with ALL, even at extremely high blast counts, because lymphoid blasts are less adherent to the endothelium compared with myeloid cells. Hyperleukocytosis related to differentiation therapy of acute promyelocytic leukemia (APL) was discussed in the section on acute myeloid leukemias in Chapter 179.

Clinically, neurologic and pulmonary symptoms usually predominate. The patient may complain of headache, blurred vision, or be confused. Ischemic stroke, often with some hemorrhagic conversion, or primary hemorrhagic stroke may occur. Hypoxia due to impaired pulmonary capillary blood flow, subendocardial ischemia, and congestive heart failure may supervene. Damage to the renal medulla may cause acute renal failure. Priapism may occur. Coagulopathy and frank *disseminated* intravascular coagulation (DIC) are common. Acute mortality is between 20% and 40%.

PREVENTION AND TREATMENT

While awaiting diagnosis, hydroxyurea (4–8 g/day orally in divided doses) for suspected myeloid leukemias or glucocorticoids for suspected lymphoid leukemias should be started. Both may be started if the differentiation between lymphoid and myeloid phenotype is not immediately clear. If oral therapy is not feasible, cytarabine or cyclophosphamide may be given intravenously. Treatment relies on prompt cytoreduction. If the diagnosis is known, the appropriate chemotherapy protocol should be started.

PRACTICE POINT

- For patients with hyperleukocytosis with leukostasis red cell transfusion should be avoided until the blast count is much lower and leukostasis symptoms resolve because they increase blood viscosity. By contrast, correction of coagulopathy is essential.

The role of leukapheresis is controversial. Limited evidence from two retrospective case series suggests a beneficial impact on early mortality but no difference in medium or long-term survival. Leukapheresis should not supplant chemotherapy but may be a valuable temporizing measure. If leukapheresis is chosen, chemotherapy should be given as soon as feasible.

Patients with hyperleukocytosis, and especially those with leukostasis, are at high risk of central nervous system (CNS) leukemia. A diagnostic lumbar puncture should be performed once peripheral blood blasts have cleared. There is a lack of evidence for or against incorporating prophylactic intrathecal chemotherapy in treatment cycles in patients with AML. High-dose IV cytarabine used for consolidation does penetrate the CNS. ALL regimens already incorporate CNS prophylaxis.

Red cell transfusion should be avoided until the blast count is much lower and leukostasis symptoms resolve because they increase blood viscosity. By contrast, correction of coagulopathy is essential. Platelet transfusion should be used liberally because the platelet count is frequently overestimated by automated cell counters due to fragments of blasts. Patients on chronic aspirin or clopidogrel therapy should be assumed to have nonfunctional platelets, and transfusion is advisable. Cryoprecipitate should be transfused to keep fibrinogen above 1 g/L. Frozen plasma should then be used to correct remaining abnormalities in the international normalized ratio (INR) and activated partial thromboplastin time (apt). Anticoagulation therapy should be reversed.

HYPERVISCOSITY

PATHOPHYSIOLOGY

Hyperviscosity is due to high levels of paraprotein causing impaired microcirculation. Waldenström macroglobulinemia with IgM levels above 50 g/L and myeloma with high IgA levels are the usual culprits; monoclonal IgG and light chain gammopathies are rarely implicated. Most symptomatic patients have a serum viscosity level greater than five times that of water (normal serum viscosity is 1.4–1.8 times that of water), while levels above 10 are invariably symptomatic. However, serum viscosity measurements are sometimes unreliable, and treatment may be appropriate at lower viscosity levels in compatible clinical circumstances.

Clinical presentations range from subtle (fatigue, headache, and dizziness) to overt (vertigo, hearing loss due to thrombosis in the inner ear, blurred vision, mucosal hemorrhage, somnolence, congestive heart failure, coma, and seizures). Patients may show nystagmus and sausage-like beading in retinal veins.

TREATMENT

For patients with severe symptoms, plasmapheresis with albumin or saline replacement should be initiated based on the patient's symptoms and not deferred pending the serum viscosity result. One plasma volume exchange should be repeated daily until symptoms subside or until serum viscosity is normal. The elevated serum protein might cause plasma volume expansion. Therefore, traditional formulas tend to underestimate plasma volume in patients with hyperviscosity. IgM is virtually entirely within the intravascular compartment, while the bulk of IgG and IgA is extravascular. Redistribution to the intravascular space may mandate more frequent (eg, twice daily) or extended exchanges over consecutive days. Treatment of the underlying malignancy must be instituted concurrent with plasmapheresis.

NEUROLOGIC COMPLICATIONS

EPIDURAL SPINAL CORD COMPRESSION

The first symptom is usually back pain, which may be exacerbated by coughing, straining, or recumbency. Motor and sensory deficits may develop subsequently with their specific nature dependent upon the anatomic location of compression but commonly include leg weakness or a sensory level. Bowel and/or bladder dysfunction are typically late features of spinal cord compression, including urinary retention as a result of autonomic dysfunction. Myeloma usually causes vertebral body destruction while non-Hodgkin lymphoma (NHL) often reaches the cord from the paraspinal soft tissue by growing through the vertebral foramina, without overt vertebral damage.

Dexamethasone 10–20 mg intravenously followed by 4–10 mg orally or intravenously every 6 hours should be instituted upon suspicion of spinal cord compromise due to the possibility of irreversible neurologic damage. Some clinicians use higher initial doses, particularly in patients with paresis or paralysis. Steroids are tapered after definitive treatment is instituted. Prompt imaging of the cord by magnetic resonance imaging (MRI) (or computed tomography [CT] if MRI is contraindicated or not immediately available) should confirm the diagnosis.

Unlike solid tumors, where neurosurgical decompression may be preferred due to the higher risks of chemotherapy and radiation-resistant disease, hematologic malignancies are often exquisitely sensitive to chemotherapy and local radiation. Surgical management may be appropriate for patients without a histologic diagnosis who present with spinal cord compression, where it can be a definitive therapeutic and diagnostic approach. Nonetheless, radiation is often the treatment of choice when a known hematologic malignancy causes spinal cord compression and should be performed as immediately as possible. Attention to pain control, deep venous thrombosis (DVT) prophylaxis, and constipation round out the supportive care. Myeloma, NHL, and granulocytic sarcomas (extramedullary AML tumors) usually respond well to radiation. Surgery is reserved for unusual cases with primary or secondary local tumor progression after radiation and systemic therapy.

Intramedullary lymphomatous masses are confirmed by gadolinium-enhanced MRI and sometimes by spinal cord biopsy. They are treated in the same fashion as extradural cord compression, but whereas spinal cord compression has little impact on the survival of NHL patients, intramedullary lesions confer poor survival, perhaps because of frequent concurrent widespread disease. AML, especially APL, rarely disseminates inside the spine.

CENTRAL NERVOUS SYSTEM DISEASE

Leptomeningeal disease

Leptomeningeal disease usually presents with cranial nerve palsies and, less frequently, with radicular pain, peripheral nerve deficits, headache, or seizures. Aggressive lymphoma, ALL, and, less often, AML are implicated. Neuroimaging to exclude impending herniation should be performed prior to the diagnostic lumbar puncture. CT is sufficient for this purpose; hence, waiting for MRI availability should not delay the diagnostic lumbar puncture (LP) and immediate instillation of intrathecal chemotherapy. MRI to assess for intracerebral deposits not causing mass effect or for intramedullary deposits can be performed after the LP, if needed. MRI frequently reveals cranial nerve thickening, communicating hydrocephalus, suspicious leptomeningeal or dural enhancement, or spinal nerve root thickening. A normal CSF cell count alone does not exclude leptomeningeal disease. The cell morphology needs to be examined. While LP is the criterion standard, the first LP is only about 70% sensitive for leptomeningeal disease so up to three LPs may be indicated, or the diagnosis may be based on the clinical picture and neuroimaging results. Flow cytometry, immunohistochemistry, or polymerase chain reaction (PCR) should be added to cerebrospinal fluid (CSF) cytology where possible to minimize the false negative rate.

Brain metastases

Lymphoma and leukemia may present with CNS involvement in the setting of a systemic malignancy or as primary CNS neoplasms. Focal neurologic deficits and seizures may result. Even if an LP or biopsy of a CNS lesion is needed to confirm the diagnosis—as for patients without a prior diagnosis of lymphoma or those with AIDS in whom CNS toxoplasmosis is considered—the symptomatic patient should receive high dose glucocorticoids while awaiting the procedure.

Treatment options for leptomeningeal disease and for intraparenchymal metastases include (1) craniospinal irradiation, (2) local radiation to parenchymal masses and symptomatic nerves along with intrathecal or systemic high-dose chemotherapy, such as methotrexate, that crosses the blood-brain barrier, or (3) high-dose systemic chemotherapy alone or with intrathecal chemotherapy. To reduce swelling, systemic corticosteroids should accompany radiation. The prognosis depends on the type of malignancy involving the CNS and on the extent of concurrent extra-CNS disease, but is generally poor.

SUPERIOR VENA CAVA SYNDROME

NHL and T-cell lymphoblastic lymphoma are the usual culprits where hematologic malignancies are responsible. Mediastinal Hodgkin lymphoma very rarely causes superior vena cava (SVC) syndrome. In patients with central lines, differential diagnosis includes SVC thrombosis, which is treated with line removal and anticoagulation.

Patients present with dyspnea and head fullness that may be worse upon bending forward. Physical exam may reveal facial plethora, facial and arm edema, dilated neck and superficial chest veins, and cervical or periclavicular lymphadenopathy. Hoarseness may be due to involvement of the recurrent laryngeal nerve. A chest X-ray confirms a mediastinal mass. Chest CT will show its relation to other mediastinal structures and provide a baseline for response assessment.

Unlike patients with SVC syndrome attributed to solid tumors, those with hematologic neoplasms benefit from upfront glucocorticoids and do not routinely require radiation or endovascular stenting. The proper chemotherapy should be started as soon as the diagnosis is established by tissue pathology. Upfront radiation risks extensive necrosis that makes a tissue diagnosis impossible if there is no other site to supply pathology. As discussed in the section on lymphoma, radiation is frequently used at the end of several cycles of chemotherapy as part of first-line treatment to minimize the risk of relapse.

PRACTICE POINT

- Examples of how treatment significantly differs from that of solid tumors include the SVC syndrome and cord compression. Hematologic neoplasms causing the SVC syndrome benefit from up-front glucocorticoids and do not routinely require radiation or endovascular stenting. Hematologic malignancies causing cord compression are often exquisitely sensitive to chemotherapy and local radiation and do not routinely require neurosurgical decompression.

THROMBOCYTOPENIC BLEEDING

Bleeding patients with thrombocytopenia due to myelosuppressive therapy or bone marrow infiltration require platelet transfusion. Adjuvant hemostatic drugs are often useful. Antifibrinolytic agents include transexamic acid (10 mg/kg intravenously or 1 gram orally every 6 hours, adjusted for renal insufficiency) and ε-aminocaproic acid (100 mg/kg intravenously over 30–60 minutes, then 1–3 g orally every 6 hours). Desmospressin (DDAVP) (3 mcg/kg up to 20 mcg intravenously) is an alternative, but tachyphylaxis develops. Precautions with DDAVP include keeping the patient supine during the infusion due to the risk of hypotension, restricting total fluid intake to 1.5 L/24 hours, using only isotonic IV fluids (including those for medication administration), and monitoring the patient closely for hyponatremia over the next 24 hours.

Splenectomy may be indicated for recurrent thrombocytopenic bleeding where the thrombocytopenia is due to splenomegaly or to idiopathic thrombocytopenic purpura (ITP) refractory to steroids, IV immunoglobulin (IVIG), and lymphoma-directed therapy. Rare patients with myeloproliferative neoplasms (MPN), although not thrombocytopenic, develop an acquired platelet function defect. Such defects can be confirmed with platelet aggregation and secretion tests. Treatment is the same as above including the use of platelet transfusion for severe bleeding. Recombinant activated factor VIIa (Niastase) is not approved for thrombocytopenic bleeding but has been used in life-threatening situations.

DISSEMINATED INTRAVASCULAR COAGULATION

Disseminated intravascular coagulation (DIC) may occur with any acute leukemia but is common in acute promyelocytic leukemia. International guidelines caution against using heparin, tranexamic acid, or other anticoagulant or antifibrinolytic therapy to treat APL-associated DIC. The mainstay of care is repletion of fibrinogen (to > 1–1.5 g/L) with cryoprecipitate followed by correction of persistently abnormal INR and PTT with frozen plasma. For suspected APL-associated DIC, platelets should be maintained $> 20 \times 10^9$/L with transfusion and ATRA (45 mg/m^2/day divided into two doses) should be started immediately, even before the diagnosis is confirmed. In patients with overt bleeding symptoms, transfusional support may need to be intensified to maintain platelet counts $> 30–50 \times 10^9$/L.

HYPERCALCEMIA

Hypercalcemia may be due to osteolysis (myeloma, some cases of NHL), 1,25-dihydroxy vitamin D production (Hodgkin lymphoma, sometimes NHL), ectopic parathyroid-related hormone peptide production (NHL, blast phase CML, or adult T-cell leukemia/lymphoma (ATLL], and acute leukemias), or elaboration of tumor necrosis factor (TNF)-α or other cytokines (ATLL, acute leukemias). Due to nephrogenic diabetes insipidus, most patients are intravascularly volume depleted.

Hypercalcemia should be specifically treated if symptomatic or if the corrected calcium is above 3.5 mmol/L (14 mg/dL). Hydration with normal saline (200–300 mL/hour intravenously, adjusted to maintain urine output 100–150 mL/hour) and bisphosphates (zoledronic acid 4 mg intravenously over 15 minutes or pamidronate 60–90 mg intravenously over 2 hours) are the cornerstones of therapy. Beyond that, a loop diuretic can be added for hypervolemic patients and calcitonin (4 IU/kg subcutaneously every 12 hours as a starting dose, up to 8 IU/kg subcutaneously every 6 hours) can be added for severe hypercalcemia, but tachyphylaxis develops. Glucocorticoids (eg, prednisone 20–40 mg/day for 2–5 days) are useful to impede 1,25-dihydroxy vitamin-D production by lymphoma or myeloma and for myeloma-associated bone pain. Treatment directed at the underlying hematologic malignancy should begin once calcium normalizes.

FEBRILE NEUTROPENIA

Neutropenic patients should be isolated from other hospitalized patients. Visitors and health care workers should observe strict hand washing protocols and wear a mask. In some hospitals, gowns are worn as well. Allogeneic transplant recipients should be placed in rooms with high-efficiency particulate air (HEPA) filters.

Febrile neutropenia is defined as a single temperature greater than or equal to 38.3°C or a temperature of at least 38.0°C sustained for 1 hour in a patient whose neutrophil count is below 0.5×10^9/L or below 1×10^9/L and expected to decline further over the next 48 hours. The history and physical exam should focus on the integrity of intravascular access devices, skin lesions, sinus and pulmonary complaints, oral lesions, pharyngitis, odynophagia, bowels (diarrhea, typhlitis), and perivaginal/perirectal infections. Digital rectal exam is relatively contraindicated, but the perianal area should be inspected and palpated for fluctuance or tenderness; if there is suspicion for a perirectal abscess, its presence can be confirmed by imaging.

The timing of fever relative to the most recent cycle of chemotherapy, prior documented infections and their antibiotic sensitivity profiles, colonization with vancomycin-resistant enterococcus or methicillin-resistant staphylococcus aureus, recent therapeutic or prophylactic antibiotic use, allergies, other reasons for immunodeficiency such as HIV infection, and exposures to sick contacts, pets, travel, tuberculosis, and blood products are all relevant to choosing appropriate empiric therapy.

Even lobar pneumonia may not be apparent on chest X-ray because profound neutropenia might prevent consolidation with pus. Aerobic and anaerobic blood cultures from two peripheral sites or one peripheral site and an indwelling central line, urinalysis, and chest X-ray are essential. The urine should be cultured if the patient is symptomatic or if she has an indwelling bladder catheter, even in the absence of an abnormal urinalysis, since profoundly neutropenic patients might not show white cells in the urine. In the presence of diarrhea, test for enteric pathogens and *Clostridium difficile*. Viral detection by direct fluorescence antigen or PCR and viral cultures should be sent from vesicular or ulcerated skin or mucosal lesions and from the throat or nasopharynx if symptoms suggest respiratory tract infection. Blood cytomegalovirus (CMV) testing (by antigen or DNA PCR methods) should be done in patients treated with alemtuzumab and in stem cell transplant recipients. Indwelling catheter sites that are clearly inflamed should also be swabbed for bacteria and fungus.

Historically, the majority of infections were due to gram-negative bacteria, although recently there has been an increase in documented gram-positive infections. Empiric coverage should follow local hospital guidelines, which take into account institutional prevalence of drug-resistant microbes. Antipseudomonal activity is mandatory. In general, empiric IV monotherapy with ceftazidime, piperacillin/tazobactam, or meropenem are recommended. The tendency now is to avoid aminoglycosides because of potential nephrotoxicity, but the addition of a split-dose aminoglycoside may be appropriate in patients with previously documented multidrug-resistant pseudomonas or suspected meningitis or endocarditis. Drugs targeting staphylococcus, like vancomycin, linezolid, or daptomycin, are not routinely added but may be considered if a catheter-related infection or cutaneous infection with methicillin-resistant *Staphylococcus aureus* (MRSA) is likely or if periorbital cellulitis is present. While most patients will be admitted to the hospital for IV antibiotics and close observation, low-risk patients can be treated as outpatients with oral combinations such as ciprofloxacin 750 mg orally twice a day with amoxicillin/clavulin 875/125 mg orally twice a day, provided the following conditions are fulfilled: quinolone prophylaxis was not employed, the patient was not hospitalized at the time fever initially developed, there is no associated acute or poorly controlled comorbidity, renal and liver function are good and stable, pneumonia or other complex infections are unlikely, mucositis is mild and the patient can tolerate oral medication, mental status is lucid and no new neurologic symptoms are present, hemodynamics and oxygenation are normal, alemtuzumab treatment was not employed, the malignancy is basically controlled, the anticipated duration of severe neutropenia is shorter than seven days, the patient has good performance status, and he or she lives less than one hour from the hospital and has a telephone from which to dial emergency medical services. Ideally, the patient would also live with a responsible adult who can keep an eye on him or her and call emergency medical services or the treating physician should the patient's condition deteriorate. The Multinational Association for Supportive Care in Cancer (MASCC) risk index may also be used to assess the advisability of treating febrile neutropenia in the outpatient setting.

Thrush should be treated with fluconazole initially. Periorbital cellulitis, nasal ulceration, unilateral eye tearing, or suspected mucormycosis should prompt sino-orbital CT or MRI and urgent ear, nose, and throat (ENT) and ophthalmologic consultation, and liposomal amphotericin B should be initiated empirically. Aspergillus and other fungi might cause typical halo signs or cavitary lesions on CT. Serial galactommanan assays are useful to corroborate suspicion for aspergillus but are not routinely available at all centers. Infectious disease consultation should be obtained. Brochoalveolar lavage is useful, but because of tissue tropism and angioinvasion, aspergillus may only be detected on bronchoscopic or transthoracic lung biopsy. Voriconzaole or posaconazole should be initiated if there is strong suspicion for mold infection. Antiviral therapy should be added if there is strong suspicion for viral infection but often can wait for the results of specific tests. Acyclovir is appropriate for herpetic mucositis and skin lesions, while ganciclovir, often with IVIG, is used for CMV pneumonia.

Broad-spectrum antimicrobials should be continued until the absolute neutrophil count recovers to 0.5×10^9/L or higher without ongoing growth factor support and fever and symptoms have resolved. Also, if a specific pathogen or site of infection is identified, a complete course of treatment directed against that organism/site should be completed, even if the neutrophil count recovers before the projected end date. For example, gram-negative bacteremia is usually treated with 10 to 14 days of antibiotics, while *S aureus* endocarditis is usually treated for 4 to 6 weeks. Indwelling vascular catheters should not be removed initially, but if a catheter-related bloodstream bacterial infection fails to clear within approximately 48 hours of appropriate antimicrobial therapy or if the bloodstream infection is caused by *S aureus,* yeast, mold, or nontuberculosis mycobacteria, catheter removal is advised.

The use of granulocyte colony–stimulating factor (G-CSF) or granulocyte-macrophage colony–stimulating factor GM-CSF during episodes of febrile neutropenia slightly shortens the duration of neutropenia and hospitalization, but has no effect on survival. Nonetheless, growth factors may be employed in complicated cases such as pneumonia, multiorgan dysfunction, or hypotension. The use of G-CSF for primary and secondary prophylaxis of febrile neutropenia will not be discussed here. Prophylactic G-CSF aims to avoid delays in the administration of chemotherapy in diseases where higher dose-intensity correlates with improved outcomes. Guidelines from several organizations consider patient age, whether the intent of treatment is curative or palliative, and the incidence of febrile neutropenia related to particular chemotherapeutic regimens in advising on the use of prophylactic G-CSF.

If fever persists for five days or longer without identifying a source of infection, empiric antifungal therapy with an echinocandin is usually initiated, the search for the culprit pathogen(s) and involved sites is repeated, and infectious disease specialists should be consulted. While uncontrolled malignancy or allergy to antibiotics themselves might induce fever, therapy should only be suspended in otherwise-well patients in whom a diligent search for a source of infection (including multiple cultures and CT of the sinuses, chest, abdomen, and pelvis) has been unrevealing.

CONCLUSION

Traditionally, hospitalists were mainly involved in the initial evaluation and stabilization of treatment-naïve patients presenting with complications related to undiagnosed hematologic malignancies. Hospitalists are increasingly called upon to manage complications that develop during treatment. Some familiarity with the different disease entities, drugs employed, and expected course is therefore necessary. While anticancer treatment is almost invariably directed by a specialist, many patients live far from tertiary care centers and many protocols are administered in the outpatient setting. Communication with the patient's primary hematologist or oncologist is always advisable

SUGGESTED READINGS

Bug G, Anargyrou K, Tonn T, et al. Impact of leukapheresis on early death rate in adult acute myeloid leukemia presenting with hyperleukocytosis. *Transfusion*. 2007;47:1843–1850.

Clark WF, Stewart AK, Rock GA, et al. Plasma exchange when myeloma presents as acute renal failure: a randomized, controlled trial. *Ann Intern Med*. 2005;143:777–784.

Coiffier B, Altman A, Pui CH, Younes A, Cairo MS. Guidelines for the management of pediatric and adult tumor lysis syndrome: an evidence-based review. *J Clin Oncol*. 2008;26:2767–2778.

Conger JD, Falk SA. Intrarenal dynamics in the pathogenesis and prevention of acute urate nephropathy. *J Clin Invest*. 1977;59:786–793.

Garcia-Carbonero R, Mayordomo JI, Tornamira MV, et al. Granulocyte colony-stimulating factor in the treatment of high-risk febrile neutropenia: a multicenter randomized trial. *J Natl Cancer Inst*. 2001;93:31–38.

Giles FJ, Shen Y, Kantarjian HM, et al. Leukapheresis reduces early mortality in patients with acute myeloid leukemia with high white cell counts but does not improve long- term survival. *Leuk Lymphoma*. 2001;42:67–73.

Kaplan JG, DeSouza TG, Farkash A, et al. Leptomeningeal metastases: comparison of clinical features and laboratory data of solid tumors, lymphomas and leukemias. *J Neurooncol*. 1990;9:225–229.

Klastersky J, Paesmans M, Rubenstein EB, et al. The Multinational Association for Supportive Care in Cancer risk index: A multinational scoring system for identifying low-risk febrile neutropenic cancer patients. *J Clin Oncol*. 2000;18:3038–3051.

Kouroukis CT, Chia S, Verma S, et al. Canadian supportive care recommendations for the management of neutropenia in patients with cancer. *Curr Oncol*. 2008;15:9–23.

Porcu P, Danielson CF, Orazi A, Heerema NA, Gabig TG, McCarthy LJ. Therapeutic leukapheresis in hyperleucocytic leukaemias: lack of correlation between degree of cytoreduction and early mortality rate. *Br J Haematol*. 1997;98:433–436.

SECTION 9
Oncology

CHAPTER 181

Overview of Cancer and Treatment

Rachel Goodwin, MD, MSc, FRCPC
Timothy P. Hanna, MD, MSc, FRCP(C)
Ralph M. Meyer, MD, FRCP(C)

Key Clinical Questions

1. What factors should be considered in determining treatment for a patient with cancer?
2. How do the outcomes of cancer clinical trials influence treatment decision making?
3. What treatment modalities exist and under what formats are these provided?
4. What are the main classes of systemic and radiation therapy?

INTRODUCTION

Cancer is a heterogeneous disease affecting all age groups, nationalities, and socioeconomic classes. Cancer patients, along with their families and friends, experience enormous social, emotional, and economic effects. In the United States, the National Cancer Institute (NCI) collects cancer-related statistics and produces the Surveillance, Epidemiology, and End Results (SEER) database (seer.cancer.gov).

It is estimated that in 2010 in the United States, 1,529,560 people will be diagnosed with and 569,490 will die of cancer. The lifetime risk of developing cancer is 1 in 2. In the United States in 2007, cancer was second to heart disease as the leading cause of death (23.2% versus 25.4%). Compared with death rates from 1975, the percentage of deaths from cardiac causes has decreased while cancer-related deaths have increased. Allowing for this, the absolute death rate among those diagnosed with cancer continues to decline. In North America, the most frequent incident cancers among men are prostate, lung, and colon and among women are breast, lung, and colon. Lung cancer is the leading cause of cancer-related deaths for both men and women. The second commonest cause of cancer deaths are prostate (males) and breast (females). Colon cancer is the third leading cause of cancer death for both sexes.

CASE 181-1

A 64-year-old woman was admitted with bowel obstruction due to metastatic rectal cancer. She has undergone many previous therapies. Some were attempts to cure the disease, and others were given with palliative intent. She was diagnosed eight years previously with stage III rectal cancer after presenting with rectal bleeding and was initially treated with curative intent consisting of 5-flurouracil and concurrent radiation therapy followed by surgery consisting of a total mesorectal resection. She then received additional chemotherapy. Three years later, her cancer recurred in the right lobe of the liver. She underwent a right hepatic lobectomy followed by further chemotherapy. She was free of disease for two years, but has recently been discovered to have peritoneal carcinomatosis and retroperitoneal lymphadenopathy. She was given radiation therapy to the lymph nodes to treat pain and followed by chemotherapy.

This case demonstrates the continuum of cancer therapy intent. At initial presentation, the goal of treatment was to cure the disease. With subsequent cancer recurrences, the goals evolved. With the first recurrence, the intent was to potentially cure the patient given the isolated liver disease. Although not cured, the surgery prolonged a disease-free state and improved quality of life. Later recurrences were associated with strategies to palliate symptoms and transition to end-of-life care. This case demonstrates use of multiple treatment modalities (systemic, radiation, and surgical) used according to different principles (neoadjuvant, adjuvant, palliative).

CASE 181-2

The approaches to management of two patients with lymphoma have been very different. The first patient was a 45-year-old man diagnosed with follicular lymphoma. His only symptoms were his finding of small lymph nodes in his right neck and left groin.

While his blood cell counts were normal, a bone marrow biopsy showed the presence of clonal lymphocytes. After thorough discussions, it was decided that he would be evaluated again in three months and that therapy would be deferred. The approach was referred to as "watchful waiting." In contrast, a 78-year-old woman presented with abdominal pain and was found to have a large mesenteric mass. A biopsy showed diffuse large B-cell lymphoma. She was treated with cyclical systemic therapy consisting of cyclophosphamide, hydroxydaunorubicin (doxorubicin or Adriamycin), vincristine (Oncovin), prednisone, and rituximab (CHOP-R). While treatment was associated with important side-effects, her oncologist now hopes that she is cured.

These two cases demonstrate how prognostic determinants influence management. Both the histologic classification of the cancer (follicular versus diffuse large B-cell lymphoma) and the extent of disease (stage) are associated with unique natural histories and the abilities to alter disease courses. Management decisions will also be influenced by patient comorbidities and preferences; these cases illustrate the caveat that patient age should not independently dominate this decision-making process.

CANCER ETIOLOGY

Four types of human cells exist: germ cells, stem cells, partially differentiated cells, and mature/specialized cells. These cells vary in their abilities to reproduce and differentiate. When cells differentiate, most eventually undergo a programmed process of cell death, referred to as *apoptosis*. Apoptosis is triggered by the cell surpassing a number of cell cycle divisions. Cancer is a disease in which cells have altered genetic processes as a result of mutations. Mutations lead to gain or loss of genetic functions that permit abnormal proliferation, failure to undergo apoptosis leading to cellular accumulation, or both. The etiology of mutations varies, with many being unknown. Factors contributing to genetic instability include inherited risks, viruses, chronic inflammation, chemical carcinogens (eg, tobacco, asbestos), radiation (eg, UVA/UVB), and lifestyle factors (eg, diet and obesity). The resulting abnormal genetic processes lead to special properties that permit cell transit, invasion, and growth at new sites, referred to as *metastases*. Increased understanding of cancer-specific genetic alterations have led to the availability of more selective therapies and the advent of the term *personalized medicine*.

PRACTICE POINT

Basic mechanism of cancer

- Think of cancer as a disease where there is an imbalance of cell proliferation and cell death. Cells become malignant when they accumulate mutations that enable escape of programmed cell death (apoptosis). Cancer therapies aim to decrease cancer cell proliferation or enhance apoptosis. New cancer therapies are increasingly directed at reversing the specific molecular process associated with a given type of cancer.

CLASSIFYING CANCER FOR TREATMENT AND PROGNOSIS

Cancer is a heterogeneous group of diseases. Three factors that assist classifying patient management strategies are cancer site, histology, and stage. *Site* refers to anatomic location (eg, breast, lung). Histology refers to pathologic cellular and tissue appearances and includes broad (eg, carcinoma, sarcoma, lymphoma) and specific (eg, squamous cell, adenocarcinoma) categorization. Histology is usually determined through pathologic evaluation of resected material or a large bore needle core biopsy. In some instances, histology can be inferred through the cytologic examination of cells obtained by fine needle aspiration (FNA). Cancers of the same site but of different histology will have different clinical behaviors, management strategies, and prognoses. *Stage* refers to the anatomic extent of disease, including anatomic regions involved with the primary tumor (T), lymph node involvement (N), and the presence or absence of distant metastasis (M); stage is often categorized using the TNM schema. Some diseases such as lymphoma and gynecologic cancers have separate staging classifications. In addition to facilitating determination of prognosis, stage has important implications for management as "local" therapies (ie, surgery, radiation therapy) are most applicable to patients with more limited stages of disease. Determination of site, histology, and stage require systematic diagnostic processes that include a comprehensive history and physical examination, obtaining diagnostic material and expert pathology review and appropriate laboratory and imaging investigations.

Recent understandings have permitted more sophisticated patient risk profile assessments that enhance abilities to determine prognosis and best management. Initially, risk categorizations were predominantly based on combining evaluations of standard clinically determined cancer-related factors such as histology, stage, and associated laboratory markers (eg, lactate dehydrogenase), patient-related factors such as age and comorbidity (see the proceeding section on Patient Factors and Goals when Determining Treatment) and general measures of health influenced by the combination of cancer- and patient-related factors (eg, the Eastern Cooperative Oncology Group [ECOG] or Karnofsky Performance Status Indices). More recently, prognostic and predictive biomarkers that include molecular markers (eg, HER2 in breast cancer, K-Ras in colon cancer) and gene expression signature profiles are either used or are being tested to determine best treatment.

PATIENT FACTORS AND GOALS WHEN DETERMINING TREATMENT

The management of individuals with cancer is highly influenced by patient-specific determinants that include their comorbidities, relative contraindications to specific treatment components, and values and preferences. As illustrated in the case descriptions at the beginning of this chapter, cancer therapy often includes the use of multiple modalities and drugs. Perhaps more than any other disease, each therapeutic component can be associated with risks of treatment-related morbidity and mortality. These risks must be balanced with the potential for benefit on a case-by-case basis. This evaluation begins with understanding global aspects of a patient's health, their functional status (which includes capacities to address basic activities of daily living), and psychosocial and socioeconomic circumstances. Understanding the need for, and availability of, caregiver support can be essential. The evaluation then proceeds to include understanding whether special risks exist with respect to specific therapies. For instance, use of anthracycline agents such as doxorubicin may not be feasible in patients with cardiac disease, platinum agents such as cisplatin must be attenuated or avoided in patients with renal disease, and radiation treatment may need to be modified in patients with a pacemaker near a thoracic tumor.

The goals of cancer therapy are to prolong life, reduce suffering, and enhance quality of life. These goals must balance the potential benefits and harms of treatment. Increasingly, treatment policies are influenced by the economic determinants of cost effectiveness and cost utility. Central to decision making is understanding whether the potential of therapy is to cure the patient and leave them with a life-expectancy that parallels that of age- and sex-matched controls, to induce a prolonged state of freedom from obvious disease and its symptoms (ie, a remission) even if eventual disease recurrence is anticipated, or to provide a temporary reduction in the burden of disease and palliation of symptoms.

The risks of the underlying cancer and treatment toxicities must be balanced with the potential benefits of the treatment intervention. This evaluation can range from the more statistically-based paradigm in which adjuvant chemotherapy (see Treatment Modalities later in this chapter) enhances the potential for cure in patients with surgically resected cancer to the trade-offs associated with palliating the symptoms created by cancer versus introducing new symptoms associated with treatment toxicity in patients with advanced disease. Decisions vary according to patient perspectives, values, and experiences. Careful communication, usually through involvement of a multidisciplinary team, is essential.

PRACTICE POINT

Making treatment decisions

- Decisions about therapy must be considered systematically and should include detailed knowledge of cancer-related risk factors and patient-specific parameters. The goals of therapy should be explicit and account for patient preferences. Communication should include the patient and their family and is facilitated by involving a multidisciplinary team.

DECIDING WHETHER THERAPY HAS BENEFITS THAT OUTWEIGH HARMS: CLINICAL AND SURROGATE ENDPOINTS USED IN CANCER CLINICAL TRIALS

The management of cancer patients has been tightly interwoven with the conduct of clinical trials. This culture continues and often clinical trials provide opportunities for patients to access therapies that may later be confirmed efficacious and become new standards of care. However, when patient care includes participation in a clinical trial, clinicians and patients need to understand the objectives of the trial and whether the endpoints used represent potential benefit to the patient. A useful paradigm is to contrast *explanatory* trials, in which a trial's objective is to determine whether an intervention is associated with a potentially efficacious causal biologic relationship (eg, treatment results in a reduction in tumor size), with *pragmatic* trials, in which the effectiveness of a therapy is demonstrated by its association with an outcome that is of clear importance to patients (eg, improved survival or quality of life). The concepts of explanatory and pragmatic trials represent a continuum. When clinicians use the data from clinical trials to determine patient management, the perspective of a "superior outcome" should be placed into an appropriate context. Clinicians need to ask whether a therapy purported to be superior was associated with benefits that are important to patients or more so represent confirmation of a biologic proof of principle. This requires an understanding of the common endpoints used in cancer clinical trials; these form the basis of everyday discussions of cancer clinicians, including during ward rounds, tumor board meetings, and patient encounters.

MAJOR VERSUS SURROGATE ENDPOINTS

The major endpoints of cancer clinical trials are overall survival, quality of life, and measures of an economic evaluation (eg, cost effectiveness, cost utility). The dominant major outcome is overall survival. Unless exceptional circumstances exist, such as a high risk of severe toxicity or extraordinary cost, treatments that lead to survival benefits are generally adopted. In contrast to how long one lives, measures of quality of life assess what the World Health Organization refers to as "physical, mental, and social well-being." In most cancer clinical trials, evaluation of quality of life is a secondary objective; trials demonstrating survival and quality of life benefits are very powerful determinants of health care practices. Assessment of quality of life is occasionally the primary objective of a clinical trial; this is particularly so in trials assessing end-of-life care. Economic evaluations are rarely the primary objective of a clinical trial but may be used when health care funding agencies consider new therapies.

Evaluation of major endpoints can be complex. Cancer patients may have long periods of survival and receive many different therapies over the course of their life, making assessments of overall survival unfeasible. The measurement of quality of life involves use of instruments and analytic principles that are associated with limitations. Economic evaluations involve extensive modeling and do not address a construct that deals directly with the health of a patient. For these reasons, surrogate or proxy endpoints are commonly used in cancer trials. Practicing clinicians face challenges in understanding whether these surrogates represent proxies for a major endpoint, such as overall survival, or emphasize assessment of a biologic proof of concept.

Common surrogate endpoints used as proxy measures for survival include disease-free survival (DFS) and progression-free survival (PFS). The definition of DFS is "the time from randomization until recurrence of tumor or death from any cause," and for PFS is "the time from randomization until objective tumor progression or death." The most frequent use of DFS is in clinical trials assessing additional therapy given after definitive surgery or radiotherapy (adjuvant treatment is discussed later under Treatment Modalities), whereas PFS is most commonly used in trials assessing patients who enter the trial with identifiable existing disease. For many cancers (eg, adjuvant therapy for breast and colon cancer, initial treatment of diffuse large B-cell lymphoma), these endpoints have been demonstrated to accurately predict overall survival and are validated surrogate endpoints. However, for other cancers, such as chronic lymphocytic leukemia, and use of some targeted therapies (see Treatment Modalities later in this chapter) to treat advanced cancer, a clear relation with survival has not been demonstrated and trials demonstrating benefits have to be more cautiously considered if the results are to be applied to patient management decisions. Clinicians need to understand whether an intervention associated with benefits that involve a surrogate endpoint warrants the risks associated with that treatment in order to "keep the cancer away." Consideration is required of the proxy power of the surrogate endpoint for major endpoints (survival and quality of life), the magnitude of improvement observed in the surrogate endpoint, and the relative risks (eg, side-effects) associated with the competing alternatives.

The benefits of a cancer treatment are also commonly expressed using language that describes whether the treatment reduces the burden of cancer. While reducing tumor burden will be necessary for a treatment to be ultimately considered efficacious, this alone may not be sufficient for adoption of the therapy, as reductions may be transient and treatment may be associated with substantial toxicity. The Response Evaluation Criteria in Solid Tumors (RECIST) criteria are often used as an endpoint in preliminary clinical trials that screen new drugs for potential efficacy and may be used as endpoints in explanatory randomized controlled trials. The RECIST criteria follow changes in the anatomic measurement of the tumor over time and include categories of *complete response* (disappearance of all lesions), *partial response* (decrease of at least 30% in the sum of diameters of lesions), *progressive disease* (increase of at least 20% in the sum of diameters of lesions or appearance of new lesions), and *stable disease* (changes that are insufficient to qualify for another response category). These endpoints emphasize biologic proof of concept, are used only under special circumstances by regulatory agencies, such as the U.S. Food and Drug Administration, to approve new treatments, and should be regarded with caution by clinicians when determining best treatments.

TREATMENT MODALITIES

With the patient assessment process completed and goals of therapy determined, details of treatment need to be considered. Traditional anticancer treatment modalities are surgery, radiation, and systemic therapy. These modalities are used separately or are combined according to four treatment formats: primary, adjuvant, neoadjuvant, and palliative. Some exceptions exist with respect to this categorization, especially when considering the hematologic malignancies.

Primary treatment is the initial therapy attempted and usually refers to intent to cure the cancer. For many solid tumors primary therapy consists of surgery. When cancer is localized but associated with highly invasive potentials, the complexity of local therapy, be it surgery or radiation therapy, may be extensive and referred to as *radical*. Increasingly, the disease extent (stage) and risk profile (often using biomarkers) are considered to determine whether primary therapy alone offers the opportunity for best outcomes or whether supplemental therapies (eg, adjuvant) are required.

Adjuvant treatment is additional treatment provided after primary treatment has attained a state of remission but a statistical risk of disease recurrence remains because of occult or micrometastatic disease. Adjuvant treatment involves use of a second modality (eg, systemic therapy after surgery or radiation therapy; radiation therapy after surgery).

Neoadjuvant treatment is given before primary treatment. Most often this consists of systemic therapy, radiation therapy, or both. Neoadjuvant therapy is used to reduce tumor size and facilitate surgery and/or to treat potential micrometastatic disease prior to surgery.

Palliative treatment involves the use of any treatment modality to reduce the tumor burden in a noncurative or nonremission-inducing situation. The intent may be to alleviate symptoms, improve quality of life, and/or extend survival. Palliative anticancer treatment should be distinguished from palliative end-of-life care. While palliative treatment is noncurative, it may be associated with life expectancies of many years (eg, in follicular lymphoma noncurative therapy is associated with five-year survivals of greater than 80%).

PRACTICE POINT

Formats and endpoints for use of anticancer therapy

- There are four formats in which surgery, radiation, and/or systemic therapy can be used: primary, adjuvant, neoadjuvant, and palliative treatments. These formats account for the intent of treatment and will be associated with the use of different clinical endpoints when evaluating the effectiveness of therapy.

MULTIDISCIPLINARY ONCOLOGY AND TREATMENT MODALITIES

A team approach is required to provide patients with optimum care. The team may include specialists representing the major anticancer treatment modalities: surgical, medical, and radiation oncology. Although it is beyond the scope of this chapter to outline the many facets of surgical oncology, it should be stressed that a successful surgical resection often results in the best chance of cure for patients with early-stage solid tumors. Other specialized health care personnel are needed for cancer care including nursing, social work, pharmacy, physical and occupational therapy, and access to specialized supports such as palliative care, supportive care units, and age-related specialized services (eg, geriatric oncology, supports for adolescents and young adults [so-called AYA population]). Involvement and ongoing communication with a primary care specialist is extremely important. Increasingly, coordination of inpatient management rests with hospitalists. A broader discussion of team roles, organization, and coordination is beyond the scope of this text. However, it is essential that the important coordinating role of the hospitalist be understood by team members and for there to be access to the resources required for multidisciplinary care.

SYSTEMIC THERAPY

Systemic therapy encompasses all drug treatment and is classified according to cytotoxic, targeted, endocrine, and immunotherapeutic. Cytotoxic treatment is synonymous with chemotherapy. Agents affect cell division or cause DNA damage. Cytotoxic agents are classified into categories based on their mechanism of inducing cell damage (**Table 181-1A**) and can be used in any of the above treatment formats. When used as adjuvant therapy, drugs from multiple categories are often used to maximize cell kill, theoretically protecting against drug resistance and minimizing risk because of nonoverlapping side-effects. When used in the palliative setting, the risk-benefit ratio of drug combinations versus single agents requires careful consideration, including how sequential "lines" of therapy may be planned. Palliative chemotherapy requires ongoing evaluations so that new regimens can be considered if patients have progressive cancer or unacceptable toxicity.

Targeted therapies have increased over the past two decades. Rather than affecting the cell division machinery, targeted agents affect specific cell proteins involved with cell signaling, cell cycle regulation, angiogenesis, tumor metastasis, apoptosis, and immune pathways. Drugs target a step in the cell proliferation pathway such as a ligand, cell receptor, an intracellular tyrosine kinase (enzymes responsible for signaling related to cell growth, death, and cellular differentiation), or other protein that propagates cell growth signals (**Table 181-1B**). Targeted agents may be combined with chemotherapy.

For patients with hormone-sensitive cancers, treatment may include hormone agonists or antagonists (**Table 181-1C**). Examples of pathways exploited include estrogen and progesterone in breast and uterine cancer and testosterone in prostate cancer. Hormonal therapy will often be provided after pathologic evaluation for the presence of a biomarker (eg, estrogen and progesterone receptors in breast cancer). Hormonal therapies include agents that block hormone production, such as aromatase inhibitors that block estrogen production and are a treatment option for patients with breast cancer.

Immunotherapy promotes an anticancer effect through enhancement of humoral- and/or cell-mediated immunity. Treatment can be specific or nonspecific. Specific therapies include monoclonal antibodies that target cancer-specific antigens (eg, CD20 is the target of rituximab in B-cell lymphoma, HER2 is the target of trastuzumab in breast cancer) or using cancer-specific antigens as vaccines to promote an immune response. Monoclonal antibodies may be conjugated with a radioactive compound, such as ^{131}I or ^{90}Y, or to an immunotoxin. Nonspecific agents activate the immune system with the intent that cancer cells will be differentially affected; examples include interferon, interleukin-2, and interleukin-21. Conceptually, allogeneic stem cell transplantation represents a special form of immunotherapy through its graft versus disease (eg, leukemia, lymphoma) effects.

TABLE 181-1A Classes of Cytotoxic Drugs, Mechanisms of Action, and Drug Examples

Cytotoxic Drug Category	General Mechanism of Action	Examples of Drugs	
Alkylating agents	Causes alkylation of DNA bases	Busulfan Melphalan Chlorambucil Cyclophosphamide	Ifosfamide Carmustin Dacarbazine Temozolomide
Platinum agents	Develops DNA adducts resulting in DNA breaks	Cisplatin Carboplatin Oxaliplatin	
Antimetabolites	Antifolate compounds that target enzyme(s) of folate metabolism	Methotrexate Pemetrexed 5-fluorouracil Capecitabine	Cytarabine Gemcitabine 6-thiopurines Cladribine
Topoisomerase Inhibitors	Inhibits either topoisomerase (Topo) I or II. These enzymes are required to decrease the torsional stress on DNA during replication and transcription by causing single and double stranded breaks.	Irinotecan Topotecan	
Anthracyclines	Inhibit Topo II enzyme and cause generation of oxygen free radicals	Doxorubicin Daunorubicin	Idarubicin Epirubicin
Antimicrotubule agents	*Taxanes*: Alter the dissociation of the microtubule *Vinca Alkaloids*: Binds tubulin and inhibits microtubule assembly	Docetaxel Paclitaxel Vincristine Vinblastine Vinorelbine	
Epipodophyllotoxins	Inhibit Topo II enzyme	Etoposide	
Anthracenediones	DNA intercalator resulting in double stranded DNA breaks	Mitoxantrone	
Antibiotic	Activated to an alkylating agent, binds DNA and creates cross links	Mitomycin C	

TABLE 181-1B Targeted Agents by Category

Targeted Agent Category	Known Target	Examples of Drugs
Small-molecule tyrosine kinase inhibitors	EGFR	Gefitinib Erlotinib
	Bcr-Abl, PDGFR, c-kit	Imatinib
	EGFR, HER2	Lapatinib
	VEGFR + multiple other kinases	Sunitinib Sorafenib
Antibodies against a signaling target	HER2	Trastuzumab
	VEGF	Bevacizumab
	EGFR	Cetuximab Panitumumab
Proteasome inhibitors	Reversible inhibitor of a large protein complex that degrades ubiquitinated proteins	Bortezomib
mTOR inhibitors	Inhibits mTOR, a protein kinase, involved in cell signaling	Temsirolimus Everolimus

EGFR, epidermal growth factor receptor; HER2, human epidermal growth factor receptor 2; mTOR, mammalian target of rapamycin; PDGFR, platelet derived growth factor receptor; VEGF(R), vascular epidermal growth factor receptor.

TABLE 181-1C Classes of Endocrine Therapy

Endocrine Agent Category	Mechanism of Action	Examples of Drugs
LHRH or GnRH agonist	Continuous treatment causes feedback to the pituitary to decrease FSH and LH. In males it decreases testosterone and in females decreases estrogen and androgen	Leuprolide Goserelin
Aromatase Inhibitor	Inhibits aromatase, an enzyme that converts androgen to estrogen	Anastrozole Exemestane Letrozole
Estrogen Modulator	Competitively blocks estrogen receptor (in some tissues it mimics estrogen [eg, bone, endometrium, fat])	Tamoxifen
Antiandrogens	Blocks testosterone at the receptor	Bicalutamide Flutamide
Progestins	Exact mechanism unknown, may interact with progesterone and glucocorticoid receptors	Megestrol Acetate Medroxyprogesterone

PRACTICE POINT

The four types of systemic therapy

- There are four general categories of systemic therapy: cytotoxic treatment that damages DNA or affects cell division, targeted therapy that affects proteins in the cell proliferation and apoptosis pathways, endocrine therapy that blocks or reduces levels of sex hormones, and immunotherapy that modulates humoral- and cell-mediated immunity.

RADIATION THERAPY

Radiation therapy is a form of localized cancer treatment that uses high-energy ionizing radiation to kill cancer cells. Radiation therapy is most often delivered from a unit that is external to the patient (external beam radiation [EBRT]). Photons produced by a linear accelerator or cobalt source ionize electrons and create free radicals that damage DNA. If this damage is not repaired, the cell dies. Radiation damages both normal cells and cancer cells, but normal cells have a greater ability to repair radiation damage than do cancer cells.

Radiation is an underutilized modality in many regions and countries. At least half of cancer patients will need radiation at some point. As radiation is directed to a specific body site, side-effects can be limited to that body region and local doses can be permitted that would be otherwise lethal. The noninvasive nature of radiation makes it particularly suited for situations where surgery would be associated with substantial morbidity (eg, head and neck cancer, cervix cancer). The focal nature of radiation makes it ideal for palliating localized symptoms, such as painful bone metastasis or bleeding.

TABLE 181-2 Modalities of Radiation Therapy

Type	Subtype	Description
Teletherapy	Conventional Radiation Therapy (2D)	Radiation with photons is planned using conventional X-ray images.
	3D conformal radiation therapy (3D-CRT)	Planning guided by CT scan. Photon beams are shaped by positioning multiple thin parallel blocks called multileaf collimators (MLC). MLC position is static during treatment.
	Intensity-modulated radiation therapy (IMRT)	A form of high-precision 3D-CRT where the intensity of radiation varies throughout each beam, improving coverage of the target and sparing normal tissues from avoidable radiation. To achieve this, MLC position is dynamic during treatment. Computer algorithms determine MLC positions. Usually combined with image-guided radiation therapy (IGRT). IGRT ensures that patient positioning is correct during treatments through regular imaging on the treatment bed. IMRT variants include Tomotherapy and Volumetric-modulated arc therapy (VMAT).
	Stereotactic radiation	Refers to radiation treatments with extremely precise assurance of patient positioning, usually through rigid frames fixed to the patient. Often involves very large single fractions of radiation (eg, stereotactic radiosurgery, Gammaknife, X-Knife, Cyberknife, stereotactic body radiation (SBRT).
	Particle therapy	Subatomic particles are accelerated to high energies for therapy (eg, protons, neutrons, carbon ions). Treatment is still largely investigational and often capable of achieving highly conformal treatments with lower dose to healthy tissues than even IMRT. Some forms have unique biological effects.
	Electron therapy	Uses high-energy electrons to treat superficial tumors such as skin cancers. Therapeutic properties are different than typical particle beams sinxe it is not useful for deep targets. Low-energy "superficial" or "orthovoltage" photons are also used for skin cancer radiotherapy.
Brachytherapy	Intracavitary brachytherapy	A sealed radioactive source is inserted into a body cavity and placed in or next to the tumor (eg, cervix cancer).
	Interstitial brachytherapy	One or more sealed radioactive sources are placed via needles directly into the target (eg, prostate cancer).
	Intraluminal brachytherapy	Sealed radioactive source placed into a lumen next to the target (eg, bronchus, esophagus).
	Mold brachytherapy	Thin catheters are placed in a mold and a sealed radioactive source is placed in multiple dwell positions along catheters to treat superficial tumors (eg, a large skin cancer).
Systemic radiation treatment	Radioimmunotherapy	A radioactive isotope is chemically linked to an antibody targeted to a specific ligand, for instance, linking isotopes to CD20-specific antibodies to treat non-Hodgkin lymphoma (Zevalin, Bexxar).
	Nonsealed radionuclides	Radionuclides without a metal housing. Usually injected intravenously for systemic treatment. Strontium-90 is avid to bone, sometimes used for diffuse bony metastasis. Iodine-131 is sometimes used for thyroid cancer.
	Whole body radiation, hemibody radiation	Rarely used. Whole body radiation may be used as part of preparation for bone marrow transplant or stem cell transplant. Hemibody radiation may be used to treat diffuse bony metastasis in the upper or lower body.

PRACTICE POINT

Radiation therapy

- More than half of all cancer patients will need radiation during their disease course. This will either be part of primary, adjuvant, neoadjuvant, or palliative therapy.

Radiation is delivered in daily doses called fractions. Palliative treatments consist of a single or a few fractions and are given in higher daily doses than curative treatments. Curative treatments often involve 20 to 35 fractions. The choice of dose and fraction number will depend on disease site, histology, stage, and risk assessment and, like all anticancer therapies, needs to account for patient specifics. The patient's ability to travel to the radiation department or stay at a hospital or lodging facility for extended time periods is an important access issue. Radiation may be concurrently administered with chemotherapy ("chemoradiation"), which may be a neoadjuvant therapy prior to surgery (eg, rectal cancer), a curative option instead of surgery (eg, head and neck cancer, cervix cancer, anal cancer, glioblastoma), or an adjuvant treatment (eg, gastric cancer).

Preparation for EBRT requires a treatment planning process. This includes simulation, where the patient is placed into his treatment position, immobilized (eg, molded plastic head mask for treating head and neck cancer), imaged (usually with a computed tomography [CT] scan), and appropriate protective devices to isolate the treatment area are constructed. Diagnostic images (CT scan) are reviewed and, using computer software, the gross tumor volume (GTV), surrounding areas suspicious for microscopic spread (clinical target volume [CTV]), and a margin for organ motion and setup error (planning target volume [PTV]) are outlined. Critical structures that should be avoided are also outlined. A graph called a dose-volume histogram (DVH) is generated, which graphically describes the dose received by parts of the outlined structures. The high precision of modern radiation therapy requires rigorous quality assurance led by medical physics specialists.

There are new and developing modalities of radiation therapy (**Table 181-2**). Brachytherapy involves insertion of live radiation sources into the patient, which treat the target from a short distance. Sometimes these sources are placed directly into the target (called interstitial brachytherapy). As compared with EBRT, brachytherapy has the advantage of delivering high doses around only the placed source. Radiation does not travel through layers of healthy tissue, meaning that toxicities might be minimized. Brachytherapy may be given as high-dose-rate (HDR) treatment that involves temporary insertion of a radiation source into the body and rapid delivery of radiation so that treatment times are short (eg, for cervix cancer) or as low-dose-rate (LDR) treatment, such as the permanent insertion of radiation sources with a low decay rate in the patient (eg, for prostate cancer).

Whether radiation is delivered by EBRT or brachytherapy, there are short- and long-term complications that will depend on disease-, patient-, and treatment-related specifics. Acute side effects usually begin one to two weeks after starting treatment and usually resolve two to three weeks after treatment completion. Just as with any cancer therapy, there are risks of chronic side effects with radiation. Chronic side effects, such as soft tissue fibrosis or cataracts, may take six months or often longer to manifest.

CONCLUSION

The scope of this chapter precludes descriptions of other important components that form part of the management of cancer patients. While the chapter has emphasized specific anticancer treatment modalities, other supports of the cancer patient require attention. These will include the important areas of symptom control, palliative care (see Chapter 215), and the evolving field of complementary and alternative medicine (see Chapter 217). Resources for the latter include the National Center for Complementary and Alternative Medicine (nccam.nih.gov) and the National Cancer Institute (www.cancer.gov/cancerinfo/treatment/cam).

SUGGESTED READINGS

Altekruse SF, Kosary CL, Krapcho M, et al, eds. *SEER Cancer Statistics Review, 1975–2007, National Cancer Institute.* Available at http://seer.cancer.gov/csr/1975_2007.

Edge SB, Byrd DR, Compton CC, Fritz AG, Greene FL, Trotti A, eds. *AJCC Cancer Staging Manual.* 7th ed. New York, NY: *Springer*; 2010.

Esther KW, Wolin KY, Colditz GA. Time course of risk factors in cancer etiology and progression. *J Clin Oncol.* 2010;28:4052–4057.

Krakoff IH. Systemic treatment of cancer. *CA-Cancer J Clin.* 1996;46:134–141.

Meyer RM, Kouroukis CT. Understanding outcome measures. *Evidence-based Oncology.* 2001;2:172–176.

Samant R, Gooi AC. Radiotherapy basics for family physicians. Potent tool for symptom relief. *Can Fam Physician.* 2005;51:1496–1501.

CHAPTER 182

Oncologic Emergencies

J. Ashley Davidson, MD
Stephen K. Chia, MD, FRCPC

Key Clinical Questions

1. What clinical presentations in cancer patients necessitate immediate action?
2. Which of these emergencies are consequences of the patient's underlying malignancy and which are caused, directly or indirectly, by antineoplastic therapy?
3. Do certain cancers confer a higher risk of developing particular oncologic emergencies than others?
4. When is it necessary for these conditions to be managed in a multidisciplinary fashion? Who are the consultants whose timely involvement is essential for optimal treatment?
5. Are there situations in which it is safe to manage these patients in the outpatient setting?
6. Are there preventive measures one can take to reduce the risk of a patient's encountering one of these acute complications of malignant disease?

INTRODUCTION

A diagnosis of cancer places patients at risk for a number of acute life-threatening complications. Such an event may herald the initial presentation of a malignant condition, represent the underlying progression of a known malignancy, or be a result of a rapid response to treatment; it may be obstructive, metabolic, or infectious in nature. Prompt recognition of these potentially lethal events is essential to timely life-sustaining intervention and preservation of organ function. Several oncologic emergencies will be outlined in this chapter, separated into those entities caused by the cancer itself and those which are related to the treatments delivered.

EMERGENCIES RELATED TO THE UNDERLYING CANCER

SPINAL CORD COMPRESSION

Carrying an imminent threat of irreversible neurologic disability, malignant spinal cord compression (MSCC) is perhaps the most dramatic of the oncologic emergencies. It is critical that one approach a new symptom of back pain somewhat differently in a patient with a current diagnosis or history of cancer from the way in which one would approach a patient without such a history.

PRACTICE POINT

- New back pain in a patient with a diagnosis of cancer may represent MSCC until this entity is ruled out by means of a thorough history, physical examination, and, if necessary, appropriate imaging.

Clinical presentation

Back pain is the initial symptom in the vast majority of patients. The pain is usually localized initially, but may later develop a radicular component, which can be unilateral or bilateral. The presence of a Lhermitte sign, parasthesias radiating down the spine on flexion of the neck, may also point to a spinal cord process.

Inquiries must be made as to symptoms of neurologic compromise, though they typically follow the onset of back pain over a period of weeks to months. If present on initial assessment, however, they significantly raise the level of urgency with which a definitive diagnosis must be pursued. These include weakness, spasticity, or loss of sensation in the lower limbs; the patient may complain of difficulty rising from a chair or climbing stairs. Motor and sensory symptoms usually precede autonomic dysfunction, but it is essential to inquire about urinary hesitancy or retention, perhaps accompanied by overflow incontinence.

Diagnosis

The targeted physical examination should focus on the evaluation of the nervous system, in particular that of the lower limbs. Most cases of MSCC involve the thoracic region, with the lumbosacral and cervical regions less commonly affected. It is critical to identify any objective weakness or spasticity, sensory deficit, or abnormal deep tendon reflexes. Examination of the perineal region is essential to identify decreased anal sphincter tone or saddle anesthesia. The latter finding, defined as decreased sensation in the region of the buttocks and posterior thighs, is indicative of cauda equina syndrome, resulting from compression of the sacral nerve roots rather than the spinal cord itself.

Any suspicion of neurologic compromise on history or physical examination should result in urgent spinal imaging to confirm or exclude MSCC. The imaging test of choice is magnetic resonance imaging (MRI). MRI offers the best anatomic definition of both the bones and soft tissues, either of which could be the cause of the suspected MSCC, and the superior anatomic detail may be useful for management decisions. It is important to image the entire spine, rather than just the area of clinical suspicion, as up to 25% of patients with MSCC have an additional focus of metastatic disease not initially evident on history or physical examination.

Management

For cancer patients without clinical evidence of neurologic compromise but still concern for MSCC, imaging need not be requested urgently but should nonetheless be investigated within 24 to 72 hours. The differential diagnosis of MSCC in these patients includes, among other conditions, osteoporotic fracture, degenerative disc disease, abscess, tuberculosis, radiation myelopathy, or leptomeningitis (infectious or neoplastic).

Time is of the essence in evaluating and treating a cancer patient with suspected MSCC as the degree of neurologic damage at the time of treatment initiation is the most important determinant of eventual functional outcome. Upon identification of any suggestion of neurologic compromise, several steps should be taken concurrently: corticosteroid therapy should be immediately initiated, imaging should be requested on an urgent basis (preferably an MRI of the total spine, though plain films could be obtained while arrangements are being made for the MRI as they may demonstrate a fracture), and consultants should be notified.

PRACTICE POINT

- The presence of any symptoms or signs of neurologic compromise in addition to back pain necessitates urgent spinal imaging and initiation of corticosteroids.

Corticosteroid therapy typically means dexamethasone, though there is little evidence to suggest superiority of a particular regimen; the specific dose or route of administration is less important than the immediacy of treatment initiation. The first dose is usually given intravenously, though the oral bioavailability of dexamethasone is excellent so it can be given orally if the establishment of intravenous (IV) access is problematic and the patient is able to swallow. A common approach is to give a bolus of 10 to 16 mg intravenously, followed by 4 to 6 mg orally or intravenously every 4 to 6 hours thereafter.

PRACTICE POINT

- In the setting of potential neurologic compromise, the dose or route of administration of corticosteroid is not as important as the rapidity of its administration.

The consulting service of choice has traditionally been radiation oncology, as radiotherapy has been the most commonly utilized modality. Not surprisingly, results have been better with this modality if the MSCC is caused by a tumor type known to be more radiosensitive (breast cancer or lymphoma) as opposed to less radiosensitive (non-small-cell lung cancer, melanoma, renal cell carcinoma). Interest in neurosurgical consultation has recently increased, however, with the results of a prospective randomized trial demonstrating superior preservation of ambulation in patients who underwent surgical decompression followed by radiation therapy compared with patients who received radiation therapy alone. Thus, patients presenting with MSCC at a single level should generally be evaluated for surgical candidacy as the initial definitive intervention. Neurosurgical consultation should also be considered for a bony collapse and compression of the spinal cord as cause of MSCC. Radiotherapy can then be administered following surgical decompression, or as the definitive modality in its own right for patients not deemed to be suitable for operative management (**Table 182-1**).

TABLE 182-1 Who should be Consulted Urgently for Suspected MSCC? Factors Favoring Surgical Decompression Versus Radiation Therapy as the Initial Definitive Treatment Modality

Factors Favoring Surgery Followed by Radiotherapy	Factors Favoring Radiotherapy
Solid tumor	Hematologic malignancy
Acceptable surgical candidate	Medical comorbidities prohibit surgery
Rapidly evolving neurological symptoms (eg, paraplegia <48 hours)	Slowly progressive neurological dysfunction (eg, paraplegia >48 hours)
Expected survival > 3 months	Expected survival < 3 months
Pathologic fracture compressing the spinal cord	Mass compressing only cauda equina or spinal roots but not cord itself
No known cancer diagnosis (unknown histology)	
Previous radiotherapy to similar region	
Spinal instability	

SUPERIOR VENA CAVA SYNDROME

A second presentation directly related to tumor expansion, superior vena cava syndrome (SVCS), results from compression of the superior vena cava, markedly inhibiting blood return from the head, neck, and upper extremities. Its presentation is usually more insidious than that of MSCC, and generally doesn't portend the same degree of irreversible functional impairment. Ultimately, obstruction of the superior vena cava tends to lead to collateral blood vessel formation, which is in turn associated with gradual improvement in the presenting symptoms. Almost all cases of SVCS are attributable to malignancy or to thrombosis associated with an indwelling vascular catheter.

PRACTICE POINT

- The most common cause of SVCS is malignancy, of which 60% to 85% of cases are lung cancers. Indwelling vascular catheters are becoming more common, and are responsible for 20% to 40% of presentations.

Culprit cancers

Lung cancer accounts for the vast majority of SVCS presentations, followed by non-Hodgkin lymphoma. The leading conditions responsible for this syndrome in young adults are lymphoma and mediastinal germ cell tumors.

Clinical presentation

The classic symptoms of SVCS are neck and facial swelling, along with venous distension of the neck and chest wall venous system. Several data series suggest, however, that the most common symptom is dyspnea; patients may also complain of headache, hoarseness, dysphagia, and cough. Urgent evaluation is required when symptoms progress to potential respiratory obstruction, such as stridor, or neurologic compromise, as evidenced by syncope, lethargy, obtundation, or even seizure activity.

Diagnosis

The diagnosis of SVCS is made on clinical and radiologic grounds, but the underlying etiology must also be pursued, particularly if the patient does not have a preexisting cancer diagnosis or an indwelling vascular catheter. Abnormalities of vital signs, or of the cardiovascular and respiratory systems on examination, such as cyanosis, indicate the requirement for more urgent workup, usually beginning with a chest X-ray. The most characteristic radiographic finding is widening of the upper mediastinum, occurring more often on the right side than the left. Pleural effusion may also be present. The absence of diagnostic abnormalities on plain film should lead one to proceed to CT scanning, which is more sensitive to mediastinal detail and better able to identify collateral vessels.

If the patient has a history of one of the malignancies mentioned above, tissue acquisition may not be necessary after obtaining a CT scan demonstrating extrinsic superior vena cava compression, but for a patient with no underlying cancer diagnosis or indwelling vascular catheter it is essential to rule out benign causes such as noncancerous tumors or fibrosing mediastinitis related to prior irradiation or infectious causes (eg, histoplasmosis). Depending on the location of the radiographic mass, this can be done using bronchoscopy, percutaneous needle biopsy, mediastinoscopy, or, in some cases, a thoracotomy.

PRACTICE POINT

- It may not be necessary to obtain tissue confirmation of malignancy in a patient with a known history of cancer, but in the absence of such a history tissue acquisition is essential to rule out a benign cause or confirm cancer subtype.

Management

Most often there is no emergent indication for intervention and therapy, for the SVCS can be directed at treatment of the underlying disease.

If the etiology is a vascular catheter, and the obstruction is detected early, treatment with a fibrinolyic agent and salvage of the catheter may be possible, otherwise catheter removal is necessary in conjunction with anticoagulation.

If it is an underlying cancer responsible for the patient's symptoms, the first step is to establish whether there is imminent airway compromise; if so, the situation is a true emergency, and the principles of resuscitation should be applied, including preparation for endotracheal intubation and intensive care unit transfer. If abnormalities of the cardiovascular or respiratory vital signs or neurologic signs are present, an intravascular stent should be considered, if appropriate expertise is available, for immediate relief of the obstruction. Subsequent therapy is dependent upon the underlying histology. Glucocorticoids can be initiated right away, and will likely result in rapid effect if the causative cancer is lymphoma, but will be less effective if lung cancer or a germ cell tumor is the culprit. Chemosensitive tumors, such as lymphoma, a germ cell malignancy, or small cell lung cancer, can be treated with rapid initiation of appropriate chemotherapy, given through a vein on the contralateral side of the body from that affected by the obstruction. A less chemosensitive histology such as non–small cell lung cancer is best treated initially with radiation.

PRACTICE POINT

- SVCS may not represent a true oncologic emergency unless there is evidence of airway compromise, vital sign abnormalities, or neurologic symptoms; these findings necessitate urgent intervention.

HYPERCALCEMIA

As many as 30% of cancer patients will present with elevated calcium levels over the course of their illness, though the incidence of hypercalcemia of malignancy (HCM) has declined substantially over the past two decades due to the introduction of routine bisphosphonate therapy for the prevention of skeletal events in various advanced malignancies. The underlying mechanisms differ depending on the primary tumor, with the most common being the secretion of humoral-related factors (humoral hypercalcemia of malignancy [HHM]) such as parathyroid hormone–related peptide (PTHrP). Other etiologies include the overproduction of vitamin D and increased osteolytic bone resorption in areas surrounding the malignant cells. Unlike PTHrP, ectopic production of parathyroid hormone (PTH) itself is rare.

Culprit cancers

The extent of bony metastatic disease is actually less important than the specific tumor histology in accounting for hypercalcemia (**Table 182-2**). Patients with HHM, resulting from PTHrP overproduction, generally harbor a squamous malignancy, most often originating in the lung, but may also be from the esophagus, cervix, ovarian, endometrial, renal, or head and neck region. Lymphoma can cause hypercalcemia through secretion of the active form of vitamin D, leading to increased resorption of calcium from bone and also absorption from the intestinal tract. Those tumors causing elevated calcium by means of direct effects on bone include breast cancer and multiple myeloma.

PRACTICE POINT

- Underlying tumor histology, especially squamous, is more important than extent of bony metastatic disease in predisposing to hypercalcemia.

TABLE 182-2 Mechanisms of Hypercalcemia of Malignancy and Underlying Tumor Histologies Associated with each Mechanism

Mechanisms of Hypercalcemia	Histologies
PTHrP production	Squamous carcinomas (lung, esophagus, head and neck, cervix); also ovarian, endometrial, renal, and breast cancers
Overproduction of 1,25-dihydroxyvitamin D	Lymphoma
Local bone effects	Breast cancer, lymphoma, and multiple myeloma

Clinical presentation

The presenting symptoms and signs of hypercalcemia are nonspecific and varied. Often, patients feel generally unwell and the physician must have a high index of suspicion to consider an elevated calcium level as a potential cause of any worsening of a patient's condition. Individual symptoms may include nausea, vomiting, anorexia, constipation, lethargy, abdominal pain, and polyuria, but ultimately, if calcium levels continue to rise, may lead to cardiac arrhythmias, acute renal failure, seizures, coma, and even death.

> **PRACTICE POINT**
>
> - The symptoms and signs of hypercalcemia are often nonspecific. Consider this diagnosis in any patient with known malignant disease whose clinical condition deteriorates without an obvious explanation.

Diagnosis

The first step is the confirmation of an elevated calcium level, ideally with an ionized calcium measurement, as the serum calcium is easily affected by changes in plasma protein concentrations.

In a patient with known disseminated malignancy, particularly of a histology frequently associated with hypercalcemia, it may be reasonable to initiate treatment while awaiting further workup. A bone scan could be performed, if not done recently, to assess for bony metastases that may be contributing to osteolytic resorption. The PTH level could also be checked, particularly in patients with a minimal disease burden or a tumor histology not often associated with hypercalcemia, as hyperparathyroidism is a frequent cause of hypercalcemia in the noncancer population and has also been reported to coexist with HCM. Measurement of PTHrP is rarely of great diagnostic value in addition to the above investigations.

Management

Not all patients with hypercalcemia require immediate or aggressive intervention. The rapidity with which one needs to initiate treatment is related to the measured calcium level, the severity of symptoms with which the patient presents, whether the elevated calcium is acute or chronic, and the prognosis of the underlying malignancy. Acute hypercalcemia is more likely to produce symptoms than a mild calcium increase in a patient with chronic hypercalcemia. An asymptomatic or mildly symptomatic patient with a calcium level below 3.5 mmol/L may only need adequate oral hydration as an outpatient and avoidance of exacerbating factors such as thiazide diuretics or a high-calcium diet and treatment of the underlying malignancy.

> **PRACTICE POINT**
>
> - Patients who are asymptomatic or minimally symptomatic with a serum calcium level below 3.5 mmol/L do not need immediate intervention. Those with prominent symptoms, or a calcium level above 3.5 mmol/L, however, require more aggressive measures with fluid hydration, adequate urine output, and, ultimately, bisphosphonates.

Hypercalcemia from any of the above mechanisms creates a vicious cycle in which patients become intravascularly volume depleted, decreasing the glomerular filtration rate and, thus, impairing the ability of the kidney to excrete excess calcium. The first step in management of the hypercalcemic patient is to interrupt this cycle and restore the ability of the nephron to eliminate calcium. Patients may require up to 4 to 6 L per day of IV normal saline, administered at up to 300 to 500 mL/h, depending, again, on the acuity of the hypercalcemia and patient comorbidities, such as cardiac compromise, which might predispose to volume overload.

Once the patient is clinically euvolemic, generally after a couple of hours of IV volume expansion, the addition of a loop diuretic (eg, furosemide 20 or 40 mg intravenously) can increase calcium excretion at the level of the loop of Henle. Thiazide diuretics may worsen hypercalcemia and thus should be avoided.

In addition to vigorous hydration, the other cornerstone of HCM management is bisphosphonate therapy. These medications inhibit bone resorption through direct and indirect effects on osteoclasts.

Among several bisphosphonates from which to choose, the best evidence exists for a single administration of pamidronate or zoledronic acid. A direct comparison suggested that the latter (zoledronic acid 4 mg intravenously) may be superior with respect to rate of complete response, duration of response, and time to recurrence of hypercalcemia.

> **PRACTICE POINT**
>
> - The cornerstone of HCM management is vigorous IV hydration, followed, in some cases, by a loop diuretic and bisphosphonate therapy.

Calcitonin can be added in the acute phase for patients who are symptomatic with markedly elevated calcium levels, but its effects are modest and short-lived due to the rapid development of tachyphylaxis. Glucocorticoids may be useful if the elevated calcium is related to a known underlying lymphoma. In the event of severe hypercalcemia (serum calcium >4.5–5.0 mmol/L) with neurologic symptoms, consultation with a nephrologist regarding dialysis should also be considered (**Table 182-3**).

EMERGENCIES RELATED TO TREATMENT OF MALIGNANCY

TUMOR LYSIS SYNDROME

Though more commonly observed as a response to treatment, the tumor lysis syndrome (TLS), a collection of serum electrolyte abnormalities resulting from the rapid breakdown of tumor cells, may also represent a direct consequence of rapid tumor growth in highly aggressive malignancies. The lysis of tumor cells releases large amounts of nucleic acid, phosphorus, and potassium into the circulation leading to potentially serious cardiac and renal compromise. Factors predisposing to TLS include intravascular volume depletion, rapidly growing malignancy, renal insufficiency, large tumor burden, and hyperuricemia.

Culprit cancers

Burkitt lymphoma and other aggressive lymphomas are the most frequently implicated, but TLS can also be seen with acute lymphoblastic leukemia, chronic leukemias, and, much less commonly, with solid tumors.

Clinical presentation

There is no typical clinical presentation for TLS, as symptoms and signs vary according to the particular electrolyte abnormality observed in a given patient. Patients at risk for TLS based on accepted stratification criteria (**Table 182-4**) require close monitoring of electrolytes during therapy. Ultimately, if such disturbances are not detected early, hyperkalemia can lead to potentially fatal cardiac arrhythmias, precipitation of uric acid can produce renal failure, and seizures can also result.

TABLE 182-3 Therapeutic Options for the Management of Hypercalcemia of Malignancy

Therapy	Usual Dose	Onset of Action	Duration of Action
Normal Saline	Infusion 100–500 mL/hour until euvolemic	Hours	During infusion
Loop diuretic (Furosemide)	20–40 mg intravenously	Hours	During therapy
Pamidronate	90 mg intravenously	24–48 hours	2–4 weeks
Zoledronic acid	4 mg intravenously	24–48 hours	2–4 weeks
Calcitonin	4–8 IU/kg subcutaneously or intravenously	4–6 hours	48 hours
Hydrocortisone	100 mg intravenously every 6 hours	2–5 days	Days to weeks
Prednisone	60 mg orally per day	2–5 days	Days to weeks
Dialysis	N/A	Hours	During treatment

Data from Stewart, and Shane, et al.

PRACTICE POINT

- The biochemical parameters that require close monitoring in patients at risk for TLS are uric acid, potassium, phosphorus, calcium, and creatinine.

Diagnosis

Identification of TLS is based, as mentioned above, on a high index of suspicion and thus, close electrolyte monitoring for patients at risk. The Cairo-Bishop criteria are generally used to establish the diagnosis of laboratory TLS (**Table 182-5**), and clinical TLS is defined as the presence of laboratory TLS in addition to either renal dysfunction (serum creatinine level greater than 1.5 times the upper limit of normal), cardiac arrhythmia, or seizure.

Management

Concerted efforts should be directed at the prevention of TLS, focusing on patients at particular risk.

For patients deemed low risk, no preventative measures are required, with electrolyte abnormalities treated as they arise.

Patients classified as intermediate risk for the development of TLS require preventive measures, however, beginning with IV hydration to maintain a urine output of approximately 100 mL/m^2/hour. Loop diuretics may be necessary to achieve the desired output. These patients may also be pretreated with allopurinol, which inhibits the enzyme xanthine oxidase, leading to decreased uric acid production from the circulating nucleic acids of lysed tumor cells. Allopurinol can be administered orally (100 mg/m^2 every 8 hours) or intravenously (200–400 mg/m^2 in 1–3 divided doses), beginning one to two days in advance of chemotherapy. Treatment is continued for three to seven days afterward, depending on the ongoing risk of TLS. The allopurinol dose may need to be adjusted for patients with underlying renal failure.

High-risk patients have traditionally been managed similarly, with allopurinol in addition to the maintenance of a vigorous urine output, but there is mounting opinion that rasburicase is the agent of choice for these patients, particularly if the uric acid level is elevated at baseline. While allopurinol can lead to the buildup of xanthine and hypoxanthine, which are poorly water soluble, rasburicase facilitates the breakdown of uric acid into allantoin, which is excreted in urine. Rasburicase is administered at a dose of 0.2 mg/kg intravenously over 30 minutes. The duration of treatment could range from one to seven days, with the U.S. Food and Drug Administration recommendation being five days. Rasburicase is contraindicated in patients with glucose-6-phosphate dehydrogenase (G6PD) deficiency.

PRACTICE POINT

- The most important element in the management of TLS is the identification of patients at risk and the institution of appropriate preventive measures. Those at intermediate risk should receive vigorous hydration and allopurinol, whereas those at high risk require the same hydration but rasburicase is preferred over allopurinol.

TABLE 182-4 Risk Stratification for the Development of Tumor Lysis Syndrome Based on a Patient's Underlying Malignancy

Type of Cancer	High Risk	Intermediate Risk	Low Risk
NHL	Burkitt, lymphoblastic	DLBCL	Indolent NHL
ALL	WBC > 100	WBC 50–100	WBC < 50
AML	WBC > 50, monoblastic	WBC 10–50	WBC < 10
CLL	N/A	WBC 10–100 treated with fludarabine	WBC < 10
Other (hematological or solid tumor malignancies)	N/A	Rapid proliferation and expected rapid response to therapy	Other patients

ALL, acute lymphoblastic leukemia; AML, acute myeloid leukemia; CLL, chronic lymphocytic leukemia; DLBCL, diffuse large B-cell lymphoma; NHL, non-Hodgkin lymphoma; WBC, white blood count (expressed × 10^9/L).
Adapted from Coiffier, et al, and Behl, et al.

TABLE 182-5 Cairo-Bishop Criteria for the Establishment of Laboratory Tumor Lysis Syndrome

Two of the following biochemical changes are required, within three days before or seven days after chemotherapy, to constitute laboratory TLS:
Uric acid >476 mmol/L (8 mg/dL) or 25% increase from baseline
Potassium >6 mmol/L (6.0 mEq/L) or 25% increase from baseline
Phosphorus >2.1 mmol/L (6.5 mg/dL) or 25% increase from baseline
Calcium < 1.75 mmol/L (7 mg/dL) or 25% decrease from baseline

From Coiffier, et al.

In the absence of prevention, if TLS develops, patients should be managed as though they were high-risk patients with hyperuricemia as described earlier. Patients should be admitted to the hospital and electrolyte abnormalities should be promptly corrected. Administration of bicarbonate is recommended for alkalinization if metabolic acidosis is present. Hyperkalemia may require calcium gluconate, insulin, and dextrose, in addition to hydration and diuresis, which are already essential components of TLS management. Hyperphosphatemia is treated with dietary restriction, oral phosphate binders, and, if refractory, dialysis. Furthermore, patients at high risk of TLS development should receive chemotherapy in a hospital equipped with dialysis capability, and it is reasonable to request a nephrology consultation for these patients prior to the initiation of chemotherapy, particularly if there is history or evidence of underlying renal compromise.

FEBRILE NEUTROPENIA

One of the most feared complications of chemotherapy is immunosuppression, and a new fever in a neutropenic patient is always a medical emergency. A patient is considered to be neutropenic if the absolute neutrophil count is below 0.5×10^9/L, or, if the neutrophil count is below 1.0×10^9/L but it is likely that the patient's nadir has not been reached and the neutrophil count is expected to fall further. An elevated temperature reaches emergent status when it has risen to 38.5°C, or two separate readings above 38.0°C are recorded separated by at least an hour.

Culprit cancers

Though some cancers can predispose to infection with certain pathogens, such as hematologic malignancies with impaired antibody generation (eg, multiple myeloma or CLL) or defective T-cell function (eg, Hodgkin lymphoma), the chance of developing febrile neutropenia is more related to the treatment (chemotherapy) the patient has received, and to the patient's age, than to the particular tumor histology.

Clinical presentation

Though fever in a neutropenic cancer patient could be due to one of several causes, such as the cancer itself, the chemotherapy or blood products the patient has received, or thromboembolic disease, the most serious potential etiology is infection, and, thus, all patients who satisfy the above definition are considered to harbor a serious systemic infection until proven otherwise. Patients can present with focal or generalized infectious symptoms of any sort, but the most common presentation is that of an asymptomatic patient with hyperthermia.

PRACTICE POINT

- Any patient presenting with febrile neutropenia is considered to harbor a serious systemic infection until appropriate investigations demonstrate otherwise.

Diagnosis

The patient encounter and workup are directed toward the search for an infectious focus. A complete review of systems is essential, paying particular attention to potential infectious sites. Physical examination should also be comprehensive with particular attention paid to any indwelling vascular device.

Investigations begin with biochemistry: complete blood count (CBC) and hepatic and renal profiles. The urine should be cultured along with blood from two different sites including one from a vascular access device, if present.

Baseline chest X-ray is generally recommended for all patients with subsequent investigations directed to particular areas of suspicion identified on history, physical examination, or laboratory testing.

Management

If ultimately identified, definitive treatment is directed at the etiology of the fever. The required investigations can take time, however, and thus the most important step in the management of the febrile neutropenic patient is the timely initiation of broad-spectrum antibiotic therapy. Treatment should not be delayed if cultures cannot be readily obtained. Traditionally, patients have been hospitalized immediately, though there are a subset of patients who can be safely managed as outpatients (**Table 182-6**). These patients also must reside close to the hospital so that they can return frequently for assessment as required. Oral treatment of choice is ciprofloxacin and amoxicillin/clavulanate, or ciprofloxacin and clindamycin if there is a penicillin allergy. The patient should return for a follow-up assessment within two to three days.

TABLE 182-6 Essential Features for the Suitability of Outpatient Management of a Febrile Neutropenic Patient

Factors favoring a low risk for severe infection among patients with neutropenia
Neutrophil count > 0.1×10^9/L
Monocyte count > 0.1×10^9/L
Normal chest X-ray
Nearly normal hepatic and renal profiles
Duration of neutropenia < 7 days
Resolution of neutropenia expected < 10 days
No suggestion of infected venous access device
No neurological or cognitive changes
Maximum documented temperature < 39.0° C
No abdominal pain
No hemodynamic or respiratory compromise
No comorbid complications (shock, hypoxia, pneumonia, vomiting, or diarrhea)

Data from Hughes, et al.

For inpatient management, the agent, or agents, of choice should include a β-lactam antibiotic with activity against *Pseudomonas aeruginosa*. The Infectious Diseases Society of America recommends either a carbapenem, imipenem or meropenem, or a cephalosporin, ceftazidime or cefepime. An antipseudomonal penicillin agent is also a reasonable option, such as piperacillin/tazobactam or ticarcillin/clavulanate. In the setting of a true β-lactam allergy, the combination of vancomycin, an aminoglycoside, and ciprofloxacin could be used. Empiric therapy can be refined appropriately once culture results are available.

Additional gram-negative coverage should be restricted to patients who are hemodynamically unstable or to centers with a high prevalence of gram-negative resistance. An aminoglycoside is a suitable choice, namely gentamycin and tobramycin, or ciprofloxacin in the setting of renal dysfunction. However, aminoglycosides are relatively contraindicated in patients who have received cisplatin as part of their cancer therapy (eg, germ cell tumours) because of concern for renal toxicity.

Additional gram-positive coverage, usually vancomycin, should be added if a catheter-related infection is suspected or documented, blood cultures demonstrate resistant gram-positive bacteria, the patient is a known colonizer of resistant gram-positive bacterium, or if there is evidence of hemodynamic compromise.

The empiric addition of antifungal treatment is indicated if a patient continues to be febrile at day four of their hospital presentation, if a new fever develops after defervescence, or if new pulmonary infiltrates are identified while under treatment with broad-spectrum antibiotics.

As survival in neutropenic patients with serious infections is related to time to neutrophil recovery, there has been interest in the routine administration of myeloid growth factors, such as granulocyte-macrophage colony-stimulating factor. Studies have shown a more rapid recovery of neutrophils and a shortening of hospitalization, but have not shown an improvement in clinical outcome. Thus, these agents could be considered for very serious infections, such as patients who are critically ill or with life threatening infections (eg, bacteremia), but are not generally recommended for routine use.

In the event that an infectious source is identified, treatment is dictated by that particular infection. If the patient defervesces and no source is found, antibiotics should be continued until the resolution of the neutropenia. At this point a hospitalized patient can be discharged. If neutropenia persists, treatment should be continued for two weeks, though the IV antibiotics can be switched to an oral regimen such as ciprofloxacin and amoxicillin/clavulanate.

PRACTICE POINT

- The most important step in the management of the febrile neutropenic patient is the prompt initiation of broad-spectrum antibiotics—preferably after cultures have been drawn, but treatment should not be withheld if cultures cannot be obtained in a timely fashion. Therapy is then adjusted based on the patient's clinical evolution and the results of investigations as they become available.

HEMORRHAGIC CYSTITIS

Cystitis is a relatively common complication of chemotherapy administration, with hemorrhagic cystitis (HC) being its most serious form. Bleeding, which can involve the entire bladder mucosa, ranges from mild oozing to hemorrhage serious enough to require continuous bladder irrigation and transfusion. In addition to chemotherapy, other causes of HC include radiation and certain infections.

Culprit cancers

HC is closely tied to two chemotherapy agents, cyclophosphamide and ifosfamide, which are used to treat a variety of solid tumors and lymphomas. Other chemotherapy agents that have been associated with HC, but not as frequently, include busulfan, thiotepa, doxorubicin, mitomycin, fludarabine, and chlorambucil.

Clinical presentation

Patients may present initially with irritative urinary symptoms while receiving one of the medications listed above, which can then progress to frank hematuria. It is important to identify patients who are hemodynamically unstable, due to profound anemia, and those who may develop urinary outflow obstruction as a result of intravesicular blood clots.

Diagnosis

If vital signs suggest that the patient is hemodynamically unstable, resuscitative measures should be undertaken such as vigorous IV fluid administration and transfusion as needed. CBC and coagulation parameters should be obtained, and all anticoagulation medications discontinued. A timely urology consult is essential.

If the patient is stable and presents with only mild bleeding, resuscitative measures may not be required but the above hematologic parameters should be measured and a urine culture sent to rule out an infectious etiology.

Management

Similar to the situation with TLS, preventive measures exist to decrease the incidence of HC during chemotherapy treatment. The first of these is vigorous IV hydration to maintain good flow through the bladder, preventing the accumulation of toxic metabolites. It is believed that the metabolite responsible for causing HC is acrolein, which can be effectively bound by a medication, 2-mercaptoethanesulfonate (mesna), which is rapidly excreted by the kidney following administration; in the urinary system, it binds acrolein and converts it to an inert molecule that can be safely excreted without damaging the bladder mucosa.

Mesna should be administered either intravenously or orally whenever ifosfamide is given, and also along with high-dose cyclophosphamide in the setting of stem cell transplantation.

PRACTICE POINT

- The chemotherapy agents most commonly associated with HC are ifosfamide and high-dose cyclophosphamide. Vigorous hydration and mesna should be preventively administered along with these medications.

In the event that hemorrhagic cystitis develops despite the recommended pretreatment with mesna, therapy has traditionally been limited to symptomatic management, namely suprahydration and continuous saline bladder irrigation, in addition to withdrawal of the offending agent. Prompt urologic consultation should be sought to initiate continuous bladder irrigation, and, in some cases, extraction of blood clots is required. In severe cases of refractory hemorrhage, vascular embolization, diversion, or even cystectomy may be necessary.

PRACTICE POINT

- Once identified, the initial management of HC includes cessation of any anticoagulant medications, hydration, and prompt urologic consultation.

CONCLUSION

Patients living with cancer are at risk for several potentially irreversible, or even fatal, acute complications of the disease and its treatment. Some of these, such as spinal cord compression, superior vena cava syndrome, and hypercalcemia, are caused by the advance of cancer itself, whereas others, such as tumor lysis syndrome, febrile neutropenia, and hemorrhagic cystitis, are more often related to antineoplastic therapy. For certain of these clinical entities, preventative measures are available and important. For all oncologic emergencies, identification of early symptoms and signs, prompt initiation of therapy, and timely involvement of the appropriate consulting services are critical to life-sustaining intervention and preservation of function.

SUGGESTED READINGS

Behl D, Hendrickson AW, Moynihan TJ. Oncologic emergencies. *Crit Care Clin.* 2010;21:181–205, 2010.

Coiffier B, Altman A, Pui CH, Younes A, Cairo MS. Guidelines for the management of pediatric and adult tumor lysis syndrome: an evidence-based review. *J Clin Oncol.* 2008;26:2767–2778.

DeVita VT, Lawrence TS, Rosenberg SA. Cancer: Principles & Practice of Oncology. 8th ed. New York, NY: Lippincott Williams & Wilkins, Wolters Kluwer; 2008.

Fauci AS, Braunwald E, Kasper DL, et al. Harrison's Principles of Internal Medicine. 17th ed. New York, NY: McGraw-Hill Medical Publishing Division; 2008.

Hensley ML, Hagerty KL, Kewalramani T, et al. American Society of Clinical Oncology 2008 clinical practice guideline update: use of chemotherapy and radiation therapy protectants. *J Clin Oncol.* 2009;27:127–145.

Hughes WT, Armstrong D, Bodey GP, et al. 2002 guidelines for the use of antimicrobial agents in neutropenic patients with cancer. *Clin Infect Dis.* 2002;34:730–751.

Major P, Lortholary A, Hon J, et al. Zoledronic acid is superior to pamidronate in the treatment of hypercalcemia of malignancy: a pooled analysis of two randomized, controlled, clinical trials. *J Clin Oncol.* 2001;19:558–567.

Patchell A, Tibbs PA, Regine WF, et al. Direct decompressive surgical resection in the treatment of spinal cord compression caused by metastatic cancer: a randomised trial. *Lancet* 2005;366:643–648.

Shane E, Dinaz I. Hypercalcemia: pathogenesis, clinical manifestations, differential diagnosis, and management. In: *Primer on the metabolic bone diseases and disorders of mineral metabolism. 6th ed.* American Society of Bone and Mineral Research 2006:176–180.

Stewart AF. Hypercalcemia associated with cancer. *N Engl J Med.* 2005;352:373–379.

CHAPTER 183

Common Issues Specific to Common Cancers

Michael Sanatani, MD, FRCPC
Eric Winquist, MSc, MD, FRCPC, FACP

Key Clinical Questions

1. Small cell carcinomas arise at what anatomical sites?
2. How do squamous cell carcinomas behave differently from small cell carcinomas?
3. How does the behavior and treatment of hormone-sensitive adenocarcinomas differ from hormone-independent adenocarcinomas?

INTRODUCTION

In the preantibiotic era of the late nineteenth century, William Osler instructed clinicians to "Know syphilis in all its manifestations and relations and all other things clinical will be added unto you." In the current era, with *Treponema pallidum* infection no longer a lifelong and endemic condition, Osler would have little objection to the application of his advice to the dozens of diseases we refer to as cancer. In this chapter, some of the more common clinical presentations and manifestations of solid cancers will be reviewed. This will include, with a deferential nod to Carl Jung, four solid cancer "archetypes," each with a distinctive character and management approaches. Molecular phenotypes may replace these histological identities in the future. To the degree that pattern recognition can expedite diagnosis and treatment, these descriptions may be of value in providing a sense of the "personality" of common cancers and their presentations and complications. That said, an open mind and high index of suspicion should always be maintained as cancer can be a fascinatingly unpredictable disease.

PRACTICE POINT

- To the degree that pattern recognition can expedite diagnosis and treatment, these descriptions may be of value in providing a sense of the "personality" of common cancers and their presentations and complications. However, an open mind and high index of suspicion should always be maintained as cancer can be a fascinatingly unpredictable disease.

Solid cancers display impressive heterogeneity, even within the same anatomical tumor sites, but a few general comments can be made. First, solid cancers that are not cured typically recur within months to a few years after completing initial therapy and have an inexorably progressive course to death over a period of months to years. Exceptions occur in clear cell renal cell carcinoma, breast adenocarcinoma, and melanoma patients who may experience recurrences decades after initial diagnosis and treatment. Interestingly, melanoma and renal cell tumors have also been observed to undergo spontaneous remission. Second, solid cancers that have metastasized to distant organs are generally not curable. There are three potential exceptions to this: (1) metastatic germ cell tumors, which typically arise in the testicle in young men (but also rarely in the ovary, pineal gland, mediastinum, or of uncertain primary origin) and are usually cured with systemic chemotherapy; (2) a portion of solid cancer patients with micrometastases treated with anticancer drug therapy added to local therapy can be cured, and this is the basis for adjuvant chemotherapy in breast, colorectal, and lung cancer; and (3) uncommonly, patients with oligometastatic disease treated surgically may be cured, for example, metastatectomy of a solitary lung or liver metastasis in a patient with a soft tissue sarcoma or colorectal cancer. If the clinical situation is at all uncertain, these possibilities should be considered before labeling a solid cancer patient incurable. Thirdly, treatment of the primary tumor in patients with incurable metastatic disease has not been shown to be of clinical benefit and is generally discouraged unless necessary to treat or avert symptoms, with the exceptions of clear cell renal cell carcinoma and ovarian carcinoma, in which surgical treatment of the primary (with cytoreductive nephrectomy and tumor debulking, respectively) have been associated with improved survival.

Cancer is a clonal cellular disease involving loss of normal controls on cell proliferation and differentiation. So the term "cancer" really describes a mechanism of disease that is the basis for more than 100 different diseases we currently classify by anatomy and histology. Cancers arise in the cells of these tissues due to acquired somatic mutations in normal cells. These in turn lead to an increase in positively acting growth cells and a decrease in negatively acting growth signals, and a decrease in activity in pathways leading to programmed cell death (apoptosis). Populations of cancer cells then survive in a hostile microenvironment and metastasize to other organs by conscripting or evading other physiological processes or defenses such as neoangiogenesis and the immune system. In contrast to antimicrobial therapy, which exploits differences in cell biology based in interspecies differences, it should not be surprising that a true "magic bullet" that destroys malignant cells without affecting a patient's normal cells has yet to be identified in any cancer. This means that current therapies using radiation and drugs attempt to exploit subtle differences between normal and malignant cells' response to cellular damage. As a result, the therapeutic index for most cancer treatments is extremely narrow. With this and the consequences of incurable cancer firmly in mind, perhaps nowhere in the practice of medicine are patients and physicians more willing to routinely accept high treatment risks in an effort to cure or even "just" control malignant disease. So it remains common for cancer patients to become seriously ill as a result of their anticancer treatment, despite advances in supportive care. Although virtually all modern solid cancer treatment is done in the outpatient setting, patients frequently require hospitalization, and the need for this may not only result from the locoregional, metastatic, or paraneoplastic effects of the disease itself, but also from treatment complications (**Table 183-1**). The identification of effective cancer drugs has been and remains largely empirical and only recently in the era of molecular biology have the mechanisms of the anticancer action of these drugs started to become truly understood. In addition to numerous hormonal therapies, several dozen cytotoxic agents are in common use for cancer treatment, and a number of "molecularly-targeted" agents have entered routine practice (**Table 183-2**). It is hoped that current efforts to improve cancer treatment toward a less empiric and more individualized approach will ultimately succeed, allowing the use of agents targeted to treat cancers identified as vulnerable while minimizing adverse effects for the patient.

SMALL CELL CARCINOMA

Small cell carcinomas, the most aggressive forms of neuroendocrine malignancies, are most common in the lung but also occur at other anatomical sites, typically "midline organs" (salivary glands, larynx, esophagus, stomach, prostate, uterine cervix, and bladder). Primary small cell carcinomas can also occur in sun-exposed areas of the skin (Merkel cell carcinoma), particularly in immunosuppressed individuals and must be distinguished from metastatic disease. The biology of small cell carcinoma is similar regardless of primary site: rapid growth (which may cause local complications due to obstruction or compression), early metastatic spread, high sensitivity to chemotherapy and radiotherapy, and low overall curability. Practically speaking, staging is binary: limited disease (historically referring to all disease encompassed in a single radiation field), associated with a small chance of cure, versus extensive disease (anatomically beyond one radiation field) and incurable. Combination chemotherapy including etoposide and a platinum analogue are typically used. Paraneoplastic syndromes are common and numerous (**Table 183-3**) with the exception of hypercalcemia, which is curiously uncommon until very late stages of disease in patients with bone metastases (Table 183-3). Hyponatremia is common, rarely requires specific treatment, and may be due to the syndrome of inappropriate antidiuretic hormone production by tumor or volume depletion. Hypernatremia is a more ominous finding, clinically suggesting diabetes insipidus (due to pituitary metastases), severe debilitation with inability to drink, or hyperosmolar nonketotic hyperglycemia. Small cell cancer is also notable for the proven value of prophylactic cranial irradiation, which should be routinely considered in all patients, although there is some debate of its value in nonpulmonary disease. Generally, the risk of brain metastases appears increased in patients with cancer involving the lungs, and may correlate with the volume of lung disease.

SQUAMOUS CELL CARCINOMA

In many ways, squamous cell carcinoma is the polar opposite of small cell carcinoma: growth is slower, it is more predictable, it spreads to nodal sites before distant organs, it has modest sensitivity to chemotherapy and radiotherapy, and it has reasonably high curability with surgery and/or radiotherapy when localized. Management is typically focused on preventing locoregional recurrence, so surgical and radiation oncologists often steer the treatment plan. The medical oncologist's role is often to provide concomitant chemotherapy with radiotherapy as either primary or postoperative adjuvant treatment in patients with locally advanced disease. Local control may be important in patients with distant metastases due to the morbidity of uncontrolled local disease in the head and neck or pelvis, so more aggressive treatment of the primary tumor may be recommended. Hypercalcemia is the most common paraneoplastic syndrome, may occur in the presence of localized disease, and is usually due to tumor production of parathyroid hormone-related peptide secretion. A high index of suspicion is required for hypercalcemia in all cancer patients with unexplained asthenia, fatigue, volume depletion, or confusion. Beyond lymph nodes, metastases typically occur in the lungs and often cavitate, leading to a mistaken diagnosis of lung abscess, a phenomenon also seen with metastatic urothelial carcinoma. These tumors may fistulize in patients with advanced or metastatic disease due to treatment response or disease progression with unfortunate effects on a patient's quality of life. Combination chemotherapy typically includes a platinum analogue combined with 5-fluorouracil and/or a taxane drug. Although tumor shrinkage is commonly seen with combination chemotherapy in untreated patients with localized disease (induction chemotherapy), squamous cell carcinomas tend to be only modestly chemosensitive, and adjuvant chemotherapy alone is generally ineffective (perhaps with the exception of lung cancers).

HORMONE-DEPENDENT ADENOCARCINOMA

Adenocarcinomas can be roughly classified based on their sensitivity to hormonal manipulation. Hormone-dependent cancers originating in the breast, endometrium, or prostate often preferentially involve lymph nodes and bone, and may behave more indolently, at least until they become refractory to hormonal manipulations. As disease progresses patients may develop a "wasting syndrome" due to cytokine-mediated effects of disease burden characterized by asthenia, weight loss, lymphedema, pain, and neurological impingement (spinal cord compression, cauda equina syndrome, radiculopathy). When bone involvement is extensive, bone marrow insufficiency may occur. Treatment usually includes exhaustive use of sequential hormonal manipulations before proceeding to sequential courses of single-agent chemotherapy with taxanes and anthracyclines along with bisphosphonates or denosumab to reduce the risk of skeletal metastatic complications. More

PART VI

Clinical Conditions

TABLE 183-1 Common Acute Complications Leading to Hospitalization in Cancer Patients

Complication	Typical Presentation	Key Management Issues
Increased intracranial pressure from CNS tumor progression	Decreased level of consciousness, confusion	Airway protection, high dose steroids, brain imaging (CT or MRI), swallowing assessment, neurosurgical and radiation oncology consultation
Hypercalcemia of malignancy	Confusion, depression, hypotension, nausea, abdominal pain, renal failure, pain crisis	Intravenous fluids, intravenous bisphosphonates, loop diuretics only if fluid overload occurs; consider calcitonin
Hyponatremia (SIADH – neuroendocrine or small cell cancer)	Confusion, nausea, weakness	Restoration, if necessary, of euvolemia with normal saline, strict fluid restriction, consider inducing impairment of renal water absorption (demeclocycline, lithium), treat underlying malignancy
Pulmonary embolism, deep venous thrombosis	Dyspnea, chest pain, tachycardia, unexplained fever, leg pain, or swelling	Anticoagulation with low-molecular-weight heparins
Malignant pleural effusion	Dyspnea, cough	Repeat thoracocenteses, pleural catheter, or chest tube with pleurodesis
Cardiac tamponade	Dyspnea, presyncope, Kussmaul sign, hypotension, muffled heart sounds, enlarged cardiac silhouette, low voltage ECG	Urgent echocardiogram and pericardiocentesis or pericardial window
Bowel obstruction	Abdominal pain, nausea, vomiting, bloating, obstipation	Surgical consultation, abdominal imaging, intravenous fluids, pain control, electrolyte management, consider octreotide injections, nasogastric or rectal tube
Hepatic failure	Jaundice, confusion or sedation, pruritus	Liver imaging, biliary stent or drain if localized tumor blockage, adjust medications for liver function, monitor sugar and temperature, bowel regime with lactulose; antihistamines, topical menthol, or cytochrome inducers for pruritus
Renal failure	Nausea, anorexia, fatigue	Urgent treatment of electrolyte derangements if necessary, renal imaging, stent or nephrostomy tube if tumor blockage present, hydration, adjust medication doses
Nausea and vomiting (severe)	Dehydration, hypotension, renal failure	Intravenous hydration, regular antiemetics appropriate to likely cause of nausea (eg, dexamethasone and neuroleptics for delayed chemo-induced nausea), rule out hypercalcemia or increased intracranial pressure
Mucositis (severe)	Oral pain, possibly infection with candida, bleeding	Intravenous hydration, treat thrush if present, consider systemic antibacterial therapy if concurrent leukopenia, empiric treatment if febrile, systemic opioid analgesia
Neutropenic fever	Fever, fatigue	Broad spectrum antibacterial therapy as per current infectious diseases febrile neutropenia guidelines, consider granulocyte growth factor support if critically ill; blood and urine cultures, admission to hospital
Pain crisis	Pain acutely reported as ≥ 7/10 when previously better controlled; unresponsive to current medication regime, new quality of pain, unable to function	Escalate doses of current regime ca. 25%, ensuring long-acting opioid and PRN breakthrough opioid given; alternatively consider trial of parenteral route or opioid rotation; assess for possible neuropathic and/or existential components, imaging of areas of pain and any areas which can cause referred pain, anesthesia or pain service consultation
Spinal cord compression, cauda equina syndrome	Back pain, bladder or bowel incontinence, extremity weakness, hypo- or hyperreflexia (depending on level), sensory level, dyspnea	Intravenous steroids, urgent imaging (MRI) of entire spine, neurosurgical and radiation oncology opinion, physiotherapy and occupational therapy consultation

TABLE 183-2 Commonly Used Drugs for the Treatment of Solid Cancers and Key Adverse Effects

Systemic Antineoplastic Agent	Common (≥ 30% incidence) or Potentially Serious (But Possibly Rare) Adverse Effects (S)
Conventional chemotherapy	*All: febrile neutropenia (S), hypersensitivity (S)*
5-Fluorouracil bolus	Stomatitis, diarrhea, cardiac ischemia (S)
5-Fluorouracil infusional Capecitabine	Palmar-plantar erythrodysesthesia, stomatitis, cardiac ischemia (S)
Bleomycin	Fever, chills, stomatitis, interstitial pneumonitis (S)
Carboplatin	Thrombocytopenia, HUS (S)
Chlorambucil	Secondary malignancy (S)
Cisplatin	Nausea, nephropathy, hearing loss, neuropathy
Cyclophosphamide	Alopecia, nausea, thrombocytopenia, pneumonitis (S), HUS (S), hemorrhagic cystitis (S)
Dacarbazine	Nausea, hepatotoxicity (S)
Docetaxel	Neuropathy, alopecia, fatigue
Doxorubicin Epirubicin	S-T changes, nausea, mucositis, alopecia, congestive heart failure (S), secondary leukemia (S)
Doxorubicin, liposomal pegylated	Palmar-plantar erythrodysesthesia, stomatitis, cardiotoxicity (S)
Etoposide	Alopecia, nausea, secondary leukemia (S), Stevens-Johnson syndrome (S)
Gemcitabine	Proteinuria, fever, HUS-TTP (S), pneumonitis (S)
Ifosfamide	Nausea, alopecia, thrombocytopenia, hemorrhagic cystitis (S), encephalopathy (S)
Irinotecan	Diarrhea, constipation, acute cholinergic syndrome, alopecia, nausea, stomatitis
Methotrexate	Nausea, stomatitis, interstitial pneumonitis (S)
Mitomycin	Thrombocytopenia, ARDS (S), HUS/TTP (S)
Mitoxantrone	Stomatitis, nausea, fatigue, cardiotoxicity (S), secondary leukemia (S)
Oxaliplatin	Neuropathy, pharyngolaryngeal dysesthesia, alopecia, fatigue
Paclitaxel	Neurotoxicity, alopecia, ECG abnormalities, nausea, fatigue, liver enzyme abnormalities, thromboembolic disease (S)
Pemetrexed	Nausea
Streptozocin	Nausea, nephrotoxicity (S)
Temozolomide	Nausea, alopecia, Stevens-Johnson Syndrome (S)
Vinblastine	Neurotoxicity, myelosuppression
Vincristine	Neurotoxicity, alopecia
Vinorelbine	Nausea, myelosuppression, neurotoxicity, liver enzyme abnormalities
Immunotherapy	
Interferon alpha	Nausea, anorexia, flu-like syndrome, diarrhea, hepatitis (S), neurotoxicity (S), depression (S)
Targeted therapy (antibodies, small molecules)	*All: hypersensitivity reactions (S)*
Bevacizumab (anti-VEGFR MoAb)	Hypertension, arterial and venous thrombosis (S), gastrointestinal perforation (S), cardiotoxicity (S)
Cetuximab, panitumumab (anti-EGFR MoAbs)	Rash, hypomagnesemia, arrhythmias (S)
Erlotinib, gefitinib (EGFR TKI)	Rash, diarrhea, hypomagnesemia, pneumonitis (S)
Everolimus (mTOR inhibitor)	Rash, cough, dyspnea, stomatitis
Imatinib (anti-*BCR/ABL* and anti-Kit TKI)	Rash, diarrhea, fatigue, myalgias, headache, myopathy (S),
Sorafenib (anti-VEGFR TKI and anti-Raf kinase)	Rash, electrolyte disturbances, anorexia, abdominal pain, palmar-plantar erythrodysesthesia, cardiotoxicity (S), hypertension (S), reversible posterior leukoencephalopathy syndrome (RPLS) (S)
Sunitinib (anti-VEGFR, anti-PDGFR and anti-Kit TKI)	Nausea, mucositis, diarrhea, anorexia, elevated creatinine, rash, elevated liver enzymes, electrolyte disturbances, palmar-plantar erythrodysesthesia, cardiotoxicity (S), hypertension (S), reversible posterior leukoencephalopathy syndrome (S)
Trastuzumab (anti-Her2/neu MoAb)	Cardiotoxicity (S), thromboembolic disease (S)
Hormonal therapy	
Tamoxifen (oral antiestrogen)	Hot flashes, thrombosis (S)
Anastrozole (and other aromatase inhibitors)	Hot flashes, arthralgias
Bicalutamide (oral antiandrogen)	Hot flashes, gynecomastia, breast tenderness
Buserelin (and other LHRH agonists)	Hot flashes

ARDS, acute respiratory distress syndrome; EGFR, epidermal growth factor receptor; HUS, hemolytic-uremic syndrome; MoAb, monoclonal antibody; mTOR, mammalian target of rapamycin; PDGFR, platelet-derived growth factor receptor; TKI, tyrosine kinase inhibitor; TTP, thrombotic thrombocytopenic purpura; VEGFR, vascular endothelial growth factor receptor.

TABLE 183-3 Selected Endocrine and Neurological Paraneoplastic Syndromes

Disorder	Associated Cancers	Diagnosis	Comments
Autonomic neuropathy	SCLC, thymoma	• Anti-amphiphysin • Anti-CRMP5 (anti-CV2) • Anti-Hu	Subacute, panautonomic neuropathy (parasympathetic, sympathetic, enteric systems)
Cushing syndrome	SCLC, bronchial carcinoid, thymoma, medullary thyroid cancer, GI, pancreatic, adrenal, ovarian	• ↓ K^+ usually < 3.0 mmol/L • ↑ Baseline serum cortisol (> 29.0 μg/dL) • Normal to ↑ midnight serum ACTH (> 100 ng/L) not suppressed with dexamethasone	Neuroendocrine lung cancers account for ~ 50–60% of cases
Hypercalcemia	Breast, multiple myeloma, renal cell, squamous cell cancers (likely lung), lymphomas, ovarian, endometrial cancers	• Hypercalcemia • Low to normal (< 20 pg/mL) PTH level; • ↑ PTHrP level	
Lambert-Eaton myasthenia syndrome	SCLC, prostate, cervical, lymphomas, adenocarcinomas	• Anti-VGCC (P/Q type)	Lower extremity proximal muscle weakness, diaphragmatic weakness, bulbar symptoms, later autonomic symptoms
Limbic encephalitis	SCLC, testicular germ-cell, breast, thymoma, teratoma, Hodgkin lymphoma	• Anti-CRMP5 (anti-CV2) • Anti-amphiphysin • Anti-Hu (typically with small cell lung cancer) • Anti-Ma2 (typically testicular cancer)	Onset days to months ~ 40–50% SCLC ~ 20% testicular ~ 8% breast
Paraneoplastic cerebellar degeneration	SCLC, gynecologic, Hodgkin lymphoma, breast	• Anti-Yo • Anti-Hu • Anti-CRMP5 (anti-CV2) • Anti-Ma • Anti-Tr • Anti-Ri • Anti-VGCC • Anti-mGluR1	
SIADH	SCLC, mesothelioma, bladder, ureteral, endometrial, prostate, oropharyngeal, thymoma, lymphoma, Ewing sarcoma, brain, GI, breast, adrenal	• Hyponatremia • Increased urine osmolality (> 100 mOsm/kg)	Euvolemia
Subacute (peripheral) sensory neuropathy	• Lung usually SCLC; breast, ovarian; sarcomas; Hodgkin lymphoma	• Anti-Hu • Anti-CRMP5 (anti-Cv2) • Anti-amphiphysin	Onset weeks to months ~ 70–80% lung Paresthesias/pain upper extremities before lower, ataxia; multifocal, asymmetric distribution

ACTH, adrenocorticotropic hormone; CGP, chronic GI pseudo-obstruction; GI, gastrointestinal; HTLV, human T-cell lymphotropic virus; nAchR, nicotinic acetylcholine receptor; PTH, parathyroid hormone; PTHrP, PTH-related protein; SCLC, small cell lung cancer; SIADH, syndrome of inappropriate antidiuretic hormone secretion.

Data from Pelosof LC, Gerber DE. Paraneoplastic syndromes: an approach to diagnosis and treatment. *Mayo Clin Proc.* 2010;85(9):838–854.

sophisticated hormonal manipulations continue to emerge, with examples including aromatase (breast cancer) and CYP17 inhibitors (prostate cancer).

THROMBOSIS IN CANCER PATIENTS RECEIVING CHEMOTHERAPY

Hospitalized patients with cancer and patients receiving active treatment for their cancer are at the highest risk of developing venous thromboembolism (VTE). Cancer increases the risk of VTE approximately 4-fold and chemotherapy 6.5-fold. The site of cancer influences risk, with stomach and pancreatic cancer having the highest risk, followed by lung, lymphoma, gynecologic, bladder, and testicular cancer. The patient's prechemotherapy leukocyte count > 11,000/mm^3, hemoglobin level < 10 g/dl or administration of red cell growth factors, prechemotherapy platelet count (≥ 350,000/mm^3), and the presence of obesity (BMI ≥ 35 kg/mm^3) also increase risk of VTE. Many of these patients have other medical conditions or require placement of a central venous catheter or surgery that further increases their risk.

HORMONE-INDEPENDENT ADENOCARCINOMA

Aggressive hormone-independent adenocarcinomas (for example, adenocarcinomas of the stomach, esophagus, bowel, lung, pancreas, and ovary) may involve lymph nodes and bone, but are also commonly associated with lung, liver, and brain metastases. Typically these patients succumb to organ failure from distant metastases. Some of these cancers may produce mucin with complications such as pseudomyxoma peritonei and an increased risk of thrombosis (increased by the use of chemotherapy) and related uncommon conditions such as marantic endocarditis. Cancer type, patient and treatment factors, and certain biomarkers are associated with thrombosis risk in cancer patients, and progress has been made in identifying the level of risk in patients receiving chemotherapy. Drug treatments historically evolved separately by site, but have gradually converged over the past decade, with platinum analogues, 5-fluorouracil, anthracyclines, gemcitabine, irinotecan, and/or taxanes commonly used. Tumor response rates are modest with progression inevitable. Molecularly-"targeted" therapies have recently made some impact on the treatment of these tumors, with the anti-HER2 monoclonal antibody, trastuzumab, in HER2 overexpressing breast cancer being the most prolific and perhaps effective example. Subsets of lung, breast, and ovarian cancer patients may benefit from the addition of the antivascular endothelial growth factor monoclonal antibody, bevacizumab, to chemotherapy. Antiepidermal growth factor receptor therapy with monoclonal antibodies (cetuximab and panitumumab) and small molecule tyrosine kinase inhibitors (erlotinib and gefitinib) appear to benefit subsets of patients with incurable colorectal and lung cancers, respectively. Specific targeted agents are also showing therapeutic promise in subsets of patients with BRCA-deficient, and EML-ALK- and BRAF-mutated adenocarcinomas.

CONCLUSION

The course of cancer and its response to treatment can be unpredictable although some patterns emerge that are typical of specific cancers. This chapter provides a general background for hospitalists who may co-manage oncology patients by reviewing the behavior of common cancers and issues that might lead to acute hospitalization.

SUGGESTED READINGS

Bremnes RM, Andersen K, Wist EA. Cancer patients, doctors and nurses vary in their willingness to undertake cancer chemotherapy. *Eur J Cancer*. 1995;31A(12):1955–1959.

Cancer Care Ontario Drug Formulary (http://www.cancercare.on.ca/cms/One.aspx?portalId=1377&pageId=10767, accessed 16 March 2011).

Connolly GC, Khorana AA. Emerging risk stratification approaches to cancer-associated thrombosis: risk factors, biomarkers and a risk score. *Thromb Res*. 2010;125 (suppl 2):S1–S7.

Flanigan RC, Mickisch G, Sylvester R, Tangen C, Van Poppel H, Crawford ED. Cytoreductive nephrectomy in patients with metastatic renal cancer: a combined analysis. *J Urol*. 2004;171(3):1071–1076.

Freifeld AG, Bow EJ, Sepkowitz KA, et al. Clinical practice guideline for the use of antimicrobial agents in neutropenic patients with cancer: 2010 update by the Infectious Diseases Society of America. *Clin Infect Dis*. 2011;52(4):e56–e93.

Gleave ME, Elhilali M, Fradet Y, et al. Interferon gamma-1b compared with placebo in metastatic renal-cell carcinoma. *N Engl J Med*. 1998;338(18):1265–1271.

Hanahan D, Weinberg RA. The hallmarks of cancer. *Cell*. 2000;100(1):57–70.

Osler W. *Familiar Medical Quotations*, first ed. Boston, MA: Little, Brown, and Co. 1968, p. 651.

Pelosof LC, Gerber DE. Paraneoplastic syndromes: an approach to diagnosis and treatment. *Mayo Clin Proc*. 2010;85(9):838–854.

Wood L, Kollmannsberger C, Jewett M, et al. Canadian consensus guidelines for the management of testicular germ cell cancer. *Can Urol Assoc J*. 2010;4(2):e19–e38.

CHAPTER 184

Diagnostic Workup of Unknown Primary

Puneet Bains, MD, FRCPC
Sharlene Gill, MD, MPH

Key Clinical Questions

1. What is the diagnostic approach to cancer of unknown primary?
2. How should patients with unknown primary be evaluated?
3. What are the common clinical presentations of cancer of unknown primary?
4. What is the management strategy of patients with no identifiable primary site?

INTRODUCTION

Cancer of unknown primary site (CUP) is described as histologically confirmed metastases with no identifiable primary site of origin. The majority of malignancies present with an obvious primary site, whereas CUP has a reported incidence of 2.3% to 7.8% in international databases. Prostate, lung, breast, and colorectal have remained the top four primary sites of cancer for most of this decade (**Figure 184-1**).

Of the over 1.5 million new cancer cases estimated to be diagnosed in the United States in 2010, 30,000 cases were reported without an identifiable source, similar to the number of new cases of pancreatic cancer diagnosed each year. After appropriate evaluation, less than 25% of these patients will have a primary site identified.

The median age of CUP patients is 60 years, with males being more affected than females. The prognosis is dismal, with median survivals ranging from 11 weeks to 11 months, a 1-year survival rate of less than 25%, and a 5-year overall survival rate of approximately 11%. However, with the advancement of diagnostic tools and techniques, the ability to identify a primary site has improved over time, allowing for treatment plans specific to the primary site.

PATHOPHYSIOLOGY

While CUP may be a distinct biologic and clinical entity, a few theories attempt to explain the biology behind CUP. There are many debatable hypotheses as follows:

- The primary tumor remains microscopic and escapes detection.
- The primary tumor spontaneously regresses after seeding the metastatic site—the "burned out primary." For example, testicular scarring is sometimes seen in metastatic germ cell tumors.
- The embryonic epithelial cells that fail to appropriately migrate may undergo malignant transformation and result in a cancer of unknown primary. Extragonadal germ cell tumors in the mediastinum and undescended testes illustrate this biologic theory.
- Aberrations in genetic and molecular profiles may also explain the origin of CUP.

Whatever the explanation, the clinical and biologic aggressiveness of cancer of unknown primary is well appreciated.

HISTOLOGY

Despite the lack of a known primary site, CUP can still be classified in histologic categories, allowing for better differentiation and treatment (**Table 184-1**).

These categories include adenocarcinoma, squamous cell carcinoma, neuroendocrine carcinoma, poorly differentiated carcinoma, and poorly differentiated neoplasm. The latter is a vague label, as the tissue does not have any defining characteristics and may include carcinoma, lymphoma, melanoma, or sarcoma. Within these histologic categories, subsets exist with favorable prognosis (**Table 184-2**).

These subsets can be managed by locoregional treatment and usually respond to systemic chemotherapy; thus, in addition to improved survival and progression free intervals, they may have the potential for cure.

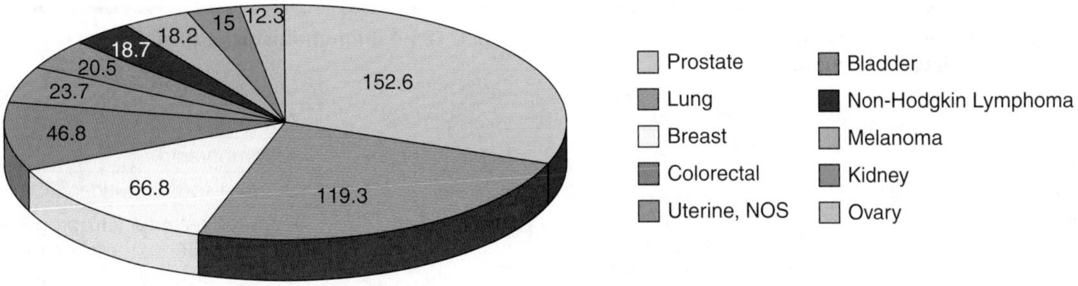

Figure 184-1 *Top ten cancer sites in 2006—males and females (per 100,000).*

DIAGNOSTIC EVALUATION

HISTORY AND PHYSICAL EXAMINATION

The clinical presentation itself will often provide the necessary information to diagnose an occult primary. Hence, the evaluation begins with a thorough history and physical. It is important to identify any possible risk factors for malignancy and any signs or symptoms suggestive of a primary site. The history should include a detailed occupational, tobacco, gynecologic, and family history.

The physical exam must also be a comprehensive and systematic head-to-toe examination. This would include a breast and pelvic exam in females, testicular and prostate exam in males, and digital rectal exam in all patients.

PRACTICE POINT

- The physical examination of any patient with an occult primary must also be a comprehensive and systematic head to toe examination. This would include a breast and pelvic exam in females, testicular and prostate exam in males, and digital rectal exam in all patients.

LABORATORY STUDIES

Laboratory studies should begin with routine blood tests to assess hematologic and end-organ function, including a complete blood count, renal and liver function tests, and lactate dehydrogenase. When appropriate, urinalysis, urine cytology, and fecal occult blood testing should also be included.

Serum tumor markers

The role of serum tumor markers has not yet clearly been established, and they have not proven to be of prognostic or diagnostic value. Although routine use of tumor markers is not recommended in the diagnostic evaluation of malignancy, they may facilitate diagnosis in the event of an unknown primary regardless of the nonspecificity of the elevation. The most commonly tested tumor markers include CEA, CA 125, CA 19-9, CA 15-3, PSA, AFP, β-HCG, and CA 15-3. CEA may be a marker for an epithelial-derived malignancy and is most commonly elevated in colorectal cancer and primary lung cancer, while CA 19-9 is typically associated with cancers of the upper abdomen. An elevated CA 125 is often associated with ovarian cancer but may also be indicative of breast cancer; in addition, elevated levels of both CA 15-3 and CA 125 may be present in benign conditions such as uterine fibroids, endometriosis, and pelvic inflammatory disease. A summary of common tumor markers is listed in **Table 184-3**.

TABLE 184-1 Histologic Variants

Adenocarcinoma	70%
Poorly differentiated carcinoma	15–20%
Squamous cell carcinoma	5%
Neuroendocrine	<5%
Poorly differentiated neoplasm	<5%

HISTOPATHOLOGY

Tissue diagnosis is of the utmost importance, both for the confirmation of malignancy and characterization of potential primary sites; thus, a biopsy of the known site of metastases is a necessity. A core or excisional biopsy is preferred because fine needle aspiration often results in insufficient tissue and histologic detail is poorly preserved. Inadequate tissue also limits the number of special studies that can be done on the pathologic sample. Limiting the number of histologic studies may impede the search for a primary site.

Light microscopy

Under light microscopy, the pathologist is able to visualize cell morphology and differentiate the tumor type. Light microscopy allows classification of the tissue into adenocarcinoma, squamous cell carcinoma, or poorly differentiated carcinoma if the distinguishing features are poorly preserved.

Immunohistochemistry

The mainstay of immunohistochemical classification for CUP involves cytokeratin (CK) staining. Cytokeratins are proteins found in epithelial cells that contain keratin intermediate filaments. Expression of these cytokeratins is often tissue or organ specific. Generally, CK 7 involves tissue from the lung, ovary, endometrium, or breast. CK 20 is usually expressed in the gastrointestinal (GI) tract, urothelium, and Meckel cells. The combination of CK 7 and CK 20 also proves to be useful in identifying a primary site, as summarized in **Figure 184-2**.

TABLE 184-2 CUP Clinical Presentations Associated with a More Favorable Prognosis

- Poorly differentiated carcinomas involving the mediastinal-retroperitoneal nodes
- Peritoneal papillary serous adenocarcinomatosis in females
- Poorly differentiated neuroendocrine carcinomas
- Isolated axillary node adenocarcinomas in females
- SCC with cervical node involvement

TABLE 184-3 Common Serum Tumor Markers and Associated Malignancies

CA 15-3	Breast
CA 19-9	Pancreatic, biliary tract
CA 125	Ovarian
Carcinoembryonic antigen (CEA)	Colorectal, non-small cell lung hepatocellular, mucinous adenocarcinomas
Prostate-specific antigen (PSA)	Prostate
Beta-human chorionic gonadotropin (β-HCG)	Germ cell, gestational trophoblastic disease
Alpha-fetoprotien (AFP)	Hepatocellular, germ cell

Following cytokeratin profiling by CK 7 and CK 20 status, additional proteins can also be informative, as listed in **Table 184-4**.

Thyroid transcription factor (TTF)-1 is an illustrative example. TTF-1 is a protein involved in regulating transcription of genes specific to thyroid and lung and is generally found in pulmonary adenocarcinomas and in thyroid malignancies. Other examples include prostate-specific antigen (PSA) staining for prostate cancer, estrogen and progesterone receptor staining in breast cancer, common leukocyte antigen in lymphomas, and chromogranin and synaptophysin in neuroendocrine tumors. The combination of positive markers can potentially narrow the differential diagnosis of the primary site of malignancy.

Electron microscopy

Light microscopy and immunohistochemistry may not always yield a diagnosis. In these circumstances, the tissue may be evaluated by electron microscopy. Poorly differentiated neoplasms are one example. Given the associated expense and the requirement for special tissue fixation, electron microscopy is not applied routinely.

Cytogenetics

Although limited, certain cytogenetic abnormalities also exist in some tumor types. In young males with a midline tumor or a poorly differentiated carcinoma, an abnormality in chromosome 12p may be the distinguishing feature for a germ cell tumor. Examples of other chromosomal aberrations include t(8;14) and t(11;22) translocations, occurring in Burkitt lymphoma and Ewing sarcoma, respectively.

TABLE 184-4 Immunohistochemical Markers

Sarcoma	Vimentin, desmin, factor VIII antigen
Lymphoma	Common leukocyte antigen
Neuroendocrine	Chromogranin
Prostate	Prostate-specific antigen (PSA)
Breast	Estrogen receptor (ER), progesterone receptor (PR), epithelial membrane antigen, gross cystic disease fluid protein-15 (GCDFP), mammaglobin
Thyroid	Thyroglobulin, calcitonin, epithelial membrane antigen
Germ Cell	Beta-human chorionic gonadotropin (β-HCG), alpha-fetoprotien (AFP)
Hepatocellular	alpha-fetoprotien (AFP)
Melanoma	S-100, Vimentin

DNA MICROARRAY

While the field of molecular gene profiling may soon allow us to readily determine the anatomic site of origin more efficiently and accurately, at present making this determination still requires an investigational strategy. DNA microarrays are able to generate gene expression profiles of unknown tissue samples. These DNA microarray databases contain known gene expression patterns of different tumor types. A comparison of CUP tissue sample with the bank of tissue in the database is made under the assumption that the CUP tissue from the metastatic site has maintained the molecular genetic profile of the primary site.

DIAGNOSTIC IMAGING

Necessary radiographic evaluation can prove to be expensive and exhaustive. This step typically begins with a computed tomography (CT) scan of the thorax, abdomen, and pelvis. Even if the primary

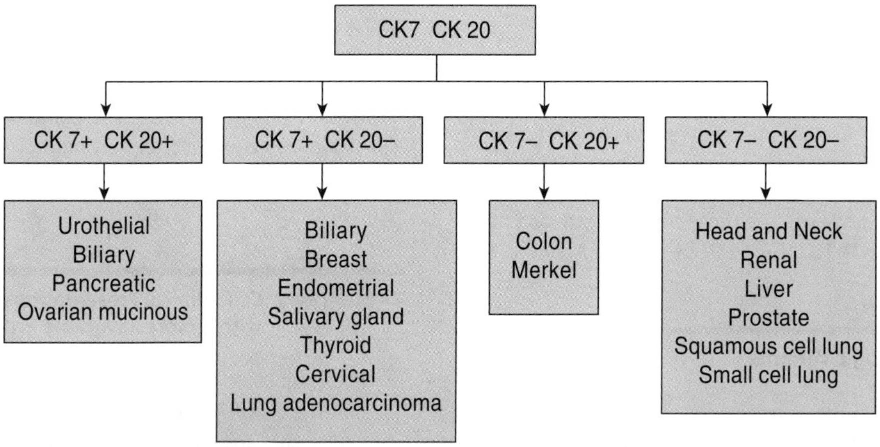

Figure 184-2 *Approach to cytokeratin staining in CUP. (Adapted, with permission, from Varadhachary GR, Abbruzzese JL, Lenzi R. Diagnostic strategies for unknown primary cancer. Cancer. 2004;100:1776–1785.)*

site has already been identified, CT can establish the extent of the metastatic disease. Further diagnostic imaging will be dictated by the clinical presentation. Isolated axillary lymphadenopathy in females should prompt an evaluation with mammography.

Positron emission tomography (PET) involves the use of a radiotracer, usually fluorodeoxyglucose (FDG). Tumors uptake FDG readily, as they are highly metabolically active, but other inflamed or infected metabolically active tissue can be falsely mistaken for a malignancy. PET scans, usually combined with CT scans (PET/CT), may reveal the primary tumor in 8% to 53% of patients, but this is also accompanied by a large number of false positives (greater than 20%). The efficacy of PET/CT in discovering a primary site is debatable. False positives increase the likelihood of further investigations that may be invasive, thereby increasing morbidity. However, a whole body PET/CT scan may be more cost effective because it can not only identify the anatomic origin of a tumor, but it can also identify metastatic sites. PET may complement conventional imaging, but current recommendations do not support its use as a replacement of conventional imaging in the diagnostic workup of a primary unknown cancer. However, an expert panel on PET, consisting of radiologists, oncologists, and nuclear physicians, deemed PET imaging to be beneficial in the workup of cancer of unknown primary. Consider local expertise and technology along with the efficacy, cost, and false-positive rate of PET/CT when making decisions about the most appropriate imaging modality.

ENDOSCOPIC EVALUATION

Endoscopy includes but is not limited to esophagogastroduodenoscopy, laryngoscopy, bronchoscopy, and colonoscopy. While not used routinely, endoscopy is increasingly employed to identify a primary tumor in the appropriate clinical circumstance. For instance, upper and lower gastrointestinal endoscopy should be considered in patients with metastatic adenocarcinoma of the liver and in patients presenting with a microcytic anemia. Rarely, more invasive procedures, such as laparoscopy, are required. These procedures come with a risk of complications, so one must consider whether the findings would result in a change in course of treatment prior to subjecting a patient to such investigations.

COMMON CLINICAL PRESENTATIONS AND SUGGESTED MANAGEMENT OF CUP

More than half of CUP cases will present with multiple sites of metastases including lymph nodes, liver, and bone. It is important to emphasize that the goal of a CUP workup is not to solve the mystery of an occult primary, but rather to identify the most appropriate empiric choice of treatment. This is critical in cases for which curative salvage options may exist even when involving distant metastases, such as germ cell tumors or lymphoproliferative malignancies. Unfortunately, the majority of CUP are due to advanced malignancy not amenable to a curative outcome.

Common clinical presentations and their recommended management are discussed below.

ADENOCARCINOMA

Adenocarcinoma of unknown primary (ACUP) represents the bulk of de novo solid tumor presentations (approximately 70%). The clinical presentation can vary but a few common scenarios do exist, often suggestive of the occult malignancy. A commonly utilized empiric systemic chemotherapy approach for ACUP involves a platinum- and taxane-based regimen with limited efficacy. However, certain subgroups may be amenable to more site-directed therapy based upon the presentations outlined below.

PRACTICE POINT

- **Adenocarcinoma:** Isolated axillary lymphadenopathy in females should prompt an evaluation with mammography. Peritoneal carcinomatosis in females may indicate an ovarian primary. Osteoblastic bone metastasis in a male patient should raise suspicion of carcinoma of the prostate and evoke a prostate examination and PSA.

Isolated axillary lymphadenopathy

Occult breast cancer can often be manifested by isolated axillary lymphadenopathy caused by metastatic adenocarcinoma. MRI may be necessary if mammography is normal. Immunohistochemical staining with estrogen and progesterone receptors should also be done on biopsy samples. These patients are treated as stage II breast cancer, regardless of whether a primary tumor is discovered. This entails a modified radical mastectomy and axillary lymph node dissection with or without radiation therapy. Treatment of the ipsilateral breast remains controversial, but the standard of care remains modified radical mastectomy. Adjuvant systemic chemotherapy after surgery is also recommended. The exact choice of the regimen relies on the tumor phenotype and will consist of chemotherapy, with or without Herceptin and/or hormonal therapy. Well-conducted studies on the role of adjuvant chemotherapy are limited, but one small retrospective cohort study reports a five-year survival benefit in those receiving adjuvant chemotherapy compared with those who did not receive any adjuvant systemic treatment (93% vs. 64%). The 5- and 10-year survival are 75% and 60%, respectively.

Peritoneal carcinomatosis

Peritoneal carcinomatosis in females may indicate an ovarian primary. Although exploratory laparotomy does not often discover a primary tumor, CA 125 is frequently elevated. These patients are treated as stage III ovarian cancer. This typically entails upfront taxane- and platinum-based chemotherapy. The role of debulking surgery in this setting is less clear.

Osteoblastic bone metastasis in a male

Osteoblastic bone metastasis in a male patient should raise suspicion of carcinoma of the prostate and evoke a prostate examination and PSA. Treatment of these patients is typically pursued as that of advanced carcinoma of the prostate, which may involve hormonal therapy with an luteinizing-hormone-releasing hormone (LHRH) agonist with or without antiandrogen therapy.

POORLY DIFFERENTIATED CARCINOMA

This is the second most common histologic variant of CUP (15% to 20%). Retroperitoneal and mediastinal disease is usually the culprit and CT of the chest and abdomen are often required. Recognizing extragonadal germ cell tumors, especially in a young male with a midline mass, is of utmost importance because of the highly curative nature of this malignancy. Serum human beta-chorionic gonadotropin (β-HCG) and alpha-fetoprotein (AFP) tests would also be warranted in the case of a midline tumour.

Young males presenting with mediastinal or retroperitoneal midline tumors should be treated with a platinum-based regimen, as with extragonadal germ cell tumors. High rates of cure are achieved in these patients—up to 40% to 50% in those with an identified chromosome 12 abnormality.

With the exception of poorly differentiated neuroendocrine carcinomas, all other poorly differentiated carcinomas are treated with empiric platinum and taxane chemotherapy. The preferred treatment for poorly differentiated neuroendocrine carcinomas is combination chemotherapy with either a platinum- and etoposide-based regimen or one that includes platinum, etoposide, and paclitaxel. The response rate achieved is greater than 50%, with a complete response rate of 15% to 25%. Long-term disease-free survival ranges from 10% to 15%.

In some circumstances, only a single metastatic site of poorly differentiated carcinoma or adenocarcinoma is identified. These cases are treated with local therapy—usually by surgical resection and, if not amenable to resection, by radiotherapy.

Squamous cell carcinoma

Squamous cell carcinoma without an identifiable primary site often presents with cervical or inguinal lymphadenopthy. An involved cervical lymph node suggests a head and neck primary, often prompting a thorough endoscopic evaluation of the nasal, oropharyngeal, and laryngeal passages. If a supraclavicular lymph node is involved, one must also search for a lung primary. An inguinal lymph node may represent a genital or anorectal primary. Female patients should undergo a careful examination of the vulva, vagina, and cervix. Males should undergo careful penile examination. A digital rectal examination should also be performed, and a sigmoidoscopy may also be necessary.

PRACTICE POINT

- **Squamous cell carcinoma:** Cervical lymphadenopthy suggests a head and neck primary; if a supraclavicular lymph node is involved, one must also search for a lung primary. An inguinal lymph node may represent a genital or anorectal primary.

If the disease site is limited to cervical lymphadenopathy, these patients should be treated as head and neck cancer. Treatment may require surgical resection, radiation, chemotherapy or a combination, depending on the extent of disease. The five-year survival rate is in the range of 35% to 50%. If the disease site involves inguinal lymphadenopathy, the recommended course of treatment requires an inguinal lymph node dissection and chemoradiation. Five-year survival rates are reported to between 15% to 20%.

CONCLUSION

Cancer of unknown primary can be a challenging diagnosis not only for the physician, but also for the patient. The primary goal of the workup is to perform a thorough yet reasonable evaluation in hope of identifying a subgroup that is treatable and potentially curable. With improved diagnostic techniques and understanding of the molecular biology of tumors, the proportion of cancers with a truly unknown primary is diminishing over time. Ultimately, the intent is to be able to provide a rationale and individualized site-directed treatment plan for the patient with the goal of optimal disease control.

SUGGESTED READINGS

American Cancer Society. *Cancer Facts & Figures 2010*. Atlanta: American Cancer Society; 2010.

Ellerbroek N, Holmes F, Singletary E, et al. Treatment of patients with isolated axillary nodal metastases from an occult primary carcinoma consistent with breast origin. *Cancer*. 1990;66:1461.

Fletcher JW, Djulbegovic B, Soares HP, et al. Recommendations on the use of 18F-FDG PET in oncology. *J Nucl Med*. 2008;49:480–508. doi: 10.2967/jnumed.107.047787.

Greco FA, Hainsworth JD. Cancer of unknown primary site. In Devita VT Jr., Hellman S, Rosenbergsa, eds. *Cancer, Principles & Practice of Oncology*. 7th ed. Philadelphia, PA: Lippincott Williams & Wilkins; 2005:2213–2236.

Gutzeit A, Antoch G, Ku H, Egelhof T, Fischer M. Unknown primary tumors: detection with dual-modality PET/CT—initial experience. Radiology. 2005;234:227–234.

Hainsworth JD, Greco FA. Treatment of patients with cancer of unknown primary site. *N Engl J Med*. 1993;329:257–263.

Hainsworth JD, Wright EP, Gray GF, Greco FA. Poorly differentiated carcinoma of unknown primary site: correlation of light microscopic findings with response to cisplatin-based combination chemotherapy. *J Clin Oncol*. 1987;5:1275–1280.

Howlader N, Noone AM, Krapcho M, Neyman N, Aminou R, Waldron W, Altekruse SF, Kosary CL, Ruhl J, Tatalovich Z, Cho H, Mariotto A, Eisner MP, Lewis DR, Chen HS, Feuer EJ, Cronin KA, Edwards BK, eds. *SEER Cancer Statistics Review*. 1975–2008, National Cancer Institute. Bethesda, MD, http://seer.cancer.gov/csr/1975_2008/.

Motzer RJ, Rodriguez E, Reuter VE, et al. Molecular and cytogenetic studies in the diagnosis of patients with midline carcinomas of unknown primary site. *J Clin Oncol*. 1995;13:274.

Pavlidis N, Briasoulis E, Hainsworth J, et al. Diagnostic and therapeutic management of cancer of an unknown primary. *Eur J Cancer*. 2003;39:1990–2005.

Pavlidis N, Fizazi K. Cancer of unknown primary (CUP). *Crit Rev Oncol Hematol*. 2005;54:243–250.

U.S. Cancer Statistics Working Group. United States Cancer Statistics: 1999–2006 Incidence and Mortality Web-based Report. Atlanta: U.S. Department of Health and Human Services, Centers for Disease Control and Prevention and National Cancer Institute; 2010. Available at www.cdc.gov/uscs.

Varadhachary GR, Abbruzzese JL, Lenzi R. Diagnostic strategies for unknown primary cancer. *Cancer*. 2004;100:1776–1785.

SECTION 10
Infectious Disease

CHAPTER 185

Fundamentals of Antibiotics

Matthew E. Falagas, MD, MSc, DSc
Ioannis A. Bliziotis, MD

Key Clinical Questions

1. What resistance patterns are associated with major nosocomial pathogens?
2. When should empiric antibiotic therapy be initiated? When is it permissible to delay empiric antibiotic therapy, if ever?
3. What impact do pharmacokinetics and pharmacodynamics have on antibiotic choice?
4. In what circumstances is combination antibiotic therapy appropriate?
5. What are the major adverse effects of antibiotics?

INTRODUCTION

In this chapter, we will use the terms antibacterial agents and antibiotics interchangeably. The term antibiotic has sometimes been defined as a substance produced by microbes that inhibits the growth of other microbes, especially bacteria. More broadly, it is used to characterize any agent with antibacterial properties, whether found in nature or synthesized artificially. Antibiotics are prescribed to approximately one-third of all hospitalized patients, and account for greater than 10% of hospital pharmacy expenditures. Up to one-half of antibiotic orders may be unnecessary, poorly chosen, or dosed incorrectly. Indiscriminant use of broad-spectrum agents is also believed to be a key contributor to emerging worldwide antimicrobial resistance. The estimated additional hospital costs associated with drug-resistant hospital-acquired bacterial infections in the United States is estimated to several billions of dollars. Hospitalists should be familiar with the currently available antibiotics, their penetration into various tissues, their major adverse effects, and their spectrum of activity relative to local patterns of antibacterial resistance. Antimicrobial prescribing should also take into account issues of cost and potential for the emergence of resistance.

ANTIBIOTIC CATEGORIES AND SPECTRUM OF ACTIVITY

Major categories, subdivisions, and some individual antibacterial agents are summarized in **Table 185-1** according to their mode of action, and side effects and drug-drug interactions are listed in **Table 185-2**. Antibacterial spectrum often overlaps between different antibiotic groups. However, few antibiotics are active against multidrug- or highly resistant bacteria. Thus, the clinician may sometimes have several choices of potentially appropriate antibiotics, but at other times may only have only one, or even none.

When choosing antibacterial therapy in the hospital setting, it is crucial to know local patterns of antibiotic susceptibility and resistance. The phenotypes of bacterial organisms with respect to resistance may be important due to their abundance, virulence, or the near absence of antibiotics active against them. Most isolates of pneumococci are still sensitive to amoxicillin and especially to ceftriaxone. However, because pneumococcal infections are very common, even a small percentage of resistant isolates results in a large absolute number of infections by them. Vancomycin-resistant enterococci (VRE) are not highly virulent, but they are important in the hospital setting because of their tendency to attack debilitated and immunosuppressed patients, and because of the limited options for therapy. Methicillin-resistant *Staphylococcus aureus* (MRSA), by contrast, is virulent and increasingly common in both the hospital and community settings. The susceptibility patterns of nosocomial strains of MRSA differ from those of strains of community-acquired *Staphylococcus aureus* (cMRSA). Hospital-acquired MRSA is usually susceptible only to vancomycin, teicoplanin (available in Europe, but not the United States), and newer agents such as linezolid, tigecycline, and daptomycin. In addition to these drugs, cMRSA is also often susceptible to trimethoprim-sulfamethoxazole, fluoroquinolones, and clindamycin.

Gram-negative rods encountered in the hospital may have characteristic susceptibility phenotypes. Resistance to ampicillin and trimethoprim-sulfamethoxazole (TMP-SMX) is rising among *Escherichia coli*, limiting the role of these antibiotics as empiric therapy for urinary tract infections (UTIs). In addition, all enteric Gram-negative rods, and especially *Escherichia coli* and *Klebsiella*

TABLE 185-1 The Main Categories, Subdivisions, and Individual Antibacterial Agents, with Spectrum of Activity and Main Modes of Action

Antibiotic Category	Subdivisions (Individual Substances)	Spectrum of Antibacterial Activity
Antibiotics acting on bacterial cell wall		
A. Beta-lactams		
1. Penicillins	Naturally occurring (penicillin G, penicillin V)	Gram-positive cocci, excluding staphylococci and most enterococci. Gram-positive rods, including anaerobes. Spirochetes.
	Penicillinase-resistant antistaphylococcal (methicillin, oxacillin, nafcillin, dicloxacillin)	Methicillin-susceptible staphylococci (MSS). Gram-positive cocci, but not many enterococci.
	Aminopenicillins (ampicillin, amoxicillin)	All the above plus enterococci, *Listeria monocytogenes, Hemophilus influenzae, Moraxella catarrhalis,* and some enteric Gram-negative rods.
	Carboxy-penicillins and ureido-penicillins (ticarcillin, piperacillin)	All the above plus *Enterobacter, Klebsiella, Pseudomonas, Acinetobacter* species, and anaerobes.
2. Cephalosporins	First generation (cefadroxil, cefazolin, cephalexine, cephradine)	Gram-positive cocci including MSS, excluding enterococci. Some strains of *Escherichia coli, Klebsiella, Proteus mirabilis.* Not active against indole-positive *Proteus* and *Serratia.*
	Second generation (cefamandole, cefaclor, cefprozil, cefuroxime, cefotetan, cefoxitin, loracarbef)	Similar to first generation, plus *Hemophilus influenzae, Enterobacter* species, indole-positive *Proteus* and *Serratia, Neisseriae.* Cephamycins (cefotetan, cefoxitin) have good anaerobic activity against *Bacteroides fragilis* but poor against Gram-positive cocci and *Enterobacter* species.
	Third generation (cefotaxime, ceftriaxone, ceftazidime, cefoperazone, cefixime)	Enhanced activity against Gram-negative rods. Ceftazidime has good, cefoperazone moderate, and the rest poor activity against *Pseudomonas aeruginosa.* Good against Gram-negative cocci. Variable activity against Gram-positive cocci, cefotaxime and ceftriaxone being excellent for pneumococci. Poor anaerobic activity.
	Fourth generation (cefepime, cefpirome)	Good activity against Gram-positive cocci, with enhanced activitiy against *Pseudomonas aeruginosa* and other Gram-negative rods.
3. Monobactams	(aztreonam)	Gram-negative rods including *Pseudomonas aeruginosa* and some strains of *Acinetobacter baumannii.* Poor against Gram-positive bacteria and anaerobes.
4. Carbapenems	(meropenem, imipenem/cilastatin, ertapenem)	Excellent activity against Gram-negative rods, including *Enterobacter* species, as well as multidrug-resistant *Klebsiella pneumoniae, Pseudomonas aeruginosa,* and *Acinetobacter baumannii* (not ertapenem). Good Gram-positive activity. No advantage over ampicillin for enterococci. Compared to imipenem, meropenem has better Gram-negative but worse Gram-positive activity. Ertapenem has narrower spectrum than the other two.
B. Glycopeptides	(vancomycin, teicoplanin)	Excellent activity against Gram-positive cocci, including MRS, highly resistant pneumococci, and enterococci.
Antibiotics acting on bacterial cell membrane		
C. Polypeptides		
1. Bacitracin		Used only topically against Gram-positive bacteria.
2. Polymyxins	(polymyxin B and polymyxin E also known as colistin)	Gram-negative microbes including multidrug-resistant *Klebsiella pneumoniae, Pseudomonas aeruginosa,* and *Acinetobacter baumannii.* Naturally inactive against *Proteus.* Poor Gram-positive activity.
D. Lipopeptides	(daptomycin)	Similar activity to glycopeptides. Good against vancomycin-resistant enterococci.
Antibiotics acting on bacterial protein synthesis		
E. Macrolides	(erythromycin, clarithromycin, azithromycin)	Good against Gram-positive cocci (excluding many staphylococci and most enterococci), *Mycoplasma* and *Chlamydia* species, *Legionella pneumoniae,* and nontuberculous mycobacteria.
F. Tetracyclines	(tetracycline, minocycline, doxycycline)	Similar to macrolides plus rickettsiae, *Brucella* species and spirochetes.

(continued)

TABLE 185-1 The Main Categories, Subdivisions, and Individual Antibacterial Agents, with Spectrum of Activity and Main Modes of Action (*continued*)

Antibiotic Category	Subdivisions (Individual Substances)	Spectrum of Antibacterial Activity
G. Glycylcyclines	(tigecycline)	Gram-positive cocci, including MRS, highly resistant pneumococci, and enterococci. Gram-negative bacteria, including multidrug-resistant *Klebsiella pneumoniae* and *Acinetobacter baumanii*, but not *Pseudomonas aeruginosa*. Good anaerobic activity
H. Aminoglycosides	(streptomycin, gentamicin, tobramycin, amikacin, netilmicin, kanamycin)	Gram-negative bacteria including multidrug-resistant *Klebsiella pneumoniae*, *Acinetobacter baumannii* and *Pseudomonas aeruginosa*. Moderate activity against Gram-positive cocci. Poor anaerobic activity.
I. Chloramphenicol		Gram-positive and negative cocci including MRS and *Neisseria meningitidis*. Enterobacteriaceae. Not active against *Pseudomonas aeruginosa* and *Enterobacter* species. Good anaerobic activity.
J. Lincosamides	(clindamycin)	Activity against Gram-positive cocci, including some MRS. Excellent anaerobic activity.
K. Mupirocin		Topical antistaphylococcal agent active against MRS.
L. Oxazolidinones	(linezolid)	Similar activity to glycopeptides. Good against vancomycin-resistant enterococci (VRE).
M. Streptogramins	(quinupristin/dalfopristin, pristinamycin)	Similar activity to glycopeptides. Good against vancomycin-resistant *Enterococcus faecium* but not *Enterococcus faecalis*. Good activity against Gram-positive anaerobes.
N. Fusidic acid		Gram-positive cocci, active against many MRS but not enterococci. Gram-negative cocci. Poor activity against Gram-negative rods except *Moraxella* and *Legionella* species.
Antibiotics acting against cell metabolism		
O. Sulfonamides	(sulfomethoxazole, sulfacetamide, sulfasalazine, sulfadiazine)	Moderate antistaphylococcal activity, also against some MRS. Poor against streptococci and enterococci. Good Gram-negative activity, including *Haemophilus influenza*, *Moraxella*, enteric Gram-negative rods, *Stenotrophomonas maltophilia* and *Acinetobacter* species. Poor anaerobic activity. Good against nocardiosis, *Pneumocystis jiroveci*, toxoplasmosis.
Antibiotics acting on DNA synthesis		
P. Quinolones		
1. First generation quinolones (nonfluorinated)	(nalidixic acid, cinoxacin,† enoxacin,† norfloxacin)	Gram-negative activity, mainly Enterobacteriaceae.
2. Second generation, fluoroquinolones	(ofloxacin, ciprofloxacin, levofloxacin*)	Wide Gram-negative activity. Additional activity against intracellular microbes. Ciprofloxacin and (to a lesser degree) levofloxacin have good anti-pseudomonal activity. Moderate activity against Gram-positive cocci.
3. Third generation, respiratory quinolones	(levofloxacin,* moxifloxacin, sparfloxacin,† gatifloxacin†)	Added good activity against streptococci, especially pneumococcus.
4. Fourth generation	(clinafloxacin,§ trovafloxacin,† prulifloxacin)	Wide spectrum of activity with additional Gram-positive (including MRS, highly resistant pneumococci, and enterococci) and anaerobic activity to the previous categories.
Q. Rifampin		Specific Gram-positive and Gram-negative microbes (staphylococci including MRS, neisseriae, brucella). First line antimycobacterial. Always used combined with other antibiotics.
R. Nitroimidazoles	(metronidazole, tinidazole)	Excellent antianaerobic activity.
Various mechanisms of action		
S. Beta-lactamase inhibitors	(clavulanic acid, sulbactam, tazobactam)	Enhance the spectrum and activity of aminopenicillins and carboxypenicillins. Sulbactam used as monotherapy against highly-resistant *Acinetobacter baumannii* in ICUs.

*Can be classified to more than one category.
†Withdrawn from U.S. market.
§Currently tested in clinical trials.

TABLE 185-2 Major Adverse Effects and Partial List of Drug-Drug Interactions of Antibiotics

Antibiotics	Major Adverse Effects	Interactions
Penicillins	Allergic and hypersensitivity reactions, including fever, rash, anaphylaxis; high intravenous doses may be associated with sodium load and edema, as well as central nervous system toxicity in patients with renal insufficiency; hepatitis (especially oxacillin)	Nafcillin decreases the effect of warfarin and cyclosporine; the combination of ampicillin and allopurinol is associated with a higher risk of rash; oral absorption of beta-blockers is diminished in patients taking amoxicillin or ampicillin; risk of anaphylaxis may be increased in patients taking beta-blockers
Cephalosporins	*C difficile* colitis; less often associated with allergy than penicillins; cefepime associated with mental status change in elderly patients with renal insufficiency	Minimal
Carbapenems	Seizures, especially when doses not properly adjusted for renal function; seizure risk is highest with imipenem, and lowest with meropenem; *C difficile* colitis	Decreased levels of valproic acid
Aminoglycosides	Nephrotoxicity, ototoxicity, neuromuscular blockade in critically ill patients	Increased risk of nephrotoxicity with use of other nephrotoxic agents, such as cyclosporine, cisplatin, NSAIDs, and vancomycin; increased ototoxicity when administered with diuretics
Sulfa drugs	Rash, fever, hyperkalemia, cytopenias, crystalluria (at high doses or with impaired renal function)	Increased anticoagulation with warfarin
Macrolides	Gastrointestinal upset, hepatitis, cholestatic jaundice, pancreatitis, QT interval prolongation	Increases the levels of many drugs by inhibiting hepatic cytochrome P450 metabolism, including cyclosporine, tacrolimus, theophylline, ergot alkaloids, carbamazepine, antihistamines, cisapride, warfarin, statins, class I antiarrthymics, and some benzodiazepines and neuroleptics
Lincosamides (eg, clindamycin)	Diarrhea, including *C difficile* colitis; rash	May potentiate the effect of warfarin
Fluoroquinolones	*C difficile* colitis; tendinopathy; mental status changes; rash	Oral absorption inhibited by antacids, ferrous sulfate, cimetidine
Tetracyclines	Diarrhea, photosensitivity, hepatitis, pill esophagitis	Oral absorption inhibited by antacids, ferrous sulfate, calcium supplements, tube feedings
Glycopeptides (eg, vancomycin)	Infusion-related flushing (red person syndrome), nephrotoxicity, ototoxicity	Use with caution when patient taking other potentially nephrotoxic agents, such as aminoglycosides, cisplatin, or colistin
Oxazolidinones (eg, linezolid)	Nausea, diarrhea, cytopenias, neuropathy	Serotonin syndrome in patients also taking selective serotonin reuptake inhibitors (SSRIs)
Lipopeptides (eg, daptomycin)	Gastrointestinal upset, creatine kinase elevations	Rhabdomyolysis in patients also taking statin therapy
Polymixins (eg, colistin)	Nephrotoxicity (20%), neuropathy (7%)	May potentiate neuromuscular blockade associated with aminoglycosides and curariform muscle relaxants
Polyene antifungals (amphotericin B)	Febrile infusion reaction (nearly universal side effect); renal tubular injury with severe potassium and magnesium wasting, metabolic acidosis, and nephrogenic diabetes insipidus; electrolyte imbalances and possibly direct cardiotoxicity may lead to life-threatening arrhythmias; cytopenias	Renal toxicity more common and severe with concomitant use of other nephrotoxins, such as cisplatin and diuretics
Azole antifungals	QT prolongation and hepatotoxicity possible with all azoles Voriconazole: transient blurring of vision (unknown mechanism) Fluconazole: generally well tolerated; less hepatotoxic than other azoles because of major renal route of excretion Posaconazole: gastrointestinal upset	Azoles inhibit the cytochrome P450 system, leading to extensive drug interactions, including cyclosporine, oral hypoglycemic agents, antiretroviral therapy, phenytoin, rifabutin, rifampin, theophylline, and warfarin; dose adjustment of other medications may be necessary

pneumoniae, may produce various types of beta-lactamases. Extended-spectrum beta-lactamases (ESBLs) are of particular significance. They confer resistance to all penicillins and commonly to all cephalosporins, and they are often accompanied by resistance to TMP-SMX, aminoglycosides, and fluoroquinolones. Carbapenems are at present the best choice for infections caused by ESBL-producing Gram-negative organisms.

Enterobacter cloacae and *Enterobacter aerogenes* commonly exhibit multidrug resistance due to the production of broad-spectrum AmpC beta-lactamase. AmpC confers resistance to second- and third-generation cephalosporins, monobactams, and many beta-lactam/beta-lactamase inhibitor combinations. However, *Enterobacter* species are often susceptible to TMP-SMX or fluoroquinolones, as well as carbapenems and fourth-generation cephalosporins, such as cefepime, which are considered the last line of antibiotics active against Gram-negative infections, and should be withheld from use as much as possible.

Pseudomonas aeruginosa and *Acinetobacter baumannii* often cause nosocomial infections in patients with multiple comorbidities, prolonged hospitalizations, prior antibiotic exposure, and intensive care unit (ICU) admission. These two bacteria are almost universally multidrug-resistant. In many countries, a large proportion of isolates are susceptible only to carbapenems, polymyxins, and tigecycline (the later being active only against *Acinteobacter*). Isolates of *Pseudomonas aeruginosa*, *Acinetobacter baumannii*, and even *Klebsiella pneumoniae* resistant to all commercially available antibiotics have been described in recent literature, primarily in ICU settings. Carbapenems, antipseudomonal penicillins, and the relatively toxic polymyxins in various combinations have been the main agents used against such isolates.

INITIATION OF EMPIRIC ANTIBACTERIAL THERAPY

PROPER DIAGNOSIS

A high degree of **clinical suspicion** for possible bacterial infection should always constitute the basis for initiation of antibiotic therapy. Unnecessary use of antibacterial agents can harm both the patient and the hospital environment. First, initiation of antibiotics without adequate documentation of infection can obscure or delay the correct diagnoses. Second, antibiotics may cause toxicity, including life-threatening *Clostridium difficile* colitis. Third, when administering an antibiotic to a patient, the clinician should consider this antibiotic inactive against future infections in the same patient for a period of time of at least three months, according to some experts. Finally, antibiotic use leads to emergence of resistance microorganisms in the hospital environment.

As with most diseases, a careful history should always be the mainstay of diagnosis. Patients should be questioned about exposure to the health care system, vaccination, living conditions, animal exposure, travel history, sexual practices, chronic diseases, immunodeficiency, recent surgery, and indwelling foreign bodies such as heart valves and joint prostheses. While the physical examination is similar to that performed in other patients, hospitalists examining patients with suspected infection should pay special attention to aspects that are often neglected, such as skin, lymph nodes, surgical wounds, decubitus ulcers, intravenous line sites, and the genital region. Helpful laboratory investigations include complete blood count, certain biochemical tests, indices of inflammation, such as erythrocyte sedimentation rate, C-reactive protein, and perhaps procalcitonin, serology, urinalysis, and pharyngeal swabs with rapid testing for group A streptococcus or influenza A. Cultures from the infected site remain the gold standard for diagnosis, definite identification of the responsible pathogen, and optimization of antibiotic therapy. Finally, clinicians should distinguish between true infection and situations mimicking infections that need only limited or no antibiotic therapy (eg, UTI versus asymptomatic bacteriuria, pneumonia versus exacerbation of chronic obstructive pulmonary disease).

TIMING OF THERAPY

Once the diagnosis of a possible infection is made, the clinician has to decide on the appropriate timing of antibiotic administration. ***Early initiation*** of antibiotic therapy should be the rule for all severe infections. There is considerable evidence that patients with sepsis have better outcomes, including reduced mortality, when antibiotic therapy is initiated as soon as possible. A large retrospective study of 2700 ICU patients with septic shock revealed that mortality was proportional to the time to initiation of appropriate antimicrobial therapy. Timely administration of antibiotics has a positive impact on a variety of serious infections. When central nervous system infection and especially meningitis is suspected, antibiotic therapy should be administered well before the definitive documentation of infection. Thus, only a few minutes delay is acceptable between the clinical suspicion of meningitis and lumbar puncture. When longer delays are expected, antibacterial therapy should be administered immediately, despite the consequent decreased diagnostic yield of lumbar puncture. Similarly, pneumonia-associated in-hospital morbidity and mortality is significantly reduced by prompt antibacterial therapy.

Delays in antimicrobial therapy are justified only in specific clinical settings. As a rule, antibiotic therapy is withheld only in hemodynamically stable patients, when the diagnosis of bacterial infection is doubtful, or when an acute or chronic infection is suspected that is best treated after identification of the responsible pathogen. Examples of clinical scenarios in which it is appropriate to delay antibiotics include a young adult with tonsillitis while awaiting the results of heterophile antibody testing, patients with possible endocarditis, in whom therapy should be delayed for at least an hour to perform three sets of aerobic and anaerobic blood cultures, and patients with suspected chronic infections due to brucellosis, syphilis, and other pathogens that mimic a wide variety of other diseases, and require specific therapy that differs from most empiric antibacterial therapies.

Antibiotic therapy initiated prior to identification of the causative infecting agent is termed ***empiric***, a Greek word meaning derived from experience. Empiric antibiotics are chosen based on knowledge of the microbes typically causing infection at a specific body site, antibiotic penetration into this site, local patterns of antimicrobial susceptibility, and antibacterial side effect profile. Empiric antibiotic therapy usually has a broad spectrum of activity, including resistant organisms prevalent in relevant clinical settings. For example, the emergence of cMRSA has led to the increasing use of vancomycin (considered a last-line antibiotic in other situations) or sophisticated, costly newer agents in the empiric therapy of skin and soft tissue infections. Similarly, the rise of multidrug-resistant Gram-negative organisms such as *Klebsiella pneumoniae*, *Acinetobacter baumanii*, and *Pseudomonas aeruginosa* has led to the use of last-line antibacterials such as meropenem or colistin as empiric therapy in certain ICUs. When culture results become available, the broad spectrum of activity of the empiric regimen should be narrowed as much as possible (step-down).

PHARMACOKINETICS AND PHARMACODYNAMICS

PHARMACOKINETICS

Antibiotic ***pharmacokinetics***, or the effects of the body on the antibiotic, depend on drug absorption, tissue distribution, metabolism, and excretion. Antibiotic ***absorption*** is most relevant to the oral administration of antibiotics. Some antibiotics, such as linezolid or levofloxacin, are nearly entirely absorbed from the gut. By contrast, oral vancomycin achieves negligible serum levels, but this route is best when high intraluminal concentrations of the drug in the gastrointestinal tract are desired, as when treating *Clostridium difficile* colitis. ***Tissue distribution*** plays a significant role in the success or failure of antibiotic therapy. For example, an antibiotic with poor distribution to the lungs is unlikely to be effective for pneumonia. Some antibiotics reach useful levels in one tissue compartment, but not another; for example, tigecycline is distributed widely in the body, but serum concentrations may be inadequate to treat bacteremias and endocarditis. In general, it is harder to achieve therapeutic antibiotic concentrations in the central nervous system, bones, pleural cavity, prostate, and poorly vascularized infected foci, such as abscesses. Fluoroquinolones often penetrate tissues that other antibiotics fail to reach, including bone and prostate. Local factors may also interfere with tissue distribution. Infections on foreign bodies often fail to respond to treatment because of the difficulty in penetrating the bacterial biofilms formed on their surfaces. Rifampin may be active in staphylococcal infections forming biofilm on foreign bodies.

Drug ***metabolism*** also affects antibiotic levels. Patients with hepatic or renal insufficiency may accumulate drugs, putting them at higher risk of toxicity, and need corresponding dose adjustment. Hepatic metabolism in particular is affected by genetic characteristics (pharmacogenetics) and drug-drug interactions. For example, isoniazid is metabolized by liver acetylation. About 50% of Europeans and Americans are slow acetylators, and will have higher isoniazid levels, increasing the risk for polyneuropathy and other toxicities. In addition, many antibiotics are metabolized by hepatic cytochrome P450 enzymes, resulting in numerous drug-drug interactions, as discussed below in the section on antibiotic toxicity.

PHARMACODYNAMICS

Antibiotic ***pharmacodynamics***, or the effect of the antibiotic on the bacteria, are related to antibiotic concentrations in blood and tissues, time, and bacterial inhibition or killing. Based on pharmacodynamic characteristics, antimicrobial agents can be divided into those that exhibit primarily ***concentration-dependent*** bacterial killing or ***time-dependent*** bacterial killing. Concentration-dependent agents, such as aminoglycosides and fluoroquinolones, achieve more bacterial killing at higher drug concentrations. Time-dependent agents, such as beta-lactams and vancomycin, accomplish maximal killing at concentrations four times higher than the minimum inhibitory concentration (MIC), with no extra bacteriocidal effects at higher concentrations.

For concentration-dependent agents, the main parameters predictive of successful clinical outcomes are the peak concentration achieved over minimum inhibitory concentration (MIC) ratio (Cmax/MIC) and the area under the concentration-time curve to MIC ratio (AUC/MIC). Thus, one or two high daily doses are considered optimal for aminoglycosides and fluoroquinolones. For time-dependent agents such as beta-lactams, the time with achieved concentrations above the MIC (t >MIC) is the pharmacodynamic parameter most predictive of bacterial killing and clinical efficacy. Thus, in theory, beta-lactam antibiotics are optimally administered in three or four doses daily, with some evidence supporting continuous administration. However, some beta-lactams antibiotics, such as ceftriaxone and ertapenem, have half-lives long enough to allow for once-daily dosing, without compromising concentrations in blood and tissues during the 24-hour period.

COMBINATION ANTIMICROBIAL THERAPY

Combination antibiotic therapy is indicated when (1) broader empiric coverage is desired than can be accomplished with a single agent; (2) infection is proven or suspected to involve bacteria such as *Mycobacterium tuberculosis* with a high potential to develop resistance against a single agent; (3) when the site of infection may interfere with the ability of certain antibiotics to reach satisfactory concentrations (eg, aminoglycosides are not used alone in pneumonia, and vancomycin is not used as monotherapy in meningitis); (4) when infections are expected to be polymicrobial, as in intra-abdominal or pelvic infections; and (5) when a drug combination results in synergy, or a decrease in the MIC of each drug when tested together against a pathogen in vitro, as seen with the use of ampicillin and gentamicin in enterococcal endocarditis. However, this in vitro increase in activity does not always translate into superior clinical results, for reasons that are not always clear. Various synergistic combinations of beta-lactams with aminoglycosides have not been shown to be better than beta-lactam monotherapy in serious infections causing sepsis, according to a large meta-analysis of 64 trials including 7586 patients. Similarly, the development of several broad-spectrum beta-lactam agents, such as antipseudomonal penicillins combined with beta-lactamase inhibitors, fourth-generation cephalosporins, and carbapenems, has led to the widespread use of beta-lactam monotherapy in febrile neutropenia, a clinical setting in which combinations of beta-lactams with aminoglycosides had once been standard.

Antibiotic combinations, especially beta-lactams with aminoglycosides, were often used to prevent the development of resistance until recently. These two drug categories have different mechanisms of action, often exhibit synergy in vitro, and provide a wide spectrum of antibacterial activity. Animal studies in the 1980s provided some evidence that this combination could forestall the emergence of resistance, but meta-analyses in patients have not shown a clear benefit. **Table 185-3** shows common indications for using antibiotic combinations in everyday clinical practice, as well as commonly used antibiotic combinations according to indication.

TOXICITY

Antibiotics toxicities may arise from impaired drug metabolism, as in renal failure or hepatic insufficiency, from direct antibiotic effects, and from drug interactions. ***Beta-lactams*** are mainly metabolized in kidneys, and thus dose adjustment is needed in renal failure. An important exception is ceftriaxone, which is primarily metabolized in the liver. Gastrointestinal discomfort and mild diarrhea are the most common side effects of beta-lactams, with severe diarrhea or pseudomembranous colitis occurring less often. Up to 10% of patients report a penicillin allergy, but the true prevalence is probably closer to 1%, as most of these patients will not have a reaction if rechallenged. Possible reactions include skin rash, drug fever, nephritis, Coombs-positive hemolytic anemia, leucopenia, and even contact dermatitis. Interstitial nephritis usually results in mild, reversible renal failure, and is mainly associated with antistaphylococcal penicillins. Seizures may occur with high doses of imipenem or penicillins. Penicillin-induced anaphylaxis occurs with approximately 1 out of 10,000 administrations. Skin testing predicts penicillin IgE-mediated allergy and anaphylaxis, but not toxic epidermal necrolysis and Stevens-Johnson syndrome. Allergic reactions are much less common with cephalosporins. Fewer than 10% of patients with penicillin allergy are also allergic to cephalosporins or carbapenems. Monobactams, such as aztreonam, do not cross react with penicillin, having a substantially different chemical structure (**Figure 185-1**).

Aminoglycosides are excreted by the kidneys, reaching high concentrations in the urinary tract. However, they are nephrotoxic in 10–25% of patients, leading to acute kidney injury from tubular necrosis, mesangial damage, and renal vasoconstriction. This is more common in elderly, severely ill, or dehydrated patients. The serum creatinine should be closely monitored in patients at risk for aminoglycoside-related nephrotoxicity. If possible, the concomitant use of other nephrotoxic agents such as loop diuretics, vancomycin, and amphotericin B should be avoided, as these may potentiate aminoglycoside nephrotoxicity. The nephrotoxicity of aminoglycosides is usually ameliorated by dose adjustment or drug withdrawal. Once-daily administration and short treatment duration (≤7 days) may reduce the risk of nephrotoxicity. Ototoxicity with sensorineural deafness is the other major adverse effect of aminoglycosides. It manifests initially with high-frequency hearing loss, which may be irreversible in some cases. It is more common with prolonged administration, as with streptomycin use for tuberculosis or brucellosis, or gentamicin use in endocarditis. Neuromuscular blockade may occur when aminoglycosides are erroneously given by rapid intravenous

TABLE 185-3 Commonly Used Antibiotic Combinations, According to Indication

Infection-Clinical Setting	Antibiotic Combinations Commonly Used	Comments
Endocarditis by staphylococci, enterococci, or relatively resistant streptococci	Beta-lactam or vancomycin *plus* an aminoglycoside	Rifampin added to the therapy in cases of prosthetic valve endocarditis
Enterococcal bacteremia	Gentamicin *plus* a beta-lactam or vancomycin	
Tuberculosis	Rifampin plus isoniazid plus ethambutol plus pyrazinamide	Various combinations are used as second-line therapy in infection by resistant mycobacteria
Brucella infections	Tetracycline plus streptomycin *or* rifampin plus doxycycline	Combinations of quionolones and rifampin have also been used
Empirical antibiotic therapy of:		
Community-acquired pneumonia	Beta-lactam *plus* a macrolide	Alternative to monotherapy with respiratory quinolones
Hospital-acquired pneumonia	Ampicillin/sulbactam *or* antipseudomonal penicillin *plus* aminoglycoside	Alternative to monotherapy with respiratory quinolones *or* antipseudomonal penicillin *or* third generation cephalosporin *or*
Meningitis	Third generation cephalosporin *plus* vancomycin	Ampicillin added to therapy in patients >50 years old at risk for infection with *Listeria monocytogenes*
Intra-abdominal infections	Beta-lactams *or* ciprofloxacin *plus* metronidazole	
Skin and soft tissue infections (especially diabetic foot)	Ciprofloxacin *plus* metronidazole *or* clindamycin	Alternatively cephalosporin *plus* metronidazole *or* clindamycin

push, or when they are administered to ICU patients receiving other inhibitors of the neuromuscular junction. Aminoglycoside use is generally avoided during pregnancy, since these antibiotics cross the placenta. Trough levels should be measured in patients receiving aminoglycosides for longer than one week, to ensure that drug accumulation is not occurring. Peak levels are usually not measured, except to ensure therapeutic levels in serious infections such as endocarditis.

Glycopeptides such as vancomycin commonly exhibit mild nephrotoxicity, which may become worse if dose adjustments are not performed based on renal clearance, similar to aminoglycosides. Serum levels of vancomycin are helpful in preventing toxicity in patients with preexisting renal failure, unstable renal function, and the elderly. There is no contraindication to coadministration with other nephrotoxic agents such as aminoglycosides, but this should be performed with great caution and only when necessary. Red person syndrome is a mild anaphylactoid reaction that causes flushing of the upper trunk and head of the patient. It is most common with the first dose of vancomycin, diminishes with subsequent doses, and can be prevented by slow administration over two hours. Some patients require premedication with antihistamines to minimize symptoms. True allergic skin rash may also occur occasionally with glycopeptide use. Ototoxicity may occur in patients with preexisting renal impairment and prolonged exposure.

Macrolides generally have mild side effects. Gastrointestinal upset due to increased motility is common. This is especially evident with erythromycin, which has been used to treat patients with gastroparesis and pseudoobstruction syndromes. Macrolides may also cause mild hepatotoxicity and QT interval prolongation. However, the most important macrolide adverse effect is drug interactions. Macrolides inhibit the CYP3A4 enzyme of the cytochrome P450 of the liver, leading to decreased metabolism and potentially toxic levels of several substances, including statins, warfarin, digoxin, carbamazepine, valproic acid, benzodiazepines, ergotamine, theophylline, vinca alkaloids, and cyclosporine. Polymorphic ventricular tachycardia (*torsades de pointes*), often preceded by QT prolongation, may occur when a macrolide is administered with other potent P450 inhibitors, such as cisapride, terfenadine, or astemizole.

Gastrointestinal upset is common with ***tetracyclines***. Esophageal irritation and ulceration may occur with oral administration; this may be minimized by drinking generous amounts of water with pills and avoiding ingestion at bedtime. Phototoxicity is very common. Hepatotoxicity may occur with large intravenous doses. Use of tetracycline, and to a lesser degree doxycycline, is contraindicated in patients with preexisting renal failure, because tetracyclines may worsen renal insufficiency. Teteracyclines should be avoided in pregnancy, as they may cause fetal skeletal deformities and dental discoloration, and maternal fulminant hepatic failure. Drug interactions with digoxin, warfarin, theophylline, and statins are similar to macrolides, but usually milder. Carbamazepine and phenytoin induce hepatic metabolism of tetracyclines, reducing their activity. Antacids, cimetidine, and milk decrease tetracycline absorption.

Diarrhea is the most common side effect of ***fluoroquinolones***. *C difficile* colitis is relatively common with respiratory fluoroquinolones such as levofloxacin and moxifloxacin, but occurs less often with older fluoroquinolones such as ciprofloxacin. All fluoroquinolones may cause QT prolongation, although this is minimal with ciprofloxacin and other older fluoroquinolones. Other important, occasional side effects include phototoxicity, tendon rupture—especially involving the Achilles tendon—seizures, and confusion. Tendinopathy and central nervous system side effects are more common in the elderly. Fluoroquinolone use should generally be avoided in patients younger than 18 years old because of their epileptogenic potential and adverse effects on developing joints. Fluoroquinolones may be teratogenic, and are contraindicated in pregnancy. Ciprofloxacin inhibits theophylline metabolism; this interaction does not occur with respiratory fluoroquinolones. Fluoroquinolones require dose adjustment in severe renal failure.

Lincosamides, such as clindamycin, most commonly cause gastrointestinal distress. Clindamycin was once considered the major cause of *C difficile* colitis, but its role in the epidemiology of *C difficile* has declined due to a rise in *C difficile* infections related to beta-lactams and fluoroquinolones. ***Sulfonamides*** may cause nephrotoxicity from crystalluria, especially with the use of high doses in the treatment of conditions such as nocardiosis and toxoplasmosis. Patients receiving high-dose sulfonamides should be

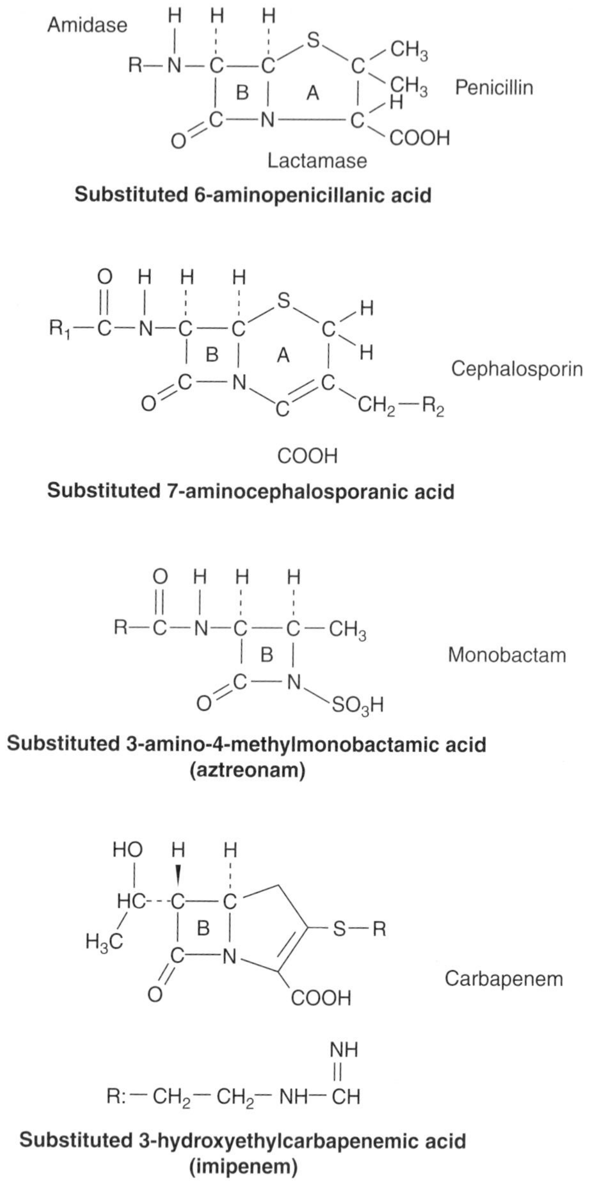

Figure 185-1 *Core structures of four beta-lactam antibiotic families. The ring marked B in each structure is the beta-lactam ring. The penicillins are susceptible to bacterial metabolism and inactivation by amidases and lactamases at the points shown. Note that the carbapenems have a different stereochemical configuration in the lactam ring that apparently imparts resistance to beta-lactamases. (Reproduced, with permission, from Katzung BG, Masters SB, Trevor AJ. Basic & Clinical Pharmacology, eleventh ed. New York, NY: McGraw-Hill; 2009. Fig. 43-1.)*

adequately hydrated, and dose adjustments should be made for patients with renal failure. Sulfa antibiotics may trigger hemolysis in patients with G6PD deficiency, and rarely lead to toxic epidermal necrolysis/Stevens-Johnson syndrome. Sulfonamides decrease the metabolism of phenytoin, warfarin, and digoxin. In combination with ***trimethoprim***, they may act as antimetabolites and cause marrow aplasia.

INTRAVENOUS VERSUS ORAL ANTIBIOTICS

Patients tolerating oral medications or nasogastric feeding may benefit from oral antibiotic administration at lower cost. For example, oral levofloxacin and metronidazole approach 100% bioavailability, and oral fluconazole is 90% bioavailable. The greater ease of administration and avoidance of adverse events associated with parenteral therapy, such as bacterial and fungal line infections or post-infusion phlebitis, may result in decreased hospital length of stay. Patients may also benefit from improved mobility. The ease of administration should not, however, lead to indiscriminate use of these and newer agents. For example, overuse of linezolid, an expensive drug active against most strains of VRE and MRSA, may promote resistance in these Gram-positive organisms.

ANTIMICROBIAL RESISTANCE AND ITS PREVENTION

In recent decades, the prevalence of nosocomial antibacterial resistance has been rising, with increased in-hospital morbidity and mortality. Acute care hospitals should take steps to reduce the inappropriate use of antibiotics. This may require developing antibiotic guidelines, educational strategies, and computer support. Specific practices are necessary to combat antibacterial resistance. Hospitals must have ***surveillance systems***, involving physicians, infection control practitioners, nurses, and the microbiology laboratory, to identify increases in the incidence of infections caused by resistant pathogens. This surveillance also includes monitoring of antibiotic consumption, and correlating usage with patterns of antibiotic resistance. When specific antibiotics appear to be linked to the emergence of resistance, ***local antibiotic policies*** may be needed to limit use. In most cases, antibiotic use is itself the main factor promoting resistance. Antibiotic use may also be reduced by ***infection control measures***, such as hand washing, isolation precautions, and immunization.

The principle of "hit hard, hit fast" or the prompt use of ***high and appropriately divided antibiotic doses*** should be applied to most hospital infections. Depending on antibiotic mode of action and pharmacodynamic characteristics, low antibiotic concentrations favor the development of bacterial resistance, mainly by means of stepwise mutations. Thus, for example, development of resistance to fluoroquinolones is linked to low areas under the concentration-time curve to MIC ratio (AUC/MIC), while beta-lactam resistance is linked to low time with achieved concentrations above the MIC ($t > MIC$). The risk of emergence of resistance is highest in organisms with MICs close to susceptibility breakpoint.

Prolonged, intense antibiotic pressure eventually selects for resistant organisms, which may heavily colonize both the affected patient and the hospital environment in general, including other hospital patients not receiving antibiotics. Thus, antibiotic therapy should be as ***brief*** as possible in order not to compromise overall efficacy, and ***de-escalation*** or narrowing the spectrum of antibiotic therapy, should be performed as soon as antimicrobial sensitivity data are available. Other suggested measures to limit antibiotic resistance, such as periodic cycling or "crop rotation" of antibiotic classes, or antibiotic combination therapy, have inadequate evidence to support their use at this time.

PRACTICE POINT

- The accelerating pace of antibiotic resistance threatens to leave clinicians with no viable therapeutic options for nosocomial infections. Measures to retard the development of antibiotic resistance in hospitals include treating infections with adequate antibiotic doses, to forestall the development of stepwise resistance mutations, tailoring therapy to narrow-spectrum antibiotics once culture results are available (de-escalation), giving antibiotics for the minimum adequate duration, restricting the use of broad-spectrum antibiotics in hospitals, monitoring and surveillance of antimicrobial resistance, and enforcing infection control measures to prevent the spread of resistant pathogens between patients.

SUGGESTED READINGS

Bliziotis IA, Samonis G, Vardakas KZ, Chrysanthopoulou S, Falagas ME. Effect of aminoglycoside and beta-lactam combination therapy versus beta-lactam monotherapy on the emergence of antimicrobial resistance: a meta-analysis of randomized, controlled trials. *Clin Infect Dis*. 2005;41:149–158.

Kasiakou SK, Sermaides GJ, Michalopoulos A, Soteriades ES, Falagas ME. Continuous versus intermittent intravenous administration of antibiotics: a meta-analysis of randomised controlled trials. *Lancet Infect Dis*. 2005;5:581–589.

Kumar A, Roberts D, Wood KE, et al. Duration of hypotension before initiation of effective antimicrobial therapy is the critical determinant of survival in human septic shock. *Crit Care Med*. 2006;34:1589–1596.

Maragakis LL, Perencevich EN, Cosgrove SE. Clinical and economic burden of antimicrobial resistance. *Expert Rev Anti Infect Ther*. 2008;6:751–763.

Paul M, Benuri-Silbiger I, Soares-Weiser K, Leibovici L. Beta lactam monotherapy versus beta lactam-aminoglycoside combination therapy for sepsis in immunocompetent patients: systematic review and meta-analysis of randomised trials. *BMJ*. 2004;328:668.

CHAPTER 186

Antibiotic Resistance

Luisa Silvia Munoz-Price, MD

Key Clinical Questions

1. What are the most frequent types of antibiotic resistance?
2. Which patients are at risk for infections with antibiotic-resistant organisms?
3. How are antibiotic-resistant organisms transmitted among patients?
4. What types of genes confer antibiotic resistance?
5. What types of isolation precautions exist, and when are they indicated?

INTRODUCTION

Antibiotic resistance was described at the dawn of the antibiotic era. In Alexander Fleming's initial report of the antibacterial action of penicillin in 1929, he noted that it was usually inactive against enteric Gram-negative bacteria. In 1940, while engaged in isolating and purifying penicillin, Edward Abraham and Ernst Chain incidentally discovered that *Escherichia coli* produced penicillinase. While the global explosion and dissemination of antibiotic resistance in recent decades is alarming, perhaps it should not be too surprising. As most antibiotics are derived from substances produced by molds and bacteria to inhibit the growth of rival microorganisms, mechanisms of antibacterial resistance evolved before humans harnessed these compounds for medicinal use.

When antibiotics reduce populations of non-resistant organisms, resistant organisms are able to proliferate. Rates of invasive infections with drug-resistant bacteria increase after recent antibiotic exposure. Conversely, reduced use of antibiotics has been shown to decrease the prevalence of antibiotic-resistant organisms. Certain bacterial infections are now resistant to all antibiotics, with a limited number of promising antibiotics in the developmental pipeline.

Highly antibiotic-resistant organisms are usually thought of as exclusively hospital-acquired pathogens. However, community acquisition of resistant pathogens is on the rise, including methicillin-resistant *Staphylococcus aureus* (MRSA) and extended-spectrum beta-lactamase-producing *Escherichia coli*. This chapter reviews resistant bacteria of importance to the hospitalist, including the ESKAPE pathogens, for which there may be no effective drug therapy in the near future (**Table 186-1**).

METHICILLIN-RESISTANT *STAPHYLOCOCCUS AUREUS* (MRSA)

The medically important staphylococci may be divided into two main groups based on the rapid coagulase test, a measure of the ability of a staphylococcal colony to produce a clot in a tube of rabbit serum. Coagulase-negative staphylococci (principally *Staphylococcus epidermidis*) have little virulence aside from biofilm production, and generally only cause infections of medical devices, such as central venous catheters and joint prostheses. By contrast, *Staphylococcus aureus* (coagulase-positive) is innately pathogenic, and is one of the few bacteria that cause severe infection in both community and health care settings.

PRACTICE POINT

- A major strategy to reduce antibiotic resistance is to prescribe the narrowest spectrum antibiotic. For example, for documented methicillin-sensitive *Staphylococcus aureus* infection, preferred drugs for intravenous therapy are nafcillin, oxacillin, and cefazolin. Drugs such as vancomycin, daptomycin, linezolid, and tigecycline should be reserved for infection with methicillin-resistant *Staphylococcus aureus*, or cases of allergy or intolerance to other antibiotics.

Although methicillin is no longer used in clinical practice, methicillin-resistance is still used as marker of staphylococcal resistance to beta-lactams. Methicillin-resistant *Staphylococcus*

TABLE 186-1 ESKAPE Pathogens: Multidrug-resistant Bacteria Most Likely to have no Effective Drug Therapy in the Immediate Future

***E**nterococcus faecium (VRE)*
***S**taphylococcus aureus (MRSA)*
***K**lebsiella pneumoniae*
***A**cinetobacter baumannii*
***P**seudomonas aeruginosa*
***E**nterobacter species*

Data from Boucher HW, et al. *Clin Infect Dis.* 2009:48:1–12.

aureus (MRSA) isolates are also resistant to oxacillin, nafcillin, cefazolin, and all other beta-lactams. Contact precautions are required for hospitalized patients with MRSA (**Table 186-2**). While many clinical isolates of coagulase-negative staphylococci are methicillin-resistant, contact precautions are not required for these organisms because of their minor clinical and epidemiological implications.

HOSPITAL VERSUS COMMUNITY-ACQUIRED MRSA

Hospital-associated MRSA (HA-MRSA) tend to cause invasive disease in debilitated or immunocompromised individuals, including pneumonia, bloodstream infections (ie, endocarditis), deep wound infections, and osteomyelitis. Patients are usually treated with vancomycin, with daptomycin and tigecycline as newer, more expensive alternatives. Tigecycline does not achieve good serum concentrations, and should not be used for bacteremias; daptomycin is inhibited by pulmonary surfactant, and should not be used to treat pneumonia. Vancomycin is sometimes combined with rifampin (for prosthetic joint infection), or with gentamicin and rifampin (for prosthetic valve endocarditis), based on somewhat limited clinical data.

Since the late 1990s, community-acquired MRSA (CA-MRSA) strains have spread across the United States and in Europe to a lesser degree. Populations at greatest risk include children, military personnel, prisoners, and athletes, although CA-MRSA infections are increasing among otherwise healthy adults. CA-MRSA most commonly causes pyogenic skin and soft tissue infection in the form of boils, deep abscesses, and cellulitis. CA-MRSA is also capable of causing potentially lethal infections, such as necrotizing fasciitis, necrotizing pneumonia, and bacteremia. When skin infection is well localized (boil < 3 cm diameter), incision and drainage seem to suffice. Antibiotic treatment with either trimethoprim-sulfamethoxazole or other active oral agents can be used for more extensive skin involvement. Clindamycin should be considered as a treatment option only if the D-test for inducible resistance is negative. If this test is not locally available, clindamycin should only be used for strains that are erythromycin-susceptible. Recurrent soft tissue infections are frequent with CA-MRSA. These patients usually require decolonization (see below).

Despite its name, CA-MRSA may be emerging as a nosocomial pathogen. It has been predicted that CA-MRSA will eventually replace HA-MRSA as the dominant hospital strain. Differentiating between CA- and HA-MRSA strains solely on epidemiological grounds may not be possible in the future. Molecular testing is definitive, but this is not practical for most clinical laboratories. The antibiogram may be helpful in differentiation: CA-MRSA strains are usually still susceptible to non-beta-lactam antibiotics, such as fluoroquinolones and trimethoprim-sulfamethoxazole.

Patients with MRSA infection or colonization at any site should be placed on contact precautions (gowns and gloves upon room entry) to prevent horizontal spread. Some institutions add droplet precautions (surgical masks) for patients with MRSA in the sputum. Active screening, using nasal cultures or rapid PCR, and reporting are currently mandatory in some states, such as Illinois; however, the impact of this intervention is still under debate. As above, decolonization can be accomplished using intranasal mupirocin (twice a day) and daily chlorhexidine baths. The length of this intervention varies depending on the study (range 3–14 days). Additionally, some patients might not respond or relapse after decolonization.

TABLE 186-2 Isolation Precautions for Hospitalized Patients with Infection, in Addition to Standard Precautions, Hand Hygiene, and use of Dedicated Medical Equipment

Type of Isolation	Components of Isolation	Most Common Examples
Contact	Gowns and gloves upon room entry	VRE MRSA ESBL-producing Gram-negatives, and other highly resistant Gram-negative bacteria *Clostridium difficile* with active diarrhea
Droplet	Surgical mask upon room entry	Influenza Meningococcal meningitis Rubella Pertussis Mycoplasma
Airborne	Negative pressure room N95 mask upon room entry	Pulmonary tuberculosis Varicella zoster Herpes zoster (shingles) or disseminated herpes simplex infection in an immunocompromised patient Measles

ESBL: extended-spectrum beta-lactamases; MRSA: methicillin-resistant Staphylococcus aureus; VRE: vancomycin resistant enterococci.

VANCOMYCIN-RESISTANT ENTEROCOCCI (VRE)

Enterococci are not highly virulent organisms, but they are important hospital pathogens because of their high degree of innate drug resistance, and their persistence and resistance to degradation in the hospital environment. The two predominant enterococci causing hospital-acquired infections are *Enterococcus faecalis* and *Enterococcus faecium*. Vancomycin-resistant enterococci (VRE) were first described in Europe in the late 1980s, and rapidly spread within the United States in the late 1990s. More than 50% of *E. faecium* in the United States are VRE. *E faecalis* tends to be susceptible to vancomycin.

Risk factors for VRE acquisition include prolonged hospitalization, prior use of antibiotics, acuity of illness, and surgery. Patients may become colonized with VRE on skin, wounds, and rectum. VRE colonization does not require treatment, and there is currently no efficacious means of eliminating the carrier state. The most frequent site of VRE infection is the urinary tract. However, some

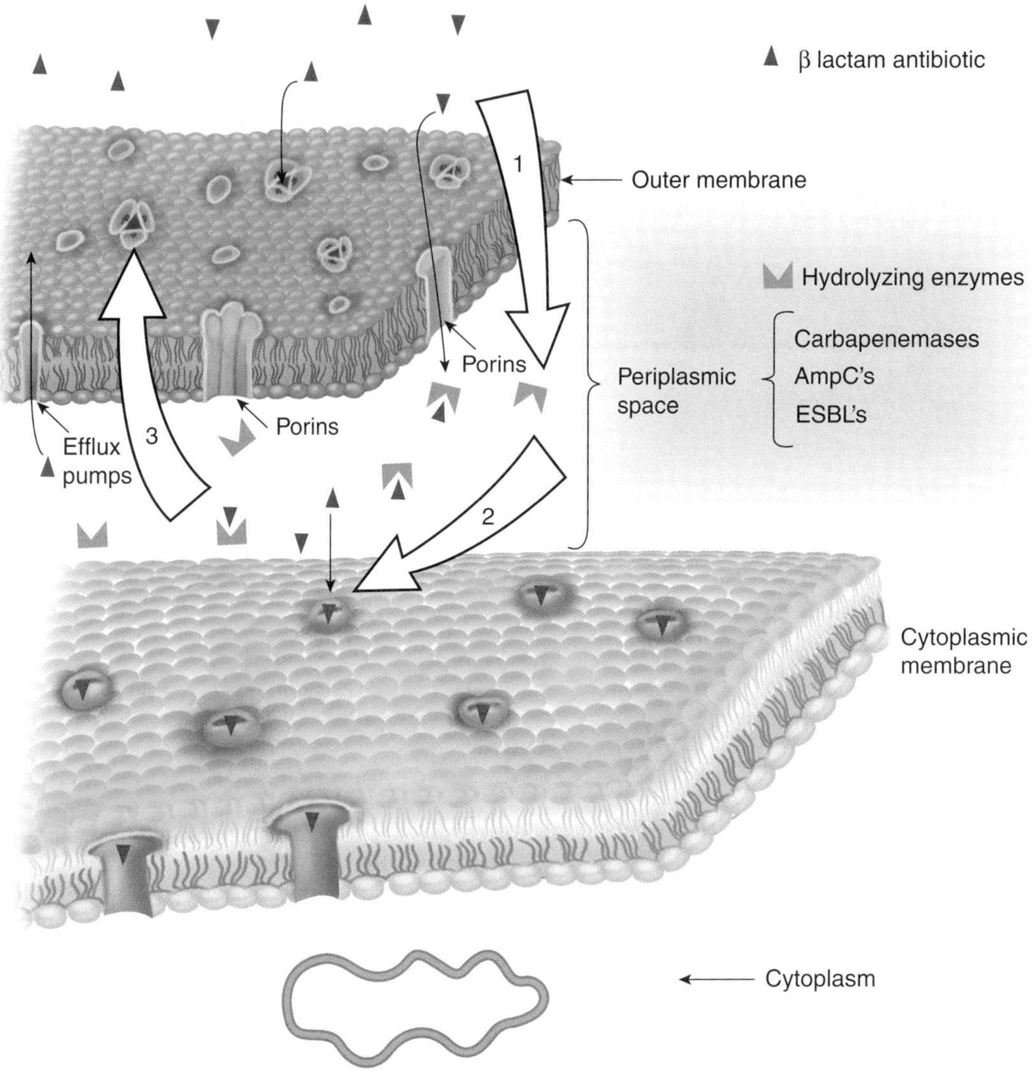

Figure 186-1 *Multiple resistance mechanisms may be present in Gram-negative bacteria, including (1) mutations leading to decreased function or loss of the porin channels that provide antibiotics with access to the periplasmic space; (2) production of inactivating beta-lactamase enzymes, or mutations in penicillin-binding proteins, leading to decreased antibiotic activity in the periplasmic space; (3) overexpression of efflux pumps, leading to rapid antibiotic expulsion via the outer membrane.*

VRE isolates in urine may represent asymptomatic bacteriuria, and do not necessarily require treatment. Other foci of VRE infection include bacteremias, especially in patients on hemodialysis, parenteral nutrition, chemotherapy, or having central venous access for other reasons, and postoperative intra-abdominal sepsis.

Treatment options include daptomycin, linezolid, and tigecycline. Susceptible strains may be treated with ampicillin, with or without aminoglycosides. Cephalosporins should not be used for treatment of VRE infections, regardless of the susceptibility reports.

Screening for VRE is performed using rectal swab cultures. Contact isolation (gowns and gloves) should be instituted if surveillance or clinical cultures are VRE-positive or if there is recent history of positive VRE cultures. Active decolonization for VRE is not standardized at this time.

Contamination of the environment with VRE (fecal patina) has been previously described. The degree of contamination increases with rectal carriage, as well as with diarrhea. A room previously occupied by a VRE-positive patient significantly increases the risk of VRE acquisition of the subsequent patient. As with MRSA, *C difficile*, and resistant Gram-negative rods, terminal room disinfection is critical to reducing nosocomial transmission.

RESISTANT GRAM-NEGATIVE RODS

Gram-negative antibiotic resistance has multiple mechanisms, including porin mutations, overexpression of efflux pumps, penicillin-binding protein mutations, and production of inactivating beta-lactamase enzymes (**Figure 186-1**). In most cases, clinical laboratories will be able to identify beta-lactamase production based on automated susceptibility testing. The two main mechanisms of high-level resistance are production of either extended spectrum beta-lactamases (ESBLs) or carbapenemases.

■ EXTENDED-SPECTRUM BETA-LACTAMASES (ESBLS)

ESBLs are a heterogenous group of enzymes that belong to different families, and thus express different phenotypes. These enzymes tend to confer resistance to most beta-lactams, including cephalosporins, without hydrolyzing carbapenems. In recent years, there has been a worldwide increase in the prevalence of

ESBLs of the CTX-M family, as well as a worrisome rise in community-acquired urinary tract infections due to CTX-M-positive *E coli*.

In most laboratories, screening for ESBL production is done by automated systems, and confirmed based on the minimum inhibitory concentrations set by the Clinical and Laboratory Standards Institute (CLSI). However, microbiologic standards for detection of ESBLs have been defined only for *Klebsiella pneumoniae, Escherichia coli,* and *Proteus mirabilis*. Therefore, although other Gram-negative rods, such as *Enterobacter* species and *Pseudomonas aeruginosa*, may express ESBLs, microbiology laboratories cannot confirm ESBL production due to the lack of defined standards for these bacteria. In these cases, the presence of ESBLs must be suspected on the basis of the antimicrobial susceptibility pattern. One clue to the presence of an ESBL-producing organism is an antibiogram showing resistance to third-generation cephalosporins, but susceptibility to cephamycins, such as the second-generation cephalosporins cefoxitin and cefotetan. (Although ESBL-producing organisms may appear sensitive to cephamycins, resistance may develop in practice.) Another clue is the partially restoration of beta-lactam susceptibility in vitro by clavulanic acid.

Severe infections due to ESBL-producers should be treated with a carbapenem, such as imipenem, meropenem, doripenem, or ertapenem. Although some strains may test susceptible to some cephalosporins in the antibiogram, these antibiotics should be considered inactive against ESBL-producing organisms. Piperacillin/tazobactam may be considered for nonlife-threatening infections, such as urinary tract infections, in apparently susceptible strains. Patients found to harbor ESBL-positive organisms should be placed on contact isolation (gowns and gloves).

CARBAPENEMASES

The prevalence of carbapenemases has risen alarmingly in recent years, probably due to the widespread use of carbapenem. The distribution of different carbapenemases varies depending on the country. In the United States, KPCs (*Klebsiella pneumoniae* carbapenemase) are the most frequently found carbapenemases. As the name suggests, these enzymes are most often expressed in *Klebsiella pneumoniae*, but may also be found in *E coli, Enterobacter* spp., *Pseudomonas* spp., and *Salmonella*. KPCs have rapidly spread across the U.S. since early 2000, and they are currently endemic in areas of New York and New Jersey. They tend to colonize and infect patients with multiple comorbidities, intensive care unit stays, and prolonged hospitalization.

PRACTICE POINT

- *Acinetobacter baumannii* has emerged as a major opportunistic pathogen, able to survive and thrive in the hospital environment because of its tolerance of a wide range of physical conditions and high degree of innate resistance to antibiotics and disinfectants. Infection has become common in intensive care units and among repatriated combat casualties, who perhaps acquired infection in contaminated field hospitals. For multidrug resistant *Acinetobacter* strains, carbapenems are preferred treatment for sensitive isolates, with ampicillin-sulbactam as a second option. Strains resistant to these antibiotics may be treated with colistin, both systemically and also by aerosol in patients with *Acinetobacter* pneumonia. Inhaled colistin is not systemically absorbed. Tigecycline is a drug of last resort. Due to concerns about inferior outcomes in patients with nosocomial pneumonia treated with tigecycline, higher doses may be considered if it must be used for lower respiratory tract infection.

Infections caused by KPC-producing Gram-negatives have 40–50% mortality. Treatment options are limited to polymyxins, and in some cases tigecycline. Patients found to carry carbapenemase-producing Gram-negative bacilli should be placed on contact isolation.

Isolates of *E coli* and *Klebsiella* producing a novel carbapenemase, New Delhi metallo-beta-lactamase 1 (NDM-1), have become prominent in India. These bacteria are resistant to all beta-lactams, fluoroquinolones, and aminoglycosides. Most isolates were sensitive to tigecycline and colistin, although a few were resistant. NDM-1 may be widespread in the community in India, where antibiotics are readily available over the counter. A few cases of infections with NDM-1 have been reported in Western travelers to India and Pakistan, often in patients seeking medical care abroad. Although the "NDM-1 superbug" has attracted much media attention, presumably because of its somewhat exotic origins, the equally resistant and increasingly endemic KPC-positive Gram-negatives represent a more imminent threat to hospitalized patients in Western countries.

PRACTICE POINT

When first-line antibiotic therapy can be avoided in normal hosts

Urinary tract infections

- Asymptomatic bacteriuria should not be treated unless patients are pregnant or undergoing urinary tract instrumentation.
- Candiduria may represent vaginal flora or colonization.
- Urine cultures are usually positive in the presence of a Foley catheter, and should not be treated in the absence of symptoms; if treatment is necessary, remove Foley and treat for seven days. Treatment of bacteriuria or candiduria with a Foley catheter in place is usually ineffective, and may select for resistant microbes.

Skin and soft tissue infections

- Drainage of abscess (< 3 cm) without cellulitis

Pulmonary infections

- Bronchitis usually does not require antibiotic treatment, with some exceptions, such as COPD exacerbation. Sputum cultures with yeast usually represent colonization or thrush.

QUALITY IMPROVEMENT

Control of antimicrobial resistance in the hospital requires multidisciplinary efforts, involving physicians, nurses, infection control practitioners, microbiologists, and pharmacists. Recommended components include both passive and active surveillance for antibiotic resistance, prompt isolation precautions for patients with proven or suspected resistant infection or colonization, and programs of antibiotic restriction and stewardship.

Working with their infectious disease colleagues, hospitalists may lead quality improvement efforts that include education about antibiotic overuse, appropriate prescribing based on local antibiotic sensitivity data, and optimal dosing and monitoring of antibiotics. Timely infectious disease consultation may facilitate changing empiric coverage to narrow-spectrum antibiotics, based on laboratory analysis of sensitivities. Hospitalists should also bear in mind that preventive measures that decrease the burden of infection, such as provision of pneumococcal and influenza vaccination, may also alleviate the spread of antibiotic resistance.

SUGGESTED READINGS

Centinkaya Y, Falk P, Mayhall G. Vancomycin-resistant enterococci. *Clin Microbiol Rev.* 2000;13:686–707.

Garnacho-Montero J, Amaya-Villar R. Multiresistant Acinetobacter baumanii infections: epidemiology and management. *Curr Opin Infect Dis.* 2010:23:332–339.

Jacoby G, Munoz-Price LS. The new beta-lactamases. *N Engl J Med.* 2005;352:380–391.

Kumarasamy KK, Toleman MA, Walsh TR, et al. Emergence of a new antibiotic resistance mechanism in India, Pakistan, and the UK: a molecular, biological, and epidemiological study. *Lancet Infect Dis.* 2010;10:597–602.

Munoz-Price LS, Quinn JP. The spread of *Klebsiella pneumoniae* carbapenemases: a tale of strains, plasmids, and transposons. *Clin Infect Dis.* 2009;49:1739–1741.

Munoz-Price LS, Hayden MK, Lolans K, et al. Successful control of an outbreak of carbapenemase-producing K. pneumoniae at a long term acute care hospital. *Infect Control Hospital Epidemiol.* 2010;31:341–347.

Pitout JD, Nordmann P, Laupland KB, Poirel L. Emergence of Enterobacteriaceae producing extended-spectrum beta-lactamases (ESBLs) in the community. *J Antimicrob Chemother.* 2005;56:52–59.

Popovich KJ, Weinstein RA. The graying of methicillin-resistant *Staphylococcus aureus. Infect Control Hosp Epidemiol.* 2009:30: 9–12.

Popovich KJ, Weinstein RA, Hota B. Are community-associated methicillin-resistant *Staphylococcus aureus* (MRSA) strains replacing traditional nosocomial MRSA strains? *Clin Infect Dis.* 2008;46: 787–794.

CHAPTER 187

Peritonitis and Intra-Abdominal Abscess

Shira Doron, MD
David R. Snydman, MD, FACP

Key Clinical Questions

1. How is spontaneous bacterial peritonitis diagnosed?
2. What is the optimal duration of treatment of spontaneous bacterial peritonitis?
3. How is secondary peritonitis diagnosed and treated?
4. When should tuberculous peritonitis be suspected?
5. How are intra-abdominal abscesses diagnosed and treated?

EPIDEMIOLOGY

Peritonitis and intra-abdominal abscesses are much feared because of the high frequency of associated septic shock and multisystem organ failure. Both primary and secondary peritonitis have an in-hospital mortality rate of approximately 20%. Intra-abdominal infections are the second leading cause of infectious death in the intensive care unit. Although the precise incidence of peritonitis is unknown, it is encountered with some regularity by physicians caring for inpatients. Spontaneous bacterial peritonitis (SBP), or primary peritonitis, occurs in up to 30% of all patients with liver cirrhosis and ascites. Secondary peritonitis and intra-abdominal abscesses are important complications of conditions commonly seen on general medical wards, such as diverticulitis, peptic ulcer disease, pancreatitis, and cholecystitis. Classic symptoms and signs of intra-abdominal infection may be blunted in older or immunosuppressed patients, increasing the challenge for clinicians.

PERITONITIS

Peritonitis is inflammation of the peritoneal surface, caused by microorganisms or irritants such as foreign bodies, bile, and barium. Peritonitis is classified as primary (or spontaneous), secondary, or tertiary. In primary peritonitis, there is inflammation of the peritoneal surface without another intra-abdominal process. Secondary peritonitis develops as a result of inflammation of another structure within the abdomen. Tertiary peritonitis refers to persistent inflammation after treatment for secondary peritonitis.

SPONTANEOUS (PRIMARY) PERITONITIS

Primary peritonitis, or spontaneous bacterial peritonitis (SBP), is most commonly seen in cirrhotic patients with ascites, and less often in patients with ascites from other causes, such as heart failure or systemic lupus erythematosus. Bacteria may gain access to the peritoneal fluid from hematogenous or lymphogenous spread, traversing the intact intestinal wall from the gut lumen or by passing through the fallopian tubes from the vagina in women.

Presentation

The classic signs and symptoms of peritonitis are fever, abdominal pain, and rebound tenderness. These may be mild or completely absent in cirrhotic patients. SBP should be suspected in all cirrhotic patients with clinical decompensation, such as the development of hepatic encephalopathy or hepatorenal syndrome.

Bacteriology

Most episodes of SBP are caused by enteric Gram-negative rods, such as *E coli* and *Klebsiella* species. An important minority of SBP episodes is caused by Gram-positive organisms, especially *Streptococcus pneumoniae*. Infections are rarely polymicrobial, and generally do not involve anaerobic bacteria. **Table 187-1** shows the relative frequencies of common organisms isolated from ascitic fluid in patients with SBP.

Diagnosis

Fluid should be obtained by paracentesis and sent for Gram stain, culture, cell count with differential, and albumin. Paracentesis is generally safe, even in the setting of grossly abnormal coagulation tests and low platelets. Peritoneal fluid should be inoculated into

TABLE 187-1 Microbiology of Spontaneous Bacterial Peritonitis

Organism	Percent of Isolates
Escherichia coli	43–49
Klebsiella pneumonia	11–20
Other enteric Gram negative rods	4–5
Streptococcus pneumoniae	3–9
Other streptococci	6–19
Staphylococcus sp.	3–6
Pseudomonas aeruginosa	1–3
Miscellaneous	8–10

Data from Heo J, et al. *Gut Liver.* 2009;3:197–204, and McHutchison JG, Runyon BA. Spontaneous bacterial peritonitis. In: Gastrointestinal and Hepatic Infections, Surawicz, CM, Owen, RL (eds), Philadelphia, PA: WB Saunders; 1995:455.

blood culture bottles at the bedside, after changing the needle on the paracentesis syringe to a sterile needle. At least 10 cc of fluid should be inoculated into the bottle if possible. A separate syringe, tube, or container of fluid should be sent for immediate Gram stain. Fluid should also be injected into purple and red top tubes for cell count and chemistries, respectively.

Gram stain is positive in only a minority of cases. In SBP, the cell count is generally greater than 300 white blood cells/mm^3, and is usually more than 1000 cells/mm^3, with neutrophils predominating on differential. An absolute polymorphonuclear (PMN) leukocyte count of greater than or equal to 250 cells/mm^3 in conjunction with a positive culture is diagnostic of peritonitis. A small percentage of patients, such as those with neutropenia, will have fewer cells with active infection. A traumatic procedure can result in entry of blood into the fluid being analyzed, artifactually raising red and white cell counts. To correct for extraneous blood, one can subtract one PMN for every 250 red blood cells present. In appropriately treated SBP, ascitic fluid cell count should start to decline within 48 to 72 hours. If a decline is not seen, an evaluation for secondary peritonitis should be undertaken, beginning with imaging of the abdomen. Repeat paracentesis is not necessary in a patient who is responding well clinically.

It can be difficult to distinguish secondary peritonitis from SBP. Some clues that the infection is secondary to an intra-abdominal process include failure to respond rapidly to antibiotic therapy, serum ascites-albumin gradient less than 1.1 g/dL, indicating the absence of portal hypertension, ascitic total protein greater than 1 g/dL, ascitic fluid glucose concentration less than 50 mg/dL, lactate dehydrogenase greater than the upper limit of normal for serum, and polymicrobial culture. If any of these findings are present, the patient should be imaged with flat and upright abdominal X-rays and an abdominal CT with oral and intravenous contrast.

Treatment

When SBP is suspected, treatment should not be delayed while awaiting the results of laboratory tests. Third-generation cephalosporins are preferred for initial therapy. It is not necessary to empirically cover *Enterococcus* or anaerobic bacteria. Historically, there has been reluctance to use ceftriaxone due to fear of worsening cholestasis in patients with liver failure, but this has not been supported by clinical experience. Due to increasing resistance, fluoroquinolones such as ciprofloxacin should not be used for empiric therapy. However, if culture results reveal a fluoroquinolone-susceptible organism, the high bioavailability of these drugs makes them a good option for oral therapy. Fluoroquinolones should never be used empirically in patients that have received fluoroquinolone prophylaxis for SBP. In patients with a good clinical response, five days of therapy is adequate. In patients with an incomplete response after five days (eg, persistent pain, fever, or altered mental status), paracentesis should be repeated. If the white blood cell count in ascitic fluid is less than 250 cells/mm^3, treatment may be stopped. If the white blood cell count is in excess of 250 cells/mm^3, but improved compared to the pretreatment value, treatment should continue, and repeat paracentesis should be considered in a few days. If the white blood cell count remains high, evaluation for secondary peritonitis is indicated. Bacteremia associated with SBP does not require a longer course of therapy, unless it is due to an organism with a robust association with endocarditis, such as *Staphylococcus aureus* or *Enterococcus*.

Prevention

Oral antibiotics are recommended as prophylaxis against SBP in patients with an ascitic fluid protein concentration less than 1.0 g/dL, any patient with a history of SBP, and patients with variceal bleeding. Ciprofloxacin, norfloxacin, and trimethoprim/sulfamethoxazole are both effective and cost-effective. Daily dosing is preferred to intermittent dosing, due to the lower likelihood for the development of antibiotic resistance.

Tuberculous peritonitis is often confused with other conditions. In alcoholic patients, it may mimic SBP, and it may be mistaken for ovarian carcinoma in women. It results from hematogenous dissemination of tuberculosis from remote foci of disease such as the lung, or from direct inoculation of bacilli into the peritoneum from intra-abdominal lymph nodes. The peritoneum becomes studded with tubercles that exude fluid, and ascites develops. Tuberculous peritonitis should be suspected in patients with the subacute onset of ascites, abdominal pain, and risk factors for TB exposure. Fever is variable. On paracentesis, there will generally be greater than 150 white cells/mm^3, with lymphocytic predominance and elevated protein. If the patient is not cirrhotic, the serum ascites-albumin gradient will be less than 1.1 g/dL, indicating the absence of portal hypertension. Ascites fluid culture is rarely positive for *Mycobacteria tuberculosis*, and peritoneal biopsy is usually necessary to make the diagnosis. Biopsy under direct visualization, ideally via laparoscopy, has a much higher yield than blind percutaneous biopsy. Therapy for confirmed TB peritonitis is the same as that given for pulmonary TB.

SECONDARY PERITONITIS

Secondary peritonitis is classified as perforation peritonitis and nonperforation peritonitis. Any ruptured gastrointestinal or genitourinary organ may result in perforation peritonitis. Causes of perforation include trauma, infection, peptic ulcer, ischemia, neoplasm, and surgery (see **Table 187-2**).

PRESENTATION

Abdominal pain is almost universal in secondary peritonitis. Nausea, vomiting, and anorexia are common. Fever and leukocytosis are frequently present. Alteration in bowel function may also be present. The specific character, location, and progression of the abdominal pain depend on the etiology of the peritonitis. Ruptured peptic ulcer pain has a sudden onset and is worse in the epigastric region, whereas appendicitis pain has a gradual onset and classically begins as a diffuse pain that localizes to the right lower quadrant, sometimes with periappendiceal abscess formation (**Figure 187-1**).

"Peritoneal signs" are used by clinicians to distinguish peritonitis that may require surgery from other types of abdominal pain. These signs include rebound tenderness, which indicates the presence of parietal peritoneal inflammation, and muscular rigidity

TABLE 187-2 Common Causes of Secondary Peritonitis by Source

Esophagus	Perforation (eg, Boerhaave syndrome, tumor)
Stomach	Perforation (eg, from peptic ulcer, tumor)
Duodenum	Perforation (eg, from peptic ulcer, tumor)
Biliary tract	Cholecystitis
	Perforation
Small intestine	Appendicitis
	Ischemic bowel
	Incarcerated hernia
	Crohn disease
	perforation
Large intestine	Diverticulitis
	Perforation
	Ulcerative colitis, Crohn disease
	Ischemic colitis
	Infectious colitis
Female reproductive organs	Pelvic inflammatory disease
Urinary tract	Perinephric abscess
Other	Necrotizing pancreatitis
	Perihepatic abscess

TABLE 187-3 Organisms in Complicated Intra-abdominal Infection

Organism	Percent of Isolates
Facultative and aerobic gram-negative	
Escherichia coli	48–71
Klebsiella species	14
Pseudomonas aeruginosa	7–14
Proteus mirabilis	5
Enterobacter species	5
Anaerobic	
Bacteroides fragilis	7–35
Other *Bacteroides* species	71
Clostridium species	29
Prevotella species	12
Peptostreptococcus species	17
Fusobacterium species	9
Eubacterium species	17
Gram-positive aerobic cocci	
Streptococcus species	4–38
Enterococcus faecalis	12
Enterococcus faecium	3
Enterococcus species	8
Staphylococcus aureus	1–4

Data from Solomkin JS, et al. *Clin Infect Dis*. 2010;50:133–164. Chen Z, et al. *BMC Infect Dis*. 2010;10:217.

of the abdominal wall (including both voluntary guarding and reflex muscle spasm). In general, peritoneal signs are specific but not sensitive for the diagnosis of peritonitis. Patients with peritonitis may lack peritoneal signs due to lax abdominal musculature (eg, postpartum women), ascites, glucocorticoid use, or the presence of an abscess that is not in contact with the anterior abdominal wall. Carnett sign may help distinguish pain arising from the abdominal wall from that of visceral origin. The patient is examined while he or she tenses the abdominal muscles by raising the head and shoulders off the bed. If the abdomen becomes tenderer during this maneuver, Carnett sign is positive, and a source of pain in the abdominal wall, such as a hernia or rectus sheath hematoma, should be suspected.

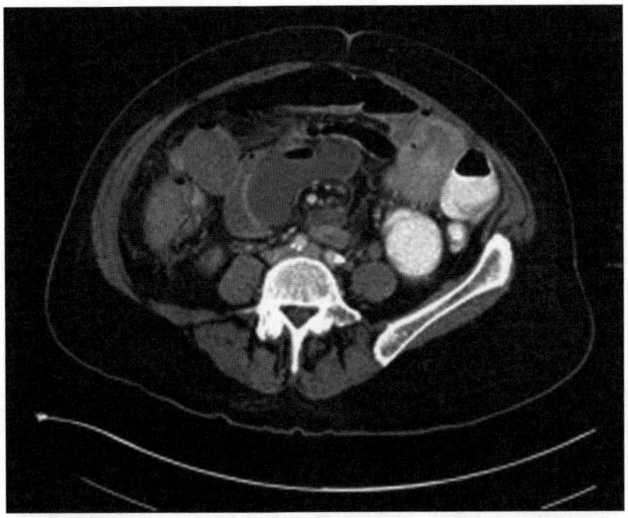

Figure 187-1 *Abdominal CT scan with oral and intravenous contrast demonstrating periappendiceal abscess in the right lower quadrant.*

BACTERIOLOGY

Infection in perforation peritonitis is usually polymicrobial, featuring *E coli*, other Gram-negative rods, and anaerobic bacteria (**Table 187-3**). The bacteria involved vary depending on the organ perforated. Different segments of the gastrointestinal tract have different microbial ecologies, and these may be further altered by hospitalization, surgery, acid blockers, or antibiotics.

DIAGNOSIS

Initial evaluation of a patient with suspected peritonitis should always include flat and upright abdominal films, and a chest X-ray. These may reveal free air in the abdomen in the case of perforated viscus (**Figure 187-2**), and also help to rule out a thoracic or pulmonary process masquerading as peritonitis.

Abdominal CT scan is the next step, unless the disease is suspected to be in the right upper quadrant, retroperitoneum, or pelvis, in which case ultrasound is often more helpful diagnostically. It is currently rare for a patient to be taken to the operating room without a CT or ultrasound. Laboratory studies that may be helpful include complete blood count, urea nitrogen, creatinine, liver enzymes, lipase, urinalysis, and pregnancy test in women of childbearing potential. Blood cultures, if positive, are helpful in determining appropriate regimen and duration of therapy in patients with health care-associated or severe infection, or those at high risk for treatment failure (**Table 187-4**).

Intra-abdominal specimens should be sent for culture in health care-associated infection and severe infection. Intra-abdominal culture should also be obtained in community-acquired infection of mild to moderate severity when there is a substantial local

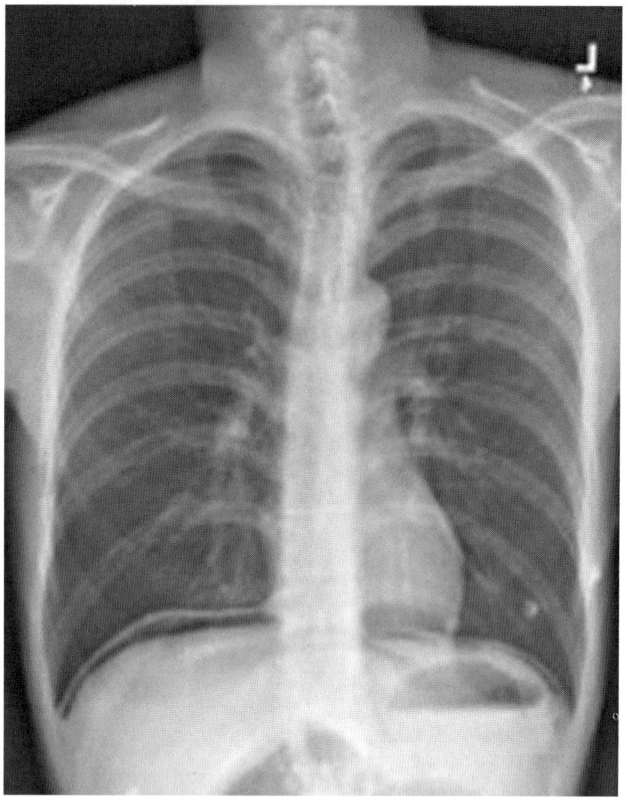

Figure 187-2 *Chest radiograph demonstrating free air under both hemidiaphragms due to perforation of a hollow viscus. (Reproduced, with permission, from Fauci AS, Braunwald E, Kasper DL, et al. Harrison's Principles of Internal Medicine. 17th ed. New York: McGraw-Hill; 2008, Fig. 121-2.)*

prevalence of antimicrobial resistance to drugs such as fluoroquinolones or ampicillin-sulbactam. At least 1 mL of fluid or tissue from the infection site should be transported to the laboratory. In order to isolate anaerobic organisms, an anaerobic transport tube should be used.

TREATMENT

In most cases, definitive therapy for secondary peritonitis involves either surgical or percutaneous drainage. Perforated organs usually need closure or removal, and fecal spillage requires wash-out. Focal collections generally are not cured without drainage. Fluid resuscitation should be initiated when the diagnosis of secondary peritonitis is made. Antimicrobial therapy should be initiated as soon as possible, while awaiting a procedure and before culture data is obtained. Many broad-spectrum antibiotics and combinations of antibiotics provide good empiric coverage for the Gram-negative enteric organisms and gut streptococci usually involved in intra-abdominal infection. Antibiotics active against obligate anaerobes such as *Bacteroides* and *Clostridium* species are needed when infection arises from the distal small bowel or colon, or from a more proximal source in the setting of obstruction or ileus. Cefotetan and clindamycin are no longer acceptable empiric agents for coverage of *Bacteroides* due to rising resistance. Empiric coverage for *Pseudomonas* is generally unnecessary in patients with mild to moderate community-acquired peritonitis. Infections arising from the biliary tract are treated similarly to proximal small bowel infections, unless they occur after a bilio-enteric anastamosis, which should be treated with regimens used for severe or high risk peritonitis. It is unnecessary to treat every organism identified on culture. *Enterococcus* and *Candida*, in particular, can often be left untreated without compromising the resolution of the infection. Therapy for these organisms should be considered if they are isolated from blood, are the predominant organism on culture, or persist as the sole organism after treatment. Acceptable antibiotic regimens are listed in **Table 187-5**. The use of ampicillin-sulbactam is discouraged in the 2010 Infectious Diseases Society of America guidelines, due to increasing resistance among *E coli*.

TABLE 187-4 Clinical Factors Predicting Treatment Failure in Intra-Abdominal Infection

Delay in initial intervention (> 12 hours)
High severity of illness (APACHE II score 15 or higher)
Advanced age
Comorbidity and degree of organ dysfunction
Low albumin level
Poor nutritional status
Degree of peritoneal involvement or diffuse peritonitis
Inability to achieve adequate debridement or control of drainage
Presence of malignancy

APACHE, Acute Physiology and Chronic Health Evaluation.
Reproduced, with permission, from Solomkin JS, Mazuski JE, Bradley JS, et al. Diagnosis and management of complicated intra-abdominal infection in adults and children: guidelines by the Surgical Infection Society and the Infectious Diseases Society of America. *Clin Infect Dis*. 2010;50:133–164.

PRACTICE POINT

- With intra-abdominal abscess, it is not necessary to target antibiotic therapy to every organism isolated. Likewise, if a patient is responding clinically to an antibiotic regimen, and culture data shows that there is an organism that is not being covered, it is not imperative to change the regimen.

In most cases, when good source control is achieved within 24 hours, only perioperative antibiotics are needed as therapy. This includes appendicitis, cholecystitis, and penetrating bowel trauma. Infections requiring a longer course are generally adequately treated after four to seven days. Patients with clinical evidence of persistent infection after four to seven days should be assessed for possible ongoing intra-abdominal infection, an extra-abdominal source of infection, or antibiotic resistance.

PREVENTION

Prevention of secondary peritonitis is limited to two principles: early and adequate treatment of intra-abdominal infections to prevent progression to rupture or abscess, and appropriate preoperative antibiotic prophylaxis and intra-operative techniques to prevent intra-abdominal contamination.

TERTIARY PERITONITIS

Tertiary peritonitis refers to recurrent intra-abdominal infection after therapy with antibiotics and drainage for secondary peritonitis. Abscess formation is expected in this setting. The predominant organisms reflect exposure to antimicrobials and the hospital environment and are therefore commonly resistant to first-line

TABLE 187-5 Antibiotic Regimens for Secondary Peritonitis

Infection	Regimen
Community-acquired, mild to moderate severity, infection of gastric or proximal small bowel source, including cholecystitis without bilio-enteric anastamosis	Cefazolin, cefuroxime, or ceftriaxone
Community-acquired, mild to moderate severity, patient not high risk (see Table 187-4), source distal small bowel or colon	Cefoxitin, ertapenem, tigecycline, or ticarcillin-clavulanic acid alone OR metronidazole plus either cefazolin, cefuroxime, ceftriaxone, cefotaxime, ciprofloxacin, levofloxacin, or moxifloxacin
Community-acquired, high risk (see Table 187-4) or severe, source distal small bowel or colon, or cholecystitis after bilio-enteric anastamosis	Imipenem-cilastatin, meropenem, doripenem, or piperacillin-tazobactam alone OR metronidazole plus cefepime or ceftazidime (in many communities resistance to the fluoroquinolones ciprofloxacin and levofloxacin is too high to make these agents acceptable for empiric therapy of severe infections)
Health care-associated	Use local microbiologic data to guide empiric therapy: Imipenem-cilastatin, meropenem, doripenem, or piperacillin-tazobactam alone OR metronidazole plus cefepime or ceftazidime Add vancomycin to cover methicillin-resistant *Staphylococcus aureus* (MRSA).

antibiotics. Examples include yeast, *Enterococcus*, and resistant Gram-negative bacteria such as *Pseudomonas* and *Enterobacter.* Most patients with tertiary peritonitis require one or more additional operative procedures to achieve control of their infection.

PERITONEAL DIALYSIS-RELATED

Many patients with renal failure prefer home peritoneal dialysis (PD). Unfortunately, peritonitis is an exceedingly common complication, and the major reason that PD patients have to switch to hemodialysis. Gram-positive bacteria cause the majority of infections, Gram-negative bacteria cause about one-quarter, and fungal peritonitis accounts for less than 5% of episodes. International Society of Peritoneal Dialysis guidelines recommend empiric coverage for both Gram-positive (including MRSA where this organism is prevalent) and Gram-negative organisms. This is usually achieved with a combination of vancomycin plus a cephalosporin or aminoglycoside. Antifungal therapy should be initiated only if the Gram stain reveals yeast. Antibiotics may be given intraperitoneally.

PD catheter removal is an important part of therapy in certain circumstances. Clinical scenarios that should prompt catheter removal include relapse of the same infection within four weeks after completing antibiotic therapy, infection not responding to appropriate antibiotics, exit site or tunnel infection, fungal peritonitis, and possibly tuberculous peritonitis.

PERITONITIS IN THE IMMMUNOCOMPROMISED PATIENT

In the immunocompromised or elderly patient, signs of peritoneal inflammation may be limited or absent, so a low threshold is needed to evaluate the abdomen for peritonitis. Many intra-abdominal conditions preferentially affect the patient weakened by drugs or disease, such as typhlitis (necrosis of the bowel wall related to breakdown of microbial defenses) in the post-chemotherapy neutropenic patient, or cytomegalovirus colitis in the post-transplant or AIDS patient. Patients who have been hospitalized or who have received antibiotic courses are at high risk of developing *Clostridium difficile* colitis.

TABLE 187-6 Visceral Abscesses

Organ	Causes	Microbiology	Other Features
Pancreas	Complication of pancreatitis Secondary infection of pancreatic pseudocyst	Polymicrobial, enteric; occasionally *S aureus*	Serum amylase frequently elevated
Liver	Complication of cholecystitis, appendicitis or diverticulitis Complication of liver transplantation Chronic granulomatous disease	Polymicrobial, enteric Increasingly monomicrobial due to *Klebsiella*, especially in Asia *Entamoeba histolytica* Occasionally *S aureus* Rarely *Yersinia enterocolitica* *Candida* in immunocompromised hosts	Alkaline phosphatase is the most frequently deranged laboratory value Amoebic abscess does not require drainage for effective treatment
Spleen	Trauma Bacteremia, especially in IV drug users Hematogenous spread to infarcted tissue in sickle cell patients Embolic from bacterial endocarditis	*S aureus* and streptococci if due to endocarditis *Salmonella* in sickle cell disease Occasionally polymicrobial, enteric *Candida* in immunocompromised hosts	May experience referred pain in left shoulder (Kehr sign) Splenic rub

PRACTICE POINT

- *Clostridium difficile* colitis without diarrhea can mimic SBP or intra-abdominal abscess. Suspect *Clostridium difficile* in any patient with abdominal symptoms and recent antibiotic use or hospitalization, especially if the serum white blood cell count is high, or if colitis is seen on CT scan.

INTRA-ABDOMINAL ABSCESSES

Abscesses can be classified by cause, like peritonitis, into primary or secondary, or by location, as intraperitoneal, retroperitoneal, or visceral. Primary abscesses develop for unknown reasons. Secondary abscesses develop near the site of an infected organ, after a perforation, traumatic injury, postoperatively, or after primary peritonitis. The location of an abscess is generally related to the site of origin of the infection and the direction of dependent drainage. Abscesses may also extend and erode. They can track from the abdomen down into the thigh or up into the pleural space. They can form fistulas, or erode into blood vessels and cause hemorrhage.

Abscesses are typically polymicrobial and involve normal bowel flora. Most have an anaerobic component, although the anaerobic bacteria are often not successfully grown on culture. Increasingly, *Staphylococcus aureus* is found as a cause of intra-abdominal abscesses. **Table 187-6** lists common associated organisms and features of abscesses in various visceral locations.

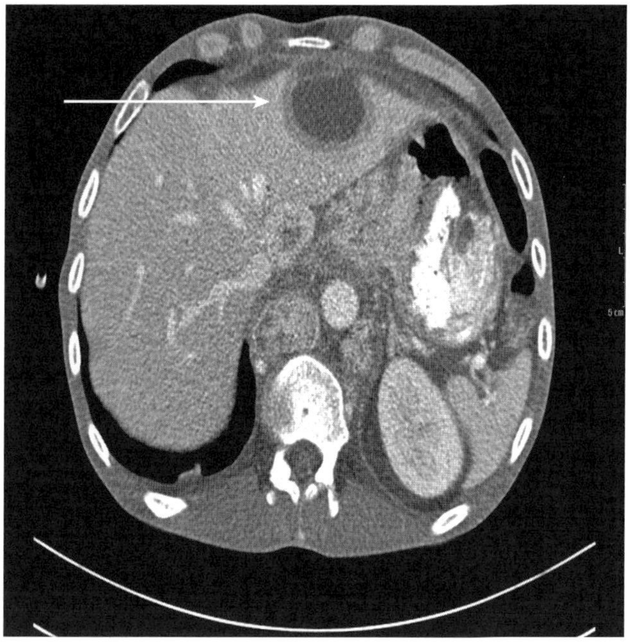

Figure 187-3 *Abdominal CT scan with intravenous and oral contrast demonstrating abscess in the left lobe of the liver; ring enhancement is present.*

TABLE 187-7 Evidence-based Medicine: Intra-Abdominal Infections

Paper	Methodology	Results	Limitations	Bottom Line
Singh O, Gupta S, Moses S, Jain DK. *Indian J Gastroenterol.* 2009;28:88–92	Comparative study of effectiveness of percutaneous catheter drainage (PCD) and percutaneous needle aspiration (PNA) in the management of 72 patients with large (> 10 cm diameter) liver abscesses	PNA was successful in 31 of 36 (86%) patients, whereas PCD was successful in 35 (97%) patients (p value not significant)	Nonrandomized study; case mix of amebic and pyogenic liver abscesses	Percutaneous catheter drainage and antibiotics are curative for many patients with very large liver abscesses
Terg R, Fassio E, Guevara M, et al. *J Hepatol.* 2008; 48:774–779	Prospective, double-blind trial in 100 cirrhotic patients with < 1.5 g/dl of total protein in ascitic fluid randomized to receive ciprofloxacin 500 mg/day or placebo for 12 months	The probability of survival at 12 months was significantly higher in patients receiving ciprofloxacin (86% versus 66%) ($p < 0.04$). Most deaths in the placebo group were due to infection	A recent Cochrane meta-analysis noted that this paper was methodologically superior to previous trials that had shown similar results	Patients with advanced cirrhosis and protein-poor ascites are at high risk of spontaneous bacterial peritonitis and other infections, and may benefit from prophylactic antibiotics
van Ruler O, Mahler CW, Boer KR, et al. *JAMA.* 2007;298: 865–873	Nonblinded controlled trial in 232 patients with severe peritonitis, confirmed at laparotomy, randomized to routine relaparotomy within 48 hours, vs. laparotomy only if clinical deterioration took place	All-cause morbidity and mortality were similar between the two groups; patients who had repeat laparotomy had longer lengths of stay in the hospital and intensive care unit (ICU)	Patients with very severe peritonitis at initial laparotomy, in whom the surgeons felt repeat laparotomy was mandated, were excluded from the trial	Routine second-look laparatomy in severe peritonitis does not improve outcomes, and was associated with longer length-of-stay in the hospital and the ICU, and higher health care costs
Basoli A, Chirletti P, Cirino E, et al. *J Gastrointest Surg.* 2008;12:592–600	Prospective, double-blind trial of three days vs. 5–14 days of ertapenem therapy in patients who required surgery for mild-moderate community-acquired peritonitis	Clinical and microbiologic cure rates were similar in the two groups	Patients were relatively young, with half having appendicitis; patients had to be afebrile for 24 hours, with a normal white count and positive bowel sounds, to stop antibiotics	Shorter courses of broad-spectrum antibiotics may be adequate for highly selected patients with mild, uncomplicated peritonitis who are doing well postoperatively

PRESENTATION

Presenting features vary widely, depending on location and source. Anorexia and nausea are common. Fever and leukocytosis are usually present. The course can be acute or subacute, or even chronic in the case of some subphrenic abscesses. There is usually tenderness and possibly fullness over the abscess. Abscesses eroding into or near the thoracic cavity may cause chest and respiratory signs and symptoms. Abscesses adjacent to the colon may cause diarrhea, and those adjacent to the bladder may cause urinary symptoms.

DIAGNOSIS

CT scan of the abdomen is usually the first step in diagnosis. Findings consistent with abscess include low-density tissue mass, capsule formation, and extraluminal gas. Oral contrast helps to distinguish intraluminal contents from abscess, and intravenous contrast helps to enhance the abscess for identification. **Figure 187-3** shows a CT scan of a liver abscess with typical ring enhancement.

Ultrasound is generally not used for diagnosis of intra-abdominal abscess, except for those in the right upper quadrant and female reproductive structures, as its sensitivity is reduced by overlying bowel gas, and it is difficult to perform in the setting of abdominal wounds and drains. Occult abscesses can sometimes be detected on radionuclide scan using radiolabeled leukocytes in a patient undergoing workup for prolonged fever or leukocytosis of unknown origin.

TREATMENT

Drainage is necessary for cure. Antibiotics are used as adjunctive therapy. Percutaneous drainage is suitable when there is only one or a few abscess cavities, ideally with communication between them, so that only a minimal number of passes with the catheter is needed for drainage; the catheter does not need to traverse bowel or other organs on its route from the skin to the abscess; and the infected fluid is not too viscous to drain through the catheter. Abscess material should always be sent for culture.

Empiric antibiotic choice should follow the same principles as in secondary peritonitis, except that anaerobic coverage is essential. Treatment should be targeted to culture results when they become available. Duration of antibiotics for intra-abdominal abscess is usually until the abscess is fully drained. If a catheter is left in for prolonged drainage, this means the antibiotics will continue for as long as the catheter is in place. When antibiotics are discontinued before fever or leukocytosis has resolved, or before complete drainage has been achieved, there is a high risk of recurrence of the infection (**Table 187-7**).

SUGGESTED READINGS

Koulaouzidis A, Bhat S, Saeed AA. Spontaneous bacterial peritonitis. *World J Gastroenterol*. 2009;15:1042–1049.

Piraino B, Bailie GR, Bernardini J, et al. International Society for Peritoneal Dialysis Guidelines/Recommendations: peritoneal dialysis-related infections recommendations: 2005 update. *Perit Dial Int*. 2005;25:107–131.

Solomkin JS, Mazuski JE, Bradley JS, Rodvold KA, et al. Diagnosis and management of complicated intra-abdominal infection in adults and children: guidelines by the Surgical Infection Society and the Infectious Diseases Society of America. *Clinical Infectious Diseases*. 2010;50:133–164.

CHAPTER 188

Clostridium difficile–Associated Disease (CDAD)

Danielle B. Scheurer, MD, MSc, FHM

Key Clinical Questions

1. Which factors are associated with an increased risk of primary or recurrent *Clostridium difficile*–associated disease (CDAD)?
2. What factors affect the accuracy of diagnostic testing of CDAD?
3. What are the most common complications of CDAD?
4. What therapies are most efficacious for primary, recurrent, or refractory CDAD?
5. What system improvements can reduce the incidence of CDAD?

INTRODUCTION AND EPIDEMIOLOGY

Clostridium difficile was first described in 1935 by pediatricians studying the acquisition of bowel flora in newborns and was termed "difficult" because of its resistance to growth on conventional media. It was not until 1978 that it was found to be associated with toxins in the stools of patients with colitis. *Clostridium difficile*–associated disease (CDAD) has now become a major nosocomial problem, affecting 3 million inpatients yearly in the United States. Acquisition of *C difficile* occurs in up to 30% of hospitalized patients, although only 30–60% have symptoms. Patients with symptomatic disease stay an average of 3.6 days longer in hospital than expected, at a cost of over $1 billion annually in the United States.

Normal gut flora confers resistance to *C difficile* colonization; only 1–4% of healthy adults carry *C difficile* in their bowel flora. Loss of normal colonic flora, usually from antibiotics, allows *C difficile* proliferation (clindamycin, cephalosporins, and fluoroquinolones are common offenders). *C difficile* colitis is also associated with other events that disturb gut flora or host immunity, such as bowel preparations, cytotoxic agents, and colonic inflammation due to inflammatory bowel disease.

CDAD was first described in frail or elderly hospitalized patients after antibiotic exposure, but it is now occurring in younger, healthy individuals with no apparent exposure to health care environments or antibiotics. Up to 20% of CDAD cases are now community acquired. *C difficile* and its spore form are easily transmitted from person-to-person or by contact with objects in the hospital environment, such as stethoscopes, clothing, and toilets. The spore form is ubiquitous in the hospital environment, resistant to alcohol-based treatment and other disinfectants, and can survive for months. Even after routine cleaning, 10–50% of room surfaces still contain spores.

PATHOPHYSIOLOGY

C difficile is an anaerobic spore-forming bacterium that produces two exotoxins (A and B) that adhere to intestinal epithelial cells, causing cell death. These toxins are transcribed from a locus composed of five genes (two toxin genes and three regulatory genes). The current epidemic strain of *C difficile* (BI/NAP1/027) has several factors that increase its virulence. A mutation in one of the regulatory genes results in a massive increase in amount of toxin production. This strain also shows high-level fluoroquinolone resistance, giving it a competitive advantage in environments where fluoroquinolone use is widespread. This strain also produces an additional toxin (binary toxin), the clinical significance of which is not clear.

Patient risk of acquiring CDAD and severity of clinical illness are variable (**Table 188-1**). The clinical spectrum of CDAD ranges from minor diarrhea to fulminant colitis with toxic megacolon. Most patients present with some combination of acute, nonbloody, watery diarrhea (although some present with obstipation), lower abdominal pain, and leukocytosis. Fever is relatively uncommon (present in less than one-third of patients). Mimickers of CDAD include bowel obstruction, fecal impaction, or toxic megacolon.

TABLE 188-1 Factors Associated with Higher Incidence and Severity of CDAD

	Host Factors	Medications	Other Factors
Higher incidence	Older age Comorbidities • COPD • Cancer • Immunosuppression • Tube feeds High colon toxin receptors Low antitoxin IgG	Antibiotics • Fluoroquinolones • Clindamycin Proton pump inhibitors H2-blockers	
Higher severity	Older age Comorbidities • COPD • Cancer • Renal failure Low cognitive score High colon toxin receptors Low anti-toxin IgG	Antiperistaltics Clindamycin Immunosuppressants	Recurrence Recent endoscopy Albumin < 3 g/dL Pain/peritonitis Hemoconcentration WBC < 1.5 K/μL WBC > 25 K/μL

COPD, chronic obstructive pulmonary disease; IgG, immunoglobulin G; WBC, white blood cell.

DIFFERENTIAL DIAGNOSIS

The differential diagnosis of acute diarrhea in hospitalized patients is extensive, and less than a third of cases of nosocomial diarrhea are due to CDAD. Non-CDAD causes of diarrhea should be considered in all patients, especially those for whom *C difficile* testing is negative, or those who do not respond to appropriate treatment. Common benign conditions causing nosocomial diarrhea include medications (stool softeners or laxatives as part of standardized order sets), foods (including tube feedings), oral contrast (from computed tomographic scans), and antibiotic-induced alterations of bowel flora. Less common microbial causes of diarrhea include *Klebsiella oxytoca*, *Klebsiella pneumoniae*, and *Staphylococcus aureus*. For a full discussion of the approach to nosocomial diarrhea, see Chapter 80.

DIAGNOSIS

The diagnosis should be made on the combination of symptoms and microbiologic data. Testing for *C difficile* is imperfect (**Table 188-2**). The cytotoxic assay is the gold standard, with excellent sensitivity (94–100%) and specificity (99%), but it is expensive and time consuming, hence most medical centers no longer routinely perform it. More commonly used are enzyme-linked immunosorbent assay (ELISA) tests for toxins. Most detect both toxin A and B, but some only detect toxin A. ELISA tests have the advantage of being quicker and cheaper but have a sensitivity of only 70–90%. Sensitivity is reduced in some strains that do not produce toxin A (or have mutant toxin A), as well as in patients that have already received antibiotic treatment for CDAD. False-positive tests are rare, and any symptomatic patient with a positive test should be treated. Culture of the organism is not routinely available, and is best reserved for outbreak investigations.

Severe colitis with pseudomembranes is virtually pathognomonic for *C difficile* (**Figure 188-1**). It is diagnosed endoscopically by the appearance of raised yellow or white plaques scattered over the colonic mucosa.

In summary, 20–30% of hospitalized patients are colonized with *C difficile*, but some strains fail to produce toxins, and some patients do not develop symptoms from the toxin when it is present. Most patients without diarrhea should not be tested for *C difficile*.

TABLE 188-2 Diagnostic Tests for *Clostridium difficile*

	What it Tests	Advantages	Disadvantages	False Positive	False Negative
ELISA	Exotoxins A, B, or both	Time (hours) Low cost High specificity	Low sensitivity (70–90%)	Rare	Prior treatment Mutant strain Toxin A deficient strain Low toxin density
Cytotoxic assay	Characteristic cytopathic effect on cell monolayer	High sensitivity and specificity	Time (days) High cost	Rare	Rare
Latex agglutination	Glutamate dehydrogenase enzyme (expressed by *C difficile*)	Time (hours) Low cost	Low sensitivity (58–68%)	Rare	Prior treatment Low *C difficile* density
Organism culture	*C difficile* organism culture on selective medium	Epidemiological tracking Genotyping Performing susceptibilities	Needs confirmation of toxigenic strain	Rare	Rare

ELISA, enzyme-linked immunosorbent assay.

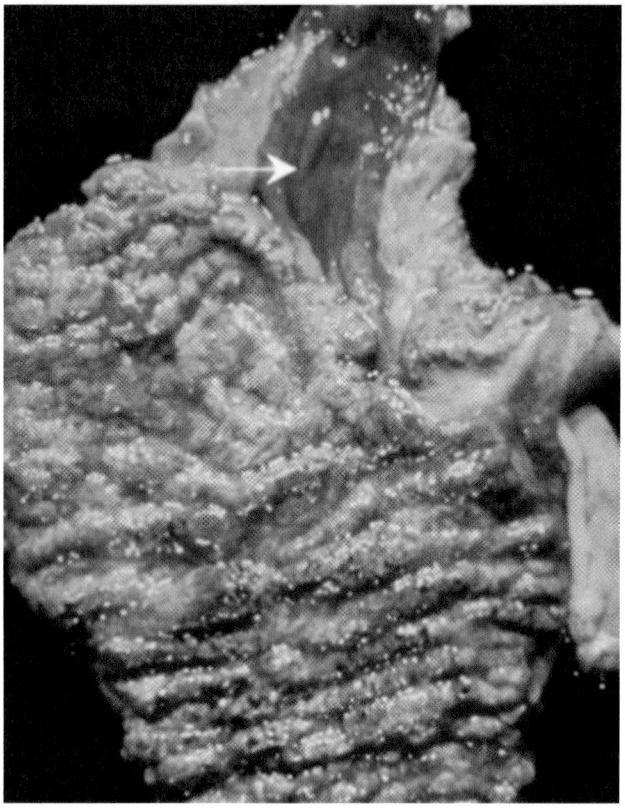

Figure 188-1 *Autopsy specimen with confluent pseudomembranes covering the cecum of a patient with pseudomembranous colitis. Note the sparing of the terminal ileum (arrow). (Reproduced, with permission, from Fauci AS, Braunwald E, Kasper DL, et al. Harrison's Principles of Internal Medicine. 17th ed. New York: McGraw-Hill; 2008, Fig. 123-1.)*

Some patients with symptomatic *C difficile* will have a negative test (20–30%) and should be treated if clinical suspicion is high. Symptomatic patients with a positive test should be treated.

TRIAGE/HOSPITAL ADMISSION

Patients with mild CDAD usually do not require hospital admission, but those with moderate to severe CDAD usually do (**Table 188-3**). Proper infection control measures should be instituted to protect other patients. Contact precautions should be instituted immediately for patients with proven or suspected *C difficile* infection. This includes gowns and gloves for each patient contact, and dedicated equipment in each room, such as blood pressure cuffs and stethoscopes. Strict handwashing before and after all patient contact is required as *C difficile* spores are resistant to alcohol-based treatment.

TREATMENT

Treatments depend on the severity of the disease at presentation and the response to initial therapy (Table 188-3). The offending antibiotic should be stopped whenever feasible. Symptomatic improvement is likely in mildly ill patients after antibiotics are ceased. It is also recommended to discontinue all antiperistaltic agents (although data for their causal link in worse outcomes are retrospective only). These include loperamide, diphenoxylate with atropine (Lomotil), bismuth subsalicylate (Pepto-Bismol), and tincture of opium.

PRACTICE POINT

- Fidaxomicin, the first agent in the new class of macrocyclic antibiotics, was approved for the treatment of *Clostridium difficile* colitis by the U.S. Food and Drug Administration in May 2011. In a randomized clinical trial of 629 patients, a 10-day oral course of fidaxomicin 200 mg twice daily produced rates of clinical cure equivalent to a 10-day course of oral vancomycin 125 mg 4 times daily. Overall, rates of relapse were lower in the fidaxomicin group. However, rates of relapse were similar in the subgroup of patients with the hypervirulent BI/NAP1/027 epidemic strain of *C difficile*. Side effects of fidaxomicin were generally mild and comparable to oral vancomycin. Rash, dizziness, elevated uric acid, and elevated liver transaminases were more common in the patients receiving fidaxomicin.

TABLE 188-3 First-line Treatment for CDAD Based on Severity of Illness and Initial Clinical Response

Clinical Categories	Clinical Criteria	Treatment
Mild CDAD	All of these criteria: • < 6 BM per day *and* • No fever *and* • WBC < 15,000 *and* • No peritoneal signs *and* • No evidence of sepsis	• Oral metronidazole 500 q 8 • If no clinical response at 48 hours, escalate to moderate CDAD treatment
Moderate CDAD	At least 1 of these criteria: • 6–12 BM per day *or* • Fever (37.5°C to 38.5°C) *or* • WBC 15,000–25,000 *or* • Visible lower GI bleeding	• Oral vancomycin 125 q 6 • If no clinical response at 48 hours, escalate to severe CDAD treatment
Severe CDAD	At least 1 of these criteria: • > 12 BM per day *or* • Fever > 38.5°C *or* • WBC > 25,000 *or* • Hemodynamic instability *or* • Evidence of sepsis *or* • Significant abdominal pain *or* • Ileus *or* • CDAD requiring ICU care	• Oral vancomycin 125 q 6 **plus** IV metronidazole 500 q 6

BM, bowel movement; CDAD, *Clostridium difficile* associated disease; GI, gastrointestinal; ICU, intensive care unit; IV, intravenous.

TABLE 188-4 Evidence-based Medicine: Key References for CDAD

Study	Methodology	Results	Limitations	Bottom Line
Nelson RL. Antibiotic treatment for Clostridium difficile-associated diarrhea in adults. *Cochrane Database of Systematic Reviews* 2007; Issue 3. Art. No.: CD004610. DOI: 10.1002/14651858.CD004610. pub3.	12 RCTs met criteria for inclusion	Table 188-5	Small sample size, heterogeneity in outcome measures, none stratified by disease severity	No single antibiotic was clearly superior to another
Pillai A, Nelson RL. Probiotics for treatment of Clostridium difficile-associated colitis in adults. *Cochrane Database of Systematic Reviews* 2008, Issue 1. Art. No.: CD004611. DOI: 10.1002/14651858.CD004611. pub2.	4 RCTs met criteria for inclusion	1 RCT found *S. boulardii* (in addition to standard treatment) reduced risk of recurrent disease (RR 0.59, CI 0.35–0.98) and increased cessation of diarrhea (RR 1.33, CI 1.02–1.74)	Small sample sizes of all the studies. Other three studies did not find a benefit to probiotics (*S. boulardii*, *L. plantarum*, or *L. rhamnosus* GG)	*S.boulardii* may modestly increase cessation of diarrhea and decrease the risk of recurrent disease when used in conjunction with standard treatment
Zar FA, et al. *Clin Infect Dis.* 2007;45:302–307.	Randomized trial of 172 patients with CDAD to oral vancomycin 125 mg four times a day or metronidazole 250 mg four times a day, stratified by risk (high or low)	Vancomycin equivalent to metronidazole in clinical cure rate (98% vs 90%) in low-risk patients. Vancomycin superior to metronidazole in clinical cure rate (97% vs 76%) in high-risk patients	Have to calculate "High risk": Patients with 2+ points: 1 point each for: Age > 60 Temp > 38.3°C WBC > 15 K Albumin < 2.5; 2 points each for: ICU Pseudomembrane	Metronidazole is sufficient for "low risk" CDAD, but vancomycin is superior for "high risk" CDAD

First-line treatment with either oral vancomycin or metronidazole is usually successful, although only vancomycin is approved for this indication. A recent Cochrane review concluded that no single antibiotic was superior in symptomatic or bacteriologic outcomes for unselected patients (**Table 188-4**). However, a more recent randomized, controlled trial of 172 patients found that vancomycin and metronidazole had equivalent cure rates in low-risk patients, but that vancomycin had higher cure rates in high-risk patients (Table 188-4). If intravenous therapy is required, metronidazole is more effective than vancomycin. Treatment should be continued for at least 14 days (or at least 10 days after the symptoms have abated).

There are few antibiotic therapies available other than vancomycin and metronidazole. In a recent Cochrane review, vancomycin and metronidazole were compared to several other agents, including teicoplanin, fusidic acid, bacitracin, rifaximin, and nitazoxanide. None of the comparisons showed a significant advantage or disadvantage, other than bacitracin appeared inferior to vancomycin for initial bacteriologic response, and teicoplanin, which is not currently available in the United States, appeared superior to vancomycin for initial bacteriologic response and cure (**Table 188-5**).

There is some evidence that adding probiotics to standard antibiotic regimens may enhance treatment of CDAD. One study found that adding the probiotic *Saccharomyces boulardii* to a standard antibiotic regimen improved symptoms and reduced the risk of recurrence compared to placebo (Table 188-4). However, these over-the-counter preparations are not regulated, and there have been case reports of fungemia in elderly and debilitated patients. Therefore, they cannot be recommended for routine use in all CDAD cases but may be appropriate for immunocompetent patients at high risk of recurrence.

Few data exist to support other therapies. The toxin binder tolevamer appeared to be equivalent to vancomycin in phase 2 studies but failed to reach noninferiority to vancomycin or metronidazole in a phase 3 study. Therapies studied in uncontrolled settings or case series include intravenous immunoglobulin, stool transplantation, vancomycin enemas, and anion binding resins, none of which can be recommended for routine use. Active and passive immunization is being studied but is not ready for clinical use.

In patients with refractory or fulminant disease unresponsive to metronidazole or vancomycin, second-line therapies should be considered, including vancomycin enemas (especially for patients with ileus), intravenous immunoglobulin, tigecycline, or subtotal colectomy.

RECURRENCE

Recurrence of CDAD occurs in about 20% of patients. Relapses probably result from persistent colonization with *C difficile* spores, which revert to toxin-producing forms after antibiotics are stopped, and not antibiotic resistance. Recurrences usually present within 5 days of cessation of treatment but can be delayed up to a month later. Risk factors include the number of prior episodes, resumption or continuation of antibiotics, poor antibody response, female gender, and diverticular disease. If the patient has more than one recurrence, the chance of another is more than 60%. Noncompliance and other causes of diarrhea should also be considered as possible explanations for continued symptoms.

The first recurrence should receive the same treatment as the first occurrence. Multiple recurrences usually require additional treatment. Tapering or pulsed antibiotics are frequently utilized. One small study used a tapering vancomycin regimen over the course of 6 weeks. The regimen started with vancomycin four times daily for a week, then twice daily for a week, then daily for a week, then every second day for a week, then every third day for 2 weeks. Of the 22 patients treated in this study, all were disease free at 6 months. Oral rifaximin (for 14 days following traditional treatment) has also been effective in reducing subsequent recurrences in uncontrolled trials.

TABLE 188-5 Randomized, Controlled Trials of Treatment for Primary CDAD

Comparison	Symptomatic Initial Response	Symptomatic Cure	Symptomatic Recurrence	Bacteriologic Initial Response	Bacteriologic Cure	Bacteriologic Recurrence
Vancomycin versus flagyl	=*	=	=	=	=	=
Bacitracin versus vancomycin	=	=	=	Inferior (RR 0.57 CI 0.35–0.94)	NA	NA
Teicoplanin versus vancomycin	=	=	=	Superior (RR 1.43 CI 1.14–1.81)	Superior (RR 1.82, CI 1.19–2.78)	=
Teicoplanin versus metronidazole	=	=	=	=	=	NA
Fusidic Acid versus vancomycin	=	=	=	=	=	=
Fusidic Acid versus metronidazole	=	=	=	=	=	NA
Rifamixin versus vancomycin	=	NA	NA	=	NA	NA
Nitazoxanide versus metronidazole	=	NA	=	NA	NA	NA
Metronidazole versus metronidazole + rifampin	=	NA	=	NA	NA	NA

*Equivalent response.
NA, outcome not available.

PREVENTION

Preventing primary or recurrent CDAD is of paramount importance, but there is little evidence that lactobacilli or other agents are effective in primary or secondary prevention. There is also no evidence that routine use of vancomycin or metronidazole in patients starting antibiotics for other conditions reduces the incidence of CDAD.

COMPLICATIONS

Refractory or fulminant CDAD develops in some patients, leading to systemic inflammatory response (characterized by leukocytosis, hypotension, anasarca, and renal failure). The most devastating complication of CDAD is toxic megacolon. In this condition the large bowel becomes massively dilated (>7 cm) with characteristic thumbprinting due to submucosal edema. These patients are at high risk of perforation and need surgical consultation to be assessed for emergent colectomy. Mortality is high, approximately 50%. Unfortunately, atypical presentations of toxic megacolon are not unusual. In one study of patients requiring colectomy, 20% had a negative *C difficile* antigen test, and almost 40% had no diarrhea. Therefore, CDAD should be entertained in any patient with colonic dilation.

DISCHARGE PLANNING

Patients can be discharged as soon as they are clinically stable (able to eat, walk, and toilet). Transitional care provisions may be needed in those unable to perform these elements of self-care. Continued infection control practices (contact isolation and hand hygiene) need to remain in effect wherever the patient is being discharged; it can be presumed that patients remain infectious (toxin-shedding) for the duration of the diarrhea. Discharge planning should ensure the completion of the full course of antibiotics prescribed, with contingency planning if the diarrhea recurs or worsens after discharge.

SYSTEMS IMPROVEMENT

Four major areas of system improvement can decrease the hospital prevalence of *C difficile*.

1. **Antibiotic stewardship.** Several studies have shown that antibiotic restrictions can decrease rates of *C difficile* infection. This should be part of a systemwide attempt to reduce unnecessary antibiotics by the use of automatic stop days and restricted formularies.
2. **Early diagnosis and isolation.** Early diagnosis, treatment, and immediate contact isolation of patients are essential in curbing the nosocomial acquisition of *C difficile*. Rapid turnaround time of diagnostic testing is essential, and immediate provider notification of positive tests should be built within the laboratory notification system. Systematic, reproducible protocols should exist for initiating contact precautions as soon as a *C difficile* test is ordered.
3. **Hand hygiene.** Hand washing is essential; *C difficile* spores are environmentally hardy and resistant to alcohol-based hand rubs. A hand hygiene program with active surveillance and provider feedback should be part of a systemwide attempt to reduce all hospital-acquired infections, including *C difficile*.
4. **Environment.** Appropriate environmental cleaning and environmental surveillance are crucial, to ensure patient and workplace areas are not contaminated.

SUGGESTED READINGS

Dubberke ER, Gerding DN, Classen D, et al. Strategies to prevent *Clostridium difficile* infections in acute care hospitals. *Infect Control Hosp Epidemiol*. 2008;29(suppl 1):S81–S92.

Kelly CP. A 76-year-old man with recurrent *Clostridium difficile*–associated diarrhea: review of *C. difficile* infection. *JAMA*. 2009;301:954–962.

Kelly CP, LaMont JT. Clostridium difficile–more difficult than ever. *N Engl J Med*. 2008;359:1932–1940.

Monaghan T, Boswell T, Mahida YR. Recent advances in *Clostridium difficile*-associated disease. *Gut*. 2008;57:850–860.

CHAPTER 189

Community-Acquired Pneumonia

Daniel M. Musher, MD

Key Clinical Questions

1. How is pneumonia diagnosed?
2. How should the decision be made to hospitalize the patient?
3. What are the major infectious causes of community-acquired pneumonia?
4. What empiric antibiotic therapies are appropriate in community-acquired pneumonia?
5. What steps should be taken for patients not responding to usual therapy for community-acquired pneumonia?

INTRODUCTION

Almost a million episodes of community-acquired pneumonia (CAP) occur each year in the United States in patients over the age of 65 years. While most clinicians are familiar with CAP, its diagnosis remains imprecise, its microbiology is often elusive, and management is usually empiric. Pneumonia is defined as a lung infection, characterized by cough, fever, and a pulmonary infiltrate, often with sputum production. If this sounds obvious, the reader is too easily deceived. Patients with pneumonia may not cough, a variable proportion have sputum, elderly patients are usually afebrile when first evaluated, and infiltrates may be hard to detect, especially in high-risk adults with chronic lung disease, the obese, or those for whom only a portable chest radiograph is available.

To complicate matters, many noninfectious illnesses are also characterized by cough, fever, and pulmonary infiltrates. Some of these are even called pneumonia, such as cryptogenic organizing pneumonia, sarcoid pneumonia, and lupus pneumonitis, and they may in every way mimic pneumonia as already defined. Taken together, all these infectious and noninfectious conditions cause what could be called a pneumonia syndrome. The more experienced recognizes the diverse etiologies of the pneumonia syndrome and should be unhappy about pigeonholing a patient under the rubric of CAP without considering other etiologies.

PATHOGENESIS

NORMAL HOST DEFENSES

An array of host factors protects the lower respiratory tract against inhaled or aspirated organisms. The predisposition to pneumonia increases to the extent that these factors are altered or bypassed.

The configuration of the upper airways ensures that a thin, laminar flow of air passes close to hairs and sticky surfaces that can trap potentially infectious particles. Secretory immunoglobulin A (IgA), which constitutes 10% of the protein in nasal secretions, neutralizes viruses. These and other immunoglobulins appear to prevent bacterial colonization, probably by blocking binding sites on bacterial surfaces. Closure of the epiglottis prevents food particles from passing into the trachea during swallowing. The larynx prevents the passage of secretions into the trachea and allows the generation of intrapulmonic pressure needed for an effective cough. When particles bypass these mechanisms, ciliary action of epithelial cells moves them steadily upward toward the larynx; the cough reflex propels them more rapidly in the same direction. Tracheobronchial secretions maintain moist surfaces, and pulmonary surfactant probably helps to prevent atelectasis, which might interfere with clearance distally.

When infective agents bypass these mechanisms and reach the alveoli, several innate (nonspecific) and specific defenses come into play. Cells that line the respiratory tract produce substances that kill microorganisms or opsonize them for phagocytosis, including lysozyme, lactoferrin, beta-defensins, and surfactant. Bacterial cell wall components, such as lipopolysaccharide in gram-negative and peptidoglycan in gram-positive bacteria, activate the alternative complement cascade, leading to opsonization and killing of bacteria. They also upregulate toll-like receptors, with subsequent enhancement of humoral and cellular immune mechanisms. Antibodies to bacterial cell wall components greatly enhance the host defense response;

serotype-specific antibodies are especially important in host defenses against the pneumococcus.

One way of putting these defense mechanisms into perspective is to consider animal models of infection. Some strains of *Streptococcus pneumoniae* are lethal if a few viable organisms are injected into the peritoneal cavity, but in order to produce infection by inhalation, an inoculum of 10^3 or 10^4 colony-forming units may be required. Other microorganisms resist all defense mechanisms. For example, a single inhaled *Mycobacterium tuberculosis* organism that lodges in the alveoli establishes infection in guinea pigs and is thought to do the same in humans.

RISK FACTORS FOR PNEUMONIA

Extremes of age may be the most important risk factor for pneumonia (**Table 189-1**).

Pneumonia is most common among children under the age of 2 and the elderly. Not only is bacterial pneumonia, exemplified by pneumococcal infection, more common in the elderly, it is also more severe, with the risk of death rising steadily through adulthood (**Figure 189-1**).

Factors predisposing the elderly to pneumonia include diminished gag and cough reflexes, poor glottal function, diminished toll-like receptor responses, and less robust antibody responses. Pneumococcal pneumonia generally does not affect perfectly healthy young adults. Most adults with pneumonia have one or more predisposing underlying conditions. Even when outbreaks of pneumococcal pneumonia occur among presumably healthy adults, as in military camps, concurrent viral infection, exhaustion, and emotional stress are all thought to play a contributory role. In contrast, viral pneumonia occurs when organisms are transmitted to immunologically naïve hosts, with the presence or absence of humoral antibody as the principal determinant of immunity, rather than age.

TABLE 189-1 Conditions Predisposing to (Bacterial) Pneumonia

A. Multifactorial: extremes of life, prior hospitalization, malnutrition, alcoholism
B. Decreased pulmonary clearance
   1. Chronic lung disease
   2. Cigarette smoking
   3. Alcohol, opiates
   4. Viral respiratory infection
   5. Pollution
C. Diminished neutrophil function (chemotaxis, ingestion, or killing)
   1. Diabetes mellitus
   2. Corticosteroids
   3. Renal insufficiency
   4. Cirrhosis
   5. Alcohol
   6. Genetic defects of neutrophil function
D. Defective IgG production
   1. Congenital
   2. Acquired: myeloma, lymphoma, common variable immunodeficiency
   3. HIV infection

Data from Fine MJ, Auble TE, Yealy DM, et al. A prediction rule to identify low-risk patients with community-acquired pneumonia. *N Engl J Med.* 1997;336:243–250.

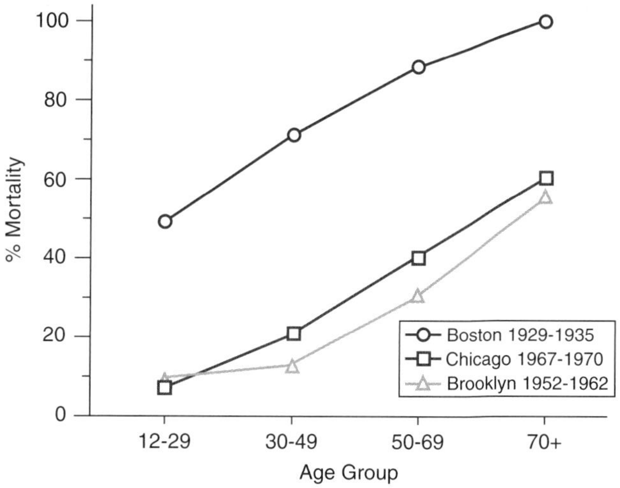

Figure 189-1 *Pneumonia mortality, although much lower than in the preantibiotic era, still rises with age. (Adapted, with permission, from Musher DM. In: Mandell GL, Bennett JE, Dolin R, eds. Principles and Practice of Infectious Diseases, 6th ed. Philadelphia, PA. Elsevier. 2004:2392–2411.)*

HOST RESPONSE

In bacterial pneumonia, the host inflammatory response causes most of the disease manifestations. The presence of bacteria and the accumulation of inflammatory cells and cytokines initiate a vicious cycle in which additional inflammatory cells are attracted and further cytokine release is stimulated. These substances cause capillary leakage with exudation of plasma into the alveoli, leading to a progressive inflammatory exudate that is detected radiologically as pneumonia.

Microorganisms other than bacteria cause pneumonia by other means. Influenza virus directly invades columnar epithelium cells, resulting in pathologic changes that range from vacuolization of some respiratory epithelial cells to desquamation of the entire epithelial layer. These changes are diffuse, leading to an interstitial pattern on chest radiograph. They also predispose to secondary bacterial invasion, which is thought to have caused the staggering death rate during the influenza outbreak of 1918–1919. *Chlamydophila pneumoniae* adheres to specific receptors and replicates within cells, producing microcolonies that stimulate an inflammatory response upon release, with a resulting focal pneumonia. Mycoplasmas also damage respiratory epithelial cells. Rather than invading cells, they adhere to the cell surface, impairing ciliary activity and generating toxic substances. Secondary bacterial pneumonia is uncommon, perhaps because mycoplasmas do not adversely affect phagocytic cells as influenza viruses do. Fungal and mycobacterial pneumonia are dealt with elsewhere in this volume.

ETIOLOGY

If pneumonia is defined as an acute or subacute condition characterized by a pulmonary infiltrate accompanied by systemic symptoms, fever, and cough, the list of possible causes is great (**Table 189-2**).

The prudent physician should give at least brief consideration to other causes before concluding that a "typical" case of CAP merits treatment with "recommended empiric" therapy.

Streptococcus pneumoniae remains the most common cause of pneumonia leading to hospitalization, causing 50–60% of cases, down somewhat from years before widespread use of the conjugate pneumococcal vaccine in infants and toddlers. Literature

TABLE 189-2 Causes of a Syndrome of Pneumonia Leading to Hospital Admission at a Large, Tertiary Care, Veterans Hospital (See Text)*

Common	Less Common	Uncommon
Streptococcus pneumoniae	*Staphylococcus aureus*	RSV,[†] adenovirus
	Influenza virus	*Nocardia*
Haemophilus influenzae	Pulmonary infarction	*Legionella*[§]
Lung cancer	*Pseudomonas*	*Chlamydophila*
Mycobacterium tuberculosis	*Klebsiella*	*Mycoplasma*
	Pulmonary edema	Anaerobic bacteria
Moraxella catarrhalis	Non-TB mycobacteria	Cryptogenic organizing pneumonia, eosinophilic pneumonia, and other noninfectious pneumonias
Pneumocystis jiroveci[¶]	*Histoplasma*	
	Cryptococcus	
		Sarcoidosis
		Kaposi sarcoma[¶]
		Q fever**
		*Coccidioides***

*From the author's long experience at the Houston Veterans Affairs Medical Center.

[†]RSV, respiratory syncytial virus; testing has not been available at this medical center for human metapneumovirus.

[§]Uncommon in Houston, Texas.

[¶]At high risk for concurrent HIV infection.

**Not endemic in Houston, Texas.

claiming that pneumococcus causes a far smaller percentage of cases is often derived from case series in which good specimens for bacterial culture were not regularly obtained, but viral cultures (which can be done from nasopharyngeal swabs) and serologic studies were done on most or all patients. Among other bacterial causes, *Haemophilus influenzae* and *Moraxella catarrhalis* are the next most common but generally cause pneumonia only in persons who have preexisting lung disease. *Staphylococcus aureus* pneumonia presents either as a segmental or lobar pneumonia or as a multiple, small cavitating emboli secondary to an intravascular infection. *Pseudomonas aeruginosa* and other gram-negative rods cause pneumonia in persons with extensive chronic lung disease or treatment with corticosteroids, as well as in immunocompromised hosts, patients with cystic fibrosis, and infrequently in severe alcoholics.

Evidence for viral infection is found in about 15% of adults hospitalized for CAP, of whom about one-half also have bacterial infection. As patients with influenza pneumonia might benefit from antiviral treatment, even if initiated >48 hours after the onset of symptoms, clinicians should consider diagnostic testing for influenza in the presence of suggestive features, such as prominent muscle aches, headache, a dry cough, and high community influenza activity. Respiratory syncytial virus and human metapneumovirus are the next most common viruses causing hospitalization for pneumonia but are currently untreatable. Although *Mycoplasma* and *Chlamydophila pneumoniae* may be common in the ambulatory setting, this author regards them as infrequent causes of pneumonia leading to hospitalization. The current literature, based entirely on serologic studies, overemphasizes their importance. Serologic diagnosis of *Chlamydophila* infection is proven to be unreliable, and diagnosis has only rarely been based on simultaneous study of paired acute and convalescent serum in the same laboratory.

Epidemiologic clues may suggest specific etiologies of a pneumonia syndrome. *Coccidioides immitis*, found in arid regions of the Americas, or *Histoplasma capsulatum*, found worldwide but especially in river basins of North America, cause a variable proportion of CAP in endemic regions. Exposure to livestock or late summer residence in a hot and dry ranching area suggests *Coxiella burnetii* (Q fever), especially if severe headache and abnormal liver enzymes are associated. Exposure to sick birds raises concern for *Chlamydia psittaci*. Prolonged cough, low-grade fever, and a pulmonary infiltrate in a parent whose children have similar symptoms suggests *Mycoplasma* or adenovirus. *Mycobacterium avium*, a well-known cause of pneumonia in patients with bronchiectasis or extensive lung scarring, has increasingly been recognized as a cause of chronic pneumonia in thin but otherwise healthy postmenopausal women. Tuberculosis should be suspected in persons from endemic areas, the immunocompromised, and those who have served time in prison or been homeless. Patients with AIDS are prone to opportunistic infection with *Pneumocystis*, *Histoplasma*, *Mycobacterium avium*, or *Cryptococcus*, which tend to present with interstitial infiltrates. They are also highly susceptible to pneumococcal disease; the age-related incidence of pneumococcal pneumonia may be increased 50- to 100-fold in young adults with HIV infection. For this reason, patients with CAP should be asked about HIV risk factors and screened if appropriate.

CLINICAL PRESENTATION

In younger patients with pneumonia, acute severe malaise and subjective fever are common, often with chills, cough, and sputum production, or at least a sensation of needing to produce sputum. When sputum is produced, it may be flecked with blood. Middle-aged men with underlying lung disease nearly always have increased sputum production. Elderly subjects tend to have much less prominent symptoms; they produce lower levels of cytokines and may respond to them less vigorously than younger adults. A common presentation of pneumonia in older adults is that they are less communicative than usual, or "not acting themselves." Much has been made of the "classical" presenting symptoms of pneumonia, as described by Osler: the sudden onset of rigors, followed by high fever, cough, pleuritic chest pain, and production of tenacious blood-tinged sputum. This presentation is uncommon today, perhaps because the incidence of CAP in otherwise healthy adults is much lower now than in the preantibiotic era. Diarrhea is common in Legionnaires disease, but it is also frequent in pneumococcal pneumonia, probably as a nonspecific gastrointestinal response to circulating cytokines. Fever, cough, and sputum production without an infiltrate are referred to as acute purulent tracheobronchitis. In those without chronic lung disease, such an illness is generally viral; in a patient who does have such chronic disease, bacterial superinfection, for example, with *Haemophilus influenzae*, may be responsible. Persistent cough of several weeks' duration without fever or sputum suggests pertussis or a postviral infection syndrome, for example, due to adenovirus. Several prediction rules for pneumonia exist, but they all have shortcomings and cannot be allowed to replace clinical judgment.

PHYSICAL EXAMINATION

Younger patients with bacterial or influenza pneumonia appear acutely ill. In contrast, elderly and frail persons may simply seem listless. Young patients nearly always have fever and cough, often with chest pain, whereas these symptoms are often absent in the elderly. Younger adults with viral, *Mycoplasma*, or *Chlamydophila* pneumonia generally do not look as acutely ill, and those with tuberculosis or other more chronic forms of pneumonia may appear chronically ill or may look relatively well. Vital signs are of great prognostic importance. Physicians should personally determine the respiratory rate and pay close attention to elevated pulse and respiratory rate or low blood pressure.

In bacterial pneumonia, crackles and increased tactile fremitus are generally present over the affected area. Dullness to percussion is detectable in about one-half of cases. Bronchial breath sounds and egophony strongly suggest pneumonia when present but are not sensitive for diagnosis. The failure to detect excursion of the diaphragm by percussion suggests that an effusion is present. Unfortunately, the overall sensitivity of the physical examination for pneumonia is fairly low, and pneumonia is usually diagnosed not by physical findings but by chest radiograph, with the absence of an infiltrate on a high-quality chest radiograph with posteroanterior and lateral views excluding the diagnosis.

RADIOGRAPHIC FINDINGS

In most cases, the radiographic appearance of a pulmonary infiltrate provides only limited insight into the etiology. Dense consolidation of a segment or lobe is usually bacterial; when due to pneumococcus, such an infiltrate tends to be associated with bacteremia (**Figure 189-2**).

When *Staphylococcus aureus* causes pneumonia via aspiration or inhalation, infiltrates resemble those caused by any other bacterial pneumonia. When hematogenous, as with endocarditis or an infected intravascular source, staphylococcal pneumonia presents with one or more round lesions, 2–3 cm in diameter, which are likely to cavitate (**Figures 189-3A**, **B**).

Subsegmental or "patchy" pneumonia may be due to bacteria, viruses, *Mycoplasma*, and *Chlamydophila*. Patchy involvement of multiple areas suggests a nonbacterial cause (**Figure 189-4**).

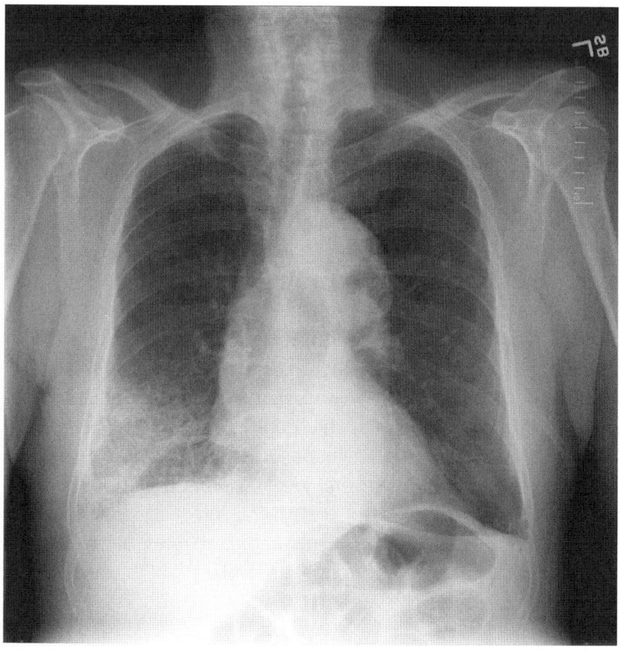

Figure 189-2 *Pneumococcal lobar pneumonia. A 78-year-old man with chronic lung disease had subjective fever, right-sided pleuritic chest pain, and greatly increased shortness of breath for 2 days. He was afebrile, and his WBC count was 10,600 with 40% band forms. Blood cultures were positive for Streptococcus pneumoniae. A sputum submitted for culture more than 24 hours after antibiotics were begun yielded no pneumococci.*

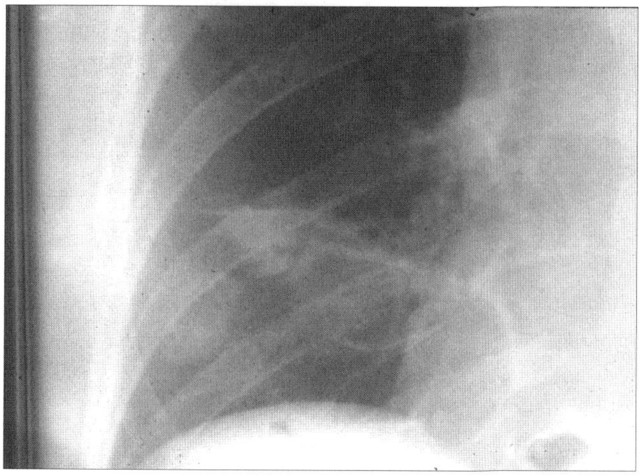

A

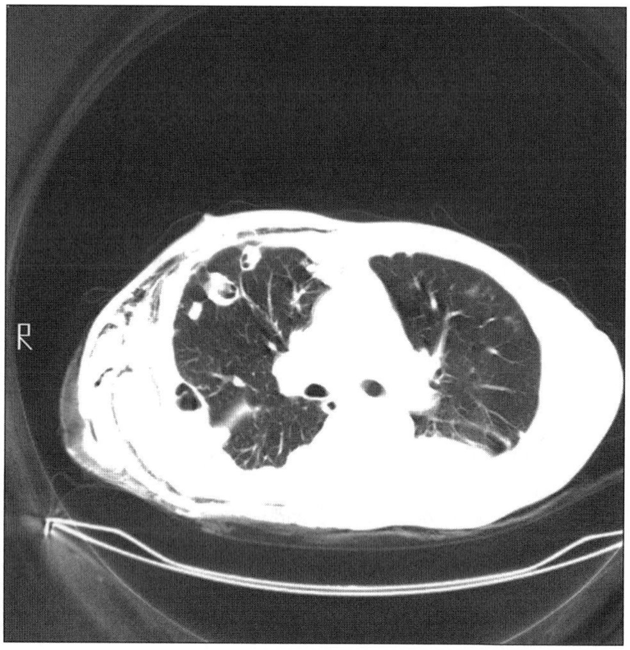

B

Figures 189-3A, B *Hematogenous Staphylococcus aureus pneumonia. A 47-year-old drug user who presented with 3 days of fever and chest pain and was found to have S aureus endocarditis. Chest radiographs showed characteristic round lesions with cavitation, confirmed by computed tomographic scan.*

Pneumocystis causes a diffuse interstitial infiltrate that may be mistaken for prominent pulmonary markings in the earlier clinical stages. Mixed anaerobic, microaerophilic, and facultative organisms may cause a lung abscess with a thick wall, a fluid level, and surrounding consolidation (**Figure 189-5**); the superior segments of a lower lobe (right more commonly than left) are the most likely places for these to appear.

Cavitary lesions of the upper lobes without a fluid level, especially if confined to the posterior segment, suggests tuberculosis. Occasionally, more acute presentations of tuberculosis may mimic CAP (**Figure 189-6**).

In one of several presentations for *Aspergillus* pneumonia, organisms grow as a mass within a cavity, causing the distinctive appearance of an intracavitary mycetoma (fungus ball) surrounded by an arc or halo of air (crescent sign).

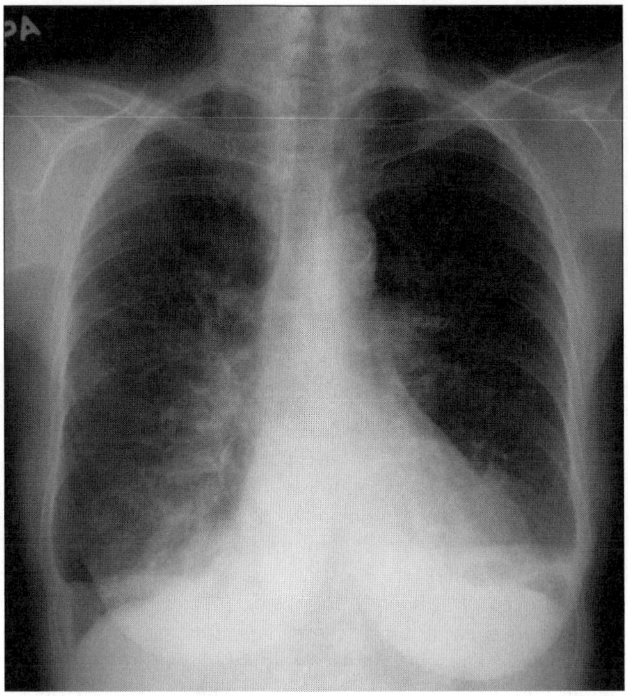

Figure 189-4 *Patient with pneumonia proven to be due to human metapneumovirus; chest radiograph shows patchy involvement of right and left lower lobes. (Courtesy of Dr. Thomas J. Marrie.)*

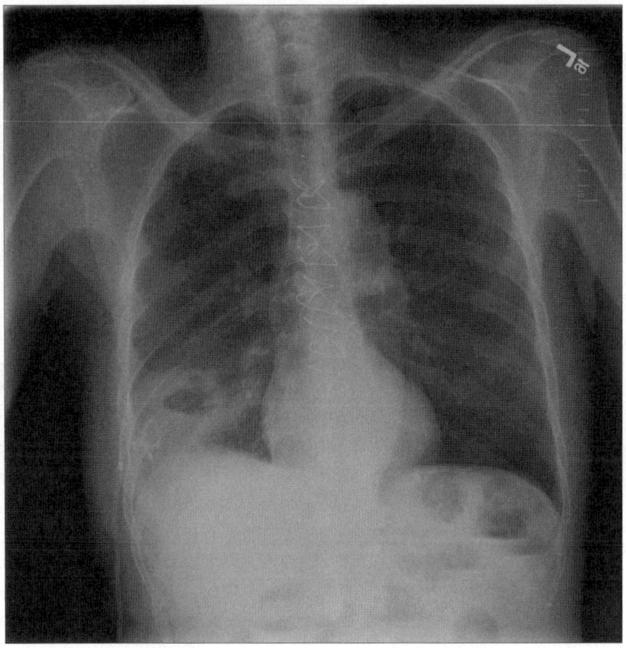

Figure 189-5 *Typical lung abscess due to aspiration of anaerobic and microaerophilic mouth organisms, generally occurring in patients with poor dentition, malnutrition, excess alcohol ingestion, and cigarette smoking.*

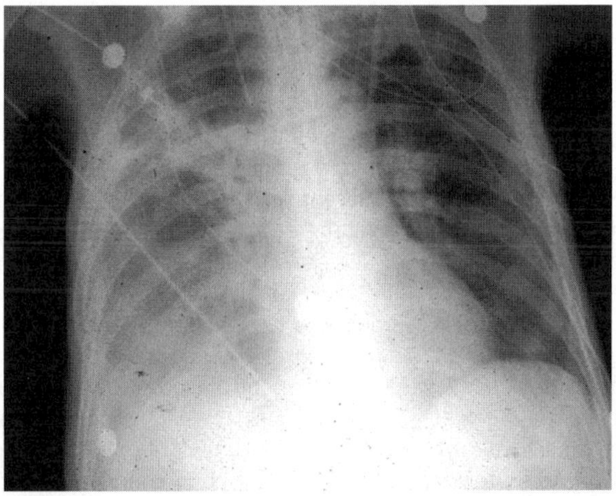

A

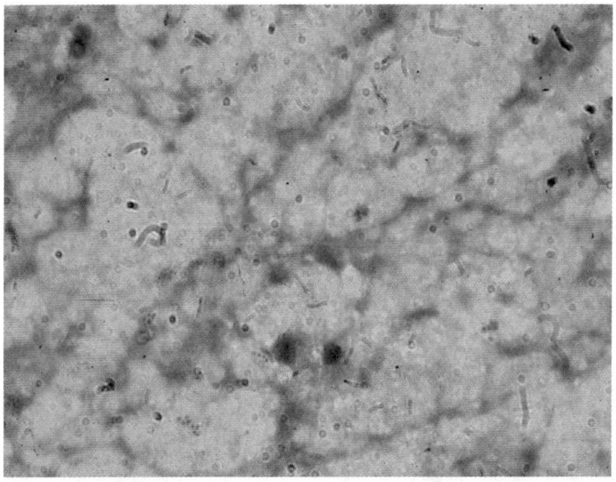

C

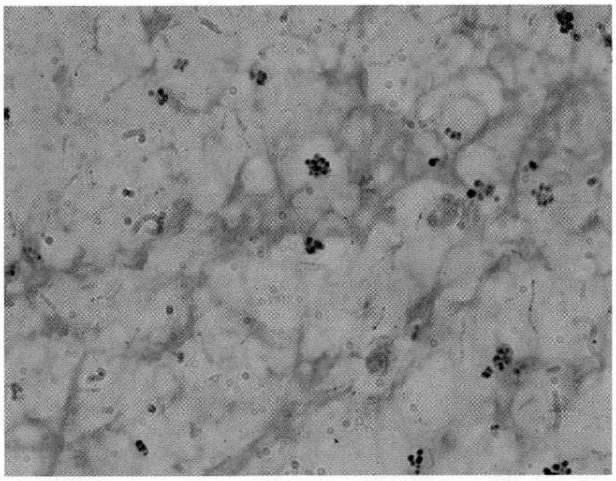

B

Figure 189-6 *(A) This homeless man was admitted to a general medical service with a diagnosis of "community-acquired pneumonia" and begun on ceftriaxone and azithromycin. No sputum sample was obtained. Blood cultures drawn on admission were negative. The patient rapidly deteriorated and was transferred to intensive care where he was intubated. (B) Microscopic examination of Gram-stained tracheal secretions showed proteinaceous material with many staphylococci and almost no white blood cells, indicating an overwhelming pneumonia. (C) Also visible on the Gram stain are faint, beaded gram indeterminate rods; acid fast stain was strongly positive for mycobacteria. The patient died, perhaps due in part to delay in diagnosis; many medical personnel were exposed to tuberculosis, which was certainly due to delay in diagnosis.*

Pneumonia of any cause, especially when rapidly progressive, may cause diffuse pulmonary infiltrates consistent with the acute respiratory distress syndrome. Although it is sometimes said that infiltrates progress after hospitalization because of correction of dehydration, animal studies suggest that the commonly observed progression of infiltrates likely reflects the ongoing inflammatory response and is not related to fluid replacement.

Chest computed tomography may help clarify the nature of an infiltrate and determine if an effusion or mass is present, but it is usually not necessary at hospital admission for patients in whom a good-quality chest radiograph can be obtained.

LABORATORY FINDINGS

Most patients with bacterial pneumonia have a white blood cell (WBC) count greater than 12,000/mm^3. In one-quarter of cases, the WBC count is within normal limits, although this should not be interpreted as reassuring. A low WBC count, for example ≤6,000/mm^3, may be seen in overwhelming infection; in patients with pneumococcal pneumonia, this finding is associated with >65% mortality. Thrombocytopenia also indicates serious infection. A serum sodium <130 mEq/L, an elevated blood urea nitrogen (BUN), or a serum glucose >250 mg/dL (13.9 mmol/L) in a nondiabetic patient is also associated with a poor prognosis. Serum bilirubin may be mildly increased, and lactate dehydrogenase (LDH) and liver transaminases may be slightly elevated. Marked elevations of LDH are seen in *Pneumocystis* and *Histoplasma* pneumonia in AIDS patients.

MICROBIOLOGIC DIAGNOSIS

The respiratory tract clears inflammatory exudate by the ciliary action of the bronchi and trachea, together with cough. Sputum is made up of this exudate, with a greater or lesser admixture of saliva. Ideally, microscopic examination of a Gram-stained sputum specimen should identify areas with inflammatory cells and few or no epithelial cells; such a sample should be a reliable indicator of the microbial flora in the infiltrate. The presence of large numbers of a single type of bacterium in an inflammatory specimen strongly suggests this organism as the etiologic agent of the pneumonia (**Figure 189-7**).

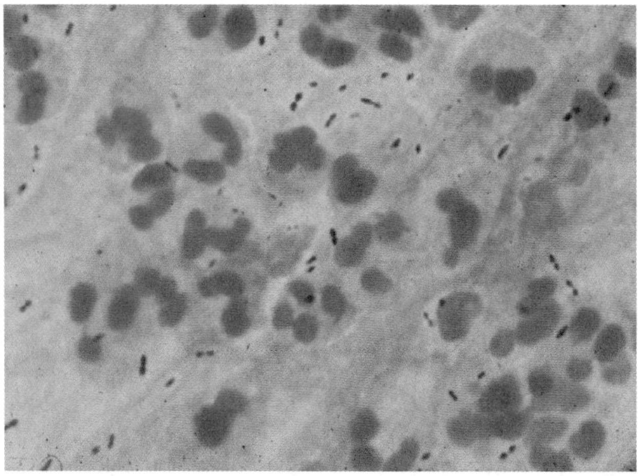

Figure 189-7 *Gram stain of sputum from a patient with pneumococcal pneumonia showing large numbers of polymorphonuclear leukocytes and many lancet-shaped gram-positive cocci with no epithelial cells, indicating that this specimen originated in the lower airways. Such a specimen is diagnostic of pneumococcal pneumonia, although it cannot, of course, exclude coexisting infection by organisms that are not seen by Gram stain, such as influenza virus.*

The absence of visible organisms in an inflammatory specimen suggests certain bacteria that do not accept Gram stain (*Legionella* or *Mycobacteria*), or other organisms such as *Mycoplasma*, *Chlamydophila*, and viruses.

Reports of the poor sensitivity of sputum to detect bacteria largely reflect the inclusion of patients who do not provide a specimen, as well as those who provide inadequate specimens or have already been treated with antibiotics. In patients with proven pneumococcal pneumonia who provide sputum that is judged to be good quality by the laboratory and who have not received antibiotics, the Gram stain is about 90% sensitive in detecting pneumococci. *Haemophilus*, *Moraxella*, and gram-negative rods are even more distinctive in their microscopic appearance. Clinicians are urged to pay more attention to Gram stain results than they have traditionally: the report of *Staphylococcus aureus* or gram-negative rods by culture when they have not been seen microscopically in a good-quality sputum suggests that these are contaminating mouth flora, perhaps explaining the overemphasis in the medical literature on gram-negative organisms as a cause of CAP.

Bacterial cultures in most laboratories will readily yield pneumococcus, *Haemophilus*, *Moraxella*, *Staphylococcus aureus*, or gram-negative bacilli when these organisms cause pneumonia. Preliminary results are likely to be available after 12–16 hours of culture, and laboratory technologists are generally happy to discuss cases with clinicians and give early results by telephone. Cultures for *Mycobacteria* and fungi take much longer.

Additional techniques are available to establish etiologic diagnoses in pneumonia. An enzyme-linked immunosorbent assay (ELISA) detects pneumococcal cell wall polysaccharide in the urine of up to 75% of patients with bacteremic pneumococcal pneumonia, and a smaller proportion of those with nonbacteremic disease. An ELISA for urinary *Legionella* antigen detects only the most common *Legionella* serotype but is positive in about 70% of cases, with greatest sensitivity in more severe disease. *Histoplasma* urine and *Cryptococcus* serum antigen tests are positive in patients with disseminated disease but less likely so in those with discrete pulmonary infiltrates.

The largest advance in recent years has been in real-time polymerase chain reaction (PCR). This can now be performed directly on sputum to detect *M tuberculosis*, or on nasal secretions to detect most respiratory viruses. Sensitivity and specificity are very high compared to culture results. PCR is not used to detect bacteria in sputum because, unlike *M tuberculosis* or respiratory viruses, most of the bacteria that cause pneumonia may also colonize the upper airways in normal adults, so a highly sensitive technique may detect colonization rather than infection. PCR for influenza virus is currently the gold standard for diagnosis. By comparison, viral culture is positive in 90–95% of cases and rapid influenza tests in 30–70%. PCR also detects respiratory syncytial virus (RSV), parainfluenza virus, and human metapneumovirus.

In the preantibiotic era, blood cultures yielded *S pneumoniae* in 20% of adult patients hospitalized for pneumococcal pneumonia. At present, blood cultures are positive in about 50% of patients diagnosed with pneumococcal pneumonia because fewer adequate sputum cultures are obtained, and the diagnosis of pneumococcal infection is more often made on the basis of blood cultures alone. Blood cultures are probably positive in 20–25% of patients with inhalation or aspiration pneumonia due to *S aureus* or gram-negative rods, in a lower proportion of those with pneumonia caused by nontypable *H influenzae*, and only rarely in pneumonia due to *Moraxella catarrhalis*. Patients with hematogenous *S aureus* pneumonia virtually always have positive blood cultures.

DIFFERENTIAL DIAGNOSIS

Many noninfectious conditions mimic pneumonia and also present with pulmonary infiltrates, leukocytosis, and fever; the most important of these are listed in Table 189-2. Lung cancer, pulmonary edema, and pulmonary infarction are the most common.

Patients with lung cancer commonly present with fever and a pulmonary infiltrate; despite the frequent diagnosis of postobstructive pneumonia, it is unclear whether infection is involved, and antibiotics are generally given, often to no avail. Patients who do not respond to the first course of antibiotics may have repeat sputum cultures, which reveal new and different flora; antibiotics selected on this basis are virtually never of benefit, and fever may persist until cancer chemotherapy is begun. Fever may also be due to tumor necrosis in this setting.

Pulmonary embolus with infarction produces pulmonary infiltrates with sputum that contains neutrophils, but few or no bacteria. Pleuritic chest pain may be a prominent clinical feature. Pulmonary edema and acute respiratory distress syndrome are often indistinguishable from pneumonia; establishing the diagnosis is especially problematic in an intensive care setting.

Cryptogenic organizing pneumonia, acute interstitial pneumonia, and other interstitial pneumonias are less common but are noteworthy because they are almost always initially misdiagnosed as CAP. Attention to the patient's history and careful review of earlier chest radiographs may reveal a longer history of symptoms and subtle prior radiologic abnormalities, more consistent with a noninfectious process.

PRACTICE POINT

- Parapneumonic effusions measuring more than 5 cm in height on lateral chest radiographs should be sampled for Gram stain and aerobic and anaerobic cultures to exclude empyema. Delays in thoracentesis for parapneumonic effusions are associated with protracted illness and longer, more costly hospitalizations.

Patients with septic pulmonary emboli should be assessed for other foci of infection, such as an infected heart valve or intravascular device. In acute aspiration of gastric contents, pneumonia results from the presence of acid; antibiotic treatment is not indicated. Pulmonary hemorrhage and vasculitis may also cause pulmonary infiltrates and fever; in vasculitis, these infiltrates may also be associated with cavitary lesions, as in antineutrophil cytoplasmic antibody (ANCA)-associated granulomatous vasculitis.

MANAGEMENT

HOSPITAL ADMISSION

Scoring systems have been designed to help the physician determine whether a patient with pneumonia requires hospitalization. The most widely cited is the Pneumonia Outcomes Research Trial (PORT) score, sometimes called the Pneumonia Severity Index (PSI) (**Tables 189-3** and **189-4**).

PRACTICE POINT

- There is great interest in the development of serum biomarkers for pneumonia, but their current role is not well defined. While high levels of C-reactive protein, procalcitonin, proatrial natriuretic peptide, provasopressin, and proadrenomedullin are predictive of mortality, they may not add to clinical predictive scores such as the Pneumonia Severity Index. There is some evidence that low procalcitonin levels may predict viral, rather than bacterial infection, thus enabling clinicians to withhold antibiotics in selected patients.

TABLE 189-3 Pneumonia Outcomes Research Trial (PORT) Severity Index*

Age (subtract 10 for women)	—
Nursing home	10
Neoplasm (active, not skin)	30
Cirrhosis or chronic hepatitis	20
CHF, CVA, chronic renal disease	10
Altered mental status	20
Respiratory rate > 30	20
Systolic BP < 90	20
Temp < 35 or > 40°C	15
Pulse > 125/min	10
Arterial pH < 7.35	30
BUN > 30 mg/dL (11 mmol/L)	20
Serum sodium < 130	20
Glucose > 250 mg/dL (13.9 mmol/L)	10
Hematocrit < 30	10
pO_2 < 60 or O_2 sat < 90%	10
Pleural effusion	10

BP, blood pressure; BUN, blood urea nitrogen; CHF, congestive heart failure; CVA, cerebrovascular accident.

*Points assigned for each criterion.

Data from Fine MJ, Auble TE, Yealy DM, et al. A prediction rule to identify low-risk patients with community-acquired pneumonia. *N Engl J Med.* 1997;336:243–250.

PRACTICE POINT

- All hospitalized patients with CAP should have sputum sent for Gram stain and culture if an adequate specimen can be obtained. Some authorities no longer recommended blood cultures for every patient with CAP, but such cultures should be obtained on those patients with higher risk of bacteremia, including those with severe pneumonia, cavitary disease, leukopenia, alcoholism, liver disease, functional or anatomic asplenia, or pleural effusion, or patients with positive urinary pneumococcal antigen.

TABLE 189-4 Pneumonia Outcomes Research Trial (PORT) Severity Index: Prognostic Value of the PORT Score

Point Score	Class	CAP*	Mortality VAMC†
≤70	II	<1%	–
71–90	III	3%	3%
91–130	IV	8%	21%
>130	V	29%	35%

CAP, community-acquired pneumonia; VAMC, Veterans Affairs Medical Center.

*Original calculation in patients with community acquired pneumonia report of PORT score.

†Results in patients with proven pneumococcal pneumonia.

Data from Fine MJ, Auble TE, Yealy DM, et al. A prediction rule to identify low-risk patients with community-acquired pneumonia. *N Engl J Med.* 1997;336:243–250.

Data from Musher DM, Alexandraki I, Graviss EA, et al. Bacteremic and nonbacteremic pneumococcal pneumonia: a prospective study. Medicine (Baltimore). 2000;79:210–221.

TABLE 189-5 CURB-65 Scoring System

One point for each of the following:
Confusion
Urea > 19 mg/dL (7 mmol/L)
Respiratory rate > 30
Blood pressure < 90/60 (either systolic or diastolic value)
≥65 years of age

Score of ≥2 indicates need for hospitalization.
Data from Lim WS, van der Eerden MM, Laing R, et al. Defining community acquired pneumonia severity on presentation to hospital: an international derivation and validation study. *Thorax*. 2003;58:377–382.

The CURB-65 score (**Table 189-5**), although easy to calculate, is less sensitive and less specific.

The immediate decision whether to hospitalize must ultimately depend upon physician judgment, but it is strongly recommended that all PORT score factors be considered in reaching a decision; before it was developed, many of these factors, such as the low serum sodium, elevated BUN/creatinine, and elevated blood sugar in a nondiabetic, were not well recognized as indicating a poor prognosis. Because the PORT score is so age dependent, a moderately elevated score in a young adult should be regarded with alarm.

A corollary decision is whether a patient needs admission to an intensive care unit (ICU). The recently described SMART-COP score (**Table 189-6**), based on systolic blood pressure, multilobar involvement, serum albumin level, respiratory rate, tachycardia, confusion, oxygenation, and arterial pH, is more effective than PSI or CURB-65 at predicting which patients will require ICU transfer for intensive respiratory or vasopressor support, being 92% sensitive compared to 74% and 39%, respectively, for the other two scoring systems. Other indicators of overwhelming infection possibly requiring ICU admission include relative leukopenia in bacterial pneumonia (WBC count ≤6000/mm^3), thrombocytopenia, and hypothermia.

TABLE 189-6 SMART-COP Scoring System*

Low systolic blood pressure (2 points)
Multilobar involvement (1 point)
Low albumin (1 point)
High respiratory rate (1 point)
Tachycardia (1 point)
Confusion (1 point)
Poor oxygenation (2 points)
Low arterial pH (2 points)

*In one study, a SMART-COP score of ≥3 points identified 92% of patients who required intensive respiratory and/or vasopressor support and correctly identified 84% of patients who did not need immediate admission to the intensive care unit. In another study, SMART-COP performed better than PSI or CURB-65 but still stratified 15% of patients incorrectly.
Data from Chalmers JD, Singanayagam A, Hill AT. Predicting the need for mechanical ventilation and/or inotropic support for young adults admitted to the hospital with community-acquired pneumonia. *Clin Infect Dis*. 2008;47:1571–1574.

ANTIBIOTIC THERAPY

Fortunately or unfortunately, guidelines have been developed for treatment of community-acquired pneumonia: fortunately, because there is now some evidence-based uniformity in the approach to treating pneumonia; unfortunately, because physicians with little interest in establishing an etiological diagnosis may reflexively adhere to guidelines without considering the full range of possible diagnoses. As a result, patients with noninfectious causes of fever and pulmonary infiltrate may receive inappropriate therapy with antibiotics, delaying correct diagnosis and appropriate treatment.

Guidelines published jointly by the Infectious Disease Society of America and the American Thoracic Society (IDSA/ATS) focus on common infectious causes of pneumonia. The full guidelines document is detailed, listing epidemiologic clues that might raise consideration of less common causes and giving approaches to evaluating and treating them, so physicians who utilize the recommendations are urged first to read the document in its entirety.

Recommended antimicrobial treatment for non-ICU hospitalized patients (**Table 189-7**) includes a respiratory fluoroquinolone (levofloxacin or moxifloxacin, but not ciprofloxacin) or a beta-lactam (cefotaxime, ceftriaxone, ampicillin, or ampicillin/sulbactam) together with a macrolide. The reasoning is that this regimen will treat pneumonia due to pneumococcus, *Haemophilus*, *Moraxella*, *Legionella*, *Mycoplasma*, and *Chlamydophila*, as well as some less common organisms. For ICU patients, a beta-lactam (cefotaxime, ceftriaxone, or ampicillin/sulbactam) should be given, plus either azithromycin or a respiratory fluoroquinolone. When *Pseudomonas* is a consideration, as in patients with gram-negative rods on Gram stain, prior failed antibiotic treatment, bronchiectasis and other structural lung disease, or chronic obstructive pulmonary disease requiring frequent antibiotics or glucocorticoids, patients should receive an antipneumococcal, antipseudomonal beta-lactam (piperacillin/tazobactam, cefepime, imipenem, or meropenem) plus

TABLE 189-7 Recommended Empiric Antimicrobial Treatment for Pneumonia, Hospitalized Patients

Non-ICU patients
Respiratory fluoroquinolone
OR
β-lactam (cefotaxime, ceftriaxone, ampicillin, or ampicillin/sulbactam) plus macrolide
ICU patients
β-lactam (cefotaxime, ceftriaxone, or ampicillin/sulbactam) plus azithromycin OR a respiratory fluoroquinolone
For *Pseudomonas*, antipneumococcal, antipseudomonal β-lactam (piperacillin/tazobactam, cefepime, imipenem, or meropenem) plus a quinolone (ciprofloxacin or levofloxacin)
OR
Antipneumococcal, antipseudomonal β-lactam as above with an aminoglycoside and azithromycin
For methicillin-resistant *Staphylococcus* aureus add vancomycin or linezolid

Data from Mandell LA, Wunderink RG, Anzueto A, et al. Infectious Diseases Society of America/American Thoracic Society consensus guidelines on the management of community-acquired pneumonia in adults. *Clin Infect Dis*. 2007;44 Suppl 2:S27–S72.

a respiratory fluoroquinolone (ciprofloxacin or levofloxacin), or an antipneumococcal, antipseudomonal beta-lactam combined with an aminoglycoside and azithromycin. Unless there is a reason to choose a quinolone instead of a macrolide, the latter should be selected because of strong evidence for a beneficial immunomodulatory effect. If methicillin-resistant *Staphylococcus aureus* (MRSA) is a consideration, as in patients with a Gram stain showing gram-positive cocci in clusters, or clinical risk factors for MRSA, such as injection drug use, chronic renal failure, influenza, or prior antibiotics, vancomycin or linezolid should be added. A newly released cephalosporin, ceftaroline, which is effective against MRSA, may be useful in this setting. Unfortunately, community-acquired MRSA is increasingly common, and patients may not have traditional MRSA risk factors.

Recommendations for empiric therapy are problematic unless they emphasize that therapy should be begun pending definitive determination of an etiologic agent, or as a fallback position if appropriate specimens cannot be obtained. The IDSA/ATS guidelines clearly recommend diagnostic testing in all hospitalized patients to help determine the etiologic agent of the infection. However, in the rush to treat empirically, many physicians tend to overlook this recommendation. In the author's experience, ICU patients who are intubated for pneumonia—thereby providing a ready source for specimen culture—are often begun on treatment with three antibiotics (eg, piperacillin/tazobactam, azithromycin, and vancomycin) *without a specimen being obtained for culture.* Thirty-six hours later, if the patient is deteriorating, the cause is unclear. If the patient has improved, it is unclear which, if any, of these drugs may be discontinued. Often, one or two drugs are arbitrarily stopped in the absence of new evidence, raising questions about the original decision to use them. Alternatively, all three drugs may be given to complete a 7–10 day course of therapy, although they may well not be needed. The administration of such broad spectrum antibiotics to ICU patients with pneumonia, which certainly contributes to the rate of *Clostridium difficile* infection, is especially ironic since pneumococcus remains the most common cause of pneumonia leading to ICU admission, perhaps followed next by viral infection. Treatment for other organisms should be considered, depending upon epidemiologic factors, medical history and index of suspicion, but is best determined by Gram stain and culture of tracheal secretions.

The time lag between arrival in the emergency department (ED) for symptoms of pneumonia and the administration of effective antibiotics has been a subject of controversy. On limited evidence, the Joint Commission, the body responsible for hospital accreditation in the United States, mandated that antibiotics be initiated within 4 hours of arrival in the ED in pneumonia patients. This policy led to possible pneumonia patients being seen before others who might have had more urgent conditions, and also to unnecessary antibiotics being administered to patients who eventually were found not to have pneumonia. The IDSA/ATS committee has dropped the 4-hour rule from its recommendations but now states that antibiotics should be given as soon as possible after the diagnosis of pneumonia is considered likely. Recognizing that long delays may occur during transfer from the ED to a hospital bed, the committee specifically recommended that the first dose of antibiotics be given while the patient is still in the ED.

The optimal duration of therapy for pneumonia is uncertain. In the case of pneumococcal pneumonia, organisms are not readily visible by microscopic examination of sputum or by culture 24 hours after the administration of an effective antibiotic. Experience from early in the antibiotic era showed that 5 to 7 days of therapy sufficed. During the Korean War, a single dose of procaine penicillin, which maintains an effective antimicrobial level for as long as 24 hours, was shown to cure otherwise healthy young adults. Nevertheless, most physicians now treat pneumonia for 10 to 14 days, despite the absence of data for additional benefit. In the author's opinion, 3–5 days of close observation with parenteral therapy for pneumococcal pneumonia and a final few days of oral treatment, in all not exceeding 5 days after the patient has become afebrile (temperature < 37.2°C), may be the best approach. The documentation of pneumococcal bacteremia need not alter this recommendation.

The proper duration of therapy for pneumonia due to other bacteria is even less clear. *Haemophilus* and *Moraxella* pneumonia probably respond similarly and are treated for 7–10 days. In contrast, pneumonia due to *S aureus* or gram-negative bacilli tends to be destructive, and concern that small abscesses have formed in the lung parenchyma might require 10–14 days of treatment. When bacteremia is documented, most authorities will treat *S aureus* pneumonia for 4 weeks. Data purporting to show that ventilator-associated pneumonia can be treated with shorter courses of antibiotics probably speak more to the uncertainty of diagnosis than to the responsiveness of true gram-negative pneumonia to therapy. Relapses of *Legionella* pneumonia have been documented when treatment is discontinued too soon; 5–10 days of treatment with the very long acting azithromycin or 14 days with a fluoroquinolone may be indicated, with 3 weeks recommended in immunocompromised patients.

FAILURE TO RESPOND TO THERAPY

The expected response to therapy includes defervescence, return of the WBC count to normal, and disappearance of the systemic signs of acute infection within 5–7 days after beginning antibiotics; cough and fatigue may persist for weeks. The failure to respond raises a number of concerns (**Table 189-8**).

If the patient simply does not improve, the antibiotic therapy may not be appropriate for the infecting organism. Admitting cultures and antibiotic susceptibilities should be reviewed to ensure that the patient has received an adequate dose of an appropriate antibiotic. The patient may have received appropriate antimicrobial therapy, but there may be a loculated infection, such as empyema, or infection behind an obstruction, such as lung cancer or a foreign body. The diagnosis of bacterial pneumonia may be incorrect; an organism from another class (mycobacterium, fungus) may be responsible, or the cause of the syndrome may be noninfectious. An initial improvement, with a partial clinical response and persistent lower-grade fever and leukocytosis strongly suggests an empyema.

TABLE 189-8 Some Reasons for Failure of Antimicrobial Therapy in Community-Acquired Pneumonia

Inappropriate antibiotic choice or dose
Organism not susceptible
Wrong dosage (eg, morbidly obese patient)
Antibiotic not given
Correct antibiotic but loculated infection
Empyema
Obstruction (eg, lung cancer)
Unidentified causative organism responsible
Non-infectious cause
Malignancy
Inflammatory infiltrate

Additional diagnostic measures that should be considered in patients with an inadequate response to initial therapy include thoracentesis of significant effusions, chest computed tomography (CT), and bronchoscopy with bronchoalveolar lavage and possibly transbronchial biopsy.

DISCHARGE CONSIDERATIONS

Patients may be switched from intravenous to oral therapy with bioavailable agents when they can tolerate oral medications and are hemodynamically stable and improving clinically. Patients may be discharged when they are clinically stable, have no other medical problems requiring continued hospitalization, and have a stable and safe discharge environment. Suggested markers of clinical stability include temperature ≤37.8°C, heart rate ≤100 beats/min, respiratory rate ≤24 breaths/min, systolic blood pressure ≥90 mm Hg, arterial oxygen saturation ≥90% or pO_2 ≥60 mm Hg on room air (for patients not previously dependent on supplemental oxygen), and mental status at baseline. It is traditional to observe patients in the inpatient setting for up to 24 hours after switching from intravenous to oral therapy, but there is no evidence to support this practice, and it is no longer considered necessary for patients who are otherwise clinically stable.

QUALITY IMPROVEMENT

The most recent IDSA guidelines target four key performance indicators for quality improvement, monitoring of guideline adherence, and educational efforts:

1. Empiric antibiotic administration that conforms to guidelines; if administered antibiotics diverge from recommended regimens, the reasons for this should be clearly stated in the medical record.
2. The first antibiotic dose should be given in the emergency room; in the current guidelines, an explicit time frame is not mandated, but the suggested range is within 6–8 hours of presentation.
3. Mortality data for all patients admitted with CAP should be collected, monitored, and compared to severity-specific norms; as well, the proportion of patients with severe CAP that are not admitted to ICUs should also be tracked.
4. The proportion of eligible patients receiving influenza and pneumococcal vaccination should be monitored (see later discussion).

The expected adherence to the key indicators is expected to be in the 80–95% range, except for influenza and pneumococcal vaccination, where adherence is expected to be >90% in patients over the age of 65 years.

PREVENTION

Pneumococcal vaccination is recommended for all patients ≥65 years, and for patients 19–64 years of age with predisposing conditions, including smoking, asthma, chronic lung disease, heart failure, diabetes, alcoholism, cerebrospinal fluid leaks, chronic liver disease, functional or anatomic asplenia, and compromised immunity. For those 19–64 years old who are asplenic or otherwise immunocompromised, a second dose of pneumococcal vaccine is recommended when 5 years have elapsed from the first dose. Patients who received pneumococcal vaccination prior to 65 years of age should receive another dose at or after age 65, provided at least 5 years have passed since the last dose. Multiple revaccinations after age 65 are not currently recommended. Patients over 50 years of age, younger patients with comorbid medical conditions at risk for influenza complications, household contacts of high-risk persons, and all health care workers should receive inactivated influenza vaccine annually. Smoking cessation guidance should be provided to smokers.

SUGGESTED READINGS

Chalmers JD, Singanayagam A, Hill AT. Predicting the need for mechanical ventilation and/or inotropic support for young adults admitted to the hospital with community-acquired pneumonia. *Clin Infect Dis*. 2008;47:1571–1574.

Charles PG, Wolfe R, Whitby M, et al. SMART-COP: a tool for predicting the need for intensive respiratory or vasopressor support in community-acquired pneumonia. *Clin Infect Dis*. 2008;47: 375–384.

Fine MJ, Auble TE, Yealy DM, et al. A prediction rule to identify low-risk patients with community-acquired pneumonia. *N Engl J Med*. 1997;336:243–250.

Johnstone J, Majumdar SR, Fox JD, Marrie TJ. Viral infection in adults hospitalized with community-acquired pneumonia: prevalence, pathogens, and presentation. *Chest*. 2008;134:1141–1148.

Mandell LA, File TM Jr. Short-course treatment of community-acquired pneumonia. *Clin Infect Dis*. 2003;37:761–763.

Mandell LA, Wunderink RG, Anzueto A, et al. Infectious Diseases Society of America/American Thoracic Society consensus guidelines on the management of community-acquired pneumonia in adults. *Clin Infect Dis*. 2007;44(suppl 2):S27–S72.

Musher DM, Alexandraki I, Graviss EA, et al. Bacteremic and nonbacteremic pneumococcal pneumonia: a prospective study. *Medicine* (Baltimore). 2000;79:210–221.

Osler W. Principles and practice of medicine. New York: D. Appleton and Co, 1892:517.

CHAPTER 190

Fever in the Returning Traveler

Serena Koenig, MD, MPH
James H. Maguire, MD, MPH

Key Clinical Questions

1. What infections should be considered?
2. What questions should be asked in the travel history?
3. What diagnostic tests should be conducted?
4. Which patients should be hospitalized?
5. What clinical factors put patients at risk for serious complications?
6. When should an infectious disease physician be consulted?

CASE 190-1

THE GREAT PRETENDER

A middle-aged male was brought in by police to the emergency room of an inner-city hospital with confusion and fever to 104°F, after being found in an incoherent state without identification. Shortly after arrival, his condition deteriorated. He became agitated, hypoxic, and hypotensive and was intubated and transferred to the intensive care unit. A chest radiograph showed diffuse infiltrates. Blood tests were most notable for a hematocrit of 18%, creatinine 2.8 mg/dL, and moderate elevations of liver enzymes. A lumbar puncture was normal. The hematology laboratory technician happened to review the patient's blood smear before going home that evening and made a diagnosis of falciparum malaria with 30% parasitemia. The patient was started urgently on intravenous quinidine and exchange transfusions. He was eventually found to be a Nigerian immigrant who had recently traveled to his native country without taking malaria prophylaxis. After a stormy hospital course complicated by acute respiratory distress syndrome and acute renal failure, he made a full recovery.

Fever in travelers is malaria until proven otherwise. Malaria has been called "the mime" for its ability to simulate a wide variety of other infectious syndromes. Hence, the diagnosis of malaria is often missed or delayed, sometimes with fatal consequences, especially when patients present for care outside of endemic areas. For example, during the Vietnam War, returning soldiers who presented with malaria to civilian hospitals had a 10-fold higher mortality than those who presented to hospitals in the Veterans Administration system, which had much greater familiarity with diagnosing and treating malaria.

INTRODUCTION

International travelers are commonly plagued by medical problems, particularly after travel to a resource-poor setting. About 8% of travelers to developing countries seek medical care while they are away or after they return. Although fever in the traveler may be caused by mild illnesses, it may also be a harbinger of potentially lethal infection. The evaluation of the febrile traveler is complicated by the wide array of possible etiologies. It is critical to consider which infections are endemic to the area visited, potential exposures, the time between exposure and the onset of symptoms, and associated clinical findings. This chapter reviews the common causes of fever in returning travelers and the appropriate initial diagnostic evaluation.

EPIDEMIOLOGY

GeoSentinel, a worldwide network of travel and tropical medicine clinics, provides the largest database for travel-related infections. From 1996 to 2004, the five most common diagnoses for patients with systemic febrile illnesses presenting to GeoSentinel clinics from the developing world were malaria, dengue, mononucleosis due to Epstein-Barr virus or cytomegalovirus, rickettsial infection, and typhoid fever.

In the GeoSentinel database, malaria was the predominant cause of systemic febrile illnesses overall, and it was one of the three top causes from each of the six regions of the developing world. Malaria was the leading cause of systemic febrile illness in travelers returning from Sub-Saharan Africa and Central America. In the United States, more than 50% of cases of imported malaria occurred among immigrant families who had made recent visits to their country of origin. Dengue was the second most likely cause of systemic febrile illnesses overall and the leading cause for fever in travelers to Southeast and South Central Asia, the Caribbean, and South America. Rickettsial infections were an important cause of fever in travelers to Sub-Saharan Africa, and they were often infected with *Rickettsia africae* (African tick-bite fever). Typhoid fever was especially common in travelers to South Central Asia, but it also occurred in travelers to other regions.

In a later GeoSentinel study of returning travelers with fever, 35% presented with a systemic febrile illness, 15% with acute diarrheal disease, and 14% with respiratory symptoms. Among those with systemic febrile illnesses, 59% were diagnosed with malaria, 18% with dengue, 6% with typhoid or paratyphoid fever, and 5% with rickettsial illness. Additional causes of febrile syndromes included mononucleosis syndromes (Epstein-Barr virus, cytomegalovirus, acute HIV infection, or toxoplasmosis), leptospirosis, amebic liver abscess, viral meningitis, and relapsing fever.

Among patients with fever and diarrhea, the most common diagnoses were traveler's diarrhea, *Campylobacter*, nontyphoidal *Salmonella* species, and shigellosis. In those with fever and respiratory symptoms, nearly half were diagnosed with bronchitis or an acute unspecified respiratory infection. Other common diagnoses were bacterial pneumonia, tonsillitis, influenza or an influenza-like illness, and sinusitis.

WHAT INFORMATION SHOULD BE ELICITED FROM THE MEDICAL HISTORY?

It is critical to identify all regions that the traveler has visited in the past year, including layovers or short stops. The Centers for Disease Control and Prevention (CDC) Web site (www.cdc.gov) has a travel site that lists common infections by each country and region, as well as reports on disease outbreaks. The World Health Organization Web site (www.who.int) also has information about disease outbreaks. It is particularly important to identify regions of travel where malaria and dengue are endemic.

It is also necessary to define the dates of travel and the timing of symptom onset, which may permit the estimation of the approximate incubation period. **Table 190-1** lists the incubation periods for several bacteria, viruses, fungi, and parasites that cause fever in returning travelers. Some infections can be excluded based on an incubation period that is inconsistent with the timing of fever. For example, a traveler presenting with a systemic febrile infection three weeks after returning would be very unlikely to have dengue, which nearly always presents within 14 days. The duration of the trip can also be helpful. Malaria is more often reported in long-term (>6 months) than short-term travelers, though 5% of patients with malaria in the GeoSentinel database had traveled for less than one week. Some infections are seasonal, but some seasonal infections (such as influenza) may present at unusual times given that peak seasons may differ in tropical climes.

TABLE 190-1 Infectious Causes of Fever and Associated Incubation Periods in Returning Travelers

Infection	Incubation Period (Range)
Bacteria	
Plague *(Yersinia pestis)*	1 to 6 days
Anthrax *(Bacillus anthracis)*	1 to 7 days
Meningococcemia *(Neisseria meningitidis)*	1 to 14 days
Meliodosis *(Burkholderia pseudomallei)*	1 to 21 days
Shigellosis *(Shigella species)*	2 to 6 days (1 to 20 days)
Campylobacter enteritis *(Camplyobacter jejuni)*	2 to 6 days (1 to 20 days)
Salmonellosis *(Salmonella species)*	2 to 6 days (1 to 20 days)
Yersinia enteritis *(Yersinia enterocolitica)*	4 to 6 days (1 to 14 days)
Legionellosis *(Legionella pneumophila)*	5 to 6 days (2 to 10 days)
Human monocytic ehrlichiosis *(Ehrlichia chaffeensis)*	5 to 15 days
Human granulocytic anaplasmosis *(Anaplasma phagocytophilum)*	5 to 21 days
Leptospirosis *(Leptospira interrogans)*	7 to 12 days (2 to 26 days)
Spotted fever *(Rickettsiae, spotted fever group)*	About 1 week (few days to 2 to 3 weeks)
Lyme disease *(Borrelia burdorferi)*	7 to 10 days (3 to 30 days)
Typhoid and paratyphoid fever *(Salmonella enterica serotype typhi* and *Salmonella paratyphi A, B, or C)*	7 to 18 days (3 to 60 days)
Bartonellosis *(Bartonella species)*	7 to 21 days
Scrub typhus *(Orientia tsutsugamushi)*	10 days (6 to 21 days)
Syphilis *(Treponema pallidum)*	10 to 90 days
Q fever *(Coxiella burnetti)*	14 to 21 days (2 to 29 days)
Brucellosis *(Brucella species)*	2 to 4 weeks (5 days to 5 months)
Tuberculosis *(Mycobacterium tuberculosis)*	Primary: weeks Reactivation: years

(continued)

TABLE 190-1 Infectious Causes of Fever and Associated Incubation Periods in Returning Travelers ***(continued)***

Infection	Incubation Period (Range)
Viruses	
Influenza virus	1 to 3 days
Chikungunya fever virus	3 to 7 days (2 to 12 days)
Viral hemorrhagic fevers (Hantavirus, Lassa fever virus, yellow fever virus, Ebola virus, Marburg virus, Rift Valley fever virus)	3 to 14 days (2 days to 2 months)
Arboviruses (many, such as Japanese encephalitis, tick-borne encephalitis, West Nile virus)	3 to 14 days (1 to 20 days)
Dengue fever	4 to 8 days (3 to 14 days)
Poliomyelitis	7 to 14 days (3 to 35 days)
Acute HIV infection	10 to 28 days (10 days to 6 weeks)
Rubella	14 days (12 to 23 days)
Cytomegalovirus	3 weeks to 3 months
Hepatitis E	26 to 42 days (2 to 9 weeks)
Hepatitis A	28 to 30 days (15 to 50 days)
Epstein-Barr virus	4 to 6 weeks
Rabies	1 to 2 months (9 days to years)
Hepatitis B	60 to 90 days (45 days to 9 months)
Fungal infections	
Acute histoplasmosis *(Histoplasma capsulatum)*	7 to 14 days (3 to 21 days)
Acute coccidioidomycosis *(Coccidioides immitis)*	10 to 14 days (7 to 28 days)
Parasites	
Trichinosis *(Trichinella spiralis)*	3 days to weeks
East African trypanosomiasis *(Trypanosoma brucei rhodesiense* and *gambiense)*	Acute: 5 to 16 days (3 to 21 days) Chronic illness: months to years
Toxoplasmosis *(Toxoplasma gondii)*	5 to 23 days
Visceral leishmaniasis *(Leishmania species)*	10 days to 6 months
Angiostrongyliasis meningitis *(Angiostrongylus cantonensis)*	2 weeks (5 days to 6 weeks)
Malaria *(Plasmodium falciparum)*	12 to 14 days (8 to 25 days)
Malaria *(Plasmodium ovale)*	14 to 16 days (10 to 20 days)
Malaria *(Plasmodium vivax)*	14 to 15 days (10 days to, in rare cases, months)
Malaria *(Plasmodium malariae)*	18 to 20 days (15 days to, in rare cases, months to years)
Acute schistosomiasis *(Schistosoma species)*	4 to 8 weeks
Fascioliasis *(Fasciola hepatica* and *gigantica)*	Acute: days to 3 months
Chronic: months to years	
Gnathostomiasis *(Gnathostoma species)*	3 weeks to months
Clonorchiasis *(Clonorchis sinensis)*	Acute: weeks to months
Chronic: months to years	
Amebic liver abscess *(Entamoeba histolytica)*	Weeks to months
Visceral leishmaniasis *(Leishmania donovani, L infantum, L chagasi,* and others)	2 to 6 months (10 days to years)
Lymphatic filariasis *(Wuchereria bancrofti and Brugia malayi)*	3 to 6 months or longer

Data from Ryan ET, Wilson ME, Kain KC. Illness after international travel. *N Engl J Med.* 2002;347:505–516; and the Travelers' Health Yellow Book of the Centers for Disease Control and Prevention.

The medical history should also elicit pertinent exposures for the traveler. Those who stay in houses may have more exposure to infection than those staying in tourist hotels. Camping, hiking, safari expeditions, and walking in grassy areas increase the risk of tick bites, which can cause rickettsial infections, Lyme disease, babesiosis, ehrlichiosis, and tickborne encephalitis. Malaria, dengue, yellow fever, and chikungunya fever are spread though mosquito bites. Fungal infections such as histoplasmosis and coccidioidomycosis can be acquired through inhalation of spores in caves or at excavation or construction sites. Leptospirosis can be acquired through exposure to freshwater, including swimming, boating, or wading. A sexual history is also important. Sexually transmitted diseases that can cause fever include acute HIV infection, hepatitis B virus, syphilis, and herpes viruses. Certain infections such as hepatitis A and acute schistosomiasis are more likely to occur among short-term travelers than immigrants or long-term expatriates, who in turn are more likely to have tuberculosis. **Table 190-2** provides a list of pertinent information that should be elicited from the febrile traveler.

TABLE 190-2 Medical History for Fever in the Returning Traveler

- Region of travel
- Duration and timing of travel, incubation period, and duration of fever
- History of impaired immunity from disease (HIV, asplenia) or medications
- History of vaccinations, pretravel immunizations, and use of malaria chemoprophylaxis and compliance with the prescribed regimen
- Description of accommodations (including whether bed nets and air conditioners were used) and whether urban or rural areas were visited
- Possible tuberculosis exposures, such as history of working in a health care center
- History of treatment at a health center, particularly if the traveler received a blood transfusion, injection, or dental or surgical procedure
- Ingestion of untreated water, contaminated food, unpasteurized milk or cheese, or raw or undercooked meat or fish
- History of bites from mosquitoes, ticks, fleas, mites, or other biting arthropods
- Exposure to animals or animal products
- History of camping, hiking, safari expeditions, or walks through grassy or shrubby areas
- Exposure to freshwater from swimming, boating, or wading
- Sexual activity while traveling (number of partners and protection used, if any)
- Exposure to caves, construction, or excavation sites
- Other unusual activities or exposures

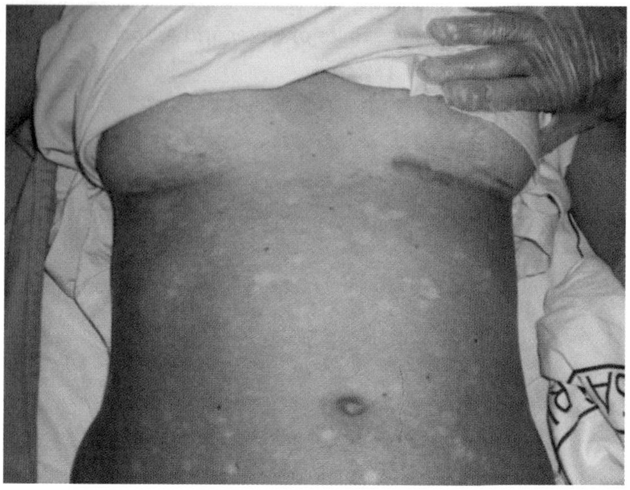

Figure 190-1 *Confluent maculopapular rash of dengue, with scattered petechiae and early bruising under the breasts. (From Pinazo MJ, Muñoz J, Betica L, et al. Emerg Infect Dis. 2008;14:1329–1330; CDC publication.)*

DIAGNOSIS: WHAT INFECTIONS SHOULD ALWAYS BE CONSIDERED?

The differential diagnosis of fever in the returning traveler is broad, as outlined in Table 190-1. The initial diagnostic evaluation of fever in travelers should focus on infections that can be rapidly life threatening, such as malaria and meningococcal meningitis, or highly contagious, such as hepatitis A, measles, and tuberculosis. *Malaria* is the most common cause of fever in travelers returning from developing countries, and, without treatment, falciparum malaria can lead to death within hours of presentation. Therefore, it is essential to consider malaria in persons with systemic symptoms who have recently traveled to an endemic area, even if they report taking chemoprophylaxis and do not complain of fever. Though most patients present with fever, rigors, and influenza-like symptoms, at least 10% of patients initially present without fever. Headache, respiratory symptoms, or gastrointestinal symptoms may predominate at presentation.

Dengue should also always be considered in febrile travelers returning from endemic areas. The prevalence of dengue has risen in many areas; reported cases increased approximately fourfold from 1995 to 2005 in South America, Central America, Mexico, and the Caribbean. Dengue fever typically presents with fever, headache, retroorbital pain, myalgia, joint pain, bone pain ("breakbone fever"), and fatigue, with or without a maculopapular or petechial rash (**Figure 190-1**). Classically, the fever has a biphasic or "saddleback" pattern, although this has been uncommon in recent series. Dengue is usually an asymptomatic or self-limited, if highly unpleasant, illness. However, patients that have previously been exposed to dengue may develop life-threatening dengue hemorrhagic fever (DHF) or dengue shock syndrome on reexposure.

Rickettsial diseases also present with fever, headache, and myalgia. In Sub-Saharan Africa, *tick bite fever* due to *Rickettsia africae*, the most common rickettsial infection, should be considered for travelers with potential exposure to tick bites (safari, camping, hiking). On physical examination, a painless eschar with regional lymphadenopathy occurs frequently at the inoculation site; in some cases, multiple inoculation eschars may be noted. A rash is usually not present.

Typhoid fever should be considered in any febrile traveler, particularly those returning from the Indian subcontinent, and those with a history of consuming unclean food or water. Typhoid presents as escalating fever, often without distinguishing features. There may be right lower quadrant pain from inflammation of Peyer patches of the ileum. Either constipation or diarrhea may be present. Rarely, rose spots are seen on the trunk of light-skinned persons. Pulmonary infiltrates, presumably arising from bacteremia, may be found in those with prolonged fever.

Noninfectious causes of fever such as *pulmonary embolism* from long flights and *drug fever* from prophylactic or empiric medical therapy for travel-related conditions are also possibilities. Febrile illnesses unrelated to travel or infections acquired after return from travel should also be considered.

WHAT DIAGNOSTIC TESTS SHOULD BE ORDERED?

A careful physical examination for the returning traveler is essential. The retina, skin, lymph nodes, heart, lungs, abdomen (in particular, liver and spleen), genital area, and extremities should be carefully examined, and the patient should have a complete neurologic exam. The initial laboratory evaluation should include complete blood count with differential, creatinine, urea nitrogen, electrolytes, liver function tests, and cultures of blood and urine. The recommended diagnostic workup for the initial evaluation of returning patients with fever is outlined in **Table 190-3**.

Malaria, dengue, rickettsial diseases, and typhoid fever should always be considered in patients with appropriate clinical and epidemiologic presentations. Thick and thin smears of peripheral blood should be performed immediately in possible malaria (**Figures 190-2** and **190-3**). Thick smears are performed on hemolyzed specimens and are more sensitive for the detection of parasitemia, but the parasite morphology is often distorted, and

TABLE 190-3 Initial Diagnostic Tests to Evaluate Fever in the Returning Traveler

All travelers:

- Electrolytes, blood urea nitrogen, creatinine, glucose
- Complete blood count and differential
- Blood and urine cultures

Travelers with relevant exposure or compatible clinical presentation:

- Thick and thin smears for malaria; rapid diagnostic test for malaria
- Acute and convalescent serology for dengue, rickettsial infections, and other infections
- HIV antibody test and/or viral load
- Stool cultures and stool studies for fecal leukocytes and ova and parasites
- Chest radiograph; consider sputum Gram stain and culture, and testing for influenza and other respiratory viruses, agents of bacterial and atypical pneumonia
- Tuberculin skin test, sputum for acid fast bacilli and mycobacterial culture
- Histoplasma antigen in urine, blood or bronchoalveolar fluid, and test for complement-fixing-type anticoccidioidal antibodies
- Consider serologic tests for *Coxiella burnetii* (Q fever) if there is hepatitis and animal exposure history
- In persons with eosinophilia: microscopic examination of stool for ova and parasites and serological tests for strongyloidiasis, schistosomiasis, and helminthic infections

speciation may not be possible. Thin smears are better for species identification and for estimating parasitemia. Giemsa stains are preferred for thin and thick smears for malaria detection. If Giemsa stains are unavailable or delayed, the Wright stain, commonly used to perform white blood cell differential counting in hematology laboratories, may be used as a somewhat inferior substitute. Rapid diagnostic tests are also available for centers without skilled microscopists. If the initial blood smears for malaria are negative but the diagnosis is still suspected, additional smears should be repeated within 12 to 24 hours.

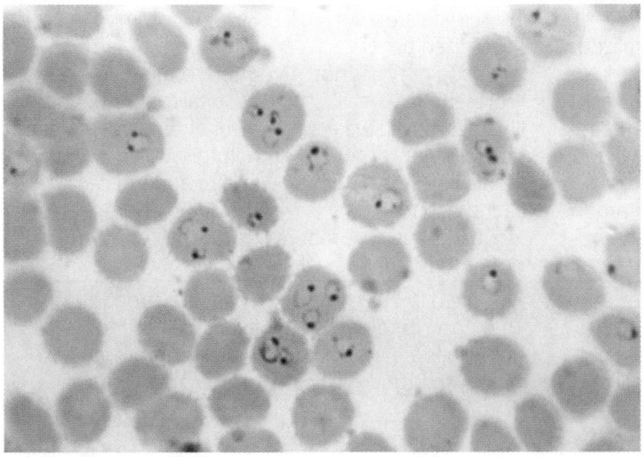

Figure 190-2 *Thin blood film with a monotonous population of small ring trophozoites, characteristic of Plasmodium falciparum; heavy parasitemia is present. Falciparum malaria is more lethal than other forms of malaria because of the high parasite burdens that may arise. Giemsa stain. (Public Health Image Library, Centers for Disease Control and Prevention.)*

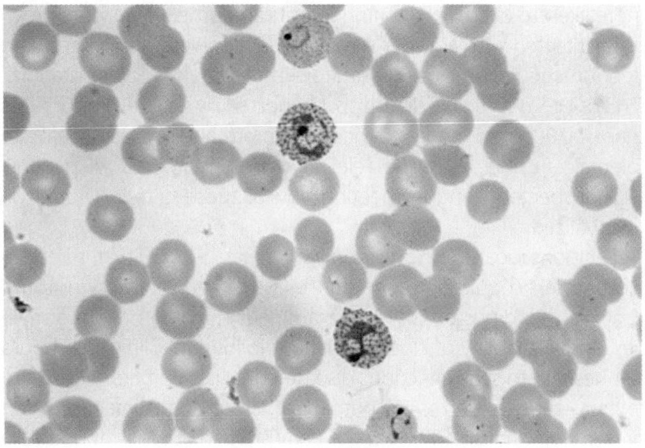

Figure 190-3 *Thin blood film with trophozoites of various ages covered in Schüffner dots, typical of Plasmodium vivax. Giemsa stain. (Public Health Image Library, Centers for Disease Control and Prevention.)*

The diagnosis of dengue infection is usually based on clinical findings. Acute and convalescent serology confirms the diagnosis, but testing is available only in specialized centers, and results do not return in time to impact decisions in care. Laboratory findings associated with dengue include thrombocytopenia, leukopenia, and elevated hepatic transaminases. The tourniquet test is a traditional diagnostic test for dengue, which indirectly measures both capillary fragility and thrombocytopenia. A blood pressure cuff is inflated to midway between systolic and diastolic pressures and left on the upper arm for five minutes. The resulting petechiae on the volar forearm just below the antecubital fossa are counted; a positive result is more than 20 petechiae per square inch. However, the tourniquet test is not very sensitive for the diagnosis of dengue, but it may indicate which patients are at risk of hemorrhagic complications.

Similarly, rickettsial infections are primarily diagnosed clinically and later confirmed by serologic tests. Typhoid fever can be diagnosed by culturing blood, stool, and urine; serology is unreliable. In some situations, serologic testing for leptospirosis, cerebrospinal fluid examination, bone marrow aspirate or biopsy, and biopsies of lymph nodes or skin lesions may be appropriate.

PRACTICE POINT

- Returning travelers with fever and hemorrhage, neurologic symptoms, respiratory distress, or other severe symptoms should be evaluated immediately. Because such infections may be rapidly fatal, urgent consultation with an infectious disease expert is advisable.

WHEN SHOULD PATIENTS BE HOSPITALIZED?

Travelers with falciparum malaria or malaria that has not been speciated should be admitted for urgent treatment and monitoring for potential complications. Patients at highest risk include nonimmune travelers, pregnant women, young children, and the elderly. Most deaths occur among patients with severe malaria within the first 48 hours after hospital admission. Those with severe malaria should be admitted to the intensive care unit.

Patients with suspected dengue should be monitored for early signs of hemorrhage and vascular permeability. DHF and dengue shock syndrome (DSS) are rare among short-term travelers, and more likely to occur among immigrants and others who were previously infected with another serotype. Nevertheless, all persons with dengue should be closely monitored for potential complications. DHS or DSS is a clinical diagnosis, suggested by a platelet count less than 100,000/mm^3 and evidence of hemorrhage or plasma leakage (pleural effusion, ascites, or elevation in hematocrit). All patients with suspected dengue meeting any of these criteria should be hospitalized.

Decisions regarding admission for other causes of fever in returning travelers should be based on the associated clinical symptoms, vital signs, findings on physical examination, laboratory abnormalities, and availability of close outpatient follow-up. Clinicians should not hesitate to seek infectious disease consultation before deciding to treat the traveler as an outpatient, since some infections can present with mild findings in the early stage of disease and rapidly progress over hours to days.

TREATMENT

MEDICAL THERAPY

Specific medications for the treatment of malaria vary based on the species of malaria, the risk of drug resistance (based on the region of travel), the age, pregnancy status, and comorbidities of the patient, and the degree of parasitemia and clinical severity of the disease. All nonimmune patients with falciparum malaria should be admitted for observation and urgent treatment, and an infectious disease specialist should be consulted for management. Consideration of hospitalization should be given even to persons who claim heavy prior exposure to falciparum malaria because it is difficult to assess acquired immunity, and immunity wanes without constant reexposure.

The World Health Organization (WHO) criteria for severe malaria include prostration, impaired consciousness, respiratory distress, repeated convulsions, circulatory collapse, pulmonary edema, abnormal bleeding, jaundice, hemoglobinuria, severe anemia, hypoglycemia, acidosis, renal impairment, elevated lactate, or hyperparasitemia. Patients meeting criteria for severe malaria should be admitted to an intensive care unit for parenteral therapy, management of volume status, identification and treatment of complications, and mechanical ventilation and dialysis if needed. Treatment of malaria is beyond the scope of this chapter but is outlined in several recent reviews (**Table 190-4**).

Patients with dengue can develop hemorrhage and hypovolemic shock due to increased intravascular permeability, thrombocytopenia, and coagulopathy. Vital signs and hematocrit should be followed for signs of dehydration and hemoconcentration. Platelet counts should be monitored, and radiographic studies such as ultrasound should be performed to detect fluid accumulation in serosal cavities. Plasma leakage typically develops four to seven days after the onset of symptoms, approximately coinciding with the resolution of fever. There is no specific therapy for dengue. Acetaminophen is the preferred agent for fever and myalgia. Nonsteroidal anti-inflammatory medications and aspirin should be avoided as they could increase the risk of bleeding. Intravascular hydration with fluids or colloids is essential for those with increased intravascular permeability. All patients with suspected dengue

TABLE 190-4 Evidence-based Medicine: Key References for Fever in the Returning Traveler

Paper	Methodology	Results	Limitations	Bottom Line
Freedman DO, et al. *N Engl J Med.* 2006;354:119–130	Clinician-based sentinel surveillance data for 17,353 ill returned travelers	There are significant regional differences in proportionate morbidity. Malaria was one of the three most frequent causes of systemic febrile illness among travelers from every region.	These data are from specialized travel clinics, and may not represent the spectrum of illness in returned travelers that would be seen in primary care practices, where milder conditions may occur with higher frequency.	Diagnostic approaches and empiric treatments can be guided by travel destination.
Wilson ME, et al. *Clin Infect Dis.* 2007;44:1560–1568	Used a large, multicenter database of returned travelers (n = 24,920) to define causes of fever by place of exposure and traveler characteristics	Of patients with fever, 26% were hospitalized, 35% had a febrile systemic illness, 15% had febrile diarrheal disease, and 14% had fever and respiratory illness. Malaria was the most common specific diagnosis.	These data are from specialized travel clinics, so they are not representative of all illnesses in all travelers. They did not capture all febrile illnesses—such as those with short incubation periods that presented during travel.	Fever is common in returned travelers, often resulting in hospitalization. Timing of fever after travel provides helpful clues. Preventing and treating malaria, and providing appropriate travel advice is critical.
Griffith KS, et al. *JAMA.* 2007;297:2264–2277	Systematic MEDLINE search from 1966 to 2006 to examine the evidence base for malaria treatment	This paper defines the important measures to reduce morbidity and mortality from malaria, including specific treatment guidelines.	Published in 2007. The most up-to-date guidelines are available at www.cdc.gov/malaria.	There is a strong evidence base to help clinicians promptly and effectively treat malaria.
Jensenius M, et al. *Clin Infect Dis.* 2003;36:1411–1417	Prospective cohort study of 940 travelers to rural Sub-Equatorial Africa to estimate the incidence, risk factors, and clinical presentation of African tick-bite fever	38 travelers (4.0% of the cohort) and 26.6% of those reporting flulike symptoms were diagnosed with African tick-bite fever.	This was a prospective study of African tick-bite fever. No data are provided on other travel-related infections.	African tick-bite fever is not uncommon among travelers returning from Sub-Equatorial Africa and presents with nonspecific findings.

should be seen in consultation with an infectious disease specialist because early signs of increased vascular permeability and coagulapathy may be subtle, and patients may develop life-threatening shock and hemorrhage.

■ POTENTIAL COMPLICATIONS

Patients infected with falciparum malaria, particularly travelers who are nonimmune, can rapidly develop the life-threatening complications of severe malaria as defined by WHO (already described). In contrast, travelers are less likely than foreign nationals to develop life-threatening dengue because severe disease is associated with a second infection with a different dengue serotype. Nevertheless, all travelers with suspected dengue should be evaluated for early signs of hemorrhage or plasma leakage.

Because the list of potential diagnoses in critically ill travelers is exceedingly long, infectious disease consultation should be urgently obtained for any traveler with danger signs, including high fever, mental status changes and other neurologic symptoms, respiratory distress, hemorrhage, and severe laboratory abnormalities, such as metabolic acidosis, renal failure, or profound anemia. Empiric treatment for possible diagnoses should be considered in such patients.

■ QUALITY IMPROVEMENT

In evaluating the febrile patient, it is critical to obtain a travel history and determine if the patient is at risk for malaria based on the region visited. For those at risk for malaria, it is essential to test immediately, and for those infected, to treat promptly with effective therapy. Severe malaria is a medical emergency, and delays in treatment increase the mortality rate. Despite this, a recent Canadian study found that the diagnosis of malaria was initially missed in 59% of patients, and the delay in treatment after presentation was 7.6 days for falciparum malaria and 5.1 days for vivax malaria. Similar results have been found in many studies of imported malaria.

Numerous resources are available for clinicians who are unfamiliar with the management of malaria. The CDC Web site (www.cdc.gov/malaria) provides up-to-date treatment guidelines. It should also be noted that malaria, dengue, typhoid fever, and other tropical and exotic diseases should be reported to public health authorities in the United States and other countries.

Dengue should be high on the differential diagnosis because it is the second most common cause of systemic febrile syndromes in travelers returning from the developing world, and it can rapidly progress in patients with severe disease. Other areas for quality improvement include performing a careful history of travel and exposures for all febrile patients, and early consultation with a travel medicine specialist for febrile patients with a recent travel history.

SUGGESTED READINGS

Centers for Disease Control and Prevention. Travelers' Health—Yellow Book 2010. Available at: http://wwwnc.cdc.gov/travel/yellowbook/2010/table-of-contents.aspx.

Freedman DO, Weld LH, Kozarsky PE, et al. Spectrum of disease and relation to place of exposure among ill returned travelers. *N Engl J Med*. 2006;354:119–130.

Griffith KS, Lewis LS, Mali S, Parise ME. Treatment of malaria in the United States: a systematic review. *JAMA*. 2007;297:2264–2277.

Kain KC, Harrington MA, Tennyson S, Keystone JS. Imported malaria: prospective analysis of problems in diagnosis and management. *Clin Infect Dis*. 1998;27:142–149.

Newman RD, Parise ME, Barber AM, Steketee RW. Malaria-related deaths among U.S. travelers, 1963–2001. *Ann Intern Med*. 2004; 141:547–555.

Ryan ET, Wilson ME, Kain KC. Illness after international travel. *N Engl J Med*. 2002;347:505–516.

Wilder-Smith A, Schwartz E. Dengue in travelers. *N Engl J Med*. 2005;353:924–932.

Wilson ME, Weld LH, Boggild A, et al. Fever in returned travelers: results from the GeoSentinel Surveillance Network. *Clin Infect Dis*. 2007;44:1560–1568.

World Health Organization. Guidelines for the Treatment of Malaria. 2nd ed. Available at: http://whqlibdoc.who.int/publications/2010/9789241547925_eng.pdf.

CHAPTER 191

Fever of Unknown Origin

David A. Oxman, MD

Key Clinical Questions

1. What are the major categories of fever of unknown origin (FUO)?
2. What basic tests should be done in evaluating patients with FUO?
3. When is more specific laboratory testing or diagnostic imaging indicated?
4. Which patients should receive empiric therapy?
5. What is the prognosis of FUO?

INTRODUCTION

The classic definition of fever of unknown origin (FUO) by Petersdorf and Beeson in 1961 was a fever greater than 38.3°C (101°F) on several occasions, persisting without diagnosis for at least 3 weeks, in spite of 1 week's investigation in hospital. In the 50 years since, medical practice has changed substantially, and much of the diagnostic evaluation for FUO can be accomplished on an outpatient basis. One proposed revision of the classic definition of FUO defines it as a febrile illness that has not been diagnosed after at least three outpatient visits or 3 days of hospitalization (**Table 191-1**). In practice, while an exact definition is difficult, FUO can be thought of as a persistent febrile illness that has eluded diagnosis despite a thorough history, physical examination, and routine diagnostic testing. Additionally, several specific categories of FUO have been proposed, including nosocomial FUO, HIV-related FUO, and FUO in the returning traveler. Over 200 different causes of FUO have been reported, but all etiologies fall into four broad groups: infectious, neoplastic, rheumatologic, and miscellaneous. The incidence of each etiology will vary with different patient populations and geographic locations.

PATHOPHYSIOLOGY

PHYSIOLOGY OF FEVER

Fever is a complex common response to disparate diseases. The febrile response includes not only elevation of core body temperature but also activation of numerous physiological, endocrine, and immunologic systems. Although the neural regulation of body temperature involves several parts of the brain, the preoptic and anterior regions of the hypothalamus have the greatest role. Pyrogens—either endogenous or exogenous—can stimulate pyrogenic cytokines such as interleukin (IL)-1, IL-6, tumor necrosis factor alpha (TNF-α), interferon gamma (IFN-γ) or act directly on hypothalamic neurons and decrease their firing rate, leading to physiological responses that decrease heat loss and increase heat production. Exogenous pyrogens include microbes and toxins, whereas endogenous pyrogens include antigen-antibody complexes, complement, tissue necrosis, and sensitized lymphocytes.

PATTERNS OF FEVER

Throughout medical history, clinicians have tried to link patterns of fever with specific diseases. In *saddleback* or *biphasic fever*, fever is present for several days, remits for a day, and then relapses for several days. This pattern has been associated with dengue, yellow fever, influenza, leptospirosis, ehrlichiosis, and tickborne relapsing fever. In *Pel-Ebstein fevers*, patients have days or even weeks of fever, followed by remission of equal duration, then another recurrence. Pel-Ebstein fevers are generally considered to suggest Hodgkin disease. However, with the exception of the tertian fever (recurring every 48 hours) of vivax malaria and the quartan fever (recurring every 72 hours) of *Plasmodium malariae*, fever patterns are not specific and are unreliable for diagnosis.

ETIOLOGIES OF FEVER OF UNKNOWN ORIGIN

MAJOR INFECTIOUS CAUSES

Since the 1950s the percentage of FUOs attributable to infections has decreased, but infection still makes up a large proportion of FUO

TABLE 191-1 Contemporary Definitions of Fever of Unknown Origin (FUO)

Type of FUO	Definition	Common Causes
Modified "classic" FUO	Fever ≥ 38.3°C (101°F) on several occasions for at least 3 weeks No diagnosis after 3 days of hospitalization or three outpatient visits	Infection, malignancy, vasculitis and other rheumatological conditions, drug fever In elderly patients in developed countries, often neoplastic; in young patients, often no diagnosis
Nosocomial FUO	Hospitalized patients with fever ≥ 38.3°C (101°F) on several occasions Fever not present or incubating at admission Diagnosis uncertain after 3 days of appropriate investigations, including 48 hours of incubating cultures	*Clostridium difficile* enterocolitis, pneumonia, infection of central line and other devices, candidemia, urosepsis, acalculous cholecystitis, drug fever, thromboembolism, sinusitis, gout, pseudogout, central fever, stroke, myocardial infarction Dressler syndrome, malignant hyperthermia
Neutropenic FUO	Fever ≥ 38.3°C (101°F) on several occasions in a patient with an absolute neutrophil count of < 500/mm^3 Diagnosis uncertain after 3 days of appropriate investigations, including 48 hours of incubating cultures	Pneumonia, central line sepsis, *Clostridium difficile* enterocolitis, mucositis, cellulitis, aspergillosis, candidiasis, fusariosis, herpes simplex virus, neutropenic enterocolitis (typhlitis)
HIV-related FUO	Patient with HIV infection and fever ≥ 38.3°C (101°F) on several occasions Duration of at least 4 weeks in outpatients or 3 days in inpatients Diagnosis uncertain after 3 days of appropriate investigations, including 48 hours of incubating cultures	Usually infectious, especially in patients not taking highly active antiretroviral therapy (HAART) Most common cause worldwide is tuberculosis; others include *Pneumocystis jiroveci* pneumonia, *M avium*, cytomegalovirus, toxoplasmosis, cryptococcosis, endemic mycoses, visceral leishmaniasis (Africa/Asia/southern Europe) Occasionally due to lymphoma, drug fever, Castleman disease, immune reconstitution inflammatory syndrome

cases. Tuberculosis—mostly reactivation of latent disease—is the most important infectious cause of FUO (**Table 191-2**). While PPD testing and chest x-ray are helpful for diagnosis, they may be falsely negative due to either anergy or extrapulmonary disease. Similarly, patients with advanced HIV disease and coinfection with tuberculosis may lack typical signs of TB infection.

TABLE 191-2 Etiologies of FUO by Category

Infectious	*Bacterial*: **tuberculosis, subacute bacterial endocarditis**, intra-abdominal abscess, osteomyelitis, brucellosis, Lyme disease *Viral*: cytomegalovirus and Epstein-Barr virus *Fungal*: endemic mycoses *Parasitic*: malaria, babesia
Neoplastic	*Hematological*: **lymphoma**, leukemia, myelodysplastic disorders *Solid organ*: renal cell cancer, hepatocellular carcinoma, atrial myxoma, breast and colon cancer
Autoimmune	**Giant cell arteritis, Still disease** (adult juvenile rheumatoid arthritis), polyarteritis nodosa, familial Mediterranean fever, polymyalgia rheumatica, **sarcoidosis**, systemic lupus erythematosus
Miscellaneous	**Drug fever, factitious fever, thromboembolic disease**, Kikuchi necrotizing lymphadenitis, hyperthyroidism

Most common causes in **bold**.

Subacute bacterial endocarditis (SBE) was once a common cause of FUO, but it is now relatively uncommon. The diagnosis can typically be made by blood culture and echocardiography, but prior antibiotics may render blood cultures sterile. The classic physical findings associated with SBE—Roth spots, Janeway lesions, and splinter hemorrhages—are late findings seen in a small proportion of cases. True culture-negative endocarditis is less common in the United States than in Europe or the developing world. Organisms that cause culture-negative endocarditis include *Coxiella brunetti* (Q fever), *Bartonella* species, *Tropheryma whipplei*, *Brucella*, and the so-called *Haemophilus parainfluenzae, Aggregatibacter aphrophilus, Aggregatibacter actinomycetemcomitans, Cardiobacterium hominis, Eikenella corrodens, and Kingella kingae* (HACEK) organisms. Special microbiological techniques to facilitate the growth of fastidious organisms, as well as polymerase chain reaction (PCR), may help identify specific pathogens. When culture-negative endocarditis is suspected, the microbiology lab should be asked to hold blood cultures for up to 21 days.

Recurrent urinary tract infection, osteomyelitis, and occult intraabdominal abscesses are other bacterial causes of FUO. Conditions that predispose to intraabdominal abscess include inflammatory bowel disease, diverticular disease, and a history of previous bowel surgery. Vertebral osteomyelitis is common in the elderly and should be considered in the patient with fever and back pain. Common viral causes of FUO causing a mononucleosis-like syndrome of fever, pharyngitis and lymphadenopathy include cytomegalovirus (CMV) and Epstein-Barr virus (EBV). Tickborne diseases such as Lyme disease, human monocytic ehrlichiosis, and human granulocytic anaplasmosis may be associated with prolonged fevers and nonspecific symptoms such as malaise, headache, and myalgias. Babesiosis often causes subclinical disease but may cause fever and in asplenic or otherwise immunocompromised patients can cause fulminant and life-threatening illness.

MAJOR NEOPLASTIC CAUSES

Fever associated with neoplasm or malignancy can result from either tissue necrosis or the release of pyrogenic cytokines. Lymphoma, myeloproliferative syndromes, and other hematopoietic malignancies are a common cause of FUO. Overall, with the advent of advanced diagnostic imaging and earlier detection, the percentage of solid-organ malignancies presenting as FUO has declined. Among solid organ tumors, renal cell carcinoma is most commonly associated with FUO, with hematuria notably absent in a large minority of patients. Other solid tumors occasionally associated with FUO are hepatocellular, breast, and colon cancer.

MAJOR AUTOIMMUNE AND INFLAMMATORY CAUSES

The relative percentage of FUOs in the developed world attributable to rheumatologic diseases has risen over time, in part due to the decline in undiagnosed infections and cancer, and also due to improved laboratory diagnostic techniques. Vasculitides, especially giant cell arteritis, are common causes of FUO in the elderly. Adult-onset Still disease is a common cause of FUO in young adults. The periodic fevers, of which familial Mediterranean fever (FMF) is the most common, are a group of inherited autoinflammatory disorders due to specific genetic mutations that cause recurrent fevers and often other symptoms such as serositis, splenomegaly, edema, and arthritis. Untreated FMF can lead to secondary amyloidosis and eventual renal failure.

PRACTICE POINT

- Giant cell arteritis (temporal arteritis) is the single most common cause of FUO in the elderly. It should be strongly suspected in any patient over the age of 50 with FUO and a high ESR. Classic manifestations include new headache, visual disturbances, tenderness and diminished pulsation of the temporal artery, and occasionally jaw claudication. However, the history and physical examination are not sensitive for giant cell arteritis (GCA). About 12% of GCA is "silent" or "masked," presenting only with fever, weight loss, fatigue, and malaise.

MAJOR MISCELLANEOUS CAUSES

Many medications have been associated with drug fever, but several have been observed to cause it more frequently (**Table 191-3**). Beta-lactam antibiotics; cardiac medications such as quinidine, amiodarone, or procainamide; antitubercular drugs such as isoniazid or rifampin; and anticonvulsants such as phenytoin and carbamazepine are common culprits. Rash and eosinophilia may also be present, but often are not. Drug fever is more often observed with recently initiated medications but occasionally may develop in a patient that has been taking the offending agent chronically. Drug fever is a diagnosis of exclusion, and can only be confirmed when the fever resolves with cessation of the suspected agent. Factitious fever may be simulated by manipulation of thermometers or self-induced by the injection of pyogenic materials. One review of FUO put the incidence of factitious fever causing FUO as high as 10%. Typically, the patient is a young adult with experience working in health care. Thromboembolic disease should be considered as a possible cause of FUO in the right clinical setting (eg, hypercoagulable state or prolonged immobilization).

TABLE 191-3 Medications Frequently Cited as Causes of Drug Fever

Antibiotics	β-lactams (penicillins, cephalosporins, carbapenems), nitrofurantoin, sulfonamides, amphotericin, isoniazid, rifampin
Anticonvulsants	Phenytoin, carbamazepine
Cardiac medications	Amiodarone, procainimide, quinidine, nifedipine, captopril, hydralazine
Anticholinergics	Phenothiazines (chlorpromazine, compazine)

THE IMMUNOSUPPRESSED PATIENT

The percentage of FUOs caused by infections is high in this group. Decreased cell-mediated or humoral immune responses lead to an increased risk of acute infection, as well as reactivation of latent infections such as tuberculosis. Impaired immune responses may also lead to an absence of typical signs on physical examination or radiography. Transplant patients on antirejection medications or patients on high-dose steroids are at increased risk of disseminated fungal infection. Febrile neutropenic patients are at high risk of bacterial sepsis and should receive empiric broad-spectrum antibiotics after appropriate cultures have been obtained. Immunosuppressed patients with FUO and pulmonary nodules should be considered for early bronchoscopy. Hepatosplenic candidiasis is typically seen after neutrophil counts have recovered and presents with abdominal pain, elevated alkaline phosphatase levels, and tiny hepatosplenic nodules on imaging studies. This condition is less often observed today because neutropenic patients receive antifungal therapy earlier in the course of illness.

THE PATIENT WITH HIV

The vast majority of FUOs in patients with advanced HIV (CD4 cell count <200 cells/mm^3) are caused by infections, with mycobacterial infection—*M tuberculosis* and *M avium-intracellulare* (MAI)—and *Pneumocystis jiroveci* pneumonia (PCP) the most common in the United States. *Cryptococcus* and other fungi are also common. Endemic mycoses should be suspected in patients from certain geographic areas—histoplasmosis in those from the Ohio and Mississippi river valleys or the Caribbean, coccidioidomycosis in patients from arid regions of the southwestern United States, Mexico, and South America. In southern Europe, visceral leishmaniasis is common. An important noninfectious cause of FUO in patients with AIDS is lymphoma, especially non-Hodgkin lymphoma. Primary HIV infection often leads to a self-limited mononucleosis-like febrile illness and should be considered as a cause of FUO with an exposure history. AIDS patients with FUO should, in addition to standard blood cultures, have isolator bottles sent for fungus and mycobacteria. Serum cryptococcal antigen and sputum stains for *Pneumocystis* should also be performed. Urine histoplasmosis antigen can be done if the patient is from an endemic area.

NOSOCOMIAL FEVER OF UNKNOWN ORIGIN

This describes a hospital-associated fever with no identifiable cause lasting for at least 3 days. These fevers often result from iatrogenic causes, such as intravascular or urinary catheter- related infections, blood transfusions, thromboembolic disease from prolonged immobilization, or drug fever. Postoperative fevers are common and are often a normal physiologic response not related to infection. *Clostridium difficile* infection is generally not subtle and is usually associated with profuse diarrhea and leukocytosis. Occasionally, diarrhea may be absent in the setting of ileus. Acalculous cholecystitis is a common cause of FUO in the critically ill patient, presenting with unexplained fever, leukocytosis, and signs of biliary obstruction. Noninfectious causes of nosocomial FUO include acute respiratory distress syndrome, postcardiac surgery pericarditis, and alcohol withdrawal.

IMMIGRANTS AND RETURNING TRAVELERS

When travelers or immigrants present with FUO, fever may be due to common illnesses such as urinary tract infection or pneumonia, but careful consideration should be given to the infectious diseases endemic to the regions of recent travel. Malaria is potentially fatal if not diagnosed early and should be suspected in any febrile traveler from an endemic area. Typhoid fever is common in most developing nations. Dengue and chikungunya are insectborne viral infections often accompanied by rash and may be seen in the returning traveler from South America, Africa, or Asia. Brucellosis—a bacterial infection transmitted by contact with animal carcasses, placentas, or contaminated milk and meat products—is very common in the Middle East, Mediterranean basin, and parts of South America. Patients may have FUO as a manifestation of acute infection or reactivation of latent disease. Arthritis, spondylitis, sacroiliitis, and hepatitis are common manifestations of *Brucella*. Q fever (caused by the bacterium *Coxiella burnetii*) is a common cause of culture-negative endocarditis in Australia, France, and Spain. Melioidosis (caused by the bacterium *Burkholderia pseudomallei*) may cause FUO in patients from Southeast Asia. Liver abscess is the most common extraintestinal manifestation of amebiasis caused by the protozoan *Entamoeba histolytica*, seen in developing countries worldwide. HIV and syphilis should be suspected in sex tourists.

TRIAGE/HOSPITAL ADMISSION

The workup of FUO is usually initiated in the outpatient setting. It is appropriate to admit patients with FUO to hospital because of severity of clinical illness and to expedite the patient's diagnostic testing.

DIAGNOSIS

HISTORY AND PHYSICAL EXAMINATION

A careful medical history and a physical examination are the most important parts of any FUO evaluation. Prior illnesses, past surgical procedures, medication lists, and vaccination histories should be thoroughly reviewed. Particular attention should be paid to travel and sexual history, recreational activities, occupational exposures, exposure to pets and other animals, and culinary habits (eg, handling and consuming raw and unpasteurized foods). Physical examination may reveal rashes, poor dentition, oral or genital ulcers, lymphadenopathy, sinus tenderness, heart murmurs, hepatosplenomegaly, or stigmata of endocarditis that may direct further diagnostic workup. A rectal examination may reveal a perirectal abscess or prostatitis. Relative bradycardia, or pulse-fever dissociation (Faget sign) suggests intracellular infection, as in typhoid fever, legionellosis, and rickettsial infection. Repeating the history and physical examination over a period of time may unearth additional clues.

ROUTINE TESTING

Diagnostic testing for FUO is summarized in (**Table 191-4**). Routine diagnostic tests that should be ordered as part of most initial evaluations include complete blood cell count with differential, serum transaminases, blood cultures (ideally three sets drawn from different sites over a period of several hours or longer), erythrocyte sedimentation rate (ESR), and C-reactive protein. Additionally, urinalysis with urine culture, tuberculin skin testing (PPD), HIV testing, and chest x-ray should be performed.

TABLE 191-4 Suggested Diagnostic Approach to FUO

All patients
Complete history and physical examination
Laboratory investigations: complete blood count and differential, erythrocyte sedimentation rate, C-reactive protein, urinalysis, liver function tests, creatine kinase, HIV antibody, rapid plasma reagin (RPR), HIV, cytomegalovirus IgM, monospot, antinuclear antibody, rheumatoid factor, serum protein electrophoresis, tuberculin skin test or interferon-gamma release assay, routine serum chemistries, serum ferritin, blood set aside for acute and convalescent serology
Microbiology: blood cultures (three sets, off antibiotics), urine culture, sputum, and other body fluid cultures as suggested by clinical scenario
Chest radiograph
CT scan of chest, abdomen, and pelvis
All patients, if above studies unrevealing or equivocal
Venous duplex imaging of lower extremities
Fluorodeoxyglucose positron emission tomographic scan, if available; if not, consider gallium-67 scintigraphy or indium-111 white blood cell scan
Selected patients
Tissue biopsy (if rash, lymphadenopathy, mass, or other target identified)
Consider temporal artery biopsy in older patients with high ESR and no other explanation for fever

Most of these studies are nonspecific, but they provide a starting point for refining the differential diagnosis and pursuing further testing. For example, lymphopenia is commonly seen with viral infections and neoplastic processes. Eosinophilia suggests a drug reaction, neoplasm, or parasitic infection, whereas basophilia, although uncommon, is associated with myeloproliferative disorders. The erythrocyte sedimentation rate (ESR) and C-reactive protein are nonspecific measures of inflammation. The ESR measures the distance that red blood cells in an upright tube fall in an hour. In inflammatory states, the liver produces fibrinogen, which increases the "stickiness" of red blood cells and makes them settle faster. C-reactive protein (CRP) is an acute phase reactant produced by the liver in inflammatory states. CRP is generally more sensitive for inflammatory states than the ESR because CRP levels in the blood rise more quickly after the onset of an inflammatory or infective process.

Given the frequency with which tuberculosis and other pulmonary processes cause FUO, all patients should undergo routine chest radiography and PPD testing. HIV testing was formerly only recommended in high-risk individuals but should be done universally in patients presenting with FUO. If acute HIV is suspected, HIV viral load testing should be performed. Autoantibody tests such as antinuclear antibody (ANA) titers and rheumatologic factor (RF) have a high false-positive rate but are useful when the clinical picture suggests rheumatological disease.

IMAGING STUDIES

Computed tomographic (CT) scans of chest, abdomen, and pelvis have become a routine and high-yield component of the FUO workup. CT scans may identify lymphadenopathy, pulmonary nodules, abdominal masses, and abscesses that are targets for biopsy or aspiration. Magnetic resonance imaging (MRI) is more sensitive for detecting central nervous system (CNS) causes of FUO, such as epidural abscess or cerebral vasculitis.

Radionuclide imaging may be a useful adjunct in FUO. Fluorine-18 fluorodeoxyglucose positron emission tomography (18F-FDG PET), sometimes performed in conjunction with CT scanning (18F-FDG PET/CT), is a particularly promising imaging modality in FUO that is able to localize sites of malignancy, inflammation, and infection. It may be more sensitive in FUO than radionuclide imaging with gallium-67 and radiolabeled leukocyte scanning with indium-111. Although nuclear medicine studies often contribute to diagnosis in FUO, lack of specificity and high false-positive rates may be a problem, and the results should be interpreted with caution.

BIOPSY

Examination of tissue is often required to diagnose an FUO. Localized abnormalities seen on physical examination or diagnostic imaging (eg, enlarged lymph nodes or pulmonary nodules) may be targeted for biopsy. In general, biopsies should be directed toward an abnormal finding and not be done routinely. The exception is in elderly patients with features suggestive of temporal arteritis, where temporal artery biopsy should be done despite the absence of physical findings. The role of bone marrow aspiration and liver biopsy in the diagnosis of FUO is debatable. We recommend pursuing bone marrow or liver biopsies only if there are suggestive abnormalities (cytopenias or abnormal peripheral smears, abnormal liver function tests) and a thorough diagnostic evaluation has been otherwise unrevealing.

TREATMENT

Specific treatment depends on the underlying cause of the FUO. Therapeutic trials without a diagnosis are generally not recommended. Undirected treatment may not only delay the diagnosis but can also cause considerable harm. Empiric antibiotics can obscure growth from blood cultures, and the routine administration of corticosteroids can worsen illness in such conditions as tuberculosis or parasitic disease. Exceptions to this rule are FUO in an immunocompromised patient or potentially septic immunocompetent patient. In these cases, empiric therapy with antimicrobials must be initiated. Similarly, when a patient is suspected to have temporal arteritis, early initiation of steroids may prevent blindness or other vascular complications and may be indicated before a definitive diagnosis can be made.

DISCHARGE CONSIDERATIONS

Discharge planning for most patients will depend on the specific diagnosis. Patients with continued fever who are otherwise stable may be discharged with close ambulatory follow-up. Up to 30% of patients with FUO are never definitively diagnosed. The prognosis in these patients is generally good. Fever resolves spontaneously in the vast majority, and mortality is low.

SUGGESTED READINGS

Blockmans D, Knockaert D, Maes A, et al. Clinical value of [^{18}F] fluorodeoxyglucose positron emission tomography for patients with fever of unknown origin. *Clin Infect Dis*. 2001;32:191–196.

Cunha BA. Fever of unknown origin: clinical overview of classic and current concepts. *Infect Dis Clin North Am*. 2007;21:867–915.

Knockaert DC, Dujardin KS, Bobbaers HJ. Long-term follow-up of patients with undiagnosed fever of unknown origin. *Arch Intern Med*. 1996;156:618–620.

Knockaert DC, Vanderschuerne S, Blockmans D. Fever of unknown origin in adults: 40 years on. *J Intern Med*. 2003;253:263–275.

Mackowiak P. Concepts of fever. *Arch Intern Med*. 1998;158: 1870–1881.

Mourad O, Palda V, Detsky AS. A comprehensive evidence-based approach to fever of unknown origin. *Arch Intern Med*. 2003;163: 545–551.

Petersdorf RG, Beeson PB. Fever of unexplained origin: report of 100 cases. *Medicine* (Baltimore). 1961;40:1–30.

CHAPTER 192

Candida and Aspergillus

John J. Ross, MD, CM, FIDSA

Key Clinical Questions

1. When should a positive urine culture for Candida species be treated?
2. When should invasive candidiasis be suspected? How is it diagnosed and treated?
3. What is the clinical significance of a positive sputum culture for Aspergillus species?
4. How useful are antigen detection tests for the diagnosis of infection with Candida and Aspergillus species?

INTRODUCTION

Mucocutaneous infection with *Candida* species is common in the hospital setting, due to the high prevalence of diabetes and the use of broad-spectrum antibiotics. Invasive infections with *Candida* species were once rare, but have become much more common in hospitalized patients, particularly among those with compromised immunity, antibiotic exposure, and central venous catheters. The increased prevalence of *Aspergillus* infections in the hospital is almost wholly due to neutropenia from chemotherapy and the use of high-dose glucocorticoids and other immunosuppressive agents in patients with organ and bone marrow transplants and rheumatological diseases.

CANDIDA INFECTIONS

EPIDEMIOLOGY

Candida species are normal flora of the oropharynx, bowel, and vagina. *Candida* overgrowth of these surfaces may arise in the setting of broad spectrum antibiotics, diabetes mellitus, or HIV infection, resulting in oral thrush, *Candida* esophagitis, and vaginal candidiasis. High estrogen states, such as pregnancy or oral contraceptive use, are an additional risk factor for vaginal yeast infection. *Candida* skin infections are often seen in moist, macerated intertrigenous folds, such as in the groin, perineum (diaper rash), pannus, axillae, and breasts.

While superficial candidiasis is common in both ambulatory and hospitalized patients, candidemia and disseminated candidiasis are usually seen in health care settings. Risk factors include critical illness, intensive antibiotic exposure, intraabdominal surgery, hemodialysis, central venous catheters, parenteral nutrition, intravenous drug use, and neutropenia.

DOES THIS PATIENT HAVE CANDIDA INFECTION?

Mucocutaneous Candida (cutaneous, thrush, esophagitis, vaginitis)

The diagnosis of mucocutaneous *Candida* infections is usually made clinically. **Cutaneous candidiasis** has a typical distribution in intertrigenous areas, with central erythema and maceration, surrounded by a collar of scale (**Figure 192-1**). Beyond this, there may be papular and pustular satellite lesions. **Oral thrush** (**Figure 192-2**) presents with painless white plaques on the mucous membranes and tongue that are easily scraped off. Fissures of the angles of the mouth (cheilitis) may also be present. Budding yeasts, hyphae, and pseudohyphae of *Candida* can be seen on microscopy when scrapings of skin or oral lesions are mixed with a drop of 10% potassium hydroxide, which digests host cells but not fungi.

Esophageal candidiasis presents with odynophagia. Oral thrush may, or may not, also be present. Endoscopy is required for confirmation in most patients. In AIDS patients with odynophagia, empiric treatment with fluconazole is reasonable. If symptoms do not subside in 3 to 4 days, endoscopy is indicated to exclude alternative causes such as herpes simplex, cytomegalovirus, and malignancy.

Vulvovaginal candidiasis presents with vaginal itching, soreness, dysuria, and dyspareunia. Vaginal discharge is often absent; when present, it may be thick and curdy, sometimes described by the patient as "cheesy." Odor is usually absent. In addition to

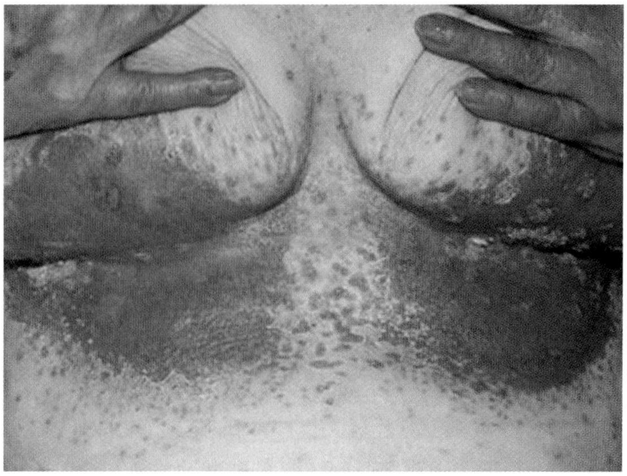

Figure 192-1 *Candida intertrigo, with prominent satellite lesions at the margins. (Reproduced, with permission, from Wolff K, Goldsmith LA, Katz SI, et al. Fitzpatrick's Dermatology in General Medicine. 7th ed. New York: McGraw-Hill; 2008. Fig. 189-4B.)*

potassium hydroxide preparations, the usual investigations for the diagnosis of vaginitis should be performed, including the "whiff" test, vaginal pH measurement, and microscopy with saline ("wet prep") for trichomonads, white cells, and clue cells. Sexually active women with vaginal discharge should also have studies to exclude chlamydial and gonorrheal infection.

Urinary tract infection

Candida species are readily grown from urine culture. Most patients with candiduria have underlying illness, such as recent surgery, diabetes mellitus, an abnormal urinary tract, or malignancy, have been treated with antibiotics in the preceding month, and have indwelling urinary catheters or other urinary drainage devices. On many occasions when candiduria is documented, urine cultures were performed for inadequate reasons, such as cloudy urine without other symptoms. The vast majority of patients with candiduria are asymptomatic, and funguria tends to clear spontaneously without treatment. Progression to candidemia is unusual, and when it does occur, it is generally seen in patients who also have central venous catheters.

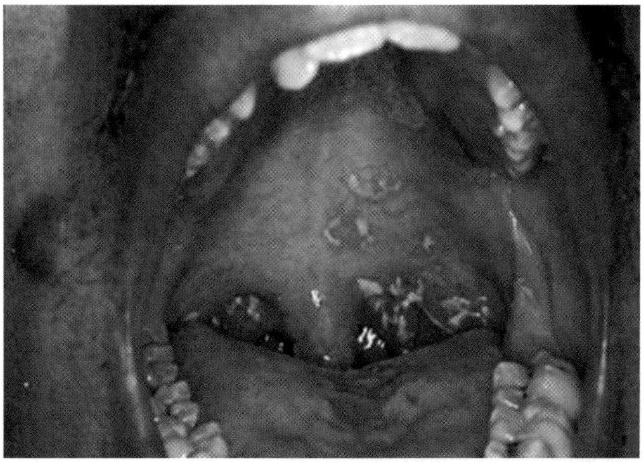

Figure 192-2 *Oral thrush, with characteristic plaques on the hard palate. (Reproduced, with permission, from Wolff K, Goldsmith LA, Katz SI, et al. Fitzpatrick's Dermatology in General Medicine. 7th ed. New York: McGraw-Hill; 2008. Fig. 189-2A.)*

TABLE 192-1 *Candida* Score for Discriminating between *Candida* Colonization and Invasive Candidiasis in Nonneutropenic Patients

Risk Factor	Points
Multifocal candidal colonization	1
Recent surgery	1
Total parenteral nutrition	1
Severe sepsis	3

A *Candida* score of ≥ 3 in a critically ill patient is associated with an eightfold increased risk of disseminated candidiasis; early antifungal administration is warranted.

Data from Leon C, Ruiz-Santana S, Saavedra P, et al. Usefulness of the "*Candida score*" for discriminating between *Candida* colonization and invasive candidiasis in non-neutropenic critically ill patients: a prospective multicenter study. *Crit Care Med.* 2009;37:1624–1633.

Candidemia and disseminated Candidiasis

Candidemia and disseminated candidiasis (*Candida* infection of usually sterile sites) should be suspected in febrile or septic patients with exposure to antibiotics, intravenous catheters, parenteral nutrition, immunosuppressive agents, or chemotherapy. *Candida* species, unlike some other fungi, are not fastidious and can be grown without difficulty from blood cultures and subcultured onto regular blood agar plates. However, the diagnosis of disseminated candidiasis may be elusive as only half of patients with disseminated candidiasis have documented candidemia. The *Candida* score (**Table 192-1**) has been proposed as a diagnostic tool to define a population of sick patients at high risk of disseminated candidiasis who would benefit from early antifungal therapy.

The serum 1,3-β-D-glucan (**Table 192-2**) is a promising, if imperfect, adjunctive test in the diagnosis of invasive candidiasis. This component of the cell wall of *Candida* and other fungi may be detected in the serum of patients with candidemia and disseminated candidiasis, sometimes at high levels. However, the 1,3-β-D-glucan test currently lacks specificity, and false-positive results are common, especially for results close to the threshold of normal.

TABLE 192-2 Usefulness and Limitations of 1,3-β-D-Glucan Assays

Fungal infections that may result in positive tests
Candidemia/invasive candidiasis
Aspergillosis
Cryptococcosis
Histoplasmosis
Blastomycosis
Coccidioidomycosis
Pneumocystis jiroveci (formerly *Pneumocystis carinii*) pneumonia
Causes of false-positive tests
Bacteremia, including *Streptococcus pneumoniae* and *Pseudomonas aeruginosa*
Antibiotics (amoxicillin-clavulanic acid, piperacillin-tazobactam)
Hemodialysis with cellulose membranes
Immunoglobulin and albumin infusion with cellulose filters
Serosal exposure to gauze

Patients with candidemia or possible disseminated candidiasis should be asked about focal complaints suggestive of metastatic *Candida* infection, such as eye pain and decreased visual acuity (endophthalmitis), back pain (vertebral osteomyelitis), and joint pain (septic arthritis). An important if rare variant of disseminated candidiasis is hepatosplenic candidiasis, or chronic disseminated candidiasis. This typically occurs in patients with persistent fever after recovery from neutropenia. Right upper quadrant pain and elevated liver enzymes may be present. Abdominal CT scan demonstrates hepatic, splenic, and renal microabscesses.

TREATMENT

Mucocutaneous Candida (cutaneous, thrush, esophagitis, vaginitis)

The treatment of **candida intertrigo** should include measures to improve aeration and drying of involved skin folds; correction of predisposing factors, such as hyperglycemia; and a topical antifungal agent, such as nystatin or an azole. Some authors argue that an antifungal cream or ointment should be used for the first several days due to their superior skin penetration, followed by several days of a drying agent, such as nystatin powder. Antifungal powders may also be used as maintenance therapy in patients at high risk of relapse. Topical glucocorticoids should be avoided, as they reduce inflammation while allowing fungal infection to persist.

Mild cases of **oral thrush** may be treated topically with clotrimazole troches 10 mg five times daily, nystatin suspension (at a concentration of 100,000 U/mL) 5 mL four times daily, or nystatin pastilles (200,000 U each) four times daily for 7 to 14 days. Moderate to severe disease is treated with fluconazole 100–200 mg orally once daily for 7 to 14 days. **Esophageal candidiasis** is treated with oral (or intravenous, in patients unable to swallow) fluconazole 200–400 mg daily for 14–21 days.

Vulvovaginal candidiasis may be successfully treated with many topical agents, including clotrimazole 100 mg vaginal tablet, or 5 g of 1% clotrimazole cream, intravaginally once daily for 7 days. Some patients prefer a single dose of 150 mg oral fluconazole for its greater ease of administration.

Urinary tract infection

Patients with asymptomatic urinary tract infection do not require antifungal treatment, with the exception of neutropenic patients, low birth weight neonates, or patients undergoing urologic procedures. Ideally, predisposing factors should be eliminated, such as indwelling urinary catheters or stents, or receipt of broad spectrum antibiotics.

For the treatment of symptomatic patients, oral fluconazole is preferred because of high urinary tract concentrations and ease of administration. *Candida* cystitis is treated with fluconazole 200 mg once daily for 14 days, and *Candida* pyelonephritis with fluconazole 200–400 mg once daily for 14 days.

Candidemia/Disseminated Candidiasis

Susceptibility patterns differ among *Candida* species. *Candida albicans* and *Candida tropicalis* are usually sensitive to fluconazole, amphotericin B, and echinocandins. *Candida parapsilosis* is sometimes resistant to echinocandins. *Candida glabrata* and *Candida krusei* may be resistant to fluconazole.

In nonneutropenic patients with candidemia and mild illness, fluconazole is reasonable initial therapy. For nonneutropenic patients with moderate to severe illness, patients with recent azole exposure, neutropenia, or infection with *C glabrata* or *C krusei*, an echinocandin is preferred. Fluconazole is preferred for *C parapsilosis* infection; echinocandins should be avoided in this setting. Amphotericin B use has become much less common due to the availability of less toxic agents.

Antifungal susceptibility testing is expensive and not routinely performed for most bloodstream *Candida* isolates, but it should be obtained in *C glabrata* isolates from blood and in other sterile site *Candida* isolates that fail to respond to therapy.

In nonneutropenic patients, candidemia should be treated for at least 2 weeks after blood cultures become negative and symptoms have resolved; longer courses are indicated in metastatic disease (eg, *Candida* endophthalmitis, meningitis, or osteomyelitis). *Candida* endocarditis usually requires valve replacement. Neutropenic patients with candidemia should be treated for at least 2 weeks after blood cultures become sterile and symptoms and neutropenia have both resolved.

Intravenous catheters should be removed from patients with candidemia who are not neutropenic. Catheter removal should be considered in neutropenic patients, although this may create intravenous access problems, and the benefit is less marked than in nonneutropenic patients, perhaps because mucositis and gut overgrowth are important sources for candidemia in the setting of neutropenia.

Infectious disease consultation is indicated in patients with suspected or proved candidemia or disseminated candidiasis.

Complications of Candidemia

As ocular dissemination and endophthalmitis are common in candidemia, ophthalmologic consultation and dilated retinal examination are recommended for all patients with candidemia. *Candida* endocarditis should be suspected in patients with persistent fever and fungemia, embolic manifestations, and cardiac murmurs. Back pain suggests vertebral osteomyelitis. *Candida* meningitis presents with fever, headache, and neck pain, although confusion may predominate in debilitated patients. Chronic renal infection may result in formation of "fungus balls" (*Candida* bezoar), which require surgical removal.

Discharge considerations

It is reasonable to discharge stable patients once they are tolerating antifungal therapy, the course of antifungal therapy has been defined, and appropriate infectious diseases follow-up has been arranged. Patients on long-term therapy with fluconazole or an echinocandin (caspofungin, micafungin, or anidulafungin) should have occasional monitoring of liver enzymes. If discharge is considered in a patient receiving amphotericin B deoxycholate or lipid formulations of amphotericin B, it should be to a facility capable of close daily attention to renal function and serum potassium and magnesium, as well as occasional monitoring of liver enzymes and complete blood counts.

Prevention

Prophylaxis with fluconazole is indicated in a few populations at high risk of invasive candidiasis, such as patients after solid organ transplantation, neutropenic patients undergoing induction chemotherapy or stem cell transplantation, and high-risk patients hospitalized in intensive care units with a high incidence of invasive candidiasis. In women with a history of recurrent *Candida* vulvovaginitis, a 150 mg dose of fluconazole at the beginning and completion of antibiotic therapy may prevent the development of symptomatic vaginal yeast infection.

ASPERGILLUS INFECTION

EPIDEMIOLOGY

Aspergillus species are ubiquitous molds that flourish in soil, decaying vegetation, and damp places, such as basements, at a wide range of temperatures. Human exposure to *Aspergillus* is common;

it is not unusual to inhale hundreds of *Aspergillus* spores on a daily basis. Despite near-universal exposure and occasional bronchial colonization, symptomatic infection is exceedingly rare in normal hosts. Most cases are seen in immunocompromised patients, especially those with neutropenia or receiving high-dose glucocorticoid therapy, and patients with underlying lung disease, especially preexisting lung cavities. Some patients with aspergillosis have low levels of mannose-binding lectin, a serum protein that is part of the innate immune system. It binds to carbohydrate residues of *Aspergillus* and other pathogens, enhancing phagocytosis by activating complement.

DOES THIS PATIENT HAVE ASPERGILLOSIS?

Aspergillus-related disease can be thought of as a spectrum ranging from hypersensitivity (allergic bronchopulmonary aspergillosis), through colonization of pulmonary cavities (aspergillomas, or fungus balls), progressing to local invasion around pulmonary cavities (chronic necrotizing or semiinvasive aspergillosis), to frankly invasive aspergillosis.

Allergic bronchopulmonary aspergillosis (ABPA) is an asthma syndrome driven by airway colonization with *Aspergillus*, which leads to severe and persistent bronchial inflammation and damage. Patients usually have a history of asthma and other atopic diseases or cystic fibrosis (CF). Clinical features of asthma or CF that should increase the suspicion of ABPA include frequent wheezing and poor responses to medical therapy, fatigue, fever, fleeting pulmonary infiltrates, hemoptysis, and expectoration of copious sputum with brown plugs. Patients with advanced ABPA may have central bronchiectasis on chest imaging. About half of patients have a positive sputum culture for *Aspergillus*. (*Aspergillus* grows on regular blood agar from sputum specimens within 1–3 days.)

PRACTICE POINT

Candida and aspergillus in sputum cultures

- *Candida* in a sputum culture rarely requires treatment. While some patients may have additional indications for antifungal therapy, such as oral thrush, or evidence of disseminated candidiasis, antifungal therapy should not be initiated on the basis of a positive sputum culture alone.
- *Aspergillus* species are occasionally isolated from sputum cultures of elderly hospitalized patients. Most of these patients have underlying lung disease or other chronic illnesses. This usually represents bronchial colonization; less than 5% of these patients are found to have invasive pulmonary aspergillosis. More aggressive evaluation is warranted in patients with fever, pulmonary infiltrates, or weakened immunity.

The screening test for ABPA is a skin prick test with *Aspergillus* antigens. A negative result rules out ABPA. A positive result (a wheal-and-flare reaction) is not specific for ABPA and should be confirmed with other tests, such as measurement of total serum immunoglobulin E (IgE) and *Aspergillus*-specific IgE or IgG.

Aspergillomas are masses of fungal material and cellular host debris in preexisting lung cavities in patients with bullous emphysema, sarcoidosis, old tuberculosis, or other lung conditions. These are sometimes asymptomatic and are picked up incidentally on chest radiography. Symptomatic aspergillomas present with cough, hemoptysis, malaise, weight loss, and occasionally fever. Bacterial superinfection may occur and may be mistaken for a primary lung abscess. The diagnosis is usually made on the basis of the typical radiographic appearance of a ball within a lung cavity. If the patient is rotated during chest computed tomographic (CT) scanning, the ball should be found to be mobile. Sputum and bronchoalveolar lavage cultures positive for *Aspergillus* species are supportive of the diagnosis, as are elevated *Aspergillus*-specific IgG. Erythrocyte sedimentation rate and C-reactive protein are usually elevated but are very nonspecific.

Chronic necrotizing aspergillosis may arise as an aspergilloma that gradually invades the surrounding lung parenchyma. Symptoms are similar to those of aspergillomas but more severe. Patients have slowly worsening cough, shortness of breath, and sometimes chest pain. Fever, malaise, and weight loss are often present. Hemoptysis may be massive and is the most usual cause of death in patients with chronic necrotizing aspergillosis. The definitive diagnosis of chronic necrotizing aspergillosis is based on the finding of fungal hyphae with tissue invasion and infarction on lung biopsy. However, the yield from percutaneous biopsy is low, and thorascopic and open-lung biopsies are hazardous in these patients because of the risk of severe bleeding. (If tissue is sent to microbiology for culture, it should be held for 4 weeks as the inoculum may be very small.) More often, the diagnosis is based on clinical findings. The radiographic findings are similar to those of an aspergilloma, but cavities tend to be larger and thicker walled. Pleural thickening may be present next to the cavity. *Aspergillus* IgG or IgE are usually elevated, but sputum cultures are only sometimes positive for *Aspergillus* species. Antigen tests (serum galactomannan and 1,3-β-D-glucan) are usually not helpful.

Invasive pulmonary aspergillosis (IPA) usually presents as an acute pneumonia in a severely immunosuppressed patient, with cough, fever, and dyspnea. *Aspergillus* species often invade blood vessels, leading to bleeding, hemoptysis, tissue infarction, and hematogenous dissemination, especially to the central nervous system. Radiologic findings are variable and nonspecific. High-resolution chest CT may show nodules, ground-glass changes, or peribronchial infiltrates. There may be low attenuation around lung nodules due to hemorrhage and infarction (halo sign), which may progress to formation of a lucent zone after recovery from neutropenia (air crescent sign). While sputum cultures are negative for *Aspergillus* in up to 70% of patients with IPA, a positive sputum for *Aspergillus* in an immunosuppressed patient with pneumonia is strongly suggestive of IPA. The yield of bronchoscopy with cultures of bronchoalveolar lavage fluid is about 50%. Tissue biopsies have a high yield but may not be feasible due to thrombocytopenia. On biopsy specimens, *Aspergillus* species appear as filamentous fungi with frequent septations and acute-angle branching (other fungi have a similar appearance, including *Pseudallescheria boydii* and *Fusarium* species).

Elevations in serum galactomannan, a cell-wall constituent of *Aspergillus* and other molds, support the diagnosis of IPA in high-risk populations, with some limitations (**Table 192-3**). At the higher cutoff values of 1.5 Optical Density Index (ODI), sensitivity is 64% and specificity is 95%. At a lower cutoff of 0.5 ODI, sensitivity rises to 78%, but specificity falls to 81%. Serial measurements of serum galactomannan may be helpful in assessing the response to therapy. Serum 1,3-β-D-glucan is less sensitive and specific than galactomannan for the diagnosis of IPA. Polymerase chain reaction for *Aspergillus* DNA is still experimental in this setting.

TREATMENT

High-dose glucocorticoids are the primary treatment of ABPA. Antifungal therapy is also helpful: oral itraconazole diminishes the burden of airway colonization with *Aspergillus*, improves clinical outcomes, and allows more rapid tapering of glucocorticoids. Anti-IgE antibody (omalizumab) is a promising experimental treatment.

TABLE 192-3 Usefulness and Limitations of Galactomannan Assays

Fungal infections that may result in positive tests
Aspergillosis
Other mold infections (*Penicillium, Paecilomyces, Alternaria, Geotrichia, Fusaria*, many others)
Cryptococcosis
Histoplasmosis
Causes of false-positive tests
Antibiotics (amoxicillin-clavulanic acid, piperacillin-tazobactam, ticarcillin-clavulanic acid)
Gluconate-containing intravenous fluids (eg, Plasmalyte)
Graft-versus-host disease of the gastrointestinal tract

Avoidance of damp areas where *Aspergillus* exposure is likely, and domestic use of high-efficiency particulate air (HEPA) filtration units, may also be beneficial.

Surgical therapy for aspergillomas and chronic necrotizing aspergillosis is potentially curative, and thoracic surgery consultation, as well as infectious diseases and pulmonology involvement, should be obtained for these patients. However, because of poor underlying lung function, surgery is risky and fraught with major complications, including bronchopleural fistulas, hemothorax, and *Aspergillus* empyema. Patients with asymptomatic aspergillomas may be observed. Patients with symptomatic aspergillomas or chronic necrotizing aspergillosis may be treated with oral itraconazole or voriconazole, or intravenous voriconazole if they are acutely ill. Patients with chronic necrotizing aspergillosis often require lifelong antifungal therapy.

The prognosis of invasive aspergillosis is poor. Antifungal therapy should be initiated as soon as the disease is clinically suspected, and infectious diseases and pulmonary consultation should be obtained. Doses of immunosuppressive drugs, such as glucocorticoids, should be minimized. Intravenous voriconazole is recommended as primary therapy, with initial doses of 6 mg/kg intravenous (IV) every 12 hours for the first day, followed by 4 mg/kg IV every 12 hours thereafter. Six to 12 weeks is the minimum duration of therapy. The oral formulation has high bioavailability, and patients may be transitioned to the oral form once they are clinically stable and tolerating oral intake. Voriconazole directly stimulates the retina, resulting in blurring, light sensitivity, and other visual disturbances in up to 30% of patients; this phenomenon is reversible and generally mild. Liver enzymes should be monitored on therapy. Patients with renal insufficiency should be treated with oral voriconazole as the IV solubilizer of voriconazole (β-cyclodextrin) may accumulate and lead to worsening renal function. Alternative agents include caspofungin, posaconazole, or lipid formulations of amphotericin B.

Complications

If it is unclear whether patients are responding to voriconazole, an echinocandin may be added or substituted. (Note that pulmonary infiltrates in patients with IPA may worsen in the first week of therapy or after recovery from neutropenia.) Clinicians should monitor patients with IPA for symptoms and signs suggestive of hematogenous dissemination of *Aspergillus* to other organs, especially the brain, eye, heart, skin, and gastrointestinal tract. Patients with metastatic lesions may benefit from surgical debridement to reduce symptoms and increase the chance of cure. Patients with IPA and major hemoptysis, or pulmonary infiltrates adjacent to the great vessels or pericardium, may need surgery to prevent exsanguination. In patients with major hemoptysis and chronic necrotizing aspergillosis, bronchial artery embolization may be useful as a temporizing measure until medical therapy has time to be effective.

Discharge considerations

Patients may be discharged on oral voriconazole therapy when medically stable, with infectious diseases and other subspecialty follow-up as indicated, and periodic monitoring of hepatic enzymes.

Prevention

In certain very high risk populations, such as stem cell transplant recipients and patients undergoing chemotherapy for acute leukemia, prophylaxis with posaconazole for invasive aspergillosis is warranted. At-risk patients should also be cared for in special units with HEPA filters and other measures to minimize fungal exposure.

SUGGESTED READINGS

Kauffman CA. Candiduria. *Clin Infect Dis*. 2005;41(suppl 6):S371–S376.

Leeflang MM, Debets-Ossenkopp YJ, Visser CE, et al. Galactomannan detection for invasive aspergillosis in immunocompromised patients. *Cochrane Database Syst Rev*. 2008;4:CD007394.

Leon C, Ruiz-Santana S, Saavedra P, et al. Usefulness of the "*Candida* score" for discriminating between *Candida* colonization and invasive candidiasis in non-neutropenic critically ill patients: a prospective multicenter study. *Crit Care Med*. 2009;37:1624–1633.

Pappas PG, Kauffman CA, Andes D, et al. Clinical practice guidelines for the management of candidiasis: 2009 update by the Infectious Diseases Society of America. *Clin Infect Dis*. 2009;48:503–535.

Soubani AO, Khanchandani G, Ahmed HP. Clinical significance of lower respiratory tract *Aspergillus* culture in elderly hospitalized patients. *Eur J Clin Microbiol Infect Dis*. 2004;23:491–494.

Walsh TJ, Anassie EJ, Denning DW, et al. Treatment of aspergillosis: clinical practice guidelines of the Infectious Diseases Society of America. *Clin Infect Dis*. 2008;46:327–360.

Wheat JL. Approach to the diagnosis of invasive aspergillosis and candidiasis. *Clin Chest Med*. 2009;30:367–377.

CHAPTER 193

Histoplasmosis, Blastomycosis, Coccidioidomycosis, and Other Dimorphic Fungi

Donald C. Vinh, MD, FRCP, FACP
John M. Embil, MD, FRCPC

Key Clinical Questions

1. What are the dimorphic mycoses, and where are they endemic?
2. What are the clinical manifestations of symptomatic histoplasmosis?
3. What is the most common extrapulmonary manifestation of blastomycosis?
4. What patients are at greater risk for disseminated coccidioidomycosis?
5. What is the most common clinical presentation of sporotrichosis?

INTRODUCTION

The dimorphic mycoses are fungi which exist in the environment as a mold, but adopt a yeast-like form in the warmer conditions of the infected host. They include blastomycosis, coccidioidomycosis, histoplasmosis, penicilliosis, paracoccidioidomycosis, and sporotrichosis. With the exception of sporotrichosis, these fungi are found only in certain geographic regions. However, they may stay dormant in the host, and reactivate when the host is no longer in an endemic area, making recognition of these infections more challenging.

HISTOPLASMOSIS

Histoplasma capsulatum is endemic to river basins of the United States and Canada, particularly the Mississippi, Missouri, Ohio, and St. Lawrence River valleys, as well as southwestern Ontario. It is also prevalent in Central America and the Caribbean, Southeast Asia (especially Vietnam, Thailand, Indonesia, and Malaysia), and the Mediterranean basin. In the environment, *H capsulatum* is found in acidic, nitrogen-rich soil, conditions provided by bird or bat guano. Infections may occur when such soil is disrupted. Certain occupations, such as farming, landscaping, demolition, and construction, or recreational activities, such as spelunking, may lead to high-inoculum exposures and outbreaks.

CLINICAL MANIFESTATIONS

In the vast majority of cases, persons infected with *H capsulatum* are asymptomatic or have only a very mild illness that is never recognized to be histoplasmosis. (These patients may be noted later in life to have pulmonary and splenic calcifications on imaging studies, consistent with remote histoplasmosis.)

A variety of clinical syndromes are seen in symptomatic patients. It is estimated that < 1% of infected patients develop symptoms, although the manifestations can be diverse (**Table 193-1**). It typically presents as a self-limited pneumonic illness, characterized by chest discomfort and dry cough, with fever, fatigue, headache, myalgias, and arthralgias. Radiographically, patchy lung infiltrates involving one or more lobes is seen, frequently accompanied by mediastinal and hilar lymphadenopathy. In most patients, improvement is prompt even without treatment, although fatigue may persist. Most patients who seek medical attention are initially misdiagnosed with community-acquired pneumonia syndrome due to atypical organisms such as *Mycoplasma* or *Chlamydophila*. These patients usually improve without antifungal treatment. A minority of patients with acute self-limited pulmonary histoplasmosis develop extrapulmonary manifestations, such as erythema nodosum, self-limited symmetrical polyarticular arthritis, or sterile exudative pleural or pericardial effusions. Severe acute pulmonary histoplasmosis may occur, especially in patients with impaired cell-mediated immunity, and occasionally in persons exposed to large inocula. It features the abrupt onset of fever, chills, cough, and dyspnea, with diffuse, bilateral reticulonodular or miliary infiltrates; intrathoracic lymphadenopathy may or may not be present. Acute respiratory distress syndrome may ensue.

Acute disseminated histoplasmosis occurs in patients with impaired cell-mediated immunity, such as AIDS. It manifests with relatively rapid onset of fever, chills, anorexia, malaise, and weight loss. Most patients also have pulmonary involvement,

TABLE 193-1 Manifestations of Histoplasmosis

Acute pulmonary histoplasmosis syndromes
Asymptomatic/mild respiratory symptoms (most common)
Acute pneumonia, mimicking community-acquired atypical pneumonia
Severe, life-threatening pneumonia
Complications of acute pulmonary histoplasmosis
Cutaneous: erythema nodosum and erythema marginatum
Rheumatologic: myalgias, arthralgias, polyarticular symmetrical arthritis
Inflammatory pericarditis with or without pleural effusion
Granulomatous mediastinitis
Fibrosing mediastinitis
Chronic cavitary pulmonary histoplasmosis
May be accompanied by "marching cavity" or pleural thickening
Disseminated histoplasmosis
Acute disseminated histoplasmosis
Chronic progressive disseminated histoplasmosis
Endocarditis/endovascular histoplasmosis
Central nervous system histoplasmosis

with dyspnea and cough, and diffuse reticulo-nodular, miliary, or interstitial infiltrates on chest imaging. Many other systems may be involved. Ulcers, nodules, or verrucous lesions may be present in the oral cavity. Patients may have skin ulcers, nodules, and umbilicated papules. There is usually hepatosplenomegaly and generalized lymphadenopathy. Bone marrow involvement may lead to pancytopenia. Granulomatous destruction of the adrenal glands may result in adrenal insufficiency. Gastrointestinal involvement is common in autopsy series, but is seldom symptomatic; it may occasionally produce abdominal discomfort and diarrhea. Culture-negative endocarditis, central nervous system infection, septic arthritis, and osteomyelitis may also occur. The presentation of acute disseminated histoplasmosis can be dramatic, manifesting as severe sepsis, acute respiratory distress syndrome, multiorgan failure, disseminated intravascular coagulation, or reactive hemophagocytosis.

PRACTICE POINT

- The presumed ocular histoplasmosis syndrome (POHS) causes vision loss and blindness due to chorioretinal scarring and macular choroidal neovascularization. Patients are typically aged 20 to 50 years, and present with sudden onset of blurred vision and loss of central visual acuity. Involvement is often bilateral. Most patients have resided in areas where histoplasmosis is endemic, and have pulmonary and lymph node calcification suggestive of past histoplasmosis infection. The histoplasmin skin test is usually positive. As antifungals are not beneficial, POHS probably represents an allergic reaction to histoplasma antigen trapped in the retina or choroidal vessels, rather than active infection. The prognosis was historically poor, but is much improved with contemporary therapies, including laser photocoagulation and monoclonal antibody to vascular endothelial growth factor.

Chronic progressive disseminated histoplasmosis typically occurs in older adults with no obvious immunosuppression. Patients present with fever, night sweats, weight loss, and fatigue over several months. Diffuse organ involvement similar to acute disseminated histoplasmosis is observed. Both forms of disseminated histoplasmosis are fatal if untreated.

Chronic cavitary pulmonary histoplasmosis presents in older adults with preexisting pulmonary disease, usually emphysema. Patients have prolonged symptoms of cough, dyspnea, sputum production, and occasionally hemoptysis, resembling exacerbations of chronic obstructive pulmonary disease, but also accompanied by fatigue, fever, night sweats, anorexia, and weight loss. Radiologically, there are unilateral or bilateral cavitary upper lobe infiltrates with lower lobe fibrosis. Histoplasmosis infection of emphysematous bullae leads to wall thickening, fibrosis, and cavity formation. Ongoing necrosis can increase the size of the cavity, leading to the so-called "marching cavity," with lobar destruction and progressive respiratory insufficiency. Pleural thickening adjacent to involved lung is usually seen. Fibrosis can lead to lung retraction and volume loss. Lymphadenopathy is uncommon, although calcified lymph nodes can be seen. This constellation of findings can be mistaken for tuberculosis or lung cancer, particularly in an older person with tobacco exposure.

Two rare chronic complications of histoplasmosis are worthy of mention. In most patients with acute pulmonary histoplasmosis, mediastinal lymph nodes enlarge but subsequently recede and calcify. However, in ***granulomatous mediastinitis***, mediastinal and hilar lymph nodes become massive, matted, and occasionally necrotic, with enlargement persisting for months to years. In most patients, cultures are negative for *H capsulatum*. Many patients are asymptomatic. Symptoms develop if the enlarged lymph nodes coalesce and compress adjacent structures, such as bronchi, causing recurrent postobstructive pneumonias, the superior vena cava, leading to the superior vena cava syndrome, or the esophagus, resulting in dysphagia, esophageal diverticula, or tracheoesophageal fistula. Fistulous tracts may result if the nodes drain spontaneously into adjacent structures, such as the airway or soft tissues of the neck. Most individuals have a protracted recovery over months to years, with ultimate calcification of the involved nodes.

Fibrosing mediastinitis is rare. Exuberant mediastinal fibrosis probably results from a reaction to *Histoplasma* antigens in predisposed individuals, rather than ongoing infection, as the organism is rarely seen in biopsies of involved tissue. Systemic symptoms are typically absent. The fibrotic response gradually encroaches on adjacent structures, compressing the great vessels, esophagus, heart, and the airways. It is often fatal.

DIAGNOSIS

The diagnosis of histoplasmosis is subject to several technical difficulties (**Table 193-2**). Definitive diagnosis requires the visualization of the yeast form in clinical specimens (**Figure 193-1**), or isolation of *H capsulatum* in microbiological culture. However, *H capsulatum* needs special media for recovery, and may take up to 4 weeks to grow. The sensitivity of culture is highest in chronic pulmonary histoplasmosis and disseminated histoplasmosis, where the fungal burden is large. Culture is less sensitive in milder forms of histoplasmosis with a low fungal burden. An additional limitation of culture is that the long turnaround time precludes its use for early diagnosis and initiation of treatment of histoplasmosis.

Nonculture methods have been developed to improve the diagnosis of histoplasmosis, primarily through antibody or antigen detection. For antibody detection, the two routine methodologies are complement fixation (CF) and immunodiffusion (ID). CF

TABLE 193-2 Diagnostic Approach for Different Clinical Manifestations of Histoplasmosis

Manifestation	Diagnostic Tests
Mild acute respiratory symptoms	Serology (complement-fixation and immunodiffusion antibodies)
Acute pulmonary histoplasmosis	Bronchoalveolar lavage with antigen detection, fungal culture and stains Urine: antigen detection Serum: antigen detection; acute and convalescent serology Consider lung biopsy
Granulomatous mediastinitis or fibrosing mediastinitis	Serology
Chronic pulmonary histoplasmosis	Respiratory secretions: fungal stain and culture Serology
Disseminated histoplasmosis	Blood: fungal culture; antigen detection Urine: antigen detection Serology Bronchoalveolar lavage: antigen detection, fungal stain and culture Consider bone marrow biopsy, if patient has pancytopenia and other tests are negative When using antigen detection to monitor disease, serial testing should be performed before treatment, at 2 wk, 1 mo, and then every 3 mo during therapy, and for at least 6 mo after treatment is stopped

antibodies are more sensitive than immunodiffusion, and are the better screening test. Complement-fixing antibodies appear 2 to 6 weeks after infection and precede the ID response. A high titer (1:32 or greater) or a 4-fold increase in titer over time indicates active histoplasmosis. However, CF antibodies are less specific, often cross-reacting to *Histoplasma*-like antigens in patients infected with other fungi, such as blastomycosis, coccidioidomycosis, aspergillosis, candidiasis, and cryptococcosis. ID measures antibodies that precipitate (precipitins) to specific *Histoplasma* antigens. These antibodies appear 4 to 8 weeks after infection. While ID is more specific for histoplasmosis than CF, it is less sensitive. Limitations to serologic testing include delays of many weeks before seroconversion occurs, and the frequent absence of seroconversion in immunosuppressed patients with disseminated histoplasmosis. Positive serology results may also represent prior resolved infection, rather than active histoplasmosis.

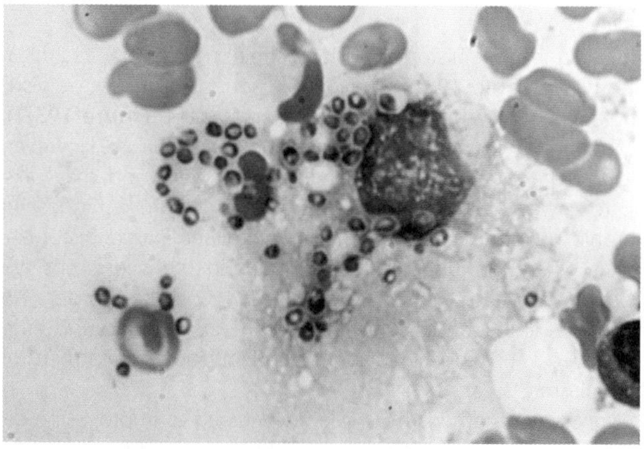

Figure 193-1 *Disseminated histoplasmosis. Bone marrow biopsy, demonstrating intracellular yeast forms in a macrophage.*

Antigen detection allows histoplasmosis to be diagnosed more rapidly than traditional methods. It is most useful in patients with disseminated histoplasmosis, where its sensitivity is 95% to 98%. In patient with early acute pulmonary histoplasmosis, its sensitivity is 75% to 90%. The sensitivity of antigen detection is higher in urine, relative to serum. Antigen may also be detected in broncho-alveolar lavage (BAL) fluid of patients with diffuse pulmonary infiltrates. Antigen levels can be serially followed to monitor response to therapy and diagnose relapse. Antigen testing is markedly less sensitive in the diagnosis of chronic cavitary pulmonary histoplasmosis.

TREATMENT

Treatment recommendations for histoplasmosis are summarized in (**Table 193-3**).

BLASTOMYCOSIS

Blastomyces dermatitidis is a thermally dimorphic fungus. In the United States, it is endemic in the states bordering the Great Lakes and in the Mississippi River basin. It is especially common in Wisconsin, Mississippi, Missouri, Kentucky, Tennessee, Arkansas, and Alabama. In Canada, blastomycosis is endemic in Manitoba and western Ontario, and is occasionally encountered in eastern Canada. It is also seen sporadically worldwide. Risk factors for blastomycosis infection include exposure to soil, especially disrupted or aerosolized soil, recreational or professional exposure to waterways, and immunosuppression.

Infections occur from inhalation of aerosolized conidia; rarely, infections result from animal bites or laboratory accidents. Inhaled conidia transform to the yeast phase at body temperature in the lungs. Initial infection may be asymptomatic or lead to symptomatic pneumonia. In either case, most patients contain *B dermatitidis* infection in non-caseating granulomas. A few persons have progressive pneumonia, or develop extrapulmonary manifestations from dissemination beyond the lungs. The most common sites of involvement in blastomycosis, in descending order of frequency, are lung, skin, bone, genitourinary tract, and central nervous system. The median incubation period is 30 to 45 days, with a longer incubation period for extrapulmonary disease.

PRACTICE POINT

- Laboratory-acquired infections with blastomycosis, histoplasmosis, and coccidioidomycosis have occurred. *Coccidioides immitis* is especially hazardous to microbiology technicians, as arthroconidia are easily dispersed and aerosolized in the laboratory. Specimens from patients with suspected coccidioidomycosis should be sent to the clinical microbiology laboratory with explicit notification of this provisional diagnosis, to minimize the risk of inadvertent exposure to laboratory workers.

TABLE 193-3 Recommendations for the Treatment of Histoplasmosis

Manifestation	Primary Treatment	Alternative Treatment	Comments
Asymptomatic	None		
Mild/self-limited disease	None		
Acute pulmonary histoplasmosis	None usually required	If patient remains symptomatic for > 1 mo: itraconazole 200 mg orally three times a day for 3 d, then 200 mg orally qd or twice a day for 6–12 wk	
Acute severe pulmonary histoplasmosis	Lipid-AmB 3–5 mg/kg IV qd for 1–2 wk, then itraconazole 200 mg three times a day for 3 d then 200 mg twice a day (for total 12 wk of itraconazole)	AmB deoxycholate 0.7–1 mg/kg IV qd in place of Lipid-AmB	If there is significant hypoxia or acute respiratory distress syndrome, consider concomitant methylprednisolone 0.5–1 mg/kg IV for the first 1–2 wk of antifungal therapy
Dermatologic/ rheumatologic complications of acute pulmonary histoplasmosis	Nonsteroidal anti-inflammatory drugs	In severe cases, consider prednisone 0.5–1 mg/kg qd (max 80 mg qd) in tapering doses over 1–2 wk	If steroids are administered, itraconazole is recommended: 200 mg orally three times a day for 3 d, then 200 mg orally qd or twice a day for 6–12 wk
Granulomatous mediastinitis	Incidental findings do not usually require therapy	If symptomatic: itraconazole 200 mg orally three times a day for 3 d, then 200 mg orally qd or twice a day for 6–12 wk	
Fibrosing mediastinitis	None	Symptomatic support (eg, intravascular stents for vessel obstruction); airways stents should be approached cautiously because of high risk of granulation tissue leading to recurrent obstruction	If findings suggest more of an inflammatory process (rather than chronic fibrosis), consider antifungal treatment. If clear distinction from granulomatous mediastinitis is not possible, consider antifungal treatment. Corticosteroids are ineffective and are discouraged
Chronic cavitary pulmonary histoplasmosis	Itraconazole 200 mg orally three times a day for 3 d, then 200 mg orally qd or twice a day for ≥ 1 y (possibly 18–24 mo)		Continue treatment until pulmonary imaging reveals no further improvement at 4–6 m intervals. Monitor for ≥ 1 y after treatment is stopped
Disseminated	Lipid-AmB (3–5 mg/kg) IV qd for 1–2 wk, then itraconazole 200 mg orally three times a day for 3 d, then 200 mg twice a day for ≥ 12 mo	AmB deoxycholate 0.7–1 mg/kg IV qd in place of Lipid-AmB; for mild-to-moderate disseminated disease, itraconazole 200 mg orally three times a day for 3 d, then 200 mg orally twice a day for ≥ 12 mo	In patients with irreversible immunocompromise, and in patients who relapse despite appropriate therapy, lifelong suppression with oral itraconazole 200 mg qd Monitor antigen level during therapy, and for 12 months after therapy is ended
Endocarditis	AmB or Lipid-AmB	Surgical valve replacement	If valve surgery is not possible, consider lifelong suppression with itraconazole
Central nervous system	Liposomal AmB (5.0 mg/kg IV qd for a total of 175 mg/kg given over 4–6 wk) followed by itraconazole (200 mg orally 2 or 3 times qd) for ≥ 1 y and until resolution of cerebrospinal fluid abnormalities, including antigen levels		

AmB, amphotericin B; Lipid-AmB, lipid formulation of amphotericin B.
Because of insufficient data, all other available azoles are deemed alternatives to itraconazole.
When using itraconazole, random blood concentration of ≥ 1 µg/mL is recommended.

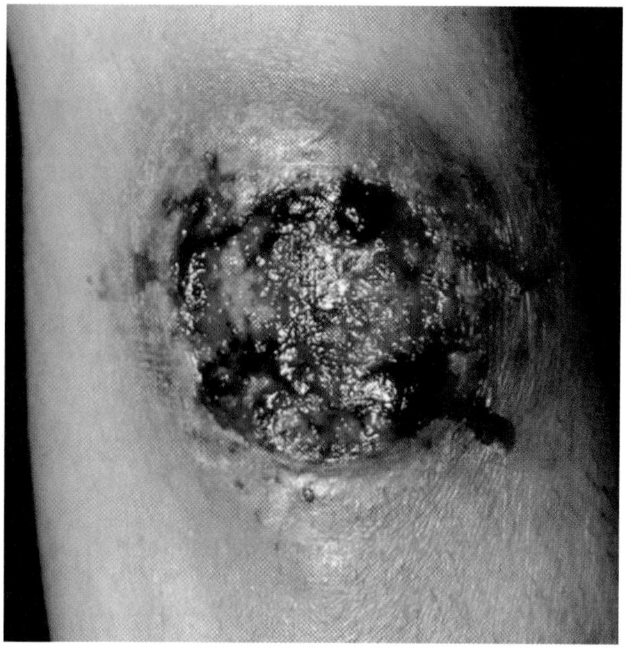

Figure 193-2 *Ulcerative cutaneous blastomycosis on a patient's calf, initially misdiagnosed as pyoderma gangrenosum. (Reproduced, with permission, from Elizabeth Spiers.)*

TABLE 193-4 Diagnostic Tests for Blastomycosis

Technique	Comments
Direct examination	A wet preparation of respiratory secretions or other tissues under light microscope may reveal characteristic forms of the pathogen, but have a low diagnostic yield; calcofluor white stains are more useful but require fluorescence microscopy
Histopathologic examination	The microorganism may be difficult to identify with standard hematoxylin and eosin stains; Gomori methenamine-silver stain should be performed if *B dermatitidis* is suspected
Culture	Diagnostic yield is approximately 86% from sputum and 92% from bronchoscopc specimens. Growth of *B dermatitidis* may require several weeks
Serology	Serology is neither sensitive nor specific
Nucleic acid detection	Detect genetic material in culture specimens where *B dermatitidis* is suspected; may reduce the time required for identification of the pathogen in culture
Antigen detection	The only currently available antigen detection assay has its greatest sensitivity in urine, although antigens can be detected in serum and other body fluids. Cross-reaction with other antigens (eg, histoplasmosis) may occur. Probably most useful in following the efficacy of treatment response
Skin testing	Not currently available for clinical use

CLINICAL MANIFESTATIONS

Blastomycosis is one of the diseases that has been termed "the great mimic." This is particularly true of ***pneumonia*** caused by *B dermatitidis*, which may cause lobar infiltrates indistinguishable from bacterial pneumonia, miliary disease that resembles pulmonary tuberculosis, nodules and mass lesions that are similar to pulmonary neoplasms, and cavities that mimic anaerobic lung abscesses or tuberculosis. Acute pneumonia presents with fevers, chills, dyspnea, and cough which is usually non-productive initially. Chronic pneumonia may develop, with the clinical presentation of a non-resolving community-acquired pneumonia. It may be associated with additional symptoms of weight loss, productive cough, and hemoptysis. Occasionally, patients may develop respiratory failure and the acute respiratory distress syndrome.

Cutaneous lesions are the most common extrapulmonary form of blastomycosis. They result from dissemination of a primary pulmonary lesion or less often from direct inoculation, and are either verrucous or ulcerated in appearance (**Figure 193-2**). Other forms of extrapulmonary blastomycosis include osteomyelitis, with the long bones and axial skeleton being most frequently affected, prostate, and central nervous system involvement, which may present with chronic meningitis, mass lesions, or brain abscess. Blastomycosis may be especially aggressive in immunocompromised hosts, who are prone to respiratory failure and disseminated disease with mortality rates of 30% to 40%.

DIAGNOSIS

(**Table 193-4**) summarizes diagnostic techniques for blastomycosis. The most reliable is recovery of *B dermatitidis* in culture. Direct observation of the pathogen with wet preparations under light microscopy, calcofluor white stains under immunofluorescence microscopy, or biopsy specimens may also be helpful. Serologic assays have limited sensitivity and specificity, and are not reliable in diagnosis. Urinary antigen assays are reasonably sensitive in diagnosis, especially when the burden of disease is high, and newer assays can distinguish blastomycosis from other fungal infections, such as histoplasmosis.

TREATMENT

Amphotericin B deoxycholate is recommended for severe blastomycosis or central nervous system involvement, based on the greater clinical experience with these agents compared to alternative drugs. Lipid preparations of amphotericin may also be effective, although clinical experience in blastomycosis is limited. After stabilization with amphotericin B, patients with severe disease or central nervous system involvement may be stepped down to oral itraconazole to complete the total duration of therapy. Although fluconazole is effective against *B dermatitidis*, experience with this agent is limited. Fluconazole has excellent penetration into the central nervous system, and may be considered in step-down therapy of central nervous system blastomycosis. Voriconazole has also been used in central nervous system blastomycosis and in refractory blastomycosis.

TABLE 193-5 Treatment Regimens for Blastomycosis

Presentation	Treatment Suggestions	Comments
Pulmonary infection		
• Moderate to severe	• Amphotericin B deoxycholate 0.7–1 mg/kg/day for 1–2 wk until stable or lipid preparations of amphotericin B 3–5 mg/kg/day for 1–2 wk followed by oral itraconazole 200 mg twice a day for 6–12 mo	• An alternative approach is to use deoxycholate amphotericin B to complete a total dose of 1.5–2.5 g, however, amphotericin B toxicity can be attenuated by minimizing the duration of therapy and switching to oral therapy when the patient is stable.
• Mild to moderate	• Itraconazole 200 mg orally once daily or twice a day for 6–12 mo	• Alternative therapies that have been suggested are ketoconazole 400–800 mg/kg or fluconazole 400 mg–800 mg/day.
Disseminated infection, not involving central nervous system		
• Moderate to severe	• Amphotericin B deoxycholate 0.7–1 mg/kg/day or lipid preparations of amphotericin B 3–5 mg/kg/day for 1–2 wk followed by oral itraconazole 200 mg twice a day to complete 12 months of therapy.	• An entire treatment course can be completed with deoxycholate amphotericin B to achieve a total dose of 2 g. To minimize toxicity, however, switching to oral therapy once the patient is stable should be considered. Bone and joint infections are usually treated for 12 months with itraconazole.
• Mild to moderate	• Itraconazole 200 mg orally once daily or twice a day for 6–12 mo	• It has been suggested that liposomal amphotericin B achieves higher central nervous system levels than other lipid formulations. Switching to oral fluconazole 800 mg orally once daily or itraconazole 200 mg orally twice a day or three times a day; or voriconazole 200 to 400 mg orally twice a day should be considered. Longer durations of therapy may be necessary for those who are immunocompromised. Bone and joint infections are usually treated for 12 months with itraconazole.
• Involving central nervous system	• Lipid preparations of amphotericin B 5 mg/kg/d for 4–6 wk followed by an oral azole for at least 12 mo	
Special populations		
• Immunocompromised	• Amphotericin B deoxycholate 0.7–1 mg/kg/day or lipid preparation of amphotericin B 3–5 mg/kg/day for 1–2 wk followed by itraconazole 200 mg orally twice a day for 12 mo	• Lifelong suppression with itraconazole 200 mg orally once daily may be required for those in whom immunosuppression cannot be reversed.
• Pregnant	• If the newborn demonstrates evidence of infection, amphotericin B deoxycholate 1.0 mg/kg/day	• During pregnancy, azoles should be avoided because of potential teratogenicity
• Children • Moderate to severe	• Amphotericin B deoxycholate 0.7–1 mg/kg/day or lipid preparation of amphotericin B 3–5 mg/kg/day for 1–2 wk followed by itraconazole 10 mg/kg/day for 12 mo	• Maximum dose of itraconazole should be 400 mg/day
• Mild to moderate	• Itraconazole 10 mg/kg/day for 6–12 mo. Maximum dose is 400 mg/day	

Data from Chapman SW, Bradsher RW, Campbell GD, Pappas PG, Kauffman CA. Practice guidelines for the management of patients with blastomycosis. *Clin Infect Dis.* 2000;30:679–683; and Chapman SW, Dismukes WE, Proia LA, Bradsher RW, Pappas PG, Threlkeld MG, Kauffman CA. Clinical practice guidelines for the management of blastomycosis: 2008 update by the Infectious Diseases Society of America. *Clin Infect Dis.* 2008;46:1801–1812.

The echinocandins, such as caspofungin, micafungin and anidulafungin, have limited activity against *B dermatitidis*, and should be avoided. Pulmonary, cutaneous, or musculoskeletal blastomycosis of mild to moderate severity may be treated with prolonged courses of oral itraconazole. Patients with irreversible immunosuppression may require lifelong suppressive itraconazole therapy at 200 mg per day, after completion of primary therapy (**Table 193-5**).

COCCIDIOIDOMYCOSIS

Coccidioidomycosis is caused by two morphologically indistinguishable but genetically distinct fungi, *Coccidioides immitis* and *Coccidioides posadasii*. *Coccidioides* species grow in nature as a mold composed of barrel-shaped arthroconidia that alternate with nonviable brittle cells. The brittle cells degenerate, allowing the arthroconidia to become airborne in the event of wind or

TABLE 193-6 Main Clinical Manifestations of Coccidioidomycosis

Acute pneumonia
Chronic progressive fibrocavitary pneumonia
Diffuse pneumonia
Pulmonary nodules and cavities
Extrapulmonary, nonmeningeal disease
Meningitis and other central nervous system disease

soil disturbance. Infection occurs after inhalation of an arthroconidial spore. Within the lung, the arthroconidia develop into large multinucleated spherical structures called spherules. These undergo internal division to release infectious endospores, which may develop into new spherules.

Unlike most fungi, which thrive in damp conditions, *Coccidioides* spp are endemic to hot, arid regions of the southwestern United States, particularly Arizona and the San Joaquin Valley of California. They may also be found in neighboring states (New Mexico, Texas, Utah, Nevada), Central America (Mexico, Guatemala, Honduras, Nicaragua) and South America (Venezuela, Colombia, Paraguay, Argentina). The incidence of coccidioidomycosis is increasing, probably because of environmental factors and population influx into endemic regions.

CLINICAL MANIFESTATIONS

The spectrum of illness due to *Coccidoides* spp is broad (**Tables 193-6** and **193-7**). While infection is common, disease is not. Determinants of disease state and severity reflect biological interactions between pathogen and host.

Asymptomatic. Approximately 60% of persons infected by *Coccidioides* spp, as evidenced by recent exposure and skin test conversion, are asymptomatic and identified primarily during epidemiological investigations. Virtually all persons with these subclinical infections are protected from second primary infections.

Symptomatic. The remaining 35% to 40% of infected patients are acutely or subacutely symptomatic. The most common presentation is a mild, influenza-like respiratory syndrome or a community-acquired pneumonia 1 to 3 weeks after exposure. Primary coccidioidal pneumonia cannot readily be distinguished from viral or bacterial pneumonia, and require high clinical suspicion, based on patient residence or travel history, and specific laboratory testing. The most common chest radiographic finding is a non-descript pulmonary infiltrate. In up to 25% of cases, there may be ipsilateral hilar or paratracheal lymphadenopathy. Mediastinal adenopathy is associated with a higher risk of disseminated disease. Pleural effusions are present in 5% to 20% of symptomatic acute primary infections; these are typically small exudates with a predominance of mononuclear cells (usually lymphocytes), and a glucose concentration similar to that of serum. A mild increase in eosinophils may also be seen in pleural fluid.

TABLE 193-7 Symptoms of Acute or Subacute Pulmonary Coccidioidomycosis

Most common
Fever
Cough, with or without sputum production
Pleuritic chest pain
Dyspnea
Systemic
Fatigue, chills, weight loss, night sweats, headache
Associated findings
Toxic erythema: diffuse, erythematous, pruritic rash
Erythema nodosum: painful, erythematous nodules
Erythema multiforme: erythematous, raised patches with a target-like appearance
Arthralgias and myalgias ("desert rheumatism")

Most cases of acute pneumonia resolve completely, either spontaneously or with treatment, within 3 weeks. However, some develop pulmonary or systemic sequelae. Approximately 5% of primary infections result in toxic erythema, erythema nodosum or erythema marginatum, with associated noninfectious arthritis; most of those patients have self-limited infection. Asthenia, or profound fatigue interfering with normal activities, is common and may last weeks to months. Approximately 5% to 10% of patients who present with respiratory symptoms, but without sepsis or extrapulmonary disease, develop residual lung complications, typically nodules or peripheral thin-walled cavities; cavities may be particularly more common in patients with diabetes mellitus. These manifestations may erroneously raise a suspicion of lung cancer, especially in nonendemic areas.

Occasionally, the pneumonic illness persists for several (≥3) months, progressing to a chronic pulmonary infection, with persistent productive cough, hemoptysis, dyspnea, fever, night sweats, fatigue, and weight loss. In association with these symptoms, biapical fibronodular lesions with retraction are commonly seen radiographically; occasionally, cavitary lesions also occur.

Although self-limiting respiratory symptoms is by far the most common presentation of pulmonary coccidioidomycosis, diffuse multilobar pneumonia may also occur. This presentation may occur during primary infection, typically from inhalation of an overwhelmingly large inoculum of arthroconidia in otherwise immunocompetent individuals. Alternatively, it may occur as a late manifestation from hematogenous dissemination in patients with underlying immunodeficiency. Typically, patients are severely ill and hypoxemic; respiratory failure or septic shock may develop. Radiographically, diffuse miliary or reticulonodular infiltrates are seen. As diffuse coccidioidal pneumonia usually results from hematogenous dissemination, patients should be evaluated for extrapulmonary disease.

Pulmonary nodules or cavities may be the residua of acute coccidioidal pneumonia in patients with longitudinal follow-up and serial radiographs. It may also be the initial manifestation of coccidioidal infection, particularly in patients who were previously asymptomatic or subacutely ill. An exposure history and specific *Coccidioides* spp testing may elucidate the cause of the nodule or cavity. However, exclusion of other etiologies may also be necessary. While most coccidioidal nodules or cavities are asymptomatic, they may also be associated with cough, pleuritic chest pain, or hemoptysis, depending on the proximity of the lesions to adjacent structures. Peripheral or pleural-based lesions may even rupture into the pleural space, resulting in a hydropneumothorax.

Disseminated disease occurs via hematogenous dissemination, usually from a primary pulmonary source, and manifests weeks to months after initial infection. Disseminated coccidioidomycosis occurs in <1% to 5% of those infected, with Filipinos, African Americans, Latinos, pregnant women, and immunocompromised patients being at highest risk. The most common sites of involvement are the central nervous system (CNS), skin, bones, joints, lymph nodes. Hepatosplenomegaly and miliary lung disease also occur. Most, but not all, patients with extrapulmonary coccidioidomycosis have disseminated disease.

Coccidioidal CNS disease primarily manifests as meningitis. The most common symptom is headache. Fever and altered mental status may or may not be present. Coccidioidal meningitis is typically basilar in location, and may lead to cranial nerve deficits. Meningismus is found in about 50% of cases. Examination of the cerebrospinal fluid (CSF) reveals lymphocyte-predominant pleocytosis, although neutrophil predominance may be seen. The presence of eosinophils, while uncommon, is highly suggestive of coccidioidal meningitis in a patient with appropriate risk factors. CSF protein is elevated and CSF glucose is depressed. Untreated coccidioidal meningitis is fatal. Even with treatment, patients are high risk for complications. Hydrocephalus is particularly common, and may be either a presenting manifestation or a late complication. Ventriculoperitoneal shunt placement is often necessary. Late-onset hydrocephalus suggests active infection, even in patients on appropriate antifungal therapy. CNS vasculitis with endarteritis obliterans is a particularly dreaded complication, presenting with the rapid development of mental status change and focal neurological deficits.

The skin is the most common site of disseminated disease. Cutaneous coccidioidal disease must be distinguished from immunologic reactions, such as erythema nodosum, accompanying primary pulmonary coccidioidomycosis. Dermatologic manifestations most commonly occur as papules, nodules, or verrucous plaques; lesions can progress to ulcers, with or without draining sinuses, and abscesses. Classically, skin lesions are seen on the nasolabial fold as well as the sternoclavicular area, although they may be seen anywhere.

Musculoskeletal involvement occurs in 20% of patients with disseminated disease. Coccidioidal osteomyelitis most commonly affects the vertebral column. Spinal disease is frequently accompanied by retroperitoneal or paraspinal masses, but spares the intervertebral disks. Affected long bones demonstrate well-demarcated lytic lesions, while smaller bones usually have a moth-eaten appearance.

DIAGNOSIS

Definite diagnosis requires visualization of the fungus in clinical specimens, or growth in fungal culture. The identification of spherules on mycological stains from tissues or fluids is pathognomonic for disease, although the sensitivity varies depending on the type of clinical specimen. Fungal culture is more sensitive than stains, but results are delayed. The availability of specific DNA probes allows earlier identification of positive cultures than traditional tests for dimorphism (mold-to-yeast conversion).

Serology is a mainstay of diagnosis, particularly when satisfactory specimens cannot be obtained for culture. Serology results are also useful for monitoring response to therapy. Two major serologic assays are used. The tube precipitin-reacting antigen detects IgM antibodies, which are detected in up to 75% of case of primary infection. These antibodies eventually disappear with resolution of the primary infection, and are not seen in chronic disease. The complement-fixing (CF) antigen detects IgG antibodies. In addition to indicating chronic infection, the IgG titer correlates with activity of disease. In coccidioidal meningitis, CSF can be tested for IgG by CF antigen to confirm diagnosis; IgG titers in CSF are useful for monitoring disease. Of note, serologic testing may produce false-negative results early in infection as well as in immunosuppressed patients.

An enzyme immunoassay (EIA) for detection of *Coccidioides* spp galactomannan antigen has been developed. This assay performs relatively well in immunocompromised patients with severe coccidioidomycosis, and antigen level correlate well with disease activity.

TREATMENT

Treatment is summarized in (**Table 193-8**).

OTHER DIMORPHIC MYCOSES

PENICILLIOSIS

Penicillium marneffei is a dimorphic fungus endemic to tropical Asia, causing disseminated infections in HIV-positive and immunocompromised travelers and residents. It is most common in Vietnam, Thailand, Taiwan, China, Hong Kong, and northeastern India. The fungus is thought to be a primary pulmonary pathogen, with infection presumably via inhalation of conidia from the environment. Penicilliosis most often affects patients with advanced HIV (CD4+ lymphocyte counts ≤100 cells/μL). Most patients present with fever, weight loss, respiratory symptoms, skin findings, generalized lymphadenopathy, and hepatosplenomegaly. Definitive diagnosis of pencilliosis due to *P marneffei* is made by identification of the fungus from smear, culture, or histopathological sections. Amphotericin B for 2 weeks, followed by itraconazole for 10 weeks, is effective primary therapy. After primary treatment, secondary prophylaxis with itraconazole is given to prevent relapse. HIV-positive patients may possibly discontinue secondary prophylaxis when there is sustained immune reconstitution.

SPOROTRICHOSIS

Sporotrichosis is caused by *Sporothrix schenckii*, a thermally dimorphic fungus with a worldwide distribution. It is ubiquitous in the environment, growing particularly well in soil, sphagnum moss, and decaying vegetation. Gardeners, carpenters, farmers, and forestry workers become infected by traumatic inoculation of fungal spores through the skin, typically from rose and other plant thorns or wood splinters. Cutaneous or lymphocutaneous sporotrichosis is the most common presenting syndrome. After fungal inoculation into soft tissues, a papulonodular lesion develops 1 to 4 weeks later, followed by secondary erythematous nodular lesions ascending proximally along lymphatic channels, a pattern as nodular lymphangitis (**Figure 193-3**). *Mycobacterium marinum* and other pathogens may also cause a similar clinical picture (**Table 193-9**). Diagnosis requires fungal isolation from tissue cultures. Itraconazole or terbinafine are used in treatment. Hot compresses may be a useful adjunctive therapy, as heat inhibits the growth of *Sporothrix schenckii*.

PARACOCCIDIOIDOMYCOSIS

Paracoccidioidomycosis is caused by *Paracoccidioides brasiliensis*, a dimorphic fungus endemic in South America, with most reported cases from Brazil, Colombia, Venezuela, Ecuador, and Argentina. It mainly affects men, and usually presents as an indolent systemic infection over several months, leading to skin nodules, mucosal ulcerations, ulcerative lymphadenitis, and chronic pneumonia of the lower lobes. Hematogenous dissemination may lead to visceral involvement, bone disease, and involvement of the CNS. Definitive diagnosis of paracoccidioidomycosis is based on the visualization of the gemmating (budding) "ship's wheel" yeast-like forms in biopsy specimens, as well as culture and serology. Prolonged treatment is required. Trimethoprim-sulfamethoxazole or itraconazole are used in non–life-threatening disease. Severe disease should be treated initially with amphotericin B.

TABLE 193-8 Management of Coccidioidomycosis

Syndrome	Antifungal Therapy: Primary	Antifungal Therapy: Alternative	Comments
Acute coccidioidal pneumonia			
Uncomplicated	Unclear if treatment necessary in most cases	Some authorities recommend treatment for all symptomatic patients: fluconazole or itraconazole 400 mg qd for at least 4–6 wk after active infection resolved	If no treatment, follow-up recommended every 3–6 mo for up to 2 y (history, physical examination, imaging, serology)
At-risk for disseminated disease*	Fluconazole (400–800 mg) or itraconazole (200–400 mg) qd for 3–6 mo		During pregnancy, amphotericin B is recommended, as azoles may be teratogenic
Severe illness†	Fluconazole (400–800 mg) or itraconazole (400–600 mg) qd for 3–6 mo		
Chronic progressive fibrocavitary pneumonia	Oral azole for at least 1 y	If no improvement with primary azole, consider alternate azole, increasing dose, or amphotericin B	For circumscribed refractory lesions, or if hemoptysis: consider resection
Diffuse pneumonia‡	Amphotericin B (0.5–1.5 mg/kg qd or alternate day) *or* lipid-formulation amphotericin B (≥2.0–5.0 mg/kg per d) or Fluconazole (400–800 mg) until clear evidence of improvement (usually weeks), then maintenance therapy	Maintenance therapy: oral azole for total duration of therapy of at least 1 y; or oral azole for duration of immunodeficiency (if one identified)	Evaluation for extrapulmonary disease should be performed
Pulmonary nodules	For stable nodules:§ antifungal therapy or resection not necessary	For completely resected lesion: antifungal therapy usually not required	For enlarging lesion, confirm diagnosis of coccidioidomycosis, exclude alternate diagnosis (eg, malignancy). Treat if active infection documented
Pulmonary cavities	If asymptomatic: no intervention	If present >2 y later, if enlargement, if adjacent to pleura, if symptomatic (eg, hemoptysis): consider resection. If rupture with pyopneumothorax: lobectomy with decortication	
Extrapulmonary, nonmeningeal disease	Oral azole, consider high-doses (eg, fluconazole up to 2000 mg qd, or itraconazole 800 mg qd)	Amphotericin B or lipid formulation amphotericin B	Consider surgical debridement or stabilization (eg, with vertebral body involvement)
Meningitis	Fluconazole 400 mg qd (up to 800–1000 mg qd)	Itraconazole 400–600 mg qd alone or with Intrathecal amphotericin B 0.1–1.5 mg /dose	Monitor for hydrocephalus, which may require shunt decompression (but not necessarily a change in antifungal agent); after resolution, lifelong azole therapy indicated

*Conditions associated with potential for severe or disseminated disease and thus warrant consideration of treatment include advanced HIV infection, diabetes mellitus, preexisting cardiac or pulmonary disease, pregnancy (especially 3rd trimester or immediate postpartum period), high-dose corticosteroids, tumor necrosis factor antagonists, and Filipino or African descent.

†Age > 55 years; weight loss > 10%; intense night sweats > 3 weeks; symptoms > 2 months; inability to work; infiltrates involving > ½ of one lung or portions of both lungs; prominent or persistent hilar lymphadenopathy; anticoccidioidal complement-fixing antibody > 1:16.

‡Bilateral reticulo-nodular or miliary infiltrates.

§Stable nodule defined as no change in size on serial radiologic imaging for 2 years.

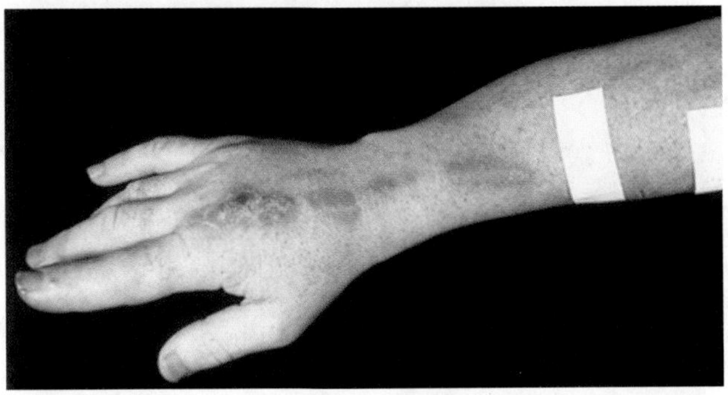

Figure 193-3 *Lymphangitic spread of nodular sporotrichosis. (Reproduced, with permission, from Wolff K, Johnson RA, Suurmond D. Fitzpatrick's Color Atlas & Synopsis of Clinical Dermatology. 5th ed. New York: McGraw-Hill, 2005. Fig. 25-44.)*

TABLE 193-9 Differential Diagnosis of Nodular Lymphangitis

Sporothrix schenckii
Mycobacterium marinum
Francisella tularensis
Nocardia spp
Leishmania brasiliensis
Other fungi: *Blastomyces dermatitidis*; *Histoplasma capsulatum*; *Cryptococcus neoformans*
Miscellaneous: *Bacillus anthracis*; cowpox virus

SUGGESTED READINGS

Assi MA, Sandid MS, Baddour LM, Roberts GD, Walker RC. Systemic histoplasmosis: a 15-year retrospective institutional review of 111 patients. *Medicine (Baltimore)*. 2007;86:162–169.

Chapman SW, Dismukes WE, Proia LA, et al. Clinical practice guidelines for the management of blastomycosis: 2008 update by the Infectious Diseases Society of America. *Clin Infect Dis*. 2008;46:1801–1812.

Galgiani JN, Ampel NM, Blair JE, et al. Infectious Diseases Society of America. Coccidioidomycosis. *Clin Infect Dis*. 2005;41;1217–1223.

Kauffman CA, Bustamante B, Chapman SW, Pappas PG; Infectious Diseases Society of America. Clinical practice guidelines for the management of sporotrichosis: 2007 update by the Infectious Diseases Society of America. *Clin Infect Dis*. 2007;45: 1255–1265.

Wheat LJ, Freifeld AG, Kleiman MB, et al. Infectious Diseases Society of America. Clinical practice guidelines for the management of patients with histoplasmosis: 2007 update by the Infectious Diseases Society of America. *Clin Infect Dis*. 2007;45: 807–825.

CHAPTER 194

Healthcare and Hospital-acquired Pneumonia

Michael Klompas, MD, MPH, FRCPC

Key Clinical Questions

1. What are common mimickers of hospital-acquired pneumonia (HAP)?
2. Is an invasive sampling procedure necessary for accurate diagnosis?
3. Which pathogens typically cause HAP?
4. Which antibiotics are indicated for treatment?
5. For how long should patients be treated?
6. What can be done to prevent HAP?

INTRODUCTION

More than 100 years ago, Sir William Osler noted the frequent mismatch between clinical and postmortem diagnoses of pneumonia. The disparity ran both ways: clinicians overdiagnosed the disease in patients without pneumonia, and failed to diagnose it in patients with demonstrable pneumonia at autopsy. Despite profound advances in the tools available to clinicians, including computed tomography scans, bronchoscopy, and advanced microbiological diagnostics, the diagnosis of hospital-acquired pneumonia (HAP), or pneumonia acquired more than 48 hours after hospital admission, continues to be elusive, partly because it has many mimickers, and partly because the population at risk tends to be very complex.

Misdiagnosis has three serious consequences: failure to treat truly infected patients early is associated with increased mortality, inappropriate use of antibiotics in uninfected patients needlessly promotes antibiotic resistant organisms including *Clostridium difficile*, and premature diagnostic closure delays detection and treatment of the patient's true cause of deterioration. Growing attention from legislators and quality improvement advocates has compounded the importance of accurate diagnosis. Some states now require hospitals to publicly report rates of ventilator-associated pneumonia (VAP), and some insurers have threatened to stop reimbursing hospitals for extra costs incurred due to VAP.

Health care–associated pneumonia is defined as pneumonia in a patient who has received health care as follows:

- Hospitalization in an acute care hospital for 2 or more days within 90 days of the infection
- Residence in a nursing home or long-term care facility
- Administration of intravenous antibiotics, chemotherapy, or wound care within the past 30 days
- Treatment with hemodialysis or attendance at a hospital-based clinic

These patients may present as outpatients, as general medical inpatients, or as ventilated patients in the intensive care unit. Although this chapter focuses primarily on VAP, since mechanically ventilated patients are at greater risk and better studied than other populations, the principles developed here are broadly applicable to all patients with health care–associated pneumonia.

EPIDEMIOLOGY

Reported VAP rates have dropped dramatically over the past 20 years. Older literature reported VAP in 10% to 15% of ventilated patients, but more recent series report VAP in 5% or fewer of ventilated patients. The risk of VAP is primarily related to the duration of mechanical ventilation. Consequently, the risk of VAP is highest in burn and trauma units where mechanical ventilation tends to be prolonged (10.7 and 9.3 VAPs per 1000 ventilator-days in burn and trauma units, respectively), and lowest in units with fewer ventilator days per patient (2.5 VAPs per 1000 ventilator-days in medical and coronary units). On meta-analysis, an episode of VAP appears to extend intensive care length of stay by about 6 days, and doubles the risk of dying. The attributable cost of VAP is approximately $10,000 per episode.

PATHOPHYSIOLOGY

The histological hallmark of HAP is heterogeneity. The lungs of ventilated patients tend to have multiple patchy areas of inflammation and infection, in various stages of recovery and progression. Cultures of these different areas often yield different organisms. These findings reveal the pathophysiology of HAP: patients tend to repeatedly aspirate small amounts of secretions into their lungs that either spontaneously heal, or progress to clinically manifest infection. In intubated patients, organisms enter the lungs through leakage around the endotracheal tube cuff. Processes that increase the risk of aspiration increase the risk of HAP. These include sedation, delirium, impaired consciousness, intubation, vomiting, and abnormal swallowing. Proton pump inhibitors are also associated with an increased risk of pneumonia, presumably because they facilitate greater microbial colonization of the upper gastrointestinal tract.

Causative organisms mirror the ecology of the mouth. The causative agents of HAP vary according to how long patients have been hospitalized. Early infections tend to be caused by the same organisms that cause community acquired pneumonia, namely *Streptococcus pneumoniae, Haemophilus influenzae, Moraxella catarrhalis,* and respiratory viruses such as influenza. Later infections are typically caused by *Staphylococcus aureus* and gram-negative organisms such as *Pseudomonas, Klebsiella, Enterobacter, Acinetobacter*. The longer patients remain in hospital, the greater the risk of colonization and infection with multi-drug-resistant bacteria, including methicillin-resistant *S aureus*, extended spectrum beta-lactamase–resistant gram negatives, and carbapenem-resistant enterobacteraciae.

DIAGNOSIS

There are no pathognomonic findings of VAP. The cardinal signs sought by clinicians (fever, hypoxemia, purulent sputum, leukocytosis, and new radiographic infiltrates) are all insensitive, with positive and negative likelihood ratios near one (**Table 194-1**). Even when present in combination, these signs have a low positive likelihood ratio.

The limited diagnostic value of these signs is due to the complexity of the patient population at risk for VAP. Hospitalized patients in general and ventilated patients in particular tend to be at risk for a wide array of complications superimposed upon underlying conditions and presenting illnesses. As such, each of the signs sought in the diagnosis of pneumonia has a broad differential diagnosis, including non-infectious aspiration pneumonitis, thromboembolic disease, sepsis, atelectasis, pulmonary edema, hemorrhage, contusion, and acute respiratory distress syndrome. Typically, only about a third of patients with the clinical syndrome of VAP (fever, purulent sputum, leukocytosis, and a new infiltrate) are confirmed to have pneumonia if they undergo intensive investigation or autopsy. Instead, two or more alternative processes are often present that alone or in combination mimic the clinical picture of VAP (for example, atelectasis and line sepsis).

TABLE 194-1 Likelihood Ratios of Clinical Signs in Ventilator-associated Pneumonia

Sign	Positive LR	Negative LR
Fever	1.2	0.86
Hypoxemia	1.1	0.91
Purulent sputum (macroscopic)	1.3	0.63
Leukocytosis	1.3	0.74
New radiographic infiltrate	1.7	0.35
Two or more of fever, leukocytosis, and/or purulent sputum	2.8	0.41

TABLE 194-2 Likelihood Ratios of Laboratory Findings in Ventilator-associated Pneumonia

Sign	Positive LR	Negative LR
>50% neutrophils in BAL fluid	2.0	0.09
Organisms seen on Gram stain		
Blind bronchial aspirate	2.1	0.60
Blinded BAL fluid sampling (mini-BAL)	5.3	0.50
Fiberoptically guided BAL fluid sampling (regular BAL)	18	0.56
Quantitative cultures		
Blind bronchial aspirate (> 10^5 CFU/mL)	9.6	0.42
Fiberoptically guided BAL fluid sample (> 10^4 CFU/mL)	1.4	0.78
Protected specimen brush (> 10^3 CFU/mL)	1.6	0.81

BAL, bronchoalveolar lavage; CFU, colony forming units.

Laboratory analysis of pulmonary secretions is critical to aid diagnosis and guide treatment, but considerable judgment is still required to make sense of microbiology results, as their predictive power is nuanced (**Table 194-2**). False-positive and false-negative cultures are common. False-positive cultures usually reflect contamination of the specimen with oral or endotracheal tube colonizers. False-negative cultures are due to sampling an uninfected lung segment, inhibition of bacterial growth by prior antibiotic exposure, or failure to cross an arbitrarily set quantitative growth threshold.

The absence of neutrophils in bronchoalveolar lavage (BAL) fluid helps rule out VAP, but their presence is not diagnostic. By extension, a sputum Gram stain with few or no neutrophils probably makes HAP very unlikely. Visualizing organisms on a BAL Gram stain is suggestive of VAP, and can provide clues about etiology. Organisms on Gram stain from blind bronchial aspirates are less reliable, since these specimens are more prone to contamination. As cultures tend to magnify small amounts of contamination, the converse is true when looking at quantitative culture data. Positive cultures from BAL specimens, which have relatively low growth thresholds for positivity, are often contaminants, but exuberant growth from a bronchial aspirate, which has a high growth threshold for positivity, is predictive of VAP, presumably because bona fide disease has a very high bioburden that is able to outgrow bystander bacteria contaminating the specimen.

A large, multicenter randomized controlled trial comparing routine BAL to endotracheal aspirates to diagnose patients with suspected VAP confirmed the balance of pros and cons between invasive and noninvasive diagnostic methods described above. The trial found no difference in mortality, length of stay, appropriateness of antibiotic choices, or total amount of antibiotic usage between the two study arms. As such, bronchoscopy should be reserved for patients failing therapy guided by endotracheal aspirates.

Radiographic studies also contribute to diagnosis, but as with clinical signs, they lack precision. Portable radiographs often suffer from technical factors that limit interpretation, such as poor inspiration, patient rotation, and obscuring of the lung fields by overlying support tubes and lines. Moreover, as these patients are prone to fluid shifts, uneven ventilation, barotrauma, and alveolar damage, new radiographic opacities may represent pulmonary edema, pleural effusions, or atelectasis, rather than infectious infiltrates. Computed tomography can help distinguish between these entities, but even this modality is imperfect. Atelectasis, pneumonitis, edema, and hemorrhage can resemble consolidation, particularly on noncontrast studies, and it is difficult to distinguish new from resolving infiltrates with a single study. Radiographic findings always need to be interpreted with the patient's clinical picture and trajectory in mind.

Given the absence of definitive signs, laboratory studies, or radiographic evidence for the diagnosis of HAP, identification and management of HAP is a dynamic process that requires repeatedly integrating findings from clinical examination, sputum analysis, and serial radiography to make a presumptive diagnosis. Both diagnosis and management therefore demand great humility, frequent revaluation, and a low threshold to alter therapy or investigate for diseases other than pneumonia if initial clinical presumptions are not borne out by the patient's course.

DIFFERENTIAL DIAGNOSIS

Most ventilated patients with fever, purulent sputum, and radiographic infiltrates do not have pneumonia. These patients often have abnormal underlying lungs and are prone to an array of complications that together or individually mimic VAP. For example, hypoxemia and an abnormal chest radiograph might be due to atelectasis or pulmonary edema, while fever, leukocytosis and purulent secretions might be due to simultaneous tracheobronchitis or infection outside the lungs (eg, sinusitis, central venous catheter-associated bloodstream infection, or intra-abdominal infection such as *C difficile*). In addition, the lungs of ventilated patients are in a state of flux due to fluid shifts, segmental variations in ventilation pressures, interference by the endotracheal tube in the clearance of normal pulmonary secretions, and mucous plugging. These changes can lead to the transient appearance of pulmonary syndromes that resemble VAP, but as often as not will resolve spontaneously without antibiotics. Note that changes in the quality or quantity of pulmonary secretions do not necessarily indicate infection, but may be due to impaired clearance of normal pulmonary secretions due to a weak cough or the disruptive presence of an endotracheal tube.

Several serious conditions also mimic VAP. Pulmonary embolism, aspiration pneumonitis, vasculitis, pulmonary hemorrhage, pneumothorax, and acute respiratory distress syndrome can all present with fever, leukocytosis, hypoxemia, abnormal pulmonary secretions, and radiographic infiltrates. True lung infections may also be secondary to other processes, such as right-sided endocarditis. Depending on the clinical scenario, clinicians may consider a variety of other tests, such as CT angiography, bronchoscopy with or without biopsy, rheumatologic tests, echocardiography, and measurement of pulmonary capillary wedge pressures.

TRIAGE/HOSPITAL ADMISSION

Outpatients with possible health care–associated pneumonia should be assessed for clinical stability. Mortality prediction scores such as the pneumonia patient outcomes research team (PORT) score were developed and validated for patients with community-acquired pneumonia; hence their applicability to patients with health care–associated infections is unknown. An important consideration is the possibility of infection with an organism resistant to oral antibiotics. It is reasonable to admit vulnerable patients for early empiric therapy with broad spectrum agents, and then revaluate the need for admission once the patient's microbiology and clinical trajectory become evident in 24 to 48 hours. Regardless of the decision to admit or not, early acquisition of blood and sputum specimens for culture and sensitivities are advised to expedite detection of antibiotic-resistant strains.

Inpatients that develop a pulmonary syndrome consistent with pneumonia merit evaluation for possible transfer to an intensive care unit. While patients that require mechanical ventilation obviously need intensive care, the decision on whether or not to transfer less acute patients is often more a function of each hospital's general level of acuity, bed availability, staffing levels, and nursing protocols than of the patient's physiological stability.

TREATMENT OPTIONS

Inappropriate or delayed treatment is associated with increased mortality. Therefore, the onus on clinicians is to begin treatment with broad spectrum agents as soon as a diagnosis of health care–associated pneumonia seems likely. The push for early treatment has to be balanced against the broad array of potential mimickers of pneumonia, the risks of antibiotic therapy, and the inadequacy of clinical signs, microbiology, and radiography to definitively diagnose pneumonia in this population. Consequently, it is critical to deliberately revaluate the patient at 24 to 48 hours after starting therapy to assess whether pneumonia still seems likely, whether investigation for other disorders are warranted, and whether antibiotics can be tailored or stopped.

Reassessment should take into account the patient's clinical course, repeat radiography, and the results of sputum or endotracheal aspirate cultures. A patient whose pulmonary syndrome has resolved or whose radiography has substantially improved in the space of a single day most likely does not have pneumonia, and antibiotics can safely be stopped. However, if the patient's syndrome is only starting to show signs of improvement, then it is reasonable to continue a full course of antibiotic therapy. The choice of antibiotics should be tailored according to culture results at this point. Patients who fail to improve or worsen despite antibiotics merit evaluation for organisms resistant to current antibiotics, the development of complications such as a lung abscess or empyema, or an alternative diagnosis such as pulmonary embolism or acute respiratory distress syndrome. Bronchoscopy and directed fungal, mycobacterial, and viral studies are also warranted in failing patients whose sputum or endotracheal aspirate cultures are unrevealing.

Initial treatment choice depends upon the timing of the pulmonary syndrome relative to admission, and the patient's risk factors for resistant organisms. Previously healthy patients who develop HAP within the first 3 to 5 days of admission (typically due to an aspiration event immediately preceding or following admission) are usually infected with the same relatively susceptible organisms that cause community-acquired pneumonia: pneumococcus, *Haemophilus, Moraxella, Legionella, Mycoplasma*, and respiratory viruses. A respiratory fluoroquinolone such as levofloxacin or moxifloxacin, or combination therapy with a third generation cephalosporin and a macrolide, is usually adequate for this population. Suggested dosing for patients with normal renal function is shown in **Table 194-3**.

These choices should be tailored in accordance with each patient's presenting history, epidemiologic risks, prior infections, recent antibiotic exposure, and the local microbial ecology. For example, patients that report a biphasic illness with a respiratory syndrome followed by transient improvement and then renewed severe symptoms may have bacterial superinfection following a respiratory virus. *S aureus* is a frequent pathogen in this setting

TABLE 194-3 Suggested Doses of Antibiotics Commonly Used to Treat Health Care–associated, Hospital-acquired, and Ventilator-associated Pneumonia

Antibiotic	Suggested Dose (Normal Renal Function)	Dose Modification for Renal Dysfunction?
Antibiotics active against MRSA pneumonia		
Vancomycin	15–20 mg/kg IV every 8–12 hours In seriously ill patients, begin with a loading dose of 25–30 mg/kg; goal trough 15–20 mg/L	Yes
Linezolid	600 mg orally or IV every 12 hours	No
Antibiotics appropriate for patients more at risk for community-acquired pathogens		
Ceftriaxone	2 g IV every 24 hours	No
Levofloxacin	750 mg orally or IV every 24 hours	Yes
Moxifloxacin	400 mg orally or IV every 24 hours	No
Azithromycin	500 mg orally every 24 hours	No
Anti-pseudomonal agents		
Ceftazidime	2 g IV every 8 hours	Yes
Cefepime	2 g IV every 8 hours	Yes
Ciprofloxacin	500–750 mg orally every 12 hours or 400 mg IV every 12 hours	Yes
Imipenem	500 mg IV every 6 hours	Yes
Meropenem	1 g IV every 8 hours	Yes
Piperacillin-tazobactam	4.5 g IV every 6 hours	Yes
Aztreonam	2 g IV every 8 hours	Yes
Gentamicin	7 mg/kg IV every 24 hours Goal trough < 1 mcg/mL	Yes
Tobramycin	7 mg/kg IV every 24 hours Goal trough < 1 mcg/mL	Yes
Amikacin	20 mg/kg IV every 24 hours Goal trough < 4–5 mcg/mL	Yes

and should be covered with the initial empiric regimen. Likewise, many communities in the United States are reporting an increased incidence of community-acquired methicillin-resistant *S aureus* (CA-MRSA). Adding CA-MRSA coverage, such as vancomycin or linezolid, is therefore prudent for patients with severe illness. Patients with structural lung disease and prior infections are more likely to be infected with antibiotic resistant nonenteric gram negatives, such as *Pseudomonas* or *Stenotrophomonas*. Patients that have recently been exposed to fluoroquinolones are more likely to be colonized with fluoroquinolones-resistant organisms.

Patients who have been in hospital for more than 3 to 5 days, who have recently been exposed to antibiotics, who have a history of drug-resistant infections, or who have a history of regular contact with health care facilities (including acute care hospitals, skilled nursing and rehabilitation facilities, dialysis and infusion centers) are at higher risk of harboring drug-resistant organisms.

PRACTICE POINT

Antibiotic selection in nursing home pneumonia

- There is a paucity of data to guide treatment of pneumonia in patients admitted to the hospital from nursing homes. According to the joint guidelines of the American Thoracic Society and the Infectious Diseases Society of America, these patients should be considered to be at risk for multidrug-resistant pathogens, such as MRSA and *Pseudomonas*, and treated accordingly. However, for many patients who acquire pneumonia while in a nursing home, the microbiology is similar to that of community-acquired pneumonia. The nursing home patients at highest risk for antibiotic-resistant pathogens are those with severe illness, immune suppression, hospitalization within the past three months, antibiotic therapy within the past 6 months, poor functional status, and who live in a locale with a high prevalence of multidrug-resistant organisms.

Empiric treatment in this population should include coverage for MRSA and multidrug-resistant gram negatives such as *Pseudomonas, E coli, Enterobacter,* and *Klebsiella*. It is wise to include two gram-negative agents in empiric therapy for patients with serious infections, given the increasing frequency of extended-spectrum beta-lactamases, carbapenemases, and other modes of resistance. Early treatment with two agents increases the likelihood that at least one agent will be active against the causative pathogen. Reasonable empiric coverage combinations include the following:

- Gram-positive coverage:
  - Vancomycin or linezolid
- Gram-negative coverage:
  - Two agents (choose one agent from each column)

Antipseudomonal cephalosporin (ceftazidime, cefepime)	Antipseudomonal quinolone (ciprofloxacin, levofloxacin)
Antipseudomonal carbapenem (meropenem, imipenem)	Antipseudomonal aminoglycoside (amikacin, tobramycin, gentamicin)
Piperacillin-tazobactam	
Aztreonam	

Suggested doses for patients with normal renal function are shown in Table 194-3. Note that aztreonam has a narrower spectrum of activity, compared to most other gram-negative agents in this list. It should therefore generally be reserved for patients with beta-lactam allergy. Daptomycin is not recommended to treat respiratory infections because it is inactivated by pulmonary surfactant.

PRACTICE POINT

Central nervous system (CNS) side effects of antimicrobials

- The elderly patients at high risk for health care–associated pneumonia are also prone to CNS side effects from antibiotics. Carbapenems lower the seizure threshold, cefepime may cause delirium, and fluoroquinolones may both cause confusion and reduce the seizure threshold.
- The risk of these side effects may be reduced by using appropriate doses for age and renal function.

Once culture and susceptibility results are available, the regimen should be trimmed to the most parsimonious regimen possible (ie, single-agent directed therapy). In most settings, there is little benefit to double coverage once antimicrobial susceptibilities of the causative pathogen are known.

COMPLICATIONS

Patients with pneumonia occasionally develop septic complications such as empyema or pulmonary abscess. These complications are best detected on computed tomography. This study is indicated for patients that fail to show signs of improvement after 48 to 72 hours of appropriate antibiotics. Some pathogens, such as *S aureus*, *Pseudomonas*, and *Klebsiella*, may cause necrotizing infections with pulmonary hemorrhage or cavitation. Anaerobes are also frequently implicated in abscesses and cavitating lesions. Patients with severe pneumonia, chemical aspiration, or barotrauma from mechanical ventilation are at risk for the acute respiratory distress syndrome. Clinicians need to be vigilant for complications of antibiotic therapy including *C difficile*, drug fever, renal toxicity, hepatitis, bone marrow suppression, hemolysis, hypersensitivity reactions, and delirium. Patients may also suffer complications from intravascular antibiotic delivery devices, such as central lines and peripherally inserted central catheter lines, since they are loci for infection and thrombosis.

DISCHARGE PLANNING

Discharge treatment considerations follow from the final antibiotic choice. If the pathogen is susceptible to an oral agent with high bioavailability, such as a fluoroquinolone or linezolid, then an oral agent to complete therapy is adequate. Otherwise, the patient will require a central line for IV therapy, with attendant implications for discharge. Follow-up should be arranged for all patients to assure resolution of their pulmonary syndrome. Chest imaging should be repeated one to three months following the infection to document clearance of lesions, and to assess the underlying parenchyma for occult lesions (this can be deferred if the patient had normal chest imaging immediately prior to developing HAP). Patients with persistent infiltrates require evaluation for endobronchial lesions causing post-obstructive pneumonia, disorders that impair ciliary clearance of secretions, immune deficits, or alternative sources of pulmonary infiltrates such as vasculitis.

QUALITY IMPROVEMENT

Hospital-acquired pneumonia has drawn substantial attention in recent years as a severe, preventable complication of care. Acid suppressants (particularly proton pump inhibitors) increase the

TABLE 194-4 Evidence-based Medicine: Key References for Nosocomial Pneumonia

Reference	Methodology	Results	Limitations	Bottom Line
Koeman M, et al. *Am J Respir Crit Care Med.* 2006;173:1348–1355.	Randomized, double-blind, placebo-controlled trial of topical oral decontamination with chlorhexidine vs chlorhexidine/colistin vs placebo, administered every 6 hours, in 385 patients requiring mechanical ventilation for at least 48 h	Topical oral decontamination reduced daily risk of nosocomial pneumonia by 65% in chlorhexidine group and 55% in chlorhexidine/colistin group	Diagnosis of VAP, based on clinical, radiologic, and microbiologic criteria, is imprecise and lacks specificity	Topical antibiotic treatment reduced daily risk of VAP, but without reductions in overall antibiotic utilization, time of mechanical ventilation, length of intensive care unit stay, length of hospital stay, and in-hospital mortality
Paul M, et al. *Cochrane Database Syst Rev.* 2006;(1):CD003344.	Meta-analysis of 64 clinical trials, including 7586 patients, comparing clinical outcomes for beta-lactam/aminoglycoside combination therapy vs beta- lactam monotherapy for sepsis	Dual beta-lactam/aminoglycoside therapy was associated with similar survival and clinical success as beta-lactam monotherapy, but with higher risk of nephrotoxicity; this also seemed to be true in subgroup with *Pseudomonas* infection	Significant heterogeneity in study population and design, making application of findings to nosocomial pneumonia problematic	No clear benefit of dual therapy with beta-lactams and aminoglycosides in patients with many serious infections, once antibiotic sensitivities are available
Chastre J, et al. *JAMA.* 2003;290:2588–2598.	Prospective, randomized, double-blind (until day 8) clinical trial, comparing 8 vs 15 d of antibiotic therapy in 401 patients diagnosed with VAP	Mortality, intensive care unit stay, duration of mechanical ventilation, and relapse rates were similar in two groups; patients in 8-d group were less likely to acquire drug-resistant infections in event of relapse, and had less total antibiotic use; however, patients in 8-d group were more likely to have relapses with nonfermenting gram-negative rods, such as Pseudomonas	Antibiotic regimen was left to discretion of treating physician; however, antibiotic prescribing patterns were similar in two groups, with most receiving initial therapy with an aminoglycoside or fluoroquinolone plus broad-spectrum beta-lactam agent	Outcomes with use of 8-d course of antibiotics in patients with VAP is similar to those who receive 15-d course of antibiotics, except perhaps for patients with infection with *Pseudomonas*

VAP, ventilator-associated pneumonia.

risk of pneumonia, so they should not be routinely prescribed for all inpatients, but rather reserved for individuals at high risk for gastrointestinal bleeding. Aspiration precautions should be ordered for patients with impaired consciousness or abnormal swallowing. Smoking cessation and vaccination against influenza and pneumococcus are long-term strategies to protect patients for the future. Hospitals should increase the likelihood of appropriate therapy by compiling and circulating antibiograms, so that clinicians may familiarize themselves with local antimicrobial resistance patterns. Hospitals should also educate practitioners about current clinical guidelines.

In the intensive care setting, quality advocates recommend (and some states mandate) a "bundle" of measures to prevent VAP. These bundles vary, but usually include some or all of the following:

- Elevation of the head of the bed above 30°
- Oral care with an antiseptic such as chlorhexidine two to 6 times per day
- Daily assessment of readiness to wean from the ventilator
- Daily cessation of sedative medications to assess patient's underlying level of consciousness
- Deep vein thrombosis (DVT) prophylaxis
- Stress ulcer prophylaxis

These recommendations are somewhat controversial, as the evidence base underlying each bundle component varies considerably. Furthermore, the connection between pneumonia and some of these recommendations is obscure in the case of DVT prophylaxis, and probably harmful in the case of stress ulcer prophylaxis. Nonetheless, there are an increasing number of case reports from hospitals reporting dramatic decreases in their VAP rates after implementation of these bundles. While these reports need to be interpreted with considerable caution since they suffer significant methodological flaws, they have nonetheless helped elevate VAP bundles to the level of de facto standard of care.

The ventilator management recommendations (daily assessment of readiness to extubate and daily sedation vacation) are probably the most powerful strategies within the bundle, since they have consistently been shown to decrease duration of mechanical ventilation and length of stay. Selective digestive decontamination with a combination of intravenous cefotaxime and topical tobramycin, colistin, and amphotericin B to the oropharynx and stomach has been associated with a small decrease in mortality, but this strategy is not currently recommended due to fears of nurturing multidrug-resistant bacteria (**Table 194-4**).

SUGGESTED READINGS

American Thoracic Society and Infectious Diseases Society of America. Guidelines for the management of adults with hospital-acquired, ventilator-associated, and healthcare-associated pneumonia. *Am J Respir Crit Care Med.* 2005;171:388–416.

Chastre J, Wolff M, Fagon JY, et al. Comparison of 8 vs 15 days of antibiotic therapy for ventilator-associated pneumonia in adults: a randomized trial. *JAMA.* 2003;290:2588–2598.

de Smet AM, Kluytmans JA, Cooper BS, et al. Decontamination of the digestive tract and oropharynx in ICU patients. *N Engl J Med.* 2009;360:20–31.

Girard TD, Kress JP, Fuchs BD, et al. Efficacy and safety of a paired sedation and ventilator weaning protocol for mechanically ventilated patients in intensive care (Awakening and Breathing Controlled trial): a randomised controlled trial. *Lancet.* 2008;371:126–134.

Heyland D, Dodek P, Muscedere J, Day A. A randomized trial of diagnostic techniques for ventilator-associated pneumonia. *N Engl J Med.* 2006;355:2619–2630.

Klompas M. Does this patient have ventilator-associated pneumonia? *JAMA.* 2007;297:1583–1593.

Society for Healthcare Epidemiology of America and Infectious Disease Society of America. Strategies to prevent ventilator-associated pneumonia in acute care hospitals. *Infect Control Hosp Epidemiol.* 2008;29(Suppl 1):S31–S40.

CHAPTER 195

Approach to the Patient with HIV

Claire Farel, MD, MPH
Paul E. Sax, MD

Key Clinical Questions

1. What conditions cause symptoms in HIV patients?
2. How are opportunistic infections diagnosed and treated?
3. What noninfectious problems are common in HIV patients?
4. When should antiretroviral therapy be started?

INTRODUCTION

More than 1 million people are HIV seropositive in the United States. As survival with HIV has increased because of antiretroviral therapy (ART), the spectrum of illness affecting this population has expanded. Opportunistic infections still occur in untreated patients and patients who do not adhere to therapy. However, in patients whose HIV infection is controlled by ART, noninfectious problems such as coronary artery disease, pulmonary hypertension, and malignancy are increasing in prevalence. This chapter uses a symptom-based approach to guide differential diagnosis in HIV, and outlines the presentation, diagnosis, and treatment of common opportunistic infections. Other aspects of HIV therapy important to the hospitalist are discussed, including medication interactions and side effects.

PATHOPHYSIOLOGY AND NATURAL HISTORY

Most patients with acute HIV infection develop symptoms from two to four weeks after exposure. Some patients are asymptomatic, but many report an acute febrile illness resembling mononucleosis. Features may include rash, anorexia, mucocutaneous ulcerations, pharyngitis, lymphadenopathy, diarrhea, myalgias, and rarely meningoencephalitis. As HIV antibody does not appear until three to four weeks after the symptoms of acute HIV syndrome develop, both HIV RNA (viral load) testing and HIV antibody should be obtained. Clinicians should bear in mind that patients with acute HIV infection may also have acquired other infections, such as viral hepatitis, syphilis, or cytomegalovirus (CMV), at the time of their HIV exposure.

HIV depletes CD4+ lymphocytes, also known as T-helper cells, leading to opportunistic infections (OIs). In acute HIV infection, CD4+ cells decline sharply, generally followed by a modest rebound, as HIV replication is brought under partial control. Over time, viremia rises, CD4+ cells are gradually depleted, and AIDS develops.

The tempo for progression to AIDS has great individual variability. Illnesses such as seborrheic dermatitis, cutaneous zoster, bacterial pneumonia, and cytopenias, while not specific to HIV, occur with increased frequency in patients with waning CD4+ cells and may be a clue to undiagnosed HIV.

TRIAGE/CONSULTATION

Admission of the patient with CD4+ count >500 cells/mm^3, suppressed viral load, and admission for a non–HIV-related reason does not necessarily require infectious diseases consultation. By contrast, newly diagnosed HIV, acute opportunistic infections, undifferentiated illness in patients with more advanced HIV, or possible modification of ART warrant review with a specialist familiar with HIV disease and its management.

DIAGNOSTIC APPROACH: GENERAL PRINCIPLES

The most recent CD4+ cell count is critical in determining the likelihood of an HIV-related complication (**Table 195-1**). If recent CD4+ counts are unavailable, there is controversy about the usefulness of CD4+ testing in the context of acute illness, which depresses the CD4+ below the patient's true baseline. Despite this caveat, we recommend measuring CD4+ cell count during hospital admissions, as markedly low values (eg, <100 cells/mm^3) almost invariably indicate severe HIV-related immunosuppression. Conversely, OIs are unusual

TABLE 195-1 HIV: Stages of Immunodeficiency and Commonly Associated Illnesses

CD4+ Count	Opportunistic Infections	HIV or AIDS-Associated Conditions
< 500 cells/mm^3	• *Mycobacterium tuberculosis* (seen at all stages of HIV infection)	• Candidal infection (oral, vaginal) • Herpes simplex infection (oral, genital) • Cutaneous zoster
< 200 cells/mm^3	• *Pneumocystis jirovecii* pneumonia • *Candida* esophagitis • Cryptococcal infection	AIDS-associated malignancies: • Kaposi sarcoma • Non-Hodgkin lymphoma
< 50 cells/mm^3	• Disseminated *Mycobacterium avium* complex • Cytomegalovirus infection • Toxoplasmosis	• AIDS-associated wasting • AIDS-associated dementia

in patients with completely normal CD4+ cell counts. Although HIV RNA values do not give as much information about a patient's immune status as CD4+ counts, they are excellent markers of ART medication adherence, as most patients faithfully taking appropriate ART will have HIV RNA levels below the limits of detection of available assays. One potential confounder to this rule is that acute infections transiently raise HIV RNA levels.

In general, admission of the HIV-positive patient on ART merits a baseline check of renal and hepatic function as well as a CBC. HIV therapy may result in signature laboratory abnormalities in some patients, such as the indirect hyperbilirubinemia seen in patients on atazanavir and the increased MCV due to zidovudine (**Table 195-2**).

For patients with excellent medication adherence, suppressed HIV RNA, and immunologic recovery with CD4+ cell counts > 200 cells/mm^3, traditional AIDS-related illnesses are vanishingly rare. Individuals with these characteristics are generally admitted for similar reasons as HIV-negative patients. However, long-term follow-up of treated HIV patients shows that they do have a higher risk of certain non-infectious complications than age-matched, HIV-negative controls. Cardiovascular, hepatic, and renal disease occurs more frequently in patients with HIV, probably due to a combination of ART-induced side effects and chronic inflammation. Malignancies also seem to be increased, perhaps as a consequence of reduced immune tumor surveillance.

TABLE 195-2 Laboratory Abnormalities Associated with Selected Antiretroviral Agents

Drug	Laboratory Abnormality
Atazanavir Indinavir	Indirect hyperbilirubinemia
Zidovudine	Bone marrow suppression, macrocytic anemia
Tenofovir	Renal dysfunction

SYMPTOM-BASED DIAGNOSTIC APPROACH

RESPIRATORY ILLNESS

Causes of respiratory symptoms in HIV include bacterial, mycobacterial, viral, and fungal pathogens, as well as malignancy and cardiovascular disease (**Table 195-3**). Clues to the etiology of the illness include the symptoms, time course, and imaging. A careful history can narrow the differential diagnosis significantly. For example, a relatively acute illness with fevers, chills, sputum production, and pleuritic chest pain is consistent with bacterial pneumonia. A subacute illness with progressive dyspnea, dry cough, low-grade fevers, and weight loss suggests *Pneumocystis jirovecii* pneumonia (PCP). The social history may elicit risk factors for endemic fungal infections and tuberculosis. Physical examination findings of cachexia or oral candidiasis should raise suspicion for more advanced HIV, as should a history of weight loss.

Initial studies in the HIV-positive patient with respiratory illness should include measurement of oxygen saturation or an arterial blood gas measurement, complete blood count with differential, two sets of blood cultures, sputum culture, chest radiograph, and serum lactate dehydrogenase (LDH), which is nonspecific, but often elevated in patients with PCP. Nasopharyngeal swab for respiratory viruses, such as influenza A and B as well as H1N1, should be sent if local epidemiology and seasonality are appropriate (**Table 195-4**). Induced sputum should be ordered and sent for PCP and AFB staining, as well as bacterial culture. Serum testing for 1,3 beta-D-glucan—a component of many fungi, including *P jirovecii*—can be quite useful, as most patients with HIV-related PCP have markedly elevated levels. A strongly positive test in a patient with a compatible clinical syndrome for PCP, therefore, can obviate the need for invasive testing such as bronchoscopy.

If the initial round of diagnostic tests is unrevealing and the patient is not improved on empiric therapy, serum cryptococcal antigen and urine histoplasmosis antigen should be considered. Other evaluation at this time may include bronchoscopy with bronchoalveolar lavage and possible transbronchial biopsy, cardiac evaluation including echocardiography, or potentially nodule or mass resection via video-assisted thoracoscopy.

CENTRAL NERVOUS SYSTEM ILLNESS

Causes of the central nervous system disease in HIV include cryptococcal meningitis, cerebral toxoplasmosis, progressive multifocal leukoencephalopathy (PML), and many others (**Table 195-5**). Advanced AIDS may be complicated by HIV-related dementia. Another important HIV-related CNS process is non-Hodgkin lymphoma, which may present as a primary mass lesion in the brain, or

TABLE 195-3 Causes of Respiratory Disease in HIV

Very Common	Less Common	Rare
• *P jirovecii* pneumonia • *S pneumoniae* • *H influenzae* • *M tuberculosis**	• Gram-negative rods, especially *Pseudomonas* • *H capsulatum* • *C neoformans* • *Aspergillus* spp • Cytomegalovirus • Pulmonary lymphoma • Heart failure • Kaposi sarcoma	• *Nocardia asteroides* • *Legionella* spp • *M avium* complex • *T gondii* • Cryptosporidia • *Rhodococcus equii* • Primary pulmonary hypertension • Abacavir hypersensivity

*Dependent on local *M tuberculosis* prevalence and patient risk factors (such as past or current residence in an endemic area).

TABLE 195-4 Diagnostic Studies for Respiratory Illness in the HIV-positive Patient

Nasopharyngeal Swab*	Bronchoalveolar Lavage
Influenza A and B (rapid testing and/or polymerase chain reaction)	Viral studies as listed under nasopharyngeal swab
H1N1 influenza	Varicella
Respiratory syncytial virus	Cytomegalovirus
Adenovirus	AFB stain and culture
Parainfluenza	Cytology
Metapneumovirus	Methenamine silver stain for *P jirovecii* pneumonia
	Bacterial culture
	Fungal culture

*Although uncomfortable for the patient, this must be inserted 1 to 2 cm into the nasopharyngeal space to ensure diagnostic yield.

as metastatic disease to the meninges in patients with high-grade lymphoma elsewhere.

Initial evaluation of the HIV-positive patient with neurologic or neuropsychiatric symptoms should include an assessment of medication adherence, possible use of illicit drugs, immunologic status, and complete physical examination with special attention to sensory-motor and mental status assessments. Brain MRI should be performed (or head CT, if MRI is not available).

Lumbar puncture is usually indicated, even in the absence of nuchal rigidity, as many of the above processes induce a relatively indolent inflammatory response. Opening pressure should be obtained in all cases. Cerebrospinal fluid (CSF) should be sent for cell count and differential, glucose, protein, Gram stain and routine culture, as well as India ink stain (for *Cryptococcus*), fungal culture, CSF cryptococcal antigen. If indicated, AFB stain and culture, and VDRL may be sent as well. Leftover CSF (at least 5 cc) should be held for other potential studies including cytology, polymerase chain reaction (PCR) testing for other pathogens such as Epstein-Barr virus (EBV), varicella zoster and herpes simplex viruses, JC virus, and HIV viral load.

TABLE 195-5 Causes of Central Nervous System Disease in HIV

Very Common	Less Common	Rare
• *C neoformans* • *T gondii** • Drug reactions • Psychiatric illness • Progressive multifocal leukoencephalopathy* • Lymphoma* • HIV	• Cytomegalovirus • *M tuberculosis*† • Bacterial brain abscess*	• *N asteroides** • *H capsulatum* • *C immitus* • *Aspergillus* spp* • *L monocytogenes* • Fungal brain abscess • Varicella zoster virus • Herpes simplex virus* • *Acanthamoeba* spp* • *T cruzi* • *T pallidum*

*Generally characterized by focal lesions on MRI or CT scan.
†Dependent on local *M tuberculosis* prevalence and patient risk factors.

Mass lesions that enhance with contrast

Mass lesions with enhancement occur more commonly in the setting of lower CD4+ counts (<200 cells/mm^3), and are most often due to toxoplasmosis (discussed below), primary CNS lymphoma or other malignancies, or rarely other infections, such as brain abscess or tuberculoma. If the patient has a history of positive *Toxoplasma* IgG serology and has multiple enhancing CNS lesions, empiric treatment for toxoplasmosis is appropriate. If the patient has a documented negative *Toxoplasma* serology and other etiologies such as tuberculoma or brain abscess are not suspected, neurosurgical consultation for brain biopsy is usually appropriate. Serum *Toxoplasma* IgM or *Toxoplasma* antibody studies of the cerebrospinal fluid are not useful in this clinical setting.

Patients with mass lesions and midline shift on imaging or evidence of increased intracranial pressure should receive adjunctive corticosteroids, usually dexamethasone. Symptoms and radiographic appearance of the lesion may improve on steroids, but this improvement should not shorten anticipated course of antibiotic treatment.

Since combination ART became the standard of care, the incidence of all AIDS-defining malignancies in the United States has decreased significantly. However, primary CNS lymphoma (PCNSL) is still over 1000 times more common in patients with HIV than uninfected controls. PCNSL may present with symptoms ranging from mental status changes to seizures, and with a single lesion or multiple lesions. PCNSL is most common in patients with more advanced disease, especially with CD4+ cell counts <50 cells/mm^3. Diagnostic workup includes MRI, CSF cytology, and, in most cases, stereotactic brain biopsy to confirm the diagnosis. CNS lymphoma in HIV usually involves B lymphocytes infected with EBV; PCR testing of CSF for EBV is sensitive, but not specific for this diagnosis.

The incidence of non–AIDS defining primary CNS malignancies is not higher in the HIV-positive patient population. However, lung cancer, which sometimes presents with brain metastases, is increased in HIV patients.

Nonenhancing mass lesions

HIV encephalopathy: HIV-related dementia, or HIV encephalopathy, is a disease of advanced immunosuppression. Characteristic findings include loss of memory, apathy, gait disturbance, and incontinence. Symptoms may be exacerbated by underlying psychiatric illness or substance abuse. There is often atrophy and nonenhancing white matter disease on MRI imaging. CSF examination may show mild lymphocytic pleocytosis, elevated protein, and detectable HIV RNA by viral load testing. Treatment with ART may lead to dramatic improvement, especially if the symptoms are of recent onset. However, the prognosis is highly variable, improvement may be delayed for months, and full recovery from severe cases is unusual. HIV encephalopathy, even when mild, may increase susceptibility of patients to the CNS side effects of antiretrovirals and other medications.

Progressive multifocal leukoencephalopathy (PML): As with HIV encephalopathy, the incidence of PML has greatly declined with the advent of ART. PML is a demyelinating disorder caused by JC virus, a common polyomavirus that is usually asymptomatic in the immunocompetent. Symptoms of PML are gradual in onset, and may culminate in hemiparesis, mental status changes, and visual field deficits, depending on the areas of involvement, which may be single or multiple. These lesions are less symmetrical than in HIV encephalopathy and are usually nonenhancing on imaging studies. The diagnosis is made on the basis of PCR testing of the CSF for JC virus. While PML is most common in patients with CD4+ counts <200 cells/mm^3, it may also be seen in patients initiating ART as an immune reconstitution inflammatory response to subclinical JC virus infection. There is currently no therapy that directly targets JC virus. One-third of patients with PML improve with effective ART; unfortunately, the remaining two-thirds have either long-term residual deficits or disease progression despite effective ART.

GASTROINTESTINAL ILLNESS

Gastrointestinal symptoms in HIV may result from infection, or, more commonly, from side effects of antibiotics and antiretrovirals, especially the protease inhibitors. Chronic diarrhea with weight loss may be due to untreated HIV itself; this HIV enteropathy is a diagnosis of exclusion, and typically responds promptly to effective ART.

Diarrhea: Causes of diarrhea in HIV are summarized in **Table 195-6**. The evaluation of the HIV-positive patient with diarrhea should consist of a careful exposure history, including travel, food, drink, and sexual activity. The medication history should include both antiretrovirals as well as antibiotics. The quality, frequency, volume, and time course of the diarrhea are important, as is the presence or absence of fevers and weight loss.

Diagnostic evaluation includes assessment of electrolyte and hematologic status, as well as a stool sample for ova and parasites, AFB and trichrome stains for mycobacteria and protozoa (*Cryptosporidium*, *Cyclospora*, *Isospora*, and microsporidia), *Clostridium difficile* toxin, and enzyme immunoassay for *Giardia*. If these studies are unrevealing, endoscopic evaluation may be required for evaluation of intraluminal pathology and biopsy, especially in patients with low CD4+ counts who are at risk for additional processes such as CMV, lymphoma, and Kaposi sarcoma.

ART-related diarrhea is usually secondary to the protease inhibitors. It is rarely associated with weight loss, and may in some cases be controlled with loperamide. For individuals with debilitating diarrhea due to this class of medications, an HIV specialist will often consider an alternative antiretroviral regimen. However, these changes should not be done without a thorough review of the patient's treatment history, including (if available) results of prior resistance testing.

Dysphagia: *Candida* esophagitis is by far the most common cause of this symptom, and is often, but not always, accompanied by visible oral candidiasis (thrush) on examination. Empiric fluconazole is reasonable (200 mg daily for 7–14 days). If the diagnosis is correct, improvement often occurs within 24 to 48 hours. For patients who fail to respond to antifungal therapy, endoscopy is indicated to exclude other possible causes of dysphagia and odonyphagia. These include idiopathic aphthous ulcers, CMV, herpes simplex, histoplasmosis, and lymphoma.

UNDIFFERENTIATED FEVER

The differential diagnosis for fever in HIV is broad and includes infection (either opportunistic or otherwise), inflammatory conditions (including immune reconstitution inflammatory syndrome), fevers from medications or malignancy, or HIV itself (**Table 195-7**).

Helpful historical information includes fever duration and severity, prior opportunistic infections and hospitalizations, medication history, including new medications and adherence to prophylaxis, domestic and international travel, sexual history, intravenous drug use, and other substance use.

Differential diagnosis is highly contingent on the stage of HIV infection, based on the most recent CD4+ count. When such information is not immediately available, inferences about immune status can often be made based on physical exam findings such as cachexia or oral candidiasis that indicate advanced HIV. Causes of fever in HIV-positive patients with CD4+ counts >500 cells/mm^3 are similar to those in immunocompetent patients. Patients with CD4+ counts between 200 and 500 cells/mm^3 are most likely to have fevers secondary to sexually transmitted infections (especially syphilis and hepatitis C among gay men) or respiratory infections, either bacterial (*Streptococcus pneumoniae* and *Haemophilus influenzae)* or viral (seasonal and H1N1 influenza). Patients with more advanced disease (CD4+ count <200 cells/mm^3) are vulnerable to both opportunistic and nonopportunistic infections. Patients with more advanced immunosuppression are also at risk for infections seen at earlier stages of disease. Diagnostic evaluation that may help to differentiate source of fever in the absence of localizing signs or symptoms is summarized in **Table 195-8**.

TABLE 195-6 Causes of Diarrheal Illness in HIV

Common	Less Common	Rare
• Cytomegalovirus • *C difficile* • *Salmonella* • *M avium* complex • *Giardia* • Protease inhibitors	• *Shigella* • *Campylobacter* • Microsporidia • Cryptosporidia • *Isospora* • *Cyclospora*	• Amebiasis • *S stercoralis* • GI lymphoma • Kaposi sarcoma • Enterotoxigenic *E coli*

GI, gastrointestinal.

TABLE 195-7 Causes of Undifferentiated Fever in HIV

Common	Less Common	Rare
• *M avium* complex • Cytomegalovirus • Drug fever* • Sinusitis • Central line infection • Early *P jirovecii* pneumonia • HIV • *M tuberculosis*†	• *Cryptococcus neoformans* • *Histoplasma capsulatum* • Endocarditis • Lymphoma • *M tuberculosis*†	• Extrapulmonary *P jirovecii* • *Bartonella henselae* • *Coccidioides immitis* • Other atypical mycobacteria • *Penicillium marneffei* • *Leishmania* spp • *Parvovirus* • *Toxoplasma gondii*

*If suspected, modification of antiretroviral regimen should be performed with the input of an expert in HIV treatment.

†Dependent on local *M tuberculosis* prevalence and patient risk factors (such as past or current residence in an endemic area).

TABLE 195-8 Undifferentiated Fever in Persons with HIV: Diagnostic Evaluation

- Blood cultures: routine for endocarditis or line infections; isolators for mycobacteria (especially *M avium*), *H capsulatum*
- Rapid plasma reagin
- Nasal swab for influenza A and B, H1N1 influenza
- Induced sputum or bronchoalveolar lavage: *P jirovecii*, *M tuberculosis*, respiratory viral panel
- Serum cryptococcal antigen, serum/urine histoplasmosis antigen (latter if patient from endemic area), legionella urine antigen
- CT abdomen/pelvis: look for adenopathy, organomegaly
- Sometimes useful: bone marrow, liver, lymph node biopsy; cytomegalovirus viral load, parvovirus polymerase chain reaction

IMMUNE RECONSTITUTION INFLAMMATORY SYNDROME

Recovery of immune function with ART is associated with a resurgence of pathogen-specific immunity. This can lead to the immune reconstitution inflammatory syndrome (IRIS), a brisk inflammatory reaction to pre-existing infections, which may have been subclinical or minimally symptomatic before ART. Virtually all HIV-related OIs have been reported in association with IRIS. The most common pathogens in IRIS are mycobacteria (both tuberculosis and atypical mycobacteria), herpes viruses, zoster, and CMV.

IRIS usually occurs in the first three months after starting ART. Rarely, delayed cases occur a year or more after starting therapy. In a typical scenario, a patient with severe immunosuppression (CD4+ cell count <100 cells/mm^3) begins ART and then presents several weeks later with fever and cervical, mediastinal, and mesenteric adenopathy. Biopsy of involved nodes reveals mycobacteria and poorly formed granulomata, with cultures eventually yielding *Mycobacteria avium* complex (MAC). Other relatively common causes of IRIS include severe herpes zoster or herpes simplex, vitritis due to CMV, and worsening of cutaneous Kaposi sarcoma.

Treatment of IRIS is directed at the underlying pathogen. ART should be continued, if at all possible. If symptoms cannot be controlled with anti-infective therapy alone, or if the IRIS is life-threatening, as can rarely occur with CNS diseases such as cryptococcal meningitis or toxoplasmosis, adjunctive corticosteroids should be given. A typical starting dose will be 60 mg of prednisone a day, with therapy continued for several weeks followed by a slow taper. Fortunately, prospective studies show that IRIS occurs in 10% of AIDS patients starting ART or less, and is rarely fatal.

NONINFECTIOUS CAUSES OF FEVER

Drug fever

HIV-positive patients have a higher rate of drug hypersensitivity than the general population, including a higher incidence of severe systemic reactions such as Stevens-Johnson syndrome and toxic epidermal necrolysis. Common offending agents include sulfonamides (including trimethoprim-sulfamethoxazole), dapsone, clindamycin, and beta-lactam antibiotics.

Some antiretroviral agents cause drug hypersensitivity. The two most important are nevirapine and abacavir. The incidence of systemic hypersensitivity reactions to nevirapine—which is often accompanied by rash and hepatitis—is significantly higher in HIV patients who are female and immunologically healthier. As a result, nevirapine is not recommended in women with CD4+ cell counts >250 and men >400 cells/mm^3. Abacavir may cause a multisystem hypersensitivity reaction shortly after initiation of the drug that may worsen after successive doses. Continued treatment, or rechallenge after cessation, may be fatal. This reaction is strongly associated with the HLA-B*5701 haplotype. Screening tests are now widely available; abacavir is contraindicated in anyone testing positive for this allele. Several protease inhibitors, including darunavir, fosamprenavir, and tipranavir, contain a sulfonamide moiety, and can rarely induce systemic hypersensitivity. However, patients with prior allergic reactions to trimethoprim-sulfamethoxazole can usually receive these sulfonamide antiviral agents safely, though they should be avoided in patients with prior life-threatening sulfa reactions.

Malignancy

The incidence of malignancies is higher in HIV-positive patients than in the general population. While AIDS-associated malignancies (including Kaposi sarcoma and non-Hodgkin lymphoma) were previously the most common causes, the range of HIV-associated malignancies has expanded due to prolonged patient survival in the ART era. Of these, non-Hodgkin lymphoma is most often associated with fever, although Hodgkin lymphoma is also more common in HIV-positive patients and may also presents with fever, night sweats, and weight loss. Malignancy should be considered in the differential diagnosis of lymphadenopathy in HIV.

SELECTED HIV-RELATED OPPORTUNISTIC INFECTIONS AND CONDITIONS

PNEUMOCYSTIS JIROVECII PNEUMONIA

P jirovecii (formerly *carinii*) pneumonia (PCP) is caused by a fungus ubiquitous in the environment, and nonpathogenic in the lungs of the normal host. Effective ART and chemoprophylaxis both markedly reduce the risk of PCP. As a result, cases today typically occur either in those who are unaware of their HIV status or not taking prescribed antiretroviral medications.

PCP most often presents as a respiratory illness progressing over weeks to months. Patients complain of dyspnea on exertion, first noticed when everyday tasks (climbing stairs, completing sentences, carrying household items) become difficult. Associated symptoms may include cough and chest tightness, and a sense that deep breathing is restricted. Constitutional symptoms including fever and weight loss are common, and physical examination may reveal other signs of immunosuppression, such as thrush, and shallow respirations. Chest radiographs often show diffuse bilateral infiltrates, with CT scanning demonstrating characteristic patchy "ground-glass" opacities.

In the presence of a subacute respiratory illness with hypoxemia, and a CD4+ count <200 cells/mm^3 is confirmed or suspected, therapy for PCP should generally be initiated, regardless of the appearance of the chest radiograph. While diffuse interstitial infiltrates are classic—often shown as "ground-glass" opacities on CT scan—lobar infiltrates, nodular or cavitary disease, or rarely, a normal chest radiograph may be observed. The diagnostic procedure of choice is sputum induction with immunofluorescence staining for PCP, but sensitivity varies depending on patient ability to provide an adequate sample and laboratory expertise. Bronchoalveolar lavage has a reported sensitivity of $>90\%$ in patients with HIV infection, considerably higher than that reported in HIV-negative patients. When microscopy is negative or difficult to obtain, serum 1,3 beta-D-glucan, a cell wall component of many fungi (including *P jirovecii*), can be a useful adjunct.

If pulse oximetry is low or the patient is tachypneic, an arterial blood gas should be performed. The degree of hypoxemia divides PCP into clinical classifications, and guides the treatment course. Mild PCP is characterized as a room air pulse oximetry of greater than 70% and an alveolar-arterial gradient (A-a gradient) of less than 35. Moderate to severe PCP is characterized as a room air pulse oximetry of less than 70% and an alveolar-arterial gradient (A-a gradient) of greater than 35. In moderate to severe PCP, corticosteroid therapy should be initiated, preferably before or at the time of antimicrobial treatment. The preferred steroid regimen is prednisone 40 mg orally twice daily for 5 days, followed by 40 mg once daily for 5 days, then 20 mg once daily for 11 days, for a total 21-day course.

Patients often worsen after starting therapy for PCP, perhaps related to an enhanced inflammatory response to dying organisms, as well as the fluid load associated with intravenous trimethoprim-sulfamethoxazole. In the setting of deterioration on therapy, adjunctive corticosteroids should be started even for patients not initially deemed candidates.

First-line treatment for PCP is trimethoprim-sulfamethoxazole (TMP-SMX) dosed at 15 to 20 mg/kg of trimethoprim daily in three divided doses. Therapy should be continued for 21 days. As TMP-SMX is well-absorbed orally, therapy can be dosed at two double-strength tablets of coformulated TMP-SMX given three times daily. For sulfa-allergic patients, second-line therapy is clindamycin 600 mg orally or intravenously given every 8 hours, along with primaquine 30 mg given orally every 24 hours. In mild disease, atovaquone oral suspension 750 mg twice daily may be considered. For moderate-severe disease only, pentamidine 4 mg/kg/day IV may also be used, but should generally be avoided due to high rates of side effects such as renal dysfunction, electrolyte abnormalities, pancreatitis, and islet cell toxicity. Of note, sulfa allergy should be confirmed in this clinical setting by a careful review of the allergy history, as TMP-SMX is the preferred treatment. Re-challenge may be considered in cases of mild sulfa allergy or sulfa intolerance.

Creatinine elevation and hyperkalemia are often associated with high-dose TMP-SMX use. Elevated creatinine in patients on TMP-SMX usually reflects inhibition of the tubular secretion of creatinine, rather than renal injury. Rarely, TMP-SMX may cause acute renal failure as a result of interstitial nephritis. TMP-SMX–induced hyperkalemia—due to an amiloride effect of trimethoprim—can be life-threatening and treated aggressively with sodium polystyrene sulfonate (Kayexalate) or by changing to an alternative PCP regimen.

If the patient is on ART, it should be continued throughout the PCP treatment course. If PCP occurs in the context of a new diagnosis of HIV, or if the patient is off ART, both prospective and observational studies have demonstrated a clinical benefit of starting ART before the completion of PCP treatment, preferably within two weeks of beginning PCP therapy.

BACTERIAL PNEUMONIA

While the incidence of bacterial pneumonia among HIV-positive patients has declined in recent years due to ART, it remains common in patients at all stages of the disease. Although vaccination against *S pneumoniae* is now standard of care in HIV-positive patients, pneumococcal pneumonias remain common. Other frequent pathogens include *H influenzae, Staphylococcus aureus*, both methicillin-sensitive and methicillin-resistant (MRSA), and gram-negative bacteria such as *Pseudomonas aeruginosa. Legionella* species, notably *L pneumophila*, do occur at a higher rate than in negative controls, and hence coverage for atypical pathogens is also warranted.

As noted above, bacterial pneumonia in HIV-positive patients presents similarly to bacterial pneumonia in HIV-negative patients: the relatively acute onset of fevers, chills, cough (often productive), anorexia, and pleuritic chest pain. As bacteremia may accompany bacterial pneumonia in HIV patients more commonly than in those without HIV, obtaining blood cultures prior to institution of antibiotics is strongly recommended. Sputum Gram stain and culture may be useful if obtained prior to antimicrobial therapy; by contrast, urinary antigen testing for *S pneumoniae* and *L pneumophila* typically remain positive for days to weeks after starting therapy.

Empiric initial therapy in most patients may be a third- or fourth-generation cephalosporin such as ceftriaxone (2 g IV daily) or cefotaxime (2 g IV every 8 hours) as well as azithromycin (500 mg daily, orally or IV). A fluoroquinolone (eg, levofloxacin or moxifloxacin, but not ciprofloxacin) may be used instead, if tuberculosis (TB) seems unlikely. If the patient has a history of pseudomonal infection, consider antipseudomonal therapy such as ceftazidime or cefepime (in place of ceftriaxone or cefotaxime) or adding ciprofloxacin. If MRSA colonization is documented, the patient is critically ill, or the pneumonia occurs during influenza season, vancomycin should be added to the regimen. Therapy should be given promptly upon evaluation, but blood and sputum cultures should be obtained prior to antibiotic administration if possible. Improvement is typically prompt, and changing to an oral regimen within days of hospitalization is usually possible. Duration of therapy is 7 to 10 days for pathogens such as *S pneumoniae* and *H influenzae,* 14 to 21 days for *Legionella* and *P aeruginosa*.

TUBERCULOSIS

Tuberculosis should always be considered in the differential diagnosis of respiratory illness in the HIV-positive patient. Although overall incidence of TB in the United States is declining gradually both in the general population and in the HIV-positive population, worldwide TB remains a major cause of mortality among HIV-positive persons. In the United States, approximately 12% of patients with TB have known HIV and another 32% have unknown HIV status.

TB has wide-ranging clinical presentations. Patients with relatively intact immune status typically present much as HIV-negative patients do, with a subacute systemic and respiratory illness featuring constitutional symptoms, cough, and cavitary infiltrates of the upper lobes on chest radiograph. By contrast, AIDS patients are more likely to have pulmonary infiltrates without cavitation, mediastinal and other lymphadenoapthy, extrapulmonary TB, and disseminated disease. Underlying tuberculosis should also be suspected in at-risk patients with slow-to-resolve pneumonia or characteristic lymphadenopathy on imaging. Diagnostic workup of TB should always include thoracic imaging, as extrapulmonary and pulmonary TB may coexist.

The diagnostic approach to suspected TB should include serial sputa for AFB stain and culture, preferably obtained in the morning to maximize bacillary yield. Sputum acid-fast stains are most likely to be positive in patients with cavitary pulmonary disease. Cultures of blood using the lysis-centrifugation technique may yield the diagnosis as well, especially in patients with advanced HIV immunosuppression and disseminated disease. Biopsies of affected sites may be required if extrapulmonary disease is suspected, and should be sent for AFB stain and culture as well as for pathologic examination.

A practical management issue is whether HIV-infected patients with pneumonia require isolation in a negative pressure room. In patients with risk factors for TB, isolation is good clinical practice until an alternative diagnosis is obtained, or there is clear clinical response to treatment of an alternative condition, such as bacterial pneumonia. TB risk factors include residence in an endemic area, homelessness or incarceration, or exposure to persons with TB (eg, a family member or in an occupational setting). Patients with prior positive purified-protein derivative (PPD) tests that do not have documented appropriate treatment should also be placed on precautions. Patients with suspected active TB should not receive a fluoroquinolone until TB is ruled out, as this drug class may have partial activity against TB, may confound diagnosis, and can limit future treatment options.

PRACTICE POINT

- Since antiretroviral drugs first became available, there has been a lively debate about the optimal timing of initiation of HIV treatment. Current U.S. guidelines recommend starting ART at CD4+ counts ≤ 500 cells/mm^3. Randomized controlled trials have shown a mortality reduction with ART in HIV-infected patients with CD4+ counts < 350 cells/mm^3. Observational data suggest that mortality is also reduced when patients start ART at CD4+ counts between 350 and 500 cells/mm^3. Early ART also decreases new HIV infections: a recent clinical trial has shown a 96% reduction in HIV transmission to HIV-negative sexual partners of HIV-positive patients who initiate ART at high CD4+ counts.

Of note, PPD testing may be falsely negative in patients with advanced immunosuppression, those on corticosteroids, or when the test is administered incorrectly (eg, intramuscularly, rather than intradermally).

CRYPTOCOCCAL MENINGITIS

Cryptococcus neoformans meningitis is usually seen in patients with low CD4+ counts (< 50 cells/mm^3). These patients often present with the gradual onset of meningitic symptoms, including headache, mental status changes, and fever. Meningeal signs and photophobia may be absent. Elevated intracranial pressure (> 200 mm H_2O) may be observed. This is an ominous prognostic finding that must be monitored during treatment. CSF pleocytosis may be minimal. Modest elevations in CSF protein and reductions in CSF glucose are often present. CSF should be sent for routine culture as well as fungal culture: *C neoformans* grows on most bacterial and fungal media within a few days. India ink stain of CSF is positive in 80% of AIDS patients with cryptococcal meningitis. CSF and serum cryptococcal antigen tests are both highly sensitive. Serum cryptococcal antigen testing has nearly 100% sensitivity, and hence a negative test virtually excludes cryptococcal meningitis even without CSF sampling.

The treatment of cryptococcal meningitis consists of both antimicrobial therapy and serial lumbar punctures to lower raised intracranial pressure. The volume of CSF removed on initial lumbar puncture should be sufficient to lower closing pressure to < 200 mm H_2O, or 50% of the opening pressure. Occasionally lumbar drains or shunts are required for refractory cases. Corticosteroids should be avoided. Cryptococcal meningitis is treated with a two-week induction period of amphotericin B 0.7 to 1 mg/kg/day IV (or the liposomal preparation of amphotericin B, dosed at 4–6 mg/kg/day), in combination with oral flucytosine (5-FC) 100 mg/kg/day divided over four doses. Flucytosine is associated with more rapid CSF sterilization and decreased risk of relapse, but may be poorly tolerated, with common side effects including nausea and bone marrow suppression. After this two-week induction period, patients who are clinically improved are switched to consolidation therapy with oral fluconazole, 400 mg daily for an additional eight weeks. After that time, the dose may be lowered to 200 mg daily for maintenance, and continued until the CD4+ cell count exceeds 200 cells/mm^3.

Timing of ART in cryptococcal meningitis is controversial. There is some data to indicate that early initiation of ART is associated with worse outcomes, perhaps because of IRIS leading to worsening intracranial pressure, although this has not been found in all studies. In the absence of definitive clinical trials, we recommend deferring ART until the initial two-week induction phase of treatment of cryptococcal meningitis is complete.

TOXOPLASMOSIS

The prevalence of toxoplasmosis infection varies by geography and diet. The major risk factors are consumption of undercooked meat (lamb, pork, and beef) and cat exposure. The prevalence of positive toxoplasma IgG in the general population (indicating past infection, often subclinical) ranges from 15% in the United States to 75% in some European countries.

Toxoplasmic encephalitis presents as a neurologic illness with systemic symptoms. Common complaints include headache, confusion, focal neurologic deficits, and fever. Imaging of the brain usually reveals multiple lesions, typically with a surrounding ring of contrast enhancement and edema (**Figure 195-1**). CD4+ cell counts are typically below 100 cells/mm^3.

Toxoplasmosis in HIV usually arises from reactivation of latent subclinical disease. Most patients have serologic evidence of prior infection, with a positive serum toxoplasmosis IgG. Serum toxoplasma IgM and CSF toxoplasma antibody studies are rarely of use. In a patient with advanced HIV-related immunosuppresion, a known positive toxoplasmosis IgG, and characteristic clinical presentation with suggestive imaging, empiric therapy directed at toxoplasmosis is warranted. In the absence of seropositivity, neurosurgical consultation should be obtained for a stereotactic brain biopsy to

A B

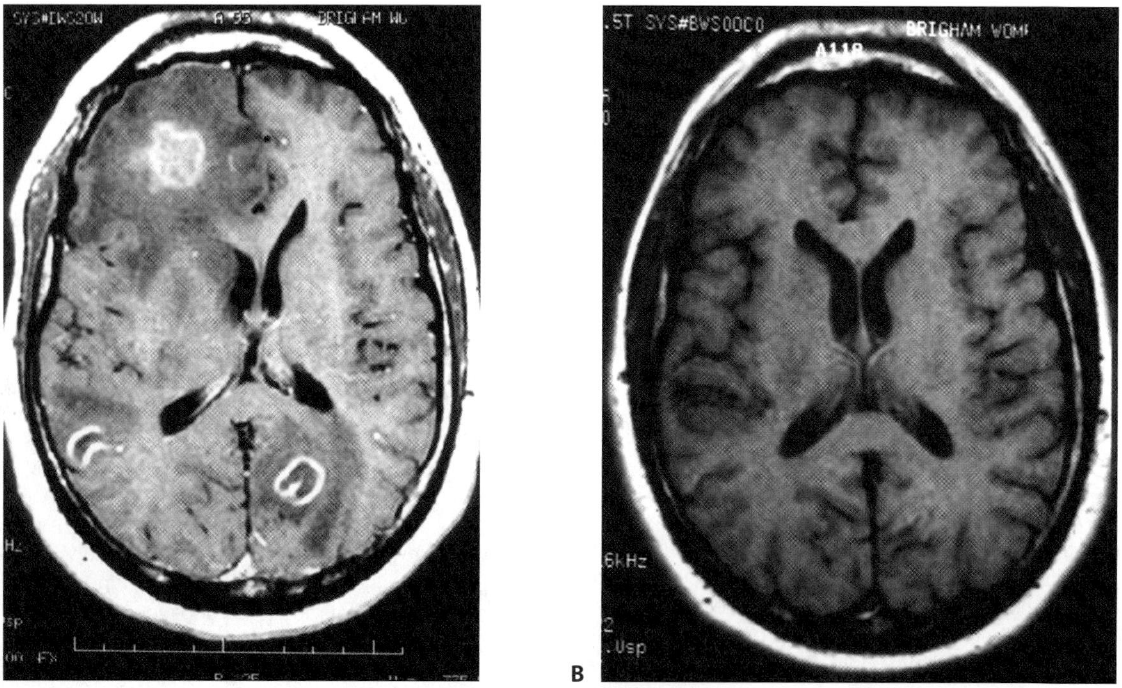

Figure 195-1 *Toxoplasma encephalitis in an AIDS patient. (A) Magnetic resonance imaging with gadolinium, demonstrating multiple ring-enhancing lesions. (B) Resolution of lesions after eight weeks of therapy with pyrimethamine and sulfadiazine. On initial presentation, the patient was also given adjunctive corticosteroids for brain edema; combination anti-retroviral therapy was initiated one week later.*

diagnosis other possible causes of enhancing mass lesions, including primary CNS lymphoma, bacterial brain abscess, tuberculosis, or other malignancies.

Recommended regimens include pyrimethamine (200 mg loading dose given orally followed by 75 mg/day), with folinic acid (10 to 25 mg/day orally) to prevent drug-induced folate deficiency, plus sulfadiazine (6–8 g/day orally in four divided doses, depending on patient weight). In sulfa-allergic patients, clindamycin (600–1200 mg IV or 450 mg orally 4 times daily) may be substituted for sulfadiazone. Small studies have also suggested that TMP-SMX, dosed at 5 mg/kg of TMP component twice daily, may also be effective; this treatment is particularly useful in patients too ill to take oral therapy. Patients who have significant mass effect and associated symptoms (depressed level of consciousness or other signs) may require dexamethasone to reduce cerebral edema. Similarly, individuals with seizures should receive anticonvulsants, but these do not need to be given prophylactically.

Clinical improvement typically occurs within 7 to 14 days, more rapidly if adjunctive dexamethasone is used. Failure to improve over this time period suggests an alternative diagnosis, and neurosurgical consultation would be indicated to obtain a stereotactic brain biopsy. Timing of ART is uncertain, given the potentially catastrophic side effect of increasing inflammation in patients with focal brain lesions. Our practice is to start ART as soon as there is clinical improvement, typically after 7 to 14 days of antitoxoplasmosis therapy.

OTHER ISSUES IN THE CARE OF THE HOSPITALIZED PATIENT WITH HIV

ANTIRETROVIRAL THERAPY

Clinicians who specialize in HIV and follow a large volume of hospitalized patients with HIV should decide when to start ART and which regimen to use. As medication adherence is critical to the success of therapy, patients receiving ART who are hospitalized are often acutely aware that these acute illnesses or surgeries may interrupt their treatment. While one to two days of missed therapy is unlikely to influence outcome, every effort should be made to continue the same ART regimen that was being received prior to admission.

DRUG–DRUG INTERACTIONS

Drug–drug interactions involving antiretroviral agents are common. Antiretrovirals have complex interactions with the cytochrome P450 enzymes of the liver. Most HIV protease inhibitors, but especially ritonavir, have a potent inhibitory effect on cytochrome P450 3A4 (CYP3A4). This property dramatically boosts the levels of some common drugs, including statins, benzodiazepines, calcium channel blockers, and digoxin. For example, simvastatin levels can be dangerously increased when given with protease inhibitors, and sedation from midazolam markedly prolonged. Another important drug–drug interaction is in the reverse direction: rifampin potently induces CYP3A4, significantly reducing plasma concentrations of all available protease inhibitors.

Because drug–drug interactions with ART are numerous and difficult to predict, some of the more important ones are summarized in **Table 195-9**. As a general rule, consultation with expertise in HIV is the best approach to identify and avoid drug–drug interactions. Clinicians are encouraged to check updated resources when considering starting new medications in patients with HIV, especially those already known to have numerous drug interactions or narrow therapeutic safety ranges. Two good sources for this issue are the drug interaction tables of the HIV treatment guidelines (aidsinfo.nih.gov) and the site run by the University of Liverpool (www.hiv-druginteractions.org).

CORONARY ARTERY DISEASE

Effective ART has led to a marked age increase among people with HIV in the United States, and it is estimated that by 2015 more than half will be over 50 years of age. People with HIV are thus increasingly at risk for diseases of aging, such as cardiovascular and renal disorders. There is also evidence that HIV itself may accelerate aging, due to chronic inflammation and immune activation.

HIV is associated with several risk factors for coronary artery disease (CAD), including hyperlipidemia, insulin resistance, a higher rate of smoking than the general population, and a chronic inflammatory state associated with the virus itself. Controlled studies consistently show that patients with HIV have higher rates of CAD

TABLE 195-9 Selected Interactions Between HIV Medications and Commonly Used Drugs

Drug	Interaction
Antacids and calcium supplements	Decreased absorption of some protease inhibitors (PIs)
Anticonvulsants	Carbamazepine, phenytoin, and phenobarbital levels may be increased or decreased; levetiracetam not affected. Levels of some antiretrovirals may also be reduced
Antidepressants	Levels of selective serotonin reuptake inhibitors may be increased or decreased by PIs; levels of trazodone and tricyclic antidepressants may be increased on PIs
Benzodiazepines	Levels ofalprazolam, midazolam, and triazolam increased by many antiretrovirals
Calcium channel blockers	Levels may be increased by ritonavir
Digoxin	Levels may be increased by ritonavir
Fluticasone	Levels increased by ritonavir; Cushing syndrome may result
H2-blockers and proton pump inhibitors	May decrease absorption of PIs, especially atazanavir
Methadone	Zidovudine increases methadone levels; abacavir, efavirenz, and ritonavir decrease ritonavir levels; ritonavir also reduces levels of other narcotics
Metronidazole	Tipranavir and lopinavir/ritonavir syrup contain alcohol, resulting in disulfiram reactions when administered with metronidazole
Oral contraceptives	Ethinyl estradiol levels decreased by ritonavir, increased by efavirenz
Sildenafil, tadalafil, vardenafil	Levels increased by PIs, decreased by efavirenz and etravirine
Statins (HMG-CoA reductase inhibitors)	Levels increased by PIs, decreased by efavirenz and etravirine; magnitude of interaction varies with statin

Adapted from Elke Backman, used with permission.

than age-matched seronegative controls. Patients with HIV and CAD should be considered for the same risk factor modifications as HIV-negative patients, although new medications (such as statins) should be checked carefully for drug–drug interactions with the patient's ART.

■ PULMONARY HYPERTENSION

The prevalence of pulmonary hypertension in patients with HIV is 0.5%, several orders of magnitude higher than the prevalence of idiopathic pulmonary hypertension in the general population. The etiology of HIV-related pulmonary hypertension may involve systemic inflammatory mediators and HIV proteins such as Nef; it does not appear to be caused or ameliorated by antiretroviral therapy. Patients present with dyspnea, fatigue, and less commonly chest pain, symptoms similar to those experienced by most patients with pulmonary hypertension. Diagnosis is made through physical examination, imaging (chest radiography, echocardiography), and more definitively via right heart catheterization. Treatment is similar to the HIV-negative patient.

■ ENDOCARDITIS

Infective endocarditis in patients with HIV is usually associated with injection drug use. *S aureus* and other gram-positive organisms are most often responsible, although a variety of organisms have been reported. The prevalence of endocarditis among HIV-positive intravenous drug users has been reported to be higher than in HIV-negative users. Patients with lower CD4+ counts have worse survival and higher complication rates.

■ MALIGNANCY

The incidence of cancer is increased in HIV-positive patients for many reasons, including lifestyle factors, faulty immune surveillance, and coinfection with cancer-causing viruses. Patients are at heightened risk for AIDS-defining malignancies such as Kaposi sarcoma, non-Hodgkin lymphoma, and cervical cancer, as well as several non–AIDS-defining cancers, including anal cancer associated with human papillomavirus (HPV), Hodgkin lymphoma, lung cancer, liver cancer, and squamous cell cancer of the head and neck. Providers should encourage risk factor reduction, such as smoking cessation and minimizing alcohol consumption, and women with HIV should have regular Pap smears.

■ PSYCHOSOCIAL ISSUES

HIV remains one of the most politically charged diagnoses in medicine. Confidentiality issues surrounding the admission and treatment of HIV-positive patients can be challenging. It may surprise inpatient clinicians to learn that an HIV-positive patient has not disclosed his or her status to a partner or family member, despite having an HIV diagnosis for years. For many patients, the threat of inadvertent disclosure is a significant stressor of hospital admission. A rule of thumb in treating HIV-positive patients is to avoid discussing HIV or treatment related to HIV in front of any other person without the patient's express permission. In addition, every effort should be made to avoid such discussions in front of a patient's roommate, if he or she is in a shared hospital room or open emergency ward. A benefit of the advent of the Health Insurance Portability and Accountability Act is the clinician's ability to cite federal privacy regulations in interactions with a patient's employer, friends, or family members. With the patient's permission, discussion of the patient's illness can and should include family members, spouses, same-sex partners, and friends.

■ FACTITIOUS HIV

Strangely, there are numerous case reports of patients claiming to have HIV infection, but ultimately found to be HIV seronegative on repeat testing. The most common explanation for this phenomenon is the secondary gain associated with an HIV diagnosis, such as eliciting a group of caring providers and access to community and health benefits. Clinicians should suspect factitious HIV whenever a patient is admitted with HIV to the hospital with a potential complication of HIV disease and found, on laboratory testing, to have a normal CD4+ cell count and undetectable HIV RNA, especially

TABLE 195-10 Prevention of Selected HIV-associated Opportunistic Infections

Pathogen	Indication	First Choice	Alternative
PCP	• CD4+ count < 200 cells/mm^3 • CD4+ < 14% or history of AIDS-defining illness	TMP-SMX • 1 DS orally daily (if *Toxoplasma* IgG positive) *or* • 1 SS daily	• TMP-SMX 1 DS orally 3 times weekly • Atovaquone 750 mg orally 2 times a day • Dapsone 100 mg orally daily or 50 mg orally 2 times a day • Dapsone 50 mg orally daily + pyrimethamine 50 mg orally weekly + folinic acid 25 mg orally weekly • Aerosolized pentamidine 300 mg via Respigard II nebulizer
Toxoplasma gondii encephalitis	• Toxoplasma IgG positive patients with CD4+ count < 100 cells/mm^3 • Seronegative patients receiving PCP prophylaxis not active against toxoplasmosis should have toxoplasma serology retested if CD4+ count decline to < 100 cells/mm^3	• TMP-SMX 1 DS orally daily	• TMP-SMX 1 DS orally 3 times weekly • TMP-SMX 1 SS orally daily • Dapsone 50 mg orally daily + pyrimethamine 50 mg orally weekly + folinic acid 25 mg orally weekly • (Dapsone 200 mg + pyrimethamine 75 mg + leucovorin 25 mg) orally weekly
Disseminated MAC disease	• CD4+ count < 50 cells/mm^3 (after ruling out active MAC infection)	• Azithromycin 1200 mg orally once weekly *or* • Clarithromycin 500 mg orally 2 times a day	• Rifabutin 300 mg orally daily (dosage adjustment based on drug–drug interactions with ART); rule out active TB before starting rifabutin

ART, antiretroviral therapy; DS, double strength; MAC, *Mycobacterium avium* complex; PCP, *Pneumocystis jirovecii* pneumonia; SS, half strength; TB, tuberculosis; TMP-SMX, trimethoprim-sulfamethoxazole.

if the patient-provided history includes multiple manifestations of advanced immunosuppression. The management strategy of choice is repeat HIV testing and, if the test is negative, psychiatric consultation.

DISCHARGE PLANNING

In clinical trials of medical drugs, 80% adherence is considered acceptable. However, in the setting of HIV, degrees of adherence of less than 100% are associated with the possibility of ART failure and drug resistance. The challenge of adherence is inflated by the nuisance side effects of ART. Hospitalists should recognize drug adherence as the major ongoing challenge of HIV patients, and provide education and resources to maximize adherence at hospital discharge. Barriers to obtaining medication at outpatient pharmacies should be reduced. As a substantial proportion of HIV patients receive government-funded ART, applications to these programs should be started while the patient is in the hospital. Adherence is increased when patients have the support of a partner, friend, or family member, but the permission of the patient is essential before initiating contact. The involvement of care managers, social workers, visiting nurses, and substance abuse counselors, if appropriate, may also provide crucial insight and assistance.

Close outpatient follow-up is essential for all HIV patients. Ideally, a member of the patient's outpatient care team, such as a clinician, a social worker, or a nurse, should visit the patient in the hospital to make a personal connection and reinforce the treatment plan and details of follow-up. Timing of outpatient follow-up should be two weeks or less for patients hospitalized with PCP or another OI, patients started on ART, or patients at risk of nonadherence to ART.

Patients should be placed on appropriate prophylaxis for OIs (**Table 195-10**). The discharge medication list should be reviewed for interactions. Inpatient vaccinations, such as pneumococcal and seasonal influenza vaccines, should be considered on discharge if indicated. In general, vaccine efficacy is diminished in patients with CD4+ counts <200 cells/mm^3, but immunizations are given and then repeated when the CD4+ count rises. Live vaccines, such as varicella zoster and nasal influenza vaccines, should be avoided in patients with AIDS.

SUGGESTED READINGS

Kaplan JE, Benson C, Holmes KH, Brooks JT, et al. Guidelines for prevention and treatment of opportunistic infections in HIV-infected adults and adolescents. *MMWR Recomm Rep.* 2009; 58(RR-4):1–207.

Lederman MM, Sereni D, Simonneau G, Voelkel NF. Pulmonary arterial hypertension and its association with HIV infection: an overview. *AIDS.* 2008;22(Suppl 3):S1–S6.

Pisculli ML, Sax PE. Use of a serum beta-glucan assay for diagnosis of HIV-related *pneumocystis jirovecii* pneumonia in patients with negative microscopic examination results. *Clin Infect Dis.* 2008;46:1928–1930.

Pulvirenti JJ, Kerns E, Benson C, et al. Infective endocarditis in injection drug users: Importance of human immunodeficiency virus serostatus and degree of immunosuppression. *Clin Infect Dis.* 1996;22:40–45.

Shelburne SA 3rd, Hamill RJ, Rodriguez-Barradas MC, et al. Immune reconstitution inflammatory syndrome: emergence of a unique syndrome during highly active antiretroviral therapy. *Medicine (Baltimore).* 2002;81:213–227.

van der Horst CM, Saag MS, Cloud GA, et al. Treatment of cryptococcal meningitis associated with the acquired immunodeficiency syndrome. *N Engl J Med.* 1997;337:15–21.

Zolopa A, Andersen J, Powderly W, et al. Early antiretroviral therapy reduces AIDS progression/death in individuals with acute opportunistic infections: A multicenter randomized strategy trial. *PLoS One.* 2009;4(5):e5575.

CHAPTER 196

Intravascular Catheter-Related Infections: Management and Prevention

Saima Aslam, MD, MS

Key Clinical Questions

1. How are catheter-related infections diagnosed?
2. What are the potential complications of catheter-related infection?
3. What is the appropriate management of catheter-related infection?
4. When is it appropriate to attempt salvage of an infected intravascular catheter?
5. How can catheter-related infection be prevented?

EPIDEMIOLOGY

Indwelling vascular catheters are the most common cause of nosocomial bloodstream infections. They are particularly common among critically ill patients, hemodialysis-dependent patients, and persons receiving chemotherapy or total parenteral nutrition. In the United States, approximately 80,000 central venous catheter (CVC)-related bloodstream infections occur each year in intensive care units (ICUs). These infections prolong hospitalization by 7.5 to 22 days, cost in excess of $20,000 per episode, and have an attributable mortality of 11.5% to 35%.

Staphylococci, including *Staphylococcus epidermidis* and *Staphylococcus aureus*, cause more than two-thirds to 90% of all catheter-related bloodstream infections (CRBSIs). Other infecting organisms include enteric gram-negative rods, *Pseudomonas aeruginosa*, and *Candida* species. Less common pathogens include *Serratia marcescens*, *Enterobacter* species, *Burkholderia cepacia* complex, and *Citrobacter freundii*.

PATHOPHYSIOLOGY

Infections of vascular catheters arise from bacterial biofilm, comprised of bacteria embedded within an extracellular polysaccharide matrix on the catheter surface (**Figure 196-1**). Bacterial biofilm may develop as early as 24 hours after catheter placement. As shown by electron microscopy, biofilm forms on the external surface of short-term catheters that have been in place for < 10 days, and may be found on the luminal surface of long-term catheters that have been in place for ≥ 10 days.

The first step in biofilm formation is the binding of free-floating, or planktonic, organisms to the catheter surface by cell wall–associated adhesins. This is facilitated by the formation of a film of host fibrin and fibronectin on the catheter surface. Other factors favoring attachment include hydrophobic and electrostatic forces, cell surface structures such as pili or fimbriae, platelet binding, and shear stress from the fluid environment. Attached organisms multiply to form microcolonies and secrete an extracellular polysaccharide matrix that forms the architectural structure of the biofilm. Bacteria embedded in biofilm typically have a lower metabolic rate, making them less susceptible to the effects of antibiotics; the minimal inhibitory concentrations of microorganisms in biofilm can be up to 1000-fold higher than for planktonic organisms. Additionally, antibiotics have difficulty penetrating biofilm. This explains why biofilm-based infections are difficult to eradicate without removal of the infected device.

Catheter infection may arise by several routes. The external catheter may become colonized by skin flora during insertion, or subsequent migration of skin organisms along the catheter surface. Luminal colonization occurs when microorganisms are introduced through the hub of the catheter. The risk of luminal infection increases with more frequent manipulation of the hub. Hematogenous seeding of the catheter may occur during bloodstream infection from another source. Uncommonly, contamination of intravenously administered fluids or drugs can cause CRBSI, sometimes leading to outbreaks. **Table 196-1** lists factors associated with development of CRBSIs.

HOW IS CATHETER-RELATED INFECTION DIAGNOSED?

The clinician must accurately make a diagnosis of catheter-related infection to appropriately treat the patient and reduce the rate of

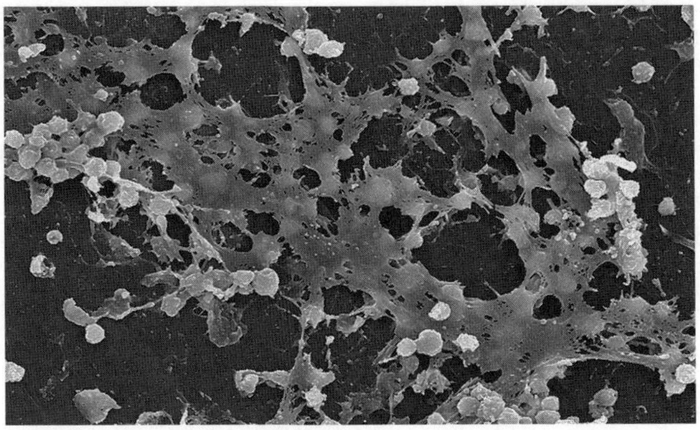

Figure 196-1 *Electron micrograph showing Staphylococcus aureus bacteria embedded in biofilm on the luminal surface of an intravenous catheter. (Public Health Image Library, Centers for Disease Control and Prevention, Rodney M. Donlan, PhD and Janice Carr.)*

unnecessary procedures. The most common presenting manifestation of catheter-related infection is fever. Erythema and purulence at the catheter site are only present in a minority of patients. Sicker patients may have hypotension and tachycardia. Leukocytosis is usually present. Diagnosis can be established by various methods for culturing the removed catheter or blood cultures with an in situ catheter.

DIAGNOSTIC TECHNIQUES NOT REQUIRING CATHETER REMOVAL

Diagnostic techniques that do not require catheter removal are not widely used. Quantitative blood cultures allow a comparison of the number of microorganisms in blood collected simultaneously via the lumen of the catheter and from a peripheral vein. A central-to-peripheral blood culture colony count ratio of 5 to 10:1 is indicative of CRBSI. Although this technique is useful in predicting CRBSIs, it is not routinely performed in most hospitals. A single bacterial count of > 100 colony-forming units (CFU)/mL in the catheter blood specimen is also suggestive of CRBSI, in the presence of a positive peripheral blood culture.

TABLE 196-1 Factors Associated with Increased Risk of Catheter-related Bloodstream Infection

Size of catheter
Greater number of catheter lumens
Frequency of hub manipulation
Type of catheter (plastic > steel)
Location of catheter (central > peripheral; jugular > femoral > subclavian; lower extremity sites > upper extremity sites
Type of placement (cutdown > percutaneous; non-tunneled > tunneled)
Duration of catheter placement (longer > shorter)
Urgency of placement (emergent > elective)
Skills of person performing venipuncture (others > IV team)
Type of skin antisepsis (povidone-iodine > chlorhexidine)
Patient factors (neutropenia, immunosuppression, end-stage renal disease)

Data from Beekmann SE, Henderson DK. Bacteremia due to percutaneous intravascular devices. In: Mandell GL, Bennett JE, and Dolin R, eds. Principles and Practice of Infectious Diseases. 6th ed. New York: Churchill Livingstone; 2005:3347–3361.

Differential time to positivity (DTP) compares the time it takes for a blood culture to become positive when drawn from the catheter versus peripheral blood. The underlying assumption is that blood drawn via the lumen of an infected catheter will have higher number of bacterial colonies than that obtained from a peripheral blood draw, and thus will become positive earlier. When catheter cultures become positive ≥ 2 hours earlier than peripheral blood, DTP is quite sensitive for the diagnosis of CRBSI. The specificity of DTP is dramatically reduced in patients receiving antibiotics at the time cultures were drawn. Most hospitals have automated blood culture machines, making information on time to positivity readily available in the microbiology laboratory.

Endoluminal brushing of the catheter while still in place and subsequent culture is very sensitive for the diagnosis of catheter-related infection in patients with peripheral bacteremia. However, adverse events such as cardiac arrhythmias, embolization, and subsequent bacteremia have been reported.

DIAGNOSTIC TECHNIQUES REQUIRING CATHETER REMOVAL

The most commonly employed method in clinical microbiology laboratories is semiquantitative culture of the catheter tip, the so-called roll-plate method. This technique consists of rolling the distal 4 cm of the catheter tip on an agar plate for culture. A yield of ≥ 15 CFU of bacteria distinguishes catheter colonization from infection. A major limitation is that only microorganisms from the external surface of the catheter are cultured, potentially underdiagnosing catheters with primarily intraluminal infection. Rapid diagnosis of CRBSI may also be achieved by direct microscopic examination of the catheter tip stained with Gram stain or acridine orange.

A more sensitive technique involves sonication of the catheter tip to dislodge biofilm-embedded organisms, with culture of the resultant sonicate. This technique is much more sensitive than the roll-plate method, with a cutoff limit for infection of $\geq 10^2$ to 10^3 CFU/catheter segment. This culturing technique retrieves organisms from both the external and internal surfaces of the catheter. A technique for the rapid diagnosis of CRBSI is direct microscopic examination of the catheter tip stained with Gram stain or acridine orange. **Table 196-2** shows the relative sensitivity and specificity of the methods outlined above.

DIFFERENTIAL DIAGNOSIS

Positive blood cultures must be distinguished from asymptomatic catheter colonization, as well as bacteremia from another source. Potentially life-threatening conditions that may masquerade as a CRBSI include infective endocarditis and septic thrombophlebitis.

WHAT ARE POTENTIAL COMPLICATIONS OF CATHETER-RELATED INFECTION?

Complicated bacteremia should be suspected in patients with persistent bacteremia or fever. Potential complications of CRBSIs include infective endocarditis, septic thrombophlebitis, osteomyelitis, septic arthritis, meningitis, epidural abscess, metastatic abscess, catheter or venous thrombosis, prosthesis infection, various embolic phenomenon, and septic shock.

S aureus bacteremia is associated with an especially high risk of complications, ranging from 25% to 43%. In one study, the strongest predictor of complicated bacteremia was a positive follow-up blood culture result at 48 to 96 hours. A scoring system based on the presence or absence of four risk factors (community acquisition, skin examination findings suggesting acute systemic infection, persistent fever at 72 hours, and positive follow-up blood culture results at 48–96 hours) accurately identified complicated *S aureus* bacteremia.

TABLE 196-2 Accuracy of Various Methods for the Diagnosis of CRBSIs

	Diagnostic Criteria	Accuracy		Disadvantages
		Sensitivity	Specificity	
Techniques without CVC removal				
Simultaneous quantitative blood cultures	Quantitative blood culture drawn through CVC yields CFU count five-fold higher or more than CFU count from simultaneously drawn blood from peripheral vein	93%	97–100%	Labour intensive, costly
Differential time to positivity	Blood culture drawn from CVC becomes positive ≥ 2 h before simultaneously drawn blood culture from peripheral vein	89–90%	72–87%	Hard to interpret when patient is taking antibiotics through the CVC
CVC-drawn quantitative blood culture	Quantitative blood culture from CVC is ≥ 100 CFU/mL	81–86%	85–96%	Cannot differentiate between CRBSI and high-grade bacteraemia
Acridine orange leucocyte cytospin	Presence of any bacteria	87% (96% if followed by Gram stain)	94% (92% if followed by Gram stain)	Not widely tested or used
Endoluminal brush	Quantitative culture with > 100 CFU/mL	95%	84%	May induce bacteraemia, arrhythmia, embolisation
Techniques requiring CVC removal				
Semiquantitative CVC tip culture, roll plate	≥ 15 CFU/mL from CVC tip	45–84%	85%	Unable to culture organisms embedded intraluminally
Quantitative CVC culture: centrifugation, vortexing, sonication	≥ 10^3 CFU from CVC tip	82–83%	89–97%	The cut-off point of ≥ 10^3 CFU vs ≥ 10^2 CFU is not well defined
Microscopy of stained CVC: Gram stain and acridine orange staining	Direct visualisation of the microorganisms	84–100%	97–100%	Labour intensive, impractical

CFU, colony forming units; CRBSI, catheter-related bloodstream infection; CVC, central venous catheter.
Raad I, Hanna H, Maki D. Intravascular catheter-related infections: advances in diagnosis, prevention and management. *Lancet Infect Dis.* 2007;7:645–657. Reprinted with permission from Elsevier.

Another study evaluated all cases of CVC-related *S aureus* bacteremia in order to determine host and pathogen factors that were associated with hematogenous complications. On multivariable analysis, symptom duration, hemodialysis dependence, presence of a long-term intravascular catheter or a noncatheter device, and infection with methicillin-resistant *S aureus* (MRSA) were significantly associated with complications. Thus, at least in patients with *S aureus* CRBSI, the above mentioned factors should prompt providers to remove the infected catheter.

Vascular catheter infections can be associated with thrombosis and septic thrombophlebitis. This may be manifested by evidence of peripheral emboli distal to the site of catheter insertion, or swelling in an extremity. In one study, thrombosis was a common complication of CVC-associated *S aureus* bacteremia (71%), with poor sensitivity of physical examination findings.

Many cases of infective endocarditis are not suspected clinically and therefore are not detected. Studies using transesophageal echocardiogram (TEE) to identify endocarditis in patients with *S aureus* bacteremia have shown high rates of valvular vegetations (25–32%). TEE is more sensitive than transthoracic echocardiogram, and is most sensitive when performed five to seven days after the onset of bacteremia. Clinically, endocarditis is seen in 17% to 20% of cases of *S aureus* bacteremia. In general, patients with *S aureus* bacteremia have a high 90-day mortality rate of 25% to 30%.

TEE should be considered in patients with CRBSI who have any of the following: a prosthetic heart valve, pacemaker, or implantable defibrillator; persistent bacteremia or fungemia, or fever more than three days after initiation of appropriate antibiotic therapy and catheter removal, as well as any case of *S aureus* CRBSI in which a duration of therapy less than four to six weeks is being considered. Depending on the clinical scenario, it may be reasonable to search for other metastatic foci of *S aureus* infection, such as vertebral osteomyelitis.

Some experts believe that a TEE is not required for patients without intravascular hardware who have rapid resolution of *S aureus* bacteremia after initiation of appropriate antimicrobial therapy.

MANAGEMENT

The Infectious Diseases Society of America recently updated their guidelines for the management of catheter-associated infections in 2009. **Figure 196-2** describes the approach to a patient with an infected catheter. Treatment of catheter infections differs depending on the type of line used.

■ PERIPHERAL CATHETER

Infection of these catheters is generally associated with local manifestations such as erythema, tenderness, or suppuration. Systemic signs such as fever or leukocytosis may be present. In general, infected peripheral catheters should be immediately removed. Local symptoms may be alleviated with warm compresses. If suppuration is present, the exudate should be cultured in order to provide appropriate therapy. Most of these infections are caused by gram-positive skin flora, and empiric therapy against these organisms may be started. In the absence of bacteremia, 7 to 10 days of oral antibiotic are recommended. The risk of bacteremia from such an infection is low.

PRACTICE POINT

Septic thrombophlebitis

- Septic (suppurative) thrombophlebitis should be suspected in patients with bacteremia or fungemia that persists despite 72 hours or more of adequate antibiotic therapy, and who have no evidence of endocarditis. The diagnosis is made on the basis of positive blood cultures plus evidence of a clot by ultrasound, CT scan, or another imaging study. At least three to four weeks of intravenous antibiotic therapy should be given. Patients are often anticoagulated, although no randomized controlled trials have been performed to support this practice. Rarely, the infected vein needs to be ligated and removed for failure to respond to conventional therapy.

NONTUNNELED CENTRAL VENOUS CATHETER

CVCs in patients with unexplained fever should not routinely be removed unless there is a local infection at the site of insertion. Catheter removal is only indicated when CRBSI is documented, local infection at the site of catheter insertion is present, or if the patient is hemodynamically unstable and the catheter is suspected as the source of infection. The tip of the removed catheter should be sent for culture. If a catheter is to be removed for suspected infection, guidewire exchange of the catheter can decrease the risk of mechanical complications. However, if culture of the removed catheter is positive, the newly inserted catheter should be replaced a second time *at a new site*. **Table 196-3** describes pathogen-specific antibiotics that can be used in the treatment of CRBSI.

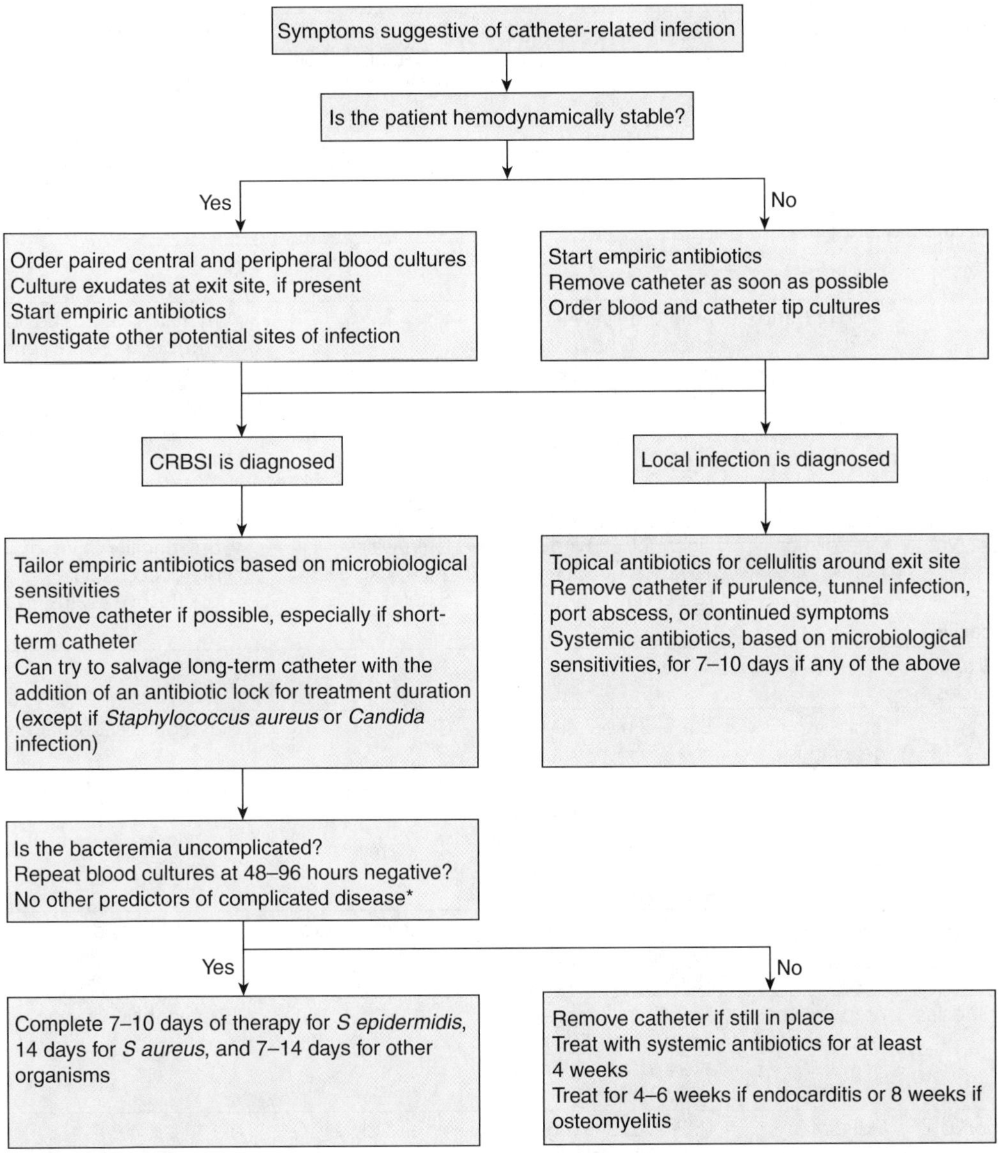

*No persistent fever, skin findings of sepsis, endocarditis, suppurative thromboplebitis, metastatic infection, or intravascular hardware, and lack of community-onset bacteremia for *S aureus*

Figure 196-2 *Approach to suspected catheter-related bloodstream infection (CRBSI).*

TABLE 196-3 Intravenous Antimicrobial Therapy for Catheter-related Bloodstream Infections

Pathogen	Preferred Antimicrobial Agent	Example, Dosage*	Alternative Antimicrobial Agent	Comment
Gram-positive cocci				
Staphylococcus aureus				
Meth susceptible	Penicillinase-resistant Pen†	Naf or Oxa, 2 g every 4 hours	Cfaz, 2 g every 8 hours; or Vm, 15 mg/kg every 12 hours	Penicillinase-resistant Pen or Csps are preferred to Vm.§ For patients receiving hemodialysis, administer Cfaz 20 mg/kg (actual weight), round to nearest 500 mg increment, after dialysis
Meth resistant©	Vm	Vm,15 mg/kg every 12 hours	Dapto, 6–8 mg/kg per day, or linezolid; or Vm plus (Rif or Gm); or TMP-SMZ alone (if susceptible)	Strains of *S aureus* with reduced susceptibility or resistance to Vm have been reported; strains resistant to linezolid and strains resistant to Dapto have been reported
Coagulase-negative staphylococci				
Meth susceptible	Penicillinase-resistant Pen	Naf or Oxa, 2 g every 4 hours	First-generation Csp or Vm or TMP-SMZ (if susceptible)	Vm has dosing advantages over Naf and Oxa, but the latter are preferred because of concerns about increasing Vm resistance
Meth resistant	Vm	Vm, 15 mg/kg IV every 12 hours	Dapto 6 mg/kg per day, linezolid, or Quin/Dalf	For adults < 40 kg linezolid dose should be 10 mg/kg; strains resistant to linezolid have been reported
Enterococcus faecalis/ Enterococcus faecium				
Amp susceptible	Amp or (Amp or Pen) ± aminoglycoside	Amp, 2 g every 4 hours or every 6 hours; or Amp ± Gm, 1 mg/kg every 8 hours	Vm	Vm may have dosing advantages over Amp, but there are concerns about Vm resistance
Amp resistant, Vm susceptible	Vm ± aminoglycoside	Vm, 15 mg/kg IV every 12 hours ± Gm, 1 mg/kg every 8 hours	Linezolid or Dapto 6 mg/kg per day	Quin/Dalf is not effective against *E faecalis*
Amp resistant, Vm resistant	Linezolid or Dapto	Linezolid, 600 mg every 12 hours; or Dapto 6 mg/kg per day	Quin/Dalf 7.5 mg/kg every 8 hours	Susceptibility of Vm-resistant enterococci isolates varies; Quin/Dalf is not effective against *E faecalis*
Gram-negative bacilli**				
Escherichia coli and Klebsiella species				
ESBL negative	Third-generation Csp	Ctri, 1–2 g per day	Cipro or Atm	Susceptibility of strains varies
ESBL positive	Carbapenem	Erta,1 g per day; Imi, 500 mg every 6 hours; Mero, 1 g every 8 hours; or doripenem, 500 mg every 8 hours	Cipro or Atm	Susceptibility of strains varies
Enterobacter species *and Serratia marcescens*	Carbapenem	Erta, 1 g per day; Imi, 500 mg every 6 hours; Mero, 1 g every 8 hours	Cefepime or Cipro	Susceptibility of strains varies
Acinetobacter species	Amp/Sulb or carbapenem	Amp/Sulb, 3 g every 6 hours; or Imi, 500 mg every 6 hours; Mero, 1 g every 8 hours	—	Susceptibility of strains varies
Stenotrophomonas maltophilia	TMP-SMZ	TMP-SMZ, 3–5 mg/kg every 8 hours	Tic and Clv	—

(continued)

TABLE 196-3 Intravenous Antimicrobial Therapy for Catheter-related Bloodstream Infections (*continued*)

Pathogen	Preferred Antimicrobial Agent	Example Dosage*	Alternative Antimicrobial Agent	Comment
Pseudomonas aeruginosa	Fourth-generation Csp or carbapenem or Pip and Tazo with or without aminoglycoside	Cefepime, 2 g every 8 hours; or Imi, 500 mg every 6 hours; or Mero, 1 g every 8 hours; or Pip and Tazo, 4.5 g every 6 hours, Amik, 15 mg/kg every 24 hours or Tobra 5–7 mg/kg every 24 hours	—	Susceptibility of Strains varies
Burkholderia cepacia	TMP-SMZ or carbapenem	TMP-SMZ, 3–5 mg/kg every 8 hours; or Imi, 500 mg every 6 hours; or Mero, 1 g every 8 hours	—	Other species, such as *B acidovorans* and *Burkholderia (Ralstonia) pickettii*, may be susceptible to same antimicrobial agents
Fungi				
Candida albicans or other *Candida* species	Echinocandin or fluconazole (if organism is susceptible)	Caspo, 70 mg/kg loading dose, then 50 mg/kg per day; micafungin,100 mg per day; anidulafungin, 200 mg loading dose followed by 100 mg per day; or fluconazole, 400–600 mg per day	Lipid AmB preparations	Echinocandin should be used to treat critically ill patients until fungal isolate is identified
Uncommon pathogens				
Corynebacterium jeikeium (group JK)	Vm	Vm, 15 mg/kg every 4 hours	Linezolid (based on in vitro activity)	Check susceptibilities for other corynebacteria
Chryseobacterium (Flavobacterium) species	Fluoroquinolone, such as Lvfx	Lvfx 750 mg every 24 hours	TMP-SMZ or Imi or Mero	Based on in vitro activity.
Ochrobacterium anthropi	TMP-SMZ or fluoroquinolone	TMP-SMZ, 3–5 mg/kg every 8 hours; or Cpfx, 400 mg every 12 hours	Imi, Mero, Erta, or Dori plus aminoglycoside	—
Malassezia furfur	AmB	—	Voriconazole	Intravenous lipids should be discontinued; some experts recommend removal of catheter
Mycobacterium species	Susceptibility varies by species	—	—	Different species have wide spectra of susceptibility to antimicrobials [256, 257]

Note: See *S aureus* section of the text regarding important antibiotic management issues concerning linezolid. AmB, amphotericin B; Amp, ampicillin; Atm, aztreonam; Cfaz, cefazolin; cfur, cefuroxime; Clv, clavulanate; Cpfx, ciprofloxacin; Csp, cephalosporin; Ctri, ceftriaxone; Czid, ceftazidime; Erta, ertapenem; Gm, gentamicin; Imi, Imipenem; iv, intravenous; Ket, ketoconazole; Lvfx, levofloxacin; Mero, meropenem; Meth, methicillin; Mez, mezlocillin; Naf, nafcillin; Oxa, oxacillin; Pen, penicillin; PenG, penicillin G; po, by mouth; Pip, piperacillim; Quin/Dalf, quinupristin/dalfopristin; Rif, rifampin; Sulb, sulbactam; Tic, ticarcillin; Tm, tobramycin; TMP-SMZ, trimethoprim-sulfamethoxazole; Vm, vancomycin.

*Initial antibiotic dosages for adult patients with normal renal and hepatic function and no known drug interactions. Fluoroquinolones should not be used for patients < 18 years of age (see the section of the text devoted to treating pediatric infection [256, 257]).

†Pen, if the strain is susceptible.

§Some clinicians will add an aminoglycoside for the first five days of therapy.

**Pending susceptibility results for the isolate.

Mermel LA, Allon M, Bouza E, et al. Clinical practice guidelines for the diagnosis and management of intravascular catheter-related infection. *Clin Infect Dis.* 2009;49:1–45. Reprinted with permission from the University of Chicago Press.

TUNNELED OR IMPLANTED CATHETER

Uncomplicated exit site infections (ie, those without systemic signs of infection, positive blood culture results, or purulence) can be managed with topical antimicrobial agents. If an uncomplicated exit site infection fails to resolve with topical therapy, or if it is accompanied by purulent drainage, systemic antibiotics should be given based on the antimicrobial susceptibility of the causative pathogen. The catheter should be removed if treatment with systemic antibiotics fails.

In the case of a CRBSI of a tunneled or implanted catheter, catheter salvage can be considered if the patient is hemodynamically stable, does not have complicated bacteremia, and is infected with an organism that is readily treatable. Catheter salvage may sometimes be achieved with systemic antibiotics, with simultaneous antibiotic lock solution (high dose of antibiotics instilled locally in the catheter lumen) for the duration of systemic therapy. If the infection is due to *S aureus* or *Candida* species, catheter salvage should not be attempted.

If other vascular sites are unavailable or the patient is at high risk for bleeding in the setting of CRBSI not complicated by an exit site or tunnel infection, then exchange of the infected catheter over a guidewire can be done. Guidewire exchange can also be considered for patients whose symptoms resolve after two to three days of IV antibiotic therapy and who do not have evidence of metastatic infection. In such situations, an antimicrobial impregnated catheter can be considered for catheter exchange.

HEMODIALYSIS CATHETER

A substantial proportion of patients with CRBSI who receive hemodialysis can be managed on an outpatient basis, given the ease of antibiotic administration and the frequency of access to the health care system. Since the risk of gram-negative infections appears to be higher in this population than in nonhemodialysis patients, empiric antibiotics while awaiting definitive culture results should always include coverage against both gram-positive and gram-negative organisms. Once a CRBSI is identified, catheter salvage can be attempted if the infection is due to an organism with low virulence and the patient is hemodynamically stable. This can be attempted using an antibiotic lock solution, in addition to systemic antibiotics. In the case of hemodialysis catheters, the antibiotic is mixed with an anticoagulant, and instilled locally within the catheter lumen when it is not in use.

An alternative to catheter exchange is replacement of the infected catheter with a new temporary catheter either over a guidewire or at a new location, or prompt catheter removal with placement of a new long term catheter once the bacteremia has resolved.

Vancomycin is less effective than nafcillin, oxacillin, or cefazolin in patients with bloodstream infection with methicillin-sensitive *S aureus* (MSSA). For example, hemodialysis-dependent patients with MSSA bacteremia treated with vancomycin are at a higher risk of treatment failure than those who receive cefazolin. In the absence of allergy to beta-lactams, vancomycin should not be continued beyond empiric therapy for hemodialysis-dependent patients with MSSA bacteremia.

COMPLICATED VS UNCOMPLICATED FEVER

In general, patients with CRBSI due to *S aureus* should receive at least four weeks of intravenous antibiotic therapy after catheter removal. However, selected patients with uncomplicated CRBSI due to *S aureus* and a negative TEE may be considered for a 2-week antibiotic course after catheter removal. However, if there is any concern for complication, or if patients have risk factors or clinical predictors of a complication, including persistent fever or positive blood cultures at 48 to 96 hours, then a more aggressive approach to identify and treat potential complications should be pursued. The catheter must always be removed in such a case due to concern for persistent seeding of the bloodstream. Delay in removing the catheter increases the risk of complications. Even if a distinct complication is not uncovered, such patients should be treated with at least four weeks of IV antibiotics.

WHEN MAY SALVAGE OF AN INFECTED CATHETER BE ATTEMPTED?

Catheter salvage may be attempted for long-term catheters with intraluminal infection in hemodynamically stable patients with uncomplicated bacteremia. In catheter salvage, systemic antibiotics are given in addition to an antibiotic lock solution (ALS). Lock therapy counters the inherent antimicrobial resistance of bacteria in biofilm by achieving a local antibiotic concentration within the catheter lumen that is 100- to 1000-fold higher than that achieved by systemically administered antibiotics. Catheter salvage without ALS is not recommended, as it is associated with poor rates of success. In small open-label trials, catheter salvage without relapse occurred in 77% of episodes with the use of ALS. However, success is much lower when the infective organism is *S aureus*. For lock therapy in hemodialysis catheters, the antibiotic is combined with heparin, and instilled into each catheter lumen at the end of each dialysis session. In small uncontrolled studies with follow-up ranging mostly from 10 days to a few weeks, the success rate was 87% to 100% for infection due to gram-negative pathogens and 75% to 84% for infection due to *S epidermidis*, but was only 40% to 55% for *S aureus* infection. A small pilot trial showed improved success rates when an antibiofilm agent, N-acetylcysteine, was added to the ALS in hemodialysis patients. Antibiotics that have been used include vancomycin, cefazolin, linezolid, tigecycline, fluoroquinolones, and aminoglycosides. Generally, these can be mixed with heparin, trisodium citrate, or sodium ethylenediaminetetraacetic acid (EDTA) as the anticoagulant.

PREVENTION

SITE OF CATHETER INSERTION

The site of catheter placement influences the subsequent risk for infection and phlebitis. This is related in part to the risk for thrombophlebitis and density of local skin flora. Internal jugular catheters are more likely to become infected than subclavian catheters due to factors such as the proximity of oropharyngeal secretions, higher skin temperature, and difficulties in immobilizing the catheter and maintaining an optimal dressing. In general, femoral catheters have rates of infection and thrombosis that greatly exceed both subclavian catheters and internal jugular catheters. However, a recent study noted that there was no difference in infection risk between the three sites when experienced operators placed CVCs with maximal sterile precautions and trained staff performed catheter care. Current guidelines recommend avoidance of femoral catheters whenever possible.

ASEPTIC TECHNIQUE

For short-term peripheral catheters, good hand hygiene before catheter insertion or maintenance, combined with proper aseptic technique during catheter manipulation, protects against infection. Good hand hygiene should be achieved through use of either a waterless, alcohol-based product or antibacterial soap and water with adequate rinsing. However, given the higher risk of infection with CVCs, more stringent antisepsis is recommended. Maximal sterile barrier precautions during insertion of CVCs, including sterile gloves, gown, cap, mask, and a large drape, lead to decreased rates of CRBSI than the use of just gloves and small drapes. Use of maximal barrier precautions prior to insertion of arterial lines has not been shown to be beneficial. The Health care Infection Control Practices Advisory Committee (HICPAC) guidelines strongly recommend the use of maximum sterile barrier precautions during the insertion of all CVCs and pulmonary artery catheters.

CUTANEOUS ANTISEPSIS PRIOR TO CATHETER INSERTION

Until recently, povidone-iodine has been the most widely used antiseptic for cutaneous antisepsis prior to insertion of arterial catheters and CVCs. However, several recent studies, and a meta-analysis of nine randomized controlled trials, demonstrated an almost 50% reduction in the rates of CRBSIs when site preparation with chlorhexidine was used, compared with 10% povidone-iodine or 70% alcohol. The alcohol-based preparation of chlorhexidine combines rapid onset of killing by alcohol and delayed antisepsis of chlorhexidine. Use of 2% chlorhexidine for skin antisepsis prior to arterial and CVC insertion is now included in the standard guidelines.

TOPICAL ANTISEPTICS AND DRESSINGS AFTER CATHETER INSERTION

Older studies demonstrated that routine use of povidone-iodine ointment at the catheter insertion site of hemodialysis catheters reduced the incidence of exit-site infections, catheter-tip colonization, and CRBSIs when compared with no ointment. Studies have also shown that mupirocin ointment applied to the catheter insertion site also decreases the rate of CRBSIs. However, there is concern for mupirocin-resistant organisms and adverse impact on integrity of polyurethane catheters. More recently, studies using topical chlorhexidine or chlorhexidine-impregnated sponges applied to the catheter site have noted about 50% reduction in the rate of CRBSI when compared with topical povidone-iodine in randomized trials. A meta-analysis and cost-effectiveness analysis of randomized controlled trials comparing chlorhexidine with povidone-iodine solutions for venous catheter site care found that the use of chlorhexidine significantly reduced the risk for CRBSIs and was cost-effective. One particular cost-benefit analysis in patients of all Philadelphia-area hospitals estimated potential annual U.S. net benefits ranging from $275 million to approximately $1.97 billion. Preventable mortality analyses showed potential decreases of between 329 and 3906 U.S. deaths annually as a result of nationwide use of chlorhexidine dressing.

Several studies including a meta-analysis have demonstrated that the use of transparent dressings versus gauze dressings does not affect the rate of CRBSI. However, transparent dressings permit continuous visual inspection of the catheter site, allow patients to bathe and shower without saturating the dressing, and require less frequent changes than do standard gauze and tape dressings. The choice of dressing can thus be a matter of preference. The data on frequency of dressing changes are not conclusive.

CATHETER SECUREMENT DEVICES

Compared with skin sutures, sutureless securement devices may help prevent CRBSI by decreasing skin trauma. One study demonstrated that use of a sutureless device to secure peripherally inserted central catheters (PICCs) decreased the rate of CRBSI versus sutures.

ANTIMICROBIAL AND ANTISEPTIC CATHETERS

Several randomized controlled trials and two meta-analyses demonstrated that minocycline/rifampin-coated catheters significantly reduced CRBSIs compared with placebo or chlorhexidine/silver sulfadiazine silver-coated catheters. Minocycline/rifampin-coated catheters have shown success in the hemodialysis population as well. In vitro studies demonstrate superior and prolonged activity of minocycline/rifampin-coated CVCs against staphylococci, compared with first-generation chlorhexidine/silver sulfadiazine-coated catheters, without the emergence of resistant organisms.

Studies involving chlorhexidine/sulfadiazine silver-coated catheters (both first-generation catheters with coating of only the external catheter surface, and second-generation catheters with coating of both the external and internal lumens) showed reduction in catheter colonization, but not in the clinical endpoint of CRBSI. A platinum/silver/carbon-impregnated catheter that allows ionic silver release has demonstrated variable decrease in catheter colonization, but no effect on the rate of CRBSIs.

The decision to use antimicrobial or anti-infective catheters should be based on the need to enhance prevention of CRBSI after standard procedures have been implemented, and balanced against the concern for emergence of resistant pathogens and the cost of implementing this strategy.

ANTIBIOTIC LOCK SOLUTIONS

Catheter lock solutions have been used not only for treatment of infections but also for prevention. A meta-analysis of seven randomized controlled trials, mainly in cancer patients, showed that the use of vancomycin lock solution with long-term CVCs reduced the risk of CRBSI by about 50%. In view of the limited activity of vancomycin against staphylococci embedded in biofilm, further data from large prospective studies are required to address concerns regarding vancomycin resistance associated with vancomycin-containing catheter lock solutions. Chelators such as EDTA or citrate have an anticoagulant activity similar to heparin, and have been found to enhance the activity of antimicrobial drugs against organisms embedded in biofilm. Other antimicrobial catheter lock solutions that may reduce catheter infection in small studies are minocycline and EDTA, gentamicin, taurolidine, or ethanol (at concentrations ranging between 25% and 40%).

A meta-analysis of randomized controlled trials showed that antibiotic catheter lock solutions in hemodialysis patients significantly reduced CRBSIs by 44% and catheter removal rates by 35%, as compared with heparin lock alone.

SCHEDULED REPLACEMENT OF CATHETERS

There are no convincing data that demonstrate decreased infection risk with scheduled changing of pulmonary artery catheters or CVCs.

EDUCATION MEASURES

Education of staff can reduce the risk of vascular catheter-related infections. A prospective, multicenter, observational study in Argentina demonstrated that education of health care workers based on the Centers for Disease Control and HICPAC recommendations, followed by feedback about compliance, significantly reduced the risk of CRBSI. The baseline infection rate significantly decreased from 45.9/1000 to 17.1/1000 device-days in the education phase, and fell further to 9.9/1000 device-days in the compliance feedback phase. Another study demonstrated that the use of a self-study module to educate physicians and nurses decreased the rate of CRBSIs by 43%.

A quality improvement initiative that included rigorous measurement, feasible interventions, and cultural change was associated with a decrease in the rate of CRBSIs by almost 50% in 103 ICUs in the United States. Interventions included handwashing, using full barrier precautions during the insertion of CVCs, skin cleansing with chlorhexidine, avoiding femoral catheters whenever possible, and removing unnecessary catheters. Both technical and cultural aspects of implementing the intervention were addressed through engagement, education, execution, and rigorous evaluation. This effect on CRBSIs was sustained to at least four years from the implementation of the protocol, and highlighted the critical role that "bundling" of various preventive approaches has on the rate of infection.

STAFFING ISSUES

Adequate nurse staffing has also been identified as a factor integral to preventing CRBSI. Additionally, several studies have found that the use of dedicated teams for placement of vascular catheters, including PICCs, decreases the rate of infection. **Table 196-4** highlights various preventive measures to decrease the rates of catheter-related infections.

TABLE 196-4 Recommendations to Decrease Rates of Vascular Catheter-related Infection

Educate health care workers regarding the indications for intravascular catheter use, and proper procedures for the insertion and maintenance of intravascular catheters.
Use maximal barrier precautions for CVC insertion.
Use 2% chlorhexidine for cutaneous antisepsis prior to catheter insertion.
Use a subclavian site (rather than a jugular or a femoral site) in adult patients to minimize infection risk for nontunneled CVC placement. Place catheters used for hemodialysis and pheresis in a jugular or femoral vein rather than a subclavian vein to avoid venous stenosis.
If adherence to aseptic technique is not ensured, replace catheter within 48 hours.
Change peripheral short-term catheters every 72–96 hours.
Topical antimicrobials only recommended for hemodialysis catheters.
Clean hubs with 70% ethanol prior to use.
Use an antimicrobial or antiseptic impregnated CVC in adults whose catheter is expected to remain in place >5 days if, after implementing a comprehensive strategy to reduce rates of CRBSI, the CRBSI rate remains above the goal set by the individual institution based on benchmark rates and local factors.
Designate trained personnel for the insertion and maintenance of intravascular catheters.
Promptly remove a catheter that is no longer required
Conduct surveillance in ICUs and other patient populations to determine CRBSI rates, monitor trends, and assist in identifying lapses in infection-control practices.

Data from O'Grady NP, Alexander M, Dellinger EP, et al. Guidelines for the prevention of intravascular catheter–related infections. *Clin Infect Dis.* 2002;35:1281–1307.

QUALITY IMPROVEMENT

Suggested performance measures include whether:

- Patients with CRBSI due to *S aureus* or *Candida* species are treated with prompt catheter removal.
- Catheters are removed from patients with CRBSI with >72 hours of bacteremia or fungemia, despite administration of antimicrobial agents to which the pathogens are susceptible.
- Patients with *S aureus* bacteremia for >72 hours after catheter removal despite appropriate antibiotic therapy receive antibiotic treatment for at least four weeks.
- Blood cultures have been obtained both percutaneously and from the catheter in patients being assessed for possible CRBSI who are not receiving hemodialysis through a catheter.
- Blood culture bottles are properly labeled, with respect to the anatomic site or catheter used to obtain the blood sample for culture.
- A beta-lactam antibiotic is used in preference to vancomycin for beta-lactam–susceptible staphylococcal CRBSI among patients without a beta-lactam allergy.

SUGGESTED READINGS

Darouiche RO, Raad II, Heard SO, et al. A comparison of two antimicrobial-impregnated central venous catheters. *N Engl J Med.* 1999;340:1–8.

Fowler VG, Olsen MK, Corey GR. Clinical identifiers of complicated *Staphylococcus aureus* bacterermia. *Arch Intern Med.* 2003;163:2066–2072.

Maki DG, Weise CE, Sarafin HW. A semiquantitative culture method for identifying intravenous-catheter-related infection. *N Engl J Med.* 1977;296:1305–1309.

Mermel LM, Allon M, Bouza E, et al. Clinical practice guidelines for the diagnosis and management of intravascular catheter-related infection. *Clin Infect Dis.* 2009;49:1–45.

O'Grady NP, Alexander M, Dellinger EP, et al. Guidelines for the prevention of intravascular catheter-related infections. *Clin Infect Dis.* 2002;35:1281–1307.

Pronovost PJ, Needham D, Berenholtz S, et al. An intervention to decrease catheter-related bloodstream infections in the ICU. *N Engl J Med.* 2006;355:2725–2732.

Raad I, Hanna HA, Alakech B, et al. Differential time to positivity: a useful method for diagnosing catheter-related bloodstream infections. *Ann Intern Med.* 2004;140:18–25.

Raad I, Hanna H, Maki D. Intravascular catheter-related infections: advances in diagnosis, prevention and management. *Lancet Infect Dis.* 2007;7:645–657.

Raad I, Hohn DC, Gilbreath BJ, et al. Prevention of central venous catheter-related infections by using maximal sterile barrier precautions during insertion. *Infect Control Hosp Epidemiol.* 1994;15:231–238.

CHAPTER 197

Infective Endocarditis

Thomas A. Owens, MD
Vance G. Fowler Jr., MD, MHS

Key Clinical Questions

1. Does the patient have symptoms consistent with infective endocarditis?
2. What tests and studies are indicated to evaluate infective endocarditis?
3. What infectious etiologies should be considered?
4. What treatments should be considered?
5. What complications should be expected?

INTRODUCTION

Infective endocarditis (IE) is a relatively common infection in the hospital setting, with an inpatient mortality rate of about 18%. The incidence of IE rises linearly with age, from around 1 case per 100,000 person-years among young adults, to over 10 cases per 100,000 person-years among those older than 75 years. The hallmark lesion of IE is the endocardial vegetation. Although the heart valves are affected most commonly, IE also may involve septal defects, mural endocardium, or prosthetic cardiac structures. Vegetations may result in valvular regurgitation or obstruction, myocardial abscess, or mycotic aneurysm. Definitive diagnosis requires identification of the causative organism in blood, cardiac structures, or emboli. Cure requires prolonged antimicrobial treatment and often valve replacement surgery, leading to substantial expense.

EPIDEMIOLOGY

Historically, IE was a disease of younger patients with rheumatic heart disease, and mainly involved viridans group streptococci. Over the last decade, however, a new form of the disease, health care–associated IE, has emerged. This new form of IE is distinct in its microbiology (predominantly *Staphylococcus aureus*) and risk factors (eg, intravenous catheters, hyperalimentation lines, pacemakers, dialysis shunts). It represents about one-third of all IE cases among noninjection drug users with native valve disease.

RISK FACTORS FOR IE

Almost any type of structural heart disease may predispose to IE, especially when the defect results in turbulent blood flow. Right-sided IE is primarily an infection of injection drug users and patients with indwelling transvenous pacemakers. In developed countries, the proportion of cases related to rheumatic heart disease has declined to 5% or less in the past 2 decades, while in developing countries, rheumatic heart disease remains the most common predisposing cardiac condition. Congenital bicuspid aortic valve is the underlying lesion in more than 15% of IE cases in patients (especially men) older than 60 years, and is associated with a poor prognosis, despite rapid valve replacement. Degenerative cardiac lesions (eg, calcified mitral annulus, calcific nodular lesions secondary to arteriosclerotic cardiovascular disease, and post–myocardial infarction thrombus) assume the greatest importance in the 30% to 40% of IE patients without any demonstrable underlying valvular disease. Marfan syndrome, when associated with aortic insufficiency, also has been associated with IE. Intravascular infections involving cardiac devices (eg, permanent cardiac pacemakers, defibrillators) also have increased significantly since the 1990s. Injection drug users are at high risk for recurrent and polymicrobial IE.

PATHOGENESIS AND PATHOPHYSIOLOGY

Mitral and aortic valvular involvement are most common in IE. Distributions of valvular involvement range from 28% to 45% of cases for isolated mitral valve IE, 5% to 36% for isolated aortic valve IE, and 0% to 35% for combined aortic and mitral valves IE. In the absence of injection drug use, the tricuspid valve rarely is involved (0–6% of cases). Pulmonary valve IE is rare (< 1%) in any clinical circumstance.

PRACTICE POINT

Valves most commonly affected by IE (in decreasing order of frequency)

- Mitral valve
- Aortic valve
- Combined mitral and aortic valve
- Tricuspid valve
- Pulmonary valve (rare)

Note: mechanical and bioprosthetic valves are affected equally

The development of IE probably requires several independent events. The normal myocardial endothelial lining is relatively resistant to infection, and constant blood flow thwarts bacteria and fungi from settling on an endocardial surface. The initiation of IE requires the simultaneous presence of both a predisposing endocardial abnormality and microorganisms in the bloodstream (bacteremia). Occasionally, massive bacteremia or particularly virulent microorganisms—especially *S aureus*—may cause IE on normal valves.

Bacteremia may occur whenever a mucosal surface heavily colonized with bacteria is traumatized, such as with dental extractions and invasive procedures, as well as gastrointestinal, urologic, and gynecologic procedures. The degree of bacteremia is proportional to the trauma produced by the procedure and to the number of organisms inhabiting the surface.

ORGANISMS RESPONSIBLE FOR IE

Many microorganisms have been identified in IE, but streptococci and staphylococci account for 80% to 90% of the cases in which an organism is isolated. The most common etiologic agents are outlined in **Table 197-1**.

S aureus is the most common cause of native valve IE, prosthetic valve IE, and injection-drug use associated IE. It is associated with aggressive disease, extracardiac metastatic infections, and a high mortality rate. **Group A, C, and G streptococci** cause aggressive IE with high mortality (up to 70%). **Group B streptococci** also lead to acute disease with high mortality, often requiring valve replacement. It is more common in elderly or immunosuppressed patients. ***Streptococcus pneumoniae*** is no longer common, but is notable for its acute and destructive course. A classical, often lethal presentation was Austrian's triad (simultaneous pneumococcal pneumonia, meningitis, and IE). ***Pseudomonas aeruginosa*** and **enteric gram-negative rods** cause acute IE, and require surgery for cure. Although traditionally thought to be primarily an infection of injection drug users, recent studies have demonstrated that the primary risk factor for gram-negative IE is health care contact.

PRACTICE POINT

Risk factors for infective endocarditis

- Previous IE with valvular damage
- Invasive vascular procedures
- Injection drug abuse
- Rheumatic heart disease (< 5% of cases of IE)
- Elderly patients with calcific aortic stenosis
- Congenital heart disease (15% of cases, bicuspid aortic valve most common)
- Prosthetic cardiac devices

Viridans group streptococci are the most common cause of community-acquired, subacute IE. **Enterococci** also usually present in subacute fashion, and comprise about 10% of IE. **Coagulase-negative *Staphylococcus* species** are typically associated with subacute disease, accounting for 20% of IE associated with prosthetic valves, and 8% of cases of native valve IE. **HACEK organisms** (*Haemophilus aphrophilus, Actinobacillus actinomycetemcomitans, Cardiobacterium hominis, Eikenella corrodens, Kingella kingae*) cause subacute disease, causing about 5% of all IE. **Fungi** are uncommon pathogens in IE, but devastating when they occur. They present subacutely, with bulky, destructive, and recaltitrant vegatations, and almost always require surgery for cure.

TABLE 197-1 Etiologic Agents in Infective Endocarditis

	Percentage of Patients		
Cause of Endocarditis	Drug Users	Nondrug Users	Prosthetic Valve
Staphylococcus aureus	68	28	23
Coagulase-negative *Staphylococcus*	3	9	17
Viridans group streptococci	10	21	12
Streptococcus bovis	1	7	5
Other streptococci	2	7	5
Enterococcus species	5	11	12
HACEK	0	2	2
Fungi/yeast	1	1	4
Polymicrobial	3	1	0.8
Negative culture findings	5	9	12
Other	3	4	7
Surgical therapy	38	48	49
In-hospital mortality	10	17	23

Data from Murdoch DR, Corey GR, Hoen B, et al. International Collaboration on Endocarditis-Prospective Cohort Study (ICE-PCS) Investigators. Clinical presentation, etiology, and outcome of infective endocarditis in the 21st century: the International Collaboration on Endocarditis-Prospective Cohort Study. *Arch Intern Med.* 2009;169:463–473.

TABLE 197-2 Clinical Admission Findings in Patients with Definitive Endocarditis

Findings	% Patients
Examination	
Fever (> 38°C)	96
New murmur	48
Worsening of old murmur	20
Vascular embolic event	17
Splenomegaly	11
Splinter hemorrhages	8
Conjunctival haemorrhage	5
Janeway lesions	5
Osler nodes	3
Roth spots	2
Laboratory studies	
Elevated C-reactive protein	62
Elevated erythrocyte sedimentation rate	61
Hematuria	26
Elevated rheumatoid factor	5

Data from Murdoch DR, Corey GR, Hoen B, et al. International Collaboration on Endocarditis-Prospective Cohort Study (ICE-PCS) Investigators. Clinical presentation, etiology, and outcome of infective endocarditis in the 21st century: the International Collaboration on Endocarditis-Prospective Cohort Study. *Arch Intern Med.* 2009;169:463–473.

CLINICAL PRESENTATION

The clinical presentation of IE is non-specific, and the differential diagnosis is broad (**Table 197-2**). The diagnosis of IE may be delayed or occasionally missed entirely because of its protean manifestations. Thus, the clinician must maintain a high index of suspicion for this potentially lethal infection. Factors contributing to the overall clinical picture of IE include local cardiac complications, embolization, which may involve any organ and is clinically underappreciated, persistent bacteremia, often leading to metastatic infection, and immunopathologic factors.

Traditionally, IE was classified as acute or subacute. Acute IE is associated with *S aureus*, *S pyogenes*, or *S pneumoniae*. Fever is almost always present. Patients often appear toxic and occasionally exhibit septic shock. Untreated cases are rapidly fatal. Although most patients with subacute IE will develop valvular dysfunction, only half of patients with acute IE will have a detectable cardiac murmur on initial examination. In right-sided endocarditis, septic pulmonary emboli may cause cough, pleuritic chest pain, and sometimes hemoptysis.

Subacute IE (death occurring in 6 weeks to 3 months) and chronic IE (death occurring later than 3 months) often occur in the setting of prior valvular disease, with viridans streptococci as a frequent pathogen. Symptoms are vague: low-grade fever (< 39°C), night sweats, fatigue, malaise, and weight loss. Chills and arthralgias may occur. Symptoms and signs of valvular insufficiency may be present. Initially, up to 15% of patients have fever or a murmur, but eventually almost all develop both.

Physical examination is often entirely normal, especially in patients with a short duration of symptoms. Findings, when present, may include pallor, fever, change in a prior murmur or development of a new regurgitant murmur, and tachycardia. Retinal emboli can cause round or oval hemorrhagic retinal lesions with small white centers (Roth spots). Cutaneous manifestations include petechiae (on the upper trunk, conjunctivae, mucous membranes, and distal extremities), nontender hemorrhagic macules on the palms or soles (Janeway lesions; **Figure 197-1**), painful erythematous subcutaneous nodules on the tips of digits (Osler nodes; **Figure 197-2**), and splinter hemorrhages under the nails. Approximately one-third of IE patients have neurologic disease which may include transient ischemic attacks, stroke, toxic encephalopathy, brain abscess, or subarachnoid hemorrhage associated with mycotic aneurysm rupture. Renal emboli may cause flank pain or gross hematuria, while splenic emboli cause left upper quadrant pain. Prolonged infection may cause splenomegaly or clubbing of fingers and toes.

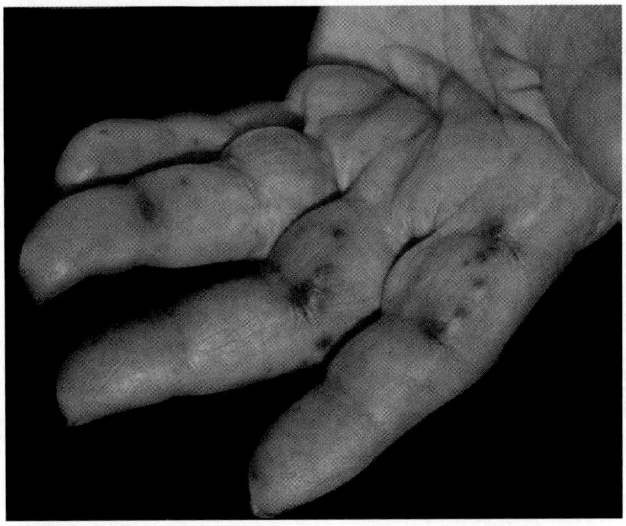

Figure 197-1 *Janeway lesions: nontender, hemorrhagic lesions on the palms and sole, from cardiac microemboli. (Reproduced, with permission, from Wolff K, Johnson RA, Suurmond D. Fitzpatrick's Color Atlas & Synopsis of Clinical Dermatology. 5th ed. New York: McGraw-Hill; 2005. Fig. 24-46.)*

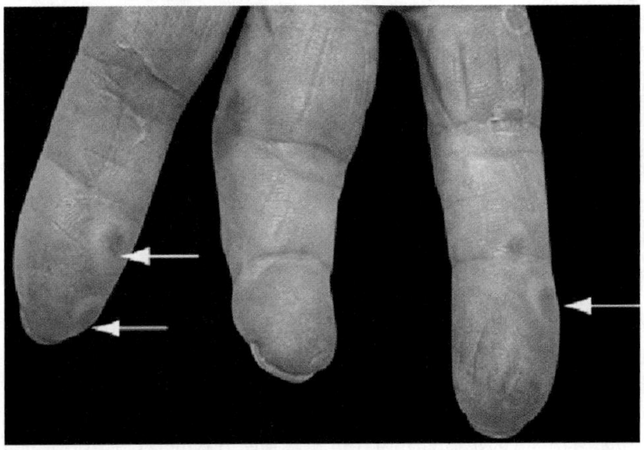

Figure 197-2 *Osler nodes: painful nodules in the fingers and toes, now rarely observed in endocarditis. Formerly thought to be immune-complex related, but probably have a similar pathogenesis to Janeway lesions, except that the microemboli are lodged in more sensitive dermal tissue. (Reproduced, with permission, from Wolff K, Goldsmith LA, Katz SI, et al. Fitzpatrick's Dermatology in General Medicine. 7th ed. New York: McGraw-Hill; 2008. Fig. 151-11.)*

This historical classification ignores the the frequent overlap in manifestations of infection by specific organisms, such as the enterococci, and the fact that most IE in the 21st century are acute infections. Therefore classification based on the etiologic causes for IE is more useful as it has implications for the expected clinical course, the likelihood of preexisting heart disease, and the appropriate antimicrobial therapy.

DIFFERENTIAL DIAGNOSIS

The differential diagnosis of IE includes other diseases with complex and varied manifestations, including noninfectious cardiac conditions such as marantic endocarditis, atrial myxoma, and other cardiac neoplasms; systemic infections such as tick-borne febrile illness, tuberculosis, brucellosis, and syphilis; and rheumatologic conditions such as antiphospholipid syndrome, polymyalgia rheumatica, reactive arthritis, systemic lupus erythematosus, and temporal arteritis.

DIAGNOSTIC TESTING

BLOOD CULTURES

The blood culture is the most important laboratory test performed in a diagnostic workup for IE. Identification of the organism and its antimicrobial susceptibility is vital to guide treatment. Documentation of continuous bacteremia (> 30 min in duration) is pivotal for establishing the diagnosis of IE. Multiple positive blood cultures, especially if *S aureus* is isolated, is an important clue for the presence of IE or other endovascular infections, such as septic thrombophlebitis or mycotic aneurysm. The presence of heart valve disorders, recent invasive procedures or intravascular catheters, or a history of injection drug use all increase the probability of endovascular infection. Patients with documented bacteremia should be examined thoroughly and repeatedly for signs and symptoms suggesting IE or other infectious complication.

Blood cultures should be obtained before starting antibiotics. To reduce false-positive blood cultures, site preparation must be carefully performed and obtained by peripheral venipuncture whenever possible. At least three blood culture sets (no more than two bottles per venipuncture) should be obtained in the first 24 hours. While three blood cultures are generally sufficient for the initial diagnosis of most forms of IE, more specimens may be necessary if the patient has received antibiotics in the preceding 2 weeks. Additional blood cultures drawn at regular intervals are important to document resolution of bacteremia. At least 10 mL of blood should be injected into each culture bottle. When IE is present and no prior antibiotic therapy was given, multiple blood cultures are usually positive because the bacteremia is continuous; at least 1 culture is positive in 99%. Premature use of empiric antibiotics are discouraged, to avoid culture-negative endocarditis. If prior antimicrobial therapy has been given, blood cultures should still be obtained, but they may be negative.

As many as 50% of positive clinical blood culture results have been estimated to be falsely positive, and one such result can lead to 4 days of unnecessary patient hospitalization. The interpretation of positive blood cultures depends on several factors, including the virulence of the organism. Positive blood cultures for *S aureus* are always significant; the risk of IE in patients with positive blood cultures for *S aureus* is 10% to 12%. Blood cultures growing *Corynebacterium* species (diphtheroids) or *Bacillus* species (except *B anthracis*) are rarely significant. Coagulase-negative staphylococci are most often contaminants, except in the setting of patients with prosthetic valves. Blood cultures have greater significance with increasing numbers of cultures positive for the same organism, a shorter time to culture positivity (implying higher bacterial load), and more severe clinical illness. The probability of IE is also increased by cardiac prosthetic material, absence of an alternative explanation for bacteremia, community acquisition, clinical evidence of IE, persistent fever, or persistent bacteremia.

Blood cultures are negative in only 5% of patients with IE confirmed by strict diagnostic criteria. In most cases, culture-negative IE is caused by the receipt of antibiotics prior to blood cultures. In a minority of patients, blood culture-negative IE is caused by fastidious organisms. The most commonly encountered true culture-negative pathogens in the United States are *Bartonella* species. Two species predominate. *Bartonella quintana* is a louse-borne infection associated with homelessness. *Bartonella henselae* is generally flea-borne, and associated with cat exposure. *Coxiella burnetti* (Q fever) is a common cause of culture-negative IE in Europe, and is associated with exposure to birthing animals. *Tropheryma whipplei*, the agent of Whipple disease, and *Chlamydia* species are rare causes of chronic IE. Although improvements in blood culture platforms have significantly increased the ability to successfully isolate yeast (eg, *Candida*) from blood, IE with molds such as *Aspergillus* continue to present with apparently sterile blood cultures. HACEK bacteria and other fastidious organisms, such as *Abiotrophia* and *Granulicatella*, formerly caused a modest proportion of culture-negative endocarditis, but these may be isolated without difficulty in most contemporary blood culture systems.

OTHER LABORATORY FINDINGS

Aside from positive blood cultures, laboratory findings in IE are nonspecific. A normocytic anemia is often seen in established infections, as are an elevated WBC count, increased erythrocyte sedimentation rate, hypergammaglobulinemia, circulating immune complexes, and rheumatoid factor, but these findings are not helpful diagnostically. Urinalysis routinely shows microscopic hematuria and, occasionally, red blood cell casts, pyuria, or bacteriuria. *S aureus* in the urine of a patient without an indwelling urinary catheter suggests staphylococcal bacteremia as the source.

ECHOCARDIOGRAPHY

Echocardiography should be performed on all patients with suspected IE. Echocardiography is unnecessary in patients in whom IE is very unlikely based on clinical features, or in bacteremia with organisms that rarely cause IE (eg, *Escherichia coli*). In most patients with suspected IE, transthoracic echocardiography (TTE) is obtained first. Due to conditions such as obesity, chest wall abnormalities, or chronic obstructive pulmonary disease, TTE may be technically inadequate in up to 20% of American adults. The sensitivity of TTE for vegetations is only about 60%, so a negative study does not rule out disease. TTE is more sensitive in right-sided IE than left-sided IE, as it visualizes the pulmonic and tricuspid valves particularly well. Specificity of TTE is excellent, and false-positive studies are rare.

In patients with at least intermediate suspicion of IE, and negative or inconclusive results on TTE, transesophageal echocardiography (TEE) should be pursued. TEE is more sensitive than conventional TTE for detecting intracardiac vegetations (95% sensitivity), particularly in prosthetic valve endocarditis. While TEE is better than TTE in the diagnosis of prosthetic valve endocarditis, both TEE and TTE are somewhat less sensitive and specific in imaging prosthetic valves, due to echogenic artifact from the sewing ring and support structures, and the difficulty of distinguishing sterile thrombus and degenerative changes from vegetations.

Patients with *S aureus* bacteremia have a high risk of underlying IE (10–12%). Cost-effectiveness studies suggest that in the setting of *S aureus* bacteremia, TEE should be the first examination in patients with suspected IE. If TEE cannot be performed for clinical reasons, or must be delayed, then TTE should be performed promptly.

PRACTICE POINT

- The risk of endocarditis in patients with *S aureus* bacteremia is high, up to 12%. A negative transthoracic echocardiogram does not exclude endocarditis in this setting. Cost-effectiveness studies suggest that it is reasonable to proceed with transesophageal echocardiogram as the initial echocardiographic study, if available.

Echocardiography is invaluable in assessing local complications of IE. Several echocardiographic findings, such as congestive heart failure (CHF), severe valvular regurgitation, paravalvular abscesses, and flail or perforated valve leaflets, indicate a need for surgical intervention. Larger and more mobile vegetations pose a greater risk of embolization. Most studies suggest that mitral valve vegetations (particularly those involving the anterior leaflet) are associated with higher rates of embolization than are noted with aortic valve vegetations. However, visualization of large vegetations by echocardiography, in the absence of clinical embolic episodes, is not sufficient to prompt early surgery. The risk of embolization drops rapidly after the first week of effective antibiotic therapy.

DIAGNOSTIC CRITERIA

The Duke criteria are the basis for establishing the diagnosis of IE. The Duke criteria use major and minor criteria to group patients as having definite or possible IE, or to reject IE in patients unlikely to have the disease. There are three ways of diagnosing definite IE: on a microbiologic basis (eg, isolation of microorganisms from cardiac tissue or a thromboembolus); on a pathologic basis (eg, evidence of active IE on histopathologic exam); and on a clinical basis (**Table 197-3A**). Major clinical criteria include echocardiographic evidence of IE (eg, vegetations or paravalvular complications of IE) and the isolation of typical IE pathogens from blood cultures. In addition, fever, predisposing cardiac conditions, physical examination findings of IE, and active injection drug use are included as minor criteria (**Table 197-3B**).

Fungal IE has a low rate of positive blood culture results. At best, only 50% of *Candida* species are associated with positive blood culture results. *Histoplasma* and *Aspergillus* are almost never retrieved from the bloodstream. Thus, fungal IE must always be considered in the clinical setting of culture-negative IE that fails to respond to appropriate antibiotic therapy.

The diagnosis of pacemaker IE may be difficult as its clinical presentation is often subtle. For this reason, fever or a positive blood culture without a primary source in patients with pacemakers or implantable cardioverter-defibrillators represents device-associated IE until proven otherwise.

TABLE 197-3A Definition of Infective Endocarditis According to the Modified Duke Criteria

Definite Infective Endocarditis
Pathological criteria
Microorganisms demonstrated by culture or histological examination of a vegetation, a vegetation that has embolized, or an intracardiac abscess specimen; or
Pathological lesions; vegetation or intracardiac abscess confirmed by histological examination showing active endocarditis
Clinical criteria
2 major criteria; or
1 major criterion and 3 minor criteria; or
5 minor criteria
Possible IE
1 major criterion and 1 minor criterion; or
3 minor criteria
Rejected
Firm alternative diagnosis explaining evidence of IE; or
Resolution of IE syndrome with antibiotic therapy for 4 days; or
No pathological evidence of IE at surgery or autopsy, with antibiotic therapy for 4 days; or
Does not meet criteria for possible IE as above

Data from Li J, Sexton DJ, Mick N, et al. Proposed modifications to the Duke criteria for the diagnosis of infective endocarditis. *Clin Infect Dis.* 2000;30:633–638.

TABLE 197-3B Definition of Terms Used in the Modified Duke Criteria for the Diagnosis of Infective Endocarditis

Major Criteria
Blood culture positive for IE
Typical microorganisms consistent with IE from 2 separate blood cultures: Viridans streptococci, *Streptococcus bovis*, HACEK group, *Staphylococcus aureus*; or community-acquired enterococci in the absence of a primary focus; or
Microorganisms consistent with IE from persistently positive blood cultures defined as follows: At least 2 positive cultures of blood samples drawn > 12 h apart; or all of 3 or a majority of 4 separate cultures of blood (with first and last sample drawn at least 1 h apart)
Single positive blood culture for *Coxiella burnetii* or antiphase 1 IgG antibody titer > 1:800
Evidence of endocardial involvement
Echocardiogram positive for IE (TEE recommended for patients with prosthetic valves, rated at least "possible IE" by clinical criteria, or complicated IE [paravalvular abscess]; TTE as first test in other patients) defined as follows: oscillating intracardiac mass on valve or supporting structures, in the path of regurgitant jets, or on implanted material in the absence of an alternative anatomic explanation; or abscess; or new partial dehiscence of prosthetic valve; new valvular regurgitation (worsening or changing or preexisting murmur not sufficient)
Minor criteria
Predisposition, predisposing heart condition, or IDU
Fever, temperature > 38°C
Vascular phenomena, major arterial emboli, septic pulmonary infarcts, mycotic aneurysm, intracranial hemorrhage, conjunctival hemorrhages, and Janeway lesions
Immunologic phenomena: glomerulonephritis, Osler nodes, Roth spots, and rheumatoid factor
Microbiological evidence: positive blood culture but does not meet a major criterion as noted above* or serological evidence of active infection with organism consistent with IE
Echocardiographic minor criteria eliminated

*Excludes single positive cultures for coagulase-negative staphylococci and organisms that do not cause endocarditis.

TEE, transesophageal echocardiography; TTE, transthoracic echocardiography.

Data from Li J, Sexton DJ, Mick N, et al. Proposed modifications to the Duke criteria for the diagnosis of infective endocarditis. *Clin Infect Dis.* 2000;30:633–638.

TREATMENT

The diagnosis of IE should be made rapidly to initiate antibiotic therapy and identify patients at high risk for complications who may benefit from early surgery. The response to antimicrobial therapy for IE is unique among bacterial infections. While organisms may exhibit exquisite in vitro susceptibility to antibiotics, eradication takes many weeks, and relapses and medical failures may occur. There are two possible explanations for these findings. First, the vegetation is a privileged site of impaired host defenses. Bacteria are encased in a fibrin meshwork which hinders the penetration of both neutrophils and antibiotics. Second, bacteria in these vegetations reach tremendous population densities, and exist in a state of diminished metabolic activity and cell division. This reduces their susceptibility to antimicrobial therapy.

General principles have been accepted that provide the framework for the current recommendations for treatment of IE.

- Parenteral antibiotics are preferred over oral drugs because of the importance of sustained antibacterial activity. Erratic and unpredictable enteral absorption with many antimicrobials makes oral therapy less desirable.
- Short-term therapy is associated with relapse, and most guidelines emphasize prolonged drug administration.
- Bacteriostatic antibiotics are less effective in the treatment of bacterial IE, and their use has been associated with relapses, a failure to control the infection, or both.
- The selection of antibiotics should be based on antimicrobial susceptibility tests, and treatment should be monitored with antimicrobial blood levels (when indicated) and clinical response to therapy.
- Blood cultures should be obtained during the early phase of therapy to ensure clearance of the bacteremia, and in the setting of persistent or recurrent fever during therapy. Surveillance blood cultures should be obtained immediately before a patient's next scheduled antibiotic dose.

A summary of recommended antimicrobial therapies are outlined in **Table 197-4**. Recommendations for antimicrobial treatment of IE caused by other pathogens may be found in the 2005 American Heart Association guidelines for diagnosis, antimicrobial therapy, and management of complications in IE. Consultation with an infectious diseases specialist is recommended in all cases of IE.

Hospitalized patients with newly diagnosed IE should be placed on cardiac telemetry and receive daily electrocardiograms to monitor for cardiac arrhythmias, myocardial infarctions (due to emboli showering the coronary artery, especially in patients with aortic IE), and myocardial abscesses or hemodynamic fistulae. An emerging atrioventricular block on ECG is an ominous finding, and suggests a paravalvular abscess eroding into the conduction system. Patients with IE may have associated myocarditis with heart failure and cardiac arrhythmias. These patients require close monitoring in an intensive care unit.

Anticoagulation during therapy for IE is controversial. Most experts agree that anticoagulants in patients with native valve IE are contraindicated, as fatal subarachnoid hemorrhage and other bleeding complications are associated with anticoagulation in this setting. In patients with *S aureus* prosthetic valve IE who have had a recent central nervous system embolic event, guidelines suggest discontinuation of anticoagulation for at least the first 2 weeks of antibiotic therapy. Anticoagulation should be reintroduced cautiously in these patients with close monitoring. In prosthetic valve IE in patients without evidence of significant vascular emboli, many clinicians continue therapeutic anticoagulation.

SURGICAL INTERVENTION

Half of all patients with IE ultimately require cardiac surgery. Generally, earlier surgical intervention has been associated with improved patient survival. A recent analysis of a large, prospectively ascertained, international cohort of patients with native valve IE revealed that early surgery was associated with significantly lower inhospital mortality than medical therapy. This benefit was most significant in patients with indications for surgical intervention, including paravalvular complications, systemic embolization, stroke, or *S aureus* infection. Patient factors such as hemodynamic status are crucial determinants of the timing of valve replacement. For example, the development of CHF in the setting of IE generally dictates valvular surgery, regardless of the acuity of infection or the amount of antibiotics already received by the patient. Patients with hemodynamic or perivalvular complications in the acute setting have a poor prognosis, and are best managed at a center with appropriate surgical and infectious diseases expertise.

Up to one-third of patients with left-sided IE will require surgical intervention during the acute stages of infection, either for valve replacement or metastatic infection. Common causes of persistent or recurrent fever despite appropriate antimicrobial therapy include paravalvular abscess, unidentified extracardiac metastatic infection, systemic emboli, or drug hypersensitivity. In patients with heart failure or persistent fever, close monitoring and early surgical consultation are essential. Most experts recommend that if evidence of active IE is present at the time of surgical valve replacement, antibiotic therapy should be continued postoperatively for several weeks at a minimum.

In contrast to left-sided IE, in which CHF is the usual indication for surgical intervention, persistent infection is the most common indication for surgery in patients with right-sided IE. Most of these patients are injection drug users with resistant or difficult to treat organisms.

COMPLICATIONS

Complications are part of the natural history of IE. Changes in clinical status or persistent signs and symptoms of active infection should prompt reassessment of the patient to evaluate for myocardial or valve abscesses, embolic phenomena, heart failure, metastatic infection, including vertebral osteomyelitis and mycotic aneurysms, conduction defects, and especially valvular dysfunction. Valvular regurgitation in endocarditis sometimes presents in abrupt and catastrophic fashion.

PROGNOSIS

Cure rates of native valve IE due to viridans streptococci are 80% to 90%, compared to 60% to 90% for *S aureus*. Cure rates are higher in injection drug users with right-sided involvement. Cure rates in fungal endocarditis are less than 50%, even with aggressive medical and surgical therapy. For prosthetic valve IE, cure rates are about 10% less for each etiology, and surgery is needed more frequently.

DISCHARGE PLANNING/TRANSITIONS OF CARE

To receive prolonged intravenous antibiotics, patients need early planning for long-term vascular access (after the initial bacteremia has cleared), home antimicrobial administration (once medically stabilized), and close medical outpatient follow-up. Peripherally inserted central catheters, which have relatively low secondary local and bloodstream infection rates, have facilitated home parenteral antibiotic therapy in many patients.

TABLE 197-4 Definitive Therapy of Bacterial Endocarditis*

Organism/Regimen	Comments
PCN-susceptible viridans streptococci (MIC ≤0.1 μg/mL) and *S bovis* native valve IE	
1. PCN 12–20 million U/24 h IV either continuously or in 4 or 6 equally divided doses × 4 wk	1. Also effective for other PCN-susceptible nonviridans streptococci
2. Ceftriaxone 2 g/24 h IV/IM in 1 dose × 4 wk	2. Uncomplicated infection with viridans streptococci, candidate for outpatient therapy; also PCN allergy
3. PCN 12–18 million U/24 h IV either continuously or in 6 equally divided doses × 2 wk or ceftriaxone 2 g/24 h IV/IM in 1 dose *plus* gentamicin 3 mg/kg IV every 24 hours × 2 wk	3. Uncomplicated infection without the following features: renal insufficiency, eighth cranial nerve deficit, prosthetic valve infection, CNS complications, severe heart failure, or age >65. Also not acceptable for nutritionally variant streptococci
4. Vancomycin 30 mg/kg per 24 h IV in 2 equally divided doses × 4 wk	4. For PCN allergy, recommended only for patients unable to tolerate PCN or ceftriaxone
Relatively PCN-resistant Viridans group Streptococci (MIC 0.12– <0.5 μg/mL) native valve IE	
1. PCN 24 million U/24 h IV either continuously or in 4–6 equally divided doses × 6 wk or ceftriaxone 2 g/24 h IV/IM in 1 dose × 4 wk *plus* gentamicin 3 mg/kg per 24 h IV/IM in 1 dose × 2 wk	
2. Vancomycin 30 mg/kg per 24 h IV in 2 equally divided doses not to exceed 2 g/24 h unless serum concentrations are low × 4 wk	2. For PCN allergy recommended only for patients unable to tolerate PCN or ceftriaxone. Goal vancomycin trough 15–20 μg/mL
Enterococci† and PCN-resistant viridans vroup streptococci (MIC >1 μg/mL)	
1. Ampicillin12 g/24 h IV in 6 equally divided doses or PCN 18–30 million U/24 h IV either continuously or in 6 equally divided doses × 4–6 wk *plus* gentamicin 3 mg/kg per 24 h IV/IM in 3 equally divided doses × 4–6 wk	1. Increase duration of both drugs to 6 wk for prosthetic valve infection or symptoms longer than 3 mo in enterococcal infection
2. Vancomycin 30 mg/kg per 24 h IV in 2 equally divided doses × 6 wk *plus* gentamicin 3 mg/kg per 24 h IV/IM in 3 equally divided doses × 6 wk§	2. Goal vancomycin trough 15–20 μg/mL. For PCN allergy; PCN desensitization is also an option. High risk of nephrotoxicity with this regimen.
Staphylococcus aureus	
1. Nafcillin or oxacillin 12 g/24 h IV in 4–6 equally divided doses × 6 wk with ***optional*** addition of gentamicin 3 mg/kg per 24 h IV/IM in 2 or 3 equally divided doses × 3–5 days	1. Methicillin-susceptible strain; omit gentamicin if significant renal insufficiency
2. Vancomycin 30 mg/kg per 24 h IV in 2 equally divided doses × 6 wk	2. PCN allergy (immediate hypersensitivity or anaphylaxis) or MRSA. Goal vancomycin trough 15–20 μg/mL
3. Nafcillin 2 g IV every 4 hours × 2 wk *plus* gentamicin 1 mg/kg IV every 8 hours × 2 wk; or daptomycin 6 mg/kg IV once daily for 2–4 wk; or nafcillin 2 g IV every 4 hours × 2–4 wk	3. Methicillin-susceptible strain; 2-wk regimen only for use in IV drug abuser with tricuspid valve only infection with no renal insufficiency and no extrapulmonary infection
4. Nafcillin or oxacillin 2 g/24 h IV in 6 equally divided doses × >6 wk *plus* gentamicin 3 mg/kg per 24 h IV/IM in 2 or 3 equally divided doses × 2 wk *plus* rifampin 900 mg per 24 h IV or orally in 3 equally divided doses × >6 wk	4. Prosthetic valve infection with methicillin-susceptible strain; use vancomycin instead of nafcillin for MRSA; Goal vancomycin trough 15–20 μg/mL
5. Cefazolin 6 g/24 h IV in 3 equally divided doses × 6 wk with ***optional*** addition of gentamicin 3 mg/kg per 24 h IV/IM in 2 or 3 equally divided doses × 3–5 days	5. PCN allergy other than immediate hypersensitivity
Coagulase-negative staphylococci, prosthetic valve infection	
Vancomycin 30 mg/kg 24 h in 2 equally divided doses × >6 wk *plus* wk *plus* gentamicin 3 mg/kg per 24 h IV/IM in 2 or 3 equally divided doses × 2 wk *plus* rifampin 900 mg per 24 h IV or orally in 3 equally divided doses × >6 wk	Can substitute nafcillin in above doses for vancomycin if isolate is methicillin susceptible, Goal vancomycin trough 15–20 μg/mL
HACEK strains	
1. Ceftriaxone 2 g/24 h IV/IM in 1 dose × 4 wk; 6 wk for prosthetic valves	
2. Ampicillin-sulbactam 2 g/24 h IV in 4 equally divided doses × 4 wk; 6 wk for prosthetic valves	2. HACEK strains increasingly may produce beta-lactamase
3. Ciprofloxacin 1000 mg/24 h orally or 800 mg/24h IV in 2 equally divided doses × 4 wk	

*Dosages for patients with normal renal function; adjustments must be made for renal insufficiency for all drugs except nafcillin, rifampin, and ceftriaxone. Gentamicin doses should be adjusted to achieve a peak serum concentration of ~3 μg/mL 30 minutes after dosing, and a trough gentamicin level of <1 μg/mL.

†Enterococci must be tested for antimicrobial susceptibility. These recommendations are for enterococci sensitive to penicillin, gentamicin, and vancomycin.

§Need for addition of aminoglycoside has not been demonstrated for PCN-resistant streptococci.

HACEK, *Haemophilus* species, *Actinobacillus actinomycetemcomitans*, *Cardiobacterium hominis*, *Eikenella corrodens*, and *Kingella* species; MIC, minimum inhibitory concentration; MRSA, methicillin-resistant *Staphylococcus aureus*; PCN, penicillin.

Data from Baddour LM, Wilson, WR, Bayer, AS, et al. Infective endocarditis: diagnosis, antimicrobial therapy, and management of complications. *Circulation.* 2005;111:e394–e433.

Careful monitoring of antimicrobial levels and renal function (when indicated), as well as other clinical signs and symptoms of infection should be arranged. Outpatient follow-up should include the primary care provider, infectious disease specialist, and cardiologist. Cardiothoracic surgery should be involved in the follow-up of patients with valvular damage which may require surgery after completion of antimicrobial treatment. Outpatient providers should be informed about diagnosis, therapeutic decisions and duration, required monitoring, and plans for possible surgical intervention. Finally, patients with newly diagnosed IE should be educated about dental prophylaxis (see below).

Active injection drug users are of special concern in discharge planning for IE. Acute infection accounts for approximately 60% of hospital admissions for this population; IE is implicated in 5% to 15% of these episodes. Nonadherance to treatment plans, central catheter care, and follow-up in this population may be particularly challenging; these patients are poor candidates for discharge home with central catheters. Secondary catheter-related bloodstream infections may be more common in this population. Successful management of IE in this population requires treatment of substance abuse and psychiatric comorbities, if present.

PRIMARY AND SECONDARY PREVENTION

Recent guidelines for the use of antibiotic prophylaxis before procedures associated with bacteremia have recommended prophylaxis for far fewer procedure types and cardiac conditions. The proportion of cases of IE that are preventable are probably few, and the risk of IE after dental procedures is probably low compared to the cumulative risk from such daily activities as tooth brushing and chewing food. As well, no large, prospective randomized trials of the use of prophylactic antibiotics prior to procedures causing bacteremia have been carried out.

The administration of prophylactic antibiotics solely to prevent endocarditis is no longer recommended for patients undergoing genitourinary or gastrointestinal tract procedures. Antibiotic prophylaxis may be considered for patients at high risk for IE who undergo an invasive procedure of the respiratory tract that involves incision or biopsy of the respiratory mucosa (eg, tonsillectomy, adenoidectomy). With regard to dental procedures, the number of cardiac conditions for which prophylaxis is still recommended was reduced to four settings:

- Prosthetic heart valves, including bioprosthetic and homograft valves
- Prior history of IE
- Certain congenital heart defects, including (a) unrepaired cyanotic congenital heart disease, including palliative shunts and conduits; (b) completely repaired congenital heart defects with prosthetic material or devices, whether placed by surgery or by catheter intervention, during the first 6 months after the procedure; or (c) repaired congenital heart disease with residual defects at the site or adjacent to the site of the prosthetic device
- Cardiac valvulopathy in a transplanted heart

The choice of antibiotics for prophylaxis was unchanged from previous iterations of the guidelines. Antibiotics should be effective against the organisms most likely to be released into the bloodstream by the procedure. Thus, primarily oral flora should be covered by antibiotics given before dental, oral, and respiratory tract procedures.

QUALITY IMPROVEMENT

Possible targets for quality improvement in IE include timely performance of blood cultures and echocardiography in suspected cases, infectious diseases consultation and appropriate antibiotic therapy in documented cases, surveillance blood cultures to document clearance of bacteremia, and removal of infected vascular catheters, without changing them over a guidewire. Central venous catheters should not be reinserted unless bacteremia has resolved. Patients should be educated about secondary prevention for endocarditis, as above. Prior to discharge, hospitalists must arrange appropriate outpatient primary care, infectious diseases, and cardiology follow-up, and monitoring for antimicrobial side effects and levels, if necessary.

SUGGESTED READINGS

Baddour LM, Wilson WR, Bayer AS, et al. American Heart Association Scientific Statement. Infective endocarditis: diagnosis, antimicrobial therapy, and management of complications. *Circulation.* 2005;111:e394–e434.

Berlin JA, Abrutyn E, Strom BL, et al. Incidence of infective endocarditis in the Delaware Valley, 1988–1990. *Am J Cardiol.* 1995;76:933–936.

Lalani T, Cabell CH, Benjamin DK, et al. Analysis of the impact of early surgery on in-hospital mortality of native valve endocarditis: use of propensity score and instrumental variable methods to adjust for treatment-selection bias. *Circulation.* 2010;121:1005–1013.

Li J, Sexton DJ, Mick N, et al. Proposed modifications to the Duke criteria for the diagnosis of infective endocarditis. *Clin Infect Dis.* 2000;30:633–638.

Murdoch DR, Corey GR, Hoen B, et al. Clinical presentation, etiology, and outcome of infective endocarditis in the 21st century. *Arch Intern Med.* 2009;169:463–473.

Task Force on the Prevention, Diagnosis, and Treatment of Infective Endocarditis of the European Society of Cardiology. Guidelines on the prevention, diagnosis, and treatment of infective endocarditis. *Eur Heart J.* 2009;30:2369–2413.

Tleyjeh IM, Abdel-Latif A, Rahbi H, et al. A systematic review of population-based studies of infective endocarditis. *Chest.* 2001;132:1025–1035.

Wilson W, Taubert KA, Gewitz M, et al. Prevention of infective endocarditis: guidelines from the American Heart Association. *Circulation.* 2007;116:1736–1754.

CHAPTER 198

Infections of the Immunocompromised Host

Sarah P. Hammond, MD
Lindsey R. Baden, MD

Key Clinical Questions

1. What is the approach to an immunocompromised patient with suspected infection?
2. What are common infectious complications in patients receiving chronic corticosteroids, or recently treated with tumor necrosis factor inhibitors or rituximab?
3. Should preventative measures be taken to prevent infectious complications in patients taking these medications?
4. What infectious complications are common among patients who have undergone splenectomy?
5. How should a transplant patient presenting with possible infection be evaluated?

INTRODUCTION

With the advent of newer immunosuppressive medications and the rise in organ transplantation internationally, the numbers of immunocompromised patients are rising. The diagnosis and management of infection in this growing population is challenging. In immunocompromised patients, the usual signs and symptoms of infection may be obscured, and they often have a higher burden of pathogens and disseminated infection, leading to worse outcomes. These patients are also prone to infection with a broad array of less familiar pathogens, including opportunists such as *Listeria monocytogenes* and *Pneumocystis jiroveci*, and latent pathogens such as cytomegalovirus (CMV), toxoplasma, and *Mycobacterium tuberculosis*, as well as typical community-acquired and nosocomial microbes.

GUIDING PRINCIPLES

Two pieces of information are essential to the care of the patient with impaired immunity: the patient's epidemiologic exposures and overall severity of immunosuppression.

The net state of immunosuppression is determined by the type, intensity, and duration of immunosuppression (including the dose and number of immunosuppressive agents or the presence of innate immunodeficiencies); anatomic factors causing a mechanical breakdown in the host defenses, such as abnormal lymphatic drainage at the site of previous surgery or radiation; and the presence or absence of immunosuppressive infections such as HIV or CMV.

Patients should be questioned about epidemiology that places them at risk for specific pathogens. These include recent events (sick contacts, animal exposure, travel, consumption of undercooked meat or unpasteurized dairy products), as well as remote residence in countries where tuberculosis is endemic, or regions of the United States where histoplasmosis, blastomycosis, or coccidioidomycosis are endemic.

MEDICATION-RELATED IMMUNODEFICIENCY

Dozens of medications, used in a wide variety of medical conditions, may impair immunologic function; an abbreviated list is shown in **Table 198-1**. Some agents, such as corticosteroids and alemtuzumab, undermine several layers of host defenses. Others have a more targeted effect, such as tacrolimus and cyclosporine, which prevent normal T lymphocyte responses to immunologic stimuli. Understanding the impact of medications on immunity helps to predict which infections the host may develop.

CORTICOSTEROIDS

Corticosteroids are prescribed for rheumatologic conditions, inflammatory bowel disease, allergic disease, asthma, among others. The immediate impact of corticosteroids on host defenses includes depletion of circulating lymphocytes (particularly T lymphocytes) and monocytes, and suppression of phagocyte migration and function. Long-term effects that increase infection risk include impaired skin and soft tissue healing.

Corticosteroid use increases susceptibility to common bacterial infections (**Table 198-2**). Reactivation of latent tuberculosis is also increased among previously exposed patients started on corticosteroid therapy. Patients should be screened for latent tuberculosis before starting corticosteroid therapy. Chronic corticosteroid use also increases susceptibility to opportunistic infections. Infrequently,

TABLE 198-1 Selected Immunosuppressive Agents

Immunosuppressive Agent	Immunologic Effect	FDA-approved Uses
Corticosteroids		
Prednisone, dexamethasone	Depletes circulating lymphocytes; suppresses phagocyte migration and function	Treatment of pulmonary and rheumatologic conditions
Antimetabolites		
Methotrexate	Inhibits dihydrofolate reductase; impairs cellular replication and repair	Treatment of RA, psoriasis, ALL, and several solid organ malignancies
6-mercaptopurine	Purine analogue; inhibits cellular DNA synthesis	Treatment of Crohn disease and ALL
Azathioprine	Disrupts purine metabolism	Treatment of RA; prevention of rejection in SOT
Mycophenolate mofetil	Inhibits inosine monophosphate dehydrogenase; inhibits B and T lymphocytes	Prevention of rejection in SOT
T lymphocyte active agents		
Tacrolimus	Inhibits T lymphocyte activation	Prevention of rejection in SOT
Cyclosporine	Inhibits T lymphocyte activation	Prevention of rejection in SOT
Sirolimus	Suppresses cytokine induction of T lymphocyte activity	Prevention of rejection in SOT
Monoclonal antibodies		
TNF-α inhibitors	Blocks effect of TNF-α, which mediates immunologic control of intracellular organisms and granuloma formation	Treatment of RA
Rituximab	Monoclonal antibody to CD20; depletes B lymphocytes	Treatment of lymphoma and RA
Natalizumab	Monoclonal antibody to alpha-4 integrins; interferes with leukocyte migration to areas of inflammation	Treatment of multiple sclerosis and Crohn disease
Alemtuzumab	Monoclonal antibody to CD52; depletes B and T lymphocytes	Treatment of CLL
Basiliximab	IL-2 receptor antagonist; prevents IL-2 mediated lymphocyte activation	Induction of immunosuppression in SOT
Daclizumab	IL-2 receptor antagonist; prevents IL-2 mediated lymphocyte activation	Induction of immunosuppression in SOT

ALL, acute lymphoblastic leukemia; CLL, chronic lymphocytic leukemia; RA, rheumatoid arthritis; SOT, solid organ transplantation.

TABLE 198-2 Corticosteroid-associated Infections

Infection	Preventative Strategy
Bacterial infections	
Increased susceptibility to all bacterial infections	Vigilance; routine vaccinations (including influenza and pneumonia vaccines)
Mycobacterial infections	
Tuberculosis	Check purified protein derivative or interferon-gamma release assay prior to steroid initiation; treat if indicated
Fungal infections	
Pneumocystis jiroveci pneumonia	Prophylaxis when appropriate
Aspergillus	A rare complication
Fusarium	A rare complication
Parasitic infections	
Strongyloides hyperinfection syndrome	Screen with *Strongyloides* antibody before steroid initiation; treat if indicated

infection with invasive fungi such as *Aspergillus* and *Fusarium* occurs with chronic glucocorticoid use.

Two infection syndromes associated with corticosteroid use deserve special mention: *Pneumocystis jiroveci* pneumonia (PCP) and *Strongyloides* hyperinfection syndrome.

PCP is associated with prolonged corticosteroid use; the risk for PCP rises with increasing steroid dose and duration. Clinically, PCP causes fever, dyspnea, and dry cough. It is characterized radiographically by diffuse bilateral pulmonary infiltrates (**Figure 198-1**). Patients with PCP may be profoundly hypoxic, particularly with ambulation. The mortality associated with PCP infection in non HIV-infected patients is high—up to 50% in some case series. Therefore, suspected PCP should be treated empirically while the diagnostic work-up is ongoing.

There are several methods of diagnosing PCP (**Table 198-3**). The gold standard is lung biopsy, with demonstration of characteristic cysts. More often, patients undergo bronchoscopy with bronchoalveolar lavage (BAL) or sputum induction, with testing of BAL fluid or sputum with direct fluorescent antigen or silver stain. A useful non-invasive test is the serum fungal marker beta-D-glucan, which may be very elevated in PCP, sometimes above the upper limit of the assay. (For the treatment of PCP in the non–HIV-infected population, see Practice Point.)

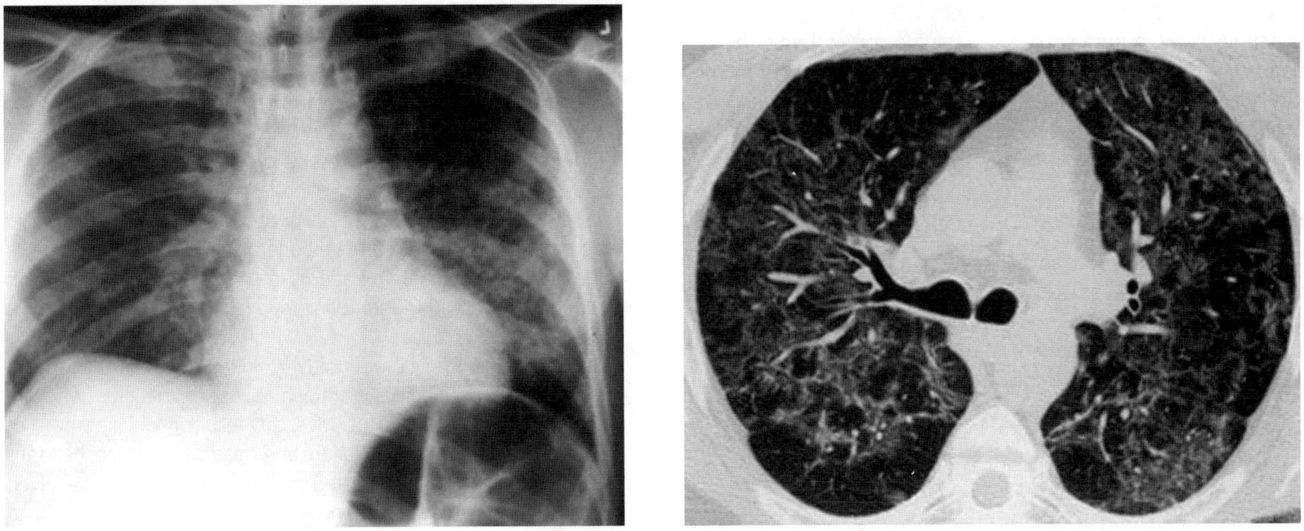

Figure 198-1 *Chest radiograph with diffuse interstitial infiltrates, and chest CT revealing ground glass infiltrates, in an HIV-positive patient with Pneumocystis carinii pneumonia (PCP). Radiographic findings in PCP may vary from impressive to quite subtle. (Reproduced, with permission, from Fauci AS, Braunwald E, Kasper DL, et al. Harrison's Principles of Internal Medicine 17th ed. New York: McGraw-Hill 2008, Fig. 200-1.)*

PRACTICE POINT

Treatment of PCP in the non-HIV infected patient

- Trimethoprim-sulfamethoxazole (TMP-SMX) is the first-line agent for treating PCP. For patients with allergy or intolerance to TMP-SMX, alternatives include combination clindamycin and primaquine or intravenous pentamidine. Pentamidine has numerous toxicities, including infusional cardiac toxicity, nephrotoxicity and hypoglycemia, and is generally a drug of last resort. Mild cases of PCP can be treated with atovaquone. No studies have assessed the use of adjunctive corticosteroids, in addition to antibiotics, to treat severe PCP infection in the non-HIV infected patient. However, in severe cases with prominent hypoxia, or in patients requiring intubation, adjunctive steroids are often used.

Risk for PCP in patients on chronic steroids is predictable and therefore should be preventable. PCP has been reported in patients on less than 20 mg of prednisone per day for fewer than 8 weeks. Unfortunately, no formal study has assessed the corticosteroid dose and duration at which prophylaxis for PCP is necessary. Many providers add prophylaxis for PCP in patients receiving between 20 to 30 mg of prednisone (or prednisone equivalent) for over 20 to 30 days. Low-dose trimethoprim-sulfamethoxazole is the first-line agent for PCP prophylaxis. Alternative prophylaxis for patients with intolerance or allergy to trimethoprim-sulfamethoxazole includes dapsone, atovaquone, and monthly inhaled pentamidine. (Of note, breakthrough cases of PCP have been reported in patients on pentamidine prophylaxis, typically in the upper lobes.)

Corticosteroids are also associated with *Strongyloides* hyperinfection syndrome. The helminth *Strongyloides stercoralis* is found in soil in many parts of the world, including the Americas; in the United States, it is endemic in the Southeast. Initial infection occurs when larvae from soil penetrate the skin of a human host (often through bare feet) and travel to the gastrointestinal tract via the venous and pulmonary systems. Infection may be clinically silent for years to decades. Eosinophilia is variably present. The hyperinfection syndrome, an accelerated phase of infection with high morbidity and mortality, can be triggered by corticosteroids. This syndrome occurs when noninfectious *Strongyloides* larvae, hatched in the intestine of an infected patient, mature into infectious larvae prior to excretion, and subsequently invade the gastrointestinal tract of the host, leading to a large increase in the parasite burden and significant clinical illness. The hyperinfection syndrome is characterized by pulmonary infiltrates and diarrhea, due to the large burden of worms in transit in the gastrointestinal tract and lungs. In addition, associated gram-negative sepsis and occasionally gram-negative meningitis may occur, as bacteria use the larvae to "hitchhike" into the bloodstream from the gut.

Hyperinfection syndrome is diagnosed by finding characteristic larvae in BAL fluid or sputum. Patients recently initiated on steroids with appropriate epidemiologic history and unexplained gram-negative sepsis, particularly meningitis, should be assessed with serum *Strongyloides* antibody testing. Hyperinfection syndrome is treated with ivermectin or albendazole. Broad-spectrum antibiotics

TABLE 198-3 Diagnosis of *Pneumocystis Jiroveci* Pneumonia

Diagnostic Method	Advantage	Disadvantage
Lung biopsy	Gold standard for diagnosis	Invasive—requires transbronchial biopsy or surgical procedure
DFA of bronchoalveolar lavage fluid	Increase sensitivity compared to induced sputum	Requires invasive bronchoscopy
DFA of induced sputum	Less invasive than biopsy or bronchoalveolar lavage	Low burden of *Pneumocystis* in sputum leads to low sensitivity
Beta-D-glucan	Noninvasive; result characteristically greater than assay	Results often not rapidly available as it is usually a send-out test; false positive results possible in patients on hemodialysis, those who have received IVIg recently, or those with other invasive fungal infections

may be required for gram-negative sepsis. To prevent *Strongyloides* hyperinfection syndrome in patients starting corticosteroid therapy, patients with eosinophilia or epidemiologic history consistent with possible exposure should be screened with serum *Strongyloides* antibody. If antibody is positive, antihelmenthic therapy should be given before steroid initiation.

TUMOR NECROSIS FACTOR-ALPHA (TNF-α) INHIBITORS

TNF-α is a cytokine produced by macrophages and T lymphocytes. It is important in granuloma formation and the immunologic control of intracellular organisms. Five TNF-α inhibitors are approved in the United States for the treatment of rheumatoid arthritis (RA), Crohn disease, and other conditions. These include infliximab, certolizumab pegol, adalimumab, and golimumab, monoclonal antibodies that bind to TNF-α, and etanercept, a soluble form of TNF-α receptor. These agents are also used in an off-label capacity to treat other inflammatory conditions.

Postmarketing studies of TNF-α inhibitors report an association between these agents and reactivation of granulomatous diseases, such as tuberculosis, histoplasmosis, and coccidioidomycosis, as well as opportunistic infection with nontuberculous mycobacteria and the intracellular pathogen *Listeria*. TNF-α inhibitors may also increase the risk of serious bacterial infection in RA patients.

The association of TNF-α inhibitors and reactivation of dormant tuberculosis has been well documented. Reactivation of latent tuberculosis has been reported mostly during the first 6 months in patients treated with infliximab, and after 6 months in patients treated with etanercept. Many patients present with extrapulmonary tuberculosis, and a large proportion have disseminated disease and bad outcomes. Therefore, patients recently treated with TNF-α inhibitors presenting with a chronic febrile illness or unintentional weight loss and an appropriate epidemiologic history should be evaluated for tuberculosis, including careful assessment for extrapulmonary and disseminated disease. To prevent reactivation of latent tuberculosis in patients treated with TNF-α inhibitors, screening purified protein derivative testing or interferon-gamma release assay should be done. Patients with positive tests should be treated for latent tuberculosis before starting a TNF-α inhibitor.

Infection with *L monocytogenes* may be more frequent in patients who have been treated with TNF-α inhibitors. Patients who have been treated with TNF-α inhibitors or other immunosuppressive drugs with signs and symptoms of meningitis or sepsis should be empirically treated with antibiotics active against *L monocytogenes*, and blood and cerebrospinal fluid cultures should be obtained for definitive diagnosis.

RITUXIMAB

Rituximab is a monoclonal antibody to CD20, a marker found on B lymphocytes. It is approved for used in non-Hodgkin lymphoma, RA, and chronic lymphocytic leukemia, and it is also used off-label for a variety of autoimmune disorders.

Rituximab depletes circulating B cells, leading to impaired antibody responses to new pathogens. In premarketing trials, there was no increased risk for infection among rituximab-treated patients, compared to those treated with other regimens for RA or lymphoma. However, since rituximab has been available commercially, it has been linked in case reports and case series to several uncommon infections, including progressive multifocal leukoencephalopathy caused by JC virus, reactivation of CMV, severe enterovirus infection, and pure red cell aplasia associated with parvovirus infection. Notably, the effect of rituximab alone is difficult to interpret in these anecdotal reports, because most of the reported patients have been treated with other immunosuppressive agents, in addition to rituximab.

Rituximab is also linked to increased risk of infection with *Babesia microti*, a tick-borne parasitic infection endemic to the northeastern United States. (Other *Babesia* species are endemic to temperate regions of Europe.) Rituximab-treated patients with babesiosis tend to have high parasite burdens and severe clinical manifestations, including adult respiratory distress syndrome. As well, prolonged or repeated courses of therapy for babesia infection with atovaquone and azithromycin may be necessary to eradicate the infection in these patients. Fever, transaminitis, anemia, and thrombocytopenia suggest *Babesia* infection in patients in endemic areas treated with rituximab, and should trigger diagnostic testing with thick and thin blood smears.

Rituximab use has been definitively linked to severe hepatitis B virus reactivation. Specifically, rituximab use in patients who are hepatitis B surface antigen positive can result in development of fulminant hepatitis, with liver failure and death. In addition, hepatitis B reactivation has been reported in patients who have received rituximab with serologic evidence of resolved hepatitis B prior to rituximab (hepatitis B surface antigen negative and hepatitis B core antibody positive). Based on this association, patients being started on rituximab should be screened for hepatitis B before treatment. Patients treated with rituximab with liver function abnormalities, including florid hepatitis, should be assessed for active hepatitis B infection.

INNATE IMNUNODEFICIENCIES

Many innate immunodeficiencies, such as severe combined immunodeficiency and chronic granulomatous disease, are uncommon, require specialized care, and are beyond the scope of this chapter. However, common variable immunodeficiency (CVID) is not rare, and these patients are often cared for by hospitalists.

COMMON VARIABLE IMMUNODEFICIENCY

While many immunodeficiencies are diagnosed at an early age, CVID usually develops in adolescence or young adulthood. It is a disorder characterized by poor production of immunoglobulins in response to antigenic stimuli. This limited humoral response to antigens leads to recurrent sinus and pulmonary infections, often caused by *Streptococcus pneumoniae* and other bacterial pathogens. Recurrent pulmonary infections over time may lead to bronchiectasis, a common complication of CVID in adults. Patients with CVID may also have chronic enteric infection with *Giardia lamblia* and chronic meningoencehphalitis due to enterovirus. Patients with CVID may also suffer from allergic and autoimmune disorders, and are at increased risk of lymphoma.

While low quantitative total immunoglobulin levels suggest CVID, the diagnosis is made by evaluation of immunologic response to new or recall antigens. Patients with CVID fail to mount an appropriate antibody response to new or booster immunizations. Regular immunoglobulin infusions in patients with CVID may prevent recurrent infections and possibly limit the respiratory tract damage that can lead to bronchiectasis.

ASPLENIA

Splenectomy may be medically necessary in patient with trauma, malignancy, refractory idiopathic thrombotic purpura, and other hematologic disorders. Patients with sickle cell anemia are often functionally asplenic. Patients with surgical or functional asplenia are at risk for overwhelming bacterial infection with encapsulated organisms, including *S pneumoniae, Haemophilus influenzae,* and possibly *Neisseria meningitides* (**Table 198-4**). Progression of bacterial infection in asplenic patients may be rapid, and historically associated with high mortality. In patients with surgical splenectomy, the risk for post-splenectomy sepsis due to an encapsulated organism

TABLE 198-4 Infections Associated with Asplenia

Infection	Preventative Strategy
Encapsulated organisms	
Streptococcus pneumoniae *Haemophilus influenzae* *Neisseria meningitidis*	Vaccinate before or 2 weeks after splenectomy
Capnocytophaga canimorsus	Thorough washing and medical evaluation for prophylactic antibiotics after dog bites
Babesia microti	Tick precautions when at risk for tick exposure in areas of risk (Northeast US)

is probably highest in the first few years after splenectomy. Sepsis may be more common after splenectomy for hematologic malignancy than after splenectomy for trauma. Asplenic patients with fever, chills, malaise, or other signs or symptoms of infection should be immediately treated with antibiotics directed at encapsulated organisms, and blood cultures must be obtained.

Asplenic patients are also at increased risk for severe infection due to *Babesia microti* and *Capnocytophaga canimorsus*. As in patients treated with rituximab, babesiosis is more severe in splenectomized patients. Treatment options include atovaquone and azithromycin, or clindamycin and quinine. Asplenic patients with babesiosis may also require multiple or prolonged treatment courses.

C canimorsus is a gram-negative organism that inhabits the oral cavity of dogs. Dog bites may lead to local inoculation, and in asplenic patients may progress rapidly to systemic infection. *C canimorsus* has been associated with severe sepsis and digital (and occasionally nasal) necrosis. Asplenic patients should be instructed to carefully wash all dog bites and seek medical assessment regarding prophylactic antibiotics after animal bites, particularly dog bites. Oral amoxicillin-clavulanic acid is useful for prophylaxis; ampicillin-sulbactam, fluoroquinolones, or third-generation cephalosporins are options for patients requiring intravenous therapy. Dog bite and animal exposure history should be obtained in all asplenic patients with sepsis.

Patients scheduled for splenectomy or who recently had an emergent splenectomy should be vaccinated for *S pneumoniae, H influenzae*, and *N meningitidis*. When the splenectomy is planned, vaccination should be carried out at least two weeks before the procedure. For unplanned splenectomies, patients should be vaccinated two weeks after the procedure or prior to hospital discharge (whichever is first), so that it is not overlooked. Patients who have undergone splenectomy should be warned about their increased risk for infection and the need to seek medical care during fever or after dog bites. Asplenic patients should also have oral antibiotics available at home for self-administration if fever develops.

TRANSPLANTATION

Recipients of solid organ transplantation (SOT) and stem cell transplantation (SCT) are at risk for infection with community and nosocomial pathogens, as well as reactivation of latent pathogens. A few distinctions between SOT and SCT are helpful when evaluating a transplant recipient with possible infection. Infections often localize to the transplanted organ and surrounding tissues in SOT recipients. For example, urinary tract infection and pyelonephritis are common after renal transplantation. Most SOT recipients require lifelong immunosuppressive therapy after transplant, and those who develop organ rejection require further immunosuppression and are at heightened risk for infection.

In contrast to SOT recipients, SCT recipients have often undergone extensive cancer treatment already, leading to immunosuppression even before the transplant procedure. Some SCT recipients have already had opportunistic infections prior to SCT. The donor stem cell type in SCT may be somewhat predictive of infectious risk after transplantation. While allogeneic stem cell recipients require immunosuppression after transplantation to prevent graft-versus-host disease (GVHD), autologous stem cell transplant recipients do not, and so are at lower risk for infectious complications after transplant. Unlike SOT recipients, allogeneic SCT recipients are often weaned off immunosuppressive medications months to years after transplantation, unless they develop GVHD, which requires increased immunosuppression analogous to rejection in SOT recipients.

When a transplant recipient presents with suspected infection, the differential diagnosis is broad. However, some infections tend to cluster during certain time frames after transplant.

During the first month after transplantation, most infections are related to the surgical procedure (in the case of SOT), the hospitalization during transplantation, conditioning chemotherapy-related neutropenia (in the case of SCT), or the donor tissue. Infections related to surgery (for SOT recipients) and hospitalization (for both SOT and SCT recipients) include wound infection, central venous catheter infection, and catheter-associated urinary tract infection. SCT recipients are also at significant risk for bacterial and fungal infection associated with neutropenia during this period of time. Bacterial infection during neutropenia often results from translocation from endogenous sources, such as the gastrointestinal tract. Mucositis from chemotherapy also increases the risk of endogenously derived bacterial infection in SCT recipients. Donor-derived infection is uncommon due to extensive donor pre-transplant screening. Exotic pathogens may sometimes be encountered in this setting, such as lymphocytic choriomeningitis virus, West Nile virus, and rabies virus. Donor-derived infection should be a consideration in SOT recipients when fever starts shortly after transplantation, and there is no evidence of nosocomial or surgical infection.

Infections in the early post-transplant period (between 2 and 6 months after transplant) are often due to opportunists, including PCP, aspergillosis, cryptococcosis, and reactivation of latent pathogens, such as CMV, varicella zoster virus (VZV), toxoplasma, and BK virus. SCT recipients with GVHD, and SOT recipients who develop rejection during this period, require aggressive immunosuppressive therapy, placing them at very high risk of infection, particularly for invasive mold infection in SCT recipients. In transplant patients with aspergillosis and other aggressive infections, reducing doses of corticosteroids and other immunosuppressive drugs should be strongly considered. PCP is also a significant risk during this time period; most transplant patients receive PCP prophylaxis for at least 3 to 12 months.

Herpes viruses, including CMV, VZV, and herpes simplex (HSV), commonly reactivate in previously exposed transplant recipients between 2 and 6 months post-transplant. CMV may cause pneumonitis, esophagitis, and colitis. CMV also has an intrinsic immunosuppressive effect, leading to increased susceptibility to other infections. Transplant recipients at risk for CMV reactivation include those who were CMV seropositive prior to transplant and those with CMV seropositive donors. Typically SOT and SCT recipients are treated with prophylactic valganciclovir for 3 to 12 months, or are monitored for CMV reactivation weekly for 3 to 6 months after transplantation to prevent CMV end organ disease. VZV and HSV infection are also common during this time period, so patients who are not treated with prophylactic valganciclovir for CMV are typically treated with prophylactic acyclovir or valacyclovir to prevent VZV and HSV reactivation.

TABLE 198-5 Evidence-based Medicine: Key References for Infections of Immunocompromised Hosts

Reference	Methodology	Results	Limitations	Bottom Line
Yale S, Limper A. *Mayo Clin Proc.* 1996;71:5–13.	Retrospective cohort study	Among 116 HIV-negative patients diagnosed with PCP, 91% received corticosteroids within the last month. Median steroid dose was 30 mg prednisone daily for 12 wk, but 25% of patients were on as little as 16 mg prednisone daily for as few as 8 wk	Examines the association between corticosteroids and PCP, but does not determine absolute risk	PCP in non-HIV infected patients was associated with corticosteroid use, even in patients on relatively low doses of prednisone for a short period of time. PCP prophylaxis should be considered in these circumstances
Sepkowitz KA, et al. *JAMA.* 1992;267: 832–837.	Retrospective cohort study	Among 142 patients diagnosed with PCP at a cancer hospital, 87% were previously treated with corticosteroids. 49% of patients diagnosed with PCP pre-mortem died	HIV testing only performed in 40 of 142 patients (all tested were negative)	PCP infection in patients with malignancy was commonly associated with corticosteroid use. Mortality was high
Cruz T, et al. *N Engl J Med.* 1966;275:1093–1096.	Case series	Description of 5 fatal cases of overwhelming *Strongyloides* infection in patients previously treated with corticosteroids. Common clinical findings included diarrhea, vomiting, abdominal pain, and shock	Uncontrolled case series	First description of overwhelming *Strongyloides* infection associated with steroids. *Strongyloides* hyperinfection can be a fatal complication of corticosteroid use
Bongartz T, et al. *JAMA.* 2006;295:2275–2285.	Meta-analysis	Meta-analysis that included 9 randomized trials of adalimumab or infliximab for the treatment of RA that found a pooled odds ratio of 2.0 for developing serious infection while on adalimumab or infliximab vs placebo	Because study is a meta-analysis, there is heterogeneity in study population in terms of RA and duration of treatment	This study suggests that there is increased risk of serious infection among patients with RA treated with adalimumab or infliximab
Keane J, et al. *N Engl J Med.* 2001;345: 1098–1104.	Retrospective cohort study	From 1998–2001, 70 cases of tuberculosis in patients treated with infliximab were reported to FDA. 57% of cases were extrapulmonary, including 17 cases (24%) of disseminated infection. The rate of tuberculosis in patients treated with infliximab was higher than background rate	Small number of cases; this study depends on accurate reporting to the FDA	Development of active tuberculosis is a significant risk after initiation of infliximab. Screening for latent tuberculosis should be undertaken in all patients prior to initiation of infliximab
Slifman NR, et al. *Arthritis Rheum.* 2003;48:319–324.	Retrospective cohort study	From 1998–2001, 15 cases of listeriosis in patients treated with etanercept or infliximab were reported to FDA. All 15 were receiving other immunosuppressive agents in addition to TNF-α inhibitor. The rate of listeriosis among patients treated with TNF-α inhibitors was higher than the general US population reported to federal programs (FoodNet)	Tiny number of affected patients; this study depends on accurate reporting to the FDA	Listeriosis may be a serious risk to patients treated with TNF- α inhibitors, particularly those treated with other adjunctive agents concurrently
Yeo W, et al. *J Clin Oncol.* 2008;27: 605–611.	Retrospective cohort study	In a cohort of 46 lymphoma patients with evidence of resolved HBV, 5/21 who received rituximab-based chemotherapy vs 0/25 who received non-rituximab based chemotherapy developed HBV reactivation	Small sample size limits interpretation	Receipt of rituximab among patient with resolved HBV treated for lymphoma predisposed to HBV reactivation
Krause PJ, et al. *Clin Infect Dis.* 2008;46:370–376.	Retrospective case-control study	Compared the immunologic status and clinical course of 14 patients with relapsing babesiosis to 46 controls with treatment-responsive babesiosis	May be limited by selection bias of cases which were from different centers	Patients with relapsing babesiosis had more complications and were more likely to have lymphoma, asplenia, or to have received rituximab

HBV, hepatitis B virus; PCP, *Pneumocystis jiroveci* pneumonia; RA, rheumatoid arthritis.

Patients more than 6 months out from transplantation remain at increased risk for infection with community-acquired pathogens, particularly from encapsulated organisms after SCT, and late reactivation of latent viruses such as hepatitis B. Transplant recipients who received prophylaxis for CMV or VZV for the first six months after transplant are also at risk for reactivation of these pathogens after prophylaxis is stopped. There is also a risk of transplant-associated malignancy, due to latent viruses such as Epstein-Barr virus and human papillomavirus, in this time period. Patients with rejection or GVHD more than 6 months after transplant may develop the same opportunistic pathogens commonly seen earlier (**Table 198-5**).

SUGGESTED READINGS

Chapel H, Cunningham-Rundles C. Update in understanding common variable immunodeficiency disorders (CVIDs) and the management of patients with these conditions. *Br J Haematol.* 2009;145:709–727.

Curtis JR, Patkar N, Xie A, et al. Risk of serious bacterial infections among rheumatoid arthritis patients exposed to tumor necrosis factor α antagonists. *Arthritis Rheum.* 2007;56:1125–1133.

Fishman JA, Rubin RH. Infection in organ-transplant recipients. *N Engl J Med.* 1998;338:1741–1751.

Padate BP, Keidan J. Enteroviral meningoencephalitis in a patient with non-Hodgkin's lymphoma treated previously with rituximab. *Clin Lab Haem.* 2006;28:69–71.

Pelosini M, Focosi D, Rita F, et al. Progressive multifocal leukoencephalopathy: report of three cases in HIV-negative hematological patients and review of literature. *Ann Hematol.* 2008;87:405–412.

Schneeweiss S, Setoguchi S, Weinblatt ME, et al. Anti-tumor necrosis factor α therapy and the risk of serious bacterial infection in elderly patients with rheumatoid arthritis. *Arthritis Rheum.* 2007;56:1754–1764.

Sharma VR, Fleming DR, Slone SP. Pure red cell aplasia due to parvovirus B19 in a patient treated with rituximab. *Blood.* 2000;96:1184–1186.

CHAPTER 199

Meningitis and Encephalitis

Karen L. Roos, MD
Jared R. Brosch, MD, MS

Key Clinical Questions

1. Is the classic triad of fever, headache, and stiff neck reliable for bacterial meningitis?
2. What signs and symptoms distinguish meningitis from encephalitis?
3. What is appropriate empiric antimicrobial therapy?
4. When should a CT scan be done before lumbar puncture?
5. What cerebrospinal fluid studies are essential, and which ones should be done if the initial studies do not yield a diagnosis?
6. When is MRI helpful in the diagnosis?
7. How soon can the patient be discharged, and how long to continue antimicrobial therapy?
8. When should a neurology consult be obtained?

INTRODUCTION

Meningitis and encephalitis may be the most terrifying diseases in medicine. Bacterial meningitis and viral encephalitis may be rapidly fatal, even in healthy persons. Survivors may suffer lasting neurological sequelae, including memory loss and seizures. Cases of meningococcal meningitis spark great anxiety in both caregivers and casual contacts. Viral meningitis, by contrast, gives patients a bad headache and a stiff neck, but uneventful recovery is the rule.

In the United States, bacterial meningitis affects 1.5 to 2.0 per 100,000 population annually, viral meningitis approximately 14 per 100,000 annually, and encephalitis 7 per 100,000 annually. Encephalitis generally refers to viral encephalitis, although bacteria, parasites, spirochetes, and fungi may all cause encephalitis. In this chapter, encephalitis refers specifically to viral encephalitis.

CLINICAL PRESENTATION

MENINGITIS

Is the classic triad reliable?

A 43-year-old woman presents with complaints of fever of 103°F, headache, nausea, vomiting, and photophobia. In the emergency department, she becomes increasingly lethargic.

The classic triad of meningitis is fever, headache, and stiff neck (nuchal rigidity). Patients with bacterial meningitis may also have an altered level of consciousness. Almost all patients with bacterial meningitis have at least two of these features, so the absence of all four makes bacterial meningitis unlikely. Patients may also complain of photophobia, nausea, and vomiting.

It is difficult, if not impossible, to exclude bacterial meningitis based on the physical examination. Findings may include nuchal rigidity (pain on passive flexion of the neck), Kernig's sign, and Brudzinski's sign. Kernig's sign is elicited with the patient in the supine position. The thigh is flexed on the abdomen with the knee flexed. Attempts to passively extend the leg cause pain when meningeal irritation is present. Brudzinski's sign is elicited with the patient in the supine position, and is positive when passive flexion of the neck results in flexion of the hips and knees. Patients with bacterial meningitis may also have focal neurological deficits or seizures.

Less than 50% of children with bacterial meningitis have nuchal rigidity. The possibility of bacterial meningitis should be considered in every child with fever, vomiting, photophobia, lethargy or altered mental status. Many cases of bacterial meningitis in children are preceded by upper respiratory tract infections or otitis media. Signs of meningitis in the neonate are nonspecific, and include irritability, lethargy, poor feeding, vomiting, diarrhea, temperature instability (fever or hypothermia), respiratory distress, apnea, seizures, and a bulging fontanel.

Patients with viral meningitis complain of fever, headache, stiff neck, photophobia, nausea, and vomiting, but are awake and alert.

PRACTICE POINT

- Patients with viral meningitis are awake and alert. They are not lethargic or confused. The patient with a febrile illness, CSF lymphocytic pleocytosis, and lethargy or confusion has encephalitis, not viral meningitis.

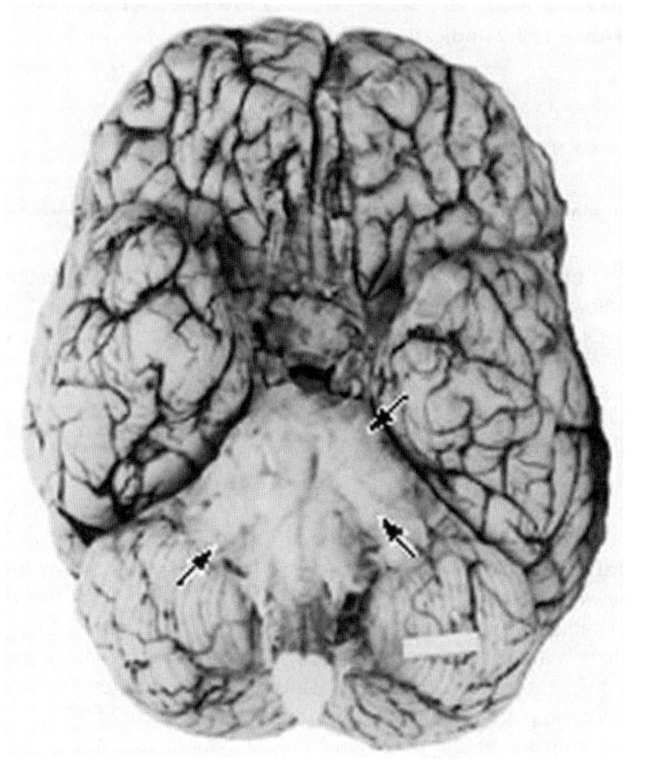

Figure 199-1 *Autopsy specimen in a patient with tuberculous meningitis, with prominent basilar exudate (arrows). (Reproduced, with permission, from Waxman SG. Clinical Neuroanatomy. 26th ed. New York: McGraw-Hill; 2010: Fig. 25-17.)*

Tuberculous meningitis presents as either a slowly progressive illness with persistent and intractable headache that has been present for weeks followed by confusion, lethargy, meningismus, focal neurological deficits and cranial nerve deficits, or an acute meningoencephalitis characterized by coma, raised intracranial pressure, seizures and focal neurological deficits. The basilar meninges are predominantly involved (**Figure 199-1**). Fungal meningitis clinically resembles tuberculous meningitis. Patients complain of headache, fever and malaise, followed by meningeal signs, altered mental status and cranial nerve palsies.

ENCEPHALITIS

Patients with encephalitis have fever and headache and at least one of the following: altered level of consciousness, confusion or abnormal behavior, new onset seizures and/or focal neurological deficits.

ETIOLOGY

BACTERIAL MENINGITIS

Pathogens causing meningitis depend upon age and predisposing or associated conditions (**Table 199-1**). *Streptococcus pneumoniae* is the most common cause of meningitis in adults older than 20 (45–50% of cases). Infection may begin with pneumonia, otitis media, or sinusitis. Meningococci are directly spread by large droplet respiratory secretions, and tend to infect adolescents who share cigarettes, cokes and kisses. *Listeria monocytogenes* (about 8% of cases) is a food-borne infection, found in sources as diverse as processed meats, unpasteurized cheeses, cheese balls, hot dogs, and raw vegetables. Neonatal bacterial meningitis infections are acquired from the maternal genitourinary tract.

TABLE 199-1 Bacterial Etiology for Meningitis Based on Predisposing Condition

Predisposing Condition	Bacterial Pathogen
Neonate	Group B streptococcus, *Escherichia coli, Listeria monocytogenes*
Healthy children and adults with community acquired disease	*Streptococcus pneumoniae, Neisseria meningitidis*
Otitis, mastoiditis, sinusitis	Streptococci sp, gram-negative anaerobes (*Bacteroides* sp, *Fusobacterium* sp), *Enterobacteriaceae* (*Proteus* sp, *E coli, Klebsiella* sp), staphylococci, *Haemophilus influenzae*
Adults over age 55 or with chronic illness	*S pneumoniae, N meningitidis,* gram-negative bacilli, *L monocytogenes, H influenzae*
Postneurosurgical or intraventricular device	Staphylococci, gram-negative bacilli
Endocarditis	Viridans streptococci, *Staphylococcus aureus, Streptococcus bovis,* HACEK group, enterococci

HACEK group, *Haemophilus* sp, *Actinobacillus actinomycetemcomitans, Cardiobacterium hominis, Eikenella corrodens,* and *Kingella kingae.*

PRACTICE POINT

- *Listeria* may cause a rhomboencephalitis, or brainstem encephalitis, often with a prodrome of several days of headache, vomiting, and fever, followed by cranial nerve palsies, cerebellar, and long-tract motor and sensory deficits. Brainstem abscess, a devastating complication, may arise. Meningitis may also be present. While most patients with *Listeria* infection are immunosuppressed, those with *Listeria* rhomboencephalitis are often immunocompetent.

VIRAL MENINGITIS

The most common etiological agent of aseptic meningitis are viruses. Enteroviruses (including coxsackievirus, echovirus, and enteroviruses 68–71) have been found in more than 75% of cases in which a specific pathogen is identified. Herpes simplex virus-2 (HSV-2) and HIV are also fairly common etiological agents of viral meningitis. Approximately 25% of women and 11% of men develop meningitis during the primary episode of genital herpes, with up to 20% of these patients having recurrent attacks of meningitis (Mollaret meningitis). Arthropod-borne viruses (arboviruses), such as West Nile, can cause meningitis or encephalitis. Lymphocytic choriomeningitis virus causes a prolonged aseptic meningitis syndrome.

VIRAL ENCEPHALITIS

Herpes simplex virus-1 (HSV-1) is the most important cause of sporadic encephalitis in immunocompetent adults, and the most common cause of viral encephalitis in developed countries. The arboviruses are viruses transmitted by the bite of a mosquito or tick. The most common arboviruses causing encephalitis in North America are West Nile virus, St. Louis encephalitis virus, and La Crosse virus.

Varicella zoster virus may cause encephalitis in association with shingles, months after shingles, and in the absence of shingles. Epstein-Barr virus may cause encephalitis as an acute complication of mononucleosis. Cytomegalovirus causes encephalitis in the immunocompromised.

DIFFERENTIAL DIAGNOSIS

BACTERIAL MENINGITIS

The differential diagnosis of bacterial meningitis includes viral meningitis, fungal meningitis, tuberculous meningitis, viral encephalitis, and an infectious mass lesion. Subarachnoid hemorrhage may also present with headache and stiff neck.

VIRAL MENINGITIS

The differential diagnosis of viral meningitis includes partially treated bacterial meningitis, fungal meningitis, tuberculous meningitis, Lyme disease, drug-induced meningitis (NSAIDs, intravenous immunoglobulin, sulfa drugs, isoniazid, and muromonab-CD3), carcinomatous meningitis, lymphomatous meningitis, and sarcoidosis.

VIRAL ENCEPHALITIS

The differential diagnosis of viral encephalitis includes the other etiological agents of encephalitis: bacteria, mycobacteria, fungi, *Rickettsia*, protozoa and parasites. Encephalitis may also be an autoimmune illness, such as nonvasculitic autoimmune inflammatory meningoencephalitis (Hashimoto encephalopathy), a paraneoplastic limbic encephalitis, or a para- or postinfectious disorder, such as acute disseminated encephalomyelitis.

DIAGNOSIS

MENINGITIS

The first step in the diagnosis of meningitis is physical examination, followed by CBC with differential, C-reactive protein, and blood for Gram's stain and culture. Antimicrobial therapy is initiated at this step. When bacterial meningitis is suspected, always start empiric and adjunctive therapy immediately after obtaining CBC and blood cultures. Do not wait for the results of spinal fluid analysis to initiate antimicrobial therapy.

Serum procalcitonin (if available) is one of the most sensitive labs for distinguishing between bacterial and viral meningitis. Serum procalcitonin and C-reactive protein (>40 mg/L) are significantly higher in patients with bacterial meningitis than in those with viral meningitis.

When is a CT scan needed before an LP?

Although every patient with suspected meningitis or encephalitis needs an LP for spinal fluid analysis, not every patient needs a CT prior to an LP. **Table 199-2** lists the indications for CT prior to LP.

Although CT scans do not diagnose increased intracranial pressure, they do demonstrate mass lesions with associated edema and brain parenchymal shifts that potentially can cause herniation following lumbar puncture. Even with a normal CT scan the risk of cerebral herniation in bacterial meningitis is not zero, and lumbar puncture is often not the cause of the herniation.

TABLE 199-2 Indications for CT Prior to LP

Abnormal level of consciousness	New onset seizure
Focal neurological deficit	Immunocompromised state
Papilledema	Poorly visualized fundi

What are the best tests on cerebrospinal fluid (CSF) to make the diagnosis?

Table 199-3 provides a list of the expected results for opening pressure, cell count with differential, glucose concentration, and protein concentration in normal and infected CSF. **Table 199-4** lists the CSF diagnostic tests for meningitis. There are several important exceptions to the expected CSF values shown in Table 199-3. In enteroviral meningitis and arboviral infections, there may be a predominance of polymorphonuclear leukocytes early in the disease. In enteroviral infection, the transition to a lymphocytic pleocytosis usually occurs over the course of 24 hours. For arboviruses, the transition to a CSF lymphocytic pleocytosis may take a week or more, and West Nile virus may never make the transition.

The CSF white blood cell count is affected by the amount of time between collection and laboratory analysis. Polymorphonuclear leukocytes have a half life of approximately 2 hours. Therefore, it is important that the spinal fluid is analyzed within 90 minutes of collection to obtain an accurate result.

In cases of suspected bacterial meningitis, CSF Gram's stain allows for rapid identification of the meningeal pathogen, and culture allows for specific identification and antimicrobial susceptibility testing. There is both a broad-range bacterial 16S ribosomal DNA PCR (polymerase chain reaction) and a meningeal pathogen-specific PCR, but their sensitivity and specificity have not been defined, and they are not routinely available. Enteroviruses grow in CSF culture; HSV-2 typically does not.

The CSF in tuberculous meningitis typically has a lymphocytic pleocytosis of 200 to 500 cells/mm^3, and a mildly decreased median glucose concentration of 40 mg/dL. The last tube of CSF collected should be sent for acid fast bacilli smear and culture. The polymerase chain reaction to detect nucleic acid of *Mycobacterium tuberculosis*

TABLE 199-3 Spinal Fluid Analysis for Meningitis

Etiology	Opening Pressure	WBC Count	Protein	Glucose	CSF/Serum Glucose Ratio
Normal	<180 mm H_2O	≤5 cells/mm^3	15–45 mg/dL	45–80 mg/dL	0.6–0.7
Bacterial	>180 mm H_2O	>100 cells/mm^3 **PMNs predominant**	>45 mg/dL	<40 mg/dL	<0.4
Viral, *Borrelia burgdorferi*, *Treponema pallidum*, *Bartonella henselae*	<180 mm H_2O	25–500 cells/mm^3 **Lymphocyte predominant**	15–45 mg/dL	45–80 mg/dL	0.6–0.7
Fungi, *Mycobacterium tuberculosis*, sarcoid, lymphoma, leptomeningeal metastases, partially treated bacterial meningitis	Normal or increased	25–500 cells/mm^3 **Lymphocyte predominant**	>45 mg/dL	<40 mg/dL	<0.6

TABLE 199-4 Cerebrospinal Fluid Diagnostic Tests in Meningitis

Stain and culture
Gram's stain and culture
India ink and fungal culture
Acid fast bacilli and *Mycobacterium tuberculosis* culture
Antibody
Coccidioides immitis complement fixation
West Nile virus CSF-IgM
Borrelia burgdorferi
Antigen
Histoplasma polysaccharide antigen
Cryptococcal polysaccharide antigen
Polymerase chain reaction
Broad-range bacterial 16S ribosomal DNA
Streptococcus pneumoniae
Herpes simplex virus types 1 and 2
Epstein-Barr virus
Mycobacterium tuberculosis
Neisseria meningitidis
Reverse transcriptase for enteroviruses
West Nile virus
Varicella zoster virus
HIV RNA
Other
Cytology and flow cytometry for metastases
IL-10 (lymphoma), IL-6 (infection, inflammation)

in spinal fluid is available, and should be sent, but the sensitivity and specificity is unknown.

Spinal fluid in fungal meningitis typically displays a normal or slightly elevated opening pressure, lymphocytic pleocytosis, elevated protein concentration, and decreased glucose concentration. The cryptococcal polysaccharide antigen is a highly sensitive and specific test, and should be performed on all CSF specimens when fungal meningitis is suspected. Histoplasma polysaccharide antigen should be performed in suspected fungal meningitis in patients who reside in or have traveled to the Ohio and Mississippi River valleys. *Coccidioides immitis* is a dimorphic fungus that is endemic to the desert areas of California, Arizona, New Mexico, and Texas. The CSF complement fixation antibody test is reported to have a specificity of 100% and a sensitivity of 75% in the setting of active disease. *Cryptococcus neoformans, Histoplasma capsulatum,* and *Coccidioides immitis* may also be identified by India ink stain of CSF, and will grow in fungal culture. If culture obtained from a lumbar puncture fails to yield the diagnosis, consider obtaining CSF from a high cervical puncture.

Aspiration or biopsy of rashes may aid the diagnosis of meningococcal disease. The rash of meningococcemia begins as a diffuse erythematous maculopapular rash resembling a viral exanthema, but the lesions rapidly become petechial. Petechiae are found predominantly on the trunk and lower extremities, but also in the mucous membranes and conjunctiva and occasionally on the palms and soles. Purpura fulminans and skin necrosis occasionally develop (**Figure 199-2**). The characteristic rash due to an enterovirus consists of erythematous macules and papules on the face, neck, trunk, and to a lesser degree the extremities.

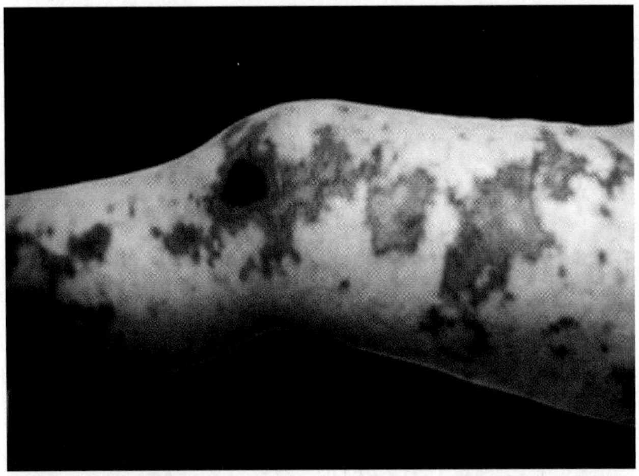

Figure 199-2 *Purpura fulminans: disseminated intravascular coagulation with cutaneous hemorrhage and necrosis in meningococcal disease. (Reproduced, with permission, from Wolff K, Goldsmith LA, Katz SI, et al. Fitzpatrick's Dermatology in General Medicine. 7th ed. New York: McGraw-Hill, 2008. Fig. 180-1C.)*

Patients with meningitis due to *Borrelia burgdorferi* complain of headache and fatigue, and often have myalgias and arthralgias. Unilateral or bilateral facial nerve palsy may be present, or a painful radiculopathy. Diagnosis typically begins with a serum ELISA (enzyme linked immunosorbent assay) for antibody to *B burgdorferi*. A positive result is confirmed with a Western blot. CSF examination demonstrates a lymphocytic pleocytosis with normal glucose and a mild to moderately elevated protein concentration. Intrathecal anti-*B burgdorferi* antibodies can be detected. Because Lyme disease antibodies can be passively transferred from blood to CSF and persist in the CSF for years, demonstration of anti-*B burgdorferi* antibodies in the CSF is not definitive evidence of neurologic Lyme disease. Instead, one must calculate the *B burgdorferi* antibody index, which is positive when > 1.3 to 1.5.

$$B\ burgdorferi\ antibody - index = \frac{anti - Borrelia\ IgG\ CSF/anti - Borrelia\ IgG\ Serum}{total\ IgG\ CSF/total\ IgG\ Serum}$$

Arboviral infection is defined by the Centers for Disease Control as a febrile illness with mild neurological symptoms during a period of likely arboviral transmission, plus at least one of the following: a 4-fold or greater increase in serum antibody titer between acute and convalescent sera, viral isolation from tissue/blood/CSF, or specific IgM antibody to an arbovirus in the CSF.

Meningitis from neurosarcoidosis is diagnosed by excluding infectious meningitis, and histologic documentation of sarcoidosis elsewhere, such as a lymph node, skin lesion, salivary gland, or from the conjunctiva. CSF angiotensin-converting enzyme is not useful.

VIRAL ENCEPHALITIS

The diagnosis of viral encephalitis is *suggested by the clinical presentation* and *supported* by spinal fluid analysis and neuroimaging abnormalities. The spinal fluid analysis has similar characteristics to viral meningitis: lymphocytic pleocytosis and a normal glucose concentration. CSF PCR has become the primary diagnostic test for encephalitis due to HSV-1. A negative test does not exclude the disease, as the PCR can be falsely negative in the first 72 hours of symptoms, and after day 10. CSF and serum should be sent to determine if there is intrathecal synthesis of HSV antibodies. A serum:CSF ratio of less than 20:1 is diagnostic of HSV encephalitis. CSF-IgM for West Nile virus is more sensitive than PCR, with PCR only being positive in approximately 60% of cases.

The characteristic abnormalities of HSV encephalitis on neuroimaging are hyperintensity in the frontotemporal, cingulate, or insular regions of the brain on T2-weighted, diffusion, and fluid attenuated inversion recovery (FLAIR) sequences. MRI may be normal in the early stages of HSV-1 encephalitis, but the majority of patients will have MRI abnormalities within 48 hours of symptom onset. In both West Nile virus encephalitis and St. Louis encephalitis, MRI may reveal hyperintense lesions in the basal ganglia and thalami on T2 and FLAIR sequences. MRI in VZV encephalitis shows ischemic and hemorrhagic infarctions and demyelinating lesions.

TRIAGE/HOSPITAL ADMISSION

Patients with suspected bacterial meningitis or encephalitis should be admitted for close observation and frequent neurological assessment, as they are at risk for the development of cerebral edema, increased intracranial pressure, and seizures. Patients with suspected viral meningitis should be monitored or admitted under a 23-hour observation with empiric antimicrobial therapy until results of the spinal fluid analysis are available.

Neisseria meningitidis is the only bacterial meningitis that requires respiratory isolation. Patients with a suggestive rash or a CSF Gram's stain showing gram negative diplococci should be immediately placed in respiratory isolation. Close contacts should be treated with chemoprophylaxis (see below).

When should a neurology consult be obtained?

Neurology consults are important for many cases of meningitis and encephalitis. Straightforward cases of viral meningitis can be managed without a consult. All patients with an altered level of consciousness, new onset seizure, or focal neurological symptoms or signs should be evaluated by a neurologist. All hospitalized patients should be followed by a neurologist and monitored closely for signs of increased intracranial pressure and the development of focal neurological deficits.

TREATMENT

EMPIRIC THERAPY

Meningitis and encephalitis are neurologic emergencies. Empiric therapy should begin within 60 minutes of arrival in the emergency room. Significant increases in mortality are found with treatment delayed more than 6 hours from presentation. Empiric therapy includes antimicrobial agents and adjunctive dexamethasone. The specific antimicrobial agents chosen depend on the patient's predisposing conditions, and the time of the year (see **Table 199-5**). In patients with suspected bacterial meningitis, dexamethasone (adult dose: 10 mg every 6 hours for 4 days; pediatric dose: 0.15 mg/kg every 6 hours) either prior to antibiotic therapy, or with the first dose of antibiotics is recommended. Acyclovir (10 mg/kg every 8 hours) is added to the empiric regimen for HSV encephalitis. Doxycycline (100 mg every 12 hours) is added for tick-borne infection if ticks are prevalent and in season in the patient's part of the country.

TABLE 199-5 Empiric Therapy

Patient Population	Empiric Treatment
Neonate	Ampicillin plus cefotaxime or an aminoglycoside
Healthy children and adults with community-acquired disease	Third- or fourth-generation cephalosporin + vancomycin [+metronidazole if otitis, mastoiditis, sinusitis are predisposing conditions]
Adults over age 55 or with chronic illness or immunosuppressed patients	Third- or fourth-generation cephalosporin + vancomycin + ampicillin
Postneurosurgical	Vancomycin + meropenem
All patients	Dexamethasone + acyclovir (if illness compatible with HSV encephalitis) + doxycycline (during tick season)

BACTERIAL MENINGITIS SPECIFIC THERAPY

Modify antimicrobial therapy based on specific bacterial pathogen antimicrobial sensitivity testing (**Table 199-6**). The length of treatment is dependent on the specific pathogen. Meningitis due to *S pneumoniae*, *H influenzae*, and group B streptococci is treated with intravenous antibiotics for 10 to 14 days. Patients with *S pneumoniae* meningitis should have repeat spinal fluid analysis, if safe to do so, after 48 hours of treatment to ensure the culture is sterile. Bacterial meningitis due to *L monocytogenes* and *Enterobacteriaceae* is treated for 3 to 4 weeks. Meningitis caused by *N meningitidis* requires treatment for 5 to 7 days. Respiratory isolation must be continued for at least 24 hours after the initiation of antimicrobial therapy. Chemoprophylaxis for meningococcal meningitis is typically rifampin 600 mg every 12 hours for 2 days (four doses total). However, a single dose of ciprofloxacin 500 mg is just as effective as rifampin, but it is only indicated for patients over 18 years of age. Neither rifampin nor ciprofloxacin should be prescribed for pregnant women or children. Instead, a single injection of intravenous or intramuscular ceftriaxone (250 mg for adults; 125 mg for children) is recommended. Meningococcal meningitis patients treated with penicillin G should also receive rifampin prophylaxis before discharge from the hospital.

Lyme meningitis is treated with either intravenous ceftriaxone 2 g per day for 14 to 28 days, or oral doxycycline, which is likely as effective, given as 200 to 400 mg twice daily for 10 to 14 days for adults and children >8 years old. There are currently no indications to treat Lyme disease for longer than 28 days, despite cases of patients with subjective symptoms beyond that point.

VIRAL MENINGITIS

Viral meningitis is treated symptomatically with antipyretics, antiemetics, and analgesics. Amytriptyline and NSAIDs are often required for months to treat headache from viral meningitis. Patients with HSV-2 meningitis can be treated with acyclovir 800 mg 5 times daily, famciclovir 500 mg 3 times daily, or valacyclovir 1000 mg 3 times daily for 7 to 14 days.

FUNGAL MENINGITIS

The treatment of cryptococcal meningitis includes a combination of either intravenous amphotericin B (0.7–1.0 mg/kg/d) or amBisome 4 mg/kg/day or abelcet 5 mg/kg/day *plus* oral flucytosine (25 mg/kg four times a day). This combination is typically used for two weeks or until the CSF culture is sterile. This induction therapy is followed by fluconazole 400 to 800 mg/day, which is continued for 8 to 10 weeks. CNS histoplasmosis is treated with intravenous amphotericin B (0.7–1.0 mg/kg/d). A total dose of 30 mg/kg is recommended. A course of amphotericin B is

TABLE 199-6 Recommended Specific Antibacterial Treatment and Dosing

Microorganism	Antibiotic	Dose
Streptococcus pneumoniae		
Penicillin susceptible (MIC < 0.1 mg/L)	Penicillin G	Neonates: 0.15–0.2 mU/kg/d (every 8–12 hours) Infants and children: 0.3 mU/kg/d (every 4–6 hours) Adult: 24 million units/d (every 4–6 hours)
	or ceftriaxone	Infant or child: 80–100 mg/kg/d (every 12 hours) Adult: 4 g/d (every 12 hours)
	or cefepime	Infants and children: 150 mg/kg/d (every 8 hours) Adult: 6 g/d (every 8 hours)
	or cefotaxime	Neonate: 100–150 mg/kg/d (every 8–12 hours) Infant or child: 225–300 mg/kg/d (every 6–8 hours) Adult: 8–12 g/d (every 4–6 hours)
Penicillin tolerant (MIC 0.1–1.0 mg/L)	Ceftriaxone *or* cefepime *or* cefotaxime	As above
Penicillin resistant (MIC > 1 mg/L or Cefotaxime/ceftriaxone MIC ≥ 1 mg/L	Cefepime (*or* cefotaxime *or* ceftriaxone)	As above
	plus vancomycin	Neonates: 20–30 mg/kg/d (every 8–12 hours) Infant and child: 60 mg/kg/d (every 6 hours) Adults: 45–60 mg/kg/d (every 6–12 hours)
Neisseria meningitidis	Penicillin G	as above
	or ampicillin	Neonate: 150 mg/kg/d (every 8 hours) Infant and child: 300 mg/kg/d (every 6 hours) Adult: 12 g/d (every 4–6 hours)
Penicillin resistant	Ceftriaxone *or* cefotaxime	As above
Listeria monocytogenes	Ampicillin	As above
Critically ill patients	*plus* gentamicin	Neonate: 5 mg/kg/d (every 12 hours) Infant and child: 7.5 mg/kg/d (every 8 hours) Adult: 5 mg/kg/d (every 8 hours)
Streptococcus agalactiae (group B streptococci)	**Ampicillin** *or* penicillin G *or* cefotaxime	As above
Escherichia coli or other Enterobacteriaceae	Ceftriaxone or cefepime *or* cefotaxime	As above
Pseudomonas aeruginosa	**Meropenem** *or*	Infant and child:120 mg/kg/day (every 8 hours) Adult: 6 g/d (every 8 hours)
	ceftazidime	
Staphylococcus aureus		
Methicillin susceptible	Nafcillin *or* oxacillin	Neonates: 75 mg/kg/d (every 8–12 hours) Infants and children: 200 mg/kg/d (every 6 hours) Adult: 9–12 g/d (every 4 hours)
Methicillin resistant	Vancomycin	As above
Staphylococcus epidermidis	**Vancomycin**	As above
	or linezolid	Neonates: 20 mg/kg/d (every 8–12 hours) Infant and child: 30 mg/kg/d (every 8 hours) Adult: 600 mg (every 12 hours)
Haemophilus influenzae	Ceftriaxone *or* cefepime *or* cefotaxime	As above

Recommended agents are in **bold**.
Intraventricular vancomycin administration: children 10 mg/d, adults 20 mg/d.

followed by oral itraconazole 200 mg twice daily for 6 months to a year. *C immitis* meningitis is treated with either high dose fluconazole (1000 mg daily) as monotherapy, or a combination of intravenous and intrathecal amphotericin B (0.25–0.75 mg/d 3 times weekly). High dose fluconazole therapy as induction therapy can be followed by lower doses of fluconazole (200–400 mg daily) indefinitely. Treatment of fungal meningitis requires frequent examination of CSF for culture.

The management of increased intracranial pressure is as critical to a successful outcome from fungal meningitis as antifungal therapy. Intracranial pressure should be measured at the initial lumbar puncture and at the completion of induction therapy, and any time during the course of the illness when the patient has a change in mental status or a change in the neurological examination. Increased intracranial pressure is best managed with a ventriculostomy during acute infection, followed by a ventriculoperitoneal shunt. The practice of daily lumbar punctures to decrease CSF pressure by 50% and maintain CSF pressure at < 300 mm/H_2O is impractical. Shunt revision should be done quickly in patients with deteriorating consciousness. The longer the duration of symptoms at presentation, the less impact shunting will have on reversing neurological complications.

TUBERCULOUS MENINGITIS

Patients with tuberculous meningitis are treated with isoniazid, rifampin, and pyrazinamide for 2 months, followed by isoniazid and rifampin for an additional 10 months. Present recommendations are that HIV-negative patients are treated with dexamethasone for the first 3 to 4 weeks of therapy, and then the patient is switched to prednisone therapy for an additional 4 weeks. Previous practice had been to use corticosteroid therapy only in patients who developed hydrocephalus or coma.

VIRAL ENCEPHALITIS

There are very few antiviral agents for viral encephalitis. Encephalitis due to HSV-1 is treated with intravenous acyclovir 30 mg/kg/day divided every 8 hours, and infused over 60 minutes. (Slow acyclovir infusion prevents renal tubular crystal formation and renal insufficiency.) Oral antivirals have not been adequately studied in this setting; therefore, patients should be maintained on intravenous acyclovir for 3 weeks. Patients who are not responding to acyclovir and those in whom a definitive agent cannot be identified can be treated with foscarnet. The recommended dose is 60 mg/kg every 8 hours. Varicella zoster virus encephalitis is treated with intravenous acyclovir.

COMPLICATIONS

MENINGITIS

The mortality rate for bacterial meningitis is between 10% to 20%. Up to 25% of survivors have serious neurologic sequelae, including hearing loss, impaired executive functioning, seizure disorders, and deficits from ischemic stroke or intraparenchymal hemorrhage. Patients with viral meningitis often complain of headache for weeks to months.

ENCEPHALITIS

Complications from HSV encephalitis include impaired memory and seizure disorder.

DISCHARGE PLANNING

MENINGITIS

Patients with bacterial meningitis should remain in the hospital during antibiotic therapy, and discharged when this is complete. Chemoprophylaxis should be provided for patients with meningococcal meningitis and their family members as outlined above. Patients with fungal meningitis and tuberculous meningitis may be discharged to continue antimicrobial therapy at home when they are stable.

ENCEPHALITIS

Patients with HSV encephalitis should remain in the hospital for the first 2 weeks of acyclovir therapy, and then if stable, can be discharged to complete a 3-week course of acyclovir therapy at home.

SUGGESTED READINGS

Hasbun R, Abrahams J, Jekel J, Quagliarello VJ. Computed tomography of the head before lumbar puncture in adults with suspected meningitis. *N Engl J Med*. 2001;345:1727–1733.

Khetsuriani N, Holman RC, Anderson LJ. Burden of encephalitis-associated hospitalizations in the United States, 1988–1997. *Clin Infect Dis*. 2002;35:175–182.

Tunkel AR, Glaser CA, Bloch KC, et al. The management of encephalitis: clinical practice guidelines by the Infectious Diseases Society of America. *Clin Infect Dis*. 2008;47:303–327.

Tunkel AR, Hartman BJ, Kaplan SL, et al. Practice guidelines for the management of bacterial meningitis. *Clin Infect Dis*. 2004;39:1267–1284.

CHAPTER 200

Osteomyelitis and Septic Arthritis

Yonatan H. Grad, MD, PhD
John J. Ross, MD, CM, FIDSA

Key Clinical Questions

Osteomyelitis

1. How does bone become infected?
2. What tests and aspects of the history and physical exam are most helpful in diagnosis?
3. What treatment options should be considered?
4. How can response to treatment be monitored?

Septic Arthritis

1. What are the components of an evaluation for possible acute bacterial (septic) arthritis?
2. When should empiric antibiotics be used to treat suspected septic arthritis, and which antibiotics?
3. What are the key elements to treatment of septic arthritis?

OSTEOMYELITIS: INTRODUCTION

Osteomyelitis is bone infection with accompanying inflammation and bone destruction. Bone resists infection under normal circumstances. Factors that influence the establishment and progression of osteomyelitis include the virulence of the pathogen, inoculum size, characteristics of the involved bone, presence of foreign objects, host immune system, and duration of infection. Bone may be infected by direct contamination during trauma or surgery, spread of infection from adjacent soft tissue, or hematogenous seeding of microbes. The diagnostic and therapeutic approach varies depending on the mode of infection. However, as treatment for osteomyelitis is long, complex, expensive, and not always successful even when management is optimal, proper diagnosis and pathogen identification is of great importance in all cases.

PATHOPHYSIOLOGY

Bacteria infect bone through trauma or surgery, spread from adjacent soft tissue, or bacteremic seeding. They then attach to host cells and extracellular matrix components, as well as implanted biomaterials, if present. Bacterial strategies to evade the host immune response include elaboration of biofilm, a hydrated matrix that establishes a physical barrier against both host defenses and antibiotics. Bacteria embedded in biofilm are also less metabolically active, making them less susceptible to antibiotics. Inflammation associated with bacterial toxins and the host immune response leads to bone lysis. Over time, as infection becomes chronic, suppuration leads to vascular congestion, raised intraosseous pressure, and ischemia of infected bone. The necrotic bone separates from healthy bone to form a sequestrum, a diagnostic finding of chronic osteomyelitis. If the dead bone cannot be resorbed, new bone may form from the surrounding healthy bone tissue, encasing the sequestrum in an involucrum. The walled-off sequestrum may become functionally similar to an abscess, with bacterial growth continuing in a pocket of necrotic tissue inaccessible to immune surveillance or antibiotics. As pressure in the sequestrum builds, infection may erupt through the involucrum, leading to subperiosteal or soft tissue abscesses, or a sinus tract through overlying soft tissue.

PRACTICE POINT

- Failure rates are high in the treatment of osteomyelitis. Except for the vertebrae and other bones containing red marrow, most adult bones are not highly vascular. Many antibiotics also have marginal bone penetration. The problem of antibiotic delivery is often exacerbated by peripheral vascular disease, especially in diabetic patients. Dead bone is present in many adult patients with osteomyelitis, and acts as a nidus for relapse after cessation of antibiotics. Cure of osteomyelitis requires debridement of dead bone and treatment of peripheral vascular disease, when present.

DOES THIS PATIENT HAVE OSTEOMYELITIS?

The evaluation for osteomyelitis begins with the history and physical exam. Patients should be asked about risk factors for osteomyelitis, such as diabetes, vascular disease, intravenous drug use, and recent trauma or surgery. Physical findings of osteomyelitis may include sinus tracts, nonhealing wounds and ulcers that probe to bone, and evidence of associated peripheral vascular disease or diabetes. However, the exam is often unrevealing, especially in hematogenous osteomyelitis of deep sites. Laboratory evaluation includes blood cultures, white blood cell (WBC) count with differential, erythrocyte sedimentation rate (ESR), and C-reactive protein (CRP) level. The WBC count is usually nonspecific and more often elevated in acute than chronic osteomyelitis. ESR and CRP can be elevated in many conditions and may also be normal early in osteomyelitis. If ESR and CRP are elevated due to osteomyelitis, they can be used to assess patient response to treatment. CRP may drop within one to two weeks of starting appropriate therapy, while ESR falls more slowly. Other serum markers associated with bone disease, such as calcium, phosphate, and alkaline phosphatase, are usually normal in osteomyelitis.

The initial radiographic study in suspected osteomyelitis should be plain films of the affected area. These may show soft-tissue swelling, narrowing or widening of joint spaces, bone destruction, and periosteal reaction. If plain radiographs suggest osteomyelitis and blood cultures are positive, a presumptive diagnosis can be made and no further evaluation is needed. When plain films are not diagnostic, MRI should be the next radiologic study to diagnose osteomyelitis. MRI and CT are both useful in revealing medullary and cortical destruction, periosteal reaction, articular damage, and soft-tissue involvement. MRI is better for diagnosing soft tissue involvement, and CT is more sensitive for detecting cortical and medullary sequestra. Overall, MRI is more sensitive than CT, and also does not expose the patient to radiation. Bone marrow edema on MRI may be seen as early as three days into the course of osteomyelitis. However, MRI is not helpful in assessing the response to therapy, as bone marrow edema persists for months after microbiological cure. Another limitation is that bone marrow edema on MRI is not specific for osteomyelitis: it may also be caused by trauma, Charcot arthropathy, and surgery. Radionuclide bone scans have similar sensitivity to MRI, but also similar problems with specificity, as well as much lower spatial resolution. They may be useful in the presence of orthopedic devices which create artifacts on CT and MRI.

Isolation of a microbial pathogen via bone biopsy, along with histologic findings of inflammation and osteonecrosis, is the gold standard for the diagnosis of osteomyelitis. Antibiotics should be held before biopsy to maximize the yield of cultures, unless the patient is prohibitively ill. Percutaneous bone sampling should be pursued when feasible, but is limited by sampling error. Larger needles increase the diagnostic yield. The biopsy should be performed through healthy tissue under direct imaging guidance. If percutaneous biopsy and blood cultures are negative, and clinical suspicion of osteomyelitis remains high, then percutaneous biopsy should be repeated, or an open biopsy performed. Open bone biopsy provides the best results, but is more morbid. In patients with overlying wounds or sinus tracts, microbes cultured from superficial samples are often nonpathogenic, and correlate poorly with those responsible for the deep osteomyelitic infection, with the significant exception that identification of *Staphylococcus aureus* usually correlates with deep infection.

OSTEOMYELITIS FROM DIRECT INOCULATION

Direct inoculation of bone tissue by pathogens may take place during surgery or orthopedic trauma. The risk of osteomyelitis after an open fracture depends on the type of fracture, degree of contamination, surrounding soft tissue injury, and timing of local or systemic antibiotics after contamination. Commonly involved organisms include staphylococci, gram-negative bacilli, and other skin flora and soil organisms. As these patients often undergo multiple surgical procedures, they are also at risk for nosocomial pathogens.

CLINICAL PRESENTATION AND EVALUATION

Acute trauma–associated osteomyelitis can often go undiagnosed, as the initial signs can be mistaken for inflammation from other causes associated with the episode of trauma. As untreated acute osteomyelitis progresses to chronic osteomyelitis, signs and symptoms indicative of chronic osteomyelitis, such as fracture nonunion, poor wound healing, and sinus tract formation, may appear. Plain radiographs are often unhelpful, as traumatic and postoperative changes confound interpretation. MRI is sensitive, but less specific in this setting. It is reasonable to pursue another imaging modality, such as CT or radionuclide bone scan, prior to surgical intervention.

TREATMENT CONSIDERATIONS

The management principles for open fracture include early treatment with surgical debridement and administration of a short course of antimicrobial prophylaxis to prevent osteomyelitis. When osteomyelitis develops, the practice principles are microbe identification, surgical debridement, and tailored antibiotic therapy. The presence of foreign objects, such as fixation devices, requires long term oral antimicrobial therapy until fracture healing and removal of the fixation devices. When oral suppression fails to result in fracture healing, definitive therapy with removal of foreign objects, further surgical debridement, and additional directed antimicrobial therapy should be considered.

OSTEOMYELITIS FROM ADJACENT SOFT TISSUE INFECTION

Individuals with diabetes and peripheral vascular disease are the population at highest risk from this type of osteomyelitis, especially in the foot. Peripheral neuropathy predisposes to soft tissue ulceration in the feet, and vascular disease impairs proper immune response and wound healing. A significant percentage of these patients ultimately require amputation due to chronic soft tissue and bone infections.

CLINICAL PRESENTATION AND EVALUATION

Patients may have no fever and few signs of inflammation. The persistence of soft tissue inflammation and ulceration for a week or longer, however, should raise suspicion for underlying osteomyelitis. Physical exam should include the evaluation of pulses and Doppler ultrasound measurement of vascular flow, as well as characterization of neuropathy. If necessary, a more detailed evaluation including arteriography and nerve conduction studies could be considered.

One of the most useful tests for osteomyelitis in patients with soft tissue wounds is the "probe-to-bone" test, which involves advancing a sterile surgical probe through the ulceration. If the probe reaches bone, then the bone is almost certainly infected. In patients with diabetic foot ulcers, an ulcer that measures more than 2 cm^2 is strongly suggestive of osteomyelitis (**Table 200-1**). If suspicion remains high in the absence of convincing data from clinical exam and plain films, MRI is a sensitive and specific tool to assist in confirming infection.

TREATMENT CONSIDERATIONS

These infections are frequently polymicrobial, and include aerobic and anaerobic gram-positive and -negative bacteria, with staphylococcal and streptococcal species commonly involved. Treatment usually requires a combination of broad spectrum antimicrobial treatment and surgical intervention, such as debridement or amputation. Often, revascularization is a critical part of the treatment plan, as debridement and antibiotics will fail to clear an infection unless the vascular supply is adequate. The duration of antimicrobial treatment should be at least six weeks. Some argue that antimicrobial therapy should continue until complete resolution of the skin and soft tissue defects.

TABLE 200-1 Likelihood Ratios (LR) for Diagnosing Lower Extremity Osteomyelitis in Patients with Diabetes Mellitus

Risk Factors/Findings	Positive LR	Negative LR
Probe to bone	6.4	0.39
Bone exposure	9.2	0.70
Ulcer area > 2 cm	7.2	0.48
Ulcer inflammation	1.5	0.84
Clinical gestalt	5.5	0.54
Erythrocyte sedimentate rate > 70	11	0.34

Adapted from Butalia S, Palda VA, Sargeant RJ, Detsky AS, Mourad O. Does this patient with diabetes have osteomyelitis of the lower extremity? In: Simel DL, Rennie D, eds. *The Rational Clinical Examination.* New York: McGraw-Hill; 2009.

HEMATOGENOUS OSTEOMYELITIS

Any bone can be seeded by hematogenous spread of microbes, but in adults the spine is most often affected. Vertebral osteomyelitis, or spondylodiscitis, commonly involves the lower thoracic or lumbar spine and less frequently the cervical spine, often presenting as lower back pain or torticollis, respectively. Vertebrae are well perfused, and neighboring vertebrae share segmental arteries. Infection therefore often involves adjacent vertebrae with their intervertebral disc (**Figure 200-1**). Epidural or psoas abscesses are common complications. The source of bacteremia may include skin and soft tissue infections, urinary tract infections, dental abscesses, and central venous catheter–associated infections, but it is often unidentified.

CLINICAL PRESENTATION AND EVALUATION

The initial presentation of back pain is associated with fever in fewer than half of cases. Neurologic symptoms of motor and sensory deficits from spinal cord or nerve root compression are present in only a small percentage of patients. As the presentation of vertebral osteomyelitis is nonspecific, a high clinical suspicion is necessary for timely diagnosis. Physical exam may reveal tenderness over the affected area of the spine, with paraspinal muscle spasm.

Most cases of vertebral osteomyelitis are monomicrobial. The most common pathogen is *S aureus*, but many organisms may be responsible, including *Mycobacterium tuberculosis* and *Brucella* in endemic areas, *Salmonella* in those with sickle cell disease, and gram-negative organisms and fungi in immunosuppressed patients and intravenous drug users. *M tuberculosis* typically involves the thoracic, rather than lumbar spine, and may produce intravertebral lesions with a radiographic appearance seen most commonly with this pathogen and *Brucella* (**Figure 200-2**). Plain radiographs are often unrevealing, but MRI has high sensitivity for disk space infection, cord compression, and paraspinal abscess. As blood cultures are positive in less than half of cases, CT-guided biopsy is the diagnostic procedure of choice. Open surgical biopsy should be considered when percutaneous biopsy fails to provide a diagnosis, or patients fail to improve on empiric or directed treatment. If blood cultures are positive, infectious endocarditis must be ruled out.

TREATMENT CONSIDERATIONS

Treatment aims to cure infection and ameliorate the sequelae of vertebral bone destruction and paravertebral soft tissue swelling, which may include pain, neurologic complications, and spine instability. The mainstay of treatment is antimicrobial therapy for at least six weeks. Many infectious diseases physicians elect to treat for eight weeks or more, depending on the extent of disease

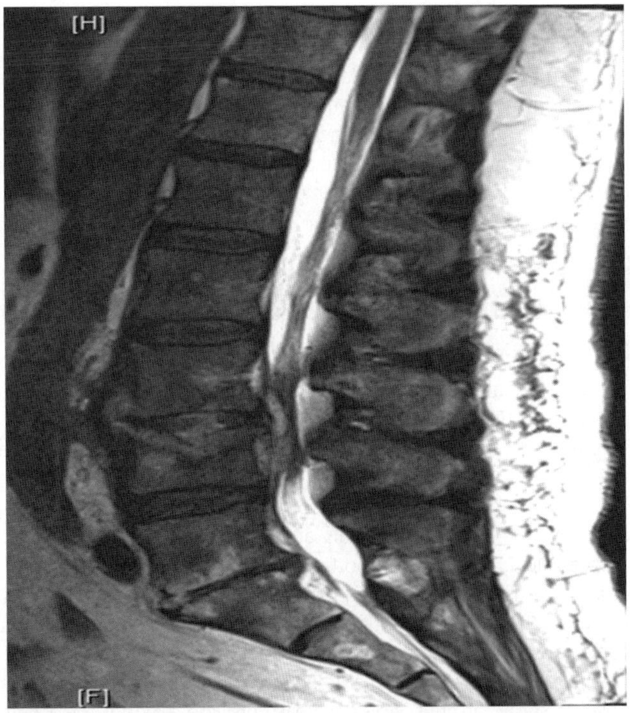

Figure 200-1 *Sagittal T2-weighted image demonstrating increased signal in the disc space and soft tissue posterior to the vertebral bodies suggestive of discitis in a patient with blood cultures positive for Staphylococcus aureus.*

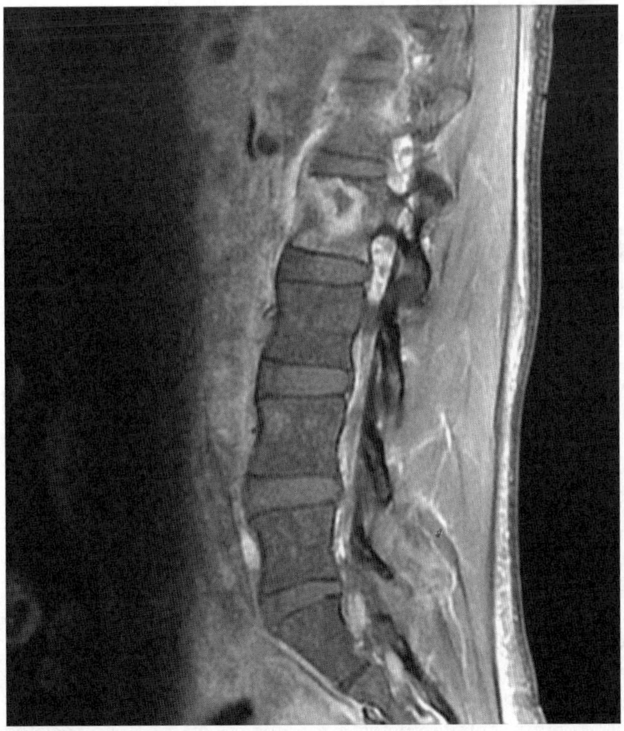

Figure 200-2 *Sagittal T1 postcontrast images demonstrating rim-enhancing lesion in the L2 vertebral body, suggestive of intraosseous abscess. Bone biopsy was positive for tuberculosis.*

and the virulence of the infecting organism. As the vertebrae are more vascular than other bones, surgical debridement is less often necessary than in other cases of osteomyelitis. However, epidural or paraspinal abscess, spine instability, neurologic symptoms, and failure to improve on appropriate antimicrobial therapy should prompt neurosurgical consultation. Clinical exam and the inflammatory markers ESR and CRP are helpful in following response to treatment. Follow-up MRI may give the impression of progression of osteomyelitis, even though there is otherwise clinical improvement, and results should be cautiously interpreted in the broad clinical context.

GENERAL PRINCIPLES OF OSTEOMYELITIS TREATMENT

In osteomyelitis, cure often requires a combination of medical and surgical intervention, with debridement of infected and necrotic bone and surrounding soft tissue, as well as accompanying prolonged courses of antibiotics. When debridement is extensive, reconstructive surgery may be necessary, including bone grafts and muscle and skin flaps. Sufficient vascular supply is a critical element to healing, and revascularization procedures may be necessary as well.

Empiric antibiotic therapy should begin after collecting samples for Gram stain, culture, and histology, or sooner if the patient's clinical status mandates immediate treatment, and should be targeted to the most common pathogens in the clinical scenario. Empiric regimens typically include vancomycin for gram-positive coverage, with a second drug, such as ciprofloxacin, ceftazidime, or cefepime, with activity against *Pseudomonas* and other gram-negative bacilli. Once culture and susceptibility data are available, empiric therapy should be narrowed as much as possible. Treatment usually lasts six weeks, but may be lengthened depending on the extent of surgical debridement, vascular supply, presence of foreign material, and overall immune function. Additionally, if evidence of infection persists through antibiotic therapy, and the antibiotic was selected based on reliable microbiological data, then complications of infection, including the formation of sequestra or abscesses, should be sought.

In cases of chronic osteomyelitis in which the patient or the clinical context favor a nonsurgical approach, oral antibiotics can be administered to treat intermittent flares. If a foreign body such as an internal fixation device is present at the area of osteomyelitis, then the goal may be to perform limited interventions and provide antimicrobial treatment until sufficient healing that the bone is strong enough to sustain definitive intervention.

TRIAGE AND HOSPITAL ADMISSION

Patients with suspected osteomyelitis should be admitted for further evaluation, including surgical and infectious diseases consultation, as indicated by the clinical context.

COMPLICATIONS

Diabetic foot infections may deteriorate abruptly and require urgent debridement or amputation. Vertebral osteomyelitis may be complicated by epidural abscess and neurologic compromise; ongoing evaluation of these patients should include periodic neurologic examination of the lower extremities. Adverse outcomes from osteomyelitis treatment include direct side effects of treatment, those that are secondary to the therapies themselves and with incomplete or failed treatment. Prolonged antibiotic treatment risks *Clostridium difficile* infection, and drug-specific reactions may include renal failure, hepatitis, and cytopenias. Use of peripherally inserted central catheters carries the risk of catheter-associated infection and thrombosis. Incomplete or failed treatment can result in recurrent local infection requiring further surgery and antibiotics and in systemic infection with sepsis.

DISCHARGE PLANNING

Patients discharged on parenteral antibiotics should have routine, usually weekly, monitoring of CBC, electrolytes, and antibiotic levels as indicated by the therapy (eg, vancomycin or gentamicin), as well as ESR and CRP to monitor response to therapy. One health care provider should be identified as responsible for review of laboratory results. Management of patients with long-term treatment plans should be pursued in conjunction with an infectious diseases specialist.

QUALITY IMPROVEMENT

Management of the osteomyelitis centers on making an accurate microbiological diagnosis and performing timely therapeutic interventions. First and foremost, all efforts should be made to hold administration of antibiotics until after a diagnostic procedure so long as permitted by the clinical scenario, as it is critical to confirm the diagnosis of osteomyelitis and identify the infectious agent and its antibiotic susceptibilities.

SEPTIC ARTHRITIS: INTRODUCTION

A painful, warm, swollen joint has many possible causes, including infection, trauma, osteoarthritis, crystal disease, or systemic disease. Of these, acute bacterial septic arthritis results in most rapid joint destruction, and it is primarily for this reason that the joint must undergo prompt evaluation. Native joint septic arthritis occurs at a rate of 2 to 10 cases per 100,000 per year in the general population, and as high as 38 cases per 100,000 per year among patients with rheumatoid arthritis. Approximately half of the cases of septic arthritis result in impaired joint function, and mortality rates range from 10% to 15% in normal hosts and up to 30% in patients with comorbidities.

PATHOPHYSIOLOGY

Bacteria enter the joint space primarily through hematogenous spread, as well as direct inoculation and spread from a contiguous infection in soft tissue or bone. Synovial capillaries lack a basement membrane, facilitating translocation of bacteria during episodes of bacteremia. The resulting inflammatory response of the synovium is intensely neutrophilic. Bacterial toxins and neutrophil proteases break down cartilage, and the increased intraarticular pressure leads to ischemic injury through vascular thrombosis and obstruction. In acute bacterial septic arthritis, injury happens quickly; significant joint damage can take place within one to two days.

DOES THIS PATIENT HAVE SEPTIC BACTERIAL ARTHRITIS?

DIFFERENTIAL DIAGNOSIS

The differential diagnosis of septic bacterial arthritis includes rheumatoid arthritis, crystal-induced joint diseases, reactive arthritis, osteoarthritis, trauma, viral arthritis, Lyme disease, and other systemic diseases.

Diagnosis begins with a thorough history concentrating on elements that place individuals at higher risk for septic arthritis (**Table 200-2**). The most important risk factor for the development of septic arthritis is preexisting joint disease, with up to half having a history of joint inflammation or injury. Systemic illness and other conditions, such as immunosuppression, diabetes mellitus, renal and liver insufficiency, and intravenous drug abuse, also predispose to septic arthritis. As skin breaks provide a portal for occult bacteremic seeding of joints, a history of skin lesions should be noted. Rheumatoid arthritis places individuals at particularly high risk through the combination of joint damage, immunosuppressive medications, and poor skin quality.

TABLE 200-2 Likelihood Ratios (LR) for Diagnosing Septic Arthritis

Risk Factors/Findings	Positive LR	Negative LR
Age >80 years	3.5	0.86
Diabetes mellitus	2.7	0.93
Rheumatoid arthritis	2.5	0.45
Recent joint surgery	6.9	0.78
Skin infection	2.8	0.76
HIV-1 infection	1.7	0.47
Fever	0.67	1.7
Abnormal WBC count	1.4	0.28
ESR >30 mm/h	1.3	0.17
CRP >100 mg/L	1.6	0.44

Adapted from Margaretten ME, Kohlwes J, Moore D, Bent S. Does this adult patient have septic arthritis? In: Simel DL, Rennie D, eds. *The Rational Clinical Examination.* New York: McGraw-Hill; 2009.

Joint warmth, pain, swelling, and restricted motion suggest septic arthritis, and mandate arthrocentesis. When bedside joint aspiration cannot be done, the procedure should be done by CT or ultrasound guidance. Synovial fluid should be evaluated for cell count and differential, Gram stain, aerobic and anaerobic culture, and crystals. Pathogen identification via Gram stain and culture of synovial fluid are the gold standard for diagnosis for septic arthritis, with cultures being informative in >90% of cases of nongonococcal bacterial septic arthritis. Arthrocentesis should be performed prior to the administration of antibiotics, unless the patient's clinical status does not allow a delay in empiric treatment. Inoculating the synovial sample into blood culture bottles offers a theoretical improvement in sensitivity. A synovial fluid white blood cell count of more than 50,000 cells/mm^3 and neutrophil predominance is traditionally taken as indicative of infection. However, this is neither specific nor sensitive for septic arthritis. Crystalline arthropathy commonly causes synovial white blood cell counts in this range, while immunosuppressed patients may not be able to mount synovial leukocytosis in response to infection. As well, atypical joint pathogens such as *M tuberculosis* or fungi may be associated with synovial white blood cell counts of lower magnitude. Synovial protein and glucose studies are neither sensitive nor specific, and should not be checked.

Gonococcal arthritis yields positive synovial fluid cultures in less than half of cases. Diagnosis is usually based on the combination of finding gonococcus in genitourinary, rectal, or oropharyngeal samples, and a clinical syndrome suggestive of disseminated gonococcal infection (**Figure 200-3**).

Serum studies should include blood cultures, peripheral white blood cell count with differential, and inflammatory markers ESR and CRP. None of these tests are specific, but a leukocytosis with left shift, or an elevated ESR and CRP, at the beginning of treatment may be helpful to track response to treatment. Serologic studies for Lyme disease should be considered in patients from endemic areas with evidence of inflammatory arthritis but negative Gram stain and culture.

Radiographic studies are not essential in uncomplicated septic arthritis, but may help to diagnose complicating factors. Plain films can demonstrate foreign bodies, adjacent osteomyelitis, periarticular soft tissue swelling in early septic arthritis, joint space loss, periosteal reaction, marginal and central erosions, and destruction of subchondral bone. CT and MRI can demonstrate nonspecific joint inflammation, effusion, subchondral cysts, and articular cartilage destruction.

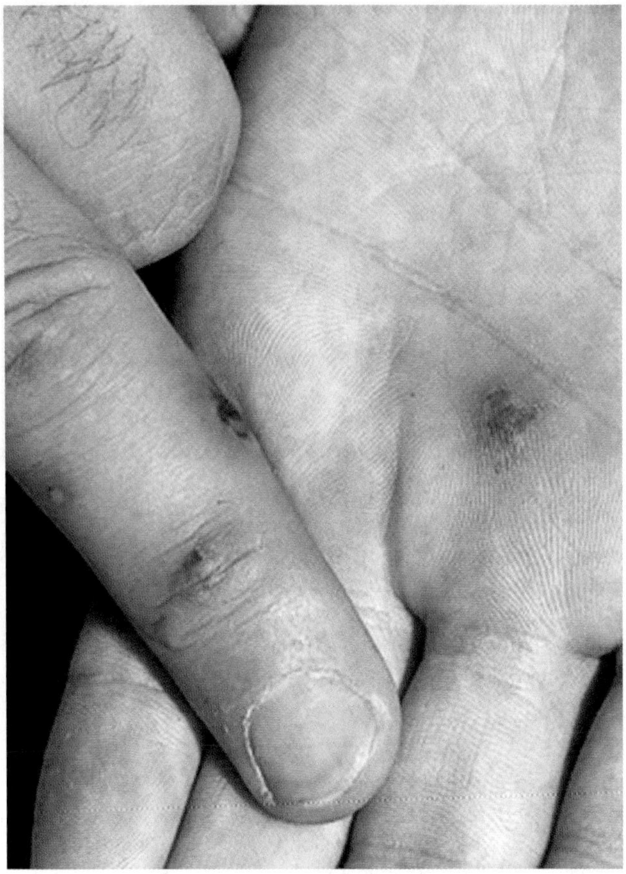

Figure 200-3 *Skin lesions of disseminated gonococcal infection (DGI): the classic triad of DGI includes urethritis, arthritis, and scattered hemorrhagic pustules, more often found on the extremities than the trunk. Most patients with DGI lack all the components of the syndrome. (Reproduced, with permission, from Wolff K, Goldsmith LA, Katz SI, et al. Fitzpatrick's Dermatology in General Medicine. 7th ed. New York: McGraw-Hill; 2008. Fig. 205-4.)*

CLINICAL PRESENTATION

Septic arthritis classically presents with a swollen, painful joint with limited range of motion. Typical features of infection, including fever and leukocytosis, are frequently absent, especially in patients with rheumatoid arthritis, renal or hepatic disease, or immunosuppression. Most cases present as monoarticular arthritis, with up to half affecting the knee; most other cases involve other large peripheral joints. Involvement of small joints of the hand usually reflects direct inoculation or bite, and involvement of the joints of the feet usually arises with progression of contiguous soft tissue infection or osteomyelitis, as commonly observed in patients with diabetes and vascular insufficiency. Intravenous drug users are more prone to sacroiliac and sternoclavicular involvement (**Figure 200-4**). Polyarticular arthritis is more common among patients with impaired immunity, and with gonococcal, pneumococcal, group B streptococcal, and gram-negative infection.

MICROBIOLOGY

All microbial pathogens can infect synovium, and selected bacteria are often correlated with particular demographics (see Table 200–2). *S aureus* is now the most common pathogen overall (**Table 200-3**). (In the 1970s, at the peak of the gonorrhea epidemic in the United States, gonococcal arthritis was the most prevalent cause of infectious arthritis in young persons, but has

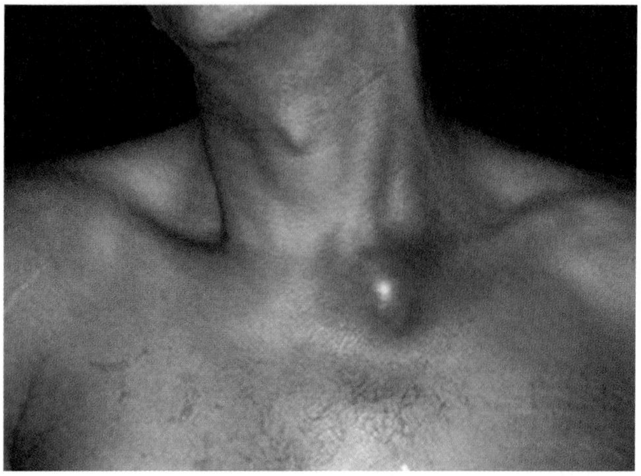

Figure 200-4 *Sternoclavicular septic arthritis accounts for 17% of septic arthritis in intravenous drug users, but only 1% of septic arthritis in the general population. Osteomyelitis, chest wall abscess, and mediastinitis are serious and common complications that require surgical debridement. Staphylococcus aureus is usually responsible. (Reproduced, with permission, from Fauci AS, Braunwald E, Kasper DL, et al. Harrison's Principles of Internal Medicine. 17th ed. New York: McGraw-Hill; 2008, Fig. 328-1.)*

since become rare.) Intravenous drug users are at risk for staphylococcal and streptococcal infections as well as pseudomonal and other gram-negative infections. Polymicrobial infections are usually seen after contaminated open injuries. Animal bites, particularly from cats, are associated with *Pasteurella* infection, and human bites with *Eikenella corrodens* and other human oral flora. Use of TNF-inhibitors predisposes to mycobacterial infections.

TABLE 200-3 Organisms Isolated in 2407 Cases of Septic Arthritis

Organism	Isolates, Number (% total)
Gram positive	
Staphylococcus aureus	1066 (44)
Staphylococci, coagulase negative	84 (3)
Streptococci	
Streptococcus pyogenes	183 (8)
Streptococcus pneumoniae	156 (6)
Streptococcus agalactiae	69 (3)
Other streptococci	104 (4)
Gram negative	
Escherichia coli	91 (4)
Haemophilus influenzae	104 (4)
Neisseria gonorrhoeae	77 (3)
Neisseria meningitidis	28 (1)
Pseudomonas aeruginosa	36 (1)
Salmonella spp	25 (1)
Other gram-negative rods	110 (5)
Miscellaneous (including anaerobes)	136 (6)
Polymicrobial	33 (1)

Adapted from Ross JJ, Saltzman CL, Carling P, et al. Pneumococcal septic arthritis: review of 190 cases. *Clin Infect Dis.* 2003;36:319–327.

TRIAGE/HOSPITAL ADMISSION

Patients with septic joints should be admitted to hospital for orthopedic and infectious diseases consultation, consideration of joint debridement and irrigation, and initiation of parenteral antibiotics.

TREATMENT

Antibiotics and joint drainage are the foundation of septic arthritis treatment. Empiric broad spectrum antibiotics can be considered once arthrocentesis has been performed, or without delay if indicated by the clinical situation, such as evidence of septic physiology. Antibiotic selection should be guided by the Gram stain of the synovial fluid and the patient's epidemiology and clinical history. In the absence of informative microbiological data, epidemiological data can assist in directing empiric antibiotic selection. Vancomycin may be used as monotherapy for otherwise healthy patients with septic arthritis. In intravenous drug users and patients with underlying illness at higher risk for infection with gram-negative rods, vancomycin plus an antipseudomonal beta-lactam or ciprofloxacin may be used. If the Gram stain shows gram-positive cocci, vancomycin alone can be used. Once culture and antibiotic susceptibility data become available, antimicrobial therapy should be tailored appropriately. If the Gram stain is negative and the patient is hemodynamically stable, antibiotic treatment should be held pending culture data and investigation of alternative diagnoses.

Antibiotics should be administered in conjunction with joint drainage. The goal of drainage is to decrease the bacterial burden, remove necrotic debris, and disrupt loculated fluid. Drainage can be performed by arthrocentesis if the joint is readily accessible and the clinical context appropriate, or by arthroscopy or arthrotomy, combined with joint irrigation. Large joints, including axial joints, shoulders, and hips, should undergo arthoscopy or open drainage. Treatment of smaller joints may include initial aspiration, followed by more invasive procedures if treatment fails. Serial drainage procedures should be repeated until resolution of effusions and demonstration of negative Gram stain and cultures.

Though definitive data guiding the duration of antibiotic therapy is lacking, common practice is to treat for three to four weeks. Antibiotics are often administered parenterally initially, followed by oral therapy in good responders with infections sensitive to oral antibiotics. Treatment duration and route of administration should be adjusted based on any local or systemic factors contributing to impairment of immune activity, the antibiotic susceptibility of the organism, concomitant bacteremia or other infection, and the overall clinical picture. Physical therapy and rehabilitation of the joint are critical to maintaining joint function, and in their absence loss of joint function may ensue.

COMPLICATIONS

Septic arthritis can result in joint destruction and immobility. The affected joint should be closely followed during treatment for recurrent signs and symptoms of infection, as infected joints may require repeated irrigation and drainage even after appropriate antibiotic therapy and initial drainage. In patients with bacteremia or polymicrobial infection, endocarditis should be considered as a possible underlying diagnosis.

DISCHARGE CONSIDERATIONS

Patients with septic arthritis may be discharged once there is significant improvement in symptoms and follow-up has been arranged with orthopedic surgery and, when comanaged, with infectious

TABLE 200-4A Evidence-based Medicine: Key References for Osteomyelitis

Study	Methodology	Results	Limitations	Bottom Line
Euba G, et al. *Antimicrob Agents Chemother.* 2009;53:2672–2676.	Randomized, open-label trial of 8 weeks of oral rifampin plus oral trimethoprim-sulfamethoxazole vs 6 wk of intravenous cloxacillin followed by 2 wk of oral cloxacillin for chronic osteomyelitis with methicillin-sensitive *Staphylococcus aureus* (MSSA)	Over long-term (10 y) follow-up, cure rates were equivalent with IV (90%) and oral (89%) therapy	Relatively small study (50 patients); all patients had surgical debridement prior to antibiotic therapy; most patients were relatively young and had no comorbid illnesses	Moderately high doses of oral antibiotics after surgical debridement may be curative in relatively healthy patients with MSSA chronic osteomyelitis
Zuluaga AF, et al. *Arch Intern Med.* 2006;166: 95–100.	Prospective study comparing bone cultures and nonbone cultures (such as wound swabs) in 100 patients with chronic osteomyelitis; patients had to be off antibiotics for at least 48 h at the time of cultures	Concordance between bone and nonbone cultures was poor; yield of bone cultures was higher (94%), compared to nonbone cultures (89%); yield for anaerobes was much higher in bone biopsies	It is not clear whether performing bone biopsies actually improved clinical outcomes	In chronic osteomyelitis, results of bone cultures differ significantly from results of nonbone cultures, such as cultures of wounds and sinus tracts

TABLE 200-4B Evidence-based Medicine: Key References for Septic Arthritis

Study	Methodology	Results	Limitations	Bottom Line
Peltola H, et al. *Clin Infect Dis.* 2009;48:1201–1210.	Randomized, open-label trial of 10 vs 30 days of clindamycin or a first-generation cephalosporin in Finnish children aged 3 mo to 15 y; IV therapy was given only for the first 2–4 days of therapy	Outcomes were similar between the 2 groups; C-reactive protein was helpful in assessing response to treatment	Patients were healthy children without any underlying illness; there were no cases of methicillin-resistant *Staphylococcus aureus* (MRSA)	Previously healthy children with septic arthritis due to organisms other than MRSA can be treated with 10–14 days of antibiotics; it is unclear if these results can be generalized to adults with septic arthritis, who usually have underlying illnesses
Frazee BW, et al. *Ann Emerg Med.* 2009;54:695–700.	Cross-sectional review from 2 urban academic emergency departments in northern California	MRSA was the commonest cause of community-onset septic arthritis; synovial fluid leukocyte counts somewhat lower than expected	Small retrospective study	Empiric antibiotics for septic arthritis should include drugs active against MRSA in communities where MRSA is prevalent
Mathews CJ, et al. *Ann Rheum Dis.* 2007;66:440–445.	Systematic literature review	Current recommendations for management of adult septic arthritis rely almost exclusively on expert opinion and retrospective data	There are no randomized, controlled trials of antibiotic duration or joint drainage in adult septic arthritis patients	Optimal antibiotic duration and methodology for joint drainage in septic arthritis are unknown

diseases service. Depending on the clinical scenario, the patient may require continued parenteral antibiotics via a peripherally inserted central catheter or, if tolerating oral medications and sufficiently clinically improved, may be discharged with oral antibiotics. All patients with septic arthritis will need aggressive physical therapy, and depending on the joint involved may require discharge to an institution to provide rehabilitation or to home.

QUALITY IMPROVEMENT

If at all possible, antibiotics should be delayed until after a diagnostic procedure, as it is critical to confirm the diagnosis of septic arthritis and identify the infectious agent and its antibiotic susceptibilities. Similarly, blood cultures should be obtained in each case of suspected septic arthritis to assist with diagnosis and management. Analysis of the synovial fluid should always include evaluation for crystals with polarizing microscopy (**Table 200-4**).

SUGGESTED READINGS

Osteomyelitis

Butalia S, Palda VA, Sargeant RJ, Detsky AS, Mourad O. Does this patient with diabetes have osteomyelitis of the lower extremity? In: Simel DL, Rennie D, eds. *The Rational Clinical Examination.* New York: McGraw-Hill; 2009.

Calhoun JH, Manring MM. Adult osteomyelitis. *Infect Dis Clin N Am.* 2005;19:765–786.

Jeffcoate WJ, Lipsky BA. Controversies in diagnosing and managing osteomyelitis of the foot in diabetes. *Clin Infect Dis.* 2004;39: S115–S122.

Lew DP, Waldvogel FA. Osteomyelitis. *N Engl J Med.* 1997;336:999.

Lipsky BA, Berendt AR, Deery HG, et al. Diagnosis and treatment of diabetic foot infections. *Clin Infect Dis.* 2004;39:887.

Septic Arthritis

Coakley G, Mathews C, Field M, et al. BSR & BHPR, BOA, RCGP and BSAC guidelines for management of the hot swollen joint in adults. *Rheumatology.* 2006;45:1039–1041.

Goldenberg DL. Septic arthritis. *Lancet.* 1998;351:197.

Margaretten ME, Kohlwes J, Moore D, Bent S. Does this adult patient have septic arthritis? In: Simel DL, Rennie D, eds. *The Rational Clinical Examination.* New York: McGraw-Hill; 2009.

Ross JJ, Saltzman CL, Carling P, Shapiro DS. Pneumococcal septic arthritis: review of 190 cases. *Clin Infect Dis.* 2003;36:319–327.

CHAPTER 201

Prosthetic Joint Infections

Geoffrey Tsaras, MD, ChB, MPH
Elie F. Berbari, MD

Key Clinical Questions

1. How can prosthetic joint infection (PJI) be distinguished from aseptic failure of the joint arthroplasty due to mechanical loosening or dislocation?
2. Which pathogens are usually responsible for PJIs?
3. What are the management strategies and treatment options for infected prosthetic joints?
4. Can an infected prosthetic joint be effectively treated with retention of the prosthesis?
5. What is the optimal antimicrobial regimen for a PJI?
6. How should patients with PJI s on long-term parenteral or oral antibiotics be monitored and followed up?

EPIDEMIOLOGY

Joint replacement surgery (arthroplasty) is one of the major accomplishments of modern medicine over the past four decades. It has provided excellent and cost-effective results in alleviating pain and improving mobility and quality of life in patients with debilitating joint disease. Most arthroplasties are performed on hips and knees, but shoulder, elbow, and other small joint replacements are not uncommon. It is estimated that over 750,000 prosthetic joints are implanted each year in the United States, with projections of over 4 million primary arthroplasties per year by 2030. Less than 10% of prosthesis recipients develop complications that require revision surgery. Fortunately, prosthetic joint infection (PJI) is less common than other forms of joint failure, such as aseptic loosening or dislocation. Nevertheless, given the exponential increase in total joint replacement surgeries, the cumulative numbers of PJI is increasing. Moreover, PJI represents the most dreaded and devastating complication of arthroplasty. Overall, about 1 to 2% of prosthetic joints become infected, with higher rates for total knee arthroplasties (TKA) compared with total hip arthroplasties (THA) (2.5% vs 1.5%). PJIs may occur at any time after arthroplasty. The risk of infection is higher after revision arthroplasty, with rates of 3.2% and 5.6% reported for revision THA and TKA, respectively. Consequences of PJI may include reoperation, potential for permanent removal of the prosthesis, large skeletal defects after surgery, prolonged courses of antimicrobial therapy, severe functional impairment, and persistent joint pain. Rarely, PJIs result in loss of limb or life. The cost of treatment of PJIs is in excess of $50,000 per episode, with an estimated total expenditure of over $250 million per year in the United States.

PATIENT RISK FACTORS

Conditions and events that predispose a prosthetic joint recipient to infection include host characteristics, index arthroplasty factors, and perioperative and postoperative factors. Host characteristics include advanced age, morbid obesity, diabetes mellitus, malignancy, HIV seropositivity, and systemic steroid use. Arthroplasties performed due to underlying rheumatoid arthritis are four times more likely to be infected compared to those for degenerative osteoarthritis. Other joint factors, such as primary arthroplasty undertaken due to trauma or fracture, revision arthroplasty, regardless of indication, and prior PJI, are independent risk factors for infection. Perioperative factors such as a National Nosocomial Infections Surveillance System surgical risk score greater than 2, American Society of Anesthesiologists greater than 2, duration of surgery greater than 75th percentile for the procedure or longer than three hours, postoperative superficial surgical site infection, wound drainage or wound hematoma, and distant nonarticular infections such as UTIs and soft tissue infection increase the risk for PJI. The use of systemic antimicrobial prophylaxis, *Staphylococcus aureus* decolonization in carriers, and the use of antimicrobial therapy in the fixation of impregnated bone cement reduce the risk of PJI in patients undergoing joint arthroplasty.

PATHOPHYSIOLOGY

Depending on the onset of infection relative to the date of implantation, PJIs are classified as early (within three months), delayed (three months to two years), or late (after two years). There are three mechanisms by which prosthetic joints become infected: colonization of the device with microorganisms at the time of index surgery or immediately thereafter; direct spread from contiguous skin and soft tissue infections, penetrating trauma, or preexisting osteomyelitis; or hematogenous spread from distant infected foci. Generally, early and delayed infections are acquired at the time of implantation, and late infections occur predominantly from the hematogenous route, although there is significant overlap. Not surprisingly, in the very few well-designed cohort studies to elucidate the risk factors for PJIs, postoperative surgical site infections have been the most significantly and consistently identified risk factor for PJIs, with an associated odds ratio of over 35 in one study. Bacteremia from infections at distant sites such as the respiratory tract, urinary tract, or the skin can secondarily seed a well-fixed prosthesis and cause a PJI. Although this is relatively rare, it is particularly true for *S aureus*. It is estimated that one-third of joint recipients with ensuing *S aureus* bacteremia will develop *S aureus* PJI.

Two unique factors combine to make prosthetic joint infection an enormous challenge to eradicate: the presence of a foreign body and the production of bacterial biofilm.

THE FOREIGN BODY

The prosthetic implant is a foreign body devoid of microcirculation. This prevents adequate delivery of antibiotics to the site of infection. Furthermore, the implant is nonphagocytosable and renders granulocytes around the prostheses functionally defective. Local immunity is thus further impaired. It is estimated that as little as 100 colony-forming units of *S aureus* are sufficient to infect 95% of subcutaneous implants.

THE ROLE OF BIOFILM

The first phase of PJI is adherence of microorganisms to the surface of the implant. These microorganisms then elaborate a glycocalyx of highly hydrated exopolysaccharides, better known as slime. Biofilm refers to slime and the bacteria embedded within. Bacteria in biofilm form organized and complex communities, with structural and functional heterogeneity, resembling multicellular organisms. Bacteria in biofilm even communicate by a signaling process known as quorum sensing. Sessile (attached) bacteria in biofilms are protected from antimicrobial agents and host immune responses, compared with free-living (planktonic) bacteria. Biofilm acts as a physical barrier to antibiotics and white blood cells (WBCs). As well, microorganisms in biofilms are in a low metabolic state (stationary phase) due to poor availability of nutrients such as glucose and oxygen. This renders them less susceptible to growth-dependent antibiotics, such as beta-lactams. Infections are therefore difficult to diagnose (low inoculum, few planktonic bacteria, mild inflammatory reaction), difficult to cure (poor access of antimicrobials to bacteria), and persist or recur after discontinuing antibiotics (revert to planktonic state after antibiotic pressure has been released).

MICROBIOLOGY OF PROSTHETIC JOINT INFECTION

The microbiology of PJIs may vary depending on time of onset, mechanism of infection, acuity of clinical presentation, and location of prosthetic joint. Gram-positive organisms, especially staphylococci, account for the vast majority of PJIs (**Table 201-1**). Infections in the early postoperative period, or those presenting with sudden onset joint pain and effusion, are commonly due to virulent organisms such as *S aureus*, gram-negative bacilli, and mixed infections. Delayed infections with subtle, chronic symptoms and signs may be caused by less virulent, more indolent bacteria such as coagulase-negative staphylococci, enterococci, and *Propionibacterium acnes*. Shoulder arthroplasties have a greater preponderance for *P acnes* infections, compared to lower extremity joints. Several *Streptococcus* species are responsible for some PJIs from contiguous pyogenic skin infections. Viridans streptococci, *Peptococcus* species, *Peptostreptococcus* species, and gram-negative rods may be recovered from PJIs following dentogingival processes or manipulations. More than one organism is recovered in about 10% to 12% of cases, and a similar proportion of patients have no organisms isolated at all (culture-negative PJI). The most common reason for the latter is prior use of antimicrobial therapy. Unusual bacteria, fungi, and mycobacteria are rarely isolated.

TABLE 201-1 Common Pathogens in Infected Joint Arthroplasty

Pathogens	% Frequency
Methicillin-sensitive *Staphylococcus aureus*	8–18
Methicillin-resistant *Staphylococcus aureus*	2–27
Coagulase-negative staphylococci	21–26
Streptococcus sp.	4–18
Enterococcus sp.	2–8
Pseudomonas	4–13
E coli	4–7
Other Gram-negative rods	4–5
Propionibacteria	3–6
Other (fungal, mycobacterial, anaerobic, mixed)	8–11

Data from Lee J, et al. *J Hosp Infect.* 2010;75:273–276; Hsieh PH, et al. *J Antimicrob Chemother.* 2009;64:392–397; Müller M, et al. *J Orthop Surg Res.* 2008;3:31.

DIFFERENTIAL DIAGNOSIS

ASEPTIC FAILURE

Joint pain and malfunction may be septic (related to infection) or aseptic (biomechanical failure). In a recent review of over 50,000 hip and 60,000 knee revision procedures from the Nationwide Inpatient Sample database, 85.2% and 74.8% of surgeries, respectively, were due to aseptic failure. A major cause of aseptic implant failure is osteolysis from particulate wear debris. Relative motion between opposed surfaces leads to loss of prosthetic material, with generation of particles that get deposited in the space between implant and bone. These are phagocytosed by macrophages, and a granulomatous reaction ensues. Inflammatory mediators are released, stimulating osteoclastic bone resorption. Biopsy specimens from tissues surrounding the osteolytic lesions may demonstrate this process, commonly referred to as "arthroplasty effect." Misalignment of the arthroplasty can also result in inappropriate (eccentric) mechanical loads, and cause implant loosening and mechanical damage to the implant material or the bone–implant interface.

SKIN AND SOFT TISSUE INFECTIONS

PRACTICE POINT

- The possibility of prosthesis infection should be considered in all patients with wound infections after implantation of a prosthetic joint. A sinus tract to the prosthesis is diagnostic of prosthetic joint infection, but this is absent in most cases.

The skin and subcutaneous tissue overlying a prosthetic joint may become infected. The pain, tenderness, differential warmth, and erythema of cellulitis are clinically indistinguishable from a PJI. However, the pain in soft tissue infection may not be worse with movement, and a joint effusion (ballotable swelling) may be absent. Nonetheless, given the very low sensitivity and specificity of clinical findings, and high risk of subsequent spread of local infection to the joint, infectious diseases and orthopedic surgeon consultation should be sought for appropriate evaluation of the joint.

STERILE JOINT INFLAMMATION

Patients with prosthetic joints and inflammatory arthroplasties such as rheumatoid arthritis or systemic lupus erythematosus occasionally experience inflammation of their prosthesis from activation of the underlying disease. Gout and pseudogout may also result in joint pain that may be clinically indistinguishable from a PJI.

DIAGNOSIS OF PROSTHETIC JOINT INFECTIONS

DOES THIS PATIENT HAVE A PJI?

Distinguishing septic from aseptic implant failure preoperatively may be exceedingly difficult, but is of great importance. Failure to recognize a PJI at or before revision surgery will lead to implantation of a new prosthesis into an infected surgical site without appropriate debridement, and inadequate local or systemic antimicrobial treatment. This might lead to persistent infection and ultimately implant failure. On the other hand, suspicion of PJI where there is none can result in delayed reimplantation, extended length of hospital stay, increased number of surgeries and anesthetic exposures (with attendant risks), prolonged patient immobilization and rehabilitation, and increase in overall costs. No single clinical feature, laboratory test, or imaging study can unequivocally establish a diagnosis of PJI before surgery. It requires careful synthesis of information from multiple investigations. The tools available to clinicians and orthopedic surgeons in making a correct diagnosis, their accuracy and reliability, is the subject of discussion in the next section.

HISTORY AND PHYSICAL EXAMINATION

The symptoms and signs of PJIs are variable, and depend to a large extent on the time of presentation and mechanism of infection. Pain at the implant site is the presenting symptom in over 90% of patients. It is of acute onset in early infections and may be associated with joint swelling, tenderness, erythema, and differential warmth. Systemic symptoms like fever, chills, rigors, and general malaise may occur, but are neither sensitive nor specific for PJI. Signs of surgical site infection, such as wound dehiscence and purulent drainage in the early postoperative period, should prompt suspicion for a PJI, as the implant is not hermetically separated from the superficial wound in the early postoperative period. Indeed, the presence of a sinus tract communicating with the device is diagnostic of PJI, although this is not a common finding. Late infections occur mostly from hematogenous seeding, and also tend to present with acute pain. Delayed infections are the most difficult to pick up, as the symptoms and local signs are subtle or absent. Joint pain, when present, is insidious in onset, is persistent and progressive, and may be associated with implant loosening and functional deterioration. Important historical information includes the type of prosthesis, date of implantation, past surgeries on the joint, comorbid conditions, current or prior antimicrobial therapies, and drug allergies or adverse effects, as these affect treatment decisions and prognosis. The elderly are disproportionately represented in total joint recipients and PJIs, and so a complete preanesthetic medical evaluation (PAME) is almost always indicated.

LABORATORY TESTS

Inflammatory markers of prosthetic joint infections

The peripheral WBC count, percentage of segmented neutrophils and band neutrophils, erythrocyte sedimentation rate (ESR), and C-reactive protein (CRP) levels are routinely used to screen for PJIs. These tests, however, are neither sensitive nor specific enough to firmly rule out or establish the diagnosis. The WBC count may be normal in indolent infections due to lack of a systemic inflammatory response, and may be elevated in concurrent nonarticular infections. ESR, a nonspecific acute inflammatory marker, is usually elevated after joint surgery, and remains high for up to three months after surgery. Therefore, a single measurement is not useful particularly in early infections. Likewise, CRP is elevated after arthroplasty, and remains elevated for up to three weeks. Various studies have evaluated the performance characteristics and accuracy of these screening tests with varying results. In a recent meta-analysis from our group, CRP was found to have the best discriminative function of the three (**Table 201-2**). Newer cytokine markers of PJI, including IL-6, procalcitonin, and TNF-alpha are being studied with promising results, but there is currently not enough evidence to justify their routine use in the preoperative diagnosis of PJI.

Synovial fluid analysis

Aspiration of the prosthetic joint under fluoroscopic or ultrasound guidance is a useful procedure that adds to the body of evidence to establish or refute a diagnosis of PJI in patients whose arthroplasties are failing. Synovial fluid samples should be sent for leucocyte cell count and differential, Gram stain, and culture. For those without underlying inflammatory joint diseases, a synovial fluid WBC count greater than 1700/mm^3 and proportion of neutrophils more than 65% have a high degree of accuracy in distinguishing PJIs from aseptic failure (Table 201-2). Joint fluid Gram stain has a low sensitivity (< 26%) but very high specificity (> 97%) for the diagnosis of PJI. Synovial fluid culture provides data that is not only diagnostic, but guides the choice of perioperative antimicrobial therapy, including antibiotics to impregnate into cement or beads during surgery. If the patient is not a candidate for surgery, these cultures will facilitate the prescription of an appropriate suppressive regimen.

RADIOLOGIC STUDIES

Conventional radiographs, CT scans and MRIs may be used as adjuncts in the diagnosis of PJI, but have serious limitations that preclude their routine use. Joint dislocations, lucency at the bone-cement interface, or bony erosions on plain radiographs are suggestive but nonspecific for PJIs (**Figure 201-1**). New subperiosteal bone growth is a more specific finding, but it is often absent in early infections. CT scans provide better contrast between normal and abnormal tissues, but imaging artefacts caused by metallic implants limit its use. MRI displays greater resolution for soft tissue abnormalities and greater anatomic detail, but can only be used safely when implants are made of titanium or tantalum.

NUCLEAR MEDICINE STUDIES

Radionucleotide imaging studies are quite sensitive and are not affected by metallic implants. However, results are limited by lack

TABLE 201-2 Diagnostic Tests in Preoperative Diagnosis of Prosthetic Joint Infections

Test	Sensitivity %	Specificity %	PPV%	NPV%	Positive LR	Negative LR
Peripheral blood*						
WBC > 11,000 cells/mm^3	45	87	—	—	2.6	0.7
ESR > 30 mm/h	75	70	—	—	2.6	0.37
CRP > 8 mg/L	88	74	—	—	3.3	0.16
Synovial fluid						
WBC > 1700 cells/mm^3	94	88	73	98	8	0.1
Neutrophil > 65%	97	98	94	99	48	0.0
Culture	56.3	98	90	88.3	—	—
Gram stain	< 26	> 97	—	—	—	—
Imaging studies						
^{67}Gal bone scan	50	78	—	—	—	—
^{99}Tc bone scan	100	< 23	30	100	—	—
^{111}Indium WBC scan	38–83	88–100	58	94	—	—
Bone and WBC scan	66	98	91	89	—	—
18-FDG PET scan	90	89	—	—	—	—

CRP, C-reacticve protein; ESR, erythrocyte sedimentation rate; LR, likelihood ratio; NPV, negative predictive value; PPV, positive predictive value; WBC, white blod cell; —, data not provided.

*Cut-off may vary with laboratory.

Data from Berbari EF, Mabry T, Tsaras G, et al. Inflammatory blood laboratory levels as markers of prosthethic joint infection: a systematic review and meta-analysis. *J Bone Joint Surg Am.* 2010;92:2102–2109.

Trampuz A, Hanssen AD, Osmon DR, et al. Synovial fluid leukocyte count and differential for the diagnosis of prosthetic knee infection. *Am J Med.* 2004;117:556–562.

Lentino JR. Prosthetic joint infections: bane of orthopedists, challenge for infectious disease specialists. *Clin Infect Dis.* 2003;36:1157–1161.

of specificity. Bone scintigraphy with technetium-99m-labeled methylene diphosphonate has an almost 100% sensitivity, but is only 5% to 23% specific because of increased periprosthetic bone remodeling that occurs up to a year after implantation. Sequential bone and gallium-67 scanning improves specificity of bone scintigraphy. Bone scans have also been combined with indium-111 oxyquinoline or 99-m Tc-hexamethylpropyleneamine oxime–labeled white cell scans, 99m-Tc-labeled antigranulocyte monoclonal bodies and 99m-Tc ciprofloxacin scans to improve specificity. The role of fluorine-18-fluorodeoxyglucose positron emission tomography (FDG PET) scans for diagnosis of PJIs is evolving. In a recent systematic review, the pooled sensitivity and specificity was reported as 82% and 86%, respectively. The utility of hybrid imaging modalities like PET/CT scans are currently being studied, but the data is insufficient at this time to influence current practice. In general, nuclear medicine studies are most useful in ruling out infections. A negative study reduces the chances of a PJI significantly, whereas a positive test requires additional investigation.

HISTOPATHOLOGY

Intraoperative frozen sections, sampled from multiple areas including bone-cement or prosthesis–bone interface and abnormal appearing areas, should be examined for evidence of acute inflammation. More than five neutrophils per high power field (hpf) at a magnification of 400×, has a sensitivity of over 82% and specificity of over 93% for diagnosis of PJI. Increasing the cut off to 10 neutrophils per hpf increases the positive predictive value. In either case, the negative predictive value is about 98%.

INTRAOPERATIVE CULTURES

The identification of microorganisms from at least three intraoperative culture samples from periprosthetic tissue is highly predictive of infection. We recommend that five or six samples be sent for aerobic and anaerobic culture to optimize diagnostic yield if culture sonication of the explanted prosthesis is not done. In vitro antimicrobial susceptibility data should always be requested. Fungal and/or mycobacterial cultures may be considered if bacterial cultures are negative in a patient with apparent infection, but should not be routinely recommended. Swab cultures from superficial wounds or sinus tracts tend to represent microbial colonization of surrounding skin, and may not be representative of the bacteriology of the deeper tissue layers. However, when deep cultures are delayed or not obtained, swab cultures may be done, and only considered significant if *S aureus* or *Pseudomonas aeruginosa* is recovered. Ideally, antibiotics should be discontinued at least two weeks (preferably four weeks) before surgery. Perioperative antimicrobial prophylaxis should also be held until culture specimens have been collected, to increase chances of isolating the culprit organism. Despite these measures, intraoperative cultures could remain falsely negative. This may be attributable to a low organism burden, inappropriate culture medium, presence of fastidious microorganisms, or prolonged transport time to the microbiology laboratory.

Novel techniques to improve the detection of microorganisms include ultrasonication of the prosthesis or amplification-based analysis of bacterial 16S ribosomal DNA by polymerase chain reaction. Sonication of explanted hip and knee prosthesis to dislodge adherent bacteria for culture has better yield than conventional tissue cultures, especially in those who have received antimicrobial therapy within two weeks of surgery. A cut off of five or more colony-forming units per agar plate growth was found to have sensitivity and specificity of 78.5% and 98.8%, respectively. These are highly specialized techniques and should be discussed in advance with the microbiology laboratory director and infectious diseases consultant before sampling and transport to the laboratory.

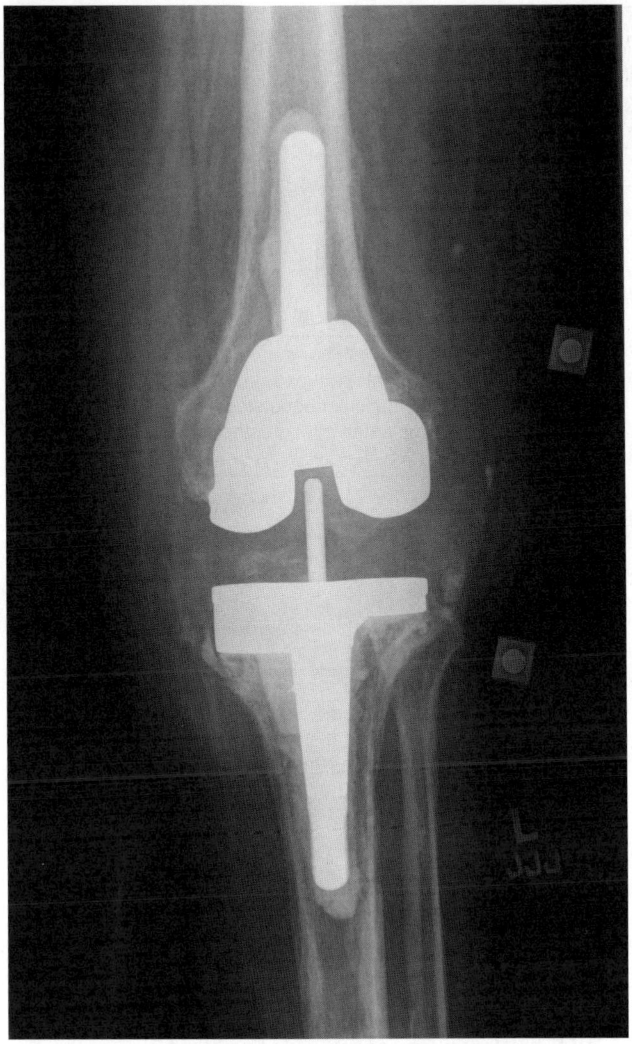

Figure 201-1 *Plain radiograph showing lucency at the bone-cement interface in a chronically infected left prosthetic knee.*

DEFINITIVE DIAGNOSIS OF PROSTHETIC JOINT INFECTIONS

There is no uniformly accepted case definition for prosthetic joint infection. Widely accepted criteria for confirming a case of PJI may include any one or a combination of the following:

1. Presence of a sinus tract that communicates with the prostheses, or
2. Purulence surrounding the prosthesis observed at the time of debridement or removal of the prosthesis, or
3. Two or more cultures from joint aspirates or intraoperative cultures that yield the same microorganism, or
4. Acute inflammation consistent with infection present on histopathologic examination in conjunction with at least one positive culture, or
5. Sonicate of joint arthroplasty growing more than 20 CFU/mL organisms

TRIAGE AND HOSPITAL ADMISSION

Initial evaluation of patients with suspected PJIs can be done either in the outpatient or inpatient setting, depending on the acuity of presentation, the extent of infection, the age of the joint, the mechanism of infection, and the immune status of the host. Patients with symptoms of less than three weeks duration, primary arthroplasty less than three months ago, or suspected infections from the hematogenous route, may be admitted for consideration of prosthesis salvage, with debridement and exchange of the acetabular polyethylene liner, and retention of the prosthesis. Immunocompromised hosts, patients with local signs of rapidly advancing infection, systemic involvement, or hemodynamic instability will also require admission for diagnostic workup and prompt initiation of empiric antibiotics. Other clinically stable patients can be meticulously evaluated as outpatients, especially if they have recently been on antibiotics, in order to allow careful planning of definitive surgical and medical strategies.

TREATMENT OF PROSTHETIC JOINT INFECTIONS

The ultimate goal in the treatment of PJIs is to retain adequate mobility through a painless, functional mechanical joint. This usually requires a combination of surgical and medical management strategies that ideally aim to eradicate (cure) the infection while preserving the prosthesis. Either or both objectives may not be achievable in many circumstances. The infected prosthesis may be retained in some instances, but may need to be removed in others, with or without eventual replacement. Palliation through conservative surgery and/or chronic suppressive antimicrobial therapy may be more realistic than cure in selected cases. Goals of treatment must be defined on a case-by-case scenario. Treatment approach is based on a host of factors including duration of symptoms, joint age and condition of the implant, status of surrounding bone and soft tissue, causative pathogen(s) and susceptibility patterns, patient comorbid conditions, technical abilities of the surgical team, and patient preference.

TREATMENT OPTIONS

Various treatment strategies have been employed in the management of PJIs. No randomized control trials comparing the different treatment options are available, or likely to become available in the future. Treatments differ considerably between individual centers, and among individual orthopedic surgeons, but certain general principles apply (**Figure 201-2**). The various surgical options, the patient characteristics that inform these choices, and their advantages and disadvantages are outlined in **Table 201-3**. Antimicrobial therapy is an integral part of treatment of PJIs, either as adjunctive therapy, or on rare occasions, as the only modality for those who can not undergo surgical intervention. Antibiotics should be targeted at the isolated organism(s), achieve high tissue concentrations, and be active against slow-growing biofilm organisms. The route of administration and duration of antimicrobial therapy depends on the associated surgical treatment or lack thereof, and is discussed below. Intraoperatively, parenteral antimicrobial therapy may need to be initiated empirically based on local prevalence of resistant organisms, if preoperative cultures were not obtained. Commonly utilized antibiotics for specific pathogens, alternative agents, and recommended dosages are outlined in **Table 201-4**.

DEBRIDEMENT AND IMPLANT RETENTION

This procedure involves debridement of all infected tissue, with removal of fibrous membranes and devitalized bone and soft tissue, large volume irrigation, and polyethylene liner exchange, with retention of the *original* prosthesis in one surgery. This is followed by a prolonged course of parenteral and oral antimicrobial therapy. In our institution, we administer parenteral antimicrobial therapy for four to six weeks, followed by lifelong oral antimicrobial suppression. If a rifampin-susceptible *Staphylococcus* species is isolated, we recommend three to six months of a rifampin-based

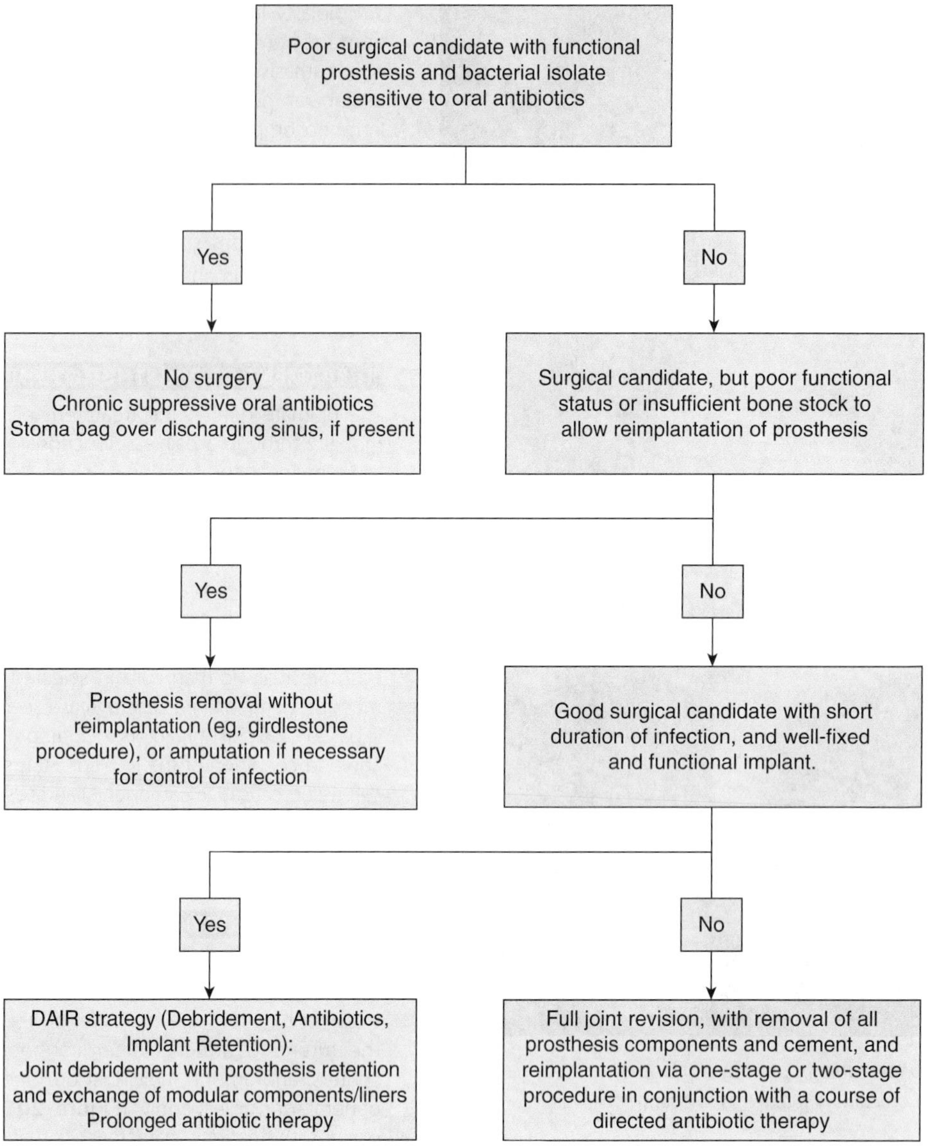

Figure 201-2 *Approach to treatment of patients with prosthetic joint infections.*

combination oral antibiotic regimen after THA and TKA infections respectively, before lifelong monotherapy (**Figure 201-3**).

ONE-STAGE VS TWO-STAGE EXCHANGE SURGERY

This procedure involves excision of all foreign material, meticulous debridement of devitalized bone and soft tissues, and reimplantation of a *new* prosthesis. Reimplantation during the *same* surgery (one-stage revision or direct exchange) is mostly performed in Europe. This is followed by four to six weeks of parenteral antimicrobial therapy. Additional oral antimicrobial therapy is optional. A delayed or two-stage replacement arthroplasty is preferred by most authorities, and is the procedure commonly employed in the United States. Following resection of prosthetic components and debridement, reimplantation is carried out at a *second* surgery several weeks later. In the intervening period, patients receive four to six weeks of IV antibiotics. Patients may be observed off therapy for a brief period for evidence of residual infection either clinically or by serial inflammatory markers before reimplantation. Confirmation of successful joint sterilization is also required by histologic or microbiologic criteria prior to prosthesis reimplantation. Repeated debridement may thus be necessary. Typically, the new prosthesis is inserted 6 to 8 weeks after removal of a TKA, and 8 to 12 weeks after removal of a THA. Antibiotic-impregnated cement is often used to fix the prosthesis at the time of reimplantation.

PERMANENT PROSTHESIS REMOVAL (RESECTION ARTHROPLASTY, ARTHRODESIS)

This procedure consists of definitive removal of the prosthesis and debridement without re-implantation. Resection is followed by four to six weeks of parenteral antibiotics. Arthrodesis of the knee (fusion of the tibia and fibula to facilitate weight bearing) can be done by external fixation at the time of resection, or delayed till completion of antibiotic course for internal fixation with intramedullary rods.

AMPUTATION

This is a procedure of last resort when all other limb salvage surgeries have failed. The infection is essentially cured by surgical removal. Antibiotics are administered perioperatively for only 24 to 48 hours to decrease surgical wound infection and perioperative bacteremia.

TABLE 201-3 Treatment Modalities for Prosthetic Joint Infections

Treatment	Patient Characteristics	Pros	Cons
Debridement and implant retention	Early postop infection (<3 mo) Hematogenous infection Short duration of symptoms (<3 wk) Well fixed stable prosthesis No sinus tract	Single surgery Preserves prostheses and bone stock Favorable response with susceptible streptococcal PJI	Leaving infected FB in place 60% failure rate with *Staphylococcus aureus* High failure rate with chronic infections
One-stage revision arthroplasty	Healthy patient Adequate bone stock Intact soft tissue Low virulence, antibiotic sensitive organism Unable to tolerate second major surgery	Avoids second surgery with additional cost Low morbidity Early mobility Can be used with draining sinuses Can be used for GNB infection 86–100% success with THA	Suboptimal for TKA infections Risk of reinfection with residual organism Poor outcomes if sinus tract present
Two-stage revision arthroplasty	Medically fit for ≥2 surgeries Adequate bone stock Compromised soft tissue	Treatment of choice for TKA Can be used for patients with draining sinus tracts 97% success with *S aureus*	Restricted mobility Expensive Time consuming Risk of further tissue damage
Permanent explantation (resection arthroplasty with or without arthrodesis)	TKA reimplantation not feasible No functional benefit with arthroplasty(nonambulatory patient) Failure of exchange arthroplasty Severely immunocompromised Poor bone stock Active IVDA	Usually a salvage procedure Arthrodesis may provide excellent pain relief and stable leg when successful	Shortened limbs Poor functional outcome Decreased success with GNB or mixed infections Risk of pin tract infections and bone fracture following arthrodesis
Amputation	Life threatening infections Recurrent PJI Failed other interventions Intractable pain Severe bone loss	Curative May be only option if arthrodesis fails	Functional limitation
Long-term suppressive antibiotics as primary therapy	Surgery contraindicated Severe coexisting illness Immobilized, does not need functional prostheses Refuses surgery	Symptomatic relief Maintain functioning joint Prevent sepsis	Success rate only 10–25% Potential toxicities of antibiotics

LONG-TERM ORAL SUPPRESSIVE ANTIBIOTICS

Indefinite, and possibly lifelong, oral antimicrobial therapy may be appropriate for patients treated with debridement and retention; in special circumstances, revision arthroplasty if residual acute inflammation is noted at the time of reimplantation; or in selected patients with significant comorbidities, where the risks of surgery outweigh the benefits.

COMPLICATIONS

Complications of PJIs may arise from surgery, antibiotics, or the infection itself. If untreated, PJIs may result in intractable pain, deformity, poor mobility, or uncontrolled sepsis. Surgical complications include hematoma formation, wound infection, prosthesis dislocation, periprosthetic fracture, venous thromboembolism, acute coronary syndromes, health care associated infections, and death. Every surgical procedure for PJIs has an inherent failure rate, and the chances of relapse or recurrence of PJIs is variable. Outpatient parenteral antibiotic therapy (OPAT) can lead to further complications. Intravascular catheter placement may result in arrhythmias, bloodstream infection, or venous thrombosis. **Table 201-5** provides a summary of the potential adverse effects of commonly used parenteral and oral antimicrobial agents.

DISCHARGE PLANNING

The practice of administering intravenous antimicrobial therapy in the home and in alternate care settings has grown rapidly over the last decade, and has become the mainstay of treatment in prosthetic joint infections. Antibiotics can be given at home by the patient or visiting nurses, at outpatient infusion centers, or in extended care facilities. Infectious diseases consultation should be obtained early to define the choice and duration of antimicrobial therapy. Hospital discharge planners or care managers should also be involved early during admission to coordinate with pharmacy, social services, and the outpatient care providers. A percutaneous intravascular central venous catheter can be placed perioperatively if the patient is not bacteremic.

TABLE 201-4 Initial Antimicrobial Treatment of Prosthetic Joint Infection Due to Commonly Occurring Organismsa*

Microorganism	Agents of Choice	Alternative Regimen(s)
Staphylococcus aureus or CoNS, oxacillin susceptible	Nafcillin sodium 1.5–2 g IV every 4 hours *or* Cefazolin 1–2 g IV every 8 hours	Vancomycin 15 mg/kg IV every 12 hours
S aureus or CoNS, oxacillin resistant	Vancomycin 15 mg/kg IV every 12 hours	Linezolid 600 mg IV or orally every 12 hours *or* Daptomycin 4–6 mg/kg every 24 hours
Enterococcus species, penicillin susceptible	Penicillin G 20–24 million units every 24 hours Continuous infusion or in six divided doses *or* Ampicillin sodium 12 g IV every 24 hours Continuous infusion or in six divided doses	Vancomycin 15 mg/kg IV every 12 hours
Enterococcus species, penicillin resistant	Vancomycin 15 mg/kg IV every 12 hours	Linezolid 600 mg IV or orally every 12 hours *or* Daptomycin 4–6 mg/kg every 24 hours
Beta-hemolytic streptococci	Penicillin G 20–24 million units every 24 hours Continuous infusion or in six divided doses *or* Ceftriaxone 2 g IV every 24 hours	Vancomycin 15 mg/kg IV every 12 hours
Propionibacterium acnes, Corynebacteria species	Penicillin G 20–24 million units every 24 hours Continuous infusion or in six divided doses *or* Ceftriaxone 2 g IV every 24 hours	Vancomycin 15 mg/kg IV every 12 hours *or* Clindamycin 600–900 mg IV every 8 hours
Pseudomonas aeruginosa	Cefepime 1–2 g IV every 12 hours *or* Meropenem 1 g IV every 8 hours *or* Imipenem 500 mg IV every 6–8 hours	Ceftazidime 2 g IV every 8 hours *or* Ciprofloxacin 750 mg orally every 12 hours *or* Ciprofloxacin 400 mg IV every 12 hours
Enterobacter species	Meropenem 1 g IV every 8 hours *or* Imipenem 500 mg IV every 6–8 hours	Ceftazidime 2 g IV every 8 hours *or* Ciprofloxacin 750 mg orally every 12 hours *or* Ciprofloxacin 400 mg IV every 12 hours

*Dose adjustment necessary for renal impairment.

CARE TRANSITIONS

The hospitalist has a unique role on the OPAT team. The physician's responsibilities include establishing the diagnosis, prescribing treatment, determining the appropriate site of care, arranging for adequate monitoring during therapy with the outpatient primary care provider, and assuring overall quality of care. Patients should be provided with oral and written instructions on adverse effects of their antibiotics. Outpatient follow-up should be arranged with the primary care physician, orthopedic surgeon, and infectious disease specialist. A list of recommended laboratory parameters and frequency of monitoring is shown in Table 201-5.

QUALITY IMPROVEMENT AND PREVENTION OF PJIS

Rates of PJI following joint arthroplasty have decreased with improvements in surgical technique, operating theatre design, and antimicrobial prophylaxis. Aseptic surgical techniques and advances in device designs have contributed to the decline in PJIs. Proper administration of preoperative intravenous antimicrobial prophylaxis have been shown in multiple prospective clinical trials to decrease the rate of subsequent PJI. First-generation cephalosporins such as cefazolin are recommended as first-line agents. Vancomycin is an alternative where there is type 1 hypersensitivity to penicillin or a high incidence of surgical site infections (SSI) attributable to methicillin-resistant *S aureus* or methicillin-resistant *S epidermidis*. These antimicrobials should be given for no longer than 24 hours. There is a growing body of evidence showing significant reduction in rates of orthopedic device infections when *S aureus* carriers are decolonized prior to surgery. In our institution, we encourage intranasal screening for *S aureus* prior to arthroplasty. We recommend a five-day course of intranasal mupirocin, and at least two days of chlorhexidine body washes

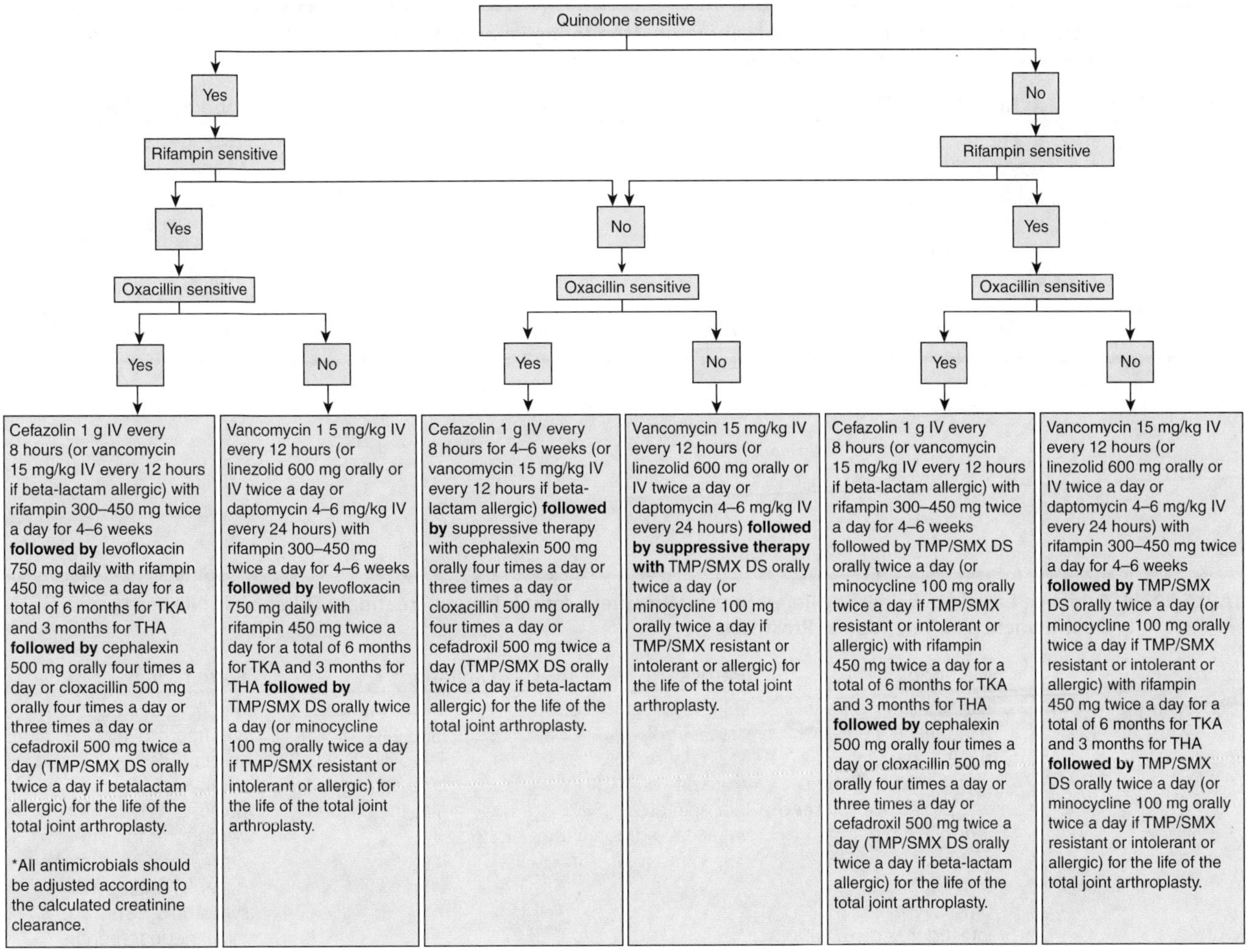

Figure 201-3 *Guidelines for the treatment of Staphylococcal species prosthetic joint infection after debridement and retention of the joint prosthesis components. *TKA, total knee arthroplasties; THA, total hip arthroplasties; TMP/SMX DS, trimethoprim-sulfamethoxazole double strength.*

TABLE 201-5 Potential Side Effects and Suggested Laboratory Monitoring Parameters for Commonly Used Antimicrobial Agents for Prosthetic Joint Infections

Antimicrobial	Notable Side Effects	Caution	Laboratory Monitoring*
Beta-lactams	Maculopapular rash, antibiotic-associated diarrhea, reversible neutropenia, hepatic dysfunction	Hypersensitivity to beta-lactams	CBC, RFTs; liver enzymes (for nafcillin, oxacillin, carbapenems)
Vancomycin	Red person syndrome, reversible neutropenia, reversible nephrotoxicity, irreversible ototoxicity (rare)	Avoid in patients with previous severe hearing loss	CBC, RFTs, vancomycin levels (goal trough 10–15 μg/mL)
Daptomycin	GI side effects, myopathy	Caution with concurrent HMG-CoA reductase inhibitors	CBC, RFTs, liver enzymes, creatine kinase
Aminoglycosides	Irreversible ototoxicity, reversible nephrotoxicity	Caution in patients with preexisting renal failure, hearing loss	CBC, RFTs,† aminoglycoside levels†
Linezolid	Myelosuppression, peripheral and optic neuropathy	Avoid tyramine-containing foods and serotonergic agents	CBC (IV or orally)
Fluoroquinolones	GI side effects, phototoxicity, tendon rupture, arrhythmias (rare)	Do not take with antacids, monitor QTc with concurrent arrhythmogenic medications	Liver enzymes
Trimethoprim-sulfamethoxazole	GI upset, dermatological reactions, myelosuppression, nephrotoxicity	Avoid if hypersensitive to any sulfa drug	CBC, RFTs

(continued)

TABLE 201-5 Potential Side Effects and Suggested Laboratory Monitoring Parameters for Commonly Used Antimicrobial Agents for Prosthetic Joint Infections (*continued*)

Antimicrobial	Notable Side Effects	Caution	Laboratory Monitoring*
Minocycline	Photosensitivity, hyperpigmentation of skin, drug-induced lupus, dizziness, vertigo	Do not take with antacids or iron, caution with concurrent anticoagulant therapy or OCP	CBC,§ liver enzymes§
Rifampin	Orange discoloration of body secretions, hepatotoxicity	Should not be used as monotherapy, caution with concurrent anticoagulant therapy or OCP	CBC,§ liver enzymes§
Clindamycin	Rash, hepatotoxicity, *C difficile* colitis	History of *C difficile* colitis	CBC, RFTs, Liver enzymes

CBC, complete blood count; GI, gastrointestinal; OCP, oral contraceptive pill; RFTs, renal function tests.
*Laboratory tests for *parenteral antibiotics* should be done weekly unless otherwise stated (Infectious Diseases Society of America guidelines).
†Twice weekly.
§Frequency as clinically indicated.

TABLE 201-6 Evidence-based Medicine: Key References for Prosthetic Joint Infection Treatment Outcomes Following Debridement and Retention of Prosthesis

Study	Methodology	Results	Limitations	Bottom Line
Zimmerli W, et al. *JAMA*. 1998;279:1537–1541.	Randomized, double blind trial to compare the efficacy of ciprofloxacin-rifampin vs ciprofloxacin-placebo long-term therapy (3–6 mo) for staphylococcal orthopedic implant infections, after initial debridement	33 patients enrolled, with stable implants, and < 21 d of symptoms. Cure rate of 100% in rifampin group, 58% in placebo group after 33–35 mo follow-up	Very small sample size (12 in each group completed study); internal fixation devices were also included in study	PJI due to rifampin and fluoroquinolone susceptible staphylococci may be effectively treated without removal of device, provided implant is stable, duration of symptoms is short, and initial debridement is performed
Marculescu CE, et al. *Clin Infect Dis*. 2006;42:471–478.	Retrospective cohort analysis for outcomes of patients with PJI treated with debridement and retention of the prosthesis (5-year, single center)	99 patients; risk factors independently associated with treatment failure were presence of sinus tract (hazard ratio, 2.84) and duration of symptoms > 8 d (hazard ratio, 1.77)	Single-center retrospective study with potential for uncontrolled selection biases; no data on rifampin-based combinations of antimicrobials	Debridement and retention of prosthesis may be reasonable alternative to staged arthroplasty, for patients with short duration of symptoms and absence of sinus tract
Byren I, et al. *J Antimicrob Ther*. 2009;63:1264–1271.	Retrospective study of a cohort of PJI patients managed with debridement, antibiotics and implant retention to determine treatment failure rates by antibiotic duration	112 patients; overall, 18% treatment failure rate during mean follow-up of 2.3 y. Rate of failure increased 4-fold after stopping oral antibiotics	Single-center retrospective observational study design; results could have been confounded by comorbidities, leading to both poor outcomes and decision to undertake less invasive procedure	Oral antibiotics after debridement and retention may only achieve suppression rather than cure in subgroup of patients, and may need to be continued indefinitely

(the night before and the morning of surgery) for carriers, in addition to the appropriate perioperative intravenous antimicrobial prophylaxis. Good hand hygiene and optimal wound care also decrease rates of SSI. There is no evidence to recommend routine antibiotic prophylaxis for patients with arthroplasties undergoing invasive dental, gastrointestinal or genitourinary tract procedures. Patients with arthroplasties, who are suspected to have bacteremia especially due to *S aureus*, should have rapid initiation of antimicrobial treatment after appropriate cultures are obtained (**Table 201-6**).

SUGGESTED READINGS

Berbari EF, Hanssen AD, Duffy MC, et al. Risk factors for prosthetic joint infection: case-control study. *Clin Infect Dis*. 1998;27:1247–1254.

Lentino JR. Prosthetic joint infections: bane of orthopedists, challenge for infectious disease specialists. *Clin Infect Dis*. 2003;36:1157–1161.

Parvizi J, Ghanem E, Menashe S, Barrack RL, Bauer TW. Periprosthetic infection: what are the diagnostic challenges? *J Bone Joint Surg Am*. 2006;88(Suppl 4):138–147.

Sia IG, Berbari EF, Karchmer AW. Prosthetic joint infections. *Infect Dis Clin North Am*. 2005;19:885–914.

Tice AD, Rehm SJ, Dalovisio JR, et al. IDSA practice guidelines for outpatient parenteral antimicrobial therapy. *Clin Infect Dis*. 2004;38:1651–1672.

Trampuz A, Hanssen AD, Osmon DR, et al. Synovial fluid leukocyte count and differential for the diagnosis of prosthetic knee infection. *Am J Med*. 2004;117:556–562.

Trampuz A, Osmon DR, Hanssen AD, Steckelberg JM, Patel R. Molecular and antibiofilm approaches to prosthetic joint infection. *Clin Orthop Relat Res*. 2003;414:69–88.

Trampuz A, Piper KE, Jacobson MJ, et al. Sonication of removed hip and knee prostheses for diagnosis of infection. *N Engl J Med*. 2007;357:654–663.

CHAPTER 202

Sexually Transmitted Infections

Clare Rock, MD
Colm Bergin, MD, FRCPI, FRCP

Key Clinical Questions

1. Which hospitalized patients should be screened for sexually transmitted infections?
2. How should patients with vaginal or urethral discharge be diagnosed?
3. What are the common causes of genital ulcers?
4. What are the benefits of universal HIV screening in health care settings?

INTRODUCTION/EPIDEMIOLOGY

In the United States, there are 15 million cases of sexually transmitted infections (STIs) yearly, including 4 million cases of *Chlamydia trachomatis* alone, and the current seroprevalence of herpes simplex virus type 2 (HSV-2) is 22%. Most, but not all, cases of STIs occur in young people, who may be oblivious or indifferent to health risks, including pelvic inflammatory disease, infertility, cervical cancer, an increased risk of HIV acquisition, and cardiac and neurologic complications of syphilis. Up to 40% of sexually active females aged 15 to 19 in the United States have an STI. The prevalence of genital chlamydia and HSV-2 is thought to be similar in Europe and in other developed nations. Worldwide, there are an estimated 90 million new cases of genital chlamydia per year, and 60 million cases of gonorrhoea per year. Syphilis has recently reemerged in many regions where it had become uncommon, including the United States, Europe, and China. All STIs increase the risk of HIV acquisition.

There are many barriers to care for patients with STIs. These include privacy concerns, fear of disclosure, lack of health care access and affordability, ongoing mental health or substance abuse problems, and denial. Adolescents are a particularly vulnerable group: symptomatic females may take up to 10 days before seeking medical attention, and many more do not present because of the absence of symptoms. For many patients, an emergency room visit or hospitalization, often for a reason other than an STI, may be the only opportunity for medical personnel to screen for HIV and other STIs, and provide point-of-care diagnosis and treatment and sexual risk reduction counselling.

SEXUAL HISTORY

The most important element in the diagnosis of an STI is a complete sexual history. The sexual history should be obtained in a professional, nonjudgmental, and thorough fashion. The interview should be in a private setting, with the patient physically comfortable and at eye level with the physician. The physician should emphasize the confidential nature of the information obtained, and that the questions asked are part of routine medical care. There should be no physical barrier, such as a desk, between the patient and physician, and the physician's body language should suggest acceptance, with arms and legs uncrossed. The physician should make eye contact with the patient, nod encouragement, and employ strategic pauses when necessary. The physician should use terminology that the patient understands, and assess for comorbid mood disorders, alcohol, and drug abuse that may increase the patient's risk of STIs. A useful format for the sexual history interview is the five Ps: partners, prevention of STIs (if any), prevention of pregnancy (if any), practices, and previous STI history.

PRACTICE POINT

The five Ps: a structured approach to taking a sexual history

Partners

- Do you have sex with men, women, or both?
- In the past 2 months, how many partners have you had sex with?
- In the past 12 months, how many partners have you had sex with?

Prevention of pregnancy

- Are you or your partner trying to get pregnant?
- If not, what are you doing to prevent pregnancy?

Protection for STDs

- What do you do to protect yourself from STDs and HIV?

Practices

- To understand your risks for STDs, I need to understand the kind of sex you have had recently.
- Have you had vaginal sex, meaning "penis in vagina sex"?
- Have you had anal sex, meaning "penis in rectum/anus sex"?
- Have you had oral sex, meaning "mouth on penis/vagina"?
- If yes, do you use condoms: never, sometimes or always?
- If never, why? If sometimes, in what situations?

Past history of STDs

- Have you ever had an STD?
- Have any of your partners ever had an STD?
- Have you or any of your partners ever injected drugs?
- Have you or any of your partners ever exchanged money or drugs for sex?
- Is there anything else about your sexual practices I need to know?

SEXUAL HEALTH ISSUES IN HOSPITALIZED PATIENTS

HIV SEROCONVERSION ILLNESS

Acute HIV infection can present to the emergency room as a mononucleosis-like syndrome. Patients have high-level viremia and are highly infectious. Clinical features may include fever, sweats, malaise, lymphadenopathy, pharyngitis, aphthous ulcers, maculopapular rash on the trunk and extremities, and aseptic meningitis. Patients may also be asymptomatic. Benefits of early diagnosis include establishment of ongoing HIV care and prevention of opportunistic infections (**Table 202-1**). The role of early antiretroviral therapy (ART) in these patients remains undefined. Knowledge of HIV-positive status also discourages risky behaviour and facilitates partner testing. Although the possibility of acute HIV syndrome is an indication for obtaining HIV serology (and viral load testing as well), clinicians should note that current guidelines recommend HIV screening in all health care settings in an opt-out capacity.

POSTEXPOSURE PROPHYLAXIS OF HIV

Postexposure prophylaxis (PEP) with a 28-day course of ART is recommended in sexual contacts of HIV-positive persons presenting within 72 hours of exposure. Receptive and insertive anal intercourse has an especially high risk of HIV acquisition. If the patient's contact is of unknown HIV status, as in sexual assault or anonymous sex, then the risk is weighed on individual basis. The possibility of surreptitious sexual assault should also be considered in patients who are brought to the hospital with alcohol or drug intoxication. A full medical and medication history should be obtained prior to commencement on PEP. Monitoring of complete blood counts and renal function on ART and outpatient HIV clinic follow-up are recommended. A full STI screen should also be performed.

TABLE 202-1 Benefits of Early HIV Diagnosis

Awareness of diagnosis can decrease onward transmission
Opportunity to engage in services and education on prevention of other STIs
Prevention of complications of HIV for index patient
Contact tracing and testing of current and previous partners

UNIVERSAL HIV TESTING

Every person presenting with a STI or suspected STI should have an HIV test. This is particularly true for high-risk groups such as sex workers, drug users, MSM, and people with multiple sexual contacts or contacts from countries of high prevalence. The benefit of screening for HIV before symptoms develop include decreased transmission, a greater likelihood of starting antiretroviral treatment in a timely manner, and a decreased risk of opportunistic infection. In 2006, the Centers for Disease Control and Prevention recommended that HIV screening be performed as part of routine medical care on all patients aged 13 to 64. The demographics of HIV in the United States have changed over the past 20 years, with a higher prevalence in persons younger than 20 years, women, racial or ethnic minorities, and heterosexual men and women. As a result, the effectiveness of risk-based testing to identify HIV-infected persons has diminished.

SEXUALLY ACQUIRED VIRAL HEPATITIS

Sexual transmission of hepatitis B represents a major mode of acquisition, particularly among men who have sex with men (MSM). In the United States and other developed countries, hepatitis B vaccine is a routine childhood vaccination. Nonimmune groups who are potentially vulnerable to hepatitis B include persons who have not been vaccinated due to lack of health care access, vaccine nonresponders, or those with waning immunity to vaccine. Acute hepatitis B can present as an influenza-like illness with anorexia, fatigue, nausea, right upper quadrant pain, and jaundice. Blood tests can show very elevated ALT and AST (often >1000 IU/L), with or without an elevated bilirubin. Fulminant disease with hepatic failure is unusual (0.1–0.5%); risk factors include concomitant acetaminophen and alcohol intake. Initial treatment is supportive, although antiviral therapy may be considered in fulminant disease. Vaccination of household members and partners and screening of contacts is also important.

STIs THAT MAY MASQUERADE AS OTHER CONDITIONS

Syphilis is known as the great pretender because of its protean manifestations and ability to mimic a wide variety of other diseases. Clinical findings may include ulcerations or heaped-up lesions (condylomata lata) involving the genitals, oropharynx, or rectum, a wide variety of psoriasiform skin rashes, lymphadenopathy, alopecia, aseptic meningitis, uveitis, hearing loss, visual loss, bone pain (periostitis), aortic regurgitation, stroke, psychiatric disease, gait disorder, and dementia. Diagnosis and treatment are discussed in further detail below.

Lymphogranuloma venereum (LGV) is caused by serovars L1, L2, and L3 of *C trachomatis*. It is endemic in Central and South America, Southeast Asia, Africa, and the Caribbean. It is uncommon in the United States and Europe, where most cases occur in MSM. Clinical manifestations include a primary stage, leading to a small, painless genital or anorectal ulcer that may not be recognized by the patient. The secondary stage of infection, occurring days to weeks later, may lead to fever and tender inguinal and femoral lymphadenopathy, which may lead to formation of abscesses (buboes) with drainage. Alternatively, patients may develop a painful anorectal syndrome with scanty rectal discharge, bleeding, pruritis, or constipation. Hemorrhagic proctitis due to LGV may be mistaken for inflammatory bowel disease, and biopsy findings in LGV proctitis may actually be similar to those of Crohn disease. Laboratory diagnosis is difficult. It is traditionally based on *C trachomatis* serology, although most tests lack specificity for the serovars causing LGV. Reference laboratories may be able to perform nucleic acid amplication tests (NAATs) on genital or rectal swab specimens. LGV is treated with doxycycline 100 mg twice daily for three weeks. When LGV is likely, presumptive treatment is recommended.

CARDINAL SYMPTOMS OF STIs

VAGINAL DISCHARGE

Vaginal discharge may be physiological or pathological. Physiologic discharge, comprised of vaginal secretions, exfoliated cells, and cervical mucus, varies with menstrual cycle, pregnancy, age, and use of oral contraceptives. It is usually minor in amount. The most common causes of vaginal discharge in premenopausal women are candidiasis, bacterial vaginosis, and trichomoniasis; trichomoniasis and perhaps bacterial vaginosis are acquired sexually. Atrophic vaginitis is a major additional cause in postmenopausal women. Other causes include allergy, chemical irritation, retained foreign body, and cervicitis from gonorrhoea or chlamydia. Vaginal candidiasis is especially common on general medical wards, due to the high prevalence of diabetes mellitus and the frequent use of antibiotics.

Helpful features of the history include a fishy odor, worse after sexual intercourse, which suggests bacterial vaginosis, and thick "cottage cheese" discharge without odor, which is consistent with vaginal candidiasis. On examination, cervicitis is suggestive of trichomoniasis, chlamydia, or gonorrhoea. Testing should include:

- Measurement of vaginal pH (vaginal pH is normally ≤ 4.5; elevated pH suggests bacterial vaginosis or trichomoniasis)
- "Whiff" test, performed by mixing vaginal secretions with 10% potassium hydroxide; a subsequent fishy odor indicates production of volatizied amines, suggestive of bacterial vaginosis
- Light microscopy of vaginal secretions, looking for white cells, yeast, mobile trichomonads, and clue cells (vaginal epithelial cells studded with bacteria)

Additional tests that may be helpful include rapid card tests for bacterial vaginosis and trichomoniasis that may be performed at the bedside. A culture system is now available for *Trichomonas vaginalis*, which is much more sensitive than wet mount testing.

Vaginal candidiasis may be treated with several topical imidazoles, with single dose treatment with oral fluconazole 150 mg being equally effective. *Trichomonas* is treated with a single 2-g dose of oral metronidazole; partners must also be treated to prevent reinfection. Bacterial vaginosis is treated with metronidazole 500 mg twice daily for 7 days.

URETHRAL DISCHARGE

Sexually transmitted pathogens associated with urethritis include *Neisseria gonorrhoeae, Chlamydia trachomatis, Mycoplasma genitalum, Trichomonas vaginalis,* and herpes simplex. If urethral discharge can be obtained, Gram stain should be performed. If more than five white blood cells are present per high-power field, patients should be empirically treated for both gonorrhea and chlamydia. Preferred therapy is single-dose intramuscular ceftriaxone 125 mg (for gonorrhea) and oral azithromycin 1 g (for chlamydia as well as gonorrhea). When no discharge is present, NAATs for gonorrhea and chlamydia should be obtained from urine specimens. These should be obtained at least two hours after last voided urine to optimize sensitivity. Empiric treatment may still be appropriate if clinical suspicion is high and adherence to follow-up uncertain. If empiric therapy is administered, culture and sensitivity testing for gonorrhea should also be obtained, due to concerns about emerging resistance (see below). Testing for *Mycoplasma* is not widely available, and is usually not necessary, as empiric treatment for chlamydia with azithromycin is also effective against *Mycoplasma*. Patients with recurrent or persistent urethritis will require evaluation and treatment for *Trichomonas* and HSV.

TABLE 202-2 Etiology of Infectious Genital Ulcers in 801 Patients in the United States, France, and the Netherlands

Herpes simplex	72%
Syphilis	20%
Chancroid	5%
Mixed	2%
Other	1%

Data from Hope-Rapp E, Anyfantakis V, Fouéré S, et al. Etiology of genital ulcer disease. A prospective study of 278 cases seen in an STD clinic in Paris. *Sex Transm Dis.* 2010;37:153–158; Bruisten SM, Cairo I, Fennema H, et al. Diagnosing genital ulcer disease in a clinic for sexually transmitted diseases in Amsterdam, The Netherlands. *J Clin Microbiol.* 2001;39:601–605; Mertz KJ, Trees D, Levine WC, et al. Etiology of genital ulcers and prevalence of human immunodeficiency virus coinfection in 10 US cities. The Genital Ulcer Disease Surveillance Group. *J Infect Dis.* 1998;178:1795–1798.

PRACTICE POINT

- Patients with gonorrhea or chlamydia should be retested three months after treatment to ensure clearance. Cotreatment for both chlamydia and gonorrhea is generally recommended, unless coinfection has been specifically excluded by laboratory testing.

GENITAL ULCERS

The most common cause of genital ulceration in the United States and Europe is herpes simplex virus (**Table 202-2**). HSV-2 predominates in genital herpes, although sexual transmission of HSV-1 has risen in recent years due to the increasing practice of oral sex. HSV-2 in particular causes painful genital ulcers and erosions, sometimes with fever and other systemic features, especially aseptic meningitis. Most patients with genital herpes do not have pustular lesions by the time they present to medical attention. Syphilis also causes genital ulceration, which is usually but not always painless. Chancroid, caused by *Haemophilus ducreyi*, is a common cause of genital ulceration in developing countries, although it is uncommon in North America and Europe. Chancroid usually produces a deep ulcer with painful inguinal lymphadenopathy.

Evaluation of genital ulcers includes culture for HSV and serologic testing for syphilis. Polymerase chain reaction for HSV may be useful in patients with older genital ulcers, in whom the yield of culture is lower. The sensitivity of syphilis serology is as low as 50% in primary syphilis. Darkfield microscopy was traditionally used to diagnose primary syphilis. However, darkfield microscopes are no longer widely available, and clinical expertise in interpreting darkfield microscopy is wanting. When no pathogen has been identified, empiric treatment for both herpes simplex (eg, valacyclovir 1000 mg twice daily for 1 week) and syphilis (a single dose of intramuscular benzathine penicillin G 2.4 million U) should be administered. As the differential diagnosis of genital ulcers encompasses a variety of noninfectious conditions (**Table 202-3**), including malignancy, skin biopsy should be performed in patients with persistent unexplained genital ulcers.

TABLE 202-3 Differential Diagnosis of Genital Ulcers
Infectious
Herpes simplex
Syphilis (*Treponema pallidum*)
Chancroid (*Haemophilus ducreyi*)
Donovanosis (*Calymmatobacterium granulomatis*)
Noninfectious
Crohn disease
Behçet disease
Contact dermatitis
Squamous cell cancer
Pemphigus vulgaris
Erosive lichen planus
Pyoderma gangrenosum
Lipschutz ulcers (immunologic reaction to a distant source of infection)
Trauma

POSTCOITAL BLEEDING

Postcoital bleeding (PCB) has many causes, including vaginitis, cervicitis, cervical dysplasia and malignancy, uterine lesions, and pregnancy. The assessment includes pregnancy testing and vaginal and cervical examination, with Papanicolaou testing, NAATs from cervical specimens for gonorrhea and chlamydia, and testing for *Trichomonas*. Diagnostic tests for vaginitis should be performed as above, in the presence of suggestive signs and symptoms. Uterine tenderness on examination suggests endometritis or adenomyosis.

ABDOMINAL AND PELVIC PAIN

The symptoms of pelvic inflammatory disease (PID) are highly variable, and include acute or chronic lower abdominal and pelvic pain, with or without fever. All women in their childbearing years presenting with abdominal pain should have pregnancy testing. Ectopic pregnancy commonly presents with acute abdominal pain; repeated episodes of PID are a major risk factor. Other causes of pelvic pain in women include endometritis, torsion or hemorrhage of an ovarian cyst, endometriosis, appendicitis, inflammatory bowel disease, urinary tract infection, and nephrolithiasis. LGV should be considered when anorectal symptoms present, particularly in MSM.

COMMON SEXUALLY TRANSMITTED PATHOGENS

CHLAMYDIA TRACHOMATIS

Chlamydia trachomatis is the most common bacterial etiology of STDs, causing 50% to 70% of nonspecific urethritis. It is an obligate intracellular organism with an incubation period of 7 to 21 days. Genital chlamydia infection is currently at epidemic levels among young people in the United States. Women are asymptomatic in 75% of cases and men in up to 40% cases, making case detection difficult and reinfection common. Symptoms in men include dysuria and urethral discharge. Symptoms in women include vaginal discharge, dysuria, postcoital bleeding, intermenstrual bleeding, dyspareunia, and abdominal pain. The major complications include pelvic inflammatory disease and sexually acquired reactive arthritis (SARA), in which urethritis is followed by polyarthritis, conjunctivitis, and mucocutaneous lesions. SARA is predominantly is disease of men. Early recognition and treatment of *C trachomatis* prevents these complications.

The most sensitive and specific test is NAAT, performed on first-void urine in males and endocervical swab in females. Recommended treatment is single-dose oral azithromycin 1 g or doxycycline 100 mg twice daily for 7 days. Patients are often treated empirically; requiring patients to return for results and treatment can result in loss to follow-up, a missed opportunity for therapy, and further propagation of infection.

NEISSERIA GONORRHOEAE

Approximately 335,000 cases of gonorrhea are reported annually in the United States, with a stable incidence over the past decade. The incubation period is three to five days. Infected men usually have urethritis with dysuria and purulent penile discharge, but infected women are usually asymptomatic. Invasive infections with *N gonorrhoeae* may lead to disseminated gonococcal infection (DGI), with oligoarthritis, tenosynovitis, and a rash with purulent hemorrhagic pustules on the extremities (**Figure 202-1**). Gonorrhea in women may result in PID, infertility, ectopic pregnancy, and chronic pelvic pain.

Diagnosis is based on Gram stains of urethral or cervical discharge showing gram-negative intracellular diplococci or NAATs

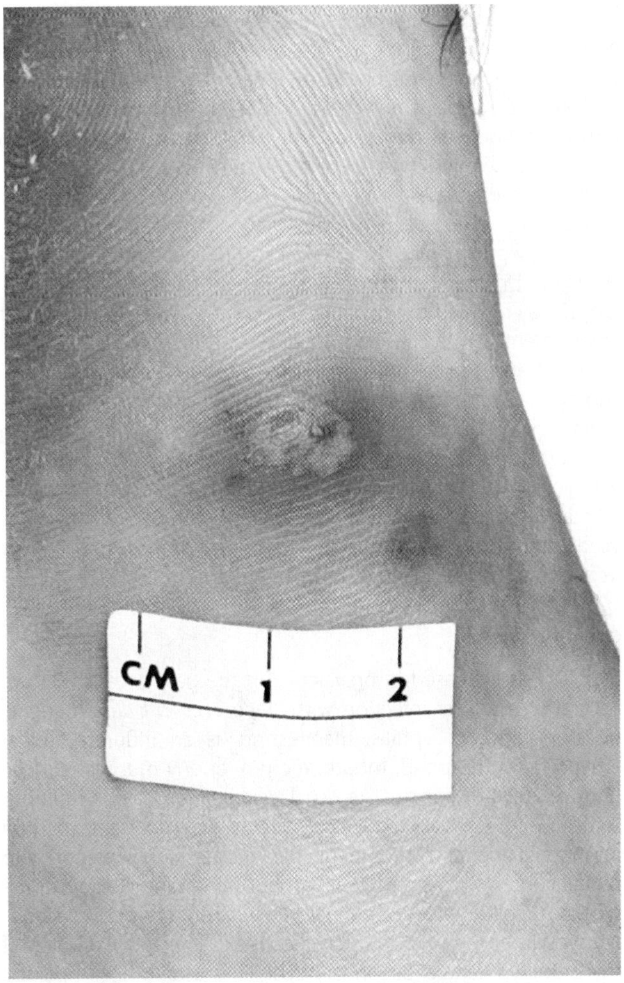

Figure 202-1 *Hemorrhagic pustule of disseminated gonococcal infection. When patients have skin lesions, only a few are typically present (Public Health Image Library, Centers for Disease Control and Prevention).*

from urine or cervical specimens. Cultures for *N gonorrhoeae* should still be obtained, as these are useful both for management of individual patients as well as epidemiological surveillance of antibiotic resistance. For MSM, pharyngeal and rectal swabs for culture should also be obtained. However, gram staining from these sites is of limited value due to the many nonpathogenic *Neisseria* species in these locations. Blood cultures should be performed in patients with suspected DGI, although the sensitivity may be as low as 30%.

Of worldwide public health concern is the rising level of antibiotic resistance in *N gonorrhoeae*. Penicillins, tetracyclines, and fluoroquinolones are no longer recommended for treatment of gonorrhea. As well, there is a serious and very worrisome problem with emerging cephalosporin resistance. This has reinforced the need for routine gonorrheal culture and sensitivity testing prior to treatment in patients with positive NAATs for gonorrhea. As of July 2011, the Centers for Disease Control recommends that patients with uncomplicated gonorrhea should be treated with intramuscular ceftriaxone 250 mg and azithromycin 1 gm. As guidelines may change rapidly, providers are advised to consult local authorities prior to providing therapy. Patients with DGI require hospitalization and treatment with intravenous ceftriaxone 1 g daily for 7 days.

HERPES SIMPLEX VIRUS

Genital herpes has been called "cold sores in a less obvious location." Patients may have associated fever, malaise, inguinal lymph adenopathy, and dysuria. While HSV-2 genital infection is currently more common, the incidence of genital HSV-1 infection has risen due to transmission via oral sex. Primary genital HSV-2 infection is more likely to be symptomatic and severe than primary genital HSV-1 infection. Recurrences of genital HSV are usually milder than the initial attack, and tend to abate over time.

Patients with primary genital HSV-2 infection are sometimes hospitalized due to extragenital manifestations. Up to 8% of patients develop aseptic meningitis, and up to 10% of women have urinary retention. Urinary retention may be due to painful vulval lesions, which may respond to sitz baths, or secondary to sacral nerve root involvement, which may require temporary urinary catherization. Systemic and topical analgesics may also be helpful. Diagnosis can be made clinically, but vesicles should be unroofed and contents sent to laboratory for viral culture. Early treatment (within 72 hours) can decrease length and severity of illness. Oral acyclovir, valacyclovir, and famciclovir are all effective. Patients with extragenital manifestations generally require therapy with parenteral acyclovir, at least initially. Patients with frequent recurrences may benefit from episodic or suppressive antiviral therapy.

SYPHILIS

Syphilis has increased in prevalence in the past decade. One to several weeks after infection with *Treponema pallidum*, patients develop primary syphilis, manifesting as an indurated ulcer (chancre) on the penis, mouth, rectum, or any mucosal surface (**Figure 202-2**). Chancres are usually single, but may be multiple. As lesions are usually painless, patients may not seek medical attention. Patients with primary chancres are highly infectious to sexual contacts. Chancres heal without treatment in about three weeks. As spirochetes disseminate throughout the body, secondary syphilis ensues, typically days to weeks after the resolution of the primary chancre. Secondary syphilis is usually accompanied by systemic symptoms, such as fever, malaise, anorexia, arthralgias, and bone pain. A prominent generalized rash may occur, classically described as a scaly, copper-colored maculopapular rash involving the trunk and extremities, including the palms and soles (**Figure 202-3**). Patients may develop alopecia and heaped-up lesions on the genitals and perineum (condylomata lata) as well as the face and oropharynx (mucous patches). Other features may include lymphadenopathy, hepatosplenomegaly, uveitis, and aseptic meningitis. Tertiary syphilis develops after a latency of years to decades. Features may include destructive lesions in soft tissue and bone (gummas), thoracic aortic aneurysm with aortic regurgitation, and a wide variety of psychiatric and neurologic syndromes, including personality change, psychosis, strokes, ocular and otic disease, and degeneration of the dorsal columns of the spinal cord.

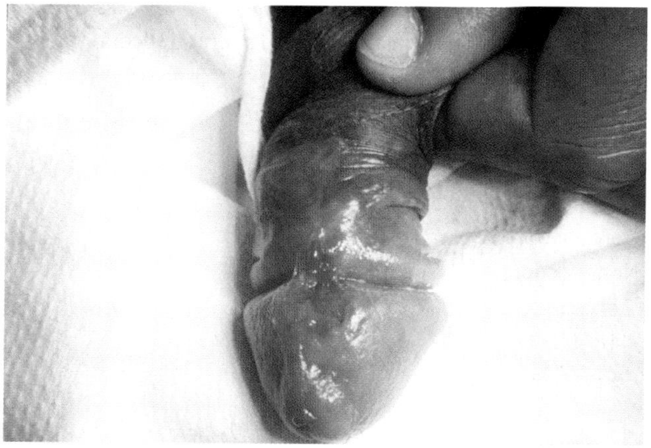

Figure 202-2 *Indurated ulcerative lesion (chancre) of primary syphilis on the ventral surface of the penis (Public Health Image Library, Centers for Disease Control and Prevention).*

PRACTICE POINT

- In secondary syphilis, titers of nontreponemal tests may be very high. In fact, titers may be so high that the flocculation reaction does not occur, leading to a false negative result. This is known as the prozone phenomenon. It may also occur with some treponemal tests. If secondary syphilis is suspected and syphilis serology is negative, the laboratory should be asked to dilute the specimen and repeat the test.

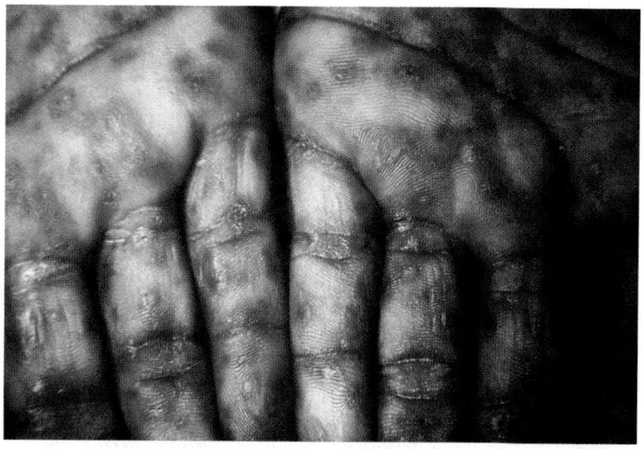

Figure 202-3 *Papulosquamous rash on the palms of a patient with secondary syphilis. Lesions are classically copper-colored in fair-skinned individuals and hyperpigmented in dark-skinned individuals (Public Health Image Library, Centers for Disease Control and Prevention).*

Diagnosis is based on serology. Traditionally, nontreponemal tests such as the rapid plasma reagin or Venereal Disease Research Laboratory were performed initially as screening tests, followed by specific treponemal antibodies. Increasingly, treponemal tests are being used as screening tests, as the treponemal enzyme immunoassay has become more widely available and may now be run in automated fashion. Nontreponemal tests are still important in assessing the response to antibiotic therapy. A major limitation of both treponemal and nontreponemal tests is their lower sensitivity in primary syphilis; treponemal tests are more sensitive than nontreponemal tests in this setting.

Primary syphilis, secondary syphilis, or early latent syphilis (patients within one year of the development of secondary syphilis) are treated with a single dose of intramuscular benzathine penicillin G 2.4 million units. A transient acute febrile reaction (Jarisch-Herxheimer reaction) may develop after penicillin treatment; this is the result of treponemal lysis, and should be distinguished from an allergy reaction. Doxycycline 100 mg twice daily for 14 days may be used in patients with true penicillin allergy. For pregnant women at risk of mother-to-child transmission, or those with neurologic involvement, desensitization to penicillin may be appropriate. Patients with late latent syphilis or cardiovascular syphilis are treated with intramuscular benzathine penicillin G 2.4 million units weekly for three weeks. Neurosyphilis requires 10 to 14 days of intravenous therapy with 18 to 24 million units of penicillin G daily. All patients with syphilis should attend specialist STD clinics where contact tracing and treatment of partners can be undertaken.

CHANCROID

Chancroid is caused by *Haemophilus ducreyi*. It is the most common cause of genital ulcerative diseases in developing countries. It is rare in the United States and Europe, but increasing travel and migration may lead to an increased incidence. It should be suspected in a returned traveler from the tropics with a painful deep undermined ulcer and tender inguinal lymphadenitis. Diagnosis is difficult. Gram stain may reveal small, pleomorphic gram-negative coccobacilli. Even with special media, the yield of culture is rather low. Polymerase chain reaction testing may be available at specialized reference laboratories. If chancroid is suspected, infectious diseases consultation is recommended to assist with diagnosis. Treatment is oral ciprofloxacin 500 mg twice daily for three days.

CONTACT TRACING

Contact tracing is the identification and diagnosis of infection in persons who have come into contact with an index case. Contact tracing of sexually transmitted diseases can be difficult due to patient reluctance to divulge contact details. As well, some sexual encounters may be anonymous in nature. Sexual partners are often asymptomatic and if not treated will reinfect the index case. Partners of patients with chlamydia, gonorrhea, and early-stage syphilis should receive empiric treatment. Referral to sexual health services facilitates appropriate counseling and tracing of previous partners.

SUGGESTED READINGS

Branson BM, Handsfield HH, Lampe MA, et al. Centers for Disease Control and Prevention (CDC). Revised recommendations for HIV testing of adults, adolescents, and pregnant women in health-care settings. *MMWR Recomm Rep*. 2006;55(RR-14):1–17.

Dowell D, Polgreen PM, Beekmann SE, et al. Dilemmas in the management of syphilis: a survey of infectious diseases experts. *Clin Infect Dis*. 2009;49:1526–1529.

Kingston M, French P, Goh B, et al. UK national guidelines on the management of syphilis 2008. *Int J STD AIDS*. 2008;19:729–740.

Miller WC, Ford CA, Morris M, et al. Prevalence of chlamydial and gonococcal infections among young adults in the United States. *JAMA*. 2004;291:2229–2236.

Workowski KA, Berman S. Centers for Disease Control and Prevention (CDC). Sexually transmitted diseases treatment guidelines, 2010. *MMWR Recomm Rep*. 2010;59(RR-12):1–110.

CHAPTER 203

Skin and Soft Tissue Infections

Cameron Ashbaugh, MD

Key Clinical Questions

1. What are the common bacterial causes of cellulitis?
2. How does the presentation help with diagnostic and therapeutic decisions?
3. What is the expected response to treatment?
4. What features suggest more complicated infection?
5. What are strategies for patients with recurrent infections?

INTRODUCTION

Cellulitis is an acute infection involving the epidermis, dermis, and subcutaneous tissues. Most cases are caused by *Staphylococcus aureus* or beta-hemolytic streptococci, although in many patients with presumed infectious cellulitis, a definite bacteriologic diagnosis cannot be made. Occasionally, cellulitis is due to nonbacterial pathogens or noninfectious inflammatory conditions. The costs to society of cellulitis are significant. Up to 2% of hospital admissions are due to cellulitis. While only 7% of patients with cellulitis are admitted to the hospital, hospitalized patients account for 80% of the total health care costs associated with cellulitis.

PATHOPHYSIOLOGY

Healthy skin is resistant to infection. Skin breakdown is usually required for cellulitis to develop. This may be obvious or too subtle to detect. Tinea pedis is an especially common portal of entry for bacteria in lower-extremity cellulitis. Other local risk factors for cellulitis include common skin conditions such as eczema and psoriasis, trauma, intravenous drug use, animal and human bites, venous stasis, and lymphedema. Medical risk factors for cellulitis include diabetes, arterial insufficiency, cirrhosis, renal insufficiency, and neutropenia.

Cellulitis occasionally causes bacteremia. Rarely, cellulitis arises from systemic bacteremia, with secondary seeding of the skin. This is more common in neutropenic patients. These infections lead to bacterial proliferation in the vessel wall, tissue ischemia, and skin necrosis. Clinically, this presents as an area of inflamed skin, with a hemorrhagic pustule that develops into a necrotic ulcer (ecthyma gangrenosum).

CLINICAL PRESENTATION

Cellulitis presents with pain, swelling, and erythema of the skin. In most patients with cellulitis, the margins of erythema are not sharply demarcated. Fever is usually present in patients admitted to the hospital with cellulitis, although it is often absent in milder forms. A minority of patients with cellulitis have enlargement of the draining lymph nodes (lymphadenitis). The bacteriology of cellulitis usually cannot be inferred from the physical examination. However, suppuration and abscess formation is strongly suggestive of *Staphylococcus aureus*. Rapid clinical evolution, lymphangitis, and features of erysipelas (discussed later), such as peau d'orange and a raised, well-demarcated border, suggest beta-hemolytic streptococci. A number of epidemiologic features in cellulitis put patients at risk for particular pathogens. These are summarized in **Table 203-1** and discussed in more detail later in this chapter. As well, several noninfectious conditions may mimic cellulitis. These are summarized in **Table 203-2**.

Bacterial cellulitis should respond to antibiotic therapy after several days of treatment. Disease progression or failure to improve usually reflects infected fluid collections or involvement of tissue deep to the skin. Involvement of deeper tissues and structures should also be suspected in cases of systemic toxicity or disproportionate pain (necrotizing fasciitis), foot ulcers in diabetics (osteomyelitis), cellulitis overlying a joint replacement (infected prosthetic joint), or cellulitis of the abdominal wall (bowel inflammation or enterocutaneous fistula) (**Table 203-3**).

TABLE 203-1 Cellulitis Pathogens Associated with Particular Epidemiology*

Exposure	Pathogen
Dog bite	*Pasteurella multocida, Capnocytophaga sp.*, mixed aerobic and anaerobic flora
Cat bite	*Pasteurella multocida*, mixed aerobic and anaerobic flora
Fish exposure	*Mycobacterium marinum, Erysipelothrix rhusiopathiae, Streptococcus iniae*
Salt water	*Vibrio vulnificus*
Fresh water	*Aeromonas hydrophilia, Edwardsiella tarda, Chromobacterium violaceum*, protothecosis
Cirrhosis	*Vibrio vulnificus* from raw seafood consumption; gram-negative rods
Intravenous drug use	*Eikenella corrodens* and other oral flora, *Pseudomonas aeruginosa* and other gram-negative rods, anaerobes including *Clostridium sp.*
Neutropenia	*Pseudomonas aeruginosa* and other gram-negative rods fungi

**Staphylococcus aureus* and group A streptococcus must be suspected in all patients with cellulitis, regardless of other exposures.

DIAGNOSTIC TESTING

The yield of blood cultures is low in healthy patients with cellulitis, but these should be performed in patients with high fever, systemic toxicity and sepsis, or compromised immunity. Wounds, pustules, and abscesses should be cultured, if present. These have a diagnostic yield of around 10% to 20%. Complete blood count, electrolytes, blood urea nitrogen, creatinine, and glucose should be performed in sicker patients or those with comorbid conditions. An elevated creatine kinase may heighten the clinical suspicion of necrotizing fasciitis or clostridial myonecrosis. Imaging studies

TABLE 203-2 Skin Conditions that Mimic Cellulitis

Condition	Distinguishing Features
Venous stasis	Erythematous, swollen, warm lower extremity with dermatitis and hyperpigmentation; typically bilateral in obese individuals, and unilateral when occurring after saphenous vein harvest or deep venous thrombosis; skin breakdown and ulceration may develop at the medial and lateral malleoli; if there is no bacterial superinfection, fever and leukocytosis will be absent, and clinical improvement occurs with limb elevation and other measures to reduce edema.
Arterial insufficiency	Nonhealing foot wounds with dependent rubor may mimic cellulitis; patients may also have claudication, rest pain, and diminished or absent pedal pulses; if suspected, noninvasive vascular studies, such as ankle-brachial index, should be performed.
Superficial thrombophlebitis	Swelling, induration, and erythema, typically at an intravenous site; palpable cord usually present; fever and leukocytosis absent if no superinfection.
Deep venous thrombosis	Unilateral swollen leg; low-grade fever may be present; superficial veins may be congested, and a cord may be palpable, but physical examination not sensitive; if suspected, obtain duplex ultrasonography.
Contact dermatitis	Weeping skin with vesicles and erythema; well-localized lesion, sometimes with pattern suggestive of irritant exposure; superinfection may occur.
Herpetic whitlow	Swollen painful finger with vesicles; patients are often health care workers, such as dental hygienists or intensive care nurses, who come into contact with the oral cavity and saliva of patients.
Pyoderma gangrenosum	Ragged undermined ulcer, typically on the lower extremity; cultures usually positive as heavily colonized with bacteria; common in inflammatory bowel disease; obtain dermatology consult and biopsy if suspected.
Insect bite	Rapid and sometimes impressive local swelling and erythema, without fever or systemic toxicity; good response to antihistamines; rarely, with spider bites, central necrosis develops.
Erythema nodosum	Hot, warm, tender plaques (panniculitis) involving the shins; seen with sarcoid, rheumatologic disease, fungal infection.
Sweet syndrome	Papules, plaques, and panniculitis involving the head, neck, upper trunk and arms; fever and neutrophilia often present; may be postinfectious syndrome in young person, or a harbinger of hematopoietic malignancy in an older one.
Gout	Exquisitely tender arthritis, often with prominent soft tissue inflammation, involving the great toe, midfoot, knee, and other joints; fever and leukocytosis often prominent; tophi may be present; may complicate hospital admission for other illness.
Calciphylaxis	Painful plaques on the extremities, which may become necrotic; typically occurs in hemodialysis patients with extensive atherosclerosis and high calcium-phosphate product.
Familial Mediterranean fever	Recurrent, brief, self-limited attacks of fever, serositis and erysipelas-like skin erythema; patients are typically of Mediterranean or Middle Eastern descent, and have a positive family history.

TABLE 203-3 Cellulitis: When to Consider Involvement of Deeper Tissues

- Assume necrotizing fasciitis if there is hypotension and cellulitis with severe site pain, especially if the pain is out of proportion to the examination.
- Evaluate for underlying osteomyelitis in diabetic patients with forefoot wounds of more than two weeks duration, or if a probe can be passed to bone.
- Evaluate for infected orthopedic hardware for surgical site cellulitis after joint replacement or fracture fixation.
- Consider underlying bowel inflammation/infection as a cause of cellulitis localized to the abdominal wall

have a limited role in the management of cellulitis. Plain radiographs may reveal a foreign body or gas in the tissues; computed tomography (CT) and magnetic resonance imaging (MRI) may assist in the diagnosis of necrotizing fasciitis.

There are important variants of cellulitis with either distinctive clinical features, bacteriology, or both. These are discussed below.

PRESENTATION PATTERNS AS GUIDES TO DIAGNOSIS

Erysipelas and recurrent cellulitis

Erysipelas and recurrent cellulitis in the absence of a wound are both generally due to streptococci. In erysipelas (**Figure 203-1**), there is skin edema with dimpling similar to the appearance of an orange peel (peau d'orange). Inflammation involving lymphatic drainage may be present as erythematous lines directed to regional lymph nodes (lymphangitic streaking). The draining nodes may be enlarged and tender. Abscesses and chronic skin ulcers are absent. The most typical laboratory abnormality is a polymorphonuclear leukocytosis. The microbiology is usually not determined; rarely blood cultures are positive. The distinctive appearance, occasional positive blood culture, molecular diagnostic studies, and the observation that penicillin is effective therapy lead to the conclusion that these infections are caused by beta-hemolytic streptococci. Group A and group G streptococci are responsible for most cases, group C and group B streptococci account for the remainder.

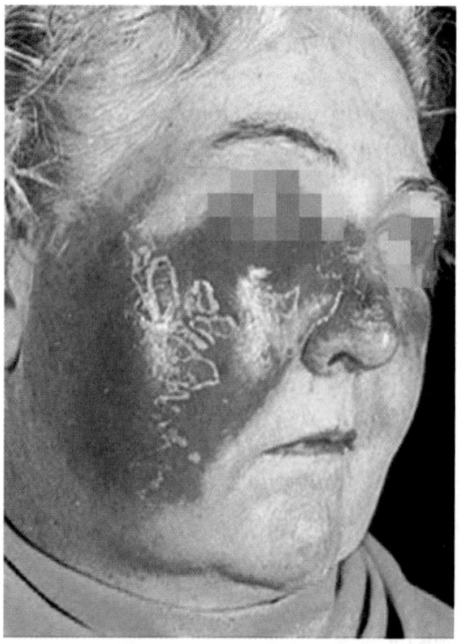

Figure 203-1 *Erysipelas with typical clinical features (superficial, fiery-red, well-demarcated, indurated dermal cellulitis with peau d'orange). Most cases involve the cheeks or extremities. Beta-hemolytic streptococci are responsible. (Reproduced, with permission, from Fauci AS, Braunwald E, Kasper DL, et al. Harrison's Principles of Internal Medicine. 17th ed. New York: McGraw-Hill; 2008, Fig. 130-4.)*

Recurrent cellulitis is often related to underlying anatomic abnormalities. The area of involvement in any given patient is consistent from episode to episode. Many patients have recurrent leg cellulitis in the setting of edema from chronic venous or lymphatic insufficiency, with morbid obesity an increasingly common underlying problem. In these patients, inflammatory changes from chronic venous stasis need to be distinguished from acute cellulitis. Other common sites are the chest wall or the ipsilateral arm after mastectomy, or in the lower extremity after saphenous vein removal for vascular grafting. Onset is sudden, with local pain and rapidly progressive erythema. Associated symptoms include fever, headache, nausea, and myalgias. The time from onset to fully developed cellulitis can be as short as a few hours. Diabetics with arterial insufficiency may also have recurrent cellulitis, often from a persistent focus of infection, such as osteomyelitis, as discussed below.

Necrotizing soft tissue infection

Necrotizing fasciitis is a rapidly progressive infection centered about the deep fascial tissues. Patients complain of severe pain at the site of involvement and frequently present with sepsis syndrome. Early in the course, the overlying skin may appear normal. Later, there is erythema with a waxy unhealthy congested appearance. In the final stages, after thrombosis of the underlying subcutaneous vessels, there is violaceous discoloration and blistering. The severe pain and ill appearance of these patients differentiate them from those with more superficial infection. In unstable patients, surgical exploration with immediate histopathologic review of a biopsy sample is standard care. When the diagnosis is uncertain and the patient is well enough to be transported, imaging may be helpful. CT is more sensitive for gas in the soft tissues (this finding is often absent in necrotizing fasciitis), and MRI is more sensitive for fascial edema. However, both imaging modalities are imprecise in this setting, and the decision to proceed with surgical exploration should be based primarily on clinical grounds.

Periorbital and orbital cellulitis

The soft tissues around the eye are separated from the orbit by the septum, a tough membrane of protective connective tissue. Preseptal, or periorbital, cellulitis is much more common than postseptal, or orbital, cellulitis. Preseptal cellulitis arises from local skin breakdown and inoculation, similarly to cellulitis elsewhere. Postseptal cellulitis may arise from sinusitis, eye surgery, trauma, periodontal infection, and occasionally preseptal cellulitis. Preseptal and postseptal cellulitis may be difficult to distinguish at the bedside. Orbital cellulitis may be diagnosed if proptosis, diplopia, vision loss, and limitation of eye movement are present. The bacteriology of preseptal cellulitis is generally similar to that of other sites. *Haemophilus influenzae* type b was once a common cause of periorbital cellulitis in toddlers, but has become rare with universal childhood vaccination. Orbital cellulitis may involve gram-negative rods and anaerobes, as well as staphylococci and streptococci, especially if it arises from a sinus or odontogenic source. In neutropenic patients or those with diabetic ketoacidosis, mucormycosis should be suspected, and urgent otolaryngology consult should be obtained. CT scan should generally be obtained to delineate the extent of orbital involvement. Ophthalmology consultation is advised if orbital involvement is suspected.

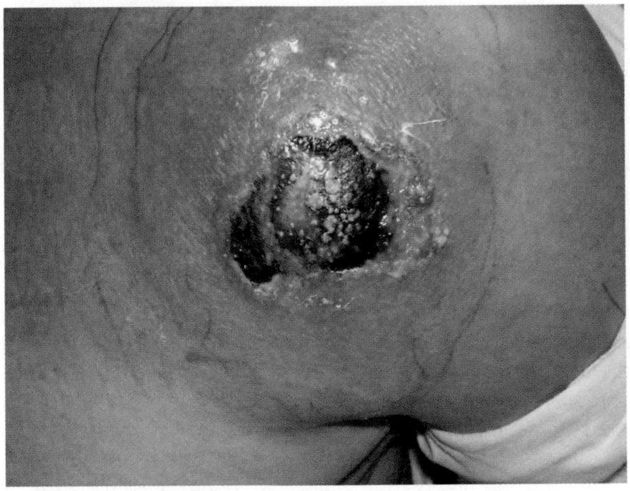

Figure 203-2 *Skin abscess (furuncle) due to methicillin-resistant Staphylococcus aureus. (Courtesy of Gregory Moran, MD.)*

Cellulitis with skin abscess

Infection that arises from a skin abscess is also common. In their simplest form, abscesses (or furuncles) develop in otherwise healthy individuals in the absence of recognized trauma. Onset is over days with progressive local swelling, erythema, and pain. Initially, there is focal induration. Later, as the abscess matures, the central area will suppurate and soften. Skin inflammation is most prominent over the abscess and extends circumferentially. Pain and tenderness are dominant features. Constitutional symptoms are unusual except with large abscesses, where fever and malaise may occur. Compared with streptococcal cellulitis, the evolution of skin abscess and skin erythema is slower, taking place over days rather than hours. *Staphylococcus aureus* causes most skin abscesses. Recurrent furuncles (**Figure 203-2**) are a typical presentation of community-acquired MRSA. Perineal abscesses are due either to *S aureus* or mixtures of aerobic and anaerobic bowel flora.

Cellulitis with wounds, diabetes, or arterial insufficiency

Wound infection with cellulitis is also common. Surgical sites, burns, bites, and lower-extremity ulcers from arterial or venous insufficiency or diabetes are damaged areas with locally impaired immunity. Bacterial infection presents with erythema of the surrounding skin and drainage from the wound. The cellulitis can be minimal or very extensive, as often seen with bite injury or infection of a pressure ulcer in a diabetic foot with arterial insufficiency. The presence of an open wound makes predicting the microbiology difficult. All wounds become colonized with multiple bacteria. All, few, or only one species present in a wound may be pathogenic in a particular patient. However, it is a mistake not to culture wounds due to the concern that these cultures will only identify colonizing species. Wound cultures should be performed to identify possible pathogens and obtain antibiotic susceptibilities to guide final therapeutic choices. In general, *Staphylococcus aureus* and gram-negative rods in wounds are more likely to be significant, and enterococci, coagulase-negative staphylococci, and *Candida* species are less likely pathogenic.

Because of neuropathic injury, arterial insufficiency, and poor neutrophil function, diabetics are at high risk of foot infection. These infections have several unique features. Because of chronic foot ulcers, osteomyelitis is present in about 20% of cases. They are typically polymicrobial, involving gram-positive, gram-negative, and anaerobic bacteria. Tissue oxygenation is often poor in these patients at baseline, and critical limb ischemia may develop quickly in the course of infection. Treatment consists of broad-spectrum antibiotics, surgical consultation for debridement of necrotic tissue and bone, and revascularization if there is clinical and imaging evidence of critical ischemia.

If foot ulcers are present, they should be cultured, but these results are not especially reliable. Cultures obtained during debridement are superior. The diagnosis and management of diabetic foot infections are described in detail in Chapter 145.

As with diabetic patients, cellulitis in the patient with peripheral vascular disease may be a limb-threatening event. These patients may have rest pain, especially in the toes and forefoot, relieved by allowing the foot to hang down over the edge of the bed. The feet are cool and pulseless, with pallor on elevation and reddish-blue discoloration when dependent. Dry, necrotic, nonhealing pedal ulcers may be present, especially on the tips of toes or pressure points such as the malleoli or metatarsal heads. The presence of infection in this setting may lead to wet gangrene and amputation. If suspected, noninvasive vascular studies should be performed, and either vascular surgery or vascular medicine should be involved.

Cellulitis associated with water exposure

Beta-hemolytic streptococci and *S aureus* remain the most common pathogens responsible for acute cellulitis that occurs after water exposure; *Aeromonas*, *Pseudomonas*, and *Vibrio* species are responsible for a significant minority of infections. Episodes typically begin after contamination of an area where there has been minor trauma. The clinical presentation is local pain and tenderness and an enlarging area of skin erythema. If a wound is present, culture can be helpful in identifying the microbiology. In the absence of a wound, a microbiologic diagnosis may not be achieved. An exceptional cause of cellulitis after water exposure is *Vibrio vulnificus* infection. This is sometimes acquired from direct exposure to seawater, but more often is acquired indirectly by eating contaminated, undercooked seafood. Ingestion results in an enteritis, with secondary bacteremia and metastatic skin involvement. Patients with impaired reticuloendothelial bacterial clearance, particularly those with advanced cirrhosis, are especially vulnerable. Inflammation is severe and extensive, often with subcutaneous hemorrhage and the development of "blood lakes" (**Figure 203-3**). Wound and blood cultures are necessary for confirmation.

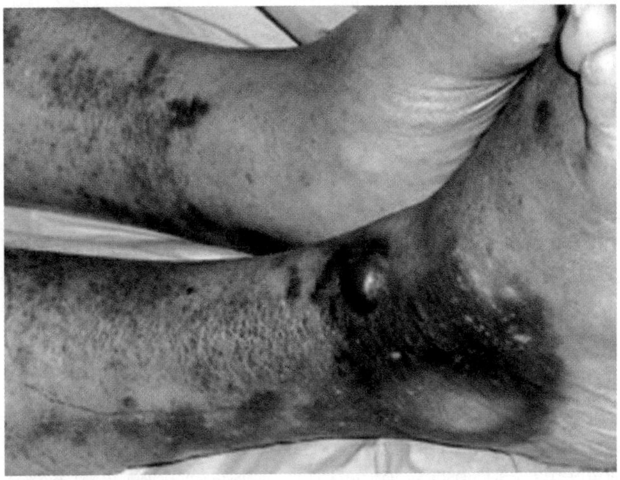

Figure 203-3 *Necrotizing cellulitis with hemorrhagic bullae due to Vibrio vulnificus in a diabetic patient with cirrhosis. (Reproduced, with permission, from Wolff K, Goldsmith LA, Katz SI, et al. Fitzpatrick's Dermatology in General Medicine. 7th ed. New York: McGraw-Hill; 2008. Fig. 183-4.)*

PART VI Clinical Conditions

Cellulitis in immunocompromised patients

Cellulitis in immunosuppressed patients poses special challenges. These patients are susceptible to the usual pathogens causing cellulitis, as well as unusual causes due to inoculation injuries (*Nocardia, Aspergillus,* atypical mycobacteria) or hematogenous dissemination after inhalation (pneumococcus, *Legionella, Cryptococcus, Aspergillus, Penicillium, Nocardia*). Faced with diverse possibilities, it is difficult to choose an empiric antimicrobial regimen with acceptable toxicities and to be certain of activity. In stable patients, particularly those where the presentation is not typical, a preferred approach is to withhold therapy pending results of skin biopsy for culture and histopathologic examination. Cultures should be sent for routine aerobic and anaerobic bacterial, fungal, and mycobacterial culture; pathology should include special stains for microorganisms.

DIFFERENTIAL DIAGNOSIS

Lyme disease

Early Lyme disease commonly presents with skin erythema extending circumferentially from the site of a tick bite. Erythema migrans is classically a target lesion with intense erythema peripherally and central pallor, but lesions with uniform erythema are common, and even central blistering with necrosis occurs occasionally. Unlike streptococcal cellulitis, the erythema is circular or ovoid. Unlike cellulitis associated with skin abscess, there is no localized fluid collection. Flu-like symptoms with fever, arthralgias, and myalgias are common in early Lyme disease, but do not help to distinguish it from cellulitis. In areas of high incidence, possible or confirmed tick exposure and a typical rash are sufficient for a clinical diagnosis and initiation of antibiotic therapy.

Noninfectious processes mistaken for infectious cellulitis

Patients with *chronic venous insufficiency* may develop dermatitis and acute inflammation, most commonly in the lower leg. Both lower extremities are usually involved, although when the venous injury is due to antecedent trauma or venous clot, inflammation may be restricted to a single limb. Critical to the development of dermatitis is chronic edema. Over time, the skin becomes indurated and develops a characteristic nodular appearance, often with bronze or purple-brown hyperpigmentation from hemosiderin deposition. Inflammation may be sufficient to appear as uniform erythema. By contrast to bacterial infection, the area of involvement is often bilateral, the site is not tender, systemic signs of infection are absent, and the erythema improves rapidly over 8 to 24 hours with limb elevation.

Gout presents as severe pain centered around a joint. The first metatarsal-phalangeal joint is the most common location, but involvement in any joint is reported. Low-grade fever and joint erythema are typical. Occasionally, joint inflammation spills over into the periarticular soft tissues. Joint localization is helpful in distinguishing gout from isolated bacterial cellulitis, but does not exclude skin infection associated with septic arthritis. Joint fluid analysis is needed to distinguish a gout attack from an infected joint.

Insect bites can induce a local hypersensitivity reaction with edema and erythema. Cases are more common in the warm and wet seasons of the year, when populations of mosquitoes and other biting insects are highest. Lesions are pruritic with circumferential erythema, and abscess formation is unusual. Modest fever is possible; high fever is unusual. Inflammation may be severe enough to merit treatment with a systemic corticosteroid.

Inflammation after *vaccine injection* can be confused with bacterial skin infection. Erythema, malaise, fever, and local tenderness are usually mild, but in the rare patient can be substantial. Localization to the upper arm and vaccination within the past 72 hours, especially with pneumococcal vaccine, are highly suggestive. Bacterial infection at the injection site must be considered, but is less common than sterile inflammation.

TRIAGE AND HOSPITAL ADMISSION

Patients presenting with fever, pain, and rapidly advancing erythema; patients failing outpatient therapy; patients with hemodynamic instability; patients with comorbidities such as peripheral vascular disease, diabetes, or chronic venous insufficiency that may complicate or delay resolution of cellulites; and patients with immune deficiency are best admitted to the hospital. Infectious disease consultation should be considered in patients who have immune deficiency, severe cellulitis, or who fail to respond to the initial antibiotic regimen. Other patients with cellulitis may be managed outside the hospital with oral antibiotics and careful observation unless the patient has cognitive, compliance, or other social issues that might jeopardize care. Necrotizing soft tissue infection is a medical emergency and requires a multidisciplinary approach, including surgical consultation at the time of presentation.

TREATMENT

In general, the first dose of the antibiotic should be promptly administered. Parenteral therapy with an antibiotic that has an appropriate spectrum of activity against the suspected organism and a long half-life is optimal for the patient likely to be discharged after a brief period of observation.

Cefazolin has good activity against both streptococci and methicillin-sensitive *Staphylococcus aureus* (MSSA) and is a reasonable first choice in patients with mild to moderate cellulitis at low risk for MRSA infection. Clindamycin is a reasonable alternative in penicillin-allergic patients. In patients with moderate to severe cellulitis, or those with risk factors for MRSA (**Table 203-4**), an antibiotic with coverage against MRSA, such as vancomycin, daptomycin, tigecycline, or linezolid, is appropriate. It is also wise to assume MRSA infection when patients have already failed outpatient treatment with a drug active against MSSA, such as cephalexin or dicloxacillin.

PRACTICE POINT

- Erythema often increases in extent in the first 24 to 48 hours after admission, despite adequate antibiotic therapy.
- Areas of cellulitis will appear more discolored when dependent or after bathing the area in warm water.
- Erythema under these conditions does not indicate treatment failure if other symptoms and signs of infection are improving.
- Avoid the temptation to modify antibiotic early in the course of therapy, particularly for erythema alone.

TABLE 203-4 Epidemiologic Risk Factors for Methicillin-Resistant *Staphylococcus Aureus* Colonization

• Prior colonization	• HIV infection
• History of boils	• Injection drug use
• Antibiotic use in the past 3 months	• Incarceration in the past year
• Health care admission in the past year	• Chronic hemodialysis
	• Men who have sex with men

> **PRACTICE POINT**
>
> - Cellulitis in the setting of venous or lymphatic insufficiency may be slow to resolve, and aggressive measures to reduce edema, such as compression stockings and elevation of the extremity above the level of the heart, may speed resolution of infection. In morbidly obese patients with cellulitis, ensure that the antibiotic dose is adequate for the patient's body mass index.

Necrotizing soft tissue infection

Patients with suspected necrotizing fasciitis require prompt surgical exploration and debridement. For streptococcal or clostridial necrotizing fasciitis, penicillin and clindamycin combination therapy is customary. Clindamycin is used because it may be more effective than penicillin against bacteria in the stationary phase of the cell cycle, and because it decreases protein and toxin synthesis. In patients with necrotizing fasciitis due to group A streptococci, intravenous immune globulin (IVIG) may decrease mortality, possibly by blunting the superantigen response in toxic shock syndrome. If MRSA is suspected as the cause of necrotizing fasciitis, vancomycin should be added. Patients with necrotizing fasciitis involving the perineum or surgical wounds should receive antibiotic therapy directed at enteric gram-negative rods and anaerobes. Possible regimens include a third- or fourth-generation cephalosporin plus metronidazole, piperacillin-tazobactam, or a carbapenem.

Erysipelas or recurrent cellulitis in the absence of a wound

All strains remain susceptible to penicillin, cephalosporins, carbapenems, beta-lactam–beta-lactamase inhibitor combinations, vancomycin, and linezolid. Most strains are susceptible to fluoroquinolones with expanded activity against gram-positive bacteria. Drug allergy, interactions with other medications, ease of administration, and cost all influence the choice of antibiotic in an individual patient. Penicillin remains appealing due to its narrow spectrum of activity. Symptomatic improvement with decrease in fever, malaise, and pain is expected in 24 hours. Skin erythema is slower to resolve and often extends for the first 48 hours. Even after improvement, erythema will be more prominent when the affected area is dependent or after bathing in warm water. The absence of a microbiologic diagnosis, the early progression of skin inflammation on therapy, and the situational changes in skin appearance commonly lead to escalation of antibiotic therapy. In this setting, drug allergies often further complicate management. The inclination to change therapy in the first few days of administration should be resisted unless there is additional evidence of clinical deterioration. Once improvement is clear, oral administration of an antibiotic can be substituted for intravenous therapy. Antibiotics are continued for 5 to 10 days. Shorter courses are acceptable if the skin appearance is at a prior baseline.

Cellulitis associated with skin abscess

Early administration of an antibiotic before lesions reach the point of suppuration may be sufficient for cure, but usually clinical improvement only begins when an abscess drains, either from spontaneous rupture or incision. Community-acquired MRSA must be assumed when making empiric antibiotic choices. Doxycycline, trimethoprim-sulfamethoxazole, and linezolid are predictably active oral agents against MRSA. Clindamycin and fluoroquinolones may be active, but should not be used in the absence of susceptibility data. Intravenous vancomycin or daptomycin are additional options for sicker patients. Antibiotic coverage for patients presenting with a perineal abscess should include agents active against MRSA as well as bowel flora. Independent of the location, incision, and disruption of internal compartments within the abscess cavity is the most effective therapy. Small abscesses may be incised at the bedside. Adequate local anesthesia is difficult to achieve, so both patient and physician need to be prepared for some patient discomfort. Abscesses wider than several centimeters are best drained in the operating room or under conscious sedation or general anesthesia. Purulent fluid recovered at abscess drainage should be cultured to provide a microbiologic diagnosis and susceptibility data. If the debridement is complete and the cellulitis is confined to several centimeters around the abscess, antibiotic therapy can be discontinued after the procedure. If pockets of infected fluid are left or the cellulitis is more extensive, antibiotics should be continued until erythema and induration improve. A typical course of antibiotic would be three to five days. Antibiotic susceptibility information is used to refine empiric antibiotic choices. Oral administration is effective, unless the pathogen is only susceptible to an antibiotic that must be given intravenously.

Cellulitis associated with wounds including bites

Prior to culture information, empiric antibiotic choices are influenced by the history of the wound and the stability of the patient. In early infection and otherwise stable patients without recent medical care, antibiotic exposure, or history of MRSA colonization (confirmed or prior boils), therapy can be directed toward streptococcal species, methicillin-sensitive *Staphylococcus aureus*, and sensitive *Enterobacteraciae*. Cefazolin or nafcillin plus a quinolone are generally active for these infections. In medically experienced patients at higher risk for infections with antibiotic-resistant bacteria or unstable patients with limb- or life-threatening infections, combinations of drugs with activity against MRSA (vancomycin, linezolid, or daptomycin) and multidrug-resistant nosocomial pathogens (cefepime, imipenem, or piperacillin-tazobactam) should be used.

Infected bite wounds should be empirically treated with agents active against beta-hemolytic streptococci, MSSA, and the oral flora of the biting species: in humans, oral anaerobes such as *Eikenella corrodens*, in cats *Pasturella multocida*, and in dogs *Capnocytophaga canimorsus*. Cefepime, ampicillin-sulbactam, and imipenem are all usually active against these pathogens. When results of wound cultures are available, complex regimens should be simplified to minimize risks of antibiotic exposure to the individual patient (drug reactions) and to the population (development of antimicrobial drug resistance). Initial therapy is with intravenous antibiotic or with oral agents that have excellent bioavailability. After clinical improvement, oral antibiotics can be substituted for intravenous agents if the susceptibility data is favorable. Duration of antibiotic is usually between 7 and 14 days, with therapy being stopped when erythema and purulent wound discharge are resolved.

Cellulitis associated with seawater exposure

Empiric treatment is directed at *Vibrio* species and other gram negatives associated with marine exposure. Combination therapy is used: doxycycline in combination with a second agent, such as cefepime, a carbapenem, or a fluoroquinolone, has demonstrated superior efficacy for *Vibrio* infection based on animal and limited human studies. In patients who are critically ill or who have risk factors for MRSA infection, an additional agent directed at MRSA is included. Empiric regimens should be simplified based on culture results. Cellulitis associated with freshwater exposure involve *Aeromonas*, *Edwardsiella*, or *Pseudomonas*. Appropriate regimens include cefepime, a fluoroquinolone, or a carbapenem.

Cellulitis in immunocompromised hosts

In stable patients with typical presentations, therapy may be identical to that described above for normal hosts. In odd presentations, therapy should be deferred until information from culture and pathology is available to guide the choice of agent. In unstable patients, antibiotic therapy directed at MRSA, streptococci, and drug-resistant enteric and nonenteric gram-negative rods is recommended (vancomycin, linezolid, or daptomycin, plus cefepime, imipenem, or piperacillin-tazobactam).

COMPLICATIONS

It is not unusual for the borders of inflammation to advance during the first 48 hours after admission despite effective antibiotic therapy. The delay often precipitates multiple medication changes. A common complication in this setting is the development of rash due to drug allergy. Except when systemic deterioration takes place, antibiotic changes within the first 72 hours of admission should be resisted.

Failure of cellulitis to improve after 72 hours is unexpected and suggests that there is either occult collection of infected fluid or that deep tissues are involved. CT or MRI are useful for exploring these possibilities. Surgical consultation should be obtained if the studies are abnormal. *Clostridium difficile* colitis may complicate any course of antibiotic therapy.

Osteomyelitis

Cellulitis with osteomyelitis is common in infected fracture repairs with draining wounds and in diabetic foot ulcers. In wounds that probe to bone or are refractory to usual antibiotics for cellulitis, bone infection should be considered. MRI helps to identify osteomyelitis in diabetic foot infection. Infected fractures usually present in the early postoperative period with cellulitis and drainage along an incision line. Wound debridement with bone biopsy for microbiologic diagnosis and prolonged antibiotic therapy are critical for optimal management of these infections.

PREVENTION OF RECURRENCE

RECURRENT STREPTOCOCCAL CELLULITIS

Patients with recurrent streptococcal cellulitis require a plan at hospital discharge to prevent future recurrence. Strategies include long-term prophylaxis or preemptive therapy. If episodes are frequent, prophylaxis with oral penicillin is effective in decreasing the number of episodes. The dose required needs to be determined empirically and may range from 250 mg twice daily to 1 g four times daily. In patients with less-frequent episodes or in those with breakthrough infection on prophylactic therapy, administration of an antibiotic at the first typical symptoms and signs is effective in preventing hospitalization. A fluoroquinolone with extended gram-positive bacteria activity or linezolid is effective. The first dose should be double the usual maintenance dose to rapidly achieve therapeutic concentrations.

RECURRENT CELLULITIS ASSOCIATED WITH BOILS

Patients who experience one episode of *S aureus* skin abscess are at risk for future episodes. Antibiotic therapy to eradicate carriage or chronic suppressive antibiotics can be helpful in patients with recurrent staphylococcal abscesses. The optimal regimen for eradication of colonization has not been established. In patients without chronic wounds or dermatitis, the combination of one to four weeks of oral doxycycline 100 mg twice daily and rifampin 600 mg once daily, with topical mupirocin to the nares twice daily and chlorhexidine skin baths twice daily during the final week of week of oral antibiotic therapy, has been successful. Isolates must be susceptible to the oral regimen for treatment to be effective. Rifampin has many problematic drug interactions and should not be used before careful review of a patient's medications. When eradication

TABLE 203-5 Evidence-based Medicine: Key References for Cellulites

Study	Methodology	Results	Limitations	Bottom Line
Siljander T, et al. *Clin Inf Dis.* 2008;43:855–861.	Case control study of 90 patients with acute cellulites and 90 matched controls. Skin, web space, throat, and blood cultures.	Group G streptococcus (GGS) grew from skin or blood in 26/90 cases. GAS recovered in 6/90 cases.	Study group was limited to hospitalized patients.	GGS and GAS are common causes of acute cellulitis.
McNamara DR, et al. *Mayo Clin Proc.* 2007;82:817–821.	Population-based survey of all diagnoses of lower-limb cellulitis.	Incidence of lower-limb cellulitis was 199 per 100,000 persons; 21.6% had a recurrence within 2 years.	Retrospective study relying on clinical diagnosis.	Acute cellulitis is common, with rate similar to hip fracture and symptomatic kidney stone.
Moet GJ, et al. *Diag Micro Infect Dis.* 2007;57:7–13.	International hospital survey from North America, Europe, and South America. Each institute sent 50 consecutive isolated cultured from pyogenic wounds.	*Staphylococcus aureus* was the most frequent isolate from skin and soft tissue infections in all 3 continents tested.	No individual patient detail.	*Staphylococcus aureus* is the dominant isolate from wounds around the world.
Ruhe JJ, et al. *Clin Infect Dis.* 2007; 44:777–784.	Retospective cohort study of 492 adult patients with community-acquired MRSA skin and soft tissue infection, comparing outcome after surgical drainage between patients receiving active (312) or inactive (190) antibiotic.	Treatment successful in 296 of 312 patients (95%) receiving active vs. 190 of 219 (87%) patients receiving inactive.	Retrospective study.	Incision and drainage for localized MRSA soft tissue infection is sufficient in the majority of, but not all, infections.

MRSA, methicillin-resistant *Staphylococcus aureus.*

is not feasible due to chronic wounds, drug interactions, or failure of therapy to eradicate colonization, then chronic antibiotic administration may decrease the number of episodes. Choice is guided by susceptibility, drug interactions, and side effects. Oral doxycycline, trimethoprim-sulfamethoxazole, fluoroquinolones, and clindamycin may all be effective. If therapy seems efficacious, it should be continued for several months and then discontinued, and the patient should be observed for recurrence.

DISCHARGE CONSIDERATIONS

Once systemic symptoms resolve, the white blood cell count falls toward normal levels, and there is some improvement in skin appearance, patients may be discharged to outpatient care. Intravenous antibiotics should be discontinued and oral antibiotic therapy should be started. The serum concentration of beta-lactam antibiotics is significantly lower after oral administration, as compared with after intravenous administration. In more severe cases of cellulitis treated initially with a beta-lactam antibiotic, it may be safer to transition to oral therapy with a fluoroquinolone, clindamycin, or linezolid if the known or predicted bacterial susceptibilities are favorable, as these agents all have excellent bioavailability. Patients should have a follow-up exam within 10 to 14 days after discharge to confirm resolution of skin infection, assess for complications of antibiotic therapy, and to be educated about preventive measures including foot care.

QUALITY IMPROVEMENT

There is little published literature on quality improvement in cellulitis management. However, there are several possible target measures for quality improvement programs. An interested infectious diseases specialist or hospitalist with special expertise could sample cellulitis admissions in real time to see if the diagnosis of cellulitis is correct, if hospitalization is necessary, and if appropriate antibiotics are being administered. Chart reviews could establish whether diabetics with cellulitis received appropriate education regarding foot care and whether appropriate follow-up and aftercare was arranged. Quality measures in patients with recurrent cellulitis should include the following as appropriate: consideration of MRSA eradication, management of comorbid diabetes and vascular insufficiency, seeking out and treating tinea pedis, and consideration of prophylactic antibiotics (**Table 203-5**).

SUGGESTED READINGS

Bernard P. Management of common bacterial infections of the skin. *Curr Opin Infect Dis*. 2008;21:122–128.

Collier DN. Cutaneous infections from coastal and marine bacteria. *Derm Ther*. 2002;15:1–9.

Eron LJ. Cellulitis and soft tissue infections. *Annals of Internal Medicine*. 2009;150:ITC–1

Goettsch WG, Bouwes Bavinck JN, Herings RM. Burden of illness of bacterial cellulitis and erysipelas of the leg in the Netherlands. *J Eur Acad Dermatol Venereol*. 2006;20:834–839.

Lipsky BA, Berendt AR, Deery HG, et al. Diagnosis and treatment of diabetic foot infections. *Clin Infect Dis*. 2004:39:885–910.

Moellering RC. A 39 year-old man with a skin infection. *JAMA*. 2008;299:79–87.

Stevens DL, Bisno AL, Chambers HF, et al. Practice guidelines for the diagnosis and management of skin and soft tissue infections. *Clin Infect Dis*. 2005;4:1373–1406.

Stevens DL. Treatments for skin and soft-tissue and surgical site infections due to mdr gram-positive bacteria. *J Infection*. 2009;59(S1):S32–S39.

CHAPTER 204

Tuberculosis

Michael Gardam, MSc, MD, CM, MSc, FRCPC
Susy Hota, MD, MSc, FRCPC

Key Clinical Questions

1. When should tuberculosis be suspected in the inpatient setting?
2. What diagnostic testing should be performed in patients with suspected tuberculosis?
3. What precautions are necessary for patients with possible tuberculosis? When may they be discontinued?
4. What treatment regimen should be begun for patients with newly diagnosed tuberculosis? What monitoring is appropriate in patients being treated for tuberculosis?

INTRODUCTION

A global pandemic of tuberculosis (TB) that began three centuries ago continues today. According to estimates from the World Health Organization, 14 million people had active TB in 2009, including 9.4 million new cases, with 1.7 million deaths. The ongoing human immunodeficiency virus (HIV) epidemic continues to fuel the spread of TB; 12% of patients with the disease are HIV positive. The incidence of TB is highest in Asia, Africa, Latin America, Russia, and Eastern Europe (**Figure 204-1**). Rates are substantially lower in North America and Western Europe, where TB is increasingly a disease of the foreign born. Other groups in developed nations with a high incidence of the disease include homeless persons, injection drug users, incarcerated persons, and some aboriginal populations. Another group at risk in developed nations is the elderly. Rates of TB in the developed world 50 years ago were similar to rates in developing countries today. Older patients born and raised in developed nations therefore have a higher likelihood of developing active TB than younger patients, due to the risk of late reactivation of latent infection.

As TB in the developed world has become uncommon, the diagnosis is often overlooked, even when in retrospect it should have been fairly apparent. Unfortunately, because pulmonary TB may be highly contagious, delays in diagnosis may have disastrous implications not only for the patient, but also for family, friends, and other close contacts, including health care workers.

PATHOPHYSIOLOGY

Tuberculosis is caused almost exclusively by *Mycobacterium tuberculosis*. Rarely, it is caused by the related organism *Mycobacterium bovis*, acquired from infected cattle or contaminated milk products. *M tuberculosis* is transmitted almost exclusively through the respiratory route by microscopic droplet nuclei. These particles are small enough to remain airborne for long periods of time and to be inhaled directly into the terminal alveoli, typically in the lower lung zones. Droplet nuclei are produced when a patient with pulmonary TB speaks, coughs, or sneezes. Rarely, they are produced from nonpulmonary sources, such as irrigation of TB-infected areas during surgery, during dressing changes of draining wounds, or while emptying of containers of infectious fluid.

M tuberculosis has adapted to survive within alveolar macrophages, the cells one would normally expect to eradicate it. Within the macrophage, the organism travels to the mediastinal lymph nodes, then disseminates throughout the body via the bloodstream, with more vascular areas receiving more organisms. Microscopic foci of live bacteria are thus deposited throughout the body, including the lung apices. Several weeks after infection, the cellular immune system walls off the bacteria in granulomas. Granulomas are not static structures; the organisms within them are alive, albeit dormant, and the cells forming the granuloma constantly turn over. At this stage, the infected individual has what is referred to as *latent tuberculosis infection*. Patients with latent infection are neither ill nor infectious to others. Roughly 85% to 90% of otherwise healthy individuals in this state never develop symptoms throughout their lifetime, despite ongoing infection. Of the 10% to 15% who do go on to develop symptoms, most do so within the first few years of becoming infected. Once symptoms have developed, the patient is referred to as having *active tuberculosis*. Although there is a predilection for disease to develop in the apices of the lungs, a

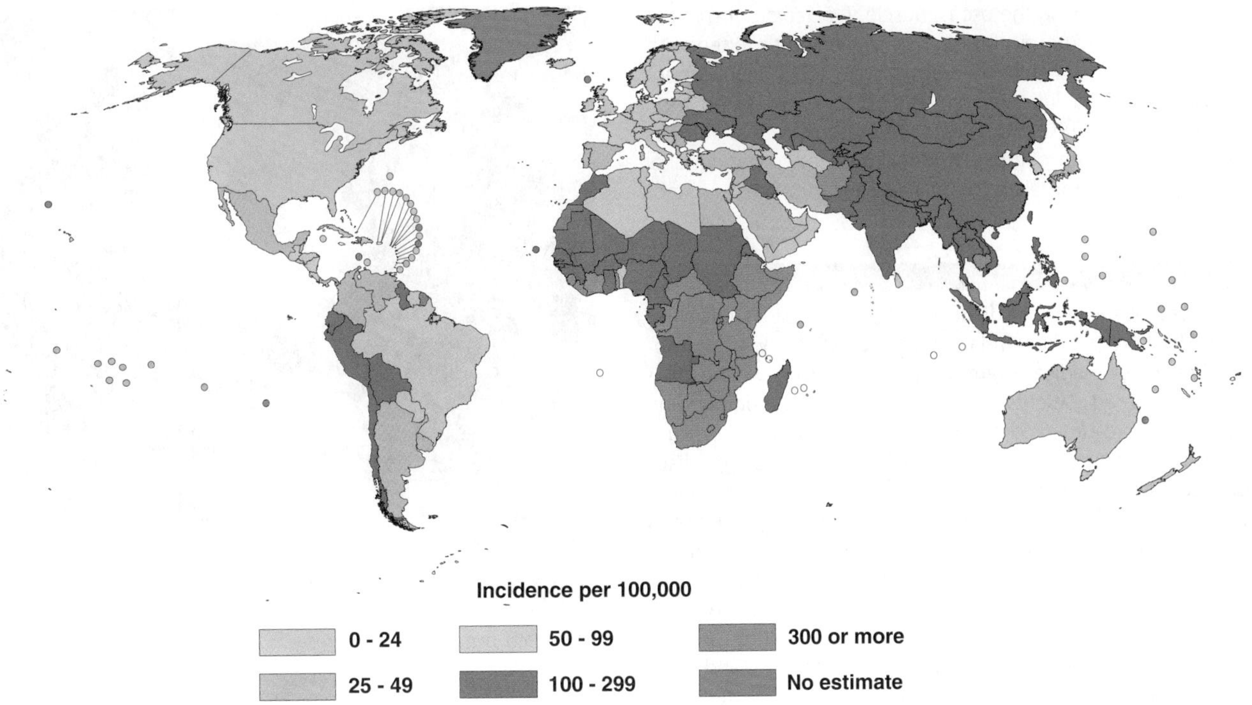

Figure 204-1 *Tuberculosis incidence in 2005, based on World Health Organization data. (Courtesy of the Stop TB Department, WHO; with permission.)*

large minority of patients will develop symptoms outside the lungs. Commonly involved extrapulmonary sites include regional lymph nodes, pleura, spine, bones and joints, and meninges. Patients with certain underlying medical conditions or receiving immunosuppressive therapy are at high risk of developing active disease if infected (**Table 204-1**).

PRACTICE POINT

- About 25% to 50% of patients with extrapulmonary TB also have active pulmonary tuberculosis. Although extrapulmonary tuberculosis is not usually contagious, chest imaging is indicated in these patients to exclude concomitant pulmonary disease.

CLINICAL PRESENTATION

Unfortunately, the symptoms of active TB are often vague and nonspecific, sometimes leading to initial misdiagnosis. It is common for a TB clinic to see patients who were initially investigated for malignancy. Patients typically report having had symptoms for weeks to months prior to being diagnosed. In some cases, symptom onset can be so gradual that patients realize the extent of their illness only after they have improved with treatment. Early cases can be entirely asymptomatic, having been detected on a chest radiograph performed for other reasons. Rarely, patients present with acute symptoms, mimicking more typical bacterial infections, or they may develop disseminated (miliary) TB, with a rapidly progressive febrile wasting illness, with or without pulmonary complaints.

Constitutional symptoms such as weight loss, fatigue, fever, night sweats, and rigors tend to be more common with pulmonary and pleural disease, together with a worsening productive cough. Although massive hemoptysis was once common in the preantibiotic era, hemoptysis is rare and, if present, is typically minor. Constitutional symptoms may be absent in cases of extrapulmonary TB, especially in patients with disease confined to lymph nodes. *Tuberculous lymphadenitis* is the most common form of extrapulmonary TB. It usually presents as painless swelling of the posterior cervical or supraclavicular lymph nodes, although patients may also develop lymph node tenderness and fistula formation. *Pleural tuberculosis* may present with fever, dyspnea, and pleuritic chest pain if the effusion is sizable enough. *Genitourinary tuberculosis* may present with dysuria, urinary frequency, flank pain, and hematuria, although it may also often be asymptomatic until hydronephrosis and severe kidney damage have occurred. *Spinal tuberculosis* (Pott disease) most often presents with back pain from infection of the thoracic or lumbar spine, often with paravertebral

TABLE 204-1 Risk Factors for Active Tuberculosis Among Persons Who Have Been Infected with Tuberculosis

Factor	Relative Risk/Odds
Recent infection (< 1 year)	12.9
Fibrotic lesions (spontaneously healed)	2–20
Comorbidity	
HIV infection	100
Silicosis	30
Chronic renal failure/hemodialysis	10–25
Diabetes	2–4
Intravenous drug use	10–30
Immunosuppressive treatment	10
Gastrectomy	2–5
Jejunoileal bypass	30–60
Posttransplantation period (renal, cardiac)	20–70
Malnutrition and severe underweight	2

Reproduced, with permission, from Fauci AS, Braunwald E, Kasper DL, et al. Harrison's Principles of Internal Medicine, 17th ed. New York: McGraw-Hill, 2008. Table 158-1.

cold abscesses involving the psoas muscle. *Tuberculous meningitis* presents as a subacute or chronic basilar meningitis, often with cranial nerve palsies; central nervous system (CNS) involvement may also produce a *tuberculoma,* leading to seizures and focal neurologic deficits. *Tuberculous peritonitis* presents with abdominal pain and ascites, with diffuse peritoneal implants on abdominal imaging; it is often mistaken for ovarian cancer or other intraabdominal malignancies.

DIAGNOSIS

The greatest obstacle to the diagnosis of tuberculosis is the failure to consider it in the differential diagnosis. Patients with pulmonary TB may seek medical attention several times before the diagnosis is considered. Patients may be treated with fluoroquinolone antibiotics for presumed community-acquired pneumonia, resulting in temporary improvement that may further delay the diagnosis and lead to potentially more contacts becoming infected. Patients with extrapulmonary TB often undergo diagnostic tests focused on detecting malignancy rather than TB. For example, patients with tuberculous lymphadenitis may have excisional lymph node biopsies to exclude lymphoma, without tissue being sent for mycobacterial culture. TB should be clinically suspected in patients who present with compatible symptoms and have epidemiologic risk factors for infection or progression to active disease. For example, pulmonary TB should be considered in a patient originally from an endemic area with chronic renal failure and a new cough. Once suspected, the diagnosis can usually be confirmed with appropriate testing without great difficulty, although there are exceptions as mentioned below.

RADIOLOGY

Basic chest radiography is useful in diagnosing pulmonary TB, especially if cavities (**Figure 204-2**) or evidence of prior TB infection is present, such as apical scarring or pleural thickening. Rarely, tiny miliary nodules are seen (**Figure 204-3**). Computed tomography (CT) and magnetic resonance imaging (MRI) scans are more appropriate for diagnosing spinal TB, meningitis, pericarditis, and TB of deep organs or organ spaces. Although radiographic findings can be typical for TB, they are rarely pathognomonic; hence the collection of fluid or tissue for histology and mycobacterial culture is essential to confirm the diagnosis.

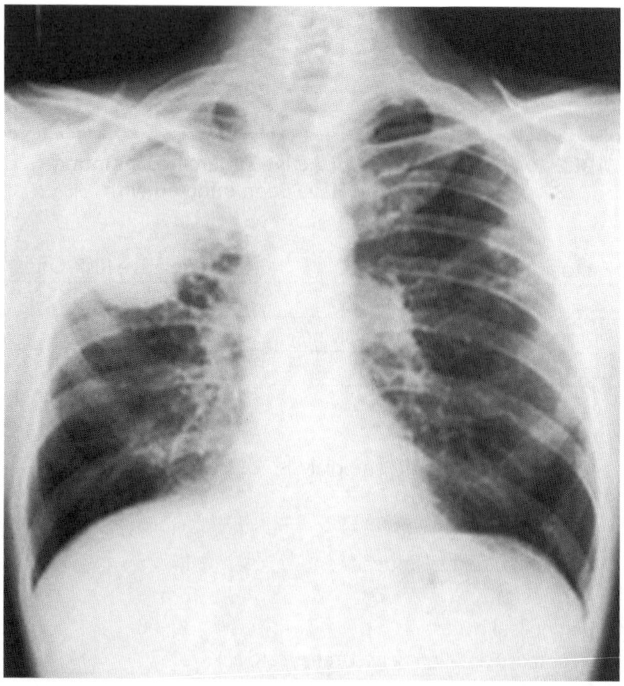

Figure 204-2 *Cavitary upper lobe tuberculosis. (Reproduced, with permission, from Tintinalli JE, Kelen GD, Stapczynski JS. Tintinalli's Emergency Medicine: A Comprehensive Study Guide. 6th ed. New York: McGraw-Hill; 2004. Fig. 70-2.)*

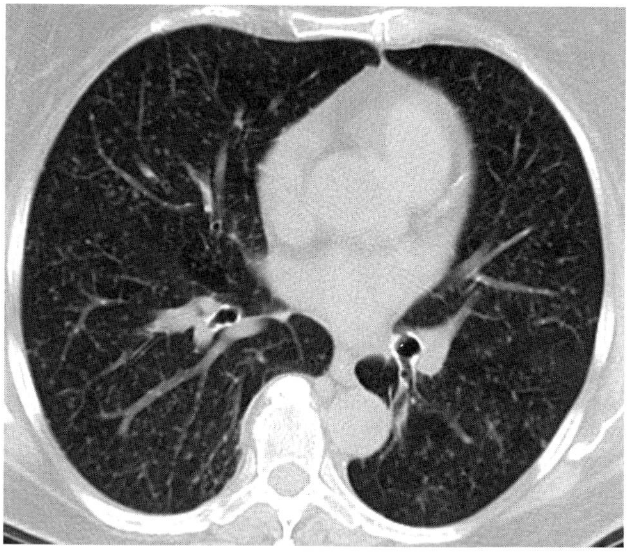

Figure 204-3 *Miliary tuberculosis: innumerable small pulmonary nodules, 1 to 3 mm in diameter, in a patient with rheumatoid arthritis treated with a tumor necrosis factor inhibitor. (Courtesy of John J. Ross, MD.)*

MICROBIOLOGIC TESTING

When a specimen arrives in the lab for TB testing, part of the specimen is concentrated, smeared on a slide, and then stained with a fluorochrome stain followed by fuchsin confirmation stain to visualize the presence of acid-fast bacilli (**Figure 204-4**). Usually, these represent *Mycobacteria* species, but *Nocardia, Rhodococcus* species are weakly acid-fast and may be detected with these stains as well. Rapid nucleic acid amplification tests (NAATs) that may be performed in three to five hours are now available to detect *M tuberculosis* complex nucleic acids on smear-positive specimens. A positive smear with a positive NAAT is presumptive evidence that *M tuberculosis* is present. A negative smear cannot rule out a diagnosis of TB, as the concentration of TB bacilli present may simply have been below the limit of detection, or the specimen may have been inadequate. In such instances, if the clinical suspicion remains, it is best to wait for the mycobacterial culture result or consider repeat sampling.

M tuberculosis takes up to eight weeks for growth and identification, using traditional solid mycobacterial culture media. Many laboratories have adopted more rapid techniques, incubating the specimen in broth and using molecular methods or analysis of mycolic acids by chromatography for species identification. In most instances, this allows for growth and identification of *M tuberculosis* within two to three weeks. Drug susceptibility testing takes an additional one to two weeks.

Microbiologic identification of TB is affected by the type and quality of specimen submitted to the lab. In pulmonary TB, the most sensitive methods of isolating the organism are induced sputum collection and bronchoalveolar lavage. Induced sputum collection involves inhalation of a nebulized hypertonic saline solution to generate a hearty cough. Unfortunately, the process

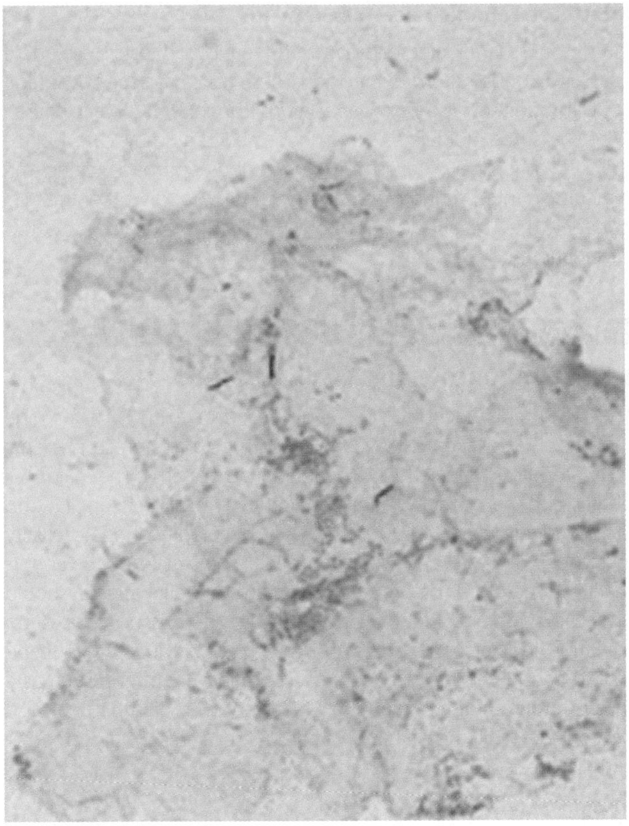

Figure 204-4 *Positive Ziehl-Neelsen sputum stain, with magenta-colored acid-fast bacilli on a blue background. (Courtesy of the Centers for Disease Control and Prevention.)*

is labor-intensive and requires the supervision of a respiratory therapist. The alternative is to collect multiple spontaneously expectorated sputum specimens, best collected on three consecutive mornings. This ensures a deeper, more concentrated sample, especially if the patient is not terribly symptomatic with cough. For those who are very symptomatic, it may not be necessary to wait a day between specimens; they can be collected every eight hours.

PRACTICE POINT

- Tuberculosis is more common at all stages of HIV disease. In HIV-positive patients with relatively normal CD4+ counts, it usually presents with upper lobe fibrocavitary lung disease, similar to that seen in HIV-negative patients. Patients with acquired immunodeficiency syndrome (AIDS) and pulmonary TB have a variety of clinical presentations, from massive hilar and mediastinal lymphadenopathy to primary pneumonia and nodular and miliary patterns. Cavitation is typically absent. Extrapulmonary TB is seen in 50% of AIDS patients, compared with approximately 40% of HIV-negative patients. Diagnosis of TB is more difficult in AIDS, as sputum smears more often negative, perhaps because of the absence of chest cavities.

Identifying *M tuberculosis* on smear and culture can be more difficult in cases of extrapulmonary TB. This is especially true for tuberculous meningitis, peritonitis, pericarditis, and pleural disease. In these cases, the smear result is typically negative, and the culture result is also often negative, but the pathology may demonstrate granulomas or even acid-fast bacilli embedded in the tissue (finding these in biopsy specimens may require a large number of tissue sections and a very dedicated pathologist, as acid-fast bacilli may be scant in extrapulmonary TB). Therefore, all biopsy specimens should be sent to both pathology and microbiology laboratories.

TABLE 204-2 Indications to Initiate Isolation for Suspected Tuberculosis

Cough and chest radiograph suggestive of tuberculosis (apical infiltrate, cavitary lesion, military pattern, infiltrate with mediastinal adenopathy)
Positive smear for acid-fast bacilli
Known tuberculosis of uncertain status (ie, adequacy of treatment uncertain)
HIV infection with undiagnosed pulmonary condition
Patients with tuberculosis risk factors and undiagnosed pulmonary infiltrates

HIV, human immunodeficiency virus.

INFECTION CONTROL

Once the diagnosis of TB is considered in a hospitalized patient, it is critically important to immediately assess the risk of the organism spreading to patients and staff. The decision to initiate airborne isolation should precede obtaining sputum samples for smear and culture in a patient with compatible symptoms and epidemiologic risk factors (**Table 204-2**). For example, an HIV-positive homeless patient with pneumonia should be housed in a negative pressure airborne isolation room while being investigated, and staff should wear appropriately fit-tested respirators when in the room.

Airborne isolation may subsequently be discontinued in patients for whom an alternative diagnosis has been ruled in, initial testing for *M tuberculosis* has been negative, and the case has been discussed with the hospital infection prevention and control department (**Table 204-3**).

The decision to discontinue airborne isolation in patients with known pulmonary TB must weigh several factors, including whether the patient is clinically improving; whether cough is still present or absent; the presence of a cavity on chest radiograph, which suggests greater contagiousness; results of repeat sputum smears; and whether drug sensitivities are known. In general, two weeks of treatment should be considered the absolute minimum duration of airborne isolation that is required. More typically, patients with pulmonary TB remain in airborne isolation for several weeks

TABLE 204-3 Indications to Discontinue Isolation for Tuberculosis

• Patients admitted to rule out tuberculosis may be taken out of negative pressure isolation when three acid-fast bacteria smears on consecutive days are negative, including one early-morning specimen, or when the diagnosis of tuberculosis seems highly unlikely on clinical grounds (ie, resolution of pneumonia with antibiotic which is not active against tuberculosis)
• Patients with known tuberculosis may be removed from negative pressure isolation when clinical improvement has occurred (improvement in cough, fever, night sweats, anorexia) and three AFB smears are negative on consecutive days are negative, including one early-morning specimen

while in the hospital. Again, removal from isolation should be done in consultation with the infection prevention and control department.

LATENT TUBERCULOSIS

By definition, latent TB produces no symptoms. Screening for latent TB is most appropriate for patients with medical risk factors for TB infection (see Table 204-1) or epidemiologic risks such as immigration from an endemic area, homelessness, intravenous drug use, incarceration, or close contact with a patient with active TB. Screening should not be performed in low-risk patients.

Tuberculin skin test

The diagnosis of latent TB has traditionally been made by demonstrating a positive response to the tuberculosis skin test (TST). Planting, reading, and interpreting the TST is deceptively simple, and misinterpretation is common. Because of this, TSTs should be performed and interpreted by experienced personnel. In general, the TST is considered to be highly sensitive and specific for latent TB infection; however, there is the possibility of both false-positive and false-negative reactions. False-positive reactions may occur due to cross-reactivity with other mycobacteria or to previous bacille Calmette–Guérin (BCG) vaccination, if the vaccine was given after the first year of life. Once a TST is positive, it should be considered positive for life and not repeated. False-negative reactions are common in the immunosuppressed, the chronically ill, and the elderly.

PRACTICE POINT

- The effects of bacille Calmette-Guérin (BCG) vaccination on the results of the tuberculin skin test (TST) depends on the age at time of vaccination. When BCG is given in infancy, as is now recommended by the World Health Organization, its effect on the TST is negligible more than 10 years after. Therefore, a TST with 10 mm or more of induration in an adolescent or adult who received BCG in infancy is indicative of tuberculosis infection. Individuals who received BCG as older children or adults are more prone to false-positive tuberculin skin test results, although this risk also diminishes with time. Use of an interferon-gamma release assay, which does not contain antigens present in BCG, may be useful to clarify the results of TST in these patients, and to exclude false positive TST results.

Interferon-gamma release assays

Interferon-gamma release assays (IGRAs) are blood tests that can be used to diagnose latent TB infection. These tests have the advantage of not producing false-positive reactions from prior BCG vaccination. Whereas some guidelines have suggested that they can replace the TST, others have taken a more cautious approach, citing the difficulty in interpreting the sizable proportion of discordant results between the TST and IGRAs that cannot all be explained by BCG vaccination.

TREATMENT

LATENT TUBERCULOSIS

The treatment of choice for latent TB is isoniazid (INH) for nine months. INH is taken with vitamin B_6 (pyridoxine), which prevents the potential adverse effect of peripheral neuropathy. The major risk of INH is hepatotoxicity. Clinical hepatitis typically occurs in < 1% of individuals; however, the chance of developing hepatotoxicity increases with age and in patients with preexisting liver abnormalities. Therefore, before starting treatment, all patients should undergo screening blood work to ensure there is no preexisting elevation in liver enzymes. In those with underlying liver disease, consideration can be made for a second-line treatment, such as a four-month regimen of rifampin. Treatment with rifampin may also be considered if the affected patient is in contact with someone with INH-resistant TB.

ACTIVE TUBERCULOSIS

Unlike latent TB infection, the treatment of active TB requires multiple drugs. Most patients with newly diagnosed TB will be started on a four-drug regimen of INH, rifampin, pyrazinamide, and ethambutol while awaiting sensitivity data, after which the regimen will be simplified (**Table 204-4**). Side effects may be significant, compounded by the need for prolonged treatment over many months. The most common adverse event is hepatotoxicity. This is most commonly associated, in order of risk, with pyrazinamide, INH, and rifampin. Asymptomatic elevations of liver enzymes above five times the upper limit of normal and symptomatic elevations above three times normal are indications for stopping treatment. Rash may develop due to sensitivity to one of the medications, usually rifampin or pyrazinamide. Rifampin may also interact with other medications metabolized by the liver, so careful attention should be paid to the patient's medication history. Patients on rifampin should be forewarned that a benign but invariable effect

TABLE 204-4 First-line Drugs for Tuberculosis, Typical Daily Dosages, and Major Side Effects

Drug	Typical Daily Dosage	Major Adverse Effects
Isoniazid (INH)	5 mg/kg, maximum 300 mg	Peripheral neuropathy, hepatitis, allergy
Rifampin	10 mg/kg, maximum 600 mg	Hepatitis, fever, rash, nausea; orange discoloration of sweat, urine, and tears, with staining of contact lenses; extensive drug interactions via hepatic cytochrome metabolism
Pyrazinamide	20–25 mg/kg, maximum 2 g	Hepatotoxicity, gout, arthralgias, rash, nausea
Ethambutol	15–20 mg/kg	Optic neuritis, typically presenting with loss of peripheral vision; periodic screening of visual fields, visual acuity, and red-green color discrimination recommended
Pyridoxine (vitamin B_6)	10–25 mg	Given to prevent INH-induced neuropathy in patients with predisposing conditions, such as diabetes, alcoholism, pregnancy and lactation, malnutrition, uremia, and HIV infection; pyridoxine supplementation also recommended in patients with seizures, as INH may increase seizure frequency

of being on this medication is an orange discoloration of tears, urine, and sweat. Finally, ethambutol can lead to optic neuropathy, resulting in decreased visual acuity, visual fields, and color vision, so vision should be assessed during every follow-up visit while on the medication.

TREATMENT REGIMENS

There are four regimens for treatment of uncomplicated active TB approved by the American Thoracic Society, Centers for Disease Control, and Infectious Diseases Society of America, with the most common regimen being INH and rifampin for six months, in combination with pyrazinamide for the first two months, as well as ethambutol until sensitivity data are available. Treating TB is not like treating other bacterial infections. The antibiotics used are quite different and for the most part are not interchangeable; each drug in the regimen fills a specific role. Because each of these drugs has significant side effects that may require changes to the initial treatment regimen, one is advised to seek expert advice when treating active TB, as inappropriate regimens can lead to treatment failure and possibly the emergence of drug-resistant bacteria.

Fully drug-sensitive pulmonary and most extrapulmonary TB can usually be cured with six months of treatment. In cases of extensive disease, treatment may be more prolonged. Meningeal and other CNS TB require longer treatment courses. Corticosteroids may be beneficial to decrease the inflammatory component of TB meningitis, pericarditis, and adrenal disease.

Drug-resistant TB is a growing problem in many parts of the world, and it is expected to become more common in developed countries. Second-line agents, such as fluoroquinolones, aminoglycosides, cycloserine, ethionamide, and clofazime, can be used to treat these cases; however, widely accepted guidelines for treatment of drug-resistant TB do not yet exist. In addition, many of these medications cause serious adverse events with prolonged use. Therefore, all cases of drug-resistant TB should be referred to and managed by a TB specialist.

DISCHARGE CONSIDERATIONS

Discharge from hospital is a critical point in the care of the patient with TB. This begins with predischarge education of the patient and family about the need for prolonged treatment, close outpatient follow-up, and screening of the patient's close contacts for TB. Potential obstacles to successful treatment, such as cultural and language barriers, denial, and perceived social stigma relating to TB, should be addressed by providers. Social work should be involved if there is any concern that the patient may not be adherent or lacks adequate social support. Public health authorities should be notified and follow-up arranged with an outpatient treating program, ideally one that uses directly observed therapy.

QUALITY IMPROVEMENT

The quality of TB care and prevention in the hospital setting should be regularly monitored. The hospital records of patients with suspected and confirmed TB should be reviewed to assess quality of care, with particular attention to the time to initiation of isolation precautions, time from admission to ordering and obtaining sputum specimens for acid-fast bacteria (AFB) stain and culture, duration of precautions, adequacy of TB treatment, and adequacy of discharge planning. Previous hospital admissions and outpatient visits prior to TB diagnosis should be reviewed to see if an assessment for TB should have been initiated earlier. Hospital workers should be screened for TB as per current CDC guidelines with tuberculin skin testing or IGRA, and this screening process should be audited periodically for completeness and adequacy of follow-up. Finally, hospitals should have training programs in place for TB, to educate health care workers about concepts of *M tuberculosis* pathogenesis and risk factors for infection, TB symptoms, indications for airborne precautions, and the rationale for TB screening of health care workers.

CONCLUSION

Although rates of tuberculosis have been declining in developed countries, it remains a significant problem in a number of populations. The diagnosis of tuberculosis is typically hampered by not considering the disease as part of the differential diagnosis. Tuberculosis can occur anywhere in the body; however pulmonary disease is the most frequently encountered and is also the most common means by which the disease is transmitted. The treatment of tuberculosis is unlike most other infectious diseases, in that multiple antibiotics in specific combinations are required for at least 6 months. Given the complex nature of the disease, the changing epidemiology of drug resistant tuberculosis, and the potential for drug toxicity and interactions, it is recommended that involvement of a tuberculosis specialist be considered when managing cases.

SUGGESTED READINGS

Blumberg HM, Burman WJ, Chaisson RE, et al. American Thoracic Society/Centers for Disease Control and Prevention/Infectious Diseases Society of America: treatment of tuberculosis. *Am J Respir Crit Care Med.* 2003;167:603–662.

Centers for Disease Control and Prevention (CDC). Updated guidelines for the use of nucleic acid amplification tests in the diagnosis of tuberculosis. *MMWR Morb Mortal Wkly Rep.* 2009;58(1):7–10.

Farhat M, Greenaway C, Pai M, Menzies D. False-positive tuberculin skin tests: what is the absolute effect of BCG and non-tuberculous mycobacteria? *Int J Tuberc Lung Dis.* 2006;10:1192–1204.

Jensen PA, Lambert LA, Iademarco MF, Ridzon R; Centers for Disease Control. Guidelines for preventing the transmission of Mycobacterium tuberculosis in health-care settings, 2005. *MMWR Recomm Rep.* 2005;54(RR-17):1–141.

Mazurek M, Jereb J, Vernon A, et al. Updated guidelines for using interferon gamma release assays to detect *Mycobacterium tuberculosis* infection—United States, 2010. *MMWR Recomm Rep.* 2010;59(RR-5):1–25.

Taylor Z, Nolan CM, Blumberg HM; American Thoracic Society; Centers for Disease Control and Prevention; Infectious Diseases Society of America. Controlling tuberculosis in the United States. Recommendations from the American Thoracic Society, CDC, and the Infectious Diseases Society of America. *MMWR Recomm Rep.* 2005;54(RR-12):1–81.

CHAPTER 205

Urinary Tract Infections and Pyelonephritis

John J. Ross, MD, CM, FIDSA

Key Clinical Questions

1. Which patients with urinary tract infections need hospital admission?
2. When should catheter-associated urinary tract infections be treated?
3. When is renal imaging indicated?
4. When should urology consultation be obtained?
5. What are the appropriate durations of therapy for uncomplicated cystitis, catheter-associated urinary tract infections, and pyelonephritis?
6. For which patients are follow-up urine cultures indicated after discharge?

INTRODUCTION

Urinary tract infections are very common, and account for a significant portion of health care costs. Over half of all women have at least one urinary tract infection (UTI) during their lifetime. In the United States, community-acquired UTIs lead to seven million office visits, one million emergency room visits, over 100,000 hospitalizations, and costs of over $1.6 billion annually. The most common nosocomial infection is catheter-associated UTI, with over one million cases yearly in the United States alone.

PATHOPHYSIOLOGY

The vast majority of UTIs arise by the ascending route. Most are caused by strains of *Escherichia coli* with surface filaments (fimbriae) that bind to urinary epithelium. UTIs occasionally arise from bacteremia. This is especially true of *Staphylococcus aureus*. Whereas *S aureus* may cause cystitis in patients with Foley catheters, when patients present with staphylococcal pyelonephritis from the community, beware of the possibility of underlying bacteremia and endocarditis.

Cystitis and pyelonephritis are 5 to 10 times more common in women, due to the short female urethra. In women under the age of 50 years, the major risk factor for UTI is frequency of sexual intercourse, which facilitates passage of bacteria into the bladder. In otherwise healthy women, UTIs are also associated with new sexual partners, reflecting sexual acquisition of uropathogenic strains of *E coli*, spermicide use, which allows periurethral *E coli* colonization, and probably genetic factors.

The normal urinary tract has robust anatomic, chemical, and immunologic defenses against infection. These are all negated by the placement of an indwelling urinary catheter. The rate of acquisition of bacteriuria after placement of a urinary catheter is 5% per day. Essentially 100% of patients have bacteriuria one month after placement of an indwelling urinary catheter. Other host abnormalities that predispose to UTI are diabetes mellitus and glucosuria, urinary stasis from obstruction, bladder diverticula, neurologic disease, vesicoureteral reflux, and urinary calculi (**Figure 205-1**), which may cause local irritation or obstruction and serve as a nidus for persistent infection.

DOES THE PATIENT HAVE A URINARY TRACT INFECTION?

ASYMPTOMATIC BACTERIURIA

Asymptomatic bacteriuria is very common. It is found in 5% of healthy women, 50% of elderly patients in long-term care facilities, and in most patients with spinal cord injury. Rates of bacteriuria are essentially 100% in patients with chronic indwelling Foley catheters or permanent ureteric stents.

Treatment

Asymptomatic bacteriuria is overtreated. Even the presence of pyuria or cloudy urine by itself does not warrant antibiotic treatment. In most groups studied, treatment of asymptomatic bacteriuria is associated with increased antibiotic side effects, increased acquisition of antibiotic-resistant organisms, and no long-term benefits. Similarly, treatment of asymptomatic candiduria has not been associated with clinical benefit, and long-term eradication rates are disappointing. Therefore, patients with asymptomatic bacteriuria should not be treated, with three notable exceptions: pregnancy,

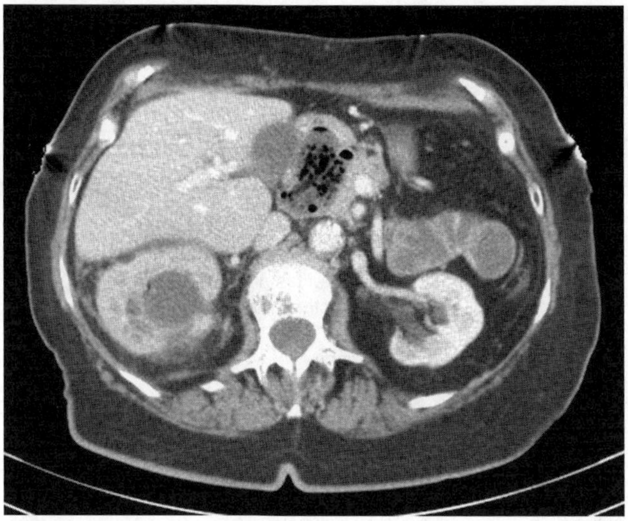

Figure 205-1 *Computed tomography scan of the abdomen showing pyelonephritis in a patient with a urinary tract obstruction from a stone at the ureteropelvic junction. The right kidney is significantly enlarged, with hydronephrosis and perinephric fat stranding.*

prior to transurethral resection of the prostate or other urologic procedures involving mucosal bleeding, and preschool children with vesicoureteral reflux. Pregnant women with asymptomatic bacteriuria should receive three to seven days of antibiotic therapy and should have urine cultures repeated later in pregnancy. Screening and treatment of asymptomatic bacteriuria have been studied and found not to be helpful in the following groups: premenopausal, nonpregnant women; diabetic women; older persons living in the community; elderly, institutionalized subjects; persons with spinal cord injuries; and patients with chronic indwelling urinary catheters.

CYSTITIS (UNCOMPLICATED URINARY TRACT INFECTION)

The diagnosis of cystitis, or infection of the urinary bladder, is straightforward in women presenting with dysuria, urinary frequency, or both, supported by the finding of positive leukocyte esterase or nitrites on urine dipstick, or pyuria on urine microscopy (defined as at least five white cells per high-power field on a centrifuged specimen). Vaginal irritation or vaginal discharge decreases the likelihood of UTI (**Table 205-1**); women with these complaints should be assessed for vaginal candidiasis and sexually transmitted diseases.

In outpatients, urine cultures need not be checked in most cases of suspected cystitis, but they should be obtained when the diagnosis is unclear and symptoms are atypical, if symptoms persist or relapse after treatment, or if pyelonephritis is suspected (ie, fever or back pain is present). In hospitalized patients, urine cultures should be obtained whenever UTI is suspected. If urine cultures demonstrate $< 10^5$ organisms/mL, patients may have bacterial urethritis without cystitis. Gonorrhea or chlamydia should be considered in this setting (**Figure 205-2**).

PYELONEPHRITIS

In healthy adults, kidney infection is diagnosed when all or most of the following findings are present: oral temperature ≥ 38°C (100.4°F) or rectal temperature ≥ 38.5°C (101.3°F), flank pain or costovertebral angle tenderness, serum leukocytosis, and nitrites or leukocyte esterase on urinary dipstick or pyuria or white cell casts on urine microscopy. These findings are usually, but not invariably,

TABLE 205-1 Likelihood Ratios for Urinary Tract Infections in Women

Symptom/Finding	Positive LR	Negative LR
Dysuria present	1.5	0.5
Frequency present	1.8	0.5
Vaginal discharge absent	3.1	0.3
Vaginal irritation absent	2.7	0.2
All of the above	23	—
Positive urine dipstick (either positive leukocyte esterase or positive nitrates)	4.2	0.3

LR, likelihood ratio.
Data from Bent S, Nallamothu BK, Simel DL, Fihn SD, Saint S. Does this woman have an uncomplicated urinary tract infection? In: Simel DL, Rennie D, eds. *The Rational Clinical Examination*. New York: McGraw-Hill; 2009.

combined with lower tract symptoms of urinary frequency and dysuria. In the geriatric patient, pyelonephritis may present with atypical symptoms, such as malaise, confusion, and vague abdominal pain. Fever is usually lower grade, and flank pain often absent. Pyelonephritis is the most common cause of gram-negative bacteremia. Up to 61% of older adults with pyelonephritis are bacteremic at presentation.

PROSTATITIS

Acute bacterial prostatitis presents with fever, rigors, perineal discomfort, dysuria, and urinary urgency and frequency. The prostate is swollen and often exquisitely tender on examination. Acute prostatitis is generally seen in older men, with *E coli* as the most common culprit. Urinalysis and urine cultures should be sent. (Urinary cultures after vigorous prostate massage have fallen out of favor, due to concerns regarding provocation of bacteremia.) In the sexually venturesome, *Neisseria gonorrhoeae* should be entertained, and urethral swabs or urinary gene probes should be sent for gonococcus. Prostatic abscess is not very common, but it should be suspected in men with persistent fever and exquisite prostate tenderness. Human immunodeficiency virus (HIV) and diabetes mellitus are predisposing factors. Pelvic computed tomography (CT) or transrectal ultrasound is diagnostic.

Chronic bacterial prostatitis presents with relapsing dysuria and other urinary symptoms. If perineal discomfort and prostatic tenderness are present, they are usually much milder than in acute prostatitis. *E coli* and other gram-negatives are usually responsible; rarely, *Cryptococcus neoformans* or other fungi are involved.

DIFFERENTIAL DIAGNOSIS

PELVIC INFECTIONS

In women with vaginal discharge, a suggestive sexual history, or a negative urinalysis, pelvic examination should be performed to exclude vaginitis, cervicitis, and pelvic inflammatory disease, with studies for gonorrhea and chlamydia. Other causes of dysuria in women include atrophic vaginitis, seen in postmenopausal women; interstitial cystitis, an enigmatic disorder most common in younger women; and irritant urethritis from tampons, contraceptive gel, and other substances.

RENAL TUBERCULOSIS

Genitourinary tuberculosis (TB) is rare in the United States. However, it is a valid diagnostic consideration in patients with urinary symptoms, sterile pyuria, calcification of the renal parenchyma, and risk

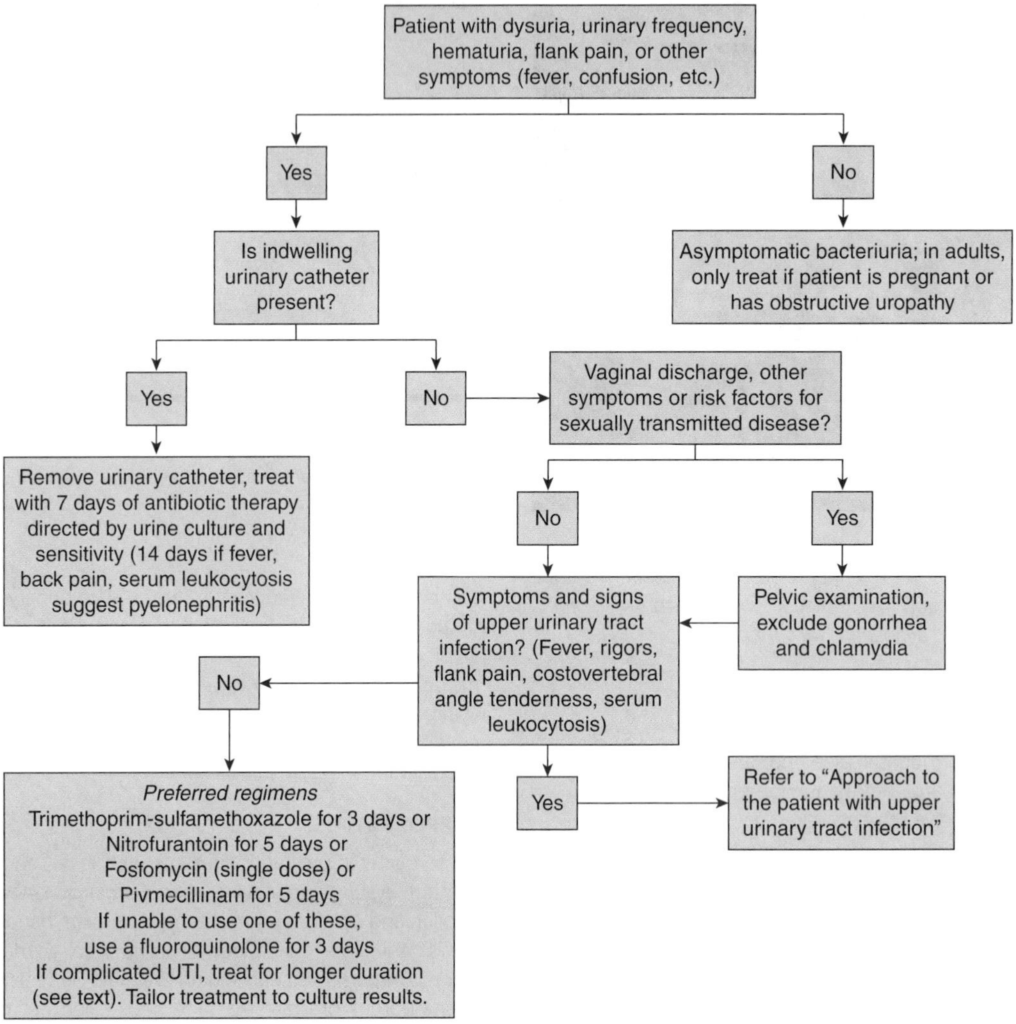

Figure 205-2 *Approach to the patient with urine culture, urine dipstick, or urine microscopy suggestive of urinary tract infection (UTI).*

factors for TB exposure. Most patients lack fever, night sweats, or active pulmonary TB. Diagnosis is made on the basis of three early morning urine cultures for acid-fast bacilli. Treatment is similar to that of other forms of TB.

TRIAGE AND HOSPITAL ADMISSION

Patients with uncomplicated cystitis (lower tract infection) do not require hospital admission unless there are other medical concerns, such as confusion, dehydration, and inability to take oral antibiotics. Reliable patients with pyelonephritis (UTI) with mild illness, good oral intake, and anatomically normal urinary tracts may be treated as outpatients with oral fluoroquinolones (**Figure 205-3**). Conversely, patients with pyelonephritis with moderate to severe illness, nausea and vomiting, renal insufficiency or structural abnormalities of the urinary tract, poor social situation, high risk for noncompliance, or who are pregnant require hospital admission and stabilization.

TREATMENT

■ CYSTITIS

According to guidelines issued by the Infectious Diseases Society of America in 2011, the preferred antibiotic regimens for acute uncomplicated cystitis are nitrofurantoin monohydrate/macrocrystals 100 mg twice daily for 5 days, or trimethoprim-sulfamethoxazole 160/800 mg (one double-strength tablet) twice daily for 3 days, or fosfomycin 3 gm in a single dose (see below), or pivmecillinam 400 mg twice daily for 5 days.

Nitrofurantoin is a time-honored urinary anti-infective, whose active metabolites damage bacterial ribosomes and DNA. Based on a recent clinical trial, 5 days of therapy seems to be as effective for cystitis as traditional 7-day regimens. Nitrofurantoin is generally active against *E coli* and *Citrobacter*, as well as many strains of vancomycin-resistant enterococci. However, it is less useful against many gram-negative rods causing urinary catheter-associated UTI, including *Pseudomonas*, *Providentia*, *Serratia*, *Proteus*, *Enterobacter*, and *Klebsiella*. Nitrofurantoin is not effective in the treatment of pyelonephritis, and it should be avoided in patients with creatinine clearances of less than 40 mL/min.

Three days of antibiotic therapy with trimethoprim-sulfamethoxazole (TMP-SMX) is still effective for acute cystitis in areas where rates of resistance are low (< 20%) among community-acquired isolates of *E coli*. Studies have shown that cystitis relapse rates are lower with TMP-SMX, compared to beta-lactam antibiotics such as penicillins and cephalosporins. In addition, TMP-SMX in associated with a substantially lower relative risk of *Clostridium difficile* colitis, compared to fluoroquinolones and cephalosporins.

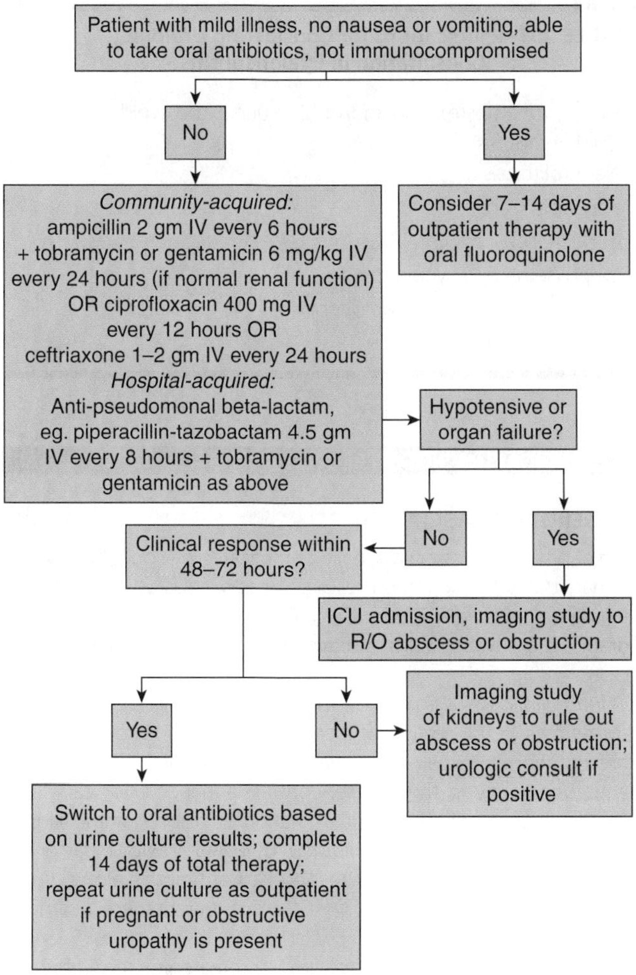

Figure 205-3 *Approach to the patient with upper UTI (ICU, intensive care unit; R/O, rule out).*

Pivmecillinam is a beta-lactam antibiotic with relatively specific action in the urinary tract. It has reasonable cure rates for acute cystitis, although somewhat lower than other first-line agents. It is not available in the United States or Canada, although it is widely used in Europe.

Fluoroquinolones are no longer recommended as first-line agents for acute uncomplicated cystitis, unless one of the above drugs cannot be used because of allergy, intolerance, or resistance. Although fluoroquinolones are still effective for the treatment of acute uncomplicated cystitis, widespread use of fluoroquinolones is associated with increasing bacterial resistance to this class of agents, threatening their use for more serious indications. As well, compared to first-line agents, fluoroquinolones have a greater propensity to cause "collateral damage", including *Clostridium difficile* colitis, colonization and infection with methicillin-resistant *Staphylococcus aureus*, and tendon rupture.

Patient with complicated UTI, or cystitis in the setting of intermittent catheterization, spinal cord injury, urinary tract abnormalities, or weakened immunity, should receive more than 3 days of antibiotic therapy. Studies support a 10-day course of conventional doses of oral ciprofloxacin (500 mg twice daily), or a 5-day course of high-dose oral levofloxacin (750 mg/day), for complicated UTI with fluoroquinolone-sensitive pathogens. Selected patients with severe illness or major urinary tract anomalies, or those treated with beta-lactam antibiotics, may require longer antibiotic courses.

TABLE 205-2 Bacteriology of Acute Pyelonephritis in 467 Patients

Pathogen	No. (%)
Gram-negative	449 (96)
Escherichia coli	418 (90)
Klebsiella sp.	13 (3)
Enterobacter sp.	10 (2)
Proteus mirabilis	6 (1)
Citrobacter sp.	2 (0.4)
Gram-positive	18 (4)
Staphylococcus saprophyticus	10 (2)
Enterococcus sp.	4 (1)
Group B streptococci	4 (1)

Data from Talan DA, et al. *JAMA.* 2000;283:1583–1590; Peterson J, et al. *Clin Ther.* 2007;29:2215–2221.

PRACTICE POINT

Cystitis

- Fosfomycin is an older, broad-spectrum urinary tract antiinfective, given as a single 3 g dose. A structural analogue of phosphoenolpyruvate, it inhibits the initial step in bacterial cell wall synthesis. It is generally less effective than TMP-SMX and fluoroquinolones. However, it may still be useful as a relatively inexpensive treatment for uncomplicated UTI due to vancomycin-resistant enterococci. Side effects are uncommon and generally mild, such as GI upset.

PYELONEPHRITIS

Patients with pyelonephritis who are ill enough to require hospital admission should generally receive 14 days of antibiotic therapy. Most, if not all, antibiotic therapy can be delivered orally. Initial therapy for patients from the community is directed against gram-negative rods, especially *E coli,* as they predominate in the microbiology of pyelonephritis (**Table 205-2**). Preferred regimens include ampicillin plus an aminoglycoside, a fluoroquinolone, or a broad-spectrum cephalosporin such as ceftriaxone. (Regimens containing ampicillin have a minor advantage in that they are usually active against enterococci; fluoroquinolones and cephalosporins are not.) Most antibiotics are excreted in the urinary tract and achieve high concentrations in urine. As aminoglycosides and fluoroquinolones display concentration-dependent killing, compared with the time-dependent killing of β-lactam antibiotics, they may be theoretically superior to β-lactams in the treatment of pyelonephritis. (Moxifloxacin has inferior urinary tract penetration, compared with other fluoroquinolones, and is not indicated for the treatment of UTIs.)

When patients with prior UTI are admitted to the hospital with pyelonephritis, antibiotic therapy should take into account prior culture and sensitivity data, and broader empiric therapy should be prescribed if the patient has a previous history of antibiotic-resistant organisms. Patients who develop pyelonephritis in the hospital or chronic care setting may also require broader empiric therapy, possibly with an antipseudomonal β-lactam in combination with an aminoglycoside or fluoroquinolone. Contrary to popular wisdom, there is no evidence that hydration is beneficial in treating or preventing UTIs unless complicated by prerenal azotemia or kidney stones. Hydration has been recommended as a means of rapidly reducing bacterial counts by dilution. However, dilutional

TABLE 205-3 Indications for Renal Imaging in Patients with Presumed Pyelonephritis

Uncertain diagnosis
Severe illness
Immunocompromise
Worsening renal function
Failure to improve after 72 hours of antibiotics
Suspected kidney stone or urinary tract obstruction
Relapsing or recurrent pyelonephritis
Male gender

TABLE 205-4 Indications for Considering Urologic Consultation in Pyelonephritis

Urinary tract obstruction and/or high urinary postvoid residual volume
Nephrolithiasis
Perinephric abscess
Intrarenal abscess
Emphysematous pyelonephritis
Xanthogranulomatous pyelonephritis
Gross hematuria

effects on antibiotics and urinary antibacterial factors, such as Tamm–Horsfall protein, probably negate this. Hydration may be useful in minimizing the potential nephrotoxicity of aminoglycosides. Urinary analgesics, such as phenazopyridine (Pyridium) are generally unnecessary, and may cause GI upset, headache, and rarely methemoglobinemia.

PRACTICE POINT

Pyelonephritis

- In healthy young women with appropriately treated pyelonephritis, fever may be impressive and sustained, taking up to four days to resolve. Older women with pyelonephritis tend to become afebrile more quickly than younger ones. This probably reflects a more vigorous inflammatory response in younger patients.

Imaging studies are not warranted in acute pyelonephritis when the diagnosis is straightforward and the patient is not critically ill. Renal ultrasound or CT should be performed in patients with presumed pyelonephritis when the diagnosis is unclear, when patients are severely ill or immunocompromised, when new or worsening renal insufficiency is present, when patients are not improved after 72 hours of antibiotics, when structural abnormalities or obstruction of the urinary tract are suspected, or when pyelonephritis is relapsing or recurrent (**Table 205-3**).

Plain films of the abdomen may also be helpful in excluding nephrolithiasis. Some authorities also recommend obtaining renal imaging in diabetics with pyelonephritis, as these patients are at high risk of papillary necrosis, renal abscess, and other complications.

PROSTATITIS

Relapses of prostatitis are common because of poor antibiotic penetration and the limited drainage of infected secretions from the prostate. Acute bacterial prostatitis is usually treated with three to four weeks of oral antibiotics, based on culture results, with needle drainage of abscesses if present. Chronic prostatitis may require 6 to 12 weeks of oral therapy; cure rates are often low because of microabscesses or small calculi, which enable infection to persist. TMP-SMX or fluoroquinolones are preferred for their superior penetration into the prostate. Prostatic abscesses should be drained transperineally or transrectally under ultrasound guidance. Men with chronic pelvic pain, sterile urine cultures, and no response to antibiotics may be suffering from the chronic pelvic pain syndrome. Alpha-blockers and nonsteroidal anti-inflammatories may be considered in these patients.

COMPLICATIONS OF PYELONEPHRITIS

GEROTA'S FASCIA

Perinephric abscess occasionally complicates pyelonephritis when urinary tract obstruction is present. The abscess is usually restricted to the perinephric space by Gerota's fascia. Percutaneous catheter drainage is now standard and avoids the need for surgery in most cases.

Intrarenal abscess is often seen as a consequence of bacteremia, sometimes in the setting of staphylococcal endocarditis. Patients present with flank pain and fever, with a slow clinical response to antibiotics. Early in the course, contrast-enhanced CT scans may show either intense focal inflammation in a lobe of the kidney (facetiously termed *lobar nephronia,* by analogy with lobar pneumonia). These patients may respond to antibiotics alone, but if frank suppuration is evident on CT scans, percutaneous catheter drainage is appropriate.

Emphysematous pyelonephritis is a life-threatening form of upper UTI in diabetics, associated with gas and tissue necrosis in the renal parenchyma and perinephric soft tissues, and is usually caused by *E coli*. Emergent nephrectomy is the traditional treatment in septic patients. However, percutaneous catheter drainage with medical therapy has been successful in less severely ill patients in case reports and in the author's experience. Kidney function is often significantly reduced on the affected side.

Xanthogranulomatous pyelonephritis is a variant of pyelonephritis in middle-aged women, associated with chronic nephrolithiasis, obstruction, and prior symptomatic UTIs. Patients present with fever, malaise, and abdominal pain. The renal calyces are dilated and the parenchyma replaced by necrotic inflammatory tissue, especially lipid-laden macrophages. Kidney stones are usually embedded in the inflammatory process. Involvement is usually unilateral. *E coli* and *Proteus* are most often responsible. As the involved kidney is usually defunct at the time of diagnosis, nephrectomy is customary. Localized disease can be treated with partial nephrectomy and antibiotics (**Table 205-4**).

INFECTIONS ASSOCIATED WITH FOLEY CATHETERS

NOSOCOMIAL CATHETER-ASSOCIATED URINARY TRACT INFECTIONS

The presence of a Foley catheter increases the risk of UTI in several ways. Bacteria are able to migrate outside the catheter and the urethral mucosa to gain entry to the bladder; less often, they ascend through the lumen of the catheter. Bacteria produce biofilm (glycocalyx) on the catheter, protecting them from antibiotics and host defenses. In time, they may also deposit biofilm directly on the bladder uroepithelium. As well, urinary catheters may damage the protective glycosaminoglycan layer of the bladder mucosa, and the presence of foreign bodies such as urinary catheters can depress neutrophil function. Errors in catheter care contribute to infection risk. These include elevating the tubing above the bladder and allowing the tubing to droop below the collecting bag.

The diagnosis of catheter-associated UTI is somewhat imprecise. Surveillance definitions use as criteria the presence of a positive urinary culture ($\geq 10^5$ colony-forming units/mL) with at least one of the following symptoms: fever > 38°C (100.4°F), urgency, frequency, dysuria, and suprapubic tenderness. As urinary symptoms are usually absent in catheterized patients, catheter-associated UTI in the hospital is usually a diagnosis of exclusion, made on the basis of fever, a positive urine culture, and the absence of another infectious source.

Although *E coli* is still the most common microbe in catheter-associated UTI, it is less predominant than it is in the bacteriology of community-acquired cystitis and pyelonephritis. Enterococci, *Pseudomonas, Enterobacter, Providentia, Citrobacter,* and *Candida* each cause significant proportions of catheter-associated UTI. Bacteremia from catheter-associated UTI is uncommon, occurring in < 1% of cases, but because of the large number of hospitalized patients with Foley catheters, up to 15% of nosocomial bacteremias may be urinary in origin.

Treatment

Removal of the urinary catheter and bag is an essential component of treatment for these infections. Ideally, the urinary catheter should be removed permanently. Condom catheterization is an alternative to the indwelling urinary catheter in men with impaired mobility and no urinary obstruction. Most men prefer condom catheters from a comfort standpoint, and the incidence of bacteriuria is less than with indwelling urinary catheters. Clean intermittent catheterization (straight catheterization) every six hours may also be considered, especially in the setting of neurologic disease such as spinal cord injury.

Data are lacking to make definitive recommendations regarding duration of therapy. However, seven days of treatment is customary, based on culture and sensitivity data. If bacteremia is documented, or flank pain is present to suggest pyelonephritis, 14 days of total therapy is indicated.

PURPLE URINE BAG SYNDROME

Elderly patients with chronic Foley catheters and drainage bags occasionally develop purple urine in the collecting system, provoking consternation on the part of patients and caregivers. The proposed mechanism is bacterial breakdown of tryptophan to indirubin and indigo. Multiple gram-negative bacteria are implicated, and urine cultures are usually polymicrobial. The condition is benign, and responds to antibiotics and removal of the urinary catheter and bag. If patients are asymptomatic, antibiotic treatment may not be necessary. However, many patients consider resolution of purple urine desirable.

BLADDER STONES AND *CORYNEBACTERIUM UREALYTICUM*

Another complication of chronic Foley catheterization, especially in elderly men with a history of bladder manipulation, is infection with the resistant diphtheroid *Corynebacterium urealyticum*. This urea-splitting gram-positive rod may cause struvite stone formation in the bladder and encrusted cystitis. Clues include the presence of alkaline urine and repeated urine cultures with gram-positive rods, often misinterpreted as normal flora. Because microbiology laboratories usually assume that urinary diphtheroids are contaminants, the condition may not be diagnosed unless the clinician requests speciation of the isolate. Treatment involves bladder stone removal and intravenous vancomycin. Linezolid is a potential option for oral therapy.

DISCHARGE CONSIDERATIONS

Patients with UTI and pyelonephritis may be discharged from the hospital once there is significant improvement in urinary and systemic symptoms, they are able to tolerate oral medications, and primary care follow-up has been arranged. Patients who are doing well do not need to be observed overnight after switching to oral medication. If patients are asymptomatic at the end of therapy, follow-up urine cultures are not required, except in pregnant women, children, and patients with chronic pyelonephritis on suppressive antibiotic therapy.

PREVENTION OF URINARY TRACT INFECTIONS

Postcoital voiding may help to prevent UTIs in susceptible, sexually active women. *Postcoital antibiotics* (single-strength TMP-SMX or ciprofloxacin 100 mg) may also be helpful and are as effective as daily prophylaxis in premenopausal women. *Continuous low-dose antibiotics* are also used as prophylaxis in women with frequent UTIs, particularly when infection is not related to coitus. TMP-SMX, fluoroquinolones, and nitrofurantoin have all been used in this setting. Clinicians should be aware that both short- and long-term uses of nitrofurantoin are associated with uncommon but potentially severe reactions, including pulmonary hypersensitivity, hepatitis, hemolytic anemia, and peripheral neuropathy.

In acidic urine, *methenamine mandelate* and *methenamine hippurate* break down to ammonia and formaldehyde, which denature proteins and act as broad-spectrum antibiotics active against gram-positive bacteria, gram-negative bacteria, and fungi. They are ineffective against *Proteus* and other urea-splitting bacteria that produce alkaline urine. Methenamine compounds may prevent UTI recurrences, and they are generally well tolerated, aside from occasional GI upset. Administration of vitamin C (ascorbic acid) may help to ensure acidic urine. Methenamines should be avoided in patients with chronic renal failure. They are also not effective in patients with chronic indwelling urinary catheters, as formaldehyde fails to achieve therapeutic concentrations in the bladder.

Cranberry juice or tablets are modestly effective in UTI prophylaxis in ambulatory women. Polyphenols in cranberry juice prevent the fimbrial adhesion of uropathogenic strains of *E coli*. Cranberry juice may potentiate warfarin. *Vaginal estrogens* in postmenopausal women reduce vaginal overgrowth with gram-negative bacteria, promote protective colonization by lactobacilli, and reduced UTIs in small clinical trials.

Impregnated urinary catheters, coated with silver alloy or minocycline and rifampin in combination, reduce the short-term risk of UTI in hospitalized patients, but the cost–benefit implications are hazy. There are no data on whether *suprapubic urinary catheters* reduce short-term infection rates in hospitalized patients, compared with Foley catheter insertion, although some patients may prefer them for reasons of comfort.

QUALITY IMPROVEMENT

Not inserting a urinary catheter and removing a urinary catheter that is not indicated are the most effective means of preventing UTIs and the many other complications of catheter insertion

(**Table 205-5**). Foley catheters are widely overused in the inpatient setting; up to 50% of urinary catheter use is inappropriate. Even when insertion is appropriate, urinary catheters are often left in for too long.

Accepted indications for urinary catheters are bladder outlet obstruction, urinary incontinence in patients with open sacral or perineal wounds, as a comfort measure in the terminally ill, at the patient's request, monitoring of urine output in the critically ill, and during prolonged surgical procedures with general or spinal anesthesia.

Physicians are often not aware that their patients have indwelling urinary catheters. Quality improvement measures to decrease hospital-acquired UTIs should focus on raising physician awareness of the presence of a urinary catheter and encouraging its removal. One effective intervention is the introduction of computer-based order entry for urinary catheters. This can require hard indications for catheter placement, set default catheter removal dates, require reordering of the catheter if it needs to stay in longer, and provide physician reminders that the catheter is still present. Nurse reminders about unneeded urinary catheters, such as during multidisciplinary patient rounds, also reduce the length of urinary catheterization (**Table 205-6**).

TABLE 205-5 Complications of Foley Catheter Insertion

Common
- Asymptomatic bacteriuria
- Urinary tract infection
- Hematuria from traumatic insertion or bladder irritation
- Bladder spasm
- Diminished patient mobility
- Encrustation and blockage by bacterial biofilm
- Retained catheter due to nondeflating balloon

Less common
- Urethral false passage
- Balloon inflation in urethra
- Urethral stricture or necrosis
- Bladder stone formation around the balloon
- Polypoid cystitis
- Bladder perforation or peritonitis
- Laceration or erosion of the glans penis

TABLE 205-6 Evidence-based Medicine: Key References for Pyelonephritis

Study	Methodology	Results	Limitations	Bottom Line
Jernelius H, et al. *Acta Med Scand.* 1988;223:469–477.	Randomized, double-blind trial of 1 vs 3 weeks of combined therapy with pivampicillin and pivmecillinam for acute pyelonephritis	61 patients enrolled; bacteriologic cure rates in 1-week group only 28%, with large number of clinical relapses of lower UTI	Relatively small study; antibiotics used are not marketed in North America	One week of β-lactam antibiotics is probably insufficient for cure of pyelonephritis
Wing DA, et al. *Obstet Gynecol.* 1998;92:249–253.	Randomized, open-label study comparing initial therapy with ceftriaxone, cefazolin, or ampicillin plus gentamicin, followed by oral cephalexin, in pregnant women with pyelonephritis	179 pregnant women enrolled; outcomes similar among all groups, including length of stay, rates of bacteriologic cure, and birth outcomes; average antibiotic duration (parenteral plus oral) 13 days total	Cefazolin no longer considered front-line therapy for pyelonephritis	In pregnant women with pyelonephritis, similar cure rates are achieved when initial therapy is either ceftriaxone or ampicillin plus gentamicin
Talan DA, et al. *JAMA.* 2000;283;1583–1590.	Randomized, double-blind trial of oral ciprofloxacin 500 mg twice daily for 7 days vs oral trimethoprim-sulfamethoxazole (TMP-SMX) twice daily for 14 days in acute uncomplicated pyelonephritis	378 women enrolled, only 255 included in analysis; higher clinical cure rates with ciprofloxacin (96%) than TMP-SMX (83%), largely due to 18% resistance rate of *E coli* to TMP-SMX	Exclusion criteria include hospital admission, sepsis, immunocompromise, pregnancy, renal insufficiency, urinary tract abnormalities	In patients with pyelonephritis who do not need hospital admission, 7 days of oral ciprofloxacin results in acceptable cure rates
Peterson J, et al. *Urology.* 2008;71: 17–22.	Randomized, double-blind trial of levofloxacin 750 mg once daily for 5 days vs ciprofloxacin 500 mg twice daily for 10 days in the treatment of complicated UTI or pyelonephritis	1109 subjects enrolled; similar outcomes in terms of clinical cure, urine sterilization, and adverse events	Only 28% of patients had pyelonephritis; almost all patients tolerated initial oral therapy; rates of bacteremia were low; patients with urinary obstruction were excluded	Short-course, high-dose therapy may cure pyelonephritis in patients who are not very ill, but the results of this study may not be generalizable to the patients with pyelonephritis treated by hospitalists

SUGGESTED READINGS

Behr MA, Drummond R, Libman MD, Delaney JS, Dylewski JS. Fever duration in hospitalized acute pyelonephritis patients. *Am J Med.* 1996;101:277–280.

Cornia PB, Amory JK, Fraser S, Saint S, Lipsky BA. Computer-based order entry decreases duration of indwelling urinary catheterization in hospitalized patients. *Am J Med.* 2003;114:404–407.

Fakih MG, Dueweke C, Meisner S, et al. Effect of nurse-led multidisciplinary rounds on reducing the unnecessary use of urinary catheterization in hospitalized patients. *Infect Control Hosp Epidemiol.* 2008;29:815–819.

Lo E, Nicolle L, Classen D, et al. Strategies to prevent catheter-associated urinary tract infections in acute care hospitals. *Infect Control Hosp Epidemiol.* 2008;29:S41–S50.

Nicolle LE, Bradley S, Colgan R, Rice JC, Schaeffer S, Hooton TM. Infectious Diseases Society of America guidelines for the diagnosis and treatment of asymptomatic bacteriuria in adults. *Clin Infect Dis.* 2005;40:643–654.

Scholes D, Hooton TM, Roberts PL, Gupta K, Stapleton AE, Stamm WE. Risk factors associated with acute pyelonephritis in healthy women. *Ann Intern Med.* 2005;142:20–27.

Warren JW, Abrutyn E, Hebel JR, Johnson JR, Schaeffer AJ, Stamm WE. Guidelines for antimicrobial treatment of uncomplicated acute bacterial cystitis and acute pyelonephritis in women. Infectious Diseases Society of America (IDSA). *Clin Infect Dis.* 1999;29:745–758.

CHAPTER 206

Viral Infections

Stephen B. Greenberg, MD, MACP

Key Clinical Questions

Infectious Mononucleosis

1. What are the major complications in Epstein–Barr virus–associated infectious mononucleosis ("mono")?
2. What other viruses cause a mononucleosis-type clinical syndrome?
3. What are the appropriate diagnostic tests for acute Epstein–Barr virus infections?
4. What are the current treatment recommendations for Epstein–Barr virus–associated infectious mononucleosis?

Varicella-Zoster Virus

1. What are the complications of adult varicella-zoster virus infection?
2. What are the treatment options for varicella-zoster virus infections?
3. What is the best way to treat postherpetic neuralgia?
4. What are the indications for the varicella-zoster vaccine in adults?

Influenza

1. When should patients with influenza-like illness be hospitalized?
2. How good are rapid virus diagnostic tests for influenza virus?
3. How is influenza infection best treated with antiviral agents?
4. What are the major complications of acute influenza?

INFECTIOUS MONONUCLEOSIS

INTRODUCTION

Viruses may infect any organ system of the body and present with common or rare clinical conditions. Viral infections may be trivial or life-threatening. Any given clinical syndrome, such as pneumonia, may have a multitude of viral causes. Additionally, some viruses, such as human cytomegalovirus (CMV), have protean clinical manifestations, including pneumonitis, colitis, encephalitis, and a mononucleosis-like syndrome. This chapter will discuss three common viruses in hospitalized patients: Epstein–Barr virus (EBV), varicella-zoster virus (VZV), and influenza virus, along with their complications.

EPIDEMIOLOGY

Infectious mononucleosis is spread by close physical contact with infected secretions, and is often referred to as "kissing disease." It is most often seen in adolescents and young adults and is not serious in most individuals. However, it can lead to significant time away from school or work, and may be associated with persistent fatigue and prolonged convalescence in some individuals.

PATHOPHYSIOLOGY

Although other viruses produce a similar clinical syndrome, infectious mononucleosis is most often caused by acute EBV infection. Most people become infected with EBV before the age of 6. When EBV infection occurs early in life, it is usually asymptomatic or subclinical. Infection in young adulthood is more likely to lead to clinical "mono," perhaps because of a more robust immune response. The major cell infected by EBV is the B lymphocyte; up to 20% of host B lymphocytes may be infected. Cellular immunity is heavily involved in containing EBV infection; the atypical lymphocytes seen in acute EBV infections are activated CD8+ T cells. The humoral immune system produces antibodies directed against the virus. For unclear reasons, antibodies are also produced against unrelated antigens found on sheep and horse red cells. These antibodies are known as heterophile antibodies, and they form the basis for the mononucleosis spot ("monospot") test.

CLINICAL PRESENTATION

Infectious mononucleosis usually presents with exudative pharyngitis, fever, and symmetrically enlarged cervical lymph nodes. Sore throat may cause severe discomfort. Tonsillitis is common; if massive, "kissing tonsils" may impinge on the airway. Fever lasts from a few days to 2 weeks. The cervical lymphadenopathy can become generalized but usually subsides over 2 to 3 weeks. Splenomegaly, usually mild, is present in ~50%. EBV needs to be distinguished from other causes of exudative pharyngitis, such as group A streptococcus, CMV, and acute human immunodeficiency virus (HIV) infection. Occasional complications (**Table 206-1**) include acute airway obstruction, spontaneous splenic rupture, rash, autoimmune hemolytic anemia, and neurologic syndromes such as meningoencephalitis, transverse myelitis, facial nerve palsy, optic neuritis, and Guillain–Barré syndrome.

TABLE 206-1 Complications of Epstein–Barr Virus–Associated Mononucleosis

- Rash, including nonallergic rash to amoxicillin and other antibiotics
- Airway obstruction
- Splenomegaly and splenic rupture
- Splenic infarct
- Autoimmune hemolytic anemia
- Thrombocytopenia
- Aplastic anemia
- Hepatitis and cholestasis
- Meningoencephalitis or Guillain–Barré syndrome
- Hemophagocytic syndrome
- Malignancy (Hodgkin lymphoma; Burkitt lymphoma in Africa; nasopharygeal carcinoma in Asia; CNS lymphoma in AIDS; lymphoproliferative disease in transplant patients)

DIAGNOSIS

Laboratory tests support the diagnosis of infectious mononucleosis but are not definitive. Most patients have an absolute lymphocyte count over 4500/mm^3 and more than 10% atypical lymphocytes on peripheral blood smear. Total white blood cell counts are often elevated. Mildly elevated aminotransferase levels are common. The monospot test is a rapid latex agglutination assay for heterophile antibodies. Up to 90% of patients have heterophile antibodies at some time in the course of infectious mononucleosis. They persist for up to 1 year after acute EBV infection.

EBV-specific antibody assays are useful in patients with negative heterophile antibodies (see **Figure 206-1**). The viral capsid antigen (VCA) antibody test measures either specific immunoglobulin G (IgG) or IgM antibodies. Epstein-Barr nuclear antigen antibody (EBNA) test measures IgG, which rises during convalescence and stays elevated for life. Early antigen antibody assay (EA–D) is usually positive during acute infection. Polymerase chain reaction (PCR) assays are available but are rarely used in diagnosing infectious mononucleosis. EBV does not grow in routine tissue culture.

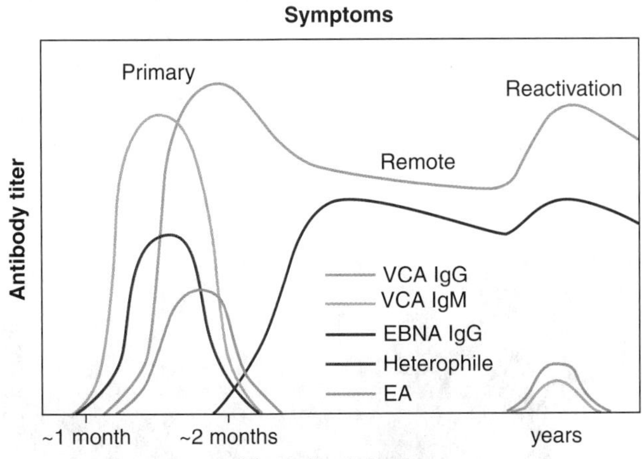

Figure 206-1 *Serologic titers distinguish primary infection from remote infection. Immunoglobulin G (IgG) anti–viral capsid antigen (VCA) and IgM anti-VCA rise in concert with symptoms of primary infection and a positive heterophile test. After symptoms resolve, remote infection is characterized by Epstein–Barr nuclear antigen (EBNA) and IgG anti-VCA without early antigen (EA), although EA and IgM may reappear with or without symptoms on viral reactivation or Epstein–Barr virus–related neoplasia. (Reproduced from Gulley M, et al. J Mole Diagn 2008;10:272–292 with permission from the American Society for Investigative Pathology.)*

TRIAGE/HOSPITAL ADMISSION

Most patients with infectious mononucleosis have a good prognosis and recover quickly. However, some cases can be severe and last for several months. A minority of patients develop chronic fatigue syndrome, which may be more common in women and in those with preexisting mood disorders. If airway obstruction or difficulty breathing is observed, tracheotomy or endotracheal intubation should be considered. If splenic rupture has occurred, admission for attempted splenic preservation or splenectomy will be necessary.

TREATMENT OPTIONS

Supportive care with rest, fluids, and moderate doses of acetaminophen, ibuprofen, or other antiinflammatories is the mainstay of care for infectious mononucleosis. Warm saltwater gargles may relieve the discomfort of sore throat. Use of steroids for EBV-associated infectious mononucleosis remains controversial. A recent meta-analysis suggests there is insufficient evidence for its use in routine cases (**Table 206-2**). Many clinicians use corticosteroids in mononucleosis complicated by impending airway obstruction, autoimmune hemolytic anemia, thrombocytopenia, aplastic anemia, or neurologic complications, but the evidence to support its use in these settings is not robust.

Impending airway obstruction, as defined by difficulty breathing, mandates admission to the hospital and close observation. Otolaryngology consult should be considered in these patients. The clinical benefit of acyclovir for treating acute infectious mononucleosis remains unclear based on published studies.

COMPLICATIONS

Airway obstruction with acute infectious mononucleosis is rare but serious. It usually requires close observation with the ability to do emergent tracheotomy or endotracheal intubation. Splenic rupture presents with acute abdominal pain (or, rarely, left-sided chest pain) and symptoms and signs of hypovolemia. Kehr sign (radiation of pain to the left shoulder) is present in 50% of cases. Splenic rupture may be spontaneous or due to trauma and usually occurs within 3 weeks after clinical symptoms have begun. Computed tomography (CT) abdomen and surgical consultation should be obtained if the diagnosis is suspected. Hemodynamically unstable patients should undergo splenectomy. In stable patients, close observation with nonoperative management or spleen-sparing interventions such as partial splenectomy, splenorrhaphy, and splenic artery embolization may be considered. Other complications that may require subspecialty consultation are autoimmune hemolytic anemia, encephalitis, and pneumonitis.

TABLE 206-2 Infectious Mononucleosis and Corticosteroids

- Randomized trials: 6
- Number of children and young adult patients: 268
- Treatment: Acyclovir/valacyclovir (2/6)
  Prednisone/prednisolone × 5 to 10 days
- Result: "Modest" clinical benefit, no significant reduction in duration of illness or days missed from school or work, no difference in relapse rate

Data from McGee S, Hirschmann J. Use of corticosteriods in treating infectious diseases. *Arch Intern Med.* 2008;168(10):1034–1046.

DISCHARGE PLANNING

Individuals who play sports should be warned against participation for at least 3 weeks, when they may resume noncontact training. Those who do weight lifting or strenuous contact sports should wait at least 1 month after their illness began. It may be useful to obtain an ultrasound to document resolution of splenomegaly, but this practice is not accepted by many individuals. Patients should be warned that fatigue may take months to resolve.

QUALITY IMPROVEMENT

Knowledge and treatment gaps exist in the current management of mononucleosis. Studies of the utility of ultrasound follow-up of splenomegaly in athletes, along with additional studies outlining the natural history of recovery, could help to define when individuals can safely return to normal activity. New antivirals need to be found and tested in the acute management of EBV-associated infectious mononucleosis. Although there is currently no EBV vaccine available, trials are under way to see if candidate vaccines are immunogenic and safe.

VARICELLA-ZOSTER VIRUS

INTRODUCTION/EPIDEMIOLOGY

Varicella (or chickenpox) is primary infection with the VZV virus. It usually occurs in childhood in temperate climates, and in adolescence or young adulthood in the tropics. Before the introduction of the varicella vaccine in 1996, there were an estimated four million cases of chickenpox in the United States each year. Since the introduction and widespread use of the vaccine in childhood, the incidence of chickenpox has been reduced in many populations by as much as 90%.

PATHOPHYSIOLOGY

Primary infection with VZV occurs in the nasopharynx with spread to lymphoid tissue and specifically to memory CD4 + T cells, with adherence to cutaneous epithelia within the first few days following infection. Cell-free virus is present in skin vesicles and can infect sensory nerve endings and epithelia and result in latency of virus and sensory ganglia. Latent VZV genomes are localized to < 10% of sensory ganglia and neurons. Herpes zoster increases with increasing age and with other causes of decreased cellular immunity. Susceptible children are more likely to develop chickenpox from exposure to virus of varicella patients than from exposure to herpes zoster lesions.

CLINICAL PRESENTATION

Primary varicella infection is an illness of 3 to 5 days in duration, associated with rash, malaise, and low-grade fever. The characteristic rash of varicella consists of macules and papules that evolve into vesicles and crust over. Lesions are usually in different stages of development at any given time. The vesicle sits atop an erythematous base and has been referred to as a "dewdrop on a rose petal" because of its appearance. Lesions may become superinfected with staphylococci or streptococci, and necrotizing fasciitis is an occasional complication. Disseminated infection occurs in the immunocompromised patient. In adults, varicella pneumonia is common, occurring in at least 1 in 400 patients; asymptomatic radiologic infiltrates are even more common.

Following recovery from chickenpox, VZV remains latent in ganglion cells. *Shingles,* or *herpes zoster,* is caused by reactivation of latent VZV. It usually appears in a dermatome distribution, but it may disseminate in immunodeficient patients once it spreads through the bloodstream. Most often, shingles involves the trunk or face. A dreaded form of shingles is *herpes zoster ophthalmicus,* or involvement of the first division of the trigeminal nerve, which may be sight-threatening if keratitis (corneal lesions) develops. Hutchinson sign in herpes zoster ophthalmicus (involvement of the nasociliary nerve, with vesicles at the tip or side of the nose) is said to predict corneal involvement. Another shingles variant is the Ramsay Hunt syndrome, with involvement of nerves of the geniculate ganglion; findings may include facial nerve palsy and other cranial neuropathies, as well as pain and vesicle formation involving some combination of the face, neck, external ear, tympanic membrane, anterior tongue, and soft palate. Vertigo, tinnitus, and hearing loss may also be present. Herpes zoster without skin lesions (*zoster sine herpete*) is sometimes invoked as a cause of acute and chronic radicular pain.

The incidence of shingles increases with increasing age. The median age for cases of herpes zoster is ~64 years. Because of the increase in individuals over the age of 60 years, the incidence of herpes zoster may well increase over the next few decades. Second episodes of herpes zoster occur in < 5% of individuals. When zoster is severe and involves multiple dermatomes in a younger patient without known immunosuppression, HIV should be considered.

DIFFERENTIAL DIAGNOSIS

The differential diagnosis of chickenpox includes smallpox, in which skin lesions in the same area are of similar clinical stage, unlike varicella, and contact dermatitis secondary to plant exposure such as poison ivy (**Figure 206-2**). Recurrent skin lesions in a pseudodermatome distribution may be due to herpes simplex virus. In these cases, there are repeated episodes of herpes simplex virus lesions on the skin in the same area. This pattern of recurrence does not occur with herpes zoster.

DIAGNOSIS

VZV infections can be identified using histologic staining of skin lesions, viral cultures, PCR, or serologic assays. Immunohistologic staining of skin scrapings is inexpensive and 90% sensitive and 95% specific for the diagnosis of infections. Although viral cultures are specific, they take several days and appear to have a sensitivity of only 60% to 75%. PCR is the most sensitive and specific test for varicella-zoster infections, but it takes at least 1 day and is expensive. Serology is only useful for screening for susceptibility to the VZV.

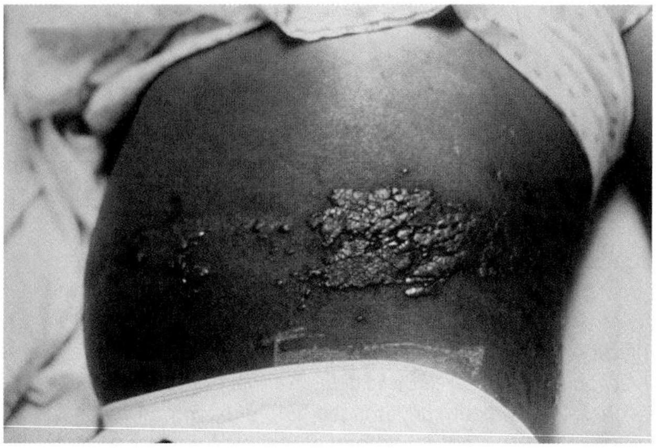

Figure 206-2 *Herpes zoster lesions in thoracic dermatome. (Courtesy of the Centers for Disease Control and Prevention, Public Health Image Library.)*

TABLE 206-3 Oral Antiviral Medications for Herpes Zoster

Medication	Dosage	Duration of Treatment, Days	Most Common Adverse Effects	Precautions and Contraindications
Acyclovir	800 mg 5 times daily (every 4–5 hours)	7–10	Nausea, headache	Dosage adjustment required for patients with renal insufficiency
Brivudine	125 mg once daily	7	Nausea, headache	Contraindicated for patients treated with 5-fluorouracil or other 5-fluoropyrimidines because of drug interaction associated with severe and potentially fatal bone marrow suppression
Famciclovir	500 mg 3 times daily (approved dosage in United States; in some other countries, 250 mg 3 times daily is approved)	7	Nausea, headache	Dosage adjustment required for patients with renal insufficiency
Valacyclovir	1000 mg 3 times daily	7	Nausea, headache	Dosage adjustment required for patients with renal insufficiency; thrombotic thrombocytopenic purpura/hemolytic uremic syndrome reported at dosages of 8000 mg daily in immunocompromised patients

Reproduced, with permission, from Dworkin RH, Johnson RW, Breuer J, et al. *Clin Infect Dis*. 2007;44:S1–S26. University of Chicago Press. © 2006 by the Infectious Diseases Society of America.

TRIAGE/HOSPITAL ADMISSION

Patients with CNS involvement, disseminated infection, or high risk for dissemination, and those who require IV medications should receive inpatient care. Patients with herpes zoster ophthalmicus should be admitted to the hospital and ophthalmology consultation obtained.

Varicella infection is highly contagious, and patients with primary varicella infection (chickenpox), disseminated herpes zoster, or immunocompromised patients with zoster at risk for disseminated infection may transmit infection via airborne virus from respiratory secretions. These patients should be placed in a negative pressure room on both airborne precautions and contact precautions until all lesions have dried and are crusted over. Only personnel who are immune to chickenpox should enter the room and care for the patient. Immunocompetent patients with uncomplicated herpes zoster and localized dermatomal involvement need only standard precautions, but they also should be cared for by health care workers who are varicella immune.

TREATMENT OPTIONS

Skin lesions of varicella and herpes zoster should be kept clean and dry. Topical antibiotics or dressings with tight adhesives should be avoided. Antivirals shorten the duration of infection in adults with primary varicella infection and shingles and probably lower the risk of complications if started within 24 to 48 hours of new vesicle development. Medications approved for use in adults include acyclovir, valacyclovir, and famciclovir (**Table 206-3**). In shingles, each appears to reduce pain and time to skin lesion resolution and may reduce the duration of postherpetic neuralgia. Famciclovir and valacyclovir are both oral prodrugs that are converted to the active form after ingestion. They have high oral bioavailability and offer the advantage of three times daily dosing in herpes zoster, compared with five times daily for acyclovir. All three agents require dosage adjustment in renal insufficiency. The use of steroids in patients with herpes zoster is controversial. Although they may help reduce postherpetic neuralgia, controlled studies are inconclusive; therefore, they are not routinely indicated in herpes zoster infections (**Table 206-4**).

Postherpetic neuralgia (PHN) is pain persisting for at least 120 days after the onset of herpes zoster. Poor quality of life, insomnia, and depression are often associated with PHN. Risk factors for PHN are older age, more severe initial pain, a more severe rash on presentation, and a painful prodrome. PHN has a variable response to treatment. There are three medications approved for treatment of PHN: gabapentin, 5% lidocaine patch, and pregabalin (**Table 206-5**). Tricyclic antidepressants and opioid analgesics are also efficacious. Antivirals alone do not appear to be effective in treating the pain of PHN. Some patients appear to be refractory to all treatments.

COMPLICATIONS

Because of the ability of VZV to replicate in nerve tissue and establish latency there, neurologic complications are not unusual. Primary varicella infection may be complicated by cerebellar ataxia (1 in 4000 cases) and encephalitis (1 in 1000 cases). Cerebral vasculitis may lead to late strokes.

TABLE 206-4 Herpes Zoster Infections and Corticosteroids

- Randomized trials: 5
- Number of patients: 780
- Treatment: Acyclovir (3/5)
- Prednisone/prednisolone × 21 days
- Result: Beneficial (3/5), failure (2/5), no effect on postherpetic neuralgia

Data from McGee S, Hirschmann J. Use of Corticosteroids in Treating Infectious Diseases. *Arch Intern Med*. 2008;168(10):1034–1046.

TABLE 206-5 Analgesic Medications Useful in the Treatment of Patients with Herpes Zoster

Medication	Beginning Dosage	Titration	Maximum Dosage	Most Common Adverse Effects
Opioid analgesics (dosages given are for oxycodone)*	5 mg every 4 hours as needed; dosage can be converted to long-acting opioid analgesic combined with short-acting medication continued as needed	Increase by 5 mg 4 times daily every 2 days as tolerated	No maximum dosage with careful titration; consider evaluation by a pain specialist at dosages > 120 mg daily	Nausea/vomiting, constipation, sedation, dizziness
or				
Tramadol*	50 mg once or twice daily	Increase by 50–100 mg daily in divided doses every 2 days as tolerated	400 mg daily (100 mg 4 times daily); for patients > 75 years of age, 300 mg daily in divided doses	Nausea/vomiting, constipation, sedation, dizziness, seizures, postural hypotension
Gabapentin†	300 mg at bedtime or 100–300 mg 3 times daily	Increase by 100–300 mg 3 times daily every 2 days as tolerated	3600 mg daily (1200 mg 3 times daily); reduce if renal function is impaired	Sedation, dizziness, peripheral edema
or				
Pregabalin†	75 mg at bedtime or 75 mg twice daily	Increase by 75 mg twice daily every 3 days as tolerated	600 mg daily (300 mg twice daily); reduce if renal function is impaired	Sedation, dizziness, peripheral edema
Tricyclic antidepressants, especially nortriptyline†	25 mg at bedtime	Increase by 25 mg daily every 2–3 days as tolerated	150 mg daily	Sedation, dry mouth, blurred vision, weight gain, urinary retention§

*Consider lower starting dosages and slower titration for frail and elderly patients (eg, 5 mg twice daily for oxycodone); dosages given are for short-acting formulations.

†Consider lower starting dosages and slower titration for frail and elderly patients (eg, 10 mg at bedtime for tricyclic antidepressants).

§Consider a screening electrocardiogram for patients ≥ 40 years of age.

As adapted from Dworkin RH, et. al. with permission from *Clin Infect Dis*. 2007;44:S1–S26. University of Chicago Press. © 2006 by the Infectious Diseases Society of America.

The most common complication of herpes zoster is PHN. Herpes zoster may be associated with aseptic meningitis. (Mild cerebrospinal fluid lymphocytosis may also be seen in herpes zoster in the absence of aseptic meningitis.) The syndrome of herpes zoster ophthalmicus with delayed contralateral hemiplegia is usually seen 6 weeks following a case of trigeminal nerve herpes zoster. Less common complications include hepatitis, pneumonitis, and myelitis (**Table 206-6**).

VZV reactivation may occur in the absence of shingles, as in CNS vasculopathy and necrotizing retinitis. VZV vasculopathy of the CNS presents with headache, fever, confusion, transient ischemic attacks, and strokes. Cerebral angiography reveals areas of arterial stenosis and occlusion. Diagnosis is made by finding VZV DNA by PCR, or VZV IgG, in spinal fluid. Necrotizing retinitis may present as acute retinal necrosis (ARN) or progressive outer retinal necrosis (PORN). Both conditions may lead to retinal detachment and blindness and are more common in AIDS. ARN is caused by both varicella-zoster and herpes simplex viruses, whereas PORN is caused almost exclusively by VZV.

TABLE 206-6 Complications of Varicella-Zoster Virus Infections

Dissemination
Hepatitis
Pneumonitis
Encephalitis/CNS and peripheral vasculopathy
Postherpetic neuralgia

DISCHARGE PLANNING

At the time of discharge, patients should be informed about the natural progression of herpes zoster. Continued pain relief will be needed in most cases as an outpatient. Patients who develop PHN must be seen at regular intervals to receive additional medical therapy and emotional support. Skin lesions take up to 3 weeks to heal and may often look worse in the second and third week as they crust over. Viral shedding from skin lesions occurs until they become crusted over. Patients should preferentially have varicella-immune caregivers until crusting occurs.

QUALITY IMPROVEMENT

Hospitalists should consider recommending the live-attenuated zoster vaccine in outpatient follow-up for their patients over the age of 60 who are not immunosuppressed and have not had shingles.

INFLUENZA

INTRODUCTION/EPIDEMIOLOGY

Influenza occurs in yearly outbreaks, mainly during winter months throughout the world. It is caused by influenza A or B viruses. When significant changes occur in both surface proteins, hemagglutinin and neuraminidase, worldwide pandemics can occur, as recently observed with the novel A/H1N1 virus.

TABLE 206-7 Pandemic H1N1 Influenza

- First reported case in Mexico, March 2009
- Pandemic declared by the World Health Organization in June 2009
- Novel H1N1 is quadruple reassortment of two swine strains, one human strain, and one avian strain of influenza
- Spread throughout the United States in fall 2009
- Monovalent vaccine developed and distributed in 2009

Once an outbreak begins, it usually spreads in a community over 8 to 12 weeks and becomes the major cause of acute upper and lower respiratory tract illnesses. Infection with epidemic strains is common in school-age children. However, increased mortality occurs primarily in the elderly. Transmission occurs by aerosols or droplets generated during coughing or sneezing. In the United States, an average of 20,000 to 40,000 deaths and 300,000 hospitalizations occur annually with influenza epidemics. In April 2009, the first case of novel H1N1 virus occurred in Mexico. Over the next few months, 41 countries had reported cases. The World Health Organization declared that a pandemic situation was in effect in June 2009 (see **Table 206-7**).

PATHOPHYSIOLOGY

There are three types of influenza viruses: A, B, and C. Only influenza A viruses have pandemic potential. Eight gene segments are surrounded by 10 or 11 coat proteins. Minor changes, or antigenic drift, occur in the surface proteins each year. Major changes, or antigenic shift, occur every 10 to 20 years in the viral surface hemagglutinin and neuraminidase. The updated yearly vaccine is based on the observed antigenic drift; the rapid emergence of an influenza strain with antigenic shift results in a virus–vaccine mismatch, as occurred in 2009 with H1N1. Influenza viruses spread by respiratory secretions to susceptible hosts. Respiratory symptoms are secondary to dysfunction of cells and release of inflammatory mediators. The incubation period is from 18 to 72 hours.

CLINICAL PRSENTATION

The acute onset of fever and cough is suggestive of influenza, but it is nonspecific, as other respiratory viruses have a similar clinical presentation. Pharyngitis and myalgias are common. Acute HIV syndrome can be mistaken for an influenza-like illness.

Primary influenza pneumonia is a serious complication in a minority of patients with acute influenza illness. Influenza can lead to secondary bacterial pneumonia or a mixed picture of both viral and bacterial pneumonia (**Table 206-8**). *Streptococcus pneumoniae* is the most common bacterial pathogen isolated following acute influenza. However, *Staphylococcus aureus* pneumonia is diagnosed with increased frequency in patients following recent influenza infection. Other potentially life-threatening conditions associated with influenza infection include myositis, rhabdomyolysis, CNS involvement, and myocarditis.

TABLE 206-8 Viral Causes of Pneumonia

- Influenza viruses A and B most common
- Respiratory syncytial virus, parainfluenza virus, and coronavirus/rhinovirus less common
- Increased frequency in elderly
- Cause up to 10% to 30% of community-acquired pneumonia

DIAGNOSIS

Influenza-like illness is associated with fever, sore throat, cough, and systemic complaints. During an outbreak of influenza in a community, acute respiratory tract illness can be assumed to be due to influenza virus. There are a number of rapid antigen tests that vary in sensitivity between 40% and 60% in adults. These rapid antigen tests more sensitive in children because of the increased viral excretion in younger patients. Other diagnostic tests are indirect fluorescent antibody (IFA) and direct fluorescent antibody (DFA), as well as PCR and viral culture. PCR is highly sensitive and specific, but it requires at least a day and is not readily available in many laboratories. Viral cultures are also sensitive and specific, but they take several days before giving a positive result. Serology for influenza is available, but it is mainly of epidemiologic utility.

Who should be tested for influenza virus? During a community-wide outbreak of influenza, patients with underlying disease and influenza-like illness (ILI) should be tested for the presence of influenza virus. In individuals who are immunocompetent and present with an ILI, testing for the presence of virus is not usually indicated. However, all hospitalized patients with ILI should be tested for the presence of influenza virus. A rapid antigen test that is positive can be used to decide about specific antiviral therapy. If a rapid antigen test is negative, and the patient is thought to have an ILI in the hospital, then sending a specimen for further testing, such as viral culture or PCR, would be indicated.

TRIAGE/HOSPITAL ADMISSION

Patients with acute respiratory tract illness during an influenza outbreak should be considered for hospital admission if they are elderly or too weak to care for themselves at home, have an underlying condition such as chronic obstructive pulmonary disease or congestive heart failure, or there is a clinical suspicion for pneumonia. During an influenza epidemic, it is important to triage as many patients as possible for care at home.

TREATMENT OPTIONS

Several antiviral agents are currently approved for use in acute influenza illness. The adamantanes amantadine and rimantadine are only active against influenza A viruses. Because there is widespread resistance to the adamantanes that has emerged among recent isolates of influenza A, these antivirals are no longer used. The neuraminidase inhibitors oseltamivir and zanamivir are active against both influenza A and B viruses. Increased resistance to the neuraminidase inhibitors has been described in recent isolates. Widespread resistance to oseltamivir has emerged in the United States and Europe in >90% of influenza A/H1N1 viruses, but the pandemic strain of novel H1N1 appears to be much more sensitive to oseltamivir (**Table 206-9**). Zanamivir resistance has been reported rarely.

TABLE 206-9 Antivirals for Influenza Virus Infections

Antiviral	Activity	Dosage (5 Days)	Side Effects
Amantadine	Influenza A only	100 mg/day orally	CNS, GI
Rimantadine	Influenza A only	100 mg/day orally	CNS, GI
Oseltamivir	Influenza A and B	75 mg twice/day orally	GI
Zanamivir	Influenza A and B	2 inhalations twice/day	Bronchospasm

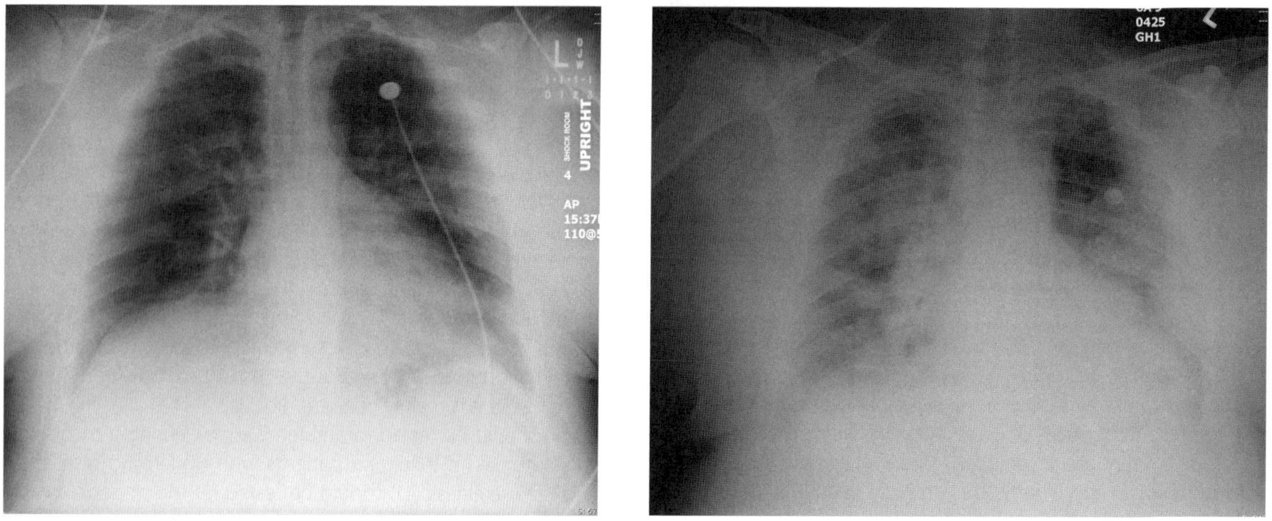

Figure 206-3 *Chest radiographs of a hospitalized patient with novel H1N1 pneumonia/acute respiratory distress syndrome over 48 hours. (Courtesy of Venkata Bandi, Ben Taub General Hospital, Houston, Texas.)*

COMPLICATIONS

Pneumonia is a serious complication of acute influenza infection. Primary influenza pneumonia, although rare, is a serious cause of increased mortality. Clinically, the patient presents with cough and dyspnea. A chest radiograph will reveal diffuse infiltrates or an acute respiratory distress syndrome (ARDS) pattern (**Figure 206-3**). Elderly patients and those with cardiovascular disease constitute the highest risk groups. The mortality rate in acute influenza pneumonia is high. Secondary bacterial pneumonia can occur 2 to 3 weeks after the onset of influenza symptoms. *S pneumoniae* or *S aureus* (including methicillin-resistant *S aureus* [MRSA]) are the two most commonly identified bacterial pathogens. A mixed viral and bacterial pneumonia has also been described following acute influenza.

Another uncommon complication of influenza infection is myositis (**Table 206-10**). This occurs more commonly with influenza B virus than with influenza A and is more often seen in children. Myoglobinuria and rhabdomyolysis have also been reported following acute influenza infection. CNS complications are also rarely reported. These include encephalitis, transverse myelitis, and Guillain–Barré syndrome.

DISCHARGE PLANNING

Patients should be cautioned that, although the prognosis is good in acute influenza, malaise and fatigue may persist for some time. If the patient comes from a nursing home, the physician will need to contact nursing home personnel to take measures to protect other residents from an outbreak of acute influenza.

TABLE 206-10 Influenza Virus–Associated Myositis

- Influenza type A > B
- Mostly in school-age children
- Calf muscles commonly involved
- Increased creatine kinase levels
- Begins during convalescence
- Self-limited
- Antivirals

QUALITY IMPROVEMENT

With the widespread use of approved influenza vaccines, the severity of outbreaks could be minimized. Medical facilities need to have contingency plans ready in case of influenza epidemics, especially during pandemics. It is important to educate communities about the detrimental effect of using the emergency room for acute ILI during outbreaks. Based on the resistance data with current antivirals, newer antivirals for the resistant strains of influenza will be needed in future outbreaks.

SUGGESTED READINGS

Asgari, MM, Begos, DG. Spontaneous splenic rupture in infectious mononucleosis: A review. *Yale J Biol Med.* 1997;70:175–182.

Dickens KP, Nye AM, Rickett K. Should you use steroids to treat infectious mononucleosis? *J Fam Prac.* 2008;57:754–755.

Dworkin RH, Johnson RW, Breuer J, et al. Recommendations for the management of herpes zoster. *Clin Infect Dis.* 2007;44(Suppl 1): S1–S26.

Gilden D, Cohrs RJ, Mahalingam R, Nagel MA. Varicella zoster virus vasculopathies: Diverse clinical manifestations, laboratory features, pathogenesis, and treatment. *Lancet Neurol.* 2009;8: 731–740.

Glezen WP. Prevention and treatment of seasonal influenza. *N Engl J Med.* 2008;359:2579–2585.

Gulley ML, Tang W. Laboratory assays for Epstein-Barr virus-related disease. *J Mol Diagn.* 2008;10:279–292.

Johnson RW, Wasner G, Saddier P, Baron R. Herpes zoster and postherpetic neuralgia: Optimizing management in the elderly patient. *Drugs Aging.* 2008;25:991–1006.

McGee S, Hirschmann J. Use of corticosteroids in treating infectious diseases. *Arch Intern Med.* 2008;168:1034–1046.

Pabbaraju K, Wong S, Wong AA, Appleyard GD, et al. Design and validation of real-time RT-PCR assays for detection of pandemic (H1N1) 2009 virus. *J Clin Microbiol.* 2009;47:3454–3460.

Putukian M, O'Connor FG, Stricker P, McGrew C, et al. Mononucleosis and athletic participation: An evidence-based subject review. *Clin J Sport Med.* 2008;18:309–315.

SECTION 11

Neurology

CHAPTER 207

The Neurologic Examination

David J. Likosky, MD, SFHM
Scott Andy Josephson, MD

Key Clinical Questions

1. What elements of the history and examination are most useful in lesion localization?
2. What elements of the neurologic examination can be assessed at the bedside without formal testing?
3. What tests can be performed on the unresponsive patient?
4. What scales and tools are used to document the findings of the neurologic exam?

INTRODUCTION

The neurologic examination is central to the evaluation of patients with neurologic complaints. It relies heavily on the history and on directed, hypothesis-driven physical testing. The neurologic examination can provide a great deal of information quickly. Even when it is not diagnostic, it guides the appropriate choice of imaging and ancillary testing. However, if it is performed in a cursory fashion, one can easily miss clues to a diagnosis that may not be apparent on imaging. This chapter reviews the essential elements of the neurologic examination in evaluating patients in the hospital.

IMPORTANCE OF THE HISTORY

The history allows the hospitalist to narrow the range of diagnostic testing and perform a more focused neurologic examination.

CASE 207-1

A 57-year-old right-handed man presents with an episode of syncope while typing a manuscript. He recalls no prior episodes but does have a history of well-controlled hypertension and hyperlipidemia. You are called by the emergency department physician to admit the patient to telemetry and rule out an arrhythmia. The patient recalls similar episodes that he has had for as long as he can remember. They were bothersome during school but are brief and infrequent now. He also notes that they were worse when he was tired.

When taking the neurologic history, the focus should be, first, on localizing the lesion and, second, on developing a differential diagnosis. Missed diagnoses are common in neurology when jumping to a conclusion before establishing where the problem may lie. Tempo is helpful: is the process waxing and waning, as in delirium, steadily progressive, as in dementia, or in a stepwise decline, as from multiple strokes? During which activities is weakness more pronounced: rising from a chair, carrying heavy loads, or brushing or washing hair, as with proximal weakness, or opening a jar, opening a car door, or turning a key in a lock, as with distal weakness? Is the sensory phenomenon negative, such as the numbness resulting from a stroke, or positive, such as tingling from nerve root compression?

CASE 207-1 *(continued)*

The patient's physical examination was unrevealing. A computed tomography (CT) scan of his brain was negative, but an electroencephalogram (EEG) showed occasional epileptiform discharges from the left hemisphere. The patient was begun on anticonvulsants at a very low dose and has had no further episodes.

Without a detailed history, this patient might have been admitted to telemetry and had extensive and inappropriate cardiac investigations. He might have been discharged with the diagnosis of unexplained syncope and gone on to have a seizure at an inopportune time. With a careful history, he leaves instead with a correct diagnosis and life-altering therapy.

LOCALIZING THE LESION

A major goal in neurology is to localize the lesion causing the patient's symptoms. Diagnosis in neurology, as in other domains of medicine, relies partly on pattern recognition. Important patterns include the hemiparesis and language deficit of a dominant middle cerebral artery stroke, the cranial nerve findings and crossed body involvement of a brainstem stroke, the distal neuropathy of diabetes, the ascending weakness of Guillain–Barré syndrome, and the diurnal variation of ptosis and diplopia in myasthenia gravis. However, many signs and symptoms in neurology are nonspecific and may be produced by lesions in more than one anatomical site.

CENTRAL VERSUS PERIPHERAL

CASE 207-2

A 27-year-old man who has previously been healthy complains of strange sensations. You note that his mental status is normal, as are his cranial nerves, with the exception of an afferent papillary defect on the right. He has full strength, with increased muscle tone diffusely, and developed a mild right-sided foot drop about a year ago, for which he never sought treatment. Sensation is normal except for much of his left hemithorax. Reflexes are mildly hyperactive, and a Babinski sign is present.

A fundamental distinction in neurologic disease is deciding whether a central or peripheral lesion is responsible. Central lesions affect the brain and spinal cord, and peripheral lesions affect the anterior horn cells, peripheral nerves, neuromuscular junctions, or muscles. Localizing a lesion to the central or peripheral nervous system avoids excessive, "shotgun" imaging, resulting in potential morbidity and inflated costs. In the case above, there are elements that are likely central (afferent pupillary defect, hyperactive reflexes, increased tone, and Babinski sign) and others that could be either (foot drop). It would be helpful to further define the abnormal sensation using dermatome and peripheral nerve maps (**Figures 207-1** and **207-2**). If the new abnormality does not conform to the distribution of a peripheral nerve or dermatome, a central lesion is probable, and neuroimaging is indicated. Ordering an electromyogram (EMG) in this setting would be inappropriate and of low yield.

In this case, the patient has lesions that are separated in space (different locations in the CNS) and time (old foot drop, new altered sensations). Magnetic resonance imaging (MRI) of the brain is ordered, which demonstrates multifocal T2 hyperintensities that particularly involve the periventricular white matter, consistent with demyelinating lesions of multiple sclerosis.

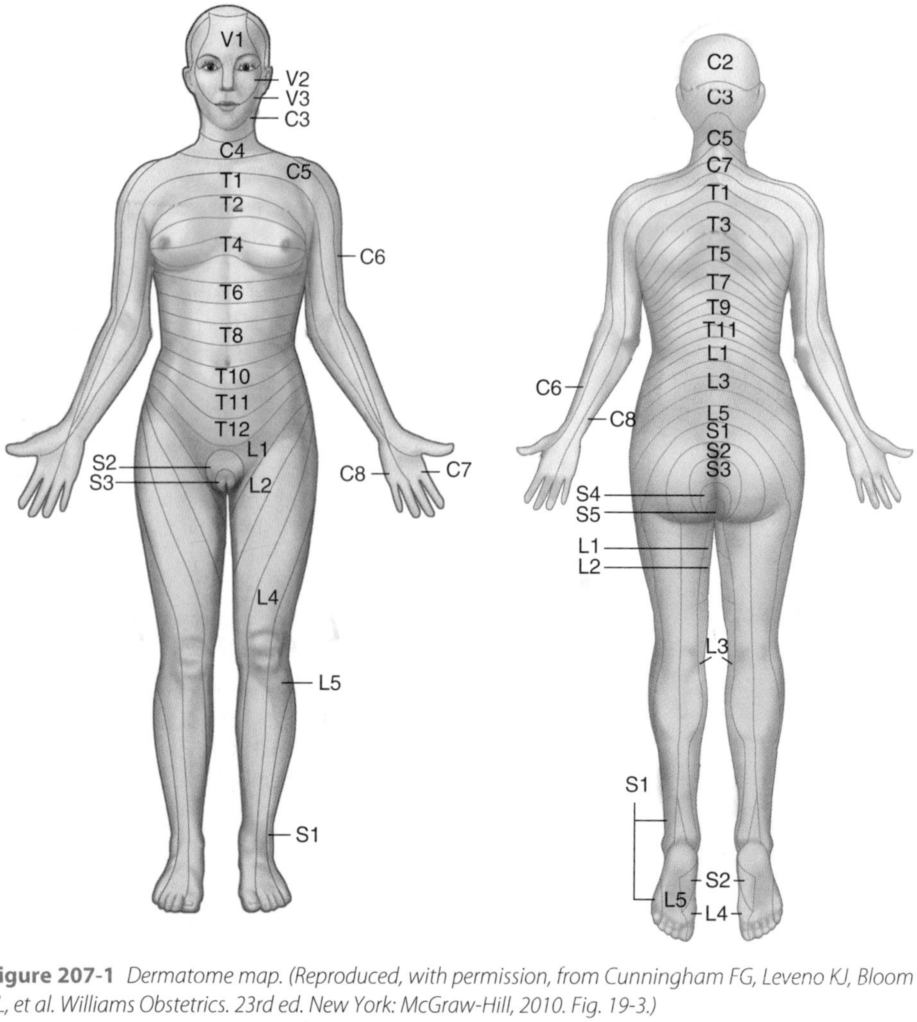

Figure 207-1 *Dermatome map. (Reproduced, with permission, from Cunningham FG, Leveno KJ, Bloom SL, et al. Williams Obstetrics. 23rd ed. New York: McGraw-Hill, 2010. Fig. 19-3.)*

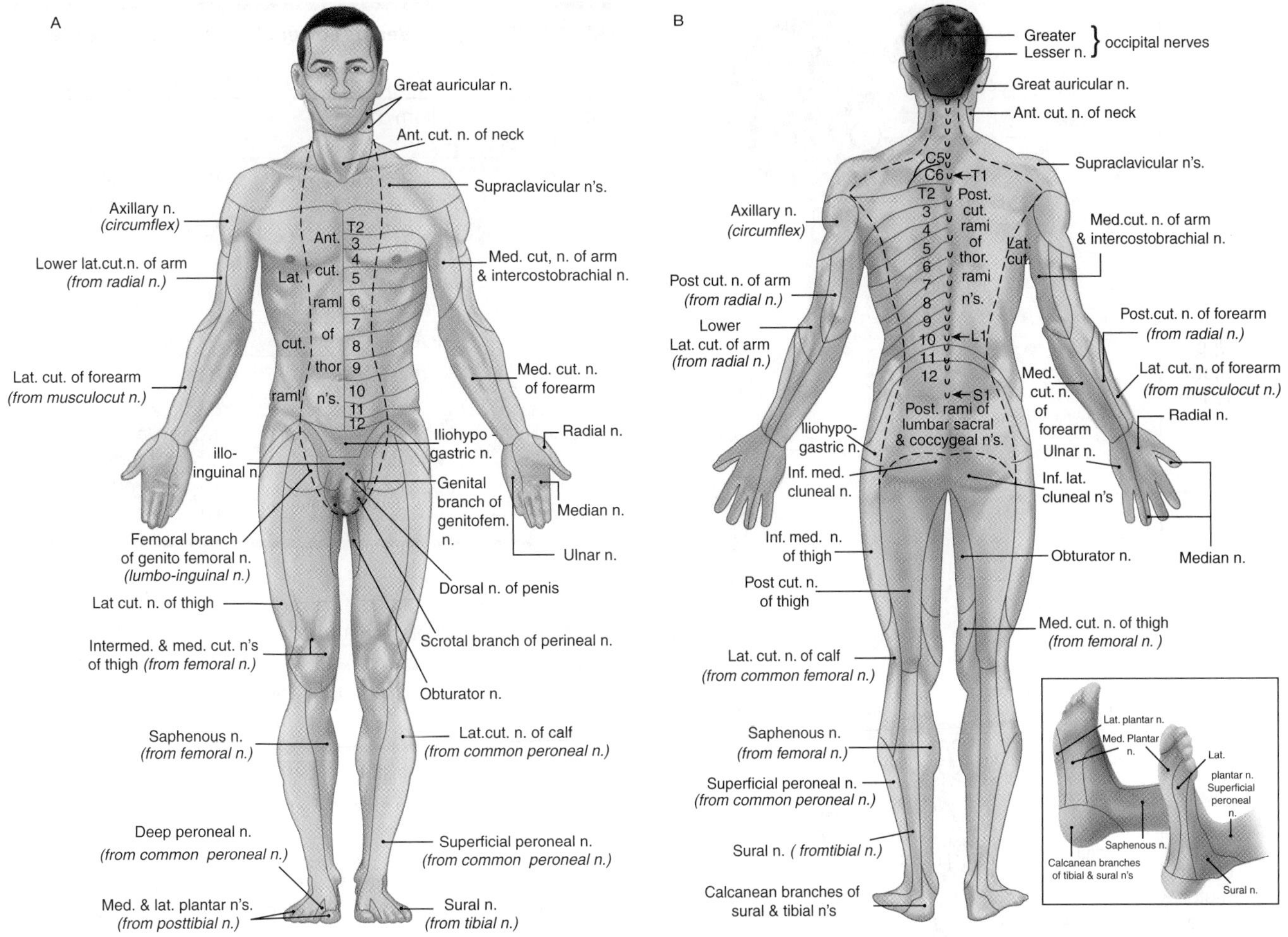

Figure 207-2 *Map of peripheral sensory nerves. Front (A). Back (B). (Reproduced, with permission, from Haymaker W, Woodhall B: Peripheral Nerve Injuries, 2nd ed. Philadelphia, Saunders, 1953.)*

UPPER VERSUS LOWER MOTOR NEURON LESION

When patients have weakness, it is helpful to localize the lesion to either the upper or lower motor neuron (**Figure 207-3**). Severity of weakness does not distinguish between these anatomical sites, but examination of tone, reflexes, and other elements of the exam do (**Table 207-1**). When upper motor neuron weakness is present, the lesion must be in the brain or spinal cord. Lower motor neuron weakness may have multiple localizations (**Table 207-2**), none of which can be discerned through imaging studies of the brain and spinal cord; key next steps may include EMG and nerve conduction studies (NCSs).

POSTERIOR FOSSA LESIONS

CASE 207-3

A 76-year-old woman is reportedly found "twitching" in the hallway of her apartment building, after having been seen to be well 1 hour prior. She is intubated for airway protection. In the emergency department, she has a recorded blood pressure of 240/130 mm Hg. On exam, her right eye is abducted in downgaze, and the right pupil is larger than the left. Cranial nerves are otherwise intact. She withdraws to painful stimulus with the right arm, which appears ataxic with movement. She is able to communicate intact sensation. She is hyporeflexic, and Babinski signs are present bilaterally.

The posterior fossa contains the brainstem and cerebellum. Due to their bony encasement, even minor amounts of swelling may result in obstruction of cerebrospinal fluid outflow and significant morbidity and mortality. In posterior fossa stroke, the time window for successful therapy is narrower than that for other areas of the brain, due to the poor natural history. Brainstem signs include abnormal cranial nerve findings, such as unequal or misshapen pupils and facial asymmetry. In addition, crossed signs—contralateral findings in face and body—may be present. Many of these are present in our case patient. Our patient had urgent neuroimaging that did not reveal a hemorrhage and recovered following thrombolysis for ischemic stroke.

ESSENTIAL ELEMENTS OF THE NEUROLOGIC EXAMINATION

An in-depth neurologic examination can take an exorbitant amount of time when not driven by a hypothesis. Many of the patients cared for by hospitalists warrant only a brief screening

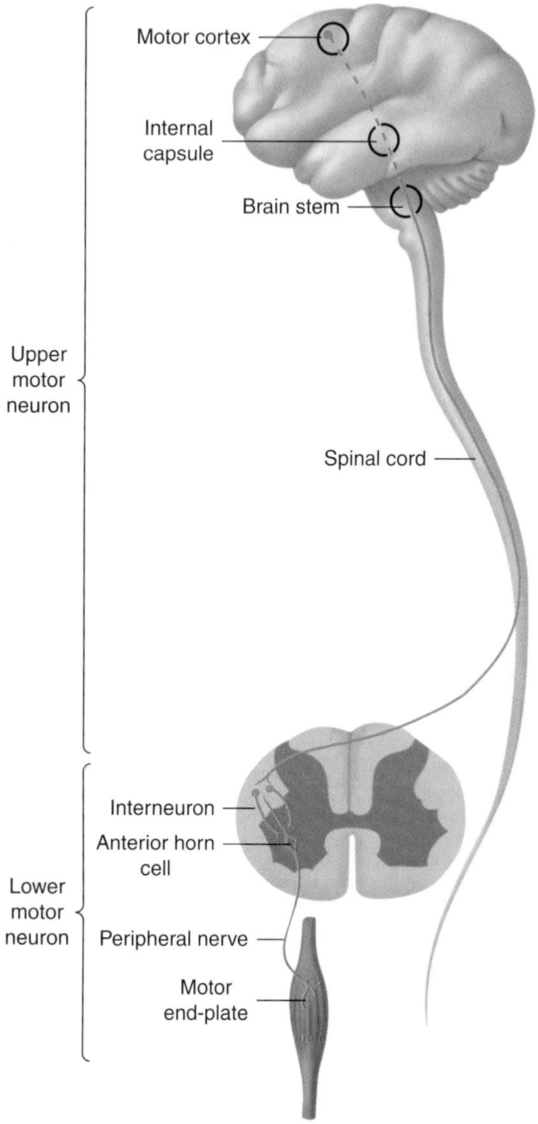

Figure 207-3 *Anatomical localization of upper and lower motor neuron lesions. (Reproduced, with permission, from Waxman SG. Clinical Neuroanatomy. 26th ed. New York: McGraw-Hill, 2010. Fig. 5-22.)*

examination. It is particularly important to assess for underlying mental frailty due to underlying dementia, as neurologic illness often becomes more apparent due to the stresses of hospitalization. This may take the form of delirium unmasking dementia or respiratory failure revealing underlying neuromuscular weakness.

TABLE 207-1 Upper Versus Lower Motor Neuron Weakness

	Upper Motor Neuron	Lower Motor Neuron
Pattern of weakness	Pyramidal	Variable
Function/dexterity	Rapid alternating movements slow and clumsy (indicates disease in cerebellar or corticospinal tracts)	Impairment of function is mostly due to weakness
Tone	Increased	Decreased
Tendon reflex	Increased	Decreased, absent, or normal
Other signs	Babinski sign, other central signs (eg, aphasia, visual field cut)	Atrophy (except with problems of the neuromuscular junction)

Fortunately, much of the neurologic examination is observational. The attentive clinician may be able to document many essential elements of the exam without formal testing:

Mental status

- Established during history taking when asking specific questions
- Language fluency is apparent during the history.

Cranial nerves

- Vision, eye movements, and sternocleidomastoid, as the patient watches the examiner walk between the sides of the bed
- Facial symmetry, lid strength, hearing, and tongue strength as the history is taken

Motor examination

- Gross abnormalities can be seen as the patient moves in bed or between the bed and a chair.
- Subtle signs, such as the external rotation of a foot, as evidence of upper motor neuron–type leg weakness
- Tremor may be noted at rest and with movement.

Coordination

- Although getting the patient to walk may be difficult, it is often very revealing.
- Observe the patient manipulating the nurse call button and moving the bedside tray, or ask the patient to retrieve a medication list from a purse or drawer.

Sensory examination and reflexes

- Usually require formal testing for assessment

TABLE 207-2 Patterns of Muscle Weakness

	Motor Neuron Disease	Neuropathy	Neuromuscular Junction	Myopathy
Weakness pattern	Variable	Distal	Diffuse	Proximal
Deep tendon reflexes	Increased, normal, or decreased	Decreased or absent	Normal or decreased	Normal or decreased
Atrophy	Yes	Yes	No	No
Fasciculations	Yes	Sometimes	No	No
Sensory symptoms and signs	No	Yes	No	No

PRACTICE POINT

The ability to test higher cognitive functions such as memory and language is limited in patients who cannot sustain attention. Inattentiveness, or the inability to concentrate, often indicates delirium, particularly when accompanied by fluctuating mental status, alteration of consciousness, and disorganized thinking. Bedside tests useful in assessing attention and delirium include:

- Assessing the level of arousal (awake, drowsy, lethargic, or comatose); speak to nurses and family members to assess whether mental status is waxing and waning.
- Assessing the level of awareness (orientation to person, place, and time). Note that an oriented patient may still be confused, and a disoriented one may have psychosis, amnesia, or aphasia instead of delirium.
- Days of the week or months of the year, forward and backward (serial 7s and spelling words backward are not good tests, particularly for patients who are illiterate or uneducated)

Have the patient play a game that requires attention. For example, if the examiner taps once, the patient taps twice on the table; if the examiner taps twice, the patient does not tap on the table. Alternatively, have the patient tap the examiner's palm every time a certain letter of the alphabet is mentioned.

Many elements do require specific attention and testing, as one may miss significant findings or leave others poorly defined. These are typically symptom-driven, as in a patient presenting with suspicion of intracranial disease, spinal cord disease, peripheral weakness or numbness, or multifocal neurologic disease. If the patient cannot pay attention, as in the case of delirium, the examiner may erroneously assume that he or she has an underlying dementia. Therefore, formal neuropsychological testing is best delayed until the patient has recovered from acute illness and the delirium has resolved.

UNRESPONSIVENESS

CASE 207-4

A 62-year-old man is found unresponsive. His cranial nerves are tested individually and are intact, with the exception of unequal pupils, corneal reflexes, and abnormal eye movements. He does not respond to painful stimuli. Babinski sign is present on the left. MRI reveals a basilar artery thrombosis.

Frequently, the exam is erroneously thought to be of little use in patients who are unresponsive or comatose. At the very least, pupillary, corneal, and gag or cough reflexes can be evaluated easily in the nonparalyzed patient. Facial strength, along with the motor and sensory systems, can be evaluated with response to painful stimuli.

Coma can result from two different localizations: bilateral cerebral hemispheric damage, as in head trauma or metabolic disturbances, such as hepatic encephalopathy or drug intoxication, and damage to the reticular activating system in the brainstem. Most cranial nerve nuclei (III to XII, except XI) are housed in the brainstem near the reticular activating system. If there are cranial nerve abnormalities, the lesion responsible for coma likely involves the reticular activating system, as in the patient vignette above. In the more common scenario where the cranial nerves are normal, bilateral hemispheric dysfunction is likely the culprit.

HEADACHE

CASE 207-5

A 45-year-old otherwise healthy woman presents with progressive headaches and left-sided weakness. She has had recent fevers. Her exam reveals bilateral papilledema, in addition to mild left-sided weakness.

Headache is a common element in patients with various underlying intracranial processes. These patients may have normal exams or relatively nonspecific exam findings. The character of the headache and nature of its onset are very important. A moderate headache of subacute onset is evaluated differently than a severe headache of acute onset. An exacerbation of a previously evaluated migraine syndrome may not warrant repeated imaging, but a sudden-onset "worst headache of my life" certainly does.

This patient has papilledema on exam, concerning for raised intracranial pressure, which may present solely with headache. Causes of high intracranial pressures include venous sinus thrombosis, cerebrovascular disease with edema, malignancy, meningoencephalitis, mass lesion, pseudotumor cerebri, and brain abscess. In these cases, historical elements such as blurred vision, diplopia, headache, and nausea will often be of more help in the differential diagnosis than the exam. Signs in patients with headaches due to focal lesions include a depressed level of consciousness, pupillary asymmetry, unilateral weakness, and pronator drift. However, even large subdural hematomas may be missed on a thorough examination, requiring a high index of suspicion from the history and communication with family members who may report a subtle personality change.

CASE 207-5 *(continued)*

Further history reveals three spontaneous miscarriages. Over the next several hours, the patient develops bilateral weakness, increasing headache, and a left-sided seizure that generalizes. Magnetic resonance venography (MRV) shows a venous clot and stroke with hemorrhagic conversion. She is subsequently found to have antiphospholipid antibody syndrome.

VERTIGO

CASE 207-6

A 54-year-old man with a history of myocardial infarction and stroke complains of vertigo. He is recovering from a recent upper respiratory infection. The emergency department physician calls you to admit the patient for a possible brainstem stroke.

Vertigo is a source of frequent consternation, as it may represent the common sequelae of an upper respiratory tract infection or a harbinger of life-threatening posterior fossa disease. Key initial steps are to determine whether the patient has true vertigo (the illusion of movement) or a different sensation, such as presyncope.

Elements of the history and exam that suggest a central cause of vertigo, such as brainstem stroke, intracranial mass lesions, or multiple sclerosis, include headache, persistent symptoms, neck pain, visual disturbances, speech difficulty, cranial nerve palsies, and ataxia. Horizontal nystagmus is common in both central and peripheral vertigo, but vertical nystagmus is more common with central rather than peripheral conditions. Hearing loss is uncommon with central disease.

CASE 207-6 (continued)

The patient's history is reassuring. The only finding on a detailed neurologic exam is two beats of horizontal nystagmus. He is sent home from the emergency department and does well.

COMPLAINTS REFERABLE TO THE SPINAL CORD

CASE 207-7

A 32-year-old woman with a distant history of tuberculosis and recent treatment with prednisone for an asthma exacerbation presents with midback pain and vague complaints of difficulty walking, along with a sensation of her legs giving way. On examination, her gait is tentative, and Babinski signs are present bilaterally.

Few areas are more important in neurologic localization than the spinal cord. Because the spinal cord is tightly confined in a bony canal, irreversible damage with profound consequences can be millimeters or minutes away. Historical features that increase the risk of spinal cord compression include recent trauma, metastatic cancer or myeloma, and systemic infection, especially with bacteremia, which increases the risk of epidural abscess. Pain at the site of compression is usually the first symptom. Patients may have radicular pain at the level of compression, often exacerbated by coughing or straining. Leg weakness and sensory disturbances are also common. Cauda equina involvement may produce bowel and bladder disturbances.

Sensory testing must be performed to help define the level of involvement. This can be performed with a safety pin or tuning fork run quickly over the patient's back. This brief examination is of immense value in determining what level should be imaged. Reflex testing may also help to define the level, as well as the affected side if disease is unilateral (**Table 207-3**). Weakness, hyperreflexia, and Babinski signs may also be present.

TABLE 207-3 Tendon Reflexes and Their Associated Nerve Root Levels

Reflex	Peripheral Nerve	Nerve Root
Biceps	Musculocutaneous	C5, C6
Triceps	Radial	C7, C8
Brachioradialis	Radial	C5, C6
Abdominal	Segmental cutaneous nerves	T8–T9 (above umbilicus); T10–T11 (below umbilicus)
Patellar	Femoral	L3, L4
Achilles	Tibial	S1, S2

TABLE 207-4 Grading of Muscle Strength (Modified Medical Research Council Scale)

Grade 0	No movement whatsoever
Grade 1	Flicker or trace contraction
Grade 2	Moves only when gravity eliminated (in the horizontal plane only)
Grade 3	Moves against gravity but not resistance
Grade 4–	Moves against gravity and light resistance
Grade 4	Moves against gravity and moderate resistance
Grade 4+	Submaximal movement against resistance
Grade 5	Full power

CASE 207-7 (continued)

The patient's sensory exam reveals a clear change in sensation below T11. Subsequent evaluation confirms Pott's disease of the spine.

MULTIFOCAL DISEASE

Multifocal disease can be difficult to diagnose. Many neurologic diseases present with ill-defined symptoms, particularly in the early stages. There is a tendency to label a patient as a malingerer in the absence of an easily discernible pattern or localizable lesion. This risk of misdiagnosis is increased in patients with vague complaints or barriers to communication.

Multifocal disease calls for an even more careful history and examination, as disease manifestations may be protean. Conditions such as polyarteritis nodosa, sarcoidosis, Sjogren syndrome, porphyria, and lead poisoning can be clinically confusing even when disparate sensory and motor symptoms are not part of the clinical picture. When these are the presenting symptoms, the difficulty in lesion localization may drive electrodiagnostic studies, as well as a wide-ranging laboratory evaluation.

DOCUMENTING THE EXAMINATION

When caring for patients with neurologic disease, documentation of the examination requires greater precision than "nonfocal" and general terms such as "weak." Whereas the sensory exam does not lend itself well to quantification, the motor strength and reflex testing do (**Tables 207-4** and **207-5**). It is important to record what areas are tested and the degree of weakness noted. This information is especially valuable when patients have fluctuating symptoms either in the hospital or after discharge.

TABLE 207-5 Grading of Deep Tendon Reflexes

4	Very brisk, often with clonus (record the number of beats)
3	Brisk
2	Normal
1	Minimal
0	Absent

Specialized instruments, such as the National Institutes of Health Stroke Scale (NIHSS), may be very helpful for the hospitalist (http://www.ninds.nih.gov/doctors/NIH_Stroke_Scale.pdf). In addition to quantifying the deficits in patients suffering acute stroke and determining eligibility for thrombolysis, the NIHSS is an excellent tool for documenting neurologic deficits. Many hospitals mandate recording of the NIHSS on admission and at intervals during a hospital stay. If the patient has a significant change, a covering physician or nurse will be able to quantify the degree of difference and determine whether additional interventions are needed. Free training courses are available online.

CONCLUSION

The neurologic examination is key in determining the etiology of neurologic complaints. While the potential range of evaluation can be daunting, a focused examination that is informed by the history has a high yield. This is no less true for patients who are poorly responsive. By using standardized tools and scales, one can more easily communicate change and intervene with more certainty. With a core set of neurologic examination skills and knowledge, the practicing hospitalist plays a central role in the care of these patients.

SUGGESTED READINGS

Biller J, Gruener G, Brazis P. DeMyer's *The Neurologic Examination: A Programmed Text*. 6th ed. New York: McGraw-Hill; 2011.

Booth CM, Boone RH, Thomlinson G, et al. Is this patient dead, vegetative, or severely neurologically impaired?. In: Simel DL, Rennie D, eds. *The Rational Clinical Examination*. New York: McGraw-Hill; 2009:215–226 [chapter 17].

Froehling DA, Silverstein MD, Mohr DN, Beatty CW. The Rational Clinical Examination. Does this dizzy patient have a serious form of vertigo? *JAMA*. 1994 Feb 2;271(5):385–388.

Goldstein LB, Simel DL. Is this patient having a stroke?. In: Simel DL, Rennie D, eds. *The Rational Clinical Examination*. New York: McGraw-Hill; 2009:627–641 [chapter 48].

Lance JW. The Babinski sign. *J Neurol Neurosurg Psychiatry*. 2002;73:360–362.

Lanska DJ, Goetz CG. Romberg's sign: development, adoption, and adaptation in the 19th century. *Neurology*. 2000;55:1201–1206.

Lindsay, KW, Bone I, Callander R. *Neurology and Neurosurgery Illustrated*. New York: Churchill Livingstone; 1997.

Owen G, Mulley GP. The palmomental reflex: a useful clinical sign? *J Neurol Neurosurg Psychiatry*. 2002;73:113–115.

Rao G, Fisch L, Srinivasan S, et al. Does this patient have Parkinson disease? In: Simel DL, Rennie D, eds *The Rational Clinical Examination*. New York: McGraw-Hill; 2009:505–514 [chapter 38].

Smetana GW and Shmerling RH. Does this patient have temporal arteritis. In: Simel DL, Rennie D, eds. *The Rational Clinical Examination*. New York: McGraw-Hill; 2009:643–656 [chapter 49].

CHAPTER 208

Stupor and Coma

Nicholas D. Schiff, MD
Joseph J. Fins, MD, FACP

Key Clinical Questions

1. How do stupor, coma, persistent vegetative state, minimally conscious state, and akinetic mutism differ?
2. What historical features and examination findings are useful in the diagnosis of acute stupor and coma?
3. How is acute coma in hospitalized patients managed?
4. What prognostic information should be given to surrogate decision makers for patients with severe alterations of consciousness?

INTRODUCTION

Alterations of consciousness are frequently encountered by hospitalists in the practice of general medicine. *Coma* is an unconscious brain state produced by several acute or chronic brain insults. The acute onset of coma is a medical emergency and requires immediate assessment and specific therapy. Coma is distinct from vegetative state, minimally conscious state, and akinetic mutism, conditions that are sometimes confused with it. The timing and probability of recovery from coma and the vegetative state differ considerably, depending on the nature of the underlying brain injury. We review diagnosis and prognosis in disorders of consciousness, address ethical challenges arising in the care of these patients, and provide a guide to discussions with surrogate decision makers for the comatose or severely brain-injured patient.

COMA AND RELATED DISORDERS OF CONSCIOUSNESS

LETHARGY, OBTUNDATION, AND STUPOR

Lethargy refers to a minor decrease in alertness and energy, whereas *obtundation* refers to a moderate decline in responsiveness. *Stupor* is applied to patients with marked impairment of arousal who nevertheless sometimes respond purposefully to vigorous physical stimuli, such as prodding, sticking with a pin, or calling out loudly. Stupor resembles deep sleep.

COMA

Coma is a brain state characterized by the total absence of patterned behavioral arousal. Comatose patients are completely unresponsive. Like stuporous patients, they appear to be in deep sleep, lying motionless with eyes closed, but without eye opening or purposeful movements induced by vigorous stimulation. Coma is produced by a variety of acute or chronic brain insults. It may be distinguished from syncope, concussion, or other forms of transient unconsciousness by its time course. The term *coma* implies duration of at least 1 hour. Although some comatose patients recover rapidly, especially when coma is due to a concurrent systemic illness, a more gradual recovery is often seen for patients with brain injuries sufficient to produce even a day of coma. In such patients, recovery will be marked by the patient's entering into a vegetative state or minimally conscious state, as defined below.

Although coma patients lack purposeful responses to internal or external stimuli, noxious stimuli may cause them to grimace or make stereotyped withdrawal movements of the limbs generated by spinal reflexes. These movements are not directed toward the external stimuli and are not organized actions consistent with purposeful avoidance. In very deep coma, even these primitive reflex responses may disappear.

In coma, normal brain arousal mechanisms that control the level of neuronal activity in the brain and the normal sleep–wake cycle are disrupted. Coma requires disruption of either bilateral hemispheric functioning or the brainstem reticular activating system (**Figure 208-1**). Causes of coma include metabolic disturbances, such as anoxia, acidosis, and hyponatremia, drug intoxication, severe bilateral injuries to the cerebral hemispheres, and injuries to a small set of regions of the upper brainstem or thalamus resulting from stroke or herniation syndromes (**Table 208-1**).

Clustered within the brainstem and basal forebrain are several neuronal populations that support wakefulness. These include glutamatergic and cholinergic neurons in the brainstem and

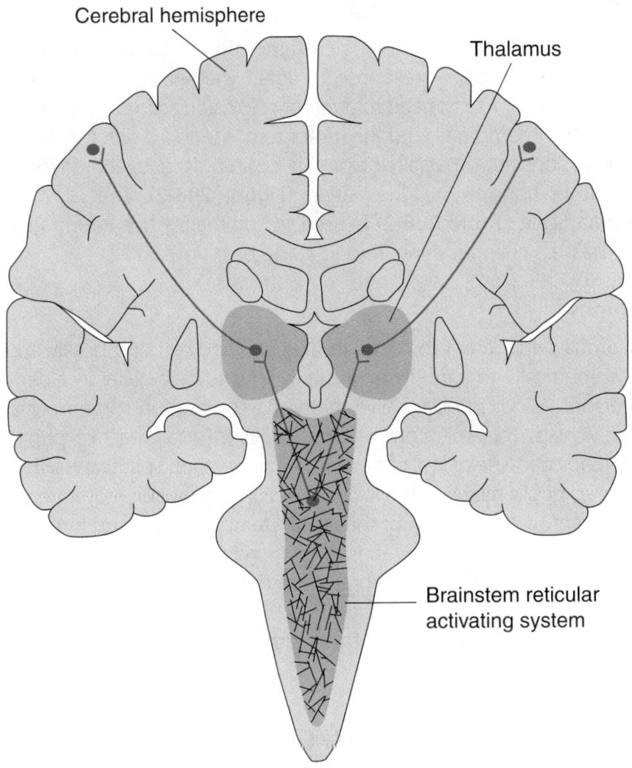

Figure 208-1 *Anatomical basis of coma. Consciousness is maintained by the normal functioning of the brainstem reticular activating system above the midpons and its bilateral projections to the thalamus and cerebral hemispheres. Coma results from lesions that affect either the reticular activating system or both hemispheres. (Reproduced, with permission, from Simon RP, Greenberg DA, Aminoff MJ. Clinical Neurology. 7th ed. New York: McGraw-Hill, 2009. Fig. 10-1.)*

TABLE 208-1 Causes of Acute Coma

Supratentorial lesions that may lead to herniation syndromes
Subdural hematoma
Epidural hematoma
Cerebral contusion
Intracerebral hemorrhage
Brain abscess
Cerebral infarction
Brain tumor
Subtentorial lesions affecting brainstem function
Basilar artery thrombosis or embolism
Pontine hemorrhage
Cerebellar hemorrhage or infarct
Metabolic abnormalities
Acid–base disturbances
Anoxia
Drug intoxications
Hepatic encephalopathy
Hyperosmolar states
Hypertensive encephalopathy
Hyperthermia
Hypothermia
Hypoglycemia
Hyponatremia
Sepsis/systemic inflammatory response syndrome
Meningitis or encephalitis
Subarachnoid hemorrhage
Seizures, status epilepticus, and postictal state

basal forebrain, serotoninergic and noradrenergic neurons of the brainstem, and histaminergic and orexin-producing neurons of the hypothalamus. Because arousal is controlled by multiple systems, relatively large bilateral injuries to the upper pons, midbrain, or central thalamus are needed to produce coma in humans. Coma arising from such focal injuries is short-lived, typically lasting only hours or a few days, and is unlikely to be encountered by the hospitalist.

Following a coma produced by severe brain injury, patients may either deteriorate, with progressive neuronal damage leading to brain death, or show signs of recovery, heralded by brief periods of eye opening without behavioral responsiveness. Comas that do not resolve quickly instead evolve into the vegetative state, minimally conscious state, and other related clinical syndromes.

VEGETATIVE STATE

In the persistent vegetative state, there is a limited recovery of arousal, with spontaneous periods of eye opening, reflecting some functional recovery of the brainstem and reticular activating system, but without evidence of awareness of self or the environment. The vegetative state frequently arises following coma, and the structural injuries producing the vegetative state strongly overlap with those that produce coma. Common causes include diffuse axonal injury from brain trauma and anoxic brain injury from cardiac arrest. Autopsies of patients in the persistent vegetative state typically show widespread disconnection of the corticothalamic system, with extensive death of thalamic neurons. Within the thalamus, the central thalamic neurons show the greatest volume loss; bilateral damage to these regions in isolation can produce coma.

MINIMALLY CONSCIOUS STATE

The minimally conscious state is differentiated from the vegetative state by inconsistent but unequivocal evidence of awareness of self or the environment. A range of subtle behaviors may indicate responsiveness in the minimally conscious state. For example, a patient might be limited to tracking of objects in the visual field or localization of auditory stimuli, such as head turning to a ringing bell. Because these behaviors may be manifested only intermittently, the patient must be assessed over multiple examinations.

Alternatively, some minimally conscious patients may have high-level responses, such as intermittent verbalization and communication. Although the bedside distinctions between the vegetative and minimally conscious states may be subtle, pathologic studies suggest that there are major differences in underlying structural pathology. Some patients in the minimally conscious state have no evidence of thalamic injury or severe diffuse axonal injury, patterns that are never seen in the vegetative state. This suggests a different anatomical substrate for residual cerebral function in many patients in the minimally conscious state. It is likely that substantial portions of the corticothalamic system are preserved in patients with the minimally conscious state, in contrast to those in the vegetative state.

AKINETIC MUTISM

Akinetic mutism is a somewhat ambiguous term. In general, it refers to conditions consistent with the minimally conscious state or a higher level of recovery. Akinetic mute patients show apparent attentiveness and vigilance, as often evidenced by deliberate visual tracking of the examiner around the room, but exhibit a paucity of behaviors, even when vigorously prompted. More specifically, akinetic mutism is a syndrome associated with bilateral damage to the anterior medial regions of the cerebral cortex, often arising from rupture of an aneurysm at the junction of the anterior cerebral arteries. These medial frontal cortical regions are closely linked and are also associated with the central thalamus and basal ganglia. Patients suffer from severe memory loss, markedly slowed behavioral responses, and an apathetic, listless appearance.

LOCKED-IN SYNDROME

Akinetic mutism may be confused with locked-in syndrome, which results from lesions ventral to the reticular activating system in the midpons. Patients are conscious but mute and quadriplegic. They usually retain control over eye opening, vertical eye movements, and ocular convergence. Causes include pontine hemorrhage, central pontine myelolysis, tumor, and encephalitis.

DIAGNOSIS AND MANAGEMENT OF COMA AND STUPOR

HISTORY

Caregivers of patients in a coma may provide useful information about the tempo of coma onset. Precipitous onset suggests a brainstem stroke, subarachnoid hemorrhage, or other vascular calamity. The rapid evolution of hemiparesis and other hemispheric findings to coma over minutes or hours suggests intracerebral hemorrhage. A more indolent progression from localizing findings to coma over days to weeks suggests tumor, abscess, or subdural hematoma. Coma preceded by delirium and lacking focal neurologic deficits suggests an intoxication or metabolic derangement.

GENERAL PHYSICAL EXAMINATION

Vital signs

The patient may have hypertension, which predisposes to intracerebral hemorrhage or stroke. The presence of severe hypertension suggests coma from hypertensive encephalopathy, or coma from intracerebral or subarachnoid hemorrhage leading to secondary hypertension. Hypothermia may be a primary cause of coma, but it may also complicate drug intoxications, myxedema, hypoglycemia, and hepatic encephalopathy. Hyperthermia may be seen in heatstroke, malignant hyperthermia from inhalational anesthetics, neuroleptic malignant syndrome, anticholinergic drug toxicity, status epilepticus, and pontine or hypothalamic lesions.

Trauma

When trauma is possible, patients should be examined for signs of basilar skull fracture, such as raccoon eyes, Battle sign (bruising over the mastoid process), hemotympanum, and cerebrospinal fluid leak from the nose or ear. Patients may have soft tissue bruising over the scalp or, rarely, a depressed skull fracture.

Meningeal irritation

Nuchal rigidity and the Brudzinski sign (involuntary flexion of the hip and knee in response to passive neck flexion) may be seen in meningitis and subarachnoid hemorrhage, but they may be absent in elderly, immunosuppressed, debilitated, or deeply comatose patients with these conditions.

Optic fundi

Papilledema and retinal hemorrhage may be present in patients with increased intracranial hemorrhage or either acute or chronic hypertension. Subhyaloid, or superficial, retinal hemorrhages suggest subarachnoid hemorrhage.

NEUROLOGIC EXAMINATION

Key elements of the neurologic examination in stupor and coma include the pupillary response to light, whether eye movements occur in response to head rotation or cold caloric stimulation of the tympanic membrane, and the motor response to a painful stimulus. These signs are especially helpful in localizing the level of involvement in transtentorial herniation (**Figure 208-2**). The Glasgow Coma Scale (**Table 208-2**) is used to summarize this information and assess changes in neurologic status over time.

Pupils

Normal pupils are 3 to 4 mm in diameter and respond briskly and symmetrically to light. Normal pupils tend to be smaller in elderly persons. Minor pupillary asymmetry may be seen in some normal individuals. Thalamic compression results in small reactive pupils, perhaps because of loss of descending sympathetic pathways. Fixed dilated pupils may be seen in compression of the oculomotor nerve, transtentorial herniation of the medial temporal lobe, and intoxication with anticholinergic and sympathomimetic drugs. Fixed midsize pupils are indicative of brainstem damage. Pinpoint pupils are seen with narcotic overdose, organophosphate poisoning, pontine damage, and miotic eye drops for glaucoma.

Extraocular movements

In comatose patients, eye movements may be tested by engaging the vestibular system, either through passive head rotation (doll's eyes) or irrigation of the tympanic membrane with ice water (cold caloric testing). If comatose patients have conjugate horizontal eye movements spontaneously (roving eye movements), with passive head rotation, or with cold caloric testing, which is expected to elicit tonic conjugate eye movement toward the irrigated ear, the brainstem pathways for conjugate eye movement are intact. Abnormalities in conjugate eye movements imply impaired brainstem function from structural lesions, metabolic disorders, or intoxications.

Motor response to pain

Noxious stimuli used to test motor responses include pressure on the nail beds, sternum, or brow ridges. When consciousness is only moderately depressed, patients may reach toward the site of painful stimuli (localization). *Decorticate posturing* entails flexion of the arms and adduction of the shoulders, with extension of the leg and ankle. *Decerebrate posturing* includes extension of the elbow, with internal rotation of the shoulder and forearm and leg extension. Traditionally, decorticate posturing has been thought to indicate thalamic damage or compression, with decerebrate posturing implying midbrain dysfunction, although neither sign is precisely localizing. Posturing may be seen in reversible metabolic disorders and intoxications, as well as mass lesions and infarcts. Unilateral posturing suggests a lesion of the contralateral cerebral hemisphere or brainstem. Pontine and medullary lesions may produce only knee flexion in response to pain.

INVESTIGATIONS AND MANAGEMENT

Urgent general steps in the diagnosis and management of the patient with coma and stupor are summarized in **Table 208-3**. Specific treatment is directed at the underlying cause.

PROGNOSIS IN COMA, MINIMALLY CONSCIOUS STATES, AND VEGETATIVE STATES

Coma is an inherently precarious condition. The short-term mortality of patients with coma after brain trauma is 40% to 50%, and 54% to 88% for patients comatose after a cardiac arrest. Patients with traumatic brain injuries have a higher likelihood of significant

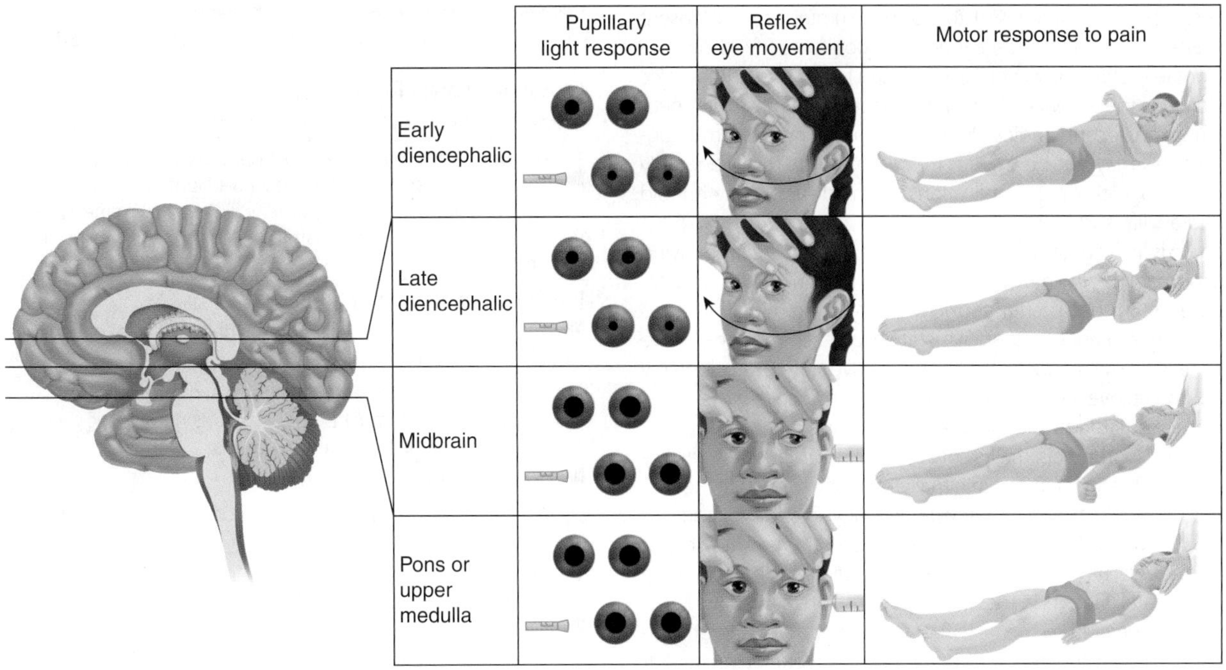

Figure 208-2 *Neurologic signs in coma with downward transtentorial herniation. In the early diencephalic phase, the pupils are small (~2 mm in diameter) and reactive, reflex eye movements are intact, and the motor response to pain is purposeful or semipurposeful (localizing) and often asymmetric. The late diencephalic phase is associated with similar findings, except that painful stimulation results in decorticate (flexor) posturing, which may also be asymmetric. With midbrain involvement, the pupils are fixed and midsize (~5 mm in diameter), reflex adduction of the eyes is impaired, and pain elicits decerebrate (extensor) posturing. Progression to involve the pons or medulla also produces fixed, midsize pupils, but these are accompanied by loss of reflex abduction as well as adduction of the eyes and by no motor response or only leg flexion upon painful stimulation. Note that, although a lesion restricted to the pons produces pinpoint pupils as a result of the destruction of descending sympathetic (pupillodilator) pathways, downward herniation to the pontine level is associated with midsize pupils. This happens because herniation also interrupts parasympathetic (pupilloconstrictor) fibers in the oculomotor (III) nerve. (Reproduced, with permission, from Simon RP, Greenberg DA, Aminoff MJ. Clinical Neurology. 7th ed. New York: McGraw-Hill, 2009. Fig. 10-2.)*

recovery than those who have sustained a cardiac arrest. The typically younger age of patients with traumatic brain injuries and the delayed mechanisms of neuronal death following brain trauma and axonal disconnection in this condition may account for the marked variation in recovery compared with nontraumatic causes. Recovery after prolonged traumatic coma is well described. Unlike coma from anoxic brain injury, unconsciousness for 1 month after trauma does not necessarily preclude significant recovery.

Traditionally, the prognosis of anoxic brain injury has been related to the duration of neurologic impairment. If brainstem functions, such as pupillary responses and corneal responses, and motor

TABLE 208-2 Glasgow Coma Scale*

I. Best motor response	
Obeys commands for movement	6 points
Purposeful movement to painful stimulus	5 points
Withdraws to painful stimuli	4 points
Abnormal flexion (decorticate posturing)	3 points
Extension (decerebrate posturing)	2 points
No response	1 point
II. Verbal response	
Oriented	5 points
Confused but able to answer questions	4 points
Inappropriate words	3 points
Incomprehensible speech	2 points
No response	1 point
III. Eye opening	
Spontaneous	4 points
To verbal stimuli, command, speech	3 points
To pain only (not applied to face)	2 points
None	1 point

*Total score is the sum of I + II + III (maximum 15 points).

TABLE 208-3 Emergency Management of the Acutely Comatose Patient

Assess the adequacy of the patient's airway, breathing, and circulation
Secure IV access and draw blood for serum glucose and electrolytes, hepatic and renal function, coagulation studies, and complete blood count.
Administer IV glucose (typically as 50 mL of 50% dextrose), thiamine 100 mg, and naloxone 0.4 to 1.2 mg.
Obtain arterial blood gas and pH measurements to assess for acid–base disturbances.
Treat seizures, if present.
Detailed physical and neurologic examination
CT scan of the head, especially if signs suggestive of mass lesion or subarachnoid hemorrhage are present
Lumbar puncture if signs of meningeal irritation are present
Blood and urine toxicology screens

responses, such as withdrawal to noxious stimuli, are still absent 3 days after cardiac arrest, there is no likelihood for recovery beyond the vegetative state. However, although this remains true for anoxic brain injury in the absence of interventions aimed at preserving neuronal function, recent studies of mild therapeutic hypothermia suggest that this may not be true for treated patients. This is a rapidly evolving area, with major implications on the decision to withhold or withdraw life-sustaining therapy.

Prognosis in vegetative state also depends on the underlying mechanism of brain injury. Patients who remain in the vegetative state for 3 months after anoxic brain injury are highly likely to remain in a permanent vegetative state. However, the time frame for recovery following posttraumatic vegetative state is considerably longer, with recovery occurring as late as 1 year. Recovery thereafter is rare and restricted to the minimally conscious state.

Prognosis in the minimally conscious state is another rapidly evolving area. Patients in the minimally conscious state for months may recover above the level of severe disability. In addition, the rare examples of very late recovery of communication in severely brain-injured patients have invariably been in patients in the minimally conscious state. Patients in the minimally conscious state have faster rates of recovery within the first year after either traumatic or nontraumatic injury compared with patients in the vegetative state. It is critical to distinguish between the vegetative and minimally conscious states when evaluating the postcomatose patient, as even small signs of consciousness identified by hospitalists on rounds may have a major bearing on prognosis.

TABLE 208-4 Criteria for the Diagnosis of Brain Death

Cessation of brain function
Unresponsiveness to all sensory input, including pain and speech
Absent brainstem reflexes: absent papillary, corneal, and oropharyngeal responses; no eye movement with oculocephalic (doll's eye) and vestibulo-ocular (caloric testing) maneuvers; no ventilatory effort when the patient's Pco_2 is permitted to rise to 60 mm Hg
Irreversibility of brain dysfunction
The cause of coma must be known, adequate to explain the clinical picture, and irreversible.
Sedative drug intoxication, hypothermia, neuromuscular blockade, and shock must be ruled out, as neurologic recovery may still be possible in these conditions.
Persistence of brain dysfunction
These criteria must persist for an appropriate length of time, as follows: 1. Six hours with a confirmatory isoelectric (flat) electroencephalogram (EEG) 2. Twelve hours without a confirmatory isoelectric EEG 3. Twenty-four hours for anoxic brain injury without a confirmatory isoelectric EEG
Additional confirmatory tests
Demonstration of the absence of cerebral blood flow confirms brain death without a waiting period. Cerebral angiography provides the most unequivocal assessment; Doppler techniques and technetium imaging are used in some centers.

ENGAGING SURROGATE DECISION MAKERS

Decisions about ongoing care or its withdrawal in patients with severe disorders of consciousness necessarily involve surrogates. A surrogate decision maker is a person, such as a spouse, partner, family member, or friend, who directs care when the patient is incapacitated. Surrogate decision makers face multiple challenges, including unfamiliarity with coma and related conditions. The hospitalist can help surrogates make informed decisions by educating them about the distinctions between these disorders of consciousness and their likely outcomes.

Although surrogates generally take loss of consciousness to be permanent and irreversible, it is not invariably a dire prognostic sign. Great skill is required to provide a balanced assessment of prospects for recovery, without either offering false hope or too quickly excluding some degree of recovery. Hospitalists should also take into account the patient's prior wishes about medical care and quality of life, if known, and be sensitive to the ability and willingness of surrogates to provide acute and chronic care, as even patients with relatively good outcomes are likely to have significant disabilities.

Discussions with surrogates can be structured around *time-delimited prognostication*. The hospitalist provides guidance on possible outcomes, based on the patient's current status and evolution over time. For example, it is justified to provide an early and definitive diagnosis of brain death when patients meet clinical criteria (**Table 208-4**). For other patients, prognostication is more difficult. Predicting outcomes for a comatose patient after out-of-hospital cardiac arrest may require considering the impact of novel therapeutic interventions, such as hypothermia. It would be

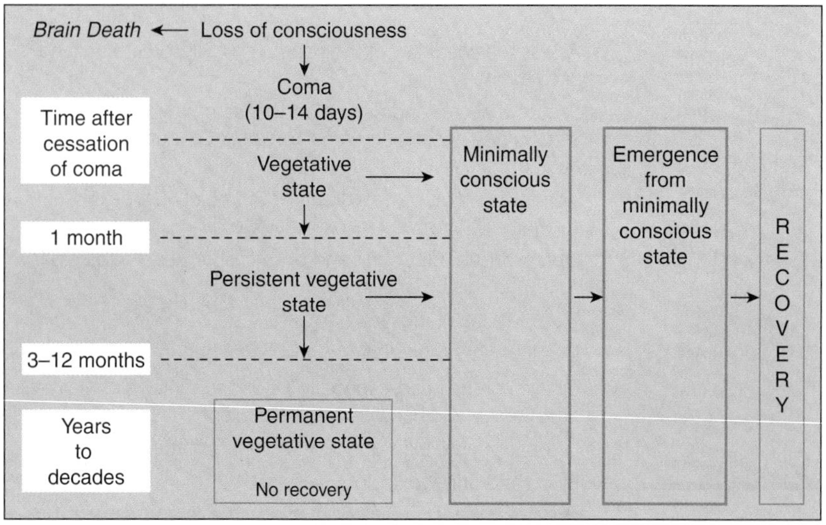

Figure 208-3 *Outcomes after the development of a vegetative state. (Adapted from Fins JJ. Neuroethics and neuroimaging: moving towards transparency. Am J Bioeth. 2008;8[9]:46–52.)*

inappropriate and premature to offer a definitive prognosis in a comatose patient with traumatic brain injury who has begun to regain brainstem function and appears to be moving quickly into the vegetative state. Patients such as these may warrant a cautiously optimistic approach. Clinicians should explain to surrogates that prognosis depends on whether the patient reaches certain milestones over time.

If patients remain in the vegetative state for 1 month, they are classified as being in a persistent vegetative state. Although some patients may still improve to the minimally conscious state and above, the prognosis for recovery becomes less favorable at this point (**Figure 208-3**). The vegetative state is considered permanent if it persists at 3 months after anoxic brain injury, 12 months after traumatic brain injury.

The minimally conscious state indicates at least some awareness and the potential to regain consistent consciousness and sometimes even the ability to communicate. The prognosis of the minimally conscious state is variable and rather ill-defined. Instances of recovery of personality and speech, albeit with persisting severe disability, have arisen even after years in the minimally conscious state. When patients enter the minimally conscious state, surrogates should be updated but cautioned to temper expectations, although not extinguish them. The distinction between the vegetative and minimally conscious states is critical during care hand-offs and transitions, such as hospital discharge, so that a patient does not become erroneously labeled as permanently vegetative, when in fact he or she is transitioning into a minimally conscious state. A failure to inform accepting physicians about ongoing evolution of brain states may adversely affect a patient's chances for improvement.

PRACTICE POINT

- Reactive pupils in the presence of otherwise impaired brainstem function suggests metabolic encephalopathy.

SUGGESTED READINGS

Adams JH, Graham DI, Jennett B. The neuropathology of the vegetative state after acute insult. *Brain.* 2000;123:1327–1338.

Fins JJ. Neuroethics and neuroimaging: moving towards transparency. *Am J Bioeth.* 2008;8:46–52.

Fins JJ, Master MG, Gerber LM, Giacino JT. The minimally conscious state: A diagnosis in search of an epidemiology. *Arch Neurol.* 2007;64:1400–1405.

Lammi MH, Smith VH, Tate RL, Taylor CM. The minimally conscious state and recovery potential: A follow-up study 2 to 5 years after traumatic brain injury. *Arch Phys Med Rehabil.* 2005;86:746–754.

Laureys S, Owen AM, Schiff ND. Brain function in coma, vegetative state, and related disorders. *Lancet Neurol.* 2004:3:537–546.

Maxwell WL, MacKinnon MA, Smith DH, McIntosh TK, Graham DI. Thalamic nuclei after human blunt head injury. *J Neuropathol Exp Neurol.* 2006;65:478–488.

Posner JB, Saper CB, Schiff ND, Plum F. *Plum and Posner's Diagnosis of Stupor and Coma.* 4th ed. Oxford: Oxford University Press; 2007.

Rossetti AO, Oddo M, Logroscino G, Kaplan PW. Prognostication after cardiac arrest and hypothermia: A prospective study. *Ann Neurol.* 2010;67:301–307.

CHAPTER 209

Intracranial Hemorrhage and Related Conditions

Alexander E. Ropper, MD
Allan H. Ropper, MD, FRCP

Key Clinical Questions

1. What are the types of intracranial hemorrhage, and how are they identified?
2. Which patients require emergent or nonemergent neurosurgical intervention?
3. How are aneurysmal and traumatic subarachnoid hemorrhage differentiated?
4. What medical treatments bear on the management of intracranial hemorrhage?
5. How is raised intracranial pressure managed?
6. Is anticoagulation safe after an intracranial hemorrhage?
7. How is brain death determined?
8. What tests should be obtained in patients with ventriculoperitoneal shunts and fever?

INTRODUCTION

Intracranial hemorrhages can be divided into three main categories. The first two, spontaneous intracerebral hemorrhage (bleeding within the brain parenchyma) and subarachnoid hemorrhage from aneurysm rupture, are considered strokes. The third category is intracranial hemorrhage from trauma, which may result in parenchymal, subarachnoid, subdural, or epidural bleeding. For ease of exposition, we use the term *intracranial hemorrhage* for all forms of bleeding within the skull and the term *intracerebral hemorrhage* for the more restricted category of bleeding within the substance of the brain.

When bleeding secondary to head trauma is excluded, intracerebral hemorrhage accounts for 10% of strokes. In the United States, rates range between 7 and 11 cases per 100,000 yearly, with a higher incidence in African Americans and Hispanics. The highest incidence globally is found in Japan, where rates are as high as 61 per 100,000 population.

SPONTANEOUS INTRACEREBRAL HEMORRHAGE

PATHOPHYSIOLOGY

The most common underlying condition in patients with spontaneous intracerebral hemorrhage is hypertension. Other associated conditions are coagulopathy, tumor, cerebral venous thrombosis, vascular malformation, amyloid angiopathy, and hemorrhagic transformation of ischemic stroke. The frequency of hypertension in patients with cerebral hemorrhage has been ~75% in many population studies. Certain subgroups of hypertensive patients are at high risk for intracranial hemorrhage, including those younger than 55 years, smokers, and especially patients who have stopped taking chronically administered antihypertensive medications. Several prospective trials have demonstrated that the risk of cerebral hemorrhage decreases with administration of antihypertensive medications. Coagulopathy has become an increasingly frequent cause of primary intracerebral hemorrhage, with both medical anticoagulation and disorders such as uremia and liver failure contributing to this increase.

PRESENTATION

Several clinical features may help distinguish cerebral hemorrhage from other forms of stroke, such as headache, nausea, vomiting, confusion, systemic hypertension, and in advanced cases, decreased level of consciousness and enlargement of the pupils. The most common location for spontaneous intracerebral hemorrhage is the basal ganglia, accounting for ~65% of cases. The presenting features, in addition to the above-described signs common to all hemorrhages, are hemiplegia and confusion. Thalamic hemorrhage presents similarly, usually with hemiplegia and often with hemianesthesia. Pontine hemorrhage causes rapid coma, quadriplegia, pinpoint pupils, and loss of extraocular movements. Cerebellar hemorrhage represents a special case that causes vomiting, vertigo, dizziness, gait ataxia, and progressive coma from hydrocephalus. Lobar hemorrhages are becoming more common with the prevalence of anticoagulant and antiplatelet therapy and cause signs referable to the region of bleeding. The differential diagnosis in all these cases includes ischemic stroke, and the distinction between ischemic stroke and hemorrhage must be made quickly.

Management of patients with intracranial hemorrhage can be separated into acute and subacute stages. Acutely, the greatest concern is for herniation, with secondary compression of the brainstem and irreversible brain damage. In addition, mass effect from a blood clot in the brain leads to elevated intracranial pressure, which in turn decreases cerebral blood flow and results in brain death. In the days following cerebral hemorrhage, a number of medical complications related to coma and immobilization become the focus of diagnosis and treatment.

DIAGNOSIS

Computed tomography (CT) scan without contrast is the primary diagnostic tool. CT angiogram or magnetic resonance imaging (MRI) may be required in special cases to establish the diagnosis of an underlying aneurysm, vascular malformations, or bleeding from an intracranial neoplasm.

All patients with suspected intracranial hemorrhage should have their coagulation parameters checked, specifically partial thromboplastin time (PTT), international normalized ratio (INR), and platelet count. Patients should be asked about anticoagulant medication, such as warfarin, aspirin, clopidogrel, and other antiplatelet agents, and recent cranial trauma.

TREATMENT

The main considerations for the hospitalist are correction of coagulopathy, blood pressure management, and seizure prophylaxis. The management of elevated intracranial pressure (ICP) results in several predictable secondary medical problems, as discussed below.

Correction of coagulopathy

Patients receiving chronic warfarin therapy require correction of the INR to a level <1.3 to 1.4. This is typically accomplished with vitamin K 10 mg, preferably IV, and with infusion of fresh frozen plasma, while sequentially measuring INR. If emergency neurosurgical intervention or other surgery is required, concentrated recombinant factor VII or factor IX may be used, with the understanding that they may subsequently increase systemic clotting risk. In our experience, these factor compounds have been effective in reversing the effects of warfarin within 20 minutes. Patients receiving antiplatelet medications, probably including low-dose daily aspirin, should receive 6 units of platelets. In thrombocytopenic patients, it is probably advisable to correct the platelet level to >100,000 if feasible. It has not been established if abnormal platelet function in patients with chronic renal failure requires platelet transfusion, but we often employ this strategy.

Blood pressure management

Most patients with cerebral hemorrhage are acutely hypertensive from the effect of raised ICP on barosensitive areas in the medulla. A reasonable approach is to keep mean arterial pressure between 70 and 100 mm Hg, which balances the risks of expansion of the clot from hypertension, and decreased cerebral perfusion from hypotension. Nicardipine and labetalol are frequently used antihypertensive drugs in neurologic practice, as they are short-acting and easily titrated. Patients who are chronically hypertensive may be maintained on their home medications. After the acute stage,β-blockers or angiotensin-converting enzyme inhibitors are generally used, but the choice is determined more by local practice and other medical factors.

PRACTICE POINT

- Mean arterial pressure at normal heart rates may be estimated as (diastolic blood pressure × ⅔) + (systolic blood pressure × ⅓).

Seizure prophylaxis

In most centers, antiseizure drugs are administered for several weeks or until resolution of the clot, although this practice has not been studied in large randomized trials. The preferred anticonvulsant varies between institutions. We use levetiracetam, as opposed to phenytoin, given the more favorable side effect profile and predictable kinetics of the former. Phenytoin use has been associated with worse outcomes after intracerebral hemorrhage in some series.

Surgical evacuation

There is evidence from one large and several small controlled trials that surgical evacuation of spontaneous intracerebral hemorrhage does not affect outcome. However, there may be exceptions depending on the clot's location, size, and proximity to the cortical surface. Hydrocephalus an accompaniment of some hemorrhages, usually mandates intraventricular drainage or surgical evacuation of the clot. Several small series suggest that corticosteroids do not improve outcome.

ANEURYSMAL SUBARACHNOID HEMORRAGE

PRESENTATION

The typical presentation is a sudden, extreme headache described as "the worst of my life," often associated with vomiting and various degrees of neck stiffness. Patients may have milder "sentinel" headaches in the days and weeks prior to presentation, perhaps as a result of small prodromal hemorrhages or aneurysmal stretch. Approximately 75% of subarachnoid hemorrhages are due to rupture of intracranial aneurysms (**Figure 209-1**), with another 10% attributed to arteriovenous malformations (AVMs). Subarachnoid hemorrhage due to AVM may cause less severe headache. Patients may be alert or suddenly become comatose. Systemic hypertension and meningismus are common on examination. The sudden rise in ICP in subarachnoid hemorrhage may produce intraocular

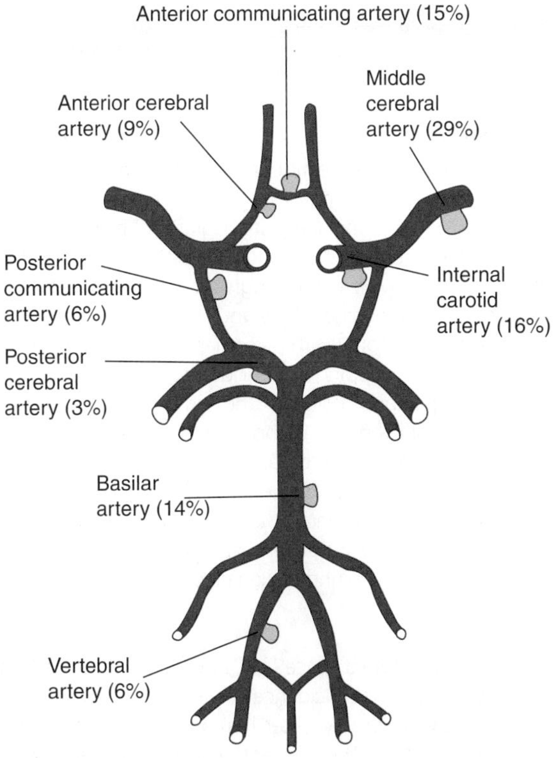

Figure 209-1 *Frequency and distribution of intracranial aneurysms. (Reproduced, with permission, from Simon RP, Greenberg DA, Aminoff MJ. Clinical Neurology. 7th ed. New York: McGraw-Hill; 2009).*

TABLE 209-1 Hunt and Hess Scoring System for Subarachnoid Hemorrhage	
Grade	**Description**
I	Asymptomatic or with slight headache
II	Moderate to severe headache, nuchal rigidity; cranial nerve palsy
III	Confusion, drowsiness, and mild focal deficit
IV	Persistent stupor or semicoma, early decerebrate rigidity
V	Deep coma and decerebrate rigidity

bleeding, or Terson syndrome, which is associated with higher mortality. The clinical state after subarachnoid hemorrhage is graded by the Hunt and Hess scale (**Table 209-1**), sometimes referred to as the "H and H" score. Complications of subarachnoid hemorrhage may be severe and include acute and delayed hydrocephalus, vasospasm with resultant ischemic stroke, and rerupture of the aneurysm, which is often fatal.

DIAGNOSIS

The best initial test is a noncontrast head CT scan, which has a sensitivity of 95% within 24 hours after aneurysm rupture but diminishes to <75% by the third day. If the CT scan fails to demonstrate hemorrhage in a case with compatible clinical features, then a lumbar puncture should be performed to detect blood and blood products. The opening pressure is high (>20 cm H_2O) in aneurysmal subarachnoid hemorrhage. Xanthochromia of the supernatant corroborates the presence of blood in the cerebrospinal fluid (CSF) space; it persists for up to two weeks but may not present in CSF collected in the first hours after hemorrhage. A substantial decline in the number of red blood cells in serial tubes is expected from a traumatic lumbar puncture, whereas the red cell count and degree of xanthochromia remain constant across tubes when it is due to subarachnoid hemorrhage. Once the diagnosis of subarachnoid hemorrhage is confirmed, a CT angiogram, MR angiogram, or conventional angiogram is used to define the site of aneurysm or other vascular malformation.

TREATMENT

General measures in the treatment of subarachnoid hemorrhage include intensive care unit monitoring, bed rest, analgesia, provision of a quiet environment, and adequate hydration. The risk of rebleeding from a single aneurysm following rupture is ~4% within the first 24 hours and 1.5% every day through the first two weeks. As the cumulative risk of rebleeding is 20%, and the outcome of rebleeding is usually poor, craniotomy with placement of titanium clips across the aneurysm neck (clipping), or endovascular obliteration of the aneurysm with platinum coils or other embolic material (coiling) is performed within the first 24 hours after presentation in most centers. The decision to clip or coil should be individualized and depends on factors such as aneurysm size, morphology, and location, as well as patient age and clinical status. As the risk of rebleeding is lower with AVMs, surgical removal, if feasible, is less urgent in these patients and can be undertaken electively at a later date.

Vasospasm

Clots in the subarachnoid space lead to delayed spasm of vessels of the circle of Willis. The incidence of vasospasm peaks between the fourth and seventh days after hemorrhage but may be seen as late as three weeks. The conventional management of vasospasm has been to induce hypertension with vasopressors such as phenylephrine, and hypervolemia and hemodilution with normal saline, referred to as "HHH" or "triple H" therapy. Because of the risk of inducing rerupture of the aneurysm with this treatment, clipping or coiling of the aneurysm is required if not already performed. Nimodipine, a calcium channel blocker, is the only medication proven to be effective as a protective agent against ischemic stroke from vasospasm. It is begun at a dose of 60 mg every four hours, orally or by nasogastric tube, as soon as feasible. If mean arterial pressure goes below 70 mm Hg, the medication is held, or the dose can be reduced to 30 mg every two hours. Nimodipine is continued for 21 days following hemorrhage or at least for the duration of the inpatient stay. The use of anticonvulsants and corticosteroids in subarachnoid hemorrhage is controversial and center dependent.

TRAUMATIC BRAIN INJURY

Traumatic brain injury (TBI) comprises a spectrum of clinical entities, some of which include intracranial bleeding. Management of patients with traumatic intracranial hemorrhages includes correction of coagulopathies, blood pressure regulation, and antiseizure medication. The clinical examination of brain-injured patients is best performed before sedation or paralytic agents are administered. The Glasgow Como Scale (GCS) is widely used to grade the severity of traumatic brain injury. It incorporates verbal response (1–5), eye opening (1–4) and best motor response (1–6).

CT scan of the head without contrast may detect skull fractures, acute or chronic hemorrhage, hydrocephalus, intraventricular blood, or intracranial masses. Neurosurgical consultation should be obtained when any intracranial blood is found. When performing the initial assessment of patients with head trauma, the cervical spine should be considered to be injured and unstable until otherwise demonstrated by imaging or examination. We typically place adult trauma patients in a hard cervical collar and perform CT of the cervical spine.

EPIDURAL HEMATOMA

Epidural hematomas usually result from rupture of the middle meningeal artery, leading to hematoma formation between the dural covering of the brain and the inner table of the skull (**Figure 209-2**). The clinical picture is traditionally described as

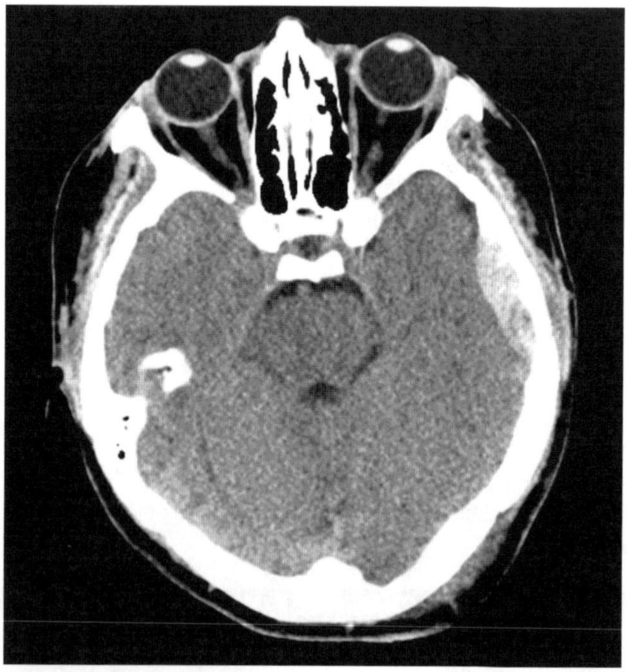

Figure 209-2 *Acute epidural hematoma in a 31-year-old woman who was hit by a truck.*

a brief loss of consciousness followed by a lucid interval, then progressive neurologic deterioration. However, this is not very common. Most epidural hematomas present with progressive hemiplegia and loss of consciousness from the time of injury. The advisability of surgical evacuation of these hematomas depends on the patient age, size of hemorrhage, and neurologic examination. Although most cases require surgery, many patients with epidural hematomas who remain awake and without focal neurologic signs for approximately six hours after the injury can be observed. Because epidural hematomas are infrequently epileptogenic, antiseizure medications are usually not given unless there is an underlying brain contusion.

SUBDURAL HEMATOMA

Subdural hematomas are most common in the elderly as a result of brain atrophy and the prevalence of anticoagulation and antiplatelet agents and a high incidence of falls. They usually result from the rupture of veins that bridge the dura. There may be acute, subacute, or chronic hemorrhage, or some combination of these. A CT scan without contrast can determine hematoma age (**Figure 209-3**). As with most other cerebral hemorrhages, the decision regarding surgery depends on the age and neurologic status of the patient, the estimated age of the hemorrhage, and its size and location.

Antiseizure medications are advised, as subdural blood or the underlying brain contusion are epileptogenic, although the duration of treatment has not been established. Levetiracetam is used most commonly, with no evidence favoring it; it does not require a loading dose or monitoring of serum concentration. The dosage is increased if the patient has posttraumatic seizures.

Correction of coagulopathy is paramount in acute subdural hematoma. Management strategies for this are as discussed in the previous section on intracerebral hemorrhage. There is no generally accepted interval after subdural hemorrhage during which previously necessary anticoagulant or antiplatelet drugs are interdicted; the risks and benefits must be weighed by the hospitalist for each patient. We generally withhold these drugs for a minimum of one month, unless there is an absolute requirement related to mechanical heart valves, recently placed stents, or other apparatus.

TRAUMATIC INTRACEREBRAL AND SUBARACHNOID HEMORRHAGE

Traumatic intracerebral hemorrhages are managed similarly to the previously discussed spontaneous intracerebral hemorrhages. They may be difficult to distinguish from a brain contusion. Traumatic brain contusions tend to occur in the anterior frontal or temporal lobes and may swell, causing secondary brainstem compression. Traumatic intracerebral hemorrhages tend to swell less than contusions but may expand rapidly in the setting of uncorrected INR and hypertension.

The most common site of hemorrhage following trauma is in the subarachnoid space (**Figure 209-4**). Traumatic subarachnoid hemorrhage is more common than aneurysmal rupture. Although it can occur anywhere in the subarachnoid space, it is most common over the convexities of the cerebral hemispheres, whereas aneurysmal rupture usually leads to a characteristic distribution of blood in the basal cisterns and sylvian fissures (**Figure 209-5**). The amount of blood resulting from traumatic hemorrhage is also generally far smaller than from aneurysmal rupture. If the history is not entirely clear, as in cases in which a patient has fallen and reports a headache before or after the fall, a CT angiogram of the cerebral vessels or other vascular imaging is performed to exclude an aneurysm.

Unresolved issues in the care of patients with traumatic subarachnoid hemorrhage include the timing of subsequent CT scanning and the need for antiseizure medications. For patients with minimal or mild TBI (loss of consciousness <5 min, Glasgow Coma Scale score of 14–15, and minimal blood on CT scan), we perform a repeat CT scan six hours following the original scan, observe patients for 24 hours, and administer levetiracetam for seven days. If the patient

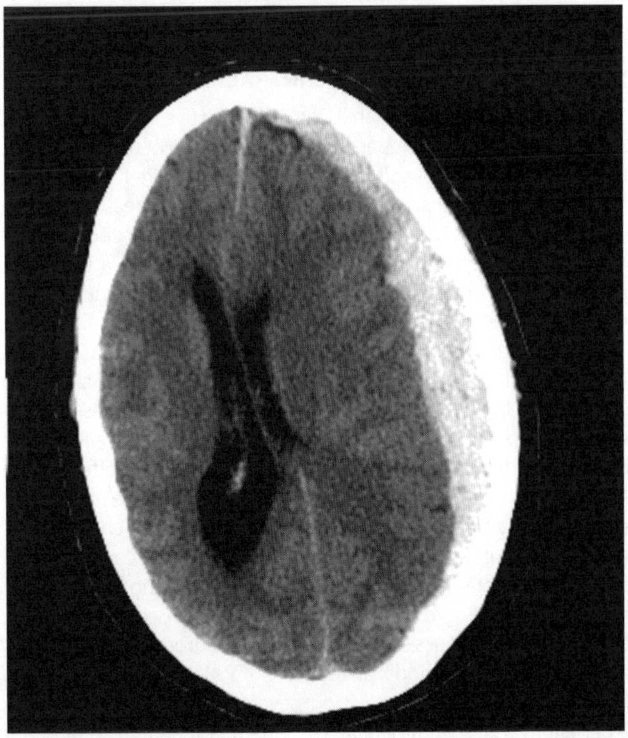

Figure 209-3 *Acute left hemispheric subdural hematoma in a 52-year-old man following a fall.*

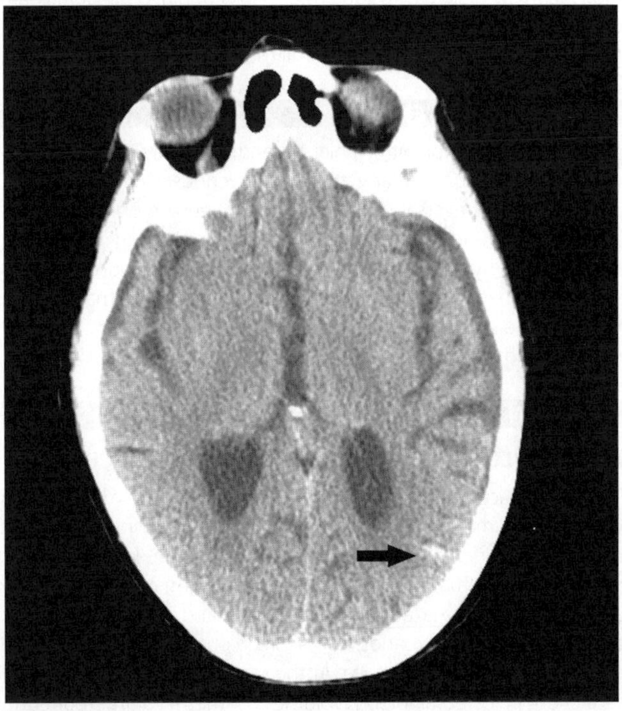

Figure 209-4 *Traumatic subarachnoid hemorrhage. Subarachnoid blood is collected in the sulci of the left parietal lobe (arrow); this is a common occurrence and does not require surgical intervention.*

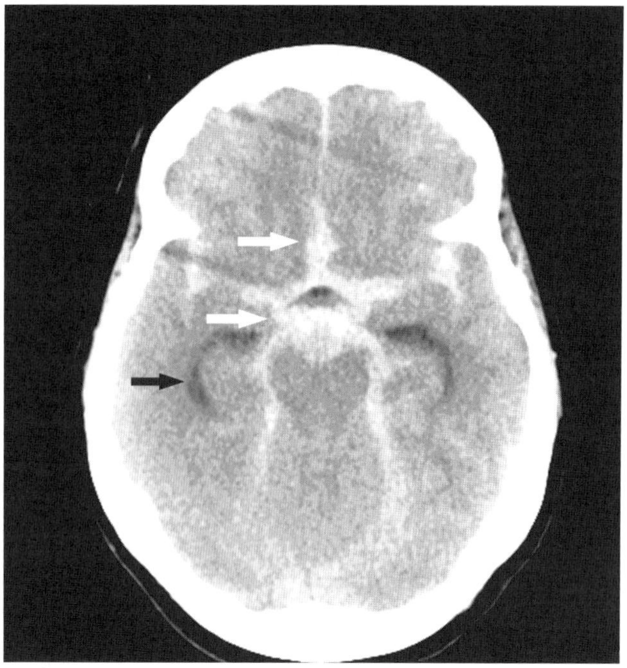

Figure 209-5 *Subarachnoid hemorrhage from a ruptured basilar artery aneurysm. Blood appears as a white signal diffusely in the subarachnoid spaces (white arrows), and incipient hydrocephalus is demonstrated by enlarged temporal horns of the lateral ventricles (dark arrow).*

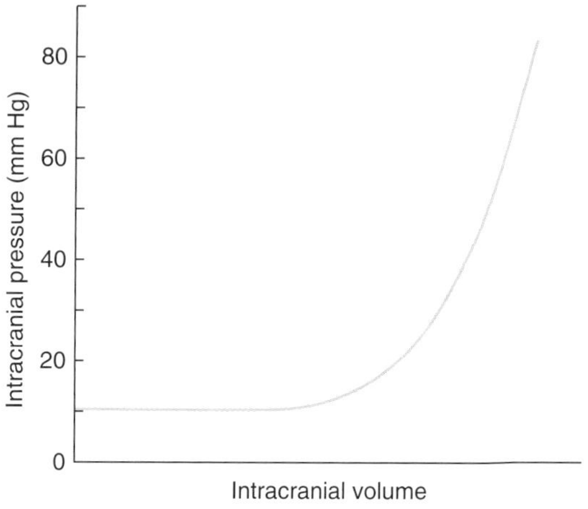

Figure 209-6 *Intracranial compliance curve. Minor changes in intracranial volume lead to alarming increases in intracranial pressure once an intracranial pressure of 20 mm Hg has been reached. (Reproduced, with permission, from Morgan GE, Mikhail MS, Murray MJ. Clinical Anesthesiology. 4th ed. New York: McGraw-Hill; 2006).*

has had a seizure, this medication or an equivalent is given for at least six months. Criteria for cessation of anticonvulsants are dominated by local practice. But generally include at least six months without a seizure and one or more normal electroencephalogram (EEG) tracings. Most patients with mild and moderate brain injury are discharged home with appropriate physical and psychological (cognitive) therapy. Repeat outpatient imaging is generally not required. Individuals with severe residual motor or cognitive difficulties are discharged to specialized units that provide comprehensive head trauma rehabilitation, including family support and instruction.

QUALITY IMPROVEMENT

Quality indicators for intracranial hemorrhage may include pneumatic compression therapy to reduce venous thrombosis from immobilization, reversal of anticoagulation, early mobilization and rehabilitation, and measures to address contributing conditions, such as falls, hypertension, smoking, and cocaine abuse. Patients with spontaneous intracranial hemorrhage should be managed in the intensive care setting to allow for intensive monitoring of blood pressure and neurologic status.

TOPICS IN NEUROCRITICAL CARE

PHYSIOLOGY OF INTRACRANIAL PRESSURE (ICP)

The fixed space of the cranial vault allows for only a small amount of added volume. Elevation in ICP is thus expected with all cerebral mass lesions, including intracerebral hemorrhage, large ischemic strokes with edema, herpes simplex encephalitis, and global brain swelling after hypoxia, acute hepatic failure, and Reye syndrome. As an intracranial mass expands, CSF is forced out of ventricles and into the spinal subarachnoid space. At the same time, there is a gradual reduction in cerebral blood volume. As these volume-buffering mechanisms fail, ICP rises exponentially and eventually reaches levels that approximate the mean blood pressure in the arteries at the base of the brain, compromising cerebral blood flow. This relationship can be approximated as cerebral perfusion pressure (CPP) = mean arterial blood pressure (MAP) − ICP. The result of reduced CPP is global brain ischemia and ultimately, brain death.

As ICP rises, brain tissue is displaced from regions of higher pressure to those of lower pressure across the midline of the cerebral hemispheres, downward through the tentorial opening, and through the foramen magnum. These tissue shifts result in fairly stereotyped herniation syndromes that include coma, unilateral and bilateral pupillary dilation, loss of reflex eye movements, and altered respiration.

ICP can be measured directly with one of several devices. The normal ICP in a resting adult is ~5 to 10 mm Hg. Elevations >20 mm Hg generally require treatment. Although pressures at this level do not compromise cerebral perfusion, the exponential shape of the intracranial compliance curve causes any additional mass to produce a marked and precarious rise in ICP (**Figure 209-6**).

TREATMENT OF ELEVATED INTRACRANIAL PRESSURE

Several treatments and maneuvers are effective in reducing ICP. Among the common ones are sedation, elevation of the head of the bed, and control of fever. Most patients who require ICP treatment are drowsy, stuporous, or unresponsive. There is no reason to withhold pain medications or sedating drugs such as benzodiazepines once a clinical examination has been performed and a treatment plan initiated. For patients who are awake, alternatives such as dexmedetomidine are used increasingly for sedation.

Elevating the head of the bed to ~30 degrees generally results in a modest reduction of intracranial pressure by maximizing venous and CSF outflow from the cranium. A few studies demonstrate a drop in blood pressure that is equal to or greater than the drop in ICP, resulting in a potentially net deleterious effect. Head elevation is nonetheless commonly practiced, and the result is assessed simply by measuring ICP and blood pressure changes.

Increases in core body temperature greatly elevate cerebral blood flow and cerebral blood volume, thereby increasing ICP. Treating febrile episodes aggressively with acetaminophen, cooling blankets, appropriate antibiotics, and, if necessary, neuromuscular paralysis are all effective methods of reducing ICP. Induced hypothermia is also effective in reducing ICP, but several trials have failed to show a benefit for TBI. The immediate hypothermia used as a component of resuscitation after cardiac arrest has, in contrast, improved neurological outcome.

Hyperventilation reduces pco_2 and causes cerebral vasoconstriction by an unknown mechanism. The resultant decrease in cerebral blood volume results in a rapid but transient drop in ICP. For this reason, hyperventilation is used mainly as a temporizing maneuver in mechanically ventilated patients during periods of clinical decompensation. Hypocarbia is accomplished by increasing the ventilator rate but maintaining the tidal volumes or in urgent situations, by manual ventilation.

The management of systemic blood pressure in the presence of a cerebral mass has long been a matter of uncertainty. In cerebral hemorrhage, as discussed above, it is considered prudent to lower extreme hypertension to minimize the risk of continued bleeding. However, excessive blood pressure reduction results in inadequate cerebral perfusion and global ischemia. Levels that are safe for each circumstance and for individual patients have not been determined. The most effective blood pressure management is guided by direct measurement of ICP, allowing calculation of cerebral perfusion pressure. In general, individuals who are chronically hypertensive are allowed to retain a degree of moderate hypertension. However, patients with mean arterial blood pressures >100 mm Hg are generally treated with rapid-acting, titratable IV medications such as labetalol and nicardipine.

The mainstay of medical treatment for raised intracranial pressure is hyperosmolar therapy. Hyperosmolarity of the blood establishes a gradient for water movement between the interstitial space of the brain and the vasculature. Almost any agent that raises serum osmolarity is effective in proportion to the level of serum concentration achieved. Either serum sodium concentration or directly measured serum osmolarity can be used as a guide to treatment.

Normal saline has an effective osmolarity of 309 mOsm/L and will therefore create mild hyperosmolarity when infused over a long period of time. High osmolarity is more quickly achieved by infusing mannitol or 23.4% saline, which acts over minutes, or 3% saline, which acts over hours. Subsequent infusion of normal saline may be used to maintain elevated osmolarity. Furosemide may also be used for this purpose but has a delayed effect. Mannitol or hypertonic saline infusions risk causing intravascular volume overload and congestive heart failure, whereas furosemide may produce intravascular volume depletion and hypotension. Several trials have indicated that corticosteroids do not improve outcome in head injury or cerebral hemorrhage, and they are generally not used.

Targets for serum sodium and osmolarity

Serum sodium concentrations of ~145 to 154 mEq/L or serum osmolarity levels of ~310 to 325 mOsm/L are appropriate targets for the empiric treatment of raised ICP. When rapidly acting hyperosmolar agents are being used, measurement of blood sodium and osmolarity every six hours is desirable. Patients should also have ongoing clinical assessments of volume status and central venous pressure to avoid congestive heart failure. Once a target level of hyperosmolarity has been achieved, a return to normal sodium levels is allowed only slowly to avoid rebound brain swelling. When syndrome of inappropriate antidiuretic hormone (SIADH) or diabetes insipidus is part of the clinical illness, management with hyperosmolar agents becomes complex, and nephrology consultation may be helpful.

ACQUIRED DISORDERS OF WATER AND SODIUM BALANCE IN BRAIN INJURY

Many types of acute and chronic cerebral disease may produce SIADH. A cause of hyponatremia that is more specifically associated with subarachnoid hemorrhage and head trauma is cerebral salt wasting. This is thought to result from the release of natriuretic peptides from either the brain or cardiac atria. Hyponatremia from either SIADH or cerebral salt wasting can exaggerate brain edema and cause convulsions; it is therefore appropriate to treat low serum sodium more aggressively in patients with cerebral injury. The distinction between the two disorders is made by assessing intravascular volume. Patients with SIADH are euvolemic, whereas those with cerebral salt wasting are volume depleted. Fluid restriction for acute hyponatremia from SIADH is usually initiated when serum sodium drops below 132 mEq/L. If unsuccessful, 3% saline is added. In salt wasting, normal saline and hypertonic solutions are used. Some centers also use fludrocortisone. Overly rapid correction of hyponatremia should be avoided, as this may lead to pontine and extrapontine myelinolysis.

Diabetes insipidus is sometimes encountered after cerebral injury from trauma or surgery. The diagnosis should be suspected in the presence of polyuria, hypernatremia, and urine that is dilute in comparison to serum. Treatment is to allow patients to drink ad libitum to satisfy their thirst, with the goal of an even fluid balance. For unresponsive patients or refractory cases, fluid and sodium replacement is given intravenously in proportion to urine output, and DDAVP (desmopressin) is added if necessary.

BRAIN DEATH

Virtually all cases of large intracranial masses that progress unchecked will lead to brain death, due to reduction in cerebral perfusion pressure to levels that cannot sustain neuronal viability. Secondary events such as hydrocephalus and herniation of brain tissue contribute to a reduction in blood supply. As conventionally defined, brain death requires the complete cessation of function of all intracranial structures, including the cerebrum and brainstem.

Clinical criteria for brain death include deep unresponsive coma, loss of brainstem reflexes, including unobtainable pupillary responses to light, corneal responses, and lack of eye movements with caloric stimulation of the external auditory canals, and apnea despite levels of carbon dioxide adequate to stimulate the brainstem, usually given as 60 mm Hg. Many institutions corroborate cerebral death in adults with an electrocerebrally silent ("flat") EEG or by the direct demonstration of completely impeded blood flow on any one of several imaging techniques. These are not obligatory if the nature of the brain injury is well defined and some reasonable period of observation has elapsed.

Beyond the technical aspects of brain death and its philosophical and theological implications, these circumstances are among the most difficult to manage. Families are often not prepared for the suddenness of death, have difficulty equating brain death with personal or religious notions of death, and are often put in the untenable position of being asked whether a ventilator and other support should cease. It is wise to prepare families for the eventuality of brain death and to explain in advance the process of testing and removal of the ventilator if brain death is demonstrated. An intermediate step involves the opportunity for transplantation, a discussion and situation that require tact, knowledge, and confidence.

ANTICOAGULATION AFTER HEAD INJURY, INTRACRANIAL HEMORRHAGE, AND NEUROSURGERY

A common question asked in the management of neurosurgical patients is the safety of prophylactic anticoagulation for the prevention of venous thromboembolism. Patients with brain lesions are at high risk for thrombosis as a result of prolonged immobility and paralyzed extremities. We use both compression stockings and sequential compression devices on the legs of operative and nonoperative patients. Early ambulation is also important, and we advocate early involvement of physical and occupational therapists.

There are few studies supporting the use of prophylactic unfractionated heparin or low-molecular-weight heparins to reduce venous thromboembolism in neurosurgical patients. The consensus has been that the overall risk of intracranial bleeding is elevated slightly and outweighed by the benefit of prevention of thromboembolism in an immobilized patient. These medications are commonly administered in the critical care setting, but the additional risk of cerebral hemorrhage is always considered, and the decision to administer prophylactic anticoagulation is patient and center dependent. It is advisable to monitor PTT and platelets to avoid excessive anticoagulation and thrombocytopenia.

VENTRICULOPERITONEAL AND OTHER VENTRICULAR SHUNTS

Placement and revision of permanent ventricular shunts are common neurosurgical procedures. Hydrocephalus is the usual indication for diverting CSF from the ventricles. Hydrocephalus results from overproduction or underabsorption of CSF or from blockage of the ventricular outflow pathways. A shunt redirects CSF from the ventricular system to the peritoneum, pleural space, or right atrium. Many of these shunts have valves that allow for adjustment of the pressure at which a valve will open and drain CSF.

Fever in patients with shunts is a common problem faced by hospitalists and neurosurgeons. Shunt infection as a cause of fever is uncommon after the immediate postoperative period, and certainly much less common than urinary tract infections and pneumonia. Attribution of fever or leukocytosis to shunt infection is a last resort. The length of time since the shunt surgery is most helpful in determining the likelihood of infection. Recently operated patients are at greater risk than those who had shunts inserted months or years previously. The workup in febrile patients with shunts includes a complete blood count, chest radiograph, urine analysis, and urine culture. A noncontrast head CT should also be obtained, as ventricular enlargement is commonly but not always seen in acute shunt malfunction, as well as a shunt series (four plain films of the skull, chest and abdomen that allow evaluation of the continuity and proper placement of shunt tubing). Patients with acute shunt malfunction generally have severe headache, nausea, vomiting, and sleepiness from worsening hydrocephalus.

When shunt malfunction is suspected, a shunt tap may be performed to assess catheter patency and obtain CSF for analysis. If CSF is needed to exclude meningitis, it is prudent to consider a lumbar puncture rather than a shunt tap because of the lower risk of shunt contamination with lumbar puncture.

SUGGESTED READINGS

Bullock MR, Chesnut R, Ghajar J, et al. Guidelines for the surgical management of traumatic parenchymal lesions. *Neurosurgery*. 2006;58(3 Suppl):S25–S46.

Epstein NE. A review of the risks and benefits of differing prophylaxis regimens for the treatment of deep venous thrombosis and pulmonary embolism in neurosurgery. *Surg Neurol*. 2005;64:295–301.

Hamilton MG, Yee WH, Hull RD, Ghali WA. Venous thromboembolism prophylaxis in patients undergoing cranial neurosurgery: a systematic review and meta-analysis. *Neurosurgery*. 2011;68: 571–581.

Mendelow AD, Gregson BA, Fernandes HM, et al. Early surgery versus initial conservative treatment in patients with spontaneous supratentorial intracerebral haematomas in the International Surgical Trial in Intracerebral Haemorrhage (STICH): A randomised trial. *Lancet*. 2005;365:387–397.

Naidech AM, Garg RK, Liebling S, et al. Anticonvulsant use and outcomes after intracerebral hemorrhage. *Stroke*. 2009;40:3810–3815.

Roberts I, Yates P, Sandercock I, et al. Effect of intravenous corticosteroids on death within 14 days in 10008 adults with clinically significant head injury (MRC CRASH trial): Randomised placebo-controlled trial. *Lancet*. 2004;364:1321–1328.

CHAPTER 210

Transient Ischemic Attack and Stroke

Galen V. Henderson, MD

Key Clinical Questions

1. How are stroke and transient ischemic attack differentiated?
2. Who is eligible for IV recombinant tissue plasminogen activator?
3. What is the best cerebral imaging modality?
4. What is the optimal blood pressure in hospitalized patients with stroke?
5. What is the best antiplatelet therapy for secondary prevention of transient ischemic attack and stroke?
6. Should every patient be started on a statin?

INTRODUCTION

Stroke is the third leading cause of death in the United States. There are more than 700,000 strokes in the United States each year, resulting in more than 160,000 deaths annually, with 4.8 million stroke survivors alive today. Although there was a 60% decline in stroke mortality between 1968 and 1996, the rate of decline began to slow in the 1990s and has plateaued in several regions of the country. The incidence of stroke may actually be increasing. From 1988 to 1997, the age-adjusted hospitalization rate for stroke grew by 19%, and total stroke hospitalizations increased by 39%. In 2004, the cost of stroke in the United States was estimated at $53.6 billion (direct and indirect costs), with a mean lifetime cost estimated at $140,048. Stroke is also a leading cause of functional impairments, with 20% of survivors requiring institutional care after 3 months, and 15% to 30% being permanently disabled. Utility analyses show that a major stroke is viewed by more than half of those at risk as being worse than death.

CAUSES OF STROKE

The most common cause of stroke is atherosclerosis of large and medium-size vessels of the neck and base of the brain (**Figure 210-1**). Risk factors for atherosclerosis include hypertension, diabetes, hyperlipidemia, cigarette smoking, and family history. Hypertension and diabetes also predispose to lacunae, which result from blockage of small perforating branches of the large cerebral arteries, with a predilection for the basal ganglia, thalamus, internal capsule, and pons. Patients with giant cell arteritis, systemic lupus erythematosus, and other vasculitides are at increased risk of stroke. Fibromuscular dysplasia is a cause of stroke in younger patients and is more common in women. Atrial fibrillation and valvular heart disease predispose to embolic stroke. Cocaine use predisposes to stroke for several reasons, including vasospasm, activating effects on platelets, and rupture of arteriovenous malformations and aneursyms in association with hypertension. IV drug users may develop embolic stroke from bacterial endocarditis. Stroke may also result from dissection of the carotid and/or vertebral arteries. Moyamoya syndrome results from bilateral narrowing of the distal internal carotids and adjacent anterior and middle cerebral arteries, with the development of fragile collateral vessels on angiography (**Figure 210-2**). It may be inherited as an autosomal recessive disorder or acquired in the setting of atherosclerosis, sickle cell disease, or basilar meningitis. Children present with ischemic stroke, whereas adults tend to develop intracranial hemorrhage. Hypercoagulability from genetic abnormalities in coagulation factors, leukemia, myeloproliferative disorders, antiphospholipid antibody syndrome, oral contraceptives, and sickle cell disease also predispose to stroke. Causes of stroke are summarized in **Table 210-1**.

CLINICAL PRESENTATION

Strokes and transient ischemic attacks (TIAs) present with the abrupt onset of neurologic deficits. In stroke, the duration of symptoms is longer than 24 hours. In TIA, symptoms resolve completely within 24 hours; in most patients with TIA, symptoms resolve within 30 minutes to 1 hour. However, if patients with clinical TIA have evidence of ischemia on magnetic resonance imaging (MRI) with diffusion-weighted sequences, the lesion is considered to be a stroke. The distinction between TIA and ischemic stroke has become

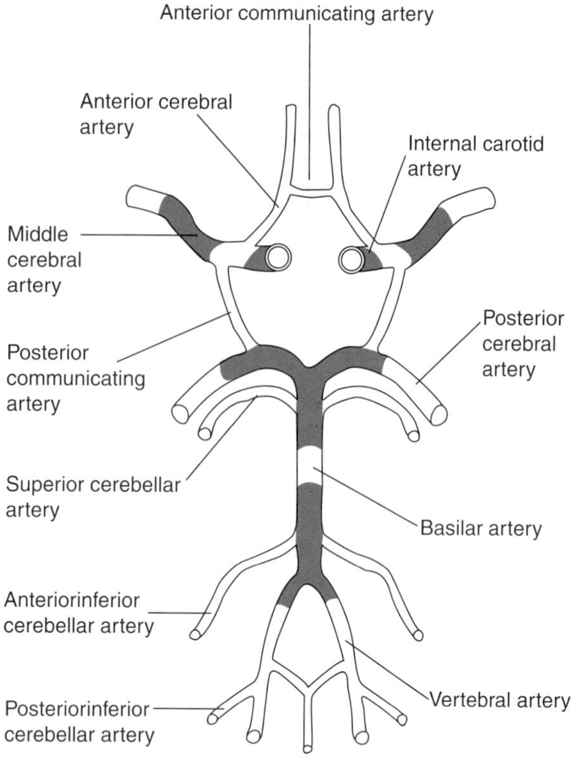

Figure 210-1 *Sites of predilection (shaded areas) for atherosclerosis in the intracranial arterial circulation. (Reproduced, with permission, from Greenberg DA, Aminoff MJ, Simon RP. Clinical Neurology. 5th ed. McGraw-Hill; 2002. Figure 9-4.)*

less important in recent years, as measures for secondary prevention are similar in each group. Moreover, TIA is a robust short-term predictor of stroke: the 90-day stroke risk after TIA is as high as 10.5%, with the greatest risk in the first week.

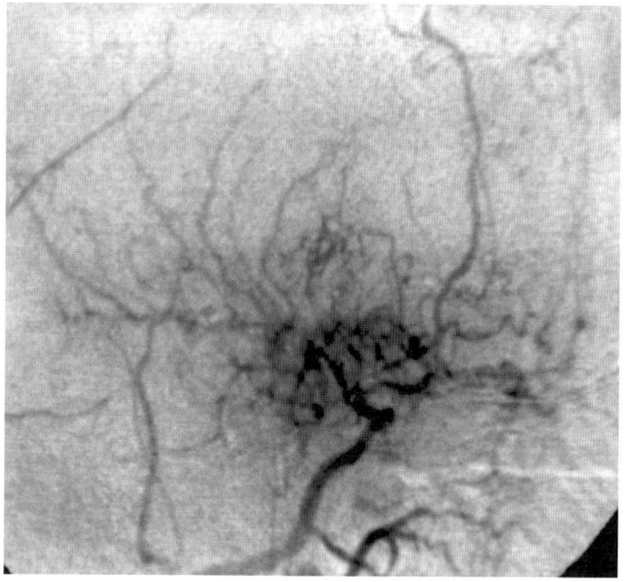

Figure 210-2 *Right carotid angiogram in moyamoya syndrome, lateral view. The middle cerebral artery and its branches are replaced by a diffuse capillary pattern that resembles a puff of smoke (moyamoya is Japanese and means "smoke" or "haze"). (Reproduced, with permission, from Greenberg DA, Aminoff MJ, Simon RP. Clinical Neurology. 5th ed. McGraw-Hill; 2002. Figure 9-7B.)*

TABLE 210-1 Conditions Associated with Stroke

Vascular disorders
Atherosclerosis
Lacunar infarction
Carotid or vertebral artery dissection
Fibromuscular dysplasia
Vasculitis and infections
Giant cell arteritis
Systemic lupus erythematosus
Behçet disease
Primary angiitis of the CNS
Syphilis
Varicella zoster
HIV/AIDS
Cocaine, amphetamines, and other drugs of abuse
Moyamoya syndrome (multiple progressive intracranial occlusions)
Venous and sinus thrombosis
Embolism
Atrial fibrillation
Mural thrombus
Prosthetic heart valves
Rheumatic heart disease
Infectious endocarditis
Marantic endocarditis
Patent foramen ovale
Atrial septal defect
Atrial myxoma
Hypercoagulable states
Antiphospholipid antibody syndrome
Thrombocytosis
Polycythemia
Sickle cell disease
Leukemia
Waldenström macroglobulinemia
Oral contraceptives
Activated protein C resistance
Deficiency of protein C, protein S, or antithrombin III
Thrombotic thrombocytopenic purpura
Disseminated intravascular coagulation
Miscellaneous
Fabry disease
CADASIL
MELAS

AIDS, acquired immunodeficiency syndrome; CADASIL, cerebral autosomal dominant angiopathy with subcortical infarcts and leukoencephalopathy; HIV, human immunodeficiency virus; MELAS, mitochondrial encephalopathy with lactic acidosis and strokelike episodes.

Stroke may be produced by thrombosis, embolism, and hemorrhage. In embolic stroke, lesions are characteristically maximal at onset, whereas the symptoms of thrombotic stroke evolve over minutes to hours. In subarachnoid hemorrhage, patients may present with the sudden onset of "the worst headache of my life"

TABLE 210-2 Conditions that Mimic Thromboembolic Stroke

Sudden onset of persistent focal deficit
Partial seizure with postictal (Todd) paralysis
Abscess with seizure
Tumor with bleeding or seizure
Toxic-metabolic insult superimposed on old cerebral lesion
Hypoglycemia
Subdural hematoma (acute)
Multiple sclerosis
Cerebritis
Sudden onset of transient focal deficit
Partial seizure
Migraine with aura
Arteriovenous malformations (may also present with symptoms of partial seizure or migraine)

or with a sudden extreme pressure sensation in the head or neck. For parenchymal hemorrhages, symptoms occur suddenly and progress over 30 minutes to 1 hour. Many conditions may mimic ischemic or hemorrhagic stroke (**Table 210-2**). It is important to determine anterior versus posterior circulation stroke to tailor imaging and intervention. In addition, posterior circulation strokes are more likely to produce complications related to altered consciousness. Large cerebellar strokes pose a risk of herniation and may require emergent neurosurgical decompression, especially if > 3 cm in size or if there is evidence of edema or hemorrhagic transformation. Recognition of progressive brainstem and cerebellar symptoms due to thrombosis of the basilar artery may allow for early intervention to prevent the devastating morbidity from infarct due to complete occlusion.

Lesions in the *anterior cerebral artery* are uncommon. Patients present with paralysis and sensory loss of the contralateral leg. Patients may have urinary urgency and incontinence from the failure to inhibit reflex bladder contractions.

The *middle cerebral artery (MCA),* the largest branch of the internal carotid artery, is the vessel most commonly affected in ischemic stroke. The clinical picture depends on the location of the damage (ie, whether all cortical branches are affected vs individual cortical branches) and whether the dominant or nondominant hemisphere is affected. Strokes affecting the *superior division* of the MCA lead to hemiparesis affecting the contralateral face, hand, and arm but sparing the leg, with accompanying sensory deficits; if the dominant hemisphere is involved, expressive (Broca) aphasia may develop, with loss of speech production but preserved speech comprehension. *Inferior division MCA* strokes may lead to contralateral homonymous hemianopia, hemineglect, loss of graphesthesia and stereognosis, and apraxias. Involvement of the dominant hemisphere also produces Wernicke, or receptive, aphasia, with speech consisting of fluent but meaningless babble. Lesions at the bifurcation of the MCA may lead to deficits in both superior and inferior vascular territories. Leg weakness may also ensue if the occlusion is proximal to the lenticulostriate branches of the MCA.

Internal carotid artery occlusion may be asymptomatic if collateral circulation is adequate, or it may produce strokes similar to middle cerebral artery syndromes if collateral circulation is poor. About 15% of cases of incipient carotid occlusion are heralded by episodes of transient monocular blindness (amaurosis fugax).

PRACTICE POINT

- In acute stroke, it is important to determine whether the patient's speech is fluent, whether the patient understands speech, and whether the patient can repeat simple phrases. In acute global aphasia, the patient will not have fluent speech, will not comprehend speech, and will be unable to repeat phases. It is not possible at this point to localize the site of damage.
- Expressive or receptive aphasia from anterior circulation strokes may present acutely as global aphasia but then become productive or receptive as the patient recovers.
- If the patient does not have fluent speech and cannot repeat phrases, but can comprehend speech, the patient has an expressive (Broca) aphasia localizing to the inferior frontal gyrus.
- If the patient's speech becomes fluent without the ability to comprehend speech or repeat phrases, the patient has a receptive (Wernicke) aphasia localizing to the superior temporal gyrus.
- It is also important to distinguish a language disorder (aphasia) from a purely motor disorder (dysarthria).

Posterior cerebral artery strokes produce contralateral homonymous hemianopia. If the vascular lesion is near the origin of the posterior cerebral artery in the midbrain, vertical gaze palsy, oculomotor (III) nerve palsy, and internuclear ophthalmoplegia may occur. If the dominant hemisphere is affected, patients may also have anomia, alexia without agraphia, or visual agnosia.

Strokes involving the *vertebrobasilar* circulation may lead to a variety of symptoms from brainstem ischemia, such as ipsilateral cranial nerve palsies with contralateral hemiplegia, ipsilateral cerebellar ataxia, nystagmus, vertigo, vomiting, dysphagia, dysarthria, Horner syndrome, and hiccup.

PRACTICE POINT

Horner syndrome is characterized by

- Ptosis, usually slight
- Miosis (pupillary constriction), more marked in the dark
- Anhidrosis (absence of facial sweating), if the lesion is proximal to the carotid arteries

Horner syndrome may result from sympathetic damage at any of the following locations:

- Brainstem, especially lateral medullary infarction (Wallenberg syndrome)
- Cervical spinal cord
- Anterior roots of C8 and T1
- Cervical sympathetic chain (carcinoma of the apex of the lung)
- Trauma, occlusion, aneurysm, or dissection of the internal carotid artery

Horner syndrome may thus result from either anterior or posterior (vertebrobasilar) cerebrovascular disease. If accompanied by vertigo and ataxia, it suggests cerebellar or medullary stroke from a vertebral artery lesion.

Lacunar infarcts occur from degenerative changes in small penetrating arteries deep in the brain from hypertension. They are often clinically silent. When symptomatic, they may have an acute or subacute onset and may produce distinctive syndromes, such as pure motor hemiparesis (the most common type of lacunar infarct), pure sensory loss, dysarthria/clumsy hand syndrome, and ataxic hemiparesis, with incoordination out of proportion to motor weakness.

PRACTICE POINT

- Patients with bilateral watershed infarcts affecting the border zone between the anterior cerebral and middle cerebral circulations may have the "man in a barrel" syndrome, with weakness of the legs and proximal upper extremities, as well as relative sparing of the hands and distal upper extremities. In the hospital setting, this may result from an episode of prolonged systemic hypotension from shock and may only be recognized when patients are transferred from the ICU to the general medical ward.
- Patients with bilateral infarcts involving the watershed regions between the MCA and posterior cerebral artery will be unable to direct voluntary gaze and may suffer loss of visual recognition due to bilateral parieto-occipital lesions (Balint syndrome). These patients may be initially misdiagnosed as confused.

ASSESSMENT

PHYSICAL EXAMINATION

Areas of special interest on general examination include vital signs (hypertension, irregular pulse); funduscopic examination, which may reveal retinal emboli (Hollenhorst crystals) in carotid disease; presence of carotid pulses or bruits; temporal arteries, which may be nodular, thickened, or pulseless in giant cell arteritis; and the cardiac examination, for evidence of atrial fibrillation, cardiomegaly, and valvular disease. Blood cultures should be obtained in febrile patients to exclude endocarditis.

NEUROLOGIC FINDINGS

The neurologic examination attempts to identify the site of the lesion and the likely culprit vessel. Certain findings are helpful in localizing a stroke to either the anterior circulation (the internal carotid artery and its major branches, the anterior cerebral, middle cerebral, and anterior choroidal arteries) or the posterior circulation (the vertebral arteries and basilar artery, their cerebellar branches, and their termination in the posterior cerebral arteries). The presence of aphasia indicates a lesion in the anterior circulation, rather than posterior, and makes lacunar infarction unlikely. Hemianopia also makes lacunar infarct unlikely. Although hemianopia may be present in either anterior or posterior circulation lesions, isolated hemianopia indicates a posterior cerebral artery lesion. Ocular palsies, nystagmus, and internuclear ophthalmoplegia indicate a posterior circulation lesion affecting the brainstem. Hemiparesis can be produced by a wide variety of lesions. However, hemiparesis of the face, hand, and arm, with relative sparing of the leg, suggests an MCA lesion. Hemiparesis that affects the face, hand, arm, and leg equally suggests a lesion in the internal carotid, stem of the MCA, a lacuna in the internal capsule or basal ganglia, or a brainstem stroke. Crossed hemiparesis (affecting the face and contralateral side of the body) suggests a brainstem lesion, as does a crossed sensory deficit. An isolated hemisensory deficit is likely due to a lacunar infarct.

The neurologic examination is discussed in detail in Chapter 207.

BLOOD TESTS

Routine blood tests in stroke should assess for potentially treatable causes of stroke: complete blood count (thrombocytosis, polycythemia, sickle cell disease, leukemia), erythrocyte sedimentation rate (giant cell arteritis and other vasculitides, endocarditis), serum glucose (to exclude hypoglycemia masquerading as stroke), serologic tests for syphilis, and lipid panel.

ELECTROCARDIOGRAM

Electrocardiogram (ECG) should occur as soon as possible after TIA or stroke to exclude atrial fibrillation or flutter. Inpatient telemetry monitoring may be useful to exclude paroxysmal atrial fibrillation.

NEUROIMAGING

Imaging of the brain is recommended before therapy for acute ischemic stroke. MRI, with diffusion-weighted imaging (DWI) and apparent diffusion coefficient (ADC) sequences, is the most sensitive imaging modality (**Figure 210-3**). Acute infarct appears bright on DWI and dark on ADC; these changes correlate with the presence of cytotoxic edema. The relative intensity of DWI and ADC change over time and are helpful in dating the infarct if this is unclear from the history. Changes may be apparent on MRI with DWI/ADC 30 minutes after the onset of symptoms, whereas noncontrast computed tomography (CT) is insensitive in the first several hours after infarction.

If MRI is not immediately available, head CT should be performed. Despite the diagnostic superiority of MRI, CT remains the most practical initial brain-imaging test. In most instances, CT

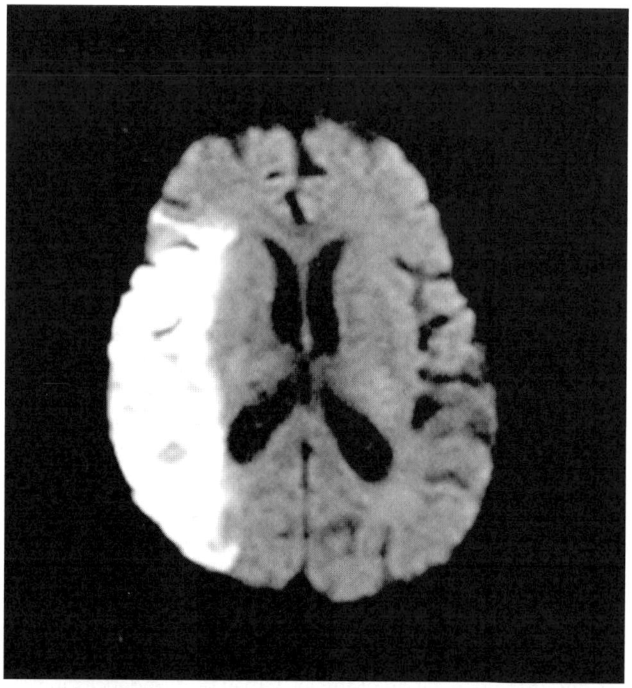

Figure 210-3 *Magnetic resonance imaging (MRI) with diffusion-weighted image (DWI) showing a large right middle cerebral artery infarction. The DWI bright signal changes are evident well before and more clearly than alterations in the computed tomography (CT) scan or conventional MRI. (Reproduced, with permission, from Ropper AH, Samuels MA. Adam's & Victor's Principles of Neurology. 9th ed. New York: McGraw-Hill; 2009. Figure 34-3A.)*

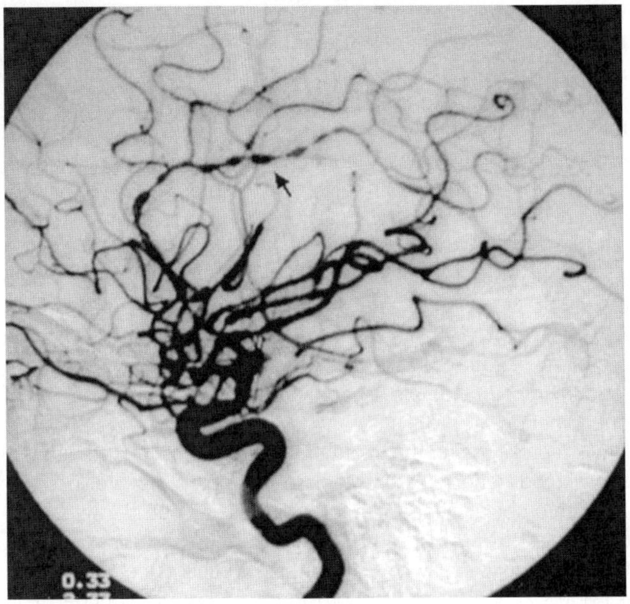

Figure 210-4 *Cerebral angiogram from a 32-year-old man with CNS vasculitis. Dramatic beading (arrow) typical of vasculitis is seen. (Modified, with permission, from Fauci AS, Braunwald E, Kasper DL, et al. Harrison's Principles of Internal Medicine. 17th ed. New York: McGraw-Hill; 2008, Fig. 364-5.)*

provides the necessary information to make decisions about emergency management, particularly thrombolysis. A physician skilled in assessing CT or MRI studies should be available to interpret the initial scan.

Echocardiography is reasonable in the evaluation of patients with TIA or stroke of possible embolic cause, especially in patients in whom no other cause has been identified. Transesophageal echocardiography is particularly useful in identifying patent foramen ovale, aortic arch atherosclerosis, and endocarditis and is reasonable when identification of these conditions will alter management.

VASCULAR IMAGING

Noninvasive imaging of the extracranial vessels should be performed routinely as part of the evaluation of patients with suspected TIA or stroke. Initial assessment may involve carotid duplex ultrasound, MR angiogram, or CT angiogram, depending on local availability and expertise. Transcranial Doppler ultrasound is especially helpful in the serial assessment of vasospasm after subarachnoid hemorrhage. Catheter angiography is the most sensitive and specific vascular imaging test; it is used to confirm abnormalities detected on noninvasive imaging or to further define unusual pathology, such as suspected vasculitis (**Figure 210-4**). Imaging of the intracranial or extracranial vasculature in the emergency assessment of patients with suspected stroke is useful at institutions providing endovascular recanalization therapies.

WHICH PATIENTS WITH TRANSIENT ISCHEMIC ATTACK SHOULD BE HOSPITALIZED?

Several studies have identified risk factors for stroke after TIA. The newer $ABCD^2$ (age, blood pressure, clinical symptoms, duration of symptoms, and diabetes) score provides a more powerful prediction standard and incorporates elements from older scoring systems. Patients presenting with TIA score points (indicated in parentheses) for each of the following factors: age ≥ 60 years (1), blood pressure 140/90 mm Hg on first evaluation (1), clinical symptoms of focal weakness with the spell (2) or speech impairment without weakness (1), symptom duration ≥ 60 minutes (2) or 10 to 59 minutes (1), and diabetes (1). In combined validation cohorts, the 2-day risk of stroke was 0% for scores of 0 or 1, 1.3% for 2 or 3, 4.1% for 4 or 5, and 8.1% for 6 or 7.

It is reasonable to hospitalize patients with TIA if they present within 72 hours of the event and any of the following criteria are present:

1. $ABCD^2$ score ≥ 3
2. $ABCD^2$ score = 0 to 2, and uncertainty that diagnostic workup can be completed within 2 days as an outpatient
3. $ABCD^2$ score = 0 to 2 and other evidence to indicate that the patient's event was caused by focal ischemia

In general, I recommend treating patients with a suspected neurovascular event with similar urgency as patients with chest pain and possible myocardial infarction. Rapid evaluation and treatment of TIA may avert the devastating consequences of stroke in many patients.

STROKE CENTERS

Ideally, patients with stroke should be cared for in certified stroke centers, which have been shown to improve patient outcomes and reduce complications. In many states, emergency medical services are directed to bring patients with suspected stroke directly to stroke centers, bypassing facilities that are not able to provide specialized care. However, this may not be feasible in some areas due to low population densities.

Key elements of *primary stroke centers* include acute stroke teams, stroke units, stroke care protocols, and an integrated emergency response system. Essential support services include the ability to obtain and interpret head CT scans 24 hours daily and rapid laboratory testing. Administrative support, strong leadership, and continuing medical education are also important elements for stroke centers. Most stroke patients may be appropriately cared for in primary stroke centers.

Comprehensive stroke centers are capable of caring for seriously ill stroke patients with complex cerebrovascular disease. The components of comprehensive stroke centers include expertise in neurosurgery, vascular neurology, and neuroradiology; advanced neuroimaging capabilities, such as MRI and cerebral angiography; the ability to perform clipping and coiling of intracranial aneurysms, carotid endarterectomy, and intra-arterial thrombolytic therapy; and specialized infrastructure elements, such as a neurologic intensive care unit and stroke registry.

WHICH PATIENTS WITH STROKE REQUIRE ADMISSION TO THE INTENSIVE CARE UNIT?

Triage to an intensive care unit (ICU) setting for monitoring and treatment is appropriate for patients with

- Cerebellar strokes > 3 cm. Because cerebral edema is usually maximal in ischemic stroke 3 to 5 days after the event, large cerebellar strokes may lead to serious delayed complications, such as brainstem compression or hydrocephalus from obstruction or compression of the fourth ventricle or the cerebral aqueduct.
- Strokes involving > 50% of the MCA circulation in patients younger than 60. These patients are at risk of malignant cerebral edema and may eventually require decompressive hemicraniectomy, with temporary removal of the overlying skull, which is either frozen or inserted in the patient's peritoneal cavity, and incision of dura to allow the brain to swell outward.

MANAGEMENT OF TRANSIENT ISCHEMIC ATTACK AND STROKE

GENERAL SUPPORTIVE MEASURES

Hypoxia and the increased metabolic demands associated with fever may be deleterious to patients with stroke, as they may lead to infarct extension. Hypoxic patients with stroke should receive supplemental oxygen. Airway support and ventilatory assistance are recommended for patients with acute stroke with decreased consciousness or bulbar dysfunction causing compromise of the airway. The source of fever should be sought and antipyretic medications given to lower body temperature in febrile stroke patients. Other factors that may reduce neuronal viability, such as hypoglycemia and decreased cardiac output due to hypovolemia and cardiac arrhythmias, should also be corrected. Cardiac monitoring should be performed to screen for atrial fibrillation during the first 24 hours after onset of ischemic stroke.

IV THROMBOLYSIS

IV administration of recombinant tissue plasminogen activator (rtPA) is the only Food and Drug Administration (FDA)-approved therapy for acute ischemic stroke. It improves outcomes for a broad spectrum of patients treated within 3 hours of stroke onset. Treatment within 90 minutes is most likely to result in a favorable outcome, although treatment at 90 to 180 minutes also is beneficial. Patients with major strokes, determined by a National Institutes of Health Stroke Scale (NIHSS) (http://www.ninds.nih.gov/doctors/NIH_Stroke_Scale.pdf) score > 22, have a very poor prognosis, but some positive treatment effect with rtPA has been documented. Patients with large strokes with substantial edema, mass effect, or midline shift on CT scan, as well as patients of advanced age, are at higher risk of hemorrhage, and the decision to treat with rtPA should be made with caution. Treatment with rtPA is associated with symptomatic intracranial hemorrhage in ~6% of cases, which may be fatal. The use of anticoagulants and antiplatelet agents should therefore be delayed for 24 hours after treatment.

IV rtPA (0.9 mg/kg, maximum dose 90 mg) is recommended for selected patients within 3 hours of onset of ischemic stroke. Physicians should review the criteria used in clinical trials to determine the eligibility of the patient (**Table 210-3**). Significant risks include bleeding complications and angioedema. Patients whose blood pressure can be lowered safely with antihypertensive agents may be eligible for treatment, and the physician should assess blood pressure stability before starting rtPA (see below). A patient with a seizure at the time of onset of stroke may be eligible for treatment as long as the physician is convinced that residual impairments are secondary to stroke and not a postictal phenomenon.

IV streptokinase for the treatment of stroke is not recommended, and ancrod, tenecteplase, reteplase, desmoteplase, urokinase, or other thrombolytic agents should not be used outside the setting of a clinical trial. American Stroke Association guidelines suggest that thrombolysis may be considered for patients between 3 and 4.5 hours after stroke onset, provided patients are younger than 80 years, have NIHSS ≤ 25, are not taking oral anticoagulants, and do not have a history of both prior stroke and diabetes, but rtPA is not FDA-approved in this patient population.

SHOULD PATIENTS BE TREATED WITH THROMBOLYSIS BEYOND 3 HOURS AFTER ONSET OF STROKE?

Thrombolysis in stroke is most effective when administered as early as possible after the onset of symptoms. Based on the European Cooperative Acute Stroke Study (ECASS-3), there is a modest benefit of thrombolysis given between 3 and 4.5 hours after stroke, although this seems to be less than the benefit observed with thrombolysis between 0 to 3 hours after stroke onset. The eligibility

TABLE 210-3 Administration of IV Recombinant Tissue Plasminogen Activator (rtPA) for Acute Ischemic Stroke*

Indications	Contraindications
Clinical diagnosis of stroke with disabling deficit	Sustained blood pressure > 185/110 mm Hg despite treatment
Onset of symptoms to time of drug administration ≤ 3 hours	Platelets < 100,000; hematocrit < 25%; glucose < 50 or > 400 mg/dL
CT scan showing no hemorrhage,	Use of heparin within 48 hours and prolonged PTT, or elevated INR > 1.7
well-established infarct, or alternative explanation for the focal deficit	Rapidly improving symptoms
Age ≥ 18 years	Prior stroke or head injury within 3 months; prior intracranial hemorrhage
Consent by patient or surrogate	Major surgery in preceding 14 days
	Minor stroke symptoms
	GI bleeding in preceding 21 days
	Recent myocardial infarction
	Coma or stupor
Administration of rtPA	
IV access with two peripheral IV lines (avoid arterial or central line placement)	
Review eligibility for rtPA	
Administer 0.9 mg/kg IV (maximum 90 mg) IV as 10% of total dose by bolus, followed by remainder of total dose over 1 hour	
Frequent cuff blood pressure monitoring	
No other antithrombotic treatment for 24 hours	
For decline in neurologic status or uncontrolled blood pressure, stop infusion, give cryoprecipitate, and reimage brain emergently	
Avoid urethral catheterization for 2 hours	

*See Activase (tissue plasminogen activator) package insert for complete list of contraindications and dosing.
CT, computed tomography; INR, international normalized ratio; PTT, partial thromboplastin time.
Modified, with permission, from Fauci AS, Braunwald E, Kasper DL, et al. *Harrison's Principles of Internal Medicine.* 17th ed. New York: McGraw-Hill; 2008, Table 364-1.

criteria for treatment are similar to those for persons treated at earlier time periods. However, patients who meet any of the following additional criteria should be excluded:

- Patients older than 80 years
- Those with a baseline NIHSS > 25
- Those with a history of both stroke and diabetes
- All patients receiving an oral anticoagulant are excluded, regardless of their international normalized ratio (INR)

The safety and efficacy of treatment with rtPA within 3 to 4.5 hours after stroke in patients with these exclusion criteria have not been established and require further study. Additionally, the relative utility of rtPA in this time window compared with other methods of thrombus dissolution or removal has not been established. Patients should be informed that use of rtPA between 3 and 4.5 hours after stroke is considered off-label or investigational by the FDA.

BLOOD PRESSURE MANAGEMENT

The management of arterial hypertension in acute stroke remains controversial, as data are inconclusive or conflicting. Many patients have spontaneous declines in blood pressure during the first 24 hours after onset of stroke. Until more definitive data are available, a cautious approach is recommended.

Patients with hypertension who are otherwise eligible for treatment with rtPA may have their blood pressure lowered so that their systolic blood pressure is ≤ 185 mm Hg and diastolic blood pressure ≤ 110 mm Hg before lytic therapy is begun. The clinician should be sure that the blood pressure is stabilized at the lower level before treating with rtPA and maintained below 180/105 mm Hg for at least the first 24 hours after IV rtPA treatment. Because the maximum interval from stroke onset until treatment with rtPA is short, many patients with sustained hypertension above the recommended levels cannot be treated with IV rtPA.

It is generally agreed that patients with markedly elevated blood pressure may have their blood pressure lowered. A reasonable goal would be to lower blood pressure by ~15% in the first 24 hours after onset of stroke. The level of blood pressure that would mandate such treatment is not known, but consensus exists that medications should be withheld unless the systolic blood pressure is > 220 mm Hg or the diastolic blood pressure is > 120 mm Hg.

Evidence from one clinical trial indicates that initiation of antihypertensive therapy within 24 hours of stroke is relatively safe. Thus, antihypertensive medications should be restarted at ~24 hours for patients with preexisting hypertension who are neurologically stable, unless there is a specific contraindication to restarting treatment.

STATIN THERAPY

Patients suffering from ischemic stroke or TIA with elevated cholesterol, coronary artery disease (CAD), and evidence of atherosclerosis should be managed with lifestyle and diet modification and medications. Statins are indicated for these patients, with a low-density-lipoprotein cholesterol (LDL-C) goal of < 100 mg/dL. An LDL-C < 70 mg/dL is recommended for patients with multiple risk factors. In the Stroke Prevention by Aggressive Reduction in Cholesterol Levels (SPARCL) trial, therapy with atorvastatin 80 mg/day also reduced the risk of stroke and cardiovascular events in patients with atherosclerotic ischemic stroke or TIA but without known CAD. In this group, it is recommended to treat to a target LDL-C < 70 mg/dL or an absolute reduction in LDL-C of at least 50%, as the greatest benefits of statin therapy were seen in patients who achieved these goals. Ischemic stroke or TIA patients with low high-density-lipoprotein cholesterol may be considered for treatment with niacin or gemfibrozil.

ANTICOAGULANTS

Urgent anticoagulation with heparin to prevent early recurrent stroke, halt neurologic worsening, or improve outcomes is not recommended for patients with acute ischemic stroke. Urgent anticoagulation should not be used in lieu of IV thrombolysis for treatment of otherwise eligible patients, and it is not recommended for patients with moderate to severe strokes because of an increased risk of serious intracranial hemorrhage. Although anticoagulation is indicated in patients with stroke due to embolism from atrial fibrillation or prosthetic heart valves, it should be avoided within 24 hours of treatment with IV administered rtPA. In contrast, anticoagulation is recommended for patients with TIA from cardiac embolism in the setting of atrial fibrillation.

ANTIPLATELET THERAPY IN ACUTE ISCHEMIC STROKE

Administration of aspirin (initial dose 325 mg) within 24 to 48 hours after stroke onset is recommended for most patients. Aspirin should not be considered a substitute for other acute interventions for treatment of stroke, including IV rtPA. Aspirin use should be avoided within 24 hours of thrombolytic therapy. The administration of clopidogrel alone or in combination with aspirin is not recommended for the treatment of acute ischemic stroke. Outside the setting of clinical trials, the IV administration of antiplatelet agents that inhibit the glycoprotein IIb/IIIa receptor is not recommended.

ANTIPLATELET THERAPY FOR SECONDARY PREVENTION

Patients with stroke or TIA are at high risk of recurrent stroke and other vascular events. In-hospital initiation of secondary stroke prevention avoids gaps in care, promotes better adherence, and leads to better short-term vascular outcomes. For patients with noncardioembolic ischemic stroke or TIA, antiplatelet agents, rather than oral anticoagulation, are recommended to reduce the risk of recurrent stroke and other cardiovascular events. Aspirin (50–325 mg/d) monotherapy, aspirin combined with extended-release dipyridamole, and clopidogrel monotherapy are all acceptable options for initial therapy. The combination of aspirin and extended-release dipyridamole is recommended over aspirin alone. Clopidogrel is preferred in patients with aspirin allergy. The combination of aspirin and clopidogrel increases the risk of major hemorrhage, and it is not routinely recommended for patients with ischemic stroke or TIA unless they have a specific indication, such as a coronary stent or acute coronary syndrome. Clopidogrel was compared with aspirin plus extended-release dipyridamole in the Prevention Regimen for Effectively Avoiding Second Strokes (PRoFESS) trial and found to have similar efficacy in the prevention of recurrent stroke. For patients who have an ischemic cerebrovascular event while taking aspirin, there is no evidence that increasing the dose of aspirin provides additional benefit. These patients are often changed to other antiplatelet regimens, although no clinical trials have been performed to validate this strategy.

HYPERGLYCEMIA

Persistent hyperglycemia (> 140 mg/dL) in the first 24 hours after stroke is associated with poor outcomes. Serum glucose concentrations > 140 to 185 mg/dL probably should trigger insulin administration. Glucose concentrations should be closely monitored, with adjustment of insulin doses to avoid hypoglycemia.

HYPERBARIC OXYGEN AND HYPOTHERMIA

Data on the utility of hyperbaric oxygen are inconclusive, and some data imply it may be harmful. Thus, with the exception of stroke secondary to air embolization, this intervention is not recommended for treatment of patients with acute ischemic stroke. Although data demonstrate the efficacy of hypothermia for improving neurologic outcomes after cardiac arrest, the utility of induced hypothermia for patients with ischemic stroke is not established.

CAROTID DISEASE

The treatment of symptomatic carotid stenosis is evolving. Best medical therapy in major published trials of carotid endarterectomy did not include statin therapy, newer antiplatelet agents, or optimized control of hypertension. Ongoing trials are comparing carotid endarterectomy (CEA) with the newer technique of carotid angioplasty and stenting (CAS) using embolic protection devices. Current recommendations are that patients with recent TIA or stroke within the past 6 months and ipsilateral severe (70–99%) carotid stenosis should undergo CEA if the estimated morbidity and mortality are <6%. CEA is also recommended for patients with recent TIA or stroke and ipsilateral moderate (50–69%) carotid stenosis, provided that estimated morbidity and mortality are <6%, although the benefit is less marked in this group, particularly in women, for reasons that are unclear but may relate to the smaller caliber of carotid vessels in women. CEA is not indicated for carotid stenosis <50%. Many patients benefit from early revascularization (performed within 2 weeks of TIA or stroke). CAS performed by experienced operators with morbidity and mortality rates known to be <6% is an alternative to CEA in patients who are not favorable surgical candidates.

PREVENTION OF COMPLICATIONS, QUALITY METRICS, AND DISCHARGE PLANNING

EMERGENCY MANAGEMENT OF ISCHEMIC STROKE

Core metrics for acute ischemic stroke patients include the following: the percentage of patients with ischemic stroke or TIA with a deficit who have an NIHSS score documented in the admission note or initial neurology consultation, the percentage of patients eligible for thrombolysis who receive it within the appropriate time window, the percentage of patients treated with IV thrombolysis who receive it within 60 minutes of arrival, and the percentage of patients with ischemic stroke who receive antithrombotic therapy by the end of hospital day 2.

DEEP VENOUS THROMBOSIS PROPHYLAXIS

Patients with an ischemic stroke or a hemorrhagic stroke who are nonambulatory should start receiving deep venous thrombosis (DVT) prophylaxis by the end of hospital day 2. Stroke patients with a paretic or paralyzed lower extremity are at very high risk of developing DVT. One study noted proximal DVT in more than a third of patients with moderately severe stroke. Nonpharmacologic approaches include early mobilization and use of intermittent pneumatic compression stockings. Pharmacologic approaches include subcutaneous unfractionated heparin, low-molecular-weight (LMW) heparins, or direct thrombin inhibitors in patients with heparin-induced thrombocytopenia.

DISCHARGE ON ANTITHROMBOTIC THERAPY

Patients with a noncardioembolic ischemic stroke or TIA should be discharged on aspirin monotherapy (50–325 mg daily), aspirin 25 mg/extended-release dipyridamole 200 mg twice daily, or clopidogrel 75 mg daily, as long as no contraindications exist. For patients with a stroke due to a cardioembolic source (eg, atrial fibrillation, mechanical heart valve), warfarin is recommended unless contraindicated. Warfarin is otherwise not recommended for secondary stroke prevention in patients presumed to have a noncardioembolic stroke.

ANTICOAGULATION FOR ATRIAL FIBRILLATION/FLUTTER AND OTHER CAUSES OF CARDIOGENIC EMBOLISM

Patients with an ischemic stroke of cardiogenic origin due to atrial fibrillation, atrial flutter, or rheumatic mitral valve disease should be discharged on lifelong anticoagulation therapy with warfarin with a target INR of 2.5 (range 2–3). Aspirin is an alternative agent for patients with contraindications to warfarin. Anticoagulation for at least 3 months is recommended for patients with stroke due to myocardial infarction with mural thrombus, with an INR target of 2.5. Antithrombotic therapy with warfarin, aspirin, clopidogrel, or aspirin–dipyridamole may be considered in patients with cardiomyopathy and a left ventricular ejection fraction ≤ 35%. Patients with mechanical prosthetic heart valves should be treated with warfarin to maintain an INR target of 3 (range 2.5–3.5). Patients with prosthetic valves who develop embolic stroke despite a therapeutic INR may be treated with low-dose aspirin in addition to warfarin. Although the risk of thromboembolism in patients with biomechanical heart valves is low, warfarin anticoagulation with an INR target of 2 to 3 may be considered if they develop otherwise unexplained ischemic stroke.

DISCHARGE ON STATIN MEDICATION

Statin therapy is recommended for patients with ischemic stroke or TIA who have atherosclerosis and an LDL-C level ≥ 100 mg/dL, with or without concomitant CAD.

DYSPHAGIA SCREENING

Patients with stroke should undergo screening for dysphagia with an evidence-based bedside testing protocol before being given food, fluids, or medication by mouth. Up to 50% of stroke patients develop dysphagia, and are at risk for increased length of hospital stay, malnutrition, and aspiration pneumonia. Patients with abnormal screening results should be referred for a complete examination by a speech and language pathologist or other qualified individual. Recent evidence suggests that pneumonia rates may be reduced when dysphagia screening and treatment are included in a comprehensive stroke management plan.

STROKE EDUCATION

During the hospital stay, patients with ischemic or hemorrhagic stroke and their families or caregivers should be educated about risk factors for stroke, warning signs of stroke, activation of an emergency medical system, need for follow-up after discharge, lifestyle modification, and medications prescribed at discharge. Family and caregivers also need guidance in planning effective and realistic care strategies appropriate to the patient's prognosis and rehabilitation potential. Health care access and affordability should also be explored with patients and families.

SMOKING CESSATION COUNSELING

Patients with stroke who smoke, have smoked, or who have caregivers who smoke should be given smoking cessation advice or counseling during their hospital stay. Smoking nearly doubles the risk of ischemic stroke. Numerous prospective investigations have demonstrated substantial decreases in coronary heart disease mortality and stroke risk for former smokers. The Framingham Heart Study concluded that smoking was a significant independent risk factor for stroke. Patients who receive even brief smoking cessation advice from their physicians are more likely to quit than those receiving no counseling at all. Avoidance of second-hand smoke should also be advocated. Nicotine products and medications such as sustained-release bupropion or varenicline may be helpful for smoking cessation and should be considered.

REHABILITATION ASSESSMENT

Patients with stroke should be assessed for rehabilitation services. Forty percent of stroke patients are left with moderate functional impairment and 15% to 30% with severe disability. More than 60% of those with stroke never receive rehabilitation. The primary goal of rehabilitation is to prevent complications, minimize impairments, and maximize function. Stroke rehabilitation should begin as soon as the diagnosis of stroke is established and life-threatening problems are under control. Patients should be mobilized and encouraged to resume self-care activities as soon as possible. Substantial evidence indicates better clinical outcomes when patients with stroke are treated in a setting that provides coordinated, multidisciplinary stroke-related evaluation and services. Effective rehabilitation interventions initiated early after stroke can enhance the recovery process and minimize functional disability.

CONTROL OF OTHER RISK FACTORS

Hypertension

Treatment of hypertension is indicated in all patients with TIA or stroke more than 24 hours after presentation. Although optimal blood pressure after stroke is uncertain, normal blood pressure has recently been redefined by the seventh report of the Joint National Committee on Prevention, Detection, Evaluation, and Treatment of High Blood Pressure (JNC 7) as $<120/80$ mm Hg. A comprehensive blood pressure reduction plan includes sodium restriction, weight loss, regular aerobic exercise, and a diet rich in fruits and vegetables. Drug therapy should be individualized, but diuretics and angiotensin-converting enzyme (ACE) inhibitors are reasonable initial choices. Reduction in stroke risk is strongly correlated with the absolute magnitude of blood pressure reduction.

Diabetes

Diabetic patients with stroke should be treated with diet, exercise, oral hypoglycemic drugs, and insulin to achieve conventional targets for glycemic control, such as hemoglobin A1c (HbA1c) $<7\%$.

Alcohol

Heavy alcohol consumption increases stroke risk, whereas light consumption of alcohol, especially wine, reduces the overall risk of stroke. However, there is a linear increase in the risk of hemorrhagic stroke with all degrees of alcohol consumption. Heavy drinkers should curtail or stop alcohol use. For those who choose to drink alcohol, consumption should be limited to a maximum of two drinks per day for men and one drink per day for nonpregnant women. Several drugs of abuse, including cocaine, amphetamines, and heroin, increase stroke risk through their effects on vessels, platelets, and the endothelium. Referral for counseling is appropriate in these patients.

Obesity

Weight loss is recommended for the obese, as increased body weight and abdominal fat are directly associated with stroke risk, and weight reduction may also assist in the control of hypertension, diabetes, hyperlipidemia, and metabolic syndrome. Obesity also increases the risk of sleep-disordered breathing, which has been independently associated with increased stroke risk. Physical activity reduces the risk of stroke. Ideally, patients should engage in aerobic exercise of at least 30 minutes' duration three times weekly. Patients with disabilities after stroke benefit from physical therapy and occupational therapy consultation for specialized exercise and rehabilitation programs.

Oral contraceptives

The incremental risk of stroke associated with low-dose oral contraceptives (OCs) in women without additional risk factors appears to be low, if it exists. It is suggested that OCs be discouraged in women with additional risk factors, such as cigarette smoking or prior thromboembolic events. For those who elect to assume the increased risk, aggressive therapy of stroke risk factors may be useful.

Hyperhomocysteinemia

Hyperhomocysteinemia is associated with a twofold increase in the risk of stroke. Following guidelines for daily intake of folate, vitamin B_6, and vitamin B_{12} by consumption of vegetables, fruits, legumes, meats, fish, and fortified grains and cereals may reduce the risk of stroke, particularly for primary prevention. However, the efficacy of folate, vitamin B_6, and vitamin B_{12} supplementation in the secondary prevention of stroke has not been demonstrated.

SUGGESTED READINGS

Amarenco P, Bogousslavsky J, Callahan A III, et al. High-dose atorvastatin after stroke or transient ischemic attack. *N Engl J Med.* 2006;355:549–559.

Arima H, Chalmers J, Woodward M, et al. Lower target blood pressures are safe and effective for the prevention of recurrent stroke: The PROGRESS trial. *J Hypertens.* 2006;24:1201–1208.

Del Zoppo GJ, Saver JL, Jauch EC, Adams HP Jr; American Heart Association Stroke Council. Expansion of the time window for treatment of acute ischemic stroke with intravenous tissue plasminogen activator: A science advisory from the American Heart Association/American Stroke Association. *Stroke.* 2009;40:2945–2948.

Easton JD, Saver JL, Albers GW, et al. Definition and evaluation of transient ischemic attack: A scientific statement for healthcare professionals from the American Heart Association/American Stroke Association Stroke Council. *Stroke.* 2009;40:2276–2293.

Furie KL, Kasner SE, Adams RJ, et al. Guidelines for the prevention of stroke in patients with stroke or transient ischemic attack: A guideline for healthcare professionals from the American Heart Association/American Stroke Association. *Stroke.* 2011;42:227–276.

Goldstein LB, Bushnell CD, Adams RJ, et al. Guidelines for the primary prevention of stroke: A guideline for healthcare professionals from the American Heart Association/American Stroke Association. *Stroke.* 2011;42:517–584.

Hacke W, Kaste M, Bluhmki E, et al. Thrombolysis with alteplase 3 to 4.5 hours after acute ischemic stroke. *N Engl J Med.* 2008;359:1317–1329.

Sacco RL, Diener HC, Yusuf S, et al. Aspirin and extended-release dipyridamole versus clopidogrel for recurrent stroke. *N Engl J Med.* 2008;359:1238–1251.

CHAPTER 211

Parkinson Disease and Related Disorders

Joseph N. Rudolph, MD
Ruth H. Walker, MB, ChB, PhD

Key Clinical Questions

1. What are the diagnostic criteria for idiopathic Parkinson disease?
2. What is the differential diagnosis of a patient with parkinsonian symptoms?
3. What is the pathophysiology of Parkinson disease?
4. What treatments are available? How do they relate to the underlying pathophysiology?
5. What side effects and long-term effects may occur in a patient with Parkinson disease who is on medication?
6. What complications may occur when a patient with Parkinson disease is admitted to the hospital?

INTRODUCTION AND EPIDEMIOLOGY

Parkinson disease (PD) develops in 12 to 20/100,000 people yearly, with a prevalence as high as 1% in those older than 65 years. With appropriate treatment, there appears to be no significant effect on life expectancy. However, quality of life is markedly reduced due to a variety of factors, some of which have only recently been recognized, such as autonomic system dysfunction.

Estimates of the economic burden of PD in various countries range from $4,000 to $20,000 per patient yearly, including roughly 33% to 40% in indirect costs, such as lost productivity. On average, PD-affected patients can no longer work full time by 3.4 years after diagnosis, and most file for disability by 5 years. In addition, PD is a risk factor for nursing home placement.

PATHOPHYSIOLOGY

PD is associated with the loss of dopaminergic neurons located in the midbrain, in the substantia nigra pars compacta (SNc). Patients who are still early in their clinical course have lost ~80% of the SNc neurons, implying that the degenerative process begins long before motor symptoms appear, and that the basal ganglia are able to compensate until there is a critical loss of dopaminergic neurons. How the loss of dopamine disrupts normal functioning of the basal ganglia is not fully understood, but it appears to result in pathologic synchronization of neuronal firing throughout the region that interferes with both voluntary and involuntary movements. PD has many nonmotor symptoms as well, suggestive of a more widespread neurodegenerative process involving neurotransmitters other than dopamine. There is increasing evidence for more extensive involvement of the brainstem and cortex, perhaps explaining the effects of PD on cognition, behavior, and sleep.

In most cases, the cause of PD is unknown. Mutations in single genes such as *parkin, DJ-1,* and *LRRK2* are responsible for only a minority of cases of PD but are more prominent in patients who develop symptoms before the age of 50. The relationship of these mutations to neuronal death is not known, but it may involve several mechanisms, including protein misfolding, defective protein degradation by proteosomes, and increased oxidative stress. Recently, an association of PD with relatively common mutations in the gene for the lysosomal enzyme glucocerebrosidase has been described.

The pathological hallmark of PD is the presence of Lewy bodies in the neurons of the SNc. Lewy bodies may be more widely distributed and are found in the cortex in the related disorder known as dementia with Lewy bodies. Lewy bodies are composed of intracellular clumps of proteins, including alpha-synuclein and ubiquitin. Alpha-synuclein is thought to be a phospholipid-binding protein that helps vesicles dock with the plasma membrane. It is not known whether Lewy bodies are toxic to the neurons in which they develop; more likely, they are a mechanism for keeping damaged proteins out of the way of normal cellular functioning.

DIFFERENTIAL DIAGNOSIS OF PARKINSONISM: PARKINSON-PLUS SYNDROMES

The term *parkinsonism* refers to the presence of signs of idiopathic PD, such as slowness of movement (bradykinesia), absence of movement (akinesia), increased tone (rigidity), resting tremor, and impaired postural reflexes. Some or all of these features may be seen in other neurodegenerative disorders, known as the Parkinson-plus syndromes, or atypical parkinsonism. The term *secondary parkinsonism* is used when another etiology has been identified, such as medication or cerebrovascular disease.

MULTIPLE SYSTEM ATROPHY

CASE 211-1

A 55-year-old man presents with gradual onset of stiffness and dizziness. When he gets up from bed or from the table, he needs to stand still for a minute or two, or he would faint. He has difficulty walking and reports that this is because he feels as if he "is on a boat." He reports loss of sexual function for 3 years with no clear cause. Examination is notable for orthostatic hypotension, limb stiffness, and ataxic gait.

Patients with multiple system atrophy (MSA) may have varying combinations of parkinsonism, cerebellar disease, and autonomic dysfunction that may resemble idiopathic PD, especially in the early stages. MSA-parkinsonism (MSA-P) involves striatonigral degeneration (rather than nigrostriatal, as seen in PD). Although MSA-P predominantly affects the neurons postsynaptic to the dopaminergic neurons, patients seem to be at least partly responsive to levodopa therapy. MSA-cerebellar (MSA-C) mostly affects the olivocerebellar connections, with disproportionate involvement of the middle cerebellar peduncles. These tracts originate in the pons and travel to the cerebellar cortex. MSA-autonomic (also called Shy–Drager syndrome) is characterized by degeneration of the locus coeruleus, the dorsal motor nucleus of the vagus nerve, and the catecholamine-producing neurons of the ventrolateral medulla.

Pathologically, alpha-synuclein inclusions are found in glial cells, rather than neurons as in PD. The locations of the inclusions determine the clinical spectrum of disease and can include the SNc, locus coeruleus, putamen, inferior olives, pontine nuclei, cerebellar Purkinje cells, and intermediolateral columns in the spinal cord.

MSA is usually not inherited, and the cause is unknown. There is no disease-modifying treatment, and treatment is symptomatic. Parkinsonian patients may have some response to levodopa, which should be increased to the maximum tolerated dose. Autonomic dysfunction is managed by giving midodrine, a vasoconstrictor, and mineralocorticoids such as fludrocortisone to increase blood pressure, with antispasmodics or catheters for urinary incontinence. Physical and speech therapy are often useful. As with all parkinsonian disorders, swallowing is often affected and should be evaluated to reduce the chances of aspiration, a major cause of morbidity and mortality.

PROGRESSIVE SUPRANUCLEAR PALSY

CASE 211-2

A 68-year-old woman presents with difficulty walking and abrupt falling. She has been falling spontaneously with increasing frequency, especially when walking down stairs. She also has been having trouble swallowing. On examination, her neck is stiff and slightly extended, with milder stiffness of the wrists. Her eye movements seem somewhat slowed, with decreased ability to look down, and her overall demeanor is muted.

In its early stages, progressive supranuclear palsy (PSP) may be indistinguishable from PD, but axial symptoms such as gait impairment and balance problems are usually prominent and severe earlier in the course. Prominent features of PSP include supranuclear palsy with early impairment of vertical gaze, mild dementia with frontal features, dysarthria, and dysphagia. PSP has been linked to genetic variants in tau, a microtubule-associated protein. Pathologically, the brain shows inclusion bodies made up of tau protein, along with tufted astrocytes and globose tangles. PSP (like most atypical parkinsonian syndromes) shows a poor response to levodopa, but this should be tried as one of the few available pharmacotherapeutic options. Early involvement of a speech therapist is important.

PRACTICE POINT

- Patients with progressive supranuclear palsy may have excessive eyelid retraction coupled with an unblinking stare, giving them a look of constant surprise, in contrast to the masked facies of the Parkinson disease patient.

DEMENTIA WITH LEWY BODIES

In dementia with Lewy bodies (DLB), patients present with features identical to idiopathic PD but have early dementia and behavioral abnormalities out of proportion to the accompanying motor symptoms. Visual hallucinations, which are usually benign and nondistressing, are a typical early feature. Pathologically, DLB resembles PD, in that the cytoplasm of affected cells has similar Lewy body inclusions, but these are more widely distributed, and the affected area includes the cerebral cortex, in addition to the SNc. Treatment is similar to that for Alzheimer disease (acetylcholinesterase inhibitors) and to the other parkinsonian syndromes.

PRACTICE POINT

- Patients with Lewy body dementia are hypersensitive to antipsychotics and may get excessively sedated or more parkinsonian when they receive them.

CORTICOBASAL DEGENERATION

Corticobasal degeneration (CBD) is a tauopathy that manifests with parkinsonian symptoms and dementia. There can be cortical symptoms, such as apraxia, aphasia, higher order sensory loss, or alien hand syndrome, where one limb may writhe or perform complex involuntary movements, such as picking at the hair or clothes. Patients may have asymmetric parkinsonism or limb dystonia. Imaging shows asymmetric atrophy of the frontoparietal cortex; pathologically, there are ballooned, achromatic neurons. Corticobasal syndromes may feature in other conditions, such as Alzheimer disease and PSP. The neurologic symptoms are related to the distribution of the tau-immunoreactive inclusion bodies in the cortex and basal ganglia.

OTHER CAUSES OF PARKINSONISM

VASCULAR PARKINSONISM

Microvascular changes and small infarcts from atherosclerosis may disrupt the fibers of the basal ganglia, leading to parkinsonian symptoms without degeneration of dopaminergic neurons. This is usually seen in patients with typical vascular risk factors, such as hypertension, diabetes, hyperlipidemia, smoking, and older age. Patients with vascular parkinsonism generally have early gait problems, including falling and freezing, and often more marked postural tremor. Patients with vascular parkinsonism warrant a trial of levodopa but are generally less responsive than patients with idiopathic PD. The mainstay of treatment is physical therapy. To reduce the risk of future events, patients should be treated aggressively for reversible risk factors and receive antiplatelet agents.

MEDICATION-INDUCED PARKINSONISM

Numerous agents block dopaminergic neurotransmission and produce parkinsonian symptoms. Classical antipsychotics used in schizophrenia, such as haloperidol, thioridazine, and perphenazine, work by blocking dopamine receptors. A predictable side effect of these medicines is the development of tremor, rigidity, and slowness of movement, indistinguishable from idiopathic PD. Elderly patients may develop parkinsonian symptoms when treated with haloperidol, risperidone, or olanzapine for nocturnal delirium in the hospital (sundowning). In some cases, patients are discharged from the hospital on these agents without a clear understanding of their nature. Drug-induced parkinsonism usually produces bilateral symptoms. Treatment begins with discontinuing the offending agent, but in some cases the symptoms persist. When symptoms persist after several months and interfere with the patient's functioning, cautious therapy with levodopa may be warranted. In this situation, it is likely that treatment with an antipsychotic unmasked underlying idiopathic PD.

If absolutely essential for the management of hospital-acquired psychosis or agitation, atypical antipsychotics with fewer parkinsonian side effects can be used, such as quetiapine and clozapine, starting at very low doses. (Patients on clozapine need to have frequent blood tests to monitor for agranulocytosis.)

Drug-induced parkinsonism may also be a side effect of antiemetic medications that block peripheral dopamine receptors, such as metoclopramide, promethazine, and prochlorperazine. These agents may cross the blood–brain barrier and lead to parkinsonism. As with the antipsychotics, these drugs may be prescribed too liberally to hospitalized patients, and even chronically to outpatients. An antiemetic with a different mechanism of action, such as ondansetron, may be an appropriate alternative.

DIFFERENTIAL DIAGNOSIS: NONPARKINSONIAN DISORDERS

Problems with walking in the older patient may have variety of causes. These include pain, orthopedic problems, arthritis of the foot and ankle, fear of falling, and peripheral neuropathy, in addition to the non–basal ganglia disorders discussed here.

ESSENTIAL TREMOR

A condition that frequently brings patients to the neurologist for evaluation for possible PD is essential tremor (ET). This was previously known as benign familial tremor, but it is not necessarily familial and is not benign for those who are impaired by it. In ET, tremor is more typically bilateral than unilateral, although it can be asymmetric. In contrast to the tremor of PD, it is absent at rest and brought on by action, such as pouring a drink, bringing a cup to the mouth, or writing. There is little stiffness or postural instability, although severe tremor can affect walking and balance. There may be tremor in the neck, causing head oscillations. Tremor is worsened by stress and improved by relaxation. Alcohol may reduce the symptoms.

PRACTICE POINT

- Head tremor is not a feature of Parkinson disease. Its presence is strongly suggestive of essential tremor. Conversely, rigidity and bradykinesia are not seen in patients with essential tremor.

The diagnosis is made on clinical grounds. About 50% of ET cases are familial; thus, the presence of an affected family member supports the diagnosis. If the tremor is not apparent on examination, the patient should be asked to do whatever brings the tremor out, such as pouring water from one cup to another or writing. Drawing a spiral is useful to bring out subtle tremor and to document tremor severity.

Reversible causes of tremor should be excluded, specifically hyperthyroidism and medications such as lithium, valproate, theophylline, cyclosporine, and caffeine. If tremor improves with alcohol intake, mild alcohol consumption may ease embarrassment during social occasions; care should be taken that the patient does not develop dependence on alcohol. The two first-line medications are primidone, an older anticonvulsant, and propranolol. Other antiepileptic medications, such as gabapentin, levetiracetam, and topiramate, have been tried, with varying success. Deep brain stimulation (DBS, surgical implantation of electrodes) in the motor nuclei of the thalamus is used in severe cases.

NORMAL PRESSURE HYDROCEPHALUS

Normal pressure hydrocephalus (NPH) is characterized by cognitive dysfunction, urinary incontinence, and gait apraxia, presumably from impaired resorption of cerebrospinal fluid (CSF). The possibility of this diagnosis may be raised by family members of the parkinsonian patient who have heard of impressive cures following ventriculoperitoneal shunt placement. The apraxic gait in NPH is characterized by a wide base, with slow, short steps, and the patient has difficulty lifting each foot off the ground, as if glued to the floor (magnetic gait). Although the gaits of NPH and PD may be similar, patients with PD usually do not freeze with each step, and the stance is not widened. Patients with NPH do not have a masked face, stooped posture, or slowed movements.

The gait disorder in NPH is caused by dysfunction or destruction of the periventricular fibers from the leg region of the motor cortex. The diagnosis of NPH is ultimately clinical but is supported by neuroimaging demonstrating ventricular enlargement out of proportion to cortical atrophy, impaired CSF flow after injection of radionuclide tracers, and alleviation of symptoms with removal of large volumes of CSF by lumbar puncture. However, placebo effects can occur with this procedure, and care should be taken to avoid false-positive interpretations, especially as placement of a ventriculoperitoneal shunt is not a benign procedure.

CEREBELLAR DISEASE

Cerebellar dysfunction causes a wide-based, ataxic gait, distinct from the shuffling gait of PD. However, the basal ganglia may be involved in cerebellar disorders, and parkinsonian symptoms may be seen, for example, in some of the autosomal dominantly inherited spinocerebellar ataxias or in the cerebellar form of MSA. The diagnosis is supported by eye movement abnormalities and limb or truncal ataxia.

SPINAL STENOSIS

Narrowing of the cervical canal with spinal cord compression can cause spasticity that interferes with walking. This may be detected as a clasp-knife increase in tone of the lower extremities, as distinguished from the lead-pipe rigidity of PD (see below). Increased activity of the deep tendon reflexes at the knees and ankles, with positive Babinski signs, will help localize the lesion to the cervical spinal cord. Atrophy of the small muscles of the hands due to cervical radiculopathy can be a sign of cervical spine disease. Clinicians should also bear in mind that spinal stenosis may complicate PD, as abnormal posture may promote spinal degeneration from increased vertebral wear and tear.

DIAGNOSIS

There is no definitive test for PD prior to autopsy. The diagnosis is clinical, based on the presence of major criteria as delineated by the United Kingdom Brain Bank, namely, bradykinesia with resting tremor, rigidity, or postural instability, not related to another known etiology. Nonmotor symptoms, such as depression, anxiety, impaired cognition, muscle aches, insomnia, daytime somnolence, impaired olfaction, and constipation, may precede the onset of motor symptoms (**Figure 211-1**).

Unilateral tremor is the most common initial motor symptom (**Table 211-1**). Despite subsequent involvement of the contralateral side, the disease usually continues to be somewhat asymmetric. The tremor is present at rest and often observed when the patient is distracted and relaxed. The resting tremor of PD may be brought out by walking or having the opposite hand perform repetitive movements. Patients may also have a component of action tremor or postural tremor, but if either of these is the major symptom in the absence of parkinsonian signs, then another diagnosis, such as ET, should be considered. The postural tremor of PD tends to manifest after patients have held their hands outstretched for a few seconds (emergent tremor), rather than immediately, as in ET. While, both PD and ET are common conditions and may coexist, there is debate regarding whether they are etiologically related.

For a diagnosis of PD, exclusion of atypical and secondary parkinsonism is required. Patients should be evaluated for features of atypical parkinsonian disorders, such as early falling (within 5 years of disease onset), prominent autonomic dysfunction, early dementia, and visual hallucinations. Use of neuroleptics or antiemetics should be excluded. A diagnosis of drug-induced parkinsonism does not exclude the possibility of concomitant idiopathic PD, although it should be noted that the effect of the medication may persist for several months after discontinuation.

The neurologic examination is targeted to highlight parkinsonian features.

The limbs and neck should be assessed for rigidity. There may be difficulty in distinguishing rigidity from spasticity; spasticity, or the increase in tone that appears following an upper motor lesion, such as a stroke or a spinal cord injury, is velocity-dependent, becoming almost minimal when the limb is moved slowly and more resistant when the force is applied suddenly (clasp-knife rigidity). In parkinsonian rigidity (lead-pipe rigidity), muscle tone is unchanged regardless of the velocity with which the force is applied.

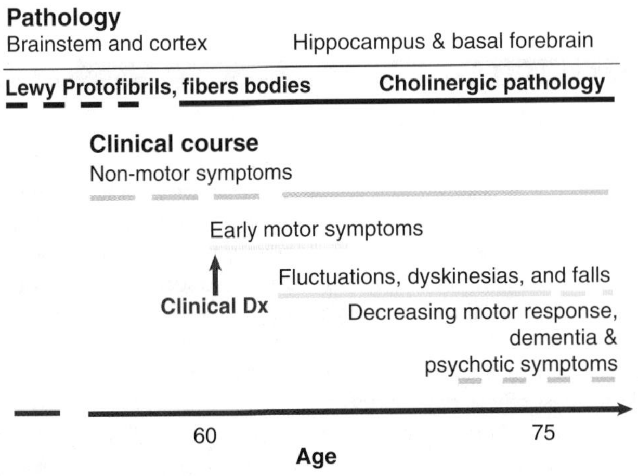

Figure 211-1 *Natural history of Parkinson disease, with neuropathologic correlation. (Reproduced, with permission, from Fauci AS, Braunwald E, Kasper DL et al. Harrison's Principles of Internal Medicine 17th ed. New York: McGraw-Hill 2008, Fig. 366-2.)*

TABLE 211-1 Initial Symptoms in Patients with Parkinson Disease

Symptom	Percentage of Patients
Tremor	70
Gait disturbance	11
Stiffness	10
Slowness	10
Muscle aches	8
Loss of dexterity	7
Handwriting disturbance	5
Depression, nervousness, other psychiatric disturbance	4
Speech disturbance	3

Modified from Ropper AH, Samuels MA. *Adams and Victor's Principles of Neurology*. 9th ed. New York: McGraw-Hill; 2009.

Bradykinesia is evaluated by having the patient perform repetitive tasks using one limb at a time: opening and closing fists, pronating-supinating the hand on the knee, tapping each heel on the ground, and finger tapping, with the index finger against the thumb (it is not necessary to tap all the fingers to the thumb in sequence, as this requires frontal lobe function and can confound the examination). There is usually an asymmetry between the speed of each side. Mild bradykinesia is often dismissed as being due to age, but it is not seen in normal aging. If possible, compare the patient's spontaneous facial movements and hand gesticulations with those of someone of similar age.

Postural stability and gait are evaluated in several ways. The patient is asked to stand up without the use of his or her arms (they may be crossed over the chest). Walking is observed, with attention to arm swing, stride length, posture (either forward or sideways tilt), and the ability to turn with a pivot. If the patient cannot pivot and instead requires multiple little steps to turn, it is referred to as turning en bloc. Patients may freeze, especially on turning or in doorways, and be unable to take a step without help. Festination (hurrying) may occur: the stooped patient takes small rapid steps, as if in pursuit of his or her shifting center of gravity, and may even topple over. Balance is tested using the pull test. The patient is told to stand with feet at shoulder width, warned that he or she is about to be pulled back, and instructed to take a couple of backward steps to stop from falling. The patient is then pulled firmly backward from the shoulders (the physician should position the hands either side of the patient to be prepared to catch him or her if necessary). If the patient requires more than two or three steps backward to restore balance or would fall if not caught by the examiner, then postural reflexes are impaired. A positive glabellar tap test, in which the patient continues to blink with repetitive tapping between the eyebrows, is seen in PD.

There are no blood tests that confirm the diagnosis of PD. At present, in the absence of molecular therapies, genetic testing is not clinically useful. Imaging of the dopamine transporter using a radiolabeled marker (DaTscan) is accepted as confirming the diagnosis of PD, but is not yet widely available. Magnetic resonance imaging (MRI) is not useful for diagnosing PD, although it may reveal features that raise the possibility of MSA, PSP, or vascular parkinsonism. Cerebellar or pontine atrophy is more consistent with MSA, whereas midbrain atrophy would indicate PSP. Iron deposition in the striatum may be seen in MSA.

The diagnosis of PD is often most evident after several years, when the clinical progression and response to medication can be observed. Although atypical parkinsonian disorders often respond partially to levodopa, a sustained motor response to levodopa over years supports the diagnosis of idiopathic PD.

The most widely used scale for evaluating the severity of PD is the Unified Parkinson's Disease Rating Scale (UDPRS), which has recently been refined and revised. This rating scale has sections dedicated to cognitive/psychiatric symptoms, activities of daily living/history, physical examination, and medication-related and autonomic symptoms. The scale is used to measure the severity of disease as well as the progression, and scores can be compared at serial visits. Disease severity may also be evaluated in the setting of a medication trial, both for clarifying diagnosis and for estimating medication effect.

TRIAGE/HOSPITAL ADMISSION

ACUTE WORSENING OF PARKINSONIAN SYMPTOMS

PD is a characterized by slow, gradual progression, and any sudden deterioration is always due to another cause. As with many neurologic conditions, any metabolic derangement can exacerbate the symptoms of the underlying disorder. The health care provider must evaluate for factors such as an acute infection, especially of the urinary tract or lungs, dehydration, or electrolyte disturbances. In addition, it should be determined if any new medication is being taken with adverse consequences. New focal, or even nonfocal, neurologic signs may indicate a stroke or a subdural hematoma following a fall.

Patients who have DBS electrodes implanted will acutely deteriorate if their DBS batteries wear out, and become extremely rigid and unable to walk. They may even have an appearance similar to neuroleptic malignant syndrome, with severe rigidity and rhabdomyolysis. These patients should be treated with aggressive dopaminergic therapy and hydration. Contact should be made with a neurosurgeon as soon as possible to schedule a battery replacement. This situation may be avoided by calculation of battery life and monitoring.

MEDICATION ADMINISTRATION

To minimize the chance of complications due to under- or overtreatment while in the hospital, it is vital that patients continue to take their medications as they did at home. Careful attention must be paid to dosage and timing. Undertreatment results in impaired mobility, with the risk of falls, aspiration, deep venous thrombosis, constipation, and decubitus ulcers. It can also worsen confusion. Overtreatment causes dyskinesia, falls, agitation, confusion, and hallucinations.

Because timing of PD medications is critical for patients with more than mild disease, it is essential that they be taken on time. In the hospital this may become difficult, as levodopa every 3 hours, or even more often, is a departure from typical medication administration schedules. If a patient with PD is admitted to the ward, the nursing staff must be educated that PD medications should be given on a schedule closest to the patient's home schedule (but that the patient should not be awakened during the night to take the next dose). In extreme cases, it may be helpful for the pharmacy to become involved. Medication errors frequently arise due to the different formulations available for carbidopa-levodopa (**Table 211-2**).

The pharmacy should be made aware of which formulation is desired, especially in the cases where different ones are taken by the same patient. Although drug holidays were once used to manage medication complications, these are now a thing of the past, with major risks and little benefit. Amantadine should never be suddenly stopped, as this can cause a withdrawal syndrome.

TABLE 211-2 Some Available Formulations of Carbidopa–Levodopa

Drug Name (Trade Name)	Comment
Carbidopa–levodopa (Sinemet)10/100*	75 mg daily of carbidopa is required to inhibit dopa-decarboxylase; thus, three times daily dosing of this formulation is inadequate.
Carbidopa–levodopa (Sinemet) 25/100	This is the most commonly used formulation. In most patients, it can be started at one half tablet three times daily and increased to one tablet three times daily.
Carbidopa–levodopa (Sinemet) 25/250	Highest strength formulation
Carbidopa-levodopa orally disintegrating (Parcopa) 10/100, 25/100, 25/250	Sublingual formulation can be useful in patients with dysphagia. There is no improvement in efficacy or release time.
Carbidopa/levodopa (Sinemet) CR 25/100 Carbidopa/levodopa (Sinemet) CR 50/200	With the controlled-release formulation, patients often report that they do not feel the medication "kicking in" as they do with regular-release tablets. Serum levels can be erratic. This formulation is most useful for overnight or early morning symptoms.

*The first number indicates milligrams of carbidopa, the second, milligrams of levodopa. An additional formulation contains entacapone (Stalevo).

DECONDITIONING

Elderly patients become deconditioned easily after even a short hospital stay. This is particularly applicable to parkinsonian patients. All parkinsonian patients admitted to the hospital should receive physical therapy as soon as possible. They may also benefit from inpatient rehabilitation in a skilled nursing facility prior to returning home.

TREATMENT OPTIONS

PHARMACOTHERAPY

The current American Academy of Neurology guidelines suggest starting patients on a monoamine oxidase type B (MAO-B) inhibitor, such as selegiline, which provides mild symptomatic benefit. When dopaminergic therapy is required, there is debate about whether patients should be started on levodopa, which is most effective in treating motor symptoms, but which may hasten the appearance of levodopa-induced dyskinesias (see below), or on dopamine agonists (ropinirole and pramipexole), which are slightly less efficacious.

The authors' preference is to use dopamine agonists in younger patients in an attempt to delay the appearance of dyskinesias. Younger patients are more likely to tolerate the necessary slow titration of these medications and have fewer side effects. When functioning is no longer adequately treated, levodopa should be added. Levodopa should be used in older patients, particularly if

TABLE 211-3 Drugs Commonly Used in the Treatment of Parkinson Disease

Medication	Starting Dose	Target Dose	Main Benefit	Side Effects
Levodopa				
Carbidopa-levodopa (Sinemet)	12.5–50 mg three times daily	Up to 50–200 mg every 3 hours	Reduction of tremor and bradykinesia; less effect on postural difficulties	Nausea, dyskinesias, orthostatic hypotension, hallucinations, confusion
Controlled release carbidopa–levodopa	25–100 mg once daily	Up to 50–200 mg every 4 hours	May prolong levodopa effects	
Dopamine agonists				
Ropinirole	0.25 mg three times daily	9–24 mg daily	Moderate effects on all aspects; reduced motor fluctuations of levodopa	Orthostatic hypotension, excessive and abrupt sleepiness, confusion, hallucinations
Pramipexole	0.125 mg three times daily	0.75–3 mg daily	As above	As above
Glutamate antagonist				
Amantadine (Symmetrel)	100 mg daily	100 mg twice or three times daily	Smoothing of motor fluctuations	Leg swelling, congestive heart failure, prostatic outlet obstruction, confusion, hallucinations, insomnia
Anticholinergics				
Benztropine (Cogentin)	0.5 mg daily	Up to 4 mg daily	Tremor reduction, less effect on other features	Atropinic effects: dry mouth, urinary outlet obstruction, confusion, psychosis, sedation
Trihexyphenidyl (Artane)	0.5 mg twice daily	Up to 2 mg three times daily	As above	As above
COMT inhibitors				
Entacapone	200 mg with levodopa	Up to 8 times a day	Prolonged effect of levodopa	Urine discoloration, diarrhea, increased dyskinesias
MAO-B inhibitors				
Rasagiline	0.5 mg	1 mg daily	Reduced "off" time, questionable neuroprotection	Hallucinations, confusion
Selegiline	5 mg	5 mg twice daily	Questionable neuroprotection Mild symptomatic effect, reduced off time, mild psychomotor stimulation, anti-depressant effect	Nightmares, agitation

COMT, catechol-O-methyltransferase; MAO-B, monoamine oxidase type B.
From Ropper AH, Samuels MA. *Adams and Victor's Principles of Neurology.* 9th ed. New York: McGraw-Hill; 2009.

gait and balance are already compromised by other factors, including normal aging, and effective treatment needs to be instituted quickly for safety reasons. (Drugs used in PD are summarized in **Table 211-3**, and a suggested treatment algorithm is provided in **Figure 211-2**.)

Levodopa

The mainstay of treatment since the early 1970s has been levodopa, the immediate biochemical precursor to dopamine. Levodopa is metabolized in plasma by dopa decarboxylase to dopamine. Dopamine, being a polar molecule, cannot cross the blood–brain barrier. As a result, only a limited amount of the ingested levodopa is transported into the brain. In addition, peripheral dopamine makes the patient severely nauseated. To combat this problem, carbidopa, a dopa decarboxylase inhibitor, is coformulated with levodopa. This reduces the peripheral metabolism of levodopa and enables more of it to cross the blood–brain barrier via the large neutral amino acid transporter. Decarboxylation to dopamine then occurs in the brain, with fewer peripheral side effects. In particularly nausea-sensitive patients, extra carbidopa can be taken.

Other side effects of levodopa are hypotension, arrhythmias, vivid dreams, hallucinations, and somnolence. There may be effects on mood, including emotional lability, increased libido, and anxiety. Confusion and loss of mental acuity can also occur with this medication. Unfortunately, decreased mental acuity and orthostatic hypotension tend to be later features of PD itself, making it difficult

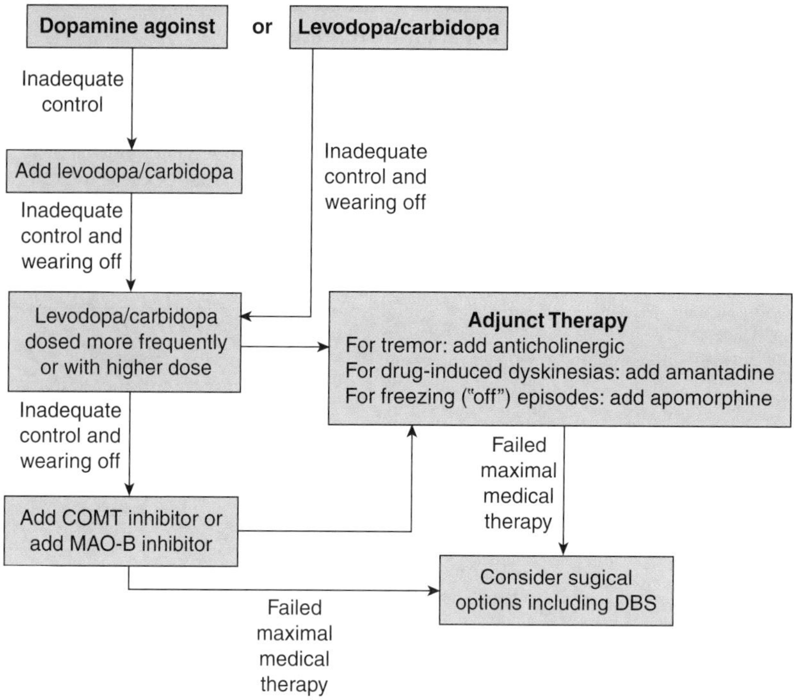

Figure 211-2 *Suggested treatment algorithm for symptomatic Parkinson disease. (Reproduced, with permission, from Fauci AS, Braunwald E, Kasper DL et al. Harrison's Principles of Internal Medicine 17th ed. New York: McGraw-Hill 2008, Fig. 366-4.)*

to distinguish between disease-related and medication-induced symptoms.

As PD progresses, higher doses of levodopa are required for functioning, and in most patients the involuntary choreiform movements known as levodopa-induced dyskinesias will appear. These are often more troubling to caregivers than to patients and do not always require dose modification, but they can occasionally be violent and disabling (see below).

The long-acting form of carbidopa–levodopa (brand name Sinemet CR) can be useful in certain situations, although the term *controlled release* is somewhat of a misnomer, given the erratic bioavailability of the drug as compared with the standard preparation of this medication. It is most useful when given at bedtime for overnight symptoms, when specific plasma levels are less important than attempting to maintain some drug in the system until morning. This formulation can also be useful for those who experience early morning foot cramps or motor difficulties prior to their first morning medication dose.

PRACTICE POINT

- Although often prescribed by nonspecialists, controlled-release carbidopa–levodopa rarely gives the same motor benefits as regular carbidopa–levodopa. It is equivalent to about two thirds of the regular dose and may not provide the same "kick" or "jump start" to improve motor symptoms.

Inhibitors of dopamine metabolism

Medications that inhibit metabolism of dopamine offer a useful therapeutic strategy to enhance dopaminergic function. MAO or catechol-*O*-methyltransferase (COMT) metabolize dopamine and other biogenic amines. MAO can be taken alone or in combination with levodopa. COMT inhibitors are only prescribed as adjuncts to levodopa. One drug from each class may be prescribed together for a synergistic effect. (This may be queried by pharmacies, but use of these medications in combination is safe and effective.) When taken as an adjunct to carbidopa–levodopa, these medicines permit the dosing interval to be lengthened slightly, improving quality of life, as the patient is less bound to the clock and does not have to take pills as frequently. It may also be possible to lower the dose of levodopa with COMT inhibitor use. The earliest COMT inhibitor, tolcapone, has a risk of liver toxicity, but it is more effective, as it inhibits both peripheral and central COMT. Liver enzymes should be monitored regularly in patients on this drug. The more recently developed COMT inhibitor entacapone is better tolerated, although less effective, as it inhibits only peripheral COMT. Entacapone is available in a somewhat costly coformulation with carbidopa–levodopa to reduce pill burden.

PRACTICE POINT

- Warning patients that entacapone will turn their urine orange may save a call to your office.

There are two versions of MAO, and both break down dopamine equally. MAO-A inhibitors have been used primarily as antidepressants. They require compliance with a low-tyramine diet to avoid increased norepinephrine levels and hypertensive crisis, as well as avoidance of selective serotonin reuptake inhibitor (SSRI) antidepressants, which can lead to serotonin syndrome. MAO-B inhibitors, which are currently used for treatment of PD, have a much lower risk of these complications, except at high doses, and dietary restriction does not seem to be required.

The MAO-B inhibitors selegiline and rasagiline may have neuroprotective effects that might slow disease progression in PD, although definitive evidence is lacking. Selegiline has a mild symptomatic effect and may improve depression and fatigue. Because its metabolic products include methamphetamine, it should be taken early in the day, at breakfast and lunch, to reduce the likelihood of insomnia and nightmares. Either of these medications may help reduce motor fluctuations in more advanced disease.

Dopamine agonists

Rather than replacing missing dopamine in the presynaptic nerve terminal, dopamine agonists act directly on the postsynaptic dopamine receptor. Pramipexole and ropinirole are the agonists in current use as oral formulations. Rotigotine is a dopamine agonist used in transdermal form. The dopaminergic ergot derivatives pergolide and bromocriptine are no longer used, as they can cause pulmonary or cardiac valve fibrosis.

This class of medications should be started at a low dose and increased slowly to reduce the likelihood and severity of side effects such as confusion, sedation, and hallucinations. They should be used with particular caution in the elderly. Other side effects of dopamine agonists include lower extremity edema, repetitive stereotyped behaviors (punding), and sleep attacks. Sleep attacks occur more frequently in people who are already sleep deprived, as is often seen in PD. Impulse control disorders (including compulsive shopping, cleaning, gambling, internet use, or hypersexuality) may occur, usually in predisposed individuals. It is important to ask patients about these behaviors, as the connection to medication use may not be recognized.

Apomorphine is an injectable dopamine agonist that can be used as rescue therapy for "off" episodes, when the patient needs a rapid response and cannot wait for the effect of carbidopa–levodopa. It may be especially useful in patients who still are part of the workforce.

Anticholinergic medications

This group of medications, which includes benztropine and trihexyphenidyl, was used prior to the discovery of levodopa. Anticholinergics are believed to have a particular role in the treatment of tremor, although studies have yet to show this unequivocally. They should be used with caution in the elderly, who are particularly prone to side effects such as hallucinations, cognitive impairment, and urinary retention. These are usually reversible with drug discontinuation.

Amantadine

The antiviral drug amantadine was noted to reduce the symptoms of PD prior to the levodopa era. It is effective both for primary PD symptoms and for levodopa-induced dyskinesias. It acts by blocking glutamatergic *N*-methyl-d-aspartate (NMDA) receptors. Glutamate hyperfunction may be seen in the setting of dopamine depletion and parkinsonism and may have a role in the pathophysiology of dyskinesias. As would be predicted from the blockade of glutamate receptors, amantadine can cause confusion and hallucinations.

NEUROSURGERY

Neurosurgical options are now state-of-the-art for the treatment of PD in select patients whose symptoms are no longer controlled by optimal medical therapy. Historically, surgical destruction of specific structures in the basal ganglia (ablative therapy) predated the development of levodopa but became obsolete after this medication was discovered. DBS of basal ganglia targets is currently preferred because it has fewer side effects and is less destructive. However, ablation may be indicated in patients who require surgery but cannot have DBS electrodes implanted for medical or logistical reasons, such as remote residence from programming sites. Patients should be evaluated for DBS by a movement disorders specialist for appropriate patient selection. DBS should be avoided in patients with multiple system atrophy, as outcomes are usually poor. Experience in other forms of atypical parkinsonism is limited.

DBS in PD delivers electrical impulses directly to a nucleus in the basal ganglia (either the subthalamic nucleus or the globus pallidus pars interna) that partially reverses the effects of dopamine depletion. It is unclear exactly how DBS works. Although the original hypothesis was that it inhibited the target area, recent evidence suggests that it may alter the excitatory outputs of the target zone. Both inhibitory and stimulatory effects have been reported. DBS may also work by normalization of pathologic hypersynchronization in the setting of dopamine depletion.

Most DBS patients have significant improvement, at least in terms of motor symptoms and side effects. The effect of DBS appears to be equivalent to the effect of levodopa, in that the optimal effect is as good as the patient's best on-medication state, but not better. Patients are able to decrease the amount of medication they take, typically by 50% to 70% and no longer experience severe motor fluctuations. DBS does not improve, and may indeed worsen, nonmotor symptoms, including depression, apathy, and impaired cognition. Speech can also be adversely affected. Some of these effects may relate to decreasing dopaminergic medication.

Brain MRI appears to be generally safe be performed in a patient with DBS with the voltage set to zero and the stimulation switched off. Patients undergoing tests involving electricity, such as electrocardiograms, should turn their DBS off temporarily, which they can do using their own remote control on/off device, which is provided to them after surgery. Any change of stimulation settings should be performed by a trained DBS programmer. More specific issues, including the safety of electrocautery for dental or surgical procedures, should be directed to the patient's neurosurgeon or to the device company.

NONMEDICAL THERAPIES

Nonpharmacologic treatments are an essential component of care for the patient with PD. Ideally, these are provided by a multidisciplinary team approach. Speech can be severely hypophonic in PD and challenging to a hearing-impaired caregiver. Speech therapists can provide exercises, such as the Lee Silverman Voice Therapy (LSVT), to improve vocal output. Swallowing evaluation should be considered in patients who have progressed to the stage of balance impairment, even if they do not report coughing when they drink water. Use of thickened liquids may reduce the likelihood of a fatal pneumonia. Severe dysphagia may eventually require percutaneous gastrostomy tube placement.

Early attention to posture and mobility, along with evaluation by physical and occupational therapists, is vital. Assistive walking devices, including canes, walkers, and wheelchairs, should be used when appropriate. Patients should be encouraged to stay active; exercise may have neuroprotective effects, in addition to benefits for overall health and mood. Music therapy can be very helpful; parkinsonian patients often move more easily to the external stimulus provided by music.

Patients with PD tend to lose weight for reasons that are not entirely explained by motor difficulties and dysphagia. Malnutrition may worsen PD symptoms and increase the risks of complications from falls and infection. Vitamin E and other vitamins may have neuroprotective effects in PD, probably due to antioxidant properties. Dietary vitamins appear to be more beneficial than vitamin supplements. Adequate calcium and vitamin D intake is important for bone health, as PD patients are at high risk of falls.

Because amino acids compete with levodopa for gut uptake, a high-protein meal can interfere with drug absorption. However, taking medication on an empty stomach can cause nausea. Some patients find it helpful to take most of their daily protein at the evening meal, when the need for motor function is decreased.

Older patients tend to drink fewer fluids to reduce urinary frequency and the risk of incontinence, especially when they have impaired mobility, putting them at risk for dehydration. Poor fluid intake may increase the risk of falling by worsening orthostatic hypotension, which may be a feature of PD, and may be exacerbated by medications such as levodopa. Constipation is a common PD symptom and is also improved with increased fluid intake, as well as a high-fiber diet and regular physical activity. Despite these measures, regular administration of a stool softener is usually required.

COMPLICATIONS

"WEARING OFF"

A common complaint of patients with advanced disease is that the levodopa wears off; for example, a dose that provided symptom relief for 4 hours now lasts for only 3. After ruling out metabolic disturbances, there are several potential strategies to follow. Two possibilities are to increase the dose of medication or to increase the frequency of doses. Another option is to prescribe an inhibitor of dopamine metabolism, such as entacapone, rasagiline, or selegiline. These choices are guided by a number of factors, including efficacy of the current dose, medication side effects, and patient preference.

LEVODOPA-INDUCED DYSKINESIAS

The other major medication complication is the development of levodopa-induced dyskinesias. These are choreiform or dystonic movements that occur usually at peak blood levels of dopaminergic medications (peak-dose dyskinesias), but they may also occur when medication is taking effect or wearing off (on-off dyskinesias). They occur more frequently with levodopa, but they may also be seen with dopamine agonists. Dyskinesias may manifest in any part of the body and may include behavior that appears to be restless fidgeting or facial twitches. More severe forms can be toe-curling dystonias, violent limb movements, and even difficulty breathing due to involvement of the diaphragm. These symptoms usually resolve as the levodopa dose wears off, and the patient is often left with a narrow window of time during which the PD symptoms are controlled and the dyskinesias are less severe. This window is soon followed by medication "off" time, as the PD symptoms return. In some cases, levodopa-induced dyskinesias have nonmotor features, such as sweating, cardiac arrhythmias, and anxiety.

For most patients, the dyskinesias are mild enough that they prefer the medicated "on" state to the undermedicated, rigid, akinetic "off" state. In many cases, the spouse or caregiver is more bothered by the abnormal dyskinetic movements than the patient. Amantadine may be helpful in controlling dyskinesias, most likely due to its antiglutamatergic actions.

DYSPHAGIA

Pharyngeal muscle dysfunction, causing dysphagia, and aspiration are common in PD. If the clinical picture is suggestive, or if the patient has advanced disease, hospitalized patients with PD should be placed on aspiration precautions, with avoidance of thin liquids and eating while reclining in bed, and should undergo formal speech and swallowing evaluation. Patients should receive their usual medications, as aspiration risk is increased by undermedication.

FALLS

Falling is a frequent symptom and cause of emergency room visits. Care should be taken, however, in attributing a recent increase in falls to the patient's PD. As discussed above, PD does not rapidly progress, and a secondary cause should be sought. These may include infections or other metabolic problems, spinal cord injury, stroke, or subdural hematoma.

PRACTICE POINT

- An important cause for emergency room visits in patients with Parkinson disease is caregiver burnout: the decompensation may not be in the patient, but rather in the home situation.

COGNITIVE IMPAIRMENT

It is increasingly recognized that PD is more than just a motor disorder. Cognition and behavior are frequently noticeably affected in moderate to advanced stages of the disease. With more sensitive testing, deficits can be detected even in relatively early stages. Typical deficits include dysfunction in executive function and decision making (frontal-type dementia) and slowing of information processing (subcortical dementia), in contrast to the memory problems, aphasia, anomia, and acalculia typical of Alzheimer disease. These may be accompanied by personality changes, such as disinhibition or apathy. Poor judgment, greater risk taking, and lack of insight increase the risk of falling. Visual hallucinations may occur in PD, especially (but not necessarily) with underlying dementia, and are usually aggravated by dopaminergic medications.

Elderly patients admitted to the hospital, regardless of diagnosis, often become more confused in the evenings and are prone to sundowning and agitation. Typical antipsychotic medications should not be used, as these may worsen parkinsonism. Atypical antipsychotics such as quetiapine may be given in very low doses (eg, 12.5 mg), with monitoring for sedation and hypotension. Benzodiazepines should be avoided, as they tend to result in worsened confusion in this population.

DEPRESSION

Depression in PD is more than a reaction to a chronic, progressive illness. It seems to be an organic depression, and responds to antidepressants. Despite their greater side effects, older, less selective antidepressants may be more effective than SSRIs. Some patients are prone to anxiety, which may worsen with disease progression, and can exacerbate motor symptoms. Anxiety may also be associated with both the "off" state, and peak-dose dyskinesias. Apathy and fatigue appear to be distinct features in PD, without good therapies at present. MAO-B inhibitors can have a mild stimulant effect in some patients.

SLEEP PROBLEMS

Patients with PD often have sleep difficulties, with nocturnal awakenings and daytime somnolence.

Patients may experience a vicious cycle, as medications increase disruption of the normal sleep cycle, and sleep deprivation exacerbates neurologic symptoms of PD. Rapid eye movement (REM) sleep behavior disorder (RBD) can occur, particularly in men with PD, and often predates the development of frank motor symptoms. In this condition, the sufferer acts out his or her dreams, often kicking and thrashing during sleep, sometimes resulting in injury to the patient or to the bed partner. RBD can be effectively treated with low doses of clonazepam, which may act through facilitation of GABAergic descending inhibitory pathways.

Night staff in the hospital should be aware of this sleep dysregulation, as the patient may request a sleeping aid. The patient may try to walk to the nurses' desk or to the bathroom if he or she cannot sleep, with the attendant risks of falling, especially if medication has not been given recently. Patients with PD and gait problems should be classified as fall risks and should be accompanied to the bathroom or instructed to use a urinal, especially at night.

AUTONOMIC NERVOUS SYSTEM DYSFUNCTION

Marked autonomic dysregulation suggests the diagnosis of MSA, but it can also occur in idiopathic PD. Orthostatic drops in blood pressure can result in unsteadiness, lightheadedness, and even loss of consciousness. Hospitalized patients with PD should be screened with postural vital signs, and use of antihypertensive medications should be reassessed. Patients with orthostatic hypotension should be encouraged to hydrate, liberalize salt intake, wear compression stockings, and sleep with the head of the bed raised by 30 degrees. If these measures do not work, a blood pressure–raising agent such as fludrocortisone or midodrine can be used. (These drugs should not be used late in the day due to the risk of nocturnal hypertension.)

Patients with PD may develop neurogenic bladder and need to urinate frequently, particularly at night. Nocturia then interferes with sleep, predisposing the patient to be tired the next day. Treatment with an anticholinergic may reduce nocturia, and also have beneficial sedative and mild antiparkinsonian effects. Unfortunately, anticholinergics may also lead to confusion and hallucinations, nocturnal falls, and urinary retention that renders the patient prone to urinary tract infections.

Patients frequently complain of excess salivation and drooling, which is due to impaired swallowing. This can be treated with peripherally acting anticholinergics, such as propantheline, with the risk of anticholinergic side effects noted above, or with botulinum toxin injections into the salivary glands. Botulinum toxin type B is preferred, as it appears to have a stronger anticholinergic effect. Chewing gum may also help by stimulating swallowing.

Constipation is very common in PD and may predate the diagnosis. Unfortunately, levodopa therapy is often unhelpful in resolving constipation, and entacapone may even make it worse. Hospitalized patients should receive aggressive bowel regimens, as limited mobility is likely to worsen their preexisting constipation. Nausea should be treated with non-dopamine-blocking agents.

DISCHARGE PLANNING

This disease, as with many neurologic disorders, brings with it a heavy burden for the caregiver. Patients with moderate to advanced PD often deteriorate during an acute medical illness and fail to recover to their premorbid baseline. As the patient becomes less able to care for himself or herself, the caregiver must assist with an increasing number of tasks, ranging from the mundane, such as buttoning a shirt, to the more physically demanding, such as helping the patient get into and out of a car. The caregiver should be asked about stress levels, frustration, and decreased social interactions. Patient and caregiver needs should be addressed, and mechanisms of support should be discussed, including home health aides and support groups. Social work involvement may be helpful. Future respite admissions should be considered.

Hospital discharge may provide an opportunity to assess the home situation. The home should be assessed for safety, ideally with a home visit from an occupational therapist. Loose carpets and rugs and cluttered floors should be cleared. Shower chairs, raised toilet seats, handrails, and transfer bars can be provided, in addition to other assistive devices, such as canes, walkers, and specialized utensils or tools.

As it becomes harder for the patient to manage at home, it may be appropriate to discuss alternate living arrangements. The range of possibilities, from assisted facilities that involve privacy and an independent apartment to a full-fledged nursing home, should be explored. Frontal lobe dysfunction may reduce the patient's insight, and decision making may be challenging. It should be made clear that the caregiver is not "dumping" his or her relative, but rather acknowledging the difficulty of the situation.

In both the inpatient and outpatient settings, a multidisciplinary team approach for PD is ideal, potentially involving the patient's primary care physician, neurologist, psychiatrist, neuropsychologist, pharmacist, social worker, visiting nurse, and physical, occupational, and speech therapists. As in the hospital, patients need to remain active. Exercise and mental and social stimulation are all important in maintaining physical condition and quality of life.

CONCLUSION

Parkinson disease is increasingly recognized as a complex multisystem disorder, causing autonomic, cognitive, psychiatric, sleep, and other symptoms, in addition to motor impairment. Recognition and treatment of these features can significantly improve patients' quality of life. A multi-disciplinary approach is ideal. Pre-emptive interventions such as swallowing evaluations; physical, occupational, and speech therapy; and neuropsychological and psychiatric evaluations can improve care during both inpatient and outpatient care. Awareness of caregiver stress is an important component of care and can lead to fewer hospital admissions.

SUGGESTED READINGS

Goetz CG, Tilley BC, Shaftman SR, et al. Movement Disorder Society-sponsored revision of the Unified Parkinson's Disease Rating Scale (MDS-UPDRS): Scale presentation and clinimetric testing results. *Mov Disord.* 2008;23:2129–2170.

Lang AE, Lees A, eds. Management of Parkinson's disease: An evidence-based review. *Mov Disord.* 2002:17:S1–S166.

Pahwa R, Factor SA, Lyons KE, et al. AAN Practice Parameter: Treatment of Parkinson disease with motor fluctuations and dyskinesia (an evidence-based review). *Neurology.* 2006;66: 983–995.

Pohar SL, Allyson Jones C. The burden of Parkinson disease (PD) and concomitant comorbidities. *Arch Gerontol Geriatr.* 2009;49: 317–321.

Reichmann H. Initiation of Parkinson's disease treatment. *J Neurol.* 2008:255:57–59.

Vossius C, Nilsen OB, Larsen JP. Parkinson's disease and nursing home placement: The economic impact of the need for care. *Eur J Neurol.* 2009;16:194–200.

Weintraub D, Comella CL, Horn S. Parkinson's disease—Part 3: Neuropsychiatric symptoms. *Am J Manag Care.* 2008;14(2 Suppl): S59–S69.

CHAPTER 212

Seizures

Susan M. Palac, MD

Key Clinical Questions

1. How can clinicians distinguish among seizures, syncopal events, and other causes of spells?
2. What historical features are helpful? What diagnostic tests are appropriate?
3. Which patients with new-onset seizures require an antiepileptic drug?
4. How should patients with status epilepticus be managed?

INTRODUCTION

A *seizure* is defined as a sudden attack of involuntary behavior or experiences resulting from abnormal cortical neuronal activity. About 5% of the population of the United States will experience one at some point during their lifetime. *Epilepsy,* the chronic disease defined by the occurrence of two or more unprovoked seizures, is seen in approximately 2 million to 4 million people in the United States alone. The World Health Organization (WHO) reports that in primary care settings worldwide, epilepsy is the second most common neurologic condition, after headache.

TRIAGE AND HOSPITAL ADMISSION

Epilepsy and seizures are also common in the inpatient setting. In a large multicenter study in both community and academic hospital emergency departments, 1.2% of 31,508 patient visits were related to seizures. Overall, 27% of these patients were admitted. Of those patients suspected of having new-onset seizures, 63% were admitted. Reasons for admission for patients with seizures include diagnostic evaluation (especially when the diagnosis of seizure is unclear), uncontrolled seizures, toxicity from antiepileptic drugs (AEDs), and injuries sustained during a seizure.

CLASSIFICATION AND CLINICAL FINDINGS

Seizures are classified into two broad categories: primary generalized and partial (**Table 212-1**). *Generalized seizures* by definition are characterized by loss of consciousness. *Absence seizures* are typically brief staring spells, lasting seconds. These usually begin in early childhood and remit in adolescence in childhood, but they may persist into adulthood. Patients with *myoclonic epilepsy* have quick jerking movements, most often in the morning after awakening. They are often not diagnosed until a generalized tonic-clonic seizure occurs. *Generalized tonic-clonic seizures,* also known as convulsions, are recognized by tonic extension of the extremities, followed by clonic jerking (**Figure 212-1**). Variations of these include generalized seizures with either a primarily tonic or clonic component. *Atonic seizures* are characterized by sudden loss of tone. These patients are especially prone to injuries as a result of falling without warning.

Partial seizures start with abnormal neuronal discharges in a limited area of the cerebral cortex. The site of the ictal focus dictates the clinical symptoms during the seizure. Any partial seizure can progress into a generalized seizure if the epileptic activity spreads to involve both hemispheres. Partial seizures are subclassified into simple and complex. During a *complex partial seizure,* the patient loses awareness of his or her surroundings. Typical symptoms in temporal lobe seizures include staring, walking aimlessly, and automatisms such as lip smacking or picking at clothes or bedsheets. Patients may experience epigastric rising or nausea, anxiety, déjà vu, visual distortion, or olfactory hallucinations. Seizures are typically one to three minutes in duration and are almost always less than 30 minutes long. Conversely, a patient with a *simple partial seizure* is awake and aware throughout the event. Clinical features may include hemibody clonic movements, déjà vu, or visual or olfactory hallucinations.

DID THIS PATIENT HAVE AN EPILEPTIC SEIZURE?

When called upon to care for a patient with a seizure, the first question the hospitalist must ask is whether the "seizure" was epileptic or not. Many types of physiologic events are characterized by episodes

TABLE 212-1 Seizure Types in Adults

Primary Generalized	Partial
Absence	Simple
Myoclonic	Complex
Tonic	Partial with secondary generalization
Clonic	
Generalized tonic-clonic	
Atonic	
Myoclonic-astatic	
Other idiopathic generalized	

TABLE 212-2 Conditions That Mimic Seizures

Cardiac syncope
Vasovagal syncope
Orthostatic hypotension
Postanoxic myoclonus
Transient ischemic attack
Panic or anxiety attack
Benign nocturnal myoclonus
Classic migraine with aura
Sleep disorders (narcolepsy, parasomnias, night terrors, somnambulism, paroxysmal nocturnal dystonia)
Transient global amnesia
Movement disorders (tremor, paroxysmal dyskinesias/choreoathetosis)
Psychogenic nonepileptic spells

of loss of consciousness or awareness. Common conditions that can mimic seizures are listed in **Table 212-2**. Answering this crucial first question begins with obtaining a clinical history. Vital points of the history include:

1. *Was the event paroxysmal?* Epileptic seizures are always sudden in onset. This is also true of some, but not all, of the mimickers of seizures, so that this information alone cannot distinguish epileptic seizures from nonepileptic spells.
2. *Was the episode provoked?* Common triggers for epileptic seizures include sleep deprivation, concomitant systemic illness, drug intoxication or withdrawal, and flashing lights. Syncope often follows a change in posture, micturition, or a sudden fright.
3. *Was there a clinical prodrome?* A seizure may begin with an aura of focal neurologic symptoms or signs. The aura may consist of obvious behavior changes, such as focal motor jerking or staring off with oral automatisms. It may also be a purely internal experience for the patient, including visual or olfactory hallucinations, focal sensory changes, déjà vu, or a subjective "feeling" that the patient cannot describe well. An epileptic aura is stereotypic for any given patient. It is typically short in duration, lasting seconds to one to two minutes. Conversely, if present, a prodrome to nonepileptic events is usually described as lightheadedness or just not feeling well. This can last minutes and sometimes even hours.
4. *What were the clinical features of the event?* The appearance and actions of the patient during the event are critical pieces of information. Certain clinical features can help differentiate epileptic seizures from nonepileptic events, as noted in **Table 212-3**. Some are more specific than others. For example, tonic posturing is often seen in focal seizures emanating from the frontal lobe, but it is rare in nonepileptic events. Tongue biting, traditionally considered a reliable sign of a generalized seizure, occurs in less than 30% of convulsions, but may also occur in psychogenic spells. Similarly, urinary incontinence is not specific to epileptic seizures. Bizarre behavior, such as flailing or thrashing movements, is often labeled psychogenic. However, this can also be seen in physiologic events, including frontal lobe epileptic seizures and some sleep disorders, as listed in Table 212–2. Fear or anxiety, the hallmark of panic disorder, is common in complex partial seizures emanating from the amygdala. Hallucinations, especially visual, are common in migraine, but they are also common auras in temporal lobe complex partial seizures. Unresponsiveness is common after both epileptic seizures and nonepileptic attacks. The duration may be helpful in making the distinction. Postevent unresponsiveness is typically shortest (seconds to one minute) with syncope, is longer in epileptic seizures (up to 30–60 minutes), and longest with psychogenic events where "unresponsiveness" can last hours. However, with prolonged unresponsiveness, subclinical status epilepticus must always be ruled out.

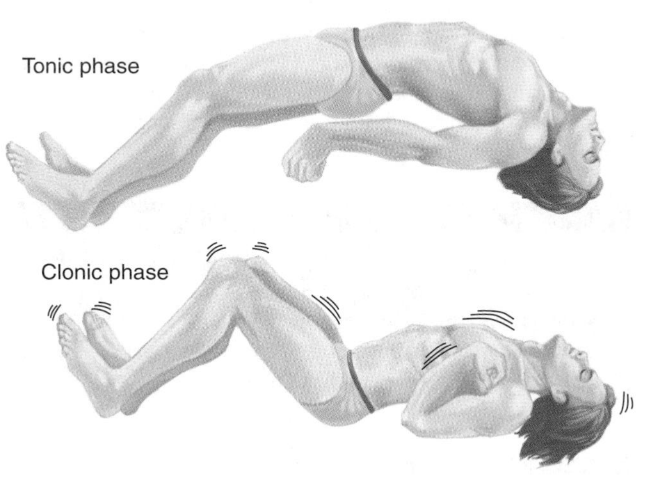

Figure 212-1 *Generalized tonic-clonic seizure. In the tonic phase (top), lasting 10 to 30 seconds, the patient has tonic muscle contractions leading to flexion, then extension, of the neck and trunk. The vocal muscles contract, and the patient may cry out and become cyanosed. Jaw contraction may lead to tongue injury. This is followed by the clonic phase (bottom), with symmetric muscle contraction and relaxation that produces limb jerking. The clonic phase diminishes in intensity and usually ends after approximately one minute. (Reproduced, with permission, from Simon RP, Greenberg DA, Aminoff MJ. Clinical Neurology. 7th ed. New York: McGraw-Hill, 2009. Fig. 8-2.)*

When trying to decide whether a spell is a seizure or nonepileptic event, remember that not all that shakes or jerks is epileptic. Myoclonus, characterized by quick, sudden jerks, is common after cerebral hypoxia and anoxia, as well as in metabolic disorders, such as hepatic and renal dysfunction. Myoclonus is seldom epileptic and should not be mistaken for primary epileptic seizures.

PRACTICE POINT

- Confusion following a spell strongly suggests seizure. Recovery of full orientation is rapid after syncope but typically takes 10 to 30 minutes after a seizure.

TABLE 212-3 Clinical Characteristics in Epileptic Versus Nonepileptic Spells

Clinical Sign or Symptom	Epileptic	Nonepileptic
Appearance	Flushed or cyanotic	Pale, diaphoretci
Motor movements	Rhythmic tonic-clonic jerks	Complex tonic posturing
	Tonic extension	Myoclonus
	Sudden onset flailing/thrashing Repetitive rocking	Nonrhythmic jerking
	Lip smacking	
	Nonpurposeful picking/slapping	Non-sudden onset flailing/thrashing
	Head turning	
	Eye deviation	
	Fencing posture	
Subjective experience	Stereotypical olfactory, gustatory,	Tunnel vision
	visual, or aural (rare) hallucination	Light-headedness
	Rising in stomach	Palpitations
	Déjà vu	
	Fear or anxiety	
Tongue biting	Can occur but < 50%	Rare but can occur
Urinary incontinence	Can occur	Can occur
Sensory changes	Positive feeling (ie, paresthesias, dysesthesias)	Negative feeling (ie, numbness)
Postevent state	Confusion	Unresponsive < 5 min
	Agitation	(prolonged unresponsiveness sometimes seen in psychogenic seizures)
	Unresponsiveness usually < 1 h	
	Headache	
	Extreme fatigue	

5. *What is the patient's medical history?* A history of diabetes, renal failure, or liver disease should raise the clinician's suspicion that the event in question was a seizure provoked by a systemic metabolic disturbance. A patient with cancer who has an episode of altered awareness should be evaluated for brain metastases causing a focal or generalized seizure. Cardiac or vascular disease favors the diagnosis of syncope. In patients with psychiatric disease, it should not be assumed that the presenting "seizure" is psychogenic in origin. Adult patients with mood disorders are 1.7 to 7 times more likely to develop epilepsy than those without a psychiatric history. In addition, some antidepressants and antipsychotic medications can provoke seizures. Thus, it is incumbent on the hospitalist to exclude all other physiologic conditions before a diagnosis of pseudoseizure is made.

The value of an accurate history and description of a seizurelike event cannot be overestimated. This information is often elusive when a patient is cognitively impaired or postictal. The hospitalist must be dogged in the pursuit of history from family or witnesses to the event in order to avoid a misdiagnosis.

PHYSICAL EXAMINATION

When evaluating a patient with a spell, the physical examination is most helpful during or immediately after the event. Ongoing subtle motor movements should lead to consideration of nonconvulsive status epilepticus. Elevated blood pressure or increased heart rate is common not only in convulsions but also in partial seizures. An irregular pulse more likely reflects a cardiovascular syncopal event, although autonomic dysfunction can also be seen with seizures. Focal neurologic deficits such as hemiparesis and hemiparesthesias are typical in focal cerebral ischemia, such as a transient ischemic attack (TIA). However, these deficits can also be seen after a partial seizure (postictal Todd paralysis). Thus, although the physical examination by itself is seldom diagnostic, in combination with the clinical history, it can help distinguish epileptic from nonepileptic spells.

PRACTICE POINT

- The falls and powerful muscle contractions associated with seizures may result in serious injury. These may include fractures of long bones or vertebral bodies, periorbital hemorrhages, subdural hematoma, and burns. Such injuries may not always be immediately obvious to clinicians.

ELECTROENCEPHALOGRAPHY

Electroencephalography (EEG) is still the gold standard used to distinguish epileptic seizures from nonepileptic events. However, it is only definitive if the patient has an event during EEG recording. Only approximately 30% of patients with chronic unprovoked seizures show epileptiform activity on routine EEG. If done within 24 to 48 hours of a seizure, some studies have shown that the yield increases to up to 70%. About 2% to 3% of healthy adults have a false-positive EEG. Overall, a positive EEG may be helpful in ascertaining whether an event was epileptic, especially if done within 24 to 48 hours of the spell. A negative study is not helpful.

TABLE 212-4 Clinical Features in Syncope Versus Seizures

Favors Syncope	Favors Seizures
Pallor, diaphoresis	Flushed, cyanotic
Lightheadedness, dizziness	Head turning
Chest pain	Unusual posturing
Palpitations	Unusual behavior
Vertigo	Tongue biting
Nausea	Limb jerking
Occurs with prolonged standing or sitting, micturition, defecation, cough	Prodromal preoccupation Prodromal hallucinations
History of hypertension	Prodromal mood changes
Orthostatic hypotension	Postevent headache
	Postevent confusion
	Lesion on brain MRI
	Focal neurologic deficit on exam

MRI, magnetic resonance imaging.

TABLE 212-5 Metabolic Disturbances and Systemic Disorders Associated with Seizures

Hypoglycemia
Hyponatremia
Hyperosmolar states, including hypernatremia and hyperosmolar nonketotic hyperglycemia
Hypocalcemia
Hypomagnesemia
Uremia
Hepatic encephalopathy
Porphyria
Drug overdose
Drug withdrawal
Global cerebral ischemia
Hypertensive encephalopathy
Eclampsia
Hyperthermia

SYNCOPE VERSUS SEIZURE

Perhaps the most vexing diagnostic problem for the hospitalist faced with a patient with an attack of altered consciousness is distinguishing a syncopal attack from an epileptic seizure. Overall, syncope is much more common than seizures, especially in elderly patients, who comprise a large portion of the hospitalist's practice. A thorough history of the paroxysmal event provides the most reliable data in differentiating seizures from syncope. Clinical features useful in making the distinction between these two types of episodes are presented in **Table 212-4**. Findings on physical exam may help in the differential diagnosis, with abnormal cardiac findings suggesting syncope and focal neurologic signs more likely associated with seizures. Beyond the history and physical, diagnostic tests are surprisingly of little yield. An electrocardiogram (ECG) is abnormal in only approximately 7% of patients who present to the emergency department with syncope. Despite this statistically low yield, it is recommended that all adult patients who present with an episode of altered consciousness have an ECG.

EEG is of less diagnostic value than ECG. When ordered as part of a syncope workup, EEGs are abnormal in up to one-quarter of patients, but most of these abnormalities are nonspecific. Less than 2% of EEG studies show epileptiform discharges, the definitive EEG finding in seizures. Based on this evidence, it is best to obtain an EEG only when clinical features of the patient's spell raise suspicion of epileptic seizures.

DIAGNOSTIC EVALUATION FOR SEIZURES

Once the hospitalist has decided that the spell in question was indeed an epileptic seizure, diagnostic testing is ordered to find the underlying etiology. Seizures can be idiopathic or may be provoked by a systemic problem, such as electrolyte disturbances, alcohol withdrawal, or infection. Provoked seizures are usually generalized tonic-clonic but may be partial, particularly in patients with a previous stroke or other focal neurologic injury. A provoked seizure is managed by treating the underlying cause. Prolonged treatment with an antiepileptic drug is usually not indicated in these instances. In unprovoked seizures, labs and neuroimaging studies are normal.

LABORATORY STUDIES

Routine laboratory studies, including electrolytes, calcium, magnesium, and glucose, are indicated in the evaluation of the seizure patient. Seizures may be seen with hypo- or hypernatremia, hypo- or hyperglycemia, hypocalcemia, and hypomagnesemia. Altered potassium levels are not associated with seizures. The yield of these studies is generally low. However, as uncorrected metabolic disturbances can cause ongoing seizures and even status epilepticus, these studies should be included in the evaluation of all patients presenting with seizures. Blood urea nitrogen and creatinine should be obtained to exclude uremia, as well as liver function tests, if hepatic dysfunction is possible. Complete blood count is of low yield. A normal or marginally elevated white blood cell count (WBC) may be seen with meningoencephalitis. Metabolic disturbances and systemic disorders that may lead to seizures are summarized in **Table 212-5**.

DRUG SCREEN AND TOXICOLOGY

Alcohol-related seizures account for up to one half of patients with new-onset seizures in some emergency departments. An alcohol level is appropriate when there is clinical suspicion of excessive use. Other recreational drugs, particularly stimulants such as methamphetamine, MDMA (3,4-methylenedioxymethamphetamine, Ecstasy), and cocaine, can cause seizures. Benzodiazepine withdrawal is another drug-related cause of seizures. A multitude of other drugs, especially when taken in excess, are associated with seizures (**Table 212-6**). Exposure to some toxins is associated with generalized tonic-clonic seizures. Carbon monoxide poisoning does not usually cause seizures unless the carboxyhemoglobin level is greater than 50%. Ethylene glycol or methanol ingestion can cause severe neurologic dysfunction, including seizures. These substances are often not included in routine toxicology screens, so the diagnosis can easily be missed.

In regard to the question of whether drug screens should be done in all patients presenting with seizures, there are no prospective studies on the yield and utility of such testing in new-onset seizures. However, missing the diagnosis of drug intoxication can lead to inappropriate and potentially harmful anticonvulsant treatment, as well as a lost opportunity for intervention in the patient's substance abuse problems. Hence, drug screens are usually recommended as part of the evaluation.

Serum AED levels may sometimes be useful, but the results must be interpreted with caution. In a patient known to have epilepsy, a low AED level does not always reflect noncompliance with

TABLE 212-6 Drugs Associated with Seizure Occurrence

Bupropion
Tricyclic antidepressants
Tramadol
Diphenhydramine
Venlafaxine
Antipsychotics
Theophylline
Metronidazole
Penicillins
Fluoroquinolones (levofloxacin, ciprofloxacin)

medications. Some patients maintain seizure control on doses of medications that result in measured "low" levels. Likewise, a high drug level is not cause for immediate reduction in medication dose, unless the patient is clinically toxic. Serum levels of many of the newer AEDs are not available for at least 48 to 72 hours and are of limited use in the acute care of the patient with seizures.

NEUROIMAGING

Brain imaging is recommended for all patients presenting with a new-onset seizure. Although studies report that 34% to 52% of computed tomography (CT) scans done in the emergency department after a seizure are abnormal, the findings led to a change in acute management in only 9% to 17% of patients. Significant abnormalities include cerebral hemorrhage, stroke, subdural hematoma, tumor, and brain abscess. Neuroimaging is more likely to be positive in patients presenting with altered mentation, focal seizures, or focal deficits on neurologic examination. This evidence has led the American Academy of Neurology to recommend that an immediate CT scan be considered for patients presenting acutely with seizures, especially in the presence of an abnormal neurologic exam or focal seizure onset.

An acute CT brain scan is indicated in a patient known to have *chronic* epilepsy if the presenting seizure (1) has different clinical signs than the patient's usual seizures, (2) is prolonged (lasting >5 minutes), or (3) is followed by a prolonged postictal period of altered mentation. New findings on neurologic exam are also a clear indication for acute brain imaging. If the CT scan is negative, magnetic resonance imaging (MRI) should be done once the patient is stable to look for a new cerebral lesion as the cause of the change in seizure presentation. When a lesion is suggested but not well defined on CT scan, follow-up imaging with MRI is required. A patient who presents with a focal seizure or has focal neurologic deficits on exam should have an MRI if the CT scan is negative.

It is important to include a brain MRI in the evaluation of a patient with human immunodeficiency virus (HIV) infection or other immunosuppressed state who suffers a seizure. MRI is more sensitive than CT in detecting opportunistic infections in the brain, such as toxoplasmosis, progressive multifocal leukoencephalopathy, cytomegalovirus (CMV), tuberculosis, Cryptococcus, and primary central nervous system (CNS) lymphoma. Seizures can be the initial presentation of these conditions. Early detection with MRI can improve the chances of response to appropriate therapy.

ELECTROENCEPHALOGRAM

For patients admitted after a first unprovoked seizure, the EEG may help estimate the risk of seizure recurrence. Epileptiform activity on EEG doubles the risk of seizure recurrence. In a meta-analysis of early studies, patients with epileptiform activity on EEG were more likely to have seizure recurrence with a relative risk of 2. Similar results were found in a more recent analysis where the probability of seizure recurrence in patients with these EEG abnormalities was 49.5% versus 27.4% in patients with normal EEGs. Common, nonspecific EEG abnormalities, such as focal or diffuse slowing, have not been shown to be associated with an increased risk of seizure recurrence. For the patient with chronic seizures, it is important to obtain an EEG when there is a concern for ongoing subclinical seizures. This is especially true for patients admitted in clinical status epilepticus, as discussed below.

TREATMENT ISSUES

PATIENTS WITH A FIRST SEIZURE

In a patient with a first unprovoked seizure, the hospitalist is faced with the difficult decision of whether to start treatment with an AED. Probably the most important consideration in this decision is the risk of a recurrent seizure. Multiple studies have examined risk factors for seizure recurrence, such as age, seizure type, time of day the first seizure occurred, and family history of seizures. Only two stand out as consistent predictors: abnormal EEG with epileptiform activity (as discussed) and an abnormal neurologic exam or underlying neurologic disorder, learning disability, or developmental delay.

Does treatment with an AED reduce the risk of seizure recurrence? The answer to this question is complicated. Large studies have shown that immediate treatment with an AED after a first seizure reduced the risk of a second seizure within the next one to two years by approximately 34%. However, after five years, there was no significant difference in seizure remission rate between groups of patients treated with an AED and patients who were untreated. Thus, after a single seizure, treatment with an AED reduces the risk of seizure recurrence in the short term but does not affect long-term prognosis for the development of epilepsy.

Given all this, the hospitalist needs to base his or decision on initiating treatment not only on the available statistical evidence, but also on patient lifestyle, occupation, anxiety level, and other personal circumstances. Choosing the optimum medication for a patient involves weighing the risk-benefit ratio. The best AED for a patient is one that is most likely to be effective for the patient's type of seizures with the fewest side effects. This will obviously vary from patient to patient.

PATIENTS WITH EPILEPSY

The most common reason for admission of patients with known epilepsy is the occurrence of breakthrough seizures. Interviewing the patient often reveals an obvious cause, such as missed medication doses or chronic noncompliance. In patients who are taking medications as prescribed, the prescribed AED dose may be inadequate. It is appropriate to titrate the AED dose upward in these patients, if tolerated. Although serum drug levels may provide some guidance, doses must always be prescribed on an individual basis for patients. Consultation with a neurologist is recommended to help the hospitalist in this task.

Breakthrough seizures in patients with epilepsy may also be due to the loss of efficacy of the prescribed AED. In this case, a change in treatment to a different AED or the addition of a second drug is usually required. These treatment decisions are complicated, and referral to an epileptologist is suggested.

MEDICATIONS

Since the mid-1990s, the number of available AEDs has doubled, providing physicians with a myriad of choices for treatment. The hospitalist needs to be familiar with the efficacy and side effect profile of these medications. **Table 212-7** lists current AEDs with

TABLE 212-7 Antiepileptic Drugs: Recommended Daily Doses for Healthy Adults and Side Effects

Drug	Daily Dose	Common Side Effects
Phenobarbital	3–5 mg/kg Once or twice daily	Sedation Incoordination Cognitive impairment Depression
Phenytoin	4–8 mg/kg Once daily	GI upset Dizziness Incoordination Ataxia Tremor Cognitive clouding Gingival hyperplasia Hirsutism Coarsening of facial features
Carbamazepine Regular Extended release	5–20 mg/kg Three times daily Twice daily	Tremor Incoordination Diplopia Weight gain Nausea
Valproic acid Regular Extended release	30–40 mg/kg Two or three times daily Once daily	Tremor Weight gain Hair thinning Nausea Incoordination Constipation
Gabapentin	600–3600 mg/day Two or three times daily	Tremor Incoordination Weight gain Somnolence Peripheral edema
Oxcarbazepine	600–2400 mg/day Twice daily	Hyponatremia Dizziness Diplopia
Lamotrigine Regular Extended release	100–400 mg/day Once or twice daily Once daily	Ataxia Incoordination Diplopia Tremor Insomnia Headache
Levetiracetam Regular Extended release	500–4000 mg/day Twice daily Once or twice daily	Irritability, agitation Somnolence Weight gain
Topiramate	100–400 mg/day Twice daily	Cognitive impairment Word-finding difficulties Somnolence Parasthesias Weight loss, anorexia Kidney stones Oligohydrosis Metabolic acidosis

(continued)

TABLE 212-7 Antiepileptic Drugs: Recommended Daily Doses for Healthy Adults and Side Effects (*continued*)

Drug	Daily Dose	Common Side Effects
Zonisamide	100–400 mg/day Once or twice daily	Somnolence Cognitive impairment Irritability Oligohydrosis Depression Weight loss, anorexia Incoordination Kidney stones Pancreatitis
Pregabalin	100–600 mg/day Two or three times daily	Somnolence Weight gain Peripheral edema Dizziness Ataxia
Lacosamide	100–400 mg/day Twice daily	Somnolence Dizziness Ataxia Tremor
Rufinamide	800–3200 mg/day Twice daily	Somnolence GI upset Dizziness
Vigabatrin	1000–3000 mg/day Twice daily	Vision loss Visual field defects Peripheral neuropathy Tremor Weight gain Fatigue

GI, gastrointestinal.

recommended daily doses and common side effects. The doses listed apply to otherwise healthy adults. Patients with renal or hepatic dysfunction may require dose adjustment. Drug–drug interactions are not addressed in the table. Several AEDs have major drug interactions, notably phenobarbital, phenytoin, carbamazepine, and valproic acid.

Two other important points are important to consider in choosing an AED for treatment. Older AEDs including phenobarbital, phenytoin, and carbamazepine are associated with low Vitamin D levels and early bone loss. There is currently insufficient data about the effect of newer AEDs on bone health. It is recommended that Vitamin D levels be followed in all patients treated with an AED so that appropriate treatment can be initiated if needed to prevent osteopenia and osteoporosis. In females of child-bearing age, the hospitalist must be aware that phenobarbital, phenytoin, carbamazepine, valproic acid, topiramate and oxcarbazepine all interact with oral contraceptives such that the effectiveness of the contraceptive is diminished. On the other hand, estrogen lowers the level of lamotrigine so that patients taking oral contraceptives require compensatory higher doses of the AED to prevent seizures.

The hospitalist is often responsible for expeditiously stabilizing a patient with acute seizures. In this setting, the choice of AEDs will be limited to those that can be tolerated in relatively high

TABLE 212-8 Antiepileptic Drug Toxicity

Drug	Symptoms of Toxicity	Drug	Symptoms of Toxicity
Phenobarbital	Sedation	Valproic acid	Tremor
	Incoordination		Confusion
	Dysarthria		Ataxia
	Megaloblastic anemia		Thrombocytopenia
	Hepatic dysfunction		Hepatic dysfunction
	Respiratory depression		Parkinsonism
Phenytoin	Nystagmus		Pancreatitis
	Ataxia	Gabapentin	Sedation
	Incoordination	Oxcarbazepine	Sedation
	Dysarthria		Hyponatremia
	Tremor	Lamotrigine	Tremor
	Confusion		Myoclonus
	Sedation		Ataxia
	Dyskinesias, chorea, dystonia	Levetiracetam	Hostility
	Peripheral neuropathy		Psychosis
	Bone marrow suppression	Topiramate	Cognitive impairment
	Hepatic dysfunction		Severe speech impairment
	Lymphadenopathy		Severe metabolic acidosis
	Increase in seizure frequency	Zonisamide	Sedation
Carbamazepine	Tremor		Aplastic anemia
	Confusion	Pregabalin	Sedation
	Psychosis	Lacosamide	Sedation
	Ataxia		PR prolongation
	Diplopia	Rufinamide	Dizziness
	Sedation		Diplopia
	Tics		Ataxia
	Myoclonus	Vigabatrin	Diplopia
	Neutropenia		Fatigue
	Aplastic anemia		Headache
	Hepatic dysfunction		Incoordination
	Change in color vision with yellow overtones		
	Cardiac conduction defects		
	Congestive heart failure		

initial doses, so that a therapeutic level is reached quickly. Current medications that best meet this criterion include phenytoin, valproic acid, levetiracetam, and lacosamide, all of which are available for IV administration, and benzodiazepines such as clonazepam and lorazepam.

■ MEDICATION TOXICITY

A frequent reason for hospital admission in patients on AEDs is drug toxicity. Symptoms of toxicity seen with commonly prescribed AEDs are listed in **Table 212-8**. The most common are gait ataxia, GI upset, and somnolence. These are usually dose related. Others are not, especially organ system dysfunction or failure. Idiosyncratic allergic reactions, including Stevens–Johnson syndrome, have been reported with all AEDs. In general, treatment of drug toxicity is discontinuation of the AED until symptoms have resolved. However, holding the medication too long results in a subtherapeutic drug level and puts the patient at risk for recurrent seizures. Managing this situation requires knowledge of the pharmacokinetics of the AEDs. AED toxicity presents a complicated treatment challenge, and the hospitalist may wish to confer with an epileptologist in this situation.

SPECIAL CONSIDERATIONS IN THE ELDERLY

The most common identifiable cause of new-onset seizures in the elderly is cerebrovascular disease, which accounts for up to one half of acute seizures in older patients. Seizures are more likely in large, hemorrhagic strokes with cortical involvement. Other causes are metabolic disturbances, trauma, and tumors. The use of antidepressants and antipsychotics in older patients lowers the seizure threshold. Alzheimer dementia and other neurodegenerative disorders are also an important cause of seizures in geriatric patients. Seizures in the elderly are often partial onset, with or without secondary generalization. Complex partial seizures in the elderly most often originate in the temporal lobe and manifest as episodes of confusion and staring into space; oral and motor automatisms are usually absent. Older patients often have prolonged postictal confusion and sedation. The geriatric patient is more vulnerable to sedation, hyponatremia, drug interactions, and other side effects of AEDs.

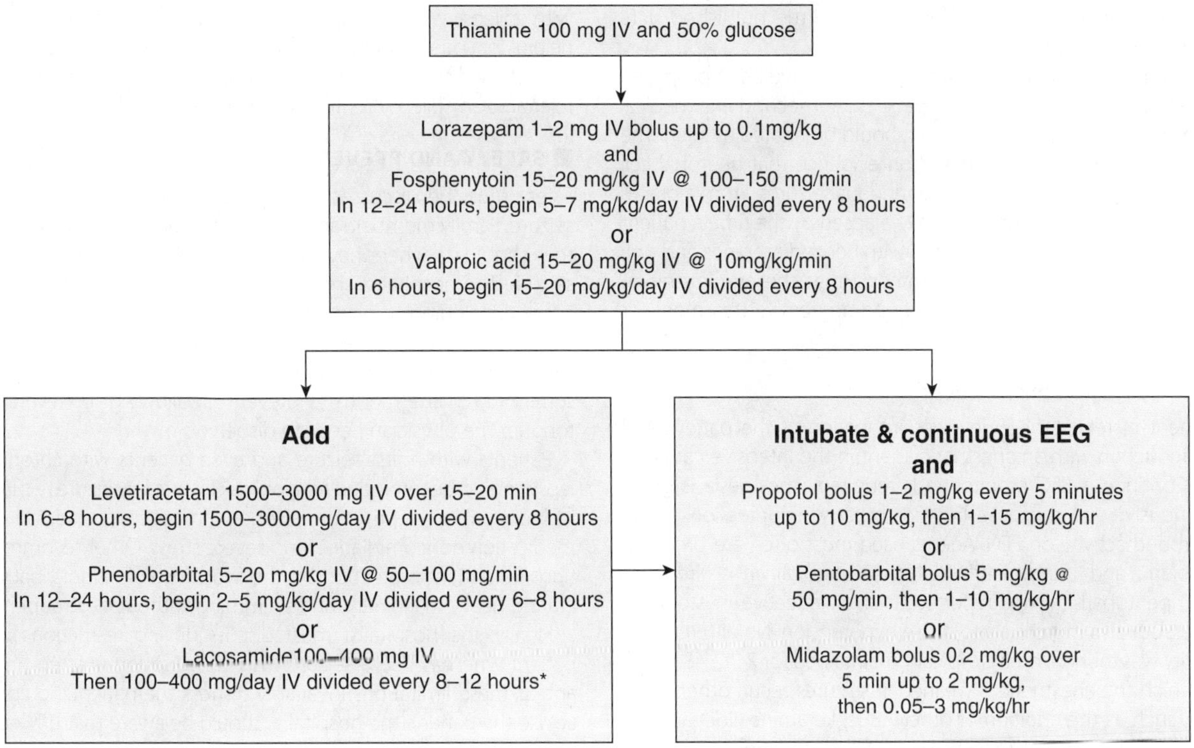

* Dose in SE not established

Figure 212-2 *Treatment protocol for status epilepticus. (EEG, electroencephalogram; SE, status epilepticus.)*

STATUS EPILEPTICUS

The traditional definition of status epilepticus (SE) is a prolonged seizure, or cluster of seizures, without a return to baseline, lasting longer than 30 minutes. A revised operational definition, proposed to lower morbidity and mortality, is any seizure lasting more than five minutes. Seizures can be generalized tonic-clonic, complex or simple partial, absence, or subclinical. Up to 50% of cases of SE occur in patients with epilepsy due to recent changes in AEDs or noncompliance. The remainder of cases in adults are most often secondary to stroke.

SE is a medical emergency, with mortality ranging from 7% to 40%. Predictors of mortality include generalized seizure, increased patient age, anoxic brain injury, stroke, CNS infection or tumor, and long duration of SE. Successful outcomes require early and aggressive treatment and collaboration between the emergency department physician, hospitalist, and neurologist. The discussion that follows provides guidelines for the treatment of generalized SE (summarized in **Figure 212-2**).

SUPPORTIVE TREATMENT

Once the diagnosis of SE is made, treatment should commence immediately. Initial treatment consists of stabilization of airway, breathing, and circulation and administration of oxygen while blood is drawn for laboratory studies. It is recommended that the patient be treated empirically with IV thiamine 100 mg and 50 mL of 50% glucose.

PHARMACOLOGIC TREATMENT

First line

IV benzodiazepines are the first-line drug treatment of SE. Diazepam, midazolam, and lorazepam have all been used successfully. Lorazepam is more effective than diazepam, with no difference in adverse events. Midazolam has not been adequately evaluated in comparative studies. Therefore, lorazepam is recommended. The initial dose should be a 1 to 2 mg IV bolus, followed by sequential boluses up to a total of 0.1 mg/kg.

Second line

While benzodiazepines are being given, a long-acting AED should also be given IV. Phenytoin was traditionally used in the past. However, fosphenytoin is now recommended, as it can be administered more quickly and has a lower risk of cardiovascular complications. The loading dose of fosphenytoin is 15 to 20 mg/kg, at a rate of 100 to 150 mg/min. Maintenance therapy can be started 12 to 24 hours after the initial load, at 5 to 7 mg/kg/day divided into doses administered every 8 hours. A reasonable alternative to fosphenytoin is IV valproic acid. The initial loading dose is 15 to 20 mg/kg given IV over ~15 minutes. A maintenance dose of 15 to 20 mg/kg/day given in 8-hour intervals should be started within 6 hours of the initial load. Serum AED levels should be followed, and extra doses should be given as necessary to maintain levels at the high end of the therapeutic range.

Third line

There is currently debate about the next line of therapy if seizures continue after treatment with benzodiazepines and an AED. Conventional algorithms recommend IV loading doses of a second AED. Choices include valproic acid, phenobarbital, levetiracetam, and lacosamide. Phenobarbital is known to be very effective in SE. However, it must be given slowly to minimize the risks of hypotension and cardiac side effects. In addition, it causes severe respiratory depression, so that most patients require intubation. These side effects make phenobarbital suboptimal at this point in the treatment of SE. Levetiracetam and lacosamide are both available in IV formulations and can be given rapidly with few adverse side effects. However, there is little published data regarding efficacy of either drug in SE.

More aggressive treatment protocols for SE have been proposed recently. In these schemes, SE that persists after second-line medical therapy is considered refractory and should be treated as such. The rationale for this proposal is based on evidence that neuronal cell death begins after 30 minutes of continuous seizures. From a practical point of view, 30 minutes will have elapsed by the time a patient in SE has been stabilized and treated with benzodiazepines and one AED. Hence, these schemes recommend that the administration of a second AED should be skipped and aggressive treatment for refractory SE started.

Refractory status epilepticus

Treatment of refractory SE involves intubation of the patient and coma induction with an anesthetic agent in the intensive care unit (ICU). Continuous EEG monitoring is required. Anesthesia is given continuously, with the dose titrated to cause suppression of the background activity on EEG. Agents used most often are propofol, midazolam, and pentobarbital or phenobarbital. In a literature review, pentobarbital was reported as most effective in stopping seizures, but also more likely to cause hypotension. No difference in mortality was found. Coma is typically maintained for 24 to 48 hours, after which the anesthetic is weaned. If seizures recur, other treatments, such as the addition of other AEDs, ketamine, lidocaine, or electroconvulsive therapy, can be tried. Overall, the prognosis in this situation is very poor.

Partial status epilepticus

Complex partial SE is not as clinically dramatic as generalized SE. Patients often present in a "twilight" state or are persistently confused. An EEG should be obtained in the evaluation of such patients to avoid a misdiagnosis of psychiatric disease. Aggressive medical therapy is recommended for complex partial SE. Simple partial SE usually manifests as repetitive focal motor seizures (epilepsia partialis continua) and typically reflects an acute cortical injury or a cerebral inflammatory process. These seizures are often resistant to treatment with AEDs. The morbidity and mortality of simple partial SE are relatively low. The risks and benefits of medical therapy must be carefully assessed when deciding how aggressively to treat this type of SE.

Nonconvulsive status epilepticus

Ongoing seizure activity on EEG in the absence of clinical seizures is termed *nonconvulsive status epilepticus (NCSE)* and is often unrecognized. NCSE is most common after clinical generalized SE appears to have resolved, with a reported incidence of 14% to 20%. It is particularly important that the hospitalist consider a diagnosis of NCSE in comatose patients in the ICU. In studies, NCSE was found on EEG in 8% to 17% of patients in coma without signs of clinical seizures during hospitalization. This evidence points out the importance of obtaining an EEG in patients with SE after it appears that clinical seizures have stopped, as well as in critically ill patients in coma of unclear etiology.

DISCHARGE CONSIDERATIONS

Patients need to follow up with their primary care provider, and generally with a neurologist as well. Referrals to other care providers, such as a psychiatrist or psychologist for counseling, may also be appropriate. Most physicians recognize the importance of these referrals for patients with psychogenic nonepileptic spells, but psychiatric referral may also be indicated because mood disorders are a common comorbidity of epilepsy. Neuropsychological evaluation may be helpful for patients with epilepsy who complain of memory loss. Social services are often helpful for patients with epilepsy and difficulty with employment and cost of medications. Finally, for the patient with recurrent seizures, referral to an epilepsy center should be considered.

SAFETY AND PREVENTION

Safety must be discussed with patients and their families after a seizure. Family members and friends often are confused about what they should do when they witness the patient having a generalized seizure. The hospitalist should inform them of how to protect the patient, including turning the patient on his or her side and cushioning the head, arms, and legs. It is surprising that some families still believe that they should forcibly restrain the patient and place something in the mouth to prevent "swallowing" or severing the tongue. The physician needs to dispel this myth.

Patients with a first seizure and even patients with chronic epilepsy should be reminded to avoid risk factors for seizure recurrence, including sleep deprivation, alcohol and other recreational drugs, medication noncompliance, and severe stress. Other recommendations for patient protection are the avoidance of heights, baths, operating heavy machinery, and swimming without close supervision.

Finally, the hospitalist must discuss driving restrictions with a patient who has had a seizure. This conversation is often unpleasant, as these limitations invariably distress the patient. To correctly advise the patient, the hospitalist should be aware that driving laws and recommendations vary from state to state. Regulations for each state can be found on the Epilepsy Foundation Web site at www.epilepsyfoundation.org.

SUGGESTED READINGS

Berg AT. Risk of recurrence after a first unprovoked seizure. *Epilepsia.* 2008;49(Suppl 1):13–18.

Claassen J, Hirsch LJ, Emerson RG, et al. Treatment of refractory status epilepticus with pentobarbital, propofol, or midazolam: a systematic review. *Epilepsia.* 2002;43:146–153.

Claassen J, Mayer SA, Kowalski RG, et al. Detection of electrographic seizures with continuous EEG monitoring in critically ill patients. *Neurology.* 2004;62:1743–1748.

DeLorenzo RJ, Waterhouse EJ, Towne AR, et al. Persistent nonconvulsive status epilepticus after control of convulsive status epilepticus. *Epilepsia.* 1998;39:833–840.

Henneman PL, DeRoos F, Lewis RJ. Determining the need for admission in patients with new-onset seizures. *Ann Emerg Med.* 1994;24:1108–1114.

Huff JS, Morris DL, Kothari RU, et al. Emergency department management of patients with seizures: A multicenter study. *Acad Emerg Med.* 2001;8:622–628.

Krumholz A, Wiebe S, Gronseth G, et al. Practice parameter: evaluating an apparent unprovoked first seizure in adults (an evidence-based review). *Neurology.* 2007;69:1996–2007.

Marson A, Jacoby A, Johnson A, et al. Immediate versus deferred antiepileptic drug treatment for early epilepsy and single seizures: A randomized controlled trial. *Lancet.* 2005;365:2007–2013.

Prasad K, Krishnan PR, Al-Roomi K, et al. Anticonvulsant therapy for status epilepticus. *Br J Clin Pharmacol.* 2007;63:640–647.

Treiman DM, Meyers PD, Walton NY, et al. A comparison of four treatments for generalized convulsive status epilepticus. *N Eng J Med.* 1998;339:792–798.

Wiebe S, Tellez-Zenteno JF, Shapiro M. An evidence-based approach to the first seizure. *Epilepsia.* 2008;49(Suppl 1):50–57.

CHAPTER 213

Multiple Sclerosis

John J. Ross, MD, CM, FIDSA
Allan H. Ropper, MD, FRCP

Key Clinical Questions

1. What are the major disease manifestations and complications of multiple sclerosis?
2. How are exacerbations of multiple sclerosis treated?
3. What are treatment options for complicating symptoms of multiple sclerosis, such as fatigue, bladder dysfunction, and spasticity?
4. What disease-modifying agents are available to treat multiple sclerosis? What are their major toxicities?

INTRODUCTION

Multiple sclerosis (MS) is an autoimmune, T-cell-driven disease of the central nervous system characterized initially by demyelination and, eventually, by axonal destruction and neuronal loss. It is the most common neurologic disease in young adults.

EPIDEMIOLOGY

The peak age of onset between 20 and 40 years, and it has a twofold higher incidence in women. It has long been observed that latitude of residence in childhood is a risk factor for the development of the disease. MS is rare in equatorial areas, and the prevalence rises sharply with increasing distance from the equator. The relation of MS prevalence to latitude and altitude suggests that increased sun exposure in childhood protects against MS, but more recent work favors a genetic predisposition to MS that is geographically clustered.

Genetic factors play a major role in the development of MS, and a family history is common. The major histocompatibility complex allele HLA-DRB1*1501 and two cytokine receptor genes, the interleukin 7 receptor alpha chain gene (IL7RA) and the interleukin 2 receptor alpha chain gene (IL2RA), have been implicated. Susceptibility to MS is likely polygenic, with the contribution of most genes to MS risk being relatively small. Clusters of MS cases have suggested an infectious trigger, although the search for a specific viral or bacterial cause of MS has been thus far fruitless.

CLINICAL PRESENTATION

SYMPTOMS

Multiple sclerosis is characteristically a relapsing and remitting disease, but there is great variation in its course. Common presenting symptoms of MS are summarized in **Table 213-1**. Weakness, numbness, or both in one or more limbs are common first symptoms. Patients may have paresthesias in the extremities or a band-like tightness around the trunk or limbs. The legs may feel heavy or difficult to control. Neck flexion may cause a sensation of electric shocks in the shoulders, back, and occasionally in the thighs. This finding, known as the Lhermitte sign, may also be present in cervical spondylosis, vitamin B12 deficiency, radiation myelopathy, and other conditions affecting the cervical spine.

Certain acute or subacute clinical syndromes are particularly characteristic of MS, although they also occur in association with other diseases of the nervous system. *Optic neuritis* most often presents with a deep aching sensation in the eye for a day or two, followed by rapid visual loss over several days or less. It is usually unilateral, but may be bilateral or sequential. Swelling of the optic nerve head (papillitis) is seen in 10% of patients, the majority of cases being retrobulbar and, therefore, having a normal disc head. In *acute myelitis*, patients develop paraparesis or paraplegia over hours to days, with extensor plantar responses, ascending paresthesias, a sensory level on the trunk, and impaired sphincter function. *Cerebellar ataxia* and *brainstem syndromes* are also frequent. Sphincter dysfunction, especially urinary urgency, is common as the disease progresses.

SIGNS

Common examination findings include hyperreflexia, extensor plantar responses, lower-extremity ataxia, impaired rapid alternating movements, and loss of vibration and proprioception. Evidence

TABLE 213-1 Predominant Presenting Symptoms of Multiple Sclerosis

Paresthesias and other sensory disturbances	37–45%
Motor weakness	20–27%
Disturbance of gait or balance	13–35%
Vision loss or optic neuritis	15–17%
Diplopia and/or vertigo	10–13%

Data from Swanson JW. Mayo Clin Proc. 1989;64:577–586; Weinshenker BG, Bass B, Rice GP, et al. *Brain.* 1989;112(Pt 1):133–146.

of optic neuropathy may be present, either obvious (visual loss) or subtle (afferent pupillary defect). Previous episodes of optic neuritis cause optic nerve atrophy. Somewhat less frequent findings include nystagmus, intention tremor, spasticity, dysarthria, and paraparesis. Unilateral internuclear ophthalmoplegia is another characteristic finding but is not common.

NATURAL HISTORY

At first, most patients (85%) fall into the category of relapsing-remitting MS, undergoing periodic symptomatic flares (relapses) with incomplete recovery (remission). Emotional stress and infections have tentatively been associated with flares. The postpartum period is another frequent time of relapse; MS often abates during pregnancy. In 10% of patients, the disease has little response to treatment and a progresses inexorably from the onset (primary progressive MS). A minority (5%) have "benign" MS, with few relapses and little disease progression 10 to 15 years after diagnosis. Most patients with relapsing-remitting MS eventually develop a secondary progressive course characterized by steady neurologic deterioration and pathologically, by a progression from demyelination to neuronal loss. The cervical cord is particularly prone to disease in these cases.

DIAGNOSIS

The diagnosis of MS requires evidence of dissemination of disease in both space and time, although the time-honored requirement for the occurrence of clinical relapses has been replaced by imaging evidence of lesions of varying ages and in several central nervous system locations (**Table 213-2**). The major diagnostic test for MS is now magnetic resonance imaging (MRI). Typical lesions on MRI are bright on T2-weighted and fluid-attenuation inversion recovery (FLAIR) images, consistent with high water content (**Figure 213-1**). Early lesions are isodense on T1-weighted images and display enhancement with gadolinium, but more advanced ones may be T1 isodense, indicating necrosis ("black holes"). Typical locations include the periventricular regions, corpus callosum, cerebellar peduncles, and spinal cord.

Lumbar puncture is helpful but not mandatory for the diagnosis of MS. The cerebrospinal fluid (CSF) may display a minimal increase in lymphocytes ($< 50/mm^3$) and total protein. Levels of myelin basic protein may be increased during disease flares. Oligoclonal bands on electrophoresis are the most sensitive CSF test for MS, but these may also be present in infectious and inflammatory conditions, such as Lyme disease, HIV, and neurosarcoidosis. Abnormal visual-evoked potentials may support the diagnosis of MS by demonstrating otherwise inevident optic nerve damage.

PRACTICE POINT

- The diagnosis of multiple sclerosis should be made with reservations if a patient's symptoms and signs can be explained by a single clinical lesion. A definitive diagnosis of multiple sclerosis requires demonstration of multiple lesions with evolution over time (dissemination in space and time).

DIFFERENTIAL DIAGNOSIS

A large number of infectious, inflammatory, vascular, and genetic conditions may mimic MS, both clinically and radiologically (**Table 213-3**). The diagnosis of MS is most difficult early in the course of the disease, when evidence for dissemination in space and time are lacking, or when the disease runs a progressive course without periodic exacerbations. Connective tissue diseases, particularly lupus and Sjögren syndrome, may cause multifocal inflammatory lesions in the cord or brain that mimic MS ("lupus sclerosis"). The presence of systemic features (eg, fever, sweats, or rigors) and involvement of other organ systems (eg, arthritis, rash, sicca syndrome, or peripheral neuropathy) suggests an underlying systemic disorder rather than MS.

TABLE 213-2 The 2010 Revised McDonald Criteria for the Diagnosis of MS

The diagnosis of multiple sclerosis requires demonstration of dissemination of lesions in both time and space, as follows:	
Dissemination in sime	Dissemination in space
≥ 2 attacks	Objective clinical evidence of ≥ 2 lesions
OR	OR
Simultaneous gadolinium-enhancing and non-enhancing lesions on MRI at any time	≥ 1 T2 lesion in at least 2 of 4 typical locations (periventricular, juxtacortical, infratentorial, spinal cord)
OR	
A new T2 and/or enhancing lesion on follow-up MRI, in addition to a previously documented MRI lesion	
The diagnosis of primary progressive MS requires one year of insidious neurological progression, plus 2 of 3 of the following:	
1. ≥ 1 T2 lesions in at least 1 area characteristic for MS (periventricular, juxtacortical, or infratentorial);	
2. ≥ 2 T2 lesions in the cord;	
3. Positive CSF (isoelectric focusing evidence of oligoclonal bands and/or elevated IgG index)	

CSF, cerebrospinal fluid; MRI, magnetic resonance imaging; MS, multiple sclerosis.
Data from Polman CH, Reingold SC, Banwell B, et al. *Ann Neurol.* 2011;69:292–302.

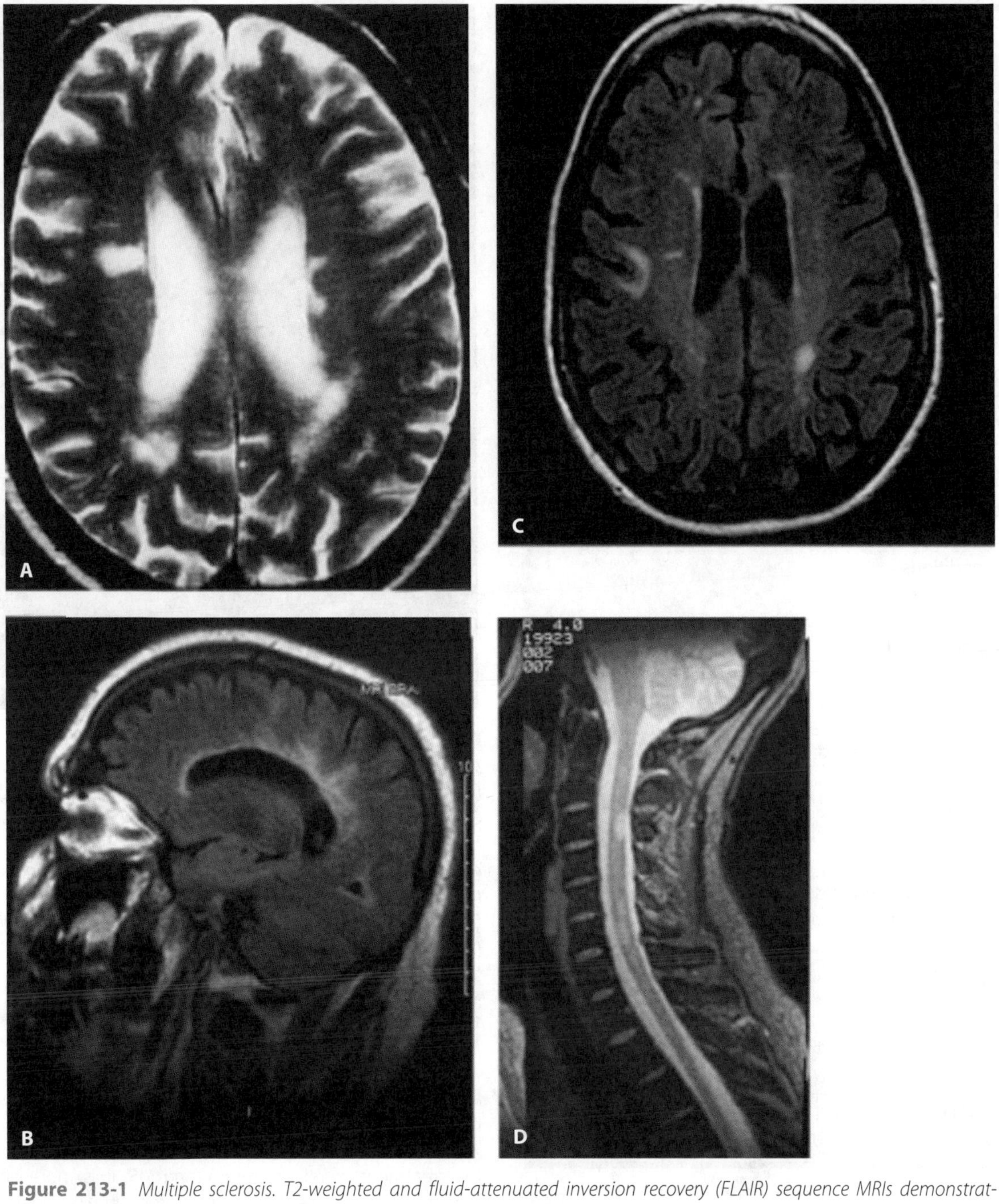

Figure 213-1 *Multiple sclerosis. T2-weighted and fluid-attenuated inversion recovery (FLAIR) sequence MRIs demonstrating multiple plaques in the periventricular white matter (A), emanating radially from the corpus callosum ("Dawson fingers"; B), a "C-like"–shaped lesion in the right subcortical white matter that is created by interruption of the lesion by the adjacent cortex (C) and cervical spinal cord (D). The radial orientation and periventricular location of cerebral lesions are typical of MS. (Reproduced, with permission, from Ropper AH, Samuels MA. Adam's & Victor's Principles of Neurology. 9th ed. New York: McGraw-Hill, 2009. Figure 36-1.)*

TREATMENT

DISEASE-MODIFYING TREATMENT

Disease-modifying agents and their major toxicities are summarized in **Table 213-4**. In the majority of patients, MS is a progressive disease that leads to disability without treatment. The current treatment paradigm is that disease-modifying therapy reduces the number of relapses and results in better long-term outcome, including retention of cognitive ability. If one treatment is not tolerated or fails as evidenced by disease progression or frequent relapses, another should be substituted. Glatiramer acetate and the beta-interferons have equivalent efficacy, reducing the yearly risk of relapse by about 30%. Glatiramer may cause anxiety and panic attacks, and the interferons may elicit depression. Both produce an acute flu-like syndrome that abates with time in most patients and can be mitigated by premedication. Intravenous monthly natalizumab is more effective, reducing relapse rates by 60%. However, its use in 0.1% of cases is complicated by progressive multifocal leukoencephalopathy (PML), caused by reactivation of the John Cunningham (JC) virus in the brain. Natalizumab is therefore currently reserved for patients who have failed or are intolerant of other disease-modifying therapies, or those who have rapid progression of MS with an abundance of active lesions on MRI. MS patients who develop new neurologic symptoms on natalizumab

TABLE 213-3 Differential Diagnosis of Multiple Sclerosis

Infections
Neurosyphilis
HIV
Lyme disease
Progressive multifocal leukoencephalopathy (PML)
Human T-cell lymphotropic virus 1 (HTLV-1, tropical spastic paraparesis)
Neurobrucellosis
Inflammatory conditions
Systemic lupus erythematosus
Sjögren syndrome
Mixed connective tissue disease
Systemic sclerosis
Behçet disease
Neurosarcoidosis
Central nervous system vasculitis
Toxic-metabolic disturbances
Vitamin B12 deficiency
Vascular conditions
Cerebrovascular disease
Vascular malformations with recurrent bleeding
Antiphospholipid antibody syndrome
Microinfarcts due to polycythemia vera or thrombocytosis
Subacute bacterial endocarditis with recurrent emboli
Cerebral autosomal dominant arteriopathy with subcortical infarcts and leukoencephalopathy (CADASIL)
Genetic disorders
Mitochondrial diseases
Spinocerebellar ataxias
Leukodystrophy
Structural conditions and mass lesions
Central nervous system lymphoma
Syringomyelia
Tumors of the foramen magnum and posterior fossa
Platybasia
Chiari malformation
Cervical spondylosis
Herniated disc
Other demyelinating diseases
Acute disseminated encephalomyelitis

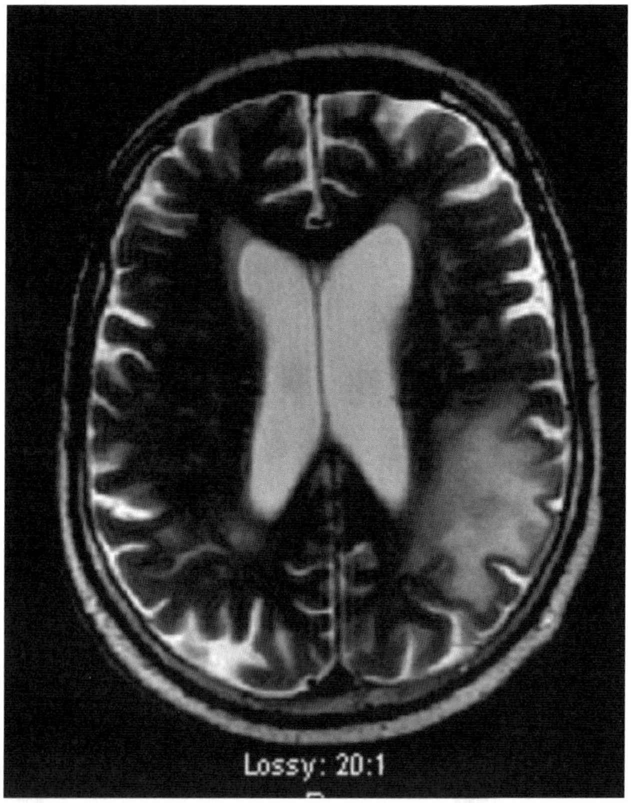

Figure 213-2 *Compared with multiple sclerosis (MS), progressive multifocal leukoencephalopathy (PML) is more likely to produce large, confluent lesions on T2-weighted magnetic resonance imaging (shown). Clinically, PML more often presents with hemiparesis and mental status changes, whereas MS is more likely to produce optic neuritis, brainstem syndromes, and spinal cord lesions. However, it is often impossible to distinguish a relapse of MS from PML based solely on clinical and radiologic findings, and a lumbar puncture with PCR for JC virus is usually required for definitive diagnosis. (Reproduced, with permission, from Ropper AH, Samuels MA. Adam's & Victor's Principles of Neurology. 9th ed. New York: McGraw-Hill, 2009. Figure 33-4B.)*

should have an MRI. If it is not possible to exclude PML based on MRI (**Figure 213-2**), a lumbar puncture should be performed, and cerebrospinal fluid should be sent for polymerase chain reaction for JC virus. PML in most clinical settings is usually fatal. However, patients with PML due to natalizumab may recover if the drug is stopped immediately and patients undergo plasma exchange, immunoadsorption, or both to remove natalizumab, which may otherwise persist for many months. Patients may experience worsening of symptoms and enlarging lesions on MRI days to weeks after cessation of natalizumab, a phenomenon that is likely attributable to immune reconstitution inflammatory syndrome (IRIS), as seen more commonly in HIV-infected patients treated with highly active antiviral therapy. Patients with IRIS benefit from corticosteroid therapy to reduce inflammation and prevent immune-inflicted neurologic damage.

Many other immunosuppressive drugs have modest activity in MS, but two monoclonal antibodies, rituximab and alemtuzumab, are moderately to highly effective in reducing relapse rates and may have benefit in cases of progressive disease.

A new oral agent, fingolimod, has recently been approved for the treatment of relapsing-remitting MS. It is more effective in reducing relapse rates than is interferon beta-1a. However, it has serious potential adverse effects, including transient bradycardia in the first few days of therapy, macular edema, and hepatitis. Rates of serious infections appear to be increased, including pneumonia, disseminated varicella zoster infection, and herpes simplex encephalitis. Additional oral agents that may be available to treat MS in the near future include cladribine, laquinimod, teriflunomide, and BG-12. Although patients may prefer these drugs to injection, each drug has specific risks that will have to be weighed by clinicians.

ACUTE RELAPSES

Acute symptomatic relapses of MS may be treated with pulses of high-dose corticosteroids. A typical regimen is methylprednisolone 1 gm intravenously daily for three to five days. Some authorities recommend following this with a short course of tapering doses of oral prednisone. Prior to treatment, MRI is generally performed to assess for new T2 and enhancing lesions. The possibility of pseudorelapse due to infection, psychoactive medications, and other medical

TABLE 213-4 Drug Therapy of Multiple Sclerosis

Drug	Dosage and Route	Mechanism	Side Effects
Primary progressive multiple sclerosis			
No therapies with proven efficacy at present			
Relapsing-remitting multiple sclerosis			
Interferon beta-1a (Avonex)	30 μg intramuscularly once weekly	Do not cross blood-brain barrier; may act by blocking peripheral T-cell activation and proliferation, and by inducing apoptosis of autoreactive T cells	Fatigue, fever, flulike symptoms, injection-site reactions, neutropenia, liver function test elevations, depression; efficacy may be hindered by the formation of anti-interferon antibodies in some patients, especially with more frequent dosing regimens
Interferon beta-1a (Rebif)	44 μg subcutaneously three times weekly		
Interferon beta-1b (Betaseron)	250 μg subcutaneously every other day		
Glatiramer (Copaxone)	20 mg subcutaneously once daily	Polypeptide mixture with structural resemblance to myelin basic protein; produces bystander suppression, activates anti-inflammatory Th2 cells, blocks autoreactive T cells, and induces anergy; onset of action is delayed for several months	Injection site reactions, flulike symptoms, chest pain, tachypnea, facial erythema, urticaria, fat necrosis at recurrent injection sites
Natalizumab (Tysabri)	300 mg intravenously every four weeks	Monoclonal antibody against the lymphocyte α4-β1 integrin receptor; prevents lymphocyte binding to vascular endothelial cells and inhibits lymphocyte migration into the central nervous system	Headache, fatigue, arthralgias, infections, and infusion reactions, including anaphylaxis; about 0.1% of patients develop progressive multifocal leukoencephalopathy (PML)
Fingolimod (Gilenya)	0.5 mg orally once daily	Sphingosine 1-phosphate receptor modulator; blocks egress of lymphocytes from peripheral lymph nodes, indirectly leading to decreased lymphocyte migration into the central nervous system	Transient bradycardia and decreased atrioventricular node conduction with first few doses, macular edema, cough, altered pulmonary function tests, headache, diarrhea, infections (especially reactivation of varicella and herpes simplex), altered liver enzymes, back pain
Secondary progressive multiple sclerosis			
Mitoxantrone	12 mg/m^2 intravenously every 3 months, to a maximum lifetime dose of 140 mg/m^2	Topoisomerase inhibitor; impairs DNA synthesis and repair; broad-spectrum immunosuppressive agent	Cardiac toxicity, nausea, alopecia, neutropenia, anemia
Agents with limited supporting evidence: Azathioprine, methotrexate, mycophenolate mofetil, cyclophosphamide			

conditions should be considered, and a urinalysis, urine culture, and chest radiograph should be performed to exclude urinary tract infection and pneumonia.

SYMPTOMS DUE TO PROGRESSION OF NEUROLOGIC DISEASE

The management of common symptoms complicating MS is summarized in **Table 213-5**. *Bladder management* is of particular relevance to the hospitalist. Urologic symptoms are present in up to 75% of patients with MS. These may result from bladder (detrusor) overactivity, leading to urgency, frequency, and urge incontinence; detrusor insufficiency, with incomplete bladder emptying; or detrusor-sphincter dyssynergia, causing hesitancy and interrupted urinary stream. It is not unusual for MS patients to suffer from all three conditions.

MS patients with urinary urgency and frequency should first be evaluated for urinary tract infection with urinalysis and urine culture. A postvoid residual volume (PVR) of the bladder should also be obtained, either by portable ultrasound or catheterization. If the PVR is greater than 100 ml, patients should be educated in clean intermittent bladder self-catheterization. Urgency often responds to urinary antispasmodics such as oxybutynin or tolterodine; patients taking these medications may need to perform intermittent self-catheterization as well, as they may aggravate concomitant urinary retention. Pelvic floor exercises and bladder retraining may alleviate urinary urgency by enhancing the ability of the pelvic floor muscles to counteract detrusor contraction. Treatment of constipation is thought to improve bladder function, although there is little data to support this contention. Patients with pure detrusor insufficiency may benefit from bethanecol to promote bladder emptying.

Although urinary tract infections (UTIs) are common in MS patients with bladder dysfunction, asymptomatic bacteriuria should not be treated. Cystoscopy and renal ultrasound should be performed in patients with frequent UTIs to assess for bladder stones, nephrolithiasis, and anatomic lesions that may predispose to infection. Cranberry juice may have modest efficacy in the prevention of UTIs.

Depression and fatigue are ubiquitous in MS and may be the most disabling symptoms in some patients. They deserve attention with both psychotherapy and medications. Changing from interferon to an alternative drug or a drug holiday, should be considered. Spasticity in the legs may be more prominent than weakness and can be treated with baclofen or tizanidine. Extreme cases benefit from an implantable intrathecal pump for infusion of baclofen. *Impotence* responds variably to phosphodiesterase inhibitors.

TABLE 213-5 Treatment of Associated Symptoms in Multiple Sclerosis

Symptom	Therapy	Possible Side Effects
Bladder urgency	Oxybutynin 5 mg two or three times daily (immediate release), 5 mg daily (extended release)	Anticholinergic side effects (dry mouth, constipation, confusion, somnolence), exacerbation of glaucoma, urinary retention
	Tolterodine 2–4 mg twice daily	
Cognitive dysfunction	No drug therapy with proven benefit; treatment of associated fatigue and depression and cognitive behavior therapy may helpful	
Depression	Selective serotonin reuptake inhibitors (SSRIs)	Generally well tolerated; may cause sexual dysfunction; possible risk of suicidality in younger patients
	Selective serotonin and norepinephrine reuptake inhibitors	Useful alternative to SSRIs in patients who suffer side effects
	Tricyclic antidepressants	Limited by anticholinergic side effects; may be useful in patients with insomnia and urinary urgency
Fatigue	Amantidine 100 mg two or three times daily	Hallucinations, ankle swelling, skin mottling, anticholinergic side effects
	Modafinil 100–200 mg twice daily	Anxiety, insomnia, anorexia, palpitations, severe dermatologic reactions
	Methylphenidate 5–10 mg/day	Anxiety, insomnia, anorexia
Pain	Gabapentin 100 mg three times daily; may be slowly titrated upward to maximum dose of 3,600 mg/day	Fatigue and somnolence are usually dose-limiting
	Carbamazepine 100 mg twice daily, titrated to a maximal dose of 400–1000 mg/day	Rash, hepatitis, drowsiness, nystagmus, nausea, cytopenias; hypothyroid patients may need higher levothyroxine doses due to accelerated T4 metabolism
	Amitriptyline 25–75 mg/day at bedtime	Anticholinergic side effects are common, including dry mouth, urinary retention, and confusion
Spasticity	Baclofen 10 mg two or three times daily, titrate to a maximal dose of 100 mg/day	Somnolence, fatigue, hypotonicity
	Tizanidine 2 mg at bedtime, titrate up to a maximum dose of 16–20 mg/day	Somnolence, fatigue
	Gabapentin 100 mg three times daily, titrate to 300–900 mg three times daily	Somnolence, fatigue

Cognitive decline has been recently recognized as a frequent accompaniment of chronic MS and correlates roughly with cerebral atrophy on imaging studies. Neuropsychological testing and cognitive rehabilitation techniques may prove helpful.

PRACTICE POINT

- The symptoms of MS may transiently worsen in response to elevated body temperature (*Uhthoff phenomenon*). This may be due to the adverse effects of heat on conduction in demyelinated nerves. Fever, infection, saunas, hot baths, and vigorous exercise may all lead to pseudoexacerbations of MS. Pseudoexacerbations or pseudorelapses may also be caused by medications, metabolic derangements, and the premenstrual phase of the menstrual cycle.

PRACTICE POINT

- Multiple sclerosis may begin as a *clinically isolated syndrome*, such as optic neuritis, acute myelitis, or acute brainstem syndrome, without definite evidence of disseminated MS. Treatment of patients with clinically isolated syndromes using disease-modifying agents such as glatiramer or the interferons may reduce the risk of evolution to clinically definite MS.

DISCHARGE CONSIDERATIONS

Primary care and neurologic follow-up should be arranged at discharge. Outcomes in MS are likely to be better if the patient is able to establish a long-term relationship with an engaged and caring neurologist. All patients with relapsing MS should be evaluated for disease-modifying therapy, either during hospitalization or shortly thereafter. Patients with disabilities are likely to benefit from the involvement of physical therapists, occupational therapists, and social work prior to discharge, and from visiting nurses and outpatient physical therapy after discharge. Pneumococcal and influenza vaccination status should be assessed before discharge.

QUALITY IMPROVEMENT

Possible targets for quality improvement in hospitalized patients with MS include the following:

- Screening for common associated symptoms, such as anxiety, constipation, depression, falls, fatigue, sexual dysfunction, and spasticity, should be performed
- As pneumonia is common in MS patients, influence and pneumococcal vaccination status should be assessed.
- A complete blood count, chest radiograph, urinalysis, and urine culture should be obtained to exclude pseudorelapse due to infection in patients with worsening MS symptoms.

- Patients should be screened for decubitus ulcers at admission, and those at high risk for decubitus ulcers due to limited mobility should be placed on a specialized pressure-reduction mattress.
- Patients should be screened for bulbar symptoms and signs, such as dysarthria, dysphagia, and absent gag reflexes. If present, a speech therapist should be consulted, and a formal swallowing assessment should be performed.
- Patients should be screened for bladder dysfunction, and postvoid residual volumes should be measured.

SUGGESTED READINGS

Cheng EM, Crandall CJ, Bever CT Jr, et al. Quality indicators for multiple sclerosis. *Mult Scler*. 2010;16:970–980.

Clifford DB, DeLuca A, Simpson DM, et al. Natalizumab-associated progressive multifocal leukoencephalopathy in patients with multiple sclerosis: lessons from 28 cases. *Lancet Neurol*. 2010;9:438–446.

Cohen JA, Barkhof F, Comi G, et al. Oral fingolimod or intramuscular interferon for relapsing multiple sclerosis. *N Engl J Med*. 2010;362:402–415.

Fowler CJ, Panicker JN, Drake M, et al. A UK consensus on the management of the bladder in multiple sclerosis. *J Neurol Neurosurg Psychiatry*. 2009;80:470–477.

Lucas RM, Ponsonby AL, Dear K, et al. Sun exposure and vitamin D are independent risk factors for CNS demyelination. *Neurology*. 2011;76:540–548.

Polman CH, Reingold SC, Banwell B, et al. Diagnostic criteria for multiple sclerosis: 2010 revisions to the McDonald criteria. *Ann Neurol*. 2011;69:292–302.

CHAPTER 214

Peripheral Neuropathy

Kaveh Saremi, MD
Annabel Kim Wang, MD

Key Clinical Questions

1. What are the symptoms and signs of peripheral neuropathy?
2. Which patients with peripheral neuropathies require hospitalization?
3. Which peripheral neuropathies are seen in the inpatient setting?
4. What are the common causes of peripheral neuropathies?
5. How are peripheral neuropathies evaluated?
6. What are the best treatment options for peripheral neuropathy?

CASE 214-1

A 31-year-old man was seen for inpatient consultation for possible polyneuropathy. His history dates back 1 year when he developed asthma for the first time. At the same time, he noted progressive paresthesias that started in his feet and then progressed to involve his hands. He was unsure when the weakness in his left leg developed. He was later found to have eosinophilia and eventually treated for Churg–Strauss syndrome. He developed sepsis and required bowel resection. After his bowel resection, he noted bilateral arm weakness, which was worse on the right side. His medical course was complicated by renal failure, malabsorption, and *Clostridium difficile* infection currently treated with metronidazole. His examination was significant for bilateral footdrop, with significant but asymmetric weakness in the left greater than the right leg, and the right greater than the left arm. Vibration sense was absent, and joint position sense was impaired in his toes. Light touch, cold, and pinprick were diminished to his knees and elbows. He was areflexic.

The new onset of paresthesias and/or weakness in an asymmetric fashion should alert the clinician to a vasculitic process. The presence of asthma and eosinophilia with multiple mononeuropathies is diagnostic for Churg–Strauss syndrome. The presence of inflammation, fibrinoid necrosis, and hemosiderin on nerve biopsy would have been diagnostic for vasculitis. Addressing the neuropathic symptoms should lead to earlier diagnosis and treatment of the underlying disorder. This patient has multiple causes for peripheral neuropathy in addition to this vasculitis: medications (metronidazole), sepsis, malabsorption leading to vitamin deficiencies, and immobility, predisposing to compressive neuropathies.

INTRODUCTION AND EPIDEMIOLOGY

Nontraumatic peripheral neuropathy is present in 2.4% of the general population and in as many as 8% of individuals over the age of 55. Diabetes is the most common cause in developed nations. At least 60% of diabetics have objective evidence for peripheral neuropathy. Overall, diabetic neuropathy ranks third behind macrovascular disease and nephropathy in lifetime expenditures associated with diabetic complications. Neuropathy is responsible for more hospital admissions than all the other diabetic complications combined and is a causative factor in up to 75% of all nontraumatic amputations.

PATHOPHYSIOLOGY AND CLINICAL FEATURES

Peripheral neuropathy is classified by the level of anatomical involvement (**Table 214-1**).

Radiculopathy affects the spinal root, leading to pain, paresthesias, and weakness in the distribution of the nerve root. It is most often caused by herniation of an intervertebral disk. Other causes include Lyme disease.

Plexopathy involves either the brachial plexus or the lumbosacral plexus, with symptoms involving multiple nerves. Causes include trauma, tumor infiltration, bony or vascular compression, radiation injury, and viral infection. Plexopathy may occur acutely in-hospital as a procedural complication, as in lumbosacral plexopathy due to groin hematoma after cardiac catheterization, or brachial plexopathy from stretch injury after cardiothoracic surgery.

TABLE 214–1 Patterns of Peripheral Neuropathy

Pattern	Example
Radiculopathy	Cervical, thoracic, lumbar, sacral
Plexopathy	Brachial, lumbosacral
Mononeuropathy	Median, ulnar, radial, axillary, femoral, peroneal, tibial, sciatic
Multiple mononeuropathies	Mononeuritis multiplex
Polyneuropathy	Motor, sensory, autonomic

Mononeuropathy is dysfunction of a solitary peripheral nerve. This is typically due to trauma (as in footdrop from peroneal nerve palsy after fibular fracture), compression (as in "Saturday night palsy," compression of the radial nerve in the axilla from falling asleep with the arm draped over a park bench or other hard surface, as seen in alcoholics), or entrapment (median nerve in carpal tunnel syndrome). Involvement of several noncontiguous individual nerves is referred to as *multiple mononeuropathies* or *mononeuropathy multiplex*; vasculitis is the most common cause.

Polyneuropathy affects many peripheral nerves simultaneously, with distal and more or less symmetric involvement. Symptoms typically begin in the feet before ascending to involve the legs and hands. It may involve sensory, motor, and autonomic nerves, either in isolation or varying combinations. Sensory symptoms may be persistent or intermittent. Positive sensory symptoms (dysesthesias or paresthesias) are described as tingling, burning, freezing, and electric-like. Negative sensory symptoms include numbness and anesthesia. Allodynia or dysesthesia occurs when innocuous stimuli are perceived as being painful. Loss of balance, incoordination, and gait difficulty may also occur with sensory neuropathies. Weakness, when present, is also generally distal and symmetric. Symptoms of autonomic neuropathy (**Table 214-2**) include lightheadedness or orthostatic hypotension, diminished sweating with heat intolerance, and diarrhea. They may be mistaken for nonneurologic illness. Autonomic neuropathy may be prominent in diabetes mellitus, Guillain–Barré syndrome, uremia, porphyria, and amyloidosis.

TABLE 214-2 Symptoms of Autonomic Neuropathy

Type	Cause	Symptom
Parasympathetic		
Pupillomotor	Lack of pupillary constriction	Glare/blurred vision
Secretomotor	Decreased lacrimation	Dry eyes
	Decreased salivation	Dry hands
GI	Dysmotility	Bloating, early satiety, diarrhea, constipation
Genitourinary	Dysfunction	Urinary retention, sexual dysfunction
Sympathetic		
Adrenergic	Orthostatic hypotension	Lightheadedness, shoulder pain
Sudomotor	Decreased sweating	Hypohidrosis, anhidrosis, heat intolerance
Vasomotor	Impaired vasoconstriction	Cold extremities

Polyneuropathy is classified by the temporal onset of symptoms (**Table 214-3**): acute (< 4 weeks' duration), subacute (4–8 weeks' duration), or chronic (> 8 weeks' duration). Polyneuropathy may further be subclassified into axonal, demyelinating, or mixed injury, based on the results of nerve conduction studies.

ACUTE POLYNEUROPATHY

Acute or subacute polyneuropathies tend to be inflammatory, infectious, or postinfectious in origin. Acute symmetric polyneuropathy with the rapid onset of ascending paralysis is usually due to *acute inflammatory demyelinating polyradiculoneuropathy (AIDP),* also known as *Guillain–Barré syndrome.* AIDP results from an autoimmune attack on peripheral nerves. It is preceded by recent *Campylobacter jejuni* infection in up to one third of cases. AIDP also occurs after viral infections, such as cytomegalovirus and Epstein–Barr virus. The diagnosis is based on the development of symmetric and ascending weakness of the limbs, hyporeflexia or areflexia, with variable sensory and cranial nerve involvement. Autonomic failure with fluctuating blood pressure and heart rate occurs in one third of patients and is a significant cause of morbidity. An elevated cerebrospinal fluid (CSF) protein without cells (albuminocytological dissociation) is diagnostic. AIDP has also been reported in the setting of recent human immunodeficiency virus (HIV) infection, viral hepatitis, Lyme disease, lymphoma, and systemic lupus erythematosus. Other causes of acute flaccid paralysis are listed in **Table 214-4**.

Other causes of acute polyneuropathy are porphyria, diphtheria, vasculitis, paraneoplastic syndromes, drugs, and toxins such as arsenic.

PRACTICE POINT

Critical illness polyneuropathy

- Critical illness polyneuropathy is a common and often unrecognized cause of hospital-acquired polyneuropathy. Risk factors include sepsis or systemic inflammatory response syndrome, prolonged ICU stay, renal failure, low serum albumin, parenteral nutrition, hyperglycemia, and hyperosmolarity; the relationship between glucocorticoid exposure and critical illness polyneuropathy is unclear. In mild cases, some improvement may occur within weeks. In more severe cases, improvement may take months, and be incomplete or absent. Therapy is supportive, and includes attention to nutritional status, early mobilization, and physical and occupational therapy to prevent contractures and maintain range of motion of the extremities.

CHRONIC POLYNEUROPATHY

Chronic symmetric polyneuropathy is the most common form of polyneuropathy. Axonal involvement is usual. Causes include metabolic, toxic, inherited, infectious, and inflammatory etiologies (see Table 214–3). In the hospital setting, diabetes mellitus, uremia, alcohol, and HIV are especially prevalent causes. Many drugs are associated with neuropathy, including cisplatin, vincristine, amiodarone, isoniazid, ethambutol, metronidazole, and nitrofurantoin. Vitamin B_{12} deficiency may cause polyneuropathy, as well as myelopathy.

TABLE 214-3 Classification of Polyneuropathies

Acute polyneuropathies	
Acute inflammatory demyelinating polyradiculoneuropathy (AIDP) or Guillain–Barré syndrome (GBS)	
Acute motor axonal neuropathy	
Acute motor and sensory axonal neuropathy	
Acute autonomic neuropathy	
Chronic polyneuropathies	**Examples**
Inflammatory	Chronic inflammatory demyelinating polyneuropathy, vasculitis
Infectious	Hepatitis C, HIV, diphtheria, leprosy
Inherited	Familial amyloid polyneuropathy, Charcot–Marie–Tooth disease, Refsum disease
Metabolic	Diabetes, hypothyroidism, uremia, liver failure
Toxic	Alcohol, amiodarone, cisplatin, ethambutol, isoniazid, lead, linezolid, metronidazole, nitrofurantoin, pyridoxine
Nutritional deficiencies	Vitamins B_6, B_{12}, and E deficiencies
Systemic disorders	Rheumatoid arthritis, sarcoidosis, Sjögren syndrome
Monoclonal gammopathy	Monoclonal gammopathy of undetermined significance, systemic amyloidosis, Waldenström macroglobulinemia, cryoglobulinemia, POEMS (polyneuropathy, organomegaly, endocrinopathy, M protein, skin), Castleman disease
Malignancies and associated treatment	Small cell lung cancer, breast cancer, lymphoma, chemotherapy
Polyneuropathies with autonomic symptoms	
AIDP or Guillain–Barré syndrome	
Paraneoplastic neuropathy (acute and chronic)	
Diabetes	
Amyloidosis (familial and systemic)	
Fabry disease	
Porphyria	
Hereditary and sensory autonomic neuropathies	
HIV-associated polyneuropathy	
Sjögren neuropathy	
Neuropathies associated with drugs (cisplatin, paclitaxel, vincristine) and toxins (arsenic, acrylamide, organophosphates)	

HIV; human immunodeficiency virus.

TABLE 214-4 Causes of Acute Flaccid Paralysis

Localization	Diagnosis
Brain	Brainstem stroke, infection
Spinal cord	Transverse myelitis, arteriovenous dural malformation, tumor, abscess
Anterior horn cell	Infection (poliovirus, West Nile virus)
Muscle	Inflammatory or necrotizing myopathy
	Hypokalemia periodic paralysis
	Hypophosphatemia
Neuromuscular junction	Botulism
	Myasthenia gravis
	Tick bite paralysis
	Lambert–Eaton myasthenic syndrome
	Industrial or biological toxins
Sodium channel blockade	Neurotoxic marine poisoning

PRACTICE POINT

Chronic polyneuropathy:

- In the hospital setting, diabetes mellitus, uremia, alcohol, and HIV commonly cause chronic polyneuropathy. Many drugs are associated with neuropathy, including cisplatin, vincristine, amiodarone, isoniazid, ethambutol, metronidazole, and nitrofurantoin. Hospitalists can take steps to educate patients, especially diabetics, about foot care and avoid drugs, if possible, that may exacerbate their problem. Measures to improve outpatient glucose control can begin in the hospital because they have been shown to have sustained effects on long-term diabetic complications such as neuropathy, nephropathy, retinopathy, and cardiovascular disease.

Chronic neuropathy is occasionally demyelinating in nature. *Chronic inflammatory demyelinating polyneuropathy (CIDP)* resembles Guillain–Barré syndrome, with predominantly motor symptoms and a progressive or relapsing course over 6 months or more. *Multifocal motor neuropathy* presents with wasting and weakness predominantly in the upper extremities and may be mistaken for motor neuron disease (amyotrophic lateral sclerosis [ALS]). *Paraproteinemia* may cause a progressive, predominantly sensory polyneuropathy, in which the paraprotein is often an immunoglobulin M (IgM) antibody directed against myelin-associated glycoprotein. Some variants of *Charcot–Marie–Tooth disease* are demyelinating. Classically, these patients have a positive family history of neuropathy, footdrop, "stork" legs or "inverted champagne bottle" legs with calf wasting, high arches, and palpable peripheral nerves, but the clinical picture is highly variable. Patients with unrecognized inherited neuropathies, such as Charcot–Marie–Tooth disease, are at risk for a devastating acute polyneuropathy after chemotherapy.

DIAGNOSIS

The evaluation of peripheral neuropathies always begins with a detailed medical history, followed by both complete physical and neurologic examinations. Past medical history, associated symptoms, medications, drug and alcohol use, toxin exposures, and family history can provide insight. The pattern of onset (eg, distal, proximal, and symmetric), the temporal onset (eg, acute, subacute, and chronic), and associated symptoms and signs are useful clues. The general physical examination may provide clues to the etiology of neuropathy (**Table 214-5**). Neurologic examination should include examination of major sensory modalities, including light touch, pinprick and temperature, deep pressure, vibration testing, and joint position. Romberg test, motor bulk, strength and tone, and deep tendon reflexes should also be documented. Mental status changes are unusual in peripheral neuropathies but may occur with West Nile virus, porphyria, and acute heavy metal poisoning.

Nerve conduction studies are helpful in delineating the relative contributions of axonal and demyelinating disease and the degree of motor and sensory involvement. However, such studies cannot evaluate the small nerve fibers that carry pain and temperature sensation, which are often involved in diabetic neuropathy. Absent sensory responses with normal motor studies are consistent with a sensory ganglionopathy. Abnormal motor responses with normal sensory studies are suggestive of motor neuropathy, such as multifocal motor neuropathy with conduction block or a motor neuronopathy, including causes such as polio, West Nile Virus, and ALS. *Needle electromyography (EMG)* is helpful in determining the chronicity of the peripheral neuropathy, but it can also identify concomitant nerve root (radiculopathy) or muscle (myopathy) involvement. Both nerve conduction studies and needle electromyography should be performed as a two-part study and are collectively referred to as EMG. Electrodiagnostic testing in the inpatient setting can often be fraught with technical difficulties, but it is helpful in the diagnosis and prognosis of AIDP, botulism, myasthenia gravis, and critical care neuromyopathy.

Small nerve fibers are preferentially affected in distal painful neuropathies. Small fiber neuropathy can be diagnosed using quantitative sensory testing of cold and heat/pain sensation, autonomic testing, or skin biopsy. *Autonomic testing*, which evaluates heart rate, blood pressure, and sweating, can provide further information about small fiber and autonomic nerve function. Autonomic testing of cardiovagal, adrenergic, and postganglionic sudomotor function may not be readily available in the inpatient setting.

Suggested initial tests in peripheral neuropathy are listed in **Table 214-6**. Common causes of peripheral neuropathy should be excluded, including hypothyroidism (thyroid-stimulating hormone), diabetes (fasting glucose and hemoglobin A1c), and vitamin B_{12} deficiency (in addition to B_{12} levels, methylmalonic acid and homocysteine may help to diagnose vitamin B_{12} deficiency in patients with low-normal B_{12} levels). Erythrocyte sedimentation rate and C-reactive protein are helpful screening tests for autoimmune disorders. Rheumatoid factor, antinuclear antibodies, antineutrophil cytoplasmic antibodies, and antibodies to Sjögren syndrome antibodies A and B (SS-A and SS-B) may be indicated in select patients. HIV antibody, hepatitis C antibody, and syphilis serology screen for neuropathy related to infection. Systemic causes of polyneuropathy can be evaluated with routine complete blood count and metabolic panel to assess for anemia, uremia, and liver disease. Monoclonal gammopathies may be excluded with serum and 24-hour urine for immunofixation.

Nerve biopsy can be useful when diagnoses such as vasculitis, amyloidosis, lymphoma, leprosy, and sarcoid are being considered. *Punch skin biopsy* may identify isolated small fiber neuropathy through diminished epidermal nerve fiber density. *Chest radiograph* is useful in screening for neoplasms, especially when there is a smoking history and a possible paraneoplastic disorder.

TABLE 214-5 Findings on Physical Examination Associated with Specific Peripheral Neuropathies

Unusual Findings	Associated Peripheral Neuropathy
Orange tonsils	Tangier disease (deficiency of high-density lipoproteins)
Retinitis pigmentosa, hearing loss, ichthyosis	Refsum disease (peroxisomal disorder/phytanic acid)
Papilledema	POEMS
Hearing loss	Inherited neuropathy, mitochondrial disorders
Bilateral facial palsy	Guillain–Barré syndrome, sarcoid, lymphoma
Enlarged tongue, petechiae	Systemic amyloidosis
Severe autonomic failure	Diabetes, amyloidosis
High arches, hammer toes, palpable nerves	Inherited neuropathy (eg, Charcot–Marie–Tooth
Angiokeratomas	Fabry disease

POEMS, polyneuropathy, organomegaly, endocrinopathy, M protein, skin changes.

TABLE 214-6 Initial Diagnostic Testing in Polyneuropathy

Complete blood count
Erythrocyte sedimentation rate or C-reactive protein
Vitamin B_{12}
Folate
Serum electrolytes, blood urea nitrogen, and serum creatinine
Serum glucose and hemoglobin A1c
Liver function tests
Thyroid-stimulating hormone
Urinalysis
Serum and 24-hour urine protein electrophoresis and immunofixation
HIV antibody
Chest radiograph (for pulmonary malignancy as a cause of paraneoplastic neuropathy)
Nerve conduction studies/needle electromyography

DIFFERENTIAL DIAGNOSIS

Disorders of the spinal cord, anterior horn cells, and neuromuscular junction can all mimic peripheral neuropathy. *Cervical spondylosis* may present as quadriparesis, whereas *thoracic or lumbosacral spinal cord lesions* may lead to paraparesis. Deep tendon reflexes may be diminished, and bladder dysfunction may occur acutely. *Transverse myelitis,* secondary to multiple sclerosis, collagen vascular disease, infections, and paraneoplastic disorders, can present with motor, sensory, and autonomic symptoms, which vary depending on the size and location of the spinal cord lesion. CSF analysis demonstrates inflammation with moderate lymphocytic pleocytosis, elevated protein, and IgG index. A spinal sensory level and a focal area of increased T2 signal on spinal magnetic resonance imaging (MRI) are often present. *Spinal dural arteriovenous malformations* may present in a similar fashion. *Subacute combined degeneration* of the spinal cord due to vitamin B_{12} or copper deficiency may present as a neuromyelopathy. Upper motor neuron signs, such as increased deep tendon reflexes, are often masked by the superimposed polyneuropathy.

The anterior horn cells of the spinal cord may be involved in degenerative conditions, such as motor neuron disease, and infections, such as poliomyelitis. West Nile virus is a mosquito-borne illness with peak transmission in late summer. Infection usually results either in no symptoms or a mild flulike illness. West Nile virus occasionally leads to meningitis, encephalitis, or a poliomyelitis-like, rapidly progressive febrile paralytic illness from damage to the anterior horn cells. Weakness is usually asymmetric and ranges from flaccid monoplegia to disabling quadriplegia. CSF and serum IgM antibodies against West Nile virus are positive. Treatment is supportive.

Pre- and postsynaptic neuromuscular junction disorders should also be considered. In *myasthenia gravis,* caused by antibodies that block the postsynaptic acetylcholine receptors, weakness is fluctuating, worse in the evening, and usually proximal and fatigable. The ocular, pharyngeal, and laryngeal muscles are often involved, leading to ptosis, diplopia, dysphagia, and a nasal voice. The diagnosis may be overlooked in the setting of acute respiratory failure. *Lambert–Eaton myasthenic syndrome (LEMS)* results from antibody-mediated blockade of presynaptic acetylcholine release. It is usually related to underlying small cell lung cancer or autoimmune disease. The hallmark of LEMS is proximal weakness of the limbs, which increases in power with sustained contraction; the ocular muscles are spared.

Botulinum toxin blocks presynaptic release of acetylcholine, leading to a descending flaccid paralysis with blurry vision, ptosis, dysphagia, dysarthria, and eventually respiratory compromise. Patients are often intubated, but careful examination may reveal dilated pupils with a normal sensory exam. *Botulism* usually occurs after ingestion of contaminated food. It may also be acquired from open wounds, use of black tar heroin, or inhalation of aerosolized toxin, as in bioterrorism. Diagnosis is made by assay of stool, serum, and food (if available) for botulinum toxin. Later in the course, neurotoxin assays are less sensitive, but anaerobic cultures of wounds and stool for *Clostridium botulinum* may still be positive. Nerve conduction studies reveal small compound motor action potential amplitudes that increase with exercise. Antitoxin therapy is most effective when administered within 24 hours. Treatment is otherwise supportive, with special attention to the respiratory status.

In patients with foot pain, it may be difficult to distinguish small fiber neuropathy from peripheral vascular disease, arthritis, and plantar fasciitis. Small fiber neuropathy is often unrecognized because the distal pain and temperature loss can be subtle, and the presence of ankle reflexes and normal nerve conduction velocities are misleading. As noted above, punch skin biopsy may be helpful in this setting.

TRIAGE/HOSPITAL ADMISSION

Peripheral neuropathy is often diagnosed in patients who are admitted to the hospital for other reasons but rarely does it justify hospital admission on its own. There are major exceptions. Sudden flaccid paralysis warrants immediate admission, with close monitoring for respiratory compromise in a step-down unit or ICU. Patients who present with the acute, asymmetric onset of weakness have vasculitis, which is potentially life-threatening, until proven otherwise.

Hospitalization for chronic polyneuropathy is unusual. Admission is reasonable for complications of chronic polyneuropathy, such as infection or threatened amputation, or for treatment of intractable pain. Patients with inflammatory or demyelinating chronic polyneuropathies may require hospital admission for IV immunoglobulin or plasmapheresis.

TREATMENT

Most forms of neuropathy have no specific treatment, aside from identification and correction of the underlying cause. For example, glucose control should be optimized in diabetics, vitamin B_{12} and thyroxine should be repleted in those who are deficient, alcoholics should receive thiamine and encouragement to abstain from drinking, and medications responsible for neuropathy should be stopped. Patients with entrapment neuropathies, such as carpal tunnel syndrome, may benefit from surgical release.

Neuropathic pain may be diminished by therapy with antiepileptic drugs (gabapentin, pregabalin, or carbamazepine), serotonin–norepinephrine reuptake inhibitors (venlafaxine and duloxetine), or a tricyclic antidepressant (amitriptyline or nortriptyline).

Patients with allodynia and dysesthesias may obtain relief from a metal frame to raise the bedclothes off the feet. Focal pain may respond to a topical lidocaine patch.

Specific treatments for acute demyelinating polyneuropathies include IV immunoglobulin or plasmapheresis. Acute flaccid paralysis requires supportive care with aggressive attention to rehabilitation. Continuous pulmonary, blood pressure, and heart rate monitoring is required. Respiratory deterioration, for example, a negative inspiratory pressure <-15 cm H_2O, should prompt intubation. Mechanical ventilatory assistance is required in about one third of patients with AIDP. Tracheostomy is recommended if mechanical ventilation will be required for more than 2 to 3 weeks. Enteric nutrition is necessary for patients on mechanical ventilation. Heparin and graduated pressure stockings should be started to prevent deep venous thrombosis (DVT). Prevention of pressure sores is important. Patients should be treated by a multidisciplinary rehabilitation team.

Patients with autonomic neuropathy and orthostatic hypotension may be managed by liberal salt and fluid intake, and small, frequent meals. Fludrocortisone or midodrine may also be helpful. At night, patients with orthostatic hypotension should sleep in a semirecumbent position, with the head of the bed elevated at 30 degrees, to facilitate salt and water retention and avoid supine hypertension. Gastroparesis may respond to prokinetic agents such as metoclopramide and erythromycin. Pressure stockings and abdominal binders may help to reduce pooling of blood.

COMPLICATIONS

Hospital complications in patients with peripheral neuropathies are related to immobility and invasive treatment and may include skin breakdown, nosocomial pneumonia, urinary tract infection, central venous catheter sepsis, DVT, and pulmonary embolism. Death may occur from respiratory insufficiency, infection, or severe dysautonomia. Complications of IV immunoglobulin may include headache, rash, stroke, renal failure, or anaphylaxis, especially in individuals with IgA deficiency. Large fluid volume shifts can lead to myocardial infarctions, and complications from line placement are associated with plasmapheresis. Superimposed compressive neuropathies may occur in immobile patients. Undertreated anxiety, depression, and pain may increase morbidity. Alcohol withdrawal may be seen in patients with polyneuropathy due to alcohol abuse. In-hospital injuries from falls or orthostatic hypotension can occur.

DISCHARGE CONSIDERATIONS

Physical therapy and occupational therapy evaluations may be very helpful in both the inpatient and outpatient setting. Patients with footdrop may benefit from an ankle/foot orthosis. Diabetics and other patients with chronic polyneuropathy should be educated about foot care, including meticulous skin and nail care and frequent self-examination to identify early skin breakdown, advised to obtain properly fitted shoes to reduce ulcer risk, and referred for outpatient podiatry evaluation.

Patients with AIDP or severe polyneuropathy require inpatient rehabilitation for strengthening and mobility. Outpatient providers and caregivers need to be aware of persisting problems in these patients, including fall risk, fatigue, pain, dysautonomia, and communication difficulties that may lead to frustration and exacerbate depression. Patients on immunosuppressive medications require monitoring for adverse effects. Patients with limited mobility at discharge need continuing measures to prevent DVT. Follow-up care by both the neurologist and primary care physician is recommended.

QUALITY IMPROVEMENT TO ADDRESS PERFORMANCE GAPS

Preventable complications in the hospitalized patient with peripheral neuropathy are primarily related to their limited mobility. These patients should be recognized at being at high risk of decubitus ulcers and placed on preventive measures. Pressure, friction, and shear forces should be minimized by frequent turning and positioning and avoidance of excessive bed rest. The use of pressure-relieving devices, such as dynamic air mattresses, should be strongly considered in patients with severe polyneuropathy. Nutritional status should be assessed. Thermal injury, as from hot water baths, should be avoided. Prevention measures should be in place for DVT, nosocomial pneumonia, and falls. Patients with diabetes should have their glycemic regimen reassessed if their hemoglobin A1c indicates suboptimal glucose control.

SUGGESTED READINGS

Brannagan TH III. Current treatments of chronic immune-mediated demyelinating polyneuropathies. *Muscle Nerve.* 2009;39:563–578.

Dyck PJ, Kratz KM, Karnes JL, et al. The prevalence by staged severity of various types of diabetic neuropathy, retinopathy, and nephropathy in a population-based cohort: The Rochester Diabetic Neuropathy Study. *Neurology.* 1993;43:817–824.

Dyck PJ, Thomas PK, eds. *Peripheral Neuropathy.* Philadelphia: Elsevier; 2005.

England JD, Gronseth GS, Franklin G, et al. Evaluation of distal symmetric polyneuropathy: The role of laboratory and genetic testing (an evidence-based review). *Muscle Nerve.* 2009;39:116–125.

Haber P, Sejvar J, Mikaeloff Y, DiStefano F. Vaccines and Guillain-Barré syndrome. *Drug Saf.* 2009;32:309–323.

Hughes R. Peripheral nerve diseases: The bare essentials. *Pract Neurol.* 2008;8:396–405.

Said G. Diabetic neuropathy—a review. *Nat Clin Pract Neurol.* 2007;3:331–340.

Tavee J, Zhou L. Small fiber neuropathy: A burning problem. *Cleve Clin J Med.* 2009;76:297–305.

Vucic S, Kiernan MC, Kornblath DR. Guillain-Barré syndrome: An update. *J Clin Neurosci.* 2009;16:733–741.

SECTION 12

Palliative Care

CHAPTER 215

Principles of Palliative Care

Rachelle E. Bernacki, MD, MS
Diane E. Meier, MD

Key Clinical Questions

1. What is the best approach for patients with serious or advanced chronic illness?
2. What do patients and families consider important at this time?
3. What signs and symptoms suggest that a patient is dying?
4. What steps can be taken to relieve symptoms in patients with advanced illness?

INTRODUCTION

Hospitalized patients with advanced illness have a high burden of symptoms including pain, nausea, and dyspnea. These symptoms can arise from the disease itself as well as from the therapies used to treat it. They can arise at any point in the course of illness and can significantly diminish quality of life. Palliative care is the field of medicine focused on symptom management and improving quality of life for patients living with a life-threatening illness (Morrison & Meier, 2004), whether the goals for care include cure, life prolongation, or living with a chronic illness. Palliative care expertise includes the assessment and treatment of pain and other symptoms, and the relief of suffering caused by thye physical, psychosocial, and spiritual aspects of disease. Unlike hospice, which requires that a physician endorse a six-month prognosis in order for a patient to qualify for service, palliative care, sometimes also referred to as supportive care, is provided in conjunction with curative treatment at any point in the disease trajectory from the time of diagnosis (**Figure 215-1**). As a patient becomes sicker, palliative care may become a greater focus either because the burden of curative treatments outweighs the benefits or they are no longer effective or because the patient no longer desires them. Palliative care is provided by an interdisciplinary team including physicians, nurses, social workers, pharmacists, psychologists, and chaplains (Morrison & Meier, 2004). Palliative care teams treat not only the patient, but also attend to the needs of the family, understanding that family can include any person the patient identifies as part of his or her support network. Palliative care is provided early in the course of illness and across multiple care settings; therefore, communication among the varied settings and continuity of care is essential to achieving quality care for patients (**Table 215-1**).

While *palliative care* refers to an approach to care focused on symptom management and improving quality of life, *palliative medicine* refers to the medical specialty focused on providing palliative care. Despite the emergence of palliative medicine as a formally recognized medical specialty in 2007, all physicians who care for patients with serious and advanced illnesses need to be able to provide appropriate pain and symptom management and identify and treat other sources of suffering in their patients. In order to achieve this goal, all physicians need training in palliative care (Block et al, 2007). Even with such training, physicians will identify some patients who have needs so complex that referral to a specialized palliative medicine team will be appropriate.

Palliative care can be provided in any setting, including hospitals, clinics, nursing homes, emergency facilities, prisons, and home (**Table 215-2**). Hospice is a common way for people in the United States to receive palliative care at home when they reach the last few months of life. To qualify for hospice benefits, a patient must have a two-physician certified life expectancy of six months or less, and the patient must agree to give up insurance coverage for medical care focused on cure or life prolongation. Hospice is covered by Medicare as well as most health insurance providers. In the United States, the vast majority (> 90%) of patients receive hospice services at home, although the number of patients receiving hospice in nursing homes is growing (Teno et al, 2004). Patients enrolled in home hospice generally have a primary caregiver who is guided by a hospice nurse who visits on an as-needed basis, typically ranging from one to three times per week depending on the patient's status. Nursing aides provide personal and custodial care typically for about four hours per day. The hospice agency can help the family arrange

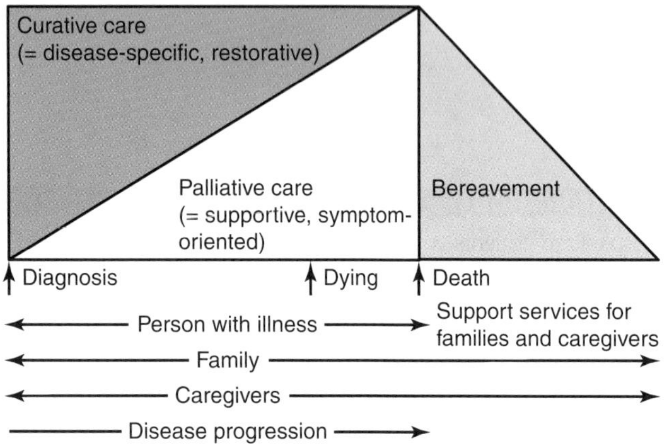

Figure 215-1 *Palliative care model. Courtesy of the United States Department of Health and Human Services. (Courtesy of the US Department of Health and Human Services.)*

TABLE 215-2 Palliative Care Models

Model	Care Setting
Consultation service team	Usually in a hospital or nursing home; often includes social work evaluations
Combined hospice program and palliative care program	Hospital, nursing home, freestanding hospice inpatient facilities
Dedicated inpatient unit	Acute hospitals, nursing homes
Hospice-based palliative care in the home	Home
Outpatient palliative care practice or clinic	Hospital or private practice

Data from National Consensus Project for Quality Palliative Care. 2009. *Clinical Practice Guidelines for Quality Palliative Care.* 2nd edition. http://www.nationalconsensusproject.org

for other (private pay) custodial care as needed by the patient. Durable medical equipment (hospital bed, wheelchair, commode, etc) and medications related to symptom management are provided at no charge to the patient under the hospice benefit. While hospice providers can manage most symptoms at home, if a crisis occurs, the patient can be admitted to an acute care facility until symptoms are under control.

PATHOPHYSIOLOGY

In patients with advanced illness, death is more often the result of sequential systemic changes rather than failure of a single organ. Despite differing courses of diverse illnesses, the dying process is remarkably similar across disease states. Altered carbohydrate, fat, and protein metabolism leads to a catabolic state, and homoeostasis is lost in association with increasing cytokine concentrations. Loss of both adipose tissue and muscle may be severe. Cytokines, including tumor necrosis factor, interleukins 1 and 6, and interferon γ, contribute directly to the weight loss, anorexia, and fatigue that characterize end-stage disease.

TABLE 215-1 Palliative Care Services

- Provides relief from pain and other distressing symptoms
- Will enhance quality of life and may also positively influence the course of illness
- Is applicable early in the course of illness, in conjunction with other therapies that are intended to prolong life, such as chemotherapy or radiation therapy
- Includes those investigations needed to better understand and manage distressing clinical complications
- Integrates the psychological and spiritual aspects of patient care
- Offers a support system to help patients live as actively as possible until death
- Affirms life and regards dying as a normal process
- Intends neither to hasten or postpone death
- Offers a support system to help the family cope during the patient's illness and in their own bereavement
- Uses a team approach to address the needs of patients and their families, including bereavement counseling, if indicated

Reproduced with permission from World Health Organization's Definition of Palliative Care. Accessed online August 28, 2009, at: http://www.who.int/cancer/palliative/definition/en.

DIAGNOSIS AND TREATMENT

PALLIATIVE CARE DOMAINS

The key aspects of palliative care can be divided into eight domains including (1) structure and processes of care; (2) physical aspects of care; (3) psychological and psychiatric aspects of care; (4) social and practical aspects of care; (5) spiritual, religious, and existential aspects of care; (6) cultural aspects of care; (7) care of the imminently dying patient; and (8) ethical and legal considerations. Specific components of these domains are outlined in **Table 215-3**.

STRUCTURE AND PROCESSES OF CARE

Care should be provided in the setting the patient chooses. If it is not possible to provide care in the patient's preferred location, the least restrictive alternate setting should provide flexible visiting hours, adequate space for visitors, and sufficient respite for care

TABLE 215-3 Palliative Care Domains

Area	Examples
Physical	Pain, shortness of breath, nausea, fatigue, weakness, anorexia, insomnia, confusion, constipation, treatment side effects, functional capacities, treatment efficacy and alternatives (and patient and family preferences)
Psychological/ psychiatric	Anxiety, depression, care-giving needs or capacity of family; stress; grief and bereavement risks for the patient and family (ie, depression and comorbid complications); coping strategies
Social	Family structure and geographic location; cultural concerns and needs; finances; sexuality; living arrangements; caregiver availability; access to transportation; access to prescription and over-the-counter medicines
Spiritual/ religious/ existential	Spiritual background, beliefs, and practices of the patient and family; hopes and fears; life completion tasks; wishes regarding care setting for death

Data from National Consensus Project for Quality Palliative Care. 2009. *Clinical Practice Guidelines for Quality Palliative Care.* 2nd edition. http://www.nationalconsensusproject.org

providers. When the patient cannot be in their setting of choice, creative measures are taken to make the alternate care setting as comfortable and familiar as possible.

A key element of palliative care is effective communication in order to elicit a patient's preferences and goals of care. Understanding the needs and goals of the patient and family is essential for providing high-quality palliative care. Palliative care teams also provide coordination of care and create plans to deal with potential crises, thereby allowing the patient to remain in their setting of choice. Palliative care providers also need good prognostication skills in order to help patients and families define goals of care and make appropriate decisions and plans (Block, 2001). For example, when a family member calls and states that a patient is eating poorly, it is important to know whether this represents a potentially reversible condition that could be relieved with a treatment or procedure or, alternatively, is a sign that the patient is approaching the final days or weeks of life. Prognostic information is important in helping patients make treatment decisions. For example, one patient may want treatment to be able to eat, drink, and survive long enough to attend a granddaughter's marriage, while a different patient in a similar clinical situation may decide that he does not want to undergo yet another procedure. When the disease progresses, communication becomes even more important to ensure that all involved have the same understanding of the prognosis and plan of care. Finally, clinician recognition of the signs and symptoms of the active dying phase of illness is crucial to completing the developmental tasks of the end of life, helping patients and families understand what is happening and what to expect, and coordinating care and logistics in the days leading up to death. Although it is impossible to know exactly what will happen to any particular patient, providers can use scored instruments (eg, the Palliative Performance scale, the Karnofsky scale, and the Eastern Cooperative Oncology Group's (ECOG) scale) along with clinical experience to offer patients and families estimates such as hours to days, days to weeks, weeks to months, and months to a year that communicate prognosis while recognizing the inherent uncertainty of such predictions (Lamont & Christakis, 2003).

Palliative medicine teams formulate and document care plans based on patient wishes, then convey this information to patients, family, and other providers (Morrison & Meier, 2004; Steinhauser et al, 2000). Care plans change according to the needs of the patient and family and should involve additional input from other specialists. Functional and cognitive status, disease trajectory, cultural and spiritual preferences, and home support must be considered in formulating care plans. For example, a patient may want to remain at home during the final days and weeks of life, but his wife, who is the primary caregiver, has trouble managing his medications due to mild cognitive impairment. In this situation, home nursing services or hospice can provide a weekly mediset and daily phone call reminders to the wife to ensure administration of the medicines. As death nears, the team may address the possibility of pursuing inpatient hospice given the wife's limitations.

PHYSICAL ASPECTS OF CARE

Physical symptoms associated with advanced illness include pain, dyspnea, nausea, vomiting, fatigue, weakness, anorexia, insomnia, anxiety, depression, confusion, and constipation. Pharmacologic, nonpharmacologic, and complementary therapies can help alleviate these symptoms (Goldberg & Morrison, 2007). Feeding and nutrition goals can be addressed early in the course of the disease in anticipation of the need to make decisions about the use of artificial nutrition and hydration in the future.

The goal of pain and symptom management is reduction of the symptoms to a level the patient defines as satisfactory. Providers should be careful not to state that all symptoms will be completely alleviated, because while that is sometimes possible, more often symptoms, such as pain and nausea, are attenuated to an acceptable level. Pain in advanced illness often requires the use of opioids, and physicians must be willing to prescribe opioids in doses sufficient to relieve pain and to acquire the appropriate management skills to predict opioid side effects such as constipation. Physicians should also anticipate and correct patients' misconceptions about the use of opioids including side effects, addiction, and somnolence.

PSYCHOLOGICAL AND PSYCHIATRIC ASPECTS OF CARE

In addition to addressing physical aspects of care, palliative care should address psychological issues and psychiatric needs and support emotional growth. Physicians should acknowledge the stress involved in caring for patients with life-threatening illness for both our colleagues and for our patient's family and other caregivers. Caregivers reporting emotional stress have a significantly increased mortality rate: physician identification of vulnerable caregivers and referral to social work and other community resources can be lifesaving. Physicians must recognize the importance of the time after referral to hospice and understand that patients and families are particularly vulnerable to feeling abandoned at this time by their physicians. Making follow-up appointments for patients and calling on the telephone can help reassure patients that a referral to hospice is not abandonment by the physician. It is important to express thanks and appreciation for the privilege of caring for the patient, and when appropriate, to say goodbye to the patient and her family members. Physicians must also be aware of normal and complicated grief, and screen and address those appropriately (Prigerson et al, 1995) (**Table 215-4**). Hospice programs provide bereavement services and follow-up for 12 months after the death of the patient. Finally, all providers can discuss and offer coping strategies to determine the most constructive approach to dealing with loss based on individual family needs and temperament.

SOCIAL AND PRACTICAL ASPECTS OF CARE

Referral to a palliative care social worker can promote access to services, community resources, and volunteers that can help patient and family in the home or with transportation. Collaboration with pharmacists can ensure that patients have access to necessary medications; home nursing agencies can ensure proper equipment is available. Family structure and living arrangements, geographic location, finances, and caregiver availability are considered and reflected in the care plan. For example, an older patient with advanced illness may have a partner who is ill and unable to provide care. In such a situation where the support system is already

TABLE 215-4 Risk Factors for Poor Bereavement Outcomes

Poor social supports
Past history of psychiatric problems, especially depression
Past history of childhood separation anxiety
High initial distress
Unanticipated death, lack of preparation for death
Other major concurrent stresses and losses
History of abuse or neglect in childhood
Lifestyle rigidity
Highly dependent relationship with the deceased
Death of a child

Data from Stroebe M, Schut H. and Stroebe, W. Health outcomes of bereavement. *Lancet*. 2007;370:1960.

at its limit, the palliative care team must develop a plan to ensure appropriate care and safety for the patient and his partner. Sending a patient home without adequate support can often lead to readmission; addressing needs early and activating community support can allow patients to remain at home as long as possible. Different teams may provide these services in differing ways. Some teams have dedicated social workers to address these issues, whereas other teams may use case managers or nurses to focus on these matters. It is important to realize the care coordination involved is more than a physician, nurse, or social worker can do alone; the interdisciplinary nature of palliative care draws upon the strengths of each field.

SPIRITUAL, RELIGIOUS, AND EXISTENTIAL ASPECTS OF CARE

Beliefs surrounding illness and death are profoundly influenced by a patient's and family's religious and spiritual values (Sulmasy, 2006). The salient spiritual needs of patients at the end of life encompass questions of meaning, value, and relationship. Physicians can play a key role helping patients express these needs by asking patients about their religious and spiritual beliefs and practices and how these impact the patient's view of illness. At a minimum, physicians should recognize these spiritual needs, inquire as to the patient's spiritual roots, and offer a referral to the hospital chaplain. Chaplains and other members of the spiritual care service can address such issues in a nonthreatening and supportive way and help facilitate religious or spiritual rituals as well as contact spiritual communities identified by the patient and family. When religious beliefs appear to be a barrier to providing good end-of-life care, spiritual engagement is the direct approach to resolution. For example, one patient and his family had a strong religious belief in a miraculous cure for metastatic cancer. The palliative care team chaplain explored this belief explicitly and negotiated a treatment plan that was respectful of the family's belief but also realistic and practical. The chaplain articulated that forgoing additional chemotherapy would not change whether a miracle was possible. The patient then accepted a referral to hospice care, where they received continued spiritual, emotional, and physical support.

CULTURAL ASPECTS OF CARE

The experience of a serious illness is deeply affected by a patient's and family's cultural values (Kagawa-Singer & Blackhall, 2001). Culture often defines how patients and families understand illness, suffering, and dying. Encounters between physicians and patients of different backgrounds are common given the diversity in the United States, and, therefore, there are many opportunities for crosscultural misunderstandings (Kagawa-Singer & Blackhall, 2001). Use of life-prolonging therapies and technology, the locus of decision making, and truth telling are all influenced by cultural norms. While autonomy is the legal basis for medical decision making in the United States, some cultures prefer that families make medical decisions as a unit. Adult children commonly wish to protect their parent from bad news and may ask the clinician not to tell the truth. Palliative medicine providers often address this issue by helping the family understand that the information will not be imposed but offered only if the patient indicates an explicit desire to know. This is done by asking the patient if they are the kind of person that prefers all the details about their illness, or if they would rather hear a general outline or leave the details of decision making to a family member. Such communication can demonstrate respect for the patient's culture without assuming that the patient will conform to cultural norms. Skilled communication, genuine curiosity, and openness to differences can increase the likelihood that patients and families are satisfied with the process and outcomes of care.

CARE OF THE IMMINENTLY DYING PATIENT

The transition to the actively dying phase should be recognized and explicitly communicated to the patient, family, and care providers. If the patient is at home, hospice nurses can be a key resource to families at this time. Many families worry about whether they will know when the person is actively dying. They are fearful of uncontrolled pain and other suffering and are greatly reassured by an explanation of the normal process of dying, which involves increasing sleepiness, gradual onset of coma, irregular respirations, and a peaceful death. In the small percentage of patients with escalating pain or agitated delirium near death, provide assurance that, when necessary, these symptoms are effectively managed by concentrated oral liquid opioids, benzodiazepines, and antipsychotics that are easy for family members to administer in the home. By understanding the signs and symptoms of impending death and knowing how to address the symptoms that do arise, physicians can explain to family members what to expect and reassure them that their loved one will receive good care.

While each person experiences the final stages differently, common symptoms exist. These terminal symptoms include progressive weakness and fatigue, loss of appetite, dehydration, and drowsiness. Family members often want to feed patients who are unable to eat. Although physicians may recognize that feeding will not help the patient and may even harm by leading to aspiration, they must also recognize that feeding is a primary means of nurturing. Physicians can encourage small sips, ice chips, easy to swallow foods such as ice cream, and promotion of other means of demonstrating human care, such as mouth and skin care. Most patients are unable to drink in their final days and many families ask about intravenous fluids. During the dying process, artificial hydration can lead to pulmonary edema and dyspnea, ascites, peripheral edema, and infections at intravenous catheter sites and should be discouraged. Symptoms including dry mouth and thirst can be addressed by attentive oral care, such as ice chips, artificial saliva, and cleansing. Because patients may become unable to take medications orally, the sublingual, transdermal, rectal, and subcutaneous routes may be used. If the patient is incontinent of urine, diapers and heavy towels may be used to avoid catheterization, but catheterization may provide comfort and skin protection and relieve a major care burden for the family.

Changes in respiratory patterns are common in imminently dying patients. Breathing usually becomes shallow as death nears and periods of apnea are common. Secretions that accumulate in the pharynx due to the patient being too weak or unresponsive to swallow or cough can produce a rattling sound that can be distressing to the family. Deep suctioning should be avoided, as it can lead to gagging and may be uncomfortable. Glycopyrrolate, atropine, or scopolamine can be effective in reducing rattle by decreasing the amount of mucus and saliva produced. Rooms should be cool and well ventilated, and a fan can aid in reducing the sensation of dyspnea. It may be appropriate to stop taking blood pressure and monitor only respiratory rate and pulse in order to avoid disturbing the patient. The pulse rate typically increases and is weak and irregular in the final hours to days of life.

Drowsiness and decreased responsiveness is common, and, rarely, patients become confused or agitated. When possible, confusion or agitation should be treated according to the cause. If the patient is experiencing agitation due to increased pain, pain should be treated with opioids as appropriate; if the pain is thought to be due to dyspnea, it should be treated with oxygen and opioids. Behavioral interventions such as brushing a patient's hair or providing music therapy can be highly effective in treating agitation. When these measures do not work and the cause is uncertain, agitation should be treated with low doses of neuroleptics, such as haloperidol (or if more sedation is needed, chlorpromazine).

ETHICAL AND LEGAL CONSIDERATIONS

Ethical and legal issues commonly arise in palliative care. Advance care planning can help communicate patient preferences across different health care settings and should be discussed early in the course of any serious or chronic illness. In such discussions, physicians should encourage patients to appoint surrogate decision makers and educate them on how to make decisions and discuss choices with their loved one. All physicians should follow accepted ethical principles including respect for autonomy, acting in the patient's best interest, avoiding harm, treating patients equally, and maintaining confidentiality. At the point when the patient is no longer able to express his wishes, the team should turn to the patient's trusted decision maker and his or her previously expressed wishes to help guide care. Palliative care teams also discuss with patients and families the need for wills, guardianship agreements, and financial documentation prior to the loss of decision-making capacity.

Some patients may make requests for their physicians to assist them to die. Such requests for aid in dying are often triggered by pain, depression, or other distress. Physicians must address these issues whenever a patient raises the matter of assisted suicide; treating pain and depression and making referrals to hospice can help to allay some of the patient's concerns. Physician aid in dying is legal in the states of Oregon and Washington, with strict and specific safeguards.

COMPLICATIONS

In palliative care, many drugs used for symptom management can cause neuropsychiatric side effects, as they either directly or indirectly affect the central nervous system. If unrecognized, these effects can generate considerable suffering and iatrogenic harm to patients. Side effects of commonly used palliative care medications include delirium, drug-induced parkinsonism, akathisia, serotonin syndrome, and neuroleptic malignant syndrome. Antiemetics such as metoclopramide and haloperidol can cause significant levels of neuropsychiatric toxicity and should be carefully monitored and the drug discontinued if necessary. Many drugs induce delirium, including anxiolytics, opioids, antidepressants, antihistamines, steroids, antipsychotics, and antibiotics (fluoroquinolones such as ciprofloxacin). Timing of administration of medications can help determine the offending agent. If the offending medication or medications remain necessary to treat other distressing symptoms such as pain, management of delirium with neuroleptics, opioid rotation, and hydration may be helpful.

DISCHARGE CONSIDERATIONS

Prior to discharge with hospice, evaluation of home safety and equipment needs is required. Necessary supplies including hospital beds, oxygen, commodes, and shower chairs should be delivered prior to patient arrival, and the hospital team must ensure that a family member or friend is at the home to accept delivery. If the patient requires ambulance transport home, the timing of arrival should be carefully considered (ie, time the ambulance arrival when young children are at school). Most transport companies allow a family member to travel with the patient if he is going home with hospice. For opioid prescriptions, the hospital team should confirm who will prescribe opioids for the patient after discharge and verify that the patient's pharmacy actually carries the medication. For opioids, a quantity must be specified (ie, cannot write "one-month supply"). Patients on opioids should not be discharged until the prescription is filled and available at home, as it is often difficult to find a pharmacy that carries these medicines, particularly in poor neighborhoods. Prior authorization from insurance companies may be required for some new medications or large quantities, therefore this should be discussed prior to discharge. Finally, it is prudent to discuss prognosis (eg, hours to days, days to weeks, weeks to months) with patient and family. Some patients and families may opt to attempt to have their loved one get home prior to death, even if death is en route. Other families may choose to remain in the hospital when death is imminent. Families should be guided in the important developmental tasks of this stage of life including conducting important conversations while the patient is still able to participate. Many teams provide family members with a written list of the "five things" to think through and discuss as applicable when a loved one is dying: thank you; forgive me; I forgive you; I love you: goodbye (Byock, 2004). Depending upon their age and wishes, children may visit after being prepared for what they will see. It may be helpful to encourage children to draw a picture or write a letter to the patient expressing their feelings toward them, as a means of saying goodbye.

QUALITY IMPROVEMENT

Health care organizations are beginning to use palliative care to improve quality because it is an effective approach to reducing symptoms and improving patient and family satisfaction. In addition, the use of palliative care services can improve transitions of care, support timely and successful discharge, avert unnecessary readmissions, and contribute to efficient use of health care resources. Many hospitals now use palliative care programs to help meet pain management and other quality accreditation standards.

CONCLUSION

Palliative care aims for the relief of suffering caused by physical, psychosocial, and spiritual aspects of disease and utilizes an interdisciplinary team to provide care. By focused symptom management and clear goals of care, patients living with advanced illness can improve quality of life and spend valuable time with friends, family, and loved ones.

SUGGESTED READINGS

Block SD. Perspectives on care at the close of life. Psychological considerations, growth, and transcendence at the end of life: the art of the possible. *JAMA* 2001;285(22):2898–2905.

Byock I. *The Four Things that Matter Most: A Book about Living.* New York: Free Press 2004.

Goldberg GR, Morrison RS. Pain management in hospitalized cancer patients: a systematic review. *J Clin Oncol.* 2007;25(13):1792–1801.

Kagawa-Singer M, Blackhall LJ. Negotiating cross-cultural issues at the end of life: "You got to go where he lives". *JAMA.* 2001;286(23):2993–3001.

Lamont EB, Christakis NA. Complexities in prognostication in advanced cancer: "to help them live their lives the way they want to". *JAMA.* 2003;290(1):98–104.

Morrison RS, Meier DE. Clinical practice. Palliative care. *N Engl J Med.* 2004;350(25):2582–2590.

Prigerson HG, Maciejewski PK, Reynolds CF, et al. Inventory of complicated grief: A scale to measure maladaptive symptoms of loss. *Psychiatry Research.* 1995;59(1–2):65–79.

Steinhauser KE, Christakis NA, Clipp EC, et al. Factors considered important at the end of life by patients, family, physicians, and other care providers. *JAMA.* 2000;284(19):2476–2482.

Sulmasy DP. Spiritual issues in the care of dying patients: "… it's okay between me and god". *JAMA.* 2006;296(11):1385–1392.

Teno JM, Clarridge BR, Casey V, et al. Family perspectives on end-of-life care at the last place of care. *JAMA.* 2004;291(1):88–93.

CHAPTER 216

Structure and Process: Communication

Amanda L. Caissie, MD, PhD
Camilla Zimmermann, MD, PhD, FRCPC

Key Clinical Questions

1. What are some practical methods of breaking bad news at any stage of disease?
2. How do you maintain hope while discussing goals of care in the context of a poor prognosis?

INTRODUCTION

Palliative care requires excellent communication skills. Clinicians navigate difficult situations including prognostication, breaking bad news, discussing hospice, and planning for the end of life, while acknowledging and addressing physical, psychological, and spiritual distress for both the patient and family. Communication strategies vary based on the individual preferences of the patient and family, cultural norms, the context of the situation, and the patient's stage of disease. The latter may be divided broadly among the time of diagnosis, the transition toward palliative care, and the time leading up to and including the patient's death. This chapter will describe approaches to communication for situations that arise commonly in the treatment of patients with life-threatening illnesses.

GENERAL COMMUNICATION SKILLS

Communication skills are essential for all physicians, as they develop rapport, gather and relay information, and help patients make informed decisions. Although communication in medicine often involves the family as well as the patient, this is particularly the case in palliative care. The parties involved often have divergent perspectives, stemming from diverse generational, educational, socioeconomic, cultural, and spiritual backgrounds, that can have a profound effect on physician–patient/family interactions. It is important not to generalize and to realize that diverse viewpoints may coexist within any one seemingly similar group. For this reason it is essential to elicit individual communication preferences, rather than assuming that these fall neatly into a specific category.

All clinical interactions have emotional as well as informational elements. Effective communication requires that clinicians recognize their own emotions in addition to those of patients and families. Likewise, communication has verbal and nonverbal components, and it is important to recognize and respond to nonverbal cues in addition to listening for verbal ones and eliciting concerns. Respect and empathy are paramount, and both can be expressed verbally or nonverbally in very little time. In contrast to entering a room looking at the chart instead of the patient, the simple gesture of making introductions to everyone present speaks volumes as one begins the clinical relationship.

Open-ended questions promote greater understanding and are used to start the "ask-tell-ask" approach, which lends itself to almost any clinical interaction (Back, et al, 2008). When first communicating with a patient about a particular issue, such as diagnosis or prognosis, start by asking what the patient understands about her illness. After assessing what the patient knows (and identifying and acknowledging any associated emotions), tell the patient any additional information and/or clarify misconceptions. Perhaps most importantly, follow up by asking another question to both ensure that the patient understands and that you have understood the emotional impact on the patient. When in doubt, it is useful at ask, "Do you have any questions?"

BREAKING BAD NEWS

The communication of bad news is difficult for both the clinician and patient. Although most studies regarding strategies for breaking bad news have focused on the time of diagnosis, there are various stages in the disease trajectory where this situation may apply. For patients with cancer, for example, this may include each successive time that the cancer progresses on a certain treatment,

TABLE 216-1 SPIKES Protocol for Delivering Bad News

Setting up the interview:
Arrange for privacy.
Involve significant others.
Sit down.
Make connection with the patient.
Manage time constraints and interruptions.
Assess the patient's *perception:*
What does the patient know?
Obtain the patient's *invitation:*
How much does the patient want to know?
Give *knowledge* and information to the patient:
Warn the patient that bad news is coming (eg, "Unfortunately, I have some bad news to tell you.")
Start at the level of comprehension and vocabulary of the patient.
Use nontechnical words.
Avoid excessive bluntness.
Give information in small portions, and check for the patients understanding.
Address the patient's *emotions* with empathic responses.
Summarize and *strategize:*
Check the patient's understanding.
Ask if the patient is ready at that time to discuss a plan.
Make a treatment plan.

Data from Baile WF, Buckman R, Lenzi R, et al. SPIKES–a six-step protocol for delivering bad news: application to the patient with cancer. *Oncologist.* 2000;5:302–311.

the news that no further chemotherapy is indicated, and the news that the prognosis is short. While each situation will be different, it is useful to develop a core communication strategy that can be tailored to the circumstances.

The SPIKES protocol is a practical method for breaking bad news at any stage of disease (**Table 216-1**). It is easy to use and applicable to almost any clinical communication situation. Addressing the patient's emotions is typically the most difficult aspect for physicians. It is important for patients to feel that the emotional impact of the news is acknowledged; this can be achieved by the use of a simple statement such as, "I know that this is very difficult news for you." A mnemonic that is helpful in this regard is NURSE: name the emotion, understand and respect the emotion, support the patient, and explore the emotion.

The dreaded phrase "nothing else can be done" is a fallacy and should not be used. In addition to supportive medical treatments, emotional and social supports can always be offered and are interventions in themselves. Indeed, one may argue that the physician–patient/family relationship is one of the most valuable components of therapy regardless of disease stage.

THE REQUEST TO WITHHOLD BAD NEWS

Requests to withhold bad news about a diagnosis or prognosis may come directly from the patient or, more often, from the family. In survey studies, most patients report that they want to know information about their disease and prognosis even if it is bad news. If a family requests nondisclosure, one should attempt to identify possible reasons for this request and whether it reflects the desire of the patient. Reasons may range from cultural norms regarding family-based decisions to beliefs that discussing a poor prognosis will make it come true or destroy a patient's hope. At times the family is concerned about disclosure, when in reality the patient already knows or would want to know if given the option.

According to the principle of autonomy, the patient should have the right to choose whether to be told information about his illness. The first step in communicating bad news is, therefore, to assess how much information a patient would like to know. For patients who do not speak English, a translator should be used, rather than relying on the family for translation. It is helpful to begin with an opening statement about information that is known to the patient such as, "As you know, we have performed a number of tests." Further dialogue may proceed as follows: "Would you like to know detailed information about your illness, or are there aspects that you would prefer not to know?" If the patient requests the information, one may wish to add a confirmatory statement such as, "I unfortunately have bad news for you. Would you like me to continue?"

The amount of information patients want may depend on social factors such as cultural background and level of assimilation, as well as individual factors such as not being ready to cope with the information. For the minority of patients who do not want to know their diagnosis and/or prognosis, one must respect this and try to understand their decision. Permission may then be obtained from the patient to discuss the situation and treatment plan with an appointed family member. It is important, however, to stress that disclosure to the patient may be necessary for informed consent for certain treatments and procedures. If there is conflict about disclosure, a hospital ethics consultation should be sought. Patients who do not want to know clinical information at a given time should be given the invitation to ask questions at any point in the future.

PROGNOSTIC DISCLOSURE

"How long do I have, Doctor?" is probably one of the most dreaded questions physicians are asked. However, it is an important question to answer, as it will help patients and families to prioritize and plan for the limited time ahead. Prognostication involves the discussion of the probable course and outcome of an illness. This is not limited to a discussion of the likely duration of survival, but includes discussion of the symptoms and situations that may occur as a result of the illness and an explanation of the goals, benefits, and risks of possible treatments.

Communication of prognosis is central to patient education and is necessary for informed consent and shared decision making. Patients may make different choices regarding investigations or active treatments if they are properly informed, rather than relying on their own preconceptions. In the Study to Understand Prognoses and Preferences for Outcomes and Risks of Treatment (SUPPORT), where explicit prognostic information was provided, patients were more likely to discuss advance directives and less likely to desire cardiopulmonary resuscitation (CPR) if they felt prognosis was "poor." Disclosure of prognosis is important not only because it respects patient autonomy in terms of medical decisions, but also because it affords the patient and family an opportunity to fulfill plans such as attending a family member's wedding, traveling to see friends or family, or saying goodbyes, and to deal with practical issues such as assigning power of attorney, making a will, and preparing funeral arrangements.

Physicians are constantly formulating a prognosis when making treatment decisions, but often do not explicitly communicate this information to the patient. Although clinical predictions are often optimistic, physicians are generally able to identify patients with less than three to six months to live. Barriers to disclosing the prognosis may include a focus on diagnosis or treatment, lack of formal education around prognostication, lack of self confidence, beliefs in a

TABLE 216-2 Discussing Prognosis

Determine the patient's understanding of the prognosis.
Ask the patient how much information she wants to know about prognosis.
Explain that any prognosis is an estimate and that exact information is not possible.
Explain that the prognosis is dynamic and changes with time.
Give a prognosis that is not too exact or too vague (eg, "measured in months" rather than "six months")
Present the information honestly while demonstrating empathy.
Discuss what may occur in the future regarding symptoms and what arrangements should be made.
Emphasize the clinician-patient connection and resources available to the patient and family.
Check understanding of the patient and encourage questions.
Book a follow-up appointment to address outstanding questions.
Document the discussion in the chart.
Ensure consistency of information communicated by various members of the clinical team.

self-fulfilling prophecy, attempts to maintain patient hope, difficulty dealing with emotional issues, time constraints, and fear regarding medicolegal implications of predictions. Given the importance that patients place on timely and empathic disclosure of prognosis, it is important to be aware of these barriers so that they may be addressed.

There are many tools available to assist with prognostication. These range from performance status scales, such as the Karnofsky performance status scale and Eastern Cooperative Oncology Group scale, to detailed tools incorporating information such as age, gender, performance status, comorbidity, symptoms, diagnosis, and laboratory results. For patients with cancer, visceral and brain metastases are poor prognostic factors, as are symptoms such as dyspnea, anorexia, and delirium and laboratory values such as hypercalcemia, leukocytosis, and hypoalbuminemia. Although these tools are useful for clinicians in determining prognosis, they must be supplemented and individualized with clinical experience and knowledge.

Communication of the prognosis is not a one-time occurrence, but a dynamic process that continues on an ongoing basis throughout the disease trajectory. The SPIKES protocol may be used as a general framework for communicating prognosis; specific guidelines are presented in **Table 216-2**.

It is likely that the patient already has some perception of the prognosis, which may be based on conversations with other clinicians or friends or on information from the Internet or other sources. Sometimes the patient has a sound understanding, and other times expectations appear to be entirely unrealistic. It is important to elicit and acknowledge the patient's understanding of the situation as well as to gauge how much prognostic information she wants to know and to what level of detail. Although some patients desire exact information, it should be emphasized that a prognosis is always an estimate and that the situation may change with time. Other patients may desire very little prognostic information and this should be respected provided that the goals of care are discussed and appropriate plans are made for the patient and family.

ESTABLISHING GOALS OF CARE

The discussion of prognosis is inextricable from the discussion of goals of care. These should be readdressed frequently throughout the patient's disease course and individualized based on the stage of disease and unique characteristics of the patient. An individual's values will influence how they prioritize goals of care, and two patients with a similar prognosis may desire very different courses of treatment. For example, whether a patient will accept or decline life-prolonging treatment will depend on how he prioritizes the goals of prolonged duration of life compared with minimization of treatment side effects, symptom control, and quality of life. Illness may also change one's perceptions and treatment preferences. One study found that patients with advanced cancer were more likely to accept second-line chemotherapy treatments with only slight potential benefit and substantial potential side effects than what oncologists or healthy counterparts imagine accepting in the patient's situation.

What physicians think they convey in terms of information is not always what the patient perceives. MacKillop and colleagues (1988) showed that while over 90% of physicians felt they had accurately conveyed the extent of disease and intent of treatment, almost one-third of patients with metastatic disease thought their disease was localized, and almost one-third of patients on palliative treatment thought the intent was curative. This may result from a misunderstanding of medical information: terms such as *curable, controlled*, or *terminal* disease need to be explained to avoid miscommunication. Other patients and families may understand the palliative nature of the medical treatment, but hope for a miracle or cure. It is important for clinicians to realize that such seemingly contradictory thinking is common and is a manner of coping with the illness. Often patients or families will ask several clinicians the same questions about prognosis; it is, therefore, important that all members of a clinical team are communicating the same information in a consistent fashion.

Many physicians are concerned about destroying hope when discussing goals of care in the context of poor prognosis. If the physician is honest in informing patients when they are passing through various stages of their disease, there is a wide spectrum of realistic hopes that patients may have depending on the situation, ranging from cure or prolonged life to finding meaning in life, quality of life, symptom control, spending time with loved ones, and dying peacefully with dignity. A clinical pearl of communication is, "Hope for the best, prepare for the worst," which acknowledges that hope can be sustained while also planning for the occurrence of clinical situations that may evolve quickly (Back, et al, 2008).

END-OF-LIFE PLANNING DISCUSSIONS

Most patients in Western countries would like to be involved in their health care decisions. Although the focus of end-of-life discussions is often on code status or on planning for a crisis situation, there are many other decisions that need to be made. These include preferences about the extent of investigations, aggressiveness of treatment, hospice enrollment, place of death, organ donation, and religious rites to be performed prior to or after death. As important as what to do in the case of incompetence is how to proceed with care while the patient is competent and able. This requires that the patient understand the nature of the underlying illness and the consequences of treatment at any given time. For example, there is a time in the course of illness when treatment of hyperkalemia can be life saving, and another when it will produce added suffering without appreciably increasing life expectancy. In order for discussions about end-of-life preferences to be effective, the patient needs to gain an appreciation for the extent of his or her underlying illness, and the physician needs to understand the cultural and individual preferences of the patient. Thus, end-of-life discussions are always conversations, rather than information sessions.

ADVANCE DIRECTIVES

Advance directives provide an opportunity for patients to state their preferences for care while they are capable of doing so. The Patient Self Determination Act (PSDA) became effective in the United States in 1991 and requires that Medicare and Medicaid providers (eg, hospitals, nursing homes, and home health agencies) provide information to patients at the time of enrollment on their rights regarding advance directives. These include the right to participate in their health care decisions, the right to accept or refuse treatment, the right to prepare an advance directive, and the right to information on providers' policies regarding these rights. Unlike other legally binding documents, advance directives can be completed without an attorney, which facilitates their implementation.

Advance directives typically consist of a living will and the assignment of a substitute decision maker, or durable power of attorney, who will make decisions for a patient in the case of incompetence. Although the number of patients with completed advance directives has increased substantially since the passage of the PSDA, approximately half of all severely or terminally ill patients still lack advance directives. This may be due to a patient's lack of understanding of his prognosis, a lack of awareness of the existence and process for completion of an advance directive, or a perceived lack of relevance to the patient's situation. Physicians should be honest with patients regarding their prognosis, inform them about the availability of advanced directives and their importance, and indicate their willingness to discuss any medical issues that arise during or after the completion of the advanced directive.

Living will

The living will states the patient's preferences for care and serves not only to maintain patient autonomy, but also to minimize the burden of decision making on families faced with the emotionally charged situation of a loved one who is near death. Typically, the directive has instructions regarding whether life-sustaining treatment should be given and may have specific directions regarding the use of CPR, mechanical ventilation, tube feeding, and use of antibiotics. In order for these directives to be meaningful, it is important to explain to patients what these various life-sustaining procedures are, and how they would or would not contribute to quality and/or quantity of life in the patient's situation. Many patients do not inform their physicians that they have an advance directive or living will, and this needs to be specifically asked about so that physicians can discuss patients' answers and clarify any misinterpretations. As the patient's situation changes, the living will may need to be updated.

Durable power of attorney

Regardless of whether a living will is completed, it is important for patients to assign a durable power of attorney. If patients have not made such an assignment, then the law in Canada and in certain areas of the United States outlines a hierarchy of substitute decision makers for patients who are incapacitated (**Table 216-3**).

However, the first person on a hierarchy list may not be the one the patient would have chosen, and may not share similar viewpoints or values. At times, a patient may want to protect his loved ones and prefers not to discuss his medical situation with them. This becomes problematic when a person who has not been involved in the care of the patient is later acting as a substitute decision maker. In addition, substitute decision makers often inaccurately predict the patient's wishes (eg, believing that a patient would want more interventions than they actually would). For these reasons, it is useful for physicians to meet with patients and their assigned power of attorney to clarify wishes for care. The documentation of these wishes in the living will as well as in the patient's chart can help avoid misunderstandings and ensure that future care proceeds as the patient desires.

TABLE 216-3 Substitute Decision Maker in Approximate Order of Priority*

1. Durable power of attorney for health care
2. Spouse
3. Legal guardian
4. Adult child (18 years or older)†
5. Parent
6. Sibling (18 years of age or older)†
7. Close friend (only in certain states)

*Order may vary from state to state; if it is not clear who should make decisions, consult with the hospital ethics board.

†If there are several family members with the same priority, then decisions are made by consensus, by majority, or by chosing one member who is responsible for making decisions on behalf of the group.

Code status

Studies have shown that physicians are concerned about futile interventions at the end of life, and that most patients want to be involved in decisions about CPR. In a study focusing on American veterans who died from cancer, families reported higher satisfaction with end-of-life care when the patient had a do-not-resuscitate (DNR) order at the time of death. However, many physicians are uncomfortable initiating discussions about code status, and patients generally do not spontaneously ask about this subject. Although the majority of patients are competent when admitted to the hospital, DNR orders are usually either not written at all or written when the patient is no longer competent to make medical decisions. Therefore, discussions regarding code status often occur with the family and with substitute decision makers rather than with patients themselves. **Table 216-4** outlines a framework for these types of discussions.

The approach to discussing code status is important and may dictate the outcome. If one approaches a code discussion with the question, "Would you want everything done in the event of…", then most patients and family members understandably request a full code. Ideally, code status preferences are already indicated in a living will, and it is important to ask on admission to the hospital whether an advance directive exists. If so, then the advance directive should be reviewed and the patient's preferences should be documented. If there is no advance directive, then a discussion needs to take place with the patient and/or power of attorney to review the patient's underlying condition and overall prognosis, explain what is involved in CPR, and outline what the outcomes typically are for patients in a similar situation. Success rates of CPR are low, with a chance of survival to discharge from hospital of approximately 15%. Conditions such as metastatic cancer, renal failure, sepsis, or reduced performance status diminish the prognosis considerably. This may not be understood by patients or families, whose impression of the outcome of CPR may be based on overly optimistic scenarios depicted in movies or on television.

At times, orders are written that are variations of the "full code" or DNR orders. This is not ideal, as confusion may arise in the midst of a code when an order such as "chest compressions, and defibrillation but no intubation" exists. The actions taken at the time of a code are stepwise and often automatic, potentially resulting in

TABLE 216-4 A Framework for Discussions of Code Status and End-of-Life Care with Families

Determine whether the patient has an advance directive.
Schedule a family meeting to discuss the patient's condition and clarify the family's understanding of the illness.
If there is no durable power of attorney, determine who is the substitute decision-maker (SDM).
Remind the SDM of his obligation to act in the patient's best interest, taking into account the patient's values rather than the SDM's own preferences.
Explain the patient's underlying condition and prognosis.
Explain the nature and outcome of cardiopulminary resuscitation.
Explain and discuss specific procedures and treatments.
Summarize what will or will not be done and answer any questions.
Assure the family that the patient's comfort and dignity will be respected and that appropriate management of symptoms will continue.
Inform the family of how to contact you if they have further questions.
Document the discussion and outcome in the patient's medical record.
Continue to review and revise the plan as needed.

unwanted interventions if DNR orders are not clear or if a variation on the order exists. Increasingly, hospitals and other health care institutions have protocols regarding code status, including exactly which order should be written. Conversely, one should not assume that because a DNR order exists, the patient does not desire any other therapeutic interventions. Specific treatments should be discussed in detail with the patient or substitute decision maker, so that a complete understanding can be reached about what is desired. This also serves to allay patients' fears that their care will be inferior if a DNR order exists. Finally, it is important to emphasize that the patient will not be abandoned and that care will continue for pain and symptom management in addition to support for the patient and family.

DISCUSSING HOSPICE AND PALLIATIVE CARE

Communicating the roles of hospice and palliative care to patients and families is a challenge in itself. When the hospice and palliative care movements were established in the 1960s and 1970s, the focus was mainly on care at the end of life. The role of palliative care has since broadened, as indicated by the most recent World Health Organization definition (**Table 216-5**).

Contemporary palliative care focuses on quality of life as well as dignity in death and is complementary to, not exclusive of, therapies directed at the underlying illness. Hospice is more limited, due to what is or is not covered by the Medicare hospice benefit. The Medicare hospice benefit was established in 1983 and is available to patients with a prognosis of six months or less to live and the desire to receive the benefits of hospice services while forgoing disease-directed treatment. Both palliative care and hospice employ an interdisciplinary approach with expertise from fields such as medicine, nursing, social work, physiotherapy, occupational therapy, and spiritual care, and provide support to both the patient and the family. Hospice also includes services such as homemakers, medications, supplies, and equipment; care may occur at home or in a hospice facility, nursing home, or hospital.

TABLE 216-5 World Health Organization Definition of *Palliative Care*

Palliative care

- Provides relief from pain and other distressing symptoms.
- Affirms life and regards dying as a normal process.
- Intends neither to hasten or postpone death.
- Integrates the psychological and spiritual aspects of patient care.
- Offers a support system to help patients live as actively as possible until death.
- Offers a support system to help the family cope during the patient's illness and in their own bereavement.
- Uses a team approach to address the needs of patients and their families, including bereavement counseling, if indicated.
- Will enhance quality of life and may also positively influence the course of illness.
- Is applicable early in the course of illness in conjunction with other therapies that are intended to prolong life, such as chemotherapy or radiation therapy, and includes those investigations needed to better understand and manage distressing clinical complications.

Reproduced, with permission, from World Health Organization's Definition of *Palliative Care*. Available at http://www.who.int/cancer/palliative/definition/en.

HOSPICE

Referrals to hospice typically occur very late, and only approximately one-third of Americans die under hospice care (Glare & Sinclair, 2008). This may be due to a lack of understanding of the prognosis on the part of the clinician or patient and/or the lack of coverage by many hospices of costly services such as palliative chemotherapy, palliative radiation, and blood transfusions. For patients who are not willing to forgo such treatments, the prognosis and goals of care should be clarified. If these are understood and a patient still refuses referral to hospice, then another option is simultaneous palliative care or a hospice bridge program, if available. The involvement of palliative care services prior to the discussion of hospice may help with the difficult communication issues that arise at this transition point. As with communicating other types of difficult news, it is important to acknowledge the emotional aspect of the discussions. Multiple discussions over time may be necessary before a patient will agree to a hospice referral.

PALLIATIVE CARE

While palliative care referrals can be placed at anytime, early referral (eg, at the diagnosis of metastatic disease for patients with cancer) can optimize management of physical and psychological symptoms, link the patient with services that will be available in acute crises, and facilitate communication regarding end-of-life planning. Some patients are able to acknowledge their prognosis and are active participants in advance care planning. Such patients are generally appreciative of early referral to palliative care services and may even initiate the referral themselves. For others who have difficulty coming to terms with their prognosis, explicit discussions about palliative care may not be possible; for these patients, the referral may be better introduced in terms of management of specific symptoms. Paradoxically, it is often the latter group of patients who benefit most from specialized palliative care, as the palliative care team is able to support them through the psychological and physical distress they are experiencing. It is important to emphasize to the patient that unlike hospice, palliative care is not restricted to those with a limited prognosis. Patients can and should receive palliative care support if needed for symptom control during disease-directed treatments such as chemotherapy.

COMMUNICATION IN THE LAST DAYS AND HOURS OF LIFE

In the last days and hours of life, the patient's desire for information inevitably diminishes compared with their need for emotional support. The family, on the other hand, requires a great deal of communication and information to prepare for the patient's death. If possible, the family will need forewarning that death is imminent in order to prepare emotionally as well as practically for issues such as time spent with the patient and preferences regarding religious or cultural practices. It is important to obtain contact information for the loved ones who would like to be with the patient in her last days to hours, so that they can be informed when death is near. If feasible, arranging for more privacy at this time will help not only the patient and family but also surrounding patients.

Even in the last days and hours of life, some families find it difficult to accept that the end of life is near. If the patient is imminently dying and the cause is irreversible, it is important to meet formally with the family to address any outstanding concerns and emphasize the goals of care. Once the patient and family have acknowledged that the prognosis is short and the goal of care is comfort, they will need explicit guidance regarding what to expect during the dying process. It is important to explain that patients will likely stop eating and drinking and that verbal communication will likely cease as sleep increases. The family may feel helpless at this point and will take comfort in knowing that they are helping simply with their presence or with small gestures such as assistance with the patient's mouth care.

A pain-free and peaceful death is an obvious goal of palliative care, but bereavement care should not be overlooked. The family is integral to the therapeutic relationship and will retain memories of the patient's illness, and of the day of death, long after their loved one has died. The support and preparation of the family by the health care team can make a large difference in rendering these memories as positive as possible.

PRACTICE POINT

1. Determine what the patient understands and how much she would like to know before telling her new information.
2. During and after clinical interactions, ensure that the patient understands the plan and that you have understood the emotional impact on the patient.
3. Avoid expressions such as, "nothing else can be done." Instead, emphasize what can be done in terms of palliation, and reassure the patient and family that they will not be abandoned.
4. Initiate conversations about advance care planning, palliative care, and hospice early in the course of illness.
5. Ensure that there is consistency in the clinical team when discussing prognosis and the treatment plan.
6. Respect a patient's hopes while encouraging plans for the future: "Hope for the best; prepare for the worst."

CONCLUSION

Communication is important in any clinical discipline but particularly in palliative care, as the information conveyed often involves bad news and evokes emotions in all participants of the clinical interaction. These emotions need to be acknowledged and addressed with empathy in order for a therapeutic relationship to ensue. This is a stage when many important decisions are made, not only for palliative treatment and advance care planning, but also for personal projects and goals. Patients and families appreciate honest, open communication that nonetheless leaves room for hope and promises nonabandonment. Despite the difficulty of these discussions, they can be very meaningful, and will have a lasting impact on all involved.

SUGGESTED READINGS

Back AL, Anderson WG, Bunch L, et al. Communication about cancer near the end of life. *Cancer*. 2008;113(S7):1897–1910.

Balmer CE, Thomas P, Osborne RJ. Who wants second-line, palliative chemotherapy? *Psychooncology*. 2001;10(5):410–418.

Covinsky KE, Fuller JD, Yaffe K, et al. Communication and decision-making in seriously ill patients: findings of the SUPPORT project. The Study to Understand Prognoses and Preferences for Outcomes and Risks of Treatments. *J Am Geriatr Soc*. 2000;48 (5 Suppl):S187–S193.

Ehlenbach WJ, Barnato AE, Curtis JR, et al. Epidemiologic study of in-hospital cardiopulmonary resuscitation in the elderly. *N Engl J Med*. 2009;361:22–31.

Emanuel EJ, Emanuel LL. Proxy decision making. *JAMA*. 1992;267: 2221–2226.

Emanuel LL, Ferris FD, von Gunten CF, et al. EPEC-O: Education in Palliative and End-of-Life Care for Oncology. Participant's Handbook Module 9: Negotiating goals of care. Chicago, IL: *The EPEC Project*, 2005.

Finlay E, Casarett D. Making difficult discussions easier: using prognosis to facilitate transitions to hospice. CA; *Cancer J Clin*. 2009;59:250–263.

Glare PA, Sinclair CT. Palliative medicine review: prognostication. *Journal of Palliative Medicine*. 2008;11(1):84–103.

Mackillop WJ, Stewart WE, Ginsburg AD, et al. Cancer patients' perceptions of their disease and its treatment. *Br J Cancer*. 1988;58: 355–358.

Saraiya B, Bodnar-Deren S, Leventhal H, et al. End-of-life planning and its relevance for patients' and oncologists' decisions in choosing cancer therapy. *Cancer*. 2008;113(S12):3540–3547.

CHAPTER 217

Domains of Care: Physical Aspects of Care

Cindy Lien, MD

Key Clinical Questions

Pain

1. How do I choose an appropriate opioid dose for my patient?
2. What adjuvant medications can I use for neuropathic pain?
3. How do I treat a patient who is experiencing a pain crisis?
4. When should I consult a palliative care or pain specialist?

Nausea

1. How do I select an appropriate antiemetic for my patient?
2. How do I treat nausea in a patient with malignant bowel obstruction?

Dyspnea

1. What nonpharmacologic strategies can I use to relieve my patient's dyspnea?
2. What is an appropriate dose of opioid for treating dyspnea?
3. What do I say to family members who are concerned that morphine may hasten the patient's death?

Secretions

1. How do I manage loud secretions ("death rattle") in a dying patient?
2. What do I say to family members who are distressed by the noisy secretions?

(continued)

PAIN

INTRODUCTION

Studies of patient perspectives on end-of-life care universally report pain control as a major priority. Nonetheless, the literature shows that many patients with life-limiting illnesses experience poor pain control. In one well-known study (SUPPORT trial: Study to Understand Prognoses and Preferences for Outcomes and Risks of Treatments), approximately 40% of hospitalized patients experienced severe pain in the last three days before death.

When the focus of care is quality of life and comfort, any poorly controlled symptom should be treated as a medical emergency for that patient. Many patients already fear that pain will be an inevitable part of their disease process and that "nothing can be done." Hospitalists play a vital role in correcting this misconception and ensuring that patients with advanced illnesses receive adequate pain control.

PATHOPHYSIOLOGY

Pain can be described as nociceptive or neuropathic in origin. In nociceptive pain, peripheral nociceptors in the skin, musculoskeletal system, or viscera detect noxious stimuli and send impulses via afferent A-delta or C fibers to the dorsal horn of the spine. These signals are transmitted through ascending spinothalamic tracts to the thalamus and then to the cortex. Neuropathic pain occurs when the peripheral or central nervous system itself suffers damage or develops pathologic changes in sensitization. Neuropathic pain is generally more difficult to control than nociceptive pain. In reality, however, any type of chronic pain can significantly alter the sensory pathways and cause pathologic activation of the nervous system even after the initial pain stimulus has dissipated. The mechanisms of activation are quite complex and can involve central sensitization pathways, including multiple neurotransmitters (substance P, amino acid ligands), receptors (mu opioid, neurokinin-1, N-methyl-D-aspartate [NMDA]), and intracellular pathways (nitric oxide, protein kinase C).

It is important to recognize that the patient ultimately experiences pain not just as a physical phenomenon, but as an emotional experience. The International Association for the Study of Pain (IASP) has defined *pain* as "an unpleasant sensory and emotional experience associated with actual or potential tissue damage, or described in terms of such damage. While it is unquestionably a sensation in part or parts of the body, it is always unpleasant and therefore, an emotional experience." Patients with life-threatening illness are especially vulnerable to emotional and cognitive factors that can influence their experience of pain.

DIAGNOSIS: HOW DO I EVALUATE MY PATIENT'S PAIN?

Assessment of pain begins with a thorough history, including location, onset, duration, intensity, quality, and aggravating or ameliorating factors. The evaluation should also include a history of any associated functional decline, a psychosocial assessment (including exploration of any associated fears and concerns about disease progression), and a careful physical exam. The clinician should formulate a differential diagnosis of the clinical etiology of pain, which may include processes unrelated to the patient's known terminal disease. For example, chest pain in a patient with breast cancer could be due to bony metastases, postradiation skin

Key Clinical Questions

Terminal Delirium

1. How do I evaluate an agitated dying patient?
2. How do I identify terminal delirium and distinguish it from other kinds of delirium?
3. What medications are useful for treating terminal delirium?

Nutrition and Hydration

1. How do I counsel family members who are upset that the patient is no longer eating?
2. Are there any clinical situations in which artificial nutrition and hydration may be helpful for patients with advanced disease?

Complementary Medicine

1. Is there data to support the use of complementary therapy to relieve common symptoms such as pain and nausea?
2. How do I advise a patient who asks me about a therapy with which I am unfamiliar?

changes, cardiac ischemia, pulmonary embolism, costochrondritis, or gastroesophageal reflux disease.

The clinician should also determine the type of pain a patient is experiencing, as this will guide the appropriate treatment strategy.

- Nociceptive pain can be categorized as somatic or visceral. Somatic pain includes skin, musculoskeletal, or bone pain. It may be described as *sharp, constant, throbbing, aching*, and *exacerbated by movement*. It is usually well localized. Unlike somatic pain, visceral pain is generally poorly localized and arises from injury to organs or the lining of body cavities. It may be described as *cramping, aching, tearing, deep*, or a *pressure sensation*. Examples of visceral pain include symptoms from bowel obstruction, cholecystitis, or cardiac ischemia.
- Neuropathic pain can result from injury to any part of the nervous system, such as the peripheral nerves or spinal cord. Examples include postherpetic neuralgia, radiation-related brachial plexus injury, postthoracotomy pain, and phantom limb pain. Neuropathic pain is frequently described as *burning, tingling, stabbing, electric*, or *shooting*. It may also be described as *aching*. Physical findings may include allodynia, which is pain caused by a normally painless stimulus such as light touch. Neuropathic pain may also radiate.
- Some pathologic processes can cause a mixed pain syndrome that includes both nociceptive and neuropathic pain. One example is bone metastases to the spine, which may incite nociceptive, somatic bone pain as well as neuropathic pain from nerve root compression.

When a patient is unable to communicate, the clinician must then rely on the family or caregiver's report and careful observation for nonverbal cues, such as guarding or grimacing with movement, to assess pain. One common misconception is that a patient who exhibits no physiologic signs of discomfort (such as tachycardia or hypertension) is unlikely to be experiencing pain. In fact, patients with chronic pain rarely show these signs of sympathetic arousal. These physiologic changes are more typically seen in acute pain, though even some patients with acute pain do not exhibit these signs.

Several pain scales have been developed to monitor pain intensity and efficacy of treatment (**Figure 217-1**). Some patients may have no difficulty with the numerical pain scale, while others find it easier to report simplified categories of mild, moderate, or severe pain. Patients with mild cognitive deficits may be able to utilize the Faces Pain Scale, which was originally developed for pediatric patients.

Diagnostic tests should be tailored appropriately to a patient's overall goals of care. Generally, if a study has good potential to result in effective therapies (such as radiation) that would enhance

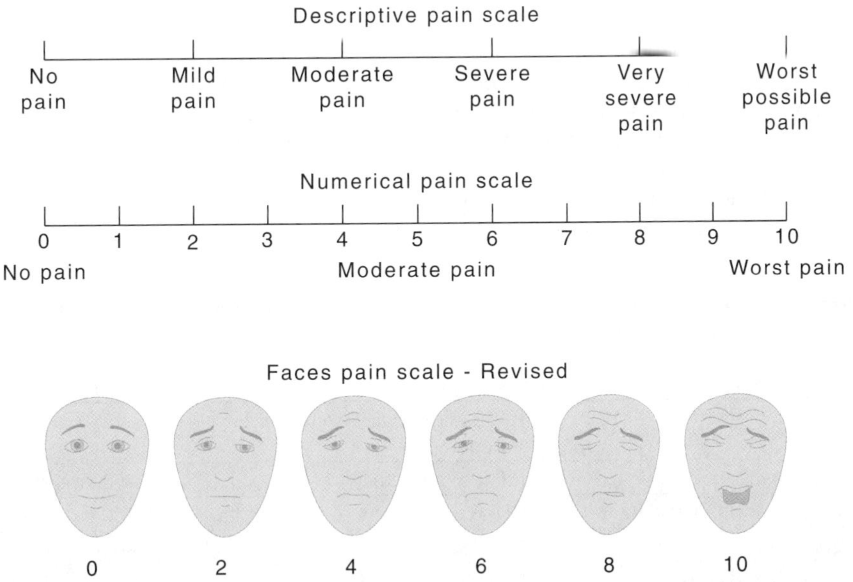

Figure 217-1 *Pain intensity scales. (From: Hicks CL, von Baeyer CL, Spafford P, van Korlaar I, Goodenough B. Faces Pain Scale-Revised: Toward a Common Metric in Pediatric Pain Measurement. Pain. 93:173, 2001. This figure has been reproduced with permission of the International Association for the Study of Pain® (IASP®). The figure may not be reproduced for any other purpose without permission. Instructions on administering the scale are available at www.painsourcebook.ca.)*

a patient's comfort, there may be reason to pursue the study even in the setting of advanced disease.

PRACTICE POINT

- New or worsening back pain in a patient with a history of malignancy warrants thorough evaluation including possible imaging.

TREATMENT

GENERAL PRINCIPLES

The World Health Organization (WHO) has developed a well-known analgesic ladder that recommends the use of nonopioid analgesics such as nonsteroidal anti-inflammatory drugs (NSAIDs) or acetaminophen for mild pain, with the addition of opioids for moderate and severe pain. The WHO ladder also recommends consideration of adjuvant therapies such as antidepressants and anticonvulsants at any level of pain if appropriate. One should keep in mind that many patients with terminal illness have at least moderate to severe pain and thus will need an opioid immediately in addition to nonopioid analgesics.

Treatment choice should also be guided by the type of pain. Opioids are generally effective for nociceptive pain, including both somatic and visceral types. Somatic pain such as musculoskeletal or bone pain may also be quite responsive to NSAID therapy. Bone pain may require a combination of additional therapies including bisphosphonates, corticosteroids, calcitonin, or radiation therapy. Visceral pain from bowel obstruction may warrant an antisecretory agent to reduce bowel distension, such as a somatostatin analogue (octreotide) or an anticholinergic (scopolamine, hyoscyamine).

Neuropathic pain is often less responsive to opioids and requires the use of adjuvant medications. **Table 217-1** shows common adjuvant medications for neuropathic pain.

The mainstays in neuropathic pain therapy include tricyclic antidepressants and anticonvulsants such as gabapentin. Other agents that may be effective for neuropathic pain include corticosteroids, autonomic drugs (clonidine, prazosin, terazosin), lidocaine patches, and capsaicin cream. NMDA receptor antagonists such as ketamine can be considered for intractable pain but would require administration by a pain specialist.

The side-effect profile may greatly influence one's choice of pain medication. NSAIDs are not recommended for those with significant risk of renal compromise, including patients who are elderly or have chronic kidney disease. Patients with multiple myeloma and a normal creatinine still carry a substantial risk for renal failure with NSAIDs. NSAIDs may also be contraindicated in patients at risk for gastrointestinal bleed or those on concomitant blood-thinning agents. Tricyclic antidepressants should be used cautiously in the elderly due to anticholinergic side effects. Nortriptyline is well studied and is generally considered the best tolerated tricyclic agent for the elderly, as it has the least anticholinergic activity. Opioids have some well-known side effects including constipation and sedation. However, because most patients with terminal illness will eventually need an opioid for adequate pain control, the clinician should become adept at dosing opioids and managing their side effects.

OPIOID ANALGESICS

Many clinicians have received little formal training in pain management and do not feel fully confident selecting and dosing opioids. This discomfort may be exacerbated by misconceptions about opioids on the part of both clinicians and patients. Opioids rarely cause respiratory depression when dosed appropriately for pain. Studies have shown that patients with underlying lung disease such as chronic obstructive pulmonary disease (COPD) can safely use opioids if dosed appropriately.

True opioid addiction is uncommon in terminally ill patients suffering from pain. Providers sometimes mistake behaviors like clock-watching or irritability as signs of addiction, but usually these are manifestations of pseudoaddiction in a patient receiving an inadequate pain regimen. These drug-seeking behaviors tend to cease when patients are given adequate doses at regular intervals.

Some patients and family members may not readily articulate their fears of opioid addiction. They may also worry that their disease is progressing or that they are "giving up" if they take opioids. Many patients directly associate morphine with dying. Clinicians should be attuned to these fears and educate their patients accordingly. It is also important to emphasize that pain medications will not advance one's disease, and may in fact improve function by reducing pain.

Selecting an opioid

Commonly used opioids include morphine, oxycodone, hydromorphone, fentanyl, and methadone. For most patients being initiated on opioids, there is not a compelling reason to choose, for example, hydromorphone over morphine. For certain patient populations, however, the choice of opioid does matter. Patients with significant renal failure should generally avoid morphine. The metabolites of morphine can accumulate in renal failure and cause neurotoxic side effects including myoclonus and delirium. Fentanyl and methadone are the safest opioids to use in renal failure patients including those on dialysis. Hydromorphone and oxycodone may be used cautiously in those with mild to moderate renal failure, with consideration of a reduction in dose or decrease in frequency. Similarly, patients with liver failure may need dose and frequency adjustments, but it is not

TABLE 217-1 Common Adjuvant Medications for Neuropathic Pain

Drug	Drug Class	Starting Dose	Usual Effective Dose
Gabapentin	Anticonvulsant	100–300 mg orally every night at bedtime*	300–1200 mg orally three times a day
Pregabalin	Anticonvulsant	150 mg orally daily	300–600 mg orally twice a day
Nortriptyline	Tricyclic antidepressant	10 mg orally every night at bedtime	50–150 mg orally every night at bedtime
Dexamethasone	Corticosteroid	4 mg orally twice a day	Variable
Lidocaine 5% patch	Topical local anesthetic	1 patch 12 hrs/day	1–3 patches 12 hours/day
Capsaicin cream	Topical substance P modulator	0.025% cream three times a day	0.025–0.075% three to four times a day

*Use low dose of gabapentin initially to minimize sedation, titrate every 3–7 days as tolerated. Maximum dose in renal impairment ~300 mg/day. Discuss dialysis dosing with pharmacy.

TABLE 217-2 Equianalgesic Opioid Doses

Drug	Oral	Intravenous
Morphine	30 mg	10 mg
Oxycodone	20 mg	—
Hydromorphone	7.5 mg	1.5 mg
Fentanyl*	—	0.1 mg (100 mcg)

*General rule of thumb for converting oral morphine equivalents to fentanyl patch: Divide the morphine oral total daily dose by 2 to calculate an approximate dose of fentanyl mcg/hr patch Example: morphine 50 mg total dose in 24 hrs ~ 25 mcg/hr fentanyl transdermal patch.

TABLE 217-3 Commonly Used Opioids: Moderate to Severe Pain in Opioid-naïve Patients

Drug	Initial Oral Dose*	Initial Intravenous Dose*
Morphine	7.5–15 mg every 4 hours	2–5 mg every 2 hours
Oxycodone	5–10 mg every 4 hours	
Hydromorphone	2–4 mg every 4 hours	0.3–1 mg every 2 hours

*Use the lower end of the dose range for elderly patients or patients with renal/liver compromise. Morphine is not recommended in patients with significant renal failure.

clear that one particular opioid is significantly safer than the others in this setting.

Studies have shown that methadone may play a useful role in patients with severe pain who have responded poorly to other opioids or who have developed intolerable side effects. Methadone has opioid receptor activity as well as some antagonist NMDA receptor activity. It has good bioavailability and no known active metabolites (thus accounting for its safety in renal failure). However, due to a long half-life and complexities in dosing ratios, it should generally be initiated by clinicians with prior training or in consultation with a specialist.

Certain opioids are almost never recommended. Both meperidine (Demerol) and propoxyphene (Darvon) should be avoided because their metabolites can accumulate with repeated dosing and cause serious neurotoxicity such as seizures. Codeine should not be used for severe pain because it has a "ceiling effect" whereby further titration results only in increased side effects without improved pain relief. Furthermore, codeine must first be metabolized to morphine to provide analgesia, and approximately 10% of the population lacks the appropriate hepatic enzyme. These patients derive no benefit from codeine.

Principles of opioid dosing

Equianalgesic doses: Different opioids have different potencies (ie, dose required to achieve a certain effect). Equianalgesic doses of two different opioids should achieve a similar degree of pain relief for most patients, although some patients may have idiosyncratic responses to different opioids due to genetically determined variations in metabolism. **Table 217-2** shows equianalgesic doses of commonly used opioids. Looking at the table, morphine 10 mg intravenously should achieve similar pain relief as morphine 30 mg orally and oxycodone 20 mg orally. Misconceptions that "morphine does not work but hydromorphone does" may arise from a lack of knowledge of equianalgesic doses. A patient who finds no relief with morphine 4 mg intravenously but responds well to hydromorphone 1 mg intravenously may have in fact needed a higher dose of morphine (hydromorphone 1 mg intravenously is equianalgesic to approximately morphine 6.6 mg intravenously).

General opioid dosing guidelines:

- **Table 217-3** lists reasonable starting doses and dosing intervals for moderate to severe pain in opioid-naive patients.
- **Figure 217-2** demonstrates opioid conversions using simple mathematical ratios.
- Patients with chronic pain will need a long-acting pain medication (eg, sustained-release oxycodone or morphine, fentanyl patch, or methadone), not just short-acting medications. If unable to use a long-acting pain medication, chronic pain patients should at least receive a standing pain regimen with as-needed availability.
- Patients on sustained-release medications should also have a short-acting medication for breakthrough pain. Each dose of breakthrough opioid should be approximately 10% to 20% of the total daily requirement of the sustained-release opioid.
- If greater than three doses of breakthrough pain medications are needed in a 24-hour period, one should consider increasing the amount of sustained-release opioid. An appropriate increase would be 50% to 100% of the total amount used for breakthrough pain in 24 hours.
- When switching between different opioids, some experts recommend a 25% to 50% dose reduction after one has calculated the equianalgesic dose. This is to account for a phenomenon called *incomplete cross tolerance*, in which a patient who has developed some tolerance to the old opioid may not have the same degree of tolerance to the new opioid. The dose reduction is intended to reduce the risk of undesirable side effects.

ACUTE PAIN CRISIS

Patients with terminal illness, particularly those with cancer, may suffer severe exacerbations of pain from bone metastases, pathologic fractures, bowel obstruction, or other manifestations of progressive disease. When a patient presents with severe, uncontrolled pain (7–10 intensity), this is considered an acute pain crisis or palliative care emergency. Clinicians should treat these symptoms aggressively while determining the underlying cause. The American Pain Society (APS) has published guidelines on rapid titration of opioids for severe cancer-related pain. **Figure 217-3** shows a treatment algorithm for severe pain that is adapted from the APS guidelines.

PRACTICE POINT

- Severe pain should be treated as a palliative care emergency.

OPIOID INFUSIONS

Infusions can be useful in certain settings but require a good understanding of basic principles.

- Opioid infusions should be used only when there is a specific indication. They should not be automatically started in a dying patient who is "comfort care" unless the patient has symptoms of discomfort.
- When using an opioid infusion to treat a patient who is not at the final stages of illness, the clinician should be attuned to patient fears that he or she may be actively dying. Many people associate a "morphine drip" with dying.

Your patient has been receiving hydromorphone 0.5-1 mg IV every two hours PRN during this hospitalization for pain due to bone metastases. You would like to initiate an appropriate oral regimen of both long-acting and short-acting medications.

Step 1: Determine the patient's total daily opioid requirement:
In this example, you review the record and calculate that your patient has been using an average of 6 mg IV hydromorphone per 24 hours for several days now.

Step 2: Convert to oral morphine equivalents using equianalgesic ratios:
You know that 1.5 mg IV hydromorphone is equianalgesic to 30 mg orally morphine. Thus, convert 6 mg IV hydromorphone to oral morphine equivalents using this ratio:

$$\frac{1.5 \text{ mg hydromorphone IV}}{30 \text{ mg orally morphine}} = \frac{6 \text{ mg hydromorphone IV}}{x \text{ mg orally morphine}}$$

$$x = 120 \text{ mg orally morphine}$$

Step 3: Reduce by approximately 25% for incomplete cross tolerance:
120 mg orally morphine – (25% x 120 mg orally morphine) → 90 mg orally morphine

Step 4: Determine a long-acting regimen that approximates the total oral morphine requirement.
A reasonable option is sustained release morphine 45 mg orally every 12 hours which will yield 90 mg orally morphine/day
(Constraints will include what doses are available commercially. Sustained release morphine is available in 15, 30, 60, 100, 200 mg tablets)

Step 5: Determine a breakthrough dose that reflect 10–20% of the total daily requirement of sustained-release opioid
15% of 90 mg orally morphine →13 mg orally morphine → select morphine immediate release 15 mg orally every 4 hours PRN

Suppose your patient is unable to take sustained release morphine due to inability to swallow whole pills (sustained release morphine is not crushable). One option is to use a fentanyl transdermal patch instead.

From Step 3: You have determined that the goal is approximately 90 mg orally morphine equivalents per day, which reflects a 25% reduction for incomplete cross tolerance.

Divide by 2 to calculate an approximate dose of fentanyl mcg/hr transdermal
90 mg ÷ 2 → approximately fentanyl 45 mcg/hr transdermal → select fentanyl 50 mcg/hr patch

An appropriate breakthrough dose is still morphine 15 mg orally every 4 hours PRN. Your patient can either crush the immediate release morphine tablets or use liquid formulations. A concentrated elixir form is also available commercially in 20 mg/mL concentration for patients who cannot swallow.

Figure 217-2 *Opioid equianalgesic conversion example.*

- Seek the advice of a pain expert before starting an infusion for a patient who is opioid-naïve.
- Patients who were previously on sustained-release oral regimens but are now unable to take pills (eg, surgery, bowel obstruction) need another means of fulfilling their baseline pain medication needs. For most inpatients, an opioid infusion is appropriate. The total daily oral need should be converted into intravenous morphine or hydromorphone equianalgesic units, then divided by 24 hours for an hourly infusion rate. Consider a 25% to 50% dose reduction for incomplete cross-tolerance if switching between opioids. Fentanyl patch (discussed later) is another option for those without intravenous access, but it is not appropriate for acute pain.
- Patients with severe pain who have required multiple IV boluses to control their symptoms are also potential candidates for opioid infusions. The initial infusion rate should be calculated based on their prior documented 24-hour needs, or if in an acute pain crisis, projected from their needs over the past 4 hours.
- Opioid infusion orders should not be written as broad ranges of "morphine 2–20 mg/hour, titrate to comfort." This type of order gives no specific guidelines for titration and places the patient at risk of overdose if titration occurs too rapidly. A more appropriate order might be "morphine 2 mg/hour and morphine 2 mg intravenously every 15–30 minutes as needed for breakthrough pain. May titrate infusion to 4 mg/hour if patient requires greater than two boluses within one hour or for poorly controlled pain."
- There should always be an additional order for as-needed boluses, either nurse-administered or through a patient-controlled analgesia (PCA). Most clinicians do not realize that it takes at least 8–12 hours to achieve new steady-state blood levels of morphine or hydromorphone after a change in the basal infusion rate. If one simply continues titrating up an infusion in a symptomatic patient without administering as-needed boluses, this patient is at risk of undertreatment of symptoms in the immediate setting as well as overdose/respiratory depression once the opioid reaches a new steady state in several hours.

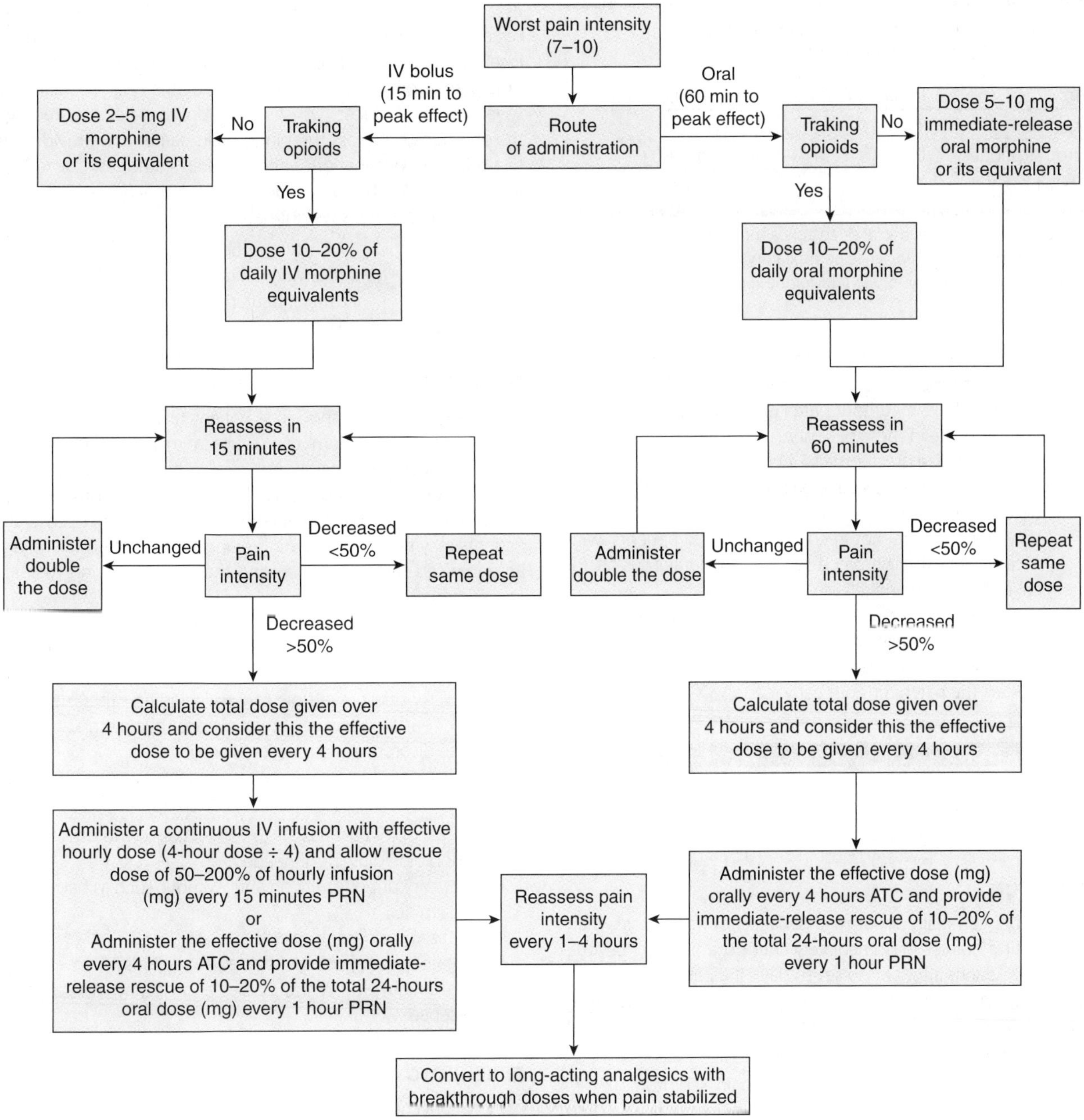

Figure 217-3 *Management of acute pain crisis. (From: Rapid Titration with Short-Acting Oral or Intravenous Opioids. In Guideline for the Management of Cancer Pain in Adults and Children. Glenview, IL: American Pain Society, 2005. This figure has been adapted with permission of the American Pain Society.)*

- Bolus orders can be rapidly titrated for poorly controlled pain. Peak effect for morphine and hydromorphone boluses occurs within 15–30 minutes. If a particular bolus dose is inadequate, the dose can be safely increased every 15–30 minutes without needing to rapidly titrate up the basal infusion rate.
- The basal infusion rate should be reassessed every 8 hours but not more frequently. The infusion rate can be increased based on the amount of boluses required, but generally should not be increased by more than 100% at a time.

PATIENT-CONTROLLED ANALGESIA

Patient-controlled analgesia may be used for patients with significant pain who are alert and able to use the equipment appropriately. PCAs should not be used in patients who have delirium, dementia, or other cognitive deficits. **Table 217-4** shows commonly used PCA doses and lockout intervals in opioid-naïve patients. Higher doses may be needed in patients who have previously been on opioids. PCA pumps can be programmed to deliver patient-controlled boluses, a basal infusion, or both, though opioid-naïve patients generally should not be started on a basal infusion without the advice of a pain expert.

FENTANYL PATCHES

The fentanyl transdermal patch is another option for patients who cannot reliably take pills, but it is important to understand appropriate dosing and limitations of use:

- Equianalgesic dosing for the fentanyl patch compared with oral morphine appears earlier in this chapter (Table 217-2). Note that the commonly used fentanyl 25 mcg/hour patch is equianalgesic to approximately 50 mg oral morphine per day.

TABLE 217-4 Patient-controlled Analgesia (PCA): Opioid-naïve Patients

Drug	Initial PCA Dose*	Typical Lockout
Morphine	1.5 mg	6 minutes
Hydromorphone	0.2 mg	6 minutes
Fentanyl	20 mcg	6 minutes

*Elderly patients or those at risk for sleep apnea should be monitored closely for symptoms of somnolence or respiratory depression. Initial PCA doses should be reduced by 25% to 50% for these patients.

Elderly or opioid-naïve patients should not be initiated on the 25 mcg/hour dose unless there is demonstrated need for this much opioid. A 12 mcg/hour patch is available, which may be more appropriate in these patients.

- The patch can take greater than 24 hours to reach peak effect. It is not appropriate for acute pain or if frequent titration is needed.
- Fentanyl patches are not recommended for patients with significant cachexia. The patch requires subcutaneous fat for effective absorption and release of drug.
- Fentanyl patches generally should not be used in febrile patients, as the uptake of medication is increased and can result in unexpected side effects (such as sedation) or poor analgesia if the patch runs out early.

COMPLICATIONS

Concerns about side effects from opioids often result in undertreatment of pain. Clinicians should make it a priority to recognize and treat opioid-induced side effects.

SEDATION

Many patients complain about mild sedation or "fogginess" when initially starting opioids or immediately after dose titration, but the effect usually wanes after two to seven days. If a patient complains of persistent symptoms and other causes of sedation have been ruled out (eg, other medications, metabolic disturbances, or central nervous system processes), one can consider several options:

- Reduce opioid dose (10% to 25%) if pain symptoms allow. Consider adding nonopioid adjuvant pain medications to facilitate dose reduction.
- Rotate to another opioid.
- Add a psychostimulant such as methylphenidate, with a starting dose of 2.5 mg orally twice a day and titrate up to a maximum of 1 mg/kg/day in divided doses. Psychostimulants should be avoided in patients with significant anxiety, arrhythmias, delirium, or psychosis.

NAUSEA

Like sedation, opioid-induced nausea usually improves after the first week. This symptom is discussed in greater detail in the nausea section of this chapter. First-line therapies for opioid-induced nausea include dopamine antagonists such as prochlorperazine and haloperidol.

CONSTIPATION

Unlike other opioid side effects, constipation does not wane with time. Patients taking opioids should be given a standing bowel regimen to prevent constipation. The combination of docusate sodium with senna is one option. There should be a low threshold to escalate the bowel regimen if symptoms persist. Some patients will need a combination of more aggressive laxatives including lactulose, polyethylene glycol, and enemas. Methylnaltrexone, a selective opioid antagonist, has been approved by the FDA for treatment of severe opioid-induced constipation. Unlike naloxone, methylnaltrexone does not cross the blood-brain barrier and provides effective relief of constipation without opioid withdrawal or reduction in analgesia. Methylnaltrexone can be given every other day as needed, and dosing is weight based:

< 38 kg:	0.15 mg/kg subcutaneously
38–61 kg:	8 mg subcutaneously
62–114 kg:	12 mg subcutaneously
> 114 kg:	0.15 mg/kg subcutaneously

DELIRIUM

Any mental status change in a patient taking opioids should be taken seriously. Delirium can cause a myriad of complications including injury, uncertainty in overall prognosis or assessment of disease progression, and a delay in discharge. Delirium can be particularly distressing because it compromises a patient's sense of self. Patients may find this quite frightening, families often struggle with an enhanced sense of loss, feeling that they are losing their loved one even before death.

However, one should not automatically blame opioids for every new mental status change, especially if a patient has been on a stable dose for some time. Workup for delirium should include an evaluation for other reversible causes, including other medications, infection, central nervous system disease, hypoxemia, metabolic/electrolyte disorders, and renal or liver failure.

If the delirium ultimately seems attributable to opioids but the patient needs continued pain control, consider the following options:

- Reduce opioid dose (10% to 25%) if pain symptoms allow. Use nonopioid adjuvants if needed.
- Treat concurrently with an antipsychotic such as haloperidol or olanzapine.
- Rotate to a different opioid.
- Use nonpharmacologic strategies, including environmental cues for day and night, glasses and hearing aids, and family presence.

NEUROTOXICITY

Patients on chronic opioids can develop neurotoxic side effects from opioid metabolites, especially in the setting of high opioid doses, dehydration, or renal failure. Myoclonus is a common manifestation of this neuroexcitatory state. Symptoms may be mild, such as an occasional jerking of extremities, but with continued opioid administration patients may develop frequent twitching of muscle groups in the extremities and face. Other signs of neurotoxicity include delirium, hyperalgesia (increased sensitivity to pain), and allodynia (pain from nonnoxious stimuli). In severe neurotoxicity, patients may even develop generalized seizures. Hyperalgesia is particularly confusing because clinicians may mistake this as worsened pain from an underlying disease process. Further opioid escalation actually worsens the hyperalgesia.

Treatment strategy depends on both the severity of symptoms and overall prognosis. In an imminently dying patient with mild myoclonus, it may be appropriate to simply monitor the patient for any worsening symptoms. For patients with ongoing need for opioids and concerning manifestations of neurotoxicity, consider several strategies:

- Reduce opioid dose (10% to 25%) if neurotoxic symptoms are mild (only occasional myoclonus). Consider adding nonopioid adjuvant pain medications to facilitate opioid dose reduction.

- Rotate to another opioid if there are signs of significant neuroexcitation, including myoclonus, allodynia/hyperalgesia, delirium, or hallucinations. The new opioid should be initiated at 25% of the equianalgesic dose. Methadone and fentanyl are particularly good options in severe neurotoxicity because they do not have active metabolites. Clinicians without specific training in pain management should consult an expert for any cases of significant neurotoxicity and when initiating methadone or fentanyl, due to complexities of dosing in this setting.
- Add medications to reduce myoclonus. Options include benzodiazepines (lorazepam, clonazepam, midazolam) and muscle relaxants (baclofen, nifedipine).

PRACTICE POINT

- Consider opioid neurotoxicity in patients with worsening pain despite rapidly increasing doses of opioids.

RESPIRATORY DEPRESSION

Though respiratory depression remains a commonly feared side effect, clinically significant respiratory depression is actually quite rare when opioids are dosed appropriately. Respiratory depression is a late effect, and patients should exhibit signs of somnolence before their respiratory function is compromised. Naloxone should be reserved for those with life-threatening respiratory depression. To prevent sudden reversal of analgesia (and almost certain pain crisis), an incremental dosing approach is recommended. Mix 0.4 mg (1 mL ampule) of naloxone into 9 mL of saline to make a diluted 0.04 mg/mL naloxone solution. Administer 1–2 mL of this diluted solution intravenously approximately every 1 to 2 minutes until respiratory depression resolves. Repeated doses may be necessary due to the short duration of naloxone and a continuous infusion may be required if the patient was given long-acting opioids.

INDICATIONS FOR CONSULT

- Uncontrolled pain or intolerable side effects from pain medications: Consider calling a pain or palliative care specialist to assist with modification of pain regimen or treatment of side effects. The consultant can also help assess whether your patient has a specific pain syndrome that may benefit from an interventional procedure such a nerve block or intrathecal pump.
- Neurologic deficits or threatened neurologic compromise: Such symptoms warrant urgent imaging and consultation from neurology, neurosurgery, or radiation-oncology. Even if a patient has advanced illness with a poor prognosis, good palliative care includes preserving function and maximizing quality of life.
- Emotional or spiritual distress that may be exacerbating pain: Consider a referral for palliative care, social work, or chaplaincy support.
- Pain symptoms from disease progression: Communication with the primary outpatient provider is especially vital when a patient presents with disease progression. The outpatient physician can help clarify priorities and overall goals of care. Consider referral to palliative care for additional support.
- Patients with unusual dosing needs due to a history of chronic opioid use, illicit drug use, or methadone maintenance: Consider a pain or palliative care consult. Such patients are at great risk of undertreatment due to high opioid tolerance and psychosocial or behavioral issues.

SUGGESTED READINGS

Guideline for the Management of Cancer Pain in Adults and Children. Glenview: American Pain Society; 2005.

Moryl N, Coyle N, Foley KM. Managing an acute pain crisis in a patient with advanced cancer: "This is as much of a crisis as a code." *JAMA*. 2008;299:1457.

Principles of Analgesic Use in the Treatment of Acute Pain and Cancer Pain. Glenview: American Pain Society; 2008.

NAUSEA

INTRODUCTION

Nausea and vomiting are common symptoms in patients with advanced illnesses, including cancer, congestive heart failure, end-stage renal disease, and AIDS. For patients and families facing a life-threatening illness, nausea and vomiting can cause substantial distress due to concerns about maintaining adequate nutrition and worries that these symptoms indicate disease progression.

PATHOPHYSIOLOGY

Nausea and vomiting can be triggered by activation of any of four general pathways:

- Cortex: Activation can occur due to meningeal irritation, increased intracranial pressure, or cognitive/emotional factors such as anxiety.
- Chemoreceptor trigger zone: This area is located in the floor of the fourth ventricle and lacks a blood-brain barrier. It is easily activated by metabolic abnormalities, toxins, and medications present in the cerebrospinal fluid (CSF). Activation of the chemoreceptor trigger zone is mediated primarily by the dopamine (D2) receptor, but others include neurokinin-1 (NK1) and serotonin (5HT3).
- Vestibular system: Motion or inner ear disease can activate the vestibular apparatus via histamine (H1) and muscarinic acetylcholine (ACh) receptors.
- Peripheral pathways: Activation can occur through mechanoreceptors and chemoreceptors in the gastrointestinal tract and heart, as well as 5HT3 receptors in the gastrointestinal tract. These signals are then transmitted along afferent tracts including the vagus, glossopharyngeal, splanchnic, and sympathetic nerves.

Each of these four pathways can then activate the vomiting center, a specific area of the medulla that coordinates the final act of vomiting via the parasympathetic system and gastrointestinal tract. Activation of the vomiting center is believed to be mediated by H1 receptors or muscarinic ACh receptors.

DIAGNOSIS AND TREATMENT

Evaluation should include a thorough history and physical exam, with careful attention to common causes of nausea in the terminally ill, including medications (chemotherapy, opioids), constipation, electrolyte abnormalities, liver and kidney failure, radiation therapy, central nervous system lesions, bowel obstruction, and anxiety. It is important to try to identify the likely mechanism or pathway responsible for a patient's nausea, as this will guide the therapeutic approach.

NONPHARMACOLOGIC TREATMENT

Nonpharmacologic strategies can be a helpful starting point for many patients. Patients should avoid strong smells and eat small, frequent meals as they are able. Relaxation techniques may be useful

TABLE 217-5 Common Causes of Nausea and First-line Pharmacologic Therapies

Etiology	Probable Mechanism and Receptors	First-line Treatment
CNS lesion	Increased ICP, meningeal irritation	Dexamethasone
Opioid-induced	Stimulation of CTZ (D2) Gastroparesis Constipation	D2 antagonists: haloperidol, metoclopramide, prochlorperazine Consider opioid rotation
Metabolic/uremia/liver failure	Stimulation of CTZ (D2)	Treat reversible causes (electrolytes, meds) D2 antagonists: see above
Chemotherapy-induced	Gut release of 5HT3 → stimulation of peripheral pathways Stimulation of CTZ (D2, 5HT3, NK1) Anticipatory nausea	5HT3 antagonist: ondansetron Dexamethasone NK1 antagonist: aprepitant Anxiolytics: lorazepam (see also guidelines from American Society of Clinical Oncology)
Radiation-associated	Gut release of 5HT3 → stimulation of peripheral pathways	5HT3 antagonist: ondansetron
Bowel obstruction	Gut mechano/chemoreceptors → stimulation of peripheral pathways Toxins, inflammatory agents → CTZ (D2)	Metoclopramide (if incomplete obstruction) or haloperidol, dexamethasone, octreotide, nasogastric tube, venting gastrostomy
Constipation	Gut mechanoreceptors	Aggressive scheduled bowel regimen
Gastroparesis	Gut mechanoreceptors	Promotility: metoclopramide
Motion, vestibular disease	Stimulation via vestibulocochlear nerve (H1, ACh)	Anticholinergic: scopolamine H1 blockers: promethazine, diphenhydramine

ICP, intracranial pressure; CTZ, chemoreceptor trigger zone; D2, dopamine type 2 receptor; 5HT3, 5-hydroxytryptamine type 3 receptor (serotonin); NK1, neurokinin type 1 receptor; ACh, acetylcholine receptor; H1, histamine type 1 receptor; CNS, central nervous system.

for patients with significant anxiety or anticipatory nausea (nausea that occurs prior to chemotherapy sessions due to a conditioned response). Patients with chemotherapy-induced symptoms may consider acupuncture, as a study by the Cochrane Database of Systematic Reviews found that acupuncture-point stimulation appears to reduce the incidence of acute chemotherapy-induced vomiting.

PHARMACOLOGIC TREATMENT

Most patients with nausea or vomiting will need some type of pharmacologic therapy. **Table 217-5** shows common clinical etiologies of nausea and recommended first-line pharmacologic therapies based on likely mechanisms and receptors. **Table 217-6** lists common antiemetics, doses, and side effects.

KEY PRINCIPLES OF PHARMACOLOGIC TREATMENT

- Determine the clinical etiology of nausea and select a first-line antiemetic based on the likely mechanism.
- Use the first-line agent on a scheduled basis initially until nausea symptoms are controlled, and then consider tapering to as-needed dosing.
- If symptoms persist, consider adding another agent in a different class while keeping the first-line agent. Nausea is frequently multifactorial and may need therapy directed at multiple sources.
- Recognize the side-effect profiles of different antiemetics and use them to the patient's advantage, not disadvantage.
  - Haloperidol can be useful in patients who are also delirious.
  - Ondansetron can cause constipation and would be inappropriate for a patient with nausea due to constipation or obstipation.
- Avoid using multiple agents in the same class simultaneously.
  - The combined use of haloperidol, metoclopramide, or prochlorperazine can cause extrapyramidal symptoms such as dystonia and akathisia.

PRACTICE POINT

- Recognize common antiemetic side effects and avoid using multiple agents in the same antiemetic class simultaneously.

OPIOID-INDUCED NAUSEA

Opioid-induced nausea warrants further discussion because it is particularly common and troublesome in this population. Opioids cause nausea through multiple mechanisms, including decreased gut motility (constipation, gastroparesis), stimulation of the chemoreceptor trigger zone via dopamine receptors, and enhanced vestibular sensitivity. Symptoms of opioid-induced nausea usually resolve during the first week of opioid use. One strategy is to use a dopamine antagonist such as prochlorperazine, haloperidol, or metoclopramide on a scheduled basis for several days. The antiemetic can subsequently be tapered as the patient develops tolerance to the opioid side effects. Another effective agent is olanzapine, which has mixed dopamine, acetylcholine, histamine, and serotonin activities. Patients with persistent nausea may require an opioid dose reduction (10% to 20%) or rotation to another opioid. Patients taking opioids should be on a scheduled bowel regimen to prevent constipation.

MALIGNANT BOWEL OBSTRUCTION

Malignant bowel obstruction is a common complication in patients with advanced abdominal and pelvic malignancies. In patients who are not surgical candidates, medical management should include several concurrent mechanical and pharmacologic strategies:

- Decompression via nasogastric tube can provide rapid relief of nausea and abdominal distension. A percutaneous gastrostomy tube may be considered in patients with persistent obstruction since patients can be transitioned home with a gastrostomy tube in place.

TABLE 217-6 Common Antiemetics

Antiemetic	Class	Dosage	Major Adverse Effects
Haloperidol (Haldol)	D2 antagonist (CTZ)	0.5–2 mg orally or intravenously every 4–6 hours	EPS
Metoclopramide (Reglan)	D2 antagonist (GI, CTZ)	5–20 mg orally or intravenously every 6 hours	EPS GI colic
Prochlorperazine (Compazine)	D2 antagonist (CTZ)	5–10 mg orally or intravenously or 25 mg by rectum every 6 hours	EPS Sedation
Olanzapine (Zyprexa, Zydis)	Multiple: D2, ACh, H1, 5HT3 antagonist	2.5–5 mg orally or sublingually every night at bedtime and every 6 hours	Sedation, dizziness
Promethazine* (Phenergan)	H1 blocker, Anticholingergic	12–25 mg orally or intravenously or 25 mg by rectum every 6 hours	EPS, sedation, delirium
Diphenhydramine* (Benadryl)	H1 blocker	25–50 mg orally or intravenously every 6 hours	Sedation, delirium, dry mouth, urinary retention
Scopolamine* (Transderm scop)	Anticholinergic	1.5 mg patch every 72 hours	Dry mouth, blurred vision, delirium, urinary retention
Ondansetron (Zofran)	5HT3 antagonist	4–8 mg orally or intravenously every 8 hours	Constipation
Dexamethasone (Decadron)	Anti-inflammatory Central activity unknown	4–20 mg orally or intravenously once or twice a day	Delirium, anxiety, insomnia, GI mucosal irritation
Lorazepam* (Ativan)	Anxiolytic	0.5–2 mg orally or intravenously every 6 hours	Sedation, delirium
Aprepitant† (Emend)	NK1 antagonist	125 mg orally (day 1), 80 mg orally (days 2–3)	Fatigue
Dronabinol* (Marinol)	Cannabinoid	2.5–10 mg orally two to three times a day	Confusion, ataxia, paranoia, hallucinations

*Use with particular caution in elderly patients due to adverse effects.
†For use primarily in chemotherapy setting in combination with ondansetron and dexamethasone
EPS, extrapyramidal symptoms; CTZ, chemoreceptor trigger zone; D2, dopamine type 2 receptor; 5HT3, 5-hydroxytryptamine type 3 receptor (serotonin); NK1, neurokinin type 1 receptor; ACh, acetylcholine receptor; H1, histamine type 1 receptor; GI, gastrointestinal.

- Pain control is a priority and generally requires the use of opioids.
- Antisecretory agents are useful for reducing abdominal distension. Hyoscyamine can be given 0.125–0.25 mg sublingually four times a day or scopolamine can be administered through a patch. Octreotide is a somatastatin analogue that can be administered subcutaneously 50–150 mcg three times a day or through continuous infusion of 300 mcg over 24 hours.
- Patients should be given a scheduled antiemetic to relieve associated nausea. Metoclopramide is recommended for patients with partial obstruction, but it should be discontinued if the patient develops worsened abdominal pain or cramping. It should not be used in patients with complete bowel obstruction. Haloperidol can be used for nausea in patients with complete obstruction or those with symptoms of colic. Dexamethasone 4 mg orally or intravenously two to three times a day can be useful for both its antiemetic and anti-inflammatory properties, including treating tumor-associated inflammation and potentially reducing the obstruction.
- Studies have demonstrated successful symptom management of malignant bowel obstruction using a combined regimen of metoclopramide, octreotide, and dexamethasone, including the recovery of bowel transit in some patients with partial obstruction.

COMPLICATIONS

Antiemetics can cause a number of side effects. Sedation is common with antihistamines and neuroleptic agents, including dopamine antagonists and atypical antipsychotics. Sedation may be a desired effect for some patients nearing the end of life, but a dose adjustment or medication change may be necessary for patients who find this problematic. Almost all classes of antiemetics can cause delirium, including antihistamines, benzodiazepines, anticholinergics, corticosteroids, and cannabinoids. The elderly are especially vulnerable and should be monitored closely. Patients on dopamine antagonists may develop extrapyramidal symptoms such as akathisia and dystonia. Management includes treatment with diphenhydramine or benztropine and discontinuation of the offending agent. Serotonin antagonists such as ondansetron can cause constipation and patients may need prophylactic laxatives.

Patients with persistent nausea and vomiting often develop dehydration and electrolyte disturbances, which can further exacerbate symptoms of nausea. It may be reasonable to consider intravenous hydration, even in patients with a limited prognosis, with the goal of relieving symptoms. Consider referring patients with persistent bowel obstruction for surgical evaluation, depending on the stage of illness and overall prognosis. Additionally, patients and families may struggle with news that disease-modifying therapies (such as chemotherapy) are no longer possible due to intractable symptoms, poor functional status, or advanced disease. Their psychosocial distress should be addressed with the assistance of the primary outpatient clinician, palliative care clinician, social worker, or chaplain.

SUGGESTED READINGS

Naeim A, Dy SM, Lorenz KA, et al. Evidence-based recommendations for cancer nausea and vomiting. *J Clin Oncol*. 2008;26:3903.

Wood GJ, Shega JW, Lynch B, et al. Management of intractable nausea and vomiting in patients at the end of life: "I was feeling nauseous all of the time…nothing was working." *JAMA*. 2007;298:1196.

DYSPNEA

INTRODUCTION

Dyspnea, defined as the subjective experience of difficult or uncomfortable breathing, is a very common and distressing symptom for patients. Dyspnea has been reported in up to 78% of cancer patients, 70% of patients with congestive heart failure, 70% of patients with dementia, 56% of COPD patients, and 62% of patients with AIDS. Of note, studies show that patients with higher dyspnea scores report decreased quality of life indices. Despite its prevalence and impact on quality of life, dyspnea often goes untreated. One study reported that over 60% of patients with advanced cancer had had dyspnea for greater than three months, yet most had not received any treatment for their symptoms.

PATHOPHYSIOLOGY

The pathophysiology of dyspnea is complex and not yet fully understood. The respiratory center, located in the medulla and pons, coordinates the movements of the diaphragm and chest wall muscles during breathing. The respiratory center receives sensory input from several sources, including pulmonary vagal afferents, peripheral and medullary chemoreceptors, and peripheral mechanoreceptors from respiratory muscles and joints. The pulmonary vagal afferents include pulmonary stretch receptors, alveolar C fibers that respond to interstitial and capillary pressure, and pulmonary irritant receptors.

Several mechanisms appear to trigger the sensation of dyspnea:

- Increased work of breathing: This can be caused by increased airway resistance, such as in COPD or asthma, or weakened musculature, as occurs in neurodegenerative disorders or severe cachexia.
- Chemoreceptor activity: Receptors in the medulla primarily detect hypercapnia, and those in the carotid and aortic bodies detect hypoxemia. Hypercapnia appears to have a greater role in triggering dyspnea than hypoxemia.
- Neuromechanical dissociation: Researchers have described an important relationship between the brain's efferent motor output for respiration and the afferent information it receives in response to these efforts. Dyspnea can occur when there is a mismatch, or neuromechanical dissociation, between what the brain desires from respiration and the sensory feedback from pulmonary vagal afferents and peripheral mechanoreceptors. A patient with amyotrophic lateral sclerosis (ALS) may experience dyspnea because the brain is not receiving the expected feedback in chest wall expansion. In another example, normal subjects became dyspneic when researchers limited the inspiratory flow rate despite no change in respiratory work or oxygenation status.

DIAGNOSIS

The gold standard for diagnosis is always the patient's report of symptoms. Studies have demonstrated that there is no clear correlation between symptoms of dyspnea and respiratory rate, oxygen saturation, and accessory muscle use. Interestingly, some patients feel dyspneic despite normal oxygen saturations, while others do not feel dyspneic even though they are hypoxemic. It is therefore important to screen all patients for dyspnea, since patients may have no obvious signs of respiratory compromise or distress.

Common etiologies should be considered, including pneumonia, pleural effusion, space-occupying lung lesions, bronchospasm, pulmonary embolism, COPD, cardiac ischemia, congestive heart failure, anemia, and ascites. Patients with cancer may also have disease-specific processes such as radiation or chemotherapy-induced pneumonitis, malignant pericardial effusion, superior vena cava syndrome, or lymphangitic spread of tumor. Patients with primary neurologic or neuromuscular disorders may have symptoms of dyspnea associated with progressive muscle weakness.

The decision of whether to pursue diagnostic studies should take into account the patient's overall goals of care, disease trajectory, and the likelihood that the study results will enhance management of dyspnea symptoms. For some patients, workup to rule out pneumonia, pleural effusion, or pulmonary embolism may still be appropriate as there are specific treatments that can help their symptoms. Sometimes no clear etiology for dyspnea can be found. The National Hospice Study, which followed terminal cancer patients during their last six weeks of life, found that 24% of patients with dyspnea had no signs of lung involvement or cardiac disease.

TREATMENT

Treatment of dyspnea should be directed at the etiology, if known. Patients with advanced illness may still be considered candidates for procedures like thoracentesis for a large pleural effusion. The ultimate goal in all cases should be the subjective relief of symptoms rather than the correction of any single parameter, such as oxygen saturation or respiratory rate. Patients may need further nonpharmacologic and pharmacologic therapies if treatment of the underlying etiology of dyspnea does not fully relieve their symptoms.

NONPHARMACOLOGIC TREATMENT

Placing patients in an upright position improves the mechanics of the intercostal muscles and lessens the work of breathing. A cool fan or moist cloth over the face can improve symptoms, possibly through stimulation of the V2 branch of the trigeminal nerve, which may then inhibit dyspnea perception centrally. The presence of a family member or volunteer at the bedside can help relieve anxiety associated with dyspnea. Cognitive and behavioral interventions, similar to those used in pulmonary rehabilitation for COPD patients, can also improve symptoms of dyspnea. Several trials of nursing-led interventions, which included relaxation techniques, breathing control, activity pacing, and psychosocial support, demonstrated a reduction in dyspnea scores.

Oxygen is frequently used in patients with dyspnea, though evidence to support its use is mixed. There is strong evidence to support oxygen use in COPD patients, for both symptomatic relief and improved survival. However, several randomized control studies of cancer patients with dyspnea have demonstrated that oxygen and air are equally effective for relief of symptoms. Some studies have suggested that a subset of cancer patients with hypoxemia have better symptom relief from oxygen, though at least one randomized controlled trial reported no difference between oxygen and air, even in hypoxemic patients whose oxygen saturations improved with therapy. In the palliative care population, a trial of supplemental oxygen is reasonable if the patient has had insufficient relief with other approaches. The potential benefits and risks of oxygen therapy should be considered before discharging a patient with home oxygen. Considerations include the degree of symptom relief, the risk of falls with tubing, the presence of smokers in the home, and the additional cost of oxygen.

PHARMACOLOGIC TREATMENT

Opioids

Opioids are the first-line agents in pharmacologic therapy for dyspnea near the end of life. Their exact mechanism is not fully

TABLE 217-7 Opioids for Dyspnea

Drug	Oral	Parenteral
Opioid-naïve patients		
Morphine	2–5 mg orally every 4 hours	1–2 mg intravenously every 2 hours
Oxycodone	2.5–5 mg orally every 4 hours	—
Hydromorphone	0.5–1 mg orally every 4 hours	0.1–0.2 mg intravenously every 2 hours
Opioid-tolerant patients		
Increase baseline opioid dose by 25%		

understood, but opioids are believed to decrease the chemoreceptor response to hypercapnia and increase preload through cardiovascular vasodilation. Opioids have been shown to reduce dyspnea in patients with advanced cancer, congestive heart failure, and COPD, and can also increase exercise tolerance in patients with COPD and congestive heart failure. Doses required to control dyspnea are usually lower than those required for pain (**Table 217-7**). A reasonable starting dose of morphine for an opioid-naïve patient is morphine 1–2 mg intravenously every 2 hours or 2–5 mg orally every 4 hours. For patients already on opioids for pain, consider a 25% increase in their usual opioid dose to treat dyspnea. Other opioids such as hydromorphone and oxycodone can be used. There is no evidence to suggest any substantial differences in efficacy between opioids in the treatment of dyspnea. Patients who require frequent opioid doses may need initiation of either long-acting opioids or an opioid infusion. Principles for ordering and titrating infusions can be found in the section on pain managment.

PRACTICE POINT

- Opioids can be used safely for dyspnea even in patients with underlying lung disease

Anxiolytics

Dyspnea can be closely associated with anxiety, with each symptom exacerbating the other. Anxiolytics can be a helpful adjunct to opioids for treating dyspnea (**Table 217-8**). Lorazepam can offer rapid relief and is available in oral concentrate form. Clonazepam can be beneficial for chronic dyspnea due to its longer half-life. One trial has shown that midazolam can improve dyspnea control when added to a morphine regimen, though in practice its use is generally reserved for severe symptoms. Midazolam can be given 0.2–0.5 mg intravenously slowly for severe dyspnea or for refractory symptoms of panic or anxiety.

TABLE 217-8 Anxiolytics for Dyspnea

Drug	Dose
Lorazepam	0.5–1 mg orally or intravenously every hour until dyspnea controlled; then every 4–6 hours scheduled
Clonazepam	0.25–0.5 mg orally every 12 hours
Midazolam	0.2–0.5 mg intravenously slowly every 15 minutes until dyspnea controlled; consider infusion

COMPLICATIONS

RESPIRATORY DEPRESSION

Some clinicians or patients may be hesitant to use opioids due to fears that they will cause respiratory depression and hasten death. These fears are largely unfounded. Many studies have shown that opioids improve dyspnea without compromising respiratory function when dosed appropriately. One meta-analysis that included COPD, congestive heart failure, cancer, and interstitial lung disease patients reported statistically significant improvement in dyspnea with no deaths attributable to opioids. It is also important to recognize that major changes in respiratory status such as apnea or periodic breathing may be indicative of imminent death from natural disease progression, rather than opioid-induced.

In the rare instance of respiratory depression due to accidental opioid overdose, naloxone can be used, but it should be diluted to avoid complete reversal of analgesia in palliative care patients. One ampule (0.4 mg in 1 mL) should be diluted with 9 mL saline to create a 0.04 mg/mL solution and then given in 1 mL doses every 1–2 minutes until respiratory depression is reversed. Further doses may be needed if long-acting opioids were used. If the only manifestation of opioid overdose is somnolence with intact respiratory function, naloxone should not be given and the patient should just be monitored closely.

INDICATIONS FOR CONSULT

Consults may be appropriate in the following situations:

- Uncontrolled symptoms of dyspnea: Consider palliative care assistance for further evaluation and titration of medications. In very severe cases, patients may need infusions of a sedative such as midazolam. Palliative sedation should be considered a last option, and a specialist in end-of-life care should be consulted first to ensure that all other potential therapies have been pursued.
- Reversible fluid collections including pleural effusion, ascites, and pericardial effusion: A single drainage procedure may be sufficient for some patients, but those with a tendency to reaccumulate may warrant pleurodesis or placement of an indwelling catheter for continued drainage.
- Significant emotional or anxiety component: Consider palliative care, social work, or chaplaincy assistance for psychosocial support.

SUGGESTED READINGS

Ben-Aharon I, Gafter-Gvili A, Paul M, et al. Interventions for alleviating cancer-related dyspnea: a systematic review. *J Clin Oncol.* 2008;26:2396.

Luce JM, Luce JA. Management of dyspnea in patients with far-advanced lung disease: "Once I lose it, it's kind of hard to catch it..." *JAMA.* 2001;285:1331.

Thomas JR, von Gunten CF. Management of dyspnea. *J Support Oncol.* 2003;1:23.

SECRETIONS

EVALUATION AND TREATMENT

As their level of consciousness diminishes, many dying patients lose the ability to clear oropharyngeal secretions and develop noisy respirations. Also known as the "death rattle," this symptom has been reported in 60% to 90% of dying patients. Some family members and providers may find the noise distressing, though patients are generally obtunded and are thought to be undisturbed by it.

Treatment strategies include placing the patient in a lateral or semiprone position to promote drainage of secretions. Gentle suctioning may be helpful for secretions that are easily accessible, but deep suctioning is generally ineffective and may cause discomfort to the patient. Intravenous fluids can increase the production of secretions and should be minimized or discontinued.

Anticholinergic agents can be used to reduce oropharyngeal secretions, though few trials have been conducted to study their efficacy. **Table 217-9** lists commonly used agents. It is important to recognize that anticholinergics can cause side effects including sedation, delirium, urinary retention, constipation, and dry mouth. Patients receiving anticholinergic agents should receive scheduled mouth care including lip balm and mouth swabs.

Noisy secretions can be difficult to control despite the above interventions. Since most patients experience the "death rattle" during the dying process, family education is paramount to minimize emotional distress. Clinicians can explain that as patients become less alert, the oropharyngeal muscles relax and patients are no longer able to swallow secretions. The loud respirations are a sign of air moving past the pooled secretions and relaxed muscles. Some family members may need reassurance that the patient is receiving adequate air and that this is not a sign of drowning. The most important point to emphasize is that these symptoms are normal and an expected part of the dying process.

SUGGESTED READINGS

Wee B, Hillier R. Interventions for noisy breathing in patients near to death. Cochrane Database of Systematic Reviews. 2008;1:CD005177.

Wildiers H, Menten J. Death rattle: prevalence, prevention, and treatment. *J Pain Symptom Manage*. 2002;23:310.

TERMINAL DELIRIUM

EVALUATION AND TREATMENT

Nearly half of all dying patients will display signs of restlessness or agitation in their last days of life due to delirium. Symptoms include grimacing, moaning, mumbling speech, hallucinations, twitching or jerking, and changes in the level of arousal. Because delirium is common in hospitalized patients both with and without terminal illness, it is important to recognize other physiologic signs that may indicate a patient is in the dying phase. Manifestations can include decreased perfusion with cool extremities or cyanosis, tachycardia or bradycardia, hypotension, respiratory changes such as Cheyne-Stokes breathing or apnea, decreased urine output, and progressive somnolence.

Many of the general principles of delirium assessment and treatment still apply in the dying patient. Medications such as anticholinergic drugs (antiemetics, antisecretion agents, tricyclic antidepressants), opioids, sedatives, and corticosteroids are common precipitants for delirium in this population. The offending medications should be discontinued or weaned if possible, keeping in mind that delirious patients should not be left with undertreated pain, dyspnea, or other symptoms. Certain drugs such as opioids may need to be rotated (ie, a patient with severe renal insufficiency and signs of opioid neurotoxicity from morphine may need to be rotated to fentanyl or methadone). Other common and reversible causes of delirium include untreated pain, full bladder, or fecal impaction. The patient's overall clinical status and goals of care should determine the extent of workup. If a patient appears to be nearing the end of life, it is very appropriate to forgo a workup for metabolic abnormalities, renal failure, or infectious causes of mental status change.

Nonpharmacologic interventions for delirium can be helpful, including family presence at the bedside, gentle reminders to help with reorientation, hearing or visual devices, and psychosocial/spiritual support. Antipsychotic medications are the primary pharmacologic treatment for terminal delirium. Common medications are listed in **Table 217-10**. Antipsychotics can cause varying levels of sedation, with haloperidol causing the least sedation and chlorpromazine causing the most sedation.

Most clinicians recognize that benzodiazepines are generally discouraged in the treatment of delirious patients due to the potential for paradoxical worsening of symptoms and agitation. One exception is the dying patient with significant agitation despite treatment with strong doses of antipsychotic medications. In this situation, benzodiazepines may be added for their sedative effect. Lorazepam can be given 0.5–2 mg intravenously, orally, or

TABLE 217-9 Anticholinergics for Secretions

Drug	Dose
Hyoscyamine	0.125–0.25 mg sublingually every 6–8 hours
Glycopyrrolate	0.1–0.2 mg intravenously every 8 hours
Scopolamine	1.5 mg patch every 72 hours*
Atropine (1% ophth)	1–2 gtt sublingually every 6 hours

*Scopolamine patch takes approximately 12 hours for onset of action (24 hours to reach steady state). Additional agents may be necessary if more rapid effect is desired.

TABLE 217-10 Antipsychotics for Terminal Delirium

Drug	Dose
Haloperidol	0.5–2 mg orally, intravenously, or subcutaneously every 6 hours and every hour as needed (maximum 20 mg in 24 hours)
Olanzapine	2.5–5 mg orally or sublingually every 12 hours and every 4 hours as needed (maximum 30 mg in 24 hours)
Chlorpromazine	25–50 mg orally, by rectum, or intravenously every 8 hours and every 4 hours as needed

subcutaneously every 2 hours as needed. Diazepam is available rectally and can be given 10 mg orally every 6 hours. If these measures prove ineffective, consider contacting a palliative care specialist to discuss the possibility of further sedating medications.

SUGGESTED READINGS

Del Fabbro E, Dalal S, Bruera E. Symptom control in palliative care–Part III: dyspnea and delirium. *J Palliat Med.* 2006;9:422.

White C, McCann MA, Jackson N, et al. First do no harm... terminal restlessness or drug-induced delirium. *J Palliat Med.* 2007;10:345.

NUTRITION AND HYDRATION

INTRODUCTION

Patients and families can experience tremendous emotional distress when a severe illness has compromised nutritional status or the ability to eat. For many, nutrition can become a symbolic battleground of the fight against death. Food can also be a medium through which many families express their love. When patients do not eat, well-intentioned family members may struggle with feelings of rejection or fear that their loved one has "given up." In many cases, clinicians can be pressed to answer questions about the role of artificial nutrition and hydration in the setting of advanced illness.

ANOREXIA-CACHEXIA SYNDROME

Patients may show signs of anorexia-cachexia, a complex wasting syndrome mediated by cytokine and neurohormonal factors. This syndrome is well recognized in cancer and AIDS patients, but is also seen in patients with advanced chronic illnesses such as congestive heart failure and COPD. It is important to explain to patients that this decline is a natural part of the disease process and not due to any deficiency on their part. Patients or family members may focus on weight loss as a sign that they have not done enough to ensure adequate calories. Although patients may appear malnourished, this catabolic condition is generally not reversible even with aggressive nutrition.

Clinicians should screen for treatable causes of poor intake that may masquerade as anorexia-cachexia. These conditions include oral mucositis or candidiasis, esophagitis, reflux disease, gastrointestinal dysmotility, constipation, nausea, chronic pain, or depression. If a reversible cause for anorexia is not found, management of the anorexia-cachexia syndrome can include behavioral and pharmacologic strategies.

Patients should be empowered to determine their own eating habits, including eating the foods that are most appealing and deciding the quantity and frequency of intake. Patients who are easily nauseated or have early satiety should eat small portions only as they are able. Families should be advised to refrain from any comments and behavior that pressure the patient to consume more. Patients can liberalize dietary restrictions, including those that were previously important for management of long-standing conditions such as diabetes or hyperlipidemia, provided that doing so will not cause uncomfortable symptoms such as fluid retention. Some patients and family members may need tremendous support and education as they make this transition. Many have spent years pursuing every measure to fight their illness, such as eating all the "right" foods while undergoing chemotherapy, maintaining their caloric intake, or carefully adhering to a diabetic diet. Patients and family members may find themselves having to acknowledge for the first time that the disease is advancing and incurable. Clinicians should be attuned to these psychosocial concerns and may need to facilitate appropriate support systems for their patients, such as social work, chaplaincy, and hospice.

TABLE 217-11 Appetite Stimulants

Drug	Dose
Megestrol*	400 mg orally twice a day
Prednisone	5 mg orally three times a day
Dexamethasone	4–8 mg daily in divided doses
Dronabinol	2.5–7.5 mg orally three times a day

*Liquid form of megestrol is associated with better compliance and ease of administration than tablets.

Patients or family members may ask if there is a role for appetite stimulants. Pharmacologic agents can be considered, but appetite stimulants have demonstrated only modest or limited benefit at best, and all have certain contraindications and side effects. Before starting an agent, it is important to discuss specific goals (such as a small amount of weight gain or increased appetite) and a clear timeframe in which to assess whether the goals are being met. If there is no obvious benefit after two or three weeks, the drug should be discontinued. **Table 217-11** lists common appetite stimulants and doses. These include the following:

- Megestrol acetate (Megace) is a synthetic progestational agent that has been shown to increase appetite and weight in randomized control trials of patients with cancer and AIDS. Weight gain manifests as increased fat stores but not lean muscle mass. The data for improved quality of life indices is less clear than the effects on appetite and weight. Potential adverse effects include fluid retention, adrenal insufficiency, hypertension, and thromboembolic events. Megestrol should not be used in patients with a history of thromboembolism and is generally not recommended for patients with congestive heart failure.
- Corticosteroids such as dexamethasone and prednisone have been shown in randomized controlled trials to improve subjective appetite and overall sense of well-being, though patients did not demonstrate any significant weight gain. Corticosteroids are most appropriate for patients with a shorter life expectancy or for those who cannot receive megestrol due to history of thromboembolism. They should not be used longer than a few weeks due to the potential for significant side effects including peptic ulcer disease, cushingoid changes, and myopathy.
- Dronabinol (Marinol) is a synthetic cannabinoid that has demonstrated modest benefit in appetite stimulation in AIDS patients, but unconvincing effect on weight gain. For cancer patients with anorexia, the evidence is weak and does not demonstrate improved appetite and weight gain. Adverse effects of dronabinol are primarily central nervous system related and include dizziness, euphoria, and confusion. Cannabinoids should be avoided in elderly patients, as they are particularly sensitive to the side effects.

ARTIFICIAL NUTRITION AND HYDRATION

When patients and families inquire about a feeding tube or TPN, clinicians should explore their specific concerns and goals. Many people hope that artificial nutrition and hydration (ANH) will improve strength or lengthen survival. Unfortunately, the literature supports the use of ANH for only specific patient populations. For the vast majority of patients with advanced illness, ANH does not improve survival or quality of life.

ANH can lengthen survival of patients with certain conditions including extreme short-bowel syndrome, amyotrophic lateral sclerosis, acute phases of stroke or head injury, and those in a permanent vegetative state. The data for cancer patients is more varied due to the heterogeneity of the population. Most clinicians would consider ANH appropriate for patients whose disease location interferes with their ability to swallow or transit food (eg, head and neck cancer, esophageal cancer, proximal bowel obstruction) but who otherwise have good functional status. Some studies suggest that ANH may be useful in patients who are actively undergoing chemotherapy or radiation, while other studies do not support this finding. Patients with cancer-related anorexia-cachexia do not gain weight even when given aggressive calories. Lastly, when a patient's disease is no longer responding to disease-modifying treatments, experts agree that the risks of ANH, such as infection, aspiration, or volume overload, generally outweigh the benefits.

The literature does not support the use of ANH in patients with advanced dementia. Enteral tube feeds have been shown to increase the risk of aspiration, diarrhea, and gastrointestinal discomfort. Patients with dementia are at risk for pulling on feeding tubes, and studies have shown that the presence of a feeding tube increases the likelihood that patients will be physically restrained. Advanced dementia patients receiving ANH and adequate caloric intake still demonstrate continued weight loss or depletion of lean body mass. There is no evidence to suggest improved healing of decubitus ulcers, either.

If a decision is made to pursue ANH, the clinician should discuss specific goals with the patient and family, such as weight gain or maintenance, and designate a timepoint at which they will reassess whether ANH is still meeting these goals. It is also important to discuss in advance that should any significant complications arise, such as infection, this would be an indication to discontinue ANH because the risks of continuing would outweigh any potential benefit.

It is important to recognize that patients, families, and clinicians may have their own deeply rooted beliefs about the role of ANH at the end of life. Cultural or religious traditions may influence an individual's beliefs, even when medical providers feel that the data does not support the use of ANH. If significant concerns arise, clinicians should consider including a chaplain or clergyperson, social worker, and ethics support staff in these discussions.

PRACTICE POINT

- Define specific and measurable goals before initiating patients on appetite stimulants or artificial nutrition and hydration.

EDUCATING PATIENTS AND FAMILIES

Clinicians play a key role in educating patients and families on nutritional issues at the end of life. Although families may express great concern that their loved one will suffer from hunger, patients in the last stage of life rarely report feeling hungry. Many patients can live comfortably for weeks with minimal food and water. Forcing patients to eat can cause emotional distress, nausea, and aspiration. Many patients and families are also unaware that artificial nutrition and hydration may cause complications including infection, aspiration, and fluid overload with worsened pulmonary edema or ascites, all of which can shorten lifespan.

Conversely, families of patients at risk for aspiration may have been instructed not to offer food or liquids. In the context of limited prognosis or imminent death, the concern about aspiration becomes less important as long as there are not obvious symptoms of discomfort. Depending on the goals of care, these patients may be offered small amounts of food or drink, as long as this contributes to comfort and quality of life. Measures such as sitting upright, tucking the chin when swallowing, and using a thickening agent with fluids, may enable patients at risk for aspiration to eat and drink small quantities for pleasure.

It is important, however, to help family members learn other ways of nurturing their loved ones at the bedside. Thirst is a common complaint at the end of life. Of note, intravenous fluids have not been shown to affect the sensation of thirst. Visitors can learn how to moisten the mouth and provide ice chips to alleviate thirst. Small sips of fluid and candy lozenges can be appropriate if patients are alert and do not show signs of discomfort. Families can also be encouraged to interact with patients through conversation, reading, or music.

SUGGESTED READING

Casarett D, Kapo J, Caplan A. Appropriate use of artificial nutrition and hydration—fundamental principles and recommendations. *N Engl J Med*. 2005;353:2607.

COMPLEMENTARY MEDICINE

INTRODUCTION

The National Center for Complementary and Alternative Medicine (NCCAM), an agency of the National Institutes of Health, has defined complementary and alternative medicine as "a group of diverse medical and health care systems, practices, and products that are not generally considered to be part of conventional medicine." The term *complementary medicine* refers to therapies that are used together with conventional medicine. *Alternative medicine* describes practices that are used in place of conventional medicine. The field of complementary and alternative medicine (CAM) includes a wide variety of practices, some of which do not conform to usual biomedical and scientific principles.

The NCCAM groups complementary and alternative medicine into several domains:

- Whole medical systems: These practices are built on complete systems of theory and practice that have evolved separately from conventional medicine. Some have existed longer than Western medical practices. Examples include homeopathy, traditional Chinese medicine, and Ayurveda (practiced on the Indian subcontinent). Systems such as traditional Chinese medicine may incorporate other domains below such as biologically-based practices (herbal therapies) and energy-based therapies (acupuncture).
- Mind-body medicine: These techniques utilize the mind to affect bodily function and control symptoms. Examples include meditation, guided imagery, music therapy, and hypnosis. Some would include patient support groups and cognitive-behavioral therapies in this category.
- Biologically-based practices: These therapies are based on substances found in nature including food, herbs, vitamins, and minerals.
- Manipulative and body-based practices: These treatments are based on movement of specific body parts. Examples include chiropractic and massage therapy.
- Energy-based therapies: These practices focus on energy fields such as electromagnetic fields or biofields, which purportedly surround and penetrate the body. Examples include qi gong, reiki, acupuncture, and magnetic therapy.

The use of CAM is very common in the general population. The Centers for Disease Control and Prevention's (CDC's) National Center for Health Statistics conducted a National Health Interview Survey in 2007 and found that an estimated 38.3% of adults had used CAM therapy in the past twelve months. Additionally, the survey reported an estimated $33.9 billion in out-of-pocket expenses for visits to CAM practitioners and purchases of CAM products, classes, and materials. CAM use appears to be particularly high in oncology patients, with studies reporting CAM use in 48% to 88% of patients. Some of these surveys also suggest that younger, higher educated, higher income, and female patients are more likely to use CAM. Herbal products, megavitamins, and minerals appear to be some of the most commonly used therapies.

ROLE OF THE CLINICIAN

Despite the widespread use of CAM in the general public, most medical providers have limited knowledge about these practices. They may not even be aware that their patients are pursuing CAM. Studies have found that most patients do not mention the use of CAM to their providers unless specifically asked. Clinicians may also struggle with how best to advise patients about certain unproven therapies without alienating those with different personal, cultural, or religious belief systems. Clinicians may encounter patients whose family members or friends are actively encouraging them to use CAM therapies. Studies have shown that friends, families, and mass media are very common sources of information for patients who decide to use CAM.

Clinicians can play a key role in advising patients who are considering the use of CAM therapies. Patients should be counseled that overall, research suggests that CAM therapies are most useful when used for alleviation of symptoms and enhancement of quality of life. There is no compelling scientific evidence at this time to support the use of alternative approaches in lieu of conventional therapies. Patients should carefully consider the potential risks and benefits of CAM therapies using reliable sources, including their medical provider and government-sponsored websites that detail current research findings and potential adverse effects.

Clinicians should advise patients and their families to consider the following questions before pursuing a CAM therapy:

- Is there research to support the use of this particular therapy?
- Does the therapy require that you stop conventional medical treatments?
- Are there substantial side effects that can interfere with your ongoing medical treatments?
- Does the treatment or practitioner make unfounded claims such as the ability to cure cancer?
- Does the treatment require travel to another country?
- Is the treatment available to the general public or is it promoted as a secret, exclusive therapy?
- Is the CAM practitioner licensed by the state to provide that specific therapy?
- Is the treatment offered by an established medical institution or is it offered only by one individual?
- How expensive is the treatment and does it require substantial out-of-pocket expense?

A full review of the different CAM therapies is beyond the scope of this discussion, but clinicians should familiarize themselves with the following:

- Commonly used therapies that might benefit palliative care patients
- CAM therapies with potential safety issues
- Resources for further education of providers and patients

COMPLEMENTARY AND ALTERNATIVE THERAPIES WITH POTENTIAL BENEFIT

There is some clinical data to support the use of CAM in palliative care patients, but the body of evidence is not extensive. Research challenges include small sample sizes, difficulty creating an appropriate control arm, difficulty standardizing the delivery of intervention, short trial duration, and limited funding.

Acupuncture has been studied for its potential role in the management of symptoms, including nausea, vomiting, and pain. There is some positive evidence to support its use in chemotherapy-induced nausea and vomiting as an adjunct to standard antiemetic treatment. Acupuncture can also be effective for postoperative nausea and vomiting. Some trials have suggested that acupuncture may be useful in the treatment of pain, but systematic reviews have concluded that further studies are still needed. The risks of adverse events from acupuncture are minimal, and most complications have been related to lack of sterility of needles. Patients should be advised to only seek treatment from qualified, licensed practitioners who use disposable single-use needles. Although bleeding events are generally minor and localized, it is probably best to advise patients with bleeding disorders or on anticoagulation to avoid acupuncture. There have been case reports of rare serious events such as pneumothorax, but in general acupuncture is a safe complementary therapy.

Massage therapy can provide relief of anxiety and fatigue, based on several trials in cancer patients, though the duration of effect is not well established. Massage therapy has also been studied for its effect on pain, with several trials showing statistically significant reductions in pain measures in the immediate setting. Of note, however, pain reduction was not sustained over time. One particular form of massage, manual lymph drainage, was found in a few limited trials to reduce symptoms of lymphedema when used with compressive measures. Massage therapy is generally safe, but clinicians should advise patients with bleeding disorders or bony metastases to exercise caution and avoid all but the gentlest massage techniques.

Mind-body therapies such as hypnosis, meditation, guided imagery, and relaxation techniques have increasingly become integrated into the care of palliative care patients. Studies of mind-body interventions demonstrate potential to improve mood, relieve emotional distress, and enhance overall quality of life. Randomized control trials of relaxation training and guided imagery support their use in the treatment of anxiety. Some mind-body interventions also show promise in the treatment of physical symptoms. Hypnosis may have a role in pain and nausea treatment, based on several small randomized controlled trials. Additionally, nursing-led interventions such as breathing and relaxation techniques reduced dyspnea scores in several studies. If a patient reports benefit from mind-body therapies, clinicians can generally support their continued use as long as there is no clear interference with conventional treatments.

SAFETY CONCERNS

Some CAM therapies are safe to pursue even if evidence for efficacy is limited, but clinicians should advise their patients that certain practices carry potential risks. Patients should not initiate any CAM therapies without carefully researching and considering the risks.

Quality control for herbal preparations is not standardized, and there is real potential for harm through inconsistencies in preparation and contamination. Clinicians should counsel patients that "natural" does not necessarily mean that a product is safe. Patients have developed renal failure necessitating dialysis and even renal transplant after taking herbal preparations containing a nephrotoxic Chinese herb, *Aristolochia fang chi*. In one series, the patients were taking an herbal remedy for weight loss and a manufacturing error resulted in the substitution of *Aristolochia fang chi* for the intended herbal preparation. Patients taking herbal remedies for ezcema also have developed end-stage renal failure due to contamination from *Aristolochia fang chi*. This same herb is implicated in the development of urothelial cancer. In another example, PC-SPES ("PC" stands for prostate cancer; "spes" means "hope" in Latin), a product containing eight herbs, initially showed promise in the treatment of patients with advanced prostate cancer including decreased serum prostate-specific antigen, but it was recalled due to toxicity and contamination with conventional medications including warfarin and indomethacin. A report of a severe acquired bleeding diathesis after PC-SPES use suggested possible anticoagulant effect from warfarin contamination. The FDA subsequently issued a warning to discontinue use of PC-SPES, and this product is no longer available.

Additionally, many agents are pharmacologically active and carry the potential to interact with important conventional therapies. St. John's wort is an inducer of cytochrome P450 (CYP3A4) and has been found to reduce levels of chemotherapeutic agents including irinotecan. Experts in CAM therapies advise against the use of St. John's wort with concurrent chemotherapy. Ginseng and ginkgo biloba can also increase cytochrome p450 activity. Green tea (polyphenols) and grapefruit juice are known inhibitors of the cytochrome p450 system. Further information about drug interactions can be found in the resources listed below.

Macrobiotic diets are mainly vegetarian, high in grains, and low in fat. Patients at risk for malnutrition should avoid macrobiotic and other highly restrictive diets. Some macrobiotic diets are also high in phytoestrogens and may pose some risk for patients with estrogen-positive breast or endometrial cancer. Similarly, the literature recommends that these patients avoid large quantities of soy products and ginseng, as some preparations of ginseng have been found to contain phytoestrogens.

Many patients take high doses of vitamins with the hope that they may slow cancer progression, but there is no reliable evidence to support this. Additionally, vitamin C has some anticoagulant effect and vitamin E can diminish platelet function. Patients who are thrombocytopenic or taking anticoagulants should avoid high doses of these vitamins.

One of the most serious indirect consequences of the use of CAM is the delay of conventional treatment in favor of alternative therapies. Clinicians should strongly caution their patients against pursuing any CAM therapies that interfere with the initiation of recommended conventional therapies.

PRACTICE POINT

- Many herbal therapies are pharmacologically active and can interact with conventional treatments such as chemotherapy.

DISCHARGE CONSIDERATIONS

- Communicate with the responsible outpatient provider to discuss clinical status, overall goals, and plan of care. Such communication is particularly important in palliative care patients because of the high likelihood of new symptoms/side effects or a change in clinical status soon after discharge.
- Anticipate future symptoms and discuss with patients and their families. Develop a contingency plan for acute or worsening symptoms. Depending on overall plan of care, advise patients whether they should contact the hospice agency, outpatient provider, or return to the emergency room.
- Communicate with patients and families about their overall understanding of the disease and plan of care, including code status. Patients who wish to avoid resuscitation will need appropriate documentation so that future caregivers are aware of their wishes, including EMS personnel who might be called in an acute situation.
- Many patients will develop difficulty swallowing pills. Consider nonoral routes of medications in advance and communicate with patient's hospice agency if applicable. Hospice agencies can be particularly helpful in determining what non-oral routes of medications can be arranged at home (sublingual, rectal, subcutaneous infusions), what medications are commercially available, and what can be compounded by local pharmacies.

QUALITY IMPROVEMENT

Studies show that common symptoms such as pain, nausea, and dyspnea remain undertreated in patients with terminal illness, despite a clear impact on quality of life indices. Many factors contribute to this problem, including inadequate assessment by providers and underreporting by patients. Patients may be reluctant to report symptoms because they do not want to be perceived as a complainer, or they may worry that their symptoms are a sign of disease progression. Many patients also fear that they will become addicted to opioids. Clinicians may need to spend time uncovering these concerns to ensure good medication adherence. Additionally, clinicians themselves may carry certain misguided fears about prescribing opioids, such as causing respiratory depression or hastening death. These fears are largely unfounded but still contribute to the undertreatment of pain and dyspnea in patients with cancer, advanced COPD, other lung diseases, and congestive heart failure.

Other barriers lie in the realm of clinical systems, including a failure to assess and treat symptoms in a timely fashion. Hospitals should already have measures in place to routinely screen for pain, but patients can still suffer through long wait times for pain medications to arrive at the bedside. Patients with chronic or ongoing pain

TABLE 217-12 Online Resources

General information on CAM
National Center for Complementary and Alternative Medicine www.nccam.nih.gov
NIH Office of Dietary Supplements www.ods.od.nih.gov
Dietary Supplements Labels Database dietarysupplements.nlm.nih.gov/dietary
Natural Standard www.naturalstandard.com
UptoDate www.uptodate.com and www.uptodate.com/patients
Cancer websites
National Cancer Institute (NCI) Office of Cancer Complementary and Alternative Medicine www.cancer.gov/cam
M.D. Anderson Cancer Center www.mdanderson.org/departments/cimer
Memorial Sloan-Kettering Cancer Center www.mskcc.org/aboutherbs
Reporting of adverse events
Any adverse events from dietary or herbal supplements should be reported to the U.S. Food and Drug Administration
FDA Medwatch: 1-800-FDA-1088 www.fda.gov/medwatch/how.htm

should not be left to advocate for themselves with inappropriate PRN regimens, when in fact a long-acting regimen or a PCA may be more appropriate.

Many patients with advanced illness do not recognize the severity of their disease until an acute event occurs and they are hospitalized. Hospitalists are in a unique position to help patients during this time of crisis. Patients may wish to evaluate their quality of life and formulate appropriate, personalized goals for their future care. It is important to recognize that in certain populations, the palliative care approach continues to be underutilized, particularly in non-cancer diagnoses such as advanced COPD, congestive heart failure, end-stage liver disease, and dementia. Patients and family members are often unaware of the natural progression of these diseases, and an acute hospitalization is an opportunity for clinicians to help them understand the anticipated disease course and discuss whether palliative care or hospice is an appropriate option.

ONLINE RESOURCES FOR PATIENTS AND CLINICIANS

Further information is available for both patients and providers on a variety of reputable websites (**Table 217-12**).

SUGGESTED READINGS

Bardia A, Barton DL, Prokop LJ, et al. Efficacy of complementary and alternative medicine therapies in relieving cancer pain: a systematic review. *J Clin Oncol.* 2006;24:5457.

Weiger WA, Smith M, Boon H, et al. Advising patients who seek complementary and alternative medical therapies for cancer. *Ann Intern Med.* 2002;137:889.

ADDITIONAL SUGGESTED READINGS

General Symptom Management

Abrahm JL. A Physician's Guide to Pain and Symptom Management in Cancer Patients. Baltimore: John-Hopkins; 2005.

Fast Facts and Concepts: End of Life/Palliative Education Resource Center. http://www.mcw.edu/EPERC/FastFactsIndex

Pantilat, SZ, Isaac M. End-of-life care for the hospitalized patient. *Med Clin N Am.* 2008;92:349.

CHAPTER 218

Psychosocial, Cultural, and Spiritual Aspects

Stephanie Grossman, MD, FHM, FAACP
Farnaz Arabshahi, RN, FNP
Debbie Gunter, RN, FNP, ACHPN
Gwendolynn Harrell, RN, CHPN
Shella Patel, ANP, BSN, MSN
Sandra Schaap, MDiv
Tammie E. Quest, MD

Key Clinical Questions

1. What steps are most likely to relieve caregiver distress?
2. What steps are most likely to address a patient's anger?
3. What questions have been found to be moderately effective in screening for health care literacy?
4. What is the FICA Spiritual History Tool?

CASE 218-1

A 62-year-old woman who is regaining function after a recent stroke was observed to be crying at each clinical visit.

INTRODUCTION

Psychosocial aspects of care influence patient outcomes, compliance, and decision making. Patients experience illness within the context of their cultural and spiritual experience and do so surrounded by a network of family and caregivers. This chapter will identify and discuss the assessment and management of cultural, spiritual, and family caregiver aspects of care.

PSYCHOSOCIAL ASPECTS OF DISEASE

EMOTIONAL DISTRESS

Response to emotional distress is an important aspect of forging the therapeutic relationship. Patient encounters may reveal intense emotions such as fear, anger, sadness, and hopelessness, especially when patients face unexpected serious or life-threatening illness. The patient may already be experiencing significant life stressors prior to hospitalization, such as divorce, death or illness of a close relative, financial worry, difficulty with family relationships, or substance use or abuse. The patient may have undiagnosed or undertreated psychological or behavioral issues including anxiety or depression. When presented with empathetic opportunities, physicians often shift their focus to biomedical explanations. Responding to emotional distress with a supportive approach can help promote an atmosphere of trust, improved patient satisfaction, and better patient outcomes (**Table 218-1**).

When clinicians encounter anger, they should determine whether the source of the anger is internalized (eg, related to fear, loss of control, being a burden, or a result of anticipatory grief of life goals not accomplished) or externalized (eg, directed at others including health care providers). Personal feelings of guilt or fear may lead to anxiety, depression, or self-neglect. Effectively addressing anger may build trust and a strong therapeutic relationship, which are essential to optimal care (**Table 218-2**).

CAREGIVER BURDEN

Similar to a chronic stress experience, care giving creates physical and psychological strain over an extended period of time. The often unpredictable and uncontrollable nature of chronic disease, such as the need to be hospitalized, can cause additional distress in multiple life domains including family and work relationships. It has been suggested that physicians should support family caregivers in five key areas (1) excellence in communication with the family, (2) advance care planning and clear decision making, (3) support for home care, (4) empathy for family emotions and relationships, and (5) attention to grief and bereavement (**Table 218-3**).

FINANCIAL BURDEN OF DISEASE

The economic impact of illness is substantial to patients, families, and our health care system. It is estimated that 16% of families spend more than one-twentieth of their income on health care. Thirty-nine

TABLE 218-1 Responding to a Patient's Emotional Distress

1. Listen to the patient
   - No interruptions
2. Listen to yourself.
   - Read your own feelings but do not act on your emotions quickly
   - Allow your emotions to cue more discovery about the patient
3. Reflect thoughts, feelings, and behavior
   - Reflection means restating what a patient has said using their own words and phrases
4. Affirmation and respect
   - Thank the patient for risking the sharing of emotions
5. Empathic curiosity
   - Don't be afraid to ask for more information about the emotions (eg, Can you share with me more about your sadness)
6. Summarize and paraphrase
   - Restate the patient's story in your own words; in contrast to reflection, paraphrase and summary involves
7. Make a plan
   - May involve changes in how you and the patient communicate
   - Set expectations for next steps
   - Offer follow-up
   - Create a time period for returning

Data from Ambuel B, Responding to Patient Emotion, 2nd Edition. Fast Facts and Concepts. August 2005; 29. Available at: http://www.eperc.mcw.edu/fastfact/ff_029.htm.)

percent of terminally ill patients reported that health care costs have caused moderate or severe financial problems for them or their families. Health care costs have the potential to leave patients and families in financial ruin. In a 2007 study, it was estimated that 62% of all bankruptcies were due to medical care. The bankrupt patients and families, typically middle class, educated, homeowners, may then join the ranks of the uninsured or underinsured as a result. It is estimated that medical end-of-life care consumes 10% to 12% of the total health care budget in the United States and 27% of the Medicare budget.

TABLE 218-2 Focused Tips for Dealing with Anger

1. Engage the patient, but do not enmesh with nor do the emotional work for the patient.
2. Maintain adult-adult communication rather than fostering the patient's dependency.
3. Do not personalize the patient's anger.
4. Adopt a patient-centered worldview by ascertaining his values, priorities, and hopes.
5. Normalize anger so that the patient can move through this stage.

Data from Houston RE. The angry dying patient. Prim Care Companion. *J Clin Psychiatry*. 1999;1:5–8.

TABLE 218-3 Responding to Caregiver Needs

1. Excellence in communication with the family
   a. Proactive guidance with data sharing
   b. Family meetings
2. Advance care planning and clear decision making
   a. Discussions of values and preferences
3. Support for home care
   a. Specific teaching of the caregiver for medication administration
   b. Referral for support for 24-hour advice
   c. Roleplaying with caregivers about how to communicate with emergency providers and patients advance care planning wishes
   d. Teaching natural course of decline and expectations
4. Empathy for family emotions and relationships
   a. Referral to supportive resources
   b. Validate caregivers feelings and frustrations
5. Attention to grief and bereavement
   a. Condolence call
   b. Normalize grief
   c. Suggest journaling, counseling, and support groups

Data from Rabow MW, Hauser JM, Adams J. Supporting family caregivers at the end of life: "they don't know what they don't know". *JAMA*. 2004;291(4):483–491.

IMPACT OF CULTURE ON DISEASE

DEFINITIONS

Culture is defined as learned behaviors, beliefs, values, practices, and customs. Race, ethnicity, nationality, language, and gender influence culture, as well as social and economic status, sexual orientation, and occupation.

Cultural diversity is defined as the variety of human societies or cultures in a specific region or in the world as a whole. The United States population has become more diverse than ever before, and this trend is expected to continue in the foreseeable future. According to the United States Census Bureau's 2003 population report, 11.7% of the population was born in a foreign country; physicians increasingly care for patients from various cultural backgrounds. In order to ensure patients receive the best possible health care, physicians must be cognizant of the diverse backgrounds they may encounter in a clinical setting and approach these patients in a sensitive manner.

Cultural competency is "the combination of similar beliefs, feelings, and guidelines used by professionals to effectively provide care in cross-cultural circumstances." The provider should appreciate that one culture is not uniformly practiced among its members and avoid making assumptions about patients' cultural preferences. Strategies for cross-cultural interviewing include directly inquiring about a patient's beliefs and thoughts toward medical care (**Table 218-4**).

THE CULTURE OF HEALTH CARE

The culture health care in the United States embraces a Western, disease-centered model, where mechanical dysfunction of an organ or an organ system in response to specific insults causes sickness. This system commonly interprets medical illness as "mechanical malfunction," whereas some other societies perceive illness as an

TABLE 218-4 Cross-cultural Interview Questions Regarding Serious Illness and End-of-life Care

"Some people want to know everything about their medical condition, and others do not. What is your preference? Do you prefer to make medical decisions about future tests or treatments for yourself, or would you prefer that someone else make them for you?"
To patients who request that the physician discuss their condition with family members: *"Would you be more comfortable if I spoke with your* [brother, son, daughter] *alone, or would you like to be present?"*
If the patient chooses not to be present: *"If you change your mind at any point and would like more information, please let me know. I will answer any questions you have."* (This exchange should be documented in the medical record.)
When discussing medical issues with family members, particularly through a translator, it is often helpful to confirm understanding: *"I want to be sure that I am explaining your mother's treatment options accurately. Could you explain to me what you understand about your mother's condition and the treatment that we are recommending? Is there anything that would be helpful for me to know about how your family, community, or religious faith views serious illness and treatment?"*
Sometimes people are uncomfortable discussing these issues with a doctor who is of a different race or cultural background: *"Are you comfortable with me treating you? Will you please let me know if there is anything about your background that would be helpful for me to know in working with you or your* [mother, father, sister, brother]*?"*

Data from Searight HR, Gafford J. Cultural diversity at the end of life: issues and guidelines for family physicians. *Am Fam Physician*. 2005;71(3):515–522.

imbalance of forces in the body. The patient's *explanatory model of illness* includes his own cultural framework. What may appear to be nonadherence may in fact be related to a conflict between the patient's or family's explanatory model of illness compared with that of the clinical team. In addition to their underlying race, religion, and socioeconomic background, health care providers' education and clinical experiences help shape their thoughts as clinicians and impact their practices. For these reasons, providers and patients may not share common beliefs in certain treatments. Clinicians should always inquire about how their patients view illness and treatments and their potential effectiveness when individualizing a disease management plan. By showing respect for patients and taking the time to have an open dialogue, clinicians may achieve compliance with a treatment that the patient may have otherwise refused.

PRACTICE POINT

- Clinicians should always inquire about how their patients view illness and treatments and their potential effectiveness when individualizing a disease management plan. By showing respect for patients and taking the time to have an open dialogue, clinicians may achieve compliance with a treatment that the patient may have otherwise refused.

OVERGENERALIZATION AND STEREOTYPING

While recognizing that there are many similarities among people from the same culture, it is important for health care providers to keep in mind the concept of individualism by recognizing uniqueness in lifestyle, personal history, belief system, communication style, education, generation, and health status. The concept of generalization can lead to stereotyping, or the notion that all people from a given group are the same. This may greatly impact an individual's attitude toward other cultures by creating conflicts and misunderstandings.

HEALTH LITERACY

Health literacy is the degree to which one can obtain, process, and understand basic health information and services needed to make appropriate health decisions. National Assessment of Adult Literacy indicates that only 12% of the American adult population has proficient health literacy skills. Low health literacy has been linked to poor health knowledge, incorrect medication use, poorer health status, and higher hospitalization rates. Physicians are often unaware of a patient's limited literacy. The most accurate tools for assessing health care literacy, the REALM (3 minutes) and S-TOFHLA (7 to 12 minutes), require several minutes to perform. Hospitalists should be able to identify patients at increased risk of low health literacy, rapidly screen these patients by asking a few simple questions, and regularly assess their recall (ie, understanding of information during their hospitalization). Clues to problems with health literacy include (1) difficulty with written materials (eg, delay in reading the materials or completing materials with incorrect responses), (2) responses to questions about medications (eg, inability to tell the provider when or how to take medications), (3) behaviors that appear to be noncompliant (eg, missed appointments may be a result of the patient not being able to read an appointment reminder card). Screening questions that have been found to be moderately effective include the following:

1. How comfortable are you filling out medical forms?
2. How often do you have someone help you read health information?
3. How do you rate your own reading ability?

Strategies for managing patients with low health literacy are identified in **Table 218-5**.

HEALTH CARE DISPARITIES

Minority Americans receive less and lower-quality health care than the majority (white) populations, and the reasons accounting this disparity are exceedingly complex. (See Chapter 3 for a more detailed discussed of disparities in health care in the United States.) The Institute of Medicine findings suggest the following: (1) Racial and ethnic disparities in health care exist even when insurance status, income, age, and severity of conditions are comparable. (2) Differences in health care occur in the context of broader historic and contemporary social and economic inequality. (3) Many sources, including entire health systems, providers, patients, and health care plan managers, contribute to racial and ethnic disparities. (4) Bias, stereotyping, prejudice, and clinical uncertainty on the part of health care providers may contribute to racial and ethnic disparities in health care. (5) Racial and ethnic minority patients are more likely than white patients to refuse treatment, but differences in refusal rates are generally small. Clinicians should be aware that these disparities exist and that solutions are complex and multifactorial. Clinicians should proactively provide additional resources through multidisciplinary teamwork to enable less-disparate care.

COMMUNICATION AND DECISION MAKING

Optimal patient care requires effective communication and informed decision making. Language barriers commonly exist when English is not the patient's first language. Clinicians should be familiar with when and how to effectively use translators during the medical interview.

TABLE 218-5 Techniques Recommended for Improving Communication with Patients who have Limited Health Literacy

Communication Method	Comment
Talk more slowly	Communication is enhanced when patients have more time to absorb what is being said.
Use nonmedical language	Unless patients have personal experience with a particular medical illness, they have no reason to be familiar with medical terms that pertain to that illness. Explain things to patients in simple terms, like you might explain them to your grandmother.
Limit information	Research shows that patients recall only a fraction of what clinicians tell them—often because clinicians give them too much information. Recall is enhanced if information is limited to two or three key points and these points are repeated.
Use "teach-back"	Ask patients to repeat what you told them about what they need to do, to verify that they understand correctly.
Encourage questions	Individuals with low literacy tend to lack self-empowerment and often will not spontaneously ask questions. You need to encourage them to do so.

Data from Searight HR, Gafford J. Cultural diversity at the end of life: issues and guidelines for family physicians. *Am Fam Physician*. 2005;71(3):515–522.

THE IMPACT OF SPIRITUALITY ON DISEASE

The word *spirit* stems from the Latin noun *spiritus*, meaning breath, and from the verb *spirare*, meaning to breathe. It is related to the experience of connectedness to the moment, to self, to others, to nature, and to the significant or sacred. It could be said that spirituality makes one "breathe" in the nonphysical sense; it provides meaning and strength and helps individuals cope with life's challenges.

Although religion expresses spirituality by defining the practices, beliefs, and texts about transcendence shared by a particular community, spirituality is not limited to religion. Illness affects the spirit; it affects what gives people strength, meaning, and direction in life and what helps them to feel rooted and connected to self, others, nature, and sometimes to God. Not just a physical event, illness disrupts all aspects of life, provokes anxiety, and can cause isolation. In addition, illness often brings about reflection on one's life and relationships, possibly causing a redefinition of self and priorities. Coping with a life-threatening illness becomes the patient's life work. Many patients and family members struggle with the existential questions:

- Meaning: Has my life mattered?
- Reflection: How will I be remembered?
- Connections with loved ones: Who do I need to forgive?

The existential questions that patients face can cause spiritual suffering, a form of pain that cannot be treated with medication. Despite this, many patients find it important that their medical providers acknowledge and show interest in their spirituality. A survey on spirituality in medicine from 2006 revealed that 62% of seriously ill patients found it "moderately" to "incredibly" important that primary care physicians (PCPs) address spiritual concerns. Only 11% were asked by PCPs if they would like to discuss spiritual concerns, and 12% were asked about importance of spirituality to them. When asked why they did not bring up spirituality with their PCP, 62% of the patients stated they did not think it was part of a physician's job, 31% did not think the PCP had time, and 17% did not think the PCP would want to discuss it (**Figure 218-1**).

What	**What** do you call the problem? **What** do you think the illness does? **What** do you think the natural course of the illness is? **What** are the most important results you hope to receive from this treatment? **What** are the chief problems your sickness has caused for you? **What** do you fear most about your sickness?
Why	**Why** do you think this illness or problem has occurred?
Who	**Who** do you turn to for help? **Who** should be involved in decision making?
How	**How** do you think the sickness should be treated? **How** severe is your sickness? **How** do you want us to help you?

Figure 218-1 *Explanatory model of illness.*

Spirituality, including beliefs about illness, health, dying, and afterlife, instructs many patients' values and norms. It also plays an important role in medical decision making and helps narrow down patients' goals for their health care.

PROVIDERS OF SPIRITUAL CARE

Patients enter the health care system to seek help with psychological or mental discomfort. While they are receiving medical care, there may be significant spiritual suffering, especially when the illness turns out to be serious and/or life threatening. The Joint Commission on Accreditation of Health Care Organizations recognizes that offering spiritual care contributes to the healing (even when there is no cure) and well-being of patients and their loved ones and, therefore, requires health care institutions to assess and address their patients' spirituality in an adequate way. Spiritual care supports the unique framework people use to give meaning to their lives, regardless of what the specific framework is.

HOSPITAL CHAPLAINS

Unlike community ministers, the training of health care chaplains includes supervised training in the clinical setting along with a degree in theology. This education enables them to assess the spiritual pain patients may be experiencing and to assist patients in using their own sources of strength to cope with illness without imposing beliefs, solutions, and values. Since most health care chaplains do not have a medical background, they approach patient care from a different angle, focusing on patients' stories and sources of strength. Sometimes chaplains are "bridges" between the medical language used by providers and the spiritual language the patient and family uses to express their fears, hopes, and beliefs. The chaplain can ask the medical provider clarifying questions during family meetings and, at the same time, make spiritual values and beliefs part of the conversation. By building relationship and trust, providing reflective listening, and using rituals and prayer when appropriate, the chaplain can assist patients with finding the spiritual healing they need.

While chaplains are the spiritual care specialists in the health care environment, they are not alone in serving this function. Handzo and Koenig (2004) describe the role medical providers have in

TABLE 218-6 FICA Spiritual History Tool

F	Do you have a spiritual belief or Faith? Do you have spiritual beliefs that help you cope with stress? What gives your life meaning?
I	Are these beliefs Important to you? How do they influence you in how you care for yourself?
C	Are you part of a spiritual or religious Community?
A	How would you like your health care provider to Address these issues with you?

addressing spirituality as "generalists in spiritual care." They propose that medical providers include a short spiritual assessment as part of the physical assessment. Medical providers need not engage in theological discussions, try to answer unanswerable questions, or reach beyond their expertise. However, understanding how a patient's religious beliefs help or hinder her ability to cope with illness and influence her health care decisions is essential to good medical care. If necessary, the medical provider can then refer a patient to the chaplain, who further explores and supports the patient's spirituality. The FICA Spiritual History Tool is an example of an effective instrument for guiding conversations in the clinical setting (**Table 218-6**).

CONCLUSION

Understanding cultural aspects of disease is integral for successful patient-provider interactions and achieving mutual goals. Providers should appreciate basic elements of culture, including Western medicine's orientation in the context of the patient's explanatory model of illness, tendencies for over generalization and stereotyping, and the importance of considering health literacy as a barrier to optimal outcomes. Proactively providing additional resources by using interpreters, social workers, chaplains, and other caregivers may enhance communication and reduce disparities in care.

SUGGESTED READINGS

Cross T, Barzon J, Dennis K, Isaacs R. *Towards a Culturally Competent System of Care: A Monograph on Effective Services for Minority Children Who are Severely Emotionally Disturbed.* Washington, DC: CASSP Technical Assistance Center, Georgetown University Child Development Center. 1989.

Emanuel ES, Fairclough DL, Slutsman J, Eamnuel LL. Understanding economic and other burdens of terminal illness: the experience of patients and their caregivers. *Annals of Internal Medicine.* 2000;132:6:451–459.

Handzo G, Koenig HG. Spiritual care: whose job is it anyway? *South Med J.* 2004;97:1242–1244.

Himmelstein DU, Thorne D, Warren E, Woolhandler S. Medical bankruptcy in the United States, 2007: results of a national study. *Am J Med.* 2009;122(8):741–746.

Hogan C, Lunney J, Gabel J, Lynn J. Medicare beneficiaries' costs of care in the last year of life. *Health Affairs.* 2001;20(4):188–195.

Institute of Medicine. *Unequal Treatment: Confronting Racial and Ethnic Disparities in HealthCare.* Washington, D.C.: National Academy Press.

Kutner M, Greenberg E, Jin Y, Paulsen C. *The Health Literacy of America's Adults: Results from the 2003 National Assessment of Adult Literacy (NCES 2006-483).* Washington, DC: National Center for Education Statistics, US Department of Education; 2006.

Merlis, M. *Family Out-of-Pocket Spending for Health Services.* New York: Commonwealth Fund, June 2002.

Nelson A. Unequal treatment: confronting racial and ethnic disparities in health care. *J Nat Med Assoc.* 2002;94(8):666–668.

Powers, BJ, Trinh, JV, Bosworth, HB. Can this patient read and understand written health information? *JAMA.* 2010;304(1):76–84.

Puchalski, Improving the quality of spiritual care as a dimension of palliative care: the report of the consensus conference. *J Palliative Med.* 2009;12(10):885–904.

CHAPTER 219

Care of the Imminently Dying Patient

Rita F. Moldovan, DNP, MS, RN
Sydney Dy, MSc, MD

Key Clinical Questions

1. How do I know if a patient is dying?
2. What should I include in a family meeting?
3. What should I consider in the withdrawal of life-sustaining treatment?

OVERVIEW

There is substantial evidence that patients with advanced chronic illness often receive inappropriate or inadequate care, have poorly managed symptoms, experience spiritual distress and financial worries, and possess incomplete knowledge about illness progression. Hospitalized dying patients frequently receive aggressive care up to and including life-sustaining treatment and resuscitation, but inadequate preparation for potential death. Since approximately 50% of deaths occur in the hospital setting, substantial numbers of patients may experience increased suffering due to futile or iatrogenic interventions, needless delays to timely discharge, and insufficient patient and family inclusion in decisions about end-of-life care.

Recent government data show the aggregate costs of dying in the hospital amount to $20 billion. The average cost of an admission ending in death is three times that of a patient who is alive at discharge ($26,000 versus $94,00). Patients who had procedures (73%) were more likely to die than those who had none (27%). Twelve percent of those who died were admitted for an elective procedure, while 72% were admitted through the emergency department. Medicare insured 67% of all the patients who died in hospitals at a cost of more than $12 billion. Although more studies are needed to show whether this is too much or too little to spend, abundant evidence suggests that there is significant room for improvement in the area of end-of-life care.

An underlying diagnosis of metastatic cancer, end-stage renal or lung disease, severe liver disease, or congestive heart failure and a decline in performance status increase the likelihood of dying in the hospital. Other factors include prolonged length of stay without evident progress and a diagnosis of frailty in elderly patients. The dying process may begin with a gradual decline in a patient initially admitted with multiple comorbidities. The decline to death may occur more rapidly with a sudden cardiac event or respiratory failure. Sometimes invasive procedures such as the placement of a percutaneous feeding tube, stent, endoscopic retrograde cholangiopancreatography (ERCP), or bronchoscopy may precipitate the decline of a compromised, frail patient.

CARE ON THE GENERAL UNIT

The dying process usually occurs over hours to weeks and should be suspected when certain signs are present (**Tables 219-1** and **219-2**).

Factors that may prolong the dying process include artificial hydration, nutrition, and supplemental oxygen as well as unresolved emotional or spiritual conflicts that include the patient's "readiness" to die, family conflict, or need for reconciliation (**Table 219-3**).

Ideally, the patient's health care team (eg, the patient's primary nurse, a social worker or care coordinator, and sometimes consultants or the hospital chaplain) periodically meet with key family members and with the patient, if appropriate, to update progress, answer questions, address issues relating to prognosis, and provide additional perspective and support. As soon as the team recognizes the dying process as more imminent, a subsequent family meeting should take place with members of the multidisciplinary care team. Clinicians should document in the medical record attendees, a summary of understanding about the disease process, the patient's values and preferences, any decisions about life-sustaining treatment, and next steps.

TABLE 219-1 Stages of Dying

Early stage
Bedbound; loss of interest/ability to eat, drink, take medications; increasing sleepiness/delirium
Middle stage
Obtunded, death rattle; inability to clear pooled secretions
Late stage
Coma, cool extremities, mottling, altered respiratory pattern, fever

Data from Weissman D. Fast Facts and Concepts. Available at http://www.eperc.mcw.edu.

In a private place, the health care team should spend more time listening to the family than speaking, soliciting, and responding to questions. The team should assure the family that the patient will not be abandoned and will be kept comfortable. The team should also empathetically respond to the stress, fears, and challenges of a family facing the death of a loved one. Honest sharing of the prognosis helps the family prepare emotionally and practically for the patient's death. Although families may not believe the prognosis, the medical team should be honest and not withhold information that may result in a false sense of hope. Disclosing a poor prognosis should include planning on the medical team's part, firing a "warning shot," and asking who the patient wants present for that conversation.

Clinicians should aggressively manage distressing symptoms. Allowing the family access to the patient by providing relaxed visiting hours and overnight stay, if possible, promotes a normal grieving process and enhanced communication (**Table 219-4**).

Palliative sedation (PS) involves inducing varying degrees of sedation to manage distressing symptoms, such as agitation, delirium, dyspnea, pain, or emotional distress, that are refractory to all other treatment modalities. Patients who are in the dying trajectory (days to weeks) with severe, irreversible illness and refractory symptoms should receive PS. The decision for PS involves deliberative evaluation and collaboration with the patient who has decisional capacity, the family or surrogate, pain and palliative care services, psychiatry, and pastoral care. The sole intent of PS, which includes the potential for future wakefulness, is to relieve suffering, not to hasten death. A do-not-resuscitate (DNR) order must be written, and informed consent must be obtained. Following death, offering the family private time to spend in the presence of the deceased patient can help facilitate the grieving process.

For the patient able to tolerate ambulance transport, practical discharge options (eg, home hospice care, inpatient hospice, or a nursing facility that provides palliative and hospice care) are based on the patient's needs, local resources, and family preference for the site of death. For an actively dying patient, the team should respect the wishes of the family who may want the patient to die at home even if there is a risk of death during transit. A required emergency medical services (EMS) DNR form, available from the hospital, hospice, or state Web sites, documents DNR and do-not-intubate (DNI) status for ambulance transport. Social workers factor local resources in their assessment of family care-giving capability. Home discharge is not always the best option, especially with limited family care-giving capabilities, complex care requirements, difficult-to-manage symptoms, and the availability of alternative solutions.

TABLE 219-2 Signs of Dying

Decreasing cardiac output
Tachycardia, hypotension, cyanosis, mottling, livedo reticularis
Renal failure
Oliguria/anuria
Neurologic dysfunction
Metabolic imbalance, reduced perfusion, decreasing level of consciousness, terminal delirium: hypo- or hyperactivity

TABLE 219-3 Family Meeting

Prepare staff prior to family meeting to establish medical facts, and voice concerns; arrange for a quiet setting; plan for adequate time; determine patient competence, or appropriate surrogate; assure all appropriate staff and family attend the meeting. *What is the patient's prognosis?* *What are the current medical issues?* *What are the current options, risks, and benefits?* *What are the team concerns about the situation?* *Are there conflicts among team about patient's treatment, goals of care, etc.?* *Are all of the consultant services on board with treatment plan?*
Establish what is known by the patient and each family member. *Tell us what you understand about the patient's condition.* *What have other doctors told you about your condition?* *What does the patient/family want to know?* *How do you want me to handle information about your illness? Some patients want to make all decisions for themselves while other patients prefer others to do this for them.*
Use simple language with sensitivity to deliver information including your opinion about the likelihood of survival. Do not be afraid to say "dying." *This is what we know about your father's condition right now (give specific details).* *I feel badly to have to tell you this, but the tests are back and it is not what we hoped for.* *We are doing X, Y, and Z. We're doing everything we can but we may find in 48 hours (or other specified time frame) that this approach is not working. Your father's heart (brain, liver, kidneys) are very damaged. If he survives this hospital stay, he will be in a coma, not able to talk to you, etc.* *I would not be surprised if [the patient] died within the next month/week/day/hours.* *I can't give you an exact time, but in my experience patients with your condition live ___ weeks/months/years to ___ weeks/months/years (give ranges).*
Respond to emotions. Give time for the information to sink in, silence is appropriate. Verbally recognize emotions. Touch the family member's hand or shoulder if appropriate. Offer water or to call someone if needed. *I wish the news were different. What worries you the most?* *Tell me more about your feelings about what I just said. Is there anyone you would like me to call?* *I'm sorry to have to tell you this. How can I help?* *You appear to be angry. Can you tell me what you are feeling?*

TABLE 219-4 Sample Comfort Care Order Set

Include
Goals of care discussion; code status: do not (re)intubate, treat dysrhythmias, or hemodynamic instability.
Discontinue
Medications, labs, transfusions, neurological exams, vital signs, pulse oximetry, monitor display, gastric tube, enteral feeds, dialysis.
Withdrawal of ventilator support
Extubate to room air, face mask, T-piece, nasal cannula.
Symptom management
Pain, dyspnea, terminal secretions, anxiety, delirium, depression, nausea/vomiting, hiccups, pruritus, dry eyes.
Psychosocial
Liberal visiting hours, bereavement packet for family
Consults
Palliative care service, social work, pastoral care

Prior to transport, the health care team should prepare the family about the signs and symptoms of dying, including decreasing consciousness, changes in respiratory pattern, decreasing urinary output, skin mottling, and coolness. Since the patient may retain the sense of hearing, both family and staff should be prudent about conversations held at the bedside. The family can take advantage of this time to express feelings of love, gratitude, asking and granting forgiveness, and saying goodbye. Final communications even as the patient loses consciousness and enters coma are important for a peaceful death outcome. Social workers can help with practical arrangements (eg, financial, funeral) and may have educational materials. An excellent online resource is The Handbook for Mortals at www.growthhouse.org/educate/flash/mortals/layouts/frameset1.html.

For patients discharged to home hospice, the health care team should provide prescriptions that can be filled on site for emergency drugs that the family may need at home. These include short-acting liquid opiate concentrates to manage pain and dyspnea, a benzodiazepine or haloperidol to manage agitation, an anticholinergic such as hyoscine or glycopyrrolate for upper airway gurgle or secretions, and prochlorperazine suppository for nausea and vomiting (**Table 219-5**).

TABLE 219-5 Standard Home Hospice Medications

Morphine oral solution 20 mg/ml. Give 5 mg. orally every 2 hours as needed for pain or shortness of breath. Dispense 30–60 cc.
Lorazepam 1 mg/1 cc solution. Give 1 mg orally every four hours as needed for restlessness or agitation. Dispense 30 cc.
If the patient is elderly or may not tolerate lorazepam, write for haloperidol.
Haloperidol 1 mg/2cc solution. Give 1 mg orally every four hours as needed for restlessness or agitation. Dispense 30 cc.
Prochlorperazine 25 mg rectal suppository. Give one suppository by rectum every 12 hours as needed for nausea and vomiting.
Hyoscine solution 0.125 mg/ml. Give 1 ml orally four times a day as needed for upper airway congestion. Dispense 30 cc.

DECELERATION OF CARE IN THE INTENSIVE CARE UNIT

Approximately 20% of deaths in the United States occur during or following an intensive care unit (ICU) admission. Palliative care remains an ongoing need in this setting due to the severity of illness, the choice of chronic and terminally ill patients for a trial of ICU care, and rising numbers of elderly patients whose numbers will double by 2030 from 35 million to 72 million.

Patients at high risk for death in the ICU include those with acute respiratory failure, multisystem organ failure with sepsis or malignancy, coma, chronic obstructive lung disease with respiratory failure, decompensated congestive heart failure, severe cirrhosis, metastatic colon cancer, non–small cell lung cancer, anoxic encephalopathy after cardiopulmonary resuscitation, and severe dementia. A predicted ICU stay greater than or equal to five days indicates a poor prognosis for survival. If the physician has reason to believe the patient will not survive, he should inform the family using dying terminology.

Patients in the ICU, even those on mechanical ventilation and sedation, often have significant symptoms and suffering due to disease and interventions. Symptoms include pain, dyspnea, anxiety, panic, delirium, and distress due to inability to communicate. Many patients can report their symptoms, and for very ill patients, even routine procedures such as turning in bed can cause severe pain.

Up to 95% of ICU patients may not be able to make their own decisions due to sedation or illness, thereby necessitating family and/or surrogate involvement. Even when the patient's wishes are known, surrogates may feel unable or unwilling to follow the patient's wishes, feel quite burdened with the task of making decisions, perceive conflict among team members and/or consultants, or need more time to make decisions. In addition, physicians frequently hesitate to make recommendations about end-of-life care even when the family looks to guidance about prognosis. Physicians have a responsibility to provide recommendations and guidance for the family to enable shared decision making so that they have sufficient time to make decisions. When signs of improvement in the patients clinical condition do not occur after a specified period of time in the ICU, then the physician should continue discussions of the goals of care, which may include transitioning to comfort care at the end of life. Although physicians are generally not obligated to offer interventions that in their best judgment will not meet mutually defined goals of care, they should try to maintain a positive relationship with the family, continue efforts to reach consensus during the course of care, and obtain ethics consultation to facilitate conflict resolution.

Intensivists should evaluate the efficacy and goals of providing antibiotics, vasoactive drugs, renal dialysis, and ventricular assist devices for patients with irreversible progression of disease. Selected interventions may be maintained for a time-limited period to allow for family visitation, spiritual services and rituals, and closure of life affairs. Physicians may recommend not escalating aggressive care such as pressors or blood products and focusing on comfort measures at the end of life. During family meetings, the multidisciplinary team should discuss withdrawal of life-sustaining treatment (LST) with the goal of maintaining patient comfort at the end of life and allowing natural death. When therapies such as dialysis or vasoactive drugs are discontinued, clinicians should carefully consider the efficacy of all other LST. Rather than offer the family a menu of possible options (antibiotics, artificial hydration/nutrition, pressors, dialysis, and other measures), clinicians should define goals in general terms for the patient's quality of life. Once the goals of care are established, the clinician team should proceed with interventions that best address the goals of care.

WITHDRAWAL OF LIFE-SUSTAINING TREATMENT PROCESS

Survival rates for in-hospital cardiopulmonary resuscitation (CPR) have not changed substantially from 1992 to 2005 and average 18% survival. Survival rates were lower among the following patients: older age, male gender, cancer or multiple comorbid conditions, or transfers from a skilled nursing facility. Patients with pneumonia, hypotension, renal failure, cancer, and homebound status were significantly less likely to survive resuscitation. In addition to ICU prognostication, scoring mechanisms such as the Glasgow Coma Scale, the Acute Physiology and Chronic Health Evaluation, and the Mortality Prediction Model, the physician's clinical judgment, experience, and philosophy of care also play a role in determining prognosis and guiding the decision to deescalate care. The chances for survival of patients in the dying trajectory who undergo resuscitation are qualitatively nonexistent or extremely low at best. Clinical judgment and knowledge about the patient's wishes guide making recommendations for the use of CPR versus allowing for natural death. The family's decision not to resuscitate is often a helpful first step in getting family members to recognize the inevitable outcome and move toward withdrawal of life-sustaining but noncurative interventions. The following steps should be taken:

1. Reassure families that the patient is not being abandoned and of the ongoing commitment to help the patient.
2. Ensure patient comfort including aggressively treating breathlessness and pain.
3. Educate families about the process of withdrawing LST, the potential for survival following extubation, and the dying process, including the presence of involuntary movements.
4. Respect the spiritual and cultural needs of families including bedside prayer services and certain rituals around the dying process.
5. Discontinue treatment and monitoring that does not promote patient comfort, remove tubes, and lower bedrails to allow family access to the patients and promote a quiet atmosphere that does not interrupt family visits.
6. Avoid neuromuscular blocking agents (eg, vecuronium, pancuronium, and atracurium), as they preclude evaluation of patient comfort; allow considerable time for such drugs to clear the system especially in patients with renal and liver failure.
7. Provide simple extubation to humidified or room air as the better option *as long as adequate sedation and analgesia are provided* because there is less risk of producing prolonged and unacceptable respiratory symptoms.
8. Use opiates rather than supplemental oxygen, which can prolong the dying process by hours or days, to relieve dyspnea, grimacing, and agitation. A suggested starting dose is morphine 5 to 10 mg and/or midazolam 2 to 4 mg via intravenous (IV) push every 10 minutes until symptoms are relieved for opiate-naïve patients.
9. Provide acute grief support through pastoral care, social work, the family advocate, and palliative care.
10. Have information available on funeral and cremation services, social security and death benefits, normal grief reactions, follow-up counseling, bereavement groups, and contacts for psychological counseling.
11. Consider writing a sympathy note to the family. A letter of condolence may facilitate closure and clinicians should not omit this practice. There may be many reasons why this practice is not commonly done, including changes in societal expectations. Writing a note generally requires all clinical staff to overcome their own sense of failure or loss or inability to express emotions when their patient dies. Hospitalists in particular may feel that they do not know their patients well enough.

PRACTICE POINT

The bereavement note

- Acknowledge the death and include the patient's name.
- Express sympathy and concern or, if appropriate, describe in detail the extent and depth of the relationship between the patient and physician.
- Avoid issues of legal liability or revisiting clinical details of illness.
- Avoid phrases such as "it was meant to be" or "I know how you feel."
- Share a personal memory of the patient; include their special qualities, such as courage during the illness, or character.
- Comment on the family's loving care for the patient.
- Remind family of their qualities that will help them cope: strength, resilience, religious faith.
- Offer your contact information if family has questions.
- Include a statement such as, "It was a privilege to have participated in your loved one's care."
- Add a sincere closing such as, "You are in my thoughts and prayers."

PRACTICE POINT

- A physician's professional responsibility for caring for a hospitalized patient does not end when the patient dies in the hospital. A letter of condolence may provide a powerful message to the bereaved family members and facilitate closure for the patient's family and physician. Failure to do this may communicate a lack of concern about their loss.

"Unlike expressions of condolence made by telephone or in person, a letter of condolence is a concrete gift that the recipient can and will review over and over" (Bedell, Cadenhead, & Graboys, 2001). It sends a powerful message that physicians recognize the privilege of our profession that allows sharing with patients and families moments of life and death.

ORGAN DONATION

If the patient is an organ donor, follow state and organization policies and procedures. Federal and Medicare regulations require hospitals to provide family members with the opportunity to authorize organ donation for their loved one; inform them that the donation will not disfigure the patient and that the primary insurer usually covers the costs associated with this process.

BEREAVEMENT

Significantly influenced by culture, bereavement encompasses both inner feelings of grief and the outward signs of mourning. The process of uncomplicated grieving includes physical, emotional, cognitive, and behavioral responses that can normally occur over months to years but gradually decline over time.

Clinicians may facilitate the normal grieving process by educating the family about the normal dying process, listening to the family's reminiscences, and allowing time during family meetings for expressions of grief that normally include a range of emotional responses. Clinician presence at the bedside for a few moments at the time of withdrawal of life support or following death provides comfort to the family, sends a sign of nonabandonment to the family, and also allows the clinician time for personal closure. The spiritual care provider or hospital chaplain may facilitate a prayer service or other rituals. Normalize the grief process through anticipatory grieving

TABLE 219-6 Risk Factors for Poor Bereavement Outcomes

Poor social supports
Past history of psychiatric problems, especially depression
Past history of childhood separation anxiety
High initial distress
Unanticipated death, lack of preparation for death
Other major concurrent stresses and losses
History of abuse or neglect in childhood
Lifestyle rigidity
Highly dependent relationship with the deceased
Death of a child

Data from Stroebe M, Schut H, Stroebe W. Health outcomes of bereavement. *Lancet,* 2007;370:1960.

(eg, thinking about what it will be like to live without the loved one and encourage the family to express their feelings).

Beetween 10% and 15% of survivors experience chronic depression, and up to 20% experience complicated grief involving persistent, disruptive yearning and pining for the loved one for at least six months with significant functional impairment in important areas of life. Signs of complicated grief include trouble accepting the death, excessive bitterness related to the death, feeling uneasy about moving on, detachment from formerly close others, feeling life is meaningless and holds no hope of fulfillment without the loved one, and feeling agitated since the death. Risk factors for complicated grief include sudden or traumatic death, suicide or homicide, the death of a child, and the experience of multiple losses (**Table 219-6**). Signs of complicated grief include severe isolation, violent behavior, suicidal ideation, and severe or prolonged depression.

Hospitals may provide resources with information on funeral homes, cremation, social security, financial and child support/care considerations, and bereavement support including bereavement groups and individual counseling services. Local hospices will usually provide bereavement care and support groups to families even if the patient did not receive hospice care (although there may be a fee). Services include risk assessment; follow-up for at least 12 months after death, including phone calls, anniversary and holiday cards, memorial services; and information on referral to bereavement counselors and specialists or support groups.

CLINICIAN GRIEF AND SELF-CARE

Caring for patients who are dying can take a toll on the providers entrusted with their care. It is natural for us to grieve the death of our patients, especially when we have developed a relationship with them, or if we have had to deal with strong grief reactions from the family. Other clinicians who cared for the patient may be grieving as well. Processing the patient's death with other members of the care team through a debriefing session can be helpful.

Physicians may feel guilty when a patient dies unexpectedly or about how the patient's care and dying were managed in the final days. As well, patient deaths remind clinicians that all of us will ultimately face our own death.

Physicians can cope with their grief by spending time with dying patients to say goodbye, visiting the funeral home or gravesite, or writing a bereavement note to the family and sharing one's thoughts about the patient. Other coping methods include keeping a journal, taking short vacations, exercising, meditating, and gardening. Some hospitals have grief rounds that provide a venue for clinician discussion of emotional reactions to caring for dying patients.

CONCLUSION

The end-of-life care team that is utilizing tools of effective communication, skills in symptom management and bereavement, encouraging rituals for closure, and acknowledging patients as human beings can be one of the most valued resources in Hospital Medicine.

SUGGESTED READINGS

Anderson M. *Sacred Dying: Creating Rituals for Embracing the End of Life.* New York: Marlowe & Company, 2001.

Bedell SE, Cadenhead K, and Graboys TB. *N Engl J Med.* 2001;344(15): 1163.

Bedell SE, Delbanco TL, Cook EF, Epstein FH. Survival after cardiopulmonary resuscitation in the hospital. *N Engl J Med.* 1983;309: 569–576.

Curtis JR, Engelberg RA. Measuring success of interventions to improve the quality of end-of-life care in the intensive care unit. *Crit Care Med.* 2006;34(11 Suppl):S341–S347.

Ehlenbach WJ, Barnato AE, Curtis JR, et al. Epidemiologic study of in-hospital cardiopulmonary resuscitation in the elderly. *N Engl J Med.* 2009;361:22–31.

Schulz R, Hebert R, Boerner K. Bereavement after caregiving. *Geriatrics.* 2008;63(1):20–22.

Schuman Z. Implementing institutional change: an institutional case study of palliative sedation. *J Palliat Med.*2005;8(3):666–676.

Truog RD, Campbell ML, Curtis JR, et al. Recommendations for end-of-life care in the intensive care unit: A consensus statement by the Academy of Critical Care Medicine. *Crit Care Med.* 2008;36(3):953–963.

Zhao Y, Encinosa W. 2009. The cost of end-of-life hospitalizations, 2007. Available at http://www.hcup-us.ahrq.gov/reports/statbriefs/sb81.jsp.

SECTION 13

Pregnancy

CHAPTER 220

Overview of Physiologic Changes of Pregnancy

Meghan Hayes, MD
Lucia Larson, MD

Key Clinical Questions

1. What are normal physiologic adaptations during pregnancy?
2. What are abnormal, concerning findings during pregnancy?
3. How does pregnancy affect laboratory values?

INTRODUCTION AND EPIDEMIOLOGY

Pregnancy and delivery require amazing maternal adaptation, with nearly every organ system altered by hormonal and/or mechanical means. Physiologic changes begin at conception and continue throughout pregnancy and the postpartum period. Such changes may impact the manifestation and course of a disease process as well as have implications for treatment. Maternal vulnerabilities, such as increased risk of thrombosis, hypertension, or diabetes, may also be revealed during pregnancy. Since any woman of reproductive age has the potential to be pregnant, their care must occur in the context of an understanding of normal and abnormal pregnancy physiology.

PHYSIOLOGY BY SYSTEM

CARDIOVASCULAR

A healthy heart adapts well to the marked demands of pregnancy, but congenital or acquired heart disease may present or worsen in the gravid woman due to the cardiovascular changes associated with increased cardiac workload. Estrogen mediates an increase in cardiac output by six weeks gestation via increased preload and stroke volume. Blood volume rises by 30% to 40% during pregnancy, peaking at the end of the second trimester. Cardiac output (CO) peaks in the third trimester, typically 30% to 50% above baseline. Total peripheral resistance declines by 20%. Systolic and diastolic blood pressures drop by 10 to 15 mm Hg in the first trimester then return to baseline in the second half of pregnancy; diastolic blood pressure declines more than systolic, so pulse pressure widens. The cardiac axis is shifted leftward, anterior and cephalad.

Blood flow distribution changes during pregnancy such that up to 25% of CO is directed to the uteroplacental unit (a new "end-organ") and up to 20% to the kidneys. An increased proportion of CO supplies breast tissue, but cerebral blood flow remains at baseline proportions.

Cardiovascular adaptations lead to common complaints in pregnant women: palpitations, decreased exercise tolerance, and dizziness. A shift of the heart toward the chest wall may contribute to the experience of palpitations by the gravida, but palpitations may also represent increased sensitivity to mild sinus tachycardia, premature atrial or ventricular systoles, or, less likely, supraventricular tachycardia. It is postulated that the increase in blood volume may be associated with stretching of the myocardium, thereby potentially increasing myocardial irritability and predisposing to arrhythmias. While this is not clearly proven, both atrial and ventricular arrhythmias may occur in pregnancy just as they occur in the nonpregnant patient. By late pregnancy there is attenuated ability to increase cardiac output with exercise, and this combined with normal weight gain of pregnancy can lead to decreased exercise tolerance. Beyond midpregnancy the gravid uterus causes aortocaval compression in the supine position, decreasing CO by 30%, and venous return, leading to dizziness and dyspnea (termed *supine hypotensive syndrome*) in some women. Pertinent exam findings include systolic flow murmur by midpregnancy, mammary soufflé, point of maximal impulse (PMI) displaced leftward and cephalad, and mild bilateral lower-extremity edema. Heart rate increases but is not generally above 100 beats per minute. While the neck veins may appear full, jugular venous pulsation is not elevated. Electrocardiograms of pregnant women often will show left axis deviation, atrial enlargement and nonspecific ST-T wave changes, but such findings should be carefully interpreted within clinical context. The cardiac silhouette may be generous on chest radiograph. Increased cardiac output and volume of distribution in pregnant women necessitate careful attention to timing of intravenous contrast dye bolus for computed tomography pulmonary angiography (CT-PA), in order to avoid radiation exposure for an inconclusive study. *Care should be taken to position pregnant woman in the left lateral decubitus (or at least with hip elevation to displace the pregnant uterus off the vena cava) when performing medical investigations or treating ill pregnant women to minimize such adverse hemodynamic effects.*

RESPIRATORY

Pregnancy contributes to mechanical changes as well as progesterone-mediated physiologic adaptations in the respiratory system. In the upper airway, hyperemia, glandular hyperactivity, increased edema, and friability occur, related to elevated plasma volume and estrogen. Chest wall circumference increases by 5 to 7 cm due to elevated relaxin levels, and, eventually, the uterus elevates the diaphragm by about 4 cm though diaphragmatic excursion remains unchanged or even increased.

During pregnancy, oxygen consumption increases by 30% to 60% due to increased metabolic demands. Elevating progesterone levels increase respiratory drive early in pregnancy with continued effect throughout. Minute ventilation (tidal volume multiplied by breaths per minute) increases by up to 50% through increased tidal volume; respiratory rate should remain unchanged. Vital capacity remains unchanged while functional residual capacity declines by up to 25%. Overall, pulmonary function testing interpretation remains unchanged, as forced expiratory volume in 1 second (FEV1), FEV1/forced vital capacity (FVC) ratio, and peak expiratory flows remain stable.

Compensated respiratory alkalosis is expected on arterial blood gas testing, with PaO_2 elevated to 100 to 105 mm Hg, and $PaCO_2$ expected at 28 to 32 mm Hg. Clinically, pregnant women may complain of mild exertional dyspnea because of increased respiratory drive and physiologic anemia; however, this should not limit activities of daily living nor worsen with progressing pregnancy. Pertinent chest radiographic findings include generous cardiac silhouette, increased anteroposterior diameter, and prominent pulmonary vasculature. *Clinical implications of respiratory anatomic changes in pregnancy include common complaints of gestational rhinitis (nasal congestion), epistaxis, and snoring, increased difficulty with intubation, and effect on needle insertion site for thoracentesis by the elevated diaphragm.*

It is recommended that the most experienced provider available perform intubation since failure rates are far higher in pregnant women. Maternal oxygen saturation of 95% or greater is desirable to maintain PaO_2 greater than 70 mm Hg for optimal placental oxygen diffusion.

RENAL/URINARY

Anatomic changes in the genitourinary system begin early in pregnancy, with kidneys increasing in size by about 1 cm in length and 30% in volume by midpregnancy, related to elevated blood volume and enlarging vasculature. The renal collecting system dilates due to progesterone and prostaglandin-mediated smooth muscle relaxation initially and mechanical obstruction by the uterus later, so that mild to moderate hydronephrosis is expected on imaging. As a standard ultrasound parameter, ultrasound imaging should visualize ureteral jets in the absence of true obstruction. Ureteral peristalsis decreases, increasing the risk for ascending infection.

Early pregnancy vasodilatation due to surging progesterone and relaxin lead to increased glomerular filtration rate (GFR) and renal plasma flow (RPF) by 6 weeks. Glomerular filtration rate increases by 50%, and RPF increased by an even greater percentage. Medication metabolism is therefore accelerated, such that medications may require more frequent dosing (eg, twice daily rather than once daily) and higher doses (eg, when using antimicrobials with dosing ranges) for efficacy. Creatinine clearance rapidly increases by 25%, so that serum creatinine values average 0.5 mg per dL and blood urea nitrogen (BUN) and uric acid levels decline. Bicarbonate excretion is accelerated, related to respiratory changes; pregnant women therefore have decreased buffering capacity and increased susceptibility to acidosis.

Altered glomerular membrane charge selectivity increases excretion of protein, albumin, and glucose. Up to 300 mg of protein on 24-hour urine collection is considered normal during pregnancy. Correlation between spot urine protein-to-creatinine ratios and 24-hour urine protein collection values have been variable, therefore only very low or very high urine protein-to-creatinine values are useful; and, although cumbersome, 24-hour urine protein collection remains the gold standard.

Progesterone markedly stimulates the renin-angiotensin system. Renin is produced by the placenta, thus there is an increase in maternal sodium absorption and potassium excretion. Between 6 to 8 liters of water are retained to sustain normal pregnancy. Erythropoietin levels also increase, in order to meet red blood cell demands.

Clinical implications of renal physiologic adaptations include increased susceptibility to urinary tract infections including pyelonephritis, nephrolithiasis, and acidosis. See Chapter 221 for a discussion of the implications of medication prescribing.

GASTROINTESTINAL

Progesterone mediates gastrointestinal (GI) smooth muscle relaxation, decreasing motility. As pregnancy progresses, the mechanical impact of the gravid uterus alters GI function. The majority of pregnant women experience nausea and vomiting early in pregnancy, attributed to high hCG levels plus estrogen and progesterone. Constipation is common, related to decreased motility and delayed gastric emptying; absorption may be delayed. Not surprisingly, gastroesophageal reflux is reported by up to half of pregnant women and is related to progressive uterine enlargement, decreased lower esophageal sphincter tone and increased intraabdominal pressure.

Hepatic physiology is generally stable during pregnancy. The high estrogen state of pregnancy may mimic liver disease findings, with palmar erythema and telangiectasias, in the absence of hepatic pathology. Alkaline phosphatase levels rise due to placental production. Dilution causes serum albumin and total protein levels to decline, which may impact pharmacokinetics of protein-bound medications. It is therefore preferable to obtain free drug levels rather than total levels when clinically indicated.

The gallbladder increases in size, although emptying capacity declines. Bile is more lithogenic during pregnancy and more saturated with cholesterol. Biliary sludge is common and may spontaneously resolve after delivery. Gallstones are more likely to be symptomatic than sludge and less likely to resolve spontaneously. Thus, there is an increased incidence of symptomatic gallstones both during pregnancy and post partum.

HEMATOLOGIC

Marked adaptation allows increased blood flow to the uterus and developing placenta and preparation for delivery's hemostatic challenge. Blood volume increases by 50% to 100% beginning by the 6th week of gestation. Plasma volume increases by 50% with an initial rapid rise, then gradual increase to peak at the 30th week. Erythrocyte mass rises less significantly, leading to the physiologic anemia of pregnancy, with typical Hgb levels of 10 to 12 g/dL by term. Neutrophilic leukocytosis may be seen, typically not beyond 16 × 10^9/L. Platelet count typically remains stable in pregnancy. Isolated mild thrombocytopenia (115 to 150 × 10^9/L) occurs in approximately 10% of pregnancies by term. Pregnant women are hypercoagulable due to increased estrogen effects on clotting factors as well as increased venous stasis. There is a marked increase in venous thromboembolic risk continuing through six to eight weeks postpartum. Levels of the following may double by the third trimester: fibrinogen, factors V, VII, VIII, X, von Willebrand factor, and thrombin activation. D-dimer increases by the second trimester and remains elevated to the postpartum period. Protein S level and activity decline during pregnancy, as does sensitivity to activated protein C (APC). Protein C level and activity and antithrombin remain stable in normal pregnancy, but decreased antithrombin may be seen in association with preeclampsia and/or proteinuria. *D-dimer is not a useful test to rule out venous thromboembolism in pregnancy since it is elevated in most pregnancies by term. Although thrombocytopenia can occur during pregnancy, it should not be forgotten that preeclampsia, sepsis, disseminated intravascular coagulation (DIC), and abruption are important causes of decreased platelet counts in pregnancy.*

ENDOCRINE

Pancreas

Early normal pregnancy is characterized by accelerated starvation, with mildly decreased fasting plasma glucose and increased ketogenesis, which leads to risk of starvation ketosis after prolonged fasting. By mid- to late pregnancy, insulin resistance increases, heralded by large volumes of dilute urine and generally tolerated unless fluid is restricted via human placental lactogen (hPL), human placental growth hormone (hPGH), and likely tumor necrosis factor–alpha (TNF-α). This adaptation supplies the fetoplacental unit with 50 to 100 grams of glucose daily by the third trimester. Insulin sensitivity returns to baseline within 48 hours of delivery. Thus, the insulin needs of type 1 and type 2 diabetics may decrease early in pregnancy (particularly if there is significant "morning sickness" causing nausea and vomiting), causing an increased risk of nocturnal hypoglycemia. Insulin doses generally need to be increased later in pregnancy in response to increasing insulin resistance. This physiology is also responsible for the development of gestational diabetes in some women. There is a higher incidence of fetal loss with diabetes, both due to an increase in congenital anomalies related to the teratogenic effect of glucose in patients with elevated hemoglobin A1C and to the renal and vascular complications of the disease itself. Management with a multidisciplinary team that includes specialists with expertise in diabetes in pregnancy is important.

Thyroid

Maternal thyroid hormone production increases by 50%. Hepatic production of thyroid hormone–binding globulin increases by two- to threefold, driven by elevated estrogen levels. Free levels of T4 and T3 remain stable but total levels rise. Maternal iodine requirements increase in order to fulfill T4 production, with increased renal iodine clearance. The fetal thyroid begins to function by 12 weeks and is fully functional by 18 weeks, so it is essential that maternal levels are sufficient for early development. Multidisciplinary collaboration enhances maternal and neonatal outcomes.

In the first trimester, b-HCG levels peak at 8 to 12 weeks and stimulate thyrocytes, which causes transient T4 production and thyroid-stimulating hormone (TSH) suppression. This may be exaggerated in molar pregnancy or hyperemesis gravidarum. If the mother is iodine replete, by the third trimester, there is a mild decrease in T4 and mild increase in TSH. *These changes often result in the need to increase levothyroxine doses during pregnancy as compared with the prepregnancy dose. Recommendations are to increase doses by 25% to 30% in all patients on thyroid replacement.*

Parathyroid

Maternal mineral hemostasis is challenged by fetal skeletal formation then further challenged during lactation. Total serum calcium declines slightly due to decline in serum albumin; ionized calcium remains unchanged. Urinary calcium levels rise by 12 weeks gestation. Parathyroid hormone (PTH) is key to calcium homeostasis in the nonpregnant state, acting directly via renal and bone effects and indirectly via intestinal absorption. Levels of PTH decline during pregnancy, and it would be expected that 1,25 $(OH)_2$ vitamin D levels would drop as well, but 1,25 $(OH)_2$ vitamin D levels rise. It is likely that the placenta may contribute 1,25 $(OH)_2$ vitamin D. Prenatal vitamins provide adequate vitamin D supplementation.

Pituitary

The size of the pituitary increases by up to 70% by the third trimester largely due to hyperplasia of lactotrophic cells in the anterior lobe. Prolactin levels increase due to estrogen and progesterone stimulation of lactotrophic cells, and the placenta also produces prolactin by late pregnancy. Adrenocorticotropic hormone (ACTH) levels rise due to placental corticotropin-releasing hormone (CRH), which is not suppressed by dexamethasone. ACTH levels rise further during labor. Oxytocin levels rise throughout pregnancy, eventually facilitating parturition. Vasopressin levels decline due to placental production of vasopressinase, which may be a cause of transient diabetes insipidus (DI) during pregnancy. *Careful monitoring of volume and electrolyte status in these patients, and confirmation that the DI is related to a benign process and not to posterior pituitary disease is important.*

LABOR AND DELIVERY-PERTINENT PHYSIOLOGY

A complex biochemical cascade, beyond the scope of this discussion, culminates in parturition. During labor, cardiac output further increases by one-third from the already augmented output of pregnancy, and systemic vascular resistance increases up to 25% with contractions. With each contraction, 300 to 500 milliliters of blood is "autotransfused" from the uteroplacental to the maternal circulation. Valsalva maneuvers while pushing increase myocardial oxygen consumption and may increase maternal blood pressure. These changes may be important in patients with underlying cardiac disease who are unable to tolerate increased volume and increased cardiac work.

Regional anesthesia for pain control during delivery, either spinal, epidural, or combined spinal-epidural, may lead to acute vasodilatation and resulting hypotension. Spinal anesthesia has been associated with greater hypotension than epidural anesthesia, however, it can be administered more rapidly if needed urgently. An epidural catheter offers the opportunity to provide continued pain relief after delivery with neuraxial opioids. Hypotension from neuraxial anesthesia may be reduced by preloading with crystalloid, or occasionally colloid, decreased dose, and slower administration.

CONCLUSION

This chapter reviews the physiologic changes that begin at conception and continue throughout pregnancy and the postpartum period, how such changes impact the manifestation and course of a disease process, and maternal vulnerabilities. An understanding of normal and abnormal pregnancy physiology is central to providing optimal care for this population of patients.

SUGGESTED READINGS

Hill CC, Pickinpaugh DO. Physiologic changes in pregnancy. *Surg Clin N Am*. 2007;88:391–401.

Rosene-Montella K, Keely E, Barbour LA, Lee RV, eds. *Medical Care of the Pregnant Patient*, 2nd ed. Philadelphia, PA: American College of Physicians, 2008.

Smith R. Parturition. *N Engl J Med*. 2007;356:271–283.

CHAPTER 221

Medication Management

Raymond O. Powrie, MD, FRCP, FACP

Key Clinical Questions

1. What key questions should the practitioner ask to ensure safe use of medication during pregnancy?
2. What are the limitations of the Federal Drug Administration drug classification?
3. How should the physiologic changes in pregnancy that affect medication clearance influence prescribing of medication?

INTRODUCTION

Until the middle of the last century there was a widespread belief among both clinicians and patients that the human fetus grew in a protected environment that minimized any potential effects of substances ingested by the mother. This misperception ended dramatically when the effects of thalidomide became widely known to clinicians and the general public in the late 1960s. Ever since this tragedy, there has been a tendency for both patients and clinicians to approach the use of medications in pregnancy with great anxiety because of fears of causing adverse fetal effects. Despite this, use of medications during pregnancy remains widespread throughout the world. Therefore, it seems that a dichotomy exists: a widely perceived fear regarding the ingestion of medication during pregnancy juxtaposed against the practical reality that medications are necessary and continue to be used during the course of gestation.

This chapter aims to provide a helpful evidence-based approach to guide hospitalists who may be asked to consult on or care for pregnant women through this challenging terrain. **Table 221-1** lists some references that discuss the safety of particular agents in pregnancy. **Table 221-2** makes some clinically-based recommendations about which medications are preferred for specific indications during pregnancy. The remainder of this chapter will provide a general approach to prescribing in pregnancy that should guide the reader in the informed use of the information contained in both the listed references and the provided summary table.

KEY CONCEPTS FOR APPROPRIATE USE OF MEDICATIONS IN PREGNANCY

MOST MEDICATIONS "CROSS THE PLACENTA"

With few exceptions, no placental barrier exists for medications that can be administered orally. Drug levels in the fetus may be the same, lower, or higher than in the mother. In general, lipophilic drugs, drugs that are nonionized at physiologic pH, and drugs of low molecular weight cross the placenta more efficiently than other drugs, but the fetus will have exposure to almost any medication that can be administered orally to the mother.

MEDICATION USE DURING PREGNANCY CAN CAUSE A WIDE RANGE OF ADVERSE EFFECTS

Teratogenesis is more than just "missing parts." Although the thalidomide tragedy drew attention to medication-associated malformations such as limb reduction defects, drugs may have other, perhaps more subtle, effects during pregnancy such as intrauterine growth restriction (eg, atenolol), intrauterine fetal demise (eg, possibly cyclophosphamide), long-term cognitive or behavioral toxicities (eg, valproic acid and mental retardation), and neonatal toxicities (eg, neonatal abstinence syndrome such as may be seen with narcotics and benzodiazepines)

PRACTICE POINT

Potential teratogenic effects of medications in pregnancy

- Malformations
- Intrauterine death due to either embryotoxicity or fetotoxicity
- Intrauterine growth restriction
- Behavioral toxicity
- Neonatal toxicities

TABLE 221-1 Resources for Helping to Determine which Medication to Use when Treating Medical Illness in Pregnancy

Publication	Authors	Publisher	Format
Drugs in Pregnancy and Lactation: A Reference Guide to Fetal and Neonatal Risk	Briggs GS, Freeman RK, Yaffe SY.	Lippincott Williams & Wilkins; 8th ed., 2008	Hardcover 2144 pages
Teratogenic Effects of Drugs: A Resource for Clinicians (TERIS).	Friedman JM, Polifka JE.	John Hopkins University Press, 2nd ed., 2000	Hardcover 793 pages
Medication Safety in Pregnancy and Breastfeeding: The Evidence-Based, A to Z Clinician's Pocket Guide	Koren G	McGraw-Hill Professional, 1st ed., 2006	Paperback 312 pages
Medication Safety in Pregnancy and Breastfeeding	Koren G	McGraw-Hill Professional, 1st ed., 2007	Hardcover 623 pages
Drugs for Pregnant and Lactating Women	Weiner CP, Buhimschi C	Churchill Livingstone, 1st ed., 2004	Hardcover 1101 pages
Drugs During Pregnancy and Lactation	Schaefer C, Peters PWJ, Miller RK	Academic Press, 2nd ed., 2007	Hardcover 904 pages
Prescribing in Pregnancy	Rubin PC, Ramsey M	BMJ Books, 4th ed., 2008	Paperback 256 pages
Catalog of Teratogenic Agents	Shepard TH, Lemire RJ	John Hopkins University Press, 12th ed., 2007	Hardcover 656 pages
Medications & Mothers' Milk: A Manual of Lactational Pharmacology	Hale T	Pharmasoft Medical Publishing, 13th ed., 2008	Conveniently sized paperback 1172 pages
Online computer databases			
REPRORISK	Produced and marketed by Thomson Reuters Micromedex Inc. Module available at http://thomsonreuters.com		Online data base or diskette contains TERIS, REPROTOX, REPROTEXT, and Shepard's Catalog of Teratogenic Agents
TERIS	Information available at http://depts.washington.edu/terisweb/teris		Online subscription or diskette
Reprotox	Thomson Reuters Micromedex Inc. Module available at www.REPROTOX.org		Online subscription or diskette PDA version available

Reprinted, with permission, from Powrie RO and Wiley-Blackwell Publishers. Prescribing in Pregnancy: A Practical Approach. In deSwiet's *Medical Disorders in Obstetric Practice*. 5th ed. London: UK, 2010:636–640. Table 30-1 and Table 30-2.

THE LIST OF KNOWN HUMAN TERATOGENS IS SHORT

Despite all the potential effects of medication use during pregnancy, there are really only about 30 known human teratogens that could be prescribed by physicians. Many of these known teratogens are not commonly used in medical practice. The most commonly prescribed human teratogens are listed in the Practice Point on page 1833.

MEDICATION EFFECTS MAY VARY DEPENDING ON THE POINT IN THE PREGNANCY WHEN THEY ARE ADMINISTERED

Human gestation can be divided into specific periods, and each of these periods may be associated with distinctive medication-use risks.

The first 14 days after conception (the two-week period between conception and the first missed menstrual period) are often called the "all or nothing period." During this time frame, drug effects are likely to be nil or result in miscarriage. At this point, the conceptus has not interfaced significantly with maternal circulation and drug exposures are likely to be only at a very low level. At this same time, all cells in the conceptus are nonspecialized (pluripotential) and are generally believed either to experience lethal effects of drugs (resulting in pregnancy loss) or no effect at all.

Between days 14 and 60 after conception (the *embryonic period*—a seven week time frame following the first missed menstrual period) organogenesis is occurring, and drug exposure during these weeks can lead to major or minor malformations. It is worth noting however, that this high-risk period accounts for only 5% of the 280-day human gestation. In fact, most human teratogens causing malformations probably have even shorter specific periods when the developing embryo is specifically susceptible to their toxicities. For example, thalidomide effects were seen only if the drug was taken between days 21 and 36. Valproic acid, which can cause neural tube defects, will not do so if taken after day 27 because the neural tube has completely closed by this date.

An important consequence of unique vulnerabilities of the embryonic period is that some significant toxicities may have already occurred before a woman gets to a doctor to confirm her pregnancy. Therefore, the onus is on all providers prescribing medication to women of reproductive age to speak to these patients about the potential effects of their medications during pregnancy and the potential for harm even before the pregnancy is clinically apparent.

During the period between days 60 and 280 of gestation, progressive fetal growth and neurologic development is occurring. Toxicities during this period may cause impaired growth (eg, atenolol), neurologic or behavioral abnormalities (eg, valproic acid and mental retardation), or specific organ toxicities (eg, angiotensin converting enzyme [ACE] inhibitors and renal dysfunction). There is, therefore, no period in a pregnancy during which a medication can be considered completely safe. Rather, each distinct period in gestation represents some unique potential vulnerabilities.

TABLE 221-2 Suggested Medications in Pregnancy by Indication

Condition or Product Type	Data Suggests Use Justifiable when Indicated	Data Suggests Use may be Justifiable in Unique Circumstances	Data Suggests Rarely Justifiable for Indication Listed	Useful Review Articles and Comments
Acne	Topical erythromycin$_{B}$ topical benzoyl peroxide$_{C}$ topical clindamycin$_{B}$	Oral erythromycin$_{B}$	Tetracycline$_{D}$ doxycycline$_{D}$ topical tretinionc$_{C}$	PMID: 2971690 PMID: 16487888
Analgesics	Acetominophen$_{A}$ codeine$_{C}$ meperidine$_{C}$ morphine$_{C}$	All NSAIDS$_{B/C}$ (Intermittent use of NSAIDs in the first two trimesters for anti-inflammatory purposes may be justifiable but repeated use after 28 weeks is to be avoided.) ASA$_{D}$ (Low-dose ASA < 100 mg per day does appear to be safe in pregnancy.)		These review article details issues surrounding the use of NSAIDs in pregnancy including case reports of constriction of the ductus arteriosus, renal dysfunction and hemostatic abnormalities in the fetus and neonate. Malformations associated with NSAIDs have not been reported however. PMID: 16638921 PMID: 16194696 PMID: 15013926
Antihistamines	Diphenhydramine$_{B}$ (but avoid in first trimester) chlorpheniramine dimenhydrinate $_{B}$ loratidine$_{B}$ cetirizine$_{B}$	Fexofenadine$_{C}$		These 2006 review articles systematically and critically review the literature on the treatment of allergic rhinitis in pregnancy. PMID: 16579874 PMID: 16443148
Antimicrobials	Erythromycin$_{B}$ base, ethyl succinate or stearate (not estolate) penicillins$_{B}$ cephalosporins$_{B}$ azithromycin$_{B}$ vancomycin$_{C}$ nitrofurantoin$_{B}$ metronidazole$_{B}$ (after first trimester) isoniazid$_{C}$ acyclovir$_{C}$ AZT$_{C}$ and other antiretrovirals except for Efavirenz$_{D}$ (sustiva)	Antifungals: (all$_{C}$ except amphotericin$_{B}$ nystatin clotrimazole and terbinafine, which are$_{B}$) The following agents are commonly used in pregnancy but are best reserved for use when alternate agents are less effective: clarithromycin$_{C}$ aminoglycosides$_{D}$ trimethoprim$_{C}$ sulfonamides$_{C}$	Tetracycline$_{D}$ Fluoroquinilones$_{C}$ despite very concerning animal data; increasing human data suggests fluoroquinolones might warrant their placement in the "use may be justified in rare circumstances" category: erythomycin estolate$_{B}$ efavirenz$_{D}$	Two 1997 and one 2006 review article on the use of antimicrobials in pregnancy are: PMID: 9266582 PMID: 9067781 PMID: 16648419
Asthma	Beta-agonists: albuterol$_{C}$ metaproterenol$_{C}$ salmeterol$_{C}$ pirbuterol$_{C}$ formeterol$_{C}$ Inhaled steroids: budesonide$_{B}$ beclomethasone$_{C}$ flunisolide$_{C}$ fluticasone$_{C}$ triamcinolone$_{C}$ Systemic steroids$_{C}$: ipatropium$_{B}$ cromolyn$_{B}$	zafirlukast$_{B}$ montelukast$_{B}$ omalizumab$_{B}$		New national recommendations for the management of asthma in pregnancy were published in early 2005 and can be obtained through the NHLBI at *http://www.nhlbi.nih.gov/health/prof/lung/asthma/astpreg.htm.* Most medications commonly used to treat asthma (aside from the leukotriene antagonists) have considerable clinical experience with their use in pregnancy that suggests their safety and particularly justifies their use to control asthma in pregnancy. PMID: 17363831 PMID: 17181448 PMID: 16946229 PMID: 16443145

(continued)

TABLE 221-2 Suggested Medications in Pregnancy by Indication *(continued)*

Condition or Product Type	Data Suggests Use Justifiable when Indicated	Data Suggests Use may be Justifiable in Unique Circumstances	Data Suggests Rarely Justifiable for Indication Listed	Useful Review Articles and Comments
Constipation	Bisacodyl$_C$ docusate glycerin psyllium sodium biphosphate magnesium hydroxide sorbitol mineral oil			PMID: 17889809
Cough	Guaifenesin$_C$ dextromethorphan$_C$ albuterol$_C$ codeine$_C$			This review article discusses the treatment of the common cold in pregnancy. PMID: 18474699
Depression	Amitriptyline$_D$ Nortriptyline$_D$ Fluoxetine$_C$ Sertraline$_C$	Sertraline$_C$ fluvoxamine$_C$ escitalopram$_C$ citalopram$_C$ venlafaxine$_C$ mirtazapine$_C$ paroxetine$_C$ (Increasing data suggests this agent may fall into the category to the right because of a small risk of both teratogenicity and neonatal syndromes.)		General review of behavioral health: PMID: 18378767 Bipolar affective disorder: PMID: 17764378 Depression: PMID: 18760228 Anxiety: PMID: 17955910 Schizophrenia: PMID: 12553132
Diabetes	Insulin (human, beef or pork, lispro)	Glyburide$_B$ has a developing role in the management of gestational diabetes as an alternative to insulin with comparable outcomes. PMID: 18622055 Metformin$_B$ *glucophage*™: Use of this agent in early pregnancies of women with polycystic ovary syndrome is increasing. PMID: 19084097	Chlorpropamide$_C$ tolbutamide$_D$ glipizide	PMID: 19104375 PMID: 18297574 PMID: 17596473
Diarrhea	loperamide$_B$ diphenoxylate/atropine			PMID: 12635420 PMID: 16673005
Dyspepsia	Ranitidine$_B$ famotidine$_B$ nazitidine$_C$ cimetidine$_B$ sulcrafate$_C$ Antacids$_B$: $Al(OH)_3$, $Mg(OH)_2$, $CaCO_3$	Omeprazole$_B$ lansoprazole$_C$ esomeprazole$_B$	Misoprostol$_X$	Despite placing proton pump inhibitors in the second category here, they are widely used in pregnancy and published data suggest they are not a major teratogenic risk in humans. We recommend their use if agents in the first column are ineffective in controlling symptoms. PMID: 12635419 PMID: 11430180

(continued)

TABLE 221-2 Suggested Medications in Pregnancy by Indication *(continued)*

Condition or Product Type	Data Suggests Use Justifiable when Indicated	Data Suggests Use may be Justifiable in Unique Circumstances	Data Suggests Rarely Justifiable for Indication Listed	Useful Review Articles and Comments
Headache	Acetaminophen$_A$ codeine$_C$ meperidine$_C$ morphine$_C$ metoclopramide$_B$ caffeine$_C$ For prophylaxis: amitryptiline$_B$ nortiptyline$_D$ beta-blockers$_{B\ and\ C}$	All NSAIDs $_{B/C}$ (Intermittent use of NSAIDs in the second trimester may be justifiable.) Butalbital$_C$ in *fioricet* and *esgic*	Sumatriptan$_C$ noratriptan$_C$ rizatriptan$_C$ zolmatriptan$_C$ A growing literature about the use of these agents (particularly sumatriptan) in human pregnancies may eventually support their use as a second line agent in pregnancy. This article reports on the data presently available from the drug manufacturer's pregnancy registry for sumatriptan and cautiously reports no demonstrable teratogenic effect at this time. PMID: 10649172 Ergotamine$_X$ (Although unlikely to be a teratogen this agent is concerning for its potent vasoconstrictive and uterotonic effects.)	These review articles summarize the data about the treatment of migraine in pregnancy. PMID: 18583683 PMID: 18345969 PMID: 18332840 An effective role for nonpharmacologic management with biofeedback, physical therapy and relaxation is suggested in this small trial. PMID: 8682668
Hypertension	Labetalol$_C$ methyldopa$_B$ Pindolol$_B$ Other beta blockers: acebutalol$_B$ all others (may want to avoid atenolol because of an association with intrauterine growth restriction) nifedipine$_C$ hydralazine$_C$	calcium channel blockers other than nifedipine$_C$ clonidine$_C$ prazosin$_C$ hydrochlorothiazide$_B$ diazoxide$_C$	ACE inhibitors D Accupril, perindopril, ramipril, captopril, benazepril, trandolapril, fosinopril, lisinopril, moexipril, enalapril Angiotensin II Antagonists D eprosartan, telmisartan, valsartan, candesartan, irbesartan, valsartan	PMID: 15805801 PMID: 18259046
Nasal Congestion	Oxymetazoline$_C$ nasal steroids nasal cromolyn$_B$ nasal ipratropium$_B$	Pseudoephedrine$_C$		PMID: 16579874 PMID: 16443148
Nausea Vomiting	Metoclopramide$_B$ prochloperazine$_C$ dimenhydrinate$_B$ promethazine$_C$ doxylamine plus pyridoxine	Ondansetron$_B$		PMID: 17967157 PMID 18077743 PMID: 17889806 Although ondansetron is commonly used o treat nausea and vomiting in pregnancy, the published experience is limited and the authors view it as a second-line agent.

(continued)

TABLE 221-2 Suggested Medications in Pregnancy by Indication (*continued*)

Condition or Product Type	Data Suggests Use Justifiable when Indicated	Data Suggests Use may be Justifiable in Unique Circumstances	Data Suggests Rarely Justifiable for Indication Listed	Useful Review Articles and Comments
Pruritus	Topical: Moisturizing creams and lotions, oatmeal cream or powder calamine lotion, topical glucocorticoids$_C$ Systemic: Hydroxyzine$_C$, chlorpheniramine$_B$ diphenhydramine$_B$			PMID: 2289340 PMID: 10396430 PMID: 12031026
Thrombosis	Heparin (both low molecular weight and unfractionated)	Fibrinolytics such as streptokinase$_C$ and tPA *altepase*$_{C8}$	Warfarin$_X$ *coumadin*™ This agent is believed by some to have a role in the management prosthetic heart valves after the first trimester as it may be associated with a lower risk of prosthetic valve thrombosis. PMID: 10647757	PMID: 1918847 PMID: 18987370
Vaccines	Diptheria$_C$ tetanus$_C$ hepatitis A$_C$ hepatitis B$_C$ influenza$_C$ immune globulin$_C$ inactivated polio vaccine$_C$ tuberculin test$_C$		Live vaccines: MMR Sabin polio vaccine (oral) varicella	General PMID: 14719841 Influenza and pertussis: PMID: 18677141 Pertussis, tetanus, diphtheria: PMID: 18509304 For travelers: PMID: 18760249

Letter designations are U.S. FDA Pregnancy Categories from individual product package inserts.

References in the final column of this table are listed by their PubMed identification number. The citation and abstract can be obtained by going to www.pubmed.gov and entering this number into the search function.

Note: Every patient and circumstance is different and the literature on medication use in pregnancy is continually evolving. This table does not constitute specific therapeutic recommendations, and the reader is referred to the resources in in this table as a guide to therapeutic decisions.

Reprinted, with permission, from Powrie RO and Wiley-Blackwell Publishers. Prescribing in Pregnancy: A Practical Approach. In deSwiet's *Medical Disorders in Obstetric Practice*. 5th ed. London: UK, 2010:636–640. Table 30–1 and Table 30–2.

MEDICATION PREGNANCY SAFETY DATA: SOURCES AND THEIR LIMITATIONS

Much of the data that exists about the effects and safety of drug use in pregnancy is on the basis of animal studies. Before drugs are released on the market in the United States and Canada, animal testing looking for drug-related malformations needs to have occurred. Human data, however, is not required. This is because new drug testing on pregnant women is felt to be unethical and (aside from the important exception of thalidomide) most human teratogens have been found to be teratogenic in laboratory animals as well. However, two major problems with the use of animal data exist. First, animal data cannot always be confidently extrapolated to humans. There is considerable variability between species and even between strains of a species regarding the effects of the medication on a developing fetus. Second, behavioral and intellectual effects of medications are very difficult to recognize in animals. Much of human gestation is a time of progressive neurologic development. Medications that do not cause gross malformations may still have effects on developmental milestones, intelligence, and behavioral health that will not be readily discernable in animal models.

In general, the best use of animal data is when it is paired with human data and the findings suggest a common and biologically plausible association. However, most of the human data we presently have has its own challenges. One of the most significant problems with human data is that there is a large background risk of congenital abnormalities making it difficult to differentiate abnormalities that are caused by medications from those due to other causes. Beetween 2% and 4% of infants are born with some defect, and of these 20% are due to chromosomal abnormalities. Five percent are due to gene mutations and 65% of these defects remain unexplained. Likely, no more than 10% of identified human malformations are due to teratogenic agents. Because most human teratogens have their effect in only 0.1% to 30% of exposed fetuses, large numbers of exposures need to be studied to clearly identify an increase against the background risk of anomalies. The best evidence for teratogenic effects would be from prospective studies in humans, but these are done infrequently because they are difficult, lengthy, and expensive. Most studies determining effects of drugs in pregnancy are either case-control or cohort studies. In case-control studies, infants with anomalies are paired with infants without a particular anomaly. The number of infants exposed to the studied agent in each group is then compared. In cohort studies, the incidence of a particular anomaly among infants exposed to a particular agent are compared with the incidence of that anomaly among infants not exposed to that agent. In a case-control study, 220 cases and 220 controls must be studied to find a relative risk of 2.5 with a power of 80%.

The problems with such retrospective data are many. Most importantly, associations attributed to medication effects may simply reflect the reason the mother was on the medication rather than the medication itself. One must be cautious about ascribing anomalies to medication effects when in fact the anomaly may be caused by the underlying maternal condition that is being treated.

Human case reports and registries are another flawed source of human data. There is substantial recall bias among women with a difficult pregnancy outcome. Women who bear children with an anomaly are much more likely to recall medication use in pregnancy and so are their providers. An illustration of this is the fact that the incidence of teratogenesis of isotretrinoin was felt to be 80% with voluntary reporting to a registry at the pharmaceutical company but has been subsequently found to be only 36% in prospective studies.

PRACTICE POINT

Some known human teratogens

Commonly used agents

- Carbamazepine
- Cyclophosphamide
- Diethylstilboestrol
- Isotretinoin
- Lithium
- Methimazole
- Methotrexate
- Mycophenolate Mofetil
- Penicillamine
- Phenobarbital
- Phenytoin
- Tetracyclines
- Valproic Acid
- Warfarin
- ACE inhibitors (eg, captopril) and angiotension receptor blockers (eg, losartan)

Less commonly used agents

- Androgenic hormones and high dose norprogesterones
- Busulfan
- Iodides
- Thalidomide

Agents generally no longer in use as medication

- Mercury
- Trimethadione
- Acitretin/etretinate

Another difficulty with human data is that there is a difference in the response of individual human fetuses to different medications much in the same way as there is in adults. A classic example of such a phenomenon is seen with phenytoin. Many teratologists believe that phenytoin can cause something known as fetal hydantoin syndrome in 10% of infants exposed *in utero*. Fetal hydantoin syndrome (FHS) is a combination of features of intrauterine growth restriction, mild mental deficiency, a large anterior fontanel, a metopic ridge, ocular hypertelorism, depressed nasal bridge, short antevertal rise, bowed upper lip, cleft lip and palate, and nail and distal phalangeal hypoplasia. The risk of this syndrome increases dramatically in subsequent pregnancies if the mother has previously borne a child with FHS. One theory for this phenomenon is that the teratogenic risk of phenytoin varies with the activity of the enzyme epoxide hydrolase in mother and fetus. Decreased activity of this enzyme in patients taking phenytoin may lead to increased levels or toxic arene oxide intermediates, which some investigators suspect may be the direct teratogen in some cases of FHS.

Another problem with human data is that most cautionary information about medication use in pregnancy is related to anatomic defects identified in newborns on the initial exam at birth. Rarely are there studies that examine behavioral, functional, developmental, and/or delayed effects. The logistics and expense of carrying out such studies are daunting. This is especially true if one considers the potential for medications to affect the offspring of offspring through toxicities of a medication on the gametes *in utero*. Such effects are very unlikely to ever be uncovered.

An illustration of the complexity of drug pregnancy safety data is found in the history of the ACE inhibitors. Captopril was the first ACE inhibitor marketed in the United States and was initially released to market as an FDA category C drug on the basis of animal studies suggesting it is unlikely to be a teratogen. (See the discussion of the FDA pregnancy drug classification later in this chapter.) Postmarketing surveillance of this drug revealed an association with ogliohydramnios, fetal calvarial hypoplasia, fetal pulmonary hypoplasia, intrauterine growth restriction, intrauterine fetal death, and neonatal anuria. Most teratologists believed that the effect of ACE inhibitors was not a direct effect on organogenesis but rather a fetal toxicity. They hypothesized that high levels of angiotensin are probably physiologically necessary to maintain glomerular filtration at the low perfusion pressure seen inside the fetus. Therefore, use of ACE inhibitors in pregnancy is associated with poor perfusion of the kidneys, followed by renal failure and atrophy of the kidneys. Poor urine output contributes to the oligohydramnios, fetal calvarial hypoplasia, and fetal pulmonary hypoplasia seen in infants exposed to the drug. Since this association was made, ACE inhibitors were classified as class C drugs for the first trimester but as class D drugs for second and third trimesters. Subsequent population-based studies of ACE inhibitors, however, have suggested that there may also be a first trimester effect on organogenesis in addition to the later effects on fetal renal function and have led to recommendations to avoid the use of these agents completely during pregnancy, although the FDA has not yet changed the pregnancy safety classification for these agents.

Another example of the complexity of drug safety data in pregnancy is metronidazole. Metronidazole was long considered a human teratogen because it was found to be mutagenic in bacteria, carcinogenic in mice, and associated with congenital anomalies in several case reports in the medical literature. Therefore this important agent for the treatment of bacterial vaginosis was often not used or used only with hesitation by obstetricians. However, this changed when a series of publications demonstrated no increased human risk associated with the use of metronidazole during pregnancy. Therefore, a drug that was withheld from pregnant women is now widely used during gestation with no evidence of untoward effects.

PRACTICE POINT

Four questions to ask in guiding medication use in pregnancy

- **Question 1:** Is the symptom to be treated self limited and/or amenable to nonpharmacologic management?
- **Question 2:** If the medication is *not* administered, what are the possible outcomes for mother and fetus?
- **Question 3:** What data is available on the safety of this medication in pregnancy and is there a similar drug with better safety data available that could be used instead?
- **Question 4:** How is the patient's (and the provider's) understanding and value system affecting decisions about the use of this medication in pregnancy?

How then should the clinician sensibly approach this flawed and limited data? Neither the clinician nor the patient should believe that any drug can be called completely safe in pregnancy any more than we would believe that any drug can be called completely safe outside of pregnancy. At the same time, the clinician and the patient should not feel that any drug is absolutely contraindicated in pregnancy. A more evidence-based approach is to consider whether benefits of a particular agent warrant any known or theoretical risks. Likewise, it is worth discarding the concept that there are any "safe" periods for medication use in pregnancy; again, a more evidence-based approach is to talk of "more vulnerable" and "less vulnerable" times during the pregnancy.

How then should the clinician approach the problem of deciding what drugs should or can be used during pregnancy? A useful approach is to address this question in four separate parts, listed in the Practice Point and discussed in the proceeding section.

QUESTION 1: IS THE SYMPTOM TO BE TREATED SELF LIMITED AND/OR AMENABLE TO NONPHARMACOLOGIC MANAGEMENT?

It is important when approaching medication use in pregnancy to have the patient (and the provider) understand that pregnancy is a time when unnecessary or unhelpful medications that do not significantly affect the course of an illness should be avoided. As well, the option of nonpharmacologic management should always be considered in pregnancy. Treatment such as biofeedback or relaxation techniques for tension headaches might be preferable to analgesics in some cases.

QUESTION 2: IF THE MEDICATION IS NOT ADMINISTERED, WHAT ARE THE POSSIBLE OUTCOMES FOR THE MOTHER AND THE FETUS?

Many providers incorrectly entertain the idea of there being a central conflict regarding medication use in pregnancy in which the fetal and maternal needs are at odds. This is rarely the case. Fetal well-being is dependent on maternal well-being, and, therefore, treatment of maternal disease to maintain maternal health is generally very much in the interest of the fetus. For this reason, when deciding whether use of a particular medication is justifiable in pregnancy, it is important to consider the possible outcomes for the mother and fetus of *not* instituting (or continuing) pharmacologic treatment. It is often the case that withholding treatment will place the fetus and mother at greater risk than any potential effects of the medication.

QUESTION 3: WHAT DATA IS AVAILABLE ON THE SAFETY OF THIS MEDICATION IN PREGNANCY, AND IS THERE A SIMILAR DRUG WITH BETTER SAFETY DATA AVAILABLE THAT MIGHT BE USED INSTEAD?

This is the question that many clinicians find the most challenging. Table 221-1 lists several of the most helpful references available to assist in the answering of this question. Table 221-2 also offers a symptom- and disease-based list summarizing which agents are generally justifiable, sometimes justifiable, and almost never justifiable for a particular indication during pregnancy.

PRACTICE POINT

Food and drug administration pregnancy drug classification

- *The US FDA Pregnancy Drug Classification system was put in place in 1979. In 1997, the FDA advised that the system be revised to address its limitations and in 2008 a proposal was put forward to eliminate the letter-based categorization and rely solely on prose summaries of available pregnancy safety data. When and if this proposed change will be adapted remains unclear.*

Category A: controlled studies show no risk

- Controlled studies in women fail to demonstrate a risk to the fetus in the first trimester, there is no evidence of a risk in later trimester, and therefore, the possibility of fetal harm appears remote.

Category B: no evidence of risk in humans

- Either animal reproduction studies have not demonstrated a fetal risk but there are no controlled studies in pregnant women, or animal-reproduction studies have shown an adverse effect (other than decrease in fertility) that was not confirmed in controlled studies in women in the first trimester (and there is no evidence of a risk in later trimester).

Category C: risk cannot be ruled out

- Either studies in animals have revealed adverse effect on the fetus (teratogenic) or appropriate animal data is not available. Drugs should be given only if the potential benefit justifies the potential risk to the fetus.

Category D: positive evidence or risk

- There is positive evidence of human fetal risk, but the benefits from use in pregnant women may be acceptable despite the risk (eg, if the drug is needed in a life-threatening situation or for a serious disease for which safer drugs cannot be used or are ineffective). There will be an appropriate statement in the "warnings" section of the labeling.

Category X: contraindicated in pregnancy

- Studies in animals or human beings have demonstrated fetal abnormalities or there is evidence of fetal risk based on human experience, or both, and the risk of the use of the drug in pregnant women clearly outweighs any possible benefit. The drug is contraindicated in woman who are or may be pregnant.

Perhaps somewhat unfortunately, the most commonly used resource in the United States with which question 3 is answered is the U.S. Food and Drug Administration's (FDA's) pregnancy categories. These classification categories are found in most prescription medication package inserts and in the Physician's Desk Reference (PDR). The categories are summarized in the Practice Point and listed as subscripts following each agent in Table 221-2. The intent of the FDA classification was to help the clinician briefly summarize available data about the potential toxicities of an agent in pregnancy. Clinicians tend to use the letter categories as an order of safety, although a drug may be in category B when there is no human data available. Problems result from the fact that the complexity of the data is not fully considered and that the classification of agents rarely change even after decades of accumulated data.

Even within medications from both the same drug class and pregnancy safety category, it is worth being cautious about the use of the newest agents during pregnancy unless there has been significant human pregnancy data. Many fetal toxicities such as the first trimester effects of ACE inhibitors have been identified in the years following release onto the market. Therefore, even an older drug with a less favorable pregnancy safety category may at times be preferable to a newer agent with an apparently more favorable pregnancy classification. An example of this would be the use of amitripytline (an FDA pregnancy category D drug) to initially treat depression rather than newer agents such as venlafaxine (an FDA category C drug) given the lack of published human data about the use of venlafaxine in pregnancy.

QUESTION 4: HOW DOES THE PATIENT'S AND THE PROVIDER'S UNDERSTANDING AND VALUE SYSTEM AFFECT DECISIONS ABOUT THE USE OF MEDICATION IN PREGNANCY?

Studies suggest that women believe that medications ingested in pregnancy end in significant malformations in a significant number of cases. Misinformation can come from media, friends, family, and even nurses, pharmacists, and physicians. Therefore, it is important for the provider to know what the patient's understanding of the potential toxicities are and work with her to clarify and address her concerns The physician should determine how the patient understands her illness, what the patient's specific fears are, and what the patient can tolerate in terms of outcome. Often irrational fears can be allayed by exploring these questions. A woman at 20 weeks may want to avoid taking medication for fear that her baby will be born with a missing arm or leg, an outcome that the provider can reassure her could hardly be attributed to any drug taken that late in gestation. These same questions should also be asked of the providers. The provider's understanding of the patient's illness, his or her own sense of the patient's capability of tolerating the symptoms, and what outcomes he or she fears may significantly effect willingness to prescribe medication in pregnancy. Providers need to be cognizant of these issues to avoid being too paternalistic or having their own fears or prejudices guide decision making that should be based on evidence and the patient's values rather than the physician's anxieties. In the end, providers should work with our patients to make a judgment based on the available data, the indication of a particular agent and an awareness of the patient's value system to determine whether the available information justifies or warrants the risk inherent in the use of all medication in pregnancy.

Once the best medication choice has been made in conjunction with the patient, the provider should consider pregnancy-related changes in pharmacokinetics that can affect drug dosing and response during pregnancy. A 30% to 50% increase in gastric emptying time during pregnancy may delay absorption of oral agents. An increase in gastric pH related to a 40% decrease in gastric acid secretion that occurs in pregnancy may also affect medication absorption. Renal clearance of medication is increased in pregnancy because glomerular filtration rates increase to 150% of nonpregnant values. Therefore, medications that are cleared renally, such as penicillin, digoxin, and lithium, may require shortened dosing intervals or significant dosage changes in pregnancy. Hepatic clearance of pharmacologic agents may be altered in pregnancy. Progesterone increases hepatic metabolism of some drugs such as phenytoin (Dilantin) but may also decrease metabolism of agents such as theophylline and caffeine through competitive inhibition of microsomal oxidases. The cholestatic effect of estrogen during pregnancy may affect clearance of drugs such as rifampin that are excreted in the biliary system.

The commonly used agent labetalol has an elimination half-life (t1/2) of 102 minutes in patients with pregnancy-induced hypertension as opposed to its t1/2 of 160 to 480 minutes in nonpregnant controls. The nifedipine elimination half-life is 1.35 hours in pregnancy versus 3.4 hours in controls.

Substantial changes in the volume of distribution also occur in pregnancy. Plasma volume increases to 150% of prepregnancy values by 24 to 28 weeks gestation so that the volume of distribution for medication is increased and drugs may require dosage increases. At the same time the physiologic dilutional hypoalbuminemia that occurs in pregnancy combined with the displacement of bound drugs by the hormones of pregnancy may lead to an increase in free drug level for a particular serum level.

PRACTICE POINT

Physiologic changes in pregnancy that can affect medication pharmacokinetics

- Increased blood volume
- Increased glomerular filtration rate
- Dilutional hypoalbuminemia
- Slowing of gastric and intestinal motility

The main practical applications of the above physiologic and pharmacokinetic changes are as follows:

1. Serious consideration should be made to monitoring of medication levels and adjustment of medication dose during pregnancy.
2. Free drug levels in general are better guides than total serum levels in pregnancy because of altered protein binding.
3. Dosing intervals may need to be shortened in pregnancy.
4. Inadequate dosing frequency always needs to be considered as a possible cause for failure of medications during pregnancy.

The last and perhaps most important issue to be aware of when prescribing in pregnancy is that medication compliance is a significant challenge. Drug labeling warnings, pharmacists, and an unrealistically high perception of teratogenic risks all contribute to this phenomenon. One small study from Wales found that 15% of women with epilepsy who claimed to be taking antiepileptic drugs in pregnancy showed no evidence of having done so on testing of their hair. One of these noncompliant patients died suddenly at 30 weeks gestation. Providers need to work with their patients to increase understanding about the important interdependence of maternal and fetal health and the justifiable and "healthful" use of indicated medications during pregnancy.

CONCLUSION

All providers prescribing medication to women of reproductive age should speak to these patients about the potential effects of their medications during pregnancy and the potential for harm even before the pregnancy is clinically apparent. The acute hospitalization presents an opportunity to evaluate all medications, adjust dosages, and educate patients and families about their indication and safety profile.

SUGGESTED READINGS

Brent RL. How does a physician avoid prescribing drugs and medical procedures that have reproductive and developmental risks? *Clin Perinatol*. 2007;34(2):233–262.

Briggs GS, Freeman R, Yaffe S, *Medication in Pregnancy and Lactation*, 8th ed. Philadelphia, PA: Lippincott Williams & Wilkins, 2008.

Buhimschi CS, Weiner CP. Medications in pregnancy and lactation: part 1. Teratology. *Obstet Gynecol*. 2009;113(1):166–188.

Buhimschi CS, Weiner CP. Medications in pregnancy and lactation: part 2. Drugs with minimal or unknown human teratogenic effect. *Obstet Gynecol*. 2009;2(1):417–432.

Cooper WO, Hernandez-Diaz S, Arbogast PG, et al. Major congenital malformations after first-trimester exposure to ACE inhibitors. *N Engl J Med*. 2006;354(23):2443–2451.

Einarson A, Ho E, Koren G. Can we use metronidazole during pregnancy and breastfeeding? Putting an end to the controversy. *Can Fam Physician*. 2000;46:1053–1054.

Friedman JM, Polifka JE. *Teratogenic Effects of Drugs: A Resource for Clinicians (TERIS)*, 2nd ed. Baltimore, MD: Johns Hopkins University Press, 2000.

Hartsfield JK Jr., Holmes LB, Morel JG. Phenytoin embryopathy: effect of epoxide hydrolase inhibitor on phenytoin exposure in utero in C57BL/6J mice. *Biochem Mol Med*. 1995;56(2):131–143.

Koren G. *Medication Safety in Pregnancy and Breastfeeding*. New York, NY: McGraw-Hill Professional, 2007.

Koren, G, Levichek, Z. The teratogenicity of drugs for nausea and vomiting of pregnancy: perceived versus true risk. *Am J Obstet Gynecol*. 2002;186(5, part 2):S248–S252.

Kyle PM. Drugs and the fetus. *Curr Opin Obstet Gynecol*. 2006; 18(2):93–99.

Pavek P, Ceckova M, Staud F. Variation of drug kinetics in pregnancy. *Curr Drug Metab*. 2009;10(5):520–529.

Prevost RR, Akl SA, Whybrew WD, Sibai BM. Oral nifedipine pharmacokinetics in pregnancy-induced hypertension. *Pharmacotherapy*. 1992;12(3):174–177.

Rayburn WF, Amanze AC. Prescribing medications safely during pregnancy. *Med Clin North Am*. 2008;92(5):1227–1237, xii.

Rogers RC, Sibai BM, Whybrew WD. Labetalol pharmacokinetics in pregnancy-induced hypertension. *Am J Obstet Gynecol*. 1990; 162(2):362–366.

Rosene-Montella, K, Keely E, Barbour LA, Lee RV. *Medical Care of the Pregnant Patient*, 2nd ed. Philadelphia, PA: American College of Physicians-American Society of Internal Medicine, 2008.

Rubin PC, Ramsey M. *Prescribing in Pregnancy*, 4th ed. London, U.K.: BMJ Books, 2008.

Splinter M, Nightingale B, Sawgraves R, et al. Medication use during pregnancy by women delivering at a tertiary university hospital. *South Med J*. 1997;90:498–502.

Schaefer C, Meister R, Weber-Schoendorfer C. Isotretinoin exposure and pregnancy outcome: an observational study of the Berlin Institute for Clinical Teratology and Drug Risk Assessment in Pregnancy. *Arch Gynecol Obstet*. 2010;281(2):221–227.

Schaefer C, Peters PWJ, Miller RK. *Drugs During Pregnancy and Lactation*, 2nd ed. London, U.K.: Academic Press.

Shehata HA, Nelson-Piercy C. Drugs in pregnancy. Drugs to avoid. *Best Pract Res Clin Obstet Gynaecol*. 2001;15(6):971–986.

Van Dyke DC, Hodge SE, Heide F, Hill LR. Family studies in fetal phenytoin exposure. *J Pediatr*. 1988;113(2):301–306.

Webster WS, Freeman JA. Prescription drugs and pregnancy. *Expert Opin Pharmacother*. 2003;4(6):949–961.

Weiner CP, Buhimschi CS. *Drugs for Pregnant and Lactating Women*. Philadelphia, PA: Churchill Livingstone, 2004.

CHAPTER 222

Critical Care of the Pregnant Patient

Meghan Hayes, MD
Ghada Bourjeily, MD

Key Clinical Questions

1. What are physiologic changes of pregnancy pertinent to critical care?
2. What are common reasons for pregnant women to require critical care?
3. What factors impact airway intubation during pregnancy?
4. What issues arise in hemodynamic monitoring during pregnancy?
5. What vasopressors can and should be used during pregnancy?
6. Are there special considerations for resuscitation during pregnancy?

INTRODUCTION

The majority of critical care admissions for pregnant and peripartum women are for obstetric disorders, primarily hypertensive complications (particularly hemorrhagic stroke) or intrapartum hemorrhage. Medical indications, such as sepsis, respiratory failure, cardiomyopathy, or ischemic stroke are less common. Maternal mortality in developed nations remains rare (10 to 16 per 10,000 births); however the proportion attributable to medical disorders has been increasing as women with underlying medical conditions and older women conceive, perhaps with assisted reproductive technology. Standard scoring systems, such as APACHE scores, overestimate mortality in pregnant and peripartum women, particularly if they have an obstetric indication for critical care. Delivery or surgery may contribute to rapid improvement. A small proportion of obstetric patients require critical care. Hospitalists and intensivists may have limited experience managing these patients.

PHYSIOLOGIC ADAPTATIONS

Virtually every organ system adapts to accommodate pregnancy and delivery. Hemodynamic alterations prepare for blood loss of one-half to one liter at delivery. Blood volume increases by 50% (**Table 222-1**).

Cardiac output increases by 30% to 50% and total peripheral resistance decreases by 20%, leading to blood pressure declining by 10 to 15 mm Hg in the first half of pregnancy, then returning to baseline in the second half. Diastolic blood pressure decreases more than systolic; pulse pressure is widened. Central venous pressure (CVP) and pulmonary capillary wedge pressure (PCWP) remain unchanged. Blood flow distribution is altered such that up to 25% of maternal cardiac output is directed to the uterus, 20% to kidneys, with an increase in breast flow. When supine, women in the second half of pregnancy experience aortocaval compression (termed supine hypotensive syndrome), in which cardiac output may drop by 30%. Left lateral decubitus positioning relieves aortocaval compression and improves venous return and cardiac output.

Maternal respiratory adaptations help optimize fetal oxygenation. Initial changes are progesterone mediated with diaphragmatic elevation contributing to changes later in pregnancy. Minute ventilation increases 30% to 60% by increased tidal volume; respiratory rate remains unchanged. Tachypnea is abnormal and warrants investigation! Diaphragmatic elevation leads to a 20% reduction in functional residual capacity by late pregnancy. Given that diaphragmatic excursion is usually unchanged in pregnancy, this drop in functional residual capacity is counterbalanced by an increase in inspiratory capacity and the resultant effect is no significant change in total lung capacity. On the other hand, oxygen consumption is significantly increased during pregnancy and rises further during labor and delivery. For those reasons, oxygen reserve is reduced in pregnancy. Arterial blood gas testing reveals a compensated respiratory alkalosis due to the above described changes and enhanced renal bicarbonate excretion. PaO_2 is typically 100 to 105 mm Hg during pregnancy and $PaCO_2$ decreases to 28 to 32 mm Hg. Maternal pulse oximetry greater than 95% is desirable in order to maintain a PaO_2 greater than 70 mm Hg and optimize placental oxygen diffusion.

Hematologic changes also occur in pregnancy with a progressive activation of the hemostatic system to prepare the parturient for the hemostatic challenge of delivery. The anticoagulant

TABLE 222-1 Cardiac, Respiratory and Hematologic Physiologic Changes in Pregnancy

	Direction of Change	Percentage of Change or Normal Range in Pregnancy
Blood volume	↑	30–40% increase
Heart rate	↑	Increases by 10–20 bpm
Cardiac output	↑	30–60% increase
Systemic vascular resistance	↓	25–30% decrease
Blood pressure	↓	10–15 mm Hg decrease in first two trimesters
Colloid oncotic pressure	↓	10–15% decrease
Total lung capacity	↓	4–5% decrease
Functional residual capacity	↓	20% decrease
Diffusion capacity	↔	No change
Tidal volume	↑	Increased
Respiratory rate	↔	No change
Minute ventilation	↑	50% increase
PaO_2	↑	Average 100–105
$PcaCo_2$	↓	Average 28–32
pH	↑	Mild respiratory alkalosis
A-a gradient	↑	Increase in late gestation to approximately 20
Protein S	↓	
Activated Protein C resistance, fibrinogen, factor V, VIII, IX, X,	↑	
Plasminogen activator inhibitor type 1 and 2	↑	
Activity of tissue plasminogen	↓	

Modified from Miller MA, Bourjeily, G. Management of the critically ill pregnant patient. Pulmonary and Critical Care Update (PCCU). April 2009, 23 (Lesson 8); with permission.

activity of protein S is reduced and activated protein C resistance rises. Procoagulant activity is increased, with higher concentrations of fibrinogen and factors V, VIII, IX, and X, leading to enhanced thrombin production. On the other hand, fibrinolysis is decreased as a result of increased activity of plasminogen activator inhibitor type 1 and type 2 and decreased activity of tissue plasminogen. Shortcomings of these changes are an increase in the risk of venous thromboembolism (VTE) antepartum until six weeks postpartum.

INDICATIONS FOR CRITICAL CARE DURING PREGNANCY/PERIPARTUM

Obstetric indications include preeclampsia and related complications: eclampsia, HELLP (hemolysis, elevated liver enzymes, low platelets), hypertensive crisis, pulmonary edema, oliguric renal failure, and cerebral hemorrhage. All of these complications would meet criteria for severe preeclampsia and would warrant urgent delivery. Close collaboration with obstetrics is essential for optimal maternal (and fetal/neonatal) outcome. Although often maternal manifestations of preeclampsia are quickly reversible with delivery and judicious fluid and blood pressure management, they may persist or even worsen in the postpartum period, requiring ongoing vigilance. While still pregnant, blood pressure goals must minimize maternal hypertensive complications, which are more likely above 160 mm Hg systolic and 110 mm Hg diastolic, while maintaining sufficient uteroplacental flow. Blood pressure reduction should be attempted promptly with caution in pregnant women given the potential for impaired uteroplacental flow and fetal compromise. Options include intravenous labetalol or hydralazine, noting that hydralazine has been associated with greater hypotension in this setting. Short-acting oral nifedipine may be useful if intravenous access is delayed but may also precipitously lower the blood pressure. Magnesium sulfate infusion is superior to phenytoin and benzodiazepines for preventing seizures in preeclampsia and reducing recurrence of eclamptic seizures. Given that most seizures are self-limited, there are limited studies comparing different drugs; however, benzodiazepines may be helpful for acute seizure treatment, noting risk of neonatal respiratory depression.

Additional obstetric conditions warranting critical care include acute fatty liver of pregnancy, peripartum cardiomyopathy, amniotic fluid embolism, and placental abruption and hemorrhage. Acute fatty liver of pregnancy (AFLP) is rare, estimated to occur in 1 in 13,000 deliveries, but carries a high mortality. Manifestations may include fulminant hepatic failure with hypoglycemia, coagulopathy, and renal failure; about half of cases are associated with preeclampsia. It may initially be difficult to differentiate AFLP from HELLP syndrome (defined as transaminases greater than twice the upper limit of normal and platelet count less than 100,000 per mm^3), but AFLP should be suspected in patients with otherwise unexplained hypoglycemia and severe hepatic dysfunction. Liver transplantation may be necessary. Recurrence rates are significant in subsequent pregnancies.

Peripartum cardiomyopathy is defined as dilated cardiomyopathy with no other known cause, with onset in the last month of pregnancy or within five months postpartum. Rates vary markedly across the world, with highest rates reported in Africa. The etiology has not fully been defined. Risk factors include advanced maternal age, multiple gestations, preeclampsia, and African descent. Treatment includes standard congestive heart failure management, including vasodilators, diuretics, and sodium restriction. Prior to delivery, hydralazine and nitrates should be used rather than angiotensin converting enzyme inhibitors, which have adverse fetal renal effects at all stages of gestation. After delivery, enalapril and captopril are considered compatible with breastfeeding. Anticoagulation should be initiated if ejection fraction is less than 35%, mural thrombus is present on imaging, or atrial fibrillation is observed, as thrombosis is a major cause of mortality in these patients. Up to half of women recover ventricular function to baseline levels within six months, with variable persistent dysfunction ranging from mild to fatal in the other half. Recurrence rates are high, and women warrant careful counseling and surveillance regarding future pregnancies.

Amniotic fluid embolism (AFE) remains exceptionally rare, described as occurring in between 1 to 8000 and 1 to 80,000 deliveries, with high maternal morbidity and mortality. Reported risk factors include prolonged labor, multiparity, increased maternal age, and oxytocin administration. The pathophysiology remains in question. Some propose terming AFE "the anaphylactoid syndrome of pregnancy," with maternal response to miniscule amounts of amniotic fluid's vasoactive and procoagulant factors. This theory remains debatable as amniotic fluid has been found in the maternal circulation in patients without signs or symptoms of AFE. Sudden decline in maternal and/or fetal status intrapartum or maternal status postpartum is the most common presentation, with hypotension, respiratory symptoms, coagulopathy, and cardiac arrest occurring in the majority. Early recognition of the syndrome and initiation of supportive measures, including aggressive blood products, are essential. If onset is antepartum, rapid delivery improves perinatal and maternal outcome. Novel interventions such as the use of recombinant factor VII administration, cardiopulmonary bypass, ventricular assist devices, and ECMO have been reported.

Medical conditions requiring critical care for pregnant and peripartum women include acute respiratory distress syndrome (ARDS), venous thromboembolism, status asthmaticus/asthma exacerbations, sepsis, pneumonia, and myocardial infarction. Pyelonephritis is of particular concern during pregnancy, with maternal complications including ARDS and sepsis due to reduced buffering capacity and decreased oncotic pressure. Pregnant women with pyelonephritis warrant inpatient management given potential maternal complications plus risk of preterm labor and premature delivery. Careful fluid administration and ongoing monitoring are essential for these women to ensure they are adequately fluid resuscitated but do not progress to fluid overload. Extensive discussion of medical conditions is outside the scope of this chapter and is reviewed in more detail in the chapter on medical disorders in pregnancy.

Trauma also leads to critical care admissions for pregnant and peripartum women, with the majority of cases due to motor vehicle accidents (MVAs). Falls, particularly in the third trimester, and domestic violence are the next leading causes in this population. Improper seat belt positioning contributes to maternal and fetal injury in MVAs; the lap belt should be placed below the gravid uterus and shoulder belt between the breasts. Obstetric complications of traumatic injuries include placental abruption, uterine rupture, and preterm delivery. The gravid uterus upwardly displaces abdominal organs so that bowel may be involved in upper abdominal trauma. Fetal instability often precedes maternal instability. Uteroplacental flow will be compromised to maintain maternal blood pressure. Multidisciplinary care for pregnant trauma patients that includes fetal monitoring will lead to optimal outcome for both mother and fetus.

AIRWAY INTUBATION

In addition to the usual causes of respiratory failure in the nonpregnant population, there are a number of pregnancy-specific conditions that might lead to acute respiratory failure. These causes include preeclampsia, amniotic fluid embolism, peripartum cardiomyopathy, and hemodynamic instability related to massive obstetric hemorrhage. Ovarian hyperstimulation related to hormonal manipulation surrounding assisted reproduction may also be associated with ARDS. Although indications are quite similar, the threshold for intubation might be different in the pregnant population since $PaCO_2$ is normally decreased and PaO_2 increased in pregnancy and a $PaCO_2$ of 38 and a PaO_2 of 70 are indications of acute respiratory failure.

Noninvasive ventilation (NIV)

The use of NIV has not been well studied in the obstetric population. Successful use of NIV has been described in pregnancy in chronic, stable settings such as in obstructive sleep apnea or chronic respiratory failure from neuromuscular disease. The use of NIV may be suboptimal in acute settings given airway edema and the increased risk of aspiration in pregnancy. However, in patients with a preserved mental status and no other contra-indications who may not require assisted ventilation for prolonged periods of time, short trials of NIV may be attempted prior to endotracheal intubation.

Endotracheal intubation

Anesthesia-related mortality ranks seventh in maternal mortality in the U.S. This is in part due to the fact that failure rate for endotracheal intubations in pregnant patients is 1 in 280 compared to 1 in 2330 in the general surgical population. Failure to intubate may be associated with a higher risk for cardiac arrest and aspiration.

A number of factors complicate endotracheal intubation in pregnancy. Reduced airway patency is one of the factors. Higher blood volume and estrogen levels in pregnancy cause capillary engorgement and mucosal edema leading to difficult visualization of the landmarks of the upper airway. Mallampati scores, a measure of upper airway patency, increase progressively in pregnancy and upper airway size as measured by acoustic reflectance method is reduced in the supine position. Airway edema may be further exaggerated in patients with a prolonged second stage of labor, excessive intravenous fluids, and preeclampsia. Preeclampsia is associated with lower oncotic pressures with possible coagulopathy worsening airway edema. Weight gain and the increase in breast size can lead to difficulty in manipulating the upper airway and reduced chest compliance. Obesity is also one of the major risk factors for maternal mortality in a review of anesthesia-related maternal mortality.

Pregnant women are also at a higher risk for aspiration related to a progesterone mediated relaxation of the lower esophageal sphincter, an increase in intra-abdominal pressure (due to the enlarging uterus), and delayed gastric emptying. The use of aspiration precautions is advisable.

An important consideration during sedation and paralysis of a pregnant woman is the reduced oxygen reserve given the 20% reduction in functional residual capacity (which is likely more pronounced in the supine position) and the increase in oxygen consumption. Sedation and paralysis eliminate the rise in minute ventilation that usually occurs to compensate for these changes/demands and rapid desaturation and hypoventilation occur.

Therefore, preoxygenation with 100% oxygen should be done before and between intubation attempts during pregnancy and lower doses of sedatives may be needed. This should be done with caution as prolonged manual ventilation may distend the stomach increasing the risk of aspiration even further. A left lateral position also helps improve venous return in patients with a tenuous hemodynamic status, since cardiac output may be reduced by 25% to 30% in the supine position in the late stages of pregnancy.

An additional complicating factor is the urgent nature of airway intubation in the obstetric population.

Because of the increased risk of morbidity and mortality associated with airway intubation in pregnancy, airway intubation should be performed by providers with the most extensive experience. Airway assessment according to the American Society of Anesthesiology practice guidelines is critical in pregnancy, even in cases of urgent intubation. The management of the difficult airway should follow the American Society of Anesthesiology practice guidelines. In this algorithm, the laryngeal mask airway (LMA) is recognized as the tool of choice for "cannot ventilate, cannot intubate" (CVCI) patients.

A chest radiograph to ensure proper placement of the endotracheal tube carries only a negligible risk of fetal radiation exposure and should be done as in the nonpregnant patient.

PRACTICE POINT

Airway intubation

1. Upper airway size smaller in pregnancy, even smaller in preeclampsia.
2. Rate of intubation failure much higher in pregnancy.
3. Airway examination should be performed prior to intubation.
4. Laryngeal mask airway should be considered as an option and made readily available.
5. Use aspiration precautions

HEMODYNAMIC MONITORING

Profound hemodynamic changes occur in pregnancy to prepare for the needs of the growing feto-maternal unit and to compensate for the expected losses during pregnancy. These changes are summarized in Table 222-1. Indications for hemodynamic monitoring specific for obstetric patients include severe preeclampsia with either refractory hypertension, oliguric renal failure, or unclear intravascular volume status. Hemodynamic monitoring may also be needed in obstetric patients with severe structural heart disease in the peripartum period, or cardiovascular collapse such as in the setting of an acute amniotic fluid embolism.

Monitoring may be done either invasively or noninvasively. Echocardiography has been shown to correlate with invasive monitoring in the measurement of cardiac output, ventricular filling pressures, stroke volume, and pulmonary artery pressures.

Echocardiography interpretation should be performed with caution in pregnancy given that physiologic chamber dilatation and the increase in flow may overestimate pulmonary artery pressures. Patients with refractory hypertension and oliguria were successfully managed in a small series with echocardiography suggesting that this test may be an effective alternative to pulmonary artery catheterization during pregnancy in specific circumstances.

Invasive monitoring may be needed in cases of severe stenotic valvular disease, severe cardiomyopathy, sudden cardiovascular collapse, ARDS/indeterminate fluid status, refractory oliguria, and unclear volume status despite fluid resuscitation and refractory septic shock. Invasive monitoring may occasionally be indicated for labor and delivery in high risk patients. Invasive monitoring has somewhat fallen out of favor with recent trials not showing any clear benefit compared to central venous catheters. There are no randomized controlled trials evaluating the clinical usefulness of pulmonary artery catheters in pregnancy in general. Available data suggest that although there is a modest correlation between central venous pressures (measured with a central venous catheter) and a pulmonary capillary wedge pressure in the management of patients with untreated preeclampsia, this correlation may lessen after initial interventions.

PRACTICE POINT

Hemodynamic monitoring

1. Indications relatively similar to nonpregnant population.
2. Providers should be aware of normal hemodynamic changes of pregnancy.

VASOPRESSORS

Acute hypotension requiring vasopressor support in the pregnant woman most commonly results from vasodilatation in the setting of neuraxial anesthesia. Additional vasodilatation on top of the physiologic vasodilatation of pregnancy is poorly tolerated. Hemodynamic compromise may also be precipitated by hypovolemia, sepsis, anaphylaxis, and cardiogenic shock. A pregnant woman has an additional end organ, the fetus, with uteroplacental flow receiving 20% to 30% of maternal cardiac output. Maternal hypotension risks fetal and neonatal acidosis. It is critical to restore intravascular volume first, as uteroplacental flow is compromised further by vasoconstriction in addition to hypovolemia.

Limited data is available comparing vasopressors during pregnancy, so physician familiarity and drug availability have roles in vasopressor choice. All vasopressors have potential to impair uteroplacental flow. There is minimal information regarding developmental toxicity. Currently phenylephrine and ephedrine are the most commonly used vasopressors in this population. Phenylephrine is a short-acting alpha agonist with potent vasoconstricting effect that may be easily titrated. It does not act on beta receptors thus does not lead to maternal tachycardia; however, reflex bradycardia due to increased venous return may occur, requiring atropine administration. Ephedrine has been used extensively by obstetric anesthesiologists. It is a direct alpha and beta agonist and also indirectly releases norepinephrine. Maternal cardiac output increases by increased heart rate and contractility. Alpha effect causes peripheral vasoconstriction and increased blood pressure. Titration is difficult due to its slow onset and tachyphylaxis develops after repeated doses.

Recent reports comparing ephedrine to phenylephrine infusion at cesarean delivery show that ephedrine is associated with more maternal nausea and vomiting, higher heart rate, and a higher incidence of fetal acidosis but comparable effects on blood pressure. A meta-analysis comparing the two drugs reported similar findings including a higher fetal pH associated with phenylephrine. In summary, if hypotension persists after an adequate intravascular volume has been restored, phenylephrine is the drug of choice in pregnant patients with circulatory collapse, unless a clear benefit in restoring hemodynamics is expected from another drug.

PRACTICE POINT

Use of vasopressors

1. Ensure adequate intravascular volume.
2. Consider the fetus an end organ.
3. Once the need for a vasopressor has been established, phenylephrine is preferred because of less fetal acidosis and lower maternal heart rate.

CARDIAC ARREST AND RESUSCITATION

The incidence of cardiac arrest in pregnancy has been estimated at 1 in 30,000, causing about 10% of maternal deaths. It remains a rare and potentially catastrophic event for mother and fetus. Outcomes for both depend on the underlying cause of arrest and rapidity of resuscitation. Causes of cardiac arrest in this setting include venous thromboembolism, preeclampsia, sepsis, amniotic fluid embolism, hemorrhage, trauma, underlying cardiac disease (either congenital or acquired), or iatrogenic (anesthetic complications or anaphylaxis).

Prompt initiation of cardiopulmonary resuscitation protocols is essential, with attention to a few additional details. Pregnant women are at increased risk of aspiration during resuscitation and desaturate rapidly, therefore immediate intubation with 100% oxygen administration and cricoid pressure is advised in this population. Position the mother in the left lateral decubitus position to relieve aortocaval compression; a wedge, roll, or team member's knee under her right hip will achieve this goal. A "Cardiff wedge" is designed for compressions on a pregnant patient but these are not widely available. Hand position for compressions may be a few centimeters higher on the sternum due to breast engorgement and diaphragmatic elevation but no studies are available to demonstrate that higher compressions result in better cardiac output. Defibrillation energy and locations are unchanged. Any fetal monitoring devices must be removed prior to defibrillation to avoid the possibility of arcing.

PRACTICE POINT

Resuscitation of the pregnant patient

1. Emphasis on oxygenation and secure airway.
2. Left lateral decubitus positioning; wedge under right hip to improve CO with CPR.
3. Remove fetal monitoring devices prior to defibrillation.
4. Vasopressin degraded by placental vasopressinase, so use epinephrine.
5. Prefer alternatives to amiodarone given potential for fetal thyroid impact.
6. If maternal resuscitation not successful within five minutes, proceed to cesarean delivery if viable fetus (approx 24 weeks) with CPR throughout.

Drug administration generally proceeds as usual, with note of potential issues with amiodarone and vasopressin. Alternatives to amiodarone, such as lidocaine and procainamide, would be preferable given concern for its fetal thyroid impact; however, if resuscitation team members are most familiar with amiodarone and it is most quickly available, antiarrhythmic administration should not be delayed as the risk of untreated ventricular arrythmias by far outweighs the risk of fetal thyroid dysfunction. The placenta produces vasopressinase, which could degrade vasopressin, thus epinephrine is preferable.

If the fetus is viable (24 weeks or greater), it is strongly recommended to perform cesarean delivery by five minutes into resuscitation to improve maternal and fetal outcomes. In 1986, Katz, et al, recommended perimortem cesarean delivery and in 2005 published data revealing intact neurologic outcome in neonates delivered within five minutes of arrest. Maternal chest compressions should continue throughout delivery efforts. Immediately after uterine evacuation, maternal cardiac output increases due to autotransfusion from uterine circulation and relief of aortocaval compression; chest compressions are more effective after delivery as well. Regular maternal cardiac arrest drills are recommended to ensure all pertinent disciplines are prepared for this uncommon event.

CONCLUSION

As women with underlying medical conditions and older women conceive, the proportion of critically ill, pregnant women with medical disorders may increase. This chapter briefly reviews common obstetric disorders that may require critical care and aspects of resuscitation that are unique to pregnancy.

SUGGESTED READINGS

Baskett TF, O'Connell CM. Maternal critical care in obstetrics. *J Obstet Gynaecol Can.* 2009;31(3):218–221.

Bourjeily G, Miller M. Obstetric disorders in the ICU. *Clin Chest Med.* 2009;30(1):89–102; viii.

Gist RS, Stafford IP, Leibowitz AB, Beilin Y. Amniotic fluid embolism. *Anesth Analg.* 2009;108(5):1599–1602.

Katz V, Balderston K, DeFreest M. Perimortem cesarean delivery: were our assumptions correct? *Am J Obstet Gynecol.* 2005;192: 1916–1920.

Katz VL, Dottes DJ, Droegemuller W. Perimortem cesarean delivery. *Obstet Gynecol.* 1986;68:571–576.

Lewis G, ed. The Confidential Enquiry into Maternal and Child Health (CEMACH). Saving Mothers' Lives- Reviewing maternal deaths to make motherhood safer 2003–2005. The seventh report on confidential enquiries into maternal deaths in the United Kingdom. London: CEMACH; 2007.

Miller MA, Bourjeily, G. Management of the critically ill pregnant patient. Pulmonary and Critical Care Update (PCCU). April 2009; 23 (Lesson 8) www.chestnet.org/education/online/pccu/vol23/lessons07_08/index.php

Reidy J, Douglas J. Vasopressors in obstetrics. *Anesthesiol Clin.* 2008; 26(1):75–88, vi–vii.

Stevens TA, Carroll MA, Promcene PA, Seibel M, Monga M. Utility of Acute Physiology, Age, and Chronic Health Evaluation (APACHE III) score in maternal admissions to the intensive care unit. *Am J Obstet Gynecol.* 2006;194:e13–e15.

Vasquez DN, Estenssoro E, Canales HS, et al. Clinical characteristics and outcomes of obstetric patients requiring ICU admission. *Chest.* 2007;131(3):718–724.

Zeeman GG. Obstetric critical care: a blueprint for improved outcomes. *Crit Care Med.* 2006;34(9 Suppl):S208–S214.

CHAPTER 223

Common Medical Problems in Pregnancy

Niharika D. Mehta, MD
Kenneth K. Chen, MD, FRACP
Carmen Monzon, MD
Karen Rosene-Montella, MD

Key Clinical Questions

1. How do common diseases and their treatment impact on pregnancy?
2. How might pregnancy impact on common illness?

INTRODUCTION

Although women of childbearing age represent a younger and generally healthy population, currently 40% of women entering pregnancy have chronic medical conditions. The rise in the rates of obesity and type 2 diabetes, combined with modern medical technology, have resulted in pregnancy in older and sicker women. It is important to consider how diseases and their treatment may impact pregnancy and how pregnancy may affect certain diseases. This chapter will focus on the most common medical problems in pregnancy.

CARDIAC DISEASES

During pregnancy, blood volume and cardiac output rise, and systemic vascular resistance decreases. Later in pregnancy the gravid uterus may compress the inferior vena cava, thereby significantly decreasing preload in the supine position. Cardiac output increases 40% by mid-pregnancy until labor and delivery when it increases further. Increased blood volume and left atrial dimensions may contribute to the increase in palpitations and supraventricular tachycardia. If the heart is damaged either by congenital heart disease or by cardiomyopathy, the increase in cardiac work cannot occur as effectively. In addition, just after delivery, with a uterine contraction a liter of blood can be shunted from the uterus into the general circulation. Cardiac lesions associated with a fixed cardiac output will not tolerate this sudden increase in volume. Hence, the most common complications in late pregnancy or immediately after delivery include pulmonary edema and, less commonly, right heart failure. In addition, the risk of a fetus developing congenital heart disease is increased if the mother has the same problem (for example, 1:4 in tetralogy of Fallot and 1:15 in atrial septal defects). Patients with severe pulmonary hypertension and/or Eisenmenger syndrome characterized by a reversed right-to-left shunt have increased mortality rates, especially during the first 48–72 hours postpartum.

Systemic vascular resistance decreases about 25%, which may improve any cardiac condition that benefits from after-load reduction such as aortic insufficiency. When compression of the inferior vena cava decreases venous return to the heart, patients with preload-dependent cardiac conditions such as aortic stenosis or poor left ventricular function may experience hypotension, especially when supine. Because the increased cardiac demands peak at 24 to 28 weeks of gestation, cardiac decompensation may become evident at the end of the second trimester.

Labor and delivery may be associated with cardiac decompensation when one to two units of blood leave the uteroplacental circulation during contraction. When the contraction ceases, the blood returns to the uteroplacental circulation.

Patients with peripartum cardiomyopathy that occurs in the third trimester and up to six months following delivery have symptoms and signs consistent with congestive heart failure. Approximately, one-third of these patients will completely recover, one-third will have chronic congestive heart failure, and one-third may have a progressive cardiomyopathy that may require cardiac transplantation in severe cases.

Postpartum fluid shifts occur during involution of the uterus and the low-resistance circulation of the placenta, postpartum blood loss, and increase in preload when the uterus no longer compresses the inferior vena cava.

Acute myocardial infarction is a rare complication during pregnancy. Coronary dissection with normal coronary arteries on angiography is more common in the peripartum or postpartum period. Patients with longstanding diabetes may develop myocardial ischemia during pregnancy. Antiphospholipid antibody-associated arterial thrombosis and arterial vasospasm and cocaine ingestion may also result in myocardial infarction.

Finally, women with artificial heart valves who receive anticoagulant treatment will need to continue to do so during pregnancy. Decision about type of anticoagulation requires a careful risk-benefit discussion, and should not include warfarin during the first trimester or toward term. Careful monitoring to achieve consistently therapeutic levels of anticoagulation is important. Ideally these patients should receive care and obstetric at a tertiary medical center that can provide combined cardiac and obstetric antenatal care.

INFECTIOUS DISEASES

THE FEBRILE PREGNANT FEMALE

Although pregnant women develop the same infections as nonpregnant individuals, there are important pregnancy-related issues that should be considered in the evaluation and treatment of these patients. Pregnant women are predisposed to certain infections and pregnancy may alter the course of some infections. Clinicians need to consider maternal-fetal transmission and the impact of some antibacterial or antiviral drugs upon the fetus.

A primary systemic infection with toxoplasmosis, rubella, cytomegalovirus, herpes simplex virus, syphilis, and parvovirus can be associated with congenital malformations and disease. Primary infection with coccidiomycoses, especially common in the southwestern United States, can be complicated by fungal meningitis, otherwise rare in a normal host.

Fever, mild uterine tenderness, and contractions may suggest chorioamnionitis or infection of the amniotic sac and fluid. The diagnosis is made by consultation with an obstetrician and consideration of amniocentesis (positive Gram stain, amniotic fluid glucose usually < 15 mg/dL). Treatment may require delivery.

Infection of the endometrium, an ascending polymicrobial infection, occurs in the postpartum period. Risk factors include prolonged rupture of membranes, delivery requiring instrumentation, and cesarean section, especially unplanned or emergent. Obstetricians can advise on the best antibiotic regimen depending on early postpartum endometritis (within the first 48 hours) and later endometritis (more than one week postpartum). Septic pelvic thrombophlebitis may be considered when a patient has persistent fevers despite an appropriately treated postpartum endometritis. If pelvic thrombosis is not seen by computed tomography (CT) or magnetic resonance venography (MRV) of the pelvis in a patient who does not appear to be ill, alternative diagnoses such as abscess, hematomas, and necrotizing fasciitis should be considered.

PYELONEPHRITIS

Incidence

Acute pyelonephritis complicates 1–2% of all pregnancies and can be associated with significant maternal and fetal morbidity. Untreated asymptomatic bacteriuria is associated with a 25% incidence of pyelonephritis. Therefore, asymptomatic bacteriuria in a pregnant patient should always be treated.

Pathophysiology

Pyelonephritis is most common during the second half of the pregnancy as a result of increased ureteral obstruction and urinary stasis, which result from both mechanical and hormonal factors. It is usually unilateral, affecting the right kidney more frequently because of uterine dextrorotation. Prior history of pyelonephritis, urinary tract malformations, and calculi put patients at a higher risk for development of an acute episode of pyelonephritis during pregnancy.

Clinical features

Pyelonephritis most commonly presents with systemic signs and symptoms including flank pain, fever, costovertebral angle tenderness, shaking chills, nausea, vomiting, and less often with features of cystitis, such as dysuria and frequency.

Diagnosis

Laboratory findings generally include a positive urine culture and pyuria on urinalysis. Additional laboratory studies should include a complete blood cell count and serum chemistry evaluation. Transient renal insufficiency with as much as 50% decrease in creatinine clearance is observed in about a quarter of all patients. Although blood cultures are often obtained in these patients, their utility is limited. Pathogens isolated from blood cultures rarely differ from those found in the corresponding urine culture. Blood cultures are recommended in cases that are complicated by sepsis, temperature of at least 39°C, or respiratory distress syndrome.

Differential diagnosis

Ovarian vein thrombosis may present as fever and flank pain and so should be considered in patients suspected of having pyelonephritis who have normal urinalysis.

Pregnancy considerations

Pyelonephritis has unique complications in pregnancy. These include development of acute respiratory distress syndrome (ARDS), which can occur in up to 10% of patients. It is more common in patients with pyelonephritis and preterm labor who are being treated with beta-agonist tocolysis. Acute pyelonephritis during pregnancy is also associated with preterm delivery, with reported incidence between 6% and 50%, depending upon gestational age at presentation.

Management

Early aggressive treatment of pyelonephritis is important in preventing complications. The current standard of care includes hospitalization and parenteral antibiotics. Initial antibiotic choice is empiric. Several equally efficacious regimens are available and are summarized in **Table 223-1**. Most patients respond within 72 hours. Therapy with the best oral agent, according to culture and sensitivity testing, should be continued to complete a two-week course. Most experts recommend that suppressive therapy should be continued until delivery for all pregnant patients with

TABLE 223-1 Suggested Antimicrobial Regimens for the Treatment of Pyelonephritis in Pregnancy

Ampicillin (+) Gentamicin 2 grams IV every 6 hours
Gentamicin 2 mg/kg load, then 1.7 mg/kg in 3 divided doses (once daily dosing is also acceptable)
Ampicillin-sublactam 3 grams IV every 6 hours
Ceftriaxone 1 gram IV/IM every 24 hours
Cefuroxime 0.75–1.5 grams IV every 8 hours
Cefazolin 1–2 grams IV every 6–8 hours
Mezlocillin 3 grams IV every 6 hours
Piperacillin 4 grams IV every 8 hours

IM, intramuscularly; IV, intravenously.

a single episode of pyelonephritis. Prophylactic regimens include nitrofurantoin 100 mg once daily or cephalexin 250 mg once daily taken by mouth.

LISTERIOSIS

Overview

Although most often reported as a mild illness, listeriosis deserves mention here because of the increased incidence in pregnancy and propensity for fatal disease in the fetus. The incidence of listeriosis in pregnancy is 12 per 100,000, compared with a rate of 0.7 per 100,000 in the general population.

CLINICAL PRESENTATION

Although severe maternal illness from listeriosis has been reported, it is rare. In most cases, maternal illness is mild and sometimes even asymptomatic. Fever, chills, back pain, and flu-like symptoms are most commonly reported. Illness can resolve spontaneously and the diagnosis be missed if cultures are not obtained. Patients with comorbidities, such as a history of splenectomy, human immunodeficiency virus (HIV) infection, steroid use, diabetes, or use of immunosuppressive medications, are at increased risk for severe maternal illness, which includes meningitis and meningoencephalitis.

Fetal and neonatal concerns

In contrast to maternal illness, fetal and neonatal infection is severe and frequently fatal, with a case fatality rate of 20% to 30%. Neonatal listerial infection can cause pneumonia, sepsis, or meningitis. A characteristic severe in utero infection, granulomatosis infantiseptica, may result from transplacental transmission, characterized by widespread abscesses and/or granulomas in multiple internal organs. Most infants with this condition are either stillborn or die soon after birth.

Diagnosis

Diagnosis of listerial infection can only be made by culturing the organism from a sterile site such as blood, amniotic fluid, or spinal fluid. Vaginal or stool cultures are not helpful in diagnosis because some women are carriers but do not have clinical disease. Gram stain is useful in only about 33% of cases, both because *Listeria* is an intracellular organism and can be entirely missed, and because the organism can resemble pneumococci (diplococci), diphtheroids (*Corynebacteria*), or *Haemophilus* species.

Treatment

Pregnant women with isolated listerial bacteremia can be treated with ampicillin alone (2 g IV every four hours). Patients who are allergic to penicillin can be skin tested and desensitized, if necessary, or treated with trimethoprim-sulfamethoxazole (5 mg/kg of the trimethoprim component IV every six hours). Vancomycin has also been used in case reports of listerial infection.

ACUTE BRONCHITIS

Overview

Acute bronchitis usually refers to a self-limited respiratory illness characterized by the predominance of a productive cough in a patient with no history of chronic obstructive pulmonary disease and no evidence of pneumonia. Most cases of acute bronchitis have a viral etiology; however, atypical bacteria including *Bordetella pertussis, Chlamydia pneumoniae*, and *Mycoplasma pneumoniae* are important causes. The etiologic pathogen is isolated from the sputum in only a minority of patients.

No studies have particularly looked at the course of acute bronchitis in pregnancy. A retrospective cohort study found an association between placental abruption and acute respiratory illnesses including acute bronchitis among white women.

Management

Most pregnant patients with acute cough syndromes require no more than reassurance and symptomatic treatment with inhaled beta-agonists. A chest X-ray should be performed if clinically indicated. Antimicrobial therapy may be considered in patients when a treatable pathogen is identified or in epidemic settings to limit transmission. **Table 223-2** includes suggested antimicrobial regimens for pregnant patients.

There are no compelling data suggesting improved outcomes of acute bronchitis as a result of treatment with antibiotics.

PNEUMONIA

Incidence

The incidence of pneumonia requiring hospitalization in pregnancy is between 2.6 to 15.1 per 10,000 deliveries, a rate comparable to that seen in nonpregnant women of a similar age. Pregnancy is associated with reduction in cell-mediated immunity, which places pregnant women at an increased risk of severe pneumonia and disseminated disease from some atypical pathogens such as herpes virus, influenza, varicella, and coccidioidomycosis.

PATHOGENESIS

The etiology of pneumonia in pregnancy is similar to the nonpregnant population, with streptococcus pneumoniae being the most commonly isolated organism. Other causes include *Staphylococcus aureus, Haemophilus influenzae, Legionella spp, Mycoplasma pneumoniae*, chlamydia and viruses. Among patients requiring admission to intensive care units, *Pseudomonas aeruginosa and Enterobacteriaceae* play an important role.

Mothers who develop pneumonia are more likely to have coexisting medical problems including asthma, drug abuse, anemia, and HIV infection. The use of corticosteroids for enhancement of fetal lung maturity and tocolytic agents has also been associated with antepartum pneumonia.

Clinical presentation

Pregnant women with pneumonia present no differently than nonpregnant women and pneumonia should be considered in any woman presenting with fever, cough, sputum production, chills, rigors, dyspnea, and pleuritic chest pain. Occasionally, nonrespiratory symptoms such as vomiting, abdominal pain, and fever may predominate.

Diagnosis

A chest radiograph should be performed in all patients suspected to have pneumonia. Laboratory data should include a complete blood count, serum chemistries for hepatic, renal, glucose evaluation, assessment of oxygenation, and two sets of blood cultures; however, blood cultures may be positive only 7–15% of the time. The American Thoracic Society does not recommend routine performance of sputum culture and Gram stain. However, if a drug-resistant pathogen or an organism not covered by usual empiric therapy is suspected, sputum culture should be obtained. HIV status should be reviewed for all pregnant women with pneumonia and testing should be offered if it has not previously been done. Testing for pneumocystis carinii infection should occur in all HIV positive women who present with pneumonia.

TABLE 223-2 Recognized Causes of Acute Bronchitis and Treatment Options

Pathogen	Comments	Treatment Options in Pregnancy
Influenza virus	Precipitous onset with fever, chills, headache, cough and myalgias	Antiviral agents recommended for treatment of influenza have either very little or concerning pregnancy safety data. With the H1N1 pandemic, pregnant women have been found to be at increased risk of complications and treatment with oseltamivir 75 mg orally twice daily is recommended.
Parainfluenza virus	Epidemic may occur in fall. Croup in a child at home suggests the presence of this organism.	No treatment available
Respiratory syncytial virus	Outbreaks occur in winter or spring. Approximately 45% of adults exposed to an infant with bronchiolitis become infected.	No treatment available
Coronavirus	Severe respiratory symptoms may occur.	No treatment available
Adenovirus	Infection is clinically similar to influenza, with abrupt onset of fever.	No treatment available
Rhinovirus	Fever is uncommon, infection is generally mild.	No treatment available
Bordetella pertussis	Incubation period is one to three weeks. Posttussive vomiting may be present. Fever is uncommon.	Azithromycin for five days (500 mg on day 1, 250 mg days 2–5) *or* Erythromycin for 14 days (500 mg 4 times daily) *or* Trimethoprim/Sulfamethoxazole for 14 days (160/800 mg twice daily)
Mycoplasma pnemoniae	Gradual onset over two to three days of headache, fever malaise, and cough. Wheezing may occur. Dyspnea is uncommon.	Azithromycin for five days (500 mg on day 1, 250 mg days 2–5) or no therapy
Chlamydia pneumoniae	Gradual onset of cough with preceding hoarseness	Azithromycin for five days (500 mg on day 1, 250 mg days 2–5) or no therapy

Data from Wenzler RP, Fowler AA. Clinical practice. Acute bronchitis. *N Engl J Med.* 2006;355(20)2125–2130.

Differential diagnosis

The differential diagnosis for a pregnant woman presenting with symptoms of pneumonia is varied. Pulmonary embolism can present identically to an acute pneumonia with dyspnea, cough, chest pain, fever, and chest X-ray infiltrates. Aspiration, chemical pneumonitis, amniotic fluid embolism, and pulmonary edema related to sepsis, tocolysis, or preeclampsia can also present similarly.

Potential maternal and fetal effects

Pregnancy increases the risk of maternal complications from pneumonia, including the need for mechanical ventilation. Respiratory failure due to pneumonia is the third leading indication for intubation in pregnancy. Other maternal complications include pulmonary edema, bacteremia, empyema, pneumothorax, and atrial fibrillation. Pregnancies complicated by acute respiratory illnesses, including viral and bacterial pneumonia have been shown to be associated with placental abruption. Increased rates of preterm labor and delivery before 34 weeks of gestation have also been described.

The neonatal mortality rate due to antepartum pneumonia ranges from 1.9% to 12%, with most mortality attributable to complications of preterm birth. Although most cases of pneumonia in pregnancy are caused by organisms that do not affect the fetus except through their effects on maternal status, some organisms, such as varicella and CMV may present specific risks to the fetus. The fetus may also be at risk from maternal conditions that predispose to pneumonia, such as anemia or HIV infection.

Management

While no specific guidelines exist to help assess severity and the need for hospitalization in pregnant women, it is best to ensure adequate maternal oxygenation (oxygen saturation ≥95% or pO_2 ≥70 mm Hg) and fetal well-being before considering outpatient treatment.

Several recommendations exist for treatment of pneumonia in pregnancy. **Table 223-3** summarizes some suggested recommendations based upon ATS guidelines. Although levofloxacin and doxycycline are often recommended in the treatment of pneumonia in the nonpregnant population, these drugs should be avoided in pregnancy. Clarithromycin has shown to have adverse effects in animal trials at doses equivalent to 2 to 17 times the maximum recommended human dose. It is therefore best avoided in pregnancy, with use limited to those cases in which no alternative therapy is appropriate.

With appropriate therapy, an improvement can be expected in 72 hours, after which the regimen can be changed to an oral medication to complete 10–14 days therapy.

■ VIRAL HEPATITIS

In general, pregnancy does not affect the diagnosis or clinical course of viral hepatitis. It has been reported, however, that acute hepatitis may be more severe with hepatitis E. The differential diagnosis includes other common causes of liver dysfunction such as biliary obstruction, drug-induced liver disease, as well as liver diseases uniquely associated with pregnancy such as acute fatty liver, preeclampsia or HELLP (hemolysis, elevated live enzymes, and low platelets), and cholestasis of pregancy.

Herpes simplex virus (HSV) hepatitis

As a form of disseminated primary herpes infection, usually Herpes simplex type 2, HSV has been reported in the second and third

TABLE 223-3 Recommendations for Treating Pneumonia in Pregnancy

Type of Pneumonia	Recommended Antibiotics Acceptable for Use in Pregnancy	Comments
Community-acquired pneumonia Organisms: *S pneumoniae* *Respiratory viruses* *M pneumoniae* *H influenza* *C pneumoniae* *Legionella* *Unknown*	Ceftriaxone (2 g IV daily) or cefotaxime or ampicillin/sulbactam (3 g IV every 6 hours) PLUS Macrolide (azithromycin, erythromycin) If concern for MRSA, add vancomycin (15 mg/kg every 12 hours)	Avoid tetracycline and doxycycline in pregnant or breastfeeding mothers. Antipneumococcal fluoroquinolone may be used in nonpregnant patient but generally avoided in pregnancy or breastfeeding mothers
Hospital-acquired pneumonia/ health care–associated pneumonia/ ventilator-associated pneumonia Organisms: Aerobic gram negatives *(P. aeruginosa, Escherichia coli, Klebsiella pneumoniae, Acinetobacter sp.)* Gram positive cocci *Staphylococcus aureus, esp. methicillin resistant (MRSA)* Oropharyngeal commensals (viridans group strep, coagulase negative staph, *Neisseria sp, Corynebacterium sp*)	Ceftriaxone(2 g IV daily) or ampicillin/ sulbactam (3 g IV every 6 hours) If concern for MDR: Ceftazidime (2 g IV every 8 hours) or cefepime (2 g IV every 8 hours) or imipenem 500 mg every 6 hours) or piperacillin/tazobactam (4.5 every 6 hours) or aztreonam (2 g every 6–8 hours) PLUS Gentamycin or tobramycin PLUS Vancomycin (15 mg/kg every 12 hours)	Efficacy of once daily dosing for gentamycin in pregnancy not well established.
Aspiration pneumonia Organisms: Oropharyngeal commensals (viridans group strep, coagulase negative staph, *Neisseria sp, Corynebacterium sp*)	Clindamycin or Penicillin	
Varicella pneumonia	Acyclovir IV 10 mg/kg every 8 hours	

trimester. Pregnant patients may have characteristic mucocutaneous lesions and anicteric liver failure due to severe hepatocyte injury with extreme elevations of serum transaminases, an increased prothrombin time, and only mildly elevated serum bilirubin. If prescribed early in the course of illness, acyclovir may be effective in ameliorating the course of illness.

PULMONARY DISEASE

SHORTNESS OF BREATH

Normal pregnancy is characterized by an increase in minute ventilation, due to an increase in tidal volume but not of respiratory rate. This results in a change in arterial blood gases with the average PaO_2 in pregnancy 100 mm Hg at sea level and PCO_2 in the range of 28 and 32 mm Hg. An ABG with a PaO_2 of 79 mm Hg and a PCO_2 of 40 mm Hg in a pregnant female is very abnormal. Because fetal hemoglobin has a different oxygen dissociation curve from adult hemoglobin, the fetus requires that maternal oxygenation remains greater than a PaO_2 of 70 mm Hg This means that maternal oxygen saturation should be greater than 95%.

Pregnant women have an increased risk for pulmonary edema due to the 50% increase in blood volume that is predominantly achieved through an increase in plasma free water and a lower oncotic pressure. Pyelonephritis, medications that are used to stop preterm labor, and preeclampsia may precipitate pulmonary edema. Pregnancy-associated pulmonary edema often responds to withdrawal of the precipitating cause and a low diuretic dose.

Dyspnea of pregnancy usually begins in the middle of gestation as the patient's increased perception of dyspnea. These patients should have a completely normal physical examination, oxygenation, chest X-rays, and pulmonary function testing.

If shortness of breath occurs at 24–48 weeks when blood volume reaches its maximum, underlying heart disease should be considered.

A rare cause of dyspnea unique to pregnancy is amniotic fluid embolism occurring during the third trimester but usually during delivery. Rapid and progressive respiratory failure may be associated with hemodynamic instability and disseminated intravascular coagulopathy. This is a diagnosis of exclusion and treatment is supportive care.

The presentation of VTE may be subtle during pregnancy due to the absence of other co-morbidities. See below.

ASTHMA

Overview

Asthma affects 3.7% to 8.4% of all pregnancies and is one of the most common serious medical complications encountered in pregnancy in the United States. Asthma may develop during gestation triggered by an upper respiratory infection with persistent bronchospasm or be triggered due to reflux or sinusitis, both increased during pregnancy.

Effect of pregnancy on asthma

The course of asthma is usually unpredictable in pregnancy and numerous studies have suggested that a third of the patients improve, a third remain the same, and another third worsen. Factors contributing to improvement may be the pregnancy-associated rise in serum cortisol or the increase in progesterone that acts as a potent smooth muscle relaxant. Several factors may be responsible for worsening. Gestational rhinitis, bacterial sinusitis, and gastroesophageal reflux disease, all of which occur at an increased incidence in pregnancy, may worsen asthma control in the gravid state.

Effect of asthma on pregnancy

Most studies have shown that well-controlled pregnant patients with asthma do not have a significantly higher rate of adverse outcomes than those without asthma. However, patients with poorly controlled asthma are more likely to have miscarriages or therapeutic abortions, infants with low birth weight, and intrauterine growth restriction, and are more likely to undergo cesarean section. Preterm delivery and maternal hypertension have also been noted in poorly controlled women with asthma, but these risks have not been shown consistently and may partly be related to use of systemic steroids in these patients. Preeclampsia has also been associated with severe asthma in some studies.

Management

Management of asthma in pregnancy does not significantly differ from the nonpregnant patient. **Table 223-4** discusses the use and safety of commonly used asthma medications in pregnancy. While dealing with an acute asthma exacerbation in a pregnant woman, it is of vital importance to recognize that normal CO_2 in pregnancy is 28–32 mm Hg, which is lower than the nongravid state. Therefore, a tachypneic pregnant patient with a $PaCO_2$ above this range might be in impending respiratory failure. **Figure 223-1** shows the recommendations for assessment and management of acute asthma exacerbation in the hospital setting. These are based on the NAEP guidelines for asthma management in pregnancy.

While asthma exacerbations are rare in labor and delivery, it is important to ensure that asthma medications are not discontinued through labor and delivery. Most drugs used for asthma treatment can be safely used in breastfeeding women. Whether breastfeeding decreases the likelihood of the development of asthma in offspring is as yet controversial, but it does appear to decrease atopy.

TABLE 223-4 Safety of Asthma Medications in Pregnancy

Medication Type	Data Suggests Use Justifiable When Indicated	Data Suggests Use Justifiable in Rare Circumstances	Data suggests Use Almost Never Justifiable	Useful Review Articles and Comments
Short-acting inhaled beta-2 adrenergic agonists	$albuterol_C$ $bitolterol_C$ $pirbuterol_C$ $metaproterenol_C$ $terbutaline_C$			Published experience with these drugs in animals and humans suggests that beta-sympathomimetics do not increase the risk of congenital anomalies. Albuterol is the most studied of these agents. Metaproterenol is the second most studied. NAEP guidelines for the management of asthma in pregnancy can be obtained through the NHLBI at http://www.nhlbi.nih.gov/health/prof/lung/asthma/astpreg.htm PMID: 16946229 PMID: 16443141 PMID: 10830999
Long-acting inhaled beta-2 adrenergic agonists	$salmeterol_C$ $formoterol_C$			Of the few studies that have examined pregnancy outcomes with prenatal exposure to long-acting beta-2 agonists, no adverse events were found. However, due to small numbers in the studies, and because animal models have shown delayed ossification, use of this agent should be reserved for patients who have failed low potency steroids and/or cromolyn alone. PMID:11945116 PMID:9746382
Xanthines	$theophylline_C$ $aminophylline_C$			These drugs do not appear to be human teratogens. The clearance of aminophylline and theophylline is increased in pregnancy but may be variable. If daily dose exceeds 700 mg, blood levels should be checked for optimal dosing. PMID: 15695974 PMID: 16443141

(continued)

TABLE 223-4 Safety of Asthma Medications in Pregnancy *(continued)*

Medication Type	Data Suggests Use Justifiable When Indicated	Data Suggests Use Justifiable in Rare Circumstances	Data suggests Use Almost Never Justifiable	Useful Review Articles and Comments
Inhaled corticosteroids	Low potency: beclomethasone dipropionate$_C$ Medium potency: trimacinolone acetonide$_C$ High potency: fluticasone propionate$_C$ budesonide$_B$ flunisolide$_B$			Beclomethasone and budenoside are the most widely studied of the inhaled corticosteroids in pregnancy and should be considered the preferred inhaled steroids in pregnancy. Relatively little of these agents are absorbed and human data has not suggested any teratogenic effects of these agents. Triamcinolone is the next most studied inhaled steroid in pregnancy, with this limited experience suggesting no adverse pregnancy effects Fluticasone has not been studied in pregnancy; however its minimal systemic absorption and the safety of the other steroids in pregnancy make its use in pregnancy generally felt to be justifiable. PMID:16004676 PMID: 16775906
Systemic steroids	prednisone$_C$ methylprednisolone$_C$ dexamethasone$_C$ hydrocortisone$_C$			Most data suggest that systemic steroids do not present a teratogenic risk in human pregnancy. In doses equivalent to prednisone 25 mg/day, they do not cross the placenta because of placental metabolism (the same is not true for betamethasone or dexamethasone). Even in higher doses, the effect of hydrocortisone or prednisone on the fetus in terms of suppression of the hypothalmo-pituitary-adrenal axis is minimal. Several case control studies have found a significant association with first trimester steroid use and oral clefts; however this was not seen in cohort studies. Even if this association is real, the risk is still small. For every 1000 embryos exposed during the susceptible days of first trimester, probably no more than three will develop an oral cleft. The background risk in the general population is 1 per 1000. Therefore, the benefits of controlling a life-threatening disease make steroid use when indicated in the first trimester still generally justifiable. PMID: 15013068
Mast cell stabilizers	Cromolyn sodium$_B$ Nedocromil$_B$			Human and animal data suggest these agents are not teratogens. These agents are virtually not absorbed through mucosal surfaces and the swallowed portion is largely excreted in the feces.
Inhaled anticholinergics	Ipratropium$_B$			Although animal studies are reassuring, no published human data exists. These drugs are poorly absorbed by the bronchial mucosa so fetal exposure is likely minimal.

(continued)

TABLE 223-4 Safety of Asthma Medications in Pregnancy *(continued)*

Medication Type	Data Suggests Use Justifiable When Indicated	Data Suggests Use Justifiable in Rare Circumstances	Data suggests Use Almost Never Justifiable	Useful Review Articles and Comments
Leukotriene inhibitors		Zafirlukast $_B$ Montelukast$_B$ Omalizumab$_B$	Zileuton $_B$	Although these agents have reassuring animal data and are widely used in pregnancy because of the FDA category B rating, published safety data in human pregnancy is limited at this point. Their use should be limited in pregnancy to those cases in which a woman has had significant improvement in asthma control with these medications prior to becoming pregnant that was not obtainable through other methods. Zileuton is different than other agents in this class as there is some animal data to suggest association with adverse pregnancy outcomes.
Antihistamines	Diphenhydramine$_B$ (but avoid in first trimester) Chlorpheniramine Dimenhydrinate$_B$	Cetirizine$_B$ Fexofenadine$_C$ Loratidine$_B$		These 2003 and 2006 review articles systematically and critically review the literature on the treatment of allergic rhinitis in pregnancy. PMID: 12921487 PMID: 16579874 While the newest generation antihistaminic agents are widely used in pregnancy and have not had any concerning animal data associated with them, we still consider them to be second-line agents in pregnancy because of the lack of published human pregnancy safety data about them.
Cough	Guaifenesin$_C$ Dextromethorphan$_C$ Albuterol$_C$ Codeine$_C$			
Nasal congestion	Pseudoephedrine$_C$ Oxymetazoline$_C$ Nasal steroids Beconase™$_C$ Rhinocort™$_C$ Flonase™$_C$ Nasacort™$_C$ Nasal cromolyn$_B$ Nasal ipratropium$_B$			These 2006 review articles systematically and critically review the literature on the treatment of allergic rhinitis in pregnancy. PMID: 16443148 PMID 16579874

PMID; Pubmed id number, for easy access to reference and abstract.

Adapted, with permission, from Mehta N, Newstead-Angel J, Powrie RO. Prescribing in Pregnancy and Lactation. In: Bourjeily G, Rosene-Montella K (eds), Pulmonary Problems in Pregnancy, Respiratory Medicine, Humana Press, a part of Springer Science+Business Media, LLC. 2009;71–88.

PLEURAL EFFUSION IN PREGNANCY

Overview

Pleural effusions can be caused by a variety of conditions, both specific and unrelated to pregnancy. Physiologic changes of pregnancy, including an increased blood volume and decreased colloid osmotic pressure, promote transudation of fluid into the pleural space. Benign postpartum pleural effusions have been noted on chest radiographs and ultrasound studies after normal vaginal delivery with an incidence of about 25%. Pregnancy-specific conditions that predispose to pulmonary edema such as preeclampsia, amniotic fluid embolism, chorioamnionitis, or endometritis, may also result in pleural effusion.

Diagnosis

Diagnostic approach is largely guided by findings on history and physical exam and conditions being considered in the differential. A diagnostic thoracocentesis should always be considered in the presence of fever, hemoptysis, weight loss, or when hemothorax or emphysema is suspected.

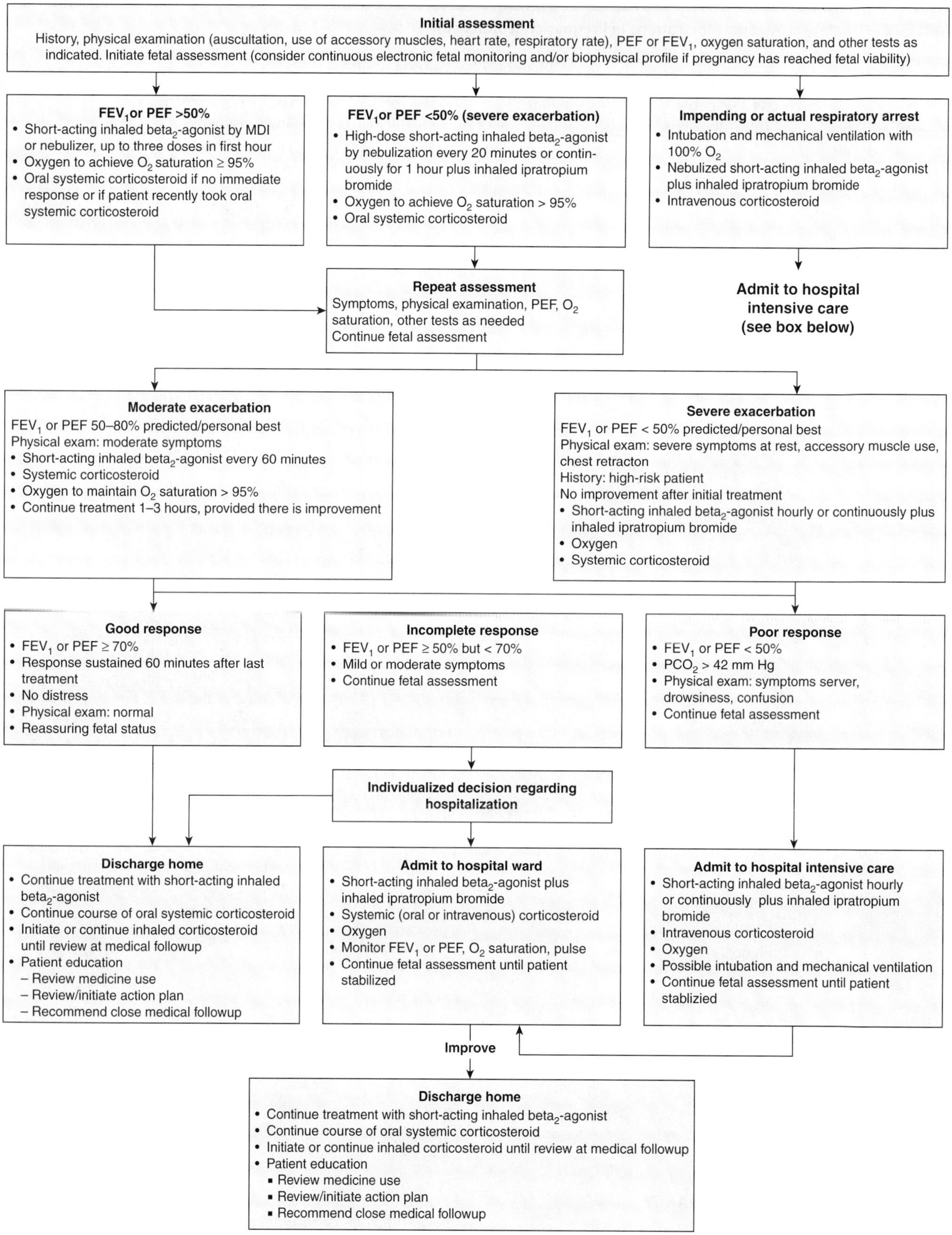

Figure 223-1 *Management of asthma exacerbations during pregnancy and lactation: Emergency department and hospital-based care. FEV_1, forced expiratory volume in 1 second; MDI, metered-dose inhaler; PCO_2, carbon dioxide partial pressure; PEF, peak expiratory flow. (From the Asthma and Pregnancy Report. NAEPP Report of the working group on Asthma and Pregnancy. NIH publication No. 93-3279. Bethesda, MD: U.S. Department of Health and Human services; National Institutes of Health; National Heart, Lung, and Blood Institute 1993. Available from URL: http://www.nhlbi.nih.gov/health/prof/lung/asthma/astpreg.txt.)*

Management

Management usually involves treatment of the underlying condition. Rarely, a therapeutic thoracentesis may be necessary, particularly in case of a large (eg, TB) or rapidly accumulating effusion (eg, malignancy). Presence of blood, pus, or chylous effusion warrants placement of a thoracostomy tube. While performing these procedures in pregnancy, it is important to remember that the diaphragm is about 4–5 cm elevated and a higher approach may be needed.

PNEMOTHORAX IN PREGNANCY

Overview

Although it is infrequently reported in literature, primary spontaneous pnemothorax (PSP) might be encountered reasonably often in pregnancy. In contrast to pneumothorax that accompanies existing lung disease (called *secondary spontaneous pneumothorax*), PSP usually resolves satisfactorily with simple observation, aspiration, or tube drainage Recurrence is a recognized feature of PSP and occurs more frequently in pregnant patients. Majority of these recurrences occur during the same pregnancy or in the postpartum period.

Management

Most patients are conservatively managed. Observation may suffice for a small pneumothorax (<2 cm) in patients without shortness of breath. Aspiration should be in patients with difficulty breathing or if the pneumothorax is larger than 2 cm. Chest tube drainage would be indicated in patients with persistent air leak. Surgical correction can be considered in the postpartum period to prevent recurrence in subsequent pregnancies.

Pregnancy concerns

Risk of recurrence may be increased in labor and delivery due to the repeated Valsalva maneuvers during vaginal birth, with resulting increase in intrathoracic pressures. Therefore in a pregnant woman with a past history of PSP, vaginal delivery should be assisted with forceps or vacuum to limit valsalva breathing. Should a cesarean section be necessary, it is best performed under regional anesthesia to avoid intrathoracic pressure increases associated with intubation and general anesthesia.

ALI and ARDS

Overview Acute respiratory distress syndrome is characterized by an acute onset of noncardiogenic pulmonary edema resulting in severely impaired oxygenation. Patients with less severe hypoxia are considered to have acute lung injury (ALI), whereas those with more severe hypoxia are considered to have ARDS.

Etiology

Eighty-five percent of all ARDS cases result from four causes, with sepsis being the most common:

- Sepsis from pulmonary or nonpulmonary sources
- Major trauma
- Multiple transfusions
- Aspiration of gastric contents

In the obstetric patient, several causes unique to pregnancy have to be considered. These are listed in **Table 223-5**.

Effect of pregnancy on ARDS

Pregnancy does not change total lung capacity, nor does it increase the A-a gradient. Noncardiogenic pulmonary edema or ALI, is known to occur more frequently in pregnant women with an estimated incidence of 80 to 500 cases per 100,000 and is responsible for 25% of transfers of obstetric patients to intensive care units.

TABLE 223-5 Causes of Acute Respiratory Distress Syndrome Unique to Pregnancy

1. Tocolytic induced pulmonary edema
2. Preeclampsia
3. Acute fatty liver of pregnancy
4. Gastric aspiration
5. Amniotic fluid embolism
6. Placental abruption
7. Obstetric hemorrhage
8. Chorioamnionitis
9. Endometritis
10. Pyelonephritis
11. Septic abortion
12. Retained products of conception

Both the normal decrease in serum oncotic pressure that occurs in pregnancy due to a physiologic dilutional hypoalbuminemia and changes in maternal endothelium may explain this pregnancy-related propensity to pulmonary edema.

Effect of ARDS on pregnancy

The effect of maternal ARDS on neonatal outcomes is not well studied, but high rates of fetal death, spontaneous preterm labor, and fetal heart rate abnormalities are reported.

Differential diagnosis

Cardiac causes of pulmonary edema such as peripartum cardiomyopathy, ischemic heart disease, or occult valvular heart disease and fluid overload should be considered in the differential diagnosis of ARDS. Other conditions such as interstitial pneumonia, acute eosinophilic pneumonia, acute bronchiolitis obliterans pneumonia, acute hypersensitivity pneumonitis, and diffuse alveolar hemorrhage may have a clinical and radiological picture similar to ARDS.

Management

Pulmonary edema in pregnancy is a medical emergency. The first and immediate goal is to maintain adequate maternal oxygenation ($PaO_2 \geq 70$ mm Hg equivalent to oxygen saturation 95%) through the use of oxygen supplementation to avoid hypoxia in the fetus. Mechanical ventilation may be needed in severe cases to ensure adequate oxygenation.

Tables 223-6 and **223-7** list the salient features of investigation and management of ARDS in the pregnant patient.

When pulmonary edema is suspected to be related to preeclampsia, initial management consists of oxygen supplementation, fluid restriction, and blood pressure control while plans are made for delivery. IV magnesium is used as a first-line agent for seizure prophylaxis and treatment in preeclampsia/eclampsia, based on two randomized controlled trials that confirm superiority over dilantin. However, its use in the setting of ALI may not be justified given the possible causative association with noncardiogenic pulmonary edema. Dilantin may be preferable for seizure prophylaxis in this setting.

Many preeclamptic patients are relatively intravascularly volume contracted, despite having massive amounts of peripheral edema and pulmonary edema. Over-diuresis of a preeclamptic patient can impair maternal renal perfusion, cardiac output, and uteroplacental perfusion, leading to fetal distress. Most patients with pulmonary edema in pregnancy will respond dramatically to doses of

TABLE 223-6 Diagnostic Tests Indicated in the Obstetric Patient with Acute Lung Injury

1. CBC with differential white blood cell count: Rule out anemia as a contributing factor and look for bandemia, suggesting infection.
2. Creatinine and BUN: Rule out renal failure.
3. PTT, fibrinogen, and FDP: Look for evidence of amniotic fluid embolism.
4. AST, uric acid, and urine protein creatinine ratio (in addition to CBC and creatinine mentioned above): Look for evidence of preeclampsia.
5. Blood and urine cultures in all patients with fever or bandemia.
6. Urine drug screen: Look for evidence of cocaine or narcotics as a cause.
7. Echocardiogram: Rule out underlying cardiac cause for pulmonary edema or evidence of cardiac compromise in preeclampsia.

AST, aspertate transaminase; BUN, blood urea nitrogen; CBC, complete blood count; FDP, fibrinogen degradation products; PTT, partial thromboplastin time.

furosemide as low as 10 mg IV especially if renal function is normal. Despite the need for careful fluid restriction and gentle diuresis, there is little evidence that central hemodynamic monitoring in these patients improves outcomes.

Whether delivery has a positive impact on maternal condition in patients with ARDS is unclear. There are case reports describing improvement in maternal oxygenation after delivery in patients with ARDS, but the mechanism for this is not well understood and may be partly related to resultant decreased cardiac work.

For the most part, patients with ARDS secondary to chorioamnionitis, placental abruption, amniotic fluid embolism and preeclampsia need immediate delivery, while those with pyelonephritis or varicella pneumonia can often recover without delivery.

TABLE 223-7 Salient Features in Management of Acute Respiratory Distress Syndrome in Pregnancy

1. Supplemental oxygen to maintain maternal oxygen saturation above 95%.
2. Consider intubation for PaO_2 < 70 mm Hg or $PaCO_2$ > 45 mm Hg on 100% oxygen.
3. Look for precipitating causes listed in Table 223-5 in addition to sepsis, massive transfusion, aspiration of gastric contents, or trauma.
4. Appropriate diagnostic testing as listed in Table 223-6.
5. Immediate discontinuation of tocolytic therapy when applicable.
6. Fluid restriction.
7. IV furosemide 10–20 mg.
8. IV antibiotics if infection suspected.
9. Echocardiogram to rule out cardiac cause for pulmonary edema.
10. Consider afterload reduction with sodium nitroprusside or hydralazine if patient is pregnant, and angiotensin converting enzyme inhibitors or angiotensin-receptor blockers in the postpartum patient.

RENAL DISEASE

NEPHROLITHIASIS

Incidence

Renal stones are commonly encountered in pregnancy, complicating about 1 in 200 pregnancies. Renal colic refers to severe pain associated with complete or partial obstruction of the ureters. However, the diagnosis of urolithiasis may be challenging in pregnancy due to the physisologic changes in the renal system in the gravid state.

Pathogenesis

Pregnancy is associated with physiologic dilatation of the ureters, resulting from smooth muscle relaxation induced by progesterone. This may occur as early as the first trimester. Furthermore, there is decreased peristalsis and anatomic dilatation resulting from mechanical obstruction of the collecting system from the gravid uterus. With the resultant urinary stasis, there is increased propensity for infection and crystal aggregation. In addition, increases in GFR lead to higher concentration of urinary calcium that further predisposes to stone formation.

Clinical presentation and diagnosis

Pregnant patients with urolithiasis present no differently from nonpregnant patients. However, modes of investigation in pregnancy do differ. Ultrasonography (USG) would be the preferred initial test, as opposed to abdominal CT scan, to avoid fetal radiation exposure. Bilateral hydronephrosis may be seen on ultrasound (US) due to physiologic changes. It is therefore important to identify the presence of ureteral jets in the bladder, which would rule out a ureteral obstruction by stone.

The sensitivity of ultrasound in confirming urolithisis ranges from 34–86%. If a stone is clinically suspected despite ultrasound findings, a single shot IVP may be performed. If diagnosis still remains in question, magnetic resonance urography may be helpful.

Management

The initial management plan for urinary stones in pregnancy is conservative (hydration, analgesics, and antibiotics if infection is present). Opioid analgesics can safely be used in pregnancy. Nonsteroidal antiinflammatory drugs (NSAIDs) should be avoided due to oligohydramnios and premature narrowing or closure of the patent ductus arteriosis. Most patients will spontaneously pass the stone with conservative management. Urology consult may be appropriate in patients with prolonged or recurrent symptoms in which ureteral stents may be needed. Indications for a diversion procedure, stenting, or percutaneous nephrostomy, include persistent pain, infection or high-grade hydronephrosis beyond normal pregnancy-related dilatation.

Pregnancy concerns

While some data suggests an increased risk of preterm labor in patients with stones, most available reports do not suggest a significant increase in obstetric complications.

ACUTE RENAL FAILURE

Definition

Acute renal failure (ARF) is rare in pregnancy, but transient mild to moderate renal dysfunction is more common. By definition, ARF is a syndrome of rapid decrease in glomerular filtration rate (GFR), increasing serum creatinine, and urea levels and oliguria or anuria. It is important to note that physiologic increase in GFR in pregnancy leads

TABLE 223-8 Severity Ranges of Creatinine in Pregnancy

Severity	Creatinine Range (mg/dL)
Mild	0.9–1.4
Moderate	1.4–2.9
Severe	3.0 or greater

to lower serum creatinine and BUN. Renal dysfunction in pregnancy is therefore defined as creatinine above 0.8 mg/dL (**Table 223-8**).

Etiology and pathogenesis

ARF in pregnancy can result from prerenal, intrarenal, or postrenal causes. **Table 223-9** lists some causes of acute renal failure in pregnancy.

TABLE 223-9 Causes of Renal Failure in Pregnancy

- Blood loss resulting from abrution, postpartum hemorrhage, placenta previa
- Volume contraction: Preeclampsia, eclampsia, hyperemesis
- Infection: Sepsis resulting from pyelonephritis, chorioamnionitis, endometritis, septic abortion
- HELLP; acute fatty liver of pregnancy, TTP; HUS; amniotic fluid embolism
- Drug reactions
- Obstruction from pelvic hematoma, damage to ureters during cesarean section, ureteral stones or strictures, compression by gravid uterus or tumor
- Related to underlying disease: Lupus nephritis, scleroderma crisis, antiphospholipid antibody syndrome

HELLP, hemolysis, elevated live enzymes, and low platelets; HUS, hemolytic uremic syndrome; TTP, thrombotic thrombocytopenic purpura.

Management

Initial management of ARF commences with identification and treatment of underlying causes. Judicious fluid management and avoidance of nephrotoxins are important. Care should be taken to adjust dosing of medications that are renally cleared. Low-dose dopamine has not been found to be effective and is not recommended. Loop diuretics may be helpful in treatment of volume overload; however, there is no data to support the use of diuretics in patients with oliguric renal failure from preeclampsia, a disease of hemoconcentration and vasospasm. Renal replacement therapy should be considered in the case of volume overload, hyperkalemia refractory to medical management, metabolic acidosis, or symptomatic uremia (mental status changes, pericarditis, neuropathy).

Pregnancy and fetal considerations

Adverse fetal outcomes associated with ARF in pregnancy are typically due to altered uteroplacental hemodynamics. It is therefore crucial to maintain volume and maternal acid-base balance and prevent further renal deterioration. In a patient with ARF, if delivery is imminent, the neonate may be subject to rapid dehydration as a result of increased solute load in fetal circulation leading to osmotic diuresis.

DIALYSIS AND PREGNANCY

Although uncommon, pregnancy does occur in women on chronic dialysis. Conversely, dialysis may become necessary in a pregnant woman with ARF from worsening underlying renal disease or de novo causes. There is no difference in outcomes with peritoneal or hemodialysis. In general, an increased dose of dialysis is recommended for pregnant patients to achieve a predialysis blood urea nitrogen of less than 50 mg/dL.

HYPERTENSIVE DISORDERS OF PREGNANCY

Hypertensive disorders represent one of the most common medical problems in pregnancy and encompass the diagnoses of chronic hypertension, gestational hypertension, and preeclampsia.

CHRONIC HYPERTENSION

Chronic hypertension in pregnancy is defined as a blood pressure of 140/90 or greater on two separate occasions before 20 weeks gestation or persisting beyond 12 weeks postpartum. It is associated with a 20% risk of developing preeclampsia. While essential hypertension is the most common cause, consideration of secondary causes is necessary in this young population.

Physiologic changes in the cardiovascular system during pregnancy allow for a decrease in blood pressure in the first two trimesters, with a return toward baseline in the third trimester. In the second half of pregnancy, inferior vena cava (IVC) compression from a gravid uterus in the supine position may falsely lower blood pressure readings, so it is important to measure blood pressure (BP) in a pregnant woman in the seated position.

Treatment of mild to moderate hypertension in pregnancy neither benefits the fetus nor prevents preeclampsia. In addition, excessive lowering of blood pressure may result in adverse fetal outcomes from decreased placental perfusion. Oral agents that are commonly used to treat hypertension in pregnancy include labetalol, nifedipine, and methyldopa. Clonidine has also been used in pregnancy without increased risk of congenital malformations; however, an effect on offspring behavior has been suspected based on human and animal studies. Other oral agents that are reasonably safe for pregnancy but with limited efficacy include hydralazine and hydrochlorthiazide. Angiotensin-converting enzyme (ACE) inhibitors and angiotensin receptor blockers (ARBs) are contraindicated at any gestational age in pregnancy. **Table 223-10** outlines the pharmacologic management of hypertensive urgency in a pregnant woman.

GESTATIONAL HYPERTENSION

Gestational hypertension is defined as elevation in blood pressure developing after 20 weeks gestation without proteinuria. Women with gestational hypertension progress to preeclampsia in 15–45% of cases and often require early delivery. Surveillance for development of preeclamsia and close fetal monitoring is recommended.

PREECLAMPSIA

Overview

Preeclampsia is a pregnancy-specific complication that occurs in 5–10% of all pregnancies. It is defined as a BP ≥ 140/90 accompanied by proteinuria of > 300 mg per 24 hours after the twentieth week of gestation in a previously normotensive patient. When it is diagnosed in a patient with preexisting chronic hypertension, it is referred to as chronic hypertension with superimposed preeclampsia. Most cases of preeclampsia occur close to term.

Pathophysiology

Risk factors for development of preeclampsia include first pregnancy or pregnancy with a new partner, age less than 18 years or

TABLE 223-10 Pharmacologic Treatment of Hypertensive Urgency in a Pregnant Woman

Medication	Onset of Action and Duration of Action	Acute Dosing for Severe Hypertension	Maintenance Dose
Labetalol	Begins to work in 5–10 minutes. Lasts three to six hours	Labetalol is given as a series of boluses until BP comes down to the desired level: • 10 mg IV push • then in 10 min, 20 mg IV push • then in 10 min, 40 mg IV push • then in 10 min, 80 mg IV push • then in 10 min, 80 mg IV push up to a total dose of no more than 300 mg total • then followed with oral labetalol or a labetalol drip	• Oral labetalol 100–200 mg 2 to 3 times a day (100–600 mg 2 to 3 times a day; maximum 2400 mg/day) • IV labetalol infusion 0.5–2.0 mg/min (Labetalol comes in vials of 100 mg/20 mL) • Put 5 vials (100 mL) of labetalol into 150 mL of IV fluid (D5W/LR/NS) to get a solution of 2 mg/mL) • Start at 15 mL/h (0.5 mg/min) • Titrate up to as high as 60 mL/h (2 mg/min)
Nifedipine	Begins to work in <30 minutes Lasts 4–5 hours	10–20 mg orally every 30 min to a maximum of 50 mg	Maintenance 10–20 mg orally 3 times a day of the short-acting or 30–120 mg once daily of long-acting formulation
Hydralazine	Begins to work in 10–20 minutes Lasts for 3–6 hours	2.5 to 10 mg IV every 30 min	Maintenance dose starts at 10 mg orally 4 times a day and can be gradually increased to 50 mg orally 4 times a day

D5W, dextrose 5% in water (solution); LR, lactated Ringer (solution); NS, normal saline.

older than 35, past history of preeclampsia, chronic hypertension, renal disease, diabetes mellitus (type I, II, or gestational), obesity, SLE, thrombophilia, multiple gestation, and molar pregnancy.

Etiology of preeclampsia is unclear. On a pathophysiologic level, preeclampsia is characterized by diffuse endothelial damage, hemoconcentration, and vasospasm.

Clinical presentation

The main symptoms of preeclampsia include headache, visual disturbance, epigastric or right upper quadrant abdominal discomfort, edema, and rapid weight gain. Signs include hypertension, retinal vasospasm, right upper quadrant tenderness, and clonus. Lab studies supporting the diagnosis of preeclampsia are outlined in **Table 223-11**.

Severe preeclampsia is defined as the presence of one of the following symptoms or signs in the presence of preeclampsia (1) systolic BP of ≥160 mm Hg or diastolic BP of ≥110 mm Hg on two occasions at least six hours apart; (2) proteinuria of more than 5 g in 24-hour period; (3) pulmonary edema; (4) oliguria (<400 mL in 24 h); (5) persistent headaches and/or seizures (eclampsia); (6) epigastric pain and/or impaired liver function; (7) thrombocytopenia; and (8) intrauterine growth restriction. HELLP syndrome characterized by hemolysis, elevated liver enzymes and low platelet count is a variant of severe preeclampsia occurring in about 20% of cases of severe preeclampsia.

TABLE 223-11 Lab Abnormalities in Preeclampsia

1. Hemoglobin >12 g/dl (normally near 10 g/dl in pregnant women near term)
2. Platelet count <150,000/mm^3
3. Elevated liver enzymes (AST and ALT)
4. Creatinine >0.8 mg/dl (normal for pregnancy 0.5–0.7 mg/dl)
5. Uric acid >0.5 mg/dl
6. 24-hour urine collection with >300 mg of protein

ALT, alanine transaminase; AST, aspartate transaminase.

Treatment

The only known treatment of preeclampsia once it occurs is delivery as soon as obstetrically feasible. Despite this, it is important to note that preeclampsia can present postpartum, and both preeclampsia and eclampsia have been reported for up to 21 days following delivery. Management of preeclampsia includes treatment of hypertension, seizure prophylaxis, and limitation of fluids due to the risk of pulmonary edema. **Table 223-12** outlines the management of a pregnant woman hospitalized with severe preeclampsia.

ENDOCRINE DISORDERS

■ DIABETES

Effect of pregnancy on preexisting type I and type II diabetes

Insulin requirements often decrease by 10% to 20% in the first trimester of pregnancy due to increased insulin sensitivity. The risk of overall and nocturnal hypoglycemia during this time is further compounded if the patient has hyperemesis or preexisting gastroparesis.

Rising human placental lactogen and human placental growth hormone levels from the beginning of the second trimester then cause an increase in insulin resistance, and insulin requirements rise gradually until approximately 36 weeks of gestation. Women with preexisting type 2 diabetes controlled with diet and exercise will usually require pharmacologic treatment by mid-second trimester. A sudden decrease in insulin requirements in the third trimester needs to be taken very seriously, as it may be a signal of placental failure, and close fetal surveillance is required.

All metabolic processes are accelerated during pregnancy and the threshold of starvation ketoacidosis occurring after a prolonged fast is much lower. This coupled with hyperemesis in

TABLE 223-12 Labor and Delivery Sample Admission Orders for Severe Preeclampsia

Bed rest with seizure precautions
Vital signs (blood pressure, pulse, respiration); deep tendon reflexes; and mental status every 15 to 60 minutes until stable, then every 60 minutes while on magnesium sulfate.
Accurate intake and output; Foley catheter if needed.
Administer lactated Ringer solution at 75 mL per hour IV to maintain urine output of 30 to 40 mL per hour; total intake (IV and oral) should not exceed 125 mL per hour or 3,000 mL per day.
Continuous fetal heart rate monitoring.
Laboratory tests:
Dipstick urine collection for protein level on admission
24-hour urine collection for total protein level
CBC with platelets, peripheral blood smear
BUN, creatinine, uric acid
AST, ALT, LDH
Fetal evaluation: nonstress test on admission; obstetric ultrasonography for estimated fetal weight, amniotic fluid volume, and umbilical artery Doppler measurements
Medications:
Magnesium sulfate
Loading dose of 4 to 6 g diluted in 100 mL of normal saline, given IV over 15 to 20 minutes, followed by a continuous infusion of 2 g per hour
Assess serum magnesium level if urine output is < 30 mL per hour or there is a loss of deep tendon reflexes, decreased respiratory rate, or altered mental status.
Therapeutic range for serum magnesium is 4 to 7 mg per dL.
Corticosteroids (if between 24 and 34 weeks of gestation and not previously administered).
Betamethasone (Celestone), 12 mg IM initially, then repeat in 24 hours
or
Dexamethasone, 6 mg IM initially, then repeat every 12 hours for three additional doses.
For systolic blood pressure > 160 mm Hg or diastolic > 110 mm Hg, one of the following should be given to achieve a systolic measurement of 140 to 155 mm Hg and/or a diastolic measurement of 90 to 105 mm Hg.
Hydralazine, 5 to 10 mg IV every 15 to 30 minutes (maximal dose: 30 mg)
or
Labetalol, 20 mg IV initially; if the initial dose is not effective, double the dose to 40 mg and then 80 mg at 10-minute intervals until target blood pressure is reached or a total of 220 mg has been administered; the maximal dose of IV labetalol is 220 mg in a 24-hour period.
Calcium gluconate, 1 g IV; keep at bedside in case of respiratory depression from magnesium sulfate use

ALT, alanine transaminase; AST, aspartate transaminase; BUN, blood urea nitrogen; CBC, complete blood count; IM, intramuscularly; IV, intravenously; LDH, l-lactate dehydrogenase.

early pregnancy and subsequent increased insulin resistance in later pregnancy increases the risk of diabetic ketoacidosis in pregnant women.

It is recommended that a baseline eye check occur as part of preconceptual counseling as preexisting diabetic retinopathy has been shown to progress more quickly during pregnancy due to the increased production of growth factors as well as the hypercoagulable state of pregnancy. Laser therapy during pregnancy is as effective as outside pregnancy and can be safely used if required.

In women with preexisting diabetic nephropathy, pregnancy may worsen the degree of proteinuria, cause progression of renal sufficiency, and aggravate hypertension. The need to discontinue ACE inhibitors before conception, together with an increase in GFR, are the main reasons for a physiologic increase in proteinuria during pregnancy. Although pregnancy may accelerate the progression of nephropathy, postpartum renal function usually returns to prepregnancy levels in most cases. However, in women with moderate renal insufficiency, pregnancy has been estimated to shorten the time to end-stage renal failure by 36 months.

Hypertension occurs in 30% of women with diabetic nephropathy in the first trimester and in 75% by the third trimester. Deteriorating renal function and superimposed preeclampsia are responsible for the high rates of preterm delivery, low birth weight, and operative delivery. Differentiating preeclampsia from worsening nephropathy can be very difficult as proteinuria and worsening hypertension occur in both situations.

EFFECT OF PREEXISTING TYPE I AND TYPE II DIABETES ON PREGNANCY

Women with preexisting types 1 and 2 diabetes are at increased risk of preeclampsia, operative delivery, and antenatal infections (such as urinary tract and respiratory). These risks are further increased if the mother has premorbid obesity as well.

The rate of early pregnancy loss or congenital anomalies is increased for women with poor preconceptual glycemic control. Glucose is a potent teratogen and there is a linear increase in rates of congenital anomalies with rising HgbA1C levels. Late pregnancy losses are also increased in women with poor glycemic control during pregnancy. It is thought that oxidative stress resulting from oxygen depletion caused by hyperglycemia is the underlying mechanism for these findings. It has been shown that the overall rate of adverse pregnancy outcome is much lower in women who receive preconceptual counseling and are euglycemic at conception and during organogenesis.

The incidence of macrosomia is increased in diabetic pregnancies. Excess fetal growth is due to fetal hyperinsulinemia in response to maternal hyperglycemia. Macrosomic babies (>4000 g) are at increased risk for traumatic or surgical delivery, shoulder dystocia, and brachial plexus injury. Neonatal hypoglycemia due to fetal hyperinsulinemia and neonatal hyperbilirubinemia are metabolic complications that are more common in babies born to diabetic mothers.

Gestational diabetes mellitus

Gestational diabetes mellitus (GDM) is defined as glucose intolerance of variable severity that is first detected during pregnancy. It is the leading endocrine condition in pregnancy and continues to rise in the face of the obesity epidemic. Pregnancy is effectively a stress-test in which the insulin-resistant hormones of pregnancy trigger overt hyperglycemia in women who have a background of previously undiagnosed insulin resistance and/or decreased pancreatic beta-cell reserve.

It is usually diagnosed at the end of the second trimester via a diagnostic glucose tolerance test. Treatment needs to begin immediately as there is only a short window of opportunity to achieve euglycemia in order to minimize its impact on the fetus. If the following targets are not met with diet and exercise therapy alone (fasting blood glucose level or BGL <5.3 mmol/L or 95 mg/dL and/or 1-hour postprandial BGL <7.8 mmol/L or 140 mg/dL and/or 2-hour postprandial BGL <6.7 mmol/L or 120 mg/dL) then insulin therapy is commenced though glyburide, or metformin therapy may be recommended if the patient refuses insulin therapy and/or the degree of hyperglycemia is only mild. Glyburide has been the preferred agent as it does not cross the placenta, but newer data is emerging regarding the safety and efficacy of metformin use beyond the first trimester. (See proceeding section for more information.)

Glucose tolerance returns to normal immediately after delivery of the placenta and so treatment can be ceased. Women with GDM are at much greater risk of developing type 2 diabetes in the future and so they should be tested for such on a regular basis by their primary care physicians.

The use of oral hypoglycemic agents, subcutaneous insulin regimes, and insulin pumps

Insulin is considered the gold standard of treatment for both preexisting and gestational diabetes. However, there has been a trend toward increasing use of glyburide and metformin in recent times. There is currently no data to suggest that the use of either in the first trimester is associated with an increase in congenital anomalies. Glyburide does not cross the placenta and can be used throughout the second and third trimesters as well.

Metformin is frequently used as an ovulation induction agent in women with polycystic ovarian syndrome and for these women, continuing its use during the first trimester has been shown to reduce miscarriage rates. Its use during the second and third trimesters had been questionable in the past given that significant placental transfer does take place (cord blood levels similar to maternal levels) but recent data suggests that there is no long-term deleterious effects on the fetus and it may in fact reduce the risk of the offspring developing type 2 diabetes in the future.

None of the other oral hypoglycemic agents currently on the market are recommended or approved for use during pregnancy.

All the insulin types available on the market are safe for use in pregnancy. These include the newer insulin analogs, which are more rapid in onset (Humalog, Novorapid) and longer in action (Lantus) compared with the traditional recombinant human insulins (Humulin-R, Humulin-NPH).

An increasing number of women of childbearing age with type 1 diabetes are using insulin pumps that provide a continuous subcutaneous infusion of insulin for glycemic control. The main caveat here is that they need to recognize potential problems such as a blockage or kink in the infusion set that can precipitate an episode of diabetic ketoacidosis (DKA) more quickly in pregnant patients.

Management of diabetic ketoacidosis

The presentation of DKA is similar in the nonpregnant and pregnant patient, but the acidosis tends to be more pronounced at a lower serum glucose level in the pregnant patient. This is due to the combination of the accelerated starvation state of pregnancy, lower buffering capacity due to the physiologic respiratory alkalosis of pregnancy that leads to lower serum bicarbonate levels, and the increased GFR in pregnancy that leads to increased renal excretion of glucose.

Treatment requires prompt recognition and maternal stabilization with rehydration, intravenous insulin therapy, and electrolyte replacement. Infections such as those of the urinary tract should be excluded. As starvation ketosis is often the main component of ketoacidosis, the mother needs to receive adequate dextrose (with the insulin infusion) in order to meet fetal-placental glucose needs until she is eating normally. Ketone bodies and glucose cross the placenta readily and so there is high fetal morbidity and mortality associated with DKA. Fetal compromise will improve once the metabolic acidosis reverses. An urgent C-section while the mother is still acidotic is not generally recommended because of high maternal risk.

Management at time of labor and delivery

It is recommended that an insulin plan for the time of labor and delivery be provided to all patients well before the expected due date so that there is no confusion between the patient and various medical and nursing caregivers on this important occasion. It is important to avoid maternal BGLs more than 9.0 mmol/L (162 mg/dL) in the intrapartum period as this has been associated with an increased risk of neonatal hypoglycemia (which may require NICU admission), but it is also important to avoid hypoglycemia for maternal safety and well-being during this strenuous process.

In early labor, subcutaneous insulin use should be continued while the woman is still eating but these doses will need to be reduced if oral intake is decreased. When the woman is in active labor and no longer eating, an intravenous insulin and dextrose infusion should be commenced to keep the BGLs in the desired range of 4.0 to 8.0 mmol/L (72 to 144 mg/dL).

For patients with active proliferative retinopathy, using the Valsalva maneuver repeatedly in the second stage of labor is a concern as there is an increased risk of retinal hemorrhage.

Management in the immediate postpartum period

With delivery of the placenta, insulin requirements rapidly decrease back to prepregnancy levels. The target range of BGLs postpartum in the preexisting diabetic is much more relaxed compared with during pregnancy, with levels between 6.0 to 10.0 mmol/L (108 to 180 mg/dL) all being acceptable. Breastfeeding will lower BGLs and having extremely tight glycemic control may increase the risk of hypoglycemia in a lactating woman. The usual postpartum insulin requirement is approximately two-thirds of the prepregnancy insulin dosage.

Women with type 2 diabetes may be able to discontinue insulin therapy and use diet and exercise and/or oral hypoglycaemic agents in the postpartum period. The two oral hypoglycaemic agents that have been documented to be safe in breastfeeding are glyburide and metformin. The former does not enter breast milk at all and infant exposure to the latter has been estimated to be only approximately 0.5% of the maternal dose.

ACE-inhibitors can also be recommenced in lactating women, though it is recommended that a preterm infant not be exposed to it until he has reached an age equivalent to full term.

THYROID

Hypothyroidism in pregnancy

Management of thyroid diseases during pregnancy requires special considerations because pregnancy induces major changes in thyroid function, and maternal thyroid disease can have adverse effects on the pregnancy and the fetus. Avoiding maternal (and fetal) hypothyroidism is of major importance because of potential damage to fetal neural development, an increased incidence of miscarriage, and preterm delivery. However, universal screening of pregnant women for thyroid disease is not yet supported by adequate studies, but case finding targeted to specific groups of patients who are at increased risk is currently strongly supported.

Both overt and subclinical hypothyroidism can have an adverse impact on the course of pregnancy or fetal development. Overt hypothyroidism should be corrected before initiation of pregnancy and preconception thyroxine (T4) dosage should bring the thyroid stimulating hormone (TSH) level < 2.6 mU/L. Women with subclinical hypothyroidism (serum TSH above the upper reference limit but free T4 [fT4] within the reference limits) should also be treated with T4 replacement. This recommendation is based on observational evidence demonstrating that women suffering from overt or subclinical hypothyroidism deliver babies with an average intelligence quotient (IQ) score 7 points below the mean IQ score of children born to healthy women and women on T4 replacement. The importance of maternal thyroid hormone replacement is emphasized by the fact that the fetal thyroid does not develop until the second trimester of pregnancy and fetal thyroid hormone production does not become optimal until mid-gestation.

Maintaining a serum TSH < 3.0 mU/L is acceptable in the second and third trimesters of pregnancy. After delivery, the dose of T4 therapy can usually be reduced back to the preconception dosage.

Hyperthyroidism in pregnancy

If a suppressed TSH is detected during pregnancy, hyperthyroidism must be distinguished from normal physiology (gestational thyrotoxicosis) and hyperemesis gravidarum because of the potential adverse effects on the mother and fetus.

Hyperthyroidism in pregnancy is not rare; estimated prevalence is 0.1–0.4% with Graves disease accounting for 85% of cases and toxic solitary or multiple nodules plus thyroiditis accounting for most of the rest. Hydatidiform molar disease is a very uncommon cause these days due to the advent of dating ultrasounds.

Gestational thyrotoxicosis presents in the mid- to late first trimester, often with hyperemesis. Classical hyperthyroid symptoms are absent or minimal apart from weight loss, which is often the result of malnutrition secondary to vomiting. The suppression in TSH is mediated by rising human chorionic gonadotropin (hCG) levels and therefore it will usually self-resolve by mid-gestation at the latest. Approximately 50% of women suffering from hyperemesis have a subnormal TSH and elevated fT4 level. In this setting, the assessment of free triiodothyronine (fT3) level and TSH receptor antibody (TRAb) titre are helpful as 90% of hyperemesis cases have normal fT3 and most cases of Graves disease will be TRAb positive.

If Graves disease or hyperfunctioning nodules are diagnosed, propylthiouracil is preferred to carbimazole because of the association with congenital abnormalities with the latter medication. Therapy should be adjusted to maintain maternal fT4 in the upper non-pregnant reference interval. Though rare, the possibility of neonatal Graves disease needs to be entertained if the maternal TRAb levels are high in the third trimester. Women with well-controlled Graves disease during pregnancy should be warned about the possibility of postpartum flare-up, which usually occurs between six weeks to six months postpartum. It is not recommended that radioactive iodine therapy be used during pregnancy and lactation.

Postpartum thyroiditis

Postpartum thyroiditis (also see Chapter 224 Postpartum Consultation for Common Complaints) may occur in up to 10% of all pregnancies, usually between six weeks and six months after delivery, but it can occur up to one year later. Because a hypothyroid phase often follows the hyperthyroid phase and is occasionally permanent, careful monitoring is necessary, as women may be hypothyroid at the time of any subsequent pregnancy.

PARATHYROID

Hypercalcemia

Primary hyperparathyroidism is usually diagnosed during pregnancy through routine blood testing following prolonged or extremely severe hyperemesis gravidarum or else the serendipitous finding of nephrocalcinosis, renal calculi, or excessive calcification of the placenta during fetal ultrasonography. It may frequently be part of the multiple endocrine neoplasia (MEN-1 or MEN-2a) syndrome. Urinary calcium excretion is typically not used as part of the diagnostic evaluation as it is increased in normal pregnancy.

Symptomatic hyperparathyroidism is best treated by minimally invasive surgical removal of the parathyroid adenoma during the second trimester, after embryogenesis is complete and before such time that premature labor may be stimulated. In skilled hands, the procedure takes no more than 30 minutes.

Surgery can also be offered in late pregnancy (after 35 weeks gestation) if the patient becomes profoundly symptomatic, as the neonatal outcome is much improved with surgery. This is due to the reduced risk of stillbirth, intrauterine growth restriction (IUGR), premature labor, and especially neonatal hypocalcemic tetany, which can frequently cause prolonged neonatal intensive care unit admissions if fetal parathyroid suppression takes a long time to recover.

Hypocalcemia

Hypoparathyroidism is very rare in pregnancy and is usually part of the autoimmune polyglandular syndrome, which would frequently be associated with mucocutaneous candidiasis and adrenal insufficiency. Maintenance of normocalcemia involves substantial oral supplementation with calcium and activated vitamin D (calcitriol). The doses of supplementation usually have to be increased, particularly in the third trimester, as there is high fetal uptake of calcium into the skeleton.

PITUITARY

Pituitary insufficiency

The differential diagnosis of pituitary insufficiency in the pregnant patient is diverse and is listed in **Table 223-13**.

The management of the pregnant woman with preexisting pituitary insufficiency centers on adequate hormonal replacement. In general, thyroid hormone and cortisol requirements increase

TABLE 223-13 Causes of Hypopituitarism in the Pregnant Patient

Preexisting before Pregnancy
Pituitary adenoma
Vasculitis
Infiltrative disorders (hemochromatosis, sarcoidosis, amyloidosis)
Hypothalamic tumors (craniopharyngiomas, germinoma, meningioma, glioma)
Eosinophilic granuloma (histiocytosis X)
Pituitary apoplexy
Prior surgical or radiotherapy treatment
During Pregnancy or Postpartum
Lymphocytic hypophysitis/infundibulohypophysitis
Sheehan syndrome (peripartum necrosis)

throughout pregnancy due to increased hepatic production of thyroxine-binding globulin (TBG) and cortisol-binding globulin (CBG). It is vital that FT4 rather than TSH level is monitored as the latter will always be low in patients with hypopituitarism. Hydrocortisone is generally the preferred glucocorticoid replacement therapy of choice as there is minimal transplacental passage to the fetus.

Mineralocorticoid replacement is not required in pituitary insufficiency as the renin-angiotensin-aldosterone axis is intact. Regular obstetrical follow-up with serial ultrasounds to detect IUGR is recommended.

Stress doses of glucocorticoids must be given at the time of labor and delivery; please refer to the section on Primary Adrenal Insufficiency for recommended doses.

Please refer to Chapter 224 for the discussion on lymphocytic hypophysitis and Sheehan syndrome.

PROLACTINOMAS

It is uncommon for pregnancy to occur in women with untreated prolactinomas because hyperprolactinemia is associated with infertility. However, the ability of dopamine agonists to reduce prolactin levels to the normal range restores ovulation in about 90% of patients, many of whom are then able to achieve pregnancy.

Rising estrogen levels during pregnancy have a stimulatory effect on prolactin secretion that can cause the growth of the lesion. The risk is much higher for macroadenomas compared with microadenomas. For this reason, dopamine agonists are always discontinued once pregnancy is confirmed in someone with a microadenoma.

With macroadenomas, dopamine agonists are frequently continued throughout pregnancy in order to prevent tumor growth. Numerous studies have shown that there are no adverse effects on the fetus with the use of bromocriptine. There is much less data on cabergoline, but it is thought to be safe as well, though it is not favored in any case due to its longer half-life.

It is recommended that prepregnancy baseline visual field testing and MRI imaging of the pituitary be done for women with macroadenoma and that they be reviewed on a regular basis (every four to six weeks) throughout gestation for evidence of tumor expansion. There is no role for measuring prolactin levels throughout pregnancy as the levels increase in any case.

In the postpartum period, lactation has not been shown to increase the size of adenomas and is strongly encouraged.

Diabetes insipidus

The development of new-onset diabetes insipidus in the third trimester is usually due to increased vasopressinase activity either due to increased placental production or decreased hepatic vasopressinase metabolism due to liver damage from various causes including preeclampsia, acute fatty liver of pregnancy, or HELLP, syndrome. This phenomenon is called transient vasopressin-resistant diabetes insipidus (DI) of pregnancy.

Preexisting central diabetes insipidus often worsens during pregnancy due to the increased clearance of endogenous vasopressin by increasing levels of vasopressinase. Subclinical central DI can also be unmasked for the first time during pregnancy due to this mechanism.

DDAVP is the treatment of choice for both central DI and transient vasopressin-resistant DI of pregnancy as it is not degraded by vasopressinase. Thiazide diuretics, which are used for the treatment of nephrogenic diabetes insipidus, are safe to be continued during pregnancy. Transient vasopressin-resistant DI of pregnancy tends to resolve a few days to weeks after delivery.

ADRENAL

Adrenal insufficiency

The most common cause is immune-mediated destruction of the adrenal cortex (Addison disease). This diagnosis should always be entertained in patients who have irretractable lethargy, nausea, and vomiting that is out of keeping with normal symptoms of pregnancy. A normal pregnancy outcome should be expected as long as the patient takes the appropriate dosages of glucocorticoids and mineralocorticoids; these doses often need to be increased slightly throughout pregnancy as rising progesterone levels act as antagonists to the glucocorticoid and mineralocorticoid receptors.

Hydrocortisone and prednisone are the preferred glucocorticoid replacement agents as their placental passage to the fetus is much lower compared with dexamethasone or betamethasone. Stress doses must always be administered in times of severe hyperemesis or physical stress as well as at the time of labor and delivery; please refer to **Table 223-14** for a suggested protocol of the latter.

Pheochromocytoma

This condition can have profound effects on both mother and fetus and so it is important that it be considered as part of the differential diagnosis for hypertension in the pregnant woman, particularly in the first half of pregnancy.

Fasting plasma metanephrine levels are the most sensitive and specific diagnostic test, though it should be noted that the levels are slightly increased in pregnancy. Falsely elevated levels can be caused by pharmacologic agents such as tricyclic antidepressants, labetalol, and methyldopa.

Anatomic localization is required for definitive treatment once a biochemical diagnosis has been made. In pregnancy, the modality of choice to achieve this is MRI. Nuclear scanning with metaiodobenzylguanidine (MIBG) is contraindicated in pregnancy.

TABLE 223-14 Stress Dose Steroids During Surgery or Delivery

1. Hydrocortisone 100 mg IV on call to operating room or at onset of labor
2. Hydrocortisone 100 mg IV every 8 hours over course of surgery or labor and delivery
3. Hydrocortisone 50 mg IV every 8 hours day 1 postoperative or postpartum
4. Hydrocortisone 25 mg orally every 8 hours day 2 postoperative or postpartum
5. Usual preadmission doses of hydrocortisone orally from day 3 postoperative or postpartum

Medical therapy in the form of alpha-blockade should be initiated once a biochemical diagnosis is made; and the patient should be counseled that the benefits of alpha-blockade in pregnancy far outweigh any potential unknown effects. Beta-blockade is then instituted after alpha-blockade is achieved to avoid tachyarrhythmias; the dose should be titrated to achieve a maternal heart rate of 80–100 beats per minute.

Surgery, in the form of laparoscopic adrenalectomy, can be considered once adequate medical therapy and localization of the lesion have been achieved. If the lesion is diagnosed during the first two trimesters, the best time to operate is during the second trimester, and if the lesion is diagnosed during the third trimester, surgery should be delayed until delivery though the timing of this will need to be brought forward if the mother remains symptomatic despite the medical blockade. An elective C-section is the delivery method of choice as the process of labor exacerbates the catecholamine surges.

Primary hyperaldosteronism

This condition is frequently unmasked in the postpartum period as the high progesterone levels during pregnancy antagonize the action of mineralocorticoids on their own receptors. Hypertension with hypokalemia is the classic presentation, though often the potassium level may be normal.

Both renin and aldosterone levels are increased during pregnancy. Therefore a suppressed renin level may be useful in diagnosing this condition during pregnancy, though it should be noted that medications such as beta-blockers and calcium channel blockers that suppress renin levels need to be discontinued for at least two weeks before formal testing of renin and aldosterone levels.

It is recommended that spironolactone not be used in pregnancy due to its antiandrogenic effects; there is a theoretical risk that feminization of a male fetus may occur. Calcium channel blockers are regarded to be the most effective antihypertensive agent, as they have some effect in reducing aldosterone synthesis and release. If the hypertension and/or hypokalemia cannot be controlled medically, laparoscopic removal of the affected adrenal gland during the second trimester may be warranted.

DEPRESSION

Depressive disorders affect at least 12% of women at some time in their lives. In the United States, depression is the leading cause of nonobstetric hospitalization among women age 18 to 44 years. The peak period for onset of depression occurs during the childbearing years and its impact extends to the offspring and the families involved. Unfortunately, perinatal depression remains underdiagnosed and undertreated in ob-gyn and primary care settings. Furthermore, the diagnosis of depression in pregnant women can be challenging because there is great overlap between the diagnostic symptoms of depression and the symptoms of normal pregnancy.

A systematic review found prevalence rates of depression that vary from trimester to trimester: 7.4% in the first, 12.8% in the second, and 12% in the third trimester. Risk factors for depression in pregnancy include a previous depressive episode, recent negative life events, adolescence, unmarried status, financial disadvantage, African American or Hispanic ethnicity, and poor social support. Untreated depression can lead to harmful prenatal health behaviors such as poor nutrition, poor prenatal medical care, smoking, alcohol, and other substance use. The fetus of untreated depressed women may demonstrate abnormal neurobehavioral responses such as altered heart rate reactivity.

Obstetric complications associated with depression include preeclampsia, preterm delivery, low birth weight, miscarriage, small-for-gestational age babies, low Apgar scores, neonatal complications, and high neonatal cortisol levels at birth. Exposure to higher cortisol levels is thought to be the mechanism of the effect on later childhood development that may include language and cognitive impairment, sleep problems, impulsivity, attention deficit disorders, behavioral dyscontrol, and psychopathology.

ANTIDEPRESSANT USE AND PREGNANCY

How can depressive symptoms be treated during pregnancy? Depression in nonpregnant patients is mostly treated with selective serotonin reuptake inhibitors (SSRIs) and serotonin-norepinephrine reuptake inhibitors (SNRI). Up to 9% of women have taken an antidepressant at some point during gestation, given that at least one-half of pregnancies are unplanned. Most of these exposures will be to one of the newer antidepressant medications. The odds ratio of 1.7 for spontaneous miscarriage with SSRI exposure, and reports of a 1.45 relative risk are within the range of the normal population.

Most meta-analyses report that newer antidepressants do not increase the risk of malformation rates above the 1–3% population baseline risk. The teratogenicity data from Denmark reports a 1.34 increased relative risk, but it does not control for underlying maternal psychiatric disorders. Small increased risk in omphalocele, craniosynostosis, and anencephaly with all SSRIs, and right ventricular outflow tract obstruction with paroxetine have been found in some other studies, but these findings were not replicated in other studies. Nevertheless, the Food and Drug Administration issued a public health advisory in 2005 regarding paroxetine and the FDA pregnancy category was changed from C to D.

Neonatal adaptation symptoms with maternal SSRI exposure have been reported. The syndrome described includes transient and usually mild jitteriness, poor muscle tone, weak or absent cry, respiratory distress, hypoglycemia, low Apgar scores, and possible seizures. The drugs with the highest association with the neonatal adaptations syndrome include paroxetine, fluoxetine and venlafaxine, with one study reporting on citalopram as well. Long-term sequelae have not been systematically studied and an accurate blinded infant assessment as well as a neonatal behavioral symptom scale should be helpful in examining this syndrome more accurately.

A case control study published in 2006 showed an increased risk of persistent pulmonary hypertension of the newborn (PPHN) from a baseline of 1–2 per 1000, to 6–12 per 1000 for infants exposed to SSRI after week 20 of gestation. The authors of the study suggest that SSRIs may promote pulmonary artery constriction after birth by inhibiting nitric oxide or by a direct effect on pulmonary smooth muscle cells. These theories have been challenged, and furthermore, SSRI use before week 20 seemed to be a somewhat protective factor against PPHN, so it is difficult to advise patients about the absolute risk.

Other psychotropic medications and pregnancy

Benzodiazepines are used during pregnancy for management of anxiety or insomnia. Meta-analyses have identified a small increased risk of oral cleft with in utero exposure, though a case-control study failed to confirm this teratogenic risk. Pyloric stenosis and alimentary tract atresias have also been reported, as well as low birth weight and floppy infant syndrome.

If benzodiazepines need to be used, consider delaying treatment until after oral cleft closure and choose medications with shorter half-lives at the lowest possible dose.

Mood stabilizers are the most widely used medications for management of mood instability (mania, depression, and psychosis in bipolar patients) and include lithium and the antiepileptic medications. The main concern with first trimester exposure to lithium is an increased risk (0.1%) in Ebstein anomaly, which has a risk of 0.05% in the unexposed population. Lithium remains one of the preferred treatments for bipolar disorder and this increased risk needs to be weighted against the risk of a mood decompensation. Stable serum levels may require increase in dosages as the pregnancy progresses due to the normal changes in blood volume in pregnancy. Careful monitoring of dosage and lithium level at delivery is recommended to avoid toxicity.

Valproate has an increased risk of neural tube defects of 5–9% with first trimester exposure and a fetal valproate syndrome that includes cardiovascular abnormalities and developmental delays, and craniofacial abnormalities have been described. There is newer information that exposure to valproate later in gestation may be associated with neurobehavioral changes as well. Toxicity at birth with valproate may include decreased fibrinogen levels, liver toxicity, hypoglycemia, deceleration in heart rate, abnormal muscle tone, and lower IQ. Women of reproductive age who are planning to have children should be switched from valproate to another agent prior to pregnancy so that the disease can be controlled by an alternative agent before gestation.

Exposure to carbamazepine in the first trimester carries an increased risk of craniofacial abnormalities, fingernail hypoplasia, growth restriction, and a risk of neural tube defect of 0.5–1%.

Lamotrigene is associated with an increased risk of congenital malformations similar to the general population (2–3%). Some studies have suggested an increased risk of cleft palate deformity, and it is worth noting that infants with antigen characteristics that differ from the mother may be at increased risk for skin rash and liver toxicity.

Haloperidol is the most commonly used antipsychotic in pregnancy because several studies have not found increased risks of congenital malformations. Chlorpromazine has a poor side-effect profile in pregnancy due to orthostasis and sedation and has an increased risk of malformations of 2.4% and so should generally be avoided.

Newer antipsychotics are better tolerated than the above mentioned medications, but the data regarding safety with these is limited. Some studies have shown no increased risk of major malformations with olanzapine, risperidone, quetiapine, and clozapin but have found lower birth weight. Side effects of these medications can also be problematic in pregnancy, particularly weight gain and glucose intolerance.

Postpartum blues, depression, and psychosis

Between 15% and 85% of normal postpartum women may experience the blues (postpartum blues), which present within the first 10 days after giving birth with a peak incidence at the fifth day. It can be difficult to distinguish from a true depressive disorder given that symptoms include mood swings, mild elation, irritability, tearfulness, fatigue, and confusion. Women who experienced postpartum blues may have a history of premenstrual dysphoria and depression, either related or unrelated to pregnancy. No treatment is required other than improved sleep and support, but it is worth noting its presence because it can be a risk factor for postpartum depression.

The DSM IV classifies postpartum depression as a major depressive disorder with a specifier of postpartum onset within one month after childbirth. Screening with a specific tool such as the Edinburgh Postnatal Depression Scale (EPDS) is important since it emphasizes clinical domains of depression and may help differentiate from normal postpartum findings. Risk factors for postpartum depression include depression during or prior to the pregnancy, previous premenstrual dysphoria, stressful life events during the pregnancy, poor social support, marital conflict, low income, immigrant status, and young maternal age. It is thought that the etiology may be related to hormonal fluctuations, either as a direct influence in mood or due to their affect on sleep patterns in the postpartum period.

Postpartum psychosis is a true psychiatric emergency that occurs in one to two per 1000 births. The onset usually occurs within the first four weeks after delivery, although manifestations of the clinical picture can be present in the first three days postpartum. The cognitive disorganization that occurs with postpartum psychosis may result in a mother's neglect of her infant's needs and unsafe practices. It is highly associated with bipolar disorder and most of the time requires inpatient psychiatric hospitalization for rapid stabilization and decreased risk of suicide or infanticide. Patients present with acute confusion, delusions, and grossly disorganized behavior.

The use of antidepressants during lactation for treatment of PPD or other psychiatric disorders such as obsessive-compulsive disorder and panic disorder is an important clinical issue. The evidence on the effects of antidepressants during breastfeeding consists of small sample studies and case reports. It is important to take into account the amount of medication present in the breast milk, the reported adverse events, and the infant serum level of the drug to discuss recommendations with patients. Pooled analyses indicate that sertraline and paroxetine tend to have undetectable infant serum drug levels. Fluoxetine and citalopram were more likely to result in elevated breast milk levels. Of the tricyclic antidepressants, nortriptyline and imipramine have the largest serum level data showing levels that are not detectable. Doxepin, on the other hand, has been associated with sedation and respiratory depression and is considered contraindicated in breastfeeding women.

Antipsychotics and breastfeeding

Studies of the safety of both first- and second-generation antipsychotics are quantitatively insufficient to make specific recommendations regarding breastfeeding. Risperidone and chlorpromazine have the lowest degree of excretion in breast milk and there is only one case report of drowsiness with chlorpromazine. One antipsychotic, clozapine, is considered contraindicated with breastfeeding due to high infant-relative dosage and reported adverse effects.

The available data suggests that the amount of medications (anxiolytics) to which newborns are exposed is not very high; it is important to note that neonates metabolize these medications more slowly than adults and accumulation may occur, causing infant sedation, nausea, and poor feeding. Therefore, long-acting medications are not recommended, and the lowest possible dose of a short-acting benzodiazepine should be used if these medications are needed while breastfeeding.

NEUROLOGY

HEADACHES

In general, pregnancy does not have a consistent impact on the frequency or severity of migraine headaches and the onset of migraines may begin during pregnancy. Migraine that presents for the first time after 20 weeks gestation should prompt an investigation for preeclampsia. Pseudotumor cerebri is an unusual cause of headache that is more frequently seen in pregnant women. The fundoscopic examination will reveal papilledema but otherwise the neurologic examination will be normal. Increased intracranial pressure on the optic nerve may cause progressive visual loss. The postpartum period (defined as six weeks after delivery) but not pregnancy is associated with an increased risk of stroke and intracerebral hemorrhage, which may be related to thrombosis and/or preeclampsia.

EPILEPSY

Seizure disorders complicate approximately 1% of all pregnancies, and up to 10% of epileptic women will present for the first time during pregnancy. It is, however, important to recognize that not all seizures result from epilepsy. Both patients with and without known seizure disorders may have seizures as a consequence of preeclampsia or eclampsia, so investigation for preeclampsia is necessary for all third-trimester seizures.

Although most antiepileptic drugs have teratogenicity of various degrees, epileptic women have an increased risk of fetal malformations even without their administration. The maternal and fetal risk of uncontrolled seizures resulting in hypoxemia and acidosis must be part of any risk-benefit assessment of withdrawing effective treatment. If a patient has been seizure free for greater than a year, holding treatment first trimester in consultation with a neurologist could be considered.

The dosage of antiepileptic medications may be influenced by the increased volume of distribution and by increases in hepatic and renal clearance.

Valproate and carbamazepine are preferred in breastfeeding women, given the low degree of excretion in breast milk and limited reported adverse effects in infants. Lamotrigene has its own particular set of concerns. Even though only 60% of the drug is transferred to the breast milk, infants present with higher-than-expected drug levels when breastfed.

GASTROINTESTINAL DISEASE

ABDOMINAL PAIN

Gastroesophageal reflux disease occurs due to delayed gastric emptying and decreased gastroesophageal sphincter tone from progesterone effects on smooth muscle. Constipation is also common and related to the effects of progesterone upon the smooth muscle of the bowel. The differential of abdominal pain is broad and includes contractions, pain from adhesions interfering with expansion of the uterus into the abdomen, urinary retention, degenerating fibroid, ectopic pregnancy, ovarian torsion, stress on the round ligaments as the uterus expands, rupture of an ovarian cyst, and bleeding into a corpus luteal cyst. Late in pregnancy, uterine contractions, abruption placentae, pelvic arthropathy, and rarely rectus hematoma may occur.

Vomiting, pyelonephritis, appendicitis, cholecystitis, and rarely vovlulus of the large bowel may also be seen during pregnancy.

CHOLELITHIASIS

Pregnancy is a risk factor for the development of cholesterol gallstones and biliary sludge. Higher estrogen levels increase biliary cholesterol secretion and higher progesterone levels decrease gallbladder smooth muscle motility. Preexisting gallstones are more likely to cause symptoms.

BUDD CHIARI SYNDROME

Pregnancy hypercoagulability is also a risk factor for hepatic vein thrombosis or the Budd Chiari syndrome. Typically, patients suddenly develop abdominal pain and ascites after delivery.

JAUNDICE

Common causes of jaundice during pregnancy include cholestasis from raised estrogen levels, acute fatty liver of pregnancy, disseminated intravascular coagulopathy, severe preeclampsia, hyperemesis, and severe septicemia in late pregnancy. Drug effects (chlorpromazine, tetracycline, steroids), chronic liver disease, gall stones, and chronic hemolysis should also be considered.

LIVER DISEASE

Pregnancy-associated changes

Some of the physiologic changes of pregnancy can simulate laboratory abnormalities seen with liver disease. For example, serum albumin concentrations typically decrease from a mean of 4.2 g/dL in nonpregnant women without liver disease to 3.1 g/dL at the end of gestation due to an increase in plasma volume. Due to leakage of placental alkaline phosphatase into the maternal blood during the fifth month, typically serum alkaline phosphatase levels rise. Hepatosplenomegaly should not be found in the normal pregnancy and bilirubin, AST, ALT, and 5'nucleotidas, and γ-glutamyl levels should be normal. Telangiectasis of the chest, back, and face and palmar erythema may occur in up to 60% of normal pregnant women but should disappear after delivery. Acute fatty liver of pregnancy (AFLP) can lead to jaundice, liver failure, and death.

Diagnosis

The week of gestation may provide an important clue to the diagnosis. Liver diseases specifically associated with pregnancy occur at certain times. In the first trimester, nausea and vomiting with jaundice is consistent with hyperemesis gravidarum and AFLP has not been reported to occur during this time. Cholestasis of pregnancy typically presents at 30 weeks, usually with generalized pruritis, malaise, and fatigue due to symptoms being worse at night. Jaundice may develop in one-third to one-half of patients after the onset of pruritis. In 5–10% of pregnancies, liver diseases may develop with preeclampsia and eclampsia in the third trimester. In approximately 1 in 13,000 pregnancies, AFLP occurs in the third trimester.

The pattern of serum liver enzyme abnormalities may be helpful in establishing the diagnosis. The jaundice of cholestasis of pregnancy is usually not severe, less than 6 mg/dl along with elevated alkaline phosphatase levels three to four times the upper limit of normal in pregnancy and elevated serum bile acids. With preeclampsia and eclampsia, the liver injury is due to hepatocellular injury or ischemia so aminotransferase levels are more elevated than alkaline phosphatase or bilirubin. When patients develop abdominal pain, hypotension, fever, leukocytosis, nausea, and vomiting with abnormal liver tests in the third trimester, hepatic infarction, subcapsular hematoma, and hepatic rupture are rare complications of preeclampsia and eclampsia. AFLP is a disease of acute hepatocyte failure so laboratory tests may be initially unimpressively abnormal. If the serum transaminases rise to more than 10 times the upper limit of normal, alternative diagnoses should be considered. The prothrombin time and rising bilirubin are the most reliable indicators of hepatic failure.

Treatment

For patients with AFLP, supportive care and early delivery are critical due to the high fetal and maternal mortality. If hepatic failure is present, patients should be referred to a transplant unit early in the course. Likewise, the preferred treatment of patients with severe preeclampsia-related liver diseases is delivery.

Effect of chronic liver disease on pregnancy

Pregnancy does not alter the progression of chronic liver disease, but the outcome of the pregnancy may be influenced by the patient's overall health, resulting in a higher incidence of miscarriage and prematurity.

HEMATOLOGIC CONDITIONS

SICKLE CELL DISEASE

Rates of severe preeclampsia, chest and urinary infections, and biliary disease are higher in pregnant patients with sickle cell disease.

Even in high-risk perinatal clinics, the perinatal mortality rate and maternal mortality rate is increased.

VENOUS THROMBOEMBOLISM IN PREGNANCY

INCIDENCE

There is a five-fold increase in the incidence of venous thromboembolism (VTE) in pregnancy that occurs at an incidence of 0.5–3 per 1000 pregnancies. VTE continues to be the leading nonobstetric cause of maternal death in the developed world. Thromboembolic events are evenly distributed throughout the three trimesters and the postpartum period, although more recent studies suggest a slightly higher incidence in the first trimester. In addition, because the postpartum period is by definition shorter (six weeks, as compared to 12 weeks in a trimester), the day-to-day risk of VTE in the postpartum period is higher. The incidence of fatal pulmonary embolism is also higher in the postpartum period.

Pathophysiology

Pregnancy is a hypercoagulable state, characterized by an increase in levels of clotting factors, decrease in anticoagulant activity (lower levels of protein S and increased activated protein C resistance), and decreased fibrinolytic activity. In addition, stasis induced by venous compression by the gravid uterus and hormonal influence on vasculature further adds to the coagulant risk.

Risk factors that may contribute to the development of VTE in pregnancy include prolonged bed rest, cesarean section, obesity, parity > 3, underlying thrombophilia, prior VTE, or preeclampsia.

The genetic predisposition to VTE may be identified by a positive family history in those patients for whom pregnancy is an additional risk factor.

Clinical presentation

Clinical features of deep vein thrombosis (DVT) include pain and swelling in the affected leg, but it is important to remember that LE edema in pregnancy is common and is often asymmetric. Anatomy of the pelvic vasculature is such that the right iliac artery crosses over the left iliac vein. With the cardiovascular changes of pregnancy, there is compression of the left iliac vein by the right iliac artery, resulting in asymmetric lower extremity edema (left greater than right) and the finding that the vast majority of DVTs occur in the left leg.

Symptoms of pulmonary embolism (PE) include dyspnea, chest pain that may be pleuritic, syncope, hemoptysis, and apprehension. Shortness of breath is a very common complaint in pregnancy, but tachypnea is always an abnormal finding. It is important to have a low threshold for investigating a dyspneic pregnant woman who is tachycardic and tachypneic so that diagnosis of PE is not missed.

Diagnosis

Clinical diagnosis of DVT and PE in pregnancy is unreliable. Compression of pelvic veins by the gravid uterus can make interpretation of results difficult. In addition, isolated iliac vein thrombosis may not be picked up by routine methods of detection. D-dimers are known to be elevated in pregnancy and may not help in decision making. Clinical prediction rules for PE have not been validated in pregnancy. Pregnant patients with PE are younger and less likely to have comorbid conditions compared with nonpregnant patients, and generally appear "well" and in more than 60% of cases have normal arterial blood gases.

Doppler ultrasound is the noninvasive test of choice in the pregnant woman with suspected DVT. In symptomatic patients with a high pretest probability but a negative test, serial Dopplers should be done and an MRV of the pelvis should be considered to look for isolated iliac clot. A recent study found that 60% of DVT in pregnancy is found in the proximal veins without evidence of calf thrombosis, suggesting that propagation from calf vein clots may not be the mechanism of proximal thrombosis in pregnancy. Chest X-ray and ECG are helpful in a patient with suspected PE to rule out other causes. Both ventilation-perfusion lung scan (V/Q scan) and CT angiogram can be safely used in pregnancy for diagnosis of PE. Fetal radiation exposure with either of these tests is minimal (**Table 223-15**). In the majority of cases of fatal PE in the U.K. Confidential Enquiry into Maternal Mortality, there was a failure to make the diagnosis because of the mistaken belief that diagnostic testing would be harmful to the fetus. Pulmonary angiogram is usually reserved for severe cases in which localization of embolus is necessary prior to embolectomy.

TABLE 223-15 Fetal Radiation Exposure with Maternal Testing

Study	Radiation Exposure (RADS)
Chest X-ray	<.001
Lung Scan	0.01–0.02 ventilation 0.01–0.03 perfusion
Pulmonary Angiogram	<.050 via brachial route 0.2–0.3 via femoral route
CT angiogram	0.2–0.3
Ultrasound	None
MRI/MRA/MRV	None
Upper GI series	0.1
Lumbar spine series	0.9
Barium enema	1
Complete IVP	0.5
Head CT	<0.01
CT abdomen	2.0–3.0

Treatment

Treatment of VTE in pregnancy involves anticoagulation with low-molecular-weight heparin (LMWH) or unfractionated heparin (UFH). Dosing is weight based, and may require increases with increasing gestation. Warfarin is a known human teratogen and its use in pregnancy is contraindicated for this indication. **Table 223-16** lists medications for treatment of acute DVT and PE in pregnancy.

Most centers maintain patients on full therapeutic anticoagulation for the rest of their pregnancy until six weeks postpartum or at least six months, whichever is longer. Trials investigating lowering the intensity of anticoagulation after 4–12 weeks are currently underway, but this practice has not yet been validated in pregnancy. LMWH is the preferred agent in pregnancy, and has been associated with less thrombocytopenia and osteoporosis. Weight gain, increased blood volume, and increased clearance with pregnancy progression may require change in dosing, but this is usually guided by checking peak anti-Xa levels, which are done monthly.

Peripartum management of anticoagulation can be challenging. Epidural analgesia for pain control during labor or spinal anesthesia may be necessary for an operative delivery. Guidelines from the American society of Regional Anesthesia and Pain management (ASRA) recommend that in patients on therapeutic doses of LMWH, regional anesthesia be delayed at least 24 hours after last dose of LMWH injection to decrease the risk of spinal hematoma. This may be possible in a patient undergoing an elective induction of labor, but in most cases, the onset of labor cannot be predicted. We

TABLE 223-16 Medications for Treatment of Venous Thromboembolism in Pregnancy

Drug	Dose	Route	Frequency
Unfractionated heparin	80 units/kg bolus, then 18 units/kg/hr	Intravenous	Continuous, with dose adjustment using aPTT values
Enoxaparin	1 mg/kg	Subcutaneous (SQ)	Every 12 hours. Due to increased clearance once daily dosing at 1.5 mg/kg may not be adequate.
Tinzaparin	175 units/kg	SQ	Every 24 hours
Dalteparin	200 units/kg	SQ	Every 24 hours

therefore switch the patient over to subcutaneous unfractionated heparin in the last month of pregnancy, two or three times a day, at a dose sufficient to keep the mid-interval aPTT approximately twice normal. The patient is instructed to stop heparin injections at the first sign of labor and aPTT is monitored closely once the patient is admitted to the hospital. Provided the aPTT is normal, regional anesthesia can be used with no contraindication. Following delivery, LMWH can be resumed 24 hours after removal of epidural or spinal catheter. In the postpartum period, warfarin can be safely used, even in breastfeeding mothers. Anecdotal evidence suggests that there is increased incidence of bleeding from surgical sites during the overlap of warfarin and LMWH. In patients who have had an operative delivery, we usually start Coumadin two weeks after delivery, to avoid the risk of surgical bleeding.

Women with prior VTE are believed to have a higher risk of recurrent VTE in a subsequent pregnancy. There is evidence to suggest that this is especially true in patients whose first event was related to pregnancy, puerperium, or oral contraceptive use. An underlying thrombophilia and a family history of VTE are considered additional risk factors. Thromboprophylaxis is therefore recommended in these patients in subsequent pregnancies. **Table 223-17** lists some anticoagulant prophylaxis regimens in pregnancy and the postpartum period. Prophylaxis needs to be continued for six weeks postpartum.

CONCLUSION

Any hospitalized patient of childbearing age contemplating children should have optimal medical management and counseling prior to becoming pregnant. Clinicians should take steps to identify coexisting diseases in the pregnant patient and complications of pregnancy before they become more severe. Optimally, management of medical problems requires prevention strategies to reduce progression of illness that would otherwise necessitate multiple medications, emergency treatment, and readmissions to the hospital. Team management of these patients with obstetric internists, high-risk obstetricians, and appropriate subspecialty consultation is recommended to achieve optimal medical status and function. Care of this unique population also requires optimal communication among team members so that it is clear who will be responsible for monitoring treatment and patient and family education.

TABLE 223-17 Suggested Regimens for Thromboprophylaxis in Pregnancy

1. Enoxaparin 40 mg SQ once daily until 20 weeks gestation, then 40 mg twice daily. At 36 weeks gestation, switch to UFH 10000 units SQ twice daily until delivery.
2. UFH 5000 units SQ twice daily in the first trimester, 7500 units SQ twice daily in the second trimester, and 10000 units SQ twice daily in the third trimester.

Suggested regimens for postpartum prophylaxis

1. Enoxaparin 40 mg SQ once daily
2. Warfarin, with target INR of 1.5 to 2

UFH 5000 units SQ twice daily

INR, international normalized ratio; SQ, suncutaneously; UFH, unfractionated heparin.

SUGGESTED READINGS

Bandi VD, Munnur U, Matthay MA. Acute Lung injury and Acute respiratory distress syndrome in pregnancy. *Crit Care Clin.* 2004; 20(4):577–607.

Bourjeily G, Paidas M, Khalil H, Rosene-Montella K, Rodger M. Pulmonary embolism in pregnancy. *Lancet.* 2010;375(9713): 500–512.

Cole DE, Taylor TL, McCullough DM, Shoff CT, Derdak S. Acute respiratory distress in pregnancy. *Crit Care Med.* 2005;33(suppl 10) S269–S278.

Cormier CM, Canzoneri BJ, Lewis DF, et al. Urolithiasis in pregnancy: Current diagnoses, treatment and pregnancy complications. *Obstet and Gynecol Survey.* 2006;61(11):733–741.

Gammill HS, Jeyabalan A. Acute renal failure in pregnancy. *Crit Care Med.* 2005;33(suppl 10) page 84.

Janakiraman, Vanitha. Listeriosis in pregnancy: diagnosis, treatment, and prevention. *Rev Obstet Gynecol.* 2008;1(4):179–185.

Knox TA, Olans LB. Liver Disease in Pregnancy. *NEJM.* 1996;335(8): 569–576.

Lal A, Anderson G, Cowen M, Lindow S, Arnold AG. *NAEP Guidelines. Chest.* 2007;(132)3;1044–1048.

Lim WS, Macfarlane JT, Colthorpe CL. Treatment of community acquired lower respiratory tract infections in pregnancy. *Am J Respir Med.* 2003;2(3):221–233.

Macejko AM, Schaeffer AJ. Asymptomatic bacteriuria and symptomatic urinary tract infections during pregnancy. Urol *Clin North Am.* 2007;34(1):35–42.

Mantel GD. Care of the critically ill parturient: oliguria and renal failure. *Best prac and res clin obstet gynecol.* 2001;15(4):563–581.

Metzger BE, Buchanan TA, Coustan DR, et al. Summary and Recommendations of 5th International Workshop-Conference on Gestational Diabetes Mellitus. *Diabetes Care.* 2007;30S(2): S251–S262.

Mittal P, Wing DA. Urinary tract infections in pregnancy. *Clin Perinatol*. 2005;32(3):749–764.

Poole JH, Thorsen MS. Acute renal failure in pregnancy. *Am J Mat Child Nursing.* 1999;24(2):66–73.

Ramsey PS, Ramin KD. Pneumonia in pregnancy.*Obstet Gynecol Clin North Am.* 2001;28(3):553–569.

Reddy SS, Holley JL. Management of the pregnant chronic dialysis patient. *Advances in chronic kidney disease.* 2007;14(2): 146–155.

Sheffield JS, Cunningham FG. Urinary tract infection in women. *Obstet Gynecol.* 2005;106(5 Pt 1):1085–1092.

The American Thyroid Association Taskforce on Thyroid Disease During Pregnancy and Postpartum. Stagnaro-Green A (Chair), Abalovich M, Alexander E, Azizi F, et al. Guidelines of the American Thyroid Association for the Diagnosis and Management of Thyroid Disease During Pregnancy and Postpartum. Thyroid. 2011;21:1–45.

CHAPTER 224

Postpartum Consultation for Common Complaints

Courtney Bilodeau, MD
Karen Rosene-Montella, MD

Key Clinical Questions

1. What are the common causes of postpartum fever?
2. What antibiotics are recommended for common postpartum infections?
3. What is the differential diagnosis for a postpartum headache?
4. When does a postpartum headache require radiologic imaging?
5. What are the common postpartum neuropathies?
6. What is the differential diagnosis for a postpartum seizure?
7. What is the postpartum course and management for autoimmune diseases including myasthenia gravis, multiple sclerosis, rheumatoid arthritis, systemic lupus erythematosus?
8. What is the postpartum management for thyroid disorders and diabetes mellitus?
9. What is the postpartum management for preeclampsia and chronic hypertension?
10. What is the long-term cardiovascular risk for patients with a history of preeclampsia?

INTRODUCTION

The postpartum period, lasting six months, is a unique time during which there is a physiological return to the prepregnancy state. Night sweats, mood disturbance, urinary frequency, perineal and vaginal discomfort, and breast engorgement are all common complaints from postpartum women. Clinicians treating postpartum patients in the hospital setting must be able to differentiate these normal changes from disease states at a time of increased risk for flares of chronic medical conditions and the onset of new conditions.

POSTPARTUM FEVER

Low grade fever frequently occurs in the first 24 hours after delivery. Postpartum fever is defined as a temperature of ≥38.0 degrees Celsius (100.4 degrees Fahrenheit) on any two of the first ten days postpartum exclusive of the first 24 hours. Infection is the leading cause of postpartum fever in the United States; the overall postpartum infection rate is around 6%, with the incidence of planned cesarean deliveries up to 10%, and higher in unplanned deliveries. Endometritis is the most common infection in the postpartum period, followed by urinary tract infection, lower genital tract infection, wound infection, pulmonary infection, thrombophlebitis, cholecystitis, and mastitis. A recent database analysis looking at readmissions within six weeks of delivery found that the cause of readmission is primarily infectious in origin, and that hypertension and uterine and wound infections were the most common causes for readmission. A surprising finding suggested that a recent pregnancy increases the risk for pneumonia, appendicitis, and cholecystitis. As expected, readmission rates were significantly higher after cesarean section than after vaginal delivery. Pregnant patients have decreased buffering capacity, increased cardiac output, and decreased systemic vascular resistance so patients with sepsis related to postpartum infection may decompensate quickly. Prompt action with close follow-up is recommended.

Postpartum endometritis

Postpartum endometritis is typically a polymicrobial infection of lower genital tract flora infecting the upper genital tract. The prevalence of endometritis has been greatly reduced with the standard use of antibiotic prophylaxis with cesarean deliveries. The risk of endometritis is increased by various factors:

- Prolonged labor
- Prolonged rupture of membranes
- Multiple vaginal examinations
- Operative vaginal delivery
- Bacterial vaginosis
- Chorioamnionitis
- Cesarean section (especially nonelective)
- Antepartum isolation of group B streptococci, Chlamydia, or mycoplasma

The criteria for diagnosis of endometritis include fever and uterine tenderness. Other signs and symptoms include foul lochia and chills. The postpartum uterus should be firm, nontender, and below the umbilicus; with endometritis a soft, subinvoluted uterus may lead to excessive vaginal bleeding.

When endometritis is suspected, laboratory or imaging data are rarely needed before initiating treatment. If despite treatment, a patient has persistent fever or unusually severe or localized pain, further studies may be helpful. A WBC with differential, blood cultures (which are positive in 10–20% of patients), and endometrial cultures may be diagnostic and can help direct antimicrobial therapy. Endometrial cultures should be acquired with a double or triple lumen technique to prevent vaginal and cervical contamination. Pelvic ultrasonography can identify retained products of conception, which need to be removed by dilatation and curettage because they are an ongoing nidus of infection. Computed tomography (CT) or magnetic resonance imaging (MRI) are used to diagnose alternative causes of persistent pain and fever including ovarian vein thrombosis, abscess, or hematoma. Please refer to a full discussion of ovarian vein thrombosis in Chapter 223 Common Medical Problems in Pregnancy.

The most common infectious agents when endometritis is suspected in the first 24 to 48 hours postpartum are Gram-positive cocci (predominantly group B streptococci, *Staphylococcus epidermidis,* and *Enterococcus* sp) or Gram-negative bacteria (predominantly *Gardnerella vaginalis, Escherichia coli, Klebsiella pneumoniae,* and *Proteus mirabilis*). After 48 hours, involvement of anaerobic bacteria (predominantly peptostreptococci, *Bacteroides* sp, and *Prevotella* sp) is likely, and by seven days, C. trachomatis is often found. The treatment regimen for postpartum endometritis includes broad spectrum parenteral antibiotics. In the first 48 hours after delivery, the recommended regimen is clindamycin (900 mg every eight hours) plus gentamicin (1.75 mg/ kg every eight hours or 5 mg/kg every 24 hours). If there is persistent fever or enterococcus is suspected, ampicillin or vancomycin in penicillin allergy should be added. Alternative regimens include cefotetan, cefoxitin, piperacillin/tazobactam, and ampicillin/sulbactam. There is a trend to use clindamycin and gentamicin for predelivery chorioamnionitis and ampicillin sulbactam for postpartum fever due to endometritis. With anaphylaxis to penicillin or cephalosporins, clindamycin and gentamcin are still preferred. Treatment continues until a patient has been afebrile for 48 hours and uterine tenderness has resolved. Oral therapy after parenteral therapy is not recommended as there is no evidence for improved outcome or decreased risk of recurrence. However, patients with bacteremia confirmed by positive blood cultures should complete a 7–10 day course of antibiotics. Late postpartum endometritis (48 hours to six weeks postpartum) may be treated with oral metronidazole and doxycycline (100 mg IV or orally every 12 hours) for 14 days.

Wound infection

Postpartum wound infections complicate 2% to 8% of cesarean sections. Risk factors for wound infection include nonelective cesarean section, preoperative fever, prolonged rupture of membranes, diabetes mellitus, and obesity. Patients with postpartum endometritis are also at increased risk for wound infection. Approximately 3% to 5% of patients with endometritis have a concurrent wound infection. On clinical examination, the infected abdominal incision is erythematous, indurated, and tender and may have purulent drainage. Frequently the incision requires opening and drainage. The fascia should be examined to ensure that it is intact and no dehiscence has taken place. Gram stain and culture of wound drainage is rarely needed before broad spectrum antibiotics are initiated. The wound should be irrigated and dressed with clean bandages two to three times daily. Antibiotics are typically required for at least a week or until signs of infection have resolved.

Episiotomy infection occurs after 1% to 2% of vaginal deliveries. The infection may be limited to the skin and superficial fascia along the incision site or may spread beyond this area. Treatment may require debridement and broad spectrum antibiotics. Some experts are recommending antibiotic prophylaxis for repair of third and fourth degree episiotomy extensions following episiotomy extensions.

Serious complications of wound and episiotomy infections include dehiscence and necrotizing fasciitis. These are more common in diabetics and severely obese women. Necrotizing fasciitis is a potentially fatal illness without aggressive medical and surgical management. Clinical signs of necrotizing fasciitis include discolored or pale wound margins without sensation, leukocytosis, metabolic derangement, disseminated intravascular coagulation (DIC) and hypotension. Discoloration that follows a facial plane in the perineum is often the first clinical clue to fasciitis. The most common bacterial pathogens to cause necrotizing fasciitis are group B streptococci, anaerobes, and nonhemolytic streptococci and staphylococci. Treatment requires immediate surgical debridement and broad spectrum antibiotics.

BREAST INFECTION

The majority of postpartum patients experience breast discomfort with swollen, firm, and tender breasts. Simple engorgement causes low grade fevers without any other clinical signs of infection and typically resolves within 48 hours. Breast infections, including mastitis and abscess, are rare in women who do not breastfeed but occur in 2% to 3% of breastfeeding women. The patient may describe chills, flu-like symptoms, and have high fevers (102° to 104°F). Mastitis causes localized erythema and swelling with a cellulitic appearance. A breast abscess is characterized by fluctuance and diffuse erythema, with a localized area of tenderness.

The most frequent pathogen in postpartum breast infection is *Staphylococcus aureus,* and toxic shock has been reported with mastitis in the postpartum period. Other less common pathogens include β-hemolytic streptococci, *H influenzae, H parainfluenzae, Escherichia coli,* and *Klebsiella pneumoniae.*

Clinical evaluation includes culture of expressed breast milk and aspirated fluid if there is a fluctuant mass. Prompt antibiotic treatment is required and should continue for seven days or until resolution of infection. Recommended antibiotic coverage includes Nafcillin 2 g IV every 4 hours or dicloxacillin 500 mg orally every 6 hours or cephalexin 500 mg orally every 6 hours. Alternative regimens include amoxicillin/clavulanate 875 mg orally every 12 hours or azithromycin 500 mg orally initially, then 250 mg orally daily. If methicillin-resistant *Staphylococcus aureus* (MRSA) is suspected then TMP-SMX-DS orally every 12 hours or vancomycin 1 g IV every 12 hours are recommended.

For mastitis, the patient should be encouraged to avoid milk stasis by continuing to nurse or pump expressed milk. Hot compresses also aid in comfort and expression of milk. Patients should be closely followed as an abscess can develop even after antibiotics have begun. If a patient has a breast abscess, then incision and drainage or needle aspiration may be warranted. Patients with breast abcesses should be advised to discontinue breastfeeding until after drainage is performed, if indicated, and signs of infection are resolved. In communities with a high rate of MRSA, it is found in up to 50% of women with postpartum breast abscesses.

POSTPARTUM HEADACHE

Hormonal fluctuations, sleep deprivation, and anxiety all contribute to the increased frequency of headaches in the postpartum period. The differential diagnosis of headache varies from minor to life-threatening causes and therefore warrants a prompt and thorough clinical evaluation. Alarm symptoms that warrant emergent evaluation with neurolgic imaging include headache of acute onset, abnormal or focal neurologic findings, seizure, and/or decreased level of consciousness. If a postpartum patient has a new Horner's syndrome, the anterior and posterior circulation should be imaged at the same time to rule out dissection. **Table 224-1** summarizes the differential diagnosis of postpartum headache along with common features, and modes of evaluation or treatment.

Migraine

Migraines have an increased predominance in the post-puberty years of females over males, suggesting a role of ovarian sex hormones in their pathogenesis. It is thought that migraines may be trigged by the decline of estrogen levels after a period of elevated estrogen, which occurs during the menstrual and postpartum periods. The majority of women who suffer from migraines have an improvement during pregnancy, and around 40% of women experience a recurrence postpartum. The postpartum migraine may be less severe than a patient's typical migraine, but usually has classical features including a bifrontal, prolonged, and pulstatile headache, and may include nausea, vomiting, and aversion to loud noise, bright light, and physical activity. Migraine or vascular headache may also be a presenting feature of preeclampsia, and so should always trigger an evaluation for preeclampsia in a peripartum patient, even in the absence of hypertension. Postpartum patients, including those who are breastfeeding, may be safely treated with most medications including acetaminophen, NSAIDS, caffeine, opioids, and triptans. Severe migraines may also be relieved with intravenous hydration, antiemetics, and steroids.

Tension-type headaches

Tension-type headaches (TTHS) are the most common type of headaches in adulthood. Similar to migraines, there is a female predominance in TTHS prevalence, suggesting a female sex hormone contribution to their pathophysiology. There are fewer studies on TTHS in pregnancy compared with migraines. In one small study, 28% of women reported remission of TTHS in pregnancy. TTHS are frequently described as bifrontal, bioccipital, or neck pain that is squeezing and aching. Nausea, light, or sound sensitivity are common, but loss of functional capacity is generally not described. The treatment methods for TTHS are similar to migraine headaches. Alternative therapies include relaxation techniques, biofeedback, and physical therapy.

Cluster headaches

Cluster headaches occur less frequently in women than men, but recent reports describe an increase in the number of female cases and a decrease in the male-to-female ratio of the disease. There is no definitive evidence for a link between cluster headaches and sex hormone levels. Data suggests only a small percent of women suffer from cluster headaches in pregnancy and the incidence is not changed in the postpartum period. Cluster headaches are unilateral, generally orbito-temporal pain that is nonthrobbing and

TABLE 224-1 Postpartum Headache

Cause of Headache	Common Features	Treatment/Evaluation
Migraine	Bifrontal, prolonged, and pulstatile Other: nausea, vomiting, and aversion to loud noise, bright light, and physical activity	Acetaminophen, NSAIDS, caffeine, opiods, triptans Severe: intravenous hydration, antiemetics, and steroids.
Tension-type	Bifrontal, bioccipital or neck with squeezing and aching. Other: nausea, light, and sound sensitivity	Acetaminophen, NSAIDS, caffeine, opiods Alternative therapies: relaxation techniques, biofeedback, and physical therapy
Cluster	Unilateral, orbito-temporal and nonthrobbing, penetrating. Other: ptosis, conjunctival injection, or lacrimation	Oxygen, intranasal lidocaine, triptans
Post-dural puncture	Severe, postural (worse with sitting up or standing)	Blood patch, intravenous fluid
Cerebral vein thrombosis	Severe headache (gradual or acute) Other: focal neurological signs (motor, sensation, aphasia), disordered consciousness, seizure, papilledema, nuchal rigidity, intracranial hypertension.	MRI/V, CT venography, cerebral angiography. Treatment may include intravenous mannitol, neurosurgical intervention, anticoagulation, or thrombolysis
Subarachnoid hemorrhage (Arteriovenous malformation or aneurysm)	Mild to severe sudden, diffuse headache Other: nausea and vomiting, confusion, focal neurologic deficit, nuchal rigidity, intraocular hemorrhages, hypertension, hypoxemia, ECG changes	Head CT or MRI, Lumbar puncture Treatment includes blood pressure and pain control, possible neurosurgical intervention
Posterior reversible encephalopathy syndrome (PRES)	Severe diffuse headache, confusion, seizure, and visual abnormalities	MRI Blood pressure management
Preeclampsia	Vascular headache Visual complaints Sudden, severe headache	PRES Intracerebral bleed Laboratory findings of preeclampsia, hypertension

penetrating. Ptosis, conjunctival injection, or lacrimation may be observed. The first-line treatment in the postpartum period is oxygen, followed by intranasal lidocaine or triptans.

Postdural puncture headaches

The accidental dural puncture (ADP) rate with epidural insertion for obstetric anesthesia is common, with reported rates as high as 6.5%. ADP may go unrecognized until a patient complains of headache. The reported incidence of headache after ADP in the obstetric population ranges from 45–80%. Patients describe a severe, markedly postural (worse with sitting up or standing) headache that can last several days. Treatment is with a blood patch, potentially repeated if relief is not given after the initial patch. Intravenous fluid may also aid in comfort.

Vascular headaches

A cerebrovascular event should always be considered in a postpartum patient with a severe headache. The incidence of cerebral vein thrombosis (CVT), subarachnoid hemorrhage, and posterior reversible encephalopathy syndrome (PRES) increases in the postpartum period. Women who are postpartum with "the worst headache of their lives" require a thorough neurologic evaluation including CNS imaging.

Cerebral vein thrombosis (CVT) In adulthood, CVT is more common in women than men, with 75% of cases found in women. The hypercoagulable state present during pregnancy and postpartum is a significant risk factor for thrombosis. Additional risk factors include cesarean section, anemia, dehydration, and infection. Headache is a frequent symptom of CVT due to increased intracranial pressure, hemorrhagic infarcts, and distention of the sinus walls on pain sensitive dura mater. The headache may be described as severe and acute or gradually worsening over several days. Other clinical findings of CVT are focal neurological signs (motor, sensation, aphasia), disordered consciousness, seizure, papilledema, nuchal rigidity, and intracranial hypertension. Radiologic imaging is required for diagnosis. CT scans are not as reliable as the highly sensitive MRI/MRV. CT venography or cerebral angiography may also be used. A multidisciplinary team including neurology and neurosurgery should be established to care for the patient, with an initial goal to stabilize the patient to prevent or reverse cerebral herniation if signs of increased intracranial pressure are present. Treatment should include anticoagulation once there is MRV confirmation of the diagnosis and no evidence of hemorrhage. Severe cases may also require intravenous mannitol, neurosurgical intervention, or thrombolysis. The majority of patients with CVT have a good outcome.

Subarachoid hemorrhage (SAH) While rare, hemorrhagic cerebral accidents are a major nonobstetric cause of mortality in pregnancy, with most due to rupture of an arterial aneurysm or arteriovenous malformation. Symptoms of SAH include mild to severe headache of sudden onset, nausea, vomiting, confusion, focal neurologic deficit, nuchal rigidity, intraocular hemorrhages, hypertension, hypoxemia, and ECG changes. CT scanning is primarily used to investigate for SAH. Intracerebral and subarachnoid bleed may also occur with preeclampsia, and so it should also be considered if there is any evidence of CNS bleed in a peripartum patient. The ability to detect hemorrhage depends on numerous factors including the amount of blood and the interval between symptoms and imaging. MRI is more sensitive if done several days from symptom onset. A lumbar puncture may also be needed for diagnosis, especially in cases of normal radiologic studies. Ideally the puncture should be performed within 12 hours after headache onset to determine if blood is present due to a SAH versus traumatic tap. SAH is more likely if after waiting 12 hours elevated bilirubin is measured, signaling erythrocyte breakdown. A multidisciplinary team including neurology and neurosurgery is recommended for management, with attention to blood pressure and pain control.

Posterior reversible encephalopathy syndrome (PRES) Since first described by Hinchey in 1996, several publications have demonstrated PRES as a cause of headache in pregnancy and postpartum. This condition of vasogenic edema, particularly in the posterior circulation territory, is likely caused by several factors including vasospasm and breakdown of the blood-brain-barrier. Pregnancy- and postpartum-specific conditions of preeclampsia and eclampsia cause vascular endothelium dysfunction and blood pressure elevations above baseline, predisposing to PRES. Clinical signs and symptoms include a severe, diffuse headache, confusion, seizure, and visual abnormalities. Diagnosis is made with MRI (findings include posterior cerebral white matter edema). Management includes strict blood pressure control and close observation.

■ POSTPARTUM NEUROPATHIES

Neuropathies that may occur in the postpartum period, include Bell's palsy, carpal tunnel syndrome, de Quervain tenosynovitis, and compression or stretch injury to the lateral femoral cutaneous, femoral, peroneal, or obturator nerves.

Bell's palsy

Bell's palsy, facial nerve palsy, is caused by compression or ischemia to the nerve. Bell's palsy is most commonly seen in the third trimester, but can be seen in the postpartum period. After careful examination, treatment includes reassurance, as the majority of patients gradually improve within three months. Corticosteroids and acyclovir should be considered for treatment to shorten the course and limit long-term sequelae. Both have been used safely in pregnancy. Bell's palsy may be a presenting feature of preeclampsia, probably related to edema. All patients with Bell's palsy are at risk for eye dryness and corneal injury, therefore artificial tears during the day and a lubricant at night is recommended.

Carpal tunnel syndrome (CTS)

The edema from fluid retention in pregnancy can predispose women to median nerve entrapment causing CTS. The symptoms can first present in the postpartum period and may last until after weaning in breastfeeding women. Due to the transient nature of CTS in the postpartum period, conservative management is recommended. This includes wrist splints, modifications of daily activities that exacerbate symptoms, and NSAIDs. As in nonpregnant patients, hypothyroidism should be excluded.

de Quervain tenosynovitis

Stenosing tenosynovitis of the first dorsal compartment of the wrist, known as de Quervain tenosynovitis, may occur during the postpartum period due to repetitive activities in newborn care. Ice and NSAIDs and physical and/or occupational therapy may be used for symptomatic relief.

Lumbosacral spine and lower extremity nerve injuries

While rare, stretch and compression nerve injuries may occur during vaginal and cesarean section deliveries. Risk of these injuries is increased by prolonged labor and fetal macrosomia or malposition. Lateral femoral cutaneous nerve injury (also known as meralgiaparesthetica) is a sensory-only deficit of the anterolateral thigh that is a common postpartum complaint. Femoral nerve injury can cause decreased sensation in the anterolateral thigh and medial calf along with impaired knee extension. Common peroneal nerve injury causes decreased sensation at the anterloateral calf and dorsum of the foot and foot drop. Obturator nerve injury causes decreased sensation to the medial thigh and decreased adduction of the leg. Prognosis from these injuries is typically good, and physical therapy may play a role in recovery.

POST PARTUM SEIZURES

Seizures that occur in the postpartum period may be due to an acute condition such as a cerebrovascuclar injury, eclampsia, or from chronic epilepsy. Regardless of cause, the initial approach to a postpartum seizure is to stabilize the patient and then promptly determine the etiology for long term management and prevention.

Eclampsia

Once a seizure occurs in a preeclamptic patient the diagnosis is changed to eclampsia. This potentially life-threatening manifestation of preeclampsia typically occurs as a grand mal tonic-clonic seizure. Eclampsia may also occur without preceding signs of preeclampsia such as hypertension and proteinuria. Eclamptic seizures may occur several weeks into the postpartum period. Magnesium sulfate, given as a 2 gm bolus, then as a 1 to 2 gm per hour IV infusion, has been shown in two randomized controlled trials to be superior to phenytoin for prevention of recurrent seizures. Benzodiazepines or rapidly-acting antiepileptic drugs (AEDs), such as phenytoin, may be needed to terminate an eclamptic seizure. If IV access cannot be achieved, magnesium can be administered intramuscularly. It is important to closely monitor creatinine and magnesium levels, since magnesium is excreted renally and eclampsia can be accompanied by progressive renal failure. Respiratory depression from magnesium toxicity can be reversed with IV calcium administration.

Epilepsy

Patients with a history of a chronic seizure disorder may have an increased frequency of seizure activity in the postpartum period due to sleep deprivation and stress. If a patient required increased doses of AEDs during pregnancy, then dosage adjustments are commonly required in the postpartum period as the mother's metabolism returns to the prepregnancy state. The increased volume of distribution and the increased renal and hepatic clearance may have required increased dosing during pregnancy. The AEDs approved by the American Academy of Pediatrics for use with breastfeeding are carbamazepine, ethosuximide, phenytoin, and valproic acid.

AUTOIMMUNE DISEASES

Management of autoimmune diseases represents unique clinical challenges in the postpartum period. Understanding their basic pathophysiology and how they are affected by pregnancy and the postpartum period may help guide their management.

Myasthenia gravis (MG)

In myasthenia gravis, autoantibodies made to acetylcholine receptors at the neuromuscular junction cause weakness and fatigue. The condition is most common in women during their childbearing years. The course of MG in pregnancy and postpartum is unpredictable with documented improvements and exacerbations in several studies. Acetylcholine receptor antibodies are IgG that cross the placenta and so can cause fetal or neonatal myasthenia. Risk factors for maternal exacerbations include a prepregnancy history of moderate to severe disease and puerperal infections. The potential for exacerbation of MG postpartum may be increased by the stress and anxiety of labor or surgery (cesarean section) with anesthesia and by postpartum exhaustion. If a patient with MG is suspected to have preeclampsia or eclampsia, magnesium sulfate should not be used for seizure prophylaxis. Magnesium sulfate can interfere with neuromuscular transmission, which can cause respiratory failure and potentially maternal death. In the postpartum period, close follow-up with enforcement of maternal rest is essential. Corticosteroids, plasmapheresis, and IV human immunoglobulins (IVIG) can be safely administered for postpartum exacerbations and is compatible with breastfeeding.

Multiple sclerosis (MS)

Multiple sclerosis is a chronic demyelinating disease of the CNS thought to involve an autoimmune response directed against myelin antigens. MS also typically presents during the reproductive years and shows a female preponderance of 3:1. The majority of patients with MS show improvement during pregnancy. After delivery, however there is a reverting of the immune system to its balance between a cell-mediated and antibody-mediated system, making MS flairs more likely. Epidural anesthesia and breastfeeding have not been shown to increase risk for a MS relapse. Corticosteroids and IVIG can be safely used for postpartum relapse.

Rheumatoid arthritis (RA)

The systemic inflammatory disease, RA, typically improves during pregnancy but flares during the postpartum period. The cause of postpartum flare is multifactorial including the return of prepregnancy immune function, cytokine production, and the proinflammatory affects of prolactin. Patients with RA should be warned about a potential increase in RA relapse with breastfeeding. Treatments of postpartum RA flairs that are safe with breastfeeding include NSAIDS, corticosteroids, hydroxychloroquine, and sulfasalazine. There is little information currently available regarding the safety of TNF-alpha antagonists and breastfeeding.

Systemic lupus erythematosus (SLE)

SLE is a chronic inflammatory condition of autoantibodies that affects multiple organ systems. Unlike other autoimmune diseases, there is less evidence for increased risk of flares during pregnancy or postpartum. Laboratory findings of a SLE flare, which differentiate it from preeclampsia include decreased complement level and increased titers of anti-DNA antibodies and other suggestive symptoms including arthritis, rash, and fatigue. There are numerous case reports of catastrophic postpartum syndromes in SLE patients, both with and without antiphospholipid antibodies. Patients with known SLE or in whom SLE is suspected who become ill postpartum may need immediate ICU level intervention for SLE pneumonitis/pleuritis, cerebritis, diffuse thrombosis, and antiphospholipid antibody syndrome. Immediate treatment with steroids, IVIgG, and biologics may be needed. Evaluation for pulmonary hemorrhage, if suspected, prior to anticoagulation, should be considered.

ENDOCRINOPATHIES

Thyroid disorders

Thyroid disease is common in women of childbearing age. Pregnant women with hypothyroidism require at least a 30%

increase in dose, and patients with Graves disease may require decreasing doses of antithyroid medications toward term. After delivery, these patients need close follow-up and readjustment of medications. Postpartum thyroiditis (PPT) is a common autoimmune disease, affecting around 7% of postpartum women. Patients with a history of type I diabetes mellitus have a higher incidence of PPT, of up to 25%. Patients with TPO antibodies independent of thyroid status may be at significant risk of postpartum thyroiditis. Patients with PPT may experience symptoms of both hyper- and hypothyroidism and are at increased risk for permanent hypothyroidism. During the hyperthyroid phase, beta-blockers may be used if a patient is symptomatic with palpitations, heat intolerance, and/or nervous or racing thoughts. The duration of this treatment is short, typically up to two months. Treatment during the hypothyroid phase depends on patient symptoms and the TSH level. All patients with a TSH greater than 10 should be treated with thyroxine. Patients with levels less than 10 who are symptomatic or whose TSH is between 4 and 10 and wish to conceive, should also be treated. Close follow-up will be needed, so that patients with permanent hypothyroidism are not lost to follow-up, and patients with subclinical hypothyroidism will conceive on adequate thyroid replacement for normal fetal brain development.

Diabetes mellitus

The incidence of diabetes mellitus in pregnancy is high, affecting about 7% of pregnancies in the United States. The majority (90%) of cases are due to gestational diabetes. In the postpartum period, the diabetic patient requires close and early follow-up. Medication regimens for gestational and preexisting (type I and type II) diabetes are typically adjusted in the immediate postpartum period. Insulin requirements rapidly decrease after delivery. Typically, one-half to two-thirds of the dose of insulin needed prepregnancy is used initially in the postpartum period. Patients with gestational diabetes who required insulin during pregnancy, rarely require insulin in the postpartum period. All patients with gestational diabetes should be counseled regarding their risk for developing type II diabetes, with the risk of up to 60% development within 15 years of delivery.

CARDIOVASCULAR AND RENAL DISEASE

With the rise of obesity and maternal age in the population of women giving birth in the United States, there has also been a steady increase in the rates of preexisting and pregnancy-induced hypertension. Women with a history of chronic hypertension are at increased risk for developing preeclampsia.

Preeclampsia

Preeclampsia is a syndrome unique to pregnancy defined as hypertension (> 140/90) occurring after the twentieth week of gestation with proteinuria (> 300 mg/24 hours). Up to one-third of preeclampsia occurs in the postpartum period, within six weeks of delivery. The management of postpartum preeclampsia is similar to the management antepartum, with attention to blood pressure control and monitoring for signs of central nervous system (seizure), renal and hepatic dysfunction, and pulmonary edema. (See Chapter 223 Common Medical Problems in Pregnancy.) Blood pressure may take several weeks to normalize in the postpartum period and proteinuria may last for several months. Preeclamptic patients should be educated on their long-term cardiovascular risks, as they are twice as likely to develop chronic hypertension, ischemic heart disease, and stroke.

Chronic hypertension

The postpartum patient typically returns to her prepregnancy blood pressure within three to five weeks, but it may take as long as three to six months to stabilize to prepregnancy levels. If a patient with chronic hypertension did not require any medication during pregnancy, due to the physiologic fall in blood pressure, she will likely need to be restarted on an agent within this timeframe. There are numerous antihypertensive agents that are compatible with breastfeeding including beta-blockers, ace-inhibitors (enalapril and captopril), and calcium channel blockers.

VTE and cardiac disease

Venous thromboembolic disease occurs with increased frequency during pregnancy, and pulmonary embolism is more common postpartum. Cesarean section, thrombophilia, prolonged bed rest, obesity, metabolic syndrome, family history, and smoking all increase the risk for postpartum PE. The use of mechanical or pharmacologic thromboprophylaxis should be considered in the postpartum depending on overall risk for a thromboembolic event. Please refer to a full discussion of VTE in pregnancy in Chapter 223 Common Medical Problems in Pregnancy.

Peripartum cardiomyopathy is defined as dilated cardiomyopathy with no other known cause, with onset in the last month of pregnancy or within five months postpartum. (See Chapter 222 Critical Care of the Pregnant Patient.) Treatment should be with vasodilators, diuretics, and sodium restriction. Prior to delivery, hydralazine and nitrates should be used rather than angiotensin converting enzyme inhibitors, which have adverse fetal renal effects at all stages of gestation. After delivery, enalapril and captopril are considered compatible with breastfeeding. Anticoagulation should be initiated if ejection fraction is less than 35%, or mural thrombus or atrial fibrillation is demonstrated, as thrombosis is a major cause of mortality in these patients.

Postpartum depression and psychosis

Clinicians face the difficult task of separating common mood disturbances in the postpartum from symptoms of depression and other severe mental health disorders. Chapter 223 Common Medical Problems in Pregnancy discusses these mental health issues and treatment.

CONCLUSION

Hospitalists are often asked to make recommendations for postpartum patients hospitalized with medical illness. It is therefore important to differentiate normal changes that occur during the six month postpartum period from disease states for which the patient may be at increased risk. In addition, clinicians need to pay particular attention to medications whose metabolism may change after delivery when there is a return to the prepregnancy state, and how these and any new medications may impact the breastfed infant. Although the list of postpartum symptoms could be extensive, this chapter reviews the most common issues the internist is likely to face when caring for postpartum patients and when a multidisciplinary approach is required. When there is uncertainly about diagnosis or the question being asked, clinicians are encouraged to consult with the appropriate specialist.

Evidence

Cardiology

Bellamy L, Casas JP, Hingorani AD. Pre-eclampsia and risk of cardiovascular disease and cancer in later life: systematic review and meta-analysis. *BMJ*. 2007;335;974–985.

Harskaqmp RE, Zeeman GG. Preeclampsia: at risk for remote cardiovascular disease. *Am J Med Sci*. 2007:334:291–295.

Yoder SR, Thornburg LL, Bisognano JD. Hypertension in pregnancy and women of childbearing age. *Am J Med*. 2009;122:890–895.

Endocrine

Abalovich M, Amino N, Barbour LA, et al. Management of thyroid dysfunction during pregnancy and postpartum: an Endocrine Society Clinical Practice Guideline. *J Clin Endocrinol Metab*. 2007;92(8 Suppl):S1–47.

Baptiste-Roberts K, Barone BB, Gary TL, et al. Risk factors for type 2 diabetes among women with gestational diabetes: a systematic review. *Am J Med*. 2009;122(3):207–214.

Gerstein HC. Incidence of postpartum thyroid dysfunction in patients with type I diabetes mellitus. *Ann Intern Med*. 118:419–423.

Kim C, Newton KM, Knopp RH. Gestational diabetes and the incidence of type 2 diabetes: a systematic review. *Diabetes Care*. 2002;25:1862–1868.

Neurology

Agostoni E. Headache in cerebral vein thrombosis. *Neurol Sci*. 2004:25(suppl 3):S206–S210.

Batocchi AP, Majolini L, Evoli A, et al. Course and treatment of myasthenia gravis during pregnancy. *Neurology*. 1999;52(3):447–452.

Confavreux C, Hutchinson M, Hours MM, et al. Rate of pregnancy–related relapse in multiple sclerosis. *NEJM*. 1998;339(5):285–291.

Coutinho JM, Ferro JM, Canhao P, et al. Cerebral venous and sinus thrombosis in women. *Stroke*. 2009;40:2356–2361.

Djelmis J, Sostarko M, Mayer D, et al. Myasthenia gravis in pregnancy: report on 69 cases. *Eur J Obstet Gynecol Reprod Biol*. 2002;104(1):21–25.

Giraud P, Chauvet S. Cluster headache during pregnancy: case report and literature review. *Headache*. 2009:136–139.

Hinchey J, Chaves C, Appignani B, et al. A reversible posterior leukoencephalopathy syndrome. *N Engl J Med*. 1996;334:494–500.

Hughes M.D. Multiple sclerosis and pregnancy. *Neurol Clin*. 2004;22:757–769.

Jurgens TP, Schaefer C, May A. Treatment of cluster headache in pregnancy and lactation. *Cephalalgia*. 2009;29:391–400.

Ko ML, Pan HS, Huang LW. Posterior reversible encephalopathy syndrome in a pregnant woman. *Taiwan J Obstet Gynecol*. 2008;47(1):98–100.

Lay CL, Broner SW. Migraine in women. *Neurol Clin*. 2009;27:503–511.

Marcus DA, Scharff L, Turk D. Longitudinal prospective study of headache during pregnancy and postpartum. *Headache*. 1999;39:625–632.

Marks DR, Rapoport AM. Practical evaluation and diagnosis of headache. *Semin. Neurol*. 1997;17:307–312.

Menon R, Bushnell CD. Headache and pregnancy. *The Neurologist*. 2008;14:2:108–119.

Noseworthy JH, Lucchinetti C, Rodriguez M, et al. Multiple sclerosis. *N Eng J Med*. 2000;343(13):938–952.

Rasmussen B. Migraine and tension-type headache in a general population: precipitating factors, female hormones, sleep patterns and relation to lifestyles. *Pain*. 1993;53:65–72.

Riviello C, Ammannati F, Bordi L. Pregnancy and subarachnoid hemorrhage: a case report. *The J Mat–Fetal and Neonatal Med*. 2004;16:245–246.

Schwartz RB, Bravo SM, Klufas RA, et al. Cyclosporine neurotoxicity and its relationship to hypertensive encephalopathy: CT and MR findings in 16 cases. *AJR Am J Roentgenol*. 1995;165:627–631.

Schwartz RB, Jones KM, Kalina P, et al. Hypertensive encephalopathy: findings on CT, MR imaging, and SPECT imaging in 14 cases. *AJR Am J Roentgenol*. 1992;159:379–383.

Stam J. Thrombosis of the cerebral veins and sinuses. *New Eng J Med*. 2005;352:1791–1798.

Stein GS. Headaches in the first post-partum week and their relationships to migraine. *Headache*. 1981;21:201–205.

Van de Velde M, Schepers R, Berends N, et al. Ten years of experience with accidental dural puncture and post-dural puncture headache in a tertiary obstetric anaesthesia department. *Int. J Ob Anesthesia*. 2009;17:329–335.

van Gijn J, Kerr RS, Rinkel GJE. Subarachnoid haemorrhage. *Lancet*. 2007;369:306–318.

Vukusic S, Hutchinson M, Hours M, et al. Pregnancy and multiple sclerosis (the PRIMS study): clinical predictors of post-partum relapse. *Brain*. 2004;127(Pt 6):1353–1360.

Wong CA, Scavone BM, Dugan S, et al. Incidence of postpartum lumbosacral spine and lower extremity nerve injuries. *Obstets & Gynecol*. 2003;101:279–288.

Rheumatology

Barrett JH, Brennan P, Fiddler M, et al. Breast-Feeding and postpartum relapse in women with rheumatoid and inflammatory arthritis. *Arthritis Rheum*. 2000;43:1010–1015.

Batocchi AP, Majolini L, Evoli A, et al. Course and treatment of myasthenia gravis during pregnancy. *Neurology*. 1999;52(3):447–452.

Confavreux C, Hutchinson M, Hours MM, et al. Rate of pregnancy– related relapse in multiple sclerosis. *NEJM*. 1998;339(5):285–291.

Djelmis J, Sostarko M, Mayer D, et al. Myasthenia gravis in pregnancy: report on 69 cases. *Eur J Obstet Gynecol Reprod Biol*. 2002;104(1):21–25.

Zoli A, Lizzio MM, Ferlisi EM, et al. ACTH, cortisol and prolactin in active rheumatoid arthritis. *Clin Rheumatol*. 2002;21(4):289–293. 2005;352:1791–1798.

SUGGESTED READINGS

Berg CJ, MacKay AP, Qin C, et al. Overview of maternal morbidity during hospitalization for labor and delivery in the United States 1993–1997 and 2001–2005. *Obstet Gynecol.* 2009;113:1075–1081.

Burrows LJ, Meyn LA, Weber AM. Maternal morbidity associated with vaginal versus cesarean delivery. *Obstet Gynecol.* 2004;103(5.1): 907–912.

Ely JW, Rijhsinghani A, Bowdler NC, et al. The association between manual removal of the placenta and postpartum endometritis following vaginal delivery. *Obset Gynecol.* 1995;86(6):1002–1006.

Eschenbach DA, Rosene K, Tompkins LS, et al. Endometrial cultures obtained by a triple-lumen method from afrebile and febrile postpartum women. *J Infect Dis.* 1986;153:1038–1045.

Gordon JD, Rydfors J, Druzin M, et al. Infectious diseases. In: *Obstetrics, Gynecology and Infertility,* 6th ed. Arlington, VA: Scrub Hill Press; 2007:306.

Katz VL. Postpartum care. In: Gabbe SG, Niebyl JR, Simpson JL. *Obstetrics: Normal and Problem Pregnancies,* 5th ed. Philadelphia, PA: Churchill Livingstone; 2007:566–576.

Rosene K, Eschenbach DA, Tompkins LS, et al. Polymicrobial early postpartum endometritis with facultative and anaerobic bacteria, genital mycoplasmas, and chlamydia trachomatis: treatment with piperacillin or cefoxitin. *J Infect Dis.* 1986;153(6): 1028–1037.

Yokoe DS, Christiansen CL, Johnson R, et al. Epidemiology of and surveillance for postpartum infectious. *Emerg Infect Dis.* 2001;7(5): 837–841.

SECTION 14

Psychiatry

CHAPTER 225

Mood and Anxiety Disorders

Martha C. Ward, MD
Steven Garlow, MD, PhD

Key Clinical Questions

Depression

1. What are the signs and symptoms of a major depressive episode (MDE)?
2. What is the pathophysiology of major depression?
3. What medications, intoxicants, and diseases cause depressed mood?
4. What is adjustment disorder?
5. What is the appropriate diagnostic workup for a patient with depressive symptoms?
6. What is the treatment for major depressive disorder (MDD)?
7. What are the complications of antidepressant use?

Bipolar Disorder

1. What are the signs and symptoms of bipolar disorder?
2. What medical conditions and substances can induce mania?
3. What is the appropriate diagnostic workup for a patient with mania?
4. How is bipolar disorder treated?

Anxiety Disorers

1. What are the signs and symptoms of anxiety?
2. What are the common anxiety disorders?
3. How does generalized anxiety disorder differ from major depression?
4. What medical conditions present with symptoms of anxiety?
5. What studies should be ordered for the acutely anxious patient?
6. What is the treatment for anxiety?

DEPRESSION

INTRODUCTION

Major depressive disorder (MDD) is widespread and devastating, with lifetime prevalence greater than17% in the general population. Total costs exceed $44 billion annually, including hospitalization, medications, and loss of productivity. In medically ill patients, mood disorders are even more common; six-month prevalence increases from 5.8% to 9.4% with at least one chronic medical condition. Despite this, many physicians fail to address depressive symptoms, believing them to be appropriate in illness ("I would be depressed too, if I were that sick"). This misconception leads to poor outcomes, as physical recovery is impeded by affective disorders. This chapter will aid the hospitalist in recognition, diagnosis, and treatment of MDD.

CASE 225-1

A 66-year-old man with a history of type-2 diabetes, hypertension, and tobacco use was admitted for non-ST elevation MI and cardiac catheterization with stent placement. During morning rounds, his care team noted that the patient ate only about 10% of his breakfast and appeared to have a blunted affect. He had a history of multiple episodes of depressed mood, insomnia, and anhedonia over the years. The patient reported feeling "worthless" and sometimes wishing that he'd "just gone ahead and died." Though initially reluctant because of worries about dependence, Mr. G agreed to try an antidepressant, sertraline. At his 6-week post-hospitalization appointment he is free of mood symptoms, engaged in cardiac rehabilitation and feels hopeful about the future.

PATHOPHYSIOLOGY

The primary etiology of major depression remains obscure. Dysregulation of CNS monoamine neurotransmitters (including norepinephrine, serotonin, and dopamine) occurs in MDD. Newer theories focus on broader neuroregulatory circuits involving cholingeric activation, GABA hypoactivity, and chronically elevated hypothalamic-pituitary-adrenal activity. Immune system abnormalities and increased inflammation likely play a role.

DIAGNOSIS

MAJOR DEPRESSIVE DISORDER

Major depressive disorder is defined by the occurrence of one or more major depressive episodes (see **Table 225-1**). Though many patients will readily admit to feeling "sad" or "down," others may initially deny dysphoria, imagining this to reflect a weakness of character. Direct confrontation may not be fruitful, though observational statements made in a neutral tone might aid with patient disclosure ("you're upset"). In such cases, mood changes can also be determined by the presence of tearfulness or blunted affect. Depressed mood may also manifest as irritability, particularly in adolescence. However, caution must be taken not to label the angry patient "depressed" in the absence of other signs of MDD. There is a distinct quality and severity of mood in MDD that differs from mere sadness, and the patient who is simply despondent should likewise not be diagnosed with this disorder.

TABLE 225-1 Major Depressive Episode

A. Five (or more) symptoms present for two weeks with either (1) depressed mood or (2) loss of interest or pleasure:
   1. Depressed mood most of the day
   2. Diminished interest or pleasure in all, or almost all, activities
   3. Significant weight loss or gain (change in 5% body weight in one month) or decrease or increase in appetite
   4. Insomnia or hypersomnia
   5. Psychomotor agitation or retardation (observable by others)
   6. Fatigue or loss of energy
   7. Feelings of worthlessness or excessive guilt (not merely self-reproach about being sick)
   8. Diminished ability to think or concentrate, or indecisiveness
   9. Recurrent thoughts of death (not just fear of dying), recurrent suicidal ideation with or without a plan, or suicide attempt

B. The symptoms cause significant distress or impairment.

C. The symptoms are not due to the effects of a substance or a general medical condition.

D. The symptoms are not better accounted for by bereavement (ie, the symptoms persist for longer than two months after the death of a loved one or are characterized by marked functional impairment, feelings of worthlessness, suicidal thoughts, psychomotor retardation, or psychosis).

Loss of interest, or anhedonia, is the most common presenting symptom in MDD (particularly in the elderly). This can be difficult to identify in the context of hospitalization, where the patient's usual pleasurable activities are curtailed. Lack of engagement with family members or other visitors, as well as refusal to participate in physical therapy, may indicate anhedonia. Anorexia, fatigue, insomnia, and poor concentration may be easily attributed to the direct effects of medical illness. However, if a patient also shows depressed mood and lack of interest, these qualities should be counted toward the diagnosis of MDD. Assessment of insomnia should focus on pattern of sleep and activities during nighttime awakening, as sleeplessness in the hospital may be due to poorly controlled pain or frequent visits by nurses. Middle insomnia (waking in the night and not being able to return to sleep) and early awakening are more typical of depression, and patients often ruminate on negative thoughts. Guilt about illness is a common symptom. Patients may express concern about not meeting financial and interpersonal obligations or about being a burden to their loved ones.

Assessment of suicidality must be direct and avoid euphemisms such as "hurting yourself." Questions should elicit increasing levels of intent. First ask about passive ideation ("do you ever feel so bad that you wish you were not alive?"). When an affirmative is given, questioning should then focus on active suicidal thoughts and designs. If the patient has access to firearms or potentially toxic medications, a plan should be made for securing them prior to discharge.

Though not explicitly delineated in the DSM criteria, somatic complaints may be a manifestation of depression. Individuals with psychiatric pathology may experience physical discomfort out of proportion to the severity of medical disease. Patients may also have functional pain, consciously or unconsciously converting depressed mood into more culturally sanctioned symptoms.

SUBSTANCE-INDUCED MOOD DISORDER WITH DEPRESSIVE FEATURES

Medications and intoxicants can both cause depressive symptoms (see **Table 225-2**). Defining the temporal relationship between onset of mood disturbance and start of a new drug can help determine this correlation. **Table 225-3** lists commonly prescribed offending medications.

Chronic alcohol use leads to depressed mood. Forty percent of patients with an alcohol-related disorder meet criteria for MDD at some point in their lives. Diagnosis of major depression in the context of active alcohol use is difficult at best, and treatment with antidepressants in this situation can be deleterious and even dangerous. Abuse of other sedative-hypnotics (benzodiazepines and barbiturates), as well as opiates, can similarly produce a mood disturbance. Stimulants (cocaine and amphetamines) potentiate monoamine neurotransmitters, leading to depletion and subsequent depressed mood. Effects of stimulants on the brain linger for months to years following cessation.

Addicts usually downplay their drug and alcohol use. Inquiries into the frequency of ingestion and the amount consumed should always be grossly overestimated, thus normalizing the patient's admission. Surrogate clues must be obtained, including collateral from friends and family. Objective measures, such as a urine drug screen and serum ethanol level, may also provide further insight.

DEPRESSION DUE TO A GENERAL MEDICAL CONDITION (GMC)

To meet criteria for depression due to a GMC, it is not necessary to have symptoms for any duration of time or to exhibit a certain number of characteristics. Patients must simply display

TABLE 225-2 Substance-induced Mood Disorder with Depressive Features

A. A prominent and persistent disturbance in mood predominates in the clinical picture and is characterized by either
   1. depressed mood, or
   2. markedly diminished interest or pleasure in all, or almost all, activities.

B. There is evidence from the history, physical exam, or lab findings that the disturbance developed within a month of substance use or substance use is etiologically related to the disturbance.

C. The disturbance is not better accounted for by another mental disorder.

D. The disturbance does not occur exclusively in the context of a delirium.

E. The symptoms cause clinically significant distress or impairment in social, occupational, or other important areas of functioning.

TABLE 225-3 Pharmacological Causes of Depression

1. Interferon and other immunomodulators
2. Corticosteroids and hormones
3. Antineoplastic agents (antiestrogens, antiandrogens; to a lesser extent, vincristine, vinblastine, procarbazine, and asparaginase)
4. Neurological agents, such as levodopa and acetylcholinesterase inhibitors, as well as antiepileptics
5. Antipsychotics
6. Sedative-hypnotics
7. Analgesics (particularly opioids and NSAIDs)
8. Antibacterials (especially sulfonamides) and antifungals
9. Cardiovascular drugs: Antihypertensives (particularly β-blockers), digoxin

anhedonia or depressed mood that interferes with function and is directly caused by medical illness. When direct causality is not definite, patients should be diagnosed with MDD. However, this is purely a semantic differentiation and should not affect treatment decisions.

Heart disease and major depression are frequently comorbid. In hospitalized patients who have suffered a myocardial infarction (MI), 65% show depressive symptoms and 30% meet criteria for MDD. Depression in the post-MI period imparts a four- to six-fold increased risk of cardiac mortality at 6 and 18 months (independent of epidemiologic factors, medications, or severity of disease). Despite this, only 10% of post-MI patients are diagnosed with MDD in the hospital. This may be due to its anomalous presentation, with hostility and withdrawal more common. Unfortunately, depressed mood may be assessed as appropriate in patients suffering an MI, with many physicians stating, "I would be depressed too if I just had a heart attack." This conclusion is not only incorrect (as not all patients have post-MI MDD), but negligent, leading to unnecessary suffering and poor patient outcomes.

Mood symptoms are common in cancer, particularly in pancreatic carcinoma and other enteric malignancies. Rates increase in those with a prior psychiatric history. Depression may precede diagnosis, potentially caused by a paraneoplastic process or proinflammatory cytokines. Alternatively, mood changes may occur after cancer is discovered. Major depression can be difficult to differentiate from the existential crisis that arises from the diagnosis. In those without depression, hopelessness generally fades within the first three months. Determination of MDD can also be complicated by its significant symptom overlap with treatment side effects and the disease process itself. Fatigue is frequently described. Lethargy due to radiation and chemotherapy is cyclical, with recovery occurring as time from treatment increases. Fatigue in major depression is akin to amotivation, with difficulty starting tasks and prominent psychomotor retardation. Appropriate diagnosis is further waylaid by the hesitancy of patients to admit to mood changes. Those with cancer often take pride in coping with their illness and do not want to disappoint their doctors by showing signs of depression.

At least a third of stroke survivors experience depressive symptoms. The association is strongest in those with left hemispheric lesions, though physicians should screen for affective changes irrespective of vascular distribution. Degree of disability does not directly correlate to prevalence of mood disturbance, although post-stroke depression imparts greater functional impairment, with less recovery in activities of daily living. Major depression also confers increased overall mortality in this population.

TABLE 225-4 Depression Due to a General Medical Condition

A. A prominent and persistent disturbance in mood characterized by depressed mood or markedly diminished interest or pleasure in all, or almost all, activities
B. There is evidence from history, physical exam, or lab findings that the disturbance is a direct physiological consequence of a general medical condition.
C. The disturbance is not better accounted for by another mental disorder.
D. The disturbance does not occur exclusively during delirium.
E. The symptoms cause significant distress or impairment in social, occupational, or other important areas of functioning.

Autoimmune disease is closely linked to affective disorders. Close to half of individuals with systemic lupus erythematosus (SLE) meet criteria for MDD. Rates increase with greater disease severity and activity. Depressive symptoms are likely due to immune dysregulation, with proinflammatory cytokines modulating neural changes. Medications (particularly steroids) may also contribute to mood disturbance. Regardless of etiology, recognition and treatment is essential, as psychological distress in SLE leads to increased physical disability.

For a list of other medical diseases associated with depressed mood, see **Table 225-4**.

ADJUSTMENT DISORDER

Adjustment disorder is a pathologic response to a specific stressor (see **Table 225-5** for DSM IV criteria). Stressors may be multiple, such as financial strain in the context of physical disease. Patients with tumultuous childhoods (loss of a parent, unstable living situation) are particularly at risk for this disorder. It is important to note that this diagnosis cannot be made if the criteria for major depression are

TABLE 225-5 Diseases Associated with Depressed Mood

A. CNS Disease
   1. Stroke
   2. Dementia: Alzheimer, Huntington, Parkinson, Binswanger
   3. Traumatic brain injury
   4. Temporal lobe epilepsy
   5. Tumor
   6. Infections: encephalitis, hepatitis C, HIV
B. Endocrine disease
   1. Hypothyroidism
   2. Cushing's syndrome
   3. Hyper- or hypoparathyroidism
C. Rheumatologic disease
   1. Systemic lupus erythematosus
   2. Multiple sclerosis
   3. Psoriasis
   4. Rheumatoid arthritis
   5. Fibromyalgia
   6. Osteoarthritis
D. Cancer
E. Cardiovascular disease

met, or if mood symptoms are directly attributable to the effects of a substance or disease process.

DELIRIUM

Hypoactive delirium may be mistaken for MDD. Both disorders involve problems with memory, but patients with major depression will have insight and complain of the deficit. Disorientation in delirium may result in complete reversal of day-night sleep-wake cycle. Sleep changes also occur with MDD, but patients have consistent insomnia or hypersomnia. Delirium has an abrupt onset and a fluctuating course. Major depression may also have a relatively discrete onset. However, it rarely has a waxing and waning course (except for melancholic depression, in which mood improves as the day progresses). Unlike MDD, delirium manifests with poor attention and altered level of consciousness.

DIAGNOSTIC STUDIES

Laboratory evaluation of a patient with depressive symptoms can help to rule out an organic cause. A basic workup should include a complete blood count with differential, a comprehensive metabolic panel (including liver enzymes), thyroid stimulating hormone, an RPR, an HIV test, B12 and folate levels, electrocardiogram, serum ethanol level, and a urine drug screen. Physical exam should direct the judicious use of further testing, including CT or MRI of the brain, electroencephalogram, lumbar puncture, blood and urine cultures, chest X-ray, ANA panel and rheumatoid factor, and directed cancer screening. The patient's medication list should be carefully reviewed for possible pharmacologic causes of depression.

TREATMENT

GENERAL TREATMENT PRINCIPLES

There is no test that confirms the diagnosis of MDD. Likewise, there is no laboratory value that can be tracked to determine treatment response. Thus, target symptoms should be identified early and be well documented. This can assist subsequent care providers in determining the patient's baseline and progress. Because of the apparent subjective nature of this data, it may be helpful to administer a standardized rating scale at regular intervals. Clinician-rated scales, such as the Quick Inventory of Depressive Symptomatology (QIDS) Clinician Report, as well as patient-rated scales, such as the QIDS Self Report and Patient Health Questionnaire (PHQ)-9, are widely available.

While medication is an important treatment modality for depression, psychosocial interventions should be adjunctively employed whenever possible. This includes referrals to psychotherapy as well as to support groups. Some patients may also benefit from meeting with the hospital chaplain. When end-of-life issues arise, palliative care teams are extremely helpful.

Patient education is essential. Physicians should discuss diagnosis, target symptoms, and treatment options. Serious side-effects should be addressed, but not overemphasized. If a patient is reluctant to start treatment, the rationale should be elicited. Many are hesitant to take antidepressants because of social stigma or misconceptions concerning drug dependence and personality changes.

Most classes of antidepressants have been shown to have roughly equal efficacy. Thus, initial selection of pharmacotherapy should focus on previous treatment success, family history of medication response, safety, tolerability, cost, and patient preference. Once a medication has been started, the goal is to titrate to an adequate dose and treat for an adequate period of time. The therapeutic dose differs based on physiology, and for the elderly may be lower than recommended doses. An adequate medication trial is usually defined as 8 to 12 weeks at the therapeutic dose. However, if there is no response after 4 to 5 weeks, a change in medication may be necessary. Duration of treatment for the first major depressive episode should be at least 12 months. In patients with recurrent episodes or depression due to a noncurable illness, lifelong treatment may be necessary. If a patient has been stable on a medication for years but decompensates when faced with a physical or emotional crisis, sudden discontinuation of the previously effective medication should be avoided. Instead, short-term interventions, such as dose increase or augmentation, should be employed.

SELECTIVE SEROTONIN REUPTAKE INHIBITORS (SSRIs), SEROTONIN-NOREPINEPHRINE REUPTAKE INHIBITORS (SNRIs), AND OTHER ANTIDEPRESSANTS

Because of their tolerability, efficacy, and ease of dosing, the SSRIs are first-line treatment for major depression. The SNRIs (venlafaxine and duloxetine) may be a good choice for individuals with chronic pain because of the inhibitory effect of norepinephrine and serotonin on descending sensory neurons.

Other treatment options include nefazodone, trazodone, mirtazapine, and buproprion. Because it lowers the seizure threshold in a dose-dependent manner, buproprion should not be prescribed for patients with epilepsy, heavy alcohol use, or structural brain anomaly. Unlike the SSRIs, buproprion does not cause sexual dysfunction or weight gain. It can also aid in smoking cessation.

See **Table 225-6** for more information on the individual characteristic of these antidepressants.

TRICYCLIC ANTIDEPRESSANTS (TCAs)

The TCAs inhibit reuptake of norepinephrine and serotonin. These medications have significant anticholinergic, antihistaminergic, and antiadrenergic actions. The tertiary amines include amitriptylene, imipramine, trimipramine, doxepin, and chlomipramine. Desipramine, nortriptylene, and protriptylene are secondary amines. The secondary amines are less sedating and have less anticholinergic activity than the tertiary amines. At therapeutic doses, these medications have good efficacy. However, their use is often limited by side effects and drug interactions. Addition of medications that inhibit cytochrome p450 2D6 may cause serum TCA levels to rise to dangerous levels. Initiation of the tricyclics should occur in consultation with psychiatry. Medically ill patients who are maintained on TCAs should have cardiac monitoring, with daily repletion of potassium and magnesium.

TABLE 225-6 Adjustment Disorder

A. The development of emotional or behavioral symptoms in response to an identifiable stressor(s) occurring within three months of the onset of the stressor(s)
B. These symptoms or behaviors are clinically significant as evidenced by
   1. marked distress, in excess of what would be expected from stressor, or
   2. significant impairment in social or occupational functioning.
C. The disturbance does not meet criteria for another Axis I or II disorder.
D. The symptoms do not represent bereavement.
E. Once the stressor has ended, symptoms do not persist for greater than six months.

MONOAMINE OXIDASE INHIBITORS

Monoamine oxidase (MAO) degrades biogenic amines in the CNS and GI tract. Phenelzine, tranylcypromine, isocarboxazid, and selegeline inhibit this enzyme. Despite their efficacy (particularly in atypical and anxious depression), these medications are considered third-line because of their adverse side effect profile as well as medication and food interactions. Monoamine oxidase inhibitors (MAOIs) can cause severe orthostasis, as well as sexual side effects, insomnia, headache, dizziness, dry mouth, and constipation. Ingestion of tyramine (present in aged cheeses, smoked or cured meats, wine, and beer) while taking an MAOI can lead to hypertensive emergency. Malignant hypertension is more likely to occur when MAOIs are taken with sympathomimetics and certain anesthetics (especially meperidine). Combination of MAOIs with other serotonergic agents can cause serotonin syndrome (see discussion below). Use of MAOIs should occur in consultation with psychiatry.

ELECTROCONVULSIVE THERAPY (ECT)

ECT consists of the delivery of electricity to a patient's scalp in order to produce seizure activity. The patient is placed under general anesthesia and a neuromuscular blocking agent is given to inhibit muscle contraction. ECT is generally indicated for treatment-resistant depression and for states when immediate results are necessary for the patient's safety, such as suicidality, catatonia, or psychosis. Side effects include headache, dysphoria, muscle aches, and memory loss. Retrograde amnesia may be permanent. There are no absolute contraindications to ECT, and most of the risk ensues from anesthesia. Unstable cardiac or cerebrovascular disease increases risk. However, ECT is an efficacious and well-tolerated procedure for medically ill patients with severe depression who do not respond to pharmacotherapy or who cannot tolerate medication side effects.

SUBSTANCE-INDUCED DEPRESSION

Necessary medications may cause depressive symptoms. When this is suspected, treatment substitutions or dose reduction (particularly with steroids) should be considered. If this is not possible, then the provider must take into account duration of treatment with the offending agent, level of dysfunction caused by mood symptoms, and patient willingness to add another medication. Certain medications (such as interferon) are notorious for inducing mood symptoms, and prophylactic treatment with an antidepressant is recommended. There are improved outcomes with administration of paroxetine prior to initiation of interferon-α for hepatitis C infection.

When depression is caused by an intoxicant, the best course of action is clearly to discontinue its ingestion. Unfortunately, this is not often so simple. Patients with addiction may be unwilling (or unable) to quit using drugs and alcohol. Treatment with antidepressants in the context of continued intoxication will provide no relief of depressive symptoms and will not prevent the patient from using. When sobriety has been confirmed, yet depressive symptoms persist, there is no clear consensus as to time until treatment initiation. One reasonable approach would be to wait about four weeks after cessation to begin treatment for depression, particularly when the mood symptoms are causing impairment of function or extreme distress.

DEPRESSION DUE TO A GENERAL MEDICAL CONDITION

If a medical condition is permanent and causes major depression, then pharmacotherapy should not be delayed. In cases in which medical illness is thought to be short-lived, the physician must consider the effects of the mood symptoms on the course of illness and the patient's quality of life. If mood symptoms cause suffering or worsen medical disease, treatment is indicated. The high prevalence of major depression in certain conditions may event merit prophylactic antidepressant use. In acute stroke survivors, there is evidence for prophylactic use of escitalopram.

TREATMENT OF DEPRESSION IN THE MEDICALLY ILL

CARDIOVASCULAR DISEASE

The tricyclic antidepressants should likely be avoided in cardiovascular disease. Like class 1A antiarrythmics, these drugs may slow ventricular conduction by blocking sodium channels. This can lead to PR, QRS, and QT prolongation, torsades de pointes, and sudden cardiac death. Tricyclics also block myocardial muscarinic receptors, which can lead to tachycardia. The TCAs, like the MAOIs and trazodone, can also cause orthostasis. Conversely, venlafaxine and bupropion may elevate blood pressure, and should likely be avoided in patients with poorly-controlled hypertension. Fluoxetine can cause bradycardia when used with β-blockers. The SSRIs and mirtazapine are likely good first-line agents for the patient with cardiovascular disease.

DIABETES MELLITUS

Fluoxetine has been shown to decrease mean blood glucose and hemoglobin A1C levels. The TCAs can worsen glycemic control. However, their modulation of descending pain tracts may alleviate symptoms of peripheral neuropathy. MAOIs can interact with oral diabetes medications to potentiate hypoglycemia, and thus should be avoided in patients taking sulfonylureas and thiazolidinediones.

HEPATIC DISEASE

Nefazodone may induce fulminant hepatic failure (albeit rarely) and carries a boxed warning to this effect. Nearly all of the antidepressants (with the exception of escitalopram and to a lesser extent sertraline) are cleared through the CYP p450 system and thus doses should be decreased in liver impairment.

RENAL INSUFFICIENCY

Renal disease may slow clearance of medications, including antidepressants. Thus, dosage adjustments may be made. SSRIs and bupropion are the treatment of choice for patients with kidney failure.

COMPLICATIONS OF ANTIDEPRESSANT USE

SUICIDALITY

The SSRIs carry a boxed warning concerning a risk of increased suicidal thinking and behavior in young adults. This is likely due to the activating properties of these medications. Patients must be warned of this possibility when starting treatment.

SEROTONIN SYNDROME

Use of serotonergic agents may cause autonomic hyperactivity (tachycardia, mydriasis, diarrhea, hyperthermia), neuromuscular abnormalities (tremor, clonus), and mental status changes (agitation, delirium). Certain drug combinations are more likely to cause toxicity, including MAOIs with SSRIs or TCAs. Meperedine, fentanyl, tramadol, ondansetron, metoclopramide, dextromethorphan, and MDMA have also been triggers of this syndrome. Once the offending medications are discontinued, treatment is largely supportive. Benzodiazepines may be given to decrease agitation. Serotonin antagonists, such as cyproheptadine, olanzapine, and chlorpromazine may also be beneficial. In extreme cases, intubation and paralysis should be initiated.

TABLE 225-7 Properties of First-line Antidepressants

Medication	Dosing	Half-life	P450 Inhibition	Side Effects and Toxicity
SSRIs				
Fluoxetine	20–80 mg	24–72 hrs, metabolite 4–16 days	2D6, 2C moderate 1A2, 3A	Initial anxiety, insomnia, sexual dysfunction
Paroxetine	10–50 mg	20 hrs	Strong 2D6	Nausea, headache, somnolence, dry mouth, constipation, dizziness
Sertraline	50–200 mg	24–26 hrs, metabolite 66 hrs	Minimal	Gastrointestinal upset, sleep disturbance, headache, sexual dysfunction
Citalopram	10–40 mg	33 hrs	Moderate 2D6	Nausea, vomiting, increased sweating, dry mouth, headache, ejaculatory failure
Escitalopram	10–20 mg	42 hrs	Minimal	Nausea, diarrhea, insomnia, dry mouth, ejaculatory failure
Fluvoxamine	50–300 mg	15 hrs	Strong 1A2, 3A, 2C	Nausea
SNRIs				
Venlafaxine	37.5–225 mg	4 hrs, metabolite 10 hrs	Minimal	Nausea, dizziness, somnolence, insomnia, nervousness, HTN
Duloxetine	40–120 mg	12 hrs	Moderate 2D6	Nausea, dry mouth, dizziness, headache, somnolence, constipation, insomnia
Other				
Trazodone	150–400 mg	5–9 hrs, metabolite 4–14 hrs	Minimal	Sedation, orthostasis, priapism in 1/6000 males, may decrease INR in patients taking coumadin
Nefazodone	200–600 mg	2–4 hrs, metabolite 18 hrs	Strong 3A	Dry mouth, sedation, dizziness, nausea, constipation, rare liver failure
Mirtazapine	7.5–45 mg	20–40 hrs	Minimal	Somnolence, increased appetite, weight gain
Buproprion	150–400 mg	21 hrs, metabolite 43 hrs	Strong 2D6	Headache, nausea, dry mouth, insomnia, agitation, lowers seizure threshold

SSRI/SNRI DISCONTINUATION SYNDROME

Abrupt discontinuation of SSRIs and SNRIs has been associated with flu like symptoms, myoclonus, electrical sensations, and psychological distress. Symptoms may last up to two weeks, and while uncomfortable, are not dangerous. This syndrome is more likely to occur with agents that have a short half-life, such as paroxetine, sertraline, fluvoxamine, and venlafaxine. It is best to taper these medications over a few weeks.

OVERDOSE

As little as 10 times the daily dose of a TCA can be fatal. Death is most frequently caused by cardiac arrhythmia, though seizures and CNS depression also occur. MAOIs can induce hypertensive emergency in overdose. SSRIs are relatively benign when taken in excess, with very low risk of cardiovascular and CNS toxicity (**Table 225-7**).

DISCHARGE PLANNING

Patients with a good response to antidepressants may be treated by their primary care physician. If there is a partial response or treatment failure after an adequate trial of more than one antidepressant, psychiatric referrals should be made. Suicidal patients require psychiatric hospitalization. The patient's cooperation with a voluntary admission is preferable, but involuntary status should be obtained for any patient who is a danger to himself or others. Additionally, patients who are unable to care for themselves due to the severity of their depression should be transferred to a mental health facility.

DISPARITIES IN HEALTH CARE

The prevalence of depression is largely uniform in African American, Latino, and Caucasian groups in the US. Despite this, African Americans and Latinos have lower odds than whites of being diagnosed and treated for depression. African Americans and Latinos more often present with somatic complaints rather than mood symptoms, and nonwhite patients have been shown to be less likely to accept therapy for depression. In the Latino population, language barriers and poor health literacy may also complicate appropriate diagnosis.

PROGNOSIS

MDD is a chronic illness. Up to 75% of patients will have a second major depressive episode within five years from their initial event, though rates decrease with antidepressant treatment. In untreated MDD, relapse becomes increasingly frequent and severe (**Table 225-8**).

BIPOLAR DISORDER

INTRODUCTION

Bipolar disorder is a catastrophic chronic illness. Despite a lifetime prevalence of just 1% in the general population, it incurs a significant financial burden with total costs exceeding $45 billion per year in the U.S. Prevention of mood cycling through stable pharmacotherapy is crucial. Mania, whether primary (in bipolar disorder) or secondary to an organic cause, is a psychiatric emergency that can complicate the course of treatment for the

TABLE 225-8 Evidence for Heart Disease and Major Depression

Study	Methodology	Results	Limitations
Depressed affect, hopelessness, and the risk of ischemic heart disease in a cohort of U.S. adults. Anda R, et al. *Epidemiology*. 1993;4:285–294.	Study of cohort of 2,832 U.S. adults age 45–77 years who participated in the National Health Examination Follow-up Study (mean follow-up = 12.4 years).	Depressed affect was associated with an increased risk of fatal ischemic heart disease [relative risk = 1.5; 95% confidence interval (CI) = 1.0–2.3].	Self-report of depressive symptoms without structured clinical interview
Symptoms of depression, acute myocardial infarction, and total mortality in a community sample. Barefoot JC, et al. *Circulation*. 1996;93:1976–1980.	Prospective, observational study of 409 men and 321 women who were residents of Glostrup, Denmark, born in 1914. Physical and psychological examinations were done in 1964 and 1974 and patients were followed for incidence of MI until 1991.	A 2-SD difference in depression score on the obvious depression scale was associated with relative risk of 1.71 ($P = .005$) for MI. Findings were unchanged after controlling for risk factors and signs of heart disease at baseline.	Homogeneous study population, self-report of depression without structured clinical interview
Precursors study. Ford DE, et al. *Arch Int Med*. 1998;158:1422–1460.	Prospective, observational study of 1190 male medical students.	The men who reported clinical depression were at significantly greater risk for subsequent coronary heart disease (relative risk [RR], 2.12; 95% confidence interval [CI], 1.24–3.63) and myocardial infarction (RR, 2.12; 95% CI, 1.11–4.06).	Self-report of depression without structured clinical interview, diagnosis of depression not based on DSM criteria, high SES and male only study population
Major depressive disorder predicts cardiac events in patients with coronary artery disease. Carney RM, et al. *Psychosomatic Medicine*. 1988;50:627–633.	Prospective cohort study of 52 patients undergoing cardiac catheterization and subsequently found to have significant coronary artery disease. Patients were given structured psychiatric interviews before catheterization and contacted 12 months after catheterization, and the occurrence of myocardial infarction, angioplasty, coronary bypass surgery, and death was determined.	Overall, 77.8% of the MDD patients and 34.9% of the non-MDD patients had at least one major cardiac event (relative risk 2.2, $p < 0.02$). Univariate analysis of cardiac risk factors and MDD was performed. MDD produced the strongest correlation ($r = 0.40$) with the occurrence of major endpoints.	Small sample size, statistically significant increased prevalence of smoking in group with MDD compared to those without MDD
Depression following myocardial infarction: impact on 6-month survival. Frasure-Smith N, et al. *JAMA*. 1993;270:1819–1825.	Prospective cohort study of 222 patients who had an MI and survived to be discharged from the hospital. Patients were interviewed for MDD between 5 and 15 days following the MI and were followed up for six months. Primary outcome was mortality at six months.	By six months, 12 patients had died. All deaths were due to cardiac causes. Depression was a significant predictor of mortality (hazard ratio, 5.74; 95% CI, 4.61 to 6.87; $P = .0006$). The impact of depression remained after control for left ventricular dysfunction (Killip class) and previous MI, the multivariate significant predictors of mortality in the data set (adjusted hazard ratio, 4.29; 95% CI, 3.14 to 5.44; $P = .013$).	Women are underrepresented (78% of participants were male), DSM requirements for duration and impairment not assessed in interviews
Depression and 18-month prognosis after myocardial infarction. Frasure-Smith N, et al. *Circulation*. 1995;91:999–1005.	Prospective cohort study of 222 patients who had an MI between August 1991 and July 1992. Patients were interviewed for MDD between 5 and 15 days post-MI and all patients and/or families were contacted at 18 months to determine survival status.	There were 21 deaths during the follow-up period, including 19 from cardiac causes. Seven of these deaths occurred among patients who met NIMH Diagnostic Interview Schedule (DIS) criteria for depression, and 12 occurred among patients with elevated Beck Depression Index (BDI) scores. Multiple logistic regression analyses showed that both the DIS (odds ratio, 3.64; 95% confidence interval [CI], 1.32 to 10.05; $P = .012$) and elevated BDI scores (odds ratio, 7.82; 95% CI, 2.42 to 25.26; $P = .0002$) were significantly related to 18-month cardiac mortality.	Women are underrepresented (78% of participants were male), DSM requirements for duration and impairment not assessed in interviews

(*continued*)

TABLE 225-8 Evidence for Heart Disease and Major Depression *(continued)*

Study	Methodology	Results	Limitations
The enhancing recovery in coronary heart disease patients (ENRICHD) randomized trial. Berkman LF, et al. *JAMA.* 2003;289: 3106–3116.	Randomized clinical trial conducted on 2481 MI patients. Major or minor depression was diagnosed by DSM criteria and severity by the 17-item Hamilton Rating Scale for Depression (HAM-D). Random allocation was to usual medical care or CBT-based psychosocial intervention. Primary end point was death or recurrent MI.	After an average follow-up of 29 months, there was no significant difference in event-free survival between usual care (75.9%) and psychosocial intervention (75.8%).	Outcomes may have been confounded by increased use of SSRIs in both control and intervention groups, treatment time may not have been sufficient to see response
Sertraline antidepressant heart attack randomized trial (SADHART). Glassman AH, et al. *JAMA.* 2002;288(6): 701–709.	Randomized, controlled double-blind study of patients hospitalized in the previous month for acute coronary syndrome (myocardial infarction, 74%; unstable angina, 26%). Those who also met criteria for MDD were randomized to 24 weeks of treatment with sertraline (50 to 200 mg/day) or placebo. The primary outcome measure was change from baseline in left ventricular ejection fraction (LVEF).	Sertraline had no significant effect on mean LVEF, increase in ventricular premature complex runs, QTc interval greater than 450 milliseconds at end point, or other cardiac measures. All comparisons were statistically nonsignificant ($P < 0.05$). The incidence of severe cardiovascular adverse events was 14.5% with sertraline and 22.4% with placebo (not a statistically significant difference).	DSM diagnoses did not require duration nor impairment criteria, many cardiac exclusion criteria may make less applicable to post-MI population
The Canadian cardiac randomized evaluation of antidepressant and psychotherapy efficacy (CREATE) Trial. Lesperance F, et al. *JAMA.* 2007;297: 367–379	Randomized, controlled 12-week trial of 284 patients with CAD and MDD by DSM criteria and HAM-D scores of 20 or higher who underwent two separate randomizations: (1) to receive 12 weekly sessions of interpersonal therapy (IPT) plus clinical management (n = 142) or clinical management only (n = 142) and (2) to receive 12 weeks of citalopram, 20 to 40 mg/d (n = 142), or matching placebo. The primary outcome measure was change between baseline and 12 weeks on the 24-item HAM-D.	Citalopram was superior to placebo in reducing 12-week HAM-D scores with a small to medium effect size of 0.33. There was no evidence of a benefit of IPT over clinical management, with the mean HAM-D difference favoring clinical management. Citalopram incurred no statistically significant adverse events when compared to placebo.	Recruitment of subjects via advertisements may limit generalizability, more women than men received IPT

medically ill. Prompt recognition is essential. This discussion will aid the hospitalist in diagnosis and treatment of mania and bipolar disorder.

CASE 225-2

A 50-year-old woman with no past psychiatric history received high dose steroids for a severe asthma exacerbation. On hospital day 2, the patient was seen naked, dancing in the hallway. She was speaking rapidly and was difficult to interrupt. She stated that she is a famous hip-hop artist and became hostile and threatening when asked to return to her room. To ensure her safety, a 1:1 sitter was requested. A psychiatry consultant diagnosed substance-induced mania and recommended stopping prednisone and prescribing olanzapine until her symptoms subside. With this intervention, her manic symptoms rapidly resolved.

PATHOPHYSIOLOGY

The etiology of bipolar disorder is not clearly defined. Alterations in cellular signaling (modulated by G proteins, protein kinase C, and calcium flux) may contribute to pathology. Abnormalities of the hypothalamic-pituitary-adrenal axis and thyroid function have been documented in bipolar patients. Monoamine neurotransmitter irregularities (particularly norepinephrine) may also play a role.

DIAGNOSIS

BIPOLAR I DISORDER

Bipolar I is diagnosed by the presence of a manic or mixed episode (see **Table 225-9**). The elevated mood of mania is enthused and often infectious, and the interviewer may be drawn to the patient's gregarious nature. Individuals may be sexually inappropriate or intimate in their disclosure of personal details. Inflated self-esteem can reach delusional proportions, with the patient claiming a special relationship to God, political leaders, or celebrities. Manic individuals have a decreased need for sleep and remain remarkably energized despite very little rest. Speech is loud, rapid, and uninterruptable, with fluid flow of ideas. Increase in goal-directed activity can manifest in an intrusive social manner in the hospital, with frequent phone calls or prolific letter writing. Expansive plans are thwarted in the hospitalized patient, possibly leading to increasing irritability, complaints, and angry tirades. Manic individuals may deny the presence of illness. Collateral information about past reckless behavior (spending sprees, gambling, sexual indiscretions) can help to confirm the diagnosis.

In a mixed episode, the symptoms of both mania and depression occur nearly every day for a week. Patients appear extremely labile, with alternating euphoria, sadness, and irritability. Agitation is common, with extreme discomfort and anxiety due to dysphoria in the context of excessive energy. A high suicide risk is associated with this state.

TABLE 225-9 Manic Episode

A. A distinct period of abnormally and persistently elevated, expansive, or irritable mood, lasting at least one week (or any duration if hospitalization occurs).
B. During the period of mood disturbance, three or more of following symptoms (four if mood is irritable) have been present to a significant degree:
1. Inflated self-esteem or grandiosity
2. Decreased need for sleep
3. More talkative than usual or pressure to keep talking
4. Flight of ideas or racing thoughts
5. Distractibility (easily drawn to unimportant stimuli)
6. Increase in goal-directed activity or psychomotor agitation
7. Excessive involvement in pleasurable activities that have a high potential for painful consequences (sexual indiscretions, shopping sprees, foolish investments)
C. Symptoms are not due to a mixed episode (characterized by the symptoms of both a major depressive episode and a manic episode occurring nearly every day for one week).
D. The mood disturbance causes marked impairment, necessitates hospitalization, or includes psychosis.
E. The symptoms are not due to the direct physiological effects of a substance or a general medical condition.

Although bipolar I is defined by the presence of a manic or mixed episode, major depression is more frequently the presenting episode (75% of the time for females and 67% of the time for males). Regardless of mood state at presentation, nearly all individuals with bipolar I will have depressive episodes, with time between episodes decreasing as the disorder progresses. This can present a diagnostic challenge in differentiating bipolar from major depressive disorder. Clinical suspicion for bipolar I should arise in mood-disordered individuals with agitated or treatment-refractory depression, a rapid response to antidepressants, a family history of bipolar I, periodic impulsivity or erratic, pleasure-seeking behavior, and episodic sleep disturbance.

BIPOLAR II DISORDER

Bipolar II is defined by the occurrence of at least one major depressive episode, as well as one hypomanic episode. Hypomania differs from mania in duration and level of severity (see **Table 225-10**).

TABLE 225-10 Hypomanic Episode

A. A distinct period of persistently elevated, expansive, or irritable mood, lasting at least four days
B. During the period of mood disturbance, three (or more) symptoms associated with a manic episode (four if mood is irritable) have been present to a significant degree.
C. The episode is associated with an unequivocal change in functioning that is uncharacteristic of the person when not symptomatic.
D. The disturbance in mood and functioning are observable by others.
E. The episode is not severe enough to cause marked impairment in functioning, necessitate hospitalization, or induce psychosis.
F. The symptoms are not due to the effects of a substance or a general medical condition.

TABLE 225-11 Medical Causes of Mania

Neurologic: Cerebrovascular accident (particularly orbitofrontal and thalamic stroke), traumatic brain injury, complex partial seizure, multiple sclerosis, Wilson disease, cerebellar atrophy
Infectious: HIV, neurosyphilis, cryptococcosis, influenza, Q fever
Metabolic: Vitamin B12 deficiency, hyperthyroidism, Cushing's syndrome
Neoplastic: Meningioma, glioma, brainstem tumor, thalamic metastasis

During hypomania, patients do not suffer significant dysfunction, nor do they have hallucinations or delusions. However, individuals with this illness may still be extremely disabled during the course of a major depressive episode, even requiring hospitalization. Bipolar II is a chronic and debilitating illness, and patients have a greater risk of attempting and completing suicide than those with either bipolar I or major depression.

SECONDARY MANIA: MOOD DISORDER DUE TO A GENERAL MEDICAL CONDITION WITH MANIC FEATURES AND SUBSTANCE-INDUCED MANIA

When mania is due to medical illness or the effects of a substance, the diagnostic criteria do not specify duration or number of characteristics. Patients must simply show elevated, expansive, or irritable mood that causes significant distress or interferes with function. Age of onset can assist in differentiating organic mania from bipolar disorder. Secondary mania is more likely the diagnosis when the initial episode occurs after age 45. Substance-induced mania should be suspected when the mood disturbance coincides with the initiation of a new medication (particularly steroids).

Neurologic insult is the most frequent medical cause of manic symptoms. Lesions in the right frontal and temporal cortices (whether vascular, neoplastic, or traumatic) impart an increased risk. CNS infection is a common source of secondary mania, with multiple case reports of temporal (particularly HSV) encephalitis inducing manic symptoms. Patients with HIV-associated neurotoxicity and dementia also have a high prevalence of mania compared to the general population. See **Table 225-11** for common medical causes of mania.

Many pharmacologic agents can induce prolonged euphoric or irritable mood (see **Table 225-12**). Corticosteroids and stimulants are the most frequent offenders. Among the antidepressants, venlafaxine and the TCAs are most likely to precipitate mania.

DIAGNOSTIC STUDIES

Onset of mania in the hospitalized patient should prompt a thorough workup to rule out medical disease or substance intoxication as a cause of symptoms. Laboratory evaluation does not differ significantly than that for major depression, with the exception that imaging of the brain should not be delayed (unless the patient has a well-documented history of bipolar disorder). Additionally, patients on mood stabilizers must have a serum level drawn.

TREATMENT

ACUTE MANIA

Patient safety may be compromised in the setting of acute mania. Treatment should be initiated immediately. Pharmacotherapy is the mainstay, though use of a 1:1 sitter and suicide precautions should be employed if necessary. Both atypical antipsychotics (olanzapine, ziprasidone, aripiprazole, risperidone, and quetiapine) and mood stabilizers (lithium, divalproex, carbamazepine) have indications

TABLE 225-12 Pharmacologic Causes of Mania

Corticosteroids (including ACTH)
Antidepressants and L-tryptophan
Sympathomimetics and methylphenidate
Thyroxine
Sedative-hypnotics (Alcohol, alprazolam, triazolam)
Levodopa
L-glutamine
Captopril
Cimetidine
Cyproheptadine
Cyclosporine
Disulfiram
Isoniazid
Muscle relaxants (cyclobenzaprine and baclofen)
Metoclopramide
Procainamide
Procarbazine
Propafenone
Hallucinogens (LSD, PCP)
Hydralazine
Opioids
Yohimbine
Zidovudine

for monotherapy in acute mania. However, if manic symptoms are even moderately severe, combination therapy is preferable. Antipsychotics have immediate effects and many can be given intramuscularly. Mood stabilizers can be given in a loading dose but take a few days to reach therapeutic levels in the blood. ECT is a good option for patients with severe or psychotic symptoms. Consultation with psychiatry is recommended.

■ MAINTENANCE THERAPY FOR BIPOLAR DISORDER

Bipolar disorder is not an insignificant illness and destabilization can be devastating. When bipolar patients are admitted, mood stabilizers must not be discontinued. A serum level should be checked to determine if a therapeutic range has been achieved. Monitoring and adjustment of dose may be necessary if new medications are started, due to the many drug interactions with mood stabilizers. Subtherapeutic dosing secondary to upregulation of cytochrome p450 can lead to catastrophic outcomes. To prevent precipitation of a manic episode, sleep schedules should be preserved and the addition of antidepressants avoided (even if an individual presents with depressed mood). If a patient is euthymic and stable on medications, psychiatry consultation is unnecessary. See **Table 225-13** for a synopsis of medications used for maintenance of bipolar disorder.

■ COMPLICATIONS

Adverse effects of the medications used for bipolar maintenance are listed in Table 225-13. Lithium has a narrow therapeutic index, with toxicity occurring at serum levels greater than 1.5 mEq/L. Injury to the kidneys accumulates with each supratherapeutic episode. Lithium overdose is usually unintentional, often caused by acute renal insufficiency or volume depletion. Mild intoxication presents with confusion, tremor, and nystagmus. Increasing lithium levels lead to nausea, vomiting, agitation, seizures, bradycardia, and hypotension. Treatment consists of fluids, supportive care, and hemodialysis. Lamotrigine, which is indicated for maintenance therapy only, can cause severe rash (particularly in those with sensitive skin). Slow titration helps to decrease this risk. Lamotrigine, valproic acid, and carbamezapine may all be fatal in overdose.

DISHCARGE PLANNING

Acute mania requires psychiatric hospitalization. Stable patients should receive referral for subsequent treatment by an outpatient psychiatrist.

PROGNOSIS

Patients with bipolar I disorder are likely to relapse. Approximately 50% of patients have a second manic episode within two years of their initial event. In the long term, only 15% of individuals are well. One-third have chronic symptoms with significant social and occupational impairment. Treatment with mood stabilizers improves outcome, but only 50% to 60% of individuals on lithium achieve remission.

DISPARATIES IN HEALTH CARE

African Americans with manic symptoms are more likely than Caucasians to be misdiagnosed with schizophrenia. This may be due to the presence of psychosis or greater prevalence of comorbid substance use in the African American population.

ANXIETY DISORERS

INTRODUCTION

Anxiety disorders are common, with one in four individuals meeting criteria for at least one DSM-IV diagnosis. Additionally, patients that enter the hospital without any previous psychiatric pathology may become acutely anxious in the face of invasive procedures and the threat of death. The following discussion will assist the hospitalist in recognition and treatment of both situational anxiety and the main anxiety disorders.

CASE 225-3

A 33-year-old woman has been evaluated three times over the past four months with chest pain, nausea, and shortness of breath. ECG, chest X-ray, and initial cardiac enzymes were unremarkable. Admitted for observation, she had further testing for myocardial ischemia, including negative cardiac enzymes and a normal persantine-thallium stress test. More detailed questioning revealed multiple similar episodes over the past year. The first time this occurred, Ms. B was driving to work and thought that she had ingested "too much coffee." Even though she had been taking the bus to prevent further attacks, she continued to have episodes that were unrelated to any stimulus. Low-dose clonezapam and fluoxetine were prescribed for panic disorder, leading to a significant improvement of her symptoms, with no further attacks or avoidant behavior. Her clonezapam was able to be successfully tapered.

PATHOPHYSIOLOGY

Fear is a stereotypical response that acts as an alarm to external threat. This reaction is mediated by the locus coeruleus and the limbic system via norepinephrine, serotonin, and GABA. Physiologic changes, such as tachycardia and tachypnea, are due to increased sympathetic activity. Cognitive symptoms include a sense of

TABLE 225-13 Maintenance Therapy for Bipolar Disorder

Medication	Dosing	Therapeutic Serum Level	Half-life	Side Effects	Drug Interactions
Lithium	900–1800 mg/day divided	1.0–1.5 mEq/L for acute mania, 0.6–1.2 mEq/L for maintenance	18–30 hrs	Ataxia, tremor, polyuria, diarrhea, weight gain, hypothyroidism, rash, leukocytosis, renal impairment, arrhythmia and T wave flattening	NSAIDs, diuretics, ACE-Is, metronidazole increase levels Acetazolamide, alkalizing agents decrease levels
Divalproex	load 20–30 mg/kg/day, then 15 mg/kg/day	50–125 μg/mL	9–16 hrs	Sedation, tremor, ataxia, diarrhea, nausea, weight gain, hepatotoxicity, rare pancreatitis	ASA, chlorpromazine, fluoxetine, fluvoxamine, topiramate, cimetidine, erythromycin, ibuprofen can increase levels Phenytoin, ethosuxamide, rifampin, carbamezapine can decrease levels
Lamotrigine	200–400 mg/day (slow titration)	n/a	33 hrs	Rash (can have Stevens Johnson syndrome), sedation, blurry vision, ataxia, GI upset, blood dyscrasias	Divalproex increases level Carbamazapine, phenobarbitol, phenytoin, primidone, and OCP decrease levels
Carbamazepine	400–1200 mg/day	4–12 μg/mL	Initial 26–65 hrs, 12–17 hrs with repeated doses	Sedation, dizziness, confusion, GI upset, aplastic anemia, agranulocytosis, SIADH, rash	Induces its own clearance phenobarbitol, phenytoin, primidone, and OCP decrease levels Nefazodone, fluoxetine, fluvoxamine increase levels
Olanzapine	10–20 mg/day	n/a	21–54 hrs	Possible metabolic syndrome, dizziness, sedation, dry mouth, constipation, rare tardive dyskinesia, rare NMS	CYP450 1A2 inhibitors increase levels CYP450 1A2 inducers (cigarette smoke, carbamazepine) decrease levels
Quetiapine	100–400 mg/day	n/a	6–7 hrs	Sedation, orthostasis, dry mouth, constipation, possible metabolic syndrome	rare
Aripiprazole	10–30 mg/day	n/a	75 hrs	Dizziness, insomnia, akathisia, GI upset, orthostasis	CYP450 3A4 and 2D6 inhibitors can increase levels, inducers may decrease levels

impending doom and dread. Behavioral reactions serve to remove the individual from harm. Acute anxiety also induces this reaction, but occurs in response to an internal threat or an external cue that is not inherently dangerous. Early exposure to trauma and genetic factors predispose individuals to these pathologic responses to stress.

Additional mechanisms are responsible for the onset of specific disorders. Infusion of carbon dioxide and sodium lactate can induce panic attacks in those with panic disorder. These substances lower systemic pH, increasing respiratory drive via the medulla. In those with panic disorder, hyperventilation and anxiety ensues. This is likely due to hypersensitivity of the central asphyxia alarm system. Obsessive-compulsive disorder (OCD) appears to involve abnormal signaling in the corticostriatal pathways. Functional neuroimaging in patients with OCD shows increased activity in the orbitofrontal cortex, caudate, and thalamus. In addition to increased noradrenergic activity, individuals with posttraumatic stress disorder (PTSD) display alterations of the endogenous opioid system and the HPA axis. These patients also have structural changes in the hippocampus and amygdala.

DIAGNOSIS

When a patient presents with the physical signs of anxiety, it is essential to inquire about emotional and behavioral responses. Many patients focus primarily on somatic complaints, delaying appropriate recognition. Undiagnosed anxiety disorders impose a heavy economic burden, with unnecessary visits to emergency rooms, hospitalizations, subspecialty consultations, and invasive procedures. Perhaps more costly is the anguish experienced by the anxious patient who goes untreated. Many patients suffer secondary depression and abuse drugs and alcohol.

■ PRIMARY ANXIETY DISORDERS

Primary anxiety disorders include panic disorder (with or without agoraphobia), specific phobia, social phobia, generalized anxiety

TABLE 225-14 Primary Anxiety Disorders

I. Panic disorder

A. Recurrent, unexpected panic attacks characterized by four or more of the following: palpitations, chest pain, diaphoresis, shortness of breath, sensation of choking, nausea, trembling, paresthesias, chills or hot flashes, dizziness, derealization or depersonalization, fear of dying, fear of losing control or going crazy

B. Persistent concern about future attacks, worry about the meaning or consequences of attacks, or significant change in behavior surrounding the about of future attacks

C. The disorder may occur with or without agoraphobia.

II. Agoraphobia

A. Fear of being in places or situations where escape may be difficult or embarrassing, or in which help may be unavailable in the event of having a panic attack

B. Fear often results in avoidance of the feared places or situations.

III. Social phobia

A. Marked and persistent fear of one or more social or performance situations in which the person is concerned about negative evaluation or scrutiny by others

B. The individual fears humiliation or embarrassment, perhaps by manifesting anxiety symptoms.

C. Feared social or performance situations are avoided or endured with intense anxiety or distress.

IV. Specific phobia

A. Marked and persistent fear that is excessive, unreasonable, and cued by the presence of or anticipation of a specific object or situation

B. Exposure to feared object or situation provokes an immediate anxiety response.

C. Individual recognizes that fear is excessive or unreasonable.

D. Avoidance, anticipatory anxiety, or distress is significantly impairing.

V. Obsessive-compulsive disorder

A. The individual experiences either

1. obsessions, defined as recurrent or persistent thoughts, impulses, or images that are experienced as intrusive and inappropriate, and/or
2. compulsions, defined as repetitive behaviors or mental acts whose goal is to prevent or reduce anxiety or distress.

B. Individual recognizes that the thoughts and behavior are excessive or unreasonable.

C. Obsessions cause marked distress, are time-consuming, or cause significant impairment.

VI. Generalized anxiety disorder

A. Excessive anxiety and worry about a number of events or activities, occurring more days than not for at least six months

B. Worry is difficult to control.

C. Worry is associated with at least three of the following: restlessness, fatigue, difficulty concentrating, irritability, muscle tension, or sleep disturbance.

VII. Posttraumatic stress disorder

A. Exposure to a traumatic event that threatens the life or body integrity of an individual or their loved ones, with response of helplessness or horror

B. Re-experience of event, including one of the following: flashbacks, nightmares, reliving experience or experiencing distress when exposed to cues associated with event

C. Avoidance behavior, including three of the following: efforts to avoid thoughts or activities associated with trauma, inability to recall events surrounding trauma, decreased interest in activities, detachment, restricted affect, or sense of a foreshortened future

D. Symptoms of increased arousal, including two of the following: sleep difficulties, irritability, poor concentration, hypervigilence, or exaggerated startle response

disorder (GAD), posttraumatic stress disorder (PTSD), and obsessive-compulsive disorder. See **Table 225-14** for diagnostic features of these illnesses.

A panic attack is an intense episode of autonomic activation accompanied by feelings of fear and impending doom. Attacks have a sudden onset, peak within 10 minutes, and usually resolve within a half-hour. In panic disorder, these episodes become autonomous and arise outside of substance use or stressful situation. The patient worries about the meaning of attacks and changes behavior to avoid them. Avoidance may progress to agoraphobia. Individuals with panic disorder frequently interpret their paroxysmal symptoms as a catastrophic medical event (such as an MI) and may present to emergency rooms multiple times before receiving an accurate diagnosis.

A phobia is an excessive fear of a particular object or situation. Exposure to the phobic stimulus induces panic. This can complicate both diagnosis and treatment of medical illness. Individuals with blood-injection-injury specific phobia may refuse phlebotomy or have a vasovagal response to seeing blood. Claustrophobia may prevent the successful completion of needed scans. Severe social phobia can be disabling in the hospital setting, where scrutiny by others is unavoidable.

Those with GAD have chronic, uncontrollable worry about multiple aspects of life. These individuals have prominent somatic complaints (headaches, muscle tension, gastrointestinal distress) and often seek medical care for symptom relief. Unless appropriately treated, hospitalized patients with GAD may aggravate staff and physicians with a seemingly exorbitant need for reassurance and explanations.

Individuals with OCD have recurrent intrusive thoughts and spend an excessive amount of time performing repetitive or ritualistic behaviors. Obsessions concerning contamination are most prevalent, and patients may wash until their skin is raw. This obsession is especially problematic in the medical setting, where germs abound. Other common patterns include pathological doubt followed by checking (to see if the door is locked or stove turned off), the need for symmetry or precision, and compulsive counting. Patients with OCD may experience intense anxiety if rituals are curtailed by hospitalization.

PTSD is a maladaptive response to a life-threatening event that results in re-experiencing of the incident, avoidance behavior, and increased arousal. While much attention has been paid to the emergence of PTSD in combat veterans, the disorder may also occur in civilians after traumatic events or natural disasters. It has also been documented after MI, CABG, and surgery performed under inadequate anesthesia. The disorder is more likely to occur in situations in which the traumatic event is perceived as uncontrollable. Thus, actions should be taken to allow hospitalized patients to maintain a sense of control over themselves and their environments.

ORGANIC CAUSES OF ANXIETY: ANXIETY DUE TO A GENERAL MEDICAL CONDITION AND SUBSTANCE-INDUCED ANXIETY

A bewildering array of medical diseases can mimic primary anxiety disorders (see **Table 225-15**). This presents a diagnostic challenge: up to 42% of all patients referred for psychiatric evaluation have underlying medical illness as a cause for their symptoms. Of the diseases presenting with anxious symptoms, 25% are endocrine disorders, 25% neurological, and 12% cardiovascular, rheumatologic, or infectious. When a patient with a known medical disease presents with complaints of anxiety, evaluation should focus on whether an exacerbation of the illness could be responsible. Family history of disorders that mimic anxiety, such as hyperthyroidism or cardiac arrhythmias, can provide important clues.

Careful examination of the patient's presentation can also aid in diagnosis. Anxiety due to medical disease generally lacks the emotional component of primary disorders. Somatic complaints may not cause as much distress or interfere significantly with overall function. Constellations of symptoms are less likely to meet criteria for any particular DSM-IV diagnosis, and warning signs (such as loss of consciousness or incontinence) may be present. Unlike those with organic syndromes, patients with primary anxiety are likely to have a childhood history of emotional trauma, a family history of mood and anxiety disorders, life stressors preceding onset of disease, and avoidance behavior. Presentation of primary anxiety after age 35 is uncommon. A lack of response to anxiolytic medications should prompt a reassessment of the diagnosis of a primary anxiety disorder.

Drugs frequently cause anxious symptoms. Stimulants, including caffeine and over-the-counter medications (such as dextromethorphan), can induce anxiety. Prescription medications (most frequently steroids and other immunomodulators) may also be responsible. Withdrawal from sedatives and opioids may lead to autonomic hyperreactivity. See **Table 225-16** for a list of frequent offenders.

TABLE 225-15 Medical Causes of Anxiety

Endocrine: Cushing disease, adrenal insufficiency, Addison disease, adrenal tumors, carcinoid syndrome, diabetes (hypoglycemia), hyperparathyroidism, hyperthyroidism, hypothyroidism, insulinoma, menopause, ovarian dysfunction, pancreatic carcinoma, pheochromocytoma, pituitary disease, PMS, testicular disease
Neurologic: tumors, tertiary syphilis, cerebrovascular disease, encephalopathy, epilepsy (especially temporal lobe foci), essential tremor, Huntington disease, migraine, MS, myasthenia gravis, polyneuritis, postconcussive syndrome, vertigo
Cardiovascular: Anemia, CHF, CAD, arrhythmias, hypovolemia, mitral valve prolapse
Respiratory: Asthma, COPD, hyperventilation, hypoxia, pneumonia, pneumothorax, pulmonary edema, PE
Rheumatologic: Anaphylaxis, polyarteritis nodosa, rheumatoid arthritis, SLE, temporal arteritis
Metabolic: Acidosis, acute intermittent porphyria, electrolyte abnormalities, hyperthermia, Wilson disease
Gastrointestinal: colitis, IBS, esophageal dysmotility, PUD
Infectious disease: AIDS, atypical pneumonia, Brucellosis, Malaria, Mononucleosis, TB, viral hepatitis

TABLE 225-16 Substance-induced Anxiety

Intoxication: Analgesics, antibiotics (penicillin, sulfonamides), anticholinergics, anticonvulsants, antidepressants, antihistamines, antihypertensives, anti-inflammatory agents, antiparkinsonian agents, aspirin, caffeine, chemotherapeutics, cocaine, digitalis, hallucinogens, heavy metal poisoning, marijuana, neuroleptics, steroids, sympathomimetics, theophylline, thyroid supplements, tobacco
Withdrawal: Ethanol, narcotics, sedative-hypnotics

CHRONIC ANXIETY VERSUS MAJOR DEPRESSION

Approximately half of all patients with MDD meet criteria for panic disorder, agoraphobia, or GAD. This significant overlap can make distinguishing diagnoses difficult, with sleep disturbance, psychomotor agitation, difficulty concentrating, irritability, and fatigue attributable to either illness. However, the presence of certain symptoms can help with differentiation. Psychomotor retardation, dysphoria, hopelessness, and thoughts of death are more specific to major depression. Unlike those suffering from MDD, anxious individuals rarely lose interest in their usual activities, though they may avoid situations because of irrational fears. The somatic symptoms of anxiety differ from those of depression, with tachycardia, palpitations, tachypnea, and diaphoresis prominent.

DIAGNOSTIC STUDIES

A wide array of illnesses and ingestions can masquerade as anxiety. Initial laboratory evaluation must rule out organic causes for anxious symptoms. Recommended studies do not differ significantly from those for depression (see earlier discussion). The organ system involved in the majority of the patient's somatic complaints may focus further testing. Patients with known anxiety disorders can present with serious medical illness, and clinicians must not delay diagnostic evaluation by prematurely narrowing the differential (ie, patients with panic disorder can still suffer an MI).

TREATMENT

SITUATIONAL ANXIETY

Medical illness, particularly when severe enough to require hospitalization, imposes significant psychological stress. Patients without any previous psychiatric diagnosis may become appropriately fearful when undergoing invasive procedures or facing life-threatening

TABLE 225-17 Pharmacology of Commonly-used Benzodiazepines

Medication	Dose Equivalent (mg)	Half-life (hrs)	Onset
Midazolam	2	1–12	Fast
Oxazepam	15	5–15	Slow
Lorazepam	1	10–20	Intermediate
Alprazolam	0.5	12–15	Intermediate-fast
Chlordiazepoxide	10	5–30	Intermediate
Clonazepam	0.25	15–50	Intermediate
Diazepam	5	20–100	Fast
Flurazepam	15	40	Fast
Clorazepate	7.5	30–200	Fast

disease. In the acutely anxious patient, delaying effective treatment is akin to withholding medication for pain. Benzodiazepines (BZDs) are first-line therapy for short-term treatment of intermittent anxiety in those without primary disorders.

Sedation is often a limiting side effect of the benzodiazepines. Medications should be started at low doses and titrated as needed to minimize this problem. In some patients, particularly the elderly, BZDs may cause paradoxical agitation and precipitate delirium. Dependence can occur with prolonged use. Because of this, they should be used with great caution (if at all) in patients with a history of addiction. The use of agents with shorter half-lives, such as alprazolam, can result in rebound symptoms with infrequent dosing. BZDs can cause withdrawal if abruptly discontinued, and a taper should be used to avoid this possibly life-threatening complication. Though all benzodiazepines are likely equally efficacious at equivalent doses, clonezapam may be the most attractive agent due to its long half-life and relatively slow onset (thereby decreasing addictive potential). See **Table 225-17** for further details on the BZDs.

ANXIETY DISORDERS

Antidepressants are first-line therapy for the anxiety disorders. Because of their tolerability and safety profiles, SSRIs are the agents of choice. Fluoxetine, sertraline, paroxetine, fluvoxamine, citalopram, and escitalopram all have indications for the treatment of panic disorder, agoraphobia, social phobia, OCD, and PTSD. Paroxetine and escitalopram are approved for GAD. Alternatively, the SNRIs duloxetine and cymbalta may be used to treat anxiety disorders. Buproprion should be avoided as it can be anxiogenic. When initiating treatment, lower starting doses and slow titration should be employed to prevent worsening of symptoms. Higher total doses may be necessary to achieve remission.

Among the other antidepressants, the tricyclics clomipramine and imipramine and the MAO-inhibitor phenelzine may be used to treat anxiety disorders. Intolerable side effects and drug toxicity often limit their use. These agents are reasonable second- or third-line choices in patients with severe, treatment resistant illness. TCAs and MAO-Is should be started with the assistance of psychiatry.

For patients newly diagnosed with an anxiety disorder, BZDs may be used in conjunction with antidepressants to temper activating symptoms associated with initiation of SSRIs and SNRIs. They also may be used in the short-term to treat patients with known anxiety disorders who were previously stable on antidepressants alone. Benzodiazepines are indicated for panic disorder, agoraphobia, social phobia, and GAD. Monotherapy with these medications may be the treatment of choice for specific phobia, and can be administered just prior to confronting the feared object or situation (before starting a procedure, or on the way to MRI). BZDs should be avoided in acute trauma and in PTSD, as they may actually be harmful.

Buspirone is a $5HT_{1A}$ partial agonist approved for the treatment of social phobia and GAD. Similar to SSRIs, buspirone must be taken for a number of weeks before maximum therapeutic benefit is attained. Clinical trials have shown promising results for this medication, but anecdotal experience is disappointing.

Antiadrenergic agents can also diminish somatic symptoms associated with anxiety. The β-blocker propranolol is indicated for social phobia and may also be a useful treatment for panic attacks, panic disorder, social phobia, GAD, and PTSD. Clonidine, an α2 agonist, may also help decrease sympathetic hyperactivity. The α1-antagonist prazosin may be used to treat PTSD. Anticonvulsants and antihistamines are sedating and may relieve feelings of restlessness, but this is an off-label use of these medications.

PSYCHOTHERAPY AND OTHER NONPHARMACOLOGIC INTERVENTIONS

Cognitive-behavioral therapy (CBT) is as effective as pharmacotherapy for certain disorders, such as social and specific phobia. For other anxiety disorders, including OCD and GAD, a combination of CBT and medication improves outcomes. Cognitive-behavioral formulations of anxiety focus on maladaptive information processing and actions. Therapy seeks to correct faulty cognition and modify escape responses. Engagement in therapy may be challenging for the hospitalized patient, though teaching symptom management (such as relaxation techniques) may be possible with the assistance of psychiatry consultation. Other psychosocial interventions, such as recruitment of family members to provide emotional support, may also be beneficial.

ORGANIC CAUSES OF ANXIETY

When medical illness is the cause of anxiety, treatment of the disease is the intervention of choice. If the illness is permanent, symptoms are causing distress, or anxiety does not remit when physical health returns, pharmacotherapy with anxiolytics (in the short term) or antidepressants (in the long term) is indicated. Behavioral modification techniques are also effective in this population. In substance-induced anxiety, addiction must be addressed.

DISCHARGE PLANNING

Psychic tension greatly increases the risk for suicide. Acutely anxious patients should be screened for both passive and active suicidal ideation and hospitalized if at risk. Patients whose anxiety is sufficiently severe to warrant sustained pharmacotherapy should likely be referred to psychiatry upon discharge.

DISPARITIES IN HEALTH CARE

In the outpatient setting, African Americans and Latinos receive appropriate care for anxiety or depression less frequently than Caucasians (odds ratios are 0.44 and 0.60, respectively). Both minorities find treatment with antidepressants less acceptable than Caucasians, but this does not fully account for the discrepancy.

PROGNOSIS

Patients with panic disorder have a fairly good prognosis, with 30% to 40% free of all symptoms long term. Those with PTSD fare even better. Fifty percent of untreated patients are in remission at one year after the traumatic event. OCD frequently has a protracted course, with 20% to 40% experiencing lifelong disabling behaviors.

CONCLUSION

Mood and anxiety disorders are common and underdiagnosed. Failure to identify and initiate appropriate treatment can cause unnecessary suffering and readmissions, and significantly affect medical outcomes. The hospitalization provides an opportunity to improve patient outcomes by properly recognizing, diagnosing, and initiating a therapeutic plan that can be transitioned to the outpatient setting.

SUGGESTED READINGS

Frances, Allen, et al. *Diagnostic and Statistical Manual of Mental Disorders*, fourth Edition. Arlington, VA: American Psychiatric Association; 2000.

Lisanby SH. Electroconvulsive Therapy for Depression. *N Engl J Med.* 2007;357:1939–1945.

Musselman DL, Lawson DH, Gumnick JF, et al. Paroxetine for the Prevention of Depression Induced by High-dose Interferon Alfa. *N Engl J Med.* 2001;344(13):961–966.

Robinson RG, Jorge RE, Moser DJ, et al. Escitalopram and Problem-Solving Therapy for Prevention of Poststroke Depression. *JAMA.* 2008:299(20):2391–2400.

Sadock, BJ, Sadock VA. *Kaplan & Sadock's Synopsis of Psychiatry*, tenth Edition. Philadelphia, PA: Lippincott Williams & Wilkins; 2007.

Stern TA, Fricchione GL, Cassem NH, et al. *Handbook of General Hospital Psychiatry*, 5th Edition. Ed. Susan F. Pioli. Philadelphia, PA: Mosby; 2004.

Schatzberg, AF, Nemeroff, CB. *The American Psychiatric Publishing Textbook of Psychopharmacology*, third Edition. Ed. Arlington, VA: American Psychiatric Publishing; 2004.

CHAPTER 226

Assessment and Management of Psychosis

Anand K. Pandurangi, MBBS, MD

Key Clinical Questions

1. What is psychosis?
2. What are the various psychotic disorders?
3. How are psychotic disorders diagnosed?
4. How is psychosis treated in the acute hospital setting?
5. What are the complications of psychosis?
6. What is an optimal discharge plan for patients who are recovering from psychosis?

INTRODUCTION

New-onset psychosis and recurring psychosis identified during the course of assessment and treatment of medical disorders, require immediate intervention. 0.5–2.5% of all (nonpsychiatric) hospitalized patients have a preexisting chronic psychosis and 5–25% of all referrals for psychiatric consultation are for a psychotic disorder. New-onset psychoses may be secondary to a general medical condition, iatrogenic or functional in nature (**Table 226-1**). Initiation of treatment for new cases and continuation (or resumption) of treatment for preexisting psychosis is of paramount importance. Neglecting or under treating the psychosis will likely lead to behavioral and medical complications. Psychosis can quickly erupt into a crisis, affecting the management of the medical disorder(s) and altering their outcome. The presence of comorbid psychiatric conditions, especially if unrecognized or under treated often increases the length of stay and cost of care.

DEFINITIONS AND TERMINOLOGY

The term *psychosis* was first used in the mid-19th century to denote an abnormal state of mind, and typically refers to a loss of touch with reality. In 1896, Emil Kraeplin dichotomized the functional psychoses into dementia precox and manic-depressive illness to denote a chronic deteriorating cognitive disorder and an intermittent mood disorder, respectively. In 1911, Eugen Bleuler renamed the former condition as schizophrenia. This dichotomization does not cover all psychotic disorders, and various other psychotic disorders have been described. These include stress-induced reactive psychosis, conditions with mixed psychotic and mood symptoms called schizoaffective psychosis, and cyclical disorders called cycloid psychoses. In the *Diagnostic and Statistical Manual of Mental Disorders* (4th edition, text revision [DSM-IV-TR]), functional psychoses are described under two broad categories, namely schizophrenia and related psychoses, and mood disorders with psychosis. Psychosis secondary to a general medical condition or substance abuse is simply described as such (eg, psychosis secondary to hypothyroidism, alcohol-induced psychosis). All other psychoses are diagnosed as psychosis, not otherwise specified.

Psychosis refers to a sustained mental state of loss or impaired touch with reality. It is manifested by one or more of the following: hallucinatory experiences, delusional beliefs, disordered communication, and disorganized, unusual, strange and/or regressed behaviors. These are also referred to as positive symptoms. Transient states of perceptual alterations such as those occurring after sleep deprivation or as part of a desired religious experience are typically not considered psychosis. Psychosis is often a manifestation of substance abuse. Many general medical conditions, especially central nervous system (CNS) disorders, may lead to the manifestation of psychosis. Finally, psychosis is frequently associated with delirium and dementia.

POSITIVE SYMPTOMS

Hallucination refers to perceptual experience(s) in the absence of an external stimulus. The source of the perception is typically placed in objective space (ie, not from inner self, ego, subconscious, mind, soul, etc). The perception may be in any sensory modality. For example, hearing voices of people who are not around or seeing images such as those of god, the devil large and small animals, dead people, or fire. Hallucinations may also occur in the olfactory,

TABLE 226-1 Key Points

- Psychosis is a sustained mental state of impaired contact with reality.
- Psychosis is manifested with one or more of the following: hallucinations, delusions, disordered communication, and unusual behaviors.
- Short-lasting functional psychotic disorders include brief psychotic disorder and schizophreniform disorder.
- Chronic or recurrent functional psychotic disorders include schizophrenia, schizoaffective disorder, delusion disorder, and severe mood disorders.
- Substance abuse may cause psychosis.
- Endocrine, immunologic, metabolic, neoplastic, and other general medical disorders may lead to the manifestation of psychosis.
- Psychosis may be seen as part of dementia or delirium, or in association with a developmental disorder such as autism or mental retardation.
- Assessment includes history of the psychotic symptoms including time course, medical review of systems, physical and mental status examinations, and laboratory tests as needed.
- Diagnosis is made by applying the DSM-IV criteria to the above information.
- Antipsychotic medications are essential to control the psychosis.
- A safe and supportive environment is necessary.
- Florid psychosis persistent for several days is best treated on a psychiatric unit, when feasible.
- Psychosis may take 3–14 days to resolve and sometimes longer.
- Education of the patient and significant others on compliance, side effects, and signs of relapse is a key ingredient of a safe discharge plan.
- Patients need follow-up care within one to two weeks of discharge.

tactile, gustatory, or proprioceptive modalities. Auditory hallucinations are more typical in functional psychosis, and visual and tactile hallucinations are more common in psychoses secondary to use of substances or from a general medical condition. However, this is not a hard and fast rule, nor is it diagnostic in and of itself.

Delusion refers to a fixed false and irrational belief. The contents are not congruent with those of the subculture to which the patient belongs and the conclusion has been arrived in an irrational manner. Delusions are categorized based on their content into persecutory, grandiose, somatic, etc Here are a few examples: (1) A man with schizophrenia believes that the FBI has stationed 360° cameras around his house, office, and car and beams these pictures around the globe to publicize his life. (2) A woman believes that surgeons enter her room in the night and replace her organs with diseased ones to spread a new type of disease. (3) A middle-aged construction worker attempts to make a million dollar bid online as a down payment for the purchase of a Caribbean island because "the next big wave was to happen as soon as I patent my new permanent roof tiles."

Thought disorder refers to impairments in the process of thinking, and is also referred to as formal thought disorder (FTD). A commonly seen type of this is "loose associations," although there are more than 18 varieties of disordered thinking. The impairment may be in the thinking process, language, speech, or communication. For example, a 25-year-old male with schizophrenia when asked during initial evaluation, "what seems to be the problem?" responded as follows: "I was driving along the expressway when the spiders appeared, looking ugly, uhh they made all the difference to god's creativity. I had to know who this was. Had seen him before. His voice had that distinct sound—you know the one's animals make when they are doing their perfunctory thing. No wonder you doctors can tell all the difference."

Disorganized behavior refers to a host of behaviors reflective of a lack of organization, cohesiveness, and purpose in one's external behavior, often reflecting the internal chaos of the mind. States of excitement, stereotypical movements, severe withdrawal and isolation, catatonic stupor, regressed behaviors including poor self-care and hygiene, etc are all subsumed under this term.

NEGATIVE SYMPTOMS

Negative symptoms refer to a set of emotional and behavioral manifestations that indicate loss of normal mental functions.

Blunted affect refers to a diminution in the tone, experience, range, and depth of emotion and is used interchangeably with the term *flat affect*. A person exhibiting a blunted affect may not show appropriate sadness, happiness, anger, etc as warranted by an event or situation.

Alogia refers to a state of reduced speech. The patient may respond minimally to questions and/or appear to have difficulty being productive with verbal expressions.

Apathy, avolition, and anhedonia describe a state of reduced interest and emotion and inability to experience pleasure.

Asociality refers to reduced social interactions including limited or no close relationships. It should not be confused with antisocial, which refers to breaking social norms and laws without a sense of remorse.

RELATED TERMINOLOGY

In the context of psychosis, terms such as reality testing, impaired capacity, poor judgment, poor insight, poor ego boundaries, etc are often used by psychiatric clinicians.

Reality testing: This is the capacity to correctly interpret internal stimuli such as thoughts, feelings, and somatic sensations, etc, and/or the external environment, such as people and events in relation to oneself. Example: A patient may believe that gurgling sounds out of one's belly are messages from his deceased mother that he is being controlled by the devil.

Poor ego boundaries: This is a disturbance in volition, ownership, and boundaries of one's thoughts, feelings, and perceptions. Thus, a patient may believe his thoughts are being heard/known by others. Patient may attribute control of actions such as eating, talking, walking, etc or emotions to others. For example, a 25-year-old woman believed that the dentist had inserted a powerful microchip into her teeth and was able to make her experience sexual feelings toward older men.

Poor insight: This is a lack of awareness of one's own behavior, especially in relation to the need for change. For example, a 35-year-old man was angry at his wife for having called the mental health crisis line for help after he had been neglecting to eat or shower and was sitting at home for several days gazing out of the window and sighing frequently. He claimed he was "just resting."

Poor judgment: This is the inability to assess the totality of one's situation, consequences, and necessary actions. For example, a 65-year-old person with suspected dementia refused to move out of the home after it had been condemned by the social service agency because "it is my mother's home and I will fix it by the weekend."

Impaired capacity: This is the inability to assess a specific condition or situation, its consequences, and actions to be undertaken. Example: A 45-year-old man with a history of traumatic brain injury, seizures, and severe cognitive impairment had developed aplastic anemia and was in isolation on the step-down medical unit with a

TABLE 226-2 Disorders with Psychosis

Disorder	Course and Duration	Features and Diagnosis	Outcome/Comments
Brief psychotic disorder	Acute, days to <4 weeks	Often precipitated by stress. Dramatic and fluctuating psychosis. Other causes ruled out.	Full remission of symptoms and return of function.
Schizophreniform disorder	Acute, >4 weeks and less than 6 months	Schizophrenia-like symptoms. Mood disorder. Substances and medical conditions ruled out as cause.	May progress to schizophrenia.
Schizophrenia	Chronic, years	>1 month of psychotic symptoms, >6 months of behavior change. Mood disorder, substance abuse and general medical conditions ruled out. Functional decline.	Persistence of symptoms in 30–60% of patients. Some recovery is possible in most.
Schizoaffective disorder	Chronic, years	Symptoms of psychosis and mood disorder are equally prominent. >2 weeks of psychosis without mood symptoms.	Outcome is better than schizophrenia.
Delusion disorder	Chronic, >1 month to years	Prominent nonbizarre delusion(s). No hallucinations or minimal.	Personality is preserved. Function often preserved.
Depression with psychosis	Intermittent >2 weeks	Depression is primary. Content of psychosis often congruent with mood.	Outcome better than schizophrenia. Responds well to electroconvulsive therapy.
Mania with psychosis	Intermittent >1 week	Mania is primary. Content of psychosis often congruent with mood.	Outcome better than schizophrenia.
Substance-induced with psychosis See Table 226-4	Variable. As long as substance is used.	Psychosis follows substance use. Visual and tactile hallucinations may often be seen. Alcohol and amphetamine psychosis may mimic delusions and hallucinations of schizophrenia.	Psychosis may persist days to weeks after abstinence.
Delirium with psychosis	Brief in duration	Disturbed consciousness. Psychosis often inferred from behavior. Fragmentary and fleeting delusions. Visual and tactile hallucinations may be seen.	May require frequent parenteral antipsychotics in small doses rather than bolus or single large dose.
Psychosis due to a general medical condition See Table 226-3.	Varies with condition	Verified by diagnosis of the underlying medical condition, and resolution with its treatment. Visual hallucinations may often be seen. May be part of delirium.	
Dementia with psychosis (Alzheimer, vascular, etc)	Intermittent or chronic	Often inferred from behavior. Delusions are fragmentary and not well elaborated.	May not be evident as much in late dementia. Low doses of antipsychotics may be sufficient.
Developmental disorder with psychosis (autism spectrum disorders, mental retardation)	Intermittent or chronic	Delusions are often poorly formed and fragmentary. Visual hallucinations may be seen. Psychosis may sometimes be understood as literal or concrete interpretation of reality, or over-learned behavior.	Higher doses of medications often not well tolerated.

fever. He consistently refused to have any blood transfusion, saying "had the flu many times, clears up in a couple of days."

DISORDERS

A brief description of each disorder is given below and **Table 226-2** lists all psychotic disorders.

■ BRIEF PSYCHOTIC DISORDER

This disorder manifests acutely, is often associated with a significant external stress, runs a short course of days to weeks, and resolves without leaving significant residual pathology. One or many positive psychotic symptoms are present. Often these are dramatic and changing. Negative symptoms are typically absent. The symptoms may reflect the stress. For example, a 17-year-old girl manifested an acute psychosis with delusions that she was pregnant with evil twins and believed that she would deliver them any day now resulting in mayhem in the world. She had been raised with strong religious values and had reluctantly participated in sexual intercourse with her boyfriend during spring break. With short-term hospitalization and antipsychotic therapy, the psychosis resolved without any residual deficits.

■ SCHIZOPHRENIFORM DISORDER

In this condition, the onset is acute with one or more positive symptoms of psychosis that tend to be well defined. Negative symptoms are absent. There may or may not be a clearly associated stress factor. The condition lasts several weeks and may resolve or progress to schizophrenia. Often the term is used as an "on-hold" diagnosis till one can establish (or rule out) the more onerous diagnosis of schizophrenia.

SCHIZOPHRENIA

This is the best-established disorder in this group. Typically, it begins between 18 and 25 years of age, although both earlier and later onset are recognized. It is a pervasive mental disorder and manifests with symptoms in multiple domains, such as thinking, perceptions, emotions, and (lack of) insight. Auditory hallucinations, persecutory delusions, disturbances in the ownership and privacy of one's thinking (thought broadcasting, thought insertion, thought withdrawal), loose associations, and negative symptoms of blunted and inappropriate affect are classic symptoms of schizophrenia. Depending on the main symptoms, it is subtyped into paranoid, disorganized, and catatonic types.

The psychosis may manifest episodically or continuously but the disorder is continuous. Behavioral changes (prodrome) such as social withdrawal and odd thinking may precede the core psychotic symptoms. The psychotic symptoms last well over a month at a minimum, and typically for several months to even years. Milder psychotic symptoms and behavior changes may remain after the major symptoms have subsided (residual). Impairment in role function accompanies the psychosis and persists chronically, making this illness one of the most disabling medical conditions. Most of the decline is seen within the first five years of the illness. The symptomatic and functional outcome is not uniform for all and is quite variable. Approximately one-third of patients have a milder form of the illness and do well, another third have moderate severity and may remain with some symptoms and disability, while unfortunately another third have a severe form of the disorder and remain with significant symptoms and severe disability.

It is important to rule out mood disorders (depression, mania) and (physical) medical causes as well as substance use as causes of psychosis before making a definite diagnosis of schizophrenia.

SCHIZOAFFECTIVE DISORDER

This condition manifests with both prominent symptoms of psychosis and mood. It is conceived of as a chronic condition, similar to schizophrenia in its course and outcome. Some classifications recognize a schizophrenia subtype and a bipolar subtype, within schizoaffective disorder.

DELUSION DISORDER

This disorder is characterized by the presence of strong delusions, typically with a common theme. Hallucinations are either not present or minimal. There is both an acute form and a chronic form. Generally, the personality is intact and function is well preserved. Here are two examples: (1) A 50-year-old South Asian non-Christian male who ran a successful business was obsessed with becoming familiar with the Vatican campus and architecture, as he firmly believed he was to be the next pope. (2) A 50-year-old community college physics professor constantly changed jobs, as he believed the CIA and intelligence services of other countries were after his discoveries, and searched his office daily in the night to copy his formula.

MISCELLANEOUS FUNCTIONAL PSYCHOSES

Certain presentations of psychosis are difficult to assign to any of the above disorders. Catatonic presentations especially do not follow a set course. While a small number follow a typical chronic schizophrenia course, others are intermittent and have a better prognosis. There is controversy as to whether they are to be grouped independently or as mood disorders. This includes the so-called cycloid psychoses. Another example is psychosis presenting in the context of epileptic disorder; while some are clearly postictal in their timing, others can be preictal, interictal, chronic, or variably intermittent, yet with a clear relation to the seizure disorder. Yet other psychotic illnesses are seen in specific cultures, such as somatic delusion of shrinking genitals, delusion of pregnancy in a male, or delusion of being possessed. All such conditions are diagnosed as psychosis not otherwise specified (NOS) in the DSM-IV or in the totality of the context, considered atypical presentations of anxiety, depression, or somatoform disorders.

DEPRESSION WITH PSYCHOSIS

This is primarily a mood disorder and is characterized by typical depressive symptoms such as sadness, low energy, lack of interest, insomnia, and poor appetite. The psychotic symptoms are typically, though not always, congruent with the mood. For example, a 35-year-old woman with depression of several months' duration expresses belief that she is dying of multiple cancers, despite no medical evidence to support this, or a 75-year-old man with severe depression expresses nihilistic beliefs that his internal organs have rotted and that he is already dead.

Assessment has to include history, examination, and tests to rule out medical causes. Treatment includes the use of antidepressants and antipsychotic medication. Electroconvulsive therapy is often indicated.

MANIA WITH PSYCHOSIS

This is a primary mood disorder and is characterized by elevated mood, hyperactivity, distractibility, grandiose ideas, and pressured speech. In the more severe forms of mania, psychosis manifests with grandiose delusions and disorganized behavior. Hallucinations may also be experienced. Here are two examples: (1) A 21-year-old man with mania for one week drove off in a brand new Cadillac without paying for it as he believed he owned the car dealership. (2) A 35-year-old woman suffering from mania for several weeks was found dancing semi-nude in a public parking lot under the belief she was a film actress playing the role of a stripper and dancing in a club.

In addition to history and examination, assessment should include ruling in or out medical causes such as HIV, endocrine disorders, space-occupying lesions, demyelinating disorders, and medications. Treatment includes the use of mood stabilizer agents such as lithium or divalproex sodium in combination with antipsychotic medications.

DEMENTIA WITH PSYCHOSIS

Psychosis is very common in patients with dementia. As core cognition declines, paranoid ideation, hallucinations, delusions, and disorganized behavior may be seen. Agitation secondary to such experiences is often the cause of disruptive behaviors and may lead to hospitalization. Another common precipitant of psychosis and agitation in dementia is the occurrence of medical disorders such as urinary tract infection, bronchitis, pneumonia, and infected decubitus ulcers.

DELIRIUM WITH PSYCHOSIS

Although delirium is defined as a disorder of consciousness, psychosis is a frequent component of delirium. The description of the various causes of delirium is beyond the scope of this chapter. Psychotic symptoms such as hallucinations, paranoia, fleeting delusions, and disorganized behavior are frequently seen and often are the presenting symptoms of the underlying delirium.

Assessment includes a standard workup of the causes of delirium with appropriate treatment. Psychosis is treated with low to medium doses of antipsychotic medications. Medicines may have to be administered parenterally in the more agitated and uncooperative patient.

TABLE 226-3 Medical Conditions that may Manifest Psychosis

System/Cause	Disorders: Common*	Disorders: Uncommon†
Endocrine	Addison, Cushing, hyper and hypothyroidism	Hyper and hypoparathyroidism, pituitary disorders including Sheehan syndrome
Infections	Lyme disease, pneumonia	Diphtheria, legionnaire disease, malaria, typhoid
Inflammatory	Acute rheumatic fever, systemic lupus (cerebritis, vasculitis), sarcoidosis	Temporal arteritis
Metabolic	Diabetic ketoacidosis, hepatic encephalopathy, hypoglycemia, hypoxia, hyponatremia, uremia	Acute intermittent porphyria, Niemann Pick, Tay-Sachs
Nutritional	Vitamin B1 deficiency (Wernicke-Korsakoff syndrome), B12 deficiency	Folic acid deficiency, niacin deficiency (pellagra)
Pharmacologic	Anticholinergics, antiobesity, antiparkinsonian: levodopa, partial agonists, sympathomimetics	Antacids: cimetdine; antihistamines; antihypertensives: clonidine, propranolol, reserpine; anti-inflammatories: cyclosporin, NSAIDs, salicylate; antineoplastics: methotrexate, 5-fluorouracil; cardiac: digoxin, antiarrhythmic drugs
Substance abuse	Alcohol, amphetamines, cocaine, cannabis	Lysergic acid diethylamine (LSD), belladonna alkaloids, phencyclidine (pcp), mescaline, psilocybin
Toxic		Carbon monoxide poisoning, industrial toxins, heavy metal poisoning (eg, lead, mercury)
Trauma	Epidural hematoma, intraparenchymal hemorrhage, subarachanoid hemorrhage, subdural hematoma	
Central Nervous System Disorders		
CNS disorders	Multiple sclerosis, normal pressure hydrocephalus, epilepsy especially partial complex	
Basal ganglia disorders	Parkinson disorder	Huntington disease, Wilson disease, Fahr disease
CNS infections	HIV encephalopathy, any encephalitis, meningitis	Herpes encephalitis, rocky mountain spotted fever, syphilis
Dementias	Alzheimer disease, Vascular dementia	Pick disease, Creutzfeld-Jacob disease
Space occupying lesions	Cerebral neoplasm	Cerebral abscess, intracranial aneurysm, angioma
Vascular	Cerebrovascular events, hypertensive encephalopathy	
Congenital Disorders		
Developmental	Autism, mental retardation, Tourette syndrome	
Genetic: other	Down syndrome (Trisomy 21)	Adrenoleucodystrophy (X-linked), Klinefelter syndrome (XXY), Marfan syndrome (Chromosomes 5, 15), mitochondrial disorders, Prader-Willi (15q), velocardiofacial syndrome (22q)

*Common: Either the condition is common or psychosis as a manifestation is common.
†Uncommon: Either the condition is uncommon or psychosis as a manifestation is uncommon.

DEVELOPMENTAL DISORDERS WITH PSYCHOSIS

Individuals with developmental disorders (DD) such as mental retardation (now known as intellectual disability) and autism are especially vulnerable to psychosis. The period of young adulthood is a critical period, and often psychosis first manifests at this stage. The onset may be acute or gradual and the course is highly variable from short lasting to chronic. In individuals with a severe form of a developmental disorder, it is often difficult to correctly ascertain the presence of psychosis, as many behaviors of psychosis seamlessly merge with those of the underlying disorder. Assessment is made difficult by unique communication impairments such as deafness, mutism, or limited speech. Together the DD and the psychosis make it very challenging to assess the medical disorder for which the patient may have been admitted to the hospital. Physicians are encouraged to obtain the services of DD specialists, especially in communication, including sign language interpreters to assist in the assessment. Congenital and genetic disorders should be considered in the medical and neurologic assessments. Treatment should emphasize the use of lower doses of medication, as such individuals are highly vulnerable to acute and long-term neurologic adverse effects. Milieu therapies are important and should emphasize familiarity. Objects familiar to the patient should be allowed to be with the patient within safety constraints (favorite dolls, pictures, clothing, etc). A family member or familiar caregiver can play an invaluable role in milieu interventions and communication.

Table 226-3 lists some of the common and better-known general medical conditions that may manifest psychosis. Visual and tactile hallucinations are often a clue to an underlying physical or pharmacologic etiology. The psychosis may virtually mimic any of the functional disorders and it is the detection of a physical cause by history, examination, or testing that establishes the medical etiology. The course of the psychosis in these conditions is highly

TABLE 226-4 Substance-induced Psychosis

Substances Known to Induce Psychosis
Alcohol
Cannabis: marijuana
Hallucinogens: ketamine, LSD, mescaline, phencyclidine (angel dust), psilocybin, etc
Inhalants: amyl nitrate, gasoline, paint, paint thinners, etc
Opioids: morphine, oxycodone, hydromorphone
Stimulants: amphetamines, metamphetamines, cocaine, methylphenidate (Ritalin), designer drugs (MDMA or ecstacy)

variable and dependent on the underlying disorder. In chronic conditions, such as lupus, multiple sclerosis, seizure disorder, and hepatic and renal failure, psychosis may manifest recurrently. An interesting although not pathagnomonic distinction between psychoses secondary to a general medical condition and schizophrenic disorders is the absence of negative symptoms (see page 2, column B) in the former.

PSYCHOSIS INDUCED BY SUBSTANCE ABUSE

Table 226-4 lists the common substances of abuse that may manifest with psychosis. It is beyond the scope of this chapter to fully discuss substance-induced psychosis. Visual and tactile hallucinations are common. Alcohol-induced psychosis may manifest with classic paranoid delusions and hallucinations and may easily be misdiagnosed as schizophrenia. In LSD psychosis, temporal lobe phenomena such as experiences of deja vu and jamais vu are not uncommon. Classic substance-induced psychosis resolves within days of abstinence. However, when the psychosis is active, it is important to treat it adequately with antipsychotic medications and supportive therapies as well as standard withdrawal protocols.

ASSESSMENT

PSYCHIATRIC HISTORY AND EXAMINATION

Assessment should start with a focus on current symptoms, their duration, severity, and impact on daily function, and then proceed to past psychiatric history, substance abuse history, and brief psychosocial history including current living situation and support network. A separate history should be obtained for unsafe behaviors including self-injurious behaviors, suicidal ideation, intention, plans and attempts, and any ideas/behaviors of aggression/violence toward people and property. Following the history, mental status examination should be conducted to assess current positive and negative symptoms of psychosis as well cognitive functions such as attention, orientation, and memory. The mini–mental status examination is a handy tool to document the latter. A complete psychiatric assessment should be performed, preferably by a psychiatrist to arrive at multiaxial diagnoses in accordance with the DSM-IV-TR.

SUBSTANCE USE HISTORY AND TESTING

A detailed substance abuse history is a necessary part of the workup of psychosis and should cover all commonly abused substances, especially those known to cause psychosis. See Table 226-4. A urine test for common drugs of abuse, and, if indicated, additional blood or urine tests for toxicology, should be ordered.

MEDICAL HISTORY, REVIEW OF SYSTEMS, AND LABORATORY ASSESSMENT

It is imperative that all patients presenting with any psychotic symptom or behavior receive a proper medical workup including medical history, review of systems, and required testing. It is not, however, appropriate to order tests without a clinical indication, for example head CT, EEG, or CSF studies. Prenatal, birth, and early developmental history needs to be gathered from patient, family, or collateral source to rule in or out genetic, congenital, and developmental conditions known to manifest with psychoses (see Table 226-3). Laboratory assessment has two main purposes: (1) to rule in or out specific medical causes suspected from the history and examination, and (2) to assess common comorbid medical conditions, such as anemia, hypertension, obesity, and diabetes. It should be remembered that patients with chronic mental illness are at a 1.5 to 2 times higher risk of having a systemic medical disorder.

NEUROLOGIC ASSESSMENT

It is appropriate for a patient having a psychotic illness to be assessed neurologically with an EEG, brain scan, and neuropsychological testing at least once in the course of his or her illness, preferably early on. In cases of new-onset psychosis and psychosis in the elderly person, such testing is more likely to yield clinically significant findings, such as neurodevelopmental abnormalities, seizure foci, or atrophic, vascular, and neoplastic lesions.

TREATMENT OF ACUTE PSYCHOSIS

The physician has the option of choosing from many available antipsychotic medications, although the evidence to date suggests they are roughly equal in efficacy but vary widely in their side effects. Effect on the comorbid medical conditions, such as obesity, diabetes, cardiac disorders, and neurologic disorders, and any information available from prior experience of the patient, can help inform this decision.

ANTIPSYCHOTIC MEDICATIONS

First-generation antipsychotics (FGA) (see **Table 226-5**), also known as *typical* antipsychotics are effective with positive psychotic symptoms but have a higher potential to cause extrapyramidal effects, such as dystonia, parkinsonism, akathisia, and tardive dyskinesia. The most widely prescribed typical antipsychotic is haloperidal (Haldol). Other available FGA medications from the phenothiazine class are fluphenazine (Prolixin), trifluperazine (Stelazine), perphenazine (Trilafon), and chlorpromazine (Thorazine). Nonphenothiazine FGA antipsychotics are thiothixene (Navane), loxapine (Loxitane), and molindone (Moban). All these agents are thought to reduce psychosis, predominantly through the blockade of dopamine-2 receptors in the midbrain-limbic circuits.

Second-generation antipsychotics (SGA) are used more widely in practice due to reduced extrapyramidal effects, and are virtually the first line of treatment. These include risperidone (Risperdal), olanzapine (Zyprexa), quetiapine (Seroquel), and ziprasidone (Geodon). Aripiprazole (Abilify) is considered an atypical SGA although its mechanism of action is different; it is a partial dopamine agonist. Clozapine is also an atypical SGA, and while being a very effective antipsychotic with proven superiority in refractory schizophrenia, it has additional toxicities and is reserved for use in refractory patients. Its use requires periodic monitoring of the white cell and absolute neutrophil count, weekly for six months, and monthly thereafter. The SGAs are moderately dopamine blocking and also evidence antagonism to serotonin-2 receptors. A scale of chlorpromazine-equivalent units (CPZ units) is available to convert the dose of one typical FGA to that of another, and can be approximated to the atypical SGAs as well (see Table 226-5).

TABLE 226-5 Commonly Available Antipsychotic Medications

Generic and Common Brand Names	Mechanism of Action & DA2 Receptor Potency	Daily Dose* in mg	Common Adverse Events	Comments
First-generation Antipsychotic (FGA) (Typical)				
Chlorpromazine (Thorazine)	D2 antagonist, low	200–1800	Hypotension, sedation, EPS, TD	First available antipsychotic
Loxapine (Loxitane)	D2 antagonist, medium	25–200	Sedation, EPS, TD	
Molindone (Moban)	D2 antagonist, medium	25–225	Activation, EPS	
Thiothixene (Navane)	D2 antagonist, medium to High	10–80	EPS, TD	
Perphenazine (Trilafon)	D2 antagonist, medium to high	8–64	EPS, TD	Used in CATIE, largest nonindustry trial
Trifluperazine (Stelazine)	D2 antagonist, medium to high	5–60	EPS, TD	
Fluphenazine (Prolixin)	D2 antagonist, high	5–60	EPS, TD	
Fluphenazine decanoate long-acting inj		12.5–100 every 3 wks		
Haloperidol (Haldol)	D2 antagonist, high	2–20	EPS, TD	Most widely used typical antipsychotic
Haloperidol decanoate, long-acting inj		25–200 every 4 wks		
Second-generation Antipsychotic (SGA) (Atypical)				
Risperidone (Risperdal)	D2 & 5 HT2 antagonist, high	1–6	Hypotension, sedation, weight gain, EPS at higher doses	
Risperidone long-acting inj (CONSTA)		12.5–50 every 2 wks		
Paliperidone (Invega) D2 & 5HT2 antagonist, high		6–18 sedation, dizziness, akathisia		Active metabolite of risperidone Paliperidone palmitate inj 17–234 every 4-weeks
Olanzapine (Zyprexa)	D2 & 5 HT2 antagonist, medium to high	5–20	Hypotension, sedation, weight gain, DM	
Olanzapine pamoate, long-acting inj, (Relprevv)		150–400 every 2–4 wks		
Quetiapine (Seroquel)	D2 & 5 HT2 antagonist, low	100–800	Hypotension, sedation	
Ziprasidone (Geodon)	D2 & 5 HT2 antagonist, medium	40–160	Hypotension, prolonged QTc	
Arpiprazole (Abilify)	Partial D2 agonist, 5-HT2 antagonist, high	5–30	Activation, nausea	
Lurasidone (Latuda)	D2, 5 HT2, medium	40–80		Somnolence, dizziness, nausea, Parkinson
Asenapine (Saphris)	D2, 5 HT2, high	5–20	Oral numbness, dizziness, somnolence, akathisia, weight gain	Sublingual
Clozapine (Clozaril)	D2 & 5 HT2 antagonist, low	100–800	Sedation, weight gain, hypotension, seizures agranulocytosis, DM	WBC monitoring required

5-HT2, serotonin 2 receptor; D2, Dopamine 2 receptor, DM, diabetes mellitus; EPS, extrapyramidal symptoms; TD, tardive dyskinesia; WBC, white blood cell count.
*Dose ranges given reflect those used in common clinical practice.

DOSING

The antipsychotic agent is started at an initial dose of approximately 100 CPZ units, for example, 2 mg of haloperidol, or 2 mg of risperidone, or 100 mg of quetiapine, and titrated up every one to two days untill sufficient control of symptoms is achieved. Additional doses of the drug may be used on an as-needed basis to supplement the regular dose. The dosing is illustrated in two cases using haloperidol and quetiapine as examples. The drug choice in the examples is arbitrary and the dosing is just one example of standard practice. Other dosing regimens may be substituted without loss of efficacy.

CASE 226-1

A middle-aged female on a medical unit for the management of diabetic ketoacidosis is evidencing acute psychosis with delusions and hallucinations. Start haloperidol by mouth, at 2 mg twice a day, and titrate up by 2 mg every one to two days, until

symptoms and behavior are controlled, or a dose of 20 mg/day is reached. Supplement the regular dose with haloperidol 2 mg as needed by mouth or injection, every four to six hours. Order diphenhydramine 25 mg intramuscularly as needed for dystonic reaction and benztropine 1–2 mg twice a day for any emergent parkinsonian symptoms.

CASE 226-2

A 25-year-old male with traumatic gun shot injury that has undergone a laparatomy is evidencing acute psychosis on the surgical unit. Start quetiapine 100 mg by mouth at night. Increase by 100 mg every day till symptoms are controlled, or a dose of 600 mg is reached. Order quetiapine 50–100 mg by mouth as needed every six to eight hours for agitation or disruptive or dangerous behavior. Note that quetiapine (Seroquel) is not available as an injection, and for parenteral use, a second antipsychotic such haloperidol (Haldol), ziprasidone (Geodon), or ariprazole (Abilify) may be used.

RESUMPTION OF TREATMENT FOR PREEXISTING PSYCHOSIS

Medical illnesses often act as stressors and escalate preexisting psychosis, and often patients become noncompliant with medications. An antipsychotic should be reinstituted at the soonest possible time. In others who remain compliant, continue the antipsychotic. In both cases, it is best to use the antipsychotic that the patient was receiving most recently. In noncompliant patients, the starting dose may have to be lower than the most recently prescribed dose and gradually titrated up to the full dose to guard against adverse effects. As treatment proceeds, the dose may need to be increased beyond the previous maintenance dose.

MANAGEMENT OF ADVERSE EFFECTS

Common side effects include extrapyramidal effects such as dystonia, treated with intramuscular diphenhydramine, and parkinsonism, treated with benztropine 1–2 mg two to three times a day. Other anticholinergics that may be substituted for benztropine include trihexyphenidyl (Artane) or biperiden (Kemadrin). Akathisia is a subjective sense of unease with objective motor restlessness that may arise a few days into treatment, and is treated with lorazepam (Ativan) 1–2 mg two or three times a day, or propranolol (Inderal) 10–40 mg two or three times a day.

MANAGEMENT OF SEVERE AGITATION

The use of as-needed antipsychotic medication has been mentioned earlier. Sometimes it is necessary to use two antipsychotics for managing acute agitation. For example, a patient may be on quetiapine and while the standing dose is being titrated up, additional as-needed haloperidol by injection (intramuscular or intravenous), such as 2–5 mg every four to six hours may be given. SGAs are also available for intramuscular injections and include ziprasidone 10–20 mg intramuscular every six to eight hours, aripiprazole 9.75 mg intramuscular every eight hours, and olanzapine 5–10 mg intramuscular every six to eight hours. Lorazepam 1–2 mg as an intramuscular or intravenous injection may also be used to control psychotic agitation. It is not recommended to use more than two antipsychotics in any form for managing most cases. The potential for greater adverse effects such as excessive sedation, orthostasis and falls, and EPS is increased with polypharmacy, while not much is added to efficacy. Soft restraints to the hand and feet may have to be used to prevent injury.

ADJUNCT MEDICATION

Patients with preexisting psychosis are often on a mood stabilizer such as divalproex sodium or lithium; antidepressant medications; benzodiazepines, such as lorazepam or clonazepam; and/or hypnotic-sedatives such as zolpidem (Ambien) and eszopiclone (Lunesta). In such cases, it is best to coordinate the care with the outpatient psychiatrist by obtaining his or her opinion on continuation or discontinuation of these medications. In the absence of any such input, it is prudent to use the lowest effective dose of these agents for active symptoms, and not blindly resume all psychotropics. The exceptions to this rule are clozapine, high-dose benzodiazepines (eg, greater than 4 mg of lorazepam per day), and selective serotonin receptor inhibitors (paroxetine, sertraline, citalopram, etc), in which the potential for withdrawal effects is high. Fluoxetine (Prozac) has a long half-life and is self-tapering.

MILIEU AND PSYCHOSOCIAL THERAPIES

Patients exhibiting psychosis are best cared for in a private room for their own safety and comfort as well as that of other patients. In case of severely agitated, destructive, and/or disruptive behaviors, the use of soft restraints may be necessary till the medications are dosed appropriately and are able to be effective. In case of unsafe behavior including self-injurious ideation and behaviors or suicidal behavior, it is recommended that the patient be on one-on-one observation, with 24/7 visual contact and arms-length supervision as warranted by the condition.

The issue of keeping the patient on a medical-surgical unit versus transfer to a psychiatric unit is often difficult. Clearly, if the acute medical-surgical issues that the patient is in the hospital for have been addressed or are subsiding, then it may be appropriate to promptly move the patient to a dedicated psychiatric unit. On the other hand, if the medical-surgical problems need active management including interventions, such as intravenous infusions, telemetry, frequent medical-neurologic examinations, postoperative surgical care, or care of extensive burns, then it is recommended to keep the patient on the appropriate unit, while initiating or continuing the psychiatric care.

Patients with psychosis should not receive too much stimulation from the environment; care should be taken to minimize this. They should be allowed to participate in self-care activities as tolerated by their medical condition. Paranoid patients may feel further threatened by loss of autonomy and control. Visits by care givers and visitors should be brief and structured. Emotionally neutral activities are preferred rather than free access to health and news channels on TV, movies, etc.

A social worker or care coordinator should work with the patient and significant others to address any external stress and environmental manipulation, as feasible. The patient's dignity should be upheld at all times. The patient should be respected and kept fully informed of all health care plans and decisions, albeit with brief and succinct information. As discussed in more detail later in this chapter, consent should be obtained for all procedures, testing, and treatment outside routine care.

PSYCHIATRIC CONSULTATION

As soon as psychosis is suspected or history of a preexisting psychotic disorder is obtained, a psychiatric consultation is recommended. However, physicians may manage a psychosis if such consultation is not available, especially if the preexisting psychosis is a chronic condition and is stable or in remission. In this case, simply continuing the previous treatment with attention to proper dosing may suffice. However, if the psychosis is new in onset or has relapsed, it is recommended that a psychiatric consultation be obtained as soon as possible. In hospitals where such consultation is not feasible and active psychosis persists beyond three days, the patient should ideally be transferred to a hospital where such consultation is available or to a psychiatric unit, as appropriate. Psychiatric consultation is also recommended in case of questions regarding capacity to make medical decisions and possible involuntary treatment. The consultation should be ongoing till the psychosis is resolved, fully stabilized, or the patient is discharged.

CAPACITY AND CONSENT

Physicians will frequently encounter situations wherein the capacity of a patient with psychosis is called into question. This may arise if and when a patient refuses or does not cooperate with routine care, specific medical-surgical procedures for testing or treatment, psychiatric treatment, and/or requests premature discharge or attempts to leave. The situation may be urgent or nonurgent and elective. In each case except the most pressing situation, it is prudent to obtain a psychiatric consultation, which should include an opinion on the capacity of the patient to make a specific medical decision. Simple instruments are available to assess key areas pertaining to capacity. In an urgent situation, the physician may initiate life-saving intervention while seeking a consultation and consent from an appropriate entity in accordance with hospital policy and local, state, and federal law. In less urgent situations, the consultation and capacity assessment and appropriate consenting should precede the intervention.

Typically, a patient is considered to have capacity unless and until assessed to be otherwise. Such assessment may be performed by any physician although it is better to have a licensed mental health professional, preferably a psychiatrist, conduct this. Although state laws vary considerably, most states allow for urgent medical treatment against the wishes of an individual, if (1) lack of treatment is likely to result in permanent injury or death, (2) the individual is assessed to not have capacity to make the decision, and (3) consent has been obtained from an appropriate third party, typically legal next of kin or a local magistrate. Continuation of the treatment and initiation of less urgent interventions including non–life-saving interventions often require an assessment of capacity, recommendation by an independent physician, preferably a mental health professional, approval by an ethics or equivalent committee, and/or consent by a magistrate. A full discussion of all the issues, such as involuntary treatment, psychiatric commitment, advanced directives, is beyond the scope of this chapter.

COMPLICATIONS AND MANAGEMENT

The complications of an active psychosis (**Table 226-6**) include behavioral and/or medical events. These include severe agitation, disruptive behavior, unsafe behaviors including suicidal ideation and attempt, aggressive and violent behavior, leaving against medical advice, elopement, and escape. These behaviors may result from psychotic experiences such as hallucinations and delusions including paranoid fears, or may be the result of independent psychiatric disorders such as substance abuse and personality disorder. When assessed to be the result of psychosis, such behavior is best treated with a combination of antipsychotic medication and supportive therapy/counseling, including education of patient/significant other. If assessed to be from factors other than the psychosis, psychosocial interventions including negotiation with the patient, liaison by a psychiatrist, or assistance by a social worker or care coordinator may be helpful, depending on the issues.

Medical complications may include compromised fluid intake, electrolyte imbalance, poor nutrition and weight loss, autonomic hyperactivity including tachycardia, hypertensive crisis, hyperthermia, muscle rigidity, increased creatine kinase, and acute renal failure. The syndrome of malignant catatonia may start as a state of psychotic excitement and progress to catatonic stupor, and many of the physical complications noted above may be part of this syndrome. Its features overlap significantly with those of neuroleptic malignant syndrome (NMS).

TABLE 226-6 Behavioral and Medical Complications of Psychosis

Behavioral	Physical/Laboratory
Neglect of self-care	Exacerbation of medical disorders such as hypertension, diabetes, seizures, and infections
Withdrawal and catatonia	Dehydration, electrolyte imbalance
Severe excitement	Autonomic arousal and hyperactivity
Injury to self and others including homicide	Injuries (from restraint): soft tissue, fractures, etc
Suicide	Muscle breakdown, increased CPK, acute renal failure
Depression	Starvation, ketosis, acidosis, and metabolic disturbances
Amotivation, social isolation, deficit states, institutionalization	Sudden death

CPK, creatine phosphokinase.

Medical complications from psychotropic medications may include adverse effects such as extrapyramidal symptoms and signs, orthostatic hypotension, excessive sedation, liver enzyme abnormalities, blood dyscrasias including leucopenia, mild leucocytosis, changes in ECG including prolongation of QT interval, seizures, and micturition difficulties including rarely distended bladder. The combination of haloperidol and lithium was reported to be associated with a toxic encephalopathic syndrome, although this entity remains controversial. All neuorleptic agents have been associated with NMS, especially those with higher D2-blocking property, such as haloperidol. Clozapine has a 0.5–1.0% risk of inducing agranulocytosis, 2–5% risk of seizure, and is rarely associated with myocarditis. Olanzapine has sometimes been reported to cause an acute ketoacidosis. Clozapine and olanzapine when combined with benzodiazepines such as lorazepam, especially when given intramuscularly have been associated with apneic episodes, and rarely death.

Medical syndromes from the withdrawal of psychotropic agents may include SSRI discontinuation syndrome manifested by motor restlessness, insomnia, nausea, and vomiting, sense of confusion, and rarely seizure. Clozapine withdrawal may manifest a similar syndrome. Withdrawal from benzodiazpines may lead to tachycardia, hypertension, and seizures. It is therefore prudent to taper these medications rather than sudden discontinuation.

CONCLUSION

Psychosis is often seen on medical-surgical units as a comorbid condition. Acute psychosis constitutes an emergency and should be assessed and treated as such. Behavioral and medical complications may result from untreated or poorly treated psychosis. Psychosis is a syndrome and depending on the underlying disorder, its course and outcome will vary. There are both acute- and short-lasting psychotic disorders and chronic disorders. Medical factors and substances of abuse should be considered in the assessment of psychosis. Antipsychotic medications are the mainstay of treatment and careful attention should be given to the selection of the agent and dosing. Antipsychotics have many side effects, which play a significant role in the choice of medication. Psychosis in the context of an acute medical condition may be successfully treated on a medical unit and most psychoses will resolve or may be controlled with proper treatment. Psychiatric consultation is recommended and can be helpful in determining the nature of the psychosis, the choice of antipsychotic medication, the capacity to consent, in detecting adverse effects and their management, and in making recommendations on after-care. Brief psychosocial interventions such as structured activity, patient counseling, involving significant others, and care coordination increases the chances of successful management and better outcomes. Follow-up care with a psychiatrist or mental health clinic is an integral part of the management of psychotic disorders.

SUGGESTED READINGS

American Psychiatric Association. *Diagnostic and Statistical Manual of Mental Disorders*, 4th ed., text revision (DSM-IV-TR). Washington, DC: American Psychiatric Association Press; 2000.

Buchanan RW. Clozapine: efficacy and safety. *Schizophr Bull.* 1995;21:579–591.

Davidson L, McGlashan TH. The varied outcomes of schizophrenia. *Can J Psychiatry*. 1997;42:34–43.

Feifel D. Rationale and guidelines for the inpatient treatment of acute psychosis. *J Clin Psychiatry*. 2000;61(14):27–32.

Freudenreich O, Stern TA. Clinical Experience with the management of schizophrenia in the general hospital. *Psychosomatics*. 2003;44:12–23.

Goff DC, Henderson DC, Manschreck TC. Psychotic patients. In Cassem NH, ed. *Massachusetts General Hospital Handbook of General Hospital Psychiatry*. St Louis, MO: Mosby; 1997, pp.149–171.

Kane JM, Leucht S, Carpenter D, et al. The expert consensus guideline series. optimizing pharmacologic treatment of psychotic disorders. introduction: methods, commentary, and summary. *J Clin Psychiatry*. 2003;64:5–19.

Lamdan RM, Ramchandani D, Schindler BA. The chronically mentally ill on a general hospital consultation-liaison service. their needs and management. *Psychosomatics*. 1997;38:472–477.

Richards CF, Gurr DE. Psychosis. *Emerg Med Clin North Am*. 2000;18:253–262, ix.

CHAPTER 227

Decision-Making Capacity

Raymond Young, MD

Key Clinical Questions

1. Who determines the competency of an individual?
2. How does a clinician determine whether a patient has decision-making capacity?
3. What are the assumptions of informed consent or refusal?
4. What are the questions a clinician should ask a patient who wants to leave against medical advice?

INTRODUCTION

In the United States, a driver's license assumes competency to drive a car despite absence of proof that competency exists and despite statistics that as many as 50,000 Americans die and many more are disabled from car accidents annually. The same is true for obtaining a license to own a gun. When patients agree with recommendations of their physicians, the issue of competency is rarely raised despite the absence of competency. It is when patients and physicians disagree—when patients make decisions that clinicians feel are detrimental to their well being—that issues of competency are raised. The issue of competency is complex. Many medical decisions are affected by personal issues, religious and spiritual beliefs, or social pressures.

Competency is primarily a legal term rather than a medical one. Informed consent implies that patients have certain rights and expectations when it comes to making decisions regarding their own medical care. Patients have the right to be informed, their decision making should be voluntary, and they must be competent to make adequate decisions. In the hospital setting, the most common question posed to consultation liaison psychiatrists relates to decision-making capacity. Psychiatrists may help in the assessment of a patient's cognitive and emotional ability to make a decision. The hospital's ethics committee may help resolve the primary issue affecting the patient, especially if it is more a moral decision involving life and death decision making rather than a clinical one. The patient's spiritual advisor or hospital chaplain may be invaluable in sorting out the relevant issues and promoting resolution of conflict when decisions are made that make the medical providers uncomfortable (**Figure 227-1**).

CASE 227-1

MECHANICAL VENTILATION

Three weeks ago a 68-year-old woman sustained a cervical spinal cord injury from a fall. Quadriplegic, she will likely die if artificial ventilation is discontinued. The patient stated that "my life as it is now is not worth living. I am not happy." The patient seems to understand the implications of discontinuing artificial ventilation. The patient's family wants her to continue mechanical ventilation and they are concerned about the patient's thought process. Is this patient competent to make such a decision?

Is this patient competent to make medical decisions relating to her care?

This patient wants to discontinue mechanical ventilation. Does this patient truly understand the choice she is making? Is this patient depressed? Could this patient's mental state impact her decision to stop mechanical ventilation? Does this patient have the right to refuse to continue mechanical ventilation? The first question to ask is whether this patient has the decision-making capacity to choose whether to continue with mechanical ventilation.

COMPETENCY AND DECISION-MAKING CAPACITY

Competency is defined as the minimal mental, cognitive, or behavioral ability, trait, or capability that is required for a person

1. Does the patient have the ability to voice a decision?

If the answer is no, the patient is typically unable to respond as the result of conditions that are associated with:

Such cognitive impairment stupor, coma, expressive aphasias, severe mental retardation, developmental disorders, traumatic brain injury that the patient cannot respond
or
Severe indecision that the patient cannot voice a decision.

If the answer is yes, then proceed to question 2.

2. Does the patient have the ability to understand relevant information?

The amount of information that a reasonable person would want to know includes:

- The medical condition or diagnosis
- Recommended tests or treatments
- Potential risks and benefits of each
- A comparison to other treatment options as well as no treatment

This step provides opportunities to clarify misunderstandings that may have arisen due to medical jargon, language barrier, or educational level.

Patients with cognitive disorders may be unable to repeat what has been heard.

If the answer is yes, then proceed to question 3.

3. Does the patient have the ability to appreciate the relevant information and its potential consequences?

In addition to cognitive disorders, denial and psychiatric illness may affect the patient's ability to process information. Psychiatric consultation may be helpful in identifying the underlying problem (severe depression, psychosis, personality disorders such as narcissism, dependency, obsession and paranoia, and borderline personality) and the best approach.

Some of these patients may not be able to develop adequate trusting relationships with the team and may see medical staff as detrimental to their care.

If the answer is yes, proceed to question 4.

4. Does the patient have the ability to make rational decisions?

Risk-taking, impulsive decision making, fear, anxiety, and hopelessness interfere in the processing of information.

If the pattern of behavior is not a deviation from previous behavior, this may be the patient's normal processing and thus rational for the patient.

Patient continues to refuse mechanical ventilation.

If the patient appears to lack decision-making capacity proceed to legal options, obtaining input from hospital legal services, pursuing guardianship, and ethics consultation. In emergent medical situations, the physician must decide on behalf of the patient. In all other situations, a substitute must be identified, and asked to consider what the patient would have decided if the patient was able to make the decision, rather than what the identified decision maker would do. A family meeting includes the health care team, social workers, and consulting psychiatrist to discuss the situation. In case 227-1 her family request aggressive treatment.

Psychiatrists, social workers, and ethicists review her condition and the need for medical treatment. An assessment is made about the patient's literacy, educational level, and ability to comprehend the information, including an assessment about the presence of delirium and other disorders that would affect decision-making capacity. Clinicians pursue alternatives to no treatment. They also obtain advance directives.

Or

If the patient now appears to have decision-making capacity, she either agrees to continue mechanical ventilation or to stick with her original decision.

Figure 227-1 *Algorithm for the patient who refuses recommended treatment.*

to perform a particular legally recognized act or to assume a legal role. Only a judge can determine the competency of an individual. A legal concept, this determination relates to a specific situation, meaning a person may be competent to perform one act but may not be competent to perform another. Applelbaum and Grisso articulate four legal standards for the determination of competency:

1. The communication of choice
2. Understanding relevant information as it applies to that choice
3. Appreciating the situation and its consequences
4. Rational decision-making.

PRACTICE POINT

- Competency is defined as the minimal mental, cognitive or behavioral ability, trait, or capability that is required for a person to perform a particular legally recognized act or to assume a legal role. A legal concept, this determination relates to a specific situation, meaning a person may be competent to perform one act but may not be competent to perform another. Only a judge can determine the competency of an individual.

In a clinical situation, the judge will factor in the clinician's assessment of a patient's decision-making capacity in his determination of competency.

In the hospital setting, all patients are assumed to be competent and on admission sign a general statement consenting to treatment. A patient may be competent to identify a health care proxy but not competent to decide whether to proceed with mechanical ventilation. In the hospital, the determination of decision-making capacity can be made by any licensed physician and does not require the evaluation of a psychologist or psychiatrist even though one is often consulted to make that determination. The determination of decision-making capacity (like competency) is task specific, meaning a specific determination cannot be generalized to other decisions being made. Similar to the concept of competency, decision-making capacity utilizes four standards:

1. An understanding of the information provided
2. Communication of choice
3. An appreciation of available options
4. Rational decision-making.

PRACTICE POINT

- The determination of decision-making capacity (like competency) is task specific, meaning a specific determination cannot be generalized to other decisions being made. Similar to the concept of competency, decision-making capacity requires an understanding of the information provided, communication of choice, an appreciation of available options, and rational decision making. In the hospital the determination of decision-making capacity can be made by any licensed physician and does not require the evaluation of a psychologist or psychiatrist.

Understanding medical information

This refers to patients being able to express a basic understanding of their medical illness, the reasons for hospitalization, and the treatment options, including noting the risk and benefits of the options presented to them. In the case example, the patient should be able to explain her situation, ie, that she is in the hospital on mechanical ventilation due to paralysis. She should be able to explain that she has one of two options, either to continue on mechanical ventilation or to stop mechanical ventilation. Her physicians need to assess her awareness of the benefits and risks of mechanical ventilation and the risks and benefits associated with termination of mechanical ventilation.

Communication of choice

The patient should be able to express a preference or decision about a specific treatment. Indecisiveness may be a clue that a patient lacks decision-making capacity.

In the case example, the patient has clearly expressed her wishes that mechanical ventilation should be discontinued.

An appreciation of the options made available to them

Does the patient have the ability to truly understand how her decisions regarding treatment apply to her? It is more than just a factual understanding of the risks and benefits of a treatment decision, but rather an understanding of how that treatment decision results in consequences that directly affect future outcomes. In the case example, can the patient truly appreciate that her decision to discontinue mechanical ventilation will most likely result in her death?

Rational decision-making

This refers to the decision process behind the communication of choice being made. Does the patient have a good explanation for why she is making her decision? If such a thought process is appropriate, then such a decision may be rational even if the clinician totally disagrees with the decision being made. If our patient is able to explain rationally why she wishes to discontinue mechanical ventilation, then the decision may be appropriate even if it results in her death.

A patient must be able to satisfy all four of these standards to have decision-making capacity. How to evaluate a patient for decision-making capacity utilizing these standards depends on the patient's illness, the treatment that is in question, and the consequences of the decision being made with respect to treatment.

In 1977, Roth proposed a sliding scale approach to the determination of decision-making capacity and therefore competency. The determination of decision-making capacity would vary according to risk-benefit ratio. In the case example, the level of determination of decision-making capacity would be high because the patient has made the decision that she no longer wants to continue with mechanical ventilation, and the discontinuation of ventilation places the patient at high risk of harm and likely death. However, if the patient was in agreement for continued mechanical ventilation, then the threshold for determining decision-making capacity would be very low because not only is she in agreement with her physicians, but the risk to the patient would be much lower than if she were to stop mechanical ventilation.

Bostwick, and colleagues suggested utilizing a three-dimensional model for determining decision-making capacity. The model looks at the benefits of the proposed treatment (high versus low); the risk of the proposed treatment (high versus low); and the patient's decision to either accept or refuse treatment. This model allows the clinician to make a quick assessment of whether or not the threshold for determining decision-making capacity will be high or low. Any physician, regardless of specialty, can make a general assessment of decision-making capacity when appropriate. This chapter will address three factors:

1. The circumstances under which the question of decision-making capacity should be asked
2. How to assess decision-making capacity
3. Indications for psychiatric consultation to assess decision-making capacity.

When should the question of decision-making capacity be asked?

The patient's refusal of treatment is the most common reason to assess decision-making capacity of a patient. In addition, it is appropriate to assess a patient's decision-making capacity to ensure informed consent or capacity to make a decision to leave against medical advice.

How should one approach assessing decision-making capacity?

There are five basic questions that the primary team can ask of the patient when assessing decision-making capacity.

1. Will you explain the treatment we recommend?
2. What is your understanding of how this treatment can help you?
3. What is your understanding of what could happen if you do not receive this treatment?
4. What alternatives would you choose instead to address the problem?
5. Why have you decided to accept or refuse the treatment suggested?

These basic questions allow the clinician to cover the four standards of assessment of decision-making capacity (understanding the illness, communication of choice, appreciation of their choice, and rational decision making).

When is it helpful to have a psychiatric consultation in assessing decision-making capacity?

The hallmark of a good physician is to ask for help when there is uncertainty about a patient's decision-making capacity. Asking for a psychiatrist's opinion may be most helpful in the following situations:

1. A patient's psychiatric history raises questions about competency
2. Cognitive impairment such as delirium may jeopardize decision-making capacity
3. A vulnerable patient defers to family members despite previously expressed core values about treatment
4. There is discord among family members, patients, or health care team members relating to aggressiveness of care and risk of treatment options.

Psychiatric history: If a patient suffers from schizophenia, is he more likely to have impaired decision-making capacity than nonschizophrenic patients? If a patient is severely depressed and refusing life-saving treatment, does she have impaired decision-making capacity?

The MacArthur Competence Assessment Study examined the decision-making capacity of hospitalized patients with mental illness, namely, each patient's ability to understand relevant information regarding his illness and treatment, his ability to express a choice and to appreciate the implications of his choice, and his ability to rationally justify his decision. The study showed three findings:

1. Hospitalized patients with mental illness were more likely to show impaired decision-making capacity compared with hospitalized patients without mental illness.
2. Patients hospitalized with schizophrenia did well on most facets of decision making. When they didn't do well, the patients had more active psychotic symptoms such as delusions and disorganization of thinking. Schizophrenic patients were shown to have decision-making capacity and would show improvement in their ability as their illness was properly treated.
3. The majority of hospitalized patients with depression retained their decision-making capacity regardless of the severity of their symptoms. Hospitalized medically ill patients with life-threatening conditions were found to perform well on decision-making abilities and performed similarly to those individuals who were healthy living in the community.

Lapid and colleagues examined the decision-making capacity of severely depressed patients. The patients were assessed on their decision-making capacity to consent to treatment of electroconvulsive therapy. Despite the severity of their depression, patients were able to retain their decision-making capacity.

A study by Cohen and colleagues examined patients who suffered from major depression and schizophrenia and looked at their decision-making capacity to consent to or refuse to participate in medical research. Depressed individuals that agreed to participate in research protocols had similar levels of decision-making capacity compared with those depressed individuals who did not agree to participate. There were also similar rates of agreement to participate in high risk studies when compared with nonpsychiatric subjects.

The majority of schizophrenic patients had decision-making capacity, and impairment in capacity was not an automatic characteristic of schizophrenia. And in those schizophrenic patients who had impaired decision-making capacity, it was not correlated to the psychopathology of the illness but rather the chronicity of the illness.

Cognitive impairment: Studies examining patients with mild Alzheimer disease show that decision-making capacity remains intact when the threshold for determining decision-making capacity is low. The more complex the determination, the more likely patients will show deficits in their ability to understand, appreciate, communicate a choice, and give rational decisions about their choice.

Okonkwo and colleagues found that decision-making capacity was most likely affected by memory, level of executive functioning, semantic knowledge, and processing speed. These cognitive domains were most likely to affect the patient's ability to understand the treatment, appreciate the treatment, and to give a rational explanation of his choice. Although the ability to offer a choice was not always affected, patients with mild cognitive impairment and mild Alzheimer's dementia were more likely to offer a poor choice.

Conflict between the patient and family: Good communication between families and the clinician can usually lead to better decision-making on behalf of the patient, leading to more positive outcomes. It is the family that is often asked to act as surrogate decision-makers for the patient when the patient lacks decision-making capacity, as for example, when a patient is critically ill in the intensive care unit. Having social support is often a requirement for some treatments such as organ transplantation. However, there are times when the patient and family disagree with one another on treatment decisions.

In the case example, the patient's family disagrees with the patient's wishes to discontinue mechanical ventilation. A family member, more likely the designated power of attorney of health care, may push to become the surrogate decision-maker despite the absence of legal precedent that rests on the premise that the patient lacks decision-making capacity.

If a family member has been awarded guardianship for a patient, then the family member may be the clinical decision-maker even if the patient is capable of expressing a choice. A guardian is an individual appointed by the court to have the legal authority to make decisions for a person with respect to the person and his or her property. A court appoints a guardian for an individual only when that person has been declared incompetent.

INFORMED CONSENT AND INFORMED REFUSAL

Informed consent and informed refusal assume competency and decision-making capacity. In order for a patient to either give informed consent or refusal of treatment they must satisfy three criteria:

1. **Information or knowledge**
   The patient must be given adequate information or knowledge about his or her medical condition and information regarding his or her treatment options. The information about such options must include not only the benefits associated with the treatment but the risks to the patient as well.
2. **Competence**
   The patient must show:
   - Capability of understanding the information given to him regarding the medical condition and an understanding of the treatment options, risk and benefits
   - Capability of expressing a choice regarding treatment, whether to agree or refuse
   - An appreciation of his or her choice, how it impacts future outcome
   - Capability of giving a rational explanation of the preferred choice of treatment.
3. **Voluntariness**
   The physician-patient role assumes influence; however, the physician should always help the patient clarify goals, give coherent options aligned with the patient's goals, and make appropriate recommendations. The patient must be able to express voluntarily his or her consent or refusal for treatment. The patient must not be negatively influenced or coerced by external sources.

All patients are required to give informed consent, although there are four exceptions to that rule:

1. **Medical emergencies**
   When a patient's medical condition is serious, posing imminent life-threatening danger and the patient is unable to give consent to life-saving treatment (due to lack of capacity or inability to communicate a choice) and has no representative or advance directives to communicate on his or her behalf, then it is generally assumed that the patient gives consent to the treatment. These exceptions do not include situations in which the patient is found to have the decision-making capacity to refuse treatment, even if such treatment is deemed necessary to prevent the patient from life-threatening injury.
2. **Incompetence**
   For patients who have been determined incompetent in a court of law, the legally appointed guardian represents the patient and consents to treatment on the patient's behalf. For those patients who during their hospitalization have been determined to lack the decision-making capacity to refuse treatment, then the clinician has to determine whether to give consent for the patient to receive treatment. If a patient has a person acting as power of attorney (POA) for health care, then that individual will make the decisions on the behalf of the patient. If the patient does not have specific advance directives and lacks a specified POA, then most states will allow family members to consent to treatment on behalf of the patient. If the decision to consent to treatment is not an emergency, the clinician and hospital may have to pursue guardianship, especially if the patient does not have family members or lacks capacity to designate a health care proxy.
3. **Waiver**
   The patient may decide to waive his right to all the information necessary to make an informed decision (whether it is to consent to treatment or refuse treatment).
4. **Therapeutic privilege**
   This exception to informed consent is the most controversial because it raises the possibility that there are certain situations in which complete disclosure of all medical information regarding the treatment, risks, and benefits may actually prove detrimental to the patient's well-being. Therefore the clinician chooses not to disclose all the information because she determines it is in the patient's best interest not to.

JEHOVAH'S WITNESS PATIENTS AND BLOOD TRANSFUSION

CASE 227-2

JEHOVAH'S WITNESS

A 27-year-old female is hospitalized for a flare up of her Crohn disease. Very concerned about her poor nutrition and significant anemia, the physicians in charge of her care maintain that it is vital that she receives a blood transfusion. The patient, a Jehovah's Witness, refuses due to her religious faith that prohibits blood transfusions. The physicians explain to her that this is a medical emergency, that she will likely die without a blood transfusion but the patient still refuses.

Does this patient have the right to refuse a blood transfusion? Can the clinician provide consent for the patient to receive a blood transfusion based on the exception that this is a medical emergency?

Patients who practice the faith of Jehovah's Witness will refuse life-saving blood transfusion based on their religious principles. The receiving of blood products is considered a violation of God's law. As clinicians we must uphold their decision based on the principles of self-determination and autonomy. The patient has a right to determine what is done or not done to her body (provided that the patient has decision-making capacity, and is thus competent), even if we as clinicians believe that a patient's decision may have life-threatening consequences.

In the above example, the determination of whether the patient will receive a blood transfusion is based on two conditions. One is being able to identify the patient's treatment preferences. The patient must be able to either communicate that she is a practicing Jehovah's Witness or if she is unable to communicate, she must have identification or advance directives indicating that she is a Jehovah's Witness. If this can be determined, then the patient cannot receive a blood transfusion based on her identified faith.

The other condition depends on the patient's ability to provide an informed decision to refuse a blood transfusion. It is very important that even if a clinician encounters a patient who may identify herself as part of a group that disagrees with some aspects of treatment (such as a Jehovah's Witness refusing blood transfusions), he or she is still obligated to give the patient a chance to provide an informed decision to refuse such treatment. The clinician must provide all the necessary information to the patient about her medical condition, care, and treatment options, and allow the patient to make her own decision about treatment and identify the patient as competent to make that decision.

There are exceptions allowing clinicians to provide consent to patients for blood transfusions who may be identified as Jehovah's Witnesses. Minor children of parents who practice as Jehovah's Witnesses are protected under the law so that parents are unable to refuse life-saving treatment on their children's behalf based on religious principles. Clinicians may provide consent for patients to receive treatment who at the time when a life-saving blood transfusion was needed could not be identified as Jehovah's Witness. In most cases, the clinician is protected from being sued for malpractice.

PATIENT SELF DETERMINATION ACT 1990

The Patient Self Determination Act, which Congress passed in 1990, gives patients the right to make choices and decisions about their medical care. Patients can specify what care they will accept and what care that they will refuse. A patient's living will and the establishment of a POA for health care must be recognized as acts of self-determination by the patient. All hospital and home health programs that receive funding from Medicare and Medicaid must recognize a patient's living will and POA for health care.

Hospital and home health care programs must comply with these actions:

1. Each patient at the time of admission must be asked if he or she has an advance directive.
2. If the patient does not have an advance directive, the patient must be given written information about establishing an advance directive.
3. If the patient does have an advance directive, then it must be documented and placed in the patient's medical record.
4. The hospital and/or home health care program must be able to demonstrate that policies and procedures regarding advance directives that meet federal and state law requirements are in place.

LEAVING AGAINST MEDICAL ADVICE

One percent to two percent of all medical admissions are prematurely terminated by the patient before the clinician decides that the patient can be safely discharged. On the one hand, clinicians have been taught to respect the autonomy of the patient and his right to refuse treatment. However, the clinician also recognizes the increased risk of readmissions, poor outcomes, medical legal ramifications, and higher health costs in patients who leave against medical advice (AMA). Sometimes adversarial input due to conflict existing between patients and the medical team result in a patient signing out AMA. When conflict occurs, the hospitalist may be able to avoid the question of competency by meeting with the involved parties and providing the patient with cohesive input.

Patients who leave AMA are more likely to be readmitted to the hospital relatively soon after leaving the hospital. For example, in a study by Hwang and colleagues, patients who were admitted to the general medical service were seven times more likely to be readmitted within two weeks of leaving the hospital AMA, and they were generally readmitted for the same initial complaint that resulted in their original hospitalization.

Patients who leave AMA are more likely to have poorer outcomes. A retrospective study of 100,000 patients hospitalized for acute myocardial infarction by Friscell and colleagues found that those patients who left AMA had a 40% higher risk of death and readmission for up to two years after leaving AMA. Other studies have found the increased mortality rate to range from 15% to 19% within six months to a year after leaving the hospital AMA.

There are common predictors for patients leaving AMA:

1. Miscommunication between the clinician and patient
2. Evidence of active substance use
3. Financial obligations such as a need to get back to work
4. Personal obligations

A study by Anis and colleagues found that 13% of patients with HIV or AIDS left the hospital AMA and that high predictors of leaving AMA in this population included leaving the day they received their welfare checks and a history of IV drug use.

Windish and Ratanawongsa identified eight questions that clinicians should ask themselves when a patient wants to leave AMA:

1. Do I have full insight into this patient's beliefs about health and illness?
2. How can I use my insight to counsel this patient in a patient-centered way?
3. What factors are making it difficult for us to communicate?
4. How can I reestablish my trust in this patient and this patient's trust in me?
5. What are this patient's concerns about remaining in the hospital?
6. How can I acknowledge those concerns and communicate empathy and respect for this patient?
7. How does this patient's desire to leave make me feel about myself?
8. How does this patient's desire to leave make me feel about my professional responsibilities toward this patient?

By answering these questions, the clinician may be able to identify factors that may be leading to the patient's decision to leave AMA and offer possible solutions that would ultimately change the patient's decision to leave AMA.

From a legal standpoint, a patient can leave the hospital AMA as long as the patient can show decision-making capacity, including an ability to understand the nature of the illness, the proposed treatment options, and the associated risks and benefits to staying in the hospital versus leaving AMA. The patient must be able to demonstrate an appreciation of how the decision to leave the hospital will impact future health and provide a rational decision for wanting to leave AMA. Physicians should document this capacity in the medical record.

INVOLUNTARY HOSPITALIZATION OF MEDICAL INPATIENTS

Patients on inpatient medical units who lack medical decision-making capacity may require involuntary hospitalization. Patients who are delirious, withdrawing from substance abuse, or suffer personality changes secondary to their medical condition may want to leave AMA but due to lack of decision-making capacity they cannot leave AMA and they are prevented from doing so.

Patients who are delirious or have personality changes secondary to their medical condition do not meet criteria for psychiatric commitment. The primary goal is to get the patient to consent to medical treatment. Steps to ensure that the patient does not leave the hospital include using the least restrictive method to keep the patient in the hospital, such as use of sitters, security, or police to help in restricting the patient to the hospital; contacting family or power of attorney of health care to obtain consent to medical treatment; and pursuing guardianship if no family or POA representative is available.

It is important to distinguish between involuntary commitment to a psychiatric facility versus involuntary hospitalization for medical patients that lack decision-making capacity. Commitment of a patient requires evidence that the patient is mentally ill with the need of psychiatric treatment and without such treatment that the patient would be at continued risk of deterioration, that the patient is either a danger to himself or a danger to others, a danger to property, or the patient is unable to care for himself due to mental illness.

THE USE OF RESTRAINTS

Restraints have been considered a part of acceptable medical practice since the 1940s. Restraints (both physical and chemical) have been used for the purpose of protecting the patients from self-harm (such as fall prevention), to prevent them from harming others, and to prevent patients from interfering with their own medical treatment.

Physical restraints are defined as any method, whether it is manually holding a patient, or utilizing a mechanical device or equipment (such as ties or belts) to reduce the ability of a patient move his body freely.

Chemical restraints are referred to medications when they are used to restrict or manage a patient's behavior by limiting the patient's ability to move freely and such use of the medication is not a standard treatment or usage of the medication. Examples include usage of antipsychotics for treatment of dangerous, agitated behavior in patients suffering from an agitated delirium.

The use of restraints has become more controversial as there is little evidence to show that restraints are effective. In fact there is evidence that the use of restraints leads to increased harm to patients. For example, studies have shown that the use of restraints for fall prevention has actually led to more serious injury from falling than those patients who were not restrained.

Chang and colleagues evaluated the use of physical restraints in patients who received mechanical ventilation in the intensive care unit. They found that the risk of unplanned extubation was three times higher in physically restrained patients. Unplanned extubation can lead to prolonged hospitalization, cardiopulmonary arrest, and death.

A study by Martin and Mathisen compared the usage of physical restraints in adult critical care units in the United States with adult critical care units in Norway and found that the usage of physical restraints was less prevalent in adult critical care units in Norway. They found this difference largely related to different nursing practices. They utilized more nurses per patient, and nurses maintained a more direct visual observation of their patients.

The Joint Commission on Accreditation of Health care Organization (JCAHO) and the Centers for Medicare and Medicaid Services (CMS) have pushed for alternatives to restraints. The goal is to utilize restraints only when less restrictive methods have not been found to be effective. The clinician must document that alternative uses to restraints have either been used or considered and they must document justification for the usage of restraints. Patients must routinely be assessed during their time in restraints to monitor their well-being and assess continued justification for usage of restraints. Routine assessments include (1) assessing hydration status, (2) vital signs, (3) mental status, (4) peripheral circulation, (5) toileting, (6) skin integrity, and (7) degree of agitation.

CONCLUSION

It is very important for the clinician to understand the concepts of competency and decision-making capacity and how they apply to broader concepts of informed consent, the right to refuse treatment, and the patient's right to leave the hospital AMA.

All patients are assumed to be competent unless they have already been deemed incompetent by a judge in a legal proceeding. Although only a judge can determine the competency of a patient, such a determination is influenced by the clinician's assessment of the patient's decision-making capacity.

All clinicians can determine the decision-making capacity of their patients. Psychiatric illness and cognitive impairment can have an impact on a patient's ability to have capacity but do not automatically exclude a patient from having decision-making capacity. Ultimately, the determination of a patient's decision-making capacity is based on his ability to understand the information about his medical condition and treatment, his ability to communicate a choice about treatment, his ability to appreciate how his choice impacts his future outcome, and his ability to give a rational decision about his choice.

Evidence

Determination of decision-making capacity

Appelbaum PS, Grisso T. Assessing patients' capacities to consent to treatment. *New England Journal of Medicine (NEJM)*. 1988;319:1635–1638.

Bostwick J, Dodd M, Magid M, Philbrick K. Is your patient making the 'wrong' treatment choice? *Current Psychiatry*. 2006;5(3):13–20.

Roth LH, Meisel A, Lidz CW. Tests of competency to consent to treatment. *American Journal of Psychiatry*. 1977;134:279–284.

Determination of decision-making capacity in patients with mental illness

Cohen B, McGarvey E, Pinkerton R, Kryzhanivska L. Willingness and compe-tence of depressed and schizophrenic inpatients to consent to research. *J Am Acad Psychiatry Law*. 2004;32:134–143.

Grisso T, Appelbaum PS. The MacArthur treatment competence study, III: abilities of patients to consent to psychiatric and medical treatments. *Law Hum Behavior*. 1995;19:149–174.

Lapid M, Rummans T, Poole K, et al. Decisional capacity of severely depressed patients requiring electroconvulsive therapy. *The Journal of ECT*. 2003;19(2):67–72.

Okonkwo OC, Griffith HR, Belue K, et al. Cognitive models of medical decision-making capacity in patients with mild cognitive impairment. *Journal of the International Neuropsychological Society*. 2008;14:297–308.

Patients who leave AMA

Anis A, Sun H, Guh D, Palepu A, Schechter M, O'Shaughnessy M. Leaving hospital against medical advice among HIV-positive patients. *CMAJ*. 2002;167(6):633–637.

Fiscell K, Meldrum S, Barnett S. Hospital discharge against advice after myocardial infarction. *Am Journal Med*. 2007;120(12):1047–1053.

Hwang SW, Li J, Gupta R, Chien V, Martin RE. What happens to patients who leave the hospital against medical advice? *CMAJ*. 2008;168(4):417–420.

Windish D, Ratanawongsa N. Providers' perceptions of relationships and professional roles when caring for patients who leave the hospital against medical advice. *J. Gen Intern Med*. 2008;23(10):1698–1707.

Physical restraints

Chang L, Wang K, Chao Y. Influence of physical restraint on unplanned extu-bation of adult intensive care patients: a case-control study. *Am J Crit Care*. 2008;17:408–415.

Martin B, Mathisen L. Use of physical restraints in adult critical care: a bicultural study. *Am J Crit Care*. 2005;14:133–142.

When a clinician determines that a patient does not have decision-making capacity, this impacts a patient's ability to give informed consent, refuse treatment, and leave AMA. Having knowledge of a patient's advance directives and power of attorney (if available) can be very useful in determining the next steps to take in the care of patients who are incapacitated.

Psychiatric consultants can be helpful in these assessments. The psychiatrist can help with the determination of decision-making capacity, treat and diagnose psychiatric conditions that may interfere with decision making, talk with the patient's outside psychiatrist, provide resources for patients and families, guidance for the health care team that may be divided over the best approach, and minimize the number of patients who choose to leave AMA.

SUGGESTED READINGS

Ai D, Owen G, McGuire H, Singh S, Chruchill R, Hotopf M. Mental capacity in psychiatric patients: systemic review. *British Journal of Psychiatry*. 2007;191:291–297.

Alfandre D. "I'm going home": discharges against medical advice. *Mayo Clinic Proceedings*. 2009;84(3):255–260.

Applelbaum PS, Grisso T. The MacArthur Treatment Competence Study, I. Mental Illness and competence to consent to treatment. *Law Hum Behavior*. 1995;2. April 19(2):105–126.

Carmen M, Joffe S. Informed consent for medical treatment and research: A review. *The Oncologist*. 2005;10:636–641.

Curtis J, White D. Practical guidance for evidence-based ICU family conferences. *Chest*. 2008;134:835–843.

Grisso T, Appelbaum PS, Mulvey E, Fletcher K. The MacArthur Treatment Compe-tence Study: II. Measures of abilities related to competence to consent to treatment. *Law Hum Behavior*. 1995;19:127–148.

Ibrahim S, Kwoh K, Krishnan E. Factors associated with patients who leave acute care hospitals against medical advice. *Research and Practice* 2007;97(12):2204–2208.

Jeste D, Depp C, Palmer B. Magnitude of impairment in decisional capacity in people with schizophrenia compared to normal subjects: an overview. *Schizophrenia Bulletin*. 2006;32(1): 121–128.

Leo R. Competency and the capacity to make treatment decisions: a primer for primary care physicians, primary care companion. *J Clin Psychiatry*. 1999;1:131–141.

Sullivan MD, Youngner SJ. Depression, competence, and the right to refuse life saving medical treatment. *American Journal of Psychiatry*. 1004;151:971–978.

CHAPTER 228

Eating Disorders

Angela S. Guarda, MD
Graham Wester Redgrave, MD

Key Clinical Questions

1. What is an eating disorder and why are eating disorders important to hospitalists?
2. What questions aid in making the diagnosis?
3. What screening tests are indicated?
4. When is emergent hospitalization warranted?
5. What are the complications of starvation and of binge/purge behaviors?
6. What is refeeding syndrome?
7. What are the evidence-based treatments for eating disorders?
8. Is there a role for enteral or parenteral nutrition in the treatment of anorexia nervosa?
9. What is the behavioral management of an eating disorder patient on a hospitalist service?
10. What ethical considerations are specific to the treatment of eating disorders?
11. What are appropriate plans for discharge and follow-up care?

INTRODUCTION

Medical morbidity associated with eating disorders is high and most hospitalists will encounter patients with these disorders, so knowledge of the presentation, natural history, complications, and medical management of these conditions is important. Patients with eating disorders may be admitted through emergency rooms in the setting of an acute event such as syncope or a seizure, or referred by their primary care provider for an abnormal electrocardiogram or for laboratory values warranting admission for medical monitoring and stabilization. The majority of patients are likely to have anorexia nervosa (AN), but some may have bulimia nervosa (BN). Others may present with an atypical eating disorder in which abnormal eating behavior is not associated with drive for thinness or fear of being fat.

Eating disorders are best thought of as disorders of motivated behavior and are similar to addictions. As with substance abuse disorders, patients exhibit a narrowing of their behavioral repertoire. They develop increasingly driven ritualized behaviors and progressive functional impairment. The vast majority of affected individuals are female with the lifetime prevalence of AN and BN in women estimated at 0.9% and 1.5% respectively. Although less common in males, it is also the case that males with eating disorders are less likely to reach medical attention, and community rates of eating disorders in men and boys are higher than the 10% male gender prevalence observed in clinical samples. Mortality for AN is one of the highest amongst psychiatric conditions, with sixfold increases in standardized mortality rates reported in a recent study.

Because eating disorders are motivated behavioral conditions, ambivalence toward and frank avoidance of treatment are common. Patients may conceal their behavior from others and avoid professional help, complicating both diagnosis and management. When they do present for treatment, they are frequently in crisis, seeking assistance in managing complications of their disorder, or because they are brought to treatment by others. Half of all community cases of AN and BN go undetected, underscoring the importance of recognizing signs and symptoms. Once identified, most patients are reluctant to engage in treatment, preferring treatment on their own terms, picking and choosing interventions that feel best, rather than those that may be best for them. Knowing how to engage patients to seek effective treatment is one of the most important challenges for the clinician.

INDICATIONS FOR EMERGENT HOSPITALIZATION

Medically unstable patients with eating disorders are ideally treated by a multidisciplinary team, on a dedicated inpatient specialty unit, using a rehabilitative approach including intensive behavioral and group therapy. Such programs are effective in restoring weight in underweight patients and in normalizing eating behavior. In AN, weight restoration to a BMI of 19–21 is necessary though not usually sufficient for recovery. Treatment should also address medical complications, interrupt unhealthy behaviors, establish a normal eating pattern, and use psychotherapeutic strategies to assist patients in challenging cognitive distortions that sustain their behavior. A focus on relapse prevention and transition to outpatient treatment are critical components of long-term rehabilitation, especially in chronically ill patients who have become functionally impaired as a consequence of their eating disorder.

Unfortunately, there are few specialized hospital-based behavioral programs capable of managing medically complex cases, and access may be limited further by insurance or financial issues. As a result, patients are often admitted to hospitalist services for initial medical monitoring and stabilization. Reasons for emergent hospitalization can include hypokalemia or other serious electrolyte imbalances, hypoglycemic coma, symptomatic bradycardia, severe hypotension, dehydration, syncope, seizure, prolonged QTc interval, severe marasmus with BMI < 14, or development of suicidal or other psychiatric instability. Single cases admitted to a general hospital ward can be difficult to manage behaviorally and present special challenges to the hospitalist.

This chapter will address the diagnosis and treatment of eating disorders with a focus on medical management of complications, approaches to blocking eating disorder behaviors on a general hospital floor, as well as appropriate guidelines for discharge planning and ethical issues specific to managing these patients.

DIAGNOSING AN EATING DISORDER

The Diagnostic and Statistical Manual of Mental Disorders (DSM-IV) distinguishes three categories of eating disorders: AN, BN, and eating disorder not otherwise specified (EDNOS). Both AN and BN are characterized by an overvalued fear of being fat and a primary preoccupation with dieting behavior. The main distinction between these disorders is one of weight, with AN trumping the diagnosis of BN for patients who are underweight.

■ ANOREXIA NERVOSA

In general, a BMI of less than 18 should raise suspicion for AN in the absence of other defined etiology for weight loss. AN is characterized by self-starvation, fear of weight gain, and denial of the seriousness of low body weight. There are two subtypes of AN, restricting and binge-eating/purging type. In restricting type AN, patients restrict food intake, especially of calorie-dense foods, sometimes combined with excessive exercise, but they do not binge or use purging behaviors. In the binge-eating/purging subtype, patients additionally engage in intermittent binge-eating, self-induced vomiting and/or the misuse of laxatives, diuretics, or enemas. Although amenorrhea is included as a diagnostic criterion for AN, it does not help distinguish more severe cases or have prognostic value, and it is likely to be dropped in the upcoming revision to DSM-IV.

■ BULIMIA NERVOSA

BN is characterized by chronic dieting with intermittent binge eating followed by compensatory behaviors to prevent weight gain. Most patients with BN are normal weight although some may be low normal weight and others may be overweight or obese. Bingeing is defined as the rapid consumption of a large amount of food, typically more than 1,000 calories, and up to 10,000 or more calories, associated with a sense of loss of control over eating. In BN, binges occur with a frequency of twice a week or more and as with AN there are two subtypes of BN: purging and nonpurging type. The more common purging type BN is characterized by compensatory self-induced vomiting or abuse of laxatives following a binge, whereas in nonpurging BN, only periodic compensatory fasting without weight loss and or excessive exercise are employed to avoid weight gain following a binge.

■ EATING DISORDER NOT OTHERWISE SPECIFIED

This third classification is a catch-all category that includes any other psychological eating disturbance resulting in clinically significant functional impairment. Examples are subthreshold variants of AN and BN or binge eating disorder (BED) in which bingeing is not accompanied by compensatory behaviors. Thus, individuals with BED tend to be overweight. Finally, the EDNOS category also includes a range of atypical eating disorders including anxiety-related eating disorders, such as fear of swallowing (globus hystericus) or idiosyncratic overvalued preoccupations with food intolerances or bowel cleansing rituals that impair an individual's function.

Clinically, eating disorders are best viewed dimensionally. There is significant overlap between syndromes and it is not uncommon for patients to move from one diagnosis to another over time or to substitute behaviors. The most common progression is from restricting subtype AN to a purging disorder, either BN purging type or AN binge-eating/purging type.

TABLE 228-1 Signs and Symptoms of Eating Disorders

Starvation-related	Binge-purge-related
• Dry skin, lanugo, alopecia • Cold intolerance, hypothermia, cyanotic extremities • Weakness, fatigue • Sinus bradycardia, hypotension • Presyncope or syncope • Early satiety, bloating, constipation • Primary or secondary amenorrhea • Peripheral neuropathy • Osteoporosis and fractures • Muscle wasting, cachexia • Bruising, nosebleeds	• Perioral acne • Parotid gland enlargement • Dental caries and erosion of lingual surface of teeth • Orthostatic hypotension and dehydration • Presyncopal and syncopal symptoms • Heartburn, gastroesophageal reflex • Muscle cramps and paresthesias (from electrolyte abnormalities) • Diarrhea and constipation (laxative abusers) • Cardiac arrhythmia • Amenorrhea or oligomenorrhea

DIAGNOSIS

Physical signs and symptoms of AN and BN are listed in **Table 228-1**. **Table 228-2** lists two brief screening questionnaires, with similar sensitivity and specificity, useful in detecting eating disorders.

TABLE 228-2 Screening Tools for Eating Disorders

SCOFF	ESP (Eating disorders screen for primary care)
• Do you make yourself SICK because you feel uncomfortably full? • Do you worry you have lost CONTROL over how much you eat? • Have you lost more than ONE stone (14 lbs) over the last three months? • Do you believe yourself to be FAT when others say you are thin? • Would you say that FOOD dominates your life?	• Are you satisfied with your eating patterns? • Do you ever eat in secret? • Does your weight affect how you feel about yourself? • Has anyone in your family ever suffered with an eating disorder? • Do you currently suffer with or in the past have you suffered with an eating disorder?
Cut off: Two or more abnormal responses has a sensitivity of 100%, specificity of 87.5% for an eating disorder.	Cut off: Two or more abnormal responses has sensitivity of 100%, specificity of 71% for an eating disorder.
Data from Morgan JF, et al. *BMJ.* 1999;319:1467–1468.	Data from Cotton MA, et al. *J Gen Intern Med.* 2003;18:53–56.

A positive screen should be followed by clarifying questions. Useful questions include desired weight ("What would you like to weigh?"), preoccupation with thoughts of food, weight, or shape ("What percent of the day are you preoccupied with thoughts of food or feeling fat?"); typical daily food intake with attention to variety of foods consumed and calorie density ("Tell me what you ate yesterday for breakfast, lunch, and dinner?"), hours spent exercising per week and frequency of bingeing, vomiting, laxative, diuretic, or diet pill use, including dose used. Recent adoption of vegetarianism or development of food intolerances as well as refusal to eat meals with others and social isolation should raise the index of suspicion for an eating disorder.

Collateral information from a family member is important since patients often underreport or deny eating disordered behaviors and preoccupations. Observing the patient can be helpful when the diagnosis is unclear. Hospital nursing staff may detect behavioral signs of an eating disorder including driven pacing, excessive standing and fidgeting despite emaciation, idiosyncratic and detailed food requests or food refusal, ritualistic eating behavior, hiding food, evidence of self-induced vomiting or diarrhea suggestive of laxative abuse and comments that suggest fear of being fat in a patient who is evidently underweight.

SCREENING TESTS

Initial laboratory tests and medical workup for an eating disorder should include serum electrolytes including calcium, magnesium, and phosphate levels and liver function tests, a complete blood count, urinalysis and toxicology screen, thyroid stimulating hormone, and an electrocardiogram. In patients with marasmus and a BMI of < 13. A chest X-ray is also indicated since these patients can on occasion present with opportunistic infections seen in severely immunosuppressed hosts.

PATHOPHYSIOLOGY

What causes eating disorders, and what factors contribute to their maintenance? The etiology of eating disorders is multifactorial. Genetic vulnerability, sociocultural pressure to engage in dieting behaviors, and environmental stressors all play a role in onset. Family studies estimate the heritability of AN and BN as 50–70%. Individual genetic vulnerability is likely to explain why despite the pervasiveness of dieting behavior among adolescents and young adults, less than 3% of young women progress to clinical AN or BN. A majority of cases report a significant stressor during the year of onset contributing to restriction of food intake. Examples of common stressors include physical illness, parental divorce, a romantic disappointment, or homesickness after leaving for college. Given the rare prepubertal incidence of these conditions and the preponderance of females affected, it is also likely that estrogen levels play a role in susceptibility and age of onset.

Most important, especially in the acute management of these conditions, is an understanding of the pathophysiological consequences of starvation and of disordered eating which in turn help sustain continued anorectic and bulimic behavior. For example, deliberate starvation in AN results in delayed gastric and intestinal transit times, obsessive preoccupation with food and hyperactivity, all of which escalate anorectic behaviors and cognitions. Similarly, patients who vomit often develop loss of the gag reflex, gastroesophageal reflux, and delayed gastric emptying. These physiological changes in turn facilitate continued vomiting.

Psychiatric comorbidity also plays a role in sustaining eating disorders. Major depression, anxiety disorders, and substance abuse are common comorbidities in these patients and starvation is associated with a syndrome of depression, reversible with refeeding, which may contribute to patients' feelings of helplessness and hopelessness regarding treatment or prospects for recovery. Amongst general medical conditions co-occurring with eating disorders perhaps the most important is type I diabetes, since intentional insulin omission or restriction is a commonly employed method of purging calories in this patient subgroup, resulting in hyperglycemia and increased risk of diabetic ketoacidosis. Patients with both diabetes and an eating disorder have higher rates of hospital admission and emergency room visits, higher levels of hemoglobin A_{1c}, and higher rates of diabetic complications, making screening for an eating disorder an important component of the workup in any case of unexplained brittle diabetes.

MEDICAL COMPLICATIONS OF STARVATION AND OF PURGING BEHAVIORS

Most physiological complications and risks associated with eating disorders arise from either starvation or from purging behaviors, placing individuals with the purging subtype of AN at highest risk for serious medical morbidity and mortality. Almost all organ systems can be involved, and knowledge of the major medical complications is important in managing patients in the acute setting and in avoiding the development of refeeding syndrome, a potentially life threatening complication of rapid nutritional restoration.

CARDIOVASCULAR

Bradycardia, prolonged QTc interval, and hypotension are frequent complications of starvation. Asymptomatic bradycardia with a heart rate below 45 or a QTc of > 500 msec warrants admission for cardiac monitoring given the increased risk of sudden death associated with these findings, especially in patients with additional electrolyte abnormalities from purging. Tachycardia in the severely anorectic patient should be cause for concern since in these normally bradycardic individuals it may signal an occult infection or impending cardiac decompensation.

Orthostatic hypotension is common in starvation and as a result of purging behaviors including vomiting and abuse of laxatives or diuretics. Furthermore, some patients intentionally fluid restrict to lower their weight. Atrophic peripheral muscles and decreased venous return to the heart contribute to postural orthostatic heart rate and blood pressure changes increasing the risk of presyncopal or syncopal episodes.

Prolonged starvation can result in reduced left ventricular mass and resultant mitral valve prolapse as well as systolic and diastolic dysfunction with decreased ejection fraction. Ipecac abuse, although uncommon, can lead to a toxic cardiomyopathy, and caffeine, commonly abused as an appetite suppressant, or ephedrine-containing diet pills, can increase risk of adverse cardiac arrhythmias.

METABOLIC

Hypokalemia and acid-base imbalances arise from vomiting, diuretic, or laxative abuse. Elevated bicarbonate and low potassium are typical of frequent vomiting behavior and hypokalemia associated with a metabolic acidosis can be seen in laxative abusers. Since hypokalemia is unusual in young women, this laboratory finding should raise suspicion for an occult eating disorder and prompt questions about eating behavior. Other less common electrolyte abnormalities include hypomagnesemia and hypocalcemia. Hypophosphatemia is one of the hallmarks of the refeeding syndrome and is discussed in the relevant section below. Some patients present with water intoxication and hyponatremia associated with excessive water intake, consumed in order to increase satiety, to falsely elevate weight for medical weigh-ins, or to "eliminate toxins." Severe hyponatremia and low serum osmolality can progress in the extreme case to cerebral edema, ataxia, coma, and even death.

Hyponatremia can also result from abuse of thiazide diuretics or prolonged purging behavior depleting total body sodium. An unexplained seizure in a patient with an eating disorder is most commonly due to hyponatremia or hypoglycemia. Care should be taken to avoid aggressive intravenous correction of hyponatremia with hypertonic solutions due to the risk of sudden pontine myelinolysis described in several AN case reports. Oral repletion of potassium, phosphate, magnesium, and calcium is preferable and safer than IV administration and should be attempted first.

GASTROINTESTINAL

Bilateral parotid gland enlargement and dental enamel erosion may be evident on exam in patients with severe vomiting behavior. Purging by vomiting is also associated with reflux esophagitis and the risk of a Mallory-Weiss tear, whereas extreme binge eating in starved individuals can lead to potentially lethal acute gastric dilatation best managed with conservative nasogastric decompression. In starvation, delayed gastric emptying and slowed intestinal motility result in frequent complaints of satiety, fullness, abdominal discomfort, bloating, or constipation which inhibit further food intake. Invasive tests to workup these complaints, including endoscopy and colonoscopy, are not necessary in the face of a clear diagnosis of AN or BN unless there is additional data to suggest a comorbid medical cause or complications such as gastrointestinal bleeding.

Studies in AN have shown that increased oral intake normalizes gut transit times within weeks and is accompanied by resolution of gastrointestinal complaints. Although prokinetic drugs such as metoclopramide may help alleviate discomfort and fullness, only with reversal of the starved state and interruption of binge/vomit behaviors do these symptoms fully resolve. It is important to stress to patients that their gastrointestinal symptoms are consequences of their disordered eating and that symptomatic treatment with medications alone will generally be ineffective. Proton pump inhibitors may provide partial symptomatic relief from complaints of reflux esophagitis, however the primary treatment here too should be behavioral, with a focus on cessation of the binge-purge behavior.

Severe laxative or enema abuse can worsen constipation and result in anorectal problems including hemorrhoids and rectal prolapse. When laxatives are discontinued patients may develop large fluid shifts with marked fluid retention and edema as a result of secondary hyperaldosteronism. Peripheral edema is best managed conservatively by elevating the legs and by the judicious use of a potassium-sparing diuretic such as spironolactone when fluid retention is severe. Laxatives need not be tapered and can be stopped on admission. Most patients do well with twice daily docusate 100 mg and a fiber bulk laxative. If this is not sufficient to regularize bowel movements, the addition of an osmotic agent such as polyethylene glycol for the initial few weeks of treatment can be helpful.

Both pancreatitis and transaminitis are occasionally seen as complications of eating disorders, and patients with AN frequently have elevated total cholesterol levels despite their very low fat intake. Some have hypothesized that this finding is due to depressed cholesterol binding proteins or to low triiodothyronine levels inhibiting cholesterol breakdown.

ENDOCRINE

Eating disorders are associated with multiple reversible endocrine abnormalities. These are secondary to malnutrition and starvation and include hypothalamic amenorrhea, hypercortisolemia, growth hormone resistance, and sick euthyroid syndrome. Women with AN, and up to 30% of those with BN, develop amenorrhea or oligomenorrhea. Disturbances in GnRH pulsatility and associated low levels of estrogen, FSH, and LH characterize the resultant anovulation. Although TSH is generally in the normal range, endogeneous T_3 levels are low and reverse T_3 levels, and T_4 levels are often depressed. All these physiologic adaptations to starvation are presumably aimed at conserving energy resources and are not an indication to treat with hormone replacement. If hyperthyroidism is detected in a patient with AN, it should raise suspicion for surreptitious thyroxine abuse in the service of weight loss.

MUSCULOSKELETAL

Musculoskeletal complications arise from starvation and include generalized muscle weakness and atrophy as well as osteopenia and osteoporosis. AN is associated with increased risk of debilitating spinal or hip fractures over time related to bone loss. More than 90% of women with AN in one study were osteopenic with close to 40% having osteoporosis. Bone loss is thought to arise as a consequence of both low estradiol and the hypercortisolemia associated with AN, with onset of osteoporosis frequently observed by DEXA scan within months of diagnosis. Growth hormone resistance and low levels of insulin-like growth factor may also contribute both to osteoporosis and to stunting of growth in adolescent patients with AN. Prospective trials of estrogen replacement in AN have not been shown to improve bone density; although oral contraceptives are often prescribed to patients, this indication is not supported by evidence-based data. Similarly, there is a lack of efficacy studies for the use of bisphosphonates in AN. One small randomized controlled trial suggests that alendronate may increase bone mineral density in these patients but its effect was significantly less than that of weight restoration. Only weight restoration and the resumption of spontaneous menstrual cycles have consistently been shown to improve, albeit not normalize, bone mineral density in AN. The prescribing of hormone replacement therapy in AN may be counterproductive in that hormone-induced withdrawal bleeding can worsen anemia and be misinterpreted as normal reproductive functioning by patients, thereby decreasing their already poor motivation for weight gain. Furthermore, use of bisphosphonates in women of childbearing age is problematic since they are stored in bone and may be teratogenic and because pregnancy is a high bone turnover state during which they may be released into the circulation. For these reasons, current recommendations are limited to long-term treatment with calcium carbonate 600 mg twice daily and vitamin D at least 1,000 i.u. daily for all low weight patients with an eating disorder.

HEMATOLOGIC

Pancytopenia with hypocellular bone marrow is seen in severe AN as a reversible complication of starvation. These patients are immunocompomised and at increased risk of infection. Since patients are often hypovolemic, hematologic parameters may be normal on admission but drop with rehydration as hemoconcentration is corrected. A repeat blood count should therefore be performed within one or two days of admission.

NEUROLOGICAL

Cerebral atrophy in AN can be severe and although brain volume increases with weight restoration, data are mixed as to whether loss of brain volume is fully reversible or whether neurocognitive changes seen in AN completely resolve with refeeding. Patients with eating disorders may present with a seizure arising from hypoglycemia or hyponatremia. Severe neurological complications can be associated with the rapid correction of electrolytes or refeeding and are discussed below under refeeding syndrome. Peripheral nutritional polyneuropathy is not unusual in severely malnourished patients.

RENAL

End-stage renal disease is a rare complication of AN and has been described in multiple case series. It appears to be more common in laxative abusers and may be the result of chronic hypokalemia. A study of 24-hour creatinine clearance in 45 patients with AN found that laxative abusers had a significantly lower creatinine clearance than restricting subtype patients.

REFEEDING SYNDROME

An awareness of the symptoms and management of refeeding syndrome is essential to the treatment of severely malnourished patients with AN. If not promptly recognized and treated this condition is life threatening. Refeeding syndrome comprises a constellation of metabolic and clinical changes resulting from rapid refeeding whether oral, enteral, or parenteral. These can include hypophosphatemia, hypoglycemia, edema and congestive heart failure, ileus, seizures, coma, and sudden death. In general, the risk is lowest with oral, and highest with parenteral nutrition.

PRACTICE POINT

- Monitor closely for refeeding syndrome during nutritional rehabilitation of starved patients including hypophosphatemia, hypoglycemia, and fluid overload.

In starved individuals, as calorie intake increases, anabolism shifts to carbohydrate metabolism from protein and fat catabolism. Blood glucose increases and there is an increase in insulin release. Depleted glycogen stores make the regulation of blood glucose unpredictable and increase the risk of reactive hypoglycemia, which is frequently asymptomatic.

Insulin secretion also stimulates the cellular uptake of phosphate for the production of adenosine triphosphate (ATP), in order to meet anabolic demands. Total body phosphate is depleted in starvation, although serum levels may initially appear normal. As phosphate moves intracellularly, hypophosphatemia manifests one to five days after initiating feeding and can be life threatening if not promptly recognized and treated. Similarly, hypomagnesemia from intracellular movement of magnesium may only be evident several days into refeeding.

Starved patients are often hypotensive and may have autonomic instability reflected in marked postural hypotension or heart rate changes. Care should be taken not to aggressively hydrate these patients since their low protein and albumin and malnourished tissues make edema and third spacing likely and can result in anasarca or congestive heart failure. The increase in insulin secretion also contributes to sodium retention, which in turn decreases renal excretion of sodium and water and worsens fluid retention. Congestive heart failure is especially a risk in patients with an occult starvation-related cardiomyopathy. If edema is pronounced and weight gain very rapid (more than 3–4 lbs per week) suggesting severe fluid retention, an echocardiogram is indicated, especially in chronic cases or those of advanced age who are at highest risk of cardiac complications following years of chronic malnutrition.

To avoid refeeding syndrome, we recommend gradual intravenous hydration if symptomatic with hypotonic saline and 5% dextrose at a maintenance rate no faster than 83 cc/hr supplemented by oral intake of no more than 1,000 cc of fluids/day. Close monitoring of finger sticks, especially postprandially, is recommended to avoid the risk of a potential hypoglycemic coma and daily electrolytes including sodium, potassium, calcium, magnesium, and phosphate should be drawn until several sequential values in the normal range are obtained. Oral repletion of phosphate, potassium, or magnesium is faster and safer than intravenous correction.

The risk of refeeding syndrome is closely tied to the amount of food ingested. Patients should initially be fed a low salt, low fat, low lactose diet of 1200–1500 calories/day. This should be gradually liberalized to a regular diet and advanced by 500 calories/day every two to three days to a daily intake of 3500 calories/day with a target rate of weight gain between 3–4 lbs/week. Mild to moderate pedal edema is common during the first few weeks of refeeding and should be managed conservatively by encouraging elevating the legs, compression stockings, and salt restriction until it resolves. In patients with a history of purging, diuretics compound the risk of hypokalemia. Since these agents are abused by some patients in order to lose weight, diuretics should be reserved for cases with severe edema when there is concern for congestive heart failure.

Other severe complications associated with refeeding include Wernicke encephalopathy and central pontine myelinolysis. Central pontine myelinolysis most commonly results from the overly rapid correction of hyponatremia and presents with altered mental state, dysarthria, or mutism appearing within days of the correction of sodium levels and progressing in some cases to worsening motor impairment and at the extreme coma or death. Thiamine deficiency can result in Wernicke-Korsakoff syndrome, a particular risk in AN patients with comorbid alcohol abuse. We recommend treatment of all patients with a BMI of 14 or less with 100 mg of IV thiamine prior to food intake or to the administration of IV dextrose in order to avoid this very serious risk.

PRACTICE POINT

- To minimize refeeding syndrome the diet in AN should "start low and go slow" with initial calorie intakes of 1200–1500 calories/day advanced to a weight gain diet of 3500 calories/day over the course of 10–14 days. This calorie level should achieve weight gain rates of 2–4 lbs/week.

TREATMENT

For AN, treatment is best thought of as composed of two phases: weight restoration and relapse prevention. Relapse, as with other behavioral conditions, is the norm rather than the exception, although most patients are able to progress further with each cycle of treatment and the majority eventually recovers. Evidence-based data on treatment of AN is limited due to cost, and to methodological and ethical issues that complicate design and feasibility of randomized treatment interventions. Most evidence therefore comes from correlational studies and clinical experience, which support weight restoration as necessary for recovery. Inpatient behavioral specialty units can weight restore the vast majority of patients at a rate of 2–4 lbs/week using oral feeding alone. These programs use a combination of behavioral, group, and family therapy. Treatment focus is on normalizing eating behavior and broadening patients' food repertoire using close nursing observation to assist patients in interrupting eating disorder behavior patterns. Group therapy is especially effective since patients with eating disorders are able to appreciate other patients' needs to change their behaviors. As with substance abuse disorders, when confronted by peers, patients are more likely to recognize the irrational logic they use to defend their own dieting. Despite the success of intensive behavioral programs in achieving weight restoration and normalizing eating behavior, relapse is common, with 30–50% of individuals who reach target weight likely to relapse within one year of discharge.

No medication has been shown to be superior to placebo in the treatment of AN. Current outpatient treatment guidelines include weekly psychotherapy and nutritional counseling with a focus on weight gain these sessions should include monitoring of the patients' weight. Involvement of close family and social supports is recommended.

Full recovery is best viewed as a protracted process often occurring over years and requiring multiple treatment interventions. Long-term outcome studies indicate recovery rates of close to 50%. There are few indicators of good versus poor prognosis. Full recovery can be seen even in patients with life-threatening AN who have been ill for decades and who present with extreme cachexia and multiple medical complications or organ failure.

For BN, several outpatient treatment interventions are effective in interrupting the restrict-binge-vomit cycle. The most well-studied of these is cognitive behavioral therapy (CBT), which maintains a behavioral focus on normalizing eating while simultaneously challenging irrational cognitive beliefs and identifying triggers and alternate coping strategies. Self-help CBT manuals are less effective than therapist-led CBT, but superior to control interventions and are an easily available, inexpensive, initial intervention that can be offered to patients. Antidepressants have also been found effective in decreasing binge-vomit frequencies in BN although they are less effective than CBT in achieving abstinence from these behaviors. Of these medications, high dose fluoxetine at 60 mg daily has been studied most extensively and is commonly employed in conjunction with CBT. Although relapse is common in the treatment of BN, over 50% of patients achieve eventual recovery with treatment.

AN is characterized by refusal to eat not by inability to eat or by a nonfunctional gastrointestinal tract. The safest and most effective form of refeeding is oral, both from a physiological standpoint and because this disorder is marked by a narrowing of the food repertoire and conditioned avoidance of high calorie-density foods. The variety of foods consumed at discharge from inpatient specialty treatment was recently shown to be inversely related to relapse rates, suggesting that exposure to diverse foods and normalization of eating patterns is an important component of treatment. Although supplemental tube feeding is used by some behavioral programs to augment poor rates of weight gain in select cases, most specialty units do not find this necessary in order to achieve optimal rates of gain in the vast majority of patients.

The situation on a medical unit is more complex, since it is difficult to reproduce the skilled nursing care and peer pressure of a specialized eating disorder program on a medical floor, thereby lessening the likelihood that patients will comply with dietary recommendations. The initial prescribed diet in AN should be oral and caloric intake should start low as outlined above, while monitoring for evidence of refeeding syndrome. A trial of supplemental enteral feeding may be reserved for patients who are failing to gain weight with oral feeding alone. The mere threat of prescribed enteral feeds may help ambivalent patients eat. Other patients may prefer enteral feeds as a way to "medicalize" their condition and avoid responsibility for their behavior. In the short term this may be acceptable to boost slow weight gain although the long-term goal is to achieve normalization of dietary intake by transitioning the patient to oral food only. We do not recommend the placement of PEG tubes or long-term enteral feeding since this approach does not tackle patients' fear of widening their food repertoire and consuming calorie dense foods. In general, most experts agree that parenteral feeding should be avoided in AN, especially in cachectic patients, given the high risk of medical complications, including life-threatening infection or refeeding complications combined with the availability of less invasive methods of nutritional restoration.

BEHAVIORAL MANAGEMENT

Eating disorder patients may be difficult to manage on a medical ward largely because of their similarity to addictions. Patients may understand the severity of their condition intellectually yet be unable or unwilling to stop their behavior. They may overtly continue to exercise, restrict or hide food, vomit, or abuse laxatives despite the severe medical consequences of these behaviors that led to their admission. Driven dieting and binge eating behaviors are experienced as compelling and the preoccupation with thoughts of food and body weight as consuming.

We recommend checking daily weight and instructing nursing staff to monitor the patient as closely as possible, if necessary by employing a professional sitter, for evidence of eating disordered behaviors. This may include tray checks and calorie counts to assess amount of food consumed, instructing patients to allow staff to check the toilet bowl before flushing for evidence of vomiting or diarrhea and curtailing time out of bed or off the unit contingent on behavior. Sitters should be instructed regarding what behaviors to watch for. The patient should be repeatedly and firmly yet supportively redirected for any noncompliant behavior and reminded of its medical risks. Patients may also engage in behaviors aimed at deliberately deceiving staff by hiding food or vomitus, water loading before weigh-ins, or wearing weights.

Staff should recognize that in most cases it is difficult to effectively treat these patients on a general medical floor and that the goal of hospitalization should be stabilization and transfer to a behavioral specialty program. As is the case with other motivated behavioral conditions including substance abuse disorders, behavioral treatment and rehabilitation is difficult to achieve outside such a specialized program. Hospital staff may experience strong negative feelings toward these patients because of their denial of illness and manipulative behaviors or may have difficulty setting limits on and redirecting the patient due to feelings of compassion for him or her. The patient may complain she is only "understood" by staff interested in talking with her about her feelings rather than on supportively and consistently stigmatizing her self-destructive behavior. As a result, the team may become "split" in their views of how the patient should be cared for. Normalizing these reactions and discussing counter-transference feelings in team meetings with staff is important in order to prevent such issues from interfering with the provision of appropriate care. A psychiatry consult should be obtained to help mediate these concerns, to establish if the patient has other comorbid psychiatric conditions that warrant treatment, as well as to facilitate transfer to a more appropriate treatment facility once the patient is medically stable.

ETHICAL CONSIDERATIONS SPECIFIC TO THE TREATMENT OF EATING DISORDERS

The three primary ethical questions that arise in the treatment of eating disorders are (1) Is the patient competent to refuse care? (2) What is the role, if any, of involuntary treatment? and (3) What are the limits of confidentiality when the patient's condition is life threatening?

Patients with AN are not grossly incompetent; however their capacity to make a rational free choice regarding whether to reject or accept treatment may be impaired. In life-threatening AN, patients are often incompetent to make treatment decisions involving their own eating and weight. Although they recognize the need for others with the same disorder to receive treatment, they demonstrate a selective defect in self-evaluation, appearing unable to appreciate their own need to gain weight. They may provide seemingly rational explanations for their behavior, arguing they are different in some fundamental way from others with the same disorder. Incompetence to refuse treatment is a state-dependent condition and is worsened by starvation. Insight usually improves gradually with weight restoration and with behavioral change.

Because dieting is driven and rewarding to patients with AN, attempts to normalize eating behavior or weight are unpleasant and patients usually enter specialty treatment not of their own initiative but under pressure from others. Pressure may range from gentle persuasion to compulsion and involuntary treatment. To be successful, however, treatment must at some point win the cooperation of the patient. Recovery is a process of conversion in belief, from seeing dieting as an idealized and necessary goal, to stigmatizing it as a negative behavior. Because treatment resistance is endemic to AN, ethical decision-making pervades the treatment of this disorder.

Civil commitment is used occasionally by few specialty centers when all other attempts to engage the patient have failed, when a patient's life is at risk, and when there is reasonable confidence that the treatment will be beneficial. Data on involuntary treatment is limited, although case control studies suggest that discharge BMIs are similar for voluntary and involuntary cases and weight restoration can be accomplished in the majority. Although long-term prognosis is worse for involuntary cases, these are correlational studies, and the involuntary group is likely to have a worse prognosis with or without treatment. Furthermore, empirical data indicating harm from involuntary treatment is absent and at least two studies have shown that close to half of patients admitted involuntarily or under pressure from others later came to view being hospitalized against their will as justified in saving their lives. Treatment setting is likely important, however, and this data comes from behavioral specialty units. There is no data on the outcome of involuntary treatment in a general psychiatric or medical unit. Presumably likelihood of a good outcome is higher in a specialty program for eating disorders.

Involuntary treatment should in our opinion only be considered if the patient's family is in support of the team. Family involvement maximizes the likelihood that the intervention will result in a therapeutic outcome. Patients with AN may refuse to allow the clinician contact with their family. Most commonly this occurs because the patient is trying to keep relatives and the medical team at arm's length in order to avoid weight gain. When AN is endangering a patient's life however, treatment should be viewed as a medical emergency. Under these circumstances it becomes appropriate to break confidentiality. Communication with close family is especially important when patients are admitted to a hospitalist service not only to apprise family of the seriousness of the patient's condition but to urge them to align with the hospitalist team and the consult psychiatrist in providing firm yet supportive pressure to encourage the patient to accept voluntary transfer to a specialty program as the next step in his or her rehabilitation.

CONCLUSION

The goal of hospitalization is to stabilize the patient medically and transfer him or her to an appropriate specialty program for the treatment of eating disorders. It is helpful to state, both to patients and family members, that AN is a motivated behavioral condition much like addiction, that recovery is always possible, and that specialty treatment often is effective in assisting patients to recover. For severely medically compromised patients, a hospital-based eating disorders program with access to medical consultants may be most appropriate. For less ill patients, outpatient treatment can be effective especially if behaviorally oriented. The most common psychotherapeutic approach is cognitive-behavioral in orientation with family involvement whenever possible. For severely underweight patients with a BMI of < 15, outpatient treatment alone is less likely to lead to weight restoration and long-term recovery than intensive treatment programs. The medical costs of treating AN are extremely high and many patients lack adequate insurance coverage. Patients may however qualify for coverage under Medicare if disabled by their condition. The importance of maintaining a firm, positive stance in recommending behavioral treatment is critical since patients and family members may feel hopeless about prospects of recovery in the light of past treatment failures.

SUGGESTED READINGS

American Psychiatric Association. Practice Guidelines: Treatment of Patients with Eating Disorders, third edition. *Am J Psychiatry.* 2006;163(suppl 4):54.

Cotton MA, Ball C, Robinson P. Four simple questions can help screen for eating disorders. *J Gen Intern Med.* 2003;18:53–56.

Goebel-Fabbri AE. Disturbed eating behaviors and eating disorders in type 1 diabetes: clinical significance and treatment recommendations. *Curr Diab Rep.* 2009;9:133–139.

Goldstein DJ, Wilson MG, Thompson VL, Potvin JH, Rampey AH, Jr. Long-term fluoxetine treatment of bulimia nervosa. Fluoxetine Bulimia Nervosa Research Group. *Br J Psychiatry.* 1995;166:660–666.

Guarda AS. Treatment of anorexia nervosa: insights and obstacles. *Physiol Behav.* 2008;94:113–120.

Guarda AS, Pinto AM, Coughlin JW, Hussain S, Haug NA, Heinberg LJ. Perceived coercion and change in perceived need for admission in patients hospitalized for eating disorders. *Am J Psychiatry.* 2007;164:108–114.

Hoek HW. Incidence, prevalence and mortality of anorexia nervosa and other eating disorders. *Curr Opin Psychiatry.* 2006;19:389–394.

Kamal N, Chami T, Andersen A, Rosell FA, Schuster MM, Whitehead WE. Delayed gastrointestinal transit times in anorexia nervosa and bulimia nervosa. *Gastroenterology.* 1991;101:1320–1324.

Lawson EA, Klibanski A. Endocrine abnormalities in anorexia nervosa. *Nat Clin Pract Endocrinol Metab.* 2008;4:407–414.

Mitchell JE, Crow S. Medical complications of anorexia nervosa and bulimia nervosa. *Curr Opin Psychiatry.* 2006;19:438–443.

Morgan JF, Reid F, Lacey JH. The SCOFF questionnaire: assessment of a new screening tool for eating disorders. *BMJ.* 1999;319:1467–1468.

Papadopoulos FC, Ekbom A, Brandt L, Ekselius L. Excess mortality, causes of death and prognostic factors in anorexia nervosa. *Br J Psychiatry.* 2009;194:10–17.

Schebendach JE, Mayer LE, Devlin MJ, et al. Dietary energy density and diet variety as predictors of outcome in anorexia nervosa. *Am J Clin Nutr.* 2008;87:810–816.

Tresley J, Sheean PM. Refeeding syndrome: recognition is the key to prevention and management. *J Am Diet Assoc.* 2008;108:2105–2108.

CHAPTER 229

The Suicidal Patient

Robert K. Schneider, MD

Key Clinical Questions

1. What terms and concepts are required for understanding suicidality?
2. What are chronic or predisposing risk factors for suicide?
3. What are acute or potentiating risk factors for suicide?
4. What are protective risk factors for suicide?
5. How does the hospitalist determine in the patient is at baseline risk for suicide or elevated risk?
6. How does the hospitalist device a plan of care for the suicidal patient?

INTRODUCTION

Suicidality (defined as one's attraction to suicide) is very common in patients with severe psychiatric disorders even though completed suicide (killing oneself) is relatively rare. The risk of suicidality is never zero. Even patients hospitalized for medical or surgical reasons, many of whom also have severe psychiatric disorders, experience suicidality but since the focus of their care is medical or surgical rather than psychiatric, their suicidality often goes unnoticed, unevaluated and untreated. Given, then, the hospitalist's high likelihood of treating patients experiencing suicidality, all hospitalists require the knowledge and skills necessary to assess and manage patients with varying levels of suicidality. Accordingly, a working knowledge of, and fluency with, terminology surrounding suicidality is required. Assessment (including screening) involves exploring the patient's overall risk profile, including chronic/predisposing factors, the acute/potentiating factors, and protective factors. Subsequently, the hospitalist must determine whether the patient's overall suicidal risk is at or above baseline. Finally, the hospitalist must devise appropriate management to address the patient's suicide risk.

ASSESSMENT OF SUICIDALITY: WHAT THE HOSPITALIST SHOULD KNOW

A hospitalist is most likely to address suicidality with patients in three distinct situations:

1. Patients who may not overtly express suicidality but are at increased risk for suicide and should be assessed
2. Patients who express suicidality while hospitalized
3. Patients admitted after a suicide attempt

Patients who are admitted after suicide attempts are the most conspicuous examples of suicidality and because of this receive the most attention in our literature. However, hospitalists will see many more patients *silently* at risk for suicide than those who are admitted for overt suicide attempts. Many hospitalists do not detect the underlying increased risk for suicide and therefore do not inquire further. This chapter addresses the practical knowledge and skills required to assess suicidality in any hospitalized patient. This information can be applied in most commonly found situations where suicidality is suspected. The hospitalist can be a first line of defense against suicide by accurately assessing and treating the hospitalized patients who are at increased risk for suicide.

WHAT KEY WORDS AND CONCEPTS ARE REQUIRED TO ASSESS SUICIDALITY?

The terminology used to describe thoughts and actions related to self-harm is often confusing for health care professionals. The following construct (**Figure 229-1**) frames the essential vocabulary and concepts, defines key terms, and describes an easily accessible construct for suicidality.

THE SPECTRUM OF SUICIDALITY

The terms *suicide, completed suicide*, or *"successful"* suicide all refer to the actual act of killing oneself. A *suicide attempt* is an act of deliberate self-harm with the intent to kill oneself. However, the act may not seem deliberate (eg, taking too many pain medications) so the degree of intent (ie, the wish to die) may be hard to ascertain from the patient. The degree of lethality (ie, the likelihood of completion) is typically not hard to determine but should be

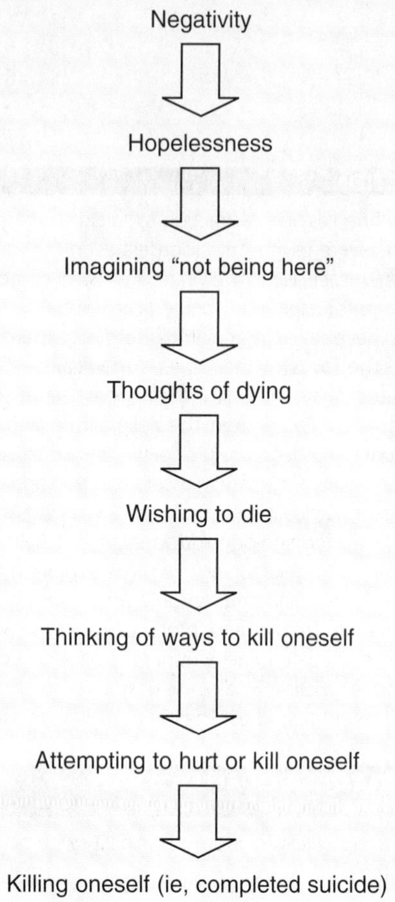

Figure 229-1 *Spectrum of suicidality.*

taken in the context of the patient's intent. The combination of the questions of intent and lethality lead to the notion that *suicidal ideation* (thoughts of suicide) or *suicidality* (attraction to suicide) are part of a spectrum of thoughts or feelings ranging from hopelessness to imagining "not being here," to specific plans for self-harm, to acting on suicidal plans. (See **Table 229-1** for a list of risk factors for suicide.) Circumstances in the life of the patient help the clinician to ascribe meaning to a suicide attempt. Obviously, if the individual says that he or she wrote a note and jumped off a bridge that is a clear attempt to *complete suicide*. However, if the individual says that he or she took a handful of ibuprofen after breaking up with a significant other, this may indicate a "cry for help" or an immature expression of pain.

Hopelessness and associated emotions are some of the most consistent markers for severity of a psychiatric disorder, particularly mood disorders. While suicidality in some form is frequently present in severe psychiatric disorders (eg, major depression), completed suicide is relatively rare. In the United States, over 15 million people suffer with depression within a given year, and many will think about suicide, but fewer than 30,000 people will actually complete suicide from the total general population. Despite decades of study documenting epidemiologic correlations with completed suicide (ie, risk factors), there is no effective screening approach that accurately predicts completed suicide. Most leaders in suicide research note that suicide is not predictable and go on to advise the clinician that the clinical goal is not to predict but to fully assess.

CHRONIC AND PREDISPOSING RISK FACTORS FOR SUICIDE

Completed suicide has a base-rate of 12 per 100,000 in the general population. The most studied predisposing epidemiologic factors related to suicide risk are gender, race, and age. These predisposing chronic risk factors are fixed and therefore establish a baseline risk for suicide. In these categories men are at least four times more likely to complete suicide than women. However, women are about 10 times more likely to attempt suicide or make suicide gestures. Whites and Native Americans have significantly higher suicide rates than African Americans, Hispanics, or Asians. In the United States, white men commit 70% of suicides. Age is also a significant risk factor. Suicide rates dramatically increase in the seventh decade of life, especially for men.

Substance abuse, especially severe alcoholism, is a chronic risk factor. For some alcoholics in later life, when the social effects of chronic use have accumulated (isolation, alienation), a sudden or significant change (medical disease, divorce, loss of a job, death of a loved one) carries a particularly high risk for suicide. On the other hand, alcohol intoxication is an acute risk that quickly passes after the patient is sober.

PSYCHIATRIC DISORDERS AS RISK FACTORS FOR SUICIDE

The presence of a psychiatric disorder can pose acute and/or chronic risk for suicide depending upon the patient's history and the acuity of the symptoms. Although a major mental disorder is associated with more than 90% of suicides, this likelihood is difficult to determine because the vast majority of the data on this subject is obtained retrospectively. However, of people with psychiatric

TABLE 229-1 Risk Factors for Suicide

Chronic/Predisposing	Acute/Potentiating	Protective
Male	Recent extreme loss	Marriage or committed relationship
Older age (>65 years)	Exacerbation of a	Religious affiliation
White or Native American	Psychiatric disorder	Children in the household
Prior suicide attempt	Medical condition	Positive social support
Psychiatric disorder	Impulsivity	
Chronic medical condition	Access to firearms	
Family history of suicide	Substance abuse	
Chronic pain		
Substance abuse		

conditions who complete suicide, depression accounts for 50%, alcohol and drug abuse 20–25%, and schizophrenia or bipolar disorder 10%. Other psychiatric disorders also increase the risk for suicide, such as posttraumatic stress disorder (PTSD), panic disorder, and personality disorders that are characterized by impulsivity. In general, all psychiatric disorders carry a greater risk for suicide when compared with the general population.

When inactive symptoms of the disorder (ie, during remission or recovery) become reactivated (ie, during relapse or recurrence), the chronically elevated baseline risk for suicide is acutely increased. Knowing where the patient falls longitudinally within the progression of their disorder also helps the clinician assess risk. For example, patients early in the course of schizophrenia carry a greater risk than later. Most suicides in people with schizophrenia (60%) occur within six years of the first hospitalization.

MEDICAL AND PSYCHIATRIC COMORBIDITY AS A RISK FACTOR FOR SUICIDE

There is a complex relationship between medical and psychiatric disorders in suicidality because medical illnesses also carry an increased risk for suicidal ideation and suicide attempts. Any concomitant medical conditions increase the lifetime risk for suicidal ideation and suicide attempts to 35% and 16%, respectively. Given that medical illnesses and depression are often comorbid, it is very important to note that the odds ratio (OR) for suicidal ideation and suicide attempts remains high, 1.82 ($P < .01$) and 2.38 ($P < .001$) when controlled for depression and alcohol use. Thus psychiatric disorders and medical illnesses contribute independently to the risks for suicidal ideation and suicide attempts.

MEDICAL ILLNESS AS A RISK FACTOR FOR SUICIDE

Medical illness of any type significantly increases the risk of a depressive or anxiety disorder, and hospitalization itself is a risk factor. Patients recently discharged from a general hospital (ie, nonpsychiatric admission) carry an increased risk for suicide too. One study placed the risk at 32/100,000, which is about three times the baseline risk of the general population. This particular study revealed the missed opportunity for psychiatric intervention—only one patient had been referred for a suicidality assessment.

Like psychiatric disorders, medical disorders pose acute and chronic risks. Much of the increased risk is attributable to co-occurring psychiatric illnesses, particularly major depression, substance-related disorders, personality disorders, and delirium. Physical illness is a profound risk factor, contributing to over 70% of suicides in those over the age of 60. Chronic medical illness is strongly associated with depression and substance abuse; however, even when the latter risk factors are accounted for, medical illness is still associated with increased suicidal risk. Higher rates of suicide have been reported in cancer, AIDS, end-stage renal disease, neurologic disorders such as multiple sclerosis, asthma, and a number of other medical conditions. Data from the U.S. National Comorbidity Survey identified a dozen general medical diagnostic categories with statistically significantly elevated odds ratios for suicide attempts, most ranging from 1.1 to 3.4, but with a much higher ratio in AIDS. Cancer and asthma patients each have a fourfold risk of attempting suicide compared with the general population, even after adjusting for demographic and psychiatric variables. Loss of or poor functional capacity and associated chronic pain may be common threads among these medical conditions that link them with suicidal risk. Some clinicians have the misperception that most terminally ill patients have a strong wish for a hastened death. On the contrary, Breitbart and colleagues' (2000) study showed only 17% of cancer patients with this desire, but depression was a strong predictor of which patients desired a hastened death.

PRIOR SUICIDE ATTEMPTS AS RISK FACTOR FOR SUICIDE

Prior suicide attempts represent a significant increased risk for both a subsequent attempt and a completed suicide in the future. A prior suicide attempt of any description is associated with an almost 40-fold increase in suicide risk. Prior attempts represent a dramatic increase in risk that is greater than the increased risk associated with any psychiatric disorder. The powerful association makes screening for prior suicide a major focus of any prevention efforts. Regrettably, of those attempting suicide, more than half complete their suicides the first time.

Extreme loss or abrupt social disruptions such as divorce or loss of a job also increase acute risk. Following a spouse's death in later life is a particularly vulnerable period. The losses and disruption of life posed by medical illness can be devastating.

Patients who carry a chronic high risk for suicide should be managed in concert with a psychiatrist. For example, a patient may have a long history of multiple drug overdoses with subsequent psychiatric hospitalizations. This patient will most likely have suicidal ideation to some degree at any time and is chronically at increased risk for suicide. In some chronically suicidal patients with personality disorders, psychiatric hospitalization is used only as a last resort because the hospitalization is unlikely to change the chronic suicidal ideation. In fact, for such patients hospitalization may reinforce the suicidal ideation by creating an escape or gratifying a regressive need for attention. Short admissions, focused on stabilization and maintaining an outpatient treatment program, are usually most effective for the patient with chronic high baseline risk for suicide. These complex patients require the active management that a mental health specialist can provide.

ACUTE AND POTENTIATING RISK FACTORS FOR SUICIDE

Exacerbation of depression with severe hopelessness, psychic pain, shame, or humiliation acutely increases risk of suicide. Depressive symptoms combined with extreme anxiety (panic or obsessions) or manic symptoms particularly increase risk. The initial treatment plan should target these exacerbated symptoms. The risk of suicide seems highest in the first few depressive episodes, especially in late-onset depression. This is also true for bipolar disorders and schizophrenia. Many of the suicides that occur early in the course of the disorder are in people who have neither been diagnosed with a disorder nor have had treatment initiated. Although suicide risk is higher early in the course of depressive illness, the risk remains higher for patients with depression than for the general population throughout the course of the illness.

When psychosis is present, suicidal ideation is very dangerous and constitutes an emergency, particularly when command hallucinations or intense persecutory delusions are present. This patient should be evaluated by a mental health professional as soon as possible and remanded for inpatient care if necessary.

PROTECTIVE FACTORS FOR SUICIDE

Increasing or augmenting protective factors is an important focus of treatment since the presence of protective factors can decrease risk, and their absence can increase risk for suicide. Often protective factors involve connection and relationships. Married people are at a lower risk than isolated people (single, divorced, and widowed). Households with children who are under 18 years old seem to provide some protection for the adults. Employment or meaningful work appears protective. Religious affiliation may have some protective value above that of social contact in general. Though difficult to study, "a reason for living" has tremendous value clinically. Discussing protective factors takes time; however, the information obtained is essential for establishing an effective management plan.

CLINICAL ASSESSMENT

PRIORITIZING AND ORGANIZING FACTORS ASSOCIATED WITH RISK FOR SUICIDE

Risk is categorized along three dimensions when genuine, significant risk for suicide is discovered:

1. Chronic and predisposing factors that affect lifetime risk for suicide
2. Acute and potentiating factors that occur in immediate proximity to suicidality
3. Protective factors that, when present, mitigate against acute or chronic risks *and the absence of protective factors increases risk*

A clinician's skills in assessing the spectrum of suicidality and accurately categorizing suicide risk are essential for managing patients with psychiatric disorders. For a hospitalist it may be helpful to know how these skills are analogous to the skills required to assess chest pain and its nuances. Because most chest pain does not represent a myocardial infarction, a clinician would not send all patients with chest pain to the emergency room for admission. Similarly, he or she should not send all patients with suicidal ideation to the emergency room for admission. In both situations, there is an informed response that depends on accurate assessment and referral or treatment.

The evidence and effective intervention surrounding suicide and suicidality are not clear cut. The following comparisons between completed suicide and cardiac sudden death may be a helpful starting point:

- Most first-time events are fatal.
- Having a prior near-fatal event defines the greatest risk for a future event and encompasses the largest population studied.
- Almost all studies are retrospective.
- The greater the number of risk factors, the greater the risk.
- The absolute number of fatal events is small relative to near-fatal events.
- Assessment combined with risk reduction is the focus of care.

SCREENING FOR SUICIDALITY

When assessing for suicidal ideation it is best to start at the less severe end of the spectrum (negativity and pessimism) and then proceed to greater degrees. While it is critical to identify patients at the more serious end of the spectrum (ie, those who have a plan and are intent on carrying it out), it is also essential to identify patients at lesser degrees of risk to permit earlier preventive interventions. Also, establishing the information on the less extreme end will typically lead to very useful information regarding the severity of the disorder and constructing a plan. For a hospitalist screening for suicidality is like screening for alcoholism. Similar to asking the blunt question, Are you an alcoholic?, the question, Are you going to kill yourself? is equally unproductive in obtaining information from the proximal part of the suicidal spectrum. When asking patients about suicidal ideation, clinicians should start at the less serious end of the spectrum of suicide risk. By determining the depth of the patient's hopelessness and helplessness (ie, suicidality), the clinician has obtained some of the best markers of severity. Additionally, when these symptoms are identified, validated, and targeted for treatment by the clinician, the patient's suicidal risk diminishes, and recovery is more promising. By assessing suicidal ideation across its entire spectrum, the clinician *and* patient gain greater insight into the severity of an underlying disorder. Also, patients are usually more willing to discuss negativity and hopelessness than suicide. The following questions demonstrate a progression from less specific questions about suicidality to very specific questions about suicide.

PRACTICE POINT

- Are you having difficulty staying hopeful?
- Have you ever felt life isn't worth living?
- Did you ever wish you would go to sleep and not wake up?
- Have you had increased thoughts about death or dying?
- Have these thoughts ever been about taking your own life?
- Have you imagined the way you would do it?
- Are you currently considering or planning to kill yourself?

This approach facilitates conversation and opens the door for further discussion when more explicit suicidal ideation is present. Some patients do not realize that hopelessness and despair themselves, let alone suicidality, may be symptoms of a disorder. If the symptoms seem related to a stressor and because the despair has a "good reason," the patient may discount the symptoms. If the patient does not associate a stressor with his painful feelings, he may think he is "going crazy." The clinician has an opportunity to educate and reassure the patient by explaining that these thoughts and feelings are symptoms of a disorder (eg, major depression) and can be expected to diminish or resolve with treatment.

CASE 229-1

MJ, a 68-year-old man, is ready for discharge tomorrow after a five-day hospitalization for chronic obstructive pulmonary disease (COPD) exacerbation and pneumonia. This is his third admission in three months and he had none prior. He has lost 15 pounds during this three-month period. His outpatient workup for weight loss was negative. During discharge planning it is discovered that his wife died four months ago. The hospitalist asks, "Are you having thoughts of harming yourself?" and the patient honestly replies, "No." The hypothetical interaction would end there, leaving much important information undiscussed.

However, if the hospitalist had started with, "How do you stay hopeful or how do you keep going?", then the hospitalist would have found a man in bereavement and possibly depression who is open to talking more about this with someone after discharge. This more sensitive approach offers a fuller communication that gives additional information about the severity of the disorder, the presence or absence of protective factors for suicide, as well as diagnostic information. The more sensitive approach suggested also gives greater confidence in the response, "I am not going to kill myself." When the patient informs the hospitalist that, although frustrated with this debilitating disease compounded by his wife's death after a long bout of cancer, he is hopeful, active, and future focused.

DISCUSSING SUICIDAL IDEATION WHEN DISCOVERED

When suicidal ideation is discovered, explicit and direct discussion about suicidal intent takes place. Unlike the gradual approach outlined previously when screening for potential suicidality (ie, when there is no overtly expressed suicidal ideation), pursuing details of the suicidal ideation (ie, onset, frequency, method, lethality of method, specificity of plan, access to means, etc) helps the hospitalist establish the intensity of the suicidal ideation. The following questions are examples that may be helpful in suicide risk assessment:

PRACTICE POINT

- When did you first notice these thoughts?
- Are they constant or episodic?
- Have these thoughts progressed to any plans?
- Do you have access to any guns?
- Have you taken any steps to advance these plans?
- Have you acted on these thoughts?

Next, to counterbalance the suicidal thoughts of the patient, the clinician should discuss the patient's reasons for living. It is helpful to look actively for future plans, people to support the patient, and direct prohibitions to suicide (eg, religious beliefs). These questions often help patients to consider their suicidal ideations from different perspectives. The following questions illustrate this approach:

PRACTICE POINT

- What keeps you from acting on these thoughts?
- Who can help you through this difficult time?
- What future plans do you have?
- How would your death impact the people around you?
- Let's figure out a plan to make you safer.

CASE 229-2

SG is a 47-year-old woman readmitted for a hypertensive crisis related to her polycystic kidney disease. Her renal failure has reached the point where she needs dialysis and then a kidney transplant. After receiving this news she says, "Well I may as well go ahead and kill myself now."

The hospitalist should ask directly, "How long have you had these thoughts?", and "Have you ever acted on those thoughts?" This patient quickly reveals no significant past history of suicidality, and a strong support system is actively involved. However, she describes a tremendous sense of defeat with her worsening medical condition: "I shoot off my mouth, but you are right, I should see someone and talk more about this."

■ CURRENT RISK FOR SUICIDE VERSUS BASELINE RISK

Management of the suicidal patient focuses on reducing the immediate risk back to baseline or lower if possible. Several assumptions are critical here: the risk is never zero; some risks cannot be mitigated (ie, gender, age, race, past history); some patients carry very high baseline risks for suicide (ie, past suicide attempts, older white males); some will commit suicide despite a full assessment and good clinical management. Sudden change in risk is often more indicative of imminent risk than the absolute level of risk. People with low baseline risks who suddenly have a major change (ie, sudden illness, death of a loved one, intoxication) may not have a very high absolute risk, but relative to their low baseline risks, have a major shift in risk. On the other hand, someone who carries a high baseline risk may actually have a higher absolute risk than the previous patient but may not be at imminent risk if no recent changes have occurred. Remember that completed suicide is rare, suicidal ideation is common in severe psychiatric disorders, and clinicians cannot always prevent suicide, but they can reduce the risks.

■ IS THERE IMMINENT RISK FOR SUICIDE (IS AN ATTEMPT LIKELY IN THE NEXT 24–48 HOURS)?

Imminent risk is easy to determine when a patient has a clear plan for suicide and intent to implement (or has just attempted). Unpredictable patients (ie, psychotic or intoxicated) are also likely to be at imminent risk because they are resistant and frequently incapable of forming a relationship with the hospitalist. However, it is typically more difficult to determine whether the risk for suicide is imminent. Often many risk factors are present but protective factors or prohibitions against suicide are also present. Neither of the last two cases had a past history of either mental illness or suicidality, which would have represented increased risk for suicide over their baseline risks. Therefore they many not appear at imminent risk. Unfortunately, when multiple risk factors are present, there is no evidence-based scale on which to weigh these complex factors. Clinical judgment is the only tool available to judge the complexities of risk.

■ ASSESS THE SUPPORT SYSTEM AVAILABLE TO THE PATIENT

Determining the patient's support system is a crucial component of fully assessing the patient's risk factors for suicide. If a patient has an actively involved well-functioning family or lives in a structured environment where observation is available, then this patient may be potentially treated as an outpatient even with relatively high risk for suicide. On the other hand, even at a lower level of risk, hospitalization may be indicated for a patient with inadequate support structure. When an active support system is present, it is ideal to include supportive others in the management plan.

■ WHAT SETTING IS REQUIRED FOR THE INITIAL STEPS OF MANAGEMENT?

Identifying the setting for implementing the management plan involves assessing the patient's economic and social support resources. Practically speaking, there are usually just two options, either home or the hospital. Legal and ethical principles require hospitalists to use the least restrictive setting to provide effective intervention and management while maintaining the safety of the patient and others. This is often a difficult balancing act. Limitations in the availability of psychiatric hospitalization have shifted the treatment of psychiatric disorders toward outpatient settings. Mobilizing complementary professional resources (ie, social workers, nurses, and community services) can help form a supportive structure for the at-risk patient. However, when the risk for suicide is imminent, inpatient hospitalization is required in a secure unit, staffed with skilled professionals.

■ MAKE THE MANAGEMENT PLAN EXPLICIT

Reviewing the details of the management plan with the patient helps to actively enlist the patient in the treatment. Documenting and communicating the plan to the support system, when available, is also important for longitudinal management and decision making. A written plan gives the patient and the support structure valuable follow-up information, including emergency contact numbers. It is not uncommon for a management plan to include a contract for safety. It is typically a simple statement that is then signed by the patient: "I, Susan Thomas, agree to call the emergency numbers and come to the ER if I have any feelings about hurting myself."

TABLE 229-2 Essential Concepts Related to—Suicide

- Many hospitalized patients are silently at high risk for suicide and should be assessed
- Suicidal thoughts are extremely common, but completed suicide is not
- The clinical goal is to fully assess the risk for suicide, not predict it.
- Screening for suicide should begin with discussing hopelessness and negativity
- If suicidality is present, then fully assess risk factors:
  - Chronic/predisposing factors (gender, family history, age, etc)
  - Acute/potentiating factors (recent loss, exacerbation of illness, access to firearms)
  - Protective factors (social support, children less than 18 in home, religious beliefs)
- Devise and communicate a plan addressing the risk factors

Though a "contract for safety" is used frequently, it is often overvalued and erroneously perceived as carrying the weight of a legal document. Contracts for safety, which are sometimes referred to as "no-harm contracts" or "suicide contracts," were originally conceived to facilitate management of the suicidal patient. These contracts are vehicles that articulate the treatment plan with parameters for increasing treatment intensity. The utility of this approach lies in the explicit nature of the communication and the explicit agreement of the patient to the plan. The absence of the patient's agreement is an indication to consider psychiatric admission. Though contracts for safety can be helpful communication tools, they alone provide little protective value for a patient who is intent on committing suicide (**Table 229-2**).

SUGGESTED READINGS

American Psychiatric Association. Practice guideline for the assessment and treatment of patients with suicidal behaviors. *Am J Psychiatry*. 2003;(suppl):160:1–60.

Block SD. Assessing and managing depression in the terminally ill patient. *Ann Intern Med.* 2000;132:209–218.

Bostwick JM, Levenson JL. Suicidality. In: *The Textbook of Psychosomatic Medicine*. American Washington, DC: Psychiatric Publishing; 2005;219–234.

Breitbart W, Rosenfeld B, Pessin H, et al. Depression, hopelessness, and desire for hastened death in terminally ill patients with cancer. *JAMA.* 2000;284:2907–2911.

Druss B, Pincus H. Suicidal ideation and suicide attempts in general medical illnesses. *Arch Intern Med*. 2000;160:1522–1526.

Harris EC, Barraclough BM. Suicide as an outcome for medical disorders. *Medicine*. 1994;73:281–389.

CHAPTER 230

The Difficult Patient

Glenn J. Treisman, MD, PhD
Joyce E. King, MD

Key Clinical Questions

1. How do you identify a "difficult patient"?
2. What strategies can clinicians use to achieve long-term clinical results and reduce unnecessary admissions to the hospital?

INTRODUCTION

The term *difficult patient* refers to a subgroup of patients that provoke unpleasant emotions—feelings of frustration, anger, helplessness, inadequacy, or irritation—in the doctors caring for them. These patients are described in the records of the earliest physicians. Thomas Sydenham wrote in his famed treatise on hysteria "All is caprice. They love without measure those whom they will soon hate without reason. Now they will do this, now that; ever receding from their purpose." These patients have a series of overlapping characteristics, shown in **Table 230-1**.

Although many authors see conflicts between clinicians and patients as specific to one dyadic relationship, most patients identified as difficult or disordered have a long history of failed medical relationships and are often dissatisfied when they arrive. They recreate the same dissatisfying relationships by repeating the behaviors that caused their previous experiences. Emotionally provoked staff members will likely behave in ways that only further confirm the patient's expectation that he or she will receive poor treatment.

Many neurologic disorders and medical conditions, including tumors, endocrine and autoimmune disorders, and medications, cause psychiatric syndromes, such as personality changes, major depression, cognitive dysfunction, and executive dysfunction. All of these can result in behaviors that make patients "difficult." The following discussion is organized around the psychiatric conditions that provoke and sustain "difficult" behaviors, and introduces the concept of a behavioral approach to managing these patients.

CASE 230-1

A 28-year-old man with HIV and hepatitis C presented to the hospital for a complicated cellulitis and abscess of hand and forearm that developed after an altercation. The emergency room physician performed an incision and drainage and admitted him to the hospital for intravenous antibiotics. The patient acknowledged occasional nasal heroin and cocaine use but denied addiction. At the time of admission, the attending ordered oxycodone 10 mg every six hours as needed. The health care team suspected that the patient was homeless when he refused to provide a telephone number or family contact.

During multiple prior admissions the patient had displayed such hostility that nurses limited their interactions with him. The nurses reported the smell of tobacco smoke near the patient's bathroom, but he declined a nicotine patch. He left the floor to smoke and often returned appearing sleepy and intoxicated. He received escalating doses of intravenous (IV) narcotic medication from cross-covering clinicians. The day team did not appreciate that his night time extra doses amounted to a significant escalation of his opiate use. His readmissions precluded follow-up with his primary care physician from another hospital network. Multiple attending physicians during his monthly hospitalizations further disrupted continuity of care.

On hospital day 2, the patient refused his dressing changes without IV narcotics. The nurse reported that she tried to coax the patient to undergo a dressing change with oral opiates but that he started yelling obscenities at her. Extremely irritable, the patient was alternately pleading and demanding

TABLE 230-1 Descriptions of Difficult Patients from the Medical Literature

High resource utilization
Test seeking
Drug seeking
Somatization
Excessive emotion
Unreasonable demands
"Borderline" personality
Dissatisfied
Unexplained symptoms
Chronic pain
Surgery seeking
Desire to direct treatment
Lack limits
Noncompliant
Unresponsive to treatment

IV pain medications. He threatened to leave if "the people here don't start treating me with respect." This patient's hostility made his primary nurse feel defensive and uncomfortable.

THE ROLE OF LIFE EXPERIENCES AND ASSUMPTIONS

At this point, a psychological and social history revealed that the patient had grown up in east Baltimore under the worst of conditions. His physically abusive father abandoned his family. His mother was largely unreliable due to substance abuse. After asking numerous questions about his past medical experiences, we determined that the patient had received medical care only in "institutional settings," and his experience with white male authority figures had been dismal.

We discussed his history of negative interactions with health care in institutional settings, and how his "assumption" that he will be mistreated leads to antagonistic behavior toward nurses and doctors, who respond in turn with hostility.

After commenting on how unfortunate these experiences must have been, we informed him that we would like to start with a clean slate. We reinforced our commitment to getting him better and to trying to make his stay as comfortable as possible while still doing what would be medically justified by the risks and benefits of treatments.

We negotiated with the patient that if he wore a nicotine patch, cooperated with dressing changes, and restrained from foul language, one of us would accompany him outside to smoke twice a day. Although he could not receive IV opiates, he would receive his preferred opiate orally, hydromorphone (Dilaudid) in equianalgesic dosing to the oxycodone he had been prescribed.

THE BENEFITS OF INITIATING TREATMENT OF DEPRESSION IN THE HOSPITAL

His behavior improved. The diagnosis of depression would not have been made had it not been for the extended exposure to the patient in the setting of walking him outside. While smoking, he described his life as miserable and meaningless. He stated that he could not sleep at night and felt "hateful" all of the time. He said he often thought he would be better off dead and admitted that he sometimes hoped someone, "like a police," will shoot him. We offered him medications for sleep and depression and described major depression to him. The treatment of his depression allowed the forging of a better relationship as we discussed the way his depression had interfered with his life.

PATIENT EDUCATION ABOUT WHAT IS GOOD AND BAD ABOUT EXTRAVERSION

We told our patient that he needed to choose between being Martin Luther King Jr., who had rules he followed even when he was angry, sad, or felt like he was not getting anywhere, and being Marion Barry, who, when he got caught smoking crack with a prostitute said "it wasn't me." I described to the patient that he had "special abilities to persuade people" so that he usually got his way, but that he was using those powers to harm himself and those around him. He was able to expand this and engage with the idea.

NONJUDGMENTAL RECOGNITION OF ADDICTION

On day 3 he was much more irritable, with nausea and flulike symptoms. We diagnosed him with opiate withdrawal and offered to treat him for his withdrawal with higher doses of opiates followed by a slow taper. We described how addiction can sneak up on people. At this point, we also introduced the idea that some people have very little emotion, most people have an average amount of emotion, but that he had a very large amount of emotion, using the term "two scoops of feelings." We explained that this was a form of being "gifted," but for him it had been a curse. We clarified that his belief that he should be having a better life was actually accurate, but that no one had helped him learn to manage his intense feelings. We offered to help him with this over the several subsequent days. We added a long-acting opiate to stabilize him on a regimen. During the remaining days of his admission, we slowly tapered his opiates and offered to refer him to an outpatient program if he wished. The medical team saw him twice a day, often confronting him gently on the way his feelings cause him problems and with suggestions on how to behave during intense feeling states in order to be more effective.

THE IMPACT OF THE DOCTOR–PATIENT RELATIONSHIP AND SYSTEM OF CARE ON OUTCOMES

Consider the example of our patient, who had multiple readmissions to a tertiary hospital outside of his network. He seemed to benefit from hospitalization as a possible way to obtain temporary shelter and food, receive intravenous narcotics that made him feel better, and perhaps experience fewer restrictions than in the city hospital where he was enrolled in care. When asked why he did not go back to the hospital of his primary care physician, he responded, "They do not treat me right." The challenge for the clinicians taking care of him was how to change the behavior resulting in monthly readmissions. We determined that the plan would be most successful if directed by one primary care physician. We ascertained through communication that his primary care physician would accept him back and manage his HIV and other medical issues as well as his substance abuse. Because he would likely benefit from the direction of one individual, he was transferred to the hospital of his primary care physician. Although not customary practice, this may have been the only way to break the cycle of readmissions so that appropriate resources could be put in place to provide him with the help he needed.

TABLE 230-2 Psychiatric Differential Diagnosis of the Difficult Patient

- Maladaptive psychological life experiences:
  Negative experiences including trauma, misuse, learned helplessness, and poor coping skills
- Psychiatric disease:
  Depression, schizophrenia, bipolar disorder and dementia
- Problematic personality:
  Uncooperative, stubborn, manipulative and maladaptive
- Behavioral disorder:
  Addiction, disorders of overvalued ideas, and maladaptive conditioned learning

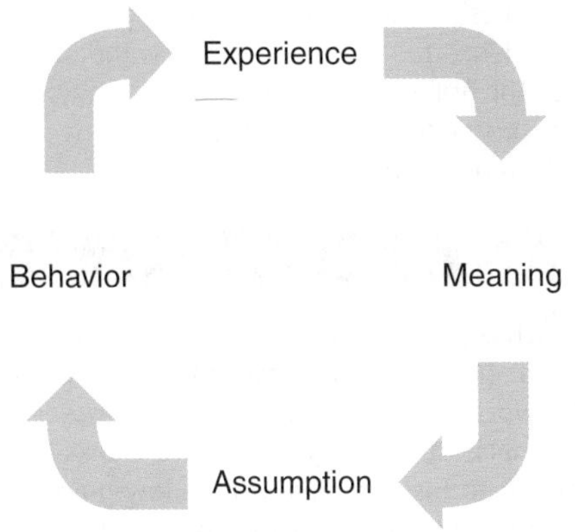

Figure 230-1 *The Cycle of life experience.*

PATHOPHYSIOLOGY

Studies of difficult patients are fraught with technical challenges but have generally found that about 15% of patients are perceived as difficult. Six psychiatric disorders had particularly strong associations with being labeled as difficult: somatoform disorder, panic disorder, dysthymia, generalized anxiety, major depressive disorder, and alcohol abuse or dependence. The presence of mental disorders accounted for a substantial proportion of the excess functional impairment and dissatisfaction of difficult patients, but not for all of it. It is not surprising that these "difficult" patients often develop symptoms that precipitate hospitalization for potentially serious symptoms, noncompliance with treatments, or, sometimes, as a result of outpatient or emergency department physicians' lack of time or patience.

Our organizational rubric is developed out of the elegant work of McHugh and Slavney in *Perspectives of Psychiatry*. We will first discuss the psychological precedents from the patient's life experiences. This is followed by a discussion of the role of psychiatric disease states, problematic personality traits, and behavioral conditioning and addictions. Patients often have more than one related condition, each exacerbating the others (**Table 230-2**).

PRACTICE POINT

- Behavior disturbances have multiple causes—those due to underlying medical illness, those due to major psychiatric illness, and those related to interpersonal styles. The management strategy begins with a history and physical examination, including a neurologic assessment, so as not to overlook delirium or other underlying medical illness that requires emergent treatment, a review of all medications and dosages, and a toxicology screen in patients suspected of substance abuse. Patients with cognitive deficits may be easily confused by a change in environment; may be susceptible to medications with anti cholinergic properties, steroids, and analgesics; and may exhibit paranoia or delusions due to a developing delirium. Patients with stroke, Parkinson disease, and traumatic brain injury may exhibit features of apathy syndromes, such as lack of motivation and inability to initiate behavior even though they are not depressed or delirious. Alcohol and other substance withdrawal may also account for the observed behavioral disturbances.

THE ROLE OF LIFE EXPERIENCES

Life experience is difficult to subject to randomized clinical trials and does not fit well into "evidence-based medicine." **Figure 230-1** illustrates the cycle of life experience and how behavior develops out of the assumptions one makes about the world. This cycle can be interrupted at any of the arrows shown. Patients must understand the psychological precedents that shape their behavior, and they need a clinician who is willing to confront their behavior and guide it toward more adaptive and successful function. (Refer to preceding case study.)

Commitment to acceptance of any goals patients bring, even unhealthy goals, undermines these patients' need for guidance and direction from the clinician, much to their detriment. To defuse this dynamic, the clinician may communicate that the patient is very important despite their misbehavior and that the health care team wants to help. Changing this cycle of hostility requires tackling some of the patient's assumptions and establishing the critical core of the doctor–patient relationship. Patients can fire you and go elsewhere, but they cannot prescribe their own treatment.

PSYCHIATRIC DISEASES

Patients with major mental illness have higher rates of mortality and medical morbidity. As a group they have poorer compliance with medical interventions and exhibit high-risk behaviors and unhealthy habits resulting in higher rates of medical complexity and comorbidity. In most health care systems the chronically mentally ill are disenfranchised from medical care. They take more time and are more challenging to treat than other patients. Frequently underinsured, they have poor access to medical care and decreased willingness to take advantage of accessible care. Specific mental disorders tend to be associated with different types of difficult behaviors.

PRACTICE POINT

- Patients with major psychiatric illness such as major depression, bipolar illness, schizophrenia, and substance abuse are at risk for receiving suboptimal care due to mental illness. The first step in treating their medical illness is to collaborate with their psychiatrists or seek hospital psychiatric consultation.

SCHIZOPHRENIA

Schizophrenia is a progressive, disabling, lifelong, chronic mental illness characterized by a stepwise deterioration of executive function, social interactions, and a paranoid psychosis without return to baseline between episodes. Patients more often focus their paranoia on outside agencies and people regularly in their lives. The so-called positive features—the auditory hallucinations, delusions, and feelings of external control—are episodic and disruptive. The "negative features" include affective flattening (or inappropriate affect), ambivalence, autism (with social withdrawal), and loose associations. The following exemplifies how physician attitudes affect their approach to patients with mental illness and the degree of difficulty inherent in treating these patients:

CASE 230-2

A man with schizophrenia had the persistent delusion that the VA in Florida was shooting radio waves into his abdomen. He presented with worsening abdominal pain and a seemingly stable 4 cm abdominal aortic aneurysm. For two weeks his complaints were attributed to his paranoia despite low-grade fevers and a rising white blood cell count. He died of massive internal hemorrhage shortly after a gallium scan correctly diagnosed his mycotic aortic aneurysm.

Physicians often approach clinical interactions with the preconceived notion that all complaints by patients with schizophrenia are generated by the illness, or that they will be unable to follow treatment recommendations—an assumption that is often incorrect.

MAJOR DEPRESSION

The term *depression* denotes a symptom, a complaint, and several conditions that are probably biologically determined syndromes caused by brain dysfunction. Depressed patients are often lumped together in studies and included or excluded by symptom scales rather than strict criteria, making the literature difficult to understand. There are at least three separate conditions to be considered when thinking about depression, namely, demoralization, chronic dysthymia, and major depression (**Figure 230-2**).

The term *demoralization* describes those patients suffering from the expected or understandable psychological state of decreased mood associated with adversity, loss, and grief. Ranging from mild to severe, demoralization can lead to suicide, social withdrawal, and serious medical morbidity. It responds to the "tincture of time," support, encouragement, and reintegration into occupational, social, and recreational activities. Most physicians do not perceive these patients as difficult; they often evoke genuine sympathy and are usually grateful for the counseling, encouragement, and guidance they receive.

Dysthymia has come to mean chronic major depression, depressive personality style, and subsyndromal major depression. The term as used here denotes a chronic pessimistic personality style, but the term is frequently used in other ways. These patients are like Eeyore in *Winnie the Pooh*, chronically negative but usually quite functional unless they encounter circumstances where their personality style interferes with their function. Their chronic pessimism can lead to frustration on the part of the physician caring for them.

Dysthymic patients latch onto doctors and try to get the doctor to make them feel better emotionally when they constitutionally resist doing so.

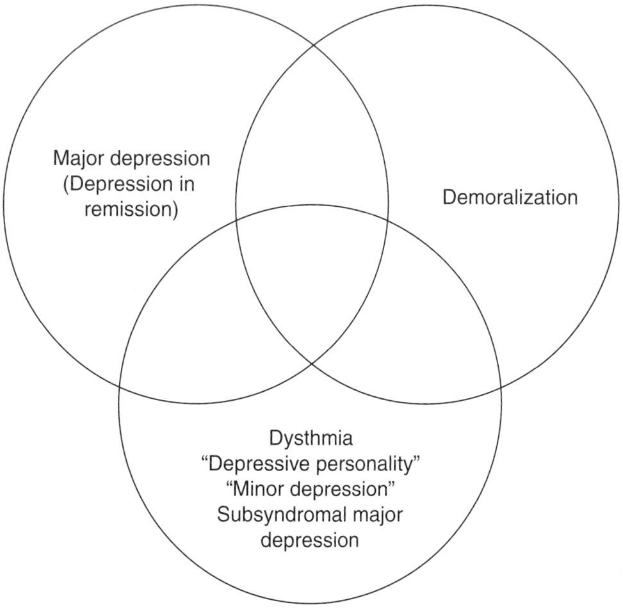

Figure 230-2 *Venn diagram of subtypes of depression.*

PRACTICE POINT

Dysthmic patients

This quote from *Winnie the Pooh* is illustrative:

(Eeyore the donkey) "Hallo, Pooh. Thank you for asking, but I shall be able to use it again in a day or two."

"Use what?" said Pooh.

"What we were talking about."

"I wasn't talking about anything," said Pooh, looking puzzled.

"My mistake again. I thought you were saying how sorry you were about my tail, being all numb, and could you do anything to help?"

"No," said Pooh. "That wasn't me," he said. He thought for a little and then suggested helpfully: "Perhaps it was somebody else."

"Well, thank him for me when you see him."

Major depression describes a biologically determined medical condition that is the result of monoamine neurotransmitter dysfunction and usually an episodic disorder, characterized by periods of illness with symptoms alternating with recovery to baseline. In addition to a genetic component, activation of the stress axis, chronic central nervous system inflammation, a variety of medical conditions including certain cancers, and some medications may provoke major depression. Depending on the type of person who has the condition, patients may experience sadness, loss of emotions, apathy, anxiety, and agitation.

Patients suffering from major depression exaggerate their personality vulnerabilities. They are caught up in an endless web of pessimism and hopelessness, often overwhelmed by their problems and feeling unable to cope. Family and friends share their pervasive opinion that they should be able to "pick themselves up by their bootstraps." The anxiety caused by major depression can give them a "clinging" quality, evoking discomfort for caregivers. The prominent symptom of anxiety can trap patients into a cycle of using benzodiazepines to relieve it, only to have their anxiety worsen dramatically as the benzodiazepines wear off.

Patients with major depression are more "difficult" due to their focus on negative thoughts and feelings; sense of hopelessness, neediness, and abandonment; increased anxiety and likelihood that they will often experience their physical symptoms in an amplified way. Depressed patients can overwhelm physicians, particularly when they resist the diagnosis of a mental illness. Committed to the idea that their depression is the result of their medical (and other) problems, they attribute all of their psychological symptoms to stress rather than to depression. If physicians are also caught up in the patients' psychological explanation for their emotional state, they may miss the diagnosis of major depression. It frequently seems reasonable that the depressive symptoms represent demoralization related to the medical condition rather than a major depression. Vital sense will be diminished in sick people, and self-attitude changes are often explained away as frustration and hopelessness because of the lack of response to previous treatment.

We have found that anhedonia is both sensitive and specific for the diagnosis of depression in medically ill patients. Patients will describe not being able to get their usual pleasure, joy, excitement, or satisfaction from activities that were previously rewarding. The following two consults only a few weeks apart for patients with almost identical prognoses illustrate anhedonia and major depression in one of the patients.

Chronic pain is frequently complicated by major depression; it has a poorer prognosis when the depression is untreated and a better prognosis when it is treated. Several antidepressants have been shown to be efficacious in the treatment of chronic pain, fibromyalgia, and chronic fatigue syndrome—diagnoses commonly seen in patients with somatization disorder. These medications may not treat depression but only the chronic symptoms that these patients experience. Accumulating evidence supports the hypothesis that depression is a medical disease state, and the effort to distinguish a "mental illness" such as major depression (a biological dysregulation of brain chemistry) from a "physical illness" such as fibromyalgia has become a completely unhelpful exercise.

CASE 230-3

Two patients with anhedonia: The first patient described that his family visits would make him forget about his illness, how he was excited about seeing his grandchildren, but as soon as they left, he would feel like giving up and just want to quit. The second patient said that he felt bad all the time, and when his family visited he would try to put a good face on it, but he wished they would just stop visiting because there was no point.

There are few activities for hospitalized patients to enjoy, and their anhedonia may not represent psychiatric pathology. However, visitors, improvement in condition, special television programs, certain foods, or even interactions with the nurses will usually brighten up hospitalized patients.

Early morning awakening with difficulty returning to sleep is a compelling symptom for the diagnosis of depression. Periodicity or a previous higher level of function should be seen as supportive of the diagnosis. In the hospital this can be difficult to assess because of the frequent awakenings patients experience, but patients may describe waking up in the early morning hours and worrying in a way that does not occur in the afternoon.

IN-HOSPITAL TREATMENT OF DEPRESSION

Patients with chronic medical illness and major depression often go untreated. Outside the hospital, physicians barely have adequate time to assess one medical problem during a problem-focused visit. Patients with depression often feel hopeless, are less likely to take their medications, and are less likely to engage in rehabilitation. They have a poorer prognosis for almost every condition studied. In the hospital, they are seen daily, offering an opportunity to slowly increase the dose of their antidepressants and make sure they are tolerating their medications. The commonly held myth that there are no rapid improvements with antidepressants is exactly that, a myth. While you cannot count on a response until you have given the drug for several weeks, many patients respond far sooner. This seems particularly true of medically ill patients, who often respond surprisingly quickly. Starting treatment also ensures that depression will be considered at follow-up. (Refer to Case 230-1)

Patients with chronic medical problems are at risk for suicide, and it is incumbent to recognize suicidal feelings and obtain timely consultation. A high-risk time for suicide is when patients first start to get a response from antidepressants, when their energy level increases before their mood actually improves. Patients should be warned about this phenomenon, but reassured that this predicts an excellent response. They should be instructed to tell you if they feel suicidal but maintain hope for the improved mood that follows the increased energy.

PERSONALITY DISORDERS

William Osler said, "It is much more important to know what sort of patient has a disease than what sort of disease a patient has." The whole area of personality and temperament is confounded by entrenched psychological theories and dogma about the developmental influences of certain kinds of trauma. The concept of borderline personality originates in psychoanalytic ideas of the early 20th century that have become doctrinaire. This chapter focuses on the branch of psychology that has attempted to measure temperament or disposition, and how to deal with the traits, regardless of origin. In the simplest terms, character can be seen as the outcome of underlying temperament or disposition interacting with learning and environment. The methods used to measure traits of personality have been consistent over time and seem to have predictive validity. The personality traits introversion–extraversion on one axis and instability–stability on another are normally distributed in a Gaussian manner in the population. The most straightforward description of this axis of personality is that introverts react to stimulation with inhibition, while extraverts react with excitation. **Figure 230-3** depicts the distribution of introversion and extraversion.

There is also a stability–instability axis (many refer to instability as neuroticism), which is orthogonal to the extraversion–introversion axis (**Figure 230-4**).

When this axis is combined with the extraversion–introversion axis, one gets the four Greek Humors of temperament.

■ INTROVERTS

As shown in the diagram, introverts are consequence-avoidant, future-directed, and function-directed. They avoid circumstances likely to lead to negative outcomes rather than seeking circumstances that will lead to positive outcomes. Their behavior is more likely to be shaped by consequences and they are less sensitive to rewards. They are concerned about illness, physical sensations, their own internal milieu, and avoiding negative consequences. They are therefore concerned about side effects of treatments, the correctness of diagnosis, and the effects of their illness, and when

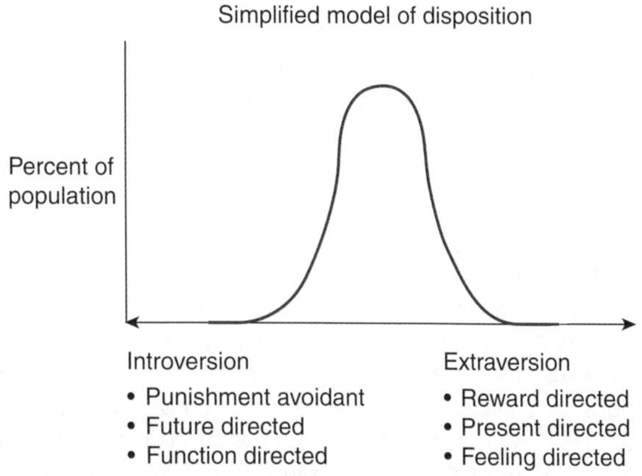

Figure 230-3 *Simplified model of disposition.*

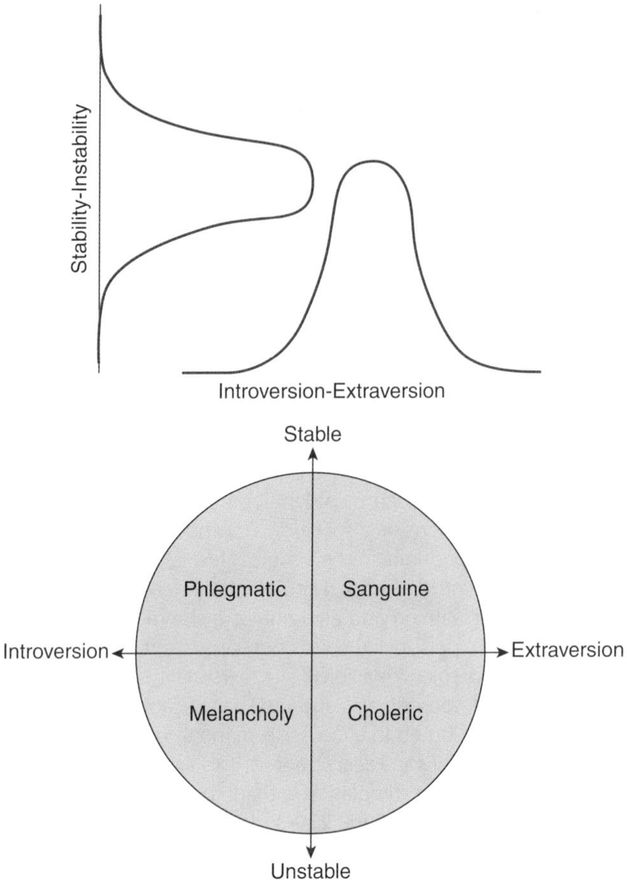

Figure 230-4 *Distribution of some personality traits and their relationship to the four humours of the ancient Greeks.*

faced with decisions tend to hesitate rather than act decisively, based on fear of making an error.

Introverts are at their best when analyzing situations that require thought and consideration before action. They are good at accounting, law, and medicine, and thinking about safety, prevention, and right and wrong. They are at a disadvantage in situations requiring action when all choices have potential negative consequences, such as embarking on treatment or accepting diagnostic labels. Ruminating patients can get trapped in endless lists of side effects, adverse outcomes, dangers related to tests and procedures, and the consequences of a particular diagnostic label. The question, What if you are wrong? can paralyze them and obstruct their treatment. They are particularly sensitive to the social meaning of certain diagnoses, such as psychiatric conditions. Physicians tend to be introverted, and therefore they often have an easier time relating to the obsessive introverts who ruminate endlessly about their illness and the decisions in treatment. Nonetheless, physicians can eventually lose patience with this process and become frustrated by a patient's relentless need for reassurance. They often struggle with the recapitulating patient and need to learn ways to push the patient forward.

Fortunately, clinical medicine has an endless list of terrible consequences that can be used to help shape the behavior of introverts. Introverts usually respond well to opportunities to avoid "bad" decisions, negative consequences, and missed opportunities. They can usually be directed to good decisions by clear clinical analysis of pros and cons of a decision in terms of risks and benefits. They often get bogged down in worries about side effects and ruminative doubts about wrong diagnoses and the need for further tests, but because physicians swim in these waters all the time they can usually lead the patient to the best choice and course of action. Clear descriptions of the "bad things that will happen if you miss your medications" are a powerful motivator for introverts and come naturally to doctors who deal with those bad things every day, as in the following case.

CASE 230-4

A patient was unable to choose a course of action despite clear communication that overall it was better to have surgery as soon as possible. He had made lists of every reason to have surgery and every reason to wait until later, including spending time with his family so he could prepare them. A careful description of how his family would be affected if he waited for the surgery and "something happened" was so distressing to him that it trumped his lists and pushed him to make a decision that was clearly the right one. Involving his daughter in this conversation facilitated decision making.

EXTRAVERTS

Extraverts are reward sensitive, present focused, and feeling focused. They actively seek positive feelings and desired emotional states, pursuing circumstances likely to provide a positive emotional outcome. They tend to want immediate relief from discomfort, and their behavior is reinforced strongly by rewards, particularly those associated with positive emotions. They are concerned about comfort, appearance, and obtaining the medication or treatment they have chosen. They will pursue a particular diagnosis or status from clinicians if it will get them what they desire and they are less concerned about ensuring that the diagnosis is correct.

Extraverts present a different paradigm for introverted doctors to manage. They are focused on feelings, rewards, and the present. This means they often demand instant relief, have an agenda for what they want, and are persuaded that they can direct their own care better than their doctor. The phrase, "I know what helps me", particularly when delivered in an impatient or irritated tone of voice, is nearly pathognomonic of the difficult extraverted patient. These patients almost always demand specific tests, treatments, and medications and hold fixed ideas about their diagnoses. They want to be made comfortable and equate comfort with wellness, while doctors usually equate function with being well. Ultimately, the central problem is that, in the words of Dr. King, "our therapeutic goals are not aligned." Extraverts' goal of feeling better often immediately leads to excessive use of benzodiazepines for anxiety, opiates for pain, sedative hypnotics for sleep, and stimulants for the inevitable accompanying sedation. Their conviction that something is wrong that can be "fixed" leads to excessive surgery and tests.

The frustration that physicians feel is in part provoked by the emotional landscape these patients inhabit. They feel things strongly and focus on the present. This leads to their changeable nature previously described in the quote by Sydenham. The patients love you when they are getting what they want, and hate you when they are not. Because they are so present focused, the things you have done for them in the past do not carry into the present. There is nothing "in the bank" in terms of trust, patience, and previous experience to help them through a difficult time. These patients are also vulnerable to seeing events as just "happening" to them, with little insight into their own role in their difficulty; this tends to make them see themselves ever as victims. In our current culture of victimhood and lack of personal responsibility, they go to the head of the line with explanations of why nothing is their fault and nothing that they can do will make things better.

STABILITY

Stable patients have emotions that are slow to change, demonstrate a small emotional response to a large emotional stimulus, and have a very consistent emotional response to a given stimulus. Unstable patients have emotions that change quickly, have a large emotional response to a small stimulus, and have an inconsistent emotional response to a given stimulus. Unstable extraverts (those of choleric temperament)—sometimes referred to as borderline personalities—may split the health care team and are difficult for most clinicians.

Fortunately, these patients are very sensitive to rewards and can be shaped by using the rewards they seek to help change their behavior to more productive modes. Most psychologists see these traits as neutral. Unstable extraverts can be very successful if they learn to modify their natural inclination in certain circumstances. We find it helpful to explain the nature of the difficulty they are having and how it interferes with the doctor–patient relationship. There are two parts to the conversation. The first is to give these patients an explanation of the difficulties they are having with many facets of their life by describing what is good about extraversion and what is bad. The description of patients as having "two scoops of feelings" has been particularly useful. The conversation leads in to the treatment for this, which is to help these patients to learn how not to let feelings run their lives. A method we use frequently is to make comparisons with people these patients are likely to admire who share their traits of intense feelings (a passionate nature) and then to contrast them with similar figures who have failed spectacularly when they let their feelings determine their behavior (such as Martin Luther King Jr. compared with Marion Barry, or Madonna compared with Britney Spears). (Refer to Case 230-1.)

Most patients of this type have been told that they are missing something (a conscience, a superego lacune, poor object relations) when in fact they suffer from too much of something. I told our patient that he was "a genius of feelings," which brought a smile to his face. These patients act entitled because they already sense that they are special. The message is that they are special, that they do deserve more, but that they will not get more until they learn to manage their feelings instead of letting their feelings manage them.

The second element of this conversation is to describe the doctor–patient relationship and the responsibilities each member holds in the relationship. This is sometimes referred to as a role induction and involves the "limit setting" part of working with patients with personality vulnerabilities. This includes the responsibility on the part of these patients to do their best to get well, to discuss the alternatives and then agree to a treatment plan, and to get a second opinion if not satisfied with the diagnosis and treatment plan. Many difficult patients with personality disorders will balk at a treatment plan that does not give them what they want, even if they acknowledge that what they want will be bad for them. This includes their desire for addictive drugs, allowing them to smoke in the bathroom, allowing them to come and go from the hospital as they wish, and allowing them to dictate their treatment. This gives the clinician the opportunity to tell the patient that she will gladly provide care if the patient changes his mind in the future, but she must decline to be a part of any treatment that might be harmful or be less than optimal for her patient. A discussion of why manipulative and suicidal behavior will be bad for the patient and his treatment is important for patients with these behaviors.

PRACTICE POINT

Patients with difficult interpersonal styles are at risk for receiving suboptimal care due to negative diagnostic labels and noncompliance. Follow a management strategy that is based on the patient's level of coping to facilitate cooperation.

- First, determine whether the problem results from miscommunication or misunderstanding between the patient and medical staff that could easily be resolved through clarification.
- Second, approach the patient with consistency and humility and maximize the patient's autonomy if the patient is paranoid. Straightforward and regular interactions should bolster the patient's adaptive defenses and strengthen the therapeutic alliance.
- Third, the health care team (nurses, residents, attending, and possibly patient relations, chaplain, or social workers) as a whole should see the patient on rounds to set limits to disruptive behavior and avoid splitting among personnel, at least initially.
- Institutional standards or a contract to contain disruptive behavior with patient negotiation and a working therapeutic relationship may prove effective, especially if the patient has previously tried to sabotage treatment, manipulate, or engage in antisocial behavior.

In working with difficult patients, many clinicians use treatment contracts to help delineate the limits and expectations for treatment. Our experience has been that such contracts may be very useful, but they can also serve as the way to "get rid" of patients who have overwhelmed the system. We have begun to advocate discharging uncooperative patients early with a smile and much encouragement to return if they decide our approach might help them. This does not mean that we think that any patient who is not completely cooperative should be discharged, it rather is directed at patients who are exhausting resources while not getting better, or more commonly, actually being harmed by the treatments that they end up getting. Any patients you would allow to leave against medical advice (AMA) can be discharged AMA if they are uncooperative, as in the following case.

CASE 230-5

The patient had been admitted for a nonhealing leg wound and uncontrolled diabetes and left AMA six times in three weeks. Each time he came in, he would receive IV hydromorphone and then decline further treatment. We told him that if he left AMA during this admission, we would only treat him with ketorolac during future admissions. Since we would allow him to leave AMA after hydromorphone, we certainly could let him leave AMA before it. He (of course) called our bluff and left AMA, and at his next admission, when we would only give him ketorolac, he immediately stormed out of the hospital. At his next admission a few days later, he complained when I showed up, asking me how I knew he was there. When I explained to him that I would always be there when he was admitted, he reluctantly agreed to stay and had successful treatment, including a buprenorphine taper when he developed withdrawal symptoms.

In circumstances where patients are so ill or cognitively impaired that they cannot be allowed to leave, we recommend simply telling them they will not be allowed to leave until stable, and treat them the same way we treat anyone who cannot cooperate but needs life-sustaining treatment. This approach also discourages patients who are uncooperative, using resources without gaining benefit, and demoralizing their doctors, but it allows them time to rethink their behavior and return to treatment when they are confronted with the need to change. Remarkably, many of these patients return. Over years they have told us in a variety of ways that they came back because we said no to them, and that we were the first doctors who thought they could actually get better.

ADDICTIONS

Poorly understood in medicine, addictions are usually categorized as diseases due to the biological nature of the abnormal appetite and drive that develop in addiction. This approach ignores the volitional component of addiction, which is essential to understanding the condition, and misses the huge number of sober addicts who remain in programs. On the opposite extreme, it has also become popular to look at drug addiction as a lifestyle or choice. This approach is not valid either. The demoralizing and dehumanizing activities in which addicts engage are repugnant and distressing to them, but they are unable to break free of the drug's hold on them. They like the drug, but they hate the addiction.

Patients suffering from addictions are frequently perceived as difficult. Doctors are not angry with patients with medical diseases such as congestive heart failure, but when their patient with alcohol addiction drinks, they become judgmental. Patients with addictions are often difficult in much the same way as extraverts. This is in part because extraverts are at increased risk for addictions, and by virtue of the fact that an addiction directs the patient's attention toward feelings, the present, and getting the drug that is reinforcing—all characteristics of extraversion. Introverts who develop addictions often look like extraverts when they are actively using drugs, adopting the style of manipulation and insensitivity to consequences that are the hallmarks of the extraverted personality disorders. They return to an introverted style as they recover. Patients have their behavior shaped by the rewarding nature of the drugs they use until the behavior becomes a loop of positive reinforcement that gradually excludes all other activities.

Addicted patients inevitably seek to maintain their addiction through manipulation, coercion, and lying. In addition, the destruction of employment and family relationships caused by substance use removes the supports most often sought by physicians caring for the difficult patient. Patients who are abusing illicit substances or misusing prescribed controlled substances present to their physicians in confusing ways. The physician is initially puzzled about the possibility of a missed diagnosis, a nagging sense that something about the interaction was "off," or why best efforts with a patient are repeatedly thwarted. These patients drain the resources of the hospital staff by asking for higher doses of opiates or requesting a specific nurse because "she understands my pain." They often wait until change of shift or evening hours when their usual physician is not available to ask for specific drugs by name or insist on intravenous opiates when the daytime plan had been made to switch to oral agents. They refuse magnetic resonance imaging scans at the last minute unless they can have a benzodiazepine of choice and some opiate during the study. They are off the floor when a procedure is scheduled and then complain that they have been in the hospital for days and nothing is happening. A high level of suspicion must be entertained for substance abuse in difficult patient encounters in order not to miss addictions, as they are associated with high morbidity and mortality and are imminently treatable.

Once the physician has diagnosed addiction, the following steps should be started in the hospital and pursued as part of the medical treatment plan:

1. **Conversion.** The patient is helped to recognize the addiction as a disorder that needs treatment. Some patients must lose nearly everything in their life before they can "hit bottom" and see the severity of their condition. Others can heed the properly presented warning of a good clinician. "Motivational interviewing" and "confrontation with a smile" are two descriptors of ways to achieve this. Essentially, in this step patients accept the diagnosis of an addictive disorder and decide that they are ready to get better.
2. **Detoxification.** Patients who are actively in the loop of using and craving are usually unable to break out of that loop without an intervention to detoxify them.
3. **Rehabilitation.** As patients become progressively more addicted, their lives become focused entirely on the behaviors involved in obtaining and using drugs, and gradually exclude all other activities. They become socially, occupationally, and recreationally disconnected. As they recover, there is little to fill their time other than craving drugs, and little to distract them from negative feelings. The activities that result in positive reinforcement of behavior in life and give life a sense of pleasure and satisfaction usually involve activities in these life domains. Rehabilitation means filling up these domains with meaningful life activities, but these must be rebuilt (or built) over time. This is often the most time-consuming element of recovery. It is not uncommon to hear people who have successfully recovered describe this phase in months and years.
4. **Treatment of comorbid conditions.** The fourth step occurs simultaneously with the third and consists of the treatment of comorbid conditions, both medical and psychiatric. Depression, personality disorders, HIV, hepatitis C, and chronic pain all act as triggers and interfere with recovery. The last step is relapse prevention. This is a long-term (indefinite) plan to prevent the elements that combined to allow the addiction to develop in the first place from allowing it to recur. Twelve-step programs, physician monitoring, and constant reminders of the danger of recurrence of addiction are needed in a long-term systematic way. (Refer to Case 230-1.)

Motivational interviewing, role induction, and detoxification can usually be initiated in the hospital, and sometimes completed. Familiarity with and referral to the outpatient network of rehabilitation services is essential for lasting success with addicted patients.

CHRONIC PAIN

The issue of the management of chronic pain is central to the role of dealing with difficult patients. Patients with acute pain are usually relatively straightforward to manage, while those with chronic pain are far more difficult. Unfortunately, the efforts to make pain a vital sign and to ensure that all pain is relieved have led to a massive overuse of narcotics and escalating problems of iatrogenic addiction. Nonmalignant chronic pain is often not relieved with chronic opiates and can be made worse by chronic opiate use.

PRACTICE POINT

- Although some patients benefit from chronic opiate administration, it is increasingly clear that many do not. Opiate-mediated hyperalgesia is common in patients with chronic pain on long-term opiates. The longer term the pain, the less often opiates are the answer. This is not the case for acute pain. If tissue is not being damaged (neuropathy, low back pain, chronic headache, fibromyalgia, and other chronic conditions), the opiates often cause real problems for patients later and can reinforce abnormal illness behaviors. Alternative methods of pain management may be more useful for chronic pain.

Pain has two components, a sensory element and an affective element. It is the affective element that produces the distress associated with pain. Patients with depression have an increased sensitivity to pain, particularly the affective component. Patients with significant extraversion or instability are more reactive to the distress associated with pain and will tolerate a lower level of function in their effort to eliminate pain. They are at increased risk for addiction and medication overuse.

In general, opiates are probably reasonable for acute pain caused by tissue damage (surgery, trauma, malignancy). Chronic pain is not usually the result of ongoing tissue damage, but rather the result of altered sensory and sympathetic nervous function (as in neuropathy, low back pain, chronic headache, fibromyalgia). While some patients benefit from chronic opiate administration, it is increasingly clear that many do not. Patients are often given opiates at ever increasing doses to try to combat their pain, and while some may benefit, many become increasingly intoxicated and exhibit more dysfunction as the dose increases. Opiate-mediated hyperalgesia is common in patients with chronic pain on long-term opiates. The longer term the pain, the less often opiates are the answer.

Patients with chronic pain are often in the "difficult patient" category and are often focused entirely on the goal of pain relief to the detriment of getting better and improving function. They arrive demanding escalating doses of opiates and are often given comfort-directed pharmacologic interventions such as benzodiazepines and other sedative-hypnotics.

A BEHAVIORAL APPROACH TO MANAGEMENT OF CHRONIC PAIN AND RELATED CONDITIONS

In the early 1900s, Ivan Pavlov described the ability to change behavior in animals by association with a particular stimulus. He was able to measure salivation in dogs in response to food, but then by pairing the food with a bell, he was able to elicit salivation in response to the bell. Described as classical conditioning, this type of passive conditioning has been observed with patients in many settings. Patients who have had several exposures to chemotherapy will often develop nausea and may even vomit when arriving at the cancer center. It is possible to condition changes in immune function, condition asthma attacks, and condition neutral stimuli to cause pain. Classical conditioning (or Pavlovian conditioning) occurs when a patient associates a behavior with a desirable or undesirable stimulus or experience.

Operant conditioning, described later by B. F. Skinner, occurs when a behavior performed by the patient is associated with a specific consequence. This type of conditioning results in increasing or decreasing the likelihood of the associated behavior. As an example, a pigeon pecks a key and receives a food reward. This results in more frequent and faster key-pecking behavior. Skinner described "shaping," where successive rewards could result in more complex behaviors. Pigeons can be shaped to peck a ball into a slot for food by first shaping the bird to peck the ball and then rewarding it only when it pecks the ball in a specific direction. Skinner described four types of conditioning, as shown in **Table 230-3**.

If the consequence of the behavior is a reward (positive reinforcement) or the removal of something noxious (negative reinforcement), behaviors increase. If the consequence of the behavior is the removal of the reward (extinction) or the delivery of something noxious (punishment—often incorrectly referred to as negative reinforcement), behaviors decrease.

All of these conditioning paradigms have been described for doctor–patient interactions. A patient who throws a tantrum on the ward and demands narcotics has probably been reinforced for that behavior by the previous delivery of narcotics in the same situation. Subtle reinforcement of illness behaviors such as limping, splinting, moaning, crying, and even falling can occur with patients who are vulnerable to the reinforcing effects of particular responses.

TABLE 230-3 Behavioral Reinforcement from Operant Conditioning

Quality of the Consequence	Positive (Rewarding)	Negative (Noxious)
Delivery of consequence	Positive reinforcement Increased Behavior	Punishment Decreased behavior
Withdrawal of consequence	Extinction Decreased behavior	Negative reinforcement Increased behavior

From Operant reinforcement as described by BF Skinner.

A caveat here is that reinforcement works only when the consequence or reward being employed to shape behavior has salience to the person being shaped. Pigeons must be hungry to work for food rewards. Patients in a given set of circumstances are more or less vulnerable to the reinforcing effects of narcotics, attention, praise, encouragement, criticism, relief from distress, and diagnostic labels. A person with a good job may be eager to return to work and may perceive an excuse from work as aversive and therefore understate her level of discomfort. A person who is unhappy at work may find a note excusing him a reward and may thus overestimate his discomfort. Physicians are constantly shaping their patients. All doctor–patient interactions subtly shape behavior. (Refer to Case 230-1.)

Patients are positively reinforced by opiate and sedative-hypnotic medications, attention from doctors, disability payments, and permission to express prohibited feelings. They are negatively reinforced by the pain relief provided by narcotics, the relief from insomnia provided by sedative hypnotics, and the relief from the expectations and demands at work and at home. This will increase medication seeking, doctor seeking, and pain-related behavior. This will also shape patients to be less committed to recovery.

Fortunately, these same behavioral tools can be used to shape recovery-related and function-related behaviors. Izzy Pilowsky described illness-related behaviors in the absence of ongoing pathology with the term *abnormal illness behavior*. Many of these behaviors are conditioned to occur. Ignoring abnormal illness behaviors will help result in their extinction. Rewarding healthy behaviors such as rehabilitation, function, and coping will encourage them to develop. Examples of this include the use of letters, forms, attention, and personal approval as positive reinforcers of specific behavior. Patients on chronic opiate treatment for pain might be required to demonstrate steady progress at physical therapy (PT) with increasing exercise duration. I have told patients that if they are too sick for PT, then they don't need the opiates because the opiates are only prescribed to make PT tolerable. It is also important to recognize that patients condition their physicians as much as we condition them. In a seminal study of prescription-writing behavior, Turk showed that nonverbal pain behaviors have a potent influence on the prescription-writing behavior of doctors. Continuous positive reinforcement leads to high rates of behavior, while intermittent reinforcement leads to long sustainable behavior. When patients "wear us down" and we "cave" and prescribe narcotics, we are ensuring that the behavior will continue a long time.

The deliberate application of behavioral techniques to treatment of difficult patients takes much of the emotional element out of the picture. We emphasize that we will focus on what the patient is doing and not on what they are feeling. Successful treatment can be described as occurring in five steps, similar to those for addictions. Prior to beginning treatment, a full evaluation for medical and psychiatric conditions must be completed. It is critical to know the case when starting treatment with difficult patients.

Treatment begins with a role induction. This consists of describing the entire formulation to the patient of what the doctor thinks is wrong. We include the medical and psychiatric elements in the discussion. We allow adequate time for patients to ask questions about each condition, why we think they have it, and how it affects them, but we do not allow patients to derail the discussion or argue about the diagnosis. When patients argue about the diagnosis, we tell them that if they disagree after we explain things fully, we will arrange for them to get a second opinion. It is important not to allow the patient to short circuit the discussion of diagnosis by leaping to treatment. The discussion of treatment begins after the patient has heard the diagnostic formulation completely. Typical formulations describe the medical problems first, then the way they are complicated by the lack of reward in major depression, the amplification of sensation due to temperament, and the lack of coping skills and aversive experiences that have made it hard to get good treatment. We finally discuss the way in which conditioning has systematically incapacitated the patient. We offer an optimistic discussion of treatments that are often contrary to the patient's requested treatments, but we explain how they will result in a better outcome. We stress the losses and indignities the patient has suffered from his illness and how important it is to try to recover his life. We finish the role induction by pointing out that we could be wrong, and that the patient will need to decide whether he wants to seek treatment elsewhere or engage in the treatment we have prescribed. This approach is paternalistic, but it also establishes the critical core of the doctor–patient relationship.

The next step involves detoxification, if needed, and the development of a set of behavioral goals with associated rewards and consequences. This is the equivalent of the detoxification step in addictions treatment, in which the sustaining behavioral rewards that maintain abnormal illness behavior are removed.

The initiation of medical and psychiatric treatments (equivalent to the treatment of comorbid conditions in addictions) is critical to the success of the overall treatment. This is done in concert with the initiation of behaviorally based rehabilitation. Treatment often includes an opiate taper, physical therapy, and comprehensive rehabilitation for chronic pain, chronic bowel dysfunction, or any other chronically deconditioned organ system. Finally, relapse prevention is provided in the form of a program to prevent the recrudescence of the pathological response to the underlying illness. Almost all difficult patients will have a chronic medical problem that will continue to need attention and treatment. Without ongoing care, the pattern of behavioral reinforcement for disability and deconditioning is likely to recur.

The current medical care system does not adequately reward clinicians for their care, nor does it provide an incentive for successful treatment. The growing emphasis on customer satisfaction, financial efficiency, and allowing patients to prescribe their own treatment has been a disservice to these patients. It is tragic to watch these patients flail against those who want to help them, and exploit every weakness in the system to ensure their own demise. Clinicians are discouraged from engaging with difficult patients by a system that can actually penalize clinicians for caring for them appropriately (eg, by prioritization of patient satisfaction and short length of stay over long-term clinical results). However, incentives may change with new reimbursement models that provide a lump sum for an extended period of care; already, hospitals are increasingly looking to hospitalists and others to develop new systems to reduce readmissions.

CONCLUSION

Difficult patients usually present with underlying illness that has been made worse by psychiatric conditions that exacerbate the illness and lead to disability. A comprehensive diagnostic formulation that includes comorbid psychiatric conditions allows clinicians to develop treatment plans that overcome the barriers to successful medical treatment. The route to success is to focus on the patient's medical treatment and behavior, and to pay less attention to the patient's feelings, emotional provocations and manipulations, and comfort. Unfortunately, these patients require more time, are less satisfied, use more resources, and are less able to pay for their treatment.

Because these patients are often conditioned to engage in self-defeating behavior, they may sabotage their own care to hurt a clinician when they are angry about something, even though, as Sydenham observed, they ever recede from their purpose. It has become politically popular to see difficult patients in terms of their rights, but a patient who is difficult may be suffering from impaired autonomy and is not necessarily making decisions in an autonomous fashion. There is also a growing literature discussing the characteristics of physicians who have difficulty with patients and on how to improve physician skills, suggesting a view that difficult patients are a product of clinician failure. Certainly, better skills are helpful in managing difficult patients, but mastery of treating the underlying problem is necessary to rehabilitate patients to full function. "Understanding" how the patient feels may be comforting but no more therapeutic than having the orthopedic surgeon "understand" your fracture. Ultimately, the best way to manage difficult patients is to help them get better, but many patients will need to hear the same message repeatedly before they are ready to accept the treatment plan most likely to succeed. Patient advocacy, oddly enough, sometimes involves advocating for something that the patient does not want but certainly needs.

SUGGESTED READINGS

Bekhit MH. Opioid-induced hyperalgesia and tolerance. *Am J Ther.* 2010;17(5):498–510.

Fordyce WE, Fowler RS, DeLateur B. An application of behavior modification technique to a problem of chronic pain. *Behav Res Ther.* 1968;6(1):105–107.

McHugh PR, Slavney PR. *The Perspectives of Psychiatry.* 2nd ed. Baltimore, MD: JHU Press; 1998.

Pilowsky I. Abnormal illness behaviour. *Br J Med Psychol.* 1969;42(4):347–351.

Poulos CX, Hinson RE, Siegel S. The role of Pavlovian processes in drug tolerance and dependence: implications for treatment. *Addict Behav.* 1981;6(3):205–211.

Skinner BF. The operant side of behavior therapy. *J Behav Ther Exp Psychiatry.* 1988;19(3):17.

Sydenham T. *The Works of Thomas Sydenham M.D.* Translated from the Latin edition of Dr. Greenhill. Printed for the Sydenham Society, London, 1850.

Treisman GJ, Angelino A. *The Psychiatry of AIDS: A Guide to Diagnosis and Treatment.* Baltimore, MD: Johns Hopkins University Press; 2004.

Turk DC, Okifuji A. What factors affect physicians' decisions to prescribe opioids for chronic noncancer pain patients? *Clin J Pain.* 1997;13(4):330–336.

William Osler A. Concise History of Medicine *Medical Standard Book Co.* 1919 available online at http://www.archive.org/details/aconcisehistory00oslegoog.

CHAPTER 231

Approach to the Patient with Multiple Unexplained Somatic Symptoms

Anne F. Gross, MD
Jeff C. Huffman, MD
Theodore A. Stern, MD

Key Clinical Questions

1. What is the psychiatric differential diagnosis for patients with unexplained physical symptoms?
2. How can factitious disorder (Münchausen syndrome) be differentiated from malingering?
3. What is conversion disorder, and how is this different from factitious disorder?
4. What are the best practices in the care of patients with Münchausen syndrome and related conditions?

INTRODUCTION

Patients who present with multiple unexplained somatic symptoms pose a significant diagnostic and management challenge for any physician. Such patients are common in medical settings, representing approximately one-third of primary care patients. The most common presenting symptoms include chest pain, fatigue, headache, and dizziness; when such symptoms go unexplained the work-up can involve unnecessary—and even dangerous—tests and procedures, as well as substantial medical cost. **Figure 231-1** provides a diagnostic algorithm to assist in the evaluation of a patient who presents with multiple unexplained somatic symptoms.

GENERAL APPROACH TO THE PATIENT WITH MULTIPLE UNEXPLAINED SOMATIC SYMPTOMS

Table 231-1 outlines the major tenets of the approach to patients with multiple unexplained somatic symptoms. Before one meets with the patient, it may be helpful to consider that the individual may be difficult to interview (eg, providing a vague and/or elusive history, or being argumentative or hostile). The specific approach to a given patient with multiple symptoms depends largely on the type of physical complaints for which the patient presents. However, regardless of the chief complaint, a thorough history is critical to the evaluation of true medical and neurologic illnesses; importantly, this interview should not be conducted while one is performing the physical examination. The medical history in such a patient helps the practitioner to determine if the patient is actually experiencing the symptom reported, if the symptom has been exaggerated or feigned (eg, as in factitious illness and malingering), if there is a pathophysiological basis for the medical or neurologic complaints, if there is a characteristic pattern of symptoms, and if the patient meets criteria for a somatoform disorder.

SPECIFIC DISORDERS ASSOCIATED WITH UNEXPLAINED PHYSICAL SYMPTOMS

SOMATIZATION DISORDER

Presentation

Somatization disorder involves a history of multiple unexplained physical complaints over many years that results in frequent treatment-seeking, high utilization of the health care system, significant functional impairment, and psychological distress. The symptoms include dysfunction in multiple body systems: sexual, pseudoneurological, and gastrointestinal (GI), as well as pain symptoms. **Table 231-2** presents the *Diagnostic and Statistical Manual of Mental Disorders*, 4th edition (DSM-IV), criteria for somatization disorder. The disorder is much more common in women of low socioeconomic status, in minorities, in those living in rural areas, and in women with a history of sexual or physical abuse. It frequently coexists with other psychiatric illnesses, including depression, anxiety disorders, substance abuse disorders, and personality disorders; roughly three-fourths of patients with somatization disorder have a personality disorder, most commonly obsessive-compulsive personality disorder. Importantly, the diagnosis of hypochondriasis and somatization disorder can be made concurrently, and up to one-third of patients with hypochondriasis meet criteria for somatization disorder.

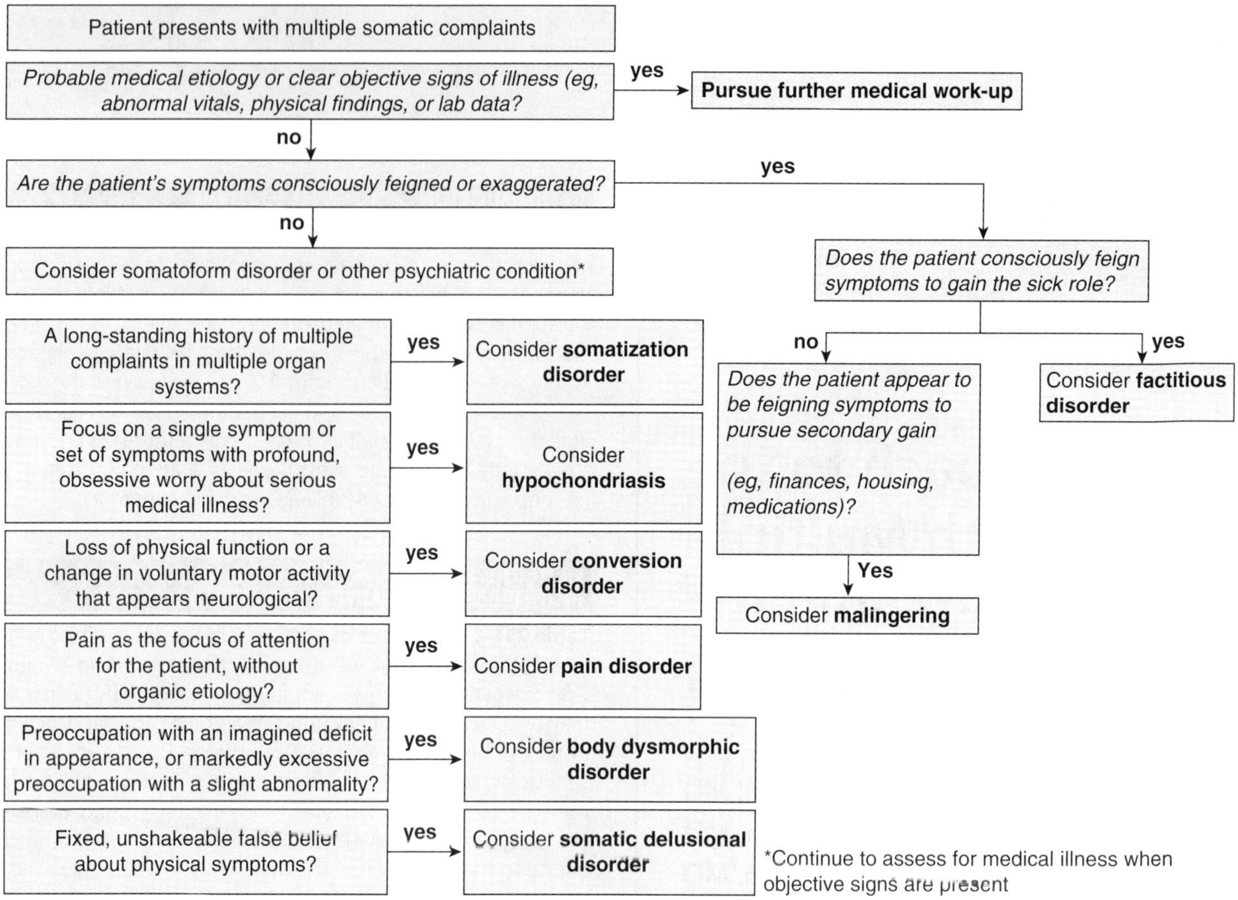

Figure 231-1 *Diagnostic considerations in the patient with multiple unexplained symptoms.*

Evaluation

Table 231-1 provides the overall approach to patients with multiple somatic symptoms. The medical history reported by patients with somatization disorder is often pan-positive, inconsistent, and disorganized; the level of patient distress is high as are their complaints of disability. Such vagueness can result from alexithymia, a difficulty identifying and describing emotions. The physical examination should be limited to the body system involved in the complaint and should focus on the objective physical findings; similarly, laboratory tests should only be obtained if there is a clear indication. Because these patients often present with menstrual and sexual complaints, the evaluation should include a thorough menstrual and sexual history; associated physical examination and laboratory testing (including pelvic examination, pregnancy test, or sexually transmitted disease testing) should be performed if indicated by the history.

Management

Table 231-3 presents an approach to managing patients with somatoform disorders, including somatization disorder. Rather than attempting to cure the patient of somatization disorder, the physician should carefully assess the medical diagnoses, decrease the patient's current distress, and help the patient to maintain or improve the level of psychosocial function. Additional treatment suggestions for somatization include the following:

- *Consideration of referral to individual psychodynamic psychotherapy.* While not a treatment for somatization disorder itself, this may help a patient who has emotional distress secondary to the physical illness or untreated symptoms secondary to sexual or physical abuse.
- *Consideration of referral to cognitive-behavioral therapy (CBT).* This treatment has proven to be beneficial by helping patients to identify cognitive distortions associated with their physical symptoms.
- *Avoidance of psychotropic medication.* Unless there is a co-occurring psychiatric condition (eg, depression, anxiety, or substance abuse) that would benefit from medication, psychotropic medications should not be prescribed.

■ HYPOCHONDRIASIS

Presentation

Hypochondriacal patients, unlike other patients within the somatoform spectrum, can complain of one recurrent symptom or have multiple manifestations during their illness. In addition, these patients' physical complaints are accompanied by three features that are essential to the diagnosis: (1) profound nondelusional fear or preoccupation and worry about their body, (2) a constant fear of disease, and (3) a conviction of illness that can be based on misinterpretation of benign physical signs or symptoms (despite reassurance from physicians and medical testing that there is no medical illness). Symptoms must persist for at least 6 months, and disease fear or conviction causes significant distress. Hypochondriasis can be a limited and transient response to stress, a primary disorder, or a part of another major psychiatric illness (including major depression).

Hypochondriasis is equally common in men and women, and it usually presents in early adulthood. The differential diagnosis of hypochondriasis includes major depression; therefore, one should screen for an episodic nature of the illness as well as for neurovegetative symptoms. In addition, hypochondriasis is highly

TABLE 231-1 A Diagnostic Approach to the Patient Who Presents with Multiple Unexplained Somatic Symptoms

History of present illness:

- Identify the chief complaint and obtain adequate detail to assess for all potential medical conditions.
- Document the influence of complaints on the patient's ability to function (eg, impact on interpersonal relationships and ability to work).
- Document recent psychosocial stressors.
- Ask: What has helped the patient cope during times of stress? What does the patient think is wrong with her? Does the patient fear something serious is wrong?
- Consider: Is the patient pursuing medical treatment for secondary gain?

Past medical and psychiatric history:

- Review past physical complaints.
- Identify existing medical diagnoses related to the presenting illness.
- Record prior invasive medical and/or surgical procedures the patient has endured to diagnose and/or treat these symptoms.
- Obtain information about current or past treaters (be mindful to obtain a release of medical records to facilitate your review of past documentation and your speaking to current providers) as well as the circumstances under which care has been provided (eg, pain contracts, legal mandates) and ended.
- Discover a history of doctor-shopping or utilizing different hospitals.
- Obtain information about current and past medications that have been prescribed for the current complaint (with an emphasis on narcotics and benzodiazepines).
- Review personal or family illnesses during the patient's childhood.
- Assess personal and family psychiatric history, with a focus on prior diagnoses, use of psychiatric treatment, and history of self-harm.

Social history:

- Review patient's psychosocial supports, marital status, employment status, and living situation.
- Obtain a history of domestic, physical, sexual, and/or emotional abuse.
- Review legal agency involvement.

Physical exam:

- Focus on the body system involved in the chief complaint.
- Review vital signs and laboratories.
- Determine if there are objective abnormalities on the physical exam that are consistent with medical/neurologic illness, to assist in determining whether additional medical work-up should be pursued.

comorbid with anxiety disorders (over three-fourths of afflicted patients suffer from an anxiety disorder, the most common being panic disorder). Of note, approximately two-thirds of patients with hypochondriasis have a co-occurring personality disorder. Overall, the prognosis of patients with hypochondriasis is often poor; it is typically a chronic condition.

Evaluation

One should be aware that patients with hypochondriasis often describe symptoms in a detailed and obsessive manner. Most commonly the patient will present with gastrointestinal or cardiovascular symptoms but may have complaints in any body system. Frequently, the patient will outline in detail the feared diagnosis associated with each symptom. Patients should be asked about the meaning of their symptoms (eg, What do you think causes your chest pain?), which may help them to discuss fears about illness. Importantly, patients with hypochondriasis often

TABLE 231-2 DSM-IV Diagnostic Criteria for Somatization Disorder

The patient must experience each of the four criteria at some point in their illness:

1. Two GI symptoms:
   - Bloating
   - Nausea
   - Vomiting
   - Diarrhea
   - Multiple food sensitivities
2. One pseudoneurological symptom:
   - Amnesia
   - Difficulty swallowing
   - Blindness
   - Blurred/double vision
   - Deafness
   - Mutism
   - Aphonia
   - Fainting or loss of conciousness
   - Seizures
   - Difficulty walking
   - Paralysis or muscle weakness
   - Urinary retention
3. Four pain symptoms:
   - Headache
   - Back pain
   - Joint pain
   - Extremity pain
   - Abdominal pain
   - Rectal/perineal pain
   - Dysmenorrhea
   - Dyspareunia
   - Dysuria
4. One sexual symptom:
   - Sexual indifference
   - Erectile or ejaculatory dysfunction
   - Menorrhagia/metrorrhagia
   - Hyperemesis gravidarum

Symptoms must begin by age 29 and result in disproportionate social and/or occupational dysfunction; the symptoms are not intentionally feigned, not caused by drugs, alcohol, or medication, and not fully explained by a known physical disorder.

TABLE 231-3 A General Approach to the Management of a Patient Who Presents with Multiple Unexplained Somatic Symptoms

1. Arrange regularly scheduled brief primary care physician appointments at 2- to 6-week intervals.
2. Set the agenda of these appointments at the outset, and pursue no further work-up unless objective findings are identified.
3. Identify psychosocial precipitants to new complaints, and avoid confrontation.
4. Discuss the role of stress on the physical symptoms the patient is experiencing.
5. Make benign recommendation when appropriate (eg, referral to physical therapy, vitamins, heating pads).
6. Contact collateral information including previous care providers and family members.
7. Assess for comorbid psychiatric illness, and refer to psychiatry as indicated, with an emphasis to the patient that psychiatry will help manage the impact that stress has on the symptoms.
8. Continue to thoughtfully rule out organic illness when objective signs are present.

become angry and dissatisfied with their medical care and typically have presented to multiple physicians with somatic complaints without any identified etiology.

Patients with hypochondriasis must also be assessed for obsessive-compulsive disorder (OCD) and psychotic disorders. All three of these disorders may present with an obsessive, ruminative pattern with attention to bodily details and intense preoccupation about illness, but the treatments for OCD, psychotic disorders, and hypochondriasis differ. Patients with hypochondriasis, while convinced that something devastating is wrong, should be able to consider alternative explanations for their symptoms; patients who are not able to be convinced otherwise may suffer from a delusional disorder. Patients with OCD—in contrast to patients with hypochondriasis—have compulsions associated with their somatic obsessions; such compulsions may include washing, counting, or performing mental acts.

Treatment

Overall management should adhere to the principles in Table 231-3. A primary goal of treatment should be to help the patient cope with and tolerate physical sensations or symptoms. Because hypochondriasis includes distorted cognitions, fears, and an unwavering conviction of illness, treatment should be focused on the psychological meaning of the symptoms and what it means to be ill, rather than on a recurrent work-up of symptoms. Additional treatment recommendations include the following:

- Providing the patient with accurate information about findings on examination, and correcting the patient's misunderstandings of previous diagnoses
- Educating the patient about cognitive distortions
- Referring for CBT to target the cognitive distortions and illness behavior
- Considering psychiatric consultation since the differential diagnosis includes OCD, anxiety disorders, and delusional disorder

CONVERSION DISORDER

Presentation

Conversion disorder differs from somatization disorder and other somatoform disorders in that it involves presentations of only pseudoneurologic symptoms. The DSM-IV diagnostic criteria for conversion disorder include (1) a loss of physical function or a change in voluntary motor or sensory function that suggests a neurologic (or other medical) condition but defies medical explanation, (2) the symptoms are not intentionally produced by the patient, (3) the onset of symptoms is associated with psychological factors, and (4) such symptoms cause significant distress or impairment in social or occupational function. The most common symptoms of conversion disorder include weakness, paralysis, sensory deficits (eg, aphonia, deafness, and blindness), seizures, gait abnormalities, or anesthesia. Often these episodes will recur and differ in their presentations.

There is often a temporal relationship between a psychologically stressful event and symptom onset. For instance, a child who witnesses her father beating her mother may suddenly develop conversion blindness. At times a patient will have experienced a prior stressful medical illness, and the patient will reexperience these symptoms when psychological stress arises. For example, pseudoseizures (a type of conversion disorder) are common in patients with epilepsy.

Conversion disorder is more prevalent in women than in men, and the presentation may differ based on cultural and sociodemographic factors. Comorbid psychiatric illness is common in these patients; the most common Axis I disorders are depression, anxiety, and schizophrenia, and it is important to rule out dissociative disorders. Often these patients suffer from Axis II pathology, including histrionic personality disorder and dependent personality disorder. Without treatment, nearly one-fourth of patients have recurrent pseudoneurological symptoms within 1 year; approximately 20% develop somatization disorder in the next 4 years.

Evaluation

A neurological examination is required for patients who present with a loss or change in voluntary motor or sensory function. Patients may appear anxious about the outcome of the examination, but they often appear indifferent (described as *la belle indifference*). The absence of confirmatory neurologic findings indicates a conversion disorder, especially if there is a temporal relationship of symptoms with a psychologically stressful event. Often, a careful neurologic examination will reveal deficits that do not correspond with an anatomic and or physiologic distribution. In addition, close observation can be used to determine whether the examination changes when the patient is not being "watched" (eg, if the patient moves his arm when he thinks the doctor is not paying attention). Provocative tests may also work: a patient with functional blindness will often show a slight smirk if the examiner makes faces at the patient.

Despite being consciously unaware of symptoms, patients with conversion disorder will often protect themselves from harm or injury. For example, in a patient who presents with upper extremity weakness, if the evaluator holds the patient's arm over her head and drops it, a patient with a conversion disorder will not let the arm fully drop, while a malingerer typically will let it hit her in the head.

Even after a comprehensive neurological examination, the physician must use care when diagnosing conversion disorder, as up to 30% of patients diagnosed with conversion disorder end up having an organic disorder as the cause of the presenting symptoms. Therefore, careful and appropriate neurological studies (eg, neuroimaging, lumbar puncture, or an electroencephalogram) should be performed, as indicated by symptoms, to rule out a general medical disorder.

Treatment

Treatment of patients suffering from conversion disorder involves provision of support and reassurance as well as noninvasive treatments (eg, physical therapy or behavioral techniques). Treatment recommendations include the following:

- Don't tell patients that there is "nothing wrong with you."
- Educate the patient that the symptoms will gradually improve with time, and that testing did not reveal any neurologic deficits.
- Work with the patient to identify psychosocial stressors that may have precipitated the illness; this may prevent future episodes and decrease the likelihood of long-term disability.
- Consider psychiatric referral to address coexisting psychiatric diagnoses and to provide psychotherapy targeting the psychological stressor associated with the development of conversion symptoms.

SOMATOFORM PAIN DISORDER

Presentation

In somatoform pain disorder (also known as pain disorder), pain is the predominant focus of symptomatology. According to DSM-IV criteria, pain occurs in one or more anatomic sites as the focus of attention of the patient; furthermore, it often causes significant impairment (including disability), high rates of family distress, inappropriate use of analgesics, and increased health care utilization. Importantly, psychological factors have a role in the onset, exacerbation, and maintenance of pain. Finally, the pain is not intentionally produced, which differentiates it from factitious pain or pain associated with malingering.

Clinical features involve severe and constant pain that may not follow an anatomic pattern; if it is associated with a medical condition, the severity of pain is disproportionate to the level expected by a physician. The most common sites of pain are the face, the back, and the pelvis, and the pain is often the focus of the patient's life (which often leads to an inability to work). Associated psychiatric conditions include depression (found in one-fourth to one-half of patients with chronic pain), substance abuse (especially of opiates and benzodiazepines), anxiety, and sleep disturbances. While the prevalence is unknown, this disorder occurs equally in men and women; however, women are more apt to complain of headaches while men tend to complain of back pain. The course of illness is variable, but it is often chronic; the prognosis is poor if a patient is given disability and pain becomes the focus of the patient's life.

Evaluation

A chief complaint of pain can be a source of frustration for the evaluating physician, especially when the complaints are vague and do not follow a neurologic distribution, and when the patient appears to be medication-seeking. Since this syndrome is often associated with comorbid medical illness, a thorough medical and neurological evaluation should be performed at the time of the initial evaluation. If there are associated neurologic symptoms (including weakness) further work-up should be pursued, including neuroimaging. In addition, because this syndrome is often associated with substance abuse, depression, and anxiety, conducting a comprehensive psychiatric review of systems is essential.

Treatment

The approach described in Table 231-3 is effective for pain disorder. Key principles of treatment include focusing on patients' function and on coping with pain, rather than aiming for resolution of pain and associated symptoms. Additional treatment suggestions include the following:

- Provide psychoeducation about pain disorder.
- Avoid the use of opiates for the treatment of chronic pain unless absolutely indicated; nonopiate alternatives should be pursued.
- Consider nonopioid analgesics, benign pain treatments (eg, heating pads), and alternative treatments for chronic pain (eg, acupuncture).
- Be wary of endorsing disability requests; a good prognosis in pain disorder is associated with the ability to maintain work and to maintain social/occupational responsibilities.

■ BODY DYSMORPHIC DISORDER

Presentation

Body dysmorphic disorder (BDD) is a preoccupation with some imagined deficit in appearance, or a markedly excessive preoccupation of a slight abnormality in appearance typically found on the face, scalp, breast, or genitals; facial blemishes and nasal shape are the most common perceived abnormalities. Common associated behaviors include camouflaging lesions, checking behaviors, compensation for a perceived abnormality (eg, stuffing one's shorts if a small penis is perceived), and grooming to cover up perceived abnormalities. Substantial time is spent performing these compensatory behaviors in a compulsive manner. Patients' distress is not alleviated by others telling them that there is no deficit or that they are attractive.

This disease affects approximately 1 to 2% of the population, and its frequency is equal in men and women; its onset is in adolescence, the presentation can be culture-specific, and it is highly comorbid with other primary psychiatric disorders (including major depressive disorder, social anxiety, OCD, and substance abuse). Many believe that BDD should be classified as an obsessive-compulsive spectrum disorder, rather than a somatoform disorder, given genetic evidence as well as the fact that BDD patients often have OCD symptoms. These patients have a high level of impairment and often chronic course, as well as high rates of suicidal ideation and suicide attempts.

Patients with BDD are typically reluctant to seek psychiatric referral and usually present to dermatologists or plastic surgeons. In fact, 7 to 9% of patients who undergo cosmetic surgery meet criteria for BDD; unfortunately, symptoms do not remit after cosmetic procedures, and the patient often continues to have difficulties with self-image even after surgical procedures.

Evaluation

Whenever a patient presents with a physical deformity and the physician either does not see the deformity or believes the deformity is much less severe than the patient perceives, assessment for BDD should be pursued. Specialists in cosmetic surgery should screen patients for this disorder given its high prevalence in this setting and the likelihood that such patients will be dissatisfied with the results of any "corrective" procedure. When a diagnosis of BDD is made, a thorough assessment for substance abuse, depression, and suicidal thoughts is appropriate given the frequent co-occurrence of these conditions with BDD.

Treatment

Key tenets in the treatment of BDD are to prevent iatrogenesis (especially via surgical procedures) and referral for psychiatric treatment. Unfortunately, referral to psychiatric care is difficult: patients are typically unwilling to see a psychiatrist (as they do not think that their difficulties stem from psychiatric illness), and the distress and social anxiety caused by their symptoms often prevent patients with BDD from keeping appointments consistently. Effective treatments for BDD include the following:

- High-dose selective serotonin reuptake inhibitors (SSRIs); as with other obsessive-compulsive-spectrum disorders, this is the treatment of choice.
- Switch to the tricyclic antidepressant clomipramine or augment the SSRI with an antipsychotic (such as olanzapine) if the patient does not respond to trials of SSRIs.
- Psychotherapy—specifically CBT—which has decreased the behavioral aspects of illness (including checking, grooming, and exposure to mirrors) and addressed cognitive distortions.

■ FACTITIOUS DISORDER

Presentation

Patients with a factitious disorder consciously feign or create symptoms to assume the sick role. This is in contrast to both somatoform disorders (where somatic symptoms are unconsciously produced) and malingering (where symptoms are feigned or produced illness for secondary gain, such as financial gain, legal avoidance, or housing).

Patients with factitious disorder, in addition to reporting symptoms and creating physical signs of illness, often undergo multiple medical and/or surgical procedures to appear sick in

TABLE 231-4 Common Presentations of Münchausen Syndrome

System	Presentation
Gastrointestinal	Acute abdominal pain; may have history of multiple surgeries and intestinal obstruction
Hematologic	Anemia and multiple bruises (from bloodletting or self-administration of anticoagulation)
Neurologic	Seizures
Dermatologic	Dermatitis artifacta (secondary to self-inflicted wounds)
Constitutional	Fevers (that are produced by heating a thermometer under a light bulb or some other heating source)
Endocrine	Hypoglycemia and hyperthyroidism
Cardiovascular	Chest pain

an often masochistic manner. The DSM-IV categorizes factitious disorder into subtypes: predominantly physical signs/symptoms, also known as Münchausen syndrome; predominantly psychological signs and symptoms; and a combined subtype.

Münchausen syndrome is the subtype most commonly seen in general medical settings. Patients—who often have prior or current true medical conditions—may present with reports of symptoms, self-induced signs of illness, or even laboratory abnormalities caused by illicit activities. For instance, a patient with type I diabetes may present with recurrent hypoglycemia and abscesses that result from putting bacteria on the tip of an insulin-filled syringe. These patients often travel from hospital to hospital trying to gain admission; they often present in the summer (when medical house staff is new and supervision is limited), at night, or on weekends. **Table 231-4** lists the most common presentations of factitious disorder. Factitious disorder by proxy (Münchausen syndrome by proxy) is a particularly disturbing disorder in which someone, often a mother, produces physical signs or symptoms in a child, to indirectly assume the sick role.

Factitious disorder with predominantly psychological symptoms is more difficult to diagnose; syndromes include pseudologia fantastica (in which patients provide extensive and false stories about their life to gain sympathy from providers), impostership (where the patient assumes the identity of a famous person), and factitious bereavement (where the patient presents with depression and suicidal ideation after a reported death).

Factitious disorder is predominantly seen in women, often under the age of 40; they almost invariably have a sophisticated medical knowledge from being a nurse or physician, from having a parent in the medical field, from having a close relative who was hospitalized for a particular illness, or from having had a true medical or psychiatric illness at a younger age. Personality disorders, especially borderline personality disorder, are also exceedingly common, and many patients have suffered from childhood abuse or deprivation that has resulted in frequent hospitalizations. Often these patients will have a normal to above average IQ and do not suffer from a formal thought disorder.

Upon presentation to the hospital, the patient will use convincing medical terminology and will present with a story of an acute illness that is plausible and that may appeal to the nurturance and knowledge of the physician as a way to get treatment. However, the patient, upon being admitted to the hospital, typically becomes more demanding, with increasing complaints about misdiagnosis and mismanagement of care. The staff may become angry, and the patient may leave the hospital against medical advice (AMA), with hopes of going to a nearby hospital for "better" treatment.

Evaluation

When one is initially evaluating a patient with suspected factitious disorder, confrontation is not helpful because the patient will adamantly deny feigning symptoms. Instead, an investigative process should be undertaken to confirm the diagnosis; this process involves gathering information from collateral sources (including past care providers, family members, and mental health professionals), and carefully observing the patient. Certain elements of the patient's history should sensitize the physician to the possibility of factitious disorder: a history of multiple hospital admissions without a primary care physician, multiple forms of identification (often from different states), a sophisticated knowledge of medical terminology, an absence of people who can verify the person's history, a history of working in the medical field or of having an illness as an adolescent, a history of personality disorder, and a complicated medical history that entails multiple symptoms as well as many medical and surgical procedures with scars. Throughout the process it is helpful to remain calm and investigative rather than being overly focused on the angry feelings from care providers that these patients almost invariably evoke.

Ultimately, as suspicion for factitious disorder grows, a room search is often necessary that may uncover hidden thermometers, containers of contaminated material (eg, sputum or feces), needles, and syringes of insulin or bottles of medications. After evidence has been discovered by the treating physician, the physician must confront the patient about the dangers of his or her behavior and suggest further psychiatric treatment to address the underlying emotional distress. This can be done by the primary treatment team, often in conjunction with a psychiatric consultation.

Treatment

Treatment relies on early identification of the disorder, before serious medical complications arise from unneeded procedures. Specific treatment strategies include the following:

- Focus on management rather than cure, by working to confirm the diagnosis and by avoiding any tests or procedures unless clearly indicated by objective findings.
- Ensure adequate observation of the patient.
- Involve staff in the patient's care: meet and discuss the different feelings that are evoked when dealing with such patients.
- Consult psychiatry to help manage the behavior and reduce the emotional distress of the patient; ultimately, referral for outpatient psychiatric care is indicated, and psychotherapy has the potential to provide relief, though these patients typically refuse such referrals.
- Contact the appropriate authorities (eg, department of children and families) and investigate the safety of the child, if Münchausen syndrome by proxy is suspected.
- Document the diagnosis in the patient's record.

MALINGERING

Presentation

Like factitious disorder, malingering involves the production of feigned signs or symptoms of medical or psychiatric illness. However, the goal in malingering is not to attain the sick role, but rather is secondary gain (avoidance of legal charges, financial gain, housing, and/or obtaining substances of abuse, especially opiates and benzodiazepines). The DSM-IV defines malingering as the intentional production of false or grossly exaggerated physical or psychological symptoms, motivated by external incentives.

Malingering is most common in men who have a diagnosis of antisocial personality disorder. Upon presentation, often to the emergency department, patients will have a clear goal or motivation for their behavior; clinical indicators for malingering include legal involvement (such as presentation for an assessment that was recommended by an attorney, or presentation directly from jail), a substantial difference between reported symptoms by the patient and objective findings (eg, patients reporting severe, acute pain but having normal vital signs and appearing comfortable when examiners are not in the room). Symptoms are often vague (eg, headache or body aches/pain) but can be more specific. Patients may also report psychiatric symptoms, such as disabling depression (to get disability), or panic attacks or insomnia (to get benzodiazepines). Patients with malingering are often uncooperative with an evaluation or suggested treatment (in stark contrast to factitious disorder, where patients are often compliant with suggested invasive tests and procedures).

Evaluation

Secondary gain, when present, may be an indicator of malingering; however, patients with secondary gain may also have a true medical or psychiatric illness that needs medical attention. If the physician believes that there is no true physiological or psychological illness to cause the symptoms, and that the patient is indeed malingering, collateral information should be obtained. For instance, talking with the patient's other providers and parole and police officers, sorting through previous medical records to look for repeated similar presentations, and talking with family members, who may be able to confirm a history of substance abuse or legal problems, often proves helpful. If the provider is seeing the patient in an outpatient setting, additional psychological testing (including the Minnesota Multiphasic Personality Inventory), may be helpful to elaborate on the presence of antisocial personality disorder.

Treatment

The treatment for malingering differs based on the setting in which the patient is seen. It is always useful to be aware of feelings that these patients can produce, and to use a calm, objective tone when speaking with patients suspected of malingering.

Specific treatment recommendations include the following:

- Avoid direct confrontation (the patient may have a history of aggressive or violent behavior that may be disinhibited by active substance abuse).
- Allow the patient to save face by suggesting that the symptoms (eg, pain, anxiety, or insomnia) will improve over time.
- Avoid iatrogenesis.

CONCLUSION

This chapter reviews the diagnostic approach to patients with multiple unexplained symptoms and specific treatment recommendations for common disorders. The acute hospitalization provides an opportunity to diagnose and optimize the management of these patients. Interdisciplinary teamwork may uncover information that would otherwise be unavailable to the outpatient providers and therefore develop a coherent care plan. As always, the inpatient care team has the responsibility to effectively communicate the results of hospitalization and recommendations of consultants to outpatient caregivers.

SUGGESTED READINGS

American Psychiatric Association. *Diagnostic and Statistical Manual of Mental Disorders.* 4th ed., text revision. Washington, DC: American Psychiatric Association; 2000.

Barsky AJ, Stern TA, Greenberg DB, Cassem NH. Functional somatic symptoms and somatoform disorder. In: Stern TA, Fricchione GL, Cassem NH, Jellinek MS, Rosenbaum JF, eds. *Massachusetts General Hospital Handbook of General Hospital Psychiatry,* 5th ed. Philadelphia, PA: Mosby; 2004:269–291.

Barsky AJ. Somatoform disorder. In: Hyman SE, Jenike MA, eds. *Manual of Clinical Problems in Psychiatry.* Boston, MA: Little, Brown; 1990:177–189.

Calabrese L, Stern TA. The patient with multiple physical complaints. In: Stern TA, Herman JB, Slavin PL, eds. *Massachusetts General Hospital Guide to Primary Care Psychiatry,* 2nd ed. New York, NY: McGraw-Hill; 2004:269–278.

Greenberg DB, Braun IM, Cassem NH. Functional somatic symptoms and somatoform disorders. In: Stern TA, Rosenbaum JF, Fava M, Biederman J, Rauch SL, eds. *Massachusetts General Hospital Comprehensive Clinical Psychiatry.* Philadelphia, PA: Mosby/Elsevier; 2008:319–330.

Rabinowitz T, Lasek J. An approach to the patient with physical complaints or irrational anxiety about an illness or their appearance. In: Stern TA, ed. The Ten-Minute Guide to Psychiatric Diagnosis and Treatment. New York, NY: Professional Publishing Group; 2005:225–238.

Stern TA. Factitious disorders. In: Hyman SE, Jenike MA, eds. *Manual of Clinical Problems in Psychiatry.* Boston, MA: Little, Brown; 1990:190–194.

SECTION 15

Addiction

CHAPTER 232

Patients with Multiple Unexplained Somatic Symptoms

Mary Eno, MD, MPH

Key Clinical Questions

1. Why don't they just stop using?
2. Why do they start using?
3. Is my patient addicted?
4. How can I help my addicted patient?
5. Why did my patient leave against medical advice?
6. What treatments are available?
7. Does addiction treatment work?

INTRODUCTION

Patients with addiction can baffle and overwhelm even the most compassionate physicians, and these patients sometimes even deceive themselves into believing there is no problem. The symptoms of drug and alcohol use can mimic or co-occur with mental illness and chronic pain, complicating the diagnosis. Families can play a role in the development of addiction and also in its treatment. Fortunately, addiction is a treatable disease of the brain. Physicians have a unique opportunity to intervene in the addictive process and shepherd our patients—and our colleagues—into treatment when needed.

The brain is hardwired to reward behaviors that enhance survival of the individual or the species. The reward is pleasure, and it happens when dopamine levels rise in the limbic system. For example, eating when you are hungry, drinking water when you are thirsty, or having sex releases dopamine, which is subjectively experienced as pleasurable. People are motivated to seek pleasure and avoid pain in order to survive. Every behavior you perform is related to pain avoidance or short- or long-term pleasure reward.

Drugs of abuse—including alcohol, nicotine, illicit drugs, and some prescription medications—are potentially dangerous because they raise the dopamine in the limbic system faster, longer, and much higher than any natural reward (such as food, sex, or seeing your family). The brain, which is motivated to seek immediate reward, drives an individual's behavior to repeat the intense pleasure as much as possible. Dopamine also enhances learning and classical conditioning, so a person with an addiction unconsciously learns the pleasurable "survival value" of the drug. If the drug use continues, it essentially hijacks the brain's motivational dopamine system, tricking it into behaving as though the individual needs the drug to survive. At this point, the individual becomes dominated by seeking and repeating drug use. Changes take place in the brain that make it extremely uncomfortable to be without the drug. Natural dopamine production downregulates, and the brain becomes less responsive to dopamine presence. This is known as *tolerance,* meaning more of the drug is needed to produce a pleasurable sensation. It also means that previously pleasurable activities are no longer gratifying. The relative absence of dopamine leads to dysphoria in the absence of reinforcing drugs. Taking the drug is the fastest and easiest way for an addicted person in withdrawal to feel "normal" again. Eventually, continuing drug use overwhelms voluntary control and crowds out other relationships, becoming more important than an individual's family, values, even food and sex. At this point, drug users isolate from other people to focus obsessively on drug use, and may use any means necessary—including manipulation, deceit, sometimes even violence—to obtain the drug of choice. Survival instincts can override judgment and moral values. This is why "drug seeking" patients can seem so difficult. The brain is motivated to survive, and following the brain changes of chronic drug use, survival equals continued use.

In late-stage addiction, a patient's body has usually become so used to the presence of the drug that the patient reports needing the drug to feel "normal." Without the drug, the patient will become increasingly uncomfortable and anxious until nothing in the environment can prevent the person from using. At that point, asking an addicted person to stop using is like asking you to stop breathing. If you were to voluntarily stop breathing, your hypoxic drive would make you increasingly anxious and uncomfortable until nothing in your environment could prevent you from taking a breath. And with the first breath you would begin to feel relief, begin to return to "normal." After derangement of multiple brain systems, stopping breathing is what it feels like for an addicted person to stop using. That is why the relapse rate is so high if the disease of addiction is not treated properly.

RECOGNIZING ADDICTION

Substance use occurs on a continuum from sporadic use to abuse to dependence and addiction. Rather than being defined by frequency of use, the hallmark of addiction is continued use despite consequences. Consequences may be social (damaged relationships), financial (money spent on drugs, or lost pay due to work absence), legal (driving under the influence or disorderly conduct), or medical (infections, overdoses, injuries while intoxicated, pancreatitis). In general, "if you've had problems because of drinking or using drugs, then you have an alcohol or drug problem." This means that some alcoholic and addicted individuals use episodically, or in a "binge" pattern—not necessarily every day. The natural history of addiction is progressive, with a variable rate—some patients progress rapidly from abuse to severe addiction; others smolder for years with less severe consequences. Very few are able to stop permanently on their own. With each relapse to substance abuse, the addiction usually returns immediately to its worst point and progresses further. Depending on the substance(s) of choice, there can be a "shotgun effect" of end-organ damage involving every organ system (see subsequent chapters 233, 234, 235, 236 for sequelae of specific drugs).

"I DON'T HAVE A PROBLEM"

Alcoholic and addicted patients are frequently in denial, meaning they honestly believe they do not have a problem; or they may desire very strongly to stop, but find they cannot because the biological motivation to use has become so strong. In addition, patients may not even remember some of the consequences of their use if they were intoxicated to amnesia ("blackouts")—particularly with alcohol. They can also misinterpret the causal relationships with their drinking, for example, believing, "I drink a lot because my wife nags me," when in fact the opposite is true. Addicted patients in denial frequently do not fully see the effects their use has on the lives around them.

SUBSTANCE USE AFFECTS DECISION MAKING

Cognitive changes occur with chronic drug use, particularly with loss of ability to make decisions and weigh future consequences against immediate gratification—this is why addicted patients sometimes baffle us by leaving the hospital against medical advice. They do not make decisions the way nonaddicted people do. When the neurochemistry of the limbic system is altered in long-term drug use, decisions about drug use are driven by craving rather than by reason. In addition, many addicted people begin using during adolescence, around age 12 to 14. Individuals who rely on drug use as their primary coping mechanism do not learn any further coping skills that foster maturity. This means that a 46-year-old patient who has been using continuously since adolescence may have the emotional maturity and coping skills of a 13-year-old.

DIFFERENTIAL DIAGNOSIS

- *Tolerance* refers to homeostatic adaptations due to the repeated presence of a drug over an extended period. It is defined by emergence of physical symptoms (a *withdrawal syndrome*) when the substance is stopped. The body adapts in this way to many prescription medications, such as antihypertensives, SSRIs, and opioid pain medications; this is why clonidine, beta-blockers, and SSRIs need to be tapered slowly rather than stopped abruptly. Both tolerance and withdrawal are expected in patients with chronic pain on long-term opioid therapy, but neither defines addiction. That is why substance use disorders are diagnosed based on *behaviors*, not just physical tolerance and withdrawal.
- *Pseudoaddiction*. Imagine for a moment that a person has chronic or acute pain from, say, a femoral fracture. Imagine that the pain was not adequately treated with the medication prescribed at discharge. What strategies could the person employ to get the pain treated? The person might take larger doses of the prescribed pain medication, refill it early, leave repeated messages for the prescribing physician, even resort to an emergency department visit for pain medication. She might borrow a few Vicodin from a friend's supply. Based on her behavior, she might correctly be labeled a "drug seeker." This is *pseudoaddiction*, when untreated pain motivates a patient to seek relief in ways that resemble addictive behaviors. It can be difficult to unravel whether pain or addiction, or *both*, are causing the behaviors; thus pseudoaddiction should always be in the differential diagnosis list.
- *Mental illness*. Acute intoxication can mimic the symptoms of anxiety, depression, mania, paranoia, psychosis, even schizophrenia (specific substances in subsequent chapters 233, 234, 235, 236). Drug rebound and withdrawal can also imitate psychiatric conditions. Only a careful history with strict attention to the timing of onset of psychiatric symptoms and drug use can begin to elucidate the diagnosis. There is a strong association between substance use disorders and major depression, dysthymia, hypomania, social phobia, panic, and generalized anxiety; close to half of substance users may have some degree of concurrent personality disorder. Sometimes people with mental illness resort to illicit drug use in order to avoid unpleasant psychiatric symptoms; mental illness and drug use can then produce new psychiatric symptoms that result in more drug use. Drugs can precipitate new psychotic breaks that persist after intoxication in previously unaffected individuals. The two can be intimately entwined and fuel each other. *Dual diagnosis* or *co-occurring disorder* refers to a coexisting Axis I or II psychiatric diagnosis as well as a substance use disorder (SUD). *Substance-induced mood disorder* refers to new mood symptoms experienced after the onset of substance use. Some sober time may be required to disentangle drug effects from underlying mental illness. Symptoms or diagnosis of mental illness prior to introduction of drugs and alcohol can be a clue. Outcomes are generally poorer for dually diagnosed patients, and once concurrent mental illness is established, addiction and mental illness must be treated *concurrently*, rather than waiting for the SUD to "clear." The patient may never achieve sobriety if the mental illness is not treated.
- *Chaotic social situation*. A patient who is homeless or has an abusive or unstable social situation may present with behaviors mimicking addiction, such as missed appointments, multiple admissions (including admissions for pain control), early refills on medications, multiple phone calls, and the like. The person may meet criteria for *problem opioid use* or *problem prescription drug use* based on behaviors that are troubling to health care personnel rather than behaviors driven by addiction.

EPIDEMIOLOGY AND RISK FACTORS

Excluding nicotine (which in itself causes 485,000 deaths in this country each year), substance use disorders have a 16% lifetime prevalence in the United States. Death rates are 50 to 100 times higher among substance users. Four out of every ten families are affected by addiction. Given the 50% genetic contribution to the etiology of addiction, an affected family member is a powerful risk factor. The 50% environmental contribution has to do with cultural and family norms that value or stigmatize drugs and alcohol, exposure at an early age, and availability of mind-altering substances. We know that perception of drugs and alcohol as dangerous and socially unacceptable are protective against experimentation and development of addiction. Point prevalence is highest among males 15 to 19, but addiction cuts across gender, race, and socioeconomic status. In women, there is a strong association between sexual/physical violence, including childhood sexual abuse, and starting to drink. As a profession, physicians have among the highest rates of substance abuse and addiction.

Impulsivity and an orientation toward immediate gratification are risk factors for SUDs. Thus adolescents are at high risk: they can be impulsive, rebellious, and novelty-seeking with poorly developed judgment. Early exposure to substances in adolescence may lead to permanent brain changes; one-third of adolescent drinkers develop alcohol abuse or dependence in adulthood, and the younger the age at first use, the greater risk of subsequent SUD. Early diagnosis makes treatment more effective, so failing to screen for substance use is like not checking blood sugar in a new diabetic, or not checking for HIV disease with suspicious infections. It is important to ask adolescents about substance use and to check urine toxicologies to confirm the history.

TWELVE-STEP PARTICIPATION SUPPORTS SOBRIETY

Alcoholics Anonymous (AA) started in 1935 when two self-proclaimed "hopeless alcoholics"—one of them a physician—came together to help each other stop drinking. They published a guide, formally titled *Alcoholics Anonymous* but better known as the "Big Book" in 1939, whereby others could retrace their steps in supporting each other to sobriety. AA is free and available in nearly every locale, currently with more than 2 million members in 105,000 groups across 182 countries. The only requirement to attend meetings is a desire to stop drinking. The 12 Steps refer to a "higher power," which some members interpret as God; however, AA is spiritual—not religious—and members may interpret "higher power" as any force stronger than themselves. For example, a group of people can be a higher power. AA specifically refutes any connection to organized religion, and the "Big Book" addresses atheism and agnosticism. Many patients are able to stop drinking or using with only 12-Step participation in the absence of professional treatment. Statistically, AA with physician visits works as well as professional therapy (cognitive behavioral therapy and/or motivational enhancement therapy), but it is impossible to know which patients will respond best to which treatment; thus it is recommended that patients start with professional treatment to learn a new bedrock of skills, and then continue with lifelong 12-Step participation.

Unfortunately, patients are unlikely to follow up with an AA telephone number provided by physicians; however, putting the patient directly in touch with an AA member while they are in the office can be tremendously effective. A *sponsor* is an individual with several years of successful recovery who can shepherd a new member, or *newcomer*, through the 12 Steps and be available to the newcomer 24 hours a day, 7 days a week should a crisis or craving emerge. The sponsor serves as a mentor and positive role model, accompanying the newcomer to meetings, and maintaining frequent contact between meetings. A newcomer can always ask the group to assign an appropriate sponsor. Physicians can demonstrate support for a patient's 12-Step "program" by inquiring what step she is working on, whether she has a sponsor, and how much "sober time" she has. It is important for the physician to listen to the patient's concerns (and complaints) about 12-Step participation, then encourage the patient to continue attending. Because every AA group is autonomous, each group develops its own personality and flavor; a patient who does not like one group should try another. The 12-Step mutual-help model has been modified to help compulsive behaviors from drug use (Narcotics Anonymous, Pills Anonymous, Marijuana Anonymous, Cocaine Anonymous, and others) to compulsive sex to hoarding and cluttering. There are also groups for alcoholics with special interests such as musicians, professionals, gay and lesbian people, nonsmokers, and various ethnic groups. AA groups for physicians include Caduceus and International Doctors in AA (IDAA).

ADDICTION IS A FAMILY DISEASE

Codependence describes a loved one's misguided attempts to protect an addicted or alcoholic individual from the consequences of his or her consumption of drugs or alcohol. It is a natural instinct to shelter loved ones from negative consequences, but in the case of addiction, this can be very harmful by allowing the addiction to continue and progress to greater severity. Unwittingly acting as an accomplice to an addiction is known as *enabling*. Enabling ranges from making excuses and explaining away behaviors to bailing an addicted individual out of jail, to providing a place to use drugs or alcohol, to joining in the use of alcohol and drugs. Codependents tend to focus on helping the addicted person manage short-term crises rather than focusing on long-term recovery from drugs and alcohol. The addicted person and the family may derive some unconscious secondary benefit from the addictive behavior that makes it difficult to stop (eg, the codependent individuals may be distracted from addressing their own problems by helping the addicted person instead). Codependents may even ally with the addicted person against physicians or others encouraging treatment and recovery. The stress of codependence, and involvement with an addicted person can be the root of somatic complaints. Thus drug and alcohol abuse should be part of the family history obtained of every patient.

Just as codependents can have a large role in enabling a person's addiction, they also can have an important role in recognizing the disease and ushering the patient into treatment. Some addicts won't stop using until they feel harm and perceive that they must stop to survive; thus the best way to expedite treatment is for codependents to stop sheltering their loved one from the consequences of their use of alcohol or drugs. The consequences can then move an alcoholic or addicted person toward accepting treatment. When families are involved in treatment with the addicted individual, outcomes improve significantly. Sometimes, codependents need therapy or treatment to gain perspective before they are able to support their addicted family member toward treatment. Family members learn they only control their own behavior, but quitting their codependent roles can ease their anxiety and may be helpful in influencing the addicted family member to seek treatment. "Love with detachment" is a goal for family members. Professional group therapy, with a focus on codependency, is often available to family members at treatment centers. Al-Anon is a mutual support group for people whose lives have been affected by another person's addiction. It is based on the 12 Steps, although its central philosophy is that members should start to focus on themselves rather than continuing to focus on their loved one's addiction. Ala-Teen, Families Anonymous, and Tough Love are other mutual support group for families.

PROCESS ADDICTIONS

Rather than abusing chemical substances, some people continue certain behaviors—such as overeating, gambling, or high-risk sex—despite disastrous consequences. Many behaviors are classified among the spectrum of impulse control disorders, such as trichotilomania (obsessive hair-pulling), kleptomania (decreased ability to overcome impulses to steal unwanted items), intermittent explosive disorder (failure to inhibit aggressive impulses that are disproportionate to the precipitating stressor), and obsessive-compulsive disorders. However, the compulsive nature of these behaviors is not mutually exclusive with addiction. These behaviors raise dopamine in the limbic system, although much less than substances of abuse, and are repeated in order to produce pleasure and decrease anxiety. Some research indicates a shared genetic vulnerability between substance abuse and impulse control disorders. Because process addictions share common threads with substance use disorders, it follows that some of the same treatments might be useful. 12-Step groups have been modified to address hundreds of different behaviors, from binge eating (Overeaters Anonymous) to compulsive shopping (Overspenders Anonymous), pornography overuse, Internet overuse, pathological gambling (Gamblers Anonymous), hoarding, pathological cluttering, and many others.

ADDICTION TREATMENT WORKS

The brain changes of addiction set the stage for a chronic, recurring illness requiring long-term ongoing treatment. Just as providers care for chronic diseases like diabetes, hypertension, and asthma, they can help manage and coordinate care for the chronic disease of addiction. The first step is recognizing and diagnosing, then referring for treatment, and following up each time you see the patient. Detoxifying an addicted person in the hospital has no more effect on the disease of addiction than treating diabetic ketoacidosis (DKA) affects the course of diabetes. Both require long-term, ongoing management and treatment. Significant research demonstrates that, with proper treatment, addiction has recovery and outcomes nearly identical to the other chronic diseases.

Detoxification means poison exiting the body—in this case, alcohol or drugs of abuse clearing from the brain and blood. When a person is physically dependent on substances, detoxification can result in symptoms known as withdrawal. Some withdrawal syndromes are exquisitely uncomfortable; others are life-threatening. Withdrawal can be medically supervised, which means symptoms are managed to keep patients as safe and comfortable as possible during withdrawal. This is only the first step in what will become lifelong treatment. Just as successfully managing a diabetic patient through DKA does not change the course of the disease, a detoxification episode will not alter the natural history of addiction unless the patient is treated. Just as the person with diabetes will need ongoing hypoglycemics, statins, and blood sugar monitoring, the person with addiction will need ongoing counseling, group participation (to defeat the isolation of addiction), and sometimes urine toxicology monitoring. Long-term management of stressors and reemergent cravings, even after sustained abstinence, is crucial to relapse prevention. If the treatment for diabetes or hypertension is stopped, the symptoms again manifest in full force. The same is true for addiction and alcoholism.

Treatment means interventions delivered by licensed professionals; *mutual help* refers to community support groups such as AA. Most treatment models employ both treatment *and* mutual help, engaging patients and their families in education and therapy whenever possible. Because multiple brain systems are disrupted with long-term substance abuse (and multiple areas of a patient's life are damaged by addiction), multiple modalities are required to strengthen impulse control, overcome learned responses, support decision making, teach new coping skills, and focus on rewards that compete with substance use. It is clear that skilled, empathic therapy styles achieve better outcomes than confrontational approaches. Many treatment programs also incorporate the use of medications to help maintain sobriety—such medications have a small but measurable benefit and should be routinely offered to patients (information on such medications is in subsequent chapters). Thus the best treatment programs have specialized physician involvement; without physician involvement, programs may not be able to offer medications or diagnose or treat comorbid psychiatric or medical disorders.

Abstinence-based means that a treatment program expects abstinence from *all* mind-altering substances, not just the patient's drug of choice (eg, a patient in treatment for alcohol dependence is expected not to use heroin or cocaine; a person in treatment for methamphetamine dependence is expected not to use cannabis or recreational Vicodin). A patient is considered to be abstinent and sober when taking medications as prescribed by a physician—including methadone or buprenorphine (Suboxone) for relapse prevention; all major 12-Step groups are in agreement. *Sobriety* (abstaining from mind-altering chemicals) is the bedrock to recovery, but recovery from addiction is more than just abstinence. It is learning new honesty and coping skills, and many times involves a spiritual transformation that can result in a new citizenship in society. Recovery is not something that is ever complete; it is evolving, never-ending growth.

No significant outcome advantage has been proven for *residential* over outpatient treatment. The treatment venue is less important than the duration of engagement in treatment. Some patients, due to the severity of their disease or the chaos of their social situation, may benefit from more highly structured treatment (residential or partial hospitalization vs outpatient). In general, more intense treatment is offered during the newly sober period, tapering off to less frequently as the patient gains stability and experience. Research shows that a minimum of 3 months of treatment is required for sustained benefit, with continued progress after 3 months. It is important for the patient to maintain some continuous connection to mutual help and/or treatment for life—otherwise relapse can occur even after years of abstinence.

When do substance users seek treatment? Some addiction experts believe that spiraling consequences and distress related to substance use, compounded by pressure from family, friends, and others can catalyze change following a specific "trigger event," when an individual realizes that she cannot manage her addiction without help. In many cases, an intervention staged by family and friends can be helpful in moving a patient toward treatment. It is important to take advantage of such opportunities, when a substance user is ready to accept help; patients can be lost if treatment is not easily available to them.

MONITORING

Patients with chronic disease underreport damaging health behaviors that may reflect poorly on them. For example, patients with diabetes may underreport dietary indiscretion, and patients with congestive heart failure may underreport their salt intake; thus it is important to check hemoglobin A1Cs and daily weights to be certain that the medical treatments are working, and to provide an objective measure of compliance with those treatments. Substance use disorders are no exception, and monitoring, usually with urine toxicology screening or breath-alcohol testing, is an important part of addiction treatment. Because relapse is a part of chronic disease, positive toxicology results (meaning the sample was positive for the presence of illicit substances), in concert with the patient's history, should be addressed with empathy and support, not with confrontational accusation.

BRIEF INTERVENTION IMPROVES OUTCOMES

Hospitalists have a unique opportunity to help motivate someone toward treatment. The admission provides a "teachable moment," and, as already mentioned, intervention outcomes are better for physicians who use an empathic approach rather than a confrontational one—this means being accepting, not *approving of* drug use. Overt persuasion results in patients' working hard to resist the persuasion; they do not want to acknowledge painful realities to themselves or others. *Motivational interviewing* (MI) is a process that allows patients to voice their own reasons for stopping or cutting back. Most substance users have some degree of ambivalence (strong feelings both ways) about continuing their use, and MI is a way to identify and amplify the desire to stop using. In its simplest form, motivational interviewing queries the patients on the benefits of continuing substance use, the disadvantages of stopping, the disadvantages of continuing, and the advantages of sobriety. Asking nonjudgmentally about all four, without criticizing or blaming, allows patients to state their own reasons for quitting and does not create resistance.

Another model for brief intervention is the four A's: ask, advise, assist, arrange. For any substance, including nicotine, the physician *asks* about length of use and consequences (family, job, financial, legal, injuries, blackouts, withdrawal, diminished self-care, etc) and then gives brief, specific, personalized *advice* about the health effects of the patient's use: "As your physician, I must advise you that smoking cigarettes is bad for your liver. Because of your elevated liver function tests, it is important that you stop smoking now. If you stop smoking cigarettes, the damage may not progress further." The physician can *assist* the patient with a referral to an addiction medicine specialist, 12-Step groups (such as Nicotine Anonymous), or a treatment center specializing in addictions; sometimes this might include prescriptions for nicotine replacement or other medications. Remember that just giving a phone number to a patient results in poor follow-up; but putting the person in touch with a 12-Step member or treatment center while in the office or hospital can have excellent results. Finally, *arrange* for patients to follow up with primary care to review any action they have taken. Some patients will not be ready to stop using immediately; physicians must remain patient, empathic, and supportive at every admission when inquiring about substance use.

CONCLUSION: ADDICTION IS A TREATABLE BRAIN DISEASE

Addiction is a multifactorial chronic brain disease with social and behavioral dimensions. The brain's limbic system is the seat of the disease, but addiction can result in end-organ damage to every system. The natural history addiction is generally chronic relapsing-remitting with overall progression over time. New discoveries in brain imaging, genetics, and neurobiology shed light on the multiple brain systems affected in addiction. While psychobehavioral treatment remains the cornerstone of treatment, medications to modulate brain functions involved with cravings are emerging to buttress patients' recovery. With proper treatment, patients with the disease of addiction have outcomes equivalent to those with other chronic diseases such as asthma, diabetes, and hypertension. The hospitalist physician can have a pivotal role in recognizing disease and directing these patients toward treatment and recovery.

SUGGESTED READINGS

Alcoholics Anonymous. www.aa.org.

Dupont R. *The Selfish Brain: Learning from Addiction*. Center City, MN: Hazelden Publishing; 2000.

Erowid. For nonmedical information about illicit drug use and paraphernalia from a drug user's perspective. www.erowid.org.

National Institute on Drug Abuse Information for Healthcare Professionals. www.drugabuse.gov/NIDAmed/.

Ries RK, Miller SC, Fiellin DA, Saitz R. *Principles of Addiction Medicine*, 4th ed. Philadelphia, PA: Wolters Kluwer Health/Lippincott Williams & Wilkins; 2009.

Substance Abuse and Mental Health Services Administration (SAMHSA). Searchable database of treatment facilities. www.samhsa.gov.

CHAPTER 233

Sedatives

Eric D. Collins, MD

Key Clinical Questions

1. How common are alcohol and sedative dependence in the general hospital setting?
2. How is alcohol withdrawal optimally managed?
3. What factors make it more likely for a patient to develop delirium tremens?
4. What are the differences in management of withdrawal from alcohol, benzodiazepines, and barbiturates?
5. What should be done with the patient dependent on alcohol or a sedative following the inpatient medical hospitalization?

INTRODUCTION

Sedatives constitute a diverse group of agents, including alcohol (ethanol, ethyl alcohol, EtOH), benzodiazepines, nonbenzodiazepine hypnotic medications (so-called Z-drugs such as zolpidem [Ambien]), barbiturates, and several other compounds, including chloral hydrate and meprobamate. The class also includes gamma hydroxybutyrate (GHB), a short-acting sedative, which is specifically addressed in Chapter 236, "Other Drugs of Abuse." The agents covered in this chapter collectively are often referred to as sedatives, sedative-hypnotics, or sometimes hypnotics. Here the term *sedatives* will be used for this class of compounds; it will not apply to all classes of medications (eg, antihistamines, various antidepressants, antipsychotics, opioids, and others) that may produce sedation. Note that while the *Diagnostic and Statistical Manual*, Fourth Edition, Text Revision (DSM-IV-TR) uses the term *sedative-hypnotic*, this chapter employs the term *sedative* for the same class of agents. While all sedatives may produce drowsiness, sleep, and a feeling of relaxation, they do not always do so, particularly when tolerance has developed. Many sedatives also produce muscle relaxation, and all may produce addiction (see Diagnosis section for definition), which will likely complicate and exacerbate the course of the underlying disorder(s) that led to hospitalization.

The sections in this chapter specifically cover alcohol, benzodiazepines, Z-drugs (zolpidem, zaleplon, zopiclone, eszopiclone), barbiturates, and others, as appropriate. All sedatives, including alcohol, have the common effect of dose-dependently depressing neuronal function, though this may occur by one or more mechanisms. Most of these agents, in overdose, may produce fatal respiratory depression, but this is rarely the primary reason for use. Human beings have used alcohol for countless millennia to produce many desired effects, including diminished anxiety, relaxation, sleep, analgesia, and intoxication. Sedating medicinal plants have also been employed for millennia, usually to facilitate sleep and less often for any of many other purposes, some of which reflect the actual pharmacology of one or more compounds present in the plant(s). It is beyond the scope of this chapter, however, to address sedating herbs and other medicinal plants.

EPIDEMIOLOGY OF ALCOHOL USE DISORDERS

Estimates of the prevalence of alcohol use disorders in the general population vary, in part depending on the country being surveyed and the diagnostic criteria used, but a recent estimate put the lifetime prevalence of alcohol dependence (according to DSM-IV-TR) at 12.5% in the United States. Estimates of the prevalence of alcohol dependence among hospitalized patients also vary, partly because studies have employed different methods to ascertain and define alcohol use disorders, and because some studies have included measures of "at risk" drinking rather than alcohol use disorders, and because different populations have been studied. One study from the 1980s suggested that as many as 25% of all admissions to a tertiary hospital center had an alcohol use disorder (sometimes quiescent, or in remission) and that most physicians did not make the diagnosis of an alcohol use disorder in those patients likely affected by one. Further, even when the diagnosis was made, there was frequently no intervention documented to address the alcohol use disorder. There are few data from the United States on the prevalence of alcohol use disorders (AUDs) among hospitalized patients, but a recentstudy from Germany suggested that 5.3% of a very large sample of patients had a current AUD, that 3.6% were currently drinking above recommended levels, with an additional 3.1% having alcohol dependence in remission. The prevalence of dependence on sedatives is difficult to estimate because of limited data, but it is almost certainly less than the prevalence of alcohol dependence and probably in the range of 1 to 5% of hospitalized patients, most of whom have co-occurring anxiety disorders or other substance use disorders (SUDs).

INTOXICATION WITH ALCOHOL OR SEDATIVES

Ingestion of sedatives or alcohol typically produces reductions in anxiety and muscle tension, and impairments in memory; intoxication may result in uncoordinated motor functioning (gait ataxia, finger to nose incoordination, positive Romberg sign), nystagmus, slurred speech, and various aberrant behaviors, including behavioral disinhibition, impairment of consciousness, reduced respirations, and drowsiness or sleep. Nevertheless, intoxication may also be difficult to detect, particularly when patients have developed significant tolerance to these agents or are medically or psychiatrically ill and not previously known to the doctors caring for them. Even individuals with high levels of tolerance, however, are not immune to the potential memory disturbances and frank amnesia associated with intoxication with alcohol and other sedatives. These periods of amnesia are frequently referred to as blackouts, and they appear to be more likely with short-acting sedatives, alcohol, or the combination of alcohol with other sedatives. Some predatory individuals attempt to take advantage of this by spiking the drink of a potential victim (of robbery, rape, or other crimes) with a sedative. This possibility should be considered in the evaluation of crime victims who appear intoxicated and/or who cannot remember the crime(s) purportedly perpetrated against them.

Overdoses with many sedatives and alcohol may produce sleep, unconsciousness, coma and even death, which results from the respiratory depression produced by all these agents. Overdoses with alcohol, often referred to as alcohol poisoning, may result in coma and death. Alcohol poisoning is the cause of about 50 deaths in the United States annually, often involving an adolescent or young adult who is not a regular drinker but who consumes a large volume of alcohol in a short period of time, producing very high blood levels of alcohol. Benzodiazepine and Z-drug overdoses by themselves are rarely, if ever, lethal, but their presence in combination with other sedative agents, including alcohol, works synergistically to produce respiratory depression. Combination overdoses of benzodiazepines or Z-drugs with nonlethal doses of barbiturates or opioids may also be lethal. Barbiturates very effectively suppress respiration and are indeed lethal in overdose, even when taken as a single agent without any other respiratory depressants. Phenobarbital doses of 6 g to 10 g may be fatal, while smaller doses of short-acting barbiturates (eg, secobarbital, pentobarbital) in the range usually of 2 g to 3 g may be fatal. The older, nonbarbiturate sedatives, chloral hydrate, meprobamate, ethchlorvynol, and glutethimide, produce effects similar to barbiturates during intoxication, and all can be fatal in overdose, even when taken without other medications or alcohol.

The history, either directly from the patient or from his or her associates, usually provides sufficient evidence to confirm intoxication with alcohol or sedatives. The smell of alcohol on the patient's breath or clothing is an obvious clue to alcohol intoxication, which may then be confirmed by the blood alcohol content (BAC, discussed in detail in the Diagnosis section), obtained directly from a serum sample or indirectly by measurement of the breath alcohol content with a breathalyzer. Urine testing for sedatives (see later discussion) will help confirm the diagnosis of sedative intoxication.

DIAGNOSIS OF DEPENDENCE ON ALCOHOL AND SEDATIVES

An old joke defines an alcoholic as someone who drinks more than his or her doctor. Fortunately, better screening instruments exist to identify those who are at risk for alcohol dependence, and to identify individuals with an AUD. The best method available to identify an individual with an AUD is eliciting a good history. For a variety of reasons, many physicians do not develop the skill and habit to take a careful and thorough alcohol use history. Many physicians simply have not learned what questions to ask beyond quantity, frequency, and duration of use questions. While these questions are important, they infrequently elicit the kind of information that helps practitioners sort out whether an individual actually has an alcohol use disorder. And these quantity, frequency, duration questions have led many to create unfortunate rules of thumb, such as, "If the patient tells you he drinks x drinks daily, double it." (Some variations on this include unreferenced and unsupportable rules such as "Multiply the amount the patient admits to drinking by 2.4"). Among the problems with these rules of thumb is that they encourage practitioners to expect patients to lie to them and thus make the practitioners less likely to ask the questions necessary to make a diagnosis of an alcohol or sedative use disorder. When this happens, of course, it reduces further the likelihood of a meaningful dialogue between physicians and patients about alcohol use. Another of the many phenomena that may make physicians less likely to screen for alcohol and other SUDs is the mistaken belief, often supported unwittingly by the press, which only publicizes celebrity relapses and never sustained sobriety, that treatment for SUDs is usually fruitless. This is very far from the truth. Substance dependence syndromes are chronic, life threatening, frequently remitting and relapsing illnesses that definitely respond to treatment (at rates similar to the chronic illnesses commonly encountered in general medicine).

Use of a few lists of questions or criteria for making substance abuse diagnoses will dramatically improve the efficiency of discussions between patients and their providers about alcohol use (and, with minor modifications, the use of other substances). Specifically, the CAGE questions (**Table 233-1**), so named because the acronym CAGE includes the first letter of the word containing the main idea of each of four questions related to alcohol effects, have been shown to be a very efficient screening instrument to identify individuals who may have an alcohol use disorder. The CAGE questions should arguably be incorporated into every clinical history, given their utility and simplicity in helping identify patients in need of additional screening to determine whether an alcohol use disorder is present. These questions also encourage a broader and more meaningful discussion about the role of alcohol in a person's life, which discussion in turn supports even brief efforts to help patients identify their own reasons to change drinking behaviors. The import of such a discussion cannot be underestimated because alcohol dependence does respond to treatment, and it directly impacts dozens of other conditions addressed by hospitalists.

To identify an individual with an alcohol or sedative use disorder, it is helpful to keep in mind both the criteria for abuse and

TABLE 233-1 CAGE Questions

Have you ever

1. felt the need to *cut* down your drinking?
2. felt *annoyed* by criticism of your drinking?
3. had *guilty* feelings about drinking?
4. taken a morning *eye* opener?

TABLE 233-2 DSM-IV Criteria for Abuse and Dependence

Dependence	Abuse
(at least three in a 12-month period)	(at least one in a 12-month period) Symptoms must never have met criteria for substance dependence for this class of substance
Tolerance (marked increase in amount; marked decrease in effect)	Recurrent use resulting in failure to fulfill major role obligation at work, home, or school
Characteristic withdrawal symptoms; substance taken to relieve withdrawal	Recurrent use in physically hazardous situations
Substance taken in larger amount and/or for longer period than intended	Recurrent substance-related legal problems
Persistent desire or repeated unsuccessful attempts to quit	Continued use despite persistent or recurrent social or interpersonal problems caused or exacerbated by the substance
Much time/activity to obtain, use, recover	
Important social, occupational, or recreational activities given up or reduced	
Use continues despite knowledge of adverse consequences (eg, failure to fulfill role obligation, use when physically hazardous)	

To make either diagnosis, there must a maladaptive pattern of substance use leading to clinically significant impairment or distress, as manifested by the above (three or more criteria for Dependence, one or more criteria for Abuse).

dependence. These are listed in **Table 233-2**. Recalling these criteria when taking a substance use history can help identify those individuals more likely to have an SUD, because the diagnostic criteria can guide a physician to explore the various consequences of and associated findings in addictive use of any substance. In addition, physicians can identify potential problem sedative use by inquiring about the following: use of sedatives for any reason other than the prescribed indication, continued use despite resolution of the target symptoms identified by a prescribing physician, continued use despite harm due to use, and acquisition of the sedatives from multiple physicians or from other illicit sources.

Laboratory testing is helpful in assessing individuals with alcohol use disorders, and it can provide important clues that may assist in making a diagnosis of alcohol or sedative dependence. First, the blood alcohol content (BAC), may be measured directly in serum, or it may be approximated, usually quite closely, by use of a breathalyzer to measure the amount of alcohol in exhaled air, using a simple, common (if somewhat variable) ratio of breath to BAC. The BAC is usually reported in units of g/dL (sometimes referred to as grams percent) or mg/dL (milligrams percent), reflecting the mass of alcohol present in 100 mL (1 dL) of blood. **Table 233-3** provides a list of common behavioral responses to alcohol in nontolerant individuals with different BAC levels. In the United States, a BAC at or above 0.08 g/dL represents the legal limit for driving under the influence of alcohol. This is a common benchmark, though it should be noted that there is considerable individual variation in the degree of impairment of reaction time and motor coordination at any BAC. Some individuals will, in fact, be impaired in their ability to operate a motor vehicle safely at a BAC less than 0.08 g/dL, while others (typically those with significant tolerance) will not show much or even any evidence of impairment. Note that a BAC level of 0.40 g/dL is lethal in approximately 50% of nontolerant individuals but, in highly tolerant individuals, it could be associated only with moderate drunkenness. When individuals have significantly elevated BAC (>0.150 g/dL) and do not seem to be impaired at all on interview, then they likely have developed significant tolerance to alcohol and/or sedatives (for which there is cross tolerance), so that regular, daily, or near daily use of one or both may safely be assumed. The window of time during which alcohol may be detected in the blood or breath depends on the peak BAC. A useful estimate of the kinetics of alcohol metabolism is that the BAC will fall 0.015 g/dL every hour after peak BAC is achieved, assuming that there is no further alcohol ingestion. Thus, an individual with a peak BAC of 0.360 g/dL should reach a BAC of 0.00 g/dL approximately 24 hours after that peak was reached.

TABLE 233-3 Common Effects at Various Blood Alcohol Concentration Levels in Nontolerant Individuals

BAC (g/dL)	Effects
0.02	Mellow, warm, less inhibited
0.05	Relaxed, less alert, early coordination impairment
0.08	Definite impairment in coordination, judgment
0.10	Noisy, decreased reaction time, mood swings, embarrassing behavior
0.15	Clearly drunk, impaired balance and movement
0.30	Many pass out
0.40	Most pass out, some die
0.50	Breathing stops, many die

Other laboratory tests for alcohol use disorders are sometimes helpful but, unfortunately, usually of limited utility. A simple urine test for alcohol in the urine has no advantage over a breathalyzer or serum alcohol test, because alcohol is only present in the urine while it remains in the serum. Recently, interest has grown in urine testing for ethylglucuronide (EtG) and ethylsulfate (EtS), two conjugation products of alcohol. The test for EtG reportedly can detect alcohol consumption for up to 80 hours following the last ingestion of alcohol. But there is potentially wide variability in the degree to which alcohol is conjugated to EtG and EtS, and incidental alcohol exposure (eg, to ethanol-containing hand gels) can result in positive test results on these assays. As such, these tests are not useful for screening purposes but may have a role in monitoring individuals who are striving to maintain complete abstinence from alcohol. Other potential laboratory markers of heavy alcohol use have been investigated and generally found inadequate as screening tests to detect alcohol dependence, because they lack either the specificity or the sensitivity to detect heavy drinking. These potential markers include carbohydrate deficient transferrin (CDT), gamma glutamyl transferase (GGT), aspartate aminotransferase (AST), and alanine amino transferase (ALT). These tests are not recommended for widespread screening to detect alcohol use disorders. The clinical history, augmented by the CAGE questions and the diagnostic criteria described earlier, remains the best means to identify individuals with alcohol use disorders.

Laboratory urine testing for benzodiazepines and barbiturates is widely available and generally very good, although various assays for benzodiazepines may be more or less sensitive to some benzodiazepines, notably clonazepam, to which many assays are relatively insensitive (and thus require a higher concentration of clonazepam metabolites in the urine for detection). Common tests for barbiturates and benzodiazepines do not detect other sedatives. Urine tests for other sedatives, including the Z-drugs and older sedatives (eg, meprobamate, chloral hydrate, ethchlorvynol), are not in widespread use in hospital settings, although these tests may be requested specially from outside laboratories when dependence on one or more of these agents is suspected.

In some instances in which dependence on barbiturate sedatives is suspected but questioned, it may also be useful to conduct a pentobarbital challenge test to confirm the presence of physiological dependence on barbiturates or other sedatives. In this test, a challenge dose of pentobarbital 200 mg orally is administered, and the patient evaluated an hour later. A patient without tolerance to sedatives will develop evidence of barbiturate intoxication (nystagmus, slurred speech, ataxia, finger to nose incoordination, positive Romberg sign, and drowsiness). The absence of any overt effect of the pentobarbital challenge is prima facie evidence of physical dependence on barbiturates, other sedatives, and/or alcohol.

WITHDRAWAL FROM ALCOHOL AND SEDATIVES

Individuals who use a sedative or alcohol on a daily basis for more than 2 weeks may experience some withdrawal upon sudden cessation of use. The likelihood of withdrawal increases with longer periods of use; sedative and alcohol withdrawal are dose-dependent phenomena not usually observed when individuals have been using small amounts of these substances. Alcohol or sedative withdrawal symptoms may also emerge in individuals who do not use the substance(s) on a daily basis, particularly among individuals who use these substances in a binge pattern more days of the week than not. A so-called hangover may include symptoms of withdrawal as well as of toxicity from binge use of the substances (note that hangover effects are most common with alcohol).

The common, mild to moderate signs and symptoms of alcohol withdrawal are shown in **Table 233-4**. Most patients who experience withdrawal complain of anxiety, sweating, headaches, insomnia, bad dreams, GI upset, nausea/vomiting, and sensory disturbances affecting the tactile, visual, and/or auditory systems and progressing sometimes to frank hallucinations (the perception of a sensory stimulus in the absence of a real sensory stimulus). Some individuals develop alcohol withdrawal seizures, once called "rum fits," which are generalized tonic-clonic seizures that usually occur in the first 24 to 48 hours following cessation of or a very significant reduction in alcohol use. Administration of sedatives may delay the onset of withdrawal seizures (so that it may occur later, following general anesthesia, for example). In general, alcohol withdrawal syndromes may range from mild to severe.

TABLE 233-4 Common Signs and Symptoms of Mild to Moderate Alcohol Withdrawal

Symptoms	Signs
Anxiety/nervousness	Tachycardia
Gastrointestinal distress	Hypertension
Headache	Tremor
Bad dreams	Sweating
Insomnia	Vomiting
Sensory disturbances	Generalized tonic-clonic seizures
Nausea	
Fatigue	

TABLE 233-5 Signs and Symptoms of Delirium Tremens (DTs)

Delirium
confusion
disorientation
behavioral agitation
waxing/waning of consciousness
Fever
Severe autonomic instability
tachycardia
hypertension
Arrhythmias
Hallucinations—visual or tactile (rarely auditory)

Some patients in severe alcohol withdrawal develop delirium tremens, also known as DTs, which is characterized by the signs and symptoms shown in **Table 233-5**. Delirium tremens is potentially fatal, with mortality commonly estimated at 1 to 5% (with some references suggesting that mortality remains as high as 15%), and its management is ultimately supportive, because the syndrome cannot be reversed once it has begun. DTs occurs more commonly in individuals who have previously had DTs, in those who have already had an alcohol withdrawal seizure in the current withdrawal episode, and in individuals with concurrent medical illness, including infection and head injury.

The most important element of the management of alcohol withdrawal is prevention of the two life-threatening consequences of alcohol withdrawal: seizures and DTs; prevention of both is usually accomplished by administering sufficient doses of benzodiazepines either to treat withdrawal early before it becomes severe or to prevent withdrawal symptoms altogether, if possible. Management of DTs commonly requires admission to an intensive care unit, where patients may require very close monitoring of vital signs and administration of high doses of benzodiazepines or barbiturates to alleviate the severe autonomic instability and behavioral agitation of DTs.

In general, withdrawal from sedatives produces similar signs and symptoms to withdrawal from alcohol, as described earlier. Barbiturates and other, older sedatives may be more likely to produce seizures and/or delirium during withdrawal. But the syndromes differ principally in their time course, which is directly correlated with the elimination half-life of the agent on which an individual has become dependent. Long-acting sedatives, such as diazepam or phenobarbital, for example, would typically present more gradually than alcohol withdrawal and with a later onset of withdrawal seizures and peak symptoms. It should be noted that long-acting sedatives may be somewhat less likely than alcohol to produce severe withdrawal symptoms, but seizures and very severe withdrawal syndromes, including delirium, do occur with these agents.

The general approach to managing alcohol withdrawal is to substitute an adequate dosage of a long-acting benzodiazepine (eg, diazepam, chlordiazepoxide, or clonazepam) to alleviate alcohol withdrawal symptoms, particularly to ensure that vital

TABLE 233-6 Common Initial Dose Ranges for Benzodiazepines in Alcohol Withdrawal

Benzodiazepine	Mild Withdrawal*	Moderate Withdrawal
Chlordiazepoxide†	25 to 50 mg every 6 hours	75 to 100 mg every 6 hours
Lorazepam	1 to 2 mg every 6 hours	3 to 4 mg every 6 hours
Diazepam†	10 to 20 mg every 6 hours	30 to 40 mg every 6 hours
Clonazepam†	0.5 to 1 mg every 6 hours	1.5 to 2 mg every 6 hours
Barbiturate		
Phenobarbital†	30 to 60 mg every 6 hours	90 to 120 mg every 6 hours

*Note that these initial doses will not be sufficient for some patients; those patients who consume large quantities of alcohol (typically > 10 to 15 standard drinks daily) may need larger doses than those listed here.

†These long-acting agents allow a more rapid taper than shorter-acting agents, so that individuals may be tapered off their medication in as little as 4 or 5 days. These long-acting sedatives can accumulate; individuals should be observed carefully for signs of oversedation if these starting doses are not tapered within a few days.

signs are in the normal range for that patient. This approach reliably and markedly reduces the risk of seizures. While some practitioners favor the use of the shorter-acting benzodiazepine, lorazepam, in alcohol withdrawal, because it is not metabolized in the liver and would therefore not accumulate in patients with severe liver disease, this is rarely necessary, because metabolic function is usually well preserved until severe end-stage liver disease is present. Lorazepam's principal advantage derives from its availability as a parenteral agent, which may be given either intravenously or intramuscularly. During the benzodiazepine induction phase, it is especially important to observe the effects of early doses of benzodiazepines very closely in the hours following each dose administration. This allows adjustments to be made to the patient's dosing schedule and shortens the time required for dosage stabilization prior to beginning the tapering process. **Table 233-6** provides a range of suggested doses of several common benzodiazepines and phenobarbital for use in mild to moderate alcohol withdrawal during the sedative induction phase. Severe alcohol withdrawal, typically manifested by marked vital sign abnormalities accompanied by at least moderate severity of many of the other signs and symptoms of alcohol withdrawal, usually requires management in an intensive care unit with large, frequent doses of intravenous diazepam or lorazepam titrated to produce moderate sedation.

There are two main approaches to establishing the benzodiazepine taper schedule: a fixed dose regimen or a symptom-triggered one. While there are some advantages to the symptom-triggered approach, particularly in terms of minimizing the total dosage of benzodiazepines utilized, in many general hospital settings the symptom-triggered approach is too labor intensive to be practical because it requires regular administration of an alcohol withdrawal rating scale to determine the need for additional benzodiazepine dosing. As such, most treatment teams prefer a fixed-flexible dose regimen in the general hospital. Following stabilization of vital signs with absence of other significant alcohol withdrawal signs and symptoms, most patients in alcohol withdrawal may be tapered off the standing benzodiazepine regimen in approximately 10 days, with dosage reductions of approximately 10% of the total daily dosage each day over the course of those 10 days, though patients generally tolerate larger percentage reductions in the first days with more gradual reductions later during the taper (a so-called geometric rather than linear taper schedule). Given the short duration of many hospitalizations, a 10-day taper schedule may require providing a continuation of the taper schedule during the early outpatient period. This may not be appropriate for all individuals, in which instances it may be reasonable to enlist the help of a significant other to control and administer the dosages during the outpatient tapering period. When a significant other is not available, long-acting benzodiazepines should be used and given for as short a period after discharge as possible.

Withdrawal from alcohol may also be managed very effectively with a long-acting barbiturate (phenobarbital), again with the need first to stabilize the patient's vital signs and eliminate other withdrawal signs and symptoms, followed by a taper schedule over approximately 10 days. There is some evidence that alcohol withdrawal may also be managed with anticonvulsants (carbamazepine, gabapentin, valproic acid, and others), either in conjunction with benzodiazepines or as a standalone therapy, although the evidence thus far for anticonvulsants in alcohol withdrawal is insufficient to support their use over benzodiazepines.

Withdrawal from sedatives is somewhat more complicated than withdrawal from alcohol. First, withdrawal from benzodiazepines and the Z-drugs may be managed using long-acting benzodiazepines, as described for alcohol withdrawal, but with the vital caveat that long-term use (for more than 6 months) of these drugs, even at modest dosages, may be associated with a greater risk of seizures and for a period of days to weeks following cessation of use. As a result, many practitioners recommend a sedative taper regimen over several months. This may best be accomplished by switching a patient to phenobarbital and tapering it gradually over several months. Adjunctive use of anticonvulsants may play a role to reduce the seizure risk, but the evidence for this is limited. Second, withdrawal from barbiturates and other sedatives cannot safely be accomplished using benzodiazepines, because benzodiazepines do not adequately reduce the risk of seizures or withdrawal delirium. As such, phenobarbital is the agent of choice for managing withdrawal from barbiturates and other sedatives not addressed specifically earlier in the chapter.

Mixed sedative dependence syndromes, in which individuals regularly ingest multiple agents, possibly including alcohol, should be managed with phenobarbital because it will safely cover withdrawal symptoms from all sedatives and alcohol.

COMPLICATIONS OF ALCOHOL AND SEDATIVE USE

Sedative overdoses

With alcohol poisoning, the management is supportive and may require a brief period of artificial ventilation until the alcohol level falls and spontaneous respiration resumes. Overdoses of barbiturates and other older nonbarbiturate medications are also managed supportively. Depending on the half-life of the agent ingested, the period of artificial ventilation (if required) may last much longer than in cases of overdoses of alcohol and/or short-acting sedatives. An overdose with benzodiazepines (including a mixed overdose of multiple sedatives and/or opioids, which is more dangerous than a benzodiazepine-only overdose) may be managed in part by administration of the benzodiazepine antagonist, flumazenil, which competitively binds but does not activate the gamma-aminobutyric acid (GABA)/benzodiazepine receptor. The use of flumazenil, however, should be considered very carefully, because flumazenil may precipitate seizures in individuals who have developed physiologic dependence on benzodiazepines. Physicians administering flumazenil should be prepared to manage seizures, should they emerge, and they should limit use of flumazenil to individuals who are in danger of severe respiratory depression.

Wernicke-Korsakoff syndrome

Chronic, heavy use of alcohol can lead to a very serious complication, Wernicke-Korsakoff syndrome, which involves a functional thiamine (vitamin B1) deficiency. The disease is associated with alcohol dependence but does not occur exclusively in heavy drinkers and has been reported in patients following bariatric surgery or on some chemotherapy regimens. Its relationship to alcohol use is well understood, as alcohol inhibits the absorption of thiamine, a necessary cofactor in the aerobic metabolism of glucose. Without thiamine, nerve cells cannot metabolize glucose aerobically. Under these conditions, consumption of carbohydrates and/or administration of glucose, particularly repeatedly to an individual with depleted thiamine stores, may precipitate an encephalopathic state known as Wernicke encephalopathy, which is characterized by the triad of confusion, ophthalmoplegia, and ataxia. In many cases, patients with Wernicke encephalopathy subsequently develop Korsakoff syndrome (also known sometimes by the misnomer Korsakoff psychosis), which is characterized by anterograde amnesia (inability to form new memories), some retrograde amnesia, decreased initiative, and confabulation. Despite the misnomer term sometimes employed, psychosis is not a regular feature of the Korsakoff syndrome. The treatment of Wernicke encephalopathy is administration of thiamine 100 mg to 250 mg intravenously, with continued thiamine dosing of at least 100 mg daily, either orally or parenterally (if GI absorption may be inadequate).

DISCHARGE CONSIDERATIONS

When the hospitalist encounters a patient with a chronic, relapsing, and remitting disorder, the usual hospital care includes initiating medications that may affect the course, morbidity, and/or mortality of the chronic illness and making aftercare arrangements to help the patient manage the illness following hospitalization. In the management of alcohol and sedative use disorders, these matters are among the most important but least addressed aspects of care. Nowhere else in medicine is so common and potentially devastating a chronic, relapsing, and remitting condition (addiction) given such relatively little attention day in and day out by the majority of health care professionals. The reasons for this are many, but they include the following: many practitioners generally fail to make the diagnosis of addiction; physicians frequently harbor unfounded or exaggerated fears about speaking with patients about a diagnosis of addiction, even when the diagnosis has been made; there is a common misperception that treatment for addiction does not work, even while the data overwhelmingly refute this belief; and the health care system fails to provide covered, affordable treatment options. This section briefly reviews the pharmacological options available to help patients maintain sobriety and some important considerations regarding aftercare referrals. Physicians who pay attention to these tasks will improve the likelihood of their patients' maintaining sobriety, which will dramatically improve the lives of those sober patients and their families. The reward for the physicians who help steer their patients toward appropriate treatment is great and pays dividends for years to come.

Medications for alcohol dependence

This section briefly reviews the use of five medications potentially valuable in the management of alcohol dependence. In the United States, there are four Food and Drug Administration (FDA)-approved treatments for alcohol dependence: disulfiram (Antabuse), oral naltrexone (ReVia), depot naltrexone (Vivitrol), and acamprosate (Campral). One other medication, topiramate (Topamax), has shown efficacy in helping individuals with alcohol dependence, but topiramate was not submitted to the FDA to obtain an indication to treat alcohol dependence. Nevertheless, it is an important, potentially valuable tool for some patients.

TABLE 233-7 Signs and Symptoms of the Antabuse–Alcohol Reaction

Flushing
Sweating
Thirst
Pulsating headache
Nausea
Copious vomiting
Tachycardia
Chest pain
Shortness of breath
Orthostasis
Vertigo
Potentially death (rare)

Disulfiram (Antabuse) was FDA-approved for alcohol dependence in 1954. It works by irreversibly inhibiting the aldehyde dehydrogenase enzyme responsible for breaking down the toxic metabolite, acetaldehyde, which is formed when alcohol dehydrogenase breaks down alcohol. When aldehyde dehydrogenase is inactivated by disulfiram, acetaldehyde accumulates and produces the constellation of symptoms shown in **Table 233-7**. The severity of the reaction is directly proportional to the amount of aldehyde that builds up, and this is directly related to the degree of enzyme inactivation and to the amount of alcohol consumed. It usually lasts from 30 minutes to several hours. In rare cases, patients on disulfiram have died after ingesting alcohol, and anyone being given disulfiram needs to be warned about all the risks of the Antabuse–alcohol reaction. Because aldehyde dehydrogenase is irreversibly inhibited by disulfiram, the reaction may persist, reportedly as long as 14 days, following the last use of disulfiram. In clinical practice, most patients are able to drink without significant reaction as early as 3 days after the last use of disulfiram, but it is impossible to know which patients will have persistent enzyme inhibition (or slower regeneration of the enzyme). Given these factors, disulfiram is not appropriate for all alcohol-dependent patients. Those who are prone to impulsive, reckless choices are not good candidates for disulfiram therapy. Nevertheless, discussing disulfiram therapy with patients may help sort out which of them are the most highly motivated to maintain sobriety, because those who are ambivalent about alcohol abstinence are frequently less enthusiastic about disulfiram. The usual initial dosing of disulfiram is 500 mg daily, which may later be reduced to 250 mg daily for maintenance therapy. Some patients need the higher dosing of disulfiram to produce adequate enzyme inhibition. The single most common reason for failure of disulfiram therapy is poor adherence to the disulfiram related to a desire to drink in moderation (rather than failure due to side effects of disulfiram, which is usually well tolerated). No patient should be started on disulfiram without further alcohol dependence treatment in place.

The relatively long acting opioid antagonist, naltrexone, was first approved in the United States for the treatment of opioid dependence. It seems to function by blocking the effects of alcohol on endogenous opioids. Several studies have shown that it reduces alcohol use among alcohol-dependent individuals, in part by making it less likely that a slip or lapse to alcohol use will lead to a relapse. The medication is generally very well tolerated, and the liver function tests of individuals treated with naltrexone for alcohol dependence actually improved, despite a black box warning in the package insert related to elevations of liver enzymes associated with naltrexone.

The difficulty some alcohol-dependent patients have with adherence to daily medication regimens led to the development of an injectable depot formulation of naltrexone, which was FDA-approved as Vivitrol. It was studied in a large trial and helped reduce drinking more than placebo and was generally very well tolerated, though there were some individuals who developed sterile abscesses at the injection site. The advantage of monthly injections is significant, though it must be weighed against the high cost of the medication.

In 2004, the FDA approved acamprosate (Campral) for the treatment of alcohol dependence. The mechanism of action is not completely understood, though those supporting its utility argue that it works through modulation of glutamatergic and gabaergic neurotransmission. Though the medication is very well tolerated and has no significant drug interactions, it requires dosing three times daily and seems to work better in those alcohol-dependent patients who have achieved at least a week of sobriety prior to induction of the medication.

The anticonvulsant medication, topiramate (Topamax), which may also modulate both glutamatergic and gabaergic action in the central nervous system, has shown efficacy to reduce drinking in a recent study of patients with alcohol dependence. The usual target dose range is 200 mg to 300 mg total daily, divided twice a day, but the medication is titrated to that dosage slowly over several weeks, as tolerated. The common side effects of topiramate include paresthesias, change in taste, decreased concentration, cognitive side effects including word-finding difficulties, and anorexia. Despite these side effects, the medication is generally well tolerated. The medication may produce a metabolic acidosis, with subsequent effects on bone density, and doses above 200 mg daily may interfere with hormonal contraceptive agents.

There are no FDA-approved medications for the treatment of sedative dependence. The most important elements of the management of sedative dependence are safe, sufficiently gradual medically assisted withdrawal (described earlier) and referral to some form of follow-up care to reduce the likelihood of relapse.

Referral to aftercare

As noted earlier, research has shown that most physicians do not discuss the diagnosis of alcohol dependence with their patients. Fewer still document that they recommended anything more than cutting down on alcohol use. Because hospitalized patients may be more likely to listen to their physicians, acute hospitalization represents an important opportunity to encourage patients not only to consider making a behavior change but to take positive steps toward achieving a sustained and meaningful change. The most effective technique for helping patients become sufficiently motivated to reduce, or ideally in most instances to eliminate their substance use, is called motivational enhancement therapy. A useful description of this technique is beyond the scope of this chapter, but it should suffice to say that motivational enhancement therapy is an evidence-based approach that increases the likelihood of behavior change by encouraging a mental process in which the patients themselves make the argument for behavior change rather than having that argument thrust upon them.

Once the discussion about behavior change has begun, the hospitalist may wish to ask for a consultation from an addiction specialist. Either the addiction physician, or when an addiction specialist is not available, the hospitalist will then inform the patient about both residential and outpatient care. Residential care has the advantage of being much more intensive than outpatient programs, and it increases the likelihood that a patient will remain abstinent during the initial and highest-risk phase of treatment immediately following detoxification, because residential care occurs in protected, highly supportive, supervised, and monitored settings. But there are a number of issues with residential care: it is not a panacea as relapse still occurs frequently, it is often expensive and inadequately covered by insurance plans, and it does not universally and optimally manage co-occurring psychiatric disorders. Outpatient care should follow either the inpatient detoxification or residential treatment, and, ideally, it will be tailored to suit the needs of each individual. Outpatient treatment is available in both individual and group modalities, and it may utilize either the Alcoholics Anonymous (AA, or 12-Step) approach and/or other evidence-based psychosocial treatments such as relapse prevention therapy (RPT) or contingency management (CM), in which initially small, often increasing rewards are offered to individuals for each confirmed day or week (or other similar time frame) of sustained abstinence. These approaches definitively do help patients maintain abstinence, and they are especially useful for the subset of individuals who feel very strongly that AA is not for them.

Although less a formal treatment and more precisely a self-help approach or movement, AA meetings are free and widely available throughout the United States and the world. Physicians who make referrals to AA do improve their patients' likelihoods of remaining abstinent. Further action to facilitate actual meeting attendance in the hospital, if meetings are available, will improve the likelihood that a patient will make a connection to AA and actually attend meetings following discharge. In addition, especially for individuals who refuse AA, efforts to facilitate direct communication between the patient and outpatient treatment providers while the patient is still in the hospital may improve the likelihood that the patient will follow up with aftercare.

CONCLUSION

Substance dependence syndromes are chronic, life threatening, frequently remitting and relapsing illnesses that definitely respond to treatment (at rates similar to the chronic illnesses commonly encountered in general medicine). Use of a few lists of questions or criteria for making substance abuse diagnoses will dramatically improve the efficiency of discussions between patients and their providers about alcohol use (and, with minor modifications, the use of other substances). These questions also encourage a broader and more meaningful discussion about the role of alcohol in a person's life, which discussion in turn supports even brief efforts to help patients identify their own reasons to change drinking behaviors. The import of such a discussion cannot be underestimated because alcohol dependence does respond to treatment, and it directly impacts dozens of other conditions addressed by hospitalists.

SUGGESTED READINGS

Anton RF, O'Malley SS, Ciraulo DA, et al. Combined pharmacotherapies and behavioral interventions for alcohol dependence: the COMBINE study: a randomized controlled trial. *JAMA*. 2006; 295(17):2003–2017.

Coder B, Freyer-Adam J, Bischof G, et al. Alcohol problem drinking among general hospital inpatients in northeastern Germany. *General Hospital Psychiatry*. 2008;30(2):147–154.

Garbutt JC, Kranzler HR, O'Malley SS, et al. Efficacy and tolerability of long-acting injectable naltrexone for alcohol dependence: a randomized controlled trial. *JAMA*. 2005;293(13):1617–1625.

Johnson BA, Rosenthal N, Capiece JA, et al. Topiramate for treating alcohol dependence: a randomized controlled trial. *JAMA*. 2007;298(14):1641–1651.

Kosten TR, O'Connor PG. Management of drug and alcohol withdrawal. *N Engl J Med*. 2003;348(18):1786–1795.

Mayo-Smith MF. Pharmacological management of alcohol withdrawal: a meta-analysis and evidence-based practice guideline. American Society of Addiction Medicine Working Group on Pharmacological Management of Alcohol Withdrawal. *JAMA*. 1997;278(2):144–151.

O'Brien CP. The CAGE questionnaire for detection of alcoholism: a remarkably useful but simple tool. *JAMA*. 2008;300(17): 2054–2056.

CHAPTER 234

Opioids

John A. Hopper, MD

Key Clinical Questions

1. Is this patient opioid dependent?
2. Is this patient in opioid withdrawal?
3. How should opioid withdrawal be managed?
4. How can pain be managed in an opioid-dependent patient?
5. What discharge planning should take place for opioid-dependent patients?

INTRODUCTION

Opioid misuse, primarily in the form of heroin, has been a longstanding problem in the urban United States. Opioids are now among the most commonly prescribed medications in the U.S. As a result, problems related to opioids are frequently seen in hospitalized patients. The admitting diagnosis may be related directly to opioids, or opioid related problems may complicate the hospital course. Regardless of the source or severity of the problem, all Hospital Medicine specialists must understand the evaluation and management of patients who are regularly taking opioids.

DEFINITIONS

The term *opiate* traditionally refers to those drugs that are naturally derived from the poppy plant, and *opioid* generally refers to synthetic and semisynthetic drugs that are structurally similar to morphine, the prototypic opiate. In this chapter, the term *opioid* is preferentially used to encompass the broad category of morphine-like analgesics (**Table 234-1**).

The clinical management of opioid-related problems requires the use of both clear terminology and clinical definitions. *Tolerance*, *dependence*, and *addiction* are sometimes used inappropriately due to lack of understanding or lack of clinical clarity. In this chapter, the terms *addiction* and *opioid addiction* refer to the pathologic syndrome of opioid dependence with uncontrolled use despite consequences. Hospitalized patients may also present with pseudo-addiction, which is drug-seeking behavior that occurs in response to inadequate treatment of pain.

EPIDEMIOLOGY

Opioid use and problems associated with opioid use have increased dramatically in the United States over the last 15 years. Although there is significant regional variation in the types of opioids used and the patterns of use, several trends are worth noting. Epidemiologic surveys from the United States indicate that over 5 million people used opioids for nonmedical purposes in 2007. U.S. data from 2005 indicate there were more than 100,000 new users of heroin that year. Given these trends, it is likely that Hospital Medicine specialists will frequently encounter patients with opioid-related problems.

HEROIN

Heroin (diacetylmorphine) is a semisynthetic derivative of morphine that is illicitly available as a crystalline white powder. Heroin can be smoked, injected, or inhaled by nasal insufflation ("snorted") to produce relaxation and an intense euphoria. Increased abuse in the United States over the last 20 years has been largely linked to greater availability, lower price, and greater purity. Increased drug purity has allowed new users to experience the euphoria of heroin by snorting rather than injecting and is partially responsible for the increase in new heroin users. Among patients entering treatment for heroin use in 2005 in the United States, approximately two-thirds of patients were injecting and one-third were inhaling.

PRESCRIPTION ANALGESICS

Opioids are prescribed for the treatment of acute and chronic pain for millions of Americans. Rates of opioid prescribing have

TABLE 234-1 Opioids

Types	Chemical Name	Brand Name(s)	Slang Name(s)
Naturally derived	Opium	Laudanum, Paregoric	Big O, Black stuff, Block
	Morphine	MS Contin, Oramorph, Duramorph, Roxanol	Duramorph, M, Miss Emma, Monkey, Roxanol, White Stuff
	Codeine	Empirin with codeine, Fiorinal with codeine, Robitussin A-C, Tylenol with codeine	C, Co-dine, School Boy, Syrup
Semisynthetic	Diacetylmorphine (heroin)		Big H, Blacktar, Boy, Brown sugar, Dope, Horse, Junk, Mud, Skag, Smack
	Oxycodone	Oxycontin, Oxy IR, Roxicodone, Percolone, Percocet, Percodan, Roxicet, Tylox	Hillbilly heroin, Killers, OC, Oxy, Oxycotton, Perc
	Hydrocodone	Vicodin, Lorcet, Lortab, Maxicodone, Norco, Vicoprofen, Zydone	Hykes, Vike
	Hydromorphone	Dilaudid	Big D, D, Dillies, Little D, Lords Pills
	Oxymorphone	Opana, Opana ER, Numorphan	
Synthetic	Methadone	Dolophine, Methadose	Dolly, Dolls, Juice
	Meperidine	Demerol, Pethidine	
	Propoxyphene	Darvocet, Darvon-N, Wygesic	Pinks, Footballs
	Fentanyl	Duragesic, Actiq, Sublimaze	Apache, China White
Partial Agonists	Pentazocine	Talwin, Talacen	T's
	Buprenorphine	Suboxone, Subutex	
Nonopioid mu-agonist	Tramadol	Ultram, Ryzolt	
	Tapentadol	Nucynta	

increased substantially over the last two decades. Abuse of and dependence on prescription analgesics in the United States have mirrored the increased use of opioids for the treatment of chronic pain. Data from the 2006 Drug Abuse Warning Network show approximately 324,000 emergency room visits involving nonmedical use of pain relievers.

HOSPITAL PRESENTATION AND ASSESSMENT

Opioid-using patients may present to the hospital for a drug-related (intoxication, withdrawal) or non-drug-related problem. Fever, dyspnea, and acute pain are common presenting complaints for opioid-using patients. Underlying infection is often the cause of these complaints, particularly among injection drug users (IDUs). Endocarditis, skin and soft tissue infections, bone and joint infections, epidural abscess, and even pneumonia are more common among IDUs than in general medicine patients. When an opioid user is seen, a key part of the evaluation is to determine if the individual is physically dependent on opioids.

PHYSICAL DEPENDENCE

A clinical diagnosis of physical opioid dependence is generally obtained through history alone, although the exam can provide a definitive diagnosis for the patient in opioid withdrawal. Physical dependence to opioids occurs at varying rates depending on the patient and the opioid (drug, dose, duration). In general, most patients will have some degree of physical tolerance after two weeks of continuous opioid use. In assessing continuous use, the clinician will need to have some understanding of the duration of opioid action and the pattern of use by the patient. Daily use of a short-acting agent may not result in physical dependence if there is significant time when the patient has no drug exposure (ie, a daily dose of hydrocodone at bedtime).

PRACTICE POINT

Physical opioid dependence

- A patient can be considered physically opioid dependent when there is daily, continuous use of an opioid for more than two weeks and when a physical withdrawal syndrome occurs in the absence of opioid use.

OPIOID ADDICTION

Diagnosing opioid addiction in the hospital setting may be straightforward, as in the patient who is enrolled in a program for addiction treatment, but frequently the diagnosis is more elusive. Patient reasons for withholding information about drug use typically occur due to past experiences with the medical system, fear of clinician prejudice about drug use, as well as fear about legal issues related to drug use. When evaluating a patient for aberrant opioid use, after assessing for tolerance and withdrawal, an initial question such as, "What problems have opioids caused for you?" may provide clues as to specific criteria for opioid addiction (**Table 234-2**). The use of state-controlled substance registries can be helpful in the evaluation of suspected prescription drug misuse.

Urine drug testing

The role of urine drug testing in the diagnosis of opioid addiction is fairly limited. Providers need to be aware of general test characteristics as well as what tests are locally available. Specific (and separate) urine radioimmunoassay screening tests are widely used by hospitals to screen for opiates, oxycodone, meperidine, propoxyphene, and methadone metabolites. When ordering a urine drug screen, providers need to be aware of which tests the hospital routinely performs and which require specific orders. A screening test in which no drugs are detected never rules out

TABLE 234-2 Criteria for Diagnosis of Opioid Addiction*

Tolerance
Increased amount of opioids needed to achieve intoxication or desired effect
Diminished effect with continued use of the same amount of opioid
Withdrawal
Characteristic withdrawal syndrome when opioids stopped
Opioids are taken to relieve or avoid withdrawal
Using more opioids or using for longer period of time than intended
Desire or unsuccessful efforts to cut down opioid use
Excessive time spent obtaining, using, recovering from opioid use
Social, occupational, recreational activities are given up because of opioid use
Opioid use continues despite knowledge of persistent problems caused by use

*Diagnosis requires three or more criteria in a 12-month period.
Data from American Psychiatric Association. *Diagnostic and Statistical Manual of Mental Disorders*, 4th ed., text revision. Washington, DC: American Psychiatric Association; 2000.

opioid addiction, and a "positive" screening test can only be used to support a clinical diagnosis. Definitive testing can be performed with gas chromatography/mass spectroscopy, but such testing is expensive and results are not immediately available.

THE OPIOID WITHDRAWAL SYNDROME

The opioid withdrawal syndrome is a constellation of findings that includes symptoms of sympathetic hyperactivity (eg, sweating, tremor, tachycardia, anxiety, pupillary dilation). Opioid withdrawal includes both subjective and objective findings and is dramatically influenced by patient characteristics. A more severe withdrawal syndrome may occur with patients who are psychologically addicted to opioids, have a high degree of opioid tolerance, or have significant concomitant pain. With a short-acting opioid such as heroin or hydrocodone, withdrawal symptoms typically begin 6 to 12 hours after the last use and will peak at 24 to 48 hours (**Table 234-3**). Peak withdrawal symptoms for a long-acting agent, such as methadone, will occur after 72 hours. Patients may report or develop a pattern of withdrawal that does not follow the prototypic syndrome.

TABLE 234-3 Opioid Withdrawal Symptoms and Timecourse (Short-acting Opioids)

Hours After Last Opioid Use	Signs and Symptoms
6–12	Lacrimation, yawning, pupil dilation, rhinorrhea, sweating
12–18	Irritability, anxiety, nausea, sleep problems
18–24	Abdominal cramps, restlessness, anorexia, piloerection, tremor
>24	Vomiting, diarrhea, muscle spasms, tachycardia, chills, hyperthermia, severe insomnia

OPIOID WITHDRAWAL SEVERITY

Many systems have been developed to grade opioid withdrawal. The Clinical Opioid Withdrawal Scale (COWS) is a widely used 11-item instrument that contains both subjective and objective elements (**Table 234-4**). It is important for clinicians to recognize that mild opioid withdrawal may be purely subjective (eg, anxiety). Patients who describe a constellation of severe subjective withdrawal symptoms (eg, nausea, anxiety, pain, restlessness) without physical withdrawal signs could represent feigned withdrawal or could occur in a patient who is in withdrawal and anxious about developing a more severe withdrawal syndrome. In either case the appropriate clinician response is continued monitoring and reassurance that appropriate treatment will be provided for relief of specific symptoms.

PRACTICE POINT

Detoxification

- Cessation of opioids in a patient with opioid addiction (detoxification) is not treatment. Patients with opioid addiction require referral to addiction treatment as part of the hospital discharge plan.

PROTRACTED WITHDRAWAL

Clinicians working with opioid-addicted patients should be familiar with protracted opioid withdrawal, also called the chronic opioid abstinence syndrome. Protracted withdrawal symptoms occur one to three weeks after the last opioid use and may persist for 12 weeks. A typical pattern of symptoms includes fatigue, poor sleep, lack of motivation, generalized malaise, anhedonia, diffuse myalgia, and poor sleep. The protracted course of these symptoms is psychologically distressing and is partially responsible for the high rate of relapse to drug use in addiction treatment.

MANAGEMENT OF THE OPIOID WITHDRAWAL SYNDROME

Management of the opioid withdrawal syndrome (OWS) will be based on patient characteristics, goals of treatment, and local resources. Patient characteristics include determination of the presence or absence of pain (acute and chronic), the presence or absence of pathologic opioid use (abuse and addiction), the type and amount of opioid being used, and the cause and severity of withdrawal. The goal of treatment will be either stabilization on an opioid or complete cessation of all opioids. Resources to consider include the availability of consultants in the assessment of pain and/or addiction, the types of medications available for withdrawal management, and the aftercare resources for posthospital management.

For opioid-addicted patients who are not currently receiving addiction treatment, the presence or absence of pain is the primary determinant of medication selection. Patients with pain will require agonist treatment with buprenorphine, methadone, or other opioid agonists. Patients without pain (other than withdrawal pain) can be managed with clonidine or buprenorphine. Clonidine can be used for the management of a mild OWS. Physicians should consider buprenorphine for the management of moderate to severe withdrawal. When buprenorphine is prescribed, patients should be evaluated for extended (beyond the hospital) treatment. If buprenorphine or other opioids will not be used after hospitalization, buprenorphine should be discontinued two or three days prior to discharge to allow the patient to undergo peak withdrawal symptoms in a controlled setting.

TABLE 234-4 The Clinical Opiate Withdrawal Scale

Resting pulse rate _____beats/min *Measure after patient is sitting or lying for 1 minute* 0 pulse rate 80 or below 1 pulse rate 81–100 2 pulse rate 101–120 4 pulse rate greater than 120	GI upset *Over last 30 minutes* 0 no GI symptoms 1 stomach cramps 2 nausea or loose stool 3 vomiting or diarrhea 5 multiple episodes of diarrhea or vomiting
Sweating *Over past 30 minutes; not accounted for by room temperature or patient activity* 0 no report of chills or flushing 1 subjective report of chills or flushing 2 flushed or observable moistness on face 3 beads of sweat on brow or face 4 sweat streaming off face	Anxiety or irritability 0 none 1 patient reports increasing irritability or anxiousness 2 patient obviously irritable/anxious 4 patient so irritable/anxious that participation in assessment is difficult
Restlessness *Observation during assessment* 0 able to sit still 1 reports difficulty sitting still, but is able to do so 3 frequent shifting or extraneous movements of legs/arms 5 unable to sit still for more than a few seconds	Bone or joint aches *If patient was having pain previously, gauge the additional component attributed to opioid withdrawal only* 0 not present 1 mild diffuse discomfort 2 patient reports severe diffuse aching of joints/ muscles 4 patient is rubbing joints or muscles and is unable to sit still because of discomfort
Tremors *Observation of outstretched hands* 0 no tremor 1 tremor can be felt but not observed 2 slight tremor observable 4 gross tremor or muscle twitching	Yawning *Observation during assessment* 0 no yawning 1 yawning once or twice during assessment 2 yawning three or more times during assessment 4 yawning several times/minute
Pupil size 0 pupils pinned or normal size for room light 1 pupils possibly larger than normal for room light 2 pupils moderately dilated 5 pupils so dilated that only the rim of the iris is visible	Runny nose or tearing *Not accounted for by cold symptoms or allergies* 0 not present 1 nasal stuffiness or unusually moist eyes 2 nose running or tearing 4 nose constantly running or tears streaming down cheeks
Gooseflesh skin 0 skin is smooth 3 skin piloerection can be felt or hairs standing up on arms 5 prominent piloerection	**Total Score:** Sum of all 11 items • 5–12 = mild • 13–24 = moderate • 25–36 = moderately severe • >36 = severe withdrawal

Data from Wesson DR, Ling W. The Clinical Opiate Withdrawal Scale (COWS). *J Psychoactive Drugs*. 2003;35(2):253–259.

OPIOID WITHDRAWAL PHARMACOTHERAPY

Clonidine, methadone, and buprenorphine are the medications most commonly used for the management of OWS in patients with opioid addiction (**Table 234-5**).

Clonidine

Clonidine is a centrally acting alpha-agonist that can ameliorate opioid withdrawal symptoms that occur as a result of sympathetic hyperactivity. The main advantage of clonidine is that it is a widely available, noncontrolled drug. Titration of clonidine is limited by the side effects of sedation, hypotension, and constipation that occur at the doses needed to provide relief. For patients with opioid addiction, clonidine does little to relieve drug craving.

Methadone

Methadone is a full-opioid agonist that can be prescribed in the hospital for the treatment of opioid withdrawal. Methadone can be used in the outpatient setting for treatment of pain in patients without addiction. The physician prescribing methadone for outpatient treatment of addiction must have a Drug Enforcement Administration license to prescribe Schedule 2 Controlled Drugs,

TABLE 234-5 Typical Medication Dosing Regimens for Treatment of the Opioid Withdrawal Syndrome

Medication	Typical Doses	Typical Dosing Intervals	Maximum Daily Dose
Clonidine	0.1–0.2 mg orally	Every 2–6 hours	1.2 mg
Methadone	10–20 mg orally	Every 6–8 hours	30–40 mg
Buprenorphine	2–4 mg	Every 2–4 hours	16 mg

and methadone can only be prescribed at the treatment program. Methadone has been associated with QT prolongation; providers should consider obtaining an electrocardiogram (ECG) prior to prescribing methadone.

Buprenorphine

Buprenorphine is a partial opioid agonist that can be prescribed for the treatment of opioid addiction by physicians who have received a waiver from the Drug Enforcement Administration. Physicians without the opiate treatment waiver can use buprenorphine for up to three days in a hospital setting. Because buprenorphine is a partial opioid agonist it can precipitate withdrawal in an opioid-dependent person who has significant drug levels of a full opioid agonist (eg, heroin). This withdrawal occurs when high affinity (but low activity) buprenorphine displaces full agonists from the mu-receptors, resulting in a relatively lower overall level of opioid activity. Because of the potential for inducing withdrawal, buprenorphine should only be used by a physician who is thoroughly familiar with the pharmacology of the drug.

Adjunct medications

In addition to the primary medication used for withdrawal treatment, other medications may be used for symptomatic treatment in a monitored setting. Patients receiving clonidine will likely need more adjunct medications for withdrawal symptoms than patients receiving opioid medications for withdrawal. Common symptoms requiring adjunct treatment include myalgia, abdominal cramps, diarrhea, and sleep problems. Anxiety is a common withdrawal symptom and is best managed by first increasing the dose of the primary treatment medication before considering anxiolytics (**Table 234-6**).

OPIOID MAINTENANCE TREATMENT

Use of an addiction treatment medication for more than 180 days is considered maintenance treatment. Maintenance treatment with methadone or buprenorphine is effective for a large proportion of patients with chronic, relapsing opioid addiction. Maintenance treatment results in significant reductions in the use of illicit opioids as well as lower morbidity and mortality, and it allows patients to engage in addiction recovery activities. There is no limit on the duration of maintenance treatment; patients should continue medication for as long as is required to abstain from illicit opioids. For patients who are admitted to the hospital and currently enrolled in maintenance treatment the goal of treatment will generally be to continue medication and ensure follow-up with the treatment provider after discharge.

TABLE 234-6 Medications for Symptomatic Treatment of Acute Opioid Withdrawal

Symptom	Medication
Sleep problems	Zolpidem, temazepam, trazodone
Myalgia	Acetaminophen, nonsteroidal antiinflammatory drugs
Diarrhea	Loperamide
Abdominal cramps	Dicyclomine

METHADONE MAINTENANCE

As noted earlier, methadone maintenance treatment must generally occur in the setting of a licensed treatment program and is regulated by the federal and state government. Depending on state regulation, physicians in rural areas can receive special approval to provide methadone maintenance. Programs are generally open six or seven days a week and provide on-site counseling, medication dispensing, and drug testing. After some time in successful treatment, patients may earn "take-home" privileges and in addition to on-site dosing will also have some doses that are dispensed and self-administered at home. Effective methadone maintenance doses are frequently in the range of 80–120 mg, although there is wide variation. Hospital providers should be aware that outpatient treatment programs dispense methadone in a liquid form and that programs may use "blind dosing" (particularly for patients on dose tapers), and doses may be titrated in increments as low as 1 mg. Hospitals will typically have methadone available as 5 and 10 mg tablets so some adjustment in dose may be needed for the hospitalized patient. For example, a patient taking methadone 62 mg daily for maintenance could receive a hospital dose of 60 mg to 65 mg a day. For patients with opioid addiction, methadone cannot be continued after hospital discharge unless the patient is enrolled in a licensed opioid maintenance program.

BUPRENORPHINE TREATMENT

Buprenorphine treatment can be provided by any physician with a DEA waiver for Office-Based Opioid Treatment. Qualified physicians can receive a waiver to provide opioid-assisted addiction treatment through a notification and approval process (http://buprenorphine.samhsa.gov). Addiction treatment utilizing buprenorphine can take place in the setting of traditional addiction treatment programs or in the office of any qualified provider. With office-based treatment, patients will typically receive prescriptions for buprenorphine, which can be filled at a local pharmacy. Buprenorphine providers must ensure that patients are involved in addiction counseling and provide appropriate monitoring of therapy.

CONFIRMATION OF TREATMENT STATUS

Patients may present with a history of opioid maintenance therapy that cannot immediately be verified. These situations include the patient who reports (1) enrollment in a methadone maintenance program at a time when the program cannot be contacted (weekend or after hours); (2) current treatment with buprenorphine by a provider who cannot be contacted; (3) treatment by a chronic pain program that is outside the immediate community and cannot be readily contacted. Treatment status can usually be determined with a single telephone call, but occasionally the clinician needs to make a treatment decision in the absence of complete information. Providers should be prepared to obtain a release of information from the patient when contacting other sources of care. Urine drug testing can be helpful in this situation, but treatment decisions should not be delayed or made solely on the basis of urine toxicology.

For patients who report current addiction treatment with a full-agonist and present in withdrawal, a single dose of a long-acting oral agent (methadone 10–20 mg or extended release morphine 15 mg) can be given at intervals of 8 to 12 hours until treatment can be verified. Patients in moderate to severe withdrawal may require an oral immediate-release opioid (morphine sulfate 15 mg) to provide some initial withdrawal treatment. For patients who are treated chronically with buprenorphine, doses of 4 mg (sublingual) can be given every 6, 8, or 12 hours to provide adequate control of withdrawal symptoms. In a hospital setting, providers can give opioid therapy in the treatment of addiction for up to three days while verifying treatment status. If it is subsequently determined that a patient is actively enrolled in maintenance addiction treatment, medication can be continued for the duration of hospitalization. For patients who are not in treatment, opioids should be discontinued unless a referral to treatment is arranged for after discharge (see Discharge Considerations).

OPIOID INTOXICATION

Initial management of acute opioid intoxication (overdose) usually occurs in the emergency room, but subsequent care may occur on an inpatient setting. Intoxication may occur in new opioid users, as part of a suicide attempt, when drug purity is unexpectedly high, and during induction on a long-acting opioid (eg, methadone). When opioid-tolerant individuals have been tapered off opioids (such as after incarceration or after abstinence-based addiction treatment) there is a risk of overdose if opioids are reinitiated at a dose to which the patient had previously been tolerant. Injection drug users are particularly vulnerable to overdose when getting opioids from a new source where drug purity is not known.

The consequences of opioid intoxication include altered level of consciousness and respiratory depression. Respiratory depression will be more pronounced in patients using additional central nervous system (CNS) depressants such as alcohol and benzodiazepines. Respiratory depression can be severe enough to result in death.

Opioids may result in psychiatric symptoms, particularly when given in high doses and when used in the elderly. Nightmares, anxiety, agitation, paranoia, psychosis, and hallucinations have all been reported. These symptoms can occur with intrathecal administration of opioids as well as oral and parenteral administration.

Initial treatment of opioid intoxication includes the use of the short-acting injectable opioid antagonist naloxone and potentially oxygen therapy. In the opioid-naïve individual with opioid overdose, full-agonist reversal generally occurs when 0.4 mg of naloxone is given (IV/IM/SQ/ET) every two to three minutes. The intravenous route provides the most predictable response. For opioid-dependent patients, smaller doses should be used and titrated to reverse respiratory depression. Giving full-reversal doses of naloxone to opioid-dependent individuals may result in a severe withdrawal syndrome. Doses of 0.1 to 0.2 mg of naloxone can be used in incremental fashion to reverse respiratory depression. Patients who have overdosed with a long-acting or high-affinity agent (eg, methadone, buprenorphine) will generally need admission for oxygen, monitoring, and intravenous naloxone infusion.

PAIN MANAGEMENT AND OPIOID DEPENDENCE

As noted, acute pain is a frequent precipitant for hospital admission of the opioid-dependent patient. Chronic pain is also a common comorbidity among patients who are opioid dependent. Patients with a history of opioid dependence, including patients in recovery from addiction, may have long-term pain from traumatic injuries, neuropathies, chronic joint infections, and venous stasis (with and without ulceration).

The basic principles of hospital pain management apply to opioid-tolerant patients, with the additional need to provide a baseline level of opioids that prevents the development of withdrawal. By following this strategy, physicians will often find the need to prescribe opioid doses that are above typically prescribed doses. The clinician can be reassured that with careful titration and monitoring effective analgesia can be obtained without inducing respiratory depression or untoward sedation.

There are some important principles of pain management that are unique to opioid-dependent patients. In general, clinicians should avoid using partial opioid agonists (eg, butorphanol, pentazocine) for pain management in opioid-dependent patients, as these drugs may precipitate opioid withdrawal. The partial agonist buprenorphine may occasionally be used for management of both pain and opioid addiction in the hospitalized patient but should only be done by a clinician with experience in such situations. Patients with opioid dependence who are maintained on full opioid agonists may have some degree of hyperalgesia, which can present as unrelenting or worsening pain despite increasing doses of opioids. Long-term management of hyperalgesia can involve discontinuing opioids, adding nonopioid adjuncts for pain management, or opioid "rotation" in which a pharmacologically different opioid is substituted for the current opioid. Opioids with active metabolites that may precipitate seizures, such as meperidine and propoxyphene should generally be avoided in the management of pain in opioid-dependent patients.

DISCHARGE CONSIDERATIONS

Clinicians will need to make a determination about the aftercare plan for the patient with opioid addiction early in the course of treatment. Medication management, particularly the use of opioids, will be determined by the expected length of stay, the presence or absence of pain, and the plan for addiction treatment after discharge. Resources for addiction assessment and referral will vary across institutions. Typical sources of clinical support include social work, case management, addiction medicine, and psychiatry/addiction psychiatry.

ADDICTION TREATMENT

Addiction treatment after hospitalization should be offered to all patients with opioid addiction. The risk of death from overdose is particularly high when opioid-dependent patients are tapered off opioids without subsequent aftercare. The United States Substance Abuse and Mental Health Services Administration maintains a Substance Abuse Treatment Facility Locator (http://findtreatment.samhsa.gov) with information on over 11,000 treatment programs in the United States. The Treatment Facility Locator includes methadone and buprenorphine treatment options for patients who need opioid maintenance treatment.

Many patients, despite years of opioid addiction, will deny the need for addiction treatment after hospitalization. Common statements include the following: "I know what to do"; "After what I've been through I would never use again"; "I'm better now." The clinician must recognize that the vast majority of long-term opioid users will relapse, and a treatment referral should be offered for all patients. Providers can support self-efficacy but still make

TABLE 234-7 Discharge Treatment Recommendations

Opioid addiction—no longer taking opioids
Addiction treatment (intake within 1 week)
Primary care follow-up (7–10 days)
Noncontrolled medications for symptomatic treatment
Opioid addiction—on maintenance treatment
Methadone—Follow-up on next business day at methadone treatment program
Buprenorphine—Prescribe buprenorphine until follow-up with outpatient treatment provider*
Opioid tolerant—chronic pain without addiction
Prescribe opioids (when indicated) for follow-up with long-term prescriber (ideally within 1 week)

*Buprenorphine can only be prescribed at discharge by a physician with a Drug Enforcement Administration waiver to prescribe opioids in accordance with the Drug Addiction Treatment Act of 2000.

a strong case for aftercare by acknowledging both patients' desire for sobriety and the likelihood of relapse without additional support.

Among patients who opt for treatment after discharge the timing of follow-up is crucial for treatment success (**Table 234-7**). Patients with both pain and addiction will likely need opioids at discharge and follow-up with an addiction medicine specialist. For patients who are enrolled in and returning to opioid maintenance treatment, coordination with the opioid treatment program (OTP) prior to discharge is essential. The OTP will need to be informed of the patient's hospitalization in order to account for the patient's absence from treatment. In addition the OTP will need to know what controlled drugs have been administered during hospitalization for subsequent drug test monitoring. The OTP will also need to know the day of return to treatment. The hospital physician will need to coordinate maintenance medication treatment to ensure there is no medication "treatment gap" after discharge. Patients on methadone/buprenorphine treatment who receive their usual treatment dose on the day of discharge will not require a discharge prescription for opioids if they can be seen the next business day. For patients enrolled in methadone treatment, a physician can legally give a prescription for up to three days of methadone at discharge. Practically speaking, it is best to limit discharge methadone due to risks of diversion, overdose, and the considerable difficulty patients can have in obtaining methadone tablets from a pharmacy. With coordination of care, patients will generally require no methadone at discharge or perhaps a one-day prescription for patients discharged on a weekend.

DISCHARGE MEDICATION

For patients who are discharged on opioid agonists, such as methadone or buprenorphine, adjunct medications are usually not required, except in the management of constipation. Patients who are not on opioid agonists will need appropriate treatment for symptom management. As described for acute opioid withdrawal, typical symptoms include bone pain, myalgia, loose stools, abdominal cramps, and poor sleep. Management of these problems is similar to inpatient management with a few modifications.

Patients receiving clonidine in the hospital for symptom management may benefit from placement of transdermal clonidine prior to discharge. The clonidine patch (typically 0.1 mg/24 h or 0.2 mg/24 h if blood pressure allows) can be removed without replacement after discharge, one week from when it was first placed. Clinicians may want to substitute trazodone as a noncontrolled drug for sleep (doses of 25–150 mg orally at bedtime) after discharge, although a short course of temazepam or zolpidem can be used.

Naltrexone is approved as a maintenance treatment for opioid addiction in patients who have been detoxified from opioids. Naltrexone is a pure opioid antagonist that can be used as part of the long-term management of an opioid-addicted patient who is not appropriate for methadone or buprenorphine maintenance. Initiation of naltrexone must be done with caution by a prescriber experienced in its use; naltrexone can precipitate severe, prolonged opioid withdrawal in opioid-dependent patients who have used any opioid in the last two weeks. Liver enzyme monitoring should be performed for patients on maintenance naltrexone.

PRACTICE POINT

- Long-term use of nonopioid controlled drugs should generally be avoided for patients with opioid addiction. Because of abuse and potential harm, benzodiazepines, hypnotics, sedatives and stimulants should only be used after appropriate evaluation, consultation and when noncontrolled medications are ineffective.

CONCLUSION

Opioid-using patients are commonly cared for by Hospital Medicine specialists. A brief but structured assessment will allow the clinician to determine which patients are opioid tolerant, as well as those with opioid abuse and addiction. A thoughtful approach to inpatient management and aftercare can lead to high levels of patient and provider satisfaction.

SUGGESTED READINGS

Alford DP, Compton P, Samet JH. Acute pain management for patients receiving maintenance methadone or buprenorphine therapy. *Ann Intern Med.* 2006;144(2):127–134.

Ballantyne JC, Mao J. Opioid therapy for chronic pain. *N Engl J Med.* 2003;349(20):1943–1953.

Collins ED, Kleber HD, Whittington RA, Heitler NE. Anesthesia-assisted vs buprenorphine- or clonidine-assisted heroin detoxification and naltrexone induction: a randomized trial. *JAMA.* 2005;294(8):903–913.

Fiellin DA, O'Connor PG. Clinical practice: office-based treatment of opioid-dependent patients. *N Engl J Med.* 2002;347(11):817–823.

Hopper JA, Shafi T. Management of the hospitalized injection drug user. *Infect Dis Clin North Am.* 2002;16(3):571–587.

Kosten TR, O'Connor PG. Management of drug and alcohol withdrawal. *N Engl J Med.* 2003.;348(18):1786–1795.

Krantz MJ, Martin J, Stimmel B, Mehta D, Haigney MC. QTc interval screening in methadone treatment. *Ann Intern Med.* 2009;150(6):387–395.

O'Connor PG. Methods of detoxification and their role in treating patients with opioid dependence. *JAMA.* 2005;294(8):961–963.

CHAPTER 235

Stimulants

Christina M. Delos Reyes, MD

Key Clinical Questions

1. What are the most commonly abused stimulants?
2. How are the acute cardiovascular complications of stimulants managed?
3. How are the acute psychiatric complications of stimulants managed?
4. What are the other medical sequelae of abused stimulants?
5. What factors should be considered when discharging a patient with complications of stimulants?

INTRODUCTION

WHAT ARE THE MOST COMMONLY ABUSED STIMULANTS?

Cocaine is a naturally occurring plant alkaloid found in the leaves of the coca bush, *Erythroxylon coca*. Cocaine for illicit use comes in two major forms, the base and the salt. Cocaine base or "crack" is smoked, while cocaine salt or powder cocaine is snorted intranasally or dissolved for intravenous injection. Amphetamine and methamphetamine are synthetic stimulants that are typically abused by the oral or intravenous route. "Ice" is crystallized methamphetamine that can be smoked or used intranasally. "Ecstasy" or MDMA is 3,4-methylenedioxymethamphetamine, and it is usually abused by the oral route. MDMA has both hallucinogenic and stimulant properties. Over-the-counter stimulants include ephedrine, phenylephrine, and pseudoephedrine. Two additional plant-derived stimulants that may be encountered in clinical settings include ephedra or "ma-huang" (from the dried branches of *Ephedraceae* species) and khat (prepared from the *Catha edulis* plant) (**Table 235-1**).

Prescription stimulants include methylphenidate, methamphetamine, dextroamphetamine, mazindol, phenmetrazine, and phentermine. Prescribed stimulants may be used therapeutically for multiple conditions, including attention deficit disorder, narcolepsy, fatigue in multiple sclerosis, and refractory depression, as well as in palliative care. When prescribed stimulants such as methylphenidate or dextroamphetamine are abused by patients who have valid prescriptions for them, clinicians may see unintended side effects such as elevation in resting heart rate or other cardiovascular complications; this may be a clue to the prescriber that unauthorized dose escalation is occurring.

Stimulants increase catecholamine neurotransmitter activity, leading to acute medical and psychological effects. Some stimulants, like cocaine, work via blockade of presynaptic neurotransmitter reuptake pumps. Other stimulants, such as amphetamines, cause presynaptic release of catecholamines. Medical effects result from overstimulation of the sympathetic nervous system leading to peripheral vasoconstriction, increased heart rate, lowered seizure threshold, and other adverse effects. Psychological effects result from stimulation of corticomesolimbic dopamine circuits in the brain, leading to desired effects (increased energy and alertness, euphoria, decreased appetite and need for sleep) as well as negative effects, including anxiety, grandiosity, impaired judgment, psychosis (paranoid delusions and hallucinations) and addiction.

Nicotine and caffeine are mild stimulants that are in widespread use. Nicotine acts at the nicotinic acetylcholine receptor and causes the release of acetylcholine (ACh), dopamine, norepinephrine, serotonin, gamma-aminobutyric acid (GABA), and glutamate. Nicotine has complex physical and psychological effects that are dose related. Physical effects include acute increases in blood pressure, heart rate, and cardiac output and cutaneous vasoconstriction (at low doses); ganglionic stimulation and adrenal catecholamine release (at high doses); and hypotension and bradycardia (at extremely high doses). On a psychological level, nicotine can cause both stimulation (when smoked under conditions of fatigue) and relaxation (when smoked under conditions of anxiety)—these effects make nicotine strongly reinforcing. Caffeine is a nonselective A_1 and A_{2A} adenosine receptor antagonist and acts by modulating dopamine and glutamate. While dietary doses of caffeine

TABLE 235-1 Commonly Abused Stimulants

Street Name	Drug(s) [Trade Name]
Amphetamines	
Bennies, peaches	Amphetamine sulfate [Benzedrine]
Black Beauties, crank, cristy, crystal, crystal meth, meth, pep pills, quartz, speed, uppers, white crosses	Methamphetamine [Methedrine, Desoxyn]
Cramming drug, R-ball, rits, vitamin R	Methylphenidate [Ritalin, Concerta]
Dexies, footballs	Dextroamphetamine [Dexedrine, Dextrostat]
Ice, crystal	Freebase (smokable) methamphetamine
Cocaine preparations	
Crack, rock, gravel, supercoke	Freebase (smokable) cocaine
Big C, blow, coke, flake, flave, nose candy, snow, sugar boogers, white lady	Cocaine HCl
Pasta, bazooka	Coca paste
Designer drugs	
Ecstasy, XTC, Adam, M&M, Stars, 007s	Methylenedioxymethamphetamine (MDMA)
Eve	Methylenedioxyethamphetamine (MDEA)
The love drug	Methylenedioxyamphetamine (MDA)
STP (serenity, tranquility, peace), sweet tart	Dimethoxymethamphetamine (DOM)
Cathinone/cathine	
African salad, Bushman's tea, chat, kat, qat	khat
Cat	methcathinone
Drug combinations	
C&M	Cocaine + marijuana
Death hit	Cocaine + strychnine
Goofball, snowball, speedball	Cocaine + heroin
Ice	Methamphetamine + freebase cocaine
Liquid lady	Cocaine + alcohol
Pineapple	Methylphenidate + heroin
Poor man's speedball	Methamphetamine + heroin
Snackies	MDMA + mescaline
Space ball, space base, space dust	Cocaine + phencyclidine
Speedboat	Freebase cocaine + marijuana + phencyclidine (all smoked together)
Speedies	MDMA + amphetamine
Super X	MDMA + methamphetamine

are generally safe and well tolerated, very high doses of caffeine may cause clinically significant negative physiologic and psychologic effects, including tolerance and withdrawal, features of a substance dependence syndrome, or discrete psychiatric disorders (eg, caffeine intoxication, caffeine-induced anxiety disorder).

EPIDEMIOLOGY

About 44% of the world's users of cocaine reside in North America, where its use has been stable for the last decade. Cocaine is the second most widely used illicit drug in the United States, after marijuana. According to the 2006 National Survey on Drug Use and Health (NSDUH), the lifetime prevalence of cocaine use is 35.3 million Americans (14%), whereas the past-month prevalence is 2.4 million individuals (1%). The lifetime prevalence of noncocaine stimulant use is 20.1 million Americans (8%), whereas the past-month prevalence is 1.2 million individuals (0.5%). Cocaine abuse or dependence occurs at a rate of 1.7 million individuals (0.7%) annually, while noncocaine stimulant abuse or dependence affects 400,000 individuals (0.2%) annually.

Cocaine is the drug most often associated with visits to hospital emergency departments (450,000 visits annually, or 31% of all drug-related visits), while methamphetamine is associated with 109,000 visits annually, or 7.5% of visits. Cocaine is associated with high mortality and has been implicated in 39% of all drug misuse deaths investigated by medical examiners.

Polysubstance abuse is the norm for stimulant users. Patients diagnosed with one substance use disorder (SUD) will often have another. Cigarette smokers or binge alcohol drinkers are each ten times more likely to use cocaine than nonsmokers or moderate drinkers. Almost one-quarter of those who use MDMA also meet the American Psychiatric Association's *Diagnostic and Statistical Manual of Mental Disorders* (DSM) criteria for another SUD, especially nicotine, alcohol, or marijuana.

Caffeine is the most widely used mood-altering drug in the world. In the United States alone, 87% of children and adults regularly consume caffeine in foods and beverages.

Around the world, 57% of men and 10% of women smoke tobacco products, primarily cigarettes. In the United States, about

TABLE 235-2 Stimulant Intoxication

Physiologic Effects	Psychological Effects	Toxic Effects
Dizziness	Grandiosity	Hyperthermia
Tremor	Restlessness	Seizures
Hyperreflexia	Hypervigilance	Rhabdomyolysis
Hyperpyrexia	Aggression	Acute renal failure
Mydriasis	Impaired judgment	Hepatotoxicity
Tachypnea	Stereotyped behavior	Increased myocardial oxygen consumption
Tachycardia		Disseminated intravascular coagulation
Hypertension		

21% of the adult population smokes. However, among individuals with severe mental illness, about 70–90% are smokers.

INTOXICATION

Stimulant intoxication includes physical changes, many of which can be severe and acute, including fulminant hyperthermia, seizures, rhabdomyolysis, acute renal failure, hypertension, and increased myocardial oxygen consumption. Stimulant intoxication may also include severe behavioral effects, including aggression, hypervigilance, acute psychotic reactions, and suicidal ideation. These acute complications of abused stimulants are due to increased sympathomimetic effects and activation of dopamine circuits (**Table 235-2**).

Treatment for acute toxicity includes stabilization of airway, breathing, and circulation; administration of activated charcoal; seizure control with benzodiazepines; aggressive management of hypertension; and management of hyperthermia. The acutely intoxicated stimulant user should be approached in a subdued manner. Do not approach the patient from behind or move quickly. Speak in a low tone of voice and try to avoid touching the patient unless you are absolutely sure it is safe to do so.

Cocaine is well-known for its cardiovascular complications. Repeated doses may result in accumulation of drug and cardiovascular toxicity even when the user is not exhibiting euphoria. Cocaine is a potent inhibitor of neuronal catecholamine uptake. In high doses cocaine blocks fast sodium channels in the myocardium; the result is depression of depolarization and slowing of conduction velocity. This is manifested on electrocardiography (ECG) as prolonged PR, QRS, and QT intervals, similar to those seen with type IA antiarrhythmics. Other effects of cocaine include coronary artery vasoconstriction that is mediated by α-adrenergic stimulation and possibly by release of endothelium-derived vasoconstrictors, such as endothelin. A procoagulant effect of cocaine may predispose to coronary artery thrombosis. The sympathomimetic effects of cocaine lead to increased myocardial oxygen demand and, in the context of both the procoagulant effect and vasoconstriction, may result in myocardial ischemia, acute myocardial infarction, and arrhythmias.

HOW ARE THE ACUTE CARDIOVASCULAR COMPLICATIONS OF STIMULANTS MANAGED?

Management depends on specific manifestations of toxicity (**Table 235-3**). Hypertension may be managed with benzodiazepines and vasodilators such as nitroglycerin and nitroprusside. Phentolamine, an α-antagonist, can also be used to counteract the vasoconstriction. Arrhythmias result primarily from β-adrenergic stimulation. β1-specific blockers, such as esmolol or metoprolol, should be selected rather than nonselective β blockers to avoid antagonizing the β2-mediated arteriolar dilation that may be opposing the α-mediated vasoconstriction. Nonselective β2 blockade can worsen the hypertension. Many experts advise that beta-blockers should not be considered first-line agents for controlling chest pain or hypertension in patients using cocaine since that would leave alpha-adrenergic stimulation unopposed, but this remains controversial.

If the arrhythmia is a wide complex tachycardia, sodium bicarbonate should be used to counteract the sodium channel blockade effect of cocaine. Lidocaine has also been used safely in this context. Other type I antiarrhythmic drugs should be avoided.

Treatment of myocardial ischemia and infarction should include oxygen, aspirin, nitrates, and benzodiazepines. Because vasospasm is a mechanism of myocardial ischemia in this context, calcium channel blockers should be used. Other treatment options for coronary vasoconstriction include phentolamine and labetalol (the latter in the presence of tachycardia). Propranolol should be avoided because of the potential harmful effects of β_2 blockade, as already discussed. The decision to administer fibrinolytics in cocaine intoxication requires extreme caution because of the risk of hypertension-related complications (ie, cerebral hemorrhage), associated trauma, and high frequency of misleading ECGs. Specifically, early repolarization variant (J point and ST elevation) is a common cause of abnormal ECG in young patients with cocaine-associated chest pain. If available, coronary angiography and revascularization with angioplasty, if required, are the preferred methods of treatment of cocaine-induced acute myocardial infarction. If these methods are unavailable, and the patient has classic symptoms and signs of acute myocardial infarction and no contraindications, fibrinolytics can be given.

Hyperthermia results from increased muscular activity due to agitation, seizures (increasing heat generation), and intense vasoconstriction (impairing heat dissipation). Immediate cooling and sedation are necessary to reduce morbidity and mortality. First-line agents are benzodiazepines, which treat both agitation and seizures. Haloperidol and other dopamine antagonists should be avoided because they may lower the seizure threshold, further impair heat dissipation, and/or potentiate cardiac arrhythmias. External cooling measures and paralysis to reduce heat generation may be necessary to control hyperthermia. Even when muscle hyperactivity is prevented by paralysis, persistent seizure activity may cause brain injury. Therefore, electroencephalograms should be used to monitor paralyzed patients, and seizures should be controlled with anticonvulsant drugs or general anesthesia, if necessary. Ventilation with high oxygen concentrations is indicated in hyperthermia to meet the resultant extreme metabolic demands on organ systems. Acute renal failure may result from hypovolemia and/or hypotension, and rhabdomyolysis with myoglobinuria; acute renal failure may be prevented by vigorous fluid replacement, alkalinization of the urine, and, possibly, the use of mannitol.

TABLE 235-3 Treatment Summary for Acute Medical and Neuropsychiatric Effects of Cocaine

Acute coronary syndrome	Oxygen Diazepam 5–10 mg IV or lorazepam 2–4 mg IV Aspirin 325 mg Nitroglycerin 0.4 mg times 3, every 5 min, followed by an infusion titrated to a mean arterial pressure reduction of 10% or relief of chest pain Phentolamine 1 mg IV; repeat in 5 min Verapamil 5–10 mg IV Heparin 60 units/kg bolus, followed by 12 units/kg/h Percutaneous intervention (angioplasty and stent placement) or fibrinolytic therapy for STEMI [ST-segment-elevation myocardial infarction] Glycoprotein IIb/IIIa inhibitors
Supraventricular tachycardia	Oxygen Diazepam 5 mg IV or lorazepam 2–4 mg IV Adenosine 6 mg or 12 mg IV Consider diltiazem 20 mg IV or verapamil 5 mg IV Cardioversion if hemodynamically unstable
Ventricular dysrhythmias	Oxygen Sodium bicarbonate 1–2 meq/kg Lidocaine 1.5 mg/kg IV bolus followed by 2 mg/min infusion Diazepam 5 mg IV or lorazepam 2–4 mg IV Defibrillation if hemodynamically unstable
Hypertension	Observation Diazepam 5–10 mg IV or lorazepam 2–4 mg IV titrated to effect Phentolamine 1 mg IV; repeat in 5 min Nitroglycerin or nitroprusside continuous infusion titrated to effect
Pulmonary edema	Lasix 20–40 mg IV Nitroglycerin infusion titrated to blood pressure Consider phentolamine or nitroprusside
Anxiety and agitation	Diazepam 5–10 mg IV or lorazepam 2–4 mg IV titrated to effect
Seizures	Diazepam 5–10 mg IV or lorazepam 2–4 mg IV titrated to effect Phenobarbital 25–50 mg/min up to 10–20 mg/kg
Intracranial hemorrhage	Neurosurgery consultation avoid β-blockers for blood pressure control
Hyperthermia	External cooling measures Paralysis to reduce heat generation Ventilation with high oxygen concentrations
Acute renal failure	Vigorous fluid replacement Alkalinization of the urine Consider mannitol

Adapted, with permission, from Hollander JE, Hoffman RS. Cocaine. In: Goldfrank LR, Flomenbaum NE, Lewin NA, et al, eds. *Goldfrank's Toxicologic Emergency.* 7th ed. McGraw Hill; 2002.

Designer drugs, especially MDMA, are stimulants with some hallucinogen-like effects, so acute physiological effects include more pronounced hypertension and hyperthermia as compared to other hallucinogens. Toxicity of designer drugs may be related to additives such as ketamine or LSD. There are numerous case reports of MDMA use resulting in hyperthermia, rhadomyolysis, serotonin syndrome, hyponatremia with cerebral edema, fulminant hepatic failure, and stroke. Other stimulant-derived hallucinogens may cause cardiac arrhythmias.

Both prescribed and illicit stimulants interact with other medications, which may result in serious adverse reactions, often cardiovascular in nature (**Table 235-4**).

HOW ARE THE ACUTE PSYCHIATRIC COMPLICATIONS OF STIMULANTS MANAGED?

The acute psychiatric complications of stimulants are generally treated with movement to a quiet environment, decrease in external stimuli, and oral or injectable benzodiazepines. In cases of extreme agitation, seclusion and/or restraint may be necessary. Haloperidol must be used with caution because of the risks of decreased seizure threshold and reduced blood pressure.

Stimulant withdrawal syndrome is unlike the withdrawal syndrome from alcohol or opioids because there are not obvious physical signs and symptoms that prompt immediate resumption of use in order to avoid withdrawal. Thus patterns of stimulant use

TABLE 235-4 Stimulant Medication Interactions

Medication	Clinical Interaction
Alcohol	Increase blood pressure
Beta-blockers	Increase heart rate
Caffeine	
Carbamazepine	
Monoamine oxidase inhibitors	
Nonsteroidal antiinflammatory medications	
Anticholinergics	Arrhythmias
Bromocriptine	
Digoxin	
Halothane anesthetics	
Calcium channel blockers	Reduced blood pressure
Haloperidol	

may more often be in the form of episodic binges, as opposed to chronic daily use for alcohol, benzodiazepines, or opioids. Therefore, the absence of a daily use pattern does not indicate less impairment.

Chronic stimulant use is associated with a withdrawal syndrome. The severity and duration of withdrawal depend upon the intensity of the preceding months of chronic abuse and the presence of predisposing psychiatric disorders, which amplify withdrawal symptoms. The "crash," or drastic reduction in mood and energy, can start 15–30 minutes after the last use. The user experiences craving, depression, irritability, anxiety, and paranoia. The craving for stimulants decreases over 1–4 hours and is replaced by a need for sleep and food. Hypersomnolence lasts between 8 hours and 4 days. Sleep is interrupted by brief awakenings during which the user experiences hyperphagia ("the munchies"). This phase is followed by a protracted dysphoric syndrome consisting of anhedonia, boredom, anxiety, panic attacks, generalized malaise, problems with memory and concentration, and occasional suicidal ideation. This induces severe craving that may lead to resumption of stimulant use and a vicious cycle of recurrent binges. Intermittent craving can last months to years after the last stimulant use and is gradually extinguished over time.

NICOTINE WITHDRAWAL

The withdrawal syndrome from nicotine is similar to that of other stimulants and includes irritability, difficulty concentrating, restlessness, anxiety, depression, increased appetite, and impairment in reaction time and attention. Withdrawal symptoms peak around 48 hours after the last use, then gradually diminish over several weeks. Symptoms of dysphoria, anhedonia, and depression may continue for several months after cessation. Symptoms of withdrawal are due to nicotine and are similar with all tobacco products, whether cigarettes, chewing tobacco, or snuff.

Nicotine replacement therapy (NRT) is used in hospitalized smokers to treat acute nicotine withdrawal symptoms as well as to promote smoking cessation. Recent research supports including NRT in interventions for hospitalized smokers, along with counseling, since pharmacotherapy and counseling may be synergistic. Nicotine replacement products include a patch, gum, lozenge, nasal spray, and inhaler; all provide similar relief from withdrawal symptoms and efficacy for smoking cessation. Even patients with hypertension and/or cardiovascular disease benefit from NRT, including in an inpatient hospital setting. Clinically significant drug interactions of NRT include reduced analgesia from opioids and reduced sedation from benzodiazepines.

Note that NRT is not routinely recommended for smokers with acute coronary syndromes because safety has not been established, and most of these patients have minimal nicotine withdrawal symptoms when they are hospitalized in a tobacco-free environment. Counseling for smoking cessation is appropriate for smokers hospitalized with acute cardiovascular complications.

EFFECTS ON MEDICAL DISORDERS

WHAT ARE THE OTHER MEDICAL SEQUELAE OF ABUSED STIMULANTS?

Use of stimulants may result in many health consequences that can bring users into the hospital or complicate existing medical and/or psychiatric conditions. Stimulants have deleterious effects on every system of the body, including the central nervous system (CNS) and the cardiovascular, pulmonary, gastrointestinal, and endocrine systems, as well as having effects on pregnancy and the fetus (**Table 235-5**).

Medical sequelae in long-term stimulant users tend to accumulate over time, although any specific complication may occur relatively quickly after initiation of use. This is in contrast to long-term consequences of alcohol, tobacco, or marijuana, which usually require years for development of serious medical problems.

The clinical features of chronic stimulant use include depression, fatigue, poor concentration, and mild parkinsonian features such as myoclonus (inappropriate, spontaneous muscle contractions), tremor, or bradykinesia (slowing of movements). Patients presenting with these signs, especially at a young age, should be suspected of stimulant abuse and screened carefully. High-dose stimulant use over long periods of time causes neurophysiologic changes in brain systems. These CNS effects can take months to resolve, and occasionally do not resolve, even after stimulant use is stopped.

Additionally, stimulant use can worsen known psychiatric disorders. Panic attacks may increase in intensity and frequency. Schizophrenia is more susceptible to exacerbation and relapse. Stimulant intoxication and withdrawal frequently mimic or exacerbate mood disorders such as major depression and bipolar disorder.

Chronic use of MDMA can lead to a paranoid psychosis that is clinically indistinguishable from schizophrenia; it is usually reversible after a prolonged drug-free state. Several studies suggest that MDMA use (possibly in conjunction with marijuana) can lead to cognitive decline in otherwise healthy young people. This neurotoxicity has been described to occur with typical recreational doses. Other persistent neuropsychiatric effects of MDMA include impairment in memory and executive functions, reduced concentration, impulsiveness, and hostility.

DISCHARGE CONSIDERATIONS

WHAT FACTORS SHOULD BE CONSIDERED WHEN DISCHARGING A PATIENT WITH COMPLICATIONS OF STIMULANTS?

The level (intensive care unit or general medical floor) and duration of medical care are dependent on the severity and duration of stimulant toxicity. If signs and symptoms of toxicity are mild to moderate and resolve after a 4- to 6-hour observation period in the ED, patients may be medically discharged. Patients with cocaine-associated chest pain who are not at high risk for acute coronary syndrome may be admitted to a 9- to 12-hour chest pain observation unit. These patients may subsequently be discharged

TABLE 235-5 Effects of Stimulant Use

Psychological	**Central nervous system**	**Pulmonary**
Emotional lability	Headache	Chronic productive cough
Irritability	Transient focal neurological deficits	Asthma exacerbation
Insomnia	Tremor	Pulmonary edema
Exaggerated startle reactions	Myoclonus	Pulmonary hemorrhage
Paranoia	Bradykinesia	Pneumothorax
Aggressive behavior	Dyskinesia	Pneumomediastinum
Aberrant sexual behavior	Cerebral vasculitis	Bronchiolitis obliterans
Anxiety	Cerebral edema	
Depression	Cerebral hemorrhage	
Hallucinations	Cerebral infarction	
Psychosis	Cerebral atrophy	
Delirium	Toxic encephalopathy	
Obstetric	**Gastrointestinal**	**Head and neck**
Placenta previa	Anorexia	Dental enamel erosion
Premature rupture of membranes	Nausea/vomiting	Gingival ulceration
Placental abruption	Diarrhea	Mydriasis
Spontaneous abortion	Intestinal ischemia	Chronic rhinitis
	Gastroduodenal perforation	Nasal septal perforation
Fetal		
Intrauterine growth retardation		
Fetal hypertension		
Cardiovascular	**Endocrine**	**Other**
Hypertension	Hyperprolactinemia	Postural abnormalities
Arrhythmias	Elevated thyroxin level	Hyperthermia
Cardiomyopathy		Rhabdomyolysis
Myocardial ischemia/infarction		Acute renal failure

with close follow-up if they "rule out" for myocardial infarction (MI) by troponin testing and cardiovascular complications do not occur during their 12-hour observation. Patients with altered mental status, persistent abnormal vital signs, nonsinus rhythms, or significant end-organ toxicity (such as rhabdomyolysis) should be admitted for further care and observation. After acute clinical issues have resolved, referral for psychiatric follow-up care may be needed. Evaluation for complications related to intravenous drug abuse (eg, endocarditis, serologic testing for viral hepatitis and human immunodeficiency virus, other sexually transmitted diseases, etc,) should be considered. Counseling for smoking cessation and consideration of longer-term treatment of nicotine dependence (including NRT, buproprion, and varenicline) are also appropriate.

CONCLUSION

The acute hospitalization provides an opportunity to address stimulant abuse and prevent complications. Because polysubstance abuse is the norm for stimulant users, these patients are also at increased risk of developing other withdrawal syndromes that may be prevented or ameliorated. This chapter reviews common abused stimulants, the signs and symptoms of withdrawal, the evaluation for complications related to abuse, and management issues that should be considered when a patient who abuses stimulants is hospitalized on the general medical service. Both prescribed and illicit stimulants interact with other medications, which may result in serious adverse reactions, often cardiovascular in nature and many patients abuse.

SUGGESTED READINGS

Freeman K, Feldman JA. Cocaine, myocardial infarction, and β-blockers: time to rethink the equation? *Ann Emerg Med.* 2008;51(2):130–134.

Hollander JE, Henry TD. Evaluation and management of the patient who has cocaine-associated chest pain. *Cardiol Clin.* 2006;24(1):103–114.

Hollander JE, Hoffman RS. Cocaine. In: Goldfrank LR, Flomenbaum NE, Lewin NA, et al, eds. *Goldfrank's Toxicologic Emergency.* 7th ed. New York: McGraw-Hill; 2002.

Ries R, Fiellin D, Miller S, Saitz R, eds. *Principles of Addiction Medicine.* 4th ed. Philadelphia, PA: Lippincott, Williams & Wilkins; 2009.

Shannon MW, Borron SW, Burns M, eds. *Haddad and Winchester's Clinical Management of Poisoning and Drug Overdose.* 4th ed. Philadelphia, PA: Saunders; 2007.

CHAPTER 236

Other Drugs of Abuse

Michael Weaver, MD, FASAM

Key Clinical Questions

1. Is this patient intoxicated with marijuana?
2. Does marijuana cause withdrawal?
3. How is hallucinogen intoxication managed?
4. How is gamma-hydroxybutyrate (GHB) overdose treated?
5. What medical problems are caused by inhalants?

INTRODUCTION

Patients may be admitted to a hospital with an overdose, intoxication, or withdrawal syndrome from drugs of abuse. More commonly, patients admitted with medical problems or trauma may be abusing illicit drugs and may develop complications of this during their inpatient stay. It is important to ask all patients about drug use. Recognition of problems due to drug abuse can help clinicians provide optimal care to hospitalized patients.

HOSPITALIZATION AND DRUG USE

There are many different drugs that may be abused. In the hospital setting, certain classes of drugs of abuse are more likely to be encountered due to the high prevalence of use outside a hospital setting or due to medical consequences of use. Alcohol abuse is widely prevalent and encountered in hospital settings due to intoxication or withdrawal. Cocaine use may result in exacerbation of angina or asthma. Other drug classes are encountered less frequently in hospital settings due to lower prevalence of overall use, as well as lower incidence of severe medical complications. It is worthwhile for practitioners to be aware of these complications, which are often related to acute intoxication but may also be due to withdrawal. This chapter covers adverse effects of marijuana, hallucinogens, other "club drugs" such as gamma-hydroxybutyrate (GHB), and inhalants.

Hospitalized patients will frequently be using more than a single drug. Polysubstance abuse is the norm, rather than the exception. Patients diagnosed with one substance use disorder (SUD) will often have another SUD. For example, nearly all patients with hallucinogen dependence also abuse alcohol. It is important to ask patients directly about all illicit drug use. Many patients are forthcoming with medical personnel if they are asked in a nonjudgmental manner. Other clues from a thorough physical examination and some common laboratory tests can help establish a diagnosis of recent drug use (**Table 236-1**).

Some patients are able to use illicit substances while hospitalized. They may bring drugs and possibly paraphernalia with them at admission (in clothing, a purse, or other possessions), or visitors may bring drugs to a patient sometime during the hospitalization. Occasionally a patient may obtain drugs from another patient or from hospital personnel. Under these circumstances, intoxication may present with altered mental status, unexpected resolution of withdrawal symptoms, or a change in patient behavior. Drug use during a hospital stay may be verified by urine drug testing, especially confirmatory testing for specific substances that have not been prescribed. Hospital security personnel may be able to search the patient's hospital room and possibly inspect the patient's belongings. The hospital's risk management department should be notified of any illicit drug use on the premises by a patient. Depending on the situation, discovery of this drug use need not result in a drastic response such as immediate discharge of the patient. It may be used as an opportunity for brief intervention to address the seriousness of the patient's addiction.

MARIJUANA

Marijuana is the most frequently abused drug in the United States, with a prevalence of around 4% of the adult population that uses regularly. This rate has remained relatively steady since the early 1990s. Marijuana is also known as cannabis, "pot," "weed," "hash," and many other names.

TABLE 236-1 **Indicators of Drug Use Disorders**

Finding	Medical Indication	Drug(s)
Conjunctival injection	Current use	Marijuana
Tachycardia	Intoxication	
Pinpoint pupils	Intoxication, overdose	Opioids
Vertical nystagmus	Intoxication	Phencyclidine
Nasal septal perforation	Vasoconstriction	Any snorted drug
Sores, hyperpigmentation around mouth and/or nose	Chemical irritation	Inhalants
New murmur	Endocarditis from injection drug use	Any injected drug
Track marks, fresh needle marks	Injection drug use	
White blood cell count low	Human immunodeficiency virus	
Transaminases (alanine aminotransferase, aspartate aminotransferase) elevated	Viral hepatitis	
Urine drug screen positive	Recent drug use	Marijuana, phencyclidine, stimulant, opioid, benzodiazepine

IS THIS PATIENT INTOXICATED WITH MARIJUANA?

The onset of acute marijuana intoxication is within minutes when smoked, and the effects last for 3 to 4 hours. Acute psychological signs of intoxication include euphoria, time distortion, and short-term memory impairment. Acute physiological signs of intoxication include elevation in heart rate, blood pressure, and respiratory rate, as well as dry mouth and conjunctival injection (bloodshot eyes). Other effects are an increase in appetite ("the munchies") and impairment in reaction time. Impairment of concentration and motor performance lasts for 12 to 24 hours due to accumulation of marijuana in adipose tissue, with slow release of tetrahydrocannabinol from fatty tissue stores and enterohepatic recirculation. Thus marijuana users may think that they are no longer impaired several hours after use when the acute mood-altering effects wear off. However, impairment of cognition, coordination, and judgment lasts much longer than the subjective feeling of being "high." Impairment is intensified by combination with other drugs, especially alcohol. This explains why fatal traffic accidents occur more often among individuals who test positive for marijuana, and industrial accidents are also more likely.

The differential diagnosis of marijuana intoxication includes intoxication with other drugs of abuse. Marijuana intoxication appears clinically similar to sedative intoxication, but marijuana intoxication may have more psychotic features and is differentiated by elevated vital signs instead of vital sign depression. On physical examination, conjunctival injection is a clue to determine marijuana intoxication.

Acute intoxication with marijuana alone rarely requires medical treatment, although dysphoria may result in distress that causes the user to seek help. First-time users, older persons, users of high-potency marijuana, or those predisposed to psychiatric illness are at higher risk of experiencing unpleasant effects during intoxication. These unpleasant effects, such as anxiety, paranoia, or palpitations, are managed with supportive treatment (**Table 236-2**). Placing the distraught user in a quiet environment and maintaining gentle contact is often sufficient until the acute effects subside. More severe marijuana effects such as paranoia or psychosis with hallucinations may result in extreme anxiety or agitation. This requires close observation with possible administration of a benzodiazepine or haloperidol for sedation.

Patients with medical comorbidities are at higher risk for adverse outcomes from marijuana intoxication. Patients with coronary artery disease may develop angina from tachycardia caused by marijuana. Immunosuppressed patients are at higher risk for infections, especially pulmonary aspergillosis from spores found in marijuana preparations. Particulate matter from unfiltered marijuana cigarettes ("joints" or "blunts") may trigger an exacerbation of asthma or chronic obstructive pulmonary disease.

DOES MARIJUANA CAUSE WITHDRAWAL?

Heavy marijuana use for more than 3 weeks results in a withdrawal syndrome after abrupt cessation. Marijuana withdrawal begins within 10 hours of the last dose and consists of irritability, agitation, depression, insomnia, nausea, anorexia, and tremor. Most symptoms peak in 48 hours and last for 5 to 7 days. Some symptoms, such as unusual dreams and irritability, can persist for weeks. The differential diagnosis for marijuana withdrawal syndrome includes major depression and viral gastroenteritis. Major depression lasts longer than the expected timeframe for resolution of marijuana withdrawal, and a viral syndrome is accompanied by fever and other changes in vital signs not seen with marijuana withdrawal. Marijuana withdrawal is uncomfortable but not life threatening. Thus treatment is entirely supportive and nearly always accomplished without the need for adjunctive medications.

HALLUCINOGENS

There are many different types of hallucinogens, which include naturally occurring plant (and even animal) derivatives, synthetic drugs, and "designer drugs" (**Table 236-3**). The prototypical hallucinogens are lysergic acid diethylamide (LSD), psilocybin, and mescaline. LSD is the most commonly abused. Designer drugs are

TABLE 236-2 **Treatment Tips for Acute Intoxication: Marijuana and Hallucinogens**

- Settle the intoxicated patient in a quiet environment.
- Establish contact with a gentle touch (hold hand) during a period of relative lucidity.
- Maintain contact through periods of anxiety and perceptual distortion.
- Administer benzodiazepine (lorazepam, diazepam) for severe anxiety.
- Consider low-dose haloperidol for severe psychotic reactions (but may lower seizure threshold).

TABLE 236-3 Hallucinogens

Chemical Name	Abbreviation	Origin	Slang Name(s)
Alphamethyltryptamine	AMT	Synthesized	Love pills, trip
Bromo-dimethoxyphenethylamine	2-CB	Synthesized	Bromo, DOB, Nexus, Spectrum
Bufotenine		Colorado river toad venom	Bufo, toad-licking
Dimethoxymethyl-amphetamine	DOM	Synthesized	STP (Serenity, Tranquility, and Peace)
Dimethoxy-propylthiophenethylamine	2C-T-7	Synthesized	7-Up, Blue Mystic, Tripstacy
Dimethyltryptamine	DMT	Canary grass, prairie bundleflower	Businessman's trip, Dimitri, Fantasia
Ibotinic acid, muscinol		Mushrooms	
Ketamine		Manufactured	Cat valium, ket, kit cat, Special K
Lysergic acid diethylamide	LSD	Synthesized	Acid, blotter, microdot
Lysergic acid hydroxyethylamide	LSA	Morning glory seeds, Hawaiian baby Woodrose	Natural high, organic high
Mescaline		Peyote cactus	Cactus, mesc, peyote
Methylenedioxy-amphetamine	MDA	Synthesized	Eve, The Love Drug
Methylenedioxy-methamphetamine	MDMA	Synthesized	Ecstasy, X
Phencyclidine	PCP	Synthesized	Angel dust, Peace Pill
Psilocybin		Mushrooms	Magic mushrooms, shrooms

synthetic derivatives of federally controlled substances, created by slight alterations in the molecular structure and produced illegally in clandestine laboratories. Many designer drugs are derived from stimulants (for example, methylenedioxymethamphetamine—also known as Ecstasy—is derived from methamphetamine) (see Chapter 235 on Stimulants). Designer drugs have some psychoactive properties and cause visual disturbances but are not true hallucinogens like LSD. Phencyclidine (PCP, Angel Dust) and ketamine (Special K) are dissociative anesthetics that produce perceptual distortions similar to hallucinogens. Ketamine is a derivative of phencyclidine that is less potent and shorter acting and is still used therapeutically in medical settings as an anesthetic in humans.

The most widely used hallucinogen is LSD, with a lifetime prevalence of use of 14% among young adults in the United States. Among club-going young adults, rates of hallucinogen use are much higher, up to 70% (see "Club Drugs" section later in chapter). Ketamine and Ecstasy use is primarily concentrated among young adults attending clubs or parties, including "raves."

Hallucinogens produce perceptual distortions and cognitive changes with a clear sensorium and without impairment in level of consciousness or attention (**Table 236-4**). The quality of the hallucinogen-induced psychedelic state, or "trip," is influenced by the mood (set) and environment of the user (setting) at the time of induction. Reactions to hallucinogenic drugs are idiosyncratic, and individual reactions vary according to the purity of the drug taken, the dose, and the setting. During a hallucinogen experience, periods of lucidity alternate with periods of intense reaction to the drug. Generally, reactions are most intense and frequent in the early part of a trip, leading to a "peak," and then longer periods of lucidity with gradual clearing of the drug.

A "bad trip" is when the user experiences feelings of extreme anxiety, and it can be caused by fear, anxiety, or anger at the time the drug is taken. It may be difficult to distinguish between a bad trip and an acute psychotic reaction. Most bad trips can be handled without medication. Support can be provided by a friend, nurse, or physician. It is important to make physical contact with the patient

TABLE 236-4 Hallucinogen Intoxication

Perceptual Distortions	Psychiatric Effects	Physiologic Effects
Light trails behind moving objects	Anxiety	Pupillary dilation
Micropsia (the sensation that the user is very large in relation to the surroundings)	Depression	Tachycardia
Macropsia (the sensation that the user is very small in relation to the surroundings)	Paranoia	Diaphoresis
Synesthesias (cross-linking of the five senses (eg, "see the sounds, taste the colors")	Impaired judgment	Tremulousness
Sensation that the body is made of wood, plastic, or rubber	Ideas of reference (getting personal messages from the television or radio)	Lack of coordination
Out-of-body experiences (sensation of floating over or outside one's physical body)	Depersonalization ("I am not real")	Hyperreflexia
Sense of profound understanding or universal connection	Derealization ("The environment is not real")	Seizures
Feeling of impending doom		Hyperthermia

(eg, holding hands) when treating a bad trip; this may be the only means of contact with someone who is having a very severe hallucinogenic reaction. However, the patient may react suddenly or violently to a touch, so the contact person should be alert for this. The physical space in which treatment takes place should be quiet, softly lit, and away from large groups of people, since excessive stimuli may overwhelm the patient. Absence of stimuli, though, may intensify the hallucinations. Deep, slow breathing may be helpful as a distraction. Try to make contact with the patient during lucid intervals and maintain this contact into the intense periods of drug reaction. Efforts to make contact with the patient during an intense period are generally not successful. As with any drug intoxication or overdose, if verbal contact can be made, ascertain what was taken, how much was taken, and when it was taken. It may be helpful to have parents or friends obtain a sample from the same batch, and to talk to others who took the same dose at the same time.

HOW IS HALLUCINOGEN INTOXICATION MANAGED?

Acute physiologic complications of hallucinogen intoxication rarely require medical treatment (Table 236-4). Up to a third of frequent ketamine users experience severe gastrointestinal cramping known as "k-cramps," but the cause is unknown and there is no known treatment. Severe agitation due to a hallucinogen may be treated with a benzodiazepine or haloperidol. Malignant hyperthermia and seizures may occur. Agitation, dry skin, and increased muscle tension are some warning signs for hallucinogenic hyperthermia.

In low-dose intoxication with phencyclidine, the patient presents with nystagmus, confusion, ataxia, and sensory impairment. Phencyclidine is the only drug of abuse that causes a characteristic vertical nystagmus (although it can also cause horizontal or rotatory nystagmus), which helps to identify phencyclidine as the cause when a patient presents with intoxication by an unknown drug. Moderate phencyclidine intake may lead to a catatonic-like picture, with the patient staring blankly and not responding to stimuli; the patient's eyes remain open, even when the patient is in a comatose state. In high doses, the drug produces seizures and severe hypertension. The hypertension should be treated vigorously since it may cause hypertensive encephalopathy or intracerebral bleeding; intravenous antihypertensive medications should be administered to reduce blood pressure. Phencyclidine can also cause life-threatening hyperthermia with temperatures over 106 degrees Fahrenheit, which may occur many hours after use; rapid cooling measures (ice packs, cooling blanket, etc) may be required. Psychotic behavior can be treated with haloperidol. If the patient is severely agitated and poses a potential threat to self or others, haloperidol or lorazepam is effective for control of agitation; barbiturates may be even more useful in this setting with this drug, according to some reports.

CLUB DRUGS

Club drugs are licit and illicit drugs from different classes that are used primarily by young adults in bars, clubs, concerts, and dance parties or "raves." The National Institute on Drug Abuse (NIDA) has identified six drugs as club drugs: LSD, ketamine, methamphetamine, methylenedioxymethamphetamine (Ecstasy), gamma-hydroxybutyrate (GHB), and flunitrazepam. The club drug scene changes rapidly and may include prescription opioids, benzodiazepines, and over-the-counter cold-and-cough preparations (**Table 236-5**). Intoxication or overdose from certain club drugs (GHB, opioids, benzodiazepines), especially in combination, may result in serious medical consequences, and even death.

GAMMA-HYDROXYBUTYRATE

GHB is a sedative that is both a precursor and a metabolite of gamma-aminobutyric acid (GABA). It has been used as a sleep aid as well as for treatment of narcolepsy. It also increases

TABLE 236-5 Club Drugs

Chemical Name	Brand Name(s)	NIDA Club Drug	Slang Names	Drug Type
Alprazolam	Xanax	No	Blue haze, X	Benzodiazepine Sedative
Dextromethorphan (DXM)	Coricidin, Robitussin	No	Dex, DXM, Robo, Triple C's	Opioid (OTC)
Diazepam	Valium	No	Downers, Mother's little helper, V's	Benzodiazepine Sedative
Flunitrazepam	Rohypnol	Yes	Mexican Valium, Roofies, rope	Benzodiazepine Sedative
Gamma-hydroxybutyrate (GHB)	Xyrem	Yes	Georgia Home Boy, Grievous Bodily Harm, Liquid Ecstasy	Sedative
Hydrocodone	Hycodan, Lortab, Vicodin	No	Hykes, Vike	Opioid
Ketamine	Ketalar	Yes	Special K, kit cat, cat valium	Arylcyclohexylamine Hallucinogen
Lysergic acid diethylamide (LSD)		Yes	Acid, blotter, microdot	Prototypical Hallucinogen
Methamphetamine	Desoxyn	Yes	Crank, crystal meth, ice, speed	Stimulant
Methylenedioxy-methamphetamine (MDMA)		Yes	Ecstasy, X	Designer Drug Stimulant
Methylphenidate	Ritalin	No	Rits, smart pills, vitamin R	Stimulant
Oxycodone	OxyContin, Percocet, Tylox	No	Hillbilly heroin, OC, Oxy, Perc	Opioid
Pseudoephedrine	Sudafed	No	Suzie	Stimulant (OTC)

episodic secretion of growth hormone, so some body builders use it to promote muscle growth. It is relatively easy to manufacture from common household products, although improper manufacture may result in unintended toxic by-products. Gamma-hydroxybutyrate is labeled a club drug by NIDA.

Desired effects of GHB last around 3 hours, and repeated use may prolong its effects, which have been likened to those of alcohol. These include euphoria, relaxation, and disinhibition. Small increases in the amount ingested may lead to significant intensification of effects, and onset of central nervous system (CNS) depression with cognitive impairment and ataxia. Alcohol and other drugs have synergistic effects with GHB, thus increasing the chance of overdose.

The clinical hallmark of GHB overdose is the rapid onset of profound coma with respiratory depression, bradycardia, and myoclonus. Overdose on GHB should be considered as part of the differential diagnosis of any patient presenting with rapid onset of coma of unknown cause. Other conditions in this differential diagnosis include head trauma, CNS infection, elevated intracranial pressure, and metabolic disorders. Because GHB is not detectable by routine drug screening, a history of use by the patient is essential. The clinical signs of GHB overdose are difficult to distinguish from those of overdose on benzodiazepines or alcohol. Death may result from GHB overdose due to respiratory failure, aspiration, pulmonary edema, or traumatic injury related to the rapid onset of coma.

HOW IS GHB OVERDOSE TREATED?

In cases of acute GHB intoxication, physicians should provide physiological support and maintain a high index of suspicion for intoxication with other drugs. Most patients who overdose on GHB recover completely if they receive proper medical attention. Management of GHB ingestion in a spontaneously breathing patient includes oxygen supplementation, intravenous access, and comprehensive physiologic and cardiac monitoring. Providers should attempt to keep the patient stimulated and awake. Atropine may be used for persistent symptomatic bradycardia. Naloxone and flumazenil are ineffective for GHB intoxication, and activated charcoal is contraindicated due to the risk of aspiration and the short half-life of GHB. These patients may be discharged (with plans for follow-up) if they are clinically well within 6 hours. If a patient is still intoxicated after 6 hours, admit the patient to the hospital for additional observation and supportive care; patients whose breathing is labored should be managed in the intensive care unit, as intubation and mechanical ventilation may be required.

The most dangerous effects of GHB use often occur with the use of other drugs. Concurrent use of sedatives or alcohol may increase the risk of vomiting, aspiration, or cardiopulmonary depression; the use of GHB and stimulants may increase the risk of seizure. Protease inhibitors used to treat HIV alter GHB metabolism via the cytochrome P-450 enzyme system, resulting in even small doses of GHB causing overdose.

Some individuals develop physiological dependence on GHB, although this requires use multiple times daily. Withdrawal from GHB is similar to withdrawal from sedatives such as benzodiazepines and alcohol. The symptoms of withdrawal start within 6 hours of the last use, then increase in intensity over several hours to days and may persist for 2 weeks after stopping the drug. Physiologic signs of withdrawal include diaphoresis, tremor, tachycardia, and hypertension. Other symptoms are nausea with vomiting, anxiety, restlessness, insomnia, and "feelings of doom." Severe withdrawal involves agitation, delirium, and psychosis.

GHB withdrawal is treated with benzodiazepines, which may require very high doses. Antipsychotics or pentobarbital may have some utility in treatment of severe GHB withdrawal, although antipsychotics may lower the seizure threshold, especially when used without a sedative.

INHALANTS

Inhalants are volatile substances that produce chemical vapors which can be inhaled for psychoactive effects. Examples of abused inhalants include glue, drycleaning fluids (carbon tetrachloride), gasoline, aerosol propellants from whipped cream cans or deodorant sprays, amyl nitrite, butyl nitrite, nitrous oxide ("laughing gas"), and some industrial solvents. Inhalants are second only to marijuana in likelihood of use by adolescents in the United States, and about 10% continue to use beyond adolescence for at least 6 years.

WHAT MEDICAL PROBLEMS ARE CAUSED BY INHALANTS?

Many of the inhalants are similar to general anesthetics and sensitize the myocardium to catecholamines; fatal arrhythmias have been reported due to inhalant abuse. Antiarrhythmic medications can be given as needed, and supplemental oxygen is administered for hypoxia as well as to enhance clearance of the inhalant.

Chronic inhalant use by industrial workers has caused peripheral neuropathies, as well as hepatic, renal, and bone marrow damage. Cases of methemoglobinemia have been reported secondary to butyl nitrite abuse. Chronic complications of abuse usually clear if the patient remains abstinent, though impairment of working memory and executive cognitive function may persist.

DISCHARGE CONSIDERATIONS

Treatment of intoxication or withdrawal from marijuana, hallucinogens, club drugs such as GHB, or inhalants is usually supportive care. (Table 236-2) The length of hospital stay is variable but is often short term. Patients presenting with GHB overdose may be discharged after 6 hours if stable. Patients with phencyclidine intoxication may be discharged if they remain stable after 12 hours of observation. In contrast, serious complications such as respiratory failure or malignant hyperthermia may result in a prolonged hospital course.

After the acute medical and/or psychiatric consequences have been addressed, the underlying addiction should also be addressed. Many users of drugs such as marijuana, hallucinogens, club drugs, and inhalants do not recognize the severity of their addiction. Hospitalization for treatment of medical consequences related to illicit drug use may provide a "teachable moment" for a clinician to help motivate the patient to make a change in behavior and start down a path toward recovery from addiction (see Chapter 232, Patients with Multiple Unexplained Somatic Symptoms). Treatment of medical consequences such as intoxication or withdrawal is only the first step in treating addiction and should always be followed by a referral to a local resource for specific long-term addiction treatment.

There are no pharmacologic agents available for long-term treatment of abuse of marijuana, hallucinogens, GHB, or inhalants. Treatment involves similar components to those of other types of substance abuse, including individual counseling, support groups, and 12-Step self-help group (Narcotics Anonymous) attendance.

CONCLUSION

Marijuana, Club Drugs such as hallucinogens or GHB, and inhalants may be used by patients admitted to the hospital. These drugs are less likely to result in users seeking medical attention than other drugs such as cocaine or alcohol. However, intoxication or withdrawal from these drugs can complicate other medical conditions and prolong the hospital length of stay. After the acute complications of abuse of these drugs are addressed in the hospital setting, patients should be referred for specific treatment of the addiction.

SUGGESTED READINGS

Strassman RJ. Adverse reactions to psychedelic drugs: a review of the literature. *J Nerv Ment Dis.* 1984;172:577–595.

Weaver MF, Jarvis MA, Schnoll SH. Role of the primary care physician in problems of substance abuse. *Arch Intern Med.* 1999;159:913–924.

Wu LT, Schlenger WE, Galvin DM. Concurrent use of methamphetamine, MDMA, LSD, ketamine, GHB, and flunitrazepam among American youths. *Drug Alcohol Depend.* 2006;84:102–113.

SECTION 16

Pulmonary and Allergy Immunology

CHAPTER 237

Allergy and Anaphylaxis

Kimberly D. Manning, MD, FACP, FAAP
Neil H. Winawer, MD, SFHM
Mandakolathur R. Murali, MD

Key Clinical Questions

1. What are the presenting symptoms of a severe allergic reaction or anaphylaxis?
2. What are the most common causes of allergic reactions?
3. How do anaphylactic and anaphylactoid reactions differ? How are they treated?
4. What conditions mimic allergic reactions?
5. What are the most common types of allergic reactions among hospitalized patients?
6. Which patients require outpatient referral to an allergist?

INTRODUCTION

Allergic reactions result from an aberrant immune response to an inciting antigen or allergen. The subsequent inflammatory state produces a wide range of clinical symptoms. Anaphylaxis, the most extreme form of allergic reaction, refers to sudden, severe, and potentially fatal hypersensitivity developing in seconds to minutes after exposure.

EPIDEMIOLOGY

It is estimated that anaphylaxis accounts for 1 in 2000 ambulance trips and is fatal in as many as 0.7 to 2% of cases. Two epidemiologic studies demonstrated that 1 out of every 2700–5100 hospitalizations can be linked to anaphylactic reactions. While the term *allergy* denotes an immediate hypersensitivity reaction involving immunoglobulin E (IgE) antibody, a large number of severe allergic reactions are not IgE mediated. These "anaphylactoid" reactions are clinically indistinguishable from anaphylaxis and include hypersensitivity to radiocontrast dye, angiotensin-converting enzyme inhibitors, and opiates.

CLINICAL PRESENTATION

Patients experiencing allergic reactions may vary widely in their clinical presentations. Factors affecting the clinical picture include the amount and persistence of antigen, its route of entry, and the end organ response to vasoactive mediators. The majority of allergic reactions manifest as skin findings, such as flushing, pruritus, and transient urticaria. In more severe reactions, a larger number of deep dermal mast cells are recruited, resulting in angioedema.

The onset of anaphylactic reactions can occur minutes to hours after exposure to an allergen and denotes the systemic activation of mast cells. Aside from the cutaneous manifestations, patients may experience respiratory manifestations (hoarseness of voice, dyspnea, wheezing, cough, and chest tightness), gastrointestinal manifestations (nausea, vomiting, colicky abdominal pain, and diarrhea), and cardiovascular manifestations (peripheral vasodilation, reflex tachycardia, and hypotension with resultant cardiovascular collapse).

PRACTICE POINT

- The onset of anaphylactic reactions can occur minutes to hours after exposure to an allergen and may manifest as cutaneous, respiratory, gastrointestinal, or cardiovascular symptoms.

PATHOPHYSIOLOGY

When the body is exposed to an antigen, a specific IgE antibody is formed that binds to high-affinity receptors, called Fc epsilon type I, located on mast cells and basophils. Upon reexposure to that allergen cross-linking of cell-bound IgE antibody occurs, resulting in Fc epsilon receptor aggregation and activation. The resultant mast cell degranulation leads to release of inflammatory mediators such as histamine, prostaglandins, tryptase, platelet activation factor, and leukotrienes, all directly contributing to the allergic response through smooth muscle contraction, bronchoconstriction, vasodilation, increased vascular permeability, and edema (**Figure 237-1**). Allergic reactions mediated by T-helper type 2 (TH2) cells (a subset of CD4+ T-cells) preferentially produce interleukins (IL) 4, 5, and 13; all powerful mediators of allergic

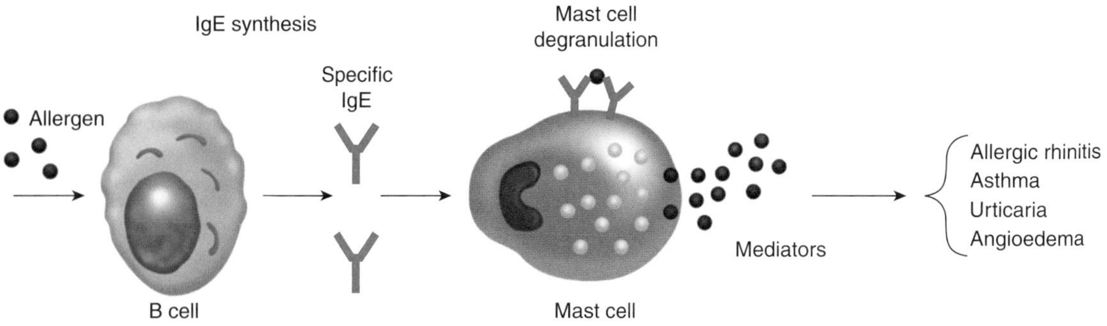

Figure 237-1 *Mechanism of allergic inflammation.*

response. IL-4 promotes B-cell activation and T-cell proliferation and is also responsible for CD4+ T-cell differentiation to TH2 cells. IL-5 recruits and activates eosinophils, contributing to the late phase of allergic inflammation. The functions of IL-13 overlap considerably with those of IL-4 and it synergizes with IL-4 in the production of IgE antibody by B cells.

DIFFERENTIAL DIAGNOSIS

Several disease processes can mimic the clinical features of anaphylaxis. Vasovagal reactions, cardiac arrhythmias, bronchoconstriction, and hypoglycemia, for example, can all be associated with hypotension, pallor, diaphoresis, dyspnea, and wheezing. Pruritis and urticaria may serve as distinguishing factors as they are absent in these mimicking conditions. Viral exanthems and enanthems, depending on their timing, can also be mistaken for hypersensitivity reactions, but they do not manifest itching.

PRACTICE POINT

- Several disease processes such as vasovagal reactions, hypoglycemia, and bronchoconstriction can mimic the clinical features of anaphylaxis (hypotension, diaphoresis, and wheezing). The cutaneous findings of pruritis and urticaria may serve as a distinguishing factor, as they are absent in mimicking conditions.

ANGIOEDEMA

Angiotensin-converting enzyme inhibitor angioedema

In addition to catalyzing the conversion of angiotensin I to angiotensin II, angiotensin-converting enzyme (ACE) breaks down bradykinin, in both tissues and plasma, into inactive peptide fragments. Patients taking ACE-inhibitors, therefore, have elevated levels of bradykinin, which stimulates cough receptors and can lead to bouts of angioedema. Most reactions occur in the first week following initiation of the drug, but up to 40% can occur months or even years after starting the drug. Typically patients present with angioedema involving the lips, tongue, uvula, soft palate, and, much less commonly, bowel, manifesting as acute abdominal pain.

Antihistamines are ineffective, and systemic corticosteroids offer limited benefit in the treatment of ACE-inhibitor-induced angioedema. Symptoms improve with discontinuation of the drug, and patients should not be rechallenged with a different ACE-inhibitor or treated at a lower dose. Most patients with ACE-inhibitor angioedema can tolerate an angiotension receptor blocker (ARB). However, treatment needs to be individualized given rare case reports of angioedema with these agents. If there is a strong indication for the ARB (eg, diabetic nephropathy, heart failure) and the episode of angioedema was non–life threatening, then an ARB can be prescribed with caution.

PRACTICE POINT

- Unlike immediate hypersensitivity drug reactions, ACE-inhibitor-induced angioedema may occur at any time while the patient is taking the drug, making it potentially overlooked as a cause of angioedema.

Hereditary angioedema

Hereditary angioedema (HAE), a rare autosomal dominant disease characterized by a low or nonfunctioning C1 esterase inhibitor can present with episodes of angioedema involving the face, larynx, lips, abdomen, genitalia, and extremities. While attacks may occur in childhood, typically the disease manifests in the second or third decade of life. Aside from prior bouts of angioedema, patients will often endorse a family history of similar attacks. If there is diagnostic uncertainty, a *C4 level* is a cost-effective screening test. A normal C4 level effectively rules out HAE since a low or nonfunctional C1 esterase inhibitor results in the activation of C4. The C2 level correlates with activity of disease.

While HAE is a rare disorder clinicians must distinguish it from anaphylaxis. During episodes of HAE the cascade produces vasoactive kinin proteins such as kallikrein and bradykinin (**Figure 237-2**); mast cells are not activated; hence patients do not manifest pruritus or concomitant urticaria. Therefore, traditional therapies with antihistamines, steroids, and epinephrine have little therapeutic utility. Acute episodes are managed with supportive care and the administration of pasteurized C1 esterase inhibitor concentrate. C1 esterase inhibitor is derived from human plasma and bears infection transmission risks similar to other blood product transfusions. A new formulation—pasteurized, nanofiltered C1 esterase inhibitor concentrate—awaits U.S. Food and Drug Administration (FDA) approval for acute attacks but is currently recommended for prophylactic use. Ecallantide, a potent inhibitor of plasma kallikrein, has FDA approval for treatment of acute attacks. Subcutaneous administration of icatibant, a peptide inhibitor of the bradykinin B2 receptor, is approved in Europe for treatment of acute attacks but is not yet FDA approved.

PRACTICE POINT

- Unlike common histamine-mediated allergic reactions, patients with bradykinin-mediated reactions—hereditary angioedema (HAE) and ACE-inhibitor angioedema—do not attain therapeutic benefit from epinephrine, antihistamines or steroids. HAE treatment may include C1 esterase inhibitor concentrate or the potent kallikrein inhibitor, ecallantide. ACE-inhibitor angioedema treatment includes supportive care and prompt removal of the drug.

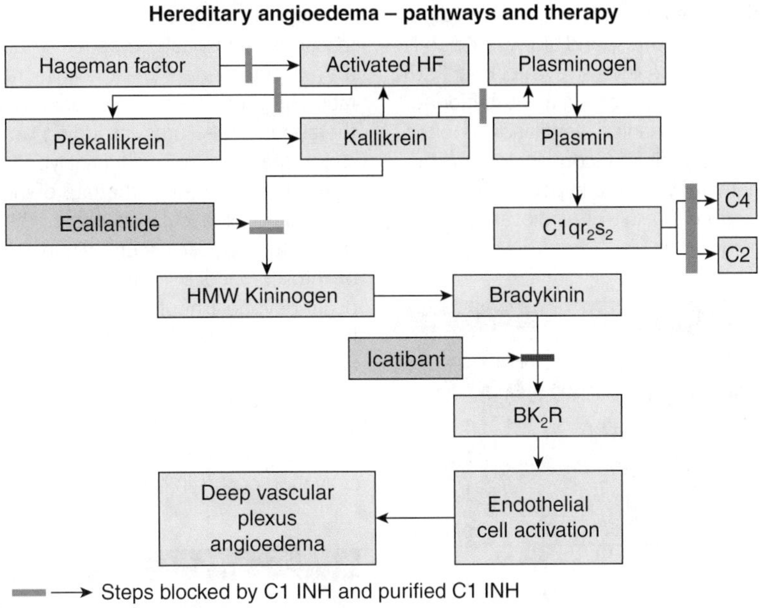

Figure 237-2 *Hereditary angioedema—pathways and therapy.*

SYSTEMIC MASTOCYTOSIS

Systemic mastocytosis, another rare disorder characterized by an overabundance of mast cells in the liver, spleen, bone marrow, skin, and gastrointestinal tract shares similarities with allergic and anaphylactoid reactions. Symptoms of flushing, pruritis, and/or abdominal pain may be seen, and hepatosplenomegaly, lympadenopathy, anemia, and/or coagulopathy may also be present. When systemic mastocytosis is considered, serum total and beta tryptase levels are useful diagnostic tests. A total tryptase level of > 20 ng/mL with an increase in the alpha subunit is suggestive of the diagnosis. The beta tryptase level is usually within normal range, unlike in *anaphylaxis wherein the beta tryptase is elevated*. The diagnosis can be confirmed by bone marrow biopsy, which reveals a multifocal dense infiltrate of mast cells, often with spindle shape morphology. Flow cytometry of bone marrow cells is typically positive for CD25+, CD2+, c-kit, or CD117+.

CARCINOID SYNDROME

Carcinoid tumors may also be associated with symptoms analogous to anaphylaxis. The constellation of skin flushing, abdominal cramping, diarrhea, and bronchoconstriction may be misleading. When carcinoid tumors are suspected, patients should have 24-hour urine levels of 5-hydroxyindoleacetic acid (5-HIAA) measured.

VOCAL CORD DYSFUNCTION

Vocal cord dysfunction may masquerade as anaphylaxis and can be substantiated by detecting an auscultatory inspiratory stridor over the trachea and confirmed by laryngoscopy as well as by a flattening of the inspiratory loop on spirometry during an attack.

DIAGNOSIS

The diagnosis of allergic reactions and anaphylaxis is based on clinical grounds and is self-evident when patients display the classic constellation of symptoms (**Table 237-1**). In these instances further diagnostic testing is rarely indicated. However, during some presentations of anaphylaxis or anaphylactoid reactions—such as perioperative anaphylaxis, unexplained syncope, or recurrent anaphylaxis—determination of serum total and beta tryptase can confirm a mast cell–mediated event because they remain elevated for 4–8 hours following symptoms.

TRIAGE/HOSPITAL ADMISSION

INDICATIONS FOR HOSPITALIZATION AND INTENSIVE CARE UNIT ADMISSION

Triage decisions in patients with allergic reactions rely upon both the severity of the reaction and the initial response to treatment. Patients presenting with mild to moderate symptoms (urticaria and/or angioedema with stable airway and hemodynamics) can generally be treated in the emergency department and discharged home. Patients with more severe reactions require hospitalization for further monitoring.

Patients with allergic reactions who present with severe wheezing, shortness of breath, hypotension, altered mentation, hoarseness of voice, or stridor should be treated as a medical emergency with early attention focused on securing the airway and cardiopulmonary

TABLE 237-1 Symptoms of Allergic Reactions and Anaphylaxis

Cutaneous • Flushing • Pruritus • Urticaria • Angioedema
Respiratory • Hoarseness • Dyspnea • Wheezing • Cough • Chest tightness
Gastrointestinal • Nausea • Vomiting • Abdominal pain • Diarrhea
Cardiovascular • Peripheral vasodilation • Reflex tachycardia • Hypotension

status. Patients who respond to therapy should be observed in the hospital for 24 hours. Patients who respond slowly or poorly to primary treatment strategies require intensive care unit (ICU) admission, particularly those requiring endotracheal intubation for life-threatening laryngeal edema. Mechanical ventilation is often indicated for patients with respiratory failure secondary to bronchoconstriction refractory to initial therapy. Severe hypotension calling for vasopressors can occur as a direct result of cardiovascular collapse and also warrants ICU monitoring.

PRACTICE POINT

Allergic reaction symptoms that should be treated as a medical emergency and prompt hospital admission include the following:

- Severe wheezing
- Shortness of breath
- Hypotension
- Altered mentation
- Hoarseness of voice
- Stridor

Early attention should focus on securing the airway and cardiopulmonary status. Patients who respond to therapy should be observed in the hospital for 24 hours. Patients who respond slowly or poorly to primary treatment strategies require intensive care unit (ICU) admission.

Reactions occurring in the hospital

While the mechanism of an allergic reaction occurring in the hospital is the same as the outpatient setting, there are specific triggers unique to the hospitalized patient. Additionally, allergic reactions that occur in the hospital have the potential to be severe, as parenteral administration of an allergen induces more frequent and severe responses than oral ingestion.

PRACTICE POINT

- Parenteral administration of an allergen induces more frequent and severe responses than oral ingestion. Therefore, allergic reactions in the hospital may occur more frequently or manifest more severely.

Medications cause the majority of anaphylactic reactions in hospitalized patients with the beta-lactam antimicrobials—specifically penicillin or penicillin analogues—causing most episodes. Because cephalosporins share structure, and up to 50% cross-reactivity, patients who have a history of *anaphylaxis* to penicillins should not be challenged with cephalosporins. The distinction between a reported history of allergy versus anaphylaxis to penicillins is important, as up to 90% of patients who endorse a history of a penicillin "allergy" (without anaphylaxis) do not exhibit IgE antibodies to penicillin. Cross-reactivity to cephalosporins in these patients is significantly lower (10–15%). Latex allergy may also pose a threat to those who have had recurrent exposure, particularly health care workers.

PRACTICE POINT

- Patients with a history of true anaphylaxis to penicillin should not be challenged with cephalosporins. However, a reported history of penicillin allergy (without anaphylaxis) bears significantly less cross-reactivity to cephalosporins.

Anaphylactoid reactions are responsible for most severe drug reactions in hospitalized patients. Radiocontrast media and opiates may directly trigger mast cell degranulation. The clinical presentation is often identical to anaphylaxis and may require similar therapeutic measures, including antihistamines, bronchodilators, steroids, and/or epinephrine. Hypersensitivity to radiocontrast dye is usually unrelated to the rate of infusion and can have either an immediate or a delayed onset. The immediate-onset hypersensitivity to contrast occurs within minutes of very small amounts of infused media. In the delayed-onset presentation, symptoms occur beyond 1 hour of infusion to as late as 1 week postexposure. Patients treated with nonsteroidal antiinflammatory drugs (NSAIDS) and aspirin may also be prone to severe anaphylactoid responses, particularly those with an underlying history of asthma, nasal polyps, or rhinosinusitis. Serum tryptase levels can be elevated in both IgE and non-immune-mediated hypersensitivity as mast cell activation occurs in both.

PRACTICE POINT

- Anaphylactoid reactions, including those due to radiocontrast media and opiates, are responsible for most severe drug reactions in hospitalized patients. The immediate-onset hypersensitivity to contrast dye occurs within minutes or, in delayed response, beyond 1 hour and as late as 1 week postexposure.

An emerging group of drugs causing an anaphylaxis-like syndrome (IgE as well as non-IgE mediated) are chemotherapeutic agents such as carboplatinum, cisplatinum, as well as the monoclonal biologicals such as cetuximab, rituximab, and others. The mechanisms incriminated include tumor lysis, cytokine storm, and hypersensitivity reactions. Some of these mechanisms can be prevented by premedication with steroids and/or antihistamines, and in recalcitrant cases desensitization has been a useful option.

ATOPY

Patients with a past medical history of atopic conditions such as asthma, seasonal allergies and eczema do not have an increased incidence of anaphylaxis to drugs. However, their reactions are more severe, and they are at greater risk for anaphylactic reactions to radiocontrast media, food or latex.

TRANSFUSION REACTIONS

Transfusion reactions to intravenous immunoglobulin (IVIG) can lead to allergic reactions in patients with IgA deficiency. These patients produce IgE and IgG autoantibodies against IgA and may experience a mast cell-mediated reaction ranging from urticaria or angioedema to anaphylaxis. Most transfusion reactions however, occur through the formation of immune complexes resulting in serum sickness (See Chapter 177, Transfusion of Blood Components, Derivatives, and Their Adverse Effects).

MANAGEMENT

INITIAL HOSPITAL TREATMENT

Successful management of severe allergic and nonallergic reactions requires prompt recognition and treatment. Patients with immediate hypersensitivity (histamine-mediated) reactions are managed with epinephrine, antihistamines and corticosteroids, whereas these treatment modalities have limited effectiveness in bradykinin-mediated reactions (ACE-inhibitor angioedema and HAE). In the acute setting the underlying mechanism may be difficult to distinguish, and patients experiencing symptoms of upper airway obstruction, acute respiratory failure or shock should be treated for an immediate hypersensitivity reaction with one or more of the medications listed below.

Epinephrine

Patients with marked upper airway obstruction, bronchospasm, or hypotension should be administered aqueous epinephrine *intravenously*: 0.1 mg (1:10,000) over 5–10 minutes or continuous infusion if necessary, 1 to 4 mcg/min. Patients with severe airway edema or stridor that is recalcitrant to initial therapy necessitate immediate intubation.

If intravenous access is not readily available or if the reaction is less severe, *intramuscular* (thigh) injection of epinephrine: 0.3–0.5 mg (1:1000) should be administered. Intramuscular (IM) thigh injections achieve much higher peak plasma epinephrine concentrations than epinephrine administered via intramuscular or subcutaneous injection into the upper arm. Racemic epinephrine via nebulizer can be administered as an adjunct or alone in cases of mild laryngeal swelling where IV/IM epinephrine is not indicated.

PRACTICE POINT

- Intramuscular thigh injections of epinephrine achieve much higher peak plasma concentrations than epinephrine administered via intramuscular or subcutaneous injection into the upper arm.

Antihistamines

An antihistamine H1 receptor antagonist, such as diphenhydramine 50mg, can be administered parenterally and repeated every 4–6 hours. H2 receptor antagonists (eg, ranitidine) should also be administered, and can provide additional benefit in controlling activation of histamine receptors in the splanchnic vascular bed.

Corticosteroids

Corticosteroids are often used in cases where antihistamines are unable to adequately control swelling. They may help to reduce inflammation and vascular permeability particularly in the late phase of the allergic response.

Beta2-adrenergic agonists

These agents, delivered via nebulizer relax bronchial smooth muscle and are commonly used in addition to oxygen in patients who present with wheezing secondary to bronchospasm. They have no effect on urticaria or angioedema.

Intravenous fluids and vasopressor therapy

Intravenous fluid resuscitation should begin immediately in hypotensive patients. Those with sustained hypotension following epinephrine and aggressive rehydration should be started on an epinephrine drip or other vasopressor agent such as phenylephrine. Patients taking beta-blockers who are refractory to vasopressor therapy should receive glucagon (1 mg in 1 L of D5W at 5–15 mL/min). Glucagon has positive inotropic and chronotropic effects mediated by cyclic adenosine monophosphate (AMP) (not beta receptors), which explains its usefulness as an adjunct therapy in hypotensive patients.

CONSULTATION

Most patients hospitalized for anaphylactic reactions should be seen by an ear, nose, and throat (ENT) specialist to assess the degree of airway edema. Outpatient referral to an allergist or pulmonologist is necessary to evaluate and assess the need for further workup. Skin testing has no utility in the hospital setting as mast cells will be refractory to an antigen challenge for several weeks. On rare occasions it may be necessary to initiate or continue therapy of a medication to which the patient has a history of severe allergy or anaphylaxis. In these instances an allergist or inpatient clinical pharmacist can oversee a desensitized protocol in which increasing increments of the drug are administered orally or intravenously. This procedure is not without risk and should be performed in an observed setting with emergency resuscitation equipment available.

PRACTICE POINT

- In patients experiencing anaphylaxis, skin testing has no utility in the hospital setting as mast cells will be refractory to an antigen challenge for several weeks.

PREVENTION

Patients with a history of anaphylactic and allergic reactions are at risk for recurrent episodes. Patient education, including avoiding allergens and self-medication, is critical to long-term prevention.

Allergy to radiocontrast media complicates management of hospitalized patients requiring important diagnostic radiographic studies. Any patient who has had a life-threatening reaction to radiocontrast media should not be given the same agent. For patients with a history of allergy to radiocontrast dye, prophylactic management should be directed to the type and severity of hypersensitivity. The classic premedication regimen involves giving those with a history of *urticaria* 50 mg of prednisone orally at 13, 7, and 1 hour prior to the procedure, and 25 mg intravenous diphenhydramine 1 hour prior to the procedure. Patients who have a history of *life threatening anaphylactoid reactions* (ie, angioedema, hypotension) should additionally be administered 25 mg of oral ephedrine and 300 mg of cimetidine orally 1 hour prior to the procedure. While premedication regimens may vary among institutions, the most important aspect is administering steroids at least 6 hours prior to the injection of contrast media. To further minimize the risk of reactions, many centers exclusively utilize nonionic low-osmolality radiocontrast media.

DISCHARGE PLANNING/FOLLOW-UP

Patient education prior to discharge should focus on the nature of the illness, severity of presentation, and precipitating factors. Patients should be able to recognize potential triggers and describe which substances may cross-react and cause allergic reactions. Patients should receive prescription instructions about self-administered autoinjectable epinephrine in the event of recurrent allergic reaction. In those patients with life-threatening anaphylaxis as well as those with food-related anaphylaxis, prescription of two doses of epinephrine has been recommended as part of the patient education process. Patients with severe reactions or reactions that affect regular activities or function should receive referral to an allergist for additional testing and/or desensitization. Lastly, the primary care physician must be notified of all adverse reactions occurring during the inpatient setting, and all such reactions should be clearly documented in the medical record. Medical alert bracelets should be ordered and worn by patients who have experienced life-threatening anaphylaxis and anaphylactoid reactions.

QUALITY IMPROVEMENT

Allergic reactions, when severe, may require prolonged ICU admission incurring significant cost. Proper triage may expedite appropriate treatment, preventing clinical decompensation and prolonged hospital stays. Consultation, both inpatient (ENT) and outpatient (allergist or pulmonologist) can help optimize therapy, elucidate etiology, and assist with critical pieces of patient and family education. Anticipatory guidance and follow-up education promote patient adherence and recognition of possible allergens and cross-reacting agents. Moreover, using premedication protocols, careful choice of radiocontrast media, and thorough documentation reduce cost by minimizing preventable adverse outcomes.

SUGGESTED READINGS

Brockow K, Christiansen C, Kanny G, et al. Management of hypersensitivity reactions to iodinated contrast media. *Allergy*. 2005;60:150–182.

Laporte JR, deLatorre FJ, Gadgil DA, et al. An epidemiologic study of severe anaphylactic and anaphylactoid reactions among hospital patients: methods and overall risk. The International Collaborative Study of Severe Anaphylaxis. *Epidemiology*. 1998:9:141–146.

Lieberman P, Comargo CA Jr, Bohlke K, et al. Epidemiology of anaphylaxis: findings of the American College of Allergy, Asthma and Immunology Epidemiology of Anaphylaxis Working Group. *Ann Allergy Asthma Immunol*. 2006;97:596–602.

Morgan BP. Hereditary angioedema—therapies old and new. *N Engl J Med*. 2010:363:581–583.

Sabroe RA, Black AK. Angiotensin-converting enzyme (ACE) inhibitors and angio-oedema. *Br J Dermatol*. 1997;136(2):153–158.

Sampson HA, Munoz-Furlong A, Bock SA, et al. Symposium on the definition and management of anaphylaxis: summary report. *J Allergy Clin Immunol*. 2005:115:584–591.

CHAPTER 238

Asthma

Fernando Holguin, MD, MPH
Jennifer E. Zora, BS

Key Clinical Questions

1. Which patients with asthma require hospital admission?
2. What are the evidence-based guidelines for treatment of asthma in the hospital?
3. What is the optimal dosing of systemic corticosteroids in the treatment of an acute asthma exacerbation?
4. Which asthma patients require admission to the intensive care unit?
5. When is intubation indicated in the case of severe asthma?
6. What conditions need to be met before discharging a patient from the hospital?

INTRODUCTION

Asthma is a chronic respiratory disease associated with reversible airflow obstruction, bronchial hyperresponsiveness (BHR), and airway inflammation that can be triggered by various stimuli including viral upper respiratory infection, environmental allergens, and occupational exposures, and can lead to recurrent episodes of wheezing, cough, and dyspnea.

EPIDEMIOLOGY

In the United States in 2009, the prevalence of asthma was 8.2% affecting 24.6 million people (17.5 million adults and 7.1 million children). Thus, asthma stands as one of the leading chronic diseases in the United States.

The prevalence of current asthma is higher in children (9.6%) compared to adults (7.7%), and in females (9.3%) compared to males (7.0%). There is considerable variation in asthma prevalence estimates across racial and ethnic groups, with African Americans having higher prevalence than Caucasians and Hispanics. However, within Hispanics, there is marked variation among different ethnic groups; for example, Puerto Ricans have the highest asthma prevalence in the U.S. population in contrast to Mexican Americans, who have the lowest prevalence rates. The reasons why there are large differences in asthma prevalence rates across races and ethnicities are poorly understood and are likely explained by multiple factors including genetic susceptibility, health care access, environmental exposures, and nutritional factors.

PRESENTATION

History and physical examination of the asthmatic patient reveal recurrent respiratory symptoms characterized by wheezing, cough, and chest tightness. Trigger exposures may exacerbate respiratory symptoms and may include exposure to airway irritants (smoke, strong fumes, air pollution, etc.), aeroallergens, respiratory infections, and cold air. Psychological stress and physical exercise are also known to trigger respiratory symptoms in the absence of any other concomitant exposures; however, in many instances trigger factors are not identified.

Respiratory symptoms may have a nocturnal predominance and are frequently more severe in the morning after waking up, when airflows are usually lower. The frequency and severity of respiratory symptoms is highly variable and may stem from sporadic to constant and from barely noticeable to life threatening.

PRACTICE POINT

- Respiratory symptoms may have a nocturnal predominance and are frequently more severe in the morning after waking up, when airflows are usually lower.

PATHOPHYSIOLOGY

Although asthma is generally regarded as a single disease entity, it is likely a syndrome composed of a heterogeneous group of pathophysiologic mechanisms (different triggers, risk factors, patterns of inflammation, and response to treatment, etc.) that cause airway obstruction and common respiratory symptoms. *Persistent adult asthma* phenotypes have been broadly divided into the following categories: clinical or physiologic phenotypes (severity defined, exacerbation prone, treatment resistant, and adult versus child onset); phenotypes related to triggers (aspirin sensitivity, environmental and occupational exposures, menses, and exercise); and inflammatory phenotypes (eosinophilic, neutrophilic, and pauci-inflammatory). Many nonallergic phenotypes and phenotypes that begin in adulthood likely have very different pathophysiologies than allergic asthma. Although this classification scheme is useful to describe the pathophysiology of asthma, considerable overlap among categories exists.

In allergic asthma, an allergen is initially exposed to dendritic cells functioning as antigen-presenting cells. These cells interact with B lymphocytes to produce immunoglobulin E (IgE) in the context of appropriate cytokine and T lymphocyte interactions. Circulating IgE binds high-affinity receptors in blood and tissue mast cells and low-affinity receptors on the surface of lymphocytes, eosinophils, neutrophils, platelets, and macrophages, thus recruiting these cells to the airways. Subsequent exposures to the same antigen will crossbridge IgE bound to mast cell receptors, facilitating mast cell degranulation and release of various cytokines and chemokines, which recruit additional inflammatory cells to the lungs.

The initial release of histamine and leukotrienes from mast cells leads to constriction of airway smooth muscle and can lead to airway obstruction. The *early phase* of inflammation encompasses the response in the first hour and is followed by a *later phase* within four to six hours, in which prolonged airway obstruction develops due to cytokine release from resident epithelial cells and inflammatory cells, as well as recruited inflammatory cells. In addition to airway obstruction, this inflammatory response leads to airway edema, mucous hypersecretion, and bronchial hyperresponsivness (BHR). Over time and in relation to the degree of underlying inflammation and disease severity, BHR becomes nonspecific; that is, BHR can be elicited through a variety of nonallergen factors such as strong fumes, air pollution, cold air, exercise, and psychological stress.

PRACTICE POINT

- The *early phase* of asthma exacerbation inflammation occurs in the first hour and is followed by a later phase within four to six hours, in which prolonged airway obstruction develops due to cytokine release from resident epithelial cells and inflammatory cells, as well as recruited inflammatory cells. This inflammatory response leads to airway edema, mucous hypersecretion, bronchial hyperresponsiveness, and consequent airway obstruction.

DIFFERENTIAL DIAGNOSIS

Many diseases present with similar respiratory symptoms to asthma, and clinicians should maintain a high index of suspicion for alternate respiratory diagnoses (**Table 238-1**). Wheezing and cough can occur with congestive heart failure, which may be associated with airway vascular congestion and peribronchial cuffing secondary to pulmonary edema, bibasilar inspiratory crackles on auscultation, and an elevated serum brain natriuretic peptide (BNP). Airway obstruction (eg, foreign body, tumor, laryngeal edema, anaphylaxis, and other) could lead to stridor, which can be mistaken for wheezing.

Paradoxical vocal fold motion disorder (PVFMD), a poorly understood disease that can mimic asthma, is characterized by abnormal adduction of the vocal cord folds during inhalation and occasionally during exhalation, which can lead to complete or partial transient laryngeal occlusion. During these paradoxical vocal cord motion events, patients experience significant respiratory distress characterized by cough, dyspnea, a choking sensation, and wheezing or stridor. Relief with short acting beta-agonists or other medications used for asthma control is minimal to none. The severity and repetitive nature of symptoms caused by PVFMD lead to high health care utilization.

TABLE 238-1 Asthma Exacerbation Differential Diagnosis

Mechanical airway obstruction (eg, foreign body)
Structural airway abnormality (eg, tumor)
Aspiration or severe gastroesophageal reflux disease
Paradoxical vocal fold motion disorder
Heart failure
Chronic obstructive pulmonary disease
Vasculitis
Bronchiectasis
Pulmonary embolism
Interstitial lung disease
Bronchial papillomatosis
Bronchopulmonary aspergillosis
Recurrent polychondritis with airway involvement
Hypersensitivity pneumonititis
Sarcoidosis with endobronchial involvement

PVFMD is commonly encountered among patients referred for difficult or refractory asthma and chronic cough evaluation. However, *among patients referred to tertiary centers for refractory asthma or cough, the prevalence of PVFMD can be as high as 40% to 50%.* Many PVFMD patients inappropriately receive chronic systemic steroids. Patients with PVFMD commonly have frequent emergency department visits and may be intubated for respiratory distress.

Differentiating asthma and chronic obstructive lung disease (COPD) can be very difficult, and at times impossible. (See Chapter 239 for a comprehensive review of COPD). Although asthmatics would be expected to have a more reversible airway obstructive process than patients with COPD, this characteristic occurs with high variability in COPD patients, as up to one-third or more of patients with COPD will have a reversible component to their obstruction. Both disorders can coexist in the same patient as a result of chronic smoking and/or airway remodeling. Emphysematous changes on chest computed tomography (CT) and/or severe airway obstruction with hyperinflation in the absence of an acute exacerbation would favor the diagnosis of COPD over asthma.

Bronchiectasis can also present with airway obstruction and symptoms compatible with asthma. However, clinical features that reduce the likelihood of asthma diagnosis include chronic sputum production at baseline, recurrent lower-tract respiratory infections, hemoptysis, and inspiratory crackles on auscultation. Chest CT should detect bronchiectasis. In approximately 1% to 2% of patients, bronchiectasis and asthma coexist with bronchopulmonary aspergillosis (ABPA). In this case, bronchiectasis occurs predominantly centrally, with areas of mucoid impaction. Patients with ABPA usually have IgE levels greater than 1000 ng/ml with peripheral blood eosinophilia more than 10% specific Aspergillous IgG or IgE antibodies. A negative intradermal test for Aspergillus antigen adequately rules out this condition.

TABLE 238-2 Triage Decision Making Based on Asthma Severity

Asthma Exacerbation Severity	Representative Symptoms	Spirometric Measurement (PEF or FEV_1)	Triage/Admission
Mild	Dyspnea with activity	> 70% predicted (or personal best)	Home
Moderate	Dyspnea limits typical daily activity	40–69% predicted (or personal best)	Often requires ED visit +/– hospital admission (if no rapid ED improvement)
Severe	Dyspnea at rest that interferes with conversation	< 40% predicted (or personal best)	Hospital or ICU admission
Life-threatening	Dyspnea significantly limiting speech	< 25% predicted (or personal best)	Hospital or ICU admission

ED, emergency department; FEV_1, forced expiratory volume in 1 second; ICU, intensive care unit; PEF, peak expiratory flow.

PRACTICE POINT

- *Nonrespiratory symptoms* may occur in conjunction with asthma syndromes, including rhinitis and eczematous rash within the "atopic triad," eosinophilia and/or vasculitis in Churg-Strauss; nasal polyps in aspirin-sensitive asthma (Samter syndrome); and pulmonary infiltrates and allergy to *Aspergillus* in allergic bronchopulmonary aspergillosis.

DIAGNOSIS

Asthma diagnosis must be confirmed by pulmonary function testing that shows evidence of airway obstruction with a bronchodilator response greater than or equal to 12% (or 200 mL) improvement of the forced expiratory volume in one second (FEV_1) after short-acting bronchodilators. Bronchodilation should only be assessed after witholding asthma medications at least 4 hours for short-acting β2-receptor agonists (SABA) and 24 hours for long-acting β2-receptor agonists (LABA).

PRACTICE POINT

Asthma diagnosis

- Pulmonary function testing (PFT) shows evidence of airway obstruction with a bronchodilator response greater than or equal to 12% or 200 cc of FEV_1 after a short-acting bronchodilator. Bronchodilation should only be assessed after withholding asthma medications (at least 4 hours for short acting β-agonists and 24 hours for long acting β-agonists).

In cases where there is no evidence of airway obstruction or bronchodilation on initial pulmonary function testing, patients should undergo testing with methacholine (a cholinergic agent used to elicit bronchial constriction) to exclude asthma. A positive test occurs when there is a reduction in FEV_1 greater than or equal to 20% (percent change 20 or PC20) from the baseline postmethacholine level. The methacholine test is very sensitive (ie, it would be unusual to have asthma with a negative test) but lacks specificity, such that a positive test can be seen in the setting of other airway diseases or allergies. Diligent assessment for presence or absence of asthma through testing and evaluation of treatment response will help eliminate the approximately 30% of patients who are incorrectly diagnosed with this disease clinically (false positive) and are unnecessarily treated with corticosteroids.

TRIAGE AND HOSPITAL ADMISSION

When patients with severe asthma exacerbations do not adequately respond to outpatient therapy, clinical assessment should include a brief history, physical examination (assess respiratory rate and heart rate, use of accessory respiratory muscles, chest retraction, neck and pulmonary auscultation, oxygen saturation), and pulmonary function testing (FEV_1 or peak expiratory flow [PEF] measurement) to help triage for possible hospital admission.

Several published guidelines aid clinicians in admission decision making. A triage system based on the history of symptoms and spirometric measurement (PEF or FEV_1) can aid triage decision making (**Table 238-2**).

Patients admitted with high risk of asthma-related death (**Table 238-3**) should receive very close inpatient monitoring, possibly in the intensive care unit (ICU), based on response to initial therapy.

If necessary, repeated assessment of severity, including signs and symptoms as well as PEF or FEV_1 measurements, help determine the need for hospital admission (**Figure 238-1**).

MANAGEMENT

INITIAL TREATMENT FOR ACUTE ASTHMA EXACERBATION

Immediate treatment of significant asthma exacerbation can start with emergency medical services (EMS) and include supplemental oxygen, inhaled SABA, anticholinergic agents, and oral systemic corticosteroids using established protocols under appropriate

TABLE 238-3 Risk Factors for Asthma-related Death

- Previous severe exacerbation (intubation or intensive care unit admission for asthma)
- ≥ 2 hospitalizations or > 3 emergency department visits in the past 12 months
- Use of > 2 canisters of short-acting beta-agonist (SABA) per month
- Reduced ability to perceive airway obstruction or worsening symptoms
- Low socioeconomic status or urban residence
- Illicit drug use
- Psychiatric disease or severe psychosocial stress
- Comorbidities, such as cardiovascular disease or other chronic lung disease

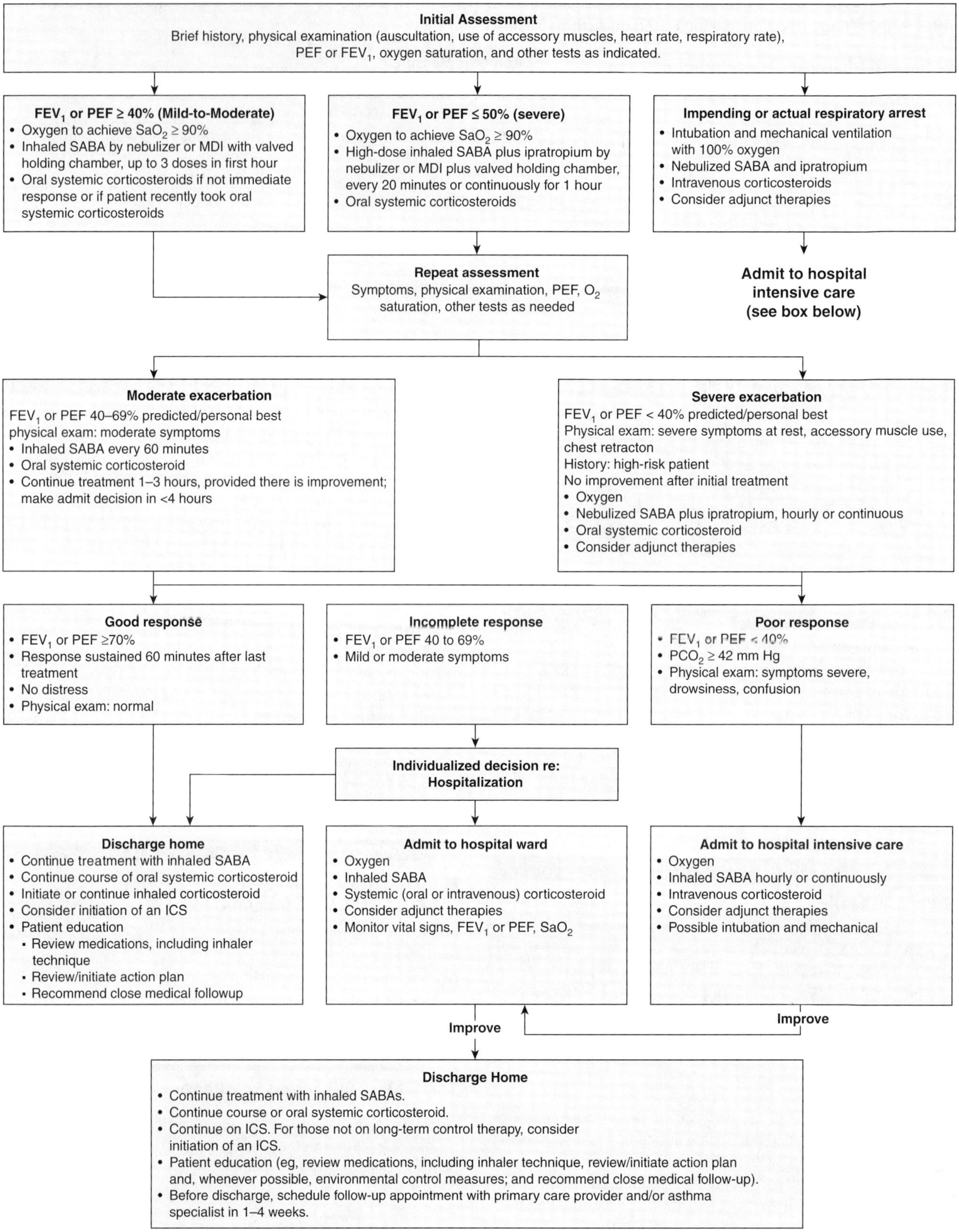

Figure 238-1 *Management of asthma exacerbations: emergency department and hospital-based care. FEV_1, forced expiratory volume in 1 second; ICS, inhaled corticosteroid; MDI, metered-dose inhaler; PCO_2, partial pressure carbon dioxide; PEF, peak expiratory flow; SABA, short-acting beta2-agonist; SaO_2, oxygen saturation. (From the Guidelines for the Diagnosis and Management of Asthma of the National Asthma Education and Prevention Program (NAEPP) Expert Panel Report 3, 2007.)*

medical supervision. Continued upon arrival in the emergency department, supplemental oxygen can correct hypoxemia in moderate and severe asthma exacerbations. Repetitive or continuous administration of SABA and ipratropium via metered-dose inhaler (MDI) or nebulizer can quickly reverse airflow obstruction, and continuous administration is more efficacious. Oral systemic corticosteroids decrease inflammation and are used to supplement treatment in asthmatics who fail to respond adequately or at all to SABA treatment. **Table 238-4** lists medications and dosages for adults with acute asthma exacerbation.

TABLE 238-4 Dosages of Drugs for Acute Asthma Exacerbations

Medication	Adult Dose	Comments (Not All Inclusive)
Inhaled Short-Acting Beta$_2$-Agonists		
Albuterol Nebulizer Solution (0.63 mg/3 mL, 1.25 mg/3 mL, 2.5 mg/3 mL, 5.0 mg/mL)	2.5–5 mg every 20 minutes for 3 doses, then 2.5–10 mg every 1–4 hours as needed, or 10–15 mg/hour continuously	Only selective beta$_2$-agonists are recommended. For optimal delivery, dilute aerosols to a minimum of 3 mL at as flow of 6–8 L/min. Use large volume nebulizers for continuous administration. May mix with ipratropium nebulizer solution.
MDI (90 mcg/puff, 200 puffs per canister)	4–8 puffs every 20 minutes up to 4 hours, then every 1–4 hours as needed	In mild-to-moderate exacerbations, MDI plus valved holding chamber (VHC) is as effective as nebulized therapy with appropriate administration technique and coaching by trained personnel.
Levalbuterol (R-albuterol) Nebulizer solution (0.63 mg/3 mL, 1.25 mg/0.5 mL, 1.25 mg/3 mL)	1.25–2.5 mg every 20 minutes for 3 doses, then 1.25–5 mg every 1–4 hours as needed	Levalbuterol administered in one-half the mg dose of albuterol provides comparable efficacy and safety. Has not been evaluated by continuous nebulization.
MDI (45 mcg/puff)	See albuterol MDI dose	
Systemic Beta$_2$-Agonists		
Epinephrine 1:1,000 (1 mg/mL)	0.3–0.5 mg every 20 minutes for 3 subcutaneous doses	No proven advantage of systemic therapy over aerosol.
Terbutaline (1 mg/mL)	0.25 mg every 20 minutes for 3 subcutaneous doses	
Anticholinergics		
Ipatropium bromide Nebulizer solution (0.25 mg/mL)	0.5 mg every 20 minutes for 3 doses, then as needed	May mix in same nebulizer with albuterol. *Should not be used as first-line therapy*. Should be added to SABA therapy for severe exacerbations. The addition of ipratropium has not been shown to provide further benefit once the patient is hospitalized.
MDI (Each puff contains 18 mcg ipratropium bromide and 90 mcg of albuterol.)	8 puffs every 20 minutes as needed up to 3 hours	
Ipratropium with albuterol Nebulizer solution (Each 3 mL vial contains 0.5 mg ipratropium bromide and 2.5 mg abuterol.)	3 mL every 20 minutes for 3 doses, then as needed	
MDI (Each puff contains 18 mcg ipratropium bromide and 90 mcg of albuterol).	8 puffs every 20 minutes as needed up to 3 hours	
Systemic corticosteroids (Applies to all three corticosteroids)		
Prednisone Methylpredisolone Prednisolone	40–80 mg/day in 1 or 2 divided doses until PEF reaches 70% of predicted or personal best	For outpatient "burst," use 40–60 mg in single or 2 divided doses for total of 5–10 days in adults. There is no known advantage for higher doses of corticosteroids in severe asthma, and there is no advantage for intravenous administration over oral therapy with a normal functioning gastrointestinal tract. The total course of systemic corticosteroids for asthma exacerbation requiring an ED visit or hospitalization may last from 3–10 days. A taper is only required for a course lasting greater than one week, and may only be necessary for a course greater than 10 days. ICS can be started at any point during treatment of an acute asthma exacerbation, but should not be used alone as therapy for an acute asthma exacerbation.

ED, emergency department; ICS, inhaled corticosteroid; MDI, metered-dose inhaler; PEF, peak expiratory flow; SABA, short-acting beta-agonist.
(From the Guidelines for the Diagnosis and Management of Asthma of the National Asthma Education and Prevention Program (NAEPP) Expert Panel Report 3, 2007.)

CONTINUED THERAPY AFTER ASSESSMENT OF ASTHMA SYMPTOMS AND SEVERITY

Management and treatment should be based on the level of asthma severity (see Figure 238-1). *Severe exacerbation is marked by an FEV_1 or PEF less than 40%,* and these patients should receive supplemental oxygen to achieve a saturation level of oxygen in hemoglobin (SaO_2) greater than or equal to 90%, administration of continuous SABA and ipratropium by nebulizer or metered-dose inhaler (MDI), and oral systemic corticosteroids. Patient drowsiness or increased blood partial pressure of carbon dioxide (pCO_2) levels may signal impending respiratory failure and the need for immediate intubation and mechanical ventilation. Following intubation, the patient should continue to receive nebulized SABA and intravenous corticosteroids.

Moderate exacerbation is be marked by an FEV_1 or PEF greater than or equal to 40% and less than 69%, and these patients should receive supplemental oxygen, inhaled SABA (up to three doses in the first hour, and then hourly), and possibly oral systemic corticosteroids if (1) there is no immediate response to therapy or (2) the patient has recently taken systemic corticosteroids.

Repeat assessment of severity and response to therapy, including assessment of symptom severity, physical examination, PEF, and oxygen saturation, should guide continued treatment. Severe exacerbation of asthma generally does not improve after initial treatment. Treatment of mild to moderate exacerbation may continue for one to three hours, and the decision of whether the patient requires admission may be made at approximately four hours following presentation.

A poor response to initial therapy requires admission to the ICU and is demonstrated by an FEV_1 or PEF less than 40%, a PCO_2 greater than or equal to 42 millimeters mercury (mm Hg), and use of accessory muscles, chest retraction, severe drowsiness or confusion on physical exam. *An incomplete response to initial therapy* comprises an FEV_1 or FEF between 40% and 69% of predicted, and requires case-specific decision making regarding hospital admission or discharge home. *A good response to therapy* is defined by an FEV_1 or PEF greater than or equal to 70% and a response that is sustained for at least an hour after the last treatment, a normal physical exam, and no signs of distress; such patients may be discharged home.

IN-HOSPITAL ASTHMA MANAGEMENT

In-hospital asthma treatment should consist of bronchodilator (BD) therapy and daily systemic steroids. Steroid therapy (oral or intravenous) at a dose ranging from 40–80 mg/day of prednisone or equivalent steroid dosing is optimal (divided into two daily doses). No data support benefit from higher steroid doses. The frequency of SABAs should be guided by the level of severity and the clinical response of the patient. BD therapy, more frequent or continuous at the beginning of hospital stay, may range from continuous therapy to every four to six hours during hospitalization. Inhaled steroids should be initiated during hospital stay prior to discharge, but are not used to manage acute asthma exacerbations.

Several treatments have limited or no utility in the treatment of acute asthma exacerbation based on available evidence. Routine antibiotic administration does not have a role in acute asthma exacerbation. Intravenous magnesium and helium-oxygen therapy (Heliox™) have limited evidence to support their use in asthma exacerbations, but may be considered as additional adjunctive therapies in patients not responding to other recommended therapies. No evidence supports continued use of anticholinergics during the hospital stay.

Frequent assessment of pulmonary function (PEF or FEV_1), in addition to symptoms and physical exam findings, is indicated to help determine continued need for inpatient stay and therapy. PEF or FEV_1 should be assessed at least daily in patients admitted (but not intubated) with asthma exacerbation. Assessments should also be made whenever there is perceived clinical deterioration during the inpatient stay, despite aggressive medical therapies.

PRACTICE POINT

- Steroid therapy (oral or intravenous) at a dose ranging from 40–80 mg/day of prednisone or equivalent steroid dosing is optimal (divided into two daily doses). No data support benefit from higher steroid doses.

CONSULTATION

Inpatient consultation

Many hospitals have limited or no availability of allergy and immunology specialists for consultation. Some hospitals have pulmonary and critical care specialists available for consultation. Hospitalists should consider inpatient specialty consultation when patients with severe or life-threatening asthma exacerbations fail to respond to initial therapies within 24 to 48 hours or require intubation. They may also consider specialty consultation when patients with asthma require frequent hospital admissions or emergency department visits despite medical regimen augmentation and adherence.

Outpatient consultation and referral

Patients classified as having severe asthma should be referred to an allergy and immunology specialist or pulmonology specialist for evaluation. Chronic asthma criteria that indicate specialty referral based on severity include at least one major criterion or at least two minor criteria (**Table 238-5**).

COMPLICATIONS AND PROGNOSIS

For each age group through age 25 to 34 years, the death rate from asthma is less than 1 per 10,000 persons with asthma. The highest at-risk-based death rate is in persons aged greater than 65 years (10.5 per 10,000 with current asthma). Females have higher at-risk-based death rates than males (2.3 per 10,000 and 1.8 per 10,000, respectively). For most age groups, males have higher rates than females; only for persons aged greater than 65 years was the rate for females (11.3 per 10,000 with current asthma) higher than for

TABLE 238-5 Indications for Outpatient Specialty (Allergy or Immunology Specialist or Pulmonary Specialist) Referral, One Major Criterion or Two Minor Criteria

Asthma severity major criteria:
- Use of high-dose inhaled steroids for more thn 50% of the preceding year
- Continuous or near-continuous oral steroids

Asthma severity minor criteria:
- Daily controller medication in addition to inhaled steroids
- Beta-agonist required daily or near-daily
- Persistant airway obstruction
- One or more urgent care visits for asthma per year
- Three or more oral corticosteroid bursts per year
- Clinical deterioration with reduction in oral steroid dose
- Near-fatal asthma event in the past

males (9.1). Blacks have higher at-risk-based death rates (3.4) than whites (1.9). This is true for males and females, adults and children, and for each age group. Among regions, the highest asthma death rate per 10,000 with current asthma occurred in the Western United States (2.5).

DISCHARGE PLANNING

DISCHARGE READINESS CRITERIA

Consensus guidelines have been published regarding objective criteria that need to be met for the appropriate discharge of an asthmatic patient. However, these guidelines represent expert opinion and have not yet been supported by clinical trials. In general, a patient may be discharged after achieving an FEV_1 greater than or equal to 70% predicted in conjunction with signs of clinical improvement, or on the basis of marked clinical improvement alone.

THE ASTHMA ACTION PLAN

Following acute asthma exacerbation, patients should continue inhaled SABA, complete a course of oral systemic corticosteroids, and continue or possibly initiate inhaled corticosteroids. Patient education during hospital stay and at discharge should include a focus on asthma precipitants, avoidance of environmental exposures that might trigger exacerbation, the prescribed medication regimen, how to control and prevent symptoms by adjusting medication dosages (if necessary), and how to properly use medications, especially inhalers.

Patients should receive counseling prior to discharge regarding their home management. A discharge *home management plan* should be prescribed and given to the patient in a written format so that she might be able to recognize and respond to signs of asthma exacerbation, including decreased PEF. The action plan should outline medication adjustments that can be done at home by the patient to respond to exacerbation, including increased used of SABA, and if needed, oral corticosteroids. Patients should be instructed to avoid or reduce contact with allergens or environmental irritants, including tobacco smoke (both primary and secondhand). The patient should monitor his/her response to treatment and communicate with a physician about signs of deterioration, such as decreased responsiveness to SABA.

To prevent relapse or additional exacerbations, in conjunction with a written asthma action plan, follow-up care should occur within one to four weeks of hospital discharge. More rapid follow-up should occur in patients with more severe exacerbations or those with more medical comorbidities. At follow-up, the patient and health care provider should review the asthma action plan, discuss medication adherence and environmental control, and address barriers to medication use and environmental control if necessary. The provider may consider step-up or step-down care based on the level of asthma control at that time and decide upon further asthma education in the form of classes or workshops, if indicated.

LONGITUDINAL AND OUTPATIENT THERAPEUTICS OR REGIMEN AUGMENTATION

Recent asthma guidelines recommend a focus on monitoring response to treatment instead of asthma severity. Two parameters help define asthma control: *impairment* and *risk*. The current (or recent) frequency and intensity of symptoms and functional limitations define *impairment* in asthma patients. *Risk* represents the likelihood of asthma exacerbations and progressive decline in lung function.

The outpatient pharmacologic treatment of asthma aims to reduce impairment (prevent chronic symptoms, maintain lung function, meet the family and patient's expectations) and risk (prevent exacerbations, prevent loss of lung function, and provide optimal therapeutics with minimal side effects).

Outpatient pharmacologic agents are prescribed based on the degree of asthma severity: intermittent, mild, moderate, or severe. The degree of asthma severity is ascertained by determining the level of impairment and risk. *Impairment* includes multiple measures such as frequency of daytime and nocturnal respiratory symptoms, use of SABAs, and lung function (FEV_1 and FEV_1/forced vital capacity [FVC]). *Risk* involves determining the number of exacerbations requiring oral or systemic steroids per year. Classification of asthma severity for persons age 12 years or older is described by a group of asthma experts working on behalf of the National Institutes of Health (NIH) and the National Heart and Lung Blood Institute (NHLBI) called the National Asthma Education and Prevention Program Expert Panel Report # 3 (EPR3) (**Figure 238-2**).

Based on asthma classification, from intermittent to persistent (mild, moderate, severe) patients may require various forms of inhaled and oral therapies (**Figure 238-3**). Stepwise management of chronic intermittent or persistent asthma includes the following stages: intermittent asthma, step 1; mild asthma, step 2; moderate asthma, step 3; and severe asthma, steps 4, 5, or 6. The medications indicated for each step include the following: step 1, SABA taken as needed; step 2, low-dose inhaled steroids (ICS); step 3, low-dose ICS + LABA; step 4, medium-dose ICS + LABA; step 5, high-dose ICS + LABA and consider omalizumab (humanized antibody that interferes with binding of IgE to the high-affinity IgE receptor FcεRI) for patients who have allergies and meet IgE-level criteria; step 6, high-dose ICS + LABA + oral corticosteroids and omalizumab if patient meets criteria. For steps 3, 4, 5, and 6, a short course of oral systemic corticosteroids should be considered.

LABA medications should be limited to patients who remain poorly controlled on medium- to high-dose ICS, as LABAs have been associated with increased mortality risk in recent large systematic reviews. LABAs should never be used as monotherapy, and the FDA has released new recommendations that include stopping LABA in patients once asthma control is achieved with ICS.

Patients deemed to be well controlled are maintained on the current step therapy with regular follow up every one to six months to maintain control, and step-down should be considered if a patient has remained well controlled for at least three months. For poorly controlled patients, the recommendation is to step-up one step and reevaluate in four to six weeks. For very poorly controlled patients, the approach is to add systemic corticosteroids, step-up one to two steps, and reevaluate in two weeks.

QUALITY IMPROVEMENT TO ADDRESS PERFORMANCE GAPS

SECONDARY PREVENTION

Strategies for secondary prevention of asthma exacerbation should be utilized in conjunction with frequent follow-up with a managing physician and education about asthma triggers and how and when to take medications to keep asthma symptoms well controlled and prevent asthma attacks.

All asthmatics should receive the influenza vaccine annually. Adults with asthma between the ages of 19 and 64 should get a single dose of Prevnar 13 pneumococcal vaccine; all asthmatics adults over age 65 should receive the Prevnar vaccine as well as a second dose five years after the first dose. Vaccinations during hospitalization for an acute asthma exacerbation are appropriate for patients who have not yet received their appropriate vaccinations. Environmental and occupational allergens and irritants should be controlled; tobacco smoking and exposure to secondary smoke should be avoided. Allergic immunotherapy and/or the administration of anti-immunoglobulin E (IgE) may be

Components of Severity		Classification of Asthma Severity ≥ 12 years of age			
		Intermittent	Persistent		
			Mild	Moderate	Severe
Impairment Normal FEV_1/FVC: 08–19 yr 85% 20–39 yr 80% 40–59 yr 75% 60–80 yr 70%	Symptoms	≤ 2 days/week	> 2 days/week but not daily	Daily	Throughout the day
	Nighttime awakenings	≤ 2 times/month	3–4 times/month	> 1 time/week, but not nightly	Often 7 times/ week
	Short-acting $beta_2$-agonist use for symptom control (not prevention of EIB)	≤ 2 days/week	> 2 days/ week but not daily, and not more than on any day	Daily	Several times per day
	Interference with normal activity	None	Minor limitation	Some limitation	Extremely limited
	Lung function	• Normal FEV_1 between exacerbations • FEV_1 > 80% predicted • FEV_1/FVC normal	• FEV_1 > 80% predicted • FEV_1/FVC normal	• FEV_1 > 60% but < 80% predicted • FEV_1/FVC reduced 5%	• FEV_1 < 60% predicted • FEV_1/FVC reduced > 5%
Risk	Exacerbations requiring oral systemic corticosteroids	0–1/year (see notes)		≥ 2/year (see notes)	
		Consider severity and interval since last exacerbation. Frequency and severity may fluctuate over time for patients in any severity category. Relative annual risk of exacerbations may be related to FEV_1.			
Recommended Step for Initiating Treatment **(See "Stepwise Approach for Managing Asthma" for treatment steps.)**		**Step 1**	**Step 2**	**Step 3**	**Step 4 or 5**
				And consider short course of oral systemic corticosteroids.	
		In 2–6 weeks, evaluate level of asthma control that is achieved and adjust therapy accordingly.			

Figure 238-2 *Classifying asthma severity and initiating treatment in youths ≥ 12 years of age and adults: assessing severity and initiating treatment for patients who are not currently taking long-term control medications.*

Notes:

- *The stepwise approach is meant to assist, not replace, the clinical decision-making required to meet individual patient needs.*
- *Level of severity is determined by assessment of both impairment and risk. Assess impairment domain by patient's/caregiver's recall of previous two to four weeks and spirometry. Assign severity to the most severe category in which any feature occurs.*
- *At present, there are inadequate data to correspond frequencies of exacerbations with different levels of asthma severity. In general, more frequent and intense exacerbations (eg, requiring urgent, unscheduled care, hospitalization, or ICU admission) indicate greater underlying disease severity. For treatment purposes, patients who had two or more exacerbations requiring oral systemic corticosteroids in the past year may be considered the same as patients who have persistent asthma, even in the absence of impairment levels consistent with persistent asthma.*

EIB, exercise-induced bronchospasm; FEV_1, forced expiratory volume in 1 second; FVC, forced vital capacity; ICU, intensive care unit. (From the Guidelines for the Diagnosis and Management of Asthma of the National Asthma Education and Prevention Program (NAEPP) Expert Panel Report 3, 2007.)

utilized in the treatment of allergic asthma. Leukotriene modifiers are useful in some patients, especially those with aspirin-sensitive asthma.

Control of comorbid disease may contribute to improved asthma and symptom control, including the following conditions.

Gastroesophageal reflux disease

Gastroesophageal reflux disease (GERD), although once thought to negatively impact asthma control, does not appear to directly influence asthma symptoms and severity. However, GERD is a known risk factor for vocal cord dysfunction (VCD), which mimics many of the respiratory symptoms associated with asthma. H2 receptor antagonists and proton-pump inhibitors may be used to help control GERD symptoms.

Rhinitis

Because patients with atopy have analogous upper and lower airway symptoms in response to similar allergen exposures, asthma and rhinitis can be closely intertwined. Also, in many patients, controlling the upper respiratory symptoms will lead to better asthma control, explained by improvements in allergic inflammation throughout the airway and/or reduced postnasal discharge,

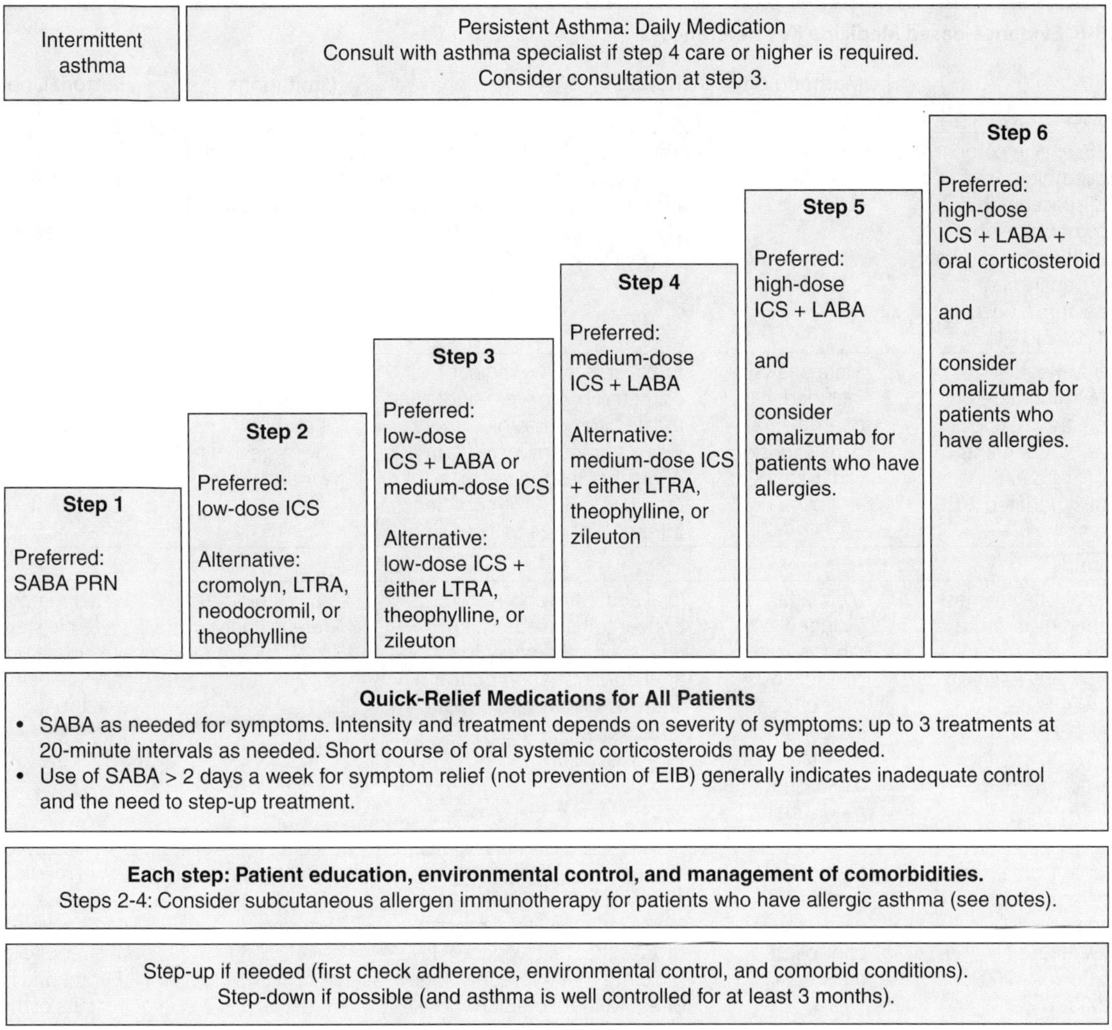

Figure 238-3 *Stepwise approach for managing asthma in adults and youths 12 years of age or older.*
Alphabetical order is used when more than one treatment option is listed within either preferred or alternative therapy.
Notes:
- *The stepwise approach is meant to assist, not replace, the clinical decision-making required to meet individual patient needs.*
- *If alternative treatment is used and response is inadequate, discontinue it, and use the preferred treatment before stepping up.*
- *Zileuton is a less desirable alternative due to limited studies as adjunctive therapy and the need to monitor liver function. Theophylline requires monitoring of serum concentration levels.*
- *In step 6, before oral corticosteroids are introduced, a trial of high-dose ICS + LABA + either LTRA, theophylline, or zileuton may be considered, although this approach has not been studied in clinical trials.*
- *Steps 1, 2, and 3 preferred therapies are based on Evidence A; step 3 alternative therapy is based on Evidence A for LTRA, Evidence B for theophylline, and Evidence D for zileuton. Step 4 preferred therapy is based on Evidence B, and alternative therapy is based on Evidence B for LTRA and theophylline and Evidence D for zileuton. Step 5 preferred therapy is based on Evidence B. Step 6 preferred therapy is based on (EPR-2 1997) and Evidence B for omalizumab.*
- *Immunotherapy for steps 2 to 4 is based on Evidence B for house-dust mites, animal danders, and pollens; evidence is weak or lacking for molds and cockroaches. Evidence is strongest for immunotherapy with single allergens. The role of allergy in asthma is greater in children than in adults.*
- *Clinicians who administer immunotherapy or omalizumab should be prepared and equipped to identify and treat anaphylaxis that may occur.*

ICS, inhaled corticosteroid; LABA, long-acting inhaled beta$_2$-agonist; LTRA, leukotriene receptor antagonist; SABA, inhaled short-acting beta$_2$-agonist. (From the Guidelines for the Diagnosis and Management of Asthma of the National Asthma Education and Prevention Program (NAEPP) Expert Panel Report 3, 2007.)

which can also lead to VCD and asthma-like symptoms. Oral loratidine and/or nasal steroids may be utilized for treatment of rhinitis.

Obesity

Obesity, reflected by body mass index (BMI) greater than 30 kilograms per meter of height squared, serves as an important risk factor in asthma severity and in adult-onset asthma. The mechanisms by which obesity affects asthma are unknown, but appear unrelated to airway or systemic inflammation.

Vitamin D deficiency

Vitamin D deficiency can lead to impaired lung function measured by FEV_1, increased airway hyperresponsiveness (AHR) measured by

TABLE 238-6 Evidence-based Medicine Key References

Study	Methodology	Results	Limitations	Bottom Line
Beta-agonists				
Newman KB, et al. A comparison of albuterol administered by MDI and spacer with albuterol by nebulizer in adults presenting to an urban emergency department with acute asthma. *Chest.* 2002;121(4):1036–1041.	Prospective, open-label study.	There was a statistically greater improvement in peak flow rates in the MDI/spacer group (126.8 versus 111.9 L/min, respectively; $p = 0.002$).	Nonrandomized, nonconcurrent study design.	SABA is at least as effective when delivered via MDI compared with nebulizer.
Cates CJ, et al. Regular treatment with salmeterol for chronic asthma: serious adverse events. Cochrane Database of Systematic Reviews 2008, updated 2010.	Meta-analysis; included controlled parallel design clinical trials, +/– blinding.	In patients taking regular salmeterol who were not taking inhaled corticosteroids, there was a significant increase in risk of asthma-related death, odds ratio (OR) 9.52 (95% confidence interval [CI]) 1.24 to 73.09).	Rare mortality and occurrence of serious adverse events warrants further study.	In patients not taking corticosteroids, there is an increased risk of asthma-related death for patients taking salmeterol.
Corticosteroids				
Rowe BH, et al. Effectiveness of steroid therapy in acute exacerbations of asthma: A meta-analysis. *Amer J Emerg Med.* 1992;10(4):301–310.	Meta-analysis; included randomized, controlled trials or quasi-experimental trials (alternate day or sequential medication administration).	Oral and intravenous steroids appear to have equivalent effects on pulmonary function after administration during acute asthma exacerbations (effect size [ES] –0.07; CI: –0.39, 0.25).	Many studies that were included were small.	Oral and parenteral systemic steroids are equally effective in acute asthma exacerbation.
Manser R, et al. Corticosteroids for acute severe asthma in hospitalized patients. Cochrane Database of Systematic Reviews 2001, updated 2008.	Meta-analysis; included randomized, controlled trials.	There were no statistically significant differences detected in % predicted FEV_1 among groups that received low-dose (≤ 80 mg methylprednisolone or equivalent), medium dose (> 80 mg and ≤ 360 mg) and high dose (> 360 mg) systemic corticosteroids (any route) after 24, 48 or 72 hours.	A small number of studies were included.	Low-, medium-, and high-dose systemic corticosteroids may offer equivalent therapeutic benefit in acute asthma.
Rowe BH, et al. Inhaled budenonide in addition to oral corticosteroids to prevent asthma relapse following discharge from the emergency department: a randomized controlled trial. *JAMA.* 1999;281:2119–2126.	Double-blind, randomized, controlled trial.	After 21 days, 12.8% of 94 patients in the budesonide group experienced a relapse (defined by symptoms and an unscheduled office visit) compared with 24.5% of the placebo group. There were pulmonary function differences between the groups at 21 days.	Use of relapse as a primary outcome may not be a consistently documented outcome.	Use of ICS in addition to systemic corticosteroids after discharge reduces the risk of relapse in patients with acute asthma exacerbation.
Adjunct Treatment				
Rodrigo GJ, et al. Heliox for non-intubated acute asthma patients. Cochrane Database of Systematic Reviews 2006, updated 2010.	Meta-analysis; randomized, single or double blinded, controlled trials were included.	No significant group differences were found.	Small studies and between-group comparisons were used for analysis.	The use of Heliox treatment does not significantly improve pulmonary function during acute asthma exacerbation.
Bradshaw TA, et al. Intravenous magnesium sulphate provides no additive benefit to standard management in acute asthma. *Respir Med.* 2008;102(1):143–49.	Double-blind, randomized, controlled trial.	Intravenous magnesium sulphate did not decrease hospital admission rates or increase % predicted peak expiratory flow (PEF) at 60 min for all patients, or for subgroups of patients with acute asthma.	Higher percentage of patients receiving inhaled corticosteroids prior to magnesium dose compared with similar studies, and number of patients in the "life-threatening" subgroup is small.	No additional benefit is provided from intravenous magnesium sulfate when given as an adjunct to standard therapy for acute asthma.

(continued)

TABLE 238-6 Evidence-based Medicine Key References *(continued)*

Study	Methodology	Results	Limitations	Bottom Line
Adjunct treatment				
Camargo CA, et al. A randomized placebo-controlled study of intravenous montelukast for the treatment of acute asthma. *JACI*. 2010;125(2):374–380.	Randomized, double-blind, controlled trial.	Montelukast significantly increased FEV_1 after 60 minutes; the difference between change from baseline was 0.10 liters (95% CI: 0.04, 0.16). Improvements in FEV_1 were seen at all time points between 10 and 120 minutes after administration ($p < .05$).	Only acute improvement measured, and secondary endpoints related to disposition are harder to accurately assess across hospital sites.	Intravenous montelukast added to standard care in adults with acute asthma produced significant relief of acute airway obstruction.

CI, confidence interval; ES, effect size; FEV_1, forced expiratory volume in 1 second; ICS, inhaled corticosteroid; MDI, metered-dose inhaler; OR, odds ratio; PEF, peak expiratory flow; SABA, short-acting beta-agonist.

response to methacholine challenge, and reduced glucocorticoid responsiveness. However, increased dietary Vitamin D does not improve clinical course of asthma in studies to date.

Stress

Increased psychosocial stressors may contribute to asthma onset through glucorticoid insensitivity and cytokine dysregulation that lead to heightened airway inflammation. Therefore, minimizing stress may lead to improved asthma control.

TRANSITIONS OF CARE

Patients should follow up with a primary provider or specialist (eg, allergy and immunology specialist or pulmonologist) within two weeks of hospital discharge, or sooner if indicated based on severity level at the time of hospital discharge compared with admission and time required for improvement while in the hospital.

DISPARITIES IN HEALTH CARE

African Americans may exhibit fewer symptoms than other racial groups, sensing air-flow obstruction to a lesser extent. Therefore, they require vigilant additional evaluation to avoid sudden death from asthma. Also, patients of Puerto Rican descent have the highest asthma prevalence and severity in the United States; in contrast, Mexican Americans have the lowest prevalence and severity. The reasons for racial and ethnic differences in asthma among persons in the United States are not well understood at this time.

COSTS AND RESOURCE UTILIZATION

Annually, an average of 11.6 million persons reported at least one asthma attack during the preceding 12 months. Among persons with current asthma, 56% had at least one asthma attack in the preceding 12 months; additionally, females with current asthma had a higher attack rate than males, and children were more likely to have had an attack than adults. From 2001 to 2003, there were a total of 2.5 hospitalizations for every 100 persons with current asthma. During this time period, the rates of hospitalization for asthma were higher in children and African Americans. Additionally, there were an estimated 8.8 emergency room visits for asthma per 100 subjects with current asthma. The emergency room visit rates were higher for African Americans and Hispanics when compared with Caucasians (**Table 238-6**).

SUGGESTED READINGS

Chowdhury BA, Dal Pan G. The FDA and safe use of long-acting beta-agonists in the treatment of asthma. *N Engl J Med*. 2010; 362:1169.

Ibrahim WH, Gheriani HA, Almohamed AA, Raza T. Paradoxical vocal cord motion disorder: past, present and future. *Postgrad Med J*. 2007;83(977):164–172. PMCID: 2599980.

Lazarus SC. Clinical practice. Emergency treatment of asthma. *N Engl J Med*. 2010;363(8):755–764.

Miller GE, Gaudin A, Zysk E, Chen E. Parental support and cytokine activity in childhood asthma: the role of glucocorticoid sensitivity. *J Allergy Clin Immunol*. 2009;123(4):824–830.

Moorman JE, Rudd RA, Johnson CA, King M, Minor P, Bailey C, et al. National surveillance for asthma--United States, 1980–2004. *MMWR Surveill Summ*. 2007;56(8):1–54.

National Center for Environmental Health. *Asthma prevalence, health-care use and mortality: United States* 2005–09. Available at http://www.cdc.gov/nchs/data/nhsr/nhsr032.pdf.

National Heart, Lung, and Blood Institute, National Asthma, Education and Prevention Program (NAEPP). *Expert Panel Report 3*. Bethesda, MD; 2007.

Raviv S, Smith LJ. Diet and asthma. *Curr Opin Pulm Med*. 2010;16(1): 71–76.

Rose D, Mannino DM, Leaderer BP. Asthma prevalence among US adults, 1998–2000: role of Puerto Rican ethnicity and behavioral and geographic factors. *Am J Public Health*. 2006;96(5):880–888. PMCID: 1470587.

Wenzel SE. Asthma: defining of the persistent adult phenotypes. *Lancet*. 2006;368(9537):804–813.

CHAPTER 239

Chronic Obstructive Pulmonary Disease

Gerald W. Staton, MD
Lewis Satterwhite, MD

Key Clinical Questions

1. What conditions can mimic an acute exacerbation of chronic obstructive pulmonary disease (COPD) and require different diagnostic and treatment modalities?
2. What inpatient therapeutic modalities can help reduce mortality or length of stay for patients with exacerbation of COPD?
3. What medications should be utilized for a patient who is being discharged after an acute exacerbation of COPD to prevent further exacerbations?
4. What are the appropriate situations for use of noninvasive ventilation for patients with an acute exacerbation of COPD?
5. Other than medications, what modalities need to be considered and discussed with a patient at the time of discharge after an acute exacerbation of COPD?

INTRODUCTION

DEFINITION AND BACKGROUND

Chronic obstructive pulmonary disease (COPD) is a group of clinical and pathological pulmonary disorders that are preventable and treatable and are characterized by airflow limitation that is not fully reversible. The most common phenotypes of COPD are emphysema and chronic bronchitis. Emphysema is generally defined by pathologic and physiologic criteria as irreversible enlargement of the airways and loss of elastic recoil. Clinically, emphysema is characterized by dyspnea along with an expanded chest, decreased breath sounds, radiographic lucency, and flattening of the diaphragms. Chronic bronchitis is defined clinically by the finding of cough and sputum production on most days of at least 3 months per year for 2 consecutive years. Pathologically, the hallmark of chronic bronchitis is large airway inflammation and the hypertrophy and hyperplasia of the mucous-secreting goblet cells. The diagnosis of COPD requires spirometry which should be obtained in patients (at a time free of exacerbation) who exhibit cough, sputum production, dyspnea or risk factors/exposure history. COPD is defined clinically by airflow limitation on pulmonary function tests that is not fully reversible. The severity of COPD is classified by the degree of limitation in the forced expiratory volume in 1 second (FEV_1) (**Table 239-1**).

Hospitalists often manage patients presenting with new symptoms consistent with COPD, patients with acute exacerbations of underlying COPD, and patients whose COPD complicates the course of care for other medical conditions. In this chapter, we will review best practices for each of these scenarios and solutions for optimizing care of these patients as they transition out of the acute care setting.

RISK FACTORS

Tobacco smoking is the single most important risk factor for the development of COPD. Cigarette, pipe, and cigar smoking account for more than 90% of cases of COPD; yet, clinically important disease is only found in 10% to 20% of smokers. Clearly there are other predisposing factors because dose-dependent exposure to tobacco does not wholly determine the onset or severity of disease in COPD. Other factors that lead to the onset (or accelerate the progression) of COPD include exposure to second-hand smoke, environmental irritants and pollutants (including biomass), occupational exposures, malnutrition, early life pulmonary infections, HIV infection, and genetic predisposition. The role of genetics is incompletely understood, but COPD is more common in the relatives of those with COPD.

PATHOGENESIS

Tobacco smoke and other exposures cause inflammatory, biochemical and anatomic changes that account for the symptoms, limitations, and complications of COPD (**Figure 239-1**). Anatomically, the central airways, peripheral airways, lung parenchyma and pulmonary vasculature are all affected. Irritant exposure and yet-to-be elucidated host factors interact to result in an inflammatory process, and an imbalance of proteinases, anti-proteinases and oxidative stress. Physiologically, ciliary dysfunction, mucous hypersecretion, loss of elastic recoil, airflow limitation, impaired gas exchange and pulmonary hypertension can all be manifestations.

TABLE 239-1 GOLD Criteria for Chronic Obstructive Pulmonary Disease Severity

GOLD Stage	Severity	Symptoms	Spirometry
0	At risk	Chronic cough, sputum production	Normal
I	Mild	With or without chronic cough or sputum production	$FEV_1/FVC < 0.7$ and FEV_1 80% predicted
II	Moderate	With or without chronic cough or sputum production	$FEV_1/FVC < 0.7$ and 50% $FEV_1 < 80\%$ predicted
III	Severe	With or without chronic cough or sputum production	$FEV_1/FVC < 0.7$ and 30% $FEV_1 < 50\%$ predicted
IV	Very severe	With or without chronic cough or sputum production	$FEV_1/FVC < 0.7$ and $FEV_1 < 30\%$ predicted *or* $FEV_1 < 50\%$ predicted with respiratory failure or signs of right heart failure

FEV_1, forced expiratory volume in 1 second; FVC, forced vital capacity; GOLD, Global Initiative for Chronic Obstructive Lung Disease.

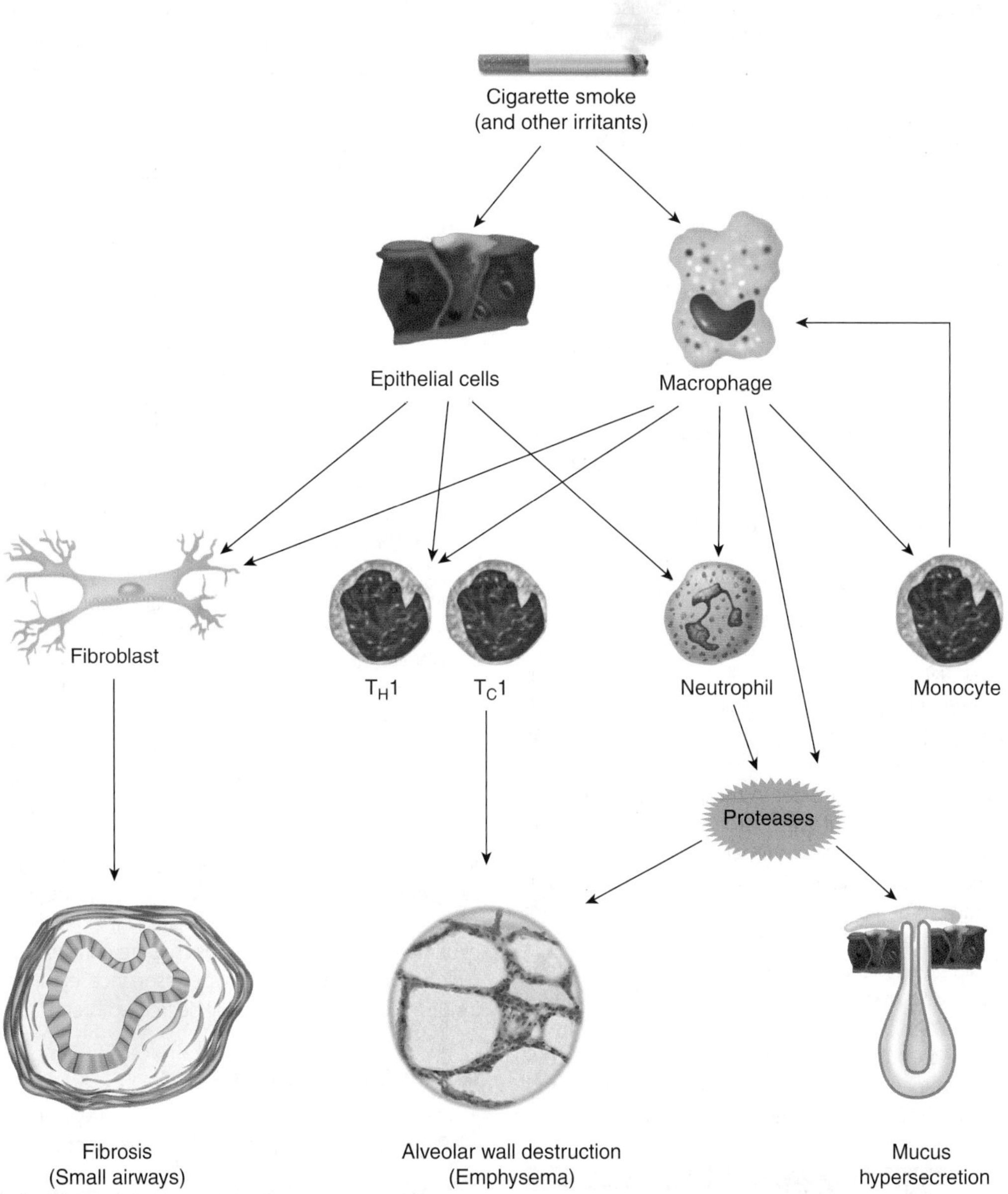

Figure 239-1 *Pathogenesis of chronic obstructive pulmonary disease. (Reproduced, with permission, from Brunton LL, Chabner BA, Knollmann BC. Goodman & Gilman's the Pharmacological Basis of Therapeutics, 12th ed. New York: McGraw-Hill, 2011. Fig. 36-2.)*

EPIDEMIOLOGY

PREVALENCE AND EXACERBATIONS

Estimates of the rates of COPD in the United States and worldwide vary widely, but data are consistent that the disease burden is large and COPD is underdiagnosed. Survey data from 2007 estimate that 10.2 million Americans have COPD. COPD accounted for 672,000 hospital admissions in 2006 and caused 127,049 deaths in 2005, according to the American Lung Association. COPD is known to be increasing among women and is the fourth leading cause of death in both the United States and Europe.

COPD COMPLICATING OTHER DISEASES

There is increasing evidence that patients with COPD have high rates of morbidity and mortality caused by extrapulmonary problems. Patients with COPD have been found to have higher rates of cardiovascular, gastrointestinal and psychiatric illnesses among others. It is estimated that COPD is a primary or contributing cause of almost 10% of all admissions to the hospital. Cardiovascular morbidity and mortality might be even higher than that of lung disease and respiratory failure.

COPD EXACERBATION: DIFFERENTIAL AND EVALUATION

An acute exacerbation of COPD (AECOPD) is defined as a change in the baseline symptoms of dyspnea, cough and/or sputum color or volume that necessitates a change in management. When a patient with COPD or risk factors for COPD presents with any of these complaints, the diagnosis of AECOPD must be considered against a number of other diagnoses that can mimic an AECOPD. Once a diagnosis of AECOPD is reached, issues of causation of the exacerbation and level of severity need to be addressed. There is no single agreed-upon system to rank severity of exacerbations, but broadly categorizing among three levels has been suggested: (1) home management; (2) hospital management; and (3) respiratory failure.

ETIOLOGY AND DIFFERENTIAL DIAGNOSIS OF AECOPD

AECOPD has many different potential causes and the specific trigger for any one event is sometimes never elucidated. It is commonly agreed, however, that various triggers cause acute inflammation superimposed on the chronic inflammation of the underlying disease. During an AECOPD, inflammatory cells of many inflammatory pathways can be found in sputum and blood. Together, all infectious agents (bacteria, virus, and other) account for up to 80% of acute exacerbations.

The differential diagnoses to consider as triggers in patients that have underlying COPD and an acute respiratory decompensation is extensive (**Table 239-2**). Many of these triggers incite the inflammatory pathway at the root of an AECOPD, but they may also require other specific therapy. When a trigger is not immediately obvious from history and physical exam, there are certain other diagnoses that must be considered. A recent autopsy study of patients that were diagnosed as having an AECOPD and that died within 24 hours of admission showed that 37% of these deaths were due to heart failure and 21% due to pulmonary embolism. Patients admitted with otherwise unexplained exacerbations of COPD are often found to have pulmonary emboli when this diagnosis is pursued.

DIAGNOSTIC EVALUATION

For patients with known or suspected COPD, any complaint consistent with a COPD exacerbation warrants a thorough investigation. The degree of diagnostic evaluation should be determined by the patient's subjective degree of discomfort, physical exam abnormalities and/or any alterations in vital signs or diagnostic studies.

TABLE 239-2 Precipitants of Acute Exacerbation of Chronic Obstructive Pulmonary Disease: Differential Diagnosis

Pneumonia
Upper respiratory tract infection
Pulmonary embolism
Reactive airways disease or allergens
Congestive heart failure
Pneumothorax (trauma, rib fracture)
Arrhythmia
Myocardial infarction
Upper airway obstruction
Sleep disordered breathing
Sedating medications
Medication nonadherence
Environmental irritants (smoke, smog, workplace irritants)
Thickened bronchial secretions (eg, dehydration)

Careful consideration of any conditions in the differential diagnosis of AECOPD (Table 239-2) must be undertaken.

KEY HISTORY AND PHYSICAL EXAMINATION

Along with questions regarding a change in dyspnea, a new or changed cough, and a change in sputum color and volume, the history helps establish the change from the patient's baseline symptoms. The history may also provide clues to other diagnoses or triggers (Table 239-2) for patients suspected of having an AECOPD.

For patients with suspected AECOPD, but without a diagnosis of COPD, questioning regarding age, smoking status, exercise tolerance and other respiratory exposures can help increase or decrease the suspicion of COPD as the underlying disease.

AECOPD is associated with increased dyspnea, increased sputum purulence, wheezing, constitutional symptoms (fever, malaise, myalgias, etc), and cough. Other past medical history and comorbid conditions can affect overall mortality and may influence patient triage for monitoring and therapy.

The physical exam can help identify undiagnosed COPD, exclude other diagnoses in the respiratory decompensation of patients with known COPD, and help triage the severity of a diagnosed AECOPD. For evaluating the severity of an exacerbation, ominous physical exam findings portending higher risk and poorer outcomes include altered mentation (agitation and/or obtundation), respiratory muscle retraction, paradoxical abdominal movement, cyanosis and diaphoresis. These findings necessitate higher levels of monitoring and expedited care. Other findings that are consistent with an AECOPD include wheezing, cough, hyperresonance, expanded lung fields on lung percussion and diffusely decreased breath sounds.

LABORATORY EVALUATION

In the initial evaluation of AECOPD, pulse oximetry O_2 saturation > 89% is evidence of acceptable oxygenation.

PRACTICE POINT

- An arterial blood gas should be rapidly obtained to evaluate any patient with an AECOPD considered for hospital admission, as recommended by international guidelines.

Arterial blood gases (ABGs) are able to more accurately determine the derangement of gas exchange by calculating an alveolar-arterial gradient, and may detect worse hypoxia than expected or evidence of hypercarbia. Importantly, the pH from the ABG may also provide valuable information helping direct management (eg, consideration of noninvasive ventilation). Arterial blood gas interpretation must take into account the patient's baseline status. Patients with more severe disease are likely to have elevated partial pressure of carbon dioxide (Pco_2) with a relatively preserved pH as the kidneys compensate for chronic hypoventilation. Ominous findings include elevated Pco_2 with a decreased pH (indicating an acute onset or worsening of hypoventilation), low partial pressures of oxygen, and severely elevated Pco_2.

Guidelines recommend hematology profiles and basic chemistry panels in the evaluation of COPD. These tests may show polycythemia associated with chronic COPD, or conversely, anemia. These basic labs are most valuable in identifying other diagnoses to be considered or comorbid conditions that may require parallel treatment. If patients are known or suspected to be treated with theophylline, the serum levels of the drug should be measured.

Routine collection of sputum for gram stain and culture is not recommended in the management of COPD exacerbation. Sputum gram stain and culture may play a role in the laboratory evaluation of patients that do not respond to initial therapy and/or have evidence of frank pneumonia.

RADIOGRAPHY AND ELECTROCARDIOGRAPHY

Chest radiography is indicated for evaluation of AECOPD. Findings on the radiograph may influence the type of care if there are findings such as pneumothorax, atelectasis, focal infiltrate or pulmonary edema. About 20% of patients thought to have an AECOPD have chest radiograph findings that influence management.

PRACTICE POINT

- About 20% of patients thought to have an AECOPD have chest radiograph findings that influence management.

Patients with dyspnea and other chest complaints need electrocardiography (ECG) evaluation to identify relevant findings including coronary ischemia or arrhythmias. The irregular rhythm of multifocal tachycardia (MAT) that is found frequently in COPD patients may be difficult to distinguish from atrial fibrillation without the ECG. MAT responds to the treatment of the underlying lung disease and rate control whereas atrial fibrillation requires additional therapeutic approaches.

SPIROMETRY

Spirometry, while a core diagnostic tool for the evaluation of outpatient stable COPD, does not have a role in the evaluation of COPD exacerbations. In fact, national and international guidelines recommend against the use of spirometry in the setting of AECOPD.

TRIAGE: DETERMINING SEVERITY, INDICATIONS FOR ADMISSION, AND LEVEL OF CARE

DETERMINING SEVERITY OF AN EXACERBATION

No single system exists to classify patient severity of illness once they are identified as having an AECOPD. The American Thoracic Society and European Respiratory Society (ATS/ERS) guidelines define severity based upon where the exacerbation is managed (home versus inpatient versus ICU) requiring clinicians evaluating patients for AECOPD to rely on previously mentioned risk factors for mortality and clinical acumen to best triage patients.

TABLE 239-3 Indications for Hospitalization of Patients with Acute Exacerbation of Chronic Obstructive Pulmonary Disease

1. Acute exacerbation characterized by increased dyspnea, cough, or sputum production, plus one or more of the following:
    - Inadequate response of symptoms to outpatient management
    - Inability to walk between rooms (patient previously mobile)
    - Inability to eat or sleep due to dyspnea
    - Conclusion by family and/or physician that patient cannot manage at home; supplementary home care resources not immediately available
    - High-risk comorbid condition, pulmonary (eg, pneumonia) or nonpulmonary
    - Prolonged, progressive symptoms before emergency visit
    - Altered mentation
    - Worsening hypoxemia
    - New or worsening hypercarbia
2. New or worsening cor pulmonale unresponsive to outpatient management
3. Planned invasive surgical or diagnostic procedure requires analgesics or sedatives that may worsen pulmonary function
4. Comorbid condition (eg, severe steroid myopathy or acute vertebral compression fractures) that has worsened pulmonary function

CRITERIA FOR ADMISSION

The Global Initiative for Chronic Obstructive Lung Disease (GOLD) and ATS/ERS guidelines for management of COPD provide criteria for hospitalization in AECOPD (**Table 239-3**). Numerous studies have tried to identify patient characteristics that successfully predict patient prognosis and lower risk patients who could be managed as outpatients, but no prediction rules have been successful. Certain findings may predict the success or failure of outpatient management. Older age, lower baseline FEV_1, hypoxemia, previous recent exacerbations and extensive comorbidities can increase risk of mortality or relapse exacerbation.

CRITERIA FOR INTENSIVE CARE UNIT ADMISSION

The best location to manage any particular patient with an AECOPD will vary based on individual hospital resources and staffing, with differences in the availability of specified inpatient respiratory units, step-down or intermediate care units and personnel. Therefore, criteria for intensive care unit (ICU) admission or monitoring is often institution specific. Nonetheless, some guidelines suggest criteria for ICU admission (**Table 239-4**).

MANAGEMENT OF AN ACUTE EXACERBATION OF COPD

INITIAL HOSPITAL TREATMENT

Bronchodilators

Short-acting beta-agonists such as albuterol are a mainstay of outpatient management of stable COPD and play a key role in the treatment of AECOPD, to improve symptoms and FEV_1. Beta-agonists induce airway smooth muscle relaxation via increased cyclic adenosine monophosphate and have their largest effect on peripheral airways. They have onset within minutes, peak action at 30 minutes and last for several hours. During exacerbations, treatments may be given as frequently as every 1 to 2 hours as the half-life of the

TABLE 239-4 Indications for Intensive Care Unit Admission of Patients with Acute Exacerbation of Chronic Obstructive Pulmonary Disease
1. Severe dyspnea that responds inadequately to initial emergency therapy
2. Confusion, lethargy, or respiratory muscle fatigue (the last characterized by paradoxical diaphragmatic motion)
3. Impending respiratory failure
4. Hemodynamic instability
5. Persistent or worsening hypoxemia despite supplemental oxygen or severe/worsening respiratory acidosis (pH < 7.30)
6. Assisted mechanical ventilation is required, whether by means of endotracheal tube or noninvasive technique

medicines can be reduced. For initial treatment of a patient being admitted to a general medical floor, beta-agonists should be given every two hours, but may be given as frequently as every 20 minutes or continuously for patients in extremis. Levalbuterol, a pure R isomer of albuterol (albuterol is a 1:1 mixture of the R and S isomers) may produce better bronchodilation in asthma exacerbations, but this effect has not been shown in COPD. There is also some thought that levalbuterol may cause less tachycardia when compared to racemic albuterol, but *scarce evidence supports this effect or its clinical significance*. Based on the multitude of conflicting data surrounding the use of levalbuterol, it is difficult to recommend its routine use, but it may be reasonable in patients that appear to have an adverse effect from albuterol or for a short time while frequent dosing of a beta-agonist is needed.

Short-acting anticholinergics, including ipratropium, are also important in the treatment of AECOPD and should be used in concert with beta-agonsists to treat acute exacerbations. They bronchodilate via inhibition of muscarinic pulmonary acethylcholine esterase receptors and have their largest effects on central airways. The onset of action is slower than that of beta-agonist with an onset of approximately 15 minutes, a peak effect at 60 to 90 minutes, and duration of 4 to 6 hours.

The optimal dose of albuterol is 2.5 to 5.0 mg via nebulizer or six to eight puffs (90 mcg each) via metered dose inhaler (MDI). For ipratropium, the optimal dose is 0.5 mg via nebulizer or 4 to 8 puffs of an MDI (at 17 mcg per puff). Inhalational technique varies widely from patient to patient, especially in times of respiratory distress. However, evidence supports delivery of drug via *MDI with a spacer* for equivalent results at a lower cost compared to a nebulizer. Long-acting bronchodilators, including long-acting beta-agnoists (eg, salmeterol) and long-acting anticholinergics (eg, tiotropium) have no role in the management of AECOPD, and have not been studied in that setting. Oral and injection bronchodilators are not as effective as inhaled route and should be avoided.

Corticosteroids

Systemic steroids are indicated for the treatment of AECOPD requiring hospitalization. More controversial, however, is the optimal route of administration and dose.

> **PRACTICE POINT**
>
> - Systemic steroids have been shown to speed recovery of FEV_1, lower the number of treatment failures and shorten hospital length of stay. A short taper of steroids, over 1 to 2 weeks, may result in a greater improvement of FEV_1 compared to a short burst.

Steroids have significant side effects, including hyperglycemia, which is the most common acute side effect. Higher doses and longer duration of exposure increase these risks. Guidelines suggest that initiating steroids at a dose of prednisone 30 to 40 mg (or equivalent), but many of the trials showing benefit of systemic steroids have used higher doses and IV administration. The initial dose of steroids should be tailored to the patient. Patients requiring hospitalization but without impending respiratory failure may be started at a dose of prednisone 30 to 40 mg daily to maximize benefit and minimize risk, whereas use of higher doses and IV route should be considered for patients in more distress or frank respiratory failure. A taper of steroids may result in a greater improvement of FEV_1 compared to a short burst. Current recommendations include oral steroid therapy for a taper of 1 to 2 weeks. No data supports use of inhaled steroids in AECOPD.

Antibiotics

Bacterial infections play an important role in AECOPD. Guideline recommendations encourage the use of empiric antibiotics for patients with AECOPD that have suspected infection. Antibiotics should be tailored to the patient risk factors as well as to community and hospital specific microbial patterns, but should always include coverage for the most common causal pathogens (ie, *Haemophilus influenzae*, *Streptococcus pneumonia*, and *Moraxella catarrhalis*). For patients with very severe airflow limitation, extended spectrum coverage should be considered as more resistant bacteria (ie, *Pseudomonas*, other gram-negative rods) can cause exacerbations. There is no consensus regarding the optimal antibiotic to choose for AECOPD, but increasing resistance among common causative agents argues for the use of a second- or third-generation cephalosporin.

Oxygen and noninvasive ventilation

Oxygen level monitoring and supplemental oxygen provision are often necessary for patients with AECOPD (**Figure 239-2**). Depending on the severity of baseline disease, these patients may have recognized or unrecognized hypoxemia and the intercurrent illness can frequently make that situation worse or create new hypoxemia. Early and frequent assessment of blood oxygen levels (via arterial blood gases or pulse oximetry) is critical for patients with an AECOPD. Oxygen can be supplied via nasal cannula, face masks, non-rebreather masks or high flow oxygen masks. Especially for patients with respiratory distress and high work of breathing, the rapid inspiration may overcome the reservoir of a non-rebreather mask. In this situation, oxygen delivered by high flow masks yields the greatest percentage of inspired oxygen. The goal of oxygen supplementation should be to achieve a goal Spo_2 of 88% to 92% and/or a Pao_2 of >60. Care must also be taken to provide adequate but not excessive levels of oxygen for patients that have baseline hypercapnea to avoid exacerbating carbon dioxide retention. Carbon dioxide binds reversibly to reduced hemoglobin, but oxygen drives the reaction to release carbon dioxide, a phenomenon known as the Haldane effect. Patients receiving supplemental oxygen need frequent assessment of blood oxygen levels and levels of alertness. The GOLD guidelines recommend rechecking an arterial blood gas 30 to 60 minutes after initiation of oxygen therapy.

Positive pressure ventilation

Noninvasive positive pressure ventilation (NIPPV) has been shown to benefit some patients with an AECOPD. Special consideration should be given for patients with a pH between 7.2 and 7.35, as this patient population has the most evidence supporting benefit. It is possible to consider NIPPV for patients with an even more severe academia with close monitoring.

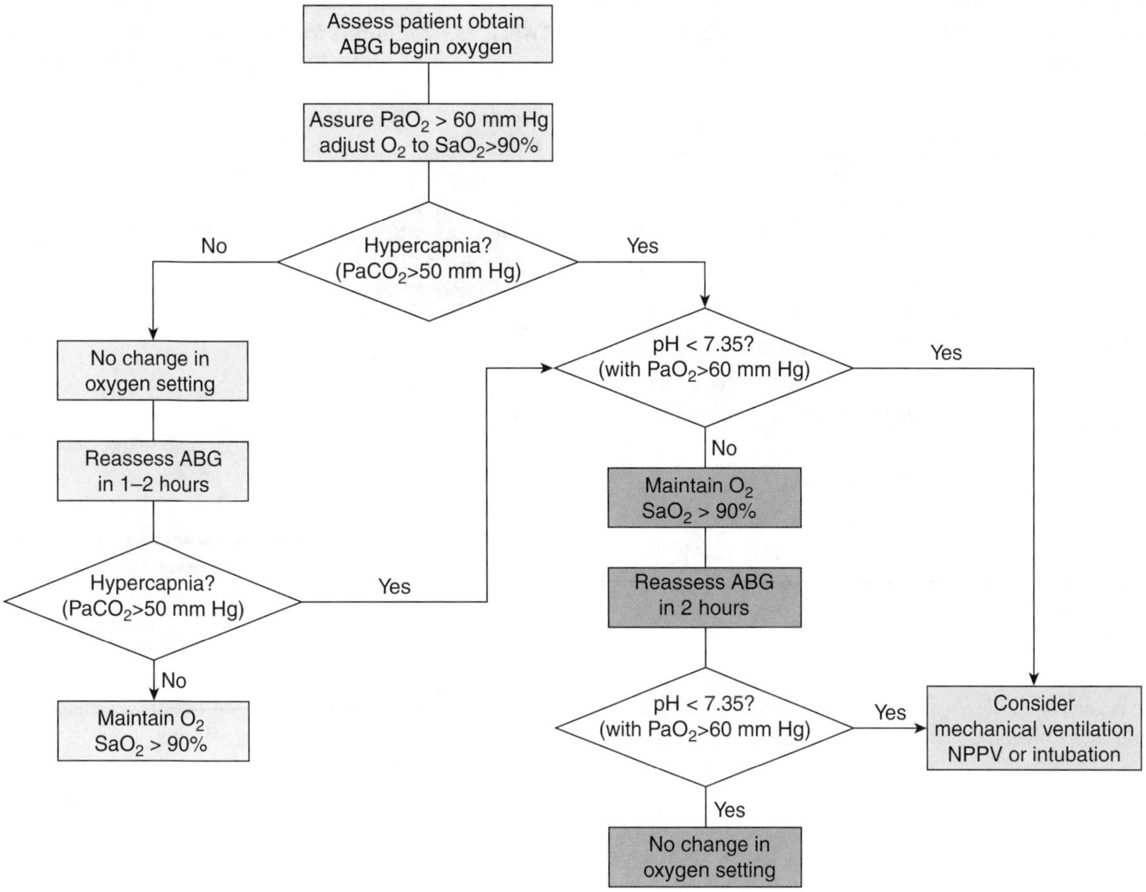

Figure 239-2 *Algorithm for oxygen and carbon dioxide assessment during an acute exacerbation of chronic obstructive pulmonary disease. ABG, arterial blood gas; O_2, oxygen; P_{ACO_2}, partial pressure of carbon dioxide in arterial blood; P_{AO_2}, partial pressure of oxygen in arterial blood; S_{AO_2}, saturation level of oxygen in hemoglobin.*

PRACTICE POINT

- Positive pressure ventilation applied at two levels during the respiratory cycle (bi-level ventilation) has been shown to decrease mortality, the need for intubation, and the length of hospital stay for patients with an AECOPD.

NIPPV should be considered for patients with mild to moderate acidemia, increased work of breathing and hypercapnea. Absolute contraindications to NIPPV include immediate need for intubation, untreated tension pneumothorax and a comatose state. Relative contraindications for use of NIPPV include severity of disease, likelihood of failure and anatomical risks (**Table 239-5**). If NIPPV is selected, patients require frequent reassessment and close observation. An ABG should be rechecked 30 minutes to 1 hour from the time of NIPPV initiation. Within the first 1 to 2 hours, there should be a clear trend toward improvement in clinical and laboratory (pH, P_{CO_2}) parameters. Without rapid improvement, strong consideration must be given to intubation and mechanical ventilation.

Invasive mechanical ventilation is sometimes required to treat severe exacerbations of COPD. The decision to intubate and mechanically ventilate a patient with an AECOPD is ultimately clinical, but guideline statements offer possible indications for intubation that include severe dyspnea, respiratory rate > 35, somnolence, severe acidosis (pH < 7.25), refractory hypoxemia and complications of comorbidities. Mortality increases significantly when patients with an AECOPD require mechanical ventilation due to greater disease severity and/or the inherent risk factors of mechanical ventilation.

OTHER THERAPIES

Methylxanthines such as theophylline and aminophylline have been used to treat COPD (both stable and during exacerbations) for decades. A systemic review of methylxanthines in AECOPD did not find significant benefits but did describe increased side effects, including palpitations and arrhythmias. While guidelines do list methylxanthines as alternate therapies for patients that do not respond to first-line therapies, they should be considered later-line therapy. If methylxanthines are used, they require monitoring for side effects and toxicity. Serum levels should be monitored every several days, and daily after a dose change until

TABLE 239-5 Relative Contraindications for Use of Noninvasive Positive Pressure Ventilation

1. Craniofacial abnormality or trauma
2. Respiratory arrest/apnea/refractory hypoxemia
3. Cardiac arrest/unstable cardiac arrhythmia
4. Hemodynamic instability
5. Inability to tolerate aerophagia (swallowing too much air), eg, recent gastrointestinal surgery
6. Inability to cooperate or protect airway
   a. Severe encephalopathy
   b. Severe upper gastrointestinal bleed
   c. High risk for aspiration

TABLE 239-6 Evidence for Specific Therapies in Acute Exacerbation of Chronic Obstructive Pulmonary Disease

Therapy	Outcomes Improved
Antibiotics	Decreased treatment failure Decreased inhospital mortality
Oral corticosteroids	Decreased treatment failure Decreased hospital LOS Increased FEV_1 after 3 days
Noninvasive positive pressure ventilation	Decreased need for intubation Decreased inhospital mortality Decreased hospital LOS
Pulmonary rehabilitation (following recovery)	Decreased readmissions Decreased mortality in follow-up Increased quality of life in questionnaires Increased exercise capacity in 6MWT

6MWT, 6-minute walk test; FEV_1, forced expiratory volume in 1 second; LOS, length of stay.

TABLE 239-7 Centers for Medicare and Medicaid Services Criteria for Oxygen Supplementation

Group I coverage

- $PAO_2 \le 55$ or $SAO_2 \le 88\%$
  - At rest
  - During sleep
- OR ↓ $PAO_2 > 10$ mm Hg or ↓ SAO_2 5% associated with symptoms or signs of hypoxemia
  - During activity

Group II coverage

- $SaO_2 = 89\%$ (not + 89%).
- Any of the following:
  - Dependent edema
  - Pulmonary hypertension or cor pulmonale
  - Hematocrit > 56%

Requires retesting between 61 and 90 days

PAO_2, partial pressure of oxygen in arterial blood; SAO_2, saturation level of oxygen in hemoglobin.

levels are relatively stable. Acute illness and medication changes at the time of admission can affect metabolism and serum levels of methylxanthines. If theophylline is used, drug levels should be adjusted to 8 to 12 mg/mL.

Other therapies that have been used to treat AECOPD include mucolytic therapy, postural drainage and chest physiotherapy. These modalities may improve symptoms, but have not been shown to improve outcomes. Guidelines do not recommend pulmonary rehabilitation during treatment for an AECOPD, but early ambulation and physical and/or occupational therapy for patients that are not in respiratory failure is advisable (**Table 239-6**).

TRIGGERS FOR CONSULTATION

Management of an AECOPD may have varying levels of complexity. The decision to consult a pulmonary or a critical care specialist will be determined by hospital and referral resources, as well as experience level of clinicians and frequency of caring for these patients. For the inpatient management of an acute exacerbation, acuity of illness, hemodynamic compromise and poor response to therapy should be the overriding considerations for consultation. The ATS/ERS guidelines for the management of COPD list the following factors as indication for outpatient specialist consultation: age of COPD onset <40 years old, two or more exacerbations per year (despite adequate outpatient management), rapidly progressive disease, severe disease (FEV_1 <50% predicted), need for long-term oxygen therapy, onset of comorbid illness (osteoporosis, heart failure, bronchiectasis, lung cancer) and/or evaluation for surgery. A consultant may also help with discharge planning and follow-up care for patients after their acute illness. Outpatient specialty referral may be indicated for most patients once they have completed their inpatient treatment.

OUTPATIENT THERAPEUTICS AND REGIMEN AUGMENTATION

SUPPLEMENTAL OXYGEN

If patients remain hypoxemic at the time of discharge, they will require home oxygen therapy. To meet the Centers for Medicare and Medicaid Services (CMS) criteria for 24 hours per day long-term home oxygen therapy, patients must have resting, room air PaO_2 of 55 mm Hg or less or PaO_2 of 59 mm Hg or less with coexisting congestive heart failure, peripheral edema, hematocrit >56%, or cor pulmonale (**Table 239-7**). Alterations of oxygen levels during sleep and/or exercise can also qualify patients for supplementation during those activities. Hypoxemia at hospital discharge following AECOPD may represent a prolonged recovery from an acute illness, a new baseline, or a new recognition of a chronic problem. Regardless, **long-term oxygen therapy improves mortality for COPD patients that have resting hypoxemia.** Patients that have a new prescription for home oxygen should be reassessed with an arterial blood gas within 3 months to determine the ongoing need for supplemental oxygen.

ORAL STEROIDS

Systemic oral steroids are indicated for the treatment of an AECOPD that requires hospitalization. At the time of discharge, completing a short course of oral steroids for a 1 to 2 week taper is suggested. Once the patient has stabilized, there is no indication for long-term treatment with steroids for COPD.

INHALED THERAPIES

Inhaled long-acting bronchodilators (long-acting beta-agonists and long-acting anticholinergics) and inhaled corticosteroids (ICS) have a significant role in the regimen augmentation when a patient with AECOPD is being discharged. Strong evidence supports that inhaled medications reduce deterioration in health status, improve lung function (FEV_1), and reduce the number of exacerbations per year. Recently, guidelines have acknowledged that combined ICS and long-acting beta-agonists (LABA) are associated with a reduction in the rate of decline of lung function. Additional data indicate that the combination of LABA and ICS plus long-acting anticholinergic for patients with more advanced COPD is associated with additional improvement in quality of life and a reduction in subsequent hospitalizations. All patients who have been hospitalized with AECOPD should be discharged on a combination of a long-acting bronchodilator and ICS, as meta-analysis data suggests mortality reduction with this regimen compared to placebo and other regimens. Some evidence shows that short-acting anticholinergic agents, used chronically, may impart increased cardiovascular risk in COPD patients, while mounting evidence suggests that long-acting anticholinergic agents may not have significant cardiovascular risks. The decisions of which medications to utilize should be made in light of clinical acumen, patient preferences and patient-provider discussions regarding treatment goals and potential adverse effects.

MUCOLYTIC AND MUCOKINETIC AGENTS

Mucolytic agents are sometimes used in the treatment of COPD, but there is not any convincing evidence that they have meaningful benefits, and they are not recommended in the guidelines.

COPD COMPLICATING ADMISSIONS FOR OTHER DIAGNOSES

Underlying COPD may complicate the care of patients admitted for other diagnoses. Complications may result from the underlying compromise of the respiratory symptom or because an exacerbation occurs at the time of, or shortly after, the onset of the original stress. Also, patients hospitalized for any reason are exposed to iatrogenic risks such as resistant microbes, painful procedures (causing splinting), sedative medications (hypoventilation), and decreased physical activity (deconditioning).

The use of beta-blockers in COPD has long been a controversial topic. A 2005 Cochrane Review demonstrated that there was no short-term decrease in FEV_1 or responsiveness to inhaled beta-agonists for patients that received cardioselective beta-blockers, regardless of the severity of COPD. Therefore, cardio-selective beta-blocker prescription is reasonable for chronic COPD patients who have a cardiac indication to receive this therapy.

While COPD can complicate any medical or surgical illness, there are certain processes where this occurs more frequently. Patients with congestive heart failure and COPD often present complaining of shortness of breath. It is difficult to decipher if the worsening of the baseline condition is because of cardiac decompensation, pulmonary exacerbation or both. Normal levels of serum brain natriuretic peptide (BNP) can significantly decrease the likelihood of cardiac decompensation, but elevated BNP is less specific and more difficult to interpret. A full physical examination and workup is often necessary and occasionally an empiric trial of treating both conditions is warranted. Patients recovering from surgical procedures need to have special consideration of postoperative activity, pain control (without over-sedation) and abdominal processes (swelling, ileus, etc).

PERIOPERATIVE EVALUATION

Large numbers of patients with recognized or unrecognized COPD have the need for surgery. Hospitalists are often asked to determine which patients represent undue risk and if there are any measures that can minimize these risks. In general, pulmonary complications are equal (in prevalence, morbidity, mortality, and length of stay) when compared to cardiac complications for moderate and high risk surgeries. Perioperative care of COPD patients includes identifying and managing any acute worsening from pulmonary baseline, risk assessment, preoperative risk minimization (ensuring proper preoperative care and medications) and postoperative risk minimization. Separate chapters describe perioperative pulmonary care (see Chapters 55 and 56).

PROGNOSIS AND END OF LIFE CARE

PROGNOSIS

COPD patients' pulmonary function progressively declines over the course of the disease. Tobacco cessation is the most important factor in slowing the progression of COPD, but even those patients that stop smoking experience continued age-related decline in lung function. Predicting the future health of a patient with COPD is important at the time of discharge to ensure all appropriate treatment modalities are considered as well as ensuring patients have the needed social support to meet the demands of daily life.

TABLE 239-8 BODE Index Scoring System

	0	1	2	3
FEV_1 (% predicted)	≥65	50–64	36–49	≤35
6MWT distance	>350 m	250–349 m	150–249 m	≤149 m
MMRC dyspnea scale	0–1	2	3	4
BMI	>21	<21		

6MWT, 6-minute walk test; BMI, body mass index; BODE, body mass index, airflow obstruction, dyspnea and exercise capacity; FEV_1, forced expiratory volume in 1 second; MMRC, modified Medical Research Council.

Once a patient is admitted for an AECOPD, morbidity and mortality are significantly different when compared to COPD patients that have not been hospitalized previously. The 1-year readmission rate for COPD patients discharged for AECOPD is as high as 59% for patients with severe disease and the 1-year mortality rate is as high as 22%. Two-year mortality approaches 50% for patients admitted with AECOPD and hypercapnea.

Increasing age, male sex, white race, prior hospitalization, weight loss, pulmonary hypertension, hypoxemia, hypercapnea, decreased FEV_1, and decreased diffusing capacity of the lung for carbon monoxide (DLCO) have all been identified as risk factors for death with COPD. Progressive decline in FEV_1 has historically been used as the primary measure of predicting the course of COPD, but it is being replaced by an indexed score, the BODE score. The BODE score (**Table 239-8**) has the advantage of taking into account multiple factors that have been shown to be predictive of respiratory and all-cause mortality. The BODE index requires a (*B*) BMI, FEV_1 as a measure of (*O*) obstruction, degree of (*D*) dyspnea on the Medical Research Council dyspnea scale, and (*E*) exercise capacity as measured by a 6-minute walk test. Patients who have a 5 or greater BODE score are appropriate for evaluation for lung transplant and/or other advanced treatment modalities.

END-OF-LIFE CARE

For patients that have not previously expressed their desires regarding invasive or life supporting treatments, difficult decisions have to be made during the time of an acute illness. It is preferable, however, to facilitate patient expression of their end-of-life wishes in a stable and less stressed state. The time of discharge from the hospital can be a "teachable moment" and discussion of what the patient would or would not want in the case of future illness and/or respiratory failure should occur.

For some patients, an emphasis on palliative care (formerly or informally) and/or hospice referral may be appropriate. Dyspnea is a key symptom that must be addressed as a source of anxiety and discomfort for the patient. Oxygenation status, respiratory rate and other objective measures are not good indicators of a patient's perception of breathlessness. When underlying causes of dyspnea can be corrected, that should be the focus of care. When the underlying causes are not reversible, opiods in low to moderate doses have good effect in relieving dyspnea. For patients who have a significant component of anxiety along with dyspnea, benzodiazepines may be added to relieve symptoms.

DISCHARGE PLANNING

For the majority of patients admitted with an AECOPD, improvement is noted within a short period from admission. For the minority of patients that do not improve, alternative diagnoses, intensified therapies, and/or palliative measures must be considered. The latter stages of an acute inpatient stay can focus on tapering the frequency of medication dosing, transitioning care to an outpatient setting, patient education, and prevention of future exacerbations.

The GOLD and the ATS/ERS guidelines provide lists of criteria that should be met for consideration of discharge to home. These include controlling or reversing the reason for admission, hemodynamic stability, return to oxygenation baseline, less frequent need for inhaled bronchodilators, ability to resume ambulating, no parenteral therapy for 12 to 24 hours, ability to eat and sleep without being disturbed by dyspnea, understanding the use of medications, and completion of arrangements for follow-up and/or home care. For patients to meet all of these criteria, length of stay might increase beyond what is reasonable or desirable. While the patient's trend should be back toward baseline, full recovery and baseline oxygenation status might take several weeks and strict adherence to the guidelines may not be practical or feasible.

QUALITY IMPROVEMENT

SECONDARY PREVENTION

Smoking cessation

Counseling regarding tobacco cessation for active smokers is essential because tobacco cessation is the best way to slow the decline in lung function. There is some limited data that counseling during an inpatient stay might increase the chance of quitting and more robust evidence that quit rates can be increased by inpatient counseling followed by continued outpatient intervention. Also, several pharmacological strategies have been shown to improve quit rates. Options include nicotine replacement, buproprion (which can be used in conjunction with nicotine replacement) and varenicline. A Cochrane Review compiled several trials of varenicline and found that relative risk of cessation was 2 to 3 times greater when compared to placebo, approximately 1.5 times greater when compared to buproprion, and approximately 1.3 times greater when compared to nicotine replacement therapy.

Vaccinations

All patients with COPD should have the 23-valent pneumococcal polysaccharide vaccine, and those patients aged greater than 65 that have not had the vaccine in the last 5 years should have it administered regardless of previous vaccination status. Also, all patients with COPD should have the influenza vaccine annually.

PATIENT EDUCATION

Efforts toward education are also vital for improving the patient's health after discharge and include education regarding proper inhaler technique, and avoidance of second hand smoke (and other respiratory irritants). Patient education regarding the ability to recognize the symptoms of an exacerbation should be emphasized.

PULMONARY REHABILITATION

Pulmonary rehabilitation is an important part of outpatient COPD care after an admission of an AECOPD, and should be considered at the time of discharge for all patients with chronic lung disease with the goal of alleviating symptoms and optimizing functional capacity. Evidence supports that entering pulmonary rehabilitation within 10 days of hospital discharge is safe. Furthermore, patients enrolled in early pulmonary rehabilitation experienced improved exercise tolerance and health status at 3 months. Beyond functional capacity, pulmonary rehabilitation programs often focus on establishing social support and care networks that are most appropriate for the patient and can have quality-of-life benefits beyond physical improvements.

PRACTICE POINT

- Evidence supports that entering pulmonary rehabilitation within 10 days of hospital discharge is safe, and patients enrolled in early pulmonary rehabilitation experience improved exercise tolerance and health status at 3 months.

SURGICAL TREATMENT OPTIONS AND TRANSPLANT EVALUATION

Surgical treatment options for COPD include lung volume reduction surgery (LVRS), bullectomy, lung transplantation and investigational approaches. LVRS involves bilateral removal of 25% to 30% of total lung volume. The NETT trial, published in 2003, demonstrated that LVRS improved exercise capacity but not survival among all patients with severe emphysema. This trial did, however, identify subgroups that did have a survival advantage. The best candidates for LVRS are patients with predominantly upper-lobe disease and a low exercise tolerance at baseline. Bullectomy has not been well studied in randomized trials, but it may be considered for patients with at least one-third of the thorax occupied by bullae.

For patients with advanced disease another therapy to consider is lung transplantation. Lung transplant referral is indicated for younger patients with COPD that have progressive symptoms despite maximal medical therapy, including smoking cessation. Lung transplant for COPD has been shown to improve quality of life, but effect on mortality has not been clearly demonstrated and is more controversial.

TRANSITIONS OF CARE

Patients transitioning from inpatient to outpatient care, whether for an AECOPD or for patients with underlying COPD admitted for other reasons, have many educational and therapeutic needs. Education needs include smoking cessation, inhaler technique and mobility prescriptions. For patients that might still have pain issues or decreased mobility, education regarding incentive spirometry is vitally important. Follow-up care should be arranged with a primary care physician, a pulmonary specialist or both. For discharges after an AECOPD, follow-up should be arranged at discharge for the patient to be seen within 2 weeks of discharge. Patients should be seen sooner if they are going to a rehabilitation facility, if they are on an oral steroid taper, have a new oxygen prescription, or have other significant changes to their care regimen.

DISPARITIES IN HEALTH CARE

COPD has long been considered a disease of white, male smokers. Data, however, shows that the epidemic is increasing most rapidly for women and African Americans. In 2000, more women died of COPD than men, and the death rate is increasing more rapidly for African Americans. To some degree, these changes represent changes in the demographics of cigarette smoking over the last decades. However, some data suggests that women and African Americans may actually be more susceptible to chronic lung disease when compared to white men. In general, women have smaller caliber central airways than similarly sized men and African Americans

TABLE 239-9 Evidence-based Medicine: Key References for Chronic Obstructive Pulmonary Disease

Reference	Methodology	Results	Limitations	Bottom Line
Calverely P, et al. *N Engl J Med.* 2007; 356:775–789. TORCH trial	Randomized, double-blind, placebo-controlled trial of placebo vs salmeterol alone vs fluticasone alone vs salmeterol plus fluticasone inhaled twice daily for 3 y. 6112 patients were active or former smokers with diagnosis of COPD, FEV_1 < 60% predicted and no significant bronchodilator response	Comparing combination therapy to placebo, there was nonstatistically significant reduction in mortality (OR, 0.825; CI 0.681–1.002). Compared to placebo, combination therapy reduced exacerbations. There were higher levels of pneumonia in both groups receiving fluticasone when compared to placebo	There was a large drop-out rate (as might be expected in a COPD trial with a placebo arm)	There is insufficient data to suggest that inhaled corticosteroids decrease mortality in patients with COPD, but addition of inhaled corticosteroid may reduce exacerbations for patients on LABAs that have recurrent exacerbations. For monotherapy in COPD, LABA should be used rather than an ICS
Taskin DP, et al. *N Engl J Med.* 2008;359:1543–1554. UPLIFT	Randomized, double-blind, placebo-controlled trial of tiotroprium vs placebo to decrease decline in FEV_1 over time (before and after bronchodilation) in 5993 patients	There was no significant difference in decline in FEV_1 over time in the tiotroprium group as compared to placebo. Tiotroprium did lead to increases in FEV_1 (but not change over time), improved quality of life scores, and fewer exacerbations	There was a large drop-out rate and short-acting inhaled anticholinergics were stopped in all patients	Tiotroprium may be prescribed to alleviate symptoms of COPD, but should not be expected to alter progression of disease
Anthonisen NR. *JAMA.* 1994;272:1497–1505. Lung Health study	Randomized, placebo-controlled trial comparing no intervention to smoking cessation counseling plus placebo to smoking cessation counseling plus inhaled short-acting anticholinergics in 5887 patients	Participants in both smoking cessation groups experienced smaller declines in FEV_1 over time. Responses to short-acting anticholinergics were not cumulative over time	There was predictably low adherence to prescribed inhalers	Smoking cessation counseling can lead to declines in rates of smoking, and FEV_1 decline was mitigated amongst patients who received counseling, and the effect was strongest in those who did abstain
Bronchard L, et al. *N Engl J Med.* 1995; 333:817–822.	Prospective randomized trial comparing use of NIPPV vs standard care for treating 85 patients admitted to ICU with COPD exacerbation	NIPPV significantly decreased rate of endotracheal intubation, hospital LOS, and in-hospital mortality	Large percentage of patients admitted to ICU with COPD exacerbation were excluded, limiting population of patients to which data can be applied	For selected patients with acute exacerbations of COPD, application of NIPPV can prevent need for endotracheal intubation and speed recovery
National Emphysema Treatment Trial Research Group. *N Engl J Med.* 2003;348:2059–2073. NETT trial	Randomized trial of 1218 patients with severe emphysema to receive lung volume reduction surgery vs continued medical care. Overall mortality and maximal exercise capacity were compared as primary outcomes	In entire study group, there was no difference in overall mortality. Surgery group had significantly higher percentage of patients who improved maximal exercise capacity when compared to nonsurgery group. In subgroup analysis, patients with mostly upper-lobe disease and low exercise tolerance, there was a mortality benefit from surgery. Amongst subgroup of nonupper-lobe emphysema and high exercise capacity, mortality was higher in surgery group. Interim analysis identified group of patients with high risk of surgical death	No difference in mortality overall. Caution must be used when results of subgroup analysis are applied	Lung volume reduction surgery may be indicated for specific group of patients who have predominantly upper-lobe emphysema and low exercise capacity. Risks and benefits must be weighed against options of doing nothing vs lung transplant. Patients with FEV_1 ≤ 20% predicted and either homogenous emphysema or DLCO ≤ 20% predicted are at high risk of death from lung-volume reduction surgery

COPD, chronic obstructive pulmonary disease; DLCO, diffusing capacity of the lung for carbon monoxide; FEV_1, forced expiratory volume in 1 second; ICS, inhaled corticosteroid; ICU, intensive care unit; LABA, long-acting beta-agonist; NIPPV, noninvasive positive pressure ventilation; OR, odds ratio.

have smaller trunk/leg ratios than whites. These differences could explain more clinically significant airflow limitation after exposure to cigarettes or other respiratory toxins. Possible differences in specific genes, proteases, and/or cytokines might also explain some differences in response to exposures.

OUTCOMES TO MONITOR

There are many possible outcomes to monitor and measure regarding quality of care for patients admitted with an AECOPD or for patients with COPD treated in the hospital for other issues. The percentage of patients provided with smoking cessation counseling would be appropriate for either group, as would vaccination rates.

For patients treated for an AECOPD, tracking the number of patients referred for pulmonary rehabilitation is another option, as is the short-term re-admission rate. Lastly, the percentage of patients with severe COPD that are referred to hospice and/or palliative services could be monitored.

COSTS AND RESOURCE UTILIZATION

While only smoking cessation and supplemental oxygen have been proven to have an impact on chronic COPD mortality, there are many other modalities that could improve quality of life and possibly decrease health care costs for patients with COPD.

Smoking cessation programs, health-maintenance case workers for patients with COPD and pulmonary rehabilitation programs each offer ways in which large institutions might decrease overall costs for the care of a population of COPD patients. Vaccinations have been shown to have significant cost-savings as well.

Another area of focus for resource utilization is goals of care and end of life discussions. A 2006 study found that COPD patients in the last 6 months of life were more likely to be admitted to an ICU and have longer length of stay when compared to patients in the last 6 months of life with lung cancer (**Table 239-9**). Total health care costs were $4000 more per patient during this time frame. Improved communication (preferably before admission, but also possibly at the time of admission) regarding goals of care and realistic expectations could prove to decrease these costs while hopefully improving quality of life for terminal patients and their families.

SUGGESTED READINGS

Almagro P, Balbo E, Ochoa de Echaguen A, et al. Mortality after hospitalization for COPD. *Chest*. 2002;121:1441–1448.

Bronchard L, Mancebo J, Wysocki M, et al. Noninvasive ventilation for acute exacerbations of chronic obstructive pulmonary disease. *N Engl J Med*. 1995;333:817–822.

Celli BR, Cote CG, Marin JM, et al. The body-mass index, airflow obstruction, dyspnea, and exercise capacity index in chronic obstructive pulmonary disease. *N Engl J Med*. 2004;350(10):1005–1012.

Celli BR, MacNee W, Augusti A, et al. ATS/ERS TASK FORCE. Standards for the diagnosis and treatment of patients with COPD: a summary of the ATS/ERS position paper. *Eur Respir J*. 2004;23: 932–946.

Connors AF Jr, Dawson NV, Thomas C, et al. Outcomes following acute exacerbation of severe chronic obstructive lung disease: the SUPPORT investigators (Study to Understand Prognoses and Preferences for Outcomes and Risks of Treatments). *Am J Respir Crit Care Med*. 1996;154(4 pt 1):959–967.

Global Initiative for Chronic Obstructive Lung Disease. Global Strategy for the Diagnosis, Management, and Prevention of Chronic Obstructive Pulmonary Disease. Updated Dec 2009. Available at: http://www.goldcopd.com. Accessed December 30, 2009.

Munafo M, Rigotti N, Lancaster T, et al. Interventions for smoking cessation in hospitalised patients: a systematic review. *Thorax*. 2001;56(8):656–663.

Nathan SD. Lung transplantation: disease-specific considerations for referral. *Chest*. 2005;127:1006–1016.

Salpeter SS, Ormiston T, Salpeter E, et al. Cardioselective beta blockers for chronic obstructive pulmonary disease (Cochrane Review). *Cochrane Database Syst Rev*. 2005(1): Issue 4. Art. No.: CD003566.

Seemungal TA, Donaldson GC, Bhowmik A, et al. Time course and recovery of exacerbations in patients with chronic obstructive pulmonary disease. *Am J Respir Crit Care Med*. 2000;161: 1608–1613.

CHAPTER 240

Cystic Fibrosis

David Tong, MD, MPH
Arlene Stecenko, MD

Key Clinical Questions

1. How do mutations in the cystic fibrosis (CF) gene relate to the clinical manifestations of the disease?
2. What criteria help determine when a CF patient should be admitted to hospital for respiratory complications of the disease?
3. What treatment modalities are most effective in restoring lung function to baseline for CF respiratory exacerbations?
4. Why is CF–related diabetes (CFRD) one of the most important comorbidities in CF and how does it alter the course of the disease?
5. What are the most effective treatment modalities for the two most common pulmonary complications of CF: massive hemoptysis and pneumothorax?

INTRODUCTION

DEFINITION AND OVERVIEW

Cystic fibrosis (CF) is an autosomal recessive disease due to mutations in the CF transmembrane conductance regulator (CFTR) gene. The CFTR gene is expressed in epithelial cells in a variety of organs including the lung, sinuses, pancreas, sweat gland, intestine, liver, and vas deferens, and thus CF is a mulitorgan disease. CF is the most common inherited life-shortening disease of Caucasians in the United States. More than 90% of the morbidity and the mortality is due to lung disease. CF lung disease is characterized by the triad of altered mucociliary clearance, chronic polymicrobial infection of the airways, and an exaggerated inflammatory response. The ultimate outcome of CF lung disease is destruction of the normal airway architecture and death due to respiratory failure.

With therapy, primarily aimed at slowing the progression of lung disease and improving nutrition, median survival is approaching 40 years of age. Unfortunately, there is no cure for CF. The average CF adult can expect to spend 2 to 3 hours a day taking a variety of inhaled medications, ingest 30 to 50 pills per day, and be hospitalized about once per year for a period of 1 to 3 weeks. Even with insurance, most CF patients have out-of-pocket health care costs approximating $10,000 per year.

However, there are a significant number of CF patients who have normal lung function, rarely require hospitalizations, and need only a few medications to control their disease. Thus, there can be tremendous variability in the severity of the pulmonary phenotype in this monogenic disease ranging from death in childhood due to respiratory failure to living to retirement and the thought of enjoyment of family and friends as old age ensues.

GENETIC EPIDEMIOLOGY—INCIDENCE AND ETHNIC DISTRIBUTION

The incidence of CF varies tremendously according to ethnicity. Also, those countries, such as the United States, that have universal newborn screening for CF will have more accurate measures of incidence than those countries that do not. CF occurs in about 1 in 3500 white births, 1 in 17,000 African Americans, and 1 in 90,000 Asians in Hawaii. Once considered a disease affecting only children, the life expectancy in CF has increased dramatically in the past 3 decades. Now 41% are over 18 years of age, and median predicted survival has increased from 28 years for those born in 1990 to 38 years for those born in 2008.

PATHOPHYSIOLOGY

The CFTR protein is a chloride channel in the apical aspect of epithelium in a variety of organs, including the lungs, sweat ducts, vas deferens, liver, pancreas, and intestines. Through unknown mechanisms, expression of mutant CFTR and the resultant failure to conduct chloride also causes marked increase in sodium import through the epithelial sodium channel, ENaC. In the lung epithelium, this results in marked reduction in the depth of the airway surface lining fluid and loss of effective mucociliary clearance.

CFTR also transports glutathione, the major antioxidant in the lung. Thus, expression of mutant CFTR results in failure to export glutathione to the extracellular compartment resulting in extremely low levels of antioxidant capacity in the epithelial lining fluid and more susceptibility to damage. Mutant CFTR also causes failure to transport

TABLE 240-1 Class of Gene Defects

Class	Mutation Example	Cellular/Molecular Phenotype
I	W1282X	Absent CFTR production due to nonsense mutations, frameshift mutations, or abnormal mRNA splicing
II	ΔF508	Improper intracellular processing of CFTR with less than normal amounts of CFTR protein at the apical plasma membrane
III	G551D	Defective regulation of CFTR channels at the apical plasma membrane
IV	R117H	Defective permeation of anions through CFTR channels at the apical plasma membrane
V	3849 + 10KbC > T	Reduced synthesis of normal CFTR
VI	Q1412X	Altered apical membrane residence time of CFTR channels with truncated c-termini

Reproduced, with permission, from Kreindler, *Pharmacology and Therapeutics.* 2010;125:219–229.

bicarbonate, contributing to the development of pancreatic exocrine insufficiency and eventual development of malabsorption.

Recent evidence suggests that CFTR may be expressed in pancreatic beta cells thus providing a potential molecular mechanism for the very high prevalence of diabetes in CF.

Expression of mutant CFTR, particularly in neutrophils and airway epithelial cells, results in an abnormal proinflammatory response characterized by an excessive and persistent production of cytokines that generates a neutrophil dominated inflammation. The CF airway shows a tremendous preponderance of neutrophils even shortly after birth. These neutrophils are a source of elastase and reactive oxygen species that destroy lung tissue. Furthermore, dying neutrophils in the CF lung do not undergo apoptosis but rather necrosis, resulting in release of massive amounts of sticky, uncoiled DNA that markedly increases the viscosity of airway secretions.

Persistent bacterial infection (particularly with *Pseudomonas aeruginosa* and *Staphyloccocus aureus*) of the airway is the hallmark of CF lung disease, and proposed mechanisms for this include defective phagocytosis, defective intracellular killing, increase in the number of receptors for bacteria on epithelial cells, and promotion of biofilm formation by the bacteria.

The CFTR gene is on chromosome 7, and there are more than 1600 disease causing mutations of this gene, within six classes (**Table 240-1**). The most common mutation, Δ508 is a three-base pair deletion in exon 10, resulting in deletion of the phenylalanine residue at position 508. This defect accounts for 66% of the CF mutations worldwide. About 15 mutations may account for 80% to 90% of the mutations seen in Caucasians.

Mutations where there is little or no full length CFTR at the outer plasma membrane are considered "severe" and those where there is a full length protein but in some way the protein has defective function are considered "mild." However, significant discordance between gene mutations and severity of lung disease suggests the importance of modifier genes and environmental interactions in disease expression, and explains why two cystic fibrosis patients with the same gene defect in the CFTR gene can present with very different disease severity and clinical course.

Cystic fibrosis can affect multiple organs but the vast morbidity and of mortality occurs due to lung disease. The triad of impaired mucociliary clearance, persistent airway infection, and exaggerated inflammatory response leads to bronchiectasis and ultimately respiratory failure and death. Lung function declines progressively in most CF patients, with an annual rate of decline in function varying from 1% to 4% decrease per year. The rate of decline may be punctuated by acute pulmonary exacerbations with precipitous drops in lung function and incomplete recovery from the exacerbation. Resetting of baseline lung function at a new lower level may occur following respiratory exacerbations. Frequent respiratory exacerbations are the hallmark of lung disease severity in CF, and significantly impact quality of life, health care costs and survival.

The cause of acute pulmonary exacerbations is currently unknown, but likely is related to increased bacterial load rather than infection by a different strain of bacteria. Other risk factors include increased exposure to particulate air pollutants and viral infections (eg, influenza virus, respiratory syncitial virus) However, nearly 20% of CF pulmonary exacerbations have no identified inciting cause.

DIFFERENTIAL DIAGNOSIS

The diagnosis of CF can be considered for patients with symptoms of COPD or asthma who are not responding as expected to treatment. Also, the isolation of mucoid *Pseudomonas* in a person with chronic respiratory symptoms should suggest the diagnosis of CF. CF patients may also present with isolated pancreatitis so patients with recurrent pancreatitis unexplained by alcohol, medications or gallstones should be considered for workup for CF. Pansinusitis is rare in healthy children and adults so this finding should prompt a screening for CF. Nasal polyps are unusual in healthy adolescents younger than 20 years old and should prompt a screening for CF.

PRACTICE POINT

Cystic Fibrosis diagnosis should be considered in people with any of the following:

- Symptoms of COPD or asthma not responding as expected to treatment
- Isolation of mucoid pseudomonas in a person with chronic respiratory symptoms
- Isolated pancreatitis or recurrent pancreatitis unexplained by alcohol, medications, or gallstones
- Pansinusitis
- Nasal polyps in healthy adolescents younger than 20 years old

DIAGNOSIS

CF may be suspected in a patient because of having one or more characteristic phenotypic symptoms, a positive history of CF in a sibling, or a positive newborn screen. The diagnosis of CF is made by two positive sweat chloride results done on separate days using quantitative pilocarpine iontophoresis in a clinical laboratory certified by the Cystic Fibrosis Foundation (**Table 240-2**). However, 2% of patients with a convincing clinical presentation for CF have a

TABLE 240-2 Pilocarpine Sweat Test Table

Chloride Concentration	Interpretation
>60 mEq/L	Positive
40–60 mEq/L	Indeterminate
<40 mEq/L	Negative

sweat chloride in the indeterminate range and some rare mutations are associated with normal sweat test results. In this situation, a CFTR genotype and sequencing can identify whether the person has two disease causing mutations.

All 50 states in the United States have now implemented newborn screening for CF. Prior to newborn screening, about 3% to 5% of CF patients were diagnosed as adults. This number will decrease with time but it will take several years to decades before diagnosis of CF in adulthood is a rarity. In addition, many states screen only for the most common mutations and thus newborn screening will not identify all CF persons.

■ PULMONARY EXACERBATION DIAGNOSTIC TESTING

Diagnostic testing in the setting of acute pulmonary CF exacerbation should include CF sputum cultures (using the Cystic Fibrosis Foundation approved methods for detecting polymicrobial isolates), complete blood count, comprehensive chemistry panel, and posterior-anterior and lateral chest x-ray. Pregnancy test should be obtained for women of childbearing age. CF patients with change in symptoms should undergo pulmonary function testing (PFTs) with spirometry to assess FEV_1 and any change from the patient's baseline level. A significant decrease in FEV_1 from baseline (even with unimpressive symptoms or physical examination) may prompt inpatient admission for IV antibiotics rather than outpatient management.

Additional testing for patients who have not responded to standard treatment of a CF pulmonary exacerbation as expected may include sputum for fungal stain and cultures, sputum for acid fast bacilli, and immunoglobulin (Ig) E level (to evaluate for allergic bronchopulmonary aspergillosis, [ABPA]).

Chest computed tomography (CT) is *not* necessary for treatment of routine acute pulmonary exacerbations. However, if suspicion for lung abscess, pulmonary embolus, or nontuberculous mycobacteria (NTM) is high, chest CT may be helpful.

Follow-up inpatient PFTs may be considered to document recovery of lung function after initiation of therapy, but acutely in the hospital setting the results may be discordant with the patient's clinical course.

For patients with cystic fibrosis-related diabetes (CFRD) who are doing carbohydrate counting to dose their insulin, 2-hour postprandial blood sugars should be obtained in addition to preprandial and bedtime blood sugars in order to determine if failure to achieve glycemic control is responsible for failure to restore lung function to baseline.

Sinus CT is only indicated based on significant new sinus symptoms during the patient presentation. They should not be ordered routinely for pulmonary exacerbation in the absence of new sinus symptoms or signs.

TRIAGE/HOSPITAL ADMISSION

Although there is currently no standard definition of an acute pulmonary exacerbation in CF, a number of different criteria have been devised for clinical trials and clinical care. The majority of definitions capture respiratory symptoms such as increased cough, increased sputum production, shortness of breath and chest pain, as well as other measures such as loss of appetite, fatigue, and missing either work or school. However, CF clinicians put the most reliance on a decrease in lung function and will diagnose a pulmonary exacerbation in the absence of any reported change in symptoms if there is a significant decrease in FEV_1. This may be particularly true in those exacerbations that develop over a period of a few weeks and the patient is simply unaware of how much symptoms have increased until lung function and symptoms return to baseline following appropriate treatment.

Treatment of the exacerbation, if not severe, begins with outpatient oral antibiotics, increase in airway clearance, and emphasis on compliance with chronic pulmonary medications. More frequent clinic visits and greater use of antibiotics is associated with better PFT results. Close follow-up, usually within a week or two, is needed to make sure lung function has returned to the patient's baseline.

If lung function does not improve despite a trial of oral antibiotics, then the standard of care is to start intravenous (IV) antibiotics. The Cystic Fibrosis Foundation recommends that home therapy may be appropriate for select patients, but that intravenous antibiotics in a nonhospital setting should not be done unless resources and support equivalent to the hospital setting can be assured for the treatment of an acute exacerbation of pulmonary disease.

Issues to consider when deciding whether to administer IV antibiotics in the outpatient setting include the severity of the exacerbation, whether adequate delivery of other treatments such as airway clearance therapies can be maintained, and the presence of comorbidites such as malnutrition and diabetes that require in hospital care. The current practice in many Cystic Fibrosis Centers is to admit patients with a pulmonary exacerbation to hospital for intensive treatment if outpatient management using oral antibiotics has not restored lung function to baseline. Once hospital treatment has been initiated, been shown to be tolerated by the patient, and the patient is clinically improving, then it may be appropriate to complete treatment in the home.

Hemoptysis, often a sign of pulmonary exacerbation, is a common presenting complaint, occurring in about 9% of CF patients and can range from slight streaking to massive bleeding. Massive hemoptysis (which occurs in 4% of patients) is defined as more than 240 mL of blood in a 24-hour period. It is due to arterial bleeding from hypertrophied bronchial arteries. There is no evidence-based data to guide triage of hemoptysis in CF patients, but current consensus-based recommendations from the Cystic Fibrosis Foundation are that patients with at least mild hemoptysis (measured as >5 mL) should contact their health care provider and scant hemoptysis (<5 mL) should contact their health care provider if it is the first ever episode or if it persists.

Scant hemoptysis may not require hospital admission if there is no other evidence of a significant acute pulmonary exacerbation, but massive hemoptysis (>240 mL) always requires hospital admission. Some centers admit for hemoptysis greater than 120 mL in a 24-hour period.

About 3% of CF patients will have a pneumothorax during their lifetime with an annual incidence of 0.64%, with attributable mortality as high as 16%. Disease severity predicts pneumothorax complication, with 75% of pneumothoraces occuring in patients with an FEV_1 <40% predicted. CF patients with a pneumothorax should almost always be admitted to hospital as the risk of progression and further respiratory compromise are high.

MANAGEMENT

■ ACUTE PULMONARY EXACERBATION MANAGEMENT

Many, if not most, of the large, multicenter, double-blind, placebo-controlled clinical trials evaluating efficacy of pulmonary drugs in CF have been for outpatient management to prevent respiratory exacerbations, rather than for the management of an exacerbation once it is severe enough to require hospitalization. Therefore, recommendations for inpatient treatment rely on limited studies of small number of patients and on expert opinion. A sample inpatient admission protocol for CF patients with an acute respiratory exacerbation includes specific details of care in addition to an educational tool.

The current mainstay of treatment for acute respiratory exacerbations consists of IV antibiotics and enhanced airway clearance. In addition, pulmonary and nonpulmonary complications of CF that may impair the ability to restore lung function to baseline require evaluation and management; and nutritional support must be addressed. *P aeruginosa* is the most frequent organism found during an acute exacerbation. However, polymicrobial infections are also common, particularly with *Staphylococcus aureus* as well as multiple strains of *Pseudomonas*, each with a different pattern of antibiotic sensitivity. More recently, organisms previously thought to be commensals, such as *Stenotrophomonas maltophilia*, are now viewed as potentially pathogenic. Early isolates of pseudomonas are nonmucoid and have a broader range of antibiotic sensitivity. However, in the CF airway the organism can mutate to a mucoid form and also can form a biofilm. Such mutations, particularly toward a biofilm, may make antibiotics less effective.

Antimicrobials

The Cystic Fibrosis Foundation guidelines—for the treatment of a respiratory exacerbation in patients whose culture grows pseudomonas—recommend using two IV antibiotics of different classes (**Table 240-3**). Depending on the antibiotic sensitivities on the sputum culture, an aminoglycoside and a beta-lactam antibiotic is the preferred combination. Dual therapy may prevent the development of resistance and may have more benefit than monotherapy. There have been some clinical trials comparing monotherapy with combination therapy, but there is insufficient evidence due to the small number of patients in each trial to recommend one over the other.

Antibiotic selection should be based initially on the most recent sputum susceptibility results and later adjusted if there is inadequate response. However, if the patient improves with initial therapy, there is no need to change antibiotics even if the admission sputum indicates inadequate sensitivity to the chosen antibiotics as there is poor correlation between antibiotic susceptibility results and clinical outcomes. Finally, if current sputum results indicate broad resistance with no good antibiotic options a previously successful regimen may be started as initial therapy.

Aminoglycosides are frequently used in the treatment of acute pulmonary exacerbations. CF patients, particularly those under 40 years of age, require higher doses than non-CF patients to achieve therapeutic blood levels. Also, once daily tobramycin dosing has been shown to be as effective as multiple daily dosing and is associated with less renal toxicity. Clinical pharmacy consultation is critical for monitoring aminoglycoside levels.

Although some cystic fibrosis centers are routinely using continuous infusions of beta-lactam antibiotics in the treatment of acute pulmonary exacerbations, there are not enough data to support this practice routinely.

The optimal duration of intravenous antibiotic treatment for an exacerbation is not known. The usual goal is to restore lung function to baseline and this can take from 10 to 21 days. However, no prospective studies have evaluated the optimal duration of antibiotic course, and therefore, this area deserves further study.

Pulmonary exacerbation prevention

Macrolides, such as azithromycin at 500 mg 3 times a week, have been shown in large, multicentered, placebo-controlled studies to reduce the rate of hospitalizations and improve FEV_1 in those patients infected with *P aeruginosa*. Recent data indicates that chronic use of azithromycin may be helpful in those CF patients with methicillin-resistant *S aureus*. During therapy for acute pulmonary exacerbations, chronic pulmonary maintenance therapies may be continued (**Table 240-4**).

Renal function and relevant monitoring of electrolytes and blood counts may be necessary, depending on the antibiotic choices and known side effects. Infectious disease consultants should assist with antimicrobial selection and clinical pharmacists, when available, should assist with antimicrobial dosing and monitoring.

TABLE 240-3 Antibiotic Recommendations and Dosing for Acute Respiratory Exacerbations*

Pseudomonas only (Recommend two-drug therapy, tobramycin plus beta lactam if pseudomonas is sensitive)
Tobramycin 10 mg/kg IV every 24 hours[†]
Amikacin 10 mg/kg IV every 8 hours[†]
Ceftazidime 50 mg/kg IV every 8 hours (max. 10 g/d)
Piperacillin-tazobactam 4.5 mg IV every 6 hours
Meropenem 2 g IV every 8 hours
Colistimethate 2.5 mg IV every 12 hours
Aztreonam 2 g IV every 8 hours (major indication is severe PCN or cephalosporin allergy)
Methicillin-sensitive *staphylococcus aureus* and *pseudomonas*. Recommend two-drug therapy: one of the following plus tobramycin 10 mg/kg/24 hr if pseudomonas is sensitive
Ticarcillin-clavulanate 3.1 g IV every 4 hours
Cefepime 2 g IV every 8 hours
Meropenem 2 g IV every 8 hours
Piperacillin-tazobactam 4.5 mg IV every 6 hours
Methicillin-resistant *S aureus*
Linezolid 600 mg IV every 12 hours
Tigecycline 100 mg bolus then 50 mg IV every 12 hours
Vancomycin 15–20 mg/kg every 8–12 hours[§]

*Dosing for normal renal function. Adjustments may be necessary when renal dysfunction is present.

[†]Pharmacokinetics or infectious diseases consultation recommended.

[§]Trough levels of 15–20 mcg/mL recommended.

TABLE 240-4 Chronic Pulmonary Maintenance Therapy

Inhaled
Dornase alpha 2.5 mg nebulized daily or twice a day
Aztreonam 75 mg nebulized three times a day for 1 month every other month—can rotate with another aerosolized antibiotic
Tobramycin 300 mg nebulized twice a day for 1 month every other month—can rotate with another aerosolized antibiotic
Colistimethate 150 mg nebulized twice a day for 1 month every other month—can rotate with another aerosolized antibiotic
Sodium chloride 7% 4 mL nebulized twice a day to three times a day for FEV_1 > 40%. Most often hypertonic saline is preceded by inhaled beta-2 agent. Can be used in patients with lower lung function but may not be tolerated. In this situation, can use lower concentrations, like 5% or 3% but these have not been studied
Oral
Azithromycin 500 mg orally Monday, Wednesday, and Friday
Airway clearance therapies
Chest physiotherapy using manuel, vest, Acapella valve twice a day
Huff cough
Exercise

Airway clearance

Airway clearance through increased chest physiotherapy (compared to home regimen, and up to 4 times per day) can improve exacerbation outcomes and improve symptoms more rapidly. Manual chest physiotherapy may be performed by respiratory care, nursing staff, physical therapists, other clinicians or family members. Mechanical chest physiotherapy using vibrating vests and Acapella devices may also be employed. In addition, aerosols aimed at improving clearance (3% or 7% hypertonic saline and/or pulmozyme) can be prescribed at increased frequencies.

Insufficient data supports continuing inhaled antibiotics if similar IV antibiotics are given during an exacerbation. Utilizing both routes of delivery could enhance antimicrobial activity in the lungs but could also increase the risk of toxicity. Therefore, the decision to do so should be made on an individual basis.

Systemic glucocorticosteroids have been used in the past as adjunct therapy for a CF respiratory exacerbation. However, two placebo-controlled studies in a small number of children showed that the addition of glucocorticosteroids to the regimen of IV antibiotics and enhanced airway clearance was no better than placebo in improving the recovery rate from the exacerbation. Glucocorticosteroids also worsen hyperglycemia which is known to contribute to oxidative stress and inflammation in the CF lung. Thus, glucocorticosteroids cannot be recommended for the routine treatment of a CF pulmonary exacerbation unless the exacerbation is due to status asthmaticus or ABPA.

PRACTICE POINT

- Glucocorticosteroids are not recommended for the *routine* treatment of a CF pulmonary exacerbation unless the exacerbation is due to status asthmaticus or ABPA.

Hypoxemic and hypercapneic respiratory failure may occur during hospitalization. Patients with poor baseline status due to chronic progression do poorly with mechanical ventilation but those with milder disease with acute exacerbations have better outcomes with mechanical intubation. Discussions regarding end-of-life care should be done before acute intervention is required.

INFECTIOUS PULMONARY COMPLICATIONS

Burkholderia cepacia

Burkholderia cepacia is a fatal necrotizing pneumonia associated with bacteremia in 20% of infected patients. *B cepacia* complex commonly is multidrug resistant and can produce a pronounced inflammatory response associated with rapid loss of lung function.

Patients with *B cepacia* complex have a very high mortality following lung transplantation as the high dose immunosuppression needed to prevent acute rejection frequently results in wide spread dissemination of the *B cepacia* and death from multiorgan failure. Consequently, many transplant centers view the presence of *B cepacia* complex as an absolute contraindication to lung transplantation.

Nontuberculous mycobacteria

Nontuberculous mycobacteria (NTM) should be considered in CF patients with unexplained fatigue, night sweats, hemoptysis or progressive decline in lung function that is not responding to usual CF pulmonary treatment. In particular *Mycobacterium abscessus* and *Mycobacterium* avium complex (MAC) infections are found in approximately 5% of CF adults. Infection is diagnosed by at least two NTM positive sputum cultures collected on different days or a positive bronchoalveolar lavage culture. MAC is treated with long-term therapy (usually daily rifampin, azithromycin, and ethambutol) for 12 to 18 months. *M abscessus* is difficult to treat and eradicate as it may only be sensitive to intravenous antibiotics.

Fungal infections

Aspergillus fumigatus can be isolated in 40% to 60% and *Candida albicans* in 20% to 30% of patients. ABPA occurs in up to 10% of CF patients. Invasive aspergillosis and aspergillomas are very uncommon. ABPA may be clinically indistinguishable from a CF exacerbation as both may present with airway obstruction, fleeting pulmonary infiltrates, bronchiectasis, and hemoptysis.

ABPA should be considered in a CF patient with deteriorating lung function that is not responding to standard CF treatment. Testing for specific IgE and IgG to A *fumigatus* can diagnose ABPA, particularly in CF patients with eosinophil counts $>1000/mm^3$ or elevated IgE >500 IU/mL.

Treatment for ABPA requires high dose glucocorticosteroid therapy (oral prednisone at 0.5–2 mg/kg, max 60 mg/d) plus itraconazole (5 mg/kg/d, max 200 mg orally twice a day). If the patient has CFRD, insulin dose usually needs to be increased. High-dose glucorticosteroids are given usually for 2 weeks before tapering. If total IgE is greater than 1000 IU/mL, glucocorticosteroids often are not tapered until the IgE level is below 1000 IU/mL. If there is no improvement with high-dose steroids, the diagnosis should be questioned and corticosteroids tapered quickly followed by stopping the intraconazole.

PRACTICE POINT

- ABPA should be considered in a CF patient with deteriorating lung function that is not responding to standard CF treatments. Testing for specific IgE and IgG to A *fumigatus* can diagnose ABPA, particularly in CF patients with eosinophil counts $>1000/mm^3$ or elevated IgE >500 IU/mL.

HEMOPTYSIS MANAGEMENT

Because pulmonary exacerbation often manifest with mild hemoptysis, >5 mL of blood should be treated with antibiotics. The affected lung should be kept dependent to prevent bleeding from affecting the other lung. Lack of consensus about continuing versus stopping chest physiotherapy with mild to moderate hemoptysis leads some to stop the therapy until 24 to 48 hours after the bleeding has ceased, while others continue this intervention. Patients with scant and mild hemoptysis most often have aerosol treatments continued, while aerosol treatments should be individualized for those with mild to moderate hemoptysis.

Bronchial artery embolization (BAE) is the treatment most often indicated for massive hemoptysis. Bronchoscopy is not appropriate before BAE as there is little evidence that bronchoscopy can localize bleeding, and it can delay a lifesaving procedure. Lung resection may be considered only after other measures such as BAE have failed to control the bleeding. Chest physiotherapy should be stopped in massive hemoptysis. Aerosol treatments are often discontinued in patients with massive hemoptysis.

PRACTICE POINT

- Massive hemoptysis often requires BAE by interventional radiology. Bronchoscopy is not considered appropriate before BAE as it can rarely localize bleeding and can delay a lifesaving procedure.

PNEUMOTHORAX MANAGEMENT

Most CF patients with a pneumothorax, regardless of size, should be admitted to hospital. However, the size does help determine the appropriate treatment. A small pneumothorax, defined as the distance between the apex and the cupola of ≤ 3 cm, can be treated with oxygen to help resorb the pneumothorax and serial examinations and chest x-rays are done to assess whether the pneumothorax is enlarging. A large pneumothorax (> 3 cm between the apex and the cupola) requires chest tube placement even in clinically stable patients.

Because 50% to 90% of CF patients with a pneumothorax will have a recurrence, pleurodesis should be considered for recurrent large ipsilateral pneumothoraces. Pleurodesis does not reduce lung transplantation candidacy, and can be performed safely. Surgical pleurodesis with video assisted thoracoscopic surgery is the preferred method, and should be done timely to avoid respiratory infections related to splinting and immobility.

PRACTICE POINT

- Because 50% to 90% of CF patients with a pneumothorax will have a recurrence, pleurodesis should be considered for recurrent large ipsilateral pneumothoraces.

Antibiotics are not prescribed routinely with pneumothorax; however, IV antibiotics may be indicated if the pneumothorax persists for more than a few days. Noninvasive positive pressure ventilation should be withheld.

Airway clearance therapies that increase positive expiratory pressure and intrapulmonary percussive ventilation should not be used in patients with large pneumothoraces, and it may be appropriate to withhold such therapies in patients with small pneumothoraces. Aerosol treatments should not be stopped routinely in either large or small pneumothoracees, but may be held if they increase coughing in a patient.

EXTRAPULMONARY MANIFESTATIONS

CF is a multiorgan disease and there are frequently extrapulmonary manifestations of the disease (**Table 240-5**). Often hospital providers need to address these issues when patients are hospitalized for an acute pulmonary exacerbation. In addition, exacerbation of disease in other organs at times requires hospital admission. Clinicians should be able to diagnose and treat common extrapulmonary manifestations of CF and maintain a low threshold to evaluate for them.

Sinusitis

Close to 100% of patients with classic CF (elevated sweat chloride, typical pulmonary and gastrointestinal manifestations) have radiologic evidence of pansinusitis. Approximately 43% of CF patients have nasal polyps with 25% having symptoms due to polyps sometime during their lifetime.

CFTR ion transport abnormalities lead to abnormalities in mucociliary clearance in the sinuses, impairing drainage into the nasal cavity. It is not known whether infection is a major contributor to the pansinusitis seen on radiologic examination. However, once nasal polyps develop, the drainage problem is worsened by blocking the openings to the sinuses, leading to increased infection and inflammation. One quarter of adult CF patients have chronic symptoms of sinusitis, which may cause headaches, facial pain, fever, purulent nasal discharge, halitosis, double vision, blurred vision, proptosis, and postnasal drip.

Nasal polyposis may results in epistaxis, rhinorrhea, mouth breathing, obstruction of nasal air flow, distortion of facial features, halitosis, and decreased sense of smell.

Nasal polyp resection provides immediate relief of nasal obstruction, but polyps will recur in 58% to 89% of CF patients.

Antibiotics should not be prescribed for asymptomatic CF patients with radiologic findings of sinusitis but are appropriate when patients become symptomatic. The possibility of coexisting allergies contributing to the development of nasal polyps should be considered. No consistent results have been demonstrated but nasal glucocorticoidsteroids and nasal cromolyn may be tried. Daily nasal irrigation and other supportive measures are often used. For particularly severe cases, intravenous antibiotics (selected based on results of sinus culture by otolaryngology) for 4 to 6 weeks in conjunction with a 2-week course of oral glucocorticosteroids may benefit patients, but well-designed studies have not been performed.

Endoscopic sinus surgery is recommended for all CF patients before lung transplant as recurrent infections in the lungs post transplant may be due to bacteria harbored in the sinuses. In contrast, because sinus surgery benefits are often transient in CF, sinus surgery may be considered for symptomatic sinusitis that has failed routine medical therapy including a course of outpatient intravenous antibiotics and oral glucocorticosteroids. Limited evidence suggests that surgical treatment of sinusitis in CF may improve some health outcomes (eg, reduced average number of annual hospital days), but improvement in lung function should not be expected.

Gastrointestinal tract

The most common GI tract complications of CF are esophagitis and ileal obstruction. Gastroesophageal reflux is exacerbated by coughing as well as the generation of larger negative intrapleural pressures leading to increased esophagitis incidence with more severe CF disease. Proton pump inhibitor therapy is usually effective.

CF can also lead to ileal obstruction (distal ileal obstruction syndrome [DIOS]) from retention of mucofeculent tenacious material in older children and adults. DIOS presents with crampy abdominal pain and relative constipation but can present acutely with abdominal obstruction. A tender right lower quadrant mass may be found on physical examination, and plain abdominal x-ray shows a speckled fecal gas pattern in the right lower quadrant. Often the entire colon is full of impacted fecal material. The differential diagnosis includes appendicitis, constipation, and intussusception.

Incidence of DIOS has decreased (now only about 4% of CF patients) with the use of enteric coated microspheric pancreatic enzyme replacement therapy. In CF patients who undergo surgery and require narcotics for postoperative pain, DIOS incidence may increase and complete bowel obstruction can occur with just a few narcotic doses. Some institutions initiate stool softeners and cathartic medications (eg, lactulose) empirically in CF patients following lung transplantation as soon as patients begin taking liquids by mouth.

PRACTICE POINT

- Distal ileal obstruction syndrome (DIOS) occurs in 4% of CF patients and presents with crampy abdominal pain and relative constipation but can present acutely with abdominal obstruction. Physical exam may reveal a tender right lower quadrant mass.
- In CF patients who undergo surgery and require narcotics for postoperative pain, DIOS incidence may increase and complete bowel obstruction can occur with just a few narcotic doses. Empiric stool softeners and cathartic medications (eg, lactulose) should be considered as soon as patients begin any oral intake following surgery.

TABLE 240-5 Extrapulmonary Manifestations of Cystic Fibrosis

Organ System	Useful Diagnostic Test	Therapeutic Approach
Pancreas (exocrine)		
Pancreatitis	Elevated amylase and lipase, exclusion of other causes	Bowel rest, pain management
Pancreatic insufficiency	Steatorrhea, elevated fecal fat or decrease fecal elastase	Enteric-coated microencapsulated enzymes containing proteases and lipases
Nutritional deficiencies	Albumin, prealbumin; levels for vitamins A, E, and D, Protime (vitamin K)	Aggressive caloric intake, including a high fat diet, replacement of vitamin A, E, D, and K
Pancreas (endocrine)		
CF-related diabetes (CFRD)	Random glucose > 200 mg/dL on two or more occasions or Fasting blood glucose (FBG) > 126 mg/dL on two or more occasions or Oral glucose tolerance test (OGTT) with FBG > 126 mg/dL and 2 hour value > 200 mg/dL or hemoglobin A_{1c} > 6.5%	Insulin with continued high calorie diet
Hepatobiliary		
Multilobular biliary cirrhosis Gallstones Microgallbladder Hepatic steatosis Hepatic congestion from cor pulmonale	Workup includes liver function tests, ultrasound, ERCP, and exclusion of other causes of liver disease; liver biopsy often not needed	Ursodeoxycholic acid (UDCA)
Gastrointestinal		
Neonatal meconium ileus Distal intestinal obstruction syndrome (DIOS)	History, examination and abdominal radiographs	Systemic hydration polyethylene glycol electrolyte (PEG) solutions by mouth or enemas, laparotomy and bowel resection (very rarely)
Clostridium difficile associated colitis	Stool cultures and toxin, colonoscopy or abdominal CT scan	Antibiotic treatment
Fibrosing colonopathy	Contrast enema	Reduced enzyme dose, occasionally colonic resection
Appendicitis	Examination, ultrasound, abdominal CF scan	Appendectomy
Bone and joint disease		
Osteoporosis	Dual energy x-ray absorptiometry (DEXA)	Calcium and vitamin D supplements, consider bisphosphonates
Arthritis	Serological analysis to exclude other causes of arthritis	Short courses of nonsteroidal and steroidal antiinflammatory medications
Hypertrophic pulmonary osteoarthropathy	Radiographs of long bones	Short courses of nonsteroidal antiinflammatory medications
Reproductive disease		
CBAVD resulting in azoospermia	Semen analysis	Reproduction possible through sperm retrieval and assisted reproductive techniques
Cervical mucus abnormalities	Fertility may be normal	Counseling on contraception options, reproductive issues, and family planning

Reproduced, with permission, from Hanley ME, Welsh CH. Current Diagnosis & Treatment in Pulmonary Medicine. New York: McGraw-Hill, 2003. Table 8-1.

Liver

Bile duct epithelial cells express CFTR leading to impairment in bile and mucus secretion. Localized stasis and obstruction generates an inflammatory response and reactive oxygen species leading to bile duct damage that is seen in nearly all CF patients. Some develop gall bladder disease, but few progress to biliary cirrhosis and liver failure.

Gall bladder disease is characterized by a small, shrunken gall bladder. Gallstones develop in 20% of CF adults but are symptomatic in only 5% of CF adults.

Cirrhosis and liver failure occur in about 2% of CF adults. CF patients with a history of DIOS have significantly higher risk of developing severe liver disease than those who have never had DIOS.

Abdominal imaging with ultrasound or magnetic resonance imaging may be indicated in CF patients with suspected liver disease.

Ursodeoxycholic acid for patients with CF–associated liver disease can often normalize serum alkaline phosphatase levels. However, the natural progression of CF liver disease may not change with such treatment. For end stage cirrhotic liver disease, liver transplantation may be the only option.

Pancreas

Mutant CFTR gene expression in the pancreatic ductal system results in failure of the normal postnatal development of the *exocrine* pancreatic gland, leading to pancreatic exocrine insufficiency and malabsorption in 85% of CF patients. Abnormally low fluid secretion but normal protein secretion into the pancreatic duct causes protein precipitation, duct obstruction, and eventual pancreatic injury severe enough to cause malabsorption.

Symptoms of malabsorption may include diarrhea, bulky foul smelling stools, voracious appetite, abdominal pain after eating, and excess gas. Diagnosis of pancreatic insufficiency occurs with finding levels of pancreatic elastase in the stool that are less than 200 mcg/g stool. Other causes of malabsorption in CF patients—lactose intolerance, celiac disease, Crohn disease, for example—can occur and should be considered in the differential if the patient does not respond to pancreatic enzyme replacement.

Pancreatic enzyme replacement therapy (PERT) dosage is individualized and should be adjusted based on symptoms. The most effective preparations are enteric-coated, acid-resistant microspheres, now with greater formulation consistency, with recently required FDA approval. The initial dose is 500 lipase units per kg per meal and half that amount for snacks. The dose can be increased to a maximum of 2500 lipase units per kg per meal. If symptoms do not improve at maximum PERT doses, intestinal contents may never reach a sufficiently high pH (~5.0) to release the enzymes from the microspheres. Histamine (H2) blockers or proton pump inhibitors may then be given in addition to the pancreatic enzymes. Other malabsorptive syndromes should be considered if patient does not respond to acid inhibition with their PERT. Increasing the enzyme dose further may lead to fibrosing colonopathy.

Enzyme replacement capsules should be taken at the very beginning of the meal or snack. However, if the meal lasts more than 30 minutes, a split dose can be given at the beginning and halfway through the meal. Enteric coated pancreatic enzyme micorspheres cannot be used with continuous feeding as they obstruct the feeding tubes. The CF community is currently awaiting FDA approval of a powdered or liquid PERT formulation.

CF–related diabetes

CFRD has some features of type 1 and type 2 diabetes mellitus, with decreased insulin production and a component of insulin resistance (especially during stress). CFRD prevalence increases with age, with 50% of CF adults over age 30 with disease.

Early in the clinical course of CFRD, postprandial blood glucose levels are elevated but most patients have normal fasting glucose levels and hemoglobin A_{1c} (HbA_{1c}) level. Yearly oral glucose tolerance testing is recommended to screen for CFRD in all CF patients 10 years and older. Standard ADA criteria for diagnosis of diabetes is used in CFRD—a fasting plasma glucose (FPG) > 126 mg/dl and/or 2 hours post-75 gm of glucose solution > 200 mg/dl—confirmed on two separate days when the patient is in stable baseline health. Additional criteria for diagnosing CFRD include HgA_{1c} > 6.5% on two occasions or random plasma glucose levels > 200 mg/dl on two separate occasions.

Often the first manifestations of CFRD are seen during acute respiratory exacerbations, only to subside when the exacerbation has completely resolved but to reappear again with the next exacerbation. Therefore, for CF patients admitted to hospital for a respiratory exacerbation, fasting and 2 to 3 hour postprandial finger stick glucose levels should be measured in the first 48 hours of hospitalization. If fasting levels are > 126 mg/dL and/or 2-hour postprandial > 200 mg/dL after the initial 48 hours of admission, finger stick monitoring should be continued, and plasma glucose levels measured. If two or more plasma glucose levels show a FPG > 126 mg/dL and/or 2-hour postprandial are > 200 mg/dL, then CFRD is diagnosed and endocrinology should be consulted for further evaluation and management.

Complications of CFRD are quite different than type 1 or type 2 diabetes. Diabetic ketoacidosis occurs exceedingly rarely in CFRD and should prompt measuring islet cell antibodies to evaluate for type 1 diabetes. *The major complication of CFRD is acceleration in the rate of decline in lung function.* CF patients with diabetes have significantly worse lung function, more frequent acute respiratory exacerbations, and reduced survival rates compared to CF patients without diabetes. CFRD patients die of progressive pulmonary disease and respiratory failure, rather than macrovascular complications of diabetes. Microvascular complications occur in 10% to 23% of patients with CFRD, including retinopathy (16% of patients after 5 years and 23% after 10 years of CFRD), neuropathy, and nephropathy; but the severity of these microvascular complications is less severe than found in type 1 or type 2 diabetes.

The primary nutritional goal in CFRD is to maintain a high energy diet that is 120% to 150% of that recommended for age because higher BMI is associated with improved outcomes. For this reason, the standard dietary restriction of type 1 and type 2 diabetes do not apply to patients with CFRD. They are encouraged to maintain a diet high in fat and protein intake with no restrictions on carbohydrates except to minimize simple sugars.

PRACTICE POINT

- Patients with CFRD should maintain a diet high in fat and protein intake with *no restrictions* on carbohydrates except to minimize simple sugars. Because CF patients have high caloric requirements and improved outcomes with higher BMI, diabetic diet restriction is not appropriate in this diabetic population.

Insulin is the preferred drug to treat CFRD. No trial has yet shown that an oral agent is superior to insulin in improving nutritional status or glucose control. *Insulin treatment in CFRD results in improvements in BMI and lung function.* Since CF adults are often advised to consume three 1000 calorie meals and two 500 calories snacks per day, the insulin regimen is tailored to their caloric intake. In addition, CF patients should exercise frequently which also requires tailoring of the insulin regimen. Finally, during a respiratory exacerbation when insulin resistance can be substantial, rapid changes in insulin dosing may be required to maintain glucose levels at target.

Long-acting insulin for patients with fasting hyperglycemia and short acting insulin for meals using a specific dose of insulin per number of carbohydrates being consumed at that meal (ie, carbohydrate counting) helps maintain proper diabetic control. In addition, fingerstick glucose readings before meals can direct additional sliding scale short acting insulin needs for blood glucose levels above 180 mg/dl. All patients with CFRD may consider an insulin pump to reduce drug injections and improve quality of life. Target fasting glucose levels in adults with CFRD recommended by the American Diabetes Association (ADA), are between 70 and 130 mg/dL and 2 to 3 hours after meals less than 180 mg/dL. Further investigation will better delineate if more strict control that this will promote better outcomes. Little evidence exists for strict inpatient glucose control in patients with CF exacerbations, and ADA recommendations for other diabetic patients (maintain blood glucose 140–180 mg/dL) should guide practice.

NUTRITION IN THE HOSPITALIZED CF PATIENT

Malnutrition and malabsorption of fat soluble vitamins are common in CF patients. Malnutrition is multifactorial and due to a combination of decreased appetite, malabsorption, and increased energy requirement, especially during acute exacerbations.

Malnutrition, as indicated by a low body mass index (BMI), continues to be a major problem in CF. In 2009, almost 60% of CF adults in this country were underweight (BMI < 22 for women and < 23 for men). For those that are underweight, the following are important considerations: attention to appropriate doses of pancreatic enzymes; maintaining adequate calories for their needs; addressing underlying diseases that may decrease their oral intake (esophagitis, chronic abdominal pain, delayed gastric emptying, and depression); diabetes screening; and if diabetic, that target glucose levels are being met. About 10% of CF patients receive enteral tube feeds for nutritional failure. They are typically supplemented at night and encouraged to eat during the day.

Levels of fat soluble vitamins (A, D, E, K) should be assessed yearly in the outpatient setting. Up to 80% of CF adults are vitamin D deficient (related to malabsorption and other factors) leading to poor bone health and lower innate immunity of the lung. High dose vitamin D3 (50,000 units once a week for 12 weeks) restores vitamin D levels in most CF patients to sufficient levels, but daily maintenance dosing of vitamin D3 is then required (2000 units/d) to maintain adequate levels.

CONSULTATION

For CF patients admitted to the hospital, hospitalists should facilitate subspecialty consultation with a pulmonologist who has expertise in CF as well as an infectious disease specialist familiar with CF management. Endocrinology consultation can assist with management of CFRD, especially since insulin requirements change rapidly with acute pulmonary CF exacerbations.

Respiratory care consultation can assist patients with inhaled therapies as well as chest physical therapy (device assisted [eg, Acapella] and manual). Floor nursing staff and physical therapy consultation should also assist with chest physical therapy to assist patient in clearing the inflamed bronchioles.

In addition, the pharmacy team can provide invaluable assistance in dosing and monitoring of high risk antibiotics. Furthermore, nutrition service consultation should assist with caloric requirements during a respiratory exacerbation.

Finally, for those patients whose baseline FEV_1 is 30% predicted or less, introduction to a member of the lung transplant team (for patients seen in transplant centers) can help during the hospital admission to stage the timing for a lung transplant evaluation.

PROGNOSIS

The decline in lung function in CF follows a chronic disease trajectory of gradual decline punctuated by acute exacerbations causing sudden drops in lung function (usually assessed as FEV_1). Often only partial recovery of lung function to a new, lower baseline follows a respiratory exacerbation. The number of exacerbations per year correlates with the rate of decline in FEV_1 and thus progression of disease. In addition, those with CFRD have significantly more respiratory exacerbations and more rapid disease progression than those CF patients without diabetes. Failure to return to baseline FEV_1 after an exacerbation is associated with female sex, pancreatic insufficiency, malnutrition, allergic bronchopulmonary aspergillosis, a larger drop in FEV_1 during the exacerbation, and infection with pseudomonas, *B cepacia* complex, and/or methicillin-resistant *S aureus*.

DISCHARGE PLANNING

If the patient is discharged before completion of the course of treatment, the patient must have close follow-up to determine when the antibiotics can be stopped. In addition, the patient should be informed that duration of treatment may be more prolonged when choosing outpatient versus in hospital treatment. However, some centers with shorter hospital lengths of stay for admitted adult CF patients have demonstrated better outcomes compared to other centers where patients complete their hospital antimicrobial course in the hospital. Inpatient versus outpatient management of acute pulmonary exacerbations of CF should be individualized based on the patient's social situation, local inpatient and outpatient resources for CF, and the patient's clinical condition.

Guidelines recommend that CF patients receive outpatient follow-up at least every 3 months at a center accredited by the Cystic Fibrosis Foundation and staffed by an interdisciplinary team consisting of pulmonologists, nurses, social workers, respiratory therapists, and nutritionists, all with expertise in CF clinical care. By far, the most frequent reason for additional clinic visits is an acute pulmonary exacerbation. Review of practices in CF Centers with the best pulmonary outcomes (as measured by median FEV_1 for the patients served by that center) indicate that these centers treat each exacerbation quickly and aggressively with the expectation of returning lung function to baseline.

QUALITY IMPROVEMENT

PREVENTION

Infection control

Even if pathogenic organisms are not found on sputum culture, all CF patients should be assumed to have transmissible organisms and *contact isolation* instituted. The Cystic Fibrosis Foundation strongly recommends that CF patients avoid physical contact with each other, and therefore CF summer camps and other gatherings of CF patients are no longer recommended and in fact are actively discouraged.

Cohorting CF patients when hospitalized to prevent nurses from taking care of multiple CF patients (when possible) will help reduce transmission of resistant organisms to other CF patients. When nurses or clinicians must care for multiple CF patients, those with less resistant organisms should be seen first each day. Providers should always see the patients with *B cepacia* **last** during the day to decrease the chances of spreading this deadly organism to other CF patients.

QUALITY IMPROVEMENT INITIATIVES

The Cystic Fibrosis Foundation maintains a national *Cystic Fibrosis Patient Registry* that has been collecting clinical data that are analyzed on a national level since 1986. Patients attending a Cystic Fibrosis Foundation–accredited center provide informed consent so that detailed clinical information on each clinic visit and hospitalization is submitted annually to the Cystic Fibrosis Foundation. Some of the measures reported include FEV_1, BMI, annual screening for CFRD, sputum culture results, number of pulmonary exacerbations, length of hospital stay, and guidelines for care consisting of quarterly clinic visits, quarterly sputum cultures, biannual lung function tests, annual influenza vaccination, use of maintenance pulmonary medications to prevent respiratory exacerbations, and annual assessment by a nutritionist and a social worker.

These data are compiled by the Cystic Fibrosis Foundation and each center then receives a center specific report each year which contains 69 different outcome measures. For each measure, the center specific information is compared to the national average, and if applicable, to the 10 best performing centers. In 2009, data on a total of 25,638 individual CF patients were collated for the Registry report.

The Cystic Fibrosis Foundation has also developed an extremely strong national quality improvement program called the *Learning and Leadership Collaboratives*. Each year, 6 to 10 CF Center teams enroll in a year-long collaborative where they learn the tools of process improvement through application on a specific theme. The themes for the 2010 collaboratives were CF diabetes and adult CF care. The Clinical Microsystems approach focuses on multidisciplinary teams and involves all members of the staff involved in the patient's care. The five Ps are then addressed: purpose, patients, professionals, processes, and patterns. The team then prioritizes which areas to focus on and develops quality improvement (QI) projects for those areas. More information and tools can be found at http://www.clinicalmicrosystem.org.

Other QI initiatives include *CF My Way*, a validated problem solving medication adherence program to improve patient compliance. Studies have documented compliance with therapy to be only around 50% in CF due to the number and complexity of their treatment with oral medications, inhaled interventions and airway clearance techniques multiple times a day. This program aims to increase compliance.

■ COST AND RESOURCE UTILIZATION

The cost of inpatient treatment for CF has been estimated to be 30% to 40% of their annual health care costs. Cost of inpatient CF care is significant for both private insurance and HMO systems. In a study of CF patient with private insurance conducted in 2006, those with CF had higher mean annual expenditures than non–CF enrollees for the 20 to 29, 30 to 44, and 45 to 64 age ranges ($52,929 vs $2261, $58,468 vs $3555, and $50,930 vs $5310, respectively). Average annuals costs for adult and pediatric CF patients combined were $16,545 for hospitalizations, $18,461 for prescriptions, and $13,092 for outpatient costs. This is compared to $1,267 for outpatient, $467 for inpatient, and $437 prescriptions costs for non–CF enrollees. In an HMO system, average annual costs averaged $13,300 for Kaiser Permanente in 1996 ranging from $6200 for mild disease to $43,300 for severe disease, with 47% from hospitalizations.

CONCLUSION

Cystic fibrosis is the most common inherited life-shortening disease of Caucasians in the United States caused by mutation in the CFTR gene. Cystic fibrosis can affect a variety of organs, but 90% of mortality is due to lung disease. However, it can present as asthma, pancreatitis, pansinusitis or nasal polyps and not be initially recognized as cystic fibrosis. Increased respiratory symptoms are indicative of an acute pulmonary exacerbation but an isolated drop in FEV1 without any reported change in symptoms is also concerning for exacerbation. The mainstay of treatment for acute pulmonary exacerbations is antibiotic therapy and enhanced airway clearance. Hemoptysis and pneumothoraces are major pulmonary complications that may require hospitalization. Nonpulmonary complications of CF such as pancreatic insufficiency, sinusitis, malnutrition and CF related diabetes are important contributors to morbidity and mortality. Consultation with appropriate subspecialists who have expertise in CF management is important. Respiratory therapists, nutritionists, and pharmacists also play vital roles in the care of the CF patient. Finally, referral for lung transplant evaluation should be considered when the baseline FEV_1 drop to 30% predicted or less. The Cystic Fibrosis Foundation is very active in quality improvement through the national Cystic Fibrosis Patient Registry as well as specific initiatives to improve the care of people with cystic fibrosis.

SUGGESTED READINGS

Flume PA, Mogayzel PJ Jr, Robinson KA, et al. Clinical practice guidelines for pulmonary therapies committee. Cystic fibrosis pulmonary guidelines treatment of pulmonary exacerbations: treatment of pulmonary exacerbations. *Am J Respir Crit Care Med.* 2009;180(9):802–808.

Flume PA, Mogayzel PJ, Robinson KA, et al. Cystic fibrosis pulmonary guidelines pulmonary complications: hemoptysis and pneumothorax. *Am J Respir Crit Care Med.* 2010;182:298–306.

Flume PA, Robinson KA, O'Sullivan BP, et al. Clinical practice guidelines for pulmonary therapies committee. cystic fibrosis pulmonary guidelines: airway clearance therapies. *Respir Care.* 2009;54(4):522–537.

Goss CH, Burns JL. Exacerbations in cystic fibrosis. *Thorax.* 2007;62:360–367.

Kreindler, JL. Cystic fibrosis: exploiting its genetic basis in the hunt for new therapies. *Pharmacology and Therapeutics.* 2010;125:219–229.

Moran A, Brunzell C, Cohen R, et al. Clinical care guidelines for cystic fibrosis-related diabetes. *Diabetes Care.* 2010;33(12):2697–2708.

O'Sullivan BP, Freedman SD. *Cystic fibrosis. Lancet.* 2009;373:1891–1904.

Sokol RJ, Durie PR. Recommendations for management of liver and biliary tract disease in cystic fibrosis. *J Pediatr Gastroenterol Nutr.* 1999;28:S1–S13.

Stallings VA, Stark LJ, Robinson KA, Feranchak AP, Quinton H. Evidence-based practice recommendations for nutrition-related management of children and adults with cystic fibrosis and pancreatic insufficiency: results of a systematic review. *J Am Diet Assoc.* 2008;108(5):832–839.

Yankaskas JR, Marshall BC, Sufian B, Simon RH. Cystic fibrosis adult care. *Chest.* 2004;125:S1–S39.

CHAPTER 241

Interstitial and Diffuse Parenchymal Lung Diseases

Sonye K. Danoff, MD, PhD
Peter Terry, MD

Key Clinical Questions

1. Does the hospitalized patient with unexplained dyspnea have interstitial lung disease (ILD)?
2. How and why should idiopathic pulmonary fibrosis (IPF) be differentiated from other forms of ILD?
3. What is an acute exacerbation of IPF, and how can it be discriminated from other causes of worsening in ILD?
4. When is bronchoscopy indicated in the diagnosis or evaluation of ILD?
5. When should a pulmonary consultation be requested for patients with ILD?
6. How can patients with high oxygen requirements be transitioned home?

INTRODUCTION: CLASSIFICATION OF INTERSTITIAL LUNG DISEASE

EPIDEMIOLOGY

The interstitial lung diseases (ILDs) are a heterogeneous group of disorders with the common feature of inflammatory or fibrotic injury to the lung parenchyma. Hence, these disorders are also described as the diffuse parenchymal lung diseases (DPLDs). There are numerous potential etiologies for ILD which can be broadly divided into five categories: idiopathic, drug/medication related, environmental/occupational, genetic/hereditary, and autoimmune associated (**Table 241-1**).

While considered rare, these diseases affect approximately 500,000 individuals in the United States each year and result in 40,000 deaths, comparable to the number of deaths from breast cancer. The exact epidemiology is difficult to determine as patients presenting with these diseases are sometimes misidentified as having more common disorders such as congestive heart failure or chronic obstructive pulmonary disease. Further the epidemiology varies based on the subtype of ILD. Thus, epidemiology is best considered in the context of the ILD subsets.

CLASSIFICATION AND PRESENTATION

Because of the diversity of diseases encompassed in ILD, the American Thoracic Society and European Respiratory Society developed a two-level classification system to facilitate the clinical evaluation of ILD (**Figure 241-1**). This system divides ILDs initially based on specific mechanisms of disease into disorders of known etiology, idiopathic interstitial pneumonia, granulomatous disease, and rare diseases. The idiopathic interstitial pneumonias (IIPs) are further classified in a second level based on histologic appearance. For the purpose of this discussion, we will focus primarily on the IIPs and mention several other ILDs of particular relevance to the hospitalist.

IDIOPATHIC PULMONARY FIBROSIS

CASE 241-1

A 75-year-old man with a history of hypertension and coronary artery disease presents with progressive dyspnea for 3 weeks following an apparent upper respiratory infection. He has had a history of worsening dyspnea over the past year with a recent negative stress test. He was told 5 years earlier that a chest x-ray done as part of a routine physical showed scarring at the lung bases. Medications include aspirin and a beta-blocker.

Idiopathic pulmonary fibrosis (IPF) is one of the most common ILDs encountered by hospitalists. This disorder primarily affects individuals over age 60 years. Recent epidemiologic studies show the prevalence increases with each successive decade from 18.7 to 23.3/100,000 in 55 to 64 year olds to 29.3 to 50.0/100,000 in 65 to 74 year olds to 48.4 to 87.9/100,000 in >85 year olds. IPF affects approximately 200,000 people in the United States and results in 20,000 deaths per year. A notable exception to the older age of onset is in patients with familial IPF. In this genetic disorder, patients may present two to three decades earlier with symptomatic disease. The median survival is 3 to 5 years from

TABLE 241-1 Etiologies of Interstitial Lung Disease by Category

Autoimmune	Common/conventional:
Scleroderma	Amiodarone
Rheumatoid arthritis	Bleomycin
Systemic lupus erythematosis	Methotrexate
Polymyositis/ dermatomyositis	Biologics:
	TNF inhibitors
Sjorgren syndrome	Genetic/hereditary
Occupational/environmental	Hermansky-Pudlak
Asbestosis	Surfactant protein A and C deficiency
Silicosis	Telomerase mutations
Berylliosis	
Bird fancier's lung	
Idiopathic	
Medication-induced	

the time of diagnosis in symptomatic patients. Diagnosis is made based on a consistent history (slowly progressive dyspnea), findings of dry, Velcro-like crackles on exam and consistent radiograph with basilar predominant interstitial changes (**Figure 241-2**). The hallmarks of IPF on chest CT are basilar predominant subpleural reticulation and honeycombing with traction bronchiectasis (**Figure 241-3**). Ground glass opacities may be seen during acute exacerbations, however, this should be a minor feature of a baseline CT study. The diagnosis of IPF mandates the exclusion of other etiologies including environmental exposures, medication and autoimmune disease.

NONSPECIFIC INTERSTITIAL PNEUMONIA

CASE 241-2

A 42-year-old woman presents with rapidly progressive dyspnea over 2 to 3 weeks. She has a history of Raynaud disease for several years, but recently noted onset of redness and cracking at the tips of her fingers. She has also noted a purplish rash above her eyes. In the past 4 weeks, she has had increasing difficulty rising from a chair and now is unable to get up without using her hands to push off. Her mother has a history of rheumatoid arthritis.

Nonspecific interstitial pneumonia (NSIP) is the form of ILD most common in patients with autoimmune disease. As a result, this form of ILD is more common in women than men and has an earlier age of onset than typical with IPF. The diagnosis is typically suspected based on the clinical symptoms and radiograph showing patchy ground glass opacities with minimal fibrosis (Figure 241-3). Open lung biopsy is necessary for definitive diagnosis. The prognosis of NSIP is generally good, with the exception of patients with evidence of fibrosis.

RESPIRATORY BRONCHIOLITIS-ILD/DESQUAMATIVE INTERSTITIAL PNEUMONIA

CASE 241-3

A 37 year-old man presents with insidious onset dyspnea and cough worsening over several months. He has no prior medical history or significant exposures. He smokes one pack a day of cigarettes and has done so for 10 years. A CT on presentation shows bilateral upper lobe ground glass opacities. Work up for autoimmune disease is negative.

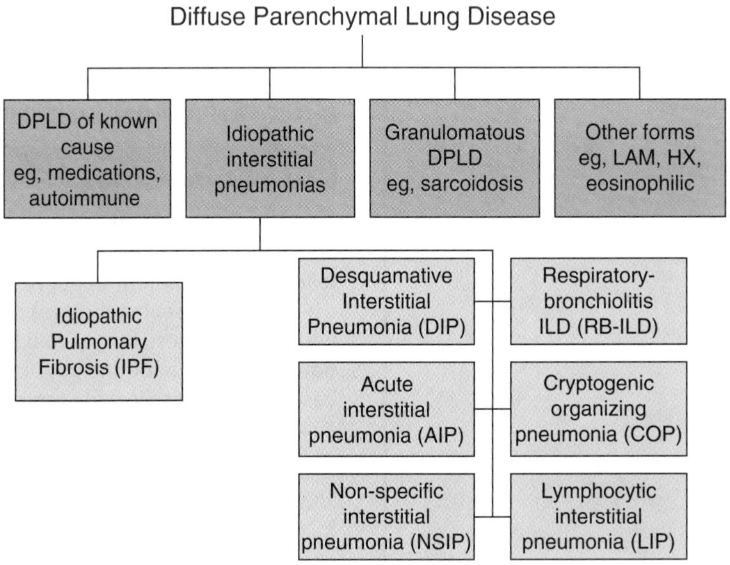

Figure 241-1 *American Thoracic Society/European Respiratory Society classification of interstitial lung disease. DPLD, diffuse parenchymal lung disease; LAM, lymphangioleiomyomatosis; HX, histiocytosis X. (Adapted from American Thoracic Society/European Respiratory Society International Multidisciplinary Consensus Classification of the Idiopathic Interstitial Pneumonias. This joint statement of the American Thoracic Society [ATS], and the European Respiratory Society [ERS] was adopted by the ATS board of directors, June 2001 and by the ERS Executive Committee, June 2001. Am J Respir Crit Care Med. 2002;165[2]:277–304.)*

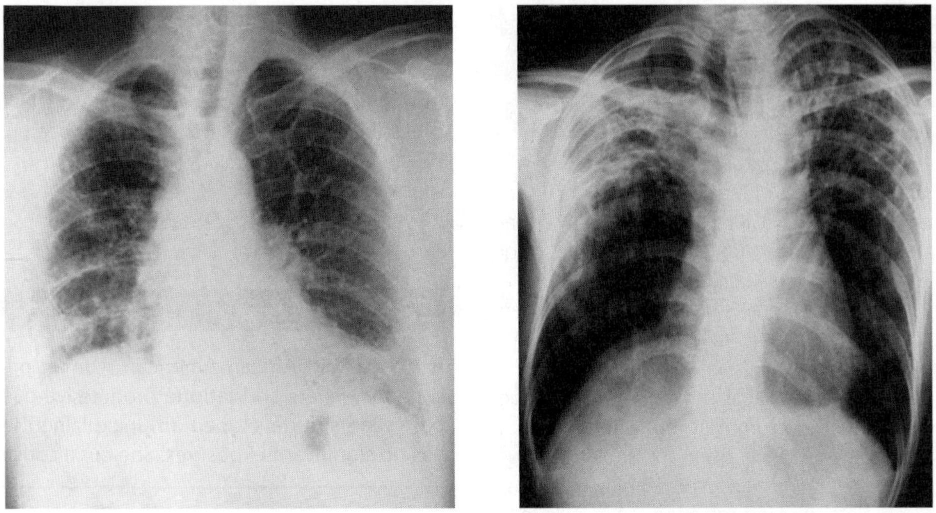

Figure 241-2 *Representative chest x-rays that can be seen in patients with idiopathic pulmonary fibrosis (IPF) and sarcoid. IPF is characterized by basilar predominant interstitial markings. By contrast, sarcoid typically shows an upper lobe distribution of fibrosis which may also be accompanied by bilateral hilar adenopathy.*

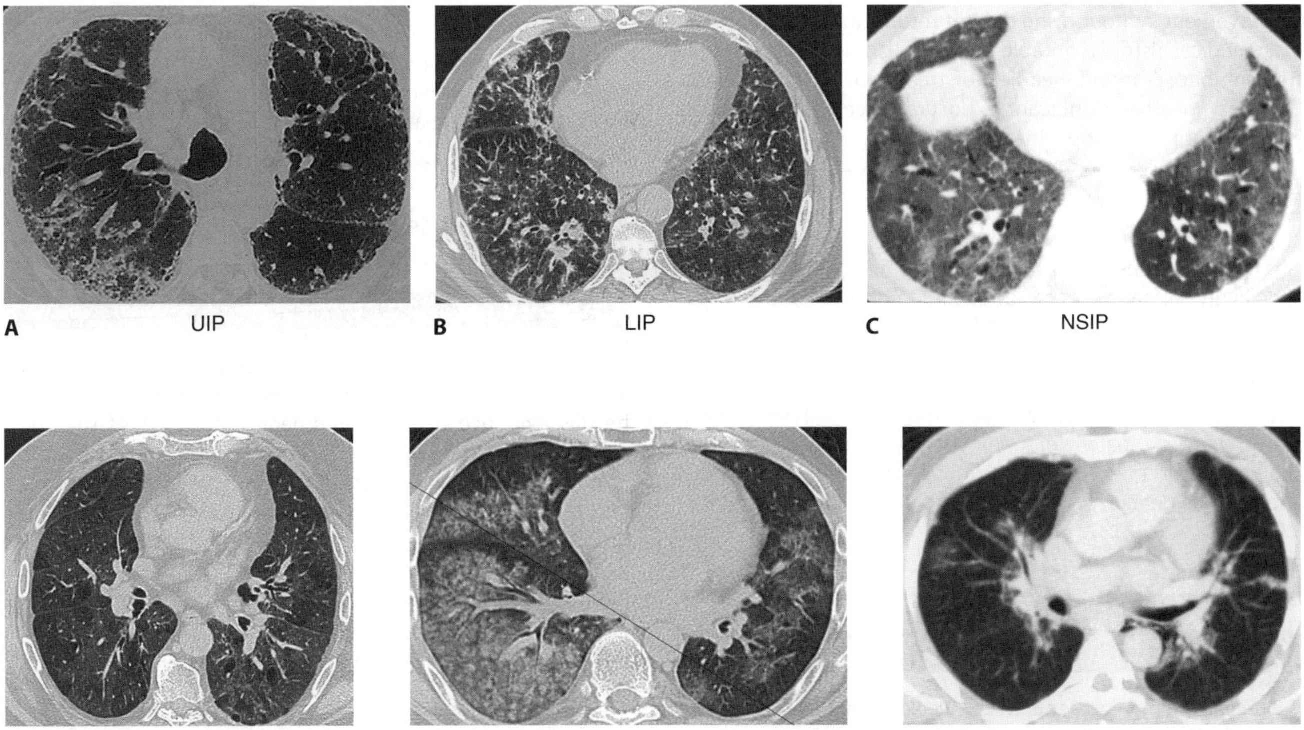

Figure 241-3 *Representative computed tomography patterns that can be seen in patients with interstitial lung disease (ILD). ILD can be characterized by many different radiographic patterns. With the exception of usual interstitial pneumonia (UIP) radiograph, there is substantial overlap among different forms of ILD. A number of the patterns are shown with the associated pathology noted. (A) UIP is characterized honeycombing, traction bronchiectasis, and increased reticular markings. (B) Lymphocytic interstitial pneumonia may demonstrate a micronodular pattern. (C) Nonspecific interstitial pneumonia (NSIP) often appears as a diffuse ground glass opacities (GGOs). (D) Hypersensitivity pneumonitis (HSP) appears as a nearly homogeneous pattern of GGO. (E) Cryptogenic organizing pneumonia (COP) appears as a patchy infiltrate which may be GGO or dense. (F) Sarcoid can present with bronchovascular infiltrates and hilar adenopathy.*

PRACTICE POINT

- RB-ILD and DIP are largely reversible with abstention from smoking.

Respiratory-bronchiolitis interstitial lung disease (RB-ILD) and desquamative interstitial pneumonia (DIP) represent a poorly appreciated spectrum of smoking-related lung disease. These disorders can occur in cigarette smokers years after starting smoking. Unlike the more commonly encountered smoking related disorders, chronic obstructive pulmonary disease (COPD), and emphysema, RB-ILD and DIP are largely reversible with abstention from smoking. The age of onset of this disorder is variable, but tends to be younger than IPF. It occurs most frequently in smokers, but can be encountered occasionally in nonsmokers. The diagnosis should be suspected based on clinical presentation. However, definitive diagnosis requires lung biopsy. Complete smoking cessation can reverse most cases of RB-ILD/DIP. Individuals who develop this disorder without apparent tobacco smoke exposure can be treated with steroids, but the response is variable.

CRYPTOGENIC ORGANIZING PNEUMONIA

CASE 241-4

A 50-year-old woman presents with recurrent fever, cough, and dyspnea. She had similar symptoms approximately 1 month previously and received a course of oral antibiotics with some improvement, although she did not return to her baseline. Her past medical history is notable for psoriasis. She began monthly TNF-inhibitor 3 months earlier for treatment of her psoriasis. She has no other significant exposures. Her CT chest shows patchy ground glass opacities in both lungs.

Cryptogenic organizing pneumonia (COP)/bronchiolitis obliterans organizing pneumonia (BOOP) is a common and nonspecific lung injury pattern which can be encountered in a number of situations including medication related, with autoimmune disease and following viral infections. The presentation may be virtually identical to that of pneumonia. Patients frequently receive one or several courses of antibiotics prior to diagnosis. Radiographically, the CT can show patchy ground glass opacities (GGOs) or dense infiltrates (Figure 241-3). The diagnosis is made by lung biopsy. Prognosis is generally good with steroids forming the mainstay of therapy.

ACUTE INTERSTITIAL PNEUMONITIS

CASE 241-5

A 60-year-old man presents with 3 weeks of rapidly progressive dyspnea. Despite outpatient antibiotics, he has become more dyspneic and is cyanotic on presentation to the emergency department. He has no significant past medical history or exposures. Chest x-ray shows diffuse, bilateral infiltrates.

Acute interstitial pneumonitis (AIP) is the most dreaded presentation of ILD. This enigmatic disorder can occur apparently in the absence of any trigger, although it can also complicate autoimmune disease. The age at onset is variable. Patients present with rapidly progressive dyspnea over a few weeks to month. Radiographs are indistinguishable from acute respiratory distress syndrome or a bilateral pneumonia. Infection must be excluded or treated empirically. The prognosis is dismal with over 70% of patients dying of respiratory failure within weeks of presentation. High-dose steroids have been used with occasional success in AIP particularly in the setting of underlying autoimmune disease.

SARCOIDOSIS

CASE 241-6

A 45-year-old African American woman presents with cough, dyspnea, fevers and fatigue progressive over 6 months. In the past year, she developed an unexplained left facial palsy. She has no significant exposures. She has a cousin with sarcoidosis.

Sarcoidosis is the most common form of ILD. The etiology remains unknown. It is more common in women, African Americans, and people of Scandinavian and Irish descent. Sarcoidosis is a systemic disorder which can manifest in skin, lung, heart, liver, marrow, or peripheral or central nervous system. The diagnosis of pulmonary sarcoidosis is suggested by upper lobe interstitial changes on chest x-ray with or without associated bilateral mediastinal and hilar lymph node enlargement (Figure 241-2). In contrast to many other forms of ILD, crackles on exam are a feature in later stage disease. Diagnosis can be made by identification of classic noncaseating granulomas on biopsy of involved tissue. Diagnosis of pulmonary sarcoidosis is typically made by transbronchial lung biopsy or transthoracic needle aspiration of effected lymph nodes. The clinical course is highly variable, with some individuals developing destructive fibrocavitary disease and others having asymptomatic lymph node enlargement.

AUTOIMMUNE-ASSOCIATED INTERSTITIAL LUNG DISEASE

CASE 241-7

A 34-year-old man presents with facial edema, a high pitched voice, and worsening dyspnea over 1 week. On chest x-ray, he has evidence of a pneumomediastinum. CT of the chest confirms an extensive pneumomediastinum with dissection into the planes of the neck. The lung parenchyma shows a diffuse ground glass pattern. The patient reports 3 months of progressive finger swelling and stiffness and worsening muscle weakness. He denies any exposures and is on no medications. Initial labs indicate an elevated creatine phosphokinase and aldolase.

Autoimmune-associated ILD should be suspected in young patients presenting with ILD in the setting of a constellation of systemic symptoms. In this case, the patient presented with pneumomediastinum in the setting of new onset polymyositis. The recognition of subtle, or not so subtle, systemic symptoms can be difficult in the context of a dramatic presentation. However, once the symptoms of weakness and arthritis were identified, biochemical and serologic testing can quickly confirm the underlying diagnosis. Obtaining a standard panel of serologies on all patients with ILD is valuable. While the sensitivity and specificity of studies may vary regionally, ANA, RF, RNP, Scl-70, and Jo-1 antibodies are useful as an initial screen.

DRUG-ASSOCIATED INTERSTITIAL LUNG DISEASE

CASE 241-8

A 75-year-old man presents with worsening dyspnea and increased cough over 3 months. His past medical history is notable for atrial fibrillation and a prior myocardial infarction. He has been on an aspirin, beta-blocker, and amiodarone for the past 3 years. Chest CT at presentation shows patchy bilateral ground glass opacities. Examination shows no evidence of lower extremity edema or elevated jugular venous pressure. He does have crackles on auscultation of the lungs.

Drug-associated ILD can be difficult to identify as the medication involved can be of many months' or years' duration. The number of medications associated with ILD is increasing rapidly. This is especially true of the many biological agents in clinical use. A useful Web-based resource for determining if a medication can be associated with the development of ILD is Pneumotox (www.pneumotox.com). The recognition of drug-associated ILD depends on ruling out other potential etiologies such as heart failure or an underlying autoimmune disease. In addition to evaluating prescription medication, patients should be asked about over-the-counter and herbal remedies as well as dietary supplements. In general, discontinuing the offending medication results in improvement of symptoms within weeks to months. Some patients may require a several week course of systemic steroids to limit lung injury while the medication is washing out.

DIAGNOSING ILD IN THE HOSPITALIZED PATIENT

CLINICAL FEATURES

While the care of a patient with known ILD can be challenging, even more challenging is diagnosing previously unrecognized ILD in a hospitalized patient (**Figure 241-4**). The presenting symptoms dyspnea, cough and fatigue are common to a number of more prevalent diseases including pneumonia, congestive heart failure, and COPD. Hence, maintaining a high level of suspicion for this diagnosis is critical. A detailed history may identify features helpful in discriminating these potential diagnoses. Have the symptoms truly been acute or has there been a more protracted period of decline? While ILD may have a fulminant acute presentation, many patients when prompted will offer a history of a more subacute decline preceding the acute illness. Have the symptoms responded appropriately to a reasonable therapeutic intervention? Patients who fail to respond to multiple courses of antibiotics or who have worsening dyspnea on exertion despite prior efforts at diuresis should raise the concern for ILD.

Ultimately the diagnosis is based on a thorough history and physical examination (Figure 241-4). The importance of the history cannot be emphasized sufficiently. Many a patient with bird fancier's lung has passed through the hands of capable physicians who neglect to ask about environmental exposures. While these patients often present in the outpatient setting, it is not unusual to find that a patient has been seen and or hospitalized repeatedly for pneumonia or bronchitis. Further in distinguishing IPF, with its very poor prognosis, from other potentially more treatable forms of ILD, this history is critical.

Physical findings on pulmonary examination can be nonspecific with crackles or squeaks or no findings at all. Perhaps the most useful finding is the basilar predominant Velcro-like crackles often heard in IPF. Clubbing is variably associated with ILD, but can occur with other disorders. Systemic signs of autoimmune disease (Raynaud disease, arthritis, rash) can help raise the suspicion for ILD.

PULMONARY FUNCTION TESTING

The role of spirometry in the monitoring of airways disease (COPD, asthma) in the hospitalized patient is well established. Less so is the role of pulmonary function testing in the patient with ILD. The classic features of ILD are restriction including forced vital capacity <80% predicted without evidence of obstruction; or total lung capacity <80% predicted. In addition, diffusing capacity (DLCO) is typically reduced, with a single breath DLCO <80% predicted. In the acute setting PFTs are often deferred; however, establishing post-treatment PFTs are invaluable in subsequent patient care. Not only do the PFTs provide a measure of disease severity which may be different from that assessed clinically, but they can also provide

History:
Symptoms (cough, dyspnea, fatigue)
Tempo of symptom development
PMH especially autoimmune
SH (smoking, work and avocation exposures, pets)
FH (ILD, cirrhosis, early gray hair, marrow dysfunction, autoimmunity)
Medications (current and past, including OTC)

Physical Exam:
Head & neck: pharyngeal crowding
Lung-crackles, squeaks, rhonchi, lung size
Cardiac-elevated P2, atrial fibrillation
Abdomen-organomegaly
Extremities-clubbing, cyanosis, edema
Skin-rashes, sclerodactyly, Raynaud phenomenon
Neuromuscular-muscle weakness, cranial neuropathies

Lab Studies:
CBC with differential
CMP
RF, CCP, ANA, Ro, La, RNP, Scl-70
Aldolase, CPK, Jo-1

Pulmonary Function Testing:
Spirogram
Lung Volumes
DLCo

Radiographs:
High resolution chest CT

Other studies which may be indicated:
Bronchoscopy
Surgical Lung Biopsy
Echocardiogram for LVF and RVSP
6 Minute Walk Test or Ambulatory Saturation
Nocturnal Oximetry or Overnight Sleep Study

Figure 241-4 *Standardized evaluation for interstitial lung disease (ILD). A standardized evaluation for a new diagnosis of ILD includes a comprehensive history and physical examination as well as pulmonary function tests, chest computed tomography, and targeted laboratory studies. In appropriate situations, bronchoscopy and/or surgical biopsy may be indicated. Assessment of oxygen requirement and cardiac function are relevant in many patients. PMH, past medical history; SH, social history; FH, family history; OTC, over the counter medication; CBC, complete blood count; CMP, comprehensive metabolic panel; RF, rheumatoid factor; ANA, antinuclear antibody; CCP, anti-citrullinated protein antibody; Ro-anti, Ro antibody; La-anti, La antibody; RNP, anti-ribonucleoprotein antibody; Scl70-anti, Scl70 antibody; CPK, creatine phosphokinase; Jo-1-anti, Jo-1 antibody; DLCO, diffusing capacity of the lung for carbon monoxide; P2, second heart sound; RVSP, right ventricular systolic pressure; LVF, left ventricular function.*

an important clue as to coexistent right heart disease if the DLCO is reduced out of proportion to the lung volumes. This can also be seen in patients who develop ILD on the background of emphysema.

RADIOGRAPHIC CHARACTERISTICS

A number of common diagnostic modalities are helpful in the detection of ILD. Radiographic studies are a mainstay of diagnosis. Chest x-rays may show increased interstitial markings or reticulo-nodular changes which provide an initial suggestion of ILD. However, high-resolution chest CT scans are significantly more helpful (Figure 241-3). Diagnosis of IPF can be made based on a characteristic radiograph and exclusion of all other etiologies.

BRONCHOSCOPY AND LUNG BIOPSY

PRACTICE POINT

- Surgical lung biopsy is the preferred method for diagnosis of IIP. However, many patients do not need biopsies. ILD presenting in the setting of a known trigger (such as medication or autoimmune disease) rarely requires a tissue diagnosis. Biopsy diagnosis should be reserved for patients with atypical presentations or who fail to respond appropriately to initial therapy.

Definitive diagnosis of IIPs other than IPF depends on lung biopsy. Bronchoalveolar lavage can be helpful in the diagnosis of infection which can complicate or mimic ILD. It is also useful for assessment of eosinophilia which is characteristic of a number of forms of ILD. Transbronchial biopsies can be diagnostic for sarcoidosis or for the excluding malignancy but have poor sensitivity for diagnosing most ILD. Surgical lung biopsy is the preferred method for diagnosis of IIP. However, many patients do not need biopsies. ILD presenting in the setting of a known trigger of ILD (such as medication or autoimmune disease) rarely requires a tissue diagnosis. Biopsy diagnosis should be reserved for patients with atypical presentations or who fail to respond appropriately to initial therapy. Many anecdotal reports suggest exacerbation of lung disease in the setting of a surgical lung biopsy. These exacerbations can be life threatening and often result in a permanent decrement in lung function. This risk should temper the decision to pursue an essentially diagnostic procedure.

Because of the potential complexity of diagnosis and the need for long-term follow-up, early involvement of pulmonary consultation in patients with suspected ILD is critical. Patients with a new diagnosis of ILD need to establish care with a pulmonologist with experience in this field. By involving a specialist early in the course, both diagnostic and therapeutic decisions can be made jointly with the hospital staff.

TRIAGE AND HOSPITAL ADMISSION

CRITERIA FOR ADMISSION

Patients with known ILD who experience significant respiratory decline frequently benefit from hospitalization for evaluation of infection, treatment of infection or cardiac comorbidity, or intensification of immunosuppression. Because the etiology of worsening dyspnea is often uncertain at admission, a thoughtful evaluation is required in all ILD patients. Because patients with ILD typically have exercise induced hypoxemia, any patient with new resting hypoxemia merits admission. Further, patients with worsening exercise desaturation require evaluation. Thus it is critical to assess patients both at rest and with exertion. Frequently, minimal exertion such as talking, standing, or walking, will reveal the desaturation.

PRACTICE POINT

- Any patient with new resting hypoxemia merits hospital admission. Patients with worsening exercise desaturation may require inpatient evaluation. Clinicians should assess patients both at rest and with exertion.

More challenging is the recognition of a new diagnosis of ILD in a patient admitted for progressive dyspnea or hypoxemia. This diagnosis requires a high level of suspicion on the part of the treating physician as symptoms and signs can be nonspecific. Any patient with a new diagnosis of ILD should undergo a standardized evaluation for possible etiology (Figure 241-4).

CRITERIA FOR ICU ADMISSION

The admission of patients with ILD to the ICU continues to be a controversial decision. For some patients, ICU care including intubation is both appropriate and life-saving. This group includes patients with pulmonary manifestations of autoimmune disease. The role of intubation is more uncertain in patients with IPF with acute exacerbations. This clinical entity, recently formally defined, occurs in patients with a decline in lung function in the absence of evident inciting event such as infection. What is certain is that the survival rate following intubation in this setting is extremely poor. Patients and their families should be appropriately advised regarding the potential for ventilator dependence. Ultimately, the benefit of ICU care is dependent on the precipitating event and the potential to reverse this event without significant long-lasting lung injury.

MANAGEMENT

GENERAL APPROACH TO TREATMENT

The appropriate management of patients admitted to the hospital for pulmonary decompensation from ILD depends on accurate identification of the precipitating event. In general, decompensations can be divided into pulmonary and nonpulmonary categories. Pulmonary etiologies include worsening of underlying ILD (acute exacerbations of IPF), infections, pneumothorax and thromboembolic disease. Nonpulmonary etiologies of ILD decompensation include cardiac dysfunction (pulmonary hypertension, right heart failure, left heart failure, or ischemia) and neuromuscular dysfunction. All patients with pulmonary decompensation should undergo chest imaging. Chest x-ray can identify significant infections; however, chest CT is often more sensitive to changes in underlying lung disease including the appearance of new GGOs. If there is a suspicion for thromboembolic disease, chest CT provides a simple method for evaluation. Because the CT image is often not adequate for differentiating infection versus inflammatory injury, consideration should be given in each patient for empiric treatment of possible infection. If the patient is febrile or exhibits cough productive of sputum, cultures including sputum and blood should be obtained. For patients with dry cough, bronchoscopy or induced sputum should be considered. Empiric antibiotics are typically appropriate given the limited pulmonary reserve. If the patient is on immunosuppression for ILD or autoimmune disease, opportunistic infections (eg, *Pneumocystis jiroveci* pneumonia [PCP]) should also be considered and ruled out.

Cardiac disease is increasingly recognized to be a major comorbidity in ILD. Thus, both pulmonary hypertension (PH) and acute coronary syndrome should be considered in the hospitalized patient with ILD. Echocardiograms in the setting of pulmonary decompensation can show transiently elevated right heart pressures; however, echocardiogram with severe PH, right ventricular enlargement or decreased right ventricular function should prompt further evaluation for PH, including thromboembolic disease. Right heart catheterization should be considered prior to starting therapy for PH in patients with ILD.

PRACTICE POINT

- In ILD decompensation, echocardiogram may show transient moderately elevated right heart pressures. However, findings of severe pulmonary hypertension, right ventricular enlargement or decreased right ventricular function should prompt further evaluation for alternate etiologies of pulmonary hypertension, including thromboembolic disease.

TREATMENT AND MONITORING

Inpatient treatment of ILD decompensation must be tailored to the etiology of decompensation. Acute exacerbation of IPF is defined by NIH–sponsored guidelines of diagnostic criteria from the IPFNet study group (**Table 241-2**). The treatment of acute exacerbations of IPF involves pulse steroids (methylprednisolone 1 g IV daily for three doses). Prednisone is then initiated at 1 mg/kg oral daily dose for 2 to 4 weeks. In the setting of high-dose steroids, prophylaxis for PCP should be started.

TABLE 241-2 Diagnosis of Acute Exacerbation of Idiopathic Pulmonary Fibrosis

Diagnostic Criteria
1. Previous or concurrent diagnosis of idiopathic pulmonary fibrosis*
2. Unexplained worsening or development of dyspnea within 30 days
3. High-resolution computed tomography with new bilateral ground-glass abnormality and/or consolidation superimposed on a background reticular or honeycomb pattern consistent with usual interstitial pneumonia pattern†
4. No evidence of pulmonary infection by endotracheal aspirate or bronchoalveolar lavage§
5. Exclusion of alternative causes, including the following: • Left heart failure • Pulmonary embolism • Identifiable cause of acute lung injury¶
Patients with idiopathic clinical worsening who fail to meet all five criteria due to missing data should be termed "suspected acute exacerbations."

*If the diagnosis of idiopathic pulmonary fibrosis is not previously established according to American Thoracic Society/European Respiratory Society consensus criteria, this criterion can be met by the presence of radiologic and/or histopathologic changes consistent with usual interstitial pneumonia pattern on the current evaluation.

†If no previous high-resolution computed tomography is available, the qualifier "new" can be dropped.

§Evaluation of samples should include studies for routine bacterial organisms, opportunistic pathogens, and common viral pathogens.

¶Causes of acute lung injury include sepsis, aspiration, trauma, reperfusion pulmonary edema, pulmonary contusion, fat embolization, inhalational injury, cardiopulmonary bypass, drug toxicity, acute pancreatitis, transfusion of blood products, and stem cell transplantation.

Reproduced, with permission, from Collard HR, Moore BB, Flaherty KR, et al. Acute exacerbations of idiopathic pulmonary fibrosis. *Am J Respir Crit Care Med.* 2007;176(7):636–643.

COMPLICATIONS AND PROGNOSIS

The most significant complication associated with pulmonary decompensations is a lasting decline in lung function. The occurrence of pulmonary exacerbations is clearly associated with poorer prognosis. Oxygen requirements may require frequent reassessment.

DISCHARGE PLANNING

Patients with ILD require thoughtful discharge planning as patients often require home oxygen. Prior to discharge patients should be evaluated for resting and exercise oxygen requirement to maintain an oxygen saturation greater than 88%. Nocturnal oxygen use is indicated for patients with nocturnal desaturation.

A common problem encountered in discharge planning is the high supplemental oxygen requirements. Patients typically can receive up to 6 L/min by nasal cannula for needs with activity. Beyond this oxygen level, patients may require face-mask oxygen at home. If the goals at discharge include rehabilitation in a recovering patient, plans to reassess oxygen requirement and decrease oxygen use should be made at discharge. Patients may also use home pulse oximetry monitoring to allow more autonomy in titrating oxygen. Patients and their families should be aware that maintaining oxygen saturation greater than or equal to 88% is the goal. Oxygen may be reduced or taken off at rest if this criterion is met. Conversely, oxygen can and should be increased with activity to maintain this goal.

For secondary prevention, patients should receive pneumonia vaccine (if not previously vaccinated or boosted) and influenza vaccine if appropriate to season of hospitalization. Follow up with a pulmonary specialist is indicated for all patients with ILD.

QUALITY IMPROVEMENT: A MULTIDISCIPLINARY APPROACH TO ILD

Care of the patients with ILD is best accomplished by a multidisciplinary approach. While definitive therapies for some forms of ILD are not available, increasing evidence supports that patients with ILD benefit from formalized pulmonary rehabilitation to improved patient quality of life. Like vaccination, this simple intervention may improve patient survival and quality of life.

In addition to active interventions aimed at prolonging life, attention to *quality of life* particularly in the end stage of ILD is critical. Patients newly diagnosed with ILD are frequently unaware of the often poor prognosis particularly with IPF. Understanding and transmitting prognosis based on diagnosis accurately and sensitively is a key component of patient care. Involving a pulmonary specialist to assist patients in understanding what therapeutic options are reasonable may be beneficial. While discussions of end-of-life decisions are often more appropriate in the outpatient setting, the propensity of patients with ILD to present with acute exacerbations, means that these discussions are also needed in the acute inpatient setting. Reassuring patients and their families regarding the ability to keep patients comfortable at the end of life is critical. Involvement of palliative care specialists and hospice care may be indicated for patients with acute exacerbations of IPF for symptom management and control or for patients in whom improvement in function is unlikely.

SUGGESTED READINGS

American Thoracic Society/European Respiratory Society International Multidisciplinary Consensus Classification of the Idiopathic Interstitial Pneumonias. This joint statement of the American Thoracic Society (ATS), and the European Respiratory Society (ERS) was adopted by the ATS board of directors, June 2001 and by the ERS Executive Committee, June 2001. *Am J Respir Crit Care Med.* 2002;165(2):277–304.

Collard HR, Moore BB, Flaherty KR, et al. Acute exacerbations of idiopathic pulmonary fibrosis. *Am J Respir Crit Care Med.* 2007; 176(7):636–643.

Cordier JF. Cryptogenic organising pneumonia. *Eur Respir J.* 2006; 28(2):422–446.

Johkoh T. Imaging of idiopathic interstitial pneumonias. *Clin Chest Med.* 2008;29(1):133–147, vi.

King TE Jr, Tooze JA, Schwarz MI, Brown KR, Cherniack RM. Predicting survival in idiopathic pulmonary fibrosis: scoring system and survival model. *Am J Respir Crit Care Med.* 2001;164(7):1171–1181.

Nakamura Y, Chida K, Suda T, et al. Nonspecific interstitial pneumonia in collagen vascular diseases: comparison of the clinical characteristics and prognostic significance with usual interstitial pneumonia. *Sarcoidosis Vasc Diffuse Lung Dis.* 2003;20(3): 235–241.

Vassallo R, Ryu JH. Tobacco smoke-related diffuse lung diseases. *Semin Respir Crit Care Med.* 2008;29(6):643–650.

Vourlekis JS, Brown KK, Schwarz MI. Acute interstitial pneumonitis: current understanding regarding diagnosis, pathogenesis, and natural history. *Semin Respir Crit Care Med.* 2001;22(4):399–408.

CHAPTER 242

Sleep Apnea and Obesity Hypoventilation Syndrome

Ashish Mehta, MD
David A. Schulman, MD, MPH, FCCP

Key Clinical Questions

1. How prevalent is sleep apnea?
2. What are the key distinguishing features between obstructive and central sleep apnea?
3. What are the consequences of untreated sleep apnea?
4. What are the indications for inpatient therapy for sleep apnea?
5. How should patients with suspected sleep apnea be managed at hospital discharge?
6. What is obesity hypoventilation syndrome and how is it best treated?

INTRODUCTION

Sleep apnea is defined by repeated transient cessations of respiration during sleep. The more common type of this disorder, obstructive sleep apnea (OSA), has a prevalence approaching 5%. The burden of disease in the hospitalized patient is even greater than the general population because inpatients carry many predisposing risk factors for OSA: obesity, congestive heart failure, coronary artery disease, hypertension, stroke, and diabetes. Epidemiologic data suggest that the majority of patients with sleep apnea are undiagnosed. In 2004, national hospital discharge codes revealed fewer than 300,000 cases of sleep apnea amongst almost 35 million inpatient stays, yielding a prevalence of *identified* disease of less than 1%.

Although sleep apnea by itself is rarely a primary indication for hospitalization, recent evidence suggests that inpatient management of this disease needs to improve. Less than 6% of those identified as having sleep apnea in the 2004 National Hospital Discharge Survey received therapy with continuous positive airway pressure (CPAP) while in the hospital. Hospital Medicine physicians can ensure that OSA patients are identified and receive treatment. The key to identifying the possible presence of sleep apnea depends largely on an appreciation of risk factors and clinical features. Goring and Collop showed in 2008 that almost 80% of patients with suspected sleep apnea referred for a sleep study after an inpatient hospitalization were confirmed to have OSA. Therefore, inpatient identification and referral for evaluation can improve diagnosis rates and reduce the percentage of affected patients left untreated. This chapter will review the fundamentals of sleep apnea, address the *management of patients with stable sleep apnea in the inpatient setting*, delineate the necessity of preoperative screening in at-risk patients, and identify which patients should undergo further testing.

PRACTICE POINT

- Almost 80% of patients with suspected sleep apnea referred for a sleep study after an inpatient hospitalization were confirmed to have OSA.

PATHOPHYSIOLOGY

Sleep-disordered breathing includes two related diseases: obstructive sleep apnea and central sleep apnea—although as many as 90% of all cases are OSA. The distinction between OSA and central sleep apnea is an important one as the treatment options and responses to therapy are quite different. Obesity hypoventilation, also known as *Pickwickian syndrome*, is a condition in which patients afflicted with sleep apnea develop diurnal hypercapnia and hypoxemia.

OBSTRUCTIVE SLEEP APNEA

The upper airway is a compliant structure that is also susceptible to collapse. Complex neurologic and musculoskeletal interactions cause a reduction in the cross-sectional area of the upper airway during sleep, which can result in a reduction or cessation of airflow in susceptible individuals. The imbalance between the forces that promote airway patency (the pharyngeal dilator muscles) and the negative inspiratory forces generated by the diaphragm (which promotes airway collapse) causes obstruction. The majority of patients with OSA demonstrate obstruction in the retropalatal or retrolingual areas as these locations carry the greatest risk of collapse when a negative pressure forms inside the airway during inspiration.

Even during wakefulness, the cross-sectional area of the upper airway is smaller in patients with OSA compared with disease-free controls, often the result of anatomic contributors, such as enlarged tonsils, large tongue, a high-arched palate, and abnormal positioning of the maxilla and mandible. At sleep onset, a decrease in neural output to the pharyngeal dilator muscles increases the risk of collapse. In addition, supine positioning during sleep promotes collapse by bringing the weight of external tissue to bear upon the anteroposterior diameter of the pharynx, which is usually its shortest axis (and thus the one along which collapse is most likely). Snoring, caused by a vibration of the upper airway, can be the earliest sign of obstruction, although it is a very common clinical finding (occurring in up to 40% of men and 20% of women) and has a low positive predictive value (approximately 50%) for the presence of frank sleep apnea in an otherwise unselected population.

As obstruction worsens, periods of time during which airflow is inadequate (hypopnea) or absent (apnea) occur. During these episodes there are transient increases in arterial carbon dioxide tension and decreases in arterial oxygen tension. Episodes of obstruction typically terminate in an arousal from sleep, precipitated by the changes in oxygen and carbon dioxide as well as marked pressure swings within the thoracic cavity, as the affected individual unconsciously attempts to pull in air past the obstruction, an effort that fails due to the negative pressure serving to further pull the airway walls inward, worsening collapse. The lack of restful sleep from repetitive arousals throughout the night is responsible for the symptom of excessive daytime sleepiness in affected patients. Notably, only about half of patients with sleep apnea report overt sleepiness; others may report symptoms of fatigue, lack of energy, or other related symptoms without frank sleepiness.

PRACTICE POINT

- Only about half of patients with sleep apnea report overt sleepiness. Others may report symptoms of fatigue, lack of energy, or other related symptoms without frank sleepiness.

CENTRAL SLEEP APNEA

Several mechanisms contribute to the pathophysiology of central sleep apnea. Central events are marked by a transient absence of respiratory effort. Affected patients fall into two main groups, those with daytime hypercapnia and those without. All human beings have a slight decline in respiratory drive during sleep, with a typical increase in pCO_2 of about 5 mm of mercury; this change is normally achieved through a transient period of hypoventilation at sleep onset. Amongst patients with daytime hypoventilation (including those with chronic obstructive pulmonary disease and a number of neuromuscular disorders), an already impaired ventilatory drive is further suppressed, causing apnea.

Normocapneic patients with central apnea have a longer period of hypoventilation than is normally present at sleep onset. Circulatory delay, common in heart failure and often associated with central apnea, increases the amount of time it takes for carbon dioxide sensors in the medulla to appreciate the effect of a change in minute ventilation. Overshoot hypercapnia and subsequent tachypnea in an effort to reduce carbon dioxide levels leads to arousal.

The other major mechanism of central sleep apnea requires that the central apnea patient demonstrate a change in minute ventilation out of proportion to that which would be needed to correct a change in the partial pressure of carbon dioxide. Affected patients will have a prolonged period of hypoventilation at sleep onset, occasionally leading to arousal from overshoot hypercarbia and associated hypoxia. In both of these cases, Cheyne-Stokes respiration (also known as periodic breathing) can occur, characterized by a fluctuation in breathing apnea and tachypnea with a crescendo-decrescendo morphology.

TABLE 242-1 Differential Diagnosis of Obstructive Sleep Apnea, Based on Symptom

Symptom	Differential Diagnosis
Frequent nocturnal arousal and daytime somnolence	Central sleep apnea
	Benign prostatic hypertrophy
	Periodic limb movement disorder
	Environmental sleep disorder
	Nocturnal pain
	Mood disorder (eg, depression) inadequately controlled
	Insufficient sleep (most common cause of daytime sleepiness)
	Narcolepsy
	Idiopathic hypersomnia
	Awakening from other endocrinologic, cardiac, pulmonary, renal, or hematologic disorders
Snoring	Primary snoring
Paroxysmal dyspnea	Congestive heart failure
	Chronic obstructive pulmonary disease
	Nocturnal gastroesophageal reflux
	Nocturnal panic attacks

DIFFERENTIAL DIAGNOSIS

When evaluating patients for possible OSA, the symptom-based differential diagnosis can be broad (**Table 242-1**). While history may be highly suggestive of OSA, several other disorders can mimic its symptoms. Central sleep apnea presents with witnessed breathing pauses at night and daytime fatigue, although the mechanism of disease and appropriate treatment is quite different. Other causes of frequent nocturnal arousals and daytime somnolence include periodic limb movement disorder, prostatism and environmental sleep disorder, in which a stimulus external to the patient causes recurrent sleep disruption. Patients with nocturnal pain and inadequately controlled mood disorders may also demonstrate frequent nocturnal arousals. Excessive daytime sleepiness can be a symptom of insufficient sleep (the most common cause of daytime somnolence), depression, narcolepsy and idiopathic hypersomnia, as well as a number of endocrinologic, cardiac, pulmonary, renal, and hematologic disorders.

Snoring does not necessarily equate to sleep apnea. Primary snoring, while a socially difficult condition, has not clearly been associated with any long-term health repercussions. Patients who awaken with paroxysmal dyspnea at night may also suffer from congestive heart failure, chronic obstructive pulmonary disease, nocturnal gastroesophageal reflux or nocturnal panic attacks. A small percentage of patients with severe sleep apnea will demonstrate diurnal hypercapnia, although the diagnoses of underlying pulmonary disease (either restrictive or obstructive) and neuromuscular disease affecting the muscles of respiration should also be entertained.

DIAGNOSIS

CASE 242-1

A 55-year-old man is admitted for an acute myocardial infarction. Comorbidities include hypertension requiring three antihypertensive medications, type 2 diabetes, and morbid obesity (BMI 32). When should you suspect OSA? What additional data are needed to diagnose sleep apnea?

Patients with OSA present to the hospital with other medical problems and the clinician must identify at-risk patients so that they might undergo appropriate evaluation. Older age, obesity, and male sex are the most significant risk factors for OSA. Because the prevalence of these characteristics in the general population is too high for them to be useful as a screening tool, history and physical examination are critical in determining which patients are appropriate referrals for sleep testing (**Table 242-2**).

A screening history for OSA includes an assessment of both nocturnal and diurnal symptoms, and the accuracy of the history improves if the patient's bed partner is available for questioning as that person can offer greater insight into events that occur when the patient is unconscious. *Snoring* is the most common symptom of obstructive sleep apnea, present in more than 90% of patients with the disease, suggesting that the absence of snoring (by history from bed partner or other witness) would have a good negative predictive value for OSA. The presence of *witnessed apneas, seen in 75% of patients with OSA,* has a positive predictive value of greater than 80% for the presence of sleep apnea, although data do not suggest their presence can indicate the severity of the disease. The absence of witnessed apneas, does not reliably exclude the diagnosis of OSA, however. Another suggestive clue in the history includes *waking up with a sensation of choking or gasping for air.* This symptom usually represents an arousal from an apneic episode, with the sensation normally subsiding within seconds of waking. Rarely, patients may complain of *insomnia* (which probably represents disturbed sleep secondary to arousal), although the majority of patients report no difficulty initiating sleep. *Nocturia* is a frequent complaint amongst patients with apnea and occurs in part because OSA patients have higher circulating levels of atrial natriuretic peptide, leading to a greater urine output. In addition, some patients who wake from apnea have no recollection of the event (as the obstruction resolves with arousal), leading them to believe that they woke to urinate.

The presence of *excessive daytime somnolence (EDS)* is very common in OSA patients, although the complaint is nonspecific and its utility in discriminating affected patients from those without the disorder is poor. A validated questionnaire to assess sleepiness, such as the Epworth Sleepiness Scale (see http://epworthsleepinessscale.com/1997-version-ess/), can quantify fatigue, although the symptom remains nonspecific. Other daytime symptoms of OSA include irritability, memory disturbance, and morning headaches (secondary to cerebral vasodilation due to transient carbon dioxide retention).

Other medical disorders have been associated with OSA (**Table 242-3**). Although most of these disorders do not have a good positive predictive value for sleep apnea, recent guidelines recommend considering the diagnosis of OSA in patients with refractory hypertension. Sleep apnea is also more common in patients with renal failure, hypothyroidism, and acromegaly. Myocardial diastolic dysfunction has been associated with sleep-disordered breathing, although a causal link has not been definitively proven. The presence of neuromuscular disease can increase the risk of both central and obstructive sleep apnea. In addition, the regular use of narcotics or benzodiazepines can cause or exacerbate OSA. Any of these risk factors should trigger more detailed questioning about symptoms of OSA.

TABLE 242-2 History and Physical Examination Findings Suggesting Sleep Apnea

Heroic snoring
Nocturia
Witnessed breathing pauses during sleep
Excessive daytime sleepiness
Tongue or tonsillar enlargement
Retrognathia
Large neck circumference (> 16 inches in women, > 17 inches in men)

TABLE 242-3 Other Comorbid Conditions Associated with Obstructive Sleep Apnea

Systemic hypertension
Pulmonary hypertension
Myocardial infarction
Stroke
Diabetes mellitus and glucose intolerance
Atrial fibrillation
Congestive heart failure
Hypothyroidism
Neuromuscular disease

PRACTICE POINT

- Guidelines recommend considering the diagnosis of OSA in patients with refractory hypertension.
- The regular use of narcotics or benzodiazepines can cause or exacerbate OSA.

Physical examination may be helpful in identifying patients at higher risk of sleep apnea, but *no exam findings can confirm or preclude the diagnosis with a significant degree of certainty.* Obesity is associated with OSA, with a prevalence of OSA as high as 70% in morbidly obese patients. Neck circumference (> 17 inches in men, > 16 inches in women) confers increased risk of OSA. Other anatomic factors conferring an increased risk include retrognathia, micrognathia, tonsillar hypertrophy, an enlarged uvula, macroglossia, and inferior displacement of the hyoid. Assessment of cross-sectional area of the pharynx using a validated tool such as the Mallampati scale can help to quantify airway crowding and OSA risk.

Several screening tools exist that attempt to integrate components of the history (and physical examination in some cases) to create a composite risk score. The Berlin questionnaire (**Figure 242-1**) has a positive predictive value approaching 90%. A combination of such tools and clinical acumen can best determine which patients should undergo further evaluation.

PRACTICE POINT

- The Berlin questionnaire has a positive predictive value near 90% for diagnosing OSA.

OVERNIGHT PULSE OXIMETRY AND IN-HOSPITAL POLYSOMNOGRAPHY IN DIAGNOSIS OF OSA

Multiple trials have evaluated the effectiveness of clinical prediction rules and other simple testing devices for making a definitive diagnosis of obstructive sleep apnea, as overnight polysomnography (PSG) can be inconvenient and expensive. Although home-based PSGs are being developed, current evaluation requires the patient to spend a night in a sleep laboratory utilizing nighttime PSG, the current reference standard test. Most insurers require this test prior to the initiation of therapy with CPAP. Even when the diagnosis is highly suspected and can be confirmed by the presence of heroic snoring and witnessed apneas during hospitalization, a formal study will be necessary in most cases.

As an alternative to PSG, some have proposed the use of overnight continuous pulse oximetry to diagnose OSA as it is comparatively inexpensive, simple to perform and can be performed in the patient's hospital room. However, the presence of nocturnal desaturation does not equate to the presence of obstructive sleep apnea and cannot reliably distinguish central from obstructive apnea as an explanation for any observed desaturation. In addition, the absence of desaturation does not exclude the diagnosis of OSA. In some cases, patients may not sleep for much of the night; the absence of significant desaturation could simply represent the absence of significant sleep. On the whole, overnight oximetry can be useful to exclude OSA in appropriately chosen patients who are at high risk, but patients would still require a full PSG prior to initiation of CPAP therapy if abnormalities are found.

In-hospital PSG for patients considered to be high-risk for sleep apnea may be considered during their inpatient stay, although this test is not usually reimbursed by insurers when performed during hospitalization. In addition, in-hospital sleep may not be representative of typical in-home sleep because of

Berlin Questionnaire
Sleep Apnea

Scoring Berlin Questionnaire

The questionnaire consists of 3 categories related to the risk of having sleep apnea. Patients can be classified into High Risk or Low Risk based on their responses to the individual items and their overall scores in the symptom categories.

Categories and Scoring:

Category 1: items 1, 2, 3, 4, and 5;

Item 1: if **'Yes'**, assign **1 point**
Item 2: if '**c**' or '**d**' is the response, assign **1 point**
Item 3: if '**a**' or '**b**' is the response, assign **1 point**
Item 4: if '**a**' is the response, assign **1 point**
Item 5: if '**a**' or '**b**' is the response, assign **2 points**

Add points. *Category 1 is positive if the total score is 2 or more points.*

Category 2: items 6, 7, 8 (item 9 should be noted separately).

Item 6: if '**a**' or '**b**' is the response, assign **1 point**
Item 7: if '**a**' or '**b**' is the response, assign **1 point**
Item 8: if '**a**' is the response, assign **1 point**

Add points. *Category 2 is positive if the total score is 2 or more points.*

Category 3 is positive if the answer to item 10 is '**Yes**' or if the BMI of the patient is greater than 30 kg/m^2.

(BMI is defined as weight (kg) divided by height (m) squared, ie, kg/m^2).

High Risk: if there are 2 or more categories where the score is positive.

Low Risk: if there is only 1 or no categories where the score is positive.

Additional Question: item 9 should be noted separately.

Figure 242-1 *The Berlin Questionnaire. (Data from the Netzer NC, Stoohs RA, Netzer CM, Clark K, Strohl KP. Using the Berlin Questionnaire to identify patients at risk for the sleep apnea syndrome. Ann Intern Med. 1999;131(17):485–491.)*

Berlin Questionnaire
Sleep Apnea

Height (m) __________ Weight (kg) __________ Age __________ Male / Female

Please choose the correct response to each question.

Category 1

1. Do you snore?
☐ a. Yes
☐ b. No
☐ c. Don't know

If you answered 'Yes':

2. You snoring is:
☐ a. Slightly louder than breathing
☐ b. As loud as talking
☐ c. Louder than talking
☐ d. Very loud – can be heard in other rooms

3. How often do you snore?
☐ a. Almost every day
☐ b. 3–4 times per week
☐ c. 1–2 times per week
☐ d. 1–2 times per month
☐ e. Rarely or never

4. Has your snoring ever bothered other people?
☐ a. Yes
☐ b. No
☐ c. Don't know

5. Has anyone noticed that you stop breathing during your sleep?
☐ a. Almost every day
☐ b. 3–4 times per week
☐ c. 1–2 times per week
☐ d. 1–2 times per month
☐ e. Rarely or never

Category 2

6. How often do you feel tired or fatigued after your sleep?
☐ a. Almost every day
☐ b. 3–4 times per week
☐ c. 1–2 times per week
☐ d. 1–2 times per month
☐ e. Rarely or never

7. During your waking time, do you feel tired, fatigued or not up to par?
☐ a. Almost every day
☐ b. 3–4 times per week
☐ c. 1–2 times per week
☐ d. 1–2 times per month
☐ e. Rarely or never

8. Have you ever nodded off or fallen asleep while driving a vehicle?
☐ a. Yes
☐ b. No

If you answered 'Yes':

9. How often does this occur?
☐ a. Almost every day
☐ b. 3–4 times per week
☐ c. 1–2 times per week
☐ d. 1–2 times per month
☐ e. Rarely or never

Category 3

10. Do you have high blood pressure?
☐ Yes
☐ No
☐ Don't know

Figure 242-1 *(continued)*

the physiologic derangement that necessitated hospitalization, as well as fragmented sleeping in the hospital environment due to noise and staff interruptions.

MANAGEMENT

MANAGEMENT OF STABLE OSA IN THE HOSPITALIZED PATIENT

Many hospitalized patients carry a prior diagnosis of OSA. Several studies have recently evaluated the prevalence and management of sleep apnea in the hospitalized patients, and found that management of OSA in the hospital setting is frequently overlooked. One study showed that less than 6% of patients received this therapy during hospital stay, despite home adherence to CPAP. Several challenges impede optimal management of OSA patients during an acute hospitalization. The burden of disease is high and resources are limited to provide CPAP machines to all affected patients, as the setup often requires significant involvement by a respiratory therapist. Many patients are not able to report the correct home setting for their CPAP machine, and the mask interface with which the patient has become comfortable may not be available at the hospital.

Patients already on treatment should be encouraged to bring in their home device for use during their hospital course. While this may not be feasible in all patients or in all facilities, it would tremendously decrease the burden on the hospital to provide devices for inpatient use. If patients are unable to retrieve their own device, contacting the patient's durable medical equipment provider can often provide information about the machine's setting and the specific mask interface used by the patient at home, so that this can be replicated during hospitalization.

PRACTICE POINT

- Patients already on treatment should be encouraged to bring in their home device for use during their hospital course.

MANAGEMENT OF HOSPITALIZED PATIENTS WITH UNTREATED OSA

CASE 242-2

A 64-year-old woman is admitted for congestive heart failure exacerbation. During her hospitalization, she demonstrates heroic snoring and witnessed breathing pauses while sleeping. How important is it to treat her with CPAP during her hospitalization?

While CPAP clearly benefits patients with various etiologies of respiratory failure, little evidence supports urgent implementation of CPAP for OSA during hospitalization. A recent trial of OSA patients admitted with acute decompensated heart failure randomized patients to receive CPAP or standard heart failure management found that acute treatment of OSA with CPAP resulted in significant improvement in cardiac systolic function after 72 hours.

Little evidence supports *inpatient* initiation of CPAP for uncomplicated OSA. Implementation of positive airway pressure for the first time to an acutely ill patient can lead to significant discomfort and noncompliance absent close supervision by a qualified respiratory therapist. In addition, inpatient respiratory therapy departments may not have resources to initiate therapy in all patients. When CPAP therapy is used during hospitalization in patients that are suspected to have OSA, a referral for outpatient testing after discharge carries benefit because coverage for CPAP therapy is difficult to arrange in those that have not undergone appropriate testing. Even if the patient is willing to pay for therapy out of pocket, PSG is preferred for therapeutic titration to prevent undertreatment (yielding residual apnea) or overtreatment (leading to discomfort and increased rates of noncompliance).

PRACTICE POINT

- Inpatient initiation of CPAP for uncomplicated OSA is not indicated. Even if CPAP therapy is used during hospitalization in patients who are suspected to have OSA, hospitalists should refer patients upon discharge for outpatient sleep study testing because it is difficult to arrange for outpatient CPAP therapy in those who have not undergone appropriate testing.

SCREENING FOR OSA IN THE SURGICAL POPULATION

Patients with sleep apnea bears high risk of perioperative complications, including postoperative ICU admission, prolonged length of hospital stay, encephalopathy and infection, particularly if they receive general anesthesia or opioids. Morbidly obese patients often desaturate rapidly during periods of apnea due to low resting lung volumes. Therefore, care during the intubation process should focus on preventing significant desaturation during the induction of anesthesia. Failure to recognize OSA patients prior to surgery may leave providers unable to anticipate possible complications and implement preventative measures. Recent American Society of Anesthesiologists guidelines recommend screening patients for OSA risk factors, as perioperative pulmonary complications increase with increasing severity of sleep apnea.

Hospitalists should identify obstructive sleep apnea preoperatively. One recent study screened all patients using the Berlin Questionnaire presenting for elective surgery and performed PSG in those that were found to be high risk. It found that the prevalence of sleep apnea in this surgical population was more than 20%, but more importantly that over 70% of these cases were undiagnosed. Therefore, preoperative screening for sleep apnea is strongly recommended, with those found to be high risk ideally undergoing testing prior to surgery. Even if testing is not feasible preoperatively, identification of high-risk patients should generate a lower threshold to intervene postoperatively and reduce pulmonary complications with active management when necessary.

TREATMENT OF OSA IN THE CPAP INTOLERANT

While continuous positive airway pressure serves as the most effective therapy for obstructive sleep apnea, its use is associated with significant noncompliance (> 50% in some studies). Efforts to improve compliance with CPAP may include the use of different facial interfaces (**Figure 242-2**) to improve patient comfort, desensitization therapy, the addition of heated humidification or a switch to bilevel positive airway pressure therapy. No single intervention improves satisfaction in all patients requiring CPAP therapy, although the involvement of a qualified respiratory therapist can help determine which to try first.

PRACTICE POINT

- Efforts to improve compliance with CPAP may include the use of different facial mask interfaces to improve patient comfort, desensitization therapy, heated humidification, or a switch to bilevel positive airway pressure therapy. No single one of these interventions improves satisfaction in all patients requiring CPAP therapy, although the involvement of a qualified respiratory therapist can help determine which to try first.

Other therapeutic options include *oral appliance therapy* (OAT), surgical treatments and supplemental oxygen. Oral appliances work either by repositioning the lower jaw (mandibular advancement) or by holding the tongue forward. Although mandibular advancement devices (**Figure 242-3**) have been better studied, both treatments are effective in patients with less-severe disease and amongst those who are not morbidly obese. Surgical treatments have also shown benefit in these groups as well as those with specific anatomic defects on physical examination. Oxygen therapy can benefit OSA patients who have significant desaturation at night. While supplemental oxygen does not have a marked impact on the frequency of obstructive events, it attenuates nocturnal hypoxemia, which is a greater predictor of cardiovascular risk than the frequency of the apneas themselves. Lastly, in affected patients who use medications that increase apnea severity (such as opiates and benzodiazepines), dose reduction or discontinuation should be considered, when possible.

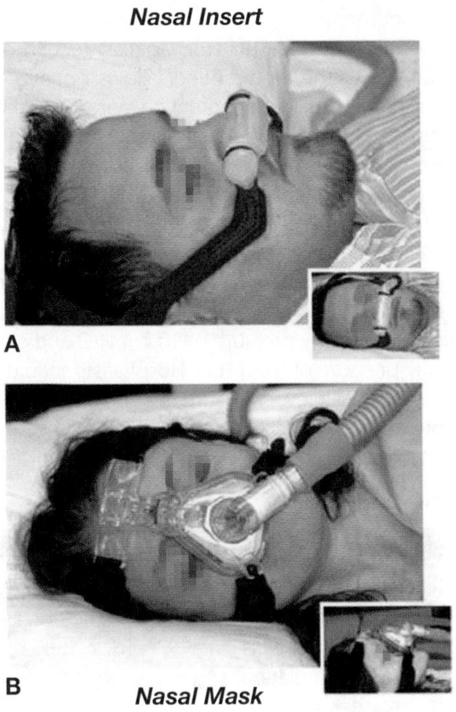

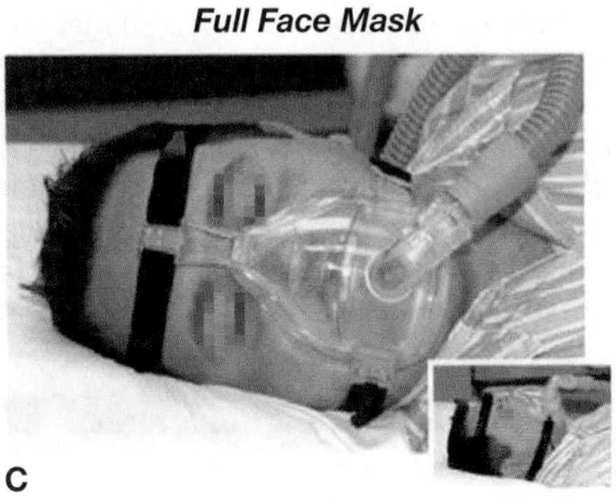

Figure 242-2 *Pictures of different continuous positive airway pressure interfaces. (A) Nasal Insert, (B) Nasal Mask, (C) Full Face Mask (Reproduced, with permission, from Pack A. Fishman's Pulmonary Diseases and Disorders. 4th ed. New York: McGraw-Hill; 2008. Fig. 97-16.)*

CONSULTATIONS

Respiratory therapy consultation for all patients for whom CPAP is prescribed during the hospitalization will allow the patient selection of interface (mask type) and appropriate fitting to minimize nocturnal mask leak and optimize patient comfort. Many respiratory therapists are also trained in desensitizing techniques for patients who complain of intolerance, although training will vary among medical centers.

Consultation from a pulmonologist or sleep specialist (when available) should be requested when CPAP nonadherence cannot be adequately addressed by a respiratory therapist. In addition, patients who require more aggressive outpatient therapy

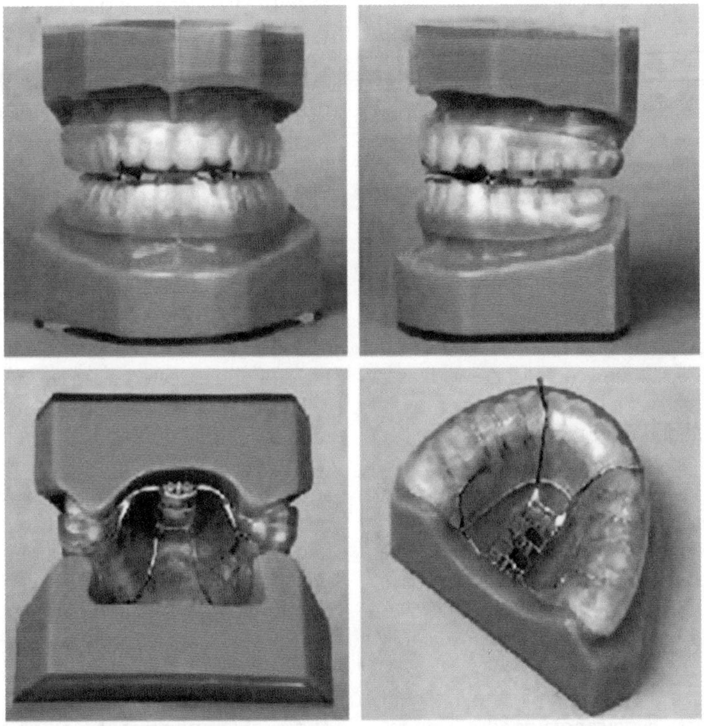

Figure 242-3 *Mandibular advancement devices. (Reproduced, with permission, from Pack A. Fishman's Pulmonary Diseases and Disorders. 4th ed. New York: McGraw-Hill; 2008. Fig. 97-22.)*

may benefit from inpatient consultation. Symptoms suggesting include persistent sleepiness despite compliance with CPAP therapy, persistent snoring on treatment, the development or worsening of cor pulmonale or the presence of obesity hypoventilation (discussed below). Lastly, consultation should be considered in all patients with predominantly *central* sleep apnea due to the complexity of this need optimizing treatment in patients with this disease.

COMPLICATIONS AND PROGNOSIS

OSA confers an increased risk of incident hypertension, coronary artery disease, atrial fibrillation, complex ventricular ectopy, cerebrovascular disease, a worsened prognosis in heart failure and increased cardiovascular mortality. While few data support an increased rate of complications during hospitalization for medical illness attributable to OSA, multiple trials of postoperative complications demonstrate a higher rate of pulmonary, cardiac, gastrointestinal, and bleeding complications in patients with sleep apnea. As a result, many anesthesiologists screen patients for sleep-disordered breathing during preoperative evaluation. However, evidence has not yet proven any attenuation of surgical risk with CPAP therapy.

OBESITY HYPOVENTILATION SYNDROME

CASE 242-3

A 44-year-old morbidly obese man is brought into the emergency department obtunded with a pCO_2 of 94 mm Hg. He is well known to your health care system; he is a never-smoker and has no previous signs of neuromuscular disease during annual evaluation by his primary care physician. What is his likely diagnosis and how should he be treated?

Obesity hypoventilation syndrome (OHS) is a disorder related to sleep apnea, defined by the presence of waking alveolar hypoventilation ($paCO_2$ >45 mm Hg) in the setting of obesity (BMI >30) with no other clear predisposing risk factors. Approximately 90% of patients with OHS have comorbid sleep-disordered breathing with OHS. It occurs in an estimated 10% to 20% of OSA patients.

The pathogenesis of OHS is not completely understood, but is likely related to physiologic derangements and consequences that occur as a result of obesity. Among these contributors are respiratory muscle dysfunction, diminished central ventilatory drive, and increased resistance to certain hormonal modulators, such as leptin. Obesity reduces respiratory system compliance, increases airways resistance and creates a state of relative respiratory muscle weakness—possibly related to fatigue from the increased work of breathing. Other as-yet-unidentified contributors must also exist, as the majority of patients with obesity do not develop OHS. In most cases, correction of obesity improves the elevated daytime $paCO_2$ and hypoventilation. CPAP therapy corrects daytime hypercapnia in a significant minority of OHS patients, although some have advocated instead for nocturnal bilevel pressure, which improves nocturnal minute ventilation and may improve diurnal respiratory muscle strength.

Patients with OHS may come to the attention in the inpatient setting after admission with severe hypercapnia or admission for other acute medical illnesses such as pneumonia. Despite obesity, these patients will not have other obvious contributors to hypercapnia (sedative use, chronic obstructive pulmonary disease or neuromuscular disease). Although they are often admitted to the intensive care unit for rapid correction of their hypercapnia, transfer to the medical floor allows optimization of care prior to discharge. Unlike patients with pure OSA, these patients do not typically require additional diagnostic testing to justify the use of home positive pressure therapy, as hypoventilation is an approved indication for this treatment. Most providers implement bilevel pressure acutely to assist with the probable underlying OSA as well as the hypoventilation with empiric choices of pressure levels based upon patient tolerance and the need to eliminate carbon dioxide. Commonly used starting pressures include inspiratory positive airway pressure of 10 cm H_2O and expiratory positive airway pressure of 5 cm H_2O. Hospitalists should refer these patients for a formal bilevel pressure titration after discharge, as the optimal pressure levels will depend upon the severity of the underlying obstructive physiology.

PRACTICE POINT

- Unlike patients with pure OSA, obesity-hypoventilation patients do not typically require additional diagnostic testing to justify the use of home positive pressure therapy, as hypoventilation is an approved indication for this treatment.

Patients with OHS use significantly more resources and have far greater medical expenses when compared with morbidly obese eucapnic patients and sleep-disordered breathing patients without hypercapnia. Additionally, OHS patients have a greater morbidity and mortality than obese subjects without OHS. These patients have higher rates of comorbid congestive heart failure, angina, and cor pulmonale, as well as a greater rate of hospitalization, need for intensive care, and need for mechanical ventilation. Timely recognition and treatment of patients with OHS can minimize the frequency of poor outcomes.

DISCHARGE PLANNING

Patients with sleep apnea who were on therapy prior to their hospitalization and who do not demonstrate any signs of inadequate treatment have no specific discharge needs. Hospitalists should ensure such patients know how to reach the durable medical equipment provider who services their positive airway pressure devices and can provide supplies, if CPAP masks or tubing are required. Even if disease is stable and well controlled, annual follow-up with a sleep specialist should be considered to ensure continued compliance with therapy and monitoring for complications of undertreated disease.

For patients without previously documented disease, ensuring rapid confirmation and implementation of therapy by arranging an outpatient polysomnogram is strongly recommended, more so if the patient was admitted with a disease that might have resulted from inadequately treated disease, such as myocardial infarction, congestive heart failure or cerebrovascular accident. The hospitalist may need to arrange nocturnal oxygen supplementation for severely affected patients if polysomnography cannot be performed soon after discharge. However, not all such patients will qualify for therapy, due to lack of definitive evidence of benefits of this treatment in patients with sleep apnea. Arranging an outpatient appointment with a sleep specialist for these patients is critical, as close follow-up after implementation of CPAP therapy is one of the best predictors of long-term compliance with treatment (**Table 242-4**).

TABLE 242-4 Evidence-based Medicine Key References

Study	Methodology	Results	Limitations	Bottom Line
Goring K, Collop N. *J Clin Sleep Med.* 2008;4(2):105–110.	Retrospective chart review of 100 polysomnographies ordered after hospitalization	High frequency of sleep disordered breathing (77%) in sample, especially with underlying cardiopulmonary disease	Retrospective; cannot determine impact of sleep-disordered breathing on acute exacerbations of cardiopulmonary disease	Patients with sleep-disordered breathing can be successfully identified during hospitalization
Finkel KJ, et al. *Sleep Med.* 2009;10(7): 753–758.	Prospective observational study of surgical patients screened for OSA	23.7% of patients screened high risk for OSA of which 81% did not have prior diagnosis of OSA; among patients tested 82% had OSA	Did not look at outcomes of patients with OSA; home studies used to make diagnosis of OSA	Undiagnosed OSA is prevalent in adult surgery population, and universal screening can help identify these patients
Hwang D, et al. *Chest.* 2008;133: 1128–1134.	Preoperative patients were screened for sleep-disordered breathing and tested with home oximetry; postoperative complications were assessed	57% of patients had evidence of sleep-disordered breathing by nocturnal oximetry; postoperative complications were much higher with greater degrees of nocturnal desaturation	Nocturnal desaturation used to identify patients with sleep-disordered breathing	Postoperative complications are much greater in patients with sleep-disordered breathing, highlighting importance of preoperative screening and testing
Khayat RN, et al. *Chest.* 2009;136(4): 991–997.	Randomized clinical trial of patients admitted with decompensated heart failure who underwent sleep study and randomized to treatment with CPAP vs usual care for heart failure	Left ventricular ejection fraction was significantly superior in intervention arm	Small study of 46 patients; unable to look at other outcomes	Early identification of OSA in patients with acute decompensated heart failure is important as treatment with CPAP can improve systolic function in this setting

CPAP, continuous positive airway pressure; OSA, obstructive sleep apnea.

SUGGESTED READINGS

Basner RC. Continuous positive airway pressure for obstructive sleep apnea. *N Engl J Med.* 2007;356(17):1751–1758.

Finkel KJ, Searleman AC, Tymkew H, et al. Prevalence of undiagnosed obstructive sleep apnea among adult surgical patients in an academic medical center. *Sleep Med.* 2009;10(7): 753–758.

Flemons WW. Clinical practice. Obstructive sleep apnea. *N Engl J Med.* 2002;347(7):498–504.

Goring K, Collop N. Sleep disordered breathing in hospitalized patients. *J Clin Sleep Med.* 2008;4(2):105–110.

Hwang D, Shakir N, Limann B, et al. Association of sleep-disordered breathing with postoperative complications. *Chest.* 2008;133: 1128–1134.

Khayat RN, Abraham WT, Patt B, Pu M, Jarjoura D. In-hospital treatment of obstructive sleep apnea during decompensation of heart failure. *Chest.* 2009;136(4):991–997.

McNicholas WT. Diagnosis of obstructive sleep apnea in adults. *Proc Am Thorac Soc.* 200815;5(2):154–160.

Mokhlesi B, Kryger MH, Grunstein RR. Assessment and management of patients with obesity hypoventilation syndrome. *Proc Am Thorac Soc.* 2008;5(2):218–225.

Netzer N, Eliasson AH, Netzer C, Kristo DA. Overnight pulse oximetry for sleep-disordered breathing in adults: a review. *Chest.* 2001;120(2):625–633.

Spurr KF, Graven MA, Gilbert RW. Prevalence of unspecified sleep apnea and the use of continuous positive airway pressure in hospitalized patients, 2004 National Hospital Discharge Survey. *Sleep Breath.* 2008;12(3):229–234.

CHAPTER 243

Pleural Diseases

Christopher Parks, MD
David M. Berkowitz, MD
Rabih Bechara, MD

Key Clinical Questions

1. What are the valuable and helpful diagnostic testing modalities available in the evaluation of a pleural effusion?
2. How is empyema diagnosed and managed?
3. When does a malignant pleural effusion deserve serial drainage versus an indwelling drainage catheter versus pleurodesis?
4. What are the indications for chest tube placement (tube thoracostomy) in patients with a small pneumothorax?
5. When can a chest tube be removed, and how is that done?

PLEURAL EFFUSIONS

INTRODUCTION

Pleural effusion complicates many different diseases making its precise incidence difficult to determine. The rate is estimated at 3.2 patients per 1000 population. The causes of effusions are varied (**Table 243-1**), with heart failure as the most common etiology. No data on hospital admission rate due to pleural effusions exists. Morbidity and mortality from pleural effusions correlates with the underlying etiology rather than the pleural effusion itself. Patients with pleural effusions secondary to malignancy or cirrhosis tend to have a poor prognosis while pleural effusions secondary to treatable or ameliorable conditions such as pulmonary emboli or surgery tend to have much better prognoses.

PATHOPHYSIOLOGY

Normally, only a small 0.1 to 0.2 mL/kg or approximately 6 to 12 cc occupies the space between the visceral pleura lining the lung and the parietal pleura lining the chest wall and diaphragm. Fluid due to filtration from microvessels and stoma in the parietal pleura moves out of the pleural space by connecting to lymphatic channels. In the normal physiologic state the rate of pleural fluid turnover is 0.15 mL/hr, and in disease states this can be increased to approximately 30 ml/hr. A pleural effusion may collect in the pleural space due to increased production or decreased reabsorption of this fluid. Potential mechanisms of abnormal fluid accumulation include increased capillary permeability of the microvessels primarily in the parietal pleura, stoma obstruction, and decreased plasma oncotic pressures (**Figure 243-1**). In addition to serous fluid (hydrothorax), blood (hemothorax), lipid (chylothorax), and pus (empyema) may occupy the pleural space. Symptoms likely result from decreased chest wall compliance and stimulation of neurogenic receptors rather than direct compression of lung tissue.

Light's Criteria classifies pleural effusions as either a transudate or an exudate (**Table 243-2**). Transudative pleural effusions indicate the presence of a systemic process, implicating organ systems other than the lungs. Volume overload medical conditions, including renal failure, heart failure, cirrhotic liver disease and hypoalbuminemia, cause transudates by overwhelming the capacity of the pulmonary lymphatics to absorb fluid. These types of effusions frequently occur bilaterally. In contrast, exudative pleural effusions indicate a local pleural process and necessitate a different diagnostic and therapeutic approach. These effusions form secondary to inflammation and obstruction of local lymphatic flow and most often occur unilaterally.

PRACTICE POINT

Light's criteria defining exudative effusions:

- Pleural fluid/serum protein ratio >0.5
- Pleural fluid/serum LDH ratio >0.6
- Pleural fluid LDH 2/3rd upper limit of normal serum LDH

PRESENTATION

The usual symptoms of pleural effusion, dyspnea and chest pain, are nonspecific and many patients are asymptomatic. If incidentally noted on chest x-ray (CXR), the history should focus on symptoms and risk factors that may elucidate an underlying disease.

TABLE 243-1 Differential Diagnosis of Pleural Effusions

System	Diagnosis
Cardiac	Heart failure
	Postcoronary artery bypass graft
	Postcardiac injury syndrome
	Pericarditis
Pulmonary	Pneumonia: parapneumonic effusion or empyema
	Pulmonary embolism
	Sarcoidosis
	Trapped lung
	Acute or chronic atelectasis
Gastrointestinal	Cirrhosis or other causes of portal hypertension
Gynecologic	Ovarian hyperstimulation syndrome
Neoplastic	Primary lung cancer
	Metastatic disease to the lung
	Meig syndrome
Rheumatologic/collagen vascular diseases	Systemic lupus erythematosis
	Rheumatoid arthritis
Renal	Uremia
	Nephrotic syndrome
Occupational	Asbestosis
Trauma/iatrogenic injury	Drug induced
	Radiation therapy
	Hemothorax
	Chylothorax
Idiopathic	Yellow nail syndrome

TABLE 243-2 Transudate and Exudate Pleural Effusions: Differential Diagnosis

Transudates	Exudates
Congestive heart failure	Pneumonia (parapneumonic effusion)
Cirrhosis with ascites	Cancer
Nephrotic syndrome	Pulmonary embolism
Peritoneal dialysis	Bacterial infection
Myxedema	Tuberculosis
Acute atelectasis	Connective tissue disease
Constrictive pericarditis	Viral infection
Superior vena cava obstruction	Fungal infection
Pulmonary embolism	Rickettsial infection
Urinothorax	Parasitic infection
	Asbestos
	Meigs syndrome
	Pancreatic disease
	Uremia
	Chronic atelectasis
	Trapped lung
	Chylothorax
	Sarcoidosis
	Drug reaction
	Postmyocardial infarction syndrome (Dressler syndrome)

Reproduced, with permission, from Collard HR, Moore BB, Flaherty KR, et al. Acute exacerbations of idiopathic pulmonary fibrosis. *Am J Respir Crit Care Med*. 2007;176(7):636–643.

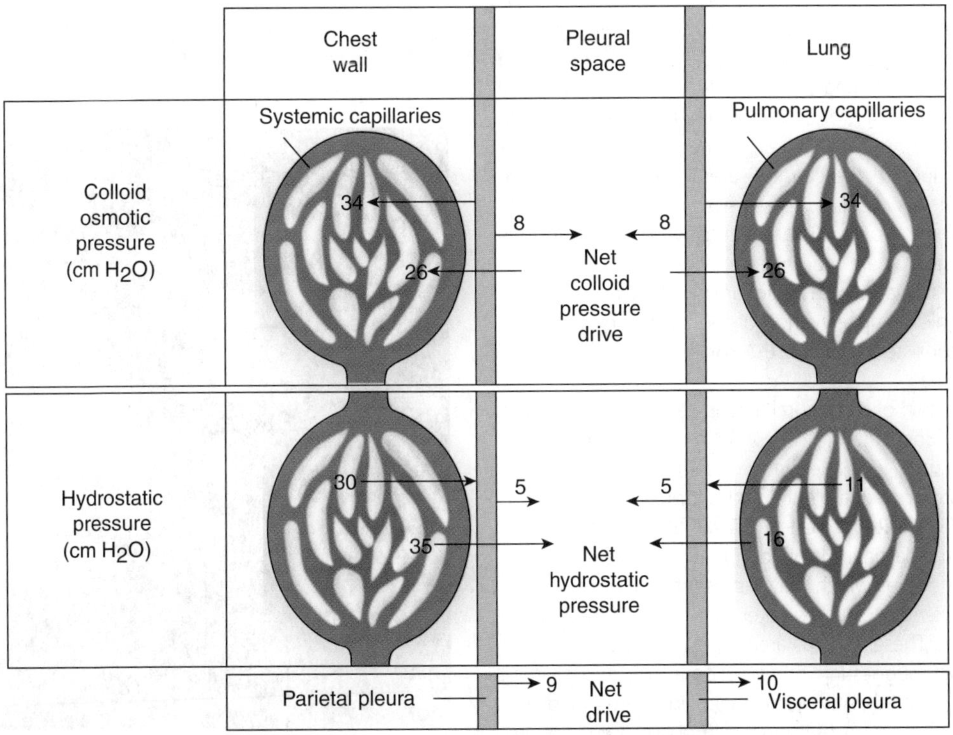

Figure 243-1 *Pathophysiology of pleural effusion genesis. (Reproduced, with permission, from Doherty GM. Current Diagnosis & Treatment: Surgery. 13th ed. New York: McGraw-Hill, 2010. Fig. 18-5.)*

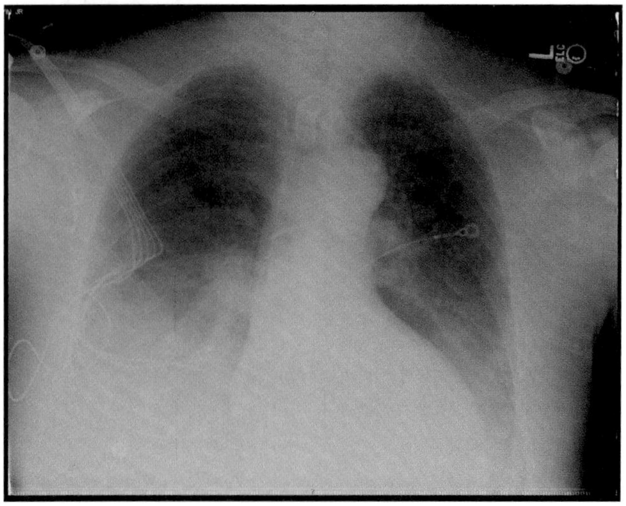

Figure 243-2 *Chest x-ray shows right pleural effusion.*

Dyspnea usually only occurs in patients with very large effusions, but can occur with smaller effusions in patients with underlying lung disease and in approximately 50% of patients with malignant pleural effusions. The degree of breathlessness does not correlate with the size of the effusion. Chest pain caused by pleural inflammation is typically described as a stabbing or shooting pain. Deep inspiration and cough exacerbate the pain commonly at the site of the inflammation but may be referred anywhere in the thorax particularly the lower thorax and back. Placing pressure over the chest wall may provide partial relief.

Dullness to percussion, *decreased* tactile fremitus, egophany (e to a changes), and decreased breath sounds may suggest any process that leads to loss of air space, including an effusion greater than 300cc. Other physical exam findings will be related to the underlying disease process.

IMAGING

A simple upright anteroposterior (AP) or posteroanterior (PA) chest radiograph will detect fluid volumes of greater than 300 cc. If a pleural effusion is strongly suspected but not seen, a decubitus film (obtained with the patient lying with the affected side down) may detect as little as 50 cc of fluid and indicate whether the fluid is free flowing (**Figure 243-2**). A CXR will help delineate the effusion size and may provide clues to the cause. Bilateral effusions are more likely to be present in systemic diseases such as congestive heart failure or nephrotic syndrome. Unilateral massive pleural effusions which fill the hemithorax are more likely malignant. In addition to massive size, signs associated with malignancy include rib crowding, lobulated pleural thickening, elevation of the hemidiaphragm and mediastinal shift consistent with obstruction of a bronchus by an underlying carcinoma.

If further visualization of the pleural fluid is necessary to evaluate for the presence of loculations, non-contrast, non-high resolution computed tomography (CT) adequately quantifies the extent of loculation or the presence of a pleural rind prior to definitive drainage procedures (**Figure 243-3**). Chest CT will also identify parenchymal infiltrates, mediastinal lymphadenopathy, or pleural abnormalities. Chest CT findings which may represent pleural metastasis include pleural thickening, usually greater than 1 cm, or mediastinal pleural involvement. These findings are very specific but not sensitive. Key CT findings suggesting mesothelioma include unilateral effusion and nodular pleural thickening with involvement of the intralobular septa. CT using a pulmonary embolism (PE) protocol will be necessary to identify the presence of PE. See Chapter 108: Advanced Cardiothoracic Imaging.

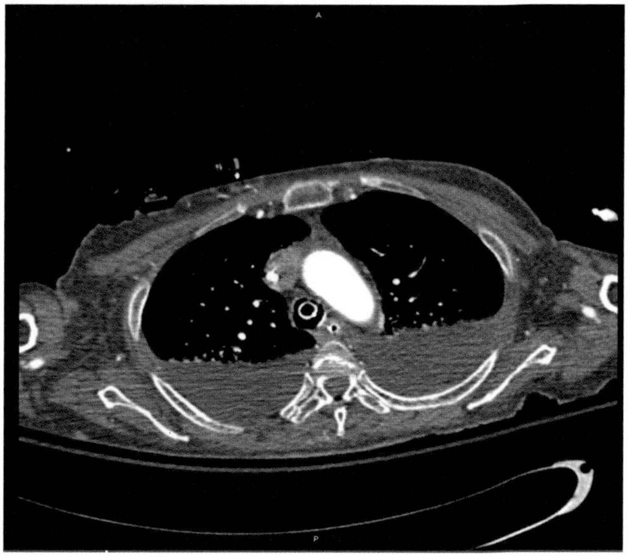

Figure 243-3 *Computed tomography showing bilateral effusions.*

Positron emission tomography (PET) CT with fluorine-18 labeled glucose has a very high sensitivity and negative predictive value (>90% for each) for the detection of malignant pleural disease. Specificity and positive predictive value are not as good. False-positives occur in other conditions with increased pleural inflammation (eg, lupus pleuritis).

MRI provides better resolution than the CT, and better visualizes certain structures such as the chest wall and diaphragm. MR is superior to CT for complex pleural effusions and effusions with masses because it can possibly better define the mass dimensions and consistency. CT is often recommended above MRI to evaluate complex pleural effusions due to added expense and limited ability of MRI to visualize the lung parenchyma compared with CT.

Ultrasound can distinguish solid from liquid pleural fluid with roughly 92% accuracy and combined with chest radiography, the accuracy increases to 98% (**Figure 243-4**).

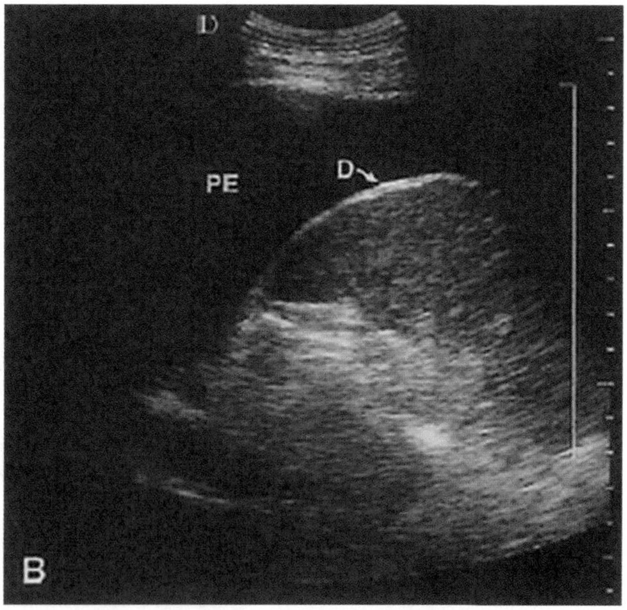

Figure 243-4 *Ultrasound image of a pleural effusion. D, diaphragm; PE, pulmonary embolism.*

TABLE 243-3 Effusion Characteristics Based on Effusion Type

Etiology or Type of Effusion	Gross Appearance	White Blood Cell Count (cells/μL)	Red Blood Cell Count (cells/μL)	Glucose	Comments
Malignant effusion	Turbid to bloody; occasionally serous	1000 to < 100,000 M	100 to several hundred thousand	Equal to serum levels; < 60 mg/dL in 15% of cases	Eosinophilia uncommon; positive results in cytologic examination
Uncomplicated parapneumonic effusion	Clear to turbid	5000–25,000 P	< 5000	Equal to serum levels	Tube thoracostomy unnecessary
Empyema	Turbid to purulent	25,000–100,000 P	< 5000	Less than serum levels; often very low	Drainage necessary; putrid odor suggests anaerobic infection
Tuberculosis	Serous to serosanguineous	5000–10,000 M	< 10,000	Equal to serum levels; occasionally < 60 mg/dL	Protein > 4.0 g/dL and may exceed 5 g/dL; eosinophils (> 10%) or mesothelial cells (> 5%) make diagnosis unlikely
Rheumatoid effusion	Turbid; greenish yellow	1000–20,000 M or P	< 1000	< 40 mg/dL	Secondary empyema common; high LD, low complement, high rheumatoid factor, cholesterol crystals are characteristic
Pulmonary infarction	Serous to grossly bloody	1000–50,000 M or P	100 to > 100,000	Equal to serum levels	Variable findings; no pathognomonic features
Esophageal rupture	Turbid to purulent; red-brown	< 5000 to > 50,000 P	1000–10,000	Usually low	High amylase level (salivary origin); pneumothorax in 25% of cases; effusion usually on left side; pH < 6.0 strongly suggests diagnosis
Pancreatitis	Turbid to serosanguineous	1000–50,000 P	1000–10,000	Equal to serum levels	Usually left sided; high amylase level

LD, lactate dehydrogenase; M, mononuclear cell predominance; P, polymorphonuclear leukocyte predominance.

Ultrasound helps determine the presence, size, extent, and location of the pleural effusion and thin echogenic bands in the effusion may suggest the presence of a complicated and loculated effusion. Ultrasound guidance for thoracentesis decreases the incidence of pneumothorax in nonventilated and ventilated patients. Ultrasound findings suggestive of malignancy include identification of either solid or hypoechoic pleural densities with irregular borders or increased cellular debris (increased density material within the pleural fluid).

THORACENTESIS

Obtaining a specimen of the fluid for analysis should be done in all patients unless a clear etiology is suggested, such as the presence of pulmonary edema in patients with heart failure, bilateral pleural effusions in patients with the nephrotic syndrome or anasarca, left-sided effusion in patients with acute pancreatitis, or effusions arising in patients having undergone certain surgical procedures. However, if the effusion does not resolve in response to therapy, then a thoracentesis should be performed. See Chapter 117 Thoracentesis, which describes the proper technique for performing a thoracentesis.

DIFFERENTIAL DIAGNOSIS

The differential diagnosis of pleural effusions includes many clinical diagnoses and systemic disorders. Disorders can be identified based on the patient's medical history, whether the fluid is a transudate or exudate (Table 243-2), and other characteristics of the pleural fluid (**Table 243-3**).

Effusions due to heart failure

Heart failure causes approximately 60% of all pleural effusions and greater than 90% of transudative effusions. Most pleural effusions due to heart failure are bilateral (75%), but they can also occur unilaterally, with right-sided effusion more common than left. Usually transudates, they may appear exudative after aggressive diuresis. They are straw colored and have low cell count with a mononuclear predominance. These effusions usually resolve with the treatment of the underlying congestive heart failure; they usually do not require diagnostic thoracentesis if a diuretic trial leads to effusion resolution over days to weeks.

Parapneumonic effusions

Most parapneumonic effusions are sterile, clear exudates that generally resolve with antibiotic treatment and rarely require chest tube drainage. However, a minority (5%) are complicated with loculations and fibrin deposits. The fluid may be infected, as suggested by a low glucose, an elevated LDH, and a low pH on fluid analysis. This stage of pneumonia will not resolve with antibiotics alone and predisposes the patient to complications such as continued pleural sepsis and empyema.

Empyema progresses through three stages: exudative, fibrinopurulent, and organizing (**Table 243-4**). In the *exudative stage*, the pleural fluid is nonviscous and freely flowing, with minimally inflamed pleural membranes, and the patient is likely to respond to antibiotics but may require drainage according to Thoracic Society Guidelines. The *early fibrinopurulent stage* is characterized

TABLE 243-4 Three Stages of Empyema

	Exudative	*Fibrinopurulent*	*Organizing*
Fluid viscosity	Free flowing	Increased	Loculations, pus
Cells	Neutrophils	Fibroblasts	Fibroblasts and debris
pH, glucose	Normal	Decreased	Low
Treatment	Antibiotics, drainage	Antibiotics, drainage	Surgery

by increasing viscosity of the fluid, thickening of the pleural membranes, and formations of intrapleural loculations. Patients may respond to antibiotic therapy alone but often require emptying of the pleural space via chest tube drainage. In the *organized stage*, the patient will likely require surgical debridement of the pleural peel that has formed.

All patients with pleural infections should be treated with antibiotics. The proper choice of antibiotics depends on the presumed site of the development of the empyema. In a community-acquired empyema, the primary organisms include streptococcal pneumonia, gram-negative organisms and anaerobic organisms. A third-generation cephalosporin plus metronidazole to cover methicillin-sensitive *Staphylococcus aureus* (MSSA), gram-negative organisms, and anaerobic organisms. Aminoglycosides should be avoided secondary to poor pleural penetration. For health care associated or hospital-acquired empyema, antibiotic coverage should be broadened to include methicillin-resistant *Staphylococcus aureus* (MRSA), but anerobic coverage is less important. Piperacillin-tazobactam plus vancomycin are reasonable initial choices.

Drainage of a parapneumonic effusion may be required to prevent progression through the three stages of empyema. Parapneumonic effusions are divided into four categories and assigned a risk for poor outcomes. *Large volume drainage intervention, usually by tube thoracostomy procedure, is generally required in three circumstances:* (1) effusion >50% of the hemithorax or loculated effusion or effusion with thickened parietal pleura; (2) fluid-positive bacterial Gram stain or culture or pus; (3) fluid pH <7.2 (see section below on Tube Thoracostomy). Other circumstances that may meet indication for pleural fluid drainage include glucose <60 or LDH >3 times upper limit of normal. Fibinolytic therapy may be considered for loculated pleural effusions, based on several uncontrolled trials showing greater fluid removal.

While parapneumonic effusions and especially empyema may commonly lead to pleural fluid with a low pH, other etiologies may be considered in patients with pleural fluid with a low pH (**Table 243-5**).

Effusions related to pulmonary embolism

Small pleural effusions occur frequently in patients with pulmonary embolism (up to 50% of patients may have blunting of costophrenic angle). Few patients (< 10%) sustain moderate sized pleural effusions, and rarely would an effusion due to PE occupy greater than 1/3 of the hemithorax. The pleural fluid is often exudative, especially when pulmonary infarction occurs, but can be transudative. The effusions appear serous or serosanguineous, and the cell counts increase moderately with a neutrophil predominance.

Effusions in AIDS patients

Pleural effusions occur very commonly in AIDS patients, with an incidence of 7% to 27% found during hospitalization. The most common causes of effusion are infectious, but up to one-third are malignant (eg, Kaposi sarcoma) (**Tables 243-6** and **243-7**). Bacterial pneumonia accounts for 30% of infectious effusions in AIDS patients. Effusions occur commonly with mycobacterial infections as well, seen with tuberculosis and the mycobacterium avium complex, accounting for approximately 10% of pleural effusions in AIDS patients.

Effusions are commonly found in patients with Kaposis sarcoma; however, the fluid is rarely positive for malignant cells, and most patients have endobronchial disease. Pleural fluid cytology is more helpful for diagnosing lymphoma and pleural effusion lymphoma. Due to poor nutritional status, patients with AIDS are also more likely to be hypoalbuminemic, which commonly causes pleural effusions. Pleural fluid analysis in patients with AIDS should include protein, LDH, cell count, culture and cytology—similar to analysis in non–AIDS patients. Finally, tuberculosis (TB) may present with pleural effusion in an AIDS patient. While pleural fluid analysis for acid fast bacilli to rule out TB is only moderately sensitive, the sensitivity improves with serial pleural fluid analysis (up to 3). However, pleural biopsy may be necessary for diagnosis in some cases.

Rheumatoid pleurisy

Pleural involvement in patients with rheumatoid arthritis (RA) is clinically evident in up to 5% of RA patients, but at autopsy 50% will have pleural involvement and pleural effusion. Effusions in RA result from immune complex deposition and disruption of the normal reuptake of fluid by pulmonary lymphatic system. Rheumatoid effusions are characterized by a triad of findings: glucose <30, pH 7, and LDH >1000. The effusions typically develop after 5 years of

TABLE 243-5 Causes of Low Pleural Fluid pH

Empyema
Esohageal rupture
Urinothorax
Malignancy
Lupus (< 20%)
Tuberculosis (< 20%)

TABLE 243-6 Common Infectious Causes of Pleural Effusions in AIDS Patients

Typical Bacteria
Pneumocystis jiroveci (formerly *Pneumocystic carinii*, *Pneumocystis carinii* pneumonia [PCP])
Mycobacteria
Cryptococcus
Nocardia
Histoplama
Toxoplasmosis

TABLE 243-7 Malignant Causes of Pleural Effusion in AIDS Patients
Kaposi sarcoma
Lymphoma
Castleman disease
Lung cancer

articular manifestations, but can occur as early as 3 years prior to and as late as 20 years after articular manifestations. The effusion is usually unilateral, and two-thirds of patients have no other lung pathology. One-third will either have pulmonary fibrosis or pulmonary nodules. Both steroids and NSAIDs have been used to treat rheumatoid pleurisy, but no controlled trials support these interventions. Once steroid treatment is instituted, the pleural effusion usually resolves within 3 to 4 months. The response to therapy, whether systemic or intrapleural, occurs independently of the articular inflammation, with half of these patients having a protracted course.

Lupus pleuritis

Among all connective tissue disorders, systemic lupus erythematosus (SLE) most commonly causes pleuritis. Pleuritis in SLE presents more often in women than men, with pleural effusions occurring in up to 30% of patients. The pleural symptoms may antedate other disease manifestations and can be bilateral, unilateral, or alternate from one side to the other. A 60- to 80-mg dose of prednisone daily produces positive results in patients with lupus-related pleural effusions. There is no data on duration of therapy or the use of DMARDs at this time.

Sarcoidosis

Pleural effusion is a rare complication of sarcoidosis (< 1% of patients). The natural history of sarcoidosis-related pleural effusions varies; some resolve spontaneously, whereas others resolve with treatment within the same time frame. While sarcoidosis remains in the differential of lymphocytic predominant pleural effusions and eosinophilic effusions, other etiologies should be considered in the differential diagnosis with these types of pleural effusions (**Tables 243-8** and **243-9**). In the individualized treatment of symptomatic patients, the dose of prednisone ranges between 20 to 40 mg/day with a taper over 3 to 4 weeks.

Postcardiac injury syndrome (Dressler syndrome)

Postcardiac injury syndrome is an immunologic entity associated with a wide array of manifestations, including pericarditis, fever, leukocytosis, elevated sedimentation rate, pulmonary infiltrates,

TABLE 243-8 Causes of Lymphocyte Predominant Pleural Effusions
Tuberculosis
Chylothorax
Lymphoma
Yellow nail syndrome
Rheumatoid pleurisy
Sarcoidosis
Lung transplant rejection
Late (> 2 mo) postcoronary artery bypass graft

TABLE 243-9 Causes of Eosinophilic Pleural Effusions
Pneumothorax
Hemothorax
Benign asbestosis
Pulmonary embolism
Parasitic disease
Fungal disease
Drug induced
Lymphoma
Carcinoma
Churg-Strauss syndrome
Tuberculous pleural effusion
Sarcoidosis

and pleural effusion. The syndrome can occur days, weeks, and even months after myocardial infarction, cardiac surgery, pacemaker placement, and angioplasty. It is seen more commonly after cardiac surgery, occurring in up to 30% of patients. The effusion is usually treated with anti-inflammatory medication and exhibits a variable time course for adequate response. Nonresponders require steroids tapered over 3 to 4 weeks.

Hepatic hydrothorax

Hepatic hydrothorax is the term for a pleural effusion arising in a patient with cirrhosis. It is usually the result of fluid transfer from the abdomen to the pleural space through defects in the diaphragm. Hepatic hydrothorax is more frequently right sided (85% of cases), but 13% are left sided only and 2% bilateral; and ascitic fluid can be absent in many patients. The first-line treatment includes diuresis and sodium restriction. This treatment works to counteract ascites caused by sodium retention in the kidney. Diuretic dosing must be managed and monitored carefully, as dose increases can precipitate hepatic encephalopathy or renal insufficiency in some patients. Recommended initial therapy includes spironolactone with furosemide. If diuretic treatment at escalated doses fails, patients may benefit from a transjugular intrahepatic portosystemic shunt procedure. Thoracentesis is reserved for large effusions in symptomatic patients or for patients with fever, to rule out a spontaneous bacterial empyema which occurs in up to 13% of patients, diagnosed based on pleural fluid absolute neutrophil count > 250/microliter or positive gram stain or culture.

Tube thoracostomy with talc pleurodesis attempts have largely been unsuccessful. Treatment failures are likely secondary to the rapid formation of fluid in the pleural space, which prevents the formation of adhesions between the visceral and parietal pleura. In the largest case series of 18 who had talc pleurodesis, 44% recurred at 3 months, and there was a 57% morbidity rate and 39% mortality rate. As morbidity can include prolonged chest tube drainage, excessive protein loss, renal failure, infection, and severe leak at the chest tube site, *pleurodesis is not recommended for hepatic hydrothorax*. Patients with hepatic hydrothorax nonresponsive to diuretic treatment constitute a difficult to treat population, and the therapeutic approach must be individualized.

PRACTICE POINT

- Tube thoracostomy with talc pleurodesis is not recommended in pleural effusions due to hepatic hydrothorax, as effusions often recur after intervention, and morbidity and mortality are high.

Hemothorax

Hemothorax, or bleeding in the pleural space, is most commonly caused by blunt or penetrating trauma. Nontraumatic causes are far less common and include malignancy, pulmonary embolism with infarction and tuberculosis. Independent of cause, large chest tube drainage constitutes the primary therapy because large volumes of blood in the pleural space rapidly form intrapleural loculations and increase the risk for empyema and fibrothorax. In some patients with retained intrapleural blood, fibrinolytic agents are instilled with good results. Most patients have either partial or complete resolution, and very few require eventual decortications or have any major complications (eg, bleeding) reported. Thoracoscopy, if performed early in the course of the injury and before pleural adhesions form, can play an important role in the management of patients who sustain traumatic hemothorax complicated by major intrathoracic vessel injury and air leaks.

PRACTICE POINT

- In hemothorax, large chest tube drainage constitutes primary therapy, as large volumes of blood in the pleural space rapidly form intrapleural loculations and increase the risk for empyema and fibrothorax.

Chylothorax

Chylothorax, defined as the appearance of lymph and emulsified fat in the pleural effusion, rarely causes pleural effusion. Clinicians should be able to distinguish chylothorax from a simple cholesterol effusion by suspected etiology, onset, and pleural fluid analysis (**Table 243-10**). The Mayo Clinic identified only 203 patients over a 21-year period. Chylothorax is due to thoracic duct injury or obstruction related to malignancy, thoracic surgical procedures, and chest trauma. A number of cases are associated with diseases such as lymphangioleiomyomatosis and lymphangiectasis. After the underlying cause is determined, specific treatment may be effective for managing the resulting chylothorax. The cornerstone of treatment involves nutritional intervention to prevent protein, vitamin, and lymphocyte loss. Success with a medium-chain triglyceride diet has been variable. Conservative management in a symptomatic patient involves drainage of the chylous effusion by thoracentesis or chest tube placement. Somatostatin has been used successfully in a few cases of chylous effusions refractory to chest tube drainage. Pleurodesis can be successful in the management of chylothorax, especially if the rate of chyle flow is not high. In refractory cases, embolization and surgical interventions such as ligation of the thoracic duct, pleuroperitoneal shunting, and fibrin glue to repair the defect in the duct are used.

TABLE 243-10 Differentiating Pleural Fluid Chylothorax from Cholesterol Effusion

	Chylothorax	Cholesterol Effusion
Causes	Surgery, trauma, lymphoma, lymphangiomatosis	Lung entrapment, tuberculosis, rheumatoid arthritis, empyema
Onset	Rapid, early	Insidious, late
Symptoms	Dyspnea	Usually none, but may have dyspnea
Cells	Lymphocyte predominant	Neutrophil predominant
Diagnosis	Cholesterol < 200	Cholesterol > 200

Malignant pleural effusions

In 2000, there were estimated to be approximately 150,000 cases of malignant pleural effusion. Seventy-five percent of malignant pleural effusions are caused by lung, breast, or ovary carcinomas (primary cell type: adenocarcinoma) or lymphoma. In men, the leading cause of malignant pleural effusion is lung cancer; while in women, the leading cause is breast cancer. A relatively unusual cause of pleural effusion is mesothelioma, but in this disease malignant effusions are very common. Seventy-five percent of patients with malignant mesothelioma will have a pleural effusion, and 60% of those effusions will be on the right side. These effusions are usually large, occupying greater than 50% of the hemithorax, and associated with pleural thickening and plaques. These effusions must be differentiated from benign asbestos pleural effusions which appear earlier in the course of the disease, are smaller and less symptomatic and do not contain malignant cells. The majority of patients with malignant pleural effusions present with dyspnea due to decreased chest wall compliance and decreased lung volume in the ipsilateral lung. Other symptoms have been more associated with specific types of cancer—for example, chest pain with mesothelioma and hemoptysis with bronchogenic carcinoma.

Pathophysiology Malignant pleural effusions can form either by direct extension of tumor cells from adjacent structures or through the spread of distant tumors through the pulmonary vasculature. Malignant cells obstruct the stoma, which are normally able to reabsorb pleural fluid and release factors such as cytokines which stimulate increased pleural fluid production.

Up to 50% of effusions in cancer patients have nonmalignant causes. Thoracentesis should be performed to distinguish malignant effusions from other causes of pleural effusions, including "paramalignant effusions"—those related to the tumor but not malignant. Paramalignant effusions can be due to local effects of the tumor: postobstructive pneumonia, obstruction of the thoracic duct with resultant chylothorax, or effusion secondary to pulmonary embolism.

Multiple treatment modalities for cancer also may lead to iatrogenic pleural effusion, including radiation therapy and chemotherapeutic agents such as bleomycin or doxorubicin. For a complete list of pulmonary toxic agents, please see www.pneumotox.com. Other nonmalignant causes of pleural effusions may develop that are unrelated to these patients' cancers as in Table 243-1.

Pleural fluid analysis All patients with either known or suspected malignancy should have a small volume thoracentesis if the patient is asymptomatic or large volume for symptom control. Usually 30–50 cc is sufficient for the lab to process all studies needed. Pleural fluid cytology has a diagnostic yield of approximately 65% that can be increased with repeat thoracentesis. Which study of fluid cytology, 48% of patients were positive on an initial fluid sample, with an additional 16% positive on a second sample, and an additional 16% were positive on a third sample. No further positives were obtained after the third sample. Increased volumes do not increase the diagnostic yield. Most malignant pleural effusions are exudates, but 3% to10% are transudates. Some authorities recommend further evaluation of the pleural space if the pleural fluid cytology is negative. Evaluation may include pleuroscopy, pleural biopsy or video assisted thoracoscopic surgery (VATS).

PRACTICE POINT

- Real-time ultrasound decreases the pneumothorax rate from 8.8% to 1.1% and the number of dry (no fluid obtained) taps decreases from 15% to 0%. Nonguided taps should only be attempted if ultrasound is not available. If bedside ultrasound is not available, marking by ultrasound radiology is an alternative, but the procedure must be performed with the patient in the same position that the ultrasound marking occurred.

Treatment Identification of a malignant effusion provides important prognostic information and may change goals of treatment to palliation of symptoms.

Meta-analysis data of patients with malignant pleural effusions suggests a median survival of 4 months (shorter for lung, ovarian, and gastrointestinal cancers; slightly longer for breast cancers and lymphomas). Depending on the severity of symptoms and rapidity of accumulation, treatment options include simple observation, minimally invasive procedures such as thoracentesis, pleurodesis, and invasive procedures such as pleurectomy. Nearly 100% of malignant effusions will recur within 30 days, and most patients will require further intervention. If the initial thoracentesis does not provide symptomatic benefit, alternate causes (eg, pulmonary embolism) of the patient's dyspnea should be aggressively sought.

PRACTICE POINT

- Nearly 100% of malignant effusions will recur within 30 days, and most patients will require further intervention following conservative management. Severity of symptoms and the rapidity of fluid reaccumulation guide treatment decisions.

Serial large volume thoracentesis In patients with slowly reaccumulating fluid (>2 months between necessary therapeutic thoracenteses) or in patients whose medical condition precludes more invasive options, repeated thoracentesis is the best therapy. Repeated thoracenteses, thus, are reserved for patients with (1) slowly reaccumulating pleural fluid; (2) cancers which respond to concurrent therapy; (3) short life expectancy; or (4) poor tolerance to more invasive therapy.

Indwelling pleural catheter This simple outpatient procedure is performed under conscious sedation for patients with rapidly reaccumulating pleural fluid (<1 month between necessary therapeutic thoracenteses). A chronically indwelling pleural catheter may be placed with one end in the pleural space and one external limb, thereby allowing for drainage of pleural fluid at home. Multiple studies have shown such a catheter device to be effective in the management of dyspnea from malignant pleural effusions. In some patients the presence of the catheter in the pleural space acts as a sclerosing agent and can provide similar results to chemical pleurodesis. For motivated patients it can be used for long-term relatively labor-intensive intermittent drainage. Complications may include bleeding or infection at the catheter site, pain, and failure to completely drain the effusion.

Pleurodesis This procedure applies either a chemical or mechanical force to abrade the pleural surfaces causing inflammation and obliteration of the pleural space. Prior to undergoing pleurodesis, complete re-expansion of the lung should be demonstrated as well as symptom relief. In the United States, talc is the most common substance used for pleurodesis, but many other substances are available including tetracycline, mitomycin, bleomycin, and silver nitrate. Mechanical pleurodesis is accomplished with either mechanical pleural abrasion or through the prolonged use of a chest tube. The use of chemical pleurodesis is generally less invasive and more effective than the use of mechanical pleurodesis. Few studies compare the respective agents head to head, but in a large meta-analysis the success rate of the nonantineoplastic agent was superior to the rate of the neoplastic agents.

Common complications to pleurodesis include fever, pain, and gastrointenstinal symptoms. Rare complications include respiratory failure, cardiovascular complications, and empyema. Because of this procedure's high cost and moderate patient discomfort, it should be reserved for patients with a life expectancy >3 months.

Pleuro-peritoneal shunts When pleurodesis fails and in patients who are not candidates for chronic indwelling catheter placement, a pleuro-peritoneal shunt directs a catheter with one end in the pleural space and one end in the peritoneal cavity. Patients who are not candidates for a chronic indwelling catheter include poor anatomy (eg, morbidly obese), low literacy (eg, unable to understand self drainage), and/or poor social or other support (eg, no home assistance). There are two systems for this procedure which is normally placed by thoracic surgery under general anesthesia. The first is an active system which requires the activation of a pump (Denver pleuro-peritoneal shunt) and the second is a passive system (Laveen shunt). The complication rate of these shunts is approximately 15%, with major complications including shunt occlusion and infection. The palliation efficacy rate is approximately 73% to 90%.

Pleurectomy The final method for control of malignant pleural effusions is pleurectomy, a morbid procedure that should be performed only for patients whose health and expected longevity permits recovery from the surgery. This procedure should be done in the operating room by a surgeon experienced in such procedures. It is used primarily in the treatment of malignant mesotheliomas and almost always effective at obliterating the pleural space.

PNEUMOTHORAX

Pneumothorax is a collection of air or gas in the pleural cavity of the chest between the lung and the chest wall. Pneumothorax can occur due to many causes: primary spontaneous, secondary spontaneous, traumatic or iatrogenic. When pneumothorax leads to rapid reduction of oxygenation and/or blood pressure due to rapidly increasing entrained air and pressure within the pleural cavity, a tension pneumothorax is diagnosed.

Symptoms of pneumothorax may include shortness of breath or chest pain. Physical examination findings in patients with pneumothorax may include the following:

- Unilateral absent breath sounds
- Unilateral chest wall movement (also seen in atelectatic lung)
- Soft tissue crepitus (chest, neck, mediastinum)
- Tracheal deviation to the opposite side of the affected lung (a sign associated with tension pneumothorax)

When patient is on a ventilator, breath sounds may be difficult to assess or unreliable due to "referred" air movement sounds from the ventilator.

TENSION PNEUMOTHORAX VS NONTENSION PNEUMOTHORAX

Patients who develop acute respiratory distress and rapidly decompensate to hypotension or respiratory failure and/or cardiac arrest (often pulseless electrical activity or asystole) may have tension pneumothorax. Management of tension pneumothorax requires

TABLE 243-11 Conditions Associated with Primary Spontaneous Pneumothorax

Family history
Thoracic endometriosis
Smoking
Marfan syndrome

maintaining a low threshold or suspicion for the condition; rapidly assessing the patient; and managing the condition based on clinical findings, as there may not be adequate time to attain CXR for diagnosis prior to instituting definitive therapy for relief and reversal of the high pressure.

Assessing patients for tension pneumothorax in rapidly deteriorating patients or patients with cardiac arrest should start with *assessment of the trachea*. If tracheal deviation is present and the patient is developing hypotension or respiratory or cardiac arrest, the clinician should manage by immediately placing a large bore needle/catheter (14 gauge) into the second intercostal space of the affected lung (side opposite to the deviated trachea position), called a needle thoracostomy. This intervention should allow immediate air release from the affected lung and rapid improvement in clinical parameters.

Following improvement of clinical parameters, the needle/catheter may need to be connected to a wall suction device; and the clinician should immediately consult a specialist who can place a tube thoracostomy (chest tube).

PRIMARY SPONTANEOUS PNEUMOTHORAX

Primary spontaneous pneumothorax (PSP) occurs without a precipitating event in a patient with no known lung disease. The incidence PSP is 7 to 18 episodes per 100,000 patients per year in men and 1 to 6 per 100,000 patients per year in women. Most patients with PSP likely have some form of underlying lung disease which results in subpleural bleb formation that can rupture. Other conditions may also be associated with PSP (**Table 243-11**). PSP may be precipitated by changes in barometric pressure; and small, ipsilateral, hemorrhagic pleural effusions are found in approximately 10% of patients. PSP most commonly occurs in tall, thin boys and men aged 10 to 30 years; and smoking increases the risk approximately 20-fold in men and less so in women. Ninety percent of PSPs occur at rest with pleuritic chest pain and acute dyspnea being the most common symptoms. These symptoms typically resolve spontaneously within 24 hours.

On physical examination decreased breath sounds and hyperresonance to percussion are common physical findings. Hypoxemia due to VQ mismatching is common, but hypercarbia is rare. The pneumothorax can be diagnosed on a standard chest radiograph when there is visualization of the visceral pleural line removed from the chest wall on an upright radiograph (**Figure 243-5**). Various treatment options are available (**Table 243-12**).

The risk of recurrence after an initial PSP is 32% to 52%, and recurrence rate increases with each subsequent pneumothorax. Patients who develop recurrent PSP should be considered for medical or surgical intervention options to prevent recurrence (**Table 243-13**).

SECONDARY SPONTANEOUS PNEUMOTHORAX

Secondary spontaneous pneumothorax (SSP) occurs in the presence of another disease (**Table 243-14**). Hyperexpansion of the distal air spaces from obstruction or inflammation in the airways

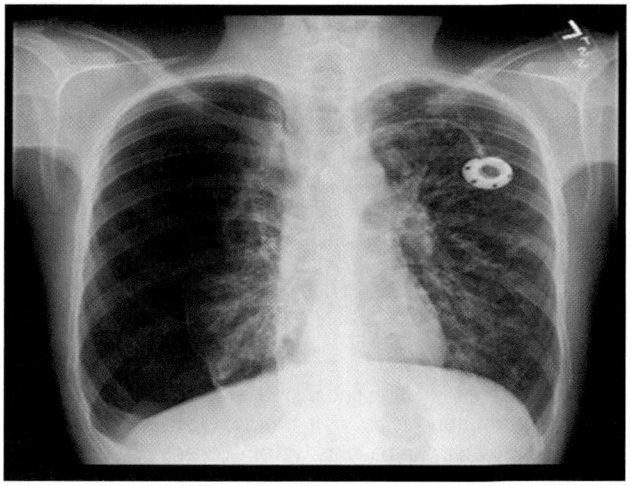

Figure 243-5 *Chest x-ray showing right-sided pneumothorax.*

can lead to alveolar rupture and retrograde movement of air along the bronchovascular bundle to the mediastinum with rupture through the mediastinal parietal pleura or direct rupture through the visceral pleura from an inflammatory parenchymal process.

Patients with SSP have more severe dyspnea than those with PSP because of their decreased pulmonary reserve. Up to 15% of patients with SSP have life-threatening hypoxemia, and hypotension. The symptoms of SSP do not resolve spontaneously. A suspicion of pneumothorax should remain heightened in the COPD patient with dyspnea and unilateral chest pain.

Underlying lung disease—hyperlucent lungs or thin walled bullae—often makes identification of the visceral pleural line problematic. A supine radiograph may show pneumothorax gas juxta-cardiac or in the costophrenic sulcus and may produce a deep sulcus sign. Chest CT may be necessary to diagnose an SSP.

Unlike PSP patients virtually all patients with SSP require hospitalization due to hypoxemia, hypercapnia, and respiratory distress. Pneumothorax less than 3 cm can usually be observed in SSP patients, while all others require chest tube placement. Patients with SSP are also more likely to have persistent air leaks requiring further therapy such as pleurodesis or VATS. Preventive measures for SSP recurrence include VATS or pleurodesis and should be performed in all patients with SSP after their *first* pneumothorax (Table 243-13).

TABLE 243-12 Treatment Options for Primary Spontaneous Pneumothorax

Patient is clinically stable and the pneumothorax is < 3 cm	Supplemental O_2	May discharge home after 6 hr if no progression on repeat CXR
> 3 cm and symptomatic	Needle aspiration	May discharge home with stopcock or Heimlich valve Follow up in 2 days
Failed 1 or 2 or if concomitant fluid on CXR	Chest tube	Small caliber < 22-Fr
Unstable	Chest tube	

TABLE 243-13 Prevention of Recurrence of Spontaneous Pneumothorax

Therapeutic Options	Comments
Chemical pleurodesis via chest tube	Reduces recurrence rate Effective agents: • Talc slurry (most effective) • Doxycycline
Video-assisted thoracoscopic surgery	Intervention options: • Stapling of large bleb with talc poudrage • Pleural abrasion
Smoking cessation	

IATROGENIC PNEUMOTHORAX

Causes of iatrogenic pneumothorax include subclavian vein catheter insertion (incidence among all users, 2.8%), thoracentesis, percutaneous pleural biopsy, transbronchial lung biopsy, and mechanical ventilation (especially with high ventilator peak or plateau pressures). Management decisions are similar in iatrogenic pneumothorax as PSP.

TUBE THORACOSTOMY (CHEST TUBE) MANAGEMENT BASICS (FIGURE 243-6)

INDICATIONS AND CONTRAINDICATIONS

Table 243-15 lists the many indications for placement of a chest tube (tube thoracostomy). There are no absolute contraindications, particularly in acute situations, but extra care should be exercised in patients with coagulapathy or who at high risk for adhesions (prior pleurodesis or chronic infection).

PROCEDURE

The size of the chest tube depends on the viscosity of the fluid. Catheter types include small, usually 8- to 18-French tubes used primarily for the drainage of pneumothorax or free flowing fluid, and larger (up to 40 French catheters) for the drainage of hemothorax.

The insertion site is based on location of the area to be drained. This can be visualized either on chest radiography (CXR or CT) or via ultrasound. A common site is the fourth or fifth intercostal space midaxillary or anterior axillary line. Alternatively, for pneumothorax, the midclavicular line in the second intercostal space may be used. The two most common techniques for placement include a- The Seldinger Technique, where insertion is performed over a guidewire b- Tunneling, where tissue dissection is than followed by tube insertion in the pleural space.

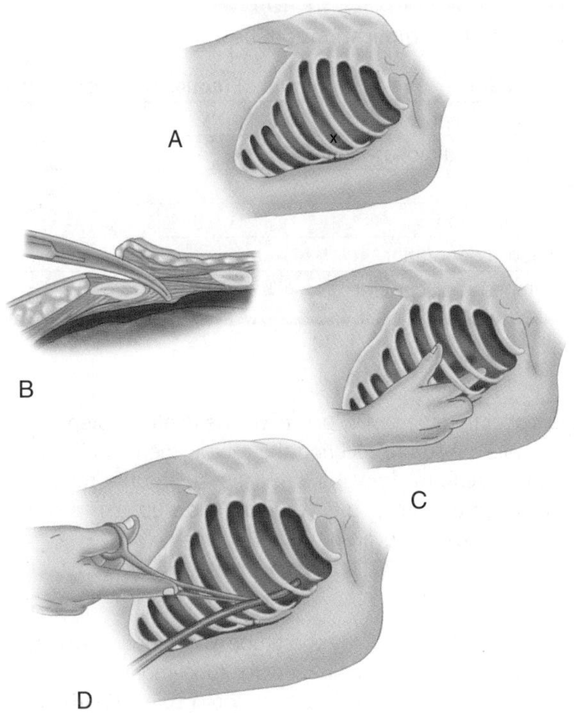

Figure 243-6 *Tube thoracostomy (chest tube) or pleural drain placement. Steps that are usually taken to perform tube thoracostomy: (A) localization of correct site; (B) entrance of probe above the rib; (C) digital probe; (D) placement of tube. (Reproduced, with permission, from Brunicardi FC, Andersen DK, Billiar TR, et al. Schwartz's Principles of Surgery. 9th ed. New York: McGraw-Hill; 2010. Fig. 7-3.)*

CHEST TUBE REMOVAL

Ultimately, the individual service that placed the chest tube is responsible for its management and removal. Hospitalists should work closely with consultants (pulmonologists, surgeons, radiologists) who have placed chest tubes to collaboratively manage and remove the tubes when indicated. Often the most challenging decision regarding chest tube management is when to remove the tube. Several criteria must be met for chest tube removal:

1. The initial reason for which the chest tube was placed has resolved.
2. The lung is fully expanded.
3. The pleural fluid output is < 200 cc/day.
4. There should be no air leak.

Once these criteria are met, the chest tube should be taken off suction and placed on water seal. Some clinicians will remove the chest tube on water seal, while some prefer to clamp the tube for 4 to

TABLE 243-14 Diseases Associated with Secondary Spontaneous Pneumothorax

Chronic obstructive pulmonary disease
Pneumocystis jiroveci pneumonia (formerly *Pneumocystis carinii* pneumonia, PCP)
Cystic fibrosis
Tuberculosis
Idiopathic pulmonary fibrosis
Lung cancer
Sarcoidosis

TABLE 243-15 Indications for Tube Thoracostomy (Chest Tube)

Pneumothorax (spontaneous, iatrogenic, tension)
Chest trauma
Hemothorax
Complicated parapneumonic effusion or empyema
Chylothorax
Malignant pleural effusions
Pleurodesis
Bronchopleural fistula

TABLE 243-16 Complications of Chest Tube Placement

Complication	Frequency of Occurrence
Chest tube malposition	20%
Reexpansion pulmonary edema	1%
Empyema	1–3%
Lung perforation	0.2–0.6%
Diaphragm perforation	0.4%
Subcutaneous placement	0.2%

6 hours prior to removal. Dry gauze with petroleum is prepared prior to removal. The suture securing the tube is then cut. The patient is asked to perform the Valsalva maneuver, and the tube is then removed and the dressing is secured. Follow-up CXR is obtained immediately post removal and 24 hours later.

COMPLICATIONS

Other than malposition of the chest tube (which occurs in up to 20% of tube placements), complications of tube thoracostomy (chest tube placement) are relatively uncommon (**Table 243-16**).

Other complications occur in only 1% to 3% of insertions. Several serious rare complications include perforation of the heart, abdominal organs, and/or mediastinal structures. Bleeding from intercostal arteries occurs very infrequently, and compression of the right ventricle leading to right heart failure occurs rarely. While infection at the insertion site and empyema rarely occur, antibiotic prophylaxis does not reduce risk. Complications do not appear to be related to the type of fluid or the volume removed. Some experts advocate limiting initial drainage to 1.5 L, but this is not a generally agreed upon limitation.

SUGGESTED READINGS

Dev SP, Nascimiento B, Simone C, Chien V. Chest-tube insertion. *N Engl J Med.* 2007;357:e15.

Haas AR, Sterman DH, Musani AI. Malignant pleural effusions: management options with consideration of coding, billing, and a decision approach. *Chest.* 2007;132(3):1036–1041.

Heffner JE, Nietert PJ, Barbieri MS. Pleural fluid pH as a predictor of survival for patients with malignant pleural effusions. *Chest.* 2000;117:79–86.

Lee YC, Davies RJ, Light RW. Diagnosing pleural effusion: moving beyond transudate-exudate separation. *Chest.* 2007;131(3):942–943.

Light RW. The undiagnosed pleural effusion. *Clin Chest Med.* 2006;27(2):309–319.

Natanzon A, Kronzon I. Pericardial and pleural effusions in congestive heart failure-anatomical, pathophysiologic, and clinical considerations. *Am J Med Sci.* 2009;338(3):211–216.

Porcel JM, Light RW. Pleural effusions due to pulmonary embolism. *Curr Opin Pulm Med.* 2008;14(4):337–342.

Porcel JM, Light RW. Diagnostic approach to pleural effusion in adults. *Am Fam Physician.* 2006;73(7):1211–1220.

Sahn SA, Jeffner JE. Spontaneous pneumothorax. *N Engl J Med.* 2000;342:868–874.

Wong CL, Holroyd-Leduc J, Straus SE. Does this patient have a pleural effusion? *JAMA.* 2009;301(3):309–317.

PRACTICE POINT

Criteria and recommendations for chest tube removal based on levels of evidence:

Level of recommendation

Level 1

- Chest tube drainage should be ≤ 2 mL/kg/day or ≤ 200 mL/day (whichever is less) before removal.

Level 2

- Chest tubes can be removed equally safely at end-inspiration or end-expiration.
- Chest tubes may be safely removed on suction.
- A brief trial of waterseal prior to chest tube removal may allow occult air leaks to become clinically apparent and reduce the need for chest tube reinsertion due to recurrent pneumothorax. Such trials, however, will generally increase hospital length of stay and the number of chest radiographs (CXRs) obtained.
- After pulmonary resection, small air leaks will resolve significantly more quickly if the chest tube is placed to water seal.

Level 3

- In nonmechanically ventilated patients, a routine CXR following removal of a chest tube is generally not indicated. The decision to obtain a CXR should be based on the individual clinical situation and the patient's signs and symptoms.
- In mechanically ventilated patients, a CXR obtained between one and three hours after removal of a chest tube is sufficient to identify a recurrent pneumothorax.
- A daily CXR is not indicated to monitor chest tubes in the intensive care unit. Routine monitoring and patient care will identify the need for CXR based on clinical necessity.

Evidence definitions

- **Class I:** Prospective randomized controlled trial.
- **Class II:** Prospective clinical study or retrospective analysis of reliable data. Includes observational, cohort, prevalence, or case control studies.
- **Class III:** Retrospective study. Includes database or registry reviews, large series of case reports, expert opinion.
- **Technology assessment:** A technology study which does not lend itself to classification in the above-mentioned format.

Devices are evaluated in terms of their accuracy, reliability, therapeutic potential, or cost effectiveness.

Level of recommendation definitions

- **Level 1:** Convincingly justifiable based on available scientific information alone. Usually based on Class I data or strong Class II evidence if randomized testing is inappropriate. Conversely, low quality or contradictory Class I data may be insufficient to support a Level I recommendation.
- **Level 2:** Reasonably justifiable based on available scientific evidence and strongly supported by expert opinion. Usually supported by Class II data or a preponderance of Class III evidence.
- **Level 3:** Supported by available data, but scientific evidence is lacking. Generally supported by Class III data. Useful for educational purposes and in guiding future clinical research.

CHAPTER 244

Pulmonary Hypertension

Allan J. Walkey, MD, MSc
Harrison W. Farber, MD

Key Clinical Questions

1. How does the classification system for pulmonary hypertension (PH) aid in understanding the pathophysiology, diagnostic evaluation, and treatments for this condition?
2. What signs and symptoms might increase the suspicion for elevated pulmonary arterial pressures?
3. What is a rational diagnostic approach to suspected PH?
4. What is the meaning of an elevated pulmonary pressure determined by echocardiography?
5. When should right heart catheterization be considered in the evaluation of suspected PH?
6. What are the key steps in the evaluation and management of acute right heart failure secondary to elevated pulmonary arterial pressure?
7. What are the common side effects of the medications used to treat PH?

INTRODUCTION

Pulmonary hypertension (PH) is simply defined as a mean pulmonary arterial pressure >25 mm Hg at rest. However, this deceptively simple definition encompasses a broad spectrum of clinical entities. In this chapter, we will present an evidence-based approach to the care of the patient with elevated pulmonary arterial pressures. **Table 244-1** lists landmark studies supporting the approach presented in this chapter.

DISEASE CLASSIFICATION, EPIDEMIOLOGY, AND PATHOPHYSIOLOGY

The first step in understanding the myriad presentations of pulmonary hypertension is to comprehend the pathophysiologic differences that divide the major groups of this disorder. These groups, as defined by the 2008 Fourth World Symposium on Pulmonary Arterial Hypertension, are shown in **Table 244-2**. Group I disease is defined as pulmonary arterial hypertension (PAH). PAH is characterized histologically by plexiform lesions occluding the pulmonary vasculature, in situ thrombosis, intimal proliferation and medial thickness, all resulting in decreased pulmonary vascular surface area, increased pulmonary vascular resistance, and functional disruptions of normal endothelial homeostasis. These perturbations are most notable in the prostacyclin, endothelin, nitric oxide, and serotonergic pathways regulating endothelial function. It is these pathways that are the targets of current PAH therapy. Group I PAH is most commonly associated with other conditions, including collagen vascular disease (most notably, systemic sclerosis), portal hypertension and HIV infection. Idiopathic pulmonary arterial hypertension (IPAH, formerly, "primary pulmonary hypertension") is rare, but life-threatening, with a prevalence of approximately 15 cases/million, an incidence of 2.4 cases/million/year, and a median survival of only 2.8 years without treatment. Group I disease also includes the distinct entity of pulmonary venoocculsive disease (PVOD), which is generally less amenable to vasodilator treatment. Recent evidence suggests that PAH in systemic sclerosis may be more similar to PVOD than IPAH, suggesting a mechanism for the poor response of SSc-associated PAH to current treatment.

Group II disease constitutes the most common cause of elevated pulmonary pressures: pulmonary venous hypertension. Pulmonary venous hypertension results from elevated left atrial pressures due to left ventricular systolic, diastolic (heart failure with preserved ejection fraction), or valvular disease. Due to the low sensitivity of traditional echocardiographic measures (eg, E/A ratio) for the diagnosis of left ventricular diastolic dysfunction, this disorder may be confused with IPAH in the absence of right heart catheterization showing an elevated pulmonary capillary occlusion pressure. Although treatment of underlying cardiac disease and diuresis are the mainstays of group II disease therapy, a small proportion of patients with long-standing pulmonary venous hypertension may develop physiology and histology consistent with group I disease; this is usually poorly responsive to traditional cardiac risk factor modification. Initial treatment of patients with pulmonary venous hypertension with pulmonary vasodilators may result in flash pulmonary edema from sudden reduction of pulmonary vascular resistance and acutely increased preload overwhelming the compromised left ventricle. This underscores the importance of right heart catheterization to correctly characterize the etiology of pulmonary hypertension prior to starting therapy.

TABLE 244-1 Evidence-based Key References: Pulmonary Hypertension

Topic	Supporting Literature
Epidemiology	Humbert M, Sitbon O, Chaaouat A, et al. Pulmonary hypertension in France: results from a national registry. *Am J Resp Crit Care Med.* 2006;173:1023–1030.
	Lam CSP, Roger VL, Rodeheffer RJ, et al. Pulmonary hypertension in patients with preserved ejection fraction: a community based study. *J Am Coll Card.* 2009;53:1119–1126.
	Badesch DB, Raskob G, Elliott G, et al. Pulmonary arterial hypertension: baseline characteristics from the REVEAL registry. *Chest.* 2010;137(2):376–387.
Classification and pathophysiology	Farber HW, Loscalzo J. Pulmonary arterial hypertension. *N Engl J Med.* 2004;351:1655–1665.
	Simonneau G, Robbins IM, Beghetti M, et al. Updated clinical classification of pulmonary hypertension. *J Am Coll Cardiol.* 2009;54:S43–S54.
	Overbeek MJ, Vonk MC, Boonstra A, et al. Pulmonary arterial hypertension in limited cutaneous systemic sclerosis: a distinctive vasculopathy. *Eur Respir J.* 2009;34(2):371–379.
Diagnosis: examination, laboratory	Rich S, Dantzker DR, Ayres SM, et al. Primary pulmonary hypertension: a national prospective study. *Ann Intern Med.* 1987;107:216–223.
	Dahlstrom U. Can natriuretic peptides be used for the diagnosis of diastolic heart failure? *Eur J Heart Fail.* 2004;6:281–287.
	Nagaya N, Nishikimi T, Uematsu M, et al. Plasma brain natriuretic peptide as a prognostic indicator in patients with primary pulmonary hypertension. *Circulation.* 2000;102:865–870.
Diagnosis: echocardiography, imaging	Aurigemma GP, Zile MR, Gaasch WH. Lack of relationship between Doppler indices of diastolic function and left ventricular pressure transients in patients with definite diastolic heart failure. *Am Heart J.* 2004;148:E12.
	Fisher MR, Forfia PR, Chamera E, et al. Accuracy of doppler echocardiography in the hemodynamic assessment of pulmonary hypertension. *Am J Respir Crit Care Med.* 2009;179:615–621.
	Chetty KG, Brown SE, Light RW. Identification of pulmonary hypertension in chronic obstructive pulmonary disease from routine chest radiographs. *Am Rev Respir Dis.* 1982;126:338–341.
	Tunariu N, Gibbs SJ, Win Z, et al. Ventilation-perfusion scintigraphy is more sensitive than multidetector CTPA in detecting chronic thromboembolic pulmonary disease as a treatable cause of pulmonary hypertension. *J Nucl Med.* 2007;48:680–684.
Treatment	Barst RJ, Rubin LJ, Long WA, et al. A comparison of continuous intravenous epoprostenol (prostacyclin) with conventional therapy for primary pulmonary hypertension. The Primary Pulmonary Hypertension Study Group. *N Engl J Med.* 1996;334:296–302.
	Jais X, D'Armini AM, Jansa P, et al. Bosentan for the treatment of inoperable chronic thromboembolic pulmonary hypertension: BENEFit. *J Am Coll Cardiol.* 2008;52:2127–2134.
	Galie N, Ghofrani HA, Torbicki A, et al. Sildenafil citrate therapy for pulmonary arterial hypertension. *N Engl J Med.* 2005;353:2148–2157.
Complications	Belenkie I, Dani R, Smith ER, Tyberg JV. Effects of volume loading during experimental acute pulmonary embolism. *Circulation.* 1989;80:178–188.
	Kallen AJ, Lederman E, Balaji A, et al. Incidence of central line infection in pulmonary hypertension patients receiving prostanoids. *Infect Control Hosp Epidemiol.* 2008;29:332–339.

Group III disease describes pulmonary hypertension due to chronic lung disease and hypoxic vasoconstriction. This group most commonly presents with known pulmonary diseases such as chronic obstructive pulmonary disease (COPD), interstitial lung disease (ILD), obstructive sleep apnea (OSA), and/or obesity hypoventilation syndromes. Treatment of the underlying lung disease and use of supplemental oxygen are the foundations of care for pulmonary hypertension associated with chronic hypoxemia. Because pulmonary vasodilators may elicit significant ventilation/perfusion mismatch and severe hypoxemia with in patients with underlying structural lung disease, these medications are currently investigational in this patient population.

Group IV disease is caused by embolic disease to the pulmonary circulation. Most commonly, the source of emboli are thrombi, generating chronic thromboembolic pulmonary hypertension (CTEPH). However, any source of emboli (tumor, parasite, foreign body) can generate group IV disease. Definitive treatment of group IV disease due to thrombotic pulmonary emboli involves pulmonary arterial thromboenderterectomy.

Group V disease is best described as a catch-all of miscellaneous causes of PH. These include diseases with multifactorial mechanisms (ie, hematologic disorders, metabolic disorders, sarcoidosis, etc) or disease states associated with external compression of pulmonary arteries, such as tumor, lymphadenopathy, or fibrosing mediastinitis (most commonly caused by radiation therapy for Hodgkin disease).

There may be overlap of disease classification in of any individual case of PH. Given the potential complications associated with improper use of pulmonary vasodilators in patients with group II–V disease, initiation of these agents (prostacyclins, phosphodiesterase inhibitors, endothelin receptor antagonists) should be restricted to specialists with experience in their use, only after a diagnostic group has been established for a particular patient.

DIAGNOSIS

As described above, obtaining a correct diagnostic classification for any patient with suspected or established PH is essential for initiating proper treatment. Therefore, an evidence-based approach to the diagnostic evaluation of suspected PH is paramount. Patients

TABLE 244-2 2008 Fourth World Symposium on Pulmonary Arterial Hypertension: Classification

Group I. Pulmonary arterial hypertension • Idiopathic (formerly "primary pulmonary hypertension") • Heritable • Drug or toxin-induced (eg, anorexigens, rapeseed oil, l-tryptophan, methamphetamine, and cocaine) • Associated conditions: collagen vascular disease, congenital heart disease, portal hypertension, HIV infection, schistosomiasis, chronic hemolytic anemias • Associated with significant venous or capillary involvement ▪ Pulmonary venoocclusive disease ▪ Pulmonary-capillary hemangiomatosis
Group II. Pulmonary venous hypertension • Left-sided systolic, diastolic, or valvular heart disease
Group III. Pulmonary hypertension associated with lung disease and/or chronic hypoxemia • Chronic obstructive pulmonary disease • Interstitial lung disease • Mixed restrictive and obstructive lung diseases • Sleep-disordered breathing • Alveolar hypoventilation disorders • Chronic exposure to high altitude • Developmental abnormalities
Group IV. Chronic thromboembolic pulmonary hypertension
Group V. Pulmonary hypertension of unclear or multifactorial mechanisms • Hematologic disorders: splenectomy, myeloproliferative disorders • Systemic disorders: sarcoidosis, pulmonary Langerhans' cell histiocytosis, lymphangiomatosis, vasculitis, neurofibromatosis • Metabolic disorders: Gaucher's, glycogen storage disease, thyroid disease • Other: tumoral compression of pulmonary vessels, fibrosing mediastinitis, chronic hemodialysis.

Adapted, with permission, from Simmoneau G, et al. Updated clinical Classification of Pulmonary Hypertension. *J Am Coll Cardiol.* 2009;54:S43–S54.

with PH most often present with nonspecific signs and symptoms, as exemplified by an average time from presentation to diagnosis of two years. The following discussion will present a general diagnostic algorithm (**Figure 244-1**) for a patient with suspected PH. Ultimately, *the diagnosis of pulmonary hypertension must be established by right heart catheterization in all patients.*

SYMPTOMS

While PH often presents in hospitalized patients as an incidental echocardiographic finding of a high-velocity tricuspid regurgitant jet, certain presenting symptoms should also trigger evaluation for pulmonary hypertension in the alert clinician. Due to their gradually progressive and nonspecific nature, PH symptoms are often misdiagnosed as asthma, cardiac ischemia, or left undiagnosed. However, *exertional* symptoms such as progressive exertional dyspnea, lightheadedness, syncope, or exertional chest pain should include pulmonary hypertension on their differential diagnosis. The presence of any of risk factors for the PH listed above (eg, exposure to toxins, anorexigens, diagnosis of systemic sclerosis, cirrhosis, HIV, congestive heart failure, COPD, sleep apnea, pulmonary embolism) should further raise suspicion for PH. In fact, echocardiographic screening for PH in high-risk populations (such as those with a known genetic mutation, a first-degree relative with PAH, systemic sclerosis, congenital heart disease, portal hypertension awaiting liver transplant) is advocated in the literature.

PHYSICAL EXAMINATION SIGNS

Examination findings for pulmonary hypertension are often subtle. Exertional oxygen desaturation may be the first sign of the diffusion limitation caused by reduction of the pulmonary arterial surface area. A prominent second heart sound is the most sensitive examination finding for pulmonary hypertension, present in more than 90% of IPAH patients, but is nonspecific. Other nonspecific findings of PH include those of right heart strain such as right ventricular heave and tricuspid murmur (an increase in tricuspid regurgitation with inspiration is called Carvahlo sign), and signs of right heart failure such as elevated jugular venous pressure, peripheral edema, and ascites. Examination should include an evaluation for signs of PH-associated disease listed above, with special attention paid to signs and symptoms of systemic sclerosis or Raynaud phenomenon, which are commonly associated with pulmonary hypertension.

LABORATORY EVALUATION

Laboratory tests may be performed to help classify PH or aid in prognosis. Limited laboratory evaluation of a patient with suspected PH may include arterial blood gas analysis to differentiate an abnormal A–a gradient from chronic hypoventilation, HIV testing, tests of liver function/disease (albumin, coagulation, hepatitis serologies), or tests for connective tissue disease (ANA with anti-centromere pattern is associated with PH in limited systemic sclerosis). Brain natriuretic peptides (BNP, pro–NT-BNT) may be elevated in right heart strain of any etiology and BNP may be falsely *negative* in chronic diastolic CHF. Thus, BNP cannot differentiate the underlying etiology of PH. However, in patients with known PH, persistently elevated BNP (> 180 pg/mL) after prostacyclin treatment is associated with poor prognosis, with median survival less than 12 months.

ECHOCARDIOGRAPHY

Echocardiography allows for the estimation of pulmonary arterial systolic pressure via application of a modified Bernoulli equation

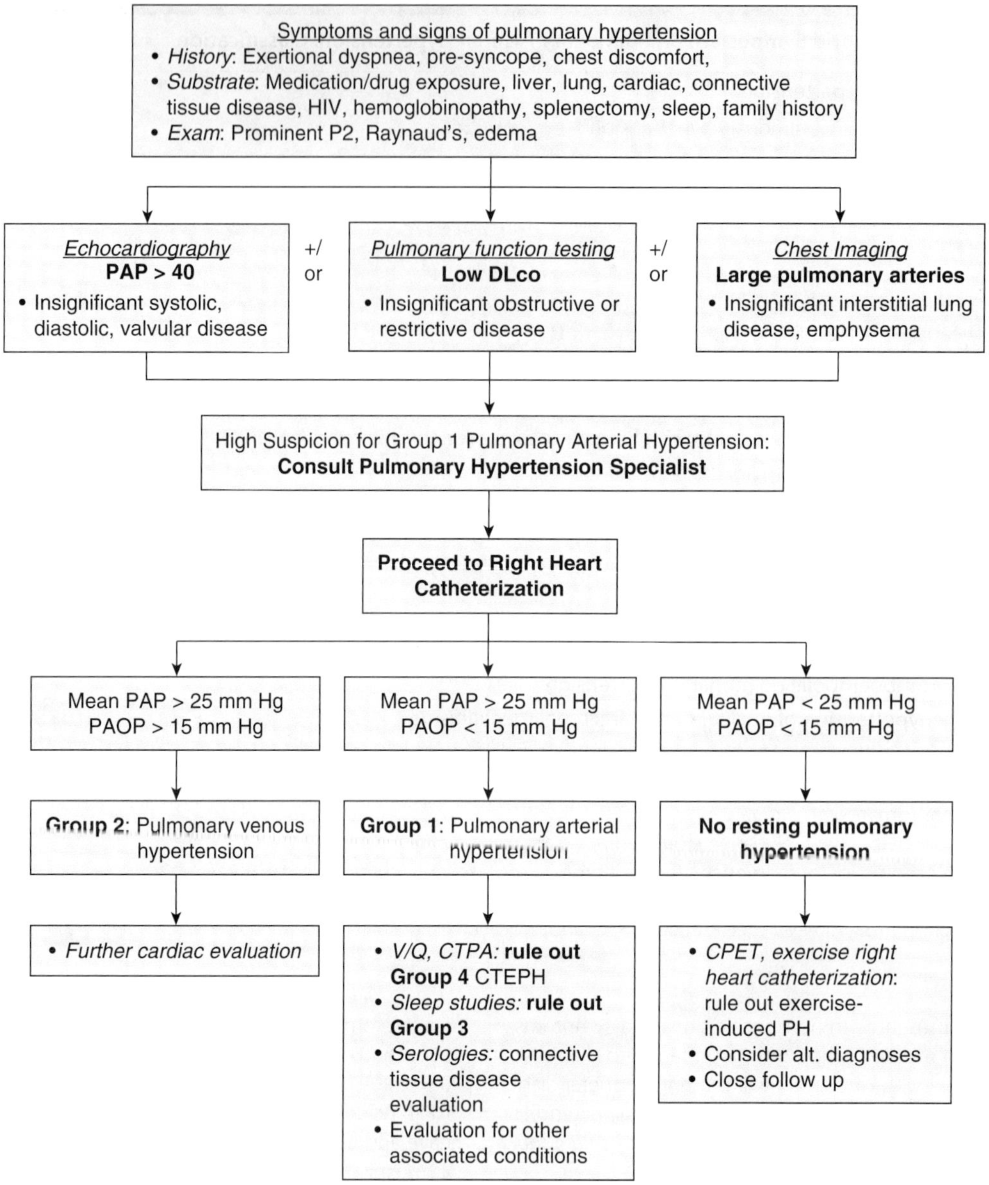

Figure 244-1 *Algorithm for evaluation of suspected pulmonary hypertension.*

to the tricuspid regurgitant jet velocity [4 × (velocity)^2]. It also provides information of left ventricular function, valvular heart disease, intracardiac shunt, and right ventricular function. The ubiquity of echocardiography in the evaluation of patients with dyspnea, syncope or chest discomfort (all symptoms associated with PH), often results in incidental detection of elevated pulmonary pressures during echocardiography. Echocardiography is recommended as the initial screening tool for pulmonary hypertension. However, it is important to understand its limitations as a diagnostic tool in PH. First, tricuspid regurgitation must be present for echocardiographic estimates of PA systolic pressures, and it is not present in approximately 25% of PH cases. Thus, absence of tricuspid regurgitation does not exclude PH. Second, the test characteristics of echocardiography for the detection of PH range widely based on the population screened (**Table 244-3**). In addition, echocardiographic estimates of pulmonary arterial systolic pressure. have been shown to be within 10 mm Hg of right heart catheterization measurements only 48% of the time. Therefore, while echocardiography is certainly a valuable tool for the evaluation of subjects with pulmonary hypertension, echocardiography can neither accurately rule in or out the diagnosis of PH. Direct measurement of cardiopulmonary parameters by cardiac catheterization must be performed in all patients with a high clinical suspicion of PH.

■ RIGHT HEART CATHETERIZATION

Right heart catheterization is the gold standard for the diagnosis of PH. PH treatment should not be instituted in the absence of right heart catheterization since it allows assessment of multiple

TABLE 244-3 Test Characteristics of Echocardiography for the Diagnosis of Pulmonary Hypertension

Associated Condition	Sensitivity	Specificity
Portal hypertension	97%	77%
Systemic sclerosis	58–90%	75–96%
Chronic obstructive pulmonary disease	60–78%	75%
Pulmonary fibrosis	77%	45%

hemodynamic factors essential in the diagnosis and treatment of PH. A full discussion of right heart catheterization is beyond the scope of this chapter; however, practice points to aid the interpretation of right heart catheterization data are shown in the sidebar. Patients with a high clinical suspicion of PH should be referred to a pulmonary or cardiology specialist with PH experience.

PRACTICE POINT

Interpretation of right heart catheterization values in the evaluation of pulmonary hypertension

- Right atrial pressure and right ventricular diastolic pressure provide an index of the degree of right heart failure; additionally a RA pressure > 20 mm Hg confers a poor prognosis.
- Filling pattern of the right ventricle provides an index of pericardial constrictive disease that can mimic PH.
- Mean pulmonary arterial pressure is used to diagnose the presence of PH (mean PAP > 25 mm Hg at rest).
- Pulmonary artery diastolic pressure-to-pulmonary artery occlusion pressure gradient is important in the analysis of the contribution of pulmonary venous hypertension (eg, CHF) to pulmonary hypertension. Pulmonary arterial occlusion pressure > 15 mm Hg with pulmonary arterial diastolic pressure-to- pulmonary artery occlusion pressure gradient < 5 mm Hg makes left heart disease the most likely etiology for elevated pulmonary pressures.
- Cardiac index < 2 L/min in pulmonary arterial hypertension is indicative of right heart failure and generally an indication for a therapy with prostanoids.
- Vasodilator testing is used to determine the potential for responsiveness to calcium channel blocker therapy; however, vasoreactivity is present in less than 5% of patients with PAH (usually only patients with IPAH or HPAH).

ADDITIONAL TESTING

Chest X-ray

Plain chest films may increase the suspicion for PH: a descending branch of the right pulmonary artery > 20 mm is often associated with pulmonary hypertension. Additionally, chest X-ray adds critical information as to the potential cause of PH. For example, a normal plain film in the setting of elevated pulmonary pressures suggests IPAH or CTEPH, or the presence of reticular opacities suggests PH secondary to interstitial lung disease or connective tissue disease.

Chest CT

Computed tomographic imaging of the chest may add additional information to the chest radiograph. Although a main pulmonary artery diameter > 33 mm may be associated with IPAH, this association does not appear as reliable in subjects with underlying parenchymal lung disease. CT scans are more sensitive than chest radiography in the diagnosis of underlying ILD.

V/Q scan

V/Q scanning has utility in the evaluation of CTEPH, where it has a greater sensitivity for the detection of chronic pulmonary thromboembolic disease than CTPA.

Electrocardiogram

ECGs of patients with PH may show signs of right heart strain and hypertrophy. These signs—right axis deviation, large R/S ratio > 1 in V1, R/S ratio < 1 in V5 or V6, P pulmonale—lack both sensitivity and specificity for routine use in diagnosis.

Pulmonary function testing

Pulmonary function testing (PFT) showing an isolated low diffusing capacity of the lung for carbon monoxide without anemia increases the suspicion for pulmonary vascular disease. In patients with known PH, PFTs may help in determining the diagnosis and severity of causes of secondary PH such as COPD and ILD.

Polysomnography

Sleep studies are indicated for the diagnosis and treatment of PH secondary to OSA.

Cardiopulmonary exercise testing

Cardiopulmonary exercise testing is valuable in the evaluation of unexplained dyspnea. Subjects with low maximum VO_2, low anaerobic threshold, low oxygen pulse, elevated ventilatory equivalent of CO_2 (VE/VCO_2), a large A–a gradient and increased dead space should undergo further evaluation for PH. This test may not be available in all centers.

Biopsy

Lung biopsy is rarely indicated after a diagnosis of PH has been established, usually only to confirm the suspicion of occult underlying causes such as pulmonary venoocclusive disease.

TREATMENT

A complete review of the pulmonary hypertension therapy is beyond the scope of this chapter. In general, treatment of group II–V disease is directed at the underlying disease pathology that has contributed to pulmonary hypertension. Evidence for use of pulmonary specific vasodilators in these groups, with the exception of bosentan for inoperable CTEPH, is currently at the case report level and is currently being evaluated in clinical trials.

Treatment of group I pulmonary hypertension is guided by findings on right heart catheterization and functional status. Multiple agents now exist in various drug classes for the treatment of group IPAH. The agents, indications, and common side effects are shown in **Table 244-4**. Below we present a brief discussion of the indications, mechanisms of action, and the major side effects of the currently approved treatments for group IPAH.

CALCIUM CHANNEL BLOCKERS

Dihydropyridine calcium channel blockers are not FDA-approved for use in pulmonary arterial hypertension and have been shown to be useful only in IPAH patients with positive vasoreactivity testing. This group encompasses < 5% of all patients with IPAH.

PROSTACYCLINS

Epoprostenol, treprostinil, and inhaled iloprost comprise the currently approved prostanoid medications for the treatment of PAH. These medications are analogues of the procystacyclins, endogenous vasodilator products of arachnidonic acid metabolism produced by the vascular endothelium. Through stimulation of intracellular cAMP, the prostacyclins inhibit smooth muscle proliferation and platelet aggregation. Intravenous epoprostenol is the only agent shown in a randomized controlled trial to confer a mortality benefit in PAH. Because of its short half-life, interruption of epoprostenol infusion may result in acute increases in pulmonary vascular resistance and hemodynamic collapse. For this reason, longer-acting medications such as treprostinil—with a half-life of hours rather than minutes—have been developed. Additionally, treprostinil may be administered subcutaneously, intravenously, or inhaled. Inhaled iloprost also allows for inhalational dosing and the theoretical advantage of improved V/Q matching compared with

TABLE 244-4 Pulmonary Vasodilators

Pulmonary Vasodilator	NYHA Functional Status Indication	Route	T 1/2	Common Side Effects
Prostacyclins				
• Epoprostenol	II–IV	Intravenous	6 min	Hypotension, jaw/leg pain, flushing, headache, diarrhea, thrombocytopenia
• Treprostinil	II–IV	Intravenous, subcutaneous Inhaled	4 hr	In addition to above, local reactions (SQ administration), bacteremia
• Iloprost	II–III	Inhaled	30 min	Bronchospasm, cough, trismus, flushing, hypotension
Endothelin Receptor Antagonists				
• Bosentan	III	Oral	5 hr	Liver toxicity, headache, anemia, edema, flushing, hypotension
• Ambrisentan	II–III	Oral	9–15 hr	Headache, edema, anemia, liver toxicity
Phosphodiesterase-5 inhibitors				
• Sildenafil	II–III	Oral	4 hr	Headache, diarrhea, flushing, hypotension, priapism, optic neuropathy
• Tadalafil	II–III	Oral	17.5 hr	Same as sildenafil

intravenous medications. In general, patients with right heart failure, NYHA functional class IV disease and cardiac index of <2 L/min generally require continuous intravenous prostacyclin therapy. Common side effects of the intravenous prostacyclins include thrombocytopenia and bleeding, jaw pain, leg pain, flushing, headache, nausea, and vomiting.

ENDOTHELIN-RECEPTOR ANTAGONISTS

Bosentan and ambrisentan represent the currently available endothelin-receptor antagonists in the Unites States. These agents are widely used due to the ease of oral administration. Endothelin A receptors are located on vascular smooth muscle cells and mediate vasoconstriction and proliferation, while endothelin B receptors, located on endothelium, promote vasodilatation. However, it appears that, in vitro, the effects of endothelin A receptors are of greater importance than endothelin B receptors. The nonselective endothelin-receptor antagonist bosentan has been the most widely studied of the endothelin antagonists; multiple randomized studies have shown improved six-minute walk distance and improvement in NYHA functional class. Liver toxicity represents the most common side effect (8–12%) of bosentan and liver function tests must be followed routinely. Other side effects include edema, anemia, decreased efficacy of oral contraceptives, and potentially, male infertility. Ambrisentan, a selective endothelin A antagonist with a lower rate of transaminase abnormalities than bosentan, was recently approved by the FDA.

PHOSPHODIESTERASE INHIBITORS

Sildenafil and tadalafil represent the FDA-approved phosphodiesterase 5 (PDE-5) inhibitors for the treatment of PAH. PDE-5 inhibition results in increased intracellular cGMP, which enhances vasodilatation. The PDE-5 inhibitors, like the ET antagonists, have been shown to improve six-minute walk time and functional status. Side effects include flushing, hypotension, headaches, and epistaxis.

ADJUNCTIVE THERAPY

Oxygen, systemic anticoagulation, diuresis, and digoxin represent adjunctive therapies for the long-term management of PAH. Although these therapies are not supported by clinical trials, they are recommended by societal guidelines.

SURGICAL THERAPY

Prior to the advent of pulmonary vasodilator therapy, lung transplantation was common for patients with severe PAH. Other surgical therapies, including atrial septostomy, may be considered for advanced cases not responsive to maximal medical therapy.

COMMON INPATIENT COMPLICATIONS OF PULMONARY HYPERTENSION

Right heart failure and complications of chronic indwelling central venous access are the common issues that arise in the inpatient care of patients with pulmonary hypertension. Triage of patients with right heart failure or complications of central venous access depends of the patient's hemodynamic stability, with hypotensive patients generally requiring ICU-level care, urgent cardiology or pulmonary consultation, and right heart catheterization to acutely assist in the management of pulmonary vasodilator therapy.

RIGHT HEART FAILURE

Patients with advanced pulmonary arterial hypertension may present with right heart failure, which may range in severity from asymptomatic volume overload to shock. Unlike a right ventricular myocardial infarction, which often responds well to volume loading, the decompensated right ventricle from pressure overload generally responds poorly to volume loading. This is due to "ventricular interdependence." The right and left ventricle share the intraventricular septum, thus right ventricular pressure overload can cause the septum to shift into the left ventricle, decreasing left ventricle filling and cardiac output. Therefore, cardiogenic shock in the patient with PH and right ventricular failure is generally managed in the intensive care unit with potent pulmonary vasodilators (eg, intravenous epoprostenol, inhaled nitric oxide), diuresis, and, if necessary, inotropic, vasopressor, and renal replacement support. Caution must be taken with the use of positive pressure ventilation and its acute reduction in preload, which may precipitate cardiovascular collapse in PH.

COMPLICATIONS OF CENTRAL VENOUS ACCESS

Patients with continuous infusions of prostacylins often present with complications of central venous access. These include loss of access (causing acute discontinuation of pulmonary vasodilators), central line puncture (and risk of air embolism), and central line infection. Loss of venous access should be considered an emergency situation, due to risk of acute increases in pulmonary vascular resistance and cardiovascular collapse. Attempts must be made to gain venous access immediately; however, peripheral intravenous access can be used emergently, with transition to central venous access after stabilization.

Central line puncture is also managed by quickly establishing alternative venous access, clamping the indwelling line proximal to the puncture, and starting the prostacyclin infusion through the new catheter. Often, the indwelling central line may be repaired by experienced nursing personnel.

Central line infection and bacteremia occur at a rate of approximately one case every five years in patients receiving intravenous prostanoids. This rate appears to be lower than reports of indwelling catheters for other conditions. However, treprostinil is associated with approximately twice the risk of bloodstream infections as epoprostenol. It is important to note that bacteremia associated with treprostinil is most often caused by gram negative organisms, unlike other line infections, and initial antibiotic coverage for gram-positive and -negative organisms, including *Pseudomonas* species, is necessary in these patients. Consultation of a surgical specialist for removal of tunneled venous lines is generally required only for staphylococcal infections or recurrent bacteremia.

PRACTICE POINT

- Central line infections associated with continuous trepoprostinil infusion are most commonly caused by gram-negative organisms, including *Pseudomonas* species.

DISCHARGE PLANNING AND QUALITY IMPROVEMENT STRATEGIES

The involvement of outpatient specialized nursing services who provide ongoing education, central venous line care, and emotional support is critical to the care of patients with advanced pulmonary arterial hypertension. These nurses, along with the pulmonary hypertension specialist, should be involved in discharge planning for all PH patients with continuous intravenous infusions. As in all patients with high risk for right heart failure, daily weight assessment and plans for excessive fluid accumulation are helpful in avoiding readmission.

CONCLUSION

Pulmonary hypertension represents a broad spectrum of diseases which result in elevation of pulmonary arterial pressures. An understanding of the pathophysiologic mechanisms involved with this array of conditions is necessary for the successful care of patients with PH.

SUGGESTED READINGS

Barst RJ, McGoon M, Torbicki A, et al. Diagnosis and differential assessment of pulmonary arterial hypertension. *J Am Coll Cardiol.* 2004;43(12 Suppl S):40S–47S.

McLaughlin VV, Archer SL, Badesch DB, et al. ACCF/AHA 2009 expert consensus document on pulmonary hypertension: a report of the American College of Cardiology Foundation Task Force on Expert Consensus Documents. *J Am Coll Cardiol.* 2009;53:1573–1619.

SECTION 17

Renal

CHAPTER 245

Acid-base Disorders

Vijay H. Lapsia, MBBS, MD
David Wiener, MD

Key Clinical Questions

1. What are common causes of increased anion gap metabolic acidoses?
2. How is the urinary anion gap used in the diagnosis of normal anion gap metabolic acidoses?
3. What are the major types of renal tubular acidosis, and how are they diagnosed?
4. How is urinary chloride used in the diagnosis of metabolic alkalosis?
5. How is the ΔGap used to diagnose complex acid-base disorders?

INTRODUCTION

Acid-base disturbances occur frequently in the acutely ill hospitalized patient. Many physicians are intimidated by the complexity of acid-base analysis, as multiple, partially offsetting disorders can be challenging to diagnose. However, in the hospital setting, especially the critically ill, it is crucial that patients with acid-base disturbances be quickly identified and the abnormality be accurately interpreted. Swift intervention to treat the underlying causes is often necessary to avoid the often lethal consequences of severe acid-base disturbances.

NORMAL ACID-BASE HOMEOSTASIS

A typical Western diet generates about 15,000 mmol of volatile acids, in the form of CO_2, and ~70 mmol (1 mmol/kg) of fixed acid each day. CO_2 is excreted by normal respiration. Fixed acids are buffered by intra- and extracellular buffers. New buffers, predominantly HCO_3^-, must be continuously produced to replace buffers consumed in titrating fixed acids. Complex acid-base homeostasis mechanisms, which include chemical buffering in conjunction with the excretion of CO_2 by the respiratory system and new HCO_3^- production by the kidneys, normally maintain the blood pH between 7.35 to 7.45.

The kidney plays a central role by reabsorbing all of the filtered bicarbonate, approximately 4000 mmol per day, and also generating new bicarbonate. The central nervous system and the respiratory systems control the arterial CO_2 tension ($PaCO_2$). Under normal steady-state conditions, the H^+ balance is preserved by intricate mechanisms which ensure that the net quantity of acid secreted and the consequent renal generation of new bicarbonate equals the rate of metabolic proton generation. A disturbance of this fine balance results in an acid-base disorder.

PRACTICE POINT

Glossary of terms for acid-base disorders

- Acidemia: serum pH < 7.36
- Alkalemia: serum pH > 7.44
- Acidosis: pathophysiologic processes which favor development of acidemia
- Alkalosis: pathophysiologic processes which favor development of alkalemia
- Hypercapnia: underexcretion of CO_2
- Hypocapnia: overexcretion of CO_2
- Anion gap: unmeasured anions in plasma
- ΔAG: prevailing minus normal AG
- ΔHCO_3^-: normal minus prevailing HCO_3^-

SIMPLE ACID-BASE DISORDERS

These disorders involve only a single acid-base disorder, and include metabolic acidosis, metabolic alkalosis, respiratory acidosis, and respiratory alkalosis. A key distinguishing feature is that the pH is always abnormal, as the compensation is never complete. Simple acid-base disorders can be classified as acute or chronic, based on the degree of compensation (**Table 245-1**).

TABLE 245-1 Expected Compensatory Responses in Simple Acid-base Disorders

Abnormality	Compensation
Metabolic acidosis	$PaCO_2 = (1.5 \times HCO_3^-) + 8 \pm 2$
Metabolic alkalosis	For each 10 mEq/L increase in HCO_3^-, $PaCO_2$ increases by 6 mm Hg
Respiratory acidosis	
Acute	For each 10 mm Hg increase in $PaCO_2$, HCO_3^- increases by ~ 1 mEq/L
Chronic	For each 10 mm Hg increase in $PaCO_2$, HCO_3^- increases by ~ 4 mEq/L
Respiratory alkalosis	
Acute	For each 10 mm Hg increase in $PaCO_2$, HCO_3^- decreases by ~ 2 mEq/L
Chronic	For each 10 mm Hg increase in $PaCO_2$, HCO_3^- decreases by ~ 4 mEq/L

PRACTICE POINT

- **Compensation:** The clinician should be able to use the pH to identify the primary disorder when a simple acid-base disorder is present. Over time, the pH approaches, but does not become normal. Renal compensation for respiratory disturbances takes 3 to 5 days. Even for chronic simple acid-base disturbances, the body does not fully compensate.
- A normal pH in the presence of abnormal HCO_3^- and $PaCO_2$ suggests a combined disturbance, and the AG and excess AG should be calculated. For example, a patient with chronic renal failure may develop an acute metabolic alkalosis which offsets his chronic metabolic acidosis if his uremia results in vomiting.
- Three independent disorders may occur concurrently, but four primary acid-base disorders cannot coexist because a patient cannot hyperventilate and hypoventilate at the same time.

MIXED ACID-BASE DISORDERS

When multiple acid-base disorders coexist independently and are not merely as compensatory responses, they are classified as mixed acid-base disorders. These are not uncommon in the critically ill patient, and can lead to dangerous extremes of pH and a poor outcome. However, the pH may also be normal or near normal when acidosis and alkalosis coexist in the same patient. A patient with diabetic ketoacidosis who also has metabolic acidosis resulting from chronic kidney disease is an example of a mixed acid-base disorder. Triple acid-base disorders are not uncommon, and are often not recognized unless until the clinician specifically considers this possibility. For example, a patient with metabolic acidosis due to lactic acidosis complicating severe sepsis may develop metabolic alkalosis from intravenous bicarbonate administration, with superimposed respiratory alkalosis due to hyperventilation from mechanical ventilation. Another example is the patient with respiratory acidosis due to altered consciousness, metabolic acidosis due to diabetic ketoacidosis, and metabolic alkalosis from vomiting may have an identical arterial blood gas. It is critical to always interpret acid-base abnormalities in the clinical context of the patient.

PRACTICE POINT

Common acid-base examples in the hospital setting

Respiratory alkalosis	Anxiety, pain, hypoxia, sepsis, acute or chronic liver disease, mechanical ventilation, pregnancy, drugs (salicylates, progesterone, catecholamines), central nervous system disease
Acute respiratory acidosis	Acute airway obstruction, narcotic analgesics, severe pneumonia, severe pulmonary edema, hemothorax, pneumothorax, flail chest, ventilator dysfunction
	Neuromuscular disorders and central nervous system depressants
Chronic respiratory acidosis	Chronic lung disease, central hypoventilation
	Chronic neuromuscular disorders
Metabolic alkalosis	Low urinary chloride: vomiting, nasogastric suction, past diuretic use, posthypercapnia
	Normal or high urinary chloride: primary or secondary hyperaldosteronism, diuretic use, excess alkali, refeeding
	Note: a PCO_2 > 55 mm Hg suggests additional primary respiratory abnormality.
Metabolic acidosis	Elevated anion gap: ketoacidosis, renal failure, lactic acidosis, rhabdomyolysis, toxins
	Excess anion gap (total anion gap – normal anion gap of 12) + measured bicarbonate concentration: If > normal serum bicarbonate range, then coexisting underlying metabolic alkalosis
	If < normal serum bicarbonate range, then coexisting underlying nongap metabolic acidosis
	Normal anion gap: posthypocapnia, GI or renal losses, hyperchloremic acidosis (as in the recovery phase of DKA, due to failure to regenerate bicarbonate from ketoacids lost in urine)
Respiratory acidosis, metabolic acidosis, and metabolic alkalosis: low pH, high PCO_2, low HCO_3	Obtunded patient (respiratory acidosis) with lactic acidosis (metabolic acidosis) and vomiting (metabolic alkalosis)

APPROACH TO ACID-BASE DISORDERS

The first step in interpreting acid-base disorders is to perform a detailed history and physical examination. Next, one should simultaneously measure arterial blood gas (ABG) and plasma chemistries. Blood gas analyzers directly measure the pH and $PaCO_2$; the

PRACTICE POINT

Stepwise approach to acid-base disorders

1. The pH is the key to initial evaluation of all acid base disorders.
2. The primary abnormality is the process which causes the pH shift.

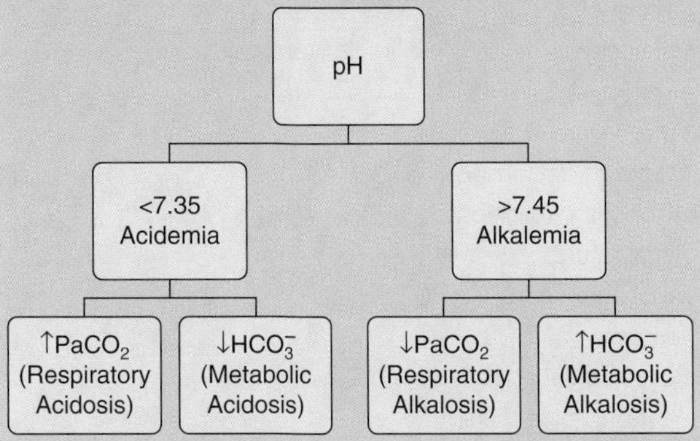

3. If respiratory acidosis or alkalosis, then determine whether acute or chronic.
4. If metabolic acidosis, then calculate the anion gap. An anion gap of > 20 is suggestive of a primary metabolic acidosis, regardless of pH or serum bicarbonate concentration.
5. Calculate the ΔGap (ΔAG – ΔHCO_3^-) to assess for a complex acid-base disorder. Remember 1 mmol of unmeasured acid titrates 1 mmol of bicarbonate. If ΔGap is substantially greater than zero, there is an underlying metabolic alkalosis; if it is substantially less than zero, then there is an underlying non-AG metabolic acidosis.

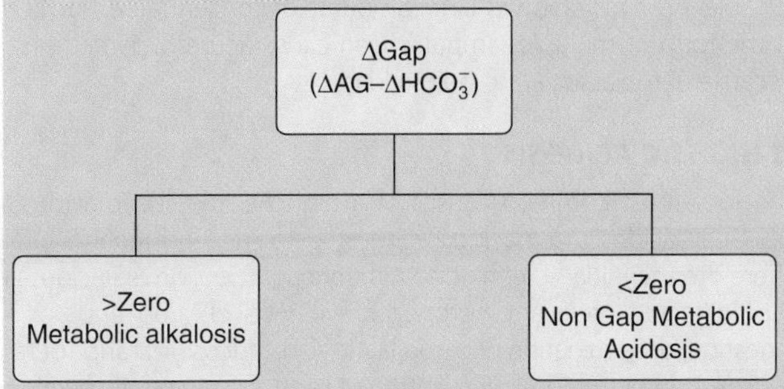

6. In patients with normal anion gap metabolic acidosis, calculate the urinary AG. In metabolic acidosis from bicarbonate loss in diarrhea, the urinary anion gap (UAG) is typically −20 to −50 mmol/L. A positive or near zero UAG indicates inappropriately low urinary NH_4^+ excretion, suggesting that renal tubular acidosis is responsible.
7. In metabolic alkalosis, measure urine chloride. A low (< 20 mmol/L) urine chloride suggests volume depletion, often from vomiting or recent diuretic use. A normal or high urine chloride, if no recent diuretic use, suggests mineralocorticoid excess or alkali loads.

bicarbonate value reported in an ABG analysis is calculated based from the pH and $PaCO_2$. Blood bicarbonate concentration is measured in the metabolic panel as total dissolved CO_2, which is ~95% bicarbonate. The samples can be validated by comparing the calculated HCO_3^- value reported on the arterial blood gas measurement with the measured HCO_3^- value on the chemistry panel. If the difference between the two values is greater than 2 mmol/L, the samples may not have been drawn simultaneously, or a laboratory error may be present. Excessive heparin in the syringe used to obtain the arterial blood sample can also cause confounding results.

TABLE 245-2 Relationships in Primary Acid-base Disorders

Condition	pH	HCO_3^- mEq/L	$PaCO_2$ mm Hg
Normal	7.4	24	40
Metabolic acidosis	↓	↓	↓
Metabolic alkalosis	↑	↑	↑
Respiratory acidosis	↓	↑	↑
Respiratory alkalosis	↑	↓	↓

Next, identify the primary acid-base disorder by looking at the arterial pH, HCO_3^- and $PaCO_2$ (**Table 245-2**). If either respiratory acidosis or alkalosis, then determine whether the condition is acute or chronic from the change in the serum bicarbonate (Table 245-1). Finally calculate the anion gap (AG) and ΔAG (see below). Further evaluation will be guided by the type of acid-base disorder.

PRACTICE POINT

Important formulae for solving acid-base problems

- Henderson-Hasselbalch equation: $pH = pK + \log [(HCO_3^-) / (0.03 \times PaCO_2)]$; pK = 6.1
- Kassirer-Bleich equation: $H^+ = 24 \times PCO_2/HCO_3^-$
- Anion gap: $Na^+ - (Cl^- + HCO_3^-)$ (represents unmeasured anions in plasma, normally 10–12 mmol/L)
- Anion gap, corrected for albumin: 12–2.5 (4.0-measured albumin)
- Winter's formula: $PaCO_2 = 1.5 \times HCO_3^- + 8\ (\pm 2)$ ($PaCO_2$ = last 2 digits of pH – chronic metabolic acidosis)
- ΔGap = ΔAG – ΔHCO_3^-
- Calculated osmolality (OSM): 2 × Na + glucose/18 + BUN/2.8 + EtOH/4.6; elevated OG (> 10 mOsm/L)
- Osmolal gap: measured OSM – calculated OSM

THE ANION GAP

The anion gap represents unmeasured anions in plasma, such as anionic proteins, phosphate, sulfate, and organic anions, and normally averages 10 to 12 mmol/L. High AG acidosis is present when excess acid anions, such as acetoacetate and lactate, accumulate in extracellular fluid.

A number of conditions can cause the anion gap to decrease, either due to a rise in unmeasured cations or a fall in anionic albumin (**Table 245-3**). The expected anion gap should be corrected for

TABLE 245-3 Conditions which can decrease the Anion Gap

Hypercalcemia
Hypermagnesemia
Hyperkalemia
Paraproteinemia
Lithium toxicity
Severe hypernatremia (> 170)
Bromide intoxication (may occur with pyridostigmine or with herbal medications)
Hypoalbuminemia

albumin levels. A fall in serum albumin by 1 g/dL from the normal value (4.0 g/dL) decreases the anion gap by 2.5 mmol/L. For example, a measured anion gap of 12 mmol/L is usually normal. However, in a patient with a serum albumin of 1 g/dL, the expected AG is 12 to 2.5 (4.0 − 1) = 4.5 mmol/L.

A normal HCO_3^- does not preclude an increased anion gap. For example, a patient who simultaneously has separate conditions causing an anion gap metabolic acidosis and metabolic alkalosis may have a normal, high or low, measured HCO_3^-. In this setting, recognizing that an elevated AG indicates the presence of AG metabolic acidosis may alert the clinician to the possibility of a mixed acid-base disorder.

ΔAG AND ΔHCO_3^-

Interpreting mixed acid-base disorders can be tricky, especially when the combination of disturbances result in a normal pH, HCO_3^- and $PaCO_2$. In such situations, comparing the change in HCO_3^- (ΔHCO_3^-) and the change in the AG (ΔAG) can be useful. The ΔHCO_3^- is calculated as $\Delta HCO_3^- = [HCO^-_{3actual}] - 24$, where is 24 is the normal serum bicarbonate concentration, and ΔAG is calculated as $\Delta AG = AG_{actual} - 12$, where is 12 is the normal AG. The normal AG should be adjusted based on the serum albumin, as detailed above. If the ΔHCO_3^- and ΔAG differ from each other by more than 3, then one should consider the possibility of multiple metabolic acid-base disorders coexisting.

PLASMA OSMOLAR GAP

The normal range for serum osmolality is 285 to 290 mOsm/L. The major molecules contributing to the serum osmolality include sodium, urea nitrogen, and glucose. Alcohol (ethanol) may certainly contribute to osmolality if present. The osmolar gap is obtained by subtracting the calculated osmolarity (see formulae below) from the measured osmolarity. A difference of more than 10 mOsm/L is abnormal (osmolar gap) suggests another solute, such as lactate, ethanol, ethylene glycol, methanol, contrast dye, and mannitol.

METABOLIC ACIDOSIS

The two major categories of clinical metabolic acidosis are high AG and normal AG; the latter is also known as hyperchloremic acidosis (**Table 245-4**). These may occur because of an increase in endogenous acid production, such as lactate and ketoacids, loss of bicarbonate, as in diarrhea, or accumulation of endogenous acids, as in renal failure. Metabolic acidosis can affect the respiratory, cardiac, and nervous systems, and in severe cases may lead to death. When the blood pH falls significantly, the tidal volume may increase, leading to the characteristic clinical finding of Kussmaul respiration.

TABLE 245-4 Causes of Metabolic Acidosis with a High or Normal Anion Gap

Elevated anion gap
Ethylene glycol
Lactic acid
Methanol
Paraldehyde
Aspirin
Renal failure
Diabetic ketoacidosis
Alcoholic ketoacidosis
Renal failure
Normal anion gap
Diarrhea
Renal tubular acidosis
Acetazolamide therapy
Ureteral diversion
Renal failure (can cause either normal or increased anion gap metabolic acidosis)
Adrenal insufficiency

TREATMENT PRINCIPLES

Metabolic acidosis indicates the presence of an important underlying condition that requires treatment. Whether metabolic acidosis should be treated with alkali depends in large part on whether acute or chronic metabolic acidosis is present. For *chronic* metabolic acidosis, the benefit of alkali treatment is clear-cut, and includes improved bone and muscle integrity, improved growth in children and preservation of renal function in patients with chronic kidney disease. For *acute* metabolic acidosis, the benefit of alkali treatment is less certain. In particular, clinical trials have shown no clinically significant effect of alkali treatment of acute metabolic acidosis on either mortality or on cardiovascular performance. However, treating acute metabolic acidosis with alkali might be considered if arterial pH is less than 7.1. Slow IV administration of 50 to 100 mEq of $NaHCO_3$, over 30 to 45 min, during the initial 1 to 2 hours of therapy can be used. It is essential to monitor plasma electrolytes during the course of therapy, since the [K^+] may decline as pH rises. Normalization of values is not recommended, and may potentially be deleterious. If alkali treatment is used, a target pH of 7.2 is reasonable. Administration of large amounts of concentrated $NaHCO_3$ in the form of multiple "ampules" can cause acute hypernatremia because of the associated sodium load.

HIGH AG ACIDOSIS

The four most common causes of a high AG metabolic acidosis are lactic acidosis, ketoacidosis, ingested toxins, and renal failure. Therefore the initial screening to differentiate the high AG acidoses should include relevant history for evidence of drug and toxin ingestion, determination of blood lactic acid, glucose, ethanol, beta-hydroxybutyrate, blood urea nitrogen, and creatinine, inspection of the urine for oxalate crystals, and identification of predisposing factors for lactic acidosis, such as hypotension, shock, cardiac failure, leukemia, cancer, unrecognized bowel ischemia, thiamine deficiency, and drug or toxin ingestion.

LACTIC ACIDOSIS

Lactic acidosis almost always indicates the presence of impaired tissue perfusion, most commonly due to hypotension, arterial disease, or sepsis. Rarely, an unsuspected neoplasm produces lactic acid and is the causative factor. Identifying and treating the underlying cause is central to therapy. Alkali therapy is usually reserved for severe acidemia (pH < 7.1). While the use of alkali in moderate lactic acidosis is controversial, it is generally agreed that attempts to return the pH or HCO_3^- to normal by administration of exogenous $NaHCO_3$ are either unhelpful or possibly deleterious.

DIABETIC KETOACIDOSIS

In diabetic ketoacidosis, treating with insulin prevents production of ketones and enables endogenous metabolism of accumulated ketones to bicarbonate, thus correcting the acidosis. Bicarbonate therapy is rarely needed except with extreme acidemia (pH < 7.1), and then in limited amounts only.

ALCOHOLIC KETOACIDOSIS

Mixed acid-base disorders are common in alcoholic ketoacidosis. The degree of ketosis and ketonuria can often be underestimated on initial presentation. Patients are often volume depleted, and respond to volume expansion. With restoration of circulation by resuscitation with isotonic saline, the preferential accumulation of beta-hydroxybutyrate is then shifted to acetoacetate. This paradoxically results in an increasingly positive nitroprusside reaction as the patient improves (the nitroprusside ketone reaction detects acetoacetic acid, but not beta-hydroxybutyrate). Patients should receive thiamine prior to administration of glucose-containing solutions.

ACIDOSIS FROM DRUGS AND TOXINS

Salicylates

Intoxication typically results in either respiratory alkalosis or a combined respiratory alkalosis and high AG metabolic acidosis, depending on the stage and level of intoxication. Treatment includes gastric lavage to remove unabsorbed salicylate, and forced alkaline diuresis to increase renal salicylate excretion. Acetazolamide administration can be useful in patients with simultaneous alkalemia.

Alcohols

In the appropriate clinical setting, identification of an osmolar gap may be the first indication of a poison-associated AG acidosis. Ethylene glycol, methanol, and isopropyl alcohol all cause an elevated osmolar gap, but only the first two cause a high AG acidosis. Ingestion of ethylene glycol, present in antifreeze, can be suspected by observing urine oxalate crystals, the presence of an osmolar gap in serum, and a high AG acidosis. Some antifreeze agents contain a fluorescent dye which may be detected by viewing the urine with the aid of a Wood's lamp. Methanol metabolism results in the formation of formaldehyde and formic acid, which can cause severe optic nerve and central nervous system damage.

Treatment of methanol and ethylene glycol poisoning includes the prompt institution of a saline or osmotic diuresis, supplementation with thiamine, pyridoxine, and folic acid to maximize metabolism by nontoxic pathways, and inhibition of alcohol dehydrogenase with fomepizole. Fomepizole therapy has replaced therapy with ethanol, as the decline in ethylene glycol level is more predictable, and fomepizole does not cause the neurological obtundation seen during ethanol infusion. Correction of systemic acidosis with sodium bicarbonate may reduce the tissue penetration of toxic metabolites. Indications for emergent hemodialysis include the presence of ocular manifestations, severe (AG > 30, pH < 7.25) or worsening metabolic acidosis, blood methanol or ethylene glycol concentrations > 50 mg/dL, renal failure, or deteriorating vital signs despite intensive supportive care.

Renal failure

Uremic acidosis is characterized by inadequate net acid excretion due to impaired ammonia and titratable acid excretion. Simultaneous hyperkalemia may further inhibit renal ammonia metabolism and contribute to type IV renal tubular acidosis (RTA). Significant loss of bone mass may occur, as the retained acid is buffered by alkaline salts released from bone. Oral alkali replacement to maintain the [HCO_3^-] at a level of ~24 mmol/L is recommended. Treating the patient with chronic kidney disease and metabolic acidosis with sodium bicarbonate appears to slow the progression of the chronic kidney disease.

TABLE 245-5 Classification of Renal Tubular Acidosis

	Proximal (Type II)	Distal (Type I)	Distal (Type IV)
Mechanism	Defective proximal tubule HCO_3^- absorption	Defective collecting duct H^+ secretion	Defective ammonia excretion
Common causes	Genetic disorders in children; myeloma, nephrotoxic medications in adults	Genetic disorders of the tubule in children; autoimmune disease, interstitial nephritis in adults	Chronic kidney disease and impairments of renin-aldosterone axis
$FE_{HCO_3^-}$	> 10%	< 3%	< 3%
Urine pH	During alkali treatment > 5.5; chronic, no alkali treatment < 5.5	> 5.5	Usually ≤ 6.0
Serum K^+	Hypokalemia; worsens with therapy	Hypokalemia; often improves with therapy	Hyperkalemia; correcting hyperkalemia can correct the RTA
Ca_2^+ excretion	Increased	Increased	Usually normal

$FEHCO_3^-$, fractional excretion of bicarbonate measured when the serum bicarbonate is normal.

NORMAL AG METABOLIC ACIDOSIS

This disorder results from failure of the kidneys to produce adequate net acid excretion to balance endogenous acid production (renal tubular acidosis) (**Table 245-5**) or from alkali loss, either from the gastrointestinal tract (diarrhea) or the kidneys (certain forms of RTA). Differentiating RTA from diarrhea can be done using the combination of history and laboratory studies, in particular the urinary anion gap.

URINARY AG

The urinary anion gap (UAG) is the sum of the urine sodium and urine potassium concentrations, minus the urine chloride concentration, all measured in mmol/L:

$$UAG = U_{Na} + U_K - U_{Cl}$$

It is used to assess indirectly urinary ammonium excretion, which is increased in patients with diarrhea, and reduced in patients with renal tubular acidosis. If the UAG is negative in a patient with metabolic acidosis, the urinary NH_4^+ level is appropriately increased. In metabolic acidosis from bicarbonate loss in diarrhea, the UAG is typically −20 to −50 mmol/L. A positive UAG indicates inappropriately low urinary NH_4^+ excretion, suggesting RTA is the cause of the acidosis.

TYPE I RTA (DISTAL RTA)

Type I RTA is characterized by hypokalemia, normal AG metabolic acidosis, low urinary NH_4^+ excretion, as reflected by a positive UAG, and a high urine pH (pH ≥ 6.5) in the presence of untreated metabolic acidosis. These patients commonly come to medical attention either because of growth retardation and failure to thrive in children, or recurrent renal stone formation in adults. Urinary citrate, an important inhibitor of urinary calcium oxalate crystallization, is decreased in distal RTA, contributing to the nephrolithiasis. Type I RTA in children is frequently caused by genetic mutations in distal tubular ion transporters. In adults, type I RTA may result from acute interstitial nephritis, or autoimmune diseases, such as systemic lupus erythematosus and Sjögren syndrome.

Oral alkali supplementation, dosed at 1 mmol/kg/d, is the mainstay of therapy. Patients typically require 50% of the alkali as potassium citrate to treat the concomitant hypokalemia. Sodium alkali salts, such as sodium citrate or sodium bicarbonate, are used to correct the remainder of the metabolic acidosis, while avoiding excessive potassium supplementation and development of hyperkalemia.

TYPE II RTA (PROXIMAL RTA)

Type II RTA is characterized by hypokalemia and normal AG metabolic acidosis. In contrast to type I RTA, urine pH in untreated type II RTA is ≤6.0. Many patients with type II RTA exhibit the Fanconi syndrome (type II RTA, glycosuria, generalized aminoaciduria, and phosphaturia). Causes of type II RTA include inherited genetic disorders, such as cystinosis, hereditary fructose intolerance, and Wilson disease, and acquired disorders, such as multiple myeloma, renal transplant rejection, and certain medications, including acetazolamide, ifosfamide, and the antiretroviral drug tenofovir. Identifying and correcting the underlying causes are central to treating acquired forms of proximal RTA. If the underlying cause cannot be reversed, oral alkali therapy is used. Large amounts of bicarbonate, typically 10 to 15 mmol/kg/d, are typically required in children with type II RTA. As the serum bicarbonate increases, renal bicarbonate losses increase, causing the need for very high doses. Similar to type I RTA, 50% of the alkali should be given as a potassium salt, typically as potassium citrate, and 50% as a sodium salt, either sodium citrate or sodium bicarbonate.

TYPE IV RTA

Type IV RTA is characterized by hyperkalemia, normal AG metabolic acidosis, and disturbances in the renin-aldosterone axis leading to impaired release or action of aldosterone. Most patients have concomitant chronic kidney disease, most commonly diabetic nephropathy and interstitial nephritis. Other causes or contributing factors include HIV, sickle cell disease, urinary tract obstruction, lupus nephritis, amyloidosis, myeloma, adrenal insufficiency, kidney transplant rejection, and a variety of medications, such as cyclosporine, ACE inhibitors, angiotensin receptor blockers (ARBs), NSAIDs, trimethoprim, heparin, and potassium-sparing diuretics. In these patients, it is important to differentiate type IV RTA from uremic metabolic acidosis. The urine pH in most patients with type IV RTA is acidic, usually ≤6.0, but may be elevated. The acidosis is usually mild, and bicarbonate therapy may not be needed. In the majority of cases, hyperkalemia causes the metabolic acidosis through its effects on renal ammonia metabolism. Accordingly, correcting the hyperkalemia with dietary modification typically corrects the metabolic acidosis. Loop or thiazide diuretics may be necessary in some patients. Sodium bicarbonate may be needed if persistent metabolic acidosis is present despite correction of the hyperkalemia. Exogenous mineralocorticoid therapy should be avoided in patients with chronic kidney disease, since mineralocorticoids can contribute to worsening of renal function. We generally do not recommend discontinuing ACE inhibitors or ARBs in patients with type IV RTA, because of the important effects of these medications to decrease cardiovascular events and to slow the progression of chronic kidney disease.

METABOLIC ALKALOSIS

Patients with metabolic alkalosis may present with delirium, cardiac arrhythmias, and neuromuscular irritability when the pH exceeds 7.55. Perhaps more often, patients come to medical attention because of compensatory hypoventilation, which may lead to hypoxia, respiratory failure, or pneumonia. Patients may have a history of diuretic use, vomiting, and poorly controlled hypertension. Laboratory values demonstrate an elevated arterial pH, increased serum HCO_3^-, and an increase in $PaCO_2$ secondary to compensatory alveolar hypoventilation.

PRACTICE POINT

- Metabolic alkalosis: Measure the urinary chloride level to assesses the circulating volume. The urinary sodium is less reliable when the renal threshold for bicarbonate is exceeded and sodium is excreted in the urine, even when a patient is volume depleted.

Metabolic alkalosis can occur secondary to exogenous administration or endogenous synthesis of HCO_3^-. However, the kidneys have an impressive ability to excrete HCO_3^-, and retain excess alkali only if volume deficiency, chloride deficiency, hypokalemia or renal insufficiency, typically stage IV/V CKD, are present. In the hospital setting, patients who receive oral or intravenous HCO_3^-, acetate in parenteral hyperalimentation solutions, citrate in transfusions or during plasma exchange therapy may develop alkalosis if hemodynamic disturbances disrupt the normal excretion of HCO_3^- by the kidneys. Gastrointestinal H^+ losses can occur from vomiting or gastric fluid aspiration. Diuretics, both thiazide and loop diuretics, can cause metabolic alkalosis as a result of a contracted extracellular fluid volume. Chronic use of these drugs activates additional mechanisms, such as secondary hyperaldosteronism, and hypokalemia, which can perpetuate the alkalosis. Metabolic alkalosis associated with vomiting, sweat, and recent diuretic use is usually associated with a low urinary chloride (**Table 245-6**).

Penicillins, hypomagnesemia, and chronic hypokalemia may lead to metabolic alkalosis by promoting urinary acid secretion. Alkali therapy during the treatment phase of severe lactic acidosis or ketoacidosis may result in metabolic alkalosis during recovery. Similarly, alkalosis will develop if the elevated $PaCO_2$ secondary to prolonged CO_2 retention is abruptly returned to normal. Increased aldosterone levels, due to autonomous primary adrenal overproduction or secondary aldosterone release due to renal overproduction of renin, increases net acid excretion and may result in metabolic alkalosis. Mineralocorticoid excess is usually associated with a urinary chloride >30 mEq/L. Other causes of metabolic alkalosis include Bartter syndrome, Gitelman syndrome, Liddle syndrome, villous adenoma, and milk-alkali (calcium-alkali) syndrome.

TREATMENT

Volume expansion with isotonic saline in combination with correction of hypokalemia, if present, usually corrects the alkalosis of chloride-responsive metabolic alkalosis. Alkalosis associated with potassium depletion promptly responds to potassium repletion. Chloride-resistant metabolic alkalosis requires treatment of the causative condition, and generally does not respond well to either NaCl or KCl administration. Rarely, acid therapy may be necessary. Intravenous acid preparations include either HCl or NH_4Cl, 100 mmol/L, and should be administered only through a central vein. NH_4Cl should be avoided in patients with liver disease because of the possible exacerbation of hepatic encephalopathy.

TABLE 245-6 Cause of Metabolic Alkalosis

Chloride-responsive (urinary chloride < 20)
GI
Nasogastric suction
Vomiting/diarrhea
Laxative abuse
Villous adenoma
Renal
Diuretics
Post-hypercapnea
Refeeding alkalosis
Cystic fibrosis (sweat losses)
Chloride-resistant (urinary chloride > 30)
Mineralocorticoid excess
Primary or secondary aldosteronism
Secondary aldosteronism (eg, CHF, renal artery stenosis, liver disease)
Cushing syndrome
Licorice ingestion
Alkali load
Citrate (transfusions)
Acetate (TPN)
Severe hypokalemia/hypomagnesemia

RESPIRATORY ACIDOSIS

Respiratory acidosis is diagnosed by an increase in $PaCO_2$ and decrease in pH. Patients may become acutely anxious, agitated, obtunded or comatose; tremor, asterixis, and myoclonic jerking may be present on examination. Cerebral vasodilation may occur, with headaches and signs of raised intracranial pressure, such as papilledema, abnormal reflexes, and focal muscle weakness.

Differentiating acute from chronic respiratory acidosis is critical for accurate diagnosis and treatment. Acute respiratory acidosis increases HCO_3^- by 1 mmol/L for every 10 mm Hg increase in $PaCO_2$, whereas in chronic respiratory acidosis (>24 hours), renal adaptation increases the HCO_3^- by 4 mmol/L for every 10 mm Hg increase in $PaCO_2$. The serum HCO_3^- usually does not rise above 38 mmol/L. General anesthetics, sedatives, head trauma, alcohol, intracranial tumors, syndromes of sleep-disordered breathing, diseases of the motor neurons, neuromuscular junction and skeletal muscle, and improperly adjusted mechanical ventilation may result in respiratory acidosis. In a stable mechanically ventilated patient, respiratory acidosis may develop secondary to a sudden rise in CO_2 production, as from fever, agitation, sepsis, or overfeeding, however it is more often due to a fall in alveolar ventilation from worsening pulmonary function, high levels of positive end-expiratory pressure in the presence of reduced cardiac output, or sudden occlusion of the upper airway.

TREATMENT

The goal of therapy is improved ventilation. Underlying respiratory conditions, such as acute exacerbations of COPD, should be aggressively treated. Sedatives and other central nervous system depressant drugs should be stopped, and the narcotic antagonist, naloxone, may need to be administered. Patients may require noninvasive positive pressure ventilation, or endotracheal intubation and assisted ventilation. Severe hypercapnia should be cautiously corrected, as a rapid fall in pH may provoke cardiac arrhythmias, reduced cerebral perfusion, and seizures.

RESPIRATORY ALKALOSIS

The diagnosis of respiratory alkalosis depends on measurement of arterial pH and $PaCO_2$. Other laboratory findings may include a reduced serum K^+ and elevated serum Cl^-. Acute respiratory alkalosis is not usually associated with increased renal HCO_3^- excretion, but within hours net acid excretion is reduced. Acutely, HCO_3^- concentration falls by 2.0 mmol/L for each 10 mm Hg decrease in $PaCO_2$. Chronic hypocapnia reduces the serum HCO_3^- by 4.0 mmol/L for each 10 mm Hg decrease in $PaCO_2$. However, it is unusual to observe a plasma HCO_3^- < 12 mmol/L from respiratory alkalosis alone.

Chronic respiratory alkalosis is usually asymptomatic due to renal compensation. Acute respiratory alkalosis ("hyperventilation") presents with lightheadedness, confusion, syncope, tachycardia, anxiety, and dyspnea. Alkalosis promotes the binding of calcium to albumin, leading to decreased serum ionized calcium, and possibly seizures, tetany, and circumoral and acral paresthesias.

Many cardiopulmonary disorders associated with hypoxia, including pulmonary embolism, pneumonia, and pneumothorax, are associated with respiratory alkalosis in their early to intermediate stages. Respiratory alkalosis is common during mechanical ventilation. Central nervous system insults, such as meningitis, encephalitis, brain tumor, or head injury, liver failure, and early gram-negative septicemia may lead to respiratory alkalosis. Some drugs, including salicylates, theophylline and aminophylline, thyroxine, and catecholamines, cause respiratory alkalosis. Chronic respiratory alkalosis is a normal finding in pregnancy and does not require treatment. Hyperventilation from anxiety or panic attacks is a diagnosis of exclusion. It is important to consider other conditions such as pulmonary embolism, acute coronary syndrome, and hyperthyroidism prior to making the diagnosis. Chronic respiratory alkalosis is particularly common in patients with acute or chronic liver disease. The associated secondary metabolic acidosis should not be treated with alkali, as increasing serum pH can worsen hepatic encephalopathy in these patients.

TREATMENT

Management is limited to correction of the underlying disorder. Acid infusions, antidepressants, and sedatives are not recommended. The respiratory alkalosis present in pregnant women does not require treatment.

CONCLUSION

Acid-base disorders are commonly identified in hospitalized patients. In almost all conditions, the presence of an acid-base disorder indicates the presence of a clinically significant underlying disease process. This underlying disease needs to be identified and aggressively treated. In specific conditions, but not all, direct treatment of the acid-base disorder with either acid or alkali therapy is also needed.

SUGGESTED READINGS

Brent J. Fomepizole for ethylene glycol and methanol poisoning. *N Engl J Med.* 2009;360:2216–2223.

Karet FE. Mechanisms in hyperkalemic renal tubular acidosis. *J Am Soc Nephrol.* 2009;20:251–254.

Kraut JA, Madias NE. Serum anion gap: its uses and limitations in clinical medicine. *Clin J Am Soc Nephrol.* 2007;2:162–174.

Laski ME, Sabatini S. Metabolic alkalosis, bedside and bench. *Semin Nephrol.* 2006;26:404–421.

Kraut JA, Kurtz I. Toxic alcohol ingestions: clinical features, diagnosis, and management. *Clin J Am Soc Nephrol.* 2008;3:208–225.

CHAPTER 246

Acute Kidney Injury

Kuyilan Karai Subramanian, MD
Ajay K. Singh, MD, MBA, FRCP

Key Clinical Questions

1. How is acute kidney injury defined?
2. What are the major causes of acute kidney injury?
3. How is acute kidney injury diagnosed and managed?
4. What role does renal replacement therapy, such as hemodialysis, have in acute kidney injury?

INTRODUCTION

Acute kidney injury (AKI) is defined as a potentially reversible sudden deterioration in renal function due to prerenal, intrarenal, or postrenal causes. AKI is frequently accompanied by dysregulation of extracellular fluid volume and electrolytes and a marked increase in the retention of nitrogenous and nonnitrogenous waste products over a period of hours to weeks. AKI may be oliguric (< 400 mL/day) or nonoliguric (> 400 mL/day). AKI can also be defined as an acute and sustained increase in serum creatinine of 0.5 mg/dL (44.2 micromol/L), if the baseline is less than 2.5 mg/dL (221 mmol/L), or an increase in serum creatinine more than 20% if the baseline is more than 2.5 mg/dL (221 mmol/L).

There have been several attempts to achieve consensus among intensivists and nephrologists on the definition of AKI. The Acute Dialysis Quality Initiative (ADQI) group published the RIFLE classification of AKI in 2004 based on three severity categories (risk, injury, and failure) and two clinical outcome categories (loss and end-stage renal disease) (**Table 246-1**). The parameters assessed in the RIFLE classification are changes in serum creatinine level or glomerular filtration rate (GFR) or urine output (UO) from the patient's baseline. The baseline serum creatinine level and GFR may not be readily available. Hence the consensus committee recommends the use of the Modification of Diet in Renal Disease (MDRD) equation to estimate GFR/1.73 m^2. The proportional decrease in GFR is calculated from 75 mL/min per 1.73 m^2, the agreed-upon lower limit of normal.

A modified RIFLE criteria schema has been proposed by the Acute Kidney Injury Network (AKIN).The AKIN diagnostic criteria (**Table 246-2**) and the classification/staging system (**Table 246-3**) for AKI are an abrupt (within 48 hours) reduction in kidney function currently defined as an absolute increase in serum creatinine of more than or equal to 0.3 mg/dL (≥ 26.4 μmol/L), a percentage increase in serum creatinine of more than or equal to 50% (1.5-fold from baseline), or a reduction in urine output (documented oliguria of less than 0.5 mL/kg per hour for more than 6 hours). The absolute increase in the serum creatinine levels (≥ 0.3 mg/dL) in this diagnostic criterion is based on epidemiologic data demonstrating that changes in serum creatinine levels of 0.3 to 0.5 mg/dL are associated with increased mortality risk. Also, the timeline of "within 48 hours" is deliberately included in the diagnostic criteria because of data demonstrating poorer outcomes within this period. The clinical utility and universal adoption of either RIFLE or AKIN criteria remain uncertain, and future studies are needed to demonstrate their validity.

EPIDEMIOLOGY

AKI IN THE HOSPITALIZED PATIENT

The prevalence of AKI has been reported to be approximately 1% of all hospital admissions in the United States. Major causes of hospital-acquired AKI include volume depletion resulting in decreased renal perfusion, major surgery, septic shock, congestive cardiac failure, contrast nephropathy, and aminoglycoside antibiotics. Acute tubular necrosis (ATN) is identified as the most frequent clinicopathologic entity in hospital-acquired AKI, followed by prerenal azotemia, acute-onset chronic renal failure, and urinary tract obstruction.

TABLE 246-1 RIFLE Classification for AKI

- Risk (R)—Increase in serum creatinine level × 1.5 or decrease in GFR by 25%, or UO <0.5 mL/kg/h for 6 hours
- Injury (I)—Increase in serum creatinine level × 2.0 or decrease in GFR by 50%, or UO <0.5 mL/kg/h for 12 hours
- Failure (F)—Increase in serum creatinine level × 3.0, decrease in GFR by 75%, or serum creatinine level >4 mg/dL with acute increase of >0.5 mg/dL; UO <0.3 mL/kg/h for 24 hours, or anuria for 12 hours
- Loss (L)—Persistent AKI, complete loss of kidney function >4 weeks
- End-stage kidney disease (E)—Loss of kidney function >3 months

AKI IN THE CRITICALLY ILL PATIENT

AKI occurs in 1 to 25% of the patients admitted in critical care units, with major causes including sepsis, multiorgan failure, hypotension, nephrotoxin administration, and prerenal factors. AKI affects mostly older patients who have chronic morbidities or are severely ill on admission to the hospital. The overall in-hospital mortality rate in intensive care unit (ICU)-associated AKI is approximately 60%.

COMMUNITY-ACQUIRED AKI

Community-acquired AKI accounts for 1% of the hospital admissions in the United States. Community-acquired AKI in developed nations mainly affects older patients, with causes including acute tubular necrosis, prerenal azotemia, acute-onset chronic renal failure, and obstructive uropathy. In the developing countries, AKI is predominantly a disease of infants and children and is due to prerenal etiologies, such as dehydration from acute diarrheal illness. Falciparum malaria, HIV/AIDS, obstetrical mishaps, dengue fever, snake bites, insect stings, botanical and chemical nephrotoxins, acute glomerulonephritis, hemolytic uremic syndrome, and alternative medical therapies are important etiological factors of AKI in the tropics. Crush injury from natural disasters such as earthquake contributes to regional epidemics of AKI.

CAUSES OF AKI

The causes of AKI can be classified under three broad categories: prerenal, renal, and postrenal (**Table 246-4**). Prerenal azotemia and ischemic ATN account for 75% of AKI.

PRERENAL CAUSES

Prerenal causes are characterized by a reversible loss of kidney function and a drop in GFR due to decreased renal perfusion, while the integrity of renal structural components is maintained. Prerenal causes account for approximately 70% of community-acquired AKI and 40% of hospital-acquired cases. Prerenal azotemia is typically due to decreased effective circulating volume, true hypovolemia, or impaired renal perfusion.

TABLE 246-2 AKIN Diagnostic Criteria for AKI

An abrupt (within 48 hours) reduction in kidney function currently defined as an absolute increase in serum creatinine of more than or equal to 0.3 mg/dL (≥26.4 μmol/L), a percentage increase in serum creatinine of more than or equal to 50% (1.5-fold from baseline), or a reduction in urine output (documented oliguria of less than 0.5 mL/kg per hour for more than 6 hours).

TABLE 246-3 AKIN Classification/Staging System for AKI

Stage	Serum Creatinine Criteria	Urine Output Criteria
1	Increase in serum creatinine of more than or equal to 0.3 mg/dL (≥26.4 μmol/L) or increase to more than or equal to 150% to 200% (1.5- to 2-fold) from baseline	Less than 0.5 mL/kg per hour for more than 6 hours
2*	Increase in serum creatinine to more than 200% to 300% (>2- to 3-fold) from baseline	Less than 0.5 mL/kg per hour for more than 12 hours
3†	Increase in serum creatinine to more than 300% (>3-fold) from baseline (or serum creatinine of more than or equal to 4.0 mg/dL [≥354 μmol/L] with an acute increase of at least 0.5 mg/dL [44 μmol/L])	Less than 0.3 mL/kg per hour for 24 hours or anuria for 12 hours

Note: This classification is modified from RIFLE (Risk, Injury, Failure, Loss, and End-stage kidney disease) criteria.

The staging system proposed is a highly sensitive interim staging system and is based on recent data indicating that a small change in serum creatinine influences outcome.

Only one criterion (creatinine or urine output) has to be fulfilled to qualify for a stage.

*200% to 300% increase = 2- to 3-fold increase.

†Given wide variation in indications and timing of initiation of renal replacement therapy (RRT), individuals who receive RRT are considered to have met the criteria for stage 3 irrespective of the stage they are in at the time of RRT.

Decreased effective circulating volume may be due to cardiac failure, aortic stenosis, nephrotic syndrome, cirrhosis, hepatorenal syndrome, acute pancreatitis, cardiac tamponade, sepsis, or systemic vasodilatation in conjunction with sepsis or anesthesia.

Intravascular volume depletion, a possible result of dehydration due to vomiting, diarrhea, poor fluid intake, fever, and diaphoresis, is the most common cause of prerenal azotemia in the outpatient setting. Excessive urination (polyuria) due to excess diuretics, diabetes insipidus, or poorly controlled diabetes mellitus can also cause AKI. Other causes of volume depletion include gastrointestinal bleeding and plasma loss due to burns, trauma, and anaphylaxis.

Decreased renal perfusion may result from renal artery stenosis or renal vein thrombosis, or more often from drugs such as nonsteroidal antiinflammatory drugs (NSAIDs), which interfere with glomerular autoregulation, especially in patients above the age of 60 with additional risk factors for prerenal azotemia, such as atherosclerotic vascular disease, preexisting CKD, hypotension, diuretic use, cirrhosis, nephrotic syndrome, and congestive cardiac failure. Immunosuppressive drugs, such as tacrolimus and cyclosporine, lead to acute kidney injury by inducing vasoconstriction of the afferent and efferent glomerular arterioles of the kidneys. Angiotensin-converting enzyme (ACE) inhibitors may cause AKI in patients with unilateral or bilateral renal artery stenosis.

INTRARENAL CAUSES

Intrarenal causes of AKI are characterized by the loss of kidney function due to structural damages to glomeruli, tubules, vessels, or interstitium and are often categorized based on the primary site of renal injury.

TABLE 246-4 Causes of AKI

Prerenal
Intravascular volume depletion: diarrhea, vomiting, hemorrhage, poor fluid intake, sepsis, overdiuresis
Decreased effective circulating volume to the kidneys: congestive cardiac failure, nephrotic syndrome, cirrhosis, or hepatorenal syndrome
Renal hypoperfusion due to exogenous agents: ACE inhibitors, NSAIDs
Renal
Acute tubular necrosis: ischemia
Toxins: drugs (eg, aminoglycosides), contrast agents, pigments (myoglobin or hemoglobin); heavy metals
Glomerular disease: rapidly progressive glomerulonephritis, systemic lupus erythematosus, small-vessel vasculitis (Wegener granulomatosis or polyarteritis nodosa), Henoch-Schönlein purpura (IgA nephropathy), Goodpasture syndrome
Acute proliferative glomerulonephritis: endocarditis, poststreptococcal infection
Vascular disease
Microvascular disease: atheroembolic disease (cholesterol-plaque microembolism), thrombotic thrombocytopenic purpura, hemolytic uremic syndrome, HELLP syndrome (*h*emolysis, *e*levated *l*iver enzymes and *l*ow *p*latelets)
Macrovascular disease: renal artery occlusion, abdominal aortic aneurysm
Interstitial disease: allergic reaction to drugs, autoimmune disease, systemic lupus erythematosus, mixed connective tissue disease, pyelonephritis, infiltrative disease (lymphoma or leukemia)
Postrenal
Benign prostatic hypertrophy or prostate cancer, cervical cancer, retroperitoneal disorders, intratubular obstruction (stones, urate crystals, myeloma light chains), pelvic mass or invasive pelvic malignancy, intraluminal bladder mass (clot, tumor or fungal ball), neurogenic bladder, urethral strictures

Acute tubular necrosis (ATN) (**Figure 246-1**), is the most common cause of intrinsic renal failure and is also the most common cause of hospital-acquired acute kidney injury. It usually results from tubular ischemia and inflammation, as in sepsis and shock, or tubular toxins such as heme pigments, for example, myoglobin

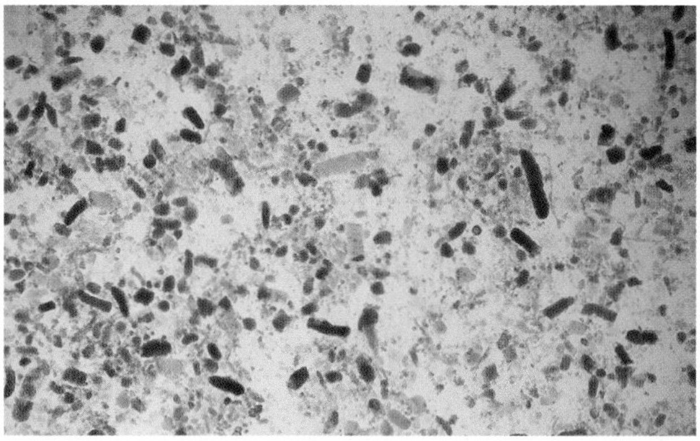

Figure 246-1 *Acute Tubular Necrosis (ATN). (Courtesy of Dr. Serban Nicolescu).*

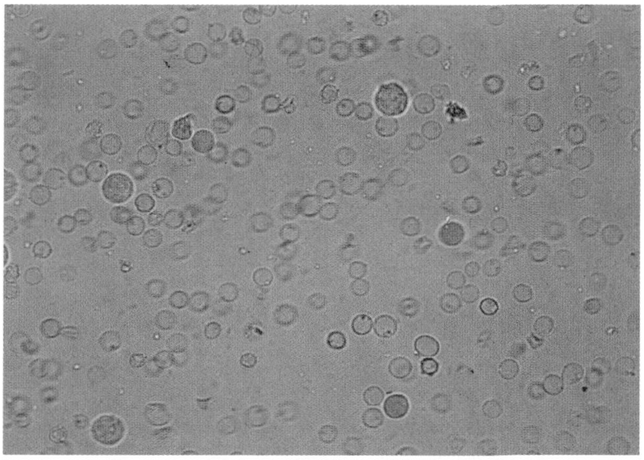

Figure 246-2 *Dysmorphic red blood cells in urine: A common finding in glomerulonephritis. (Courtesy of Dr. Richard Dion).*

from rhabdomyolysis or hemoglobin from intravascular hemolysis, cisplatin, ethylene glycol, and myeloma light chains. Ischemic tubular necrosis may occur in patients with sustained prerenal azotemia. Ifosfamide, a chemotherapeutic agent is known to cause acute tubular dysfunction in the proximal tubule.

Hospital-acquired ATN is often multifactorial. For example, it may occur in a septic patient exposed to a potentially nephrotoxic drug, such as an aminoglycoside or amphotericin, or after the administration of a radiocontrast agent in a hypovolemic patient with preexisting renal dysfunction.

Patients with severe renal ischemia may develop cortical necrosis with injury to both tubules and glomeruli. Causes include severe sepsis, dehydration, snake bites, obstetrical catastrophes, thrombotic microangiopathies, and malaria. The prognosis for recovery is less favorable than for ATN.

Glomerular disease in the form of rapidly progressive glomerulonephritis (RPGN) and acute proliferative glomerulonephritis may cause AKI (**Figure 246-2**). RPGN may be primary or secondary in origin, the latter being associated with systemic diseases like systemic lupus erythematosus, Wegener granulomatosus, polyarteritis nodosa, Henoch-Schönlein purpura, and Goodpasture syndrome. RPGN can also progress to end-stage renal disease (ESRD) in days to weeks. Acute proliferative glomerulonephritis occurs in patients with bacterial endocarditis, poststreptococcal infection, and postpneumococcal infection.

Vascular disease (ie, microvascular and macrovascular renal arterial disease) can cause AKI. Thrombotic thrombocytopenic purpura, hemolytic uremic syndrome, HELLP syndrome (hemolytic anemia, elevated liver enzymes, low platelet count), glomerular capillary thrombosis, and atheroembolic disease may all cause AKI. Patients undergoing interventional or invasive procedures involving the major vessels and those with arrhythmias are at an increased risk for AKI from atheroemboli (**Figures 246-3** to **246-5**).

Interstitial disease, such as acute interstitial nephritis (AIN) often result from an allergic reaction to an offending agent (**Table 246-5**). Withdrawal of the offending agent frequently results in reversal of AKI. AIN may also occur in systemic inflammatory conditions like sarcoidosis, systemic lupus erythematosus (SLE), Legionnaires' disease, and hantavirus infection.

POSTRENAL CAUSES

Postrenal AKI is characterized by loss of kidney function due to intrinsic or extrinsic masses obstructing the urinary collecting system, from the tip of the papillae to the urethral meatus. The most

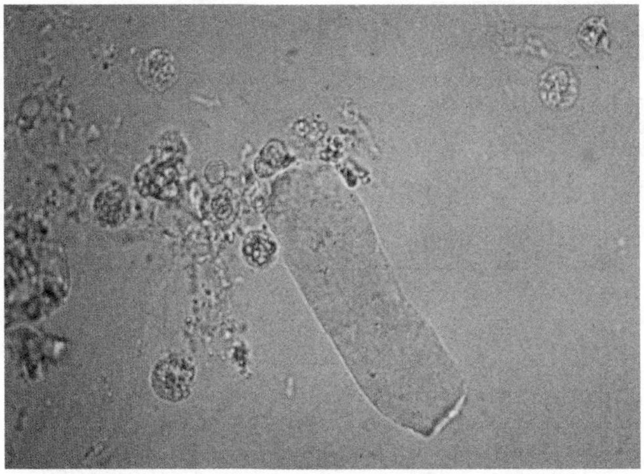

Figure 246-3 *Hyaline cast: a common finding in pre-renal acute kidney injury; may also be seen in normal individuals with concentrated urine. (Courtesy of Dr. Richard Dion).*

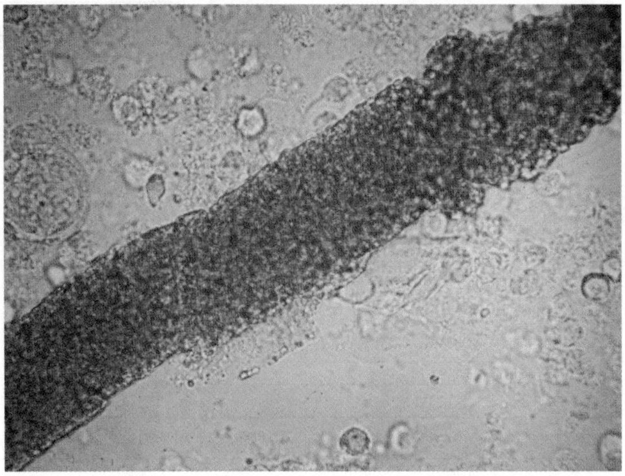

Figure 246-5 *Red blood cell cast: a common urine microscopic finding in glomerulonephritis. (Courtesy of Dr. Richard Dion).*

common causes are prostatic hypertrophy or carcinoma cervical cancer and other causes contributing to bladder neck obstruction. Less common causes include bilateral renal stones, bladder carcinoma, retroperitoneal fibrosis, colorectal cancer, blood clots in the urinary tract, papillary necrosis, and neurogenic bladder.

PATHOPHYSIOLOGY

Figure 246-6 depicts the interaction of hemodynamic, immunological, and inflammatory factors in mediating AKI.

EVALUATION

HISTORY AND PHYSICAL EXAMINATION

A comprehensive history and physical examination is recommended in patients with AKI. Patients should be asked about nonspecific symptoms of azotemia, such as anorexia, nausea, vomiting, malaise, fatigue, pruritus, metallic taste in the mouth, and dyspnea. Bone pain may suggest AKI from multiple myeloma. The patient's daily fluid intake and output records, daily weights, inpatient and outpatient medications, including NSAIDs and other over-the-counter medications, and outpatient laboratory data should be reviewed. Recent radiology studies should be assessed to determine if the patient has a history of recent contrast use in angiography or computed tomographic (CT) imaging.

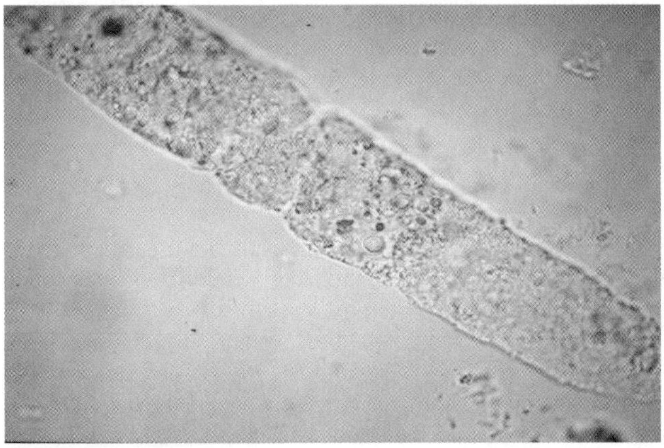

Figure 246-4 *Granular cast with a waxy margin: a common finding in pre-renal azotemia and acute tubular necrosis. (Courtesy of Dr. Richard Dion).*

On physical examination, patients should be assessed for signs of volume overload, such as peripheral edema, pulmonary rales, and elevated neck veins. Physical findings of advanced renal failure include asterixis, myoclonus, and pericardial or pleural rubs. A minority of patients with acute interstitial nephritis have fever and rash. Muscle pain, bluish discoloration of the toes, livedo reticularis, and loss of foot or ankle pulses suggest atheroembolic renal failure. Palpable purpura, mononeuritis multiplex, hemoptysis, or prominent upper respiratory tract symptoms, such as sinusitis or otitis, suggests glomerulonephritis associated with systemic vasculitis. Other clinical clues for the diagnosis of AKI are listed in **Table 246-6**.

TABLE 246-5 Drugs Associated with Acute Interstitial Nephritis

Beta–lactam antibiotics • Methicillin • Ampicillin • Oxacillin • Penicillin • Nafcillin • Cephalosporins Other antibiotics • Sulfonamides • Rifampin • Polymyxin • Ethambutol • Tetracycline • Vancomycin • Erythromycin • Ciprofloxacin • Acyclovir • Indinavir • Alpha-interferon Diuretics • Thiazides • Furosemide • Chlorthalidone • Triamterene	NSAIDs • Fenoprofen • Indomethacin • Naproxen • Ibuprofen • Tolmetin • Diflunisal • Piroxicam • Ketoprofen • Diclofenac Other drugs • Proton-pump inhibitors • Diphenylhydantoin • Cimetidine • Sulfinpyrazone • Allopurinol • Aspirin • Carbamazepine • Phenindione • Clofibrate • Phenylpropanolamine • Aldomet • Phenobarbital • Azathioprine • Diazepam • Captopril • Cisplatin

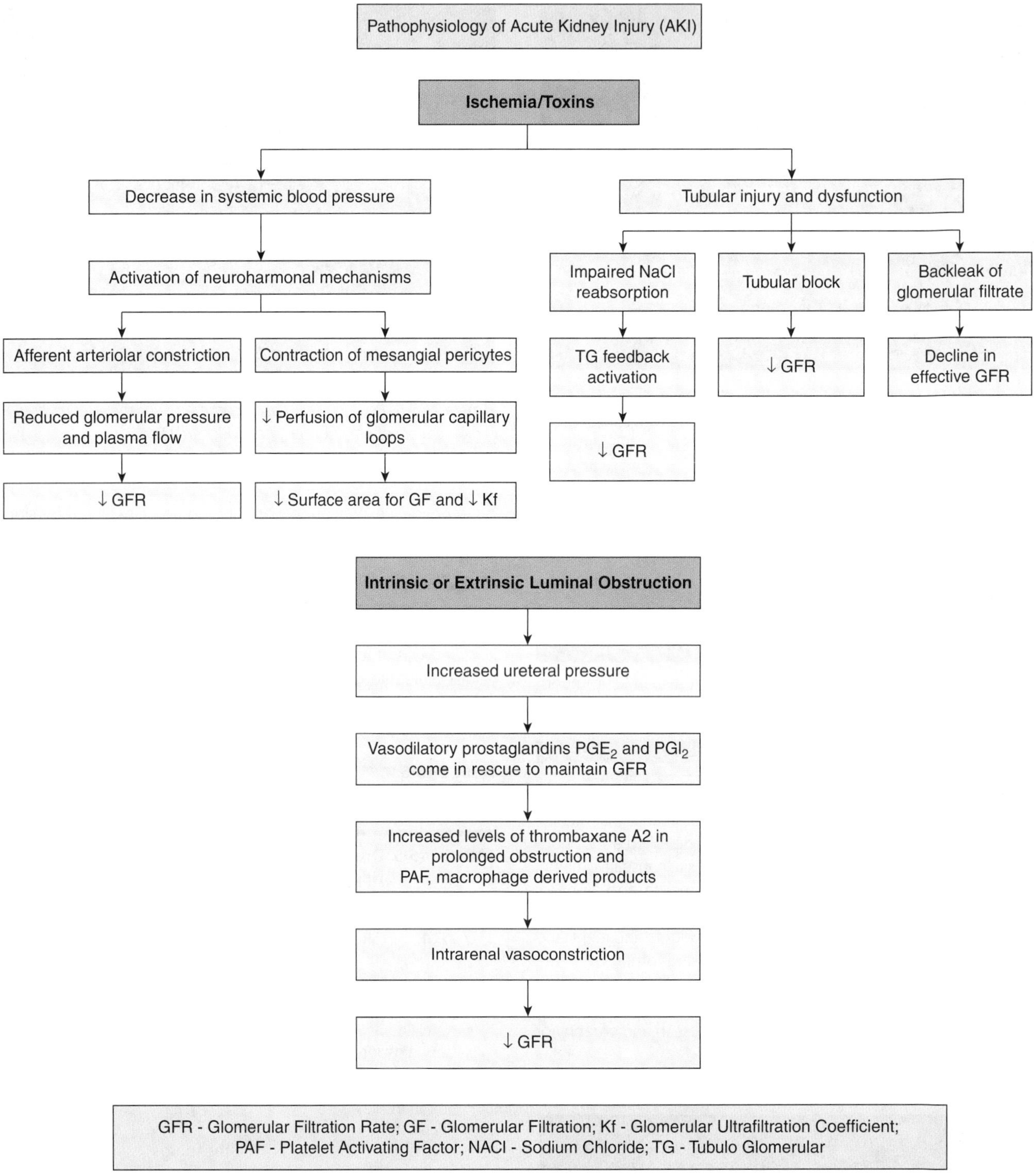

Figure 246-6 *Pathophysiology of AKI.*

URINE EVALUATION

A urine specimen should be collected for dipstick, microscopic sediment analysis, culture, and urine chemistries such as sodium, protein, creatinine, and osmolality. Heme-positive urine with few erythrocytes on microscopy suggests myoglobinuria or hemoglobinuria, as in rhabdomyolysis and transfusion reactions. Eosinophiluria, once thought to be diagnostic of AIN, is neither sensitive nor specific for this condition as it may be seen in pyelonephritis, prostatitis, glomerulonephritis, atheroembolism, and transplant rejection. In ethylene glycol ingestion, double-pyramid, ovoid, or dumbbell-shaped oxalate crystals are usually present in the urine. Amber-colored rhomboid uric acid crystals may be found in urine in tumor lysis syndrome.

Urine indices help to differentiate prerenal azotemia from ATN. The fractional excretion of sodium (FE_{Na}) is the percentage of sodium filtered by the glomeruli that is excreted in the urine. Patients that are volume depleted are sodium-avid and have a low FE_{Na}. It is calculated as follows:

$$FE_{Na} = \frac{[\text{Urine Na} \times \text{Plasma creatinine}]}{[\text{Plasma Na} \times \text{Urine creatinine}]} \times 100$$

TABLE 246-6 List of Clinical Features and Diagnostic Clues

1. Pre-renal AKI		Absolute or postural hypotension
		Low jugular venous pressure
		Dry mucus membranes (dehydration)
		Decreased effective circulatory volume (eg, heart failure or liver disease)
2. Intrinsic AKI		
	Diseases of the large renal vessels	Flank or abdominal pain (renal artery thrombosis)
		Retinal plaques, palpable purpura, livedo reticularis (atheroembolic disease)
		Flank pain (renal vein thrombosis)
	Diseases of small vessels and glomeruli	New cardiac murmur (post-infectious glomerulonephritis), skin rash or ulcers, arthralgias (lupus), sinusitis (anti-GBM disease), lung hemorrhage (anti-GBM, ANCA-associated vasculitis, lupus)
		Fever, neurologic abnormalities (HUS-TTP)
		Headache, papilledema, heart failure with LVH (malignant hypertension)
	Acute tubular necrosis	Postictal state, trauma or prolonged immobilization (rhabdomyolysis)
		Fever, transfusion reaction (hemolysis)
		Bone pain, fatigue, malaise in individuals > 60 years (multiple myeloma)
		History of alcohol abuse, altered mental status (ethylene glycol ingestion)
	Tubulointerstitial disease	Fever, rash, arthralgias (allergic interstitial nephritis)
		Fever, flank pain, tenderness (acute bilateral pyelonephritis)
3. Post renal AKI		Palpable bladder, flank, or abdominal pain

In prerenal azotemia, urine osmolality is usually > 500 mOsm/kg, the urinary sodium concentration is < 20 mmol/L, and the fractional excretion of sodium (FE_{Na}) is < 1%, whereas in tubular necrosis and urinary obstruction the urine osmolality is < 350 mOsm/kg, the urine sodium concentration is > 40 mmol/L, and the FE_{Na} is > 1% (in ATN, the FE_{Na} is usually, but not always, > 2%). There are exceptions: the FE_{Na} may be < 1% in acute tubular injury due to radiocontrast exposure or heme pigment, especially early and also in acute glomerulonephritis; in early urinary tract obstruction, the urinary sodium concentration and FE_{Na} can be low. The FE_{Na} is also not reliable in the setting of chronic kidney disease, where a high FE_{Na} may be seen in patients with prerenal azotemia, especially early in the clinical course. Typical urine findings in different causes of AKI are listed in **Table 246-7**.

PRACTICE POINT

- The fractional excretion of sodium (FE_{Na}) aids in differentiating prerenal azotemia from acute tubular necrosis. However, in patients who have recently received diuretics, sodium excretion is enhanced, and the FE_{Na} is not reliable. In this setting, the fractional excretion of urea (FE_{Urea}) may be helpful as urea excretion is not enhanced by diuretics. It is calculated as follows:

$$FE_{Urea} = \frac{[\text{Urine urea} \times \text{Plasma creatinine}]}{[\text{Plasma urea} \times \text{Urine creatinine}]} \times 100$$

- Normally, the FE_{Urea} is 50–65%, while in prerenal azotemia, it is usually less than 35%.

  Patients with metabolic alkalosis and prerenal azotemia have a falsely elevated FE_{Na}, because of bicarbonaturia with obligate losses of sodium in urine. In these patients, the fractional excretion of chloride (FE_{Cl}) may be used instead:

$$FE_{Cl} = \frac{[\text{Urine Cl} \times \text{Plasma creatinine}]}{[\text{Plasma Cl} \times \text{Urine creatinine}]} \times 100$$

- A FE_{Cl} < 1% is consistent with prerenal azotemia.

BLOOD TESTS

Serum blood urea nitrogen (BUN), creatinine, electrolytes, calcium, phosphorous, and albumin should be obtained in all patients. Serum creatinine concentration typically rises by 1 to 1.5 mg/dL daily when there is a marked decrement in kidney function. Other useful blood tests include uric acid, creatinine kinase, serum immunoelectrophoresis, serum osmolal gap, and complete blood count with differential. In malignancies, serum urate and calcium levels are often high. Eosinophilia suggests allergic interstitial nephritis. Elevated serum creatine kinase is present in rhabdomyolysis. Abnormal serum electrophoresis is present in

TABLE 246-7 Urine Findings in AKI

Condition	Dipstick Test	Sediment Analysis	Urine Osmolality mOsm/kg	Fractional excretion of sodium
Prerenal azotemia	Trace or no proteinuria	A few hyaline casts possible	> 500	< 1
Intrarenal azotemia				
Tubular injury ischemia	Mild-to-moderate proteinuria	Pigmented granular casts	< 350	> 1
Nephrotoxins	Mild-to-moderate proteinuria	Pigmented granular casts	< 350	> 1
Acute interstitial nephritis	Mild-to-moderate proteinuria; hemoglobin; leukocytes	White cells and white-cell casts; eosinophils; red cells	< 350	> 1
Acute glomerulonephritis	Moderate-to-severe proteinuria; hemoglobin	Red cells and red-cell casts; red cells can be dysmorphic	> 500	< 1
Postrenal azotemia	Trace or no proteinuria; can have hemoglobin, leukocytes	Crystals, red cells, and white cells possible	< 350	> 1

multiple myeloma. In alcohol ingestions such as ethylene glycol or methanol, there is high osmolal gap.

EVALUATION FOR OBSTRUCTION

Urinary tract obstruction should be excluded in patients presenting with AKI. Renal ultrasonography is the preferred imaging technique, with a sensitivity of 80 to 85% and a specificity approaching 100% for the diagnosis of obstruction. Ultrasonography also helps identify kidney stones and kidney size. To locate the exact site of obstruction and correct it, percutaneous anterograde urography (via percutaneous puncture of the renal pelvis under fluoroscopy) and retrograde urography (via cystoscopy and ureteral catheterization) may be necessary. In patients with retroperitoneal fibrosis, obstruction of the urinary tract may be difficult to visualize by sonography, and computed tomography or magnetic resonance imaging may be necessary. Bladder catheterization can be useful in ruling out urethral obstruction.

RENAL BIOPSY IN AKI

Percutaneous renal biopsy has a limited role in the immediate evaluation and treatment of AKI. However, it is valuable in diagnosing primary renal diseases, such as glomerulonephritis and AIN, after prerenal and postrenal causes of AKI have been excluded. Renal biopsy also plays a role in the evaluation of early allograft dysfunction in renal transplant patients, and in management decisions related to subsequent use of immunosuppressive therapy.

NOVEL BIOMARKERS OF AKI

The definition of AKI is still based on a rise in serum creatinine and fall in urine volume and GFR. However, serum creatinine is not an optimal marker of renal function as it is influenced by age, sex, race, diet, exercise, and lean muscle mass. Moreover, secretion of creatinine may account for 10–40% of its excretion, potentially masking a drop in GFR. The development of novel, sensitive, and specific biomarkers of renal function and injury has been a recent area of intense research. Serum cystatin C, a cysteine protease inhibitor produced by all nucleated human cells and freely filtered into the glomerulus, appears to be a more accurate marker of renal function and a more robust predictor of all-cause mortality in elderly persons than serum creatinine. Potential urinary biomarkers of early AKI are under investigation, such as kidney injury molecule-1, shed by proximal tubular cells after ischemic or nephrotoxic damage; interleukin-18, generated in the proximal tubule in AKI; osteopontin, a cytokine involved in kidney inflammation and repair; and the cytoprotective proteins clusterin, fatty acid–binding protein, and neutrophil gelatinase–associated lipocalin, which are overexpressed by tubular cells undergoing injury and oxidative stress. However, their precise role in the diagnosis and management of AKI has yet to be defined.

MANAGEMENT OF AKI

The management of AKI is directed at identifying and treating the underlying cause and preventing and treating complications. This may involve reversal of hemodynamic instability, elimination of nephrotoxins and avoidance of additional insults, and correction of electrolyte disturbances, uremia, and acid–base disorders.

Maintenance of euvolemic status is central to the management of ischemic acute renal failure. Assessment and correction of volume status are based on careful physical examination, and at times by invasive monitoring. Composition of the fluid replaced should match that of the fluid lost. Minor to moderate hemorrhagic loss is treated with normal saline (0.9% NaCl), whereas severe blood loss is best managed by transfusing packed red blood cells. Repletion of fluid is usually done with normal saline in hypovolemic patients; however, most patients with AKI will have volume overload.

Distinguishing true hypovolemic AKI from hepatorenal syndrome (HRS) is a challenge in patients with cirrhosis and ascites. A gentle fluid challenge should be performed in these patients, with slow administration of fluids titrated to jugular venous pressure or central venous/pulmonary artery pressure. In true hypovolemia, urine output increases and the serum creatinine falls, whereas in HRS, a fluid challenge is usually ineffective. In patients with AKI and volume overload, loop diuretics such as furosemide, dosed between 20 and 100 mg, should be administered as an intravenous bolus, initially every 6 hours. The dose can be increased if an adequate response is not achieved. If bolus dosing of furosemide is ineffective, a continuous infusion of furosemide may be initiated, although evidence for its efficacy compared to intermittent diuretic dosing is limited. When oliguria or anuria persists despite conservative management, dialysis is indicated.

Treatment of intrarenal AKI depends on the underlying pathology. Immunosuppressive agents may be beneficial in treating acute glomerulonephritis or vasculitis. Angiotensin-converting enzyme (ACE) inhibitors are helpful in treating AKI associated with hypertension and scleroderma renal crisis. AKI due to malignant hypertension should be treated by vigorous control of blood pressure. Possible culprit drugs should be stopped in patients with possible AIN. The role of corticosteroids in the management of AIN remains unclear as no randomized, controlled trials have been performed, and retrospective studies have shown conflicting results.

Obstruction of the urethra or bladder neck can be relieved temporarily by insertion of a transurethral or suprapubic catheter. Obstructive lesions of the ureter are treated by stenting, either by anterograde percutaneous or retrograde cystoscopic placement. Patients often undergo a postobstructive diuresis for several days following relief of the obstruction, and care should be taken to avoid dehydration. Transient salt wasting syndrome occurs in approximately 5% of patients and requires administration of intravenous normal saline to maintain blood pressure.

The most common electrolyte disturbance in AKI is hyperkalemia. Initial treatment should include the use of calcium chloride if the potassium level is >6 mEq/L, or if electrocardiographic changes of hyperkalemia are seen. Potassium may be transiently shifted into cells with intravenous insulin (10 units) and glucose (25 g) as a bolus infusion. As acidosis favors hyperkalemia by promoting extracellular movement of potassium, intravenous sodium bicarbonate (three ampules in 1 L of 5% dextrose) leads to translocation of potassium into cells and may also facilitate renal potassium excretion. Sodium polystyrene sulfonate (Kayexalate) given orally (25 to 50 g mixed with 100 mL of 20% sorbitol) or as enema (50 g in 50 mL of 70% sorbitol and 150 mL of tap water) is a more definitive therapy that leads to excretion of potassium from the body. (Kayexalate enemas with 70% sorbitol are rarely associated with colonic necrosis, especially in critically ill patients, and should be avoided if other therapeutic options are available.) Dialysis remains an important option if hyperkalemia is severe or is refractory to treatment.

Acidosis may be corrected by administering sodium bicarbonate when the pH level is less than 7.2, or the serum bicarbonate level is less than 15 mEq/L. Bicarbonate may be administered orally (a 300 mg tablet contains 3.6 mEq of sodium bicarbonate) or intravenously. Ampules for intravenous administration are provided as 7.5% sodium bicarbonate (44.6 mEq/50 mL) or 8.4% sodium bicarbonate (50 mEq/50 mL). The required bicarbonate dose is measured by the following equation: bicarbonate deficit (mEq) = (lean body weight, LBW) (0.5) (desired HCO_3 – actual HCO_3). If acidosis cannot be corrected, dialysis is performed.

Diet plays an important role in patients with AKI who become nutritionally deficient. The daily caloric intake should be 30 to 45 kcal (126 to 189 kJ) per kg per day. In nondialysis patients, protein intake should be restricted to 0.6 g per kg per day. Patients receiving dialysis should have 1 to 1.5 kg/day.

RENAL REPLACEMENT THERAPY (RRT) IN AKI

Dialysis as a treatment modality in AKI is most useful in the elimination of metabolic wastes and uremic toxins, but it is also effective in the maintenance of fluid, electrolyte, and acid–base status. There is limited consensus among nephrologists regarding choice of dialysis, timing of initiation, frequency and intensity of dialysis, and impact on patient outcomes, due to lack of definitive evidence from studies conducted thus far in the setting of AKI (**Table 246-8**).

CONTINUOUS RENAL REPLACEMENT THERAPY VERSUS HEMODIALYSIS

In critically ill patients, continuous renal replacement therapy (CRRT) is now a popular and frequently preferred alternative to intermittent hemodialysis, especially in hemodynamically unstable patients.

CRRT can be either arteriovenous or venovenous. Continuous arteriovenous hemofiltration (CAVHF), continuous arteriovenous hemodialysis (CAVHD), and combination hemodiafiltration (CAVHDF) or continuous venovenous hemofiltration (CVVHF), continuous venovenous hemodialysis (CVVHD), and combination hemodiafiltration (CVVHDF) are the different technical modalities of CRRT. CVVHD is preferred over CAVHD because of the high ultrafiltration rate, predictable blood flow rate, avoidance of arterial puncture, ease of vascular access (either femoral or internal jugular vein, via a double lumen catheter), and reduced risk of heparin-induced bleeding.

Compared to intermittent dialysis, CRRT has several advantages, including lower risk of hemodynamic instability, ease of administration of nutritional support, and more accurate control of the fluid and metabolic status. Disadvantages include prolonged anticoagulation, nursing burden, cost, and limited mobility.

TABLE 246-8 Renal Replacement Therapy in AKI

- Refractory hypervolemia, hyperkalemia ($K^+ > 6.5$ mEq/L), acidosis (pH < 7.1), azotemia (BUN > 100 mg/dL), uremic signs, and severe dysnatremias ($Na^+ > 155$ mEq/L or < 120 mEq/L) are absolute indications for dialysis
- Hemodialysis (HD) is more effective than peritoneal dialysis (PD) in the management of AKI because solute clearance and control of metabolic abnormalities are usually better in HD
- Hemodialysis can be intermittent dialysis, slow low-efficiency dialysis (SLED), or continuous renal replacement therapy (CRRT)
- In patients with hemodynamic instability, SLED or CRRT is recommended over HD
- Peritoneal dialysis (PD) is useful when hemodialysis is unavailable or vascular access cannot be obtained and is the mainstay of treatment in resource-limited settings. The major disadvantages are risk of peritonitis and visceral injury during catheter placement
- The optimal timing for the initiation of dialysis is still unclear
- The dialytic modality of choice depends on the availability of resources in the health care institute, technical expertise of the clinicians, and the clinical status of the patient

Sustained low-efficiency dialysis (SLED) or extended daily dialysis (EDD) is another increasingly popular dialytic modality of choice for critically ill patients and has the benefits of both continuous and intermittent dialysis methods. The advantages of SLED are good hemodynamic tolerability, high clearance levels of even small solutes, convenient treatment schedules, and cost-effectiveness.

PERITONEAL DIALYSIS

Peritoneal dialysis (PD) is not a favored therapeutic modality for AKI. However, it is the preferred mode of renal replacement therapy in resource-limited settings and the developing world. Advantages include easy portability and access placement, better hemodynamic stability among patients, and the avoidance of systemic anticoagulation and its associated complications. Disadvantages include the risk of injury to the viscera during catheter placement, low levels of solute clearance, metabolic instability in critically ill patients, and the high risk of peritonitis.

DIALYSIS-RELATED COMPLICATIONS

Dialysis-induced complications include hypotension and complement cascade activation during the blood–dialyzer interaction. Hypotension worsens existing AKI because of impaired renal autoregulatory mechanisms. The upregulation of neutrophil adhesion molecules due to blood–dialyzer membrane interaction result in further damage to renal tissues. Unlike cuprophane, biocompatible membranes like polymethylmethacrylate or polyacrylonitrile do not activate complement to any great extent, and the use of biocompatible membranes is associated with improved recovery of renal function and reduced mortality among AKI patients requiring dialysis.

PROGNOSIS

The mortality rate of AKI ranges from 20 to 50%, and up to 70% in the ICU and surgical setting. Advanced age, severe underlying disease, preexisting poor nutritional status, and multisystem organ failure are associated with increased mortality. About 10–20% who suffer AKI will require maintenance dialysis. Infection, cardiorespiratory complications, and underlying disease states are the major causes of death in patients with AKI, rather than AKI itself. The availability of health care in a given country greatly influences the prognosis for AKI.

CONSULTATION

Nephrology consultation is appropriate in AKI when the cause is unclear after initial testing has been performed; if assistance is required with assessment and management of volume status; if intrinsic renal disease, such as glomerulonephritis or AIN, is suspected, and renal biopsy may be needed for diagnosis; and if an indication for dialysis is present, such as refractory fluid overload, severe metabolic acidosis, hyperkalemia, pericarditis, mental status changes, or overdose with a dialyzable toxin or drug.

DISCHARGE CONSIDERATIONS

Hospitalized patients who suffer AKI have a higher mortality both in-hospital and after discharge, even when compared to otherwise similar control populations. Patients who survive AKI should have close outpatient follow-up, with clinical assessment and measurement of serum creatinine and electrolytes. Patients should be warned to avoid dehydration and drugs that may worsen renal function, such as NSAIDs. Drug doses should be adjusted for estimated GFR. Patients who appear likely to need dialysis in the near future should be told to avoid phlebotomy and intravenous placement in one arm to preserve it for graft or fistula creation.

QUALITY IMPROVEMENT

When reviewing the care of patients who develop AKI in the hospital, an assessment should be made of the adequacy of preventive measures. Was there untreated hypovolemia, hypotension, or infection? Was renal function evaluated before surgery? Were nephrotoxic drugs used when there were alternative agents? If radiocontrast agents were given, was their use essential? Did the patient receive prophylactic measures for radiocontrast nephropathy, such as aggressive hydration, N-acetylcysteine, and bicarbonate? Was the diagnosis of AKI recognized in a timely fashion?

Suggested quality measures in the management of AKI include whether a urinalysis, renal ultrasonography, urine creatinine, and electrolytes were obtained; whether volume status was properly assessed and managed; whether nephrology consultation was obtained, if appropriate; whether dialysis was initiated when necessary; whether drug dosing was adjusted for renal function and nephrotoxic medications discontinued; and whether appropriate nutritional support was provided.

CONCLUSION

AKI is associated with significant morbidity and mortality and accounts for 1% of all hospital admissions in the United States. AKI can occur due to pre-renal, intrinsic renal or post-renal causes. Maintenance of the volume status, identification and elimination of nephrotoxins, correction of electrolytes, uremia and acid-base disorders are the salient therapeutic goals in the management of AKI. Prompt nephrology consultation is required when these goals become challenges in treating AKI. Renal replacement therapy should be considered and initiated in consultation with the nephrologist when needed. In summary, early clinical diagnosis and interventions are the key objectives for achieving optimal outcomes in AKI.

SUGGESTED READINGS

Anderson S, Eldadah B, Halter JB, et al. Acute kidney injury in older adults. *J Am Soc Nephrol.* 2011;22:28–38.

Himmelfarb J, Ikizler TA. Acute kidney injury: changing lexicography, definitions, and epidemiology. *Kidney Int.* 2007;71:971–976.

Lafrance JP, Miller DR. Acute kidney injury associates with increased long-term mortality. *J Am Soc Nephrol.* 2010;21:345–352.

Molitoris BA, Levin A, Warnock DG, et al. Improving outcomes from acute kidney injury. *J Am Soc Nephrol.* 2007;18:1992–1994.

Pisoni R, Wille KM, Tolwani AJ. The epidemiology of severe acute kidney injury: from BEST to PICARD. *Nephron Clin Pract.* 2008;109:c188–c191.

Vaidya VS, Ferguson MA, Bonventre JV. Biomarkers of acute kidney injury. *Annu Rev Pharmacol Toxicol.* 2008;48:463–493.

Waikar SS, Liu KD, Chertow GM. Diagnosis, epidemiology and outcomes of acute kidney injury. *Clin J Am Soc Nephrol.* 2008;3:844–861.

CHAPTER 247

Calcium Disorders

Elizabeth H. Holt, MD, PhD
John P. Bilezikian, MD

Key Clinical Questions

1. How is serum calcium normally regulated?
2. What are the causes of hypercalcemia in hospitalized patients?
3. How is hypercalcemia diagnosed and managed?
4. What causes hypocalcemia in hospitalized patients? How is it diagnosed and managed?

INTRODUCTION

Abnormalities of calcium metabolism are common in hospital practice. Hypercalcemia has a prevalence of 0.1% in the general population and 1% among hospitalized patients. In the inpatient setting, hypercalcemia often portends serious illness, especially malignancy. Hypocalcemia is also common in the hospital, especially in patients with chronic renal failure or sepsis. Hypocalcemia may also be a manifestation of vitamin D deficiency, which has a prevalence of up to 80% on specialized geriatric inpatient units.

CALCIUM METABOLISM

Precise regulation of calcium homeostasis is essential because calcium is critically involved in many physiological activities. It is the major mineral of bone. It also plays major roles in neuronal transmission, muscle contraction, and blood coagulation. Calcium is also required for the functioning of many enzymes, endocrine secretory processes, and biochemical signaling pathways.

NORMAL SERUM CALCIUM LEVELS

A typical laboratory range for serum total calcium concentration is between 8.4 and 10.2 mg/dL. Approximately half of this total amount is bound to albumin, with the remainder in free (ionized) form. The normal free calcium concentration range is 4.5 to 5.3 mg/dL. A small fraction (10%) of circulating calcium is complexed with anions, such as citrate and phosphate.

REGULATION OF CALCIUM HOMEOSTASIS

The three organ systems that together regulate serum calcium are the gastrointestinal tract, kidneys, and skeleton. The two principal regulatory hormones are parathyroid hormone (PTH) and 1,25-dihydroxyvitamin D_3. PTH is a peptide hormone that is secreted from the parathyroid glands in its active full-length configuration, known as PTH(1-84). Its half-life in plasma is very short, on the order of 3 to 5 minutes. The major regulator of PTH secretion is the free calcium concentration in extracellular fluid. Elevated levels of free or ionized calcium promptly block secretion of PTH, while reduced serum calcium levels promptly increase secretion of PTH. 1,25-dihydroxyvitamin D_3 is produced by a sequence of activation steps (**Figure 247-1**). It starts with the generation of cholecalciferol (vitamin D_3) through exposure of skin to ultraviolet light of a specified wavelength (90–315 nm). Cholecalciferol or its plant analogue, ergocalciferol (vitamin D_2) can also be obtained by dietary sources or in nutritional supplements. Cholecalciferol or ergocalciferol is converted in the liver to a hydroxylated form, 25-hydroxyvitamin D_3 or 25-hydroxyvitamin D_2. The hydroxylated forms of vitamin D are further activated to their final products by a second hydroxylation step in the kidney leading to 1,25-dihydroxyvitamin D_2 or D_3. Both dihydroxylated forms of vitamin D are active in human subjects, although there is controversy over whether vitamin D_3 is more potent than vitamin D_2. PTH maintains serum calcium concentrations by conserving calcium that has been filtered at the kidney glomerulus and by mobilizing calcium from bone. 1,25-dihydroxyvitamin D maintains serum calcium by facilitating absorption of calcium from the gastrointestinal tract and, like PTH, mobilizing calcium from bone. Under normal conditions, the amount of calcium absorbed in the gut (approximately 150–200 mg/d) is matched by the amount of calcium eliminated by the kidney. At the dynamic

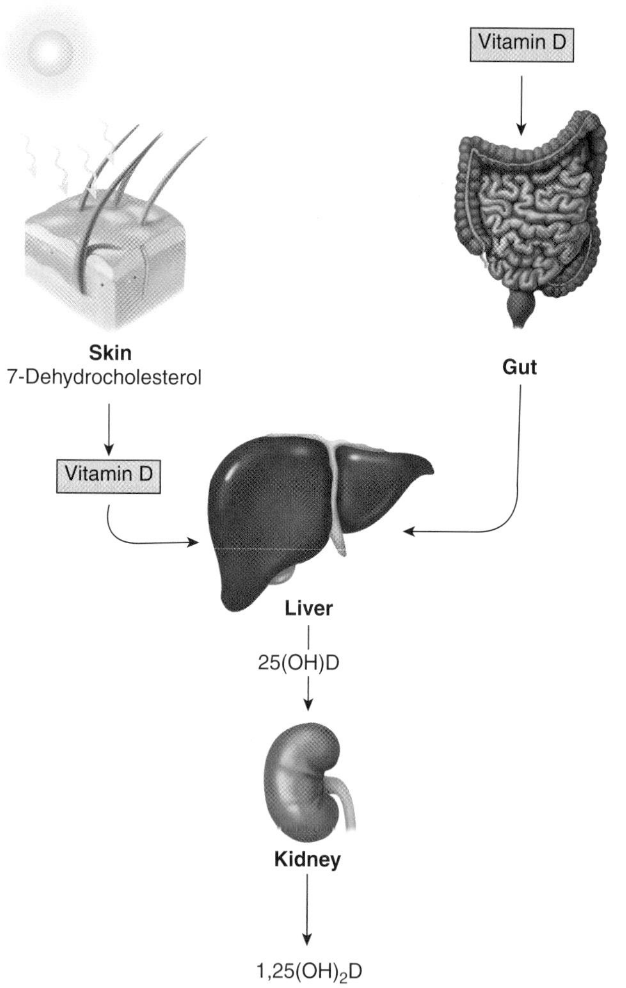

Figure 247-1 *Vitamin D synthesis and activation. Vitamin D is synthesized in the skin in response to ultraviolet radiation and is also absorbed from the diet. It is then transported to the liver, where it undergoes 25-hydroxylation. This metabolite is the major circulating form of vitamin D. The final step in hormone activation, 1-hydroxylation, occurs in the kidney. (Reproduced, with permission, from Fauci AS, Braunwald E, Kasper DL, et al. Harrison's Principles of Internal Medicine. 17th ed. New York: McGraw-Hill; 2008, Fig. 346-4).*

skeletal interface, as much as 500 mg of calcium is turned over daily. This process is in a steady state, with net calcium neither gained nor lost. Thus, under normal circumstances, there are no significant fluctuations in body calcium stores, nor is there any major change in circulating serum calcium concentrations.

Changes in free or ionized calcium concentration are registered virtually instantly by parathyroid cells via the calcium-sensing receptor (CaSR). The receptor is located on the parathyroid cell surface, where its extracellular domain senses binding of calcium ions. The Ca^{2+}-CaSR complex uses a G-protein coupled pathway to transmit the signal to the interior of the cell. Subsequent fluctuations in intracellular calcium stores regulate PTH gene transcription. If the circulating calcium concentration rises, the Ca^{2+}-CaSR complex leads to a rise in intracellular calcium, inhibiting both PTH secretion and synthesis. If the serum calcium concentration falls, the Ca^{2+}-CaSR complex sends a reduced signal to the cell, leading to an increase in PTH secretion and synthesis.

1,25-dihydroxyvitamin D decreases PTH production, although not as powerfully as does the ionized calcium signal. There is a stronger interaction between levels of 25-hydroxyvitamin D and PTH. Their relationship is an inverse one, with PTH levels rising when 25-hydroxyvitamin D levels fall below approximately 25–30 ng/mL. In turn, increased PTH stimulates the 1-alpha hydroxylase enzyme in the kidney that is responsible for the conversion of 25-hydroxyvitamin D to 1,25-dihydroxyvitamin D (**Figure 247-2**). When PTH levels are elevated (ie, primary hyperparathyroidism), 1,25-dihydroxyvitamin D levels increase. When PTH levels are low (ie, hypoparathyroidism), 1,25-dihydroxyvitamin D levels are typically low. The three organ systems (bone, gastrointestinal tract, and kidneys) and the two calcium-regulating hormones (PTH and 1,25-dihydroxyvitamin D) work together to maintain normal calcium homeostasis. When they are not perturbed by disease or by the aging process, they are an exquisitely sensitive and effective servomechanism.

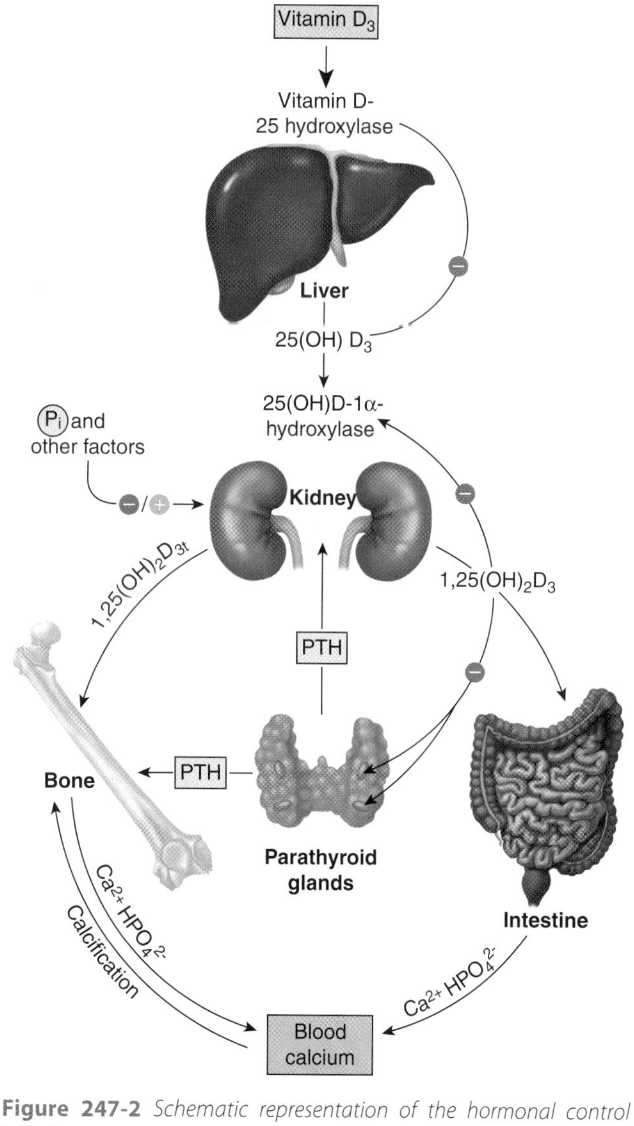

Figure 247-2 *Schematic representation of the hormonal control loop for vitamin D metabolism and function. A reduction in the serum calcium below 2.2 mmol/L (8.8 mg/dL) increases secretion of parathyroid hormone (PTH), mobilizing additional calcium from bone. PTH promotes the synthesis of 1,25(OH)2D in the kidney, which, in turn, stimulates the mobilization of calcium from bone and intestine, and regulates the synthesis of PTH by negative feedback. (Reproduced, with permission, from Fauci AS, Braunwald E, Kasper DL, et al. Harrison's Principles of Internal Medicine. 17th ed. New York: McGraw-Hill; 2008, Fig. 346-5).*

LABORATORY MEASUREMENT OF BLOOD CALCIUM

The measurement of serum calcium may be helpful when a disorder of calcium metabolism is suspected. However, there are many disorders of calcium metabolism, such as osteoporosis or Paget disease of bone, in which the serum calcium concentration is typically normal. Serum measurements may be performed by spectrophotometry or by atomic absorption spectrophotometry, with the latter yielding more accurate measurements. Spuriously high readings may occur if the tourniquet is in place too long before blood is drawn and hemoconcentration occurs. Under these circumstances, the measured serum calcium value can rise by as much as 0.4 mg/dL. On the other hand, the sample can read falsely low if the blood sample is obtained from a central, high-flow site via a central venous catheter. For most clinical situations, the total serum calcium is measured. This may need to be corrected for the circulating albumin concentration. For every 1 g/dL reduction in the serum albumin, the total calcium is adjusted upward by 0.8 mg/dL. This may be calculated as follows:

$$\text{Corrected total calcium} = \text{measured total calcium} + 0.8\,(4.0 - \text{serum albumin})$$

In theory, free or ionized serum calcium is a more accurate physiological measurement than the adjusted total serum calcium concentration, but the sampling technique (the blood has to be free-flowing and not impeded by a tourniquet) and strict anaerobic collection conditions are problematic. Moreover, the measuring instrument has to be in regular use and properly calibrated. Samples have to be measured immediately. These technical issues somewhat limit the clinical utility of the ionized calcium measurement.

HYPERCALCEMIA

Signs and symptoms of hypercalcemia may be absent or subtle, except when calcium is significantly elevated or has increased rapidly. The diagnostic workup of hypercalcemia is usually straightforward (**Figure 247-3**) because two causes, primary hyperparathyroidism and malignancy-associated hypercalcemia, account for approximately 90% of cases. In addition, most individuals with primary hyperparathyroidism are asymptomatic and discovered on routine biochemical screening tests, while most individuals with malignancy-associated hypercalcemia have a known advanced malignancy at the time that hypercalcemia occurs. If the malignancy is not known, it is generally quickly apparent. When neither of these

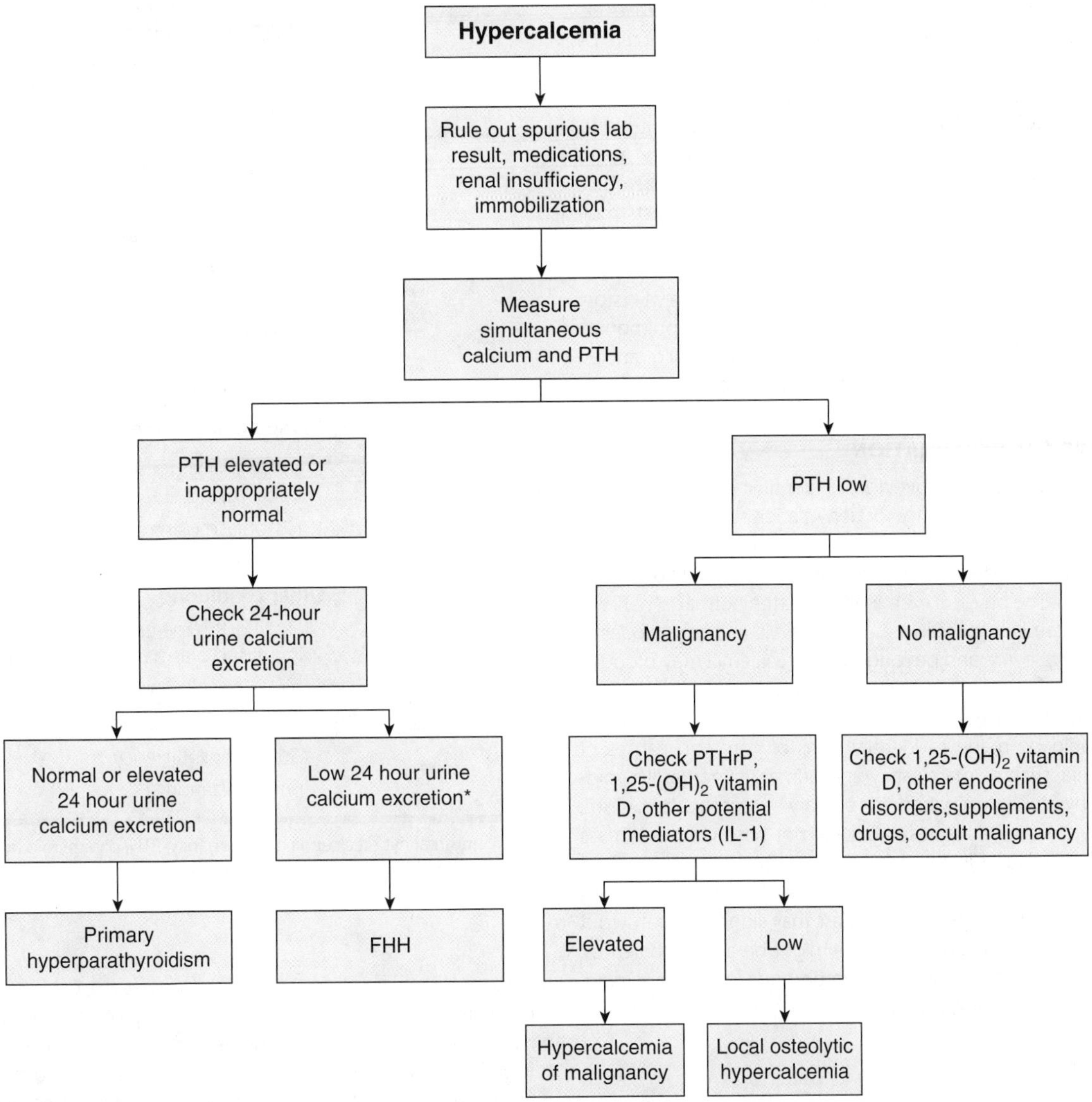

Figure 247-3 *Diagnostic approach to hypercalcemia. FHH, familial hypocalciuric hypercalcemia; PTH, parathyroid hormone; PTHrP, parathyroid hormone-related protein. *A low 24-hour urinary calcium does not necessarily rule out primary hyperparathyroidism.*

two etiologies is readily apparent, identification of the other potential etiologies requires a comprehensive history, physical examination, laboratory tests, and, occasionally, diagnostic imaging studies.

PRESENTING SYMPTOMS AND HISTORY

Many individuals with mild hypercalcemia (serum calcium level < 11 mg/dL) are asymptomatic, although some may report mild fatigue, vague changes in cognitive function, depression, or constipation. Symptomatic manifestations of hypercalcemia become more apparent when the serum calcium concentration is between 12 to 14 mg/dL. These symptoms include anorexia, nausea, weakness, and depressed mental status. As hypercalcemia may induce polyuria and nephrogenic diabetes insipidus, dehydration can occur should the compensatory polydipsia not be able to match urinary water losses. When serum calcium levels rise above 14 mg/dL, profound dehydration, renal dysfunction, and central nervous system changes, such as progressive lethargy, disorientation, and coma, may develop.

In addition to the absolute magnitude of the serum calcium elevation, the rate of increase in serum calcium also influences symptoms. Individuals who are chronically hypercalcemic may have relatively few symptoms, even with serum calcium values up to 15 to 16 mg/dL. In contrast, those whose calcium level has risen abruptly may have symptoms at much more modest calcium levels. Elderly or debilitated patients are more likely to be affected by hypercalcemia than younger individuals.

The medical record may contain clues to etiology. Prescription medications (**Table 247-1**), foods, and vitamin and nutritional supplements should be reviewed. A careful family history might uncover a familial endocrine condition. A history of family members with endocrine tumors of the pituitary or pancreas suggests multiple endocrine neoplasia type 1 syndrome (MEN-1). A family history of pheochromocytoma or medullary thyroid cancer is consistent with MEN-2 syndrome. Patients with sarcoidosis may have a history of unexplained fever, lymphadenopathy, skin rashes, or pulmonary symptoms. Bone pain suggests myeloma or other malignancies, although it may also be a nonspecific finding of hypercalcemia.

TABLE 247-1 Causes of Hypercalcemia

PTH mediated	**Primary hyperparathyroidism**
	Parathyroid adenoma
	Parathyroid hyperplasia
	Parathyroid carcinoma
	Tertiary hyperparathyroidism
	Familial hypocalciuric hypocalcemia
	Lithium
	Thiazide diuretics
PTH-independent	**HHM: PTHrP mediated**
	Squamous carcinoma of the lung, oropharynx, nasopharynx, larynx, and esophagus
	Gynecologic (cervical, ovarian)
	Urologic (renal, transitional cell of bladder)
	Pheochromocytoma
	Pancreatic islet cell tumors
	T-cell lymphoma
	Others
	HHM: 1,25-$(OH)_2$-D_3 mediated
	B-cell lymphoma
	Local osteolytic hypercalcemia
	Multiple myeloma
	Breast carcinoma metastatic to bone
	Lymphoma
	Others
	Medications/supplements
	Vitamin D
	Vitamin A
	Thiazide diuretics
	Calcium-containing antacids (in milk-alkali syndrome)
	Granulomatous diseases
	Sarcoidosis
	Tuberculosis
	Histoplasmosis
	Leprosy
	Other conditions
	Factitious hypercalcemia (due to increased plasma protein levels)
	Acute renal failure
	Severe thyrotoxicosis
	Adrenal insufficiency
	Immobilization

HHM, humoral hypercalcemia of malignancy; PTH, parathyroid hormone; PTHrP, parathyroid hormone-related protein.

THE PHYSICAL EXAMINATION

The physical examination is directed at identifying signs or symptoms of hypercalcemia. Evidence for dehydration such as orthostasis or dry mucous membranes may be present, although hypercalcemia has to be quite marked and prolonged for these physical findings to be appreciated. The physical examination is often normal in patients with hypercalcemia, especially if calcium levels are only modestly elevated. Rarely, severe and prolonged hypercalcemia may produce a visible horizontal deposit of calcium salts on the cornea, a finding called band keratopathy.

Effort should be made to identify signs of common causes of hypercalcemia, such as malignancy and primary hyperparathyroidism. The physical examination in primary hyperparathyroidism, like most hypercalcemic states, is usually not noteworthy. A mass is virtually never found in the neck, because enlarged parathyroid glands are still too small to be felt. However, when the serum calcium is markedly elevated, a neck mass may signify a parathyroid carcinoma. Symptomatic kidney stones might be accompanied by costovertebral tenderness. Enlarged lymph nodes suggest sarcoid, lymphoma, or metastatic carcinoma.

DIAGNOSIS

Laboratory studies

The first step in evaluating hypercalcemia is adjustment for serum albumin. If the corrected serum calcium is elevated, it should be repeated. Renal function should also be assessed, because hypercalcemia may develop or worsen in the setting of acute renal failure. If hypercalcemia is confirmed, the next step is measurement of serum PTH. The PTH level is the most important test for distinguishing between the two most common causes of hypercalcemia, primary hyperparathyroidism and malignancy-associated hypercalcemia (Table 247-1). The so-called "intact" immunochemiluminometric assay for PTH assay primarily measures the intact molecule,

PTH(1-84), and a large circulating fragment that is foreshortened at the amino terminus, PTH(7-84). A more specific assay that measures only PTH(1-84), the "bio-intact" assay, is also available, but it has not shown any clear advantages over the older assay, which has been in clinical use for over 20 years. When the creatinine clearance falls below 60 mL/min, these assays may begin to show elevations in PTH due to the accumulation of inactive fragments, and also perhaps due to increased secretory activity of the parathyroids (secondary hyperparathyroidism).

When the parathyroid glands are functioning normally, hypercalcemia should suppress PTH levels. Hypercalcemia is said to be PTH-mediated if serum calcium is elevated, and the PTH level is high or inappropriately normal. In this latter situation, one is usually dealing with primary hyperparathyroidism, although familial hypocalciuric hypercalcemia (FHH) and medication-induced hypercalcemia, as from thiazide diuretics or lithium, can also be associated with elevated PTH levels. When PTH levels are appropriately suppressed in hypercalcemia, the differential diagnosis includes malignancy, granulomatous disease, medications, milk-alkali syndrome, thyrotoxicosis, and adrenal insufficiency.

Other recommended tests in the evaluation of hypercalcemia include serum electrolytes and 25-hydroxyvitamin D. Levels of 25-hydroxyvitamin D typically exceed 150 ng/mL in vitamin D toxicity due to excess intake. Levels this high cannot be achieved by sun exposure alone. High 1,25-$(OH)_2D$ levels may be seen in any granulomatous disease, particularly sarcoidosis or certain lymphomas. Inorganic phosphorus measurement may be helpful, as a low-normal serum phosphate is often seen in primary hyperparathyroidism, while high phosphate may be seen in vitamin D intoxication. An elevated serum creatinine may indicate dehydration, or true renal dysfunction due to renal deposition of calcium salts or other causes. An elevated alkaline phosphatase level suggests elevated bone turnover. This may be confirmed by a bone-specific alkaline phosphatase measurement, or other indices of bone turnover, such as serum osteocalcin, serum C-terminal collagen peptide measurement, or urinary N-terminal collagen peptide. Most forms of hypercalcemia are accompanied by hypercalciuria (24-hour urine calcium excretion >4 mg/kg/24 h). However, in primary hyperparathyroidism, renal calcium excretion is lower than expected for the degree of hypercalcemia, because PTH conserves filtered calcium in the distal renal tubule.

Additional tests

Other diagnostic studies are dictated by clinical circumstances. A shorted QT_c interval can be seen on the electrocardiogram, particularly if the hypercalcemia has occurred over a short period of time. Bone mineral density (BMD) by dual energy x-ray absorptiometry (DXA) can be helpful. In primary hyperparathyroidism, there is a typical pattern of BMD with relative preservation of cancellous bone, as in the lumbar spine, and preferential reduction in cortical bone, as in the femoral neck and distal third of the radius. Abdominal imaging studies (CT or ultrasound) may identify renal stones or nephrocalcinosis. Serum and urine protein electrophoresis should be obtained if myeloma is suspected. Skeletal radiographs may reveal lytic lesions of multiple myeloma or other malignancies. Skeletal radiographs in primary hyperparathyroidism may show subperiosteal bone resorption or brown tumors of bone, but are rarely needed for diagnosis at present.

CAUSES OF PTH-MEDIATED HYPERCALCEMIA

Primary hyperparathyroidism

Elevation of both the serum calcium and PTH concentrations, in the absence of lithium use or low urinary calcium excretion as seen in familial hypocalciuric hypercalcemia, supports a diagnosis of primary hyperparathyroidism. In this condition, PTH levels are usually within 1.5 to 2.0 times above the upper limit of normal. Extremely high levels of PTH raise the specter of parathyroid carcinoma. Typically, primary hyperparathyroidism is associated with mild hypercalcemia, within 1 mg/dL above the upper limit of normal. The PTH level may be elevated, but may also fall in the upper portion of the normal range, which is inappropriate in hypercalcemia. Normocalcemic primary hyperparathyroidism is a new diagnostic entity applied to patients whose total and free serum calcium levels are normal, but in whom the PTH level is consistently elevated. In the absence of a secondary cause for elevated PTH levels, it is felt that these individuals have an early form of primary hyperparathyroidism.

Primary hyperparathyroidism is the most common cause of hypercalcemia in outpatients. The incidence of primary hyperparathyroidism is estimated to be approximately 21.6 per 100,000 person-years. The mean age at diagnosis is in the sixth decade of life, and there is a female-to-male ratio of 2:1. The clinical manifestations of primary hyperparathyroidism depend largely on the severity of the hypercalcemia. When primary hyperparathyroidism was first described more than 80 years ago, most patients presented with biochemically advanced disease, and overt radiographic abnormalities of bone (osteitis fibrosa cystica) or kidneys (nephrolithasis or nephrocalcinosis). Since the introduction more than 40 years ago of automated multichannel auto-analyzers for measuring serum chemistry, primary hyperparathyroidism is most often diagnosed by routine blood testing, well before the development of other signs or any symptoms. It also may be uncovered during the evaluation of osteoporosis or during the workup of renal stone disease. The most common clinical presentation today is mild asymptomatic hypercalcemia. In 75% to 80% of cases, a solitary, benign parathyroid adenoma is present. Hyperplasia involving multiple parathyroid glands is found in 15% to 20% of cases, and parathyroid carcinoma is present in less than 0.5%. On occasion, double adenomas are found. Patients with MEN-1 or MEN-2 usually have parathyroid hyperplasia involving all parathyroid glands.

Parathyroid surgery is always indicated in symptomatic primary hyperparathyroidism, unless there are medical contraindications. The role of parathyroid surgery in asymptomatic primary hyperparathyroidism is more controversial. According to the guidelines of the Third International Workshop on the Management of Asymptomatic Primary Hyperparathyroidism, indications for surgery in asymptomatic patients include a serum calcium >1 mg/dL above the upper limit of normal; creatinine clearance <60 mL/min; T-score <−2.5 at lumbar spine, hip, or distal third of the radius; and age <50. Patients who do not meet these guidelines can be followed expectantly. Thiazide diuretics and lithium should be avoided. Dietary calcium should not be restricted, because such restriction may promote further elevation of PTH, and possibly have adverse effects on bone mass. In patients who are vitamin D deficient, cautious replacement of vitamin D is advised. Patients should maintain hydration. Bisphosphonates increase lumbar spine BMD in primary hyperparathyroidism, without a major effect on the serum calcium concentration. The calcimimetic, cinacalcet, reduces the serum calcium in primary hyperparathyroidism without having a major effect on BMD. Neither alendronate nor cinacalcet has been approved by the Food and Drug Administration (FDA) for use in primary hyperparathyroidism. Cinacalcet has been approved by the FDA for use in parathyroid cancer.

Lithium can change the set point for the calcium-sensing receptor on the parathyroid gland, such that a higher serum calcium concentration is needed to inhibit PTH secretion. This can lead to mild biochemical abnormalities, such as high levels of calcium and high-normal to elevated PTH levels, that mimic primary hyperparathyroidism, but do not require medical intervention.

Thiazide-associated hypercalcemia also occurs. Many patients with hypercalcemia on thiazides probably have primary hyperparathyroidism. When thiazide therapy is discontinued, the hypercalcemia often persists, and the diagnosis of primary hyperparathyroidism is made.

Familial hypocalciuric hypercalcemia

Familial hypocalciuric hypercalcemia, also known as benign familial hypercalcemia, is a rare genetic condition caused by inactivating mutations in the CaSR. This results in insensitivity of the parathyroid cell to ambient serum calcium, a higher set point for the extracellular ionized calcium concentration, and inappropriately normal to mildly elevated PTH levels. Patients with FHH have chronic asymptomatic hypercalcemia, associated with very low urinary calcium excretion. The relatively low urinary calcium excretion in FHH helps distinguish it from primary hyperparathyroidism, although low urinary calcium excretion may also occur in individuals with primary hyperparathyroidism. A family history of asymptomatic, stable mild hypercalcemia, especially in individuals younger than 40 years, is suggestive of FHH. Other evidence for FHH includes the presence of a very low urinary calcium to creatinine clearance ratio (< 0.01), or a history of family members who have undergone noncurative parathyroidectomy for presumed primary hyperparathyroidism. When FHH is suspected, further evaluation is necessary, such as screening of other family members for hypercalcemia. Genetic testing for FHH is available at select centers and may be appropriate in some cases. Sometimes it can be exceedingly difficult to distinguish FHH from primary hyperparathyroidism.

Tertiary hyperparathyroidism

Conditions that are associated with low serum calcium are usually also associated with chronically elevated PTH levels, which is an appropriate physiological response. This is called secondary hyperparathyroidism. The rise in PTH may be sufficient to restore the serum calcium to normal, or calcium may remain low or in the low normal range. Secondary hyperparathyroidism is not a hypercalcemic state. Common causes of secondary hyperparathyroidism include vitamin D deficiency, intestinal malabsorption of calcium or vitamin D, renal-based hypercalciuria, severe nutritional calcium deficiency, and especially chronic renal insufficiency. Correction of the underlying cause usually returns serum PTH concentrations to normal. The return of the PTH to normal may be relatively rapid, if the inciting condition is of relatively recent onset, or it can be protracted, if the associated condition has been longstanding. In patients with prolonged secondary hyperparathyroidism, the reactive state can become semiautonomous, leading to hypercalcemia. This is known as tertiary hyperparathyroidism. It is most often seen in patients with poorly controlled chronic kidney disease. Tertiary hyperparathyroidism is usually associated with hyperplasia of multiple glands, but may also be caused by a parathyroid adenoma from a single clone of parathyroid cells.

Further investigations

Most patients with primary hyperparathyroidism have a serum calcium concentration below 11 mg/dL. The serum phosphate tends to be in the low normal range (2.5–3.2 mg/dL). A non-anion gap hyperchloremic acidosis from a PTH-induced defect in bicarbonate resorption is rarely seen. Urinary calcium excretion tends to be in the upper range of normal. Nevertheless, hypercalciuria in primary hyperparathyroidism does not always predispose to renal stones, an interesting observation in view of the fact that in euparathyroid subjects, hypercalciuria is a risk factor for kidney stones. Bone turnover markers tend to be at the upper limit or normal, but occasionally can be frankly elevated.

Once the diagnosis of primary hyperparathyroidism is made, it should be determined whether or not the patient meets guidelines for parathyroidectomy. If the clinical situation is appropriate, consideration should be given to the possibility of one of the MEN syndromes, particularly if the patient is young, or has a personal or family history of a related endocrinopathy. A diagnosis of MEN-1 or MEN-2 should prompt a search for multiple parathyroid gland disease.

CAUSES OF PTH-INDEPENDENT HYPERCALCEMIA

If the serum calcium concentration is elevated but the PTH level is appropriately suppressed, the patient has hypercalcemia due to causes other than hyperparathyroidism, or PTH-independent hypercalcemia. Cancer is the most common cause. When PTH is suppressed and the patient does not have a malignancy, diagnostic considerations extend to other causes of PTH-independent hypercalcemia, including thyrotoxicosis, vitamin D intoxication, sarcoidosis, immobilization, Addison disease, and various drugs and supplements.

In ***hypercalcemia of malignancy***, calcium is usually moderately or severely elevated, and PTH is low or undetectable. Significant dehydration and generalized debility are usually evident, along with other cancer-related symptoms. Usually, the diagnosis of malignancy has already been established when patients become hypercalcemic. Hypercalcemia of malignancy has two forms: humoral hypercalcemia of malignancy (HHM) and local osteolytic hypercalcemia. HHM results from tumor production of a circulating factor with systemic effects on calcium metabolism, acting at the level of skeletal calcium release, renal calcium handling, or intestinal calcium absorption. The usual cause of HHM is parathyroid hormone-related protein (PTHrP). Normally, PTHrP serves as a paracrine factor in tissues such as bone, skin, breast, uterus, placenta, and blood vessels, where it is involved in cellular calcium handling, smooth muscle contraction, and growth and development. The amino terminus of the PTHrP peptide is closely homologous with native PTH, and they share a common receptor. When PTHrP circulates at supraphysiologic concentrations, it induces metabolic effects similar to PTH, activating osteoclasts to resorb bone, decreasing renal calcium output, and increasing renal phosphate clearance.

Tumors that produce HHM by secreting PTHrP are typically squamous cell carcinomas, arising from the lung, esophagus, head and neck, or cervix. Other tumors that may elaborate PTHrP include adenocarcinoma of the breast or ovary, renal carcinoma, transitional cell carcinoma of the bladder, islet cell tumors of the pancreas, T-cell lymphoma, and pheochromocytoma. As tumors that produce PTHrP do so in relatively small amounts, the syndrome typically develops in patients with a large tumor burden. It is therefore unusual for HHM to be the presenting feature of a cancer. The diagnosis may be confirmed by a commercially available radioimmunoassay for PTHrP. Care should be taken to ensure that blood for PTHrP levels is drawn and handled correctly to avoid spurious low results. Rarely, HHM is caused by the unregulated production of 1,25-dihyroxyvitamin D, usually by B-cell lymphomas, or other mediators that interfere with calcium homeostasis.

The other major mechanism of malignancy-associated hypercalcemia is the direct invasion of bone by tumor, associated with lytic destruction and calcium release. While this was formerly thought to be a mechanical process, it now appears to be driven by the local elaboration of cytokines leading to osteoclast-mediated bone resorption. In local osteolytic hypercalcemia, PTHrP and calcitriol are within normal limits. Bony metastases are usually obvious on imaging studies. The classic tumor associated with this syndrome is multiple myeloma, although breast cancer and certain lymphomas may also be responsible. Local osteolytic hypercalcemia may be perpetuated by a positive feedback loop, whereby factors produced by bone promote the growth and survival of metastases, and the tumor induces osteoclasts to produce factors promoting tumor growth, bone resorption, and hypercalcemia. Interruption of this positive feedback loop is the rationale for the use of bisphosphonates in the treatment of multiple myeloma.

PTH-independent hypercalcemia also occurs in sarcoidosis, tuberculosis, and other granulomatous diseases. Macrophages in the granuloma convert 25-hydroxyvitamin D to 1,25-dihydroxyvitamin D, via an unregulated 1-α hydroxylase enzyme. 25-hydroxyvitamin D levels are typically not elevated. When serum 25-hydroxyvitamin D levels are elevated, excessive vitamin D intake becomes the more likely etiology. Endocrine conditions that may occasionally lead to hypercalcemia include severe hyperthyroidism, which stimulates bone resorption, and Addison disease, where volume depletion reduces calcium clearance and control of calcium absorption is mitigated by glucocorticoid deficiency.

Immobilization is a stimulus for bone resorption and may increase serum calcium levels, particularly in bedbound hospitalized patients. This is usually seen in persons with high bone turnover, such as adolescents and patients with unrecognized hyperparathyroidism or Paget disease of bone. Drugs and dietary supplements may be associated with hypercalcemia. Vitamin D intoxication and excessive intake of vitamin A, which activates bone resorption, are occasional culprits. Thiazide diuretics may cause hypercalcemia due to enhanced renal retention of calcium. In many cases, this develops in individuals with underlying mild primary hyperparathyroidism.

If investigation of these diagnoses proves fruitless, the rare possibility of occult malignancy should be considered, especially if PTHrP is elevated. Further imaging studies would then be needed for tumor localization, including a plain chest radiograph or a computed tomographic scan of the chest to rule out lung malignancy. If these are unrevealing, consideration should be given to otolaryngoscopic examination, esophagoscopy, or CT of the abdomen, followed by radiographic or endoscopic evaluation of the genitourinary tract if necessary.

PRACTICE POINT

- In the early 20th century, the Chicago physician Bertram Sippy grew rich and nationally famous because of his "Sippy diet" for peptic ulcers—a regimen of milk, cream, eggs, and cereal 3 times a day, punctuated by aggressive antacid therapy with hourly sodium bicarbonate and magnesium hydroxide. This may or may not have been very effective for ulcers, but some patients certainly did develop severe hypercalcemia, in what became known as milk-alkali syndrome. Patients developed a metabolic alkalosis, which favors renal reabsorption of calcium, and the resulting hypercalcemia would produce renal vasoconstriction and a drop in GFR, leading to further increases in serum calcium. Up to one-third of these patients had chronic renal failure. Milk-alkali syndrome became rare with the introduction of H2-blockers and proton pump inhibitors for peptic ulcer disease. However, a similar disorder is seen increasingly in postmenopausal women who consume large amounts of supplemental calcium carbonate and vitamin D for the prevention of osteoporosis. Pregnant or bulimic women with metabolic alkalosis from emesis who are taking calcium and vitamin D are also at risk. It has been suggested that the disorder be renamed the calcium-alkali syndrome. Treatment is volume expansion with saline, cessation of alkali intake, and limitation of calcium supplementation.

TABLE 247-2 Treatment of Hypercalcemia

Intravenous fluids
Normal saline
Loop diuretic
Furosemide intravenous (titrated to response, if necessary)
Medications
Bisphosphonates
• Pamidronate (30–90 mg IV)
• Zoledronic acid (4 mg IV)
Calcitonin (4 IU/kg SC every 12 hours)
Prednisone (20–100 mg orally daily or equivalent)—in selected situations
Plicamycin (15–25 μg/kg IV)—no longer used
Gallium nitrate (200 mg/m^2/day infusion over 5 days)—no longer used
Other interventions
Decrease calcium and vitamin D intake (if causative)
Maintain adequate oral hydration
Primary therapy directed at tumor
Chemotherapy
Radiation
Surgery

TREATMENT OF HYPERCALCEMIA

Hypercalcemia that requires urgent management is usually due to malignancy, rather than a parathyroid disorder. However, primary hyperparathyroidism occasionally can present with severe hypercalcemia against a background of mild, asymptomatic disease. Urgent management of hypercalcemia includes aggressive rehydration, bisphosphonate therapy to decrease bone resorption, and elimination of contributing factors, such as calcium or vitamin D supplements, thiazide diuretic therapy, and immobilization. Second-line therapies include calcitonin to increase renal calcium excretion, and glucocorticoids to diminish intestinal calcium absorption.

Saline hydration

Most patients with emergent hypercalcemia are dehydrated due to anorexia and polyuria. Intravascular volume should be aggressively restored with intravenous normal saline, with an initial bolus of 500 to 1000 mL, followed by maintenance fluids at a rate of 200 mL per hour or more, depending on the patient's renal function and cardiac reserve (**Table 247-2**). Typically, patients require 3 to 4 L for rehydration in the first 24 hours. Patients need careful monitoring of fluid intake and output to prevent fluid overload. Normal saline dilutes serum calcium, and facilitates calciuresis by increasing glomerular filtration rate and the amount of filtered calcium, and decreasing tubular calcium reabsorption. Administration of furosemide or other loop diuretics to further promote calcium excretion may be considered after intravascular volume is restored. However, the use of loop diuretics to treat hypercalcemia has not been studied in randomized controlled trials, and may not be superior to vigorous use of saline alone. Thiazide diuretics should be avoided, as they enhance calcium reabsorption.

Bisphosphonates

The major target of medical management in hypercalcemia is osteoclast-mediated bone resorption. In severe hypercalcemia, a pharmacologic approach to inhibit osteoclast action is warranted. First line therapy is an intravenous bisphosphonate, such as pamidronate or zoledronic acid. Pamidronate is administered in a dosage of 30 to 90 mg intravenously over several hours. Serum calcium levels should decline in 24 to 48 hours, although the maximal effect may not be evident for several days. Zoledronic acid is given at a dosage of 4 mg intravenously over no less than 15 minutes. It appears to have a greater potency and a longer duration of action than pamidronate. The need for repeat treatment with either pamidronate or zoledronic acid depends on the aggressiveness of the underlying malignancy. The first dose of intravenous bisphophonates may be associated with fever, headache, arthralgias, and myalgias. Intravenous bisphosphonates should be used with caution in the setting of renal dysfunction. Dose reduction of zoledronic acid is recommended for creatinine clearance below 60 ml/min, and its use in patients with creatinine clearance below 30 ml/min is not recommended. Pamidronate may be used with caution in patients with renal insufficiency, but the dose should be infused slowly, over 4 to 6 hours. The newer bisphophonate ibandronate may be associated with a lower risk of nephrotoxicity than other intravenous agents.

Other approaches to emergent hypercalcemia

The action of intravenous bisphosphonate is not immediate. If there is a need to reduce the serum calcium quickly, the combined use of subcutaneous calcitonin (4 IU /kg every 12 hours) and intravenous bisphosphonate has become popular. Although rather weak, calcitonin acts rapidly, probably by facilitating urinary calcium excretion. The combination of a short acting and long acting anticalcemic can be very effective in managing these patients. In severe or refractory cases, hemodialysis against a low-calcium bath may be employed. Plicamycin and gallium nitrate are treatments of largely historical interest, because of either toxicities (plicamycin) or ineffectiveness (gallium nitrate).

Glucocorticoids

In multiple myeloma, vitamin D intoxication, or disorders associated with the ectopic production of 1,25-dihydroxyvitamin D, such as sarcoidosis and lymphoma, the use of glucocorticoids can be very effective. Glucocorticoids impair vitamin D action, inhibit intestinal calcium absorption, and may have a direct antitumor effect.

Addressing the underlying disorder

Successful management of acute hypercalcemia also requires treating the underlying etiology. When primary hyperparathyroidism is the cause, parathyroid surgery is indicated when the patient is stable enough to undergo the procedure. In malignancy-associated hypercalcemia, surgery, radiotherapy or chemotherapy may be appropriate. However, because hypercalcemia is often an end-stage complication of malignancy, such interventions may not be warranted.

DISCHARGE CONSIDERATIONS

The discharge plan should include short-term repeat measurements of calcium, creatinine, and other electrolytes in the outpatient setting, and a long-range plan should be in place to prevent recurrence of hypercalcemia, such as repeat bisphosphonate dosing when needed. Patients should be told to seek prompt care if recurrent symptoms of hypercalcemia develop, such as nausea, vomiting, malaise, and polyuria. Patients should be educated as to their underlying condition, particularly if this is a malignancy, in which case outpatient oncology follow-up should be arranged. Consideration should be given to hospice care if hypercalcemia arises in the setting of advanced malignancy with poor prognosis.

HYPOCALCEMIA

Hypocalcemia is a serum calcium level below normal, when corrected for the albumin concentration. As with hypercalcemia, a free (ionized) calcium determination on a correctly collected sample can be useful to confirm hypocalcemia.

PRESENTING SYMPTOMS AND HISTORY

Chronic hypocalcemia, unless severe, is usually asymptomatic. When albumin-adjusted serum calcium levels fall below 7.5 to 8 mg/d, however, signs and symptoms become more likely. They include numbness, paresthesias, and muscle spasms. Severe symptomatology can be manifest as carpal, pedal, or laryngeal spasm and seizures.

A careful history may suggest the cause of hypocalcemia. Important historical features include low dietary calcium and vitamin D intake, minimal sun exposure, gastrointestinal tract disease that may reduce vitamin D absorption, such as chronic pancreatitis, celiac disease, and inflammatory bowel disease, and alcohol, which decreases parathyroid hormone secretion both directly, and also indirectly, by causing magnesium depletion. A family history of hypocalcemia suggests a genetic cause of hypoparathyroidism or an inherited abnormality of vitamin D metabolism. Prior neck surgery or neck irradiation may lead to hypoparathyroidism. A history of adrenal insufficiency and mucocutaneous candidiasis suggests autoimmune polyendocrine syndrome type 1. Acute pancreatitis, rhabdomyolysis, and tumor lysis may lead to tissue precipitation of calcium, and massive blood transfusion may lead to intravascular precipitation of calcium with citrate.

PHYSICAL FINDINGS AND DIAGNOSTIC TESTING

The physical examination is not very sensitive for hypocalcemia. There may be a positive Chvostek sign (ipsilateral contraction of the facial muscles, induced by tapping on the facial nerve at a point about 1 cm below the zygomatic arch and 2 cm anterior to the earlobe). Trousseau sign may be elicited by inflating a blood pressure cuff on the arm above systolic pressure for three minutes. It is considered positive if carpopedal spasm develops, with flexion of the wrist, metacarpophalangeal joints, and thumb, and hyperextension of the fingers (**Figure 247-4**). Patients with these signs of neuromuscular

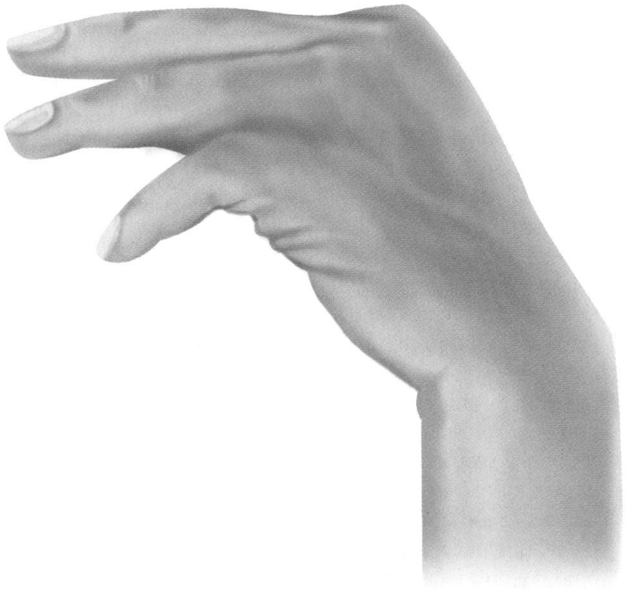

Figure 247-4 *Position of fingers in carpal spasm due to hypocalcemic tetany. (Reproduced, with permission, from Gardner DG, Shoback D. Greenspan's Basic & Clinical Endocrinology. 8th ed. New York: McGraw-Hill; 2007. Fig. 9-18).*

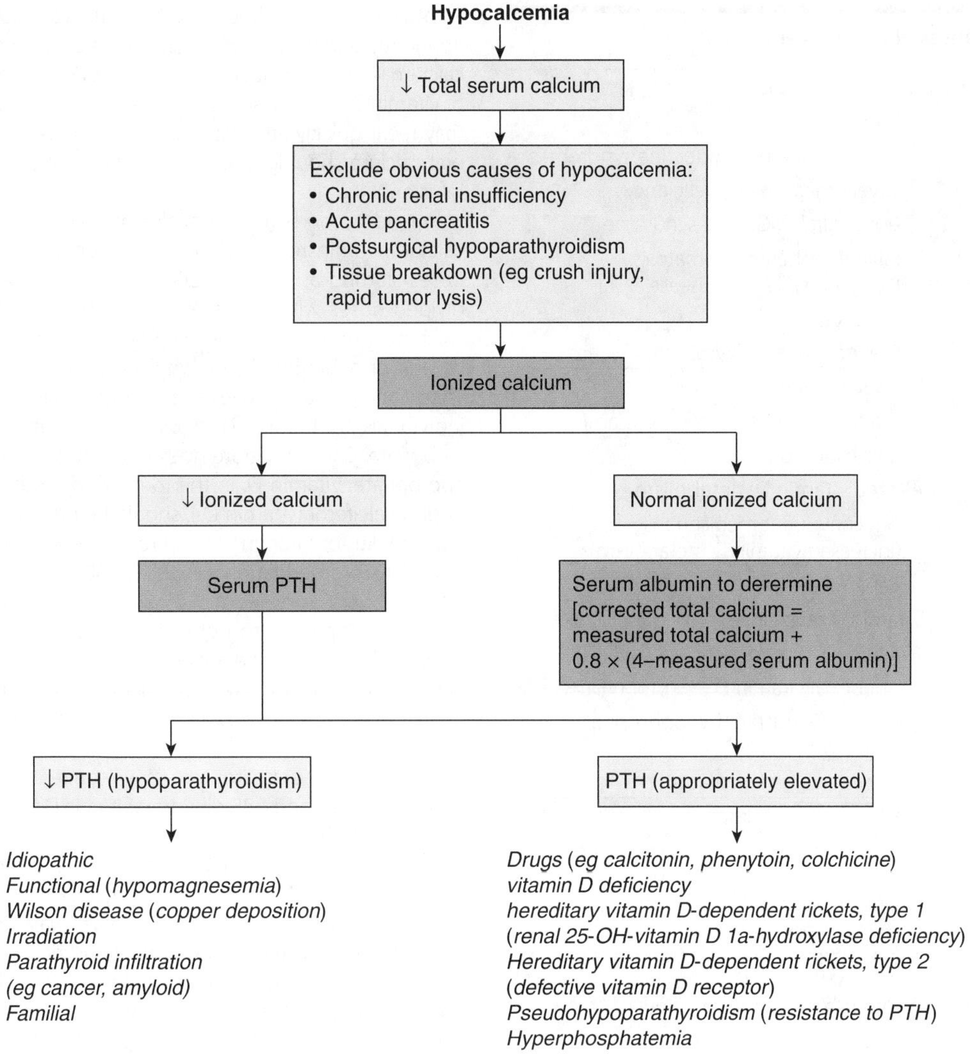

Figure 247-5 *Diagnostic algorithm for hypocalcemia. (Reproduced, with permission, from Nicoll D, McPhee SJ, Pignone M, et al. Pocket Guide to Diagnostic Tests. 5th ed. http://www.accessmedicine.com/pocketDiagnostic.aspx).*

irritability are at risk of frank tetany or seizures. Prolongation of the QT_c interval may be evident on the electrocardiogram.

The serum calcium must be adjusted for albumin, as above, and a low value confirmed with a measurement of serum ionized calcium. Levels of phosphate, magnesium, creatinine, PTH, and 25-hydroxy-vitamin D should be determined. 24-hour urinary calcium may be occasionally helpful. It is low in hypoparathyroidism and vitamin D deficiency, and high in patients with familial hypocalcemia with hypercalciuria, due to activating mutations in the calcium-sensing receptor. Genetic testing is available for some inherited disorders leading to hypocalcemia.

DIFFERENTIAL DIAGNOSIS

After confirming that calcium levels are truly low, exclusion of ***hypoparathyroidism*** by checking the level of PTH is central to the diagnostic workup of hypocalcemia (**Figure 247-5**). The most common causes of hypoparathyroidism are as a complication of thyroid, parathyroid, or other neck surgery, and autoimmune destruction (**Table 247-3**). Autoimmune damage to the parathyroid glands may occur in isolated fashion, or in connection with failure of other endocrine glands, such as premature ovarian failure, hypothyroidism, and Addison disease, and mucocutaneous candidiasis. Infiltration of the parathyroid glands, as may occur in hemochromatosis, Wilson disease, and metastatic cancer, can lead to hypoparathyroidism. Congenital absence of the parathyroid glands may be seen in DiGeorge syndrome. Functional hypoparathyroidism may result from severe hypomagnesemia, because magnesium is necessary for both PTH release and PTH action. This is commonly seen in hospitalized alcoholic patients who are often markedly hypomagnesemic.

The other major category of hypocalcemia includes conditions in which the parathyroid glands respond appropriately to hypocalcemia, and PTH is elevated. In ***vitamin D deficiency***, serum calcium concentrations may be low or in the low normal range, because of compensatory increases in PTH, with secondary mobilization of skeletal calcium and reduction in renal calcium excretion. Clinical manifestations of vitamin D deficiency include osteomalacia, pathologic fractures, falls, and muscle weakness. Vitamin D deficiency has also been linked to autoimmune disease, cancer, and cardiovascular disease. Dietary vitamin D deficiency in the elderly is common, but often overlooked. Other adults at risk for vitamin D deficiency include darker complexion and low sun exposure. Recent reports suggest that vitamin D deficiency may be widely prevalent.

Other causes of hypocalcemia include ***pseudohypoparathyroidism***, a genetic disorder of PTH resistance associated with elevated parathyroid hormone levels, moon facies, short stature, and short fourth metacarpals. In ***acute pancreatitis***, fatty acids released

TABLE 247-3 Causes of Hypocalcemia

PTH deficiency or resistance	**Hypoparathyroidism**
	Postsurgical
	Autoimmune polyendocrine syndromes
	Severe magnesium deficiency
	Congenital: DiGeorge syndrome
	Infiltrative: hemochromatosis, thalassemia, Wilson disease
	PTH resistance
	Pseudohypoparathyroidism
Vitamin D deficiency or resistance	**Nutritional deficiency**
	Insufficient dietary intake of vitamin D
	Malabsorption
	Altered vitamin D metabolism
	Anticonvulsant medications (increased vitamin D metabolism)
	Renal failure
	Vitamin D resistance
	Vitamin D pseudodeficiency (VDDR I)
	Abnormal vitamin D receptor (VDDR II)
	Vitamin D-resistant hypophosphatemic rickets/osteomalacia
	Oncogenic osteomalacia
Iatrogenic	Phosphate supplements
	Bisphosphonates (mainly seen with intravenous preparations in patients who are vitamin D deficient)
	Plicamycin
Miscellaneous conditions	Sepsis, critical illness
	Hypoalbuminemia (factitious)
	Calcium malabsorption
	Hyperphosphatemia
	Acute pancreatitis
	Rhabdomyolysis
	Multiple transfusions of citrate-containing blood products
	Osteoblastic metastases (prostate or breast carcinoma)

PTH, parathyroid hormone.

through the action of pancreatic enzymes complex with calcium. Hypocalcemia due to the formation of calcium phosphate complexes occurs in severe ***hyperphosphatemic states***, such as renal failure, rhabdomyolysis, and tumor lysis. Hypocalcemia may also be seen in patients given ***multiple red blood cell transfusions*** to which calcium chelators have been added to prevent clotting. In patients with ***critical illness***, hypocalcemia is probably multifactorial, arising as a consequence of the release of procalcitonin and other acute phase reactants, hypoalbuminemia, hypomagnesemia, and impaired PTH secretion

TREATMENT OF HYPOCALCEMIA

When hypocalcemia is severe and symptomatic, calcium gluconate should be administered by slow intravenous infusion. A typical calcium infusion is prepared with 10 ampules (100 mL) of 10% calcium gluconate (93 mg elemental calcium/ampule) in 1 L of D_5W, administered at 50 mL/h. For an average-sized person, this is equivalent to 15 mg calcium/kg of body weight. Serum calcium should be tested frequently, and the rate of infusion adjusted accordingly to maintain calcium levels in the low–normal range. Deficiencies in magnesium or vitamin D should also be corrected. In severe cases, hypocalcemia may recur quickly after discontinuation of the calcium infusion, so oral calcium should be administered concurrent with tapering the infusion.

In mild or moderate hypocalcemia, patients may be given oral calcium, adminstered as calcium carbonate or calcium citrate, in doses starting at 1000 to 1500 mg of elemental calcium daily in divided doses with meals. Patients should be instructed to take calcium with a protein meal, particularly patients with hypochlorhydria or achlorhydria, or who are on proton pump inhibitors. The protein meal supplies the acid that may be missing in these individuals, and which is required for the absorption of calcium carbonate. Calcium citrate does not require acid for absorption. If appropriate, vitamin D, in the form of cholecalciferol (vitamin D_3) or ergocalciferol (vitamin D_2), should be provided. Recommended daily intake for vitamin D is currently being revised upward. The official recommendation for adults 50 years and older, 400 to 600 IU/d, is acknowledged by most experts to be inadequate. A popular approach to normalizing vitamin D levels in deficient individuals is to provide a weekly capsule of 50,000 IU for 8 to 12 weeks. This approach requires a prescription for ergocalciferol, because cholecalciferol is currently unavailable by prescription in the United States in this form.

Chronic hypoparathyroidism may require long-term administration of vitamin D and 1,25-dihydroxyvitamin D as needed to maintain normal levels. The goal of therapy is to maintain the serum calcium at a level at which the patient is asymptomatic. To avoid hypercalciuria, serum calcium levels are often maintained in the lower range of normal. Periodic monitoring for hypercalciuria and nephrocalcinosis in these patients may be appropriate. Hypoparathyroidism is the last classic endocrine deficiency disease for which the missing hormone is not available as an approved therapy. However, recent studies have shown promise in the use of recombinant parathyroid hormone (teriparatide) for hypoparathyroidism.

DISCHARGE CONSIDERATIONS

Patients should have repeat measurements of calcium, creatinine, and other electrolytes within 1 to 2 weeks of hospital discharge. Outpatient endocrinology follow-up is appropriate for patients with hypoparathyroidism.

SUGGESTED READINGS

Bilezikian JP, Khan AA, Potts JT Jr. Guidelines for the management of asymptomatic primary hyperparathyroidism: summary statement from the third international workshop. *J Clin Endocrinol Metab.* 2009;94:335–339.

Fraser WD. Hyperparathyroidism. *Lancet.* 2009;374(9684):145–158.

Holick MF. Vitamin D deficiency. *N Engl J Med.* 2007;357:266–281.

Patel AM, Goldfarb S. Got calcium? Welcome to the calcium-alkali syndrome. *J Am Soc Nephrol.* 2010;21:1440–1143.

Perazella MA, Markowitz GS. Bisphosphonate nephrotoxicity. *Kidney Int.* 2008;74:1385–1393.

Shoback D. Clinical practice: hypoparathyroidism. *N Engl J Med.* 2008;359:391–403.

Stewart AF. Clinical practice: hypercalcemia associated with cancer. *N Engl J Med.* 2005;352:373–379.

Wermers RA, Kearns AE, Jenkins GD, Melton LJ 3rd. Incidence and clinical spectrum of thiazide-associated hypercalcemia. *Am J Med.* 2007;120:911.e9-911.e15.

CHAPTER 248

Chronic Kidney Disease and Dialysis

Ursula C. Brewster, MD
Mark Perazella, MD, FACP, FASN

Key Clinical Questions

1. How are the stages of chronic kidney disease defined?
2. What are the different dialysis modalities, and how do patients choose one over another?
3. What is the difference between an arteriovenous fistula and an arteriovenous graft? What are their associated complications?
4. When is it appropriate to initiate dialysis?
5. How are hemodialysis and peritoneal dialysis performed? What are their common complications?
6. What complications are common in hospitalized patients with chronic kidney disease?

INTRODUCTION

Over 26 million Americans, or approximately one in nine adults, have chronic kidney disease (CKD). These patients require special attention from hospitalists because of a high incidence of acute kidney injury (AKI) and other complications during hospitalization. These patients are at risk of AKI not only from known nephrotoxins, such as contrast agents and nonsteroidal anti-inflammatory drugs (NSAIDs), but also from other commonly prescribed agents. Other major issues in the hospital care of these patients include preservation of venous access, electrolyte and acid-base correction, and anemia management. As many of these patients advance to end-stage renal disease (ESRD) requiring dialysis, hospitalists should have a basic understanding of the principles of renal replacement therapy (RRT).

CHRONIC KIDNEY DISEASE

The National Kidney Foundation has defined a staging system for CKD (**Table 248-1**) based on glomerular filtration rate (GFR) as the best marker of kidney function. CKD is defined as an absolute GFR less than 60 cc/min, or structural or functional kidney abnormalities eg, hematuria, proteinuria, abnormal imaging) with a preserved GFR (> 90cc/min). Serum creatinine concentration (sCr) is a poor marker of kidney function, as normal values vary with age, gender, and muscle mass. It is especially inadequate in the setting of AKI. In the early stages of serious kidney injury, the sCr may be falsely reassuring, as it may only rise well after the initial insult. GFR is a better marker of kidney function and is used as the basis for the staging system.

As GFR is not readily measured, mathematical formulae are used to estimate it. Both the Cockcroft-Gault and the Modification of Diet in Renal Disease (MDRD) formulas are commonly used, with many laboratory reports listing estimated GFR (eGFR) (**Table 248-2**). The Cockcroft-Gault formula is simple, but often overestimates kidney function. The MDRD is a more arduous calculation, but is more accurate in patients with advanced CKD. However, it underestimates GFR in patients with near-normal sCr. These formulas are only useful when sCr is in a steady state. When the sCr is rapidly changing, as in acute kidney injury, they are completely inaccurate and should not be used. In that case, a 24-hour urine collection for creatinine clearance (CrCl) is a better indicator of kidney function. A 24-hour urine collection is recommended whenever renally excreted drugs possessing significant toxicity need to be administered.

Despite optimal medical care, patients with advanced CKD often progress to ESRD. When feasible, ESRD is best treated with transplantation. When donors are available, this is done preemptively, and dialysis is avoided. If dialysis seems unavoidable, preparation and discussion should start at least one year in advance, involving the patient, primary care physician, family, nephrologist, and other caregivers. However, some patients require acute dialysis in the hospital, with quick education by hospitalists and nephrology teams.

PREPARATION OF PATIENTS FOR DIALYSIS

DIET EDUCATION

Patients with advanced CKD need instruction about the importance of dietary adherence. Diets for stage 5 CKD are restricted in sodium, potassium, and phosphorus. In the past, CKD patients were told to dramatically limit protein intake, as it was thought that this would slow progression of proteinuric kidney disease. Most experts now

TABLE 248-1 Chronic Kidney Disease Staging System

Stage	Description	GFR (ml/min/1.73 m²)
0	At increased risk	>90
1	Kidney damage with normal or increased GFR	≥90
2	Kidney damage with mild decrease in GFR	60–89
3	Moderate	30–59
4	Severe decrease in GFR	15–29
5	Kidney failure	<15 or dialysis

GFR, glomerular filtration rate.

agree that a modest protein restriction (0.7 g/kg/day) is likely safe, but more restricted diets pose too great a risk of malnutrition. Salt restriction in patients with CKD cannot be overemphasized. Potassium restriction is also important in advanced disease.

DIALYSIS MODALITY CHOICE

Modalities of dialysis that hospitalists should be familiar with include peritoneal dialysis (PD), traditional in-center hemodialysis (HD), home HD, and nocturnal HD (**Table 248-3**). These modalities are discussed in detail in the proceeding section. The choice should be based on dialysis access options, patient lifestyle, and patient support network.

HEMODIALYSIS ACCESS PLANNING

When the need for HD is urgent, dual-lumen dialysis catheters can be placed at the bedside or radiology suite by nephrologists, surgeons, or interventional radiologists. These may be used immediately after confirmation of placement by radiography. The internal jugular and femoral veins are preferred sites. Catheters should not be placed in the subclavian vein, because central venous stenosis may develop, precluding the later use of that upper extremity for surgically created fistulae and grafts. Catheters may be untunneled, or tunneled with subcutaneous cuffs. Tunneling the catheter subcutaneously prior to vein entry decreases the likelihood of skin bacteria reaching the bloodstream and causing infection, and allows these catheters to remain in place for longer periods of time. Catheters are not preferred for long-term vascular access. They have high rates of malfunction and infection (approximately 2 to 4 episodes per 1000 patient days) and are associated with increased patient mortality compared with fistulae or grafts.

Ideally, access for HD is established well in advance of the need to start dialysis, as an arteriovenous fistula (AVF) may need months to mature before it is viable. Patients with CKD should be referred to an experienced access surgeon when their estimated GFR is 20 ml/min/1.73 m², or when they are expected to require dialysis in the next three to six months.

TABLE 248-2 Estimation Formulas of Glomerular Filtration Rate

Cockcroft-Gault equation:

$$\frac{(140 - \text{age}) \times (\text{IBW})}{S_{Cr} \times 72}$$

MDRD equation:

$$170 \times (S_{Cr})^{-0.999} \times (\text{Age})^{-0.176} \times (0.762 \text{ if female}) \times (1.80 \text{ if black}) \times (\text{BUN})^{-0.170} \times (\text{albumin})^{0.318}$$

BUN, blood urea nitrogen; IBW, ideal body weight; MDRD, modification of diet in renal disease; S_{cr}, serum creatinine.
Units: Age in years; Albumin in g/dl; BUN in mg/dl; IBW in kg; S_{Cr} in mg/dl.

TABLE 248-3 Dialysis Modalities

Modality	Description
In-center hemodialysis	Patient goes to a dialysis clinic for treatment, typically three times a week
Home hemodialysis	Patient or partner needles the patient's access, and runs his or her treatments on a compact hemodialysis machine, either daily or a scheduled number of treatments per week
Nocturnal hemodialysis	Patient goes to a dialysis clinic at night, and undergoes longer hemodialysis treatments by skilled nurses overnight during sleep
Continuous ambulatory peritoneal dialysis	Patient does 4 to 6 manual exchanges of dialysate into the abdomen over the course of a 24-hour period
Automated peritoneal dialysis	Peritoneal dialysis is done via an automated machine that cycles fluid in and out of the abdomen over a set period of time (usually 8 to 10 hours), often during sleep

Long-term vascular access for HD requires identification and preservation of suitable veins over time. Fistula require veins greater than 0.3 mm in diameter on ultrasound mapping. *The importance of vein preservation cannot be overemphasized.* Many CKD patients will require HD access and should have their veins protected, particularly while hospitalized. To this end, one upper extremity (usually the nondominant arm) should be spared from blood draws, sphygmomanometers, and intravenous catheters (including peripherally inserted central catheter [PICC] lines). Scarring of veins occurs rapidly, often making future access creation impossible.

Arteriovenous fistulae are preferred over synthetic arteriovenous grafts because of their longer lifespan and lower infection rate. An AVF is made by surgically anastamosing a native artery to a native vein, usually in the forearm or upper arm (**Figure 248-1**). Over time, the vein will "arterialize," so it can withstand thrice-weekly cannulation. Fistula maturation usually requires 6 to 12 weeks. Surgical or percutaneous interventions may be required when maturation is delayed. A successful fistula can last over a decade with low thrombosis and infection rates.

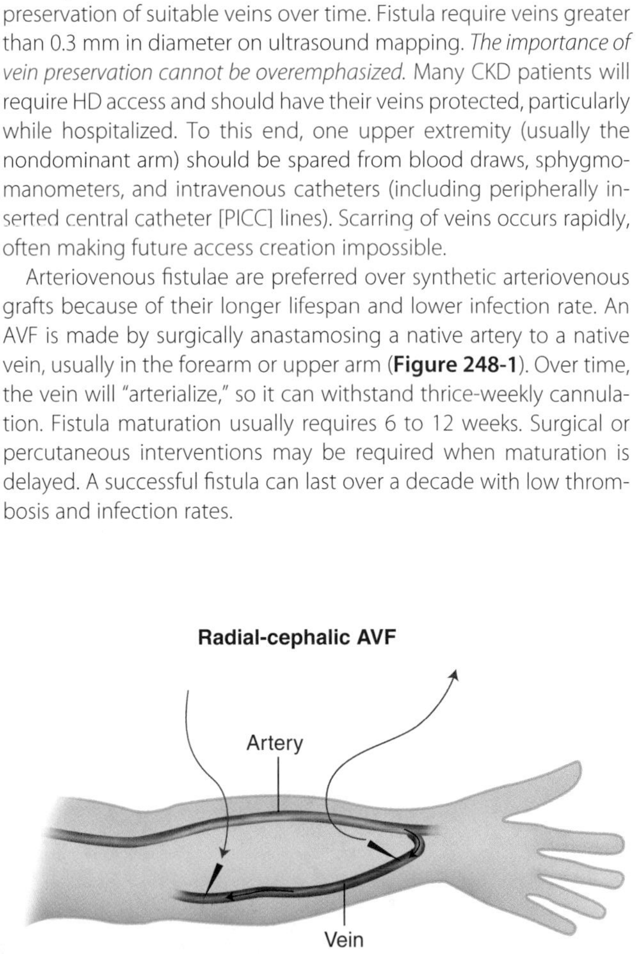

Figure 248-1 *Arteriovenous fistula showing the direct anastamosis between artery and vein in the upper extremity.*

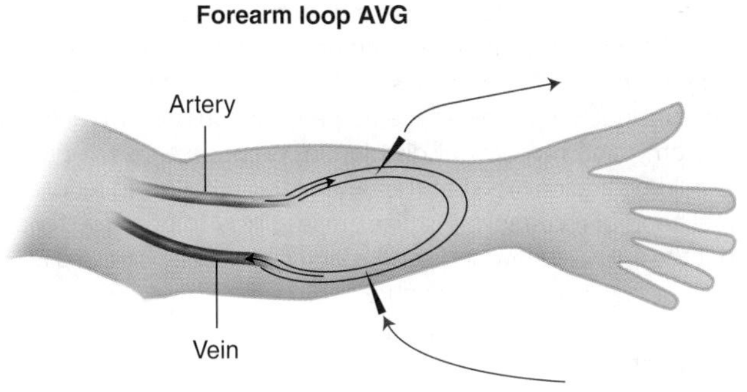

Figure 248-2 *Arteriovenous graft showing artificial graft material (black) placed as a conduit between artery and vein in the upper extremity.*

PRACTICE POINT

- Because many CKD patients will require HD access, clinicians should take the following steps to protect their veins during hospitalization. This means ensuring that one upper extremity (usually the non-dominant arm) is spared from blood draws, sphygmomanometers, and intravenous catheters (including PICC lines). Scarring of veins occurs rapidly, often making future access creation impossible.

If a suitable vein for creation of an AVF is unavailable, an arteriovenous graft (AVG) made of polytetrafluoroethylene (PTFE) or other synthetic material may be interposed between native vessels as an alternative (**Figure 248-2**). An AVG can be used for HD two to four weeks after placement. Unfortunately, synthetic PTFE grafts are not as durable as an AVF. On average, grafts thrombose more often and have lower patency rates. Additionally, because these grafts are made of synthetic material, infection usually requires surgical excision and abandoning the access.

INITIATION OF DIALYSIS

In some patients, CKD slowly progresses and dialysis can be initiated in a predictable fashion. For others, AKI necessitates urgent initiation of treatment.

ACUTE INITIATION

There are several life-threatening scenarios that warrant urgent nephrology consultation and initiation of dialysis, with immediate placement of a double-lumen dialysis catheter for access (**Table 248-4**). These catheters are most often untunneled. In addition, these temporary dialysis catheters are preferred in patients with bacteremias or other endovascular infections. If there are no infectious issues, a tunneled dual-lumen catheter can be placed for dialysis, with lower long-term infection risks.

TABLE 248-4 Acute Indications for Dialysis

Severe metabolic abnormalities (hyperkalemia, hypercalcemia)
Severe acidosis not responsive to bicarbonate therapy
Intoxications and overdoses (ie, methanol, ethylene glycol, lithium, theophylline, salicylates, metformin)
Severe volume overload not responsive to diuretics
Uremia in the setting of chronic renal failure

CHRONIC INITIATION

Dialysis in progressive CKD is undertaken to avoid complications of advanced uremia. Current guidelines (and Medicare reimbursement) recommend the initiation of dialysis when creatinine clearance drops below 10 ml/min. Diabetic patients seem more susceptible to the side effects of uremia, and may require dialysis when the creatinine clearance falls below 15 ml/min. In patients with CKD, physiologic derangements begin well before the need for dialysis. Spontaneous decreases in protein intake, anemia, and altered calcium, phosphorus and PTH homeostasis may begin when creatinine clearance is as high as 30 to 40 ml/min. Early nephrology referral helps manage these early complications of CKD and allows for a smooth transition to dialysis. Patients who have been actively managed by a nephrologist well prior to dialysis have better outcomes than patients seen later in the disease process.

Uremia results from high levels of nitrogenous wastes and other toxins in the blood. Gastrointestinal symptoms such as nausea, vomiting, and anorexia are prominent. Central nervous system (CNS) symptoms include fatigue, confusion, tremors, seizure, and coma. Abnormal platelet function, with a prolonged bleeding time and high risk of hemorrhage, is also common. Classic physical exam findings, such as a pericardial friction rub, asterixis, and wrist or foot drop, may signal the need for more urgent dialysis.

HEMODIALYSIS

Hemodialysis (HD) is based on the diffusion of solutes across a semipermeable membrane down a concentration gradient (**Table 248-5**). Heparinized blood is pumped through a synthetic dialyzer at 300 to 500 cc/min, while individualized dialysate is run countercurrently at 500 to 800 cc/min (**Figure 248-3**). The dialyzer is made of a semipermeable membrane that separates blood and dialysate, and across which solutes and water diffuse. Dialysis replenishes bicarbonate, removes nitrogenous wastes, and balances electrolytes and divalent ions. The dialysis circuit consists of a heparin pump, a blood pump, an air leak detector, and arterial and venous pressure monitors. The dialysis machine alerts staff if it detects blood or air leaks, blood clots, or variability in patient blood pressure and heart rate. Because 30 to 40 gallons of water are used during each dialysis treatment, water purification systems are used to remove bacteria, endotoxin, trace metals, and other contaminants.

The major constituents of the dialysis solution are listed in **Table 248-6**. These are adjusted in the dialysis prescription, depending on the patient's serum potassium, serum calcium, and acid-base balance. The length of the dialysis session is based on measurement of "dialysis adequacy" to ensure the patient is achieving adequate clearance. Solute clearance, determined by the reduction of urea per treatment, is measured regularly by calculating Kt/V,

TABLE 248-5 Definitions

Dialysis	The clearance of small molecules and toxins using diffusion across a native (peritoneal) or synthetic semipermeable membrane
Ultrafiltration	Fluid removal across a semipermeable membrane during dialysis by convection
Hemofiltration	Continuous dialysis therapy in which large amounts of fluid are removed by convection from blood, with concurrent reinfusion of an electrolytic solution
Hemodiafiltration	The combination of hemodialysis and hemofiltration

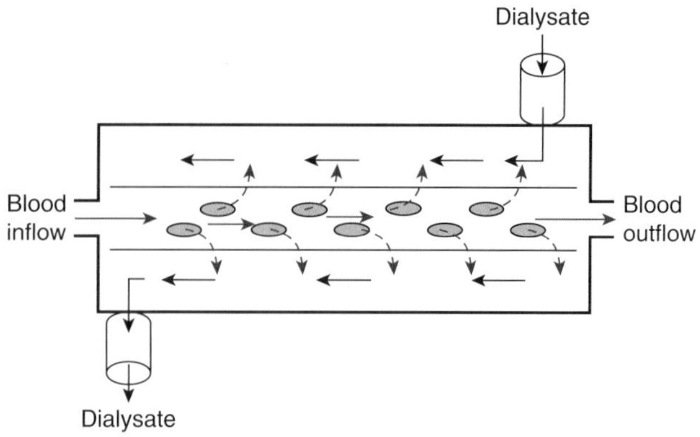

Figure 248-3 *Hemodialysis cartridge.*

where K equals the clearance coefficient, t equals duration/time of each dialysis treatment, and V equals volume of distribution of urea. This is regularly calculated in every HD patient, with a targeted goal of 1.4 or greater. If a patient's value falls short, often time, the numerator of the equation, is increased to improve clearance. In general, patients require between three and four hours of dialysis per treatment for adequate clearance. Larger patients need more time. Dialysis adequacy is also influenced by inadequate blood flow through a vascular access, small dialyzer surface area, and missed or early termination of dialysis sessions by patients. Before HD can be initiated, vascular access that will provide adequate blood flow (300 to 500 cc/min) must be in place.

VASCULAR ACCESS COMPLICATIONS

Bleeding

Hemorrhage from HD access can be caused by needle laceration or intrinsic access problems. Outflow stenosis can increase pressure within the access and predispose patients to prolonged bleeding after needle removal. Needles repeatedly placed at the same site in the access can weaken it, leading to an aneurysm in a fistula or a pseudoaneurysm in a graft. These defects may rupture, leading to exsanguination. Therefore, needle sites must be rotated within the access. Bleeding also occurs in the setting of infection, particularly in AVGs. Spontaneous bleeding from an AVG requires surgical repair or excision to prevent recurrent bleeding. If a fistula is lacerated and bleeds, it can sometimes be salvaged with rest, unlike an AVG. Repair will be necessary if an aneurysm is present. Immediate surgical consultation is mandatory in any case of access site bleeding.

Thrombosis

Clot formation is the most common cause of arteriovenous access loss. Sluggish blood flow from acquired venous stenosis is the usual cause. AVGs are especially prone to thrombose, as they often develop neointimal hyperplasia and venous stenosis at anastomosis sites. Access salvage in the setting of thrombosis is most successful early, in the first 24 to 48 hours. Treatments for established thrombosis include thrombolytic agents, percutaneous or surgical thrombectomy, and mechanical dissolution. Venous stenosis, if present, should be angioplastied at the time of thrombolysis to reduce the likelihood of recurrence. Fistulae are less likely to become stenotic, but the arterial inflow and venous outflow must be assessed at the time of the declotting procedure.

TABLE 248-6 Common Components of Dialysate Bath on Hemodialysis

	Concentration	
Component	Range	Typical
Sodium (mEq/L)	135–155	140
Potassium (mEq/L)	0–4	2
Calcium (mEq /L)	0–3.5	2.5
Bicarbonate (mEq/L)	25–40	35
Glucose (mg/dL)	100–200	200

Infection

Dialysis catheters have high rates of infection and bacteremia. Empiric antibiotic therapy should include vancomycin and a second intravenous antibiotic active against gram-negative bacilli. However, antibiotics alone are not effective at curing catheter infections. This is particularly true of dialysis catheters infected with *Staphylococcus aureus, Candida* species, and *Pseudomonas*. These should always be removed, and a nontunneled catheter should be inserted at another site. (If no other viable access sites exist, the catheter should be exchanged over a guidewire as a last resort.) Patients with *Staphylococcus aureus* bacteremia are at high risk of metastatic infection, and they should be monitored for the development of complications such as endocarditis, epidural abscess, osteomyelitis, septic arthritis, endophthalmitis, and meningitis.

Patients with catheter infection with less virulent organisms, such as coagulase-negative staphylococci, can be treated with intravenous antibiotics initially. If symptoms do not resolve in 48 to 72 hours, the catheter should be removed. If the patient improves clinically, the infected catheter can be exchanged over a guidewire, and intravenous antibiotics can be continued. Alternatively, in those patients who improve rapidly with antibiotics, the catheter can be left in place and intravenous antibiotics can be continued, together with adjunctive antibiotic lock therapy (antibiotic solutions left in the catheter lumen after dialysis).

Arteriovenous graft infections require total excision of the graft and intravenous antibiotic therapy. Arteriovenous fistulae are less common, as native vessels are more resistant to infection. If infections do occur, they may often be cured with intravenous antibiotics alone.

Duration of intravenous therapy for catheter infection is at least two weeks. Surveillance blood cultures should be obtained one week after stopping antibiotics if the infected catheter has been retained. If these are still positive, the catheter should be removed. Patients with persistent bacteremia and fungemia after catheter removal should receive at least four to six weeks of antibiotic therapy.

Arterial steal syndrome

Grafts and fistulae divert arterial blood into the venous system and away from distal tissues, resulting in digital ischemia. Symptoms include coldness or cramping of the hand, numbness, tingling, pain, or overt ischemia with discoloration. Patients with new grafts and fistulae should be carefully monitored for these symptoms, particularly in those with peripheral vascular disease. This syndrome can also present late, as a fistula matures, enlarges, and steals larger volumes of blood. In extremely large fistulae, high-output cardiac failure can occur, but this is rare.

PROCEDURAL COMPLICATIONS OF HEMODIALYSIS

Hypotension is the most common adverse event associated with HD, occurring during 25% to 55% of treatments. Dialysis removes urea from the extracellular space, creating an osmolar gradient from the extracellular to the intracellular space. Fluid shifts to the intracellular space lead to extracellular volume depletion. In addition, when patients are noncompliant with fluid restriction, removal of large volumes is sometimes required to reach a target "dry weight" in a single 3- to 4-hour dialysis session. Rapid removal of volume often results in hypotension, as fluid does not have time to reequilibrate from the interstitial to the intravascular space. Boluses of saline, albumin, or mannitol are given to transiently increase blood pressure. Strategies to prevent episodic hypotension include reduced dialysate temperature, high sodium dialysate, and medications such as the alpha-agonist midodrine.

The symptoms of *dialysis disequilibrium* include headache, nausea, confusion, restlessness, blurred vision, asterixis, and seizures. It is most common in chronically uremic patients beginning dialysis. The osmolar gradient resulting from rapid reduction in serum urea leads to water entry into neurons and cerebral edema. Dialysis disequilibrium is prevented by conducting the first several dialysis treatments at low blood flows and short duration.

Cardiac arrhythmias may occur in the setting of dialysis and are related to rapid fluctuations in potassium, calcium, and magnesium. ESRD patients with underlying cardiac disease are at higher risk. *Quality-of-life complications* associated with HD include nausea, cramping, headache, chest pain, and itching. Individual patients may be plagued with these symptoms to the point of intolerance.

PERITONEAL DIALYSIS

In peritoneal dialysis (PD), the patient's peritoneum is used as a semipermeable membrane through which diffusion, convection, and ultrafiltration occur. Many patients prefer PD over HD because of the greater flexibility and control that PD allows. Unlike HD, residual renal function is often necessary for adequate solute clearance, so efforts should be made to preserve it in these patients, even if it is minimal. Patients with prior major abdominal surgery may have adhesions that could limit the flow of dialysate, and therefore may not be candidates for PD. Laparoscopic PD catheter placement allows assessment of the suitability of the peritoneum in these patients. As PD is usually a home modality, an evaluation of social supports is essential. Morbidly obese patients or brittle diabetics are less than optimal candidates for PD because of high glucose exposure. However, many well-controlled diabetics do well on PD with aggressive adjustment of insulin regimens.

The basic continuous ambulatory peritoneal dialysis (CAPD) system consists of a bag of dialysis solution, a transfer set that serves as a conduit for fluid, and an indwelling silastic catheter. Dialysis solutions for PD contain physiologic concentrations of sodium, magnesium, and calcium, with lactate usually added as a buffer. During PD there is an exchange of solutes and fluid between the peritoneal capillary blood supply and the dialysis solution; the blood vessel wall, interstitium, and peritoneal mesothelium compose the semipermeable membrane. A volume of fluid, typically between 2 and 2.5 liters, is infused through the catheter into the peritoneal cavity and allowed to dwell for a prescribed number of hours. The volume of fluid varies by patient comfort and body habitus. The number of hours the fluid is allowed to dwell depends on the innate characteristics of the patient's peritoneal membrane. Patients are generally categorized as either rapid or slow transporters of solutes and fluid. Solutes transfer across the peritoneal membrane, equilibrate with the infused dialysate, and are subsequently drained out of the peritoneal cavity.

Dextrose is used as the primary osmotic agent, and standard solutions of 1.5%, 2.5%, or 4.25% are used to facilitate movement of fluid into the peritoneal cavity and achieve ultrafiltration. Higher dextrose–containing dialysate solutions (4.25%) generate higher osmotic gradients and remove greater volumes of ultrafiltrate. However, high-dextrose infusions increase the production of advanced glycosylation end products (AGEs), leading to oxidation and peritoneal membrane damage. This may lead to eventual failure of the peritoneal membrane and inability to adequately transfer solutes, necessitating a switch to HD. In diabetic patients, higher dextrose–containing solutions will increase serum glucose concentrations and worsen glycemic control. In patients with acute volume overload, large ultrafiltration volumes can be achieved with 4.25% dextrose solutions for short dwells (< 1 hour) repeatedly, until the patient's symptoms improve.

Automated PD is an alternative to conventional CAPD. In contrast to manual infusion and drainage of PD solutions, a machine performs the exchanges. The PD cycler consists of a scale and a dialysate warmer, and infuses, dwells, and drains peritoneal fluid. Patients usually undergo automated PD while asleep, allowing greater mobility during the day. The length of time each exchange dwells in the peritoneal cavity is often shorter than with CAPD, but the total volume of fluid infused is often much greater.

Children are usually treated with PD because the large extracorporeal blood volume required by the HD tubing and dialyzers can be hemodynamically prohibitive. Patients with severe cardiovascular disabilities also tend to tolerate the gentler daily ultrafiltration of PD better than intermittent HD.

PERITONEAL DIALYSIS ACCESS

A silastic (Tenckhoff) catheter is inserted into the peritoneal cavity by a qualified surgeon, interventional radiologist, or nephrologist and tunneled beneath the skin to exit on the anterior abdominal wall. After placement, it should be immediately flushed with low volumes of dialysate and then capped off. Two weeks are required for wound healing and anchoring of the catheter in the subcutaneous tissue. It may sometimes be used cautiously before this two-week timeframe with low fluid volumes and maintenance of the supine position, to prevent increased intraabdominal pressure and peritoneal leaks. Patients are carefully trained in how to access the catheter in a sterile fashion. Both patient and provider should be masked, and sterile technique is mandatory. Peritoneal fluid samples for laboratory analysis should only be obtained with proper technique by trained providers. Catheters may develop cracks over time; these can often be repaired by trained PD staff.

PERITONEAL DIALYSIS COMPLICATIONS

Peritonitis is the most serious complication of PD. Patients develop abdominal pain and have cloudy dialysate effluent. Dialysate sampling will demonstrate more than 100 white blood cells, with over 50% polymorphonuclear cells. On average, peritonitis occurs once every 15 to 20 months (a much lower rate than HD catheter infections). The most common organisms are gram-positive bacteria. Growth of multiple organisms, including gram-negative bacteria, should prompt an evaluation for an intestinal or intraabdominal source. Nearly 80% of episodes may be managed at home, with the addition of antibiotics to the dialysate. Patients receiving antibiotics should also receive fungal prophylaxis (oral nystatin or fluconazole) to avoid fungal overgrowth and peritonitis. Fungal peritonitis is devastating and requires the removal of the peritoneal catheter and either temporary or permanent conversion to HD.

Other complications of PD include malnutrition from loss of albumin and amino acids into the dialysate. Diabetics may struggle with weight gain and hyperglycemia from dextrose in the dialysate solution. After years of PD and the frequent use of high-dextrose solutions, the peritoneal membrane may develop scarring and adhesions, which limit solute clearance and ultrafiltration. In these cases, it is often necessary to switch to HD.

CONTINUOUS RENAL REPLACEMENT THERAPY

For critically ill patients who are hemodynamically unstable, continuous renal replacement therapy (CRRT) is often employed. Several modalities exist, including continuous venovenous hemofiltration (CVVH), continuous venovenous hemodialysis (CVVHD), continuous venovenous hemodiafiltration (CVVHDF), sustained low-efficiency dialysis (SLED), and extended daily dialysis (EDD). They all require a double-lumen catheter, a blood pump with safety devices similar to conventional HD, and a dialysis filter. All forms of CRRT must be done in an intensive care unit setting with properly trained staff. CRRT allows for very slow fluid removal, resulting in excellent hemodynamic tolerance, even in patients with shock or severe fluid overload. In addition, because the therapy is continuous, fluid removal and correction of metabolic abnormalities can be modified at any time, allowing for rapid adjustment in critically ill patients. CRRT can also compensate for the large fluid volumes required for parenteral nutrition. The data on CRRT benefit over conventional HD is not conclusive, but it continues to be employed in critically ill patients who may not tolerate conventional HD, and in those with fulminant hepatic failure who are at risk for cerebral edema.

COMMON PROBLEMS IN HOSPITALIZED CKD PATIENTS

GASTROINTESTINAL BLEEDING

ESRD patients, regardless of dialysis modality, are at increased risk of gastrointestinal bleeding from acquired platelet dysfunction and may also be receiving medications such as aspirin and heparin that increase bleeding risk. Dialysis patients are also prone to bleeding from angiodysplasia, for unclear reasons. Azotemic patients with severe bleeding should be dialyzed. Subcutaneous or intravenous desmopressin, at dosages of 0.3 μg/kg body weight, may be therapeutic in uremic bleeding by releasing von Willebrand factor from storage sites. There is also evidence to support the use of conjugated estrogens or cryoprecipitate in uremic bleeding. The decision to transfuse a CKD patient who is a transplant candidate should be carefully considered, as transfusion is often associated with antibody formation, perhaps hindering the matching of a future kidney allograft.

HYPERTENSION

Hypertension is common in CKD and ESRD patients. Most of these patients should be on renin-angiotensin-aldosterone system inhibitors, such as angiotensin-converting enzyme (ACE) inhibitors or angiotensin receptor blockers (ARB), as these improve cardiovascular outcomes and survival and preserve residual renal function. In hospitalized patients, these medications are problematic because they may increase the risk of AKI and hyperkalemia. They should certainly be stopped in the setting of AKI and in CKD patients undergoing intravenous contrast exposure. When these medications are held in the setting of AKI, practitioners should be sure to restart them once the sCr approaches baseline, to allow for the long-term benefits of these drugs.

BONE DISEASE

Patients with CKD and ESRD suffer from a complex spectrum of bone diseases. Osteomalacia may be seen with isolated vitamin D deficiency. Hyperphosphatemia, hypocalcemia, skeletal resistance to parathyroid hormone (PTH), and impaired renal production of 1, 25-dihydroxyvitamin D may lead to high-turnover bone disease and osteitis fibrosa cystica. Parathyroid gland hyperplasia may develop and may be difficult to reverse. Patients with secondary hyperparathyroidism may develop bone pain, muscle weakness, and erythropoietin-resistant anemia. Medical treatment to prevent hyperparathyroidism includes oral calcium, active vitamin D preparations, and calcimimetic drugs such as cinacalcet. Parathyroidectomy is still sometimes required. However, if PTH is oversuppressed by medical or surgical therapy, adynamic bone disease may develop. Management of serum phosphorus concentration is critical to the regulation of PTH.

PHOSPHORUS CONTROL

Phosphorus clearance falls with declining GFR, and hyperphosphatemia is common in CKD. It may cause hypocalcemia and tetany in the short term and renal osteodystrophy and cardiovascular disease over the long term. Serum phosphorus levels should be controlled by dietary restriction as well as oral phosphorus binders (both calcium and noncalcium based) at mealtimes. Calcium-based binders (calcium carbonate or calcium acetate) are less expensive then noncalcium-based binders (sevelamer or lanthanum). In larger doses, they promote positive calcium balance, which appears to contribute to cardiovascular calcification. Aluminum-based phosphorus binders should be avoided because of their association with dementia and adynamic bone disease in renal failure. Medications that can worsen phosphorus control, such as phosphorus-containing bowel preparations, should be avoided in hospitalized CKD patients. These have been associated with acute kidney injury from phosphate overload and should certainly be avoided in patients with stages 3 to 5 CKD.

USE OF CONTRAST AGENTS

Iodinated radiocontrast causes contrast nephropathy, particularly in patients with stages 3 to 5 CKD and diabetes mellitus. It should generally be avoided in these patients, and even patients with ESRD on dialysis, as they benefit from preservation of even minimal residual renal function. When use of radiocontrast agents is essential in CKD or ESRD, prophylaxis with intravenous fluids (NaCl or $NaHCO_3$) and N-acetylcysteine should be used. Using low or isoosmolar radiocontrast and limiting contrast volume may also be helpful. Current data do not suggest HD prevents contrast nephropathy. Gadolinium contrast in patients with CKD stages 4 and 5 (GFR < 30 cc/min) must be avoided because of its devastating association with nephrogenic systemic fibrosis.

ACID-BASE DISORDERS

Chronic metabolic acidosis is common in advanced CKD, as the kidney cannot excrete the daily ingested acid load. CKD may be complicated by type 4 renal tubular acidosis, further worsening acid-base balance. CKD patients are less able to handle an acute acid load, as might occur with lactic acidosis, and may develop severe metabolic acidosis quickly. Oral $NaHCO_3$ and furosemide may be therapeutically effective, but dialysis may be required in severe cases.

MYOCARDIAL INFARCTION

Patients with CKD are at higher risk of cardiovascular events, including acute coronary syndrome (ACS). Serum troponin levels (troponin T and I) can be mildly elevated in CKD and ESRD patients. To diagnose ACS in renal insufficiency, a single troponin is not helpful, but rising troponins over time suggest acute cardiac injury. Therapy for ACS remains the same as in the general population.

ANEMIA MANAGEMENT

Anemia is a nearly universal complication of CKD. Increased blood loss with recurrent blood draws, higher risk of gastrointestinal (GI) bleeds, and decreased erythropoietin production promote anemia. Limiting packed red cell transfusions is important to avoid immune sensitization for patients who are candidates for kidney transplantation. Iron, B12, and folate deficiency should be excluded as contributing factors. The side effects of oral iron often necessitate the use of intravenous iron. Newer formulations of parenteral iron, such as iron sucrose and iron gluconate, have a lower anaphylactic risk than iron dextran. Recombinant erythropoietin therapy is critical in the management of anemia in CKD patients. These agents (erythropoietin and darbepoietin) are administered subcutaneously in outpatients with advanced CKD, and either intravenously or subcutaneously in ESRD patients on dialysis.

ACUTE KIDNEY INJURY

Patients with CKD are vulnerable to acute kidney injury (AKI) in the hospital, most often due to drug toxicity or ischemia. All medications prescribed to CKD patients must be reviewed for possible nephrotoxicity and dose adjusted for renal function. Patients with CKD need careful monitoring and follow up after hospital discharge; renal function often does not return to baseline after acute injury occurs. ACE inhibitors and ARBs should be stopped in the setting of AKI, but restarted upon its resolution, as these agents prevent progression of kidney diseases and have important cardiovascular benefits.

HYPERKALEMIA

Patients with CKD are at risk of hyperkalemia because of dietary indiscretion, medication effects, or transfusion. Patients with ESRD will likely need dialysis to correct severe hyperkalemia, but the other treatment modalities still have a role, such as intravenous calcium for myocardial stabilization and beta-2 agonists and infusions of glucose and insulin to shift potassium into cells. Bicarbonate therapy may be helpful in the setting of a nonanion gap metabolic acidosis. Potassium resin binders may be used as adjunctive therapy in CKD and ESRD patients, but are not a substitute for other therapies.

PRACTICE POINT

- ADEs occur in as many as 50% of hospitalized patients with CKD. Commonly misdosed drugs included antibiotics, acetaminophen, narcotics, beta-blockers, digoxin, ACE inhibitors, diuretics, oral hypoglycemics, metformin, lithium, allopurinol, colchicine, famotidine, and ranitidine. Clinicians should review all medications including those prescribed as needed with attention to indication, safety, and dosing. Regarding narcotics it is preferable to administer medications that are not primarily excreted by the kidneys if the patient can tolerate alternatives. Likewise, certain antihypertensives ordinarily considered "short-acting" such as hydralazine may have unpredictable and prolonged antihypertensive effects due to altered metabolism.

ADVERSE EVENTS FROM DRUG MISDOSING

In one sample of patients with CKD admitted to community hospitals, adverse drug events (ADEs) related to improper dosing for renal function occurred in over 50%, with half of these being classified as serious. Commonly misdosed drugs included antibiotics, acetaminophen, narcotics, beta-blockers, digoxin, ACE inhibitors, diuretics, oral hypoglycemics, metformin, lithium, allopurinol, colchicine, famotidine, and ranitidine.

CONCLUSION

Chronic Kidney Disease is in the backdrop of many hospitalized patients. These patients are increasingly prone to AKI overlying CKD and sometimes progress to ESRD while in the hospital. Patients on dialysis require special attention and care to avoid metabolic complications discussed and to preserve vascular access options that may one day be needed for dialysis. A basic understanding of their dialysis modality and its more common complications is critical to provide high level care.

SUGGESTED READINGS

Adams JE. Dialysis bone disease. *Semin Dialysis.* 2002;15:277–289.

Allon M. Dialysis catheter-related bacteremia: treatment and prophylaxis. *Am J Kid Dis.* 2004;44:779–791.

Forni LG, Hilton PJ. Continuous hemofiltration in the treatment of acute renal failure. *N Engl J Med.* 1997;336:1303–1308.

Himmlefarb J. Success and challenge in dialysis therapy. *N Engl J Med.* 2002;347:2068–2070.

Hug BL, Witkowski DJ, Sox CM, et al. Occurrence of adverse, often preventable, events in community hospitals involving nephrotoxic drugs or those excreted by the kidney. *Kidney Int.* 2009;76:1192–1198.

Levey AS, Bosch JP, Lewis JB, et al. A more accurate method to estimate glomerular filtration rate from serum creatinine: a new prediction equation. *Ann Intern Med.* 1999;130:461–470.

Madhukar M. The basics of hemodialysis equipment. *Hemodial Internat.* 2005;9:30–36.

Paulson WD, Ram SJ, Sibari GB. Vascuar access: anatomy, examination, management. *Semin Nephrol.* 2002;22:183–194.

Stenvinkel P. Pecoits-Filho R, Lindholm B. Coronary artery disease in end-stage renal disease: no longer a simple plumbing problem. *J Am Soc Nephrol.* 2003;14:1927–1939.

Stevenson KB, Hannah EL, Lowder CA, et al. Epidemiology of hemodialysis vascular access infections from longitudinal infection surveillance data: predicting the impact of NKF-DOQI clinical guidelines for vascular access. *Am J Kidney Dis.* 2002;39:549–555.

Teitelbaum I, Burkart J. Peritoneal dialysis. *Am J Kidney Dis.* 2003; 42:1082–1096.

Wang AY, Lai K. Use of cardiac biomarkers in end stage renal disease. *J Am Soc Nephrol.* 2008;19:1643 –1652.

CHAPTER 249

Disorders of Sodium and Water Balance

Elwaleed A. Elhassen, MD
Robert W. Schrier, MD

Key Clinical Questions

1. What is the difference between sodium and water balance and the regulation of each?
2. How is volume depletion assessed in patients with normal heart function and in those with underlying cardiac failure?
3. Which fluids are best for volume repletion?
4. How do diuretics work, and what are their side effects? How can resistance to their action be overcome?
5. How should hyponatremia and hypernatremia be assessed and safely corrected?

INTRODUCTION

Sodium and water disturbances are among the most commonly encountered disorders in hospitalized and critically ill patients. Sodium and water balance are independently regulated by mechanisms that are designed to maintain circulatory integrity and plasma osmolality, respectively. Sodium balance is regulated by changes in sodium intake and excretion, whereas plasma osmolality is regulated by changes in water intake and water excretion.

Water is the predominant constituent of the human body. In healthy individuals, it makes up 60% of a man's body weight and 50% of a woman's body weight. Body water is distributed between two compartments: the intracellular fluid compartment, containing 55% to 65%, and the extracellular fluid compartment, containing the remaining 35% to 45%. The extracellular fluid compartment is further subdivided into the interstitial space and the intravascular space. The interstitial space comprises approximately 75% of the extracellular fluid compartment, whereas the intravascular space contains 25%. Total body water diffuses freely between the intracellular space and the extracellular space in response to solute concentration gradients. Therefore, the amount of water in each compartment depends entirely on the quantity of solute in that compartment. The major extracellular solute is sodium, while potassium is the major intracellular solute. This solute distribution is maintained by active transport, via the Na^+/K^+-ATP-dependent pumps found on cell membranes.

PATHOPHYSIOLOGY OF SODIUM BALANCE

The extracellular fluid compartment depends on the total body sodium content as well as the integrity of the mechanisms responsible for its maintenance. Sodium content is normally tightly regulated by modulating renal retention and excretion in situations of deficiency or excess extracellular fluid. The operative homeostatic mechanisms include an afferent sensing limb and an efferent effector limb. Disorders of either sensing or effector mechanisms can lead to failure to adjust renal sodium handling, resulting in hypertension and edema in positive sodium balance or hypotension and hypovolemia with negative sodium balance.

EFFECTIVE ARTERIAL BLOOD VOLUME

Effective arterial blood volume refers to the blood volume detected by baroreceptors in the arterial circulation. The effective arterial blood volume can change independently of the total extracellular fluid volume, leading to sodium and water retention in different clinical situations.

Afferent limb sensing sites include low-pressure cardiopulmonary receptors (atrial, ventricular, and pulmonary stretch receptors), high-pressure arterial baroreceptors (carotid, aortic arch, and renal sensors), and central nervous system and hepatic receptors. Activation of these afferent sites engages several *effector mechanisms*. Activation of the sympathetic nerves stimulates proximal tubular sodium reabsorption. Renin release from the renal juxtaglomerular apparatus stimulates the formation of angiotensin II, a potent vasoconstrictor. Angiotensin II also stimulates the adrenal gland to secrete aldosterone, which increases tubular sodium reabsorption. Other effector mechanisms include prostaglandins that modulate renal blood flow and sodium handling, natriuretic peptides that enhance renal sodium excretion in response to atrial stretching, and pituitary secretion of arginine vasopressin (AVP), a modest vasoconstrictor that also enhances renal water retention.

REGULATION OF WATER BALANCE

Osmoregulation is the regulation of water intake and excretion to maintain constant body osmolality (tonicity). Disorders of water homeostasis result in hypo- or hypernatremia, whereas disorders of total body sodium content result in extracellular volume depletion or overload. Since osmolality in all body fluids is essentially equal, it can be estimated by measuring the plasma osmolality. The normal plasma osmolality is 275 to 290 mOsm/kg. It is kept within this range by hypothalamic osmoreceptors, which are capable of sensing a 1% to 2% change in tonicity. Osmoreceptors influence thirst and the release of the antidiuretic hormone AVP. The combined effect of AVP stimulation and thirst results in water intake and retention, which lowers plasma osmolality and sodium concentration by dilution, whereas suppression of thirst and AVP secretion leads to the contrary.

DISORDERS OF SODIUM BALANCE

EXTRACELLULAR FLUID VOLUME CONTRACTION

Extracellular fluid (ECF) volume contraction is caused by loss of sodium or water in excess of intake. These losses may be a result of renal or extrarenal losses or sequestration in potential spaces, such as the peritoneal cavity, retroperitoneum, pleural spaces, or muscles, which are not in hemodynamic equilibrium with the ECF ("third-spacing").

Extrarenal causes

The gastrointestinal tract is the most common extrarenal source of fluid loss. Vomiting or nasogastric suction may cause volume loss with metabolic alkalosis. Diarrhea may result in volume depletion with metabolic acidosis. Third-space sequestration, excessive sweat production, and loss of skin barrier from burns or exudative skin lesions may lead to significant ECF volume depletion. Hemorrhage, as from gastrointestinal bleeding or trauma, may lead to significant volume loss.

Renal losses

Diuretics may cause renal sodium wasting, volume contraction, and acid-base disturbances if abused or inappropriately prescribed. Genetic and acquired tubular disorders can result in renal sodium wasting and volume contraction. Mineralocorticoid deficiency and resistance often lead to renal sodium wasting. This may occur in the setting of primary adrenal insufficiency (Addison disease) or hyporeninemic hypoaldosteronism secondary to diabetes mellitus or other chronic interstitial renal diseases. Severe hyperglycemia or high levels of blood urea after relief of urinary tract obstruction can lead to obligatory renal sodium and water loss secondary to glucosuria or urea diuresis, respectively.

Clinical manifestations

The symptoms of hypovolemia are nonspecific and can range from mild postural symptoms, thirst, muscle cramps, and weakness, to drowsiness and disturbed mentation with profound volume loss. Physical examination may reveal tachycardia, cold clammy skin, postural or recumbent hypotension, and reduced urine output depending on the degree of volume loss (**Table 249-1**). Rarely, diminished skin turgor may be seen. Reduced jugular venous pressure (JVP) noted at the base of the neck is a useful parameter of volume depletion and may roughly estimate the central venous pressure (CVP). However, an elevated CVP does not exclude hypovolemia in patients with underlying cardiac failure or pulmonary hypertension. The absence of symptoms or obvious physical findings does not preclude volume depletion in an appropriate clinical setting, and hemodynamic monitoring or administration of a fluid challenge may sometimes be necessary.

TABLE 249-1 Clinical Evaluation of Extracellular Fluid Volume Depletion

Mild to moderate volume loss
• Thirst • Delayed capillary refill • Postural dizziness and weakness • Dry mucous membranes and axillae • Cool clammy extremities and collapsed peripheral veins • Tachypnea • Tachycardia with pulse rate > 100 beats per minute or postural pulse increment of 30 beats per min or more • Postural hypotension (systolic blood pressure decrease of > 20 mm Hg with standing) • Low jugular venous pulse • Oliguria
Severe volume loss and hypovolemic shock
• Depressed mental status or loss of consciousness • Peripheral cyanosis • Reduced skin turgor (in young patients only) • Marked tachycardia, low pulse volume • Supine hypotension (systolic blood pressure < 100 mm Hg)

Laboratory findings consistent with volume depletion include hemoconcentration and increased serum albumin concentration. However, anemia or hypoalbuminemia may confound interpretation of these laboratory values. In healthy individuals, the ratio of blood urea nitrogen (BUN) (mg/dL) to serum creatinine (mg/dL) approximately equals 10. In volume depletion, this ratio increases because of a differential increase in the tubular reabsorption of urea. Several clinical conditions confound this ratio. Upper gastrointestinal hemorrhage and administration of corticosteroids increase urea production and the ratio of BUN to creatinine. Malnutrition and underlying liver disease diminish urea production, and thus the BUN-to-creatinine ratio is less useful in these clinical settings.

In the absence of renal salt wasting or diuretics, elevated urine osmolality and specific gravity may indicate hypovolemia. Hypovolemia normally triggers avid renal sodium reabsorption, resulting in low urine sodium concentration and low fractional excretion of sodium. The fractional excretion of sodium (FE_{Na}) is calculated using the following formula: $FE_{Na} = [U_{Na} \times P_{creat} / U_{creat} \times P_{Na}] \times 100$, where U_{Na} and U_{creat} are urinary sodium and creatinine concentrations, and P_{Na} and P_{creat} are plasma sodium and creatinine concentrations, respectively. Decreased FE_{Na} (less than 1%) is consistent with ECF volume depletion. However, arterial underfilling due to low cardiac output or systemic arterial vasodilatation, as in cirrhosis, is also associated with an FE_{Na} less than 1%, in spite of increased ECF and edema.

Treatment

Volume depletion is treated by replacing fluid deficits and ongoing losses with a replacement fluid closely resembling the lost fluid. Clinical parameters help to distinguish mild to moderate from severe volume loss (Table 249-1), but invasive monitoring may be needed in some patients. Mild volume contraction can usually be corrected via the oral route. In hypovolemic shock with evidence of life-threatening circulatory collapse or organ dysfunction, intravenous fluid must be given as rapidly as possible until clinical parameters improve. A slow, more judicious approach is warranted in the elderly and those with underlying cardiac conditions in order to avoid overcorrection with subsequent pulmonary edema.

Crystalloid solutions are effective, as they distribute primarily in the ECF. Colloid-containing solutions, such as 5% and 25% albumin and hetastarch (6% hydroxyethyl starch), remain within the vascular compartment by virtue of their large molecular sizes. As studies have not shown an advantage for colloid-containing solutions in the treatment of hypovolemia, they are best reserved for hemodynamically unstable patients in whom rapid correction is needed, such as trauma and burn victims. Otherwise, isotonic saline is usually the initial replacement fluid of choice in volume-depleted patients.

Hypovolemic shock may be accompanied by lactic acidosis due to tissue hypoperfusion. Fluid resuscitation restores tissue oxygenation and decreases the production of lactate. Correction of acidosis with sodium bicarbonate has several potential adverse effects, including increasing tonicity, overexpanding ECF volume, and worsening intracellular acidosis. Therefore, its use to manage lactic acidosis in the setting of volume depletion is not recommended, unless the arterial pH is below 7.1.

■ EXTRACELLULAR FLUID VOLUME EXPANSION

Excess extracellular fluid accumulation usually results from sodium and water retention by the kidneys. Renal sodium retention may be primary or a compensatory response to reduced effective arterial blood volume. It manifests clinically with edema and weight gain, commonly in response to congestive heart failure (CHF), cirrhosis with ascites, or the nephrotic syndrome.

Renal sodium and water retention in CHF involves activation of the renin-angiotensin-aldosterone system (RAAS), as well as nonosmotic AVP stimulation, which drives the hyponatremia associated with CHF. Arterial underfilling is also responsible for water and sodium retention in cirrhosis. Unlike CHF and cirrhosis, in which the kidneys are structurally normal, the nephrotic syndrome is characterized by kidneys that are functionally impaired. Rarer causes of edema include drug-induced edema, which may be seen with ingestion of systemic vasodilators, such as minoxidil and diazoxide, dihydropyridine calcium channel blockers, and thiazolidinediones. Nonsteroidal anti-inflammatory drugs (NSAIDs) can exacerbate volume expansion in CHF and cirrhotic patients by decreasing vasoregulatory prostaglandins in the kidneys.

Clinical manifestations

Patients with left heart failure may present with exertional dyspnea, orthopnea, and paroxysmal nocturnal dyspnea, whereas patients with predominant right heart failure or biventricular failure may exhibit weight gain and lower-limb swelling. Physical examination may reveal JVP elevation, pulmonary crackles, a third heart sound, or peripheral edema in the ankles or sacrum. Nephrotic patients classically present with periorbital edema because of their ability to lie flat during sleep. Patients with severe nephrotic syndrome may exhibit marked generalized edema with anasarca. Cirrhotic patients present with ascites and lower-limb edema consequent to portal hypertension and hypoalbuminemia. Physical examination may reveal stigmata of chronic liver disease, such as jaundice, spider angiomata, palmar erythema, Dupuytren contractures, and splenomegaly.

Therapy

Management of ECF volume expansion consists of treating the underlying cause and achieving negative sodium balance with dietary sodium restriction and diuretics. Moderate dietary sodium restriction (2 to 3 g/day; 86 to 130 mmol/day) should be instituted. Restriction of total fluid intake is usually only necessary for hyponatremic patients. Medications that promote sodium retention, such as NSAIDs, corticosteroids, estrogens, and androgens, should be eliminated, if possible. Diuretics are the cornerstone of therapy to remove excess volume. Other measures can be used when the response to diuretics is inadequate. Extracorporeal fluid removal by ultrafiltration can be utilized in patients with acute decompensated heart failure with renal insufficiency or diuretic resistance. In cirrhosis, large-volume paracentesis with albumin infusion (8 grams per liter of ascitic fluid removed) can be employed to remove large volumes of ascitic fluid. Interventional maneuvers to shunt ascitic fluid to a central vein can also be considered in refractory ascites, and they may result in improvement of the GFR and sodium excretion.

Diuretics are the mainstay of therapy for edematous states. As ECF volume expansion in CHF and cirrhosis may be a compensatory mechanism for arterial underfilling, a judicious approach is necessary to avoid a precipitous fall in cardiac output and tissue perfusion. Diuretics can be classified into five classes, based on their predominant sites of actions along the nephron (**Figure 249-1**). They inhibit the reabsorption of sodium and an accompanying anion, usually chloride. The resultant natriuresis decreases the ECF. However, the time course of natriuresis is limited because renal mechanisms attenuate the sodium excretion.

The most serious *adverse effects of diuretics* are electrolyte and acid-base disturbances. Loop diuretics increase the excretion of potassium, magnesium, and calcium. Thiazide diuretics have similar effects on potassium and magnesium, but unlike loop diuretics, they decrease urinary calcium losses. Thiazide diuretics interfere with urine-diluting mechanisms, and may therefore pose a risk of hyponatremia. Patients on diuretic therapy require electrolyte monitoring, and may need oral supplementation of potassium and magnesium. Addition of a potassium-sparing diuretic may need to be considered in patients with severe or recurrent hypokalemia. The volume depletion caused by thiazides and loop diuretics leads to increased tubular urate reabsorption, promoting hyperuricemia and gout. Ototoxicity may occur with large intravenous doses of loop diuretics, particularly when an aminoglycoside is coadministered. Gynecomastia may develop with spironolactone therapy.

Long-term *loop diuretic tolerance* occurs as a consequence of hypertrophy of the distal nephron segment and enhanced sodium reabsorption from increased exposure to solutes not absorbed proximally. This can be addressed by combining loop and thiazide diuretics, as the latter blocks reabsorption distal to the loop of Henle.

Diuretic resistance refers to edema that is or has become refractory to a given diuretic. Diuretic resistance has several causes. Chronic kidney disease is associated with decreased secretion and tubular delivery of diuretics, reducing their concentration at the active site in the tubular lumen. Arterial underfilling in cirrhosis and CHF is associated with diminished nephron responsiveness to diuretics because of increased proximal tubular sodium reabsorption, leading to decreased delivery of sodium to the distal sites of diuretic action. Nonsteroidal anti-inflammatory drugs block prostaglandin-mediated increases in renal blood flow, leading to sodium retention.

Treatment of diuretic resistance includes salt restriction, increasing the dose of loop diuretic, administering more frequent doses, and using combination therapy to sequentially block more than one site in the nephron, as that may result in a synergistic interaction between diuretics (**Figure 249-2**). In patients who respond poorly to intermittent doses of a loop diuretic, a continuous intravenous infusion can be tried and has been associated with greater overall diuresis and a better safety profile. Ultrafiltration may be necessary in highly resistant edematous patients. **Table 249-2** lists effective diuretic doses in patients with CHF, nephrotic syndrome, advanced cirrhosis, and renal failure.

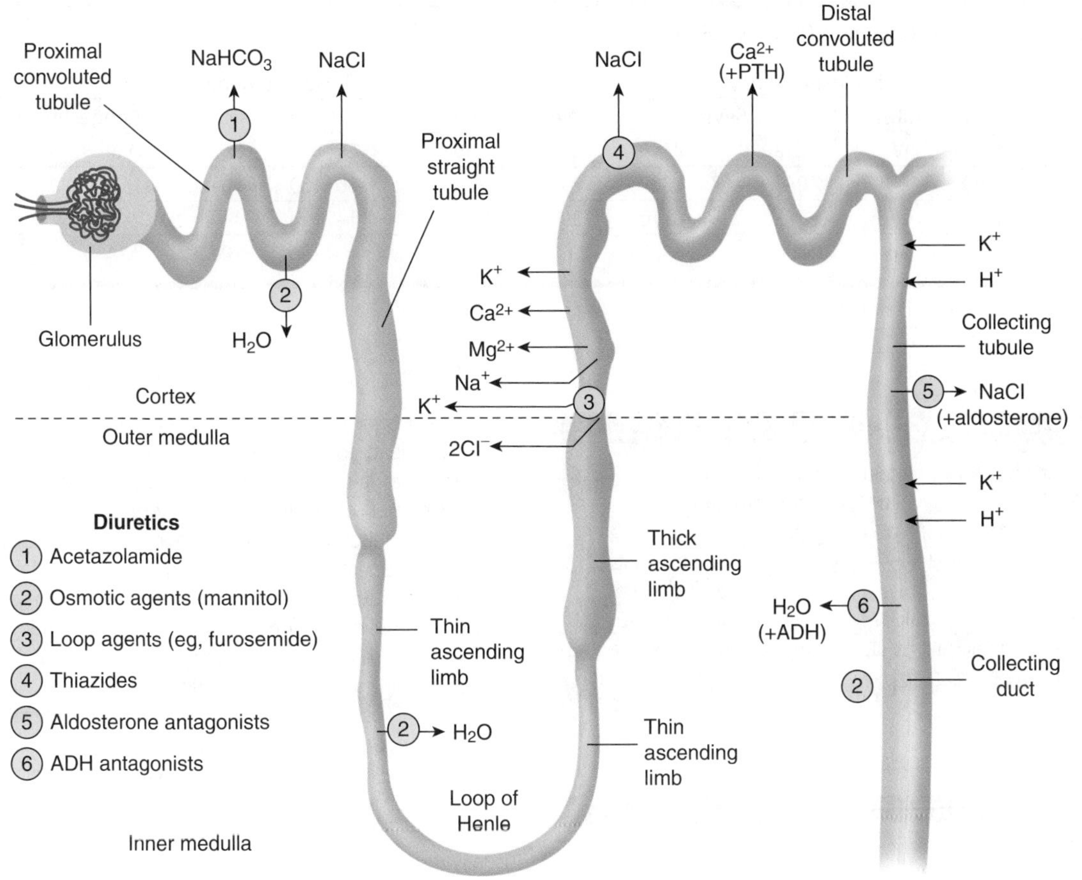

Figure 249-1 *Tubule transport systems and sites of action of diuretics. (Reproduced, with permission, from Katzung BG, Masters SB, Trevor AJ. Basic & Clinical Pharmacology. 11th ed. New York: McGraw-Hill; 2009. Fig. 15-1.)*

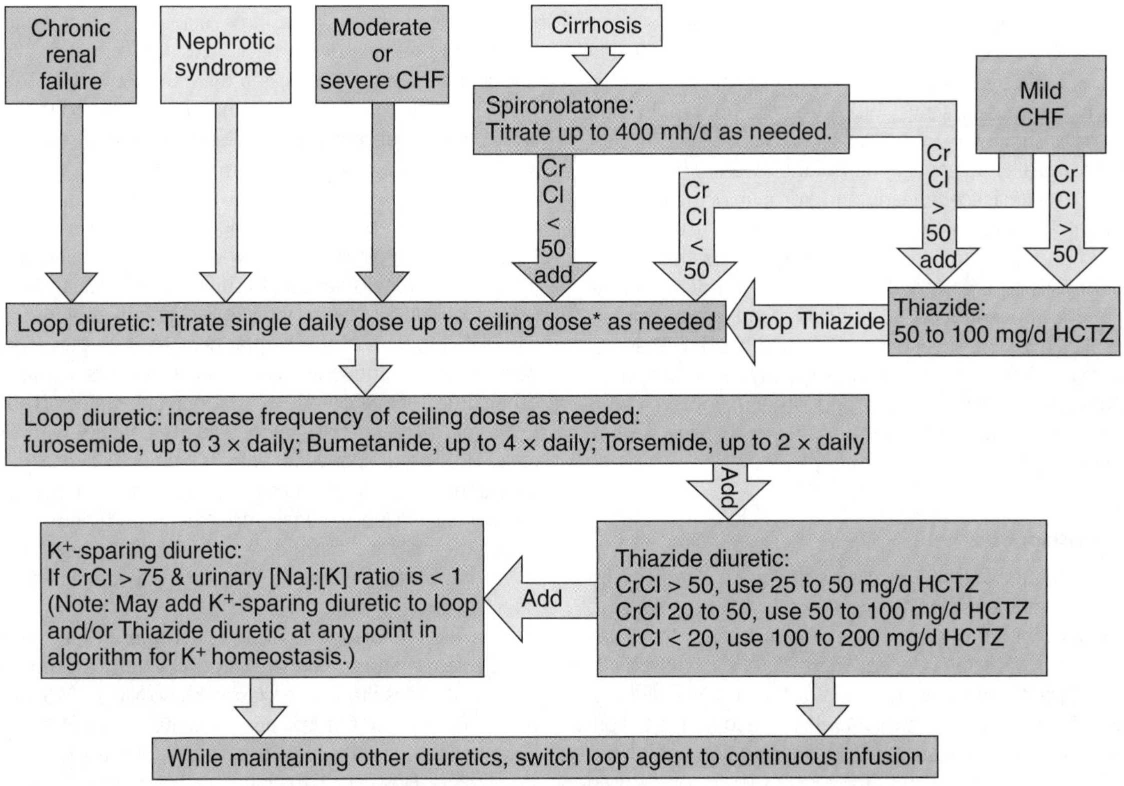

Figure 249-2 *Algorithm for diuretic therapy in patients with edema caused by renal, hepatic, or cardiac disease. (*For dosing details, see Brater DC. Diuretic therapy. N Engl J Med. 1998;339:387–395.) (Reproduced, with permission, from Brunton LL, Lazo JS, Parker KL. Goodman & Gilman's The Pharmacological Basis of Therapeutics. 11th ed. New York: McGraw-Hill; 2006. Fig. 28-12.)*

TABLE 249-2 **Therapeutic Regimens for Loop Diuretics in Milligrams/Day**

	Renal Insufficiency				Preserved Renal Function					
	Moderate		Severe		Neprotic Syndrome		Cirrhosis		Congestive Heart Failure	
	Oral	IV	Oral	IV	Oral	IV	Oral	IV	Oral	IV
Furosemide	80–160	80	240	200	240	120	80–160	40–80	160–240	40–80
Bumetanide	2–3	2–3	8–10	8–10	3	3	1–2	1	2–3	2–3
Tursemide	50	50	100	100	50	50	10–20	10–20	50	20–50

GFR, glomerular filtration rate; IV, intravenous.

PRACTICE POINT

- Edema in cirrhosis may be controlled by alcohol cessation, sodium restriction, and diuretic therapy. The diuretic combination of furosemide and spironolactone, given in a ratio of furosemide 40 mg and spironolactone 100 mg daily to maintain optimal electrolyte balance, is more effective than either drug administered alone. These drugs may be gradually titrated upward to a maximal dosage of furosemide 160 mg and spironolactone 400 mg daily.

DISORDERS OF WATER BALANCE

HYPONATREMIA

Hyponatremia (plasma sodium concentration below 135 mmol/L) is the most common electrolyte abnormality in hospitalized patients, occurring in 15% to 30% of medical inpatients, with over half of cases being acquired during hospitalization. Most patients with hyponatremia have hypoosmolar or hypotonic hyponatremia, with excess water in relation to solute. However, hyponatremia does not always signify a hypotonic state. Rarely, patients have *hypertonic hyponatremia*, or *translocational hyponatremia*, due to osmotically active solutes that do not readily penetrate into cells, such as mannitol, contrast media, and sorbitol. To equalize osmolality across cell membranes, water shifts out of cells to the extracellular space, leading to a drop in plasma sodium concentration. The most common cause is excess extracellular glucose, as in poorly controlled diabetes mellitus. Plasma sodium concentration falls by 1.6 mmol/L for every 100 mg/dL rise in the plasma glucose concentration. In *pseudohyponatremia* (isotonic hyponatremia), hyponatremia occurs when the solid phase of plasma, primarily lipids and proteins, is greatly expanded, as in hypertriglyceridemia and myeloma and other paraproteinemic disorders, leading to an artifactual decrease in plasma sodium concentration.

Etiology and diagnosis

Hypotonic hyponatremia is the most common plasma sodium disorder in the hospital setting, indicating an excess of water relative to sodium in plasma. This can occur with a decrease in total body sodium, or hypovolemic hyponatremia; a near-normal total body sodium, or euvolemic hyponatremia; or an excess of total body sodium, or hypervolemic hyponatremia (**Figure 249-3**). Since sodium is the primary cation in the ECF compartment, its concentration determines ECF volume. A careful history and a physical examination focused on the evaluation of the ECF volume allows for the classification of the hyponatremia into one of three categories: hypovolemic, euvolemic, or hypervolemic.

In *hypovolemic hyponatremia*, deficits of both total body sodium and water lead to ECF volume depletion, with consequent AVP secretion and decreased solute-free water excretion.

Renal causes of solute-rich fluid loss include diuretics, mineralocorticoid deficiency, salt-losing nephropathy, such as polycystic kidney disease and interstitial nephritis, and partial urinary tract obstruction. Fluid losses may also be extrarenal, especially gastrointestinal, such as gastroenteritis, peritonitis, pancreatitis, and ileus, as well as hemorrhage or excessive sweating. Historical features may include vomiting, diarrhea, diuretic use, thirstiness, or hyperglycemia with glucosuria. Physical examination may reveal tachycardia, orthostatic hypotension, and flat neck veins. Helpful urinary studies include urine sodium and the Fe_{Na}, which are typically less than 10 mmol/L and 1%, respectively, with extrarenal fluid losses. Urine sodium and Fe_{Na} greater than 10 mmol/L and 1%, respectively, usually indicate renal losses, such as secondary to diuretic use and osmotic diuresis.

In *euvolemic hyponatremia*, total body sodium content is generally normal, but there is hypoosmolality from a relative gain of water. Physical examination is notable for the absence of both features of volume overload, such as peripheral edema, ascites, pulmonary edema, and features of volume depletion, such as tachycardia, low blood pressure, or flat neck veins. Concentrations of BUN and uric acid are normal or low, and the urine sodium is usually greater than 20 mEq/L. In this setting, hyponatremia is often due to the syndrome of inappropriate antidiuretic hormone secretion (SIADH), attributable to release of AVP from the pituitary or, rarely, an ectopic source such as lung carcinoma. This leads to impaired water excretion, while the regulation of sodium balance is virtually unaffected. Ingestion or administration of water is also required, since a high level of AVP alone is not usually sufficient to produce hyponatremia. Causes of SIADH include infectious, inflammatory, neoplastic, and vascular disorders of the central nervous and respiratory systems, pain, narcotics, anticonvulsants, antidepressants, neuroleptics, and other drugs active on the central nervous system (**Table 249-3**). However, in many hospitalized elderly patients with SIADH, the cause is obscure. Several entities should be considered prior to diagnosing SIADH. These include profound hypothyroidism, adrenal insufficiency, renal impairment, and primary polydipsia. Hyponatremia may also be seen in excessive beer consumption (beer potomania), as beer is rich in carbohydrates and water, but poor in solutes and electrolytes.

To make the diagnosis of SIADH (**Table 249-4**), patients must be euvolemic, and the urinary osmolality must exceed 100 mOsm/kg of water despite a low plasma osmolality (<275 mOsm/kg of water). Because of the low urine volume in SIADH, the urinary sodium concentration is high, usually greater than 40 mmol/L in the steady state. However, if the patient is volume depleted or on a salt-restricted diet, the urine concentration may be lower. Expanding the ECF volume with normal saline or normal salt intake increases urinary sodium, but does not correct the hyponatremia. Supportive

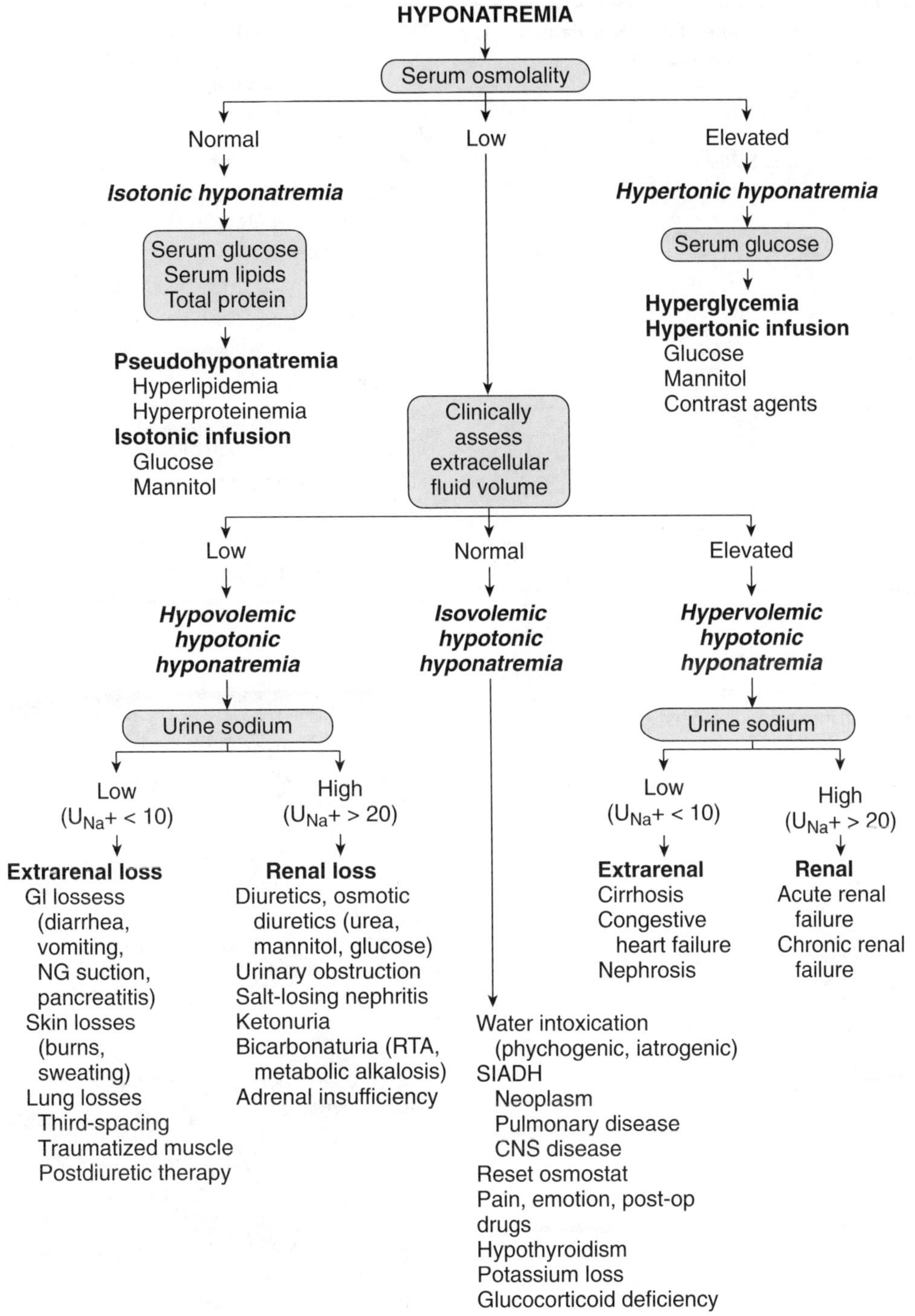

Figure 249-3 *Diagnostic algorithm for hyponatremia. (Adapted, with permission, from Johnson RJ, Freehaly J, eds. Comprehensive Clinical Nephrology. 2nd ed. St. Louis, MO: Mosby; 2003.)*

laboratory tests for SIADH include hypouricemia (serum uric acid <4 mg/dL) and low BUN (<10 mg/dL). When the diagnosis is still uncertain, ECF volume depletion can be ruled out by infusing 2 L of normal saline over 24 to 48 hours. Correction of hyponatremia, along with a drop in urinary osmolality, suggests volume depletion rather than SIADH. Caution must be exercised when administering saline to hyponatremic patients, because in a subset of patients this can induce brisk water diuresis and a rapid rise in serum sodium. Osmotic demyelination, with severe neurologic morbidity and even death, may occur with rapid correction of plasma sodium concentration (greater than 10 mEq/L rise in 24 hours) in patients with chronic hyponatremia.

Careful monitoring of serum and urinary electrolytes is therefore warranted. If rapid overcorrection occurs, administration of hypotonic fluid or even AVP may be needed to halt the progressive rise in serum sodium.

In *hypervolemic hyponatremia*, both total body sodium and water are increased, but water is comparatively more so. Underlying causes include cardiac failure and liver cirrhosis, in which the kidneys are intrinsically normal, but respond to decreased effective arterial perfusion with increased AVP levels and activation of RAAS. Acute and chronic kidney disease may be associated with hyponatremia if water intake exceeds the ability to excrete equivalent volumes. Hyponatremia is a risk factor for diminished survival in cardiac failure

TABLE 249-3 Causes of the Syndrome of Inappropriate Antidiuretic Hormone Secretion

Drugs
• **Antipsychotics**
• **Antidepressants (tricyclics and SSRIs)**
• **Narcotics**
• **Anticonvulsants**
• Cytotoxic drugs (vincristine, cyclophosphamide, ifosfamide)
• Nicotine
• Clofibrate
• Nonsteroidal anti-inflammatory drugs
• MDMA (ecstasy)
Pulmonary disorders
• **Bacterial and viral pneumonia**
• Lung abscess
• Bronchiectasis and cystic fibrosis
• Tuberculosis
• Aspergillosis
• Mechanical ventilation with positive pressure
Central nervous system disorders
• **Subdural hematoma**
• **Subarachnoid hemorrhage**
• **Stroke**
• **Tumors**
• Meningitis, encephalitis, brain abscess
• Vasculitis and other inflammatory disorders
• Multiple sclerosis
• Guillain-Barré syndrome
• Hydrocephalus
Malignancies
• **Small cell lung cancer**
• **Head and neck cancer**
• Non–small cell lung cancer
• Mesothelioma
• Gastrointestinal adenocarcinoma
• Genitourinary tract cancers
• Leukemia
Others
• **Postoperative stress**
• **Pain**
• **Nausea and vomiting**
• Endurance exercise
• AIDS
• Hereditary gain-of-function mutation in the V2 receptor

Note: The most common causes are listed in **bold**.

TABLE 249-4 Criteria for the Diagnosis of the Syndrome of Inappropriate Antidiuretic Hormone Secretion Secretion

Key features
Decreased effective osmolality (< 275 mOsm/kg of water)
Inappropriately elevated urinary osmolality > 100 mOsm/kg of water despite hypotonicity
Clinical euvolemia
Urinary sodium > 20 mEq/L with normal dietary sodium intake
Normal thyroid, adrenal, pituitary, and renal function
No recent diuretic use
Supplemental features
Plasma uric acid < 4 mg/dL
Blood urea nitrogen < 10 mg/dL
Fractional excretion of sodium > 1%; fractional urea excretion > 55%
Failure to correct hyponatremia after infusion of normal saline
Correction of hyponatremia through fluid restriction

and cirrhosis. In the absence of diuretics, Fe_{Na} should be less than 1% in both conditions. However, a Fe_{Na} greater than 1% is seen in the hypervolemic hyponatremic patient with acute or chronic kidney disease with tubular dysfunction leading to suboptimal sodium and water absorption.

The clinical manifestations of hyponatremia are mainly neurologic and caused by intracellular fluid shifts, leading to brain swelling and edema. The severity of symptoms depends on the rate of decline of serum sodium concentration, because the adaptive mechanisms to protect brain cell volume require a longer time to be fully functional. These mechanisms involve a gradual loss of potassium and organic solutes to restore cell volume to normal. Symptoms include nausea, vomiting, headache, lethargy, seizures, and a progressively decreased level of consciousness, ending in coma and death. Neurologic signs of severe acute hyponatremia may include depressed deep tendon reflexes, hypothermia, pseudobulbar palsy, and Cheyne-Stokes respirations.

PRACTICE POINT

- Psychiatric patients are at risk for hyponatremia for many reasons, including the thirst-producing anticholinergic side effects of antidepressants and antipsychotics; SIADH from typical and atypical antipyschotics; tricyclic antidepressants, and selective serotonin reuptake inhibitors; obsessive-compulsive behavior; and pseudosatiety from water consumption in patients hospitalized for alcoholism or anorexia. Schizophrenic patients are particularly at risk; up to 14% have hyponatremia and up to 25% have polydipsia. This predisposition may be multifactorial, relating to a decreased osmotic threshold for AVP release, an enhanced renal sensitivity to AVP, and a defect in the osmoregulation of thirst. SIADH and psychogenic polydipsia may be differentiated based on the urine osmolality: in SIADH, urine osmolality is ≥ 100 mOsm/kg, while in psychogenic polydipsia it is < 100 mOsm/kg. Fluid restriction is the main treatment for psychogenic polydipsia, but is difficult to enforce in practice. Clozapine may have a lesser tendency to cause polydipsia and hyponatremia than other antipsychotics. Unfortunately, it has uncommon but severe adverse effects, including agranulocytosis, seizures, myocarditis, and orthostatic hypotension. The antibiotic demeclocycline, which blocks the activity and action of AVP, may have some utility in treatment of psychogenic polydipsia.

Therapy

Hypovolemic hyponatremia is treated with volume repletion with isotonic saline to expand ECF volume and interrupt AVP release. Volume expansion should be continued until blood pressure is restored and the patient demonstrates clinical euvolemia. When the initial volume estimate is equivocal, a fluid challenge with 0.5 to 1 L of isotonic saline can be both diagnostic and therapeutic.

Hypervolemic hyponatremia: The treatment of hyponatremia in the context of volume overload requires management of the underlying cardiac failure or liver cirrhosis. Sodium and water restriction as well as diuretics should be employed as necessary. When hyponatremia occurs, fluid restriction to amounts less than insensible losses plus urine output is necessary to cause a negative solute-free water balance, but is often difficult to achieve. Diuretic-resistant cases of CHF and liver cirrhosis may be treated with ultrafiltration and large-volume paracentesis, respectively.

Euvolemic hyponatremia: The treatment of hyponatremia in euvolemic patients depends on the degree of symptoms and on whether it has developed acutely (within hours) or chronically (over more than 48 hours). Acute hyponatremia with onset in the hospital is most often related to hypotonic solutions. The rapid development of hyponatremia with very low sodium values (< 110–115 mmol/L) may cause fluid to shift into brain cells, possibly leading to cerebral edema and death, as the adaptive changes cannot keep pace with intracellular fluid shifts leading to brain swelling within the confined skull space.

In acute severe hyponatremia with neurologic symptoms, the treatment of choice is 3% hypertonic saline, infused initially at 1 to 2 ml/kg/hour (**Table 249-5**). For each 100 ml of 3% hypertonic saline, the serum sodium concentration will increase approximately by 2 mmol/L. This should be continued until a less severe level of hyponatremia has been attained (ie, 125–130 mmol/L) or symptoms resolve. Furosemide may be added to enhance solute-free water excretion and hasten return to normal serum sodium. If seizures, obtundation, or coma are present, hypertonic saline may be infused at 4 to 6 ml/kg/hour for a short period of time.

When hyponatremia develops over several days, brain cells extrude organic solutes from their cytoplasm, allowing intracellular osmolality and plasma osmolality to equalize without a large increase in cell water. Because of this rapid normalization of chronic hyponatremia may also lead to cerebral edema. Hyponatremia should be corrected very gradually when it is has been present for more than 48 hours, or the duration is unknown. Serum sodium should be corrected by no more than 12 mmol in 24 hours and 18 mmol in 48 hours. It should be corrected even more slowly in high-risk patients with severe malnutrition, alcoholism, or advanced liver disease, who have an impaired ability to protect their intracellular volume by generating osmotically active molecules such as glycine, taurine, and myoinositol.

Too-rapid correction of chronic hyponatremia, outpacing the brain's ability to recapture lost organic osmolytes, may result in osmotic demyelination syndrome, which especially effects glial cells of the brainstem. Patients improve initially as hyponatremia resolves, but within days develop new, progressive, and sometimes permanent neurologic deficits, including fluctuating level of consciousness, quadriparesis, pseudobulbar palsy, ataxia, dysarthria, and locked-in syndrome. Magnetic resonance imaging (MRI) may show T2-weighted hyperintensities in the brainstem, especially the pons, consistent with demyelination.

In patients with chronic asymptomatic hyponatremia, hypothyroidism and secondary adrenal insufficiency should be sought and treated appropriately if present. Potentially responsible medications should be discontinued. Ideally, SIADH is treated with therapy directed against its underlying cause. However, if the cause cannot be identified or expeditiously treated, hyponatremia should be treated conservatively with fluid restriction. To achieve negative water balance, daily fluid intake must be significantly limited to less than the 24-hour urine output plus insensible losses. The maximum tolerated fluid intake is proportional to the oral osmotic load, so adequate intake of dietary protein and salt should be encouraged. Many patients will find the recommended degree of fluid restriction intolerable and difficult to comply with. Oral medications that may be helpful include urea (30 grams per day), demeclocycline (300–600 mg twice daily), or lithium, but these therapies have poor tolerability, inconsistent responses, and significant toxicities.

Recently, vasopressin receptor antagonists (vaptans) have been introduced for the treatment of hyponatremia. These agents act by increasing electrolyte-free water excretion (aquaresis) and hence raising serum sodium concentration. Conivaptan, a combined V1 and V2 receptor antagonist, has been approved by the United States Food and Drug Administration (FDA) for four-day intravenous use in the hospital setting to treat euvolemic and hypervolemic hyponatremia. However, there are insufficient data to use conivaptan in the treatment of acute symptomatic hyponatremia at this time. Conivaptan might be considered particularly for those with moderate to severe hyponatremia and symptoms, but not seizures, delirium, or coma, which would warrant the use of hypertonic saline. The Selective V2 receptor antagonist, tolvaptan, is orally active and has been approved by the FDA for euvolemic and hypervolemic hyponatremia.

TABLE 249-5 Using Hypertonic Saline to Treat Acute Symptomatic Hyponatremia with Neurologic Symptoms

- Infuse 3% hypertonic saline initially at 1–2 ml/kg/hour.
- For each 100 ml of 3% hypertonic saline, the serum sodium concentration will increase approximately by 2 mmol/L.
- Monitor serum Na^+ level frequently.
- Discontinue hypertonic saline as soon as the patient is asymptomatic or less severe degree of hyponatremia has been attained (125–130 mmol/L).

Discharge considerations

Chronic asymptomatic hyponatremic patients rarely need to be hospitalized and they can be worked up and treated on an outpatient basis. Patients with severe symptomatic hyponatremia who require hypertonic saline are best monitored in an intensive care setting. Once symptoms resolve, hypertonic saline should be discontinued because its main objective is to alleviate cerebral edema rather than to correct the serum sodium concentration. This may be followed by restricting water, liberalizing dietary salt intake (except in edematous states), and possibly using V2 receptor antagonists. The decision of discharge depends on other patient comorbidities and the underlying cause of the hyponatremia.

HYPERNATREMIA

Although not as common as hyponatremia, hypernatremia is not infrequent in hospitalized patients, particularly those in intensive care units. Hypernatremia is always associated with hyperosmolality, as sodium salts are the major extracellular solutes. Hyperosmolality leads to an exodus of water from cells to the extracellular compartment to maintain osmotic equilibrium, with a loss of intracellular volume and shrinkage of brain cells. The major defense against sodium elevation is the stimulation of thirst and AVP, leading to increased water intake and retention. While AVP is important, thirst provides greater protection against hypernatremia. Thus, hypernatremia due to water loss occurs mainly in vulnerable patients with altered mental status and those who are unable to obtain water, such as infants, the elderly, and the severely ill.

The causes of hypernatremia are grouped into three categories, according to the total body sodium content as estimated by extracellular volume (**Figure 249-4**). Thus, the diagnostic approach to the hypernatremic patient hinges on the assessment of extracellular volume. The history should include a review of recent and current medications, vomiting, diarrhea, increased urinary losses (polyuria), recent fluid intake, and the presence or absence of thirst. Physical examination must assess volume and neurologic status.

In *hypovolemic hypernatremia*, there is a predominant loss of solute-free water leading to elevation in the serum sodium

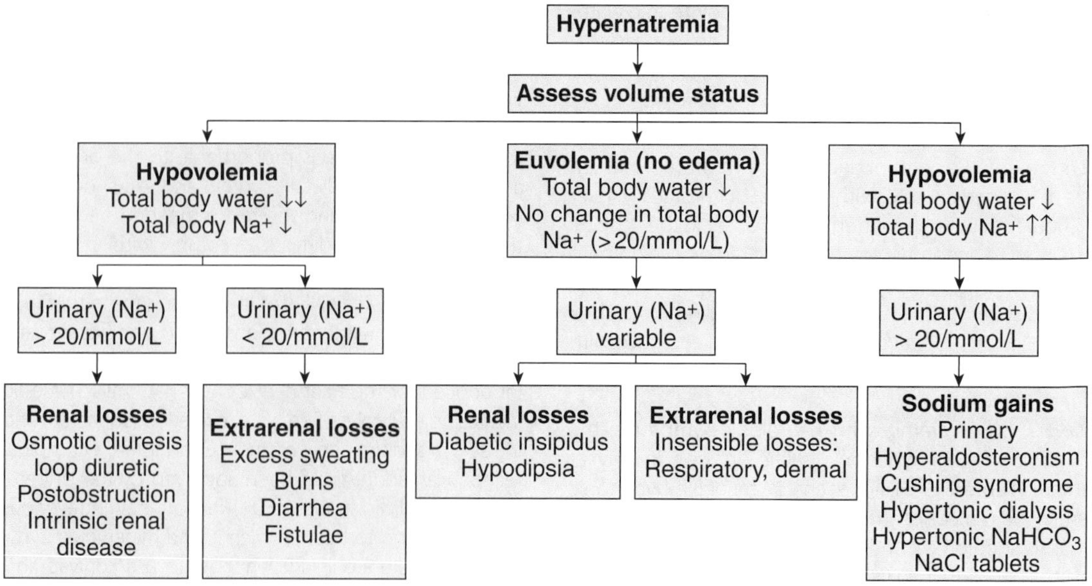

Figure 249-4 *Diagnostic approach to hypernatremia. (Reproduced, with permission, from Lerma EV, Berns JS, Nissenson AR. Current Diagnosis & Treatment: Nephrology & Hypertension. New York: McGraw-Hill; 2009. Fig. 3-4.)*

concentration. This can occur either from renal or extrarenal sources. Extrarenal losses include gastrointestinal causes, with diarrhea being more likely than vomiting to cause hypernatremia. Osmotic diarrhea, as induced by lactulose, malabsorption, and some infectious diarrheas, may result in water being lost in excess of sodium and potassium, leading to hypernatremia. Secretory diarrhea, in contrast, produces fluid with an electrolyte content similar to plasma, leading to volume and potassium loss, but not hypernatremia. Insensible salt and water losses through evaporation from the respiratory tract and sweat, as in fever or strenuous exercise in hot temperature, may lead to hypernatremia, because of the hypotonic nature of the lost fluid.

The most common renal causes of sodium and water loss are loop diuretics and osmotic diuresis. Loop diuretics may lead to hypernatremia because they provoke loss of isotonic or hypotonic fluid. Excessive hypotonic urinary loss of nonelectrolyte solutes, such as urea and glucose, causes hypernatremia by impairing tubular reabsorption of sodium and water. Most hypotonic fluid losses do not cause hypernatremia, unless inadequate free water is ingested or infused to replace the ongoing losses. Hence, these disorders usually also involve some component of inadequate fluid intake.

In *hypervolemic hypernatremia*, there is excess sodium in the extracellular compartment with evidence of extracellular volume expansion. This is usually seen in hospitalized patients who receive excessive amounts of saline or sodium bicarbonate to treat metabolic acidosis, or those receiving enteral or parenteral feedings without adequate free water administration.

Euvolemic hypernatremia

Loss of water without sodium increases fluid tonicity, but usually does not result in clinically evident volume depletion because water is mainly distributed in the intracellular compartment. *Euvolemic hypernatremia* occurs when there is loss of fluid that is low in sodium and potassium salts. The classic example is diabetes insipidus (DI) from either defects in AVP production or release (central DI), a failure of renal response to AVP (nephrogenic DI), or, rarely, from rapid degradation of AVP by vasopressinase during pregnancy. Most patients with DI present with polyuria and polydipsia; hypernatremia is not present unless fluid intake is inadequate.

Central DI can be partial or complete. Causes include head trauma, brain surgery, and inflammatory, neoplastic, and infiltrative disorders of the hypothamalus and pituitary. However, no cause is identified in about half of the cases. Nephrogenic DI is usually a congenital or acquired defect of vasopressin V2 receptors or the vasopressin-dependent water channel (aquaporin 2). Acquired causes include medullary or interstitial renal disease, such as interstitial nephritis, polycystic kidney disease, partial urinary tract obstruction, and advanced chronic kidney disease. Hypercalcemia and hypokalemia may also cause nephrogenic DI, as well as various drugs that impair response to AVP, such as lithium. The various forms of DI must be differentiated from primary polydipsia in patients who present with polyuria.

Urine sodium, volume, and osmolality should be measured to determine the integrity of the AVP-renal axis. The normal response to hypernatremia is to increase AVP release, resulting in urine osmolality that can reach a maximum of 1000 mOsm/kg in normal young individuals, and above 500 mOsm/kg in elderly patients who usually have reduced responsiveness to AVP. Reduced urine osmolality indicates either impaired AVP release (central) or action (nephrogenic).

The various forms of DI may be differentiated from primary polydipsia in patients with polyuria by performing the water deprivation test, along with administration of AVP. An increase in urine osmolality with exogenous AVP is consistent with central DI, whereas lack of response suggests nephrogenic DI. With fluid restriction leading to a 3% weight loss, patients with primary polydipsia should spontaneously increase their urine osmolality and will not increase their urine osmolality more with exogenous vasopressin. With partial central DI, fluid restriction will not maximally stimulate AVP, thus a further increase in urinary osmolality (> 10%) will occur with exogenous vasopressin.

Clinical manifestations

Patients without perturbed neurologic status and with normal thirst mechanisms should complain of thirst. If allowed to progress, hypernatremia becomes associated with confusion, restlessness, irritability, and other neurologic manifestations of cellular dehydration and brain cell shrinkage. Clinical signs may include muscular twitching, hyperreflexia and ataxia. Severe elevations of serum sodium may lead to focal and grand mal seizures, intracerebral hemorrhage, and death. More severe symptoms and signs occur in patients with a more rapid rise of serum osmolality, patients with extreme elevations of serum osmolality, especially above 325 mOsm/kg, and patients at extremes of age, with the very young and the very old being most vulnerable to severe manifestations. Hypernatremia developing over a longer period of time enables brain cells to undergo osmotic adaptation by generating idiogenic osmoles to guard against cell shrinkage. While protective, they may nonetheless predispose the brain to edema if hypernatremia is corrected rapidly by favoring intracellular fluid shifts.

Therapy

In hypernatremia with extracellular volume depletion, restoration of ECF volume is the primary therapeutic target. Isotonic saline is the fluid of choice, and the volume and rate of administration should be guided by clinical parameters including pulse rate, orthostatic blood pressure measurements, and urine output. Once euvolemia is established, further fluid therapy should be delivered to gradually correct tonicity in the form of hypotonic (0.45%) saline.

In rare patients who develop hypernatremia with extracellular volume expansion, loop diuretics may be employed. Ultrafiltration may sometimes be needed to treat hypernatremia in patients with advanced renal impairment.

In patients with hypernatremia without extracellular volume depletion or expansion, the total body sodium is unchanged, but there is a deficit of total body water. Water can be replaced either orally or parenterally with 5% dextrose in water (D5W) or 0.45% NaCl (half-normal saline). The estimated fluid deficit can be estimated by a formula that uses total body water (TBW) because sodium concentration reflects tonicity in all body compartments. For example, a 75 kg man with a serum sodium concentration of 157 mmol/L would need water as estimated by the following:

$$\text{Actual TBW} = \text{body weight} \times 60\% \ (50\% \text{ in women})$$
$$\text{TBW} = 75 \times 0.6 = 45 \text{ L}$$

Then, desired body water is calculated from the following formula:

$$\frac{\text{Actual serum sodium} \times \text{TBW}}{\text{Desired serum sodium}} = \frac{157 \text{ mmol/L} \times 45/\text{L}}{140 \text{ mmol L}} = 50.5 \text{ L}$$

The estimated water deficit is the difference between desired body water and actual body water. In this example, the administration of 5.5 L (50.5 L – 45 L) should correct the water deficit and normalize the serum sodium concentration. In addition to estimated water deficit, estimated ongoing water losses during the time of repletion should be added. This includes at least a liter per day of insensible losses, with greater amounts in febrile or mechanically ventilated patients.

Water replacement should be carried out gradually over hours to days, unless there is evidence that hypernatremia has evolved quickly. This is because water replacement needs to keep pace with the osmotic adaptation process by which the brain cells keep from shrinking. Replacement also has to be tailored to the presence of neurologic symptoms and signs, which call for more rapid serum sodium correction. Acute symptomatic hypernatremia that developed over hours may be rapidly corrected, as the risk of cerebral edema is minimal. In patients with acute symptomatic hypernatremia, serum sodium should be lowered by 1 mmol/L per hour. Once the patient is no longer symptomatic, the correction rate can be slowed to 0.5 mmol/L per hour. Hypernatremia that has developed over more than 24 hours or of unknown duration should be corrected with a maximal rate of 0.5 mmol/L per hour. Half of the water deficit should be replaced over the first 24 hours, with the remainder over the following 24 hours or longer. The cornerstone of central DI treatment is desmopressin (dDAVP), administered either nasally, intravenously, or subcutaneously. Patients with nephrogenic DI do not respond to exogenous desmopressin. Salt restriction and thiazide diuretics produce mild volume contraction, which helps to decrease urinary output. Nonsteroidal anti-inflammatory drugs also help reduce urine output. Patients with lithium-associated nephrogenic DI may benefit from amiloride.

Discharge considerations

Water replacement can be carried out orally once neurologic symptoms resolve, taking ongoing fluid losses into consideration. Discharge planning needs to be tailored according to the underlying cause of hypernatremia and the clinical stability of the patient. Patients on gastric tube feedings who develop hypernatremia should be discharged on free water supplementation via the tube several times daily.

QUALITY IMPROVEMENT

Hyponatremia developing in the hospital setting may be due to administering hypotonic fluids (D5W, D5 0.45% saline or 0.45% saline), particularly in patients with hypovolemia or in the postoperative period, when AVP is stimulated. Educational efforts should emphasize the need for clinicians to prescribe isotonic maintenance fluids.

Hypernatremia developing in the hospital is usually due to the administration of hypertonic intravenous fluids, such as sodium bicarbonate or 3% saline. Compromised renal function aggravates this problem by impairing solute-free water excretion. Other patients who may manifest hypernatremia in the hospital include those with increased insensible losses from fever or hyperventilation, particularly when they cannot express their desire for water. Quality measures to address those issues include restricting the administration of hypertonic solutions unless clearly clinically indicated, as well as meticulously monitoring the fluid and electrolyte profiles of hypernatremia-prone patients.

CONCLUSION

Disorders of sodium and water homeostasis are involved in virtually all critically ill patients, thus a knowledge of the pathophysiology, diagnosis and management is pivotal for excellent patient care.

SUGGESTED READINGS

Adler SM, Verbalis JG. Disorders of body water homeostasis in critical illness. *Endocrinol Metab Clin North Am*. 2006;35:873–894.

Brater DC. Diuretic therapy. *N Engl J Med*. 1998;339:387–395.

Ellison DH, Berl T. Clinical practice. The syndrome of inappropriate antidiuresis. *N Engl J Med*. 2007;356:2064–2072.

Finfer S, Bellomo R, Boyce N, et al. A comparison of albumin and saline for fluid resuscitation in the intensive care unit. *N Engl J Med*. 2004;350:2247.

Salvador D, Rey N, Ramos G, Punzalan F. Continuous infusion versus bolus injection of loop diuretics in congestive heart failure. *Cochrane Database Syst Rev*. 2004;1:CD003178.

Schrier RW, Bansal S. Diagnosis and management of hyponatremia in acute illness. *Curr Opin Crit Care*. 2008;14:627–634.

Upadhyay A, Jaber BL, Madias NE. Incidence and prevalence of hyponatremia. *Am J Med*. 2006;119(7 Suppl 1):S30–S35.

Verbalis JG, Goldsmith SR, Greenberg A, Schrier RW, Sterns RH. Hyponatremia treatment guidelines 2007: expert panel recommendations. *Am J Med*. 2007;120(11 Suppl 1):S1–S21.

CHAPTER 250

Potassium and Magnesium Disorders

Steven M. Gorbatkin, MD, PhD
Lynn Schlanger, MD
James L. Bailey, MD

Key Clinical Questions

1. What are the causes of potassium and magnesium disorders?
2. What are the potential consequences of potassium and magnesium disorders?
3. How are potassium and magnesium disorders treated?
4. How are potassium disorders treated in clinical situations with rapid potassium shifts, such as diabetic ketoacidosis, hyperglycemic hyperosmolar state, and periodic paralysis?

INTRODUCTION

Potassium and magnesium disorders are common in the hospital setting. About 12% of hospitalized patients have hypokalemia, 3% have hyperkalemia, and 11% have hypomagnesemia. Potassium disorders are a particular challenge for hospitalists, as the first clinical manifestation of a severe potassium abnormality may be a cardiac arrhythmia.

Potassium (K^+) is the most abundant intracellular cation. In a 70 kg adult, the total body K^+ is approximately 3500 mmol (50 mmol/kg). About 98% is located in the intracellular compartment, with the majority localized in muscle (70%). Because only 2% of the total body K^+ is in the extracellular compartment, laboratory results correlate poorly with total body K^+. Normal levels of extracellular potassium are between 3.5 and 5.0 mmol/L, while intracellular K^+ levels range between 140 and 150 mmol/L.

Similarly, plasma magnesium (Mg^{2+}) accounts for only 1% of the total body magnesium stores, and plasma Mg^{2+} correlates poorly with total body magnesium. Plasma magnesium is normally 1.7 to 2.3 mg/dL (0.70–0.95 mmol/L). Magnesium abnormalities can also have major clinical consequences, such as torsades de pointes. Hypokalemia is often accompanied by hypomagnesemia, which renders potassium repletion less effective.

POTASSIUM BALANCE

Dietary K^+ is excreted mostly in the urine (90%), with a minor component of fecal excretion (10%). In severe chronic kidney disease, stool losses may exceed 25% to 50% of dietary intake. Under normal conditions, the kidney can adjust potassium excretion over a wide range depending on K^+ intake. The recommended daily K^+ for patients with normal renal function is 4700 mg (120 mmol). If K^+ control mechanisms are intact, an increased daily intake of 400 mmol can be tolerated with < 1 mmol/L increase in plasma K^+ values. Daily K^+ intake for patients on hemodialysis or with severe chronic kidney disease is typically 2000 mg (51 mmol) per day. Conversely, many patients on peritoneal dialysis can tolerate a normal daily intake of K^+ due to losses of potassium in the urine and peritoneal fluid.

PRACTICE POINT

Potassium unit conversion

- 25.6 mmol of elemental potassium is equivalent to 1 g of potassium. Since the charge of the potassium cation is 1^+, 1 mmol = 1 mEq.

HYPERKALEMIA

ETIOLOGY

Hyperkalemia is defined as a plasma K^+ > 5.0 mmol/L. Hyperkalemia can result from redistribution, reduced K^+ excretion, or increased K^+ intake. Medications may lead to hyperkalemia by affecting either potassium redistribution or excretion (**Table 250-1**).

Pseudohyperkalemia is a laboratory artifact due to potassium release from cells prior to laboratory measurement. It should be suspected when hyperkalemia is reported in the setting of red blood cell hemolysis, leukocytosis (> 70,000/mm^3) or thrombocytosis (> 500,000/mm^3), and no ECG changes are present. It has become less common with the increased use of plasma for potassium

TABLE 250-1 Medications Associated with Hyperkalemia

Mechanism	Medications
Increased potassium load	KCL, penicillin G
Renin release inhibition	Beta-blockers, NSAIDs, COX-2 inhibitors
Angiotensin I to II conversion inhibition	ACE inhibitors
Angiotensin II receptor blockade	ARBs
Aldosterone synthesis inhibition	Heparin
Aldosterone receptor blockade	Spironolactone, eplerenone
Renal epithelial Na channel; (ENaC) blockade	Triamterene, amiloride, Trimethoprim, pentamidine
Inhibition of Na-K-ATPase	Digoxin, calcineurin inhibitors (cyclosporin, tacrolimus)
Drug-induced rhabdomyolysis	Statins, cocaine
Drug-induced tumor lysis	Selected chemotherapy agents
Transcellular shift	Succinylcholine

ACE, angiotensin-converting enzyme; ARB, angiotensin receptor blocker; NSAIDS, nonsteroidal anti-inflammatory drugs.

measurement, rather than serum. Plasma is the supernatant collected from heparinized whole blood, whereas serum is the supernatant remaining after centrifugation of a clotted whole blood sample. Serum K^+ is normally 0.3 mmol/L above the plasma K^+, but may be higher if K^+ is released from the clot formed in the tube. If pseudohyperkalemia is suspected, the plasma potassium should be measured instead of the serum potassium. Pseudohyperkalemia can also occur due to potassium release from muscle cells following prolonged constriction with a tourniquet or limb exercise while a tourniquet is in place.

Redistribution of potassium

Redistribution of potassium from the intracellular to the extracellular space can occur in severe acidosis due to nonorganic acid metabolic acidosis, hyperosmolar states, tissue breakdown, and hyperkalemic periodic paralysis. Organic acids such as lactic acid and ketoacids are less likely to cause hyperkalemia than non-organic acids. These organic acids have greater transmembrane mobility, allowing movement into cells with H^+, rather than movement of K^+ out of cells in exchange for H^+. Hyperkalemia in diabetic ketoacidosis usually results from insulin deficiency and hyperosmolality, rather than acidosis. Hyperglycemia increases extracellular osmolality, drawing water from cells down the osmotic gradient. Potassium follows the water movement (solvent drag), and hyperkalemia results.

Tissue breakdown may liberate large amounts of intracellular potassium, resulting in rapid, life-threatening increases in extracellular potassium. Rhabdomyolysis, tissue necrosis, tumor lysis with chemotherapy, and large hematomas are common causes. For rhabdomyolysis, hypokalemia may precede hyperkalemia because of vasoconstriction and decreased blood flow to the involved muscle.

Hyperkalemic periodic paralysis is an autosomal dominant disorder involving the muscle cell sodium channel. During these episodes, potassium moves from the intracellular to extracellular space, accompanied by movement of sodium and water into the cell. The hyperkalemia is accompanied by weakness or paralysis.

Decreased potassium excretion

Potassium excretion in the distal nephron depends upon adequate urine flow, aldosterone, and activity of the basolateral Na^+/K^+-ATPase. The reabsorption of luminal Na^+ through aldosterone-sensitive epithelial sodium channels (ENaCs) creates an electrochemical gradient for K^+ excretion in the urine. Hyperkalemia can occur in aldosterone-resistant or -deficient states by attenuating the electrochemical gradient for K^+ secretion. Acquired mineralocorticoid resistance from diabetes mellitus, obstructive uropathy, chronic tubulointerstitial disease, sickle cell anemia, lupus nephritis, and medications, as well as decreased mineralocorticoid production (including medication induced), are commonly associated with a type IV renal tubular acidosis (RTA). Type IV RTA is characterized by hyperkalemia, normal anion gap hyperchloremic acidosis with serum HCO_3 values ranging between 16 and 22 mmol/L, and decreased urinary NH_4^+ production, causing a positive urine anion gap [Urine (Na^+) + (K^+) − (Cl^-)]. In acute and chronic tubular injury, a decreased responsiveness to aldosterone can contribute to hyperkalemia. For acute kidney injury associated with prerenal azotemia or hypovolemic states, decreased urinary flow to the distal tubule and a reduction in sodium-potassium exchange can contribute to hyperkalemia.

Excessive potassium intake

Excessive intake of K^+ rarely causes hyperkalemia in the setting of normal renal function. Renal secretion of potassium is typically adequate at glomerular filtration rates (GFR) above 20–30 ml/min/1.73 m^2. Patients with end-stage renal disease (ESRD) on hemodialysis usually tolerate a daily K^+ intake of 2000 mg (51 mEq). Upregulated gut potassium excretion and shifts in transcellular K^+ prevent hyperkalemia between dialysis sessions. Loss of these mechanisms may result in the rapid development of hyperkalemia, especially with large exogenous loads of potassium, such as massive blood transfusions. Irradiation of blood and increased age of the blood increase the amount of free potassium that is released during the blood transfusion. Seven-day-old blood has approximately 23 mmol/L of K^+, while 42-day-old blood has approximately 50 mmol/L of K^+.

PRACTICE POINT

- In the setting of acute kidney injury, hyperkalemia associated with rapid transcellular potassium shifts from the intracellular to extracellular compartment can be seen with rhabdomylosis, tissue necrosis, tumor lysis, and large hematomas. Hyperkalemia in this setting may progress rapidly to cause life-threatening arrhythmias. Emergent nephrology consultation for possible dialysis is required.

SIGNS AND SYMPTOMS

Clinical effects of hyperkalemia relate to altered membrane excitability due to changes in the transcellular potassium gradient. Severe hyperkalemia leads to cardiac arrhythmias and conduction abnormalities. It may also cause weakness of the lower extremities, progressing superiorly to cause flaccid paralysis and respiratory failure. This presentation may mimic Guillain-Barré syndrome, but is easily differentiated by the response to potassium correction. Hyperkalemia may also contribute to metabolic acidosis by interfering with renal ammonium excretion.

EVALUATION OF HYPERKALEMIA IN THE HOSPITALIZED PATIENT

In the hospital setting, the initial evaluation of hyperkalemia includes monitoring for life-threatening arrhythmias, checking for pseudohyperkalemia, eliminating exogenous sources of potassium, evaluating renal function, and evaluating for rapid transcellular shifts of potassium (**Figure 250-1**).

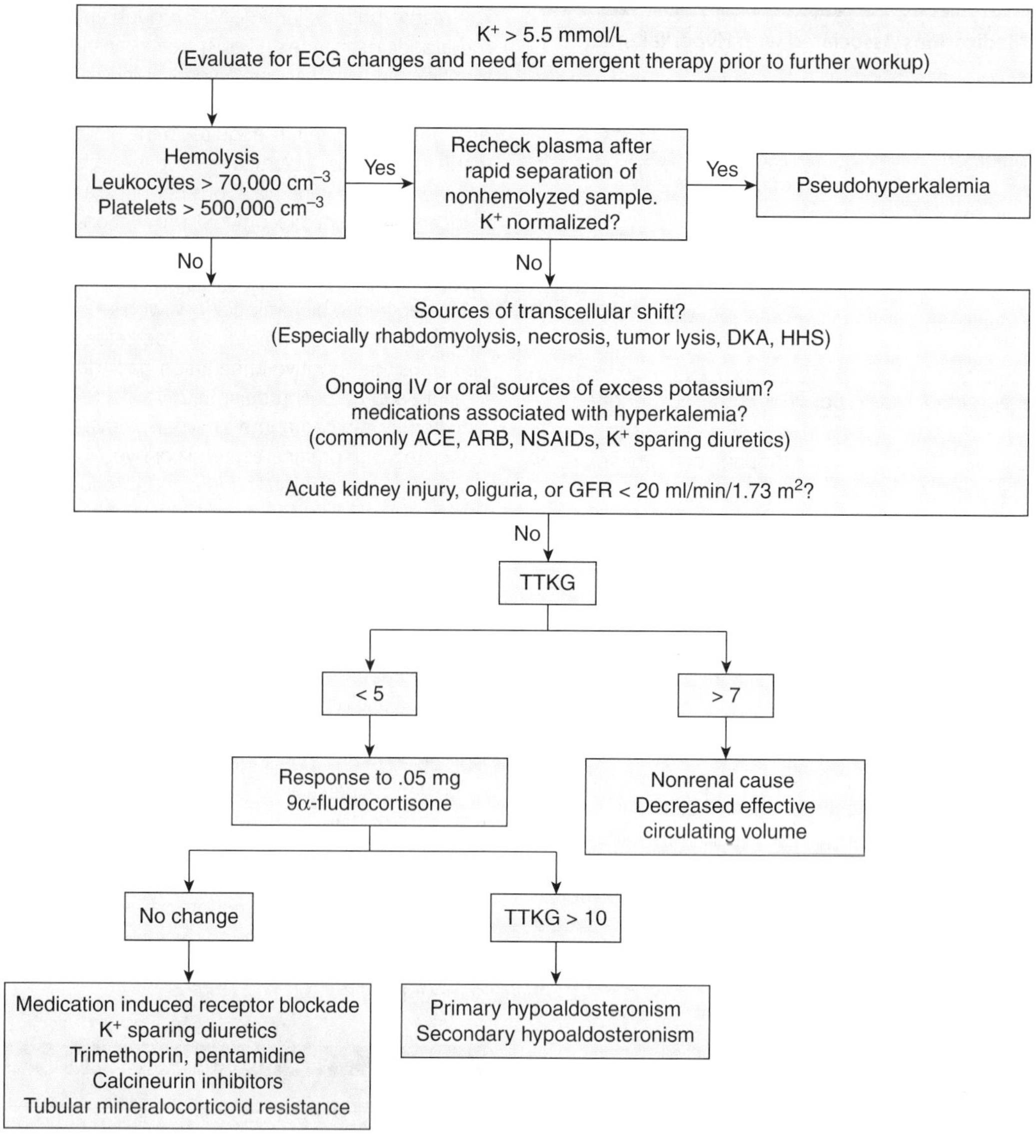

Figure 250-1 *Diagnostic assessment of hyperkalemia. (ACE, angiotensin-converting enzyme inhibitor; ARB, angiotensin receptor blocker; DKA, diabetic ketoacidosis; ECG, electrocardiogram; GFR, glomerular filtration rate; HHS, hyperosmolar hyperglycemic state; NSAIDs, nonsteroidal anti-inflammatory drugs; TTKG, transtubular potassium gradient.)*

ECG changes

Even mildly elevated K^+ levels may be associated with ECG changes, especially in the setting of rapid rises in plasma K^+ values. If ECG changes from hyperkalemia are found or if the plasma K^+ value is ≥7.0, continuous telemetry is indicated and should continue until the plasma K^+ value is ≤5.8 and there are no hyperkalemic ECG changes. Frequent chemistry checks are indicated for plasma K^+ greater than 5.8 or for hyperkalemia associated with ECG changes, severe hyperglycemia, or any clinical condition which predisposes the patient to rapid changes in plasma K^+.

Plasma potassium levels do not correlate with specific ECG changes. A symmetric increase in T wave height may be seen initially. Hyperkalemia-induced peaked T waves may be difficult to distinguish from the hyperacute T waves of myocardial injury. As potassium levels rise further, flattening of the P waves, prolongation of the PR interval, and prolonged QRS duration occur. Eventually, atrial standstill and a sine wave ECG pattern may be seen (**Figure 250-2**).

Urine potassium and transtubular potassium gradient

A 24-hour urine K^+ measurement can help differentiate between renal and nonrenal causes of hyperkalemia. With hyperkalemia, urinary excretion of K^+ should exceed 40 mmol/d. Alternatively, the transtubular potassium gradient (TTKG), a measurement of potassium secretion by the distal nephron corrected for urine osmolality, can be used:

$$TTKG = (K_U/K_S) \times (S_{Osm}/U_{Osm})$$

K_U and K_S are the concentrations of K^+ in the urine and serum, and S_{Osm} and U_{Osm} are the osmolalities of the serum and urine, respectively. Plasma potassium and osmolality can be used instead of serum values to estimate TTKG with minimal effect on clinical interpretation.

Patients with normal renal function and normal potassium intake have a TTKG of 8 to 9. In hyperkalemia, a low TTKG (<5–7) suggests an inappropriately low secretion of potassium. A high TTKG with hyperkalemia suggests normal aldosterone action and an extrarenal

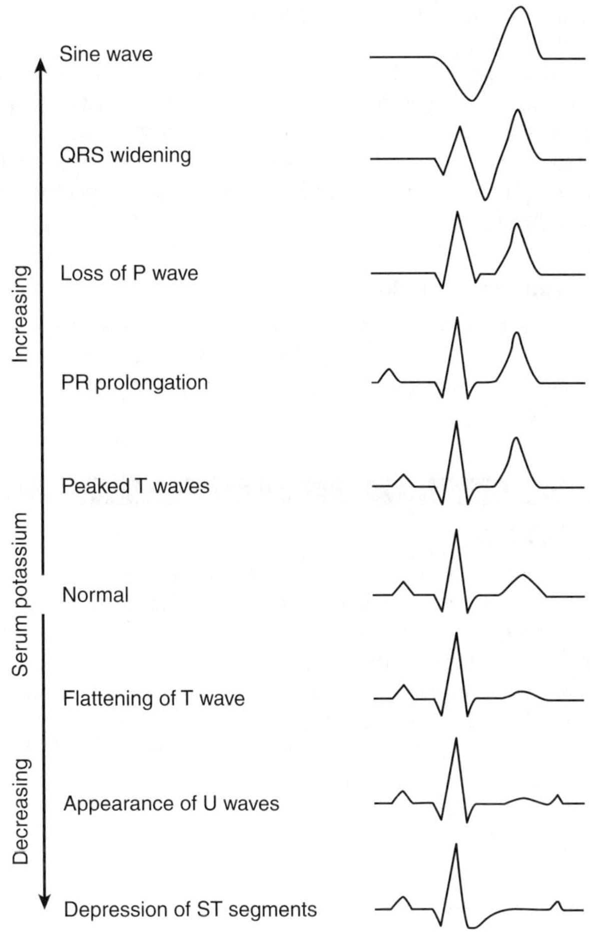

Figure 250-2 *ECG changes associated with hyperkalemia and hypokalemia. (Reproduced, with permission, from Flomenbaum N, Goldfrank LR, Hoffman R, et al, eds. Goldfrank's Toxicologic Emergencies. 8th ed. New York: McGraw-Hill; 2006: Figure 5-11.)*

cause of hyperkalemia, except in cases of volume depletion where aldosterone secretion is enhanced with a TTKG >7, but total renal potassium excretion is limited by low urine flow.

When the TTKG is inappropriately low in the setting of hyperkalemia, an increase in the TTKG to >10 after the administration of 0.05 mg of fludrocortisone suggests hypoaldosteronism. If fludrocortisone has no effect on the TTKG, drug-induced or intrinsic renal resistance to aldosterone are likely.

TREATMENT OF HYPERKALEMIA

Definitive treatments for hyperkalemia, such as gastrointestinal resins and laxatives or hemodialysis, enhance the elimination of potassium. As these therapies may not act immediately or may involve logistical difficulties, they are often used in conjunction with short-acting temporizing measures, such as cardiac membrane stabilization with calcium, and agents such as insulin that cause transcellular potassium shifts (**Table 250-2**).

Cardiac membrane stabilization

Intravenous calcium stabilizes the cardiac membrane by inhibiting membrane depolarization. It is the most important initial treatment for severe hyperkalemia. Two forms of calcium are commonly available: calcium gluconate and calcium chloride. Calcium gluconate is preferred because it can be administered through a peripheral intravenous line, whereas calcium chloride requires a central venous line to prevent tissue necrosis. A 10 mL ampule of calcium gluconate contains 90 mg (2.3 mmol) of elemental calcium, and a 10 ml ampule of calcium chloride contains 272 mg (7.0 mmol) of elemental calcium.

The initial dose of calcium gluconate is 10 mL of 10% solution infused over 2 to 3 minutes. 3.3 mL of 10% calcium chloride contains the same amount of elemental calcium. The onset of action is 1 to 3 minutes, and duration is 30 to 60 minutes. Calcium cannot be mixed with bicarbonate solutions because precipitation of $CaCO_3$ occurs.

Administration of intravenous calcium to patients taking digoxin requires extreme caution, as calcium has been shown

TABLE 250-2 Treatment of Hyperkalemia

Mechanism	Treatment	Dose	Onset	Duration	Comments
Cardiac membrane stabilization	Calcium	Calcium gluconate 10 ml of 10% solution infused over 2–3 minutes.	1–3 min	30–60 min	Do not mix with bicarbonate. Extreme caution if on digoxin. Calcium chloride alternative but risk of tissue necrosis and requires central line.
Redistribution	Insulin	10 units regular insulin IV. If BG < 250 mg/dl, give 50 ml of 50% dextrose.	10–20 min	4–6 hr peak 30–60 min	Most reliable treatment to induce redistribution.
Redistribution	Beta-2 agonist	Albuterol 10–20 mg nebulized	30 min	2–4 hr peak 90 min	Dose is significantly higher than dose for respiratory treatments. Caution for patients at risk for side effects such as tachycardia, ischemia
Removal	Kayexalate	30–60 grams oral in 20% sorbitol or 60 grams in 250 ml water by retention enema	1–2 hr	Variable	Risk of colonic necrosis if used in post-operative patients. Do not use sorbitol for enema
Removal	Hemodialysis	—	Immediate	Same as dialysis duration	Intermittent or continuous.

to potentiate the effects of digoxin toxicity in animal models, especially at very rapid infusion rates. The risk of calcium administration in this setting can be reduced by infusing the calcium gluconate over 20 to 30 minutes. Another option is to administer digoxin immune fab to neutralize the effect of the digoxin.

PRACTICE POINT

- In the setting of digoxin toxicity, mild levels of hyperkalemia (serum $K^+ > 5.0$ mmol/L) have been linked to significant mortality and digoxin immune fab may be indicated.

Potassium redistribution

Insulin is the most reliable means of inducing transcellular potassium shifts. The usual dose is 10 units of regular insulin intravenously, followed immediately by 50 mL of 50% dextrose (25 g of dextrose). For a blood glucose > 250, insulin can be administered alone with close glucose monitoring. The effect begins in 10 to 20 minutes, peaks at 30 to 60 minutes, and lasts 4 to 6 hours. Potassium levels typically drop by 0.5 to 1.2 mmol/L. An infusion of 10 units of regular insulin can also be administered over one hour in 10% dextrose.

Beta-2 agonists have an additive effect with insulin in transiently reducing plasma potassium by redistribution. High doses of nebulized albuterol are used, typically 10 to 20 mg of nebulized albuterol in 4 ml of normal saline over 10 minutes. Plasma potassium levels usually fall by 0.5–1 mmol/L. The effect begins in 30 minutes, peaks at 90 minutes, and lasts 2 to 4 hours. Intravenous albuterol has also been used, but it is not available in the United States. As some patients, including those with renal failure, have a reduced response to albuterol, it should not be the only agent used. Caution should be exercised for individuals at risk for side effects such as cardiac ischemia from the resulting increase in heart rate.

Sodium bicarbonate ($NaHCO_3$) does not reliably lead to the redistribution of potassium, and it should not be considered as first-line therapy for hyperkalemia. This is especially true in high anion gap acidosis, where hyperkalemia is usually not a direct consequence of the presence of organic acids. If intravenous or oral $NaHCO_3$ is used to treat metabolic acidosis caused by nonorganic anions, which is usually associated with a normal anion gap, plasma potassium may fall, but it is not preferred treatment even in this setting. Oral $NaHCO_3$ is useful for chronic treatment of type IV renal tubular acidosis.

Potassium removal

Sodium polystyrene sulfonate (Kayexalate) exchanges Na^+ for K^+ in the gastrointestinal tract. When taken orally, sorbitol is typically added to the resin to speed passage through the gastrointestinal tract. Each gram of resin binds 0.5 to 1.2 mmol of K^+. Oral doses of 15 to 60 g are typical. Sodium polystyrene sulfonate can also be administered rectally as a retention enema, at a dose of 30 to 60 g in 250 mL of water every 6 hours. Doses as high as 100 g have been used, but safety data is lacking. The solution should be introduced by gravity, flushed with an additional 50 to 100 mL of nonsodium containing fluid, retained 30 to 60 minutes or longer, and cleansed with 250 to 1000 mL of nonsodium containing solution at body temperature. Sorbitol should not be used rectally due to risk of colonic necrosis. Oral or rectal Kayexalate should not be used in postoperative patients for the same reason.

Dialysis is required for treatment of refractory hyperkalemia. Intermittent hemodialysis removes potassium most rapidly. Continuous renal replacement therapy is an option for patients who have ongoing causes of severe hyperkalemia, such as tissue necrosis or rhabdomyolysis. Peritoneal dialysis provides a gradual removal of potassium, but it is rarely used when the other modalities are available.

Diuretics are unreliable for the acute treatment of hyperkalemia in the setting of compromised renal function. In patients with adequate renal function, the combination of a loop and thiazide diuretic is more effective for potassium removal than either alone. Of the loop diuretics, torsemide and bumetanide have higher bioavailability than furosemide.

Potassium intake reduction

The typical daily potassium intake for a patient with end-stage renal disease is 2000 mg (51 mmol) of potassium per day, but patients with acute kidney injury may require even more stringent potassium restriction.

HYPOKALEMIA

ETIOLOGY

Hypokalemia can result from redistribution, increased potassium excretion from renal and nonrenal sources, or decreased potassium intake. Medications, especially loop and thiazide diuretics, frequently cause hypokalemia. Hypokalemia is common with tubular toxins such as amphotericin B and cisplatin. High doses of penicillin or semisynthetic penicillins such as ticarcillin and carbenicillin occasionally cause renal potassium wasting in the distal nephron due to an impermeant anion effect. Inhalation of toluene (glue sniffing) may cause distal renal tubular acidosis with associated hypokalemia.

Pseudohypokalemia

Falsely low serum or plasma potassium values may occur in conditions such as acute leukemia due to time-dependent uptake of potassium by the increased abnormal white cell mass. Rapid analysis of the sample, or storing the sample at 4°C prior to analysis, can prevent the potassium uptake and confirm the diagnosis of pseudohypokalemia.

Redistribution

Insulin directly stimulates potassium entry into cells by increasing the activity of the Na^+/K^+-ATPase pump. This mechanism is independent of stimulation of cellular glucose entry. Beta-2-adrenergic activators stimulate Na^+/K^+-ATPase mediated cellular potassium uptake by a slightly different cellular mechanism. Thus, insulin and beta-2-adrenergic activation may act synergistically to cause hypokalemia. Aldosterone stimulates direct cellular uptake and redistribution due to increased Na^+/K^+-ATPase activity. It also acts in the distal renal tubule to enhance potassium excretion.

Thyrotoxic periodic paralysis causes severe hypokalemia by redistribution, in conjunction with extremity and limb girdle weakness, hypophosphatemia, and hypomagnesemia. It is more common in patients of Asian and Hispanic origin. Attacks often occur during rest after vigorous physical activity, and can also be precipitated by carbohydrate-rich meals. Other rare genetic forms of hypokalemic periodic paralysis also exist.

Nonrenal potassium losses

Common nonrenal causes of hypokalemia include intestinal loss of potassium from diarrhea, celiac disease, ileostomy, and chronic laxative abuse. Potassium loss from vomiting and nasogastric suctioning can result in hypokalemia, although renal potassium losses from aldosterone activation may be more important in this setting. Potassium losses through the skin are usually low, except in the setting of extreme physical exertion. Severe burns may lead to hypokalemia by multiple mechanisms.

Renal potassium loss

Hyperaldosteronism, as in aldosterone-producing adenoma (Conn syndrome), causes hypertension and hypokalemia by acting on aldosterone receptors in the distal renal tubule. Cortisol also activates the aldosterone receptor. Normally, cortisol is converted to cortisone by 11-beta-hydroxysteroid dehydrogenase-2 (11βHSD-2) before it can reach the aldosterone receptor. At very high levels, such as in Cushing syndrome, cortisol overwhelms the ability of 11βHSD-2 to degrade it to cortisone, and the nondegraded cortisol activates the aldosterone receptor in the distal tubule and precipitates hypokalemia. Similarly, glycyrrhizinic acid, found in some types of chewing tobacco or black licorice, inhibits 11βHSD-2, preventing cortisol degradation and causing hypertension and hypokalemia. With vomiting and nasogastric suctioning, potassium wasting in the urine occurs through aldosterone secretion in the setting of volume depletion, as noted above.

Hypokalemia can be associated with an RTA, due to disease of either the proximal (type II RTA) or distal (type I RTA) renal tubules. Either can result from autoimmune, genetic, endocrine, medication-induced, toxin-induced, or idiopathic causes. Rare causes of hypokalemia associated with metabolic alkalosis involve defects in the thick ascending limb of Henle transport proteins (Bartter syndrome), mutations in the thiazide-sensitive Na^+/Cl^- cotransporter in the distal convoluted tubule (Gitelman syndrome), or increased activation of ENaC in the distal tubule (Liddle syndrome).

Decreased potassium intake

Decreased potassium intake is rarely a cause of hypokalemia, except in individuals who are severely malnourished. For a patient with normal renal function who consumes the recommended 4700 mg (120 mmol) of potassium per day, 90% (108 mmol) is excreted in the urine. When intake is sharply reduced, urinary potassium loss decreases to < 15–20 mmol/d in order to conserve potassium.

SIGNS AND SYMPTOMS

Individuals with serum potassium levels between 3.0 and 3.5 mEq/L are often asymptomatic. However, there is a risk of cardiac arrhythmias for individuals with predisposing conditions, such as coronary artery disease. At serum potassium levels between 2.5 and 3.0 mEq/L, patients report generalized weakness and constipation. When serum potassium levels drop below 2.5 mEq/L, there is an increased risk of muscle necrosis and rhabdomyolysis. At serum potassium levels less than 2.0 mEq/L, ascending paralysis and respiratory failure can occur.

EVALUATION OF HYPOKALEMIA

An algorithm for the diagnosis of hypokalemia is presented in **Figure 250-3**. Pseudohypokalemia and transcellular shifts should be excluded. Magnesium levels should be measured early in the workup of hypokalemia. Many disorders, such as diarrhea and excess diuresis, deplete both potassium and magnesium. Moreover, hypomagnesemia may lead to renal potassium wasting via potassium channels in the distal tubule, and make hypokalemia more refractory to treatment.

The next step is to determine whether hypokalemia arose from a renal or nonrenal source. An obvious cause may be apparent, such as profuse diarrhea or escalating doses of a loop or thiazide diuretic. When the source of hypokalemia is unclear, a 24-hour urine potassium measurement may differentiate between renal and nonrenal losses. In the setting of hypokalemia, urinary K^+ losses should fall to less than 15 to 20 mmol/d. Potassium excretion above this level suggests a renal contribution to hypokalemia. The TTKG (see above) may also help to establish the diagnosis. An inappropriately high TTKG (>4) in hypokalemia suggests increased distal potassium secretion and renal potassium loss. A low TTKG can occur with nonrenal potassium wasting, with urinary potassium losses from osmotic diuresis, or with hypokalemia secondary to diuretics which were discontinued at the time of TTKG measurement.

Patients with renal potassium wasting and TTKG >4 should be further classified by acid-base status. Patients with acidosis may have RTA, diabetic ketoacidosis, or tubular dysfunction from drugs such as amphotericin B or acetazolamide. Patients with alkalosis and hypertension may have mineralocorticoid excess or Liddle syndrome. Hypokalemia with alkalosis and normal or low blood pressure may be caused by vomiting, diuretics, and Bartter or Gitelman syndrome. The spot urine chloride is a useful diagnostic tool in evaluating the etiology of hypokalemia in the setting of metabolic alkalosis, with a spot low urine chloride (< 10 mmol/L) suggesting volume depletion and a chloride-responsive state.

ECG changes

ECG changes in hypokalemia are shown in Figure 250-2. U waves appear following the T waves, and become progressively more prominent in comparison to the T waves as potassium levels decrease. Ultimately, the U wave merges with the T wave, and the QT interval appears prolonged.

TREATMENT OF HYPOKALEMIA

Potassium repletion is the cornerstone of therapy for hypokalemia. As extracellular potassium comprises a fraction of the total body potassium store, relatively large amounts of potassium are required to correct the total body potassium deficit. A plasma K^+ 1 mmol/L below normal corresponds to a total body potassium deficit of approximately 200–400 mmol, and a drop in plasma K^+ to 2 mmol/L below normal requires 400 to 800 mmol for repletion. Underlying disorders such as metabolic alkalosis that are causing or perpetuating hypokalemia must also be addressed. Continuous telemetry and frequent electrolyte checks should be performed in severe hypokalemia, or in conditions in which the serum potassium may decline rapidly, such as diabetic ketoacidosis (DKA) and hyperosmolar hyperglycemic state (HHS).

Oral repletion

If there is no immediate threat to life, oral potassium can be used to treat hypokalemia. Generally, potassium chloride (KCl) is indicated for hypokalemia associated with diuretic use or volume depletion. A typical initial dose in a patient with normal renal function is 40 to 100 mmol (40–100 mEq) per day, in 2 to 3 divided doses. Liquid, wax matrix, and microencapsulated forms exist. Compliance is poor with the liquid form due to the strong taste. Although the wax matrix form is easier to swallow, it has been associated with erosions of the gastrointestinal tract. The microencapsulated formulation is associated with the fewest complications.

Other potassium preparations are available for different indications. Oral potassium phosphate is found in many foods, and is indicated for combined potassium and phosphorus depletion. Terminology may mislead. For example, Neutra-Phos actually has more potassium than K-Phos. Potassium bicarbonate is useful for the treatment of both metabolic acidosis and hypokalemia, while potassium citrate may prevent renal stones.

Intravenous repletion

KCl is preferred for intravenous repletion. Potassium phosphate may be used for dual phosphorus and potassium depletion. Potassium

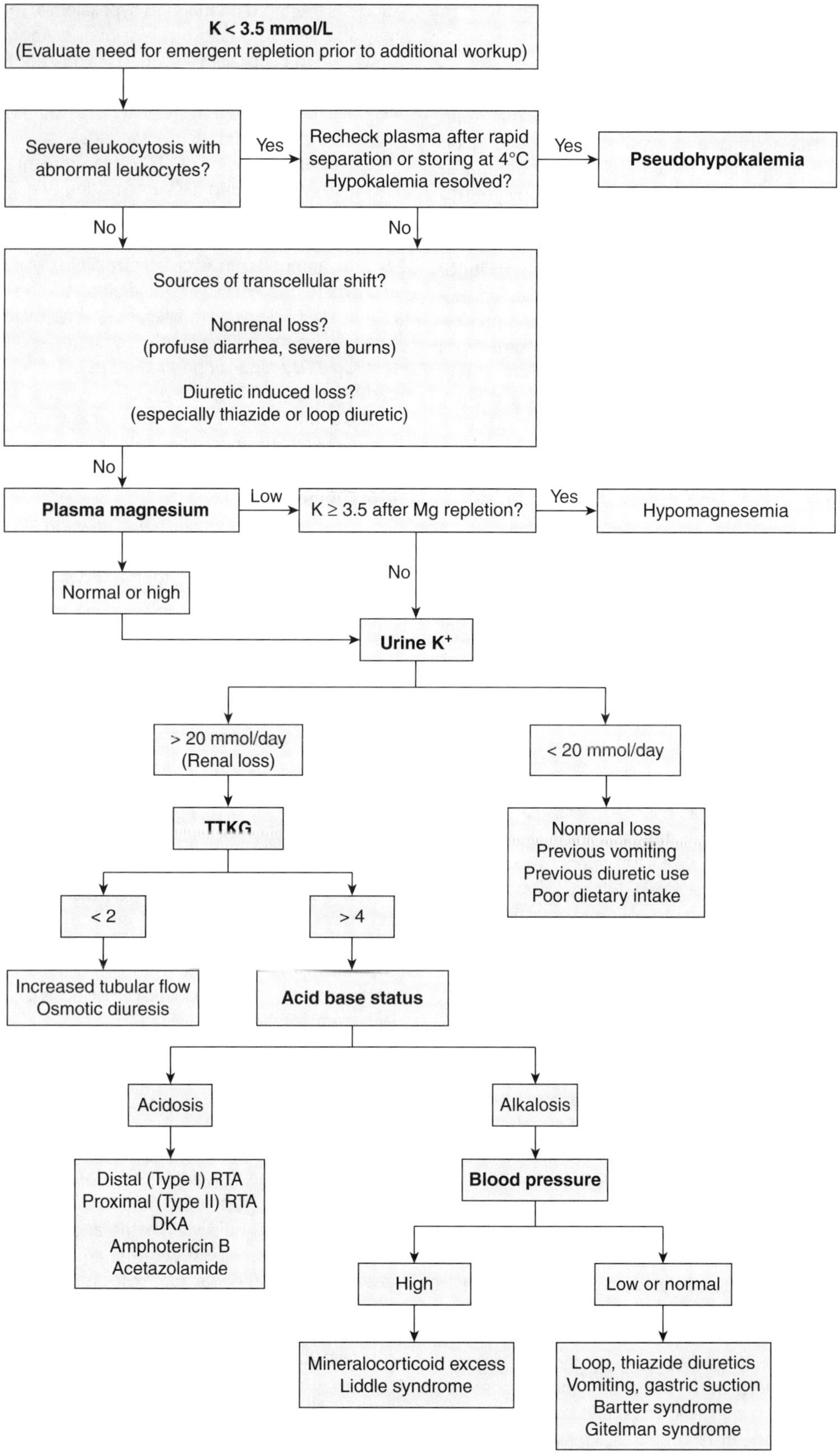

Figure 250-3 *Diagnostic assessment of hypokalemia. DKA, diabetic ketoacidosis; RTA, renal tubular acidosis; TTKG, transtubular potassium gradient.*

can be infused through a peripheral intravenous line at a maximum rate of 10 mmol/hour, and a maximum concentration of 60 mmol/L. Higher rates require a central venous line and continuous ECG monitoring. Infusion rates of 20 to 40 mmol/hour are reserved for cases of life-threatening hypokalemia requiring emergent correction.

Intravenous potassium is a common cause of iatrogenic hyperkalemia. A typical intravenous dose with normal renal function is 20 to 40 mmol (20–40 mEq). Although 20 mmol of intravenous KCl might increase plasma K^+ by 0.25 mmol/L, transcellular shifts make it difficult to predict the effect of therapy. Renal potassium clearance generally decreases significantly at a GFR below 20 to 30 mL/min/1.73 m^2, and requires reduction in potassium dosing and additional monitoring.

Hypokalemia in DKA and HHS

The use of insulin in DKA and HHS drives potassium into the intracellular space, and also decreases the hyperglycemia-induced osmolar driving force for movement of potassium from the intracellular to the extracellular space. Rapid and sometimes life-threatening potassium shifts may result. In 2004, the American Diabetes Association recommended that insulin should not be started until the serum potassium is known. If the serum potassium is < 3.3 mmol/L, insulin therapy is held until the potassium is repleted to 3.3 mmol/L or above. For patients with acceptable renal clearance of potassium, intravenous potassium can be given in the form of two-thirds KCl and one-third potassium phosphate. If the serum potassium is ≥ 3.3 mmol/L, insulin therapy can be initiated, and for potassium ≥ 3.3 and < 5.0 mmol/L, intravenous fluids should contain two-thirds KCl and one-third potassium phosphate, with a total of 20 to 30 mmol/L of potassium, until the patient can tolerate oral potassium supplements. The goal is to achieve serum potassium values between 4 to 5 mmol/L. Potassium supplementation is initially held for serum potassium values ≥ 5 mmol/L, but is often required, as total body stores of potassium are usually depleted and insulin and intravenous fluid therapy eventually unmasks the total body potassium deficit.

PRACTICE POINT

- Extreme caution and frequent monitoring are required in the treatment of hyperkalemia in diabetic ketoacidosis and hyperosmolar hyperglycemic state. Generally, these patients have a total body potassium deficit. Administration of insulin drives potassium intracellularly through direct stimulation of Na^+/K^+-ATPase, while both insulin and intravenous fluids reduce the glucose-induced hyperosmolality that drives solvent drag. These two interventions can lead to a rapid decrease in plasma potassium.

PRACTICE POINT

- Potassium should not be mixed with glucose-containing solutions, because the glucose will stimulate insulin secretion and drive potassium from the extracellular to the intracellular space.

Thyrotoxic hypokalemic periodic paralysis

Oral propranolol (3 mg/kg) is first-line treatment for thyrotoxic periodic paralysis because it rapidly reverses hypokalemia, hypophosphatemia, and hypomagnesemia, and is not associated with rebound hyperkalemia. Aggressive potassium repletion for this disorder is associated with a 25% incidence of hyperkalemia.

MAGNESIUM BALANCE

A typical American diet contains 300 to 400 mg/d of elemental magnesium. Approximately 30% to 40% of dietary magnesium is absorbed in the gut. Additionally, 40 mg/d of magnesium is secreted in the small intestine, of which 20 mg/d is reabsorbed in the colon and rectum. Approximately 100 mg appears in the urine each day, which is 5% of the filtered load. Specific cutoffs for hypomagnesemia and hypermagnesemia are difficult to establish because of the poor correlation between extracellular concentration and total body stores. Plasma magnesium levels of 1.7 to 2.3 mg/dL (0.70–0.95 mmol/L) are considered normal, but a normal serum level may be present with total body magnesium depletion.

PRACTICE POINT

Magnesium unit conversion

- 41.2 mmol of elemental magnesium is equivalent to 1 g of magnesium (24.3 mg = 1 mmol). Since the charge of the magnesium cation is 2^+, 1 mmol = 2 mEq. For a common preparation used for IV magnesium repletion, 1 g of magnesium sulfate ($MgSO_4 7H_2O$) contains 8.1 mEq (98.6 mg) of elemental magnesium.

HYPOMAGNESEMIA

ETIOLOGY OF HYPOMAGNESEMIA

Hypomagnesemia results from low dietary intake, gastrointestinal losses, and renal losses. Poor intake of magnesium is common in alcoholics and hospitalized patients receiving inadequate magnesium supplementation in parenteral nutrition or intravenous fluids. Causes of impaired gastrointestinal absorption include diarrhea, inflammatory bowel disease, laxative abuse, proton pump inhibitors, and small bowel resection.

Osmotic and loop diuretics provoke urinary losses of magnesium. Acutely, thiazide diuretics increase magnesium absorption in the distal convoluted tubule, but long-term use can reduce magnesium reabsorption and cause hypomagnesemia. Urinary wasting of magnesium is also seen in alcoholics. Many nephrotoxic drugs, such as amphotericin B, aminoglycosides, cisplatin, foscarnet, and cyclosporine, interfere with magnesium reabsorption in the thick ascending limb or distal convoluted tubule and cause magnesium wasting. Rare familial disorders, such as Gitelman syndrome, are also associated with urinary magnesium losses.

Miscellaneous causes of hypomagnesemia include acute pancreatitis, in which magnesium and calcium are saponified in necrotic fat, hungry bone syndrome, where magnesium, calcium, and phosphate are absorbed by bone after parathyroidectomy for hyperparathyroidism, and diabetic ketoacidosis, where magnesium levels fall due to osmotic diuresis and insulin-related transmembrane shifts.

HYPOMAGNESEMIA AND OTHER ELECTROLYTE ABNORMALITIES

Hypokalemia

Hypomagnesemia and hypokalemia often coexist due to similar common underlying etiologies, such as excess gastrointestinal losses and diuretics. Hypokalemia is often difficult to correct without magnesium repletion.

Hypercalcemia

Elevated ionized serum calcium levels induce renal Mg^{2+} wasting. Hypomagnesemia is common in hypercalcemia of malignancy.

However, in hypercalcemia secondary to hyperparathyroidism, magnesium deficiency is rare due to the parathyroid hormone (PTH)-induced stimulation of renal Mg^{2+} reabsorption.

Hypocalcemia

Hypomagnesemia may cause hypocalcemia due to inhibition of PTH secretion and by induction of skeletal resistance to PTH. Hypocalcemia may be present in up to half of patients with hypomagnesemia.

CLINICAL MANIFESTATIONS

Mild hypomagnesemia may be asymptomatic. Severe hypomagnesemia leads to neuromuscular, neurologic, and cardiovascular symptoms. Neuromuscular abnormalities include hyperreflexia, carpopedal spasm, delirium, seizures, and tetany. Chvostek and Trousseau signs may be present. ECG manifestations include torsades de pointes, premature ventricular contractions, ventricular tachycardias, and ventricular fibrillation. There is also an increased risk of digitalis cardiac toxicity. As serum magnesium levels do not always correlate with total body magnesium stores, normomagnesemic magnesium depletion may be considered in patients with unexplained hypocalcemia and hypokalemia and clinical risk factors for magnesium deficiency.

EVALUATION OF HYPOMAGNESEMIA

Urine studies

Urine studies are useful to evaluate renal vs nonrenal causes of hypomagnesemia. The fractional excretion of magnesium (Fe_{Mg}) is given by:

$$Fe_{Mg} = \frac{\text{(Urine Mg) (Plasma Creatinine)}}{0.7\ \text{(Plasma Mg) (Urine Creatinine)}}$$

The 0.7 in the denominator is a correction factor for the 30% of plasma magnesium bound to plasma proteins. A Fe_{Mg} of >3% in a patient with normal GFR indicates renal magnesium loss. A 24-hour magnesium collection can also be obtained and is normally 3 to 5 mmol (75–125 mg)/24 hours. In the presence of hypomagnesemia, normal kidneys should be able to reduce the 24-hour urinary excretion of magnesium even further, to 1 mmol or less.

TREATMENT OF HYPOMAGNESEMIA

Oral repletion

The most popular formulation for oral replacement is magnesium oxide (242 mg = 20 mEq Mg^{2+} per 400 mg tablet), with a typical dose of 400 mg two to three times per day. Magnesium chloride, magnesium gluconate, magnesium lactate, and magnesium L-aspartate are other options. Diarrhea is a common side effect. It may be reduced with the use of a sustained release formulation, such as magnesium chloride (64 mg per 535 mg tablet). The potassium-sparing diuretics triamterene and amiloride, which block ENaC in the distal renal tubule, can assist in treatment of hypomagnesemia refractory to oral supplementation.

PRACTICE POINT

- Refractory hypokalemia and hypocalcemia occur with severe Mg^{2+} deficiency and Mg^{2+} repletion is necessary for correction.

Intravenous repletion

Symptomatic or severe hypomagnesemia should be treated with intravenous magnesium. For active seizures or cardiac arrhythmias, an initial dose of 8 to 16 mEq of Mg^{2+} (1–2 g of $MgSO_4 7H_2O$) is administered over two minutes. For nonemergency repletion, 64 mEq of Mg^{2+} (8 g of $MgSO_4 7H_2O$) can be given over the first 24 hours, followed by 32 mEq of Mg^{2+} daily for six additional days. Since magnesium is renally cleared, the dose should be reduced by 25% to 50% and the plasma magnesium level monitored after each dose for GFR < 20–30 mL/min/1.73 m^2.

HYPERMAGNESEMIA

ETIOLOGY

Hypermagnesemia usually results from iatrogenic causes, such as magnesium treatment for preeclampsia or eclampsia, or inadvertent administration of excessive doses of magnesium-containing supplements, laxatives, Epsom salts, enemas, or antacids. The risk of hypermagnesemia is particularly high for patients with severely impaired renal function.

CLINICAL MANIFESTATIONS

Clinical manifestations are unusual with plasma magnesium levels <4.5 to 5 mg/dL. Above this range, nausea, vomiting, cutaneous flushing, hyporeflexia, and mild hypotension can be seen. For plasma magnesium levels >7 to 10 mg/dL, there may be loss of tendon reflexes, muscle weakness, and hypotension. Respiratory muscle paralysis occurs when magnesium levels exceed 12 to 15 mg/dL. ECG changes with plasma magnesium values >5 mg/dL include prolonged PR interval, an increased QRS interval, prolonged QT interval, and bradycardia. Complete heart block is seen for plasma Mg^{2+} >10 to 15 mg/dL, and cardiac arrest for levels >15 mg/dL.

TREATMENT

In mild cases, stopping magnesium administration may be sufficient. Dialysis can be performed for extreme cases. Intravenous calcium (100–200 mg of elemental calcium given over 5–10 minutes) can be used to temporarily antagonize the effects of magnesium until dialysis can be performed. Details regarding intravenous calcium administration can be found in the section on treatment of hyperkalemia. Intravenous volume infusion may be helpful in promoting magnesium excretion in patients who are not volume overloaded and who have adequate renal function.

SUGGESTED READINGS

Bosch X, Poch E, Grau JM. Rhabdomyolysis and acute kidney injury. *N Engl J Med.* 2009;361:62–72.

Gennari FJ. Disorders of potassium homeostasis: hypokalemia and hyperkalemia. *Crit Care Clin.* 2002;18:273–288.

Kim HJ, Han SW. Therapeutic approach to hyperkalaemia. *Nephron.* 2002;92(Suppl 1):33–40.

Kitabchi AE, Umpierrez GE, Murphy MB, et al. American Diabetes Association. Hyperglycemic crisis in diabetes. *Diabetes Care.* 2004;27(Suppl 1):S94–S102.

Palmer BF. A physiologic-based approach to the evaluation of a patient with hypokalemia. *Am J Kidney Dis.* 2010;56:1184–1190.

Regolisti G, Cabassi A, Parenti E, Maggiore U, Fiaccadori E. Severe hypomagnesemia during long-term treatment with a proton pump inhibitor. *Am J Kidney Dis.* 2010;56:168–174.

Topf JM, Murray PT. Hypomagnesemia and hypermagnesemia. *Rev Endocr Metab Disord.* 2003;4:195–206.

CHAPTER 251

Kidney Stones

Victor F. Seabra, MD
Orfeas Liangos, MD
Bertrand L. Jaber, MD, MS

Key Clinical Questions

1. How do you diagnose nephrolithiasis?
2. How should kidney stones be managed in the inpatient setting?
3. What medical therapy facilitates stone passage?
4. When is urology or nephrology consultation indicated?
5. What follow-up and further testing is appropriate after discharge?
6. What drugs and dietary therapies are helpful in the secondary prevention of kidney stones?

INTRODUCTION

Kidney stones are one of the most common and most painful disorders of the urinary tract. This chapter reviews the epidemiology of kidney stones, the pathophysiology and risk factors for their development, the typical clinical presentation, the initial diagnostic evaluation, the acute, often hospital-based symptomatic treatment, followed by the outpatient management focusing on secondary preventive measures.

EPIDEMIOLOGY

Nephrolithiasis is a common disorder that inflicts recurrent pain and significant morbidity onto a substantial portion of the population, including many young and otherwise healthy individuals. In the United States, approximately 5% of women and 10% of men experience a symptomatic episode before the age of 70, and the cumulative 10-year recurrence rate is estimated at 40% for women and 60% for men.

Regional variations in the frequency and nature of kidney stone disease exist within the United States, with an increased prevalence in the southeastern region of the country. This variation may be related to differences in climate and sunlight exposure, as well as dietary habits and beverage consumption. Kidney stones develop more frequently among Caucasians than African Americans. Stones in the upper urinary tract are frequently seen in industrialized countries and are associated with a more affluent lifestyle, including high animal protein consumption, gout, and traits of the metabolic syndrome, including hypertension, impaired glucose tolerance, increased waist circumference, high triglycerides, and low-high-density lipoprotein (HDL) cholesterol. Bladder stones are more commonly seen in developing countries and more frequently affect individuals with a poor socioeconomic status.

Patients with kidney stones typically present with renal colic, characterized by severe pain and autonomic symptoms such as lightheadedness, diaphoresis, nausea, and vomiting. The severity of symptoms often results in a visit to a hospital emergency room, frequently requiring hospitalization and absenteeism from work. In the United States, kidney stones account for more than 2 million outpatient visits, over 600,000 emergency room visits, and approximately 0.4% of hospital admissions. Additional costs may arise from complications, such as ureteral obstruction, pyelonephritis, and the need for stone removal by instrumentation, surgery, or extracorporeal shock wave lithotripsy (ESWL). Patients with recurrent stone disease also have a heightened risk of chronic kidney disease. The annual cost of kidney disease in the United States, including hospitalizations, professional charges, and lost productivity, exceeds $2 billion.

PATHOPHYSIOLOGY AND RISK FACTORS

Kidney stones can form from a variety of substances excreted in the urine and frequently consist of two or more different substances (**Table 251-1**). Calcareous (calcium oxalate or phosphate) stones are by far the most common, accounting for over 80% of kidney stones. Metabolic defects leading to stone formation include hypercalciuria in over 65% of cases, and less frequently, hyperuricosuria, hyperoxaluria, hypocitraturia, or some combination thereof.

For a kidney stone to form, the concentration of a dissolved salt has to exceed its solubility in urine, a condition known as super-

TABLE 251-1 Composition of Kidney Stones

Type	Frequency (%)
Calcium	70–88
• Calcium oxalate	36–70
• Calcium phosphate	6–20
• Mixed	11–31
Magnesium ammonium phosphate (struvite)	6–20
Uric acid	6–17
Cystine	0.5–3
Miscellaneous	1–4

saturation. Supersaturation is favored by increased urinary excretion of stone-forming salts, optimal urinary pH (**Table 251-2**), and decreased urinary volume, which leads to increased urinary concentration. The presence of crystallization facilitators in the urine, such as uric acid, or the absence of crystallization inhibitors, such as citrate, also contributes to stone formation.

Risk factors for kidney stone formation can be divided into diet, stone-provoking conditions, stone-provoking drugs, and anatomic abnormalities. Dietary factors promoting nephrolithiasis include low fluid intake, which promotes urinary supersaturation, high sodium and animal protein intake, which promote hypercalciuria, and high oxalate intake, which promote hyperoxaluria. In addition, a family history of kidney stones and a personal history of gout also confer an increased risk of kidney stone disease.

Table 251-3 displays a selected list of stone-provoking conditions, stone-provoking drugs, and anatomic urologic abnormalities that have been associated with stone disease. Of note, roux-en-Y gastric bypass surgery, a common bariatric surgical procedure, is associated with increased intestinal absorption of oxalate and hyperoxaluria, resulting in a long-term risk of kidney stone formation. Major stone-provoking drugs include the antiretroviral agent indinavir, which crystallizes in the urine, and the anticonvulsant topiramate, which inhibits carbonic anhydrase.

Oxalobacter formigenes is an intestinal bacterium that produces an oxalate-degrading enzyme. The resulting increased intestinal degradation of oxalate may protect against stone formation. Lack of intestinal colonization with *Oxalobacter formigenes* is prevalent in recurrent calcium oxalate stone formers and is associated with hyperoxaluria.

CLINICAL PRESENTATION

Patients with kidney stones most often present to the hospital with renal colic. Others present with a urinary tract infection, impaired renal function from obstructive uropathy, or chronic kidney damage. Increasingly, incidental kidney stones are diagnosed on imaging studies in patients admitted to the hospital for other reasons.

TABLE 251-2 Solubility of Stone-forming Salts According to Urinary pH

Solute	Acid pH	Alkaline pH
Urate	↓	↑
Oxalate	↓	↑ or ↓
Phosphate	↑	↓
Cystine	↓	↑

TABLE 251-3 Risk Factors for Kidney Stone Disease

Stone-provoking conditions
Calcareous stones
Hypercalciuria
Primary hyperparathyroidism
Milk-alkali syndrome
Sarcoidosis
Prolonged immobilization
Hyperoxaluria
Crohn disease
Short gut syndrome
Roux-en-Y gastric bypass surgery
Hypocitraturia
Laxative abuse
Polycystic kidney disease
Medullary sponge kidney
Renal tubular acidosis
Urate stones
Hyperuricosuria
Gouty diathesis
Myeloproliferative disorders
Ulcerative colitis
Struvite stones
Paraplegia
Neurogenic bladder
Recurrent urinary tract infections
Stone-provoking drugs
Vitamin C (high dose)
Vitamin D (high dose)
Uricosuric agents
Triamterene
Acetazolamide
Sulfadiazine
Indinavir
Topiramate
Anatomic abnormalities
Medullary sponge kidney
Horseshoe kidney
Pyelocalyceal diverticulum
Megacalyces
Hydrocalyces
Ureteropelvic junction obstruction
Megaureter
Bladder outlet obstruction
Bladder diverticulum
Urethral diverticulum

Typical renal colic is characterized by the acute onset of severe pain that awakens the patient from sleep. Colic typically lasts for one to four hours, followed by gradual improvement. The patient may move ceaselessly, looking for a comfortable position, and may also suffer from nausea, vomiting, and sweating.

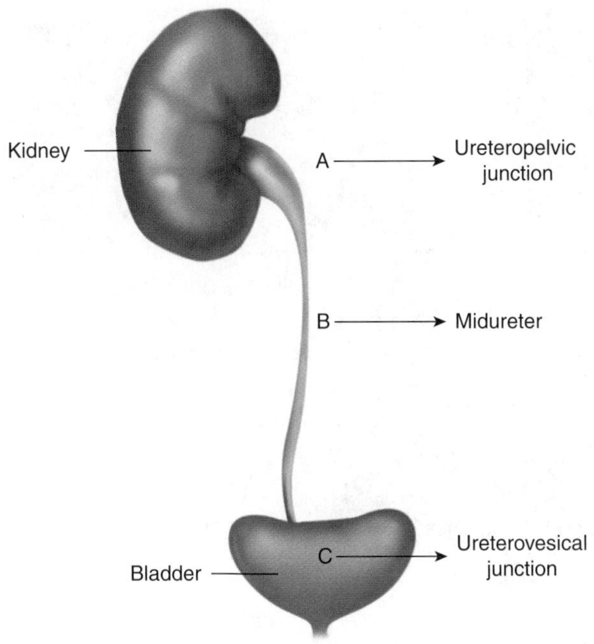

Figure 251-1 *Characteristics of renal colic according to stone location. (A) Stone at the ureteropelvic junction; mild dull to excruciating sharp pain in the flank, often radiating to the upper ipsilateral abdominal quadrant. (B) Stone in the midureter; pain radiating caudally and anteriorly toward the mid- and lower abdomen in a curved band-like fashion, initially parallel to the lower-costal margin, but then deviating caudally toward the bony pelvis and inguinal ligament. (C) Stone in the distal ureter; pain radiating into the scrotum or the tip of the penis in men, and associated with urinary frequency and urgency, dysuria, and gross hematuria.*

As shown in **Figure 251-1**, the anatomic site of the stone in the urinary tract influences the location and radiation of the pain to different locations. Several conditions of the genitourinary, musculoskeletal, gastrointestinal, and cardiovascular systems may produce hematuria, back pain, or abdominal pain, mimicking kidney stones (**Table 251-4**).

TABLE 251-4 Differential Diagnosis of Kidney Stone Disease

Conditions associated with pain	
Genitourinary system	Acute pyelonephritis, testicular torsion, epididymitis, cystitis, urethritis, prostatitis, menstrual pain, pelvic inflammatory disease, ruptured ovarian cyst, ovarian torsion
Musculoskeletal system	Abdominal muscular pain, rib pain
Gastrointestinal system	Biliary colic, cholecystitis, gastritis, acute pancreatitis, peptic ulcer disease, appendicitis, acute diverticulitis
Cardiovascular system	Acute myocardial infarction, aortic aneurysm
Miscellaneous	Retroperitoneal fibrosis, herpes zoster, pleural pain
Conditions associated with hematuria	
Acute glomerulonephritis, arteriovenous malformations, anticoagulant use, cystitis, prostatitis, neoplasia	

INITIAL DIAGNOSTIC EVALUATION

The initial workup of a patient presenting with suspected renal colic includes a urinalysis, urine culture, limited blood work, and an imaging study. The urinalysis may reveal an acid pH (<5.5), suggesting uric acid or cystine stones, or an alkaline pH (>7.5), suggesting infection with urea-splitting bacteria and struvite stone formation or renal tubular acidosis complicated by calcium phosphate stones.

Microscopic examination of the urinary sediment may reveal specific crystals (**Figure 251-2**).

Urate crystals can be rhomboid, needle shaped, or amorphous in shape (Figure 251-2*A–C*). Oxalate crystals can be dumbbell or cigar shaped (Figure 251-2*D*, calcium oxalate monohydrate) or envelope shaped (Figure 251-2*E*, calcium oxalate dihydrate). Phosphate crystals can be in the form of triple phosphate (typical "coffin-lid" structure, Figure 251-2*F*) or amorphous phosphate (Figure 251-2*G*). Cystine crystals are hexaedric and flat (Figure 251-2*H*), and pathognomonic for cystinuria. A cyanide-nitroprusside test resulting in purple-red discoloration of the urine confirms the presence of cystine crystals. A urine culture should be obtained to rule out concomitant urinary tract infection, particularly with the urea-splitting bacteria such as *Proteus* that lead to struvite stones.

A limited blood work panel for the evaluation of kidney stone disease includes serum electrolytes to evaluate for renal tubular acidosis; blood urea nitrogen and creatinine to assess kidney function; calcium, albumin, and phosphorus to evaluate for primary hyperparathyroidism; and uric acid to evaluate for gout. An elevated serum creatinine may reflect acute kidney injury as a consequence of bilateral obstructive uropathy, unilateral obstruction in the setting of a single kidney, preexisting chronic kidney disease, or extracellular fluid volume depletion or infection. Fever should trigger a more thorough investigation for pyelonephritis and sepsis.

The imaging modality of choice is a nonenhanced helical computed tomography (CT) scan, conferring 96% sensitivity and 100% specificity for the diagnosis of kidney stones. Ultrasonography, which has the advantage of no radiation exposure, can only visualize the kidney and proximal ureter. It can only detect stones equal or greater than 3 mm, and consequently, suffers from a sensitivity and specificity of 24% to 61% and 90% to 100%, respectively.

TREATMENT OF AN ACUTE EPISODE

INITIAL EMERGENCY ROOM MANAGEMENT

The symptomatic treatment includes the administration of intravenous or oral fluids to facilitate stone passage, adequate pain control with nonsteroidal anti-inflammatory drugs or opioids, and antiemetics. Although parenteral ketorolac has been shown be as effective as opioids for the treatment of renal colic, this drug should be used cautiously among patients with impaired kidney function, as repeated doses may precipitate acute kidney injury. Nonsteroidal anti-inflammatory drugs have the added benefit of reducing ureteral inflammation surrounding the stone, thus facilitating stone passage. Antibiotics are not routinely recommended for kidney stone disease, unless there is concomitant infection. To facilitate stone passage, both calcium channel blockers (eg, nifedipine) and alpha-blockers (eg, tamsulosin) have been shown to increase the likelihood of stone passage and may be considered. In one study, 63% of physicians practicing in an emergency department used alpha-blockers for medical expulsive therapy.

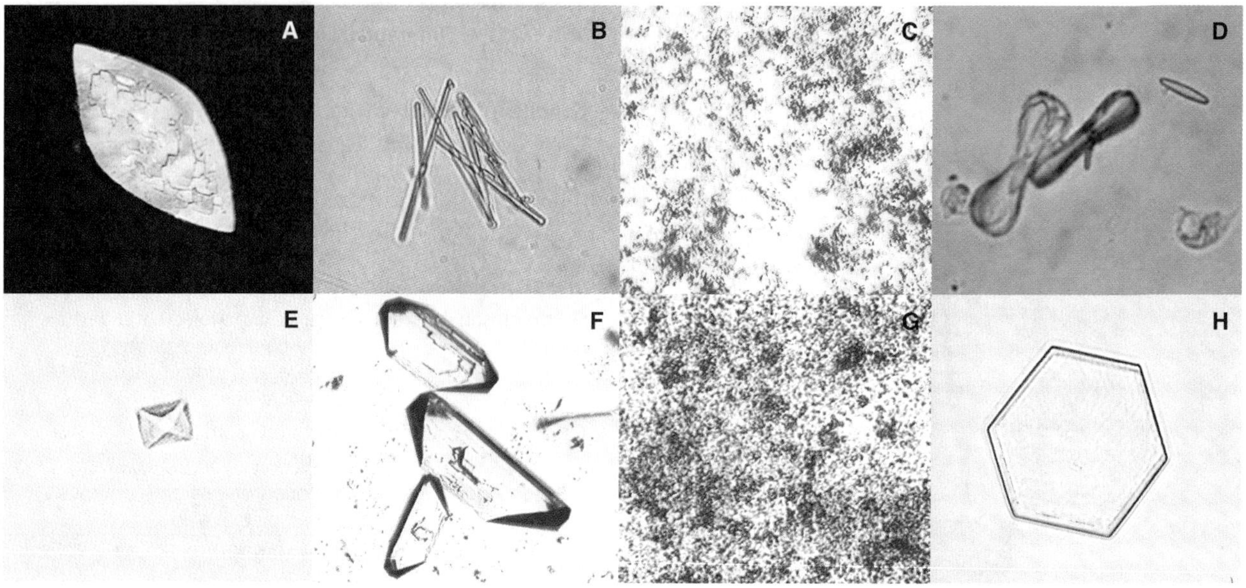

Figure 251-2 *Urinary crystal identification. Rhomboid (A), needle-shaped (B), or amorphous (C), urate; dumbbell-shaped or cigar-shaped calcium oxalate monohydrate (D), envelope-shaped calcium oxalate dihydrate (E), coffin lid–shaped triple phosphate (F), or amorphous phosphate (G). (A–C, E–H Reproduced, with permission from Graff L. A handbook of routine urinalysis. Philadelphia: Lippincott, Williams & Wilkins, 1983.) (D: Reproduced from Morfin and Chin. Urinary calcium oxalate crystals in ethylene glycol intoxication. N Engl J Med. 2005;353:e21. With permission from the Massachusetts Medical Society. Copyright © 2005 Massachusetts Medical Society, all rights reserved.)*

PRACTICE POINT

Medical expulsive therapy for kidney stones

- Kidney stones irritate the lining of the ureter, producing pain and spasm. Ureteral spasm interferes with peristalsis and decreases the likelihood of spontaneous stone passage. Calcium channel blockers and alpha-blockers at appropriate doses relax the distal ureter without abolishing peristalsis altogether. This leads to a reduction in symptoms of colic and allows a greater chance of stone passage. The best-studied agents are the calcium channel blocker nifedipine, given at relatively low doses (30–40 mg daily), and the alpha-blocker tamsulosin, dosed at 0.4 mg daily. A four-week trial of either agent may be reasonable for stable patients with distal ureteral stones measuring less than 10 mm. Nifedipine and tamsulosin may both cause orthostatic hypotension. Tamsulosin may be more effective than nifedipine, but causes the additional side effect of abnormal ejaculation in men. Corticosteroids and anticholinergics confer little additional benefit in patients already taking an alpha-blocker or calcium channel blocker.

INDICATIONS FOR HOSPITALIZATION

Failure to control the pain, impaired renal function in the setting of obstructive stones, and suspected pyelonephritis with sepsis should trigger hospitalization. If the patient is likely to require a urologic intervention, the decision for hospitalization might be made on an individual basis in conjunction with the urology service.

UROLOGY CONSULTATION

Stones larger than 5 mm are less likely to be expelled spontaneously than smaller ones (**Table 251-5**). Consequently, urologic consultation is warranted if the stone does not pass spontaneously, is larger than 5 mm in diameter, causes urinary obstruction, or is associated with urosepsis. If endourologic intervention becomes necessary, a variety of approaches can be employed, depending on the stone location. These include ureteroscopy with placement of a double J-stent tube for stones in the proximal ureter, basket stone retrieval for those in the distal ureter, and extracorporeal shock-wave lithotripsy for stone in the renal pelvis. **Figure 251-3** displays a proposed urologic treatment algorithm according to size, location, and type of stone.

NEPHROLOGY CONSULTATION

In-hospital nephrology consultation is advised in the setting of nonresolving acute kidney injury or advanced preexisting chronic kidney disease. Outpatient nephrology referral may be warranted for secondary prevention, particularly among recurrent stone formers, or first stone formers who have conditions or who take medications known to provoke stone formation. (See the proceeding section, Subsequent Outpatient Management, for a more detailed discussion.)

TABLE 251-5 Likelihood of Passage of Ureteral Stones According to Size

Size of the Stone	Mean Days Until Passage	Likelihood of Need for Intervention (%)
≤2 mm	8	3
3 mm	12	14
4–6 mm	22	50
>6 mm*	–	99

*Unlikely to pass spontaneously.

(Reproduced from Teichman. *Acute renal colic from ureteral calculus. N Engl J Med*. 2004;684–693. With permission from the Massachusetts Medical Society.)

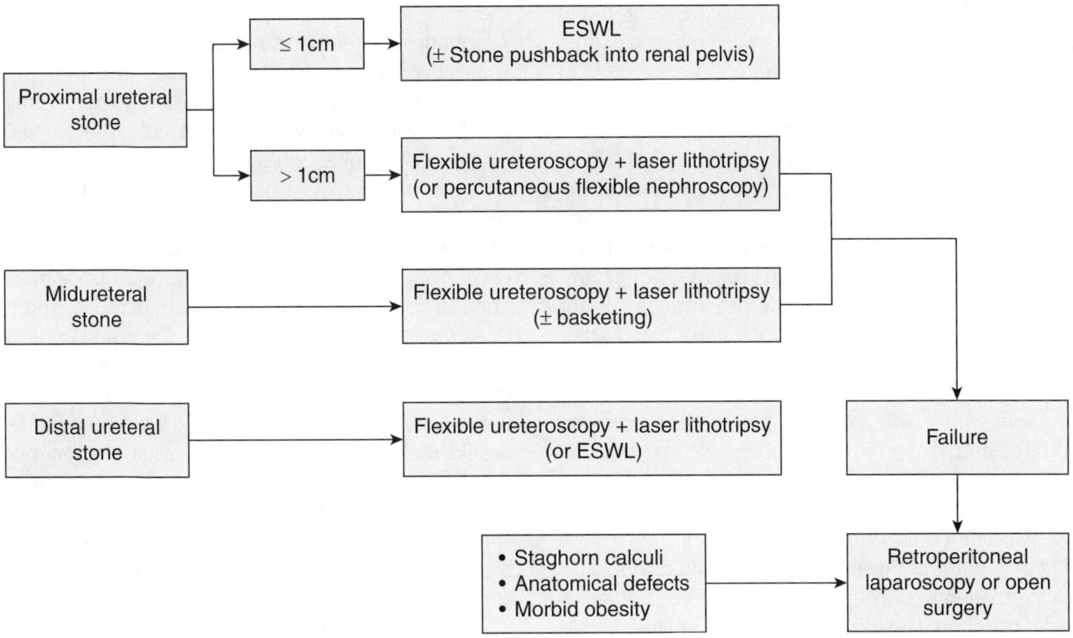

Figure 251-3 *Urologic treatment algorithm according to size, location, and type of kidney stone. ESWL, extracorporeal shock-wave lithotripsy.*

HOSPITAL DISCHARGE PLANNING

As soon as pain control is achieved, renal function recovers and a decision regarding the need for urologic intervention has been established, patients may be considered for hospital discharge. Patients who have not passed a stone at the time of hospital discharge should be given a strainer to retrieve a stone, in case of spontaneous expulsion. Outpatient follow-up with urology is usually indicated, especially if an outpatient procedure is being contemplated. Recurrent stone formers and patients at high risk of recurrence should be referred to a nephrologist at discharge.

SUBSEQUENT OUTPATIENT MANAGEMENT

GENERAL CONSIDERATIONS

In patients without risk factors for recurrent stone formation (see Table 251-3), a simplified evaluation is usually sufficient. This consists of a dietary and medical history, review of the urinalysis, urine culture, helical CT scan and blood tests obtained during hospitalization, and a stone analysis, if available. Serum levels of parathyroid hormone and angiotensin-converting enzyme may be indicated if hypercalcemia is present. However, patients with recurrent stones and those with a positive family history of stones or medical conditions associated with stone recurrence should have further evaluation.

Comprehensive evaluation includes keeping a dietary journal and completing a food frequency questionnaire. A 24-hour urine collection should also be performed, with measurement of creatinine (to confirm adequacy of collection), volume (to assess fluid intake), calcium (to rule out hypercalciuria), oxalate (to exclude hyperoxaluria), uric acid (to assess for hyperuricosuria), citrate (to rule out hypocitraturia), and cystine (to exclude cystinuria). Additional 24-hour measurements include excretion of urinary sulfate, which reflects animal protein intake, and urinary sodium, which promote hypercalciuria if elevated, and magnesium excretion rate, which promotes stone formation if low. Several 24-hour urinary collection kits are commercially available in the United States to assist in this metabolic evaluation. These also provide supersaturation indices pertaining to calcium oxalate, urate, and calcium phosphate precipitation in the urine.

SECONDARY PREVENTION

Recommendations for secondary prevention of kidney stones are based largely on observational studies and a handful of randomized controlled trials.

Diet and lifestyle modification

Every kidney stone patient should have a high fluid intake, at least 3 liters per day, allowing for excretion of dilute urine throughout the entire day and night. To ensure dilute urine at night, patients must drink one to two eight-ounce glasses of water at bedtime, followed by another eight-ounce glass during the night, as after voiding. Unfortunately, frequent nocturia limits adherence to this regimen, and daytime access to water during work hours might be difficult for some patients. In addition to the total fluid consumed, the type of beverage might also play a role. In middle-aged women, coffee, tea, and wine intake has been shown to be independently protective, whereas grapefruit juice has been shown to promote kidney stones. These findings were confirmed in men, with the additional finding that the risk of kidney stones was reduced by beer and increased by apple juice. While strongly hopped beers such as European lagers may contain significant amounts of oxalate, which increases kidney stone risk, beer consumption also increases urinary flow and dilution, likely explaining their neutral or even beneficial effects in observational studies. Dietary sodium restriction to less than 150 mEq per day should also be recommended to all patients, as high sodium intake increases urinary calcium excretion and facilitates calcium stone formation.

Dietary calcium intake has variable effects on stone formation. Excess calcium intake, especially if combined with vitamin D3 supplementation, invariably leads to increased calcium absorption and hypercalciuria. However, dietary calcium restriction reduces enteral chelation of dietary oxalate, facilitating oxalate absorption and subsequent urinary excretion, and increasing the risk of recurrent calcium oxalate stones. Calcium restriction also leads to loss of bone mass and a higher likelihood of osteoporosis. We recommend avoidance of extremes of calcium intake, and remaining within the recommended daily allowance (RDA) for calcium of 800 to 1000 mg/day.

Patients with calcium oxalate stones should limit daily intake of animal proteins to 0.8 gm per kg of body weight, which is the RDA. High-protein diets increase urinary calcium excretion because the amino acids methionine, cysteine, and cystine oxidize sulfur to sulfate, which is excreted with calcium to maintain electroneutrality.

Dietary oxalate restriction is recommended in oxalate stone formers. Foods with high oxalate content include peanuts, tea, instant coffee, rhubarb, beets, beans, berries, chocolate, spinach and other dark leafy greens, oranges, tofu, sweet potatoes, and draft beer. (The high oxalate content of coffee, tea, and beer is negated by their diuretic effects). Foods with a high purine content, such as red meat, organ meats, beer, and cruciferous vegetables, such as broccoli and cauliflower, increase urinary uric acid excretion and should be restricted in those with uric acid stones.

For indinavir-associated kidney stones, which occur in 10% to 15% of patients after six months of therapy initiation, the drug should be temporarily or permanently discontinued and vigorous hydration above 3 liters per day should be instituted. On urine sediment, indinavir crystals have a starry appearance. Indinavir stones tend to be radiolucent on CT scan and are best detected by ultrasound.

Drug therapy

In recurrent stone formers, specific pharmacologic therapies should be added for secondary prevention. For calcareous stones, if hypercalciuria is present, high dose thiazide diuretics have been shown to be consistently effective, in conjunction with a low-sodium diet. Options include hydrochlorothiazide (up to 50 mg twice daily) and chlorthalidone (12.5–100 mg per day). Amiloride combined with hydrochlorothiazide (10 mg/50 mg combination pill twice daily) has been used in an effort to minimize hypokalemia. Patients with calcium oxalate stones who have hyperuricosuria and normocalciuria have been shown to benefit from the use of allopurinol (300 mg daily).

Unproven therapies to prevent calcium oxalate stones include magnesium and pyridoxine (vitamin B6). Magnesium enhances the solubility of urinary oxalate. In clinical trials, magnesium oxide and magnesium hydroxide are ineffective in stone prevention, but there may be a benefit of potassium magnesium citrate. Pyridoxine supplementation may reduce oxalate production, and large doses are associated with a reduced risk of stone formation in women in observational studies. Another promising therapy for calcium oxalate stone formers with hyperoxaluria is oxalate-metabolizing probiotic microorganisms, such as *Lactobacillus* species or *Oxalobacter formigenes*.

In enteric hyperoxaluria due to malabsorption, as in inflammatory bowel disease, dietary oxalate restriction should be initiated. If this is unsuccessful, a low-fat diet, calcium carbonate supplements, medium-chain fatty acid supplementation, and enteral-binding therapy with cholestyramine can be attempted alone or in combination.

Hypocitraturia warrants potassium citrate supplementation, at a minimum dose of 40 to 60 mEq per day in two to three divided doses. Sodium-based citrate formulations should be avoided, due to their high sodium content. In calcium phosphate stones, citrate supplementation should be used with caution, since excessive urinary alkalinization might promote calcium phosphate precipitation.

In hyperuricosuria, in addition to reducing purine intake, potassium citrate supplementation is useful to alkalinize the urine and maximize urate solubility. If citrate alone cannot consistently raise the urine pH, an evening dose of acetazolamide may be added. Allopurinol is effective in preventing recurrent calcium-containing stones in patients with hyperuricosuria.

Cystinuria is a rare inherited tubular disorder of amino acid transport that leads to increased excretion of cystine, as well as ornithine, lysine, and arginine, which do not form stones. This autosomal recessive disorder has a prevalence of 1 in 7000. Patients develop symptoms from cystine stones beginning in the second and third decades of life. Cystine stones are extremely hard and resistant to ESWL. Patients are also prone to develop calcium oxalate stones, from associated hypercalciuria, hyperuricosuria, and hypocitraturia. Urinary cystine solubility is pH dependent, and urine alkalinization is the mainstay of treatment. In mild to moderate cystinuria, treatment consists of mild sodium restriction, potassium citrate supplementation to alkalinize the urine pH, and high fluid intake. The patient should keep a log of urinary pH results to self-monitor therapy. Captopril or tiopronin, which form soluble complexes with cysteine, should be given in more severe cystinuria.

In recurrent struvite stones, the chronic use of suppressive antibiotics or urease inhibitors such as acetohydroxamic acid may be considered.

All dietary and pharmacologic interventions should be followed up with a repeat 24-hour urine collection three to six months after the intervention in order to monitor treatment success and adherence.

CONCLUSION

Kidney stone disease is a common and debilitating urinary tract disorder, with a lifetime risk of 10% and a recurrence rate of 50%. First-time stone formers not displaying risk factors for recurrence require a limited evaluation. However, recurrent stone formers as well as first-time stone formers with risk factors for recurrence require a more extensive evaluation. Dietary interventions and lifestyle changes are uniformly recommended, but the remainder of the therapy is often tailored to specific metabolic and urinary abnormalities identified in the diagnostic evaluation. The long-term commitment and adherence to dietary and lifestyle changes and pharmacologic treatment remains a challenging task.

SUGGESTED READINGS

Curhan GC, Willett WC, Speizer FE, Stampfer MJ. Beverage use and risk for kidney stones in women. *Ann Intern Med.* 1998;128:534–540.

Graff L. A handbook of routine urinalysis. Philadelphia, PA: Lippincott Williams & Wilkins; 1983.

Hollingsworth JM, Rogers MA, Kaufman SR, et al. Medical therapy to facilitate urinary stone passage: a meta-analysis. *Lancet.* 2006;368(9542):1171–1179.

Morfin J, Chin A. Images in clinical medicine. Urinary calcium oxalate crystals in ethylene glycol intoxication. *N Engl J Med.* 2005;353(24):e21.

Pearle MS, Roehrborn CG, Pak CY. Meta-analysis of randomized trials for medical prevention of calcium oxalate nephrolithiasis. *J Endourol.* 1999;13:679–685.

Qiang W, Ke Z. Water for preventing urinary calculi. *Cochrane Database Syst Rev.* 2004(3):CD004292.

Sheafor DH, Hertzberg BS, Freed KS, et al. Nonenhanced helical CT and US in the emergency evaluation of patients with renal colic: prospective comparison. *Radiology.* 2000;217:792–797.

Teichman JM. Clinical practice. Acute renal colic from ureteral calculus. *N Engl J Med.* 2004;350:684–693.

CHAPTER 252

Hypertensive Urgencies

Marcos Lepe, MD
Joseph Varon, MD, FACP, FCCP, FCCM

Key Clinical Questions

1. What is hypertension?
2. What is the prevalence of hypertensive crises?
3. What causes hypertensive crises?
4. What are key differences between a hypertensive urgency and emergency?
5. How can one diagnose a hypertensive crisis?
6. What is the treatment for a hypertensive crisis?

INTRODUCTION AND EPIDEMIOLOGY

Hypertension is the most common reason for patients to seek medical attention in the United States. It affects over 70 million people in the United States, with global numbers approaching one billion. The annual costs of hypertension, both direct and indirect, are estimated to be $50 billion in the United States alone.

The most popular classification of hypertension is that of the Seventh Report of The Joint National Committee on Prevention, Detection, Evaluation, and Treatment of High Blood Pressure (JNC 7). Blood pressure is classified as normal, prehypertension, stage 1 hypertension, and stage 2 hypertension (**Table 252-1**).

Patients with untreated or inadequately treated hypertension are prone to sudden elevations in blood pressure and the development of *hypertensive crises*. Up to 1% of all hypertensive patients will have a hypertensive crisis in their lifetime. Hypertensive crises come in two forms. In a *hypertensive emergency*, a surge in blood pressure is accompanied by end-organ damage. *Hypertensive urgency* is an acute elevation in blood pressure without end-organ damage. There is no blood pressure threshold that defines a hypertensive crisis. Most patients have pressures that exceed 180/120 mm Hg, with diastolic blood pressures over 120 mm Hg being most strongly associated with end-organ damage. Patients who develop a hypertensive crisis in settings other than chronic essential hypertension may develop end-organ damage at lesser degrees of blood pressure elevation, as they lack the vascular smooth muscle hypertrophy that provides some protection against the effects of uncontrolled hypertension.

PATHOPHYSIOLOGY

NORMAL BLOOD PRESSURE CONTROL

Many elements are involved in blood pressure regulation, such as the renin angiotensin-aldosterone system (RAAS) of the kidney. Renin is released by the juxtaglomerular apparatus in response to low kidney perfusion, elevated sympathetic response, low dietary sodium, and other stimuli. Renin cleaves circulating angiotensinogen to form angiotensin I, which in turn is cleaved to angiotensin II by angiotensin-converting enzyme (ACE). Angiotensin II is a potent arteriolar constrictor that increases both systolic and diastolic blood pressure. It also signals the adrenal cortex to secrete aldosterone, which increases the reabsorption of sodium from urine, sweat, saliva, and bowel.

Catecholamines from the sympathetic nervous system greatly affect blood pressure, especially epinephrine. Binding of epinephrine to α1 receptors leads to vasoconstriction and increased peripheral vascular resistance, causing blood pressure to rise. Binding to β_1 receptors increases heart rate and cardiac output, which also raises blood pressure. The endothelium also locally produces vasoactive substances that affect blood pressure, such as the vasodilators nitric oxide, prostacyclin, and bradykinin, and the vasoconstrictor endothelin-1.

Arterial baroreceptors are mechanoreceptors in the carotid sinuses and aortic arch. When blood pressure rises, the mechanoreceptors are stretched, decreasing their firing rate. This decreases central sympathetic outflow and increases parasympathetic tone, lowering blood pressure. Conversely, when blood pressure falls, decreased stretching of mechanoreceptors increases their firing rate, stimulating sympathetic and inhibiting parasympathetic outflow. This

TABLE 252-1 Blood Pressure Classification Based on Guidelines from the Seventh Report of the Joint National Committee on Prevention, Detection, Evaluation, and Treatment of High Blood Pressure

	Normal	Prehypertension	Stage I	Stage II
Systolic blood pressure (in mm Hg)	< 120	120–139	140–159	> 160
Diastolic blood pressure (in mm Hg)	< 80	80–89	90–99	> 100

Data from Chobanian AV, Bakris GL, Black HR, et al. *JAMA*. Seventh Report of the Joint National Committee on Prevention, Detection, Evaluation, and Treatment of High Blood Pressure. 2003;289:2560–2572.

feedback loop is sensitive to acute fluctuations in blood pressure, but in chronic essential hypertension, the set point rises and a higher basal blood pressure is tolerated.

PHYSIOLOGIC DERANGEMENTS IN HYPERTENSIVE CRISES

In general, hypertensive crises result from a breakdown in arterial adaptation to chronic hypertension, leading to a vicious cycle of vascular injury. The endothelium adapts to high blood pressure by smooth muscle hypertrophy and vasoconstriction. Prolonged smooth muscle contraction eventually leads to endothelial dysfunction, diminished nitric oxide production, and a failure of autoregulation. Focal vasodilation, endothelial damage, and increased vascular permeability result, with leakage and deposition of fibrinogen and plasma proteins in blood vessel walls. The coagulation cascade is activated and fibrinous clot is formed, leading to ischemia, further endothelial injury, inflammation, and release of vasoconstrictive mediators, perpetuating the cycle of injury.

Under normal conditions, the brain autoregulates cerebral blood flow (CBF) to ensure that the high metabolic demands of neuronal cells are met, despite fluctuations in blood pressure. Normally, CBF is maintained at 50 mL blood per 100 g of brain tissue per minute (Strandgaard 1973) (**Figures 252-1** and **252-2**). The upper limit of autoregulation is a mean arterial pressure (MAP) of > 120 mm Hg for normotensive patients and > 180 mm Hg for hypertensive patients. (The higher threshold in hypertensive patients is due to vascular hypertrophy and other morphologic changes from chronic elevations in blood pressure.) If the upper limit of autoregulation is surpassed, endothelial dysfunction and damage may occur, the blood-brain barrier may break down, and cerebral edema and microhemorrhages may develop, giving rise to hypertensive encephalopathy.

The lower limit of CBF autoregulation also differs between hypertensive and normotensive patients. Hypertensive patients may show signs or symptoms of cerebral hypoxemia, including loss of consciousness, coma, or seizures, at MAP levels of 50 ± 5 mm Hg and below, whereas normotensive patients will show these symptoms at a MAP of 40 ± 5 mm Hg and below. This has important implications for the management of hypertensive emergencies: too rapid lowering of blood pressure in these patients poses a risk of cerebral hypoperfusion.

CAUSES

The most common causes of hypertensive crises are inadequate adherence to antihypertensive therapy and previously undiagnosed essential hypertension. Patients who stop taking some antihypertensive drugs may develop severe rebound hypertension, especially those who abruptly discontinue beta-blockers or clonidine. Chronic renal failure and sleep apnea are common medical causes of poorly controlled hypertension. Cocaine, amphetamines, phencyclidine, aminophylline, phenylephrine, diet pills, and other sympathomimetic drugs may cause hypertensive crises. Patients who take monoamine oxidase inhibitors (MAOIs), including the antibiotic linezolid and over-the-counter drugs with MAOI activity, such as St. John's wort, are at risk for developing hypertensive crisis with confusion if they also ingest selective serotonin reuptake inhibitors, tricyclic antidepressants, meperidine, tramadol, methadone, dextromethorphan, or tyramine-containing foods such as red wine, aged cheeses, smoked or pickled meats, and avocado. Bevacizumab, a monoclonal antibody against vascular endothelial growth factor that is approved for use in several advanced adenocarcinomas, may lead to hypertensive crisis.

Although most patients with a hypertensive crisis do not have a secondary cause of hypertension, such as renal artery stenosis, acute glomerulonephritis, preeclampsia, pheochromocytoma, scleroderma renal crisis, or Cushing syndrome, an evaluation for secondary hypertension should be considered, especially in the presence of compatible signs and symptoms, as described elsewhere in this volume.

In the hospital, hypertensive crises may develop after surgeries. Postoperative hypertension is arbitrarily defined as systolic blood pressure ≥ 190 mm Hg or diastolic blood pressure ≥ 100 mm Hg

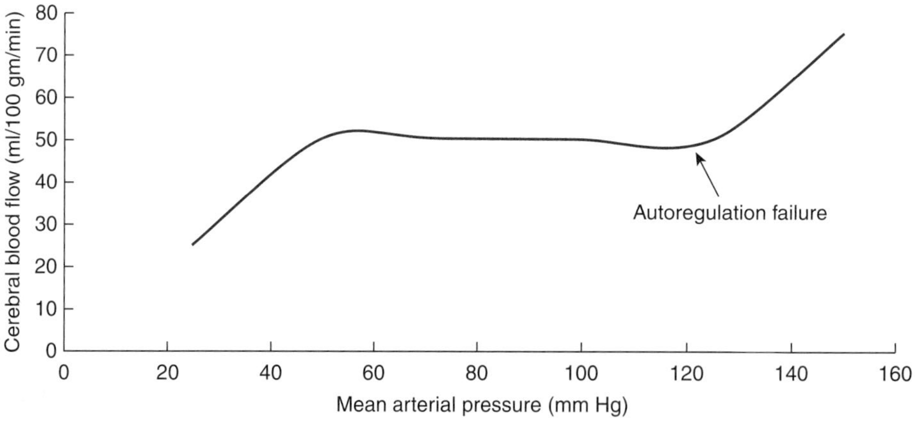

Figure 252-1 *Autoregulation of cerebral blood flow in response to changing mean arterial pressure in normotensive patient. (Data from Strandgaard S, Olesen J, Skinhoj E, et al. Br Med J. 1973;1(5852):507–510.)*

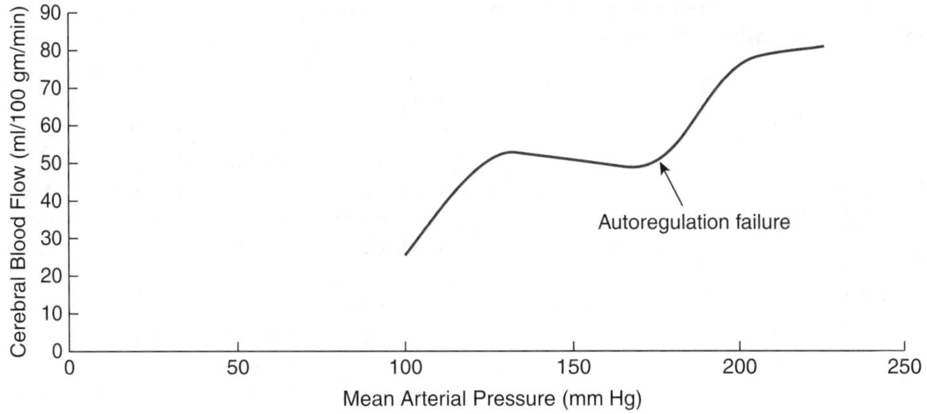

Figure 252-2 *Autoregulation of cerebral blood flow in response to changing mean arterial pressure in hypertensive patient. (Data from Strandgaard S, Olesen J, Skinhoj E, et al. Br Med J. 1973;1(5852):507–510.)*

on two consecutive readings following surgery. More than 50% of patients have a history of hypertension prior to surgery. Postoperative hypertension is most common after cardiac surgery, major vascular surgery (eg, carotid and aortic procedures), head and neck surgery, neurosurgery, trauma, and organ transplantation. Increases in sympathetic tone and vascular resistance are thought to underlie the condition.

CLINICAL MANIFESTATIONS

Clinical characteristics of the hypertensive crisis are summarized in **Table 252-2**. End-organ damage in hypertensive emergency is summarized in **Table 252-3** and discussed later in this chapter.

NEUROLOGIC

The central nervous system is the organ system most often involved in hypertensive emergency. Clinical events may include stroke, hypertensive encephalopathy, intracranial hemorrhage, and subarachnoid hemorrhage. Cerebral edema often develops, particularly in the white matter of the parietooccipital regions, leading to the reversible posterior encephalopathy syndrome (**Figure 252-3**). Although patients with this syndrome may develop severe symptoms, including headache, nausea, delirium, visual disturbances, and focal neurologic findings, as the name suggests, many patients make a good clinical recovery as the cerebral edema resolves with treatment. The reason for the parietooccipital predominance is unknown, but may involve a relative paucity of sympathetic innervation in these regions.

CARDIAC

Myocardial ischemia is common, because of high myocardial oxygen demand, high-end diastolic pressures, endothelial damage, and previous myocardial hypertrophy, in patients with underlying essential hypertension. Congestive heart failure and pulmonary edema are common. Aortic dissection is a dreaded complication and should be suspected in those with sudden tearing or ripping chest pain radiating into the back, discordant upper-extremity pulses, and new diastolic murmurs. It should be borne in mind that neurologic symptoms in hypertensive crises may also be caused by aortic dissection disrupting the cerebral circulation.

RETINOPATHY

Visual disturbances in hypertensive crisis may be due to hypertensive encephalopathy and the reversible posterior encephalopathy syndrome, but they may also be due to malignant hypertensive retinopathy, characterized by swelling of the optic disc as well as retinal hemorrhages and soft exudates (cotton-wool spots).

RENAL

The kidney, like the brain, has a capacity to autoregulate its blood supply, but in the setting of a hypertensive crisis, this ability may be overwhelmed and a vicious cycle of kidney damage may ensue, characterized by vascular damage, endothelial dysfunction, fibrinoid necrosis, inflammation, and ischemic injury.

DIAGNOSIS OF HYPERTENSIVE URGENCIES AND EMERGENCIES

The initial assessment should include a thorough medical history, including the duration and severity of hypertension, comorbid cardiovascular and renal disease, all current prescription and nonprescription medications, and recreational drugs, especially cocaine and other stimulants. Patients should be questioned in a nonjudgmental way about adherence to antihypertensive medications and possible obstacles to adherence.

TABLE 252-2 Clinical Characteristics of the Hypertensive Emergency

Blood Pressure (mm Hg)	Neurologic Status	Cardiac Findings	Funduscopic Findings	Renal Symptoms	Gastrointestinal Symptoms
Not needed for diagnosis but usually ≥ 180/120 mm Hg	Headache, confusion, somnolence, stupor, visual loss, seizures, focal neurologic deficits, coma	Prominent apical pulsation, cardiac enlargement, congestive heart failure	Hemorrhages, exudates, papilledema	Azotemia, proteinuria, oliguria	Nausea, vomiting

Data from Vidt DG. Hypertensive crises: emergencies and urgencies. *J Clin Hypertens*. 2004;6:520–525; and Chobanian AV, Bakris GL, Black HR, et al. Seventh Report of the Joint National Committee on Prevention, Detection, Evaluation, and Treatment of High Blood Pressure. *JAMA*. 2003;289:2560–2572.

TABLE 252-3 Examples of Hypertensive Emergencies

Acute aortic dissection
Acute ischemic or hemorrhagic stroke
Subarachnoid hemorrhage
Hypertensive encephalopathy
Acute myocardial ischemia/infarction
Acute heart failure
Beta-blocker or clonidine withdrawal
Catecholamine excess states
Cocaine, phencyclidine hydrochloride use
Eclampsia
Head trauma
Hemorrhage
Pheochromocytoma crisis

Data from Hebert C, Vidt D. Hypertensive Crises. *Primary Care: Clinics in Office Practice.* 2008;35:475–487.

The review of systems should focus on symptoms that might indicate end-organ damage from hypertension, such as chest pain, shortness of breath, severe headache, changes in vision, dizziness, altered mental status or somnolence, oliguria, or anuria.

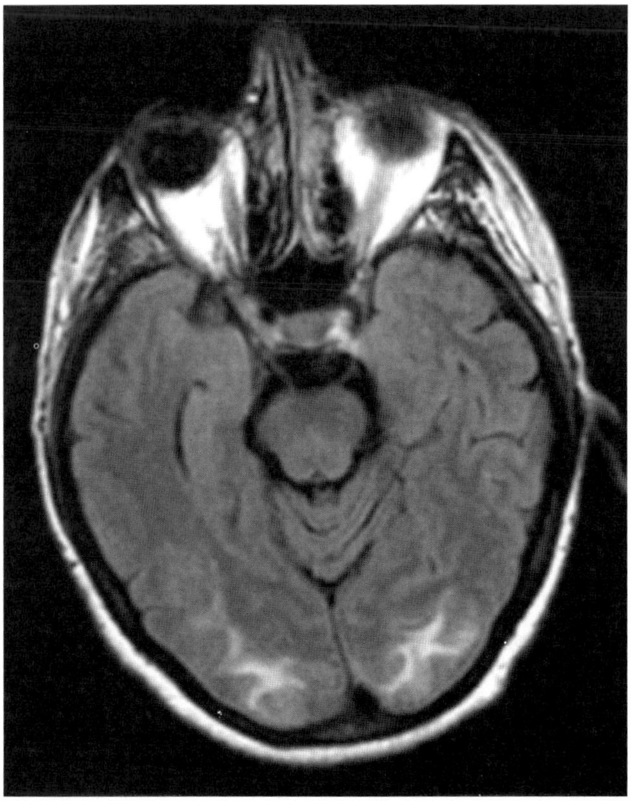

Figure 252-3 *Axial FLAIR MRI showing increased signal (white) in the occipital subcortical white matter and cortex bilaterally. These findings are typical of the reversible posterior leukoencephalopathy syndrome (RPLS) in the setting of hypertensive emergency, and probably represent reversible vasogenic edema. Other causes of RPLS include preeclampsia, cancer chemotherapy, and cyclosporine, tacrolimus, and other immunosuppressive drugs. (Reproduced, with permission, from Simon RP, Greenberg DA, Aminoff MJ. Clinical Neurology, 7th ed. New York: McGraw-Hill, 2009. Fig. 1-10.)*

On examination, the first step in diagnosing a hypertensive crisis is accurate blood pressure measurement. This should be repeated at least twice, taking precautions to properly position the patient and use an adequately sized cuff. Blood pressure should be checked in both arms and in the lower limbs. A blood pressure difference of more than 20 mm Hg between arms suggests aortic dissection, but unfortunately is not a sensitive finding. The examiner should also focus on detecting end-organ damage. On funduscopic examination, hypertensive patients often have chronic findings, such as widening of the arterial stripe ("copper-wire" and "silver-wire" changes) and arteriovenous nicking. Greater significance is attached to acute changes, such as new hemorrhages, cotton-wool retinal exudates, and papilledema. Signs of heart failure, such as elevated jugular venous pressures, S3 heart sounds, and pulmonary rales, should be sought on cardiopulmonary examination. A new diastolic heart murmur suggests aortic insufficiency from aortic dissection.

TREATMENT

Excessive blood pressure lowering should be avoided in hypertensive crisis, as many patients have chronic hypertension with vascular changes and are at risk for cerebral ischemia if blood pressure falls too quickly; this is especially true of older patients. An approach to triage in patients with hypertensive crisis is summarized in **Table 252-4**. In patients with hypertensive urgency, blood pressure lowering may usually be accomplished with oral medications over a 24- to 48-hour period. These patients do not necessarily require hospital admission. They may be observed and treated with oral agents for several hours prior to discharge with close outpatient follow-up, assuming that their blood pressure falls into an acceptable range. However, if patients with hypertensive urgency are symptomatic or if there are concerns about adherence, it is reasonable to admit these patients.

Patients with hypertensive crisis often benefit from being in a quieter and less stressful environment, if such can be provided in the inpatient setting. There are no large randomized controlled trials of therapy in hypertensive crisis. In hypertensive urgency, a reasonable approach is to restart oral antihypertensives in patients who have been nonadherent, or to increase doses of current therapy in adherent patients. In patients not previously taking antihypertensive therapy, initial choices for drug therapy include an ACE inhibitor, beta-blockers, or a calcium channel blocker. These patients are likely to require more than one agent for blood pressure control. Loop diuretics may be helpful in edematous patients. Sublingual nifedipine was once commonly used in the treatment of hypertensive crisis, but has fallen out of favor because of the risks of reflex tachycardia and hypotension.

Patients with hypertensive emergencies should be admitted to an intensive care unit for continuous monitoring of hemodynamics, neurologic status, urine output, and other manifestations of end-organ damage. Hypertensive emergencies are typically managed with short-acting titratable antihypertensive agents (**Table 252-5**). In the first hour of therapy, the goal is to lower mean arterial blood pressure by no more than 15% to 20%, with a diastolic blood pressure in the range of 100–110 mm Hg. Blood pressure is further reduced to 25% to 30% of the initial value within the next 4 to 8 hours. Oral antihypertensive agents should replace intravenous agents only when stable blood pressure control has been achieved, and there is no evidence of continuing end-organ damage.

Sodium nitroprusside has long been preferred as a first-line agent for hypertensive emergency, given its rapid onset of active, easy titration and rapid cessation of action when infusions are halted. Because sodium nitroprusside is a vasodilator, some authors caution against its use in patients with increased intracranial pressure, but its effects on cerebral vasodilation may be negated by the drop

TABLE 252-4 Algorithm for Triage Evaluation

	Severe Hypertension (Urgency)		
Parameter	Asymptomatic	Symptomatic	Hypertensive Emergency
Blood pressure (mm Hg)	< 180/120	< 180/120	Usually > 180/120
Symptoms	Headache, anxiety; often asymptomatic	Severe headache, shortness of breath	Shortness of breath, chest pain, nocturia, dysarthria, weakness, altered consciousness
Examination	No target organ damage, no clinical cardiovascular disease	Target organ damage; clinical cardiovascular disease present, stable	Encephalopathy, pulmonary edema, renal insufficiency, cerebrovascular accident, cardiac ischemia
Therapy	Observe at least 1–3 hours; initiate, resume medication; increase dosage of inadequate agent	Observe at least 3–6 hours; lower blood pressure with short-acting oral agent; adjust current therapy	Baseline laboratory tests; intravenous line; monitor BP; may initiate parenteral therapy in emergency room
Plan	Arrange follow-up within 3–7 days; if no prior evaluation, schedule appointment	Arrange follow-up evaluation in less than 72 hours	Immediate admission to intensive care unit; treat to initial goal BP; additional diagnostic studies

Data from Vidt DG. Hypertensive crises: emergencies and urgencies. *J Clin Hypertens*. 2004;6:520–525.

in systemic blood pressure. Thiocyanate toxicity, manifesting as confusion and lactic acidosis, is possible with nitroprusside infusions, especially when high doses are given in the setting of renal insufficiency. For this reason, nitroprusside infusions are usually not continued beyond 24 to 48 hours.

Other agents include labetalol, which should be used with caution in the setting of bradycardia, atrioventricular block, heart failure, and bronchospasm, and the calcium channel blocker nicardipine, which is associated with reflex tachycardia, headache, and flushing. Fenoldopam is a selective dopamine receptor antagonist and short-acting vasodilator. It seems as effective as sodium nitroprusside in hypertensive crisis, with the advantages of improved renal perfusion and promotion of diuresis. Tachyphylaxis develops after 48 hours. Although high doses of intravenous nitroglycerin are required to lower blood pressure, this drug may be especially helpful in the management of hypertension with myocardial ischemia. Headache is common with both fenoldopam and nitroglycerin.

Clevidipine is a recently approved, short-acting dihydropyridine calcium channel blocker that selectively inhibits the influx of extracellular calcium through the L-type channel. It has little effect on myocardial contractility. Side effects include headache, reflex tachycardia, nausea, and possibly atrial fibrillation. Hydralazine is currently less often used in the treatment of hypertensive crises because of its prolonged and unpredictable antihypertensive effects.

TABLE 252-5 Dose and Administration of Intravenous Agents Used in Hypertensive Emergencies

Drug	Dose and Administration
Clevidipine	Loading dose of 1–2 mg, followed by repeated incremental doubling of the dose at 90-sec intervals until the desired blood pressure is achieved. As blood pressure approaches goal, increase the dose by less than double and lengthen the time between dose adjustments to every 5–10 min. An approximately 1–2 mg/hour increase will generally produce an additional 2–4 mm Hg decrease in systolic pressure. The desired therapeutic response for most patients occurs at doses of 4–6 mg/hour. Patients with severe hypertension may require doses up to 32 mg/hour.
Enalaprilat	IV injection of 1.25 mg over 5 min every 6 hours, titrated by increments of 1.25 mg at 12- to 24-hour intervals to a maximum of 5 mg every 6 hours.
Esmolol	IV loading dose of 500–1000 μg/kg over 1 min, followed by an infusion at 25–50 μg/kg/min, which may be increased by 25 μg/kg/min every 10–20 min until the desired response to a maximum of 300 μg/kg/min.
Fenoldopam	An initial IV dose of 0.1 μg/kg/min, titrated by increments of 0.05–0.1 μg/kg/min to a maximum of 1.6 μg/kg/min.
Hydralazine	5 mg bolus then 5–10 mg IV every 20–30 min as needed.
Labetalol	Initial bolus 20 mg, followed by boluses of 20–80 mg or an infusion starting at 1–2 mg/min and titrated up to until the desired hypotensive effect is achieved. Bolus injections of 1–2 mg/kg have been reported to produce precipitous falls in blood pressure and should therefore be avoided; maximum cumulative dose is 300 mg over 24 hours.
Nicardipine	5 mg/hour; titrate to effect by increasing 2.5 mg/hour every 5 min to a maximum of 15 mg/hour.
Nitroprusside	0.5 μg/kg/min; titrate as tolerated to maximum of 2 μg/kg/min.
Phentolamine	Sympathetic crisis: IV 5–20 mg. Treatment of pralidoxime-induced hypertension (unlabeled use): IV 5 mg. Surgery for pheochromocytoma/hypertension: IM, IV 5 mg given 1–2 hours before procedure and repeated as needed every 2–4 hours.

IM, intramuscular; IV, intravenous.
Data from Varon J. Treatment of acute severe hypertension: current and newer agents. *Drugs*. 2008;68:283–297.

PRACTICE POINT

Hypertensive crisis from cocaine

- Acute and chronic effects of cocaine on the cardiovascular system include tachycardia, hypertensive crisis, myocardial infarction, stroke, aortic dissection, and cardiomyopathy. Hypertension in patients with cocaine intoxication relates to central stimulation of the sympathetic nervous system, as well as inhibition of neuronal catecholamine reuptake. Beta-blockers are contraindicated in cocaine intoxication, as they may lead to paradoxical worsening of hypertension via the unopposed alpha-adrenergic vasoconstrictive effects of cocaine. Although labetalol has both beta- and alpha-blocking properties, it should also be avoided in this setting, as it is a more effective beta-blocker than alpha-blocker. Therapeutic options for cocaine-induced hypertension include the alpha-blocker phentolamine, benzodiazepines such as diazepam or lorazepam, continuous infusions of nitroglycerin or nitroprusside, or calcium channel blockers.

DISCHARGE CONSIDERATIONS

In patients with hypertensive urgencies and emergencies, a reasonable goal of hospital care at the time of discharge is to have the patient transitioned to oral antihypertensives, with blood pressure consistently $\leq 160/100$ mm Hg. The patient should be followed closely as an outpatient over the succeeding days and weeks, in order to encourage adherence and to further titrate the patient's medications to achieve the target blood pressure (generally $< 140/90$ mm Hg, but as low as $< 130/80$ mm Hg in certain populations, including diabetics and patients with chronic renal disease). Every effort should be made to enlist family members, friends, and outside resources, such as visiting nurses and pharmacists, in optimizing medication adherence. Consultation with a nutritionist is useful for education about dietary sodium avoidance. Prior to hospital discharge, barriers to outpatient care should be addressed, such as lack of health insurance, financial problems, poor home situation, knowledge gaps, comorbid psychiatric conditions, and untreated substance abuse. The involvement of social work providers may be very helpful in this regard.

CONCLUSION

Considering the relatively short window between the onset of symptomatology and end-organ dysfunction, more than basic knowledge on identifying and treating hypertensive crises is required. This short window of time could be paramount in preventing cardiac arrest, progressive end-organ damage and long-term consequences. Proper management should include titratable agents within the ICU, and long-term management of hypertension should include oral pharmacological treatment. Finally, if we speculate on the relatively high number of cases of severe uncontrolled hypertension there are in every emergency department, we should always look for signs of end-organ damage in presence of high blood pressure and be prepared to treat it.

SUGGESTED READINGS

Aggarwal M, Khan I. Hypertensive crisis: hypertensive emergencies and urgencies. *Cardiol Clin*. 2006;24:135–146.

Chobanian AV, Bakris GL, Black HR, et al. Seventh Report of the Joint National Committee on Prevention, Detection, Evaluation, and Treatment of High Blood Pressure. *Hypertension*. 2003;42:1206–1252.

Varon J, Marik P. The diagnosis and management of hypertensive crises. *Chest*. 2000;118:214–227.

Varon J. Treatment of acute severe hypertension: current and newer agents. *Drugs*. 2008;68:283–297.

Vaughan C, Delanty N. Hypertensive emergencies. *Lancet*. 2000; 356:411–417.

Vidt DG. Hypertensive crises: emergencies and urgencies. *J Clin Hypertens (Greenwich)*. 2004;6:520–525.

Zampaglione B, Pascale C, Marchisio M, Cavallo-Perin P. Hypertensive urgencies and emergencies: prevalence and clinical presentation. *Hypertension*. 1996;27:144–147.

CHAPTER 253

Secondary Hypertension

William J. Elliott, MD, PhD

Key Clinical Questions

1. Which patients should be evaluated for secondary causes of hypertension in the inpatient setting?
2. What are the most common secondary causes of hypertension in hospitalized patients?
3. What screening and diagnostic tests are best for each?
4. What specific therapy or therapies are currently recommended?
5. What follow-up should be recommended after discharge?

INTRODUCTION

Hypertension affects 29% of the American public. Its prevalence among hospitalized patients is much higher. Hospitalized patients are older than the general population, and the prevalence of hypertension is 67% in those aged 60 years and older. In addition, hypertension is a major risk factor for the cardiovascular and renal diseases that lead to inpatient admission. Poorly controlled hypertension among general medical inpatients is most often related to other conditions, such as pain, agitation from delirium, and substance withdrawal. Secondary hypertension has a prevalence of less than 5% in the general population, but is more common among inpatients. This is due to three types of selection bias: (1) negative screening for secondary hypertension in outpatients, who are seldom hospitalized for the evaluation and are at low risk of hospitalization for other causes; (2) patients admitted for hypertensive emergencies; and (3) patients with secondary hypertension admitted for diagnostic and therapeutic procedures, often for other diagnoses. For example, 13% of patients undergoing cardiac or peripheral arterial catheterization have a documented stenosis in a renal artery (discovered during "drive-by angiograms"). Secondary causes of hypertension should at least be considered in hypertensive inpatients, especially younger ones. This ensures that these patients are assessed at least once for secondary hypertension during their lifetime. In addition, some causes, such as pheochromocytoma, Conn adenoma, and fibromuscular dysplasia, are amenable to cure, or at least long-term amelioration. This obviates the need to take antihypertensive medications over a long period of time, improving the cost-effectiveness of screening young patients.

CRITERIA FOR HOSPITAL ADMISSION

The major circumstance in which secondary hypertension leads to hospital admission is a hypertensive emergency (severely elevated blood pressure and acute, ongoing target-organ damage). These patients have a high prevalence of secondary hypertension, and the hypertensive emergency is often the first real clue to the presence of a secondary cause. After stabilization of these patients with short-acting, intravenous antihypertensive drugs, attention should be focused on developing an appropriate antihypertensive drug regimen and excluding secondary hypertension.

PRACTICE POINT

- There are many reasons why a hospitalized patient may have severe hypertension, including pain, fluid overload, a discrepancy between home and hospital antihypertensive regimen, as well as withdrawal from alcohol, prescription medication, and other substances. Clinicians should recognize precipitating factors that commonly augment blood pressure in the acutely ill and require a different approach from simply prescribing antihypertensive medications.

Less commonly, patients are admitted electively for diagnostic or therapeutic procedures related to secondary hypertension. Many of these are "23-hour admissions," and do not require major attention from hospital-based physicians, except those directly involved in the procedure. Examples include patients with possible hyperaldosteronism and bilateral adrenal nodules admitted for adrenal venous sampling, claustrophobic patients with possible pheochromocytoma admitted for magnetic resonance imaging of the abdomen after intravenous sedation, and patients with a high probability of fibromuscular renovascular hypertension sent for renal angiography with possible angioplasty.

Occasionally, secondary hypertension becomes an issue in patients admitted for diagnostic or therapeutic procedures only indirectly related to hypertension. Examples include hypertensives undergoing evaluation of incidentally discovered adrenal masses, individuals who have incidental or "drive-by" renal angiograms after a planned coronary or carotid catheterization, and patients who have an increase of greater than 25% in serum creatinine after administration of an angiotensin-converting enzyme (ACE) inhibitor or angiotensin receptor blocker (ARB). Hospitalists caring for these patients should pursue appropriate diagnosis and treatment of secondary hypertension before discharge.

PRACTICE POINT

- A primary diagnosis of hypertensive crisis—a surge in blood pressure accompanied by end-organ damage—or a hypertensive urgency—a surge in blood pressure without end-organ damage—may be the first clue to the presence of secondary hypertension. After stabilization of these patients with short-acting, intravenous antihypertensive drugs and initiating an appropriate antihypertensive drug regimen, secondary causes of hypertension should be considered, especially in younger patients.

CLINICAL SYNDROMES

The most common secondary causes of hypertension in hospitalized patients are listed in **Table 253-1**. Despite a perennial enthusiasm in internal medicine for esoteric diseases, it should be noted that the most common type of hypertension in hospitalized patients is still primary (formerly *essential*) hypertension.

CHRONIC KIDNEY DISEASE

This secondary cause of hypertension differs from the others in at least two respects: it is usually not remediable, and it may be both a cause and a consequence of hypertension. Chronic kidney disease is defined as three months or more of either an estimated glomerular filtration rate (*e*GFR) of less than 60 mL/min/1.73 m^2, or kidney damage defined as pathologic abnormalities, abnormal imaging studies, or elevated blood or urine markers of kidney injury (usually albuminuria > 30 μg/mg creatinine in a first-morning voided urine specimen). In large population-based studies, more advanced stages of chronic kidney disease are linked to greater risks of death and hospitalization. As a result, this secondary cause of hypertension is thought to be about 5- to 10-fold more common in hospitalized patients than in the general United States population.

Testing for chronic kidney disease is part of the admitting process for essentially every inpatient, with a serum creatinine (and in most hospitals, a calculated *e*GFR, based on the most recent update of the Modification of Diet in Renal Disease equations) and a urinalysis. Occasionally, the urinalysis can be falsely negative for protein if performed on a very dilute sample. If this is suspected, a first-morning voided urine specimen should be obtained to measure the albumin-to-creatinine ratio.

Intensive lowering of blood pressure is an effective means to prevent or delay the progression of chronic kidney disease to end-stage renal disease. Most authorities recommend that patients with chronic kidney diseases should have frequent urinalyses and determinations of *e*GFR, a lower-than-usual blood pressure goal (< 130/80 mm Hg), and an ACE inhibitor or an ARB as part of their medication regimen, if possible.

PRIMARY HYPERALDOSTERONISM

CASE 253-1

A 43-year-old man was admitted for observation after the car he was driving ran into the median, landing on its roof. He was not injured aside from minor abrasions and lacerations. Physical examination was unremarkable, except for blood pressure of

TABLE 253-1 Common Secondary Causes of Hypertension in Hospitalized Patients

Diagnosis	Key Features	Risk Factors	Relative Prevalence	Screening Tests
Chronic kidney disease	*e*GFR < 60 mL/min/1.73 m^2, albumin/creatinine ratio > 300 μg/mg	Hypertension, diabetes	~90%	Serum creatinine, first morning voided urine for albumin-to-creatinine ratio
Primary hyperaldosteronism	Hypokalemia, sleep apnea symptoms, resistant hypertension	Sleep apnea	~6%	Aldosterone/renin ratio
Renovascular hypertension	Abdominal bruit, "bump" in serum creatinine after ACE inhibitor or ARB	Young women (fibromuscular disease); atherosclerotic disease in older smokers	~3%	Doppler ultrasound
Cushing syndrome	Hypertension, hyperglycemia, abdominal striae, proximal muscle weakness, hirsutism	Women (Cushing disease); men (ectopic corticotropin production)	< 1%	Urinary free cortisol; midnight serum cortisol
Pheochromocytoma	Hypertension, hyperhydrosis, headache (often in paroxysms)	Phakomatoses, multiple endocrine neoplasia syndromes	< 1%	Plasma metanephrines vs. 24-hour urine for VMA and metanephrines
Coarctation of the aorta	Blood pressure differences across limbs; systolic murmur posteriorly	Turner syndrome; other congenital arterial anomalies	< 1%	Echocardiogram (especially the sternal notch view)

ACE, angiotensin-converting enzyme; ARB, angiotensin receptor blocker; VMA, vanillylmandelic acid.

168/106 mm Hg, a body-mass index of 35 kg/m^2, and an 18-inch (46-cm) neck circumference. Laboratory studies and a computed tomography (CT) scan of the head were remarkable only for serum potassium of 3.1 mEq/L. The nurses noted that his snoring could be heard from 40 feet (12 meters) away and that he had frequent apneic spells. After discharge, his blood pressure remained elevated (158–172/98–110 mm Hg) and a formal polysomnographic study verified obstructive sleep apnea. His aldosterone-to-renin ratio was 86, which decreased to 22 after 2 liters of intravenous saline. After 4 weeks of treatment with spironolactone, his blood pressure decreased to 132/76 mm Hg, serum potassium increased to 3.8 mEq/L, and both have remained controlled for over 4 years.

Primary hyperaldosteronism is more commonly recognized now than in the past. In older series, it was found in only 0.1% to 0.5% of hypertensive patients, with most patients having hypokalemia and aldosterone-producing adrenal adenomas (Conn syndrome). While the exact prevalence and significance of primary hyperaldosteronism in hypertension remains unclear, this is almost certainly an underestimate. Some studies have found primary hyperaldosteronism in up to 5% to 10% of hypertensive patients, and in patients with resistant or refractory hypertension, the prevalence may be as high as 11% to 23%. In recent series, 35% of cases were due to aldosterone-producing adenomas, 60% were due to bilateral adrenal hyperplasia, and the remainder were due to adrenal carcinoma, unilateral adrenal hyperplasia, glucocorticoid-remediable hyperaldosteronism, and other causes. Most patients did not have hypokalemia.

The renewed interest in primary hyperaldosteronism also stems from the availability of new therapies, such as laparoscopic adrenalectomy, and evidence that primary hyperaldosteronism has morbidities in addition to hypertension. Compared with patients with essential hypertension and similar levels of blood pressure elevation, patients with primary hyperaldosteronism may be at greater risk of left ventricular hypertrophy, reduced diastolic dysfunction, myocardial infarction, atrial fibrillation, stroke, albuminuria, and the metabolic syndrome. Hyperaldosteronism seems to be especially common in the setting of obesity and sleep apnea. Possible explanations include renin release during sympathetic nervous system activation during apneic episodes, adipocyte production of angiotensinogen, and aldosterone release driven by oxidized fatty acids.

The currently recommended initial screening test for primary hyperaldosteronism is the plasma aldosterone-to-renin ratio, or ARR (**Figure 253-1**). A sample is drawn from a patient who has been seated quietly for at least 15 minutes. Generally no changes are necessary in dietary salt intake or antihypertensive medications, except aldosterone antagonists, which should be stopped. Inhibitors of the renin-angiotensin system (including β-blockers) can improve the diagnostic performance of the test and may account for some of the controversy surrounding its use. In properly selected patients, an ARR of 20 to 40 (when the plasma renin activity is expressed in ng of angiotensin II/mL/hour, and the aldosterone level in ng/dL) raises the suspicion of primary hyperaldosteronism. Similarly, the utility of the ARR is inversely proportional to the plasma-renin activity, as very low levels (eg, < 0.2 ng/mL/hour, as a possible consequence of a high-sodium diet, or "low-renin hypertension") increase the ARR exponentially.

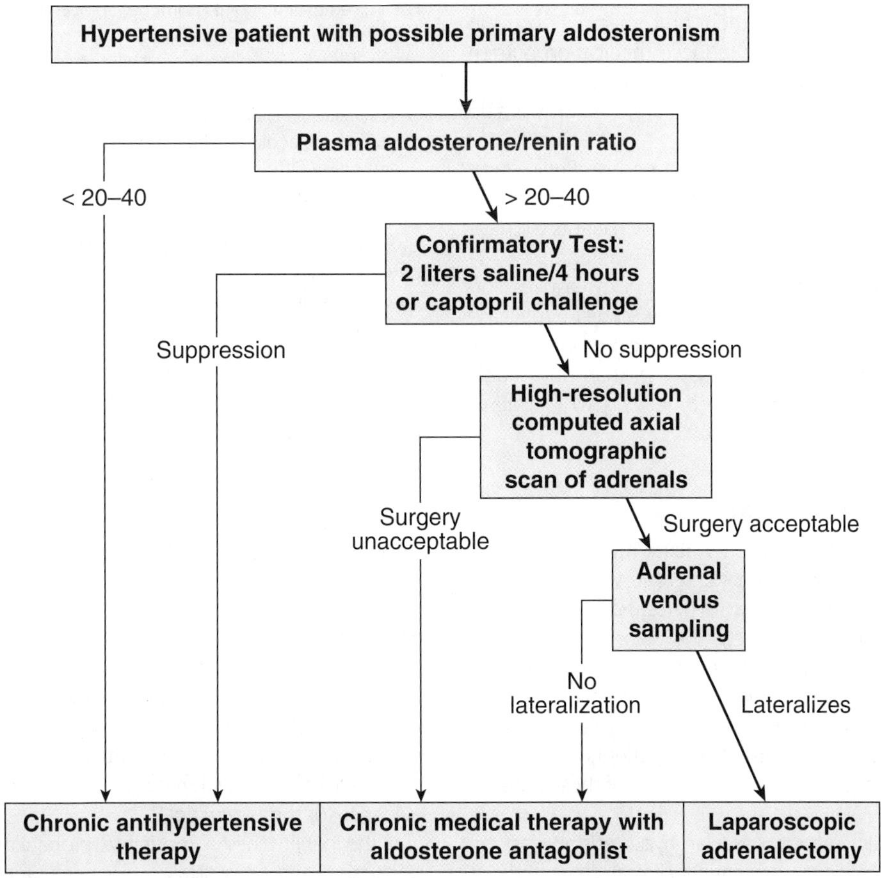

Figure 253-1 *Suggested diagnostic algorithm for most patients with suspected primary aldosteronism.*

An elevated ARR is typically followed by one of four confirmatory tests, usually on the next hospital day. Hospitalists generally prefer measuring plasma aldosterone before and after either saline infusion (2 liters over 4 hours), or oral captopril (25 mg given 2 hours earlier), because both the fludrocortisone suppression (0.1 mg every 6 hours for 4 days) and oral sodium loading (12 gm daily for 4 days) tests require too long a preparation period. The challenges with these tests involve the risk of hypotension (captopril) or volume overload (particularly troublesome in patients with heart failure). If the patient is young or has a family history of hyperaldosteronism, a morning sample of plasma for 18-hydroxycortisol and 18-oxocortisol levels may be helpful, as low or normal levels effectively rule out glucocorticoid-remediable aldosteronism (which accounts for less than 1% of primary hyperaldosteronism in most series).

If the confirmatory test shows no evidence of aldosterone suppression, a decision must be made about the risks and benefits of possible surgery. Many favor simply treating such patients with aldosterone antagonists, as most (about two-thirds) will not have surgically remediable tumors. Should laparoscopic surgery be available and the patient and physician are agreeable, an adrenal CT scan may be performed. If there is a unilateral hypodense (< 10 Hounsfield units) nodule larger than 1 cm, most patients under the age of 40 years are offered surgery. If the patient is older than 40 years or has a high clinical probability of a tumor and either normal adrenals, micronodularity, or bilateral masses, adrenal venous sampling is first performed to localize the aldosterone-producing adrenal adenoma, before surgery. Otherwise, the patient is treated with an aldosterone antagonist. Spironolactone is less costly, but eplerenone has fewer adverse effects.

Laparoscopic adrenalectomy is the surgical approach of choice because of lower rates of morbidity and shorter hospital stays. Cure rates of 56% to 77% have been cited, although eukalemia may be delayed for several days, and complete normalization of blood pressure (< 140/90 mm Hg without drug therapy) occurs in only about one-third. Because of the reduced medication burden (including side effects and potassium supplementation and its monitoring), and improved blood pressure, adrenalectomy is said to be less expensive than medical therapy.

For patients with hyperaldosteronism and a positive Berlin questionnaire, suggestive of sleep apnea, referral to a sleep center for polysomnographic testing is appropriate. Many of these patients will have improved blood pressure control on an aldosterone antagonist.

Follow-up testing for primary hyperaldosteronism requires surveillance of blood pressure, serum potassium, and, in the case of glucocorticoid-remediable hyperaldosteronism, monitoring of glucose, cholesterol, and bone density (as higher than physiologic doses of corticosteroids are often needed, leading to iatrogenic Cushing syndrome).

RENOVASCULAR HYPERTENSION

As the population ages and survival after acute myocardial infarction as the first manifestation of atherosclerotic vascular disease becomes more common, renovascular hypertension is becoming more widely recognized. Unfortunately, the diagnosis and treatment of this condition are still controversial. Recent clinical trials have shown little (if any) benefit to routine angioplasty compared with chronic antihypertensive drug therapy. The prevalence of renal artery stenosis on angiography in hospitalized patients undergoing cardiac catheterization is as high as 39%, but many of these patients were not hypertensive.

The pretest probability of renovascular hypertension can be calculated based on a patient's presenting clinical characteristics (**Table 253-2**). This clinical prediction rule correctly identifies most patients with either a very high (> 70%) or very low (< 15%) probability of renovascular hypertension who do not require additional testing (**Figure 253-2**). Before embarking on a series of diagnostic tests, two important questions should be answered. If the patient refuses vascular surgery, as might become necessary in the event of renal artery perforation during angioplasty or stenting, no further diagnostic evaluation is recommended. The more difficult question is whether an invasive intervention is indicated. Because several trials comparing percutaneous angioplasty and medical therapy have shown no long-term differences, many authorities reserve a diagnostic evaluation for a patient who cannot tolerate an ACE inhibitor or ARB (typically because of hyperkalemia, or a rise in serum creatinine > 25% over baseline), or whose blood pressure cannot be controlled to < 140/90 mm Hg with maximal medical therapy. Some would add patients with recurrent flash pulmonary edema, but the evidence for this is anecdotal.

If the patient has a moderate probability of renovascular hypertension and an indication for percutaneous intervention, one of four screening tests is recommended, based on local availability and expertise (**Table 253-3**). Centers with very experienced

TABLE 253-2 Calculation of the Pretest Probability of Renovascular Hypertension

Clinical Characteristic	Never Smoked	Current or Former Smoker
Age (in years)		
20–29	0	0
30–39	1	4
40–49	2	8
50–59	3	5
60–69	4	5
70–79	5	6
Female gender	2	2
ASCVD*	1	1
Hx HTN† ≤ 2 years	1	1
BMI < 25 kg/m²	2	2
Abdominal bruit	3	3
Serum creatinine		
0.5–0.75 mg/dL	0	0
0.75–1.0 mg/dL	1	1
1.0–1.2 mg/dL	2	2
1.2v1.65 mg/dL	3	3
1.7–2.2 mg/dL	6	6
≥ 2.3 mg/dL	9	9
Hypercholesterolemia (> 250 mg/dL, or on treatment)	1	1

For a given patient, points from the table are summed; if > 15, the probability is ≥ 70% and angiography is recommended as the initial test; if < 10, the probability is < 15% and screening tests are unlikely to be warranted.

*ASCVD, signs, symptoms, or clinical evidence of atherosclerotic cardiovascular disease; BMI < body mass index (weight in kg/[height in cm]²); Hx HTN, history of hypertension.

Data from Krijnen P, van Jaarsveld BC, Steyerberg EW, Manin't Veld AJ, Schalekamp MA, Habbema JD. A clinical prediction rule for renal artery stenosis. *Ann Intern Med*. 1998;129:705–711; and Krijnen P, Steyerberg EW, Postma CT, Flobbe K, de Leeuw PW, Hunink MGM. Validation of a prediction rule for renal artery stenosis. *J Hypertens*. 2005;23:1583–1588.

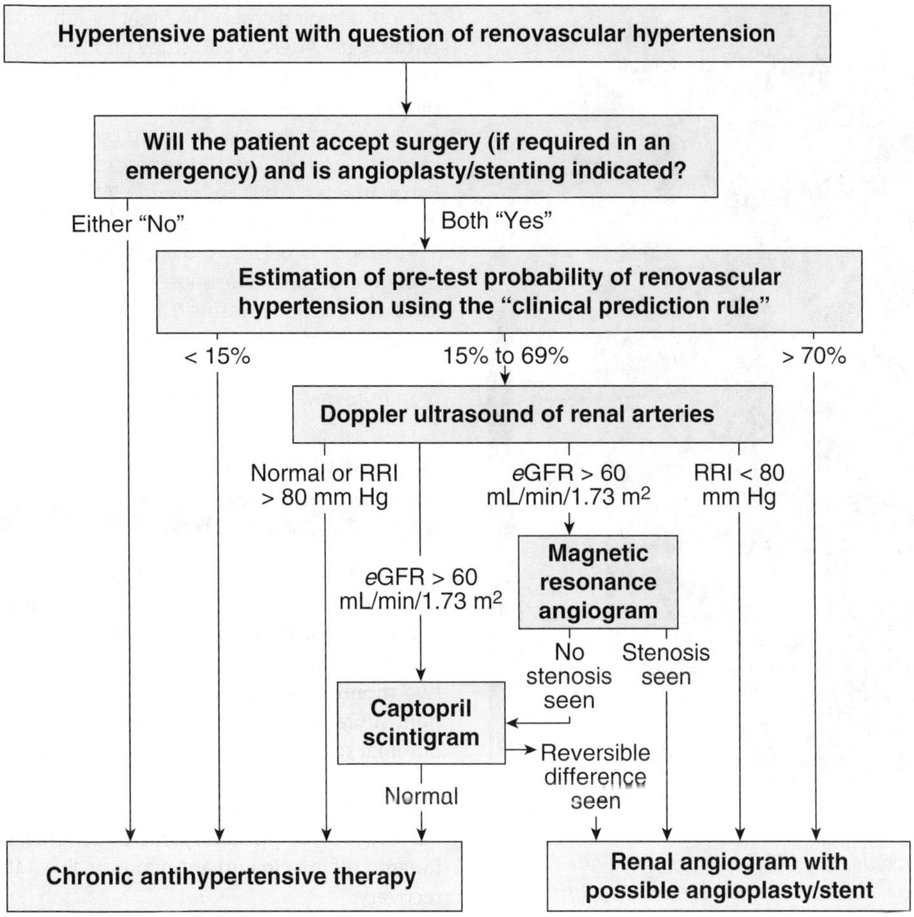

Figure 253-2 *Suggested diagnostic algorithm for most patients with renovascular hypertension. RRI, renal resistance index.*

TABLE 253-3 Summary of Advantages and Disadvantages of Screening Tests for Renovascular Hypertension

Screening Test	Doppler Ultrasound	Captopril Scintigraphy	Magnetic Resonance Angiogram	Computed Tomographic Angiogram
Number of publications (1990–2006)	47	69	30	14
Number of patients/ arteries	2653	5282	1623	1225
Sensitivity (range)	0.83 (0.17–1.00)	0.79 (0.27–1.00)	0.88 (0.54–1.00)	0.86 (0.63–1.00)
Specificity (range)	0.82 (0.63–1.00)	0.82 (0.44–1.00)	0.88 (0.23–1.00)	0.94 (0.63–1.00)
Advantages	Noninvasive, inexpensive, may predict BP results after revascularization	Noninvasive, not expensive, may predict BP results after revascularization	No iodinated contrast needed; excellent image quality	Excellent image quality
Disadvantages	Operator dependent; less useful in obesity, bowel gas, branch lesions, FMD	Less accurate in renal impairment, bilateral disease, obstructive uropathy	Expensive, poor images with stents or distal stenoses (eg, FMD), overcalls moderate stenoses; risk of gadolinium-associated fibrosing dermopathy	Expensive, time-consuming to process and interpret; not widely available; large amount of contrast sometimes needed

BP, blood pressure; FMD, fibromuscular dysplasia.

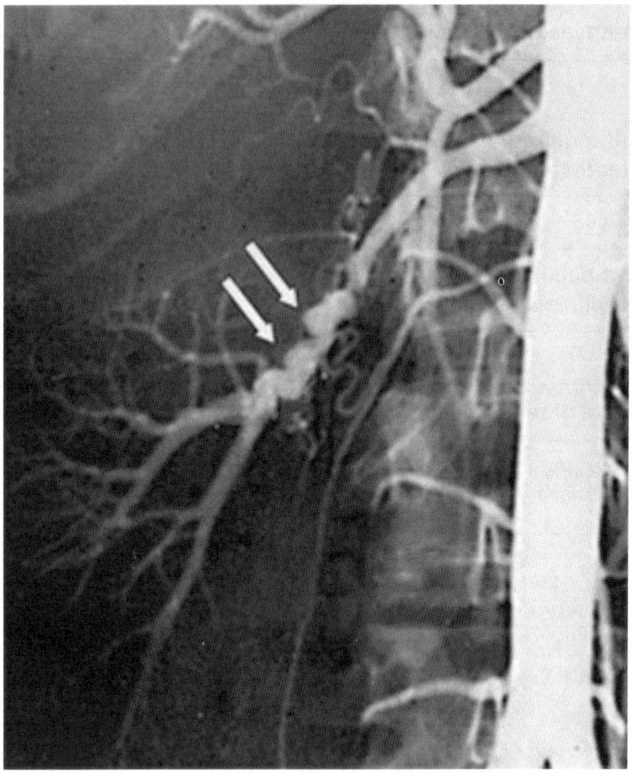

Figure 253-3 *Abdominal aortogram revealing left renal artery fibromuscular dysplasia (arrows) with a characteristic "string-of-beads" appearance. (Reproduced, with permission, from Brunicardi FC, Andersen DK, Billiar TR, et al. Schwartz's Principles of Surgery. 9th ed. New York: McGraw-Hill, 2008. Fig. 23-44.)*

Doppler ultrasound laboratories have reported excellent performance characteristics and the ability to predict a blood pressure response after intervention (renal resistive index < 80 mm Hg) with this noninvasive and relatively inexpensive test. High-resolution CT angiograms are highly sensitive for diagnosis, but they involve radiation exposure and injection of potentially nephrotoxic contrast medium. Magnetic resonance angiograms are quite sensitive and specific, and avoid exposure to iodinated contrast or radiation. However, they are generally not performed if the *e*GFR is less than 60 mL/min/1.73 m^2 because of the risk of irreversible gadolinium-associated nephrogenic fibrosing dermopathy. Conventional catheter angiography allows for treatment immediately following the discovery of a stenosis, but has the same risks of contrast and radiation exposure as CT angiogram and is also invasive (**Figure 253-3**). Although the captopril scintigram is relatively inexpensive, has been validated in large numbers of patients, and helps predict the results of angioplasty, the American Heart Association no longer recommends its use as a screening test, citing its limited utility in patients with significant azotemia, bilateral renal artery stenosis, or renal artery stenosis limited to a single kidney.

In the past, angioplasty was often delayed until the results of hormonal or hemodynamic measurements were obtained, but this has fallen into disfavor, as longer or repeated procedures were usually required. Advances in angiography, stent placement, and protection of distal circulation have improved the success rates of percutaneous renal artery revascularization. This procedure is now the treatment of choice for most types of fibromuscular dysplasia, but its role in atherosclerotic disease is controversial. The Dutch Renal Artery Stenosis Intervention Cooperative (DRASTIC) trial showed no benefit of angioplasty, although a careful reading of the 12-month data shows significantly better blood pressure control in the instrumented group. The Stent for Atherosclerotic Ostial Stenosis of the Renal Artery (STAR) study and the Angioplasty and Stent for Renal Artery Lesions (ASTRAL) study have also shown no significant differences across randomized arms, suggesting that the results of earlier meta-analyses showing no benefit to the invasive procedure might be correct. The NIH-sponsored Cardiovascular Outcomes in Renal Atherosclerotic Lesions (CORAL) trial will be larger and longer in duration; results are expected in January 2012.

Postprocedure follow-up is critical for patients with renovascular hypertension, as the diagnosis is made retrospectively, by showing lower office blood pressure 6 to 12 weeks after opening the stenosis. Adjustment of medications for blood pressure, serum potassium, lipids, and monitoring serum creatinine are all needed for several months following revascularization.

CUSHING SYNDROME

CASE 253-2

A 34-year-old woman was admitted to the hospital with a plasma glucose of 700 mg/dL. She had gained 25 pounds (11 kg) in the past six months, and developed amenorrhea, depression, and muscular weakness, particularly walking upstairs, in the last two months. Her blood pressure was 168/102 mm Hg; prominent supraclavicular and dorsocervical fat pads and purple abdominal striae were noted. A 24-hour urine contained 180 μg of free cortisol, and her serum cortisol was suppressed only after high-dose dexamethasone. Twelve months after trans-sphenoidal resection of a pituitary microadenoma, she was successfully tapered off insulin and antihypertensive agents and made a full recovery.

Most patients with signs and symptoms of glucocorticoid excess can be correctly diagnosed with an initial urinary free cortisol level > 100 μg/day, a morning or evening cortisol level (sometimes now obtained from saliva, rather than blood), and the classical low-dose and high-dose dexamethasone suppression tests. When these are inconsistent, repetition of the tests or endocrinology consultation is often helpful. The ability to assay both corticotropin-releasing hormone and corticotropin (formerly known as adrenocorticotropic hormone, or ACTH) has also simplified the hormonal diagnosis. Radiologic studies to localize the tumor to the left or right side of the pituitary or left or right adrenal are often performed before the surgeon will operate.

PHEOCHROMOCYTOMA

CASE 253-3

A 44-year-old man was hospitalized for a severe headache and a blood pressure of 260/140 mm Hg. He noted such episodes for the last two months, increasing in frequency and severity. Most lasted about 10 to 20 minutes and resolved spontaneously. Physical examination included a subungual fibroma and a 0.7 × 2 cm "ash-leaf patch" on the left at L3. Admitting laboratory studies were within the reference ranges, but a 24-hour urine contained seven times the upper limit of normal of metanephrines. His blood pressure was treated successfully with intravenous phentolamine in an intensive care unit. Oral phenoxybenzamine was begun after MRI showed an enhancing T2-weighted 2 × 3 cm lesion in the left adrenal, removed surgically four weeks later. Family studies were negative for tuberous sclerosis. He has had no recurrent symptoms five years later.

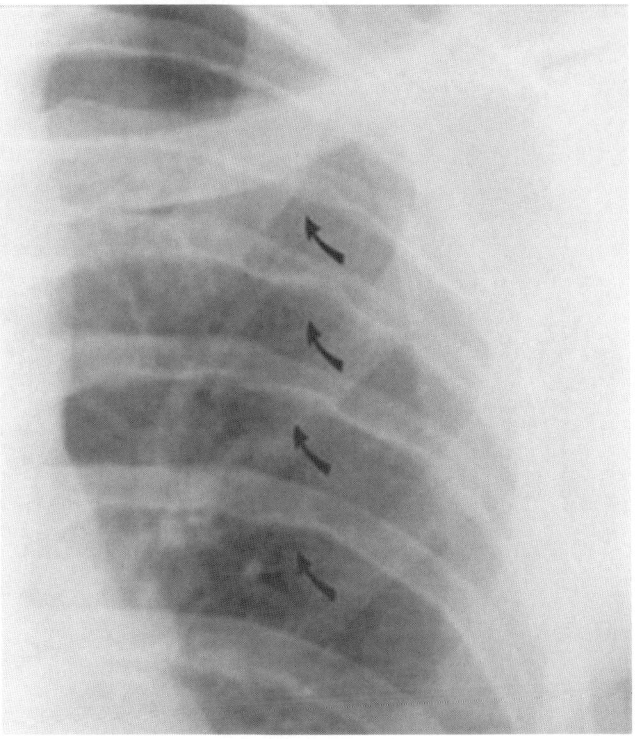

Figure 253-4 *Rib notching (arrows) caused by dilation of intercostal collaterals in a patient with coarctation of the aorta. (Reproduced, with permission, from Fuster V, O'Rourke RA, Walsh RA, et al. Hurst's the Heart. 12th ed. New York: McGraw-Hill, 2008. Fig. 15-1B.)*

The initial step in diagnosis of pheochromocytoma is demonstration of overproduction of catecholamine metabolites. Either plasma-free metanephrines or 24-hour urinary fractionated metanephrines may be used as a screening test; plasma-free metanephrines are somewhat more sensitive and logistically easier to obtain. If either is elevated, MRI or CT of the abdomen should be obtained. If these are negative and pheochromocytoma or paraganglionoma is still suspected, the tumor may be localized with either ^{131}I-metaiodobenzylguanidine (MIBG) scan or positron emission tomographic (PET) scan. Alpha-blockers are used for preoperative blood pressure management, traditionally with oral phenoxybenzamine or intravenous phentolamine when urgent control is required; postural hypotension is a troublesome side effect. Beta-blockers may paradoxically worsen blood pressure and should be given only after full alpha-blockade has been achieved. A laparoscopic approach is becoming more common for solitary adrenal pheochromocytomas. Genetic testing for pheochromocytoma-associated syndromes, such as multiple endocrine neoplasia type 2, is generally recommended.

COARCTATION OF THE AORTA

Although most patients with this disorder are diagnosed and treated as children, many with less severe coarctations remain undetected until adulthood. Clinical clues include difference in blood pressure of > 15/10 mm Hg between arms, a lower BP in a leg than the unilateral arm, or "rib notching" on chest X-ray (**Figure 253-4**). Many diagnostic techniques have been employed, but transthoracic echocardiography with suprasternal notch views is quite sensitive and probably the least expensive. Catheter-based interventions have been successful in many adults, but most remain hypertensive after relief of the coarctation.

CONCLUSION

Evaluation and treatment of secondary hypertension is most often performed in the outpatient setting. However, remediable forms of hypertension should at least be considered in hospitalized hypertensive patients, especially in those who are admitted for hypertensive urgency and emergency. An inpatient assessment for secondary hypertension ensures that the patient does not miss an opportunity for better blood pressure control, or even cure of hypertension in some patients. However, further research is necessary to determine the optimal and most cost-effective test sequence for evaluation of primary hyperaldosteronism, pheochromocytoma, and Cushing syndrome. Renovascular hypertension may not need not be considered except in patients with uncontrollably high blood pressure, or those in whom renal function deteriorates during treatment with an inhibitor of the renin-angiotensin system.

SUGGESTED READINGS

Calhoun DA, Jones D, Textor S, et al. Resistant hypertension: diagnosis, evaluation, and treatment. A scientific statement from the American Heart Association Professional Education Committee of the Council for High Blood Pressure Research. *Hypertension.* 2008;51:1403–1419.

Catena C, Colussi GL, Nadalini E, et al. Cardiovascular outcomes in patients with primary aldosteronism after treatment. *Arch Intern Med.* 2008;168:80–85.

Douma S, Petidis K, Doumas M, et al. Prevalence of primary hyperaldosteronism in resistant hypertension: a retrospective observational study. *Lancet.* 2008;371:1921–1926.

Elliott WJ. Secondary hypertension: renovascular hypertension. *J Clin Hypertens (Greenwich).* 2008;10:522–533.

Findling JW, Raff H. Cushing's syndrome: important issues in diagnosis and management. *J Clin Endo Metab.* 2006;91: 3746–3753.

Funder JW, Carey RM, Fardella C, et al. Case detection, diagnosis, and treatment of patients with primary aldosteronism: an Endocrine Society Clinical Practice Guideline. *J Clin Endocrinol Metab.* 2008;93:3266–3281.

Gus M, Goncalves SC, Martinez D. Risk for obstructive sleep apnea by Berlin Questionnaire, but not daytime sleepiness, is associated with resistant hypertension: a case-control study. *Am J Hypertens.* 2008;21:832–835.

Lenders JW, Eisenhofer G, Mannelli M, Pacak K. Phaeochromocytoma. *Lancet.* 2005;366:665–675.

Mattsson C, Young WF Jr. Primary aldosteronism: diagnostic and treatment strategies. *Nature Clin Pract Nephrol.* 2006;2: 198–208.

Newell-Price J, Bertagna X, Grossman AR, Nieman LK. Cushing's syndrome. *Lancet.* 2006:367:1605–1617.

Reisch N, Peczkowska M, Januszewicz A, Neumann HP. Pheochromocytoma: presentation, diagnosis and treatment. *J Hypertens.* 2006;24:2331–2339.

Rocha-Singh KJ, Eisenhauer AC, Textor SC, et al, for Writing Group 8. Atherosclerotic peripheral vascular disease symposium II: intervention for renal artery disease. *Circulation.* 2008;118: 2873–2878.

SECTION 18

Rheumatology

CHAPTER 254

Rheumatologic Emergencies

Paul F. Dellaripa, MD
Derrick J. Todd, MD, PhD

Key Clinical Questions

1. What are the signs and symptoms of cervical spine involvement in rheumatoid arthritis and the spondyloarthropathies?
2. What tests should be ordered in patients with suspected pulmonary-renal syndrome?
3. Which patients with interstitial lung disease are most likely to respond to corticosteroids?
4. What are common and uncommon clinical signs and symptoms associated with giant cell arteritis?
5. What factors portend an impending renal crisis in a patient with known scleroderma?
6. What are the risk factors for Raynaud digital crisis? What treatments reduce morbidity?

INTRODUCTION

Rheumatologic disease rarely presents with acute emergencies, but when it does it may reflect rapidly progressive disease or a delay in diagnosis that leads to significant morbidity and mortality. The most important and common examples of this include recognition of the protean presentations of giant cell arteritis so as to avoid and prevent permanent visual loss and to recognize the clinical pattern of the pulmonary renal syndrome which if not recognized can lead to acute respiratory failure and renal failure requiring dialysis.

THE CERVICAL SPINE IN THE RHEUMATIC DISEASES

Catastrophic neurologic injury and even death may result from cervical spine disease in patients with rheumatoid arthritis (RA) or spondyloarthropathy. Early recognition of the signs and symptoms and appropriate diagnostic evaluation are critical to avoid these complications.

ATLANTOAXIAL INSTABILITY

Up to 30% of patients with severe RA have some degree of subluxation of the atlantoaxial joint (C1-C2). In normal patients, the odontoid process of the axis (C2) is secured in front by the anterior arch of the atlas (C1) and posteriorly by the transverse ligament of the atlas. The normal distance between the odontoid process and the anterior arch of the atlas is 3 mm. Inflammation in the small joints that make up the atlantoaxial joint, or tenosynovitis of the transverse ligament of the axis, may weaken the transverse ligament, as well as lead to bony erosions in the odontoid process. As a result, the space between the odontoid and the anterior arch of the atlas widens (**Figure 254-1**), and the atlantoaxial joint becomes unstable. Most commonly, anterior subluxation, when the atlas slides forward relative to the axis, leads to cord compression and cervical myelopathy. Less commonly, posterior subluxation occurs when the odontoid is badly damaged or fractured. Rarely, vertical subluxation occurs, with C1-C2 impaction, migration of the odontoid into the foramen magnum, brainstem compression, and death. Atlantoaxial instability may also produce vertebrobasilar insufficiency by impairing blood flow in the vertebral arteries, which travel through the transverse foramina of the cervical spine.

Physical signs may include occipital or retroorbital headache, tingling in the fingers, and electric shocks in the upper extremities with neck flexion. Physical findings include hyperreflexia, a positive Babinski test, and sensory loss in the hands and feet. Unfortunately, the neurologic examination may be confounded by muscle wasting, severe joint deformities, and entrapment neuropathies, all of which are very common in RA. Ominous symptoms and signs include a sensation of the head falling forward during neck flexion, syncope, respiratory irregularities, loss of sphincter control, dysphagia, hemiplegia, or nystagmus.

Lateral radiographs of the cervical spine in flexion are the most useful initial diagnostic studies. These are diagnostic if the space between the anterior arch of the atlas and the odontoid is 9 mm or more, with an interval between the odontoid and the posterior arch of the atlas of less than 14 mm in the flexed position. In symptomatic patients, flexion films should only be performed if standard films have excluded odontoid fracture and severe subluxation. When cervical spine radiographs are not diagnostic, magnetic resonance imaging (MRI) with neck flexion and extension should be performed. MRI is especially useful in delineating the extent of cord

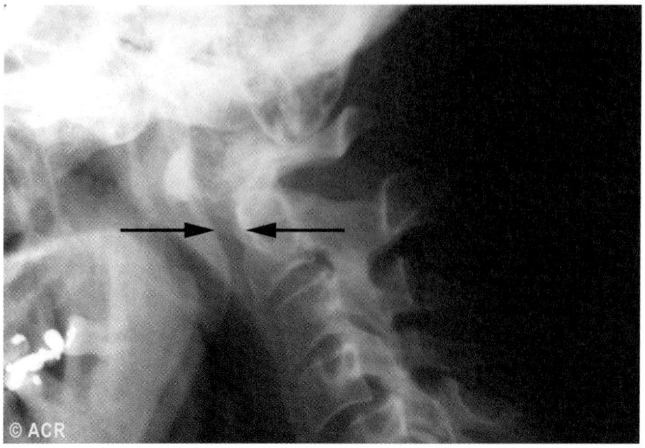

Figure 254-1 *Cervical spine in rheumatoid arthritis, showing atlantoaxial subluxation. A lateral view of the upper cervical region shows posterior displacement of the odontoid process. The preodontoid space measures approximately 8 mm (arrows). Normally this measurement should not exceed 2.5 to 3 mm in an adult, although in a child 4 to 5 mm may be within the normal range. The measurement is made at the base of the anterior aspect of the dens with the neck held in flexion. There is also anterior displacement of C4 on C5. Associated disc-space narrowing and erosion are not present. Atlantoaxial subluxation also occurs in ankylosing spondylitis. (Reproduced from the American College of Rheumatology Image Bank. © 2009 American College of Rheumatology, used with permission.)*

compression, the relationship of the odontoid to the brainstem, and in planning surgical stabilization. However, compared with plain radiographs, it may underestimate the degree of subluxation.

In the setting of progressive symptoms of cord compression, urgent neurosurgical consultation should be obtained for stabilization of the cervical spine. The role and timing of surgery in patients with atlantoaxial instability without cord compression is uncertain. The utility of medical therapy, such as rigid cervical collars and isometric neck strengthening exercises, is also unclear.

In patients with RA undergoing general anesthesia, cervical spine lateral radiographs with flexion and extension views should be obtained to exclude significant subluxation. Preoperative anesthesia consultation is mandatory in the RA patient with cervical instability. Fiberoptic intubation should be considered to limit neck manipulation.

SPINAL INVOLVEMENT IN THE SPONDYLOARTHROPATHIES

Neurologic disease is common in the spondyloarthropathies, particularly in ankylosing spondylitis. In longstanding disease, the spine is rigid, fused, osteoporotic, and brittle. Spinal fracture may occur with mild trauma, or even spontaneously. The most dreaded outcome is an acute cervical fracture, generally presenting as acute neck pain with or without neurologic compromise. Cord compression with quadriplegia may ensue unless the spine is promptly stabilized. Neurosurgical involvement is requisite. Ankylosing spondylitis may also be complicated by atlantoaxial subluxation, as in RA. Arachnoiditis may lead to scarring of sacral and lumbar nerve roots and cauda equina syndrome, with saddle anesthesia, paraparesis, and bowel and bladder disturbances.

AIRWAY INVOLVEMENT IN THE RHEUMATIC DISEASES

Airway involvement is a rare but significant source of morbidity and mortality in the rheumatic diseases. In Wegener granulomatosis (WG), a systemic vasculitis characterized by upper and lower respiratory granulomatous inflammation and glomerulonephritis, inflammation may occur in the subglottis and proximal trachea. Tracheobronchial WG often does not respond to systemic therapy and may run a course independent of the other manifestations of WG, leading to recurrent infections or ventilatory obstruction. Tracheobronchial involvement should be suspected when a patient with known WG presents with sore throat, cough, and difficulty with secretions. Chest radiography and spirometry are helpful initial tests, which may be confirmed with laryngoscopy or computed tomography scan. When this complication is suspected, otolaryngologic consultation is mandated. Treatment involves intralesional steroid injection and dilatation of obstructive lesions. When severe, stenting and tracheostomy may be necessary.

Relapsing polychondritis is characterized by episodes of inflammation of the cartilaginous structures of the outer ear, nose, larynx, and tracheobronchial tree. Tracheobronchomalacia may result from the loss of the supporting cartilage of the upper airway, resulting in either fixed airway obstruction or hyperdynamic collapse. Concerning symptoms include progressive dyspnea, stridor, hoarseness, sore throat, and chest discomfort. The flow-volume loop is a useful screening test. It may reveal extrathoracic obstruction, intrathoracic obstruction, or both. This may be confirmed with bronchoscopy or dynamic CT scanning. Treatment options include stenting, balloon dilatation, or tracheostomy.

PULMONARY-RENAL SYNDROMES

Patients may present to hospital with both pulmonary infiltrates and renal insufficiency, and no obvious cardiac or infectious cause. This should raise consideration of several diseases leading to pulmonary-renal syndromes, especially when these patients have proteinuria or active urinary sediments consistent with nephritis. Pulmonary-renal syndromes may be immune complex related, as in systemic lupus erythematosus (SLE) and cryoglobulinemia, or mediated by direct antibody binding, as in antiglomerular basement membrane (anti-GBM) disease, also known as Goodpasture syndrome. It may also be pauci-immune, characterized on biopsies by a relative lack of immunoglobulin and complement. These include the vasculitides associated with antineutrophilic cytoplasmic antibodies (ANCA), such as Granulomatosis with Polyangiitis (Wegener granulomatosis), microscopic polyangiitis (MP), and Churg-Strauss syndrome (CSS). Clinical clues may suggest a specific diagnosis, such as the arthritis, pleurisy, and photosensitivity of SLE; upper respiratory symptoms, such as sinusitis or otitis, suggestive of WG; or mononeuritis multiplex often seen in the ANCA-associated vasculitides.

Laboratory evaluation in this setting should include ANCA, antinuclear antibody (ANA), anti-GBM antibody, and cryoglobulin. Biopsy should be considered. In the face of undifferentiated disease and clinical deterioration, empiric therapy including high-dose corticosteroids and even cyclophosphamide or rituximab may be necessary, pending the results of testing or biopsy.

INTERSTITIAL LUNG DISEASE

Interstitial lung disease is an uncommon but feared complication in a variety of rheumatic diseases including scleroderma, dermatomyositis/polymyositis (DM/PM), rheumatoid arthritis, SLE, and mixed connective tissue diseases. It affects up to 50% of patients with scleroderma, 30% of patients with DM/PM, and 10% of patients with RA. While parenchymal lung disease is often insidious, in some cases it may be explosive and necessitate hospitalization. Patients may present with progressive dyspnea, dry cough, and desaturation with exercise oximetry.

High-resolution chest CT is very useful in characterizing interstitial lung disease. It may reveal ground glass opacities, seen in many conditions including acute interstitial pneumonia, nonspecific interstitial pneumonia, desquamative interstitial pneumonia, *Pneumocystic* pneumonia (PCP), viral pneumonia, pulmonary edema and acute respiratory distress syndrome. Honeycombing and traction bronchiectasis are seen in fibrotic lung disease and usual interstitial pneumonia and consolidative inflammatory lung disease is seen in cryptogenic organizing pneumonia. However, there is much overlap in the radiographic appearance of different forms of interstitial lung disease. Lung biopsy may be diagnostic, although the potential utility of a pathologic diagnosis must be balanced against the hazards of lung biopsy in patients with tenuous respiratory status.

Treatment for inflammatory lung disease involves high-dose corticosteroids with immunomodulating agents such as cyclophosphamide, azathioprine, mycophenolate, or calcineurin inhibitors, such as cyclosporine and tacrolimus. Fibrotic lung disease may require lung transplantation in suitable patients. In patients with worsening respiratory symptoms already on immunosuppressive regimens, bronchoscopy should be strongly considered to exclude opportunistic infection. In patients on high-dose steroids for interstitial lung disease (ILD) with or without a second agent, prophylaxis for pneumocystis jirovecii (PCP) should be considered.

VISION LOSS IN GIANT CELL ARTERITIS

Giant cell arteritis (GCA) is a large-vessel vasculitis that most often affects branches of the external carotid arteries. GCA must be recognized and treated promptly, as patients may suffer irreversible vision loss if the ophthalmic artery is involved. Although patients may be as young as 50 years old, most are age 65 or older. In addition, most patients are of Northern European ancestry. GCA is the most common systemic vasculitis, but it is still relatively rare. Among patients age 50 or older, incidence rates are reported at 20 to 30 cases per 100,000 patients in Northern European countries. GCA occurs at an even lower frequency in nonwhite patients, with estimates as low as 1 case per 100,000. *Temporal arteritis* is a term used to describe vasculitis of the temporal artery, which is common in GCA. Cranial symptoms of GCA include headache, scalp tenderness, jaw claudication, and visual disturbances. Involvement of the thoracic great vessels may cause upper-extremity claudication. Aortitis may present years after the initial diagnosis and treatment of GCA, with signs and symptoms of aortic dissection. GCA may sometimes present as a chronic cough, failure to thrive, and fever of unknown origin in an elderly patient. Most patients also experience fatigue, anorexia, and weight loss.

GCA may coexist with polymyalgia rheumatica (PMR), a condition that causes achiness and stiffness of the shoulder and hip girdle, worse in the morning, and associated with fatigue. Patients with established PMR have an approximately 10% risk of developing GCA at some point in their lives.

In patients with suspected GCA, ophthalmologic evaluation is the most important element of the physical examination. It may reveal evidence of anterior ischemic optic neuropathy, retinal artery occlusion, or choroidal infarction. The remainder of the physical examination may reveal subtle clues of arteritis. The presence of tender, tortuous temporal arteries is a classic but unreliable finding. A chest bruit, aortic insufficiency murmur, or discrepant upper-extremity blood pressures are signals of thoracic vessel involvement. Patients with concurrent PMR may have bursitis of the shoulders and hips with painful limited range of motion in these joints.

The diagnosis of GCA is based on the clinical presentation, with corroborative pathologic findings of arteritis. The temporal artery is the most easily accessible extracranial artery for biopsy.

TABLE 254-1 Conditions Associated with Erythrocyte Sedimentation Rate Greater Than 100 mm/hour

Polymyalgia rheumatica
Giant cell arteritis and other vasculitides
Adult-onset Still disease
Infectious endocarditis
Osteomyelitis
Septic arthritis
Multiple myeloma

Temporal artery biopsy is a high-yield, low-risk procedure. There is no single blood test that is diagnostic for GCA. Markedly elevated acute-phase reactants are suggestive, but nonspecific. The erythrocyte sedimentation rate (ESR) may be as high as 100 mm/hour, a value found in few other disease states (**Table 254-1**). However, acute phase reactants may be normal in up to 10% to 20% of patients with GCA. Anemia of chronic disease and thrombocytosis may be present.

Classification criteria exist for GCA (**Table 254-2**), designed primarily as inclusion criteria for clinical studies, rather than for use in everyday clinical practice. Certainly, there are patients with GCA who do not meet these criteria. The diagnosis of GCA should be considered in any elderly patient who presents with recent-onset headaches, visual complaints, and unexplained elevated acute phase reactants. In these instances, empiric corticosteroid treatment should be started *immediately*, and temporal artery biopsy should be arranged expeditiously. Empiric corticosteroids do not alter pathologic findings, provided that the artery in question is sampled within 10 to 14 days of initiating treatment. Neither visual disturbances nor abnormal ophthalmologic exam need to be present to warrant immediate action. The retina is exquisitely sensitive to ischemia, and patients with GCA are unlikely to recover vision once it is lost. Treatment consists of corticosteroids in the equivalent of prednisone 1 mg/kg daily. Intravenous (pulse) corticosteroids have not been proven more effective for patients with GCA, but are an option for patients with threatened vision. Likewise, since luminal thrombosis of the ophthalmic artery is thought to be the event that precipitates blindness in GCA, low-dose aspirin may also be added to the therapeutic regimen. Once a patient starts treatment with corticosteroids, vision is often spared if it has not already been affected. Threatened vision is the most common emergency situation that may arise in GCA. In addition, aortitis may require emergent corticosteroids or even surgical intervention to reduce the risk of dissection or rupture. All cases of suspect or proven GCA warrant rheumatologic consultation for long-term management of disease.

TABLE 254-2 Classification Criteria for Giant Cell Arteritis

Age 50 or older
New-onset headache
Temporal artery tenderness
Erythrocyte sedimentation rate 50 mm/hour or greater
Pathology showing arteritis

Classification of GCA is met if patient has three or more of the above criteria.

COMPLICATIONS OF SCLERODERMA

Scleroderma encompasses both localized scleroderma (morphea or linear scleroderma) and systemic sclerosis. Localized scleroderma is not discussed here, however, and the term *scleroderma* will be used interchangeably with the term *systemic sclerosis*. Scleroderma is characterized by vasculopathy and systemic fibrosis. Vascular complications include pulmonary hypertension, cutaneous calcinosis, and telangiectasia of the skin or gastrointestinal (GI) tract. Progressive fibrosis may involve the skin, GI tract, lungs, and heart. This section focuses on two emergencies in patients with scleroderma: scleroderma renal crisis and Raynaud crisis (often seen in, but not limited to, scleroderma).

SCLERODERMA RENAL CRISIS

Scleroderma renal crisis (SRC) usually develops within five years of diagnosis of scleroderma. It may even be the presenting feature of scleroderma, often in patients with other signs of scleroderma that have eluded diagnosis, such as Raynaud syndrome, cutaneous fibrosis, organ fibrosis, and telangiectasia. Rapidly progressive skin disease and prior corticosteroid usage are major risk factors for renal crisis. SRC usually presents as hypertension and progressive renal insufficiency in a patient with known scleroderma. Patients may have symptoms of malignant hypertension: headache, visual disturbances, pulmonary edema, and encephalopathy. Progression to hypertensive crisis, overt renal failure, and death is rapid without prompt recognition and treatment.

SRC is a microangiopathy of the renal vasculature, not a form of glomerulonephritis. Urinalysis may reveal proteinuria, but red blood cell casts are typically absent. The renal vasculopathy causes endothelial shearing of erythrocytes that may be detected as a microangiopathic hemolytic anemia (MAHA), with schistocytes on peripheral blood smear analysis and mild thrombocytopenia. As SRC may be the presenting feature of scleroderma, it should always be considered part of the differential diagnosis in a patient with unexplained renal dysfunction and MAHA features (**Table 254-3**). Renal biopsy does not distinguish SRC from other microangiopathies, but it may be useful to exclude glomerulonephritis. Ultimately, the diagnosis of SRC is a clinical one based on progressive hypertension, renal dysfunction, proteinuria, and MAHA in a patient with systemic features of scleroderma.

Angiotensin-converting enzyme (ACE) inhibitors are the mainstay of treatment. This is the only condition in which overt renal failure is treated with aggressive ACE inhibitor therapy, so one must have reasonable diagnostic certainty before initiating treatment. While any ACE inhibitor is likely to be effective, captopril has the largest body of supportive evidence, it is rapidly effective, and doses can be escalated rapidly. Enalapril has the advantage of intravenous dosing in exceptional circumstances. The goal of therapy should be normalization of blood pressure within a few days of starting treatment. This often requires hospitalization for close monitoring and dose adjustment of drugs. Often, serum creatinine values will lag in their improvement, and ACE inhibitor therapy should continue undeterred by rising creatinine values. There is far less experience with angiotensin receptor blockers (ARBs) in SRC, and ACE inhibitors should be used whenever possible. In patients with ACE inhibitor–induced angioedema, allergy consultation should be sought for possible desensitization.

Despite these measures, upwards of 40% of patients with SRC require dialysis treatment for progressive renal failure. Concurrent pulmonary or cardiac scleroderma often precludes renal transplantation for SRC-related end-stage renal disease. Notably, it is not unusual for renal function to recover in patients with SRC after months or even years of dialysis, provided that ACE inhibitor therapy is continued unabated. Even so, patients with SRC have a five-year mortality rate that approaches 40%, mostly because SRC portends aggressive extrarenal scleroderma.

TABLE 254-3 Causes of Microangiopathic Hemolytic Anemia with Renal Failure

Scleroderma renal crisis
Antiphospholipid antibody syndrome
Hemolytic uremic syndrome
Thrombotic thrombocytopenic purpura
Heparin-induced thrombocytopenia
Malignant hypertension
Diffuse intravascular coagulation
HELLP syndrome
Transfusion reactions
Chemotherapeutic agents

HELLP, a syndrome characterized by hemolysis, elevated liver enzyme levels, and a low platelet count.

RAYNAUD CRISIS

Raynaud phenomenon (RP) is a common, usually benign, condition of cold-induced pain, pallor, and cyanosis of the digits. It represents an exaggeration of normal physiologic vasoconstriction in response to cold. Rarely, RP may lead to Raynaud crisis, an episode of ischemia that continues despite rewarming, lasts longer than 30 minutes, and threatens the viability of one or more digits. It is a medical emergency that requires prompt intervention to reverse vasoconstriction and restore blood flow.

RP affects upwards of 20% of young women and is much less common in men and the elderly. A typical episode involves a classic series of color changes. Digits first turn white in a demarcated fashion, as digital arteries vasoconstrict in response to cold (**Figure 254-2**). With prolonged vasoconstriction, digits become blue or purple because of tissue cyanosis. Finally, digits turn pinkish-red, as blood flow is restored and the episode resolves. RP may also be triggered by stress or rapid changes in ambient air temperature,

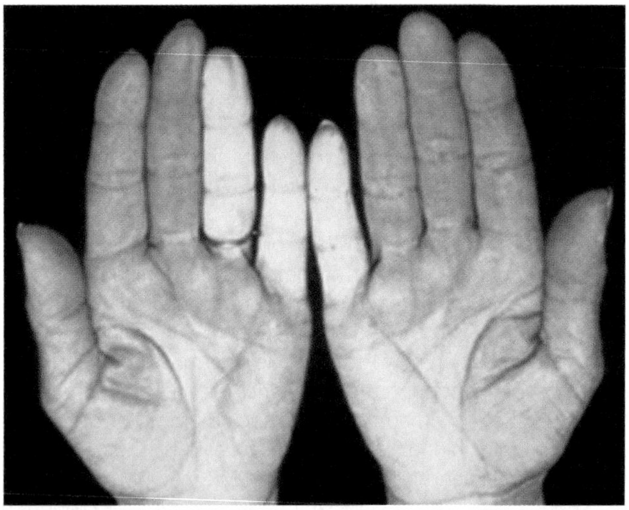

Figure 254-2 *Raynaud phenomenon, with digital pallor and cyanosis. (Reproduced, with permission, from Wolff K, Goldsmith LA, Katz SI, et al. Fitzpatrick's Dermatology in General Medicine. 7th ed. New York: McGraw-Hill, 2008. Fig. 171-1.)*

as upon entering an air-conditioned room on a warm day or reaching into a refrigerator or freezer. Of note, patient self-reporting of "cold hands" without color changes fails to satisfy the clinical diagnosis of RP. In patients with RP, episodes may involve all the digits or may be limited to a single digit (or part of a digit). Involved digits are often achy, numb, or even painful. Prolonged ischemia can lead to digital ulcerations or even a threatened digit.

RP is classified as primary or secondary. Primary RP is much more common, occurs in the absence of an underlying disease, and rarely has major sequelae. In contrast, secondary RP is associated with one or more of the conditions listed in **Table 254-4**. Many of these conditions are connective tissue diseases (CTDs) associated with vasculopathy and endothelial dysfunction. These factors contribute to the aggressiveness of secondary RP, which is more likely to require treatment because of severe symptoms, digital ulcers, or Raynaud crisis. Common drugs, such as caffeine, cocaine, amphetamines, pseudoephedrine, nicotine, and beta-blockers, can exacerbate arterial vasoconstriction in either primary or secondary RP. Patients with RP should be advised to avoid these drugs, and educated about signs and symptoms of a Raynaud crisis and the need to seek medical attention if it develops.

PRACTICE POINT

- Acquired distal tubular acidosis is found in about 30% of patients with Sjögren syndrome, probably due to loss of the luminal H(+)ATPase pump from the intercalated cells of the collecting duct. This is clinically silent in most patients. However, it may sometimes lead to potassium wasting and weakness, and even be severe enough to present with hypokalemic paralysis, quadriparesis, and respiratory failure. The prognosis is good with aggressive potassium replacement in the short term and oral supplementation of potassium and bicarbonate in the long term.

History and physical examination is often sufficient to distinguish primary RP from secondary RP. In the absence of previously identified CTD, secondary RP is suggested by ischemic episodes lasting longer than 30 minutes, recurring RP isolated to a single digit, features of scleroderma or CREST syndrome, or pitting digital scars. Positive serologic tests for ANA or other autoantibodies and an abnormal nailfold capillary microscopy help to secure a CTD diagnosis. Nailfold capillary microscopy can be performed without special instruments. For example, an ophthalmoscope may be used to inspect a nailbed that has been coated with a drop of mineral oil or even a clear bactericidal hand cleanser. Abnormal findings include dilated capillary loops, tortuous vessels, hemorrhage, or vessel dropout.

TABLE 254-4 Diseases and Conditions Associated with Secondary Raynaud Phenomenon

Category	Disease Entity
Rheumatologic diseases	Scleroderma
	Systemic lupus erythematosus
	Rheumatoid arthritis
	Sjögren syndrome
	Dermatomyositis/polymyositis
	Mixed connective tissue disease
	Vasculitis, including cryoglobulinemia
	Behçet disease
	Thromboangiitis obliterans
Other forms of vascular injury	Vibration-induced vasculopathy
	Radiation-induced vasculopathy
	Paraneoplastic vasculopathy
	Frostbite
	Chemotherapy
	Ergotamines

Raynaud crisis must be distinguished from other causes of digital ischemia, such as vascular trauma, vasculitis, proximal vessel stenosis, thromboangiitis obliterans, antiphospholipid antibody syndrome, atherosclerosis, and microembolic disease. An Allen test may be used at the bedside to assess for patency of both radial and ulnar arteries. Examination of pulses with Doppler ultrasound may help exclude proximal vascular occlusion. In selected instances, magnetic resonance angiography or even traditional vascular angiography may be necessary to confirm that the arterial stricture is at the level of the digital arteries, and not more proximal. Even then, it may be difficult to exclude digital microemboli, and proximal sources of emboli may sometimes need to be sought.

The goal of management in a Raynaud crisis is to reduce vascular contractility and restore blood flow to ischemic digits. Patients should be kept in a warm, stress-free environment to minimize further vasomotor stimuli. Affected digits should be reheated in tepid water; hot water should be avoided, as it may further damage ischemic tissue. Oxygen levels should be optimized, bearing in mind that pulse oximetry of a digit affected by RP is unreliable. Narcotic analgesia may reduce physiologic vasoconstriction induced by pain. Aspirin and sometimes heparin may reduce the risk of thrombosis within vasospastic vessels. Initial vasodilator therapy typically consists of dihydropyridine-class calcium channel blockers, such as short-acting or extended-release nifedipine or amlodipine. These may not be acutely effective, and hypotension may be dose limiting. Oral hydralazine and transdermal nitroglycerin placed proximal to the part of the extremity involved may provide temporary relief, but tachyphylaxis and rebound vasospasm may occur. Anesthesia consultation may be required for chemical block of sympathomimetic nerves locally or cervically. Endothelin receptor antagonists (eg, bosentan and ambrisentan) improve the healing rate of digital ulcers in patients with RP, but their role in Raynaud crisis has not been definitively established. In severe, refractory cases, epoprostenol infusions or sildenafil therapy may be attempted. Potential toxicities include refractory hypotension and death. Despite these efforts, patients may still experience digital necrosis and require surgical intervention; it is advisable to involve vascular surgery whenever a patient presents with a Raynaud crisis.

DRUG TOXICITY IN THE RHEUMATIC DISEASES

Allopurinol hypersensitivity syndrome ranges from a minor rash to a life-threatening systemic illness with Stevens-Johnson syndrome. It typically starts several weeks after drug initiation. In addition to rash, it may also involve fever, eosinophilia, hepatitis, and renal insufficiency. Treatment includes administration of corticosteroids and cessation of allopurinol. Rarely, allopurinol can cause a severe vasculitis associated with high titers of ANCA. This generally improves upon cessation of the drug, although in some cases such an occurrence must be treated similarly to the ANCA-associated vasculitides. Allopurinol also inhibits the metabolism of azathioprine, increasing the risk of azathioprine toxicity. The combination of allopurinol and azathiprine should be avoided if at all possible; if not, azathioprine dosing should be reduced to 25% of normal when using these agents concomitantly.

Methotrexate (MTX) is among the most commonly used medications in rheumatology. Toxicity may involve the liver, kidneys, mucous membranes, and, in less than 1% of cases, the lungs. Pulmonary toxicity associated with MTX usually presents in the first year of use, with dry cough, dyspnea, fever, and, in severe cases, hypoxemia and respiratory failure. Alveolar or interstitial infiltrates may be seen on chest radiography or CT, although imaging may be negative early in the course. The differential diagnosis includes community-acquired pneumonia, opportunistic infection, and progressive interstitial lung disease from underlying rheumatic disease. Bronchoscopy or induced sputum is often necessary to exclude opportunistic infection. Treatment in mild cases entails withdrawal of the drug. Corticosteroids may be necessary in severe cases.

Cyclophosphamide (CYC) is an alkylating agent frequently used in the treatment of vasculitis and severe lupus. Major side effects include neutropenia and lymphopenia, which may lead to overwhelming infection, especially with fungi and *Pneumocystis* pneumonia. CYC may lead to hemorrhagic cystitis and increases the lifetime risk of bladder cancer. The dose should be adjusted in the elderly and for renal function to avoid toxicity.

Azathioprine is a purine analogue used in a variety of rheumatic syndromes. It may cause severe neutropenia, infection, and transaminitis. Patients with low or absent activity of the enzyme that metabolizes azathioprine (thiopurine methytransferase, or TPMT) are at high risk for cytopenias and other toxicities. Genetic testing for TPMT is now available and should be obtained in patients who may begin azathioprine. Azathioprine has a number of problematic drug interactions, including ACE inhibitors, allopurinol, and other immunosuppressive drugs. It should be dose-adjusted in the elderly and in those with renal insufficiency.

SUGGESTED READINGS

Brown KK. Rheumatoid lung disease. *Proc Am Thorac Soc.* 2007;4: 443–448.

Chifflot H, Fautrel B, Sordet C, Chatelus E, Sibilia J. Incidence and prevalence of systemic sclerosis: a systematic literature review. *Semin Arthritis Rheum.* 2008;37:223–235.

Denton CP, Lapadula G, Mouthon L, Muller-Ladner U. Renal complications and scleroderma renal crisis. Rheumatology (Oxford). 2009;48(30):32–35.

Ernst A, Rafeq S, Boiselle P, et al. Relapsing polychondritis and airway involvement. *Chest.* 2009;135:1024–1030.

Fathi M, Vikgren J, Boijsen M, et al. Interstitial lung disease in polymyositis and dermatomyositis: longitudinal evaluation by pulmonary function and radiology. *Arthritis Rheum.* 2008;59: 677–685.

Helfgott SM, Kieval RI. Polymyalgia rheumatica in patients with a normal erythrocyte sedimentation rate. *Arthritis Rheum.* 1996;39: 304–307.

Hunder GG. Epidemiology of giant-cell arteritis. *Clevel Clin J Med.* 2002;69(2):79–82.

Kim DH, Hillibrand AS. Rheumatoid arthritis in the cervical spine. *J Am Acad Orthop Surg.* 2005;13:463–474.

Specks U. Diffuse alveolar hemorrhage syndromes. *Curr Opin Rheumatol.* 2001;13:12–17.

Tashkin DP, Elashoff R, Clements PJ, et al. Cyclophosphamide versus placebo in scleroderma lung disease. *N Engl J Med.* 2006;354: 2655–2666.

CHAPTER 255

Gout, Pseudogout, and Osteoarthritis

Robert T. Keenan, MD, MPH
Svetlana Krasnokutksy, MD
Michael H. Pillinger, MD

Key Clinical Questions

1. Why do patients have acute flares of crystal arthropathies?
2. How is gout distinguished from other monoarthropathies?
3. What are the appropriate therapies for acute and chronic gout and pseudogout?
4. What are the pathophysiologic features of osteoarthritis (OA), and how do these relate to clinical manifestations?
5. How is OA differentiated from other types of arthritis?
6. What are the nonpharmacologic, pharmacologic, and surgical treatment options for OA?

INTRODUCTION

Gout, pseudogout, and osteoarthritis make up perhaps the largest portion of the rheumatic diseases that affect primarily joints. Although these three disease entities are quite different, they share a number of features in common: all tend to be diseases seen at older ages; all three are not uncommonly seen in overlap with each other; and all three are characterized primarily by inflammatory and/or mechanical abnormalities, rather than autoimmune ones. Whereas gout and pseudogout constitute diseases of abnormal crystal formation and its resultant responses, osteoarthritis is primarily a disease of cartilage loss and autodestruction. In the following sections, we discuss these three important diseases, their pathogenesis, and management.

GOUT

Gout currently affects more than 3 million Americans, usually presenting with severe acute episodic arthritis, which may evolve into chronic destructive tophaceous disease. It is more common in men than women, and more common in African-Americans than whites. The prevalence of gout rises with age, from 17 per 1000 among individuals 45 to 64 years old, to as high as 41 per 1000 in those 75 years and older. When hospitalized for other conditions, elderly patients with gout are more likely to have their hospital discharge delayed than those without gout. The annual incidence of gout rose from 45 per 100,000 in 1977–1978 to 64 per 100,000 in 1995–1996, and is estimated to have continued to rise over the last decade. Overall, the prevalence of gout has nearly quadrupled over the past half-century. Despite being the most common inflammatory arthropathy, gout is frequently misdiagnosed and mistreated.

PATHOPHYSIOLOGY

The most important risk factor for gout is hyperuricemia, or an excess of serum uric acid, the end product of purine metabolism. Serum concentrations are determined by the balance between urate production and elimination. Hyperuricemia may be caused by either overproduction or underexcretion of urate, or a combination of both. Consumption of meat or seafood promotes hyperuricemia and gout, a phenomenon related to the high purine content of these foods. Alcohol has been known to predispose to gout since the days of Hippocrates. Alcohol consumption increases urate production through multiple mechanisms, including generation and turnover of ATP, diuresis and dehydration, production of lactic and ketoacids (which block renal urate excretion), and the consumption of purines in alcoholic beverages. Beer and ale ingestion are most strongly correlated with the presence of hyperuricemia and gout (presumably because of their higher purine content), while hard liquor increases serum urate and gout risk to an intermediate degree. Moderate wine consumption has a lesser effect on serum urate and the risk of gout, possibly because of other compounds present in wine. (Historically, the high prevalence of gout in affluent drinkers of wine and port may be related to the illicit use of lead acetate by wine merchants as a preservative and sweetener; chronic lead poisoning causes tubulointerstitial kidney disease that promotes hyperuricemia.)

PRACTICE POINT

- In a postoperative or postdiuresis patient with an acute inflammatory arthropathy, with or without fever, consider gout or another crystal arthropathy in the differential diagnosis.

More than one hundred years ago Osler suggested that sugar intake might increase the risk of gout. Recent studies show that Osler was very likely correct. The prevalence of gout has increased over the last 50 years, concomitantly with obesity and diabetes, and the introduction and rising consumption of high-fructose corn syrup. Human metabolism and degradation of fructose generates uric acid to a greater degree than seen with other sugars. In addition, fructose may have other hyperuricemia-inducing effects by virtue of its ability to modulate urate transport in the kidney. Milk consumption appears to be protective against gout, perhaps because of the uricosuric effect of milk proteins such as casein.

Uric acid is eliminated from the body by both gastrointestinal and renal routes. Approximately one-third of urate elimination occurs through the gastrointestinal system, in saliva, gastric juices, pancreatic secretions, and direct loss from the bowel. The remaining two-thirds of urate excretion is renal, via glomerular filtration and a complex balance of tubular secretion and reabsorption. Tubular handling of urate is carried out via several organic anion transporters (OATs), including URAT1. A number of agents that stimulate renal urate excretion act by inhibiting URAT1 (**Table 255-1**).

Hyperuricemia may be either primary or secondary. Primary hyperuricemia accounts for the vast majority of gout patients. About 90% of these patients are *primary underexcreters*, with genetic molecular defects in renal urate secretion. Most of these patients have otherwise normal renal function. *Primary overproducers* account for the remaining 10% of primary hyperuricemia. A few of these patients have rare neurobehavioral syndromes, such as complete hypoxanthine phosphoribosyltransferase (HPRT) deficiency (Lesch-Nyhan syndrome) or partial HPRT deficiency (Seegmiller Kelley syndrome), that result in increased biosynthesis of purines and gout.

Secondary gout occurs when preexisting conditions result in decreased uric acid excretion or increased purine turnover. Acute or chronic renal insufficiency may impair urate excretion. Diseases of cell turnover, such as malignancies and hemolytic anemia, result in abnormally increased urate production. Gout can manifest in the early teens due to a group of autosomal dominant diseases, which include familial juvenile hyperuricemic nephropathy (FJHN) and medullary cystic kidney type II disease. These diseases feature a mutant gene that interrupts the tertiary structure of uromodulin, also known as Tamm-Horsfall protein. The clinical presentation of these diseases not only includes early-onset gout, but also progressive renal failure and polyuria.

TABLE 255-1 Substances That Affect Urate Levels

Urate-Increasing Agents	Urate-Decreasing Agents
Pyrazinamide	**Uricosurics**
Nicotinate	Probenecid
Lactate, β-hydroxybutyrate, acetoacetate	Sulfinpyrazone
Salicylates (low dose)	Salicylate (high-dose)
Diuretics	Losartan
Cyclosporine	Benzbromarone
Tacrolimus	Fenofibrate
Ethambutol	Amlodipine
β-blockers	**Xanthine oxidase inhibitors**
	Allopurinol
	Febuxostat
	Uricase (rasburicase, pegloticase)

NATURAL HISTORY

The clinical evolution of gout generally occurs in four stages. In *asymptomatic hyperuricemia*, the risk of an acute gout attack increases as the level of uric acid rises past its solubility point (>6.8 mg/dL). Once solubility is exceeded, monosodium urate crystals may precipitate in joint spaces and lead to *acute gouty arthritis*. During this stage, the innate immune system initiates a cascade of events, including activation of complement and resident joint tissue macrophages, and recruitment of neutrophils from the bloodstream. Recent studies have implicated the inflammasome, an intracellular assembly of macrophages and monocytes that activates interleukin-1β (IL-1β), in the inflammatory response to uric acid crystals. IL-1β stimulates the production of other inflammatory mediators, including tumor necrosis factor (TNF)-α, IL-6, IL-8, and prostaglandin E2. This results in severe local inflammation as well as systemic response to cytokine release, such as fever and elevated acute phase reactants. These attacks are exquisitely painful but typically self-limited, even without therapy, perhaps because of immune autoregulation.

The asymptomatic interval between acute gouty attacks is known as *intercritical gout*. Over time attacks tend to come more frequently, the intercritical period dwindles, and *chronic tophaceous gout* may develop. Tophi are aggregates of urate crystals, typically accompanied by a low-level chronic inflammatory state. They are actually complex structures, consisting of a mix of monosodium urate crystals and cellular debris surrounded by activated macrophages. Although tophi are most obvious when they occur in the periarticular soft tissues, they may also develop in cartilage and bone. Radiographic images of tophi in periarticular bone characteristically reveal the pathognomonic finding of punched-out erosions with sclerotic margins and overhanging edges (**Figure 255-1**).

DIAGNOSIS AND DIFFERENTIAL DIAGNOSIS

The gold standard for diagnosing all forms of gout is needle aspiration of acutely or chronically inflamed joints or tophi, followed by polarized light microscopy to identify negatively birefringent, needle-shaped crystals (uric acid crystals). The presence of such crystals, particularly when seen intracellularly within infiltrating neutrophils, confirms the diagnosis of an acute attack and helps to distinguish gout from septic arthritis, pseudogout, and other causes of inflammatory joint disease. (Extracellular crystals alone are not diagnostic of an acute gouty attack. In patients with established gout, extracellular crystals may persist even after inflammation has resolved, residing as "innocent bystanders" in the setting of other acute joint pathologies.) The sensitivity of synovial fluid analysis for demonstrating negatively birefringent crystals in patients with acute gouty arthritis is at least 85%, with a specificity approaching 100%. In contrast, the specificity of a clinical diagnosis of gout is significantly lower, and septic arthritis and pseudogout may be misdiagnosed as gout. *Therefore, in almost all circumstances, diagnostic arthrocentesis should be performed.*

As acute gout may coexist with other joint pathology, a wider evaluation is warranted, even in the presence of intracellular, negatively birefringent crystals. In addition to crystal analysis, synovial fluid should always be sent for cell count with differential, Gram stain, and culture. Grossly, synovial fluid is typically straw colored and varies from translucent to opaque. Synovial fluid cell

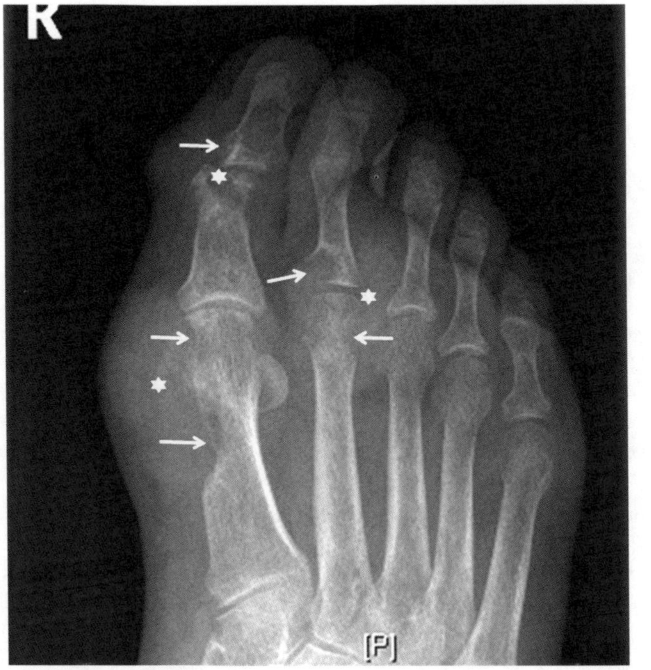

Figure 255-1 *Tophaceous gout causing an erosive arthropathy. Note the large tophi (stars) and "rat-bite" erosions with overhanging edges (arrows).*

counts in gout usually range from 2000 to 100,000 per mm^3, with greater than 50% neutrophils (usually approaching 90%). Serum uric acid can also be obtained during an acute attack. A high serum urate supports the diagnosis of gout. However, levels may be paradoxically normal or low during an acute attack due to an increase in renal excretion, rising again two weeks after the attack. Erythrocyte sedimentation rate (ESR) or C-reactive protein (CRP) are often high, but this finding is very nonspecific. Urinary urate collections should not be obtained during gout attacks; they are neither useful nor reliable in the acute period.

Radiographs in the acute setting are not generally helpful, but radiographic evidence of erosions indicates chronic disease. Ultrasound is gaining popularity in the evaluation of musculoskeletal disease, including crystal-induced arthropathy. Musculoskeletal ultrasound (MSUS) has the capacity to visualize intraarticular crystal deposits, with a characteristic hyperechoic enhancement of the outer surface of the hyaline cartilage, known as the *double contour sign*. MSUS may prove to be an alternative method for the diagnosis of the crystal arthropathies, but limitations include the inability to distinguish the presence or absence of infection.

The differential diagnosis for acute gout includes not only conditions generally associated with acute monoarthritis, such as pseudogout and septic arthritis, but also conditions leading to oligoarthritis and polyarthritis, such as reactive arthritis, psoriatic arthritis, and even rheumatoid arthritis. Ideally, a crystal diagnosis of gout should be the goal; if this is not possible, the diagnosis of acute gouty arthropathy should be made by a combination of historical and clinical criteria. A thorough history will help distinguish an acute gout attack from other causes of acute arthritis. Some of the previously proposed clinical, radiographic, and laboratory criteria include (1) a history of one or more episodes of monoarticular arthritis, followed by intercritical periods completely free of symptoms (may not be applicable in the hospital setting); (2) maximum inflammation within 24 hours of onset of the attack; (3) rapid resolution after initiation of colchicine or a nonsteroidal anti-inflammatory drug (NSAID); (4) unilateral first metatarsophalangeal joint attack

TABLE 255-2 Musculoskeletal Manifestations of Crystal-induced Arthropathy

Acute monoarthritis or polyarthritis
Bursitis
Tendonitis
Tophaceous deposits (including vertebrae)
Enthesitis
Synovial osteochondromatosis
Pseudoankylosing spondylitis
Carpal tunnel syndrome
Tendon rupture
Joint destruction
Pseudorheumatoid arthritis
Spinal stenosis
Crown dens syndrome
Inflammatory osteoarthritis

(podagra), especially if it is the first event; (5) hyperuricemia; and (6) subcortical bone cysts on plain radiograph.

Acute attacks most often affect the first metatarsophalangeal joint (up to 50% of first attacks). The tarsal joints, ankles, knees, elbows, and interphalangeal (IP) joints are also commonly affected. In elderly patients with osteoarthritis (OA), Heberden nodes or Bouchard nodes are potential targets for inflammation, and red, swollen proximal and distal IP joints may be the first manifestation of gout. Episodes of acute gouty arthritis frequently begin suddenly at night or in the early morning with dramatic pain and swelling. The joint rapidly becomes warm, red, and tender, often mimicking cellulitis. Without treatment, most acute attacks resolve in 3 to 10 days (range, 2 days to 2 weeks). Most patients, at least initially, do not have residual symptoms once an attack is complete (**Table 255-2**).

HOSPITAL ADMISSION

Acute gout

While acute attacks of gout can usually be managed in the outpatient setting, patients may need to be admitted to the hospital to facilitate workup or to rapidly and definitively rule out the possibility of infection. Patients with severe disability from their acute attack and inadequate home support may need to be admitted until they are able to ambulate or otherwise function. More often, patients at risk may develop acute gouty attacks while hospitalized for other problems. In the hospital setting, attacks may be precipitated by illness-related issues (eg, metabolic acidosis), diuretics or other medications, or disruptions in volume status or renal function.

Chronic gout

Fluctuations in serum urate levels are associated with acute gout attacks. For this reason, patients with chronic gout should have their urate-lowering medications or other prophylaxis continued during the hospital stay, unless otherwise contraindicated (eg, in the setting of acute kidney injury). For example, stopping allopurinol in hospitalized patients may precipitate acute gout and increasing allopurinol doses during an acute attack could exacerbate the existing flare and prolong the clinical course.

TREATMENT OF ACUTE GOUT

Colchicine is effective in the acute setting, and, if initiated sufficiently early, may abrogate an acute attack. It is typically less effective after the attack is established. The traditional dosing of colchicine for acute attacks (0.6 mg by mouth every one to two hours) until onset of relief; nausea, vomiting, or diarrhea; or a maximum of 10 doses frequently incurred undesirable side effects. Recent studies suggest that a more limited regimen—colchicine 1.2 mg, followed by 0.6 mg one hour later—is equally effective as the old regimen, with much less toxicity. It has now been adopted as standard of care. Patients with renal insufficiency may receive this regimen, but should subsequently temporarily discontinue any use of low-dose daily colchicine for future prophylaxis; patients without renal disease may continue their prophylaxis unabated. Intravenous colchicine curtails gastrointestinal side effects but carried a much higher risk of toxicity and even death; its use has been discontinued by the U.S. Food and Drug Administration.

PRACTICE POINT

- Treatments for acute gout, such as NSAIDs, colchicine, and corticosteroids, work best when administered within minutes to hours of the attack.

For many patients, *NSAIDs* are preferred agents for acute gout. Indomethacin is the traditional choice at 50–75 mg initially, then 50 mg every 6 hours, not exceeding 200 mg in a 24-hour period. However, clinical trials have shown that many NSAIDs, including COX-2 selective agents, are as effective as indomethacin. NSAIDs have the advantage of both nalgesic and anti-inflammatory effects, but may be relatively contraindicated in patients with gastritis, renal insufficiency, hypertension, and heart failure. In order to maximize response time while minimizing side effects, some clinicians treating acute gout add an intermediate dosing regimen of colchicine (0.6 mg every 6 to 8 hours) to their patients' NSAID regimens.

Glucocorticoids are potent anti-inflammatory agents that can be highly effective at abrogating acute gouty attacks. Intraarticular corticosteroids may be particularly useful in treating acute gout in a single joint or bursa and when systemic glucocorticoid use is undesirable. Care must be taken to establish the diagnosis and rule out infection prior to injecting steroids into the joint. As a practical matter, this means performing joint aspiration and injection as separate procedures, which may unfortunately add to the patient's discomfort. Oral and intravenous glucocorticoids are very effective, especially in patients with polyarticular attacks, and may be the agents of choice in patients with contraindications to colchicine and NSAIDs, such as renal insufficiency. Moderately high doses of oral corticosteroids are needed to treat acute gout. Most clinicians recommend a starting dose of approximately 40 mg/day of prednisone, with a slow taper to avoid rebound attacks after steroid withdrawal. Although treatment periods with oral steroids are typically brief (less than a week), relative contraindications such as diabetes, hypertension, and heart failure must be considered.

A single intramuscular injection of depot *adrenocorticotropic hormone*, or ACTH gel (25 to 80 IU, repeated 24 to 72 hours later if needed) can also terminate attacks very effectively. This treatment may be more effective than oral corticosteroids. In addition to stimulating the adrenal cortex to produce corticosteroids, ACTH may also reduce the acute inflammatory response by activating melanocortin receptor-3. Follow-up treatment using low-dose (one to two times daily) colchicine is typically recommended to prevent rebound attacks as the ACTH wears off. Unfortunately, access to ACTH gel in the United States is currently limited.

TREATMENT OF CHRONIC GOUT

The goal of chronic gout treatment is to prevent acute attacks and to decrease tophi burden. This is achieved by lowering serum urate to less than 6 mg/dL and requires a multipronged approach. *Lifestyle changes* such as weight loss, avoidance of fructose-rich foods and high-purine foods such as organ meats and shellfish, and eliminating or reducing alcohol consumption should be the first step, with the addition of one or more urate-lowering agents being necessary for most patients with chronic gout. (In milder cases, as-needed treatment of acute attacks or long-term use of a daily low dose of colchicine may be sufficient.) *A medication review* may identify agents that may be contributing to hyperuricemia. For example, thiazides and loop diuretics reduce uric acid excretion and raise serum urate. Therefore, these should be used at the lowest effective dose. Hydrochlorothiazide at a dose of 12.5 mg/day is as efficacious for hypertension as 25 mg/day, but is less likely to increase serum urate. Some patients have other medical conditions that may benefit from alternative drugs. Both losartan (for hypertension) and fenofibrate (for hyperlipidemia) have uricosuric properties and may be useful options for treatment of these conditions in patients who also have gout.

Urate-lowering agents commonly used to treat chronic gout include purine and nonpurine inhibitors of xanthine oxidase, such as allopurinol and febuxostat, and uricosuric agents such as probenecid, sulfinpyrazone, and benzbromarone.

Long considered a first-line agent for chronic gout management, *allopurinol* is a purine analog of hypoxanthine. Along with its active metabolite oxypurinol, allopurinol competitively inhibits xanthine oxidase, decreasing urate production and serum uric acid levels. Appropriate allopurinol use requires dose titration to achieve a prespecified serum urate target, most commonly less than 6 mg/dL. The average dose is about 300 mg/day. Lower doses may be sufficient in some patients, but doses as high as 800 to 1000 mg/day may be required. Side effects are uncommon but may be serious and include rash, cytopenias, and hypersensitivity syndromes, such as toxic epidermal necrolysis and Steven-Johnson syndrome. Although most serious side effects occur within the first six to eight weeks of use, long-term monitoring is required. The European League Against Rheumatism currently recommends dose adjustment in chronic kidney disease; such patients should be started on lower doses, with titration to the minimal effective dose needed to achieve the target urate level. As azathioprine is metabolized by xanthine oxidase, allopurinol use may raise azathioprine levels and result in bone marrow toxicity. Concomitant use of allopurinol and azathioprine should therefore be avoided.

Febuxostat is a potent, orally administered, nonpurine, selective inhibitor of xanthine oxidase that primarily undergoes hepatic metabolism. Dosing is limited to 40 to 80 mg daily, and dose adjustment is not needed in patients with mild to moderate kidney impairment. Febuxostat does not chemically resemble allopurinol and thus far appears to be safe for patients with allopurinol sensitivity. Some data suggest that febuxostat may be more effective than allopurinol at reducing tophaceous deposits.

Uricosuric medications such as probenecid, sulfinpyrazone, and benzbromarone (the latter two are not available in the United States) increase renal urate excretion by inhibiting the URAT1 transporters in the proximal tubule. To prevent uric acid kidney stones, patients should drink generous amounts of fluids and avoid high doses of vitamin C and other drugs that may acidify the urine. Humans, unlike most other mammals, are at risk of gout because of our loss of uricase in the course of primate evolution. A novel therapeutic approach to gout is to replace uricase. *Pegloticase* is a newly developed pegylated recombinant mammalian (porcine/bovine) urate oxidase. It is given by intravenous infusion and can rapidly and dramatically decrease serum urate levels. Pegloticase has been approved by the Food and Drug Administration for patients with gout who have failed or are intolerant of other therapy.

Although there continues to be debate about when to start urate-lowering therapy, most experts do so when the patient exhibits any of the following: two or more attacks per year, tophaceous disease, uric acid kidney stones, or excessively elevated serum urate levels of greater than 13 mg/dL in males or greater than 10 mg/dL in females. Since pharmacologic lowering of uric acid paradoxically increases the risk of gout for a period of three to six months, patients starting any of these drugs must be prophylaxed against acute attacks—typically with colchicine 0.6 mg once or twice daily beginning several days before the initiation of urate-lowering therapy, and continuing for at least several months after the target urate level has been achieved.

■ CONSULTATION

Rheumatology consultation should be obtained when the diagnosis is unclear or the presentation seems atypical for a patient with known gout. Consultation should also be obtained when synovial fluid cannot be obtained easily, when expertise is required in fluid analysis or interpretation, or when contraindications to traditional therapies complicate patient management.

PSEUDOGOUT AND CHONDROCALCINOSIS: CALCIUM PYROPHOSPHATE DEPOSITION DISEASE

Although pseudogout is frequently seen as the "poor cousin" of gout, it is a common condition that can be acutely incapacitating and chronically destructive. Like gout, pseudogout is a disease in which crystal formation leads to inflammation and mechanical damage. Unlike gout, in which a systemic metabolic derangement promotes crystal deposition, in most cases pseudogout derives from metabolic abnormalities intrinsic to chondrocytes, resulting in crystal deposition in cartilage. However, the result is similar: activation of innate immune responses by the formed crystals leads to local hyperemia, joint effusion and neutrophil influx, and the four cardinal signs of inflammation: heat, redness, pain, and swelling.

Although pseudogout may occur in familial, early-onset forms, most cases are sporadic and acquired. Acquired pseudogout is a disease of aging, rarely presenting before the age of 50. Exceptions include patients with cartilage derangement from prior injury and patients in whom the development of pseudogout is secondary to other medical conditions, such as hypomagnesemia, hypothyroidism, acromegaly, hemochromatosis, or hyperparathyroidism. Both men and women may contract pseudogout. Although the condition appears to affect women more commonly than men, the extent of this bias has not been fully established.

■ PATHOPHYSIOLOGY

In pseudogout, the offending crystal is calcium pyrophosphate, and the perpetrating cell appears to be the articular cartilage chondrocyte itself. Chondrocytes in healthy articular cartilage prevent calcification and maintain the flexible articular surface. However, in pseudogout, chondrocytes go awry and promote calcium pyrophosphate deposition (**Figure 255-2**). That chondrocytes are able to lay down calcium crystals should not be surprising, as growth plate chondrocytes direct bone formation during fetal development.

Chondrocyte dysregulation in pseudogout is associated with a local oversupply of inorganic pyrophosphate (PPi), leading to a risk of precipitation with inorganic calcium. Abnormalities in several enzymes have been implicated, such as nucleotide pyrophosphatase phosphodiesterase 1 (NPP1), which liberates PPi from adenosine triphosphate (ATP) and other nucleotide triphosphates, and the ankylosis human protein (ANKH), a transmembrane protein

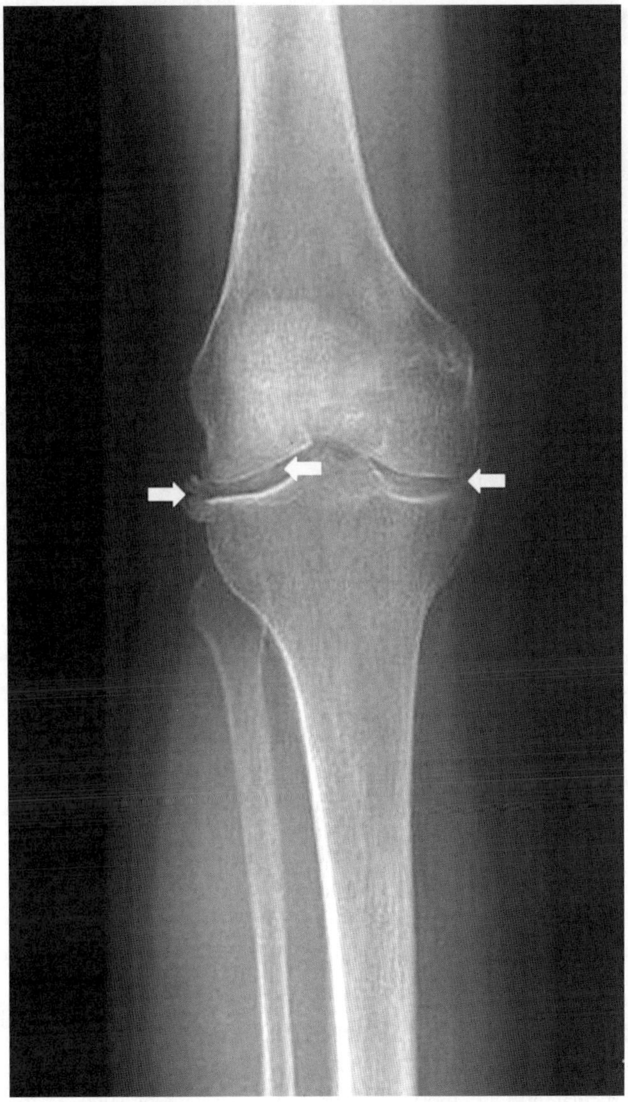

Figure 255-2 *Severe pseudogout, with linear deposition of calcium pyrophosphate throughout the meniscus (arrows).*

that transports PPi from inside to outside the cell. Mutations increasing ANKH activity have been detected in some cases of familial pseudogout. In sporadic pseudogout, ANKH may be normal in structure, but its expression upregulated.

Extracellular precipitation of calcium pyrophosphate results in crystal deposition in cartilage (chondrocalcinosis), which can often be detected on plain radiographs. The typical appearance of chondrocalcinosis is a linear or stippled radiodense deposit under the surface of cartilage. Chondrocalcinosis alone usually is insufficient to promote acute inflammation, presumably because crystals in cartilage are sequestered from the immune system. Indeed, chondrocalcinosis is frequently diagnosed as an incidental finding on radiographs taken for other reasons. However, when crystals appear in joint fluid, either from shedding from cartilage or precipitation in the joint space, they promote the same sorts of inflammatory processes seen in gout. Like uric acid crystals, calcium pyrophosphate crystals may activate complement, promoting neutrophil chemotaxis, and interact with synovial macrophages to induce production of IL-1 and other cytokines. The clinical presentation may also mimic gout, with a rapid onset of joint inflammation sometimes precipitated by trauma or metabolic derangements, and is typically self-limiting after many days of inflammation.

PRACTICE POINT

- Chondrocalcinosis (radiologic evidence of calcium pyrophosphate deposition in cartilage) is indicative of overproduction of calcium pyrophosphate. However, chondrocalcinosis frequently exists without pseudogout, and pseudogout can occur in the absence of visible choncrocalcinosis.

Calcium pyrophosphate deposition disease (CPPD) may also be associated with chronic pain and joint damage. In these cases, it may strongly resemble osteoarthritis, in that inflammation is mild, the progression slow, and radiographs are characterized by joint space narrowing (ie, cartilage loss) and osteophyte formation. In many cases, it is difficult to distinguish this condition from true osteoarthritis, or from the overlap of osteoarthritis (OA) and CPPD. Indeed, rheumatologists continue to argue over whether OA promotes CPPD disease, vice versa, or both. When arthritis is limited to joints not usually seen in OA, it can be presumed that CPPD is the driving process.

Other medical conditions have been associated with chondrocalcinosis or pseudogout. While the exact relationship between these conditions and calcium crystal deposition is not always clear, they tend to fall into several overlapping groups, which include features of tissue destruction, metabolic abnormalities, or electrolyte disruptions. Among these are hemochromatosis, in which chondrocalcinosis typically affects the second and third metacarpophalangeal joints; gout, which can coexist with pseudogout; hyperparathyroidism, with its attendant disruptions of calcium and phosphate metabolism, as well as direct chondrocyte effects; hypophosphatasia (in which PPi degradation by the nonspecific tissue enzyme alkaline phosphatase is diminished); and hypomagnesemia, which may alter pyrophosphatase activity.

DIAGNOSIS AND DIFFERENTIAL DIAGNOSIS

The typical presentation of pseudogout is that of acute monoarticular arthritis, most commonly of a large joint such as the knee, sometimes with a violent onset indistinguishable from gout. Although some clinicians aver that pseudogout is typically slower of onset and less severe than gout, these distinctions are not sufficiently rigorous to permit any speculation on whether a specific acute monoarthritis is gout or pseudogout. Compared with gout, pseudogout less commonly affects the big toe and is unrelated to dietary or bibulous indiscretion. Moreover, gout is more likely than pseudogout to be polyarticular, and since pseudogout appears to depend upon the actions of chondrocytes, it is unusual to see pseudogout in a cartilage-free structure such as a bursa. The most important consideration in the differential diagnosis of pseudogout is septic arthritis. Other crystal diseases, including hydroxyapatite and calcium oxalate deposition (the latter most common in dialysis patients), also deserve consideration. Although osteoarthritis is less inflammatory than pseudogout, patients with severe osteoarthritis occasionally have flares that may be confused with acute pseudogout. Reactive arthritis and other forms of inflammatory arthritis may appear in joints typically associated with acute pseudogout and may be clinically indistinguishable from it, though these will more often present in a chronic and polyarticular fashion.

The evaluation of a patient with pseudogout is as important for what it rules out as for what it rules in. In addition to history and physical examination, initial workup should include serum white blood cell count, electrolytes, creatinine, uric acid, and ESR or CRP. Plain radiographs of the involved joint may increase suspicion for pseudogout or another diagnosis, but will not be definitive. The presence of chondrocalcinosis supports the possibility of pseudogout, but many patients with chondrocalcinosis never develop pseudogout, and many patients with pseudogout have no radiologic chondrocalcinosis. Accordingly, the diagnosis of acute pseudogout, and the exclusion of other etiologies, is best made by inspecting fluid from a joint aspiration using a compensated polarizing microscope. *As in gout, in almost all circumstances, arthrocentesis should be performed;* in the hands of an experienced physician, the procedure is quick, relatively painless, and of high yield. The presence of positively birefringent crystals, either needle-like, rhomboid, or both, is pathognomonic of calcium pyrophosphate deposition. The presence of these crystals within neutrophils confirms that inflammation is directed at CPP crystals. In addition, the physician should obtain a cell count, Gram stain, and culture, and also examine the fluid for negatively birefringent and needle-like urate crystals. Both pseudogout and gout can coexist with infection, and also with each other, so that the presence of one does not rule out the possibility of the other. Indeed, since synovial fluid Gram stains are of fairly low sensitivity, a patient with a synovial fluid white count of 100,000/mm^3 should be presumed to have an infection pending culture results, even if evidence of acute pseudogout or gout is also seen.

Patients with CPPD disease may, either instead of or in addition to acute pseudogout, experience progressive cartilage degeneration as in osteoarthritis. When this occurs in joints not typical for osteoarthritis, a crystal-based etiology may be presumed. In addition, patients may experience CPPD as a low-level inflammatory arthritis in almost any joint. When this occurs in the small joints of the hands, it may mimic rheumatoid arthritis (pseudorheumatoid arthritis). In these individuals, plain radiographs may reveal a combination of osteoarthritis-like joint narrowing, chondrocalcinosis, and erosive disease. Patients with pseudogout as well as osteoarthritis in the second and third metacarpophalangeal joints should be assessed for hemochromatosis. Patients with atypical but crystal-proven pseudogout, or those who develop CPPD before the age of 50, should be assessed for an underlying etiology. The workup may include levels of calcium, phosphate, magnesium; iron studies, including serum ferritin; levels of parathyroid- and thyroid-stimulating hormone; and levels of insulin-like growth factor (IGF)-1 in patients with features of acromegaly. In most cases, these evaluations are not fruitful.

TREATMENT

As with gout, acute pseudogout should be treated with whatever anti-inflammatory is most likely to be both effective and benign for the particular patient. Most patients with acute pseudogout respond well to NSAIDs, with selective COX-2 inhibitors probably being a reasonable option as well. Oral or intraarticular corticosteroids are also effective. Care must be taken to confirm that the joint is not infected before injecting steroids, requiring both diagnostic and then therapeutic procedures. ACTH is also an option, although availability may be limited. For unclear reasons, the response of acute pseudogout to oral colchicine is less than in gout, and oral colchicines should probably be considered a second-line therapy. However, despite conventional wisdom to the contrary, the divergent response to colchicine between gout and pseudogout is insufficiently distinct to provide a basis for diagnosis.

Long-term management of pseudogout includes attempts at prophylaxis, using low-dose colchicine (more effective than in the acute setting, and generally quite well tolerated), and perhaps NSAIDs or low-dose steroids in some cases. When underlying etiologies for pseudogout are identified, these should be treated, although data is slender as to whether this ameliorates the outcome of the associated pseudogout. For patients with chronic smoldering inflammation, the aforementioned agents remain the first choice, but recent studies have suggested that some immunosuppressives, such as hydroxychloroquine, methotrexate, or anakinra, may also be of value. In contrast to gout, there is no proven approach to prevent or reverse crystal formation.

OSTEOARTHRITIS

Osteoarthritis is the most common of the arthritic conditions, affecting nearly 30 million people in the United States alone. Although it is considered a disease of the elderly, osteoarthritis may affect individuals of almost any age, particularly when specific risk factors lead to early onset. OA can affect any joint, but most frequently involves the hands, hips, and knees. The current management of OA is largely palliative or surgical, although recent advances increase the possibility that disease control of OA may be possible in the future.

■ PATHOPHYSIOLOGY

The hallmark of OA is loss of articular cartilage, most often in joints that are subject to stress. This feature of OA led to the long-standing conclusion, still held in some circles, that OA represents wear-and-tear of cartilage alone. However, metabolic abnormalities of cartilage in OA probably accelerate its progressive deterioration. While OA may be driven by biomechanical factors, those stressors eventually lead to a catabolic state in articular cartilage. Changes in subchondral bone and synovium are also profound, suggesting that OA is a disease that involves all joint tissues.

Old age is the most robust risk factor for OA. This may relate to cumulative wear, but intrinsic aging of the cartilage may also contribute; OA cartilage in the nonelderly has features of prematurely aged tissue. Individuals with *obesity* are 5 to 10 times more likely to develop knee OA, and 2 to 3 times more likely to develop hip OA. This may be partly due to mechanical stress, but adipose tissue is also metabolically active, and secretes inflammatory cytokines that might play a role in OA. (The frequent occurrence of OA in non-weight-bearing distal interphalangeal joints of the hands also suggests the involvement of systemic factors.) *Improper joint alignment*—whether hereditary or from injury—also appears to increase the risk for OA, as does *direct trauma*, as in sports injuries. Rarely, *genetic abnormalities* in cartilage biochemistry may increase susceptibility.

The earliest pathologic features in OA are microscopic fissures on the cartilage surface. This induces chondrocyte alterations that are initially reparative, but later contribute to cartilage degradation. At first chondrocytes respond to cartilage damage by hypertrophying and producing structural cartilage elements, such as type II collagen and aggrecan; this is manifested on magnetic resonance imaging (MRI) by increased cartilage thickness. As the disease progresses, chondrocytes develop unusual features, such as cellular clustering, and secrete metalloproteinases and aggrecanases that cause intrinsic destruction of the joint cartilage. Over time, this results in loss of articular cartilage thickness, increased susceptibility to further mechanical destruction, and progressive deterioration of the cartilage surface.

Bone, bone marrow, and synovium are also involved in OA. Plain radiographs often demonstrate subchondral sclerosis and osteophytes, bony ridges that extend the joint surface and may progress to bony hypertrophy (**Figure 255-3**). It is unclear whether these are compensatory or pathologic features; however, surgical removal of osteophytes generally does not relieve the symptoms of OA. MRI studies have identified bone marrow lesions under the affected joints as a hallmark of OA. On pathology, these represent fibrotic and necrotic tissue, and possibly microfractures. Although OA has long (and incorrectly) been called a noninflammatory disease, imaging advances with MRI and ultrasound have now confirmed that most OA individuals have frank synovitis, although more mild than seen in patients with rheumatoid or psoriatic arthritis. Other studies have confirmed that in OA both synovial cells and chondrocytes produce a wide range of inflammatory cytokines.

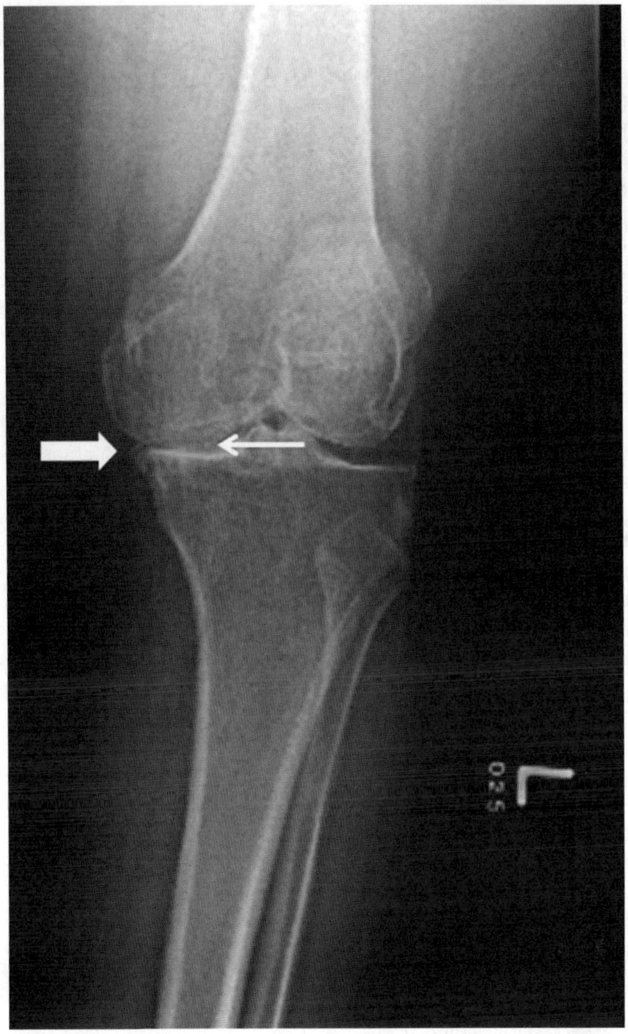

Figure 255-3 *Knee joint, showing osteophyte (broad arrow) and medial joint space loss (narrow arrow).*

■ CLINICAL FEATURES AND DIAGNOSIS

Symptoms may come on insidiously and intermittently over a number of years. The most common feature of OA is pain in weight-bearing joints, such as the knees and hips. Involvement of the shoulders, elbows, and hands is not uncommon. Any joint that has suffered abuse is susceptible, with one dramatic example being the metacarpophalangeal joints of a boxer. Unlike rheumatoid arthritis, joint involvement in OA may be monoarticular or oligoarticular, but is not typically polyarticular, and need not be symmetrical.

Pain from OA is most likely to occur during joint use. For example, knee pain tends to be exacerbated with walking, and some patients can characterize their use limitations with a high degree of accuracy. Many patients report that OA pain is worse during cold or rainy weather, a phenomenon that remains incompletely understood. OA pain may also be nocturnal. Morning stiffness may be present in OA patients but tends to be of short duration, typically lasting no more than 15 to 60 minutes, in contrast to rheumatoid arthritis, where morning stiffness may persist for over an hour. As OA progresses, the patient may notice limitation in the range of motion of the joint, due to cartilage defects, joint effusions, and osteophytes. The joint may become swollen and slightly warm. Over a long period of time, joint mobility may become profoundly limited and disability may ensue. For the patient with knee or hip OA, this may mean an inability to walk more than short distances. Patients with shoulder OA may be unable to reach into kitchen cabinets or perform basic dressing, washing, and toileting functions. Pain in one joint not infrequently results in pain in another joint of the same or the opposite limb, possibly relating to the additional stress resulting from compensation for the OA joint. Spinal involvement may lead to spinal stenosis and nerve root impingement by osteophytes.

Physical examination of the osteoarthritic joint typically reveals crepitus—palpable grinding with joint motion that reflects the fraying and roughening of the cartilage surface. Crepitus is a sine qua non of OA and is usually present in its earliest stages. Its presence, in the setting of characteristic joint pain, may be sufficient to diagnose OA, even in the absence of radiographic findings. As OA progresses, joint examination may reveal not only crepitus, but other evidence of OA, including limited range of motion, pain with motion, effusions, and bony hypertrophy. In the knee, OA is frequently accompanied by deterioration and tearing of the menisci and other adjacent structures; testing for meniscal tears using techniques such as the Apley compression test may also yield positive results.

Radiographic studies in OA have characteristic features. In weight-bearing joints, the first and most obvious finding is narrowing of the joint space, reflecting loss of radiolucent cartilage. In the knee, this results in the preferential loss of joint space in one compartment, such as the medial or lateral tibiofemoral compartment, or patellofemoral compartment, more than the others, although eventually all compartments may be affected. In the hip, the superior, weight-bearing surface of the joint is most often affected. With disease progression, other characteristic findings may appear. Subchondral sclerosis may be seen as a linear increase in bone density just below the joint surface. Although osteophytes are actually circumferential ridges, on the two-dimensional views presented by plain radiographs they will appear as bone spicules off the margins of the joints. Bone cysts—discrete, circular or ovoid regions of decreased bone density located just below the joint surface—are common, though their importance remains unclear. In the spine, OA findings may include those described above, but the different anatomic nature of the spine may also result in disc-space narrowing, foraminal narrowing, and other unique features. MRI and ultrasound are seldom if ever needed to diagnose an OA joint, but if obtained may demonstrate bone marrow edema, synovitis, and cartilage and meniscal degradation.

Laboratory studies are mainly useful to rule out other alternative diagnoses. For example, a normal ESR or CRP helps to rule out inflammatory arthritis. In patients with features suggestive of rheumatoid arthritis, a serum rheumatoid factor and anticyclic citrullinated peptide antibody (anti-CCP) titer may be useful. Serum urate levels may help stratify the patient's risk for gout. Joint fluid analysis may be the most useful laboratory investigation. In OA, synovial fluid should contain a modest number of leukocytes (less than 2000/mm^3); higher counts suggest a different or additional condition. Urate or calcium pyrophosphate crystals indicate gout or pseudogout, respectively, although these conditions and OA are not mutually exclusive. Although acute joint swelling only occasionally occurs in OA, aspiration of the joint fluid is generally needed to rule out the presence of infection in this setting. Serum and joint fluid markers of cartilage turnover, such as N-telopeptide and C-telopeptide, may have some utility in determining the rate of cartilage damage, but they are currently used only in the research setting.

As noted above, calcium pyrophosphate deposition disease (CPPD) and OA often coexist in the same patient. It is unclear whether calcium pyrophosphate deposition predisposes to OA, the cartilage damage of OA predisposes to calcium pyrophosphate deposition, or both. The finding of both diseases in several joints not normally expressing OA, such as the second and third metacarpophalangeal joints, suggests at least an element of the former. Patients with hemochromatosis are predisposed to both calcium pyrophosphate deposition and OA; once again, metacarpophalangeal OA may be a clue. Patients with gout also have a high incidence of OA, though it is unclear if this is due to cause and effect or merely coexpression in an older population. Much more rarely, ochronosis, with cartilaginous deposition of homogentisic acid, predisposes to severe OA. Patients with acromegaly also frequently have OA, presumably owing to abnormal forces across the enlarged bone. Recent studies suggest that diabetics also have a higher incidence of OA because of the buildup of advanced glycation end products (AGEs) in cartilage matrix, which may make cartilage more brittle and stiff, impair normal turnover and repair, and have local proinflammatory effects.

TREATMENT

Most OA management is palliative and conservative. Clinicians should educate their patients and provide them with a greater understanding and sense of control over their condition. Physical therapy helps to preserve muscle strength and proprioception and improve joint stress. (Muscle weakness and capsular and ligamentous damage may hinder joint proprioception in OA patients, increasing their fall risk.) For the knee, evidence suggests that regular adherence to a quadriceps-strengthening exercise regimen helps reduce pain and maintain function. Bracing is another underutilized option; even simple bracing with a neoprene sleeve may assist with joint proprioception and reduce pain with ambulation, with essentially no adverse effects. More sophisticated braces may fully stabilize the joint, or even reduce the weight across the cartilage surface. The use of a cane in the opposite hand also reduces joint stress and contributes to a sense of well-being. Other therapeutic modalities, such as heat, cold, and ultrasound, may have analgesic benefits in individual patients.

For analgesia, the American College of Rheumatology recommends the initial use of *acetaminophen* for all patients who can tolerate it. While many patients have failed acetaminophen prior to presenting to a physician, in most cases they have not used it at the maximum dose of 3 grams daily. Long-acting formulations reduce the dosing frequency and may improve compliance. Care should be taken to avoid the use of acetaminophen with combination agents that also include acetaminophen, thus pushing the dose beyond acceptable limits. Acetaminophen is well tolerated but unfortunately has a narrow therapeutic window, with an LD50 for a single dose of approximately 10 grams. Patients should be warned to avoid exceeding the maximal daily dose and to also avoid excess alcohol use.

NSAIDs may be effective in patients for whom acetaminophen is inadequate. Because NSAIDs are both analgesic and anti-inflammatory, they may be particularly useful for OA patients with a more inflammatory clinical phenotype (eg, patients with significant joint effusions). For OA, NSAIDs should be used at the lowest efficacious dose, on either an as-needed or standing basis. While all NSAIDs work by cyclooxygenase inhibition, they may differ in potency, half-life, and side effects. Most physicians should have expertise in three or four NSAIDs and be able to tailor their use to a particular patient. All NSAIDs should be considered to have potential for renal toxicity, hypertension, heart failure, gastritis, ulcers, and possibly ischemic heart disease. Selective COX-2 inhibitors reduce gastrointestinal toxicity; their relative cardiovascular risk remains controversial, but there is little evidence that the sole COX-2 inhibitor currently remaining on the market in the United States, celecoxib, has any increased cardiovascular risk relative to other NSAIDs. Patients on chronic NSAIDs other than selective COX-2 inhibitors should receive GI protection, specifically a proton pump inhibitor or misoprostol. H2 blockers have not been shown to provide sufficient protection. Extra care should be taken in patients already on low-dose aspirin for cardiovascular purposes.

Another option for OA is the use of oral *opiates*. Most rheumatologists approach the use of opiates with great caution. As OA is a chronic disease, the use of opiates is likely to become long-term, with a potential for dependency. There is also evidence that all-cause mortality is increased in older patients taking opiates for arthritis. One alternative is tramadol, with mixed opiate and antidepressant properties, and a somewhat lower abuse potential.

Topical agents are used for OA treatment, with variable degrees of supportive evidence. Capsaicin, the active ingredient in chili peppers, may be applied topically to deplete presynaptic supplies of substance P, a pain-mediating neurotransmitter. It must be applied regularly several times a day, or an initial period of discomfort will occur when it is restarted. Topical diclofenac has been approved by the FDA. It appears to be about as effective as oral diclofenac, with similar serum levels. Older preparations such as topical salicylates and counterirritants are available over the counter and may provide some relief.

If oral and topical therapies do not provide adequate relief, or are otherwise undesirable, *intraarticular treatment* may be considered. Aspiration of the joint by itself frequently relieves pressure and provides some pain relief. Glucocorticoid injection (eg, methylprednisolone 40 to 80 mg) is frequently effective, providing relief that may last for several months. Studies suggest that treatment with glucocorticoid injections every three months has no adverse effect on cartilage, at least over the first few years. When glucocorticoids are ineffective, it is reasonable to consider injection of a hyaluronic acid preparation. Although marketed as a lubricant, hyaluronic acid is biologically active and may provide benefit for many months, long after its presence in the joint has dissipated. Various hyaluronic acid preparations are available; all involve three to five serial injections, one week apart. The superiority of one preparation over the others has not been established. Given the small (1 in 1,000–10,000) but definite risk of infection resulting from joint injection, these procedures should only be performed by experienced operators.

Several alternative therapies have been proposed. A large number of small studies, some from Europe, suggest the benefit of oral ingestion of glucosamine or chondroitin sulfate, two cartilage components, for analgesia and possible joint protection. However, a large, well-blinded study found ambiguous benefit at best. Until further data is available, these agents are probably best used by enthusiastic patients on a trial-and-error basis. They appear to pose little if any risk. Several studies suggest benefit for acupuncture in the treatment of OA, although like all acupuncture studies, they are plagued by issues of blinding.

Surgical options include arthroscopy, total joint replacement, partial joint replacement, and other surgical techniques. In most cases, the goal of arthroscopy is to remove debris and to smooth roughened cartilage and menisci. Although still a very common procedure, a well-blinded study has shown no benefit over sham surgery. Another well-conducted study showed no benefit for OA symptoms of arthroscopic knee surgery over standardized physical therapy. Accordingly, arthroscopy for OA should be reserved for those with specific and unequivocal indications, such as joint locking in the presence of loose bodies. By contrast, the benefits of total joint replacement are well established in the treatment of OA. The indications for total joint replacement are failure to manage pain by medical means and/or loss of mobility. As radiographic studies do not correlate well with pain or disability, their role in surgical decision making is supportive only. Total joint replacement is highly effective at relieving pain and maintaining or restoring function; it is probably underutilized, owing to cost and patient hesitancy to undergo surgery. At the present time, replacement of the hip and knee are the best-established procedures; the procedures for the replacement of other joints, such as the shoulder, elbow, ankle, and wrist, are improving steadily. In some cases, surgeons may recommend partial joint replacements. Partial approaches may reduce operating time, but at present are mainly recommended for specialized indications.

PRACTICE POINT

- Management of osteoarthritis is currently palliative; treatment options include analgesics, anti-inflammatories and intraarticular hyaluronan. Weight loss, physical therapy, and bracing are important adjuncts to pharmacologic treatment, and may sometimes be sufficient on their own. For knees and hips, total joint replacement is indicated when medical management fails or the patient's ambulation is inappropriately limited; total joint replacement is an effective means to relieve pain and restore motion.

CONCLUSION

Arthritis of various forms is the cause of significant morbidity and mortality, and its personal and economic costs are high. Among the arthritides, osteoarthritis, gout, and pseudogout are the most common. Of the three, gout is currently the most treatable, yet patients with gout frequently experience inadequate management. Treatment of osteoarthritis and pseudogout is directed primarily at symptoms rather than at underlying causes, but research is likely to yield new and potentially effective therapies. In the meantime, optimal management of gout, pseudogout, and osteoarthritis, employing both pharmacologic and non-pharmacologic management, can reduce pain and suffering, and help patients live unimpeded, productive lives.

SUGGESTED READINGS

Choi HK, Mount DB, Reginato AM. Pathogenesis of gout. *Ann Intern Med.* 2005;143:499–516.

Jordan KM, Arden NK, Doherty M, et al. EULAR Recommendations 2003: an evidence-based approach to the management of knee osteoarthritis. Report of a Task Force of the Standing Committee for International Clinical Studies Including Therapeutic Trials (ESCISIT). *Ann Rheum Dis.* 2003;62:1145–1155.

Liote F, Ea HK. Recent developments in crystal-induced inflammation pathogenesis and management. *Curr Rheumato Rep.* 2007;9:243–250.

Nuki G. Colchicine: its mechanism of action and efficacy in crystal-induced inflammation. *Curr Rheumatol Rep.* 2008;10:218–227.

Pay S, Terkeltaub R. Calcium pyrophosphate dihydrate and hydroxyapatite crystal deposition in the joint: new developments relevant to the clinician. *Curr Rheumatol Rep.* 2003;5:235–243.

Schumacher HR Jr, Chen LX. The practical management of gout. *Cleve Clin J Med.* 2008;75(5):522–525.

Solomon DH, Rassen JA, Glynn RJ, Lee J, Levin R, Schneeweiss S. The comparative safety of analgesics in older adults with arthritis. *Arch Intern Med.* 2010;170:1968–1978.

Thiele RG, Schlesinger N. Diagnosis of gout by ultrasound. Rheumatology (Oxford). 2007;46:1116–1121.

CHAPTER 256

Systemic Lupus Erythematosus

Lisa Criscione-Schreiber, MD
Marcy B. Bolster, MD

Key Clinical Questions

1. Does this patient have systemic lupus erythematosus (SLE)?
2. Has SLE disease activity led to this patient's hospitalization?
3. How should flares of SLE be managed?
4. How does treatment of other diseases affect the status of SLE?
5. What are possible adverse consequences of the treatment of SLE?
6. How should medications for SLE be managed upon hospital discharge?

INTRODUCTION AND EPIDEMIOLOGY

Systemic lupus erythematosus (SLE) is an autoimmune disease that affects about 1 in 2000 individuals. Women of childbearing age are most commonly affected. SLE can manifest in any organ system, and disease activity varies over time. Phenotypically, SLE is highly variable and may affect some organ systems but not others in certain individuals. Both the incidence and severity of SLE are increased in individuals of African or Caribbean descent, as well as in Hispanic populations within the United States.

In the past, SLE had relatively high mortality and morbidity rates. Recent estimates place 5-year survival rates around 95% and 20-year survival rates around 80%. As survival rates have improved in individuals with SLE, so have hospitalization rates. Most hospitalists care for individuals with active SLE during the course of a year. In one retrospective analysis, more than half the patients in a lupus cohort were hospitalized at some point over the previous two years. The most common reason for hospitalization in patients with SLE is disease flare. Patients are also commonly admitted for complications of SLE or its treatment, such as infections and cardiovascular and thromboembolic disease. Individuals with SLE are at high risk for premature atherosclerosis and may be admitted with chest pain, acute coronary syndromes, or cerebrovascular accidents. As well, patients may be first diagnosed with SLE when hospitalized for a severe disease manifestation, such as pericarditis, glomerulonephritis, or neurologic disease.

PATHOPHYSIOLOGY

Autoimmune diseases are thought to occur when an environmental trigger, such as infection, sunlight, or smoking, activates an abnormal immune response in a genetically susceptible individual. Abnormalities in nearly every aspect of immune system function have been demonstrated either in humans or in animal models of SLE.

The serologic hallmark of SLE is the presence of serum autoantibodies, generally against nuclear proteins. The pathogenesis of autoantibodies may relate to defective clearance of apoptotic cells. When cells undergo apoptosis, internal proteins are displayed on surface blebs. If the apoptotic cells are not cleared, nuclear material is exposed to the immune system, which may become sensitized. Certain complement component deficiencies, namely of C4 and C1q, are associated with SLE; this may relate to the role of complement activation in clearing apoptotic cells and foreign antigens.

Autoantibodies can cause tissue damage through direct binding and subsequent immune system activation, or via formation and deposition of immune complexes in tissues. Autoantibodies are implicated in multiple manifestations of SLE, including glomerulonephritis, cutaneous lupus, cytopenias, and thrombosis. Anti–double stranded DNA (dsDNA) antibodies are associated with lupus nephritis, though glomerulonephritis can also occur in the absence of anti-dsDNA antibodies, likely mediated through other autoantibodies. Pathologic findings in the kidney in lupus nephritis include mesangial, subepithelial, and subendothelial deposits of immunoglobulin G (IgG), IgM, IgA, and complement components (the "full-house" immunofluorescence staining pattern). Cutaneous manifestations of SLE also are mediated by immune complexes, as shown by positivity of the lupus band test in involved and uninvolved skin (**Figure 256-1**). Ultraviolet light causes DNA damage and keratinocyte apoptosis, which can activate and perpetuate an immune response as described above. Autoantibodies against blood

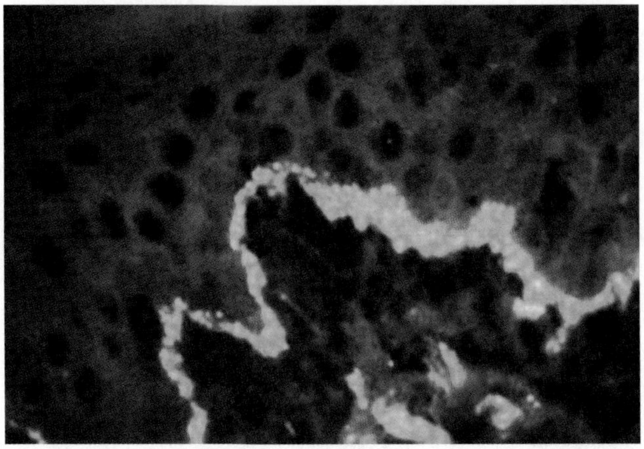

Figure 256-1 *Immunopathology of lupus erythematosus–specific skin disease: positive lupus band test. Direct immunofluorescence examination of a discoid lupus erythematosus lesional skin biopsy showing a continuous band of granular fluorescence at the dermal-epidermal junction as a result of staining with fluorescein isothiocyanate–conjugated goat anti-immunoglobulin G. (Reproduced, with permission, from Wolff K, Goldsmith LA, Katz SI, et al. Fitzpatrick's Dermatology in General Medicine. 7th ed. New York: McGraw-Hill; 2008. Fig. 156-13.)*

cell components may lead to Coombs-positive hemolytic anemia, thrombocytopenia, and neutropenia, and antiphospholipid antibodies may induce thrombotic events and recurrent pregnancy losses.

Patients with SLE also demonstrate abnormal B- and T-cell activation. B-cell hyperactivity may be present, partly due to increased levels of B-lymphocyte stimulator (BLyS); biologic therapy against BLyS, belimumab, was approved in 2011 for the treatment of adult patients with active, antibody-positive SLE despite standard therapy. Interferon-alpha probably also plays a role in abnormal immune activation; most lupus patients have a peripheral blood *interferon signature* of gene expression patterns consistent with interferon-alpha stimulation.

The pathogenesis of lupus serositis, arthritis, and neuropsychiatric disease are not well understood. Pleural effusions in active SLE are exudative, with decreased pleural fluid complement levels. Synovial fluid in lupus arthritis is generally mildly inflammatory, usually less than 2000 cells/mm^3. Certain autoantibodies have been implicated in central nervous system (CNS) lupus (such as anti-N-methyl-D-aspartate [NMDA] antibodies), but neuropsychiatric lupus is also characterized by a bland vasculopathy of cerebral vessels. The vasculopathy of lupus is increasingly appreciated as a cause of morbidity and mortality in this disease, especially as a cause of accelerated cardiovascular disease.

DIFFERENTIAL DIAGNOSIS

There are two scenarios that require the hospitalist to consider SLE in the differential diagnosis: patients with symptoms that may represent new-onset SLE, or patients with known SLE and recent symptoms that might be due to SLE, its treatment, or other causes.

NEW SYSTEMIC LUPUS ERYTHEMATOSUS

SLE should be considered in the differential diagnosis of a young person with serositis, cytopenias, or glomerulonephritis. A wide range of other diagnostic considerations are relevant in patients with these findings. New pleural and pericardial effusions are commonly caused by infection and malignancy. Pleural effusions are also caused by heart failure, liver disease, nephrotic syndrome, chylothorax, esophageal rupture, rheumatoid arthritis, and hypothyroidism; other causes of pericarditis include uremia, hypothyroidism, and radiation therapy.

Pancytopenia is common is SLE, but may also be caused by bone marrow infiltrative processes such as lymphoma, sarcoidosis, or infection. Isolated thrombocytopenia can result from SLE, as well as idiopathic thrombocytopenic purpura (ITP), thrombotic thrombocytopenic purpura (TTP; may appear concurrently with SLE), medications, infections, or liver disease. SLE is more likely to cause lymphopenia than neutropenia. Lymphopenia should prompt consideration of human immunodeficiency virus (HIV) infection and may also be caused by glucocorticoid therapy. SLE is one of many illnesses that can cause anemia of chronic disease. SLE is also associated with autoimmune hemolytic anemia, which may be associated with leukemia, lymphoma, *Mycoplasma pneumoniae* infection, and infectious mononucleosis.

In addition to SLE, other causes of new-onset glomerulonephritis include nonlupus nephritic syndromes such as acute and rapidly progressive glomerulonephritis, crescentic glomerulonephritis, or systemic necrotizing vasculitides such as Wegener granulomatosis or Goodpasture syndrome. New-onset nephrotic syndrome may be caused by SLE, as well as idiopathic membranous glomerulopathy, diabetic glomerulosclerosis, focal segmental glomerulosclerosis, or minimal change nephropathy.

Certain neurologic syndromes suggest the possibility of SLE. Transverse myelitis can be a forme fruste of SLE, and if seen in a young woman then SLE should be ruled out. New seizures may also be a presenting manifestation of SLE.

Inflammatory arthritis and rashes occur in up to 90% of individuals with SLE and support the diagnosis of SLE when present. Acute inflammatory arthritis may represent rheumatoid arthritis, parvovirus B19 infection, or reactive arthritis from infections such as *Salmonella*, *Shigella*, *Campylobacter*, and *Chlamydia trachomatis*. Mucocutaneous manifestations account for 4 of the 11 classification criteria for SLE. Certain variants of cutaneous lupus have a more robust link to systemic disease (**Figure 256-2**).

ESTABLISHED SYSTEMIC LUPUS ERYTHEMATOSUS

When patients with SLE are admitted to the hospital, two questions should be asked: Does this patient actually have SLE? If so, is SLE responsible for the patient's presentation? As noted above, disease flare is the most common reason for hospital admission in patients with SLE, followed by infection, cardiovascular disease, and thrombosis.

Hematologic manifestations, including anemia and thrombocytopenia, may require hospital admission. Anemia in SLE is often multifactorial. Patients may have anemia of chronic disease or

Clinical class	Manifestation	Risk of developing systemic disease
CCLE (Chronic Cutaneous Lupus Erythematosus)	Discoid lupus Lupus profundus Chilblain lupus	Low
ICLE (Intermediate Cutaneous Lupus Erythematosus)	Tumid lupus	Low
SCLE (Subacute Cutaneous Lupus Erythematosus)	Papulosquamous lesions Psoriasiform lesions	Intermediate
ACLE (Acute Cutaneous Lupus Erythematosus)		High

Figure 256-2 *Forms of cutaneous lupus erythematosus and their association with systemic disease.*

autoimmune hemolytic anemia related to SLE, but lupus patients often take medications that can cause gastrointestinal bleeding, including aspirin, nonsteroidal anti-inflammatory drugs (NSAIDs), and anticoagulants. The large number of lupus patients who are young women are also at risk for iron deficiency anemia from menstrual blood loss. Finally, patients with lupus nephritis may have anemia related to renal disease. Thrombocytopenia may be multifactorial as well, but immune-mediated thrombocytopenia or TTP must always be considered.

Neuropsychiatric lupus (NPSLE) can present in many ways. A new seizure may be a manifestation of NPSLE, but can also occur with accelerated hypertension from acute nephritis or noncompliance with antihypertensive therapy. In addition, posterior reversible encephalopathy syndrome (PRES) has been reported in patients with SLE, with or without significant hypertension. The causes for this syndrome and relationship to active SLE are incompletely understood. NPSLE can also present as acute delirium. Drugs and opportunistic infection of the CNS must also be considered. NPSLE can also manifest with severe depressive symptoms, even catatonia. This can be difficult to differentiate from primary depression.

Respiratory infection with typical or unusual pathogens must be considered in patients with SLE and serositis, dyspnea, or pulmonary infiltrates. Such individuals may be taking chronic glucocorticoids or other immunosuppressive medications that not only increase the risk of infection, but also blunt its symptoms when it occurs. Pulmonary infiltrates in patients with SLE may also represent life-threatening alveolar hemorrhage.

Premature cardiovascular disease is a major source of morbidity and early mortality in SLE. A 40-year-old woman with SLE is likely to have an equivalent atherosclerotic burden to a 70-year-old woman without SLE. SLE imparts a cardiovascular risk similar to that of diabetes mellitus. Chest pain and dyspnea may be manifestations of pericarditis or pleurisy, but they may also be the presenting symptoms of pulmonary embolism or pulmonary arterial hypertension. Patients with dyspnea and pericarditis should be assessed for possible tamponade. Nonbacterial thrombotic endocarditis (Libman-Sacks endocarditis) is rare, but it should be considered in any patient with SLE with dyspnea, chest pain, and signs of peripheral emboli. Accelerated hypertension suggests new glomerulonephritis.

DIAGNOSIS

SLE is a clinical syndrome, diagnosed by thorough history and physical examination with appropriate laboratory and other diagnostic testing. While the American College of Rheumatology (ACR) classification criteria for SLE were designed to improve homogeneity of individuals enrolled into clinical trials, they are also helpful for making a clinical diagnosis of SLE (**Table 256-1**). However, many

TABLE 256-1 American College of Rheumatology Classification Criteria for a Diagnosis of Systemic Lupus Erythematosus

System	Criterion	Description
Mucosal findings	Malar rash	Flat or raised erythema over the malar eminences. Malar rashes generally spare the nasolabial folds.
	Discoid rash	Early discoid rashes are erythematous and raised patches. Biopsy findings include adherent keratotic scale and follicular plugging. Older lesions become atrophic and scarred.
	Photosensitivity	Patient-described rash in reaction to sunlight.
	Oral ulcers	Ulcerations in the mouth or nose that are observed by a physician. These ulcers are frequently painless.
Organ system–specific manifestations	Arthritis	Tenderness, swelling, or effusion of 2 or more joints.
	Serositis	Pleuritis is defined as pleuritic pain or a rub heard on examination or evidence of pleural effusion. Pericarditis is defined by presence of a rub or characteristic ECG findings or evidence of a pericardial effusion.
	Renal disorder	For classification, defined as 0.5 grams or more of proteinuria or the presence of cellular casts.
	Neurologic disorder	The presence of seizures or psychosis that can not be otherwise explained.
Laboratory findings	Hematologic disorder	Hemolytic anemia with reticulocytosis *or* Total WBC count $<4{,}000/mm^3$ total on 2 or more occasions *or* Lymphopocyte count $<1500/mm^3$ on 2 or more occasions *or* Platelet count $<100{,}000/mm^3$
	Immunologic disorder	The presence of anti-DNA antibody *or* The presence of anti-Sm antibody *or* The presence of antiphospholipid antibodies defined as elevated IgG or IgM anticardiolipin antibodies or a lupus anticoagulant or a false-positive RPR
	Antinuclear antibody	At any point in time, in the absence of drugs that cause drug-induced lupus.

*A patient must meet four of these criteria for inclusion in clinical trials. Many other findings also support the diagnosis of SLE in clinical practice (see text).
ECG, electrocardiogram; Ig, immunoglobulin; RPR, rapid plasma regain; WBC, white blood cell.
Data from Tan EM, Cohen AS, Fries JF, et al. The 1982 revised criteria for the classification for systemic lupus erythematosus. *Arthritis Rheum.* 1982;25:1271–1277.
Data from Hochberg MC. Updating the American College of Rheumatology revised critieria for the classification of systemic lupus erythematosus. *Arthritis Rheum.* 1997;40:1725.

signs, symptoms, and laboratory findings seen in individuals with SLE are not included in the classification criteria. These include Raynaud phenomenon, interstitial lung disease, and hypocomplementemia.

The history should elicit whether the patient has experienced typical lupus manifestations such as arthralgia, rash, mucosal ulcers, or serositis. More than 90% of individuals with SLE have musculoskeletal manifestations, including arthritis, defined as two or more swollen or tender joints. The most commonly involved joints include the small joints of the hands, wrists, elbows, and knees; these joints should be palpated for swelling and tenderness. Most individuals with SLE have mucocutaneous lesions at some point during the course of their disease. These manifestations range from generally painless oral and nasal ulcerations to photosensitive rashes, malar rash, and discoid lupus rash. Photosensitive rashes more typically occur on sun-exposed skin, but may also occur in non-sun-exposed regions. Discoid lesions are associated with complete loss of hair, central atrophy, and hypopigmentation. The face and scalp should be carefully examined for discoid lupus rashes, including the pinnae and external auditory canals. Patients may wear wigs or have hair glued over bald patches, so the patient should be asked about prior hair loss. The skin of the fingers and hands must be carefully examined, as both erythema between the interphalangeal joints and subcutaneous nodules on the fingers are common. Periungual infarcts can often be appreciated with the naked eye if observed carefully. Blanching livedo reticularis on the extremities is also common in individuals with SLE and can predict the presence of antiphospholipid antibodies.

Before autoantibody results return, other tests may suggest SLE (**Table 256-2**). A complete blood count is one of the most useful single tests in evaluating for SLE. Leukopenia, thrombocytopenia, and anemia are all consistent with a diagnosis of SLE. The erythrocyte sedimentation rate is generally increased in active SLE. Urine should be examined for cells or cellular casts; urine protein quantitation is recommended. Serum chemistries can be helpful as well. The serum total protein may be elevated in SLE and other autoimmune diseases because of high levels of autoantibodies. Serum albumin may be low, reflective either of chronic disease or of proteinuria associated with glomerulonephritis.

Serologic studies support the diagnosis of SLE (**Table 256-3**). Almost 100% of individuals with SLE have a positive antinuclear antibody (ANA) test. Although a negative ANA test essentially rules out a diagnosis of SLE, a positive ANA test is not diagnostic; up to 15% of the general population has a positive ANA. Antinuclear antibodies may be measured three different ways, each with different sensitivities and specificities. The fluorescent antinuclear antibody assay (FANA) is highly sensitive. The FANA is performed by applying progressively more dilute patient serum to standardized cells on microscope slides, then observing the pattern of immunofluorescence by microscopy. The FANA is reported as the dilution (titer) at which nuclear fluorescence is seen. A high-titer positive ANA means antinuclear antibody activity is present even when the patient's serum is very dilute. Some laboratories use enzyme-linked immunosorbent (ELISA)-based autoantibody testing. Such testing can be automated and performed more quickly than the traditional FANA. However, ELISA testing tends to be less sensitive, as the only nuclear antibodies detected are those specifically sought by the assay. Thus, the results may be more specific for the autoantibodies associated with clinical disease. Finally, many laboratories now use multiplex immunoassays. In these assays, the patient's serum is mixed with beads coated with a variety of autoantigens. Each autoantigen bead has a specific fluorescent dye. An immunoassay analyzer determines the identity and quantity of the reacting autoantigen beads. Like ELISA-based methods, this test only detects predefined autoantibodies. ANA-negative lupus is exceptionally rare; the ANA is occasionally negative in individuals with positive anti-Ro (SSA) antibody, because the antigen may result in a cytoplasmic staining pattern. ANA tests may become negative during the course of the disease.

Several autoantibodies are more specific for SLE, including anti-dsDNA, anti-Sm, and anti-RNP. Only anti-Sm and anti-dsDNA are included in the ACR classification criteria for SLE. Anti-Ro and anti-La are common in SLE, and are also seen in Sjögren syndrome and rheumatoid arthritis. Low-complement C3 and C4 levels are not included in the ACR classification criteria for SLE, but are consistent with the presence of SLE and predict disease activity. In addition, complement component deficiencies predispose individuals to develop SLE.

TABLE 256-2 Useful Laboratory Tests for Evaluating Systemic Lupus Erythematosus*

Test	Features Consistent with SLE
CBC	Anemia
	Thrombocytopenia
	Lymphopenia
CMP	Elevated serum creatinine
	Elevated serum total protein
	Decreased serum albumin
ESR	Elevated
C-reactive protein	Elevated
Quantitative immunoglobulins	Elevated IgG
	Elevated IgM
	Elevated IgA
Urinalysis	Proteinuria
	Microscopic hematuria
	Red blood cell casts
	White blood cells in the absence of bacteria, leukocyte esterase, nitrites
Complement levels	Low C3, C4, or CH50 (whole hemolytic complement)

*These features are not seen in all patients with SLE, but when seen in the appropriate clinical context, support a diagnosis of SLE.

CBC, complete blood count; CMP, comprehensive metabolic panel; ESR, erythrocyte sedimentation rate.

PRACTICE POINT

- Antinuclear antibody (ANA) testing is very sensitive for the diagnosis of systemic lupus erythematosus (SLE). Virtually all patients with SLE have positive ANA tests. However, ANA testing is also very nonspecific. Up to 15% of healthy women test positive for ANA, and the positive predictive value of ANA testing for SLE is as low as 11%. High titers of ANA, the presence of multiple symptoms and signs of SLE, and positivity for more specific antibody tests such as anti-dsDNA increases the likelihood of a clinically significant positive ANA. Clinicians should also be aware that many other rheumatologic conditions are associated with positive ANA tests, including rheumatoid arthritis, Sjögren syndrome, dermatomyositis, drug-induced lupus, systemic sclerosis, and Raynaud phenomenon.

TABLE 256-3 Autoantibodies in Systemic Lupus Erythematosus

Antibody	Prevalence (%)	Antigen Recognized	Clinical Utility
Antinuclear antibodies	98	Multiple nuclear	Best screening test; repeated negative tests make SLE unlikely
Anti-dsDNA	70	DNA (double-stranded)	High titers are SLE specific and in some patients correlate with disease activity, nephritis, vasculitis
Anti-Sm	25	Protein complexed to 6 species of nuclear U1 RNA	Specific for SLE; no definite clinical correlations; most patients also have anti-RNP; more common in African Americans and Asians than Caucasians
Anti-RNP	40	Protein complexed to U1 RNA	Not specific for SLE; high titers associated with syndromes that have overlap features of several rheumatic syndromes including SLE; more common in African Americans than Caucasians
Anti-Ro (SS-A)	30	Protein complexed to hY RNA, primarily 60 kDa and 52 kDa	Not specific for SLE; associated with sicca syndrome, subacute cutaneous lupus, and neonatal lupus with congenital heart block; associated with decreased risk for nephritis
Anti-La (SS-B)	10	47-kDa protein complexed to hY RNA	Usually associated with anti-Ro; associated with decreased risk for nephritis
Antihistone	70	Histones associated with DNA (in nucleosome, chromatin)	More frequent in drug-induced lupus than in SLE
Antiphospholipid	50	Phospholipids, beta$_2$ glycoprotein 1 cofactor, prothrombin	Three tests available: ELISA for cardiolipin and beta$_2$G1, sensitive prothrombin time (DRVVT); predisposes to clotting, fetal loss, thrombocytopenia
Antierythrocyte	60	Erythrocyte membrane	Measured as direct Coombs test; a small proportion develops overt hemolysis
Antiplatelet	30	Surface and altered cytoplasmic antigens in platelets	Associated with thrombocytopenia but sensitivity and specificity are not good; this is not a useful clinical test
Antineuronal (includes antiglutamate receptor)	60	Neuronal and lymphocyte surface antigens	In some series a positive test in CSF correlates with active CNS lupus
Antiribosomal P	20	Protein in ribosomes	In some series a positive test in serum correlates with depression or psychosis due to CNS lupus

CNS, central nervous system; CSF, cerebrospinal fluid; DRVVT, dilute Russell viper venom time; ELISA, enzyme-linked immunosorbent assay.
Reproduced, with permission, from Fauci AS, Braunwald E, Kasper DL, et al. *Harrison's Principles of Internal Medicine.* 17th ed. New York, NY: McGraw-Hill; 2008, Table 313-1.

SPECIFIC DISEASE MANIFESTATIONS

CUTANEOUS DISEASE

The clinical classes of cutaneous lupus are acute cutaneous lupus (ACLE), subacute cutaneous lupus (SCLE), and chronic cutaneous lupus (CCLE). ACLE includes the classic malar rash (**Figures 256-3** and **256-4**), as well as bullous lupus and toxic epidermal necrolysis (TEN)-like ACLE. Patients with subacute cutaneous lupus (SCLE) have papulosquamous lesions and psoriasiform plaques (**Figure 256-5**). The SCLE rash is associated with the presence of anti-Ro antibodies. Neonatal lupus, which is associated with maternal anti-Ro antibodies, is clinically and histologically indistinguishable from SCLE. CCLE includes discoid lupus (**Figure 256-6**), lupus profundus (panniculitis), and chilblain lupus. A fourth clinical subtype is intermittent cutaneous lupus erythematosus (ICLE), or tumid lupus. Skin biopsy can help determine whether a rash is related to SLE. A lymphocytic infiltrate at the dermal-epidermal junction (interface dermatitis) is characteristic of SLE, as well as dermatomyositis. Lymphocytes also cause mild perivascular and periadnexal inflammation in SLE rashes. ACLE may contain a dermal neutrophilic infiltrate, but interface, perivascular, and periadnexal changes should also be present. As noted above, immunofluorescence microscopy reveals the lupus band, a linear array of deposited immunoglobulins and complement

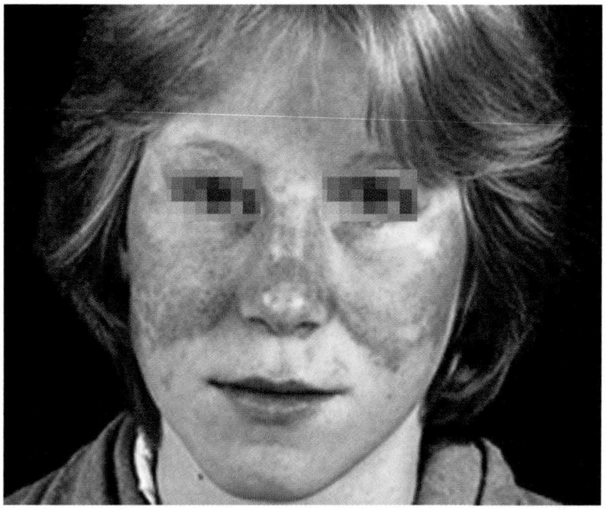

Figure 256-3 *Classic malar rash of acute cutaneous lupus erythematosus. Bright red, sharply defined erythema with slight edema and minimal scaling in a butterfly pattern on the central face. (Reproduced, with permission, from Wolff K, Johnson RA. Fitzpatrick's Color Atlas & Synopsis of Clinical Dermatology. 6th ed. New York: McGraw-Hill; 2009. Fig. 14-20.)*

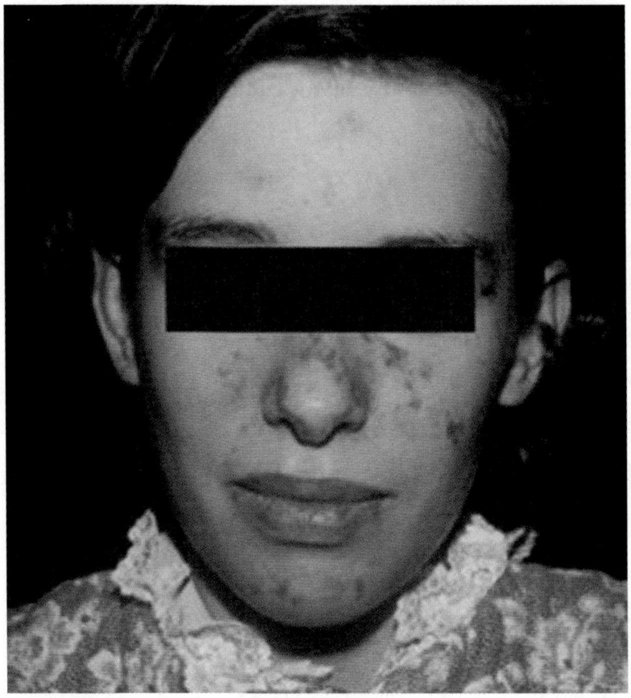

Figure 256-4 *Acute cutaneous lupus erythematosus with malar rash, in milder form. (Reproduced, with permission, from Fuster V, O'Rourke RA, Walsh RA, et al. Hurst's the Heart. 12th ed. New York: McGraw-Hill; 2008. Fig. 12-22.)*

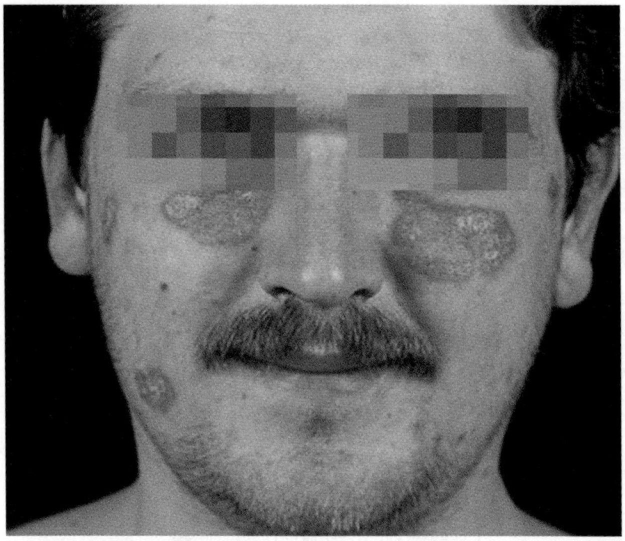

Figure 256-6 *Chronic cutaneous lupus erythematosus. Well-demarcated, erythematous, hyperkeratotic plaques with atrophy, follicular plugging, and adherent scale on both cheeks. This is the classic presentation of chronic discoid lupus erythematosus. (Reproduced, with permission, from Wolff K, Johnson RA. Fitzpatrick's Color Atlas & Synopsis of Clinical Dermatology. 6th ed. New York: McGraw-Hill; 2009. Fig. 14-23.)*

at the epidermal basement membrane that is present in both normal-appearing skin and rashes in patients with SLE.

HEMATOLOGIC INVOLVEMENT

SLE-related cytopenias generally result from peripheral destruction of cells rather than bone marrow suppression. Autoimmune hemolytic anemia, which can be Coombs positive (associated with complement or antibody on red cell membranes) or Coombs negative, affects 10% of patients with SLE. Evidence of hemolysis includes elevated lactate dehydrogenase levels, elevated reticulocyte count, decreased haptoglobin concentration, and hyperbilirubinemia. Ferritin is an acute-phase reactant, and it is not a reliable measure of total iron stores in individuals with autoimmune disease; serum iron and total iron-binding capacity are more specific. Leukopenia is seen in more than half of patients. Lymphopenia is more common than neutropenia, though antigranulocyte antibodies (not to be confused with antineutrophil cytoplasmic antibodies) can cause neutropenia in lupus patients. Severe thrombocytopenia is unusual in SLE. When thrombocytopenia exists, the blood smear should be examined for schistocytes, as thrombotic thrombocytopenic purpura (TTP) is associated with SLE. ADAMTS-13 (a disintegrin and metalloproteinase with a thrombospondin type 1 motif, member 13) level is useful for diagnosing TTP in individuals with SLE.

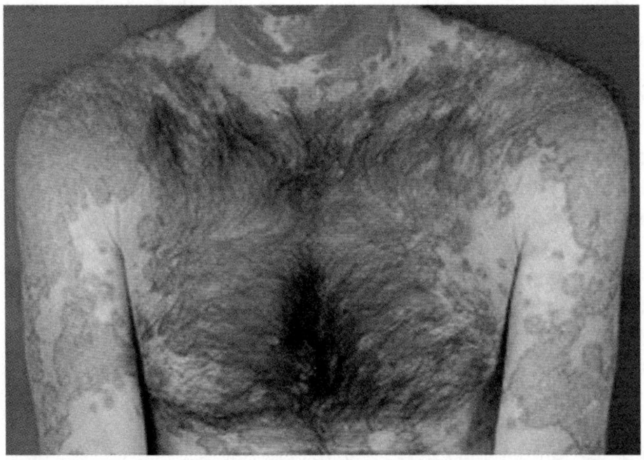

Figure 256-5 *Subacute cutaneous lupus erythematosus. Widely scattered, erythematous-to-violaceous, scaling, well-demarcated plaques on the trunk, neck, and arms, mimicking the clinical appearance of psoriasis vulgaris. (Reproduced, with permission, from Wolff K, Johnson RA. Fitzpatrick's Color Atlas & Synopsis of Clinical Dermatology. 6th ed. New York: McGraw-Hill; 2009. Fig. 14-22.)*

SEROSITIS

About 30% of individuals with SLE develop pleuritic involvement; pleuritis is more common than pericarditis in SLE. Mild serositis is clinically detected as pleural or pericardial friction rubs. Pleural effusion is suspected when there are decreased basilar breath sounds or dullness to percussion, and can be confirmed by chest X-ray or other imaging. On thoracentesis, lupus pleural effusions are exudative. Cytology of the pleural fluid may reveal lupus eythematosus (LE) cells, though this assay is infrequently performed. Significant pericardial effusions can be clinically detected through measurement of a pulsus paradoxus or by the presence of Kussmahl sign. In pericarditis, the electrocardiogram (ECG) may show characteristic low amplitude, diffuse ST-segment elevation, and PR depression or electrical alternans.

LUPUS NEPHRITIS

Renal involvement affects more than half of lupus patients. Lupus nephritis should be suspected when there is proteinuria or an active urinary sediment. Although renal involvement can be estimated clinically, renal biopsy is definitive. In 2004, the pathologic classification of lupus nephritis was updated by the International Society of

TABLE 256-4 International Society of Nephrology and Renal Pathology Society 2003 Classification of Lupus Nephritis

Class I	Minimal mesangial lupus nephritis
Class II	Mesangial proliferative lupus nephritis
Class III	Focal lupus nephritis (A): active lesions: focal proliferative lupus nephritis (A, C): active and chronic lesions (C): chronic inactive lesions with scars
Class IV	Diffuse lupus nephritis IV-S (A): active lesions: diffuse segmental proliferative lupus nephritis IV-G (A): active lesions: diffuse global proliferative lupus nephritis IV-S (A/G): active and chronic lesions: diffuse segmental proliferative and sclerosing lupus nephritis IV-G (A/G): active and chronic lesions: diffuse global proliferative and sclerosing lupus nephritis IV-S (C): chronic inactive lesions with scars: diffuse segmental sclerosing lupus nephritis IV-G (C): chronic inactive lesions with scars: diffuse global sclerosing lupus nephritis
Class V	Membranous lupus nephritis
Class VI	Advanced sclerotic lupus nephritis

Data from Weening JJ, D'Agati VD, Schwartz MM, et al. The classification of glomerulonephritis in systemic lupus erythematosus revisited. *Kidney Int.* 2004;65:521–530.

Nephrology and Renal Pathology Society (**Table 256-4**). Treatment choices for lupus nephritis are based on the International Society of Nephrology and Renal Pathology Society (ISN/RPS) disease classes.

NEUROPSYCHIATRIC DISEASE

Neuropsychiatric manifestations of SLE (NPSLE) are challenging to diagnose. The ACR has identified 19 distinct clinical syndromes of the central and peripheral nervous systems seen in SLE (**Table 256-5**). Lumbar puncture with cerebrospinal fluid analysis is necessary when evaluating acute mental status changes in lupus patients. Cerebrospinal fluid (CSF) studies that should be performed to evaluate for NPSLE include cell count, glucose, protein, IgG index, and oligoclonal bands, as well as cultures and serologies to exclude infectious causes. Pleocytosis and elevated CSF protein may be present in active CNS SLE. Oligoglonal bands reflect the presence of autoantibodies in the CSF. Tests to rule out infection include bacterial and fungal cultures, cryptococcal antigen, and the Venereal Disease Research Laboratory (VDRL) test. Magnetic resonance imaging (MRI) with and without contrast is the preferred imaging modality in NPSLE, although it may occasionally be normal. As antiphospholipid antibodies are associated with NPSLE, anticardiolipin antibodies, anti-beta-2 glycoprotein 1 antibodies, and lupus anticoagulant should be obtained, as well as a blood smear to evaluate for schistocytes that would suggest TTP. The antiribosomal P autoantibody may be associated with psychosis as a manifestation of NPSLE, and there are numerous other investigational autoantibodies that have been reported in patients with CNS involvement from SLE.

TABLE 256-5 Nineteen Clinical Syndromes Recognized as Possible Manifestations of Neuropsychiatric Lupus

Central Nervous System (CNS)	Peripheral Nervous System
Syndromes diagnosed by laboratory or radiographic testing including: • Aseptic meningitis • CNS demyelination • Cerebrovascular disease • Myelopathy Symptoms indicating CNS dysfunction including: • Headache (steroid responsive) • Chorea • Cognitive dysfunction • Psychosis • Delirium • Anxiety • Mood disorder	• Autonomic dysfunction • Myasthenia gravis • Neuropathies including: ▪ Mononeuropathy ▪ Cranial neuropathy ▪ Plexopathy ▪ Polyneuropathy ▪ Acute demyelinating polyneuropathy

Data from Ad Hoc Committee on Neuropsychiatric Lupus Nomenclature. The American College of Rheumatology nomenclature and case definitions for neuropsychiatric lupus syndromes. *Arthritis Rheum.* 1999;42:599–608.

TRIAGE AND HOSPITAL ADMISSION

Most patients with SLE flares are not hospitalized. However, several lupus manifestations are best managed in an inpatient setting due to the risk of life- or organ-threatening complications. Some of these include desquamating rashes, severe cytopenias, symptomatic pericardial or pleural effusions, accelerated hypertension, acute dyspnea, accelerated proteinuria and nephritis, and many neurologic presentations. Below, we discuss types of SLE flares that warrant admission, including thrombotic complications. Infections must frequently be considered in individuals with SLE and will not be specifically discussed here.

Most lupus-related rashes are managed comfortably at home. However, an individual with SLE and an acute, rapidly progressive desquamating rash should be admitted. Acute desquamating rashes may start as peripheral erythematous macules that progress to vesicles, and are associated with a diffuse burning sensation. The differential diagnosis of a desquamating rash includes bullous lupus, toxic epidermal necrolysis (TEN), or Stevens-Johnson syndrome. TEN-like acute cutaneous lupus is occasionally seen in SLE. All desquamating lupus rashes progress rapidly and place the patient at risk for fluid shifts and infections. Severe mucous membrane involvement is common. Skin disease may also result from SLE treatment. Hydroxychloroquine has been associated with acute generalized exanthematous pustulosis (AGEP), a cutaneous hypersensitivity reaction that presents as a desquamating rash on the face and chest.

Patients with cytopenias may need admission for evaluation and management. Individuals with SLE and the new onset of less than 50,000 platelets/mm^3 should be considered for inpatient evaluation and management, especially if bleeding is present. Patients with symptomatic anemia also warrant admission.

Pericarditis is the most common cardiac manifestation of SLE. Cardiac tamponade can occur with effusions in active SLE. The presence of dyspnea with a large pericardial effusion, pulsus paradoxus on examination, or tamponade physiology on echocardiogram necessitates admission. Large pleural effusions associated with dyspnea require admission for diagnostic and therapeutic thoracentesis. Empyema must be ruled out in any large pleural effusion in a person with SLE.

Individuals with SLE may present with accelerated hypertension (systolic blood pressure [BP] ≥180 mm Hg or diastolic BP ≥110 mm Hg). Hypertensive emergency and hypertensive urgency are defined the same in individuals with SLE as in other individuals, and considerations for admission are similar. In hypertensive patients with SLE, it may be difficult to determine whether additional findings, such as confusion and microangiopathic hemolytic anemia, are the product of hypertensive crisis or are directly related to lupus disease activity. Glomerulonephritis must always be excluded in any patient with SLE with severe hypertension.

Acute dyspnea or a new oxygen requirement in an individual with SLE warrants admission. Cardiac causes of acute dyspnea in SLE include acute coronary syndromes, pericardial effusion, cardiac valvular disease related to SLE, and congestive heart failure. Valvular disease with fibrotic growth on valves, known as Libman-Sacks veruccous endocarditis, is common. Libman-Sacks endocarditis most commonly involves the tricuspid and mitral valves. Valve thickening or cardiac valve vegetations in SLE are associated with antiphospholipid antibodies. A new murmur or peripheral emboli are both indications for hospital admission. SLE may cause myocarditis, cardiomyopathy, and congestive heart failure. Pulmonary causes of dyspnea in SLE include pleural effusions, new interstitial lung disease, pneumonia, pulmonary embolism, and pulmonary hemorrhage. An elevated D-dimer in a patient with dyspnea and SLE should prompt hospital admission. Finally, acute coronary syndromes or myocardial infarction must always be considered in any dyspneic patient with SLE. SLE itself is a risk factor for cardiovascular disease; myocardial infarctions in the absence of traditional risk factors can occur even in very young women with SLE. ECG findings suggestive of ischemia or elevated serum biomarkers are absolute indicators for admission in this population.

Worsening hypertension and peripheral edema associated with proteinuria can be signs of lupus nephritis. Admission is indicated in suspected lupus nephritis if hemodialysis may be necessary to treat volume overload or electrolyte disturbances, to expedite renal biopsy, or to start pulse treatment with methylprednisolone for three to five days after renal biopsy has been performed. Additionally, individuals failing outpatient management of known lupus nephritis (eg, worsening microscopic hematuria, worsening proteinuria, inability to control blood pressure) may also be admitted for pulse therapy with methylprednisolone.

A patient with SLE with a first seizure should be admitted for further evaluation. Individuals with SLE have a higher incidence of cerebrovascular disease and can present with stroke at a young age. Stroke in SLE may result from thromboembolism or can be hemorrhagic, especially in the setting of hypertension or thrombocytopenia. Neuropsychiatric SLE has protean manifestations, which may include acute delirium and decreased responsiveness. Individuals with SLE with acute weakness in one or more extremities should be admitted for further evaluation and management; diagnostic considerations include transverse myelitis, mononeuritis multiplex, mixed sensorimotor polyneuropathies, and cranial and peripheral neuropathies.

TREATMENT

ACUTE DISEASE FLARES

Glucocorticoids are the cornerstone of therapy for acute lupus flares requiring hospitalization. Steroid dosing should be based on disease severity. There are no accepted published guidelines for treatment with steroids in SLE. Dosing schemes for corticosteroids include pulse dosing (500–1000 mg intravenous methylprednisolone equivalent at daily intervals), high dose (1 mg prednisone equivalent per kilogram of body weight), moderate dose (prednisone 0.5 mg/kg), and low dose (prednisone 5–10 mg) daily for disease maintenance or mild flares. Tapers are highly variable in dosing and duration; alternate-day dosing is an option for tapering steroids.

Hydroxcyhloroquine reduces the frequency of SLE flares. It has favorable effects on lipids and may reduce the risk of blood clots in individuals with SLE and antiphospholipid antibody syndrome. If dosed at less than 6.5 mg/kg daily, retinal toxicity occurs in less than 1% of users. The usual dose of hydroxychloroquine is 400 mg once daily or divided twice daily. Gastrointestinal side effects are uncommon, but may be reduced by taking the medication after a meal. As it is not immunosuppressive, hydroxychloroquine can be continued during acute infection. Hydroxychloroquine has not been shown to impair healing and should be continued perioperatively. The management of allergic reactions to hydroxychloroquine is complicated by its half-life of several weeks.

Several promising agents for the treatment of SLE are currently in development. Most are biologic therapies targeting specific immune functions implicated in lupus activity. Epratuzamab (anti-CD22 antibody) is currently in late-phase clinical trials. Rituximab failed to meet clinical endpoints when tested in randomized clinical trials for both generalized SLE and lupus nephritis. The recently approved biologic therapy, belimumab, will likely not have a significant role in the management of the hospitalized patient with an acute flare of SLE.

NEPHRITIS

Lupus nephritis is unique among SLE manifestations in that there are several published randomized clinical trials. Despite this, there is no consensus on optimal treatment, and a knowledgeable rheumatologist or nephrologist should be consulted to recommend appropriate therapy. Class II (mesangial) lupus nephritis generally improves with corticosteroids alone. Proliferative glomerulonephritis (class III or IV) merits aggressive therapy to prevent progression to end-stage renal disease. Many patients have simultaneous pathologic and clinical features of proliferative and membranous (class V) glomerulonephritis. Aggressive treatment is generally most effective for proliferative glomerulonephritis, though individuals with class V nephritis were included in many of the pivotal lupus nephritis trials.

There are three major published regimens for induction treatment of class III, IV, and V lupus nephritis. The first major protocol (NIH protocol) is 6 monthly pulses of intravenous cyclophosphamide (500–750 mg/m^2), followed by maintenance pulses every 3 months, for a total of 2 years of therapy. Prednisone is also administered, starting at 1 mg/kg daily for 8 weeks and weaned over 12 months. This regimen carries a high risk of serious infection, as well as infertility and malignancy. In the search for equally effective and less toxic treatments, two other regimens have emerged. In the Euro-lupus protocol, 3 daily pulses of 750 mg methylprednisolone are administered with cyclophosphamide 500 mg intravenously every 2 weeks for 6 doses, followed by oral azathioprine (AZA) for maintenance therapy. Prednisone is dosed similarly to the NIH protocol. This regimen was shown to be noninferior to the NIH protocol in a European trial. In the third induction regimen, oral mycophenolate mofetil (MMF) 1500 mg twice daily is given with oral corticosteroids, starting at 1 mg/kg and tapered over approximately 6 months. Oral MMF and monthly intravenous cyclophosphamide for 6 months (both with the same steroid regimen) were compared, and oral MMF was shown to be noninferior to monthly intravenous cyclophosphamide. Subgroup analysis of this trial suggests that oral MMF may provide improved renal survival in African American patients. After induction therapy, as described earlier, maintenance therapy is usually oral AZA or MMF, though the ideal duration of maintenance therapy is not known.

Class V lupus nephritis is notoriously challenging to treat. A recently published clinical trial demonstrated one-year clinical remission rates of 83% with daily cyclosporine and 60% with intravenous cyclophosphamide every other month for six doses. Both regimens were accompanied by alternate day prednisone starting at 40 mg/m^2 for eight weeks, then tapered over a year, as well as angiotensin-converting enzyme (ACE) inhibitors and daily oral statins. Another recently reported pooled analysis of two clinical trials found no difference in remission rates between intravenous cyclophosphamide and mycophenolate mofetil for pure class V nephritis. All classes of nephritis convey a significantly increased risk of cardiovascular disease; up to half of patients with nephritis eventually die from cardiovascular or cerebrovascular disease. The risk of thrombotic disease related to antiphospholipid antibodies and nephrotic syndrome is around 20% in this patient population. ACE inhibition is considered essential adjunctive treatment to reduce proteinuria. Combination antihypertensive therapy to a target of 120/80 is recommended. Statin therapy should be considered, with a target LDL of less than 100.

SEROSITIS

Data regarding the treatment of large (>10 mm) pericardial effusions are published as case series. These suggest that oral prednisone 0.5 to 1 mg/kg daily, with immediate placement of a drainage catheter, results in resolution in about half of patients, with the other half requiring pericardial window. If a large pericardial effusion is accompanied by other severe manifestations of SLE, one can consider a pulse of methylprednisolone 1000 mg for three daily doses at the beginning of treatment. Colchicine 0.6 mg twice daily is useful for the management of small to moderate symptomatic pericardial effusions, as are NSAIDs in patients with normal renal function. There is minimal data to guide treatment of symptomatic pleural effusions in SLE. Thoracentesis should be performed to rule out infection. Patients should be treated with oral prednisone at the doses suggested earlier for pericardial effusions. With recurrent pleural or pericardial effusions, steroid-sparing agents such as AZA, MMF, cyclosporine, or methotrexate (MTX) should be considered. Other pulmonary manifestations such as interstitial lung disease and shrinking lung syndrome are less common, and scant data is available to guide treatment. Considerations include immunosuppressive regimens listed above; the choice of therapy is also based on individual patient presentations and comorbidities.

CUTANEOUS LUPUS

Cutaneous lupus requiring hospital admission is usually either bullous lupus or cutaneous vasculitis with ulcerations. Bullous lupus improves rapidly with dapsone, but the diagnosis must be certain, as TEN and Stevens-Johnson syndrome do not respond to dapsone. Severe mucocutaneous involvement from SLE may necessitate intravenous corticosteroid treatment and hydration. When intravenous steroids are used for cutaneous lupus, they are generally dosed at or above the equivalent of 1 mg/kg/day prednisone. Cutaneous vasculitis from SLE should be proven by biopsy if possible, then treated initially with daily oral prednisone 1 mg/kg, as well as a second immunosuppressive agent, usually AZA (2–3 mg/kg divided twice daily), methotrexate (15–25 mg orally weekly), or MMF (up to 1500 mg twice daily). Any patient with cutaneous lupus should be treated with hydroxychloroquine unless there is a known allergy.

HEMATOLOGIC

Hemolytic anemia is treated with high-dose intravenous steroids, between 500 and 1000 mg of methylprednisolone daily for one to five days. Once the anemia stabilizes, conversion to oral prednisone 1 mg/kg daily is started and tapered over a few months. Oral immunosuppressives should be considered in recurrent or refractory cases. Thrombocytopenia is treated similarly, and intravenous immunoglobulin (IVIG) is often used when hemorrhagic complications occur. IVIG dosing is 400 mg/kg/day for five consecutive days. Oral immunosuppressives are started in recurrent or refractory cases. TTP in patients with lupus is treated the same as in patients without lupus: daily plasma exchange with high-dose intravenous steroids until the platelet count reaches a safe level and measures of hemolysis activity normalize. For adjunctive therapy in refractory cases, cyclophosphamide is usually given to patients with lupus (vincristine is more commonly administered outside the setting of SLE). Although rituximab showed no benefit in a randomized clinical trial for treatment of active SLE, a small case series suggested potential benefit of rituximab for SLE-associated TTP. Rituximab is approved for treatment of ITP and is often successfully used to treat patients with SLE, thrombocytopenia, and bleeding. Although plasma exchange has been used for nearly every manifestation of SLE, it has thus far only been shown to be beneficial for TTP, neuromyelitis optica (optic neuritis with segmental transverse myelitis, associated with IgG anti-NMO syndrome antibodies), and catastrophic antiphospholipid antibody syndrome (CAPS).

NEUROPSYCHIATRIC DISEASE

In lupus patients with seizures, first exclude infection, hypertensive urgency, PRES, and medication side effects. If these are absent, patients should be treated with anticonvulsants and three to five daily pulses of 1000 mg methylprednisolone, followed by a prednisone taper beginning at 1 mg/kg/day. A steroid-sparing oral immunosuppressive is often used. For most manifestations of NPSLE, intravenous cyclophosphamide is given as steroid-sparing therapy, but the optimal duration of treatment is not determined by randomized controlled trials. Many case series describe the use of MMF and AZA for NPSLE as well. IVIG is frequently used for NPSLE, especially when the peripheral nervous system is involved.

SLE-associated inflammatory myopathy is treated with prednisone 1 mg/kg daily for at least a month while starting a steroid-sparing agent such as MTX or AZA. IVIG is used in severe cases and is effective in non-SLE-associated myositis. Rituximab is a promising therapy for inflammatory myopathy, but there is little specific experience with SLE-associated myopathy.

ARTHRITIS

Not all manifestations of SLE must be treated with high-dose (1 mg/kg prednisone equivalent or greater) corticosteroids. Inflammatory arthritis flares can be treated with NSAIDs. If a patient requires hospitalization or has severe functional limitation due to inflammatory arthritis, prednisone can be started at 0.5 mg/kg or less, and tapered over two to three weeks. Alternatively, up to 120 mg of depot intramuscular steroid, such as triamcinolone, can be administered, an approach that decreases the cumulative lifetime dose of steroids if used for moderate flares of SLE. Inflammatory arthritis refractory to hydroxychloroquine is usually treated with MTX or AZA.

HEART BLOCK

IVIG is currently being studied as a salvage treatment for congenital heart block given to pregnant women with anti-Ro (SSA) or anti-La (SSB) antibodies and a fetus with cardiac conduction abnormalities. Clinical trial results are pending for this indication, and this treatment should not be undertaken without contacting a rheumatologist.

COMPLICATIONS

In the hospital, the major complications of lupus are caused by treatment rather than the disease itself. These include complications

TABLE 256-6 Therapy Monitoring for Drugs Commonly Used to Treat Systemic Lupus Erythematosus

Agent	Testing	Frequency
Hydroxychloroquine	Dilated funduscopic and visual field testing	Every 6–12 months
NSAIDs	CBC, Cr	Every 12 months
Corticosteroids	Bone Mineral Density	Every 1–2 years
	Glucose	Yearly
	Cholesterol panel	Yearly
Azathioprine	CBC, Cr, AST	Every 1–2 weeks after dosage change, then every 4–8 weeks
	Skin cancer screening	Yearly
Mycophenolate Mofetil	Pregnancy test	At drug initiation
	CBC	Every 4–8 weeks
Methotrexate	Chest X-ray	At drug initiation
	Hepatitis B, C	At drug initiation
	Pregnancy test	At drug initiation
	CBC, Cr, AST, albumin	Every 4–8 weeks

AST, aspartate aminotransferase; CBC, complete blood count; Cr, creatinine.

of high-dose corticosteroids, such as hyperglycemia, hypertension, and psychiatric manifestations, such as mania, delirium, and agitation. Many patients require sleep aids or anxiolytics while taking glucocorticoids. In patients with severe neuropsychiatric lupus, it can be difficult to differentiate the effects of the disease from those of its treatment; rheumatology, neurology, and psychiatric consultation may be helpful in this regard.

Cyclophosphamide can cause hemorrhagic cystitis; this risk may be reduced by coadministration with mesna. A white blood cell count should be checked 10 to 14 days after high-dose intravenous cyclophosphamide, as that is when the white cell nadir occurs.

Up to 25% of deaths in SLE are attributable to infections. These may present in atypical fashion, as high-dose corticosteroids minimize fever and other symptoms. Infection is most often due to common pathogens, such as *E coli*, *Staphylococcal aureus*, and *Streptococcus pneumoniae*, although lupus patients are also at substantial risk of tuberculosis. Higher SLE disease activity and greater immunosuppressive treatment are correlated with a higher infection risk; there is some evidence that antimalarials may protect against infection. Lupus patients should receive pneumococcal vaccine; patients at risk of latent tuberculosis should have appropriate screening.

Progressive multifocal leukoencephalopathy (PML) has been reported in patients with SLE treated with rituximab, as well as other immunosuppressive regimens including corticosteroids alone. It has also been reported in individuals taking mycophenolate mofetil. PML should be considered in all patients with SLE with neurologic symptoms.

Corticosteroids impair wound healing and increase the risk of infection in patients with SLE undergoing surgery. Other oral immunosuppressives (MTX, AZA, MMF) have not been specifically studied in patients with autoimmune diseases undergoing surgery. However, many groups have suggested holding these medications for 10 to 14 days both before and after surgery to diminish the risk of perioperative infection.

Most nonrheumatologic drugs given to patients with SLE do not affect the disease itself. Although tetracycline antibiotics and other agents are implicated in the development of drug-induced lupus, these medications have not been shown to cause disease flares in lupus patients. However, lupus patients are at risk of drug interactions and other consequences of polypharmacy.

DISCHARGE PLANNING

Stability for discharge from an SLE flare must be determined on an individual basis. As a general rule, the flare should be improving before discharge. A patient with pericardial effusion should not be discharged until the risk for pericardial tamponade has passed. In thrombocytopenia, discharge can be considered once the platelet count has stabilized and bleeding has ceased; in TTP, it is standard to wait for the platelet count to stabilize over 150,000/mm^3 before discharge. Hypertension should be well controlled on an oral regimen before discharge. Patients with corticosteroid-induced diabetes should be in good glycemic control at discharge, and should be given education and instructions in the case of high or low readings prior to discharge.

Individuals with severe SLE will often have initiated immunosuppressive therapy in the hospital that must be continued in the outpatient setting upon discharge. If an infusion medication such as cyclophosphamide is prescribed, then a site for drug delivery should be identified and the insurance approval process should be started to ensure that treatment continues without interruption.

Most immunosuppressive medications require interval toxicity monitoring. Recommended laboratory studies and their frequency are included in **Table 256-6**. Levels of thiopurine methyltransferase (TPMT) can predict whether leukopenia will result from azathioprine or 6-MP treatment. If TPMT testing is pending, a patient newly started on azathioprine should have a complete blood count (CBC) every two weeks as dosage is advanced. Individuals started on ACE inhibitor therapy require serum electrolyte checks soon after discharge. Patients taking high-dose corticosteroids should be prescribed a glucometer and instructed in its use, with instructions on whom to contact in the event of significant hyperglycemia. A responsible physician must be identified to follow up the above laboratory measures and to treat steroid-induced diabetes if it occurs. Medications should be reviewed before discharge to assess for the possibility of drug interactions.

Physical and occupational therapy are important, especially after prolonged hospitalization. Unfortunately, severe SLE disproportionately affects underserved populations, and many patients are uninsured or underinsured. Involving social work–based discharge planners can help ensure treatment plans are continued after discharge.

Patients may need help with arranging transportation to and from follow-up appointments. In-home therapy and nursing aides should be considered if indicated.

QUALITY IMPROVEMENT

Everyone who takes care of patients with SLE must remain acutely aware of the high risk of cardiovascular disease and the need to implement primary and secondary prevention strategies. We recommend following similar guidelines as for diabetes mellitus, with a blood pressure target of less than 120/80 mm Hg and goal LDL cholesterol of less than 100 mg/dl. Addressing behavioral issues such as obesity, diet, exercise, and smoking cessation is also essential.

Complications of corticosteroid therapy are rampant in patients with SLE, so consideration of corticosteroid-sparing agents in the hospital is recommended. Prevention of glucocorticoid-induced osteoporosis (GIOP) should be started while patients are hospitalized. Patients should be counseled to participate in weight-bearing exercise and to avoid smoking. Serum 25-hydroxyvitamin D should be measured in patients with SLE. Most people with SLE are photosensitive, so they should both avoid the sun and use sunscreen. Studies have shown that vitamin D levels are consistently low in patients with SLE. Thus, dietary guidelines for intake of calcium and vitamin D should be reviewed with patients. Individuals taking more than 5 mg of daily prednisone (or equivalent) should consume at least calcium 1500 mg daily, in addition to vitamin D 800–1000 international units daily. Bisphosphonate therapy should be considered for males or females who are not planning future pregnancies or are beyond child-bearing age. The algorithm in **Figure 256-7** summarizes the ACR guidelines for the prevention of GIOP.

Avascular necrosis is another dreaded complication of glucocorticoid therapy. The hips, shoulders, and knees are most commonly affected. Of course, the best way to prevent complications of steroid therapy is to minimize the dose and duration of treatment. As noted earlier, not all manifestations of SLE must be treated with high-dose steroids.

Patients with SLE should receive appropriate immunizations. Live vaccines should be avoided in individuals treated with more than 10 mg of daily prednisone or its equivalent. Infectious diseases consultation is appropriate if live vaccination seems necessary.

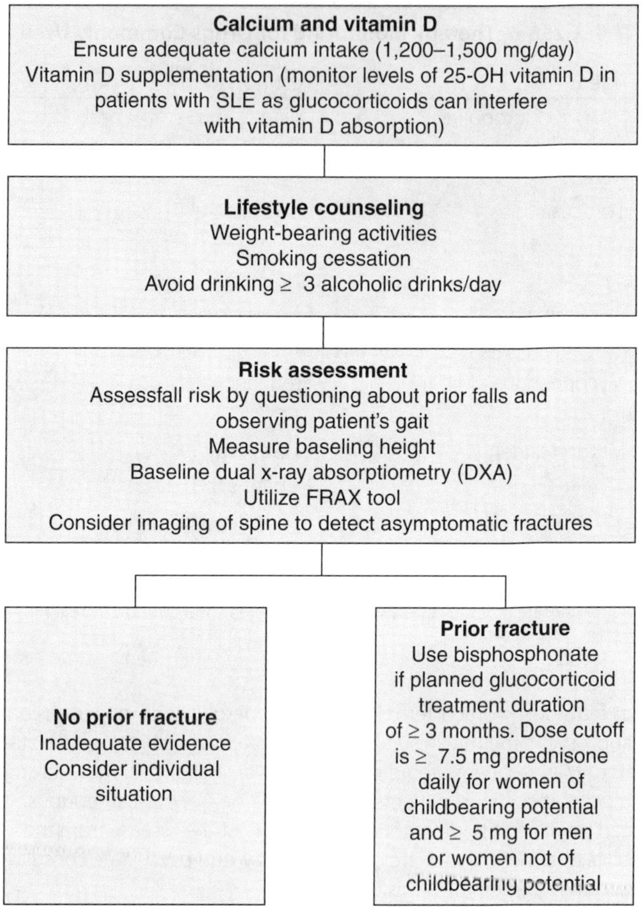

Figure 256-7 *Summary of recommendations for the prevention of glucocorticoid-induced osteoporosis in premenopausal women and men under age 50. These recommendations place a large focus on assessing fracture risk. The American College of Rheumatology task force concluded there were inadequate data to make recommendations for individuals who have not experienced a prior fragility fracture in these age groups. (Data from Grossman JR, Gordon R, Ranganath VK, et al. American College of Rheumatology 2010 recommendations for the prevention and treatment of glucocorticoid-induced osteoporosis. Arthritis Care Res. 2010;62:1515–1526.)*

SUGGESTED READINGS

Bertsias G, Ioannidis JP, Boletis J, et al. EULAR recommendations for the management of systemic lupus erythematosus. *Ann Rheum Dis*. 2008;67:195–205.

Mosca M, Tani C, Aringer M, et al. European League Against Rheumatism recommendations for monitoring patients with systemic lupus erythematosus in clinical practice and in observational studies. *Ann Rheum Dis*. 2010;69:1269–1274.

Ortega LM, Schultz DR, Lenz O, Pardo V, Contreras GN. Lupus nephritis: pathologic features, epidemiology and a guide to therapeutic decisions. *Lupus*. 2010;19:557–574.

Rahman A, Isenberg DA. Systemic lupus erythematosus. *N Engl J Med*. 2008;358:929–939.

Ruiz-Irastorza G, Cuadrado M, Ruiz-Arruza I, et al. Evidence-based recommendations for the prevention and long-term management of thrombosis in antiphospholipid antibody-positive patients. *Lupus*. 2011;20:206–218.

CHAPTER 257

Rheumatoid Arthritis and Other Inflammatory Arthritides

Lisa Criscione-Schreiber, MD
Marcy B. Bolster, MD

Key Clinical Questions

1. Does this patient have rheumatoid arthritis or another inflammatory arthritis?
2. What are the extra-articular manifestations of rheumatoid disease?
3. Is one responsible for this patient's hospitalization?
4. Is this hospitalization due to medication toxicity?
5. How should the patient's disease-modifying antirheumatic drugs be managed during the hospitalization, including perioperatively?
6. What tests and studies are useful to evaluate this patient's presentation?
7. What treatments are available?

INTRODUCTION/EPIDEMIOLOGY

Rheumatoid arthritis (RA) affects 1% of the population worldwide, with women being more commonly affected. In the recent past, there were only a few disease-modifying antirheumatic drugs (DMARDs), which were not prescribed until after joint damage had occurred. Patients were frequently admitted to the hospital for arthritis treatment, including administration of ACTH, rest, and intra-articular corticosteroid injections. Today, early, aggressive DMARD therapy, including biologic DMARDs, has dramatically improved patient outcomes. Most patients with RA are treated exclusively as outpatients, and are never hospitalized due to the disease itself. However, RA is a systemic disease with numerous potential extra-articular manifestations, including cardiovascular disease. A hospitalist must be alert to these manifestations, as they may lead to hospitalization.

PRACTICE POINT

- Early, aggressive DMARD use is a cornerstone of current RA management. The duration of rheumatoid arthritis prior to DMARD therapy is one of the most robust predictors of disease outcome. Longer delays in initiation of DMARDs are associated with greater long-term functional impairment. DMARDs may also attenuate the risk of cardiovascular disease.

Most other common inflammatory arthritides fall into the category of seronegative spondyloarthropathies, which affect up to 2% of individuals, with an equal male to female ratio. They include psoriatic arthritis (PsA) (population prevalence 0.3–1.0%), ankylosing spondylitis (AS) (prevalence 0.1–6.0%, depending on the population studied), inflammatory bowel disease–associated arthritis, reactive arthritis, and undifferentiated spondyloarthropathy. These illnesses are seronegative for rheumatoid factor, and are associated with the presence of human leukocyte antigen (HLA)-B27. The presence of HLA-B27 varies by ancestry. In general, up to 15% of the population is HLA-B27 positive. However, among individuals with spondyloarthropathies, up to 90% are HLA-B27 positive. Spondyloarthritis is characterized by axial arthritis with a predilection for the sacroiliac joints, oligoarthritis, especially of the lower extremities, and enthesitis, or inflammation of ligaments and tendons at attachments to bone. Inflammatory arthritis may be just one manifestation of a systemic disease that may include psoriasis and psoriasiform skin lesions, genital inflammation, inflammatory bowel disease, and inflammatory eye disease, such as uveitis or scleritis.

This chapter reviews articular and extra-articular manifestations of RA and the spondyloarthropathies. We will also review the indications, mechanisms, and most frequent complications of the DMARDs used to treat RA and other inflammatory arthritides, with recommendations for management of DMARD therapy in hospitalized patients with other illness, as well as during the perioperative period.

PATHOPHYSIOLOGY

Rheumatoid arthritis is thought to result when an environmental factor stimulates an aberrant immune response in a genetically susceptible host. Several genes are associated with susceptibility to development of RA. Most significantly, RA is associated with HLA-DRB1. A short amino acid sequence within this gene, known

PRACTICE POINT

- Patients with ankylosing spondylitis (AS) may have physical findings related to loss of mobility of the spine, chest, and sacroiliac joints. Decreased range of motion is from the combined effects of bony ankylosis and muscle spasm from pain and inflammation. Involvement of the costovertebral and costosternal joints in AS may lead to chest pain and *restriction of chest expansion* with maximal inspiration, which should normally be at least 5 cm measured at the fourth intercostal space. Therefore, patients with advanced AS develop restrictive lung disease and rely solely on diaphragmatic expansion for respiration. In addition, some form of interstitial lung disease may occur in up to 70% of patients with AS. The combination of restrictive lung disease and ILD can impede recovery from pulmonary infections in individuals with AS. Extra attention to pulmonary toilet is necessary to enable recovery in affected individuals.
- Pain from sacroiliitis can be elicited by direct palpation or the *Patrick test*, in which the supine patient crosses an ankle over the contralateral knee. When the examiner stabilizes the contralateral pelvis and places downward pressure on the flexed knee, pain is experienced in the contralateral SI joint. In advanced AS, patients develop abnormal *occiput-to-wall* distance measured with the scapulae and heels against the wall (this test is often abnormal in osteoporotic patients with spinal kyphosis). The *Schober test* assesses lumbar spine expansion on full forward flexion (this test is abnormal in individuals with lumbar degenerative disease) and is most useful in assessing young individuals with inflammatory back pain.
- Psoriatic arthritis is strongly associated with the metabolic syndrome. As in individuals with RA, patients with PsA are at increased risk for accelerated cardiovascular disease.

as the "shared epitope," is associated with increased risk of severe RA and development of anti-citrullinated peptide antibodies. Within proteins, the amino acid arginine can undergo posttranslational modification, mediated by peptidylarginine deaminases, into citrulline. Autoantibodies against citrullinated peptides appear to be quite specific for rheumatoid arthritis. Identification of these autoantibodies is now part of routine diagnostic testing for RA via the anti-CCP antibody test. An immune reaction against these peptides may initiate an inflammatory response in the joints. With regard to environmental exposures, cigarette smoking is the strongest proven risk factor for rheumatoid arthritis. Cigarette smoking may lead to citrullination of proteins in the lungs, rendering them immunogenic. Citrullinated peptides have been identified in the joints of RA patients, and antibodies against citrullinated peptides are also present in the joints. Up to 70% of patients with RA have anti-CCP antibodies in the serum. Rheumatoid factor (RF), or IgM anti-IgG antibodies, is detected in approximately 80% of patients. When rheumatoid factors are deposited in joints as immune complexes, they may initiate complement-mediated inflammation within the joint. The combination of a positive RF and anti-CCP antibody are highly specific for the diagnosis of RA. However, levels of rheumatoid factor and anti-CCP do not correlate with disease activity in RA.

In RA, the synovium becomes inflamed and hypertrophied, and develops into an invasive tissue known as a pannus. The pannus, composed primarily of synovial fibroblasts, secretes matrix metalloproteinases and other enzymes that erode cartilage and stimulate osteoclasts to erode bone. These processes produce the characteristic appearance of RA on plain radiographs of joint space narrowing and marginal erosions (**Figure 257-1**). Several cytokines, including

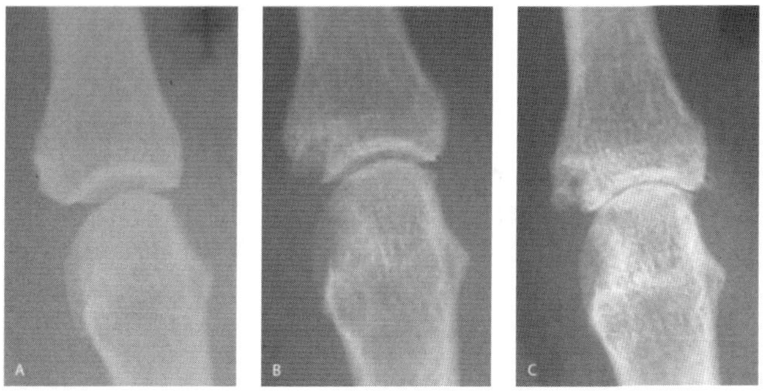

Figure 257-1 *Progressive destruction of a metacarpophalangeal joint by rheumatoid arthritis. Shown are sequential radiographs of the same second metacarpophalangeal joint. (A) The joint is normal one year prior to the development of rheumatoid arthritis. (B) Six months after the onset of rheumatoid arthritis, there is a bony erosion adjacent to the joint and joint space narrowing. (C) After three years of disease, diffuse loss of articular cartilage has led to marked joint space narrowing. (Reproduced, with permission, from Imboden J, Hellmann DB, Stone JH. Current Rheumatology Diagnosis & Treatment. 2nd ed. New York: McGraw-Hill, 2007. Fig. 15-3.)*

tumor necrosis factor-alpha (TNF-α), interleukin (IL)-1, IL-6, and IL-12, are elevated in rheumatoid arthritis joints. Each of these cytokines has been or is being studied as potential therapeutic targets for RA. Costimulation of T cells and B cells is important for maintenance of inflammation in RA, and drugs are approved to target this interaction. The mechanisms behind extra-articular manifestations of RA such as rheumatoid nodules, pulmonary, cardiac, and ocular involvement are not as well understood.

Spondyloarthropathies share some similar pathogenic mechanisms, as they are also responsive to agents that block TNF-α. These arthritides also feature erosion of bone at the joints. However, spondyloarthropathies are also characterized by bony proliferation in involved joints and the spine. In these diseases, there is significant dysregulation of bone remodeling, such that erosion and proliferation of bone may occur in different locations within the same joint. While the mechanisms of joint inflammation, pannus formation, and bone erosion in spondyloarthropathy are probably similar to those in RA, the bone proliferation is less well understood. Recent observational studies have shown that while TNF-α inhibitors decrease symptoms and inflammation in spondyloarthropathies, they do not halt bony ankylosis, which must therefore be mediated via different pathways.

DIFFERENTIAL DIAGNOSIS

NEW POLYARTHRITIS

Polyarthritis may be inflammatory or noninflammatory. In general, polyarthritis that warrants hospital admission is inflammatory. The differential diagnosis of new inflammatory polyarthritis includes not only rheumatic diseases, but also infections, neoplastic or paraneoplastic conditions, and drug reactions. Rheumatic diseases in the differential include RA, PsA, AS, undifferentiated spondyloarthropathy, polyarticular gout, pseudogout, sarcoidosis, and systemic lupus erythematosus (SLE).

Several infectious agents cause polyarthritis, either directly or indirectly (reactive arthritis). Bacterial infections with *Staphylococcus aureus*, group A and B streptococci, pneumococcus, and *Neisseria gonorrhoeae* may present with polyarthritis, usually in the setting of symptomatic or asymptomatic bacteremia with seeding of joints. Group A streptococcus can also cause poststreptococcal reactive arthritis, or less often acute rheumatic fever. Lyme arthritis due to *Borrelia burgdorferi* may present with intermittent inflammatory polyarthritis, or more commonly with persistent, usually monoarticular, inflammatory knee arthritis. Several viruses are associated with arthritis. Polyarthritis may be a presenting manifestation of hepatitis B, often with an urticarial rash. Hepatitis C and parvovirus B19 may mimic RA, presenting with symmetric polyarthritis and a false-positive RF. Tropical alphaviruses, such as Ross River virus, O'nyong-nyong, and Chikungunya, cause joint symptoms in most infected individuals that may persist for months. HIV may be associated with arthralgias and reactive arthritis. Bacteria can cause reactive arthritis as well, most commonly including *Chlamydia trachomatis*, *Ureaplasma urealyticum*, *Salmonella*, *Shigella*, *Yersinia*, and *Campylobacter* species; clinical features may include arthritis, urethritis, and uveitis.

Do not be fooled into thinking a hospitalized patient has RA based solely on a positive RF. Many infectious and inflammatory conditions, including infective endocarditis, tuberculosis, sarcoidosis, malignancies, and systemic lupus erythematosus and other autoimmune disorders also activate the immune system, and may result in a positive rheumatoid factor. In one study, 20% of patients with either untreated tuberculosis or *Klebsiella* bacteremia had positive IgM RF. Additionally, up to 55% of patients with hepatitis C infection have positive RF.

Some systemic findings may be seen in RA, although these are also seen in other conditions. Fever and leukocytosis can occur in RA, as may pulmonary and cardiac complications, including pleural effusions, pericardial effusion, and interstitial lung disease. Rheumatoid nodules occur in about 25% of RA patients, although they may not be present at the onset of RA. When present, rheumatoid nodules are associated with extra-articular disease. Fever and leukocytosis with polyarthritis may also occur with septic arthritis, viral-associated arthritis, crystal-induced arthritis, RA, adult-onset Still disease, and rare autoinflammatory conditions such as TNF receptor–associated periodic syndrome. Polyarthritis, high spiking fevers, pericarditis, neutrophilia, and an evanescent rash suggest adult-onset Still disease. Acute HIV infection or EBV infection can present with polyarthritis, fever, rash, and anemia. Systemic lupus erythematosus can cause polyarthritis; a complete blood count can help differentiate SLE from RA, as SLE is associated with cytopenias, while RA is associated with thrombocytosis and leukocytosis (and anemia). A positive antinuclear antibody (ANA) test is present in up to 30% of patients with RA. Polyarthritis accompanied by rapidly progressive interstitial lung disease, myositis, hyperkeratotic, fissuring rash, and Raynaud phenomenon is characteristic of the antisynthetase syndrome, a subset of dermatomyositis. Polyarthritis with fever may also be the presenting symptoms of sarcoidosis, which may be accompanied by erythema nodosum and hilar adenopathy.

Neoplastic processes should also be considered in the differential diagnosis of polyarthritis. Hematologic malignancies, chronic lymphocytic leukemia in particular, can induce secondary autoimmune phenomena.

DISTINGUISHING EXTRA-ARTICULAR DISEASE FROM COMPLICATIONS OF THERAPY

The patient's inflammatory disease history is somewhat predictive of the risk of extra-articular disease. A patient with well-controlled isolated articular disease in the past is less likely to have extra-articular disease than a patient with prior extra-articular disease. The intensity of immunosuppressive medication is also relevant. Several infectious processes can mimic extra-articular manifestations of RA, and vice versa.

The most common extra-articular manifestations of RA are rheumatoid nodules, secondary Sjögren syndrome, and pleural effusions. Less commonly, patients can develop pulmonary fibrosis, pulmonary nodules, and pericardial effusions. Felty syndrome (RA, neutropenia, and splenomegaly) used to occur in 1% of RA patients, and is now even rarer. Patients with RA are at increased risk for lymphoma. The risk of lymphoma correlates with the severity of RA disease activity, with an incidence ratio of 1.8 in individuals with RA compared to the general population. The risk does not appear to be significantly different among patients treated with different DMARD regimens. For many patients with seronegative spondyloarthropathies, arthritis is only a part of the disease. Many have associated inflammatory bowel disease, inflammatory eye disease, or psoriasis. Aortic insufficiency and apical pulmonary fibrosis are less common complications.

Febrile patients with RA should be aggressively investigated for infection. Fever related to active RA is generally low grade (≤ 38.5°C). Prior joint damage places RA patients at increased risk for septic arthritis: a tense effusion in one or more joints or a joint effusion accompanied by fever mandates diagnostic arthrocentesis. Treatment with TNF-α inhibitors increases the risk of skin infections, bacterial pneumonia, hepatitis B reactivation, and septic arthritis. Because TNF-α has a particular role in maintaining granuloma integrity, latent tuberculosis infection, and fungal infections such as histoplasmosis and coccidioidomycosis can reactivate in individuals treated with TNF-α inhibitors. In these patients, tuberculosis is often disseminated or extrapulmonary, and may present in an unfamiliar manner, as with septic arthritis or central nervous system involvement. The largest number of cases of TB in patients receiving biological agents has been reported in individuals receiving infliximab, followed by adalimumab, then etanercept. The risk of serious infection, including tuberculosis, also seems substantial with certolizumab. There are no reported cases of TB in individuals receiving abatacept or rituximab for treatment of RA. Although patients should be screened for TB before anti–TNF-α therapy, screening for TB is imperfect, and false-negative tests are common in patients with RA. Patients should also be screened for hepatitis B and C prior to starting TNF-α blockers or other DMARD therapy.

Pleural and pericardial effusions are occasionally seen in patients with RA. A pleural effusion should always be evaluated for infection, especially if the patient is taking DMARD therapy. TNF-α inhibitors can cause drug-induced lupus, usually manifesting as a rash with pleural or pericardial effusion.

Direct drug toxicity is a rare cause for admission of a patient with inflammatory arthritis. Methotrexate can cause significant anemia or other cytopenias in the setting of renal insufficiency. Mild elevations in transaminases occasionally occur with methotrexate, leflunomide, and other DMARDs. If significant elevations in aspartate aminotransferase or alanine aminotransferase are observed, both viral and autoimmune hepatitis must also be considered. More commonly, transaminase elevations in patients with inflammatory arthritis are attributable to NSAID use. Methotrexate may also cause hypersensitivity pneumonitis in up to 0.1% of treated patients. It is an idiosyncratic reaction that may occur any time during the course of therapy, most often during the first few months of therapy. The pneumonitis must be distinguished from pneumonia by bronchoscopy and biopsy, as it presents with dyspnea, cough, fever, and bilateral infiltrates on chest X-ray. There are case reports of hypersensitivity pneumonitis with leflunomide and sulfasalazine treatment.

DIAGNOSIS

NEW POLYARTICULAR ARTHRITIS

Even with advances in diagnostic testing and imaging, RA remains a clinical diagnosis, based on symptoms and examination findings, with laboratory and imaging studies as supporting evidence. Untreated patients with RA complain of morning stiffness involving numerous joints and muscle groups, lasting for at least an hour. RA is classically symmetric and leads to swelling and tenderness of the small joints of the hands, primarily the wrists, metacarpophalangeal joints, and proximal interphalangeal (PIP) joints (**Figure 257-2**).

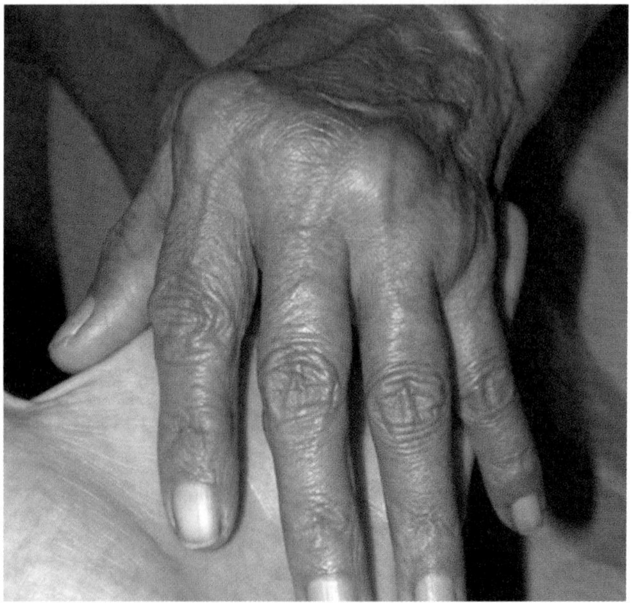

Figure 257-2 *Rheumatoid arthritis, with synovitis and ulnar deviation at the metacarpophalangeal (MCP) joints and atrophy of the interosseous muscles. (Used with permission from Richard P. Usatine. In: Usatine RP, Smith MA, Mayeaux EJ Jr, et al. Color Atlas of Family Medicine. New York: McGraw-Hill, 2009.)*

Other commonly involved joints include the knees, shoulders, ankles, hips, and metatarsophalangeal joints. If arthrocentesis is performed, the synovial fluid is inflammatory, generally with 2000 to 20,000 white blood cells/mm^3. Classification criteria for the diagnosis of RA were published in 1987 by the ACR. Although the 1987 criteria provided a helpful framework for clinicians to identify patients with RA, improved treatment modalities and initiation of treatment earlier in the disease meant that many individuals who received the diagnosis and were treated by rheumatologists never fulfilled four of the seven 1987 ACR criteria. Therefore, the ACR and EULAR (European League Against Rheumatism) in collaboration published new classification criteria in 2010 (**Table 257-1**). These criteria, like the 1987 criteria, were designed to identify patients with RA for inclusion in clinical trials. The 2010 criteria utilize a points system; an individual with ≥6 points is classified as having RA. Points are given based on number and distribution of involved joints, presence of RF or anti-CCP, elevated acute phase reactants, and duration of symptoms. The 2010 criteria include positive antibodies against citrullinated proteins (anti-cyclic citrullinated peptide or anti-CCP), which have a sensitivity of 67% and specificity of 95% for the diagnosis of RA. A specificity of 97% for the diagnosis of RA has been reported in patients with early inflammatory arthritis and both positive RF and anti-CCP antibody. Rheumatoid nodules and radiographic erosions are not part of the 2010 criteria, as patients with RA are ideally identified and treated before either of these manifestations occur.

RA is distinguished from osteoarthritis (OA) by history and physical examination. Patients with osteoarthritis classically experience less than an hour of morning stiffness in affected joints. They may have similar stiffness after prolonged recumbency (inactivity gel phenomenon). Osteoarthritis has a predilection for distal interphalangeal (DIP) joints, PIPs, and the first carpometacarpal joint (base of the thumb). Large joints including hips, knees, and shoulders are frequently involved, as is the lumbar spine. RA, in contrast, classically involves the synovial joint of C1-C2, sparing the remainder of the spine. On physical examination, patients with OA display bony enlargement with less synovial swelling in the small joints of the hands. Effusions of larger joints reveal noninflammatory synovial fluid (white blood cell [WBC] count < 2000/mm^3).

Seronegative spondyloarthropathy should be considered if the RF and anti-CCP are negative, or if polyarthritis is associated with sacroiliitis, urethritis, uveitis, psoriasis skin lesions, or a family history of HLA-B27 associated disorders. An international group has published criteria for the classification of PsA (**Table 257-2**), and the European Spondylarthropathy Study Group has published criteria

TABLE 257-1 Comparison of the 2010 American College of Rheumatology/European League Against Rheumatism (ACR/EULAR) and the 1987 ACR Classification Criteria for Rheumatoid Arthritis

2010 Criteria (points)	1987 Criteria
Synovitis of • 2–10 large joints (1) • 1–3 small joints (2) • 4–10 small joints (3) • > 10 joints (5)	• Arthritis of three or more joint areas • Arthritis of hand joints • Symmetric arthritis
Presence of rheumatoid factor or antibodies against citrullinated peptides • Either in low titer (2) • Either in high titer (3)	Presence of rheumatoid factor
Elevated sedimentation rate or c-reactive protein (1)	Not included
Duration of symptoms ≥ 6 weeks (1)	*Patient could not be classified as having RA unless symptoms present for more than 6 weeks*
Not included	Rheumatoid nodules
Not included	Morning stiffness
Not included	Radiographic changes (erosions, periarticular osteopenia)

Data from Aletaha D, et al. 2010 Rheumatoid arthritis classification criteria. *Arthritis Rheum.* 2010;62(9):2569–2581 and Arnett FC, et al. The American Rheumatism Association 1987 revised criteria for the classification of rheumatoid arthritis. *Arthritis Rheum.* 1988;31:315–324.

TABLE 257-2 Classification Criteria for Psoriatic Arthritis Study Group (CASPAR) Criteria for Psoriatic Arthritis

Criterion	Definition
1. Current psoriasis, personal history of psoriasis, or family history of psoriasis	Family history includes a first- or second-degree relative
2. Psoriatic nail changes	Onycholysis, pitting, or hyperkeratosis at the time of physical examination
3. Negative rheumatoid factor	According to local laboratory reference range
4. Dactylitis	Current swelling of an entire digit or history of dactylitis observed by a rheumatologist
5. Juxtaarticular new bone formation	Nonosteophytic, ill-defined ossification seen on plain radiographs of the hand or foot

Data from Taylor W, et al. Classification criteria for psoriatic arthritis: development of new criteria from a large international study. *Arthritis Rheum.* 2006;54:2665–2673.

TABLE 257-3 The European Spondyloarthropathy Study Group Criteria for Spondyloarthropathy

Inflammatory Spinal Pain *OR* Synovitis (asymmetric or primarily lower extremity)	
In the presence of one or more of the following:	
Manifestation	**Definition**
Family history	First- or second-degree relative with ankylosing spondylitis or psoriasis or uveitis or reactive arthritis or inflammatory bowel disease
Psoriasis	Previous or current
Inflammatory bowel disease	Ulcerative colitis or Crohn's disease
Urethritis/cervicitis or acute diarrhea	Non-gonococcal urethritis or cervicitis. Diarrhea ≤ 1 mo of arthritis onset
Alternating buttock pain	Pain in both right and left gluteal regions at different times
Enthesopathy	Tenderness at insertion of Achilles tendon or plantar fascia
Sacroiliitis	Unilateral or bilateral on plain radiograph

Data from Dougados M, et al. The European Spondylarthropathy Study Group preliminary criteria for the definition of spondylarthropathy. *Arthritis Rheum*. 1991;34:1218–1227.

for the classification of spondyloarthropathy (**Table 257-3**). These disorders resemble RA, in that morning stiffness lasts more than one hour and improves with activity. The spondyloarthropathies are all associated with sacroiliitis, which clinically manifests as buttock pain that improves with activity. Psoriatic arthritis generally involves peripheral joints with swelling, tenderness, and erythema. About 25% of people with psoriasis develop PsA, and the arthritis may precede skin disease. With current therapies, some patients with PsA never develop psoriasis, so it may be necessary to consult a rheumatologist if this diagnosis is in question. Clinical subsets of PsA presentations (from most to least common) include oligoarthritis, symmetric polyarthritis similar to RA, DIP-predominant disease, arthritis mutilans, and spondylitis (which may complicate each of the other types). While psoriatic arthritis, reactive arthritis, and other spondyloarthropathies classically involve unilateral sacroiliac joints, ankylosing spondylitis involves bilateral SI joints. An anterior-posterior view of the pelvis performed with the camera tilted 30° cephalad (Ferguson view) is the appropriate imaging study to evaluate for sacroiliitis.

KNOWN INFLAMMATORY ARTHRITIS

Pleural effusion

The most common extra-articular manifestation of RA requiring hospitalization is *pleural effusion*. Pleural disease in RA is more common in men than women, and is associated with seropositive disease. The annual incidence of pleural effusions in RA patients is 0.34% in women and 1.54% in men. About 25% of cases of pleural effusion with RA occur at the onset of joint disease. Pleural effusion is unilateral in more than 70% of cases; the left side is affected more often than the right. Clinically, affected patients may complain of pleuritic chest pain, dyspnea, and about a third have fever. Large pleural effusions must be distinguished from infectious or neoplastic effusions via thoracentesis. In RA, pleural effusions are exudative, with elevated LDH and a glucose level <60 mg/dL. Occasionally, these pleural effusions can mimic empyemas with pH <7.24, very low glucose (<40 mg/dL), LDH >Â700 U/L, but cultures are sterile. Pathology of pleural tissue shows a nodular appearance, sometimes characterized by multinucleated giant cells, but the pathology also resembles that of typical rheumatoid nodules, with palisading histiocytes around necrotic centers. RA is also associated with nodular lung disease, with rheumatoid nodules within the lung parenchyma; this must be distinguished from malignancy. RA is associated with slowly progressive pulmonary fibrosis. Rarely, patients develop pneumonitis that rapidly progresses to pulmonary fibrosis. Such presentations must be distinguished from drug-induced pneumonitis, which has been reported with methotrexate (up to 0.1–2% of treated patients), and less often leflunomide and sulfasalazine.

Rheumatoid vasculitis

Rheumatoid vasculitis historically affected about 1% of patients with seropositive RA. With the effectiveness of current therapies for RA, it has become even more unusual. Skin lesions of rheumatoid vasculitis include purpura, ulcers, and digital necrosis. Visceral organ involvement may include ischemic bowel, glomerulonephritis, myocardial infarction, cardiomyopathy, and pulmonary hemorrhage. Corneal ulcers and scleromalacia of the eye may occur. Patients may also present with rapidly progressive peripheral neuropathy or mononeuritis multiplex, which must be differentiated from other systemic necrotizing vasculitides such as polyarteritis nodosa or cryoglobulinemic vasculitis. Granulomatosis with polyanglitis (Wegener's) and microscopic polyangiitis must be considered when a patient presents with vasculitis and polyarthritis. When cutaneous manifestations are present, skin biopsy is helpful in diagnosis. With neuropathy, nerve conduction studies and nerve biopsies, particularly sural nerve biopsies, are useful diagnostic tools.

Inflammatory eye disease

Secondary Sjögren syndrome with dry eyes is common in RA, and in severe cases keratoconjunctivitis sicca may occur. Episcleritis and scleritis, including nodular scleritis, can also be manifestations of RA. Shirmer's test, a bedside measurement of tear production with filter paper, can be performed to screen for dry eye, but if keratoconjunctivitis sicca or corneal lesions are suspected, an ophthalmologist may perform rose bengal staining or a slit lamp examination.

HLA-B27 positivity is associated most commonly with uveitis (20–30%), and much less often with aortic insufficiency and apical pulmonary fibrosis.

Infection

With advances in the treatment of RA and spondyloarthropathies over the past two decades, hospitalization for disease activity is quite rare. More commonly, patients are admitted with infection. When pneumonia is detected in a patient with DMARD-treated inflammatory arthritis, both usual and unusual organisms should be considered. TNF-α inhibitors predispose patients to infections, most notably *Mycobacterium tuberculosis*, histoplasmosis, coccidioidomycosis, and aspergillosis, as well as typical and atypical bacterial pneumonia. DMARDs, particularly TNF-α inhibitors, methotrexate, and corticosteroids, also seem to increase susceptibility to *Pneumocystis jiroveci* pneumonia. Thus, especially when a patient fails to improve with treatment of usual community-acquired organisms, atypical infection should be considered in the differential diagnosis, and bronchoscopy pursued to identify the offending organism. Measurement of the serum beta-D-glucan is useful in the diagnosis of *Pneumocystis* in patients with suspicious interstitial infiltrates.

TRIAGE AND HOSPITAL ADMISSION

Hospital admission for treatment of inflammatory arthritis or disease complications is distinctly unusual. Rarely, an individual may be admitted for acute pain management during an arthritis flare if the patient or patient's family is unable to care for him or her at home. More often, patients present with complications that may relate to either the disease or its therapy. Pulmonary symptoms are a common reason for admission, as pneumonia is a frequent complication of DMARD therapy. Any inflammatory arthritis patient with a new oxygen requirement, rapidly progressive illness, failure to improve with oral antibiotic treatment, or a pleural effusion all warrant admission. With immunosuppressive therapy, atypical infections are an additional consideration, and a common infection may be more severe than in the general population.

Premature cardiovascular disease is characteristic in patients with inflammatory arthritis. Although this risk seems to be decreasing with TNF-α blocker therapy, this complication remains an important consideration. Recently, an association between psoriasis and metabolic syndrome, and thus cardiovascular disease, has been recognized. As with RA, the presence of psoriasis or other chronic inflammatory conditions may be independent risk factors for cardiovascular disease. Chest discomfort or exertional dyspnea should be thoroughly evaluated for possible cardiovascular etiologies in this patient population.

Any patient with a fused spine due to AS is at high risk for spinal fracture with trauma. Plain radiographs are insufficiently sensitive to detect fracture in this population, and computed tomography or magnetic resonance imaging must be used. Spinal fusion (**Figure 257-3**) may also result in cauda equina syndrome or atlantoaxial disease.

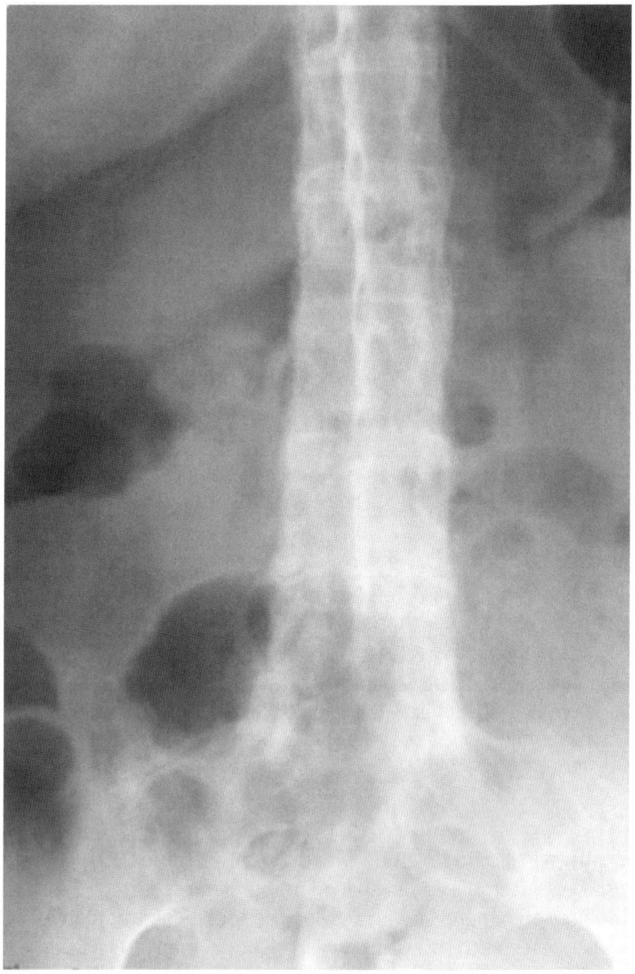

Figure 257-3 *Frontal view of the thoracolumbar spine showing the classic "bamboo" appearance of the spine in ankylosing spondylitis, resulting from fusion of the vertebral bodies and posterior elements. (Reproduced, with permission, Chen MYM, Pope TL Jr, Ott DJ. Basic Radiology. New York: McGraw-Hill, 2011. Fig. 7-45.)*

TREATMENT

INFLAMMATORY ARTHRITIS

The hospitalist should be familiar with the most common drugs used to treat inflammatory arthritis, their toxicities, and recommended monitoring. Although *nonsteroidal anti-inflammatory drugs (NSAIDs)* are less central to RA management than in the past, they are still used for breakthrough joint pain as needed. NSAIDs are associated with gastrointestinal tract bleeding, especially when combined with corticosteroids. NSAIDs may also exacerbate inflammatory bowel disease. Because of evidence linking NSAIDs to stroke and myocardial infarction, these drugs should be prescribed with caution in patients with RA due to the substantial baseline risk for cardiovascular disease in this population.

Low-dose corticosteroids (eg, prednisone 5–10 mg daily) are frequently taken by patients with RA when other DMARDs either fail to control the disease or are contraindicated. Due to complications such as hyperglycemia, osteoporosis, and cataracts, the lowest possible dose is desirable. Moderate doses can be used to treat flares of inflammatory arthritis; prednisone 20 to 30 mg daily for three to five days is usually sufficient to control an acute exacerbation of RA. This dose can then be tapered in 5 to 10 mg decrements over about two weeks.

Most patients with RA are treated with DMARDs (**Table 257-4**). *Methotrexate* is the most common initial therapy prescribed worldwide for moderately to severely active RA. Methotrexate is also an anchor therapy for PsA, and is used for other spondyloarthropathies and inflammatory bowel disease. However, it has not been shown to be effective for isolated axial disease in AS. Methotrexate is usually prescribed in doses between 10 and 25 mg as a single weekly dose for autoimmune and inflammatory diseases. Folic acid (1 mg) is concurrently administered daily. Folic acid minimizes side effects, such as oral ulcers and nausea, and may also decrease the risk of methotrexate hepatic toxicity. For patients with moderate to severely active arthritis, *leflunomide* may be used as an alternative to methotrexate, and occasionally in combination with methotrexate. Leflunomide is approved for use in rheumatoid arthritis, but has also been studied for PsA and psoriasis, and shown to be effective for both conditions. Leflunomide is Category X for pregnancy, and is thus rarely prescribed for women of childbearing potential. Other oral DMARDs, such as *azathioprine* and *cyclosporine*, are currently infrequently used for RA due to the improved efficacy and better side effect profile of biologic DMARDs. Cholestyramine is an antidote to leflunomide, and is administered at 8 mg three times daily for 11 days. Levels of leflunomide are reduced substantially within 48 hours of cholestyramine treatment.

Patients with mild to moderate RA are often treated with *hydroxychloroquine* or *sulfasalazine*. There are also often effective for the spondyloarthropathies, particularly for peripheral joint disease. These medications are taken daily, and are anti-inflammatory but not immunosuppressive. They may be given in combination with other oral or biologic DMARDs in more severe disease.

Today, there are nine *biologic therapies* approved for the treatment of moderately to severely active RA (**Table 257-5**). Five of these are anti–TNF-α therapies. Infliximab, adalimumab, and golimumab are all monoclonal antibodies against TNF-α. Infliximab is a chimeric antibody (murine variable region and human constant region), while

TABLE 257-4 Disease-Modifying Antirheumatic Drugs

Agent	Potential Toxicities	Monitoring
NSAIDs	GI bleeding, renal failure	Yearly CBC, Cr, LFTs
Hydroxychloroquine	Macular damage	Funduscopic exam and visual fields every 6–12 mo
Sulfasalazine	Myelosuppression, especially if G6PD deficient	CBC every 2–4 wk first 3 mo, then every 3 mo
Methotrexate	Myelosuppression, hepatic fibrosis, pneumonitis	CBC, LFTs, Cr every 4–12 wk
Leflunomide	Myelosuppression, acute hepatic failure	CBC, hepatic function, Cr every 4 wk for first 6 mo, then every 8–12 wk
Corticosteroids	Hyperglycemia, hypertension, osteoporosis, cataracts	Yearly urinalysis for glucose. DXA every 2 y if doses ≥ 5 mg daily

CBC, complete blood count; Cr, creatinine; DXA, bone mineral density measured by dual-energy X-ray absorptiometry scan/bone mineral density; G6PD, glucose-6-phosphate dehydrogenase; LFTs, liver function tests including aspartate aminotransferase, alanine aminotransferase, albumin.

adalimumab and golimumab are humanized antibodies. Infliximab is given by infusion at four to eight week intervals, adalimumab is administered subcutaneously at one to two week intervals, and golimumab is given subcutaneously every four weeks. Certolizumab pegol is a variable region of a humanized anti–TNF-α that is PEGylated to increase the biologic half-life. It is given by subcutaneous injection every four weeks. Etanercept is a dimeric fusion protein of a region of the human TNF-α receptor complexed to human immunoglobulin heavy chains. It is given subcutaneously once or twice weekly. Infliximab, adalimumab, etanercept, and golimumab are approved for treatment of RA, PsA, and AS. Infliximab, adalimumab, and certolizumab pegol are also approved for Crohn disease, which can be associated with spondyloarthropathy. Anti–TNF-α therapy is contraindicated in patients with acute systolic dysfunction, and must be used with extreme caution in patients with heart failure.

The four other approved biologic therapies each have different mechanisms of action. Anakinra is IL-1 receptor antagonist. Abatacept is a chimeric protein consisting of an immunoglobulin fused to the extracellular domain of cytotoxic T-lymphocyte antigen 4 (CTLA4). It acts by binding to antigen-presenting cells, and blocking the co-stimulatory signal necessary for T-cell activation. Rituximab is an anti-CD20 antibody, which is thought to act in RA by decreasing B-cell stimulation of T-cell–mediated inflammation in RA. Tocilizumab is an antibody against the IL-6 receptor, thus blocking the activity of IL-6, a cytokine important in the inflammatory response in RA.

SYSTEMIC MANIFESTATIONS

A rheumatoid pleural effusion that requires hospitalization and thoracentesis is generally treated with oral prednisone at 0.5 to 1 mg/kg daily for one to two weeks, then tapered over the next two to three months. Recurrent rheumatoid pleural effusions are sometimes treated with intrapleural corticosteroids. Small pleural effusions may not require any therapy.

Inflammatory eye disease is initially treated with topical steroids. In uveitis related to spondyloarthropathy, oral NSAIDs may be effective if no contraindications exist. Refractory or severe cases may be treated with oral prednisone in high doses (0.5–1 mg/kg daily), intravitreal corticosteroid injection, or DMARD therapy such as methotrexate, azathioprine, or mycophenolate mofetil. Infliximab is also used for inflammatory eye disease in the spondyloarthropathies.

Rheumatoid vasculitis is generally treated first with pulse-dose methylprednisolone (1 g intravenously daily for 3–5 days), followed by oral prednisone 1 mg/kg divided twice daily. Such treatment is generally accompanied by cyclophosphamide, as used for other forms of systemic necrotizing vasculitis.

PERIOPERATIVE MANAGEMENT

Many patients with inflammatory arthritis are treated chronically with corticosteroids. Patients taking more than the equivalent of 7.5 mg of prednisone daily for more than two weeks are at risk for adrenal insufficiency. A recent meta-analysis examined the question of whether stress doses of corticosteroids were necessary when patients treated chronically with corticosteroids (up to 15 mg prednisone daily) undergo surgery. The analysis found that acute adrenal insufficiency did not occur if the usual dosage of steroids was given daily, including on the day of surgery. The authors recommended that patients receiving long-term, low-dose corticosteroid therapy be carefully monitored intraoperatively, with "rescue" intravenous hydrocortisone given if the hemodynamic status declines.

TABLE 257-5 Biologic Disease-Modifying Antirheumatic Drugs

Agent	Description	Disease Indication	Administration
Adalimumab	Anti–TNF-α antibody	RA, JIA, PsA, PsO, AS, CD	Subcutaneous every 2 wk
Etanercept	Anti–TNF-α fusion protein	RA, PsA, AS, JIA, PsO	Subcutaneous weekly
Golimumab	Anti–TNF-α antibody	Ra, PsA, AS	Subcutaneous monthly
Infliximab	Anti–TNF-α antibody	RA, JIA, PsA, PsO, AS, CD, PCD, UC	Intravenous every 4–8 wk
Certolizumab pegol	PEGylated anti–TNF-α variable region	RA, CD	Subcutaneous monthly
Anakinra	IL1 receptor antagonist	RA	Subcutaneous daily
Abatacept	CTLA4-Ig	RA, JIA	Intravenous every 4 wk
Rituximab	Anti-CD20 antibody	RA, NHL, CLL	Intravenous, 2 doses 14 days apart, repeated in 6 mo
Tocilizumab	Anti–IL-6 antibody	RA	Intravenous monthly

AS, ankylosing spondylitis; CD, Crohn disease; CLL, chronic lymphocytic leukemia; JIA, juvenile idiopathic arthritis; NHL, non-Hodgkin lymphoma; PCD, pediatric Crohn disease; PsA, psoriatic arthritis; PsO, plaque psoriasis; RA, rheumatoid arthritis; UC, ulcerative colitis.

Regarding other DMARDs, a primarily European multinational group recently published a compilation of recommendations, based on literature review and expert opinion. The group recommends continuing methotrexate during the perioperative period, as a grade B recommendation with level 1b evidence (Oxford levels of evidence). There are no firm guidelines for the perioperative management of anti–TNF-α therapy. As the incidence of perioperative infection for orthopedic surgical procedures is low, it is probably not feasible to answer this question in an adequately-powered randomized controlled trial. In arthritis patients, the risk of withdrawing biologic therapy is that the inflammatory arthritis will flare, impeding rehabilitation and potentially requiring corticosteroids for treatment (perioperative corticosteroids are known to impair wound healing and increase the risk of wound infection). The risk of continuing biologic therapy is of perioperative infection, and skin infections in particular are increased with use of anti–TNF-α therapies. In inflammatory bowel disease, a recent cohort study did not find any difference in the risks of perioperative complications whether infliximab was given more or less than 12 weeks before surgery. For arthritis patients, practices vary by site, but many practitioners err on the side of caution, presuming that the risk of substantial morbidity resulting from perioperative infection outweighs the risk of flare of RA. Many practitioners hold anti–TNF-α therapy for one to two weeks prior to surgery and restart treatment after the skin has healed.

Individuals with RA may have atlantoaxial (C1-C2) inflammatory arthritis of the spine. Plain radiographs of the cervical spine in flexion and extension should be obtained preoperatively to ensure stability at this joint. Instability puts the patient at risk for spinal cord injury during cervical hyperextension, so an experienced anesthesiologist should perform intubation. Similarly, a patient with AS requiring surgery will require careful intubation and positioning to protect the spine.

COMPLICATIONS

As noted above, patients with RA are at high risk of cardiovascular disease, which is the most common cause of death in these patients, and they are also predisposed to congestive heart failure. Chest pain, exertional symptoms, or other symptoms suggestive of cardiovascular disease must be investigated in all hospitalized patients with a history of inflammatory arthritis.

The primary disease-related complications of RA are anemia of chronic disease, secondary Sjögren syndrome, ocular inflammation, pleural disease, atlantoaxial subluxation, and atlantoaxial impaction (cranial settling). Most other complications are related to treatment, rather than the disease itself. Complications of spondyloarthropathies include associated inflammatory bowel disease, uveitis, aortic insufficiency, or pulmonary fibrosis (in HLA-B27 positive patients), as well as treatment-related complications.

Many patients with RA are treated with glucocorticoids. If used during hospitalization, hyperglycemia should be anticipated and blood glucose levels monitored. When planning anti-hyperglycemic therapy, recall that blood glucose peaks about six to eight hours after an oral dose of prednisone. Patients should be given clear instructions for insulin dosing during corticosteroid tapers to avoid hypoglycemia as well.

Glucocorticoid-induced osteoporosis is a potentially avoidable complication of RA therapy. Bone loss occurs very rapidly with glucocorticoids. RA itself is an independent risk factor for osteoporosis, and glucocorticoids worsen this risk. All patients treated with oral steroids should receive calcium plus vitamin D (600 mg/400 IU) twice daily. A 25-hydroxyvitamin D level should be checked, and vitamin D supplemented as indicated. The ACR recommends that all patients who will receive glucocorticoids be assessed for their risk of osteoporosis. Lifestyle factors must be addressed first, and preventive pharmacotherapy begun if indicated.

There is currently inadequate data to guide the use of prophylaxis against *Pneumocystis jiroveci* pneumonia (PCP) in patients with rheumatologic disease. The only definite recommendation for routine prophylaxis is during treatment of granulomatosis with polyanglitis (Wegener's). There are reports of individuals with RA developing PCP in the setting of low-dose methotrexate therapy, but the exact incidence is unknown. Most reports are in association with biologic therapies, including infliximab, adalimumab, and rituximab. One report described 84 cases of PCP in RA patients treated with infliximab reported through the FDA Adverse Event Reporting System over a five-year period. Most cases occurred within the first one to two months after starting infliximab therapy. However, this report did not recommend routine prophylaxis. Instead, PCP should be in the differential diagnosis when a patient treated with DMARD therapy presents with bilateral pulmonary infiltrates and dyspnea.

Amyloidosis was seen in years past as a complication of chronic inflammation in RA, but with early, effective DMARD therapy, this is now rare. It is generally only seen in older patients with very advanced disease.

DISCHARGE PLANNING

How DMARD therapy will be managed upon discharge is crucial. Most DMARDs, including biologic therapies, have long biologic half-lives. It is an error to assume that since the patient's arthritis did not flare during hospitalization, the patient does not require DMARD therapy. Due to the long half-life of DMARD therapy, patients do not usually experience disease flare until medications have been held for more than two weeks. Thus, one should plan for either reinitiation of therapy after discharge, or commencement of an alternative therapy. For many patients, hydroxychloroquine may be considered during hospitalization as a nonimmunosuppressive DMARD. However, hydroxychloroquine takes several weeks to start having a noticeable anti-inflammatory effect. If restarting DMARD therapy is a significant concern, the patient should follow up with his or her rheumatologist within one to two weeks of hospital discharge to reassess disease activity and plan future arthritis treatment.

In the rare circumstance of a patient admitted for treatment of RA, physical therapy is an important component of care during and after the hospitalization. Even if a patient is hospitalized for a complication of RA therapy, continuing physical therapy to ensure that they are undertaking supervised activity while in the hospital is prudent.

In patients who undergo joint replacement or other surgery, restarting interrupted DMARD therapy is very important. The patient should follow up with the surgeon regarding wound healing, and DMARD therapy should be restarted within two weeks after surgery except in unusual circumstances. If DMARD therapy cannot be restarted due to problems with wound healing, then the patient should follow up with the rheumatologist to ensure that the patient's joint pain is adequately managed until DMARD therapy can be restarted.

QUALITY IMPROVEMENT

Suggested targets for quality improvement in hospital-based RA care include the following:

- **Prevention of glucocorticoid-induced osteoporosis:** Ensuring that patients are started on a bisphosphonate with appropriate calcium and vitamin D supplements when starting glucocorticoid therapy.
- **Prevention of atherosclerotic disease:** Ensuring that antihypertensive therapy is titrated to maintain blood pressure at

levels under 130/80 during hospitalization; initiating or adjusting cholesterol lowering therapy to meet a target LDL of less than 100 mg/dL; helping patients develop a smoking cessation strategy that may help reduce their risk of cardiovascular disease, and improve their quality of life through improved arthritis control (active cigarette smoking impairs the response to therapy in RA).

- **DMARD therapy:** Ensuring that each patient has a plan for ongoing management of RA or other inflammatory arthritis, including timely resumption of DMARD therapy if this is stopped because of acute infection or surgery.
- **Preventing infections:** Obtaining an immunization history and arranging appropriate immunizations; administering pneumovax and annual influenza vaccines (patients on DMARDs should not receive live vaccines, such as the nasal live attenuated influenza vaccine). Some studies have shown decreased responsiveness to vaccinations in patients treated with anti–TNF-α therapy, but that should not be seen as a deterrent to giving appropriate immunizations.

CONCLUSION

Since current DMARD therapy is so effective, patients with RA and other inflammatory arthritides are rarely admitted to the hospital for management of articular disease. Occasionally a patient develops an extra-articular manifestation of disease that requires hospitalization, usually a pleural effusion associated with RA. Immunosuppressive DMARD therapies are very effective for controlling inflammation, and also predispose individuals to infections. Such infections may be atypical and can present in unusual ways, so the clinician must have a high suspicion for infection in these patients. In the hospital setting, it may be most appropriate to withhold DMARD therapy from acutely ill patients. DMARD therapy should also be held perioperatively when possible. In order to avoid flares of inflammatory arthritis that might require glucocorticoid treatment, a plan must be made in coordination with patients' rheumatologist to manage the underlying inflammatory disease upon discharge.

SUGGESTED READINGS

Balbir-Gurman A, Yigla M, Nahir AM, Braun-Moscovici Y. Rheumatoid pleural effusion. *Semin Arthritis Rheum.* 2006;35:368–378.

Bongartz T. Elective orthopedic surgery and perioperative DMARD management: many questions, fewer answers, and some opinions. *J Rheumatol.* 2007;34:653–635.

Bongartz T, Cantaert T, Atkins SR, Harle P, Myers JL, Turesson C, et al. Citrullination in extra-articular manifestations of rheumatoid arthritis. *Rheumatology (Oxford).* 2007;46:70–75.

Nishimura K, Sugiyama D, Kogata Y, Tsuji G, Nakazawa T, Kawano S, et al. Meta-analysis: diagnostic accuracy of anti-cyclic citrullinated peptide antibody and rheumatoid factor for rheumatoid arthritis. *Ann Intern Med.* 2007;146:797–808.

Taylor W, Gladman D, Helliwell P, Marchesoni A, Mease P, Mielants H. Classification criteria for psoriatic arthritis: development of new criteria from a large international study. *Arthritis Rheum.* 2006;54:2665–2673.

Watts RA, Mooney J, Lane SE, Scott DG. Rheumatoid vasculitis: becoming extinct? *Rheumatology (Oxford).* 2004;43:920–923.

Wolfe F, Caplan L, Michaud K. Treatment for rheumatoid arthritis and the risk of hospitalization for pneumonia: associations with prednisone, disease-modifying antirheumatic drugs, and anti-tumor necrosis factor therapy. *Arthritis Rheum.* 2006;54: 628–634.

Wolfe F, Michaud K. The effect of methotrexate and anti-tumor necrosis factor therapy on the risk of lymphoma in rheumatoid arthritis in 19,562 patients during 89,710 person-years of observation. *Arthritis Rheum.* 2007;56:1433–1439.

CHAPTER 258

Physical Therapy and Rehabilitation

Thomas E. McNalley, MD
Christopher J. Standaert, MD

Key Clinical Questions

1. What are the roles of physical and occupational therapy in the inpatient setting?
2. When should I consult a physical or occupational therapist?
3. What is a physiatrist? What role does he or she play in the care of hospitalized patients, and how does it differ from the role of the hospitalist?
4. How can rehabilitation services assist in discharge planning?

INTRODUCTION

Physical therapists (PTs) and occupational therapists (OTs) address the functional needs of patients through mobilization, conditioning, and training in self-care, and other specific tasks. PTs and OTs practice in many settings, including the hospital, clinic, skilled nursing facility (SNF), long-term care facility, freestanding inpatient intensive rehabilitation center, and home. A smaller number also practice in emergency departments in the assessment and treatment of musculoskeletal injury. Less heralded is the role that PTs and OTs play in minimizing specific in-hospital complications, and optimizing successful transitions to outpatient care. Given the growing economic pressures on hospitals, including nonpayment for some nosocomial complications or for rapid readmission to the hospital after discharge ("bounce-backs"), PTs and OTs are not only crucial in helping patients regain functional capacity, but are also vital to the financial well-being of inpatient hospitals. Unfortunately, the scope of practice of PTs and OTs often lies beyond the focus of physicians. Medical education often underemphasizes the role of allied health providers and their contributions to restoring health and function. This chapter attempts to correct this underexposure by delineating the roles and responsibilities of these therapists, and indicating their impact on specific diagnoses commonly encountered by the hospitalist.

CASE 258-1

AN ICU TRANSFER TO THE MEDICAL SERVICE AFTER A DEBILITATING MEDICAL ILLNESS

A 53-year-old previously healthy male, with a past medical history of stage 1 hypertension, developed a febrile illness over several days, and collapsed at his small business. The emergency medical technicians successfully resuscitate him and he is admitted to the intensive care unit. Over a period of four weeks he has a complicated course including prolonged intubation necessitating tracheostomy placement due to respiratory failure from community-acquired methicillin-resistant *Staphylococcus aureus* (MRSA) pneumonia, encephalopathy attributed to delirium from the acute illness, acute renal failure requiring dialysis, and demand ischemia characterized by an elevated troponin without ECG changes. Ultimately, the patient stabilizes and is transferred to the general medical service after tracheostomy and placement of a percutaneous endoscopic gastrostomy (PEG) tube for nutrition. Communication is difficult due to the tracheostomy. Overnight he becomes agitated and receives haloperidol. He requires suctioning every one to two hours, and is not yet ready for discharge to a hospital-level rehabilitation facility. On rounds he appears agitated when he requires suctioning. Assessing mental status is difficult due to tracheostomy, and he does not appear to respond to commands optimally.

Although this patient clearly requires acute medical treatment, how can you improve this individual's level of functioning within the framework of his illness? What steps can you take to fast track him to a rehabilitation facility so that he can receive the complex multidisciplinary care he needs to ultimately return home to his family and maybe even return to work?

If available, early consultation with a physiatrist can be instrumental to:

- Reduce the complications that he has already experienced during his hospitalization
- Improve physical and social function
- Identify cognitive and emotional complications of traumatic brain injury (even if not physically apparent by head CT)
- Concentrate coordinated therapy
- Improve the likelihood that this patient may eventually go home.

For this patient, a physiatry consultation assisted the team in properly diagnosing and treating his agitation, which was initially assumed to be due to a combination of delirium and inability to communicate when he needed suctioning. The physiatrist, however, identifed that he had cognitive and emotional complications analagous to patients who had suffered traumatic brain injury while he was in the intensive care unit. The physiatrist made specific pharmacologic recommendations, engaged the family who had not visited him, coordinated the care of physical therapy, occupational therapy, speech therapy, and communicated with a rehabilitation facility best able to meet his complex needs. Due to the physiatrist's intervention, the patient was fast-tracked to a rehabilitation center, which gave him the greatest chance of achieving functional recovery.

PHYSICAL THERAPY

Physical therapists have completed four years of postgraduate training, with a focus in musculoskeletal assessment and treating impairments of mobility and safety. Although they most actively provide care for orthopedic and neurosurgical patients, they also clinically assess patients with medical problems such as breathing dysfunction, the need for cardiac rehabilitation, and chronic vertigo. For example, patients with respiratory disease often are readmitted due to exacerbations of their chronic disease. PTs focus on breathing, posture, mobility, range of motion of joints, and strengthening of the respiratory muscles, and they use physical modalities for those patients with musculoskeletal derangements in the thoracic or rib area. On a busy medical service, PTs can guard against the sequelae of long-term hospitalization by improving the patient's ability to move within a bed, and progress from supine to sitting, sitting to standing, and finally to ambulation. PTs use a review of the medical record, the history provided by the patient and family, and a focused musculoskeletal examination to identify deformities, atrophy, limitations in range of motion (ROM), weakness, and functional impairments that can be addressed with various interventions. They also provide a wide range of tests and measurements.

Hospitalists find PTs helpful in many areas, but may not request their services until the time of discharge, when the therapist is urgently requested to "assess for home safety." Involving the therapist as early as possible is ideal, since early interventions may decrease the length of hospital stay and increase the likelihood of the patient being discharged directly to home. As well, the patient's mood, appetite, sense of well-being, and general medical condition may all benefit from increased activity.

PT interventions may be educational, such as teaching a patient how to safely roll in bed to allow nursing care, or they can be more complex, including moving from supine to sitting, evaluating and improving sitting balance, and progressing to standing while monitoring for hemodynamic changes. Once upright, the patient may be able to ambulate, and the therapist can recommend assistive devices such as canes or walkers. For those patients with neurologic or musculoskeletal disorders, new impairments of gait may require further training, and occasionally the use of lower-extremity bracing with orthoses. If the patient is unable to reliably stand or walk or lacks adequate endurance, he or she may need a wheelchair. The power wheelchair and the much-promoted power scooter allow greater mobility, with the loss of the aerobic challenge of self-propulsion. In the United States, Medicare will often cover part of the cost of powered mobility devices in patients who meet certain criteria.

A common concern in patients with neuromuscular dysfunction is the risk of joint contractures. Up to 39% of patients who stay in the intensive care unit (ICU) for longer than two weeks develop at least one joint contracture. A stay of eight weeks in the ICU increases the odds ratio of contracture to 7.09, compared with patients staying two to three weeks. Joint contractures may result in pain, permanent deformity, gait abnormality, and loss of mobility. Contractures also predispose the patient to skin breakdown. Prevention is again best facilitated by early PT consultation. Stretching, strengthening, and protective splints all reduce the likelihood of plantar flexion deformity and other lower-extremity contractures. OTs usually address concerns with the upper extremity, as discussed below.

The PT may help prevent and treat skin injury by ensuring adequate movement to reduce the risk of decubitus ulcers, protect surgical incisions and skin grafts, and reduce discomfort from malpositioning or immobility. The therapist may also instruct the patient about the avoidance of faulty transfer techniques or seating arrangements that may lead to shear injuries to the skin.

Falls, and the fear of falling, contribute to morbidity both in and out of the hospital. In the debilitated elderly, falls may lead to fractures, especially of the hips and forearms, or intracranial pathology, including subdural hematomas. Fear of falls may lead to a downward spiral of immobility and progressive weakness that actually increase the risk of falls. Prevention should begin in the hospital. The PT can assess fall risk using the Berg Balance Scale, and intervene as needed. For some patients, simple reminders and strengthening are adequate protection; for others, an assistive device may suffice. Still others may require intervention in an intensive, interdisciplinary rehabilitation environment. Patients in the latter group usually need evaluation by a physiatrist prior to transfer to in-patient rehabilitation.

OCCUPATIONAL THERAPY

The title "occupational therapist" may confuse both patients and other health care professionals. An occupation is defined as a job or profession, but in OT it is defined as a task or activity fulfilled in daily life. OTs focus on restoring patients to their basic self-care, and ideally to independent living. Like the PT, OTs have completed four years of postgraduate training, but with a special focus on assessing, preserving, and restoring upper-extremity strength, function, and ROM. Some undergo additional training to become certified hand therapists. OT interventions include stretching and ROM exercises. Bracing and splinting may be recommended for patients with increased upper-extremity tone from neurologic disease, or scarring from burns that place them at risk for joint contracture. OTs participate in identifying postdischarge needs, and in some hospitals, they perform home-safety evaluations by observing patients in typical tasks done at home, such as cooking a meal. As with physical therapy, the wise clinician will involve OT early in the hospitalization.

SPEECH THERAPY

The ability to swallow or eat affects nutritional status and also quality of life. Many conditions increase the risk of swallow disorders, which are more common in the elderly (**Table 258-1**).

As part of the functional assessment of patients at admission, hospitalists should evaluate for the possibility of a dysphagia disorder. Family members may be the first to suspect a problem. Recurrent pneumonias, malnutrition, and social isolation may be important clues that a problem exists (**Table 258-2**).

TABLE 258-1 Risk Factors for Dysphagia

Complications of Hospitalization
• Intubation • Deconditioning • Medications (including anesthesia, opioids, sedatives, some antibiotics, carbidopa-levodopa) • Delirium
Disorders
• Cancer (especially head and neck) • Stroke, neurodegenerative • Burns and trauma • Diabetes • Cardiac dysfunction • Chronic obstructive pulmonary disorder • Cervical hypertrophic osteoarthropathy (encroachment of osteophytes at the C-6 cricoid cartilage)

Adapted from Cynthia J. Brown, Claire Peel, "Rehabilitation", in *Hazzard's Geriatric Medicine and Gerontology*, 6th ed. New York, McGraw-Hill, 2009.

The role of the speech and language pathologist is to diagnose swallowing disorders, make treatment recommendations, and coordinate an interdisciplinary approach with the health care team, including nurses, respiratory therapists, physical therapists, and nutritionists, as well as educating the patient and family. The speech therapist performs a bedside swallowing assessment unless there are contraindications. Examples that would require postponement of an evaluation include inability to cooperate because of an unstable medical condition such as active gastrointestinal bleeding or respiratory distress, inability to maintain upright or side-lying at 90 degrees, unexplained sudden change in temperature, active ventilator weaning, or altered mental status. If the bedside evaluation is inconclusive, nothing by mouth is recommended until a complete evaluation can be performed under video-fluoroscopy. This study examines the oral, pharyngeal, and esophageal stages of ingestion, and should be able to identify if there is aspiration, or significant risk of aspiration, below the level of the vocal cords. It may also evaluate whether the compensatory swallowing techniques are effective in preventing aspiration. Speech and language pathologists may recommend specific techniques to reduce the risk of aspiration such as head posture (chin tuck, turning head to weaker or stronger side, tilting head backward), body posture (upright at 90 degrees, lying on one side between feedings rather than supine), and manner of oral intake (rate, consistency, sizes, liquids by spoon).

PHYSIATRY

A rehabilitation physician, or physiatrist, is a specialist in physical medicine and rehabilitation (PM&R). Physiatry has been recognized as a specialty by the American Medical Association since 1946. The original impetus for growth of the field was the demand for sophisticated rehabilitation techniques for the large influx of injured soldiers returning from World War II. Physiatrists concentrate on the ability of patients to function optimally within the limitations placed upon them by disease processes for which there may not be a cure. A team approach to chronic conditions is emphasized to coordinate care by building on and strengthening the resources of the person and family, providing for a facilitating environment, and developing performance goals in that environment.

TABLE 258-2 Indications for Swallowing Evaluation

Any patient with:
• Past medical history of reported dysphagia symptoms • Observed dysphagia • Suspected aspiration • Decreased oral feeding, dehydration, malnutrition • Parenteral or enteral feeding • Intubation, tracheostomy, or ventilator weaning • Vocal cord paresis, paralysis, or laryngospasm • Deconditioning

TABLE 258-3 Common Indications for Physiatry Consultation

Amputation
Spinal cord injury
Stroke, in conjunction with speech therapists, recreational therapists, physical therapists, and occupational therapists
Traumatic brain injury
Medical patients requiring complex rehabilitation
Musculoskeletal syndromes: low back pain, fibromyalgia
Chronic pain management, in conjunction with psychologists, physical therapists, occupational therapists, chiropractors, and anesthesiologists with expertise in pain management and interventional procedures

A PM&R residency includes training in spinal cord injury, brain injury, stroke, neuromuscular disease, and musculoskeletal injury, as well as the performance of electrodiagnostic studies and the assessment of neuromusculoskeletal impairment. A physiatrist can help determine why a patient is weak, distinguishing between critical illness neuromyopathy, steroid myopathy, and other causes of debility in a patient. They can evaluate patients with specific impairments and can recommend orthoses, bracing, or other assistive devices to improve mobility, and provide recommendations for formal physical or occupational therapy, as well as weight-bearing and fall precautions. Physiatrists work closely with PTs, OTs, speech-language pathologists, and allied providers in the coordinated delivery of multidisciplinary care. They often oversee the rehabilitation process, and work with hospitalists to ensure that care is appropriate for the medical context (**Table 258-3**).

REHABILITATION

The definition of *rehabilitation* by the World Health Organization is "the use of all means aimed at reducing the impact of disabling and handicapping conditions and at enabling people with disabilities to achieve optimal social integration."

Acute rehabilitation refers to treatment that occurs within the first month of illness once the patient has been resuscitated or received definitive care, and by definition involves more acute medical or surgical issues than postacute rehabilitation.

Rehabilitation begins with improving mobility by getting the patient out of bed. Depending on the underlying condition of the patient, this may begin immediately, or be delayed for weeks with patients with spine injuries. Patients with upper-extremity injuries will need to learn how to get out of bed without using that arm, and require forearm supports on ambulatory assistive devices. If the lower extremity is affected, the patient must learn how to get out of bed while elevating the injured leg. Walking with a walker or crutches for patients with reduced or no weight-bearing requires 30–50% more energy compared with normal walking. For patients with decreased cardiopulmonary reserve, this can be especially challenging. For patients with preexisting impaired mobility, the goal of rehabilitation is to return the patient to functional status prior to the injury. As the patient regains mobility, rehabilitation also addresses motion of the affected joint(s) with the goal of regaining range of motion. The next step of rehabilitation is to improve motor control and coordination so that the patient will eventually be able to exercise. Strengthening exercises with progressive resistive exercises can then begin. Finally, rehabilitation helps patients and families adapt to permanent impairments.

Rehabilitation is provided at different levels with a hierarchy of interventions depending on the complexity of the patient's problems and needs. The lowest level of consultation in the hospital setting is a single therapeutic intervention by PT or OT, such as a PT safety assessment for home discharge, or to identify postdischarge needs for PT and OT. Other patients with complex needs may require continued acute hospitalization for active and potentially unstable conditions. Still other patients who have complex disabilities as a consequence of an acute injury, stroke, or medical conditions or an acute event in a patient with prior disabilities, such as multiple sclerosis, benefit from high-level rehabilitation. Complex rehabilitation requires the involvement of at least three specialists such as gait retraining, continence management, and speech therapy.

To qualify for a rehabilitation hospital, patients generally carry a "rehab diagnosis"—stroke or traumatic brain injury or spinal cord injury, among many—and must demonstrate the ability to perform over three hours of therapy daily or require complex treatment such as vent care, wound care, physical therapy, OT, and speech therapy (**Table 258-4**).

TABLE 258-4 Rehabilitation Providers and Typical Methods Used for Evaluation and Treatment

Provider	Methods of Evaluation and Treatment
Physical therapist	Assessment: • Joint range of motion, muscle strength, motor skills, coordination • Gait and mobility, including ability to perform ADLs • The need for appropriate assistive devices Educational goals: • Relieve discomfort • Regain, maintain, or improve function Treatment: • Active and passive exercise training to increase range of motion, strength, endurance, balance, coordination, and gait • Physical modalities (heat, cold, ultrasound, massage, hydrotherapy, and electrical stimulation)
Occupational therapist	Assessment: • Self-care skills and other activities of daily living • Home environment • The need for assistive technology Education: • Self-care skills training • Training in use of assistive technology Treatment: • Fabrication of splints • Upper extremity deficits
Speech therapist	Assessment: • All aspects of communication • Swallowing disorders Education: • Alteration of diet to reduce aspiration risk • Maneuvers to reduce aspiration risk Treatment: • Communication deficits
Nurse	Assessment: • Self-care skills • Family and home-care factors Education: • Self-care training • Patient and family regarding ADLs, IDLs, medications, underlying medical problems, preventive measures Treatment: • Primary focus on cure of acute medical issues or palliation if patients are terminal • Liaison with community

(continued)

TABLE 258-4 Rehabilitation Providers and Typical Methods Used for Evaluation and Treatment (*continued*)

Provider	Methods of Evaluation and Treatment
Social worker	Assessment: • Family and home care factors • Psychosocial factors Education: • Patient and family rights Treatment: • Counseling • Liaison with community
Dietician	• Assess nutritional status • Recommend dietary alterations to maximize nutrition • Monitor TPN
Recreation therapist	• Assess leisure skills and interests • Involve patients in recreational activities to maintain social roles
Prosthetist	• Makes and fits prosthetic limbs
Orthotist	• Makes a variety of orthotics including braces, ankle–foot orthoses, splints, and shoe inserts • Assesses fit of orthotics

Adapted from Cynthia J. Brown, Claire Peel, "Rehabilitation", in *Hazzard's Geriatric Medicine and Gerontology*, 6th ed. New York, McGraw-Hill, 2009.

The term *rehab* is often applied to SNFs that offer therapy services, but do not provide hospital-level or more formal inpatient interdisciplinary rehabilitation. Many elderly patients, in particular, primarily need physical therapy for endurance training so that they can safely perform ADLs and go home. Despite having a "rehab diagnosis," these patients are not candidates for intensive rehabilitation because of low endurance, weight-bearing precautions, or other factors such as inability to participate due to dementia. These patients may be more appropriate for "subacute rehab," often delivered in a SNF, with a less intensive schedule of rehabilitation services. Rehabilitation providers can generally make recommendations for the proper level of intensity in the patient's ongoing recovery, and assist with the process of establishing an appropriate discharge location.

Homebound individuals may qualify for home-health physical or occupational rehabilitative therapies, with an eye toward eventually transitioning to outpatient therapies. In general, patients receive two to three days of therapy per week in SNFs, outpatient clinics, or at home.

COMMON INPATIENT CONDITIONS THAT BENEFIT FROM REHABILITATION CONSULTATION

MUSCULOSKELETAL IMPAIRMENTS

Although rarely the primary cause of a patient's admission, osteoarthritis (OA) and other joint complaints are frequent in hospitalized persons. Joint complaints impair mobility through pain, restricted movement or contracture, and weakness from disuse. Low back pain is a particular source of limitation, and is highly prevalent in older populations. Knee osteoarthritis is also common, particularly in the obese and the elderly. Mobilization frequently requires adequate pain control. Both acetaminophen and nonsteroidal anti-inflammatory drugs (NSAIDs) are effective in osteoarthritis pain, although the risks of bleeding, renal damage, and hypertension limit use of NSAIDs. For acute flares of joint pain, intraarticular injections may reduce pain and improve mobility and function. Splinting and bracing may also contribute to pain relief and mobility. Opiates are generally reserved for the final stages of OA, and should be used with restraint.

PTs are of great value to patients with back and knee pain, as they can help to alter gait mechanics, strengthen weak muscles around painful joints, and provide assistive devices for joint protection and stability, reducing pain, and thereby allowing faster mobilization of a hospitalized patient. In the order for physical therapy, the physician should detail specific joints known to be affected. The PT should also know about upper-extremity limitations, especially when use of crutches or a walker may be required. OTs are helpful for patients with upper-extremity dysfunction related to OA or other causes.

JOINT REPLACEMENT

PTs and OTs are an integral component of care for patients undergoing joint replacement surgery, assisting in tasks ranging from mobilization, education, and self-care to home safety and modifications. Refer to Chapter 66 Rehabilitation of the Orthopedic Surgical Patient for specific information. Surgeons involve these providers early in the care process to individualize exercises depending on the patient's condition. In the immediate postoperative period, patients are educated about the importance of early mobilization to optimize function of the new joint, movements to avoid or are contraindicated to protect the prosthetic joint, exercises to perform to avoid thrombophlebitis, and when to call for assistance. Weight-bearing progresses based on the surgical technique and materials and the patient's ability to participate. PTs facilitate better outcomes, shorter hospital stays, fewer medical complications, and more successful transitions to home or rehabilitative care.

OSTEOPOROSIS

Risk factors for osteoporotic fractures include age, female gender, tobacco use, corticosteroid treatment, caffeine intake, low body weight, and inactivity. As inactivity is common in hospitalized patients, early mobilization, strength, and gait training are important strategies to mitigate the risk of worsening osteoporosis, in addition to drug therapies such as calcium and vitamin D supplementation, bisphosphonates, and teriparatide.

STROKE

There is now evidence that the best results for functional recovery occur for young patients and when PT and OT are involved early after the stroke occurs. Outcome measures include mortality, secondary prevention of complications of hospitalization, impact of other comorbidities, and tertiary prevention (rehabilitation outcomes). In the early phase of stroke, individuals often have a flaccid paralysis and are at high risk for pressure palsies and joint injury. Proper positioning and support are essential at this juncture. The speech-language pathologist has an equally important role. Death from aspiration and pneumonia is common after stroke, and a speech-language pathologist can assess aspiration risk and devise an appropriate diet or approach to feeding.

Loss of bladder control is a troubling complication of stroke that may be aggravated by simultaneous problems with muscle control, speech, and cognition. Improving mobility, attention, and communication through physical, occupational, and speech therapy interventions can greatly improve bladder management. This may lessen the risk of urinary tract infections during hospitalization and lead to more successful home discharge. Depression is another significant and common complication of stroke; roughly 30% of stroke patients develop clinical depression. In addition to psychological and pharmacologic intervention, the role of rehabilitation services in enhancing functional independence may also be helpful in managing depression.

Although neurologic impairments older than four to six months are unlikely to be completely reversed by therapy, functional performance may benefit from skilled therapies. Thus, the patient with an older stroke who is readmitted to the hospital may enjoy a better outcome if PTs, OTs, and speech therapists are consulted early in the hospital stay.

CRITICAL ILLNESS NEUROMYOPATHY

Persons who have had sepsis, hypotension, or hypoxemia may develop critical illness neuromyopathy. An electrodiagnostic study may clarify the diagnosis and provide prognostic information. Patients with more profound axonal damage generally have a worse outcome. Patients with critical illness neuromyopathy may need weeks to months to recover from their neurologic impairment; some never do. Weakness predisposes the individual to loss of joint movement and contractures. Decubitus ulcers are a threat. These individuals frequently require a high level of care upon discharge. Mobilization with a therapist can improve blood flow, encourage cardiovascular fitness, and contribute to better pulmonary hygiene. With true muscle atrophy (loss of muscle fibers), there is unlikely to be an improvement in muscle bulk through short-term interventions by therapists. However, neuromuscular control and improved recruitment of extant fibers likely contribute to improved performance. Similarly, function can improve with adaptive techniques and equipment provided by therapists.

DEBILITY

For deconditioning related to bed rest or inactivity, also known as debility, the loss of strength in healthy young men is about 1% per day, or roughly 10% per week. In elderly patients, this process is accelerated significantly, and the recovery time may exceed the duration of the initial hospitalization. In the general medical inpatient setting, debility can be compounded by medical illness, poor nutrition, orthopedic problems, and contractures. The cardiopulmonary system also declines with inactivity. Ferretti and colleagues found that after 42 days of bed rest, VO_2 max was reduced by 16%, cardiac output by 30%, and oxygen delivery by 40%. Maintenance of muscle strength during immobility can be accomplished by muscle contractions of 30% to 50% of maximal tension for several seconds each day. Studies have shown an improvement in ability to perform activities of daily living in elderly patients who had an exercise program while in the hospital.

CARDIAC CONDITIONS

Formal cardiac rehabilitation (CR) programs may benefit a wide range of patients: those recovering from myocardial infarction, those with stable heart failure, and those who have had coronary artery bypass grafting, heart transplantation, valve surgery, angioplasty, and pacemaker placement. Studies have demonstrated the value of CR in reversing coronary artery disease, reducing lipoprotein levels, and increasing physical work capacity. In the hospital setting, CR focuses on the identification of risk factors, the patient's previous and current performance status, and referral for outpatient activity. For those recovering from surgeries, this phase of CR also includes education on protecting sternal incisions. Education on safe activities to resume after discharge, risk factor modification, and vocational counseling may complete the acute CR process. Both PTs and OTs should be part of the CR team.

PULMONARY REHABILITATION

Rehabilitation programs in patients with chronic obstructive pulmonary disease and other chronic lung diseases have been shown to improve exercise capacity and quality of life, and reduce dyspnea and hospitalization. The main focus of pulmonary rehabilitation is exercise, including strength training for the upper and lower extremities, as well as respiratory muscle-specific training. Patients with chronic sputum production benefit from chest physical therapy. Patients receive education about medications, energy conservation, work simplification, and breathing techniques, such as pursed-lip breathing, posture, and diaphragmatic breathing. Nutritional interventions and psychosocial and emotional support are also provided. Pulmonary rehabilitation may be carried out in inpatient and outpatient settings.

PRACTICE POINT

Strategies to minimize negative consequences of bedrest

- Minimize duration of bedrest.
- Avoid strict bedrest.
- Allow bathroom privileges.
- Have patient stand 30–60 seconds when transferring from bed to chair.
- Encourage family to ambulate patient, engage patient with meals, and walk to hospital testing.
- Encourage daily exercises adapted to individual patient (such as ankle exercises to prevent venous thromboembolism).
- Involve physical therapy, occupational therapy, and nursing to encourage mobilization, optimize feeding, use of protective splinting, and pain management.
- Avoid physical or pharmacologic restraints.
- Daily reassessment of the need for tethers such as Foley catheter, supplement oxygen, IVs, and other devices that confine the patient to bed.

OTHER CONDITIONS

Other conditions less commonly seen in the standard inpatient setting require rehabilitation services. These include closed head injury, spinal cord injury or infection, burns, amputation, polytrauma, and

TABLE 258-5 Evidence-based Medicine: Rehabilitation Medicine

Paper	Methodology	Results	Limitations	Bottom Line
Suaya JA, Stason WB, Ades PA, et al. *J Am Coll Cardiol.* 2009;54:25–33.	Retrospective study, looking at five-year mortality in 601,099 U.S. Medicare beneficiaries hospitalized in 1997 for coronary artery disease or revascularization procedures	Five-year mortality was reduced from 21–34%, depending on the matching technique used	Retrospective study; however, the observed mortality reduction was similar to that seen in prior randomized, controlled trials and meta-analyses	Cardiac rehabilitation reduces five-year mortality after hospitalization for coronary artery disease or revascularization procedures
Puhan M, Scharplatz M, Troosters T, et al. Cochrane Database Syst Rev. 2009;(1):CD005305.	Meta-analysis of six trials of 219 patients who had either inpatient or outpatient pulmonary rehabilitation after hospitalization for an exacerbation of chronic obstructive pulmonary disease (COPD)	Pulmonary rehabilitation significantly reduced hospital admissions (pooled odds ratio 0.13) and mortality (pooled odds ratio 0.29), and improved quality of life and exercise tolerance	Only a relatively small number of randomized controlled trials and patients were available for analysis	Pulmonary rehabilitation improved exercise tolerance in all studies reviewed, and appears to improve quality of life and reduce the risk of readmission and death after COPD exacerbation
Mudge AM, Giebel AJ, Cutler AJ. *J Am Geriatr Soc.* 2008;56:630–635.	Randomized controlled trial in 124 hospitalized patients older than 65 of usual care vs. early physiotherapy review, individualized exercise program, encouragement of functional independence by nursing staff, and cognitive stimulation sessions	Participants in the intervention arm had a significantly higher functional status at discharge, as well as a significant reduction in episodes of delirium (19.4% vs. 35.5%, P = .04)	Study was underpowered for secondary outcomes such as delirium, falls, and length of stay	An intensive program of physical therapy, encouragement of functional independence, and cognitive stimulation improves functional status at discharge and prevents delirium
O'Connor CM, Whellan DJ, Lee KL, et al. *JAMA.* 2009;301:1439–1450.	Randomized controlled trial of exercise training in 2331 adults with heart failure and reduced ejection fraction	After adjustment for severity of illness, exercise training decreased all-cause mortality, all-cause hospitalizations, and cardiovascular mortality and heart failure hospitalizations	Power of the study may have been affected by the large numbers of crossovers from the usual care to the exercise group	Exercise training in patients with heart failure is safe and reduces the risk of death and readmission

the Guillain-Barré syndrome (acute inflammatory demyelinating polyneuropathy). In acute trauma, patients are frequently taken to level I trauma centers where rehabilitation services are ingrained into the provision of health care services. When trauma patients are cared for in settings with less formal infrastructure, it may be helpful to proactively involve PTs, OTs, physiatrists, and other rehabilitation providers in the care process. Many of the same issues of concern described above, such as contractures, immobility, and skin breakdown, are present in these other processes. Additionally, rehabilitation providers may also be particularly aware of the potential for medical complications in specific conditions (eg, heterotopic ossification after burns, autonomic dysreflexia after spinal cord injury, pulmonary aspiration, or bladder dysfunction associated with neurologic injury).

CONCLUSION

Hospitalists can enlist numerous professionals in the acute treatment of impairment and in discharge planning. Involving PTs and OTs early in a patient's hospital course may reduce length of stay, minimize inpatient complications, and lead to a more successful discharge at a higher level of independence. Physiatrists can assist in the diagnosis and management of neurologic and musculoskeletal conditions, and recommend appropriate levels of therapy upon discharge. Other providers, such as speech-language pathologists, psychologists, vocational counselors, and therapeutic recreation specialists, contribute to the restoration of function after illness or injury. Understanding the role of these providers and utilizing their services in an effective and timely manner are essential skills for the hospitalist (**Table 258-5**).

SUGGESTED READINGS

Altman R. Recommendations for the medical management of osteoarthritis of the hip and knee: 2000 update, American College of Rheumatology Subcommittee on Osteoarthritis Guidelines. *Arthritis Rheum.* 2000;43:1905–1915.

American Physical Therapy Association. *Guide to Physical Therapist Practice*, 2nd ed. Alexandria, VA: American Physical Therapy Association; 2001.

Brandstatter M. Stroke rehabilitation. In: *Physical Medicine and Rehabilitation, Principles and Practice*. DeLisa J, ed. Philadelphia, PA: Lippincott, Williams and Wilkins, 2005;2:1655–1676.

de Morton NA, Keating JL, Jeffs K. Exercise for acutely hospitalised older medical patients. Cochrane Database Syst Rev. 2007;(1):CD005955.

Ferretti G, Antonutto G, Denis C, et al. The interplay of central and peripheral factors in limiting maximal O2 consumption in man after prolonged bed rest. *J Physiol*. 1997;501(Pt 3):677–686.

Mueller E. Influence of training and of inactivity on muscle strength. *Arch Phys Med Rehabil*. 1970;51:449–461.

Siebens H, Aronow H, Edwards D, Ghasemi Z. A randomized controlled trial of exercise to improve outcomes of acute hospitalization in older adults. *J Am Geriatr Soc*. 2000;48:1545–1552.

SECTION 19

Vascular Medicine

CHAPTER 259

Diagnosis of Venous Thromboembolism

Lori-Ann Linkins, MSc, MD
Clive Kearon, MB, MRCPI, FRCPC, PhD

Key Clinical Questions

1. Why are objective tests needed to diagnose venous thromboembolism (VTE)?
2. Which tests can be used to diagnose a first DVT?
3. Which tests can be used to diagnose recurrent DVT?
4. Which tests can be used to diagnose PE?

INTRODUCTION

In 800 BC, Susruta, an Indian healer wrote about a patient with "a swollen and painful leg, which was difficult to treat." Centuries later, Virchow, a Prussian physician, coined the term "embolism" after discovering the relationship between a blood clot that formed within a blood vessel (thrombus), and a blood clot that breaks loose from the original and travels through the bloodstream to occlude the pulmonary vessels (embolus). The concept of venous thromboembolism was born from these early descriptions and today it remains one of the most important health problems in Europe and North America and is the third leading cause of vascular death after myocardial infarction and stroke.

The risk of VTE increases by approximately twofold per decade of age, rising from an annual incidence of 30/100,000 at 40 years of age, to 90/100,000 at 60 years, and 260/100,000 at 80 years. Approximately half of patients with untreated, symptomatic proximal DVT will develop symptomatic PE, and about 10% of symptomatic PE incidents are fatal within an hour of onset. Left untreated, one-third of patients with initially nonfatal PE will have a fatal recurrence, generally within a few weeks or months of the original event. Even with optimal treatment, 0.4% of patients with DVT and 5% of patients with PE will die from fatal PE, and about 25% with proximal DVT will develop postthrombotic syndrome, a chronic condition that is debilitating for patients.

VTE is now recognized as the leading cause of preventable death in hospitalized patients. Almost all hospitalized patients have one or more risk factors for VTE and 40% will have three or more risk factors. Since screening these patients for asymptomatic VTE is neither efficacious nor cost-effective, VTE prophylaxis (addressed in chapters 58, 59, and 60) forms the cornerstone for preventing these deaths. In addition, although 75% of venous thromboembolic events are diagnosed in the outpatient setting, about half of all episodes of VTE are associated with recent surgery or hospitalization. These findings stress the importance of having a low threshold to perform diagnostic testing in patients who present with signs and symptoms compatible with VTE within three months of hospitalization.

Therefore, VTE is both an acute and a chronic disease that causes substantial patient morbidity and mortality, and it is a major burden on the health care system. Costs for VTE include not only the expense of initial diagnosis and treatment, but also the cost of the complications of VTE (ie, postthrombotic syndrome, venous ulceration, chronic thromboembolic pulmonary hypertension, recurrent VTE) and its treatment (ie, bleeding). It is currently estimated that VTE costs the U.S. health care system $1.5 billion/year.

NOMENCLATURE

Proximal deep vein thrombosis is defined as a DVT that involves the popliteal vein or more proximal veins of the leg (most also involve the calf veins).

Distal deep vein thrombosis is defined as a DVT that is confined to the calf veins (including the calf trifurcation).

PRACTICE POINT

The natural history of VTE

- DVT typically starts in the calf (distal) veins
- 80% of symptomatic DVT are located in the proximal veins
- 80% of distal DVT will resolve without anticoagulation
- 20% of distal DVT will extend to the proximal veins within one week
- Propagation of calf DVT is more likely to occur in patients who have ongoing risk factors for VTE (eg, malignancy, immobility)
- Non-extending calf DVT rarely causes PE, but proximal DVT frequently does
- 60% of patients with symptomatic DVT will have asymptomatic PE
- 70% of patients with symptomatic PE will have asymptomatic DVT

PATHOPHYSIOLOGY

Virchow triad for the pathogenesis of thrombosis is as relevant today as it was when it was originally described in the 18th century: venous stasis, vessel wall damage, and hypercoagulability. A summary of common risk factors for VTE is given in **Table 259-1**.

VENOUS STASIS

DVT is more likely to occur in the paralyzed leg following stroke, and in the left leg during pregnancy because of extrinsic compression of the left iliac vein by the pregnant uterus and the right common iliac artery.

TABLE 259-1 Risk Factors for Venous Thromboembolism (VTE)

Patient factors
Age over 40
Previous VTE
Inherited hypercoagulable states
Underlying condition and acquired factors
Hospitalization
Acute medical illness (eg, congestive heart failure, COPD exacerbation)
Surgery
Surgery requiring general anaesthesia > 30 minutes
Lower limb orthopedic surgery
Major trauma
Nursing home
Prolonged immobility (eg, limited ambulation for > 48 hours within past 30 days)
Paralysis
Lower limb injuries
Obesity
Pregnancy, puerperium
Estrogen therapy (eg, oral contraceptive, hormone replacement therapy)
Malignancy
Cancer chemotherapy
Central vein catheterization, transvenous pacemaker
Inflammatory bowel disease
Nephrotic syndrome
Systemic lupus erythematosus
Antiphospholipid antibodies
Heparin-induced thrombocytopenia

VESSEL WALL DAMAGE

Manipulation during surgery (eg, hip replacement), iatrogenic injury, and use of indwelling venous catheters all markedly increase the risk of DVT.

HYPERCOAGULABILITY

Inherited or acquired changes in the balance of naturally occurring coagulation and fibrinolytic factors and their inhibitors predispose to thrombosis. The inherited hypercoagulable conditions that are considered strong risk factors for thrombosis, antithrombin deficiency, protein C deficiency and protein S deficiency, are rare (< 1% prevalence). Conversely, the most common inherited hypercoagulable conditions, activated protein C resistance caused by the Factor V Leiden mutation (5% prevalence in Caucasians), and the prothrombin gene mutation that leads to a 25% increase in prothrombin levels (2% prevalence), are weak risk factors for thrombosis. Common acquired hypercoagulable states are listed in Table 259-1. If VTE is suspected or confirmed in inpatients or shortly after discharge from the hospital, it is important to consider the possibility of heparin-induced thrombocytopenia (HIT).

CASE 259-1

A 63-year-old male noticed the edema of his leg following his left knee arthroplasty 10 days ago, but it had been slowly improving until 2 days ago. Now, his leg seemed to be as big as it had been the day after his surgery. He had been doing more physiotherapy lately and wondered if he might have over-exerted his leg.

On physical examination, he was in no apparent distress and his vital signs were normal. His left leg was 42 cm in circumference when measured 10 cm below the tibial tuberosity compared with his right leg which was 37 cm. There was obvious ecchymosis in the popliteal fossa and down by his medial malleolus. His incision was dry with no significant erythema or induration. He had no tenderness on palpation over the deep veins.

What is this patient's risk for VTE?
What diagnostic tests would you order?
How would your choice of diagnostic tests change if he also told you he had a history of a DVT in the same leg 2 years ago?

DOES THIS PATIENT HAVE A DVT?

Edema, pain, tenderness, and erythema are signs and symptoms of DVT, but they are also commonly found in patients who do not have DVT (ie, nonspecific). Only 15% of ambulatory patients who are suspected of having DVT will have this diagnosis confirmed on objective testing. Alternate causes for these clinical features include muscle injury, Baker cyst, cellulitis, extrinsic compression of veins, anasarca or low albumin states, and venous insufficiency.

Hospitalized patients are more likely than ambulatory patients to have DVT confirmed when it is suspected (prevalence of 30–40%). However, hospitalized patients are also more likely to have asymptomatic DVT (only 6% of patients diagnosed with DVT in a prophylaxis study in medical patients were symptomatic). This finding stresses the importance of preventing VTE instead of relying on clinical surveillance to detect and treat it early.

PRACTICE POINT

- 1 out of every 20 recurrent PE are fatal (5%)
- 1 out of every 11 major bleeds in patients receiving anticoagulant therapy are fatal (9%)

TABLE 259-2 The Wells Clinical Prediction Rule for DVT

	Points
Active cancer (treatment ongoing or within previous 6 months or palliative	1
Paralysis, paresis, or recent plaster immobilization of the lower extremities	1
Recently bedridden > 3 days or major surgery within the previous 12 weeks requiring general or regional anesthesia	1
Localized tenderness along the distribution of the deep venous system	1
Entire leg swollen	1
Calf swelling 3 cm > asymptomatic side (measured 10 cm below tibial tuberosity)	1
Pitting edema confined to the symptomatic leg	1
Collateral superficial veins (non varicose)	1
Previously documented deep-vein thrombosis	1
Alternative diagnosis as likely or greater than that of DVT	−2
Total points (pretest probability for DVT): Score > 2: High; Score 1–2: Moderate; Score ≤ 0: Low	

Data from Wells PS, Anderson DR, Rodger M, et al. Evaluation of D-dimer in the diagnosis of suspected deep-vein thrombosis. *N Engl J Med.* 2003;349:1227–1235.

Failure to diagnose DVT exposes patients to the risk of fatal PE; however, inappropriate use of anticoagulant therapy exposes patients to the risk of fatal bleeding. Because clinical assessment alone is unreliable, objective testing to confirm the diagnosis must always be performed when DVT is suspected.

CLINICAL ASSESSMENT

For the reasons outlined above, clinical assessment alone is an unreliable test for diagnosing DVT. However, clinical prediction rules have been developed that can help to stratify patients as having a low (5% prevalence), moderate (25% prevalence), or high (60% prevalence) probability of DVT (**Table 259-2**).

Hospitalized patients are less likely to have a low probability score, and low probability patients are more likely to have a DVT compared to outpatients (10% prevalence of DVT). Such classification of pretest probability is helpful when used *in combination* with other diagnostic tests (**Figure 259-1**).

If there is a moderate or high risk clinical suspicion for DVT (or PE) and patients are not at high risk for bleeding, it is recommended that anticoagulant therapy is started before diagnostic testing is performed.

IMAGING TESTS FOR DVT

Venography

Venography is the reference standard test for DVT, but it is rarely performed because it is invasive (painful), technically difficult, and exposes the patient to the risks of contrast dye (eg, nephrotoxicity, anaphylaxis) and radiation. An intraluminal filling defect (ie, section of a vein that remains dark when surrounded by white contrast dye) seen on at least two views is considered diagnostic for DVT.

Compression venous ultrasound

Ultrasonography is the first-line imaging test used to diagnose or exclude DVT. When pressure is applied to the proximal veins with an ultrasound probe, the veins should fully compress. If they do not, acute or chronic DVT is present. In symptomatic patients, when the ultrasound probe is applied to the proximal veins, the sensitivity of ultrasound for proximal DVT is 97% and the specificity is 94% when compared with venography (for both inpatients and outpatients). The sensitivity and specificity of compression ultrasound is lower in the calf veins, and the clinical significance of isolated calf vein thrombosis is controversial. For these reasons, many centers do not examine the calf veins with ultrasound; instead, if the initial assessment (eg, low clinical suspicion and negative ultrasound of the proximal veins) cannot exclude the presence of DVT, a follow-up ultrasound of the proximal veins is done after a week to exclude the possibility of calf vein thrombosis with early extension into the proximal veins. Compression venous ultrasound is frequently combined with assessment of Doppler flow; however, change in Doppler flow alone is not a sensitive or specific test for DVT.

Limitations include the factors listed below.

- Operator dependent
- Limbs with casts that cannot be removed
- Morbid obesity
- Massive edema
- Isolated pelvic DVT
- Lower sensitivity and specificity in the absence of symptoms.

The sensitivity of compression ultrasound for proximal DVT in asymptomatic patients is only 60% and the positive predictive value is also lower than in symptomatic patients; therefore, screening asymptomatic high risk patients for DVT with venous ultrasound is not recommended.

Computed tomographic venography (CTV)

CTV has been shown to have sensitivity of 89–100% and specificity of 94–100% compared with ultrasonography. This method offers the advantage of imaging for isolated pelvic DVT and can be combined with CT pulmonary angiography (CTPA) to scan for DVT and PE in one examination. However, studies have shown that the

- Incremental benefit of adding CTV to CTPA in patients with suspected PE is minimal (5% additional VTE diagnosed on CTV).
- Diagnostic accuracy of CTV in combination with CTPA is equivalent to CTPA combined with Wells assessment of pretest probability, or CTPA combined with leg ultrasonagraphy. Importantly, CTV is more expensive than the latter two methods, requires a larger dose of contrast, and substantially increases radiation exposure.

Limitations include the factors listed below:

- Use of contrast
- Radiation exposure
- False positive results due to streak artifacts
- Too expensive to use as a first-line test for DVT.

Magnetic resonance venography (MRV)/Direct thrombus imaging

Data on these methods are currently limited and like CTV, they are too expensive to use as first-line tests for DVT. A meta-analysis reported the sensitivity and specificity of MRV for proximal DVT compared with conventional venography as 92% and 95%, respectively. Although the absence of contrast gives MRV an advantage over CTV, a warning has been issued about an increased risk of nephrogenic systemic fibrosis in patients with severe renal

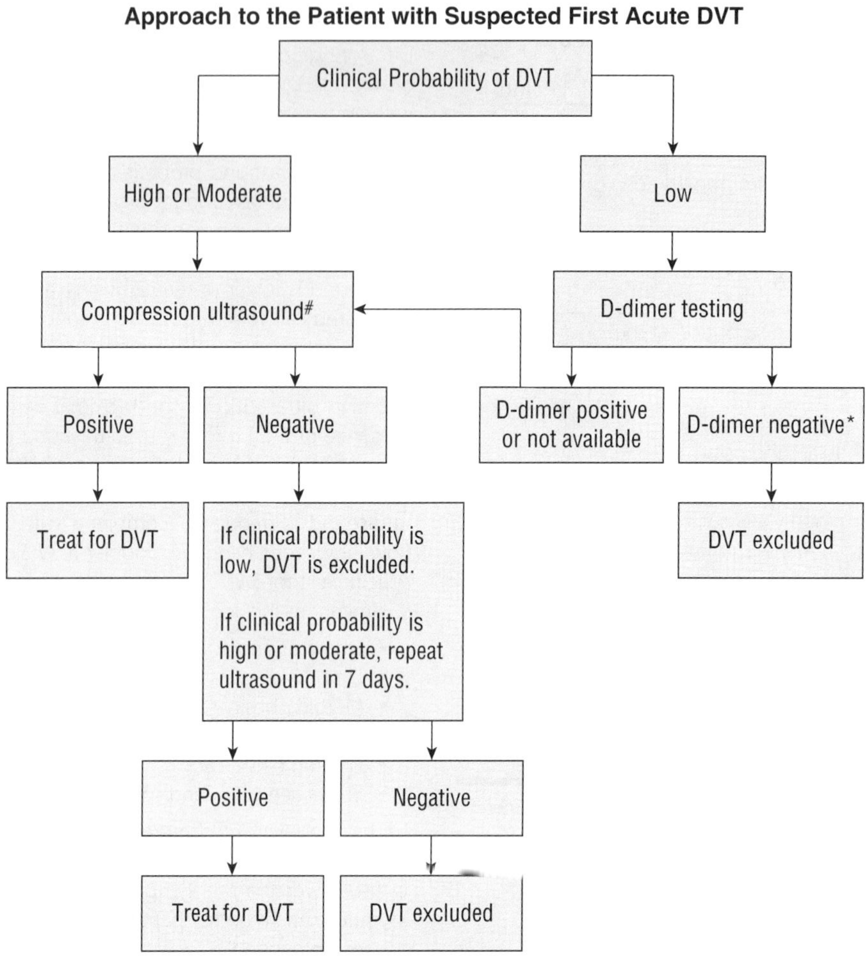

Figure 259-1 *Approach to the patient with suspected first acute DVT. *If D-dimer assay has a sensitivity of greater than or equal to 85% of proximal veins.*

insufficiency (glomerular filtration rate < 30 mL/min) when exposed to gadolinium during MRV.

> **PRACTICE POINT**
>
> Don't waste time and money by ordering a D-Dimer for the following patients:
> - Postoperative
> - Acute infection
> - Active malignancy
> - Pregnancy
>
> It is unlikely the result will be negative and a positive result is completely unhelpful.

D-dimer blood testing

D-dimer is formed when cross-linked fibrin is broken down by plasmin. Normal levels can help to *exclude* DVT, but elevated D-dimer levels are common with other conditions (eg, malignancy, disseminated intravascular coagulation, acute infection, normal pregnancy, renal disease, cardiovascular disease). D-dimer levels are also elevated after surgery and may take up to 50 days to return to baseline, depending on the type of surgery. Consequently, a positive D-dimer is *NEVER* diagnostic for DVT! A negative D-dimer can still be used to exclude DVT in a hospitalized patient with a low clinical probability for DVT, but negative results in this patient population are so uncommon (less than 10%) that the utility of the test is very poor. *Beware that there are many different types of D-dimer assays and many are not suitable for diagnosis of VTE.* The higher the sensitivity of the assay, the more likely it will be positive in a patient who truly has a DVT and the higher the negative predictive value. However, the price of high sensitivity is lower specificity, so the assay will be positive in a higher proportion of patients who do not have DVT, which limits the utility of the test.

DOES THIS PATIENT HAVE RECURRENT DVT?

Approximately 30% of patients with DVT will experience recurrent DVT during the 10 years following the initial diagnosis. Unfortunately, diagnosing recurrent DVT is much more difficult than diagnosing a first acute DVT. To begin with, the signs and symptoms experienced by patients with recurrent DVT (ie, increased edema and/or pain) are also seen in patients with postthrombotic syndrome, a chronic condition that affects approximately 25% of patients with previous DVT. Secondly, diagnostic tests for recurrent DVT are not as reliable as they are for first acute DVT. (**Figure 259-2**)

CLINICAL ASSESSMENT

Clinical prediction rules for diagnosing recurrent DVT are less well developed and validated than for a first episode of DVT and they have not been widely used.

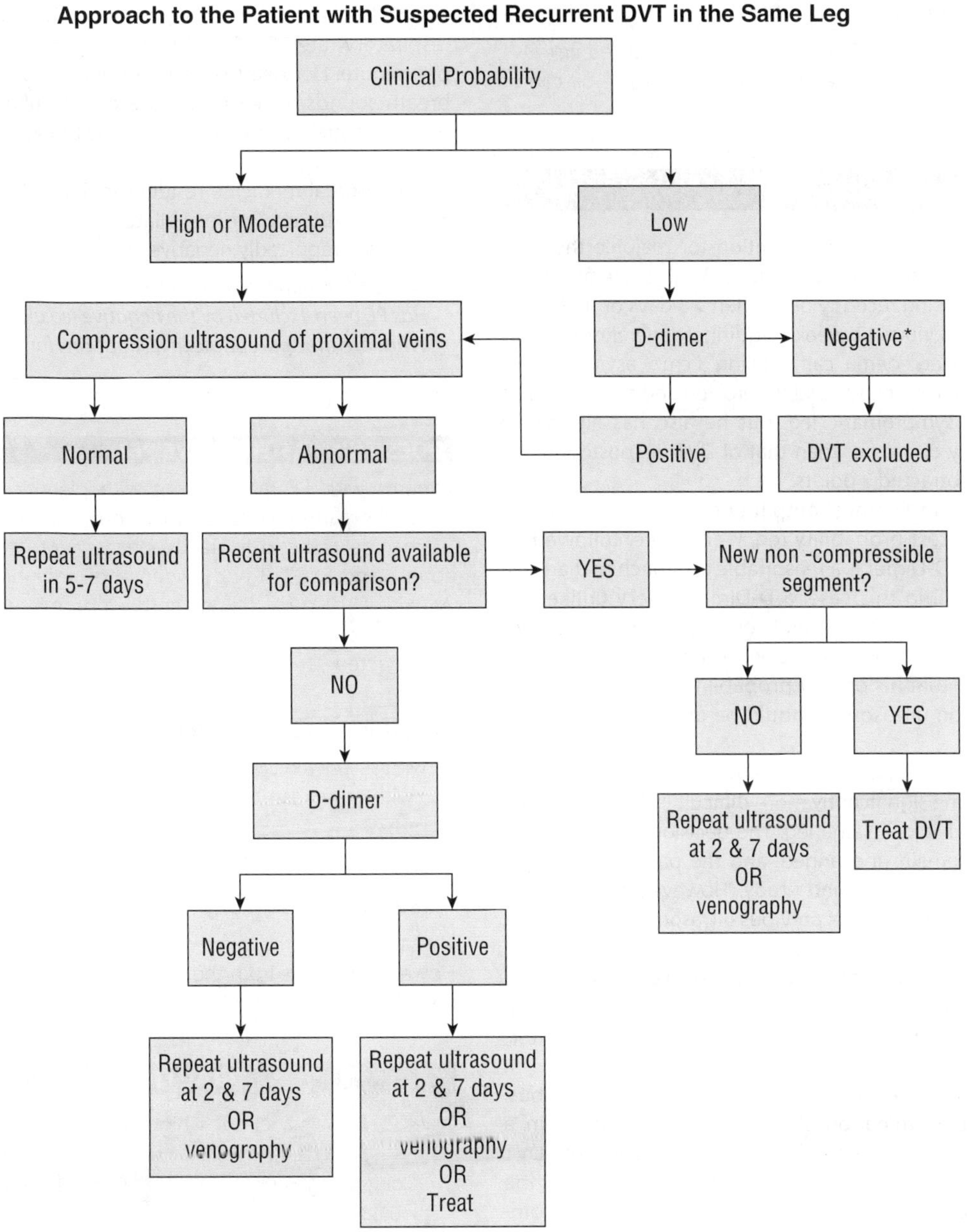

Figure 259-2 *Approach to the patient with suspected recurrent DVT in the same leg. *If D-dimer assay has a sensitivity of greater than or equal to 85%.*

IMAGING TESTS FOR RECURRENT DVT

Venography

As with first acute DVT, this method is considered the reference standard test for recurrent DVT. However, veins previously affected by DVT may not fill with contrast dye, resulting in nondiagnostic findings.

Compression venous ultrasound

In patients with a recent ultrasound that demonstrated (1) limited extent of the previous DVT or (2) complete resolution of the previous DVT, the presence a new noncompressible segment of the proximal veins (eg, popliteal or common femoral vein) on ultrasound examination is diagnostic for recurrent DVT. However, it is important to remember that *50% of patients with first acute DVT will still have incomplete compressibility on ultrasound examination one year after diagnosis despite adequate anticoagulant therapy.* Consequently, without clear evidence of a new noncompressible segment, it can be difficult to tell the difference between residual chronic DVT and new acute DVT.

One ultrasound method that has been proposed for diagnosing recurrent DVT is evidence of an increase in residual vein diameter of greater than 4 mm (when a vein is compressed with an ultrasound probe) when two ultrasound examinations are compared. However, a recent ultrasound (prior to the episode of suspected recurrence) is required for comparison, and there is evidence that the reproducibility of this measurement is only moderate. Other ultrasound features such as Doppler flow and thrombus echogenicity have not been validated as reliable methods for diagnosing recurrent DVT.

Magnetic resonance venography/Direct thrombus imaging

Preliminary studies suggest that this method may be able to distinguish between acute and chronic thrombus; however, further studies are needed before it can be recommended.

D-dimer blood testing

Although less studied than in patients with a suspected first DVT, recent clinical trials indicate that a negative D-dimer result can be used to help exclude recurrent DVT.

CASE 259-1 *(continued)*

This patient's risk of VTE: Hospitalization for major orthopedic surgery is a strong risk factor for DVT. His Wells score for DVT is 2 with points for being recently bedridden > 3 days or major surgery within the previous 12 weeks requiring general or regional anesthesia, entire leg edema, calf swelling 3 cm > asymptomatic side (measured 10 cm below tibial tuberosity) and pitting edema confined to the symptomatic leg, but he also has alternative diagnosis as likely or greater than that of DVT (ie, postoperative edema) which subtracted 2 points.

Diagnostic testing: For most outpatients with suspected DVT, calculation of pretest probability (eg, Wells score) followed by performance of a D-Dimer is a reasonable approach to diagnosing/excluding DVT. In this case, a D-Dimer is very unlikely to be negative given that this patient recently underwent major surgery. As a D-Dimer is only helpful when it is negative, it is not requested. Given that his pretest probability for DVT is moderate, a compression ultrasound should be ordered to check for DVT.

Diagnostic testing in patients with a prior history of DVT: This case would become significantly more difficult if this patient had a history of a DVT in the same leg. The decision not to order a D-Dimer would remain unchanged, and the patient would still have a compression ultrasound study. However, his clinicians would also want to try to find a previous ultrasound report which described the extent of his previous DVT.

If he was documented to have complete resolution of his previous thrombus, the finding of any noncompressible segments on the current ultrasound examination would be interpreted as representing new acute DVT.

If he had incomplete resolution of his previous thrombus, and the current examination showed incompressibility in a previously unaffected segment, he likely has a new acute DVT (eg, his previous DVT extended from the calf trifurcation to the midsuperficial femoral vein, but today's exam shows incompressibility of the common femoral vein). If today's ultrasound examination shows incompressibility in the same segments as his previous DVT, his clinicians cannot be certain that the findings represent new acute DVT. They have 3 choices in this situation:

(1) Not to treat, but to repeat the ultrasound at 2 and 7 days (to look for clear evidence of progression which would indicate acute DVT) (2) Arrange for a venogram or (3) Treat the patient as an acute DVT for 3 months.

CASE 259-2

A 72-year-old woman has been in hospital for 4 days with pneumonia. She is afebrile and her cough is no longer productive of purulent sputum, but she continues to be tachypneic and hypoxic with minimal exertion. The right lower lobe infiltrate seen on her chest x-ray on admission has not significantly changed. Her white blood cell count is slowly decreasing, but she continues to have anemia and mild thrombocytosis. All blood cultures have been negative. Her creatinine is elevated due to chronic renal insufficiency. An ECG shows sinus tachycardia.

On physical exam, her oxygen saturation is 91% on room air, respiratory rate 25, BP 120/85 mm Hg and heart rate 100 beats per minute. Her heart sounds are normal, but she has bronchial breath sounds at her right base on auscultation. She has mild bilateral pedal edema, but denies any tenderness on palpation of her legs.

The internal medicine resident looking after her is concerned about DVT/PE and orders bilateral leg ultrasounds. The ultrasounds are reportedly negative.

What is this patient's risk for VTE?
Has PE been excluded by the negative leg ultrasounds?
What are the appropriate investigations for PE?

DOES THIS PATIENT HAVE PE?

Patients with PE may present with pleuritic chest pain, shortness of breath, palpitations, hemoptysis, and syncope. Signs of PE include tachycardia, tachypnea, accentuated pulmonic heart sound, and S1Q3T3 and evidence of right heart strain on ECG. As with DVT, clinical signs and symptoms are nonspecific, and objective diagnostic testing must always be performed when PE is suspected.

CLINICAL ASSESSMENT

As with suspected DVT, clinical assessment can be used *in combination* with other tests to diagnose PE (**Table 259-3**).

IMAGING TESTS FOR PE

Pulmonary angiography

This method is the reference standard test for diagnosing PE. However, it suffers from the same limitations as venography and it is rarely used.

PRACTICE POINT

- CTPA delivers a relatively high dose of radiation to breast tissue which increases the risk of breast cancer. It should be avoided in women less than 50 years of age unless absolutely necessary.
- 1 CTPA is equivalent to 100 chest x-rays with respect to radiation!

Computed tomographic pulmonary angiography (CTPA)

CTPA (also known as spiral or helical CT) is the current first-line imaging test for PE. CTPA technology has rapidly advanced from single detector scanners to progressively larger numbers of detectors (termed multidetector CT), which enable more detailed examination of the pulmonary arteries. CTPA has the additional advantage of detecting alternate causes for symptoms in about one-third of patients with suspected PE (eg, pneumonia, lung mass). Recent studies suggest that less than 2% of patients with a negative CTPA who are not treated with anticoagulant therapy will return with symptomatic VTE during three months of follow-up.

Multidetector CTPA has a sensitivity of 83% and a specificity of 96% for PE when compared with pulmonary angiography. However, accuracy varies according to the size of the largest pulmonary artery involved. The probability that an intraluminal filling defect is due to a PE is 97% for defects in the main or lobar artery, 68% for segmental arteries, and 25% for subsegmental arteries (which

TABLE 259-3 The Wells Clinical Prediction Rule for PE

	Points
Clinical signs and symptoms of deep vein thrombosis (minimum of leg swelling and pain with palpation of the deep veins)	3.0
An alternative diagnosis is less likely than pulmonary embolism	3.0
Heart rate > 100 beats/min	1.5
Immobilization or surgery in the previous 4 weeks	1.5
Previous deep vein thrombosis/pulmonary embolism	1.5
Hemoptysis	1.0
Malignancy (treatment ongoing or within previous 6 months or palliative)	1.0
Total points (pretest probability for PE): Score < 4: PE unlikely; Score ≥ 4: PE likely	

Data from Wells PS, Anderson DR, Rodger M, et al. Derivation of a simple clinical model to categorize patients probability of pulmonary embolism: increasing the models utility with the SimpliRED D-dimer. *Thromb Haemost.* 2000;83:416–420.

means that as many as 75% of abnormalities seen in subsegmental arteries are not due to PE). Accuracy of CTPA is also influenced by clinical assessment of pulmonary embolism; the higher the clinical probability of PE, the more likely the defect that is seen on CTPA is actually due to PE (**Table 259-4**).

Limitations include the factors listed below.

- Requires use of contrast dye
- Exposure to radiation
- Subject to technical difficulties (approximately 6% of CTPA are nondiagnostic)
- Expense

Ventilation-perfusion lung scanning (V/Q)

This was the first-line test used to diagnose PE before the advent of CTPA, and V/Q scanning is still used, particularly when CTPA is contraindicated (ie, patients with renal failure, young women due to a concern about breast cancer induced by radiation exposure). Perfusion defects are nonspecific; only about 33% of patients with perfusion defects have PE. The probability that a perfusion defect is due to PE increases with the size and number of defects, and if they are mismatched. A *mismatch* refers to a perfusion defect that is not associated with a corresponding defect on the ventilation scan. Lung scan findings are highly age dependent with a relatively high proportion of normal scans in younger patients, including pregnant women, and a low proportion in those with other acute and chronic cardiorespiratory conditions (**Table 259-5**).

Limitations include the factors listed below:

- Large proportion of nondiagnostic scans
- Inability to identify alternative causes for symptoms.

TABLE 259-4 Interpretation of Findings on CTPA

Location of Pulmonary Artery Defect on CTPA	Clinical Probability of PE	Interpretation
Lobar or larger	Any	Very likely PE
Segmental	Moderate or high	Likely PE
Segmental	Low	Nondiagnostic
Subsegmental	Any	Nondiagnostic

TABLE 259-5 Interpretation of Findings on V/Q

Mismatched Perfusion Defects on V/Q Scanning	Clinical Probability of PE	Interpretation
≥ 1 segmental	Moderate to high	Very likely PE
≥ 1 segmental	Low	Nondiagnostic
≥ 1 subsegmental	Moderate to high	Nondiagnostic
≥ 1 subsegmental	Low	Unlikely PE
None	Any	PE excluded

Magnetic resonance angiography (MRA)

As with MRV, gadolinium-enhanced pulmonary MRA offers advantages over CTPA in that it can be performed on patients with an allergy to iodinated contrast dye and it avoids exposure to radiation. However, only a limited number of small studies have evaluated MRA for diagnosis of PE and it cannot be used in patients with renal insufficiency (CrCl < 30 ml/min).

D-dimer blood testing

As with suspected DVT, a negative D-dimer result can exclude PE (on its own, if it is a very sensitive assay or in combination with other tests, if it is less sensitive) (**Figure 259-3**).

What if the tests I ordered to exclude PE were nondiagnostic?

If initial testing is nondiagnostic, there is still a 20–30% chance that your patient could have a PE and further investigations are required. One approach to management of such patients is to perform ultrasonography and withhold anticoagulation if there is no DVT of the proximal veins. Ultrasonography of the proximal veins is then repeated after one and two weeks to exclude evolving VTE. See algorithm Figure 259-3.

CASE 259-2 *(continued)*

This patient's risk of PE: Hospitalization with acute infection is a strong risk factor for VTE. In addition, this patient is over age 40 and has likely been immobile while in hospital. Hypoxia that is more severe than expected, based on the patient's x-ray findings should raise suspicion of PE.

Diagnostic Testing: PE has not been excluded. If her leg ultrasounds had been positive for DVT, further investigations for PE would not be necessary because it would not change her management (ie, the treatment for DVT and PE is the same). However, in this case, proximal DVT has been excluded by negative ultrasounds, but PE has not been excluded.

Currently, CTPA is the most common first-line imaging test used to diagnose PE. However, this woman is known to have chronic renal insufficiency so this test may not be appropriate for her (ie, you need to calculate her creatinine clearance first). A reasonable alternative is a VQ scan, especially if she had a normal CXR.

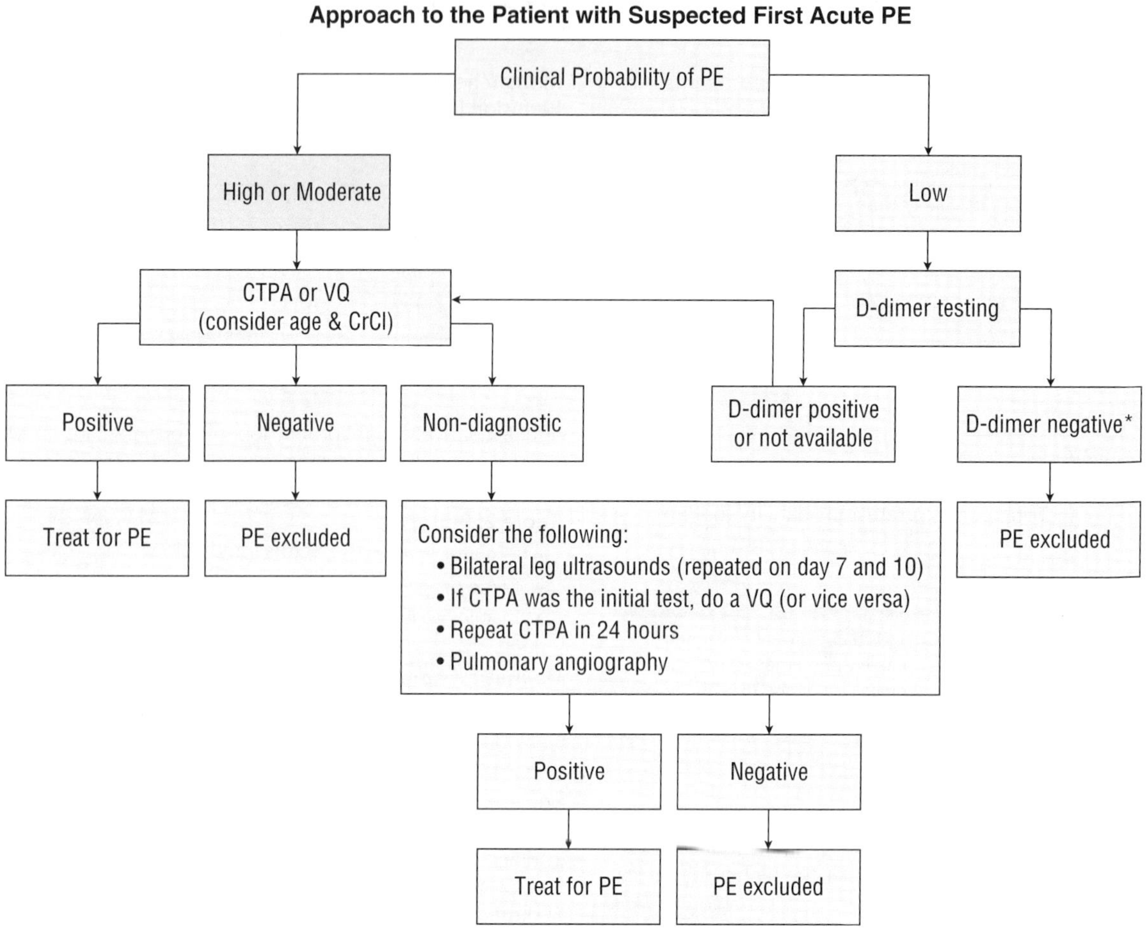

Figure 259-3 *Approach to the patient with suspected first acute PE. If D-dimer assay has a sensitivity of greater than or equal to 85%.*

CONCLUSION

Given the challenges of the clinical diagnosis of VTE and the unpredictability of sudden fatal PE as the initial manifestation, appropriate VTE prophylaxis is required to minimize morbidity and mortality from hospital-acquired VTE. In contrast to the community setting, clinical prediction rules and D-dimer testing may be less likely to discriminate between hospitalized patients who have and those who do not have VTE because the majority of patients will have moderate or high pretest probability of VTE and will have other reasons for a positive D-dimer. Since clinical assessment alone is unreliable, objective testing to confirm the diagnosis must always be performed when VTE is suspected.

SUGGESTED READINGS

Anderson FA Jr, Spencer FA. Risk factors for venous thromboembolism. *Circulation.* 2003;107:I9–I16.

Douketis JD, Kearon C, Bates S, et al. Risk of fatal pulmonary embolism in patients with treated venous thromboembolism. *JAMA.* 1998;279:458–462.

Geerts WH, Bergqvist D, Pineo GF, et al. Prevention of venous thromboembolism: American College of Chest Physicians Evidence-Based Clinical Practice Guidelines (8th edition). *Chest.* 2008;133:381S–453S.

Kearon C. Natural history of venous thromboembolism. *Circulation.* 2003;107:I22–I30.

Kearon C, Julian JA, Newman TE, Ginsberg JS. Noninvasive diagnosis of deep venous thrombosis. McMaster Diagnostic Imaging Practice Guidelines Initiative. *Ann Intern Med.* 1998;128:663–677.

Roy PM, Colombet I, Durieux P, et al. Systematic review and meta-analysis of strategies for the diagnosis of suspected pulmonary embolism. *BMJ.* 2005;331:259.

Stein PD, Fowler SE, Goodman LR, et al. Multidetector computed tomography for acute pulmonary embolism. *N Engl J Med.* 2006;354:2317–2327.

Stein PD, Hull RD, Patel KC, et al. D-dimer for the exclusion of acute venous thrombosis and pulmonary embolism: a systematic review. *Ann Intern Med.* 2004;140:589–602.

Wells PS, Anderson DR, Rodger M, et al. Evaluation of D-dimer in the diagnosis of suspected deep-vein thrombosis. *N Engl J Med.* 2003;349:1227–1235.

Wells PS, Anderson DR, Rodger M, et al. Derivation of a simple clinical model to categorize patients probability of pulmonary embolism: increasing the models utility with the SimpliRED D-dimer. *Thromb Haemost.* 2000;83:416–420.

CHAPTER 260

Treatment of Venous Thromboembolism

Lori-Ann Linkins, MSc, MD
Clive Kearon, MB, MRCPI, FRCPC, PhD

Key Clinical Questions

1. Which patients with venous thromboembolism (VTE) can be treated as outpatients?
2. What is the treatment for acute VTE deep vein thrombosis and/or pulmonary embolism (PE)?
3. What is the role of thrombolytic therapy in the treatment of PE?
4. How are patients with acute VTE and bleeding managed?
5. How is the duration of treatment of VTE determined?
6. Should I perform a thrombophilic workup?
7. What is the risk of bleeding associated with long-term anticoagulant therapy?

INTRODUCTION

The foundation of treatment of venous thromboembolism (VTE) is anticoagulant therapy. The objectives of anticoagulant therapy are: (1) to prevent extension and potentially fatal embolization of the initial thrombus and (2) to prevent recurrent VTE.

Proximal deep vein thrombosis is defined as a deep vein thrombosis (DVT) that involves the popliteal and more proximal veins of the leg. *Distal deep vein thrombosis* is defined as a DVT that is confined to the calf veins (including the calf trifurcation).

TRIAGE AND HOSPITAL ADMISSION

Patients who are hemodynamically stable with a low bleeding risk and normal renal function, and who are likely to be compliant with anticoagulant therapy, can be safely treated as outpatients. Patients with DVT and severe intractable pain or phlegmasia cerulea dolens (blue, painful leg due to complete venous obstruction leading to impaired arterial flow) should be admitted to hospital for initiation of treatment. Patients with pulmonary embolism (PE) and severe symptoms or abnormal vital signs should be admitted to the hospital and those with signs of hemodynamic compromise (eg, low oxygen saturation, low systolic blood pressure, persistent tachycardia) should be considered for thrombolytic therapy (discussed later). Validated prognostic scores are available to help physicians select which patients with PE can be treated as outpatients.

CASE 260-1

A 40-year-old male underwent a craniotomy for glioblastoma multiforme (GBM) on hospital day #1. His preoperative platelet count was 244,000/mm^3. Postoperatively, he received mechanical VTE prophylaxis and UFH 5,000 U subcutaneously twice a day. On postoperative day #11 he became acutely short of breath. CT-PA protocol imaging identified multiple bilateral PE and a common femoral DVT.

What treatment should this patient receive? If this patient had thrombocytopenia (or a 50% drop in his platelet count), would you recommend a different treatment?

CASE 260-2

A 58-year-old female with a past medical history of asthma was seen for shortness of breath on three occasions in the outpatient setting. Despite therapy for asthma, her symptoms progressed and on the day of admission she developed chest pain that radiated to her left shoulder. Routine admission testing revealed an abnormal ECG showing deeply inverted T waves in her anterior precordium without reciprocal changes in other leads and slightly abnormal liver function tests. Her vital signs were normal and stable. She had elevated troponin and brain naturetic hormone levels that did not increase on repeated testing. CT-PA protocol imaging revealed extensive pulmonary emboli, including a saddle embolus involving the right pulmonary artery, an enlarged right ventricle, and bilateral common femoral DVT.

How should this patient with a significant clot burden and evidence of right heart strain be treated?

Should she undergo testing to identify risk factors for VTE?

TABLE 260-1 Antithrombotics for Treatment of Acute Venous Thromboembolism

Antihrombotic	Dose and Administration	Advantages	Disadvantages
LMWH	Weight-based subcutaneous injection daily or twice daily	Laboratory monitoring not required Allows for outpatient treatment	Contraindicated in pts with CrCl < 30 ml/min Protamine sulphate is only partially effective in reversing anticoagulant effect Moderate risk of HIT
Fondaparinux	Weight-based subcutaneous injection daily	Laboratory monitoring not required Allows for outpatient treatment Low risk of HIT	Contraindicated in pts with CrCl < 30 ml/min No reversal agent available
Heparin	333 U/kg subcutaneous injection followed by 250 U/kg twice daily	Laboratory monitoring not required Allows for outpatient treatment	Half-life too short to be given subcutaneously only once daily
	80 U/kg intravenous (IV) bolus followed by 18 U/kg/min (aPTT titrated to plasma heparin levels from 0.3 to 0.7 IU/mL anti-Xa activity)	Short half-life if bleeding occurs Can be reversed with protamine sulphate Can be used in pts with renal failure	Requires laboratory monitoring if given intravenously Highest risk of HIT

CrCl, creatinine clearance; HIT, heparin-induced thrombocytopenia; LMWH, low-molecular-weight heparin.

TREATMENT OF ACUTE VENOUS THROMBOEMBOLISM

The first step in treating acute VTE is preventing further thrombus formation by starting an agent that rapidly inhibits thrombin. The agents approved for treatment of acute VTE in Europe and North America are low-molecular-weight heparin (LMWH), fondaparinux, and heparin (**Table 260-1**).

PRACTICE POINT

- Vitamin K antagonists will not rapidly inhibit thrombin and should not be used alone to treat acute VTE.

Patients with VTE who have heparin-induced thrombocytopenia (HIT) or a past history of HIT should receive danaparoid, lepirudin, or argatroban instead of the agents listed in Table 260-1. The agents in Table 260-1 should be given for a minimum of five days and until the INR is greater than or equal to 2.0 on two consecutive measurements. A vitamin K antagonist (VKA) (eg, warfarin) with a target INR of 2.0 to 3.0 is typically started at the same time as the parenteral antithrombotic agent. Dosing algorithms for VKAs are available. Observational studies have shown that lower VKA maintenance doses are required in older patients, women, those with impaired nutrition, and vitamin K deficiency. Optimal VKA management requires a systematic approach to obtaining INR measurements, adjusting VKA dose, and communicating these instructions to patients. Anticoagulation clinics, and use of computer programs to schedule appointments, adjust VKA dose and maintain records, can facilitate this process.

A randomized trial of patients with DVT established the need for anticoagulant therapy beyond the first week by showing a much higher risk of recurrent VTE in patients who received low-dose heparin instead of warfarin after initial treatment with full-dose heparin for 10 days. The options for ongoing anticoagulant therapy include a VKA at a target INR 2.0–3.0, high-dose subcutaneous heparin, and LMWH (at 50–75% of acute treatment dose).

New antithrombotic agents (eg, dabigatran, rivaroxaban, apixaban) are in the advanced stages of development for treatment of VTE, but are not yet approved for this indication.

THROMBOLYTIC THERAPY FOR DEEP VEIN THROMBOSIS

Thrombolytic therapy, administered systemically or directly into the thrombus (catheter directed thrombolysis), can achieve thrombus removal, improve acute symptoms, and reduce the risk of developing the postthrombotic syndrome. Catheter directed thrombolysis can be combined with mechanical thrombus disruption to further increase thrombus removal and shorten the procedure. The increase in bleeding associated with thrombolytic therapy is expected to be less with catheter directed therapy than with systemic therapy because smaller dose and shorter durations of therapy are uses. The risks and benefits of thrombolytic therapy are uncertain and it is not indicated in most patients with DVT. Catheter directed thrombolytic therapy, however, is reasonable in patients with extensive DVT (eg, involves the iliofemoral vein) of recent onset (eg, symptoms ≤ 14 days) that is associated with severe symptoms, provided the patient does not have risk factors for bleeding, resources and expertise is available to perform it optimally, and it is the patient's preference to receive such therapy.

THROMBOLYTIC THERAPY FOR PULMONARY EMBOLISM

Patients with acute PE and signs of hemodynamic compromise should be considered for systemic thrombolytic therapy. This recommendation is based on the premise that rapid lysis of PE will reduce mortality in high-risk patients. However, thrombolysis also significantly increases the risk of major bleeding compared to heparin alone (including a 2% rate of intracranial hemorrhage) and, therefore, the use of thrombolytic therapy in patients with submassive PE and no evidence of hemodynamic instability is not recommended.

Data from cohort studies have shown that right ventricular dysfunction on echocardiography, right ventricular dilatation on echocardiography or CTPA, elevated troponin levels, and elevated brain naturetic hormone levels are associated with increased early mortality in patients with acute PE. Whether these criteria should be used to select patients with hemodynamically stable PE to receive thrombolysis is uncertain. Catheter-based treatments (ie, thrombolytic therapy or mechanical removal of thrombus) require further evaluation before they can be recommended.

PRACTICE POINT

- Various thrombolytic regimens have been studied. The most widely used is rt-PA 100 mg given over two hours by intravenous infusion followed by heparin infusion with no initial bolus.

BLEEDING IN PATIENTS WITH ACUTE VENOUS THROMBOEMBOLISM

Management of a patient with acute VTE and bleeding is difficult. The first step is to ensure the patient is hemodynamically stable. After that, the following questions can help to guide management: How severe is the bleeding? Which anticoagulant is the patient receiving (and when was the last dose given)? How acute is the VTE? Can the source of the bleeding be treated?

Moderate to severe bleeding

If the bleeding is moderate to severe, the anticoagulant should be reversed (if possible), and the source of the bleeding treated. If the source of the bleeding cannot be treated, and the VTE is less than one month old, consideration should be given to inserting a permanent inferior vena caval filter. If the source of the bleeding can be treated, but requires surgery or time to heal, a temporary inferior vena caval filter should be considered and then removed if it becomes safe to resume anticoagulant therapy. If the source of the bleeding cannot be treated, and the VTE is older than three months, anticoagulants should be permanently discontinued. For reasons outlined later in this chapter, inserting an inferior vena caval filter is not recommended unless the patient has acute VTE (less than three months old).

Mild bleeding

If the bleeding is mild and likely to be transient (eg, hematuria in a patient with a urinary tract infection), the anticoagulant should be held for 24 to 48 hours and resumed once the bleeding has stopped. If the bleeding continues, consideration should be given to fully reversing the anticoagulant, and the source of the bleeding should be treated. If the bleeding resolves and the VTE is less than one month old, anticoagulants should be reintroduced with careful monitoring and/or lower doses. If bleeding persists, and the VTE is older than three months, anticoagulants should be permanently discontinued.

PRACTICE POINT

Rule #1: Do not anticoagulate a bleeding patient.
Rule #2: All effective anticoagulants increase the risk of bleeding.

Inferior vena caval filters

No randomized trial or prospective cohort study has evaluated inferior vena caval filters as sole therapy in patients with DVT (ie, without concurrent anticoagulant therapy). Permanent inferior vena caval filter insertion as an adjunct to anticoagulant therapy has been evaluated in a single large randomized controlled trial of patients with acute DVT who were considered to be at high risk for PE. The findings of this study, which were reported after two years and eight years of follow-up, indicated that filters decreased the rate of PE, increased the rate of DVT, did not change the overall rate of VTE, and had no clear influence on mortality. Indirectly, this study supports the use of vena caval filters to prevent PE in patients with acute DVT and/or PE who cannot be anticoagulated (ie, actively bleeding), but does not support more liberal use of filters. Patients who have a vena caval filter inserted should receive anticoagulant therapy if and when it becomes safe to do so, and for the same duration as for similar patients who do not have a filter.

DURATION OF ANTICOAGULANT TREATMENT OF VENOUS THROMBOEMBOLISM

Optimal duration of anticoagulant treatment of VTE is based on three factors: (1) the increase in the risk of recurrent VTE if anticoagulants are stopped, (2) the increase in the risk of bleeding on anticoagulant therapy, and (3) patient preference. The factors that determine the risk of recurrence are outlined below, while the risk of anticoagulant-related bleeding is addressed in the following section.

First, the risk of recurrence depends on whether the acute episode of VTE has been adequately treated. Studies evaluating different durations of anticoagulant therapy have shown that *all patients with VTE should receive a minimum of three months of anticoagulant therapy*. Patients who receive less than three months of anticoagulant therapy have double the risk of recurrent VTE during one to two years of follow-up.

Second, the risk of recurrence is dependent upon the patient's intrinsic risk of having a new episode of VTE. The risk of recurrence is highest in patients who have no risk factors for VTE (ie, idiopathic or unprovoked) or have a VTE provoked by a strong persistent risk factor (eg, active malignancy), and lowest in patients with a VTE provoked by a strong transient risk factor (eg, surgery). The risk of recurrence in patients with VTE provoked by a transient risk factor is one-third of the risk of recurrence for patients with unprovoked VTE. Extending the duration of anticoagulant therapy for unprovoked VTE to 6 months or 12 months protects the patient from recurrence while they are taking the anticoagulant, but does not reduce the risk of recurrence once the anticoagulant is discontinued (**Table 260-2**).

Two trials have compared long-term conventional-intensity anticoagulant therapy (INR 2.0–3.0) with low-intensity anticoagulant therapy (INR 1.75) and placebo, respectively, in patients with unprovoked VTE after a minimum of three months of anticoagulant therapy. These studies showed that treatment with extended duration conventional-intensity anticoagulant therapy reduces the risk of recurrence by about 90% whereas low-intensity anticoagulant therapy reduces this risk by about 70%. Surprisingly, the lower intensity of anticoagulant therapy did not significantly reduce the risk of bleeding compared with conventional-intensity therapy.

TABLE 260-2 Annual Risk of Recurrent Venous Thromboembolism after Anticoagulant is Stopped

	At 1 Year	At 5 Years
Transient risk factor for VTE	3%	10%
Unprovoked VTE	10%	30%

Two other factors connected with a patient's intrinsic risk of VTE that currently influence the duration of anticoagulant therapy include the number of previous episodes of VTE, and the presence of active malignancy. Patients with a second episode of unprovoked VTE have a 50% increased risk of recurrence and therefore should be considered for indefinite anticoagulant therapy. Patients with VTE and active cancer have a three-fold higher rate of recurrent VTE than patients with VTE who do not have cancer. The risk of recurrent VTE during and after anticoagulant therapy increases with more advanced stages of disease and with antineoplastic treatments such as chemotherapy. In addition, data from one large randomized trial has shown that treatment of cancer-associated VTE with extended duration LMWH reduced the risk of recurrent VTE by 50% compared with warfarin without significantly increasing the risk of bleeding.

PRACTICE POINT

- VTE should generally be treated for 3 months (or until risk factors resolve) or indefinitely
- VTE provoked by a transient risk factor is treated for 3 months
- a first unprovoked isolated distal DVT is treated for 3 months
- a first unprovoked proximal DVT or PE is treated for at least 3 months or indefinitely, depending on risk of bleeding and patient preference
- a second unprovoked VTE is generally treated indefinitely
- VTE associated with active cancer is generally treated indefinitely

Inherited thrombophilias increase the risk of a first VTE, but their influence on the risk of recurrent VTE is controversial. The risk of recurrence is reported to be highest in patients with antithrombin deficiency, patients homozygous for the Factor V Leiden mutation, and patients who are double-heterozygotes for thrombophilic states (eg, patients heterozygous for both the Factor V Leiden mutation and the prothrombin gene mutation). However, these combinations are rare. The most common inherited hypercoagulable conditions, activated protein C-resistance caused by the Factor V Leiden mutation (5% prevalence), and the prothrombin gene mutation (2% prevalence), have not been shown to significantly increase the risk of recurrence. Overall, thrombophilia screens identify an abnormality in only about 30% of patients with unprovoked VTE. A negative thrombophilia screen does not exclude an inherited thrombophilia; it just excludes the thrombophilic abnormalities that we are able to test for at this time. Consequently, the pros and cons of thrombophilia screening should be carefully weighed before the tests are ordered (**Table 260-3**).

Lupus anticoagulant and anticardiolipin antibodies (antiphospholipid antibodies) are acquired thrombophilic disorders, which may support indefinite anticoagulant therapy because of a higher risk of recurrent VTE and arterial events. However, testing for these disorders is not well standardized. It is important to be aware that antithrombin levels can be falsely low immediately following an acute VTE and that warfarin will interfere with testing for protein C deficiency, protein S deficiency and lupus anticoagulants.

PRACTICE POINT

- Don't order a test (eg, thrombophilia screen) if you don't know what you are going to do with the result!

TABLE 260-3 Pros and Cons of Thrombophilia Screening

Pros for Thrombophilia Screening	Cons of Thrombophilia Screening
Antithrombin deficiency, homozygous Factor V Leiden mutation, double-heterozygous Factor V Leiden and prothrombin gene mutation may lead to extension of duration of anticoagulant therapy.	These abnormalities are rare. Thrombophilia screening for the vast majority of patients does NOT alter management.
Informs patient of reason for developing VTE.	A negative thrombophilic screen can offer false reassurance. Patients with a family history of VTE and a negative screen likely have a thrombophilic disorder that has yet to be identified. A positive thrombophilic screen for a common abnormality can cause anxiety for the patient and potential insurance complications in the future. Thrombophilic screening is costly.
Stress importance of prophylaxis in high risk situations (eg, postoperatively, postpartum) in asymptomatic family members.	Family members should be advised of need for thromboprophylaxis in high-risk situations even if the thrombophilic screen is negative.
Can help female family members decide whether or not to use an oral contraceptive or hormone replacement.	If the index patient has a negative thrombophilic screen, a negative thrombophilic screen in a family member does not exclude the possibility of an inherited thrombophilia.

Factors that are connected with a patient's intrinsic risk of VTE, but are considered controversial with respect to their influence on the duration of anticoagulant therapy include gender, presence of residual DVT on ultrasound, elevated D-dimer after discontinuation of anticoagulant therapy, presence of postthrombotic syndrome, and thrombophilia. A recent meta-analysis reported that males have about a 50% higher risk of recurrent VTE than females. Currently, these factors do not have clear implications for duration of treatment.

BLEEDING IN PATIENTS ON LONG-TERM ORAL ANTICOAGULANT THERAPY

Risk of bleeding on anticoagulants differs markedly among patients depending on the prevalence of risk factors (eg, age greater than 75, previous gastrointestinal bleeding or stroke, renal failure, anemia, antiplatelet therapy, malignancy, poor anticoagulant control). Approximately 13% of episodes of major bleeding during the first three months of anticoagulant therapy are fatal and greater than 50% of intracranial bleeds are fatal. The risk of major bleeding in younger patients (eg, less than 60 years) who do not have risk factors for bleeding and have good anticoagulant control (target INR 2.0 to 3.0) is about 1% per year. The risk of major bleeding is expected to be as much as 10-fold higher in patients with multiple risk factors for bleeding.

CASE 260-1 *(continued)*

The safety of therapeutic anticoagulation for postoperative patients should always be discussed with their surgeons. Inferior vena cava filters are reserved for patients whose bleeding risks prohibit this approach. An inferior vena cava filter does not prevent DVT and may result in extensive thrombosis below the filter. Full dose heparin—either a continuous infusion of UFH or subcutaneous injections of LMWH—should overlap with warfarin for a minimum of 5 days until the target INR is within the desired therapeutic range of 2–3 for two consecutive days, at which point heparin can be discontinued. For UFH, this requires monitoring of the partial thromboplastin time (PTT) to reach a target range of at least 1.5 times the mean of the normal range, commonly 60–80 seconds. Laboratory monitoring of LMWH is not necessary; however, it is reasonable for patients with renal dysfunction, an elevated or very low BMI, those undergoing long-term therapy, and in pregnancy. The platelet count should be obtained at least every 3 days throughout the duration of therapy; in hospitalized patients the platelet count is commonly measured daily. These patients should remain on warfarin for at least three months. If this patient is still considered to have malignancy due to incomplete resection of his GBM, extended duration LMWH would be the preferred treatment over warfarin.

If this surgical patient had developed thrombocytopenia or a 50% drop in his platelet count, the diagnosis of HIT would be a consideration. In addition to the presence of thrombocytopenia and thrombosis, the timing of the fall of the platelet count (at least 5 days after first exposure to UFH) and whether there was another apparent cause of the thrombocytopenia (drug, sepsis, etc) would determine the pretest probability. Other clues to the development of HIT include systemic reactions to intravenous UFH, skin lesions at the site of heparin administration, or thrombosis while receiving treatment with heparin. If there is a high pretest probability of HIT, heparin should be discontinued and appropriate anticoagulation with a direct thrombin inhibitor (DTI) initiated while awaiting laboratory confirmation. For patients who develop HIT from UFH, LMWH cannot replace UFH due to cross-reaction with HIT-associated antibodies. The patient's platelet count would be expected to recover within 4 to 14 days after discontinuation of heparin. A DTI should be administered for at least 3 to 5 days and the platelet count should increase to at least 100,000/mm^3 before warfarin is initiated.

CASE 260-2 *(continued)*

The use of thrombolytic therapy for patients with submassive pulmonary embolism has not been shown to improve survival and is not currently recommended. This patient appropriately received UFH for 7 days and was discharged to home on therapeutic warfarin (target INR 2–3) with recommendations to continue warfarin indefinitely.

Given this patient's abnormal liver function tests, she was scheduled for further testing at the time of her follow-up appointment with her primary care physician. A right upper quadrant ultrasound revealed metastatic cancer to her liver, and she was subsequently diagnosed with pancreatic cancer. Idiopathic VTE should lead to consideration of underlying malignancy (age-appropriate screening), especially since presentation with bilateral leg DVT is far more likely to be found in patients with very aggressive hypercoagulable states (eg, malignancy, HIT). Extended duration LMWH should be considered once the diagnosis of cancer is established.

CONCLUSION

The majority of patients with VTE will require anticoagulation that extends beyond hospitalization. Clinicians need to ensure that care transitions include identification and communication with the receiving providers who will monitor anticoagulation. Discharge information includes drug, dosing (including last dose), timing of next dose and identification of who will advise patient of any dosage adjustment.

SUGGESTED READINGS

Ansell J, Hirsh J, Hylek E, et al. Pharmacology and management of the vitamin K antagonists: the Eighth ACCP Conference on Antithrombotic and Thrombolytic Therapy. *Chest.* 2008; 133:160S–198S.

Decousus H, Leizorovicz A, Parent F, et al. A clinical trial of vena caval filters in the prevention of pulmonary embolism in patients with proximal deep-vein thrombosis. Prevention du Risque d'Embolie Pulmonaire par Interruption Cave Study Group. *N Engl J Med.* 1998;338:409–415.

Hirsh J, Bauer KA, Donati MB, et al. Parenteral anticoagulants: the Eighth ACCP Conference on Antithrombotic and Thrombolytic Therapy. *Chest.* 2008;133:141S–159S.

Kearon C, Crowther M, Hirsh J. Management of patients with hereditary hypercoagulable disorders. *Annu Rev Med.* 2000;51: 169–185.

Kearon C, Kahn SR, Agnelli G, et al. Antithrombotic therapy for venous thromboembolic disease: American College of Chest Physicians Evidence-Based Clinical Practice Guidelines (8th Edition). *Chest.* 2008;133(suppl 6):454S–545S.

Lee AY, Levine MN, Baker RI, et al. Low-molecular-weight heparin versus a coumarin for the prevention of recurrent venous thromboembolism in patients with cancer. *N Engl J Med.* 2003; 349:146–153.

Linkins LA, Choi PT, Douketis JD. Clinical impact of bleeding in patients taking oral anticoagulant therapy for venous thromboembolism: a meta-analysis. *Ann Intern Med.* 2003;139:893–900.

Wan S, Quinlan DJ, Agnelli G, Eikelboom JW. Thrombolysis compared with heparin for the initial treatment of pulmonary embolism: a meta-analysis of the randomized controlled trials. *Circulation.* 2004;110:744–749.

CHAPTER 261

Anticoagulant Therapy

John Eikelboom, MBBS, MSc, FRACP, FRCPA, FRCPC
Magda Sobieraj-Teague, MBBS
Jeffrey S. Ginsberg, MD, FRCP(C)

Key Clinical Questions

1. What are the most important pharmacologic characteristics of specific parenteral and oral anticoagulants that are licensed for use in Europe and North America?
2. What determines the choice of anticoagulant in the prevention and treatment thromboembolism?
3. What determines the choice of anticoagulant in the management of patients with acute coronary syndromes?

INTRODUCTION

Unfractionated heparin and coumarins were discovered more than 60 years ago and for more than 40 years they were the only anticoagulants available to hospitalists. Now in 2011, several new anticoagulants have been licensed for clinical use and many more are under development. The increase in the number of licensed anticoagulants has expanded the choices available for physicians and patients but has also created new challenges in selecting the optimal therapeutic strategy. Anticoagulant drugs differ in their route of administration, speed of onset and offset of anticoagulant effect, half-life, reversibility, route of excretion, and availability of an antidote, and hospitalists need to be familiar with the properties of individual anticoagulant drugs in order to select the best agent for a particular clinical situation.

The first part of this chapter briefly reviews the most important pharmacologic characteristics of parenteral and oral anticoagulants that are licensed for use in Europe and North America. The second part of this chapter considers the choice of anticoagulant in the prevention and treatment of thromboembolism and management of patients with acute coronary syndromes and illustrates these choices using selected patient scenarios.

ESTABLISHED AND NEW ANTICOAGULANT DRUGS

Rapidly acting parenteral drugs, such as heparin, have been used for the prevention and initial treatment of thromboembolism during revascularization procedures, whereas the slower-acting oral vitamin antagonists (eg, warfarin) have been used for long-term use. Low molecular weight heparin, fondaparinux and bivalirudin have replaced heparin for many indications, and new oral anticoagulants, including the direct thrombin inhibitor dabigatran etexilate, and the factor Xa inhibitors rivaroxaban and apixaban have begun to replace vitamin K antagonists for long-term use. Dabigatran has been licensed for treatment of atrial fibrillation in Europe and North America and both dabigatran and rivaroxaban have been approved in North America and Europe for the prevention of venous thromboembolism. Apixaban has been approved in Europe for the prevention of venous thromboembolism but is not yet approved for this indication in North America.

PARENTERAL ANTICOAGULANTS

Figure 261-1 lists the parenteral anticoagulants, subdivided according to their pharmacologic target, that are licensed for use in Europe and North America. The pharmacologic properties of these agents are summarized in **Table 261-1**.

Unfractionated heparin

Heparin has important limitations because it has an unpredictable anticoagulant effect. Thus it requires routine coagulation monitoring, and it causes heparin-induced thrombocytopenia, which can result in life-threatening thrombotic complications, including limb ischemia, stroke, or death. Nonetheless, heparin retains several important advantages over more recently introduced parenteral anticoagulants such as low-molecular-weight heparin and fondaparinux. Heparin is not cleared by the kidneys, which means that it can be used in patients with renal insufficiency, and the anticoagulant effect of heparin can be neutralized by protamine, a basic protein that binds to heparin to form a stable salt that is cleared

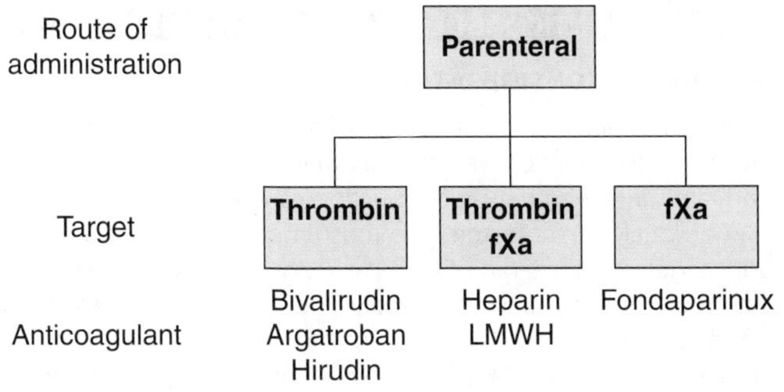

Figure 261-1 *Parenteral anticoagulants that are licensed for use in Europe and North America, subdivided according to their pharmacological target. (LMWH, low-molecular-weight heparin.)*

from the circulation. Thus, heparin remains widely used in critically ill patients and in those undergoing invasive procedures.

Low-molecular-weight heparins

Low-molecular-weight heparins (dalteparin, enoxaparin, nadroparin, reviparin, tinzaparin) are chemically or enzymatically derived from longer heparin chains. Because of their shorter chain length, low-molecular-weight heparins are much less likely than heparin to bind nonspecifically to cells and proteins and have a longer half-life (three to six hours) and a more predictable anticoagulant effect. Low-molecular-weight heparins can be given subcutaneously in fixed doses without routine coagulation monitoring and are less likely than heparin to cause immune heparin-induced thrombocytopenia or osteoporosis. The anticoagulant effect of low-molecular-weight heparins can be partially reversed with protamine.

Fondaparinux

Fondaparinux is a synthetic pentasaccharide that selectively inhibits factor Xa. Fondaparinux does not bind nonspecifically to cells or proteins, has a half-life of 17 hours, and has a predictable anticoagulant effect. Fondaparinux can be given in fixed doses by subcutaneous injection once daily, does not require routine coagulation monitoring, and it is renally excreted. Fondaparinux has been associated with the formation of anti-heparin/platelet antibodies, but there is no evidence that it causes heparin-induced thrombocytopenia. Fondaparinux does not have an antidote.

Bivalirudin

Bivalirudin is an intravenous direct thrombin inhibitor that blocks the interaction between thrombin and its substrates. Bivalirudin has a half-life of 25 minutes after intravenous injection, making the lack of an antidote less problematic than for longer-acting anticoagulants. It is about 20% renally cleared and the half-life of bivalirudin is prolonged in patients with renal impairment. Bivalirudin does not cause heparin-induced thrombocytopenia or osteoporosis.

Other parenteral direct thrombin inhibitors

The direct thrombin inhibitors, hirudin and argatroban, are less widely used than bivalirudin. Hirudin has a half-life of one to two hours and is 90% renally cleared. Argatroban has a half-life of about 40 minutes and unlike both bivalirudin and hirudin it is nonrenally cleared, making it suitable for use in patients with severe renal insufficiency.

ORAL ANTICOAGULANTS

Figure 261-2 lists the oral anticoagulants, subdivided according to their pharmacologic target, that are licensed for use in Europe and North America. The pharmacologic characteristics of the oral anticoagulants are summarized in **Table 261-2**.

Vitamin K antagonists

For more than 50 years, vitamin K antagonists, such as warfarin, were the only orally active anticoagulants that were licensed for long-term clinical use. Warfarin is an effective anticoagulant but has numerous limitations, including a slow onset and offset of action, variable dose requirements reflecting the effect of food and drug interactions and genetic polymorphisms that influence drug metabolism, and a narrow therapeutic window. As a result, routine coagulation monitoring is necessary to achieve a therapeutic anticoagulant level. Two important advantages of the vitamin K antagonist over newer oral anticoagulants are that warfarin's anticoagulant effect can be readily reversed with the administration of vitamin K, fresh frozen plasma, or prothrombin complex concentrates, and that warfarin is nonrenally cleared, making it suitable for use in patients with severe renal impairment.

Dabigatran etexilate

Dabigatran etexilate is a prodrug of dabigatran, a specific, competitive, and reversible direct inhibitor of thrombin. Dabigatran etexilate is given orally, has a bioavailability of about 6%, and is rapidly converted to its active form after absorption via the gastrointestinal tract by esterases. Dabigatran has a half-life of 12 to 14 hours in patients with normal renal function, it is 80% renally cleared, and it does not have an antidote. Dabigatran etexilate is a substrate of the P-glycoprotein transporter in the

TABLE 261-1 Comparison of the Pharmacologic Characteristics of the Parenteral Anticoagulants, Unfractionated Heparin, Low-molecular-weight Heparin, Fondaparinux, and the Direct Thrombin Inhibitors, Bivalirudin and Argatroban

Characteristic	Unfractionated Heparin	LMWH	Fondaparinux	Bivalirudin	Hirudin	Argatroban
Target	Xa and thrombin	Xa and thrombin	Xa	Thrombin	Thrombin	Thrombin
Dosing	SC, IV	SC, IV	SC, IV	IV	IV	IV
Half-life	40 minutes	3 to 6 hours	17 hours	25 minutes	1–2 hours	40 minutes
Renal clearance	Minimal	100%	100%	20%	90%	None
Routine coagulation monitoring	Yes	No	No	No	Yes	Yes
Antidote	Yes, protamine	Partial, protamine	No	No	No	No

IV, intravenous; SC, subcutaneous.

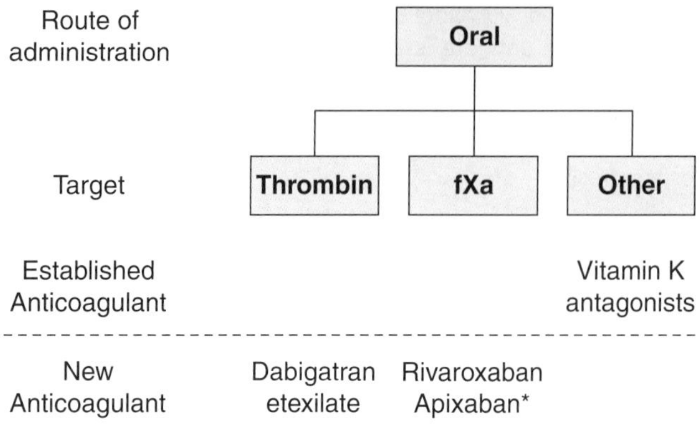

Figure 261-2 *Oral anticoagulants that are licensed for use in Europe and North America, subdivided according to their pharmacologic target. *Apixaban is licensed in Europe but is not yet licensed in North America.*

gut that is involved in the transport of drug from the cell into the lumen of the gut. The coadministration of drugs that inhibit the P-glycoprotein transporter, such as amiodarone, significantly increases drug levels of dabigatran in the blood. Dabigatran is given once or twice daily.

Rivaroxaban

Rivaroxaban is an oral factor Xa inhibitor that is rapidly absorbed via the gut and is two-thirds renally excreted. The half-life of rivaroxaban is 7–11 hours, and it does not have an antidote. Potent inhibitors of cytochrome P-450 (CYP) 3A4 and P-glycoprotein elevate drug levels of rivaroxaban by reducing its metabolism and excretion. Rivaroxaban is given once or twice daily.

Apixaban

Apixaban is an oral factor Xa inhibitor that is rapidly absorbed by the gut and is 25% renally excreted. The half life of apixaban is about 12 hours and, like rivaroxaban, it does not have an antidote. Potent inhibitors of CYP-3A4 elevate drug levels of apixaban by reducing its metabolism. Apixaban is given twice daily.

CHOICE OF ANTICOAGULANT

GENERAL CONSIDERATIONS

Selection of anticoagulant drugs is based on considerations of efficacy, safety, and convenience as well as cost, local availability, and familiarity with the drug. Selection can be tailored according to individual patient factors. The most important complication of anticoagulants is bleeding. The most serious nonbleeding complication of heparin is immune heparin-induced thrombocytopenia, which occurs in about 1% of patients undergoing cardiac surgery who receive heparin during cardiopulmonary bypass. Immune heparin-induced thrombocytopenia usually does not occur until at least five days after heparin exposure and is much less common outside of the critical care setting and in patients treated with low-molecular-weight heparin. Several direct thrombin inhibitors (hirudin, bivalirudin, argatroban) are licensed for use in patients at risk of or with established immune heparin-induced thrombocytopenia, and fondaparinux is increasingly being used for this indication.

PRINCIPLES OF ANTICOAGULANT DRUG SELECTION IN HOSPITALIZED PATIENTS

Prevention of venous thromboembolism

Drug efficacy and safety: Multiple parenteral and oral anticoagulants have been shown in randomized controlled trials to be effective and safe for the prevention of venous thromboembolism in hospitalized patients (**Table 261-3**). In general, efficacy and safety differences between the anticoagulants for venous thromboembolism prevention are modest and the choice of agent is determined primarily by convenience, cost, pharmacokinetic properties of the drug, as well as patient factors.

Patient factors: The most important patient factors that determine the choice of anticoagulant for venous thromboembolism prevention are renal function and the risk of bleeding. The potential for drug accumulation or need for drug reversal is low in patients receiving prophylactic doses of low-molecular-weight heparin. Nevertheless, low dose heparin is generally preferred over drugs that are partly or entirely renally cleared (low molecular weight heparin, fondaparinux, new oral anticoagulants) in patients with severe renal impairment, and is preferred over drugs with a longer half life (low

TABLE 261-2 Comparison of the Pharmacologic Characteristics of the Oral Anticoagulants, Vitamin K Antagonists (Warfarin), Dabigatran Etexilate, Rivaroxaban, and Apixaban

Characteristic	Warfarin	Dabigatran Etexilate	Rivaroxaban	Apixaban
Target	Vitamin K epoxide reductase	Thrombin	Factor Xa	Factor Xa
Dosing	Variable, once daily	Fixed, once or twice daily	Fixed, once or twice daily	Fixed, twice daily
Half-life	40 hours	12 to 14 hours	7 to 11 hours	12 hours
Renal clearance	None	80%	66%*	25%
Routine coagulation monitoring	Yes	No	No	Not required
Antidote	Yes, vitamin K	No	No	No
Drug interactions	Multiple	Potent inhibitors of P-gp†	Potent inhibitors of CYP3A4 and P-gp†	Potent inhibitors of CYP-3A4§

CYP-3A4, cytochrome p-450 3A4; P-gp, P-glycoprotein.
*One-half of renally-cleared rivaroxaban is cleared as unchanged drug and one-half as inactive metabolites.
†Potent inhibitors of P-glycoprotein include quinidine and amiodarone. Potent inhibitors of both CYP3A4 and P-glycoprotein include azole antifungals (eg, ketoconazole, itraconazole, voriconazole, and posaconazole) and protease inhibitors, such as ritonavir.
§Potent inhibitors of CYP-3A4 include azole antifungals, macrolide antibiotics (eg. clarithromycin) and protease inhibitors (eg. Atazanavir).

TABLE 261-3 Indications for Parenteral and Oral Anticoagulants in the Prevention and Treatment of Venous Thromboembolism*

	VTE Prevention				VTE treatment	
Agent	Hip or Knee Arthroplasty	Hip Fracture	General Surgery	Medical	Initial	Long-term
Parenteral agents						
sc, heparin		X	X	X	X†	
iv, heparin					X	
LMWH	X	X	X	X	X	X§
Fondaparinux	X	X	X	X	X	
Oral agents						
VKAs	X	X				X
Dabigatran etexilate	X¶					
Rivaroxaban	X¶					
Apixaban	X¶**					

LMWH, low-molecular-weight heparin; VKAs, vitamin K antagonists.

*Unless indicated otherwise, the 2008 American College of Chest Physicians Guidelines for Antithrombotic Therapy give all the agents listed in the table a strong recommendation over no therapy (benefits of the treatment outweigh the risks, burden, and costs) based on high or moderate quality evidence.

†Monitored or fixed weight-adjusted subcutaneous heparin

§Cancer patients

¶Dabigatran etexilate, rivaroxaban, and apixaban are not yet included in the American College of Chest Physicians Guidelines because they were licensed after publication of the guidelines.

** Apixaban is not yet approved for the prevention of venous thromboembolism in North America.

molecular weight heparin, fondaparinux, new oral anticoagulants, warfarin) and over drugs that lack an antidote (low molecular weight heparin, fondaparinux, new oral anticoagulants) in patients at high risk of bleeding and in unstable patients who may require surgery. In other settings, low molecular weight heparin and fondaparinux are generally preferred over heparin because of their excellent efficacy and safety profile and the new oral anticoagulants are preferred over parenteral agents because of their greater convenience.

Convenience: Parenterally administered anticoagulants are widely used in hospitalized patients for the prevention of venous thromboembolism but are less convenient for outpatient use because of the need for patient self-injection or for a nurse to visit the home to administer the injections. Warfarin is also effective for the prevention of venous thromboembolism in patients undergoing elective hip and knee arthroplasty and hip fracture surgery but is inconvenient because of the need for routine coagulation monitoring. The recent licensing in Europe and North America of new oral anticoagulants, dabigatran etexilate, rivaroxaban and apixaban, for the prevention of venous thromboembolism provides the opportunity to streamline out-of-hospital prophylaxis for patients undergoing hip and knee arthroplasty.

Treatment of venous thromboembolism

Drug efficacy and safety: All patients with acute venous thromboembolism should receive initial treatment with a rapidly acting parenteral anticoagulant for the first four to five days overlapped with warfarin and continued until the INR is above 2 on two occasions at least 24 hours apart. Intravenous heparin, fixed weight-adjusted or dose-adjusted subcutaneous heparin, low-molecular-weight heparin, and fondaparinux are effective and safe for the initial treatment of venous thromboembolism, and warfarin is effective for long-term treatment (Table 261-3). In high risk patients with cancer-related thromboembolism, low-molecular-weight heparin is recommended over warfarin for at least the first three months because of its superior efficacy for the prevention of recurrent venous thromboembolism.

Patient factors: Patient factors that influence the choice of anticoagulant for the initial treatment of venous thromboembolism include renal function and bleeding risk. Both low-molecular-weight heparin and fondaparinux are renally excreted and are contraindicated in patients with severe renal impairment; whereas heparin is suitable for use in patients with renal failure because it is nonrenally cleared. Intravenous heparin is also preferred in the initial treatment of patients at high risk of bleeding because its anticoagulant effect can be readily reversed with protamine.

Convenience: In the majority of patients, low-molecular-weight heparin and fondaparinux are preferred over intravenous heparin for the initial treatment of venous thromboembolism because these drugs can be administered by subcutaneous injection, once or twice daily, without routine coagulation monitoring, thereby allowing the majority of patients to be treated out of hospital. Fixed-dose twice daily subcutaneous heparin is less widely used but it is an inexpensive and acceptable alternative.

Acute coronary syndromes

Drug efficacy and safety: Heparin, low-molecular-weight heparin, bivalirudin, and fondaparinux are effective for the management of patients with acute coronary syndromes (**Table 261-4**). The choice of anticoagulant is primarily determined by the management strategy. Heparin and bivalirudin are generally recommended in patients who are invasively managed or undergoing primary percutaneous coronary intervention, whereas low-molecular-weight heparin and fondaparinux are indicated in noninvasively managed patients and in those receiving fibrinolytic therapy.

Patient factors: Patient factors that influence the choice of anticoagulant for the initial treatment of acute coronary syndrome patients are similar to those that influence treatment decisions in patients with venous thromboembolism. Intravenous heparin is generally preferred over other parenteral agents in patients with renal impairment and in those at high risk of bleeding.

TABLE 261-4 Indications for Parenteral and Oral Anticoagulants for Indications Other Than Venous Thromboembolism*

Agent	ACS	Post-MI	Revascularization (eg PCI, CABG)	"Bridging"	Atrial Fibrillation	Mechanical Heart Valves	HIT
Parenteral agents							
Unfractionated heparin	X		X	X[†]			
LMWH	X		X	X[†]			
Fondaparinux	X						X[§]
Hirudin							X
Bivalirudin	X		X				X[§]
Argatroban							X
Oral agents							
VKAs		X[¶]			X	X	
Dabigatran etexilate					X**		

ACS, acute coronary syndrome; CABG, coronary artery bypass grafting; HIT, heparin-induced thrombocytopenia; MI, myocardial infarction; PCI, percutaneous coronary intervention.

*Unless indicated otherwise, the 2008 American College of Chest Physicians Guidelines for Antithrombotic Therapy give all the agents listed in the table a strong recommendation over no therapy (benefits of the treatment outweigh the risks, burden, and costs) based on high or moderate quality evidence.

[†]For patients considered to be at high risk of thromboembolic complications.

[§]Grade 2 recommendation over no therapy (individual patient values may lead to different choices) based on low-quality evidence.

[¶]Grade 2 recommendation over no therapy (individual patient values may lead to different choices) based on high- or moderate-quality evidence.

** Dabigatran etexilate is not yet included in the American College of Chest Physicians Guidelines because it was licensed after publication of the guidelines.

Other indications

Outside of the settings of venous thromboembolism and patients with acute coronary syndromes, anticoagulant treatment options are much more limited (Table 261-4). Heparin is the preferred anticoagulant in patients undergoing revascularization procedures, and dialysis and heparin or low-molecular-weight heparin are used to "bridge" anticoagulant therapy in patients at high risk of thromboembolism who require temporary discontinuation of vitamin K antagonist therapy. Vitamin K antagonists are the only recommended anticoagulants for long-term prevention of thromboembolic complications in patients after myocardial infarction, patients with atrial fibrillation who are at risk for stroke, and in those with mechanical heart valves.

CLINICAL SCENARIOS

■ HOW DO I ANTICOAGULATE A PATIENT WITH RENAL IMPAIRMENT?

General considerations

All patients who require anticoagulation should undergo measurement of serum creatinine and (lean) body weight to enable calculation of an estimated creatinine clearance, for example, by using the Cockcroft-Gault equation. Patients with renal impairment achieve similar drug levels following a single dose of anticoagulant than those with preserved renal function, but renally cleared drugs accumulate after repeated dosing in patients with renal impairment. Thus, continuous intravenous infusion or repeat doses of anticoagulants that are renally cleared should generally be avoided in patients with an estimated creatinine clearance of less than 30 ml/min or the dose of the drug should be appropriately adjusted. A 50% reduction in the dose of low-molecular-weight heparin is recommended in patients with a creatinine clearance of less than 30 ml/min. Laboratory monitoring of anti-Xa levels can also be performed.

Choice of anticoagulant

Anticoagulants that may be considered for use in patients with renal impairment are listed in **Table 261-5**. The only licensed parenteral anticoagulants that are nonrenally cleared are heparin (minimal renal clearance) and argatroban. The advantages of heparin over argatroban include its widespread availability, the potential for subcutaneous as well as intravenous administration, the availability of an antidote, and low cost. Argatroban must be given by intravenous infusion, it is expensive, and its use is generally restricted to patients with renal impairment who cannot receive heparin because they are at risk of or have been diagnosed with immune heparin-induced thrombocytopenia. Low-molecular-weight heparin and bivalirudin can also be used in patients with renal impairment but the doses must be appropriately adjusted. Warfarin and other vitamin K antagonists are nonrenally cleared and are suitable for long-term use in patients with renal impairment.

■ HOW DO I ANTICOAGULATE A PATIENT WITH LIVER DISEASE?

General considerations

Anticoagulants should be used with caution in patients with impaired hepatic synthetic function because these patients are at increased risk of bleeding. The liver is the site of synthesis of the majority of coagulation proteins, including the vitamin K–dependent proteins factor II, VII, IX, and X and proteins C and S. Serum albumin and the prothrombin time are measures of the synthetic function of the liver but do not always reflect the presence of liver dysfunction. Hypoalbuminemia can also occur in patients with inflammatory conditions, malnutrition, and protein-losing states (eg, nephrotic syndrome), whereas a prolonged prothrombin time can also occur in patients with congenital coagulation factor deficiency, vitamin K deficiency, consumptive states, and patients treated with anticoagulants. The prothrombin time does not accurately reflect the coagulation state in patients with impaired hepatic synthetic function.

TABLE 261-5 Anticoagulants That May be Considered for Use in Patients with Renal or Hepatic Impairment

Setting	Route of Administration	Suitable for Use	Use with Caution/ Dose Modification
Renal impairment			
Creatinine clearance <30 ml/min	Parenteral	Heparin Argatroban	LMWH Bivalirudin
	Oral	Warfarin Dabigatran*	
End-stage renal failure	Parenteral	Heparin Argatroban	
Severe hepatic impairment			
(Impaired synthetic function)	Parenteral	Heparin LMWH Fondaparinux Bivalirudin	Argatroban
	Oral	Dabigatran etexilate Rivaroxaban Apixaban	Warfarin

LMWH, low-molecular-weight heparin.
*The Food and Drug Agency of United States approved dabigatran at a dose of 75 mg twice daily for stroke prevention in patients with atrial fibrillation with a creatinine clearance of 15–30 ml/min.

Choice of anticoagulant

Anticoagulants that may be suitable for use in patients with severe liver dysfunction are detailed in Table 261-5. The parenteral direct thrombin inhibitor, argatroban, and the orally active vitamin K antagonists are metabolized by the liver and can be very difficult to manage in patients with reduced hepatic synthetic function. Monitoring of individual coagulation factor levels may be required with patients with an abnormal international normalized ratio (INR) due to liver disease.

HOW DO I ANTICOAGULATE A HOSPITALIZED PATIENT WHO IS AT HIGH RISK FOR BLEEDING?

General considerations

Patients who are at high risk for thromboembolic events are often also at risk for bleeding because many risk factors are common to both conditions. Thus, patients who require anticoagulation are often older and have impaired renal function and other major comorbidities that increase their risk of bleeding. The decision to treat with anticoagulants should carefully weigh the risks of bleeding against the risk of thromboembolism, and the intensity and duration of anticoagulation should be minimized while still ensuring that patients receive effective treatment. It may be appropriate to admit patients at very high risk of bleeding to the hospital for monitoring during the initiation of anticoagulation, although there is no evidence that this approach reduces the risk of bleeding or improves clinical outcomes.

Choice of anticoagulant

The selection of an appropriate anticoagulant in patients who are at increased risk of bleeding because of renal or hepatic dysfunction is discussed above. Intravenous heparin remains an attractive option for the initiation of anticoagulation in patients at high risk of bleeding because of its short half-life and reversibility. Vitamin K antagonist therapy must be very carefully monitored during long-term treatment to maximize the time that the INR is in the target range, as poor quality INR control is a risk factor for bleeding.

HOW DO I REVERSE ANTICOAGULATION IN A PATIENT WHO IS BLEEDING?

General considerations

Decisions concerning reversal of anticoagulation should take into account the location and severity of the bleeding, the anticoagulant drug and the timing of the last dose, comorbid conditions including the indication for anticoagulant therapy, and the risk of thromboembolism when anticoagulation is stopped. In cases of urgent or life-threatening bleeding, reversal of the anticoagulant or removal of the drug takes precedence over concerns about the risk of thromboembolic complications.

Drug reversal

Table 261-6 lists general and specific strategies for the reversal of anticoagulant drugs. Most of the newer anticoagulants lack an antidote, making urgent reversal of their anticoagulant effect problematic. Infusion of fresh frozen plasma and fibrinogen concentrates and platelets is unlikely to significantly reverse the anticoagulant effect of selective factor Xa inhibitors, such as fondaparinux, rivaroxaban and apixaban, or direct thrombin

TABLE 261-6 Management of Patients Treated with Anticoagulants Who Are Bleeding

General measures	
Stop the anticoagulant	
Mechanical measures	
General hemostatic agents	
• Antifibrinolytic therapy	
• DDAVP	
• Activated prothrombin complex concentrates	
• Recombinant factor VIIa	
Removal of anticoagulant	
• Activated charcoal	
• Hemodialysis	
• Hemofiltration	
• Plasmapheresis	
Specific measures	
Anticoagulant	Reversal
Unfractionated heparin	Protamine sulphate
LMWH	Protamine sulphate*
Warfarin	Vitamin K Fresh frozen plasma Activated prothrombin complex concentrate Recombinant factor VIIa

DDAVP, Desmopressin acetate; LMWH, low-molecular-weight heparin.
*Partially reverses the anticoagulant effect of LMWH.

TABLE 261-7 New Anticoagulants in Advanced Stages of Development

	Parenteral		Oral	
Pharmacologic Target	Drug	Indications	Drug	Indications
Factor IIa (Thrombin)			AZD0837	Atrial fibrillation
Factor Xa	AVE5026 Otamixaban	VTE prevention Acute coronary syndrome	Edoxaban	VTE treatment VTE prevention VTE treatment Atrial fibrillation
Factor IX	RB006*	Percutaneous coronary intervention		

VTE, venous thromboembolism.
*Specific antidote available.

inhibitors, such as bivalirudin or dabigatran etexilate. Prothrombin complex concentrates and recombinant factor VIIa may have a role in these settings, but, with the exception of vitamin K antagonists, their efficacy for anticoagulant drug reversal in patients who are bleeding or require urgent surgery is unproven. Hemodialysis or filtration is likely to be most effective for reversal of the anticoagulant effect of drugs, such as dabigatran etexilate, that are not highly protein bound.

NEW ANTICOAGULANTS

A large number of anticoagulants have been introduced into clinical practice over the past two decades and many more are presently in advanced stages of clinical development (**Table 261-7**). Most of the new anticoagulants are small molecules designed to block the activity of individual coagulation proteins. Because of their specific mechanism of action, the new anticoagulants can generally be given in fixed doses without routine coagulation monitoring and have few off-target side effects, thereby potentially improving their benefit-risk profile. Because of their improved convenience, the new oral agents are likely to replace warfarin for many indications, but this also raises the potential for inappropriate use, for example in patients with impaired renal function, which could increase bleeding. Hospitalists will continue to play a key role in ensuring that existing and new anticoagulants are optimally used during hospitalization and at the time of hospital discharge.

SUGGESTED READINGS

Ansell J, Hirsh J, Hylek E, Jacobson A, Crowther M, Palareti G. Pharmacology and management of the vitamin K antagonists: American College of Chest Physicians Evidence-Based Clinical Practice Guidelines. 8th ed. *Chest*. 2008;133(suppl 6): 160S–198S.

Eriksson BI, Quinlan DJ, Weitz JI. Comparative pharmacodynamics and pharmacokinetics of oral direct thrombin and factor xa inhibitors in development. *Clin Pharmacokinet*. 2009;48(1):1–22.

Geerts WH, Bergqvist D, Pineo GF, Heit JA, Samama CM, Lassen MR, Colwell CW. Prevention of venous thromboembolism: American College of Chest Physicians Evidence-Based Clinical Practice Guidelines (8th Edition). *Chest*. 2008;133(6 Suppl): 381S–453S.

Goodman SG, Menon V, Cannon CP, Steg G, Ohman EM, Harrington RA. Acute ST-segment elevation myocardial infarction: American College of Chest Physicians Evidence-Based Clinical Practice Guidelines. 8th ed. *Chest*. 2008;133(suppl 6): 708S–775S.

Harrington RA, Becker RC, Cannon CP, et al. Antithrombotic therapy for non-ST-segment elevation acute coronary syndromes: American College of Chest Physicians Evidence Based Clinical Practice Guidelines. 8th ed. *Chest*. 2008;133(suppl 6): 670S–707S.

Hirsh J, Bauer KA, Donati MB, Gould M, Samama MM, Weitz JI. Parenteral anticoagulants: American College of Chest Physicians Evidence-Based Clinical Practice Guidelines. 8th ed. *Chest*. 2008;133(suppl 6):141S–159S.

Hirsh J, O'Donnell M, Eikelboom JW. Beyond unfractionated heparin and warfarin: current and future advances. *Circulation*. 2007;116(5):552–560.

Kearon C, Kahn SR, Agnelli G, Goldhaber S, Raskob GE, Comerota AJ. Antithrombotic therapy for venous thromboembolic disease: American College of Chest Physicians Evidence-Based Clinical Practice Guidelines. 8th ed. *Chest*. 2008;133(suppl 6):454S–545S.

Warkentin TE, Greinacher A, Koster A, Lincoff AM. Treatment and prevention of heparin-induced thrombocytopenia: American College of Chest Physicians Evidence-Based Clinical Practice Guidelines. 8th ed. *Chest*. 2008;133(suppl 6):340S–380S.

Weitz JI, Buller HR. Direct thrombin inhibitors in acute coronary syndromes: present and future. *Circulation*. 2002;105(8):1004–1011.

Weitz JI, Hirsh J, Samama MM. New antithrombotic drugs: American College of Chest Physicians Evidence-Based Clinical Practice Guidelines (8th Edition). *Chest*. 2008;133(suppl 6):234S–256S.

CHAPTER 262

Diseases of the Aorta

Tareck Nossuli, MD, PhD
Nicholas Tsapatsaris, MD

Key Clinical Questions

1. What is the normal size of the aorta, common femoral artery, iliac artery, and popliteal artery?
2. What do the American College of Cardiology and American Heart Association Guidelines recommend for abdominal aortic aneurysm screening?
3. What is the preferred classification system for aortic dissection?
4. When should large vessel vasculitis be suspected?
5. What are the causes of blue toe syndrome and what is the diagnostic modality of choice?

INTRODUCTION

Acute and chronic aortic syndromes have been the subject of intense investigation by physicians for centuries. These examinations have yielded a wealth of knowledge about the pathology, pathobiology, and pathophysiology of diseases of the aorta. More recent technological advancements have significantly improved our understanding of aortic syndromes at the molecular level, and have also helped in their accurate and timely initial diagnosis and long-term management. In addition, large clinical databases have elucidated the epidemiology and furthered the understanding of the natural history of many different aortic syndromes. However, despite the current armamentarium of knowledge and technology at the physician's disposal, the accurate diagnosis of acute aortic syndromes is not always apparent, sometimes with disastrous consequences. This chapter will focus on the presentation, diagnosis, and management of the various forms of acute and chronic aortic diseases, including aortic dissection and its variants, abdominal and thoracic aneurysms, multiple atheromatous embolization, giant cell and Takayasu arteritis, and blue toe syndrome (**Figures 262-1** and **262-2**).

ACUTE AORTIC DISORDERS: AORTIC DISSECTION AND ITS VARIANTS

PATHOPHYSIOLOGY

Acute aortic disorders include acute aortic dissection and its variants of intramural hematoma and penetrating atherosclerotic ulcer. All of these represent disruptions of one or more of the three layers of the aorta: the innermost intimal layer; the middle layer, or media; and the outermost adventitial layer. The intima is a very thin, endothelial-lined layer in its luminal portion, and it is prone to traumatic insults. The media is thick walled and contains multiple layers of elastic laminae (elastin, fibrin, collagen) and smooth muscle cells. The adventitia is primarily composed of collagen that helps to anchor the aorta to it surroundings, and also contains the vasa vasorum that functions to deliver blood to the outer aortic wall and to the media. The common pathway in all three acute aortic syndromes is a preceding weakening of the layers of the aorta that may lead to a tear in the intima, as in the case of dissection; rupture of the vasa vasorum, which leads to aortic infarction but with intact intima, as in the case of intramural hematoma; and atherosclerotic ulcer, which penetrates into the adventitia with surrounding hematoma. The weakening of the aortic layers occurs via various mechanisms including atherosclerosis, inflammation, cystic medial necrosis (deposition of mucoid material), disruption of the elastic lamellae, fibrosis of collagen, and medionecrosis and apoptosis of vascular smooth muscle cells.

EPIDEMIOLOGY AND RISK FACTORS

The incidence of aortic dissection is approximately 2.6–3.5 cases per 100,000 person-years, or approximately 2000 cases per year in the United States. In a review of the International Registry of Acute Aortic Dissections (IRAD), most affected individuals were male, with peak incidence in the sixth and seventh decades of life. Women who present with an acute dissection are usually older (mean age 67) than their male counterparts (mean age 63). In contrast, patients with intramural hematoma and atherosclerotic penetrating ulcers (which occur almost exclusively in the abdominal aorta) are even older (mean age 77), reflecting long-term atherosclerotic damage of the aortic wall. The mortality for aortic dissection depends on the location of the

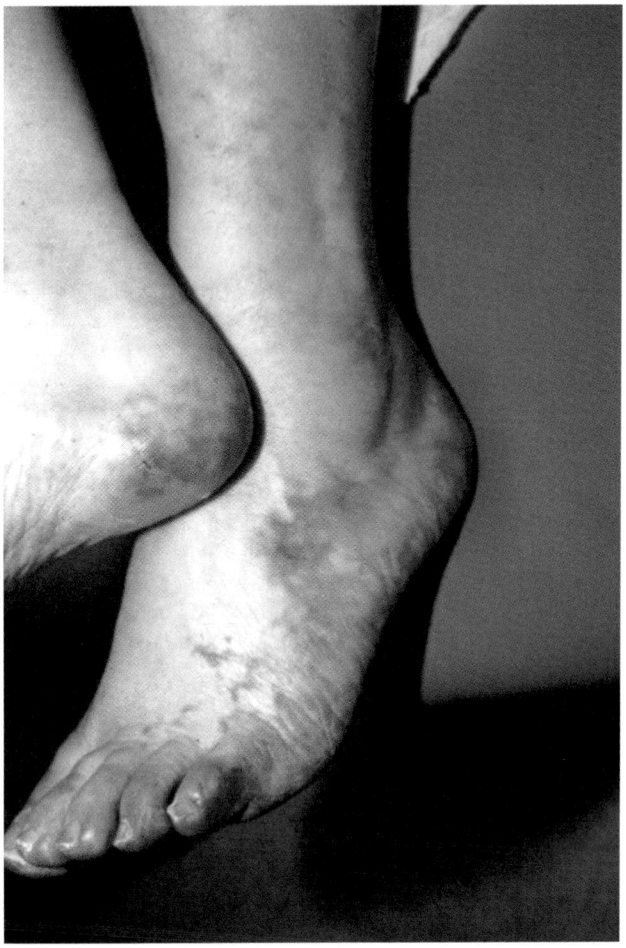

Figure 262-1 *Livedo Reticularis of Blue Toe Syndrome.*

dissection, but overall mortality for untreated acute aortic dissection is approximately 1–2% per hour from onset, within the first 48 hours. The most common origin of aortic dissection occurs in the ascending aorta (65%), with subsequent 20% occurring in the descending aorta, 10% in the aortic arch, and the rest in the abdominal aorta.

The most common risk factor for both aortic dissection and intramural hematoma is chronic hypertension, with approximately 75% of patients presenting with acute dissection reporting a history of hypertension. Increased age, smoking, hyperlipidemia, blunt trauma, cocaine use, and atherosclerosis are also important risk factors Pregnancy is a significant, under-recognized risk factor for aortic dissection insofar as up to 50% of dissections that arise in women less than 40 years old occur in the third trimester of pregnancy or in the early postpartum period. The mechanism for dissection is believed to be linked to pregnancy-related hemodynamic changes, pregnancy-induced hypertension, changes in the hormonal milieu with the release of relaxin, and underlying hypertension or connective tissue disorders. Young patients (< 40 years of age) who present with dissection are more likely to have genetically inherited conditions such as Marfan syndrome (defect in the fibrillin gene resulting in breakdown of elastic components of aortic wall), Ehlers-Danlos syndrome (defect in type III collagen in the aortic wall), Loeys-Dietz syndrome, aortic coarctation, or bicuspid aortic valve. A previous history of cardiac surgery occurred in 18% of patients presenting with dissection in the IRAD registry. In addition, disorders that are associated with vascular inflammation that leads to medial necrosis, such as giant cell arteritis, Takayasu arteritis, syphilis and Behcet, can also predispose to aortic dissection. Iatrogenic causes of aortic dissection include instrumentation of the aorta due to cardiac catheterization, intraaortic balloon pump placement, and cardiac surgery.

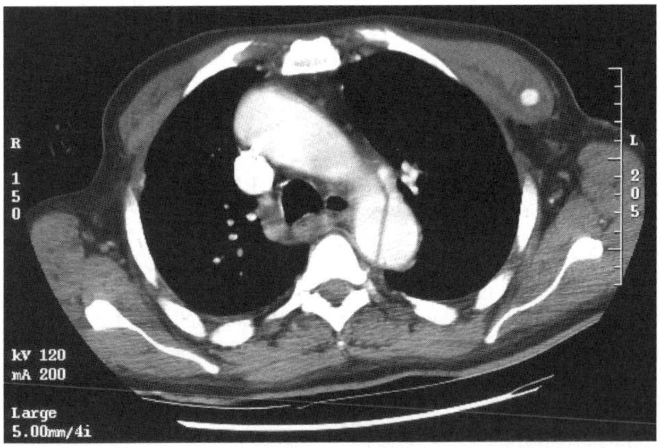

Figure 262-2 *CT image showing aortic dissection intimal flap in descending aorta.*

CLASSIFICATION OF AORTIC DISSECTION

Aortic dissection is characterized by a tear in the intima and the development of an intimal flap, thus creating a true and a false lumen. There are two common classification schemes of aortic dissection: DeBakey and Stanford. Within the DeBakey scheme, type I dissection describes a dissection that involves the full span of the aorta, originating in the aortic root, and propagating to the abdominal aorta. Type II dissection originates in and is confined to the ascending aorta through the level of the origin of the innominate artery. The management and treatment of Types I and II are identical, as they both involve the ascending aorta. Type III dissection originates in the descending aorta, distal to the left subclavian artery, and extends either distally down the aorta or retrograde to the aortic arch. Within the Stanford scheme, type A dissection is any dissection that involves the ascending aorta, regardless of site of origin. Type B dissection is any dissection that does not involve the ascending aorta. The DeBakey types I and II are equivalent to Stanford type A, and the DeBakey type III is equivalent to the Stanford type B. Since the management of DeBakey types I and II are the same, the Stanford classification system has become the preferred nomenclature.

CLASSIFICATION OF AORTIC INTRAMURAL HEMATOMA

Aortic intramural hematoma is a variant of aortic dissection and presents in an identical manner clinically, but is characterized pathologically by the absence of a detectable intimal tear. The false lumen is usually caused by rupture of the vasa vasorum into the media of the aortic wall, thus causing aortic infarction. The second cause of intramural hematoma is a penetrating atherosclerotic ulcer, which will be described below. Aortic intramural hematoma is considered to be a precursor of aortic dissection, accounting for 5–20% of patients presenting with symptoms of aortic dissection. In addition, intramural hematomas can result in classic aortic dissection, with the aortic wall infarct that can cause a secondary intimal tear. Aortic intramural hematomas have a natural history that is similar to aortic dissections, although up to 10% have been noted to resorb spontaneously. Aortic intramural hematomas are classified according to the Stanford scheme of aortic dissections. Therefore, type A intramural hematomas occur in the ascending aorta. More commonly, intramural hematomas occur in the descending aorta and are classified as type B.

CLASSIFICATION OF PENETRATING ATHEROSCLEROTIC ULCER

Penetrating atherosclerotic ulcers are atherosclerotic plaques that ulcerate into the media, leading to intramural hematomas and potential dissection. Atherosclerotic ulcers are almost exclusive to the abdominal aorta, and are associated with a higher rate of progressive disease (rupture, hematoma expansion, dissection) with medical treatment compared to aortic hematoma without ulcer. Separation of intramural hematoma, penetrating atherosclerotic ulcers, and classic aortic dissection on clinical grounds is not possible since all three entities present in the same fashion. Therefore the diagnosis is made on the basis of imaging techniques.

CLINICAL PRESENTATION OF AORTIC DISSECTION AND ITS VARIANTS

Signs and symptoms

Patients with aortic dissection, intramural hematoma, and atherosclerotic penetrating ulcer present with similar symptoms and have a variety of clinical manifestations. According to the IRAD registry, the most common symptom is sudden onset of sharp chest and/or back pain, in contrast to the classic teaching of tearing or ripping pain. The pain is severe at its onset and stays constant, as opposed to the pain of myocardial infarction, which is less severe at onset and gradually intensifies. Chest pain is more commonly reported with Stanford type A dissections and intramural hematomas, whereas back or abdominal pain is more commonly associated with Stanford type B dissections and penetrating atherosclerotic ulcers. Less common presentations include heart failure, most commonly secondary to acute aortic regurgitation in Stanford type A dissections, and syncope, which occurs in up to 13% of proximal dissections. The etiology of syncope may be due to rupture into the pericardial space causing tamponade, activation of cerebral baroreceptors, cerebrovascular accident, paraplegia (due to involvement of intercostal arteries causing spinal cord infarct), or cardiac arrest. An important point for clinicians is that up to 30% of patients are misdiagnosed as having other potentially fatal conditions such as myocardial infarction, since Stanford type A lesions can dissect most commonly into the right aortic cusp and the right coronary artery, thus causing inferior ST elevations and a rise in cardiac biomarkers. Consequences of branch artery dissection include stroke, renal and mesenteric infarction, and limb ischemia.

PHYSICAL EXAMINATION

Although hypertension is the most common predisposing factor for dissection and intramural hematoma, its absence does not exclude the diagnosis; at presentation, hypertension occurs in 36% of patients with type A and 70% of type B dissections. Hypotension is most commonly seen in proximal dissections with aortic root involvement, hemopericardium, and tamponade. Pulse deficits are helpful in diagnosis of acute aortic syndromes, but according to the IRAD registry, they occur in up to 30% of patients with type A and up to 21% of type B dissections. A diastolic murmur of aortic regurgitation, which reflects aortic root involvement with incomplete aortic valve coaptation, occurs in up to 44% of type A and 12% of type B dissections. Therefore, performance of a complete physical exam is essential in the evaluation of patients with chest pain.

DIAGNOSTIC STRATEGIES

An electrocardiogram, to help differentiate from acute myocardial infarction, and chest X-ray should be performed in all patients. A chest X-ray can demonstrate a widened mediastinum or displaced calcification in up to 85% of patients. Magnetic resonance imaging is the test with the highest sensitivity and specificity, but it is utilized in less than 5% of patients according to IRAD, as it has limited availability and takes longer to perform when compared with other modalities. The most common diagnostic tool is spiral computed tomography (CT), as it is fast and readily available in most centers in the United States. It has a sensitivity exceeding 95% and a specificity of 87–100%. In addition, CT can help with a "triple rule-out," with evaluation of dissection, pulmonary embolus, and proximal coronary artery disease all at once. However, administration of iodonated contrast makes patient selection important when kidney disease is present. Transthoracic echocardiography is of limited use, as technical considerations such as mechanical ventilation, patient body habitus, and emphysema reduce its sensitivity to 59–85%, and specificity to 63–96%. Transesophageal echocardiography (TEE) has a sensitivity of 99% and a specificity of 89%, and has the advantage of being performed quickly. However, it does require conscious sedation, making patient selection important. Aortography is more technically challenging than other diagnostic modalities, and should be performed when diagnosis is not obtained with other tools or when evaluation of coronary anatomy directly impacts surgical considerations.

MANAGEMENT

Along with admission to the intensive care unit, the major principles of initial management of both Type A and Type B lesions are decreasing the heart rate to <60 beats per minute and decreasing the arterial blood pressure to between 100 and 120 mm Hg. This decreases the rate pressure product and thus reduces the impact of shear stress on the aortic vessel wall, which then decreases the extension of dissection and reduces the possibility of rupture. Initial therapy includes intravenous (IV) infusion of beta-blockers. Labetolol is the most frequently used beta-blocker, as it also has alpha-blocking properties that result in decrease in left ventricular contractility as well as systemic blood pressure. Esmolol, a beta-blocker with short half-life (0.13 hours) can be utilized in patients going to immediate surgery, or who have chronic obstructive pulmonary disease (COPD). In patients with absolute contraindications to beta-blocker therapy (eg, COPD with severe bronchospasm), IV calcium channel blockers such as verapamil or diltiazem are appropriate alternatives, but dihydropyridines alone should be avoided. If beta-blockers are not sufficient to reach target heart rate and blood pressure goals, IV vasodilators such as sodium nitroprusside are appropriate add-on therapy. However, these should not be used as monotherapy, as they can cause a reflex increase in heart rate thus increasing shear stress on the aortic wall. Pain control with IV morphine sulfate is an important part of initial management, and is frequently overlooked.

THERAPY OF TYPE A DISSECTIONS AND INTRAMURAL HEMATOMA

Patients with type A dissections should be taken emergently to surgery upon diagnosis since mortality increases 1–2% per hour upon initial symptom onset, and carries a mortality rate of 30% by 48 hours with medical management alone. The primary goal of surgery is to prevent the major complications of proximal dissections including myocardial infarction, aortic regurgitation, and cardiac tamponade. Some of the factors that contribute to higher in-hospital mortality include advanced age (>70), hypotension, neurologic impairment, previous infarction, or valve surgery. Long-term treatment of these patients is similar to long-term treatment of patients with type B dissections, described in the next section.

THERAPY OF TYPE B DISSECTIONS AND INTRAMURAL HEMATOMA

Long-term treatment of most patients with type B lesions involves aggressive medical therapy. In a series of 384 patients from IRAD, 73% were managed medically, with a 10% in-hospital mortality. Aggressive blood pressure control (goal <120/80 mm Hg) is achieved with oral agents such a beta-blockers or nondihydropyridine calcium channel blockers. If blood pressure is not at goal, vasodilators such as hydralazine or dihydropyridines may be effective add-on therapy. However, these should not be used as monotherapy as they also have the potential to cause a reflex increase in heart rate with subsequent increase in rate-pressure product. Surgical intervention is indicated for patients who have persistent or recurrent pain, uncontrolled hypertension, develop end-organ damage, dissection progression, or aortic expansion. Endovascular repair (percutaneous stent-grafts or aortic fenestration) has been utilized for treatment of unstable type B dissections, with the goal of closing the entry of blood into the false lumen, thereby causing its decompression and thrombosis.

LONG-TERM FOLLOW-UP

Thirty percent of late deaths arise due to rupture of a secondary aneurysm that occurs within two years of initial treatment, or due to progression of dissection. Indeed, 20–30% of patients develop aneurysmal dilatation of type B dissection. Therefore, serial imaging of the aorta is mandatory. Magnetic resonance imaging (MRI) is the test of choice for follow-up imaging, although CT is an acceptable alternative. The current practice is to have imaging performed at 1, 3, 6, and 12 months after discharge, and annually thereafter. Surgery is indicated for aneurysmal expansion.

In our opinion, management of all patients with dissection, hematoma, and ulcers should include aggressive blood pressure lowering, goal LDL<70, and antiplatelet therapy.

Vascular medicine specialists are ideally suited to provide long-term follow-up for patients with aortic dissection given their expertise in cardiovascular risk modification.

ABDOMINAL AORTIC ANEURYSMS

INTRODUCTION

The abdominal aorta is the most common site of arterial aneurysms, which occur most often in the segment between the renal and inferior mesenteric arteries. An abdominal aortic aneurysm (AAA) is defined as an aortic diameter at least one and a half times the diameter measured at the level of the renal arteries, with a diameter greater than 3 cm considered to be aneurysmal. Abdominal aortic aneurysms involve all layers of the aorta and do not create a false lumen or intimal flap, as in the case of dissection.

PATHOPHYSIOLOGY

Atherosclerosis has been considered one of the primary underlying factors that lead to weakening of the media of the aortic wall, and allows for the development of AAA. Recently, it has been proposed that endovascular proteases, which degrade the elastic lamellae of the aortic wall, play an important part in the development and subsequent rupture of AAA. In particular, matrix metallopreoteinases (MMP)-2, 9, and 14 have been identified in the aortic walls of patients with AAA, as have cathepsin S and K. In addition, patients with AAA have elevated circulating levels of MMP-9, which decrease after repair. Inflammation has also been found to play a role in the pathophysiology of aortic wall deterioration and AAA development, as increased circulating levels of Interleukin-6 (IL-6) and C-reactive protein (CRP) are identified in AAA patients. A significant genetic factor has been identified, with up to 28% of patients having a first-degree relative with AAA. A family history of AAA increases the risk of developing the disease 4.3-fold.

RISK FACTORS FOR AAA DEVELOPMENT AND RUPTURE

In addition to the risk factors of family history and atherosclerosis delineated above, there are a number of other risk factors that significantly increase the risk of development of AAA, as well as increasing the risk of rupture. As demonstrated in the Veterans Affairs Cooperative Study group, smoking was the risk factor most strongly associated with AAA (odds ratio 5.07). Also, the association with smoking was directly related to number of years smoking, and decreased with number of years after smoking cessation. Hypertension and hyperlipidemia are also associated with AAA. Moreover, the incidence of AAA increases after the age of 55 in men, and 70 in women, with a male to female ratio of 9:1. In contrast, diabetes plays a protective role against the development of AAA, possibly due to the negative remodeling associated with diabetes. The Veterans Affairs Cooperative Study also noted that AAA occurred twice as frequently in white males compared with black males. COPD is also associated with expansion and increased risk of rupture of AAA, possibly due to the lack of alpha-one antitrypsin activity, which inhibits elastases that weaken the aortic wall. One of the most important risk factors for rupture is aneurysm size. Large population-based studies have consistently demonstrated that the risk of rupture significantly increases when AAA diameter exceeds 5 cm, which has led to the recommendation that all aneurysms greater than 5.5 cm should be automatically referred for surgery. For instance, one of these studies estimated the risk of rupture per person-years as 0% for AAA less than 4 cm in diameter, 1% for AAA between 4–4.99 cm in diameter, 11% for AAA between 5–5.99 cm in diameter, and 25% for AAA between 6–6.99 cm in diameter Importantly, the rate of aneurysm expansion (>1 cm/yr) over time is also associated with increased risk of rupture. These population-based studies have had a direct impact on guidelines for surgical versus medical management of AAA that are smaller than 5.5 cm in diameter, as will be described below.

CLINICAL PRESENTATION OF AAA

Signs and symptoms

The majority of patients with AAA are asymptomatic, and aneurysms are often detected incidentally on imaging studies that are performed for other reasons. Aneurysms that produce symptoms are at increased risk of rupture. The predominant symptom associated with rapid enlargement or rupture is severe back or flank pain, which is described as sudden onset, constant, not affected by movement, and may radiate to the buttocks, legs, or groin. Aneurysm rupture is associated with a clinical picture of shock, coupled with severe abdominal or back pain, and a pulsatile abdominal mass. Upper gastrointestinal tract bleeding from duodenal mucosal hemorrhage can demonstrate the presence of an enlarging aneurysm, and aortoduodenal or aortoesophageal rupture may occur with or without external bleeding. The survival rate for patients who experience a ruptured AAA is less than 50%.

PHYSICAL EXAMINATION

A palpable pulsatile mass, with or without tenderness, may be felt on exam from the epigastric to the suprapubic areas. Physical examination, which has a sensitivity of 22–96% is severely limited by patient body habitus, making palpation extremely difficult in obese individuals. Aneurysms may be palpable when they reach 4.5 cm in diameter in thin individuals, but are felt at 6 cm of diameter in moderately obese patients. If the aneurysm is tender to palpation, this may signify recent aneurysm expansion or impending rupture. Tenderness to palpation may also reflect an aneurysm with a significant inflammatory component. Evidence of associated vascular disease such as decreased peripheral pulses may be present, as well as evidence of thromboembolism, such as blue toes, livedo reticularis, or renal insufficiency.

PRACTICE POINT

- An aneurysm is defined as a dilatation of the blood vessel of interest greater than 50% of its normal diameter, which includes the intima, media, and adventitia.
- An upper limit of normal of 2.1 cm/m^2 is established at the level of the aortic sinuses. Therefore, the normal internal diameter of the aorta is < 2 cm, common femoral artery 1–2 cm, common iliac artery 1 cm, and popliteal artery < 0.7 cm.

IMAGING STUDIES

The most commonly used tool for screening (as discussed below) is abdominal ultrasound, which has sensitivity and specificity that approach 100%. The advantages of ultrasound are that it can accurately measure aneurysm size to within +/– 0.3 cm, is low cost, does not involve radiation, and is readily available in most U.S. centers. If obesity or intestinal gas pattern hinders an adequate ultrasound study, abdominal CT is an excellent alternative that is slightly more accurate with spatial resolution to within +/– 0.2 cm. In addition, CT allows for better assessment of extravasated blood, of anatomy of the aneurysm, and of the surrounding arterial tree. In patients with acute kidney injury or chronic kidney disease, CT without contrast is very useful for defining size of the AAA. Aortography is now largely supplanted by noninvasive techniques for AAA evaluation, as intraluminal clot may mask the true extent of the surrounding arterial dilatation. However, aortography is still used in some centers for planning of surgery. MRI allows for exceptional definition of aneurysm size and extension, but it lacks sensitivity to define renal vessel obstruction, it is expensive, and it is of limited availability in many U.S. centers.

SCREENING FOR AAA

The efficacy of population-based screening (which includes physical examination and ultrasound evaluation) for AAA has been evaluated by a number of large randomized trials. One of these, the Multicenter Aneurysm Screening Study (MASS) demonstrated that screening reduced AAA-related mortality in men. A later study from the MASS trial with seven year follow-up data showed a sustained benefit from screening, as well as a reduction in all-cause mortality. One study evaluated the efficacy of population-based screening in women, and determined that there was no effect on either AAA-related mortality or all-cause mortality. This may have been due to the low prevalence of AAA in women, and therefore a low event rate. From these studies, the American College of Cardiology and American Heart Association (ACC/AHA) have delineated screening guidelines for populations at high risk for AAA. These guidelines have also been adopted by the American College of Physicians (ACP) and the U.S. Preventative Services Task Force (USPSTF). Class I guideline recommends screening for men who are 60 years of age or older who are either siblings or offspring of patients with AAA. Class IIa guideline recommends a one-time ultrasound screening for detection of AAA for men who are between 65 and 75 years old who have ever smoked. Screening for men is currently reimbursed by Medicare. Screening for women is not currently recommended given the low prevalence of disease, and is therefore not reimbursed. For in-hospital patients, these screening measures may be undertaken as part of outpatient follow-up.

PRACTICE POINT

ACC/AHA Guidelines for AAA screening:

- Class I: Men 60 years of age or older who are either siblings or offspring of patients with AAA should undergo physical examination and ultrasound screening for detection of AAA.
- Class IIa: Men who are 65–75 years of age and have ever smoked should undergo a physical examination and one-time ultrasound screening for detection of AAA.

Data from Hirsch AT, Haskal ZJ, Hertzer NR, et al. ACC/AHA guidelines for the management of peripheral arterial disease. *J Am Coll Cardiol.* 2006:47:1239.

The diagnosis of AAA may be incidental to the work-up for other conditions. If an incidental diagnosis of AAA is made, this counts as part of the patient's AAA screening as recommended above, and results may be given to the patient.

MANAGEMENT OF AAA

Aggressive risk factor modification is an ACC/AHA class I recommendation, with rigorous blood pressure and lipid control as delineated for patients with atherosclerotic disease, as well as smoking cessation. Beta-blockers are a class IIb recommendation as they have been shown in a small trial to reduce the rate of aneurysm expansion, although this has not yet been reproduced. Importantly, mural thrombus is a component of all AAA, and it is not an indication for anticoagulation.

Surgical or endovascular repair is indicated for all patients with AAA of greater that 5.5 cm in diameter, or that expands at a rate greater than 1 cm/year on ultrasound or CT evaluation. In addition, repair should be performed in patients with symptomatic AAA, regardless of size, as well as those patients who present with signs and symptoms of rupture.

Two major trials have compared surgery to conservative medical management with regular ultrasound follow-up to evaluate expansion. Both of these trials demonstrated that for aneurysms between 4–5.4 cm, early surgery conferred no survival benefit over watchful waiting. Serial ultrasound or CT surveillance is indicated every two to three years for patients with aneurysms between 3–4 cm (ACC/AHA class IIa). For patients with aneurysms between 4–5.4 cm, the ACC/AHA recommends imaging every 6–12 months (class I).

SURGICAL AND ENDOVASCULAR THERAPY

All patients being referred for intervention need a preoperative risk assessment, given that there is high correlation between AAA and coronary artery disease, and that chronic kidney disease (creatinine > 3 mg/dl), chronic lung disease (forced expiratory volume < 1), and liver cirrhosis with portal hypertension may triple the risk of repair. Many studies have compared endovascular stent-grafts to open surgery, and have concluded that there is less operative mortality from endovascular compared to open repair. However, after four-year follow-up, there is no mortality benefit between the two types of repair. Thus, the role for endovascular grafts remains unclear as there is a lack of data on long-term outcomes. Therefore, current ACC/AHA guidelines recommend open repair for patients who are low or average operative risk (class I). Endovascular repair is reasonable in patients at high operative risk (class IIa), and may be considered in patients at low or average risk (class IIb). The major disadvantage of endovascular repair is the development of endovascular leaks, which require continuous monitoring and long-term serial imaging. The technical procedures and complications are beyond the scope of this text.

Consultation with a vascular medicine specialist is helpful for helping patients choose between open and endovascular repair.

THORACIC AORTIC ANEURYSMS

EPIDEMIOLOGY, PATHOPHYSIOLOGY, AND RISK FACTORS

Aneurysms that involve the aortic root to the diaphragm are termed thoracic aortic aneurysms (TAA), and are much less common than AAA (incidence of 5.9 per 100,000 person-years). The pathophysiology of TAA is similar to that described above for AAA, and includes cystic medial necrosis of the aortic wall that leads to its weakening, in addition to annuloaortic ectasia, which refers to elastolysis of the aortic annulus causing aneurysm and dissection of the ascending aorta. The risk factors for TAA are also similar to those of AAA and include smoking, COPD, hypertension, trauma, atherosclerosis, syphilis and infectious/inflammatory aortitis, as well as increased age. Family TAA syndrome is a strong predisposing factor for future development and progression of TAA. However, congenital bicuspid aortic valve, which is one of the most common congenital heart abnormalities, is more common in TAA. Some studies have demonstrated that as many as half of all of these patients will develop dilatation of the ascending aorta. Other genetically inherited conditions such as Marfan syndrome are also important risk factors for TAA development. Loeys-Dietz syndrome is a variant of Marfan syndrome, which is caused by mutations of the genes encoding transforming growth factor-beta (TGF-beta) receptors 1 and 2, and is also a significant risk factor for development of TAA. As in AAA, one of the most important risk factors for rupture is aneurysm size, thus making optimal timing for surgical correction essential.

CLINICAL PRESENTATION OF TAA

Signs and symptoms

Similar to AAA, TAAs are primarily asymptomatic and are incidental discoveries on imaging performed for other reasons. The most common cause of death in patients with TAA is rupture, and the clinical presentation is similar to acute dissection. Patients may present with acute aortic regurgitation and congestive heart failure, myocardial infarction, or thromboembolic phenomena. Patients may develop symptoms secondary to TAA compression of surrounding structures. For instance, patients may develop superior vena cava (SVC) syndrome due to SVC compression, or dyspnea, cough, and wheezing due to tracheal compression. TAA may also cause compression of the esophagus or recurrent laryngeal nerve, which produces dysphagia and hoarseness, respectively. As with AAA rupture or acute aortic dissection, patients with TAA rupture present with sudden onset of severe, sharp chest or back pain.

PHYSICAL EXAMINATION

Similar to type A dissections, the murmur of aortic regurgitation may be present at the right lower sternal border. In patients with compression secondary to TAA, SVC syndrome or unilateral jugular venous distention may be present, with lower extremity edema secondary to inferior vena cava compression, or with stridor due to compression of the bronchial tree. A pulsatile mass in the suprasternal notch may occur, and pulse deficits may also be present. Evidence of thromboembolic events may be seen upon examination of the digits.

DIAGNOSTIC MODALITIES

The diagnostic modalities for TAA are similar to those used for aortic dissection although CT and MRI are preferred. CT is the favored strategy for serial follow-up after repair, whereas MRI is chosen when visualization of the aortic root is required. As in aortic dissection, aortography is utilized for preoperative evaluation and to establish branch vessel patency.

THERAPY

Similar to AAA, beta-blockers are recommended for patients with TAA as they have been shown to slow the rate or progression of dilatation. Angiotensin receptor blockers may be important in the prevention of aneurysm development in Marfan and Loeys-Dietz syndromes, as these have been shown to arrest TGF-beta activity that has been implicated in structural destabilization of aortic media. In addition, aggressive risk factor modification is an essential part of initial therapy, with smoking cessation, lipid goals of LDL< 70 mg/dL, and hypertension management. Most experts advocate CT or MRI follow-up every six months to assess aneurysm expansion, with subsequent surgical intervention when the aneurysm becomes larger than 5.5 cm in diameter or grows at a rate or more than 1 cm/yr. Importantly, however, patients with Marfan syndrome, familial TAA syndrome, or bicuspid aortic valve are referred for surgery sooner, (when diameter exceeds 4.5 cm in diameter) because the patients have an increased risk of rupture or dissection at smaller aortic sizes.

Surgical repair involves resection of the aneurysm and its replacement with a prosthetic graft. If the aortic root is involved, a Bentall procedure is performed in which the aortic valve is replaced with a prosthetic valve, along with the aortic Dacron graft. Endovascular stent grafts have been compared to open surgery, and early evidence indicates that the endovascular approach may improve perioperative complications and mortality and decrease length of stay. However, at two year follow-up survival was not different in the endovascular group compared to the open surgery group.

MULTIPLE ATHEROMATOUS EMBOLIZATION

Aortic atherosclerotic plaques are manifestations of systemic atherosclerosis. When these plaques become large and complex, they develop into an important source of arterial thromboembolism, resulting in stroke and ischemia/infarction of other downstream organs and vascular beds. A complex atheromatous plaque (AP) is defined as a plaque having a thickness >4 mm, ulceration, or having a pedunculated portion of the plaque. Each of these three characteristics is associated with a high risk of embolic events. Rupture of the AP promotes superimposed thrombus formation, which may become a large, mobile pedunculated component of the plaque, as a result of release of multiple inflammatory mediators. In addition, analysis of the Stroke Prevention in Atrial Fibrillation-III (SPAF-III) trial demonstrated that complex AP was identified in 25% of patients presenting with AF, and was a significant independent risk factor for stroke if they occurred in the ascending aorta or aortic arch. However, in the absence of severe aortic regurgitation, descending thoracic AP are not as strongly associated with stroke.

Fifty percent of patients with atheromatous thromboembolism were noted to have a clinical presentation of stroke, with symptoms of transient ischemic attack and peripheral emboli being less common. In this same study, mortality secondary to stroke associated with AP was as high as 20%.

The diagnostic modality of choice for detection of complex AP is TEE, with sensitivity 91%, and specificity of 90%, which may be ordered as part of the initial workup for patients presenting with cryptogenic stroke.

As with the previously mentioned diseases of the aorta, initial therapy is aimed at risk factor prevention with aggressive lipid and blood pressure control, in addition to smoking cessation. According to the 2008 American College of Chest Physician guidelines, patients who are at low risk of major bleeding who have complex AP with or without a stroke are recommended to initiate heparin as well as warfarin therapy (goal international normalized ratio [INR] range 2–3), and high-dose statin therapy. The IV heparin may be stopped after INR range approaches it goal. The role of surgery has not been well defined, and is currently not recommended as first-line approach.

GIANT CELL ARTERITIS

Giant cell arteritis (GCA) is one of the primary diseases characterized by granulomatous inflammation of medium- and large-sized vessels. Its prevalence is approximately 18 in 100,000 people in the U.S., exclusively affecting those greater than 50 years of age, with women being more commonly affected than men (3:1 ratio). The inflammation induced during granuloma formation in GCA is transmural, potentially causing luminal occlusion of the affected vessels through intimal hyperplasia that subsequently produces end-organ ischemia. As a result, clinical manifestations include sudden onset of headaches, stroke, temporal artery tenderness, visual loss, and jaw claudication. GCA is strongly associated with polymyalgia rheumatica, and patients also present with symptoms due to systemic inflammation such as fever, weight loss, and generalized myalgias. GCA may produce clinically evident aortitis in up to 15% of patients, which can lead to aortic aneurysm (more commonly ascending) and rupture.

Physical examination may reveal a number of findings, depending on the location and extent of granulomatous inflammation. These may include pulse deficits, temporal artery thickening, and decreased large joint range of motion. In addition, bruits may be auscultated in the axillary, carotid, and supraclavicular areas, and the murmur or aortic regurgitation may be heard if the aortic root and valve are prominently involved.

Diagnosis is based primarily upon high clinical suspicion due to history and physical examination. All patients suspected of GCA should undergo temporal artery biopsy, which is positive in up to 80% of patients with a sensitivity of 88% and a negative predictive value of 91%. In addition, highly abnormal acute phase reactants (erythrocyte sedimentation rate or C-reactive protein levels approaching 100 mm/hour) are seen in more than 80% of cases of GCA. Treatment, which is aimed at reducing the inflammatory component of the disease, should not be withheld if temporal artery biopsy cannot immediately be performed. Prednisone (1 mg/kg/day) reduces symptoms within the first few days of initiation, and after four weeks, acute phase reactants have usually returned to normal, although this is not a reliable marker to guide therapy. In addition, low-dose aspirin may be started to reduce the risk of visual loss, transient ischemia attack, and stroke.

Importantly, there also appears to be a very strong association between GCA and future development of aortic aneurysms. A population-based study of Olmstead County residents who developed GCA between 1950 and 1985 demonstrated that compared to age- and sex-matched controls, patients with CGA were 17.3 times more likely to develop thoracic aneurysms, and 2.4 times more likely to develop abdominal aneurysms. This may be because treatment of GCA does not eliminate T-cell–mediated immune reactivity, which leads to continued inflammation within the aortic wall and eventual loss of intimal and medial structural integrity. As a result, we agree with the recommendation of Evans and colleagues, who propose that all patients with a history of GCA undergo an annual physical examination with palpation of the aorta, as well as an annual chest X-ray with lateral view for evaluation of thoracic aortic aneurysm development.

TAKAYASU ARTERITIS

Similar to GCA, Takayasu arteritis (TA) is a large-vessel vasculitis whose primary pathophysiology is inflammatory granuloma formation. Its incidence is 1–3 per million people in the U.S., with the highest prevalence in Japan. TA, or pulseless disease, affects young women (up to 90% of cases) much more commonly than men, and may involve any or all portions of the aorta along with its primary branches. The inflammation induces thickening of the walls of the affected vessels, which causes scarring and obliteration of the vessel lumen. The inflammatory process may also lead to significant weakening of the vessel wall, thus leading to development of aneurysmal dilatation.

Clinical manifestations on presentation are varied, ranging from asymptomatic to severe end-organ damage. Claudication of the upper extremities is the most common complaint, with asymmetry (a difference of greater than 10 mm Hg in each arm) or absence of pulses being the most common physical exam finding. Aneurysms occur primarily in the aortic root and can lead to aortic regurgitation. Hypertension is secondary to renal artery stenosis, and other presenting symptoms are also secondary to vessel occlusion including chest pain, abdominal pain, stroke, and headache as well as skin lesions. As in GCA, patients may present with generalized symptoms due to systemic inflammation, such as fever, malaise, arthralgias, and weight loss. In addition, acute phase reactants such as ESR and CRP are also significantly elevated, which helps with diagnosis. There are no specific diagnostic tests for TA, but use of arteriography as well as CT or MRI may demonstrate luminal narrowing of the aorta and its central branches, which help confirm the diagnosis. Approximately 50% of patients respond to steroid therapy, with relapses occurring in up to 40% of these patients. Those who are nonresponders to steroids, or who have recurrences are treated with daily cyclophosphamide and/or weekly methotraxate.

BLUE TOE SYNDROME

Blue toe syndrome is an entity that should be included in the differential diagnosis of patients who develop sudden onset of painful and cold areas of the foot and legs, or who develop sudden onset of abdominal pain or renal failure. This syndrome is characterized by small, cold, cyanotic blue or purple areas on the legs and/or feet that are painful and tender to the touch. Tissue necrosis from superficial ulceration to frank gangrene may develop. It is important to recognize that this syndrome primarily develops in the presence of normal or bounding peripheral pulses (Figure 262-1).

The primary pathophysiology of this syndrome is development of tissue ischemia secondary to occlusion of small distal arteries due to thrombosis, embolism, obstruction, and/or inflammation. Microemboli, which are primarily composed of cholesterol crystals, most commonly arise from ulcerated or stenotic plaques or from aneurysms in the peripheral circulation. Once these crystals are lodged in the microcirculation, they incite a vigorous inflammatory reaction, which further contributes to microvascular obstruction. Sixty percent of emboli originate in the femoropopliteal arteries, with the remaining 40% coming from the aortoiliac arteries. There are many causes of blue toe syndrome, including atheroembolism, cardiac embolism, hyperviscosity syndromes, hypercoagulable states, vasculitides, and induction of warfarin anticoagulation. Livedo reticularis is the most common cutaneous finding, and is characterized by a lacelike pattern of blue-red mottling of the skin. As described above, discreet areas of cyanosis in digits are also a common presentation. Cholesterol emboli can shower to various distal sites with the most common of these being the kidneys (74.5%), followed by the pancreas (52%), gastrointestinal tract (31%), and the adrenal glands (20%). Therefore, presenting signs and symptoms may include renal failure, pancreatitis, abdominal/back/flank pain, and accelerated hypertension.

Medical management is focused on eliminating nonatheromatous causes and defining the embolic source and eliminating it if possible. Unilateral symptoms suggest a source distal to the aortic bifurcation. Bilateral findings have to be caused by lesions proximal to the aortic bifurcation.

The diagnostic modality of choice to identify an embolic source is CT angiography. This obviates the theoretical concern associated with standard angiography of dislodging further emboli downstream. Both of these methods are able to identify atherosclerotic plaque, ulcerations of the plaque, and presence of aneurysm. Echocardiography should be performed in patients suspected of having cardiac disease, and ultrasound should be performed in all patients to determine proximal arterial occlusion and aneurysmal disease.

Patients with operable and hemodynamically significant lesions should undergo surgical intervention as the treatment of choice. Medical treatment, including antiplatelet therapy or anticoagulation may be sufficient in patients with less severe disease and no evidence of cholesterol embolism. However, recurrence of embolism is an indication for surgery.

CONCLUSION

Hospitalized patients with acute aortic diseases require multispecialty assessment and management. Front line clinicians should having a working knowledge of these diseases and of the capability of their practice environments so that they can mobilize multidisciplinary team care or if necessary transfer these patients to tertiary care hospitals. They also have a responsibility to communicate "incidental" radiographic findings such as a small aortic aneurysm to primary care physicians during care transitions so that secondary prevention and appropriate follow-up studies in the outpatient setting are arranged.

SUGGESTED READINGS

Aortic Dissection and Its Variants

Erbel R, Alfonso F, Boileau C, et al. Diagnosis and management of aortic dissection. Eur *Heart J.* 2001;22:1642.

Evangelista A, Mukherjee D, Mehta RH, et al. Acute intramural hematoma of the aorta: a mystery in evolution. *Circulation.* 2005;111:1063.

Ganaha F, Miller DC, Sugimoto K, et al. Prognosis of aortic intramural hematoma with and without penetrating atherosclerotic ulcer: a clinical and radiological analysis. *Circulation.* 2002;106:342.

Hagan PG, Nienaber CA, Isselbacher EM, et al. The International Registry of Acute Aortic Dissection (IRAD): new insights into an old disease. *JAMA.* 2000;283:897.

Meszaros I, Mórocz J, Szlávi J, et al. Epidemiology and clinicopathology of aortic dissection. *Chest.* 2000;117:1271.

Nienaber CA, Eagle KA. Aortic dissection: new frontiers in diagnosis and management: Part I: from etiology to diagnostic strategies. *Circulation.* 2003;108:628.

Nienaber CA, von Kodolitsch Y, Petersen B, et al. Intramural hemorrhage of the thoracic aorta. Diagnostic and therapeutic implications. *Circulation.* 1995;92:1465.

O'Gara PT, DeSanctis RW. Acute aortic dissection and its variants. Toward a common diagnostic and therapeutic approach. *Circulation.* 1995;92:1376.

Sommer T, Fehske W, Holzknecht N, et al. Aortic dissection: a comparative study of diagnosis with spiral CT, multiplanar transesophageal echocardiography, and MR imaging. *Radiology.* 1996;199:347.

Tsai TT, Nienaber CA, Eagle KA. Acute aortic syndromes. *Circulation.* 2005;112:3802.

Abdominal Aortic Aneurysms

Ashton HA, Buxton MJ, Day NE, et al. The Multicentre Aneurysm Screening Study (MASS) into the effect of abdominal aortic aneurysm screening on mortality in men: a randomised controlled trial. *Lancet.* 360:1531, 2002.

Kim LG, Scott RA, Ashton HA, et al. A sustained mortality benefit from screening for abdominal aortic aneurysm. *Ann Intern Med.* 2007;146:699.

LaRoy LL, Cormier PJ, Matalon TA, et al. Imaging of abdominal aortic aneurysms. *Am J Roentgenol.* 1989;152:785.

Lederle FA, Johnson GR, Wilson SE, et al. The aneurysm detection and management study screening program: validation cohort and final results. Aneurysm Detection and Management Veterans Affairs Cooperative Study Investigators. *Arch Intern Med.* 2000;160:1425.

Multiple Atheromatous Embolization

Amarenco P, Cohen A, Tzourio C, et al. Atherosclerotic disease of the aortic arch and the risk of ischemic stroke. *N Engl J Med.* 1994;331:1474.

Salem DN, O'Gara PT, Madias C, et al. Valvular and structural heart disease: American College of Chest Physicians Evidence-Based Clinical Practice Guidelines, 8th ed. *Chest.* 2008;133(suppl 6):593S.

Transesophageal echocardiographic correlates of thromboembolism in high-risk patients with nonvalvular atrial fibrillation. The Stroke Prevention in Atrial Fibrillation Investigators Committee on Echocardiography. *Ann Intern Med.* 1998;128:639.

Tunick PA, Nayar AC, Goodkin GM, et al. Effect of treatment on the incidence of stroke and other emboli in 519 patients with severe thoracic aortic plaque. *Am J Cardiol.* 2002;90:1320.

Tunick PA, Rosenzweig BP, Katz ES, et al. High risk for vascular events in patients with protruding aortic atheromas: a prospective study. *J Am Coll Cardiol.* 1994;23:1085.

Giant Cell Arteritis

Liozon E, Herrmann F, Ly K, et al. Risk factors for visual loss in giant cell (temporal) arteritis: a prospective study of 174 patients. *Am J Med.* 2001;111:211.

Mykelbust G, Gran J. A prospective study of 287 patients with polymyalgia rheumatica and temporal arteritis: clinical and laboratory manifestations at onset of disease and at the time of diagnosis. *Br. J. Rheum.* 1996;35:1161.

Salvarani C, Hunder GG. Giant cell arteritis with low erythrocyte sedimentation rate: frequency of occurrence in a population-based study. *Arthritis Rheum.* 2001;45:140.

Takayasu Arteritis

Kerr GS, Hallahan CW, Giordano J, et al. Takayasu arteritis. *Ann Intern Med.* 1994;120:919.

Kissin EY, Merkel PA. Diagnostic imaging in Takayasu arteritis. *Curr Opin Rheumatol.* 2004;16:31.

Weyand CM, Goronzy JJ. Medium- and large-vessel vasculitis. *N Engl J Med.* 2003;349:160.

Blue Toe Syndrome

Appelbaum RM, Kronzon I. Evaluation and management of cholesterol embolization and the blue toe syndrome. *Curr Op Cardiol.* 1996;11:533.

O'Keefe ST, Woods BO, Breslin DJ, et al. Blue toe syndrome: causes and management. *Arch Intern Med.* 1992;152:2197.

CHAPTER 263

Peripheral Arterial Disease

Catherine McGorrian, MB, BCh, LRCP&SI, MRCPI
Sonia Anand, MD, PhD, FRCP(c)

Key Clinical Questions

1. Who is at risk for developing peripheral arterial disease (PAD)?
2. How do you screen for asymptomatic PAD?
3. What are the symptoms and signs of PAD?
4. How do you diagnose PAD?
5. How do you treat PAD?

INTRODUCTION

Peripheral arterial diseases (PAD) refer to arterial pathologies that affect the vasculature outside the heart and likely affect at least 8 million people in the U.S. The prevalence of disease depends on the methodology used to define PAD. Intermittent claudication (IC) can be defined as an exertional pain, soreness, or fatigue involving a group of muscles that causes the patient to stop during walking and usually resolves within five minutes of rest. The symptoms do not cease during exertion and do not begin at rest. The prevalence of IC varies from 1% to 5% of the U.S. population. Studies using the ankle-brachial index (ABI) to screen for PAD describe a much higher prevalence of PAD than those relying on symptoms of IC, with PAD measured by an abnormal ABI affecting as many as 12% of people age 65 years or older compared to only 2% of participants in one survey with classic symptoms of IC.

CASE 263-1

A 64-year-old woman developed "sore legs" during walking, worse on her right side. At first she attributed the discomfort to her "arthritic hip" but over the last six months she noticed that she can hardly walk to the end of her apartment corridor and walking up inclines is particularly difficult. Stopping to rest relieves the discomfort, and she has had no pain during sitting or while sleeping. Her past medical history includes a first myocardial infarction (MI) at 56 years of age, hypertension, Type II diabetes, and hyperlipidemia. She has a past history of smoking.

Analysis

This patient has classic symptoms of IC. A complete physical examination including a vascular examination should be performed. She does not have symptoms consistent with critical limb ischemia or acute limb ischemia, which would require either referral to a vascular specialist or admission for emergency evaluation and limb salvage.

Diagnostic workup starts with a rest ABI +/– pulse volume recordings and/– segmental limb pressure examination.

For secondary prevention, she should be educated about symptoms of cardiovascular and cerebrovascular disease and receive the same secondary prevention as patients with coronary artery disease. Her doctor should emphasize the importance of not resuming smoking. She should be prescribed aspirin or clopidogrel taking into consideration patient specific factors such as comorbidity, cost, and tolerability. The target LDL is the same as for cardiovascular disease, the target LDL is < 100 mg/dL, and < 70 mg/dl in the highest risk patients. Because aggressive BP management reduces cardiovascular events in the highest risk patients (including those with diabetes), her target BP should be < 120/80 mm Hg starting with an ACE inhibitor. Beta-blockers are not contraindicated in patients with PAD, and she should receive a beta-blocker given her prior MI. Resistant hypertension should be evaluated because patients with PAD may have atherosclerosis elsewhere, including the renal arteries. Diabetic patients with PAD are especially likely to develop nonhealing ulcers and require amputation. The patient should receive instructions about foot care and examine her feet daily. Glycemic control should be measured to optimize her Hg AIC. Statins, aspirin, beta-blockers, and ACE inhibitors have been associated with improved survival in patients with PAD.

5-year natural history of PAD

Of 100 patients with a new diagnosis of PAD and intermittent claudication:

- Local events:
  - o One-quarter (25/100) will develop worsening claudication
  - o Of whom, 10 will require a revascularization procedure
  - o Of whom, 2 will require a major amputation procedure
- Systemic events:
  - o Non fatal myocardial infarction or stroke will affect 10 to 20 patients out of 100
  - o FATAL cardiovascular events will occur in one-quarter of patients, with 15 fatal myocardial infarctions and 5 other fatal cardiovascular events
  - o A further 10 patients will suffer non cardiovascular deaths

Figure 263-1 *The five-year natural history of peripheral arterial disease patients. (Data from Dormandy JA, Hospital Update, 1991.)*

Treatment

Ideally, she should participate in a supervised exercise rehabilitation program that may improve her pain-free walking distance by up to 180% of baseline. In conjunction with exercise, cilostazol and pentoxifylline are approved pharmacology treatments by the U.S. Food and Drug Administration. Cilostazol has been shown to improve symptoms and increase walking distance and would be the first choice unless the patient has a reduced ejection fraction or has major risk of significant bleeding.

The risk of developing PAD increases with age, with a reported prevalence of disease in the U.S. population of between 15–20% in the over-70 age group, compared with 3–10% in the general population. Men are more commonly affected than women, although with the greater longevity of women, increasing numbers of women are surviving to develop this problem. Chronic lower limb ischemia can be a significant clinical problem for patients due to limitation of mobility and impaired exercise tolerance, poor wound healing and potential ulceration, and ultimately the risk of critical limb ischemia with gangrene and amputation. However, this traditional schema of the natural history of PAD does not describe the most common morbidity risk for patients with PAD: death or disability from systemic atherosclerotic disease. PAD is an ominous risk marker for atherosclerotic disease elsewhere, and the major adverse cardiovascular event rate (myocardial infarction, ischemic stroke, and vascular death) in PAD patients is 5–7% per year, with a five-year probability of a major nonfatal or fatal cardiovascular complication of 30%35%. **Figure 263-1** shows the five-year risks of both limb-related ("local") and systemic events in a patient with PAD, from a 1991 report.

PRACTICE POINT

Association with coronary artery disease

- PAD is frequently asymptomatic; yet, the mortality of patients with PAD is two to three times that of age- and gender-matched controls with 75% of patients dying of coronary or cerebrovascular disease. Diagnosing PAD, whether in the clinic or during hospitalization, is important because physicians can take steps to institute appropriate treatment for preventing cardiovascular morbidity and mortality, and improve functional impairment, thereby preventing further functional decline.

The value of identifying PAD in our patients goes beyond institution of appropriate management of the PAD itself. It should also encompass a holistic cardiovascular risk review, with emphasis on identifying and treating the modifiable atherosclerosis risk factors, including preventive pharmacological management as appropriate. Patients with PAD have substantial functional decline compared to patients without PAD. This chapter will primarily focus on atherosclerotic conditions of the lower limb arteries. We will examine the practical aspects of screening for PAD, how to make a diagnosis of PAD, and consider the management options. Refer to other chapters for carotid and abdominal atherosclerotic pathologies.

PATHOPHYSIOLOGY

PAD arises when an obstruction (typically an atherosclerotic plaque within the arterial lumen) limits blood flow to the lower limbs. A hemodynamically significant stenosis decreases both blood flow and blood pressure distal to the stenosis, and this pressure drop is present regardless of whether the patient is resting or exercising. The patient's distal arterioles dilate to ameliorate the reduction in flow distal to the stenosis, so that the patient may be asymptomatic at rest. However, when the patient exercises, the peripheral muscles require an increase in arterial blood flow, but the arterial flow may be insufficient due to the stenosis, thereby causing symptoms.

Atherosclerotic disease most commonly affects major arterial bifurcations in areas of acute angulation and turbulent blood flow, such as the distal superficial femoral artery in the Hunter canal, the common femoral artery extending into the superficial femoral artery, and the distal aorta and aortic bifurcation. PAD may be initially asymptomatic, but can progress to a complicated spectrum of symptoms and signs, with gangrene and limb loss as the most serious limb-related adverse outcome. Primarily an atherosclerotic condition, PAD has risk factors similar to those for other atherosclerotic cardiovascular diseases; notably, advanced age, tobacco use, diabetes mellitus, hypertension, and hyperlipidemia. Smoking is also implicated as the primary insult in thromboangiitis obliterans (Buerger disease). This condition typically affects men in their 30s or 40s, and they present with a history of tobacco smoking and a rapidly progressive vasculopathy with stenoses and occlusions of multiple arteries. Other risk factors include race and ethnicity, elevated levels of inflammatory markers such as C-reactive protein, fibrinogen, leukocytes, and interleukin-6, impaired renal function, hypercoagulable states such as abnormal levels of D-dimer, homocysteine, and lipoprotein(as), other genetic factors, and abnormal waist-to-hip ratio. In addition, the presence of atherosclerosis in the coronary tree is associated with increased PAD risk. Obese patients with PAD who have elevated levels of inflammatory markers (C-reactive protein, fibrinogen, serum amyloid A, and

TABLE 263-1 Systemic Conditions that may be Associated with Peripheral Arterial Disease

Disease Group	Specific Conditions
Atherosclerosis	Associated with CVD risk factors; also Buerger disease (thromboangiitis obliterans)
Degenerative diseases	Marfan syndrome, Ehrler Danlos syndrome, cystic medial necrosis, neurofibromatosis
Vasculitides	Small vessel vasculitides, such as those associated with systemic connective tissue or automimmune diseases, eg, rheumatoid arthritis, systemic lupus erythematosis
	Medium vessel vasculitides, such as giant cell arteritis, polyareteritis nodosa, Wegener syndrome, Churg-Strauss syndrome, Kawasaki disease
	Large vessel vasculitides, such as Takayasu disease, Behcet syndrome, relapsing polychondritis, vasculitis associated with arthropathies
Thrombosis and thromboembolism	Thrombosis in situ (eg, due to disposing factors: thrombophilia, trauma, dissection) or thromoboembolism due to arterial emboli
Dysplastic diseases	Fibromuscular dysplasia

D-dimer) and do not exercise are more likely to suffer a significant decline in physical function. Less commonly, PAD may be associated with other systemic conditions such as collagen vascular diseases and the vasculitides. A more complete list of associations is seen in **Table 263-1**.

Localized PAD can also be due to such diverse causes as an aneurysm, trauma, congenital causes, and entrapment syndrome. Intermittent claudication without arterial obstruction may be seen in patients with severe anemia, pheochromocytoma, and amyloidosis.

PRESENTATION

ASYMPTOMATIC PATIENTS WITH PAD

As already described, PAD as diagnosed by ABI measurement can be asymptomatic. Especially in the elderly, other comorbidities such as severe heart or lung disease may limit their physical activity and delay the presentation of PAD. Furthermore, some patients severely limit their walking to avoid exertional leg symptoms, and present therefore with progressive functional decline rather than typical IC. The presence of atherosclerotic risk factors should alert the clinician to the possibility of PAD and to proceed with an examination looking for evidence of PAD.

SYMPTOMS OF IC

Symptoms of IC occur distally to the obstruction at times of higher oxygen and blood flow demand. Classically, patients describe exercising to their usual limit, at which time they experience calf pain. Patients cannot "walk through" the pain of IC, and ultimately have to rest for up to five minutes before resuming exercising. Symptoms of intermittent claudication do not always manifest as "pain." However, ischemic symptoms whether pain, cramping, aching, or fatigue should always arise in a functional muscle group, be reproducibly precipitated by exercise, and relieved by rest. The clinician should note both the claudication distance (how far the patient can walk before the onset of any pain) and the absolute claudication distance (the distance at which the pain becomes so severe as to necessitate stopping).

Symptoms may suggest the location of the obstruction at one of three levels: aortoiliac, femoropopliteal, and tibial artery (crural, below-the-knee, or infrageniculate) segments.

> **PRACTICE POINT**
>
> **Clinical clues to origin of ischemic symptoms**
>
> Arterial disease in the lower extremity
>
> Aortoiliac disease
> - Typical age of onset earlier in fifth and sixth decade
> - Usual risk factors of cigarettes, hyperlipidemia, hypertension
> - Pain, aching discomfort or weakness in hip, buttock, or thigh
> - Presence of impotence in males
> - Although total occlusion usually detectable by physical examination, assessment of less severe disease often grossly inaccurate
> - Decreased or absent femoral pulses and/or femoral bruits
> - Distal pulses may be present at rest due to collateral circulation
> - Normal peripheral ABI at rest and in response to exercise with reduced penile pressure consistent with isolated internal iliac disease
>
> Femoropopliteal disease
> - Calf pain
> - Extensive nature
> - Symptom progression more common than aortoiliac disease
>
> Tibioperoneal disease
> - Foot pain
> - Older patients, diabetic, often sedentary with limited life expectancy
> - Alone or in combination with SFA and popliteal disease
> - Trophic skin changes common due to extensive, distal atherosclerosis

Thigh or buttock pain on exertion, sometimes associated with impotence, should alert the clinician to the possibility of Leriche syndrome due to internal iliac arterial disease. The initial presentation and course of PAD in diabetic patients typically differs from PAD in patients with atherosclerosis.

Both smoking and diabetes accelerate the course of PAD with a higher projected five-year mortality and likelihood of requiring surgical intervention.

Patients with IC are more likely to have single-level disease, and patients with rest pain or skin ulceration are more likely to have multilevel obstruction. Because patients with PAD may have involvement of multiple arterial segments with symptoms throughout the leg, the vascular laboratory can be helpful in localizing the hemodynamically significant stenosis or stenoses.

> **PRACTICE POINT**
>
> **Intermittent claudication (IC)**
>
> Intermittent claudication
>
> - An inability to increase blood flow to meet the metabolic demands of exercising skeletal muscles causes symptoms of intermittent claudication
> - The most common areas affected are the major arterial bifurcations (areas of acute angulation) where there is the most turbulence:
>   - Most frequently, distal superficial femoral artery (SFA) in the Hunter canal
>   - Next most frequent, common femoral artery extending into SFA, distal aorta, and aortic bifurcation
> - Triad of symptoms include
>   - Pain, cramps, aching, or fatigue always in a functional muscle group
>   - Reproducibility precipitated by exercise, distance may vary depending on speed of walking, incline, type of terrain
>   - Relieved by rest by standing, with faster relief if patient sits
>
> **Pseudo-claudication (from spinal stenosis)**
>
> - Symptoms of numbness, aching, pain, and sometimes weakness in hips, thighs, buttocks, precipitated by extension of lumbar spine and weight-bearing activities such as standing for long periods and walking
> - Distinguishing features from IC include
>   - Positional nature (upright position further narrows spinal canal, causing symptoms)
>   - More variable level of activity that induces symptoms (upright position at rest); pain may be elicited during a straight-leg test during examination
>   - Relief usually requires more time (sitting for 15–20 minutes) and changing position (sitting with forward flexion of hips and not merely standing still).
>
> **Venous claudication (from venous hypertension in obstructed veins)**
>
> - Exercise worsens venous hypertension in patients with chronic venous insufficiency and in those with the chronic postthrombotic syndrome
> - Symptoms of a tight pressure in the limb, limiting activity
> - Distinguishing features from IC include
>   - Symptoms usually worse in thigh than calf
>   - Associated with venous leg edema
>   - Total resolution takes longer than with IC (much greater than 10 minutes) and may necessitate leg elevation

DIFFERENTIAL DIAGNOSIS

Comorbidities such as knee or hip arthritis, spinal disc disease, and spinal stenosis are more prevalent in patients who describe limb pain but who do not have classic symptoms of IC. Osteoarthritis of the hip or spinal canal narrowing can also cause hip and buttock pain and may coexist with PAD. Similarly, pain from venous disease, nerve root compression, or spinal cord stenosis can cause calf pain.

The history and physical examination should be able to differentiate other causes of exercise-induced lower extremity pain such as the chronic compartment syndrome, peripheral nerve pain, and hip and knee osteoarthritis.

SYMPTOMS OF CRITICAL LIMB ISCHEMIA

In more severe cases of PAD, critical limb ischemia may occur. Critical ischemia refers to chronic and severe obstruction of blood flow to the point that basal metabolic needs of the limb are not met. Patients first describe "rest pain," in which they experience troublesome ischemic pain at rest or at night when lying down. Unlike neuropathic pain, it may be relieved by placing the foot in a dependent position. Patients may describe hanging their affected foot out of bed at night in the search for some relief of their pain. The pain will likely be diffuse foot pain that may extend distally to the metatarsals. It may be accompanied by painful paresthesias and/or aching. Patients may have painful ischemic skin ulcers that typically form after minor trauma (shins, toes), or even frank gangrene. Arterial ulcers are pale to black in color, punctate, and well-circumscribed, unlike venous ulcers, which have thickened, brawny, hyperpigmented skin typically located in the region above the medial malleolus. Arterial ulcers should not be confused with diabetic ulcers. The latter typically arise over weight-bearing areas, have surrounding hypertrophic callus formation, and likely have associated infection. Unlike IC, patients with critical limb ischemia require either percutaneous or open surgical intervention to improve blood flow and to avoid major amputation.

> **PRACTICE POINT**
>
> **Diabetic patients**
>
> Compared to nondiabetics, diabetic patients have
>
> - Earlier age of onset of PAD
> - More rapid progression
> - Different distribution involving the popliteal, tibial, profunda femoris with the aorta, and iliac arteries largely disease free
> - Increased vulnerability to foot lesions (neuropathic and distal PAD)
> - Absence of ischemic pain and if pain present, may be neuropathic
> - ABI unreliable (vessels virtually incompressible due to calcific medial sclerosis)

ACUTE LIMB ISCHEMIA

When an acute arterial occlusion causes acute limb ischemia, the patient classically develops the six "Ps": pulselessness, pain, pallor, poikilothermy (coldness), paresthesia, and paralysis. Some of these features may not be present; both paresthesias or numbness and paralysis may have a later onset during the presentation, and while the foot may feel cold, it may also reflect the ambient temperature. A cold foot with a warm knee may suggest an acute popliteal occlusion with collateral circulation around the knee by the geniculate arterial system. Sometimes the enlarged geniculate vessels will be palpable on the side of the knee joint. Similarly, the skin of the medial lower aspect of the thigh may be warmer in limbs with occlusion of the superficial femoral artery. Failure to restore blood flow to the affected extremity may lead to major tissue loss or permanent nerve damage because the patient does not have time to form adequate collateral circulation.

DIAGNOSIS

THE PHYSICAL EXAMINATION

The physical examination of asymptomatic patients must be considered in conjunction with atherosclerotic risk factors to improve diagnostic accuracy of PAD. Clinical examination in the early phases may be unremarkable, and indeed the earliest sign of PAD can be an abnormal finding on an ABI test. In the asymptomatic person who is over age 70, or over 50 with an established atherosclerosis risk factor (tobacco use, diabetes, hypertension, or hypercholesterolemia), the 2006 American Heart Association/American College of Cardiology (AHA/ACC) guidelines suggest that inquiring as to the presence of calf pain should be asked as a routine part of the clinical history review of symptoms, and palpation of the lower limb vessels should be a standard component of the clinical examination. The clinician should therefore note the presence of all the major arteries in the leg (femoral, popliteal, anterior tibial, posterior tibial) and record whether the pulses are normal, reduced, absent, or possibly aneurysmal.

The examiner should listen for any iliac, femoral, or popliteal artery bruits. Bruits may also be noted over the adductor canal (also known as Hunter canal), on the medial aspect of the thigh, one-third of the way above the knee, where the superficial femoral artery runs under an aponeurosis. The presence of a bruit implies a stenosis at or proximal to the site auscultated. In the asymptomatic patient, the finding of an arterial bruit or pulse abnormality carries a strong positive likelihood of PAD. If there is no bruit but a reduced pulse, the patient may have collateral circulation or a very severe stenosis. In the person with claudication symptoms, clinical findings such as a cool extremity and/or the presence of an arterial bruit or a pulse abnormality (such as a reduced or absent pulse) are strong positive predictors of peripheral arterial disease. It is relatively unlikely to find moderate to severe PAD in a patient with no pulse abnormality and no history of claudication (likelihood ratio 0.21, 96% confidence interval 0.12 to 0.38).

PRACTICE POINT

The vascular examination

Pulses (scale 0–2: absent, diminished, or normal)

- Palpate limb pulses of both extremities simultaneously at the end of the examining table so that reduced pulses of the left or right side may be appreciated. Be careful not to mistake your own digital pulse for the patient's pulse.
- The absence of a DP is of no clinical significance unless unilateral and may be absent bilaterally in 10% of the normal population. The DP may not be appreciated if the ankle is excessively flexed. Although it usually arises from the anterior tibial artery, in some patients, the DP may arise from the peroneal artery and take a more lateral course on the dorsum of the foot.
- Do not compare proximal pulses in the lower extremity with distal pulses in the upper extremity because the arterial pressure wave is more peaked during distal propagation, the upstroke time shortens, and the amplitude increases, mainly due to an increase in systolic pressure. This is why a normal ABI (ankle brachial index) > 1. Compare femoral and popliteal pulses with the brachial pulse. Compare pedal pulses with radial and ulnar pulses.
- If pulses are present but there is uncertainty whether decreased, exercise the patient. If proximal stenosis, distal pulses will decrease further and the foot may become pale due to diversion of blood flow from skin to skeletal muscle.
- Aortic iliac disease may have reduced femoral, popliteal, pedal pulses; absent pulses suggest aortic-iliac occlusion.
- Superficial artery stenosis will have normal femoral pulses but reduced popliteal and pedal pulses on the affected limb; superficial artery occlusion will have normal femoral pulses but absent popliteal and pedal pulses on the affected limb.
- Distal disease will have normal femoral, popliteal pulses but reduced pedal pulses. Occlusion notable for normal femoral, popliteal pulses but absent pedal pulses.

Bruits (stenosis at or proximal to site auscultated)

- Avoid excessive pressure with the diaphragm of the stethoscope. Artifactual bruits may be noted over superficial vessels such as the common femoral artery and popliteal artery.
- Bruits over the flanks, lower abdominal quadrants, and adductor canal are rarely functional.
- A femoral bruit may be a sign of aortic-iliac stenosis.
- A popliteal bruit may be a sign of superficial femoral artery stenosis.

Elevation Pallor (Elevation of legs 60 degrees from horizontal for one minute)

- Look for a change in color. A severely anemic patient may also have pale legs but the color should not change with elevation.
- "Deathly pallor" indicates severe arterial obstruction.

Venous Filling time (VFT): time it takes for venous filling from elevation to dependency

- VFT can be misleading in the presence of venous insufficiency; often normal in presence of significant disease.
- Normal VFT is usually < 20 seconds but can be > 20 seconds if vasoconstriction is present secondary to cold, anxiety, or other conditions. The difference between limbs is normally < 5 seconds.

Advanced PAD

- Scattered, irregular cyanotic areas resembling livedo reticularis
- Dependency rubor (reddish to cyanotic hue of feet when hanging over the edge of the bed)
- Pallor on elevation
- Skin atrophy; loss of sweat glands; hair loss of the affected limb, especially toes; thickening of the nails (none of which are specific to PAD but common signs of the presence of PAD)
- Ischemic ulceration over affected segments
- Coldness apparent in affected area

In patients with PAD search for evidence of atherosclerotic disease elsewhere

- Check blood pressure in both arms. A hemodynamically significant stenosis will result in lower BP in the affected limb. A subclavian stenosis is most common in left arm.
- Auscultate for carotid, subclavian, and renal arteries for bruits.

The clinician should observe the leg for arterial ulcers, which may be punctuate and located along the shin or more distally. Although any loss of hair may be a possible sign of chronic PAD, this sign is neither sensitive nor specific. In patients in whom chronic moderate to severe PAD is suspected, a Buerger test can be helpful. With the patient in the recumbent position, the clinician raises one leg to at least 45 degrees, and observes for increasing leg pallor and venous guttering (Buerger sign). The clinician will also note that on restoring the leg to the flat position, reperfusion of the pale leg is sluggish, but ultimately returns to a more pronounced erythema than was initially noted (reactive hyperemia). The capillary refill time can be assessed by gently pressing the great toe until pallor is noted. When released, the great toe should become pink and healthy again within three seconds. However, a longer capillary refill time is not specific for PAD, because it may be influenced by both local factors and the presence of vasoconstriction.

THE ABI

Frequently used in epidemiological studies of PAD, the ABI is a simple noninvasive clinical test that can be undertaken in the office. It requires a blood pressure cuff and a handheld 5- or 10-mHz Doppler ultrasound (though some authors suggest that the use of a stethoscope is acceptable, as long as the methods are consistent over time). With the patient in a supine position for 5–10 minutes, the brachial systolic pressure is taken in both arms, and the highest pressure recorded. Then the systolic pressure in both the anterior tibial and dorsalis pedis arteries in the ankle are determined using a 10–12 cm sphygmomanometer cuff, and the highest pressure is recorded (**Figure 263-2**).

The ABI is the ratio of the ankle pressure to the brachial pressure. In healthy individuals the ABI should be similar in both limbs and exceed the brachial pressure by 10 to 15 mm Hg as a result of higher peripheral resistance at the ankles. The ABI typically correlates with severity of PAD (**Table 263-2**).

An ABI < 90% has a sensitivity of 95% and a specificity of 100% for detecting an obstructive lesion of > 50% in an extremity compared to the gold standard of contrast angiography.

The ABI is also not a foolproof identifier for PAD in patients with highly calcified vessels that cannot be compressed—most commonly, patients who are old, diabetic, receiving dialysis, or on chronic steroids. Measurements of an ABI greater than 1.30 suggest a noncompressible artery. If the ankle arteries are noncompressible, the toe-brachial index can be a more informative test of PAD, because small arteries are less likely to become calcified. Normal toes pressures are lower than ankle and brachial pressures; hence, a toe-brachial index of < 0.70 indicates PAD. The resting ABI may correlate with future cardiovascular events with a higher all-cause and cardiovascular mortality in patients with ABIs < 0.90 and in patients with ABIs > 1.40. What was previously defined as a "low-normal" ABI of 0.90 to 0.99 has recently been found to be associated with a significantly higher prevalence of subclinical atherosclerosis (increased carotid intima-media thickness and coronary calcium as defined by computed tomography), and is therefore a significant clinical finding in itself.

In some persons, a compelling history of IC may be elicited, and yet the ABI may appear normal. The clinician should then consider pathology in the internal and external iliac arteries, as the abnormality in patients with this pathology may only become apparent on exercise, as the inflow velocity through the stenosis increases. A treadmill or plantar flexion test may be helpful here, with the ABI measurement repeated after exercise. For nonambulatory patients, active pedal plantarflexion is a reliable alternative to the treadmill. The patient must perform 50 repetitions, only stopping when symptoms occur. In a patient without PAD the ABI will not change or only slightly increase due to peripheral vasodilation from exercise. In a patient with PAD, exercise-induced vasodilatation causes a significant blood pressure gradient and a drop in the ABI. A decrease in ABI after treadmill testing of 15–20% is diagnostic of PAD.

There are no randomized controlled trials that examine wider, population-based screening with ABI testing. However, because PAD is a relatively common condition with acceptable treatments and a long latency period and ABI is a relatively easy and acceptable test, many of the criteria for an appropriate screening program are fulfilled. The Walking and Leg Circulation Study (WALCS, 2009) has demonstrated that even with an ABI 1.00 to 1.09 individuals can have an increased risk of mobility loss at five years follow-up (hazard ratio for mobility loss 2.61, 95% confidence interval 1.08 to 6.32). The severity of the reduction in ABI has a graded association with risk of adverse CVD events (**Table 263-3**).

Despite the lack of evidence at this time, screening with ABIs has an inherent appeal, particularly in at-risk groups.

SEGMENTAL LIMB PRESSURE EXAMINATION AND PULSE VOLUME RECORDINGS

Other useful noninvasive tests include segmental Doppler pressure measurement, which uses a cuff method to identify pressure drops along the lower limbs to isolate the pressure drop across the stenotic lesion. A 20 mm Hg gradient between adjacent levels indicates underlying arterial stenosis. However, there are some weaknesses of this test, including the possibility of missing iliac lesions, and the difficulty in interpreting results in patients with noncompressible vessels.

Pulse volume recordings, usually obtained at the same time as segmental limb pressures, increase the reported diagnostic accuracy to 97%. Using a pneumoplethysmograph to detect changes in volume of the limb during the cardiac cycle, the cuff system records arterial waveforms. A normal arterial waveform has a steep upstroke, a narrow pulse width, a dicrotic notch, and a downslope returning to baseline. In the presence of arterial disease the slope and amplitude of the upstroke is reduced, the dicrotic notch is no longer seen, and the pulse width widens.

IMAGING OF THE ARTERIAL LESION

Once PAD has been confirmed, further investigations may be indicated to localize the site of the lesion, especially if the disease is severe or restrictive and surgical or percutaneous intervention is contemplated. Duplex scanning combines high resolution β-mode imaging with pulsed Doppler ultrasound. Arterial duplex ultrasonographic examination combines Doppler waveform analysis and velocities to diagnose PAD, determine the location of disease, delineate stenotic and occlusive lesions, and note changes in pulsatility and turbulence. Doppler frequencies are increased at the site of stenosis and the Doppler spectrum is broadened beyond the stenosis where flow is disturbed. There is a decrease in effective perfusion pressure roughly proportional to the severity of the occlusive process. Beyond a critical stenosis, there is a rapid fall in both distal pressure and flow. Waveform analysis and measurement of peak systolic velocity define the degree of stenosis: normal (0% stenosis), 1–19% stenosis (waveform changes without a change in peak systolic velocity relative to the proximal normal segment), 20–49% stenosis (waveform changes with an increase of peak systolic velocity by 30–100%), 50–99% stenosis (waveform changes with loss of flow reversal and increase of peak systolic velocity > 100%), and occlusion (no arterial flow).

The gold standard imaging modality has traditionally been angiography, which allows optimal visualisation of the arterial tree

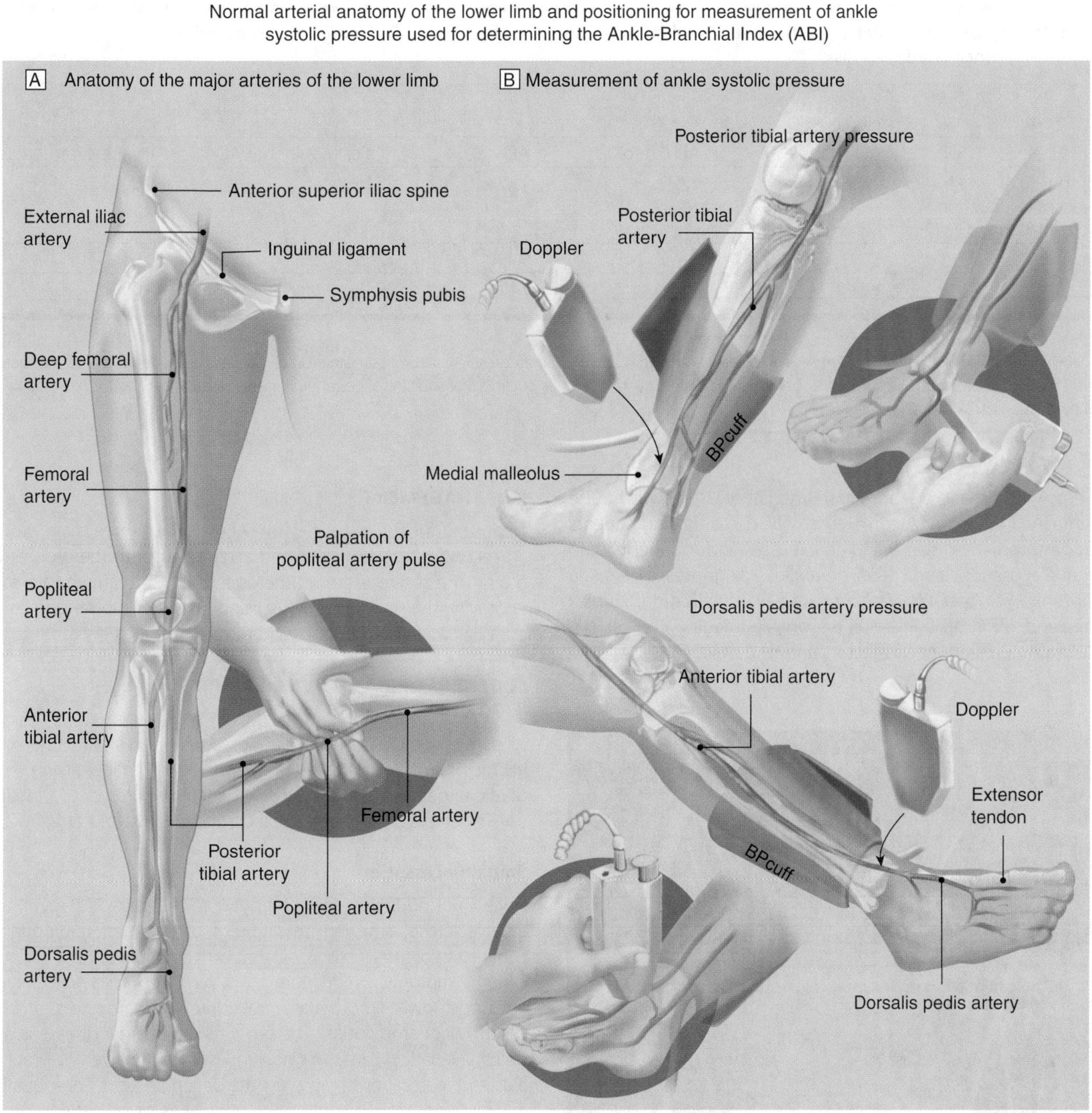

Figure 263-2 *Normal arterial anatomy of the lower limb, with suggested positioning for the measurement of the ankle systolic pressure for use in determining the ankle-brachial index. This figure shows the normal distribution of the lower limb arteries and the recommended method of palpation of the popliteal artery, with the clinician's hands tucked into the popliteal fossa. The positions in which to place the hand-held Doppler probe are shown on both the posterior tibial (shown above) and the dorsalis pedis arteries (shown below). (Reproduced, with permission, from the Journal of the Americal Medical Association 2006;29(5):536–546. Copyright © 2006 American Medical Association. All rights reserved.)*

TABLE 263-2 ABI = Lower Extremity Systolic Pressure/Brachial Artery Systolic Pressure

Incompressible Vessel	≥ 1.30 at rest
Normal	1.00–1.29 at rest
Borderline	0.91–0.99 at rest
Mild to moderate PAD	0.41–0.90 at rest
Severe PAD	0.00–0.40 at rest
Diagnostic of PAD	↓ ABI 15–20% during exercise

Reproduced from Ostergren J, et al, Impact of ramipril in patients with evidence of clinical or subclinical peripheral arterial disease. *Eur Heart J.* 2004;25:17–24, by permission of Oxford University Press.

and direct measurement of hemodynamic parameters. However, due to the invasive nature and inherent risks associated with contrast angiography, multidetector computed tomography (MDCT) scanning and magnetic resonance imaging (MRI) scanning have emerged to replace this imaging modality for most patients (**Figure 263-3**).

Table 263-4 describes the relative merits and limitations of these imaging studies.

In summary, the preferred imaging modality depends on the indications for the study, patient-specific factors (such as the presence of critical limb ischemia and renal failure or an implantable defibrillator), and institutional availability and expertise in image acquisition and interpretation. According to the ACC/AHA practice guidelines, consider an ABI for screening asymptomatic

TABLE 263-3 Association Between the Ankle Brachial Index and Adverse Clinical Outcomes in a Population at Increased CVD Risk

	Persons without clinical PAD				
Clinical event	ABI > 0.9	ABI 0.6 to 0.9	ABI < 0.6	Clinically evident PAD	P value for trend
Composite of stroke, myocardial infarction and death due to CVD	13.8%	18.7%	19.2%	23.1%	0.0003
Death due to CVD	5.3%	8.6%	9.4%	12.1%	< 0.0001
All cause mortality	8.8%	12.8%	14.7%	18.1%	0.0002

P value for trend from a Cox regression model adjusted for other CVD risk factors.
The HOPE-PAD study of n = 1715 patients age > 55 years with either established atherosclerosis, or a combination of diabetes and one other CVD risk factor.
Reproduced from Ostergren J, et al. Impact of ramipril in patients with evidence of clinical or subclinical peripheral arterial disease. *Eur Heart J.* 2004;25:17–24, with permission of Oxford University Press.

patients with risk factors; an ABI, segmental pressures with pulse volume recordings, and/or an exercise ABI for diagnosing patients with symptomatic disease; and an exercise ABI for patients who may have pseudoclaudication or unclear diagnoses to explain symptoms. For patients who require revascularization, duplex ultrasound, MRA, or CTA are all reasonable imaging choices depending on patient-specific factors and test availability.

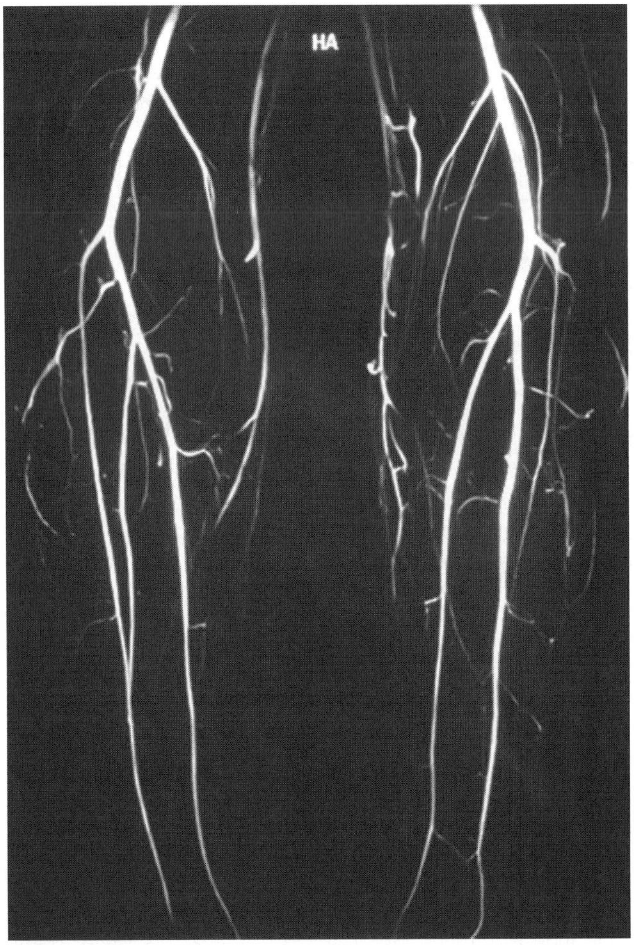

Figure 263-3 *Gadolinium contrast-enhanced magnetic resonance angiogram of the lower limbs. Contrast MR angiography is noninvasive, and findings with this imaging method are highly correlated with those found at invasive digital subtraction angiography.*

MANAGEMENT

Treatment for the patient with PAD falls into three main groups: (1) secondary prevention aimed at delaying both the progression of and the sequelae from atherosclerosis; (2) treatment aimed at improving the symptoms of PAD; and (3) acute limb-salvage procedures in cases of acute limb ischemia.

GENERAL PREVENTIVE MEASURES FOR ALL PATIENTS WITH PAD

All patients who have been diagnosed with PAD should undergo a risk factor and lifestyle assessment, with a view to identifying therapeutic targets that have a survival benefit with respect to tobacco use, hypertension, diabetes mellitus, and cholesterol status.

Smoking cessation

Since smoking is a major contributor to the genesis of peripheral atherosclerosis, smoking cessation is of paramount importance. Elimination of tobacco is associated with an improvement in claudication symptoms, a reduction in rest pain, improved graft patency rates post lower limb bypass procedures, and a decreased risk of death, MI, or amputation. The prognosis in Buerger disease is grim unless the patient can stop smoking. Use of adjunctive stop-smoking aids and medications may assist the patient in achieving cessation, and clinicians should continue to enquire as to the patient's smoking status on a regular basis, as many ex-smokers can lapse back to their smoking habit.

Blood pressure management

Clinicians should aim to achieve a blood pressure of < 140/90 mm Hg in their patients. Diabetic patients have traditionally been urged to achieve very low blood pressure targets (< 130/80 mm Hg). However, 2010 data from the Action to Control Cardiovascular Risk in Diabetes (ACCORD) study has shown that these very low targets in the diabetic group (target blood pressure < 120/80) do not improve prognosis. Beta-blockers are not contraindicated in patients with PAD, and the current guidelines from the Seventh Joint National Committee on Prevention, Detection, Evaluation, and Treatment of Blood Pressure (JNC 7) and the AHA/ACC groups propose that all antihypertensive agents are suitable in PAD. There is evidence to suggest that ACE inhibitor agents have particular value in secondary prevention in symptomatic patients with PAD. The Heart Outcomes Prevention Evaluation (HOPE) substudy on PAD patients identified a significant relative risk reduction (RRR) in fatal CVD events, nonfatal MI, and nonfatal stroke in 1715 persons with symptomatic PAD treated with ramipril, with a RRR of 0.75 (95% CI 0.61 to 0.92).

TABLE 263-4 Imaging Modalities that may be Used by the Clinician in Establishing the Diagnosis of PAD, and in Planning any Interventional Therapies

Imaging Modality	Sensitivity and Specificity	Advantages	Disadvantages	Contraindications
Duplex ultrasonography	High: may be up to 94% in detecting a stenosis > 50%.	Noninvasive and no ionizing radiation. Relatively inexpensive. Functional measurements relating to flow can be obtained.	Highly operator-dependent. Poor imaging of the crural vessels. Difficult to image calcified vessels and ↓ sensitivity for significant stenosis in tandem lesions; ↓ accuracy in assessing aortoiliac vessels due to gas, body habitus	None
MDCT	High. Compared with DSA, Computed tomography angiography (CTA) showed sensitivity and specificity of detecting an arterial stenosis of > 50% of 92% and 93%, respectively.	With technical improvements, better image acquisition at higher speeds, providing a "road map" of the vasculature from suprarenal aorta to ankles and flow information from axial cuts, imaging plaque morphology. In contrast to MRI, CT images show calcification well.	Need for ionizing radiation and iodinated contrast. Calcium in vessel walls can give rise to scatter and artefact	Patients with renal impairment or contrast allergy
Contrast MRI	Similar accuracy to duplex ultrasound and to digital subtraction angiography, with sensitivity and specificity for arterial stenoses of > 50% of greater than 90% when using 3D-gadolinium enhanced methods.	Provides a "road map" of the vasculature from suprarenal aorta to distal calves. Pedal arteries may require separate staging. No radiation exposure.	Image interpretation is operator dependent. Expensive, and image acquisition is lengthy. May overestimate degree of stenosis. Cannot reliably detect arterial calcification.	Any contraindications to MRI imaging, such as intracranial shunts, or noncompatible pacemakers.
Digital subtraction angiography (DSA)	Considered the gold standard	Provides a "road map" of the vasculature. Can make direct hemodynamic assessments.	Expensive. Risks for the patient include hemorrhage, dissection, embolism, and aneurysm formation at the puncture site.	Patients with renal impairment or contrast allergy

Lipid-lowering therapy

Lipid lowering therapy with HMG-coenzyme A inhibitors is a Class 1 indication in patients with PAD (AHA/ACC guidelines), with data from the Heart Protection Study showing that in 6748 PAD patients randomized to simvastatin or placebo, simvastatin was associated with a significant 6.3% absolute reduction in major adverse vascular events.

Antiplatelet therapy

Lifelong antiplatelet therapy has been a standard of care for patients with PAD, including those patients who may have undergone percutaneous or surgical repair of their disease. Aspirin has been shown to both reduce secondary events, and to help maintain vessel patency. Recently, a meta-analysis of 5269 patients with PAD showed that aspirin was not associated with a statistically significant reduction in all-cause or cardiovascular mortality; however this study was not powered to detect a 20% difference between the two groups (aspirin and control), and much of the study data were collected prior to 1995. Therefore, the recommendation for the use of aspirin for secondary prevention in PAD based on the Antithrombotic Trialists' Collaboration meta-analysis results should still stand at this time. Combination antiplatelet therapy (ie, aspirin and a second agent such as dipyridamole of clopidogrel) has not been established as superior to single agent therapy, and it is not advised in routine chemoprophylaxis (AHA/ACC guidelines). There is no clear role at this time for routine use of oral anticoagulation agents in patients with chronic PAD but no other compelling reason for anticoagulation (from data from the WAVE study).

Control of diabetes

The American Diabetes Association suggests that a target HbA1C of < 7.0% should be applied to manage risk of complications. However, this advice must be tempered with the current data from the ACCORD study, which suggests that very low HbA1C targets (<6.0%) are associated with an increased risk of hypoglycemic events and weight gain, with a trend toward an increase in a composite of nonfatal myocardial infarction, nonfatal stroke, and death of CVD.

TREATMENTS AIMED AT IMPROVING THE SYMPTOMS OF CHRONIC PAD

Exercise

Often neglected by clinicians, an important therapeutic tool in patients with PAD is an exercise prescription or program. Regular graded exercise can optimize patients' walking ability and maximal walking time. In our clinics, we advocate simple walking therapy to near-maximal pain threshold for 30 minutes at least four times a week. Such a regimen over six months has been shown in a 1995 meta-analysis to increase the distance to onset of claudication pain by 179% (225.3 m), and the distance to maximal claudication pain by

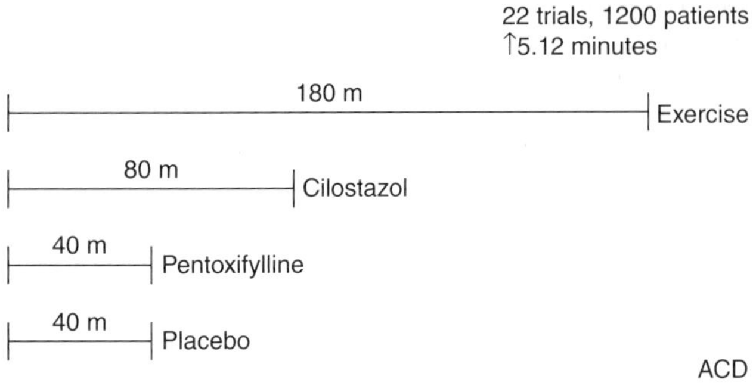

Figure 263-4 *Improvements in maximal walking distance (absolute claudication distance) in patients with intermittent claudication.*

122% (397.5 m). Furthermore, an exercise regimen can induce other benefits such as decreased adiposity, dyslipidemia, diabetes risk, and hypertension. Although PAD patients are often reluctant to undertake such a walking program, they should be positively encouraged to do so, and educated about the benefits of a simple exercise prescription over pharmacological therapy (**Figure 263-4**).

If available, supervised programs under the care of a cardiac rehabilitation or exercise physiology specialist are typically more successful than home-based programs.

Medical therapies

Drug therapies to improve the symptoms of chronic PAD are somewhat limited, and the most recent TASC guidelines suggest roles for two drugs only: cilostazole and naftidrofuryl. Cilostazole (Pletal) is a phosphodiesterase III inhibitor agent, which decreases vascular smooth muscle tone and inhibits platelet activation. Pooled data suggest that cilostazole is associated with an improvement in both initial claudication distance and absolute claudication distance in patients with symptoms of IC. There is also emerging evidence that cilostazole may be beneficial in promoting vessel patency after femoro-popliteal percutaneous angioplasty (PCA) and stenting. Cilostazole is contraindicated in patients with congestive cardiac failure. Naftidrofuryl (Praxilene) is a serotonin antagonist, which reduces platelet and red blood cell aggregation, and which may also promote aerobic metabolism in oxygen-depleted tissues. Naftidrofuryl has also been shown to increase pain-free walking distance in patients with intermittent claudication. However, in common with the studies of cilostazole, the absolute increases in walking distances achieved with naftidrofuryl are small (**Table 263-5**).

Other drugs such as pentoxifylline, buflomedil, and calcium channel antagonists have also been proposed for use in IC. While pentoxifylline, an agent which is thought to act by decreasing blood viscosity and increasing red blood cell flexibility, has been promoted as a second-line agent to cilostazole in IC, there remains limited evidence for its efficacy. At this time, neither the Inter-Society Consensus for the Management of Peripheral Arterial Disease (TASC II), nor the AHA/ACC guidelines endorse the use of these agents.

Revascularization therapies

Apart from medical therapies, persons with intermittent claudication may benefit from a revascularization procedure, either performed by open surgery or via the percutaneous route. Such patients must however undergo careful preprocedural evaluation, to ensure their suitability for such procedures. Expert opinion should always be sought. Surgical or percutaneous revascularization should only be performed in patients who have disease that is severe and/or significantly limiting their activities, and whose symptoms have proved refractory to conventional lifestyle and medical therapies. For a percutaneous angioplasty (PCA) procedure to be performed, the target lesion should preferably be focal and well-defined, and many patients will have lesions that are not suitable for such a procedure. Iliac lesions are often the most successful targets for PCA, but run a high risk of periprocedural arterial dissection, and primary stenting (ie, without prior balloon dilatation) is usually recommended. Experience in stenting lesions in the superficial femoral and popliteal arteries is increasing, with a growing literature on the use of antiproliferative drug usage in combination with either a balloon or stent delivery system. It is likely that PCA and stenting for PAD is a therapy that will continue to improve and broaden its indication. Surgical revascularization is also most efficacious in the case of more proximal disease, with distal lesions and procedures being associated with relatively more postoperative morbidity and tissue loss.

■ TREATMENT OF ACUTE LIMB ISCHEMIA

The acutely ischemic limb is a medical and surgical emergency that requires the clinician to rapidly diagnose the condition in order to put in place measures to restore arterial flow. Without an intervention to restore flow, irreversible tissue damage can occur within 6 to 12 hours of vessel occlusion. Acute and total vascular occlusion is typically due to vascular embolic disease to the lower limb. More commonly, patients will present with subacute or incipient limb ischemia, most often due to thrombosis of an atherosclerotic plaque, on a background of chronic PAD. Other precipitants of local thrombosis include trauma, low-flow states, thrombophilias, vascular grafts, and aortic dissection.

Management of the acutely ischemic limb includes immediate anticoagulation with heparin, and urgent notification of the vascular surgical team of the patient's status. Rarely, patients with heparin-induced thrombocytopenia with thrombosis (HIT) may present as an acute arterial embolism and for these patients heparin products would be contraindicated. It is therefore critical to have a high index of suspicion and treat patients with HIT with surgical embolectomy and direct thrombin inhibitors. The severity of the acutely ischemic limb may be classified using the Rutherford criteria (**Table 263-6**).

These criteria help the clinician determine the optimal treatment path: conservative management (in Stage I), and endovascular or surgical revascularisation (in Stage II). In Stage III, if the duration of ischemia is short, surgeons may consider a reperfusion strategy. However, if the limb is nonviable, delayed amputation may be the treatment of choice. Stage II management for acute ischemia due to an embolic event may include embolectomy, with or without adjunctive catheter-directed thrombolysis (CDT). If a thrombotic cause of disease is suspected, the surgeon may elect to perform surgical bypass, with or without adjunctive CDT.

All persons involved in the postreperfusion care should be aware of the possibility of an ischemia-reperfusion injury, with the possibility of sequelae such as myocardial dysfunction, electrolyte abnormalities, systemic inflammatory response syndrome, acute respiratory distress syndrome, compartment syndrome, rhabdomyolysis, and acute renal failure. The medical clinician may also be asked to offer recommendations about secondary prevention of further embolic sequelae for patients who have suffered an embolic event. The majority of systemic emboli originate in the heart, and the clinician should consider etiologies such as atrial fibrillation and left atrial appendage thrombus, valvular masses or vegetations, left ventricular thrombus, or paradoxical embolism through an atrial septal defect. Other vascular sources of emboli include proximal aneurysms (aortic, popliteal) with thrombus formation, and aortic plaque. Much

TABLE 263-5 Evidence-based Medicine: Key References for the Medical Literature-based Evidence Relating to the use of Pentoxifylline and Cilostazole in PAD

Reference	Methodology	Results	Limitations	Bottom Line
Girolami B, Bernardi E, Prins MH, et al. Treatment of intermittent claudication with physical training, smoking cessation, pentoxifylline, or nafronyl: A meta-analysis. *Arch Intern Med.* 1999;159:337–345.	Meta-analysis of randomized (n = 12) and nonrandomized (n = 1) trials that compared patients with stage II intermittent claudication treated with pentoxifylline vs. placebo. Duration of follow-up varied from 1 to 12 months.	Pooled estimates suggest an increase in pain-free walking distance with pentoxifylline (n = 6 trials, common difference of the means 21.0 m, 95% CI 0.7 to 41.3 m), and an increase in total walking distance (n = 7 trials, common difference of the means 43.8 m, 95% CI 14.1 to 73.6 m). No change was seen in resting or postexercise ABI.	Data synthesized were for differing doses of pentoxifylline, for differing follow-up periods. Data were not reported on side effects or drop outs.	Pentoxifylline is associated with significant, but small improvements in walking distances in patients with stage II intermittent claudication.
Dawson DL, Cutler BS, Hiatt WR, et al. A comparison of cilostazol and pentoxifylline for treating intermittent claudication. *The American Journal of Medicine.* 2000;109:523–530.	Randomized, placebo controlled, double-blind multicenter study of pentoxifylline (400 mg three times daily), or cilostazole (100 mg twice daily), or placebo. Population was patients with stable but at least moderate IC (ABI≤ 0.90), treated for 24 weeks with study therapy. Analysis was intention-to-treat.	In all three study groups, walking distance improved over the study period. There was no difference in improvement in maximal walking distance between the pentoxifylline group and the placebo group. The cilostazole group had a significantly greater improvement in maximal walking distance (increase of 107 m, SD 158 m, p value for comparisons with placebo and cilostazole < 0.001)	Drop-out burden in both active therapy groups: 27% of cilostazole patients and 26% of pentoxifylline patients, compared with 16% of placebo patients. Higher frequency of side effects in both active treatment groups.	No benefit seen in the pentoxifylline group with respect to walking distances. Cilostazole is beneficial in increasing walking distances, but minor side effects are common (86% of patients having at least one side effect event, eg, headache, diarrhea, pains).
Robless P, Mikhailidis DP, Stansby GP. Cilostazol for peripheral arterial disease. *Cochrane Database of Systematic Reviews* 2008, Issue 1. Art. No.: CD003748. DOI: 10.1002/14651858. CD003748.pub3.	Cochrane standardized meta-analysis of double-blind RCTs of cilostazole vs. placebo or antiplatelet therapy, in patients with IC or undergoing PAD surgery. Data were synthesized on seven RCTs that compared cilostazole with placebo, and one that compared cilostazole with pentoxifylline and placebo. All RCTs included a cilostazole group with a dose of 100 mg twice daily. Data on up to 1,579 patients were synthesized.	Cilostazole 100 mg twice daily was associated with an increase in absolute claudication distance of 49.70 m (95% CI 24.23 to 75.18), and an increase in initial claudication distance of 31.14 m (21.34, 40.93)	No data on cardiovascular event rates.	Cilostazole is associated with better walking distances in persons with intermittent claudication.
Pande RL, Hiatt WR, Zhang P, Hittel N, Creager MA. A pooled analysis of the durability and predictors of treatment response of cilostazol in patients with intermittent claudication. *Vascular Medicine.* 2010.	Meta-analysis of patient-level data from nine randomized, double-blind, placebo controlled studies comparing cilostazole with placebo. Patients were aged ≥ 40, with a 3+ month history of stable IC, and an ABI ≤ 0.90 in eight trials, and ≤ 0.80 in one trial. Data were available on n = 2591 participants.	Cilostazole was associated with a pooled mean difference in maximal walking distance of 42.1 m (95% CI 20.7 to 63.5 m, p < 0.0001). Effects were sustained throughout the study period. There was no increase in all-cause mortality in the cilostazole group compared with placebo (RR 0.95, 95% CI 0.68 to 1.35, p = 0.79).	Some statistical heterogeneity in the pooled models.	Cilostazole is associated with improvements in walking distance in persons with IC, and there was no evidence of an increase in mortality with the active therapy in this meta-analysis.

rarer causes include fat embolism, amniotic fluid embolism, air embolism, and iatrogenic causes such as intra-arterial catheters.

CONCLUSION

The prevalence of PAD increases with age and in persons with atherosclerotic risk factors. Despite its association with a significant increase in cardiovascular and cerebrovascular mortality and functional impairment and decline, PAD is underdiagnosed. Although the case of a middle-aged woman with risk factors and classic symptoms of IC is straightforward, the majority of hospitalized patients may have multiple comorbidities and/or have atypical symptoms of PAD. Hospitalists have an opportunity to detect PAD and to implement prevention therapies that will enhance survival and improve quality of life.

TABLE 263-6 Clinical Categories of Acute Limb Ischemia

Category		Description/Prognosis	Clinical Findings		Doppler Signals	
			Sensory Loss	Muscle Weakness	Arterial	Venous
I. Viable		No immediate threat	None	None	Audible	Audible
II. Threatened	a Marginally	Salvageable if promptly treated	Minimal or none (affecting toes)	Mild	Inaudible	Audible
	b Immediately	Salvageable if immediately revascularized	Affecting more than toes, with rest pain	Mild or moderate	Inaudible	Audible
III. Irreversible		Major tissue loss, permanent nerve damage inevitable	Profound	Profound, paralysis	Inaudible	Inaudible

Reprinted from Rutherford RB, et al. Recommended standards for reports dealing with lower extremity ischemia. Revised version. *J Vasc Surg*. 1997;26:517–538. Printed with permission from Elsevier.

SUGGESTED READINGS

Berger JS, Krantz MJ, Kittelson JM, Hiatt, WH. Aspirin for the prevention of cardiovascular events in patients with peripheral artery disease. A meta analysis of randomized trials. *JAMA*. 2009;301(18):1909–1919.

Gardner AW, Poehlman ET. Exercise rehabilitation programs for the treatment of claudication pain. A meta-analysis. *JAMA*. 1995;274:975–980.

Hirsch A, Criqui M, Treat-Jacobson D, et al. Peripheral arterial disease detection, awareness, and treatment in primary care. *JAMA*. 2001;286:1317–1324.

Hirsch AT, Haskal ZJ, Hertzer NR, et al. ACC/AHA 2005 Practice Guidelines for the Management of Patients With Peripheral Arterial Disease (Lower Extremity, Renal, Mesenteric, and Abdominal Aortic): A Collaborative Report from the American Association for Vascular Surgery/Society for Vascular Surgery, Society for Cardiovascular Angiography and Interventions, Society for Vascular Medicine and Biology, Society of Interventional Radiology, and the ACC/AHA Task Force on Practice Guidelines (Writing Committee to Develop Guidelines for the Management of Patients With Peripheral Arterial Disease): Endorsed by the American Association of Cardiovascular and Pulmonary Rehabilitation; National Heart, Lung, and Blood Institute; Society for Vascular Nursing; Trans Atlantic Inter-Society Consensus; and Vascular Disease Foundation. *Circulation*. 2005;113:e463–465.

Khan N, Rahim S, Anand S, Simel D, Panju A. Does the clinical examination predict lower extremity peripheral arterial disease? *JAMA*. 2006;295:536–546.

McDermott MM, Guralnik JM, Tian L, et al. Associations of Borderline and Low Normal Ankle-Brachial Index Values With Functional Decline at 5-Year Follow-Up. The WALCS (Walking and Leg Circulation Study). *J Am Coll Cardiol*. 2009;53:1056–1062.

Norgren L, Hiatt WR, Dormandy JA, Nehler MR, Harris KA, Fowkes FGR. Inter-society consensus for the management of peripheral arterial disease (TASC II). *European Journal of Vascular and Endovascular Surgery*. 2007;33:S1–S75.

Rutherford RB, Baker JD, Ernst C, et al. Recommended standards for reports dealing with lower extremity ischemia: Revised version. *J Vasc Surg*. 1997;26:517–538.

Seminars in Vascular Surgery. *Issue*. 22, 2009. Special issue focusing on acute limb ischemia.

The Warfarin Antiplatelet Vascular Evaluation Trial Investigators. Oral anticoagulant and antiplatelet therapy and peripheral arterial disease. *N Engl J Med*. 2007;357(3):217–227.

CHAPTER 264

Vasculitis

Paul A. Monach, MD, PhD
Peter A. Merkel, MD, MPH

Key Clinical Questions

1. When should a diagnosis of vasculitis be considered?
2. How is a diagnosis of vasculitis made or excluded?
3. What are the appropriate strategies for triage, consultation, and follow-up for vasculitis?
4. What treatment and staging for vasculitis should be initiated in the hospital?
5. In a patient with established vasculitis, how should new symptoms of illness be evaluated?

INTRODUCTION

The diagnosis of vasculitis is considered far more often than these diseases are actually seen—appropriately, since these rare diseases have diverse presentations, are dangerous and often rapidly progressive, yet are treatable. All vasculitides feature inflammation of the walls of blood vessels, with symptoms and findings attributable to the size(s) and locations of the involved vessels. Vessel size, epidemiology, and/or a constellation of typical clinical features have proved useful for classifying the vasculitides, with key points summarized in (**Table 264-1**).

The classification of vasculitis remains imprecise with more than one system in use. "Primary" systemic vasculitides are further sorted by the sizes of the predominant arteries involved, leading to sets of small, medium, and large vessel vasculitides. There are also several "secondary" forms of vasculitis associated with infections, drug exposure, or another form of systemic disease such as systemic lupus erythematosis or rheumatoid arthritis.

All of the primary, idiopathic vasculitides are rare diseases, each categorized as an "orphan" disease in the United States (prevalence of < 200,000 persons). However, as a group, and especially among patients with initially unexplained systemic disease who are ill enough to be hospitalized, vasculitis is common enough that hospitalists will likely encounter cases.

PATHOPHYSIOLOGY

The pathophysiology of the primary vasculitides is poorly understood. They are all considered immune mediated, based on histologic and serologic studies and by analogy to the many cases of vasculitis that have occurred secondary to infections or drug exposure. Since no pathogens have been found, the primary vasculitides are suspected to be autoimmune, with the humoral and cellular branches of the adaptive immune system involved to different degrees in different diseases.

NOTES ON INDIVIDUAL FORMS OF VASCULITIS

It is impractical to describe each of the vasculitides in detail in a single chapter, but short summaries of most of the vasculitides are provided as reference points for the subsequent discussion.

Giant cell arteritis

Giant cell arteritis (GCA) only affects adults over the age of 50, and incidence markedly increases with age, to about 1:2000 per year among Caucasians of Northern European descent by age 80. Headache is the most common symptom (80%), with scalp tenderness, jaw claudication, constitutional symptoms, and polymyalgia rheumatica (pain and stiffness in the shoulders, hips, and/or neck) each seen in 40% to 70% of patients. The presentation of GCA is often insidious and diagnosed during outpatient care, but sometimes is acute and leads to hospitalization. GCA has also been reported to be an important cause (about 10%) of fever of unknown origin in the elderly, and since the aorta and its major branches are involved in more than 15% of cases, GCA is also an important consideration in cases of claudication, loss of pulse, and asymmetric blood pressure measurements in the elderly. (See the section on laboratory testing [acute phase reactants], imaging [angiography, ultrasound], and biopsy [temporal artery]).

TABLE 264-1 Classification of the Major Primary Vasculitides, with Some Key Features (Nonexhaustive List)

Vessel Sizes and Associated Diseases	Key Diagnostic Tests	Common Clinical Features
Largest arteries: aorta and branches		
Giant cell arteritis	Temporal artery biopsy Ophthalmologic exam	Headache, visual loss, arthralgias, malaise
Takayasu arteritis	Angiography	Claudication, pulselessness
Aortitis in Cogan syndrome	Angiography	Hearing loss, vertigo, ocular inflammation
Isolated aortitis	Angiography	
Medium-sized arteries		
Kawasaki disease	Coronary artery imaging	Prolonged fever, coronary artery aneurysms
Polyarteritis nodosa	Hepatitis B virus Angiography	Purpura, hypertension, abdominal pain, neuropathy
Small arteries		
Granulomatosis with polyangiitis (Wegener)	ANCA, urinalysis Sinus and chest CT Lung or renal biopsy	Pulmonary nodules or hemorrhage, sinonasal disease, renal impairment, neuropathy, arthralgias, skin lesions, ANCA
Microscopic polyangiitis	ANCA, urinalysis Lung or renal biopsy	Pulmonary hemorrhage, renal impairment, neuropathy, purpura, ANCA
Churg-Strauss syndrome	Total eosiniophil count Sinus and chest CT Lung or renal biopsy	Asthma, eosinophilia, pulmonary infiltrates, neuropathy
Antiglomerular-basement membrane disease (including Goodpasture syndrome)	Anti-GBM antibodies Renal biopsy	Pulmonary hemorrhage, glomerulonephritis
Henoch-Schöenlein purpura	Skin biopsy	Purpura, arthritis, abdominal pain, IgA nephropathy
Cryoglobulinemic vasculitis	Cryoglobulins Hepatitis C virus Skin or renal biopsy	Purpura, neuropathy, glomerulonephritis
Primary angiitis of the CNS	Brain biopsy	Headache, multiple strokes
Arteries and veins of various sizes		
Behçet disease	Ophthalmologic exam	Oral and genital ulcers, uveitis
Relapsing polychondritis	Ophthalmologic exam	Auricular, nasal, and tracheal inflammation, ocular inflammation

ANCA, antineutrophil cytoplasmic antibodies; CNS, central nervous system; CT, computed tomography.

Takayasu arteritis

Takayasu arteritis is a rare disease (prevalence < 1:100,000), usually presenting in young adults, and 90% of patients are female. Patients often present with claudication, dizziness, abnormal blood pressure readings, and/or bruits. Diagnosis is confirmed by angiography. The types of presentation more likely to lead to hospitalization (eg, symptoms of coronary artery disease or cerebrovascular disease) carry a broad differential diagnosis, so suspicion for or against Takayasu may initially be gained by checking pulses and blood pressures and listening for bruits. (See the section on laboratory testing [acute phase reactants] and imaging [angiography, ultrasound]).

Granulomatosis with polyangiitis (Wegener's) and microscopic polyangiitis

Granulomatosis with polyangiitis (Wegener's) (GPA) and microscopic polyangittis (MPA)—grouped by some authors as antineutrophil cytoplasmic antibody (ANCA)-associated vasculitis (AAV)—are small-vessel vasculitides that together affect ~1:20,000 persons. AAV is high in the differential diagnosis of patients presenting with pulmonary hemorrhage, acute renal disease, or acute peripheral neuropathy, and is also an important consideration in patients with palpable purpura, inflammatory eye disease (scleritis or episcleritis), acute sensorineural hearing loss, cutaneous ulcers, or digital ischemia. Renal disease in AAV often leads to elevated creatinine and urinary RBC casts but in the early stages patients may only have microscopic hematuria and modest proteinuria. GPA usually (70–80%) also features granulomatous inflammation of the upper airway, with nasal discharge and crusting, epistaxis, facial pain, and/or hearing loss, and the presence of these symptoms often facilitates the diagnosis of GPA. GPA is an important consideration in cases of subglottic stenosis, orbital mass with proptosis, or pulmonary nodule(s). However, many patients with AAV present only with nonspecific symptoms of malaise, myalgias, and arthralgias. The role of testing for ANCA in diagnosing AAV is discussed in detail below. (See section on laboratory testing [autoimmune serologies, acute phase reactants, tests of renal function], imaging [chest imaging, sinus imaging], and biopsy [skin, nasal cavity and sinuses, kidney, lung, peripheral nerve and muscle]).

Churg-Strauss syndrome

Churg-Strauss syndrome (CSS) is worth considering in a patient who is ill with what might be vasculitis, has a history of asthma (often severe or poorly controlled), and has eosinophilia. The presentations of CSS most likely to lead to hospitalization are asthma exacerbation, pulmonary infiltrates, or acute peripheral neuropathy, but constitutional symptoms, nasal polyps, rash, and arthralgias are also common. Myocarditis, gastrointestinal ischemia, stroke, renal involvement (similar to AAV), and eye inflammation are less common but important presentations. Positive tests for ANCA may be present in 30% of patients and some consider CSS part of the spectrum of ANCA-associated vasculitis. (See section on laboratory testing [autoimmune serologies, acute phase reactants, tests of renal function, complete blood count], imaging [chest imaging, sinus imaging], and biopsy [skin, nasal cavity, and sinuses, kidney, lung, peripheral nerve and muscle]).

Antiglomerular-basement-membrane disease

In contrast to AAV, symptoms of antiglomerular-basement-membrane (GBM) disease are limited to the kidneys and/or lungs (if both = Goodpasture syndrome), with rapidly progressive glomerulonephritis and/or pulmonary hemorrhage as manifestations. A blood test for anti-GBM antibodies is diagnostic, as is kidney biopsy. Testing for anti-GBM antibodies should be obtained rapidly for any patient for whom anti-GBM disease is possible, since the disease can lead to irreversible kidney damage or death from pulmonary hemorrhage. (See section on laboratory testing [autoimmune serologies, tests of renal function], and imaging [chest imaging], biopsy [kidney, lung]).

Polyarteritis nodosa

The most common features of polyarteritis nodosa (PAN) are livedo reticularis (a lacy pattern of cutaneous blood vessels on extremities that is more commonly due to benign conditions rather than vasculitis), painful cutaneous nodules or ulcers, hypertension, abdominal pain, myalgias, peripheral neuropathy, testicular pain, and digital ischemia. There is a strong association between hepatitis B virus infection and PAN; the incidence of PAN has markedly declined in countries with high rates of hepatitis B vaccination. PAN is probably the most challenging type of vasculitis to diagnose, because (1) it is particularly rare (in regions where the hepatitis B virus infection is also rare), (2) it features the most nonspecific array of symptoms and findings among the vasculitides, and (3) there are no helpful diagnostic blood tests analogous to ANCA, cryoglobulins, or eosinophil count. Biopsy or angiography is usually required for the diagnosis of PAN. For all of these reasons, PAN is contemplated much more often than it is diagnosed. (See section on laboratory testing [acute phase reactants, tests of renal function, selected testing for infectious diseases], imaging [angiography], and biopsy [skin, kidney, peripheral nerve and muscle, other organs]).

Behçet disease

The manifestations of Behçet disease (BD) that may lead to hospitalization are extraordinarily diverse: visual loss or a red and painful eye, deep vein thrombosis (including dural sinus thrombosis or Budd-Chiari syndrome), colitis resembling inflammatory bowel disease, meningoencephalitis, or pulmonary artery rupture leading to massive hemorrhage. Considering the diagnosis of BD in these settings requires recognition of the various milder but more common features of BD that may be concurrently present or reported by the patient, including recurrent oral ulcers (required for diagnosis), genital ulcers, erythema nodosum, acneiform skin lesions, inflammatory arthritis, and superficial thrombophlebitis. The diagnosis or exclusion of BD is always made on clinical grounds since there are no specific blood tests or biopsy features of the disease.

Primary vasculitis of the central nervous system

This rare disease is limited to the central nervous system (CNS) and presents with symptoms of encephalopathy, multiple small strokes, and often headache. Angiography may be normal since the disease affects small vessels. Furthermore, angiography cannot easily distinguish vasculitis from atherosclerosis or from cerebral vasospasm (which usually presents with a severe headache of sudden onset). Thus, diagnosis of CNS vasculitis is ideally made by brain biopsy. (See section on imaging [angiography], and biopsy [brain]).

Cryoglobulinemic vasculitis

Cryoglobulinemia encompasses a variety of clinical syndromes associated with circulating immune complexes that precipitate at cold temperatures. The majority of cases of cryoglobulinemia are associated with chronic hepatitis C virus infection, with plasma cell malignancies and systemic rheumatic diseases accounting for most other cases. Cryoglobulinemia associated with chronic hepatitis C virus infection or systemic rheumatic disease causes a small-vessel vasculitis that typically involves skin (palpable purpura and/or ulcers), commonly involves peripheral nerves or kidneys (glomerulonephritis), and less commonly involves a wide range of internal organs. (See section on laboratory testing [tests of renal function, paraproteins, selected testing for infectious diseases], and biopsy [skin, kidney, peripheral nerve and muscle]).

Henoch-Schönlein purpura

Henoch-Schönlein purpura (HSP) is much more common among children than adults. It is usually self-limited and presents with palpable purpura, often in association with inflammatory arthritis and abdominal pain. A minority of patients has severe renal involvement, and the presence or absence of significant proteinuria or elevated creatinine is often used to determine whether to treat with immunosuppressive agents; however, the usefulness of such treatment has not been established. (See section on laboratory testing [tests of renal function] and biopsy [skin, kidney]).

Kawasaki disease

Kawasaki disease (KD) is almost exclusively a disease of young children, and it is not rare in its characteristic age group (incidence 1:10,000 in the U.S.). The syndrome classically includes fever persisting for at least five days, erythematous rash with desquamation in the hands and feet, conjunctivitis, oral mucosal inflammation, and lymphadenopathy. However, many patients present without all of these features and, since a consequence of untreated KD is life-threatening coronary artery aneurysms, the diagnosis is considered in almost any young child with a fever lasting five days.

Vasculitis associated with other autoimmune diseases

Systemic lupus, rheumatoid arthritis, Sjögren syndrome, and inflammatory bowel disease have all been associated with vasculitis, mostly involving small vessels (palpable purpura, ulcers, neuropathy), but occasionally medium-sized vessels (analogous to PAN). Inflammatory bowel disease, relapsing polychondritis, and Cogan syndrome are each rarely associated with large-vessel vasculitis similar to Takayasu arteritis. (See section on laboratory testing [autoimmune serologies and tests of renal function]).

DIAGNOSIS: DOES THIS PATIENT HAVE VASCULITIS?

Vasculitis is commonly in the differential diagnosis for any patient with an unexplained systemic illness or any patient with one or more specific findings suggestive of vasculitis. However, it is important to realize that vasculitis is rare. Nonetheless, being open

TABLE 264-2 Red Flags that Should Prompt Consideration of Vasculitis and Vasculitis Mimics

Red Flag	Disease(s) to Consider	Nonvasculitic Causes ("Mimics") to Consider	Comment
Palpable purpura	HSP, AAV, Cryo, infection-associated, drug reaction	Atheroembolic disease, bacteremia, cardiac myxoma	Biopsy may show vasculitis but does not reveal the exact cause/type
Pulmonary hemorrhage	AAV, GBM	SLE, pneumonia, coagulopathy	Bronchoscopy establishes hemorrhage but not the cause
Acute renal failure (especially glomerulonephritis)	AAV, GBM, Cryo	SLE, acute interstitial nephritis, noninflammatory causes	Presence of other characteristic features raises suspicion
Destructive nasal inflammation (septal perforation, saddle-nose)	GPA	Cocaine use	Presence of other characteristic features raises suspicion
Mononeuritis multiplex	PAN, AAV, Cryo	Diabetes, HIV, other causes	Vasculitis is a common cause of wrist or foot drop; other peripheral neuropathies are also common in vasculitis
New headache in the elderly	GCA	Many other causes	ESR helpful for initial triage
Absent pulse or blood pressure	Large-vessel vasculitis, especially TAK or GCA	Atherosclerosis	TAK if age < 50, GCA if > 50
Acute monocular visual loss	GCA	Embolic disease	Presence of other characteristic features raises suspicion
Inflammatory eye disease (uveitis, scleritis, episcleritis)	Behçet, AAV	Also common with other rheumatic and infectious diseases	Presence of other characteristic features raises suspicion
Encephalopathy, multiple strokes, especially in a young person	CNSV	CNS vasospasm Embolic disease	Angiographic appearance similar; biopsy usually required
Thoracic aortic aneurysm	Large-vessel vasculitis, especially TAK or GCA	Syphilis, Marfan, atherosclerosis	Aortitis can occur as an isolated manifestation of vasculitis
Digit ischemia or gangrene	PAN, AAV, Cryo	Thrombotic and vasospastic disorders	Nonvasculitic causes are more common
Mesenteric ischemia or bowel infarction	PAN, AAV	Thromboembolic disorders, atherosclerosis	Nonvasculitic causes are more common
Fever > 5 days in a young child	Kawasaki	Numerous infectious and noninfectious causes	Presence of other characteristic features raises suspicion
Eosinophilia and asthma	CSS	Hypereosinophilic syndromes	Extrapulmonary symptoms and degree of eosinophilia raise suspicion
Fever of unknown origin in the elderly	GCA	Many infectious, malignant, and autoimmune causes	GCA is a common etiology

AAV, ANCA-associated vasculitis (granulomatosis with polyangiitis (Wegener) GPA; microscopic polyangitis, and Churg-Strauss syndrome [CSS]); CNSV, primary central nervous system vasculitis; Cryo, cryoglobulinemia; GBM, antiglomerular-basement-membrane disease; GCA, giant cell arteritis; HSP, Henoch-Schonlein purpura; PAN, polyarteritis nodose; SLE, systemic lupus erythematosis; TAK, Takayasu arteritis.

to the possibility of vasculitis is critical for reducing delays in diagnosis. There are many "red flags" that should alert clinicians that vasculitis must be considered (**Table 264-2**). Some of these findings merit urgent diagnostic testing and sometimes even empiric treatment for vasculitis, pending the results of testing.

Not shown in Table 264-2 are syndromes that could be caused by vasculitis but have other causes in the vast majority of cases such as fever of unknown origin, lower extremity ulcers, abdominal pain, arthralgias, myalgias, and other nonspecific symptoms.

MIMICS OF VASCULITIS

Since vasculitis is rare, nonvasculitic causes of red-flag symptoms remain more common than vasculitis in many cases. A broad range of infectious, autoimmune, toxic, malignant, thromboembolic, vasospastic, and atherosclerotic disorders can mimic many of the characteristic features of vasculitis, as outlined in general terms in Table 264-2.

DIAGNOSTIC TESTING FOR SUSPECTED VASCULITIS

The method for diagnosing vasculitis generally depends on the size of vessels involved. Small-vessel vasculitis is usually diagnosed by biopsy, but sometimes the combination of a typical clinical syndrome and a laboratory test (see proceding section) is sufficient. Medium-vessel vasculitis (PAN) is diagnosed by biopsy or angiography. GCA is usually diagnosed by biopsy (temporal arteritis) but occasionally by angiography if the aorta or its major branches are involved. Takayasu is diagnosed by angiography. CNS vasculitis is diagnosed by biopsy. Behçet disease and Kawasaki disease are diagnosed based on the clinical syndrome.

The uses of laboratory testing, diagnostic imaging, and biopsy for diagnosing vasculitis are outlined below.

LABORATORY TESTING FOR EVALUATION OF SUSPECTED VASCULITIS

Although individual laboratory tests on their own are almost never diagnostic for vasculitis, such tests are essential in the evaluation of a patient in whom vasculitis is being considered for several reasons: (1) in the proper setting, selected serologic tests may confirm a diagnosis of vasculitis; (2) laboratory testing may identify organ systems involved in the disease process (especially for renal disease); (3) laboratory tests may establish a diagnosis *other* than vasculitis.

Autoimmune serologies

Testing for various autoantibodies plays a key role in the evaluation of patients suspected of having vasculitis, but over-reliance on such testing often leads to delayed or missed diagnoses.

Antineutrophil cytoplasmic antibodies

The widespread availability of antineutrophil cytoplasmic antibodies (ANCA) testing has had a striking impact on the evaluation of patients with suspected small-vessel vasculitis. The current standard of care for ANCA testing includes combining tests for ANCA by immunoflourescence (IF) and tests for ANCA by ELISA. Only two combinations of test results constitute a truly "positive" ANCA test: the cytoplasmic (C-ANCA) IF pattern combined with antiproteinase 3 (PR3) antibodies by ELISA, or the perinuclear (P-ANCA) IF pattern combined with antimyeloperoxidase (MPO) antibodies by ELISA. In the proper clinical settings, positive ANCA testing (C/anti-PR3 or P/anti-MPO) is highly specific for the diagnosis of AAV (>95%) and may preclude the need for biopsy or at least support initiation of treatment with glucocorticoids pending a biopsy. However, ANCA testing is presumed to have lower specificity in the setting of nonspecific symptoms such as malaise, myalgias, and arthralgias—a relatively common initial presentation of AAV. The sensitivity of ANCA testing is considerably lower (70–90%), so a patient may still have GPA or MPA even if the ANCA test is negative. Thus, ANCA testing is extremely useful diagnostically but *must* be used in the context of supportive clinical and other data.

Antiglomerular-basement membrane antibodies

In the setting of renal insufficiency and/or pulmonary hemorrhage, antiglomerular basement-membrane (anti-GBM) antibodies are highly specific for the diagnosis of anti-GBM disease/Goodpasture disease as long as the initial anti-GBM antibody screening test is confirmed by Western blot. Because the treatment of choice for anti-GBM disease is the combination of high-dose glucocorticoids and plasma exchange, it is crucial to establish the diagnosis as early as possible. Antibody testing can play a central role in this process, but sometimes IF staining of a kidney biopsy can make the diagnosis more rapidly.

Antinuclear antibodies

Testing for antinuclear antibodies (ANA) is quite useful when there is suspicion of systemic lupus erythematosus (SLE), either underlying vasculitis or as an alternative diagnosis for pulmonary hemorrhage and/or acute renal failure. ANA testing is >95% sensitive for the diagnosis of lupus; therefore, a negative test essentially rules out lupus as a diagnosis, unless a patient has clear pathognomonic features.

Acute phase reactants

Although the erythrocyte sedimentation rate (ESR) and C-reactive protein (CRP) are usually elevated in patients with untreated vasculitis, and ESR and CRP are often ordered when evaluating patients with suspected vasculitis, these tests have a surprisingly low value diagnostically. ESR or CRP are neither sensitive nor specific enough to be considered as screening tests to make or exclude a diagnosis of vasculitis, except, in a limited way, as part of a diagnostic algorithm for GCA. Even for new-onset GCA, the ESR may be normal in up to 10% of cases, so a normal ESR is only helpful in ruling out GCA and avoiding the need for a temporal artery biopsy in a low-probability patient (atypical headache only), but not in a patient with additional cranial, arthritic, or constitutional symptoms. These tests may have selected roles in evaluation for persistent or recurrent disease but still must be interpreted cautiously. Furthermore, ESR and/or CRP are often elevated in the major mimics of vasculitis, especially infections (either acute or chronic) and malignancies.

Tests of renal function and other chemistry laboratory testing

Prompt assessment of renal function is an essential part of the evaluation of any patient suspected of having vasculitis. Renal disease can be either insidious or fulminant, and renal injury is usually asymptomatic even with near end-stage renal disease. Serum creatinine with estimate of glomerular filtration rate should be done immediately in all patients and compared with prior measurements. Even subtle rises in creatinine levels within the "normal" range may be indicative of serious disease.

If urinary dipstick testing demonstrates the presence of any blood or protein, then a microscopic examination of the urine sediment on a freshly collected specimen *must* be performed for any patient suspected of having vasculitis. However, it is essential that the urinalysis be performed by someone experienced in evaluating patients with glomerulonephritis, usually a nephrologist or rheumatologist. It is the norm for hospital-based and reference laboratories to miss evidence of an "active" urinary sediment since casts are often destroyed by the time the specimens are processed, and diagnostic laboratory personnel are simply not trained to detect these changes. The presence of red blood cell casts and, to a lesser extent, "dysmorphic" red cells in a urine specimen are strong indicators of glomerular disease. However, patients can still have highly active glomerulonephritis or other renal disease in vasculitis (eg, aneurysms in PAN) and not have urinary casts present.

Other routine chemistry panels, including electrolytes and liver function tests, are of limited value in diagnosing vasculitis per se and provide more useful information about nonvasculitic conditions.

Urine or serum toxicology screens for commonly used legal and illegal drugs of abuse may be appropriate for some clinical situations in which vasculitis is suspected. For example, both cocaine and methamphetamines have been associated with vasculitis and/or arterial vasospasm, and levamisole is now a common adulterant of cocaine and can cause a form of AAV.

Complete blood count

A complete blood count (CBC) should be conducted on all patients suspected of having vasculitis but is usually of limited diagnostic value. Many, but by no means all, patients with active vasculitis have anemia and/or thrombocytosis, but neither finding is sensitive or specific for the diagnosis. The one diagnostic use of the CBC in vasculitis concerns CSS; although an elevated eosinophil count is nonspecific, a normal eosinophil count (in a patient who has not received glucocorticoids) usually rules out this diagnosis.

Paraproteins (abnormal immunoglobulins)

Abnormal immunoglobulins that can be associated with vasculitis include both those that precipitate at room temperature (cryoglobulins) and other clonal immunoglobulins that may cause small-vessel vasculitis. Cryoglobulins resulting in vasculitis are most closely associated with chronic infection with hepatitis C virus. Testing for cryoglobulins requires careful attention to specimen handling and processing with incorrect practice at any of several steps resulting in uninterpretable findings (ie, high false-negative rate due to poor processing). Similarly, standard serum protein electrophoresis testing (SPEP) may not pick up some immunoglobulin clones; immunofixation electrophoresis (IFE) is a more comprehensive screen for clonal immunoglobulins. Similar issues exist for urine protein electrophoresis (UPEP) vs. urine immunofixation electrophoresis (UFE). The great majority of patients with cryoglobulinemic vasculitis tests positive for rheumatoid factor (RF), and the majority has low levels of circulating complement proteins (C4 more so than C3). RF has poor specificity, but results are obtained faster and more reliably than are tests for cryoglobulins.

Selected testing for infectious diseases

Hepatitis B, hepatitis C, and HIV virus infections are associated with vasculitis and tests for these viruses should be sent for all patients suspected of having a small- or medium-vessel vasculitis. Blood cultures are appropriate when bacteremia may be a possible cause of vasculitis. Several other infections may cause signs and symptoms mimicking vasculitis and serologic tests or cultures specific to those diseases are useful on a case-by-case basis.

DIAGNOSTIC IMAGING FOR EVALUATION OF SUSPECTED VASCULITIS

Chest imaging

The major forms of vasculitis that involve the lung are AAV (including GPA, MPA, and CSS) and anti-GBM disease. A chest X-ray is therefore prudent in any patient with acute renal failure and an active urine sediment, and one should have a low threshold for performing a computed tomography (CT) test (noncontrast, but ideally with high-resolution cuts). However, the appearances of AAV on CT imaging—solitary or multiple nodules, multifocal or diffuse infiltrates—are not sufficiently specific to be diagnostic. For a patient with known vasculitis, comparison of abnormal findings on chest imaging to prior studies is essential.

Sinus imaging

A patient in whom GPA or CSS is being considered due to prominent symptoms of nasal inflammation should have a CT (noncontrast is usually sufficient) performed to assess for sinus, mastoid, and retro-orbital involvement.

Angiography

Angiography, whether conventional or performed using CT (CTA) or magnetic resonance (MRA) techniques, is essential for the diagnosis of large-vessel vasculitis (Takayasu arteritis, GCA, and others) and many cases of medium-vessel vasculitis (PAN). For Takayasu and GCA involving the major branches of the aorta, either MRA or CTA is often sufficient. Angiography (CTA or conventional) is usually unable to differentiate between CNS vasculitis, vasospasm, and atherosclerosis.

Catheter-based conventional angiography is still considered the "gold standard" for arterial imaging and is considerably more sensitive for disease of smaller arteries. Furthermore, catheter-based angiography allows for measurement of blood pressures and selective sampling of specific arterial areas.

Ultrasound

Ultrasound of certain large arteries (particularly the carotids) can be helpful in diagnosing large-vessel vasculitis (GCA or Takayasu), since wall thickness as well as luminal diameter can be measured. Ultrasound of the temporal arteries for diagnosis of GCA has performed well in research studies at specialized centers but is not yet recommended for routine clinical use. Echocardiography, which allows visualization of the major coronary arteries in children, has an important role in the diagnosis and management of Kawasaki disease.

Positron emission tomography

Positron emission tomography (PET) scanning has been reported to identify areas of inflammation in large-vessel vasculitis in small studies, but the diagnostic usefulness of this modality for vasculitis has not been established.

BIOPSY FOR EVALUATION OF SUSPECTED VASCULITIS

Biopsy is required for the diagnosis of vasculitis in many cases, although there are important exceptions. Behçet disease and Henoch-Schönlein purpura (in children) are diagnosed on clinical grounds. Kawasaki disease is diagnosed on clinical grounds, often with confirmation by imaging showing evidence of coronary artery aneurysm(s). Large-vessel vasculitis is diagnosed by angiography in patients with Takayasu and a subset of patients with GCA. Some patients with small-vessel vasculitides (GPA, MPA, CSS, and cryoglobulinemia) can be diagnosed confidently on the basis of symptoms, signs, and laboratory and imaging findings but biopsy remains the best evidence for these diseases.

The usefulness of biopsy either in diagnosing vasculitis or in diagnosing a particular type of vasculitis depends on the organ system. Consideration of the need for biopsy is one of the main reasons for prompt consultation of the appropriate specialist.

Skin biopsy

Skin biopsies are simple, have low morbidity, and should be strongly considered in any patient with new-onset purpura or other lesions suspected to be due to vasculitis. Assuming lesions are due to vasculitis is a common clinical error. Cutaneous small-vessel vasculitis usually presents as palpable purpura, but other presentations include flat and angular (retiform) purpura, nodules, ulcers, and bullae. Vasculitis is probably the most common cause of palpable purpura, but there are others, and thus biopsy is usually indicated. The typical pathologic finding is leukocytoclastic vasculitis (LCV), which is quite helpful for confirming the presence of vasculitis but does nothing to address the many potential causes of this pathology. Immunofluorescent staining can be of additional value, especially if HSP is suspected.

It is important to realize that patients with LCV on skin biopsy may have one of the named primary vasculitides or any of several other conditions, including another named systemic rheumatic disease, a concurrent or recent infection, or drug/toxin exposure. Some patients will have vasculitis apparently limited to the skin and without any clear exposure. Thus, it is important to interpret the skin biopsy in the context of a compulsive search for other findings by history, exam, laboratory tests, and imaging.

A full-thickness skin biopsy that includes larger vessels and subdermal tissue may be necessary for some forms of vasculitis or related disease, such as PAN, panniculitis, and others.

Nasal cavity and sinuses biopsy

Although the sinonasal mucosa is frequently involved in either GPA or CSS, biopsies of these readily accessible tissues are of limited diagnostic value since the characteristic features of granulomatous inflammation, necrosis, and vasculitis are often not present; however, if seen in the right setting, then such biopsy findings are supportive of a diagnosis of vasculitis. Sinonasal biopsies and cultures may be useful to establish a diagnosis of infection or malignancy.

Temporal artery biopsy

Biopsy of the temporal artery is safe and at least 85% sensitive for diagnosing GCA, so one should have a low threshold for having it performed in an elderly patient who has either a new and persistent headache and a high ESR, or a constellation of features suggestive of GCA regardless of the ESR. Performing bilateral biopsies only modestly improves sensitivity. The specificity of finding vasculitis in temporal arteries is high for a diagnosis of GCA; however, other forms of vasculitis can involve the temporal arteries.

Kidney biopsy

Kidney biopsy is quite valuable for diagnosing AAV and remains the gold standard for the diagnosis. However, in some settings of acute renal insufficiency with an active urine sediment, other features suggestive of GPA or MPA, and a positive test for anti-MPO or anti-PR3 antibodies, kidney biopsy may not be necessary. Kidney biopsy is also quite valuable for diagnosing anti-GBM disease. Kidney pathology in HSP (IgA nephropathy) and cryoglobulinemia (MGPN) is distinct from the other vasculitides and is therefore usually diagnostic. Kidney biopsy is rarely helpful in diagnosing PAN involving the kidneys since the vessels involved are often too large and/or too patchily distributed to be detected on biopsy, and PAN does not cause glomerular disease. Of course, kidney biopsies are extremely helpful in diagnosing nonvasculitic causes of renal disease or a coexisting second pathology in patients with vasculitis.

Brain biopsy

Brain biopsy is considered to be essential for the confident diagnosis of CNS vasculitis, since vasospastic disease has a similar angiographic appearance, and a variety of infectious and inflammatory diseases can cause the type of multifocal small abnormalities that are usually seen on brain MRI in CNS vasculitis.

Lung biopsy

Lung biopsy has a high diagnostic yield for AAV for nodules or infiltrates (including eosinophilic infiltrates in CSS). Similarly, small-vessel vasculitis with capillaritis can be diagnosed by lung biopsy, but the bronchoscopic evidence of diffuse alveolar hemorrhage in the right clinical and laboratory setting often makes biopsy unnecessary. Lung biopsy can also be important in a patient with known GPA who develops a new lung lesion to help differentiate vasculitis from infection or malignancy.

Peripheral nerve and muscle biopsy

Peripheral nerves are frequently involved in PAN, CSS, GPA, and MPA, and biopsy of the sural nerve, particularly with simultaneous biopsy of the nearby muscle, has fairly good sensitivity for diagnosing vasculitis. Nerve biopsy is rarely performed on a clinically uninvolved sural nerve and probably has lower sensitivity. However, sural nerve biopsy leaves the patient with a permanent sensory deficit in the innervated area, and occasionally with neuropathic pain.

Biopsy of other organs

Vasculitis has been reported to occur in almost every organ either as part of a named systemic vasculitis or in cases of "isolated" vasculitis. Thus, biopsy of organs other than those listed above may be useful. More common is the situation in which vasculitis is found in surgical specimens for patients thought to have other medical problems. Such findings then appropriately stimulate a full evaluation of possible systemic vasculitis.

ILLNESS IN A PATIENT WITH KNOWN VASCULITIS

A new illness in a patient already diagnosed with vasculitis still frequently presents diagnostic and therapeutic challenges. Many of the vasculitides involve diverse symptoms and findings, and the features during flare do not always resemble the features at initial diagnosis. Patients receiving immunosuppressive medications for vasculitis are at risk for both conventional and opportunistic infections. Noninfectious side effects of medications are also common. Importantly, permanent damage from prior episodes of vasculitis (eg, from neuropathy, nasal septal perforation, or stenosis of a large artery) can produce chronic symptoms that fluctuate in severity and mimic active vasculitis or infection.

An example of the complexity of evaluating new clinical problems in a patient with vasculitis is that of dyspnea in a patient with GPA. This problem could indicate pulmonary hemorrhage, subglottic stenosis, pulmonary nodules (with or without superinfection), pericarditis, pulmonary embolism, bacterial pneumonia, atypical pneumonia (particularly pneumocystis jeruvicii [carinii]), or glucocorticoid-induced myopathy, all problems for which a patient treated for GPA would be at relatively high risk. Distinguishing a manifestation of recurrent vasculitis from an infection or a medication side effect can be quite difficult, so the most appropriate general advice is to think broadly: resist the temptation to assume that vasculitis is the cause of symptoms, consider the possibility that infection may coexist with active vasculitis, consider the possibility that the original diagnosis of vasculitis may have been wrong, and have a low threshold for hospitalization and consultation.

PRACTICE POINT

Here are points for distinguishing a manifestation of recurrent vasculitis from an infection or a medication side effect.

Think broadly:

- Do not assume that vasculitis is the cause of symptoms.
- The original diagnosis of vasculitis may have been wrong.
- Infection may coexist with active vasculitis.
- Have a low threshold for hospitalization and consultation.

TRIAGE AND CONSULTATION

The decision whether to hospitalize a patient who has or may have vasculitis depends on the severity of illness. Sometimes the need for admission is obvious: pulmonary hemorrhage, hematuria with elevated creatinine, or visual loss. Admission may also be indicated for other manifestations that may appear less serious but are often indicators of severe disease with the potential to cause permanent organ damage (peripheral neuropathy, hematuria, or new hypertension with normal creatinine), or to facilitate rapid evaluation. In patients who appear safe to return home, arrangement for close outpatient follow-up remains critical. For example, a patient with a moderate or high probability of having GCA may be discharged from the emergency room after receiving a first dose of glucocorticoids, but only with a prescription for prednisone (40–80 mg per day) and scheduling within one week for a temporal artery biopsy and follow-up with a primary care provider or rheumatologist.

Urgent rheumatologic consultation on either an inpatient or outpatient basis is usually indicated for patients suspected of having vasculitis and is influenced by the organ system(s) involved and the need for biopsy or advanced imaging. Consultations with specialists with expertise in particular clinical skills and diagnostic procedures (eg, ophthalmology, otolaryngology, pulmonary, nephrology, gastroenterology, dermatology, or neurology) may well also be indicated. Since syndromes that include vasculitis in the differential diagnosis often include infectious diseases and/or malignancies, it is common, and usually appropriate, for a patient with a severe illness of mysterious cause to require "pan-consults". In such situations, the hospitalist has the challenge of facilitating and prioritizing the evaluations and communicating to the patient and concerned family members the recommendations of numerous specialists.

TREATMENT

Clinicians should expect their consultants, particularly rheumatologists or nephrologists, to guide treatment for vasculitis. Hospitalists may, however, be faced with the decision of whether to start high-dose glucocorticoids in advance of consultation, and play an important role in monitoring for the many potential side effects of treatment.

Glucocorticoids are the cornerstone of treatment for all severe forms of vasculitis and are often started in the hospital. If suspicion is high for organ-threatening vasculitis (eg, GCA or acute renal failure with active sediment), then it is often wise to start glucocorticoids while the diagnostic workup is in progress. For less urgent clinical situations in which vasculitis is one of several considerations, particularly if severe infection is a possibility, then it is advisable to forgo glucocorticoid treatment until the diagnosis is confirmed. Vasculitis causing compromise to vital organs (eg, pulmonary hemorrhage, glomerulonephritis, acute peripheral neuropathy, visual loss, angina, or digital ischemia) is often treated with high-dose IV methylprednisolone, 1000 mg daily for one to three days, followed by oral prednisone 1 mg/kg/day. Starting with oral prednisone is usually appropriate for disease that is potentially severe but not actively damaging organs such as GCA with headache, Takayasu with new arterial lesions, or GPA with nasal disease and a pulmonary nodule.

The other urgent inpatient treatment decision is whether the patient requires plasma exchange. This procedure is considered standard care in anti-GBM disease. Plasma exchange is also used in some centers for treatment of fulminant AAV, particularly with rapidly progressive renal failure, but the value of this approach is under active investigation. The decision for or against plasma exchange is always an urgent one and is a major reason why it is appropriate to push for renal biopsy with immunofluorescence staining and rapid serologic testing for anti-GBM, anti-PR3 ANCA, and anti-MPO ANCA.

Additional immunosuppressive drugs are widely used in vasculitis, with the choice of agent dependent on the disease and its severity. Cyclophosphamide, azathioprine, methotrexate, and rituximab are all used for various types and stages of vasculitis. Unlike glucocorticoids or plasma exchange, the effects of these other drugs are not rapid, and the decision to start them can await evaluation by a consultant with expertise in vasculitis and in the use of these medications.

Physicians caring for patients being treated for vasculitis should be attentive to common side effects of glucocorticoids including diabetes mellitus, osteoporosis, osteonecrosis, glaucoma, cataracts, psychosis and mania, myopathy, infection, and other problems. Prophylaxis against pneumocystis jeruvicii (carinii) is widely considered indicated for any patient receiving cyclophosphamide or for any patient receiving both high-dose glucocorticoids and another immunosuppressive agent. Trimethoprim-sulfamethoxazole, either a double-strength tablet three times per week or single-strength tablet daily, is considered the drug of choice for such prophylaxis for patients who are not sulfa-allergic; dapsone (first screen for G6PD deficiency) and atovaquone are alternatives.

DISCHARGE CONSIDERATIONS

Patients with vasculitis or those in whom results of key diagnostic tests such as temporal artery biopsy are pending need to be seen quickly after hospital discharge by a rheumatologist and/or another specialist, rather than relying on the patient's primary care provider. Patients may leave the hospital with multiple new medications, often including high doses of prednisone that have a diverse range of side effects. One should also anticipate that the receipt of a new diagnosis of a dangerous and previously unheard-of disease will likely produce understandable psychological stress for both the patient and family members.

QUALITY IMPROVEMENT

Hospitals need systems to allow for rapid processing of selected tests that can establish a diagnosis of vasculitis and lead to initiation of time-critical therapies, including ANCA and anti-GBM antibody tests, measurement of cryoglobulins, temporal artery biopsies, and angiography.

Hospitals should develop a multidisciplinary team comfortable with the many aspects of the evaluation and management of these challenging multisystem diseases.

CONCLUSION

The major factor that delays the correct diagnosis of vasculitis is a delay in even considering the diagnosis. Efforts must be made to educate clinicians that the presence of any of the red flags mentioned in this chapter should rapidly prompt evaluation for possible vasculitis and initiation of appropriate consultations.

SUGGESTED READINGS

Kissin EY, Merkel PA. Diagnostic Imaging in Takayasu's Arteritis. *Current Opinion in Rheumatology.* 2004;16:31–37.

Merkel PA. Drug-Induced Vasculitis. *Rheumatic Disease Clinics of North America.* 2001;27:849–862.

Mukhtyar C, Guillevin L, Cid M, et al, for the European Vasculitis Study Group. EULAR Recommendations for the management of large vessel vasculitis. *Annals Rheum Dis.* 2009;68:103–106.

Mukhtyar C, Guillevin L, Cid M, et al, for the European Vasculitis Study Group. EULAR Recommendations for the management of primary small and medium vessel vasculitis. *Annals Rheum Dis.* 2009;68:310–317.

SECTION 20

Wartime Medicine

CHAPTER 265

Hospital Disaster Emergency Preparedness

Steven B. Deitelzweig, MD, MMM, SFHM
Richard D. Guthrie Jr., MD
Grant L. Walker, MA

Key Clinical Questions

1. What leadership principles should be followed by hospitalists and key leaders of the organization during a disaster?
2. How should an emergency command center be designed and operated while conveying an environment of safety for your staff and other essential personnel?
3. What are some significant considerations for hospitalist and organizational staffing and planning models during a disaster?

INTRODUCTION

Despite the best preparations and planning, many aspects of managing an organization and a hospitalist practice change rapidly, and many new, often unanticipated, problems arise during the peridisaster and recovery period. We present our management learnings as a large hospitalist program within a tertiary-care referral center during an unprecedented disaster in Hurricane Katrina and extend preparedness principles to other types of man-made, natural, planned, and unplanned emergencies.

LEADERSHIP

ORGANIZATIONAL

The ability to lead others through change and adversity and to sustain an effective team with a unified purpose is required during a disaster, not only within the hospitalist program level, but also at an organizational level.

All top leaders in an organization need to be present during and/or in the aftermath of a disaster. This includes not only the CEO and COO, but also the CFO, VP for human resources, and so on. In a severe disaster, issues like how to pay employees if major electronic systems are down, how to prepare an insurance claim for business interruption insurance (documentation needs to start during the actual disaster), access to significant cash reserves in order to function, and how to manage employees who have neglected their responsibilities will be among the multitude of issues for which leaders will be needed. A leadership structure with the appropriate scope of responsibilities and number of direct reports needs to be functional, and on-field promotions will likely be required. Assigning responsibility for conducting every detail of your plan is essential. It will be necessary to ask unofficial leaders to step up and help manage particular functions or groups of individuals and they must be given the authority to do so with appropriate levels of support. They need to have the traits of selfless dedication, courage, decisiveness, compassion, and optimism. The failure to quickly create new leadership structures to fill in for leaders who cannot be present will lead to an unmanageable situation.

A few key leadership principles

A strong sense of purpose with optimism: "We will make a difference in this disaster. We will care for our patients who depend on us to manage through this difficult time. Here are our challenges and we'll face them together and get through this fine." Employees (or at least all key managers) need to hear this and be updated with the status of the organization and challenges twice a day with the expectation that they drive it down into the institution. A sense of unaffordable failure can be a self-fulfilling prophecy.

Stopping rumors is one of leadership's first priorities. Rumors can quickly supplant the appropriate focus of employees. Managers should immediately report rumors to the highest level of leadership and, to the extent possible, all activities in which executive leadership are involved at the time should stop so that the rumor can be addressed.

In a disaster situation, strict rules are important. In our situation, without water pressure, fire represented our most significant threat. Smoking anywhere around campus became an immediately terminable offense. Everyone must understand the rules in a disaster. Do not hesitate to be clear. In a disaster, rules that are explained will be followed.

In a disaster, everyone's job becomes whatever they can do. If a physician is not busy, he or she can help in the cafeteria. Make this expectation clear: people will surprise you and the positive effects of acts such as this will last long past the disaster.

Emotional support in a disaster is critical for many employees. Usually, this is with a friend or colleague. It should be a stated understanding that anyone might and perhaps most people will have to step away for a moment and compose themselves in order to return to duty capable of performing their job. It is normal during a crisis. Formal counseling should also be available. Psychiatrists and/or psychologists should be essential personnel in a disaster in order to provide regular group and individual counseling as needed.

In planning for a disaster, there is no such thing as a "doomsday scenario." There is no situation that should be described in planning as "if this should happen, it would be so bad that we really couldn't plan for it." This is a fallacy. A whole city flooding was a scenario that easily could have been seen to fit in this category. However, those organizations that planned as best as they could for such a severe event did far better than those that did not. Even for events with a high likelihood for significant mortality, such as a terrorist attack or severe flu pandemic, those organizations that plan will be far better off, and no matter how bad the disaster, there will be many survivors looking to those most prepared for needed help.

HOSPITALIST

As a key component of any hospital's disaster response, it is important for the department chairperson or group leader of the hospitalist team to be involved in disaster planning. Strong leadership is crucial to maintaining a sense of confidence and an optimistic outlook in times of uncertainty.

Our past hurricane experience led us to develop a two-team system for all disasters. The number of hospitalists on Team A was determined by anticipating at least a 15–20 census per physician. These physicians are required to stay on campus. Team B is composed of individuals who have an expectation of being available within a week to relieve Team A. For predictable disasters, such as hurricanes, discharge and transfer protocols based on time until landfall can assist in volume and census management.

After Hurricane Katrina, it was uncertain how many patients would require medical care in the community. From the Hurricane Ivan experience in Pensacola, we were advised that in the 10 days after the disaster, one could anticipate a doubling of the highest emergency department volume for several weeks. The group leader must plan for surge capacity.

Included in the Hospital Medicine disaster plan would be the consideration of closure of other health care facilities and the absorption of those patients into the organization. To offer quality and safe clinical care and remain able to perform under such conditions, our hospitalists unanimously agreed to care for our patients 24/7 in weekly rotation. Our hospital census during this period was at 60% of usual, and our admission rate was running at 40% of normal. We decreased the residents staffing from three members per team to two in order to provide a five-day rotation of three teams. If possible, a staging center in a facility outside the disaster area to organize the faculty and resident staff and provide transportation is very helpful.

We experienced a sense of camaraderie after seeing all our colleagues participating in activities beyond the boundary of usual roles. For example, you should consider eliminating exclusive service functions. Our skilled nursing physician might care for the acute stroke victim, and so forth.

EMERGENCY COMMAND CENTER

Like governmental agencies, emergency command centers must be created and predesignated before a disaster. This might simply be a centralized location where administrative support and executive leadership would meet and plan. Ideally, it would be a location for the various communication devices and other equipment needed to communicate with external agencies—a central repository of key information available 24 hours a day.

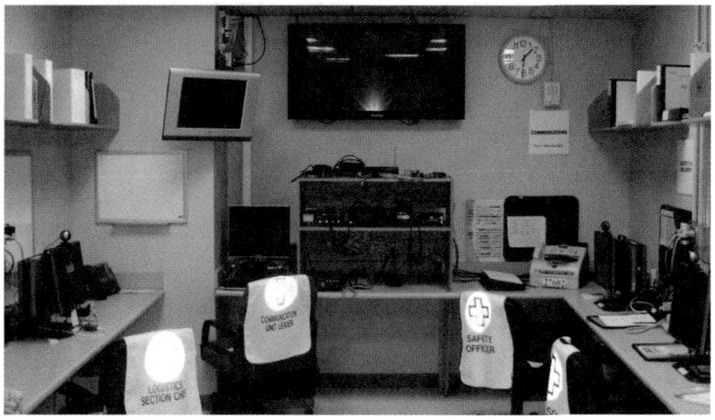

Figure 265-1 *Ochsner Command Center.*

Your command center should be located in a secure area of your safest building and ideally would have no external windows. The location of the command center (and other essential functions) would depend on the likelihood of different disasters. In our case, flooding is the major concern; hence all essential functions are moved to the second floor. It needs to be 100% self-sufficient with stand-alone emergency power, food, water, toilet facilities, heating, and air conditioning. This will be your communication hub with satellite TVs, satellite Internet stations, fixed antenna satellite phones, hospital emergency administrative radio (HEAR), emergency communication radios, and ham radios. Connection to all facility security cameras, including zoom cameras, covering all approaches to the facility is required. In the likely event communication networks fail, this will be your lifeline to the world (**Figure 265-1**)!

COMMUNICATIONS

Organizational

Effective communications within the facility and with external agencies, vendors, and so on will be critical. Numerous emergency communication tools and redundancies should be built into the plan. Communication failures led to many of the untoward events following Katrina.

Satellite phones with fixed antennas mounted through an elevator shaft to the roof with a detachable antenna on the roof and ham radios (with operators) are important when regular service fails. Cell phones become useless (even if towers stay up) since the circuits are simply overloaded. Two things that did work better were cell phones with out-of-state area codes (we now keep some of these at all times) and text messaging. We were fortunate to have an internal phone system (Spectralink phones) that allowed for rapid communication internally. Given that most people will be on the run and not in their usual location, as many leaders as possible should have these phones (and regular meetings twice a day within each department or unit can provide updates for everyone else). It is virtually impossible to over-communicate.

In shifting from internal communications to external communications, it should be stressed that public relations staff form an important component of your essential personnel. External agencies and the public need to be aware of the organization's status, capabilities, and limitations, including any needs for philanthropic support, which should be made known as early as possible after a disaster. A plan should be in place with a central person to lead this important effort. The efforts to raise philanthropic funds should be initiated early while the disaster has the attention of the local, regional, and national community.

All messaging should go through one central individual or small group of individuals to ensure appropriate messaging. For employees not on the premises in a disaster, one-way teleconferencing with a message from leadership that employees can dial into is helpful. On these calls, hundreds of employees dialed in and received important information that was able to be relayed. We had a message for physicians and one for all employees during Katrina. Multiple telecommunication line connections are the key to maintaining your Internet and telephone operations. Most cities have more than one telephone line feed. New Orleans has three such lines. Ochsner was connected to all three lines. Two lines failed, the third line from the Westbank remained operational. You need only one feed to remain operational. If you are really committed to maintaining cell phone communication, talk to your cell phone provider about installing a protected cell phone tower at your facility. Connect the tower to your emergency power. All towers have the capability to be set up to operate as a stand-alone tower. This is a minor expense and will allow all phones from this cell phone company to operate in push-to-talk mode within a two to seven mile radius, which is determined by terrain and weather.

HOSPITALIST

Fortunately, Ochsner Clinic Foundation had invested in Spectralink phones in the past few years; this internal, antenna-based phone system continued to function. We were even able to dial long distance intermittently. Our information system also went down, but we kept generator power for the Internet to allow our employees to access information and have contact with the outside world. As for a hospitalist program, we started to meet twice daily immediately after the hurricane to address concerns of emergency department volumes, maintain open communications, provide mutual psychological support, and foster a spirit of teamwork. During these meetings we believed that our department had cemented a bond that could not be created in normal circumstances. Our efforts through the storm and the unimaginable adversity were nothing short of extraordinary.

Essential personnel lists of physicians, house staff, and administrators should be developed for the entire organization. For the essential physicians in your organization, the department can decide the exact individual who will stay to be the staff physician on call at the time a severe weather or disaster plan is enacted. If alternative arrangements are desired, the plan of who would be responsible for covering these positions is retained on file in medical administration. It is critically important that these individuals be on site.

Certain essential house staff should also be required to remain on campus. The decision regarding who should remain should be coordinated among medical administration, graduate medical education, and the department chairman.

KEY FUNCTIONS OF FACILITIES MANAGEMENT

A good facilities management team with a well-thought-out disaster plan is critical. You need seasoned professionals who know your infrastructure equipment.

A key principle is that regardless of the state and national response, there will be a period of time when the organization will be on its own and needs to be self-sustaining; this could likely be two to seven days. During Katrina, we were self-sufficient for more than a month. We were able to provide supplies, food, and shelter to Federal Emergency Management Agency (FEMA) medical teams.

It is important to plan ahead of time for the number of people who might be on the premises. Decide if the organization is able to function as a shelter as well as carry out its patient care mission. For us, the answer to this question was no; this has to be clear if a disaster has significant advance warning to allow people (including family members of employees who can) to evacuate to another area of safety so that the resources in the organization can be used for essential personnel and patients.

Well before any disaster, decisions must be made regarding how much food and water (in days for the number of people expected to be present) must be available at all times for adequate preparation. We were fortunate enough to have a well for a disaster that would cut off the city water supply. In addition to drinking water, attention needs to be paid to dialysis patients' needs, as well as water for bathing and flushing toilets. Plans should be made for handling these functions if emergency water is not available without city water. An example would be having adequate plastic garbage bags and kitty litter for human excrement if toilet water is not available. Alternatively, portalets could be another option in certain circumstances. Fill all tubs, waste baskets, swimming pools, etc, with water; the water can be used for flushing or washing. Emergency power is essential to your survival. Ensure that you have enough emergency power to run your HVAC. If these are destroyed by the disaster you will need small backup generators, the same size as those used to power a house. You will need enough generators to power life-support equipment, fans, and spot air conditioners or heaters, depending on your circumstances. You will use this equipment to provide cool or warm rest/sleep areas for your patients and employees.

It is essential to keep a minimum of one week's supply of fuel to run all of your generators. Remember the small generators run on gasoline. If you are in a pinch for gasoline, use your parking lot filled with cars and fuel as a resource. If you do not have fuel tanks, purchase fuel bladders that come in various sizes up to 20,000 gallons. They are like large rubber pillows that you fill up with diesel fuel. The military uses them for combat and field operations.

All essential medical equipment must be connected to emergency power: key laboratory, X-ray, operating room, emergency room, and water treatment for dialysis.

Negotiate deals with the water company, sewage plant, power plant, county rescue police, and others to have their emergency personnel housed with you during the disaster so they can get back to work immediately to recover vital city systems.

HOSPITALIST: CONTINUITY OF OPERATIONS

The expansion of the essential personnel team list to include social workers and discharge planners is crucial to focus on the unique and unconventional logistical challenges postdisaster. Intense focus on group dynamics was essential to avoid physical and emotional burnout. Frequent and predictably scheduled face-to-face communication was also important in disseminating accurate, unadulterated information because our decision making changed hour to hour immediately after Hurricane Katrina and day to day for weeks after the event.

An initially unanticipated lesson emanated from a general knowledge of physical capabilities and liabilities. With no working elevators, navigating 11 floors of a hospital was a challenge for several people. Our survival tactics included not just adequate fluid hydration, but electrolyte replacement and knowing our people.

Not knowing the capability of our facility in this time of extreme uncertainty, we proceeded to discharge and move patients to other centers, such as Memorial Hermann Hospital in Houston and Summit Hospital in Baton Rouge via both helicopter and ambulance. Simultaneously, we focused on patients who were stable and ready for discharge to increase our organization's capacity to create a plan for providing resources for both the east and west banks of the Mississippi River.

Of course, the ailments confronted will vary based on the disaster.

We saw patients with:

- Severe dehydration
- Exhaustion caused by the lack of use or incorrect use of their medications for days resulting in exacerbation of chronic conditions such as chronic obstructive pulmonary disorder (COPD)
- Water-borne illnesses from prolonged immersion in toxic water
- Reactive airway diseases from environmental allergens
- Cellulitis from cuts and bruises by evacuees, as well as people attempting home repairs
- Carbon monoxide poisoning from generators used incorrectly inside homes
- Withdrawals from illicit drug use.

STAFF AND VOLUNTEER MANAGEMENT

An advance plan for the essential personnel required in a disaster must be developed and reviewed by multiple constituencies to make sure it is as complete as possible.

While family members are encouraged to not accompany their essential personnel employees, invariably, there will be situations where this is not possible. Expect to provide a child care function. There should be clarity on the absolute number of family members allowed (with exceptions made only by directors, etc), as well as clarity about what to expect: self-sufficiency with water and food, sleeping on the floor of an office or waiting area, and the possible lack of electricity or working toilets and showers.

Also, expect there to be pet care needs. Invariably, we found many employees who would not leave their pet at home during a disaster. To have them report to duty, we needed to be able to accommodate their pet. It is important to think through where pets can be located and who would help supervise this function.

ORIENTATION

We had developed, before the storm, the concept of a Team A and Team B. Team A would stay in-house and Team B would be expected to evacuate as needed but be able to return within a few days to relieve Team A. We recommend this approach so that in addition to essential personnel being designated, it is clear to your employees whether they need to be ready to relieve the first team or not.

As new employees arrive to assist in the disaster and/or relieve Team A, it is important to orient them. Newly arriving personnel will not be aware of experiences shared by those who have been there from the beginning. It is important to discuss these experiences as well as to review the rules in place related to the disaster.

VENDOR RELATIONSHIPS

Even with a commitment to self-sufficiency, supplies will be needed during or after a disaster. It is critical to have, prior to a disaster, a contract with vendors ensuring availability of supplies. In a disaster, many organizations may need the same supplies. Advance preparation for these needs will help you get the supplies you need as well as help the vendor think through the processes necessary to get them to you (and others).

Prepare for the worst, assuming you will not have access to supplies indefinitely. Identify food warehouses, large grocery stores, home repair stores, medical supply warehouses, pharmacies, equipment rental stores, construction sites, and any place that would have things you need to function post disaster. If these organizations plan to evacuate, ask them how to break in and how they want you to account for what you take. During Katrina, our organization had access to a food distribution warehouse that had more than a six months' supply of food and water.

Reestablishing distribution for food, fuel, medical supplies, and pharmaceuticals is essential. Contact your vendors immediately and determine what it will take to reconnect. Avenues of transportation will need to be explored immediately after danger passes to ensure trucks can deliver needed supplies. One should consider having motorcycles and all-terrain vehicles (ATVs) on site for deployment post disaster, along with chainsaws to clear a path to safety. Then communicate the route to your vendors. If you are in an earthquake zone, be sure to have access to bulldozers or backhoes.

Supplies need to be coordinated in advance and delivered at least 48 hours in advance. New Orleans hospitals that waited until 48 hours prior to Katrina were unable to get any supplies because all vendors had evacuated.

It is important to explore with state and local governments whether supply trucks will be allowed to travel in the disaster areas and under what circumstances. This was a common problem after Katrina. Since then, we have made thorough plans with the state related to travel into the area by our vendors, and we don't anticipate future problems in this regard since we have a predisaster plan that addresses these issues. Outlined below are some of the successful supply considerations.

- **Food and water on site:** Two weeks on-site; access to an additional 90 days
- **Medical and pharmacy:** Two weeks on site; free access to local distributors' warehouses
- **Construction:** Plywood, sand bags, cordless tools; access to Lowe's or Home Depot
- **Cleaning supplies:** Pallets of plastic bags, hundreds of mops and buckets, cargo containers for infectious waste; establish trash dump
- **Linen:** Two weeks' supply on hand; all laundry equipment on backup power and water
- **Toilet service:** Portalets as backup; used when we opened clinics in the community
- **Fans and air mattresses:** One per patient, employee, and visitor.

SAFETY AND SECURITY

Ensuring the safety of your workforce is an important organizational duty and will be a key factor in employees being comfortable to report to duty. Survival requires an assessment of your resources and threats. Ideally, you would have your own armed (with appropriate advanced training) security staff. In the worrisome days after Katrina, having armed security personnel present and eventually National Guard members with M-16 rifles was amazingly reassuring for personal security and met the need to establish order. All hospitals without armed security had to evacuate even if the facilities were not flooded or compromised. If an armed security force is not logistically possible, having a contracted company that can provide this quickly is helpful.

Establish agreements with local law enforcement and firemen and provide them with protected space for their vehicles, air conditioned space to sleep, free hot meals, and working showers. The more uniformed officials in your facility, the safer your staff will feel. Secure the perimeter of your facility and keep a traffic log to know who is entering and leaving. Ochsner had 50 armed security officers during Katrina and had to hire 75 contract security officers 48 hours after the storm to secure the perimeter of the facility.

Essential personnel would be expected to wear their ID. It is important to armband or otherwise identify approved family members with essential personnel, and so on. Included in the plan should be the method by which this can be done when essential personnel report to work. We found that one of the best ways to make sure we identified individuals on campus (and addressed their ability to be present, sleeping arrangements, etc) was to require the armband identification in order to get meals. This identification is important for security, for possible rapid contact with the family if a nonemployee were to become ill, and for certain types of insurance claims.

DISASTER PLAN

In addition to the infrastructure, certain predetermined algorithms should be brought into effect.

PATIENT MANAGEMENT AND CARE

An excerpt from our plan related to patient severity and timing of disasters that was set up beforehand and that is similar to a best practice order set is provided.

ORGANIZATIONAL AND HOSPITAL MANAGEMENT

Seventy-two hours prelandfall (coordinated with implementation of emergency plan) for anticipated advanced disaster (ie, Level IV or V storm):

I. Evacuation of these patients:
   - Patients awaiting organ transplantation in the hospital
   - Oscillating ventilated patients or extracorporeal membrane oxidation (ECMO) patients in pediatric intensive care unit (PICU) (note: Little Rock has Mobile echo unit)
   - Left ventricular assist device (LVAD), patients (VAD specific sites: Texas Heart, University of Alabama (UAB), depends on type)
   - Pediatric/congenital heart patients anticipating emergent surgery
   - Unstable cardiac patients requiring eminent surgery
   - Pediatric neurosurgery patients

Attending MDs evaluate all in-house patients for discharge (per usual protocol/procedure) and prioritize patients by service line based on the triage evaluation form for physicians to determine who should be transported out first if the need arises.

II. Discontinue elective surgeries and transplant surgeries.
III. Hospital medical director and/or designee is ultimately responsible for triage coordination and decisions.
IV. The operational VP's assigned role is in coordination of all activities.

POSTDISASTER MANAGEMENT

Depending on the postdisaster situation, patients may be transported out of the medical center. Which patients are transported will be determined on a case-by-case basis by medical team leaders and the medical director and coordinated through the operational VP and flight care.

"Worst-case" scenario

In the event that there is no power, no supplies, or in a situation necessitating a complete evacuation, the triage methodology should be developed prior to the disaster—ideally, depending on availability of transport, equipment, personnel, and so on. The order we selected is listed.

- Mothers and newborns
- Children
- ICU patients
- Dialysis patients
- Surgical patients
- All other medical patients
- Psychiatry
- DNR
- Hospice/terminally ill

This would probably vary based on the capabilities of the specific health systems. The plan should also include (1) plans for tracking patients, including the deceased; and (2) plans for modification of normal clinical activities (including specialized care) as related to disaster response.

CONCLUSION

We shared from our direct experience and research some of the key elements for hospital disaster emergency preparedness. Leadership's ability to guide frontline professionals using common-sense intuition, courage, selfless dedication, and compassion to make decisions at every level will be critical. Having a stand-alone infrastructure, highly trained security, and phenomenal teamwork will serve our health systems well during these times of extreme ambiguity. Planning for the modification of normal activities is a critical item and encompasses the notion that it is not "business as usual" during times of emergency.

SUGGESTED READINGS

Guin CC, Robinson LC, Boyd EC, Levitan ML. Healthcare and disaster planning, understanding the impact of disasters on the medical community. Louisiana State University, copyright Louisiana State Medical Society. www.healthcaredisasterplanning.org. Access date 7-19-11.

NIMS 700: National Incident Management System: An Introduction

The National Incident Management System (NIMS) was developed to provide a system that would help emergency managers and responders from different jurisdictions and disciplines work together more effectively to handle emergencies and disasters.

The NIMS provides a set of standardized organizational structures such as the Incident Command System and standardized processes, procedures, and systems. These processes and procedures are designed to improve interoperability among jurisdictions and disciplines in various areas such as command and management, resource management, training, and communications.

Link to the FEMA Course.

http://ochweb/page.cfm?id=2441

http://training.fema.gov/emiweb/is/is700a.asp

Link to the Safety & Security web page containing all NIMS courses.

CHAPTER 266

Bioterrorism

Daniel S. Shapiro, MD

Key Clinical Questions

1. What epidemiologic clues should heighten suspicion of a bioterrorism attack?
2. What is the appropriate organizational response to a suspected bioterrorism event?
3. What clinical syndromes are associated with possible agents of bioterrorism?

INTRODUCTION

EPIDEMIOLOGIC FEATURES SUGGESTIVE OF BIOTERRORISM

Several disease entities should raise the suspicion that a bioterrorist attack is occurring, especially when clusters of similar cases are seen. These include:

- A life-threatening, apparently infectious illness in a young, otherwise healthy person, not due to toxic shock syndrome, meningococcus, or Rocky Mountain spotted fever
- A serious pneumonia in a young, otherwise healthy adult
- Influenza outbreaks occurring during the offseason
- A febrile illness with a widened mediastinum on chest radiography (as seen in inhalation anthrax)
- The characteristic vesicular rash of smallpox
- The capillary leak syndrome of viral hemorrhagic fevers
- Laboratory suspicion or diagnosis of infections due to glanders (*Burkholderia mallei*), anthrax, smallpox, hemorrhagic fevers
- Plague (*Yersinia pestis*) or tularemia (*Francisella tularensis*) outside of endemic areas
- Neurologic findings compatible with botulism

THE INSTITUTIONAL RESPONSE TO A BIOTERRORIST EVENT

After a proven or suspected bioterrorist attack, a tremendous surge of patients may affect, and potentially overwhelm, many areas of the hospital, including the emergency department, microbiology laboratory, outpatient clinics, and inpatient medical wards. This may include many persons seeking medical evaluation who are unaffected by the bioterrorist agent. It may be problematic to differentiate the "worried well" from patients in the early stages of infection due to a bioterrorist agent. For example, anthrax (and many other infections) may first present as a "flu-like illness." If there is a recognized bioterrorism event due to the intentional release of *B. anthracis* spores during a busy influenza season, many people who would otherwise remain at home with influenza are likely to seek medical attention out of fear of inhalation of anthrax.

A bioterrorism event requires an organized, prompt response to mobilize all available resources. Hospitals should have an approved infectious disease emergency management and response plan (as in **Figure 266-1**) in place for potential bioterrorism agents, as well as for other highly virulent infections, including SARS and pandemic influenza. If the hospital does not have such a plan in place, hospitalists should contact specific services:

- *Infection control/hospital epidemiology*, to ensure that patients are placed on the proper precautions to prevent nosocomial transmission of infection. These vary with the suspected agent. For some, such as anthrax and botulism, there is no risk of person-to-person transmission. For others, such as plague pneumonia and smallpox, the risk is substantial.
- *Public health authorities*, to report possible cases (usually done by infection control/hospital epidemiology), and to engage their clinical expertise and laboratory resources.
- *The clinical microbiology laboratory*, to ensure that appropriate specimens are properly collected and transported, and to ensure that the dangers to laboratory workers are minimized. Bioterrorism agents such as *Francisella tularensis*, *Brucella* species, and viruses (including smallpox, SARS, and viral

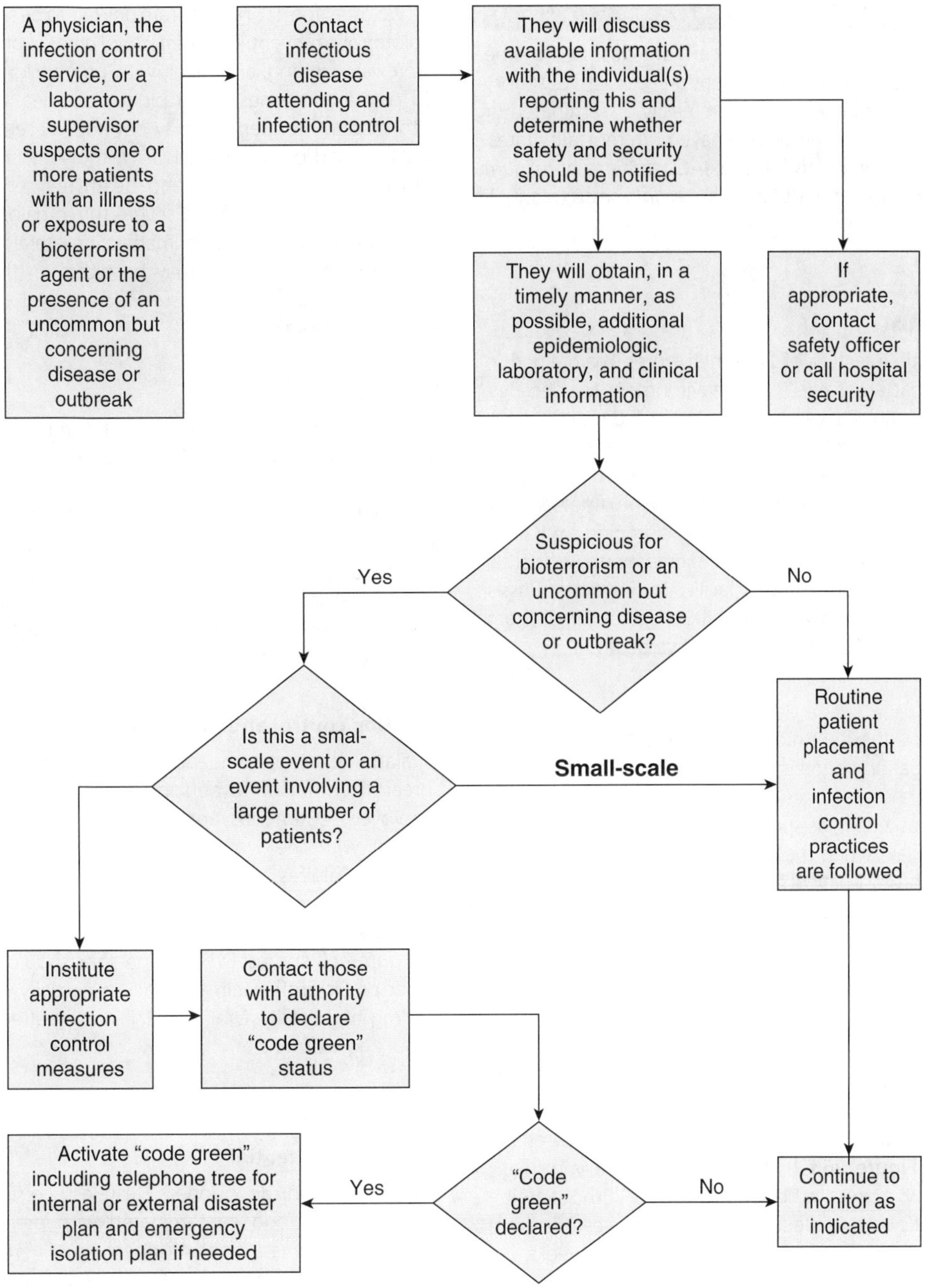

Figure 266-1 *Organizational response flowsheet for possible bioterrorism events.*

hemorrhagic fevers) are each associated with a major risk of laboratory-acquired infection.

- *The anatomic pathology department*, in the event that tissue or fluid from a patient is sent for diagnostic purposes. As with microbiology, direct communication with pathology can help optimize diagnostic testing and ensure that proper handling and safety measures are used. This may also assist in contingency planning, such as establishment of a temporary morgue.
- *The medical examiner* should be alerted in the event of patient deaths, as these may be investigated as criminal acts.
- *The infectious disease service* is essential in the diagnosis and management of the victims of bioterrorism.
- *Hospital administration*, to coordinate internal responses and deal with the flow of information both inside and outside the hospital, including dealing with news media.
- *The inpatient pharmacy*, to locate specific treatments for hospitalized patients and to maximize supplies for additional patients who may present to the hospital (this may require activation of the National Antibiotic Stockpile by federal authorities).
- *The critical care service*, since affected patients may need ICU admission. Mechanical ventilation may be necessary for pneumonia (as in plague and tularemia), acute respiratory distress syndrome (as in ricin poisoning), and neuromuscular disease (as in botulism).
- *Other clinical services* may include dermatology for evaluation and possible skin biopsy for suspected cases of smallpox and cutaneous anthrax, ophthalmology for oculoglandular tularemia, and neurology for suspected botulism.

SPECIFIC PATHOGENS AND TOXINS

The bioterrorism agents of greatest concern are classified by the U.S. Centers for Disease Control and Prevention (CDC) as "Category A" agents, so designated because they are easily disseminated or transmitted from person to person and have high mortality rates. These include *Bacillus anthracis* (anthrax), *Clostridium botulinum* (botulism), *Francisella tularensis* (tularemia), *Yersinia pestis* (plague), smallpox, and viral hemorrhagic fevers.

ANTHRAX

Bioweapon potential

Anthrax is a zoonotic infection of large herbivores, maintained in nature by spores that are viable in the environment for decades. *Bacillus anthracis* infections have a high morbidity and mortality due mainly to their production of two toxins, edema factor and lethal factor, which lead to tissue necrosis and hypotension. Cultures of *B anthracis* may be weaponized by drying, milling into fine particles, and adding an agent to counter electrostatic clumping and allow airborne dispersal. Anthrax is a proven bioweapon. Accidental release of spores from a bioweapons facility in Sverdlosk, Russia in 1979 caused at least 66 deaths. The 2001 U.S. outbreak from contaminated mail led to 22 cases, including five deaths.

Clinical features

Inhalational anthrax is the form most likely to result from a bioterror attack. The incubation period is usually from one to seven days, but may be longer; the exact incubation period in any given case may be difficult to ascertain, as spores may settle on surfaces and become airborne again when the environment is disturbed. After initial "flu-like" symptoms, patients develop high fever, respiratory distress, and shock within one to five days. Chest radiography may reveal pulmonary infiltrates and pleural effusions; widening of the mediastinum from hemorrhagic mediastinitis is a frequent and characteristic finding. The death rate of inhalation anthrax in the 2001 U.S. attack was 45%, lower than the historical mortality of 85%.

Cutaneous anthrax is the most common form of naturally-acquired anthrax, and comprised about half of cases in the 2001 attack. It begins as a pruritic papule, and evolves into a hemorrhagic vesicle. Tissue necrosis results in the formation of a black eschar within 7–10 days (**Figure 266-2**). The eschar is usually painless, and is surrounded by impressive nonpitting edema. Without antibiotics, 20% will die of systemic infection. In the rest, the eschar eventually sloughs off, with symptom resolution in two to six weeks.

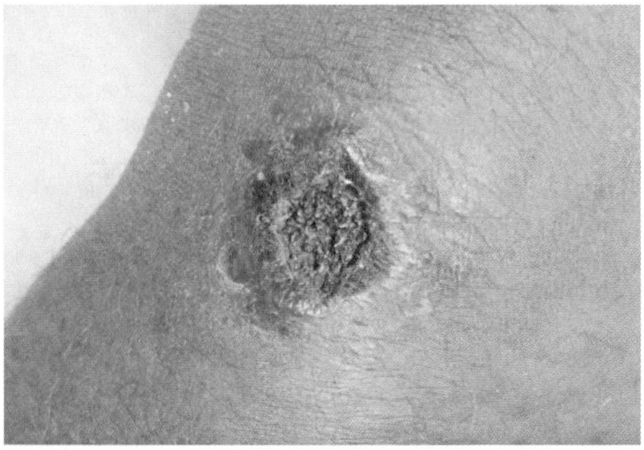

Figure 266-2 *Cutaneous anthrax, with central black eschar and surrounding brawny edema. (Public Health Image Library, Centers for Disease Control and Prevention.)*

Two other forms of anthrax are unlikely to be seen in the context of a bioterrorism event. *Gastrointestinal anthrax* presents with nausea, anorexia, vomiting, and fever, with progression to severe abdominal pain, hematemesis, and bloody diarrhea. An acute abdomen with rebound tenderness may develop. Mesenteric adenopathy is usually found on abdominal CT. Within two to five days of symptom onset, ascites, shock, and death may ensue. *Oropharyngeal anthrax* presents with fever, severe throat pain, and dysphagia. On examination, patients have marked unilateral or bilateral cervical lymphadenopathy. There may be ulcers on the tonsils, posterior pharynx, or hard palate. Tissue necrosis and edema may lead to airway compromise.

Treatment

Inhalational anthrax, oropharyngeal anthrax, and gastrointestinal anthrax in adults are treated with intravenous ciprofloxacin 400 mg every 12 hours, or intravenous doxycycline 100 mg every 12 hours. Many authorities recommend the addition of one or two additional antibiotics, such as penicillin or ampicillin, clindamycin, or rifampin. Cutaneous anthrax with systemic symptoms is treated similarly to inhalational anthrax. Otherwise, a prolonged course (60 days) of oral ciprofloxacin 500 mg twice daily or oral doxycycline 100 mg twice daily is recommended.

Infection control and prevention

Inhalational, oropharyngeal, and gastrointestinal anthrax are not spread from person to person, and standard precautions may be employed. Cutaneous anthrax may rarely be transmitted from contact with the wound or its drainage; contact precautions, including gloves and gowns, should be used, and dressings should be autoclaved or incinerated. Long courses of post-exposure prophylaxis are given, because of the extended survival of *B anthracis* spores. Exposed persons should receive 60 days of either oral ciprofloxacin 500 mg twice daily or oral doxycycline 100 mg twice daily. Oral amoxicillin is an alternative in pregnant or nursing women.

BOTULISM

Bioweapon potential

Botulinum toxin, an odorless, tasteless compound, is naturally acquired from food contaminated with preformed toxin (such as home-preserved goods), ingestion of *Clostridium botulinum* in food or environmental dust, with toxin production in the gut (most commonly seen in infants), or by wound colonization with *C botulinum,* with local toxin production. Aerosolization is the most likely method of dispersal of botulinum toxin in a bioterrorism event. Botulinum toxin could be added to water supplies, but would be degraded by the chlorine disinfectant used by most water utilities. The toxin could also be added to food, but is similarly inactivated by cooking.

Clinical features

The toxin irreversibly blocks the neuromuscular junction by inhibiting presynaptic acetylcholine release. Neurologic symptoms usually begin 12–36 hours after exposure. There is a progressive symmetric involvement of cranial nerves, with blurred vision, diplopia, ptosis, dysphagia, and dysarthria. Descending flaccid paralysis follows. This may involve the respiratory musculature, and require intubation and mechanical ventilation. Sensation is preserved, and mental status is clear. Recovery from severe cases requires sprouting of new presynaptic nerve terminals, which takes up to six months.

Treatment

Therapy is botulism antitoxin and supportive care. Except for wound botulism, antibiotics have no role in treatment.

Infection control and prevention

Botulism is not transmitted from person to person. Isolation is not required for affected patients. No postexposure prophylaxis is currently available. Due to limited quantities, antitoxin is reserved for symptomatic individuals.

TULAREMIA

Bioweapon potential

Francisella tularensis, the agent of tularemia, is a small gram-negative coccobacillus. It may be naturally acquired from tick, deerfly, or mosquito bites, contact with infected mammals or their meat and hides, ingestion of contaminated food or water, or inhalation, as from mowing a contaminated lawn. Tularemia is endemic in parts of North America, Europe, and Asia. The inoculum for pneumonia may be as low as 10 inhaled organisms, making it an attractive candidate for aerosol dispersal for bioterrorism.

Clinical features

After a typical incubation period of three to five days, fever, chills, and malaise develop, with local signs at the exposure site. In *ulceroglandular tularemia*, an ulcer forms at the site of inoculation with enlarged regional lymph nodes. Regional adenopathy may also occur without an ulcer at the inoculation site (*glandular tularemia*). In *oculoglandular tularemia*, there is involvement of the inoculated conjunctiva and the draining lymph node or nodes. If the organism is swallowed, patients may develop pharyngeal tularemia, with exudative pharyngitis or tonsillitis, sometimes ulcerative, and regional adenopathy.

Pneumonic tularemia has a significant mortality rate even with appropriate therapy. It is most commonly due to inhalation of the organism, but it can also occur secondary to seeding of the lung from another infected site. *Typhoidal tularemia* is not associated with adenopathy or any other obvious portal of entry. In addition to fever, chills, and malaise, severe disease can result in multiple end organ dysfunction, including pneumonia. Mortality is high.

Treatment

The mainstay of treatment is streptomycin. Gentamicin can be used if streptomycin is unavailable, but it is associated with higher rates of failure and relapse than streptomycin. Intravenous doxycycline and chloramphenicol are also used, but are associated with higher relapse rates than either streptomycin or gentamicin. Chloramphenicol is useful in tularemic meningitis. The clinical experience with ciprofloxacin is limited and somewhat ambiguous.

Infection control and prevention

Tularemia is not transmitted from person to person, and infected patients may be placed on standard precautions. A 14-day course of either oral doxycycline or oral ciprofloxacin may be used as postexposure prophylaxis in those exposed to aerosols of *F tularensis*. Tularemia is a major laboratory hazard, as so few organisms are required for infection. If tularemia is suspected, the microbiology laboratory should be warned immediately. Serologic testing does not carry the risks of culture, but it may be unrevealing early in the course of illness.

PLAGUE

Bioweapon potential

Plague is caused by the gram-negative rod *Yersinia pestis*. Humans acquire plague from flea bites, handling sick or dead mammals, especially cats and rodents, or inhalation of respiratory secretions from patients with pneumonic plague. Plague is endemic in the United States west of the Mississippi River, and in parts of South America, Africa, and Asia. Plague is potentially an excellent agent of bioterrorism, given its high mortality and person-to-person transmission.

Clinical features

Bubonic plague, the most common naturally-occurring type, results from infected flea bites. An eschar may form at the bite site. After two to six days, there is rapid and painful swelling of regional lymph nodes ("buboes"), with fever, chills, headache, and malaise. Bacteremia is common. In *primary septicemic plague*, patients have massive bacteremia, with multisystem organ failure and septic shock, but without buboes. Gangrene of the extremities may occur (the probable origin of the term "the Black Death"). *Pneumonic plague* is acquired from bacteremic seeding of the lungs in bubonic plague, or from inhalation of infectious aerosols from patients with plague pneumonia. It would likely be the most common presentation after a bioterrorist attack involving dispersal of aerosols of *Y pestis*. It is difficult to distinguish from other causes of bacterial pneumonia, aside from its high propensity to progress to septic shock.

Treatment

Streptomycin is the antibiotic of choice for plague. Gentamicin may be used when streptomycin is not available. Tetracyclines and chloramphenicol are also effective. Close contacts of a plague patient, particularly patients with plague pneumonia, should be identified and evaluated. In a bioterrorist event, clinicians should be alert to the possibility of antibiotic resistance, either due to the use of a naturally occurring resistant strain or an engineered strain. Cultures of blood, aspirates of buboes, and cultures of other affected areas (including cerebrospinal fluid in cases of meningitis) should be obtained prior to the initiation of antibiotic therapy.

Infection control and prevention

Respiratory droplet precautions (gloves, masks, gowns, and protective eyewear) are required for at least 48 hours after antibiotics are initiated or sputum cultures are negative. All clinical specimens should be placed in doubly sealed containers. Prophylactic antibiotic therapy with seven days of oral doxycycline or oral ciprofloxacin should be considered for persons exposed to aerosols of *Y pestis* or patients with plague pneumonia.

SMALLPOX

Bioweapon potential

The World Health Organization declared smallpox eradicated in 1980. However, the Soviet Union manufactured weaponized smallpox during the Cold War, and some of this material may have been smuggled out of the country after the fall of the Communist regime. Routine immunization with vaccinia virus ended in 1972 in the United States and at similar times in other nations, leaving most of the world's current population susceptible to smallpox. Smallpox is highly contagious and frequently lethal. Variola major, the most common and virulent strain of smallpox, has an overall mortality of 25%.

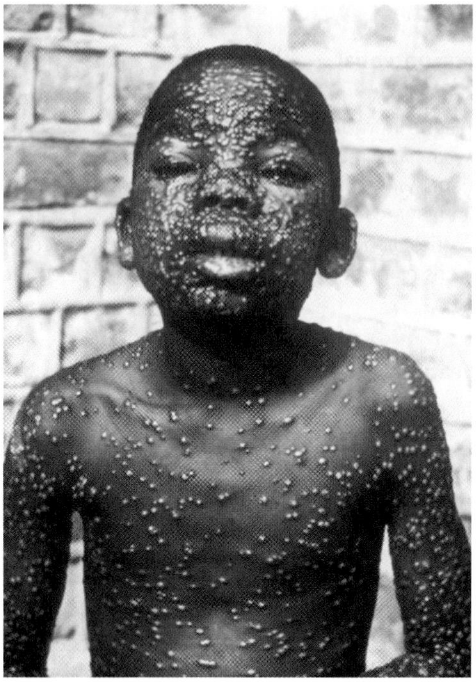

Figure 266-3 *Smallpox patient with pustular rash. Lesions are more dense on the face and extremities than the trunk, and all are in similar stages of development. (Public Health Image Library, Centers for Disease Control and Prevention.)*

Clinical features

Prodromal symptoms begin after an incubation period of 7–17 days. After two to four days of headache, malaise, fever, and body aches, a macular rash appears, usually starting in the mouth. The rash spreads to the face, moves rapidly to the arms and legs, and then the hands and feet. The entire body is usually involved within 24 hours (**Figure 266-3**). The fever may remit, and the patient feels somewhat better. The rash becomes papular by the third day. The papules then fill with a thick, opaque fluid, becoming round, firm, and raised pustules with a central depression. The fever may worsen. The pustules gradually crust over. By the end of the second week of the rash, most of the sores have scabbed over, and the fever has subsided. The scabs begin to fall off and heal to leave pitted scars. Most scabs will have fallen off three weeks after the rash appears.

Clinically, it is important to be able to differentiate the rash of smallpox from that of chicken pox, caused by varicella-zoster virus (**Table 266-1**). A large outbreak of monkeypox, which is related to smallpox, occurred in the United States in 2003 following the importation of infected animals. Clinically, monkeypox is very similar to smallpox, except that marked lymphadenopathy is more common in monkeypox.

Variola major has a hemorrhagic variant with a mortality rate of 90%. It evolves rapidly, with an average time from prodromal symptoms to death being six days. As a result, the first patients presenting after a bioterrorist attack may have hemorrhagic smallpox, which may easily be misdiagnosed as meningococcemia or other illnesses. Hemorrhagic smallpox is more common in pregnant women than in other patients.

TABLE 266-1 Differences Between Rashes of Smallpox and Chicken Pox (Varicella)*

Smallpox (Variola)	Chicken Pox (Varicella)
Pox lesions are all in the same stage	Pox lesions are in several different stages
Slow development	Rapid development
More pox on arms and legs	More pox on trunk
Pox are often present on palms and soles	Pox are usually absent from palms and soles

*Early hemorrhagic smallpox and flat smallpox, each of which has a very high mortality rate, have different rashes.

Treatment

There is currently no antiviral agent approved for the management of smallpox. Treatment is supportive.

Infection control and prevention

Smallpox is spread by large respiratory droplets and less efficiently by contact with sloughed skin matter. While smallpox is contagious during the prodrome, it is most infectious immediately after the rash develops. Patients are contagious until all of the scabs are gone. Hospitalized patients should be cared for in negative pressure rooms by vaccinated providers wearing gowns, gloves, and N95 respirators. In a large outbreak, home care and quarantine should be strongly considered for less ill patients, as the supply of negative pressure rooms is likely to be inadequate.

Vaccination with vaccinia virus within 96 hours of exposure to the index case, or to the point of aerosol attack, is part of a concerted public health response to a smallpox outbreak. Vaccinia is a live virus, with occasional major side effects, including myopericarditis, eczema vaccinatum, and disseminated infection. However, for those exposed to smallpox, there are no absolute contraindications to vaccination. Complications of vaccination can often be managed with vaccinia immune globulin.

VIRAL HEMORRHAGIC FEVERS

Bioweapon potential

The viruses that cause hemorrhagic fever in humans include filoviruses (Ebola virus and Marburg virus), arenaviruses (Lassa virus, Junin virus, and Machupo virus), bunyaviruses (Crimean-Congo hemorrhagic fever, Rift Valley fever virus, Hantaan virus, Seoul virus), and others. Some have exceptionally high mortality rates and are efficiently transmitted from person to person, especially Ebola, Marburg, and Crimean-Congo hemorrhagic fever virus.

Clinical features

These RNA viruses, while biologically diverse and having different animal or arthropod reservoirs, share important clinical manifestations. These include nonspecific signs and symptoms such as fever, malaise, muscle aches, pharyngitis, and rash, as well as increased vascular permeability, disseminated intravascular coagulation, and shock.

Patients who have returned from endemic areas with an illness compatible with viral hemorrhagic fever (VHF) should be assessed for other illnesses that may have overlapping symptoms, such as malaria, meningococcemia, and rickettsial disease.

Treatment

Specific therapy with ribavirin is available for the arenaviruses. Convalescent serum may also be efficacious for arenavirus infection. For the other VHF agents, therapy is supportive.

Infection control and prevention

Isolation precautions for suspected VHF include barrier precautions and isolation in negative pressure rooms. High-efficiency particulate air (HEPA) filter masks should be used in patients with respiratory or gastrointestinal symptoms. Blood draws should be minimized when VHF is highly suspected, and all specimens should be double bagged. Patients with suspected VHF should not be transferred from one hospital to another. Autopsies should only be performed with maximal protection, and prompt cremation of cadavers is recommended.

CONCLUSION

Hospitalists and emergency physicians may be the first to encounter bioterrorism and should be ready to respond appropriately. This chapter reviews the clinical presentation, treatment, infection control and prevention of infectious etiologies that the CDC considers of greatest concern because of ease of dissemination or person-to-person transmission and high mortality rates.

SUGGESTED READINGS

Bartlett JG. Mobilizing professional communities. *Public Health Rep.* 2001;116(suppl 2):40–44.

Centers for Disease Control and Prevention. Bioterrorism agents/diseases. HYPERLINK /exchweb/bin/redir.asp?URL=http://emergency.cdc.gov/agent/agentlist-category.asp (accessed July 19, 2011).

Lutwick LI, Lutwick SM (eds.). *Beyond anthrax: The weaponization of infectious diseases*. New York, NY: Humana Press; 2009.

Shapiro DS, Sharp SE. Sentinel laboratory guidelines for suspected agents of bioterrorism: clinical laboratory bioterrorism readiness plan. American Society for Microbiology. 2006; Available at http://www.asm.org/ASM/files/LeftMarginHeaderList/DOWNLOADFILENAME/000000001206/BTtemplateRevised 8-10-6.doc.

CHAPTER 267

Combat Stress and Related Disorders

Harold Kudler, MD

Key Clinical Questions

1. Why should we care about combat stress and related disorders?
2. How do you define cultural competence regarding military service members, veterans, and their families?
3. What are the medical problems associated with military service and deployment stress?
4. How would you describe point-of-care strategies to improve the care of military service members, veterans, and their families?
5. What resources are available to provide information, support, and access needed by military service members, veterans, and those who care for them and about them?

INTRODUCTION

An estimated 2.2 million American military members have served in Operation Enduring Freedom (OEF) in Afghanistan and/or Operation Iraqi Freedom (OIF) since the first of these wars began in 2001. As of November 2006, these two conflicts have exceeded the duration of World War II. The attention rightfully paid to OEF in Afghanistan and/or OIF war fighters should also alert the public that there are 23.4 million living American veterans, three-quarters of whom served during an official period of conflict. Approximately one in every four Americans is eligible for benefits from the United States Department of Veterans Affairs (VA) because they are either veterans or the dependents of veterans. Yet only one in four veterans is enrolled for VA health services. The remaining 75% of veterans and all their dependents receive health care outside of VA.

The composition of those currently serving is described:

- 12% of those serving in a combat area of operations are women.
- 58% of the military forces are 29 years of age or younger.
- 63% are active duty (AD) component members, and 37% are the Reserve component (RC) including Reservists and National Guard Members.

AD component members have the support of a strong military community due to their serving a continuous "hitch" on a military base. The RC "Citizen Soldiers," however, move back and forth between military and veteran status. They may live hundreds of miles from the nearest military community and thousands of miles from the troops with whom they are deployed. Spouses may be the only person in their workplace who has had a wife or husband deployed in the military. Their children may be the only ones in their school to have a parent serving overseas.

The nature of our volunteer military requires multiple deployments per member. Each time a military member deploys, the individual's risk of developing a postdeployment mental health problem increases. When a service member deploys, a family serves too. As yet, there has been little research on how the health of military family members may be affected in the course of the deployment cycle.

At the time of this writing, there are still two dependents of American Civil War Veterans receiving VA benefits. Going to war is a very long-term investment. Yet, despite the large number of veterans and their dependents and an enduring obligation to serve those who have served our country, few health care providers routinely enquire about military history or about the effects of deployment on military families. Providers are often ill prepared to recognize or treat health problems associated with military service and/or deployment stress. This chapter will focus on postdeployment mental health and articulate a public health approach that requires the development of Department of Defense (DoD)/VA/state and community partnerships in service to military service members/veterans and their families.

SCOPE OF THE ISSUE

A November 2007 study from the Walter Reed Army Institute of Research followed 88,235 U.S. Soldiers returning from Iraq. Each soldier completed both a Post-Deployment Health Assessment (PDHA) and then, an average of six months later, completed a Post-Deployment Health Reassessment (PDHRA). These global health screening tools include standard screens for posttraumatic stress disorder (PTSD), major depression, alcohol abuse, and traumatic brain injury (TBI).

While the Milliken study contained the good news that about half of those who reported significant PTSD symptoms upon arrival home had improved at the six month mark, the bad news was that *twice* as many *new* Soldiers screened positive for PTSD at that six month follow-up. During those first six months postdeployment, the depression rate doubled among the AD component and tripled among the RC. The self-report rate for alcohol abuse was 12% for the AD and 15% for the RC; yet only 0.2% of those who screened positive were referred for treatment (likely because they had the option of not being referred and feared the impact of referral upon their military careers). Respondents also reported a fourfold increase in concern about losing control of their anger.

Overall, 20.3% of the AD component and 42.4% of the RC were identified as requiring further mental health assessment and/or treatment by the six month mark. Little is known about the health status of their family members and significant others.

The health burden of returning service members and their families is by no means confined to mental health issues. Consideration of the full health impact of service in OEF/OIF is well beyond the scope of this chapter but it should be noted that a 2009 study by Cohen and colleagues found that veterans with mental disorders had 42% to 146% greater utilization in VA nonmental health settings than those without a mental disorder. Those with PTSD had the highest utilization in all categories. Female gender and lower rank were also independently associated with greater health care utilization. Comparison data is not available for non-VA settings but these findings strongly support the importance of screening for military history as a routine component of medical intake within all health care systems.

MILITARY CULTURE

Medical providers are increasingly sensitive to the importance of cultural competence, but few recognize that the military is a unique culture in itself. The clinician's understanding of military life, the deployment cycle, and the stresses of living and working in a war zone are critical to establishing credibility with patients who are either military members, veterans, or their significant others. Being in the military or in a military family is not like any other kind of life. There is strong support within a well-defined, coherent social system, but there is also little privacy. Military families may truly get to "see the world," but they rarely have much choice about where they will live or for how long. Above all, military life is defined and structured by a high standard of discipline. Few outside of the armed services understand that military culture is primarily rooted in a professional ethos of loyalty and self-sacrifice. This is necessary to maintain order during battle.

A distinct set of military ceremony and etiquette reinforces shared rituals and common identities. An enduring emphasis on group cohesion and esprit de corps connects service members to one another. Above all, military members and their families understand that the mission must come first. As a corollary to this, nonmilitary clinicians need to understand that the purpose of military medicine is to preserve the fighting force. This is distinctly different than the goal of providing patient- and family-centered care.

Military customs and concerns can generate tension in the doctor-patient relationship when military members and their dependents are seen in nonmilitary health care settings. Patients and their family members may hesitate to report postdeployment health problems because of concern that what they say may get back to the commanding officer. While such breach of medical privacy is unlikely, even in military health care settings, confidentiality is a serious concern among military members and their families that should be addressed openly and early. The stigma associated with mental health problems may be the single greatest barrier to accurate assessment and timely care of deployment-related health concerns.

It is not necessary for a clinician to become an expert on military history or military life in order to achieve the cultural competency needed to be effective in working with this population, but it is critically important to remain aware and respectful of the military way of life. For example, calling a Marine a Soldier may convince that Marine that you have no interest in either him personally or the Corps. What might feel like a small slip may be taken as a clear sign that "My doctor doesn't get it," after which important information may be left unsaid.

Clinicians who understand the nature of military training and deployment will routinely enquire about exposure to head trauma, travel-related disease, and physical or psychological trauma. Providers must be willing to ask questions and show interest when specific places or military events "pop up" in a conversation or when military "lingo" is suddenly injected. Veterans often drop such clues to see if their provider "gets it" before sharing their military experiences. It is unfortunate that some medical professionals are hesitant to ask about terms outside their own expertise. Genuine, expressed interest in the patient's military experiences is essential if the necessary bridges of trust and respect are to be built.

MENTAL HEALTH FINDINGS AMONG THE NEWEST GENERATION OF COMBAT VETERANS

As of this writing, more than 1.2 million OEF/OIF veterans are eligible for VA health care services. Although only about 23% of American veterans receive their health care through the VA, an impressive 50% of all OEF/OIF veterans eligible to use VA have already presented for at least one episode of care. Because the VA has a national electronic database, it is possible to draw some conclusions about the health issues of the 625,384 veterans. Large as this help-seeking sample is, this information cannot be reliably extrapolated to those OEF/OIF veterans who have not sought health care or who are seeking it in the community.

VA records show that the three most common health issues among OEF/OIF veterans are, in descending order, musculoskeletal, mental health, and "symptoms, signs, and ill-defined conditions." The most common musculoskeletal injuries are knee and back problems rather than the grievous injuries seen in news coverage from the war zone or military treatment facilities. Only 3% of all OEF/OIF veterans return home by way of the medical evacuation system and the remainder comes home at the appointed time with less obvious injuries. Rather than expect to *treat the war as seen on television*, it is important to realize that most combat veterans who come to your office will look pretty much like anyone else. This makes it all the more important to routinely take a military history.

Although the Gulf War Syndrome, which appeared among those who served in the early 1990s, is still under careful study, there is no evidence of a particular Gulf War Syndrome among those serving in OEF or OIF. Veterans and their family members will, however, often express concern about possible long-term health risks that might arise from health risks indigenous to the combat area or related to inoculations or toxic exposures that may have occurred during deployment. Such concerns should be respected, discussed, recorded, and evaluated. While clear answers may not always be available, sincere listening and appropriate documentation will strengthen the bond between patient and provider.

More than 50% of OEF/OIF veterans who have presented to VA have received at least one provisional diagnosis of a mental health disorder (**Table 267-1**). The most frequent among these is PTSD, which has been diagnosed in 27% of those who have presented to VA. Many clinicians, patients, and family members think of PTSD as the final common denominator in deployment-related mental health, but more OEF/OIF veterans have been diagnosed with a

TABLE 267-1 Possible Mental Health Diagnoses among 625,384 Eligible OEF/OIF Veterans who Presented to VA as of September 2010

• Provisional MH diagnoses include:	
▪ PTSD: (27% of all who presented to VA)	167,295
▪ Depressive disorder:	122,175
▪ Affective psychoses	72,972
▪ Neurotic disorders:	102,767
▪ Nondependent abuse of drugs: (Plus 85,671 with a tobacco use disorder)	27,714
▪ Alcohol dependence:	33,660

mood disorder than they have with PTSD. Note that the number with other anxiety disorders (including panic disorder and generalized anxiety disorder) is not far behind. The high rate of nondependent abuse of drugs and tobacco use disorder may be a marker for severe stress and/or psychological trauma. The take-home message is that postdeployment mental health is not just about PTSD and that a significant number of people who have PTSD may have one or more comorbid mental health problems.

Family members and significant others are also under significant stress in the course of the deployment cycle. When they present to their health providers, they may report new medical problems or exacerbation of old problems that express that stress. Family members frequently report depression, lack of sleep, irritability, concentration problems, and substance abuse problems. Clinicians should be aware of age-specific presentation of stress among military children. Toddlers may regress from previous developmental achievements and present with enuresis or encopresis. Food allergies, asthma, or digestive difficulties may flair. School-aged children may develop new-onset academic difficulties that may be taken for a learning or behavioral disorder or attention deficit. Teenagers may become withdrawn, oppositional, and promiscuous and/or abuse substances.

Different problems may surface at different points in the deployment cycle. During predeployment, each family member may respond in his or her own way to hearing that the service member has orders to deploy. Memories about problems during past deployments may stir new worries. The common, protracted training prior to actual service in the Gulf further extends the separation and places additional stress on the entire family. During deployment, families often complain of having too little contact with consequent worry about the service member's safety. On the other hand, the availability of instantaneous communication via telephone and e-mail sometimes ignites anxieties and arguments that can be more troubling to everyone involved than the events of daily life in a combat zone. After the service member returns home, he or she may experience problems that concern everyone in the family. Even when they fail to meet criteria for a formal diagnosis, problems with concentration, irritability, inability to sleep, emotional withdrawal, chronic pain, or substance abuse may have a powerful impact on all involved. Clinicians need to understand that deployment-related stress may propagate to disrupt the entire web of family life.

Deployment-related problems may be more functional than clinical, but even so, it is important for clinicians to inquire about them. They can include frequent arguments, separation, child abuse or neglect, trouble at work, unemployment, financial stress/bankruptcy, legal problems, incarceration, and ultimately, homelessness. As the saying goes, "If you don't take the temperature, you can't find the fever."

Ideally, all postdeployment health problems would be picked up somewhere within the continuum of DoD and VA care, but if only 50% of all OEF/OIF veterans eligible for VA care have come for that care, *where are the other 50%?* Clearly, many of OEF/OIF veterans do not come to VA. Some among them may not seek help at all. Still others will be seen in public or private settings.

It is possible that the 50% of OEF/OIF veterans who have not presented for VA care are, in fact, doing just fine and do not need medical attention. On the other hand, findings from the 1990 National Vietnam Veterans Readjustment Study (NVVRS) raise concerns about the silent majority. NVVRS documented that only 20% of Vietnam veterans who actually *had* a confirmed diagnosis of PTSD had *ever* sought VA mental health care. Further, those researchers found that 62% of all Vietnam veterans with PTSD *had* received mental health care at some point after the deployment. In other words, over two-thirds of Vietnam veterans with PTSD chose to seek mental health care *outside* of the VA. These findings strongly suggest that many OEF/OIF veterans might seek mental health services outside of the VA. Family members must, of necessity, seek help outside of VA even if their health issues are also related to deployment stress. The question is: Are public and private sector providers prepared to diagnose and treat postdeployment health problems among OEF/OIF veterans and their families?

SPECIFIC MENTAL HEALTH ISSUES AMONG COMBAT VETERANS

PTSD

While a full discussion of postdeployment mental health problems and their treatment is beyond the scope of this chapter, certain issues deserve mention. Chief among these is the importance of screening for PTSD and traumatic brain injury (TBI) among combat veterans encountered in practice. As mentioned, 27% of all OEF/OIF veterans who have presented for VA health care have been diagnosed with PTSD. A 2008 Rand Corporation report estimated a 19% incidence of TBI among OEF/OIF veterans. The Rand investigators also found that 57% of veterans diagnosed with a TBI in the course of the study had not previously been assessed for TBI by a physician. These findings indicate that clinicians should screen for PTSD, major depression, TBI, and substance abuse among veterans.

Validated screening tools for PTSD and TBI are readily available and in the public domain. Refer to **Table 267-2** for the Primary Care PTSD Screen (PC-PTSD). Developed by VA's National Center for PTSD, the PC-PTSD has been validated to screen for PTSD in

TABLE 267-2 The Primary Care PTSD Screen (PC-PTSD)

In your life, have you ever had any experience that was so frightening, horrible, or upsetting that, in the past month, you:

1. Have had nightmares about it or thought about it when you did not want to?

   (YES/NO)

2. Tried hard not to think about it or went out of your way to avoid situations that reminded you of it?

   YES/NO

3. Were constantly on guard, watchful, or easily startled?

   YES/NO

4. Felt numb or detached from others, activities, or your surroundings?

   YES/NO

Current research suggests that the results of the PC-PTSD should be considered "positive" if a patient answers "yes" to any three items.

primary care settings. Note that while the threshold has been set at three positive responses in military and VA settings, a cut-off of two positive answers may be more appropriate in civilian settings where the prevalence of PTSD is likely to be lower. The PC-PTSD can be incorporated into a self-assessment battery or it can be administered by a clinical team member.

A positive screen is not a diagnosis and should be followed up with a validated diagnostic tool and a clinical interview. The 17-item PTSD Checklist (PCL), another product of the VA National Center for PTSD that is in the public domain, measures the presence and intensity of each diagnostic criterion for PTSD. Self-administered or read to a patient, the PCL can be used to validate the diagnosis and measure treatment response, symptom by symptom, over time. The PCL can be obtained at the Web site for the VA/DoD Clinical Practice Guideline for the Management of Traumatic Stress (http://www.healthquality.va.gov/ptsd/ptsd_full.pdf). The PCL-C (or civilian version) is recommended in the VA Guidelines because it may be used in considering traumatic events that may have occurred before, during, or after deployment. Note that in applying the PCL, it is important to be sure that you and the patient are both referring to the same traumatic event(s).

TBI

Moderate or severe traumatic brain injuries (20%) will be obvious to clinicians, but mild traumatic brain injuries (mTBIs) may be more difficult to recognize and assess. The injury may involve closed head trauma, axonal shearing, intracranial bleeding, and/or penetrating fragments. Many clinicians have been trained to believe that anyone who has endured a TBI, even mTBI, must have experienced at least a momentary loss of consciousness, but current thinking is that some will simply feel dazed, see stars, or otherwise report having felt stunned and confused.

Patients with mTBI often report a history of headache, dizziness/balance problems, insomnia, impaired memory, ringing in the ears or hearing loss, and/or decreased tolerance for noise and light. Most people suffering from mTBI return to their previous level of function within three to six months, and it is important to reassure patients and their family members about this. On the other hand, 10% to 25% of patients will go on to develop chronic postconcussive symptoms. These enduring problems may be grouped into three categories: *somatic* (headache, tinnitus, insomnia, etc.), *cognitive* (memory, attention and concentration difficulties), and *emotional/behavioral* (irritability, depression, anxiety, behavioral dyscontrol) (**Table 267-3**).

Patients with mTBI may be at increased risk for PTSD, major depression, and/or Substance Use Disorder (SUD). There is considerable diagnostic overlap between mTBI and PTSD, and it is sometimes difficult to determine if a given patient has one, the other, or both.

The Defense and Veterans Brain Injury Center (DVBIC), the primary TBI program of the U.S. Defense Centers of Excellence, has developed and validated a three-question screening tool for mTBI that is available at http://dvbic.gbkdev.com/images/pdfs/3-Question-Screening-Tool.aspx and in the public domain. The three-question DVBIC TBI screening tool, also known as The Brief Traumatic Brain Injury Screen (BTBIS), can be self-administered or reviewed with a staff member. Screening is recommended for service members/veterans who were injured during combat operations, training missions, or other activities. Endorsement of at least one item within each of the three questions indicates a positive screen but diagnosis can only be based on a more thorough diagnostic interview and appropriate physical examination.

Screening for PTSD, mTBI, or other postdeployment health problems is of limited value if it does not lead to more comprehensive assessment and evidence-based treatment. VA/DoD Clinical Practice Guidelines (CPGs) are available for the management of traumatic stress, major depressive disorder, substance use disorder,

TABLE 267-3 Three-question Defense and Veterans Bran Injury Center Traumatic Brain Injury Screening Tool

1. Did you have any injury(ies) during your deployment from any of the following?

(check all that apply):

A. Fragment
B. Bullet
C. Vehicular (any type of vehicle, including airplane)
D. Fall
E. Blast (improvised explosive device, Rocket-Propelled Grenade (RPG), land mine, grenade, etc)
F. Other specify: ______

2. Did any injury received while you were deployed result in any of the following?

(check all that apply):

A. Being dazed, confused, or "seeing stars"
B. Not remembering the injury
C. Losing consciousness (knocked out) for less than a minute
D. Losing consciousness for 1–20 minutes
E. Losing consciousness for longer than 20 minutes
F. Having any symptoms of concussion afterward (such as headache, dizziness, irritability, etc)
G. Head injury
H. None of the above

3. Are you currently experiencing any of the following problems that you think might be related to a possible head injury or concussion?

(check all that apply):

A. Headaches	E. Ringing in the ears
B. Dizziness	F. Irritability
C. Memory problems	G. Sleep problems
D. Balance problems	H. Other specify: ______

NOTE: Confirm F and G through clinical interview.

NOTE: Endorsement of A–E meets criteria for positive TBI Screen.

RPG, rocket-propelled grenade.

postdeployment health and medically unexplained symptoms. Each can be accessed at http://www.healthquality.va.gov and all are in the public domain. A VA/DoD CPG on traumatic brain injury is available at that same site. Each VA/DoD CPG can be downloaded as a PDF or for use on a personal computer or personal digital assistant (PDA).

Clinical practice guidelines are designed to improve clinical outcomes and/or reduce inappropriate variations in care. They are not, however, meant to constrain clinical judgment. VA/DoD CPGs are educational tools expressed as clinical algorithms that present a full range of options and assist in decision making. They are evidence-based, but when no applicable research is available, offer expert consensus recommendations.

The basis for each recommendation is provided along with an explicit grading of its strength of evidence. While CPGs for PTSD are also available through the American Psychiatric Association and other organizations, the VA/DoD CPG may be particularly helpful because it was developed by and for a multidisciplinary group of providers for use across a broad range of clinical settings. Practice guidelines from the International Society for Traumatic Stress Studies (ISTSS), published as *Effective Treatments for PTSD* (Foa, Keane, Friedman & Cohen, 2008), are recommended because of their multidisciplinary nature and their detailed discussions of PTSD assessment and treatment. The comprehensive ISTSS guidelines provide a useful complement to the more schematized VA/DoD CPG. The VA/DoD CPG can be applied in real time in the office. The ISTSS guidelines can be studied afterward for greater depth and broader perspective.

THE HOSPITALIST'S ROLE IN A PUBLIC HEALTH RESPONSE TO POSTDEPLOYMENT MENTAL HEALTH ISSUES

At a March 2005 DoD/VA conference on deployment mental health in Alexandria, Virginia, then-Navy Surgeon General Richard Carmona observed that "... *most* war fighters *will not* develop a diagnosable mental illness but *all* war fighters and their families *will* face important readjustment issues in the course of the deployment cycle." Rather than attempting to sort OEF/OIF veterans and their families into oversimplified categories of either "sick" or "well," Admiral Carmona's insight requires clinicians to adopt a population-based *public health approach* focused on helping individuals and families retain or, when necessary, regain a healthy balance despite the stress of deployment.

The public health approach requires a progressively engaging, phase-appropriate integration of services. This program must be driven by the needs of the service member/veteran and his/her family rather than by the often bureaucratic structures of traditional systems of care. It must meet prospective users where they live rather than wait for them to find their way to the right mix of services. It should increase access and reduce stigma for all members of the military, veterans, and their family members.

Hospitalists can help build an effective public health system for OEF/OIF veterans and their families when they take time to find out who among their patients has served in the military or has "kept the home fires burning" for a deployed service member. Rather than reduce their patients to one or more diagnoses, hospitalists should step back to see their patients as members of a unique culture who are coping with the stress of deployment as best they can. They should realize that Guard and Reserve members may officially be veterans right now, but may still deploy again. This can create new strain for the service member and family. Evidence-based psychotherapy and psychopharmacologic interventions as laid out in clinical practice guidelines have great efficacy, but what is essential in the care of these patients is that the clinician understands deployment stress in human terms.

Hospitalists must also make sure that such patients are not allowed to fall between the cracks as they transition between DoD, VA, public, and private systems of care. They should, whenever possible, promote DoD/VA/state and community partnerships in support of service members/veterans and their families. Refer to **Table 267-4** for resources.

TABLE 267-4 Resources

A number of important resources can provide the glue that holds such partnerships together:

- *VA OEF/OIF Program Managers*: Each of the nation's 153 VA Medical Centers has an OEF/OIF program manager (usually a social worker or nurse) dedicated to helping veterans and their family members understand and connect with the benefits and services available to them. OEF/OIF program managers will literally walk a veteran through the VA system and ensure a smooth transfer to appropriate care. They will also help veterans smoothly transition between DoD/VA and or private and public medical programs. They should be part of the discharge plan for any OEF/OIF veteran. To contact the nearest OEF/OIF care manager, check your local VA medical center Web site. You can find that Web site by using the VA facility locator that can be found at http://www2.va.gov/directory/guide/home.asp?isflash=1.
- *Vet Centers:* VA has established 278 Vet Centers in towns and cities across America. Vet Centers are primarily staffed by mental health professionals who are, themselves, veterans. They provide readjustment counseling and outreach services to all veterans who served in any combat zone. They also provide services for family members for military-related issues including bereavement counseling. Veterans need not be enrolled in VA health care to use Vet Center services and there is never a charge to the veteran or the family. A Vet Center locator is available at http://www2.va.gov/directory/guide/vetcenter_flsh.asp.
- *Military OneSource*: A 24/7 Web site (http://www.militaryonesource.com) and telephone-based resource (1-800-342-9647), Military OneSource is an employee assistance program available to all service members and their families. Help can be provided in a variety of areas ranging from how to connect with appropriate clinical services to how to balance a checkbook. Military OneSource provides up to 12 sessions of free face-to-face counseling per family member per problem and can help providers access needed resources for their patients including housing and legal assistance.
- *The National Resource Directory*: This online tool for wounded, ill, and injured service members, veterans, their families, and those who support them (http://www.nationalresourcedirectory.gov) provides access to more than 11,000 services and resources at national, state, and local levels that support recovery, rehabilitation, and community reintegration. Maintained by the Departments of Defense, Labor, and Veterans Affairs, the National Resource Directory links to federal and state government agencies, veteran service and benefit organizations, nonprofit and community-based organizations, academic institutions, and professional associations in order to provide assistance to wounded warriors and their families.
- *Sesame Workshop Talk, Listen, Connect*: Sesame Workshop, the corporation behind Sesame Street, developed its Talk, Listen, Connect (TLC) series in support of military children and their families. Videos and information, available at http://www.sesameworkshop.org/initiatives/emotion/tlc, were developed by a multidisciplinary team of experts, writers, and performers to guide families through multiple challenges including deployment, homecoming, and changes that occur when a parent comes home. TLC provides advice from military families about how to deal with long separations and with visible or invisible injuries. Free kits containing DVDs and program guides for parents and professionals can be ordered at the TLC Web site.
- *Treating the Invisible Wounds of War*: This free, accredited, on-line training for health professionals, available at http://www.aheconnect.com/citizensoldier was jointly developed by the Citizen Soldier Support Program (a federally funded program based at the University of North Carolina at Chapel Hill's Odum Institute for Research in Social Science, which seeks to improve access to services for Reserve Component combat veterans and their families), VA's Veterans Integrated Service Network 6 Mental Illness Research Education and Clinical Center (which focuses on postdeployment mental illness), and the North Carolina Area Health Education Centers (AHEC) Program. It is an online tutorial that addresses the training needs of a wide range of medical and behavioral health providers with respect to OEF/OIF veterans and their families. Of particular value is the included "boots on the ground" interview with a military couple that brings home the day-to-day realities of the deployment cycle and its profound and varied effects on family life.
- Defense and Veterans Brain Injury Center Web site: http://www.dvbic.org/
- VA National Center for PTSD Web site: http://www.ptsd.va.gov.

CONCLUSION

Hospitalists have an opportunity to enhance identification of and outreach to OEF/OIF veterans, their families, increase the rate of appropriate referral, smooth transitions in care, reduce the stigma currently associated with these problems, promote healthy outcomes and greater resilience, and strengthen families and communities. In the process, they can help reduce military attrition and chronic disability. The goal here is not merely to improve postdeployment care, but to transform it into a rational system in which there is *no wrong door* to which OEF/OIF veterans or their families can come for genuine understanding and effective help.

SUGGESTED READINGS

Cohen BE, Gima K, Bertenthal D, Kim S, Marmar CR, Seal KH. Mental Health Diagnoses and Utilization of VA Non-Mental Health Medical Services Among Returning Iraq and Afghanistan Veterans. *J Gen Intern Med.* 2010;25(1):18–24.

Foa E, Keane TM, Friedman MJ, Cohen, JA. (eds). *Effective Treatments For PTSD: Practice Guidelines from the International Society for Traumatic Stress Studies. Second Edition.* New York, NY: Guilford Publications, Inc.; 2008.

Kulka RA, Schlenger WE, Fairbank JA, Hough RL, Jordan BK, Marmar CR, et al. *The National Vietnam Veterans Readjustment Study: Tables of findings and technical appendices.* Vol. 1. New York, NY: Brunner/Mazel; 1990.

Milliken CS, Auchterlonie JL, Hoge, CW. Longitudinal Assessment of mental health problems among Active and Reserve Component Soldiers returning from the Iraq war. *JAMA.* 2007;298 (18):2141–2148.

Schwab KA, Baker G, Ivins B, Sluss-Tiller M, Lux W, Warden D. The Brief Traumatic Brain Injury Screen (BTBIS): Investigating the validity of a self-report instrument for detecting traumatic brain injury (TBI) in troops returning from deployment in Afghanistan and Iraq. *Neurology.* 2006;66(5)(supp. 2):A235.

Tanelian T, Jaycox LH. Invisible Wounds of War: Psychological and Cognitive Injuries, Their Consequences, and Services to Assist Recovery. Santa Monica, CA: Rand Monographs; 2008.

U.S. Department of Veterans Affairs. Environmental Epidemiology Service. VA Web site. Available at: http://www.publichealth.va.gov/research/epidemiology/index.asp.

VA/DoD Clinical Practice Guidelines for the Management of Traumatic Stress. Available at: http://www.healthquality.va.gov/Post_Traumatic_Stress_Disorder_PTSD.asp.

CHAPTER 268

Blast-induced Traumatic Brain Injury and Polytrauma

Ricky Kue, MD, MPH, FACEP
Gabor D. Kelen, MD, FACEP, FAAEM, FRCP

Key Clinical Questions

1. How are blast-induced injuries classified?
2. What organ systems are typically affected in blast-induced polytrauma?
3. Are there strategies to predict which patient might experience delayed onset of primary blast injuries?
4. What are current management strategies for specific primary blast injuries?
5. How are blast-induced traumatic brain injuries classified?
6. How does blast-induced traumatic brain injury (TBI) differ from other types of traumatic brain injuries?
7. How can secondary insults to TBIs be avoided?
8. What are the current diagnostic and management strategies for mild, moderate, and severe TBI?

INTRODUCTION AND EPIDEMIOLOGY

The incidence of explosive blast injuries is on the rise. From 1996 to 2006, it is estimated that blast-related events have risen fourfold. Although there have been a number of explosive blast events worldwide, the actual number of mass casualty blast events occurring on United States soil have been relatively few. In 1995, a large explosive device composed of fuel oil and fertilizer was detonated in front of the Alfred P. Murrah Federal Building in Oklahoma, which resulted in 518 injuries and 168 deaths. More recently, the 2001 World Trade Center terrorist attack has resulted in more focus on homeland security and disaster preparation for these events. A civilian physician may have to respond to domestic terror events such as bombings in subways, trains, public gatherings, and nightclubs. The National Counterterrorism Center reported in 2007 that approximately 14,000 terrorist attacks have occurred worldwide, resulting in about 44,000 injuries and more than 22,000 deaths. This represented a 20% to 30% increase since 2006.

Operation Iraqi Freedom (OIF) and Operation Enduring Freedom (OEF) in Afghanistan have greatly increased our knowledge and experience in treating blast injuries. A recent study of the Joint Theater Trauma Registry (JTTR) revealed that explosive blasts accounted for almost 80% of all combat casualties from October 2001 through January 2005. The most common explosive weapon employed in OIE/OEF is the improvised explosive device (IED), which broadly describes any makeshift incendiary device constructed to injure, incapacitate, harass, or distract. Most IEDs utilize conventional military weapons (ie, artillery shells, plastic explosives, etc.) with various detonating triggers (ie, pressure plate, cellular phone, remote control) and are employed almost anywhere (ie, roadside, suicide bomber, vehicle-borne). Typical injuries seen from an IED blast have concentrated mainly on extremity and head injuries. This is likely due to advanced body armor systems currently used that afford good protection from blast injuries in the torso region.

PATHOPHYSIOLOGY

The complex physics of an explosive blast can result in a myriad of injuries on multiple victims. An explosion results in sudden and near instantaneous expansion of gas that results in a shockwave also known as a *blast wave*. As this blast wave travels, it begins to lose its pressure and velocity with distance and time (**Figure 268-1**). A blast wave is made of two components: a shockwave of high pressure, followed closely by a blast wind. Blast winds can be strong enough to propel people or objects, thus resulting in secondary injury. As the explosive shockwaves dissipate, a "negative-pressure" phase occurs as a result of the void created by dissipated air. These rapid pressure fluctuations have a destructive effect on the human body, particularly in organs at the air-tissue or air-fluid interface. These include organs such as the lungs and bowel. Two main types of energy are created by a blast that enter the body, specifically stress waves and shear waves. Stress waves are longitudinal pressure forces that result in a spalling effect occurring at air-tissue interfaces, whereas shearing waves are transverse pressure forces that result in movement along tissue planes and possible disruption along attachment sites.

Blast injuries are traditionally classified into four categories: primary, secondary, tertiary, and quaternary (**Table 268-1**). *Primary*

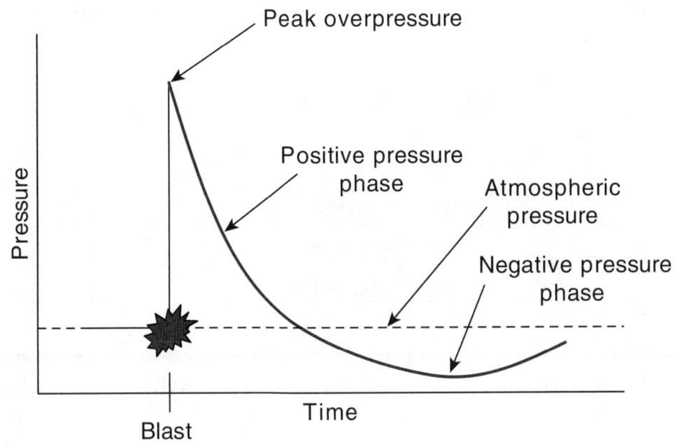

Figure 268-1 *Blast overpressure waveform.*

blast injuries occur as a result of the overpressure forces from the blast shockwave itself, thus representing true barotrauma to the body. Organs that are air-filled or contain air-fluid interfaces are typical of primary blast injuries. These include the lungs, ears, intestines, and colon. *Secondary* blast injuries are typically penetrating in nature and a result of ballistic trauma from fragments of the explosive device itself or other objects propelled into the body as a result of blast overpressure or blast winds. *Tertiary* blast injuries describe injuries sustained as a result of being thrown into stationary objects as a result of the peak overpressure or blast wind. It also includes injuries sustained from building or structural collapse, resulting in crush injuries. *Quaternary* blast injuries include all other forms of injury not falling into the first three classes, which include burns, toxic substance exposures, inhalation injuries, and radiation injuries. There is some debate over the use of a fifth classification known as *quinary* blast injuries, which are described mainly as having a hyperinflammatory state sometimes seen in blast patients developing sometime after initial insult. Some authors have attributed this to the exposure of bacteria or radiation material from a blast and thus at times classify these injuries as quaternary.

TABLE 268-1 Classification of Blast Injuries

Category	Definition	Example Injury
Primary	Injuries produced as a direct effect from blast wave and pressure changes	Rupture of tympanic membrane Pulmonary injury Rupture of hollow viscera
Secondary	Injuries from explosive fragments or other objects propelled by overpressure and blast winds	Penetrating trauma Traumatic amputations Lacerations Traumatic brain injuries
Tertiary	Injuries produced from being thrown into a stationary object or from collapse of buildings and structures	Blunt injuries Crush syndrome Compartment syndrome Traumatic brain injuries
Quaternary	Other explosion-related injuries, illnesses, or diseases	Burns Toxic gas and other inhalation injuries Exposure to hazardous materials, ionizing radiation, chemicals
"Quinary"	Delayed/remote hyperinflammatory state induced after an explosive blast or exposure to radiation or bacteria	Sepsis Multiorgan dysfunction or failure

Two important factors affect the magnitude of injury from an explosive blast. The first is the distance a person is from an explosion. The closer a person is to the explosion, the greater the blast overpressure is experienced. Individuals who are positioned further away from a blast will probably not experience the consequences of primary blast injuries due to the degradation of the pressure forces created by the blast over time. A second factor that amplifies the magnitude of a blast pressure is if detonation occurs within an enclosed space. The pressure forces generated from open-space detonations dissipate over unlimited space. In an enclosed space, however, the overpressure waves become amplified as they reflect off walls and solid surfaces, resulting in increased force. Immediate death from primary blast injuries (ie, blast lung) occurs more often with enclosed space blasts rather than open air blasts. This is supported from recent JTTR data (2004–2006) from OIF/OEF, which revealed the incidence of primary blast injuries at only 12.2%, of which 75% were tympanic membrane rupture. Blast overpressure was the cause of death in only 1.5% cases, which underscores the fact that IED blasts typically occur in open spaces and that most injuries and deaths are due to fragments.

DOES THIS PATIENT HAVE A BLAST-INDUCED TRAUMATIC BRAIN INJURY OR POLYTRAUMA?

TRAUMATIC BRAIN INJURY

Explosive blasts are a rare mechanism of traumatic brain injury (TBI) in the United States. Most TBIs occurring in the U.S. are a result of direct blunt-force trauma from falls and motor vehicle crashes. Data from the Centers for Disease Control and Prevention show an annual incidence of emergency department visits and hospital admissions for TBI to be 403 per 100,000 and 85 per 100,000 respectively. The cost for direct TBI medical care is estimated at more than $56 billion per year. Current operations in Iraq and Afghanistan have yielded significant experience in the understanding and management of blast-induced TBI. The incidence of head injuries has not substantially increased in these wars compared with others. A major difference, however, is the high survival of combat-injured soldiers including those injured from TBI, compared to previous wars. Much of this success has been attributed to advanced body armor systems. Conservative estimates for returning U.S. service members indicate that approximately 20% of the deployed force potentially suffered some form of TBI.

Traumatic brain injury has classically been categorized based on severity of symptoms: mild, moderate, and severe. Patients with *mild* TBI usually have a Glasgow Coma Scale at time of medical evaluation (GCS, **Table 268-2**) of 14 to 15 and experience brief if any loss of consciousness (LOC). Typical complaints include headaches, confusion, and amnesia. Mild TBI is frequently referred to as a "concussion" in lay-person terms. Following an acute period, most patients with mild TBI may continue to experience nonspecific symptoms such as headache, dizziness, anxiety, difficulty with concentration, depression, and insomnia lasting from a few weeks up to a year. This is known as the "postconcussive" syndrome. Patients with *moderate* TBI on initial medical evaluation will have a GCS of 9 to 13 and usually experience a longer period of unconsciousness.

Neurologic deficits become apparent with this level of TBI and typically warrant computed tomography studies as well as hospital

TABLE 268-2 Glasgow Coma Scale

Best Motor Response (M)		Best Verbal Response (V)		Best Eye Opening (E)	
Follows commands	6				
Localizes pain	5	Oriented, alert	5		
Withdraws from pain	4	Confused, appropriate	4	Opens eyes spontaneously	4
Flexor posturing	3	Disoriented, inappropriate	3	Opens eyes to voice	3
Extensor posturing	2	Incomprehensible sounds	2	Opens eyes to pain	2
No response	1	No response	1	No response	1

The Glasgow Coma Scale (GCS) is the summation of the patient's best response to motor commands, verbal answers to questions, and eye opening. A GCS score of 15 is considered "normal," whereas a GCS score of 3 is considered the lowest possible score.

admission for observation. These patients are more likely to have abnormalities found on neuroimaging studies and may require specialty consultation. Patients with *severe* TBI will have a GCS score of 8 or less and significant neurologic deficits on physical exam. These patients routinely have some abnormality present on neuro-imaging (ie, intracranial hemorrhage, skull fracture, cerebral edema, etc.) and require intubation for airway protection as well as admission to an intensive care unit for further monitoring and critical care. Mortality is closely tied to the severity of TBI with mild TBI patients having better outcomes and reduced mortality compared with severe TBI patients. Mortality for patients admitted with a presenting GCS < 13 is approximately 30%. This number rises to greater than 50% mortality for patients presenting with a GCS of 8 or less. Prognostic factors of poor TBI outcomes include age 65 and older, penetrating mechanism of injury, and bilaterally fixed pupils on initial presentation. The actual injury inflicted on the brain has been described in two distinct phases: *primary* and *secondary*, regardless of clinical severity. The primary injury is the result of the initial mechanical forces resulting in direct injury of brain parenchyma. The cerebral damage is most often completed by the time medical care can be completed and not amenable to treatment. Secondary injuries, however, refer to neuronal injury and death as a consequence of other physiologic derangements such as hypoxia and hypoperfusion. The injured brain is more susceptible to hypoxic-ischemic states due to its impaired cerebral vascular autoregulation. Studies have shown worse outcomes in severe TBI patients with even a single episode of hypotension (systolic blood pressure < 90 mm Hg). Thus, the goal of initial treatment intervention is to prevent secondary injury to an already injured brain.

PULMONARY INJURIES

The lungs are the organs that are second-most susceptible to primary blast injury. "Blast lung" is probably the most discussed and feared injury, given it is the most common fatal injury found in initial survivors of explosions. Typical pressures needed to injure visceral organs such as a lung or bowel are 40 to 75 psi above atmospheric pressure. Evidence of primary blast injuries to the lungs are present in 17% to 47% of those who die from explosions, and up to 44% of hospitalized patients and 71% of critically ill patients show evidence of pulmonary injury. Military studies from Joint Theater Trauma Registry (JTTR) data have shown that this entity has been a relatively uncommon cause of death in OIF/OEF and is more likely encountered in enclosed-space blast mechanisms. The pulmonary alveolar bed represents a significant size air-tissue interface that injures easily to the sudden pressure changes seen after an explosion. Cellular disruption, hemorrhage, and pulmonary contusions are common injuries sustained after a blast. Pulmonary barotrauma resulting in pneumothorax, hemothorax, hemopneumothorax, and pneumomediastinum is also seen in primary blast injuries.

The blast lung syndrome is classically described as the presence of dyspnea, hypoxia, and cough and represents impaired gas exchange due to vascular shunting with ventilation-perfusion mismatching. Hypoxia (room air oxygen saturations < 90%) typically reaches its nadir at 24 hours. The most common finding on chest radiograph is a bilateral central "bat-wing" or "butterfly" infiltrate similar to the one seen in patients with noncardiogenic pulmonary edema.

GASTROINTESTINAL INJURIES

Primary blast injury can occur to the gastrointestinal (GI) tract due to the many air-tissue interfaces throughout the small and large intestines. The incidence of gastrointestinal primary blast injuries is variable, with rates reported from as low as 0.3% in one series to as high as 24% in another. GI blast injuries occur more often after underwater blast injuries or in enclosed space explosions owing to heightened blast overpressure or prolonged positive-pressure phase experienced. The most common regions affected in the GI tract are at the colon and ileocecal region. Immediate intestinal perforations are the result of significant pressure forces, whereas delayed perforations result from edema and hemorrhage due to microthromboses and ischemia in the contused bowel wall.

Patients will complain of abdominal pain, nausea, vomiting, gastrointestinal bleeding, or frank peritoneal signs. Significant contusion and hemorrhage can result in hemodynamic instability typically warranting further investigation with computed tomography (CT). Imaging may reveal pneumoperitoneum, free fluid, or blood either intraabdominal or retroperitoneal as well as bowel wall thickening. The liberal use of serial focused abdominal sonography for trauma (FAST) should be considered to monitor the development of intraabdominal free fluid since its sensitivity increases with serial examinations.

AUDITORY INJURIES

The auditory system is considered the most susceptible organ to blast overpressure and thus the most common primary blast injury. As little as 5 psi of pressure above atmospheric pressure is all that is needed to injure the tympanic membrane. Recent studies coming out of the OIF/OEF experience have found that as many as 9% of blast-injured patients had tympanic membrane rupture. Other studies have published an incidence rate as high as 47%. Blast waves oriented perpendicular to the tympanic membranes will likely result in more damage than parallel blast waves. Factors that influence the severity of injury include the presence of an enclosed space blast, cerumen impaction within the auditory canals, as well as the use of hearing protection devices. Injury to the auditory symptoms will result in common auditory dysfunction symptoms such as tinnitus, hearing loss, pain, and dizziness.

Depending on the setting of the blast, as high as 94% of those with primary blast injuries will have tympanic membrane rupture. Asymptomatic patients with intact tympanic membranes have a low likelihood of occult pulmonary or gastrointestinal blast injuries. Some authors have suggested the presence of a ruptured tympanic membrane as a convenient predictor of serious primary blast injury; however studies from recent blast events suggest that survivors both with and without blast lung injuries had ruptured as well as intact tympanic membranes with one case series reporting a sensitivity of 29% for associated pulmonary blast injuries. Therefore, patients with signs or symptoms suggestive of pulmonary or gastrointestinal injury, regardless of tympanic membrane rupture after blast exposure, should prompt search for more serious injuries.

OCULAR INJURIES

The eyes represent an extremely delicate organ system highly susceptible to blast overpressures as well as projectile fragments. Some studies estimate as many as 10% of all blast survivors experience some type of eye injury. Any ocular complaints should be seriously considered and evaluated. Change in visual acuity, loss of vision, or severe ocular pain out of proportion to exam should warrant further investigation. Foreign bodies that typically cannot penetrate the skin can easily penetrate the globe. CT of the face and orbits should be considered in any patient with an ocular foreign body, evidence of entrapment, or significant facial fractures. Blast forces as well as other blunt force trauma may result in underlying facial fractures. Extraocular muscle entrapment may result in limited gaze or diplopia. Significant trauma may also result in retroorbital hemorrhage, which in turn produces a "compartment" syndrome–type process to the globe known as retrobulbar hematoma. This may result in permanent optic nerve and retinal damage. Signs include significant eye pain, changes in visual acuity, or proptosis.

SOFT-TISSUE INJURY

Extremity and musculoskeletal injuries can be seen with all classes of blast injuries. In current OIF/OEF operations, extremity trauma constitutes more than half of all combat trauma (54%) and likely represents the successful use of centrally located body armor and head protection. Soft tissue injuries as a result of explosive blasts are typically a result of crush or blunt-force trauma. Soft tissue injury as a result of blast overpressure represents a significant amount of blast force exposure and is typically fatal. Some laboratory studies investigating the likelihood of primary blast pressures as a mechanism for traumatic amputation have shown that these injuries are more likely attributed to significant fragment injury and are not explained by blast overpressure alone (**Figure 268-2**). The presence of significant soft tissue injury such as traumatic amputation should raise clinical suspicion for the presence of pulmonary, gastrointestinal, or central nervous system injuries as well (**Figure 268-3**).

TRIAGE AND HOSPITAL ADMISSION

Initial triage of blast injury patients typically involves management of a mass casualty incident, since it is infrequent to only encounter a single patient after an explosion. On-scene triage and casualty care is beyond the scope of this chapter and typically involves the use of an incident command system that prioritizes transport and treatment based on injury severity and likelihood of survival. Criteria for hospital admission will be based on severity of presentation and likelihood for delayed presentation of primary blast injuries based

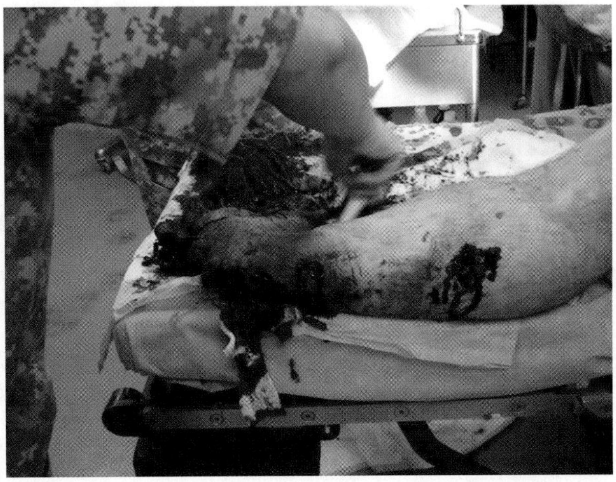

Figure 268-2 *Typical blast injuries sustained by U.S. soldiers after an IED blast. Note the significant amount of soft tissue damage and traumatic amputation of the foot. Other concurrent wounds suggest fragment damage as well as significant underlying skeletal injuries. (Courtesy of MAJ Ricky Kue, MD, MPH).*

on history. As noted earlier, otoscopic examination for tympanic membrane can be used to help risk stratify patients for the likelihood of blast injury. In the asymptomatic patient without clinical signs or symptoms to suggest injury, absence of tympanic membrane rupture may conditionally exclude the presence of other primary blast injuries. The presence of tympanic membrane rupture, however, should prompt the hospitalist to consider evaluating for the presence of other primary blast injuries in the setting of specific symptoms or prolonged observation for four to six hours for the development of delayed primary blast injuries even in the asymptomatic patient (**Figure 268-4**). Hospital admission should be based on history of mechanism, likelihood of subsequent injury (ie, enclosed space blast history, severity of injuries sustained by others nearby, type of explosive device employed), as well as presenting symptoms. Presence of signs and symptoms suggestive of organ

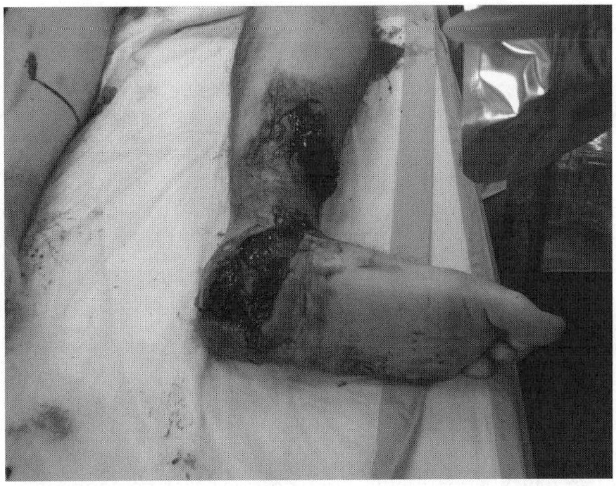

Figure 268-3 *Soft tissue blast injury sustained by a soldier while on a convoy struck by an IED. Note that there is significant soft-tissue swelling as well as fragment injuries. The IED blast wave was directed through the floor of the vehicle and into the soldier's legs. (Courtesy of MAJ Ricky Kue, MD, MPH).*

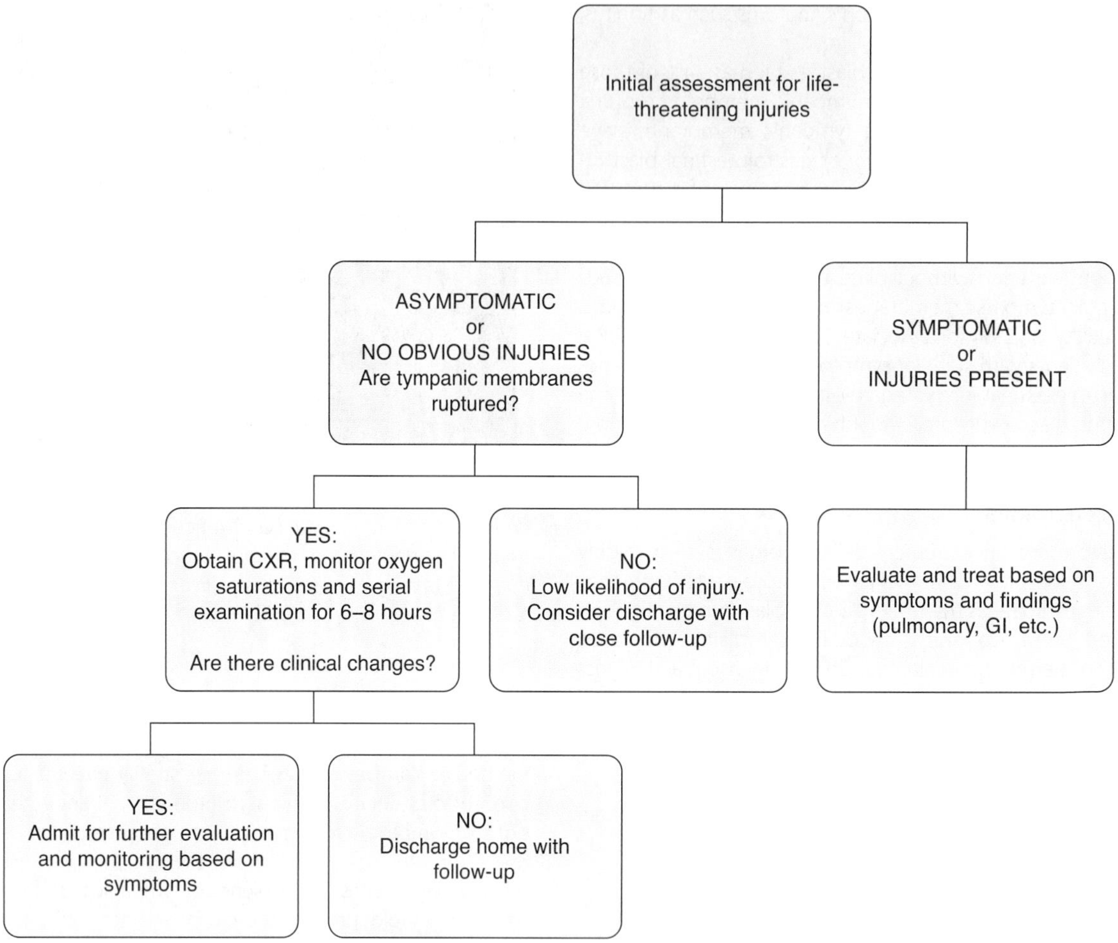

Figure 268-4 *Initial evaluation decision tree for primary blast injuries.*

injury such as hypoxia or tachypnea in pulmonary injury, or abdominal pain in gastrointestinal injury should warrant further investigation and admission for observation. Evidence of specific blast injuries should also trigger hospital admission, though most diagnosed blast injuries will typically require admission to an intensive care or trauma surgery setting.

TREATMENT OPTIONS

Provider safety is a general concept more applicable to the physician facing patients at the point of injury; however, it is more likely the hospitalist will encounter the patient in the safety of a medical care facility. The hospitalist should also be cognizant of other potential injuries from chemical or radiation exposure, if also present in the explosive device. Initial treatment priorities should concentrate on patient stabilization. Attention should be paid to the A-B-Cs of resuscitation: airway management, assuring adequate breathing, and supporting circulation. Most training courses provide a stepwise format to patient resuscitation using an A-B-C approach. Consider the American Heart Association Advanced Cardiac Life Support course as well as the American College of Surgeons Advanced Trauma Life Support courses. Recent experiences with blast injuries in OIF/OEF have supported a modified approach known as X-A-B-C, in which X represents stopping significant hemorrhage. This approach is quickly being adopted in the tactical and operational medicine environment since exanguinating hemorrhage has been a major factor in postblast mortality. During the A-B-C resuscitation, it is common to lose significant amounts of blood from an exanguinating wound sustained in a blast. Recent experiences in OIF/OEF have supported this approach, since most blast-injured patients die from their wounds and not airway loss. Bleeding should initially be controlled with direct pressure and elevation. The resurgence of tourniquet use is supported in the literature and can be used to control severe hemorrhage. Realistically, many of these treatment priorities will occur simultaneously when multiple providers are available. Specific management of critical injuries is beyond the scope of this chapter since many of these injuries will likely require surgical interventions and subsequent critical care monitoring.

Clinical management of blast-induced TBI starts with the prevention of secondary injuries by assuring adequate oxygenation, cerebral perfusion, and maintaining euglycemia. Due to the alteration in level of consciousness, most cases of moderate and severe TBI will require tracheal intubation to maintain airway patency and allow further evaluation. Oxygen saturation should be maintained at >90%. Hemodynamic status should be immediately addressed to maintain a systolic blood pressure of >90 mm Hg. It is unusual for moderate and severe TBI patients to present as hypotensive unless a concurrent source of blood loss is present. Patients with significant TBI will typically present with hypertension due to increased intracranial pressure (Cushing response). Paramount during the resuscitation phase is recognition of signs that suggest a surgical lesion amenable to immediate neurosurgical intervention. The goal is to rapidly relieve intracranial pressure and minimize further cerebral insult. Noncontrast head CT is an important part of diagnosing surgically amenable lesions. Indications for immediate neurosurgical consultation are listed in **Table 268-3**. The clinician should also consider the possibility of concurrent cervical

TABLE 268-3 Indications for Immediate Neurosurgical Consultation in Patients with Traumatic Brain Injury

Depressed skull fracture
Evidence of increased intracranial pressure
• Midline shift on CT
• Cerebral edema
Epidural hematoma
Subdural hematoma
Cerebral hemorrhage
Subarachnoid hemorrhage
Any penetrating trauma with breech of calvarium

spine injuries based on mechanism. Since patients with altered mental states cannot reliably be ruled out for cervical spine injuries based on history or physical exam. These patients should undergo concurrent cervical spine imaging concurrent with CT of the brain.

Patients with mild TBI only require thorough history and physical examinations based on symptoms. Symptoms such as headache, persistent nausea and vomiting, focal neurologic deficits, alteration in mental status or intoxication, posttraumatic seizures, or amnesia should trigger computed tomography of the brain. Cervical spine imaging should also be obtained if there is any posterior midline tenderness on palpation, focal neurologic deficits, other significant distracting injuries, alteration in consciousness or intoxication, or any limitations in range of motion. By definition, a significant alteration in mental status is incompatible with only mild TBI being present. Most of these patients will be discharged with close follow-up to monitor for any postconcussive symptoms.

Treatment of primary blast injuries will depend on location and clinical suspicion of the specific organ system involved. As mentioned earlier, the use of otoscopy alone as a screening exam lacks adequate sensitivity to rule out primary blast injuries. However, presence of tympanic membrane injury can be used as a marker to identify a subset of blast victims that may benefit from a period of observation for latent primary blast injuries, specifically blast lung. Severe pulmonary blast injury will likely require intensive care. If hypoxia is present, supplemental oxygen should be provided. For patients with severe hypoxia, consideration should be made for tracheal intubation and positive pressure ventilation (PPV). There is some controversy with ventilation strategies in blast lung injuries since these patients may respond adversely to further positive pressure as a result of iatrogenic barotrauma and subsequent pneumothorax. If PPV is necessary, consideration should be made for lung-protective strategies similarly employed with adult respiratory distress syndrome (ARDS) patients. This includes permissive hypercapnia, low-volume/high-frequency settings, or other pressure-limited/volume-controlled ventilator settings to maintain a peak inspiratory pressure below 30 to 35 cm H_2O, judicious use of positive end-expiratory pressures (PEEP) for oxygenation, nitric oxide or high-frequency oscillator ventilation. Patients with respiratory symptoms should have radiographs performed (CXR, CT, etc.) with admission to monitor oxygen saturations and progression of symptoms to respiratory failure. Aggressive intravenous fluid resuscitation should also be avoided unless hypotension requires it, since overhydration can result in worsening of underlying pulmonary contusions. Pneumothorax or hemothorax on imaging will warrant surgical consultation and tube thoracostomy.

Auditory injuries are the most common type of after-blast exposure but typically result only in expectant management. Spontaneous healing of tympanic membrane rupture typically occurs in 78% to 88% of patients. Treatment will be based on otolaryngology consultant recommendations depending on initial symptoms complaints. Patients with evidence of inner ear dysfunction should undergo neuroimaging. All patients with tympanic membrane rupture should have otolaryngology evaluation. Primary gastrointestinal blast injuries are suggested by related symptoms described earlier in this chapter. Any evidence of hemodynamic instability with abdominal complaints should trigger CT imaging and surgical consultation. Hypotension should be managed initially with isotonic crystalloid fluids followed by blood transfusion if the patient remains hypotensive. Diagnosis by abdominal CT will usually diagnose intra-abdominal or retro-peritoneal injury. Patients with significant symptoms should be admitted for serial abdominal exams with repeat imaging since the development of radiographic findings for mesenteric injury can be delayed.

Ocular injuries that occur after blast exposure include corneal abrasions, corneal lacerations, ocular foreign body, ruptured globe, orbital fractures, and retrobulbar hematoma formation. Essentially, any ocular complaint should be further evaluated by ophthalmology. Specific findings of concern include sudden visual loss or acuity change, severe pain out of proportion to exam or light, blood in the anterior chamber, abnormal gaze to suggest entrapment, abnormal papillary response to light, proptosis, or an irregular papillary shape to suggest a ruptured globe. Seidel sign refers to a stream of aqueous humor from a globe defect visible under fluorescein examination. A ruptured globe should be immediately bandaged and covered with an eye shield. Tetanus status should be updated if needed and prophylactic antibiotics administered. A fluoroquinolone antibiotic such as moxifloxacin provides adequate microbial coverage.

Soft tissue injuries from an explosive blast should be managed with direct pressure over bleeding sites with elevation and compressive dressing if needed. Tourniquet use for arterial bleeding not controlled with direct pressure has been used with success in the combat and tactical environments. The experience with tourniquet use is more limited in the civilian hospital setting since these types of injuries are not commonly encountered, but it should be considered in cases in which uncontrollable exsanguination threatens the patient's life. Tourniquet placement should occur as close to the wound as possible and tight enough until the loss of distal pulses. This ensures both hemorrhage control and prevents the development of a compartment syndrome. The time of tourniquet placement should also be noted. Significant soft tissue injuries should be radiographed to rule out underlying fracture. If a fracture is identified and considered open, prophylactic antibiotics with adequate skin flora coverage should be administered. Any significant soft tissue injury will require surgical and/or orthopedic consultation.

COMPLICATIONS

Certain complications based on specific organ systems involvement deserve mentioning. Most blast injuries by nature result in soft tissue contusion, hemorrhage, and tissue destruction. For example, with soft tissue injury, the development of compartment syndrome, particularly in the lower leg compartments, is a common complication from an explosive blast. The hospitalist should maintain a high index of suspicion and monitor for signs such as paresthesias, pallor, and pulselessness (late finding), as well as symptoms such as pain out of proportion to exam and with passive muscle stretch (early finding). These findings warrant emergent orthopedic or surgical evaluation for fasciotomy.

Sepsis and infection from significant wound contamination, burn wound infection, and tissue injury as well as the systemic inflammatory response syndrome (SIRS) after blast trauma should be anticipated complications in blast patients with significant injuries. These complications differ from quinary blast injuries, which are poorly understood and thought to be due to overwhelming release of inflammatory mediators after an explosive blast exposure resulting in a hyperinflammatory state. These patients manifest hyperpyrexia, diaphoresis, low central venous pressures, and a positive fluid balance. This injury class was based on a case series of blast patients after a bombing incident in Israel. Further studies will help better define this injury category.

One could argue that primary pulmonary blast injury appears clinically similar to ARDS. Although this is true, determining a blast exposure by history is sufficient to confirm that injuries are blastrelated.

The postconcussive syndrome is worth mentioning, since many patients experiencing mild TBI after blast exposure may have persistent neurologic and physical complaints up to one year postblast. Symptoms such as persistent headache, nausea, dizziness, vertigo, short-term memory loss, difficulties in concentration, insomnia, depression, or irritability are commonly reported. Further follow-up with neurologic testing is indicated. It is important to instruct patients on the second-impact syndrome, which can worsen outcome and mortality if a second significant brain injury is sustained without allowing enough time for recovery from the initial injury.

One specific consideration is the inappropriate diagnosis of posttraumatic stress disorder (PTSD) in patients in which mild TBI is more appropriate. It would not seem surprising to consider PTSD in blast patients, since the mere involvement with any sort of explosive blast event can be a significant emotional event. A patient well removed from the epicenter of a blast site with headaches, dizziness, anxiety, and memory difficulties may inappropriately be diagnosed with mild TBI, whereas a patient positioned well within a blast zone experiencing the same symptoms may be inappropriately diagnosed with PTSD. The point is that care should be taken in making the correct diagnosis since the subsequent treatment can differ vastly.

CONCLUSION

Explosive blasts can result in significant injury to the body. Factors such as proximity to the blast and occurrence within an enclosed space can amplify the destructive damage. Understanding the basics of blast mechanics will aid the hospitalist in predicting injury patterns such as blast lung or tympanic membrane rupture. The hospitalist should maintain a high index of suspicion for traumatic brain injury in the blast victim with altered mental status or focal neurological deficits. The key to maximizing clinical outcomes in these patients is to provide supportive care, avoid secondary insults, and recognize the need for appropriate specialty consultation when particular injuries are identified.

SUGGESTED READINGS

Butler FK, Holcomb JB, Giebner SD, et al. Tactical combat casualty care 2007: evolving concepts and battlefield experience. *Mil Med.* 2007;172:S1–S19.

Champion HR, Holcomb JS, Young LA. Injuries from explosions: physics, biophysics, pathology and required research focus. *J Trauma.* 2009;66:1468–1477.

DePalma RG, Burris DG, Champion HR, et al. Blast injuries. *N Engl J Med.* 2005;352:1335–1342.

Ling GSF, Marshall SA. Management of traumatic brain injury in the intensive care unit. *Neurol Clin.* 2008;26:409–426.

Ling GSF, Bandak F, Amonda R, et al. Explosive blast neurotrauma. *J Neurotrauma.* 2009;26:815–825.

Maas A, Stocchetti N, Bullock R. Moderate and severe traumatic brain injury in adults. *Lancet Neurol.* 2008;7:728–741.

McHugh GS, Doortje CE, Butcher I, et al. Prognostic value of secondary insults in traumatic brain injury: results from the IMPACT study. *J Neurotrauma.* 2007;24:287–293.

Moppett IK. Traumatic brain injury: assessment, resuscitation and early management. *Br J Anaesth.* 2007;99:18–31.

Owens BD, Kragh JF, Wenke JC, et al. Combat wounds in Operation Iraqi Freedom and Operation Enduring Freedom. *J Trauma.* 2008;64:295–299.

Ritenour AE, Baskin TW. Primary blast injury: update on diagnosis and treatment. *Crit Care Med.* 2008;36:S311–S317.

Wolf SJ, Bebarta VS, Bonnett CJ, et al. Blast injuries. *Lancet.* 2009;374:405–415.

CHAPTER 269

Hospitalists in the Veterans Health Administration: An Integrated Health Care System

Peter J. Kaboli, MD, MS
Thomas Barrett, MD
Sondra Vazirani, MD, MPH
Lars Osterberg, MD
Andrew Auerbach, MD, MPH

Key Clinical Questions

1. What are the reasons behind the growth of hospitalists in the Veterans Administration System?
2. How can an integrated health system serve as a conduit for disseminating best practices across facilities?

INTRODUCTION

Since the term *hospitalist* was coined more than 10 years ago the field of Hospital Medicine has seen dramatic growth. The Society of Hospital Medicine (SHM) has more than 10,000 members and estimates that there are 30,000 hospitalists nationwide, with that number likely to grow to 40,000 by 2015. The rapid growth of the field was driven by a number of factors. Initial studies comparing hospitalists and nonhospitalists revealed that care by hospitalists was associated with reductions in length of stay (LOS) by roughly one day and costs by 10–15%. A review of these earlier reports concluded that "hospitalists improve inpatient efficiency without harmful effects on quality or patient satisfaction." These improvements in efficiency stimulated hospitals to hire hospitalists, thus driving supply. With a new crop of graduating residents every year who were comfortable caring for sick hospitalized patients, the field expanded.

Following studies that showed improvements in efficiency, studies emerged showing improved clinical outcomes for mortality, readmissions, and disease-specific outcomes for congestive heart failure and pneumonia. However, a more recent multicenter trial of hospitalists in six academic centers found that hospitalist care was *not* associated with lower LOS, costs, or mortality. Regardless, growth of hospitalists has continued and may be impacted by other institutional and/or physician needs. Hospitalists have been champions of quality improvement initiatives for institutional priorities such as deep venous thrombosis prophylaxis and initiation of rapid response teams. In academic medical centers, hospitalists have improved inpatient teaching and may have expanded roles due to residency work hour reform. Physicians are also choosing this field as a career in greater numbers, especially at the completion of residency.

The growth of hospitalists in an integrated health care system has not been well described. The Veterans Health Administration (VHA) is the largest single provider of health care in the U.S. with more than 125 hospitals providing acute medical care. Due to the rapid expansion of hospitalist models of care in the private sector, describing the growth and drivers of expansion of Hospital Medicine in VHA could provide insights for hospital leadership and help new hospitalist programs learn from the experience of more seasoned programs.

SURVEY OF HOSPITALIST GROWTH IN THE VETERANS ADMINISTRATION

In order to better understand the roll of hospitalists in the Veterans Administration (VA), a survey of inpatient medical services was sent to chiefs of medicine or chiefs of staff at 129 Veterans Administration Medical Centers (VAMCs) that provide inpatient medical care. Survey results were tallied and responses reported for all respondents as well as by academic and nonacademic-affiliated VAMCs. This designation was due to the close relationship that academic-affiliated VAMCs have with residency training programs and the potential impact this could have on the adoption of hospitalist models of care.

The survey consisted of 24 multiple choice and free text questions including four domains: (1) structure of inpatient general medical services, (2) structure of medical intensive care unit (MICU) services, (3) existence of a hospitalist program, and (4) impact of residency work hour reform on inpatient general medical services. To query the existence of a hospitalist program, respondents were

TABLE 269-1 Features of VAMC Medicine Services at all VAMCs and by Academic and Nonacademic Affiliation

	All VAMCs N = 118	Academic Affiliated N = 98	Nonacademic Affiliated N = 20
General medicine services			
Have hospitalists programs	76/118 (64.4%)	61/98 (62.2%)	15/20 (75%)
Staff with resident teams	84/118 (71.2%)	84/98 (85.7%)	0/20 (0%)
Staff only teams	30/118 (25.4%)	13/98 (13.3%)	17/20 (85.0%)
Subspecialty teams	26/118 (22.0%)	25/98 (25.5%)	1/20 (5.0%)
Midlevel providers	23/118 (19.5%)	19/98 (19.4%)	4/20 (20%)
Participate in "100,000 Lives"*	97/113 (85.8%)	79/94 (84.0%)	18/20 (90%)
24-hour in-house coverage	114/118 (96.6%)	96/98 (98%)	18/20 (90%)
24-hour coverage provided by†			
Residents	76/114 (66.7%)	73/96 (76.0%)	3/18 (16.7%)
ER physicians	49/114 (43.0%)	45/96 (46.9%)	18/18 (100%)
Moonlighters	44/114 (38.6%)	30/96 (31.3%)	14/18 (77.8%)
Hospitalists	13/114 (11.4%)	10/96 (10.4%)	3/18 (5.6%)
Intensivists	9/114 (7.9%)	9/96 (9.4%)	0/18 (0%)
Midlevels	3/114 (2.6%)	3/96 (3.1%)	0/18 (0%)
MICU services			
Have MICU	114 (96.6%)	98 (100%)	16 (80%)
Staffed by intensivists	73.7%	81%	20%
Total # of intensivists	364	359.5	5
Total FTEs of intensivists	265	260.9	4.4
Mean # of intensivists	4.45	4.61	1.25
Mean FTE of intensivists	3.24	3.35	1.10
% VA employed	62.7%	60.8%	100%
24-hour in-house coverage	12.1%	12.6%	0%
Open ICU policy	57 (50.0%)	41 (41.8%)	16 (80%)
Staffed by:*			
Cardiologists	63.2%	73.1%	37.5%
Pulmonary (noncritical care)	56.1%	65.9%	31.3%
Surgeons	56.1%	58.5%	50.0%
Hospitalists	54.4%	49.8%	68.8%
Primary care providers	43.9%	36.6%	62.5%
Other specialists	21.1%	24.4%	12.5%

*100,000 Lives Campaign was promoted by the Institute for Health care Improvement to reduce hospital deaths in U.S. hospitals.
†Total is greater than 100% as more than one category could be selected.

asked, *"Does your VAMC have a 'hospitalist' service?"* The following definition of hospitalists was provided: *"Hospitalists have been defined as physicians who spend all or the majority of their clinical, administrative, educational, or research activities in the care of hospitalized patients. This could include a formal hospitalist program or physicians who would consider themselves hospitalists based upon their proportion of inpatient medicine service."* The year of initiation of the hospitalist program was asked and if the reported date was prior to 1996, the year the term *hospitalist* was introduced, the year 1995 was assigned to the response. The size of the hospitalist program was assessed using three questions: (1) how many hospitalists worked at the VAMC, (2) how many total full-time equivalent (FTE) hospitalists there were, and (3) an estimate of the percentage of medical patients who are cared for by hospitalists.

DESCRIPTION OF VA HOSPITALIST SERVICES

FEATURES OF VAMC MEDICAL SERVICES

Of 129 surveys sent, complete surveys were returned by 118 respondents (91.5%). Hospitalist programs were reported at 76 VAMCs (64.4%), including 62% of academic-affiliated VAMCs and 75% of nonacademic-affiliated VAMCs. Of all respondents, 71% had teaching services with resident physicians, 25% had staff-only services, and 20% utilized midlevel providers. Twenty-four hour in-house coverage was available in 97% of VAMCs with resident physicians providing coverage at 67% and hospitalists at 11%. A medical intensive care unit (MICU) was available at 97% of hospitals with 74% staffed by board-certified intensivists. Half were "open" and allowed noncritical care physicians to admit patients, most commonly by cardiologists (63%); 54% allowed hospitalists. A description of the general medicine and MICU services, categorized by academic and nonacademic VAMCs is detailed in **Table 269-1**.

FEATURES OF VAMC HOSPITALIST SERVICES

Of the 76 hospitalist programs, the year of initiation is diagramed in **Figure 269-1** showing a steady increase in both academic- and nonacademic-affiliated VAMCs. At the time of initiation of the programs, a mean of 2.89 hospitalists (2.65 FTEs) was reported and 56% of all general medical patients were cared for by hospitalists. In 2006, this increased to a mean of 4.3 hospitalists, or 3.95 FTEs,

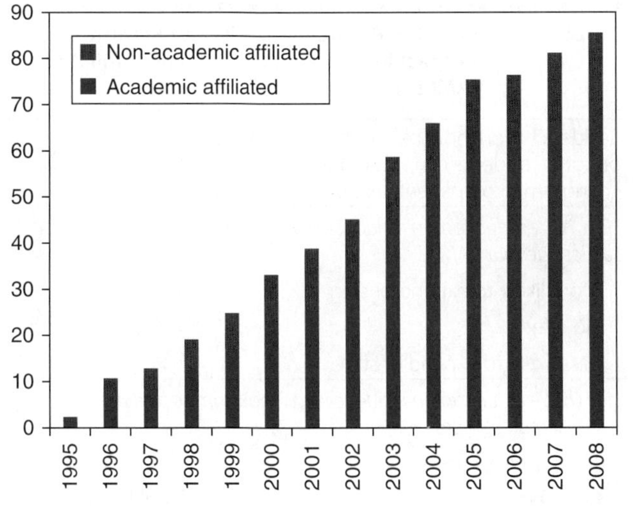

Figure 269-1 *Growth of hospitalist programs in VHA hospitals (1995–2008).*

who cared for an estimated 67% of all general medical patients. In 2008, the rate continued to increase to a mean of 5.11 hospitalists (4.87 FTEs) caring for 73% of all general medical patients. Based upon these responses, we estimated there are approximately 327 hospitalists in VHA, with 280 at academic-affiliated VAMCs and 47 at nonacademic affiliated hospitals. Twenty-four-hour in-house coverage was provided by only 13% of the hospitalist programs (**Table 269-2**).

Of the 42 VAMCs that did not have hospitalists, 10 (24 %) anticipated they would hire hospitalists within the next two years. Of these ten, reasons given for starting hospitalist programs included compliance with residency work hour reform (4), to provide relief to primary care providers to improve clinic efficiency (4), and to provide better ward team coverage (2). Of the remaining 32 VAMCs, one reported a "nocturnist" program of night time coverage that would not consider a hospitalist program, one used a hospitalist to help with resident work hour rules, and one VAMC experimented with a hospitalist program for one year, but abandoned it due to poor staff satisfaction. The remaining 29 had no intentions of starting a program in the next two years.

When asked how reductions in residency work hours impacted hospitalist services, 42% stated they were more likely to start or expand a hospitalist program, 33% were more likely to use nonteaching services, and 35% were more likely to use nonphysician providers. When asked if residency work hour reform has made it more difficult to provide high-quality care in a safe environment for hospitalized *medical* patients, 51% agreed/strongly agreed; 49% agreed/strongly agreed that work hour reform has made it more difficult to provide high-quality care in a safe environment for hospitalized *surgical* patients. In the free-text comment section, Accreditation Council for Graduate Medical Education (ACGME) residency work hour reform and related rules were the predominant reason for the initiation and/or expansion of hospitalist models, attending only services, and midlevel provider use on inpatient services.

Finally, when queried about how reductions in residency work hours has affected the ability of the medicine service faculty to provide inpatient care, 59% felt it made it harder, 62% felt it was harder

TABLE 269-2 Features of VAMC Hospitalist Services at all VAMCs and by Academic and Nonacademic Affiliation

	All VAMC Hospitalist Services N = 76	Academic-Affiliated Hospitalist Services N = 61	Nonacademic-Affiliated Hospitalist Services N = 15
When program started			
Total # of hospitalists	205	167	38
Total FTEs of hospitalists	189	150.5	38
Mean # of hospitalists	2.89	2.93	2.71
Mean FTE of hospitalists	2.65	2.64	2.71
Percentage of general medicine admits	56.1%	50.5%	80.4%
In 2006			
Total # of hospitalists	327	280	47
Total FTEs of hospitalists	300	252.7	47
Mean # of hospitalists	4.30	4.59	3.15
Mean FTE of hospitalists	3.95	4.14	3.15
Percentage of general medicine admits	67%	62.1%	88.6%
In 2008			
Total # of hospitalists	388	334	54
Total FTEs of hospitalists	370	315.9	54
Mean # of hospitalists	5.11	5.48	3.6
Mean FTE of hospitalists	4.87	5.18	3.6
Percentage of general medicine admits	73.0%	68.9%	91.1%
Percentage VA employed	94.7%	93.4%	100%
24-hour in-house coverage	13.2%	11.5%	20%

FTE, full-time equivalent.

to teach medical students, and 78% felt it was harder to teach medical residents; 55% felt it was harder to expose residents to enough patients (**Table 269-3**).

DISCUSSION

The expansion of hospitalist models of care has been dramatic over the past decade and projected to continue. The Veterans Health Administration (VHA) has also grown in parallel with the private sector and academic medical centers. We estimate VHA is one of the largest single employers of hospitalists in the U.S. with more than 325 employed hospitalists in an integrated health care system. The size and format of the 76 programs demonstrate considerable variation and represent large academic-affiliated as well as smaller, nonacademic-affiliated VAMCs.

Historically, reasons given for the adoption of the hospitalist model of inpatient care were varied and included physician preference, improved efficiency, hospital demand, and enhanced quality. The drivers in VHA may be similar, but our results suggest that ACGME work hour limits on residents has been a significant contributor to this growth, especially over the past few years. In addition, limitations in federal budgets and recent increased demand for VHA services may have been a factor in spurring the growth of hospitalist programs in VHA. This was supported by the comment section of our survey in which a number of facilities that did not have hospitalist programs were starting them in order to free up primary care providers to improve clinic efficiency.

The impact of residency work hour reform is complex, yet half of respondents felt that reductions have *"made it more difficult to provide high quality care in a safe environment for medical patients."* This perception may be due to fewer residents available on VA medicine teams, fewer hours leading to increased patient handoffs, increasing patient volume, or a combination of these and other factors. Regardless, VHA provides training opportunities for 31,290 resident physicians and 17,289 medical students annually, including a substantial proportion of salary support. Ultimately, hospitalists play an important role in medical education and the safe delivery of care to hospitalized patients.

A number of concurrent factors may also be contributing to the growth and/or evolution of hospitalist programs in VHA that were not specifically queried in our survey, but emerged through the comment sections. Inpatient efficiency or "throughput" has become an important issue in VHA, much like the private sector. The inpatient general medicine service is often the "bottleneck" slowing down the admission of patients from the emergency department leading to backlogs of patients waiting for a bed. It also can slow admissions from clinics and transfer of patients out of the ICU. Hospitalists have been charged with improving this bottleneck both within and outside VHA.

VHA and the private sector also both face a shortage of critical care physicians. Although care by board-certified intensivists is associated with 25% to 50% reductions in mortality and ICU intensivist staffing standards have been shown to be cost effective, an intensivist shortage exists. This is especially evident in smaller nonacademic-affiliated VAMCs in which only 20% of MICUs were staffed by intensivists and nearly 70% relied upon hospitalists to provide MICU coverage. Although not a solution to a shortage of critical care providers, hospitalists may be a reasonable alternative.

Another area of potential growth for hospitalists is in the provision of 24/7 in-house coverage of patients. Although 97% of VAMCs provide 24/7 coverage, hospitalists only provided that coverage 11% of the time behind residents, emergency room physicians, and moonlighters.

This survey study is limited in that it was only administered in VHA, which may limit the generalizability to the private sector and

TABLE 269-3 Impact of Residency Work Hour Reform on Teaching Services at Academic-Affiliated VAMCs (N = 98)

Residency work hour reform has limited the number of hours residents can work. What impacts have these changes had on patient care in your VAMC?	
How have reductions in residency work hours impacted hospitalist services at your VAMC?	
More likely to expand or start	41/98 (41.8%)
No effect	56/98 (57.1%)
Less likely to expand or start	1/98 (1.0%)
How have reductions in residency work hours impacted use of nonteaching services?	
More likely to use	32/98 (32.7%)
No effect	66/98 (67.3%)
Less likely to use	0/98 (0%)
How have reductions in residency work hours impacted use of midlevel providers (PA/NPs)?	
More likely to use	34/98 (34.7%)
No effect	64/98 (65.3%)
Less likely to use	0/98 (0%)
Reductions in residency work hours have made it more difficult to provide high quality of care in a safe environment for hospitalized medical patients.	
Strongly disagree/disagree	26/98 (26.5%)
Neutral	16/98 (17.4%)
Agree/Strongly agree	50/98 (51.0%)
Don't know	4/98 (4.1%)
Reductions in residency work hours have made it more difficult to provide high quality of care in a safe environment for hospitalized surgical patients.	
Strongly disagree/disagree	13/98 (13.3%)
Neutral	17/98 (17.4%)
Agree/Strongly agree	48/98 (49.0%)
Don't know	20/98 (20.4%)
How have reductions in residency work hours affected the ability of the medicine service FACULTY at your VAMC to:	
provide inpatient care	
Unchanged	40/98 (40.8%)
Harder	58/98 (59.2%)
Easier	0/95 (0%)
teach inpatient care to medical students	
Unchanged	37/98 (37.8%)
Harder	61/98(62.2%)
Easier	0/95 (0%)
teach inpatient care to residents	
Unchanged	21/98 (22.5%)
Harder	76/98 (77.5%)
Easier	0/95 (0%)
expose residents to enough patients	
Unchanged	44/98 (44.9%)
Harder	54/98 (55.1%)
Easier	0/95 (0%)

TABLE 269-4 Summary of Selected Prior Hospitalist Studies

Author	Outcome	LOS/Costs	Comment
Wachter RM, et al. *JAMA.* 1998;279(19):1560–1565.	No mortality or readmission difference	Costs ↓ 10% LOS ↓ 12%	Adjusted; quasi-randomized; university-based
Diamond HS, et al. *Annals of Internal Medicine.* 1998;129(3):197–203.	Readmission ↓ 54%	Costs ↓ 12% LOS ↓ 17%	Not adjusted; historical controls; community-based
Bellet PS. *Pediatrics.* 2000;105(3 Pt 1):478–484.	No mortality difference; Higher readmissions	Charges ↓ 9% LOS ↓ 11%	Adjusted; historical controls; university pediatrics service
Kearns PJ, et al. *Archives of Internal Medicine.* 2001;161(2):235–241.	No mortality or readmission difference	No Cost/ LOS difference	Unadjusted; no concurrent controls; community-based
Tingle LE, Lambert CT. *Family Medicine.* 2001;33(7):511–515.	No mortality or readmission difference	No Cost/ LOS difference	Not adjusted; concurrent controls; family practice program; community-based
Meltzer DO, et al. *Annals of Internal Medicine.* 2002;137(11):866–874.	Mortality R.R. 0.65 (95%CI 0.44–0.96)	Costs ↓ 9% LOS ↓ 12%	Adjusted; quasi-random; university-based; difference in second year only
Auerbach AD, et al. *Annals of Internal Medicine.* 2002;137(11):859–865.	Mortality H.R. 0.71 (95% CI 0.54–0.93)	Costs ↓ 12% LOS ↓ 13%	Adjusted; community physician controls; difference after 2nd year
Kaboli PK, et al. *AJMC.* 2004;10:561–568.	No mortality or readmission difference	Costs ↓ 10% LOS ↓ 16%	Adjusted; quasi-randomized; university-based

LOS, length of stay.

academic medical centers and we did not ask about other services provided by hospitalist programs such as consultation services, surgical comanagement, preoperative evaluations, and quality improvement work by hospitalists.

What are the implications for the growth of hospitalist services in VHA as it relates to non-VA hospitals? First, VHA physicians are salaried with various types of incentive programs. As non-VA hospitals expand their use of hospitalists, salaries and workload will need to be compared in order to be competitive. Second, the expanded role of hospitalists in the area of quality improvement and systems redesign will likely continue, as this role will continue to be of significant value to employers and hospitals. Third, academic-affiliated VAMCs will need to learn from one another how best to integrate "teaching" and "nonteaching" hospitalists into the patient care and educational missions of the hospital. Lastly, hospitalists across both the private and public sectors of care will need to work collaboratively to learn best practices from one another and how to better manage patients across both systems of care (**Table 269-4**).

CONCLUSION

In summary, our survey highlights the growth of hospitalists in VHA and reasons behind this growth. As in any health care system, hospitalists have an important role in the continued improvement in the quality and efficiency of the care provided to our patients. As a model of high-quality health care, VHA may provide an ideal environment for collaborative relationships of hospitalists across medical centers. VHA has recognized this and has established a Hospitalist Field Advisory Committee to both inform the VA Central Office on inpatient issues and serve as a conduit for disseminating best practices across facilities. As health care evolves and inpatient care is challenged with changes such as residency work hours, pay-for-performance, and national quality standards, hospitalists are uniquely qualified to meet these challenges and initiate change.

SUGGESTED READINGS

Angus DC, Kelley MA, Schmitz RJ, et al. Caring for the critically ill patient. Current and projected workforce requirements for care of the critically ill and patients with pulmonary disease: can we meet the requirements of an aging population? *JAMA.* 2000;284(21):2762–2770.

Ewart GW, Marcus L, Gaba MM, Bradner RH, Medina JL, Chandler EB. The critical care medicine crisis: a call for federal action: a white paper from the critical care professional societies. *Chest.* 2004;125(4):1518–1521.

Hauer KE, Wachter RM, McCulloch CE, Woo GA, Auerbach AD. Effects of hospitalist attending physicians on trainee satisfaction with teaching and with internal medicine rotations. *Arch Intern Med.* 2004;164(17):1866–1871.

Jha AK, Perlin JB, Kizer KW, Dudley RA. Effect of the transformation of the Veterans Affairs Health Care System on the quality of care. *N Engl J Med.* 2003;348(22):2218–2227.

Wachter RM, Goldman L. Hospitalist movement 5 yrs later. *JAMA.* 2002;287(4):487–494.

Wachter RM, Goldman L. The emerging role of "hospitalists" in the American healthcare system. *N Engl J Med.* 1996;335(7):514–517.

INDEX

Note: Page numbers followed by *f* indicate figures; and page numbers followed by *t* indicate tables.

B

C

INDEX

E

F

G

INDEX

N

O

Q

INDEX

Z

INDEX